Brief Contents *(Continued)*

D0081138

UNIT 10
Hematologic Disorders 1445

51 Structure and Function of the Hematologic System 1447

52 Assessment of Clients with Hematologic Disorders.. 1461

53 Nursing Care of Clients with Hematologic Disorders 1469

UNIT 11
Urinary Disorders..1533

54 Structure and Function of the Urinary System.................... 1535

55 Assessment of Clients with Urinary Disorders 1547

56 Nursing Care of Clients with Disorders of the Ureters, Bladder, and Urethra..................................... 1571

57 Nursing Care of Clients with Renal Disorders 1625

UNIT 12
Gastrointestinal Disorders...1683

58 Structure and Function of the Gastrointestinal System 1685

59 Assessment of Clients with Gastrointestinal Disorders 1698

60 Nursing Care of Clients with Ingestive Disorders.................. 1719

61 Nursing Care of Clients with Gastric Disorders 1748

62 Nursing Care of Clients with Intestinal Disorders................. 1787

UNIT 13
Liver, Biliary Tract, and Exocrine Pancreatic Disorders.........1833

63 Structure and Function of the Liver, Biliary Tract, and Exocrine Pancreas 1835

64 Assessment of Clients with Liver, Biliary Tract, and Exocrine Pancreatic Disorders............................. 1843

65 Nursing Care of Clients with Liver Disorders 1858

66 Nursing Care of Clients with Biliary Tract and Exocrine Pancreatic Disorders................................. 1907

UNIT 14
Metabolic Disorders...1933

67 Structure and Function of the Endocrine System.................. 1935

68 Assessment of Clients with Endocrine Disorders 1948

69 Nursing Care of Clients with Endocrine Disorders of the Pancreas.. 1955

70 Nursing Care of Clients with Thyroid and Parathyroid Disorders 2005

71 Nursing Care of Clients with Adrenal, Pituitary, and Gonadal Disorders 2041

UNIT 15
Musculoskeletal Disorders 2071

72 Structure and Function of the Musculoskeletal System............ 2073

73 Assessment of Clients with Musculoskeletal Disorders............ 2083

74 Nursing Care of Clients with Musculoskeletal Disorders........... 2098

75 Nursing Care of Clients with Musculoskeletal Trauma or Overuse.. 2129

UNIT 16
Integumentary Disorders 2171

76 Structure and Function of the Integumentary System 2173

77 Assessment of Clients with Integumentary Disorders.............. 2180

78 Nursing Care of Clients with Integumentary Disorders 2197

79 Nursing Care of Clients with Burns 2233

80 Nursing Care of Clients Undergoing Plastic Surgery............... 2267

UNIT 17
Reproductive Disorders..2291

81 Structure and Function of the Reproductive System 2293

82 Assessment of Clients with Reproductive Disorders............... 2307

83 Nursing Care of Men with Reproductive Disorders.. 2350

84 Nursing Care of Women with Gynecologic Disorders 2386

85 Nursing Care of Clients with Breast Disorders..................... 2481

86 Nursing Care of Clients with Sexually Transmitted Diseases 2459

UNIT 18
Multisystem Disorders...2477

87 Substance Abuse 2479

88 Basic Concepts of Emergency Care 2501

89 Nursing Care of Clients with Medical-Surgical Emergencies....... 2517

APPENDIX A: Religious Beliefs and Practices Affecting Healthcare 2544

APPENDIX B: A Health History Format that Integrates the Assessment of Functional Health Patterns 2552

APPENDIX C: Laboratory Values of Clinical Importance in Medical-Surgical Nursing 2555

APPENDIX D: Clinical Pathways............................2566

Discussion of "Thinking Critically" Exercises TC–1

INDEX...I–1

MEDICAL-SURGICAL
NURSING

CLINICAL MANAGEMENT FOR CONTINUITY OF CARE

FIFTH EDITION

Joyce M. Black, M.S.N., R.N., C.P.S.N.
Nursing Specialist
College of Nursing
University of Nebraska Medical Center
Omaha, Nebraska

Esther Matassarin-Jacobs, Ph.D., R.N., O.C.N.
Associate Dean, Director Undergraduate
  Program
Associate Professor, Medical/Surgical Nursing
Marcella Niehoff School of Nursing
Loyola University of Chicago
Chicago, Illinois

W.B. SAUNDERS COMPANY
A Division of Harcourt Brace & Company
Philadelphia London Toronto Montreal Sydney Tokyo

W.B. SAUNDERS COMPANY
A Division of Harcourt Brace & Company

The Curtis Center
Independence Square West
Philadelphia, Pennsylvania 19106

NOTICE

Library of Congress Cataloging-in-Publication Data

Medical-surgical nursing: clinical management for continuity of care. / [edited by] Joyce M. Black, Esther Matassarin-Jacobs.—5th ed.

    p.   cm.

  Rev. ed. of: Luckmann and Sorensen's medical-surgical nursing. 4th ed. c1993.

    Includes bibliographical references and index.

    ISBN 0–7216–6399–0 (single vol.)
    ISBN 0–7216–7484–4 (2-vol. set)
    ISBN 0–7216–7475–5 (vol. 1)
    ISBN 0–7216–7476–3 (vol. 2)

    1. Nursing. 2. Surgical nursing. 3. Psychophysiology.
I. Black, Joyce M. II. Matassarin-Jacobs, Esther. III. Luckmann,
Joan. IV. Luckmann and Sorensen's medical-surgical nursing.
    [DNLM: 1. Nursing Care. 2. Perioperative Nursing. WY 150 L9412
1997]

RT41.L87 1997   610.73—dc20

DNLM/DLC   96–7419

                                        ISBN 0–7216–6399–0 (single vol.)
                                        ISBN 0–7216–7484–4 (2-vol. set)
MEDICAL-SURGICAL NURSING: Clinical Management   ISBN 0–7216–7475–5 (vol. 1)
for Continuity of Care, 5th Edition   ISBN 0–7216–7476–3 (vol. 2)

Last digit is the print number: 9   8   7   6   5   4   3   2

To Steve, Jon, Katy, and Tricia. Sometimes I work far too hard and forget to enjoy you, the most wonderful people in my life. To the students—tomorrow's nurses. My hope is that you will enjoy nursing as much as I have.

J.M.B.

To my husband, Philip, without whose love and support I would never have taken on or completed this mammoth task. To the memories of my beloved mother and father, Grace Matassarin, R.N., and F.W. Matassarin, M.D. Thank you both for your love and support—I miss you.

E.M.J

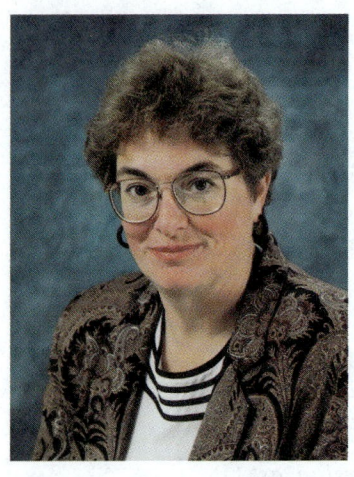

Joyce M. Black, M.S.N., R.N., C.P.S.N., is a Nursing Specialist with the Adult Health and Illness Department of the University of Nebraska Medical Center. There she teaches medical-surgical nursing to both sophomore and senior students. She is also working on her dissertation, which focuses on patient wound treatment and healthcare system risk factors in pressure ulcer healing. Ms. Black received her master's degree from the University of Nebraska Medical Center and her undergraduate degrees from Winona State University in Winona, Minnesota, and Rochester Community College in Rochester, Minnesota.

Joyce Black has also had several years of experience as a medical-surgical nurse at Saint Mary's Hospital, which is affiliated with the Mayo Clinic in Rochester, Minnesota. Her practice has included critical care, burns, respiratory disorders, orthopedics, and plastic surgery. Ms. Black is certified by the American Society of Plastic and Reconstructive Surgical Nurses, and she currently serves as editor of *Plastic Surgical Nursing.*

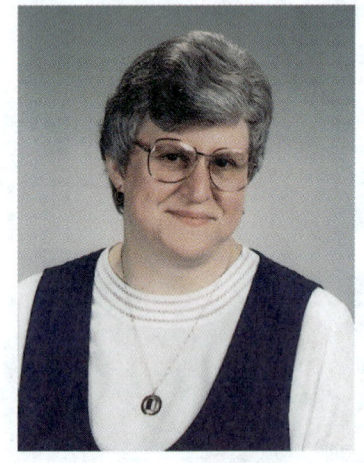

Esther Matassarin-Jacobs, Ph.D., R.N., O.C.N., is Associate Dean, Director Undergraduate Program, and Associate Professor of Medical/Surgical Nursing at the Marcella Niehoff School of Nursing, Loyola University of Chicago. Besides directing the undergraduate program, she is in charge of the oncology graduate major and has served on numerous dissertation committees. Dr. Matassarin-Jacobs received her B.S.N. from Case Western Reserve University, her M.Ed. from Wichita State University, her M.S.N. from Loyola University, and her Ph.D. from Northwestern University.

Esther Matassarin-Jacobs has worked in and taught medical-surgical nursing for more than 25 years, including teaching at Loyola for the past 19 years. She is also an NLN Accreditation Site Visitor. For the past 18 years she has been very active in preparing graduate nurses nationwide for licensure examination, including publishing two successful NCLEX review books. Her areas of research include success on the NCLEX, critical thinking in undergraduates, and assessment and management of pain.

Contributors

Leigh G. Anderson, M.A., B.S., R.N.
Administrator, The Centre for Plastic Surgery, San Bernardino, CA

Margaret M. Andrews, R.N., Ph.D., C.T.N.
Chairperson and Professor, Nazareth College of Rochester, Rochester, NY

Carol Birch, R.N., M.S.
Instructor, Medical-Surgical Nursing, South Dakota State University College of Nursing, West River Campus, Rapid City, SD

Joyce M. Black, M.S.N., R.N., C.P.S.N.
Nursing Specialist, Doctoral Candidate, College of Nursing, University of Nebraska Medical Center, Omaha, NE

R. B. Boley, Ph.D.
Professor, Biology Department, University of Texas at Arlington Arlington, TX

Elizabeth Carlson, R.N.C., Ph.D.
Assistant Professor, Department of Medical-Surgical Nursing, Niehoff School of Nursing, Loyola University Chicago, Chicago, IL

Lynne C. Carpenter, R.N., M.S., Ph.D., A.O.C.N.
Clinical Nurse Specialist, University of Michigan Breast Care Center, Ann Arbor, MI

Gretchen J. Carrougher, R.N., M.N.
Clinical Research Nurse, University of Washington Burn Center at Harborview Medical Center, Seattle, WA

Paula Carson, Ph.D., R.N.
Associate Professor, South Dakota State University, Brookings, SD

Linda Carman Copel, Ph.D., R.N., C.S.
Associate Professor, Villanova University, Villanova; Psychotherapist, Lower Merion Counseling Services, Ardmore, PA

Sherill Nones Cronin, Ph.D., R.N., C.
Associate Professor of Nursing, Bellarmine College, Lansing School of Nursing; Nurse Researcher, Jewish Hospital, Louisville, KY

Jean Elizabeth DeMartinis, Ph.D., R.N.
Assistant Professor, Program Director, Cardiac Rehab, Creighton University School of Nursing, Omaha, NE

Peggy Doheny, Ph.D., R.N., O.N.C.
Associate Professor, School of Nursing, Kent State University, Kent, OH

Patricia E. Downing, M.N., R.N.
Clinical Nurse Specialist, Formerly of School of Nursing, University of California, San Francisco, CA

Ken W. Edmisson, N.D., Ed.D., R.N.C., F.N.P.
Assistant Professor of Nursing, Graduate Studies in Nursing, School of Nursing, Belmont University, Nashville, TN

Mary Jane Garrett, Ph.D., R.N.
Assistant Professor of Nursing, University of Nebraska Medical Center, Omaha, NE

Peggy Gerard, D.N.Sc., R.N.
Associate Professor, Purdue University—Calumet, Hammond, IN

Kerry H. Greear, R.N., M.S.N., C.N.P.
Instructor, Graduate Program, South Dakota State University College of Nursing, West River Campus, Rapid City, SD

Margie J. Hansen, M.S.N., Ph.D.
Assistant Professor of Pharmaceutical Sciences, North Dakota State University, Fargo, ND

Barbara Harrison, B.S.N., M.Ed., M.S.N., Ph.D.(c).
Assistant Professor of Nursing, Bellarmine College, Lansing School of Nursing, Louisville, KY

Jane Hokanson Hawks, D.N.Sc., R.N.C.,
Assistant Professor, Associate Editor, *Urologic Nursing,* Midland Lutheran College, Fremont, NE

Beverley E. Holland, B.S.N., M.S.N., R.D.
Assistant Professor, Gerontology/Community Health/ Rehabilitation, Bellarmine College, Lansing School of Nursing, Louisville, KY

Cynthia Hromek, Ph.D., R.N.
Associate Professor, College of Saint Mary, Omaha, NE

Esperanza Villanueva Joyce, Ed.D., C.N.S., R.N.
Associate Professor, Department of Nursing and Health Sciences, Texas A&M University/Corpus Christi, Corpus Christi, TX

Annabelle M. Keene, B.S.N., M.S.N.
Associate Professor, College of Saint Mary, Omaha, NE

Beverly Kopala, Ph.D., R.N. (B.S.N., M.S., M.A., Ph.D.)
Associate Professor, Loyola University Chicago, Niehoff School of Nursing, Chicago, IL

Louise Nelson LaFramboise, M.S.N., R.N.
Assistant Professor, University of Nebraska Medical Center College of Nursing, Omaha, NE

Joan Lappe, Ph.D., R.N.
Associate Professor, Creighton University School of Nursing;
Nurse Scientist, Creighton University School of Medicine,
Osteoporosis Research Center, Omaha, NE

Anne M. Larson, R.N.C., Ph.D.
Assistant Professor of Nursing, Midland Lutheran College,
Fremont, Nebraska

Linda Lorraine Armstrong Lazure, Ph.D., R.N.
Associate Professor, Creighton University School of Nursing;
Staff Nurse, Emergency Department, Alegent Health, Bergan
Mercy Hospital, Omaha, NE

Donna W. Markey, R.N., M.S.N.
Nurse Coordinator, Surgical Services University of Virginia,
Health Science Center, Charlottesville, Virginia

Karen S. Martin, R.N., M.S.N., F.A.A.N.
Health Care Consultant, Editor, Home Health FOCUS, Omaha,
NE

Esther Matassarin-Jacobs, Ph.D., R.N., O.C.N.
Associate Dean, Director Undergraduate Program, Associate
Professor, Medical/Surgical Nursing, Marcella Niehoff School of
Nursing, Loyola University of Chicago, Chicago, IL

Cynthia McCurren, B.S.N., M.S.N., Ph.D.
Associate Professor, Adult/Gerontological Nursing, University of
Louisville School of Nursing, Louisville, KY

Cleda L. Meyer, R.N., M.S.N.
Assistant Professor of Nursing, Baker University School of
Nursing, Topeka, KS

Noreen Heer Nicol, M.S., R.N., F.N.P.
Clinical Senior Instructor, University of Colorado, School of
Nursing; Director of Nursing, Dermatology Clinical Specialist/
Nurse Practitioner, National Jewish Center for Immunology and
Respiratory Medicine, Denver, CO

Barbara B. Ott, R.N., Ph.D., C.C.R.N.
Assistant Professor, Villanova University College of Nursing,
Villanova, PA

Judith Ozuna, B.S.N., M.N.
Clinical Assistant Professor, Biobehavioral Nursing and Health
Systems, University of Washington; Clinical Nurse Specialist in
Neurology, VA Puget Sound Health Care System (Veterans
Affairs Medical Center), Seattle, WA

Joann Petty, R.N., M.S.N., O.C.N.
Bone Marrow Transplant Case Manager, Loyola University
Medical Center, Maywood, IL

Bonita Ann Pilon, B.S.N., M.N., D.S.N.
Associate Professor, Vanderbilt University School of Nursing;
Vice President for Clinical Affairs and Chief Nursing Officer,
Saint Thomas Hospital, Nashville, TN

Arlene L. Polaski, M.Ed., M.S.N., R.N
Instructor, York Technical College/University of South
Carolina–Lancaster Cooperative Program in Associate Degree
Nursing, Rock Hill, SC

Marlene Reimer, R.N., M.N.
Associate Professor, Faculty of Nursing, The University of
Calgary; Director, Wellness and Lifestyle Division, Canadian
Sleep Institute, Calgary, Alberta, Canada

Kathleen A. Ringel, D.N.Sc., C.F.N.P.
Family Nurse Practitioner, Women Veterans Coordinator,
Department of Veterans Affairs Medical Center, Omaha, NE

Sally Strong Schnell, R.N., M.S.N., C.N.R.N.
Clinical Instructor Medical Surgical Nursing, Loyola University
Chicago, Chicago; Tertiary Nurse Practitioner, Department of
Neurological Surgery, Loyola University Medical Center,
Maywood, IL

Carol Sedlak, R.N., Ph.D., O.N.C.
Assistant Professor, School of Nursing, Kent State University,
Kent, OH

Carol Sharkey, B.S.N., M.S.N., Ph.D.
Associate Professor, Regis University, Department of Nursing,
Denver, CO

Ruth Plotkin Shumaker, R.N., B.S.N., C.N.O.R.
Clinical Education Consultant, Advanced Sterilization Products/
JJMI, Canton, MS

Pamela Shumate, R.N., M.S.N.
Education Specialist, Providence Hospital, Washington, DC

Barbara Sigler, R.N., M.N.Ed., C.O.R.L.N
Adjunct Clinical Instructor—University of Pittsburgh Schools of
Nursing and Medicine, University of Pittsburgh; Clinical Nurse
Specialist—Otolaryngology and Head-Neck Oncology,
University of Pittsburgh Medical Center, Pittsburgh, PA

Dianne Smolen, Ph.D., M.S.N., R.N.
Associate Professor, Adult Health Nursing, Director, Continuing
Nursing Education, Medical College of Ohio School of Nursing,
Toledo, OH

Peter J. Ungvarski, M.S., R.N., F.A.A.N.
Clinical Director, Clinical Nurse Specialist, HIV, AIDS, AIDS
Project, Visiting Nurse Service of New York, New York, NY

Linda A. Vader, B.S., R.N.
Head Nurse, University of Michigan Kellogg Eye Center, Ann
Arbor, MI

Amy Verst, M.S.N., R.N., C.P.N.P., A.T.C.
Assistant Professor, Bellarmine College, Lansing School of
Nursing, Louisville, KY

Mary Vorder Bruegge, B.S.N., M.S.
Clinician IV, Nerancy Neuro ICU, University of Virginia Health
Sciences Center, Charlottesville, VA

Bernadette White, R.N., M.S.N.
Assistant Professor, Creighton University School of Nursing,
Omaha, NE

Reviewers

Therese Alexander, R.N., M.S.N., C.R.R.N.
Rehabilitation Institute of Chicago, University of Illinois,
Chicago, IL

Pamela A. Andreson, R.N., Ph.D.
Loyola University of Chicago, Chicago, IL

Joanna Avolio, R.N., B.S.C.N., B.Ed.
Fanshawe College, London, Ontario, Canada

Susan Anita Baker, R.N., M.S., O.C.N.
H. Lee Moffit Cancer Center and Research Institute,
Tampa, FL

Pamela Bannell, R.N., M.S.
Dominican College, San Rafael, CA

Elisa Bianchi-Smak, R.N., B.S.N., M.S.
Charles E. Gregory School of Nursing, Raritan Bay Medical
Center, Perth Amboy, NJ

Pamela J. Bolton, M.S., R.N., C.C.R.N.
Ohio State University Medical Center, Columbus, OH

Clara Boyle, R.N., M.S., Ed.D.
Salem State College, Salem, MA

Elizabeth Brady-Avis, R.N., M.S.N., C.C.R.N.
Thomas Jefferson University Hospital, Philadelphia, PA

Janet Burton, R.N., B.S., M.S.N.
Bob Jones University, Greenville, SC

Pat Bush, R.N., M.S.N.
Hopkinsville Community College, Hopkinsville, KY

Tonya Buttry, R.N.C., M.S.N.
Southeast Missouri Hospital College of Nursing, Cape
Girardeau, MO

Dorothy Calabrese, M.S.N., R.N., C.U.R.N., O.C.N.
Cleveland Clinic Foundation, Cleveland, OH

Valerie Miller Capallo, R.N., B.S.N., M.S.
The Union Memorial Hospital School of Nursing, Baltimore,
MD

Cheryl Cassis, R.N., M.S.N.
Belmont Technical College, St. Clairsville, OH

Esther Chipps, R.N., M.S., C.S.
Ohio State University, College of Nursing, Columbus, OH

Marcia Chorba, R.N., M.S.N.
Mercy Hospital School of Nursing, Pittsburgh, PA

Ann O'Rourke Cloutier, M.S.N., R.N., O.C.N.
H. Lee Moffitt Cancer Center and Research Institute,
Tampa, FL

Connie Cooper, R.N., M.S.N.
School of Nursing and Health Professions, University of
Southern Indiana, Evansville, IN

Barbara Coslow, M.S., R.N.C.
William Beaumont Hospital, Royal Oak, MI

Cheryl Terea Crenshaw, R.N., M.S.N.
North Carolina Baptist Hospital, Winston-Salem, NC

Judy Davidson, B.S.N., M.N., R.N., C.S.
Columbus College, Columbus, GA

Deborah Deierlein, M.S., R.N., A.N.P., C.S.
SUNY Medical Center at Stony Brook, Stony Brook, NY

Helen Noyes Downey, R.N., M.A., M.S.N., Ed.D.
Thomas Jefferson University, Philadelphia, PA

Diane M. Fesler, R.N., M.S.N.
College of Nursing, University of Illinois, Chicago, IL

Mary Kay Flynn, R.N., M.A., C.C.R.N.
Grand Canyon University, Phoenix, AZ

Cheryl Furchuk, R.N., B.A., M.Sc.N., Ph.D.
Victoria Hospital Research Institute, University of Western
Ontario, London, Ontario, Canada

Loree C. Francis-Felsen, Ph.D., R.N.C.
University of Florida, Gainesville, FL

Pamela R. Gaines, R.N.
Allegant-Bergan Mercy Hospital, Omaha, NE

Roberta P. Gates, R.N., M.S.N., C.S.
Darton College, Albany, GA

Andrea Georeno, B.S.N., R.N.
University of Pennsylvania Medical Center, Philadelphia, PA

Carol Goff, R.N., M.S.N.
Warren County Area Vocational-Technical School,
Warren, PA

Beth Ann Golden, R.N., M.S.N.
Broward General Medical Center, Ft. Lauderdale, FL

Joanne M. Gordon, R.N., Ph.D.
Southwest Missouri State University, Springfield, MO

Marcia Grant, R.N., D.N.Sc., F.A.A.N.
City of Hope National Medical Center, Duarte, CA

Brenda Greene, R.N., M.S.N.
Good Samaritan Hospital School of Nursing, Cincinnati, OH

Claudette J. Heddens, R.N., C.S., M.A., A.N.P.
Massachusetts General Hospital, Boston, MA

Barbara Livingston Henk, R.N., M.N.
University of California at Davis, Sacramento, CA

Susan Dawkins Herring, R.N., M.N., C.C.R.N., C.N.R.N.
Emory University Hospital, Atlanta, GA

Barbara Betz Hobbs, M.S.N., R.N.
South Dakota State University, Rapid City, SD

Dorothy Houston, R.N., M.S.Ed., M.S.N.
Shadyside Hospital School of Nursing, Pittsburgh, PA

Christopher Hubbard, Ph.D.
Northern Illinois University, De Kalb, IL

Tomasita Jacobowitz, M.S.N., R.N., C.S., N.P.
Bowman Gray School of Medicine, Winston-Salem, NC

Gail Juleff, R.N., M.S.N.
William Beaumont Hospital, Royal Oak, MI

Gloria Kersey-Matusiak, R.N., M.S.N., C.R.R.N.
Holy Family College, Philadelphia, PA

Joan Klemballa, R.N., B.S., M.A., Ph.D.
The College of West Virginia, Beckley, WV

Anita Andrews Kovalsky, R.N., B.S.N., M.N.Ed.
Community College of Allegheny County
Monroeville, PA

Helene J. Krouse, Ph.D., R.N., C.S., A.R.N.P.
University of Florida, Jacksonville, FL

Lynne Laird, R.N., M.S.
South Dakota University, Rapid City, SD

Maureen Lancellot, M.B.A., M.S.N., R.N.
University of Miami, Miami, FL

Susan K. Leach, R.N., M.S., M.B.A.
North Central Technical College, Mansfield, OH

Yolande Lockett, Ph.D., R.N., C.S., P.N.P.
Rhode Island College, Providence, RI

Pamela McKintuck, R.N., B.A.
Humber College of Applied Arts and Technology, Toronto, Ontario, Canada

Ann Butler Maher, R.N., M.S., C.N.S.C., O.N.C.
County College of Morris, Randolph, NJ

Barbara D. Manz, D.N.S., R.N.
University of Nebraska Medical Center, Omaha, NE

Marty Martin, R.N., M.S.N.
Jackson Community College, Jackson, MI

Carole Massey, M.S.N., Ed.D., R.N.
Armstrong State College, Savannah, GA

Donna Massey, R.N., M.S.N., T.N.S., T.N.C.C., C.C.R.N
Good Samaritan Hospital, Downers Grove, IL

Joan C. Masters, R.N., M.A., M.B.A.
Bellarmine College, Louisville, KY

Sandra G. Mattox, R.N.P., B.S.N., O.C.N.
University of Arkansas for Medical Sciences, Arkansas Cancer Research Center, Little Rock, AR

Marjorie Matzen, B.S.N., M.S., R.N.
Jennie Edmundson Hospital School of Nursing, Council Bluffs, IA

Karen Megivern, R.N., M.A., C.C.R.N.
University of Iowa Hospitals and Clinics, Iowa City, IA

Sharon Elaine Melberg, R.N., B.A., M.P.A.
University of California, Davis Medical Center, Sacramento, CA

Emily N. Meyer, R.N., B.S., M.S.N., C.N.O.R.
Tennessee Technological University School of Nursing, Cookeville General Hospital, Cookeville, TN

Deborah Panozzo Nelson, R.N., M.S., C.C.R.N.
EMS Nursing Education, Tinley Park, IL

Margot Nelson, R.N., Ph.D., C.S.
Augustana College, Sioux Falls, SD

Sharon O'Donoghue, M.S., R.N.
Beth Israel Hospital, Boston, MA

Netha O'Meara, R.N., B.S., M.S.N.
Wharton County Junior College, Wharton, TX

Janet Peele, R.N., M.S.N.
North Carolina Baptist Hospital, Winston-Salem, NC

Phyllis Gayden Peterson, R.N., B.A., M.N., O.C.N.
Our Lady of Holy Cross College, New Orleans, LA

Jeanette Black Pletcher, R.N., M.S., C.C.R.N.
Alta Bates Medical Center, Berkley; Critical Care Transport Division, American Medical Response West, Fremont, CA

Marilyn J. Prevatt, M.S., R.N., F.N.P.C.
Indiana Wesleyan University, Marion, IN

Margaret Prydun, R.N., M.S.N.
Alvin College, Alvin, TX

Lois Rafenski, Ed.D., R.N.
SUNY College of Technology, Farmingdale, NY

Priscilla W. Ramsey, Ph.D., R.N., C.S.
East Tennessee State University, Johnson City, TN

Donna Anne Redding, R.N., M.S.
Methodist Hospital School of Nursing, Peoria, IL

Donna Roddy, M.S.N., R.N.
Chattanooga State Technical Community College, Chattanooga, TN

Roberta Ronayne, R.N., B.Sc.N., M.Sc.
University of Ottawa, Ottawa, Ontario, Canada

Thomas Roth, Ph.D.
Henry Ford Hospital, Detroit, MI

Vincent Rudan, R.N., B.S.N., M.A., C.N.A.A.
Manhattan Eye, Ear, and Throat Hospital, New York, NY

Mary Ellen Savage, M.N., R.N., C.S.
Baylor University Medical Center, Dallas, TX

Adrienne Lois Schrader, R.N., B.S.Ed., M.S.N., C.D.E.
Tri-County Technical College, Pendleton, SC

Theresa Schumacher, R.N., M.S.N.
Good Samaritan Hospital School of Nursing, Cincinnati, OH

Lynn Simko, M.P.H., M.S.N., R.N., C.C.R.N.
Duquesne University, Pittsburgh, PA

Cheryl Smith, R.N.C., A.A.N., M.S.N.
Dekalb County Board of Health, Decatur, GA

Jennifer Smith, M.S., R.N.C.
Ohio State University Medical Center, Columbus, OH

Kathryn Stanak, R.N., B.S.N.
Felician College, Lodi, NJ

Mary Dixon Still, R.N., M.S.N., C.C.R.N.
Emory University, Atlanta, GA

Patricia Teasley, M.S.N., R.N., C.S.
Columbus College, Columbus, GA

Linda Thurby-Hay, M.S., R.N., C.S.
Henrico Doctors' Hospital, Richmond, VA

Andrea Walton, M.A., M.S.N., R.N.C.
Mid-Atlantic AIDS Education and Training Center, Medical Center of Delaware, Wilmington, DE

Barbara Wiltshire, R.N., M.S.N., C.C.R.N., C.N.S., E.T.
Henrico Doctors' Hospital, Richmond, VA

Kathryn Wirtz, R.N., M.S.N., C.C.R.N., C.N.R.N.
Northwestern Memorial Hospital, Chicago, IL

Beatrice M. Wolf, M.S.N., R.N., C.S.
Sacred Heart Medical Center, Spokane, WA

Thomas Worms, R.N., M.S.N., C.C.R.N.
Truman College, Chicago, IL

Emily Zabrocki, R.N., M.S.N., Ph.D.
Joliet Junior College, Joliet, IL

Michele K. Ziglar, R.N., M.S.N.
University of North Carolina Hospitals, Chapel Hill, NC

Helen Zimmerman, M.S.N., C.C.R.N., C.E.N.
Milton S. Hershey Medical Center, Pennsylvania State University, Hershey, PA

Publisher's Foreword

Welcome to the fifth edition of a classic nursing textbook. Books that go through multiple editions have a developmental life that must change with the times. The first three editions of this book, edited by Joan Luckmann and Karen Creason Sorensen, were called **Medical-Surgical Nursing: A Psychophysiologic Approach.** They emphasized a holistic view of the person; the theories describing connections between the mind and body in states of health and illness; and the importance of stress as a concept in understanding disease and illness—hence the subtitle. These editions were published in an era when some chose to emphasize the dichotomy between "medical model" and "nursing model" in nursing education and in textbooks. With pathbreaking comprehensiveness, the first three editions of **Medical-Surgical Nursing: A Psychophysiologic Approach** offered a synthesis of both medical and nursing models in combining detailed explanations of pathophysiology with a steady attention to nursing care of the whole person and not just the disease.

It can be argued that healthcare as practiced today is based neither on a nursing model nor on a medical model, but rather on a cost-efficiency or for-profit model. Added to the psychosocial and cultural nuances that nurses have always tried to weave into the fabric of their caring, new and sometimes alarming complexities of cost, reimbursement, resource management, and ethical quandaries affect the practice of every health professional. Many of the tasks that once were part of "direct patient care" by the nurse are now being delegated to ancillary personnel under the registered nurse's supervision. Mergers of hospitals into healthcare corporations, and diversification of these corporations into multiple delivery settings such as home care, rehabilitation, and extended care, have transformed the landscape of healthcare so that it is more accurately called a business or industry than a system.

Perhaps such consolidations may in future promise greater coordination and integration of the care delivered to an individual. For the moment, however, it seems that the task falls ever more heavily on nurses—as it always has—to help the client achieve something like a coherent passage through the maze of what the North American population experiences as managed care. More than ever, as Lewis Thomas discovered as both an eminent physician and as a patient, "the institution is held together, *glued* together, enabled to function as an organism, by the nurses and by nobody else."

Nurses need to keep the whole person in mind today no less than they did 20 years ago. But today, in addition, they must try to understand the whole spectrum of an individual's encounter with healthcare. This was recognized by Joyce Black and Esther Matassarin-Jacobs when they assumed the editorship of the fourth edition of **Medical-Surgical Nursing: A Psychophysiologic Approach.** They inaugurated features called Bridges, both to home care and to critical care, to address the nurse's need to think about the client's passage across settings. The editors and publishers have developed this focus even further in the fifth edition now in your hands, so much so that we have changed the subtitle to **Clinical Management for Continuity of Care.** Through the structure of the text headings as well as numerous innovative text features, this book shows the student how nursing care is given when the acute care hospital is no longer the normative setting. While containing the authoritative base of current medical and nursing knowledge for which this book has always been renowned, the fifth edition also reflects the realities that nurses must face in this transitional era. We intend that this and future editions of **Medical-Surgical Nursing: Clinical Management for Continuity of Care** will meet the knowledge needs of nurses as nursing itself continues to meet the challenges of healthcare in our society.

Preface

It is our conviction that a book is not a static document. Certainly, a book—bound and printed—portrays healthcare only at a given moment in time. This edition of *Medical-Surgical Nursing* is our best attempt to provide instructors and students with a guide to delivering safe and appropriate nursing care. To that end, we see this book as a "work in progress." Future editions will only improve, and we appreciate your comments, questions, and corrections to guide our future work. We can improve only with your input. We also realize that educators and students must share in the task of bringing the book to life.

PHILOSOPHY AND APPROACH

This text grows out of the belief that nurses and physicians do not compete with each other, but rather they collaborate for the benefit of the client. Nevertheless, nursing and medicine are still separate disciplines. In this text, nursing and medical content are therefore not intermingled. However, because nursing and medicine are collaborative efforts, it is often difficult for nursing students to understand one without having an understanding of the other. We therefore present thorough coverage of both nursing management and medical management.

At one time, the term *medical-surgical nursing* was almost synonymous with acute-care hospital nursing. Today, medical-surgical nursing is increasingly taking place in a variety of settings: acute-care facilities, subacute care facilities, school-based clinics, community clinics, the home, and others. To reflect that shift, this edition classifies the management of major disorders under one or more of the following headings: Emergency Care, Critical Care, Acute and Subacute Care, and Community and Self-Care. Under those headings reflecting the level of acuity of care, we present Medical Management, Nursing Management of the Medical Client, Surgical Management, and Nursing Management of the Surgical Client, as appropriate.

In this text we use the nursing process to describe nursing management, but we do not apply the nursing process to every disorder. Instead, we have elected to use the nursing process for major or prototypical disorders. Within the presentation of the nursing process for those disorders, we have developed nursing diagnoses and collaborative problems, as appropriate, with their own expected outcomes and interventions. Collaborative problems define those client problems that are not resolvable through independent nursing actions. Collaborative problems are potential complications that a client may develop because of a disorder, surgery, or nonsurgical treatment. They complete the picture of nursing care and eliminate the need to force-fit every client problem into the framework of nursing diagnosis. We have written Expected Outcomes and Implementation sections for *each* nursing diagnosis and collaborative problem because we have found from our teaching experience that students cannot easily tease apart lists of diagnoses, followed by lists of expected outcomes and interventions, and rebuild them into care plans.

ORGANIZATION

As in the fourth edition, we use a head-to-toe body systems approach in this edition. That is because this approach is more easily adapted to a variety of conceptual frameworks than is the use of a conceptual framework that would be unique to this book.

The fifth edition is divided into 18 units. The first three units are devoted to content that is applicable to all medical-surgical clients or to their significant others. The material in this first portion of the book will help the student learn to provide comprehensive care regardless of the specific diagnosis or problem. Concepts that span medical-surgical practice, such as pain, perioperative care, oncology, shock, and chronic conditions, are found in this portion of the book. The remainder of the text is divided by body systems. Most of these units begin with a "Structure and Function" chapter, followed by an "Assessment" chapter. Then, one or more "Nursing Care" chapters present the nursing care of clients with specific disorders in that body system.

Unit 1 presents an overview of nursing and healthcare today. Chapter 1 describes the "stakeholders" in healthcare delivery, because medical-surgical nurses in all areas of practice (not just managers) must be increasingly aware of how healthcare is financed. Coverage of culture, spirituality, sexuality, and the family is now condensed into a single chapter: Chapter 4. Because many medical-surgical disorders occur with greater frequency in the elderly, we have added a chapter on aging (Chapter 5) to this edition. Also new to this edition are separate chapters on acute care (Chapter 7), ambulatory care (Chapter 8), and home healthcare (Chapter 9).

Unit 2 covers health promotion, health assessment, physical examination, and diagnostic testing. The format for health assessment and physical examination that is introduced in Chapters 11 and 12 is carried through in the Assessment chapters for each body system. This structure helps the student learn one form of thorough assessment and then apply it in a focused way for clients with specific disorders. New to this edition is a separate chapter on diagnostic testing (Chapter 13).

Unit 3 looks at concepts that are common to many medical-surgical clients. Included are chapters on the cell (Chapter 14), fluid and electrolyte disorders (Chapter 15), acid-base disorders (Chapter 16), pain (Chapter 17), sleep and sensory disorders (Chapter 18), infectious disorders (Chapter 19), wound healing (Chapter 20), perioperative nursing (Chapter 21), shock (Chapter 22), and neoplastic disorders (Chapters 23 and 24).

Units 4 through 8 focus on immunologic disorders, neurologic disorders, eye and ear disorders, respiratory disorders, and cardiac disorders. New to this edition is a separate unit (Unit 9) covering peripheral vascular disorders. Units 10 through 17 cover hematologic disorders; urinary disorders; gastrointestinal disorders; liver, biliary tract, and exocrine pancreatic disorders; metabolic disorders; musculoskeletal disorders; integumentary disorders; and reproductive disorders.

Unit 18 presents care of clients with substance abuse and during emergency situations. Chapter 87 discusses the effects of substance abuse on major body systems. It also identifies populations at risk for substance abuse and presents strategies for care. Chapter 88 discusses the basic concepts of triage, maintaining the chain of custody of medicolegal evidence, and psychosocial issues in emergency nursing. It also discusses the issue of violence in the emergency department. Chapter 89 examines the management of client problems often "seen and discharged" from the emergency department, as well as the management of multiple trauma.

SPECIAL FEATURES

Bridging the gap between classroom instruction and clinical nursing care is difficult. We find that students often think, "I learned that for a test last year," and question how the material is relevant to the clinical situations that they face today. To address those questions, Joyce Black devised a method of clinical teaching in which the pathophysiology of a disorder is presented graphically and is then overlaid with corresponding clinical manifestations and treatments. The overlays allow students to visualize for themselves how changes in pathophysiology lead to various manifestations, and how a particular treatment is designed to block the progression of the pathophysiologic changes into the development of clinical manifestations. Underlying this teaching method is the assumption that it is easier to "transfer" material if you can visualize the links among pathophysiology, clinical manifestations, and interventions. The fifth edition incorporates this teaching method in special features called **Pathophysiology/Treatment Algorithms.** These features are presented on such topics as "Understanding Asthma and Its Treatment" and "Understanding Diabetes Mellitus and Its Treatment." Instructors are welcome to apply this teaching method, in which the level of pathophysiology can be adjusted to meet the needs of any curriculum, to their own programs. Any feedback would be greatly appreciated.

As another way to help students—particularly upper-level students—to integrate material that they have learned in many courses over the span of a number of years, we have included several **Case Studies** in this edition. The Case Studies, some of which are illustrated, present complex client scenarios that are typical of the situations that students will encounter in clinical practice. Following each scenario is a series of questions for students to consider.

More and more, students are recognizing the importance of providing quality nursing care to clients with backgrounds different from their own. To help them, this edition includes **Diversity in Healthcare** features on such topics as "Diabetes in Native Americans," "Coronary Artery Disease in Women," and "HIV and AIDS in Minority Populations."

Because more and more nursing care is being directed toward health promotion, in this edition we have highlighted content on risk factors and prevention in features called **Risk Factors and Levels of Prevention.**

One of the most significant recent changes in hospital nursing is the use of unlicensed assistive personnel to provide direct client care. Although we in nursing did not support the advent of using minimally trained people to provide direct client care, we recognize it as a reality that we must deal with. We also recognize that few nursing students have had the opportunity to learn how to delegate care safely. In this edition, we have therefore introduced features called **Management and Delegation.** These features discuss assessments and interventions that can, under certain circumstances, be delegated to assistive personnel. They also provide guidance about how to decide whether a particular aspect of care is safe to delegate, and they emphasize that in all cases the responsibility for client care, analysis of client data, and the safety of the client rest squarely on the nurse.

Case management is another area of ongoing change in hospital nursing, and one of the hallmarks of case management is the use of clinical pathways. Many textbooks now incorporate clinical pathways. In this book we have gone a step further by including a group of **Clinical Pathways** carefully selected by an expert in case management as among the best in use today. They are presented in Appendix D. Because the process of development of a clinical pathway is considered by many to be as important as the pathway itself, we have included discussions of these pathways with the nurses who created and use them in practice. These discussions appear as **Case Management** features in the fifth edition.

Critical Monitoring features highlight for the student those clinical manifestations that must be reported to the physician without delay. **Nursing Research** features summarize recent research and suggest implications for practice. **Care Plans** summarize the nursing diagnoses, collaborative problems, interventions and rationales, and evaluation criteria for selected disorders.

We have found that students often struggle with how to record normal findings. This edition therefore includes **Normal Physical Assessment Findings** features, which serve both to remind students of the relevant normal findings for each body system and to demonstrate how to chart those findings with clinical precision.

In addition to a separate chapter on ethics (Chapter 3), this edition, like the last, includes features called **Ethical Issues in Nursing,** many of them new to this edition and written primarily by a nurse ethicist. Each of these features presents an ethical dilemma, not necessarily for resolution but for reflection.

Bridging the distance from the theoretical to the practical, and from the hospital to the home, is essential in nursing today. To that end, we have asked practicing home care nurses to write new **Bridge to Home Healthcare** features for this edition. These features provide practical suggestions on the ever-more-critical skill of adapting medical-surgical care to the home.

Another feature, the **Bridge to Critical Care,** highlights common treatment modalities and assessments performed in critical care. Rather than attempt to discuss all of critical care nursing in these features, we have tried to impart through them a basic understanding of hospital-based critical care treatments as they are used in inpatient care. Some examples are the use of pulmonary pressure monitors, ventilators, and arterial lines.

Finally, in recognition of the need to help the client collaborate in the plan of care, we have included **Client Education Guides** with instructions in client-oriented language. Many of these Client Education Guides now include *side-by-side Spanish translations* to facilitate the teaching of Spanish-speaking clients and families.

Because of the prevalence of many diseases in the elderly, and because of the special needs of elderly clients, we have included sections called Modifications for Elderly Clients for many disorders. Because it is often difficult to differentiate normal signs of aging from pathologic conditions in the elderly, we have also included content on normal aging for each body system.

Because of the growing importance of being able to "think critically" as a nurse, we have concluded each nursing care chapter in the book with a series of **Thinking Critically** exercises. Each of these exercises presents a typical client scenario and poses some questions about what actions to take. To give the student clues about how to think through these clinical problems, each exercise includes one or more *Factors to Consider.* At the end of the book we provide a brief discussion of each of these exercises. Because there is no one right answer to a *Thinking Critically* question, these are *discussions* rather than hard-and-fast answers.

Perhaps the most immediately striking feature of the fifth edition is its use of color. In addition to the use of color throughout the book's design, we have commissioned or added full color to more than 400 illustrations for this edition.

SUPPLEMENT PACKAGE

Pocket Companion

This conveniently sized paperback handbook, fully referenced to the text, is perfect for student use in clinical settings. The alphabetical listing of diseases and disorders outlines essential content in a format that complements that of the text.

Study Guide

The *Study Guide* is designed to improve understanding of each chapter of the textbook. Learning objectives are provided for each chapter to help the student focus on critical content. In addition, *Study Guide* chapters include the following sections, as appropriate:

Learning the Language
Critical Thinking: Understanding Rationales
Thinking Clinically: Knowing What to Do and Why
Client Education: Knowing What to Teach and Why
Putting It All Together
Diagnostic Tests: Knowing Why You Do What You Do
At-a-Glance Worksheets

Included free with each copy of the *Study Guide* is a **Study Disk** containing approximately 560 NCLEX-style questions in an easy-to-use self-testing program. The program provides immediate feedback; when the user has answered a question incorrectly, the program explains why the answer is incorrect and guides the user back to specific textbook content for review.

Instructor's Manual

The *Instructor's Manual* is designed to help faculty develop lectures, assignments, and clinical assignments based on the content of the textbook. Included for each chapter are learning objectives that match those in the *Study Guide.* In addition, chapters include the following sections, as appropriate:

Facilitating Student Learning
Critical Points to Emphasize

Transparencies

More than 200 transparency masters and acetate transparencies (many in full color) provide exciting visual aids to help the instructor with classroom presentations. This transparency set, which can be used with both *Luckmann's Core Principles and Practice of Medical-Surgical Nursing* and this text, is available free of charge to adopters.

Testbank

ExaMaster, a computer testbank, is also available free to adopters. It provides approximately 2000 NCLEX-style questions from which instructors can automatically or manually generate exams. Provided for each question is the correct answer, the rationale for the correct answer (cross-referenced to the textbook page from which the question was drawn), the cognitive level according to Bloom's taxonomy, and the corresponding learning objective in the *Study Guide* and *Instructor's Manual.* These questions are also available to adopters in printed form.

ACKNOWLEDGMENTS

We have been asked several times, "Isn't a revision a lot less work than a new book?" You would think so, but it's amazing—a revision is no less work than a new book.

A project of this size certainly could not be accomplished without the collaboration of many people. First and foremost, we recognize the importance of the clinical expertise of our many contributing authors, which enables us to present a new edition that continues to be the "gold standard" in textbooks of medical-surgical nursing.

We also want to thank Margaret M. Andrews, R.N.,

Ph.D., C.T.N., who wrote the Diversity in Healthcare features; Jane Hokanson Hawks, D.N.Sc., R.N.C., and Anne M. Larson, R.N.C., Ph.D., who wrote the Case Studies; Esperanza Villanueva Joyce, Ed.D., C.N.S., R.N., who provided Spanish translations for many of the Client Education Guides; Annabelle M. Keene, M.S.N., R.N.C., who coordinated all of the assessment content and wrote the Normal Physical Assessment Findings features; Donna W. Markey, R.N., M.S.N., who wrote the Management and Delegation features; Karen S. Martin, R.N., M.S.N., F.A.A.N., who coordinated the Bridges to Home Healthcare; Barbara B. Ott, R.N., Ph.D., C.C.R.N., who wrote new Ethical Issues in Nursing features for this edition; Bonita Ann Pilon, D.S.N., R.N., C.N.A.A., who selected the Clinical Pathways that appear in Appendix D and who wrote the Case Management features; and Arlene L. Polaski, M.Ed., M.S.N., R.N., who finalized several chapters, coordinated the discussions of the Thinking Critically exercises, and reviewed proofs.

The excellent photographs used as unit-opening illustrations are the work of Lissa Clark, B.S.N., R.N., and Dan Brick, medical photographer, Biomedical Communications, University of Nebraska Medical Center, Omaha.

There are also many people at W.B. Saunders Company who have made this monumental task a "do-able" task. Thank you, Thomas Eoyang, Vice-President and Editor-in-Chief, Nursing Books, for your ongoing encouragement, help, and support. Thank you, Lee Henderson, Senior Developmental Editor; without your help and day-to-day management, we would still be behind on the deadlines. Your organization made this project move well. Thank you, Ceil Roberts and Rita Martello, for your meticulous coordination of a massive art program. Thank you, Sharon Iwanczuk, Mechanical Artist, for bringing your astute artist's eye to the development of the new illustrations for this edition. We know that the students will learn better because of your efforts. Thank you, Publication Services, for your stunning new full-color illustrations. Thank you, Gene Harris, Designer, for your fresh, appealing, full-color design. Thank you, Deborah Thorp, Copy Editing Supervisor, for finding just the right words when we couldn't, for coordinating the work of other copy editors, and for fielding countless changes, additions, and deletions with unfailing grace. Thank you, Mike Carcel, Production Manager, for keeping the book on schedule against overwhelming odds. Thank you, Rachel Hubbs and Melanie Nordlinger, for coordinating the peer reviews of the book and for handling the countless administrative tasks associated with the publication of the book. Thank you, Elizabeth Byrd, for developing and producing the book's supplement package.

Finally, we want to thank *you*—educators and students—for allowing us to join you in the teaching and learning of medical-surgical nursing. We trust that you will find the fifth edition of *Medical-Surgical Nursing: Clinical Management for Continuity of Care,* a valuable asset.

Joyce M. Black, M.S.N., R.N., C.P.S.N.

Esther Matassarin-Jacobs, Ph.D., R.N., O.C.N.

There are several people at the University of Nebraska who lifted me up and made my workload lighter while this project went on. Thank you, Dr. Lani Zimmerman, Dr. Nancy Bergstrom, Janet Cuddigan, Louise LaFramboise, and Barbara Manz. I must also thank my family for their ongoing understanding of the considerable strain on Mom's time and energy.

J.M.B.

I want to thank Frank Hicks, who helped me with the editing. I also want to thank my many colleagues at the Niehoff School of Nursing, Loyola University of Chicago, who helped in many ways they may not even have realized. They offered words of support when I was down, and they helped me stay focused.

E.M.J.

Contents

UNIT 1

Nursing and Healthcare 1

1. The Context of Medical-Surgical Nursing 3

Bonita Ann Pilon

Major Stakeholders in the U.S. Healthcare
    System....**3**
Variations in the Financing of Healthcare
    Services....**6**
The Richness and Diversity of Nursing
    Practice....**11**
Variations in Client Populations....**14**

2. Theories of Health and Illness **18**

Joyce M. Black

Theories of Illness....**20**
The Role of the Brain in Illness....**26**
Mediators of the Stress Response....**28**
Multifactorial Aspects of Chronic Disease
    Today....**29**
The Concept of Health....**36**
The Experience of Illness....**37**

3. Ethics **39**

Beverly Kopala

A Framework for the Study of Ethics....**39**
The Terminology of Ethics....**40**
Principles of Ethics....**40**
Guidelines for Ethical Nursing
    Practice....**41**
Theories to Guide Ethical Decision Making....**42**
Applying Ethical Models: The Murphy
    and Murphy Model....**43**
Research in Ethics....**45**
Ethical Concerns for Nurses....**46**
Ethical Concerns for Clients....**47**
Autonomy....**47**
Truth Telling....**48**
Resolving Ethical Problems in Nursing
    Practice....**48**

**4. Psychosocial Dimensions of Medical-Surgical
    Nursing** **50**

Ken W. Edmisson

Nursing and the Family....**50**
Cross-Cultural Nursing....**59**

Spirituality....**67**
Grief....**73**
Suffering....**74**
Sexuality....**74**

5. Aging **81**

Beverley E. Holland
Cynthia McCurren

Nursing and the Study of Aging....**81**
The Older Population....**82**
Health Promotion in the Elderly....**84**
Functional Status of the Elderly....**86**
Mental Health Disorders in the Elderly....**90**
Medication Use in the Elderly....**92**
Government Support for the Elderly....**93**
Healthcare Resources and Services for the
    Elderly....**96**
Housing Options for the Elderly....**100**
Ethical and Legal Issues Affecting the
    Elderly....**100**

6. Chronic Conditions **105**

Mary Jane Garrett

The Stages of a Chronic Condition....**105**
The Process of Adaptation....**106**
Management....**112**

7. Acute Care **120**

Joyce M. Black

History of Hospital Nursing....**120**
Acute Care Hospitals....**120**
Subacute Care....**121**
Home Healthcare....**123**
Roles and Responsibilities of Nurses in
    Hospitals....**123**
Nursing Care Delivery Systems....**124**
Ensuring Quality Healthcare Delivery....**125**
The Future of Acute Care Hospital Nursing....**131**

8. Ambulatory Care **135**

Leigh G. Anderson

Development of Ambulatory Care....**135**
Studies of Ambulatory Care Nursing....**137**
Settings for Ambulatory Care....**137**
Certification and Accreditation....**138**

9. Home Healthcare **146**

Karen S. Martin

Trends....**146**
The Specialty in Perspective....**147**
Community-Focused Philosophy....**148**
Providing Care....**151**

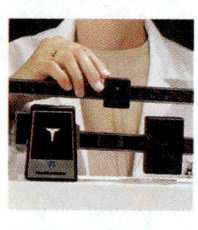

UNIT 2
Health Promotion and Health Assessment 159

10. Health Promotion 161

Esther Matassarin-Jacobs

Definitions....**161**
Understanding Health Promotion....**161**
Levels of Prevention....**165**
Risk Factors....**167**
Healthy Life-Styles....**167**
Motivating Clients....**170**
Nutrition and Exercise in Health
   Promotion....**170**
Stress Management....**171**
Health Promotion and the Older Adult....**173**
Nursing Careers in Health Promotion....**175**

11. Health Assessment 179

Annabelle M. Keene

The Health History....**179**
Guidelines for the Health History
   Interview....**185**
Components of the Health History....**186**
Organizing the Health History Interview....**206**
Recording the Health History Interview....**211**
Applying the Nursing Process to Health
   Assessment....**211**

12. Physical Examination 213

Annabelle M. Keene

The Purpose of Physical Examination....**213**
Types of Physical Examination....**213**
The Accuracy of Physical Examination....**225**
Physical Examination and the Nursing
   Process....**225**
Techniques of Physical Examination....**225**
Guidelines for Physical Examination....**231**
Preparation of the Environment....**231**
The Adult General Screening Physical
   Examination....**233**
Processing the Data....**237**
Terminating the Health Assessment....**239**
Recording Physical Examination Findings....**240**
Health Assessment, Nursing Diagnosis, and
   Nursing Process....**240**

13. Diagnostic Testing 242

Cynthia Hromek

General Nursing Management of the Client
   Undergoing Diagnostic Testing....**242**
Specificity and Sensitivity of Diagnostic
   Tests....**243**
Measurements Used to Report Laboratory Test
   Results....**243**
Laboratory Diagnostic Testing....**243**

Microbiologic Studies....**243**
Blood Studies....**245**
Urine Studies....**248**
Diagnostic Imaging....**248**
X-Ray Studies....**249**
Computed Tomography....**251**
Magnetic Resonance Imaging....**252**
Positron Emission Tomography....**253**
Ultrasonography....**253**
Angiography....**254**
Radionuclide Scanning....**254**
Endoscopy....**255**
Arthroscopy....**255**
Bronchoscopy....**256**
Gastrointestinal Endoscopy....**256**
Cytologic Studies....**257**

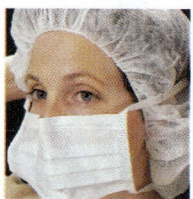

UNIT 3
Foundations for Medical-Surgical
Nursing Practice 259

14. The Cell 261

R. B. Boley
Arlene L. Polaski

Structure and Function of the Cell....**261**
Cell Replication....**261**
Cell Organelles....**262**
Tissues and Organs....**266**
Alterations in Structure and Function of the
   Cell....**266**

15. Fluid and Electrolyte Disorders 273

Bernadette White

Fluids....**273**
Fluid Balance....273
Fluid Imbalances....277
Extracellular Fluid Volume Deficit....**277**
Extracellular Fluid Volume Excess....**284**
Extracellular Fluid Volume Shift: Third-
   Spacing....**289**
Intracellular Fluid Volume Excess: Water
   Intoxication....**291**
Intracellular Fluid Deficit....**293**
Electrolytes....**293**
Action Potentials....293
Measuring Electrolytes....294
Using Collaborative Problems....295
Electrolyte Imbalances....295
Sodium Imbalances....**295**
Hyponatremia....296
Hypernatremia....300
Potassium Imbalances....**304**
Hypokalemia....305

Hyperkalemia....**310**
Calcium and Phosphorus Imbalances....**314**
Hypocalcemia and Hypophosphatemia....**315**
Hypercalcemia....**320**
Hyperphosphatemia....**322**
Magnesium Imbalances....**322**
Hypomagnesemia....**323**
Hypermagnesemia....**324**

16. Acid-Base Disorders 328

Margie J. Hansen

Regulation of Acid-Base Balance....**328**
Disorders of Acid-Base Balance....**333**

17. Pain 342

Esther Matassarin-Jacobs

Definition of Pain....**342**
The Process of Pain....**342**
*Therapeutic Implications of the Pain
  Process*....**350**
Theories of Pain....**350**
Types of Pain....**351**
Pathologic Pain Syndromes....**354**
Assessment....**360**
Nursing Intervention....**365**

18. Sleep and Sensory Disorders 397

Marlene Reimer

Sleep and Sleep Pattern Disturbances....**397**
Chronobiology....**397**
Physiology of Sleep and Arousal....**398**
Sleep Disorders....**400**
Dyssomnias....**400**
Intrinsic Sleep Disorders....**400**
Extrinsic Sleep Disorders....**402**
Circadian Rhythm Sleep Disorders....**403**
Parasomnias....**403**
Arousal Disorders....**403**
Sleep-Wake Transition Disorders....**403**
Parasomnias Associated with REM Sleep....**403**
Other Parasomnias....**403**
Sleep Disorders Associated with Medical and
  Psychological Disorders....**404**
Neurotransmitter Imbalances....**404**
Head Injury....**404**
Hormonal Imbalances....**404**
Respiratory Disorders....**405**
Cardiovascular Disorders....**405**
Gastrointestinal Disorders....**405**
Other Disorders....**405**
Hospital-Acquired Sleep Disturbances....**406**
Sleep Onset Difficulty....**406**
Sleep Maintenance Disturbance....**406**
Early-Morning Wakening....**406**
Sleep Deprivation....**406**
Diagnostic Assessment....**407**
Nursing Management....**407**
Sensory Disturbances....**409**

Classification....**409**
Sensory Overload....**409**
Sensory Deprivation....**409**
Prevention....**410**

19. Infectious Disorders 413

Carol Sharkey

The Process of Infection....**413**
Agent....**413**
Environment....**414**
Host....**415**
The Risks of Hospitalization....**417**
Urinary Tract Infections....**418**
Surgical Wound Infections....**418**
Pneumonia....**418**
*Device-Associated Infections and
  Bacteremias*....**419**
Other Nosocomial Infections....**419**
Preventing and Controlling Infection....**419**
Immunization Programs....**420**
Infection Control Programs in Hospitals....**422**

20. Wound Healing... 426

Joyce M. Black

The Body's Defense Mechanisms....**426**
Normal Wound Healing....**426**
Phases of Wound Healing....**427**
Wound Healing Intention....**432**
Nutrition and Wound Healing....**433**
Management of the Client with
  Inflammation....**434**
Management of the Client with Chronic
  Inflammation....**437**
Management of the Client with Incisions....**437**
Management of the Client with Open
  Wounds....**437**
Disorders of Wound Healing....**443**
Delayed Wound Healing....**443**
Wound Infection....**445**
Wound Disruption....**446**
Altered Collagen Synthesis....**446**

21. Perioperative Nursing................................. 449

Ruth Plotkin Shumaker

The Philosophy and Practice of Perioperative
  Nursing....**449**
Basic Concepts of Perioperative Nursing....**450**
Preoperative Nursing....**452**
Intraoperative Nursing....**466**
Postoperative Nursing....**480**

22. Shock... 497

Louise Nelson LaFramboise

Etiology and Risk Factors....**497**
Hypovolemic Shock....**498**
Cardiogenic Shock....**499**
Distributive Shock....**500**
Stages of Shock....**502**
Systemic Effects of Shock....**503**

Clinical Manifestations and Diagnostic
    Findings....**510**
General Clinical Manifestations of Shock....**510**
*Clinical Manifestations of Specific Types of
    Shock*....**512**
Emergency Care....**514**
Community and Self-Care....**528**
Multiple Organ System Failure/Systemic
    Inflammatory Response Syndrome....**528**

23. Basic Concepts of Neoplastic Disorders....... 533

Joann Petty

Overview....**533**
The Terminology of Cancer....**533**
The Challenge of Cancer Nursing....**533**
Epidemiology....**534**
Incidence....**534**
Mortality....**535**
Survival....**535**
Trends....**535**
Pathogenesis....**537**
Etiology....**539**
Predisposing Factors....**540**
Impact.....**541**
Research....**544**
Prevention and Assessment....**544**
Characteristics of Normal Cells....**544**
Growth of Cancer Cells....**545**
*Neoplastic Cell Division and
    Differentiation*....**546**
Growth of Malignant Tumors....**546**
Classification of Neoplasms....**548**
Prevention....**551**
Diagnosis....**552**

24. Treatment Modalities for Neoplastic
Disorders 562

Joann Petty

Psychosocial Aspects of Cancer....**562**
Phases of the Cancer Continuum....**562**
Diagnosis and Treatment....**562**
Survivorship....**564**
Recurrent Disease and Palliation....**566**
Terminal Illness....**566**
Treatment and Nursing Care of Clients with
    Cancer....**568**
Goals of Intervention....**568**
Surgery....**568**
Diagnostic Surgery....**569**
Staging Exploratory Surgery....**569**
Curative Surgery....**569**
Palliative Surgery....**569**
Reconstructive Surgery....**569**
Preventive Surgery....**570**
Radiation Therapy....**570**
How Radiation Therapy Works....**570**
Types of Radiation Therapy....**571**
Side Effects of Radiation Therapy....**572**
The Role of Radiation in Cancer Research....**572**
Radiation Safety....**572**
Chemotherapy....**573**

Drug Development and Clinical Trials....**573**
Objective of Chemotherapy....**575**
How Chemotherapy Works....**575**
Classification of Chemotherapy....**576**
Administration of Chemotherapy....**576**
Toxic Effects of Chemotherapy....**580**
Nursing Management of the Client Undergoing
    Chemotherapy....**584**
Bone Marrow Transplantation....**584**
Biologic Response Modifiers....**585**
Second Malignancies....**587**
Ethical Issues....**588**

UNIT 4
Immunologic Disorders 591

25. Structure and Function of the Immune
System 593

R. B. Boley
Arlene L. Polaski

Resistance....**593**
Surface Defenses....**593**
Inflammation....**594**
The Acute Phase Response....**594**
The Natural Killer Cell System....**594**
Immunity....**595**
Categories of Acquired Immunity....**595**
Anatomy of the Immune System....**595**
The Primary Immune Response and the Immune
    Cascade....**598**
The Secondary Immune Response....**599**
Immunoglobulins....**599**
Monoclonal Antibodies....**601**
Complement and Amplification of Antibody
    Function....**601**
T Lymphocytes and Cell-Mediated
    Immunity....**602**
The Role of Cytokines....**603**
Factors Affecting Immunity....**604**

26. Assessment of Clients with Immune
Disorders 607

Esther Matassarin-Jacobs

History....**607**
Biographical and Demographic Data....**607**
Current Symptoms....**607**
Past Health History....**608**
Family Health History....**608**
Psychosocial History....**608**
Review of Systems....**609**
Physical Examination....**609**

*Inspection....*609
*Palpation....*610
Diagnostic Tests....611
*Acquired Immunodeficiency Syndrome (AIDS) Tests....*611
*Tests of Immunologic Status....*611
*Tests of Bone Marrow and Lymphatics....*611
*Lymphangiography....*611
*Tests for Allergies and Autoimmune Disorders....*612

27. Nursing Care of Clients with Altered Immune Systems 614

Peter J. Ungvarski
Esther Matassarin-Jacobs

Human Immunodeficiency Virus Infection....614
Hypersensitivity Disorders....636
Organ Transplantation....641

28. Nursing Care of Clients with Connective Tissue Disorders 653

Cleda L. Meyer

Autoimmunity....653
Rheumatoid Arthritis....655
Systemic Lupus Erythematosus....674
Progressive Systemic Sclerosis....677
Ankylosing Spondylitis....678
Sjögren's Syndrome....678
Fibromyalgia Syndrome....679
Polymyositis and Dermatomyositis....679
Vasculitis....680
Reiter's Syndrome....680
Polymyalgia Rheumatica and Cranial Arteritis....680
Mixed Connective Tissue Disease....681
Lyme Disease....681
Secondary Arthritis....681
*Whipple's Disease....*681
*Other Disorders Causing Arthritis....*681

UNIT 5

Neurologic Disorders 683
Unit Editor: Bernadette White

29. Structure and Function of the Nervous System 685

Bernadette White

Cells of the Nervous System....685
*Structure....*685
*Neurons....*685

*Neuroglia....*687
Function and Impulse Conduction....687
*Resting Potential....*687
*Nerve Impulse....*688
*Refractory Period....*688
*Myelin....*689
*Saltatory Conduction....*690
*Receptors....*690
Structural Divisions of the Nervous System....690
*Central Nervous System....*690
*Peripheral Nervous System....*701
Effects of Injury and Aging on the Nervous System....705
*Regeneration....*705
*Changes Related to Aging....*705

30. Assessment of Clients with Neurologic Disorders 709

Mary Vorder Bruegge

History....709
*Biographical and Demographic Data....*709
*Past Health History....*714
*Family Health History....*714
*Psychosocial History....*714
*Review of Systems....*715
Physical Examination....715
*Vital Signs....*715
*Mental Status....*715
*Head, Neck, and Back....*718
*Cranial Nerves....*718
*Motor System....*721
*Sensory Function....*723
*Reflex Activity....*724
*Autonomic Nervous System....*728
*Functional Assessment....*729
*Clinical Applications....*729
Diagnostic Tests....730
*Noninvasive Tests of Structure....*730
*Invasive Tests of Structure....*733
*Noninvasive Tests of Function....*738
*Invasive Tests of Function....*740

31. Nursing Care of Comatose or Confused Clients 743

Sally Strong Schnell

*Disorders of Consciousness....*743
*Organ Donation....*753
*Confusional States....*763

32. Nursing Care of Clients with Cerebrovascular Disorders 771

Sally Strong Schnell

Increased Intracranial Pressure....771
Cerebrovascular Accident....784
Transient Ischemic Attacks....808
Intracranial Hemorrhage....812
Other Cerebrovascular Disorders....816

Arteriovenous Malformations....**816**
Lesions of Cerebral Veins and Sinuses....**816**
Headaches....**817**

Migraine Headaches....**818**
Classic or Typical Migraines....**819**
Atypical, or Common Migraines....**819**

Cluster Headaches....**819**
Tension Headaches (Muscle Contraction
   Headaches)....**820**
Head Pain Related to Other Structures....**820**
Traumatic Brain Injury....**820**
Secondary Brain Injuries....**830**

Epidural Hematoma....**830**
Subdural Hematoma....**830**
Acute and Subacute Subdural Hematoma....**831**
Chronic Subdural Hematoma....**831**

Intracerebral Hematoma....**831**

33. Nursing Care of Clients with Cerebral Disorders **834**

Sally Strong Schnell

Seizure Disorders....**834**
Epilepsy....**834**
Seizures....**842**
Status Epilepticus....**843**
Intracranial Tumors....**843**
Neurologic Infections....**856**
Bacterial and Pyogenic Infections....**856**
Bacterial Meningitis....**856**
Bacteria Toxins....**857**
Brain Abscess....**857**
Viral Infections....**858**
Viral Meningitis....**859**
Viral Encephalitis....**859**
Acute Anterior Poliomyelitis....**860**
Fungal Infections....**860**
Bulbar Disorders....**861**

34. Nursing Care of Clients with Degenerative Neurologic Disorders **863**

Judith Ozuna

Alzheimer's Disease....**863**
Creutzfeldt-Jakob Disease....**872**
Multiple Sclerosis....**873**
Guillain-Barré Syndrome....**877**
Parkinson's Disease....**878**
Huntington's Disease....**883**
Myasthenia Gravis....**883**
Eaton-Lambert Syndrome....**886**
Amyotrophic Lateral Sclerosis....**886**

35. Nursing Care of Clients with Disorders of the Spinal Cord, Peripheral Nerves, and Cranial Nerves **890**

Paula Carson

Disorders of the Spinal Cord....**890**
Disorders of the Peripheral Nerves....**926**
Disorders of the Cranial Nerves....**929**

UNIT 6
Eye and Ear Disorders **933**

36. Eye Disorders **935**

Linda A. Vader

Structure and Function of the Eye....**935**
Structure of the Eye....**935**
Structure of the Ocular Adnexa....**935**
Structure of the Internal Eye....**936**
Function of the Eye....**939**
Effects of Aging on the Eye....**939**
Assessment of Clients with Eye Disorders....**940**
History....**941**
Biographical and Demographic Data....**941**
Current Symptoms....**941**
Past Health History....**942**
Family Health History....**942**
Psychosocial History....**942**
Review of Systems....**943**
Physical Examination....**943**
External Eye Examination....**943**
Internal Eye Examination....**947**
Diagnostic Tests....**950**
Nursing Care of Clients with Eye Disorders....**952**
Glaucoma....**952**
Cataracts....**958**
Retinal Disorders....**961**
Retinal Detachment....**961**
Diabetic Retinopathy....**964**
Retinitis Pigmentosa....**965**
Age-Related Macular Degeneration....**965**
Retinal Artery Occlusion....**966**
Corneal Disorders....**966**
Corneal Dystrophies....**966**
Keratoconus....**968**
Sympathetic Ophthalmia....**970**
Tumors of the Eye....**970**
Malignant Ocular Tumors....**970**
Benign Lid Tumors....**971**
Malignant Lid Tumors....**971**
Eyelid, Lacrimal, and Conjunctival
   Disorders....**972**
Dacryocystitis....**972**
Hordeolum....**972**
Chalazion....**972**
Blepharitis....**973**
Conjunctivitis....**973**

*Episcleritis....***973**
*Entropion....***974**
*Ectropion....***974**
*Ptosis....***974**
*Lagophthalmos....***974**
*Blinking Disorders....***974**
*Dry Eye Syndrome....***974**
Refractive Disorders....**975**
*Myopia....***975**
*Hyperopia....***976**
*Astigmatism....***976**
Surgical Management of Refractive
*Disorders....***976**
Ocular Manifestations of Systemic
Disorders....**976**
*Endocrine Disorders....***976**
Rheumatoid and Connective Tissue
*Disorders....***977**
*Neurologic Disorders....***977**
*Circulatory Disorders....***977**
*Immunologic Disorders....***977**
*Lyme Disease....***978**

Hearing Impairment....**1001**
Otosclerosis....**1002**
Acoustic Neuroma....**1003**
Tinnitus (Head Noises)....**1003**
*Otalgia....***1003**
Ear Infections....**1003**
*Otitis Externa....***1003**
*Tympanic Membrane Infection....***1005**
*Otitis Media....***1005**
*Mastoiditis....***1006**
Ear Obstructions....**1006**
*Cerumen Impaction....***1006**
*Foreign Bodies....***1007**
Ear Trauma....**1007**
External Ear Trauma....**1007**
Tympanic Membrane Trauma....**1007**
Eustachian Tube Disorders....**1009**
Ear Masses....**1009**
*Cholesteatoma....***1009**
*Other Masses....***1009**
Balance Disorders....**1010**

37. Ear Disorders **980**

Joyce M. Black

Structure and Function of the Ear....**980**
*Structure of the Temporal Bone....***980**
*Structure of the External Ear....***980**
External Auditory Canal or Ear Canal....**981**
Tympanic Membrane....**981**
Function of the Temporal Bone and External
*Ear....***981**
Sound Wave Conduction....**981**
Wax Production....**982**
*Structure of the Middle Ear....***982**
Ossicles....**982**
Windows....**982**
Eustachian Tubes....**982**
*Mastoid Bone....***983**
Function of the Middle Ear....**983**
*Structure of the Inner Ear (Labyrinth)....***983**
Function of the Inner Ear....**984**
Hearing....**984**
Balance....**984**
Assessment of the Ear....**985**
History....**985**
*Current Symptoms....***985**
*Past Health History....***985**
*Family Health History....***986**
*Psychosocial History....***986**
*Review of Systems....***987**
Physical Examination....**987**
*Inspection and Palpation....***987**
*Tests for Auditory Acuity....***988**
*Tests for Vestibular Acuity....***989**
Diagnostic Tests....**989**
*Tests for Structure....***989**
*Tests for Function....***991**
*Laboratory Tests....***992**
Disorders of the Ear....**993**

UNIT 7
Respiratory Disorders...................................... **1019**

**38. Structure and Function of the
Respiratory System** **1021**

Joyce M. Black

*The Airways....***1021**
Upper Airway....**1022**
*Structure....***1022**
*Function....***1023**
Lower Airway....**1024**
*Structure....***1024**
*Function....***1025**
Thorax, Diaphragm, and Pleura....**1026**
*Structure....***1026**
*Function....***1027**
*The Lungs and Alveoli....***1027**
*Structure....***1027**
*Function....***1029**
Effects of Aging....**1034**

**39. Assessment of Clients with
Respiratory Disorders**............................. **1035**

Amy Verst

General Respiratory Assessment....**1035**
*History....***1035**

Biographical and Demographic Data....**1035**
Current Symptoms....**1035**
Past Health History....**1038**
Family Health History....**1039**
Psychosocial History....**1039**
Review of Systems....**1040**
Physical Examination....**1040**
Inspection....**1040**
Palpation....**1043**
Percussion....**1044**
Auscultation....**1045**
Assessment of Nose, Pharynx, and
    Sinuses....**1047**
History....**1047**
Current Symptoms....**1047**
Past Health History....**1048**
Physical Examination....**1048**
Nose....**1049**
Nasopharynx....**1050**
Paranasal Sinuses....**1050**
Smell....**1050**
Diagnostic Tests....**1050**
Tests to Evaluate Respiratory Function....**1051**
Tests to Evaluate Anatomic Structures....**1058**
Specimen Recovery and Analysis....**1062**

**40. Nursing Care of Clients with Upper
    Airway Disorders**.................................. **1067**

Barbara Sigler

Tracheostomy....**1067**
Hemorrhagic, Infectious, and Inflammatory
    Disorders....**1076**
Epistaxis....**1076**
Sinusitis....**1077**
Pharyngitis....**1079**
Tonsillitis....**1079**
Chronic Tonsillitis....**1080**
Peritonsillar Abscess....**1080**
Rhinitis....**1080**
Laryngitis....**1081**
Diphtheria....**1081**
Neoplastic Disorders....**1082**
Benign Tumors of the Larynx....**1082**
Cancer of the Larynx....**1082**
Obstructions of the Upper Airway....**1100**
Acute Airway Obstruction....**1100**
Chronic Airway Obstruction....**1101**

**41. Nursing Care of Clients with Disorders
    of the Lower Airways and Pulmonary
    Vessels** **1105**

Sherill Nones Cronin

Disorders of the Lower Airways....**1105**
Asthma....**1105**
Chronic Obstructive Pulmonary Disease....**1111**
Tracheobronchitis....**1124**
Bronchiectasis....**1125**
Disorders of the Pulmonary Vasculature....**1126**
Pulmonary Embolism....**1126**
Pulmonary Hypertension....**1129**

**42. Nursing Care of Clients with Disorders
    of the Lung Parenchyma and Pleura**.......... **1133**

Sherill Nones Cronin

Atelectasis....**1133**
Infectious Disorders....**1133**
Influenza....**1133**
Pneumonia....**1134**
Lung Abscess....**1138**
Pulmonary Tuberculosis....**1139**
Extrapulmonary Tuberculosis....**1144**
Nontuberculous Mycobacteria Infection....**1145**
Fungal Pulmonary Infections....**1146**
Restrictive Lung Disorders....**1147**
Cystic Fibrosis....**1148**
Interstitial Lung Disease....**1149**
Sarcoidosis....**1149**
Occupational Lung Diseases....**1150**
Neoplastic Lung Disorders....**1151**
Malignant Lung Tumors....**1151**
Benign Lung Tumors....**1166**
Disorders of the Pleura and Pleural Space....**1166**
Pleural Pain....**1166**
Pleural Effusion....**1166**
Primary Pleural Effusion....**1167**
Recurrent Pleural Effusion....**1167**
Bronchopleural Fistula....**1167**
Metastatic Pleural Tumors....**1167**
Disorders of the Diaphragm....**1168**
Subdiaphragmatic Abscess....**1168**
Diaphragmatic Paralysis....**1168**
Acute Pulmonary Disorders....**1169**
Noncardiogenic Pulmonary Edema....**1169**
Acute Respiratory Failure....**1169**
Adult Respiratory Distress Syndrome....**1170**

UNIT 8
Cardiac Disorders **1189**

43. Structure and Function of the Heart.......... **1191**

Barbara B. Ott

The Layers of the Heart....**1191**
The Chambers of the Heart....**1191**
The Pericardium....**1193**
The Cardiac Valves....**1193**
The Cardiac Blood Supply....**1194**
Electrophysiologic Properties of the Heart....**1195**
The Cardiac Conduction System....**1197**
The Cardiac Cycle....**1198**
Mechanical Properties of the Heart....**1199**
Regulation of Cardiac Function and Blood
    Pressure....**1202**
Effects of Aging....**1204**

44. Assessment of Clients with Cardiac Disorders 1205

Pamela Shumate

History....**1205**
Chief Complaint....**1205**
*Chest Pain....**1205***
Shortness of Breath....**1206**
Fatigue....**1206**
Palpitations....**1207**
Syncope....**1207**
Weight Gain....**1207**
Past Health History....**1207**
*Childhood and Infectious Diseases....**1207***
*Major Illnesses and Hospitalizations....**1207***
*Medications....**1207***
*Psychosocial History....**1210***
*Review of Systems....**1210***
Physical Examination....**1211**
*General Appearance....**1211***
*Level of Consciousness....**1211***
*Blood Pressure....**1211***
Postural Blood Pressure....**1211**
Paradoxical Blood Pressure (Pulsus Paradoxus)....**1211**
*Pulse....**1212***
*Edema....**1212***
Respirations....**1212**
*Head and Neck....**1212***
Examination of Neck Veins....**1212**
Examination of Carotid Arteries....**1213**
*Chest....**1213***
Inspection and Palpation of the Precordium....**1213**
Auscultation of Heart Sounds....**1214**
Examination of the Lungs....**1217**
*Abdomen....**1217***
Inspection and Palpation....**1217**
Auscultation....**1217**
Diagnostic Tests....**1217**
*Laboratory Tests....**1219***
Complete Blood Cell Count....**1219**
Cardiac Enzymes....**1219**
Blood Coagulation Tests....**1219**
Serum Lipids....**1220**
Serum Electrolytes....**1220**
Blood Urea Nitrogen....**1220**
Blood Glucose....**1220**
*Electrocardiogram....**1220***
Continuous Electrocardiogram Monitoring....**1221**
Electrocardiogram Tracings....**1222**
Electrocardiogram Variations....**1223**
*The 12-Lead Electrocardiogram....**1223***
*Signal-Averaged Electrocardiogram....**1224***
*Holter Monitoring....**1224***
*Exercise Electrocardiogram (Stress Testing)....**1225***
Electrophysiologic Studies....**1227**
Chest X-Ray Studies....**1227**
Magnetic Resonance Imaging....**1227**
Positron Emission Tomography....**1228**
Echocardiography....**1228**

Transesophageal Echocardiography....**1228**
Phonocardiography....**1229**
Myocardial Scintigraphy....**1229**
*Thallium 201 Scintigraphy....**1229***
*Dipyridamole Thallium 201 Test....**1230***
*Technetium 99m Ventriculography (Multiple Gated Acquisition Scanning)....**1230***
*First-Pass Cardiac Study....**1230***
Cardiac Catheterization....**1230**
*Right-Sided Catheterization....**1231***
*Left-Sided Catheterization....**1231***
*Complications....**1231***
Angiography....**1232**
Hemodynamic Studies....**1233**
*Central Venous Pressure....**1233***
*Pulmonary Artery Pressure....**1234***
*Cardiac Output Measurement....**1236***
*Intra-Arterial Pressure Monitoring....**1236***

45. Nursing Care of Clients with Disorders of Cardiac Function 1238

Peggy Gerard
Kathleen A. Ringel

Coronary Artery Disease....**1238**
Angina Pectoris....**1251**
Acute Myocardial Infarction....**1258**
Heart Failure....**1276**

46. Nursing Care of Clients with Disorders of Cardiac Rhythm.................................. 1295

Kathleen A. Ringel
Peggy Gerard

*Dysrhythmias....**1295***
*Atrial Dysrhythmias....**1297***
*Sinus Tachycardia....**1297***
*Sinus Bradycardia....**1298***
*Sinus Dysrhythmia....**1299***
Disturbances in Conduction: Sinoatrial Node Conduction Defects....**1299**
Disturbances in Impulse Generation....**1300**
*Premature Atrial Contractions....**1300***
*Paroxysmal Atrial Tachycardia....**1301***
*Atrial Flutter....**1301***
*Atrial Fibrillation....**1301***
*Atrioventricular Junctional Dysrhythmias....**1302***
Disturbances in Automaticity....**1302**
*Premature Junctional Contractions....**1302***
*Paroxysmal Junctional Tachycardia....**1302***
Disturbances in Conduction....**1303**
*First-Degree Atrioventricular Block....**1303***
*Second-Degree Atrioventricular Block....**1304***
*Third-Degree Atrioventricular Block....**1304***
*Ventricular Dysrhythmias....**1304***
Disturbances in Automaticity....**1305**
*Premature Ventricular Contractions....**1305***
*Ventricular Tachycardia....**1305***
*Ventricular Fibrillation....**1305***
*Torsades de Pointes....**1309***
*Preexcitation Syndromes....**1309***
Disturbances in Conduction....**1310**
*Bundle Branch Block....**1310***
*Ventricular Asystole....**1310***

Pulseless Electrical Activity....**1310**
Management of Life-Threatening
    Dysrhythmias....**1310**

47. Nursing Care of Clients with Disorders of Cardiac Structure 1327

Barbara B. Ott

Infectious Disorders....**1327**
Rheumatic Fever....**1327**
Infective Endocarditis....**1331**
Myocarditis....**1334**
Pericarditis....**1335**
Acute Pericarditis....**1335**
Acute Pericarditis with Effusion....**1336**
Chronic Constrictive Pericarditis....**1337**
Cardiac Tamponade....**1337**
Cardiomyopathy and Valvular Disease....**1338**
Cardiomyopathy....**1338**
Dilated Cardiomyopathy....**1339**
Hypertrophic Cardiomyopathy....**1340**
Restrictive Cardiomyopathy....**1341**
Valvular Heart Disease....**1342**
Mitral Valve Disease....**1342**
Aortic Valve Disease....**1347**
Tricuspid and Pulmonic Valve Disease....**1349**
*Nursing Management of the Client with Valvular
    Heart Disease*....**1349**
Congenital Disorders....**1350**
Cardiac Surgery....**1350**

UNIT 9
Peripheral Vascular Disorders 1367

48. Structure and Function of the Peripheral Vascular System 1369

Joyce M. Black

Components of the Vascular System....**1369**
Structure of the Blood Vessels....**1369**
Function of the Blood Vessels....**1372**
Blood Flow Through the Large Arteries....**1372**
Blood Flow Through the Tissues....**1374**
The Role of the Lymphatic System....**1376**
The Effects of Aging on the Vascular System....**1376**
Effects of Aging on the Lymphatic System....**1376**
Introduction to Disorders of the Vascular
    System....**1376**

49. Assessment of Clients with Peripheral Vascular Disorders 1377

Barbara Harrison

History....**1377**

Biographical and Demographic Data....**1377**
Current Symptoms....**1377**
Past Health History....**1378**
Family Health History....**1379**
Psychosocial History....**1379**
Physical Examination....**1379**
Inspection....**1379**
Palpation....**1381**
Auscultation....**1382**
Diagnostic Tests....**1383**
Noninvasive Techniques....**1383**
Invasive Techniques....**1384**

50. Nursing Care of Clients with Peripheral Vascular Disorders 1387

Barbara Harrison

Hypertension....**1387**
Syncope....**1404**
Arterial Disorders....**1405**
Chronic Arterial Occlusion....**1405**
Acute Arterial Occlusion....**1424**
Arterial Ulcers....**1424**
Aneurysms....**1425**
Classification of Aneurysms....**1425**
Abdominal Aortic Aneurysms....**1425**
Aortic Dissection....**1428**
Thoracic Aortic Aneurysms....**1429**
Peripheral Aneurysms....**1430**
Subclavian Steal Syndrome....**1430**
Thoracic Outlet Syndromes....**1430**
Vasculitis....**1430**
Thromboangiitis Obliterans (Buerger's
    Disease)....**1430**
Raynaud's Syndrome....**1431**
Venous Disorders....**1432**
Acute Venous Disorders....**1432**
Chronic Venous Insufficiency....**1436**
Venous Stasis Ulceration....**1436**
Varicose Veins....**1438**
Lymphatic Disorders....**1439**
Lymphedema....**1439**
Lymphadenitis....**1441**
Acute Lymphadenitis....**1441**
Chronic Lymphadenitis....**1441**

UNIT 10
Hematologic Disorders 1445

51. Structure and Function of the Hematologic System 1447

R. B. Boley
Arlene L. Polaski

Characteristics of Blood....**1447**

Hematopoiesis: Formation of Blood Cells....**1447**
Blood Groups and Blood Typing....**1455**
Hemostasis....**1456**
Abnormalities of the Hematologic System....**1458**
Effects of Aging....**1459**

52. Assessment of Clients with Hematologic Disorders 1461

Esther Matassarin-Jacobs

History....**1461**
*Biographical and Demographic Data....**1461***
*Chief Complaint....**1461***
*Past Health History....**1461***
*Family Health History....**1462***
*Psychosocial History **1462***
*Review of Systems....**1462***
Physical Examination....**1463**
Diagnostic Tests....**1463**

53. Nursing Care of Clients with Hematologic Disorders 1469

Esther Matassarin-Jacobs

Disorders Affecting Red Blood Cells....**1469**
*The Anemias....**1469***
*Acquired Anemias....**1471***
*Congenital Anemias....**1481***
*Polycythemias....**1485***
Disorders Affecting White Blood Cells....**1486**
*The Leukemias....**1487***
*Agranulocytosis....**1497***
*Multiple Myeloma....**1498***
Disorders of the Lymphoid System....**1500**
*Hodgkin's Disease....**1500***
*Non-Hodgkin's Lymphoma....**1503***
*Infectious Mononucleosis....**1503***
*Splenic Rupture and Hypersplenism....**1504***
Disorders of Platelets and Clotting Factors....**1506**
*Hemorrhagic Disorders....**1506***
*Purpura....**1506***
*Coagulation Disorders....**1509***
Congenital Disorders....**1512**
*Sickle Cell Anemia and Sickle Cell Trait....**1512***
*The Hemophilias....**1515***
Blood Transfusions....**1518**
*Preparing for Transfusion....**1518***
*Beginning the Transfusion....**1525***
*Monitoring During the Transfusion....**1527***
*Delayed Transfusion Complications....**1527***

UNIT 11
Urinary Disorders 1533

54. Structure and Function of the Urinary System 1535

Esther Matassarin-Jacobs

Structure....**1535**
*Kidneys....**1535***
*Ureters....**1537***
*Bladder....**1538***
*Urethra and Meatus....**1539***
Function....**1539**
*Kidneys....**1540***
*Ureters....**1544***
*Bladder....**1544***
*Urethra and Meatus....**1545***
Effects of Aging....**1545**

55. Assessment of Clients with Urinary Disorders 1547

Esther Matassarin-Jacobs

History....**1547**
*Biographical and Demographic Data....**1547***
*Current Manifestations....**1547***
*Past Health History....**1549***
*Family Health History....**1550***
*Review of Systems....**1552***
Physical Examination....**1552**
*Urinary Tract Organs....**1552***
*Related Body Systems....**1553***
Diagnostic Tests....**1555**
*Laboratory Tests....**1555***
*Radiologic Studies....**1562***
*Urodynamic Studies....**1565***
*Direct Visualization....**1567***

56. Nursing Care of Clients with Disorders of the Ureters, Bladder, and Urethra 1571

Esther Matassarin-Jacobs

Infectious and Inflammatory Disorders....**1571**
*Urinary Tract Infection (Cystitis)....**1571***
*Interstitial Cystitis....**1579***
*Urosepsis....**1581***
*Urethritis....**1581***
*Ureteritis....**1581***
*Genitourinary Tuberculosis....**1581***
Obstructive Disorders....**1582**
*Bladder Neoplasms....**1582***
*Ureteral Tumors....**1595***
*Urinary Calculi....**1595***
*Urinary Reflux....**1599***
Voiding Disorders....**1600**
*Urinary Retention....**1600***
*Urinary Incontinence....**1604***
*Neurogenic Bladder Dysfunction....**1612***
Traumatic Disorders....**1619**

Bladder Trauma....**1619**
Urethral Trauma....**1620**
Ureteral Trauma....**1620**
Congenital Anomalies....**1620**
Congenital Anomalies of the Bladder....**1620**
Congenital Anomalies of the Urethra....**1620**
Congenital Anomalies of the Ureters....**1620**
Ectopic Ureter....**1620**
Duplicate Ureters....**1621**
Abnormal Dilation of the Ureter
　(Megaureter)....**1621**
Congenital Ureteropelvic Obstruction....**1621**

57. Nursing Care of Clients with Renal Disorders

**57. Nursing Care of Clients with Renal
Disorders** **1625**

Esther Matassarin-Jacobs

Renal Disorders Associated with Extrarenal
　Conditions and Nephrotoxins....**1625**
Extrarenal Conditions....**1625**
Diabetes Mellitus....**1625**
Hypertension....**1626**
Hypotension....**1626**
Cardiovascular Disease....**1626**
Peripheral Vascular Disease....**1626**
Sepsis....**1626**
Pregnancy....**1626**
Nephrotoxins....**1627**
Acquired Disorders....**1628**
Pyelonephritis....**1628**
Acute Glomerulonephritis....**1630**
Chronic Glomerulonephritis....**1632**
Tubulointerstitial Disease....**1633**
Membranoproliferative
　Glomerulonephritis....**1633**
Rapidly Progressive Glomerulonephritis....**1634**
Idiopathic Membranous
　Glomerulonephritis....**1634**
IgA Nephropathy....**1634**
Lipoid Nephrosis....**1634**
Focal Glomerular Sclerosis....**1634**
Nephrotic Syndrome....**1634**
Hydronephrosis....**1636**
Uremic Syndrome....**1636**
Acute Renal Failure....**1636**
Renal Transplantation....**1660**
Renal Calculi....**1665**
Renal Cancer....**1671**
Renal Candidiasis....**1673**
Renal Abscess....**1673**
Perinephric Abscess....**1674**
Renal Trauma....**1674**
Renal Tuberculosis....**1675**
Renal Vascular Abnormalities....**1676**
Renal Artery Disease....**1676**
Renal Vein Disease....**1677**
Congenital Disorders....**1677**
Anomalies Involving Kidney Form and
　Size....**1677**
Anomalies Involving Cystic Disease....**1678**
Polycystic Kidneys....**1678**
Adult-Onset Medullary Cystic Disease....**1679**
Medullary Sponge Kidney....**1679**
Other Hereditary Renal Disorders....**1679**

UNIT 12

**UNIT 12
Gastrointestinal Disorders** **1683**
Unit Editor: Betty Blake

58. Structure and Function of the Gastrointestinal System

**58. Structure and Function of the
Gastrointestinal System** **1685**

Esther Matassarin-Jacobs

The Gastrointestinal Tract....**1685**
The Mouth....**1685**
Structure....**1685**
Chewing and Its Functions....**1685**
Saliva and Its Functions....**1686**
Swallowing (Deglutition)....**1687**
The Esophagus....**1687**
Structure....**1687**
Function....**1687**
The Stomach....**1689**
Structure....**1689**
Function....**1689**
The Small Intestine....**1690**
Structure....**1690**
Function....**1692**
The Large Intestine....**1694**
Structure....**1694**
Function....**1695**
Effects of Aging....**1696**

59. Assessment of Clients with Gastrointestinal Disorders

**59. Assessment of Clients with
Gastrointestinal Disorders** **1698**

Jane Hokanson Hawks

History....**1698**
Biographical and Demographic Data....**1698**
Chief Complaint....**1698**
Past Health History....**1699**
Family Health History....**1705**
Psychosocial History....**1705**
Review of Systems....**1706**
Physical Examination....**1706**
Assessing the Oral Cavity....**1706**
Assessing the Abdomen....**1707**
Assessing the Anus and Rectum....**1709**
Diagnostic Tests....**1710**
Laboratory Tests....**1710**
Fecal Analysis....**1711**
Ultrasonography....**1713**
Magnetic Resonance Imaging....**1713**
Radiographic Tests....**1713**
Endoscopy....**1714**
Exfoliative Cytologic Analysis....**1716**
Gastric Analysis....**1717**
Acid Perfusion Test (Bernstein Test)....**1717**

60. Nursing Care of Clients with Ingestive Disorders 1719

Jane Hokanson Hawks

Dental Disorders....1719
Dental Plaque....**1719**
Dental Caries....**1719**
Periodontal Disease....**1720**
Dental Emergencies....**1722**
Oral Disorders....1723
Stomatitis....**1723**
Aphthous Stomatitis (Canker Sores)....**1723**
Herpes Simplex....**1724**
Vincent's Angina (Necrotizing Ulcerative Gingivitis, Trench Mouth)....**1724**
Candidiasis (Moniliasis)....**1725**
Tumors of the Oral Cavity....**1726**
Benign Tumors of the Oral Cavity....1726
Premalignant Tumors of the Oral Cavity....1726
Malignant Tumors of the Oral Cavity....1727
Disorders of the Salivary Glands....1732
Inflammation....**1732**
Calculi....**1732**
Tumors....**1732**
Disorders of the Esophagus....1732
Dysphagia....**1732**
Dysphagia Caused by Mechanical Obstructions....1732
Dysphagia Caused by Cardiovascular Abnormalities....1732
Dysphagia Caused by Neurologic Diseases....1732
Dysphagia from Other Causes....1732
Regurgitation....**1733**
Pain....**1733**
Heartburn....**1733**
Achalasia....**1733**
Diffuse Esophagel Spasm....**1737**
Gastroesophageal Reflux Disease....**1737**
Hiatal Hernia....**1740**
Diverticula....**1741**
Esophageal Neoplasms....**1743**
Vascular Disorders....**1746**
Trauma....**1746**

61. Nursing Care of Clients with Gastric Disorders 1748

Jane Hokanson Hawks

General Clinical Manifestations of Gastrointestinal Disorders....**1748**
Pain....1748
Anorexia....1748
Nausea....1748
Diarrhea....1749
Belching and Flatulence....1749
Dyspepsia....1749
Gastrointestinal Intubation....**1749**
Types of Tubes....1749
Inserting Gastrointestinal Tubes....1750
Nutritional Support....**1752**
Enteral Nutrition....1752
Parenteral Nutrition (Total Parenteral Nutrition or Hyperalimentation)....1754

Eating Disorders....**1756**
Anorexia Nervosa....1756
Bulimia Nervosa....1759
Inflammatory and Neoplastic Disorders....**1761**
Peptic Ulcer Disease....1764
Gastric Cancer....1781
Congenital Disorders: Esophageal Atresia with Tracheoesophageal Fistula....**1784**

62. Nursing Care of Clients with Intestinal Disorders 1787

Jane Hokanson Hawks

General Clinical Manifestations....**1787**
Disorders of the Large and Small Bowel....**1788**
Inflammatory Disorders....1788
Infections and Infestations....**1788**
Appendicitis....**1791**
Peritonitis....**1793**
Inflammatory Bowel Disease....**1794**
Neoplastic Disorders....1808
Benign Tumors of the Bowel....**1808**
Neoplastic Disorders of the Bowel....**1808**
Cancer of the Small Bowel....1808
Colon Cancer....1808
Other Disorders of the Large and Small Bowel....1816
Herniations....**1816**
Diverticular Disease....**1818**
Meckel's Diverticulum....**1819**
Obstruction....**1820**
Irritable Bowel Syndrome....**1823**
Disorders of the Anorectal Area....**1825**
Hemorrhoids....**1825**
Pilonidal Cyst....**1828**
Anal Fissure....**1828**
Anal Fistula....**1828**
Anorectal Abscess....**1828**
Tumors....**1828**
Blunt or Penetrating Trauma....**1829**
Congenital Disorders....**1830**
Hirschsprung's Disease....**1830**

UNIT 13
Liver, Biliary Tract, and Exocrine Pancreatic Disorders 1833
Unit Editor: Betty Blake

63. Structure and Function of the Liver, Biliary Tract, and Exocrine Pancreas 1835

Esther Matassarin-Jacobs

Structure....**1835**
Liver....**1835**
Biliary Tract....**1835**
Pancreas....**1836**
Function....**1837**
Liver....**1837**
Biliary Tract....**1840**
Pancreas....**1840**
Effects of Aging....**1841**

64. Assessment of Clients with Liver, Biliary Tract, and Exocrine Pancreatic Disorders **1843**

Dianne Smolen

History....**1843**
Chief Complaint....**1843**
Past Health History....**1844**
Family Health History....**1844**
Psychosocial History....**1844**
Review of Systems....**1845**
Physical Examination....**1845**
General Health Status....**1845**
Nutritional Status....**1845**
Abdominal Assessment....**1845**
Diagnostic Tests....**1848**
Laboratory Studies....**1849**
Ultrasonography....**1849**
Radiologic Studies....**1849**
Radionuclide Scanning....**1853**
Paracentesis....**1854**
Peritoneoscopy....**1854**
Biopsy....**1854**
Portal Pressure Measurements....**1856**
Analysis of Duodenal or Biliary
    Drainage....**1856**

65. Nursing Care of Clients with Liver Disorders **1858**

Dianne Smolen

Jaundice....**1858**
Hepatitis....**1861**
Viral Hepatitis....**1861**
Toxic Hepatitis....**1871**
Chronic Hepatitis....**1872**
Alcoholic Hepatitis....**1872**
Cirrhosis....**1872**
Complications of Cirrhosis....**1883**
Portal Hypertension....**1884**
Ascites....**1889**
Hepatic Encephalopathy....**1891**
Fatty Liver....**1895**
Liver Neoplasms....**1895**
Liver Transplantation....**1898**
Liver Abscess....**1902**
Hemochromatosis....**1902**
Amyloidosis....**1902**
Congenital Conditions....**1903**
Wilson's Disease....**1903**
Caroli's Syndrome....**1903**
Congenital Hepatic Fibrosis....**1903**
Liver Trauma....**1903**

66. Nursing Care of Clients with Biliary Tract and Exocrine Pancreatic Disorders.... **1907**

Dianne Smolen

Biliary Tract Disorders....**1907**
Cholelithiasis....**1907**
Acute Cholecystitis....**1915**
Acute Acalculous Cholecystitis....**1918**
Chronic Cholecystitis....**1918**
Choledocholithiasis and Cholangitis....**1918**
Sclerosing Cholangitis....**1920**
Carcinoma of the Gallbladder....**1920**
Disorders of the Exocrine Pancreas....**1921**
Acute Pancreatitis....**1921**
Chronic Pancreatitis....**1929**
Pancreatic Pseudocysts....**1929**
Pancreatic Cancer....**1930**
Pancreatic Transplantation....**1931**
Pancreatic Trauma....**1931**
Cystic Fibrosis....**1932**

UNIT 14
Metabolic Disorders **1933**

67. Structure and Function of the Endocrine System **1935**

Esther Matassarin-Jacobs

The Endocrine System....**1935**
Structure....**1935**
Hormones and Their Functions....**1935**
The Endocrine Glands....**1941**
Pituitary Structure and Function....**1941**
Thyroid and Parathyroid Structure and
    Function....**1943**
Adrenal Structure and Function....**1944**
Pancreatic Structure and Function....**1945**
Hormonal Factors Regulating Carbohydrate
    Metabolism....**1945**
Insulin and Glucagon....**1945**
Other Hormonal Factors....**1946**
Ovaries and Testes....**1946**
Effects of Aging....**1946**

68. Assessment of Clients with Endocrine Disorders **1948**

Carol Birch
Kerry H. Greear

History....**1948**
Biographical and Demographic Data....**1948**
Chief Complaint....**1948**
Past Health History....**1949**

Family Health History....**1949**
Psychosocial History....**1950**
Review of Systems....**1950**
Physical Examination....**1950**
General Appearance....**1950**
Vital Signs....**1950**
Integument....**1950**
Head....**1950**
Eyes....**1950**
Nose....**1950**
Mouth....**1950**
Neck....**1950**
Extremities....**1951**
Thorax....**1952**
Abdomen....**1952**
Genitalia....**1952**
Diagnostic Tests....**1952**
Tests of Pancreatic Function....**1952**
Tests of Thyroid Function....**1952**
Tests of Adrenal Function....**1953**
Tests of Pituitary Function....**1954**

69. Nursing Care of Clients with Endocrine Disorders of the Pancreas **1955**

Carol Birch
Kerry H. Greear

Diabetes Mellitus....**1955**
Acute Complications of Diabetes Mellitus....**1981**
Hyperglycemia and Diabetic Ketoacidosis....**1981**
Hyperglycemic, Hyperosmolar, Nonketotic Coma....**1987**
Hypoglycemia (Insulin Reaction)....**1988**
Other Hypoglycemic Disorders....**1990**
Hypoglycemic Unawareness....**1990**
Hypoglycemia with Rebound Hyperglycemia (Somogyi Effect)....**1990**
Dawn Phenomenon....**1992**
Chronic Complications of Diabetes Mellitus....**1992**
Macrovascular Complications....**1993**
Coronary Artery Disease....**1993**
Cerebrovascular Disease....**1993**
Hypertension....**1994**
Peripheral Vascular Disease....**1994**
Infections....**1995**
Microvascular Complications....**1996**
Diabetic Retinopathy....**1996**
Other Ocular Disorders....**1996**
Nephropathy....**1996**
Neuropathy....**1999**
Special Situations in the Care of Clients with Diabetes....**2000**

70. Nursing Care of Clients with Thyroid and Parathyroid Disorders............. **2005**

Carol Birch

Thyroid Disorders....**2005**
Hypothyroidism....**2005**
Hyperthyroidism....**2016**
Thyroiditis....**2025**
Thyroid Cancer....**2027**

Parathyroid Disorders....**2030**
Hyperparathyroidism....**2030**
Hypoparathyroidism....**2036**

71. Nursing Care of Clients with Adrenal, Pituitary, and Gonadal Disorders.............. **2041**

Carol Birch

Adrenocortical Disorders....**2041**
Adrenal Insufficiency....**2041**
Chronic Primary Adrenal Insufficiency....**2041**
Secondary Adrenal Insufficiency....**2047**
Adrenocortical Hyperfunction....**2049**
Hypercortisolism....**2049**
Adrenomedullary Disorders....**2056**
Pheochromocytoma....**2036**
Anterior Pituitary Disorders....**2060**
Hyperpituitarism and Hyperprolactinemia....**2062**
Sexual Disturbances....**2065**
Hypopituitarism....**2065**
Posterior Lobe (Neurohypophyseal) Disorders....**2066**
Gonadal Disorders....**2066**

UNIT 15
Musculoskeletal Disorders **2071**

72. Structure and Function of the Musculoskeletal System... **2073**

Joyce M. Black

Structure of the Skeletal System....**2073**
Function of the Skeletal System....**2075**
Structure and Function of the Articular System....**2075**
Structure and Function of the Muscular System....**2077**
Cartilage....**2079**
The Role of the Musculoskeletal System in the Homeostasis....**2079**
Effects of Aging on the Musculoskeletal System....**2080**
Disorders of the Musculoskeletal System....**2081**

73. Assessment of Clients with Musculoskeletal Disorders **2083**

Peggy Doheny
Carol Sedlak

History....**2083**
Biographical and Demographic Data....**2083**
Current Symptoms....**2083**

Family Health History....**2085**
Psychosocial History....**2085**
Review of Systems....**2086**

Physical Examination....**2086**

General Musculoskeletal Examination....**2086**
Neurovascular Assessment....**2088**

Diagnostic Tests....**2092**

Noninvasive Tests of Structure....**2092**
Invasive Tests of Structure....**2094**
Laboratory Tests....**2096**

74. **Nursing Care of Clients with Musculoskeletal Disorders**........................ **2098**

Joan Lappe
Cleda L. Meyer

Metabolic Bone Disorders....**2098**

Osteoporosis....**2098**
Paget's Disease....**2104**
Osteomalacia....**2106**
Gout and Gouty Arthritis....**2107**

Connective Tissue Disorders....**2108**

Osteoarthritis....**2108**
Scoliosis....**2120**
Osteomyelitis....**2121**

Bone Tumors....**2122**

Primary Bone Tumors....**2122**
Metastatic Bone Tumors....**2122**

Disorders of the Hand....**2124**

Dupuytren's Contracture....**2124**
Ganglion....**2124**

Disorders of the Foot....**2124**

Hallux Valgus....**2124**
Hammer Toe....**2124**
Morton's Neuroma (Plantar Neuroma)....**2125**

Muscular Disorders: Muscular Dystrophy....**2125**

75. **Nursing Care of Clients with Musculoskeletal Trauma or Overuse**.......... **2129**

Joyce M. Black

Fractures....**2129**

Intertrochanteric Hip Fractures....**2153**
Intracapsular Hip Fractures....**2159**
Femoral Neck Fractures....**2159**
Subtrochanteric Femoral Fractures....**2159**
Femoral Shaft Fractures....**2160**
Condyle Fractures....**2160**
Pelvic Fractures....**2160**
Patellar Fractures....**2160**
Tibial and Fibular Fractures....**2161**
Foot Fractures....**2161**
Upper Extremity Fractures....**2161**

Sports Injuries....**2161**

Overuse Syndromes....**2161**
Strains....**2163**
Sprains....**2163**
Dislocations and Subluxations....**2164**
Rotator Cuff Tears....**2164**
Anterior Cruciate Ligaments Injuries....**2166**
Meniscal Injuries....**2166**

Repetitive Motion Injuries....**2167**
Remobilization After Traumatic Injury....**2167**

UNIT 16
Integumentary Disorders **2171**

76. **Structure and Function of the Integumentary System** **2173**

Noreen Heer Nicol
Joyce M. Black

Structure of the Skin....**2173**

Epidermis....**2173**
Epidermal Appendages....**2173**
Dermis....**2176**
Subcutaneous Fat....**2176**

Function of the Skin....**2176**

Protection....**2177**
Homeostasis....**2177**
Thermoregulation....**2177**
Sensory Reception....**2177**
Vitamin D Production....**2177**
Processing of Antigenic Substances....**2177**
Cosmetic Adornment....**2177**

Effects of Aging....**2177**

Adolescence....**2177**
Adulthood....**2178**
Older Adulthood....**2178**

77. **Assessment of Clients with Integumentary Disorders** **2180**

Noreen Heer Nicol

History....**2180**

Current Symptoms....**2180**
Past Health History....**2180**
Family Health History....**2181**
Psychosocial History....**2181**
Review of Systems....**2182**

Physical Examination....**2182**

Terminology....**2182**
Types of Lesions....**2182**
Examination Environment....**2184**
Depth of Examination....**2185**
Inspection and Palpation....**2185**
Skin Self-Examination....**2194**

Diagnostic Tests....**2194**

78. **Nursing Care of Clients with Integumentary Disorders** **2197**

Noreen Heer Nicol

General Principles of Dermatologic Nursing....**2197**

Topical Medications....**2197**

Topical Therapy....**2197**
Topical Vehicles....**2197**
Topical Corticosteroids....**2201**

Wound Dressings....**2201**
Soaks and Wet Wraps....**2202**

Skin Lubricants....**2202**
Ultraviolet Light Therapy....**2203**
Ultraviolet B Therapy....**2203**
Photochemotherapy....**2203**
Combination Therapies....**2203**
Psychosocial Aspects of Skin Disorders....**2204**
Common Skin Disorders....**2204**
Pruritus....**2204**
Eczematous Disorders....**2205**
Atopic Dermatitis....**2206**
Xerotic Eczema....**2207**
Stasis Dermatitis....**2207**
Contact Dermatitis....**2209**
Intertrigo....**2210**
Psoriasis Vulgaris....**2212**
Acne Vulgaris....**2212**
Acne Rosacea....**2213**
Pressure Ulcers....**2213**
Bullous Disorders: Pemphigus....**2220**
Infectious Disorders....**2222**
Erysipelas and Cellulitis....**2222**
Herpes Zoster....**2223**
Nail Disorders....**2223**
Cancer of the Skin....**2224**
Precursors to Cancer....**2224**
Sunburn....**2224**
Actinic Keratosis....**2225**
Skin Cancer....**2225**
Cutaneous T-Cell Lymphoma (Mycosis Fungoides)....**2230**
Kaposi's Sarcoma....**2230**

79. Nursing Care of Clients with Burns............ **2233**
Gretchen J. Carrougher

Etiology....**2233**
Risk Factors....**2234**
Pathophysiologic Response....**2234**
Psychological Response....**2236**
Inhalation Injury....**2236**
Classification of Burn Severity....**2237**
Management....**2241**

80. Nursing Care of Clients Undergoing Plastic Surgery......................................**2267**
Joyce M. Black

Basic Principles of Plastic Surgery....**2267**
Achieving Minimal Scarring....**2267**
Selecting Clients....**2268**
Understanding Motivations for Surgery....**2269**
Determining Realistic Expectations....**2269**
Documentation Through Photography....**2270**
Rhytidectomy....**2271**
Blepharoplasty....**2272**
Chemical Facial Peeling....**2273**
Collagen Injection....**2274**
Dermabrasion....**2274**
Rhinoplasty....**2274**
Body-Contouring Surgery (Lipectomy)....**2275**
Suction-Assisted Lipectomy....**2275**
Abdominoplasty....**2276**
Panniculectomy....**2276**
Reconstructive Plastic Surgery....**2276**

Reconstructive Modalities....**2277**
Breast Surgery....**2283**
Breast Augmentation....**2283**
Postmastectomy Breast Reconstruction....**2284**
Reduction Mammaplasty....**2285**
Mastopexy....**2286**
Subcutaneous Mastectomy....**2286**
Repair of Traumatic Injuries....**2286**
Facial Injuries....**2286**
Traumatic Amputations....**2288**
Modifications for Elderly Clients....**2288**

UNIT 17
Reproductive Disorders **2291**

81. Structure and Function of the Reproductive System...............................**2293**
Esther Matassarin-Jacobs

Gonadal Development....**2293**
Structure and Function of the Female Reproductive System....**2293**
Female Reproductive Structure....**2293**
External Female Genital Structures....**2293**
Internal Female Genital Structures....**2294**
Pelvic Blood Supply, Innervation, and Lymphatic Drainage....**2296**
Breast Structure and Function....**2296**
Female Reproductive Function....**2298**
Female Sexual Differentiation....**2298**
Female Hormones....**2298**
Menarche....**2298**
Menstrual Cycle....**2299**
Menopause....**2301**
Structure and Function of the Male Reproductive System....**2302**
Male Reproductive Structure....**2302**
Penis and Related Structures....**2302**
Scrotum and Testes....**2302**
Prostate and Related Structures....**2304**
Sperm....**2304**
Male Reproductive Function....**2304**
Male Sexual Development....**2304**
Spermatogenesis....**2304**
Prostatic Fluid....**2305**
Semen....**2305**

82. Assessment of Clients with Reproductive Disorders **2307**
Elizabeth Carlson
Esther Matassarin-Jacobs
Lynne C. Carpenter

Assessment of Clients with Gynecologic Disorders....**2307**

Approach to Gynecologic Care....**2307**
History....**2307**
Gynecologic History....**2308**
Physical Examination....**2312**
Diagnostic Tests....**2320**
Diagnostic Tests for the Breast....**2327**
Assessment of Men with Reproductive and Urinary
    Tract Disorders....**2329**
History....**2330**
Physical Examination....**2332**
Diagnostic Tests....**2336**
Prevention of Male Reproductive Problems....**2340**

83. Nursing Care of Men with Reproductive Disorders 2350

Esther Matassarin-Jacobs

Psychosocial Disorders Affecting Male
    Reproduction....**2343**
Physical Factors Affecting Male
    Reproduction....**2343**
*Environmental and Occupational Agents....**2344***
*Pharmacologic Agents....**2344***
*Systemic Conditions....**2345***
Infertility....**2346**
*Prostate Disorders....**2350***
Benign Prostatic Hyperplasia....**2350**
*Testicular Disorders and Procedures....**2370***
Testicular Cancer....**2373**
Testicular Torsion....**2377**
Orchitis....**2377**
Hydrocele, Hematocele, and Spermatocele....**2377**
Varicocele....**2377**
Vasectomy....**2378**
Undescended Testes....**2378**
Eunuchoidism....**2378**
Other Testicular Problems....**2378**
*Penile Disorders....**2378***
Urethritis....**2378**
Urethral Stricture....**2379**
Phimosis....**2379**
Paraphimosis....**2379**
Priapism....**2379**
Penile Cancer....**2380**
Peyronie's Disease....**2380**
Posthitis and Balanitis....**2380**
Urinary Extravasation....**2380**
Penile Injury....**2380**
Epispadias....**2380**
Hypospadias....**2380**
*Scrotal Disorders....**2381***
Infections....**2381**
Injuries....**2381**
Edema....**2381**
*Disorders of the Reproductive Ducts....**2381***
*Disorders of the Seminal Vesicles....**2382***

84. Nursing Care of Women with Gynecologic Disorders 2386

Elizabeth Carlson

Menstrual Disorders....**2386**
Dysmenorrhea....**2386**
Premenstrual Syndrome....**2388**

*Abnormal Uterine Bleeding....**2389***
Amenorrhea....**2389**
Menorrhagia....**2391**
Metrorrhagia....**2392**
Menopause....**2392**
*Surgical Menopause....**2392***
*Menopausal Difficulties....**2392***
Postmenopausal Bleeding....**2395**
Pelvic Inflammatory Disease....**2395**
Endometrial (Uterine) Cancer....**2404**
Cervical Cancer....**2406**
Uterine Prolapse....**2409**
Polyps....**2411**
Ovarian Disorders....**2412**
Benign Ovarian Tumors....**2412**
Ovarian Cancer....**2412**
Vaginal Disorders....**2413**
Vaginal Discharge and Pruritis....**2413**
Vaginitis....**2414**
Atrophic Vaginitis....**2414**
Vaginal Fistulas....**2414**
Vaginal Cancer....**2416**
Vulvar Disorders....**2418**
Vulvitis....**2418**
Vulvar Cancer....**2418**
Bartholinitis....**2422**
Other Vulvar Disorders....**2422**
Other Gynecologic Disorders....**2422**
Fallopian (Ovarian) Tube Cancer....**2422**
Genital Tract Sarcomas....**2422**
Gestational Trophoblasic Disease....**2423**
*Hydatidiform Mole....**2423***
*Invasive Mole and Choriocarcinoma....**2423***

85. Nursing Care of Clients with Breast Disorders 2431

Lynne C. Carpenter

Public Attitudes and Knowledge About Breast
    Lesions....**2431**
Breast Cancer....**2431**
*Metastatic Breast Cancer....**2450***
*Breast Cancer in Men....**2451***
Benign Breast Disease....**2451**
*Fibrocystic Breasts....**2451***
*Hyperplasia and Atypical Hyperplasia....**2452***
*Fibroadenoma....**2452***
*Papilloma....**2452***
*Duct Ectasia....**2452***
*Fissure of the Nipple....**2452***
*Lactation Mastitis....**2452***
*Breast Abscess....**2453***
*Mastodynia and Mastalgia....**2453***
*Gynecomastia....**2453***
Mammaplasty....**2453**

86. Nursing Care of Clients with Sexually Transmitted Diseases 2459

Patricia E. Downing

Sexually Transmitted Diseases: An
    Overview....**2459**
Gonorrhea....**2465**

Chlamydial Infections....**2469**
Syphilis....**2470**
Genital Herpes....**2472**
Genital Warts (Condylomata Acuminata)....**2473**
Acquired Immunodeficiency Syndrome....**2473**
Trichomoniasis....**2473**
Bacterial Vaginosis....**2474**
Vulvovaginal Candidiasis....**2475**
Lymphogranuloma Venereum....**2475**
Granuloma Inguinale....**2475**
Hepatitis B....**2475**
Pediculosis Pubis and Scabies....**2475**
Sexually Transmitted Enteric Infections....**2475**

UNIT 18
Multisystem Disorders **2477**

87. Substance Abuse.............................. **2479**

Linda Carman Copel

*Frameworks for Explaining Addictive
    Behaviors....**2479***
Biologic Framework....**2480**
Psychological Framework....**2480**
Sociocultural Framework....**2480**
*Definitions and Terminology of Substance
    Abuse....**2480***
*General Assessment for Substance Use....**2480***
*Assessment and Management of Substance-Abusing
    Clients....**2485***
Alcohol....**2486**
Amphetamines....**2488**
Caffeine....**2490**
Cannabis....**2490**
Cocaine....**2491**
Hallucinogens....**2491**
Inhalants....**2491**
Nicotine....**2492**
Opioids....**2492**
Phencyclidine (PCP)....**2492**
Sedatives, Hypnotics, and Anxiolytics....**2492**
*Nursing Care of Substance-Abusing Clients....**2494***
*Drug and Alcohol Intervention....**2494***
Confrontation on Drug Abuse....**2495**
Treatment Options....**2495**
Prevention of Relapse....**2495**
Surgery and Substance Abuse....**2497**
*The Impaired Healthcare Professional....**2497***

88. Basic Concepts of Emergency Care........... **2501**

*Linda Lorraine Armstrong Lazure
Jean Elizabeth DeMartinis*

*Ethical and Legal Considerations....**2501***
Consent to Treatment....**2501**
Right to Privacy and Confidentiality....**2502**

Mandatory Reporting....**2502**
Physical Evidence and Chain of Custody....**2502**
Bullets....**2502**
Specimens....**2503**
Laws Governing Client Transfer....**2503**
Emergency Nursing Care....**2503**
Initial Nursing Assessment....**2503**
Establishing Priorities: Triage....**2504**
Documentation....**2504**
Priority Nursing Interventions....**2504**
Airway Patency....**2505**
Supplemental Oxygen....**2506**
Spinal Precautions and Immobilization....**2507**
Cardiopulmonary Resuscitation....**2507**
Brief Neurologic Examination....**2507**
Secondary Nursing Assessment....**2507**
Discharge Teaching....**2507**
Psychosocial Needs in Emergencies....**2508**
Death and Dying in Emergency Settings....**2510**
Organ Donation....**2511**
Medical Examiner's/Coroner's Jurisdiction....**2513**

**89. Nursing Care of Clients with
Medical-Surgical Emergencies**................... **2517**

*Linda Lorraine Armstrong Lazure
Jean Elizabeth DeMartinis*

Altered Level of Consciousness....**2517**
Multiple Trauma....**2518**
Penetrating Injuries....**2518**
Blunt Injuries....**2519**
Respiratory Emergencies: Near Drowning....**2522**
Chest Trauma....**2522**
Chest Pain....**2528**
Neurologic and Neurosurgical Emergencies....**2528**
Head Trauma....**2528**
Concussions....**2528**
Skull Fractures....**2529**
Spinal Injuries....**2529**
Abdominal Emergencies....**2529**
Acute Abdominal Pain....**2529**
Gastrointestinal Bleeding....**2530**
Abdominal Injuries....**2531**
Alleged Sexual Assault....**2532**
Ocular Emergencies....**2533**
Chemical Eye Burns....**2533**
Ocular Foreign Bodies....**2533**
Ocular Avulsions....**2533**
Musculoskeletal Emergencies....**2533**
Traumatic Amputations....**2533**
Soft Tissue Emergencies....**2534**
Heat Emergencies....**2534**
Cold Emergencies....**2535**
Hypothermia....**2535**
Frostbite....**2536**
Bites....**2536**
Snake Bites....**2536**
Animal Bites....**2536**
Human Bites....**2536**
Insect Bites and Stings....**2537**
Poisoning and Overdose....**2537**
Domestic Violence....**2539**

Appendix A Religious Beliefs and Practices Affecting Healthcare **2544**

Appendix B A Health History Format that Integrates the Assessment of Functional Health Patterns........................**2552**

Appendix C Laboratory Values of Clinical Importance in Medical-Surgical Nursing........**2555**

Appendix D Clinical Pathways **2566**
    CVA/TIA....**2567**
    Lumbar Laminectomy....**2570**

    COPD....**2572**
    Pneumonia....**2575**
    CAG/PTCA....**2578**
    CABG....**2581**
    Pacemaker....**2584**
    GI Hemorrhage....**2586**
    Diabetic Ketoacidosis....**2588**
    Total Hip Replacement....**2590**
    Total Knee Replacement....**2593**
    TURP....**2596**
    Orchiectomy....**2600**
    Mastectomy....**2603**

Discussion of "Thinking Critically" Exercises **TC–1**

Index **I–1**

Special Features

Bridges to Critical Care

Chapter

32	Intracranial Pressure (ICP) Monitoring	776
42	The Ventilator-Dependent Client	1185
44	Swan-Ganz Monitoring	1234
45	Arterial Lines	1263
47	Intra-aortic Balloon Pumping (IABP)—Counterpulsation	1360

Bridges to Home Healthcare

Chapter

5	Detecting Elder Abuse	90
5	Helping Clients Manage Multiple Medications	96
9	Finding Financial Help	147
9	Medicare and Medicaid Coverage of Home Health Services	148
10	Making the Most of Health Fairs	166
15	Managing IV Therapy at Home	284
17	Controlling Pain	367
21	Recovery from Surgery	493
24	Helping Clients Cope with Cancer Treatment After Returning Home	565
24	Helping Clients Cope with the Reality of a New Diagnosis of Cancer	587
27	Following Universal Precautions at Home	626
28	Promoting Independence in Clients with Rheumatoid Arthritis	667
32	Managing Swallowing Difficulties	804
34	Safety Solutions for People with Alzheimer's Disease	868
34	Respite Care for Caregivers of People with Alzheimer's Disease	870
35	Managing the Immobile Client	913
36	Coping with Failing Vision	964
37	Living with a Severe Hearing Loss	999
40	Supporting the Client at Home After a Laryngectomy	1099
41	Conserving Oxygen	1125
42	Living with a Ventilator	1183
45	Rehabilitation After Coronary Artery Surgery	1252
45	Myocardial Infarction: Convalescence and Home Care	1265
50	Managing Peripheral Vascular Disease	1437
53	Managing Immunosuppression and Nutrition	1494
56	Caring for an Ileal Conduit at Home	1591
56	Inserting Urinary Catheters	1602
57	Living with Peritoneal Dialysis	1659
61	Managing Tube Feedings	1755
62	Adjusting to Life with an Ostomy	1804
69	Diabetic Foot Care	1999
75	Managing Casts and Braces	2152
78	Managing Pressure Ulcers	2220
79	Burn Rehabilitation	2262
83	Intermittent Self-Catheterization for Men	2351
86	Teaching About Sexually Transmitted Diseases	2464
87	Detecting Substance Abuse	2484

Care Plans

Chapter

5	The Older Client at Risk for Relocation Stress Syndrome	89
37	The Client with Vertigo	1014
41	The Client with Chronic Obstructive Pulmonary Disease (COPD)	1120
42	The Client Undergoing Thoracic Surgery	1159
42	The Mechanically Ventilated Client	1180
45	The Client with a Myocardial Infarction	1270
47	The Client with Cardiomyopathy	1343
50	Postoperative Care of the Client Who Has Had Arterial Bypass Surgery of the Lower Extremity	1416
65	Management of the Client After Liver Transplant	1900
69	Foot Infections in the Client With Diabetes	1998
74	The Client with Osteoporosis	2105
75	The Client in Traction	2143
78	The Client with Atopic Dermatitis	2208
79	The Burn-Injured Client	2244
85	The Woman with a Modified Radical Mastectomy	2440

Case Management Features

Chapter

1	Clinical Pathways	13
32	CVA/TIA	784
35	Lumbar Laminectomy	922
41	COPD/Asthma	1124
42	Pneumonia	1139
45	Percutaneous Transluminal Coronary Angioplasty and Arteriography	1247
45	Coronary Artery Bypass Graft	1249
46	Pacemaker	1315
61	GI Hemorrhage	1771
69	Diabetic Ketoacidosis (MICU)	1985
74	Total Hip Replacement	2116

74 Total Knee Replacement 2119
83 (TURP) Transurethral Resection of the Prostate 2369
83 Simple Orchiectomy (Prostatic Cancer) ...2371
85 Breast: Mastectomy 2437

Case Studies

Chapter
32 Meningioma, Fractured Hip, and Possible Cerebrovascular Accident 794
45 Cardiogenic Shock, Tachycardia, and Heart Failure 1268
61 Perforated Ulcer Managed Surgically 1774
65 Cirrhosis 1880
69 Diabetes and Pneumonia 1972
70 Hyperthyroidism and Postmenopausal Osteoporosis 2021

Client Education Guides

Chapter
17 Transcutaneous Electrical Nerve Stimulation (TENS) Units 389
18 Living with Obstructive Sleep Apnea Syndrome (OSAS) 402
22 Shock 527
24 Skin Care Within the Treatment Field 571
28 Using Topical Pain Relievers 668
31 When a Loved One Is in an Altered State of Consciousness 762
32 Transfer from Bed to Wheelchair by a Hemiplegic Client 801
32 Transient Ischemic Attacks 808
32 Migraine Headache 818
32 Monitoring Family Members After Head Injury 829
33 Status Epilepticus 840
34 Caring for Family Members with Alzheimer's Disease 867
34 Parkinson's Disease 881
35 Use of a Halo Vest 906
35 Low Back Care 918
35 Home Care After Cervical Laminectomy or Fusion 926
35 Home Care After Carpal Tunnel Release 928
36 Care After Cataract Removal 961
36 Insertion and Removal of an Ocular Prosthesis 972
37 Infection of the Tympanic Membrane, Middle Ear, or Mastoid Cavity 1008
37 Precautions After Ear Surgery 1009
40 Swallowing Technique After a Partial Laryngectomy 1091
40 Care of the Tracheoesophageal Puncture 1094
40 Exercises After Radical Neck Surgery 1096
41 Asthma 1112
42 Pulmonary Tuberculosis 1146
44 Stress Testing 1226
46 The Client with a Permanent Pacemaker 1322
47 Infective Endocarditis 1334
50 Low-Sodium Diet 1400
50 Low-Fat, Low-Cholesterol Diet 1402
50 Calorie-Restriction Diet 1403
50 Foot Care 1410
50 Stump and Prosthesis Guide 1423
56 Learning to Care for a Urinary Diversion 1593
56 Preventing Recurrence of Urinary Stones 1598
57 Acute Renal Failure 1641
57 Chronic Renal Failure 1657
61 Diet for Dumping Syndrome 1780
62 Ostomy Supplies 1803
62 Colostomy Irrigation 1815
65 Care After Liver Transplant 1899
69 Self-Injection of Insulin 1980
69 Visual Complications of Diabetes 1999
69 Sick Day Management for Diabetes Mellitus 2002
70 Thyroid Supplements 2016
74 Discharge Instructions for the Client After a Total Hip Replacement 2116
78 Skin Self-Examination 2205
78 Simple Guidelines to Help Protect You from the Damaging Rays of the Sun 2224
83 Application of Testosterone Patches 2348
84 Preventing Vaginitis 2415
84 Recovering from Radical Vulvectomy 2421
85 Arm Care After Axillary Lymph Node Dissection 2445
86 Sexually Transmitted Diseases 2465
86 How to Use a Condom 2466
89 Care of Sutured Lacerations 2535

Critical Monitoring Features

Chapter
15 Fluid and Electrolyte Imbalance Secondary to Any Etiology 325
16 Acid-Base Imbalances 337
22 Worsening Shock 511
28 Postoperative Brachial Plexus Compromise 673
31 Manifestations of Changes of Neurologic Status 756
34 Respiratory Distress with Guillain-Barré Syndrome 878
35 Autonomic Dysreflexia 909
41 Asthma 1110
47 Cardiac Tamponade 1337
56 Postoperative Monitoring After Urinary Diversion Procedures 1590
60 The Client with a Percutaneous Endoscopic Gastrostomy or Percutaneous Endoscopic Jejunostomy Tube 1731

65 Esophageal Bleeding Secondary to
    Portal Hypertension.............................1885
66 Manifestations of Adult Respiratory
    Distress Syndrome Secondary to
    Acute Pancreatitis 1927
69 The Rehydration Process.....................1985
70 Hypothyroidism...................................2015
70 Hyperthyroidism..................................2018
70 Hyperparathyroidism and
    Hypoparathyroidism 2031
71 Does Your Client Have an Antidiuretic
    Hormone (ADH) Imbalance? 2064
75 Compartment Syndrome.......................2140
75 The Client in a Cast.............................2149
80 Musculocutaneous Reconstruction..........2279

Diversity in Healthcare Features

Chapter
 2 Biocultural Aspects of Disease.................. 30
 4 Death and Dying 70
 5 Ethnopharmacology............................... 94
17 Cultural Perspectives on Pain..................347
27 HIV and AIDS in Minority Populations 616
45 Coronary Artery Disease in Women 1240
51 Blood Groups and Rh Factor in
    Diverse Cultures.................................1456
59 Nutrition and Culture 1700
69 Diabetes in Native Americans................1957
77 Biocultural Variations in the
    Integumentary System 2188
84 Women's Healthcare 2424
87 Flunitrazepam (Rohypnol) Use in
    Health Care 2489

Ethical Issues in Nursing Features

Chapter
 1 Can the Underinsured Client Be
    Cared for Adequately?..............................9
 4 What Happens When the Nursing
    Care Plan Is in Conflict with a
    Specific Cultural Practice?....................... 65
 4 Should Spiritual Beliefs that Are in
    Opposition to Modern Medical
    Practices Be Respected?......................... 68
 5 How Can You Be a Client Advocate
    to the Elderly? 101
 6 Who Should Make Decisions for
    Clients with a Chronic Illness? 118
 7 Is Whistleblowing Ever the Right
    Thing to Do? 127
 9 How Should Nurses Respond to
    Conflicts Between Patients and Family
    Members in the Home Healthcare
    Setting?..150

10 Do People Have an Obligation to
    Avoid Activities Known to Cause
    Illness that, in Turn, May Burden
    Society? 163
10 What Values Are Represented in the
    Nurse-Client Relationship? 170
11 What Should Nurses Do with
    Confidential Information?.........................189
15 Should Hydration Measures Be Used
    on All Clients?.....................................281
17 Pain: Who Is the Expert?.......................343
17 Is it Ethical to Give a Client a Placebo?....360
17 What Should the Nurse Do About an
    Incompetent Colleague?..........................378
21 Should Clients Who Have a "Do Not
    Resuscitate" Order Undergo Surgery? 460
21 Is It Your Job to Protect the Client's
    Dignity?..467
22 Are Healthcare Workers Required to
    Continue Life-Supporting Interventions
    Until the Client's Body No Longer
    Responds? 499
22 Is There a Moral Difference Between
    Withholding and Withdrawing
    Treatments? 513
23 Bioethical Questions Generated by
    Genetic Advances 552
23 Who Should Be Screened for Cancer,
    and What Tests Should Be Used? 554
24 Who Should Decide to Continue or
    End Cancer Treatment? 567
27 Do Transplant Clients Have an
    Obligation to Comply With Their
    Post-transplant Self-Care? 647
31 Should Organ Procurement and
    Donation Be Discussed with the
    Dying and Their Families?.......................754
31 What Are the Ethical Concerns
    Surrounding the Use of Physical
    Restraints?...761
31 How Can Nurses Serve as Advocates
    for Confused Clients?.............................768
34 In Revealing Information About
    Huntington's Disease, Which Should
    Take Precedence: Client Confidentiality
    or Beneficence? 884
35 What Is the Government's Obligation
    to Put Care for Its Citizens Above
    Care for Non-citizens, Given Scarce
    Resources?...915
40 What Type of Client Education Is
    Needed for Informed Consent to
    Radical Procedures? 1095
42 How Should the Federal Government
    Regulate Testing for Tuberculosis?.........1141
42 What Is the Nurse's Moral Obligation
    When Neuromuscular Blocking Agents
    Are Used? 1172
42 How Should the Decision to End
    Continuous Mechanical Ventilation Be
    Made?..1184

45 What Is Your Role in a "Do Not Resuscitate" Decision?..........................1244

53 Should Parents Who Are Jehovah's Witnesses Have the Right to Refuse a Lifesaving Transfusion for Their Child?..1519

56 What Can You Do to Prevent a Premature Hospital Discharge?...............1589

57 Do Clients with Renal Failure Have an Unconditional Right to Dialysis?............1648

62 Short-Staffing.......................................1816

65 Do Nurses Have an Obligation to Care for a Client with a Life-Style Disease?....1883

69 How Do Nurses Teach Compliance to Diabetic Clients? 1980

71 How Can You Ensure the Ethical Use of Educational Materials for Clients?......2060

79 Should the Severely Burned Client Be Allowed to Refuse Treatment?...............2249

82 Should Pregnant Women Who Engage in Substance Abuse Be Held Liable for Damage to the Fetus?......................2309

83 Should a Client's Sexual Life-Style Influence His Nursing Care?..................2344

84 How Can Nurses Ensure that Patients Have Given Their Informed Consent?.....2403

85 Are Silicone Implants a Safe Alternative for Breast Reconstruction? 2438

85 Communication Problem or Ethical Dilemma?..2442

86 Does the Right to Privacy of Clients with STDs Supersede the Right-to-Know of Potentially Infected Partners?....2463

87 What Considerations Should Be Made for Substance Abusers Who Are Being Treated for Other Medical Problems?......2485

87 What Ethical Issues Surround Your Relationship to an Impaired Nurse?........2498

88 Are Emergency Personnel Obliged to Honor Clients' Advance Directives? 2502

Management and Delegation Features

Chapter

12 Measuring and Recording Vital Signs and Other Client Data 234

13 Performing Specimen Collection and Testing..244

15 Care of Clients with Fluid Volume Deficit..282

31 Preparing Enteral Nutrition.....................759

40 Assisting with Respiratory Care 1073

62 Stoma Care and Application of Ostomy Appliances......................................1806

75 Application of Heat and Cold 2165

78 Care of Clients with Pressure Ulcers.......2216

80 Care of Clients Recovering from Plastic Surgery 2276

Normal Physical Assessment Findings Features

Chapter

26 Immune System.....................................609

30 Neurologic System.................................717

36 The Eye 940

39 Respiratory System 1042

44 Cardiovascular System..........................1206

49 Peripheral Vascular System 1378

52 Hematologic System...............................1463

55 Urinary System.....................................1556

59 Gastrointestinal System..........................1699

68 Thyroid Gland......................................1951

73 Musculoskeletal System 2086

77 Integumentary System 2182

82 Female Reproductive System.................2312

82 Male Reproductive System.....................2332

Nursing Research Features

Chapter

2 What Are the Characteristics of Women with Resilience?......................34

4 What Are the Needs of the Family of a Critically Ill Client?.............................58

4 How Can Cultural Beliefs of People Be Incorporated into Nursing Care?...........65

4 How Can Nurses Provide Spiritual Care? ...69

5 Do the Elderly Promote Their Own Health Differently than Do Younger Persons?...85

6 What Types of Health-Promotion Activities Are Used by People With Disabilities? 108

7 What are the Effects of Nursing Errors?....132

15 Which Indicators of Dehydration Are Reliable in the Elderly? 283

15 Can Clinical Predictors Reduce the Need for Costly Electrolyte Studies?.........296

18 How Well Do Clients Sleep in Critical Care Units?...............................407

18 How Does Progressive Relaxation Affect the Sleep of Older Men and Women?..409

22 Are Fingerstick Measurements of Blood Glucose Accurate in Clients with Decreased Peripheral Tissue Perfusion?.....515

22 Does the Modified Trendelenburg's Position Improve Cardiac Output and Blood Pressure?...................................518

28 What Can Healthcare Workers Do to Encourage People to Develop an "Exercise Habit"? 666

28 Are Community Water Exercise Programs Effective? 670

31 Does Coma Stimulation Affect Prognosis? 752

31 How Does Client Confusion Affect Intervention and Discharge Choices?.........754

31 Can Training Help in the Management of Sundown Syndrome Behaviors? 769

32 Is Intracranial Pressure Influenced by the Comatose Client's Awareness of Bedside Conversation?............781

32 How Does Stroke Affect Marriage?..........790

33 How Can You Support a Client with a Brain Tumor?.....................852

34 How Do Clients With Multiple Sclerosis View Their Health?...................875

35 How Is Immobility Related to Pressure Ulcer Formation in Clients with Spinal Cord Injuries?......................903

35 How Can Quality of Life Be Improved for Quadriplegic Clients?........................903

35 Can Pressure Be Relieved by Position Changes in Seated Clients with Spinal Cord Injuries?.........................906

36 Does Cataract Surgery Improve the Client's Quality of Life?.........................960

37 How Does Hearing Impairment Affect the Quality of Life in Older Clients?......1000

39 Is the Pulmonary Functional Status and Dyspnea Questionnaire a Valid Measurement of Dyspnea and Activity Intolerance in Clients With Chronic Obstructive Pulmonary Disease?............1037

40 What Is Life Like After a Laryngectomy?.....................1038

41 What Clinical Indicators Can Be Assessed in Dyspneic Clients?...............1108

41 How Does Chronic Obstructive Pulmonary Disease Affect Quality of Life?..................................1127

45 What Are the Needs of Families of Clients Having Cardiac Catheterization?.....................1248

45 Are Factors that Predict Physical Activity After Bypass Surgery Different for Women and Men?.............1251

46 What Is the Influence of CPR as Seen on Television on the Public's Perception of the Use of and Outcomes from CPR?.....1313

47 How Do Different Methods of Measuring Temperature Compare?..........1358

56 Is There a Simple, Accurate Way to Determine Whether Kegel Exercises Are Making a Difference in Pelvic Muscle Strength?................................1609

59 Do Annual Tests for Fecal Occult Blood Really Make a Difference?...........1712

60 Should Hydrogen Peroxide Rinses Be Used for Oral Care?............................1725

60 What Does the Appearance of Aspirates from Feeding Tubes Indicate?....................................1743

61 Can the pH Value of Aspirated Fluid Indicate Feeding Tube Placement?..........1751

61 Can a Pressure Gauge Help to Distinguish Gastric from Pulmonary Placement of Nasoenteral Tubes?..........1751

61 How Does Caring for Clients Who Are Dependent on Total Parenteral Nutrition Affect the Family?.................1757

61 Does Childhood Sexual Abuse Affect Women's Medical Problems Later in Life?.................................1757

61 Does Jaw Relaxation, Music, or Both, Relieve Pain After Surgery?.................1781

62 How Does Clostridium difficile Affect Hospitalized Clients?............................1789

62 How Does Inflammatory Bowel Disease Affect Daily Life?...................1801

62 How Does Dietary Fiber Affect Gastrointestinal Symptoms?...................1825

69 How Do Conventional Therapy and Intensive Therapy Compare in Their Effect on Clients with Diabetes?..............................1966

70 Could Recent Development of Thyroid Swelling Be Related to AIDS Treatment?.........................2027

71 Adrenal Insufficiency and AIDS.............2042

74 What Is the Relationship Between Coping Strategies and the Health of Women with Osteoarthritis?.................2118

75 How Do Older Clients with Hip Fractures Fare Once They Leave the Hospital?................................2159

78 How Well Do Healthy Elderly Adults Tolerate an Every-2-Hour Turning Schedule?..............................2218

79 How Do Victims of Home Fires React to Their Losses?.........................2263

83 Is Education About Testicular Self-Examination Effective?...................2375

85 Does Ability to Concentrate Differ Between Women Who Have Undergone Mastectomy vs. Breast-Conserving Surgery?...........................2439

88 How Should Violent Behavior in the Emergency Department Be Handled?......2509

88 How Should the Family Be Told of the Client's Death?.............................2511

Pathophysiology/Treatment Algorithms

Chapter

20 Understanding Inflammation and Its Treatment.................................431

28 Understanding Rheumatoid Arthritis and Its Treatment................................656

41 Understanding Asthma and Its Treatment.................................1107

42 Understanding ARDS and Its Treatment...1171

45 Understanding Myocardial Infarction and Its Treatment................................1259

53 Understanding DIC and Its Treatment.....1511

57 Understanding Chronic Renal Failure and Its Treatment...............................1642

65 Understanding Cirrhosis and Its Treatment..1876

69 Understanding Diabetes Mellitus and Its Treatment................................1958

Risk Factors and Levels of Prevention Features

Chapter
15	Extracellular Fluid Volume Deficit 279
15	Extracellular Fluid Volume Excess 285
15	Third-Spacing 290
15	Hyponatremia....................................298
15	Hypernatremia...................................302
15	Hypokalemia.....................................306
15	Hyperkalamia....................................311
15	Hypocalcemia and Hypophosphatemia.......316
15	Hypercalcemia...................................320
20	Delayed Wound Healing 434
22	Shock 501
23	Common Cancers 542
28	Rheumatoid Arthritis...........................655
31	Injury Secondary to Confusion...............766
32	Increased Intracranial Pressure 772
32	Stroke..786
32	Cerebral Hemorrhage 813
32	Head Injury 822
33	Seizures..835
34	Multiple Sclerosis 873
35	Spinal Cord Injury 891
36	Glaucoma..954
37	Hearing Loss.....................................995
40	Laryngeal Cancer...............................1084
41	Asthma 1106
41	Pulmonary Embolism 1128
42	Pneumonia.......................................1135
42	Tuberculosis.....................................1140
42	Lung Cancer 1152
45	Coronary Artery Disease......................1239
46	Dysrhythmias 1296
47	Rheumatic Valvular Disease 1329
47	Infective Endocarditis..........................1332
47	Cardiomyopathy 1339
56	Cystitis...1573
56	Bladder Cancer..................................1582
56	Urinary Calculi..................................1596

56	Urinary Incontinence 1606
57	Pyelonephritis 1628
60	Dental Caries and Periodontal Disease 1720
60	Oral Cancer 1727
60	Gastroesophageal Reflux Disease...........1738
60	Esophageal Cancer.............................1743
61	Acute Gastritis 1762
61	Peptic Ulcer Disease 1765
62	Gastroenteritis and Dysentery 1789
62	Colon Cancer....................................1809
62	Diverticular Disease 1819
62	Irritable Bowel Syndrome 1824
65	Hepatitis...1863
65	Cirrhosis...1873
66	Cholelithiasis (Gallstones) 1909
66	Acute Cholecystitis 1916
66	Acute Pancreatitis 1922
69	Type II Diabetes Mellitus.....................1956
70	Hypothyroidism.................................2006
70	Hyperthyroidism................................2017
70	Thyroiditis.......................................2026
70	Thyroid Cancer 2029
70	Hyperparathyroidism 2030
70	Hypoparathyroidism 2036
71	Primary Adrenal Insufficiency...............2042
71	Cushing's Syndrome 2050
71	Pheochromocytoma 2058
74	Osteoporosis 2102
75	Fractures 2132
83	Prostate Cancer 2366
83	Testicular Cancer...............................2374
84	Pelvic Inflammatory Disease..................2396
84	Endometrial Cancer............................2404
84	Cervical Cancer.................................2406
84	Ovarian Cancer 2412
84	Vaginitis 2414
84	Vulvitis...2418
84	Vulvar Cancer...................................2419
85	Breast Cancer....................................2432
86	Sexually Transmitted Diseases 2460

Nursing and Healthcare

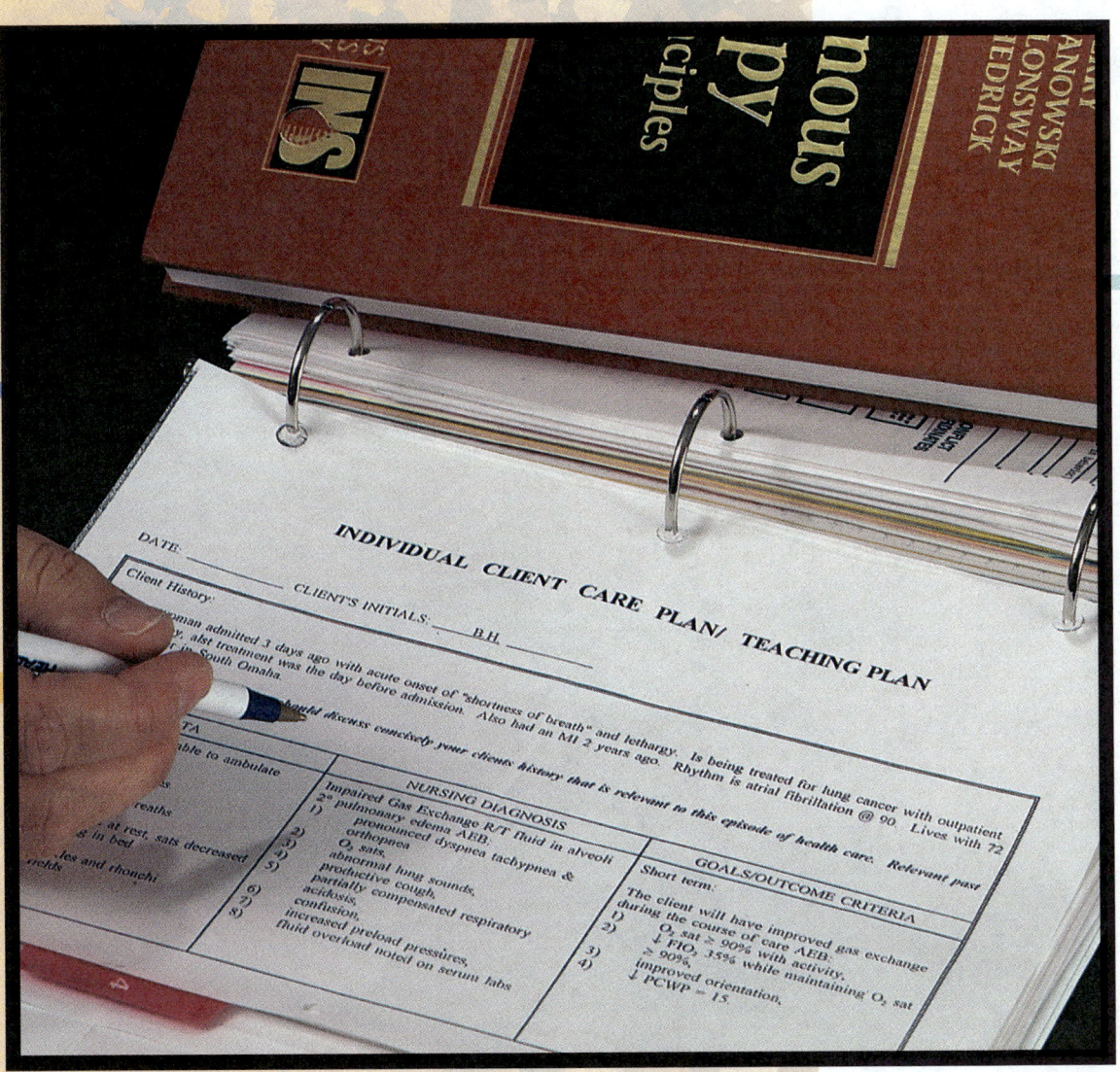

The Context of Medical-Surgical Nursing

Bonita Ann Pilon

In the United States, nurses practice within a diverse and complex healthcare system. During the 1980s, the system experienced dramatic growth in scientific knowledge, coupled with an explosion of technology. This was also a period of increased competition and regulation. Finally, the financing of healthcare was revolutionized when prospective payment was introduced. These events have had a profound impact on the practice of nursing. Understanding who the major stakeholders are within the field of healthcare and understanding recent healthcare history are critical to the practice of professional nursing. The purpose of this chapter is to inform beginning practitioners of these changes and trends to prepare professional nurses for active roles in shaping the healthcare system of the 1990s and beyond.

The chapter is divided into four sections. The first presents an overview of those groups and institutions that are most concerned with the structure and function of the healthcare industry. In the second section, the various mechanisms for funding healthcare are defined and the industry's history in the United States over the past 75 years is reviewed. The third section highlights the richness and diversity of nursing practice, and the fourth section depicts some of the special client populations that nurses serve.

Major Stakeholders in the U.S. Healthcare System

Government

The role of government in the administration of healthcare in the United States cannot be overestimated. By the mid-1980s, over 40% of healthcare dollars spent in the United States were funded by government programs. Most (27%) were funded through Medicare (a federal program) and Medicaid (a joint federal-state initiative). Other important sources of U.S. federal government fund-

ing are the Department of Veterans Affairs (VA), which oversees the VA healthcare system, and the Department of Defense, which funds healthcare for members of the armed forces and their dependents. In addition, state and local governments support local indigent care through various mechanisms.[9]

As the major payor, the U.S. federal government has been active in regulating the healthcare industry. Approximately 40% of hospital beds are occupied on any given day by Medicare recipients. Therefore, hospitals have great incentive to comply with regulations promulgated by the federal government, because they can be fined or "decertified" as a provider of care to Medicare clients if they fail to do so. This could result in the loss of millions of dollars of income for the hospital.

Government regulation is frequently opposed by the healthcare industry in the United States because it often affects the healthcare practitioner's autonomy. In 1991, for example, the U.S. Supreme Court upheld the right of the federal government to restrict healthcare providers in family planning clinics that receive federal funds from informing pregnant women about abortion options (Rust vs. Sullivan). Since the Supreme Court ruling, healthcare workers in the clinics must alter their practice or be subject to penalty. Strong condemnation of this restriction was voiced by the American Nurse's Association (ANA) and the American Medical Association (AMA), among others. Congress has considered legislation to overturn the regulation.

The U.S. federal government is also the biggest source of funding for biomedical research and public health programs, such as the Centers for Disease Control and Prevention (CDC). By the late 1980s, more than $21 billion were spent on these programs annually.[9] This represents almost 5% of every healthcare dollar spent. The growth of scientific knowledge related to healthcare is highly dependent on government funding. Nurse researchers are recipients of research grants through various U.S. government agencies, most notably the National Institute for Nursing Research at the National Institutes of Health

(NIH). Research funds are an important source of revenue for major medical centers and university-affiliated hospitals.

Physicians

The role of physicians in the healthcare system in the United States is an important one. Physicians provide direct medical services to clients in a variety of settings, including offices, clinics, hospitals, and freestanding centers. In addition, physicians control 60% to 80% of hospital costs through their decisions about the use of resources. As gatekeepers to inpatient care, physicians decide which clients to admit, where to admit them, length of stay, quantity of ancillary services, whether to perform surgery, when to initiate and to discontinue treatment regimens, and which medications to prescribe.[19] Because physicians strongly influence healthcare use, healthcare agencies and consumers are often dependent on physicians. Agencies such as hospitals rely on their medical staffs to admit clients who generate income for the hospital. Therefore, physicians are customers of the hospital just as clients are. As a result, physicians and their lobby groups, such as the AMA, usually have strong political influence within hospital organizations, the healthcare system, legislatures, and U.S. government regulating agencies.

Many physicians have perceived a decline in their dominance and control of healthcare during the 1980s and 1990s. This perceived and real loss has created anxiety and defensive tactics among some members of the profession toward a restructured healthcare system. The traditions that define medical practice, such as autonomy, professional control, solo medical practice, and fee-for-service entrepreneurialism, are being questioned and reformed. Some contend that physicians will enjoy less control in a restructured healthcare environment than they have in the past.[11]

Hospital Administrators and Governing Boards

The chief executive and chief financial officers and the governing boards of hospitals strongly influence healthcare delivery in their institutions. In addition, a majority of hospitals in the United States are members of the American Hospital Association (AHA), which represents the industry's efforts to influence legislation, regulation, judicial decisions, and health policy. Recently, the AHA filed suit to stop the National Labor Relations Board from implementing new collective bargaining rules. The suit went to the Supreme Court, where the rules were upheld.[5] The AHA is also working to block new regulations from the Health Care Financing Administration (HCFA), which will effectively decrease reimbursement for capital costs to hospitals from Medicare.[26] In late 1995, the AHA worked diligently to halt Medicare spending cuts proposed by the Republican-dominated Congress.

Business and Industry

As healthcare costs rose in the past decade (about 8% per year),[9] the influence of business and industry increased as well. Health insurance programs, such as Blue Cross/Blue Shield and commercial insurance, are purchased predominantly through employee benefit programs. As the cost of healthcare rises, insurance costs rise as well, forcing businesses to assume greater financial burdens to insure the health of employees and their dependents. Nationally, health benefit costs amount to 26% of corporate earnings; corporate medical care costs rose 21.6% in 1990, and 20.4% in 1989.[27] One major reason for the increase is the healthcare industry's practice of increasing charges to offset underpayment by Medicare, Medicaid, and other contracted payors. The result is that the private sector, insured clients, and employers pay more for care. During the past decade, business and industry leaders protested the increased costs and began to take collective action to drive costs down. Some of the strategies used have been increased deductibles, larger and more frequent copayments, reduced benefits and services, initiation of managed care programs, mandatory second opinions, precertification of admission, and increased contracting of care to health maintenance organizations (HMOs) and preferred provider organizations (PPOs). (See Box 1–1 for definition of these terms.)

In some areas of the United States, industry leaders have formed coalition groups that lobby state government for laws to restrict healthcare spending and provide major reform for the healthcare system. Increasingly, large businesses have contracted for healthcare services directly with hospitals and physician groups demanding—and receiving—significant discounts for care. The influence of large employers is expected to remain strong within the healthcare industry.

The Public

The U.S. public has a stake in healthcare from several perspectives. First, members of the public are consumers of healthcare services. As consumers, they are concerned with quality, cost, and access to care. Many U.S. citizens believe that healthcare is a right and should be universally available to all citizens, regardless of cost. Paradoxically, however, most do not want to pay these costs in the form of increased taxes. The reality is, however, that those citizens who are uninsured (approximately 37 million) or underinsured do not have equal access to healthcare services that income and insurance provide.[12] Women and children are among those who suffer the most from this problem. Because people have not reached a consensus as to the model for healthcare reform or the role government should play, a number of ideas are being explored by various interest groups.

The public also is composed of voters who can elect representatives to enact laws protecting their healthcare interests. Often, citizens band together in organized groups to influence the passage of health-related legislation that is favorable to their interests. In 1990, AIDS activist groups strongly lobbied Congress to ensure passage of the Ryan White bill (PL 101–381), which provided funds for AIDS education, service, and research. The American Association of Retired Persons (AARP) is another prominent group that actively supports healthcare legislation targeted to the elderly. Although many other consumer groups are concerned with healthcare issues, AIDS activist groups and the AARP represent two of the larger and more vocal constituencies that are currently influencing the healthcare industry.

Overall, public values regarding healthcare are changing. Consumers are interested in receiving quality healthcare at a reasonable cost. In addition, the public has a more positive view of health promotion and illness prevention than in the past. The focus on a healthy life-style is in conflict with an illness-driven healthcare system, which creates another impetus for change.[11]

Box 1–1. Major Healthcare Funding Programs in the United States

Medicare—a federally funded, federally administered national health insurance program for citizens age 65 and older, and available for certain other clients, such as those with end-stage renal disease, regardless of age. Medicare began in 1966 and is paid for through payroll taxes of all workers (a portion of social security deductions) and through monthly premiums paid by recipients. The program covers both hospitalization and physician costs; however, deductibles and restrictions apply. The federal government instituted major changes in the way hospitals were reimbursed for Medicare clients in 1983. Previously, hospitals had been reimbursed costs plus an additional amount. Since 1983, hospitals have received compensation on a prospective basis. Under prospective payment, hospitals are paid one predetermined sum for a given diagnosis. Similar types of diagnoses and conditions are grouped together, weighted for severity or intensity of illness, and assigned a dollar value for compensation. These are called diagnostic related groups, or DRGs. If the client's care for a diagnosis (acute myocardial infarction, for example) costs the hospital *more* than Medicare's payment, the hospital *loses* money. If the costs are less than the reimbursement amount, the hospital can keep the profit. This system has caused dramatic changes in the process of care, as hospitals struggle to survive financially.

Medicaid—a joint federal-state program administered by the state governments. This insurance program provides limited funding for certain low-income citizens' hospital costs and some medical care costs. Each state sets the income levels that determine eligibility for the Medicaid program. As a result, some states provide more services to more citizens than others can afford. The state must budget money from its own revenues for the program that the federal government matches by using a ratio. The federal portion is always larger than the state portion.

Blue Cross and Blue Shield—private not-for-profit health insurance companies set up through special legislation in the 1930s. The "blues" are the largest single insurer outside of the federal government. Businesses and industry can purchase healthcare insurance for their employee groups from Blue Cross and Blue Shield. Both hospitalization and medical care insurance are available.

Commercial Insurance Companies—such as Aetna, Traveler's, and Metropolitan Life, that are for-profit businesses. These agencies usually sell a host of insurance packages, health insurance being just one. Businesses or individuals may opt to buy health insurance from a commercial carrier.

Self-Insurance—businesses that develop their own insurance programs for employees. An increasing number of companies are setting aside monies (which can be millions of dollars) to cover the risk of their self-insurance program. Often, the company hires Blue Cross and Blue Shield or a commercial insurer to administer (receive, review, and pay out claims) the program for them.

HMO—a health maintenance organization, which is a system of bundled services. The client pays a monthly premium to the HMO, which entitles him or her to checkups and preventive care, medical care, prescriptions, and hospitalization if needed. The HMO employs its own physicians, may own or manage its own hospitals, and employs other healthcare providers. Some HMOs charge the client a co-payment for some services, such as prescriptions. The client is restricted in an HMO to using only HMO facilities and physicians. If clients choose to go outside the system, they must pay for some or all of their expenses. (There are specific exceptions for emergencies and for people who travel.)

PPO—a preferred provider organization, which is a group of physicians, usually at least one hospital, and sometimes ancillary providers as well, that link together to form a system of care. This care system is marketed and sold, contractually, to employers. In this system of care, the physicians, hospital, and others remain independent agents who agree to treat certain clients (those who join the PPO) at discounted prices.

Workers' Compensation—a federally mandated, state-funded and -administered insurance program available to workers injured on the job. Each employer is assessed a payroll tax, which funds the plan. Claims are filed through the employer to secure funds for treatment.

Private Pay—a term used to describe clients who have no insurance and are themselves responsible for payment of the entire healthcare bill.

Uncompensated Care—the healthcare delivered that cannot be or is not paid for by an insurance program or by clients themselves. Many private pay clients contribute to the amount of uncompensated care when they are unable to pay for the high costs of healthcare. Other sources of uncompensated care include the differences between what the care costs and what Medicare or Medicaid pays the provider. By law, providers cannot bill for the difference.

Capitation—a form of payment for healthcare services between the purchaser of care and the provider, which is often used when a large organization contracts for health services from a provider, such as a hospital or home health agency. The provider can get paid in one of two ways: (1) a flat fee is paid per incident of care (no care, no payment) or (2) the provider receives a flat fee per person enrolled in the health plan for a defined level of care, whether the enrollee seeks care or not. If few enrollees use the service, the provider does well financially. If not, the provider must care for every enrollee who seeks care regardless of whether the total money received covers the cost of the care provided.

Nurses

Nurses outnumber physicians, dentists, pharmacists, and every other single group of healthcare providers in the United States. As of March 1992, there were 2,239,816 licensed professional nurses in this country, of whom 1.85 million were employed in nursing. Among those 1.85 million registered nurses (RNs), slightly fewer than two thirds worked in hospitals, which is a distribution that has remained constant for more than a decade. Even as the supply of RNs has increased 35% since 1980, the percentage employed in hospitals has been stable at 67%. In a 1992 study, the percentage dipped slightly for the first time, to 66.5%. About 69% spend at least half of their work time on patient care activities.[24] Although these numbers seem dated, the U.S. government Department of Labor collects data every 4 years. They were collected in 1996 and will be published in early 1998.

The influence of such a large group of healthcare providers should be felt. In the past, however, the greatest impact, and the most frequently discussed aspect, of nursing within the industry has had to do with the shortage of RNs. The voice of nursing has been heard lately as thousands protest the downsizing of hospitals, the replacement of RNs by less-skilled workers, and layoffs. The epidemic of shortages since the late 1970s that generated the study and attention of various healthcare organizations, private foundations, and two federal commissions on nursing appears to be over. However, the collective expertise and leadership of nurses has not yet been fully utilized to shape the reform era. Nursing's response to rapid market changes has been largely reactionary.

Nursing influence within healthcare is felt in other important ways as well. Nurses and other healthcare groups formed a coalition to successfully defeat a recent proposal from the AMA for a new health care worker, the registered care technician (RCT). Under the leadership of organized nursing, the coalition represented more than 100 professional and citizen groups opposed to the RCT.

In 1991, the ANA, in collaboration with the National League for Nursing, the American Organization of Nurse Executives, the American Association of Colleges of Nursing, and other organized nursing groups, introduced *Nursing's Agenda for Health Care Reform*. The authors stated that "Nurses provide a unique perspective on the health care system. Our constant presence in a variety of settings places us in contact with individuals who reap the benefits of the system's most sophisticated services, as well as those individuals seriously compromised by the system's inefficiencies. . . . America's health care system is . . . very costly, its quality inconsistent, and its benefits unequally distributed. . . . In short, health care is neither fairly nor equitably delivered to all segments of the population."[2] Nursing's healthcare reform proposal attempts to address the cost-quality-access dilemmas facing the nation. This endeavor is a very proactive attempt by the nursing profession to significantly alter existing health policy.

Variations in the Financing of Healthcare Services

Funding Mechanisms

Healthcare is paid for in various ways in the United States. The major funding programs are defined in Box 1–1.

The healthcare industry has evolved through significant phases over the past 75 years with regard to quality-cost-access. To understand current issues, it is useful for nurses to understand the past, which was characterized by two major periods: (1) the period of expansion and (2) the period of regulation and cost containment. The current climate is known as the period of reform.

The Period of Expansion*

During the late 1920s, a congressional committee studied various facets of healthcare organization and financing. Findings from that committee demonstrated that the cost of healthcare per illness had substantially increased with emergence of hospitalization as the appropriate method for treating illness.[16] These rising costs, coupled with the financial problems created by the economic depression of 1929, led to financial difficulties for community general hospitals. Consequently, the need to spread financial risk across the community was recognized. Prepayment plans for hospital care spread slowly during the 1930s and evolved into the Blue Cross system.[19]

There were two objectives of the Blue Cross plans: (1) to provide a stronger financial base for community hospitals, and (2) to move the risk of economic loss due to hospitalization away from single individuals to larger groups of people. These objectives were considered socially desirable, and as a result, Blue Cross and later Blue Shield organizations benefited from favorable legislation exempting them from some of the more stringent requirements for commercial insurance companies.[19]

Evolution of Blue Cross/Blue Shield plans and their availability to the average worker signaled the beginning of an era in which the actual cost of healthcare became separated from the person who consumed the care (the insurance effect). Such a separation causes the cost of healthcare to appear artificially low to the consumer, who, in turn, can afford to purchase more services.

Demand for healthcare services because of insurance grew very rapidly in the 1940s and 1950s. Owing to economic wage and price controls during and after World War II, salary increases to workers were very limited. Fringe benefits came into vogue as a means of attracting and retaining workers. Unions began bargaining for fringe benefits in lieu of unobtainable salary increases. As a consequence, health insurance became widely available to

---

* This subsection and the one following were developed under Federal Contract (to the Division of Nursing in 1988 as part of a larger project). Grateful acknowledgment is made to the Division of Nursing for their funding support.

American workers and their families. Consumption of healthcare services, in turn, increased.

Another event of importance during the 1930s was the passage of the Social Security Act of 1935. This piece of legislation established as social policy the right of the aged to financial security. Although healthcare was not affected by this law at the time of its passage, the Social Security Act would later become the vehicle through which healthcare needs of the aged and the poor would be addressed.

After World War II, it was apparent that the nation's hospitals were obsolete and poorly distributed to meet the needs of the population. There had been great shifts in population from rural to urban areas during the war, and immediately after the war, the population began its "baby boom." The private sector had difficulty in meeting the need for improvement.[3] Congress responded by passing the Hospital Survey and Construction Act of 1946, which is more generally known as the Hill-Burton Act.

The overt purpose of the Hill-Burton Act was to eliminate shortages of hospitals, especially in rural and economically depressed areas. Ratios of beds-to-population were used to measure shortage. Funds generated by the Hill-Burton Act were dispersed over a 28-year period (1946 to 1974). The act was amended over that time period to include not only construction of new facilities, but modernization of existing facilities and, later, construction of emergency rooms and neighborhood health centers.[3]

Implicit within this legislation was the social policy of ensuring all people access to healthcare. The solution to the social problem of inadequate access was to construct more healthcare facilities. To ensure that individuals with limited ability to pay were actually served by the agencies receiving Hill-Burton Act money, the legislation stipulated a unique pay-back scheme. Each facility had to provide care to indigent clients, on an annual basis, that was equal in dollar value to the amount of money received by the hospital, prorated over a specified time period, usually 20 years. Much like a mortgage payment, the hospital provided free care each year equal to its annual repayment amount. These health services were provided, in lieu of payment, to individuals with limited access because of poverty.

The Hill-Burton Act's approach to indigent care was a noble one, but it was not successful in providing access for all indigent clients. During the long pay-back period, the cost of healthcare increased dramatically as a result of increased technology and inflation. Many hospitals began meeting their obligations for free care in a few weeks' time each year. After those obligations were met, the hospital was not legally bound by the Hill-Burton Act to treat indigent clients. By the early 1970s, the bed shortage addressed by Hill-Burton legislation had reversed itself, and an oversupply was thought to exist. In 1974, the act was allowed to expire.

The early 1950s include continued wage and price controls, growth of health insurance coverage among workers, and increased discussion of a national health insurance program. National health insurance was viewed as a means of insuring every U.S. citizen against economic loss due to the high cost of illness, regardless of employ-ment status, age, or health status. This concern repeatedly asserted itself during Truman's administration. The medical and hospital lobby successfully fought such legislation as late as 1952.[17]

By the middle of the next decade, a new social problem was identified as the nation's priority: poverty. The War on Poverty during the Johnson Administration (1963 to 1968) provided the impetus for passage of the first national health insurance plans, for which the federal government was both the insurance carrier and the payor of a large portion of the premium. These insurance programs, known as Medicare and Medicaid, were passed as amendments to the Social Security Act in 1965. The social problem of poverty was translated more specifically into limited access to healthcare services by the elderly and the nonelderly poor as the result of inability of pay. The social policy expressed by both pieces of legislation implied that access to health care for all citizens was a right. Government had an obligation to ensure that right.

Funding for the Medicare hospitalization plan (Part A) is provided by a payroll tax collected from every worker who pays Social Security taxes. The medical payment component (Part B) for physician care is paid by the enrollee through monthly premiums. The Medicare program is administered by the federal government through the Department of Health and Human Services' Health Care Financing Administration.

Administration of Medicaid is delegated to the states, which must provide certain core services but are free to tailor other services to meet specific population needs. The states also determine eligibility requirements, and these vary considerably from state to state. Funding for Medicaid is provided by a matching formula specific to each state. The federal funds are always the greatest portion of each Medicaid dollar spent. States receive differing amounts of federal money (and, therefore, provide different ranges of care) because some states are able to match more federal dollars than others through larger state tax revenues.

Implementation of Medicare and Medicaid substantially increased the federal government's (and to a lesser extent, the state governments') role in the healthcare market. The federal government became the single largest purchaser of healthcare services. Subsequently, the government played a growing role in regulation of the healthcare industry relative to both cost and quality.

The Period of Regulation and Cost Containment

In 1974, Congress passed the National Health Planning and Resources Act (PL 93–641), which required states to develop a statewide health plan for the use of resources. This act also required states to review providers' requests to initiate or expand health services.[3] This review process is known as certificate of need (CON) review and is still in force today. If the provider cannot demonstrate sufficient need for the service, the request is denied. This piece of legislation represents the first federal government effort to combine health planning and regulation in one program. It is also the first significant attempt to control healthcare costs through elimination of duplicate services and facilities. It was designed to curb the oversupply of facilities that arose during the period of expansion.

Results of the CON regulation program demonstrated in research studies have been disappointing. Steinwald and Sloan reviewed eight empirical studies and concluded that "the current evidence . . . suggests that certificate-of-need controls, initiated by the states and mandated by PL 93–641, may be regarded as a classic example of regulatory failure."[21]

Some state governments undertook their own regulatory programs during the 1970s. Rate controls were in place in at least eight states by the end of the decade. According to Steinwald and Sloan, such programs "all respond to the evils of cost-based reimbursement—they seek to counteract the unrestrained nature of hospital reimbursement by superimposing constraints that the market cannot provide."[21]

The states with mandatory rate-setting programs represented the most stringent group of prospective reimbursement programs operating during the late 1970s. "Rates of increase in total hospital expenses in the eight mandatory states were 9.7% and 8.6% for the years of 1976–1977 and 1977–1978, respectively, versus 15.8% and 14.0% for the other states and the District of Columbia"[21] These data and other studies clearly indicated that prospective rate-setting was more effective in controlling health care costs than were the CON controls. Reimbursement for Medicaid patients also had moved to a prospective system in many states, whether or not the state had mandatory rate setting.

The federal government, very much aware of the rising cost of healthcare and continuing as the nation's largest purchaser of care, began to look at methods of prospective reimbursement that could be used by the Medicare program. Research studies were under way at Yale University and other centers to develop a system of prospective payment. These studies were closely followed and sometimes funded by the Department of Health and Human Services, previously called the Department of Health, Education, and Welfare.

The hospital industry adopted its own form of regulation in December 1977. Known as the Voluntary Effort (VE), it consisted of "joint activities at the state level by the American Hospital Association, the American Medical Association, and the Federation of American Hospitals (the for-profit hospitals' trade organization) to control the rate of growth of hospital costs."[21] The results of the VE were mixed. A study by the Congressional Budget Office indicated a small, nonsignificant negative effect on hospital expenditures. A second study found a significant negative effect on cost per admission and cost per patient day. However, the study indicated that the cost savings were not passed on to the consumers, because hospital profits increased during the same period (1978 to 1980).[21]

The inability of various regulatory programs to control the rising cost of healthcare (from 9% of the gross national product in 1978 to 13% by 1992) became a priority issue with Congress. The nation was trying to recover from economic recession, and inflation in all sectors of the economy was of grave concern. In addition, the popu-

lation was aging and the ratio of workers (who paid Medicare taxes for hospitalization insurance) to the aged (who consumed the dollars paid in by using hospital services) was shrinking. There were projections that the Medicare Trust Fund would be bankrupt by the mid-1980s.[1] (That did not occur; however, HCFA and Congress continue to take strong regulatory action to control spiraling Medicare costs.)

Not surprisingly, when Congress passed the Tax Equity and Fiscal Responsibility Act (TEFRA) in July 1982, it contained temporary caps on Medicare payments, and it directed the Secretary of Health and Human Services to develop a prospective payment system (PPS) for the Medicare program. The Secretary was instructed to report back to Congress by December 1982 on the status of such a system.

In December 1982, Secretary Richard Schweiker recommended to Congress that a PPS based on diagnosis-related groups (DRGs), developed by researchers at Yale University, be used for all Medicare patients. In March 1983, Congress passed amendments to the Social Security Act authorizing such a system. This system was to replace the cost-based retrospective payment system used to determine Medicare payments to hospitals. All hospitals serving Medicare clients were to switch to PPS except for certain sole community providers, specialty hospitals, and some psychiatric units within general hospitals.

The program became operational on Oct 1, 1983. Hospitals were phased into the system over the next 11 months, when their fiscal year began. A formula was calculated for each hospital to determine its initial reimbursement rate under DRGs. Data were gathered from the hospital's own cost history (using a base year), and from a cost history by geographic region; additionally, a national rate was established. These rates were weighted and blended to determine the exact rate of reimbursement per DRG. Several adjustments have been made in the blending since PPS was initiated. The goal is to move all hospitals toward one national rate; however, that has not yet occurred.

Government was not the only entity concerned with rising healthcare costs during the early 1980s. Business and industry also were very concerned because they paid the majority of health insurance premium costs for employees. Coalitions of local and regional business leaders were formed to discuss and to try to remedy the worsening situation. With the implementation of PPS for Medicare clients, these business coalitions were joined by Blue Cross Organizations and other commercial insurers. These new groups held a common fear: that hospitals would shift uncompensated costs generated by Medicare patients to patients who were still reimbursed retrospectively on a cost-plus basis. As a result of that fear, Blue Cross and other insurers have begun to restructure their payment systems to protect themselves from potential or actual cost shifting. These fears were warranted, because cost shifting became and remains a reality.

PPS has yielded other results as well. Hospitals and other healthcare providers increasingly compete for non-Medicare clients who are more favorably reimbursed. Hospitals also compete for certain Medicare clients whose DRG rate has been profitable for the hospital. Much traditional inpatient care has been shifted to the outpatient system or to the client's home, where the cost of care is less. Insurers and providers have teamed up in creative arrangements designed to hold down costs and yet remain competitive. Such arrangements have caused alternative delivery systems to emerge, based on greater efficiency and decreased costs. Among those alternative systems are HMOs, PPOs, and independent practice associations (IPAs), among others. The number of outpatient surgical centers, freestanding and hospital-based, has increased rapidly, as have the numbers of freestanding emergency clinics.

Providers have turned increasingly to marketing to sell their system of health services to businesses and consumers. HMOs and PPOs, for example, seek to contract with employers to be the sole insurer or provider for employee groups. Capitation has emerged as a popular form of prospective payment within these contractual arrangements. Capitation is one method of financing healthcare service. It is a per-member per-month fee for a specified set of healthcare services. This money is given to providers up front, whether clients use services or not. Likewise, the healthcare provider must provide care even if all of the fees provided have been used. Medicare also is interested in capitation as a means of payment for its enrollees. In some regions of the country, Medicare enrollees already receive care through an HMO that receives capitation payments from the federal government. The American Hospital Association projected that the majority of Medicare clients would be covered by capitation by the early 1990s.[8]

The Period of Reform

By 1992, the United States had begun serious efforts at reforming its healthcare financing system. With the election of President Clinton from the Democratic Party, and with continued control of Congress by the same party, passage of major, national healthcare reform legislation seemed inevitable. President Clinton introduced the Health Security Act in early 1994, after almost a year of deliberation by a select group of economists, businesspersons, and healthcare providers. First Lady Hillary Rodham Clinton chaired the panel, which attempted to examine the current system's problems with access and cost and to identify the national priorities for healthcare delivery, including a new emphasis on prevention. Much controversy surrounded this ad hoc group. No representation was allowed from organized medicine or other provider organizations. Testimony was sought from these groups, but the actual crafting of the reform plan and ensuing legislation was carried out by the task force. The plan that emerged was so complex that when it was published as a book it contained more than 100 pages. The legislation that was sent to Congress to enact the plan was more than 1000 pages in length.

President Clinton's plan had opposition from within his own party as well as from outside. Everyone publicly agreed that the system needed to be reformed, but serious disagreement existed about how much reform was needed or could be afforded. At one point in 1994, at least six different pieces of healthcare reform legislation were being considered by Congress. The main points of contention centered on universal access and how to pay for it and on employer mandates, which require all employees to be covered by insurance provided by the employer. As a result of these issues and of a general lack of political support by Congress for the President, federal healthcare reform initiatives failed to pass. In fact, no bill was moved out of committee for a vote.

The support for reform, however, did not die in Washington. A number of states have moved through legislation and policy directives to halt the escalation of costs and to provide increased access to services for citizens regardless of ability to pay. On Jan 1, 1994, the State of Tennessee moved all Medicaid recipients into a managed care plan, with capitation paid to managed care companies, which in turn must provide a full range of healthcare services to recipients. After 1 year, this managed care approach has covered all Medicaid-eligible clients and enrolled additional "working poor" people, who otherwise would be unable to afford health insurance. By early 1995, 94% of Tennesseans had healthcare coverage. The goal is universal coverage. This coverage has been accomplished using the same dollars that previously would have taken care of only the Medicaid population.

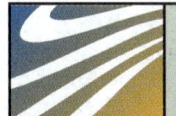

ETHICAL ISSUES IN NURSING

Can the Underinsured Client Be Cared for Adequately?

A large percentage of the U.S. population is uninsured or underinsured for healthcare. The insurance situation in the United States has thus created a two-tiered system of healthcare. One tier serves the more financially stable (private insurance, HMO/PPO plans, and the like), whereas the second tier serves the less financially stable (Medicare and Medicaid).

The dilemma with which healthcare workers are faced regarding this two-tiered system of health coverage has to do with the principle of justice. If access to healthcare services is fair, then all persons must be served equally, regardless of their ability to pay. Is the healthcare industry in the United States just? Do all persons have equal access to healthcare?

Nurses work in a variety of settings. Settings include private hospitals, public hospitals, nursing homes, private offices, home health agencies, and homeless shelters. A client's economic background often determines the type of healthcare facility at which she or he may be treated. Nurses in the facilities must show respect for each client, as a fundamental guiding principle of treatment. Nursing may not always be involved in the medical treatment decisions dictated by financial considerations; however, nursing practice can always strive for justice within the context of care.

An additional 300,000 people are now insured using the managed care capitation approach.

Reform is also being driven by the healthcare industry itself. During 1994, Columbia Health Care System, based in Dallas, acquired Hospital Corporation of America and Health Trust, both based in Nashville, to form the largest for-profit healthcare delivery system in the United States. In addition to owning hospitals, this corporation has aggressively pursued the acquisition of primary care practices of physicians in rural markets as well as in urban centers. Using such a strategy, Columbia is creating a network of integrated delivery systems that focuses on primary care as the most desirable and least costly level of care, with the availability of secondary and tertiary care when needed. With such a network in place in numerous markets across the United States, Columbia actively seeks managed care contracts from large employers, generally paid on a capitation basis, although discounted reimbursement mechanisms are still mixed with fee-for-service in most markets.

The response by the not-for-profit sector has varied. In some very competitive markets, the not-for-profit hospitals have banded together to form their own networks to compete for managed care contracts. In other areas, some not-for-profits have entered into joint venture arrangements with the for-profit sector; or in some cases, not-for-profit hospitals have been purchased by large for-profit systems. The situation has not yet stabilized, and it is expected to remain highly volatile through 1996 as the industry attempts to position itself to provide low-cost, high-quality services across the lifespan.

The healthcare system in the United States has undergone rapid change since the early 1980s. The system is still in the midst of evolution, however, and the end product is difficult to foresee. Scarcity of and competition for human and financial resources are the dominant forces operating at present. This situation creates a dilemma with regard to social values of the past: healthcare as a right versus scarcity. Nurses must recognize and grapple with these forces and with the dilemmas involved to play an active part in shaping the nation's future healthcare system (see Ethical Issues in Nursing).

What direction will the healthcare system in the United States take next? An interview with a nurse expert in health policy outlines priorities for the remainder of this decade and beyond (Box 1–2).

Box 1–2. The Future of the U.S. Healthcare System

The following is an interview with Virginia Trotter Betts, M.S.N., J.D., R.N., President, American Nurses' Association, and former Robert Wood Johnson Health Policy Fellow (1987–1988). Questioner is Bonita Ann Pilon, D.S.N., R.N., C.N.A.A., Associate Professor, Vanderbilt University, and Chief Nursing Officer, St. Thomas Hospital, Nashville, Tennessee.

Q: When we review the history of our healthcare system over the past 70 years, we see it has been characterized by a period of expansion and then a period of regulation and cost containment. The current era is focused on reform. Where is the nation heading next?

A: After the hotly debated efforts of our nation to address the need for comprehensive healthcare reform during 1993 and 1994 (which ultimately failed in Congress) our country is left with the very same factors that pointed to a growing crisis in healthcare. These problems include: (1) delivery based on episodic illness interventions, (2) the highest aggregate and per-person health care costs in the world, (3) increasing numbers of Americans without healthcare coverage, and (4) poorly understood or distributed processes and outcomes for quality care. Since we have not solved these problems through federal policy channels, they will either be addressed through state law or through private markets. The nation will continue to focus on **cost,** and only when effectiveness initiatives and quality measures have an impact on cost will we move forward on quality and access.

Q: So you believe that effectiveness is going to have to be tied to cost, that we are going to be looking at these together?

A: There was a belief that the next trend in health policy would be to go from expansion to concerns about costs to concerns about quality. We have never put to rest the myriad of cost issues. Quality is being assumed (inaccurately, I believe) because the chief interest of the current system drivers—payors and the rapidly forming care conglomerates—is cost containment. As providers we will experience this cost driver for the next few years in fairly draconian ways, I fear.

Q: President Clinton initiated major healthcare reform with the introduction of the Health Security Act in late 1993. Congress failed to act on that legislation in 1994. Now that the Republicans have taken over leadership in both houses, what will happen to the healthcare reform movement?

A: The President's plan reflected a belief that comprehensive, systematic reform was what the nation needed—a belief that was espoused since 1991 by the American Nurses' Association (ANA). The Democratic-led Congress did not act to pass the President's plan or any other plan. Now with Republican leaders in the Congress, healthcare is not at the top of their agenda; therefore, federal comprehensive reform will not even be addressed these next 2 years. After that, who knows? As I said before, the underlying problems remain and will continue to grow. Thus, states may address reform on a more local level. Private sector changes, however, are happening with dramatic speed—hence the unprecedented growth of managed care companies and the transformation of large indemnity insurance companies toward "health plans."

Q: *Nursing's Agenda for Health Care Reform* is ambitious

The Richness and Diversity of Nursing Practice

The discipline of nursing offers a wide variety of career opportunities across diverse settings. This section highlights the breadth of professional practice.

Hospital Practice

Eighty-three percent of the total RN population is employed in nursing. Of those 1.85 million nurses, the large majority (66%; more than 1 million nurses) work in hospitals. Between 1984 and 1992, the number of nurses working in hospitals increased by more than 100,000, although the percentage remained essentially unchanged from previous years.[24] It is predicted, however, that as many as 300,000 RNs may no longer have jobs in hospitals as managed care drives inefficiencies out of healthcare. Over time, most of these nurses will shift their practices to home health and long-term care.[13]

Hospital practice offers a wide variety of options to nurses. The majority of hospital nurses work in staff nurse positions, giving direct, hands-on care to clients. Most staff nurses work with medical-surgical (adult and pediatric) clients. Other common areas of practice include critical care (cardiac, neonatal, pediatric, medical-surgical, perinatal), operating room, labor and delivery, recovery room, postpartum and newborn areas, emergency department, outpatient department, hospital-based home healthcare, and inpatient hospice.

The variety and intensity of experiences available to nurses in hospital practice have traditionally attracted new graduates. In addition, other employment settings often require nurses to have several years of hospital nursing practice before they can be hired. The familiarity with care requiring high technology systems and acutely ill clients has been viewed as an asset when practicing elsewhere, particularly in the home health field, in which increased technology and skilled nursing care have allowed very sick clients to remain at home.

Among hospital nurses, more than 14% work in a leadership position. These positions include nurse executive, assistant administrator, supervisor, head nurse and nurse

---

and visionary. How will the ANA develop this agenda given the change in political climate in Washington?

A: The ANA remains committed to the principles of nursing's agenda—universal access, cost containment, improvement of quality, and restructuring the delivery system to balance health and illness services. However, we acknowledge that having comprehensive federal legislation passed to achieve these principles by the 104th Congress is unrealistic. Therefore, we are trying to use our resources of staff and volunteers to achieve incrementally some key changes, such as reimbursing advanced practice nurses under Medicaid and Medicare, increasing the numbers of advanced practice nurses, protecting public and community health programs, and preventing discrimination against nurses as providers as new health plans grow. ANA and ANA PACs (political action committees) are bipartisan organizations, and we nurses have a lot of support for these and other federal initiatives.

Q: Two major venues for opportunities for health system change right now are state health reform and private market innovations. What are the incremental reform initiatives going on at the state and local levels, and how does nursing interact with these initiatives?

A: The ANA will work closely with its 53 state nurses associations on legislation and regulatory initiatives that will further nursing's agenda. I am proud, for example, of the Tennessee Nurses Association work on the Tenn Care program—a statewide managed care initiative that expanded coverage to Tennessee's uninsured and includes advanced practice nurses as primary care providers. Nurses must get out and tell their stories to the private marketplace also—the story that nursing is the

best buy in healthcare—because we are! Private systems will orient toward value. Value in healthcare is quality outcomes plus cost effectiveness. Value and nursing are synonymous. Nursing organizations, especially the state nurses associations, are going to be so essential to nursing's success. Every nurse needs to be involved now in order to influence change.

Q: It is less than 5 years until the next century. Will healthcare reform be accomplished before then?

A: Healthcare reform as a comprehensive piece of federal legislation seems a long way off after the 1994 Republican takeover of Congress. However, the healthcare needs of the nation continue to mount, and the private market is spinning ahead to take advantage of the public policy vacuum. Healthcare delivery as we knew it yesterday is gone, and yet the tomorrow of healthcare is uncertain. We nurses need to insist that universal access to affordable, quality healthcare services remain on the public agenda.

Q: What is the future going to be like for nurses?

A: The future for nursing and for healthcare will be fraught with dramatic change. Nurses who are flexible, adaptable, and in nursing for the long haul—as a career, not a job—will do very well. They will seek positions that are unique, they will further—both formally and informally—their knowledge base, they will find the community of interest with their employers and their patients that allows for moving toward a mutually preferred future. What the nation needs is what the well-educated nurse has to offer—care, commitment, consistency, partnerships, and cost savings. If we tell our story, our future is bright.

manager, and assistant nurse managers. These nurses are accountable for the day-to-day operation of the nursing department. They develop plans for and monitor resource use; they hire, train, and evaluate staff; and they monitor the quality of client care and take action to improve quality. Head nurses and their assistants typically manage the delivery of nursing care to clients on one or more nursing units or service areas. Nurses in higher leadership positions are responsible for increasingly larger systems of care, such as all critical care areas, women and children's services, all medical-surgical units, or mental health services. Ultimately, the nurse executive is accountable for nursing practice throughout the institution. In addition, he or she is the link between professional practice within the hospital and the expectations, standards, and regulation of practice that originate from outside the hospital.

Nursing administration is an area of advanced practice within the discipline of nursing. Although the description in the preceding paragraph focuses on the role of hospital-based nurse administrators, the reader should be cognizant that nurses manage the practice of nursing and delivery of healthcare services within and across all settings.

Ambulatory Practice

One prevalent arena for nursing practice outside hospitals is ambulatory care. Ambulatory care nurses provide a diversity of services to clients. The largest number of ambulatory care nurses work in solo or group practice in physicians' offices.[24] Other areas of practice include free-standing emergency clinics, ambulatory surgery centers, occupational health positions, residential centers for senior citizens, dialysis centers, and rehabilitation centers. The term "ambulatory care" is applied to systems that serve "walk-in" clients, who return to their homes at the end of the visit.

Nurses in ambulatory practice offer a number of services to clients. Education, health counseling, health maintenance, and prevention and primary care are components of their role. In some settings, nurses regularly administer hands-on, high technology care similar to that found in hospitals, for a limited period of time. This occurs most frequently within ambulatory surgery centers and emergency clinics and in dialysis centers.

Occupational health nursing is a rapidly expanding area of ambulatory care. The focus of the occupational nurse's practice is a safe, healthy worker who contributes to the productivity of the company. The nurses are also concerned with health maintenance, health promotion, and health education.[7]

Community Practice

Public health departments, visiting nurses' associations, and home health agencies are the prime settings for community practice. Public health nurses are employed by tax-supported health departments. Because of the tax support, client services are provided free, or for a very reduced fee. Nurses carry a caseload of families that includes a range of ages and conditions across the health-illness continuum. These nurses are challenged to deliver health services in many settings: the home, school, and clinics (which often include providing care or advice on family planning, prenatal and new baby care, and sexually transmitted diseases). The nurse must draw from a broad knowledge base in nursing as well as in community resources and in the use of political processes to affect public policy.[13] The goals of public health nursing are health maintenance and client independence.[26]

Home healthcare is a rapidly growing segment of the healthcare industry and is expected to continue its growth in the 1990s. Since 1972, the number of Medicare-certified home healthcare agencies has grown from 2212 to 5800.[14] Factors such as an aging population and rising costs of inpatient care have influenced the growth of this industry. The opportunity for nursing practice continues to expand as the number of agencies increases and more clients are cared for at home rather than in the hospital.

Home health clients require care of different intensity. Maintenance home care is used for clients who need assistance with personal care or homemaking and whose underlying medical condition is stable. Such care is not provided by registered nurses. Intermediate home care is used for clients with a relatively stable medical condition, but who require professional level care to promote rehabilitation or other improvement. Intensive-level home care is required by clients who have unstable, serious illnesses that require skilled nursing care. Such clients would likely be hospitalized if such care were not available. Registered nurses provide care in the home for clients in the last two categories.[6]

Community and public health nursing has also shown more growth in employment of nurses than hospitals in the last decade (a 38% increase since 1988). The primary growth was among those nurses employed in non–hospital-based home healthcare agencies (other than visiting nurse associations).[24]

Nurses in community practice make independent assessments and decisions. The community setting promotes a highly autonomous practice.

Advanced Practice

Nurses in advanced practice are skilled specialists who usually work with specific client populations both in the hospital and in the community. These specialists have acquired advanced education and experience in their area of practice.

Clinical nurse specialists (CNSs) are the largest group of advanced practice nurses. Employed primarily in hospitals, these nurses have multifaceted roles that are performed differently in different settings, even within the same institution. The five components of the CNS role are educator, practitioner, researcher, consultant, and manager. Some CNSs work primarily in the practitioner role, often in collaboration with a group of physicians, providing highly skilled care to a specific group of clients (such as high-risk perinatal clients or heart transplant patients). The type of care provided by the CNS encompasses and surpasses that provided by the staff nurse.

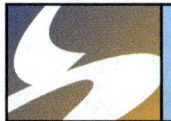

CASE MANAGEMENT

One major role for most hospital-based nurse case managers is to develop and implement *clinical pathways*. These pathways outline the client care tasks and activities that are expected for each day of hospitalization. Clinical pathways are also used for a wide range of conditions and procedures, even in such clinical areas as emergency departments and ambulatory surgery centers, where the unit of time for care is often hours rather than days. The nurse case manager leads a team of experts in the development of a pathway, which outlines the care provided by all clinicians for a certain diagnosis or procedure. Client progress toward specified outcomes is monitored to help achieve those clinical outcomes in a short time.

Throughout this book you will find Case Management features, which are linked to clinical pathways found at the end of the book (Appendix G). These are actual pathways in use in medical centers that are at the forefront of the development of clinical pathways. In the Case Management features, the nurse case managers who helped to develop the pathways and who work with staff nurses daily to help manage client care according to the pathways discuss how the pathways were developed and how they have made an impact on nursing practice at their institutions.

Other CNSs focus more strongly on the educator role, teaching and role modeling expert skills to staff nurses, thus supporting client care more indirectly. All CNSs work in a consultant role at least part of the time. Nurses, physicians, and other healthcare providers frequently seek their input for solving complex care dilemmas for specific patients or groups of clients. CNSs are expected to be knowledgeable about the latest research developments within their area of practice and to add to the development of healthcare's knowledge base through research of their own.

The manager role of the CNS has traditionally been focused on the development of specific clinical programs within the hospital. For example, the CNS for cardiac surgery clients might be asked to develop a proposal for the care of pediatric open heart surgery clients, whom the hospital anticipates admitting very soon. Such a proposal would both specify the care needs and equipment support required based on the CNS's clinical expertise and identify the education and training required for all staff involved in the care of the clients. The CNS would be expected to develop an educational program to prepare

staff for the clients, to implement the program, and to evaluate the results.

A new type of advanced practitioner emerged in the late 1980s in response to changes within healthcare delivery. To improve the process of delivering inpatient care, many hospitals initiated a case management system of care. Nurse case managers work with specific client populations and with the physicians treating those clients as well as with the staff nurses managing the day-to-day client care. Their role is to improve the coordination of care for clients across nursing units, hospital departments, and into the community. Using pre-established collaborative case management plans and clinical pathways for specific diagnoses, case managers work to keep the client moving toward a discharge within an acceptable time frame while maintaining or enhancing quality care.

Nurse case managers are found at different levels of the hospital organization. In some settings, CNSs function as case managers and, therefore, are not involved in direct client care activities on a specific unit. In other settings, most notably at the New England Medical Center (Boston), staff nurses function in a case management group practice across nursing units. Certain staff nurses in key units where specific types of clients reside during hospitalization form networks with one another and with the attending physicians. Nurses in these networks meet weekly to coordinate the caseload of patients not only during the hospital stay, but through return to the community.

A third type of nurse case manager also emerged at the end of the 1980s. At Carondelet St. Mary's Hospital (Tucson), case managers are primarily based in the community, although they are employed by the hospital. These nurses follow a caseload of frail elderly clients, multiple sclerosis clients, and others who are at risk for repeat admissions to the hospital because of both medical and social situations. The nurse case managers strive to support the client toward independent living in the community and provide symptom management while monitoring patients for signs of exacerbations of chronic illnesses. One of the goals of the program is to facilitate hospital admission early in the exacerbation period in order to avoid the most costly (and potentially the most devastating) portion of a hospital stay, such as emergency room admission and intensive care.

Nurse practitioners (NPs) are another type of nurse in advanced practice. NPs have advanced education in the diagnosis and treatment of common, recurrent illnesses as well as in health maintenance and promotion. NPs are trained in advanced pharmacology and have prescription-writing authority in many states. Nurse practitioners work in community clinics, private practice, and in group practice with physicians. Licensure requirements vary from state to state, but NPs are required to be certified in their area of practice (e.g., family nurse practitioner, pediatric nurse practitioner, and geriatric nurse practitioner), and they work under protocols established in collaboration with a precept physician. The certification process is administered by the American Nurses Association and by some specialty organizations. Nurse anesthetists (CRNAs) and nurse midwives (CNMs) are two types of advanced practitioners who are certified through specialty organizations (i.e., Council on Certification of Nurse Anesthetists and the American College of Nurse Midwives).

Some advanced practice nurses establish an independent practice. Psychiatric–mental health specialists may open their own psychotherapy practice. Family nurse practitioners may choose to own and operate their own office practice. The laws governing the scope of practice and reimbursement vary across states. Some states have enacted legislation favorable to independent nursing practice, whereas others have not.

Advanced practice nurses, though practicing in a variety of settings, have a common foundation for their practice: advanced educational preparation. Most of the roles described in this section require a master's degree in nursing (MSN). These include the clinical nurse specialist and nurse practitioner. An MSN is also required for psychiatric nurses in independent practice who seek reimbursement from third-party payors. The nurse case manager role has not yet demanded master's preparation.

However, institutions employing case managers set their own employment criteria; some agencies require an MSN, whereas others do not at this time.

Variations in Client Populations

Nurses work with clients who have diverse social, economic, and cultural backgrounds, all of which have an impact on the types of healthcare needs that clients may experience. In this section, some of the special populations that nurses serve are described.

Variations in Age

From before conception in a family planning clinic or infertility practice to hospice care in the home, the presence of nurses is vital to the individual, the family, the

---

Box 1–3. A Comparison Between the U.S. Healthcare System and the Canadian Healthcare System

As discussion and debate regarding healthcare reform continue, there is increasing comparison of the U.S. healthcare system with the Canadian system. Some stakeholders suggest the Canadian model be adopted in the United States. Others are very much opposed to such a transformation. A brief overview of the Canadian system and selected comparisons to the system in the United States are described here.

The Canadian healthcare program is universal, comprehensive, publicly funded (with no financial access barriers for care), and privately delivered. All citizens are covered for all medically necessary services through a federal-provincial health insurance system. The U.S. system is not universal, comprehensive, or publicly funded, except for Medicare and Medicaid enrollees (31 million and 19 million, respectively). These enrollees are subject to financial means tests (Medicaid) and copayment/deductible access barriers (Medicaid and Medicare). The majority of United States citizens (180 million) have private health insurance, largely financed through employers (82%). Coverage varies widely, from minimal to comprehensive. Premium rates, copayments, and deductibles also vary by policy type.[18] An estimated 37 million Americans have no health insurance whatsoever.[23]

The Canadian system has evolved over more than 45 years, beginning at the provincial level. In the past 5 years, provincial governments have tried to control costs by increased emphasis on community-based care. (A similar movement is under way in the United States, driven by market forces rather than government.) The federal-provincial funding arrangements vary across provinces, and administration and control of the program is unique within each province and the two territories. Provinces are single-source payers for both hospital and physician expenditures. There is a centralized locus of control, and the role of private insurance companies is limited by law. In the United States, private insurers are highly influential in the healthcare system, covering more than 77% of the population.[22] The locus of control in the United States is dispersed over multiple-payer sources, making control of resources much more difficult.

Using a centralized control approach, each Canadian province (and territory) prospectively determines each hospital's global budget for the coming year. A global budget is the total or lump sum amount that the hospital will receive for its services. Hospitals themselves determine the distribution of allocated funds within the institution. No deficit spending is permitted; hospitals must live within their budgets. Methods for adjusting the global budget vary by province. In Ontario (the most populated province), the Ministry of Health makes adjustments based on inflation, workload, approved new programs or expansion of existing programs, and increases in cost or volume related to certain services, such as dialysis, oncology, neonatal intensive care, and cardiovascular surgery.[23] Within these constraints, hospitals must serve all patients who seek care.

Provincial governments also negotiate reimbursement rates with medical associations, and the fees are set prospectively. Aggregate physician expenditures are controlled in five provinces (which contain 80% of the population) through a threshold approach. If physician expenditures within the province exceed what was budgeted due to increased volume of client services delivered, provinces can recoup their losses by adjusting future reimbursement rates downward or by paying current fees at a discount. This approach affects the total amount of money available to the medical profession for reimbursement and indirectly affects individual physician income.[18]

Like other provinces, Quebec negotiates expenditure targets for the total physician group; however, individual physician income targets are set as well. There are imposed ceilings on the quarterly gross billings of individual physicians, and if a physician exceeds the ceiling, he or she is reimbursed at only 25% of the allowable rate for additional care delivered. The Ministry of Health also reimburses new physicians in rural areas at a higher rate than those opening practices in urban areas, thereby influencing the geographic distribution of care.[18]

Clearly, the Canadian government at the provincial level has much tighter control over healthcare expenditures than is found among the multiple payers in the United States.

community, and the nation. Nurses have special concerns for groups that are especially at risk for poor health outcomes. Nurses provide critical services to prenatal and perinatal clients, particularly those who are adolescent, living in poverty, single, and unemployed. Case finding, screening, referral, followup, and education are among the services that nurses provide to this at-risk group. These nursing services take place primarily in the community.

Among the neonatal-pediatric population, nurses again provide important services. Public health nurses follow at-risk neonates in the home after discharge from the hospital. They are most concerned with the stability of the family unit and its capacity to care for the preterm or otherwise compromised infant. Ongoing education and support are provided by the public health nurse.

Nurses in other ambulatory and community agencies monitor and support the growth and development of children. School nurses provide primary care and counseling

to school-age children. These nurses are concerned with proper nutrition, prevention of substance abuse, and child abuse recognition and intervention.

Nurses across various settings care for adult clients from the early 20s through old age. Most younger adults come in contact with nurses through occupational health programs or in acute care hospitals when accident or illness threatens the individual's health. Women in their childbearing years, a special segment of the adult population, are followed by nurses in community health practice and in hospital practice.

Middle-aged and older adults are cared for by nurses skilled in chronic care, acute-critical care, home care, and long-term care. The nurse plays a vital part in assisting this population with health promotion, disease prevention, symptom management, performance of activities of daily living, independent living to the fullest extent possible, and support for a dignified death. The number of frail elderly is increasing; nurses in geriatric practice provide

Other systemwide comparison data are displayed in the following table.

Selected Comparisons of U.S. and Canadian Healthcare Systems

	Canada	United States
Healthcare as % of GNP	8.7 [1988]	11.2 [1987]
Per capita expenditures (U.S.$)	$1,556 [1989]	$1,973 [1987]
Length of stay (days)	8.1 [1988]	7.1 [1987]
Cost per hospital stay (U.S.$)	$2,014 [1988]	$3,532 [1987]
Cost per day (U.S.$)	$243 [1988]	$500 [1987]
Beds per 1000 population	7.1 [1986]	5.4 [1986]
Occupancy rate	83.8% [1988]	68.4% [1987]
Physicians per population ratio	486 [1985]	418 [1985]

GNP, gross national product

Satisfaction surveys have indicated that 95% of Canadians surveyed preferred their own healthcare system over a U.S. model, whereas only 37% of United States citizens surveyed preferred the U.S. system over the Canadian model.[4] Health status indicators for 1982 to 1984 reveal that Canada's infant mortality rate and age-standardized death rate for all causes were lower than those for the United States, and that life expectancy at birth for males and females was slightly higher in Canada.[18] All expenditure and health status outcome data provide support for the apparent success of the Canadian model.

Can or should the United States replicate such a model? There is strong debate as to the feasibility of replicating the Canadian system in the United States. Canada has only one tenth the population (25 million versus 241 million) and only seven provincial and two territorial government structures in addition to that at the federal level. In contrast, there are 50 state governments with which the federal government would have to negotiate funding formulas. Moreover, the culture in the United States is substantially different with regard to government's role in the lives of citizens. Among Canadians, government is expected to design, implement, and support social programs.[18] In the United States there is much more emphasis on individual accountability and noninterference by government. The second critical factor that may prevent adoption of a Canadian-type model in the United States is the political environment. Congress and state legislatures are heavily influenced by special interest groups. A movement toward a centralized, single-payer system in the United States would likely produce intense opposition from hospital, physician, and health insurance lobbies, among others.

Finally, barriers to change may arise from among U.S. citizens who are adequately insured and enjoy healthcare "on demand." Shifting from the current open-ended system to a resource-controlled system would mandate care delivery on an "as-needed" basis. Citizens would wait for elective services in some cases. Currently, only uninsured (37 million) and underinsured U.S. citizens (19 million Medicaid plus unknown numbers of privately insured persons) are denied services or subject to delay. Under a single-payer, centralized control system, all citizens would be treated equitably within the healthcare system. Ability to pay would no longer separate the "haves" from the "have nots." Although many from both groups would welcome such a redistribution of health care resources, U.S. citizens would have to modify their expectations relating to healthcare services. As in Canada, there may be a gradual evolution to the single-payer system, and this evolution may begin at the state level. The decade of the 90s is the period in which the United States must resolve these issues.

multiple services to these clients at home, in the hospital, and in long-term facilities.

Variations in Geography

Nurses work with clients who live in a variety of settings, from the inner city to rural communities. The challenges, as well as the resources to meet those challenges, are often different in each area.

The rural nurse must be a skilled generalist who is able to assess and refer patients for secondary and tertiary care, which usually is many miles away. This nurse has limited resources to call on for consultation. There are relatively few clinical nurse specialists or other advanced practitioners working in rural areas. Many rural communities have no hospital, and some do not have physicians. It is incumbent on the rural community health nurse to recognize abnormalities early in the course of illness, to make timely referrals to far-away centers, and to follow up clients to ensure they were treated. One of the greatest challenges for the rural population can be transportation to the city for care. Rural nurses work to facilitate the client and family's transition to the urban area and their return to the community.

Nurses practicing in inner city clinics and hospitals face other challenges. Public health clinics serve clients who have a limited ability to pay but who are in dire need of family planning services, prenatal care, pediatric services, and general healthcare. Nurses in both the clinic and the public hospital must be knowledgeable about the health practices and beliefs of many ethnic groups, which may have an impact on the client's ability to comply with the prescribed plan of care. Although nurses practicing in inner cities often have access to many healthcare experts for consultation, tax-supported hospitals and clinics are often underfunded, resulting in a chronic insufficiency of medical supplies, personnel, and beds. Nurses in these areas become expert at conserving and improvising to attain treatment goals.

Variations in Life-Style

Nurses work with clients who have different life-styles, which are also often different from the life-style of the nurse. Homeless clients and substance abusing clients are two examples of such populations.

Homeless clients are cared for in many ways across the country. The primary initiative among healthcare providers is to make healthcare accessible to these patients. In some cities, mobile healthcare vans travel from site to site offering primary care and referral. In other regions, walk-in clinics are open in areas frequented by the homeless population. Homeless people have special healthcare needs that range from diseases of the feet and legs (as a result of walking and perpetual shoe-wearing) to mental health conditions. Nurses, particularly nurse practitioners and community health nurses, are critical to the provision of healthcare to these individuals and families.

People who abuse drugs, alcohol, or both, also have special healthcare needs. In addition to problems of ad-

diction, the lives they may lead to procure illegal substances and alcohol (e.g., prostitution, theft, violent crime) put them at considerable risk for illness, disease, and injury. They are also members of families and of other communal groups, and therefore are at risk of transmitting their addiction to unborn children and of transmitting infectious diseases to others (such as hepatitis, AIDS, or other sexually transmitted diseases). Nurses may encounter substance abusers in several settings. Nurses are active in the treatment of substance abuse at both inpatient and outpatient centers. They support and monitor the individual's acute detoxification and recovery period. Nurses in the community often confront clients who show signs of substance abuse, in an attempt to gain client interest in referral for treatment. Among persons who are not in recovery, nurses screen for and treat the undesirable health conditions that result from substance abuse. Community-based nurses also educate and counsel clients and their significant others about the dangers of addiction and ways to prevent the spread of infectious disease.

HIV Infection

One of the biggest challenges facing nursing and the healthcare community in general is the care of persons infected with human immunodeficiency virus (HIV, also known as the AIDS virus). Nurses from across the country have risen to meet the challenge in clients' homes, in the community, and in acute care hospitals.

Nurse case managers work with AIDS clients in many large cities, coordinating and procuring necessary medical and social services. Clinic nurses in various sites across the United States give aerosol pentamidine treatments to prevent respiratory complications to outpatients. Nurse practitioners follow HIV clients from the onset of infection, for primary healthcare needs. Acute care nurses care for clients hospitalized for exacerbations, and hospice nurses assist AIDS clients in preparing for a dignified death. Nurses provide direct client care, emotional support, education, prevention counseling to friends and family, and self-care support to AIDS clients. Wherever the need has arisen, nurses have come forth with compassion and concern to meet these needs.

Conclusions

The healthcare system in the United States is large and complex, with many stakeholders (see Box 1–3 for a comparison between the U.S. healthcare system and the Canadian healthcare system). It is also a system under considerable pressure to change as a direct result of rising costs and lower accessibility to basic care for a growing number of citizens. This is the environment in which nursing practice takes place. This chapter has acquainted the reader with the political challenges facing the United States; it has also demonstrated that nurses are in the mainstream of service to both advantaged and disadvantaged client populations. Nurses play a critical role in delivering healthcare to the U.S. population. Many believe that nurses may be the key to revamping the healthcare system to one that provides access to basic primary care for all citizens. The contribution of the nursing profession to the nation's health has never been so important, as we move into the 21st century.

Bibliography

1. Aiken, L. H., & Bays, K. D. (1984). The medicare debate—round one. *New England Journal of Medicine, 311,* 1196–1200.
2. American Nurses' Association (1991). *Agenda for health care reform.* Kansas City, Mo.: American Nurses' Association.
3. Bice, T. W. (1980). Health services planning and regulation. In S. J. Williams & P. R. Torrens (Eds.), *Introduction to health services* (pp. 267–321). New York: John Wiley.
4. Blendon, R. J. (1989). Three systems: A comparative survey. *Health Management Quarterly, 11,* 2–10.
5. Burda, D. (1991). Hospital industry regroups after Supreme Court upholds NRLB rule. *Modern Healthcare, 27*(17), 2–3.
6. Cherskov, M. (1987). Capitated payment will dominate by 1995: A study. *Hospitals, 61*(6), 83–84.
7. Clemen-Stone, S., Eigsti, D. G., & McGuire, S. L. (1995). Clients with long-term care needs: Home health, hospice, and other services. In S. Clemon-Stone (Ed.), *Comprehensive community health nursing* (4th ed.) (pp 770–816). St. Louis: Mosby–Year Book.
8. Clemen-Stone, S., Eigsti, D. G., & McGuire, S. L. (1995). Occupational health nursing. In S. Clemon-Stone (Ed.), *Comprehensive community health nursing* (pp. 666–701). St. Louis: Mosby–Year Book.
9. Division of National Cost Estimates. Office of the Actuary, Health Care Financing Administration (1990). In P. Lee & C. Estes (Eds.), *The Nation's Health* (pp. 207–221). Boston: Jones & Bartlett.
10. Ethridge, P. (1991). A nursing HMO: Carondelet St. Mary's experience. *Nursing Management, 22*(7), 22–27.
11. Garner, J. S., et al. (1990). Strategic nursing management. Rockville, MD: Aspen.
12. Lewin, L. S. & Lewin, M. E. (1987). Financing charity care in an era of competition. *Health Affairs, 6*(1), 47–60.
13. "Major Job Losses Foreseen in Shift to Managed Care" (1995). *American Journal of Nursing, 95*(1), 73–75.
14. National League for Nursing (1990). Improving the performance of nurse managers in home care. In *A white paper.* New York: National League for Nursing.
15. Oberg, C. (1990). Medically uninsured children in the United States: A challenge to public policy. *Journal of School Health, 60* (10), 493–500.
16. Pilon, B. A., & Davis, S. (November, 1988). Healthcare delivery cost containment practices: History, current status, future directions. In N. Sanders (project director), *Cost management education for nurses.* Washington, D.C.: U. S. Department of Health and Human Services, Health Resources and Services Administration, Bureau of Health Professions, Division of Nursing (contract number 240–86–0064).
17. Poen, M. (1979). Politics, then health: The medicare compromise. In *Harry S. Truman versus the medical lobby* (pp. 174–209). Columbia, MO: University of Missouri Press.
18. Rakich, J. S. (1991). The Canadian and U.S. health care systems: Profiles and policies. *Journal of the American College of Healthcare Executives, 36*(1), 25–42.
19. Richardson, W. C. (1990). Financing health services. In S. J. Williams, & P. R. Torrens (Eds.), *Introduction to health services* (pp. 286–321). New York: John Wiley.
20. Rice, D. P. (1990). The medical care system: Past trends and future projections. In P. Lee, & C. Estes (Eds.), *The Nation's Health* (pp. 72–93). Boston: Jones & Bartlett.
21. Steinwald, B., & Sloan, F. (1981). Regulatory approaches to hospital cost containment: A synthesis of the empirical evidence. In M. Olsen (Ed.), *A new approach to the economics of health care* (pp. 272–307). Washington, D.C.: American Enterprise Institute.
22. U.S. Department of Commerce, 1989. Statistical abstract of the United States, 1989. Washington, D.C.: Author.
23. U.S. Department of Health and Human Services, 1989. National medical expenditure survey: A profile of uninsured Americans, research findings 1. Publication No. PHS 89-3443. Washington, D.C.: Author.
24. U.S. Department of Health and Human Services, Public Health Service, Health Resources and Services Administration, Bureau of Health Professions, Division. (1994). *1992: The registered nurse population.* Washington, D.C.: Department of Health and Human Services.
25. White, J. (1991). Hospitals object to changes in capital payment policy. *Health Progress, 74*(4), 10–13.
26. Williams, C. A. (1992). Community-based population-focused practice: The foundation of public health nursing. In M. Stanhope & J. Lancaster (Eds.), *Community health nursing: Process and practice for promoting health* (3rd ed.) (pp. 245–252). St. Louis: Mosby–Year Book.
27. Winslow, J. (January 29, 1991) Medical costs soar, defying firm's cures. *Wall Street Journal* p. B1.

2

Theories of Health and Illness

Joyce M. Black

Who gets sick and why? Who stays healthy and why? These continue to be common questions. This chapter focuses on some theories of disease development and introduces the more recent theories on health and health promotion. Chapter 10 describes the theories of health promotion in more detail.

The History of Healthcare

Early Humans

Early records of human history address illness and its effects on the body and the mind. Consider the Book of Job in the Old Testament, which details his multiple afflictions, including boils and leprosy. Paleontologists have revealed signs of injury and disease in early cave dwellers. Fossil remains show evidence of arthritis, tuberculosis, wounds incurred in fighting, and parasite infestation. Powerless, early man had to stand by and watch his fellow beings as they were stricken and killed by unknown forces. He grew convinced that these illnesses were sent from the angry spirits of dead animals or people.

Sorcerers claimed to have knowledge of the stars and the spirits and to have the ability to placate evil spirits with herbs and potions. Sorcerers were the first to practice trephining, or perforation of the skull, on living subjects. The holes supposedly enabled evil spirits to leave the body (Fig. 2-1).

Early Civilizations

When early civilizations developed in Mesopotamia, one of them, the Sumerians, based their medicine on astronomy. Sumerian people believed that a person's destiny was told in the stars and that blood was the center of life. They also believed that a horde of demons infested the earth. The demons produced jaundice, heart disease, fever, stroke, plagues, venereal disease, and arthritis. Doc-

tors at that time were priests, who treated disease by exorcism. A wide range of drugs, obtained from plants, fruits, animals and minerals, was also used. In addition, animal excreta was a common treatment to drive out demons. Horse dung was still listed as a treatment for pleurisy in a textbook on medicine published in London in 1718!

The Egyptians also managed health by ridding people of demons. All cures for diseases were put forth by the gods and kept protected by "doctors" who were priests. Instructions for treating open wounds, fractures and dislocations have been found in Egyptian ruins. The Egyptians thought respiration was the center of life, but supposed that circulation depended on respiration. They studied anatomy by examining animals. Egyptians are best known for embalming the dead. Their embalming techniques were so perfect that microscopic examination of tissue sections shows evidence of disease. Sadly, they provided better care for the dead than for the living. As centuries passed, the Egyptians would be known for their organization and world power, but not for advancing healthcare.

Asian Civilizations

Asian civilizations were also developing. Ancient Indian medicine described the physician's role in battle as having concern for food, water, fuel, and sites for the army to camp. This early awareness that poisons in the food and water could be lethal can be considered an early form of health promotion. Illness was described as an imbalance in three physical humors: spirit, bile, and phlegm. Besides defining these three physical qualities, the Eastern Indians recognized the role of psychosomatic disorders (or the mind's influence on the body). Interestingly, plastic surgery was a field in which Indians were centuries ahead of other civilizations. Rhinoplasty, the reshaping of the nose, was widely practiced. It was not done for aesthetic reasons, but for reconstruction. At the time, adultery was punishable in India by cutting off the nose, and

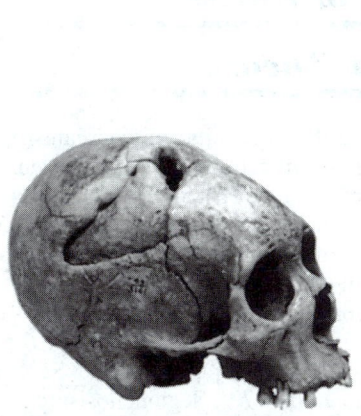
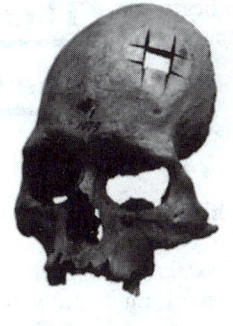
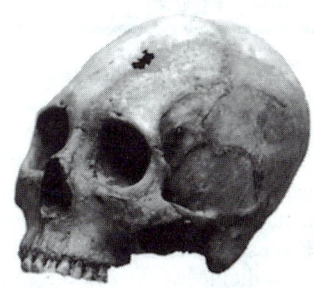

Figure 2–1. Skull with trephine holes. Holes were surgically made in skulls in an attempt to treat disease by enabling evil spirits to leave the body. Ancient skulls show that people survived even though very large trephine holes were made. In fact, some skulls show multiple large holes that had healed. The practice still exists among primitive people in parts of Algeria and Melanesia, although it is fast becoming obsolete. (Courtesy of the American Museum of Natural History.)

surgeons devised an operation to restore the normal contour of the amputated nose.

Whereas the pharaohs of Egypt were focused on building pyramids, the Chinese were focused on healthcare. Chinese medicine was based on the principle of balance between yin and yang: yang is positive, active, and masculine; yin is negative, passive, and feminine. Yin and yang were vital substances that flowed with blood throughout the body. Illness was thought to be the result of an imbalance in these two substances. Death occurred when they ceased to flow. The Chinese were the first people to immunize against smallpox and to prescribe iron for anemia. Acupuncture was developed in China many years ago, and its use has spread beyond China.

Israelite Civilization

For the Israelites, illness was not due to demonic possession; rather, it represented a visible sign of God's wrath on sinful man. Faith alone brought health to the body and salvation to the soul. The Israelites had extensive health laws (Mosaic Laws), which were recorded in the Hebrew Scriptures. People were considered "unclean" for a multitude of reasons: for example, if they touched dead animals, had gonorrhea or leprosy, or were menstruating. Unclean people were often isolated from others. In addition, very exact laws were given about foods that could and could not be eaten. For example, eating pork was forbidden. Now we know that improperly cooked pork contains *Trichinella spiralis,* an infectious organism that causes trichinosis.

Greek Civilization

Hippocrates, the Father of Medicine and author of the Hippocratic Oath, lived in Greece. In the 5th century B.C., Hippocrates wrote, "If sick men fared just as well eating and drinking and living exactly as healthy men do, and no better on some different regimen, there would be little need for the science (of medicine). But the reason why the art of medicine became necessary was because sick men did not get well on the same regimen as the healthy."

Hippocrates set healthcare on a new course by using proven cures and by breaking away from religious and demonic explanations of illness. He had a profound understanding of human suffering and taught that suffering could be reduced by hygiene and not by magic. He also believed that the body had the means to cure itself, and the healing power of nature is often discussed in his writing. Hippocrates described the body as being composed of blood, phlegm, yellow bile, and black bile; as in the humoral theory that had been propounded by several other civilizations, health and illness were thought to be due to balance or imbalance of these four elements. Fever, inflammation, boils, or diarrhea were seen as the body's way of purging itself, and no treatment was felt to be needed. As strange as Hippocrates' philosophy may seem today, the concepts set forth by Hippocrates still were in practice in the first half of 19th century in America. Just before Hippocrates' death, Aristotle was born. Aristotle and his followers did anatomic dissections, which had been illegal during Hippocrates' life, and they provided very elaborate descriptions of the body's organs.

Roman Civilization

When the center of civilization shifted to Rome, superstition and magic continued to be central to healthcare philosophy. Especially common was the use of animal liver to cure various ailments. Various gods were called on to help the people through specific troubles; for example, the goddess Opigena was summoned to assist women in childbirth. Romans also introduced the concept of sewers: the water supply was transported through an elaborate system of aqueducts.

Galen is a giant in the history of healthcare. At the height of the Roman empire, Galen wrote 22 massive volumes of material on health, illness, and healthcare. He described anatomy, physiology, diagnostic reasoning, and treatments.

The Dark Ages

During the Dark Ages, plagues of smallpox, scarlet fever, cholera, and other diseases were rampant. The bubonic plague, which was caused by the bacterium *Pasteurella pestis*, killed about one fourth of the population of Europe in the 6th Century. Smallpox, resulting in death or disfigurement, infected three fourths of the population of Europe. Plagues killed millions of people, and the powerlessness of medicine to do anything cast a dark light on doctors and moved society away from reason and back to superstition.

During the Middle Ages, virtually no progress was made in understanding the science of health or illness. Bloodletting to rid the body of bad humors was common practice. Most physically or mentally ill people were shunned from society. More medicines were being used, some of which were imported from the Orient.

The Renaissance

With the end of the Middle Ages, the culture reawoke and science began again. We call this period the Renaissance. An interest in learning developed and Greek and Roman writings were restudied. All aspects of life were changing; instead of believing that illness was due to demons, direct observation of the natural world led to knowledge. The diagnosis of illness was made by analysis of urine and bloodletting. Physicians were educated in universities. Within the next few centuries, remarkable discoveries were made. Leonardo da Vinci described the muscles and arteries, Vesalius described human anatomy, Paré developed principles of surgery, and Harvey discovered how blood circulates.

The Battle Over Infection

Armies have been defeated as often by epidemic diseases as by battle wounds. Battle wounds are easily contaminated, which exacerbates the spread of infection. Military hospitals were established at the end of the 18th century, but tremendous loss of life ensued from terrible hospital hygiene standards. Florence Nightingale's work resulted from the unnecessary death she saw on the battlefield in the Crimean War; her work led to the establishment of the profession of nursing. It was not until the later part of the 19th century that scientists began to unravel the basic causes of infectious disease. Semmelweis became convinced that puerperal fever was contagious and ordered handwashing and disinfection with calcium chloride, after which the death rate from infection dropped dramatically. Lister, expanding on the work of Pasteur, introduced disinfection into hospitals and operating rooms. Our study of the theories of illness will begin with the battle over bacteria. It is a battle which is still fought today.

Theories of Illness

The Germ Theory

Pasteur proposed that a specific microorganism was capable of causing an infectious disease. Pasteur's idea is called the germ theory. Pasteur's theory was a critical development in medical care and helped reduce deaths from infection. Infections are still a significant health problem. Poliomyelitis terrorized the United States in the 1940s and 1950s. Poliomyelitis killed many people and left many others paralyzed. Identification of the causative organism led to the development of the Salk and Sabin vaccines. In the mid-1970s, legionellosis (called legionnaire's disease), a previously unknown pneumonia-like infection, killed 29 people in Philadelphia. A causative organism was found, which led to treatment. In the early 1980s, some women who used superabsorbent tampons developed toxic shock syndrome. Again, the organism was identified and treatment methods were instituted. The most recent widespread infection that constitutes a significant public health threat is acquired immunodeficiency syndrome (AIDS). The causative virus has been identified, and intense research for treatment has been under way.

The Biomedical Model

Obviously, the germ theory does not explain all diseases. The biomedical model explains disease as a result of malfunctioning organs or cells. Within this model, conditions can be classified as diseases if they have a recognized cause, if a change occurs in structure or function of an organ, and if a group of clinical manifestations is consistently identifiable. For example, diabetes mellitus is a disease caused by a malfunctioning pancreas. The manifestations of uncontrolled diabetes mellitus are polydipsia (increased thirst), polyuria (frequent urination), and polyphagia (increased hunger). The manifestations of diabetes are directly related to an alteration in a physiologic process in the pancreas: an insufficient amount of insulin to carry glucose into the cells. Diabetes is managed with a fairly strict diet, frequent determination of blood glucose levels, administration of insulin, and regular exercise.

A concern with the biomedical model is that the model focuses on cause-and-effect relationships but tends to ignore the psychosocial components of diseases. Let us compare and contrast two cases of diabetes mellitus. John is a 45-year-old businessman who develops diabetes mellitus in midlife. He is willing to change his life-style, give himself daily insulin injections, reduce his weight, and follow his diet more closely. John's wife will prepare most of his meals following a diabetic meal plan. John will be able to check his blood glucose level at his office. In contrast, Jim is a 19-year-old college student with the same manifestations of diabetes and the same blood glucose levels as John. Both men need to make the same changes in order to manage the diabetes, but the changes Jim needs to incorporate will not be as easy for him. He eats irregularly because of his class schedule, drinks on weekends with his friends, and cannot envision being able to monitor his blood glucose levels during the daytime hours. The biomedical model classifies both John and Jim as diabetics, yet the theory cannot explain the varying reactions to the disease that are affected by age, personality, and likelihood of compliance with the therapy.

This medical orientation also defines disease as observable and quantifiable. Most of the findings are objective and are called *signs*. In our two example cases, the elevated blood glucose levels would be a sign of diabetes. *Symptoms*, are the subjective report of a disease; perhaps these two men would have reported nausea. When diseases are being diagnosed by physicians, symptoms are often noted but are not considered primary data. It may appear that the reliance on signs renders the client's symptoms unimportant. Subjective information is difficult to quantify, may be related to other factors that are not related to the disease (e.g., anxiety), or may be contrived (made up). When a common presentation of a disease exists, both signs and symptoms, it is called a clinical *syndrome*.

Some earlier research defined how clients perceive their illness and at what point health problems are considered an illness by laypersons. Findings suggested that for middle-class Americans, being ill meant *having an ailment that interfered with usual activities*. Some people also felt that disease was *an object or thing that invaded the body*. This depersonalized feeling about illness can be seen in some infectious illness that do indeed invade the body. It is important to realize that most diseases today are not infectious.

Multicausal Theories

Neither the germ theory nor the biomedical model can explain the widespread increase in noninfectious chronic diseases that affect modern civilizations. In the past, the high death rate from epidemics of infectious diseases meant that many people did not live long enough to develop chronic illnesses, especially conditions that are associated with aging. Even today, underdeveloped countries with high death rates from infectious diseases are less concerned with heart disease and cancer—ailments that plague industrialized nations.

The disorders that contribute to morbidity figures in developed nations today are ones in which a client's behavior, life-style, and genetic background play an underlying role in the development of disease. For example, essential hypertension and coronary artery disease cannot be well explained through the biomedical model. The genetic background, life-style, diet, and stress response of the client are aspects of the disease. It is becoming more common to probe the etiology of disease by examining the interrelationship of the client with the internal and external environment. Even infectious disease can be examined in a new light. Why does one person "catch a cold" when another person living in the same environment does not? Newer theories of illness causation help to explain some of these issues. These new theories can be called *multicausal* approaches to illness, because many factors specific to each client are examined.

Bernard and Cannon's Theory of Homeostasis

Claude Bernard, a 19th century physiologist, laid the foundation for homeostatic theories. Bernard was the first scientist to describe the internal milieu or environment of the body. He hypothesized correctly that if an organism is to live, it must have the capacity to maintain its internal environment. Bernard described some of the mechanisms that regulate the balance of internal body processes. He also saw health and illness in a new and enlightening way. Bernard defined health as the ability of the human organism to maintain its internal environment in a constant state despite the demands placed on it by the external environment. He postulated that illness was the result of an imbalance in the body's internal environment or in a disruption in the body's ability to communicate with the external environment. Bernard also defined disease as an adaptive effort by the body to restore its balance. He saw these adaptive efforts as appropriate to the illness but incorrect in magnitude. For example, the client with diabetes who cannot use glucose for energy uses proteins and fats instead. When fats are used for energy, an acid is produced that alters the body's acid-base balance. So, according to Bernard's theory, the diabetic client has attempted to adapt to the lack of sugar but has created a new problem—metabolic ketoacidosis.

Walter Cannon, a 20th century physician, developed the concept of feedback mechanisms to explain Bernard's theory of regulation of the internal environment. He recognized that the body's coordinated self-regulating, physiologic processes are needed to maintain a steady state. Cannon coined the term *homeostasis*, which comes from the Greek *homoios* (like) and *stasis* (standing). Cannon described homeostasis as a dynamic equilibrium, as opposed to a static equilibrium. A dynamic equilibrium is a flexible, ongoing process that maintains certain factors within a given range. He cited in his theory the body's ability to maintain temperature, blood pressure, fluid and electrolyte balances, and serum glucose, blood oxygen, and carbon dioxide levels.

Cannon also developed the concept of *fight or flight* to explain the body's reactions to emergencies. The fight-or-flight response prepares the body for muscular activity (e.g., running away) in response to a perceived or actual threat. The adrenal medulla is the pivotal organ for this response. It produces epinephrine (adrenalin) and norepinephrine, which increase the heart rate, respirations, blood pressure, and blood glucose levels and changes circulation to shunt (divert) blood from the intestines into the muscles of the legs, heart, and lungs. All of these processes prepare the body to move quickly away from danger.

Selye's Theory of the General Adaptation Syndrome

Hans Selye continued and built on Bernard's work on the body's adaptation to dangers. Selye developed a framework to describe how people respond to stress, based on observations he made while caring for sick people. He noted that regardless of the diagnosis, most clients presented certain common manifestations. These clinical manifestations included a loss of appetite, weight loss, feeling and looking ill, and various muscle aches and pains. Selye called this response to illness a *general adaptation syndrome* (GAS) because it involved generalized changes that affected several body systems. The changes were mediated by the sympathetic nervous system and adrenal cortices. Selye believed that the response to stress was measurable and described evidence of actual body changes. He noted that there was enlargement of the adrenal glands; shrinkage of the thymus, spleen, and lymph nodes; and development of gastric and duodenal ulcers. These responses occur following any stressor, which led Selye to describe stress as the nonspecific response of the body to any demand placed on it. Selye suggested that the entire body responds to stress in an attempt to maintain or adapt to the circumstances of the event creating stress. But if the demand or the stressor continues, the adaptive capacity of the body may be exceeded and disease may result. Examples of stressors of events causing stress include extreme heat and cold, physical injury, intense physical exertion, infection, and anxiety. He also recognized that each person has a limited amount of energy to use in dealing with stress. When stress is continuous, the adaptive capacity of the body may be exceeded and disease many result. Unrelenting stress may result in death. Selye believed that controlling stress is necessary for survival and that the individual must distinguish between stressors that are and are not worthy of a response.

In addition to the general adaptation syndrome, Selye described a *local adaptation syndrome* (LAS). The LAS takes place in a single organ or a specific section of the body. An example of LAS is inflammation, which is discussed in Chapter 20.

Stages of the General Adaptation Syndrome.
Selye suggested that both the GAS and the LAS develop in three distinct stages: (1) the alarm reaction, (2) the stage of resistance, and (3) the stage of exhaustion. For example, stage 1 is the arousal of the central nervous system: catecholamines (epinephrine and norepinephrine) are excreted, heart rate increases, the strength of heart contraction increases, and blood glucose levels rise. This is commonly called the *fight-or-flight response*. Cortisol is also released to increase glucose levels from stored glucose. If the stressor remains, the body cannot stay in stage 1 without experiencing pathologic changes. Changes occur in the thymus, spleen, and lymph nodes, and gastric ulcers develop. The thymus, spleen, and lymph nodes atrophy in response to the cortisol. Gastric ulcers occur because of the lack of production of protective mucus from shunted blood and the increased gastric acid production from cortisol. Stage 2 occurs when the body starts to react and to return to a homeostatic state. If the stressor is halted in this stage, the body should be able to return to a normal state. Stage 3 is the stage of exhaustion that occurs when the stressor continues and the body cannot continue to produce hormones as in stage 1 or when damage has occurred to other organs.

For example, people with severe head injury can develop bleeding gastric ulcers during the first few days after injury. This is due to the prolonged stimulation of the sympathetic nervous system and to lack of parasympathetic stimulation that provides blood flow to the gastrointestinal organs. Figure 2-2 describes the physical and psychological responses during the GAS.

Regulation of the General Adaptation Syndrome and the Local Adaptation Syndrome.
The most important regulators of the GAS and LAS are the central and autonomic nervous systems and the pituitary and adrenal glands. The pituitary and adrenal glands release hormones that inhibit or stimulate the body's stress response and defense mechanisms. Selye called the adrenal and pituitary hormones *adaptive hormones*. Adaptive hormones that inhibit excessive defense activities by the body include the glucocorticoids, which reduce inflammation, increase gluconeogenesis (production of glucose from other body sources), increase the circulation of white blood cells, and increase blood pressure. The other group of adaptive hormones are known as *proinflammatory corticoids* or *mineralocorticoids*. An example of a mineralocorticoid is aldosterone, which is secreted by the adrenal cortex and reduces the excretion of sodium for fluid balance.

Selye's theory that stress causes disease was based on the idea that excessive stress produces high levels of hormones. These hormones lower the body's resistance to disease and cause organ damage. Such hormonal activity, when pronounced and prolonged, does seem to cause serious side effects, but a new question arises. Does the stress that a person experiences automatically cause distress when the person is repeatedly exposed to the same stressor?

The body's ability to resist stress and to adapt to stressors depends on the proper balance of epinephrine, norepinephrine, and cortisol. In turn, the effect of these hormones on the body's resistance to stress depends on the individual's conditioning factors. Conditioning factors are circumstances that influence the GAS without being part of it. These factors can enhance or diminish the response to a stressor and include genetic predisposition, experience, mental attitude, diet, climate, and life-style. Because of the variability of the conditioning factors, different people respond differently to stressors. Conditioning factors help to strengthen the coping strategies through previous experiences with a stressor. Once a person has experienced a stressor, it may be easier to develop an "I've-been-through-this-before-and-it-will-be-OK" response.

Psychosocial Theories

Psychosocial theories of disease integrate physiologic, psychological, and social factors that explain disease development. They provide a different understanding of why some people get sick when exposed to microorganisms whereas others remain healthy, and they have revised popular concepts of what causes illness.

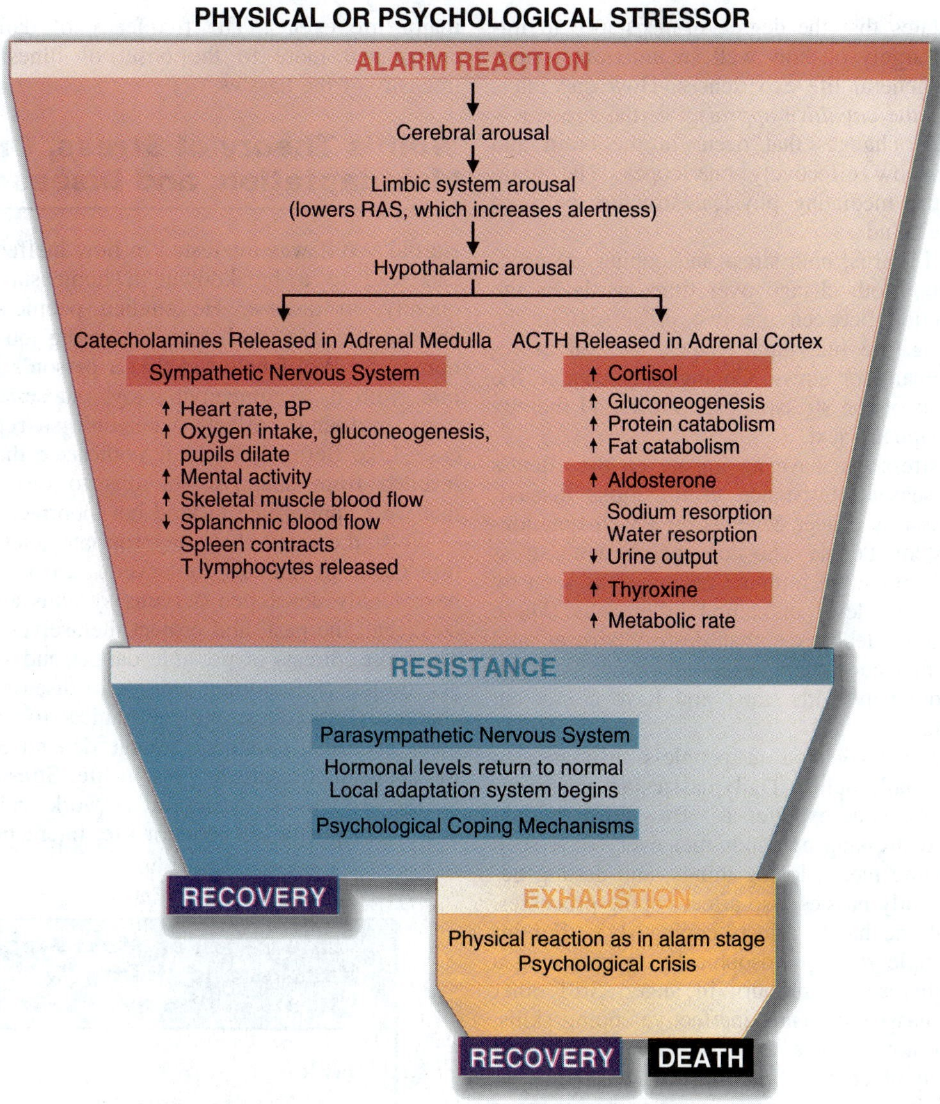

PHYSICAL OR PSYCHOLOGICAL STRESSOR

Figure 2–2. The general adaptation syndrome. Limbic system arousal (lowers reticular activating system, which increases alertness).

Mason's Theory of Specificity of the Stress Response

John Mason reexamined Selye's concept of stress and proposed that both a specific physiologic response and a nonspecific psychological response exist. He also stated that the nonspecific response, as described by Selye, is actually a psychological reaction. Mason theorized that the stress response is dependent on psychological factors (e.g., the person's perception of the stressor rather than the stressor itself). He concluded that stress is primarily a psychological phenomenon rather than a physiologic one. The physiologic response, if one occurs, develops secondary to the psychological response.

Mason also studied hormonal response to stressors. He found that cortisol, epinephrine, and norepinephrine were released in response to specific stressors (e.g., heavy exercise and exposure to cold and heat) rather than in response to nonspecific stressors, as Selye had proposed. Mason found that cortisol increases at three times: (1) in response to an individual's first experiences with new

stimuli, (2) when an individual learns to avoid noxious stimuli, and (3) when an individual receives punishment. One of Mason's studies found that levels of cortisol increased during periods of sleep deprivation and in pilots during prolonged flights. He also found a decrease in cortisol levels during weekends for people who worked Monday through Friday. Mason also demonstrated that humans can *modify* the cortisol response by coping effectively with a stressor. Research with parachute trainees over a 2-month period revealed that neuroendocrine responses to fear decreased only in those trainees who had mastered the technique of jumping. For this group, the stressor was no longer perceived as stressful because the person had dealt with it effectively.

Lazarus's Theories of the Stress Response

A newer understanding of why some people get sick when exposed to microorganisms whereas others remain healthy is revising popular concepts of what causes illness. Lazarus states that the degree of resistance to microbes depends largely on how well an individual copes with stress and general life experiences. How one interprets problems—the *cognitive appraisal* of the stressor—and the chemical changes that occur in the brain and body determine how effectively one copes. The brain appears to be the mediating physical structure between the body and the mind.

According to Lazarus, both stress and coping are processes, not events. Both change over time, partly as the result of interaction between the two processes. In the process of coping, the individual shapes, as well as responds to, a demand or stress. Coping may change the person's appraisal of the stressful experience and thereby influence what happens next.

Response to stress can have an impact on the client's resistance to diseases. Resistance to infectious disease, allergies, and possibly cancer depends on a well-functioning immune system. People who cope poorly with stress have significantly impaired immune responses as seen by a diminished activity level in natural killer cells. These cells are a type of leukocyte that destroy viruses and cancer cells on first encounter. Likewise, people who are healthy cope positively with stress and have competent immune function.

Lazarus specifically looked at people's responses to daily hassles and daily uplifts. Daily hassles are the minor life events that everyone experiences. They are irritating, frustrating, and distressing demands met every day, such as preparing routine meals, losing things, and getting delayed in traffic. Daily hassles also affect coping processes. The appraisal of the hassle affects coping style. For instance, some people react philosophically to receiving a traffic ticket, whereas others burn in anger. Still other people generate hassles by using ineffective coping skills. People who do not manage time effectively may feel pressured and out of control, with no time for family or recreational activities. Self-generated hassles due to poor coping are more harmful to a person's health than are hassles resulting from chance circumstances. This is because self-generated hassles tend to *recur* and are always *chronic* in nature. The student who always waits until the last minute to write a term paper suffers much more from this self-generated hassle than does the student who is occasionally late to class due to traffic congestion.

Lazarus also defined daily uplifts as buffers to the daily hassles. They provide relief from the daily hassles and come in three types. Daily uplifts act as *breathers* because they interrupt the intensity or frequency of the hassles. For example, reading a novel or seeing a movie provides a welcome escape from life's tiring demands. Other daily uplifts act as *sustainers* that provide people with the daily psychological nourishment needed to continue coping with life. An example of a sustainer is spending time with well-loved friends and family. Uplifts can also act as *restorers* that replenish the resources that have been depleted through harm or loss. Examples of restorers are prayer and meditation, resolving inner conflicts, and talking out problems with friends. Table 2–1 lists frequent hassles and uplifts as reported by a sample of 100 people. Lazarus's studies concluded that daily hassles are more significantly related to illness than are the major life events. The frequency of daily hassles also contributed more to the onset of illness than did the intensity of the hassles.

Wolff's Theory of Stress, Organ Maladaptation, and Disease

Harold Wolff was interested in how ineffective adaptation can lead to a breakdown in homeostasis and, subsequently, to disease. He studied people's responses to chronic stressors, such as a frustrating job or an unhappy home life. Wolff believed that a person's *total life situation,* with its accompanying joys, successes, and frustrations, profoundly affects a person's susceptibility to disease. Like Bernard, Wolff hypothesized that disease often resulted from adaptive attempts to restore homeostasis that were appropriate in kind but incorrect in magnitude.

Wolff theorized that inappropriate attempts at adaptation occur in humans for several reasons. First, humans have highly developed nervous systems and can symbolize, recall the past, and project themselves into the future. Therefore, threats of possible danger and symbols of danger are just as important a cause of disease as are noxious chemicals, microbes, and mechanical forces. Second, humans are tribal creatures; people depend on other people for many of the satisfactions in life. Stressors are created by the need to be successful at work and in association with other people. In modern life, interaction with people

Table 2–1. Ten Most Frequent Hassles and Uplifts (N = 100) (Items Listed by Frequency)

Hassles

1. Concerns about weight
2. Health of a family member
3. Rising prices of common goods
4. Home maintenance
5. Too many things to do
6. Misplacing or losing things
7. Yard work or outside home maintenance
8. Property, investment, or taxes
9. Crime
10. Physical appearance

Uplifts

1. Relating well to spouse or lover
2. Relating well to friends
3. Completing a task
4. Feeling healthy
5. Getting enough sleep
6. Eating out
7. Meeting our responsibilities
8. Visiting, phoning, or writing someone
9. Spending time with family
10. Home (inside) pleasing to you

Adapted from Kanner, A., et al. (1981). Comparison of two modes of stress measurement: Daily hassles and uplifts versus major life events. *Journal of Behavioral Medicine, 4,* 14.

of different races, religions, outlooks, and cultural values can be sources of stress to some people. A person may respond inappropriately to other individuals because of unrealistic and distorted perceptions of human relationships. The basis for this distortion again lies in the human ability to symbolize and to consider both the past and future.

Wolff's research indicated that certain individuals consistently respond to frustrating situations through a response by a particular body system or organ, perhaps the stomach, muscles of the back, colon, or nasal mucous membranes. Mucous membranes (whether in the nose, stomach, rectum, bladder, or vagina) seem to be particularly susceptible to stress. This is probably because these membranes serve as one of the primary defense mechanisms against bacterial and viral invasion. Mucous membranes exhibit several stress reactions: edema, ischemia, increased friability, malabsorption, ulceration, inflammation, and altered reactions to chemical substances. Such pathologic changes occur frequently in response to traumatic emotional situations. Pathologic changes that occur regularly and are combined with other chemical, biologic, or physical stressors can eventually lead to tissue damage, such as bleeding gastric ulcers.

Holmes and Rahe's Theory of Life Change and the Onset of Illness

Changes in life can create havoc. Change is a form of stress to which people must learn to adapt, both psychologically and physically. Some life changes are universal and affect all people (e.g., the effects of aging, the experience of pain, changes in self-concept). Other life changes are personal and affect fewer people (e.g., the birth of a child, an accident, or a change in job responsibilities). Adaptation to the change requires energy. If the person is required to adapt to many significant changes over a short period of time, the person will become overextended and expend too much energy trying to adapt, which may result in illness.

Disease and life changes are strongly linked. A psychiatrist in the 1930s began charting life events as a component of medical history. In the late 1960s the first attempt to quantify these changes was made by Holmes and Rahe.

Holmes and Rahe used a questionnaire to ask respondents to list major life changes based on their significance. Holmes and Rahe found that despite differences in life-style, education, culture, and economic status, people tended to agree on the significance of the stress of various life events. A numerical weight, called a *life change unit*, was assigned to each of the events. Once life events were weighted, they were ranked (Table 2–2). The death of a spouse ranks as the highest stressor.

Holmes and Rahe explored the relationship between the amount of change in a person's life and subsequent illness. They discovered that the higher a person's life change score, the greater the likelihood that an illness would develop. The research appeared to indicate that people with a sufficiently high score of life change units suffer major illnesses within a relatively short period of time, and that recent life events are precipitating factors

that influence the timing of onset of illness but not the type of illness. Minor ailments, serious disease, depression, and suicide attempts typically follow a cluster of both positive and negative life change units.

Some problems have been evident with this approach to illness development. For the most part, studies have been performed on subjects who have a disease, such as myocardial infarction. Subjects have been asked to retrospectively review the number of life events that occurred

Table 2–2. Social Readjustment Rating Scale	
Life Change Units	Major Life Events in Past 12 Months
100	Death of spouse
73	Divorce
65	Marital separation
63	Detention in jail institution
63	Death of close family member
53	Personal injury or illness
50	Marriage
47	Fired from job
45	Marital reconciliation
45	Retirement
44	Change in health behavior of family member
40	Pregnancy
39	Sexual difficulties
39	Gain of new family member
39	Business readjustment
38	Change in financial state
37	Death of close friend
36	Change to a different line of work
35	Change in number of arguments with spouse
31	Mortgage or loan over $10,000
30	Foreclosure of mortgage or loan
29	Change in responsibilities at work
29	Son or daughter leaving home
29	Trouble with in-laws
28	Outstanding personal achievement
26	Spouse began or ceased work
26	Began or ceased formal schooling
25	Change in living conditions
24	Revision of personal habits
23	Trouble with boss
20	Change in work hours or conditions
20	Change in residence
20	Change in schools
19	Change in recreation
19	Change in church activities
18	Change in social activities
17	Mortgage or loan less than $10,000
16	Change in sleeping habits
15	Change in number of family get-togethers
15	Change in eating habits
13	Vacation
11	Christmas
11	Minor violations of the law

From Holmes, T. H., & Rahe, R. H. (1967). The social readjustment rating scale. *Journal of Psychosomatic Research, 2,* 214. Reprinted with permission of authors and Pergamon Press, Ltd.

in the time period preceding the illness. This approach may alter the validity of the data because of recall bias. Some people cope with illness by trying to find its cause. Therefore, they may have a bias in their recall of recent life events and life changes. In addition, more than one third of these events involve either marriage or work, and the instrument is therefore focused toward younger, married, and working people. A study of men admitted to a Veteran's Administration hospital clearly revealed this bias. These men, for the most part, were unemployed, unmarried, and often homeless. They had major illness and major life stressors, but they scored low on the life change units scale. Finally, the scale does not take into consideration the stressfulness of non-events, "off-schedule" events, or chronic occurrences. For example, not getting a desired promotion (non-event) can be stressful. An unexpected *off-schedule* event, such as a pregnancy in a 45-year-old woman who believed that she was done raising her family, could not be marked on the scale. It should also be noted that the death of a child is not listed on the scale. Finally, anticipation of an event could be as stressful as the event itself, and chronic occurrences of even minor life changes could create a great impact of stress. The impact of monotony on illness is also not covered in the Holmes and Rahe scale.

In healthcare, stress can be seen in acute and chronic stages. Most commonly stress is seen in clients in acute care settings, because they are coping with such events as sudden hospitalization, sudden illness, and a new diagnosis. Clients in other settings, such as community health or home health settings, may have to learn to cope and to adapt to chronic stress, such as changes in environment, chronic disability, and loss of friends and family.

It is useful to distinguish four types of stressful events, based primarily on their duration:

● Acute, time-limited events (e.g., awaiting the results of a diagnostic test)
● Stress event sequences, in which a particular event initiates a series of stress events that occur over an extended period of time (e.g., bereavement)
● Chronic intermittent stressors, situations that occur and recur periodically (e.g., conflicts with family members)
● Chronic stress situations (e.g., chronic disability)

In stress event sequences and chronic stress conditions, stress reactions may occur over a long period. Further research is needed to determine the psychological and physiologic impact of these types of stressors. Most studies have been performed on acute stress response and measured autonomic nervous system and hormonal responses. Levels of hormones such as cortisol rarely show chronic elevations, which suggests that an equilibrium may be reached and that constant coping efforts are not needed. It is also not known if different coping efforts are more effective with acute versus chronic stressors.

The Role of the Brain in Illness

An expanded view of disease states that it is a *biopsychosociospiritual* process, means that a person's body, mind, and environment all function together to determine whether illness develops. Using this theory, illness is seen as a result of complex interactions involving multiple factors. Some factors that affect the development of disease include attitude, appraisal of stress, diet, and heredity. The biopsychosocial risk factor concept of disease is a marked departure from the germ theory. Disease is not always seen as a pathologic change caused by a foreign force. Instead, tissue damage is seen as resulting from normal bodily processes that have gone awry or been disrupted. These processes include the activity of neurotransmitters in the brain, the stress hormones of the adrenal glands and nervous system, and the helper and suppressor cells of the immune system. For example, excessive stress hormones (corticosteroids and catecholamines) can lead to artery damage or can suppress the action of antibodies and natural killer cells, which protect the body from foreign invaders and tumor development. Deficient suppressor cells may permit overaction of the immune system to the point at which the body starts attacking itself, such as in rheumatoid arthritis. These disorders are discussed in full in Chapters 28 and 74.

The knowledge of how the brain profoundly affects the function of the neurotransmitter (chemical messengers) has greatly expanded current views about health and illness. In 1975, the endogenous analgesics, enkephalins and endorphins, were discovered. Since that time, other neurotransmitters have been discovered. Equally important to the development of illness is the knowledge that the function and balance of these transmitters can be influenced by drugs, viruses, bacteria, poor nutrition, defective genes, aging, or the perception of stress.

Illness is simply not an "either-or" matter. One aspect of illness is the recognition that people are not either emotionally ill or physically ill. Ultimately, illness involves a combination of mind-body factors. These factors interact to produce symptoms experienced by the person. It is not uncommon to experience depression with physical illness or to have physical signs and symptoms of mental or emotional illness.

Historic Mind-Body Views

To fully understand the mind-body concepts we need to step back in time. Apart from the treatment of wounds and broken bones, the folklore of medicine is the most ancient aspect of the art of healing because primitive physicians showed their wisdom by treating the whole person, soul as well as body. In early times, no division was made between physical illness and mental illness. Methods of treatment were passed on by word of mouth, or *oral tradition*.

Various views on the body-mind relationship have evolved. At times the mind and body were viewed as interrelated, and at other times they were seen as divided and separate. Hippocrates, late in the 5th century B.C., taught that both the mind and body were involved in illness. He said "It is more important to know what sort of person has a disease than to know what sort of disease a person has." This connection of the mind to the body was considered important until the Renaissance.

During the Renaissance, René Descartes, the father of modern philosophy, developed a doctrine that postulated a division of reality between the mind and the body. He believed that the mind contained the essence of thinking, consciousness, and the soul, whereas the body was just a machine. Therefore, the previous connections of the mind and body were rejected. Religious and philosophical teachings were to focus on the mind and soul, whereas medicine concentrated on the physical body. This splitting of the mind from the body had significant impact on medical care. This dichotomous mind-body model of Descartes, called *cartesian dualism*, had tremendous impact on western thought. It was not until the work of Freud and others, which described an unconscious element to the human mind, that Descartes' model was seriously challenged. Freud's work helped healthcare providers develop an awareness of the significance of the emotions in mental and physical illness.

The task of reuniting the divided person in western culture has been difficult and is by no means complete. Various mind-body therapies have been developed in recent years. Biofeedback, autogenic training, and focused thought are some examples.

Wolf's Concept of Disease as a Way of Life

Stewart Wolf's theoretical approach focused on the role of the brain in regulating bodily processes and in causing disease. The brain helps maintain an internal milieu and helps the body adapt to the external environment. The response can markedly affect the body's functioning. The body needs high levels of epinephrine, blood glucose, and other hormones during times of physical threat when people must literally fight or flee. When these responses occur inappropriately or chronically, the excess hormones can cause harm. The way the brain defines any situation can evoke chemical and nervous system reactions. When people habitually respond to every frustration, disappointment, or loss as if it is a matter of life and death, then the endocrine, musculoskeletal, and autonomic nervous systems are called to respond. Wolf believed that if people view life as requiring constant domination of things and people, they can have an excessive outpouring of cholesterol, triglycerides, norepinephrine, adrenocorticotropic hormone (ACTH), and insulin. This type of attitude may contribute to deficient levels of pituitary growth hormone.

Wolf found that people who define their situation as hopeless may elicit an excessive conservation of oxygen, as if they were trying to hold their breath or "play dead" until hope returns. Breath-holding can stimulate the vagus nerve and cause cardiac dysrhythmias. Disease, then, can arise from evoked reaction patterns that are meant to be protective when the person is physically threatened but that are destructive when used inappropriately to fight symbolic battles. Wolf believed that disease could not be separated from the total person, including the person's way of life and interpretation of what life means. He suggested that "disease is a way of life, the end result of a way that people react to life's problems."

Schwartz's Model of the Brain as an Adaptive Regulator

Schwartz describes the brain as an adaptive system for regulation of the body. The central nervous system is sensitive to the external and internal environment. It processes information, and through a *feedback* system with the peripheral organs, it maintains a stable internal environment. A common example of this process is the changes seen in the body when it is cold—shivering occurs, and the skin becomes pale as blood is shunted away from the skin to prevent further loss of body heat.

Schwartz also describes a model of self-regulation and disregulation. According to the model the normal or usual response is attention, connection and self-regulation. *Attention* by the brain to external and internal environmental and psychophysiologic demands results in *connection* and *self-regulation*. The feedback loop stabilizes output and maintains homeostasis. Schwartz sees the correct functioning of the system as promoting ease or health. However, if the brain fails to pay attention to these demands (*disattention*), the result is *disconnection*. Disconnection results when the relationship between output and input or between the body and the brain becomes unbalanced and the feedback loop fails to stabilize output. The resulting disconnection of regulatory processes causes disregulation and disease. Thus, disattention is one condition that can lead to a disconnection between the brain and the body.

Consider the following example: Beth is a junior nursing student and has been under stress most of the semester, trying to work and to go to school. She has felt tired lately, but has ignored the symptoms (disattention) and has continued to work and to attend class and clinical laboratory (disconnection). Midterm arrives and the stress of studying for examinations causes Beth to become very ill (disregulation), and she cannot take an examination. Had Beth paid attention to the early warning signals of growing fatigue and intervened to slow down her commitments and to rest more frequently, she might have avoided becoming seriously ill and missing an examination.

Several implications about health and illness can be drawn from Schwartz's work. First, a degree of self-responsibility is involved in maintaining health. This does not mean that people are necessarily responsible for becoming ill. Instead, individuals are responsible for detecting the bodily feedback that indicates that an imbalance has occurred. They also need to regulate themselves to correct the imbalance. Finally, people need to seek assistance to regain self-regulation.

The role of the brain in health and illness is fairly clear in Schwartz's work. The brain is central to any change in health because it is the mediator between the external and internal environments. Through the brain's interpretation, a person can change an environment, leave it, or engage in it, or he or she can decide to rest, to exercise, or to diet. Clearly people have the ability to regulate themselves and move toward health on the healthcare continuum.

Mediators of the Stress Response

There is a growing consensus among stress researchers that to understand the relationship between stress and illness outcomes, the factors that modify or mediate the relationship must be clarified. Although stressors may produce temporary physiologic and psychological changes, most stressors are not followed by long-term illnesses. A stressor may produce an extreme reaction in one person and no reaction in another, or the same stressor may produce variable reactions in the same individual at different times. This suggests that factors exist that alter the responses to stressors. One factor that can alter a stress response is the environment, such as social supports, physical setting, and organizational factors. Social supports tend to buffer individuals from the potentially negative effects of stressors, and those people who have strong social supports may live longer and have a lower incidence of physical illness. Other factors are internal, such as personality, personal resources, temperament, history, and genetic variables. (Within the personal aspect of stress response is how the stressor is appraised and how the person copes with the stressor.) The expression of emotion, especially anger is one coping style that has been studied with interesting results. One might think that the expression of anger would have a negative effect on illness outcome, but, surprisingly, the outcome after expression of negative emotions depends on the disease. Frequently, expressing hostility and anger were shown to increase survival in people with cancer. But in people with lung disease, the expression of anger and other negative emotions increased their manifestations, and they had adverse physiologic changes (e.g., hypoxia).

Behavior Patterns

The relationship of behavior patterns, life-style, and stress to disease has been examined. An important study by Friedman and Rosenman described two behavior types: A and B. The original studies were performed to examine risk factors for coronary artery disease. Prior to these studies, it was believed that heart disease resulted from a diet that was too high in fat and cholesterol, lack of proper rest and exercise, excessive smoking, and a family history of heart disease. This theory focused on the hypothesis that heart disease can also evolve as a consequence of certain behavior types. Type A personality is characterized by constant mobilization of inner resources to combat real or imagined stresses. People with type A personality are described as aggressive, often hostile, hard-driving, and deadline-ridden, with a chronic sense of urgency. The type A person feels somewhat guilty when relaxing. Also, this person characteristically moves, walks, and eats rapidly and frequently does or thinks about two or more things at once. Job position does not appear to be a factor, because type A behavior can be seen in all occupations.

In sharp contrast is the type B personality. This person characteristically takes life with all of its stresses in stride. Although this person often is intelligent and ambitious, the type B personality does not allow activity to become self-destructive. The person can relax without feeling guilty and work without a sense of time urgency. The basic attitude toward life is calm, optimistic, and self-confident.

It is possible to see a pure type A or type B person, but people more frequently have some characteristics of both types. It is preferable to describe people as being *predominantly* type A or B.

Friedman and Rosenman's research determined that the type A person between the ages of 35 and 60 was almost three times more likely to develop coronary artery disease than was the type B person. In fact, the researchers concluded that the type B personality appeared to be almost immune to the onset of coronary artery disease. Although type A behavior patterns have a significant association with coronary heart disease, conclusions about a direct relationship cannot be made. In other words, a person with type A personality cannot be told that he will develop coronary artery disease, nor can the person with type B personality be assured that he will not develop coronary heart disease. The exact relationship of type A personality to coronary artery disease is not clear. One possible explanation is that the continuous stress placed on the sympathetic nervous system results in increased fatty acid circulation. The fatty acids may begin to occlude arteries, which leads to coronary artery disease.

Hardiness

Hardiness has recently emerged as another variable that influences a client's response to stress. Hardiness is viewed as a personality component that moderates or buffers the response to stress. Clients who are hardy can remain healthy under stressful situations. They can also view the stressor as an opportunity to practice mastery and undergo personal growth.

Concepts of hardiness have been associated with health maintenance in the following three areas:

● *Control:* the sense of mastery or self-confidence needed to appropriately appraise and interpret health stressors
● *Commitment:* the presence of active involvement in efforts to maintain or improve health
● *Challenge:* the presence of flexibility and persistence in coping with health stressors

Tools to measure or assess hardiness are being developed. Control is assessed by examining the client's sense that health and illness can be controlled (locus of control). Commitment is assessed by examining commitment to self and to one's health. Challenge is assessed by examining the client's usual response to problems and illnesses.[13]

Social Support

Scientists have noted for a long time that a relationship exists between social relationships and health. More socially isolated or less socially integrated people are less healthy, psychologically and physically, and are more likely to die. But the actual cause and effect is less clear. Are unhealthy people less likely to have and maintain social relationships? Or does the lack of social relationships cause people to become ill and die? Do people in a social network provide a basis of health? As we learn more about chronic illnesses, the role of social support seems even stronger. Physiologic studies have shown a link between the amygdala and the hypothalamus in the brain and positive social relationships. Social contact decreases hormones such as cortisol, epinephrine, and norepinephrine. From a psychological standpoint, social relationships provide a sense of meaning or coherence that promotes a healthy life-style. Social support may assist with adherence to medical treatment and appropriate seeking of medical care. Marriage is one of the most widely studied areas of social support. Marriages may be simultaneously a source of stress and support. Interestingly, it has also been suggested that regardless of the quality of the interaction, marriage provides some form of support. Frequently, a quick deterioration in the health of a survivor is seen after the death of a spouse.

Healthcare providers must seek to make use of a client's social support network. It is important to include the social network in the treatment regimen and to assess the impact of the illness on the partner.

Self-Help Groups

Self-help groups are on the rise in industrialized nations. It is estimated that there are at least 500,000 to 750,000 self-help groups in the United States, with at least 10 to 15 million members. Different forms of self-help groups can be found in non-industrialized countries. For example, some groups are organized and sanctioned by various societies. Reach for Recovery is an organized group for

women that have had a mastectomy. It is approved by the American Cancer Society. Informal groups also exist, such as people caring for older, infirm parents in their home, who meet to discuss common problems. Self-help groups are becoming a recognized and accepted form of assistance to meet people's needs. The largest groups are formed to help people with mental illnesses and the second largest groups have formed for people with AIDS.

There are two types of self-help groups. One is the 12-step program, of which Alcoholics Anonymous is the prototype. The other is a group whose members share common experiences. Characteristics of both groups include the following: help with the cognitive restructuring of an event or experience, instruction in adaptive skills, and fostering of emotional support, personal disclosure, socialization, taking actions together, empowerment, self-reliance, and self-esteem.

Multifactorial Aspects of Chronic Disease Today

As mentioned earlier, a century ago our ancestors fought infectious and communicable diseases. Although serious infectious diseases are still a public health threat, today's most life-threatening diseases are those that become chronic as a result of metabolic abnormalities induced by such factors as genetics, aging, nutrition, and environment (Fig. 2–3).

The Role of Heredity in Disease

In addition to research on the biopsychosocial aspects of diseases, there has been much medical research in other

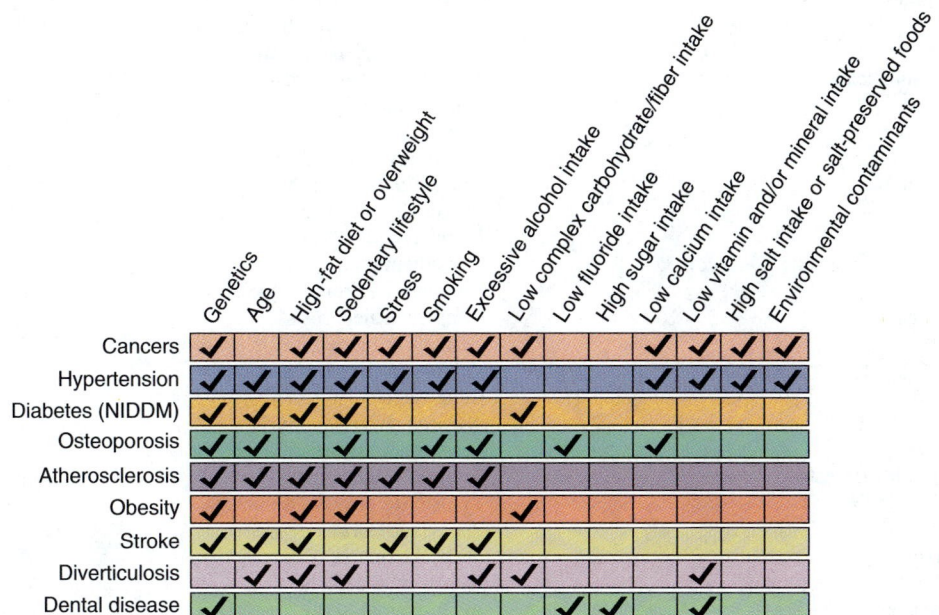

Figure 2–3. Multiple risk factors have been linked to most of the chronic diseases. (Reprinted by permission from p. 553 of *Understanding nutrition* (6th ed.) by Whitney, E. N., & Rolfes, S. R.; Copyright 1993 by West Publishing Company. All rights reserved.)

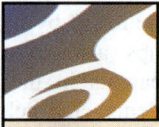

DIVERSITY IN HEALTHCARE

Biocultural Aspects of Disease

Genetic Disorders

Although sickle cell disease is a well-known disorder that has a profound impact on blacks and other groups having a distinct predilection to this serious blood disorder, it is just one of many genetic conditions linked to cultural diversity. As indicated in the Table, research has revealed that members of certain ra-

cial, ethnic, or population groups have a statistically higher probability of carrying selected genetic traits or disorders. The nature of these disorders affects virtually every body system—hematologic, respiratory, musculoskeletal, renal, gastrointestinal, integumentary, endocrine, and neurologic.

Biocultural Factors in Disease

In many disorders, multiple, and frequently interrelated, factors are responsible for differing susceptibilities to conditions. Among those factors that are examined here are variations in natural and acquired immunity, intermarriage, geographic and climatic conditions, ethnicity, race, hereditary predispositions, and

Distribution of Selected Genetic Traits and Disorders by Population or Ethnic Group

Ethnic or Population Group	Genetic or Multifactorial Disorder Present in Relatively High Frequency
Aland Islanders	Ocular albinism (Forsius-Erikkson type)
Amish	Limb girdle muscular dystrophy (IN—Adams, Allen counties)
	Ellis-van Creveld (PA—Lancaster county)
	Pyruvate kinase deficiency (OH—Mifflin county)
	Hemophilia B (PA—Holmes county)
Armenians	Familial Mediterranean fever
	Familial paroxysmal polyserositis
Blacks (African)	Sickle cell disease
	Hemoglobin C disease
	Hereditary persistence of hemoglobin F
	G6PD deficiency, African type
	Lactase deficiency, adult
	β-thalassemia
Burmese	Hemoglobin E disease
Chinese	Alpha-thalassemia
	G6PD deficiency, Chinese type
	Lactase deficiency, adult
Costa Ricans	Malignant osteopetrosis
Druze	Alkaptonuria
English	Cystic fibrosis
	Hereditary amyloidosis, type III
Eskimos	Congenital adrenal hyperplasia
	Pseudocholinesterase deficiency
	Methemoglobinemia
French Canadians (Quebec)	Tyrosinemia
	Morquio syndrome
Finns	Congenital nephrosis
	Generalized amyloidosis syndrome, V
	Polycystic liver disease
	Retinoschisis
	Aspartylglycoasaminuria
	Diastrophic dwarfism
Gypsies (Czech)	Congenital glaucoma
Hopi Indians	Tyrosinase positive albinism
Icelanders	Phenylketonuria
Irish	Phenylketonuria
	Neural tube defects
Japanese	Acatalasemia
	Cleft lip/palate
	Oguchi disease

religious practices. Some researchers have attempted to explain differences in susceptibility solely on the basis of cultural heritage, but they have not succeeded in doing so.[1-4]

Immunity. Perhaps one of the most frequently cited examples of the connection between immunity and race is that of malaria and the sickle cell trait in blacks, which has already been discussed in the chapter. Other malaria-specific variants are thalassemia, glucose-6-phosphate dehydrogenase, and Duffy blood group. Although they provide some protection from malaria, they also produce less advantageous effects.

Intermarriage. Intermarriage (i.e., marrying among one's family, tribe, or clan) among individuals from certain cultural groups has led to a wide variety of disorders. For example, an increased incidence of ventricular septal defects has been noted among the Amish and an increase in mental retardation is evident in a number of other groups. In the extreme, intermarriage among groups having few members can lead to total extinction. The number

Ethnic or Population Group	Genetic or Multifactorial Disorder Present in Relatively High Frequency
Jews	
Ashkenazi	Tay-Sachs disease (infantile)
	Niemann-Pick disease (infantile)
	Gaucher disease (adult type)
	Familial dysautonomia (Riley-Day syndrome)
	Bloom syndrome
	Torsion dystonia
	Factor XI (PTA) deficiency
Sephardi	Familial Mediterranean fever
	Ataxia-telangiectasia (Morocco)
	Cystinuria (Libya)
	Glycogen storage disease III (Morocco)
	Dubin-Johnson syndrome (Iran)
Orientals	Ichthyosis vulgaris (Iraq, India)
	Werdnig-Hoffmann disease (Karaite Jews)
	G6PD deficiency, Mediterranean type
	Phenylketonuria (Yemen)
	Metachromatic leukodystrophy (Habbanite Jews, Saudi Arabia)
Lapps	Congenital dislocation of hip
Lebanese	Dyggve-Melchior-Clausen syndrome
Mediterranean people (Italians, Greeks)	G6PD deficiency, Mediterranean type
	Beta-thalassemia
	Familial Mediterranean fever
Navajo Indians	Ear anomalies
Polynesians	Clubfoot
Poles	Phenylketonuria
Portuguese	Joseph disease
Nova Scotia Acadians	Niemann-Pick disease, type D
Scandinavians (Norwegians, Swedes, Danes)	Cholestasis-lymphedema (Norwegians)
	Sjögren-Larsson syndrome (Swedes)
	Krabbe disease
	Phenylketonuria
Scots	Phenylketonuria
	Cystic fibrosis
	Hereditary amyloidosis, type III
Thai	Lactase deficiency, adult
	Hemoglobin E disease
Zuni Indians	Tyrosinase positive albinism

From Cohen, F. L. (1984). *Clinical genetics in nursing practice* (pp. 23–24). Philadelphia: Lippincott–Raven. Reprinted by permission.

Continued on following page

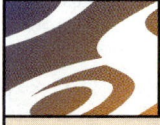

of Samaritans in Israel, for example, has been reduced to a handful of surviving aging members.

Geography/Climate. The influence of geography and climate may be illustrated by the example of a common communicable disease, rubeola (measles). Because of either the mutation of the virus or the increased individual resistance to the virus, measles became a virtually universal, though relatively benign, childhood disease in many parts of the world in the 19th and early 20th centuries. Although the majority of affected individuals experienced few ill effects from measles, certain populations, such as children in the Hawaiian Islands and parts of Africa, were severely or even mortally affected when explorers and missionaries brought the virus to their lands. Similarly, large numbers of Native Americans died from smallpox and other communicable diseases brought to North America by European explorers.

Ethnicity. Although the role of socioeconomic factors in tuberculosis cannot be disregarded, ethnicity also appears to be a factor in this disease. Groups with relatively high incidences of tuberculosis are American Indians residing in the Southwest, and Southeast Asian and Latin American immigrants. Ethnicity also is linked to several noncommunicable diseases. For example, Tay-Sachs disease, a neurologic condition affecting Ashkenazic Jews of northeastern European descent, and phenylketonuria (PKU), a metabolic disorder primarily affecting Scandinavians, are congenital abnormalities linked to specific ethnic groups.

Race. In addition to the inherited blood disorders discussed in this chapter, an estimated 70% to 90% of blacks have lactose intolerance, an enzyme deficiency that results in difficulty with the digestion and metabolism of milk.

Hereditary Predisposition to Disease. Extensive research has documented the link between predisposition to certain disease and cultural influences. For example, certain American Indian tribes including the Pima, Papago, and Seminole have a high incidence of diabetes mellitus, whereas the condition is extremely rare among Alaskan Eskimos. Culturally related dietary factors, exercise and activity patterns, and other life-style influences in combination with genetics are believed to provide a multifactorial explanation for the hereditary predisposition.

Religion. Growing evidence suggests that religious practices account for the relatively lower incidence of selected diseases among practicing members of certain religious groups. For example, research supports the notion that members of religions that prohibit smoking, such as Seventh Day Adventists and Mormons (Church of Jesus Christ of Latter-Day Saints), have a lower incidence of lung cancer and heart disease. There also is a lower incidence of breast cancer among Mormon women. For members of religions that advocate a vegetarian diet, such as Hinduism and Seventh-Day Adventism (encouraged but not required), preliminary studies suggest a variety of health benefits including lower cholesterol levels. The reported incidence of alcoholism and drug abuse is significantly lower in groups that prohibit their use, such as Baha'is, Muslims, and Mormons. Thus, religious practices may serve as a positive force in overcoming a genetic predisposition to some disorders and may result in longer, healthier lives for observant members.[4]

Culture-Bound Syndromes

Although all illness may be culturally defined, the term *culture-bound syndrome* is used when referring to disorders restricted to a particular culture or group of cultures. Culture-bound syndromes are thought to be illnesses created by personal, social, and cultural reactions to malfunctioning biologic and/or psychological processes. These syndromes can only be understood within defined contexts of meaning and social relationships.[1]

Perhaps the most widespread culture-bound syndrome is *mal ojo,* or evil eye. The belief that the gaze of the human eye can bring misfortune to people and their property is found among people from Latin American, Mediterranean, South Asian, Near Eastern, and some African cultures. The phenomenon is believed to be an extension of the religious and cultural beliefs concerning the dichotomy between good and evil. Although *mal ojo* has a core of cross-cultural similarities, many intercultural variations exist.

When illness is experienced, someone who is envious is believed to be the cause. It should be noted that *mal ojo* provides an explanatory model of illness that explains *why* the person is sick. In addition, the germ theory, accident, or other causes are cited to explain *how* the victim became afflicted. By categorizing certain illnesses as *mal ojo,* prevention and treatment are possible.

Prodromal symptoms may include uncontrollable yawning, hiccups, and eye twitching. Within 1 to 5 days, victims experience nervous tension, confusion, depression, headache, stomach cramps, diarrhea, fever, and/or exhaustion. Symptoms usually run their course in 3 to 7 days. If self-treatment is unsuccessful, a folk healer is often consulted. Folk healing varies widely among ethnic groups but

areas of disease causation. Genetic aspects of diseases have been recognized for many years, but recent technology has allowed medical researchers to identify the actual gene that is faulty in some disorders. And in the past 5 years, therapy has been developed to treat the altered gene structures.

More than a fifth of the genes that exist in humans differ in form from one person to another. This remarkable degree of genetic variation among normal people is what accounts for the naturally occurring variations in such attributes as height, hair color, intelligence, personality, and blood pressure. These genetic differences also

usually involves rituals performed by the healer. Although preventive measures exhibit a great deal of cross-cultural variation, they frequently involve wearing a talisman or amulet and use of objects such as beads or charms, which are believed to attract good or prevent harm. It should be noted that patients may consult multiple healers and combine interventions recommended by folk healers and professional healthcare providers.

More than 50 culture-bound syndromes have been documented by anthropologists and healthcare providers. The Table summarizes some of the more prevalent culture-bound syndromes.

Selected Culture-Bound Syndromes

Group	Disorder	Remarks
Blacks, Haitians	Blackout	Collapse, dizziness, inability to move
	High blood	Blood that is too rich in certain nutrients due to ingestion of too much red meat or rich food.
	Low blood	Not enough blood or weakness of the blood caused by dietary deficiencies
	Thin blood	Condition affecting women, children, and the elderly; individual is susceptible to disease and becomes sick easily
	Diseases associated with hex, witchcraft, or conjuring	Sense of being doomed by spell; gastrointestinal symptoms include nausea, vomiting; hallucinations are sometimes experienced
Hispanics	*Empacho*	Food forms a ball and clings to the stomach or intestines, causing cramping and pain
	Fatigue	Asthma-like symptoms
	Pasmo	Numbness and tingling of face or limbs; relieved by massage
	Susto	Anxiety, trembling, phobias resulting from sudden fright
Japanese	*Wagamama*	Apathetic childish behavior with emotional outbursts
Korean	*Hwa-byung*	Somatic and psychological symptoms including "pushing up" sensation in chest; palpitations, flushing, headache, epigastric mass, dysphoria, irritability, and difficulty concentrating; married women most frequently afflicted
Native Americans Various tribes	Ghost	Terror, hallucinations, sense of danger
Navajo	*Tadidiin* (corn pollen)	Allergic rhinitis and reactive airway disease; caused by allergy to corn pollen placed in the mouth for ceremonial purposes
Whites	Anorexia nervosa, bulimia	Excessive preoccupation with thinness; self-imposed starvation

1. Andrews, M. M., & Boyle, J. S. (1995). Transcultural nursing care. In M. M. Andrews & J. S. Boyle (Eds.), *Transcultural concepts in nursing care* (pp. 49–96). Philadelphia: Lippincott-Raven.
2. Giger, J. N., & Davidhizar, R. E. (1995). *Transcultural nursing: Assessment and intervention.* St. Louis: Mosby–Year Book.
3. Overfield, T. (1985). *Biologic variation in health and illness: Race, age, and sex differences.* Menlo Park, CA: Addison-Wesley.
4. Andrews, M. M., & Hanson, P. A. (1995). Religion, culture, and nursing. In M. M. Andrews & J. S. Boyle (Eds.), *Transcultural concepts in nursing care* (pp. 353–409). Philadelphia: Lippincott-Raven.

have an impact on each person's ability to handle environmental challenges, including those that produce disease. There is some degree of genetic interaction with the environment in every disease. For example, many smokers, but not all, develop lung cancer. In 1990, medical researchers identified a single gene linked to lung cancer risk. Perhaps a person's genetic makeup allows his or her body to kill early cancer cells. More than 5000 diseases are known to have a genetic component.

In certain diseases, however, the genetic component is so overwhelming that the disease occurs in a predictable manner. Such diseases are termed *genetic disorders*, and include diseases such as Huntington's chorea, which is a progressive neurologic disease.

New approaches to the treatment of genetic disease includes gene therapy. Gene therapy is the injection of DNA fragments into cells. The fragments find their way to the nucleus and repair enzymes to restore normal function to the cell. In the 1990s, research is being conducted on the use of gene therapy in the treatment of Alzheimer's disease, muscular dystrophy, cystic fibrosis, and some forms of primary and secondary epilepsy. Gene therapy remains a rapidly evolving form of treatment.

The Role of Aging in Disease

Older clients are more prone to injury, acute infections (especially respiratory infections), and other acute illnesses than are younger clients. Contributing to this are the increased occurrences of chronic illness, decreased reserve of energy, and decreased ability to respond physiologically to stress. It is common to see the aged client who is mentally competent become confused during the stress of acute illness. Recovery from acute illness takes longer than in a younger client, and a risk is present that the previous level of functioning will not be regained.

Common problems in the care of the aged client include promotion of physical safety, prevention of alterations in skin integrity, promotion of social interactions, and promotion of adequate nutrition. Nurses should not presume that all elderly clients are weak and debilitated. Qualities such as resilience help many elderly clients through losses (see Nursing Research feature). A full discussion of the aged and nurses' roles with the elderly is included in Chapter 5.

The Role of Nutrition in Disease

The ten leading causes of death are shown in Box 2–1. Four of these causes, including the top three, have some relationship to diet. The role of diet in these diseases is discussed, and more information about the actual diseases is presented later in the text.

Lipids. Lipids are fats, of which there are three types: triglycerides and their counterpart fatty acids, phospholipids and sterols. Triglycerides are used for an energy source and stored fat is used as body insulation. Triglycerides contain one molecule of glycerol and three fatty acids. The fatty acids can be saturated, monounsaturated, or polyunsaturated. The polyunsaturated and monounsaturated fats lead to a lower blood cholesterol level. Fatty acids are used as starting points for the manufacture of hormonal regulators. Phospholipids and sterol are used to build cell membranes and to manufacture hormones, vitamin D, and bile.

Lipoproteins. As fats are digested, they must be "packaged" for transport in the blood because they are

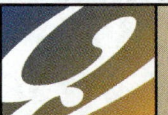

NURSING RESEARCH

What Are the Characteristics of Women with Resilience?

Waglid, G., & Young, H. (1990). Resilience among older women. Image, 22 (4), 252–255.

Many women survive the death of their spouse and live for several years alone. What qualities exist in these women?

A qualitative method was used to identify attributes of resilience that characterize elderly women who have adjusted successfully to major losses. Analysis of the data revealed five major qualities that reflected the attitude of these women. These qualities included:

- A balanced perspective of life experiences (equanimity)
- Persistence despite adversity and discouragement (perseverance)
- Belief in oneself and one's capabilities (self-reliance)
- Realization that life has a purpose
- Value of one's contribution to life and society (meaningfulness)
- Realization that each person's life path is unique, some of which must be walked alone (existential aloneness).

Not all women can sustain a loss and survive. Some women, feeling helpless and vulnerable, withdraw.

Implications for Practice

Nurses are in a strategic position to promote resilience. You can help clients through the initial reactions of shock and disbelief to a point of acceptance, with a commitment to live, not just to survive. Assist the client by promoting a positive image of the client to herself, a belief in herself, a determination to go on, humor, and spirituality.

Box 2–1. Ten Leading Causes of Death

1. Heart disease
2. Cancer
3. Stroke
4. Unintentional injuries
5. Chronic obstructive lung disease
6. Pneumonia and influenza
7. Diabetes mellitus
8. Suicide
9. Chronic liver disease and cirrhosis
10. Homicide

not soluble in water. Fats cluster together with special proteins, forming lipoproteins. There are four types:

Chylomicrons. Chylomicrons are extremely low density lipoproteins composed mostly of triglycerides. They transport diet-derived fats from the intestine to the rest of the body.

Very Low Density Lipoproteins. Very low density lipoproteins (VLDLs) are composed of 50% triglycerides. As VLDLs travel through the body, cells remove triglycerides to use for energy. VLDLs pick up cholesterol and eventually become LDLs.

Low-Density Lipoproteins. Low-density lipoproteins (LDLs) are composed of 50% cholesterol, hence their implication in heart disease. Like the VLDLs, these cells travel through the body and deliver triglycerides and cholesterol for the production of cell membranes. The liver removes LDLs from circulation to keep serum cholesterol levels low.

High-Density Lipoproteins. High-density lipoproteins consist of 50% protein. They pick up cholesterol and lipids from the cells and return it to the liver for recycling or disposal. High levels of these "scavenger" lipoproteins can reduce the risk of heart disease.

Cholesterol. Cholesterol is carried in several lipoproteins; chief among them is LDL. High cholesterol carried in LDL is correlated directly with atherosclerosis. A direct correlation means that as one factor rises, so does the other; in this case, the higher the cholesterol and LDL the higher the incidence of heart disease from atherosclerosis. High blood cholesterol in HDL correlates *inversely* with risk of heart disease.

Cholesterol becomes oxidized (combines with oxygen) and readily makes foam cells. These cells line the walls of arteries, where they harden and thicken into plaque. Antioxidants (see material under oxygen free radicals) decrease the oxidation of cholesterol into foam cells. Vitamins A (beta-carotene) and E, which are antioxidants, are carried in LDLs.

Alcohol. Alcohol intake plays several roles in health. Research indicates that moderate alcohol intake (one glass of wine per day) raises HDL levels and reduces the risk of heart disease in men and women. A high intake of alcohol is associated with hypertension, stroke, and liver disease.

Obesity. Obesity has been associated with increased risk of heart disease, stroke, and hypertension. The exact relationship is not fully understood, although the following explanation is fairly certain. When stored fat is mobilized it goes directly to the liver rather than emptying into the general circulation, as other fats do. The liver then "packages" the fat into cholesterol-carrying LDLs. This process interferes with the liver's ability to clear insulin from the blood. As a consequence, serum insulin levels

rise. Then the body's cells become insulin resistant, and blood glucose levels rise, setting the stage for diabetes.

The Role of Nutrition in Cancer

Cancer is a disease of multiple origins, such as heredity, smoking, and environmental exposure. Some cancers have dietary links. Many people fear that food additives are carcinogens. In fact, food additives have little to do with cancer. Contaminants of food, things that get into foods by accident, may be powerful carcinogens, such as pesticides and bacteria. Fat has been implicated in cancer. Fat does not cause cancer; however, animals that have been exposed to a carcinogen and are on a high-fat diet develop additional tumors and greater numbers of tumors than do animals on a low-fat diet. Thus, fat appears to be a cancer promoter, perhaps by the following mechanisms:

● Causes the body to secrete more hormones, such as estrogen
● Promotes the secretion of bile into the intestine where organisms can convert the bile into compounds that cause cancer
● Incorporates into cell membranes and changes them so they offer less resistance to carcinogenic invaders

Fiber and vegetables might help reduce the risk of some forms of cancer by speeding excretion of bile from the body, increasing transit time of food through the colon, and reducing exposure.

Beta-carotene (vitamin A) regulates cellular differentiation, which goes awry in cancer. Some people think that if they take vitamin A supplements, their risk of cancer will be reduced. This area is still being researched, but it appears that the fiber in foods that contain vitamin A is more important than the vitamin itself. Other antipromoters of cancer include vitamin B6, folate, pantothenic acid, vitamin B12, vitamin E, iron, zinc, and selenium. Some non-nutrient compounds are found in foods from the cabbage family. These foods produce chemicals that activate enzymes that destroy carcinogens. Dietitians recommend consuming various foods to dilute the effects of harmful cancer promoters, eating vegetables, and not taking vitamin supplements.

The Role of Oxygen Free Radicals in Disease

Oxygen free radicals, or superoxide radicals, are by-products of energy production. The superoxide radicals are atoms or molecules that have one or more pairs of unpaired, free electrons. These unpaired electrons are reactive and commonly bind to oxygen for stabilization. The oxygen then binds to hydrogen for stabilization. The product of this reaction is hydrogen peroxide, which is toxic to cells. The most unbalanced form of free radicals are free hydroxy radicals. They bind to polyunsaturated fatty acids, which are commonly found in cell membranes and membranes of organelles within the cell. If the free radical binds to the lysosome, the cell is destroyed (Fig. 2–4).

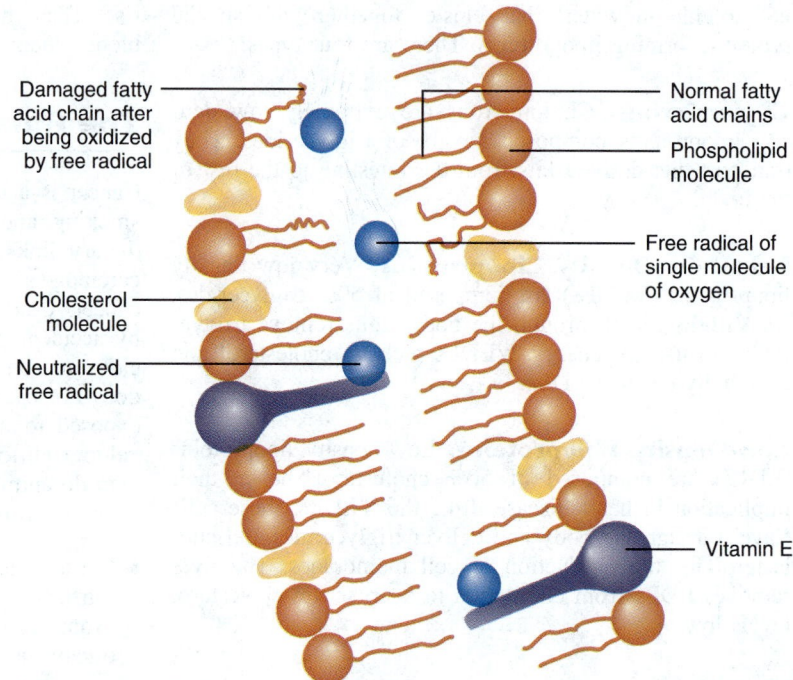

Figure 2–4. Oxygen free radicals bind to fatty acids in the cell membranes and in membranes of organelles. This damages the cell and can destroy the cell if it binds to the lysosome. Antioxidants (vitamins A, E, and C) slow this process by binding to the free radicals and preventing cell damage.

Our body is equipped to handle some of these radicals with antioxidants for the conversion of the radical back to usable oxygen. The oxidants include vitamin C and E, and beta-carotene (vitamin A). Vitamin E and selenium in cell membranes are oxidized by the free radicals, much as was just described for fatty acid. The vitamin E neutralizes the free radical and prevents it from attaching to a fatty acid. In the process, vitamin E is damaged. The damaged vitamin E is restored by vitamin C. The role of beta-carotene (vitamin A) is not clear in free radical antioxidation. Vitamins A and E are carried by the LDLs.

The Role of the Environment in Disease

Studies in cancer causation have revealed that chemicals in the workplace were responsible for specific cancers. Such discoveries have left the impression that most human cancers are associated with enviromental chemical contamination. This opinion has led to public pressure on government to control chemical contamination as a key means of cancer prevention. In most of today's industrialized world, however, work-related cancer is rare and should remain infrequent if regulations are followed. A careful analysis of the causative elements in each type of cancer has shown that prevailing life-styles in a given population—in particular tobacco use, nutritional variations, and physical activity—account for the incidence of cancer.

There are a few rarer problems that are worth mentioning. Epidemiologic studies have shown that the incidence of cancers vary by geographic area. For example, Japanese people living in Japan develop more stomach cancer and fewer colon cancers than people in the United States. However, when Japanese people move to the United

States, their children's risk of bowel and stomach cancer is equal to that of Americans. Therefore, an environmental factor must be affecting disease risk.

Sun exposure increases the risk of skin cancers. The most senstive people to the sun's effects are those with fair skin, such as people of Celtic descent. The chief cause of skin cancer is damage to DNA from ultraviolet light. An allegedly healthy look—tanned skin—can have unhealthy consequences. The view that sun exposure is needed for vitamin D absorption is now obsolete in most countries, because milk is supplemented with vitamin D. Children who have no sun exposure and do not drink milk can be at risk of rickets from low vitamin D levels. Adults who do not have adequate vitamin D develop osteomalacia. Arabic women constitute a high-risk group because they shield their skin from the sun and do not drink milk.

Air and water pollution can lead to disease. Water pollution has caused endemic infections with various microorganisms throughout the world. Air pollution increases the risk of asthma and lung cancer. Exposure to low doses of radiation or electricity is intermittently implicated in cancer development (especially childhood cancers). The exact association is not known.

The Concept of Health

The concept of health is relatively new. The word *health* as it is commonly used today did not appear in writing until about 1000 A.D. Being healthy was considered the norm, and sick people were ostracized. Shunning people who were ill was due in part from fear that the diseases were contagious. The idea of mental health, as we know it today, did not exist until the latter part of the 19th century. People who acted strangely were also ostracized. It was assumed that they were demon-possessed.

With the birth of the scientific era in the 19th century, more and more discoveries led to a better understanding of human physiology and the origins of disease. At the same time, society began to treat illness with less disgust. Health during these years was defined simply as the absence of disease. The notion that health and illness were two ends of a continuum existed for many years. In fact, it may still be used today. Some people still assume that if you have no disease you are healthy. This idea may be far from true. A seemingly healthy person may have an early form of a disease that does not yet have clinical manifestations. For example, young people in our society have heart disease, such as atherosclerosis (commonly known as hardening of the arteries). They may be only 20 years old, and no evidence of disease is present. Although they appear healthy, without proper diet and exercise the heart disease will continue to develop until clinical manifestations appear.

In 1974, the World Health Organization (WHO) proposed a definition of health that emphasized several holistic qualities of health. They said "Health is a state of complete physical, mental and social well-being and not merely the absence of disease and infirmity." There has been criticism of this definition, but it was a step in the advancement of health rather than just the treatment of illness. Since this definition was put forth, many theorists have proposed alternate definitions of health. Some of them include ideas on self-actualization, stability, growth, and development. You may want to read the definition of health that is supported by the faculty in your nursing program.

Among the theorists, Halbert Dunn is a leading proponent of a definition of health that includes self-actualization. His work was a precursor to the health promotion movement that is evident today. He coined the term *high level wellness*, which he defined as the following:

An integrated method of functioning which is oriented toward maximizing the potential of which the individual is capable. It requires that the individual maintain a continuum of balance and purposeful direction within the environment where he is functioning.

Dunn identified nine areas in which high level wellness can be promoted. Many nursing and health theorists have advanced the definitions of health. They are fully explained in Chapter 10.

The Experience of Illness

Obviously, it is important for the nurse to understand the various theories of illness causation, but perhaps it is more important for the nurse to understand how a client may respond to illness.

Illness usually refers to a group of symptoms (we will call these *clinical manifestations* in this text) or a condition underlying the symptoms. Illness behavior, however, describes the manner in which clients monitor their bodies, define and interpret their symptoms, take remedial action, and use the healthcare system. Clients perceive, evaluate, and respond to illness differently. The nurse may encounter clients who deny their symptoms, exaggerate their symptoms, or minimize their symptoms. Reac-

tions to clinical manifestations are influenced by the client's culture, knowledge base, definition of health, and previous interactions with the healthcare system. For example, if a client's definition of health is "not having cancer," then he or she is not as likely to comply with a treatment plan for diabetes, because he or she may not realize the seriousness of the disorder.

Many studies have been performed on illness behavior. For example, many studies of illness show that women report symptoms more frequently and use the services of physicians and psychiatrists more frequently than do men. Many explanations have been offered for these differences. Some researchers suggest that there may be an increased incidence of disease in women, others suggest that women have a more sensitive perception of symptoms, and still others believe that women are more willing to acknowledge their symptoms and to seek care.

Conclusions

Diseases and illness have plagued humans since the beginning of time. Early theories on illness focused on demonic possession and imbalances of body fluids. Scientific concepts of disease and illness are relatively new ideas. Today we know that diseases have multiple causes. Healthcare providers more fully understand the role of stress response, cognitive appraisal, coping, and social support. Comprehensive healthcare today encompasses a more complete understanding of what type of disease the client has and what type of client has the disease.

Bibliography

1. Andrews, M. M. (1992). Cultural perspectives on nursing in the 21st century. *Journal of Professional Nursing, 8*(1), 7–15.
2. Apple, D. (1960). How laymen define illness. *Journal of Health and Social Behavior, 1*, 219–225.
3. Bandura, A. (1982). Self-efficacy mechanisms in human agency. *American Psychologist, 37*, 122–147
4. Burman, B., & Margolin, G. (1992). Analysis of the association between marital relationships and health problems: An interactional perspective. *Psychological Bulletin, 112*(1), 39–63.
5. Caplan, G. (1964). *Symptoms of preventive psychiatry.* New York: Basic Books.
6. Cassel, E. J. (1976). Disease as an "it": Concepts of disease revealed by patients' presentation of symptoms. *Social Science Medicine, 10*, 143–146.
7. Elliott, G., & Eisdorfer, C. (Eds.). (1982). *Stress and human health.* New York: Springer.
8. Friedman, M., & Rosenman, R. (1971). Type A behavior pattern: Its association with coronary heart disease. *Annals of Clinical Research 3*, 300–308.
9. Greenberg, E. R., et al. (1994). A clinical trial of antioxidant vitamins to prevent colorectal cancer. *New England Journal of Medicine, 331*(3), 141–147.
10. Holmes, T., & Rahe, R. (1967). The social readjustment rating scale. *Journal of Psychosomatic Research, 11*, 213–217.
11. Holmes, T., & Rahe, M. (1974). Subjects' recent life changes and the onset of myocardial infarction and coronary death. In E. Gunderson & R. Rahe (Eds.). *Life stress and illness.* Springfield, IL: Charles C. Thomas.
12. House, J., Landis, K. R., & Umberson, F. (1988). Social relationships and health. *Science, 241*, 540–544.

13. Jenkins J., Wheeler, V., & Albright, L. (1994). Gene therapy for cancer. *Cancer Nursing, 17*(6), 447–456.

14. Katz, A. H. (1993). *Self help in America.* New York: Twayne Publishers.

15. Klatsky, A. L. (1995). Can a "drink a day" keep a heart attack away? *Patient Care, July 15,* 39–54, 74.

16. Locke, S., & Heisel, J. (1977). The influence of stress and emotions on human immunity. *Biofeedback Self-Regulation, 2,* 320.

17. Merz, B. (1990, Aug 17). Taking more steps toward gene therapy. *American Medical News,* p. 16.

18. Parsons, T. (1951). *The social system.* New York: Free Press.

19. Pender, N. J. (1987). *Health promotion in nursing practice.* Norwalk, CT: Appleton & Lange.

20. Pollock, S., & Duffy, M. (1990). The health-related hardiness scale: Development and psychometric analysis. *Nursing Research, 39*(4), 218–222.

20. Reed, D., et al. (1984). Psychosocial processes and general susceptibility to chronic disease. *American Journal of Epidemiology, 119*(3), 356–370.

21. Stampfer, M. J. (1988). A prospective study of moderate alcohol consumption and the risk of coronary disease and stroke in women. *New England Journal of Medicine, 319,* 267–273.

22. Temoshok, L., et al. (1983). *Emotions in health and illness.* New York: Grune & Stratton.

23. Varmus, H. (1995). NIH review of gene therapy protocols. *Science, 267,* 5206.

24. Waglid, G., & Young, H. (1990). Resilience among older women. *Image, 622*(4), 252–255.

25. Whitney, E. N., & Rolfes, S. R. (1993). *Understanding nutrition.* Minneapolis: West Publishing Co.

26. Wu, R. (1973). *Behavior and illness.* Englewood Cliffs, NJ: Prentice Hall.

27. Wyngaarden, J., Smith, L., & Bennett, J. (1992). *Cecil textbook of medicine* (19th ed.). Philadelphia: W. B. Saunders.

Ethics

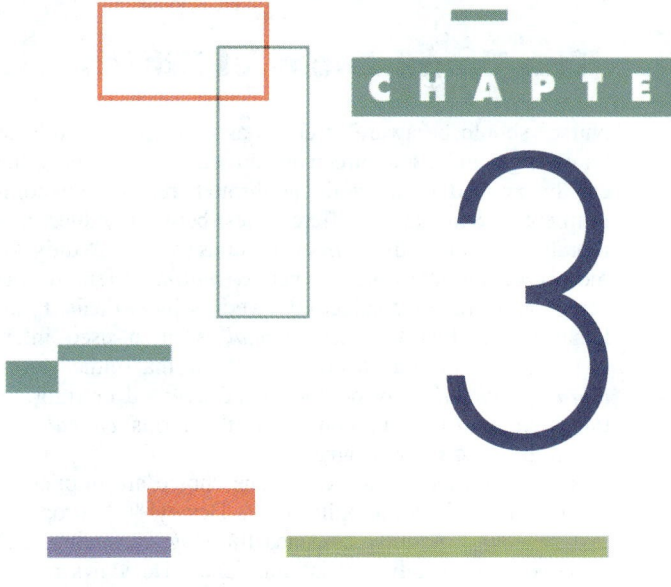

CHAPTER 3

Beverly Kopala

Nurses make judgments every day. They may give or withhold a medication based on a client's condition. They may institute interventions if a client's status deteriorates. They may take an unscheduled temperature because the client's skin feels warm to the touch. Such judgments usually do not create moral or ethical conflicts. These nursing judgments are based on knowledge and experience.

Certain situations, however, should cause the nurse involved to ask, "What is the good, the right, the morally correct thing to do?" These situations, and the moral judgments they demand, must be recognized and addressed using a systematic method of decision making.

Judgment is a cognitive process of valuing. In nursing, many factors influence your decision-making process. They include personal, professional, and societal values. Your beliefs and attitudes also exert an influence. Rules, standards, past experiences, previous choices, and habits of action also have an impact on your decision-making process. Philosophic theories, concepts, and principles affect ethical decision making as well.

At times, ethical decisions must be made by individuals, without consultation. In most cases, however, problematic ethical decisions should not be made in isolation. Nurses have a responsibility to engage in shared decision making, particularly when moral uncertainty exists about the correct or ethical course of action in a client care situation.

A Framework for the Study of Ethics

Ethics, or moral philosophy, is one branch of philosophy. Ethics involves the exploration and analysis of moral standards, judgments, choices, beliefs, and problems. As

defined by McFadden,[23(p 1)] ethics is "that science which studies the morality of human acts through the medium of natural reason. It is that science which is directive of the moral acts of man's will according to basic rational principles. . . . Ethics teaches us how to judge accurately the moral goodness or badness of any human action." McFadden incorporates critical elements of moral philosophy in the definition: the need for rational thought and the need for guiding principles in judging a human action as being morally right or wrong, or good or bad. Ethical judgments surrounding birth, death, and preservation of life issues are among those that face healthcare providers. Guiding principles, theories, and decision-making frameworks applicable to client care situations are very useful to nurses who face ethical dilemmas in nursing practice.

Many people continue to refer to their basic beliefs, values, and ideals as guides for decision making. Rarely are these factors rationally examined in terms of their impact on decisions. A feeling of uneasiness may ensue as the nurse begins to question, examine, and clarify values that have been fostered over a lifetime. Situations that appeared to be clear in the past may suddenly seem cloudy. This serves to reinforce the need for a formalized process for examining ethical issues and concerns.

When confronted with moral dilemmas and the need to make moral judgments, nurses need to engage in reflective thinking before, during, and after the decision-making process. Since ethical decisions cannot be proved correct in the traditional scientific sense of the term, the decision-maker must be able to justify the decision. Justification involves presenting sufficient reasons and a relevant basis for beliefs and actions.

Even when the decision is reached, all people involved may not be pleased with the outcome. Occasionally, a nurse may not be able to participate in an action because it violates the nurse's integrity. The best solution is not necessarily the perfect solution. Despite these difficulties, nurses who understand what the ethical decision-making process entails will be better able to effectively participate in that process.

This chapter incorporates material written for the fourth edition by Minerva I. Applegate.

The Terminology of Ethics

Nurses should be aware of ethics as a systematic body of knowledge and as a directive and practical science that can be applied to daily living through reason and commitment.[23] Sahakian[29] differentiates between ethics and morals in noting that *ethics* pertains to the "study of morals or moral issues," whereas *morals* refers to the actual standards of conduct observed by individuals. Frankena[15] states that the term *ethical* is often used interchangeably with the word *moral*, and that either term, *moral* or *ethical*, may be considered as good or right. In this chapter, to avoid confusion, the terms *ethical* and *moral* are used interchangeably.

Reflective thought and conscious choice are implied in the conduct of moral philosophy. Dewey[13(p 3)] proposes that reflective morality demands thinking, reasoning, and an appeal to an individual's conscience. He views reflection as the process through which the moral decision maker seeks dependable principles when faced with an ethical dilemma.

An *ethical dilemma* is a "problem that involves two (or more) morally correct courses of action, *but you can't do both*."[27(p 39)] It is a situation in which "*each* alternative course of action can be justified by fundamental moral rules or principles."[7(p 4)] The nature of an ethical dilemma is that it is difficult to determine the right decision or action.

Not all situations that require ethical decisions are dilemmas. Purtillo,[27(p 37)] for example, defines an *ethical issue* as "one in which one or more moral norms or principles are present, but do not create a problem" and an *ethical problem* as "one in which two or more moral norms or principles create a challenge about what to do." Problems can create a sense of distress when the nurse knows what ought to be done in a situation but a barrier exists that interferes with his or her doing so.[27]

Principles of Ethics

A number of principles serve as the foundation for ethical decision making. Beauchamp and Childress[6] identify four basic principles: justice, respect for autonomy, nonmaleficence, and beneficence. The preamble to the American Nurses' Association's (ANA) *Code for Nurses*[2] identifies one fundamental guiding principle, respect for persons, and seven basic principles flowing from the fundamental principle:

Beneficence (doing good)
Nonmaleficence (avoiding harm)
Autonomy (self-determination)
Justice (treating people fairly)
Fidelity (keeping promises)
Veracity (truth telling)
Confidentiality (respecting privileged information)

These principles, along with concern for the consequences of your actions, can be used as the foundation for directing and justifying your nursing actions. The ANA *Code for Nurses* can serve as a guide for ethical decision making and can assist in determining what to do in a particular situation.

Beneficence and Nonmaleficence

On the basis of *beneficence* and *nonmaleficence*, the nurse should do or promote good (beneficence) and do no intentional harm (nonmaleficence). It is the duty of the health professional to "produce and provide good, but not if the provision of that good also produces an equal or greater harm."[27(p 83)] The principle of nonmaleficence is the basis for most nursing as well as medical codes of ethics. Intentional harm is never permitted. But some treatments or procedures do bring with them some associated risk. One ethical question that needs to be asked is, "What level of risk is morally acceptable?" The principles of beneficence and nonmaleficence play a major role in the trusting relationship that develops between the healthcare consumer and the healthcare provider.

Autonomy

This principle supports the client's right to know, to be informed, and to be able to act on autonomous decisions. Healthcare providers are not entitled to coerce clients into decisions and actions that do not reflect the client's beliefs, values, choices, or life plans. Clients are given opportunities to make decisions, and informed consent is designed to protect autonomous choice in those healthcare decisions. Respect for *autonomy* means that the nurse will support the client's freedom of choice, independence, and self-determination. However, autonomy is not without limits.

Justice

Another principle, *justice*, implies choosing the action that is most fair and equitable after reflecting on the claims or rights of the individuals involved in the decision. As social beings, persons have certain obligations and commitments to other social beings. Part of this commitment includes the distribution of goods and services in ways that most benefit others without discrimination or bias. This principle, when upheld, prevents unfair treatment of the sick, disabled, handicapped, indigent, or other groups of individuals. It is applicable to the allocation of scarce resources and development of an optimal level of care for all clients. The current health plan in Oregon is based on this principle: a basic level of care is distributed to all eligible citizens of the state.

Fidelity and Veracity

The principles of *fidelity* and *veracity* are closely associated. Fidelity means that the nurse acts in good faith to keep promises made to the client and does not make promises that cannot be kept. Fidelity also refers to loyalty to the client–care provider relationship. Because nurses have obligations of fidelity to clients, employing institutions, and other healthcare providers, obligations may sometimes conflict. Veracity means truthfulness. Clients expect that nurses, indeed all healthcare professionals, will be truthful in their communications. Truthful communications are necessary to establish and maintain trusting relationships.

Confidentiality

The principle of confidentiality means that the nurse respects all privileged information about a client. A client must be able to assume that information given to a healthcare professional will be respected and not shared inappropriately. If the client is not able to trust that any such information will remain confidential, the client might not seek healthcare. It is not a breach of confidentiality, however, to share information with other healthcare providers who are also caring for the patient "as long as the information has some relevance regarding that case."[27](p 98)

In practice, the nurse will find that these principles occasionally conflict. For example, a situation may arise in which a client who has not been told a diagnosis asks the nurse if that diagnosis is known. If the nurse does not have the authority to reveal this information, the nurse may be faced with a dilemma—whether to inform the client on the basis of respect for autonomy or to not tell the truth and violate the principle of veracity. Competing principles must be weighed, consequences examined, and a decision made as to how to proceed.

Guidelines for Ethical Nursing Practice

Parameters for nursing practice are found in the ANA *Standards of Nursing Practice,*[3] the ANA *Code for Nurses with Interpretive Statements,*[2] the American Hospital Association's (AHA) *A Patient's Bill of Rights,*[1] and nurse practice acts of individual states.

Nurse practice acts and *Standards of Nursing Practice* primarily address the nurse's use of the nursing process in providing care that is based on sound principles and substantive knowledge and that incorporates health teaching and counseling with a focus on health promotion, maintenance, and restoration. *Standards of Nursing Practice*, in particular, indicate that nursing is client centered. Both nurse practice acts and *Standards of Nursing Practice* reflect the need for nursing judgment that is ongoing and continuous in the nurse-client interaction.

The ANA *Code for Nurses* (Box 3–1) and the AHA *A Patient's Bill of Rights* also serve as guidelines for the nurse.

The *Code for Nurses* addresses the following:

- Client dignity and uniqueness
- Privacy and confidentiality

Box 3–1. ANA Code for Nurses

1. The nurse provides services with respect for human dignity and the uniqueness of the client, unrestricted by considerations of social or economic status, personal attributes, or the nature of the health problems.
2. The nurse safeguards the client's right to privacy by judiciously protecting information of a confidential nature.
3. The nurse acts to safeguard the client and the public when health care and safety are affected by the incompetent, unethical, or illegal practice of any person.
4. The nurse assumes responsibility and accountability for individual nursing judgments and actions.
5. The nurse maintains competence in nursing.
6. The nurse exercises informed judgment and uses individual competence and qualifications as criteria in seeking consultation, accepting responsibilities, and delegating nursing activities to others.
7. The nurse participates in activities that contribute to the ongoing development of the profession's body of knowledge.
8. The nurse participates in the profession's effort to implement and improve standards of nursing.
9. The nurse participates in the profession's efforts to establish and maintain conditions of employment conducive to high quality nursing care.
10. The nurse participates in the profession's effort to protect the public from misinformation and misrepresentation and to maintain the integrity of nursing.
11. The nurse collaborates with members of the health professions and other citizens in promoting community and national efforts to meet the needs of the public.

From American Nurses Association. (1985). *Code for nurses with interpretive statements*. Washington, DC: Author.

- Client protection
- Nursing accountability and responsibility
- Maintenance of competence
- Informed judgment
- Participation in inquiry
- Implementation and improvement of standards of care
- Enhancement of employment conditions to foster the quality of care
- Enhancement of nursing's integrity and image
- Collaboration for the promotion of public health needs

A Patient's Bill of Rights addresses the clients' and families rights and responsibilities. Client's rights and responsibilities have implications for nursing care.

Both of these documents can serve as guidelines for the nurse who is confronted with situations that demand decision making. As the nurse becomes familiar with these documents, the commonalities begin to surface with respect to nursing obligations, judgments, and accountability. Box 3–2 summarizes some guidelines that could be drawn from these documents.

Box 3–2. Selected Nursing Guidelines for Ethical Nursing Practice

- Make sure that nurses and clients are adequately informed.
- Implement care systematically.
- Maintain your nursing knowledge and competence.
- Protect and safeguard your clients.
- Maintain your professional integrity.
- Uphold the rights of your clients.
- Treat clients with dignity.
- Administer individualized care.
- Administer client-centered care.
- Incorporate health teaching and counseling into your plans of care.
- Make sure that all data are recorded appropriately and communicated clearly.
- Maintain continuity of care.
- Extend your nursing goals to families and the broader public through collaborative efforts.

Nurses must know and work within the laws that govern practice. However, if the nurse believes that a particular law is unethical, the nurse can work to bring about a change in that law.

Theories to Guide Ethical Decision Making

Even with the availability of principles, codes, and professional guidelines for ethical nursing practice, it can be difficult to determine the most ethical course of action in a specific situation. A number of ethical theories provide frameworks that you can use to examine the goodness or worth of various courses of action. Among these are rule-based theories, consequence-based theories, and the ethics of care. All of these theories have value, though they are also subject to criticism. Use these theories when your usual pattern of action or professional guidelines conflict, or when you need a new social rule or guide. It is useful to be able to specify the theoretical approach used in moral thinking because it will help you to justify why you've decided on one alternative instead of another.

Consequence-based theories are also called *teleological* or *utilitarian* theories. A *consequentialist* identifies all available alternatives and evaluates them on the basis of their results. The right action is one that brings about the best overall consequences, or the greatest benefit and least harm, for all parties affected by the decision. If consequences are all undesirable, then the right action is one that brings about the least harm. To determine whether your decisions tend to be consequence based, see Table 3–1.

In rule-based theories, also called *deontological* theories, the right action is one that conforms to fundamental moral rules or duties such as "tell the truth" or "keep promises." Wrong actions are those that violate such rules. The best known deontological theory is that of the philosopher Immanuel Kant. Kant held that whether an act is morally right depends on whether the rule on which the action is based meets a certain standard of acceptability. For Kant, that standard, which he called the "categorical imperative," states, "Act only according to that maxim whereby you can at the same time will that it should become a universal law."[19(p 30)]

This means that for an act to be judged right it would be logically consistent for every other rational person in a similar situation to act in the same way. For example, Kant wrote that a lie is always a wrong act, even if the person lying thinks that doing so will bring about good consequences. If everyone lied when it seemed beneficial to do so, communications among people would become incoherent and self-defeating. For an act to be morally worthy, a person must act from a sense of duty or obligation, rather than out of fear of reprisal or for monetary gain or a sense of enjoyment or satisfaction. In addition, one should not "use" another person as a means of achieving an end or goal. To determine whether your decisions tend to be rule based, see Table 3–2.

Traits important in close personal relationships, such as

Table 3–1. Identifying Consequence-Based (Teleological) Decision Making	
Selected Concepts or Characteristics	**Questions**
Consequence orientation	Do you believe that what makes an action right or wrong is the outcome or the consequences of the action?
Greatest good	Do you ask yourself "What is the greatest 'good' or the most important value in this situation?"
Calculation of good over harmful effects	Do you believe that the right action is that which produces the greatest value, benefit, advantage, pleasure, good, or happiness or the least disvalue, harm, pain, evil, or unhappiness?
Greatest number	Do you believe that the consequences of the decisions/actions should produce the greatest value/least disvalue for as many people affected by the decision/action as possible?
Impersonal stance	Do you believe that the needs/interests of all involved parties should be given equal weight?

Table 3–2. Identifying Duty-Based (Deontological) Decision Making

Selected Concepts or Characteristics	Questions
Duty orientation	Do you evaluate actions on the basis of your duties/obligations?
The primary focus for decision making is not on the consequences of an action	Do you consider factors other than the outcomes or consequences when making decisions?
Some actions are simply known to be right or wrong	Do you believe that some actions are known to be right or wrong, no matter what the consequences?
Application of rules	Do you have basic rules that guide you in your decision making? Do you believe that some rules should be upheld without exception?
Never use a person solely as a means to an end	Do you believe that persons should not be used merely for the benefit of others?
Concern for the individual	Do you focus primarily on the needs of the individual rather than the needs of the community/society or others?

compassion, trust, and fidelity, are stressed in an ethics of care. *Caring* in these accounts refers to care for, emotional commitment to, and willingness to act on behalf of persons with whom one has a significant relationship.[6] (p 85) Emphasis is given to the actions, how they are performed, underlying motivation, and whether positive relationships are enhanced or hindered.[6]

Although the preceding provides only a brief and incomplete overview of three theories, it is useful to be able to identify the theory base that guides your ethical decision making. Most people use aspects of more than one theory in making such decisions. But conflicts may arise because people may have thought about the ethical problem in different ways. For example, if one healthcare provider approaches a situation primarily from a duty-based viewpoint and another approaches it from a consequence-based perspective, conflicts can arise that may not be resolved without mediation or negotiation.

If you can recognize some of the characteristics described here in your personal beliefs, then you can better comprehend how your beliefs influence decision making and how values and beliefs arise. Values and beliefs develop as a result of our interactions with parents, family members, friends, teachers, and others. They are also affected by education, religion, and life experiences. The values you hold affect whether a particular situation will be interpreted as one that requires a moral judgment or creates an ethical dilemma. As healthcare providers, nurses encounter situations that may cause conflicts in personal and professional values and beliefs. For example, if a terminally ill client requests advanced life support, the nurse may experience conflict over the possibility of participating in providing it. The nurse's first instinct is usually to preserve life, frequently with less concern for financial cost. A conflict may arise when the nurse reflects on the situation and considers all of the facts. On the one hand, the nurse respects client autonomy and values preservation of life. On the other hand, the nurse also considers the cost, financial and otherwise, to the family and to society. The nurse may be faced with conflicting values and a possible dilemma.

Applying Ethical Models: The Murphy and Murphy Model

Once familiar with the principles, codes, guidelines, and theories that can supply needed knowledge for ethical decision making, you can apply an ethical decision-making model. These models are designed to guide thinking and assist in problem resolution. A number of models have been used by nurses to help solve ethical dilemmas, including those proposed by Murphy and Murphy,[24] Curtin,[11] and Levine-Ariff and Groh[21] (Table 3–3). These somewhat similar models offer the nurse a systematic way to examine ethical dilemmas.

The Murphy and Murphy model clearly identifies concern for consequences in the process of ethical decision making. It requires assessment, problem identification, identification of the decision makers, exploration of alternatives, decision-making evaluation, and identification of possible modifications arising from the evaluation. Table 3–4 compares the steps of the Murphy and Murphy model to the steps of the nursing process and shows the similarity between the two problem-solving methods.

Initially, the nurse must be aware that a health problem exists. This must be clear to all involved before proceeding with the decision-making process.

The next step involves identification of an ethical problem. You may have questions about what to do in a situation, experience uneasiness because of conflicting values, or feel uncertain as to what the best decision should be.

You must then identify the persons who would be involved in making a decision related to the perceived problem. These people might be the client, family, significant others, physician, nurse, other team members, clergy, or even hospital administration or legal counsel.

The role of the nurse must be identified. Professional obligations or hospital policies and procedures, for example, will affect nurses' roles as caregivers, client advo-

Table 3–3. Comparing Models for Ethical Decision Making

Step	Murphy and Murphy Model	Curtin Model	Levine-Ariff and Groh Model
1	Identify the health problem	Get background information about the problem	Define the dilemma
2	Identify the ethical problem	Identify the ethical parts of the problem	Identify the medical facts
3	State who is involved in making the decision	Identify the ethical agents (people involved in making the decision)	Identify the nonmedical facts: ■ Patient and family ■ External factors
4	Identify the nurse's role	Identify all possible choices and the outcomes of those choices	Separate assumptions from facts
5	Consider as many alternatives as possible	Apply the relevant ethical theories, principles, and rules	Identify items needing clarification
6	Consider the long-range and short-range consequences of each alternative decision	Resolve the dilemma	Identify the decision makers
7	Reach a decision	Act on the decision	Review the underlying ethical principles
8	Consider how this decision fits into your general philosophy of patient care		Define alternatives
9	Follow this situation until the actual results of the decision are visible and use this information to help make future decisions		Follow up

Data from Murphy, M. A., & Murphy, J. (1976). Model for ethical decision making. *Nursing 76,* (8), 13–14; Curtin, L. L. (1978). A proposed model for critical ethical analysis. *Nursing Forum, 17,* 14; and Levine-Ariff, J., & Groh, D. H. (1990). *Nursing managers' bookshelf: Creating an ethical environment* (pp. 41–61). Baltimore: Williams & Wilkins.

Table 3–4. Comparing the Nursing Process with the Murphy and Murphy Model

Nursing Process	Murphy and Murphy Model
1. Assessment	1. Identify the health problem 2. Identify the ethical problem 3. State who is involved in making the decision
2. Analysis (diagnosis)	4. Identify your role
3. Planning	5. Consider as many alternatives as you can 6. Consider the long-range and short-range consequences of each alternative
4. Implementation	7. Reach your decision
5. Evaluation	8. Consider how this decision fits into your general philosophy of patient care 9. Follow this situation until you can see the actual results of your decision, and use this information to help you in making future decisions

cates, or educators. In a particular situation, the nurse's role may or may not be that of decision maker.

Those involved in making the decision must explore the available alternatives and the short- and long-term consequences of each alternative. Some alternatives will likely bring about more desirable consequences than others. Certain alternatives will support specific principles.

Once the alternatives have been fully explored by the appropriate people, a decision must be made. Some resolution of the problem is needed. A decision requires the "weighing" or ranking of the alternatives to determine which provides the best outcome. Additionally, justification must be provided as to why a particular alternative has been chosen. The nurse should then reflect on *whether or not the decision is consistent with the nurse's philosophy of client care.*

As a final step, you will need to evaluate the outcome of the decision to provide additional data for future decision making. If, on reflection, the alternative chosen did not produce the anticipated outcome, if the process of data gathering was found to be incomplete, or if some other problem was recognized, evaluation will provide the opportunity to reexamine the process and to make attempts to avoid the problem in the future. If resolution of the problem proved satisfactory, then the effectiveness of the process will be reinforced and the outcome data may be useful in future decision making. An ethical decision-making model is an important and useful tool for any nurse who is confronted with complex problems or dilemmas.

As you begin to analyze ethical problems, a set of your own personal principles will begin to emerge. Sigman[32] has described the complexity of ethical choice in nursing and addresses the need for nurses to be responsible, accountable, and committed. She also notes that the nurse sometimes has to take a risk and that choices may involve issues of freedom, change, and justice. Nelson,[25] addressing the issue of authenticity, supports Sigman and notes that if the nurse is free to act in support of self-determination, the nurse must act in a way that will not violate the freedom or rights of others.

Given basic knowledge, principles, and guidelines for ethical decision making, the nurse can apply this information in a way that will enhance decision making in nursing practice. When confronted with conflicts, either internal or external, the nurse can refer to guidelines and norms to assist in problem resolution. Assessment, observation, and communication skills enhance the nurse's ability as an ethical decision maker. Reflective thought and conscious choice enable the nurse to make informed conclusions and to act on choices as a rational decision maker.

Research in Ethics

In an International Council of Nurses publication, Tate[33] reported data gathered from nurses and nursing students in 25 countries. The study results indicated that nurses perceived common problems across many cultures and languages. Of particular note was the feeling of being alone when confronted with ethical dilemmas. The fact that ethical problems were encountered daily in nursing practice also was noted in studies by Chinn[10] and Sigman.[32]

In Scotland, Schrock[30] surveyed 131 nursing students and graduate nurses to explore ethical issues that they encountered or expected to encounter in clinical nursing practice. Some of the concerns the nurses identified included abortion, resuscitation, euthanasia, organ transplantation, and psychosurgery. Schrock noted the absence of everyday moral issues, such as truth telling and confidentiality.

Applegate[4] explored ethical issues and decision-making patterns in 60 nurses employed in hospitals. Issues identified by the nurses involved relationships, standards of care, terminal illness, congenital anomalies, setting priorities, and rights concerns. Methods used by each nurse included the following:

- Communicating ethical opinions and judgments and/or seeking higher authority

- Discriminating between right and wrong
- Intervening despite opposition
- Intervening without opposition
- Making no intervention

One major conclusion was that these nurses were functioning beyond the ethical and legal parameters of nursing practice.

Mayberry[22] also explored methods of ethical decision making used by 167 hospital-based nurses. Kohlberg's levels of moral reasoning were assessed through administration of the Defining Issues Test. The identified levels of moral reasoning were correlated with the nurses' education, age, amount of time in nursing practice, and the size of the employing hospital. Study results indicated that nurses were more apt to use an intuitive approach than to use critical inquiry or principled reasoning when solving ethical problems. Moral development, as well as principled decision making, were powerfully and consistently related to the nurses' level of education. The number of years in practice after formal schooling also affected the nurses' ability to engage in principled reasoning. The fewer the years in practice, the greater was the nurse's ability to engage in principled reasoning.

This suggested to the researcher that formal education is significant in its contribution to principled reasoning. The data also suggested that an individual's moral judgment may be strongly influenced by the work environment. Personal factors, such as respect for authority within a hierarchy that represents a conventional level of reasoning, were frequently found to characterize the reasoning of head nurses. Increasing age and experience were considered by the researcher to be factors that contribute to the development of loyalty to peers and to the institution and to commitment to the organization's aims. The researcher recommended that nursing administrators promote an environment in which nurses have opportunities to engage in systematic ethical decision making. Selected strategies were suggested to enhance nurses' ethical problem-solving skills.

Gold and co-workers[17] conducted a series of semistructured interviews with 12 nurses who provided direct patient care in various settings. Their study explored the nurses' ability to identify ethical issues encountered during their most recent work shifts. Several themes emerged from these interviews, including conflicts surrounding truth-telling, access to care, allocation of resources, and rule breaking and "whistle-blowing." Although in the course of the interviews the nurses mentioned situations that created ethical dilemmas, they had difficulty describing what an ethical decision or ethical dilemma was. None described using an ethical decision-making model or engaging in joint decision making.

Selected nursing studies have identified ethical issues confronting nurses in various clinical practice settings. Ethical decision-making patterns, as well as patterns of moral reasoning, continue to be explored. Some of the questions that deserve further study appear in Box 3-3. Ethics-focused nursing research will help to expand our body of knowledge about nursing.

Ethical Concerns for Nurses

Whether or not you are aware of them, ethical concerns in nursing are numerous. Relationships with colleagues, clients, and families, as well as issues related to allocation of resources and nonintervention, are among these concerns.

Relationships with Colleagues

Nurses work closely with one another and with other healthcare providers. Healthy working relationships with colleagues and peers are important in providing quality client care. But in the course of maintaining these relationships, the nurse may observe behaviors or actions of others that raise problems or dilemmas and require ethical decisions. For example, a dilemma may involve whether or when to report the questionable or unsafe behavior of a healthcare provider who also happens to be a friend. This behavior could relate to a lack of skill, substance abuse, poor judgment, violation of standards, lack of emotional stability, lack of interpersonal skills, or a variety of other problems. Or you may be asked to "cover" for another nurse's medication error or for repeated late arrival to work. These are only a few of the relationship problems that may arise.

Relationships with Clients and Families

When the client and/or family and health team members agree on the plan of action, satisfactory working relationships are usually maintained. Even if no obvious conflict exists among those involved, determining the correct action may require much deliberation. When the client and/or family and health team members differ in their choices about what should be done, or when mixed messages are sent, an ethical dilemma can arise. For example, if a seriously ill client repeatedly indicates, at the urging of family members, that he wants to be resuscitated in case of cardiac arrest, but he tells the nurse when family members leave that he is only requesting resuscitation because of his family, the right action needs to be determined. If the client should experience cardiac arrest, the nurse will need to make a decision about what should be done. Client and/or family meetings with multidisciplinary members of the healthcare team can enhance communication, may resolve differences, and can assist in determining what ought to be done. If this approach is unsuccessful, further resources, such as an ethics consultation, may be needed.

Some of the many ethical questions that nurses face in their relationships with clients include whether to share information that the client has revealed in confidence, whether deception is justified, how to balance personal risks against professional responsibilities, and whether to participate in the withholding of food and fluids.

Terminal Illness

Terminal illness often presents complex dilemmas for healthcare providers. Issues may involve, for example, the client's right to refuse treatment, recognition or nonrecognition of a living will and/or durable power of attorney for healthcare, questions about initiating or withdrawing life support systems, resuscitate versus do not resuscitate (DNR) orders, and disagreements about quality of life versus sanctity of life. These are issues for which nurses should be prepared for uncertainty on the part of client, family, and health team members. Support of the client as an autonomous, unique individual is required on the part of the nurse as the primary caregiver. The nurse's level of maturity, experience, philosophic orientation, and preparedness for ethical decision making have an impact on the ability to be supportive to a client in making the often complex decisions related to terminal illness.

Allocation of Scarce Resources

Nurses are becoming more involved in decisions about allocation of scarce resources. These resources may include personnel, space, equipment, facilities, funds, and other entities, such as organs available for transplantation. Healthcare resources are not unlimited. In this highly technologically capable society, it soon becomes apparent to the nurse that it is neither possible, nor may it be appropriate, to meet all clients' needs or requests for health services. At times, basic principles may be in conflict, such as the commitment to the preservation of life versus the costs of treatment to the client, family, and society.

Nonintervention

One concern that has been reported by nurses in clinical practice regards nonintervention.[4] The ANA *Code for Nurses*[2] can provide guidelines for this type of situation. Nurses should remember that not to intervene when one has a professional responsibility to do so is a conscious decision, and the outcome may be catastrophic for the client. One example is a "slow code," in which the nurse is intentionally slow to respond or to initiate resuscitation efforts when such resuscitation is appropriate. Another example is inaction when a colleague's pattern of mistakes is placing clients at serious risk of injury. The nurse has an ethical obligation to protect the client from inappropriate nonintervention. The *Code for Nurses* addresses this obligation.

Ethical Concerns for Clients

Many issues have significant implications for clients as healthcare consumers and for nurses as healthcare providers. Included among these are clients' rights, informed consent, advocacy, confidentiality and privacy, and truth telling. The following discussion includes several of these issues.

Clients' Rights

Consumers are becoming increasingly aware of their right to make healthcare decisions, including the refusal of treatment, and are becoming more involved in decision making. Their rights in this regard are being protected by the development of state and federal legislation and professional and institutional guidelines. The AHA *A Patient's Bill of Rights* provides clients with information about their rights and responsibilities as recipients of healthcare in the hospital. The living will and durable power of attorney for healthcare are legal documents called *advance directives*. They enable clients to designate, in advance, the types of medical treatments they would or would not want in specific instances (living will) or to identify one person to make treatment decisions when the client is not capable of doing so (durable power of attorney for healthcare). These legal documents foster client autonomy in decision making.

In December 1991, the federal government enacted a law, the *Patient Self-Determination Act*, mandating that persons admitted to hospitals and nursing homes receiving Medicare and Medicaid funds be asked whether they have or wish to prepare an advance directive. Institutions are required to ensure that the implications of these documents, including pertinent state laws, are explained to clients. Institutions have advance directive forms that can be completed by those who wish to do so. Once completed, the advance directive becomes part of the client's healthcare record. This law should make more people aware of options available for determining their own care. States have various provisions, however, and not all clients have completed these forms. Nurses need to maintain an awareness of policies, procedures, guidelines, and regulations that affect clients' involvement in the decision-making process.

Autonomy

By promoting clients' rights to choose freely and to act on their choices, the nurse shows respect for the client as a person and supports client rights. However, the client's right to autonomy is not absolute. The priority of client autonomy is limited to courses of action that are medically acceptable in regard to the client's well-being. This means that the client's autonomous decision must be weighed against the healthcare provider's professional judgment. A nurse does not harm or let people harm themselves while under the nurse's care. The ranking of values that determines our practice judgments will not be violated simply for the sake of the client's autonomy.

A client may engage in a wide range of autonomous actions that do not involve serious harm. For example, a client may tell the nurse that he refuses to take medication before speaking with his physician and expect the decision will be respected. However, a postsurgical patient who refuses to walk can expect that nurses will attempt to motivate him or her to do so because of the risk of harm that inactivity raises. This example shows how conflict can arise between the principles of beneficence and respect for autonomy.

Informed Consent

Informed consent means that a person who is capable of making a decision has freely and voluntarily agreed to a medical treatment or procedure or has agreed to participate as a subject in a research study. Being informed implies that specific and thorough information about the medical intervention, including options and risks, or research program is given and that the information is understood by the client. At times, questions arise about the client's ability to make an informed choice or about the adequacy of the information disclosed to the client. In addition, clients, even when given the opportunity to be fully informed, may choose "not to know." For example, an elderly client may ask that information be given to a son or daughter to evaluate. The client may then ask the son or daughter to make a decision about what should be done. Nurses should have clear guidelines to assist them in implementing their appropriate role in the consent process.

Truth-Telling

To make a decision that is most in agreement with personal beliefs, goals, and values, the client must have adequate, truthful information on which to base the decision. Indeed, clients trust that healthcare providers will be truthful in their communications. However, "nondisclosure, deception, and lying will all occasionally be justified when veracity conflicts with other obligations."[6(p 397)] In other words, on occasion, veracity may be outweighed by another competing, stronger obligation.[6] Determining whether, or when, such a situation arises is part of the complexity of the ethical decision-making process.

Resolving Ethical Problems in Nursing Practice

Nurses need to be attentive to current ethical issues and problems that confront them in clinical practice and learn to anticipate ethical questions or problems that might arise. Some of these problems are readily found in the nurse's daily practice. Others may arise as a result of dialogue with colleagues, attention to the media and to professional and lay literature, and participation in continuing education, both informal and formal.

Try to clarify the beliefs, attitudes, and values that influence your ethical decision making. Take opportunities to discuss ethical issues with other healthcare providers. Doing so will help you recognize and clarify how your personal and professional beliefs, attitudes, and values affect your decision-making process. Use this knowledge to reflect on and to improve your decisions.

Policies or guidelines can assist nurses and other healthcare providers in managing complex ethical problems that are frequently encountered in clinical practice. Such documents should be developed with provider input and be readily available to healthcare providers. Appropriate channels of communication should be identified and resources made available to nurses who are confronted with ethical problems. For example, if a nurse thinks that a colleague has acted in an unethical manner, the nurse should be aware of the mechanisms that will assist with problem resolution.

Protocols and guidelines have been developed to implement the laws associated with documents such as the living will and durable power of attorney for healthcare. You should be familiar with these documents and with the hospital policies and procedures necessary to implement them.

Criteria for instituting and withdrawing life support systems have been established in many healthcare settings and even in some state legislatures. Protocols have been developed for documenting and recording healthcare decisions, such as handling code versus do not resuscitate orders, and criteria have been developed for the selection of healthcare providers and personnel who will have input into these critical decisions. If an institution does not have these policies, the nurse must work for their development. As appropriate, policies and procedures related to ethical problems should be developed, reviewed, and revised as needed, on an ongoing basis.

Ethics committees exist in many institutions to help in the resolution of complex ethical problems. Institutional ethics committees are typically charged with staff education, consultation, and review of ethically problematic cases. Additionally, they make recommendations to policy-making bodies. Nurses should consider becoming active members of these committees. They also need to know how to request an ethics consultation to obtain appropriate guidance if confronted with difficult dilemmas in nursing practice.

Nurses, physicians, and other healthcare providers should take advantage of learning experiences, such as ethics rounds. Depending on how the rounds are structured, one can gain familiarity with various ethical problems and/or listen to or participate in case presentations and discussions with a multidisciplinary group.

Nurses should seek every opportunity to engage collaboratively, when appropriate, in systematic, ethical decision-making processes, because of the valuable input others can provide. Nurses are accountable for their moral judgments and actions in these situations as elsewhere.

When confronted with ethical problems in nursing practice, the nurse may experience a sense of uncertainty in problem resolution. As nurses become better prepared to engage in ethical decision making, some of these feelings of uncertainty may be alleviated.

Conclusions

Professional nursing demands accountability for nursing decisions and actions. When confronted with problems in practice that demand ethical decisions, you need to know how values, attitudes, and beliefs influence the decision-making process. You should also be familiar with standards, guidelines, theories, and models that guide ethical nursing practice. Be sure to uphold clients' rights, but recognize that healthcare providers also have rights. Remember that rights are accompanied by corresponding obligations. Within the clinical practice setting, support systems should be available for clients and families, nurses, and other healthcare providers who are confronted with ethical issues. Mechanisms should be available for resolving problems; these mechanisms should be developed with input from healthcare providers. Ethical decision making should be collaborative, when appropriate, and communication channels clearly delineated.

When confronted with ethical dilemmas that need immediate resolution, you will need to consciously engage in a rational, systematic decision-making process. When you have limited time for reflection, when norms have not been established or are unclear, and when time is not available for consultation or collaboration with others, make the best judgment possible in that situation. Later, reflect on and critically examine your decision to determine whether it was the best choice in that situation. The ability of the professional nurse to systematically gather data from a variety of sources and to make comprehensive judgments based on that data, while attending to client rights and maintaining respect for persons, may be the key to ethical nursing practice.

Bibliography

1. American Hospital Association. (1992). *A patient's bill of rights.* Chicago: Author.
2. American Nurses' Association. (1985). *Code for nurses with interpretive statements.* Washington, DC: Author.
3. American Nurses' Association. (1973). *Standards of practice.* Washington, DC: Author.
4. Applegate, M. I. (1981). *Moral decisions in selected clinical nursing practice situations.* Unpublished doctoral dissertation, Columbia University, New York.
5. Aroskar, M. A. (1977). Ethics in the nursing curriculum. *Nursing Outlook, 25*(4), 260–264.
6. Beauchamp, T. L., & Childress, J. F. (1994). *Principles of biomedical ethics* (4th ed.). New York: Oxford University Press.
7. Benjamin, M., & Curtis, J. (1992). *Ethics in nursing* (3rd ed.). New York: Oxford University Press.
8. Bok, S. (1978). *Lying: Moral choice in public and private life.* New York: Pantheon Books.
9. Burnard, P., & Chapman, C. M. (1988). *Professional and ethical issues in nursing.* New York: John Wiley & Sons.
10. Chinn, P. L. (1979). Issues in lowering infant mortality: A call for ethical action. *Advances in Nursing Science, 4*(1), 63–78.
11. Curtin, L. L. (1978). A proposed model for critical ethical analysis. *Nursing Forum, 17,* 14.
12. Curtin, L. L. (1986). Autonomy, accountability, and nursing practice. In P. L. Chinn (Ed.), *Ethical issues in nursing* (pp. 11–20). Rockville, MD: Aspen.
13. Dewey, J. (1960). *Theory of the moral life.* New York: Holt, Rinehart, & Winston.
14. Fowler, M. D. (1989). Ethical decision making in clinical practice. *Nursing Clinics of North America, 24*(4), 955–965.
15. Frankena, W. K. (1973). *Ethics* (2nd ed.). Englewood Cliffs, NJ: Prentice-Hall.
16. Fromer, M. I. (1986). Solving ethical dilemmas in nursing practice. In P. L. Chinn (Ed.), *Ethical issues in nursing* (pp. 81–87). Rockville, MD: Aspen.
17. Gold, C., et al. (1995). Ethical dilemmas in the lived experience of nursing practice. *Nursing Ethics, 2*(2), 131–142.
18. Green, M. (1973). *Teacher as stranger.* Belmont, CA: Wadsworth Publishing Co.
19. Kant, I. (1993). *Grounding for the metaphysics of morals.* J. W. Ellington (Trans.). Indianapolis: Hackett Publishing.
20. Kilpack, K. Y. (1986). Ethical issues and procedural dilemmas in measuring patient competence. In P. L. Chinn (Ed.), *Ethical issues in nursing* (pp. 111–122). Rockville, MD: Aspen.
21. Levine-Ariff, J., & Groh, D. H. (1990). *Nursing manager's bookshelf: Creating an ethical environment* (pp. 41–61). Baltimore: Williams & Wilkins.
22. Mayberry, M. A. (1986). Ethical decision making: A response of hospital nurses. *Nursing Administration Quarterly, 10*(3), 75–81.
23. McFadden, C. J. (1967). *Medical ethics* (6th ed.). Philadelphia: F. A. Davis.
24. Murphy, M. A., & Murphy, J. (1976). Making ethical decisions systematically. *Nursing '76, 6*(5), CG13–14.
25. Nelson, M. J. (1986). Authenticity: Fabric of ethical nursing practice. In P. L. Chinn (Ed.), *Ethical issues in nursing* (pp. 89–94). Rockville, MD: Aspen.
26. Ozar, D. T., & Sokol, D. J. (1994). *Dental ethics at chairside: Professional principles and practical applications.* St. Louis: Mosby–Year Book.
27. Purtillo, R. (1993). *Ethical dimensions in the health professions* (2nd ed.). Philadelphia: W. B. Saunders.
28. Rhodes, A. M., & Miller, R. D. (1984). *Nursing and the law* (4th ed.). Rockville, MD: Aspen.
29. Sahakian, W. S. (1974). *Ethics: An introduction to theories and problems.* New York: Harper & Row.
30. Schrock, R. A. (1980). A question of honesty in nursing practice. *Journal of Advanced Nursing, 5*(2), 135–145.
31. Sher, G. (Ed.). (1979). *Utilitarianism.* Indianapolis: Hackett Publishing.
32. Sigman, P. (1986). Ethical choice in nursing. In P. L. Chinn (Ed.), *Ethical issues in nursing* (pp. 21–36). Rockville, MD: Aspen.
33. Tate, B. L. (1977). *The nurses' dilemma: Ethical considerations in nursing practice.* Geneva, Switzerland: International Council of Nurses.

Psychosocial Dimensions of Medical-Surgical Nursing

Ken W. Edmisson

This chapter discusses some of the psychosocial dimensions of nursing care that are relevant to the practice of medical-surgical nursing. The term *psychosocial dimensions* differs from *psychosocial nursing* in two primary ways. First, *psychosocial dimensions* depicts specifically selected topics of concern, whereas *psychosocial nursing* tends to encompass the entire realm of content. Second, *psychosocial dimensions* primarily addresses general content and practices, whereas *psychosocial nursing* focuses heavily on an in-depth approach to the practice of psychosocial nursing. (A psychosocial assessment guide is located in Appendix B.)

This chapter focuses on four major psychosocial topics: the family, cross-cultural nursing, spirituality, and sexuality. A major theme throughout is the nurse's self-awareness of personal attitudes, beliefs, and feelings in relation to all aspects of psychosocial nursing care. The nurse-client relationship is affected by various factors, which include similar or different cultural practices, gender, and spirituality. Likewise, families of clients, too, are affected by and affect the care provided the client by the nurse. Although nurses are becoming more knowledgeable and comfortable with cultural practices, gender, and spirituality with respect to nursing care, these topics need to be discussed continually to provide new information and to correct misinformation.

Nursing and the Family

The family is an excellent example of the adage that nothing happens in isolation. In this chapter, we use system theory to examine the family and the impact that illness has on the family. According to system theory, change in one part of a system may lead to change throughout the system. Application of this concept to the family makes it apparent that whenever illness strikes one

This chapter incorporates material written for the fourth edition by Michele J. Upvall, Joyce M. Black, Lynn Keegan, Jane Hokanson Hawks, and Bonnie Angelo.

family member, all family members are affected in some way. Depending on the circumstances, families may be required to make minor adaptations or to completely reorganize their way of living.

The contemporary American family system should be viewed as a semiclosed system that is interactive and interdependent with changing social, economic, political, and cultural systems. Because of changes in systems outside the family, families are always facing both significant threats to their survival and opportunities for growth. Analysis of the various changes influencing an individual family allows greater likelihood for understanding and support of the unique strengths or weaknesses of a given family.

Major Changes Affecting the American Family

Change is evident today in the wide range of alternatives available to American families regarding life-style choices. Change is also necessary to survive. Today's middle-aged Americans are called the "sandwich generation" because they are caught between caring for their children and caring for their aging parents. Statistical data from the U.S. Census Bureau provides some insight into these trends.

The average life expectancy, which rose from 69.7 years in 1960 to 75.0 years in 1987, is projected to increase to 77.9 years in 2010. The proportion of the U.S. population older than 65 has increased, and this trend is predicted to continue. Between 1960 and 1987, the percentage of the population older than 65 increased from 9% to 12.2%. Furthermore, by the year 2030, it is projected that the elderly will account for 22% of the total population. With changes in payment for healthcare, many elderly are cared for by grown children. This change has introduced new stressors to many families.

The number of marriages has decreased from 11.1 (per

1000 population) in 1950 to 9.9 (per 1000 population) in 1986. The age of spouses at the time of first marriage has increased. For women, the median age at first marriage has increased from 20.6 years in 1970 to 23.3 years in 1986. During the same period, the increase for men has been from 22.5 years to 25.1 years. Evidence of a change in traditional attitudes toward marriage also may be inferred from the increasing proportion of adults choosing to remain single. In 1970, 16.2% of adults in the United States were single; in 1988, that percentage had increased to 21.9%.

Nearly half of all marriages eventually end in divorce; the median duration of a marriage is less than 7 years. The annual divorce rate almost doubled between 1950 (2.6 divorces per 1000 population) and 1988 (4.8 divorces per 1000 population). Consequently, the number of divorced people in the United States has increased from 4.3 million in 1970 to 13.9 million in 1988.

The proportion of American families composed of a legally married couple has declined from 75% of the population in 1960 to 55% in 1988. During the period between 1970 and 1988, the number of unmarried couples of the opposite sex sharing the same household increased 63%.

Changes in the American family are also seen in the increasing proportion of single-parent families, most of which are headed by women. In 1986, one of every five children in the United States lived in a single-parent home; this represents a twofold increase in the number of single-parent families since 1970. The movement away from a "traditional" two-parent family creates a lot of stress on a single parent. This stress may lead to stress-related disorders.

In 1988, 10.8 million single-parent families were headed by a female and 2.8 million were headed by a male. The median family income of single-parent families headed by women was $15,346, whereas it was $26,827 in single-parent families headed by men. A lack of money to pay for healthcare often leads to underreporting of manifestations of disorders and prolonged self-treatment.

Concepts of Family

The concept of family has been defined differently by a variety of theorists. The definition you choose should depend on your client's situation as well as your personal perspective. Do not assume that all families operate as your family of origin does, but instead recognize the differences between your perspectives, values, and beliefs and those of your client. In general, the family system is considered to involve people related in a traditional or nontraditional sense by marriage, blood, adoption, or friendship. In the most inclusive sense, family can be defined as a dynamic system of two or more people who are emotionally involved with each other and who live near one another. However, distance is often not of such importance with respect to being considered family. The term *emotional involvement* assumes reciprocal obligations and responsibilities within the context of a caring and committed relationship.[6] A major theoretical framework underlying a definition of family is the structural-functional perspective.

The structural-functional perspective arises from a social systems approach and focuses on analysis of the structure and functions of family units within a social context. Although this perspective is often criticized for seeming rigid or narrow in scope, it provides a firm and necessary foundation from which to build a more dynamic and comprehensive understanding of the family.

A family's structure refers to the general scheme of organization that results in patterned interactions among its members (internal structure) as well as relationships with other family systems (external structure). Family functions refer to the tasks performed by the family system for maintenance of the family unit, for individual members, and for society.

Family Structures

Because of the pressures and demands created by complex, constantly changing internal and external environments, the structural patterns of families vary considerably among cultures and societal groups. Common family structures in the United States include the following:

- Nuclear family
- Family of origin
- Extended family
- Blended family
- Single-parent family
- Social contract family
- Communal family

Family of Origin

The family of origin refers to the family into which an individual is born. This may also be called the *family of orientation*. The family of origin is highly significant for the transmission of culture and expectations regarding health and illness of its members. Nurses should be aware of potential role conflicts and confusion when a marked difference exists between a client's family of origin and present family structure.

Nuclear Family

The nuclear family, also referred to as the *family of marriage* or the *conjugal family*, is composed of husband, wife, and their immediate children (natural or adopted). Historically, nuclear families have tended to have the highest income, to maintain relatively close generational ties, and to function according to traditional gender roles. Although this traditional structure was once the predominant family structure in the United States, it is no longer. Besides the number of nuclear families having declined, significant changes have also taken place within contemporary nuclear families relative to traditional gender roles and expectations.

Extended Family

The extended family includes the nuclear family as well as other relatives (e.g., adopted individuals, in-laws, and ex-spouses) who also may be members of the family of origin of the husband or wife. A typical extended family unit might include a nuclear family plus grandparents, uncles, aunts, or cousins who share household arrangements and responsibilities. Although the extended family has never been common in the United States, American families often maintain kin relationships through frequent contact and exchange of information and resources.

The extended family has the potential to be very cohesive, effective, and supportive in times of crisis. However, the relationships between family generations also can be a source of strain. Unfortunately, for the "sandwich generation," this can translate into an added stressor, which may be undetected unless deliberate attempts are made to evaluate this possibility. Given the increase in life expectancy, the possible strain on the "sandwich generation" should receive greater attention in the future.

Blended Family

The blended family, also called a *reconstituted* or *stepfamily*, refers to a family composed of an adult and at least one child from one marriage and an adult with or without children from a different marriage. The number of blended families is increasing dramatically to the extent that one of every three marriages in 1985 included at least one spouse who had been married before.

Blended families face complex and unique problems. Members do not share a common family history; thus, different expectations for health maintenance and different strategies for coping with stress or illness may exist. Additionally, if one or both spouses perceived a sense of failure in a previous marriage, they may show greater-than-expected role strain and conflict in response to a family member's illness.

Single-Parent Family

The single-parent family consists of one parent and one or more children. These families are created when a single person adopts a child, when a child is born to an unmarried mother who chooses to raise the child alone, or when one spouse leaves the marriage relationship as a result of divorce, separation, or death.

When dealing with a family member's illness, single-parent families often face problems associated with inadequate financial or emotional resources for coping with the actual illness. For example, single-parent families typically have fewer funds available for preventive healthcare and less time available for visits to clinics or physicians' offices.

It is interesting to note that research has shown that the absence of a dual-parent household does not necessarily contribute to dysfunctional behavior for the individuals involved. The manner in which individuals cope with their situation is more important than is the lack of a spouse within a household.

Social Contract Family

Social contract families are also increasing; this family structure includes unmarried couples of the same or opposite sex who live together and who may have children. These families exist because of an emotional commitment that is expressed in a social contract rather than a legal one. Because of social, financial, or external pressures, these relationships are sometimes temporary. According to the United States Census Bureau, the number of couples cohabiting (including gay and lesbian couples) doubled between 1970 and 1980. In 1985, social contract families represented 2.3% of all couple households.

Communal Family

Communes may be one of two different types. The first type encompasses more than one monogamous couple with children; such households share facilities, resources, experiences, and child socialization responsibilities. The second type may consist of a household of adults and children in which all adults are "married" to each other and all are parents to the children. When illness strikes one member, the potential exists to have support of many members in responding to the crisis. Communes are declining in popularity.

Family Functions

In general, the particular structure of a family is less significant than is a family's ability to perform functions considered necessary for growth of the family system and the individual members. Wright and Leahey[73] have described the family's functioning within five broad areas:

1. Management functions
2. Boundary functions
3. Communication functions
4. Education and support functions
5. Socialization functions

Management Functions

Management functions refer to the decision making of adult members regarding resource allocation, use of power, establishment of rules, negotiation with other systems, provision of financial support for members, and planning for the future. More important, management functions should be the responsibility of adult members rather than of children. Nurses should be alerted to the need for further evaluation when someone other than an adult is primarily responsible for family management during an extended period.

Boundary Functions

The boundary function involves maintaining clear distinctions among the roles of individuals within a family, among generations, and with other systems. Studies demonstrate that when clear generational boundaries (the boundaries between children and their parents) are present, the likelihood of dysfunctional behavior is less than when these boundaries are not present.

Communication Functions

Communication functions emphasize the patterns of interactions within families. Healthy communication patterns involve direct, clear communication styles that allow all members full and appropriate expression of either affection or conflict. However, dysfunctional communication styles may be rigid or of limited range.

Education and Support Functions

Education and support functions involve the degree of genuine affection and support expressed in families. This may be likened to the concept of social support, which is defined as "information leading the subject to believe that he is loved and cared for."[18]

Social support is an extensive area of research on the benefits of families in promoting and maintaining health. In 1976, Cobb described social support as information leading to feelings of being loved or cared for, belief of self-esteem and value, and belonging to a network of communication and obligation. Today nurses see the need for social support to prevent loneliness in elderly homebound persons, to provide tangible emotional and informational support, to mediate stress, and to promote health maintenance. Social support has also been shown to improve resistance to diseases by bolstering the immune system. Social support is crucial in promoting adaptation to illness situations and in preventing crisis development.

Socialization Functions

The socialization function focuses on transmission of culture and role behavior to facilitate a member's functioning both in the family and in society. In addition to societal expectations, socialization also relates to appropriate role behavior within the family. Each member has an identified position with accompanying role responsibilities and expectations.

Levels of Family Functioning

When general family functioning is healthy, coping and adaptation to changes required by situational or developmental crises are effective. However, several factors are associated with a lower level of functioning that ultimately inhibits a family's ability to meet the needs of its members. Awareness of these factors allows nurses to plan for potential problems and to develop appropriate intervention strategies.

One of the most useful frameworks for assessing a family's functional level has been developed by Tapia. According to this perspective, families are viewed along a continuum of five levels ranging from a dysfunctional to a highly functional level:

1. Chaotic family
2. Intermediate family
3. Family with problems
4. Family with solutions to its problems
5. Ideal independent family

Chaotic Family

The *chaotic family* is highly disorganized and has difficulty meeting the basic needs of its members. The chaotic family is at high risk for ineffective coping and dysfunctional behaviors in response to illness of any member.

Intermediate Family

Compared to the chaotic family, the *intermediate family* is less disorganized and better able to meet the members' basic needs. Although this family may sometimes be suspicious of outsiders, the intermediate family is generally more willing to accept offers of assistance than is the chaotic family.

Family with Problems

The third level, the *family with problems*, might be considered "normal" despite the presence of problems. Although this family is generally able to meet basic needs, role ambiguity and confusion between the parents often exist because of differences in their maturity levels. Compared to the intermediate family, this family is much less hostile and less suspicious of those outside the family system. With support and guidance, this family is able to recognize its problems and to accept assistance or suggestions for necessary changes.

Family with Solutions

The *family with solutions to its problems*, the fourth level, is able to meet basic needs and has clear role definitions for family members. Interventions planned with this family should be directed toward the changes imposed by illness rather than toward assessment and interventions related to dysfunctional family patterns.

Ideal Independent Family

The *ideal independent family*, the fifth level, functions at a much higher level in fulfilling all members' physical, emotional, and social needs. These families communicate needs clearly, are highly receptive to health maintenance or health promotion strategies, and frequently are independent in identifying a problem area and in seeking appropriate assistance.

Nursing Process in Family Nursing

Assessment

Family assessment is the evaluation of interaction within a family system. The two major tools used in family assessment are the genogram and the ecosystems map. Family members should be encouraged to participate actively with the health professional during the development of these tools. Ideally, this procedure should be begun during admission and orientation to the healthcare agency.

Genogram

The genogram is a schematic depiction of the intergenerational relationships of at least three family generations.[40] It is similar to a conventional genealogy chart or family tree. In this system, generations are placed on horizontal lines and children are denoted through vertical lines. The symbols used in genograms vary, but generally each person's name, age, date of birth, and any health problems should be noted. If a family member is dead, both the

cause and date of death should be indicated on the genogram (Fig. 4–1).

Comprehensive Summary

After collection of data from a genogram, ecosystems map, and family interviews, the findings should be analyzed and integrated in a meaningful manner. An appropriate system should be developed for each healthcare agency or setting, depending on philosophy, relevance, and practicality. Obviously, the system used in an emergency room is different from the system used in a long-term care facility.

Despite the actual style used, the nursing assessment of the family in medical-surgical nursing practice should be viewed as an ongoing process that is integral to professional nursing care. Initially, nurses in a medical-surgical setting should focus on a general macrolevel assessment of the family relative to structure, function, and developmental status. If problems are detected, then microlevel assessment of that area may be warranted. Depending on the experience and philosophy of the nurse, the microlevel assessment may be conducted by the staff nurse during subsequent family sessions or the family may be referred to a nurse specialist in the appropriate area. For example, if a macrolevel assessment indicates that a family is functioning at a low level (the chaotic family) and is likely to need further assistance following discharge, it may be appropriate to refer this family to a community health nurse for further evaluation. A family assessment tool is shown in Box 4–1.

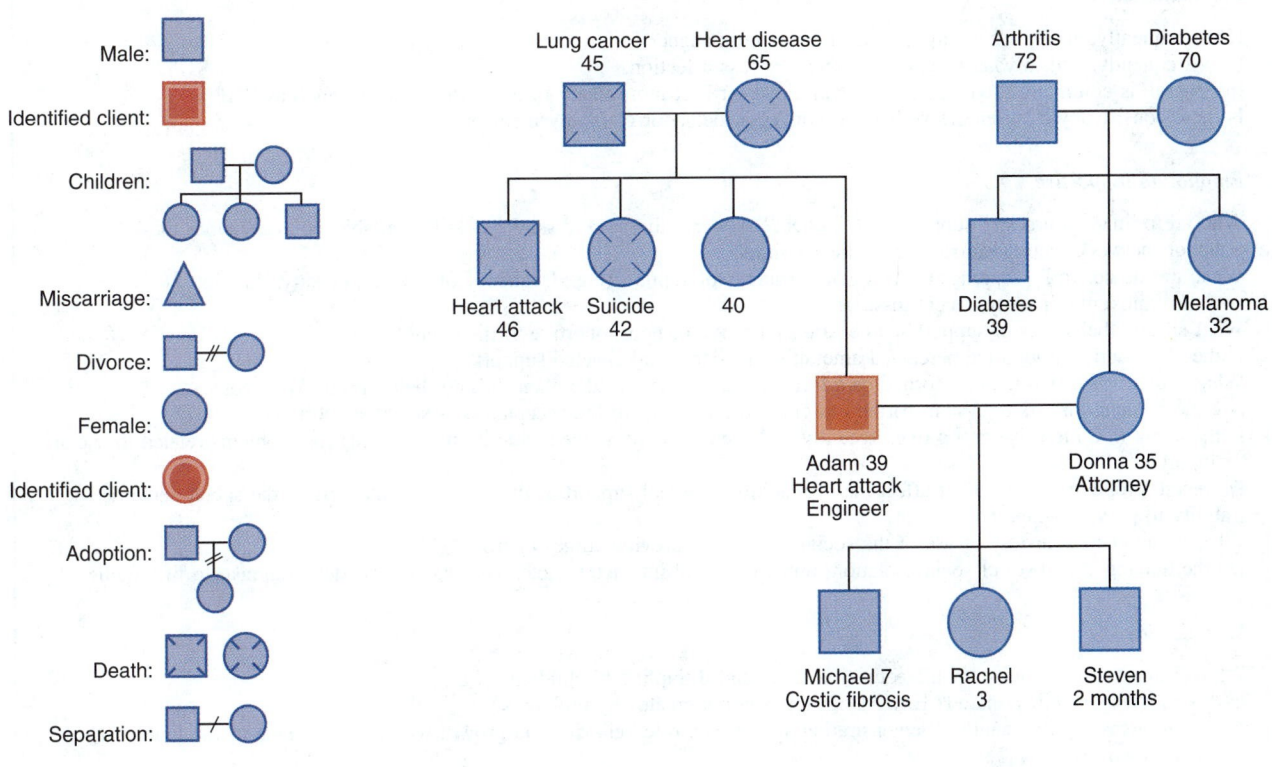

Figure 4–1. *A,* Symbols used to construct a genogram. *B,* Example of a genogram.

Box 4–1. Family Assessment Guidelines

Family Demographics

Demographic data: family name, address, telephone number

Family Structure

(The basis for assessing family structure may be a genogram or a chart that lists relevant data for each family member.)

Name	Age	Sex	Family Role	Occupation	Education
1.					
2.					
3.					
4.					

Family Functions

Management

How are decisions made? (give examples).
Who is responsible for providing economic income?
Has this changed because of a family member's illness?
How are the available family resources allocated?
Does one member require/receive more of the available resources than any other member?
How are home maintenance tasks divided?

Boundary (The ecosystems map may be used as a basis for discussion in this area.)

Who initiates and maintains relationships with the extended family, friends, and community agencies?
What, if any, are the problems in these relationships?

Communication

How frequently, and in what way, do members express anger?
How frequently, and in what way, do members express affection?
In general, is communication clear, open, and direct, or is it more likely to be evasive, covert, and circular?
Is there consistency between the verbal and nonverbal behavior of family members?

Emotional-Supportive

Who are primary sources of support for the client? Who are the more distant, yet still available, sources? Does the size of the
  support network seem adequate to the client's situation?
What are the network properties of the client's sources of support (e.g., frequency of contact, density, duration of
  relationships, multiplexity, recent losses)?
What specific behaviors of support sources are supportive or nonsupportive to the client?
Is the client satisfied with the perceived amount of available and enacted support?
What sources of support, either formal or informal, are available to the client but not being used? Why not?
Are there client barriers or system barriers to either the delivery or the acceptance of social support?
Is the client in a high-risk group (e.g., recently widowed, recently moved, elderly, mentally ill) for problems related to social
  support?
Do health problems of the client affect the availability of social support to the client? Do they affect the social network's
  ability to provide support?
What is the client's history of use of the social network in previous times of trouble?
Do the nursing diagnoses of social isolation, impaired social interaction, and/or social support deficit appear to fit the client?

Socialization

Who assumes responsibility for the education, care, and discipline of children?
Is this role/responsibility shared? How? Does this sharing create any problems?
Are each of the family members demonstrating appropriate role behavior and growth within and outside of the family? How
  is this growth exhibited?

Box 4–1. Family Assessment Guidelines *(Continued)*

Developmental Status

What is the family's stage in the life cycle?
What are the expected developmental tasks?
In what ways is the family meeting the stage-related tasks?
In what ways is the family having difficulty in this?
In what ways is the family meeting the stage-related health concerns?
In what ways is the family having difficulties with this?
What additional resources might be needed?
What are the individual developmental tasks for each member? (List each member separately.)
To what degree does the family foster or inhibit the individual members in meeting these tasks?
How has the illness situation influenced the development of individuals? of the family?

Summary

On the basis of assessment in all of the above-mentioned areas, list any identified problems and indicate the family's
  strengths and weaknesses for coping with the problem. In addition, indicate the type and availability of resources that will
  be needed to assist this family.

Nursing Diagnosis

A comprehensive family assessment leads to formulation of nursing diagnoses within two major areas: those that focus on the family unit and those that emphasize the individuals within the family.

Nursing Diagnoses Related to the Family System

Nursing diagnoses that focus on the family unit may involve Altered Family Processes or Ineffective (Disabling) Family Coping. The related factors of either diagnostic statement may be situational or developmental crisis, and the defining characteristics may vary considerably. The diagnostic statement of Altered Family Processes should be used for a normally healthy family unit that is challenged by the stress of acute or chronic illness. Some of the family behaviors that might indicate the appropriateness of this diagnostic statement include verbal outbursts, interference with necessary treatments, absence of family interaction, inappropriate communication patterns, and verbalization of fear, anxiety, or anger.

The nursing diagnostic statement of Ineffective (Disabling) Family Coping should be used when the behavior of the family is considered to be destructive, not merely lacking in support. An example of a destructive family situation is one in which the family interferes with the provision of care. Some of the defining characteristics for this diagnosis include neglect or abuse of a family member (see Bridge to Home Healthcare), depression, agitation, hostility, distortion of reality, and aggression.

Nursing Diagnoses Related to Individual Family Members

Nursing diagnoses that emphasize an individual family member's responses to the illness of a family member are generally related to fear, powerlessness, grieving, social isolation, and knowledge deficit. Even though the nursing diagnosis may focus on individual family members, they should also be viewed for their effect on the functions of the family unit and on other family members.

Nursing Diagnoses Related to Special Client Populations

Some nursing research has been completed on how families respond to various illnesses. The findings are discussed here. Although a great deal of research is still needed on the role of the family in the illness experience of family members, strides have been made within certain populations of patients. Two special populations of patients (critically ill patients and head-injured patients) have received special attention within adult medical-surgical nursing. Although commonalities exist between these groups relative to their needs, significant differences also exist; nurses should be cognizant of these to provide high-quality nursing care (see Nursing Research).

Nursing Intervention

Once appropriate nursing diagnoses and goals with measurable outcomes have been formulated, interventions should be planned, keeping in mind the possibility of a considerable variation between the needs of the family structure and the needs of individual members. For example, while the identified client is attempting to cope with terminal cancer, the spouse may be coping with an acute myocardial infarction, an adolescent daughter with an unwanted pregnancy, and a preschool-aged son with diabetes. Competing needs may also exist based on differences in developmental transitions and tasks. Interventions for any family should always begin with understanding of therapeutic family communication techniques. Therapeutic communication with families facilitates effectiveness in

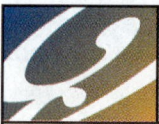

NURSING RESEARCH

What Are the Needs of the Family of a Critically Ill Client?

Fife, B. (1985). A model for predicting the adaptation of families to medical crisis: An analysis of role integration. *Image: The Journal of Nursing Scholarship, 18* (4), 108–112.

According to Fife, the major needs of families of critically ill patients are for the relief of anxiety, the provision of information and support, proximity to the patient, a feeling of helpfulness to the patient, and various personal needs of family members. Consequently, nurses should be aware of the need to assist families of critically ill patients in their coping strategies as they seek to understand the illness and treatments, gain awareness of their feelings, and develop a realistically hopeful perspective.

When caring for families of head-injured patients, nurses should be aware that the major problem is often social isolation. A perceived or actual sense of social isolation may be due to a sense of embarrassment related to the ill family member's inappropriate behavior in public settings, the lack of time or finances to participate in social activities, and drastic changes in previous family and social relationships. In addition, the actual care required by some patients can be so physically and emotionally draining to family members that not enough energy is left for negotiating social relationships and activities.

using other strategies, such as anticipatory guidance, networking, referral, and health teaching activities.

The manner in which families respond to changes imposed by illness is related to the nature of the illness, the timing of the illness relative to individual or family developmental stages, and the functional level of the family. When families are successful in their adaptation to changes imposed by illness, a buffering effect may take place that diminishes the perceived severity of the disease and supports the ill member in coping with life-style changes and treatment restrictions. However, when families are unable to adapt, resultant role confusion, conflict, and feelings of isolation may significantly compromise supportive efforts.

Therapeutic Family Communication

Therapeutic family communication comprises a four-stage process: (1) engagement, (2) assessment, (3) intervention, and (4) termination.[96]

■ Engagement

The first stage, engagement, focuses on establishing and maintaining a trusting nurse-client relationship. The ease with which trust is attained depends in large part on the family's functional level.[44] When working with families that function at a low level, nurses should emphasize trust building by being consistent in their actions, setting clear limits, adhering to promises made, and developing patience when faced with negative behavior. As a trusting relationship develops, nurses can be less directive and more collaborative in their communications.

During the engagement phase, nurses should attempt to remain essentially neutral and to avoid confrontation and power struggles. Each family member should be encouraged to express particular areas of concern or interest without fear of reprisal or argument.

■ Assessment

The second stage, assessment, focuses on exploration and identification of problem areas. During this stage, the nurse should avoid the obvious extremes of reaching a conclusion prematurely or of collecting irrelevant information. Communication patterns should be individualized to the functional level and maturity of the family members.

■ Intervention

The third stage, intervention, is the working phase of therapeutic communication with families. During this phase, communication patterns may be directive or collaborative as needed to assist the family to make changes in their approaches to the identified problem.

■ Termination

The final stage, termination, focuses on ending the relationship between the family and the nurse in a manner that will facilitate independent problem solving by the family in the future. Again, the degree to which this stage is possible is dependent on the level of family functioning and on the illness situation.

Anticipatory Guidance

One of the most useful interventions available to all nurses working with families is that of anticipatory guidance or preparation for expected occurrences. Anticipatory guidance should be provided in relation to two types of changes: those associated with illness and those associated with developmental transitions. When the family knows what is expected, the possibility is greater that the response will be positive and adaptive rather than harmful and counterproductive.

For example, when working with the family of a middle-aged man before major surgery, the nurse should provide anticipatory guidance for the family about possible behavioral changes that are likely to occur postoperatively. If a family is able to anticipate a short-lived depression following surgery, then less energy will be spent on inappropriate strategies and anxiety. Consequently, more of the family's energy and resources will be available for meeting needs of other family members or the family system itself.

Networking

In addition to anticipatory guidance, networking sessions should also be part of the plan when working with families of medical or surgical clients. A network may be defined as a type of kinship bond that occurs when people share an experience. The actual process of networking involves gathering the immediate and extended family along with friends and community associates to identify problems, generate possible solutions, and provide the necessary resources. Networking should be initiated with the client's entry into the healthcare system and continued into the community if necessary. Nurses should facilitate the development of networks that will continue following discharge without the intervention of health professionals. Networking allows others to become aware of potential problems and provide support that otherwise might not be provided.

An example of the network effect is frequently seen when families spontaneously discuss their members' illness in the hospital waiting areas adjacent to emergency rooms, intensive care units, or operating room suites. In effect, families who share their mutual concerns under such stressful conditions are providing support to each other as they attempt to understand and adapt to the various illness changes. The nurse can plan networking strategies that will provide more lasting and substantive support for the family faced with long-term changes. It has been shown that planning for respite care allows the family to renew its energy and better support the ill member.

Referral

Part of the concept of networking involves referral to community agencies. Referral is indicated whenever it is likely that the client will continue to need assistance following discharge. It should be noted that the process of referral requires more than merely supplying names and addresses of agencies regarded by the nurse as appropriate for the family's needs. For the outcome of a referral to be productive, two additional factors need to be considered: the meaning of the referral to the client and the family, and the receptivity of the responding agency. Obviously, referrals that a nurse considers appropriate may actually be resisted by a family if the community agency is seen as threatening or too inconvenient. Even when the family concurs on the necessity of a referral, the eventual outcome may be jeopardized if the receiving agency responds poorly. Therefore, a means for following up with families after a referral should be planned, so that alternative strategies may be developed when necessary. As is apparent, collaboration between families and all members of the health team is essential for effective care.

Teaching

The advent of diagnosis-related groups and subsequent early discharge from hospital settings makes the need for teaching more critical today than ever before. The nurse should be fully aware of a family's abilities to understand and to provide care before family members are released from hospital care. Although many teaching activities planned with the families of medical-surgical clients necessarily focus on providing information regarding the illness and the treatments encountered in the hospital, nurses should also focus on health promotion and health maintenance activities to be implemented following discharge. It is crucial to assess the client's and the family's willingness and ability to learn as well as their present knowledge level. Often, other issues such as anxiety and grief have a major impact on teaching and on the nurse-client relationship. Therefore, intervention strategies must be planned accordingly.

Cross-Cultural Nursing

The second component of psychosocial nursing that we discuss is the concept of cross-cultural nursing. Culture has a strong influence on health and health behaviors. It is imperative that all nurses appreciate the culture and cultural diversity of their clients.

A great influx of people immigrating to the United States continues (Fig. 4–2). As they undergo a necessary process of assimilation into the larger population, immigrants of all cultures bring with them a pride in their culture and a determination to preserve that culture. For us they offer rich cultural perspectives and traditions that encompass issues of health, happiness, and human existence.

All health professionals are finding themselves faced with an increasing number of clients from other cultures. A natural tendency exists to discount or belittle the attitudes, beliefs, and behaviors of others that appear alien or bewildering. However, with some effort at openness and understanding, the nurse can learn to appreciate the cultural differences that clients may present. The nurse may also learn how to be responsive and to work with the client and his or her beliefs and practices to maximize care.

Cross-Cultural Concepts

Culture and Cultural Diversity

Culture, by definition, refers to components and concepts of a people that are multifaceted, complex, and dynamic by nature. Culture's components and concepts are the culmination of beliefs, values, patterns of behavior, customs, tradition, and language of a people. Furthermore, culture is learned and transmitted from one generation to another and serves to guide thoughts, actions, and sentiments. Culture not only affects a person's decisions and actions, but culture also affects one's healthcare practices.

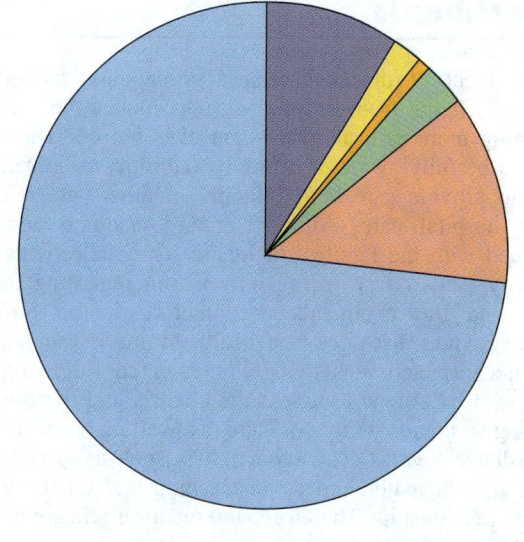

Selected Populations of the United States, 1990

■ White	199,686,070	
Percent of total population	**73.3**	
■ Black	29,986,060	
Percent of total population	**12.1**	
■ American Indian, Eskimo, or Aleut	1,959,234	
Percent of total population	**0.8**	
■ Asian or Pacific Islander	7,273,662	
Percent of total population	**2.9**	
■ Other race	9,804,847	
Percent of total population	**1.9**	
■ Hispanic origin (of any race)	22,354,059	
Percent of total population	**9.0**	

Figure 4–2. Selected population percentages for the United States: 1990. (From U.S. Department of Commerce, Bureau of the Census. [1990]. *1990 Census*. Washington, DC: Author.)

Cultural diversity is the overt and covert differences among people of different population groups with respect to their values, beliefs, language, customs, traditions, physical characteristics, and general patterns of behavior. Cultural differences affect the client's choice of healthcare as well as the response to the healthcare team. The nurse must be aware of the client's cultural orientation without stereotyping the client. Treating all clients alike regardless of culture is unsafe. For example, some groups of clients express pain openly and others are stoic in pain. If the nurse derived conclusions about the degree of pain based on behavior, one client could be overmedicated and another undermedicated. Appreciation of another's culture begins with an understanding of one's own culture.

Uprooting

Uprooting is the movement or migration of people from one country to another. The United States has been described as a nation of immigrants, because only the Aleuts and Native Americans are indigenous to America. People cross geographic boundaries for many reasons. War may force some to be refugees. Religious differences may encourage people to seek others with similar beliefs. Some people choose to move in an attempt to improve their financial status or to seek job opportunities. Finally, epidemics and disease may cause people to leave their homes in search of relief. The acquired immunodeficiency syndrome (AIDS) epidemic is a modern example of uprooting. Communities in developed and underdeveloped countries may reject a person with AIDS, which forces the individual into social isolation or results in uprooting.

On a smaller scale, hospitalization has been considered a situation of uprooting. With hospitalization, a client suddenly becomes dependent and is labeled a *patient*. Additionally, communication patterns, vocabulary, customs, and surroundings have changed.

Culture Shock

Culture shock is the reaction of people to an unfamiliar situation in which former patterns of behavior are no longer appropriate. Culture shock occurs when people are abruptly moved from one culture to another. Culture shock is also said to occur when non-American clients are brought into the American healthcare system. Initially, the person tries to learn about the new culture by asking questions. The person may feel inadequate or alone. Eventually, the person develops new behaviors and is able to function effectively. Returning to one's former culture after an extended time away might also produce culture shock.

Taboos and Myths

All societies have taboos and myths. Taboos are proscribed acts that are thought to be harmful to self or others. Myths are stories that explain why people engage in specific actions, and provide the basis for a groups' belief system. Interestingly, myths make sense to the people who believe them, but are difficult to explain to outsiders.

Many taboos also exist in Western societies. For example, it is taboo to eat cats and dogs in Western societies, but beef is readily eaten. In India, the reverse is true. Some cultures forbid the discussion of certain topics, such as mentioning the name of a person who has recently died, or the exposure of certain body parts (genitalia).

Any number of myths also exist in Western healthcare. For example, Americans believe that eating worms, snakes, and lice can cause illness, yet these foods are commonly eaten in many other parts of the world. One culture's delicacy can be another culture's taboo.

Cultural Imposition

Nurses must recognize that their own values, which are based on the Western healthcare system, are not superior, and that they do not have the right to impose cultural practices on other people. Nurses must celebrate rather than condemn cultural diversity. It is hoped that as nurses are exposed to people from other cultures, they can appreciate and value the differences.

Sadly, though, a true appreciation for difference seldom occurs. Instead, a tendency exists for the dominant cultural group (by virtue of size, perceived status, or other factors) to impose its beliefs on a less dominant cultural group. This process is called *cultural imposition*. Cultural imposition is based on ethnocentrism, in which one group is totally convinced that it possesses the right cultural ways and knowledge.

Theories of Health and Illness

Anthropologists have developed a variety of frameworks to classify various theories of health and illness. For ease of discussion, we can group these frameworks into two broad categories: Western societies and non-Western societies.

Before we discuss the specific theories of Western and non-Western societies, it is important to recognize that these are just general guidelines; not every member of these societies believes in these theories. The nurse must clarify each client's specific beliefs.

Western Belief Systems

Western societies generally believe that illness has a known cause that is not supernatural, and if that cause can be identified, the disease can be treated or cured. In Western societies, illness develops from genetic transmission, exposure to toxic substances (e.g., tobacco, cocaine), excessive dietary intake of harmful substances (e.g., fat, alcohol), and infection with bacteria, fungi, and viruses. It is a Western belief that diseases are treatable and sometimes curable. Western medicine is also focused on risk reduction and prevention. The ill client may be seen in two ways: as being somewhat responsible for his or her own health conditions as a result of practicing risky behaviors, or as being a victim of the disease.

Western definitions of health used to be simply "the absence of illness." In recent years, health and wellness have come to be seen to exist on a continuum. Theory recognizes that the client's perception of health is an important component of health.

Non-Western Belief Systems

Generally, non-Western societies subscribe to two main theories of disease and health: personalistic and naturalistic medical systems. Personalistic medical systems contain the belief that illness is caused by a sensate agent, such as a deity, ghost, ancestor, evil spirit, witch, or sorcerer.

The individual affected is a victim of aggression or is being punished. In the naturalistic system, illness is explained impersonally through the concept of equilibrium. All body elements, such as hot and cold humors, or yin and yang, are in harmony with the individual's natural and social environment. Illness occurs when equilibrium is disturbed. The following paragraphs present a short description of various peoples' beliefs about health and illness. Data such as these are not meant to prejudice healthcare providers but to assist them to understand the possible beliefs of their clients.

Contained within the beliefs of naturalistic medicine are the concepts of humors and disease. Humoral pathology is a common belief in Latin America and India. There are four humors or fluids in the body—blood (hot and moist), phlegm (cold and moist), black bile (cold and dry), and yellow bile or choler (hot and dry). The major organs of the body (heart, brain, and liver) are thought to have certain quantities of dry, moist, hot, and cold fluids. Healthy people have adequate heat and moisture, and illness is attributed to excess hot or cold. Often, the terms *hot* and *cold* are used metaphorically and may not indicate a specific temperature. For example, pregnancy is considered to be a hot experience, so the pregnant woman must not eat foods classified as hot, such as pork. Only cold foods can restore equilibrium.

A similar system of belief exists in India. The three humors, or *dosha*, are phlegm, bile, and wind. Health is a manifestation of balance of the three humors. Illness occurs when an individual experiences an imbalance.

The traditional Navajo Indians believe that disease is the result of a disharmony that is caused by violating a taboo or is an attack by a witch. They also believe that following elaborate rituals can prevent illnesses. Health is demonstrated by harmony between the individual, earth, and the supernatural, as well as by the ability to survive difficult circumstances.

Likewise, traditional Hispanic cultures teach that illness is a punishment from God for wrongdoing as well as an imbalance between hot and cold properties. Health is a gift from God or good luck. Illness can be prevented by praying, being good, eating well, wearing medals, and working.

Traditional Chinese people believe that health is a balance between yin and yang factors and that health is a gift from one's parents and ancestors. Illness is caused by an imbalance of yin and yang, and may be due to overexertion or to prolonged sitting. Illness can be prevented through better adaptation to nature. Illness is treated with foods, herbs, and curing methods that are thought to have hot or cold qualities. For example, acupuncture is considered a cold treatment for diseases that result from excess yang. Moxibustion is a hot treatment for illness that results from excess yin.

Healthcare Provision

The goal of any healthcare system is to mobilize the resources of the client, family, and society in resolving the client's problem. Additionally, healthcare systems provide an explanation of illness, a rationale for treatment, and provide sanction for cultural norms.

Western Healthcare Values

The major difficulty in studying cultural differences is that a person tends to be too close to his or her own culture to be objective. It is important, however, to examine one's own culture, because it is the view from which others see us. In this light, we focus here on the American healthcare system.

As it has evolved, the American healthcare system advocates the following values:

- Optimal health
- Democracy
- Individualism
- Achieving and doing
- Cleanliness
- Time
- Automation

■ Optimal Health

Having optimal health is viewed as a right for all citizens. The eradication of illness and deformities and the provision of many health services are now spoken of as both human rights and civil rights in the United States. This emphasis on optimal health for all citizens is in sharp contrast to that of many cultures in the world. In many cultures, health is not a major concern, and very little financial, social, or political support is given toward health promotion by these governments.

■ Democracy

With a democratic form of government, concerns about and programs to support health services and nationally sponsored health programs, such as Medicare, have come about. Again, this is in sharp contrast to cultures in which the government is autocratic, with less direct concern for the citizens.

■ Individualism

The individual in American society has always been more important than the social group. Other cultures value the group, and the individual is subordinate and given much less respect and consideration.

■ Achieving and Doing

Americans are urged to work hard and to be successful. Many Americans believe that they should continually strive to earn more money, get a better job, and climb the ladder of success. People in some other cultures have learned to enjoy what they have without continually working toward a goal, material possessions, or money.

■ Cleanliness

For Americans, cleanliness "is next to godliness" and is critical to social success. Cleanliness is seen as being related to having optimal health. Much time is spent on bathing, washing clothes, and keeping homes germ free. Some Americans seem compulsive about cleanliness. Few cultures emphasize cleanliness the way American culture does. Some people in other cultures are comfortable with clutter and dirt around them and with having only an occasional bath.

■ Time

Americans are extremely conscious of time and schedules. For Americans, time is extremely valuable, and a lot of guilt ensues if time is lost or wasted. Some cultures do not have an instrument to keep time. Some evidence suggests that the mental and physical health of these people is better than that of Westerners.

■ Automation

Automation and technology have a sharp impact on the American life-style. Machines are often able to do things instantly for us. Americans often expect instant health services, the finest technology, and instant recovery from illness. Most other cultures have a willingness to accept illness, deformity, and even death as a natural part of life.

■ Western Practitioners

The most common Western health primary care provider is the physician. Other healthcare professionals who provide care can be sought out by the client. These people include nurse practitioners, nurse midwives, physician assistants, doctors of osteopathy, and chiropractors.

Non-Western Healthcare Values

Various terms have been applied to healers practicing within personalistic and naturalistic systems. Titles such as *native healer, traditional healer, primitive healer,* and *witch doctor* have been given to healers, but they have often been used in a negative sense, to mean not as good as Western practitioners. Many prefer the term *indigenous healer* to refer to non-Western medical practitioners who are "of the culture."

■ Indigenous Healers

A comprehensive definition of indigenous healers has been developed by the World Health Organization:

A person recognized by the community in which he lives as competent to provide healthcare by using vegetable, animal, and mineral substances and certain other substances based on the social, cultural, and religious background as well as on the knowledge, attitudes, and beliefs that are prevalent in the community regarding physical, mental and social well-being and the causation of disease and disability.[72]

Indigenous healers can be classified into four major categories:

1. Those who have received integrated training in modern and traditional systems of medicine, such as Hindu and Chinese medicine

2. Practitioners trained mainly in traditional medicine but who also have some knowledge of modern medicine, such as the village health worker
3. Indigenous practitioners with no formal training but who have obtained diplomas in some particular system, such as that of India, after participating in correspondence courses
4. Those without institutional training who practice after a period of apprenticeship with an established indigenous healer

The last category of indigenous healers can be further classified into herbalists, diviners, surgeons, bonesetters, and traditional birth attendants and spiritualists. All of the indigenous healers operate at various levels of complexity, with the traditional birth attendants and herbalists performing at the most basic levels and the diviners and spiritualists treating problems of greater levels of complexity.

Nursing Process in Cross-Cultural Nursing

Leininger[41] defined cross-cultural, or transcultural, nursing as "a humanistic and scientific area of formal study and practice in nursing that is based on differences and similarities among cultures with respect to human care, health (or wellness), and illness originating from the person's cultural values, beliefs, and health practices and [the use of] this knowledge to provide cultural[ly] specific and culturally congruent nursing care to all people."[53] The concepts of cross-cultural nursing can be combined with the nursing process to provide care.

Developing Cultural Sensitivity

Before beginning any form of assessment of a client from another culture, the nurse must be certain that the client can be approached in an objective manner. Therefore, a prerequisite to assessment is to develop cultural sensitivity. (See Box 4–2 for a list of suggested readings on global cultures.)

Cultural sensitivity is defined as becoming aware of and accepting of diversity among clients and peoples throughout the world. There are differences in languages, social behavior, belief systems, and manner of dress. All too often, people look for differences between themselves and others, and not for similarities. Differences are usually seen as threatening. Prejudice and interpersonal tension decrease when people realize that they are more alike than they are different. Identifying commonalities among people of various cultures can serve as the first step in developing a greater sensitivity toward clients and families. Nurses must convey respect for the client's values, beliefs, and customs.

Assessment

Certain cultural components are present in all clients. Both subtle and obvious differences exist. Some people

---

Box 4–2. Additional Readings on Specific Cultural Groups

Ailinger, R. (1985). Beliefs about treatment of hypertension among Hispanic older persons. *Topics in Clinical Nursing*, 7(3), 26–31.

Boyle, J. (1991). Transcultural nursing care of Central American refugees. *Imprint*, 38(2), 73–77.

Boyle, J. (1989). Constructs of health and wellness in a Salvadoran population. *Public Health Nursing*, 6, 129–134.

Capers, C. (1985). Nursing and the Afro-American client. *Topics in Clinical Nursing*, 7(3), 11–17.

Egan, M. (1985). A family assessment challenge: Refugee youth and foster family adaptation. *Topics in Clinical Nursing*, 7(3), 64–69.

Foreman, J. (1985). Susto and the health needs of the Cuban refugee population. *Topics in Clinical Nursing*, 7(3), 40–47.

Giger, J., et al. (1991). Biologic variations in the black patient. *Imprint*, 38(2), 95–105.

Hamilton, C. (1991). Nursing on the Navajo reservation. *Imprint*, 38(2), 121, 174.

Kelly, K. (1991). A nursing student's experience in Haiti. *Imprint*, 38(2), 69–72.

Louie, K. (1985). Providing healthcare to Chinese clients. *Topics in Clinical Nursing*, 7(3), 18–25.

Luna, L. (1989). Transcultural nursing care of Arab Muslims. *Journal of Transcultural Nursing*, 1(1), 22–26.

Orque, M., et al. (1983). *Ethnic nursing care: A multicultural approach.* St. Louis: C. V. Mosby.

Pachter, L. M. (1994). Culture and clinical care. *JAMA*, 271(9), 690–694.

Roberson, M. (1985). The influence of religious beliefs on health choices of Afro-Americans. *Topics in Clinical Nursing*, 7(3), 57–63.

Sobralske, M. (1985). Perceptions of health: Navajo Indians. *Topics in Clinical Nursing*, 7(3), 32–39.

Wenger, A. (1991). Culture-specific care and the older Amish. *Imprint*, 38(2), 80–93.

---

may follow a cultural pattern very closely, and others may have chosen to deny it. It is important not to assume that any client has a prescribed cultural behavior pattern, as this would constitute stereotyping. To determine the degree of cultural variation in a client, an assessment should be performed.

Fong[25] and Orque[53] have identified cultural assessment guidelines. Fong developed a model called the CONFHER model. The letters stand for *c*ommunication, *o*rientation, *n*utrition, *f*amily relationships, *h*ealth beliefs, *e*ducation, and *r*eligion. Bloch developed a list of questions to elicit information about the client. The models are combined in Box 4–3.

History

Once a basic cultural assessment is performed on the client, the nurse can ask specific questions about the illness. The nurse should determine the client's beliefs about the cause of the illness. Does the client believe the disorder was caused by germs, life-style risks, spirits,

Box 4–3. Cross-Cultural Assessment

Communication Style

Is the interviewer in the correct proximity to the client (e.g., intimate or social zone)?

Are there nonverbal communication styles that need to be followed (e.g., bowing, speaking softly, touch restrictions)?

Which language does the client speak most frequently? Is an interpreter needed? Does the client speak English at all, have limited use of English, read and write in English?

Is there a need to vary the technique used to communicate with client (i.e., tempo of conversation, eye-body contact, topic restrictions, such as sexual matters, inclusion or exclusion of family members)?

Orientation

Does the client identify with a particular racial group (e.g., Asian, African, Native American) or ethnic group (e.g., Chinese, Japanese, Mediterranean)?

Where was the client born? Where has the client lived recently?

How closely does the client adhere to traditional habits and values from his or her parents' cultural system?

What is the accepted behavior of the cultural group regarding the expression of emotions and feelings, religious concerns, and responses to illness and death?

Are there restrictions related to discussion of sexual matters, exposure of body parts, certain types of surgery (e.g., hysterectomy), discussion of dead relatives, and discussion of fears of the unknown? What does the client value or desire from the healthcare system?

Nutrition

Are there preferred ethnic foods?

Are there foods that are encouraged to be eaten or discouraged from eating while ill?

What is the usual style of food preparation?

What is the frequency of eating and time of eating, and what utensils are used?

What are the implications of the usual diet for the disease process?

Family Relationships

Who is in the family? What are their roles?

What is the family order (e.g., patriarchal, matriarchal)?

What is the position of women and children in the family structure? What is their role in decision making?

Are there key family members who need to be involved in healthcare decisions?

How is the family valued during illness (e.g., present all of the time, provides baths, brings food)?

Where does the family live? Will this environment be conducive to healing and recovery?

Health Habits

What cultural healing system does the client follow predominantly (medicine men, herbalists, spiritualists, ministers)?

What religious system does the client follow (Christian Scientist, Seventh Day Adventist)?

How is illness explained (e.g., presence of evil spirits, imbalance of yin and yang, germ theory, inheritance)?

How does the client respond to pain and hospitalization?

Are there some disorders to which the client is more prone based on ethnic group (e.g., sickle cell anemia, hypertension)?

Education

What is the highest level of education the client has attained? Do the level of education and ability to read allow comprehension of verbal and written materials on healthcare?

What is the client's learning style (e.g., trial and error, didactic)?

Religion

Does the client's religion have a strong impact on how he or she relates to health and illness?

Do religious beliefs, sacred rites, and talismans play a role in the treatment of disease?

Are there religious restrictions that must be followed?

What is the role of significant religious persons during illness?

Developed from information in Fong, C. (1985). Ethnicity and nursing practice. *Topics in Clinical Nursing*, 7(3), 1–10; and Orque, M., et al. (1983). *Ethnic nursing care: A multicultural approach* (pp. 63–69). St. Louis: C. V. Mosby.

punishment for past deeds, a curse, or an imbalance of nature's forces? From this discussion, the nurse can determine the client's sense of control over the illness. This sense of control, called *locus of control*, can be internal or external. A client with an external locus of control believes that disease just happens, and that nothing can be done to prevent it from occurring. A client with an internal locus of control believes that a portion of disease could be managed personally. For example, the client may believe that he or she can control the risk of heart disease by weight control and dietary management. The issue of locus of control has an impact when planning intervention. The following are specific questions that should be asked:

What do you think caused your problem?
Has the problem become better, worse, or remained the same?
What problems has your illness caused you?
What are your fears concerning this problem?
What have you been doing for this problem?
What treatment do you think you need now?
How should family members help in the treatment of the problem?

Physical Assessment

When performing a physical assessment, the nurse should be aware of cultural preferences for limiting bodily exposure or for removing certain garments, and male-female relationships. At times, to obtain a complete examination, the client may need to accept a culturally forbidden practice. As often as possible, however, the nurse should work within the cultural parameters.

Certain physical differences may occur between people of various cultures, such as bone length, pelvic size, and number of vertebrae. These variations are discussed in the chapters in this text that focus on physical assessment of the various body systems.

Health Risk Appraisal

People of various cultures are at increased risk for various illnesses due to their cultural and genetic background. The nurse should be aware of these risks and examine the client's history and physical assessment findings for these risks. Chapter 11 discusses the risks of illness in various cultures.

Nursing Diagnosis

Nursing diagnoses are specific and are relevant to each client. They indicate type, possible cause, and obvious manifestations of the client's condition. In addition to the many diagnoses that might be applicable to a client from the same or similar culture as that of the nurse, a client from a different culture might warrant additional nursing diagnoses. These additional nursing diagnoses should attempt to address the cultural impact on the client's health. An example of such nursing diagnosis is *Social Isolation related to separation from cultural ties as evidenced by lack of family visits, inadequate food consumption, and refusal of medical regimen.*

Planning: Expected Outcomes

When planning care, the nurse must consider the client's cultural practices and how they correlate with the Western healthcare system (see Nursing Research). For example, if the client is a dying Muslim, the family would stay with the

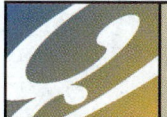

NURSING RESEARCH

How Can Cultural Beliefs of People Be Incorporated into Nursing Care?

Goldstein, D. (1987). A traditional Navajo medicine woman...A modern nurse-midwife...Healing in harmony. *Frontier Nursing Service, 62*(6): Winter.

On the Navajo Reservation in Arizona and New Mexico, certified nurse-midwives are incorporating indigenous beliefs with biomedical obstetric nursing care. Families are encouraged to seek indigenous healers as they desire, and healers are welcomed in the hospital. Certified nurse-midwives wear necklaces made of juniper seeds, which are believed to promote a safe passage of the fetus from the uterus to the outside world. Birthing rooms in the hospital are equipped with traditional Navajo woven belts suspended from the ceiling. These belts are used during the second stage of labor as the client pushes. All client teaching, antepartum through postpartum, has been modified to include traditional Navajo beliefs and dietary preferences. Maternal hygiene and infant care teaching take into consideration living arrangements that often consist of one-room hogans that do not have water or electricity. Clients have reacted favorably to the culturally sensitive care given by the certified nurse-midwives. They have been accepted into the community and participate in Navajo healing ceremonies as well.

client, wash the body before prayer time, turn the client to face Mecca, and pray five times a day. These practices are certainly outside of the normal routine for a Western hospital, but they should be allowed. Ultimately, it is imperative that the nurse bring the cultures together, in a manner of speaking, so that the client both feels comfortable with the nursing and medical care and feels that he or she has not abandoned the family members (see Ethical Issues in Nursing).

Nursing Intervention

Sometimes, clients from various countries come to the United States for treatment of very serious illnesses or conditions. They may have saved money for years to allow a lifesaving operation to be performed. Because of the cost, the client often comes alone or with just one other person. In these cases, few support systems are available to the client and the significant other. The nurse should attempt to link the client and the significant other to people in the area who are from the same culture or who are willing to work with such people.

Dietary practices vary greatly around the world. At times, the client's diet and the prescribed diet to facilitate healing are different. For example, Chinese clients often

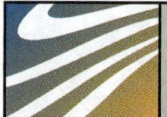

ETHICAL ISSUES IN NURSING

What Happens When the Nursing Care Plan Is in Conflict with a Specific Cultural Practice?

Nurses who care for certain client populations need to become aware of the customs, beliefs, and ideals pertaining to the healthcare of those populations. Situations may occur in which healthcare providers need to be sensitive to a specific cultural practice of their clients (such as a spiritual ritual or a dietary request).

Problems arise in cross-cultural nursing when cultural differences are not understood or respected by those involved. Nurses who care for clients who are culturally different from themselves have an obligation to their clients to allow them the freedom to express their cultural diversities. These diversities may cause the nursing care plan to be altered to fit into the particular cultural habitat. Some cultural habits may be in total opposition to the health of a client (dietary restriction, for example). Once the nurse recognizes that a cultural change needs to occur, education may begin for the client and family to help them see that the change is not a threat to their specific cultural life-style.

The nurse's obligation is to carefully explain the suggested interventions and to emphasize the importance of these interventions to the client's health. The nurse can recommend alterations in specific culturally related practices and suggest interventions for the client to consider. After that, it is the client's decision whether or not to follow the advice of the healthcare team or to continue to follow cultural practices.

eat rice for every meal. Because it is not always possible to get rice for all three meals in a Western hospital, the nurse could work with the hospital dietitian to obtain the rice. However, if that amount of rice does not meet the client's needs for protein and fat, other food sources that are culturally acceptable should be considered. But it would be possible for the nurse to serve the Chinese client hot liquids, such as tea, rather than cold beverages.

If the client does not speak English, an interpreter can be used to facilitate conversation. The nurse should be certain that the client understands what is said, especially if a new medical treatment or surgery is planned. Nonverbal communication is commonly understood and can be used. If the client can read his or her own language, a list of terms in the primary language can be written alongside the terms in English. The nurse can also communicate with the client using the same tool.

Evaluation

Evaluation of goal attainment of a client from a different culture is very similar, if not identical, to that of a client

from the same culture as that of the nurse. It is the nurse's responsibility to evaluate the selected client goal(s) for evaluation. It is also important that the client understand the process.

International Nursing

International nursing focuses on developing national health policies, curriculum development in nursing education, the promotion of primary healthcare as directed by the World Health Organization, and international research efforts.

International nursing can be defined as any nursing care activity carried out by a nurse from a donor country in a host nation. The nurse providing the care was educated and has practiced nursing in the donor country. However, the nursing services are requested by and practiced in a host country. These services are contracted for a specific time period, and can range from a matter of days to many years.[28]

Terms such as *cross-cultural, multicultural, transcultural,* and *transnational nursing* have been used as synonyms for international nursing.[8, 22, 55, 77] However, international nursing is a unique specialty, although it is related to transcultural nursing. As a specialty in nursing, international nursing reflects the different nursing needs in other countries. It requires the nurse to work within a system in which definitions of health may differ and unique skills are necessary for combining nursing knowledge and practice from both countries.

International nursing can be distinguished from transcultural nursing in a number of ways, although some overlap also occurs. Two themes emerge from this international nursing focus. First, international nursing becomes fully realized within the practice realm, although it may be based on transcultural nursing, anthropologic research, or both. Second, a national perspective or *macroperspective* is evident in international nursing.[41] This macroperspective implies that nurses must be involved in policy making and health planning, because healthcare is affected not only by cultural forces, but also by economic, political, educational, and historical forces. It is not enough to assess individuals. Sociopolitical and economic structures must also be evaluated.

Another feature that distinguishes international from transcultural nursing is the importance attached to primary healthcare in international nursing. Ministries of health in many countries have committed their countries to primary healthcare, at least philosophically. Primary healthcare is an ideology for practice that includes accessibility to healthcare services, involvement of individuals at the community level, health promotion, prevention and cure, appropriate technology, and integration of health with social and economic development.

An individual working within an international nursing framework must be cognizant of the relationship and comprehensiveness of nursing and primary healthcare. This nurse may actively collaborate with individuals involved in agriculture, natural resources, sanitation, nutrition, and textiles as well as members of the community in which healthcare services are being provided.

Although international and cross-cultural nursing are both concerned with health beliefs and practices of different cultures,[28] collaboration is crucial within international nursing. Collaboration in international nursing exists at different levels. First, collaboration takes place between the nurse from the donor country and the nurse from the host country. Second, national collaboration occurs with ministries of health and their representatives. Finally, community collaboration exists as the international nurse secures the cooperation of the community for any healthcare project.

Global Organizations

The World Health Organization (WHO) is part of the United Nations. Created in 1948, WHO is concerned with international and public health problems.

A turning point for WHO occurred with the 1978 International Conference on Primary Healthcare in Alma-Ata, in the former U.S.S.R. During this conference, members were challenged to make health services equitable through primary healthcare. The slogan from the conference became "Health for All by the Year 2000." Although it was viewed as an ambitious goal, WHO has made progress, and insight has been gained from programs that were not successful.[95]

To increase the impact of nurses working with WHO, global strategies were initiated. The Network of Collaborating Centers for Nursing Development was formally established in March 1987, in Bangkok. The goal is the creation of 30 centers throughout the world, with regional representation. Already, 14 centers have been established, which include the regions of Africa, the Americas, Europe, Southeast Asia, and the Western Pacific. These centers are creating a network of nursing leaders who are committed to successfully implementing WHO's primary healthcare philosophy.[72]

The International Council of Nurses was initiated in 1900. According to its charter, member nurses make the following pledge:

We, the nurses of all nations, sincerely believing that the best good of our profession will be advanced by greater unity of thought, sympathy and purpose, do hereby band ourselves in a confederation to further the efficient care of the sick and to secure the honor and interests of the Nursing Profession.[44]

Thus, the concept of a global nursing community was developed nearly a century ago through the International Council of Nurses. Nurses worldwide gather to share new ideas and research, and networking is facilitated. Also, the International Council of Nurses has been committed to preparing nurses in primary healthcare since 1979. Between 1983 and 1985, the International Council of Nurses conducted seven regional workshops to prepare nursing leaders for primary healthcare.[3] Their commitment continues through developing guidelines for implementing primary healthcare. In turn, these nursing leaders will educate other nurses, and so facilitate the growth of primary healthcare's philosophy from country to country.

Spirituality

As you can see, clients of different cultures may have different beliefs about health or healthcare. Likewise, persons of differing religions and beliefs may also differ. We will explore some of these variations. Again, none of the belief systems or religions are perceived as right or wrong, but instead are approached with respect and acceptance.

Concepts of Spirituality

Spirituality is a broad concept encompassing values, meaning, and purpose. It is experienced when one turns inward to explore the human capacities of honesty, love, caring, wisdom, imagination, and compassion.[26] Spirituality can be described as a human need to search for the meaning and purpose of life.[83]

Spirituality comes from *spirit*, which has several cultural and historical sources. The Latin root meant "breath." The Greeks evolved the term from the root word "wind." Biblical sources describe spirit as the breath of God flowing through us. The definition of spirit found in *Webster's Dictionary* gives us the concept of spirit as the breath of life. Buddhists think of spirit in terms of inner light or truth. In contemporary times, we have come to think of spirit as divine animation, an inner guide, something greater than ourselves, something within ourselves, and in a variety of other ways.

Spirit can be seen as a multitude of animations, present at every level of existence from the simplest material to the divine. In pure matter, spirit is perhaps that which makes the electrons spin around their nucleus, affecting both animate and inanimate life. Spirit in human beings is elevated to a higher plane, where it contains the animating principle seen in the lower forms of matter and life, but it also incorporates the principle of the divine that many call the soul.

Religion

Religion is an organized set of beliefs and practices that express those beliefs. Religion is not a synonym for spirituality, although the words overlap in meaning.

It is common for clients who are ill, suffering, or dying to question their God and to call on their religion for support. The religious practices of many clients offer support through periods of illness and at the time of death. Therefore, it is important for nurses to be aware of the impact of various religious beliefs and to not interfere with the client's practice (see Ethical Issues in Nursing). We will look at two instances in which spirituality typically assumes a major role for clients and families, that is, during grieving and suffering.

ETHICAL ISSUES IN NURSING

Should Spiritual Beliefs that Are in Opposition to Modern Medical Practices Be Respected?

A person's beliefs about his or her spiritual self are a very private and reflective matter. Some people follow spiritual guidelines accepted through organized religious institutions. Other people incorporate spiritual identities from sources including mysticism, new age phenomena, or naturalism. Personal beliefs, from whatever source, may have a great impact on a person's concept of health, illness, grief, and loss.

Spiritual healing through prayer, repentance, and positive thoughts is a practice demonstrated by certain religious groups. Christian Scientists, for example, believe that the healing of many of the body's ills should come only through prayer. They also believe that certain illnesses that their children experience are caused by their own fears and errors of thought. The Christian Science church discourages parents from seeking medical treatment for their children (from medical practitioners other than their own Christian Science practitioners). There have been several cases in the recent past in which children of Christian Science parents have died from conditions that could very easily have been treated medically (bacterial meningitis, for example).

Freedom of religion is a right that should always be protected, but should spiritual beliefs that are in opposition to common modern medical practices be respected in an industrialized nation such as the United States? Do parents have the right to impose their own spiritual guidelines on their minor children when such guidelines could cause physical impairment or possibly death?

Nurses are human beings, with human values and spiritual beliefs. During day-to-day nursing care, the spirituality of patients is not always assessed or considered as part of their care. It is important to be able to separate one's own beliefs from the beliefs of others so as not to impose one's own beliefs onto another. It is also important to be aware of one's own attitudes toward those who possess different spiritual ideas so that those attitudes do not interfere with the responsibilities of a healthcare professional.

Relevance of Spirituality to Nursing Practice

Nursing models (Newman, Rogers, Travelbee, and Watson) address spirituality directly in terms of human needs. Watson[70] states that the future of nursing belongs to caring more than curing, and that the entire profession is in the process of redefinition. We are emerging from a traditional practice of objective, rational detachment into something far greater. Part of that greatness includes the renaissance of a holistic approach. As nursing redefines

itself, it will reincorporate some of the forgotten aspects of our heritage: the role of spirit.

Watson[70(p176)] further states that "human caring theory allows the commitment and consciousness of the nurse to transcend (or at least attempt to transcend) the physical material surface and reach beyond to touch the human center of the person." When this occurs, we are less inclined to objectify persons and are more inclined to see new caring and healing possibilities. The human caring process has an energy field of its own that exceeds the sum of each individual. We must remember that caring occurs in the metaphysical realm. We cannot see this realm, we can only experience it.

Meeting the spiritual needs of clients has become a recognized part of nursing care. Nursing care is not only intended to make clients well or to prevent illness, "but to help those in health or illness to use the power within themselves as they evolve toward higher levels of consciousness."[59] Dennis[15] conducted one of the first empirical studies of nurses' spirituality. Data suggested that spiritual care is not a separate part of nursing, but that it is integral to nursing, as evidenced by the range of comments supporting spirituality in practice (see Nursing Research).

Nurses must be aware of their own spirituality to assist others in fulfilling their spiritual needs. People are not unidimensional in scope; they are at least tridimensional. They are composed of body, mind, and spirit. When the physical domain of an individual is compromised, the mind and spirit are also involved. Guided by this understanding, the nurse can more easily facilitate the harmonious interconnections within and between persons. The nurse may aid the client to incorporate a spiritual perspective in the delivery of healthcare. Additionally, there is a stronger appreciation by the individual for the interpersonal and physical environments and for the Ultimate Other or God as understood by the individual.

Spirituality and Nursing Process

Those who suffer or those in spiritual crisis need nurses who allow and, on occasion, even encourage anger, tears, and the expression of sorrow. Such people need sensitive caregivers who can say, "Yes, what happened to you is terrible, and may make no sense to you," rather than, "Cheer up, it's not that bad." If this type of care is to be offered, nurses must be supported as they learn how to call forth their inner power.

Assessment

Spiritual calls for help seldom take the form of overt statements. Instead, they appear as subtle signs. Learning to recognize these signs will better prepare you to recognize and encourage clients' expression of thoughts and feelings about their religious beliefs. These signs may be statements such as, "Do you go to church? I have not been to church in a long time. What do the chaplains do in this hospital?" On the other hand, the questions may be profound and include philosophical inquiries about your perception of life after death or the meaning of life.

How Can Nurses Provide Spiritual Care?

Dennis, P. (1991). Components of spiritual nursing care from the nurse's perspective. *Journal of Holistic Nursing, 9*(1), 27–42.

The purpose of this exploratory study was to discover and describe the components of spiritual care by nurses who provide such care. A qualitative approach was used with Watson's work on the spiritual aspect of human beings as a framework. Ten nurses who said they provided spiritual care from a nonreligious perspective were the sample. Data were analyzed by examining the interviews for incidents and facts, and then grouping the data into Watson's categories.

The study found that spiritual care for these nurses was not a separate part of nursing but an integral portion of nursing care. The nurses believed that the human spirit is at the core of every client's existence and is the power that heals. Their goal was to bring forth the inner powers and nourish the subdued spirit.

Nurses who provide spiritual care need to be committed, fully prepared to use self as a healing tool, "able to stay within the moment," and willing to be seen as "different" from other nurses.

The process of providing such care includes the nurse honoring the client's uniqueness and setting up a safe environment for discussion, therapeutic touch, or quiet time. Significant others may or may not be helpful and may block spiritual care. Nurses noted that after such care was given, the clients expressed deep gratitude and the room was quieter. The hospital was generally not conducive or supportive to providing spiritual care. The nurses generally reported having encounters with clients that were an intimate exchange and similar to a soul-to-soul union that transcended the roles of nurse and client. For some nurses, this union occurred quickly; for others, it only happened after many visits.

The study's implications are that if this type of care is to be offered, nurses need to be taught how to give such care. Nurses who work in hospital settings need empowerment if this type of care is to be given.

A second area of spiritual assessment involves the specific religious practices of a client. The nurse needs to question what these practices mean now during this time of stress and crisis. Some clients become more religious when they are in crisis and other coping mechanisms fail. Sometimes clients first explore their spiritual practice in the face of a new event (e.g., a serious illness, death of a loved one, or childbirth) that causes them to think about the hereafter. Many clients think of themselves as immortal until they are confronted with surgery or illness and are faced with their own mortality. These events trigger questions such as, "What is the meaning of life? Is there a heaven or hell? Why am I here?" In addition to collecting subjective data, the nurse may observe the environment for objective data (Box 4–4).

Nursing Diagnosis

Spiritual Distress is the problem statement used. The etiology may flow from various sources, including separation from religious or cultural ties, a change in beliefs or value systems, intense suffering during severe stress, or prolonged treatment. The defining characteristics include anger against the deity or questions about the meaning of the suffering that is being experienced. The client may joke in a macabre fashion, have nightmares, cry, act in a hostile or apathetic manner, express anger or resentment against religious figures, and cease participation in religious practices.

Box 4–4. Spirituality Assessment Guide

Subjective Data

Does the client:

- Talk about spiritual needs or concerns?
- Verbalize feelings about God, faith, prayer?
- Feel that the illness affected feelings about God?
- Find any particular religious practices helpful?
- Belong to any specific religious group or faith community?
- Have someone or something to turn to for help and hope?
- Feel lonely, depressed, abandoned?
- Feel separated from spiritual connections?
- Express bitterness, self-belittling thoughts? Project blame for illness?
- Question the validity of faith? Verbalize inner conflicts about beliefs? Question the credibility of the religious system?
- View illness as a form of punishment from God?
- Have a form of belief that fosters or weakens faith and trust? Fosters or weakens self-esteem?
- Express a preoccupation with thoughts of faith and illness?
- Have access to spiritual resources?

Objective Data

Does the client:

- Pray before meals?
- Read religious material?
- Have religious materials nearby (e.g., rosary, religious medals)?
- Express a reluctance to participate in spiritual or religious rituals?
- Express anger or resentment toward religious or spiritual leaders?
- Sleep restlessly, have disturbing dreams?

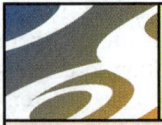

DIVERSITY IN HEALTHCARE

Death and Dying

Cultural Attitudes Toward Death

By their very nature, people are sociocultural beings who need to develop attachments with others. When these attachments threaten to become permanently severed by death, cultural explanations help people make sense of their loss. One's culture also provides guidelines for expected attitudes, beliefs, and practices before, during, and after death—one's own death and the deaths of others. In some Native American and Hispanic cultures, for example, people may believe that omens such as the appearance of an owl or a message in a dream warn of approaching death.[1]

Some elderly clients of black and Hispanic descent believe that psychics, spiritual leaders, and folk healers have the power to predict, and in some cases prevent, impending death. Older adults who know how to manipulate spiritual forces believe that they may be able to extend their lives. The nursing literature contains reports of incidents in which clients have blamed nurses for breaking taboos, thus becoming the agents responsible for death. For example, an incident was reported in which a nurse removed a necklace and its curative attachments from an elderly Native American woman to keep them in a safe place with other valuables.[2] After the client died, the family attributed the cause of her death to the nurse's behavior.

Voodoo beliefs and practices persist in North America, especially among Haitians and people from other circum-Caribbean nations. Recent immigrants from Africa and predominantly black areas of South America also may practice voodoo. Incidents of sudden death or minor injuries following hexes have been attributed to the power of suggestion and to total social isolation. The harmful effects of voodoo hexes are believed to result, in part, from autonomic nervous system responses to perceived fears. When these fears are intense, they may trigger fatal physiologic responses, such as a heart attack or stroke. When inter-connected with feelings of guilt over past or present moral transgressions, the recipient of voodoo hexes may become depressed and engage in suicidal behavior.

The acceptance of sudden, violent death is difficult for most people, irrespective of culture. Many ethnic and religious groups have therefore developed beliefs and practices concerning sudden, violent death, including suicide. Stereotypes such as the stoicism of Japanese, for whom suicide is motivated by duty to their country during times of war or by a need to atone for dishonorable behavior, have been depicted liberally in the U.S. media. Palestinian, Israeli, Iranian, Iraqi, and other terrorists, often professing to embrace fundamentalist religious beliefs, make headlines by carrying out suicide-bombings. The intended victims may be political, military, or religious figures or innocent bystanders chosen at random. it should be noted that suicide is strictly forbidden by Islamic law, but members of rebel factions of Islam have modified their interpretation of the Koran to allow them to commit suicide in certain situations.

By far, the majority of religions condemn suicide. Suicide is strictly forbidden by the tenets of Roman Catholicism, Buddhism, and other religions, which view the taking of one's own life as morally wrong. Even when an elderly person is afflicted with a painful terminal condition, suicide (and euthanasia) are prohibited.

Northern Cheyenne Indians believe that suicide or any death resulting from a violent accident disturbs the person's spiritual balance. This disharmony is called a *bad death* and is believed to render the spirit earthbound in its wanderings, thus preventing it from entering the spirit world.[3] A bad death occurs unexpectedly and violently, leaving the victim without a chance to settle his affairs or say good-bye. Suicides, heart attacks, strokes, homicides, and other causes of sudden death are categorized as bad deaths. A *good death,* however, comes at the end of a full life, when a person is prepared for death. Paradoxically, among the Tohono O'odham (Papago) tribe, the premature death of an older adult from diabetes may be viewed as a good death. Because diabetes most often affects people of more advanced years, and because of its slow progress, the client is able to prepare for death. In the healthcare community, the death would be termed *excess* or *premature,* but culturally it is not considered a bad death.[3, 4]

Older adults who follow the Buddhist religion may approach death in the following holistic manner. Illness is inevitable and is a consequence of events and actions taken. These may not necessarily occur in this life, but they also can have occurred in previous lives. There is an acceptance of death, which means that the choice has been made to anticipate the grief and accept the inevitability of death. It does not mean resignation or the denial of conventional healthcare. It does mean moving peacefully into the next existence from the presence of loving family and friends.[5]

Awareness of Dying

Physicians, nurses, members of the clergy, and others have debated extensively about whether a person should be made aware of his or her impending death. In a study by Kalisch and Reynolds,[6] 71% of whites, 60% of blacks, 49% of Japanese-Americans, and 37% of Mexican-Americans said that they believed that a person should be told if he or she is dying. These cultural groups agreed that the physician is the most appropriate person to convey the information, and that a family member is the second most appropriate choice. Among all groups, respondents said that individual preferences concerning whether to be informed about death should be respected.

Preparation of the Body for Burial and Funerals

Although most families will pay a state-licensed mortician to handle the details of preparing the body of a deceased loved one for burial, ask family members about their cultural or religious practices surrounding preparation for burial. Customs for disposal of the body after death vary widely. Muslims have specific rituals for washing, dressing, and positioning the body. In orthodox Judaism, cosmetic restoration is discouraged, as is any attempt to hasten or delay the decomposition by artificial means. As part of their lifelong preparation for death, Amish women sew white burial garments for themselves and for their family members. Members of the Church of Jesus Christ of Latter-Day Saints (Mormons) are dressed in white temple garments for final viewing and burial. Believing that the spirit or ghost of the deceased person is contaminated, some Navajo Indians refrain from touching the body after death. In preparation for burial, the body is dressed in fine apparel, adorned with jewelry and money, and wrapped in new blankets. Traditional Navajos believe that after death the structure in which the person dies must be burned.[1, 7]

Funerals vary from short, simple rituals, to long, elaborate displays. The Amish rely on family members, neighbors, and close friends for a short, quiet ceremony. Many Jewish families use unadorned coffins and stress simplicity in burial services. Some Jewish families fly the body to Jerusalem for burial in ground that they consider sacred. Some groups believe in lavish and costly funerals as a final tribute to loved ones, no matter what economic constraints the families might be facing.

Bereavement, Grief, and Mourning

Bereavement refers to the status and role of the survivors of a death. *Grief* is an affective response to a loss, whereas *mourning* is the culturally patterned behavioral response to a death. What differs between races and cultural groups is not the feeling of grief that follows

the loss of a significant other, but the forms of expression or mourning.

Although nurses frequently encourage clients and those significant to them to express their grief openly, many people are reluctant to do so in the institutional healthcare setting. Three-fourths of the black, Japanese, and white clients surveyed in one study stated that they would try hard to maintain control of their emotions in public, whereas fewer than two-thirds of Mexican-Americans said that they would try to control their expression of grief. When asked about crying, either publicly or privately, 88% of Mexican-Americans, 71% of Japanese, 70% of whites, and 60% of blacks said that it was acceptable, particularly in private. When asked whom they would seek for comfort and support in time of bereavement, these groups most frequently named someone in the family or a member of the clergy.[8]

Although the experience of grief is a universal phenomenon, it is important to recognize that the expression of grief is strongly influenced by cultural factors. How, when, how long, and for whom one grieves are culturally determined. For example, in matrilineal societies (societies in which lineage is traced through the women in the family), a woman may be expected to grieve for male members of her maternal family, such as fathers and brothers, but not for her spouse. Some mourning rituals are highly structured and lengthy, where others are relatively simple and short. In the Orthodox Jewish tradition, five successive stages of mourning extend for a year and include practices that influence virtually every aspect of life.[1, 6, 8]

The following discussion of cross-cultural bereavement behaviors of traditional Chinese-Americans, Puerto Ricans, and urban blacks is intended to show cross-cultural differences in bereavement. Because the minority groups delineated by the U.S. government are composed of dozens of cultures and subcul-

tures, and because individual expressions vary widely, cultural stereotypes about specific groups are seldom helpful.

Chinese-Americans

In general, Chinese-Americans tend to internalize their grief and refrain from expressing their emotions overtly. When faced with terminal illness and death, many Chinese-Americans are stoic and fatalistic. Traditional Chinese society recognizes that the family is the basic social unit and has codified family relationships in laws that govern degrees of kinship. *Wu-fu*, which means "five kinds of clothing," defines degrees of relationships and determines the severity of mourning in terms of the closeness of the deceased to the mourner.[9, 10]

Traditionally, Chinese people follow a double system of burial. The initial burial in a coffin lasts for 7 years. During the seventh year, the body is exhumed, and the remains are stored in an urn. The urn is kept for whatever period the family members desire. Reburial in an elaborate tomb marks the second burial. It is believed that following the second burial the person's ancestors are capable of exerting an influence on family affairs. These influences are usually positive and include the ability to protect descendants from disease and injury. It should be noted that many Chinese-Americans have adopted American burial customs and are unfamiliar with these traditions. When a Chinese-American client dies, it is therefore important to identify the closest relatives to determine what funeral and burial arrangements they prefer.[9, 10]

Puerto Ricans

Of the 17.4 million Spanish-speaking respondents to the latest U.S. census, 59% identified themselves as Mexican-American; 15%, Puerto Rican; 6%, Cuban; and 20%, other

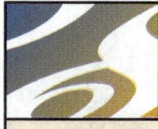

Hispanic origin. Although little is known about the specific bereavement patterns of each group, the Puerto Ricans have been studied extensively.[6, 8–10] As we look at bereavement patterns among Puerto Ricans, do not assume that all members of this group mourn in exactly this way, and do not assume that mourning will be the same for people from other Hispanic groups.

Some Puerto Ricans believe that a person's spirit will not be free to enter the next life if that person has left something unsaid before death. For this reason, it is important for family and friends to complete their relationships with a dying person. With sudden death, such closure is obviously impossible. In the case of chronic illness, however, those close to the dying person should be given the privacy necessary to accomplish this task.

Following the death, family members usually meet together to comfort one another and to pray for the dead in a *wake.* The wake provides an opportunity for mobilizing community support and for expressing grief. Although Puerto Ricans may be members of various religions, most are Roman Catholic. Religious rituals such as the anointing of the sick, Eucharistic liturgies (sometimes referred to as *masses*), and recitation of rosaries, novenas, and other prayers are intended to benefit both the deceased and the surviving family members. In North America, time restrictions for wakes are often imposed by funeral directors, but traditional Puerto Rican wakes last for several days.[9, 10]

Grief is sometimes expressed in a syndrome called *el ataque,* which is characterized by seizurelike behavior, hyperkinetic episodes, a display of aggression, and, sometimes, stupor. Such behavior is accepted and sanctioned socially in Puerto Rican culture as a way for bereaved people to displace their anger over the loss of a loved one. Although some males may display symptoms of *el ataque,* it is more common among women. *Machismo,* the cultural norm for Puerto Rican males that

encourages that feelings of suffering be kept inside, may predominate for bereaved men. White nurses sometimes erroneously construe *el ataque* and *machismo* as abnormal behaviors. However, it is important to allow family members to express grief in culturally meaningful ways without conveying judgment. Bereaved Puerto Ricans often prefer to seek support from other members of their Spanish-speaking community rather than participate in grief counseling or bereavement programs sponsored by hospice or other groups.[1]

Economic stress may add a burden to the bereaved. Many Puerto Rican families try to accompany the body of the deceased to Puerto Rico for burial. Members of the extended family, community, and church may provide financial assistance to the spouse and immediate family for the trip.[6, 9, 10]

Urban Blacks

Urban blacks are a heterogeneous group representing dozens of cultures and subcultures that originated in Africa. The way people handle the issues and challenges surrounding death usually reflects the manner in which they deal with life. There are very few new resources available to an elderly black person who faces critical illness and death. The decision-making process used to cope is likely to be patterned after responses to other stressful events throughout life.

Blacks are less likely to express grief openly and publicly than whites. Patterns of coping with death vary widely among urban blacks and are interrelated with education and socioeconomic background. One stereotype is that, when faced with a crisis, urban blacks can look after themselves and require little assistance. In reality, the urban black family is seldom capable of supporting the bereaved person. In the urban black community, a preponderance of households are headed by single women, and so it is often necessary to mobilize support from neighbors, church

members, and friends.[6, 11] Besides the cultural idiom of bereavement, older blacks may experience different modes of death or die at an earlier age than their white counterparts.[12]

1. Andrews, M. M., & Hanson, P. A. (1995). Religion, culture and nursing. In M. M. Andrews & J. S. Boyle (Eds.), *Transcultural concepts in nursing care,* (pp. 353–409). Philadelphia: J.B. Lippincott.
2. Halfe, L. B. (1989). The circle: Death and dying from a native perspective. *Journal of Palliative Care, 5*(1), 37–41.
3. Kozak, D. L. (1991). Dying badly: Violent death and religious change among the Tohono O'odham. *Omega, 23,* 207–216.
4. Huttlinger, K., Krefting, L., & Drevdahl, D. (1992). Doing battle: A metaphorical analysis of diabetes mellitus among Navajo people. *American Journal of Occupational Therapy, 46,* 706–712.
5. Chapman, A. (1991). The Buddhist way of dying. *Nursing Praxis in New Zealand, 6*(2), 23–26.
6. Kalisch, R. A., & Reynolds, D. K. (1981). *Death and ethnicity: A psychocultural study.* New York: Baywood.
7. Nagel, J. K. (1991). Unresolved grief and mourning in Navajo women. *American Indian and Alaska Native Mental Health Research, 2*(2), 32–40.
8. Ross, H. M. (1984). Societal/cultural views regarding death and dying. *Topics in Clinical Nursing, 3*(3), 1–16.
9. Eisenbruch, M. (1984). Cross-cultural aspects of bereavement: I. A conceptual framework for comparative analysis. *Culture, Medicine, and Psychiatry, 8,* 283–309.
10. Eisenbruch, M. (1984). Cross-cultural aspects of bereavement: II. Ethnic and cultural variations in the development of bereavement practices. *Culture, Medicine, and Psychiatry, 8,* 315–347.
11. Jacobs, C. F. (1990). Healing and prophecy in the black spiritual churches: A need for reexamination. *Medical Anthropology, 12*(4), 349–370.
12. U.S. Department of Health and Human Services, Public Health Service. (1992). *Healthy people 2000: Summary report.* Boston: Jones & Bartlet.

Planning: Expected Outcomes

The expected outcome for the client is decreased manifestations of spiritual distress with behaviors that may include the ability to experience forgiveness, connection to religious or cultural ties, a reaffirmation of faith or commitment to internal values, decreased feelings of guilt over past actions, or internal peace.

Nursing Intervention

Accepting others as they are, where they are—without the traditional concern for defining, controlling, and changing—permits the spirit to expand and express itself. So many people have lived a life of control, definition, and judgment, and the spirit has been driven far below the surface.[79] Nurses who have awakened their own spirituality are inclined to encourage the expression of spirit in others.

Clients in spiritual distress need the nurse to offer support through active listening, to demonstrate concern and care, and to be available and sensitive to the expressed needs.

When the nurse is asked personal questions about beliefs, she or he should attempt to give thoughtful answers and to provide an environment for the client's self-exploration and self-expression. The nurse should not force her or his religious values onto the client. The nurse healer is like a tuning fork through which the client can begin to resonate with the consciousness of the universe.[63] Entering a client's room or walking through his or her front door, being open and available, without definitions and judgments, is sometimes just what is needed to assist another within the spiritual domain.

Evaluation

Several approaches can be taken to evaluate the effectiveness of interventions for spiritual distress. These include (1) the relief-of-symptoms approach and (2) the values clarification approach.

Relief-of-Symptoms Approach

Is there a change in the client's verbalization, attitude, or both? Have the manifestations such as anger, guilt, depression, anxiety, and crying changed? If so, consider that the client may be progressing through the stages of grief and loss.

Values Clarification Approach

With use of values clarification tools, nurses can help clients identify their values. From these expressed values, short- and long-term goals consistent with the client's values and beliefs are formulated. From these written goals, then, the nurse and the client can determine if goals were met and can reformulate new goals.

Grief

Common areas for nursing intervention are helping clients and families through grief and with suffering. We will examine these dimensions of psychosocial nursing in detail.

Grief is one of the most common human responses. It can be initiated by many things; death and illness are the most common. However, any loss, even the loss of a dream or life plan, can initiate a grief response. Consider the woman who has a miscarriage; not only has she lost the child but she has also the dreams she had harbored, perhaps since her own childhood, for her child. Other losses of life plans may occur with forced or medically necessary retirement, institutionalization, divorce, or loss of a job.

Grief can be seen in clients, families, and even in other healthcare providers in many clinical settings. Grief occurs in all ages and across all cultures. Whether it is offering support to a woman with a new diagnosis of breast cancer, caring for a client who is dying of AIDS, or helping a client after an amputation, nurses are frequently faced with the task of recognizing grief as well as providing appropriate interventions.

Grief engenders many emotional reactions, which are generally influenced by cultural background, socialization, and family structure. In 1969, Kubler-Ross[36] was one of the first to write about the process of dying and, thereby, the process of grief. Her landmark work opened the doors for much improved understanding of the process of dying and much improved care of the dying person and the family. Kubler-Ross described five stages that all persons go through during the process of dying: (1) denial and isolation, (2) anger, (3) bargaining, (4) depression, and (5) acceptance. Other reactions may occur, however, such as fear, hostility, and retreat. Each of these responses should be recognized by the nurse as the client's attempt at coping and as part of the grief response.

A more contemporary concept of grief focuses on the fact that this process is not composed of a rigid set of stages with a predictable pattern of responses; the grief process is dynamic. The nurse cannot say, "Well, if Mr. Thompson is in denial today, by tomorrow he will be angry." The grief process is not that predictable. Some of the stages may be internal and may not be visible to the nurse. Other stages may never appear. Still other clients may clearly go back and forth between one stage and another.

A recent description of the grieving process recognizes some different aspects from those identified by Kubler-Ross. It is apparent that not only is grief dynamic but also that it is individualized, pervasive, and normative. Every client does not have the same grief response when faced with the same medical condition. Many factors have an impact on grief, such as the nature of the loss, the relationship of the grieving person to the individual or object lost, and the presence of support systems.

Grief is also pervasive, affecting every aspect of the client's existence. Reported responses to grieving include physical (alterations in heart rate and blood pressure, crying, and gastrointestinal disturbances), social (withdrawal from social groups and difficulty forming new relationships), cognitive (preoccupation with thoughts of the lost object or person, thoughts of personal mortality, and inability to concentrate), affective (depression, sleeplessness), behavioral (inability to carry out daily activities), and spiritual (questioning religious beliefs or faith and questions about an afterlife).

Finally, grief has been described as normal. Despite the great variations in the grief response, grief is an expected response to loss. What constitutes a normal length of time for the grieving process is another question. Many years ago, a widow was expected to be in mourning for a year, and to wear black during that time. Grieving has time limits, beyond which it becomes inappropriate or unacceptable. The boundaries of this period are dictated by culture and socialization. Grief that goes on after this acceptable period of time is called *unresolved grief*.

Stages of Grief

Four stages of the process of grief have been described:

1. Shock and numbness
2. Searching and yearning
3. Disorientation and disorganization
4. Resolution and reorganization.

Shock and numbness may leave one feeling as though time has stopped and an engulfing fog or cloud has descended. During this time, the griever may forget things, feel confused, or have a difficult time making decisions.

The stage of searching and yearning usually follows the initial period of shock. During this time, anger is usually present. The anger may be directed toward others or even toward the one who is lost. In many instances, guilt surfaces. The mourner can become convinced that if things had been done differently, the tragedy might have been averted. Feeling guilty is one way of grappling with the question "Why?" The search for answers may help resolve the feelings of guilt.

Other feelings occurring during the second stage include difficulty concentrating, physical symptoms, or feelings of emptiness and exhaustion. Sometimes, people even feel as though they are losing their minds because they cannot concentrate on anything. This stage may last for months and requires the sensitivity of a nurse who understands the grieving process.

The third stage involves disorientation and disorganization. This time is marked with more difficulties in concentration or with difficulty in starting or continuing routine projects. Physical problems may appear as a result of sublimated emotions.

In time, energy levels increase and the ability to make decisions returns. The body and mind prepare to move forward toward the fourth stage: resolution and reorganization. This period is easier if there are others to encourage and support the griever. This is why support groups are so valuable. When the griever joins a support group, he or she meets others who have gone through similar circumstances and have the strength to help newcomers.

Suffering

Suffering is submitting to or being forced to submit to and endure a particular set of circumstances not under one's control. Suffering may be physical, psychological, spiritual, or social. It is in response to suffering that many, perhaps all, of us define ourselves, take on character, and develop an ethos (a guiding belief system). To the person involved, though, suffering seems to be pointless.

To see the value of suffering we only have to ask, "How would people behave if they did not have the capacity to suffer?" Such people could not bear grief, loss, or misfortune and, in effect, would give up much of the measure of their humanness. Our capacity to feel grief and to identify with the misfortune of others is the basis for our ability to recognize, empathize with, and care for our fellow human beings.

It is important to be careful about how we conceptualize suffering. It is seldom a means for character building, but is rather a test for character already built. Our reactions to suffering may reveal us as better or worse than we had thought ourselves to be. Suffering can just as easily destroy a person's ego structure as it can make a person more resolute. In that respect, it is useful to reflect on our reaction to someone else's suffering. Suffering has the potential to make another person a stranger. To the uninitiated, the first response may be repulsion. Suffering makes people's otherness stand out in strong relief, but that otherness is exactly the condition necessary to force recognition of them and of ourselves. It is the obligation of those who care for suffering people to know how to minister to them in such a way as to include rather than exclude them from the human condition. One of our challenges as nurses is to bind the suffering and the nonsuffering into the same community. Our role is not to eliminate suffering and death but to soothe unnecessary suffering and untimely death.

Sexuality

The final section in our discussion of psychosocial components of healthcare is human sexuality. This area of humanness is an area of mystery to some and an area of controversy to others. Again, the nurse accepts and respects the client's views of himself or herself.

Concepts of Sexuality

Sexuality is an intrinsic part of being human. Sexuality has been variously described as the quality of being human,[32] the most intimate feelings of the human heart,[10] the totality of the human being,[42] and the ongoing process of recognizing, accepting, and expressing oneself as a sexual being.[82] Therefore, the term *sexuality* represents a much broader concept than the word *sex*, which, in one of its meanings, represents the physiologic act of sexual intercourse. Sexuality is a deep pervasive aspect of the total human personality and is present in some degree from birth to death.[32]

Psychological Elements of Sexuality

Gender Identity

Gender identity is the individual's sense of being male or female, and describes one's internal sense of masculinity or femininity. Gender is a part of a person's identity. Society has a substantial role in the development of gender identity. As soon as an infant is born, he or she is labeled as a boy or girl and given gender-related toys and colors of clothing. Adults respond differently to female and male children depending on their own upbringing and personal parenting style. For example, it would be nontraditional for girls to be given trucks and cars to play with. Likewise, it would be nontraditional for boys to have lace trimming on their jeans.

As children grow, they encompass the information from society and their own knowledge of their bodies to develop their own sense of gender identity. By the age of 3 years, children have a concept of themselves as boys or girls. They also know that they cannot change their sex by changing their outward appearance with clothing or make-up.

Gender Role

Gender role is the public expression of gender identity. Most social theorists believe that social influence (parents, peers, media) is the major developmental force in teaching or shaping gender roles. Gender roles are learned in school and at home. Formal learning typically includes specific information about sexual organs, changes in the body with puberty, and the need to delay sexual intercourse until "one is old enough to be in love." The most influential learning comes from the sexual value system of the family and community. Children acquire these attitudes at an early age. Often, the pattern involves repression and avoidance of sexual topics, and sexuality may be perceived as a negative experience. Another influential source of learning includes the gestures, cues, and discussions that take place within the peer group.

All gender role behavior cannot be fully attributed to society, however, since a difference is seen in the behavior of boys and girls, even at an early age. It has been suggested that the sex hormones have an influence on the brain, which also influences behavior.[11] Gender role is one area of sexuality that overlaps to include psychological, biologic, and sociocultural components.

Sexual Orientation

Sexual orientation is the preference for intimate relationships with a person of the opposite sex or the same sex. The vast majority of adults identify themselves as heterosexual (i.e., having a clear, sustained, and erotic desire for a person of the opposite sex). About 10% of adults define themselves as homosexual (i.e., having a clear, sustained, and erotic desire for a person of the same sex). Men who

desire intimate relationships with men are called *homosexuals*, or *gay*, and women who desire intimate relationships with women are called *lesbians*.

A very small number of people are bisexual (i.e., they prefer intimate relationships with both sexes). Transsexual people (transvestites) are dissatisfied with their physical body because it does not match their feelings of gender identity. They often feel that they are really trapped in the wrong body.

Over the years, society has intermingled homosexuality and transvestism; however, they are not the same phenomenon. It is a common misconception that lesbians are women who want to be men, and homosexuals are men who want to be women. Some homosexual men do have effeminate behavior, and some lesbians have masculine behavior. But most homosexual men and lesbian women are satisfied with their male or female gender.

Sociocultural Elements of Sexuality

Sociocultural components reflect the beliefs of a culture or society. These beliefs shape the development of a person as a sexual being. Social interaction is important to this process because role behaviors are modeled and social expectations learned. Religious and legal systems attempt to control or prescribe sexuality.[31] Sociocultural components also influence male and female sexuality and gender role behavior.

Male and Female Roles

Culture influences gender roles. Some cultures have clear distinctions of the appropriate roles for males and females. For example, the male role may be one of providing money to support the family (breadwinner) and the female role may be one of rearing children and caring for the household. Other cultures do not hold such sharp distinctions.

The feminist movement of the 1970s has changed many gender role behaviors in North America. It is now more common for women to work outside the home, and it is becoming more acceptable for men to stay home to care for children. However, this role reversal is not without conflict. Many women and men have a difficult time switching roles. Women report feelings of overwork when trying to balance home, family, and work responsibilities. Likewise, some men appreciate having social approval to be more involved with child care; others resent the extra demands.

Feminism is a belief pattern about the role of women that challenges the conventional ideas about gender. Feminism is not a new concept that began in the 1980s; the ideas of feminism have been expressed for more than 300 years.[78] Regardless of the time frame in which feminist thought was established, it has consistently turned the spotlight on a complex system of inequality for women in present society. Areas that have been explored include disadvantages in the workplace, including reduced pay for equal job responsibility; corporate "glass ceilings," which have prevented women from being promoted to the top levels of management; exploitation as housewives and brutality as sexual objects; exclusion from political life; discrimination in areas such as religion, education, and athletics; and general silence in history about the accomplishments of women.[51, 78] Feminists have pushed society to obliterate sexism by legalizing changes to equalize economic disadvantages and to produce equal political and educational opportunities.

Sexual Practices

Societal attitudes about sexual practices range from the nontraditional view of sex, which holds that each person must make an individual choice of appropriate behavior, to a traditional view, which holds that sex must occur only after marriage. The risk of acquiring a sexually transmitted disease or becoming pregnant, as well as religious beliefs, may also influence a person's decisions about sexual practices. When a person acts outside of the socially prescribed behaviors by having sex, and acquires a sexually transmitted disease or becomes pregnant, much guilt and internal conflict over the behavior often result. Nurses may frequently work with these clients; they need to be able to put aside personal views and beliefs to assist the client. If the nurse has religious beliefs that prohibit involvement with certain clients, such as assisting in surgery during an abortion, the nurse should make these personal issues known to the nursing administrator.

Because gender identity, gender behavior, and sexuality norms differ from culture to culture and have changed over the years, it must be understood that the norms themselves are not what is important. It is more critical that the norms are understood and accepted by the persons in that culture or society. It is equally important that healthcare professionals work within the social norms and help clients without judging them against personal norms.

The Nurse's Role in Promoting Sexual Health

The World Health Organization (WHO) developed the following definition of sexual health: "Sexual health is the integration of the somatic, emotional, intellectual, and social aspects of sexual beings in ways that are positively enriching and that enhance personality, communication, and love."[71] In other words, sexual health is the physical and emotional state of well-being that enables us to enjoy and act on sexual feelings. These definitions provide a basis for delivery of nursing care.

Nurses care for the whole person as they assess and treat human responses to actual and potential health problems. Because sexuality is a quality of being human, the sexual aspects of clients should be addressed. Nurses who are knowledgeable about and comfortable with the topic of sexuality and comfortable with their own sexuality have the opportunity to promote sexual health. All nurses can integrate sexuality into client care by focusing on preventive, therapeutic, and educational interventions that help attain and maintain sexual health.

The following four areas of competence are required of a nurse to promote sexual health:

● Knowledge of subject matter related to sexuality
● Skill in assessing and intervening with the client and family
● Personal awareness of beliefs, attitudes, and values
● Awareness of how personal beliefs, attitudes, and values affect delivery of care to clients.[42]

Competence in these four areas involves three levels of learning. First, the nurse must overcome any sexual embarrassment, which can be done by talking with other nurses, taking human sexuality courses, or through values clarification exercises.[31] Second, the nurse must be able to identify and understand sexuality problems. Third, the nurse must be able to assist clients in dealing with sexual problems.

Because the subject of sexuality is complex, basic knowledge about human relationships, sexual development, reproduction, sexual expression, sexual dysfunction and disease, and sociocultural aspects of sex, marriage, and the family is needed.[42] Knowledge of moral, legal, and religious issues related to sexuality is also important. Table 4–1 provides a concise description of changes in sexuality with aging.

Assessment Skills

To assess and intervene, the nurse must be able to discuss sexuality in a candid, unembarrassed, unbiased manner, using effective communication skills and creating a nonthreatening environment. Skill in the techniques of questioning, clarification, and validation is necessary so that the nurse can accurately determine what the client is verbalizing, symbolizing, expressing, and feeling about sexuality.

A brief sexual history can be incorporated into a total health history. Woods suggested three questions that aid the nurse in gathering information about the client's sexual roles, views of the self as a sexual being, and sexual functioning:

● Has anything, such as illness, pregnancy, or surgery, interfered with your being a mother/wife/father/husband?
● Has anything, such as illness, medical treatment, or surgery, changed the way you feel about yourself as a man/woman?
● Has anything, such as surgery, medication, or disease, altered your ability to function sexually?

Additional questions may be asked about premarital sexual activity, current sexual activity, frequency of sexual intercourse, contraceptive practices, fertility, past or present genital infections, or the presence of pain with intercourse. Questions for men should focus on the ability to maintain an erection, ejaculatory control, and problems with the urinary system. For women, additional questions might relate to arousal and the ability to reach orgasm, menstrual history, obstetric history, or menopause if the client is beyond childbearing years. The nurse may con-

Table 4–1. Changes in Sexuality with Aging

	Men	Women
Middle-aged adult	Prolonged erection Decreased premature ejaculation Greater emphasis on touch Fertility intact Sexual arousal may diminish, usually due to stress or illness Some men develop increased prostatic size	Cessation of menses, fertility varies Thinning of vaginal mucosa Sexual arousal peaks due to effects of androgens May be a fear of pregnancy
Older adult	Decrease in size of penis and testes Increased refractory time after orgasm Decreased penile sensation Decreased force of ejaculation Slowed arousal Fertility varies Interferences due to the side effects of medications and illness	Loss of vaginal lubrication, decreased fat pad over the symphysis pubis, and friable mucosa due to loss of estrogen Infertile Interferences due to the side effects of medications and illness

clude the interview by asking whether the client has any questions or problems to discuss with the nurse.

Intervention Skills

Once the problem is identified, the nurse must be able to offer the client help in an understanding, reassuring manner. The nurse creates an environment that supports sexual health by minimizing guilt and anxiety. Interventions may take the form of sex education, anticipatory guidance, or counseling. The intervention may involve initiating a referral for the client with a complex problem, offering suggestions for the problem, or simply listening to the client and offering reassurance. The nurse's goal is to facilitate the client's sexual adaptation to enhance or maintain health. Specific interventions that relate to specific disorders, such as mutilating surgery, cancer, and neurologic and musculoskeletal problems, are discussed in other chapters.

Annon developed the PLISSIT Model for Sexual Health Interventions.[2] The model is based on principles of learning theory and uses a behavioral approach to treatment of sexual problems. The model consists of the following four levels:

1. *P*ermission. Provides reassurance that sexual feelings are normal. Permission to continue what he or she has been feeling.
2. *L*imited *I*nformation. Limited information is given to avoid overwhelming the client and to allow the client to ask questions. The nurse acknowledges concerns that are common experiences.
3. *S*pecific *S*uggestions. Suggestions are offered that may change or add to sexual approaches used by client.
4. *I*ntensive *T*herapy. The client is referred to appropriate specific therapy from trained professionals.

At times, friends and family members withdraw emotionally from the client. For example, a woman may withdraw from a husband who has had a stroke, because she is not able to accept his paralysis or aphasia. Actually, she often is expressing deeper feelings. Perhaps she is angry that she has to assume all of his former responsibilities in the home, such as paying bills. Or his illness may remind her of the loss she would feel if he died, so she feels safer not getting close. The husband realizes his wife's reactions; he, in turn, internalizes a negative self-image. The nurse encourages the client and spouse to discuss these feelings with the team of healthcare providers or with each other.

Coping with outward effects of cancer treatment, such as alopecia (hair loss), weight loss, and loss of muscle mass during chemotherapy, may require some disguise. Wigs can cover hair loss, and wearing clothes that fit well may disguise weight loss. Infusion catheters can be hidden by clothing with high necks or long sleeves.

The nurse encourages the client to resume sexual activity slowly and not to feel rushed to perform. Many clients plan for sexual intercourse at certain times of the day, when their energy level is higher. For example, the client with lung disorders may have more energy in the late morning. If one client is weak or in pain, variations in the position for intercourse are suggested. Some clients may be unable to have physical intercourse, but experience pleasure from caressing.

The nurse advises the clients in the treatment of specific concerns. Women may need to use vaginal lubrication to reduce pain with intercourse. Condoms or spermicides can be used to reduce the risk of sexually transmitted disease. Men may have difficulty obtaining an erection or forceful orgasm. Various devices exist to facilitate erection. External pneumatic pumps are available that draw blood into the penile shaft for erection. Implantation of a penile prosthesis for erection is another treatment for impotence in men. Feelings of weakened orgasm are common, for which there is no specific treatment.

Personal Awareness of Beliefs, Attitudes, and Values

A nurse's beliefs, attitudes, and values may affect the way a nurse delivers care. Certainly, the nurse is entitled to these beliefs, values, and attitudes, but the nurse must be aware of what they are and remain objective when providing care that involves any aspect of the client's sexuality.

Assessment of personal attitudes toward sexuality involves deciding whether the attitudes are positive or negative. Self-examination may be necessary to determine the root of negative attitudes and beliefs. If negative attitudes cannot be overcome or if a nurse is uncomfortable in discussing sexuality, other nurses should be asked to care for the client so that the negative attitudes are not communicated.

Some of the topics that should be considered when evaluating feelings, attitudes, beliefs, and values include reproduction, masturbation, dating, sexual activity (e.g., petting and kissing), sexual intercourse in marriage, sexual intercourse outside of marriage, childbearing, contraception, sterilization, abortion, sexually transmitted diseases, homosexuality, bisexuality, transsexuality, and transvestism. Not only should you try to identify the feelings, but you should try to understand their origins. No right or wrong answers exist when it comes to these topics. However, it is important that the nurse be very familiar with personal values, beliefs, and attitudes so that their effect on practice can be determined.

Effects of Beliefs, Attitudes, and Values on Delivery of Care

Once beliefs and attitudes are assessed, it is important for the nurse to determine how they might affect the delivery of nursing care. For instance, do the attitudes and beliefs deny, inhibit, or allow for the sexuality of the client? Becoming open, nonjudgmental, and accepting of others' sexuality and developing comfort in interviewing in the area of sexuality may be a difficult task for the nurse. The nurse should not attempt to help another person with sexual problems until comfort with acceptance of others' sexuality and interviewing skills is accomplished.

Illness and Sexuality

Perhaps most clients and many healthcare professionals do not think about sexual activity occurring following surgery or illness. In fact, the mass media commonly portray sex as an act between two healthy young adults, not in people who have been injured or are debilitated. This portrayal has influenced many healthcare providers not to think about sexuality as a component of the whole being. Sadly, it is often ignored in planning care.

If the client is wondering whether sexual activity would interfere with treatments or be permissible after surgery, the client should ask the physician. Unfortunately, many clients are uncomfortable with such questions, and do not ask. Likewise, many healthcare professionals do not view seriously ill clients as sexual people and fail to teach the client about sexual guidelines.

Sexuality and Chronic Conditions

The client with a chronic illness that interferes with oxygenation, such as pulmonary or cardiac disorders, may not have the physical stamina to have intercourse. These clients may find intercourse possible if they plan it around periods of increased energy, such as in the middle of the day. Medications such as nitroglycerin prior to intercourse may decrease the fear of angina. Following myocardial infarction, many clients have concerns about sexual intercourse. Fear of dying during sex is common. The nurse should facilitate discussion of concerns with the client, even if the nurse has to initiate the conversation.

Diabetes and other vascular disorders interfere with blood supply to the genitals, and may reduce erection and orgasm. Clients with these conditions may benefit from surgery to restore the erectile tissues (see Chapter 83). If surgery is not feasible, the client may find satisfaction through touch and caressing.

Spinal cord injury results in the lack of sensation and inability to have an erection in men. Some clients can be taught methods to enjoy physical intercourse (see Chapter 35). There are others who are overwhelmed by the injury and psychologically do not feel whole enough to participate. These clients and their partners may benefit from counseling.

In clients with musculoskeletal disorders, such as arthritis, contracture may be too extensive or pain may be too great to assume positions to facilitate intercourse. These clients can often be helped by experimenting with new positions.

Clients with cancer may feel alterations in their sexuality from alopecia, loss of body mass, loss of energy, nausea and vomiting, or pain. Young clients may not be able to have a child as a result of surgery, chemotherapy, or radiation therapy. These clients should be advised about the possibility of sperm or egg banking to preserve their procreative functions.

For most clients with cancer, sexual activity is not dangerous to health. In a few situations, however, sex can be hazardous. During recovery from surgery, sexual intercourse can strain an incision or cause bleeding. Intimate contact may also increase the risk of contracting infection, especially in clients who are being treated with radiation and chemotherapy, which suppress the immune system.

Sexuality and Surgery

Some surgical interventions may have a profound impact on the client's sexuality. Surgery to remove organs related to sexual intercourse or reproduction, such as the uterus, ovaries, external genitalia, penis, testes, or breasts, may leave the client feeling asexual. Also, extensive lower abdominal surgery and surgery on the pelvic floor in men decrease erectile function and ejaculation. Prostate surgery for cancer also decreases erectile function. Newer surgical techniques are being developed that spare nerves and allow partial or complete erection. Clients need assistance to build a new self-image that does not include these body parts. This process takes months to years to develop. Sometimes, reconstructive surgery can assist to restore form and function, such as breast reconstruction (see Chapter 80). Surgery that alters the physical appearance of other body parts not so clearly associated with reproduction can also have an impact on feelings of sexuality. Surgical removal of the bowel or bladder with the creation of a new external opening on the abdominal skin commonly has an impact on sexuality.

Sexuality and Hospitalization

Anyone who has ever been hospitalized can appreciate a client's sense of loss of control in this situation. Equal to this loss is often a loss of the sense of wholeness, of which sexuality is a part. Consider the 90-year-old woman who has never married and now is hospitalized. When she was young, skirts were ankle length. Perhaps she joined the ranks of "promiscuous" women in the 1920s who showed their lower legs and knees in public! She is asked to submit to a physical examination, a bath, being only partly dressed, and perhaps being catheterized. Nurses take these activities for granted, yet this woman has never revealed her body to anyone. Although this type of client is not common, her case best exemplifies the asexual treatment that many clients receive. Nurses need to be aware of a client's need for privacy and control of his or her body.

On the contrary, some clients act out their sexual frustrations by using gestures, and obscene language or by pinching or touching the staff. This behavior can occur for many reasons. Perhaps the client is confused, has lost a sense of control, feels asexual, feels a need for attention, or needs to test established limits. The nurse needs to be firm with the client and to tell the client that the behavior is not acceptable. Psychiatric treatment may be required.

Conclusions

Psychosocial aspects of healthcare address those aspects of humanness, family structure, culture, spirituality, and sexuality that a client brings with him or her into the hospital or healthcare setting. The nurse must respect the client's beliefs and practices and take them into account when planning and providing teaching and other interventions.

Bibliography

1. American Holistic Nurses' Association. (1986). *Standards for holistic nursing care*. Raleigh, NC: Author.

2. Annon, J. S. (1976). The PLISSIT model: A proposed conceptual scheme for the behavioral treatment of sexual problems. *Journal of Sex Education Therapy, 2*, 1–15.

3. Boyle, J., & Andrews, M. (1989). *Transcultural concepts in nursing care*. Glenview, IL: Scott Foresman.

4. Branch, M., & Paxton, P. (1976). *Providing safe nursing care for ethnic people of color*. Englewood Cliffs, NJ: Prentice-Hall.

5. Brink, P. (1984). Value orientations as an assessment tool in cultural diversity. *Nursing Research, 35*, 198.

6. Bullough, B., & Bullough, V. (1990). *Nursing in the community*. St. Louis: Mosby–Year Book.

7. Carpenito, L. (1995). *Nursing diagnoses: Application to clinical practice* (6th. ed.). Philadelphia: J. B. Lippincott.

8. Carson, V. (1989). *Spiritual dimensions of nursing practice*. Philadelphia: W. B. Saunders.

9. Carter, B., & McGoldrick, M. (1989). *The changing family life cycle: A framework for family therapy* (2nd ed.). Boston: Allyn and Bacon.

10. Chenitz, W. C., et al. (1991). *Clinical gerontological nursing*. Philadelphia: W. B. Saunders.

11. Clemen-Stone, S., et al. (1991). *Comprehensive family and community health nursing* (3rd ed.). St. Louis: Mosby-Year Book.

12. Comos-Dias, L., & Griffith, E. (1988). *Clinical guidelines in cross-cultural mental health*. New York: John Wiley & Sons.

13. Copp, L. (1990). The spectrum of suffering. *American Journal of Nursing, 90*(8), 35–39.

14. Cowles, K., & Rodgers, B. (1991). The concept of grief: A foundation for nursing research and practice. *Research in Nursing and Health, 14*(2), 119–127.

15. Dennis, P. (1991). Components of spiritual nursing care from the nurses' perspective. *Journal of Holistic Nursing, 9*(1), 27–42.

16. DeSantis, L. (1988). The relevance of transcultural nursing to international nursing. *International Nursing Review, 35*, 110.

17. Dossey, B. (1991). Awaking the inner healer. *American Journal of Nursing, 91*(8), 31–33.

18. Dossey, B. (1989). Foreword. *Journal of Holistic Nursing, 3*(3), vii.

19. Dossey, L. (1990). *Recovering the soul*. New York: Bantam.

20. Douglas, M., & Mobius, A. (1985). International nursing: Challenges and consequences. *Mobius 5*, 84.

21. Ferszt, G., & Taylor, P. (1988). When your patient needs spiritual comfort. *Nursing '88, 18*(4), 48–49.

22. Fife, B. (1985). A model for predicting the adaptation of families to medical crises: An analysis of role integration. *IMAGE: The Journal of Nursing Scholarship, 18*(4), 108–112.

23. Fogel, C., & Lauver, D. (1990). *Sexual health promotion*. Philadelphia: W. B. Saunders.

24. Fonesca, J. D. (1970). Sexuality: A quality of being human. *Nursing Outlook, 18*(11), 25.

25. Fong, C. (1985). Ethnicity and nursing practice. *Topics in Clinical Nursing, 7*(3), 1–10.

26. Friedman, M. (1992). *Family nursing: Theory and assessment* (3rd ed.). Norwalk, CT: Appleton-Century-Crofts.

27. Gillis, C., et al. (1990). *Toward a science of family nursing*. Menlo Park, CA: Addison-Wesley.

28. Glittenberg, J. (1990). Global network of World Health Organization collaborating centers for nursing. *Journal of Professional Nursing, 6*(3), 137.

29. Good, C. (1987). *Ethnomedical systems in Africa*. New York: Guilford Publishers.

30. Groer, M. (1991). Psychoneuroimmunology. *American Journal of Nursing, 91*(8), 33.

31. Herth, K. (1989). The root of it all. *Journal of Gerontological Nursing, 15*(12), 32–73.

32. Ho, M. (1987). *Family therapy with ethnic minorities*. Beverly Hills, CA: Sage Publishers.

33. Jowett, B. (1937). Charmides. In *The dialogue of Plato*. New York: Random House.

34. Keegan, G., & Keegan, L. (1987). Spirituality and the technological crisis. *Healing Currents, 11*(2).

35. Kennison, M. M. (1987). Faith: An untapped health resource. *Journal of Psychosocial Nursing, 25*(10), 28–33.

36. Kubler-Ross, E. (1969). *On death and dying*. New York: Macmillan, Inc.

37. L'Abate, L., Ganahl, G., & Hansen, J. (1986). *Methods of family therapy*. Englewood Cliffs, NJ: Prentice-Hall.

38. LaFargue, J. (1985). Mediating between two views of illness. *Topics in Clinical Nursing, 7*(3), 70–77.

39. Lengermann, P., & Wallace, R. (1985). *Gender in America: Social control and social change.* Englewood Cliffs, NJ: Prentice-Hall.

40. Leininger, M. (1991). Transcultural nursing: The study and practice field. *Imprint, 38*(2), 55–66.

41. Leininger, M. (1988). Leininger's theory of nursing: Cultural care, diversity and universality. *Nursing Science Quarterly, 1*(4), 152–160.

42. Leininger, M. (1970). *Nursing and anthropology: Two worlds to blend.* New York: John Wiley & Sons.

43. Leininger, M. (1978). *Transcultural nursing: Concepts, theories and practices.* New York: John Wiley & Sons.

44. Levine, R., & Campbell, D. (1972). *Ethnocentrism: Theories of conflict, ethnic attitudes, and group behavior.* New York: John Wiley & Sons.

45. Lipson, J., & Melies, A. (1985). Culturally appropriate care: The case of immigrants. *Topics in Clinical Nursing, 7*(3), 48–56.

46. Louie, K. (1985). Transcending cultural bias: The literature speaks. *Topics in Clinical Nursing, 7*(3), 78–84.

47. Malone, R. (1990). The challenge of third world nursing. *American Journal of Nursing, 90*(7), 32–37.

48. Mason, D. J., Backer, B., & Georges, C. A. (1991). Toward a feminist model for the political empowerment of nurses. *IMAGE: The Journal of Nursing Scholarship, 23*(2), 72–77.

49. Nagai-Jacobson, M., & Burkhardt, M. (1989). Spirituality: Cornerstone of holistic nursing practice. *Holistic Nursing Practice, 3*(3), 18–26.

50. Newman, M. (1989). The spirit of nursing. *Holistic Nursing Practice, 3*(3), 6.

51. Norbeck, E., & Lock, M. (1987). *Health, illness and medical care in Japan.* Honolulu: University of Hawaii Press.

52. North American Nursing Diagnosis Association. (1989). *Taxonomy I revised—1989.* St. Louis: North American Nursing Diagnosis Association.

53. Orque, M., et al. (1983). *Ethnic nursing care: A multicultural approach.* St. Louis: C. V. Mosby.

54. Peel, R. (1987). *Spiritual healing in a scientific age.* San Francisco: Harper & Row.

55. Peterson, E., & Nelson, K. (1987). How to meet your client's spiritual need. *Journal of Psychosocial Nursing, 25*(5), 34–39.

56. Rankin, S., & Weeks, D. (1989). Life-span development: A review of theory and practice for families with chronically ill members. *Scholarly Inquiry for Nursing Practice: An International Journal, 3*(1), 3–22.

57. Reed, P. G. (1986). Religiousness among terminally ill and healthy adults. *Research in Nursing and Health, 9*, 35–42.

58. Reed, P. G. (1987). Spirituality and well-being in terminally ill and hospitalized adults. *Research in Nursing and Health, 10*, 335–344.

59. Rogers, M. (1970). *An introduction to the theoretical basis of nursing.* Philadelphia: F. A. Davis.

60. Rothenburger, R. (1990). Transcultural nursing. *AORN Journal, 51*(5), 1349–1363.

61. Salmon, M. (1988). Health for all: A transnational model for nursing. *International Nursing Review, 35*, 107.

62. Sampselle, C. (1990). The influence of feminist philosophy on nursing practice. *IMAGE: The Journal of Nursing Scholarship, 22*(4), 243–247.

63. Schunior, C. (1989). Nursing and the comic mask. *Holistic Nursing Practice, 3*(3), 16.

64. Shaffer, J. (1991) Spiritual distress and critical illness. *Critical Care Nurse, 11*(1), 42–45.

65. Shippee, R. (1979). *Touching and pleasuring behaviors in a well elderly population.* Master's thesis, University of Rochester, Rochester, NY.

66. Spradley, B. (1990). *Community health nursing: Concepts and practice* (3rd ed.). Glenview, IL: Scott Foresman/Little, Brown Higher Education.

67. Spradley, B. (1991). *Readings in community health nursing* (4th ed.). Philadelphia: J. B. Lippincott.

68. U.S. Bureau of the Census, Current Population Reports, Series P-25, No. 1018. (1989). *Projections of the population of the United States, by age, sex, and race: 1988–2080.* Washington, DC: U.S. Government Printing Office.

69. U.S. Bureau of the Census, Statistical abstract of the United States. (1990). *The national data book* (110th ed.). Washington, DC: U.S. Department of Commerce, Bureau of the Census.

70. Watson, M. J. (1988). New dimensions of human caring theory. *Nursing Science Quarterly, 1*(4), 175–181.

71. World Health Organization. (1975). *Education and treatment in human sexuality: The training of health professionals* (Report of a WHO meeting, Technical Report Series, No. 572) .

72. World Health Organization. (1976). *African traditional medicine.* Brazzaville, Congo Republic: World Health Organization.

73. Wright, L., & Leahy, M. (1984). *Nurses and families: A guide to family assessment and interventions.* Philadelphia: F. A. Davis.

Aging

Beverley E. Holland
Cynthia McCurren

Why is a separate chapter on late adulthood included in this textbook of medical-surgical nursing? The phenomenon of the aging of the U.S. population and related issues provide the answer. According to the U.S. Bureau of the Census,[69] 31 million Americans were age 65 years and older in 1991. This number will increase to approximately 33.5 million by 2005. The elderly are currently the fastest growing population segment in the country. Among all hospital admissions in the United States, nearly 60% involve individuals over age 65. Concern for rapidly increasing aging populations is an international dilemma as well.

The aging of America has profound implications for nursing practice in all settings, including acute care, community settings, and long-term care facilities.[54] Nurse experts on aging agree that nurses need much information to provide appropriate care to elders. Nurses involved in caring for the elderly must be aware of the unique physical, psychosocial, legal, ethical, and economic issues surrounding the aging process. An understanding of the resources available for elders at the federal, state, and local level is also essential.

Nurses must understand the normal aging process and be prepared to care for elderly clients with chronic disorders and with complex acute conditions. Normal aging causes many changes in the structure and function of the various organ systems. Pathologic processes frequently present and progress differently in the elderly person, often necessitating unique adaptations of planned interventions. A specific focus on aging needs to be evident in all nursing curricula. Selected effects of aging as they relate to assessment, disease presentation, and nursing interventions are presented throughout this book in discussions of the different body systems and their disorders. This chapter examines late adulthood and the implications for nursing practice from a holistic perspective. The focus is on important issues associated with the well-being of elders. Throughout this text information can be found on assessment and care plan modifications for specific health problems in the elderly.

Nursing and the Study of Aging

Patrick[56] provided a discussion of two terms often used in the study of aging: *geriatrics* and *gerontology*. Geriatrics comes from the Greek words *gēras* (old age) and *iatrike* (medical), and is the branch of medicine concerned with medical problems and care of elderly people. Geriatrics does not pertain just to the practice of medicine but is included in all healthcare disciplines. All professionals who care for elders should be familiar with the illnesses that affect them. Therefore, nurses, physicians, dentists, physical therapists, and other members of the healthcare team are all practitioners of geriatrics. Gerontology, in contrast, takes a broader perspective. It is the scientific study of the process and problems of aging. It focuses on the biologic, sociologic, and psychological aspects of normal aging.

Ebersole and Hess[21] have explained the study of aging within the discipline of nursing. They assert that geriatric nursing occurs primarily with the ill elderly in a medical setting. For these authors, a more acceptable role definition is the term "gerontic nursing," defined as the specialized nursing care of elderly persons that occurs in any setting in which nurses use their knowledge, expertise, and caring abilities to promote optimal functioning among elders. Inherent in the gerontic nursing concept is a comprehensive understanding of aging within a holistic perspective. This includes more than the medical or scientific approach and encompasses nursing's concept of the spiritual biopsychosocial person.

In 1973, the American Nurses' Association (ANA) identified standards for care of older adults. These were revised in 1976 and 1987 and defined as standards of gerontological nursing practice. *Gerontological nursing* is the term used by the ANA for nurses specializing in the care of older adults. Included in these standards are practice guidelines related to health promotion, health maintenance, disease prevention, and self-care, with a goal of restoring/maintaining optimal physical, psychological, and social functioning. In addition, organizational standards regarding nursing service, research, ethics, and professional development are included as they relate to care of elders. The *Standards of Gerontological Nursing Practice*[2] define what gerontological nurses can do and outlines their unique contributions. The standards describe and prescribe professional nursing practice related to care of elders.[11]

Nurses can become certified in gerontological nursing. The ANA provides three examinations: gerontological nurse, gerontological clinical nurse specialist (GCNS), and gerontological nurse practitioner (GNP). Advanced practice nurses, including gerontological nurse practitioners and gerontological clinical nurse specialists, have diverse opportunities for practice. These nurses can manage most of the health problems that occur among residents in skilled nursing facilities, retirement communities, day-care settings, ambulatory care settings, hospitals, and even in private practice. The nurse who specializes in the care of elders can expand into a variety of potential roles: inservice educator, counselor and health educator, case manager, telephone advice nurse, and long-term care administrator.

The Older Population

Aging trends have profound implications for nursing practice trends and for the delivery of healthcare, as supported by the following demographic data and information about aging.

Trends Among the Elderly

The 1991 Pew Health Professions Commission report, *Healthy America: Practitioners for 2005*,[63] summarized the aging population growth trend. The 65-and-older group will increase by 2.5 million between 1995 and 2005. After 2010, it will grow rapidly to 52 million in 2020 and to 65.6 million in 2030, as members of the baby boom cohort (those born between 1946 and 1964) age. Figure 5–1 depicts this rapid rise. Expressed as percentages, the proportion of the total population consisting of people older than 64 years will be 13% in 2000, and 21.8% by 2030. Not only is the total U.S. population aging, the elderly are aging, too. In 1987, 9.6% of the elderly population was older than 85 years; by 2010, this percentage will increase to 15.5%. There are now 36,000 centenarians in the United States. If present trends continue, there may be 266,000 centenarians by the year 2020.[17]

Ethnicity Among the Elderly

Percentages of ethnic groups within the United States are as follows: blacks, 12.1%; Asians and Pacific Islanders,

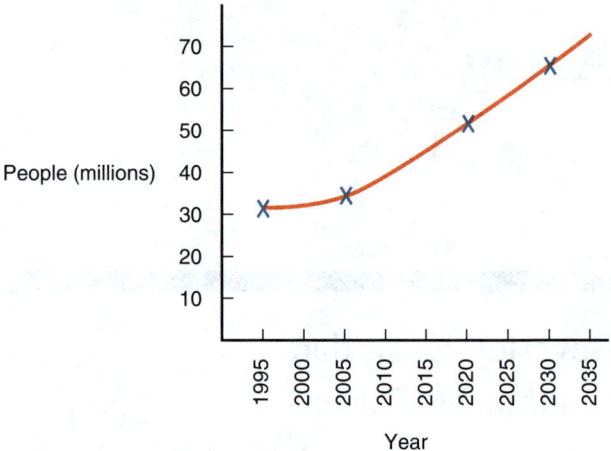

Figure 5–1. Projected rise in America's 65-and-older population.

2.9%; Native Americans 0.8%; and Hispanics, 9%.[21] Within these ethnic groups, elders compose approximately 8% of the blacks, 6% of Asians, 5.5% of Native Americans, and 5% of Hispanics.[65] Clearly, older people make up the fastest-growing age segment of the U.S. population. Equally relevant is the fact that ethnic elders are increasing at even higher rates. By the year 2050, more than 20% of all people older than 65 will be nonwhite.[68] Tripp-Reimer and co-workers[68] stress the importance of considering an elder's ethnic origin in relation to health and illness issues, family and social support, and interaction within the healthcare system.

Aging, Sex, and Marital Status

The ratio of men to women in the 65-and-older category has been on a steady decline since 1940, when the ratio was 95.5 : 100. Current census data reveal a ratio of 68.9 : 100 for the same age category (Fig. 5–2).[21, 69] Life expectancy for men is 72.7 years, and it is 79.6 years for women. Among people 65 years and older, 74.3% of men live with their spouses, compared with only 40.1% of women.[21] Implications for nursing practice in these numbers are evident. Elderly women living alone represent an at-risk population who frequently encounter discrimination (e.g., access to and quality of healthcare). Traditionally, women assumed dependent roles and let others make their decisions, including treatment choices. In general, these women represent a vulnerable population; nurses need to ensure that they receive their share of medical resources and a high standard of healthcare.[32]

Economic Forces

The largest single source of income for the elderly is Social Security benefits. These benefits constitute about 40% of an elder's income. Other contributing sources include earnings, property income, and pensions. In 1993, the median yearly income for older men was $14,983; for older women it was $8,499. The poverty rate was 12.2% among all elderly in 1993.[57] Among minority ethnic

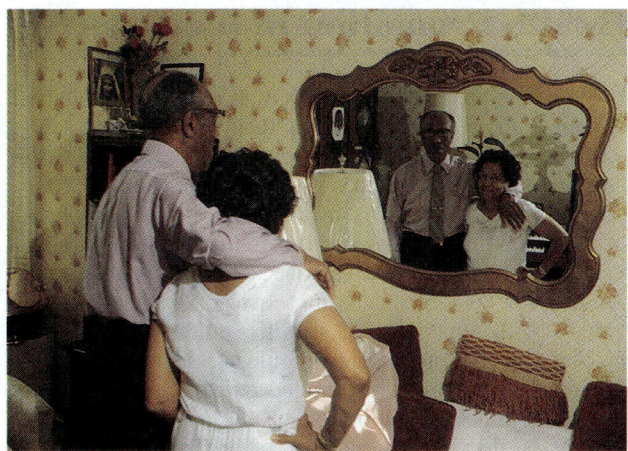

Figure 5–2. Women older than 65 are much less likely to live with a spouse than they were 50 years ago.

groups, the poverty levels are even higher. Approximately 36% of elderly black Americans currently fall below the federal poverty line, compared with 14% of elderly white Americans.[68] Eighty percent of older black women live in poverty. Hispanic, Native American, and Asian/Pacific Islander elderly generally have lower incomes than whites. More than 1 of 5 Asian/Pacific Islander older adults have incomes below the poverty level. Nearly 51% of Native Americans over the age of 65 receive incomes below the poverty level.

Although most elders receive Medicare benefits, Medicare does not provide comprehensive coverage of total healthcare expenses. Medicare does not cover most preventive care, including vision, hearing, and dental needs.[32] For an individual who is living at or near the poverty level, supplemental health insurance policies are not an option. Medicare does not reimburse for most of the services delivered by home healthcare agencies nor does it pay for a large part of nursing home costs.

Educational Issues

In 1987, Eliopoulos[22] noted that less than half of the elderly population, approximately 46.2%, had graduated from high school. Current trends indicate that by the year 2000, 63.7% of all elders will have completed high school, and more of the elderly will have advanced degrees than ever before. The nurse must be aware that there is great disparity in educational levels among various ethnic groups. Many blacks older than 65 have not had a formal education; approximately 17% of this group has completed high school. Hispanic elderly have the least amount of formal education. Asians are the most educated minority. About 12% of Native American elders have had no formal education.[56]

Cultural Aspects of Aging

Diverse Definitions of Elderly

Culture defines who is old, establishes rituals for identifying the elderly, sets socially acceptable roles and expecta-

tions for behavior of older adults, and influences attitudes toward aged members of society. The definitions of functional and chronological aging indicate that there are no arbitrary or widely accepted markers for old age. Although the prevailing definition of old age in the dominant culture frequently is considered to be age 65, there are diverse perceptions of old age in various cultures. Persons may be recognized as elders as early as age 40 among Southeast Asian and Native American groups. Social changes, such as becoming grandparents, retirement, or changes in functional status, rather than chronological age, mark entrance into old age in different cultures.[76] Nurses may provide care to aged clients who are defined chronologically as old but who, in functional terms, are active and productive.

Family Support

Nurses who care for older clients and families from different cultural backgrounds will notice that family relationships vary widely and are dependent on a cultural context. The availability of physical and personal supports from family members can facilitate the elderly person's ability to maintain independence, cope effectively with acute and chronic illnesses, remain functional and productive despite disability, and experience a peaceful death.

Some older adults from culturally diverse backgrounds who have given material and social support to children and grandchildren may expect reciprocity during their aging years. In many Hispanic, Native American, Asian American, Amish, Arab-American, and first-generation immigrant ethnic groups, the cultural norm is to provide significant care for aging parents, grandparents, and extended family members.

The importance of family support is compounded for older refugees. In instances of forced migration, the traditional family structure may have been altered or destroyed in the country of origin, sometimes in extremely violent ways. When older refugees arrive in the new host country, they may be isolated for several reasons. Older refugees may have limited or absent English-language skills, and they may have lost their social status, their country, and their home. The psychological stress related to cultural change is more intense for older refugees. The older refugee is more likely to rely on younger family members for economic and social support, housing, and access to health services.[49]

However, older adults from cultures in which independence and self-reliance are highly valued may refuse offers of assistance from their children, grandchildren, and extended family members. Depending on their personal finances, these individuals may have planned carefully for their aging in ways that rely on personal resources. They may seek assistance on a fee-for-service basis from various organizations that provide services and homes for the elderly, but refuse help from relatives.

A national sample of older Hispanics revealed that 30% reported providing child care to younger family members, 50% reported assisting in family decisions, and 12% provided financial assistance to family members. This compares with a national average of 19% of older

Americans providing child care regularly, and 15% occasionally caring for their grandchildren. More grandparents in Japan and France (51%) provide regular care than do grandparents in Great Britain (19%).[49] In black American households, the grandmother often takes a direct role in childrearing. More than twice as many young blacks live in households headed by elderly family members compared with whites.

Nursing Home Versus In-Home Care

Historically, a higher proportion of elders among minority ethnic groups have been cared for in home environments than have elderly white Americans. White elderly persons constitute 23% of the nursing home residents aged 85 and older in the United States. Hispanic and Asian/Pacific Islander elderly persons constitute 10% of the nursing home population aged 85 years and older.[76] Research indicates that family care of the elderly in other cultures is supportive for several reasons: as a substitute for formal services, as a more affordable alternative, as a caring option that is consistent with cultural values and preferences, and as an effective strategy for overcoming language barriers. In large extended families, more siblings are likely to be available to provide partial services and care for an elderly family member.[49]

Economic Issues Associated with Healthcare

National health data indicate that socioeconomic status varies among older adult whites, blacks, Native Americans, and Hispanics. The work histories of members of cultural groups, including long careers in agricultural labor, have precluded coverage within the Social Security or Medicare systems. For this reason, many elderly members from diverse cultural backgrounds face out-of-pocket healthcare expenses on limited incomes.

Most older adults from culturally diverse backgrounds have difficulty paying healthcare costs. Nurses assessing healthcare costs of the elderly and working with aged clients in their homes often find that these clients are unable to afford personal healthcare costs. Eighty-three percent of elderly Hispanics have Medicare coverage, compared with 96% of all elders. Only 21% of older Hispanics purchased supplemental Medicare insurance, compared with 65% of all elders. In many cases, family members of older adults from diverse cultural backgrounds bear the burden of paying healthcare expenses of their loved ones.[49]

Elderly who have made major adjustments in their lifestyles from their homelands to the United States and from rural to urban settings may be unaware of healthcare alternatives (e.g., preventive programs, healthcare benefits, and screening programs) for which they are eligible. Nurses should assist elderly clients from diverse backgrounds in evaluating their social networks, seeking assistance for healthcare needs, activating social contacts for support, and developing culturally competent care plans.

Health Promotion in the Elderly

Older adults are much more likely to suffer from multiple chronic and disabling illnesses than are younger adults. Approximately 80% of elderly people in the United States have one or more chronic diseases. The chronic conditions result in limitations in activities of daily living for 50%, major limitations in activities for 18%, and confinement to home for 5%. Heart disease, cancer, and strokes account for 80% of deaths in people older than 65. Individuals with hypertension, arthritis, pulmonary disorders, diabetes, visual and hearing problems, dementia, and depression require ongoing care and rehabilitation.[21]

A traditional definition of health as the absence of disease or disability is clearly not applicable to most of the older population. A more appropriate focus is on health as a state of mind and on the ability to live and function effectively in society. Health emerges as an idea that encompasses an interaction of physical, functional, and psychosocial factors. Health promotion goals must therefore include individual and group efforts related to spiritual, emotional, psychosocial, and physical concerns. Desired outcomes of health promotion programs should include maximizing functional independence, thereby reducing dependency; decreasing mortality; decreasing morbidity, including impairment; maintaining or improving quality of life; promoting behavioral change when necessary; and increasing productivity.[46]

Individually, elders can make efforts to control aspects of their health and move toward a sense of wellness (see Fig. 5–1). In fact, many elders do so, as described in the Nursing Research feature. Nursing has a prominent role in assisting elders to practice health promotion, which includes the following four aspects of wellness: self-care, physical fitness, nutritional awareness, and stress management.

Self-Care

As older adults become better informed and their awareness of the "self-help" movement increases, healthcare expectations also increase. There is an increasing desire to be in control of the body, mind, and spirit, and to assume responsibility for one's own wellness. This does not mean that traditional healthcare providers are ignored. Instead, strategies are taught that enable individuals to be responsive to their body signals and to seek action accordingly. Nurses can help the aging person understand this shared role (between the individual and healthcare professionals) for maintaining wellness. Counseling elders about factors that create an alteration in wellness and providing information about available alternatives is an important role of the nurse. Given adequate information, elders can practice effective self-care through a process of examining choices and making informed, meaningful decisions.

Most elders want to have as much control as possible over their own bodies, minds, and spirits. Assessments of elders should include an evaluation of self-care abilities, with an emphasis on abilities rather than disabilities. Sug-

- Improved oxygen transport
- Decreased blood pressure and pulse rate
- Increased vital lung capacity
- Decreased body fat and increased lean body mass
- Reduced osteoporosis
- Increased muscle strength and joint flexibility

Positive psychological changes occur as well, including improved cognitive functioning and a heightened sense of well-being.

A physical examination, which may include an exercise stress test, should be completed by the elder's physician before an exercise program is initiated. As shown in Figure 5–3, one of the best exercises for an older adult is walking, progressing to 30-minute sessions three to five times each week. Swimming and dancing are also beneficial. Age alone does not preclude elders from pursuing the whole range of possible physical activities; the issue is simply one of physical tolerance. Elders confined to a chair or with limited mobility can perform adaptive exercises. Many senior centers, wellness programs, and fitness clubs have consultants, instructors, or physical therapists who can help the elder establish an individualized exercise program.

Nutrition

Nutritional status is important to the elder's ability to mount an immune response to foreign antigens, maintain

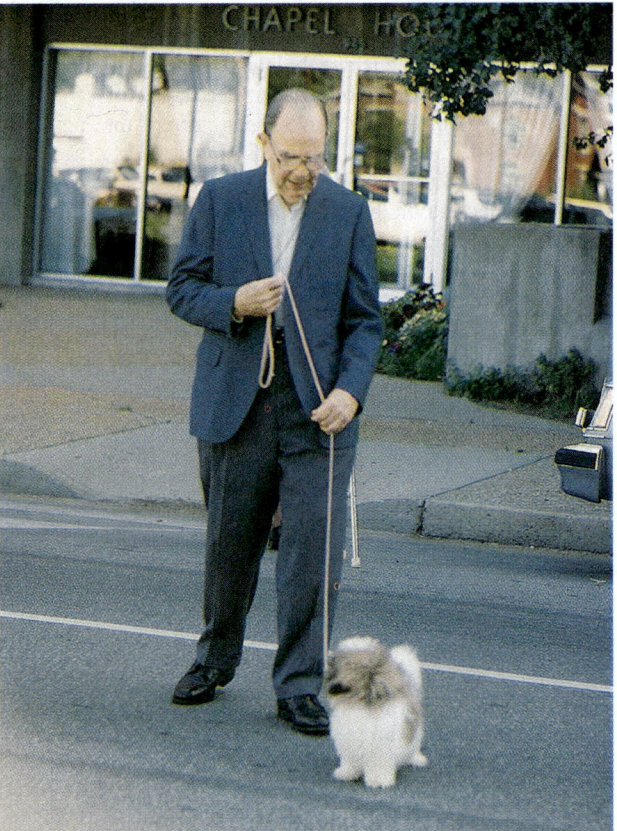

Figure 5–3. Walking provides a multitude of physiologic benefits for older people.

NURSING RESEARCH

Do the Elderly Promote Their Own Health Differently Than Do Younger Persons?

Walker, S. N., et al. (1988). Health-promoting life styles of older adults: Comparisons with young and middle-aged adults, correlates and patterns. *Advances in Nursing Science, 11*(1), 76–90.

Considerable resources in the United States have been directed toward the medical care of older persons who are ill; relatively little attention has been given to enhancing their health or to preventing illness. Little is known about the practices older adults engage in to protect or to enhance their health.

In this study, Walker and colleagues compared the health-promoting behaviors of older adults with those of young and middle-aged adults. They used the Health-Promoting Life-style Profile (HPLP) to collect data. The HPLP assesses health responsibility, nutrition, stress management, exercise, interpersonal support, and self-actualization.

Results showed that older adults had significantly higher scores for the total health-promoting life-style scale and three of the subscales (health responsibility, nutrition, and stress management) than their younger counterparts. Scores did not differ significantly for the health-promoting life-style dimensions of self-actualization, exercise, and interpersonal support.

Implications for Practice

Although many older adults in this study followed healthy life-styles, many practiced only selected components. Nurses should capitalize on the apparent trend for older adults to seek health-promoting behaviors. Programs should be initiated to provide information and opportunities to practice healthy activities. In particular, emphasis may be placed on teaching the value of exercise and providing structured exercise classes.

gested preventive practices are discussed in Chapter 10. In addition, physical fitness, nutrition, and stress management are also factors in wellness.

Physical Fitness

Exercise and activity are essential for health promotion and maintenance in the older adult and to achieve an optimal level of functioning. Approximately half of the physical deterioration of the elderly is caused by disuse rather than by the aging process or disease. Monicken[53] noted the following positive effects of exercise on health: increased energy, improved eating and sleeping, decreased discomfort and stress, and decreased smoking and alcohol use. Physiologically, benefits to the cardiopulmonary, vascular, and musculoskeletal systems result in the following:

anatomic and structural normality, think clearly, and possess the necessary energy to engage in social and fitness activities. Several expected physiologic changes related to aging that can affect nutritional status include the following:

- Decreased olfactory sensitivity and diminished taste
- Degrees of dental deterioration
- Reduced saliva production to approximately one-third the amount of younger years
- Weaker gag reflex
- Less fat tolerance
- Decreased colonic peristalsis
- Reduced gastric hydrochloric acid production, which leads to decreased digestion and absorption of vitamins, iron, zinc, and calcium[22]

Socioeconomic factors can also result in malnutrition. With reduced incomes, some elders may restrict their food intake to near-starvation levels, as might be necessitated by decisions such as choosing rent and medicine over food. Diets may be unbalanced due to the expense of fresh fruits, vegetables, and meats. Lack of transportation and the inability to carry heavy quantities of groceries can prohibit some elders from obtaining food. Living alone can also be associated with poor nutrition, since many elders may lose the motivation to prepare a balanced diet for just themselves.

Psychologically, depression and stress can affect nutritional status. Both conditions can lead to overeating or undereating. Medications can have a major influence on nutrition due to such side effects as increased or decreased appetite, constipation, nausea, or decreased absorption. Additionally, medications such as diuretics can affect fluid and electrolyte balance, leading to problems with dehydration and constipation. Risk factors for malnutrition in the elderly have been given the acronym DETERMINE, as shown in Box 5–1.

Physiologically, energy requirements lessen with aging due to a decline in basal metabolic rate and often to a decline in physical activity. The recommended daily allowance (RDA) for caloric intake is 2,300 kcal for people between 65 and 75 years and 2,050 kcal for those older than 75 years. More than 58% of the calories should come from complex carbohydrates, fewer than 30% from fat, and the remaining 12% from protein.[33] The elderly have an increased need for vitamin D, vitamin B6, and calcium to protect against osteoporosis. Twenty to 35 g/day of fiber is recommended to reduce the risk of some forms of cancer and to promote normal bowel function.

Community resources related to food and dental care should be considered for elders with alterations in nutrition.

Stress Management

Any real or perceived threat to one's physical, emotional, and social well-being can create stress. The later years of life can include such stressful events as acute or chronic illness, retirement, death of significant others, financial hardship, or relocation. Although the sources of stress may vary, the physiologic outcomes are similar. Stimulation of the sympathetic nervous system results in the release of epinephrine, norepinephrine, and adrenal glucocorticoids. Prolonged stress can result in serious consequences, including heart disease, hypertension, cerebrovascular accident, cancer, gastric ulcers, skin problems, complications of underlying disorders, and numerous social and emotional problems.

The way in which an older person adapts to stress is influenced greatly by personality traits and coping strategies used throughout life. Fostering opportunities to make new friends and maintaining old friendships is especially important. Friendships provide support to the elder in times of stress, reinforce a sense of self-worth, and provide confidence to overcome obstacles. The elderly should be encouraged to respond to stress in a healthy manner, maintaining a balance of good nutrition, rest, and exercise. Methods of relaxation should be encouraged. These can include yoga, meditation, relaxation exercises, or involvement in any activity that provides respite from stressful demands.

Teaching

Encouraging health promotion and disease prevention among elders requires effective teaching. Teaching elders is really similar to teaching members of any age group in that the unique characteristics and learning needs of the individual must be considered foremost. General guidelines for teaching older adults are listed in Box 5–2.

Functional Status of the Elderly

Assessment of functional status of the older adult is important when considering the individual's ability to function within the environment. Often, an environment can be adapted to enhance the person's ability to function and to remain as independent as possible. Research related to functional assessment has found that functional impairments (both physical and psychosocial) are good early indicators of active illness in older people.[9]

Box 5–1. Risk Factors for Malnutrition in the Elderly

Disease
Eating poorly
Tooth decay or oral pain
Economic hardship
Reduced social contact
Multiple medications
Involuntary weight loss or gain
Needs assistance with self-care
Elderly person older than 80 years

From the Nutrition Screening Initiative in conjunction with the American Academy of Family Physicians, the American Dietetic Association, and the National Council on the Aging.

Box 5–2. Guidelines for Effectively Teaching Older Adults

Vision

Provide large, easy-to-read typeface
Emphasize contrasting colors: black and white
Avoid blues and greens
Use non-glare paper
Write short, simple paragraphs
Make sure glasses are in place and clean

Hearing

Speak slowly
Enunciate clearly
Lower the pitch of your voice
Eliminate background noise
Face the learner
Use nonverbal cues
Make sure client's hearing aid is in place and working
  properly

Energy Level/Attention

Use short teaching sessions
Offer liquid refreshment and bathroom breaks
Promote comfort

Information Processing/Memory

Present most important information first
Clarify information with use of examples (one's elders
  can relate to)
Motor Skills: Teach one step at a time, demonstrate,
  allow for return demonstration
Encourage association between items
Be concrete and specific
Eliminate distractions
Encourage verbal interactions
Correct wrong answers/reinforce correct answers
Offer praise and encouragement

Compiled from Beare, P. G., & Graveley, E. (1995). Health teaching and compliance. In M. Stanley & P. Beare (Eds.), *Gerontological nursing* (pp 63–96). Philadelphia: F. A. Davis; and Burnside, I. (1988). *Nursing and the aged.* New York: McGraw-Hill.

Activities of daily living (ADLs) are activities that are essential to personal care. ADLs include toileting, feeding, dressing, grooming, bathing, and getting about. The assessment of ADL is important in deciding the level of assistance needed on a daily basis and in planning long-term care for older adults. Instrumental activities of daily living (IADL) are more complex activities that are essential to community living situations. IADLs include all the personal care activities of ADL, shopping, meal preparation, housekeeping, laundry, telephone use, use of transportation, ability to correctly take medications, and money management. The evaluation of IADLs is important in deciding the level of assistance needed by people in independent or semi-independent settings. IADLs are less important in institutional settings than in community settings, although the assessment is important for dis-

charge planning. When an older adult cannot do IADLs independently, caregivers often provide the assistance that enables the person to remain in a community setting, or referrals can be made to various community resources to help meet these needs.

Functional assessment instruments generally include scales for measuring ADLs and IADLs. The Barthel,[44] Katz,[37] and OARS[36] are used most commonly. Psychosocial functioning can be assessed by observation, interview, and a mental status screening examination (e.g., Folstein).[23] This provides information about cognitive functioning, perceptual-motor skills, insight and reasoning, and contact with reality. (See Chapter 30 for further information on mental status assessment.)

Physiologic Factors Influencing Functional Status

Sleep

Elders fall asleep with more difficulty, awaken more readily and more frequently, spend more time in the drowsiness stage, and spend less time in deep sleep than do younger adults. Functionally, these changes have little impact on the daily life of the older adult. However, adverse reactions can occur when these changes coincide with illness, stress, daily demands, or certain medications, such as hypnotics, antidepressants, diuretics, and some antihypertensives. Sleep is discussed in Chapter 18.

Sensory Impairments

Normal aging results in some sensory impairment. Vision and hearing are senses that individuals rely on to communicate and to perform activities in the environment. Sensory impairments can affect safety, communication with others, performance of daily activities, and quality of life. Assessments of elders suggest that limitations in ADL are more likely to occur in older people with sensory impairments than in those without sensory loss. Vision changes can affect the performance of a variety of daily activities: driving a vehicle; shopping for groceries; going up and down stairs; maneuvering safely in dark or unfamiliar environments; seeing markings on clocks, radios, thermostats, appliances, and televisions; and reading newspapers, signs, directories, and labels on food items and medication containers. Besides influencing daily activities, the individual with impaired vision has an increased risk of falling. Vision and hearing are discussed in Chapters 36 and 37.

Mobility

Mobility is an important aspect of physiologic functioning because it is essential for maintaining independence. Serious consequences occur when mobility declines. Mobility depends most directly on the musculoskeletal system. Decreased functioning of various body systems can place individuals at greater risk for loss of mobility. These could include decreased sensory ability (impaired vision and hearing), cardiovascular disorders (dysrhythmia, postural hypotension), neurologic disorders (parkinsonism and problems that affect gait, balance, sway, and reaction time), and depression. Various side effects of medication can also increase risk of loss of mobility, particularly the side effects of hypovolemia, postural hypotension, excessive sedation, decreased cognitive functioning, and loss of postural control.[66] Some disorders that increase with age and can have an impact on the individual's functional ability include osteoporosis, osteoarthritis, and rheumatoid arthritis (see Chapters 27 and 74).

Psychosocial Factors Influencing Functional Status

Although the physiologic changes and chronic illnesses associated with older age may affect a person's functional abilities, the psychosocial changes are often the most challenging and demanding. Some of these psychosocial challenges arise from physical changes, but many are caused by changes in roles, relationships, and living environments. These changes tax coping abilities and energies.

Ageism

"Ageism" is a term coined by Butler that refers to the prejudices and stereotypes applied to older people purely because of their age.[15] Ageism, like racism and sexism, is a way of pigeonholing a group of people and of not allowing them to be individuals with unique ways of living. Prejudice toward the elderly is an attempt by younger generations to shield themselves from their own eventual aging and death. Such stereotyping allows younger individuals to see the elderly as different from themselves, and they ultimately cease to identify with elders as human beings.[15] A shocking awakening comes when these younger people themselves grow old and find themselves the victims of the same stereotypes and attitudes.

The significance of the phenomenon of ageism is considerable. Ageism affects the well-being of older adults by influencing the attitudes of healthcare providers and political powers. Typically, reduced aggressiveness is seen in diagnosis and treatment of disease in the elderly; programs to help elders are generally underfunded; and the ability of elders to remain a contributing force as perceived by society is reduced simply due to chronological age.

This negative attitude can have a devastating effect on the older person. Realizing a negative label has been applied can cause the elder to adopt modes of dependency, helplessness, and a negative self-image, which may lead to increased vulnerability to biopsychosocial stressors.[46] Images of older persons as dependent, deteriorating, beyond rehabilitative efforts, and physically and mentally unappealing can lead to a lack of desire among professionals to care for older persons and a lack of attention to the quality of care delivered.

Nursing is in a unique position to address the issue of ageism and to develop ways to combat its pervasiveness.

Professionals should seek to gain information about aging and the aging process; to balance experiences with the ill elderly with equal time among healthy, hearty elders; and to spend time with happy and successful geriatric role models. The nurse must always realize that each elderly person has a potential for rehabilitation, treatment, self-actualization, and/or improvement in quality of life and well-being.

Multiple Losses

Many losses inevitably occur in later life. Assessing the impact of the losses and supporting the elder are major goals of nursing practice. Aging persons experience personal, social, and economic losses. Perhaps the most devastating losses are "people" losses—parents, friends, spouse, or children, as depicted in Figure 5–4.[25] Other typical losses that elders face include loss of one's home, possessions, pets, employment, social position, and/or financial security. Individuals can reach an "overload" state when losses become multiple. The emotional upheaval precipitated by many losses and changes can result in mental confusion, withdrawal, helplessness, and depression.

McCracken[47] reported on the impact of possession loss. Among 75 subjects, it was found that possessions were often valued for their association with valued persons, events, or roles in a subject's life. Parting with the pos-

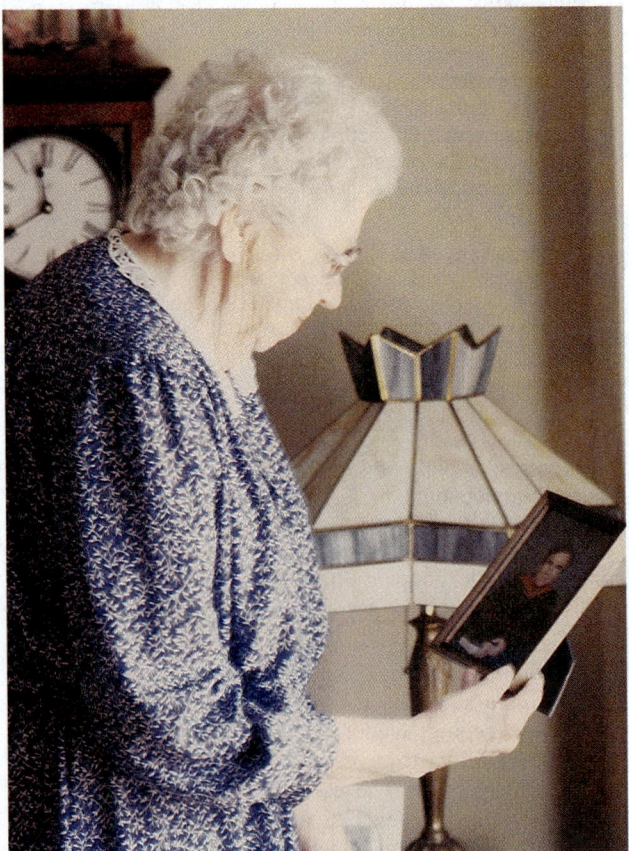

Figure 5–4. Loss of loved ones may create an emotional burden with accompanying mental and physical effects.

sessions was therefore very difficult and contributed to a loss of continuity with life history. Important possessions included clothing, photographs, linens, pictures, and selected items of furniture (cedar chest, bedroom furniture). Whenever possible, the author suggested retaining and moving with individuals those possessions that support memories, facilitate continuation of roles, and are particularly useful.

King and co-workers[38] examined the loss of one's traditional dwelling and the effect of relocation. Integral to the reaction to relocation was whether the move was voluntary or involuntary. Individuals at high risk for poor adjustment to a relocation were those with low self-esteem, no confidante, many worries, high levels of alienation, poorer self-perception of health, and depression. Nursing interventions suggested by these authors to help an elder with relocation include assessing for risk factors, empathizing with the difficulties of the move, and suggesting positive resources to effectively cope. The Care Plan offers additional related information.

Garrett[25] listed nine coping strategies for elders who were dealing with multiple losses.

- Helping others
- Making new friends
- Joining groups
- Setting goals
- Maintaining independence
- Adopting a pet
- Maintaining a sense of humor
- Sustaining family ties
- Avoiding isolation and self-pity

Garrett noted that adjustment to a loss is a challenge at any age. For elders, resolution of grief may not always be achieved, but may be integrated into their life without causing dysfunction.

Neglect and Abuse

Elder neglect and abuse are complex and serious issues affecting older adults. Instances are neither rare nor isolated in U.S. society. Research suggests that elder abuse is widespread, occurs among all subgroups of the population, and affects 4% to 10% of older people.[71] Elder abuse includes physical and psychological abuse, misuse of property, and violation of rights. Neglect includes self-neglect and neglect by caregivers.

CARE PLAN

The Older Client at Risk for Relocation Stress Syndrome

Nursing Diagnosis. Risk for Relocation Stress Syndrome related to changes associated with healthcare facility transfer or admission to long-term care facility

Planning: Expected Outcomes. The client will request information on the upcoming move, will communicate an understanding of the relocation, will utilize the available resources, and will express satisfaction with his or her adjustment to the new environment. The client and family members will take steps to prepare for the relocation.

Implementation	Rationales
Assess for low self-esteem, low confidence, many worries, high degree of alienation, poor perceived health, and depression.	These are risk factors associated with poor adjustment to a relocation.
Help the client and family members prepare for the relocation. Conduct group discussions to provide images of the new setting and communicate any additional information that will ease the transition.	These steps will help the client to cope with the new environment.
If possible, allow the client and family to visit the new location; provide introductions to the staff.	The more familiar the environment, the less stress the client will experience during the relocation.
Assess the client's needs for additional health services before the relocation.	These assessments will help to ensure that the client receives appropriate care in the new environment.
Communicate all aspects of the client's discharge plan to appropriate staff members at the new location.	This communication will help to ensure continuity of care.
Educate family members about relocation stress syndrome and its potential effects.	Encourage family members to provide needed emotional support throughout the transition period.
Encourage the client to express emotions associated with the relocation.	Allowing the client to express his or her emotions provides an opportunity to correct misconceptions, answer questions, and reduce anxiety.
Reassure the client that family members and friends know the new location and will continue to visit.	This reassurance helps to reduce feelings of abandonment and anxiety.
Assign a primary nurse to new clients.	Assignment of a primary nurse provides a consistent caring environment that enhances the client's adjustment and well being.

Evaluation. Accomplishment of expected outcomes may require considerable time. Reassessment is important.

The typical abuse victim is a woman of advanced age with few social contacts and at least one physical or mental impairment that limits the ability to perform ADL. In addition she lives alone or with the abuser and depends on the abuser for care.[5, 12, 20, 40, 54, 75]

Elder abuse has emerged as a significant aspect of family violence for several reasons. One is the increased number of older adults. With more individuals living to advanced ages, more adult children are having to assume the caregiver role. If the adult child is not prepared for this responsibility, abuse and neglect may occur. Because an older person's needs increase with time, the stress and burden of caregiving also increases, raising the risk of elder abuse.[64] The passage of state elder abuse and adult protective service laws has led to increased reporting of mistreatment and self-neglect. This has resulted in greater recognition of the problem in all communities and segments of the elderly population.

Mental Health Disorders in the Elderly

Dementia, Delirium, and Depression

Dementia (specifically Alzheimer's disease) and delirium (referred to as *confusion*) are discussed in Chapter 34. Pathophysiology, clinical manifestations, assessment parameters, and management are addressed. The focus of this discussion is on three conditions of significance to the elderly: dementia, delirium, and depression. Clinically, it is important to realize that presenting clinical manifestations of these conditions in elderly clients can be very similar. A differential diagnosis is essential.

Disorders associated with cognitive decline are among the most common and frightening problems faced by the elderly.[43] It is a common myth that older adults inevitably experience cognitive decline as a consequence of aging. This is simply not true. Serious difficulties with thinking clearly and remembering are not normal consequences of aging but are manifestations of medical illness or alterations in psychosocial well-being.

Still, the stereotypical view of cognitive decline as being a normal part of aging prevails. For this reason, an acute deterioration in cognition is frequently overlooked by many physicians and nurses: undetected cases of cognitive disorders have ranged from 16% to 72%.[26, 55] Because many older adults believe that cognitive decline is part of aging, they do not seek medical attention when they notice changes in processing stimuli or in responses to stressful life events. Family members may react to acute cognitive changes as the "beginning of the end," and quickly plan for alternative living arrangements and entertain other actions and thoughts that would likely prove unnecessary.[6]

Dementia

Dementia is a clinical syndrome characterized by intellectual deterioration that is severe enough to interfere with the ability to cope with daily life. It is gradually progressive in nature and is *irreversible*. Deficits occur in memory, language, perception, praxis, learning, problem-solving, abstract thinking, and judgment. Approximately 3% of people age 65 to 74 have dementia; the prevalence increases to 47.2% for those older than 85 years.[35] Dementia can be primary in nature, as with Alzheimer's disease, multi-infarct dementia, alcoholism, and Pick's disease, or secondary to other causes, as with Parkinson's

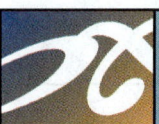

BRIDGE TO HOME HEALTHCARE

Detecting Elder Abuse*

In the home care setting, factors beyond the physical condition of the patient—such as the environment of care, relationships, and support systems—are fundamental to the achievement of positive outcomes. This is especially true when abuse of a patient is suspected. When you suspect patient abuse, you must incorporate the client, family, and caregiver into your total assessment and care plan.

When caring for clients at home, it is important to listen carefully to the client and to observe overt and covert behaviors. In addition to completing a history and physical assessment related to the client's current condition, you must confirm the caregiver's report of the client's condition. For example, if the caregiver attributes bruises to a fall, you must determine whether gait instability is consistent with the client's physical condition.

It may be difficult for a client to admit that a caregiver is abusive. Many times, abusive caregivers provide assistance with activities of daily living (ADLs), financial assistance, or emotional support, which allows the client to continue to live in the community.

Situations can appear to indicate abuse when, in reality, a caregiver is simply uninformed about client care. Client and family education must be adequate in such areas as nutrition, transfers, ambulation, and positioning, so that caregivers can adequately meet client needs.

When you suspect abuse, a multidisciplinary plan of care is essential. Inform the physician of the client situation and of any clinical manifestations. A social worker can coordinate family counseling, make referrals to community resources, and facilitate day care. Homemakers and home health aides can help to relieve the burden of care. Volunteers can provide respite for the caregiver. (The frustration of providing care can contribute to abuse. Encourage caregivers to arrange for regular absences from care.)

Do not be reluctant to confront suspicious situations for fear of jeopardizing rapport with the client and family. Although maintaining a relationship is important, client advocacy is your first priority.

---

*By Bridget Young, R.N., B.S.N., M.B.A., Visiting Nurse Association of Omaha, Omaha, NE.

disease and trauma. Causes of dementia can vary, but the clinical presentation is similar regardless of cause. Therefore, the descriptive term *dementia of the Alzheimer's type* (DAT) is generally used. Before a diagnosis of dementia is made, all potential physical and psychosocial causes of cognitive decline should be ruled out. The onset and progressive nature of the cognitive decline should be documented, and serial neuropsychological testing should be performed. The diagnosis can be complicated when delirium, depression, or both, are superimposed on dementia.

Delirium

Delirium is a syndrome characterized by global cognitive impairment of abrupt onset that is *reversible*. This condition becomes irreversible only if underlying causes go undetected or are treated unsuccessfully to the point of irreversible damage. Many synonyms are used in the literature to refer to delirium (reversible dementia, pseudosenility, acute brain failure, clouded states). Acute confusion is used widely in the nursing literature to refer to this phenomenon. Attention deficits are considered the most salient feature of delirium. Other diagnostic criteria include disorganized thinking, reduced level of consciousness, perceptual disturbances, disturbances of the sleep-wake cycle, increased or decreased psychomotor activity, disorientation, and memory impairment.

Delirium is one of the most important and prevalent cognitive disorders among hospitalized elders, with reported incidence ranging from 15% to 80%.[24] Delirium is associated with higher mortality,[58] prolonged hospital stays,[10] nursing time greater than necessary for the admitting diagnosis, and nursing home placement.[41, 42] Delirium is often the presenting symptom of physical illness in an older person, exceeding the more common indicators of fever, pain, or tachycardia. Among elders, it has been associated with a variety of conditions, especially adverse drug reactions, metabolic disorders (e.g., electrolyte disorders, renal failure, respiratory failure, and endocrinopathies), cardiac failure, cerebrovascular disorders, infection (especially pulmonary, renal, or neurological), anemia, and surgery. Many psychosocial factors can also cause or contribute to a delirious state. These might include bereavement, relocation, and sensory deprivation or overstimulation. In a study by McCurren, looking at acutely confused versus nonconfused hospitalized elders, the mean age of the confused group was 82, while the mean age of the non-confused group was 76.[48] Advancing age is highly correlated with the development of delirium.

The key to differentiating between delirium and dementia is the assessment of the onset of the cognitive manifestations. Onset of delirium is rapid, usually occurring within hours to days, whereas dementia has a slower, more gradual onset. It is imperative that reversible delirium not be classified as dementia. A comprehensive investigation for all possible physical and psychosocial factors that might cause an alteration in cognition must be conducted. Table 5–1 contrasts the primary clinical features of delirium and dementia.

Depression

Research studies suggest that significant manifestations of depression occur in approximately 10% to 15% of all community-dwelling elders over 65 years; among institutionalized elders, the prevalence rate increases dramatically to 50% to 75%.[13] Depression is a complex syndrome that manifests itself in a variety of ways in the elderly. The most common manifestations of depression are vegetative symptoms, which include insomnia, fatigue, weight loss, constipation, preoccupation with physical health, or thoughts of death. Elders suffering from depression may also exhibit sadness, crying, anxiety, irritability, or paranoia.

Depression can also lead to cognitive impairment. It is estimated that a depression-associated cognitive disorder occurs in 10% to 29% of depressed elderly patients.[59] Therefore, bedside differentiation of depression-related cognitive alteration versus dementia may be difficult. Depressed patients often look and act demented, and even do poorly on mental status tests. However, the vegetative signs of depression are generally not seen in demented individuals. Features supporting a diagnosis of depression versus dementia would include recent onset of depressive symptoms and inconsistencies with actual functional performance and cognitive testing.

Treatment Strategies

Several strategies are available for nurses to use to help elders who are suffering from dementia, delirium, or depression. The following four strategies are commonly used by gerontological nurses:

● Reality orientation
● Validation therapy
● Remotivation therapy
● Reminiscence therapy

The reader is encouraged to explore these treatment modalities and their specific application in literature for gerontological nursing and psychiatry (for example, refer to Chapter 21 in Ebersole and Hess[21]).

Substance Use Disorders

Substance use disorders refer to ingestion of any compound in quantities that may be harmful to health or well-being. This includes overindulgence in alcohol, nicotine, caffeine, over-the-counter (OTC) drugs and preparations, prescription drugs, controlled drugs (such as meperidine or codeine) and illegal drugs (see Chapter 87). Dependence on alcohol and drugs is far more common among elders than is generally thought. The addictive experience includes alterations in mood and sensation, immediate gratification, and enhanced sense of control and power. These are elements that may be missing in the lives of some elders.[27]

Valanis and colleagues[73] found that 10% to 15% of elders in the community and 20% of hospitalized elders have serious problems related to alcohol use. Older indi-

Table 5–1. Clinical Features of Delirium and Dementia

	Delirium	Dementia
Description	A reversible, acute confusional state	A gradually progressive irreversible cognitive decline
Onset	Rapid, acute, often at night	Slow, gradual
Duration	Days to weeks, but usually less than 1 month	Continuous, ongoing
Disorientation	Present, especially for time; tendency to mistake unfamiliar for familiar persons, place	May be absent in mild states of dementia
Thinking	Slow or accelerated; may be dream-like, impoverished	Impoverished; poor abstracting ability
Memory	Short-term memory impaired	Short-term memory impaired; long-term memory may be affected
Attention	Consistently impaired; easily distracted; fluctuates	Typically intact
Alertness	Reduced or increased, but awareness always affected	Typically normal; may be reduced
Perception	Invariably affected, especially at night; often have hallucinations	May be intact; usually no hallucinations
Sleep	Sleep-wake cycle altered	Usually normal for age
Course	Typically fluctuates with lucid intervals and exacerbations	Relatively stable over course of a day
Affect	Intermittent fear, perplexity, bewilderment	Flat or indifferent
Cause	Multiple potential causes (e.g., surgery, infection, drugs)	Unknown, possible environmental, hereditary, chemical
Treatment	Remove or treat the cause	Guided by signs and symptoms
Nursing interventions	Reorient the client to reality; protect from injury	Reorientation does not work for advancing dementia; use validation therapy (e.g., one technique is to agree with the client, don't argue, while maintaining his or her safety); ensure safety

Data from DSM–IV,[3] Davies,[19] Levkoff et al.,[40] and Lipowski.[41]

viduals who drink are at risk for injuries and accidents because of decreased tolerance to alcohol and the normal changes in dexterity, balance, and proprioception associated with aging. Problems commonly seen in elders who consume excessive quantities of alcohol include the following:

● Intellectual deterioration
● Gastrointestinal problems, including gastritis, hemorrhage, malnutrition, hypoglycemia, and ulcers
● Heart problems, such as cardiomyopathy, arrhythmia, and peripheral edema
● Vulnerability to liver and cerebrovascular disease

Elders may use alcohol to cope with the acute stresses, grief, and bereavement that are common to this age group. In a study of bereaved elderly, Valanis and associates[73] found that 73% of study subjects used alcohol to cope with the loss of a spouse.

It is difficult to determine the extent of prescription drug abuse by elders. Chastain[16] contends that thousands of older Americans are hooked on their prescription drugs in an "inadvertent addiction." The cycle of addiction usually begins benignly with a medication or a drink for pain or anxiety. Physicians often are unaware of the problem. They may also be unaware of the number of medications that the individual may be taking because the prescriptions may be issued from several different physicians.

Medication Use in the Elderly

In the United States, 16% of adults older than 60 years take nearly 40% of all medications prescribed.[21, 29] A comparable number of elders take OTC medications in addition to those prescribed. Elders who live in long-term care facilities take an average of four to seven different medications.[29] The trend of multiple drug use will continue as research produces more sophisticated drug therapies. When used properly, drugs can benefit the individual; when used inappropriately they threaten the individual's functional abilities and health.

Age-related changes also affect the action of the medication in the body. This can result in alterations in drug absorption, drug distribution, drug metabolism, drug excretion, and drug activity. Drug absorption rate is the time required for a medication taken orally, parenterally, or rectally to enter the general circulation. Maximum absorption of oral medications occurs in the small intestine. Age-related changes in stomach emptying, changes in gastric pH, and gastrointestinal motility may influence absorption. Drug distribution or transport depends on the adequacy of the circulatory system. Altered cardiac output and sluggish circulation delay the arrival of medication at the target receptors and retard the elimination of the drug or its by-products from the body. Changes in body composition during aging influence drug distribution. Total body water decreases with age, altering cellular distribution of drugs that are water-soluble, which results in higher than usual blood levels of water-soluble drugs. Adipose tissue or fat content increases and results in storage of lipid-soluble drugs in the fatty tissue, thus extending and possibly elevating the drug effect.

Drug metabolism occurs primarily in the liver. Due to an age-related decrease in blood flow to the liver, hepatic clearance is decreased. This slowed metabolism results in the drug remaining in the body longer and in prolongation of its half-life. Although drug excretion occurs primarily through the kidneys, some excretion also occurs through bile, feces, sweat, and saliva. Age-related changes in renal function affect both the length of time the drug is in the body and its half-life, with the potential result of drug toxic effects. The sensitivity of the central nervous system (CNS) also affects drug activity. One result is an exaggerated or idiosyncratic reaction to hypotensive drugs.

Adherence to a medication regimen depends on several factors:

- Motivation
- Understanding about the purpose of the medication
- Fine-motor movement and coordination necessary to remove medications from containers
- For oral agents, the ability to swallow the particular form of medication

In addition, the elder must be able to do the following:

- Obtain correct amounts of medication
- Distinguish the correct container
- Read directions
- Hear and remember verbal instructions
- Understand the correct timing for medication administration
- Follow the dosage schedule

These consumption factors often become important and are frequently overlooked in discussing adherence to a drug regimen.

Darnell and co-workers[17] noted that 90% of the elderly took an average of three OTC drugs and five prescription drugs daily. The most commonly prescribed and used drugs are cardiovascular drugs, anti-infective drugs, antipsychotic drugs, antidepressant drugs, and diuretic drugs.[7, 29] Analgesics, laxatives, and antacids are the most frequently used OTC drugs, followed by cough products, nonsteroidal topical preparations for arthritis-type pain, milk of magnesia, bismuth subgallate for upset stomach, eyewashes, and vitamins.[18, 29, 67]

Drug interactions are the result of two or more medications given simultaneously or in close sequence. Drug intereactions have an outcome response of drug potentiation (one drug enhances the effect of the other drug), antagonism (one drug blocks the anticipated effect of the other drug), or synergism (the combined effect of the two drugs is greater than expected when the drugs are taken together). Drug interactions increase with the age of the user and the number of drugs prescribed. Polypharmacy stems from the existence of multiple chronic conditions, the prescribing methods of physicians, the beliefs and practices of the elderly, and the increasing practice of seeing more than one primary care provider, each of whom prescribes similar drugs. Issues to consider when working with older adults and their medications are as follows:

- Use of multiple pharmacies
- Use of OTC prescriptions without informing the physician
- Sharing of drugs with neighbors, relatives, and friends
- Misuse of drugs, including overuse, underuse, erratic use, and contraindicated use

Government Support for the Elderly

The major influence on programs for older adults has been the Older Americans Act passed by Congress in 1965. The basic purpose of the Older Americans Act is to "help older persons" by providing funds to the states for services, training, and research. All of these activities are coordinated at the federal level through the Administration on Aging. Each state has an Area Agency on Aging to develop comprehensive and coordinated services at the local level. A unique element of the Older Americans Act has been that all authorized programs and services are free of charge to the client.

The Older Americans Act has had frequent amendments. Current objectives focus on a wide range of programs: healthcare services, nutrition programs, senior centers, transportation, housing assistance, residential repairs, an ombudsman program, legal services, in-home services, crime prevention, job counseling programs, and case management.

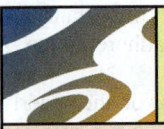

DIVERSITY IN HEALTHCARE

Ethnopharmacology

Metabolic, Genetic, and Environmental Factors

Cultural differences in drug response and metabolism have been identified by numerous researchers. The majority of studies providing evidence for transcultural differences in pharmacokinetic and pharmacodynamic properties of various drugs have compared individuals of Asian, black, Hispanic, and Native American descent to whites.[1–6]

Differences in pharmacokinetics may be genetic or may be due to environmental influences. Among blacks and whites, only about 9% are considered to be slow metabolizers, whereas 32% of Asians are.[1,6] There also is evidence of variability in protein binding based on ethnicity. Habits such as smoking and drinking alcohol are known to speed the drug metabolism, whereas a low-protein, high-carbohydrate diet is known to slow the metabolism. The fact that whites and blacks drink significantly more alcohol than Asians and eat differently may provide an environmental explanation for the greater drug impact experienced by Asian clients.[1, 3, 4, 6]

Cultural Considerations and Dosage

Because wide variations occur in the size of older adults from diverse cultures, the nurse should be aware that dosages may need to be modified. For example, the average Asian American is markedly shorter, weighs less, and has a smaller body frame than older adults from white, black, Hispanic, or Native American backgrounds. By age 65, black women carry an average of 9.1 kg (20 lb) more than their white counterparts.

Black older adults are significantly misdiagnosed as psychotic, viewed as more violent by staff, and spend more time in seclusion than whites, Hispanics or Asian Americans.[3] Thus, the actual dose of medication prescribed for blacks may be more a function of staff perception than a decision based on serum levels or clinical observations. Asians in general, and Chinese-American clients in particular, require significantly smaller doses of neuroleptics, tricyclic antidepressants (TCAs), and lithium than do whites (sometimes half the dose). Similar differences have been reported between Indian

or Pakistani clients and white older adults.[4]

Perception of Side Effects

Research indicates that Asian-Americans are more sensitive to neuroleptics than are whites. In a study by Keltner and Folks,[1] Asian-American clients began experiencing extrapyramidal effects at dosages approximately half those for whites. At equivalent doses, 95% of Asians experienced extrapyramidal effects, whereas only 67% of whites and blacks experienced those side effects. Hispanic clients taking tricyclic antidepressants experienced side effects at half the dosage observed in whites. Blacks are more susceptible to tricyclic antidepressant delirium than are whites.

Culture and Issues of Compliance

In a study of three subgroups from Southeast Asia (Hmong, Cambodian, Laotian), Kroll and others[2] determined that the client's failure to take the medication as prescribed accounted for changes in plasma levels for approximately half of the subjects. As a result of these and other study findings, cultural influ-

Social Security

Social Security legislation was enacted in 1935 during the Depression, when poverty was rampant in the United States. Although the original intent was not to provide the total income for an elderly person, for many it has become the only source of income. Social Security benefits are based on an individual's average earnings over a defined period of years before retirement.

Supplemental Security Income

Supplemental Security Income (SSI) ensures a minimum monthly income to persons with limited income who are blind, disabled, or elderly. Eligibility varies from state to state. Programs can include food stamps, social service, and Medicaid programs.

Healthcare for the Elderly

In the United States, elderly people have not always used as many formal healthcare services as they do today. Before Medicare and Medicaid, only a minute proportion of the federal budget went toward healthcare for older people. Formal government agencies gave little attention to the health and medical needs of the elderly. Now the pendulum has swung in the other direction. Older people are the largest group of healthcare consumers, and it is projected that the federal government will pay for about one-third of their healthcare costs by the year 2000.[41, 72]

In this period of healthcare reform, the political climate is one of change. Legislatures are looking for ways to reduce government spending. Government health insurance (Medicare) and government health assistance (Medicaid) programs will likely see changes that have ramifications for Americans of all ages.

ences have been identified as the cause for a significant degree of "noncompliance." Members of some cultural groups may perceive that medication should have a short-term effect and are not culturally conditioned to continue medication that does not produce an immediate response. Similarly, clients from some cultural backgrounds may refuse to take medication for conditions in which no obvious symptoms can be perceived by the client. Perhaps one of the most potentially dangerous asymptomatic disorders is hypertension, which has been called the "silent killer." Clients frequently are unaware of the deadly threat posed by hypertension until it is too late. Anecdotally, the author has observed black men discarding antihypertensive medication in the trash receptable outside a large urban hospital immediately after their clinic visits. When asked why they had discarded the medication, most individuals said that they believed in taking medicine only when they felt sick.

A less empirical but real consideration is the issue of the client's confidence and trust in the healthcare provider. Based on a combination of historical fact and myth, some Hispanic, Native American, black, and Asian/Pacific Islander clients neither trust nor have confidence in white healthcare providers. Similarly, some Arab-American clients find it difficult to trust Jewish healthcare providers because of long-standing historical and political rivalries in the Near and Middle East. The converse also is true (i.e., low levels of confidence and trust by Jewish clients have been reported when healthcare is provided by Arab Americans).

Other cultural considerations influence "compliance" with drug regimens. For example, factors such as traditional beliefs and practices; advice given by traditional, folk, or indigenous healers; religious beliefs and practices; and other factors may determine whether a client will take medicine prescribed by physicians and nurse practitioners. The nurse is encouraged to consider research findings in ethnopharmacology when administering, prescribing, or evaluating medications for clients from culturally diverse backgrounds. Obvious physical characteristics of the client need to be considered, such as weight-related dosage modifications for the smaller average size of Asian American clients. The nurse also needs to be cognizant of many metabolic, genetic, and environmental factors that influence culture-specific nursing care for older adults from diverse backgrounds.

1. Keltner, N. L., & Folks, D. G. (1992). Psychopharmacology update: Culture as a variable in drug therapy. *28*(1), 33–36.
2. Kroll, J., et al. (1990). Medication compliance, antidepressant blood levels, and side effects in Southeast Asian patients. *Journal of Clinical Pharmacology, 10*(4), 27–29.
3. Lefley, H. (1990). Culture and chronic mental illness. *Hospital and Community Psychiatry, 41,* 277–286.
4. Lin, T. (1986). Multiculturalism and Canadian psychiatry: Opportunities and challenges. *Canadian Journal of Psychiatry, 31*(7), 681–690.
5. Mendoza, R., et al. (1991). Ethnic psychopharmacology: The Hispanic and Native American Perspective. *Psychopharmacology Bulletin, 27*(4), 449–461.
6. Wood, A. J., & Zhou, H. H. (1991). Ethnic differences in drug disposition and responsiveness. *Clinical Pharmacokinetics, 20,* 1–24.

Medicare

Medicare (Title XVIII) was an amendment to the Social Security Act in 1965. It is a program of government health insurance designed to provide medical care to individuals age 65 or older, whatever their financial situation. It also covers disabled persons younger than 65 who meet specific Social Security criteria and people with renal failure.

Medicare has two parts. Hospital Insurance (Part A) covers inpatient hospital care, skilled nursing home care (up to 100 days/year), and some home care services. Part A is available to everyone who receives Medicare. Supplemental Medical Insurance (Part B) covers all or part of the cost of approved physician services and of other outpatient services, such as durable medical equipment. Part B is optional and is paid for in part by a monthly deduction from Social Security benefits.

A limitation of Medicare is the lack of coverage for preventive services. It does not cover most routine or preventive services, medications (except those given when a client is in the hospital), dental care, most vision care, and nonskilled long-term care. This is of particular concern, because these are the very services that are most important in delaying the onset of chronic illnesses and in improving the health and functioning of older adults.

Medicaid

Medicaid (Title XIX) legislation was passed at the same time as Medicare. Medicaid is a government health assistance program whose original intent was to meet the health needs of low-income people younger than 65. It is now an important program for older people who require long-term care. Medicaid is a federal and state govern-

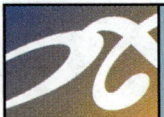

BRIDGE TO HOME HEALTHCARE

Helping Clients Manage Multiple Medications*

Clients who take several drugs often need help in understanding the best procedures and in following instructions as closely as possible. Failure to take the right drug at the right time and in the proper way often results in relapses, rehospitalizations, or nursing home placement.

Nurses have a crucial role in fostering client independence and in assessing and facilitating the client's ability to follow a prescribed medication regimen. Review all prescription and nonprescription medications, and carefully explain the administration schedule to the client and family members.

Tailoring the schedule to the client's life-style increases the likelihood that the instructions will be followed. For example, if the client goes to bed at 7:00 PM, be sure that the last dose is scheduled before that hour.

Some people need minimal help in organizing their drugs and dosages. They may benefit from any number of compliance aids that can be purchased at pharmacies, such as containers with separate compartments for each day of the week. The challenge is greater when the client has a complex medication program; reduced strength and dexterity; or a visual, hearing, cognitive, or other impairment in functional status. These people may need to purchase an automated medication dispenser that emits visual cues, such as flashing strobe lights, or audible cues, such as beeps. Dispensers that beep are ideal for people with visual impairments, while dispensers that flash a strobe light are good for people with hearing impairments.

Although units vary, an automated dispenser must above all be simple to use. One such dispenser can be programmed easily to provide a reminder at the right time for up to four times a day for a week. Not only can it manage complex schedules, but it is also tamperproof, and it dispenses only the pills needed from a supply cassette into a removable drawer. Other automated dispensers have LED screeens on which preprogrammed messages, such as "Take with food," or "Take 30 minutes before food," serve as additional reminders.

Determine how and when the client will obtain refills. If the client has no transportation, perhaps a pharmacy has a delivery service or a family member can obtain them. A social service referral is needed if the client cannot pay for prescriptions.

Monitoring the client for side effects is another important nursing intervention. Many people stop taking essential medications because of unpleasant side effects, which can sometimes be effectively managed just by changing the times of doses, for example, or by taking the medication with food.

Storage is also an important concern. Some drugs are sensitive to light; others must be secured to decrease the risk of overdoses. All medications must be safely kept away from any children who visit or live in the household.

Simplicity is the key to successful medication management. Regularly evaluate the client's regimen and household routines, and discuss with the client, family or physician any changes that would make things easier.

*By Kaye Dietrich, M.S., R.N., C.S., Midwest CompuMed, Kiel, Wisconsin.

---

ment partnership, and coverage varies across states. To qualify for Medicaid, individuals must have very limited income and assets or must be spending most of their income on medical expenses. Each state decides the specific income and asset limits. In 1973, the federal government mandated that Medicaid pay for nursing home care for all eligible adults, thus establishing Medicaid as an important source of payment for long-term care.

Healthcare Resources and Services for the Elderly

An outgrowth of the healthcare specialization of gerontology has been the recent development of innovative programs and services designed to address the unique needs of the older population (Box 5–3). The following provides information about selected community resources. For a description of continuum of care, see Table 5–2.

Acute Care

A majority of nurses who care for older adults provide that care in hospital settings. Hospitals are developing new ways of delivering care to older adults to improve both its quality and efficiency. Some hospitals are establishing geriatric units with specially trained staff who work together as an interdisciplinary team.[31] The team typically includes nurses, a geriatrician, a pharmacist, a social worker, various rehabilitation therapists (e.g., speech, physical, and occupational therapists), and mental health professionals (e.g., psychologists or psychiatrists). The focus of these programs is to help older adults with complex problems to remain at their highest possible level of functioning. Geropsychiatric and geriatric rehabilitation programs are other new models of hospital-based geriatric care that are evolving to address the unique needs of older people. Geriatric evaluation teams serve as a resource for physicians who have elderly clients who are in need of comprehensive physical and psychosocial evaluations.

Box 5–3. Resources

American Association of Homes for the Aging
1129 20th St. N.W.
Suite 400
Washington, DC 20036
(202)296–5960

American Association of Retired Persons
601 E St. N.W.
Washington, DC 20049
(202)434–2277

Gray Panthers
311 S. Juniper St., #601
Philadelphia, PA 19107
(215)545–6555

National Association of State Units on Aging
600 Maryland Ave. S.W.
Suite 208, West Wing
Washington, DC 20024
(202)484–7182

National Council on the Aging
600 Maryland Ave. S.W.
Suite 100, West Wing
Washington, DC 20024
(202)479–1200

Legal Counsel for the Elderly
601 E St. N.W.
Washington, DC 20049
(202)434–2120

National Senior Citizens Law Center
2025 M St. N.W.
Suite 400
Washington, DC 20036
(202)887–5280

Long-Term Care

Long-term care refers to a continuum of services, including medical, nursing, social, and personal care in a variety of settings. Long-term care services provide care for people at varying levels of dependence who will require care for an extended period. As their functional abilities change, elderly people use different services according to their level of dependence and availability of social support. Table 5–2 outlines some of these services.

Nursing Home Care

The close association between nursing home care and long-term care arises from the late 1970s, when nursing homes were the primary resource (and usually the only resource) for people who needed long-term care. Nursing homes are licensed by the state. Many are certified for Medicare and/or Medicaid reimbursement. About 5% of the population of people older than 65 years is in nursing homes at any given time. People in this age group have a 50% chance of being in a nursing home at some point in their life.[45] The following are characteristics of typical nursing home populations:

- Average age of 82 years
- No living spouse
- Women outnumber men by a ratio of 3:1
- Over half have a progressive dementing condition and/or arthritis, cardiovascular disease, or both
- One third have impaired vision and/or impaired hearing
- Most require assistance in several or all ADL
- Twenty percent return home, and 70% stay for longer than 1 year[52, 71]

Three levels of nursing care are provided in nursing homes, with many facilities offering all three levels. Skilled care is for persons who require highly skilled nursing care. These residents may have feeding tubes, tracheotomies, extensive wounds, infections, or medications that require 24-hour-a-day supervision and treatment by a registered nurse under the direction of a doctor. Intermediate care is a moderate level of nursing care that is suitable for persons who need supervision and moderate assistance with ADL and medications. Personal care is the third level and is suitable for individuals who cannot live alone and need a low level of nursing care. It provides supervision and minimal assistance with ADL and medications.

Subacute Care

Many hospitals and nursing homes have added subacute care units to their facilities. People in subacute units typically have short-term stays. They are generally either chronically ill or are recuperating from an illness or from surgery and need skilled nursing care and other health services, but do not require hospitalization. Subacute units usually provide rehabilitation programs, social activities, and supervision. The goal is to discharge the individual back to home. The recent dramatic changes in the delivery of healthcare to older adults have resulted in increasing numbers of people being admitted to nursing homes from hospitals for short-term subacute nursing care. Thus, the picture of the "typical" nursing home resident would accurately depict a long-term client, but it is not applicable to the many older people who are in nursing homes for subacute short-term care.

Home Care

Home care is a range of health and supportive services provided in the home for people who require assistance in meeting their healthcare needs. Services include skilled nursing, physical therapy, occupational therapy, speech therapy, social work, nutritional counseling, and provision of some medical supplies and equipment. Also included are personal care services, such as assistance with bathing, dressing, and toileting, meal preparation, and housekeeping. Services are delivered by registered and licensed practical nurses, therapists, and certified homemaker–home health aides. Most of these services are covered by

Table 5–2. Continuum of Care: Community Resources/Housing Options*

Functional Level of Care	Community Resources and Services		Living and Housing Options
	In the Home	*In the Community*	
Older adults of all functional levels		Support groups (e.g., for illness or bereavement) Advocacy services Outpatient clinics Mental health clinics Private physicians	
Older adults who are functionally independent	Gatekeepers	Senior centers Meal sites	Own home Retirement apartment House sharing
Older adults who need some help with IADL	Chore services Housekeeping Escort Transportation Emergency response system Home modifications Home-delivered meals Friendly visitors Telephone reassurance Gatekeepers	Senior centers Meal sites Adult day care Case management Respite care	Retirement facilities Assisted-living facilities Board-and-care homes Congregate housing
Older adults who need some help with IADL and ADL	All of the above, plus: Personal care services Home health aides Public health nurse Respite care at home	Adult day care Case management Respite care	Assisted-living facilities Board-and-care homes
Older adults who need help with most IADL and ADL	All of the above	Adult day healthcare Case management	Nursing homes
Older adults who are acutely ill, need rehabilitation, or are dying	All of the above, plus: Visiting nurse Visiting rehabilitation therapist Hospice care at home	Adult day healthcare rehabilitation Case management	Hospitals Rehabilitation facilities Nursing homes

* Availability of services varies from community to community.
Data from Ebersole, P. & Hess, P. (Eds.). (1994). *Toward healthy aging*. St. Louis, Mosby–Year Book; and Miller, C. A. (1995). Nursing care of older adults, theory and practice (2nd ed.) (pp. 553–565). Philadelphia: J. B. Lippincott.

Medicare and other health insurance for people who meet the specific criteria.

Hospice Care

Hospice care is a program of care for the terminally ill and their families that emphasizes alleviation of pain rather than medical cure. The goal of hospice care is to keep the individual as comfortable and pain-free as possible. Physical, psychological, social, and spiritual care are given to the dying person and the family by a team of doctors, nurses, social workers, clergy, and volunteers. Although hospice services may be provided in special hospice settings, most hospice care is provided in the individual's home.

Respite Care

Respite care provides short-term relief for family members who care for an older person at home. The elderly may receive respite care at home or at locations such as day-care centers and healthcare facilities. Trained individuals care for the older persons while the family member is away for a few hours, several days, or even several weeks.

Case Management

Case management is becoming an accepted method for providing comprehensive, individualized, and economic care of elders with complex health needs. The case manager functions as the primary care agent and coordinates acute and long-term care services. The manager serves as a client advocate who has a comprehensive view of the situation and can help solve problems as they arise.

Adult Day Care

Community-based adult day-care centers have a goal of maintaining or improving the functional abilities of impaired older persons. Typically, participants need supervision or assistance in several areas of functioning. Although most suffer from a dementing illness and are cognitively impaired, others are primarily affected by depression or functional impairments. These individuals cannot be left alone during the day when family members are at work or are unavailable. They come to day-care programs and return home in the evening. Adult day care offers a variety of services ranging from healthcare to social programs. Centers usually emphasize either rehabilitation or social activities. Few health insurance policies cover adult day-care programs, leaving most of the cost to be paid by families.

Community Programs and Services

A variety of services are available to help people maintain independence and to live in their chosen environment as long as possible. As the individual's functional levels change, many services can be made available in the individual's home; or they may be available in the community (see Table 5–2). Some services are covered by Medicare, whereas others require a fee or payment based on a sliding-fee scale.

Senior Centers

Senior centers offer a variety of social, health, nutritional, educational, and recreational services. They give older people the opportunity to gather for social activity. Transportation is often provided by centers between home and the center and to other activities in the community. Besides being meeting places, senior centers offer counseling, special trips, legal services, and advice on financial matters.

Nutritional Services

Nutritional services provide inexpensive, nutritious meals in communal settings, such as senior centers, housing projects, churches, synagogues, and schools. This service helps to promote social contact among older people. Transportation is often provided to and from meal sites.

Meal Delivery Services

Hot, nutritious home-delivered meals are provided once (and sometimes twice) a day, 5 days a week, to persons who are unable to cook for themselves. Special diets are available.

Visitation Services

Various services provide regular visits to either homebound or institutionalized elderly people who may be lonely and need companionship. Volunteers stop in regularly to do whatever a concerned friend might do: sit and chat, write letters, run local errands, and, equally important, just listen.

Telephone Services

Telephone services, often staffed by volunteers, provide daily telephone calls to people who live alone. A daily telephone call by a regular caller at a prearranged time can serve as the best reassurance that all is well. If the older person does not answer the phone, neighbors or police are alerted.

Gatekeeper Programs

Gatekeeper programs are frequently initiated as a public service by local agencies. If people who visit an elderly person's house routinely (e.g., utilities company employees, U.S. Postal Service employees, paper delivery persons, home-delivered meal volunteers) notice newspapers piled up by the door, mail overflowing the mailbox, or other possible signs of trouble, they notify their supervisor. The supervisor, in turn, notifies appropriate social service workers, who check to see if help is needed.

Chore Services

Chore service offers help in and around the home, including minor repairs, heavy housecleaning, and yard work. This service is especially beneficial to elders who are independent in most areas, but who require help with unique tasks.

Transport and Escort Services

Transport and escort services are available through various community programs. Transportation for disabled or handicapped elderly can be arranged for medical visits or for shopping trips. Frequently, an escort can be provided to ride and remain with the elder throughout the trip.

Emergency Response Systems

Emergency response systems (ERSs) provide a link between the elder living alone and emergency services. The ERS, when activated, can dispatch police, an ambulance, or other appropriate services to the individual's home. ERS alarms may be worn as jewelry (necklaces and bracelets), may be attached to the telephone, or may be placed next to the bed or in the bathroom. This service usually requires a fee that is not covered by Medicare or Medicaid.

Housing Options for the Elderly

A time often comes when maintaining the family home grows difficult for an elderly person, or when the individual no longer has the choice. A variety of options are available that, with thought and planning, can allow the older adult to remain active and to maintain a comfortable life-style in a more manageable setting.

House Sharing

The older person may share a house or apartment with an adult child or with one or more unrelated people. Each occupant has a private bedroom and shares the rest of the dwelling, expenses, and chores.

Congregate Housing

Congregate housing offers individual apartments within a specially designed, multi-unit dwelling. It offers older persons the support services they need to continue an independent life-style. The unit provides private living quarters and may provide meals in a central dining room, transportation, and social and recreational activities. Housekeeping and assistance with bathing, dressing, or other personal care may be arranged.

Board-and-Care Homes

Board-and-care homes are appropriate for elders who are not in need of professional nursing but who need personal care and assistance. These homes usually serve six to eight residents in a homelike setting.

Assisted-Living Facilities

The assisted-living option allows older adults to live in their own apartment but share a common area for meals and social activities. Assistance with laundry, housekeeping, transportation, personal care, and medication supervision is provided, as is some degree of protective supervision or 24-hour care.

Life-Care or Continuing-Care Retirement Communities

Older adults reside in a housing development designed to provide a full range of services and accommodations to meet each resident's changing needs. The development includes independent housing, congregate housing, assisted living, and nursing home care. Continuing care communities may require a lump sum entrance fee and monthly fees. Lifetime housing and a full range of healthcare and other services, including nursing care when needed, is guaranteed.

Ethical and Legal Issues Affecting the Elderly

Residents' Rights

The rights of individuals in institutions of all types are mandated by federal and state laws and the Constitution. Legal rights vary according to the setting and individual competence. In nursing homes, residents' rights are posted in a place visible to all, and they are reviewed with the individual soon after admission to the facility.

Ombudsman Organizations

Advocacy organizations for nursing home residents began between 1975 and 1979. Activities of these organizations include complaint resolution, confrontation and/or negotiation with nursing home staff, community education, legal intervention, and legislative reform. The nursing home ombudsman program is mandated by the Older Americans Act, with each state having an Office of the State Ombudsman to which all programs report.

The Omnibus Budget Reconciliation Act (OBRA)

In 1986, Congress mandated a comprehensive evaluation of nursing homes in response to cited examples of poor quality of care in nursing homes. Recommendations from this study resulted in the Omnibus Budget Reconciliation Act (OBRA), which was passed in 1987 and implemented in 1990. OBRA required that each resident in a long-term care facility be at his or her highest level of physical, mental, and psychosocial well-being, and that the facility accomplish this in an atmosphere that emphasizes residents' rights. Delivery of care and quality of care have changed dramatically since 1990.

Competence

According to Miller,[52] competence is the ability to adequately fulfill one's role and handle one's affairs. Although adult patients are presumed to be competent to make decisions concerning their own treatment, the patient's family or other caregivers may not agree with the treatment choice and may seek to have the patient declared incompetent. Before a guardian can be appointed, a competency hearing is held. If the person is declared by the court to be incompetent, the judge may assign either partial or full guardianship. With partial guardianship, the incompetent person is permitted to make limited deci-

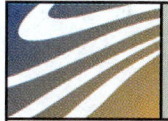

ETHICAL ISSUES IN NURSING

How Can You Be a Client Advocate to the Elderly?

Mr. Tupman is an 84-year-old Ozark native and retired carpenter who has been admitted to the surgical service for evaluation of necrotic changes in his right foot. He is a widower of 10 years and has been residing in a rural nursing home in the Ozarks for the past 3 years. It was decided that he would reside there when his only living relatives, a son and his family, moved to Arizona for a job advancement.

Although Mr. Tupman had been able to walk with assistance, his motivation to perform any activities for himself over the past year has declined markedly. Within the past few months he has required assistance with eating, dressing, and personal care. Medications have included insulin, Digoxin, Lasix, and Paxil. He has evidence of occasional short-term memory losses, and frequent crying spells have been reported; he expresses feelings of loneliness, worthlessness, and being a financial burden, and he looks forward to dying. He misses not being able to see his son and grandchildren.

Mr. Tupman's work-up reveals a progressive gangrenous lesion of the right foot secondary to severe peripheral vascular disease. The surgeon indicates that an above-the-knee amputation must be performed as soon as possible. When approached to sign the operative permit, he refuses and informs the physician that it would be foolish for him to go through such an ordeal when he has been praying to die.

His son arrives from Arizona and attempts to convince his father that surgery must be done. The son appeals to his father saying, "I cannot live with myself if I allow you to just lie there and die!" Mr. Tupman quietly assures his son that he has chosen to die as a whole person, that he is ready to be with his wife, and that this is a personal choice, not a guilt-laden choice for the son to make.

Consultation between the surgeon and the son results in a decision to proceed with the amputation with the signature of the son. The reason for circumventing Mr. Tupman's decision is that his age and physical and mental condition prevent him from making a rational decision in a life-or-death matter. Mr. Tupman appeals to the nurse to help him; she responds that she will try to help him do what he wants to do. The nurse contacts the surgeon to try to intervene, but is told the decision has been made.

The major ethical issue in this situation is the client's expressed desire to die by refusing the amputation, and that desire being denied through the action of the surgeon and Mr. Tupman's son. The subject of ethics revolves around decision-making (right versus wrong values) and determining what is behind judgments that people make. Nurses are often required to face ethical dilemmas. Ethical beliefs develop from one's morals, integrity, and values. That belief system becomes part of the unique relationship between the nurse and the patient involved in a decision-making process. In this case, the nurse's relationship to the patient is that of an advocate. The goal is to help the patient become clear about what he *wants* to do. The nurse advocate aids the patient to distinguish and clarify his values and, after sufficient self-examination, to reach decisions that represent reaffirmed or new values. Through this process, the patient's decision is truly self-determined.

Relating this to Mr. Tupman, the nurse should have intervened more persistently. The nurse has the opportunity and responsibility to know and observe the strengths, weaknesses, and complexities unique to the client. This allows an understanding of his ways and beliefs by knowing him in a holistic manner. Fragmentary knowledge of a patient does not foster successful advocacy.

Some issues the nurse should have explored are as follows:

1. What does the aging process mean to Mr. Tupman? Despite society's traditional negative view of the elderly, means are available to enhance the value of living, regardless of the aging process. Mr. Tupman needs to be aware of this. Perhaps just being in a nursing home in Arizona, where periodic family visits would be possible, could make life worth living for Mr. Tupman.

2. What does Mr. Tupman consider quality of life to be? Perhaps living with an amputation is the final insult to an already apparently dehumanized life-style. One's view of the quality of life is very much what determines the desire to live or die.

3. Is Mr. Tupman aware of the physical ramifications of the decision to forgo surgery? Gangrenous lesions are frequently very painful, progress slowly, and could eventually cause a systemic outcome.

4. What is the son's understanding of his father's reaction? The son needs to understand that his father may simply need a sufficient reason to live, to see aging as a valuable human experience rather than just a period of slow deterioration. Old age should not be a factor in this ethical decision; rather, what is the meaning that aging and life have, or can have, for Mr. Tupman?

5. What does Mr. Tupman believe his treatment will be with or without the surgery? The nurse should support the client and ensure that he realizes her support, regardless of his decision. Should he refuse surgery, he must be assured that his care will be continuous and supportive and that he will be as pain-free as possible.

To be caring practitioners, we must believe in the dignity and worth of the person and understand fully the meaning of values, choices, and priority systems from which individual decisions are made. As an advocate for patients, we must uphold the belief in self-determination through informed decision-making. The conflict between self-determination and our own personal values and technological advances must be reduced. The dignity of the human being must be upheld.

sions. When full guardianship is assigned, the person loses all his or her rights to make decisions. Frequently, the nurse is called on to participate in these hearings.

Autonomy

Autonomy is the personal freedom to direct one's own life as long as it does not impinge on the rights of others. An autonomous person is capable of rational thought and can recognize the need for problem solving. This individual can identify problems, search for alternatives, and select solutions that allow continued personal freedom, as long as the rights and property of others are not harmed. Loss of autonomy, and therefore independence, is a very real fear among the elderly. When issues concerning personal autonomy arise, nurses should refer older people to the appropriate community agencies for further evaluation.

The Self-Determination Act

The Patient Self-Determination Act (PSDA) is designed to protect the healthcare consumer by requiring all providers of Medicare and Medicaid services to inform patients of their right to refuse treatment, provide information about their state's provisions concerning advanced directives, and include documentation of patients' advanced directives in their medical records. This act is binding for hospitals, nursing homes, home health agencies, hospices, and health maintenance organizations.

Advance Directives

Advance directives is an umbrella term for legally binding documents that allow competent people to document the medical procedures that they would want to have done should they become unable to make such decisions. These documents include the living will and the durable power of attorney for healthcare. Studies have shown that most older people expect and anticipate that "someone" will know what to do when such a time comes, and they prefer family members, rather than healthcare providers, to be surrogate decision makers.[43, 50, 52, 60]

Nurses have an obligation to patients and their surrogate decision makers to help in making these decisions. Nursing interventions include providing accurate information on rights and statutes. Legislation regarding advanced directives varies from state to state, and healthcare providers need to be aware of the law in their state, listen to patient and family needs, act as liaison with physicians when necessary, or refer individuals to proper resources. Nurses can encourage older people to talk to their families to relay their wishes before a crisis occurs. When an advance directive does exist, it is the nurse's responsibility to inform other members of the healthcare team and to make certain that it is readily accessible on the chart. The nurse also should make certain that the older person's family, especially the designated surrogate, is aware of the document and its contents.

Living Wills

Living wills evolved as part of right-to-die statutes, and many changes have been made since the first legislation was enacted in the 1970s in California. In most states, a living will is in effect until the writer creates a new one or destroys the document. It can be used only for terminal illness or when death is imminent.[52]

Living wills are legal documents, now recognized in the District of Columbia and in nearly every state.[50] Their purpose is to allow a person to specify what type of medical treatment is desired if the individual becomes incapacitated. People must be competent to initiate a living will. The individual retains the right to revoke the document after it is written.

Durable Power of Attorney for Healthcare

Durable power of attorney for healthcare is an advance directive that names a surrogate to make healthcare decisions if the individual cannot make them. The document usually provides the surrogate with written guidelines stating the person's wishes, such as withholding or withdrawal of life support. Like other powers of attorney, the durable power of attorney for healthcare must be initiated when the person is competent. It can go into effect immediately, and the person does not have to be terminally ill.

Conclusions

Opportunities to care for elders exist in all settings. The number of elderly people requiring medical and surgical treatment is considerable. The proportion of all hospital patient days accounted for by people over 65 years of age was 38% in 1980 and is expected to rise to 58% by 2000.[19] Many of these hospitalized elders will be discharged to their homes with continued care needs. The role of the nurse in acute care and community settings—to act as an advocate and to promote the physical and mental well-being of elders—will be extremely important.

Given that the elderly are the fastest growing segment of the population in the country, every nurse involved with adult healthcare will undoubtedly at some point be challenged to meet the unique needs of elderly patients. It is essential that a holistic perspective be used in the consideration of the physiologic, psychological, and sociologic needs of elders.

Bibliography

1. Allen, J. E. (1992). *Key federal requirements for nursing facilities.* New York: Springer Publishing.
2. American Nurses' Association. (1987). *Standards of gerontological nursing practice.* Kansas City, MO: Author.
3. American Psychiatric Association. (1994). *Diagnostic and statistical manual of mental disorders* (4th ed., rev.). Washington, DC: Author.
4. Anderson, M. A. (1994). A challenge to nursing education. *Geriatric Nursing, 15*(5), 237.
5. Anetzberger, G. J. (1990). Abuse, neglect and self-neglect: Issues of vulnerability. In Z. Hanel, P. Ehrlich, & R. Hubbard (Eds.), *The vulnerable aged: People, services, and policies* (pp. 140–148). New York: Springer Publishing.
6. Batt, L. (1989). Managing delirium: Implications for geropsychiatric nurses. *Journal of Psychosocial Nursing and Mental Health Services, 27*(5), 22–25.
7. Baum, C., et al. (1988). Prescription drug use 1984 and over time. *Medical Care, 26*(2), 105–114.
8. Beare, P. G., & Graveley, E. (1995). Health teaching and compliance. In M. Stanley & P. Beare (Eds.), *Gerontological nursing* (pp 63–96). Philadelphia: F. A. Davis.
9. Besdine, R. W. (1983). The educational utility of comprehensive functional assessment in the elderly. *Journal of the American Geriatrics Society, 31*, 651–656.
10. Binder, E., & Robins, L. (1990). Cognitive impairment and length of hospital stay in older persons. *Journal of the American Geriatrics Society, 38*, 759–766.
11. Bliesmer, M. (1990). Gerontological nursing practice standards: Achievement and importance. *Clinical Nurse Specialist, 4*(1), 10–14.
12. Block, M. R., & Sinnott, J. D. (Eds.). (1979). *The battered elder syndrome: An exploratory study.* College Park, MD: University of Maryland, Center on Aging.
13. Buckwalter, K. (1995). Depression and suicide. In M. Stanley & P. Beare (Eds.), *Gerontological nursing* (pp. 383–399). Philadelphia: F. A. Davis.
14. Burnside, I. (1988). *Nursing and the aged.* New York: McGraw-Hill.
15. Butler, R. N., & Lewis, M. I. (1977). *Aging and mental health.* St. Louis: C. V. Mosby.
16. Chastain, S (1992). The accidental addict: Are you hooked on your prescriptions? *Modern Maturity, 35*(1), 39–42.
17. Darrach, B. (1992). The war on aging. *Life, 15*(10), 32–45.
18. Darnell, J. C., et al. (1986). Medication use by ambulatory elderly: An inhome survey. *Journal of the American Geriatrics Society, 34*(1), 1–4.
19. Davies, H. (1991). Dementia and delirium. In W. C. Chenitz, J. T. Strone, & S. A. Salisbury (Eds.), *Clinical gerontological nursing* (pp 455–489). Philadelphia: W. B. Saunders.
20. Douglass, R. L., & Hickey, T. (1983). Domestic neglect and abuse of the elderly: Research findings and systems perspectives for service delivery planning. In J. I. Kosberg (Ed.), *Abuse and maltreatment of the elderly: Causes and interventions* (pp. 115–133). Littleton, MA: John Wright.
21. Ebersole, P., & Hess, P. (Eds.). (1994). *Toward healthy aging.* St. Louis: Mosby–Year Book.
22. Eliopoulos, C. (1987). *Gerontological nursing.* Philadelphia: J. B. Lippincott.
23. Folstein, M. F., Folstein, S., McHugh, P. R. (1975). Mini mental state: A practical method for grading the cognitive states of patients for the clinician. *Journal of Psychiatric Research, 12*, 189–198.
24. Foreman, M. (1989). Confusion in the hospitalized elderly: Incidence, onset, and associated factors. *Research in Nursing and Health, 12*, 21–29.
25. Garrett, J. (1987). Multiple losses in older adults. *Journal of Gerontological Nursing, 13*(8), 8–12.
26. Gehi, M., et al. (1980). Is there a need for admission and discharge screening for the medically ill? *General Hospital Psychiatry, 3*, 186–191.
27. Hatcher, A. (1989). From one addiction to another: Life after alcohol and drug abuse. *Nurse Practitioner, 14*(11), 13–16.
28. *Healthy people 2000.* (1991). Washington, DC: U.S. Government Printing Office.
29. Hogstel, M., & Wooten, P. (1995). Mental health wellness strategies for successful aging. In M. Stanley & P. Beare (Eds.), *Gerontological nursing* (pp. 17–27). Philadelphia: F. A. Davis.
30. Hogstel, M. O. (Ed.). (1992). *Clinical manual of gerontological nursing.* St. Louis: Mosby–Year Book.
31. Inouye, S. K., et al. (1993). The Yale Geriatric Care Program: A model of care to prevent functional decline in hospitalized elderly patients. *Journal of the American Geriatrics Society, 41*, 1345–1352.
32. Jecker, N. (1995). Ethical issues in gerontological nursing. In M. Stanley & P. Beare (Eds.), *Gerontological nursing* (pp. 51–62). Philadelphia: F. A. Davis.
33. Jeffrion, L. & Seuszler, L. (1995). The gastrointestinal system and its problems in the elderly with nutritional considerations. In M. Stanley & P. Beare (Eds.), *Gerontological nursing* (pp. 241–245). Philadelphia: F. A. Davis.
34. Johnson, J., Sullivan, E., & Gottlieb, G. (1987). Delirium in elderly patients on internal medicine services. *Journal of the American Geriatrics Society, 35*, 972.
35. Johnson, L. H. & Johnson, M. A. (1995). Dementia in the elderly. In M. Stanley & P. Beare (Eds.), *Gerontological nursing* (pp. 493–504). Philadelphia: F. A. Davis.
36. Kane, R. A., & Kane, R. (1981). *Assessing the elderly* (pp. 59–64). Lexington, MA: Lexington Books.
37. Katz, S., et al. (1963). Studies of illness in the aged. The index of ADL: A standardized measure of biological and psychosocial functions. *Journal of the American Medical Association, 185*, 915–919.
38. King, K., Diamond, M., & McCanie, K. (1987). Coping with relocation. *Geriatric Nursing, 8*(5), 258–261.
39. Lau, E., & Kosberg, J. (1979). Abuse of the elderly by informal care providers. *Aging, 299–300*, 10–15.
40. Levkoff, S., Besdine, R., & Wetle, T. (1986). Acute confusional states (delirium) in the hospitalized elderly. In C. Eisdorfer (Ed.), *Annual review of gerontology and geriatrics* (vol. 6, pp. 1–26). New York: Springer.
41. Lipowski, A. (1983). Transient cognitive disorders (delirium, acute confusional states) in the elderly. *American Journal of Psychiatry, 140*, 1426–1436.
42. Lipowski, Z. (1984). Acute confusional states (delirium) in the elderly. In M. Albert (Ed.), *Clinical neurology of aging* (pp. 277–297). New York: Oxford University Press.
43. Madson, S. K. (1993). Patient self-determination act: Implications for long-term care. *Journal of Gerontological Nursing, 19*(2), 15–18.
44. Mahoney, F. I., & Barthel, D. W. (1965). Functional evaluation: The Barthel index. *Maryland State Medical Journal, 14*, 61–65.
45. McConnel, C. E. (1984). A note on the lifetime risk of nursing home residency. *The Gerontologist, 24*, 193–198.
46. McConnell, E. S., & Matteson, M. (1988). Psychosocial problems associated with aging. In M. Matteson & E. McConnell (Eds.), *Gerontological nursing: Concepts and practice* (pp. 482–527). Philadelphia: W. B. Saunders.
47. McCracken, A. (1987). Emotional impact of possession loss. *Journal of Gerontological Nursing, 13*(2), 14–19.
48. McCurren, C. (1991). Hospitalized elders: Attention deficits and confusion. Doctoral dissertation, University of Kentucky, Lexington.
49. McKenna, W. A. (1995). Transcultural perspectives in nursing care of the elderly. In M. M. Andrews, & J. S. Bole (Eds.), *Transcultural concepts in nursing care* (pp. 203–234). Philadelphia: J. B. Lippincott.
50. Meyer, C. (1993). "End-of-life" care: Patients' choices, nurses' challenges. *American Journal of Nursing, 93*(2), 40–47.
51. Mikulencak, M. (1993). The 'graying of America'—changing what nurses need to know. *The American Nurse, 25*(7), 1,12.
52. Miller, C. A. (1995) *Nursing care of older adults, theory and practice* (2nd ed.). (pp. 553–565). Philadelphia: J. B. Lippincott.
53. Monicken, D. (1991). Immobility and functional mobility in the elderly. In W. C. Chenitz, J. T. Stone, & S. A. Salisbury (Eds.), *Clinical gerontological nursing* (pp. 233–245). Philadelphia: W. B. Saunders.
54. O'Malley, J., et al. (1979). *Elder abuse in Massachusetts: A survey of professionals and para-professionals.* Boston: Legal Research and Services for the Elderly.

55. Palmateer, L., & McCartney, J. (1985). Do nurses know when patients have cognitive deficits? *Journal of Gerontological Nursing, 11*(2), 6–7, 10–12, 15–16.

56. Patrick, M. (1993). Characteristics of older people and introduction to theories of aging. In D. Carnevali & M. Patrick (Eds.), *Nursing management for the elderly* (3rd ed.) (pp. 87–98). Philadelphia: J. B. Lippincott.

57. Program Resources Development, American Association of Retired Persons. (1994). *A profile of older Americans: 1994* [brochure]. Washington, DC: Author.

58. Rabins, P., & Folstein, M. (1982). Delirium and dementia: Diagnostic criteria and fatality rates. *British Journal of Psychiatry, 140,* 149–153.

59. Ramsdell, J., et al. (1990). Evaluation of cognitive impairment in the elderly. *Journal of General Internal Medicine, 5,* 55–64.

60. Sapp, M., & Bliesmer, M. (1995). Health promotion/protection approach to meeting elders' healthcare needs through public policy and standards of care. In M. Stanely & P. Beare (Eds.) *Gerontological nursing* (pp. 3–12). Philadelphia: F. A. Davis.

61. Shanas, E., & Maddox, G. L. (1985). Health, health resources and the utilization of care. In R. H. Binstock & E. Shanas (Eds.), *Handbook of aging and the social sciences* (pp. 696–726). New York: Van Nostrand Reinhold.

62. Shawler, E., et al. (1992). Clinical considerations: Surrogate decision making for hospitalized elders. *Journal of Gerontological Nursing, 18*(6), 5–11.

63. Shugars, D. A., O'Neil, E. H., Bader, J. D. (Eds.). (1994). *Health America: Practitioners for 2005.* Durham, NC: The Pew Health Professions Commission.

64. Steinmetz, S. K. (1988). *Duty bound: Elder abuse and family care.* Newbury Park, CA: Sage Publications.

65. Stewart, R. B., et al. (1991). Changing patterns of therapeutic agents in the elderly: A ten-year overview. *Age and Aging, 20*(3), 182–188.

66. Tideiksaar, R. (1990). Falls in the elderly: Etiology and prevention. In G. Bosker, et al. (Eds.), *Geriatric emergency medicine*. St. Louis: Mosby–Year Book.

67. Trainor, P. A. (1988). Over the counter drugs: Count them in. *Geriatric Nursing, 9*(5), 298–299.

68. Tripp-Reimer, T., Johnson, R., & Tios, H. (1995). Cultural dimensions in gerontological nursing. In M. Stanley & P. Beare (Eds.), *Gerontological nursing* (pp. 28–36). Philadelphia: F. A. Davis.

69. U.S. Bureau of the Census (1991). *Statistical abstracts of the U.S.* (111th ed.). Washington, DC: U.S. Government Printing Office.

70. U.S. House Select Committee on Aging. (1986). *The rights of America's institutionalized aged: Lost in confinement* (Committee Publication No. 99–543). Washington, DC: U.S. Government Printing Office.

71. U.S. House Select Committee on Aging (1990). *Elder abuse: A decade of shame and inaction.* Washington, DC: U.S. Government Printing Office.

72. U.S. Senate Special Committee on Aging. (1989). *Developments in aging: 1988* (Committee Publication No. 101–4). Washington, DC: U.S. Government Printing Office.

73. Valanis B., Yeaworth, R., & Mullis, M. (1987). Alcohol use among bereaved and nonbereaved older persons. *Journal of Gerontological Nursing, 13*(5), 26–32.

74. Williams, M., et al. (1985). Predictors of acute confusional states in hospitalized elderly patients. *Research in Nursing and Health, 8,* 31–40.

75. Wolf, R. S., Godkin, M. A., & Pillemer, K. A. (1984). *Elder abuse and neglect: Final report from three model projects.* Worcester, MA: University of Massachusetts Medical Center, University Center on Aging.

76. Wray, L. A. (1992). Health policy and ethnic diversity in older Americans: Dissonance or harmony? *Western Journal of Medicine, Special Edition, 157,* 357–361.

Chronic Conditions

Mary Jane Garrett

Chronic conditions constitute a major challenge to healthcare providers and healthcare delivery systems. The number of clients with chronic conditions is increasing with the ever-growing number of elderly people and the increasing number of people who survive major illness. Because chronic conditions are long-term, often lifelong, the client needs to learn to adapt to the condition. Helping a client adapt to a chronic illness challenges the healthcare system, healthcare providers, and society as a whole. Adaptation to chronic conditions is a complex and ongoing process that involves physiologic, social, psychological, technological, and time factors.

Chronic conditions have been defined as "long-term health problems due to an irreversible disorder, an accumulation of disorders, or a latent disease."[18] Chronic conditions have also been seen as permanent disabilities that interfere with a person's ordinary physical, psychological, or social functioning.[15] The term "chronic condition" is the preferred term to describe these problems. "Chronic conditions" is consistent with the concept of health as multidimensional, with some dimensions of health existing until death. Using this broad definition it is apparent that chronic conditions are very prevalent. Whether you practice in an acute care setting, ambulatory setting, long-term settings, or in the community, you will be providing nursing care to clients with chronic conditions.

Chronic conditions are a major cause of morbidity (disease) and mortality (death). Recognition of chronic conditions as a major health problem, changes in social and professional values, and a growing body of knowledge related to chronic conditions are contributing to a paradigm shift in healthcare. The shift involves changes in philosophies about health, chronic illness, disability, and the roles of healthcare professionals, clients, and families in the management of chronic conditions. Increased emphasis is being given to prevention of chronic conditions and finding ways to help persons live with and shape the course of their chronic conditions.

Planning nursing care that strengthens the abilities of the client and family to live with and shape the course of the client's chronic condition is facilitated by knowledge of (1) the time pattern of chronic conditions; (2) commonalities in physical, psychological, and social adaptation to different chronic conditions; (3) general information related to applications of nursing in the care of people with chronic conditions; and (4) patterns of healthcare delivery addressing problems of people with chronic conditions. This chapter addresses each of these aspects.

The Stages of a Chronic Condition

In general, chronic conditions evolve in a typical pattern. Various terms are used to describe this process. It can be called the *course of illness,* the *trajectory,*[4] or *time phases.*[37] Awareness of the effect of time on chronic disease creates an appreciation for the challenges experienced by clients and their families living with chronic conditions. Awareness of the pattern also promotes appreciation of the fact that management of chronic conditions is carried out largely by clients and families in the home environment. Knowledge of the time pattern of chronic conditions is helping to broaden the focus of healthcare to include all levels of prevention and to increase the percentage of healthcare dollars allocated to prevention.

The general course of a chronic condition is depicted in Table 6–1. The three stages of the pattern seen in all chronic conditions are the (1) prediagnostic, (2) diagnostic, and (3) chronic stages. Some chronic conditions also have a terminal stage.

Prediagnostic Stage

In the prediagnostic stage, manifestations of chronic conditions are vague or absent. Risk factors common to one or more chronic conditions may be present. You will find, later in this book, chapters devoted to specific

Table 6–1. The Stages of a Chronic Condition	
Stage	**Clinical Manifestations**

Prediagnosis	None or vague
	Risk factors present:
	  Diet high in salt, fat, sugars
	  Diet low in complex carbohydrates
	    (fruits and vegetables)
	  Genetic predisposition
	  Increased age
	  Cultural risk factors
	  Life-style factors (inactivity, diet,
	    stress, smoking, alcohol, drugs,
	    risky behaviors)
	  Environmental threats

Diagnosis	Vague to life-threatening Onset gradual or sudden
Chronic	Mild, moderate, or severe (controlled) Remission or exacerbation Changes in physical function may be progressive or stabilized
Terminal	End-stage body system(s) failure Death expected within 6 months

chronic conditions. In this chapter, a brief overview of chronic conditions in general is presented.

Some risk factors are modifiable and others are not. Modifying personal and environmental risk factors can prevent the development or extend the prediagnostic phase of some chronic conditions. For example, not smoking or stopping smoking is a behavior under the individual's control that decreases the risk of developing chronic conditions in the respiratory, cardiovascular, and other systems. These chronic conditions include asthma, emphysema, bronchiectasis, coronary artery disease, angina, myocardial infarction, hypertension, and cancer. A low fat diet decreases the risk of obesity, coronary disease, diabetes, hypertension, stroke, and cancer. Seat belts protect against injury in the event of a vehicular accident. Reducing high levels of stress may help to reduce the risk of cardiovascular disease, peptic ulcers, asthma, ulcerative colitis, multiple sclerosis, cancer, and accidental trauma. Immunization against specific health problems can prevent the development of other diseases.

Diagnostic Stage

In the diagnostic stage, the client recognizes that something is wrong, seeks medical attention, and is diagnosed with a disorder. In some cases, chronic conditions occur as sequelae to acute illness, trauma, or treatment. In these instances, the healthcare provider may simply inform the client that he or she has a given disorder. This stage is seen in clients of all ages, because chronic disorders affect all ages.

Clinical manifestations range from vague to severe or even life-threatening. The reason manifestations differ is

that the client may have ignored early warning signs, may have been able to cope with early clinical manifestations, or the condition's course may be slow or fast. Consider the problem of hypertension. Hypertension is called a "silent killer" because most persons have no clinical manifestations. Thus, hypertension may only be diagnosed incidentally when a client is undergoing a routine physical examination or receiving treatment for another problem, or has suffered a stroke from untreated hypertension.

A medical diagnosis is established during the diagnostic state. Diagnoses of common chronic medical conditions according to age and body system are listed in Table 6–2.

Chronic Stage

The chronic stage has been referred to as the "long haul" since this is the stage during which the individual must live with the condition for a prolonged time. In fact, this stage may last for the rest of the client's life.

Clinical manifestations may be controlled or out of control. Changes in function may be stabilized, marked by remissions and exacerbations, or progressively decline. If the condition has an acute onset (i.e., stroke, spinal cord injury, myocardial infarction) the greatest return of function frequently occurs within the first 6 months. Remissions and exacerbations may be frequent or infrequent. Progressive decline may be rapid or slow. Changes in function and the rate of change are more predictable for some chronic conditions than for others. Acute episodes of illness during this stage frequently relate to exacerbations, sudden decline in body system function, or to side effects or complications of treatment. Some acute episodes can be managed at home, while others must be managed in the hospital. When death occurs at this stage it is sudden and unexpected.

Terminal Stage

Transition to the terminal stage occurs for two reasons. The terminal stage occurs when changes in body systems become irreversible and when the loss of these functions is incompatible with life, or when death is expected within 6 months.

Many chronic conditions (e.g., arthritis) do not have a terminal stage, and death for these clients is due to other causes. Technological advances have eliminated the terminal stage for other chronic conditions. For example, organ transplants in clients with organ failure may reverse this stage to the chronic stage. Recent cure for some types of childhood cancers has changed the time pattern from terminal to an "at risk" stage.

The Process of Adaptation

Adaptation to chronic conditions is a complex and continuous process that involves physiologic, psychological, social, technological, and time factors. Knowledge related to the different factors involved in adaptation has been gen-

Table 6–2. Common Chronic Medical Conditions

Body System	Onset Prior to Adulthood	Adult Onset
Neurologic	Epilepsy	Epilepsy
	Cerebrovascular accident	Cerebrovascular accident
	Cancer	Cancer
	Blindness	Blindness
	Deafness	Deafness
	Head injury	Head injury
	Spinal cord injury	Spinal cord injury
	Aneurysm	Aneurysm
	Cerebral palsy	Multiple sclerosis
	Spina bifida	Migraine headache
	Muscular dystrophy	Amyotropic lateral sclerosis
		Huntington's chorea
		Myasthenia gravis
Cardiovascular/ hematopoietic	Congenital cardiac disease	Hypertension
	Sickle cell anemia	Coronary artery disease
	Hemophilia	Myocardial infarction
		Congestive heart failure
		Chronic anticoagulation
		Chronic lower extremity ischemia
		Angina
		Cardiomyopathies
Pulmonary	Asthma	Asthma
	Antitrypsin deficiency	Chronic obstructive pulmonary disease
	Cystic fibrosis	Leukemia
		Cancer
Digestive	Deficiencies	Gastric ulcer
	Cystic fibrosis	Lactose deficiency
	Hepatitis	Colitis
		Crohn's disease
		Cirrhosis
		Cancer
		Hepatitis
Renal and urinary	Neurogenic bladder	Neurogenic bladder
	Chronic renal failure	Chronic renal failure
		Chronic urinary tract infection
		Cancer
Metabolic	Diabetes	Diabetes
		Hyperlipidemia
Musculoskeletal	Juvenile arthritis	Arthritis
	Paralysis or absence of limbs (congenital, traumatic, surgical)	Paralysis or absence of limbs
		Low back pain
		Sarcoma
		Osteoporosis
Immune	Immune deficiencies	Asthma
		Lupus erythematosus
		Scleroderma
		Arthritis
		AIDS
		Tuberculosis
Other		Alcoholism

erated by the disciplines of nursing, physiology, sociology, psychology, social work, and medicine. One nursing study is shown in the Nursing Research profile. Adaptation is pivotal in the care of any person with a chronic condition. In this chapter, we use the word "adaptation" to mean the body's or mind's response to a chronic condition. Keep in mind that some adaptations are not positive, and make the client's condition worse. We also review adaptive challenges that arise for the client and family. The nurse's role is to monitor and prevent any adaptations that are not beneficial and to assist the client and family to adapt their life-styles to the condition.

NURSING RESEARCH

What Types of Health-Promotion Activities Are Used by People with Disabilities?

Stuifbergen, A.K., & Becker, H.A. (1994). Predictors of health-promoting lifestyles in persons with disabilities. *Research in Nursing & Health, 17,* 3–13.

Most research that has been completed on health-promotion activities has not included people with chronic health problems (called disabilities in this article). Most research has been addressed to exercise, smoking cessation, and the like.

A survey was sent to people with various disabling conditions. The survey asked respondents questions relating to their definition of health, self-efficacy (the perceived ability to perform various tasks), perceived health status, barriers to health promotion, and information about their disability.

The survey was returned by 131 persons with partial paralysis, cerebral palsy, post-polio syndrome, and arthritis. Almost half of the group needed personal assistance with day-to-day activities; the other half needed no help. The group perceived themselves to be in poor health, with some problems in their perceived ability to complete health-promotion tasks. Health promotion using exercise was ranked very low, followed by nutrition and stress management.

Implications for Practice. Variation in the group studied makes generalization difficult. But we can say, in general, that people with disabilities need health-promotion activities at least as much as people without them. Those with cognitive impairments probably need much more assistance to develop some mastery of skills for health promotion. Those with painful conditions may need pain management to enable activity. For everyone, you must be certain that the client can carry out the prescribed health-promotion activities.

Physiologic Adaptation

Adaptive Changes

Chronic conditions can interfere with physiologic functions. The body's intake, transformation, and expenditure of physical energy for cellular metabolism and protein synthesis can be altered.

When the physical energy demands of chronic conditions exceed the intake and processing of physical energy, the client's general resistance to physiologic stressors is impaired. Neuroendocrine responses to psychological distress have been implicated as a factor in adaptations to anorexia, pain, fatigue, shortness of breath, and decreased immune response; progressive decline or exacerbations of chronic conditions; and delayed recovery from acute episodes of illness during the chronic stage. Over time, adaptive energy from neuroendocrine sources is believed to become exhausted.

Some changes in physiologic structure or function associated with chronic conditions are reversible. Others are not. Management and life-style changes can slow the rate of some physiologic changes. Technology may be available to compensate or substitute for some types of physical functioning. While the body can compensate for some irreversible changes, over time these compensatory mechanisms may fail.

Another adaptation seen with physiologic adaptation is the loss of coordinated function of various body systems. Clients whose levels of mobility become limited because of self-imposed inactivity, progression of chronic health problems, surgery, trauma, or acute episodes of medical treatment are at high risk of developing changes in body system functions. Collectively, these adaptive responses are commonly referred to as "hazards of immobility" or the "disuse syndrome." It should be clear that these adaptive responses increase levels of disability. Adaptive changes in body systems related to the nursing diagnosis *Risk for Disuse Syndrome* are identified in Table 6–3.

Adaptive Challenges

Adaptive challenges common to the chronic stage of illness include:

- Learning about illness and treatment
- Learning about techniques and devices that can substitute for lost function
- Acquiring skills in using these techniques and devices
- Managing the prescribed medical regimen
- Controlling manifestations
- Monitoring the body's response to therapies
- Capitalizing on physical and psychological strengths
- Maintaining or increasing energy level
- Preventing adaptive changes that occur secondary to high levels of immobility
- Preventing and handling acute health crises

Psychological Adaptation

Adaptive Changes

Psychological adaptation to a chronic condition is a difficult and demanding process. This form of adaptation is

Table 6–3. Adaptive Changes in Body Systems Related to the Nursing Diagnosis *Risk for Disuse Syndrome*

Body System	Physiologic Change
Neurologic	Decreased ability to concentrate Reduced stimulation of reticular activation system Visual and auditory hallucinations Sleep disturbance
Cardiovascular	Decreased stroke volume Increased heart rate Hypovolemia Postural hypotension Increased procoagulants Shortened thromboplastin time; thromboembolism Compression of blood vessels of calves of leg
Pulmonary	Abdominal contents pushing against diaphragm Stress on inspiratory muscles Stasis of secretions Decreased lung volume Decreased intake of oxygen
Digestive	Diminished appetite Decreased metabolism Changes in insulin release pattern and effectiveness Decreased peristalsis
Integumentary	Larger surface area of skin bearing weight Evaporation of perspiration less efficient than when exposed to air Exposure to moist bed linens Pressure perfusion impairs skin
Renal	Stasis of urine in kidneys; urinary tract infection Increased excretion of calcium (formation of urinary calculi) Increased excretion of nitrogen
Musculoskeletal	Loss of muscle tone Loss of muscle mass Contractures Heterotrophic bone disease Osteoporosis
Immune	Decreased immunity

an ongoing process that overlaps other biologic and psychosocial processes associated with gains, losses, and challenges throughout the remainder of the client's life span.

As with other ongoing processes, psychological adaptation to a chronic condition is characterized by periods of changing demands and transitions. Some of these are predictable; others are not. Predictable periods of changing psychological demands and transitions include onset and diagnosis, hospitalizations for treatment of the condition, exacerbation of illness, failure of treatments, and loss of self-care abilities. Expect these times to be especially stressful. Some of these periods will be marked by depression, when clients realize they probably will not get better and may get worse. The client and family must redefine their roles, expectations, perhaps even their goals in life. Clients in the terminal stage must adapt to their shortened life span and the process of dying.

Psychological adaptation does not seem to differ among clients with various conditions or over varying lengths of time. Therefore, we can make some general statements. Findings about the incidence of clinical depression in persons living with chronic conditions range from no different from to higher than that of community-dwelling adults without chronic health problems. Risk factors for depression have been identified as biologic changes, medications (e.g., digoxin, droperidol, ethanol), and psychological vulnerability. Thus, some cases of depression may be resolved with medical treatment or by changing medication. If these interventions are not effective, the client should receive psychiatric evaluation and treatment.[1]

Clients adapt to the same diagnosis and stage of illness in individual ways. During the diagnostic stage, one client may appear overwhelmed and assume a lower level of physical, psychological, or social functioning than the physical condition warrants. Another client may evidence minimal distress and regain or maintain a high level of physical, psychological, and social functioning.

A General Pattern of Adaptation

A general pattern of psychological adaptation to personal change perceived as a loss or threat of loss has been described by sociologists, psychologists, physicians, and nurses. Phases of this pattern have been labeled differently by different authors. The pattern has been referred to as the grief process and the mourning process.

Disbelief. The first phase of the pattern is commonly referred to as disbelief or resistance. Denial of the changes or the need for personal change is characteristic of this phase. This phase is similar to the "fight-or-flight" response and is believed to protect the client from being psychologically overwhelmed.

Developing Awareness. The second phase, most commonly referred to as the anger phase, is developing awareness. This phase is characterized by clients' withdrawal, preoccupation with self, crying, depression, expression of anger toward others, feelings of guilt for having brought the disease on themselves, anger, being different, and being alone. In this phase, the client experiences acute awareness of what has been lost and grieves for what has been lost.

Integration. The third phase of integration is characterized by a rational acceptance that a physical or psychological change has occurred and an attempt to keep emotional distress within manageable limits. Other cognitive behaviors associated with this phase are reestablishing a sense of self and meaning and purpose; revising goals in life; learning to live with uncertainty; and acquiring new strategies for coping with one's environment.

Some people describe experiencing intermittent chronic sorrow. Triggers of sadness include the anniversary of the date of onset of the condition, special events, birthdays, and losses in physical function. Knowledge that feelings of sorrow are commonly felt may help mitigate the distress associated with the experience.

Coping Behaviors

Clients with the same medical diagnosis and in the same phase of chronic illness use a variety of physical, cognitive, and verbal behaviors to manage distress. The type of behaviors used and their effectiveness are highly individual. Some coping behaviors are passive; others are active. The behaviors are frequently categorized as emotion-focused (affective) or problem-focused. *Emotion-focused behaviors* have been defined as thoughts or actions that make a person feel better but do not alter the situation causing the distress. *Problem-focused behaviors* are efforts taken to change or resolve situations causing distress. A number of behaviors fall into both categories. The prevailing assumption is that problem-focused behaviors are more efficacious than emotion-focused behaviors. However, some research suggests that a combination of both behaviors may be most efficacious, especially when the problem cannot be resolved and needs to be managed.

Interestingly, some clients report that talking about their illness helps them cope. Others report that *not* talking about their illness helps them cope. Strategies clients have reported as effective in managing distressful situations include avoiding, ignoring, accepting, thinking out, or changing the situation. Shopping, driving, going out to eat, and exercising are types of activities some find helpful in relieving stress. Other strategies clients have reported as helpful include taking naps; seeking information and advice; changing values, attitudes, and goals; imagining the worst; hope; prayer; putting the problem in God's hands; humor; positive thinking; positive self-talk; taking anger out on others; trying to maintain some control over the situation; trying to look at the problem objectively; drawing on past experiences; blaming someone else; and taking drugs, eating, smoking, or drinking alcohol.[29]

Adaptive Challenges

A number of general psychological adaptive challenges arise from having and living with a chronic condition. These adaptive challenges include the following:

- Coping with emotional responses of oneself and significant others to the illness experience
- Coping with the uncertainty of diagnosis and treatment
- Coming to terms with having a chronic condition
- Restructuring one's life around the chronic condition
- Restructuring schedules, priorities, and plans for the future

- Negotiating new and altered relationships with self, family, friends, and the healthcare system
- Developing attitudes, knowledge, and skills that enable active participation in regimen management
- Dealing with genetic concerns and issues in reproductive decision-making
- Adapting to changes in physical abilities and appearance

Personal resources that assist clients in accomplishing these adaptive tasks include life experiences, interests, memories, and the capacity to learn, change behavior, relate to others, solve problems, and express and change feelings. The ways in which clients interpret physical, social, and psychological changes during the course of their illness, and the methods they find effective in adapting to these changes are important parts of adaptation. Psychological factors believed to influence positive adaptation include denial, hope, confidence, hardiness, and sense of control.

Different numbers and types of physiologic, psychological, and social events are appraised as distressful by clients having the same chronic condition for the same period of time. A number of concerns, fears, and events of personal change are common to a variety of chronic conditions; these problems are listed in Box 6–1. Consider sharing this list with clients to facilitate communication about concerns, fears, and events of personal change they may be experiencing.

Box 6–1. Common Concerns, Fears, and Events of Personal Change Associated with Chronic Conditions

Concerns and Fears

Loss of sense of self
Loss of control and predictability
Heightened sense of mortality
Loss of productivity
Loss of valued roles
Loss of relationships
Loss of opportunity or ability for sexual expression
Uncertainty about the future
Loss of purpose and meaning in life
Fear of procedures
Fear of death

Events of Personal Change

Life plans and goals
Established roles and patterns of interacting within family and outside the home
Relationships with others
Daily routines
Loss of gratifying behaviors
Changes in health maintenance and management behaviors
Activity and sleep patterns
Financial resources
Appearance

Psychological adaptive challenges common to persons during the onset or diagnostic stage are the following:

- Coping with the anxiety of not knowing
- Coping with fantasies and fears about what might be wrong
- Coping with feelings of guilt that the disorder was self-induced
- Tolerating the physical and emotional strain of tests and painful procedures
- Balancing hopefulness and the possibility of a feared diagnosis
- Adapting to the healthcare system and different healthcare providers

Although the diagnostic stage is a crisis period for the majority of clients, adaptive behavior varies. Some clients may deny the diagnosis, or accept the diagnosis but deny the feared implications. Other clients who have experienced manifestations over a period of time may experience a sense of relief that a diagnosis has been established. Two reasons given for this sense of relief are that a diagnosis validates the existence of the problem, and that it increases the potential for alleviation.

Social Adaptation

Adaptive Changes

The roles of clients with chronic conditions overlap social roles related to age, sex, family, work, and recreation. The impact of health and illness roles on social roles ranges from minimal to severe, with health and illness roles being dominant. The degree to which clients adapt socially is influenced by changes in physical appearance, ability to communicate, ability to navigate the physical environment, social resources (e.g., people, money, and community services), and societal values and attitudes. Society responds more favorably to clients with less visible and apparent chronic conditions than to those with more visible signs of illness. Social acceptance is influenced by beliefs and values of oneself and others related to attractiveness, productivity, independence, self-reliance, normality, individual rights, and health and illness. These beliefs and values also influence the availability of social resources and health services, as well as job, recreational, and housing opportunities.

In the United States, changing social beliefs about individual rights and normality have influenced state and federal legislation (Box 6–2). This legislation has contributed to a decrease in attitudinal and architectural barriers to social integration, as well as increased availability of healthcare, housing, employment, recreation, and transportation for people with chronic conditions.

Social beliefs and expectations about behavior appropriate for people experiencing physical illness have changed over the past 40 years, since Talcott Parsons described the "sick role" in our society. Parsons stated that the individual is not responsible for his or her illness. This pattern of thinking has shifted to a belief that the individual has an active role in the development of some illnesses. Parsons also stated that society believed the

Box 6–2. The Americans with Disabilities Act

The 1990 passage of the Americans with Disabilities Act (PL 101–336) makes it illegal to discriminate against people who have chronic conditions. The Act addresses four areas:
1. Employment
2. Telecommunications
3. Public services provided by federal and state governments, and
4. Public accommodations and services operated by private entities

The Act also makes provision for private and federal enforcement of the law.

Disability is defined in the Act as "physical or mental impairment that substantially limits one or more of an individual's major life activities." This definition includes persons with functional limitations secondary to chronic conditions.

This was the first disability legislation that held the private sector accountable for the cost of compliance and provides tax incentives for making environmental adaptations. Under this law, employers of 15 or more people cannot deny employment to a disabled person who can perform essential job functions with or without reasonable accommodation. The law also mandates that policies, practices, and the physical structure of federal, state, and private facilities providing public services make it possible for people with disabilities to enjoy their services. Passage of the Act was motivated by economic as well as altruistic concerns. Equal access will increase opportunities for achieving social independence and contributing to society.

individual should be released from the usual role responsibilities. Thoughts today are shifting to beliefs that the individual should maintain responsibility for personal, family, and social activities that he or she is capable of doing or learning. The expectation that an individual should view illness as undesirable and try to get well is shifting to an expectation that cure is not possible for all illnesses and the individual should maintain an active role in managing physical health problems that cannot be cured. The expectation that the individual should seek medically competent help persists. However, individuals are more actively involved in decision-making related to care options and management of their health problems than they were 40 years ago. Differences in beliefs and expectations about clients with chronic conditions and how they respond to their "sick role" have been identified as a frequent source of conflict between caregivers and their clients and families.

Communication Patterns

Communication patterns between healthcare professionals and clients with chronic conditions and their families have been described as changing over time and tending to move through three phases. Initially, clients and families have a naive trust in healthcare workers. A characteristic of this phase is the belief that healthcare professionals will provide a cure or do what is best for the client. This naive trust is followed by a phase of mistrust and anger. A major source of anger is lack of involvement in decision-making. Over time, the second phase is replaced by trust in some healthcare workers and not in others. Healthcare providers should be aware of these phases and work with the client, providing factual information without denying hope.

Social Change Events

Social change events commonly associated with having a chronic condition relate to roles and interaction patterns, mobility patterns, employment, living arrangements, recreation, finances, time and place for vacations, and health insurance.

Adaptive Challenges

Common sociological adjustment tasks include the following:

- Preventing or adjusting to social isolation
- Normalizing
- Managing clinical manifestations and treatments in social environments
- Maintaining physical mobility in the environment
- Changing structure in present housing or locating new housing
- Dealing with rejection and discrimination
- Developing new social skills and social networks
- Teaching others about the chronic condition and how it interferes or does not interfere with abilities
- Learning about community

Family Adaptation

Because of the long-term nature of chronic conditions and the role of the family in maintaining the health of its members, a chronic condition is also a family condition. Families must cope with unusual ongoing adaptive challenges related to the presence of a chronic condition.

Some families are more effective than others in accomplishing adaptive challenges. Types of physical impairments, family resources, family perception, the developmental stage of family members and the family unit, behaviors of the client, the healthcare environment, and society are interrelated factors that have an impact on family adaptation. Some family units become stronger, whereas others disintegrate.

Challenges to family adjustment differ with different stages of the condition. Adaptive challenges during the diagnostic stage are the same as those related to acute illness. They include pulling together, learning to cope with the acute care environment and treatment, and establishing relationships with caregivers.

Other challenges include identifying the meaning of the illness, assessing potential changes in the family, moving toward integration of temporary and permanent changes while maintaining a sense of continuity between past and present, and developing an attitude of flexibility toward future personal and family goals.

Adaptive challenges during the chronic stage include maintaining a sense of normality; adjusting to changing expectations of each family member; striving to balance family resources; and maintaining autonomy of all family members despite the pull toward mutual dependency, caretaking, or focus on the family member who has the chronic condition. Some adaptive demands during the chronic stage result from treatment; for example, changing work schedules to accommodate treatment, or loss of strength due to side effects of treatment. Likewise the roles of the client may have to be assumed by other family members or friends. If the client is the breadwinner, the tasks of earning a living may have to be assumed by another. Initially, the condition may generate a lot of support from extended family members and friends. After several months, support declines. When a family has a member with a long-term disabling condition and limited financial resources, they will need to manage these complex issues. Some persons have gotten a divorce so that they can qualify for funding to care for a family member. If the family member has impaired judgment or ability to conduct personal business, another family member may need to obtain power of attorney. If the chronic condition is terminal, families must also manage issues related to the family member's death and resumption of normal individual and family lives after the death.

Management

Healthcare management after the diagnostic stage includes rehabilitation centers, units, and programs; home healthcare; long-term healthcare facilities; nurse-managed clinics; case management; and hospice care. During the other phases of chronic conditions, care may be provided in acute care hospitals, rehabilitation units, nursing homes, or the client's home.

Medical management varies with the type and stage of the chronic condition and the technology available. Management and outcomes of management are more defined for some conditions than others. Medical management includes prevention, diagnosis, treatment of acute episodes, and helping clients manage and shape the course of their chronic condition. Multidisciplinary approaches are employed in promoting maximal use of the client's functional abilities and adaptation to deficits. Increasingly, goals for management are established in conjunction with other health team members, the client, and family.

Funding Issues

Many clients with physical disabilities benefit from assistive devices and techniques that compensate or substitute for lost function. Acquiring skills in using these devices and techniques improves their functional levels. Unfortunately, many clients and families who would benefit from these services are not referred because some healthcare professionals lack knowledge about rehabilitation services, or third-party payors may not provide reimbursement for these services.

Rehabilitation Centers

Rehabilitation centers employ a multidisciplinary approach to assisting clients with high levels of physical disability. They help clients regain functional abilities and acquire knowledge and skills that maximize their ability to live with cognitive or physical disabilities. Most of these clients have recently survived life-threatening neurologic damage (stroke, paralysis, head injury), musculoskeletal trauma (accident, joint replacement), or illness. Their families are also provided with knowledge, skills, and support that facilitate adjustment to the demands of the chronic condition and enable them to assist their family member in reintegration into home and social environments. Members of the multidisciplinary team include physiatrists (physicians who specialize in physical medicine rehabilitation), nurses (many of whom have certification in rehabilitation nursing), physical therapists, occupational therapists, speech therapists (some of whom specialize in swallow therapy), nutritionists, respiratory therapists, psychologists, neuropsychologists, and recreational therapists. Some multidisciplinary teams also include a clergy member.

Rehabilitation units, both inpatient and outpatient, incorporate a multidisciplinary approach and physical conditioning for clients with specific health problems, such as cardiac disease, chronic obstructive pulmonary disease, AIDS, and chronic pain. Exercise does not reverse pathophysiologic changes, but is believed to condition muscles so that they work more efficiently and use less oxygen. Exercise also stimulates the production of endorphins that promote feelings of well-being, increases production of high-density lipoproteins, assists in weight control, and increases exercise tolerance.

Home Healthcare

Home healthcare agencies provide care to clients in the chronic and terminal stages of chronic conditions, as well as to clients recovering from acute illness. Services include laboratory monitoring, intravenous therapy for antibiotics and chemotherapy, pump-driven feedings, parenteral nutrition, respiratory support, peritoneal dialysis, physical therapy, and a wide range of nursing services. This pattern of multidisciplinary care began in New York in the late 1950s because of a shortage of hospital beds. Home healthcare experienced a tremendous spurt of growth in the late 1970s when the government instituted financial reimbursement for care based on diagnostic groupings (DRGs). (See Chapter 9.)

Long-Term Care Facilities

Long-term care facilities provide interim or long-term inpatient care to persons with levels of physical or cognitive disability that pose barriers to self-care and healthcare management in the home. Basic services include nursing care, physical therapy, and recreational therapy. Some long-term care facilities also provide day-care services. Subacute care is described in Chapter 7.

Nurse-Managed Clinics

The majority of nurse-managed clinics focus on primary prevention. Some address physical and psychosocial needs of clients in the chronic stage of chronic illnesses with well-defined treatment (e.g., hypertension, diabetes) and less well-defined treatment (e.g., multiple sclerosis, myasthenia gravis, Parkinson's disease). Changes in cost reimbursement will promote expansion of this pattern of care. This pattern of care is a revival of a concept of care that dates back to the early 1900s.

Case Management

Case management incorporates concepts of continuity and efficiency in addressing the long-term physical, psychological, and social needs of clients with chronic conditions. The primary goals of case management are promotion of self-care, promotion of quality of life, and efficient use of resources. A healthcare professional, usually a nurse or social worker, assesses and monitors client needs and the availability of services. The type of monitoring may be intermittent or continual. The case manager negotiates directly with the client, family, healthcare institutions, insurance companies, and businesses for health and social services needed by the client.

Hospice Care

Hospice care programs address healthcare needs of clients in the terminal stage of a chronic condition. Services provided are pain control, palliative and supportive care for clients, and supportive and bereavement care for significant others. Care is provided in the home or in long-term care agencies, and still others are operated by community groups. This pattern of care was implemented in the United States in the late 1960s.

Nursing Management

Chronic conditions have varying degrees of impact on physiologic, psychological, and social functioning over time. Psychological and social functioning affect physiologic functioning. Nursing assessment should address each. The focus of assessment will vary with the type and stage of the chronic condition and the healthcare setting. The overall goals of assessment and care are to facilitate client and family adaptation to the condition and help shape the course of the chronic condition. These goals are accomplished by identifying and promoting maximal use of functional abilities; determining challenges to physical, psychological, and social adaptation; identifying the personal and social resources needed to meet these challenges; and assisting the client in using these resources and obtaining additional resources, as needed.

Assessment

The focus of the health history varies with the stage of the chronic condition. In the prediagnostic phase emphasis is on obtaining the history, determining the client's current health status, and identifying risk factors. In the diagnostic phase the emphasis is on manifestations and the client's experiences related to them (e.g., When did they start? What makes them better or worse? To what degree are they interfering with sleep and the activities and demands of daily living?).

In the chronic phase, assessment should focus on several aspects of the major manifestations: change or stability; frequency and severity; what triggers; and what relieves. Manifestations common to a number of chronic conditions are anorexia, fatigue, pain, shortness of breath, and sleep disturbances. In addition, ask about facilitators and barriers encountered in carrying out prescribed healthcare regimens in the home; recreational and work environments; general energy level; sleep pattern; activity level and amount of assistance needed in conducting activities; and demands of daily living. Levels of mobility and self-care are on a continuum ranging from complete or modified independence to modified or complete dependence. The client should also be assessed for treatment-related and environmental and psychological factors, as well as illness-related factors that may be contributing to physical symptoms and immobility. Self-reported symptoms are better predictors of functioning than objective measurements of physical function.

Physical Assessment. All body systems should be assessed since chronic conditions involve one or more body systems and the number of body systems involved increases over time.

Psychological Assessment. A variety of psychological attributes of functioning have been addressed in the literature related to chronic illness. However, there is no universally accepted approach for assessing psychological functioning of persons with chronic conditions.

Psychological assessment in the prediagnostic stage addresses developmental stage and client perceptions of health and the role of self and the healthcare team in health promotion. It includes psychosocial development before diagnosis; prior experience and knowledge related

to the condition; concerns, fears, and perceived personal changes related to the condition; meaning attributed to having the condition; expectations related to treatment and course; and motivation and ability to acquire knowledge and skills for self-management.

Psychological assessment during the chronic stage should focus on the phase of psychological adjustment to transitions; the meaning the client attributes to the condition; perceived demands of the condition; concerns, fears, and events of personal change the client is experiencing; type and perceived effectiveness of coping methods; knowledge and experience related to the chronic condition; expectations related to treatment and course; and sources of hope.

The listing of concerns, fears, and events of personal change identified in Box 6–1 can be shared with clients to elicit communication about perceived concerns, fears, and the events of personal change the client is experiencing. Sharing information about coping behaviors used by others can assist the client in identifying and evaluating the effectiveness of his or her coping behaviors.

Social Assessment. Social assessment considers the impact the condition has on family and social roles and resources. Family assessment should include communication pattern with the healthcare team; developmental stage of family members and family unit; the meaning the family attributes to the chronic condition; fears, concerns, and additional adaptive tasks, demands, and challenges they are experiencing related to their family member having a chronic condition; knowledge and experience related to the chronic condition; expectations related to treatment and course; and the roles of self and family members in managing the condition. Social assessment also considers the fit of the client with his or her home and social environments, the client's social activities, and the strategies the client uses to normalize interactions with others.

Assessment Tools. A variety of tools for assessing aspects of physical, psychological, and social functioning of persons with chronic conditions are available in the literature. Some of the tools found to yield reliable data about functional abilities of clients with chronic conditions are described in Table 6–4. The Functional Independence Measure and the Rancho Los Amigos Scale are commonly used in physical rehabilitation centers to quantify functional gains during rehabilitation. These assessment tools can be used to quantify physical or cognitive abilities of clients in other settings. For example, the Rancho Los Amigos Scale (Table 6–5) is useful in quantifying changes in cognitive functioning resulting from conditions that alter brain function.

Levels of cognitive functioning in the Rancho Los Amigos Scale are based on clinical observations of physical and cognitive behaviors evidenced by clients recovering from severe head trauma. The scale contains indicators of changing abilities related to taking in, processing, and responding to information. Literature exists identifying nursing interventions for different levels of cognitive functioning.

Table 6–4. Assessment Tools for Clients with Chronic Conditions

Physical Function

Barthel index	Nine categories: feeding, transfers, grooming, toileting, bathing, walking, climbing stairs, bowel and bladder control
PULSES	Six categories: *P*resence of medical conditions, *U*pper extremity (self-care), *L*ower extremity (walking), *S*ensory, *E*limination (bowel and bladder control), *S*ocialization
Index of activities of daily living (ADL)	Six categories: bed activities, transfers, hygiene, dressing, feeding, and locomotion
Functional Independence Measure (FIM)	Eighteen categories: eating, grooming—upper body, dressing—lower body, toileting, bladder management, bowel management, transfers (bed, chair, wheelchair), transfers—toilet, transfers—tub or shower, locomotion, stairs, comprehension, expression, social interaction, problem solving, memory

Cognitive Function

Rancho Los Amigos Scale	Eight levels of responses: none, generalized, localized, confused-agitated, confused-inappropriate, confused-appropriate, automatic-appropriate, purposeful-appropriate

Pain

McGill Pain Questionnaire	Comprehensive and modified versions: modified—20 sets of sensory, affective, evaluative, and miscellaneous descriptors of pain; includes pain intensity scale, and body location of pain
Visual analog scales	Numbers or faces for rating intensity of pain

Coping

Ways of Coping Scale	Fifty cognitive and behavioral strategies used in managing distress
Jaloweic Coping Scale	Forty coping behaviors used to manage distress rated according to helpfulness

Table 6–5. Rancho Los Amigos Scale of Cognitive Functioning

Level of Response	Behavior
I None	Unresponsive to auditory, visual, or tactile stimuli.
II Generalized	Reacts inconsistently and nonpurposively to stimuli. Delayed and limited responses.
III Localized	Reacts specifically but inconsistently to stimuli. Responses are related to type of stimuli presented, such as visually focusing on an object or responding to sounds.
IV Confused-agitated	Extremely agitated and in a high state of confusion. Nonpurposeful and aggressive behavior. Unable to fully cooperate with treatments owing to short attention span. Requires maximal assistance with self-care.
V Confused-inappropriate, nonagitated	Alert and can respond to simple commands on a more consistent basis. Highly distractible. Needs constant cuing to attend to an activity. Memory is impaired, with confusion regarding past and present. Can perform self-care activities with assistance. May wander, and needs to be watched carefully.
VI Confused-appropriate	Shows goal-directed behavior, but still needs direction. Follows simple tasks consistently, and shows carryover for relearned tasks. More aware of his or her deficits, and has increased awareness of self, family, and basic needs.
VII Automatic-appropriate	Appears oriented in home and hospital, and goes through daily routine automatically. Shows carryover for new learning, but still requires structure and supervision to ensure safety and good judgment. Able to initiate tasks in which he or she has an interest.
VIII Purposeful-appropriate	Totally alert, oriented, and shows good recall of past and recent events. Independent in the home and community.

Box 6–3. Physiologic, Psychological, and Social Nursing Diagnoses Commonly Associated with Chronic Conditions

Physiologic Diagnoses

Activity intolerance
Constipation
Disuse syndrome, risk for
Fatigue
Fluid volume deficit
Fluid volume excess
Health maintenance, altered
Impaired physical mobility
Incontinence, bowel
Infection, risk for
Injury, risk for
Nutrition: less than body requirements, altered
Nutrition: more than body requirements, altered
Pain
Pain, chronic
Self care deficit (bathing, hygiene, dressing, grooming, feeding, toileting)
Urinary elimination, altered

Psychological Diagnoses

Anxiety
Body image disturbance

Decisional conflict (specify)
Fear
Grieving, anticipatory
Grieving, dysfunctional
Growth and development, altered
Hopelessness
Knowledge deficit (specify)
Powerlessness
Self esteem disturbance
Spiritual distress

Social Diagnoses

Communication, impaired verbal
Diversional activity deficit
Family processes, altered
Parenting, altered
Role performance, altered
Sexuality patterns, altered
Social interaction, impaired
Social isolation

Nursing Diagnosis

A number of interrelated physiologic, psychological, and social nursing diagnoses are commonly associated with chronic conditions (Box 6–3). Related factors contributing to the diagnoses differ according to individual characteristics, stage of chronic condition, changes in physiologic structure or function, treatment, and environment.

Planning: Expected Outcomes

The expected outcomes for the client with a chronic condition are directly related to the specific diagnosis, physiologic changes, treatment, and adaptive energy. In general, a cure is not expected and some outcomes are more predictable than others. Long-term outcomes are usually written with months allowed for achievement. Short-term outcomes that are achievable and measurable provide positive feedback to clients, families, and caregivers. This feedback is believed to decrease the potential for burnout. The client, family, and other health team members should be involved in determining long- and short-term outcomes. When clients and families identify goals that seem unrealistic to you, tell them you cannot say for sure they will not achieve them but most people with similar problems have not done so. Then, identify incremental goals you can help them achieve. For example, for the spinal cord–injured person who has a goal of walking, you can help work on maintaining range of motion, which is necessary for walking. As clients and families work toward more modest goals, they will, with time, readjust their goals. In some cases, clients and families have achieved goals that were perceived as unrealistic by others.

Implementation

Interventions for the client with a chronic condition vary depending on the condition and its stage. Many times, interventions require the collaboration of several healthcare providers. Regardless of the disorder, there are some general adaptive challenges that every client is confronted with. Client education plans during the diagnostic and chronic stage of the condition should address these challenges.

Nursing interventions should strengthen the client's and family's ability to live with and shape the course of the chronic condition. General strategies used in the care of clients with chronic conditions include direct care, teaching, counseling, working things out, making arrangements, and advocating. Interventions must be specific to the client and the setting.

Providing Client Education. Most chronic illnesses exist in a balance of control and crisis. As part of your client education effort, you will teach the client how to determine when an illness is becoming out of control, how to treat it, and when to contact the healthcare provider. For example, teach the diabetic client to recognize early the clinical manifestations of hyperglycemia and hypoglycemia, how to begin treatment, and when to notify the healthcare provider. Teach the diabetic client to carry a blood glucose testing device, sugar, and insulin at all times. Likewise, teach the asthmatic client to carry a bronchodilator and the client with angina to carry nitroglycerin.

Most chronic illnesses require some degree of daily treatment. These treatments can range from taking medication to giving multiple injections to running a home dialysis unit. Assess the client's and the family's ability to follow the treatment guidelines. Ask them what problems they have experienced in carrying out the treatment regimen. Consider these characteristics in formulating your questions:

Degree of difficulty in learning the regimen. Are there several steps involved? What complications could result from using equipment or giving medications incorrectly? Does the client or family member have the dexterity required to complete the regimen successfully? Does the client or a family member have limitations that could interfere with performing tasks?

Amount of time required to implement the regimen. How much time does the treatment regimen require? How many times each day must the regimen be applied?

Amount of discomfort and exertion associated with the regimen. How painful or inconvenient is the treatment? Do you believe the client will comply, or that a family member will be persuasive enough to ensure compliance?

Visibility of the regimen to other people, and its social acceptance. Will the client need to take equipment everywhere, as with oxygen? Does the client have a disfiguring condition, such as a tracheostomy or fistula?

Effectiveness and speed of the regimen in controlling the condition or its manifestations. How patient will the client or family members have to be in waiting for results of the treatment regimen?

Based on these and other questions, develop a comprehensive teaching plan to help the client apply the treatment regimen successfully.

Controlling Clinical Manifestations.
In addition to applying a treatment regimen properly, the client and family may need to learn other ways to control the chronic condition's influence on their lives. Some clients must plan ahead so that needed items will be available. For example, they may need to buy adequate supplies before leaving on a trip. The client may need to carry supplies on an airplane rather than checking them in baggage. Consider whether the client needs special equipment. Arthritic clients, for example, may benefit from using Velcro closures rather than zippers or buttons.

Restructuring Time.
Assess your client's time requirements. Some clients with chronic conditions have too much time; others have too little. For example, a client unemployed because of a chronic condition may have too much free time. In contrast, a client who spends hours each day undergoing a medical regimen may have little time to enjoy life.

Focus your teaching plan on helping the client maintain enough free time to enjoy a high-quality life. Examine areas of the client's life that include wasted time. A hobby or a support group may help build a support system and cultivate interests. Consult a recreational therapist at a local physical rehabilitation center for information about recreational activities in the home or community.

Adjusting to Changes in the Disorder.
Your teaching plan can provide invaluable assistance in helping clients cope with the course of a chronic disorder. Some disorders have a stable course; others are unpredictable. For example, chronic ulcerative colitis usually is quite stable, whereas multiple sclerosis can be erratic.

If your client's condition has predictable flares, inform the client and the family about them. For example, depression is common 4 to 6 months after a cerebrovascular accident or myocardial infarction. Warn and educate the client and family ahead of time, so they can watch for signs of depression and consult a healthcare provider if necessary. Support groups exist for many chronic conditions; be sure to include them in your teaching plan.

Promoting Physiologic Adaptation.
The client's physical adaptation to a chronic condition can be improved by changing medication and dosages or schedules, diet, and activity patterns. Identifying environmental or behavioral factors that trigger manifestations, reduce sleep, increase energy levels, or substitute for lost function can increase feelings of wellness. Early detection of complications also facilitates adaptation. Knowledge about the condition and its management and how to substitute and compensate for changes in physical function will facilitate physiologic adaptation.

Promoting Psychological Adaptation.
Interventions to enhance psychological adaptation during the diagnostic stage include encouraging the client's active involvement in the diagnostic process and treatment decisions (Ethical Issues in Nursing), facilitating expressions of feelings, and providing clients with or helping them to seek appropriate information.

Hospitalization during the chronic stage may be perceived as a crisis episode by some clients. Other clients may view hospitalization during this stage as a reprieve from day-to-day hassles and concerns or as a period of hope because new treatments may be available. In the terminal stage, one client may fear death and another client may view death as a preferable alternative to suffering and disability. Personal factors that are believed to contribute to the individual nature of psychological adaptation include hope, commitment, confidence, appraisal of changes, perception of the effectiveness of management, coping strategies, and personal and social resources. Appraisals of change are based on an individual's beliefs, knowledge, skills, previous losses, and threat of loss. The ability to manage loss, the threat of loss, and challenges also differs among individuals.

Promoting Social Adaptation.
Interventions that promote social adaptation include teaching and counseling related to management of the chronic condition in home, work, and recreational environments and assisting the client and family in locating professional and community resources to lower barriers to social integration. Vocational rehabilitation and job skills training may help in gaining employment. Interventions that foster and support role changes include role-playing in anticipated situations, imaginative role-taking, in which the client imagines how

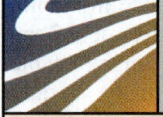

ETHICAL ISSUES IN NURSING

Who Should Make Decisions for Clients with a Chronic Illness?

Caring for clients who have chronic illnesses can be very challenging for nurses. You are called on to deliver many aspects of care to these clients, including helping ease the pain of their illness, listening to the client regarding feelings about his or her illness, assisting in the technological care of their disease process (e.g., dressing changes, tube feedings, IV infusions), and perhaps in helping patients work through their decisions about treatment options. Clients who are in the chronic stages of their illness may come to rely on you for care that may go beyond the realm of nursing practice. When decisions become overwhelming, clients might prefer that their healthcare providers make all the healthcare decisions for them. On the other hand, are healthcare decisions ever made for clients with chronic conditions without their input or consent simply because the client is thought to be unable to make the best choices for himself or herself?

There are three ethical principles involved here, the first being autonomy. All clients who are competent have the right to decide what medical treatments they want and do not want. Chronic illness may cause a client to become incompetent, but each client should be assessed carefully before deciding that he or she is truly not competent. Chronic illness is not always followed by incompetence.

The second and third principles, beneficence and paternalism, are closely related. You act beneficently in many ways, that is, you perform activities that benefit the client, but these actions are not seen as taking away a client's autonomy. For example, crushing a pill for a client who has dysphagia and cannot crush his or her own medications is of benefit to the client but is hardly seen as a dilemma regarding autonomy. On the other hand, paternalism in its extreme form allows healthcare providers to make decisions for their clients, on their behalf, without their input.

It is sometimes the wish of clients that you or a doctor make decisions for them. Perhaps the client feels overwhelmed and simply does not know what to do, or perhaps the client feels that you or a doctor would make a better decision. Is this any reason to act out of extreme paternalism? Clients with chronic illnesses are probably more vulnerable when it comes to making healthcare decisions. You should be aware of this so that you do not exercise extreme paternalism when beneficence may be more appropriate. Clients should always be allowed to make their own informed decisions. You may be able to help clients gain the knowledge they need in order to do so, which is a very important act of beneficence.

another person would respond to behaviors, and role-modeling, in which the individual is introduced to another person who has the same chronic condition and has adapted positively to the changes he or she was faced with. With use of role-modeling the client may gain practical tips about hunting for a job, finding accessible housing, and meeting new friends.

Role clarification is a strategy in which the client is provided information about behaviors necessary to play a particular role. Reference group interaction brings groups with similar problems and concerns together. These groups are helpful for exchanging ideas for solving problems and relieving feelings of isolation and helplessness.

Encourage clients to normalize their lives and resume activities with others. Some visible deformities can be disguised with scarves or make-up to reduce self-consciousness. Likewise, clients with dyspnea, by looking in a store window, can disguise the fact that they are stopping to catch their breath.

Some conditions cannot be disguised. In these cases, prepare the client to be the object of rude stares and comments by strangers and children. Eventually, the client will become inured to these boorish responses.

Evaluation

Expected outcomes for clients living with chronic conditions are achieved over time. Evaluation is used to exam-ine outcome achievement and movement to another level of care. For example, a client in acute care may become physiologically stable and be discharged to home, home care, skilled or long-term care, or to an acute rehabilitation center.

When gains in physical function are stabilized with or without assistive devices, the client can be moved to less skilled areas of care or discharged to home. Of course, the original goals may not have been met. In these instances, the cause should be determined, keeping in mind that the condition may have worsened and the expected outcome and interventions may require revision.

Conclusions

Chronic conditions transcend all care settings. Chronic conditions are characterized by a trajectory that changes its path over time. Some commonalities exist in the ongoing physical, psychological, and social adaptive challenges presented to the client living with a chronic condition. Time is an important factor to consider in assessing the client and in planning care. Consider the past and future of the condition, as well as the present. Knowledge of the temporal pattern and the task of social adaptation will provide an empathic understanding of the human experience of living with a chronic condition. A broad understanding of chronic conditions will widen the compass of your nursing role. It will assist you in providing holistic nursing care that will facilitate client and family adaptation and ameliorate the course of the condition they must live with.

Bibliography

1. Agency for Health Care Policy and Research (1993). *Clinical practice guidelines #5—Depression in primary care.* Rockville, MD: U.S. Department of Health and Human Services.
2. Baker, C., & Stern, R. (1993). Finding meaning in chronic illness as the key to self care. *Canadian Journal of Nursing Research* 25(2), 23–36.
3. Boland, S. L., & Sims, S. (1996). Family care giving at home. *Image, 28*(1), 55–58.
4. Bronstein, K. S., et al. (1991). *Promoting stroke recovery.* St. Louis: Mosby–Year Book.
5. Corbin, J., & Strauss, A. (1991). A nursing model for chronic illness management based upon the trajectory framework. *Scholarly Inquiry for Nursing Practice, 5*(30), 155–174.
6. Felton, B., et al. (1984). Stress and coping: An explanation of psychological adjustment among chronically ill adults. *Social Science Medicine, 18*(10), 889–898.
7. Felton, B., & Revenson, T. (1987). Age differences in coping with chronic illness. *Psychology and Aging, 2*(2), 164–171.
8. Flavo, D., et al. (1982). Psychosocial aspects of invisible disability. *Rehabilitation Literature, 43*(1–2), 2–6.
9. Folkman, S., & Lazarus, R. (1988). Coping as a mediator of emotions. *Journal of Personality and Social Psychology, 54*(3), 466–471.
10. Foxall, M., et al. (1985). Adjustment patterns of chronically ill middle-aged persons and spouses. *Western Journal of Nursing Research, 7*(4), 425–444.
11. Frank, R., et al. (1987). Differences in coping styles among persons with spinal cord injury: A cluster-analytic approach. *Journal of Consulting and Clinical Psychology, 55*(5), 727–731.
12. Gass, K. (1987). The health of conjugally bereaved older widows: The role of appraisal, coping, and resources. *Research in Nursing and Health, 10*(1), 29–47.
13. Gurkles, J., & Menks, E. (1988). Identification of stressors and use of coping methods in chronic hemodialysis patients. *Nursing Research, 37*(4), 236–239.
14. Hickey, S. (1986). Enabling hope. *Cancer Nursing, 9*(3), 133–137.
15. Hymovich, D., & Hagopian, G. (1992). *Chronic illness in adults and children.* Philadelphia, W.B. Saunders.
16. Kirk, K. (1992). Confidence as a factor in chronic illness. *Journal of Advanced Nursing 17*(10), 1238–1242.
17. Lambert, C., et al. (1989). Social support, hardiness and psychological well being in women with arthritis. *Image, 21*(3), 128–131.
18. Lancaster, L. (1988). Impact of chronic illness over the life span. *American Nephrology Nurses Association Journal, 15*(3), 164–168.
19. Lee, R., Graydon, J., & Ross, E. (1991). Effects of psychological well-being, physical status and social support on oxygen-dependent COPD patients' level of functioning. *Research in Nursing & Health, 14,* 323–328.
20. Leidy, N. (1990). A structural model of stress, psychological resources and symptomatic experience in chronic illness. *Nursing Research, 39*(4), 230–251.
21. Leidy, N., et al. (1990). Psychophysiological processes of stress in chronic physical illness. A theoretical perspective. *Journal of Advanced Nursing, 13,* 478–486.
22. Lindgren, C., et al. (1992). Chronic sorrow: A life span concept. *Scholarly Inquiry for Nursing 6*(1), 27–42.
23. Loomis, M., & Conco, D. (1991). Patients' perceptions of health, chronic illness and nursing diagnoses. *Nursing Diagnosis, 2*(4), 162–170.
24. Mailick, M. (1987). The impact of severe illness on the individual and family: An overview. *Social Work in Health Care, 5*(2), 117–128.
25. McNett, S. (1987). Social support, threat, and coping responses and effectiveness in functionally disabled. *Nursing Research, 36*(2), 98–103.
26. Miller, C. (1993). Trajectory and empowerment theory applied to care of patients with multiple sclerosis. *Journal of Neuroscience Nursing, 25*(6), 343–355.
27. Miller, P., et al. (1985). Coping methods and societal adjustments of cardiovascular clients. *Health Values: Achieving High Level Wellness, 9*(4), 10–13.
28. Miller, P. Sr., et al. (1990). Stressors and stress management one month after myocardial infarction. *Rehabilitation Nursing, 15*(6), 306–310.
29. Morse, J. M., & Doberneck, B. (1995). The concept of hope. *Image, 27*(14), 277–286.
30. Pollock, S. (1993). Adaptation to chronic illness: A program of research for testing nursing theory. *Nursing Science Quarterly, 6*(2), 86–92.
31. Reed, P. (1986). Religiousness among terminally ill and healthy adults. *Research in Nursing and Health, 9,* 35–41.
32. Resnick, B. (1996). Motivation in geriatric rehabilitation. *Image 28*(1), 41–46.
33. Robinson, L., et al. (1993). Operationalizing the Corbin & Strauss trajectory model for elderly clients with chronic illness. *Scholarly Inquiry for Nursing Practice, 7*(4), 253–264.
34. Rolland, J. (1987). Chronic illness and the life cycle: A conceptual framework. *Family Process, 26,* 203–221.
35. Rubin, M. (1988). The physiology of bedrest. *American Journal of Nursing, 88*(1), 50–55.
36. Segall, A. (1976). The sick role concept: Understanding illness behavior. *Journal of Health and Social Behavior, 17*(6), 163–170.
37. State University of New York Research Foundation. (1990). *Functional independence measure.* Buffalo, NY: Author.
38. Stuifbergen, A. K., & Becker, H. A. (1994). Predictors of health-promoting lifestyles in persons with disabilities. *Research in Nursing and Health, 17,* 3–13.
39. Sutton, T., & Murphy, S. (1989). Stressors and patterns of coping in renal transplant patients. *Nursing Research, 38*(1), 46–49.
40. Taylor, C. (1995). Medical futility and nursing. *Image 27*(4), 301–306.
41. Turner, J., et al. (1987). Relationship of stress, appraisal and coping to chronic low back pain. *Behavioral Research Therapy, 25*(4), 281–288.
42. Weinberger, M., et al. (1987). In support of hassles as a measure of stress in predicting health outcomes. *Journal of Behavioral Medicine, 10*(1), 19–31.
43. Zola, I. (1989). Toward the necessary universalizing of a disability policy. The *Milbank Quarterly, 67*(Suppl. 2) 401–427.

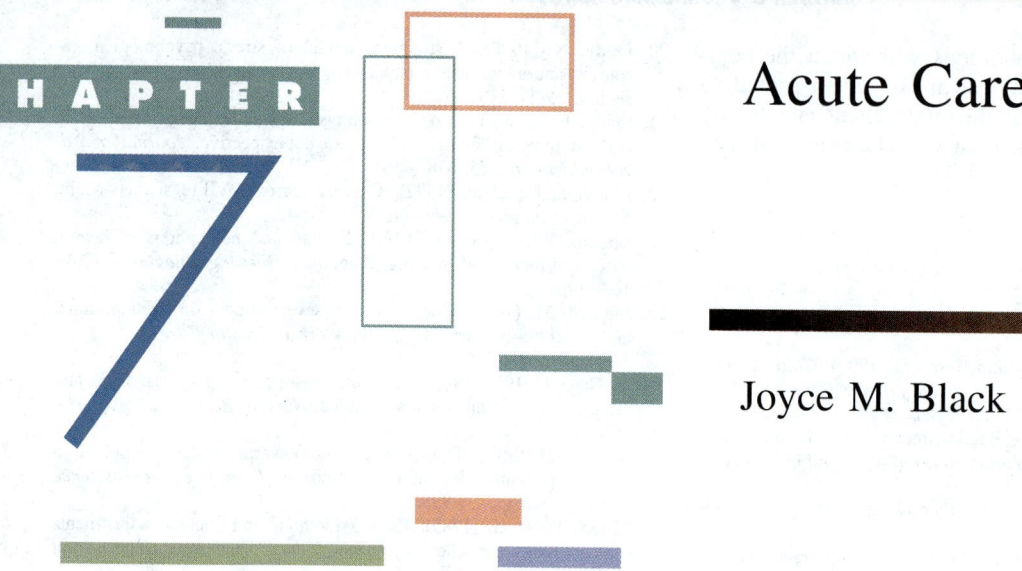

Acute Care

Joyce M. Black

If you talk to a nurse who has worked in a hospital setting for the past 15 to 20 years, you are likely to hear about how much hospitals have changed. It is true. Today's hospitalized clients are sicker than they were years ago, due in part to advances in healthcare technology. We can keep many people alive who would have died of the same diseases years ago. In addition, the hospital has very few clients who are nearly well enough to go home. In the past, some of the nurse's workload included clients who were nearly well. Today, clients who are not acutely ill are being treated in outpatient settings and by their families or significant others at home. Therefore, the workload for nurses today consists of clients who are very ill. Chapter 1 discusses the many reasons for this change; this chapter addresses what it is like to work in a hospital today.

History of Hospital Nursing

Professional nursing in the United States is only about 100 years old. Although nursing is a young profession, it is an indispensable one. The need for nursing care is the major reason for hospitalization.

At the turn of the century, most nurses were employed by affluent clients, and they worked for the clients in their homes. They worked on a fee-for-service basis and were paid by the client or the client's family. A nurse worked with only one client all day long. This early form of nursing care was called *private duty nursing*. Private duty nurses became well versed in the total care of a person, because they provided physical, psychological, and social care. When care of the ill moved into the hospitals, many nurses moved into a hospital setting.

During the Great Depression, many nurses were no longer able to find employment in clients' homes. They were forced to work in hospitals, and in many instances they worked for room and board rather than for a salary. The Blue Cross plan, developed in 1929, offered a form

of prepayment of insurance to help people pay their hospital bills. During the 1930s and 1940s, more and more people purchased such insurance to protect themselves against hospital costs. The fact that hospitals could be more assured of payment put them on a sounder financial footing. The demand for hospital-based nurses rose dramatically. Private duty nurses also moved into the hospital and provided one-to-one care for the hospitalized client at the client's request. Home-based private duty nursing care dwindled. Today, private duty nurses can still be employed by hospitalized clients, but these nurses are usually employed elsewhere and agree to care for the client on a short-term basis. Hospitals keep the names of nurses who will work as private duty nurses on a list, called a *registry*.

In the 1970s and 1980s the demand for hospital nurses continued to soar. Many schools of nursing met the demand by increasing the number of students they enrolled and graduated. Times have certainly changed. As healthcare costs have risen, third-party payors have begun to look at hospital costs and to attempt to control soaring debts. Early discharge and the use of outpatient treatments now places the client back home quickly. Although clients go home after surgery, they are just as ill as they were when they were cared for in the hospital. It should not be surprising that home healthcare nursing is increasing. Nurses still work in hospitals, but a rising percentage of nurses are caring for people in their homes.

Acute Care Hospitals

Clients who require nursing care or monitoring require hospitalization. Some examples of clients who are commonly hospitalized include those who are acutely ill, are victims of trauma, have a potentially critical condition, need intensive monitoring, need complex diagnostic studies, need surgery or complex treatments, or have an exacerbation of a chronic disorder.

The American Hospital Association defines a hospital as an institution with the primary function of providing diagnostic and therapeutic patient services for a variety of medical conditions, both surgical and nonsurgical. Hospitals are of three types: government-owned, voluntary, and for-profit. Other features of hospitals are also discussed.

Government-owned hospitals are official agencies designed to provide care for people who receive local, state, or federal government support. Their services are often provided at no cost or at a reduced cost to the client. Many of the clients have no healthcare benefits. The clients are often employed, but their employer does not provide healthcare insurance programs. Government-owned hospitals can be federally, state, or locally funded. Examples of federally supported hospitals include the Army, Navy, Veteran's Affairs, Public Health Service, and Department of Justice prison hospitals. State-supported hospitals include psychiatric hospitals, state university hospitals, and state prison hospitals. Locally supported hospitals include county or city hospitals.

Voluntary health agencies are nonprofit, tax-exempt organizations designed to meet healthcare needs of the general public. Because it operates as a nonprofit organization does not mean that a hospital does not need to be concerned with its financial status. Although no stockholders are interested in profit, the hospital must plan to have adequate profit to meet its expenses, plan for expansion, and be sustainable during economic depressions. Examples of these types of hospitals include church-affiliated, community, union, and Kaiser-Permanente hospitals. It also includes hospitals owned by special interest groups such as the Shriners, and hospitals for treatment of cancer or other chronic disorders.

For-profit hospitals, also called *proprietary hospitals*, have the same goal as businesses: to generate profit. They serve the general public like voluntary hospitals. The hospitals are privately owned by large corporations, are parts of chains of hospitals, or are owned by single owners. These hospitals have stockholders. An advantage to the larger chains of hospitals is that they can purchase medical supplies in greater volume and therefore at less cost. They also have a slight advantage when contracting for third-party payment because of their ability to reduce costs.

Magnet hospitals are medium to large urban medical centers that have a reputation for providing excellent nursing care and for having good medical outcomes. These hospitals often provide medical services for complex problems that require a team of healthcare providers who would be too expensive to replicate in multiple sites. For example, clients who require organ transplantation or care after a serious injury are commonly cared for in these institutions. The hospitals have a high retention of their staff due to high morale and good payment systems. Most magnet hospitals employ very competent, experienced nurses who need little direct supervision.

Hospitals continuously assess their outcomes and financial health by reviewing cost-benefit and clinical analysis data from their service lines. Service lines can be defined as care given to groups of clients with similar problems. For example, care of clients with heart disease or heart surgery could make up one service line. Many communities with two or more hospitals collaborate and then delineate service lines for each institution. For example, one hospital might provide all psychiatric services, another might provide acute service, and another might provide rehabilitation service. This is a cost- and resource-effective method of providing care, because duplication of effort is eliminated. Clinical outcomes are generally improved when the volume of cases increases because the staff become familiar with typical responses of clients and can detect complications earlier. In addition, equipment used to provide care can be purchased at lower costs when purchased in larger quantities.

In recent years, many hospitals have merged with others in efforts to reduce cost, combine services, and attract third-party payment contracts. Some of the mergers are collaborative, in which both parties are served by the merger. Some mergers are done to rescue ailing hospitals; other mergers are contested or surprise mergers. The environment of the hospital during a merger can be very volatile. Many persons realize that jobs could be lost in an effort to redesign the work environment and delivery systems, and morale often falls. It is important for nurses to keep client care foremost in their minds and to continue to provide high-quality care during the turmoil.

Clients can be admitted to a hospital in several ways (Box 7–1). Once the client is admitted, a primary physician (also called the *attending physician*) will oversee the client's care. Consultants may be used to diagnose problems outside of the physician's speciality. Acute care is a costly service that relies on technology and the expertise of the healthcare team to arrive at a diagnosis, begin treatment, stabilize the condition, and prepare for a transition to a less costly level of healthcare. Many people are involved in a client's care (Box 7–2).

Subacute Care

Subacute care is designed to fill the gap between acute care hospitals and long-term care. The Joint Commission for the Accreditation of Healthcare Organizations defines *subacute care* as

---

Box 7–1. How Clients Are Admitted to a Hospital

Direct—A client is seen in a physician's office and it is determined that the client needs nursing care and specialized monitoring.

Emergency—A client is seen in the emergency department and it is determined that the client needs surgery, nursing care, and/or specialized monitoring. The disease that has been diagnosed or considered likely cannot be taken care of on an outpatient or self-care basis.

Scheduled—A client has elected to undergo surgery or special diagnostic testing that requires specialized monitoring or nursing care during recovery.

Box 7–2. Personnel and Departments in a Hospital

Professional Services

Medical Staff—Consists of private practice or group practice physicians who have their own offices and use the hospital services for care of specific problems. Also made up of physicians who may work for the hospital in departments such as surgery, laboratory, radiology, or emergency.

Nursing Service—Largest group of client care providers in the hospital. Nurses are employed by the nursing service department and provide client care on one unit or ward in the hospital. Nurses are also employed in areas where no direct client care is given, such as administration and hospital-based education programs.

Pharmacy—Consists of pharmacists and assistants who dispense medications prescribed by physicians. Pharmacy staff also monitor the use of regulated medications, such as narcotics. Many pharmacists also teach clients about their medications.

Rehabilitation Services—Physical therapists treat diseases and injuries by restoring, improving, or maintaining the client's functional ability or status to increase musculoskeletal strength to prevent further problems. Occupational therapists teach clients ways to overcome or reduce the problems in activities of daily living that are a result of their disabilities.

Support Services

Administration—Several people on the hospital staff who are accountable for the operation of the entire hospital or institution. Administration can include, for example, the hospital president, vice-presidents, and nurse-managers who supervise client care on a given nursing unit.

Business Departments—Several departments manage the business of the hospital based on both client income and outgoing expenses (salaries, purchasing, operation of the building). The admitting office collects information on insurance and assigns a room to the client. The business office lists each client's charges, prepares the hospital bill, submits it to insurance companies, and records payments received. Payroll departments monitor hours worked, disperse salaries to the employees, and keep records. Purchasing departments disperse money for the purchase of new supplies.

Central Service/Material Management Department— Maintains needed supplies for client care. Provides stock supplies of routinely used items on the nursing units. Cleans and resterilizes reusable supplies.

Dietary—Prepares food for client and staff daily. Dietitians assess and manage nutritional needs of hospitalized clients.

Engineering Department—Maintains the elaborate equipment in the hospital to ensure safe and proper functioning and to adhere to government regulations

Environmental Services—Clean the hospital, including client rooms

Information Technology—Computer support staff is growing in most hospitals because of the increasing use of computers. Staff members focus on design and support mechanisms for electronic data retrieval and storage.

Laboratory—Conduct diagnostic tests to help diagnose illness. Technicians commonly work in radiology and the various laboratories. Laboratory technicians usually collect blood samples from clients; nurses often collect all other specimens and may collect blood from some clients.

Laundry—Launder, sort, and press several hundred pounds of linen each day. New linen is delivered to each nursing unit daily.

Medical Records—Store medical records for all clients. If a client is rehospitalized, former medical records are often important in diagnosing new problems. Also compile data for retrieval for reimbursement, service trending, and outcomes research.

Personnel/Human Resources Department—Hire new employees and concentrate on employee relations. Hospitals may also have people in human resources departments who serve in public relations roles to inform the hospital staff, clients, media, and the public about the hospital and its operations.

Volunteer Services—Operate coffee shops and gift shops, deliver mail to clients, and often raise funds for various hospital projects.

"comprehensive inpatient care designed for someone who has had an acute illness, injury, or exacerbation of a disease process. It is goal oriented treatment rendered immediately after or instead of acute hospitalization to treat one or more specific, active, complex medical conditions or to administer one or more technically complex medical treatments, in the context of a person's underlying long-term conditions and overall situation."

Subacute care is more intensive than traditional nursing home facility care and less acute than acute care hospital. The use of subacute care cultivates a seamless integrated healthcare system. The client should not feel a dramatic change as he or she progresses through levels of care and, most important, should be able to provide his or her own care prior to returning home.

Several factors in healthcare have made subacute care facilities one of the fastest growing segments of healthcare today. Subacute care provides healthcare for clients with complex problems at a fraction of the cost. One estimate is that subacute care is provided at 30% of the cost of the acute care general hospital. Reimbursement is more lucrative for these care settings, so many hospitals have augmented their physical structure to add subacute care units. In some hospitals, nursing units or beds on a given unit or actual beds can serve a dual purpose. These beds are called *swing beds* and can be used either as an acute care bed or as a subacute care bed, depending on the circumstances.

Subacute care areas are designed for clients who are out of the fragile phase of their illness and need routine monitoring and rehabilitation. Typical candidates are clients with diagnoses of stroke, cancer, acquired immunodeficiency syndrome (AIDS), head injury, total hip replacement, wounds needing care, vascular diseases, chronic obstructive pulmonary disease, and renal failure. These clients do not require surgery or other invasive procedures, but they do require frequent assessment and longer stays. Subacute care provides coordinated services to clients by a team of nurses, nursing assistants, physicians, specialized therapists, social workers, and dietitians. Outcomes after subacute care stays are the same as or better than those after hospital stays, so the number of subacute care areas is burgeoning.

Subacute care areas have attracted nurses from the hospital setting because nurses feel they have more time, less pressure, and a more interdisciplinary approach to client care. Another attractive feature of most subacute units is that the environment seems more like home to the client and family.

The four categories of subacute care units are as follows:

1. *Transitional subacute care* provides for short stays (5 to 30 days) with high levels of nursing care. This type of unit serves as a hospital step-down unit, which serves as an alternative to continued hospitalization and thereby reduces the number of days in an acute care setting. Typical clients in transitional subacute care include those recovering from myocardial infarction (heart attack) or open heart surgery; those who must be weaned from a ventilator; those who need wound management after burn injury or for multiple pressure ulcers; those who require more rehabilitation after stroke, orthopedic surgery, or burn injury; or those who have medically complex problems such as diabetes or digestive or renal problems.
2. *General subacute units* have some overlap with transitional units; the key difference is the acuity level of the clients. Many clients in these units are Medicare beneficiaries, because younger clients with the same level of disability tend to receive home care. These units are used for clients who require about 3.5 hours of nursing care and 1 to 3 hours of therapy daily. Typical clients are the same as those on transitional units, although the stay is longer (10 to 40 days). The goal of care is to send clients home or to a less expensive level of care, such as to long-term care or assisted-living centers.
3. *Chronic subacute units* manage clients with little hope of ultimate recovery and functional independence. Typical clients include those who cannot be successfully weaned from a ventilator, are in a long-term comatose state, or have progressive neurologic disorders. Nursing intensity is similar to that in general subacute care units. The goal of care is to stabilize the clients' conditions so they can be transferred to home or to a long-term care center. The average length of stay is 60 to 90 days.
4. *Long-term transitional subacute facilities* provide care for clients with medically complex problems or who are ventilator dependent. Average length of stay is around 25 days, but it can be more. The units are staffed primarily by RNs, and each client requires about 6 to 9 hours of care per day.

Home Healthcare

Home healthcare is not new. It is a pattern of healthcare delivery that began in New York during the 1950s, during a shortage of hospital beds. Home healthcare had a resurgence during the early 1980s, when payments to hospitals were capped on the basis of length-of-stay estimates for categories called *diagnosis-related groups* (DRGs). Hospitals needed to discharge clients quickly to home to reduce the cost of hospitalization. Home healthcare continues to be a vibrant area for practice, and nurses provide an extensive range of care in the home. Home healthcare is discussed in Chapter 9.

Roles and Responsibilities of Nurses in Hospitals

Nursing is a service provided both to individual clients and to aggregates of people (e.g., families, groups, communities, populations). To fulfill nursing's commitment to contribute to the healthcare of people, professional nurses assume multiple roles and responsibilities. Although these roles tend to overlap, they are important to distinguish. They include provider of direct care, educator, and manager.

Provider of Direct Care

Most people are familiar with nurses as providers of direct care. Nurses assess, care for, educate, and comfort clients. Nurses provide direct care in all settings and along all dimensions of the health-illness continuum, from health promotion to critical care and death.

Indirect care consists of the processes that go on in support of the actual bedside nursing care given. Sometimes this level of care is labeled *interdependent*. The nurse interprets physicians' orders, administers medication, and provides treatment for the client when performing interdependent care.

Educator

Professional nurses provide formal and informal education to their clients, individually and in groups. Informal education goes on almost continually, as clients are taught about medications while the medications are being administered, about the importance of eating a balanced diet when they choose their menu selections, and so on. The importance of informal education should not be underestimated.

Formal education is usually provided to groups of clients and their families. The nurse may use a classroom or bring videotapes or audio tapes into the client's room. Advantages to formal education are that the client is usually readied for learning, significant others are included, and the material presented is consistent from client to client. Many hospitals have formal educators on their staff for clients with complex learning needs. Certified diabetes educators, certified lactation specialists, oncology nurse specialists, and enterostomal therapists are examples of these nurses who provide education to clients in the hospital and often follow-up with the client when he or she is back in the community.

Finally, some nurses who specialize in education and rehabilitation. These nurses often work in cardiac and pulmonary rehabilitation and may subspecialize in physical therapy or exercise physiology. Their role is to assist in the rehabilitation of clients after myocardial infarction, congestive heart failure, or chronic air flow limitations (chronic obstructive lung diseases).

Manager

The term *manager* in this discussion means the effective use of human and material resources in providing care to clients. Human resources include (1) the client, (2) the nurse, (3) the family or significant others, (4) professional colleagues, (5) support groups (e.g., the American Cancer Society), and (6) resource groups (e.g., Vocational Rehabilitation). Material resources include equipment and supplies. Time is also an important resource. Finally, outcome is an important consideration in healthcare management. Outcomes are examined in more detail in the next section.

The first episode of client management that you will encounter is your provision of timely care to one client. Effective time management of only one client is difficult at first, due to interruptions and lack of familiarity with equipment and procedures. Even while caring for only one client, it is important to stay on time with assessments, medications, and treatments. Most of these aspects of nursing care are scheduled more than once every 24 hours; if you are late, the next treatment or medication may have to be delayed. As you become more experienced, care of one client will become efficient. As you care for more than one client, time management becomes more important.

Nursing Care Delivery Systems

We need to look at how client care is delivered on any nursing unit. Several techniques are in use today, and each has its advantages and disadvantages.

Total Care Nursing

Total care nursing is the oldest of the care delivery systems. One nurse is assigned to one client and provides all care. The one-to-one pattern is common in critical care, with student nurses, and with private duty nurses. The advantage is that the client only needs to work with one nurse and that one nurse can focus on meeting all the biopsychosocial needs of the client and family. Disadvantages are that this system requires that any given nurse be proficient at all nursing tasks and problem-solving areas.

Functional Nursing

Functional nursing is a system of care borrowed from industry that concentrates on duties. This pattern of care can be seen as an assembly line of care. It began during World War II, when the demand for patient care outstripped the supply of nurses. The registered nurse may coordinate the care for an entire unit or team. Other nurses may be assigned to pass medications and perform treatments. Less-trained personnel are often assigned to provide more basic care (e.g., giving baths, making beds). An advantage of this system is that care can be provided at a lower cost. Disadvantages are that the client interacts with several people; psychosocial needs are seldom met; the RN seldom cares for the client and must rely on other people's assessments of the client's problems. In addition, each member of the working group is highly dependent on the other members, and the nurse is in a very autocratic position. Functional nursing is still commonly used in skilled nursing and long-term care facilities.

Team Nursing

Team nursing is a system of care by which the RN leads a group of healthcare personnel in providing care for a team of 10 to 20 clients. Team nursing was developed in the 1950s because of social and technological changes. World War II drew many nurses from hospitals, causing gaps in the nursing population. In addition, several technological advances required specialized knowledge. Team nursing was felt to be one approach to using people's skills more effectively. Its advantages are that an RN is head of the team and generally knows the clients. In addition, the team leader is usually a more experienced nurse and can provide guidance to new or inexperienced nurses. As in functional nursing, the talents and abilities of each member of the healthcare team are used. Disadvantages to team nursing are that it is fairly expensive because the care is fragmented; a lack of delegation skills by RNs may reduce efficiency; and some redundancy may occur if each team leader has to perform several managerial tasks, such as making assignments.

Primary Nursing

Primary nursing is both a model of care delivery and a model of organizing care to achieve high-quality care outcomes. This style of care delivery emerged during the 1980s to meet the needs of increasingly complex clients. The goal is for each client's care to be comprehensive and coordinated, from admission to discharge. Each client is assigned an RN as the primary nurse, and that nurse always provides care for that client when he/she is working. In addition, associate nurses provide care when the primary nurse is absent. Advantages are obvious: the client has the same nurse, the client's psychosocial needs can be met, communication with the physician is improved, and the nurse feels very autonomous. Disadvantages are the increased cost in hiring a large RN staff; possible role confusion between primary and associate nurses; and many calls to physicians from one nursing unit. When a charge nurse system is used, the charge nurse makes telephone calls and often handles several issues in one telephone call.

Case Management

The nurse can serve a pivotal role in coordinating all of the events required for a timely recovery. Many hospitals have developed sophisticated guides, called *critical pathways* or case management plans, to direct client care and recovery from predictable problems. Case management is a care delivery mode that incorporates concepts of continuity and efficiency in addressing long-term physical, psychological, and social needs of clients. The primary goals of case management are promoting self-care, upgrading the quality of life, and using resources efficiently. Case managers are nurses who coordinate care of a group of clients, monitor the implementation of interdisciplinary care plans, and maintain communication with third-party payors and referral sources. A key distinction in the nurse's role in the case management system is that it transcends nursing unit and physician service (e.g, cardiology) boundaries. The nurse follows the client through the entire stay in the healthcare system and back into the community.

Appendix D (Clinical Pathways) contains several case management plans for you to refer to as you read about the care of a particular client. When you refer to them pay attention to the multidisciplinary care guided by the plans. Notice the detail provided so that predictable discharge dates can be met. Most of the case management plans in Appendix D were created for one hospital, and they probably cannot be used without modification to provide care for clients in other facilities. You may work with case managers and with case management plans for your own clients or in your own institution.

Management and Delegation

Today, in an effort to control costs, almost all hospitals have hired unlicensed assistive personnel (UAP) to provide care. Other than on-the-job training, UAP receive little formal training. The use of less trained and educated personnel to perform nursing duties is changing the face of nursing staffing in hospitals. The use of UAP is increasing despite the inconclusive amount of research demonstrating their effectiveness on client outcomes.

Different terms are used for nurse extenders, which may include unlicensed assistive personnel. These terms include *unit assistant, primary practice partner,* and *unit hostess*. Nurse extenders with more advanced skills might be called *clinical technicians*. Assistive personnel may help with clinical duties, nonclinical duties, or both. Some of the duties that may be delegated include giving baths, taking vital signs, serving food and collecting trays, performing unit-based laboratory tests (e.g., finger sticks for blood glucose assessment), 12-lead electrocardiograms, and skin care. Nurses need to learn when to delegate. For example, the nurse may delegate a bed bath and linen change for a client who is stable and do the bath herself on an unstable or new client. This book offers examples of appropriate delegation to unlicensed assistive personnel throughout (see the Management and Delegation features in Chapters 11, 13, 21, 31, 40, 46, 62, 74, and 75).

Box 7–3. Critical Questions for Planning Nurse Extenders

What are the appropriate core duties of an RN?
Who should perform which tasks?
What can be delegated?
What is an appropriate and cost-effective staff mix?
What is the risk management and liability at each level of caregiver?
Who can substitute for whom?
Who is the least expensive worker to do each task?
How much management or supervision is needed?
What is the philosophical commitment to the provision of total patient care by the RN here?
Will lowering the qualification of staff add further stress and frustration to our staff?
How will this affect recruitment?
What is the impact on collective bargaining?

From Gardner, D. L. (1991). Issues related to the use of nurse extenders. *Journal of Nursing Administration, 21*(10), 40–45.

In planning the use of nurse extenders, nurse managers and their staff must be aware of their specific responses to many key questions (Box 7–3). Two issues that demand particular attention are the role functions that only an RN can perform and the minimum level of RN staffing that is required to provide safe client care.

Nurses may have been taught that only RNs can or should perform certain clinical duties, and they may therefore have difficulty delegating them to less qualified personnel. As the pressure mounts to delegate tasks to lower-paid workers, nurses will need to develop managerial skills, especially those of leadership, delegation, and supervision. Nurses will remain professionally accountable for client outcomes whether or not the specific tasks that contribute to those outcomes were performed by the nurses or nurse extenders. Each nurse must clearly understand what the agency defines as the role and duties of the RN, the licensed practical/vocational nurse, and the various nurse extenders employed by the agency.

Ensuring Quality Healthcare Delivery

Amid the fast-paced changes occurring in healthcare delivery, healthcare professionals remain responsible for ensuring quality client care. Quality client care is the outcome of the integrated healthcare team approach that involves the corporate and hospital or agency administration, medical staff, board of trustees, employees, the community, and the client. Contract services, community resources, transfer agreements, and expertise from social workers or case managers enable client transitions to alternate levels of care in a continuous, coordinated, and almost seamless fashion. Through work-redesign and skill-mix reallocation, institutions are focusing goals on achieving efficient client outcomes. Work-redesign involves studying a job over a fixed period to discover if and how a certain job function could be made more efficient. Skill-mix is determined by studying the ratio of registered nurses to licensed practical/vocational nurses and nursing assistants on a unit. The best skill-mix delivers quality care while also controlling costs.

The "one-level-of-care" philosophy ensures that clients receive optimum care in all areas of an institution. For example, when intravenous conscious sedation is administered in the endoscopy unit, the same monitoring should be performed as is done when sedation is administered in the operating room or emergency department.

Great importance is placed on facilitating entry into the system and into the appropriate type of care (e.g., service or setting), as well as on the proper transition to various levels of care that the client later requires.

Clients' Rights to Quality Care

Clients have an increased awareness of the quality-of-care issue. They are demanding and receiving more information prior to the initiation of treatments. Increasingly, clients' requests for information about costs, risks, benefits, and alternatives to suggested therapies are being honored. No longer submissive to the suggested care, the client is becoming a participant and partner in healthcare, with the expectation of receiving quality care from all healthcare professionals.

Client rights have reached a new level of importance for the healthcare consumer. Regulating agencies, insurance carriers, third-party payors, and providers are responding to ensure that these fundamental rights are maintained and that clients receive quality services.

Providing Quality Client Care

Any plan for provision of client care involves the following aspects:

- Budgeting process, to assist the institution in studying, spending, and using the information to cut costs or maintain them at the present rate
- Strategic planning, to serve as a guideline for the continued and/or expanded services provided by the healthcare agency
- Performance improvement plan, to show the steps taken to improve performance based on monitoring and evaluation of staff performance
- Risk management input, to identify and eliminate potential injuries to staff and clients
- Utilization review data, to explore items such as acuity levels, outcomes, and costs, to discover what is effective care and what is not
- Client satisfaction survey results, with data gathered from clients at various stages of their stay in the agency (e.g., preprocedure, admission procedure, discharge)
- Physician input, to incorporate professional input into client care planning

- Census data, to plot current and future trends of healthcare in the organization
- Acuity levels (as designated by the healthcare organization), to plan an appropriate skill-mix for staffing

Changes in client population, diagnoses, programs, or staffing that would necessitate changes in the type, level, or amount of care are reviewed on an ongoing basis.

Other factors contributing to quality care include the adherence to, monitoring of, and evaluation of care given according to professional standards, JCAHO and Department of Health criteria, and input from other regulatory agencies. In addition, clinical pathways, clinical practice guidelines, standards of practice and care, and competence standards serve as models for professional delivery of client care.

Staffing for Quality Care

Healthcare institutions use a combination of methods to ensure a staff of caregivers who can deliver quality care to clients. Two methods include

- Daily collection of census data (a count of the number of clients occupying beds on any given day)
- Determination of acuity levels (a degree of severity of illness that affects the amount and complexity of care the client requires)

Staff are assigned or reassigned to units that have the greatest need for their expertise and experience. Staffing adjustments caused by the fluctuation of census data and acuity levels are accomplished by using per diem staff and other creative measures to ensure safe client care.

Although staffing adjustment decisions in the past were typically made at higher levels of administration, now service line leaders and empowered directors and managers are instrumental in adjusting strategies based on the many shifting variables that affect client care. These individuals are closer to the actual care setting (clients and staff) and can use their expertise to make informed decisions about staffing for quality care.

Input from the employees who actually provide care is helpful in redesigning and improving the quality of care given to clients. Because caregivers are directly involved with client care, they can contribute in significant ways by reporting problems that can be addressed in a timely fashion. Such input, especially when acted on by management, contributes to staff members' feelings of being valued.

Unfortunately, adequate staffing is not always ensured. In the spring of 1995, nurses marched on Washington, D.C., to protest clinical staffing shortages that had already endangered and could further endanger client care (see Ethical Issues in Nursing).

In an attempt to make the most effective use of available nursing staff, cross-training has evolved in hospitals. Whereas in the past a nurse was typically assigned to one unit, where she or he could become familiar with the other personnel and the unit routine, today's hospital nurse may be cross-trained to work effectively in two or more units (e.g., a surgical unit and a cardiac intensive care unit). The nurse is assigned to the unit where she or

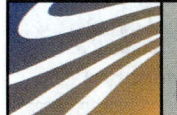

ETHICAL ISSUES IN NURSING

Is Whistleblowing Ever the Right Thing to Do?

Your hospital is experiencing troubling financial times. In an effort to cut expenses, many nurse positions have been cut. Patient care needs remain very high and the nurses on your unit are having difficulty giving good nursing care. Frequently, you believe the nursing care has become unsafe. The nurse-manager reports that there will be more nursing cuts on the unit. She seems unable to do anything about the nurse shortage on the unit.

After 2 months, the situation is getting much worse. The nurse-manager reports that three other nurse-managers were fired because they refused to cut staff. Patients on your unit are not getting adequate care. The nurses are very upset and do not know what to do.

In most healthcare settings today, the nurse is frequently not the person with the most power or control. Usually, the physician or administration has significantly more power and control. This sometimes causes ethical problems arising from power inequities.

It is your responsibility to be sure of the facts surrounding this issue. Understanding the context of the situation is essential. The ability to see a problem clearly can help to determine the nurse's actions and responsibilities.

In cases like this, it is imperative that you exhaust all relevant internal channels and procedures first. This involves contacting the nurse-manager directly to see if anything else can be done. If this meeting is not satisfactory, you may want to consider talking to the director of the nursing department.

Sometimes, calling public attention to the problem, or "whistleblowing," is the action needed. This may involve contacting the local TV station or newspaper. It should, however, be used when all other options have failed. This action may not be without consequences. There are substantial risks involved. You can lose your job even if others evaluate your position as correct and the administration's action as morally wrong. So, careful thought and evaluation are essential.

he is most needed that day, and may arrive for work not knowing in advance the work assignment for that day. This new scenario is often stress-producing for nurses and other staff members.

Nursing Intensity Classification

To ensure that staffing is adequate, it is important to understand how ill any given group of clients is and how much nursing care they will require. Hospitalized clients are classified using several systems in an attempt to determine *nursing intensity*. Nursing intensity is a combination of the amount of care and skill level at which care is provided. Usually, physical care and psychosocial or teaching skills are included. For example, a stable comatose client might require a large amount of low-complexity care that could be provided by unlicensed assistive personnel. In contrast, a newly diagnosed diabetic teenager with several personal and family problems may require less time for care, but the care should be provided by an RN.

Any patient classification system has several purposes; among these are the following:

● *Staffing*. The system will establish a unit of measure for nursing time. The unit of measure will be used to determine the number of kinds of healthcare providers that are needed for any given shift.
● *Cost*. The system can be used to determine the cost of nursing care. Profits and losses can then be calculated.
● *Tracking changes*. The acuity of care needed may change as the case mix changes or during certain times of the year.

Two methods are generally used to determine acuity. Using a factor evaluation method, each client is rated on independent elements of care; each element is scored (weighted); scores are summarized, and the client is placed in a category based on the total numeric value obtained. Using a prototype evaluation, each client is categorized according to a broad description of care requirements. The prototypes usually have four categories which describe (1) the client's ability to perform activities of daily living (ADL), (2) general health, (3) emotional support, and (4) treatment modalities (Table 7–1).

Monitoring Healthcare Outcomes

New ideas are coming into play about healthcare outcomes. The shift in healthcare was originally focused on cost reduction. Fortunately, a growing realization has developed that cost reduction may equate to losses in quality of care. New ideas are emerging that speak to the *value* of healthcare. The value of healthcare will consider what the cost of care was for any given procedure or health problem as well as the outcome of the care. This is a needed change in the direction of quality healthcare. Third-party payment contracts in the future will likely consider the value of healthcare provided at various institutions before signing contracts. We will look at some of the ways healthcare outcomes are monitored in an effort to track outcomes and value.

Broad-Based Indicators

Patient Satisfaction Surveys

As in business, healthcare providers have learned that it is easier to keep customers than to find new ones. Patient satisfaction surveys are commonly given to the client on discharge or sent to the client's home shortly after discharge. The basic question being asked is, "Would you

Table 7–1. Patient Care Classification Using Four Levels of Nursing Care Intensity

Area of Care	Category 1	Category 2	Category 3	Category 4
Eating	Feeds self or needs little food	Needs some help in preparing; may need encouragement	Cannot feed self but is able to chew and swallow	Cannot feed self and may have difficulty swallowing
Grooming	Almost entirely self-sufficient	Needs some help in bathing, oral hygiene, hair combing, and so forth	Unable to do much for self	Completely dependent
Excretion	Up and to bathroom alone or almost alone	Needs some help in getting up to bathroom or using urinal	In bed, needs bedpan or urinal placed; may be able to partially turn or lift self	Completely dependent
Comfort	Self-sufficient	Needs some help with adjusting position or bed (e.g., tubes, IVs)	Cannot turn without help, get drink, adjust position of extremities, and so forth	Completely dependent
General health	Good—in for diagnostic procedure, simple treatment, or surgical procedure (D & C, biopsy, minor fracture)	Mild symptoms—more than one mild illness, mild debility, mild emotional reaction, mild incontinence (not more than once/shift)	Acute symptoms—severe emotional reaction to illness or surgery, more than one acute illness, medical or surgical problem, severe or frequent incontinence	Critically ill—may have severe emotional reaction
Treatments	Simple—supervised ambulation, dangle, simple dressing, test procedure preparation not requiring medication, reinforcement of surgical dressing, x-pad, vital signs once/shift	Any category 1 treatment more than once/shift, Foley catheter, care, I & O, bladder irrigations, sitz bath, compresses, test procedures requiring medications or follow-ups, simple enema for evacuation, vital signs every 4 hr	Any treatment more than twice/shift, medicated IVs, complicated dressings, sterile procedures, care of tracheotomy, Harris flush, suctioning, tube feeding, vital signs more than every 4 hr	Any elaborate or delicate procedure requiring two nurses, vital signs more often than every 2 hr
Medications	Simple, routine, not needing preevaluation or postevaluation; medications no more than once/shift	Diabetic, cardiac, hypotensive, hypertensive, diuretic, anticoagulant medications, prn medications, more than once/shift, medications needing preevaluation or postevaluation	Unusual amount of category 2 medications; control of refractory diabetics (need to be monitored more than every 4 hr)	More intensive category 3 medications; IVs with frequent, close observation and regulation
Teaching and emotional support	Routine follow-up teaching; patients with no unusual or adverse emotional reactions	Initial teaching of care of ostomies, new diabetics, tubes that will be in place for periods of time; conditions requiring major change in eating, living, or excretory practices; patients with mild adverse reactions to their illness (e.g., depression, being overly demanding)	More intensive category 2 items; teaching of apprehensive or mildly resistive patients; care of moderately upset or apprehensive patients; confused or disoriented patients	Teaching of resistive patients, care and support of patients with severe emotional reaction.

From Marquis, B. L., & Huston, C. J. (1996). *Leadership roles and management functions in nursing* (p. 266). Philadelphia: J. B. Lippincott.

return to our institution for healthcare in the future?" Clients are often asked about their perception of medical care, nursing care, ancillary care, the environment, and follow-up care. Sometimes patient satisfaction surveys are discounted because of the fact that the patient has limited knowledge of what would constitute reasonable care. To overcome this feeling of helplessness by the client, some hospitals inform clients of the services they can reasonably expect while hospitalized. For example, clients are informed that they can reasonably expect adequate pain relief. Then clients are asked to evaluate if the outcome was met during the stay. This excellent change reminds all healthcare providers that the client's opinion of the care provided should always be one indicator of quality of care.

Measurement of Functional Status

Several tools exist that can measure functional status; these include general perception of health, limitations in physical ability because of health problems, ability to engage in social activities (including work), general mental health, pain, energy, fatigue, and depression. Some hospitals are using these measures to monitor how an intervention affected the functional status. For example, it is hoped that functional status would improve after coronary bypass surgery. Valid data to show improvement in a group of clients served by the hospital provides excellent evidence of healthcare value.

Access Issues

Because people are mobile, the location of the hospital and access to the agency are important factors. Hospitals are concerned about convenience, location, wait time, and lead time needed to find a primary care provider, arrange an outpatient procedure, or schedule a diagnostic procedure.

Meeting Regulatory Requirements

Regulatory agencies have the primary goal of enhancing the public's ability to secure adequate healthcare. Healthcare agencies are surveyed periodically to ensure compliance with specific rules and regulations. A survey is an in-depth study of a healthcare institution (e.g., a hospital or a long-term care facility) according to specific criteria set forth by the regulating agencies involved. All aspects of the institution's services are inspected. Important performance areas include client assessment, medication administration, use of restraints, client and family education, staff training, information management, and organizational performance. After the survey is completed, a report of findings is compiled, and the institution is notified of its satisfactory status. If a criterion is not met satisfactorily, the institution is notified, given time to correct the deficiency, and reevaluated at a later date.

Public disclosure of survey findings has begun. For hospital surveys completed after Jan 1, 1994, a status report (on 28 performance areas) is made available to the public, including media sources, insurance companies, third-party payors, clients, and competing institutions. Other healthcare delivery services function under the same disclosure rules for compliance with regulations of the inspecting agencies.

Regulatory Agencies and Statutes

Several regulatory agencies have statutes that must be met by hospitals. These laws govern hiring and employment, quality controls, and conditions of the work site to reduce hazards. The full description of these laws is beyond the scope of this book; we will only look at a few of them. Employment laws include the equal employment opportunity laws that ensure equal rights in the workplace for racial and ethnic minorities, women, the elderly and the handicapped. A worker from the 1920s might be shocked to see contemporary changes in workplace rights for everyone.

The Civil Rights Act of 1964 laid the foundation for equal employment in the United States. The thrust of Title VII of the Civil Rights Act is twofold: (1) it prohibits discrimination based on factors unrelated to job qualifications and (2) it promotes employment based on ability and merit. The areas of discrimination specifically mentioned are race, color, religion, sex, and national origin. The Equal Employment Opportunity Commission is responsible for enforcing Title VII of the Civil Rights Act. When a charge of discrimination is proven, the agency attempts to mediate the problem through persuasion and conciliation.

In 1967, Congress enacted the Age Discrimination and Employment Act (ADEA). Its purpose was to promote employment of older people based on their ability rather than their age. In early 1978, the ADEA was amended to increase the protected age to 70 years. Although people feared that this act would have serious consequences for labor-intensive occupations, such as nursing, many people are opting for earlier retirement and problems have not been reported.

The Rehabilitation Act of 1973 required all employers with government contracts of more than $25,000 to take affirmative action to recruit, hire, and advance handicapped people who are qualified. In 1990, Congress passed the Americans with Disabilities Act to eliminate discrimination against Americans with physical or mental disabilities in the workplace and in social life. Disability is defined as "any physical or mental impairment that limits any major life activity." This includes not only all individuals with obvious physical disabilities, but also individuals with cancer, diabetes, human immunodeficiency virus (HIV), AIDS, and recovering alcoholics and drug users. The act not only prohibits discrimination, but also delineates clear, enforceable standards.

The Occupational Safety and Health Act (OSHA) is broadly written legislation that requires a place of employment to be free from recognized hazards and developed environmental safety laws for the safety of the employees. The Department of Labor enforces this act. Since the inception of OSHA, many companies have vehemently criticized the act, specifically its administration. Companies have charged that the costs of meeting OSHA standards have excessively burdened American business. However, unions have asserted that the federal government has never adequately staffed or funded the Occupational and Health Administration. They have charged that OSHA has been negligent in setting standards for toxic substances, carcinogens, and other disease-producing agents.

Finally, quality assurance standards must be met by several areas of the hospital. Laboratories must test control solutions of known substances routinely to ensure that test results are accurate. Equipment used for sterilization of instruments and other supplies must be tested daily. These precautions are critical to safe care.

Legal Issues

Nurses have more responsibility than they used to. Expanded roles of nurses open the doors to greater legal risk. The nurse's employer is obligated to carry malpractice insurance for its employees. The nurse should know what is covered in the policy. In addition, the nurse should carry individual malpractice insurance.

Proper documentation is critical to serve as evidence of the quality of nursing care provided. The court still assumes that if something was not noted in a chart, it was not done. It is important to be specific and to document nursing actions taken and the client's response (e.g., pain relief). If unusual events occur, an incident report should be completed. The benefit of incident reports is that they allow the analysis of adverse client events. They should not be treated as a punitive activity but rather as a method of promoting quality care and risk management. Errors are examined to determine if the error was due to

a system problem (e.g., a faulty electrical outlet that leads to a fire or an improperly mounted siderail that allows a client to fall). If a lawsuit is filed, incident reports are usually not revealed; instead the court system relies on the information in the medical record.

Performance Improvement

Hospitals and other healthcare organizations have been challenged by their goal of attaining a planned, systematic, multidisciplinary, nationwide approach to designing, measuring, assessing, and improving performance. These institutions generally seek to enhance their measurement activities as they relate to institutional quality indicators (Box 7–4). These indicators generally include the following:

● Results of basic clinical indicators
● Continuous quality improvement
● Access to care issues
● Consumer satisfaction and judgment input
● JCAHO indicators
● Human resource management
● Organization performance

Healthcare organizations are in the midst of a transition to performance improvement from traditional quality assurance. Relevant goals include the following:

● Enhancing clinical leaders' abilities to set expectations, develop plans, and manage processes to assess, improve, and maintain the quality of the organization's clinical and support activities
● Enhancing healthcare outcomes and the perception of these outcomes and expectations by all consumers
● Measuring outcomes to determine priorities for improvement
● Systematically improving performance of important functions and maintaining stability of these functions

---

Box 7–4. Clinical Indicators with a Focus on High-Volume, High-Risk, and Problem-Prone Issues

The community/clinic focus includes the following:

▪ Communicable diseases (e.g., TB, HIV)
▪ Low birth weight as a percentage of live births
▪ Births to mothers 10 to 17 years of age as a percentage of all live births
▪ Percentage of women receiving prenatal care during the first trimester
▪ Breast cancer rates and mammography statistics
▪ Immunization rates
▪ Return visits to the same level of care or visit within 72 hours to a higher level of care
▪ Accessibility, availability, and acceptability of care
▪ Appropriateness and relevance of care (e.g., based on diagnostic laboratory work, symptomatology)

▪ Appropriateness of treatment frequency
▪ Intake system
▪ Provision for information on an emergency or after-hours basis
▪ Client education
▪ Consultation
▪ Documentation including, for example, transfers and advance directives
▪ Availability of emergency carts/equipment
▪ Use of leasing for expensive/alternative resources
▪ Client record
▪ Client rights, including advance directives, informed consent, and special concern for abuse victims and for those with cultural diversity

From Polaski, A., & Tatro, S. (1996). *Luckmann's core principles and practice of medical surgical nursing.* Philadelphia: W. B. Saunders.

Box 7–5. Qualities that Enhance Performance of Services in Healthcare Settings

- Efficacy: The degree to which the care and intervention for the client have been shown to accomplish the desired or projected outcomes
- Appropriateness: The degree to which the care and intervention provided are relevant to the client's clinical needs, given the current state of knowledge
- Availability: The degree to which appropriate care and intervention are available to meet the needs of the client
- Timeliness: The degree to which the care and intervention are provided to the client at the most beneficial or necessary time
- Effectiveness: The degree to which the care and intervention are provided in the correct manner, given the current state of knowledge, to achieve the desired or projected outcome for the client
- Continuity: The degree to which the care and intervention for the client are coordinated among practitioners, among organizations, and over time
- Safety: The degree to which the risk of an intervention and the risk in the care environment are reduced for the client and others, including healthcare providers
- Efficiency: The relationship between the outcomes and the resources used to deliver client care
- Respect and caring: The degree to which the client or a designee is involved in his or her own care decisions and to which those providing services do so with sensitivity and respect for the client's needs, expectations, and individual differences

From Polaski, A., & Tatro, S. (1996). *Luckmann's core principles and practice of medical surgical nursing.* Philadelphia: W. B. Saunders.

- Implementing quality improvement activities that optimally affect client outcomes and cost of services, and then measuring the ongoing effect of these changes on the services provided
- Instituting a flexible performance improvement plan so that new or changed services and clinical practices serve as triggers for new indicator development
- Enhancing reporting and communication mechanisms of performance improvement results so that the greatest benefit is realized
- Strengthening the client education component as a result of quality assurance and improvement of information
- Supporting performance by improving existing processes
- Designing improvement activities for new processes
- Supporting client advocacy and customer response functions by responding to complaints at the closest level of client care
- Using readily available resources to produce all-inclusive information and to minimize data collection by staff
- Exploring automated methods of improving the performance of clinical information systems

Qualities that enhance the important dimensions of performance are listed in Box 7–5.

Risk Management

Risk management follows the current trend of adapting business strategies to healthcare systems. Risk management is a planned program of loss prevention and liability control. Its purpose is to identify, analyze, and evaluate risks followed by a plan of reducing the frequency of accidents and injuries. Risk management requires a team of people from all departments in the institution. The risk manager administers the program and serves as the liaison among the hospital administration, the risk management committee, and others. They also serve as a liaison among insurance company representatives, institution attorneys, and others. Risk managers are of no typical profile and can be, for example, nurses, administrators, lawyers, or, former insurance representatives.

Nursing personnel are crucial to a successful risk management program. The five areas of highest risk in the hospital are (1) medication errors, (2) complications from diagnostic or treatment procedures, (3) falls, (4) patient or family dissatisfaction, and (5) refusal of treatment or refusal to sign consent for treatment. Medical records and incident reports serve as documents of accountability. Incident reports are used to analyze problems within the five categories and to plan for corrective actions (see Nursing Research feature).

The Future of Acute Care Hospital Nursing

Acute care nursing is changing, but a bright future exists. We will continue to see major changes in healthcare delivery and it will be essential that nurses take a primary position to help ensure that client care remains a priority. Since healthcare costs continue to rise, cost containment will also remain a major concern. As a result of cost containment, goals for acute health providers include the following:

- Increase the efficiency of care to speed transfer to a less costly level of care
- Streamline care to ease movement into capitated services or managed care contracts
- Monitor clinical pathways for variances and then implement quality improvement strategies to correct the variances

NURSING RESEARCH

What Are the Effects of Nursing Errors?

Biordi, D. L. (1993). Nursing error and caring in the workplace. *Nursing Administration Quarterly, 17* (2), 38–45.

As nurses, none of us like to make mistakes. Mistakes violate our ethic to "do no harm." Still, mistakes happen. The purpose of this study was to examine the formal and informal work processes in organizations that are used to manage errors.

The study was conducted over 1 year on two nursing units. The units were almost completely staffed by RNs and known to provide high-quality care. A participant-observational method was used.

Errors were categorized into three major progressively intense categories.

1. *Technical error* is an honest error of technique. When technical errors occurred, senior nurses (more experienced, more tenured) tended to be low-key, even good-natured, about it. They expected new and inexperienced nurses to make mistakes. Junior nurses were not so sanguine about their own errors. They worried about the mistakes and pondered over them for a while. When good faith exists and prompt disclosure occurs, honest technical errors can be repaired or prevented from recurring.
2. *Judgmental error* is an honest error in which the nurse chose the wrong strategies. Typically, nursing care is private work: each nurse works alone with clients and makes individual choices. Judgmental errors were felt to decrease after about 2 years in the work setting. Because a judgmental error is a flaw in strategic action, rather than in the person, the control of error is expressed in terms of the action itself. Nurses corrected these errors by seeking authorities for advice.
3. *Normative error* is the most serious of all errors. This error is a breach of honesty, trust, or responsibility that raises serious doubts about the ability of the person to be a nurse. These serious errors violate the core of nursing and show a lack of caring and a lack of full disclosure. Nurses who committed these errors often blamed others for the mistakes.

Implications for Practice. The analysis of error allows nurses to interpret the true basis of the mistake and its likely consequences. Nurses need to take risks with clients, but the process of safe risk-taking must be learned through clinical practice.

- Enhance client understanding of the disease and its management through education and early discharge planning
- Target high-risk, problem-prone, high-volume client care activities for quality improvement endeavors
- Act on client satisfaction concerns to promote client advocacy
- Extract applicable client, physician, and employee satisfaction data to allow a realistic focus on pertinent issues
- Support institutional quality indicators and quality-improvement team endeavors to increase the value of healthcare
- Enhance the dimensions of performance through the use of appropriateness, availability, timeliness, effectiveness, continuity, safety, efficiency, respect, and caring.

Conclusions

Acute care hospital-based nursing has changed. Years ago, the client could stay in the hospital until he or she felt well enough to go home. Cost-containment issues have demanded that clients today spend as little time as possible in acute care and quickly move to less expensive areas for care. Professional nurses have become more pivotal in the provision of high-quality care during these shortened stays. All healthcare providers are trying to maintain healthcare with excellent value during these changing times.

Bibliography

1. Alfred, C. A., et al. (1995). A cost-effectiveness analysis of acute care case management outcomes. *Nursing Economics, 13*(3), 129–136.
2. Barter, M., & Furmidge, M. L. (1994). Unlicensed assistive personnel: Issues relating to delegation and supervision. *Journal of Nursing Administration, 24*(4), 36–40.
3. Biordi, D. L. (1993). Nursing error and caring in the workplace. *Nursing Administration Quarterly, 17*(2), 38–45.
4. Coward, R. T., et al. (1995). Job satisfaction of nurses employed in rural and urban long-term care facilities. *Research in Nursing and Health, 18*(3), 271–284.
5. Douglas, L. M. (1996). *The effective nurse: Leader and manager* (5th ed.). St. Louis: Mosby–Year Book.
6. Gardner, D. L. (1991). Issues related to the use of nurse extenders. *Journal of Nursing Administration, 21*(10), 40–45.
7. Huber, D. G., Blegen, M. A., & McCloskey, J. C. (1994). Use of

nursing assistants: Staff nurse options. *Nursing Management, 25*(5), 64–68.

 8. Huber, D. (1996). *Leadership and nursing care management.* Philadelphia: W. B. Saunders.

 9. Joint Commission on Accreditation of Healthcare Organizations. (1995). *Accreditation manual for hospitals,* volume I. Author: Oak Brook Terrace, IL.

10. Johnson, K. (1994). A practical approach to patient classification. *Nursing Management, 25,* 50–55.

11. Krapohl, G. L., & Larson, E. (1996). The impact of unlicensed assistive personnel on nursing care delivery. *Nursing Economics, 14*(2), 99–108, 122.

12. Marquis, B. L., & Huston, C. J. (1996). *Leadership roles and management functions in nursing* (2nd ed.). Philadelphia: J. B. Lippincott.

13. Lengacher, C. A., & Mabe, P. R. (1993). Nurse extenders. *Journal of Nursing Administration, 23*(3), 16–19.

14. Moore, B. W., et al. (1996). Patient care leadership within an emerging integrated delivery network. *Nursing Administration Quarterly, 20*(2), 54–64.

15. Munroe, D. J. (1990). The influence of registered nurse staffing on the quality of nursing home care. *Research in Nursing and Health, 13*(4), 263–270.

16. Prescott, P. A., et al. (1991). The patient intensity for nursing index: A validity assessment. *Research in Nursing and Health, 14*(3), 213–221.

17. Prescott, P. A., Soeken, K. L., & Griggs, M. (1995). Identification and referral of hospitalized patients in need of home care. *Research in Nursing and Health, 18*(1), 85–95.

18. Salmond, S. (1995). Models of care using unlicensed assistive personnel: I. Job scope, preparation and utilization patterns. *Orthopaedic Nursing, 14*(5), 20–30.

19. Salmond, S. (1995). Models of care using unlicensed assistive personnel: II. Perceived effectiveness. *Orthopaedic Nursing, 14*(6), 47–58.

20. Schaefer, J. A., & Moos, R. H. (1996). Effects of work stressors and work climate on long-term care staff's job morale and functioning. *Research in Nursing and Health, 19*(1), 63–73.

21. Sowell, R. L., & Meadows, T. M. (1994). An integrated case management mode!: Developing standards, evaluation and outcome criteria. *Nursing Administration Quarterly, 18*(2), 53–64.

22. Stahl, D. A. (1994). Subacute care: Creating alternatives. *Nursing Management, 25*(10), 34–38.

23. Swansburg, R. C. (1996). *Management and leadership for nurse managers* (2nd ed.). Sudbury, MA: Jones and Bartlett Publishers.

24. Wyld, D. C. (1996). The capitation revolution in health care: Implications for the field of nursing. *Nursing Administration Quarterly, 20*(2), 1–12.

Ambulatory Care

CHAPTER 8

Leigh G. Anderson

Many voices are predicting the imminent demise of America's hospital-based healthcare system. A June 20, 1995, *Los Angeles Times* front-page article appears to support this notion.[64] The article reported that every 6 weeks during the previous 4 years, June 1992 through June 1995, a Southern California hospital closed. Why all the closures? Was it because Southern Californians are healthier, living longer, having fewer babies, experiencing less trauma? Surely not. Healthcare payors simply refused to reimburse the hospitals for many previously covered procedures.

Driven by this need to control healthcare costs, physicians, hospitals and other healthcare providers are turning to the less expensive ambulatory care setting in which to treat patients. A survey by the American Hospital Association (AHA), for 1994 to 1995, confirms this shift with revealing statistics. During the period studied, AHA members reported conducting 436 million outpatient visits while making only 33 million hospital admissions. Of the 23 million surgical procedures they performed, 13 million (57%) were performed in ambulatory surgery centers.

It is estimated that by the year 2000, more than 700,000 nurses will be working in some type of ambulatory care setting.[15]

Ambulatory healthcare offers a personalized, easily accessible, cost-effective, time-efficient alternative to traditional hospital-based healthcare. Working women can stop by a neighborhood women's clinic for their annual physical examination during a break at work. An executive experiencing right lower quadrant pain can have a endoscopic appendectomy performed at an ambulatory surgicenter and be back at work in 24 hours. A terminally ill patient can remain with his or her family while receiving treatment at a free-standing oncology center.

Emerging technologies are offering ambulatory care providers exciting new tools for safe and efficient delivery of healthcare. Examples of new technologies include short-acting anesthetic drugs that are quickly metabolized, laboratory tests that are easy to perform, computerized patient record-keeping, and more. In the past, patients suffering from renal disease had a poor diagnosis. Now, neighborhood dialysis units provide easily accessible treatment. Elective procedures like radial keratotomy to correct nearsightedness and eliminate the need for eyeglasses, laser therapy for smoothing facial lines, and fetal ultrasonography are all possible because of new, safe technology that can be used in the ambulatory care setting.

Cost control measures tend to be compatible with ambulatory patient care. This is because many ambulatory care agencies are staffed by lean teams, are located in space-efficient settings, and maintain just-in-time inventories. Tasks are assigned to staff according to their skill and experience. Unlicensed employees are used to perform nontechnical tasks. Team members tend to like their work and to stay put. This limits turnover expenses. Critical pathways are carefully developed and followed, resulting in consistent, cost-effective client services. Because of the size of its operation, a governing body can be close to its clients and providers. This ensures that fiscal outcomes are easily monitored.

Development of Ambulatory Care

The two world wars dramatically thrust American medicine into the 20th century. Thousands of hospital beds were needed overnight. Trained physicians and nurses were in short supply. In an effort to meet this need, many new hospitals and medical personnel training centers were established. These wartime challenges were met with proverbial American ingenuity. An example of this creativity was the emergence of the specialty of plastic and reconstructive surgery. It restored form and function to thousands of injured military personnel.

The Korean and Vietnam wars followed, providing a continuing stream of acute and chronically ill patients. Once again, science and medical research produced incredible advances. Radiation therapy was refined, microvascular surgery and organ transplantation were developed, and the ability to maintain life indefinitely with the help of mechanical support systems became common practice. Daily, the place of large, labor-intensive healthcare centers was reaffirmed . . . with an ever-increasing price tag.

In 1991, recognizing that America's healthcare system was heading for financial disaster and that something needed to be done to preserve basic healthcare services, the National League for Nursing (NLN) and the American Nurses Association (ANA) published a public statement titled *Nursing's Agenda for Health Care Reform.* The statement was endorsed by 50 professional nursing organizations. It recognized the benefits of hospital-based healthcare during the previous 70 years, but challenged nurses to look to the future, a future where safe, cost-effective client services could be provided in a variety of ambulatory settings. It emphasized primary healthcare services—activities that promote, restore, and maintain client health.

The notion of providing health services to people in their neighborhoods has always been a part of nursing. Visiting nurses' associations have promoted health, prevented illness, provided home care, and offered health teaching and support services since the 1800s. They were the forerunners of public health nurses who today provide services to specific populations. In time, these two services evolved into community nursing centers run by nurses.

One of the earliest nursing centers was the Henry Street Nurses Settlement in New York City, founded by Lillian Wald in 1893. Some 23 years later, in 1916, Margaret Sanger opened the first birth control clinic, also in New York City. In the 1920s, Mary Breckingridge established the Frontier Nursing Service in Kentucky. The Loeb Center, which was established by Lydia Hall in 1963 at Montefiore Hospital in New York City, distinguished itself as being one of the earliest facilities in which professional nurses were the sole client care providers. In 1965, as the need for more skilled nursing care providers became apparent, the role of nurse-practitioner (NP) was developed. Then, in the 1970s, nursing schools initiated community-based teaching centers to serve as sites for training nursing students and advanced-practice nurses (APNs).

The success of these nursing centers stimulated the proliferation of similar clinics run by hospitals, philanthropic organizations, the state, and the federal government. By 1980 the scope of care provided by nurse-run centers began evolving once again. For the first time, APNs received reimbursement for providing primary care services. As soon as reimbursement was added to this system, a number of outside parties immediately took note. Some important issues were raised, including the need to:

● Define core care dimensions (scope of care) and clinical practices in the ambulatory care setting
● Assign level(s) of complexity to care provided
● Identify basic ambulatory nursing competencies (nursing skills) and rank them
● Establish baselines for licensure and certification of am-

bulatory care and advanced-practice ambulatory care nurses
● Develop fee schedules for advanced practice ambulatory care nursing providers
● Obtain recognition from payors for reimbursement of ambulatory care nursing service(s)

In 1987 (rev. 1993) the American Academy of Ambulatory Care Nursing (AAACN) published *Ambulatory Care Nursing Administration and Practice Standards.*[2] This publication included a brief history of the AAACN, ambulatory care values, current practice standards, and a glossary (see Box 8–1). It was written with the help of AAACN members and was reviewed by the Joint Commission on Accreditation of Healthcare Organizations (JCAHO). It provides valuable data from which ambulatory care nurse job descriptions, core dimensions for clin-

---

Box 8–1. Ambulatory Care Terminology

The American Academy of Ambulatory Care Nursing, in its *Ambulatory Care Nursing Administration and Practice Standards,*[2] provides the following glossary of ambulatory care terminology.

Ambulatory care. Care delivered to patients whose institutional episodes of care are less than 24 hours.

Ambulatory care nursing. Nursing practice in an ambulatory care setting. Nursing care provided to patients with institutional episodes of care of less than 24 hours.

Family. Family members are defined by the patient in his or her own terms. May include individuals related by blood or marriage, or in self-defined relationships. (This definition is intended to be used by nursing when providing patient care. It is not intended as a legal definition of family.)

Healthcare team. The healthcare team includes the patient, family, and other members of the healthcare system who are involved in the development and implementation of the care plan.

Nursing care. Direct care given to individual patients and families by a nursing staff member (registered nurse, licensed practical nurse, or ancillary staff member). Care involves patient assessment, care planning or organization, delivery of care, and evaluation of patient response. Care is given or supervised by a registered nurse.

Nursing services. Organized services delivered to groups of patients by nursing staff. Includes nursing care as well as services to support or facilitate direct care, such as referral and coordination of care.

Nursing staff. Staff members who participate in delivering nursing care. These staff are either registered nurses or are supervised by a registered nurse.

Patient. An individual who requests or receives nursing services. Also called client, consumer, member, or customer in many settings.

Plan of care. An individualized approach to nursing care developed by a professional nurse for a specific patient or group of patients. It may include standard treatment approaches such as protocols, guidelines, etc.

Professional nurse. Registered nurse.

ical practice, clinical ladders and critical pathways, levels of nursing acuity, and quality improvement programs can be developed.

In the mid 1990s, several important studies on the role of the nurse in the ambulatory care setting were conducted. These studies yielded statistically valid answers to some of these questions. This research will help carry ambulatory care nursing into the 21st century and beyond.

Studies of Ambulatory Care Nursing

Nurses, along with other members of the healthcare team, are expected to document their part in the process and outcome of client care. This documentation can only be obtained by careful, scientifically controlled studies. During the last 15 years, a small group of forward-thinking nurse-researchers have been collecting and analyzing data about ambulatory nursing practice. They have enlisted the help of professional statisticians and researchers, constructed and tested measurement tools, and developed a uniform taxonomy.

Early efforts to articulate ambulatory care nursing activities were undertaken by several nursing research teams. In 1980 Hooks and colleagues[30] outlined barriers to ambulatory care practice. The next year, Verran[77] delineated seven areas of ambulatory nursing responsibility using Delphi methodology and ambulatory nurse expert opinion, then published several papers on this subject.

Additional research to define ambulatory care nursing activities was undertaken in 1984 by two other teams: Genovich-Richards and Tracy,[18] and Henninger and Daily.[27] The next year, Tighe and co-workers expanded on Verran's description of ambulatory nursing, adding a planning dimension. This study had a relatively small sample and was limited to nurses in the oncology ambulatory care setting. In 1988 Parrinello et al.[58] tested another ambulatory care patient classification instrument. Two additional studies by Joseph[33] and by Kirsch[35] were reported in 1989 and 1990. These studies further evaluated assessment and classifications of ambulatory client care. The most recent ambulatory care studies were reported by Schade and Austin in 1992,[67] and by Hackbarth and associates in 1995.[23]

The 1995 study of Hackbarth et al. identified specific practice areas in which ambulatory care nurses can maintain their competitive edge. The study identified the scope and dimension of ambulatory care nursing practice, the degree of complexity of each practice, and the frequency of performance of each practice. These items are concrete and credible, something that financial officers and managed care contract agents understand.

Settings for Ambulatory Care

In 1978 Loebs[44] described ambulatory care as services provided by individual practitioners in private offices and suburban hospital and tertiary care settings. Back then the scope of client care was simple by current standards.

Today, ambulatory care clients may include truly sick people requiring complex nursing care.

Several terms are used interchangeably by clients and healthcare professionals when referring to ambulatory care. *Outpatient care* is one of the oldest terms used to describe patient care settings outside of the hospital. This term was commonly used in the 1960s and 1970s to identify clinics provided by hospitals for indigent clients. They offered a variety of services, including well-baby checks, glaucoma testing, and sexually transmitted disease (STD) treatment at no change or at reduced rates. A variation of the outpatient clinic was the community health clinic, which was usually run by nurses. Both of these settings provided physicians and nurses in training a practice site.

The 1980s saw these clinics renamed as *freestanding* and *same-day care centers*. Their client population gradually shifted from the indigent to the well-heeled middle class. This came about because managed care organizations saw these sites as cost-effective venues for providing contracted services. A new industry emerged to support the needs of these centers.

This evolution continued into the 1990s as *23-hour* and *urgent care centers* appeared in many neighborhoods. The 23-hour organizations are a special category of ambulatory care providers. If they provide a client with more than 23 hours of consecutive service, the organization technically becomes a hospital. These facilities offer many services that were formerly provided by hospital emergency rooms. In the mid 1990s, some religious organizations began providing healthcare for their members and the larger community through *parish nursing* programs.

Features Common to All Ambulatory Care Settings

All ambulatory care settings have two features in common: (1) They do not provide client sleeping accommodations. (2) They are not occupied by persons incapable of self-care after a procedure.

Independently owned and operated recovery care centers, community birthing centers, and hospital-run 23-hour step-down units come very close to compromising these two features. All three of these facilities provide short-term recovery care for clients who have had procedures that require immediate postprocedure professional monitoring. When a client satisfactorily meets the facility's predetermined discharge criteria, he or she is discharged. Discharge criteria may vary widely from facility to facility depending on the client's procedure and preprocedure condition. Common discharge criteria include the following:

- Recovery from anesthetic agents
- Orientation to time and place
- Ability to move extremities
- Ability to void
- No allergic reactions (to dyes and other contrast media)
- Ability to ambulate safely.

Specific Ambulatory Care Settings

An ambulatory care facility may be found anywhere that people gather. Areas with significant population density, such as high-rise apartment complexes, college campuses, and large industrial parks, are likely locations. Rock concerts, ballparks, ski resorts—virtually any public site imaginable—may be a setting for an ambulatory care facility. A list of the more common ambulatory care settings is provided in Box 8–2.

Some ambulatory care centers provide a diverse array of services, at times in very creative ways. Highly technical services, such as cardiac catheterization and diagnostic imaging procedures, are now being housed in mobile units that can be scheduled to visit community ambulatory care centers. Physicians are grouping together, five or more, and providing complete patient care. General and specialty ambulatory surgicenters, which perform the majority of this country's surgical procedures, are adopting late hours so that they can accommodate working people. These efforts to consolidate medical and surgical services outside the traditional hospital setting have been encouraged by Medicare and other payors. Special segments of the population who too often tend to fall through the cracks in the hospital-based healthcare system (e.g., migrant workers, prison inmates, veterans) are now able to access healthcare through ambulatory care centers.

Box 8–2. Ambulatory Care Settings

Ambulatory surgery centers
Birthing centers
Corporate health services
Dental centers
Endoscopy centers
Group Practices—single- or multispecialty
Hemodialysis centers
Infusion therapy centers
Lithotripsy units
Managed-care organizations
Migrant health services
Mobile cardiac catheterization units
Ophthalmology surgery centers
Oral and maxillofacial centers
Podiatric centers
Private practice physicians' offices
Prison health services
Public health departments
Radiation and oncology treatment centers
Recovery care centers
Rehabilitation centers
Research centers
Rural health clinics
Student health services
Urgent and emergency care centers (freestanding)
Veterans' Administration Clinics (freestanding)
Women's health centers

Controls and Standards

The ambulatory healthcare system is not without controls. All ambulatory care providers are required to comply with certain uniform state and federal standards. These standards were developed to ensure client and caregiver safety. The four most important sources of standards are as follows:

1. Occupational Safety and Health Administration (OSHA) (state and federal). Area of concern—to protect patients and caregivers from infectious agents, hazardous materials, and other environmental risk factors
2. Americans with Disabilities Act (ADA) (federal). Area of concern—to ensure unbiased client access to services, to provide environmental enhancements that promote passage to care, prevent injury, and encourage individual self-sufficiency
3. Safe Medical Devices Act (SMDA) (federal). Area of concern—the reduction of device (external mechanical devices and internally implanted devices)-related incidents
4. National Fire Protection Association Life Safety Code 101 (federal). Area of concern—the prevention of fire in the ambulatory care center.

With the help of these guidelines, nurses working in ambulatory care centers can create and maintain a hazard-free, safe, comfortable, and therapeutic environment for clients, their families and friends, and fellow staff members.

Certification and Accreditation

Independent consumer advocates, state and federal agencies, and special interest groups associated with the legal and insurance industries are keeping a watchful eye on the evolution of ambulatory care practice. Their interest has motivated individuals and facilities providing ambulatory care services to be proactive and voluntarily seek certification (individuals) and accreditation (institutions).

Certification

The type of certification required of an ambulatory healthcare worker depends on the worker's geographical location, the community's standard of practice, and the care facility's organizational structure. General credentialing requirements are listed in Box 8–3.

Currently, according to the American Nurses Credentialing Center (ANCC), there are 26 nursing specialties that credential specialty-prepared nurses; unfortunately, there is no certification specific to ambulatory care nursing. As this area of practice becomes more established, specialty certification for ambulatory care nurses is sure to be developed.

According to the National Federation for Specialty Nursing Organizations (NFSNO), of the 42 nursing specialty organizations, 2 focus specifically on ambulatory care nursing:

Box 8–3. General Credentialing Requirements for Ambulatory Care Nurses and Other Staff

■ *Nursing assistants* may be registered with the state board of nursing or be nonlicensed. Need certificate of basic training. Encouraged to receive additional certification in special practice areas such as reading monitoring equipment, etc.

■ *Vocational and practical nurses* must be licensed by the state in which they work. Need additional certification in special procedures such as venipuncture, etc.

■ *Nurses-in-training* may have an interim permit (IP) from a local state board of nursing. Encouraged to obtain certification in many special procedures, including advanced cardiac life support (ACLS), interpreting cardiac arrhythmias, working with long-term catheters (e.g., Swan-Ganz).

■ *Staff nurses* (AA-, diploma-, or bachelor's degree–prepared nurse with current state license) need certification in quality assurance and quality improvement, risk management, and various nursing skills, as listed under nurses-in-training.

■ *Nurse-managers and administrators* (bachelor's- or higher degree–prepared nurse with current state license) should have certification in area of clinical specialty.

■ *Licensed physician assistants* (bachelor's degree with advanced training and current state license) should have certification in advanced practice activities (e.g., physical assessment).

■ *Advanced-practice nurses and nurse-practitioners* (bachelor's degree with advanced training and current state license) need certification in advanced practice activities (e.g., nurse first surgical assistant).

American Academy of Ambulatory Care Nursing (AAACN)
East Holly Ave., PO Box 56
Pitman, NJ 08071-0056
(609) 256–2350

Society for Ambulatory Care Professionals (SACP)
1 N. Franklin St.
Chicago, IL 60606
(312) 422–3900

These organizations provide a forum, national meetings, and publications, in which ambulatory care nurses can discuss, accept, modify, or reject topics common to their practice. In this way ambulatory care nurses are continuing to define the specialty.

Accreditation

Accreditation is the standard to which ambulatory care facilities aspire. Increasingly, healthcare payors expect organizations providing healthcare services to furnish measurable assurance that clients are receiving the agreed-upon contracted services. Many states are requiring that ambulatory care providers be licensed by them, accredited by a recognized accrediting body, or be Medicare-certi-

fied. This has stimulated a boom in accreditation-associated businesses. Ambulatory care nurses are expected to be familiar with the standards to which their organizations are accountable. These standards are spelled out in each accreditation body's manual. They may include some or all of the following items:

● Quality of care, quality assessment, and improvement
● Medical records
● Rights and responsibilities of patients
● Governing body
● Administration
● Plant, technology, and safety management
● Infection control
● Educational activities
● Surgical and anesthesia services
● Pharmaceutical services
● Radiology services
● Emergency services
● Teaching, research, and publication activities

Two major organizations offer accreditation for ambulatory care facilities:

Accreditation Association for Ambulatory Health Care, Inc. (AAAHC)
9933 Lawler Ave.
Skokie, IL 60077–3708
(708) 676–9628

Joint Commission on Accreditation of Healthcare Organizations (JCAHO)
1 Renaissance Blvd.
Oakbrook Terrace, IL 60181
(708) 916–5600

Their criteria, inspection processes, and costs are similar.

Two other organizations offer specialty ambulatory care accreditation: the American Association for Accreditation of Ambulatory Surgery Facilities, Inc. (AAAASF) and the NLN's Community Health Accreditation Program, Inc. (CHAP).

Scope of Ambulatory Care Nursing

An ambulatory care nurse's particular duties may vary from setting to setting. This is because ambulatory care centers can be patterned after one of two organizational models: the medical—diagnosis-related group (DRG)—model or the nursing—wellness and caring—model. Which model an organization follows depends on its structure, goals, and strategic plan.

In the *medical model,* nurses assume a subordinate role to the physician. Their activities may complement or be in collaboration with the physician. An example of a complementary relationship is a nurse and physician working in a chemotherapy center, with the nurse setting up and starting a client's intravenous (IV) lines and the physician then administering the chemotherapy agent(s). When a nurse functions in collaboration with a physician, she or he monitors a known condition or provides a prearranged treatment. An example of collaboration is when the nurse sees routine well and sick children, while the physician treats children with more serious conditions. In the medical model, the nurse has less autonomy; consequently, the complexity of the nursing process is diminished. When this model is in effect, the organization seldom bills for the services provided by the nurse. Also, under the medical model, nursing liability may be reduced, because the nurse provides care under a physician's direct supervision.

In ambulatory care centers organized around the *nursing model,* nurses assume a leadership role and provide primary client care. The nurse's tasks may include educating individuals or population groups, acting as a gatekeeper and resource manager, monitoring specific populations for healthcare needs, and following up outcomes. The nurse may consult with physician associates as needed. In some states, nurses providing care may be reimbursed for direct client visits, client education, and specific technical procedures. Because of their increased level of responsibility, these nurses have increased practice liability.

As nurses assume increased levels of responsibility in the ambulatory care setting, they are encouraged to work diplomatically with other community resource persons and agencies. This is best accomplished by respecting these individual's professional skills, seeking their input when making decisions affecting clients, and being personally available as a resource to others in the community. Marketing is another component of community relations. Maintaining a steady or growing client population (productivity) results in profitability, which business managers and payors want to see.

Ethics, the principles of proper professional conduct, are central to the nurse's role in the ambulatory care setting. Ambulatory care nurses must have a clear picture of their duties (comprehensive job description), to whom they report (organization plan), and their client population (mission statement). Understanding clients' rights, including the right to confidentiality, and respecting clients' efforts for self-determination (advance directives) are central to ethical nursing practice. Recognizing the place of family and significant others in the life of each client and how they contribute to client outcomes is also a component of ethical client care. In the end, all aspects of client care are affected by the caregivers' ethics.

Ambulatory care nurses can be greatly assisted in their work by computers. Computers can track appointments, file patient histories and laboratory test results, list caregivers and the services they have performed, track expenses, and project outcomes. Computers cannot make client care decisions, however. Decision-making remains solely in the hands of the caregiver. Understanding how to input and retrieve data in the computer is increasingly an expected part of the ambulatory care nurse's role.

Roles of the Ambulatory Care Nurse

Historically, the ambulatory care staff nurse's primary role was to help clients participate in their care so that they could achieve the highest level of wellness possible. Family members or significant others were included in this participation, as appropriate. This goal was achieved by direct or integrated activities that included client teaching and specific nursing procedures. In the early 1980s, researchers attempted to codify the various dimensions of ambulatory care nursing. These lists were made obsolete in the early 1990s, when managed-care programs reassigned many hospital-based activities to ambulatory care nurses. Thus, the scope of ambulatory care nursing grew tremendously in a relatively short time.

In 1992, a group of nurse-researchers from Loyola University accepted the challenge to redefine the dimensions of ambulatory nursing.[24,25] They produced a survey tool containing 91 closed-ended marker ambulatory care activities. The instrument also contained open-ended items which allowed for identification of additional marker activities. Responses were made on a Likert-type scale. The survey was completed by 606 ambulatory care staff nurses working in a variety of ambulatory care settings throughout the United States. Their combined responses resulted in the most accurate description of ambulatory care nursing currently available. The researchers classified the responses into two roles: (1) the clinical practice role, with eight core dimensions, and (2) the quality improvement and research role, with three core dimensions (see Box 8–4).

Core Dimensions of the Clinical Practice Role

Enabling Operations. Locating charts, directing patient traffic, and providing secretarial support are typical management tasks. To perform these tasks successfully, the nurse needs tenacity and endurance. Calling for test results, setting up and cleaning up after procedures, and taking vital signs are examples of traditional nursing activities. A strong sense of organization, an ability to prioritize, and most important, a good sense of humor are prerequisites. The how-to of enabling activities is specific to each setting. A nurse can quickly learn how to perform these activities by becoming familiar with his or her work environment, observing how other team members do things, asking questions, and reflecting on past experiences.

Technical Procedures. Giving injections, changing dressings, catheterizing patients, reviewing instructions with clients before a procedure, and witnessing consents are examples of routine nursing activities. Special skills such as starting IV drips, giving inhalation therapy treatments, or performing certain laboratory tests may require advanced training. These skills can be learned on the job, by attending a workshop, or through independent study.

Nursing Process. The nursing process is the heart and soul of ambulatory care nursing practice. It involves seeing each client in the context of his or her medical

Box 8–4. Dimensions of the Ambulatory Care Staff Nurse Role

Eight Core Dimensions of the Current Clinical Practice Role

Factor I

Enabling Operations

Maintain safe work environment
Maintain traffic box
Search for space and equipment
Set up room
Locate records
Order supplies
Transport clients
Provide emotional support
Take vital signs

Standardized alpha = .7985

Factor II

Technical Procedures

Assist with procedures
Prepare client for procedures
Chaperone during procedures
Inform client about treatment
Witness signing consent forms
Administer oral/IM medications
Collect specimens

Standardized alpha = .8206

Factor III

Nursing Process

Develop nursing care plan
Use nursing diagnosis
Complete client history
Assess client learning needs
Conduct exit interview
Evaluate client care outcomes
Chart each client encounter

Standardized alpha = .6826

Factor IV

Telephone Communications

Telephone triage
Call pharmacy with prescription
Call client with test results

Standardized alpha = .8178

Factor V

Advocacy

Make clients aware of rights
Promote positive public relations
Act as client advocate
Triage client to appropriate provider

Standardized alpha = .7136

Factor VI

Teaching

Instruct client on medical-nursing
  regimen
Instruct client on home and self-care

Standardized alpha = .8455

Factor VII

Care Coordination

Long-term supportive relationship
Act as a resource person
Coordinate client care
Assess needs and initiate referrals
Find resources in the community
Instruct on health promotion

Standardized alpha = .8289

Factor VIII

Expert Practice Within Setting

Expertise in advanced nursing practice
Function as advanced nurse resource
Serve as preceptor for students
Design and present in-service education

Standardized alpha = .7157

Three Core Dimensions of the Current Quality Improvement (QI) and Research Role

Factor I

Quality Improvement

Implement professional standards
Participate in preparation of QI plan
Collect and analyze QI data
Use QI plan in practice
Participate in interdisciplinary QI teams
Develop expected client outcomes

Standardized alpha = .8086

Factor II

Research

Participate in research of others
Follow guidelines to protect human
  subjects

Standardized alpha = .7006

Factor III

Continuing Education

Participate in one-site continuing
  education
Participate in off-site continuing
  education

Standardized alpha = .5429

Reliability alpha for entire 59-item clinical scale = .9163
Reliability alpha for entire 16 QI-research scale = .8647
Chi-square statistic for the hypothesized eight-factor solution for the clincal scale = 2969.29 with 791 d.f. (P = .000)
Goodness of fit index for the hypothesized eight-factor solution for the clinical scale = .787
Chi-square statistic for the hypothesized three-factor solution for the QI-research scale = 87.38 with 32 d.f. (P = .000)
Goodness of fit index for the hypothesized three-factor solution for the QI-research scale = .971

Modified from Nursing Economics, 1995, Volume 13, Number 2, p. 92. Reprinted with permission of the publisher, Jannetti Publications, Inc., East Holly Ave., Box 56, Pitman, NJ 08071–0056; telephone (609) 256–2300; FAX (609) 589–7463.

diagnosis, social setting, and physical environment. How this process is implemented by nurses is separate and different from the efforts of other healthcare professionals. It involves skills unique to nursing. By assessing, diagnosing, planning, intervening, and evaluating the scope of each patient's care, the nurse can help each client achieve his or her highest level of wellness.

Telephone Communications. Communicating with clients by telephone can provide continuity of care, efficiently preventing or resolving problems, and be a lifeline in the event of an emergency. Every conversation must be documented. Documentation tools include flow sheets, checklists, telephone carbon ledgers, computerized notes, and dictation that can be transcribed later. Communicating with clients by telephone raises some new issues. Are words enough to determine a client's condition? What if the words are misunderstood? Can confidentiality be ensured? Special training in telephone communication is needed before nurses assume this responsibility. Algorithms specific to the area of practice must be in place. Legal issues associated with telephone patient communications need to be worked out with each facility's legal counsel.

Advocacy. Both patients and facilities have rights. The nurse is frequently called upon to mediate between these two entities. If a client believes a service was not provided correctly he or she will most often speak to the nurse about the problem. Conversely, the nurse is expected to support his or her facility when talking with patients, their families, or significant others. Ambulatory care facilities count on their nurses to be diplomatic while communicating clearly. Strong public relations skills are a must for ambulatory care nurses.

Teaching. In an effort to ensure that clients have the greatest degree of control over their lives, nurses may have to teach them new ways to achieve autonomy. Bulletin boards, patient information brochures, posters, and audiovisual presentations can all be powerful educational tools. The effectiveness of a teaching activity is measured by how students respond. A client with diabetes who learns to test his or her blood glucose levels accurately, a paraplegic client who lifts and shifts every 15 minutes and does not have recurrence of a pressure ulcer, and a post–coronary bypass client who lowers his or her cholesterol level to below 200 mg/dl are all teaching success stories.

Care Coordination. Whether running a clinic smoothly or implementing a complicated client treatment plan, attention to detail and the successful direction of events is an important part of the ambulatory care nurse's work. Developing a plan, determining how to implement it, making it happen, and finally evaluating the outcome, all are a part of the coordination process. Critical path-

ways are valuable tools for guiding caregivers in providing consistent, coordinated care.

Expert Practice Within Setting. Ambulatory care clinics are frequently run by nurse-managers. They supervise staff, client, and facility activities. When a problem arises they are expected to provide a solution. Typical examples include improvising a solution when a piece of equipment breaks down, teaching an employee a procedure for the first time, and conducting an interview with a new client. Skill in this area may be developed by attending focused continuing education classes or doing outside reading on management topics. Time and experience, of course, also contribute to acquiring expert practice.

Core Dimensions of the Quality Improvement and Research Role

Quality Improvement. Quality improvement tasks are not optional nursing activities. Their outcomes provide evidence of compliance with various authorities. A facility's administration, client reimbursement providers, and the state and federal government all want assurance(s) that they are receiving service for the fees they pay. Quality improvement activities require skill in documenting events, tabulating outcomes, initiating interventions, and reevaluating the corrective actions. An example of a quality improvement activity in an ambulatory surgicenter would be performing admission-to-surgery time studies. With profit margins shrinking, surgicenter managers are motivated to provide client services as safely and efficiently as possible. This study would show the amount of unoccupied time between surgeries and at what points things could be tightened up. Special training is required to develop quality improvement studies and to implement them.

Research. Research activities are often overlooked by nurses. They tend to believe that research takes place only in an academic setting. This is a very narrow view of research. Observing that certain patient outcomes occur predictably is research. Trying various approaches to solve a client's problem is research. Reporting these experiences to other nurses is responsible behavior. Research activities must be guided by a uniform structure if the results are to be accepted as valid. Applying the steps of the scientific method and understanding basic statistics are mandatory nursing skills. These may be developed by attending a class or through independent study.

Continuing Education. Ambulatory care nurses are encouraged to continue growing professionally. This can be accomplished by joining a specialty nursing association, attending state and national meetings, writing papers, and reading professional journals. All of these activities contain elements of pleasure for the progressive nurse. Nurses who practice in an ambulatory care setting must actively seek continuing education experiences because their practice area is subject to rapid change.

The Nursing Process in Ambulatory Care Settings

The nursing process—assessing, diagnosing, planning, intervening, and evaluating—can be used in any setting where nurses care for clients. It is particularly useful to ambulatory care nurses because they are frequently called on to provide independent patient care. Examples of independent patient care include performing assessment histories and physical examinations, providing crisis management, and initiating emergency care. The following scenario illustrates application of the nursing process in an ambulatory care setting.

> Sue arrived late for her first in a series of hyperbaric oxygen (HBO) treatments for a brown recluse spider bite. She reported not feeling very well and questioned whether it was a good idea to begin her HBO treatments that day. It was not the first time that Bill, the registered nurse in charge of ambulatory wound care, had seen this behavior before in patients beginning HBO treatment. A few pointed questions revealed that Sue's condition had not taken a turn for the worse (assessment) but that instead, she suffered from claustrophobia (diagnosis). Bill sat down and explained how the HBO tank's ventilation, communication, and locking systems worked. Sue was unimpressed, remaining very apprehensive. Finally, she agreed to lie in the tank with the door open provided she could be in charge of closing the door when she was ready (plan). Then she allowed Bill to help her into the tank. Her breathing grew strained. Bill stayed close by and rested his hand on her shoulder. They continued talking. Gradually Sue lowered the door and then allowed Bill to lock it in place. The tank was then brought up to pressure (intervention). Needless to say, that first treatment was short, but in time Sue was able to master her fear and tolerated six full-length treatments. Her wound healed beautifully and did not require surgical intervention (evaluation).

The duration of care in ambulatory care settings depends on each patient's need. A patient undergoing an annual physical examination and laboratory work-up may be seen only once. In contrast, a couple whose baby is delivered at a neighborhood birthing center may be seen several times before labor and delivery and then several times afterward. A patient undergoing cancer chemotherapy may be seen weekly or more frequently for months on end.

Regardless of the term of care, the nursing process must remain dynamic. Sometimes this process can be implemented by a team of caregivers. When this occurs, a team leader should be chosen. This person then coordinates the group's various efforts. An example of this is the treatment of a stroke patient by a team of allied healthcare providers at a rehabilitation center. Whether a nurse works in an ophthalmology surgery center, cardiac rehabilitation unit, or home health agency, accurate record-keeping, patient confidentiality, safety, and quality care are expected. They are all the result of effectively implementing the nursing process.

Conclusions

Ambulatory care nursing has been thriving since the 1800s. The two world wars, rapid advances in technology, and changes in provider reimbursement have all had an impact on its evolution. In the 1990s managed-care providers mandated that many procedures previously performed only in a hospital be performed in ambulatory care facilities. Consequently, millions of patients flocked to ambulatory care centers for routine care. This change is being imposed on all segments of society regardless of a person's sex, ethnicity, income, and education level.

Ambulatory care is currently provided in over 26 settings by nurses who are members of more than 42 nursing specialty organizations. At present there is no certification program for ambulatory care nurses. Several ambulatory care nursing journals are available. Payors are mandating that ambulatory care facilities be accredited by one of several accrediting agencies.

Recent nurse-initiated research has defined eight core dimensions of ambulatory care nursing and a list of supporting nursing tasks. An additional three core dimensions specific to quality improvement, research, and continuing education have also been defined.

Bibliography

1. American Hospital Association, Division of Ambulatory Care. (1992). *Ambulatory care trendlines 1992. Prevention and health promotion trends.* Chicago: American Hospital Association.
2. American Academy of Ambulatory Care Nursing Standards Committee. (1993). *Ambulatory care nursing administration and practice standards.* Pitman, NJ: Anthony J. Jannetti.
3. Anderson, H. (1991). Convenient care a top priority for new center. *Hospitals, 65*(8), 66, 68, 1991.
4. Arbitman, D. (1986). A primer on patient classification systems and their relevance to ambulatory care. *Journal of Ambulatory Care Management, 9*(1), 58–81.
5. Ashley, B. W., & Cross-Skinner, S. (1992). Oncology nursing care delivery issues in the ambulatory setting. In S. M. Hubbard, P. E. Greene, M. T. Knobf, (Eds.), *Current Issues of Nursing Practice Updates, 1*(1), 1–10.
6. Barger, S., Nugent, K., Bridges, W. (1993). Schools with nursing centers: A 5-year follow-up study. *Journal of Professional Nursing, 9*(1), 7–13.
7. Barker, L. R., et al. (1991). *Principles of ambulatory care medicine* (3rd ed.). Baltimore: Williams & Wilkins.
8. Barnett, A. E. (1992). *Ambulatory care.* Rockville, MD: Aspen Publishers.
9. Beck, L. C. (1990). Let paraprofessionals boost your practice. *Medical Economics, 67*(25), 97, 101–104.
10. Beddar, S. M., & Aikin, J. L. (1994). Continuity of care: A challenge for ambulatory oncology nursing. *Seminars in Oncology Nursing, 10*(4), 254–263.
11. Behrend, S. W. (1994). Documentation in the ambulatory setting. *Seminars in Oncology Nursing, 10*(4), 264–280.
12. Brooks, N. R. (1995). Bringing home a new level of care. *Health horizons. Los Angeles Times,* Business, Pt. II, June 5, 1995; pp. 8–10.
13. Cooley, M. E., Lin, E. M., & Hunter, S. W. (1994). The ambulatory oncology nurse's role. *Seminars in Oncology Nursing, 10*(4), 245–253.
14. Crabtree, R., & Cummings, S. H. (1995). Nurses in ambulatory

care: Multiple roles and opportunities. *Seminars for Nurse Managers, 3*(2), 72–75.

15. Curran, C. R. (1992). An interview with Mary Ann Moore. *Nursing Economics, 10*(2), 87–93.

16. Doherty, V., O'Donovan, T., & Hill, G. (1988). Current status of ambulatory surgery in the United States. In G. Hill (Ed.), *Outpatient surgery* (3rd ed.). Philadelphia: W. B. Saunders.

17. Flory, J. (1990). *Ambulatory care: A management briefing.* Chicago: American Hospital Publishing.

18. Genovich-Richards, J., & Tracy, R. (1984). An assessment process for nursing staff patterns in ambulatory care. *Journal of Ambulatory Care Management, 7*(2), 69–79.

19. Gloss, E., & Fielo, S. (1987). The nursing center: An alternative for health care delivery. *Family and Community Health, 10*(2), 49–58.

20. Haas, S. A., & Hackbarth, D. P. (1995). Dimension of the staff nurse role in ambulatory care: Pt. III—Using research data to design new models of nursing care delivery. *Nursing Economics, 13*(4), 230–241.

21. Haas, S. A., Hackbarth, D. P. (1995). Dimensions of the staff nursing in ambulatory care: Pt. IV—Developing nursing intensity measures, standard, clinical ladders, and QI programs. *Nursing Economics, 13*(5), 285–294.

22. Haas, S. A., et al. (1995). Dimensions of the staff nurse role in ambulatory care: Pt. II—Comparison of role dimensions in four ambulatory settings. *Nursing Economics, 13*(3), 152–165.

23. Hackbarth, D. P., et al. (1995). Dimensions of the staff nurse role in ambulatory care: Pt. I—Methodology and analysis of data on current staff nurse practice. *Nursing Economics, 13*(2), 89–98.

24. Hastings, C. (1987). Classification issues in ambulatory care nursing. *Journal of Ambulatory Care Management, 10*(3), 50–64.

25. Hastings, C., & Muri-Nash, J. (1989). Validation of a taxonomy of ambulatory nursing practice. *Nursing Economics, 7*(3), 142–149.

26. Health Care Financing Administration. (1987). National health care expenditures: 1986–2000. *Health Care Financing Review, 8*(4), 1–36.

27. Henniger, D., & Dailey, C. (1983). Measuring nursing workload in an outpatient department. *Journal of Nursing Administration, 13*(9), 20–23.

28. Hermann, C. E. (1993). Diversified nursing practice in ambulatory care. *Nursing Economics, 11*(3), 176–179.

29. Hoffmann, F., & Wakefield, D. (1986). Ambulatory care patient classification. *Journal of Nursing Administration, 16*(4), 23–30.

30. Hooks, M., Dewitz-Arnold, D., & Westbrook, L. (1980). The role of the professional nurse in the ambulatory care setting. *Nursing Administration Quarterly, 4*(4), 12–17.

31. Horn, S., Buckle, J., & Carver, C. (1988). Ambulatory severity index: Development of an ambulatory case mix system. *Journal of Ambulatory Care Management, 11*(4), 53–62.

32. Johnson, J. M. (1989). Quantifying an ambulatory care patient classification instrument. *Journal of Nursing Administration, 19*(11), 36–42.

33. Joseph, A. C. (1989). Ambulatory care: An objective assessment. *Journal of Nursing Administration, 20*(11), 18–24.

34. Kepnes, L. J. (1984). Professional nursing practice in ambulatory care. *Nursing Management, 15*(5), 28–30.

35. Kirsch, E. (1990). Outpatient and short-stay patient classification systems. *Nursing Management, 21*(9), 118–122.

36. Knauth, D. G. (1994). Community nursing centers: removing impediments to success. *Nursing Economics, 12*(3), 140–145.

37. Koerner, B. (1987). Clarifying the role of nursing in ambulatory care. *Journal of Ambulatory Care Management, 10*(3), 1–7.

38. Lamkin, L. (1994). Outpatient oncology settings: A variety of services. *Seminars in Oncology Nursing, 10*(4), 229–236.

39. Lane, L. (1992). National and regional trends in outpatient hospital care 1980–1990. In *Ambulatory Care Trendlines.* Chicago: American Hospital Association, Division of Ambulatory Care.

40. Lanigan, J. M., Dodds, L., & Mechanic, J. (1994). The ambulatory treatment unit: An innovative model. *Journal of Nursing Administration, 24*(4), 41–44.

41. Lawrence, K. (n. d.; updates published annually). *Ambulatory care—forms, checklists and guidelines.* Aspen Research Group, Inhouse Publication, 2 vols.

42. Liebman, M. C. (1994). How do you facilitate the flow of patients through your ambulatory clinic? *Oncology Nursing Forum, 21*(6), 1091–1092.

43. Loebs, S. (1978). The pressure and problems for organized ambulatory services in the next decade. *Journal of Ambulatory Care Management, 1,* 1–10.

44. Lundeen, S. (1989). *Survival strategies for community nursing centers.* New York: National League for Nursing.

45. Maraldo, P., & Fagin, C. (1992). The nurses' national health plan. In C. Aiken & C. Fagin (Eds.), *Charting nursing's future: Agenda for the 1990s.* Philadelphia: J. B. Lippincott.

46. Martin, V. R. (1994). Administrative issues in ambulatory oncology care. *Seminars in Oncology Nursing, 10*(4), 296–305.

47. Matson, T. A. (1990). *Restructuring for ambulatory care: A guide to reorganization.* Chicago: American Hospital Publishing.

48. Mayer, G. (1992). Work sampling in ambulatory care nursing. *Nursing Management, 23*(9), 52–56.

49. Medvec, B. R. (1994). Productivity and workload measurement in ambulatory oncology. *Seminars in Oncology Nursing, 10*(4), 288–295.

50. Miller, P. L., & Folse, G. H. (1989). Patient classification and staffing in ambulatory care. *Nursing Management, 2*(8), 29–31.

51. Mitchell, M. K., & Storfjell, J. L. (1989). *Standards of excellence for community health organizations* (p. 139). New York: National League for Nursing.

52. Mitchell, M. K., & Storfjell, J. L. (1989). *Standards of excellence for home care agencies* (p. 262). New York: National League for Nursing.

53. Mohl, D. (1991). Establishing telephone triage protocols for ambulatory care practice. *American Academy Ambulatory Nursing Administrators Views, 13*(4), 1–2.

54. Moore, M. A., & Geving, A. R. (1990). Nursing's role in the ambulatory care setting. *MGM Journal,* March–April, pp. 18–24.

55. National League for Nursing. (1992). *Community nursing centers: A promising new trend in American health care.* New York: Author.

56. Palmer, R. (1983). *Ambulatory health care evaluation, principles and practice.* Chicago: American Hospital Association.

57. Parkman, C. A. (1995). Understanding the impact of nursing job redesign. *Nurse Week, 8*(12), 8, 9.

58. Parrinello, K., Brenner, P., & Vallone, B. (1988). Refining and testing a nursing patient classification instrument in ambulatory care. *Nursing Administration Quarterly, 13*(1), 54–64.

59. Parrinello, K. M., & Witzel, P. (1988). Analysis of ambulatory nursing practice. *Nursing Economics, 8*(5), 322–328.

60. Phillips, M., & Hokans, C. (1994). A review of ambulatory care analysis. *Nursing Economics, 12*(2), 88–92.

61. Pinkney-Atkinson, V. J., & Robertson, R. B. (1993). Ambulatory nursing: The handmaiden/specialist dichotomy. *Journal of Nursing Administration, 23*(9), 50–57.

62. Riesch, S. (1992). Nursing centers: An analysis of the anecdotal literature. *Journal of Professional Nursing, 8*(1), 16–25.

63. Ross, A., et al. (1991). *Ambulatory care management* (2nd ed., p. 407), Albany, NY: Delmar Publishers, 1991.

64. Rutten, T., Shuit, D. P., & Gilonna, J. M. (1995). County-USC in web of bitter dispute. *Los Angeles Times,* Sec. A, June 20, 1995, pp. 1, 16.

65. Safriet, B. (1992). Health care dollars and regulatory sense: The role of advanced practice nursing. *Yale Journal on Regulation, 9*(2), 417–488.

66. Sandrik, K. (1990). Oncology: Who's managing outpatient programs? *Hospital, 4,* 33–36.

67. Schade, J. G., & Austin, J. K. (1992). Quantifying ambulatory care activities by time and complexity. *Nursing Economics, 10*(3), 183–192.

68. Schneider, D., & Kilpatrick, K. (1994). A medical classification system for ambulatory care manpower planning. *Health Services Research, 9*(3), 221–233.

69. Scott, M. P., & Packard, K. P. (1990). *Telephone assessment with protocols for nursing practice.* Philadelphia: W. B. Saunders.

70. Smith, K. S. (1990). Telephone triage offers help and advice for patients in need. *American Medical Writers Association Journal, 5*(1), 18–22.

71. Smith, S., & Elesha-Adams, M. (1989). Allocating nursing resources in ambulatory care. *Nursing Management, 20*(1), 61–64.

72. Smyth, K. (1987). Justice and cooperation: Moving ambulatory care practice into the 21st century. *Journal of Ambulatory Care Management, 10*(3), 76–81.

73. Sullivan, E., et al. (1993). Nursing centers: The new arena for advanced nursing practice. In M. Mezey & D. McGivern (Eds.), *Nurses, nurse practitioners: Evolution to advanced practice.* New York: Springer-Verlag.

74. Tennenhouse, D. J. (1991). Minimizing liability for telephone advice. *California Nurse, 87,* 24–27.

75. Tighe, M. G., et al. (1985). A study of the oncology nurse role in ambulatory care. *Oncology Nursing Forum, 12*(6), 23–27.

76. Verran, J. A. (1981). Delineation of ambulatory care nursing practice. *Journal of Ambulatory Care Management, 4*(2), 1–13.

77. Verran, J. A. (1982). Development of the ambulatory care client classification instrument (University Microfilms No. ADG82-17479). *Dissertation Abstracts International, 43*(3), 681.

78. Verran, J. A. (1986). Patient classification in ambulatory care. *Nursing Economics, 4*(5), 247–251.

79. Verran, J. A. (1986). Testing a classification instrument for the ambulatory care setting. *Research in Nursing and Health, 9,* 279–287.

80. Walter, J. M., & Robinson, S. H. (1994). Nursing care delivery models in ambulatory oncology. *Seminars in Oncology Nursing, 10*(4), 237–244.

81. Walter, J. R., & Hubenet, K. S. (1991). The emergency and after-hours care system at Group Health Cooperative. *HMO Practice, 5,* 80–83.

82. Weir, R., & Browne, G. (1989). A study of role performance in specialty outpatient clinics. *Canadian Journal of Nursing Research, 21*(4), 45–61.

83. Weisman, E. (1990). Observation units hold promise for outpatient care. *Hospitals, 64*(12), 66.

84. Wilkinson, J. M., Sansby, S., & Leaning, J. (1991). After-hours telephone triage: Recruitment, training and retention of personnel. *HMO Practice, 5,* 90–94.

85. Young, C. M. (1990). The post-operative follow-up phone call: An essential part of the ambulatory surgery nurse's job. *Journal of Post-Anesthesia Nursing, 5,* 273–275.

86. Xistris, D. M., & Houlihan, N. G. (1994). Impact of reimbursement and health care reform on the ambulatory oncology setting. *Seminars in Oncology Nursing, 10*(4), 281–287.

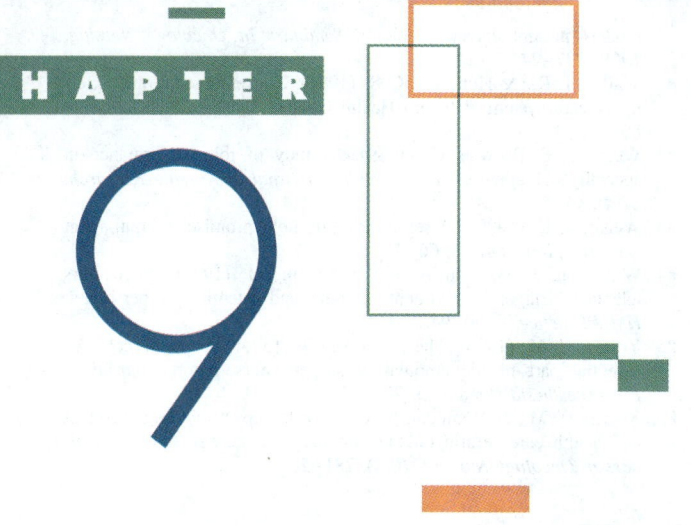

Home Healthcare

Karen S. Martin

This chapter is designed to serve as a bridge from the inpatient or long-term care setting to the home healthcare and community-focused service setting. By covering the trends, general philosophy, risks, and practice of home care, it is intended for the student or clinician whose primary or recent clinical experience has been in hospitals or nursing homes. *Community health nursing* is defined as a synthesis of nursing and public health practice that is comprehensive and is intended to promote and preserve the health of populations.[16] In this chapter, community health nursing is used as an umbrella term to cover all the diverse types of home healthcare and community-focused services, settings, and providers. Thus, community health settings where nurses practice include home healthcare agencies that are hospital-based, visiting nurse associations, tax-supported agencies, and privately or corporately owned agencies. Also included are tax-supported public health agencies, nursing centers, school nursing, wellness and occupational health, parish nursing, homeless clinics, case management, and other diverse programs that offer nursing services.

Scattered throughout this book are features called Bridge to Home Healthcare, written by nurses and other community-focused professionals to describe details of their practice. These features address environmental, psychosocial, physiologic, and health-related behavior concerns experienced by clients and their families and noted by nurses. For example, in Chapter 36, Bernadette Mruz in Coping with Failing Vision (Bridge to Home Healthcare) shares ideas that you might use with clients who continue to have vision problems but are leaving your facility to return to the challenges of their homes. You will gain insight into the roles and responsibilities of home healthcare as it is practiced with clients and families every day. You can use this information as you consider and make referrals for follow-up care. Note the references in this chapter if you want more extensive information about home care, public health, and related topics. After reading this chapter, you may discuss what community-focused opportunities you will have as a nurs-

ing student during your educational program. If you are a staff nurse, you may consider making an appointment to accompany a colleague who practices in a home care, public health, clinic, or school setting to learn more about the specialty. Together, this chapter and the Bridge to Home Healthcare features provide a review or introduction to the world of home healthcare and community-focused practice.

Trends

The status of home healthcare and community-focused services has had an explosive growth as a result of consumer demands, the advent of managed care, and escalating healthcare costs.[12] A definite shift is occurring with delivery of services moving from the hospital to the community, from a fragmented to a more ideal healthcare system where providers work together in the interest of their patients and clients, and from an inconsistent approach to the delivery of care to a greater degree of provider accountability and a more systematic, outcome- and data-driven delivery model. A "seamless healthcare system" is the term being used to describe that new model, a system which includes a wide array of services and providers who work together as a team in the interest of the client.

Today, community health nurses face challenges and opportunities unlike any they have faced before. The number of clients and complexity of their needs are increasing dramatically, as are the number and types of community health staff members and agency programs. At the same time, consumer demands for comprehensive, economical services are increasing as the availability of staff and reimbursement is decreasing. The number of clients receiving Medicare-certified home health services more than doubled between 1991 and 1994. Circulatory system diseases and diabetes were the most common medical diagnoses for these clients.[21] These trends are expected to continue, or even escalate, in the next century.[16]

Although the recipients of various community-focused services are diverse, the elderly constitute the largest single group. Population trends in the United States suggest this will continue:

- Since 1900, the percentage of people over 65 has tripled. More than 35 million people will be over 65 by the year 2000.
- Those over 65 account for one third of the healthcare consumption and may consume one half of the total healthcare dollars by 2040.
- Almost 50% of all hospital admissions nationally involve the elderly.
- Up to 60% of the elderly fail to take medications properly.
- The 3 million men and women over age 85 make up the fastest growing subset of the elderly, with a growth rate nearly three times that of the overall elderly population.[20]

Reimbursement is a challenge and responsibility that frequently confronts the staff nurse practicing in home health and community-focused settings (see Bridge to Home Healthcare: Finding Financial Help). In contrast, the staff nurse in the hospital or nursing home may not know the cost of service or supplies and may not need to discuss charges with clients and their families. When a home healthcare agency accepts a referral, financial data are usually collected by nurses. The nurse may be an intake staff member or the person who provides the initial services. Data include (1) the source of payment, (2) verification of eligibility for Medicare, Medicaid, or other programs providing payment, (3) preauthorization approval from a managed-care or other third-party payor, and (4) other pertinent concerns. Many home health services are reimbursed by third-party payors; Medicare is the largest single payor. In addition, some clients pay for services themselves (private pay) or receive services that are paid for by taxes, United Way, foundations, or grants. Often, reimbursement regulations are very complicated and involve extensive paperwork for both nurses and clients. Clients may ask their nurses for assistance as they try to deal with these regulations. The Bridge to Home Healthcare: Medicare and Medicaid Coverage of Home Health Services summarizes eligibility, requirements, and coverage information that home health nurses must know.

The Specialty in Perspective

The specialty of home healthcare and community-focused nursing has a long and distinguished history in the United States, even though it received little attention from the public or the nursing profession until recently. In 1877, Frances Root was employed in New York City as the first home visit nurse. In 1893, Lillian Wald and Mary Brewster established the Henry Street Settlement in the same city. Their goal was to offer public health nursing and community-wide programs to people of all ages who were at high risk of developing health problems and to those with acute and chronic health problems. Lillian

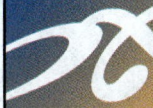

BRIDGE TO HOME HEALTHCARE

Finding Financial Help

Cindi Leo-Gofta, R.N., B.S.N.
Visiting Nurse Association of Omaha
Omaha, Nebraska

June McAtee, L.C.S.W.
Childrens' Memorial Hospital
Omaha, Nebraska

Finding financial help and support services for the chronically ill client requires patience and perseverance. By using a multidisciplinary approach and creative problem solving, patients may receive help with locating and utilizing services. New strategies should be introduced gently to help patients and families adjust to the idea of having unfamiliar service providers in their lives, or to interacting with agencies in a way that they have never anticipated.

Waiting periods for federal, state, county, and local services such as Medicare, Medicaid, Social Security Disability, and county assistance make early referral essential. Applications to these agencies can be initiated while the client is still hospitalized. A complete assessment should be made of the client's present and future needs. The assessment should address not only physical but also financial, environmental, and emotional concerns. Evaluation should include information on the client, family, and community and their ability to provide needs and what it takes to mobilize those resources. The home healthcare team should be sensitive to the ethnic, cultural, privacy, and value issues of the client by affirmation of the client's choices and goals.

A tentative approach may provide temporary relief for the client's problem, but a more permanent or long-term solution is preferable and prevents having to deal with the problem again. An example of this approach would be the client who has no money to purchase medication. Finding a resource to help purchase several days of medication may require only a telephone call to a local philanthropic group. However, a long-term solution will require creative problem solving.

When you brainstorm for a solution, remember to include all members of the healthcare team. Team members in addition to nursing personnel may be familiar with resources that are frequently used and with the staff members or volunteers who serve as gatekeepers for those resources. Local churches, human service agencies, clubs, community action groups, and health service organizations can provide numerous resources for supportive care.

Wald had the vision to (1) initiate programs and group activities at the settlement to meet the community's health-related, educational, social, and employment needs, (2) send nurses from the settlement to make home visits and provide care to new mothers, infants, and the sick, and (3) forge alliances with business and political leaders

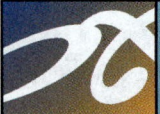

BRIDGE TO HOME HEALTHCARE

Medicare and Medicaid Coverage of Home Health Services

Nancy Scheet, R.N., M.S.N., Visiting Nurse Association of Omaha, Omaha, Nebraska

Program	Eligibility	Requirements	Coverage
Medicare	1. 65 years or older and established entitlement to Social Security or Railroad Retirement benefits 2. Endstage renal disease (waiting period applies) 3. Under 65 years and established eligibility for Social Security or Railroad Retirement disability benefits (waiting period applies)	1. Physician-prescribed plan of care 2. Services "medically necessary" 3. Requires intermittent skilled nursing, physical therapy, or speech-language pathologist 4. Homebound	1. Skilled nursing, physical therapy, speech-language pathologist 2. Skilled occupational therapy if service is initiated in conjunction with coverable skilled nursing, physical therapy, or speech-language pathologist 3. Medical social services and home health aide if provided in conjunction with skilled service 4. Medical supplies and equipment
Medicaid	1. Recipients of Aid to Families with Dependent Children (AFDC) 2. Recipients of Aid to Aged, Blind, and Disabled (AABD) who meet specific income guidelines 3. Others who meet federal or state income and categorical guidelines	1. Physician-prescribed plan of care 2. Services "medically necessary" 3. Homebound; requirements vary by category 4. Additional requirements may be established by each state and may include case management and prior authorization for services	*Required:* 1. Intermittent nursing service 2. Home health aide 3. Medical supplies and equipment *Optional:* 1. Physical therapy 2. Speech-language pathologist 3. Occupational therapy 4. Private duty nursing 5. Personal care services

to obtain support for her programs. This comprehensive approach to health can be called community health nursing and represents a true blend of public health and home care practice. Collaboration between the Henry Street staff and the New York City Mission home visit staff followed, and led to the formation of the Visiting Nurse Service of New York, the largest provider of home healthcare services in the United States. Soon, organized home visit programs were established in populated areas along the East Coast. Lillian Wald spread her vision of preventive, curative, and social services for the entire community throughout New York City and the rest of the country. By 1912, 2500 nurses were employed by 900 independent visiting nurse associations.[5]

By 1963, there were 1100 home health and home care aid organizations and hospices in the United States that employed professional registered nurses. The enactment of national Medicare legislation in 1966 accelerated the rate of agency growth. More than 15,000 home care agencies now offer services to 7 million clients and account for expenditures of over $23 billion nationally.[21] Approximately 200,000 community health nurses are employed by home care and public health agencies, school

systems, and industry. That number is expected to escalate dramatically in the next 10 years.

Interdisciplinary collaboration, teamwork, and communication are necessary in home healthcare and community-focused settings. Nurses make up the largest group of clinicians, although most home health agencies also employ or contract with home health aides and other paraprofessionals as well as other professionals. Physical therapists, occupational therapists, social workers, and speech pathologists are usually on staff, and nutritionists, pharmacists, dentists, physicians, and clergy may also be part of the team. Agency staff also need to coordinate referrals and communicate about client services with various community providers.

Community-Focused Philosophy

Clients may be individuals, families, groups, or the community.[1,2,16,27] Because home healthcare and community-focused clinicians have had the opportunity to work with clients over time, they have espoused a number of core values which influence their practice. Interdisciplinary collaboration and a seamless healthcare environment have already been mentioned. In addition, community health nurses have frequently conducted prevention and health promotion programs involving immunizations, smoking cessation, breast self-examination, and similar concerns.[23,27]

Nurses in home healthcare and community-focused settings refer to those they serve as clients, patients, consumers, or customers. Note the variety of terms used in the Bridge to Home Healthcare features. Regardless of the term they use or whether they use the terms interchangeably, they tend to base their practice on the beliefs related to the consumer movement. Included are beliefs that people have both rights and responsibilities, and that they must be knowledgeable about their own healthcare, and actively involved in decisions. These beliefs are linked to issues of access, cost, and quality, as well as the concepts of primary healthcare applicable at a national and international level. For international use, the World Health Organization[29] defined *health* as a state of complete physical, mental, and social well-being, and not merely the absence of disease or infirmity; the definition further states that health is a fundamental human right and that the attainment of the highest possible level of health is an important worldwide social goal.

The power of the client is an important core value for home healthcare and community-focused providers.[24,26,27] When a clinician enters a client's home, it is the client, not the clinician, who is in charge. In the hospital or nursing home, the nurse gives the client medications and changes dressings. In the home, nurses assist clients to provide their own care or assist family or informal caregivers to provide that care.[11] The family and other informal caregivers are critical members of the healthcare team. Their beliefs about healthcare practice and treatment, the extent of their skills, and their availability influence or even determine if the client can remain at home and the outcome of the client's care.

Staff members who provide service to clients, their families, and other informal caregivers in their homes are human bridges to home healthcare. This is true whether the staff member be a nurse, another professional, or a paraprofessional. To maximize client outcomes of care, every member of the home healthcare and community-focused team should follow some basic principles as they practice their specialty:

- Remember that you are a guest in someone's home and neighborhood. Your behavior and your manners need to convey that you completely recognize that role.
- Respect the client's cultural, religious, and ethnic heritage. Hesitate before contradicting that heritage. The client may not follow your advice.
- It is possible that the client will not respect *your* cultural, religious, and ethnic heritage. If you are a male nurse, the client may expect, and even request, a female nurse. Develop interpersonal skills—and a tough skin.
- Almost every home health client has family members or significant others who will also offer advice and

serve as your advocate or foe. Try to enlist them to be your advocates (see Ethical Issues in Nursing).
- The client owns the health-related problem that initiated your services. That problem is just one part of the client's past, present, and future. Thus, it is the client who experiences, learns to understand, and ultimately solves the problem. It is your goal to help clients and their families become as independent as quickly as possible. Talk to your peers and supervisors if you sense you are losing that perspective.
- Enjoy the unique autonomy and challenges of providing highly complex care in the home and community setting. Home health practice requires integration of high-technology skills, teaching, case management, and monitoring. Remember the necessity of communication with other members of the healthcare team. Because the nurse is usually responsible for judging whether or not the client can safely remain at home, other team members need to share this information through oral and written means.
- Maintain your sense of humor. You will need it!

Risks

The Boy Scout motto "Be Prepared" needs to be practiced by all home healthcare staff and students at all times. Preparedness is essential regardless of the nurse's responsibilities, the size of the agency or organization, or its geographical location. When a nurse works in a hospital or nursing home, colleagues, technology, supplies, and references are nearby. When a nurse makes a visit to a home, school, clinic, or other site, the nurse is often alone. The nurse is her or his own primary resource. Help and information are available via extra supplies in the trunk of the car, telephone, beepers, or faxes; help may not be available immediately.

The safety of the client and of the nurse must always be considered. Thoughtful planning to minimize the risks of accidents or violence and knowledge of the agency's disaster plan are essential. When accidents or violence occurs, interventions need to be immediate and appropriate. For example, when selecting individuals, families, or groups for a student assignment, it is necessary to evaluate the client's needs, the student's educational and life experiences, the faculty member's skills and availability, where the clients are located, the timing of the visit, the availability of other sources of help, and the student's method of transportation to, and familiarity with, the neighborhood. It is also important to establish a working relationship between the students and faculty and agency and service to enhance safety and the quality of the experiences for all. Some agencies have developed student learning centers for this purpose.[13,28] As another alternative, faculty use nursing centers as sites for some student experiences.[8,10] To increase safety for both clients and students, the Nightingale Tracker System and other communication methods are being developed to increase the links between nursing students and their instructors; the tracker is described later in this chapter.

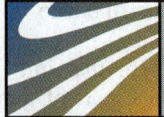

ETHICAL ISSUES IN NURSING

How Should Nurses Respond to Conflicts Between Patients and Family Members in the Home Healthcare Setting?

As a nurse caring for clients in the home, you are faced with a serious ethical problem. Your client, Mr. Samson, is an elderly, frail gentleman who has cancer and is dying. He feels quite strongly that he wants to live in his own home until he dies. Most of his physical care is provided by his only child, Susan. Susan and her father have not been able to get along well for many years. Even now, there is frequent bickering and yelling. Susan does a good job with Mr. Samson's physical care even though some aspects of it are complex. (Mr. Samson has a painful abdominal wound that has not healed and requires sterile irrigations and dressing changes.) Susan occasionally becomes overwhelmed by the stressful situation and feels like running away. Mr. Samson is aware of Susan's stress. He would like to make things easier for her but is unable to do so.

As time passes, Mr. Samson is becoming more and more depressed and angry. Because he has been allowing Susan to make all of the care decisions, Mr. Samson feels that he has maintained control of nothing in his life. He does not like the way Susan changes the dressing; he has requested several times that she give him pain medication 1 hour before the dressing change, but she usually forgets to do it. On several occasions, Mr. Samson has told his daughter of his concerns. However, he has not been forceful in his discussion because he is afraid that Susan will leave him and he would be forced to go into a nursing home. As Mr. Samson's home healthcare nurse, you would like to help.

Delivering good healthcare at home is a challenge for nurses. Since clients are being discharged from hospitals "quicker and sicker," the nurse is challenged to coordinate multidisciplinary care at home that in the past was only achievable in the hospital setting. Mr. Samson's care is quite complex. You have spent many hours teaching both Mr. Samson and Susan, helping them gain the understanding they need.

Mr. Samson is quite distressed. The conflict between him and Susan is especially troubling because Mr. Samson is unable to change or withdraw from the situation. He is completely dependent on Susan.

To help alleviate this problem the nurse can try to enhance the lines of communication between Mr. Samson and Susan. By encouraging them to voice their concerns in a quiet and respectful manner, many unsatisfactory situations can be alleviated.

Sometimes, the client's distress is not alleviated by discussions with caregivers. It is occasionally necessary to bring in help from the outside (counselor, clinical director, social worker, clergy, ethics committee). Discussions with others can sometimes bring fresh perspectives and help all involved think through issues and values. These outside facilitators can help all concerned see how values can affect behavior toward one another.

The ultimate goals are to ensure that Mr. Samson's needs are met and that his relationship with his daughter is improved.

Resources

The home healthcare student and staff nurse have valuable resources which contribute to their ability to provide high-quality care: education, experience, and common sense. These resources need to be used consistently when making home visits.

Education

Regardless of the stage of a student's nursing education or the length of time since a staff nurse graduated, faculty and texts provide valuable professional information. Formal and informal education beyond the professional program are very important for practicing home health nurses; many educators are increasingly interested in partnerships with practitioners and agencies.[25] Consider courses in first aid, cardiopulmonary resuscitation (CPR), computers, cultural awareness, community resources, current affairs, and political, legal, financial, and ethical issues. Read relevant publications and attend relevant conferences. Remember what you learned and keep updating your knowledge.

Experience

Your professional and life experiences contribute to your technical and interpersonal skills. Know where you are, and take action in those areas where you need to improve.[3] Discuss your career goals and opportunities with a trusted friend. Take every opportunity to observe a colleague providing care or completing other responsibilities such as documentation. Learn how to organize your practice and avail yourself of excellent practice pointers such as the Bridge to Home Healthcare features in this book.

Common Sense

Practice in community-focused settings is not the same as practice in the acute care setting. Develop and use your intuition and listen to it.[19] Expert home healthcare clinicians are known for their caring, flexibility, persistence, and ability to improvise. They use their judgment to alter everything from their schedule to their interventions based on the circumstances and the available resources. Expert clinicians have more than a plan A as they begin to work with a client; they can initiate plan B or plan C at a moment's notice.

Providing Care

The concepts and principles involving home healthcare and other community-focused practice are closely related to nursing practice in the hospital, outpatient departments, and other areas. The assessment, problem identification and diagnosis, plan, intervention, and evaluation steps of the nursing process provide an important foundation for that practice. Figure 9–1 illustrates the concepts of the nursing process as they relate to the Omaha System. The Omaha System is one of the four vocabularies recognized and disseminated by the American Nurses Association.[9] A circular model was chosen to depict the dynamic, interactive nature of the nursing process, the nurse-client relationship, and related theories of diagnostic reasoning and clinical judgment, sometimes referred to as analytic reasoning or expert knowledge. The Omaha System is a research-based nursing diagnosis, intervention, and outcome measurement classification or taxonomy developed by practicing community health nurses.[15,16] The Problem Classification Scheme, the Intervention Scheme, and the Problem Rating Scale for Outcomes are the components of the system. The relationships among the nursing process, the Omaha System, and home healthcare practice are described in the following paragraphs.

> A community health nurse begins service to a client following an intake or referral process. During a nurse's initial visit and all other visits, the vital importance of establishing and maintaining a positive nurse-client relationship is recognized. Freeman and Heinrich[7] emphasized that a positive relationship is developed, not discovered. Such a relationship promotes quantity and quality of data and enhances the potential for success and client progress in relation to all components of the nursing process.
>
> A nurse's initial activities include data collection, assessment, and analysis (i.e., Problem Classification Scheme). This process involves gathering, clustering, combining, summarizing, and validating diverse subjective and objective information relative to each family member, the family as an interacting unit, and the sociocultural and physical environment. A community health nurse uses principles of epidemiology to enhance systematic data collection and assessment and to identify patterns within client data. . . . The conclusion and logical end product of the data collection and assessment process is problem identification or diagnosis, which involves interpretation of the acquired data.
>
> Planning and intervening are two of the most important concepts of the model to both a client and a nurse (i.e. Intervention Scheme). Campbell[4] described a broad interpretation of planning and intervention involving nurse and family collaboration:
>
> - set priorities.
> - identify client status and expected outcome(s) criteria or goals relative to specific nursing problems and time frames.
> - delineate alternative courses of action.
> - choose and take action.
>
> Identification of admission, interim, and dismissal ratings quantifies the evaluation process (i.e., Problem Rating Scale for Outcomes). Each rating provides a baseline for comparison with later ratings during the period of client service. The evaluation component of the Omaha System allows a nurse to compare a client's health status at different points in time to determine the degree of nursing effectiveness. Through evaluation, a nurse has feedback that can be used to revise and modify plans and interventions with an individual, family, or group. Thus, evaluation is both ongoing and terminal.[16]

The Omaha System

The Problem Classification Scheme, the Intervention Scheme, and the Problem Rating Scale for Outcomes follow principles of taxonomy and consist of terms and codes arranged from the general to the specific. Terms are intended to be simple, clear, and concise. The system can be used by members of various disciplines in multiple settings. The system was developed and refined during three Visiting Nurse Association (VNA) of Omaha research projects funded by the Division of Nursing, U.S. Department of Health and Human Services, between 1975 and 1986. Further research focusing on reliability, validity, and usability was funded by the National Institute for Nursing Research, National Institutes of Health, through a 1989–1993 RO-1 grant.[14,16,18] The Omaha System exists in the public domain, so it is readily accessible to students, faculty, and other potential users.

The Omaha System is designed to facilitate nursing practice, documentation, and information management. It is a series of cues or feedback loops which help remind the user about possible client problems and intervention options and about ways to evaluate the effect of the care provided. The structured language and codes enhance pre-

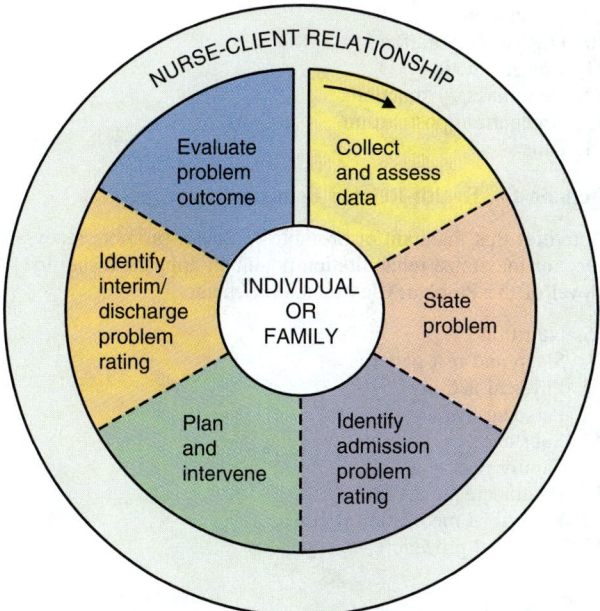

Figure 9–1. The steps of the nursing process as they relate to the Omaha System. (From Martin, K. S., & Scheet, N. J. [1992]. *The Omaha system: Applications for community health nursing* [p. 34]. © 1992 by W. B. Saunders Company. Reprinted with permission.)

cision of recording and ease of communication. Users can communicate their conclusions orally, through printed paper forms, or electronically. The Omaha System provides a clinical data framework for agencies or programs that use manual or automated versions of client records; the number of Omaha System users is increasing. The national trend among all types of healthcare providers is to automate clinical data.[9,22,30] Establishing a clinical database that is valid and reliable enables a user to generate reports that contribute to program evaluation, long-range planning, regulations required by accreditation organizations and third-party payors, and outcome statistics required as part of managed-care contracts. Many home health and community-focused agencies are making progress in their efforts to improve their client records and develop integrated clinical and financial management information systems. The time and cost required for development of such information systems, however, are significant constraints.

The Problem Classification Scheme

The Problem Classification Scheme is a taxonomy of client problems or nursing diagnoses that was developed from actual client data (Box 9–1). It consists of four levels: domains, problems, modifiers, and signs/symptoms. Domains are the four general areas that represent community health practice and provide organizational groupings for client problems: Environmental, Psychosocial, Physiological, and Health Related Behaviors. Problems are the 40 nursing diagnoses that represent matters of difficulty and concern that adversely affect any aspect of the client's well-being. Examples of client problems are Caretaking/parenting, Integument, and Nutrition. Modifiers and signs/symptoms are at the third and fourth levels.[16]

A review of the Problem Classification Scheme can

Box 9–1. Domains and Problems of the Problem Classification Scheme

Domain I. Environmental

The material resources, physical surroundings, and substances both internal and external to the client, home, neighborhood, and broader community; appears at the first level of the Problem Classification Scheme.

1. Income
2. Sanitation
3. Residence
4. Neighborhood/workplace safety
5. Other

Domain II. Psychosocial

Patterns of behavior, communication, relationships, and development; appears at the first level of the Problem Classification Scheme.

6. Communication with community resources
7. Social contact
8. Role change
9. Interpersonal relationship
10. Spirituality
11. Grief
12. Emotional stability
13. Human sexuality
14. Caretaking/parenting
15. Neglected child/adult
16. Abused child/adult
17. Growth and development
18. Other

Domain III. Physiological

Functional status of processes that maintain life; appears at the first level of the Problem Classification Scheme.

19. Hearing
20. Vision
21. Speech and language
22. Dentition
23. Cognition
24. Pain
25. Consciousness
26. Integument
27. Neuromusculoskeletal function
28. Respiration
29. Circulation
30. Digestion-hydration
31. Bowel function
32. Genitourinary function
33. Antepartum/postpartum
34. Other

Domain IV. Health-Related Behaviors

Activities that maintain or promote wellness, promote recovery, or maximize rehabilitation potential; appears at the first level of the Problem Classification Scheme.

35. Nutrition
36. Sleep and rest patterns
37. Physical activity
38. Personal hygiene
39. Substance use
40. Family planning
41. Healthcare supervision
42. Prescribed medication regimen
43. Technical procedure
44. Other

Data from Martin, K. S., & Scheet, N. J. (1992). *The Omaha System: A pocket guide for community health nursing.* Philadelphia: W. B. Saunders.

assist the reader to understand the wide range of client concerns that the home healthcare or other community-focused provider addresses. These include physical, emotional, social, religious, and economic concerns. Thus, the Problem Classification Scheme is used as a framework for assessment during a home or clinic visit and for documentation of the service provided. In that way, the scheme constantly reminds the provider that the client needs to be viewed holistically, and not as a colostomy or drug user.

The problem Integument, a problem from the Physiological domain, appears in Box 9–2. Integument has 10 signs/symptoms, including lesion and drainage. If the nurse provides care to a client who requires cleaning and a dressing change for an infected wound, that nurse may record the (1) problem, Integument; (2) signs/symptoms, lesion and drainage; and (3) more specific descriptive and quantitative clinical data on the client's form or automated record.[17] The problem Caretaking/parenting, from the Psychosocial domain, also appears in Box 9–2. It has nine signs/symptoms, including difficulty providing physical care/safety and expectations incongruent with the stage of growth and development. The nurse may visit a 14-year-old mother and her newborn and provide information about infant growth, development, and care. The nurse may record the (1) problem, Caretaking/parenting; (2) signs/symptoms, difficulty providing physical care/safety, and expectations incongruent with stage of growth and development; and (3) more specific descriptive and quantitative clinical data on the client's manual or automated record. Table 9–1 illustrates these two examples of assessment and nursing diagnosis documentation as well as terms and codes from the other two Omaha System schemes. Note that Table 9–1 depicts part of the client record documentation for two nurse-client visits, not complete record entries.

The Intervention Scheme

The Intervention Scheme is a systematic arrangement of nursing actions or activities designed to help users identify and document plans and interventions in relation to specific client problems and other concepts of the nursing process (Box 9–3). It represents a research-based effort to link the effectiveness of interventions with diagnoses, an effort not yet accomplished within the nursing profession.[16,17]

The first level of the Intervention Scheme comprises four comprehensive categories: (1) Health Teaching, Guidance, and Counseling; (2) Treatments and Procedures; (3) Case Management; and (4) Surveillance. One or more categories are used to develop a plan or document an intervention specific to a client problem. The second level of the scheme is an alphabetical listing of 62 targets. *Targets* are defined as objects of nursing intervention or nursing activities that serve to further describe problem-specific intervention categories. For the problem Integument, and the category Treatments and Procedures, useful targets include dressing change/wound care and signs/symptoms—physical. For Caretaking/parenting and the category Health Teaching, Guidance, and Counseling, possible targets are anatomy/physiology, bonding, and growth/development. The third level of the scheme is designed for client-specific information. Pertinent, concise words or phrases are generated by users as they develop plans or document care provided to a specific client. Although not part of the research projects, VNA of Omaha staff organized their suggestions into care planning guides.[15]

Table 9–1 depicts the use of intervention categories, targets, and client-specific information to describe and document a plan or intervention category specific to client

---

Box 9–2. Problems from the Problem Classification Scheme

14. Caretaking/parenting:
    Health promotion
    Potential impairment
    Impairment
    1. difficulty providing physical care/safety
    2. difficulty providing emotional nurturance
    3. difficulty providing cognitive learning experiences and activities
    4. difficulty providing preventive and therapeutic health-care
    5. expectations incongruent with stage of growth and development
    6. dissatisfaction/difficulty with responsibilities
    7. neglectful
    8. abusive
    9. other

26. Integument:
    Health promotion
    Potential impairment
    Impairment
    1. lesion
    2. rash
    3. excessively dry
    4. excessively oily
    5. inflammation
    6. pruritus
    7. drainage
    8. ecchymosis
    9. hypertrophy of nails
    10. other

Data from Martin, K. S., & Scheet, N. J. (1992). *The Omaha System: A pocket guide for community health nursing.* Philadelphia: W. B. Saunders.

Client Data	Problems and Signs/Symptoms	Problem Rating Scale for Outcomes	Intervention Categories	Intervention Targets
Psychosocial Domain				
Jane Doe: 14-year-old new mother with 2-day-old infant boy. Says she is "scared." Has not cared for infants; asking how to hold and feed. Wants son to sleep at least 6 hr. No family in area.	14. Caretaking/parenting: actual/family 01. difficulty providing physical care/safety 05. expectations incongruent with stage of growth and development	Knowledge = 2 Behavior = 3 Status = 2	I. Health teaching, Guidance, and Counseling III. Case Management	01. Anatomy/ physiology 04. Bonding 08. Caretaking/ parenting skills 59. Support group
Physiological Domain				
John Brown: 82-year-old just discharged after hemicolectomy. Has infected incision. Recalls some of discharge instructions.	26. Integument: actual/ individual 01. lesion 07. drainage	Knowledge = 4 Behavior = 3 Status = 3	I. Health teaching, Guidance, and Counseling II. Treatments and Procedures	14. Dressing change/ wound care 50. Signs/symptoms—physical 14. Dressing change/ wound care 50. Signs/symptoms—physical

Table 9–1. Omaha System Example

problems such as Integument and Caretaking/parenting. Again, note the definitions and diversity of community-focused interventions. Nurses and other providers must develop competent hands-on bedside care and technical skills, as well as educational, referral, monitoring, and motivational skills. Recall the previous comments about the client owning the health-related problem and that the client is the only one who can ultimately solve the problem.

Problem Rating Scale for Outcomes

The Problem Rating Scale for Outcomes is a framework for measuring problem-specific Knowledge, Behavior, and Status relative to a client. The scale is intended to measure client progress and to provide both a guide to practice and a method of documentation (Table 9–2). The scale was designed for use throughout the time of client service. When establishing initial ratings for client problems, the user creates an independent data baseline, capturing the condition and circumstances of the client at admission. This admission baseline is used to compare the client's condition and circumstances with ratings completed later and at dismissal. The comparison or change in ratings over time can be used to identify client progress in relation to interventions and the effectiveness of the care plan.[16,17]

The Problem Rating Scale for Outcomes is comprised of the Knowledge, Behavior, and Status subscales. Knowledge is the ability of the client to remember and interpret information. Behavior is the observable responses, actions, or activities of the client fitting the occasion or purpose. Status is the condition of the client in relation to objective and subjective defining characteristics. The scale for each of the concepts has five categories or degrees of response. For example, for the problems Integument and Caretaking/parenting, the nurse would identify baseline Knowledge, Behavior, and Status ratings during the first home or clinic visit (see Table 9–1).

The Nightingale Tracker System

The Omaha System has been described as a model of practice, documentation, and information management. It was noted that it is being automated by healthcare providers for use in a variety of agencies and institutions. The critical need to generate, store, analyze, and distribute clinical data with the help of automated information systems exists in all healthcare settings. The presence of instructors and nursing students in service settings, especially students who are just beginning their nursing education, introduces additional challenges related to practice, documentation, and information management. One of these involves communication.

Box 9–3. Intervention Scheme

Categories

I Health Teaching, Guidance, and Counseling

Health teaching, guidance, and counseling are nursing activities that range from giving information, anticipating client problems, encouraging client action and responsibility for self-care and coping, to assisting with decision-making and problem solving. The overlapping concepts occur on a continuum with the variation due to the client's self-direction capabilities.

II Treatments and Procedures

Treatments and procedures are technical nursing activities directed toward preventing signs and symptoms, identifying risk factors and early signs and symptoms, and decreasing or alleviating signs and symptoms.

III Case Management

Case management includes nursing activities of coordination, advocacy, and referral. These activities involve facilitating service delivery on behalf of the client, communicating with health and human service providers, promoting assertive client communication, and guiding the client toward use of appropriate community resources.

IV Surveillance

Surveillance includes nursing activities of detection, measurement, critical analysis, and monitoring to indicate client status in relation to a given condition or phenomenon.

Targets

1. Anatomy/physiology	22. Finances	43. Rehabilitation
2. Behavior modification	23. Food	44. Relaxation/breathing techniques
3. Bladder care	24. Gait training	45. Rest/sleep
4. Bonding	25. Growth/development	46. Safety
5. Bowel care	26. Homemaking	47. Screening
6. Bronchial hygiene	27. Housing	48. Sickness/injury care
7. Cardiac care	28. Interaction	49. Signs/symptoms—mental/emotional
8. Caretaking/parenting skills	29. Lab findings	50. Signs/symptoms—physical
9. Cast care	30. Legal system	51. Skin care
10. Communication	31. Medical/dental care	52. Social work/counseling
11. Coping skills	32. Medication action/side effects	53. Specimen collection
12. Day care/respite	33. Medication administration	54. Spiritual care
13. Discipline	34. Medication set-up	55. Stimulation/nurturance
14. Dressing change/wound care	35. Mobility/transfers	56. Stress management
15. Durable medical equipment	36. Nursing care, supplementary	57. Substance use
16. Education	37. Nutrition	58. Supplies
17. Employment	38. Nutritionist	59. Support group
18. Environment	39. Ostomy care	60. Support system
19. Exercises	40. Other community resource	61. Transportation
20. Family planning	41. Personal care	62. Wellness
21. Feeding procedures	42. Positioning	63. Other

Data from Martin, K. S., & Scheet, N. J. (1992). *The Omaha System: A pocket guide for community health nursing.* Philadelphia: W. B. Saunders.

The Nightingale Tracker System is a portable, sophisticated computer with software which offers the exciting possibility of linking home health and community-focused practice and education, technology, and the Omaha System. It was introduced in 1993 with a videotape, *Nursing: One View of the Future*[6] by the Helene Fuld Health Trust, an educational foundation. The trust board members concluded that nursing education would need to change because healthcare delivery was shifting from the acute care to the community setting. When instructors supervise students in hospitals, they are usually in the same area. In contrast, community health instructors may remain at the college or service setting while their eight or more students leave to make independent visits and see clients at homes, clinics, schools, or other sites. These instructors and students, especially students in their early semesters of education, need the ability to communicate during the student's travel time and while the student provides client care. Students may need to communicate with instructors quickly and often for the safety of both client and student.

The staff of FITNE, Inc. (formerly the Fuld Institute for Technology in Nursing Education) developed the Nightingale Tracker System to include an interactive system capable of linking students with their instructors and clinical agency staff through real-time voice, image, and data messaging. The Omaha System was selected as the clinical vocabulary for the tracker, and will be used by students as they complete clinical assignment activities. Such activities include assignment generation, preplan, client visit, postclinical documentation, and evaluation and follow-up. When the tracker is completed in the late 1990s, it will be available to the 1500 colleges and schools of nursing in the United States, as well as to

Table 9–2. Problem Rating Scale for Outcomes

Concept	1	2	3	4	5
Knowledge: the ability of the client to remember and interpret information	No knowledge	Minimal knowledge	Basic knowledge	Adequate knowledge	Superior knowledge
Behavior: the observable responses, actions, or activities of the client fitting the occasion or purpose	Not appropriate	Rarely appropriate	Inconsistently appropriate	Usually appropriate	Consistently appropriate
Status: the condition of the client in relation to objective and subjective defining characteristics	Extreme signs/symptoms	Severe signs/symptoms	Moderate signs/symptoms	Minimal signs/symptoms	No signs/symptoms

Data from Martin, K. S., & Scheet, N. J. (1992). *The Omaha System: A pocket guide for community health nursing*. Philadelphia: W. B. Saunders.

schools abroad (V. L. Elfrink, personal communication, May 17, 1995).

Conclusions

Home healthcare and community-focused service settings are experiencing unprecedented growth. Growth brings both advantages and disadvantages. Increases in client case load and services, staff, and budget can be very exciting. At the same time, when the internal systems of agencies experience extra pressure and become overloaded, employees are more likely to become frustrated, stressed, and to make errors. Teamwork and the development and improvement of existing systems are critical. Clinicians, administrators, students, and faculty need to use a variety of methods to communicate efficiently and work together to provide effective, high-quality services. There is only one reason for home health and community-focused agencies to exist—to provide services to the client.

Bibliography

1. Anderson, E. T., McFarlane, J. M. (1996). *The community as partner* (2nd ed.). Philadelphia: J. B. Lippincott.
2. Association of Community Health Nursing Educators. (1995). *Perspectives on theory development in community health nursing*. Skokie, IL: Author.
3. Benner, P. (1984). *From novice to expert*. Menlo Park, CA: Addison-Wesley.
4. Campbell, C. (1984). *Nursing diagnosis and intervention in nursing practice* (2nd ed.). New York: Wiley.
5. Dolan, J. A., Fitzpatrick, M. L., & Herrmann, E. K. (1983). *Nursing in society: A historical perspective* (15th ed.). Philadelphia: W. B. Saunders.
6. FITNE, Inc. (1994). *Nursing: One view of the future*. Videotape. Athens, OH: Author.
7. Freeman, R., & Heinrich, J. (1981). *Community health nursing practice* (2nd ed.). Philadelphia: W. B. Saunders.
8. Frenn, M., et al. (1996). Symposium on nursing centers: Past, present, and future. *Journal of Nursing Education, 35,* 54–62.
9. Lang, N. M. (Ed.). (1995). *Nursing data systems: The emerging framework*. Washington, DC: American Nurses Association.
10. Lundeen, S. P. (1994). Community nursing centers: Implications for health care reform. In J. C. McCloskey and H. K. Grace (Eds.), *Current issues in nursing* (4th ed., pp. 382–387). St. Louis: Mosby–Year Book.
11. Magnan, M. A. (1989). Listening with care. *American Journal of Nursing, 89,* 219–221.
12. Martin, K. S. (1995). Past, present, and future. *Home Health FOCUS, 1* (12), 1.
13. Martin, K. S. (in press). The Omaha System: A model for practice, documentation, and information management. In P. Brabec, S. MacKay (Eds.), *Applied community health nursing*. Albany, NY: Delmar.
14. Martin, K. S., Leak, G. K., & Aden, C. A. (1992). The Omaha System: A research-based model for decision making. *Journal of Nursing Administration, 22,* 47–52.
15. Martin, K. S., & Scheet, N. J. (1992). *The Omaha System: A pocket guide for community health nursing*. Philadelphia: W. B. Saunders.
16. Martin, K. S., & Scheet, N. J. (1992). *The Omaha System: Applications for community health nursing*. Philadelphia: W. B. Saunders.
17. Martin, K. S., & Scheet, N. J. (1995). The Omaha System: Nursing diagnoses, interventions, and client outcomes. In N. M. Lang (Ed.), *Nursing data systems: The emerging framework* (pp. 105–113). Washington, DC: American Nurses Publishing.
18. Martin, K. S., Scheet, N. J., & Stegman, M. R. (1993). Home health clients: Characteristic, outcomes of care, and nursing interventions. *American Journal of Public Health, 83,* 1730–1734.
19. Mattox, D. B. (1995). Stay safe. *Home Health FOCUS, 2* (1), 4.
20. Mikulencak, M. (1993). Facts you should know. *American Nurse, 25,* (7), 13.
21. National Association for Home Care. (1994). *Basic statistics about home care 1994*. Washington, DC: Author.
22. National Center for Nursing Research. (1992). *Patient outcomes research: Examining the effectiveness of nursing practice*. NIH Publication No. 93-3411. Bethesda, MD: National Institutes of Health.
23. Pender, N. J. (1994). *Health promotion in nursing practice*. Norwalk, CT: Appleton & Lange.
24. Reif, L. J., & Martin, K. S. (1996). *Nurses and consumers: Partners in assuring quality in the home*. Washington, DC: American Nurses Publishing.
25. Rothert, M. L., Talarczyk, G. L., & Awbrey, S. M. (1994). Partnerships in nursing education: Expanding the boundaries. In J. C. McCloskey & H. K. Grace (Eds.), *Current issues in nursing* (4th ed., pp. 170–176). St. Louis: Mosby–Year Book.

26. Smith, C. M., & Maurer, F. A. (1995). *Communty health nursing: Theory and practice.* Philadelphia: W. B. Saunders.
27. Stanhope, M., & Lancaster, J. (Eds.). (1996). *Community health nursing: Promoting health of aggregates, families, and individuals* (4th ed.). St. Louis: Mosby–Year Book.
28. Tully, M., & Bennett, K. (1992). Extending community health nursing services: The student learning center. *Journal of Nursing Administration, 22,* 38–42.
29. World Health Organization/UNICEF. (1978). *Primary health care: Alma-Ata Conference.* Geneva: Author.
30. Zielstorff, R. D., et al. (1993). *Next-generation nursing information systems.* Washington, DC: American Nurses Association/National League for Nursing.

Health Promotion and Health Assessment

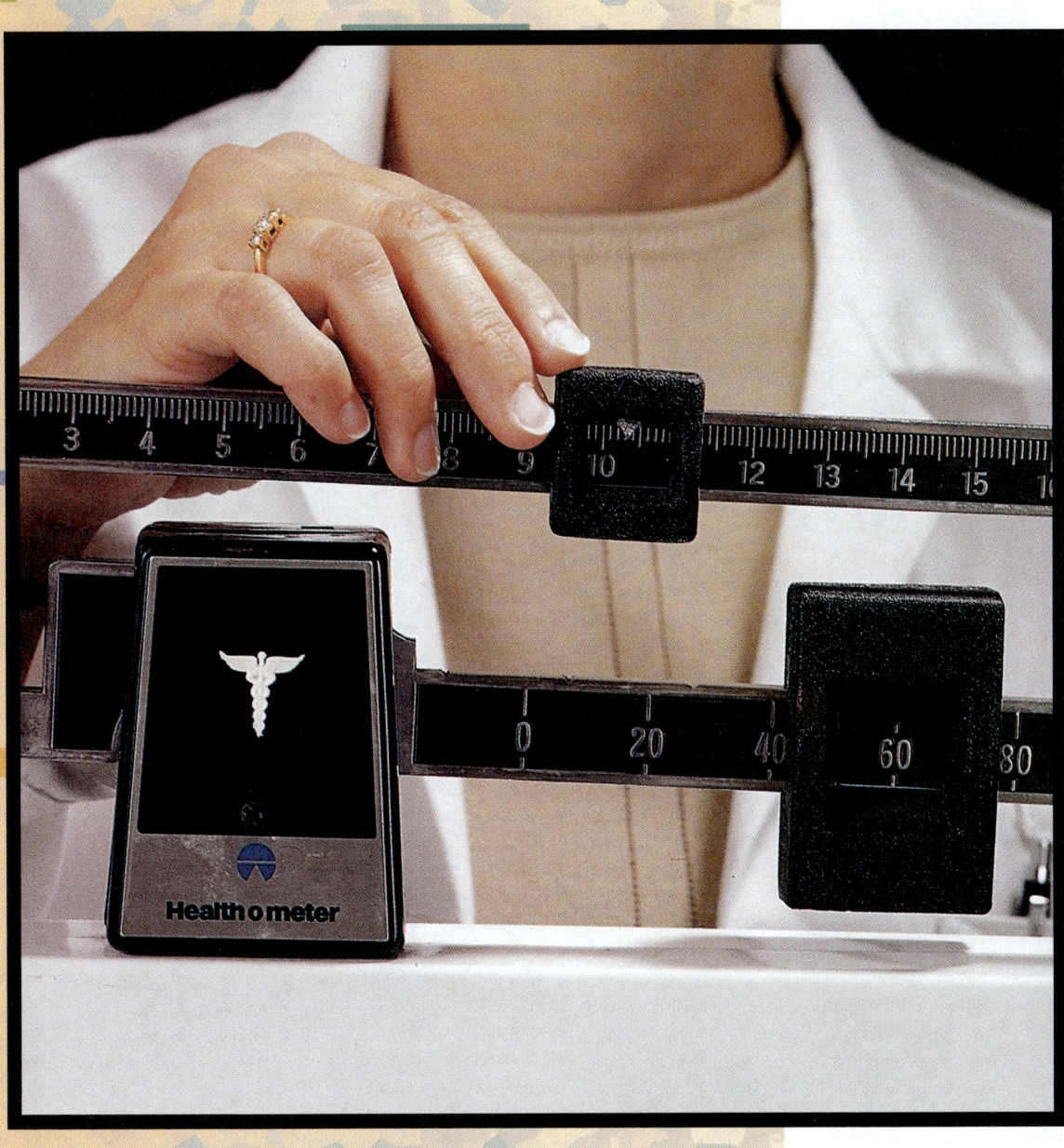

Health Promotion

Esther Matassarin-Jacobs

Health promotion is about joyful living, actualizing our potentials, and being the best we can be. It is about cleaning up and caring for our air, our water, our cities, and ourselves. It is for the well-being of the individual and for humanity. It is for and about creating a healthier internal and external environment for all living creatures on Earth. Health promotion has to do with the acquisition of mental, physical, and spiritual assets to protect and buffer us from disease as well as to move us along a continuum toward high-level wellness.

Definitions

The term *health* has been defined in a variety of ways in a variety of sources. The most widely accepted definition is the classic 1947 World Health Organization (WHO) description that health is "a state of complete physical, mental, and social well-being and not merely the absence of disease or infirmity."[81(p 1)] A variety of nursing models also offer definitions of health. These range from complex definitions (e.g., health is a pattern of expanding consciousness) to Nightingale's definition (e.g., health is an absence of disease and the ability to use one's power to the fullest). A variety of definitions are given in Table 10–1. Definitions today reflect a more holistic and subjective view of health. Individuals are asked to define what health means to them.

Likewise a variety of definitions for *wellness* have been proposed. A synthesized definition is that wellness is the quality or condition of being well, especially of being robust, healthy, and fit. Wellness is not simply the absence of manifestations; it incorporates positive mental, physical, and spiritual well-being.

Health promotion is the process of fostering awareness, influencing attitudes, and identifying alternatives so that individuals can make informed choices and change their behavior to achieve an optimal level of physical and mental health and improve their physical and social environment.

This chapter incorporates material written for the fourth edition by Lynn Keegan.

Health promotion programs are designed to improve the health and well-being of individuals and communities by providing people with the information, skill, services, and support they need to undertake and maintain positive life-style changes. *Self-responsibility* means developing the awareness and ability to take action to achieve or maintain individual freedom, health, and well-being.

Risk factors are genetic, environmental, or life-style factors that increase the probability of developing an illness or disease. A healthy life-style is a manner of day-to-day, positive, action-oriented living that works in a cumulative way to promote health and well-being.

The WHO defines *community* as a social group determined by geographic boundaries and/or common values and interests. Community members know and interact with one another. The community within a particular social structure creates norms, values, and social institutions.[80]

Understanding Health Promotion

Awakening to the importance of both individual and collective health-promoting behaviors is part of the paradigm shift of this age. Ferguson described the social transformation that is occurring concomitantly with the alteration in health behavior. Because of the popularity of a holistic approach that began during the 1970s and continues to gain support today, people are focusing attention on a search for patterns of occurrence and causes for their manifestations.

Human beings are open systems in which the sum of the parts is greater than the whole. Thus, humans are holistic, and each system has a direct or indirect effect on every other system. These patterns of action occur within the client and also between the client and the ever-changing environment. These ever-changing patterns provide an opportunity to constantly renew all areas of our being.

Table 10–1. Definitions of Health	
Nursing Model	**Definition of Health**
King's goal attainment theory	Health is a dynamic life experience. Dynamic implies a continuous adjustment to stressors in internal and external environments and the use of one's resources to achieve maximum potential.
Leininger's transcultural model	Health refers to "beliefs, values, and action patterns that are culturally known and used to preserve and maintain personal or group well-being, and to perform daily role activities."[42]
Levine's conservation principles	Health defined in terms of Anglo-Saxon word meaning "whole." Patterns of wholeness change with growth and development. Health and disease patterns reflect adaptive change.
Neuman systems model	Health is a condition in which the parts and subparts of the whole person are in harmony.
Orem's self-care model	Health is a state of wholeness, including the person's parts and modes of functioning.
Roger's unitary person model	Health and illness are seen as expressions of the interaction of a person and the environment in the process of unfolding consciousness.
Roy's adaptation model	Health is a process or state of being and a process of becoming an integrated whole.
Watson's model of human caring	Health is more than the absence of disease. It is a harmony within the mind, body, and soul.
World Health Organization definition	Health is a "state of complete physical, mental, and social well-being and not merely the absence of disease or infirmity."

Dunn was the first person to define and describe wellness, a term and an ideal that was the precursor to the health promotion movement.[17] His now-classic definition of what he termed "high-level wellness" is "an integrated method of functioning which is oriented toward maximizing the potential of which the individual is capable within the environment where he is functioning." Dunn stressed that wellness is an ongoing process directed toward higher potential, not a static goal, and that high-level wellness is a feeling of being "alive to the tips of the fingers, with energy to burn, tingling with vitality."[17] He postulated that health professionals tend to focus on disease rather than on wellness because their training is disease focused rather than wellness or prevention oriented. It is easier to fight against disease than to fight for a condition of greater wellness.

Dunn's work may have been stimulated by the work of Sigerist, a medical historian and the first person to describe the promotion of health as one of the four functions of medicine. The other three functions were defined as (1) prevention of illness, (2) restoration of the sick, and (3) rehabilitation. Sigerist believed health included a certain standard of living, good labor conditions, education, physical well being, and rest and recreation. Health requires coordinated efforts of large groups, not only those of the individual.

Travis, a pioneer in the field of wellness, popularized the theoretical concept of wellness through development and teaching of the model illustrated in Fig. 10–1. The impact of this model resulted in the recognition that wellness requires attention; it does not happen automatically. The medical model represented on the left side of the figure brings the client back from illness or disease to a neutral point. The right side represents the potential for high-level health and wellness. It is this aspect that is addressed by the field of health promotion. The objective of this model is to demonstrate how people can move from the point of illness or neutrality (no discernible illness or wellness) into the realm of high-level wellness, and to reduce the occurrence or recurrence of illness and disease.

The Evolution of the Concept of Health Promotion

The field of health promotion grew alongside the emerging ideology and practice of wellness that developed during the 1970s and 1980s. Initially, it found expression in Canada, with the publication of the Lalonde Report, and in the United States, in the Surgeon General's Report *Healthy People*. Both of these documents discuss the significance of environmental factors in influencing health and do not limit themselves to a discussion of individual life-style or personal behavior issues, which are hallmarks of the wellness movement. The Lalonde Report made recommendations in four equally weighted areas: (1) human biology, (2) environment, (3) life-style, and (4) healthcare organization. The Surgeon General's Report differed from the Lalonde Report in that it did not weight these four areas equally. Rather, life-style was noted as having a much greater influence on health than the other three categories. The Surgeon General's Report argued that we are killing ourselves, not only by careless habits but also by polluting the environment and permitting harmful social conditions to exist. For the first time, attention was directed toward environmental concerns with issues such as toxic-agent control and occupational health and safety. This report was followed by the clearly articulated and measurable *Healthy People 2000: Health Pro-*

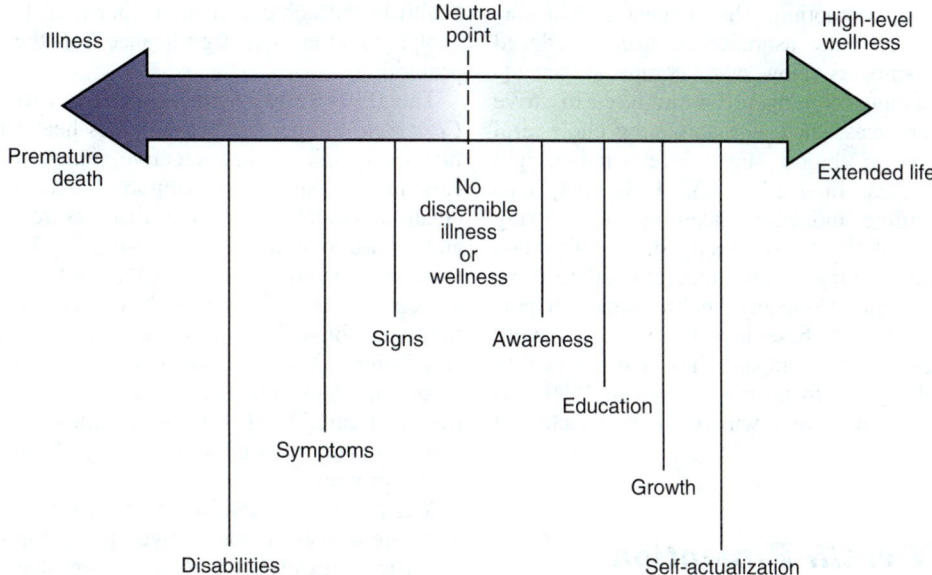

Figure 10–1. Travis's wellness model.

motion/Disease Prevention: Objectives for the Nation. This report listed specific activities for achieving each objective as proposed in *Healthy People 2000.* These publications also prompted agencies to focus on prevention and promotion through strategies of institutional change, legislation, and public policy, and not merely the realm of personal behavior change. Labonte, a health educator, believes that the ultimate challenge is to create social and health conditions that allow all of the world's citizens to achieve a state of good health.[39]

As data continue to grow in this field, evidence demonstrates that poverty is a major risk factor for development of illness and disease. Poverty is the greatest risk factor for morbidity and mortality. Social class and life-style behavior are so interrelated that they must be addressed together. Broad-based interventions that target all aspects of living, such as life-style behavior and social, economic, political, and environmental factors, are now under way (see Ethical Issues in Nursing).

Offering incentives in the workplace is the most recent

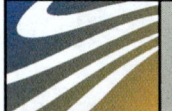

ETHICAL ISSUES IN NURSING

Do People Have an Obligation to Avoid Activities Known to Cause Illnesses that May Burden Society?

Every day we find something in the news about health maintenance or disease prevention. Research constantly tells us which foods, unsafe practices, or environmental substances cause cancer or disease. It can be a very confusing task to keep up with what can be done to prevent disease. Sometimes, people even become ill from something unknown to them, such as contaminated water or industrial waste. People can, however, do many things to stay healthy and perhaps to prevent illness.

Healthcare professionals are faced with a dilemma: Do people have an obligation to avoid activities (e.g., smoking, alcohol abuse, eating high-cholesterol foods) known to cause illnesses that may burden society? And, if they do not avoid such activities and illness occurs, does society have the obligation to care for them?

Modern research provides us with much information about the risk factors for disease. Members of the public today are the most well-informed consumers ever. Even so, people still choose to engage in activities that cause ill health. Should persons be denied the freedom to choose activities that cause them harm? Should the government impose sanctions on certain activities to prevent potential illness or disease, such as banning cigarette smoking (everywhere) or prosecuting pregnant women who drink alcohol? Should persons be held responsible for their own health-risking behaviors?

To hold persons responsible for their unhealthy behaviors is to hold them responsible for illnesses that are directly related to such behaviors. Should society have to pay for healthcare resources used by persons whose illnesses stem from their own irresponsible actions? Should healthcare workers have an obligation to care for these clients when others with no responsibility for their illness also need care?

There are no easy answers to these questions. Society will decide on its obligations by enacting public policy to direct the use of healthcare resources. The nurse's role as an educator can be invaluable here by influencing clients to avoid activities known to cause illness; thereby finite healthcare resources can be saved. Education remains the primary intervention to decrease the burden to society.

innovation in health promotion. The concept started during the 1980s, when some insurance companies reduced premiums for nonsmokers. Now other companies are offering similar discounts contingent on promises to strive for health in other areas, such as maintaining cholesterol count, blood pressure, blood sugar level, and weight within healthy ranges. In 1991, 1,053 U.S. companies were polled regarding monetary incentives for staying well. Nine percent of the firms already offered financial rewards for healthy living, with numerous other firms ready to institute them. Company health-promotion personnel are confident that these investments will benefit both the employee and the company. The average healthcare bill for employees with no risk factors in 1989 was $1,273, whereas for employees with three risk factors it was $2,284.[83]

Models of Health Promotion

In a landmark social policy statement, the American Nurses' Association (ANA) defined nursing as, "the diagnosis and treatment of human responses to actual or potential health problems."[3] Therefore, a focus on health behaviors is consistent with nursing's focus on a person's health in the context of his or her total life. It is the term "potential" that has significance for the area of health promotion.

The 1991 ANA document *Nursing's Agenda for Health Care Reform* specifically addresses health promotion. The first paragraph of the executive summary states, "America's nurses have long supported our nation's effort to create a healthcare system that assures access, quality, and services at affordable cost. . . . We call for a restructured healthcare system that will focus on the consumers and their health, with services to be delivered in familiar, convenient sites, such as schools, workplaces, and homes. We call for a shift from the predominant focus on illness and cure to an orientation toward wellness and care."[53] The entire document lists specific goals and strategies to accomplish the goals directly related to health promotion.

Many social scientists have worked on models of health-related behavior change or health-promotion behavior. These models look at the factors that have an impact on an individual's readiness to take health action. These factors include (1) perceived susceptibility to a problem, (2) perceived seriousness of a problem, (3) perceived benefits and barriers to taking action, and (4) cues to action. The Health Belief Model states that beliefs that identify readiness are both cognitive and emotional and that indi-

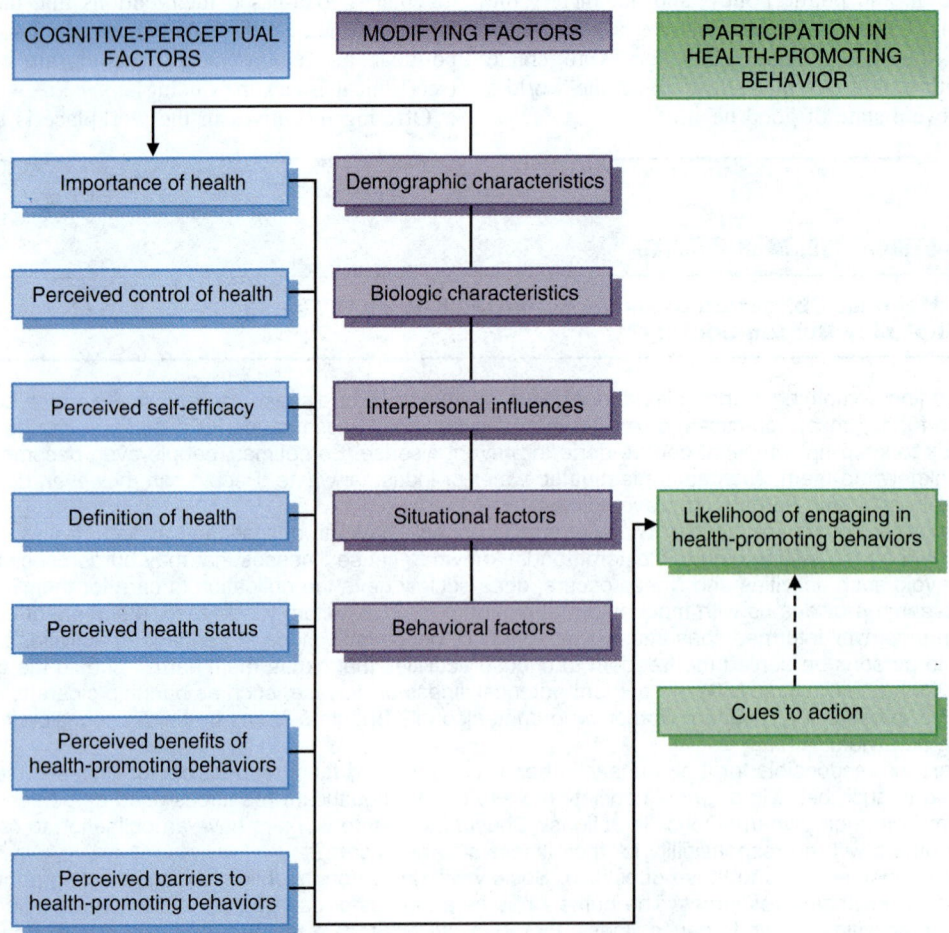

Figure 10–2. Pender's model of health promotion. (Redrawn from Pender, N. C. [1987]. *Health promotion in nursing practice* [2nd ed., p. 58]. Norwalk, CT: Appleton & Lange.)

viduals define their own motivational variables leading to health promotion.[65]

Pender developed the Health Promotion Model from earlier work on health promotion. Pender's model of health promotion is directed toward developing individual resources that enhance well-being (Fig. 10–2).[59] This model demonstrates that cognitive-perceptual factors are the primary determinants of behavior, especially health-seeking behavior.

Self-initiated activities with goals directed toward the wellness end of the continuum reflect true health promotion. This activity is one of always becoming, or of moving toward self-actualization, and is characteristic of a process that occurs over an entire lifespan. An understanding of health promotion is necessary for client goal setting, outcomes, and the development of different patterns of health-related behaviors. Laffrey and associates[40] agree that the focus on health promotion behavior "logically fits within the scope of nursing."

To promote health, nurses must understand the complex social, political, and economic forces that shape clients' lives. Nurses are charged with the responsibility of altering client attitudes toward health rather than altering the system itself. However, the nurse life-style active in the social and political arenas is in line with the ANA social policy statement that delineates involvement in social reform as being within the realm of nursing practice. The policy states, among other concerns, the "provision for the public health through use of preventive and environmental measures and increased assumption of responsibility by individuals, families, and other groups."[3]

Levels of Prevention

Preventive healthcare is more dynamic than health maintenance. This approach to healthcare has to do with health enhancement and promotion, whereas health maintenance is concerned with maintaining the status quo. When we think about the levels of prevention, a philosophical consideration embraces a commitment to wellness and a conscious desire to prevent illness and disease. The levels of prevention are primary, secondary, and tertiary. Selected behaviors associated with these levels are identified in Table 10–2.

Primary Prevention

Primary prevention is concerned with health promotion activities that prevent the actual occurrence of a specific illness or disease and specific protection (e.g., immunization). A program of health promotion or enhancement activities can be developed to increase immunity and strengthen the body and mind. Everyday life-style behavior can be examined by an individual or by the nurse, who guides the client in primary prevention. The objective is to achieve maximum functioning in each health potential.

For example, impaired mobility usually is a preventable problem. If a client is at risk for impaired mobility, many

Table 10–2. Behaviors Associated with Each Level of Prevention	
Level of Prevention	**Type of Behavior**
Primary prevention	Stop smoking or do not start smoking
	Avoid overexposure to the sun
	Support antipollution legislation
	Practice safe sex, monogamy, or abstinence
	Obtain genetic counseling
	Design and follow a regular exercise plan
	Maintain ideal body weight
	Maintain low-cholesterol, low-fat, nutritious diet
	Wear seat belt and helmet
	Identify and eliminate stressors
	Limit alcohol intake, and never drink and drive
Secondary prevention	Obtain genetic counseling
	Screening for tuberculosis
	Obtain tonometry yearly after 40 for glaucoma screening
	Get yearly Papanicolaou smears
	Get biannual eye examinations
	Practice monthly self-breast or self-testicular examinations
	Get a physical examination yearly after age 40
Tertiary prevention	Have CBC drawn before chemotherapy
	Have speech therapy after a stroke
	Participate in cardiac rehabilitation
	Have breast reconstruction
	Participate in stroke/coma rehabilitation

nursing interventions can prevent the impairment. Consider the client with arthritis who may be at risk for impaired mobility. Nursing interventions such as application of heat, a balance of exercise and rest, and administration of prescribed anti-inflammatory drugs can help prevent a serious mobility problem. Encouraging the client to eat a well-balanced diet and to engage in specific exercises may help delay the development of mobility problems.

Secondary Prevention

Secondary prevention refers to health behavior that promotes the early detection (screening) and treatment of disease and limitation of disability. It is also known as health maintenance. When working with a client, the nurse first identifies the risk factors that cannot be modified but that leave the client vulnerable to disease. Using

BRIDGE TO HOME HEALTHCARE

Making the Most of Health Fairs

Kathy Moritz Byrnes, B.S., M.P.A., *Health Fair of the Midlands, Inc., Omaha, Nebraska*

A health fair offers an opportunity to combine health screenings and health education in a casual setting. There is enormous potential to attract a large number of individuals interested and concerned about their health. The desired outcome of the event should dictate the components included in the health fair. For example, if early detection of disease is a goal of the fair, a variety of health screenings, ranging from blood pressure and vision to oral cancer, glaucoma, and pulmonary function, can be included. If the desired goal is to raise awareness of individual health, health education displays provided by local nonprofit organizations and hospitals are excellent opportunities to provide information on a wide variety of health topics. Most often, health fairs include a combination of both health screenings and education to the community.

Blood sampling is another component often included in health fairs. The method and results offered can vary from a total cholesterol reading with instant results performed with a simple finger-stick method to a fasting blood chemistry/coronary risk profile performed by venipuncture. Attention should be given to ensure compliance with state and federal laboratory regulations. To maintain confidentiality, results may be mailed directly to the participant's residence. Generally, a fee is assessed if laboratory work is included, reflecting the cost of the profile.

There is the potential that health fairs will attract the least needy people, sometimes referred to as the "worried well." Barriers for other individuals often include language, transportation, event hours convenient for working people, and cost. Extra creativity and attention may be required to increase attendance of those hard-to-reach people. To overcome barriers, offer culturally sensitive health education materials, such as items written in English and a second language. Also, involve people who are bilingual. Consider the advantages and disadvantages of where the event is held. For example, holding the event in a centrally located part of town with adequate parking, possibly close to a public transportation route, may make a difference. Grass roots publicity such as posters and fliers at local grocery stores, churches, and in newspapers may generate excellent sources of support for the event.

Most communities are rich with human and financial resources to include when planning a health fair. A network of nonprofit agencies, hospitals, physician's offices, community groups, and major corporations can play an important role in the successful health fair. Television and radio stations may also become involved in the event by providing media support and advertising. Health fairs are a positive and upbeat way to blend existing resources to celebrate the health of any community.

secondary prevention, the nurse analyzes assessment data for the purposes of deriving nursing diagnoses and identifying problems common to target populations who exhibit risk factors that are not modifiable. Emphasis is on the ranking of intervention priorities, identifying nursing management approaches within the secondary prevention mode, and evaluating outcomes. Data are obtained by interview, observation, and physical examination. The nurse then proceeds to work with the client to develop a means of early detection, such as screening for the disease.

Using the immobility example to examine secondary prevention, consider subconcepts that emerge if immobility is thought of as the prescribed or unavoidable restriction of movement in any area of the client's life. Types of immobility include physical, emotional or psychological, intellectual, and social. Causes of physical immobility may be (1) decreased energy from ischemia, hypoxia, malnutrition, and electrolyte imbalance; (2) lack of innervation, as in central nervous system or peripheral nerve impairment; (3) decreased musculoskeletal strength, as in endocrine diseases, disuse syndrome, and scar tissue formation; and (4) pain, which inhibits movement and the desire to move. Individual norms of mobility need to be considered when the nurse looks at problems of immobility. These complications may not be preventable, but

manifestations of immobility can be detected early and, therefore, complications can be prevented.

Tertiary Prevention

Tertiary prevention is directed toward rehabilitation after a disease or condition has already developed. In tertiary prevention, the nurse incorporates creative problem-solving approaches in the design, implementation, and evaluation of nursing intervention to support the client's achievement of successful adaptation to known risks, optimal reconstitution, and/or establishment of high-level wellness.

Continuing with the use of the immobility example, when a client remains immobile for any length of time, a risk exists of developing related disabilities, such as muscle and joint degeneration and metabolic and circulatory disturbances. The nurse who identifies immobility as a diagnosis will quickly develop a plan for prevention of disuse syndromes. The plan would implement (1) active exercise, (2) passive mobilization, and (3) frequent change of position. The nurse will develop outcome goals of optimal reconstitution within parameters that the client can achieve.

Risk Factors

Risk factors can generally be classified according to six categories: genetic, age, biologic characteristics, personal health habits, life-style, and environment. The purpose of risk appraisal is to provide clients with a means of evaluation of health threats to which they may be vulnerable prior to the manifestations of illness or disease. This information will help the nurse work with the client to promote health and prevent disease.

Risk factors are a key to health promotion. Once identified, risk factors can be individually addressed, and a primary prevention program can be initiated. Numerous risk factors, when left unattended or unacknowledged, can become life threatening. It is possible to uncover one or more of these risk factors during assessment. Some of the more common risk factors are as follows:

- Dietary indiscretion, deficiencies, and overindulgence (obesity)
- Fatigue and lack of sleep
- Pollution, such as noise, air, and environment
- Sedentary life-style
- Smoking
- Socioeconomic disadvantaged status
- Stress factors, such as chemical, environmental, and psychological
- Substance abuse
- Unprotected intercourse

An example of risk factor analysis is detailed in Table 10–3. This assessment of risk factors for cardiovascular disease will help you understand the concept of risk factor analysis.

Healthy Life-Styles

Health promotion, like charity and other laudable virtues, should begin at home. Friedman believes that the family is the basic system in which health behavior is first learned. Pratt finds that when families make commitments to improve and maintain their health through life-style modification, the health of all the individual members improves. Pender acknowledges the importance of family as one of many interpersonal influences on health.[59]

The development of healthy life-style behaviors as early in life as possible usually results in higher levels of health and longevity for all family members. Benjamin Spock, author, political activist, and pediatrician, cites specific problems that have had a deleterious effect on the

Table 10–3. Risk Factor Analysis for Cardiovascular Disease		
Risk Factor	**High Risk**	**Highest Risk**
Sex/age	Women after menopause	Men over age 60
Family history of high blood pressure	Two blood relatives	Three of more blood relatives
Family history of heart attack	One relative, before age 60	Two relatives, before age 60
Family history of diabetes	One or more relatives with NIDDM	One or more relatives with IDDM
Blood pressure† (degree of control somewhat modifiable)	Systolic: 160–200 mm Hg Diastolic: 90–110 mm Hg	Systolic: >200 mm Hg Diastolic: >110 mm Hg
Diabetes† (degree of control somewhat modifiable)	NIDDM uncontrolled or IDDM controlled	IDDM uncontrolled
Weight*	30% to 40% overweight	50% or more overweight
Cholesterol level†	240 to 280	Over 280
Serum triglycerides, fasting†	400 to 1000	Over 1000
Percent of fat in diet†	30% to 50%	Over 50%
Frequency of recreational exercise*	Minimal	No activity
Frequency of occupational exercise*	Minimal	Sedentary occupation
Cigarette smoking*	20 to 40 a day	Over 40 a day
Stress at home*	High	Extremely high
Stress at work†	High	Extremely high
Behavior pattern (especially men)†	Type A	Type A
Use of oral contraceptives (women)†	Under 40 and use oral contraceptives	Over 40 and use oral contraceptives
Air pollution†	Moderate	High
Sleep patterns*	More than 8 hours sleep a night	4 to 6 hours sleep a night

*Modifiable risk factors.
†Possibly modifiable risk factors.
Abbreviations: NIDDM, non–insulin-dependent diabetes mellitus; IDDM, insulin-dependent diabetes mellitus.

health of our young and, consequently, on the health of our nation as a whole (Box 10–1).

Because of these social and economic problems, it becomes difficult to focus on health-promotion behaviors. If we do not address these social situations, the result will be a continued deterioration of the nation's general health and well-being. We must emphasize the importance of the family unit in preparing children for a healthy future. Spock's recommendation is to teach children to develop an assertive sense, which, in turn, helps them to become intrinsically motivated. By age 19, only about one-quarter of children maintain the skills and talents (e.g., music, imagination, and interest in reading) they had at age 13. Spock found the difference between those who maintained their abilities and those who did not was whether or not they became intrinsically motivated. The family is the significant determinant, and this is the setting in which the initial teaching and learning process occurs. The family needs two characteristics to promote the development of intrinsic motivation and to foster a psychologically and physically healthy child: (1) the consistent offering of emotional support and (2) providing challenges and opportunities. Teens need an emotionally secure environment to which they can return from the increasingly complex world outside the home. In addition, parents need to stimulate their children and to offer them new opportunities for education and development. Children learn from behaviors modeled by their parents.

Developing Human Potential

Current definitions of health refer to the achievement of maximum potential, or self-actualization (see Table 10–1). It is within the domain of health promotion that we spend time developing and maintaining our life potentials

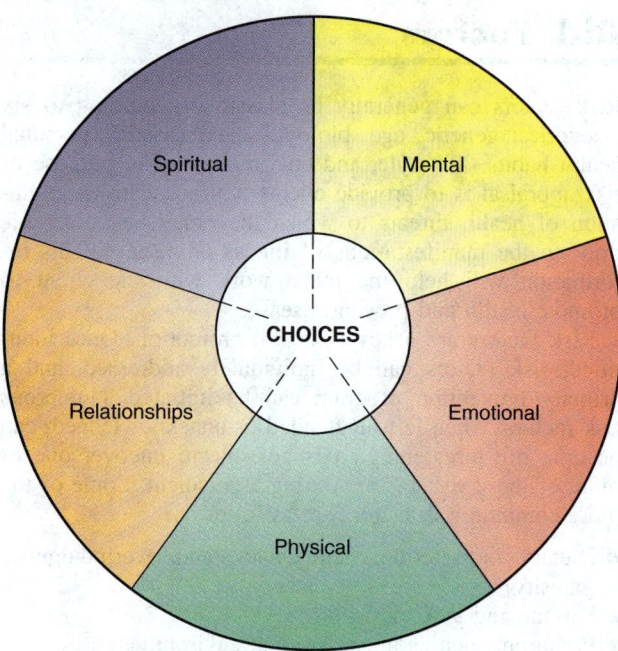

Figure 10–3. The circle of human potentials.

or becoming the best and healthiest people that we can be. The more time and energy we devote to developing our strengths, the less likely we are to develop problems. Two of the physical potentials, nutrition and exercise, are discussed later in the chapter.

Figure 10–3 represents the circle of human potentials, each of which needs to be developed to maximize health. Each physical body is unique. Through our senses of sight, touch, taste, and smell, we gather experience of the world. When the body is nurtured, it increases in strength, vitality, energy, sexuality, and the capacity to communicate and connect with other potentials.

Our picture of the world is created uniquely from mental stimuli. It is through the logical process that one learns to fully understand, enjoy, and appreciate many of life's greatest pleasures. Growth is possible when one opens up to information, suggestions, and help.

Emotions are our feelings, the inner and outer responses to the events encountered in life. One of our greatest challenges is to acknowledge, own, express, and understand our emotions. Increasing attention to the development and balancing of this potential allows our spontaneity and positive zest for living to emerge.

Spirit comes from our roots. It is related to the universal need to understand the human experience of life on Earth. Where did we come from? Where are we going? What is our purpose? Why do good and evil exist? What occurs after death? Who or what put this life form together? Development of the spiritual potential allows for the transcendence of the experience of oneness, peace, harmony, and connection with the universe.

We cannot live purposeful lives without meaningful relationships. We may not share a house with anyone, but many of us live in neighborhoods, and all of us are part of communities, cities, and states. Our relationships extend to our nation and even to the whole of planet Earth.

Box 10–1. Social Problems that Affect Health and Well-Being

Demise of the extended family

The increasing disappearance of the small, tightly knit community

The numbers of mothers in the workplace. The National Center for Health Statistics (1990) reports that in 1988, 13.3 million children—60% of all those age 5 or younger—were in a regular day care arrangement; this included half of all those children younger than age 2. This statistic does not address the children cared for by friends, neighbors, and extended family members

Dissatisfaction with so many jobs. The primary gratification is the money, an extrinsic motivation, which adds to an increasing mercenary attitude

Divorce

Excessive competitiveness in all areas of American life

Jobs being more important than family

An increasingly materialistic society

Data from Spock, B. "A Healthy Life," Lecture at Scott and White Clinic and Hospital, Temple, Texas, October 24, 1990.

The challenge in relationships is to extend ourselves and to learn how to exchange our feelings of honesty, trust, intimacy, compassion, openness, and harmony. When we share our feelings and experiences, true interchange occurs. It is through our attitude and orientation that we affect the outcome of all our encounters.

People have enormous capacity for making choices. These choices can be conscious or unconscious. Health and balance occur when the skill of effective choice making is used. Each of us is responsible for assessing our values and desires. No one else can make decisions for us.

Milio contends that the focus on choice is paramount in shaping the overall health for the person as well as for the society as a whole. The range of choices is affected by personal resources, including awareness, knowledge, one's own beliefs, and one's family's beliefs. Time, money, support of family and friends, and the urgency of other priorities all influence what choices are made. Milio states that "most human beings, professional or nonprofessional, provider or consumer, make the easiest choices available to them most of the time."[47] Nurses must be savvy to this tendency when working with clients. Lifestyle behavior patterns are not isolated choices unrelated to social, personal, or economic circumstances.

Protecting the Environment

Environment is one of the four primary determinants of health. It is not enough to think solely in terms of ourselves or of our immediate surroundings when we think of health promotion. At present, we are not just members of families, communities, states, or regions, but we are intertwined with one another and linked as a global family. What affects one of us now has a ripple effect and affects us all. Because of the massive population explosion and congested urban living conditions, it is easy to affect another person's living environment. For example, it is possible to individually pollute the air by driving a car with a defective exhaust pipe, impinge on another person's auditory air space by playing loud music, or litter another person's visual space by discarding trash where it does not belong. In a larger, collective sense, we can cumulatively do much worse and pollute the environment to such a great degree that life itself is threatened.

Health promotion, because it addresses the whole self and the whole human family, must also address the protection of the environment. It is not within the scope of this chapter to delineate ways to do this; this chapter is meant simply to awaken our awareness to the fact that each of us can play a role in cleaning, maintaining, and striving to improve the conditions of the environment to the best of our ability.

Wellness experts Callander and Travis[9] give us a number of areas to examine as we consider the health of our relationship to the planet. They are recognizing/believing, conserving, water, consuming, eating, moving, and stepping forward.

Recognizing/Believing. We need a shift in consciousness. We must awaken to the fact that we are all interdependent and begin to think and act in an integrated and synergistic fashion, rather than in the old way, which is characterized by fragmentation and competition.

Conserving. We routinely turn on lights and energy-consuming equipment without thinking of the environmental impact of our actions, such as more acid smoke billowing from coal-fired electric plants, additional spent nuclear fuel rods awaiting disposal, greater risk of coastlines damaged by oil spills, and more wild rivers being dammed up, diminishing wilderness habitats. We must practice energy conservation.

Water. More than 10 million deaths worldwide result each year from waterborne diseases. Clean, safe drinking water, even in our industrialized nation, is rapidly becoming one of our scarcest commodities. The average American uses 60 gallons of water per day. Three-fourths of it is used in the bathroom, and as much as 40% is wasted. Thirty percent to 80% of residential water is used for lawn watering.

Consuming. Americans generate 160 million tons of garbage a year, which is 3.5 lb per person per day. The irony of this situation is that we have fewer places to put it. Since the early 1980s, two thirds of our landfills have been closed, and one third of those remaining will likely be filled to capacity and closed during the next 4 years. We keep toxic substances, such as furniture polishes, plant sprays, and oven cleaners, in our homes and dispose of them through the sewer systems, often contaminating domestic water supplies. Industry uses approximately 50% of its paper, 8% of its steel, 75% of its glass, 40% of its aluminum, and 30% of its plastics for packaging. Every hour, Americans go through 2.5 million plastic beverage bottles, which may take years, or forever, to disintegrate.

Eating. Although 16 lb of feed and 2,500 gallons of water are required to produce 1 lb of meat, only 25 gallons of water are needed to produce 1 lb of wheat. Insecticides and pesticides cause a danger to our health through indirect ingestion. The United States uses an estimated 2.5 billion pounds of pesticides per year, at a cost of $6.6 billion. Up to 60% of the pesticides used on fruit and vegetables are used solely to improve the appearance of the produce.

Moving. Our dependence on the automobile exacts a great cost on the planet. Burning 1 gallon of fuel produces almost 20 lb of carbon dioxide as well as nitrogen and sulfur oxides, hydrocarbons, and lead, causing air pollution, acid rain, and lead pollution.

Stepping Forward. Global problems are complex and pervasive. Nurses need to be knowledgeable and ready to speak out on behalf of our world's well-being. It is the ideals, skills, and knowledge of each of us that, when recognized and applied, can make a positive difference in the health of the planet. We must act individually and collectively. Vote for your political candidates of choice, lobby for what you think is right, and garner legislative support for health promotion programs. By accepting the attitude that each of us can make our own little piece of the planet cleaner and healthier, Mother Earth will fare better and the likelihood of becoming healthier will increase.

Motivating Clients

Nurses encounter clients during major health changes and, therefore, are in key positions to help them make decisions and adopt behaviors that significantly alter health.[79] If we are to effectively assist others in making healthy decisions and changes, we must function as role models and have an understanding of the concepts of motivation.

Both practice and research have demonstrated that giving information to clients does not, in itself, bring about healthy behaviors.[23] Nurses frequently give up trying to teach because of a lack of client motivation. When this occurs, clients are frequently labeled as noncompliant or difficult. Orem suggests that we alter our perspective and view this seeming lack of motivation in the light of the self-care deficit theory of nursing. According to this theory, motivation is described as one of the power compo-

nents that nurses can use to help people harness their energies. Through this approach, the nurse capitalizes on the client's strengths and empowers him or her to promote health. Pender also emphasizes the importance of the helping relationship to empower the client with self-determination.

To motivate others to change health behaviors, several areas are involved. These areas include the following:

- The client must believe that the problem is solvable.
- The client must view the solution as attractive.
- The client must feel competent to successfully carry out the behavior.
- The client must feel able to overcome barriers to change.
- The client must experience positive feedback and consequences.

The role of the nurse, then, is to use multiple skills to empower clients to engage in healthy behaviors. Approaches include helping clients to identify their values and to explore feelings about themselves, with emphasis on identifying strengths. Helping clients set their own goals (developing intrinsic motivation) greatly enhances the likelihood of achieving the desired and articulated behavior changes. We need to assist our clients in differentiating between perceived and actual barriers and to promote behaviors to overcome the actual barriers. Whenever possible, nurses should act as models of health with a joyful zest for living; in this way, we teach by providing a living example.

Nutrition and Exercise in Health Promotion

Nutrition and exercise are addressed together because they work synergistically to promote high-level wellness. The lack of good nutrition and sedentary living contribute to major risk factors, such as hypercholesterolemia, obesity, and muscular atrophy. When people begin to work on one of these two areas, the other area often receives attention at the same time.

Nutrition

Nutrition has moved into the forefront as a prominent component of health promotion and disease prevention. A correlation exists between what we eat and how we feel; our potential for development of diseases is also correlated with nutrition. Cardiovascular disease, cancer, and osteoporosis are three common afflictions that are directly related to nutrition to some degree. Scores of other conditions exist that are related to poor nutrition; these may be less crippling, but they clearly affect how we feel (e.g., dental caries, constipation, and acne). The United States Department of Agriculture (USDA) has altered the dietary recommendations that were formerly based on the four basic food groups and created the new food pyramid (Fig. 10–4), which not only includes groupings but provides suggested servings from each group.

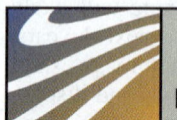

ETHICAL ISSUES IN NURSING

What Values Are Represented in the Nurse-Client Relationship?

Helping clients reach their health-related goals is the role of the nurse. While attending to that role, values of the nurse-client relationship are expressed.

You value and protect the client's ability to make autonomous decisions. You help the client collect the essential factual information, opinions, and recommendations needed to make treatment decisions. These treatment decisions are then respected by you even if you disagree with the client's choices.

You are committed to safe, effective, and compassionate nursing care. This care is delivered fairly and equally to those in need. Care and interventions must be planned by you in coordination with the client's goals.

The nurse-client relationship is founded on trust and confidence. You are a trustee of the client's healthcare goals. Because of nursing's sustained relationships with clients, you and your fellow nurses are sometimes more aware of problems surrounding the attainment of a client's goals than other healthcare providers. This heightens nursing's obligations of trust and truthfulness. Your fidelity to clients remains of utmost importance.

Because of the highly technological and interdisciplinary approach to healthcare, you must take on the role of client advocate. A strong commitment to client advocacy and professional collaboration is necessary to help the client attain his or her healthcare goals.

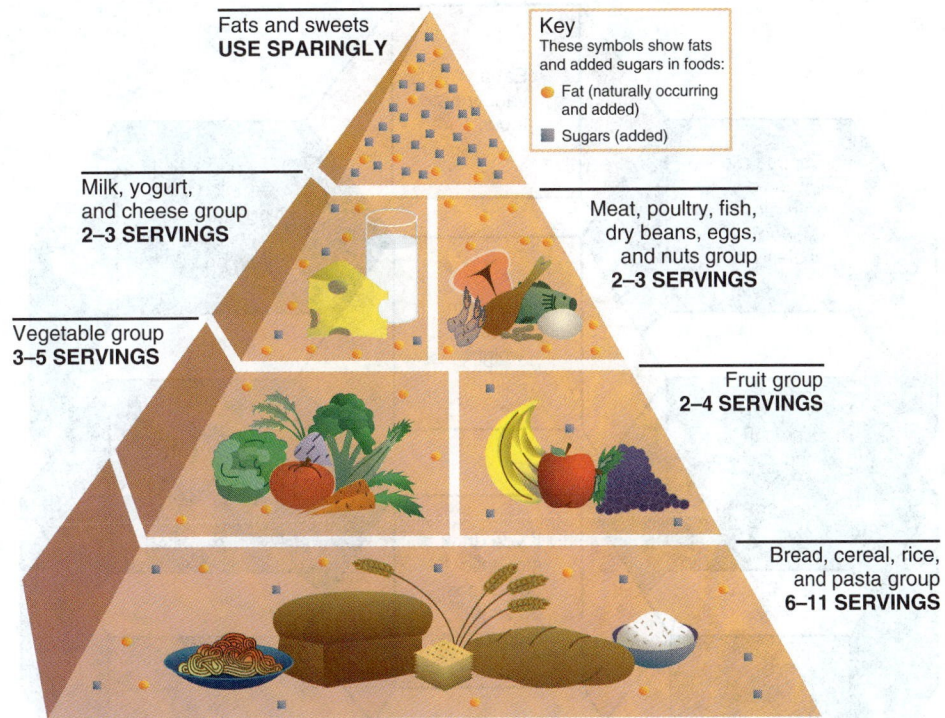

Figure 10–4. The USDA food guide pyramid. (From the U.S. Department of Agriculture, U.S. Department of Health and Human Services, Washington, DC)

Nutritional Deficits. Deficits in nutritional intake can result in stunted growth, reduced metabolic function, and delayed or premature cessation of reproductive function and can put the body at risk for many less serious illnesses. Homeostatic mechanisms protect the body from temporary deficits, but chronic nutritional deprivation creates a susceptible host for the diseases of malnutrition. Three classic deficiency diseases are scurvy (vitamin C deficiency), beriberi (thiamine deficiency), and pellagra (niacin deficiency). Malnutrition also increases susceptibility to infection and decreases wound-healing ability.

Nutritional Excesses. Overeating, or eating too many of the wrong foods, can also cause illness and disease. A large segment of our population, especially clients in the lowest socioeconomic group, eat foods that are high in fat, sugar, protein, simple carbohydrates, caffeine, and alcohol. Over a period of time, diseases of overconsumption or malconsumption appear. Obesity, atherosclerosis, alcoholism, constipation, hypertension, cardiorespiratory disorders, and some cancers are, to some extent, related to nutritional imbalance.

Balanced Nutrition. Healthy nutrition is the proper balance of nutrients, fiber, fluids, vitamins, and minerals. Whenever possible, foods should be free of chemicals, additives, preservatives, and toxins. Eat fresh foods, fruits, vegetables, legumes, and lean meats; avoid high-fat, overprocessed, and fried foods. The U.S. government recommends a decreased intake of fat and an increased consumption of complex carbohydrates (Fig. 10–5). Cli-

ents who are beginning to assess their own food intake can use a food diary, as illustrated in Figure 10–6.

Exercise

Physical fitness is beginning to take on a whole new meaning. Until recently, fitness was directed primarily toward building muscle groups for the purpose of preparing for competition. A new way of thinking about fitness is depicted in Table 10–4.

Exercise, like nutrition, should be balanced and done on a regular basis. It cannot be effective if it is performed sporadically. The purpose of exercise is to tone and strengthen internal organs and the circulatory, respiratory, and musculoskeletal systems. Exercise is more than calisthenics. The components of fitness are multiple, and all aspects should be part of a routine (Box 10–2).

A physical exercise program coupled with a wise nutritional diet is the most effective way to actualize physical health promotion. When eating and exercising wisely, one will develop improved strength and endurance, a more youthful appearance, increased vitality, good posture, and improved general physical stamina.

Stress Management

All of us have experienced stress, but each of us has different perceptions and thoughts about it. What are your perceptions? Think of a recent stressful event at home or at work that involved you and someone else. How did you react? How did the other person react? Was there a different reaction to the same event? You realize that

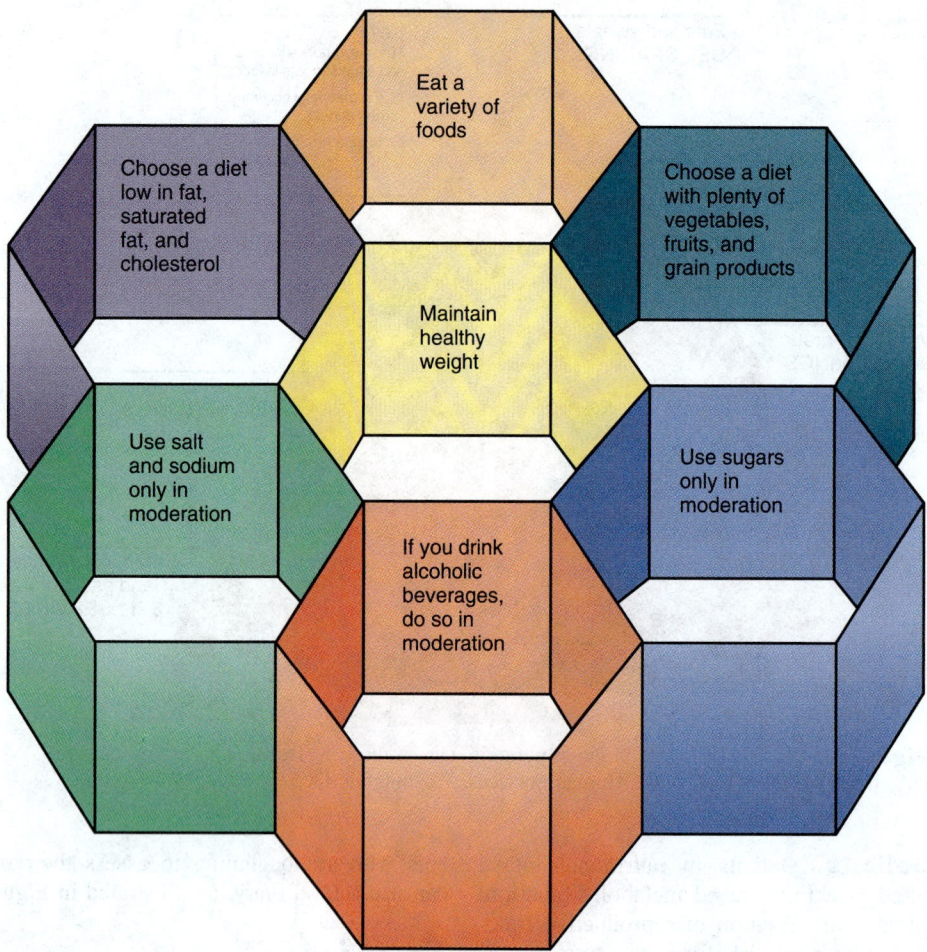

Figure 10–5. The seven guidelines for a healthy diet. (From the U.S. Department of Agriculture. U.S. Department of Health and Human Services [1990]. *Dietary guidelines for Americans.* Washington, DC: U.S. Government Printing Office.)

stress is an individual matter. No two people respond in completely the same manner. In a given situation, one person may perceive a challenge whereas the other perceives a serious stressor. The way in which you perceive each situation both directly and indirectly affects your health.

Developing Coping Skills

Many practical methods exist to cope with stress. Planning is one effective way to reduce adverse effects. For example, we prepare for predictable life changes, such as marriage, job change, or retirement. We plan by establishing goals. Through planning, we develop a belief system that allows us to dictate our own life and our own experience. Setting goals facilitates this belief system because it serves as a reminder that we have the power to create new experiences in our own lives. Goals should include areas such as meaning and purpose, fun and play, exercise, nutrition, work, and relaxation.

The most widely practiced and possibly the most effective exercise for immediate stress reduction is to evoke the relaxation response. When first learning to do this, remove yourself from the source of stress, assume a re-

laxed posture, and begin taking deep breaths through your nose. Then consciously and progressively relax all of your muscles. Begin thinking of your strengths and imagining a successful outcome. Realize that, in the great scheme of things, this event, whatever its nature, is only a minor event. Evoking the relaxation response induces a decrease in sympathetic nervous system activity and produces an altered, quieted state of consciousness. As you begin to appreciate the effects of the simple progressive relaxation technique you may want to explore and develop more long-term stress management techniques, such as biofeedback training, yoga, tai chi, meditation, and guided imagery.

Identifying Strengths

Everyone has both strengths and weaknesses. It is important to recognize this fact and to take the necessary time to identify them. When using introspection by yourself or with a client, consider the such questions as the following:

● What do I like best about myself?
● What are my personal strengths?

Record *all* foods and drinks that you had during the day and during the night.

Day of the Week (Mon   Tues   Wed   Thurs   Fri   Sat   Sun)

Breakfast
   Foods and Drinks   Amounts (cups, tbsps)

Lunch
   Foods and Drinks   Amounts (cups, tbsps)

Dinner
   Foods and Drinks   Amounts (cups, tbsps)

Snacks
   Foods and Drinks   Amounts (cups, tbsps)

Do you take vitamin or mineral supplements?   Yes_____   No_____
Please list kind and how many per day.

Figure 10–6. A food diary form. (From U.S. Senate Select Committee on Nutrition and Human Needs. [1977]. *Dietary goals for the United States.* Washington, DC: U.S. Government Printing Office.)

- Do I set goals for myself?
- Am I able to complete goals I set for myself?
- How do I perceive my personal strengths as a way of understanding these patterns?

The time taken to evaluate the source of strengths can help an individual build a belief system. Gaining knowledge of strengths and weaknesses can help us develop a sense of personal worth, which may be severely tested or even destroyed during periods of stress or crisis. People's thoughts affect their life patterns. When you work on acknowledging your strengths, you can call them to consciousness during periods of stress. Positive cognitive thoughts connect with all the human potentials so that the body responds positively. When you activate and act from your strengths, you are more likely to develop posi-

tive attitudes. The development of positive attitudes creates a better chance of effectively coping with stress during the inevitable everyday life struggles that confront us all. Some of these interventions, such as recognizing strengths, provide active techniques that enable individuals to call up inner resources to combat stress on the journey toward becoming healthy people.

Health Promotion and the Older Adult

Since the turn of the century, the elderly population of the United States has multiplied approximately eight times. At present, there are approximately 25 million peo-

Table 10–4. A New Way of Thinking About Fitness

Old Fitness Paradigm	New Fitness Paradigm
Emphasis exclusively physical	An integration of the body and mind
Compared self with others	Noncomparative
Regulated calisthenics	Aerobic dancing to motivational music. Individually paced build-up with machines that provide feedback. Motivation and subliminal tapes for individual challenge.
Competitive with others	Competition with self
Rigorous and punitive	Exhilarating and fun
Muscle building	Health building

Data from Keegan, L. (1988). Nutrition, exercise, and movement: Nourishing the bodymind. In B. Dossey, et al. (Eds.), *Holistic nursing* (p. 163). Rockville, MD: Aspen.

ple over the age of 65; there is a distinct trend toward the "graying of America." Life expectancy has risen from 47 years in 1900 to approximately 77 years, primarily as a result of effective control of smallpox, tuberculosis, diph-

Box 10–2. The Components of Fitness

Flexibility: the ability to use a joint throughout its full range of motion and to maintain some degree of elasticity of major muscle groups

Importance:

▪ Provides increased resistance to muscle and joint injury
▪ Helps prevent mild muscle soreness if exercises are performed before and after vigorous activity

Muscle strength: the contracting power of a muscle

Importance:

▪ Daily activities become less strenuous as muscles become stronger
▪ Strong abdominal and lower back muscles help prevent lower back problems
▪ Appearance improves as muscles become firmer

Cardiorespiratory endurance: the ability of the circulatory and respiratory systems to maintain blood and oxygen delivery to the exercising muscles

Importance:

▪ Increases resistance to cardiovascular diseases
▪ Improves the ability to maintain activity levels
▪ Allows for a high-energy return for daily activities

Data from Spock, B. "A Healthy Life," Lecture at Scott and White Clinic and Hospital, Temple, Texas, October 24, 1990.

theria, and other infectious diseases. Consequently, an entire segment of the population has lived to an old age and is now ripe for participation in health promotion programs. For seniors, health promotion is not just for fun, cosmetic improvement, or to prevent some distant risk factor; it is vital for enhancement and maintenance of current daily health.

Women are particularly vulnerable to problems of old age because they have a longer life expectancy (78.9 years) than men. Women are more likely to become widowed, whereas men usually remain married up to the time of their death. Also, because there are more elderly women than men, women are less likely to remarry than widowers. Consequently, women have a lesser chance of retaining supportive relationships with spouses than do males.

Health promotion programs for the elderly can be designed to address specific diseases or problems common to a particular population, or they can be more global in design. An example of a broad health promotion program is one that addresses maintenance of the following:

● Self-responsibility
● Nutritional intake
● Physical stamina, strength, and flexibility
● Control of one's own environment
● Intellectual capacities
● Financial self-reliance
● Stress control

Specific programs target particular problems such as hypertension, cancer screening, weight control, foot care, physical fitness, and other concerns. *Healthy People: The Surgeon General's Report on Health Promotion and Disease Prevention* recommends the use of health promotion programs to improve the overall health and quality of life for older adults and to reduce the average annual number of days of restricted activity due to acute and chronic conditions by 20%, to fewer than 30 days per year for people aged 65 and older.

One of the most widely known health promotion programs that focuses on the problems of older people is the Wallingford Wellness Project that operates in the suburbs of Seattle. Initially, this program was a federally funded project used to document and evaluate programs that focused on life-style changes. The program demonstrated that a comprehensive health promotion program for older people is effective, appropriate, and exciting. The outcome of the Wallingford Wellness Project program was a book by Fallcreek and Mettler,[21] entitled *A Healthy Old Age*, which includes specific guidelines and detailed steps for establishing and operating community-based health promotion programs. The other significant outcome of this program is the fact that after federal pilot funding ran out, the program continued operations and even grew in scope and design. Graduates from the Wallingford Wellness Project and other health promotion programs tend to move on to lead classes themselves in the same program or to help develop new programs closer to home. Housing projects, high-rise apartment buildings, and neighborhood centers are prime sites for health promotion programs.

Several features of the Wallingford Wellness Project are distinctive and may contribute to its long-term success. These factors should be considered when developing new programs. They include a participant-oriented focus, an intergenerational focus, individual and community empowerment, education, communication skills, and assertiveness training.

Participant-Oriented Focus. Participants and potential participants should be involved in all phases of the project, from the development of the original plan to delivery and evaluation of the content.

Individual and Community Empowerment. The long-range goal of the training program is individual and community empowerment. The focus is on helping participants develop maximum self-responsibility for their overall well-being.

Intergenerational Focus. About one quarter of the participants in the Wallingford Wellness Project are younger than 60 years. The ages of the participants to date range from 13 to 84 years.

Education. The educational component emphasizes common sense health-related information and skills that are well within the grasp of most people. The need for extensive involvement of experts in the training program is minimized. This suggests that nurses are best used as guides, organizers, and resource people, but not as the key program instructors.

Communication Skills and Assertiveness Training. Training in communication skills and assertiveness is a key program component. The Wallingford Wellness Project, a course that was originally conceived as an environmental awareness and assertiveness course, evolved to incorporate and emphasize a variety of communication skills. The development and application of these skills resulted in improvement of relationships with healthcare providers, friends, and family members; placement of desired products at local shopping places; and influencing of local legislation to enhance traffic safety provisions for older people.

Nursing Careers in Health Promotion

Nurses who want to work in the area of health promotion can seek positions with companies, schools, colleges, senior centers, municipalities, and healthcare agencies. Steps to develop programs should include

- Establishing goals and objectives
- Performing needs assessment and garnering participant involvement
- Creating a participative learning climate
- Facilitating interaction among participants

> **Box 10–3. Resources for Health Promotion**
>
> SAGE (Senior Actualization and Growth Exploration)
> 1713 Grove St.
> Berkeley, CA 94709
>
> SAGE began in 1974 and offers health-promotion programs to older people, both in institutions and in the community. It makes use of a variety of approaches. The program offers books for purchase and a videotape for purchase or rental.
>
> American Hospital Association
> 840 N. Lake Shore Dr.
> Chicago, IL 60611
>
> Publishes coordinated activity program for the elderly: A how-to manual.
>
> Growing Younger
> Healthwise, Inc.
> P.O. Box 1989
> Boise, ID 83702
>
> This program works with neighborhood groups of older adults. Healthwise, Inc., markets a training program and materials to assist other organizations in implementing similar programs.
>
> The Arthritis Self-Management Program
> 701 Welch Rd., Suite 2208
> Palo Alto, CA 94304
>
> This program is located at Stanford University and has developed many materials specifically related to arthritis and self-care.
>
> National Self-Help Clearinghouse
> Graduate School and University Center/CUNY
> 33 W. 42nd St., Room 1227
> New York, NY 10036
>
> This organization provides information on various self-help programs across the country. It publishes a highly informative bimonthly newsletter entitled "Self-Help Reporter" as well as other publications of interest.
>
> National Clearinghouse on Aging
> SCAN Social Gerontology Resource Center
> P.O. Box 231
> Silver Spring, MD 20907
>
> The organization offers bibliographies on a variety of health promotion topics.

- Developing teaching tools, such as handouts and audiovisual aids
- Developing independent teaching strategies, such as symposia, panels, brainstorming sessions, readings, discussion sessions, demonstrations, case studies, interviews, role playing, problem solving, and field trips

Nurses working in the area of health promotion will be on the cutting edge of future healthcare roles. Wellness nursing made its impact in the 1980s; health promotion nurses will be leaders into the next century.

Conclusions

Health promotion is a key watch phrase for the 21st century. Nurses are encouraged to develop a consciousness that includes attention to the social, political, and economic aspects of the environment. Through reviewing health promotion, nurses will understand that human responses to health and illness "are related to the structure of the social world, the economic and political policies that govern that structure, and the human, social relationships that are produced by the structure and the politics." Once we recognize that establishing health-promoting behaviors can alter the presence or absence of good health, then specific interventions must be delineated and disseminated to the subsets of the population that can benefit. Portnoy and co-workers[60] believe that dissemination of programs generally lags behind their development.

The process of dissemination can best be implemented and measured for effectiveness through research, practice, and evaluation. Nursing needs to strengthen its conceptual foundations to enable practitioners to better understand the parameters of, and the means to promote, health. If nurses are to enact changes at the social level, they need theoreical frameworks that are consistent with social, economic, and political forces.

Bibliography

1. Alford, D. M., & Futrell, M. (1992). Wellness and health promotion of the elderly. *Nursing Outlook, 40,* 221–226.
2. Allan, J. D., & Hall, B. A. (1988). Challenging the focus on technology: A critique of the medical model in a changing health care system. *Advances in Nursing Science, 3*(1), 22–34.
3. American Nurses' Association (1980). *A social policy statement.* Kansas City, MO: Author.
4. Angelucci, P. (1995). Notes from the field: Cultural diversity: Health belief systems. *Nursing Management, 26*(8), 72.
5. Bigbee, J. L., & Jansa, N. (1991). Strategies for promoting health protection. *Nursing Clinics of North America, 26,* 895–913.
6. Briody, M. E. (1984). The role of the nurse in modification of cardiac risk factors. *Nursing Clinics of North America, 19,* 387–395.
7. Brown, S. J. (1989). Perceived self-efficacy and recovery from cardiac illness. *Research Review: Studies for Nursing Practice, 5*(4), 2.
8. Butterfield, P. (1990). Thinking upstream: Nurturing a conceptual understanding of the societal context of health behavior. *Advances in Nursing Science, 12*(2), 1–8.
9. Callander, M., & Travis, J. (1990). *Global wellness inventory.* Mill Valley, CA: Wellness Associates.
10. Caserta, M. S. (1995). Health promotion and the older population: Expanding our theoretical horizons. *Journal of Community Health, 20*(3), 283–292.
11. Champion, V. (1995). Development of a benefits and barriers scale for mammography utilization. *Cancer Nursing, 18*(1), 53–59.
12. Clark, C. (1986). *Wellness nursing.* New York: Springer.
13. Clemen-Stone, S., Eigsti, D., & McGuire, S. L. (1991). *Comprehensive family and community health nursing* (3rd ed.). St. Louis: Mosby–Year Book.
14. Connelly, C. E. (1993). An empirical study of a model of self-care in chronic illness. *Clinical Nurse Specialist, 7*(5), 247–253.
15. Ditto, P. H., et al. (1988). Appraising the threat of illness: A mental representational approach. *Health Psychology, 7*(2), 183–201.
16. Donnelly, E. (1990). Health promotion, families, and the diagnostic process. Family Community Health, *12*(4), 12–20.
17. Dunn, H. (1961). *High-level wellness* (pp. 5–6). Arlington, VA: R. W. Beatty.
18. Dunn, H. (1980). *High level wellness.* Thorofare, NJ: Charles Slack.
19. Elipoulos, C. (Ed.). (1990). *Health assessment of the older adult* (2nd ed.). Menlo Park, CA: Addison-Wesley.
20. Eubanks, P. (1991). Hospitals offer wellness programs in effort to trim health costs. *Hospitals, 5*(32), 42–43.
21. Fallcreek, S., & Mettler, M. (1984). *A healthy old age.* New York: The Haworth Press.
22. Ferguson, M. (1980). *The aquarian conspiracy.* Los Angeles: J. P. Torcher.
23. Feuerstein, M., et al. (1986). *Health psychology: A psychobiological perspective.* New York: Plenum Press.
24. Fitzpatrick, J. J., & Whall, A. L. (1989). *Conceptual models of nursing: Analysis and application* (2nd ed.). Norwalk, CT: Appleton & Lange.
25. Fleury, J. D. (1991). Empowering potential: A theory of wellness motivation. *Nursing Research, 40,* 286–291.
26. Frauman, A. C., & Nettles-Carlson, B. Predictors of a health-promoting life-style among well adult clients in a nursing practice. *Journal of the American Academy of Nurse Practitioners, 3*(4), 174–179.
27. Friedman, M. M. (1962). *Family development.* Philadelphia: J. B. Lippincott.
28. Fuller, J., & Schaller-Ayers, J. (1994). *Health assessment: A nursing approach* (2nd ed.). Philadelphia: J. B. Lippincott.
29. Girdano, D. A., & Dusek, D. E. (1988). *Changing health behaviors.* Scottsdale, AZ: Gorsuch Scarisbrick Publishers.
30. Green, L. W., et al. (1980). *Health education planning: A diagnostic approach.* Palo Alto, CA: Mayfield Publishing Co.
31. Hann, M., et al. (1987). Poverty and health. *American Journal of Epidemiology, 125,* 989–998.
32. Harrison, J. A., Mullen, P. D., & Green, L. W. (1992). A meta-analysis of studies of the health belief model with adults. *Health Education Research, 7*(1), 107–116.
33. Heidrich, S. M. (1993). The relationship between physical health and psychological well-being in elderly women: A developmental perspective. *Research in Nursing and Health, 16,* 123–130.
34. Herron, D. G. (1991). Strategies for promoting a healthy dietary intake. *Nursing Clinics of North America, 26,* 875–884.
35. Holmes, T., & Rahe, R. (1967). Social readjustment rating scale. *Journal of Psychosomatic Research, 11,* 216.
36. Hyman, R. B., et al. (1994). Health belief model variables as predictors of screening mammography utilization. *Journal of Behavioral Medicine, 17*(4), 391–406.
37. Jensen, J., Counte, M. A., & Glandon G. L. (1992). Elderly health beliefs, attitudes, and maintenance. *Preventive Medicine, 21*(4), 483–497.
38. Kitagawa, E. M., & Hauser, P. M. (1973). *Different mortality in the U.S.: A study in socio-economic epidemiology.* Cambridge, MA: Harvard University Press.
39. Labonte, R. (1986). Social inequality and healthy public policy. *Health Promotion, 1,* 314–351.
40. Laffrey, S. C., et al. (1986). Health behavior: Evolution of two paradigms. *Public Health Nursing, 3*(2), 92–100.
41. Lalonde, M. (1974). *A new perspective on the health of Canadians.* Ottawa: Government of Canada.
42. Leininger, M. *Qualitative research methods in nursing* (p. 196). New York: Grune & Stratton.
43. Lenihan, A. A. (1990). A challenge for nursing: Promotion of self-care among the elderly. *Journal of Gerontological Nursing, 16,* 3–5.
44. Marmoi, M. G. (1978). Employment grade and coronary heart disease in British civil servants. *Journal of Epidemiology and Community Health, 32,* 244–249.
45. McAllister, G., & Farquhar, M. (1992). Health beliefs: A cultural division? *Journal of Advanced Nursing, 17*(12), 1447–1454.
46. Melnyk, K. A. C. (1990). Barriers to care: Operizationalizing the variable. *Nursing Research, 39,* 108–112.
47. Milio, N. (1976). A framework for prevention: Changing health damaging to health-generating life patterns. *American Journal of Public Health, 66,* 435–439.
48. Milio, N. (1981). *Promoting health through public policy.* Philadelphia: F. A. Davis.
49. Minkler, M. (1989). Health education, health promotion and the open society: A historical perspective. *Health Education Quarterly, 16*(1), 2–19.

50. Monk, A. (1979). Family supports in old age. *Social Work, 24*(6), 534.

51. Nightingale, F. (1969). *Notes on nursing: What it is and what it is not.* New York: Dover (originally published, 1859).

52. Norman, P. (1993). Predicting the uptake of health checks in general practice: Invitation methods and patients' health beliefs. *Social Science and Medicine, 37*(1), 53–59.

53. *Nursing's agenda for health care reform.* (1992). Kansas City, MO: Author.

54. *Nursing's agenda for health care reform: Executive summary.* (1991)(p. 1). Kansas City, MO: Author.

55. O'Donnell, M. (1986). Definition of health promotion. *American Journal of Health Promotion, 1,* 4–5.

56. Orem, D. E. (1990). *Nursing: Concepts of practice* (4th ed.). New York: McGraw-Hill.

57. Palank, C. L. (1991). Determinants of health-promotive lifestyle. *Nursing Clinics of North America, 26,* 815–832.

58. Peddicird, K. (1991). Strategies for promoting stress reduction and relaxation. *Nursing Clinics of North America, 26,* 867–874.

59. Pender, N. J. (1987). *Health promotion in nursing practice* (2nd ed.). Norwalk, CT: Appleton & Lange.

60. Portnoy, B., et al. (1989). Application of diffusion theory to health promotion research. *Family Community Health, 12*(3), 63–71.

61. Pratt, L. (1976). *Family structure and effective health behavior.* Boston: Houghton Mifflin.

62. Pruitt, R. H. (1992). Effectiveness and cost efficiency of interventions in health promotion. *Journal of Advanced Nursing, 17,* 926–932.

63. Robinson-Whelen, S., & Storandt, M. (1992). Factorial structure of two health belief measures among older adults. *Psychology & Aging, 7*(2), 209–213.

64. Ronis, D. L. (1992). Conditional health threats: Health beliefs, decisions, and behaviors among adults. *Health Psychology, 11*(2), 127–134.

65. Rosenstock, I. M. (1966). Why people use health services. *Milbank Quarterly, 44,* 94–127.

66. Schwab, T., Meyer, J., & Merrell, R. (1994). Measuring attitudes and health beliefs among Mexican Americans with diabetes. *Diabetes Educator, 20*(3), 221–227.

67. Sigerist, H. E. (1946). *The university at the crossroads: Addresses and essays.* New York: Henry Schuman.

68. Spellbring, A. M. (1991). Nursing's role in health promotion. *Nursing Clinics of North America, 26,* 805–814.

69. Spock, B. (1990). *A healthy life.* Lecture at Scott and White Clinic, Temple, TX, October 24.

70. Standhope, M., & Lancaster, J. (1992). *Community health nursing: Process and practice for health promotion.* St. Louis: Mosby–Year Book.

71. Stolte, K. (1996.) Welness: Nursing diagnosis for health promotion. Philadelphia: J. B. Lippincott.

72. Syme, S. L., & Berkman, L. (1976). Social class—susceptibility and sickness. *American Journal of Epidemiology, 104,* 1–8.

73. Tanner, E. K. W. (1991). Assessment of a health-promotive lifestyle. *Nursing Clinics of North America, 26,* 845–854.

74. Thomas, L. W. (1995). A critical feminist perspective of the health belief model: Implications for nursing theory, research, practice, and education. *Journal of Professional Nursing, 11*(4), 246–252.

75. Thorne, S. (1993). Health belief systems in perspective. *Journal of Advanced Nursing, 18*(12), 1931–1941.

76. Tones, B. K. (1986). Health education and the ideology of health promotion: A review of alternative approaches. *Health Education Research, 1,* 3–12.

77. U.S. Department of Health and Human Services, Public Health Service. (1990). *Healthy people, 2000: National health promotion and disease prevention objectives* (Publication No. PHS 91–50212). Washington, DC: US Government Printing Office.

78. U.S. Surgeon General. (1979). *Healthy people: The Surgeon General's report on health promotion and disease prevention.* Washington, DC: Department of Health, Education and Welfare.

79. U.S. Surgeon General. (1980). *Health promotion/disease prevention: Objectives for the nation.* Washington, DC: Department of Health and Human Services.

80. Utz, S. (1990). Motivating self-care: A nursing approach. *Holistic Nursing Practice, 4*(2), 13–21.

81. World Health Organization. (1974). *Community health nursing: Report of a WHO expert committee* (WHO Technical Report Series, No. 558). Geneva, Switzerland: Author.

82. World Health Organization. (1986). World Health Organization report on concept and principles of health promotion. *Health Promotion, 1*(1), 73–76.

83. Who Cares for Kids Depends on Their Status. *The Wall Street Journal,* November 29, 1990.

84. Workplace: Paying workers for good health habits catches on as a way to cut medical costs. *Wall Street Journal,* Nov. 26, 1991.

Health Assessment

Annabelle M. Keene

The nursing process hinges on thorough assessment of the client, which provides baseline data. Assessment enhances the nurse's ability to identify the client's specific needs, both physical and psychosocial. The amount, depth, and level of assessment skills vary with the nurse's knowledge and expertise. Some assessment skills are basic, such as taking a temperature. Advanced assessment skills are learned and practiced so that the nurse may use them to provide interventions and to evaluate both sick and healthy clients' health maintenance and promotion practices.

The nurse must be familiar with the parameters of human behavior and physiology before being able to recognize abnormal situations. Normal ranges for psychosocial behavior may be quite variable, whereas many physiologic manifestations have narrowly defined limits. For example, cell death occurs if body temperature becomes either too high or too low; the defined parameters are a matter of a few degrees. In contrast, symptoms of depression in survivors following the death of a loved one are expected, but prolonged depression may signal mental illness. Thus, skillful assessment requires careful observation combined with the ability to decide whether an observation is or is not normal. The nurse also considers the client's unique circumstances when comparing assessment findings to standardized norms.

The nurse evaluates how the client reacts to the assessment process itself, as well as the implications assessment findings may have for the client and significant others. Keeping these considerations in mind, the following nursing diagnoses are common to clients experiencing health assessment procedures:

Anxiety
Fear
Knowledge Deficit
Pain
Powerlessness
Situational Low Self Esteem

Each of these nursing diagnoses is followed by a related factor that identifies the specific cause leading to the problem. For example, a woman undergoing a breast examination may have anxiety related to never having experienced such an examination before or to fear of a lump being found.

Assessment requires both skill and judgment. Chapters 11 and 12 provide basic information to begin developing expertise in health assessment. Extensive practice is necessary for proficiency. The beginning nurse should also seek guidance from a skilled, competent practicing nurse. A broad knowledge base, repeated practice, and access to a mentor will assist the nurse in developing the ability to discriminate normal from abnormal.

Health assessment focuses on the individual. It is divided into two portions. The health history contains subjective information, whereas the physical examination is the objective information about a client's health status. The client is a unique entity whose spheres of interaction with physical and psychosocial environments are complex. The health history interview is free from bias, prejudice, and stereotyping. For example, an elderly client with several chronic health problems may or may not have actual health care needs that require immediate intervention. Yet the potential for complex health problems exists. Conversely, a young adult in relatively sound physical health may appear "healthy" to the casual observer when he or she may in fact have overwhelming psychosocial problems or needs affecting both current and future health status. An individualized approach to health assessment provides a valid database for further nursing care.

The Health History

The Accuracy of the Health History

Assess the accuracy and completeness of the information the client provides throughout the health history interview. Validation is important so that accurate nursing diagnoses can be formulated. Determine whether or not the client is an accurate historian, capable of and willing to provide the necessary information. The client may be unconscious or disoriented and therefore incapable of co-operating; he or she may be willing to cooperate but may be hindered by circumstances, such as a language barrier, or anxiety; or he or she may be unwilling and mistrustful about cooperating because of anger or depression. If the client cannot provide the necessary information, second-ary sources of information should be sought, such as significant others or an interpreter. However, be aware that the content and accuracy of information may be in-fluenced by the perceptions and biases of the secondary sources as well as by the sources' knowledge of the problem and recall ability.

Stereotyping during the health history interview jeop-ardizes the ability to collect accurate data. False as-sumptions and generalizations about a client may lead the nurse to pursue avenues of questioning that alienate the client and interfere with development of client trust. The mistrustful client is reluctant to divulge sensitive in-formation, perhaps fearing rejection or ridicule, resulting in inaccurate or missed nursing diagnoses.

Similarities among people result in their being grouped. People may be of the same age, sex, or ethnic back-ground, or they may share a common occupation, recre-ational activity, health risk behavior, or health problem. Each person within a group is also an individual who possesses differences that constitute uniqueness. It is valid to identify reliable research findings concerning a group's characteristics or similarities and to apply those findings to a specific client who belongs to that group. For exam-ple, blacks have a higher incidence of hypertension than do whites; regular blood pressure screening should be included at every visit to a health care provider. Generali-zations, particularly those grounded in assumptions or prejudice or based on limited experience, have the poten-tial to be harmful.

Physical appearance or presenting signs and symptoms may bias the nurse's perception of a client. Similar physi-cal manifestations may have different origins. For exam-ple, a nurse might assume that a client with an uneven, lurching gait and garbled speech is intoxicated or under the influence of a controlled substance. In fact, the client could have sustained a head injury in a motor vehicle accident and had a residual neurologic deficit. The nurse's initial inaccurate judgment may be costly in both wasted time and effort and may result in a strained nurse-client relationship. See Box 11–1 for guidelines that may re-duce stereotyping during health assessment.

Computerization has affected the health history assess-ment process in some clinical settings, particularly in am-bulatory care. Computer programs for history taking re-sult in accurate, reliable, and legible data displays when data are entered correctly. Data are recorded directly, by either the client or the nurse, by means of interactive programs. Data also may be entered from a client-com-pleted questionnaire, which is reviewed and validated by a nurse who is skilled in health assessment. Computerized health histories tend to be complete because pertinent

Box 11–1. Guidelines That May Reduce Stereotyping During Health Assessment

- Do not manipulate a client's information to make it congruent with a cultural image.
- Do not assume that a client's reported symptoms all stem from the identified medical diagnosis.
- Do not classify a client based on appearance or behavior.
- Do not ignore any aspect of the client's presentation.

assessment areas are included in the programs. Branching programs direct the nurse to collect additional data when the client responds with significant information.

The Depth of the Health History

Many factors influence the depth or level of assessment. Ideally, all data are collected at one time and in sufficient depth to allow identification of problems. But this may not always be practical. The setting for an interview may be less than ideal (e.g., the scene of a motor vehicle accident). The client's reason for seeking healthcare may preclude in-depth interviewing (e.g., a ruptured appendix). The client's attention span, energy, and comfort level may affect the ability to participate in an interview (e.g., pain). In an acute situation, the nurse collects data perti-nent to the immediate problem and assesses the client's present health status. The nurse tailors the health history interview to include the pertinent data while striving to be thorough. The database is updated and enlarged as indi-cated by the client's condition.

In clinical practice, many agencies provide specific for-mats for collecting the health history. These formats are designed to meet each agency's purposes and may vary considerably in depth and level. The nurse is responsible for tailoring the health history interview based on the needs of the client and the agency. For example, the nurse may arrange to meet several times for brief periods with clients who have limited abilities or special needs (e.g., impaired hearing or limited intellectual capacity). Or an interpreter may be required when a language barrier exists.

The health history model presented in this chapter is an *exhaustive,* or *long* format (Box 11–2). This holistic ap-proach, although time consuming, elicits a wealth of data and allows for thorough assessment of how the client functions within all aspects of the environment. The ex-haustive approach may be impractical in an acute care setting, especially if it is to be done in one sitting. How-ever, to make accurate nursing diagnoses and to identify their causes, the nurse must be knowledgeable about each component of the history. It is therefore important to learn how to collect a complete database, and to gather it over time if necessary. Students often learn history-taking skills in a laboratory setting using the exhaustive model, and they must also learn to modify the technique to an actual setting and a client's ability.

Text continued on page 185

Box 11–2. An Exhaustive Health History Format

Interview date (included as a baseline for later reference)

Biographical and Demographic Data

Full name (include aliases, if applicable)
Age
Sex
Race
Nationality or ethnic background
Primary language
Date and place of birth
Significant others and relationship to client
Home address (and alternate contact address, if applicable)
Phone number(s)
Occupation (usual and current)
Social Security number
Religion
Emergency contact or next of kin
Legal guardian (if necessary)
Source of information and reliability as a historian (note use of an interpreter, if needed)
Source of referral to agency and/or usual primary healthcare provider
Health insurance information
Advance directive information

Physical Health History

Current Symptoms

Reason for seeking healthcare, or chief complaint (recorded in client's own words)
Symptom analysis (in-depth analysis of symptoms):

- Last time client was well (discriminate between onset of symptom and when client became concerned about it)
- Date and time of onset, including time period during which symptom evolved (slow? abrupt?)
- Setting (what was client doing and where was the client when symptom began?)
- How was client feeling before problem's onset?
- Duration or how long symptom lasts (minutes? hours? days? intermittent? constant? goes away completely?)
- Frequency or how often symptom occurs (daily? weekly? monthly?)
- Location (localized? diffuse? radiating?)
- Quality (description) of symptom's characteristics (burning? piercing? stabbing? dull? aching? throbbing?)
- Quantity or severity rated by client using an analog scale such as 1 to 10, with 1 being the least and 10 being the most or worst)
- Does symptom interfere with client's usual daily activities? Do interferences cause problems for the client? What types of problems? (sleeping? eating? activity tolerance?)
- Factors that seem to precipitate (bring on) the symptom
- Factors that seem to worsen (aggravate) the symptom (activity? weather? eating? medication? position? fatigue? time of year or day?)
- Factors that relieve symptom (rest? sleep? medication [name, strength, amount and frequency taken]? heat? cold?)
- Associated factors or symptoms in other body systems that seem concurrent—review the associated body system at this time instead of later

Past Health History

Developmental (may not be appropriate for all adults)

- Any known problems with growth and development including prenatal or birth history (for example, premature delivery or low birth weight) or delay in language, speech, motor skills, etc.?

Immunizations

- Record childhood immunizations and whether kept up to date (tetanus, diphtheria, pertussis, measles, mumps, rubella, chickenpox, polio, *Haemophilus influenzae* b conjugate, hepatitis B)
- Note last dates of tetanus booster and influenza vaccination
- Note if inoculated with pneumococcal vaccination if client age 65 or over, or has a history of chronic illness

Past illnesses (childhood and adulthood)

Ask about measles (rubeola), mumps, rubella, chickenpox (the preceding are often collectively called usual childhood diseases), whooping cough (pertussis), scarlet fever, strep throat, rheumatic fever, poliomyelitis, asthma, tuberculosis, pneumonia, and any sequelae or residual effects

Serious or chronic illnesses

- Note the presence of diabetes mellitus, heart disease, hypertension, kidney problems, ulcers, thyroid problems, migraine headaches, seizure disorders, stroke (cerebral vascular accident), arthritis, Lyme disease, cancer, anemia, sickle cell anemia, bleeding tendencies, or HIV

Hospitalizations

- Date and reason for each admission
- Summary of treatment, length of hospitalization
- Name of primary care physician(s)
- Reaction to these events and their outcomes

Surgeries

- Date and type of procedures performed
- Name of surgeon(s)
- Note if performed on inpatient or outpatient basis
- Client's reaction to each procedure and its outcome

Serious injuries or accidents

- Date and type of injuries or accidents
- Ask specifically about head injuries, fractures, burns, or other trauma
- Note client's reaction to each and their outcomes

Obstetric history (if applicable)

- For completed pregnancies: number; course of each pregnancy, labor, delivery, and postpartum period; delivery date; birthweight, sex, and infant's health
- For incomplete pregnancies: number; duration of pregnancy; date and circumstances of termination (spontaneous or induced abortion, stillbirth)
- Complications (describe)

Box continued on following page

Box 11–2. An Exhaustive Health History Format (Continued)

Last visit(s) to healthcare providers

▪ Record most recent dates for dental, physical, vision, and hearing examinations. Identify provider if different from primary care provider

▪ Date and results of screening or diagnostic tests performed such as electrocardiogram (ECG), radiology studies, laboratory tests, Papanicolaou (Pap) smear, purified protein derivative (PPD) or tuberculosis tine test

Allergies

▪ Description of allergens and reactions (rash, urticaria, pruritus, watery or itching eyes, nasal congestion, running nose, breathing difficulty including asthma, pulse irregularity, convulsions, collapse)

▪ Include medications (true allergic reactions only and not side effects), food, contact agents (fabric, nickel), and environmental agents (dust, dander, pollens, cigarette smoke)

Medications currently taken including prescriptive, nonprescriptive over-the-counter, and recreational (street) drug use

▪ Ask about common over-the-counter medications by name (such as aspirin, vitamins, antacids, birth control pills, cold and allergy preparations, topical creams and lotions—many people do not think of these as medications)

▪ For all medications ask for: name; dose; route; frequency and time of day taken; reason for taking; are there problems with taking; who prescribed each drug and when

Family Health History

▪ Include members' ages, cause of death, and age at death

▪ Ask specifically about heart disease, hypertension (high blood pressure), cerebral vascular accidents (stroke), epilepsy (seizures), migraines or headaches, mental illness, Alzheimer's disease, Huntington's chorea, alcoholism, tuberculosis, asthma, allergies, diabetes mellitus, thyroid problems, eating disorders (overeating, undereating, self-induced vomiting), obesity, kidney disease, arthritis, cancer (type), sickle cell anemia, anemia, hemophilia, HIV, developmental delay

▪ Data may be displayed in a diagram of the family tree (see Fig. 11–1 later in this chapter)

Psychosocial History

Explore history of psychosocial problems

▪ Personal history
▪ Family history

Assess psychologic components

▪ General appearance

Dress
Hygiene and grooming
Posture
Motor activity
Facial expression

▪ Behavior

Verbal
Nonverbal
Reaction to interview

▪ Recent level of stress

Current perceived level of stress
Adjustment to past stressors
Signs of response to stress
Usual coping pattern

▪ Mental status and level of understanding

Level of consciousness
Orientation
Mood and affect
Speech and communication (language)
Thought process and content
Attention span
Memory
General fund of knowledge
Calculation ability
Ability to reason and think abstractly
Perception
Judgment
Insight

▪ Personality style
▪ Motivation
▪ Personal strengths
▪ Values and beliefs

Self-concept, self-esteem
Body image
Locus of control

▪ Spirituality
▪ Psychosocial risk factors (including coping ability, suicidal ideation)

Assess sociologic components

▪ Psychosocial level of development
▪ Social network and support systems (including pets)
▪ Socioeconomic status
▪ Life-style (including habits, recent travel within and outside of country)
▪ Sexuality

Assess cultural components (see Table 11–1 later in this chapter)

Review of Systems

General

Do the following symptoms occur? fever, chills, sweats, night sweats, weakness, weight loss or gain (in past 6 months), fatigue, malaise, nausea or vomiting, headaches, mood changes?

Nutrition

Describe the kinds of food usually eaten including likes and dislikes. Describe everything eaten during the last 24 hours. How much of each food was eaten? Is the client on a special type of diet such as avoiding salt, sugar, fats, or caffeine? Does the client take vitamin or mineral pills, or anything else believed necessary in the diet? Does the client have an appetite? Has it changed recently (describe)? Has the client ever had an eating problem or disorder such as anorexia or bulimia nervosa (describe)? What is the client's usual weight? Does the weight vary (ask client to describe

Box 11–2. An Exhaustive Health History Format (*Continued*)

his or her maximum and minimum weights)? Has the client gained or lost weight recently (how much weight? over how long a time period did this happen?)? Who does the food shopping in the household? Who usually prepares meals? Does the client usually have someone to share meals with? Does the person who plans and prepares food use a system such as the food guide pyramid? Does food have a special meaning for the client? Are there foods that the client looks forward to eating on special occasions (such as a religious holiday)? Are there any foods that cannot be eaten because of allergies or for other reasons? Are there any problems with following a special diet (describe)? Are there any problems with being able to swallow or chew food (describe)?

Integument

■ Skin

Inquire about past skin problems (e.g., scars; birthmarks; moles; burns). Ask if the following problems occur: dryness; pruritus (itching); rashes or other skin eruptions; odor; a change in skin color, texture, or temperature; a change in any skin lesion; growths; a sore that does not heal; easy bruising; psoriasis; eczema. Has the client had any skin lesions removed (describe)? Does the client have any tattoos or pierced body parts? Ask the client to describe his or her skin care habits (e.g., use of soap, lotions, skin oils, etc.) that may affect skin texture and moisture. How much sun exposure has the client had (e.g., sunbathing, tanning salon, severe sunburns)?

■ Hair

Are there any problems with alopecia (hair loss), dryness, brittleness, or dandruff? Does the client use hair dyes or have a permanent wave? Ask the client to describe his or her hair care habits (frequency of shampooing, use of conditioner, combing versus brushing, etc.) that may affect hair texture.

■ Nails

Are there any problems with brittleness, cracking, or splitting? Has there been a change in nail texture? Does the client bite his or her nails? Does the client wear nail polish? Have artificial nails?

Hematopoietic

Are there any problems with fatigue, unusual bleeding, easy bruising, ecchymoses (bruises), anemia, or leukemia? Has the client ever been exposed to radiation or toxic agents (describe)? Has the client ever had a transfusion of blood or a blood product (were there any problems?)? Does the client know his or her blood type (if Rh negative and has been pregnant, does the woman recall receiving *RHoGAM*)? Does the client know if he or she has any unusual type of antibodies (describe)?

Endocrine

Have there been past problems with diabetes, goiter or thyroid, or growth and development? Has the client ever been treated with hormones (describe)? Has the client ever had

neck surgery (describe)? Are there problems with: polydipsia, polyuria, or polyphagia (increased thirst, urination, or hunger); heat or cold intolerance; weakness; tremors; nervousness; dry skin or hair; excessive sweating; change in hair distribution or hirsutism (excess hair growth in unusual places); impotence or a change in sexual activity or libido?

Head

Has the client ever had a blow, trauma, or injury to the head? Ask about problems with headaches (unusual or severe), dizziness or lightheadedness, syncope (fainting or loss of consciousness), vertigo, seizures

Eyes

Has the client had past problems with eye infections (conjunctivitis or pink eye), chalazion (eyelid cyst), hordeolum (stye), glaucoma, cataracts, amblyopia (lazy eye), detached retina, or strabismus? Has the client ever received a blow to the eye? Has the client ever had eye surgery (describe)? Does the client wear an eye prosthesis (ask the client to describe how he or she cares for it)? Are there problems with a change in vision (either in general or in part of the visual field, or in night vision), failing vision or blindness, blurred vision, diplopia (double vision), spots or floaters, redness, pain, itching, lacrimation (excess tearing), dryness, discharge or drainage, swelling around the eyes, unusual sensations or twitching, photophobia (light sensitivity)? Is there difficulty reading or seeing distant objects? Do vision problems interfere with daily activities? Does the client wear eyeglasses or contact lenses (when was the last prescription change)? When was the last eye examination (results)? Last glaucoma check (results)?

Ears

Inquire about past problems with ear infections or earaches; diminution or loss of hearing. Are there problems with difficulty hearing; deafness; increased sensitivity to sound; tinnitus (ringing), crackling, buzzing, or other sounds in the ears; feeling of fullness in the ear; ear pain; discharge or drainage (describe); vertigo? Does the client have problems with excess cerumen (ear wax)? Ask how the client cleans his or her ears (is a cotton-tipped swab, hairpin, or other sharp, foreign object used that may damage the ear canal or tympanic membrane?). Does the client wear a hearing aid? When was the last ear and hearing examination performed (results)?

Nose and Sinuses

Ask if there is a history of frequent colds, sinus infections, nasal stuffiness, allergies, hay fever, or nasal trauma or fracture. Are there current problems with sneezing, postnasal drip, rhinitis (runny nose), difficulty breathing through the nose, pain over the sinuses, or epistaxis (nosebleed)? Has there been a change in the sense of smell? Does the client use a nasal spray or other cold, allergy, or sinus medication (type, amount, frequency)?

Mouth and Pharynx

Does the client have a history of sore throats or oral infection such as strep throat, herpes (cold sores), or *Candida*

Box continued on following page

Box 11–2. An Exhaustive Health History Format (*Continued*)

(thrush)? Are there problems with: mouth or tongue lesions (sore, abscess, ulcer); bleeding gums; increased saliva or dry mouth; mouth pain; sore throat; hoarseness or voice change; difficulty chewing or swallowing (dysphagia); change in taste; halitosis? Does the client use tobacco products (describe type, amount, frequency, and current use patterns)? Does the client have any dentures or bridges (do they fit well? are they worn most of the time?)? Ask the client to describe his or her dental hygiene practices (brushing, flossing, use of fluoride dentifrice). Has the client ever had oral or dental surgery (describe)? When was the last dental examination and the results (if known)? Were x-rays taken at that time?

Neck

Have there been past problems with neck injury, goiter, pain, limited movement, or swollen glands? Does the client currently have stiffness, tenderness, pain, swelling, or lumps in the neck?

Breasts and Axillae

Ask the client about a history of fibrocystic breast disease and cancer of the breast (is there a family history of breast cancer?). If the client is a woman with children, ask if she breast fed her infants. Are there current problems with breast pain, tenderness, or swelling; gynecomastia (enlargement); pruritus (itching); nipple discharge; breast lumps; dimpling or change in breast skin texture or color; change in appearance of the nipples? Does the client perform breast self-examination (if so, ask for a description of when it is done and the technique used)? If the client is a woman, has she had mammograms (when? results, if known? how often done)? Does the client take any estrogen (e.g., birth control) or corticosteroid medications (describe)? Is there a history of breast surgery (describe)?

Lungs

Inquire about a past history of breathing problems such as asthma, emphysema, wheezing, pleurisy, pneumonia, or bronchitis. Has the client ever had tuberculosis (describe any treatment received) or whooping cough? Has the client smoked or used tobacco products (describe type, amount, length of time used, attempts to stop)? If a former smoker, ask how long it has been since the client quit. Current problems include: chronic cough, sputum production (describe), hemoptysis (blood in sputum), night sweats, dyspnea (shortness of breath) with or without exertion, ability to tolerate exercise or activities of daily living without becoming short of breath, orthopnea (difficulty breathing without elevating the head when supine), pain with breathing; cyanosis (blue-tinged nail beds or lips). Has the client ever had a chest x-ray (results)? Has the client ever had a skin test for tuberculosis (results)?

Heart

Ask the client about a history of rheumatic fever, congenital heart problems, heart murmur, myocardial infarction, coronary artery disease, cardiac surgery, hypertension, or thyroid problems. Is there a family history of hypertension or myocardial infarction before age 50? Are there current problems

with: chest discomfort or pain, syncope, vertigo, palpitations, paroxysmal nocturnal dyspnea (PND [sudden awakening at night with difficulty breathing]), dyspnea on exertion (DOE), orthopnea, sudden weight gain, edema of hands or feet, hyperlipidemia or hypercholesteremia? Has the client ever had any cardiac tests, such as an electrocardiogram (ECG), stress ECG, coronary angiograms, echocardiogram, or electrophysiologic studies (results)?

Peripheral Vascular

Has the client had previous problems with varicose veins, diabetes, hypertension, pain in the extremities, injury to an extremity (describe), or edema of the hands or feet? Are there problems with lymph node swelling or tenderness, claudication (pain in legs with walking relieved by resting), numbness or coldness of an extremity, discoloration or ulceration on extremities (especially feet and ankles), hair loss over an extremity; nail changes? Has the client ever had any vascular tests, such as Doppler studies (results)? Ask what type of hose the client wears (e.g., support hose). Does the client use garters or other means of securing the hose? Does the client spend prolonged periods of time standing?

Gastrointestinal

Inquire about a history of ulcers, indigestion, heartburn, hernia, liver disease, hepatitis (type if known), gallbladder disease, pancreatic disease, appendicitis, and use of alcohol. Is there a family history of alcohol abuse or cancer of the stomach, liver, pancreas, intestines, or colorectal area? Ask the client to describe the usual bowel pattern and characteristics. Are there problems with: weight loss or gain, a change in appetite or taste, food intolerance, belching, nausea or vomiting, hematemesis (blood in emesis), pain or indigestion with eating, difficulty swallowing, diarrhea or constipation, bowel incontinence, flatulence (excess gas), changes in bowel habits or stool characteristics (e.g., clay-colored or blood in stool, ribbon-like stools), hemorrhoids (is there any pain or bleeding especially with defecation), rectal pain or itching, pain in the abdomen, ascites (swelling of the abdomen) or jaundice? Does the client use digestive aids, laxatives, enemas, or suppositories (describe)? Has the client had tests of the gastrointestinal (GI) system, such as a barium swallow, upper GI series, barium enema, sigmoidoscopy or colonoscopy, Hemoccult test, gallbladder x-rays or ultrasound, or liver scan (results)?

Urinary

Does the client have a history of bladder infection, kidney problems, urinary tract stones, or sexually transmitted disease (STD)? Is there a family history of renal disease? Ask if there are current problems with: a change in the urinary patterns, hesitancy, frequency, dysuria (pain), pyuria (pus in the urine), urgency, weak stream, dribbling or incontinence, stress incontinence, nocturia, polyuria or oliguria (increased or decreased amount of urine), flank or low back pain, a change in the color of the urine, foam in the urine (proteinuria), or discharge from the urethra? Has the client ever had tests of the urinary system such as urinalysis, cystoscopy, or intravenous pyelogram (results)?

Box 11–2. An Exhaustive Health History Format *(Continued)*

Genitoreproductive

■ General

Is there a history of genital lesions, sores, or ulcers; urethral discharge; odor; pain, burning, or pruritus; STDs (identify); infertility; problems with sexual performance? Has the client ever had surgery involving the genitoreproductive system (describe)? Does the client use a contraceptive (type)? Is he or she satisfied with the type used or is a change desired? Is the client knowledgeable about STD preventive practices or is information wanted?

■ Female

Ask about a history of pelvic inflammatory disease, endometriosis, or abnormal Pap test results. Is there a personal or family history of reproductive cancer (e.g., cervix, uterus, ovary, breast)? Review the menstrual cycle history for age at menarche and menopause (if applicable), duration and amount of menstrual flow, and last menstrual period (LMP). Are there problems with: premenstrual bloating, weight gain, fatigue, or mood changes; irregular menstrual periods; menorrhagia (excessive menses); dysmenorrhea (painful menses); amenorrhea (absence of menses); metrorrhagia (bleeding other than with menses); dyspareunia (painful intercourse); postcoital pain or bleeding? Ask when the woman's last pelvic examination and Pap test were done (results).

■ Male

Inquire about a history of inguinal hernia, prostate problems, or impotence. Is there a family history of reproductive cancer (e.g., penis, testis, prostate)? Does the man have current problems with testicular pain or mass, or blood in the ejaculate? Ask when the man's last examination was, including checking the prostate and for hernia (results?). Does the man know how to perform testicular self-examination (how often?)? Has the man had a prostate specific antigen (PSA) test (results)?

Musculoskeletal

Ask about past problems with sprains, strains, fractures, dislocations, arthritis, gout, backache, bursitis, osteomyelitis, scoliosis, or flat feet. Is there a family history of arthritis, gout, or muscular dystrophy? Are there current problems with: muscle twitches, cramps, spasms, involuntary movements, pain, or weakness; muscle atrophy; joint pain, stiffness, swelling, redness, deformity, or limited movement; crepitation (noise or grating with joint movement); backache; spinal deformity; limitation in walking, gait, running, sports activities, or activities of daily living? Has the client ever had tests involving the musculoskeletal system such as skeletal x-rays or electromyography (results)?

Neurologic

Is there a history of loss of consciousness, fainting, seizures, paralysis, paresthesia (numbness or tingling), trauma to the nervous system, cerebral vascular accident (CVA)? Is there a family history of CVA, seizures, or neurologic disease such as Huntington's chorea? Are there current problems with: vertigo, syncope, paresthesia, paralysis, headache, loss of balance, seizures, uncoordinated or involuntary movements (e.g., tics, tremors, spasms, clumsiness), speech problems, memory problems (short or long term)? Are there interferences with the activities of daily living from neurologic problems (describe)? Has the client ever had neurologic tests, such as electroencephalography, lumbar puncture, or computed tomography of the head (results)?

Psychiatric

Ask about a history of depression, bipolar disease, schizophrenia, obsessive-compulsive tendency (does it interfere with the client's activities of daily living?); sleeping problems; eating disorders (e.g., anorexia or bulimia nervosa); memory problems; or anxiety attacks. Is there a family history of mental health problems, such as depression, bipolar disease, or schizophrenia? Has the client ever been treated for mental or emotional health problems or taken psychotropic substances (describe)? Is there a history of suicide attempts? Does the client currently have problems with: mood swings; sleeping problems, such as insomnia; anxiety, especially that interferes with activities of daily living; nervousness; increased or decreased appetite; memory lapses; inability to concentrate; change in energy level or inability to complete tasks; phobias; delusions; hallucinations? Has there been a change in relationships with significant others recently (describe)? Has there been a change in living arrangements or housing recently (describe)? Has there been a change in jobs recently (describe)?

Episodic health history assessment often suffices when a client presents with an uncomplicated, short-term health problem, such as an earache. The nurse uses a systematic approach to collect data significant to the problem (Box 11–3). Proficiency in all areas of health history assessment, which are discussed in this chapter, is necessary to conduct an accurate episodic assessment.

Guidelines for the Health History Interview

The health history interview process is affected by external (environmental and interpersonal) and internal (intrapersonal and physiologic) factors. The quality and quantity of data elicited are enhanced by the nurse's sensitivity to the client and skill level with the interview process. The following guidelines are meant to assist in conducting a health history interview.

Preparation of the Environment

When possible, the interview takes place with the client in a comfortable position and setting. A quiet room with a door that closes decreases interruptions. If the client cannot leave a setting that is not private (e.g., a multibed room or an emergency room cubicle), screen the area by

---

Box 11–3. An Episodic Health History Format

Include these elements in an episodic health history:

- Client's statement of the problem (i.e., chief complaint)
- Symptom analysis
- Review of the body system to which the symptom belongs
- Exploration of the symptom's relationship to other body systems (including a review of the associated body systems)
- Investigation of the current problem's relationship to the client's past health and health maintenance and promotion practices

---

drawing the privacy drapes. Reduce or eliminate distractions (e.g., turn off the television) and inform colleagues to avoid interruptions. Use of comfortable chairs that face each other helps establish rapport. Adjust their distance to the client's preference and sense of personal space. A moderate room temperature promotes comfort. Indirect lighting avoids glare and strong shadows that may distort the nurse's observation of the client's nonverbal cues.

Preparation of the Client

After introductions, explain the nature and purpose of the health history interview to the client. Speak in a moderate tone of voice, calmly and patiently. Nonprobing, client-centered questions and remarks help put the client at ease. As the interview progresses, use more focused questions and therapeutic communication techniques to assist the client to identify problem areas. The interview technique varies between open-ended and closed questions, depending on the nature of the data being elicited. Throughout the interview, observe the client's nonverbal communication for signs of discomfort with topics under discussion. These areas may need gentle, further exploration (with the client's permission), either during the interview or at a later time. Respect the client's wishes to decline to discuss a topic. Be aware of your own interview style and skills. An interviewer's nonverbal behavior can either facilitate or inhibit a client's responses and affect the quality of the health history data.

Preparation of the Interviewer

To reduce repetitious questioning, the interview proceeds in a structured yet flexible manner. Until the nurse is comfortable with the interview format, a pocket-sized outline of the health history may be used as an aid. The nurse may take *brief* notes during the interview; if this will be done, the client is informed in advance so as not to disrupt the flow of the interview. Extensive note taking is discouraged because it suggests that the nurse is not listening attentively. The written history is compiled after the interview is completed. Terminate the interview by

summarizing highlights and allowing the client to add or clarify information. Inform the client about how the physical examination will proceed.

Components of the Health History

The health history includes the client's subjective data regarding (1) biographic and demographic information, (2) a review of the client's physical health history including the review of systems (ROS), (3) family health history, (4) psychosocial assessment, and (5) appraisal of the client's health maintenance and health promotion behaviors to assess health risks.

Sometimes a health history assessment is organized according to a nursing theory (e.g., Orem's theory of self-care) or by health behavior patterns (e.g., Gordon's functional health patterns). The format is a tool that the nurse uses to collect comprehensive data. In this chapter the health history format is an extended health database model (see Box 11–2). A health history format that integrates the assessment of functional health patterns is found in Appendix B.

If data are available in other forms, the nurse may compile them, thereby enhancing and expediting the interview. A single complete database is preferable for reference and retrieval of information.

Biographical and Demographic Information

The extent and type of information recorded in the biographical and demographic data vary, depending on the specific healthcare agency's protocol. Data include the client's full name, address and telephone number, an emergency contact person or next of kin, date and place of birth, age, sex, race, ethnic and cultural background, primary language spoken, religious preference, marital status, occupation, Social Security number, legal guardian (if necessary), type of health insurance coverage and policy number, name of primary health care provider, source of referral to the agency, source and reliability of the history information (note use of an interpreter), existence of an advance directive, and date of the health history interview (see Box 11–2).

The date of the health history interview is noted because the information constitutes the client's baseline assessment. Should the client's health status change, the health history and physical examination will reflect the extent of the change over time.

Biographical and demographic data provide clues about personal health risk. For example, some health risk may be ascribed to the client's age, sex, family history, and location of residence. Various health screening procedures are performed or recommended on the basis of the client's age, sex, or other background data. Examples of recommended procedures include periodic pelvic examinations and monthly breast self-examinations for women, periodic prostate examinations and monthly testicular self-examinations for men, and regular screening of visual acuity and testing for glaucoma as a person ages.

Physical Health History

Physical health history is integrated throughout the health history. It includes the client's current and past health status and portions of the psychosocial history and health risk assessment. In addition, the nurse conducts a head-to-toe review of body systems.

Current Symptoms

■ Chief Complaint

The physical health history begins with the client's subjective statement of the reason for seeking healthcare (also called the *chief complaint*). The response may indicate possible concerns or anxiety on the part of the client or significant others and may reveal the client's perception of the present health problem. The client may provide information about what the problem means and how he or she is coping. Allowing the client to elaborate perceptions can assist the nurse in avoiding generalizations. When the client reports a health problem, either past or current, the nurse proceeds with a *symptom analysis* (see Box 11–2).

■ Symptom Analysis

Symptom analysis is the client's description of the health problem's characteristics. Areas included are: timing, location, quality, quantity, precipitating factors, aggravating or relieving factors, and associated manifestations. In addition, the nurse asks the client to provide an opinion about the cause of the symptom or problem. Clients often have insight as to the nature and the cause of their problems, and they sometimes express fears and concerns while discussing health problems. These fears and concerns are explored to diagnose and treat clients' responses to health problems.

Timing. Description of a symptom's timing includes onset, duration, and frequency. *Onset* refers to when a symptom was first noticed (e.g., hours, days, months). *Duration* is how long the symptom lasts (e.g., minutes, hours, days, weeks). The symptom may occur continuously, intermittently, regularly, or irregularly. *Frequency* refers to how often a symptom occurs (e.g., every morning, once a week, every month).

Quality. The nurse assists the client to discriminate the quality of a symptom by using adjectives such as sharp, stabbing, dull, aching, cramping, cold, searing, burning, numb, tingling, loose, solid, soft, hard, tight, crushing.

Quantity. The nurse assists the client to describe the size, amount, number, or extent of the symptom or symptoms as well as the severity or intensity. Severity of pain is quantified by asking the client to rate the symptom on a scale, such as 1 to 5 or 1 to 10. The extent of a

symptom's effect is assessed by asking the client to describe how the symptom has altered usual daily activities. For example, "Describe how the pain has interfered with what you usually do during the day. Does it keep you awake at night?" "Has it affected your appetite?"

Location. The nurse asks the client to show where a symptom, such as pain, is located on the body, and whether it moves or is stationary. For example, "Does the pain stay in one place or does it move to another part of your body?" Asking the client to point helps define a symptom's location.

Precipitating Factors. The nurse asks what the client was doing at the time the symptom was first noticed. Does the client know what may have led to the symptom's occurrence?

Aggravating and Relieving Factors. The client is asked to recall whether any factors alleviate the symptom or make it worse. For example, "Is there anything that makes the symptom go away or be less uncomfortable?" "Is there anything that makes the symptom get worse?"

Associated Manifestations. The nurse inquires specifically whether the client has noticed anything that happens in conjunction with the symptom. For example, "Does the symptom ever occur at other times or only when _____?"

When the client reports a symptom, the nurse assesses all of the physiologic areas associated with the symptom or problem. For example, a client who reports epigastric pain will have a review of gastrointestinal, endocrine, and psychological systems. The epigastric pain may be related to problems in any of these body systems. If the client reports a symptom such as urinary incontinence, the symptom analysis includes timing, quality (e.g., are incontinent episodes accompanied by dysuria?), quantity (e.g., amount of urine leakage per occurrence, effect of episodes on daily activities), precipitating factors (e.g., obesity, pregnancy, vaginal delivery), aggravating factors (e.g., coughing, sneezing, straining, lifting, caffeine intake), relieving factors (e.g., frequent toileting, medication, pelvic muscle toning exercises), and associated manifestations (e.g., urgency, urinary retention, constipation). Location does not apply in this example. The review of body systems (see discussion later in this chapter) should include the urinary (renal), reproductive, and gastrointestinal systems as well as a careful diet history.

Past Health History

A client's past health history may be significant for both current and future health risk status. For example, the client who has not had chickenpox during childhood may be at risk for it when a community outbreak occurs, or when exposed to someone who has herpes zoster (shingles). The nurse should further assess the client's risk status and provide information about the varicella vaccination. Box 11–2 lists the data to assess for the past health history. Throughout this part of the health history interview, be alert for areas to explore.

Family Health History

The purpose of the family health history is to identify familially linked diseases that affect the client's health status and risk of potential health problems. The nurse inquires about family members' relationship to the client, their age (if currently living), the age at which they died and the cause of death (if known), and the presence of significant illnesses or health problems. The data may be displayed in a diagram (Fig. 11–1) that serves as a visual display to assist tracking the client's health risk status. A summary statement includes health problems that exist in the family. Box 11–2 lists the health problems that are of most importance in the family health history.

Psychosocial History

Psychosocial assessment is an important part of the health history. A complete psychosocial assessment, although lengthy, is essential to a client-centered approach. Psychosocial assessment is integrated throughout the history interview as the nurse gathers both subjective and objective data. If extensive assessment is indicated, the nurse may opt to pursue this following the assessment of the physical health history, after rapport has been established. Psy-

chosocial assessment also may come earlier (see Box 11–2), following the family health history.

Psychological status affects multiple areas vital to human development and behavior, such as intellectual development and capability, motivation, perception and insight, decision making, speech and communication, motor ability, sleep and rest patterns, and nutrition and elimination patterns. It is impossible to separate a human being into discrete components. Multiple dimensions that include the psychological, sociologic, and physiologic interact and affect the individual's behavior and responses to the environment. Interrelationships among the dimensions are neither static nor always predictable. Human physiologic responses to health problems are usually more predictable and are objectively observed, whereas two individuals faced with identical problems may not react the same way emotionally. For this reason, psychosocial assessment may be less reliable than objective assessment of physical findings. However, it is possible for the nurse to develop skill and expertise in psychosocial assessment by collecting both subjective and objective data.

Psychosocial assessment assists in understanding a client's response to circumstances and events, which in turn influences the client's ability to function. This understanding enables the nurse to provide comprehensive care to clients and their significant others based on accurate nursing diagnoses. Approximately two thirds of the disorders that nurses independently diagnose and treat are psychosocial. When applied to the medical-surgical client, accurate assessment of the client's responses to physical

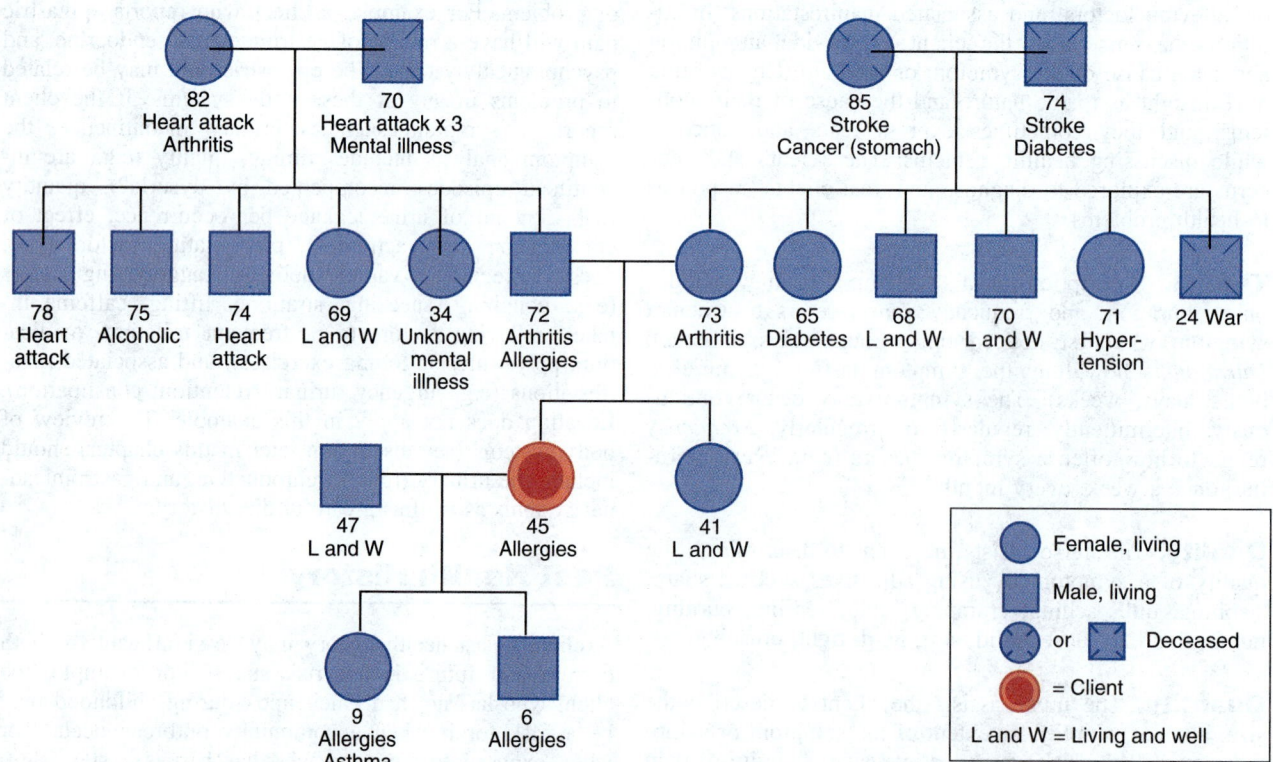

Figure 11–1. Family history diagram. A diagram such as this one assists in determining a client's risk for various disorders. This woman has an increased inherited risk of cardiovascular disease (heart attack and stroke) and arthritis.

health problems is used to help the client return to an optimal level of function, both physiologic and psychological.

Psychosocial assessment requires sensitivity and interpersonal skills. The nurse's ability to establish a therapeutic relationship directly affects the quality and usefulness of the data collected. Because many of the topics in a psychosocial assessment are of a highly personal nature, it is imperative that you be tactful and nonjudgmental and handle confidential information in a professional manner (see Ethical Issues in Nursing). An atmosphere of trust between the client and nurse encourages the client to feel free to divulge sensitive information. The nurse conveys interest to the client by listening attentively, making eye contact, and using skillful interview techniques. The nurse's personal value system may influence or bias perception of a client's behavior and experiences. Self-awareness helps the nurse to be nonjudgmental. Free from bias, the nurse is likely to establish a trusting relationship with the client and to receive relevant information. The nurse's ability to make accurate observations and to share them with the client allows the client opportunity to validate the nurse's perceptions and inferences.

The Nature of the Psychosocial Assessment

Psychosocial assessment encompasses gathering information about a client's psychological patterns and social experiences. *Psychological patterns* are the nonphysical components of a client, such as thoughts, feelings, motivations, mental status, personal strengths, and weaknesses. *Social experiences* are the parts of a client's life that are affected by or dependent on others. The term *"psychosocial"* denotes the melding of the two dimensions because it is impossible to separate the effects of psychological factors from those of social factors. Similarly, the psychosocial dimension intertwines with the physiologic dimension. All dimensions interact to produce a unique individual.

Psychosocial Risk Factors

During the healthy history interview, you will assess for factors that indicate that the client is at risk for or has a psychosocial problem. See Box 11–4 for guidelines for identifying psychosocial risk factors. If risk factors are present, you will proceed with a detailed psychosocial assessment. Table 11–1 is an interview guide that you may use for in-depth assessment of selected areas of a client's psychosocial status. Included in Table 11–1 are examples of questions that you may ask during a cultural assessment.

Psychological Assessment

The psychological dimension includes the client's perceptions about mood, thoughts, feelings, motivations, stressors, personal strengths and weaknesses, values and beliefs, and spirituality. The client's responses

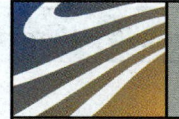

ETHICAL ISSUES IN NURSING

What Should Nurses Do with Confidential Information?

What should nurses do with confidential information? The information gained through client interviews and assessments forms the basis for the plan of care. In order for a person to feel comfortable in verbalizing personal information, a sense of trust must be reached. This sense of trust may take a while to establish (over several office visits, days in the hospital, or home visits). Because of this, it is important that communication between healthcare providers and their clients be as open and nonthreatening as possible. The healthcare provider must be astute to verbal and nonverbal information. Client information, as a rule, should remain confidential, just as the medical record is confidential.

What happens when confidential and perhaps sensitive information discloses situations that place confidentiality in an ethical dilemma? For example, a dilemma occurs when a client comes in for treatment of a sexually transmitted disease (STD) and does not want the spouse informed because the client has engaged in an extramarital affair. On one hand, confidentiality should be protected. On the other hand, perhaps the spouse needs to be examined for possible STD infection as well. Another example centers around information gained from a client regarding illegal drug use. What obligation do healthcare providers have in keeping illegal activities confidential?

Issues of confidentiality can place the nurse in some very sensitive positions. When the client reveals information of illegal practices or practices that may be harmful to others, the nurse must decide what action to take. A client's right of confidentiality should always be respected, but when such confidentiality places a nurse in a legal dilemma, the nurse must inform the client that a dilemma exists and that he or she must report the information. Clients do have a right to confidentiality, but they do not have the right to involve nurses in legal dilemmas. It is the nonlegal dilemmas, such as the STD example given above, that place nurses in uncomfortable positions. In these situations, the nurse may respect confidentiality by simply referring inquiries about the client back to the client and/or physician. The nurse may also help clients understand the possible consequences that the confidential information may have for themselves and others.

interpretations are reflected in his or her thought processes and in what is said and done. The nurse observes the client's appearance and behavior throughout the health history interview. Observations, when validated by the client, assist the nurse in understanding the client's psychological status. Data are recorded both in the health history (subjective) and physical examination report (objective).

Box 11–4. Guidelines for Identifying Psychosocial Risk Factors

Social History

Social history includes information about the client's family members, social network, and life-style. Ask if others are available to provide emotional support to the client during stressful times. This support system may include pets.

Personal and Family History

A personal or family history of psychosocial problems increases a client's risk of having problems. A client may fear recurrence of an emotional or mental health problem or worry that he or she has inherited a family-linked illness, such as schizophrenia.

Level of Stress

Change and loss are two major influences that produce stress in individuals. Clients who have experienced stressful events within the past year are at risk for developing health problems. Assess the client's present stress level compared to his or her response to previous stressful events.

Usual Coping Pattern

The usual coping pattern refers to how the client copes with a serious problem or manages high levels of stress. Ask the client to describe a particularly stressful situation and how it was managed. Assess whether the client's usual coping style is adequate and appropriate for the current situation. Other coping strategies may be necessary. Psychosocial reactions to health problems are highly individual and usually occur as the client and significant others cope with the effects of illness.

Changes in Neurophysiologic Function

Neurophysiologic changes include physical manifestations of psychological stress. The stress response, regardless of its cause, results in altered neurotransmitter levels, such as norepinephrine and serotonin, which then affect the sympathetic and parasympathetic nervous systems (see Chapter 2). The client's usual body functions, such as sleep and rest patterns, appetite, energy level, sexual function, and elimination patterns, can be affected.

Level of Understanding about Health Problem

Explore the client's level of understanding. The client may not comprehend what has happened or could happen as a result of a health problem. The client may have unrealistic expectations of the healthcare team. The nurse determines how threatening a particular health problem is and whether the client has been able to prepare psychologically for its effects.

Mental Status

Mental status refers to the client's current emotional, intellectual, and perceptual functioning. If a dysfunction is evidenced, describe the problem.

Personality Style

Personality style is the way a client usually interacts with others. Examples include dependent, independent, controlled, relaxed, dramatic, suspicious, accepting, self-sacrificing, superior, inferior, uninvolved, involved, mixed (a combination of two predominant styles), or no predominant style.

Major Psychosocial Reactions

Reactions include disruption in the ability to trust, maintain self-esteem, retain feelings of control, cope with loss and guilt, and maintain intimacy.

General Appearance. Appearance and behavior reflect the client's mental status and comfort level with the interview process. The nurse observes the client's posture, nonverbal behavior, facial expression, manner of dress with regard to the climate and occasion, grooming and hygiene, and attitude toward the assessment interview (e.g., cooperative, hostile, withdrawn). For example, "The client is dressed neatly, sits back in the chair, and answers questions without hesitation."

Motor Activity. The client's motor ability, gait, coordination, reaction time, unusual body movements (e.g., gestures, tics, tremors, foot tapping, hand wringing, grimacing, or other repetitive movements) are noted. For example, "The client drummed his fingers on the table before answering."

Behavior. The client's activities that are observed by others constitute behavior. Behavior is verbal or nonverbal. *Verbal behavior* is what the client says and includes voice tone. *Nonverbal behavior* is everything the client does that may be observed, such as posture, movement, and facial expression. The nurse observes and records both verbal and nonverbal behavior.

The client's behavior is central to psychological assessment. Accurate assessment dictates that the nurse describe observed behavior rather than interpret it. "The client is crying" is an observed behavior, whereas "The client is depressed" is a judgmental statement. Without further assessment, the nurse does not know why the client is crying. If the client tells the nurse, "I feel depressed," then the recorded statement reads, "States she feels depressed."

Mental Status. Mental status assessment consists of evaluating the client's behavior (verbal and nonverbal) and asking the client a series of questions. The purpose is to discover any problems that may require further assessment and intervention. The level and depth of questioning will vary depending on the client and the individual circumstances. The nurse can assess a client who is alert and cooperative adequately by listening and observing carefully during the health history interview. The client's responses provide information about orienta-

Text continued on page 194

Table 11–1. Interview Guide for Assessment of Selected Areas of a Client's Psychosocial Status

Assessment Area	Key Questions or Issues to Include*
Values and beliefs	What things in your life are important to you and help you want to live each day (e.g., health; respect for others; happiness; loving relationships with significant others; time to spend with your loved ones; friendships; religious beliefs; financial security; having a job or work to do)?
	How important is your health to you? to your family or significant others? (Ask person to rate importance on a scale of 1 to 10, with 10 being of most importance and 1 being of least.)
	What do you hope to accomplish in your lifetime (e.g., rear children successfully; become rich or famous; have a satisfying job or career)?
	Have you accomplished what you set out to do in your life? Are you satisfied/dissatisfied?
	If you were to come into a lot of money (win a lottery, receive an inheritance), what would you do with it?
	Do specific factors influence you when you have to make important decisions (e.g., being fair/honest; getting a fair deal; examining all sides of the issue)?
	Have any of your beliefs or values been challenged recently? Are you uncomfortable that this has happened?
	Have you changed any of your values or beliefs recently? Has this change put a strain on your relationship with significant others? Are you comfortable with the change?
Self-concept, self-esteem, body image	Describe yourself as you believe others see you and as you see yourself (e.g., emotional health; usual mood and what affects it; ability to cope with daily stressors; physical appearance; stamina; intelligence)
	Describe your major strengths and areas that you would like to improve
	What do you like about yourself? What do you wish you could change about yourself?
	Has anything happened recently to change your feelings about yourself (e.g., change in health status or physical agility; a loss of some kind; a role change)? Do you feel more positive or negative about yourself because of this change?
	Describe how you feel when you become ill or in some way incapacitated and are unable to carry on your daily activities.
Locus of control	Do you feel that you can control or manage factors that affect your state of health or illness (e.g., whether or not you smoke or exercise; what you do/do not eat; getting regular checkups)?
	Do you feel that you can control or manage factors that affect your life (e.g., your job; where you live; who your friends are)?
	Is there anything or anybody that you believe is responsible for what happens to you in your life (e.g., a supreme being; fate; luck; people who are more powerful than you)?
Spirituality	Do you have a preferred religion or religious beliefs?
	Is your religion an important influence in your life? Does it give you guidance in your daily life?
	Are there other things besides religion that are important to you as you go about your daily life?
	How often do you attend worship services? Does it bother you if you are ill or unable to attend worship services? What do you do if you cannot attend services?
	Is there someone you consider to be your spiritual advisor? Do you need to talk to this person regularly?
	Is there anything special that you do when you feel a need for spiritual support? Do you need help to practice your beliefs at this time?
	Do you have any religious or spiritual beliefs about health and illness (e.g., illness as a punishment; certain foods to eat or avoid, or practices that should be done or avoided) that the healthcare team should be aware of?
	Can the healthcare team be of spiritual help to you?
Social network and support system	Describe your family: What are its members and what are their relationships to you?
	What roles do you and your family members have (e.g., parent, child, spouse, sibling, other relative, teacher, provider, role model, best friend, authority figure, peacemaker)?
	Who in your family do you feel closest to?

Table continued on following page

Table 11–1. Interview Guide for Assessment of Selected Areas of a Client's Psychosocial Status *(Continued)*

Assessment Area	Key Questions or Issues to Include*
	Are there other people not related to you whom you consider important (i.e., significant others)?
	Do you and your family members (or significant others) get along with one another?
	Are there any problems within your family or with significant others that have strained your relationships with one another (e.g., change in living space; marital problems; arguments)?
	Are friendships important to you?
	Are you satisfied with the friendships that you have now?
	Whom would you identify as your best friend?
	Are your friends accepted by your family and significant others?
	Describe your relationships with your friends and coworkers
	What types of groups, clubs, or organizations do you belong to?
	If you had a problem or were in a crisis, whom would you turn to for help? Is this person available?
	Is there someone at work whom you confide in?
	Are there other things that help you when you need support during stressful times (e.g., a pet or inanimate object)?
	Do you have a pet or animals that are important to you? Is there someone who will take care of them for you if you are unable to do so?
Sexuality	Are you satisfied with being a man (or a woman)? Have you ever wished you were of the opposite sex?
	Are you satisfied in your sexual relationships with your spouse, significant other, or other sexual partners (e.g., frequency and quality of interactions)? Has there been a change in your sexual function? If so, describe what is different and how long it has been this way. Is this change for the better or worse?
	Have you experienced any problems with sexual activity (e.g., impotence, pain, premature ejaculation, bleeding, lack of privacy, infertility, other)? Do you feel that this may be related to a health problem or some other cause? If so, have these problems affected your relationship with your sexual partner?
	How long have you been sexually active?
	How long have you been in your current relationship?
	Can you recall the number of sexual partners you have had?
	Do you use contraceptives? If not, are you interested in information about this? Do you have any questions about the method you are using now?
	Do you use any type of protection against venereal diseases (e.g., condoms)? Have you ever been treated for a venereal disease?
	Do you have reason to believe that you have been exposed to a venereal disease such as syphilis, gonorrhea, or HIV?
Cultural components	***Identification with a cultural group:***
	How do you identify yourself to others when you are asked to what nationality or what ethnic group you belong?
	Describe how strongly you feel about your ethnic roots. Do you see yourself as a member of your ethnic group first, or do you think of yourself as a/an _____ (American, Canadian, or other) first?
	How do you identify yourself when you are asked about your racial background (e.g., black, white, Native American, Hispanic, Asian)?
	Where were you born? Where were your parents born?
	What countries (or regions of this country) have you lived in and when?
	Communication:
	What language do you speak at home? Do you speak or read other languages? Do you prefer to speak in a language other than English? Is there someone (e.g., friend, relative) whom you want to act as an interpreter for you? Do you want a professional interpreter? Is there anyone (e.g., someone of the opposite sex; a person who is older/younger than you; a person you see as a rival or enemy) who should not act as an interpreter?
	Whom do you prefer to take care of you when you need healthcare (e.g., a person of the same cultural background/same sex/same age as you)?

Table 11–1. Interview Guide for Assessment of Selected Areas of a Client's Psychosocial Status (Continued)

Assessment Area	Key Questions or Issues to Include*

Values, beliefs, and attitudes:

Can you identify any special beliefs or practices of yours that are influenced by your ethnic or cultural background? For example, are there things that you or your significant others do when a baby is born? When someone dies? When you or your family members are ill?

Is there anything special that you or your family do to stay healthy (e.g., eat or avoid certain foods; use herbs; call in someone who has special powers or gifts to help you stay well or get well)?

Is leisure time important to you? Do you take time to relax and have fun? Describe what you do when you want to relax.

Cultural sanctions and restrictions:

Is there anything the healthcare team should know about when taking care of you? For example, do you need to keep parts of your body covered to prevent others from seeing them?

Are there certain types of procedures that are forbidden for you to have done (e.g., hysterectomy, vasectomy)?

If you were to have a serious operation in which part of your body had to be removed (amputation) or cut out (excision), how should this body part be handled (e.g., preserved, buried, cremated, no special treatment)?

Are there any topics or subjects that you do not wish to talk about because it is not allowed by your beliefs (e.g., discussing people who have died)?

Health-related beliefs and practices:

Is there anything in your beliefs that you feel helps you to be (or to stay) healthy? For example, do you believe certain foods, herbs, or beverages (potions) are good for you?

Is there anything special that you do or wear to help you stay healthy or bring you luck (e.g., an amulet; prayers to ancestors; praying to a saint, supreme being, or other being; certain rituals)?

Is there anything that you believe is not good for your health or that causes illness or sickness (e.g., illness is a punishment for doing something "wrong"; you are under a spell or curse; your body is not in harmony or balance with nature; there is an imbalance between good/bad [positive/negative] forces within your body such as yin/yang or hot/cold)?

Is there anything in your religious beliefs that influences what you believe about health and illness? Describe.

Do you believe in or use other types of people to help you get better or heal when you are sick (e.g., curandero; shaman; minister, priest, or other spiritual adviser)? How do you know when to contact this person?

Are there any types of healing practices or beliefs that you have or feel you need (e.g., use of herbal remedies or potions; massage or other type of special touch; wearing a special charm or talisman to ward off evil spirits; special prayers or incantations; specific healing practices or ceremonies)?

When you are ill or sick, does your family and significant others expect you to act in a certain way (e.g., to play a particular "sick role")?

Who decides when you are sick or when you are no longer sick?

Who usually helps take care of you when you are sick?

Nutritional beliefs and practices:

Do you have any special beliefs that certain foods are better for you and help keep you healthy? Are there specific foods that you believe should be eaten if you have a certain kind of illness?

Identify foods that you believe are healthy for you to eat and foods that you believe you should avoid because they are unhealthy.

Describe how food is prepared in your home (e.g., frying; steaming; use of cooking oils [type]; how long foods are cooked; what types of seasonings are used or avoided; what foods may/may not be served together at the same meal; use of special cookware or dishes to serve food).

Table continued on following page

Table 11–1. Interview Guide for Assessment of Selected Areas of a Client's Psychosocial Status (*Continued*)	
Assessment Area	**Key Questions or Issues to Include***

Do you have certain religious beliefs that control the type of foods you eat/should not eat (e.g., kosher diet) or how food is prepared? (Also see previous question.)

Do you fast or abstain from specific foods at certain times during the week or year because of religious beliefs?

If you believe in "fasting" for religious reasons, describe what this means to you. Do you avoid certain foods or beverages? Do you eat only at specified times during the day?

Are you ever allowed to break your religious rules of diet or fasting if you are ill? Who makes this decision and who would tell you that it is acceptable to break a dietary rule?

Socioeconomic issues:

Is there anyone in your circle of family, friends, significant others, or spiritual advisers (i.e., social network) who you feel influences your health or illness status?

Are there special things that the members of your social network and support system do to help you when you are sick or to help you get better? Describe how these people would help take care of you if you were ill (e.g., stay by your side continuously; do things for you or your family; help your family).

Describe the roles that your family members play when one of the members is ill.

Do you expect your family members to help take care of you when you are sick? Describe what types of activities they might do (e.g., give you a bath; prepare your food; help to feed you; be with you).

Will your illness put a financial strain on your family? Who is the main wage earner in the family? Does anyone else help contribute to the family's income? Are there other sources for the family for financial income?

Educational background:

Can you read and write in English, or do you feel more comfortable with another language?

How much education have you had in schools?

When you learn about new things, is there a special way that you prefer to learn? For example, do you like to read information first, or do you like to watch someone do a new skill and then try to repeat it? Does it help for you to talk to someone and ask questions?

Religious beliefs and practices:

Do your religious beliefs or practices influence you in how you feel or act when you are sick or when you are well?

Are there special practices or healing rituals that you believe help to keep you well or to get better faster when you are ill?

Is there someone special who performs healing rituals for you (e.g., shaman, priest)?

Is it important to you to have a special religious person with you when you are sick or who comes to visit you (a priest or elder; imam; monk)? If so, describe how this person helps you feel better.

* The items in this section are representative but not inclusive for each assessment area.

Adapted in part from Barkley, R. A. (1990). *Attention deficit hyperactivity disorder: A handbook of diagnosis and treatment.* New York: Guilford Press.

tion, mood, memory, attention span, general knowledge, language abilities, thought processes, judgment, and insight.

If a client demonstrates impaired cognitive function, the nurse performs a Mini-Mental State Examination (see Chap. 30). Disturbances in mood or thought processes (such as suicidality) require a complete, detailed mental status examination. Areas included in a mental status ex-amination are level of consciousness, orientation, affect, mood, speech and communication, thought processes and content, attention span, memory, general fund of knowledge, calculations, ability for abstract reasoning and thinking, perceptual distortion, judgment, and insight. Even though most mental status examination data are collected during the health history, they are usually recorded with the physical examination data.

Level of Consciousness. Level of consciousness (LOC) is the client's state of awareness. The client must be alert, not just awake, for the nurse to assess mental status (see also Chap. 30). The nurse should cue the client that the questions may seem "silly" but to please answer them.

Orientation to Person, Place, Time, and Circumstances. The nurse asks the client to explain the reason for seeking healthcare. If the client's reply is unclear or digresses from the question, the nurse asks the client to state his or her name and identify where he or she is. Ability to recall the date and time are also assessed.

Mood and Affect. *Mood* is the client's subjective description of a personal emotion that is pervasive and sustained. The nurse records whether or not the described mood is congruent with the client's present situation. For example, "The client stated she was 'happy and going to celebrate' when informed that the results of her tests were negative."

Affect consists of the observable, outward demeanor that depicts the client's current emotional state, such as fear, anger, resentment, depression, anxiety, or elation. A flat affect is a lack of any facial expression or emotional response and is accompanied by a monotonous voice. A blunted affect is one that is greatly reduced in intensity but still appropriate to the situation. In addition, the nurse notes whether or not the observed affect is congruent with the client's immediate circumstances. For example, "When informed that dismissal from the hospital was postponed because of an infection, the client first cried, then shouted at the nurse to leave the room." This indicates the client first was upset and then became angry that the dismissal was delayed because of a complication. Both reactions are understandable, given the situation.

Speech and Communication (Language). The nurse evaluates the client's physical ability to speak and communicate by focusing on *how* the client talks, not the topic of the client's speech. The nurse observes the client's tone of voice, pitch, rate of speech, articulation, length of responses, pauses, and pauses before replying to questions (latency).

Thought Processes and Content. The nurse assesses whether the client's speech progresses logically and whether the client's stream of thought is spontaneous, natural, organized, logical, relevant, coherent, and goal directed. What the client says should be consistent.

Attention Span. The nurse assesses the client's ability to focus or concentrate on a task or activity over time, such as completing history forms or answering questions. If the nurse is uncertain about the client's ability, attention span can be further evaluated with the following tests. *Digit span* is a test of attention span in which the client repeats a series of five to seven numbers forward and up to five numbers backward that have been identified by the nurse. The use of *serial 7s and 3s* tests the client's attention span as well as the calculation ability. The client is asked to subtract 7 (or 3) from 100 and continue to subtract by 7 (or 3) until unable to go any further.

Memory: Immediate, Recent, and Remote. Assessment of memory usually begins with the client's recall of the past health history. The client is asked to recall information: within seconds (e.g., repeat a series of numbers); within several minutes to hours (e.g., recall specific words later during the interview; recall what was eaten yesterday); and within hours, months, or years (e.g., identify where the client grew up). The nurse should be able to verify the client's answers.

General Fund of Knowledge. The nurse asks the client to identify commonly known places, events, and people. This can be done casually during conversation.

Calculations. The nurse asks the client to perform simple arithmetic calculations (addition, subtraction, multiplication, division) without the aid of pencil or paper. See the previous discussion about serial 7s.

Ability for Abstract Reasoning and Thinking. The client's answers to general questions (e.g., explaining the reason a course of action was taken for a health problem) are usually sufficient to assess abstract reasoning. If reasoning is impaired, the client is asked to think beyond the concrete dimension by explaining a common proverb or by explaining similarities or differences between selected concepts. For example, "A bird in the hand is worth two in the bush." "What is the difference between a tree and a bush?"

Perceptual Distortion. The client should be able to discriminate reality from misperceptions. The nurse asks the client to describe any illusions or hallucinations by asking specifically about each of the senses. For example, "Do you ever feel that you are hearing sounds that other people do not?"

Judgment. Judgment (or decision-making ability) may be assessed within the context of the health history interview as the client discusses actions and decisions made in daily living. To assess further, ask the client about a realistic, rather than hypothetical, situation. For example, what would the client do in a given situation such as when a prescribed medication has run out?

Insight. Insight is assessed throughout the interview as the client explains in his or her own words what the nature of the current health problem is and what the expectations are for the healthcare team. The nurse evaluates whether the client demonstrates ability to perceive the self realistically and accurately.

When assessing mental status, the nurse individualizes questions to the client's circumstances. Variables affecting a client's ability to respond to specific questions include level of education, cultural background, degree of exposure to knowledge and information, familiarity with the nurse's language and vocabulary, and perceived acceptance of the client by the nurse. For example, it may be revealing to ask a teenager the name of a current popular singer but inappropriate to ask the same question of someone elderly. A client who has not progressed beyond a third-grade level of education may be incapable of performing complicated arithmetic calculations. A proverb widely known in one culture may have no meaning to someone from a different cultural background. Last, the nurse must have access to correct answers for the questions asked, particularly those relating to the client's personal circumstances, such as the location of his or her home, date and place of birth, and names of family members.

Other Psychological Factors. The nurse assesses additional psychological factors, such as personality style (see also Box 11–3), motivation, personal strengths, values and beliefs, spirituality, and formal psychological test results, while interacting with the client and significant others. The nurse does not usually participate in formal psychological testing of clients. However, the nurse may use data from formal testing to supplement psychosocial data collected in nurse-client interactions and in the health history.

Motivation. Motivation is highly individual and is influenced by personal needs and desires, goals, hopes, and aspirations. The nurse attempts to determine the client's motivation for seeking healthcare and, if the client is ill, the motivation for returning to an optimal level of wellness.

Personal Strengths. The client's strengths are used by the nurse when planning care. *Resources,* both internal and external, are personal elements that determine an individual's capability to adapt to challenges and threatening stressors. *Internal resources* are physiologic (e.g., immune system, nutritional state, physiologic defense systems, genetic predisposition to health, current state of each body system) and psychological (e.g., defense mechanisms, interpersonal style, usual conscious coping ability, current coping ability, and spiritual state, such as the will to live). *External resources* include the social environment (e.g., usual coping style of the family, availability of social support, and the assessment skills of the healthcare givers) and the physical, economic, and cultural environments.

Values and Beliefs. The client's value system and beliefs determine whether or not the client views healthcare as worthwhile to pursue. The client's values and beliefs may be different from those of the nurse. However, the nurse accepts them as being valid for that particular client because they help provide insight into the client's behavior.

Spirituality. Spiritual beliefs have implications for the client's well-being, such as sustaining hope or assisting with coping during periods of stress. The nurse includes spirituality assessment as part of the health history and explains to the client the purpose for asking about it (see Chap. 4). This portion of the history is usually addressed at the end of the interview after a trusting relationship is established. Because spirituality is very personal, the nurse respects a client's wish not to discuss this topic. However, the nurse asks whether there is someone special that the client prefers when spiritual support is needed.

Sociologic Assessment

The *sociologic dimension* includes information about the client's social roles and functions. The nurse assesses the client's psychosocial development, social network, socioeconomic status, lifestyle, and sexuality. The client is viewed both as an individual and as a member of a social network.

Psychosocial Development. *Psychosocial development* is the client's level of growth and development. It includes the life developmental processes and phases of growth and maturation. Psychosocial development occurs across the lifespan and includes components that are physical, emotional, psychological, social, and cognitive. These components are not necessarily distinct from one another nor is the client's progress through life's stages and phases always predictable or inflexible. An understanding of human growth and development provides a foundation from which to assess the client (See Chap. 5 for a discussion of adult growth and development.)

Social Network. A *social network* is the group of people that surrounds, interacts with, and sustains the client with intimacy, social integration, nurturing, reassurance, and assistance. The nurse becomes part of a client's social network when the client enters the healthcare system. However, the client continues to receive support from the established social network.

Social network data are collected by observing the client during interactions with family and visitors, asking questions about the client's interpersonal relationships, and determining whether there are certain individuals with whom the client prefers to maintain contact. The nurse does not assume that only family members are the most significant people to the client. When planning care, the nurse includes the significant others who may be experiencing stress along with the client. (See Chapter 4 for a discussion of family assessment.)

Socioeconomic Status. An individual's economic position within society is referred to as *socioeconomic status.* The nurse asks about factors that affect the client's financial and social well-being because they have implications for planning individualized healthcare. These include occupation, current employment status, work-related concerns, financial concerns, effect of the client's health status on the ability to work and on finances, perceived effect that the client's socioeconomic status has on access to the healthcare system, educational background, and hopes and goals for the future.

Life-Style. The client's usual daily patterns of living are referred to as *life-style*. Life-style is closely associated with socioeconomic status but also includes relationships with others. The nurse assesses the following as they apply to health: the client's usual roles and functions, work and study habits, leisure and relaxation activities, type and location of residence, living arrangements, usual manner of transportation, proximity of close friends, importance and influence of cultural beliefs on diet and health-seeking behavior or treatment, health habits (e.g., use of alcohol, medications, nicotine, recreational drugs), stress level, coping methods used to relieve stress and their effectiveness, usual sleep pattern, and degree of satisfaction with current status.

Sexuality. *Sexuality* is the behavioral expression of one's sexual identity. It involves sexual realtionships between people as well as the perception of one's maleness or femaleness. Many aspects of sexuality affect health status and have significance in relation to nursing care and client outcomes. Aspects include physical health problems that affect sexual behavior (e.g., mastectomy, colostomy, skin lesions, venereal diseases, paralysis, physical deformities), concerns with sexual performance (e.g., impotence, premature ejaculation, inability to achieve orgasm, infertility), issues of sex role function (e.g., homosexuality, bisexuality, sexual ambiguity, transsexual surgery), and effects of environmental restrictions on sexual performance (e.g., residency in a long-term care facility) (see Chapter 4).

Sexuality and sexual behavior remain sensitive topics for clients to discuss. Clients may want to discuss issues of sexuality and look to the nurse for permission and encouragement to do so. The nurse should be comfortable with sexuality issues and not allow personal beliefs and values to interfere with professional care. The nurse accepts and interacts with clients without judging them or their behavior.

Cultural Assessment

Cultural assessment is a systematic examination of the client's cultural beliefs, values, and practices as they apply to determining healthcare needs. These needs, and any culture-based interventions, must be viewed from the client's cultural context. Cultural assessment tends to be broad because it seeks information about group values, beliefs, and behaviors. The nurse must also assess what the larger group's tenets mean to the individual. Table 11–1 includes guidelines for assessing cultural components as part of the psychosocial assessment.

A Guide to Psychosocial Assessment

Although discussed separately, psychological and sociologic assessments are often combined (see Box 11–2). The nurse may collect psychosocial data that indicate a client has a psychiatric disorder. If this situation occurs, the nurse consults with other healthcare professionals

such as a psychiatric clinical nurse specialist and the client's physician.

Review of Systems

The review of systems (ROS) is a head-to-toe review of the physical health history (see discussion earlier in this chapter) for each body system. The ROS provides focus for the physical examination. Box 11–2 presents the type of information assessed. These data often are collected by having the client complete a checklist form that is then reviewed, and expanded as necessary, by a healthcare professional. In an episodic health history, the nurse focuses on those systems pertinent to the problem.

Health Promotion and Health Risk Appraisal

Health risk appraisal examines factors that affect a client's potential for developing a particular health problem. Risk factors are genetic or biologic (e.g., race, family history, personal history), behavioral (e.g., health habits such as smoking), or environmental (e.g., living in a locale with smog). Determining a client's health risk status identifies high-risk clients who may benefit from timely intervention. The nurse explains the difference between *being at increased risk* of developing a health problem and the inevitability of *actually developing* a health problem. In health risk appraisal, the nurse assesses the client's willingness to modify or reduce his or her risk status. For example, a client who smokes is at higher risk of developing pulmonary diseases than is a non-smoker. The nurse may believe that the client *should* stop smoking. However, if the client has no desire to stop, teaching will be ineffective. This client may be labeled "noncompliant" by the healthcare team when the client is only adhering to a personal decision to keep smoking.

However, a female client who is at risk of developing osteoporosis tells the nurse that she is concerned and desires to reduce her risk. This client is receptive to teaching about increasing dietary calcium intake and engaging in regular weight-bearing activity.

Health risk factors are categorized for assessment purposes. Some risk factors are potentially hazardous for many people (e.g., ground water pollution in a community dependent on wells for the water supply). Other risk factors may adversely affect a limited group of individuals (e.g., particle inhalation in workers who install insulation materials). And other risk factors are significant for a family group (e.g., genetic diseases, such as Huntington's chorea). Risk factor categories include race and genetic or family-related factors, age-related factors, biologic factors, personal habits, life-style, environmental and occupational factors, and socioeconomic factors.

Table 11–2 summarizes examples of health risk factors, their commonly associated health problems, and suggested health promotion behaviors or screening procedures that may reduce a client's potential risk or facilitate early detection. Awareness of health risk factors may motivate a client to seek screening procedures and to prac-

Text continued on page 205

Table 11–2. Health Promotion and Risk Management

Risk Factor	Potential Health Problem	Screening and Preventive Measures	
		Self-Care	*Professional Level*
Race			
Black	Hypertension	Self-monitor BP Avoid salt in diet Maintain IBW Seek professional care if systolic BP > 140 or diastolic BP > 90	Monitor if BP is elevated or client is taking antihypertensive medications
White (fair skin tones)	Skin cancer	Limit exposure to sun Wear protective clothing Use sunscreen with SPF 15 or above Perform monthly head-to-toe skin inspection Seek professional care if change noted in any moles or birthmarks, or new growths or patches do not heal	Monitor skin lesions Skin biopsy or excision and follow up treatment
	Osteoporosis	See self-care and professional level measures listed under "Personal Habits—Inadequate calcium intake"	
Japanese	Stomach cancer	Know suspicious GI symptoms: pain, hematemesis, melena, weight loss, nausea, etc.*	Follow up for laboratory tests and special diagnostic procedures
Hispanic	Diabetes mellitus	Regular exercise and weight control Consume balanced diet of no more than 30% fats with complex carbohydrates Know symptoms of hyperglycemia: polydipsia, polyuria, polyphagia, and delayed wound healing*	Diet counseling Follow up for laboratory tests, diagnostic procedures, and blood glucose monitoring and control
Native American	Alcohol abuse and related diseases	Abstinence Limit alcohol intake to 1 oz/day or less if personal tendency (e.g., 1 to 2 mixed drinks or cans of beer) Know symptoms of alcoholism* Join self-help support group such as Alcoholics Anonymous (AA)	Assessment of history and physical condition Referral to a detoxification program Counseling for client and family
Genetic or Family Related			
Overweight	Obesity-related disease	Monitor weight once per week Perform regular, sustained exercise Consume balanced diet (no more than 30% fats, and calories should not exceed metabolic needs) Join self-help group such as Weight Watchers	Diet counseling Follow up for moribund obesity (>100% over IBW)
Diabetes mellitus	Diabetes mellitus or glucose intolerance	Regular exercise and weight control Consume balanced diet Know symptoms of hyperglycemia: polydipsia, polyuria, polyphagia, and delayed wound healing*	Follow up for laboratory tests, special diagnostic procedures, and blood glucose monitoring and control
Hypertension	Cardiovascular disease Renal disease Retinopathy Cerebrovascular accident	Regular, sustained exercise Consume balanced diet Avoid excess salt intake Maintain IBW Regular BP checks (self or professional) Take BP medication daily	Regular follow up for diagnostic studies and laboratory work Monitor compliance
Heart disease (onset before age 50)	Cardiovascular disease	See "Hypertension" Know symptoms of heart disease: chest pain, dyspnea, cyanosis*	Annual physical examination, including ECG and laboratory tests

Table 11–2. Health Promotion and Risk Management (Continued)

Risk Factor	Potential Health Problem	Screening and Preventive Measures	
		Self-Care	**Professional Level**
		Stop smoking Monitor resting pulse rate Low saturated fat diet Regular exercise	Refer to smoking cessation clinics Diet counseling
Breast cancer (in mother or sister)	Breast cancer	Learn to perform BSE Perform BSE monthly	Regular professional breast examination as indicated for age and personal history Regular mammography as indicated for age
Age Related			
Vision changes	Strabismus	Monitor for difficulty focusing, especially on near objects See ophthalmologist if symptoms occur Schedule regular eye examinations as indicated for age	Follow up for complete eye examination and possible neurologic examination
	Visual acuity changes, cataracts, glaucoma, or macular degeneration	Monitor visual acuity See ophthalmologist if vision is "fuzzy," or seeing halos around lights Schedule regular eye examinations	Complete eye examination to screen for cataracts, glaucoma, and macular degeneration as indicated for age
	Injury or trauma	Wear protective eye gear when engaging in activity likely to result in projectiles or blunt trauma See ophthalmologist if injury should occur	Provide prompt diagnosis and treatment if injury occurs
Falls	Injury or trauma	Keep environment illuminated Remove loose scatter rugs Use a night-light Install handrails and grab bars Wipe up spills immediately	Provide prompt diagnosis and treatment if injury occurs
Self-medication errors	Overmedicating or undermedicating	Request and use prepackaged unit dose medications Prepare medicines in a well-lit area Wear corrective lenses when preparing medicines	Careful assessment of medication history; monitor for toxic response
Hearing problem	Presbycusis	Avoid exposure to loud noises Wear ear plugs when exposed to loud noise levels and limit lengths of exposure	Complete audiometric screening as appropriate for age and personal history
	Injury or trauma	Avoid putting sharp objects into ear canals Know symptoms of ear infections: pain, discharge from ear canal, vertigo, and fever*	Follow up for prompt diagnosis and treatment if injury or infection occurs
Inadequate dental hygiene	Dental caries Periodontal disease Premature loss of teeth	Brush teeth regularly after meals and at bedtime Floss teeth daily Have damaged teeth repaired or replaced promptly Follow recommendations for fluoride treatments; use fluoridated toothpaste Schedule regular dental checkups	Provide complete dental checkups, and follow up annually Fluoride treatments as indicated for age and locale
Impaired immune system integrity	Community-acquired infections	Keep immunizations current as recommended for age Receive vaccinations for influenza yearly and pneumococcus on time Seek professional care if symptoms of infection occur	Provide prompt diagnosis and treatment if a contagious disease or infection is suspected

Table continued on following page

Table 11–2. Health Promotion and Risk Management (*Continued*)

Risk Factor	Potential Health Problem	Screening and Preventive Measures	
		Self-Care	*Professional Level*
Impaired mobility	Falls	See self-care measures listed under falls related to vision changes Use mobility-assistance devices (e.g., cane or walker) Avoid hazardous surfaces, such as wet floors and icy pavements	Provide prompt diagnosis and treatment if injury occurs
Biologic			
Hyperlipidemia, hypercholesteremia	Cardiovascular disease	Consume balanced diet low in saturated fats Exercise regularly Avoid or stop smoking Have blood lipid and cholesterol levels monitored periodically as recommended	Regular follow up for monitoring serum levels
Hyperglycemia	Diabetes mellitus	Consume diet low in fats and simple carbohydrates Include complex carbohydrates Exercise regularly Have blood glucose levels monitored periodically as recommended Self-monitor blood glucose levels if diabetic and following a prescribed medical regimen	Regular follow up for monitoring control of blood glucose levels Adjustment of medical treatment as indicated by laboratory results
Hypersensitivity reactions	Allergic reactions, including rhinitis, bronchospasm, asthma, eczema, and atopic dermatitis	Avoid known allergens Seek prompt medical treatment if self-care measures are ineffective Discuss with physician whether allergen sensitivity testing and treatment for desensitization is indicated Wear a Medic-Alert tag Learn to use and carry an emergency kit (e.g., adrenalin) if indicated	Provide prompt diagnosis and treatment if severe reactions or complications occur Initiation of desensitization therapy if indicated
Personal Habits			
Inadequate rest and sleep	Fatigue Lowered resistance to illness	Obtain sufficient sleep to feel rested on awakening (amount varies with individual need) (Also see Chapter 18) Avoid sedatives, caffeine, alcohol Seek professional care if chronic fatigue interferes with activities of daily living	Complete history and physical examination Evaluation in a sleep laboratory
Irregular diet habits	Obesity, diabetes, hypertension, cardiovascular disease, irritability, depression, and hyperactivity or hypoactivity	Consume meals at regular times each day Eat three balanced meals per day Limit intake of salt, caffeine, refined sugar, and fats Perform regular exercise Monitor weight weekly See self-care measures listed under obesity, diabetes, hypertension, and cardiovascular disease	Regular follow up to monitor existing health problems Provide prompt diagnosis and treatment if a health problem arises
Inadequate calcium intake	Osteoporosis	Consume 800 mg of calcium per day in elemental form (men and menstruating women). In premenopausal women, 1000 mg/day. In postmenopausal women, 1500 mg/day	Follow up for periodic physical examination Possible estrogen hormone replacement therapy, when indicated

Table 11-2. Health Promotion and Risk Management (Continued)

Risk Factor	Potential Health Problem	Screening and Preventive Measures	
		Self-Care	**Professional Level**
		Limit milk products as source of calcium; include other sources of dietary calcium, such as broccoli, carrots, green beans, spinach, collard greens, and rhubarb Consume 400–800 IU/day of vitamin D Engage in daily, weight-bearing activity such as walking	Diet counseling
Excess fat intake	Colon cancer Possible breast cancer	Consume diet low in saturated fats, such as that found in beef. Substitute with fish, poultry, and beans Limit milk products and eggs Include fiber in diet such as from grains and cereals Know symptoms of colon cancer (blood in stool, change in bowel habits) and breast cancer (lump, discharge, pain)* Have stool specimen tested for occult blood Perform BSE monthly	Follow up for laboratory tests and possible diagnostic procedures Diet counseling
Low fiber intake	Colon cancer	Consume diet high in fiber, including cereals and grains, especially bran Know symptoms of colon cancer (see earlier)* Have stool specimen tested for occult blood	Follow up for laboratory tests and diagnostic procedures Supplemental fiber to include in diet
Alcohol abuse	Alcoholism Cancer of mouth, throat, esophagus, larynx, and liver Accidents, including those that result in death Cirrhosis Esophageal varices Pancreatitis Dementia	Abstinence, if high risk for alcoholism Limit alcohol intake to 1 oz or less per day if no personal tendency (e.g., 1 to 2 mixed drinks or cans of beer) Know the symptoms of alcoholism* Join self-help support group, such as Alcoholics Anonymous, if alcohol consumption interferes with performance of job or interpersonal relationships	Careful assessment of history and physical condition Referral to a detoxification program, if indicated Provide counseling Family counseling and support are often necessary (e.g., Al-Anon, Ala-Teen)
Drug abuse	Harmful side effects Drug interactions Allergic reactions Hepatitis HIV	Use prescribed medications only as directed Discard outdated medications Limit use of over-the-counter drugs to only those necessary Avoid recreational drug use Know symptoms of substance abuse* If using intravenous drugs, do not share needles or syringes	Careful assessment of history and physical condition Referral to a detoxification program, if indicated Provide counseling Family counseling and support are often necessary Screening for HIV
Tobacco use	Cancer of mouth or lung Cardiovascular disease Respiratory disease	Avoid tobacco use in any form Limit use, if unable to quit Know symptoms of tobacco-related health problems: persistent cough, oral sore that does not heal, hoarseness that persists, blood in sputum* Have regular health checkups Avoid exposing others to sidestream smoke Attend support group to help stop smoking, such as Smokers Anonymous	Follow up for laboratory tests and special diagnostic procedures Counseling for help to stop smoking Referral of family members (if indicated) for health assessment if exposed to sidestream smoke
Safety	Unintentional injury or death	Use safety equipment as indicated (seat belts, helmet, eye shield, life vest)	Thorough teaching about medications and their side effects

Table continued on following page

Table 11–2. Health Promotion and Risk Management *(Continued)*			
Risk Factor	**Potential Health Problem**	**Screening and Preventive Measures**	
		Self-Care	*Professional Level*
		Learn how to swim Never drink and drive. Appoint a designated driver Do not operate equipment or engage in hazardous activity if taking medication that causes drowsiness Develop safety awareness, e.g., learn to identify unsafe situations and avoid them or take corrective action	Provide prompt diagnosis and treatment if an injury occurs
Sun exposure	Sunburn Skin cancer	See self-care measures listed under skin cancer related to race	See measures listed under skin cancer related to race
Life-Style			
Lack of regular exercise	Obesity Cardiovascular disease	Engage in regular aerobic exercise (brisk walking, biking, jogging, swimming) at least 3 times/week for 30 to 40 minutes each Warm up prior to exercising to increase flexibility and reduce chance of injury Do not begin an exercise program until evaluated by healthcare professional for a baseline health assessment Follow professional advice regarding type of exercise program and intensity of training Wear appropriate gear for activity as protection Consume a balanced diet Know warning signals of when to stop exercising (e.g., dizziness, chest pain)*	Baseline health assessment prior to beginning exercise program Provide prompt diagnosis and treatment if complications or injury occurs Periodic assessment of cardiovascular status and endurance
Stress and coping ability	Many health problems are related to high stress levels and inadequate coping	Decrease level of stress whenever possible Develop a variety of coping skills Practice relaxation techniques (e.g., biofeedback, imagery, meditation, self-hypnosis) Recognize effects of stress on self Develop a support network* Modify life-style to reduce stress	Provide counseling for stress management Refer to appropriate support system as indicated by the individual circumstances Teach regarding relaxation techniques Carefully assess and treat if psychosomatic health problems develop
Lack of self-care activities to promote health	Cancer of breast, testis, or prostate	Monthly practice of BSE or TSE Regular professional examination as indicated for age	Periodic, regular examination
	Cancer of the cervix	Obtain regular pelvic examination and Papanicolaou (Pap) test as indicated for age and sexual activity status	Periodic, regular examination with follow up as necessary
	Vision and hearing problems	See self-care measures under age-related health problems	See measures listed under age-related health problems for vision and hearing
	Dental and gum disease	See self-care measures under age-related health problems	See measures listed under age-related health problems for dental hygiene
	Tetanus Influenza Pneumonia	Keep immunizations current*	Provide prompt diagnosis and treatment if an infectious disease occurs

Table 11–2. Health Promotion and Risk Management (Continued)

Risk Factor	Potential Health Problem	Screening and Preventive Measures	
		Self-Care	Professional Level
	Cancer	Know the seven warning signs: change in bowel or bladder habits, a nonhealing sore, unusual bleeding or discharge, lump or thickening in breast or other area, difficulty swallowing or indigestion, change in mole or wart, and persistent cough or hoarseness* Know and follow current recommendations for prevention and early entry into the healthcare system	Follow up for laboratory tests and special diagnostic procedures Provide prompt diagnosis and treatment
High-risk sexual activity	Unplanned pregnancy	Use contraceptive method acceptable to self and partner Prenatal care	Provide counseling regarding options for contraceptives Provide counseling regarding pregnancy outcome options
	Cervical cancer	Abstain from early, frequent sexual activity Limit number of sexual partners Limit number of childbirths Schedule regular Pap test as recommended for age	Regular professional pelvic examinations and Pap tests as indicated by health behavior profile
	STDs, such as HIV and herpes	Limit number of sexual partners Avoid anal intercourse Use condoms Avoid oral-genital intercourse Avoid oral contact with body fluids (semen, blood, feces, urine) Seek professional care for regular, periodic assessment if engaging in high-risk sexual activity Know symptoms of STDs, e.g., sore on genitals or mucous membranes, discharge from penis or vagina, abnormal bleeding, dyspareunia Refrain from sexual activity if symptoms of STDs develop	Follow up for prompt diagnosis and treatment should STD be suspected Provide counseling regarding safe sex practices Refer to public health for contact and follow up of possible infected partners
Travel	Diseases prevalent to locale	Obtain necessary vaccinations before departure Seek prompt treatment if illness develops while traveling or after return	Provide prompt diagnosis and treatment if illness occurs
Environmental and Occupational			
Sports	Fractures, sprains, and strains	Have a baseline health assessment prior to beginning a sport Wear protective gear to avoid injury (e.g., eye shield, helmet, padding)* Follow recommendations for warm-up and cool-down exercises Limit mobility of injured body part until rehabilitation begins	Provide prompt diagnosis and treatment of injuries Rehabilitation
Outdoor activity	Sunburn Skin cancer Frostbite Hypothermia or hyperthermia	Wear protective gear appropriate for the weather Use sunscreen with an SPF of 15 or above Limit exposure to extremes of heat or cold Learn survival tactics relative to activity Know early signs of hypothermia (disorientation) and hyperthermia (dry, hot skin)	Provide prompt diagnosis and treatment if a problem occurs See measures listed under skin cancer related to race

Table continued on following page

Table 11–2. Health Promotion and Risk Management (Continued)

Risk Factor	Potential Health Problem	Screening and Preventive Measures	
		Self-Care	Professional Level
		Attempt to seek medical treatment as soon as possible if a problem arises Avoid future exposure to extremes of heat or cold because of increased vulnerability	
Loud noise	Hearing loss	Limit exposure to loud music and machinery Wear protective ear plugs Have regular screening of hearing and seek professional care if hearing loss is evident	Regular, complete audiometric screening, as appropriate
Chemical fumes, airborne particle exposure	Respiratory diseases Cancer	Provide adequate ventilation Wear protective gear (goggles, respirators) Limit exposure when possible (chemicals, dry cleaning fluid, film processing, mining, asbestos exposure, household cleaners) Evaluate occupational risks Reduce exposure by changing jobs, if necessary Know symptoms of possible disease, such as hoarseness, persistent cough, hemoptysis, chronic dyspnea* Avoid smoking	Prompt diagnosis and treatment if disease should occur
Stress-provoking activity	Many stress-related health problems may occur	See "Stress and coping ability" under Life-Style	Provide counseling regarding stress management
High-accident risk activity (also see Safety under Personal Habits)	Unintentional injury or death	Avoid high-accident-risk activities Learn safety measures Practice safety measures so they become habitual Use safety equipment such as goggles, helmets Get sufficient rest Avoid alcohol, drugs, or medications known to cause drowsiness when engaging in high-risk activity Obtain treatment if injury occurs	Provide prompt diagnosis and treatment if an accidental injury occurs
Low-level electromagnetic radiation exposure	Cancer of brain or eye Leukemia Sarcoma Possible birth defects	Limit exposure Monitor immediate environment for radiation levels Promptly seek health assessment and treatment for possible problems	Provide prompt diagnosis and treatment if a health problem occurs
Socioeconomic			
Recent immigration	Diseases common to locale of origin or where traveled	Obtain necessary immunizations before departure Seek professional care if symptoms of disease occur, especially during or after recent travel	Careful assessment of history and physical examination Provide prompt diagnosis and treatment if a health problem occurs
Lack of adequate health insurance coverage	Delayed or postponed treatment of health problems Undetected health problems	Use free walk-in health care facilities	Refer client to social services or welfare agency for assistance with applying for available healthcare, such as Medicaid or Medicare

* Seek professional care if symptoms are present.
ECG, electrocardiogram; HIV, human immunodeficiency virus; BP, blood pressure; BSE, breast self-examination; GI, gastrointestinal; IBW, ideal body weight; SPF, sun protection factor; STDs, sexually transmitted diseases; TSE, testicular self-examination.

tice health promotion behaviors, particularly for health problems that are treatable or manageable through timely intervention. Environmental and occupational risk factors are linked with specific health problems and may be susceptible to change. Socioeconomic risk factors are less easily eliminated; however, their effects may be modified through skillful case finding and risk management.

The client's risk profile is assessed throughout the health history interview. A client with multiple risk factors linked to specific health problems is at greater risk for developing those problems than is the client with fewer or no risk factors. Persons in hazardous occupations include firefighters, police, miners, heavy equipment operators, lumber and construction workers, factory and textile workers, musicians, and people who use chemicals or pesticides, such as farmers, landscapers, gardeners, painters, and artists. Risk for accidental injury or trauma has been linked to multiple stressors, inadequate coping ability, mental and physical fatigue, decreased reaction time, and substance abuse. Stressors include strained interpersonal relationships, physical or psychological abuse, inadequate financial resources, recent change in life-style, sensory stimulation overload, nutritional deficits, and hazardous environments. Life-style and personal habits affect one's health status significantly and many are modifiable.

After assessing a client's risk profile, the client's health risk status is evaluated. Each identified risk factor is examined with the client to determine whether or not its effects can be modified. If the client is interested in reducing health risks (e.g., stopping smoking or wearing seatbelts), the nurse intervenes either directly or indirectly. Approaches to behavior changes are discussed with the client. Direct interventions include teaching sessions to provide information and counseling or to reinforce client behavior. Indirect interventions include referral to an appropriate community resource or other healthcare professional (e.g., nutritionist, smoking-cessation program, counselor, support group for substance abusers, dieters's support programs). The goals for the client are (1) to take responsibility for modifying factors that can affect health and (2) to strive for optimal health. Box 11–5 provides a clinical example of how to integrate health risk appraisal into the history interview.

Health Promotion Across the Lifespan

Health promotion needs change with age and sex. For example, after age 50, a client's risk of developing cancer

---

Box 11–5. Example of Integrating Health Risk Appraisal into the History Interview

Biographical and Demographic Data

S. W. is a 28-year-old, single, white, female, self-employed fashion clothes designer. Self-insured. Admitted to nursing unit after surgical repair of the right knee.

Health Maintenance Activities

Annual examinations for teeth, vision, Pap smear. No breast self-examination. Last physical examination 18 months ago.

Personal Habits

Denies smoking. Consumes one to two alcoholic drinks or glasses of wine most days. Uses own automobile frequently, wears seatbelts "when [she] remembers to put them on." Uses tanning room at health spa twice a week for 30 minutes.

Diet

No restrictions, likes most foods. Prefers to limit sugar and salt intake. Typical 24-hour diet includes food guide pyramid groups. Usually eats breakfast and dinner; lunch consumed "on the run." Dines out often with clients at restaurants.

Exercise

Jogs once per week for 2 to 3 miles and performs step aerobics once per week at health spa. Tripped and fell while jogging 3 weeks ago; twisted right knee.

Stress Management

Feels "moderate" pressure to succeed in business. Life becomes "hectic" when new fashion lines shown. Uses im-

agery for relaxation (usually effective). Denies current problems with stress management.

Sleep and Rest

Gets approximately 6 to 7 hours' sleep per night and feels rested.

Sexuality

Sexually active since age 18. Admits to five or six partners in past 10 years, with one partner for past 2 years. Prescribed oral contraceptive for 6 years. Partner does not use condoms.

Past Health History

No previous illness, injury, or surgery. No allergies.

Family Health History

Mother diagnosed with breast cancer at age 42; treated with surgery and is currently healthy. No other known family-linked health problems.

Health Risk Appraisal

S. W. is at risk for (1) breast cancer, (2) possible skin cancer, (3) automobile-related injury or death, (4) possible sexually transmitted diseases, including HIV, and (5) recurrent injury to the right knee. She also is at risk for health problems related to alcohol consumption, inadequate nutrition, inadequate exercise patterns, and a stress-producing life-style. There may be concerns about financial security that can be explored with S. W. during further questioning.

of the bowel or breast increases compared with that of someone younger.

Specific screening procedures are performed during a complete health assessment to determine potential and actual health problems. For example, after age 40, glaucoma screening is recommended every 2 years. For health maintenance and prevention, specific health management behaviors are recommended based on age. For example, routine childhood immunizations for contagious diseases are administered according to a schedule that correlates with the development of the immune system as well as to periods when exposure is most likely to occur. Adults may be deficient in routine immunizations or previous exposure to childhood contagious diseases. These clients are recommended to have screening titers and immunizations.

Recommendations for common screening procedures and health management behaviors across the lifespan are listed in Table 11–3. Recommendations change periodically as research and epidemiologic studies reveal new information about occurrence and newer, easily applied, sensitive screening methods are developed. The nurse is familiar with the most current recommendations.

Refer to Chapter 23 for a discussion of risk factors for developing the common types of cancer (p. 542), as well as primary risk factors and secondary type of cancer prevention (see p. 542). Also see Table 23–6, the American Cancer Society Guidelines for early detection in asymptomatic populations.

Screening Tests and Procedures

Screening tests and procedures are used to assess if a client has a health problem (e.g., a skin test for tuberculosis) or is at risk for future health problems (e.g., serum cholesterol screening as a risk factor for atherosclerosis). When the nurse inquires if the client has had a *specific screening test or procedure,* such as an eye examination or mammograms, the client also is asked when the test was last performed and what the results were. The nurse uses this information to assess the client's health risk status and to recommend further follow-up or screening procedures.

Organizing the Health History Interview

Data collected during the health history interview are organized by topical areas. The nurse uses a comprehensive, flexible approach to collect data while allowing for in-depth focus assessment in areas of particular concern. The nurse's approach includes a head-to-toe assessment of the client. Various formats are helpful for conducting a health history interview. Gordon's functional health patterns (FHPs) are presented as an example.

FHPs may be used to collect health history data. This approach to assessment assists the nurse in identifying the client's health patterns, deviations from these patterns, and actual or potential nursing diagnoses. Each of the 11 patterns has its own assessment criteria, which are listed in Appendix B.

Health Perception and Health Management Pattern. The health perception and health management pattern describes the client's perception and understanding of the health status. This includes the client's life-style and behaviors to promote, maintain, and restore health and well-being.

Nutritional-Metabolic Pattern. The nutritional-metabolic pattern describes the client's food and fluid consumption in relationship to the body's metabolic needs. Adequacy of nutrient supply to local tissues is included. Multiple factors influence the client's behavior, such as physiologic (e.g., dehydration), pathophysiologic (e.g., peptic ulcer), psychosocial (e.g., the emotional significance of food), and socioeconomic (e.g., financial ability to purchase food).

Elimination Pattern. The elimination pattern focuses on the client's patterns of excretory function, including the bowel, bladder, and skin. Habits for excretory regularity and perceived difficulties are assessed.

Activity-Exercise Pattern. The activity-exercise pattern describes the client's activities of daily living requiring energy expenditure. These include self-care measures, physical exercise, stamina, and leisure and recreational activities.

Sleep-Rest Pattern. The sleep-rest pattern refers to the client's usual habits for sleep, rest, relaxation, and energy level. Patterns are assessed for a 24-hour period to consider circadian rhythmicity.

Cognitive-Perceptual Pattern. The cognitive-perceptual pattern describes the client's ability to perceive, comprehend, and use information as well as the sensory functions. Pain is included in this pattern.

Self-Perception and Self-Concept Pattern. The self-perception and self-concept pattern includes the client's view of self, including attitudes, identity, body image, sense of self-worth, and self-esteem.

Role Relationship Pattern. The role relationship pattern describes the client's roles in society and interpersonal relationships.

Sexuality-Reproductive Pattern. The sexuality-reproductive pattern refers to the client's satisfaction or dissatisfaction with sexuality and reproductive functions. These include sex role behavior and identification, physiologic and biologic functions, and sociocultural aspects of sexual behavior.

Coping–Stress Tolerance Pattern. The coping–stress tolerance pattern describes the client's general coping strategies and effectiveness in managing stress.

Text continued on page 211

Table 11–3. Recommendations for Common Screening Procedures and Health Management Behaviors Across the Lifespan*

Potential Health Problem	Recommended Preventive/ Screening Examination†	Birth to 18 Months	2 to 6 Years	7 to 12 Years	13 to 18 Years	19 to 39 Years	40 to 64 Years	65 Years and over
Growth and developmental concerns	History—re: developmental disorders	Parent/family dysfunction. Physical, mental, emotional, and social growth. Behavioral and learning disorders	Discipline, school readiness		Sexual practices	Relationships with significant others. Parenting behaviors. Job satisfaction.		Retirement planning; declining mental acuity
	Nutrition history	Breastfeeding, iron intake	Sweets, between-meal snacks, fats (saturated), cholesterol, sodium, iron, calcium			Fats (saturated). cholesterol, complex carbohydrates, fiber, sodium, calcium		
				Caloric balance and selection of exercise program		Iron for women until menopause		
	Complete physical examination	Birth and 2, 4, 6, 15, and 18 months	Every year until age 5	Every 2 years	Every 2 years	Every 5 years	Every 3 years	Every year
Vision Problems	Strabismus check, amblyopia	Every Visit						
	Assessment of visual acuity		Every year beginning at age 3	One time	One time	Every 2 to 4 years to include glaucoma screening		Every 1 to 2 years to include glaucoma screening
Hearing problems	Audiometry	18 months	Every year	One time	One time		Every 3 years	Every year
Dental problems	Assessment of teeth/cleaning	Every visit (baby bottle tooth decay)	Every 6 months beginning at age 3	Every 6 months to 1 year				
	Fluoride	+	+	+	+			
	Brushing and flossing		+	+	+	+	+	+

Table continued on following page

Table 11-3. Recommendations for Common Screening Procedures and Health Management Behaviors Across the Lifespan* (Continued)

Potential Health Problem	Recommended Preventive/Screening Examination†	Birth to 18 Months	2 to 6 Years	7 to 12 Years	13 to 18 Years	19 to 39 Years	40 to 64 Years	65 Years and over
Infectious diseases	Routine immunizations	DTP, OPV, MMR, Hib, HBV, VZV per protocol	DTP, OPV, MMR per protocol			MMR if not given at 4 to 6 years		
	PPD or tine test	At age 1	One time	One time	One time	One time	One time	One time
	Tetanus-diphtheria booster		One time between 4 to 6 years		One time between 14 to 16 years	Every 10 years		
	Influenza vaccine			Every year if high risk under age 65				Every year
	Pneumococcal vaccine							One time
Accidents and injuries	Automobile restraints	Car seats	Car seats until age 4; seat belts	+	+	+	+	+
	History—re: risk factors	Burns, falls, choking, poisoning	Poisoning, drowning, burns, bicycle accidents	Bicycle accidents, burns, poisoning, firearms	Bicycle accidents, burns, firearms, drinking while driving, suicide	Drinking while driving, firearms, back injury, burns, suicide	Drinking while driving, burns, back injury, falls	Falls
Substance abuse	History—re: use of tobacco, drugs, alcohol			+	+	+	+	+
Birth defects	Rubella titer				Unimmunized female			
	Amniocentesis					Over age 35		
Unplanned pregnancy	Sex education			+	+	+	+	
	Contraceptive information			+	+	+	+	
Anemia	Hemoglobin and hematocrit	One time, early infancy	Age 3 and 5 years	Ages 8, 10, and 12	Ages 15 and 18	One time	Every 3 years	Every year
Bacteriuria	Urinalysis		One time at age 3	One time	One time	Every 1 to 3 years		Every year

Condition	Screening/Examination						
Bowel cancer	Rectal examination						Every year
	Stool examination for occult blood						Every year beginning at age 40
	Sigmoidoscopy						Every 3 to 5 years after two negative tests taken 1 year apart, beginning at age 40
Breast cancer	Breast self-examination (BSE)				Every month		
	Professional examination				Every 3 years		Every year
	Mammogram				One time between ages 35 and 39 if high risk		Every 1 to 2 years until age 50; then every year until age 75
Cervical cancer/gynecologic problems	Papanicolaou (Pap) smear			Every 1 to 3 years if sexually active	Every year until 3 exams in a row are negative; then decrease frequency		
	Pelvic examination				Every 1 to 3 years		Every year
Heart disease	History—re: exercise program or physical activity	Every visit		Every visit			
	Electrocardiogram					One time	
Hypertension	Blood pressure	Every year beginning at age 3	Every 1 to 2 years				Every year
Hyperlipidemia	Blood cholesterol level	Age 3 if family history	+		Every 5 years	Every 5 years	Every 3 to 5 years
Obesity	Height and weight	Every visit	+	+	+	+	+
Oral cancer	Professional examination				Annually	Annually	Annually
Scoliosis	Back examination	Every year beginning at age 8	Every visit				

Table continued on following page

Table 11–3. Recommendations for Common Screening Procedures and Health Management Behaviors Across the Lifespan* (Continued)

Potential Health Problem	Recommended Preventive/ Screening Examination†	Birth to 18 Months	2 to 6 Years	7 to 12 Years	13 to 18 Years	19 to 39 Years	40 to 64 Years	65 Years and over
Sexually transmitted diseases (STDs)	VDRL/RPR				One time if sexually active	One time	One time	One time
	Chlamydial testing Gonorrhea culture HIV counseling and testing				+ + +	+ + +	+ + +	+ + +
Testicular/ prostate problems	Testicular self-examination (TSE)					Every month	Every month	Every month
	Professional examination					Every 5 years	Every 2 to 3 years between 40 and 50/then every year	Every year
Prostate cancer	Prostate specific antigen (PSA)						Every year between 50 to 70 years	

* Recommendations are subject to change, based on the most current information available. Recommendations in this table are based on guidelines from the American Academy of Family Physicians, the American Academy of Ophthalmology, the American Academy of Pediatrics, the American Cancer Society, the American College of Obstetricians and Gynecologists, the American College of Physicians, the National Cancer Institute, the National Heart, Lung, and Blood Institute, Centers for Disease Control and Prevention, and the U.S. Preventive Services Task Force.
† The list of preventive/screening services is not exhaustive nor are all services listed indicated for every client at every visit. Type and frequency of visits and services is determined by individual and family health history and personal habits.

DTP, diphtheria and tetanus toxoids combined with pertussis vaccine; DPV, oral polio vaccine; HBV, hepatitis B vaccine; Hib (or HbCV), *Haemophilus* b conjugate vaccine; HIV, human immunodeficiency virus; MMR, measles, mumps, and rubella vaccine; OPV, oral polio vaccine; RPR, rapid plasma reagin test for syphilis; VDRL, Venereal Disease Research Laboratory test (a test designed to detect syphilis); VZV, varicella zoster virus vaccine; +, ongoing preventive behavior (these items should be assessed during each contact with the client).

Included are the client's perception of stressors and their effect on the client.

Value-Belief Pattern. The value-belief pattern focuses on the values, beliefs (including spiritual), and goals that guide the client's choices and decisions, particularly in healthcare. Sources of strength and meaning for the client are identified.

Appendix B presents a health history interview guide organized according to functional health patterns including an ROS. Note areas already discussed and reduce repetitive questioning so as not to fatigue the client.

Recording the Health History Interview

Interview data are recorded in the client's record according to specific agency protocol. The format is organized and may be a narrative, outline, or checklist with written supplementary comments. All pertinent data (both positive and negative findings) are recorded. Data are clear, concise, comprehensive, and consistent, with no gaps or areas of ambiguity. The nurse uses approved agency abbreviations and terminology whenever possible to promote communication among healthcare team members.

Applying the Nursing Process to Health Assessment

In health assessment, the nurse seeks to gather as much data about the client as possible, both subjective and objective. These data are analyzed to determine the client's needs and responses to potential and actual health problems. The nurse considers the client's preferences when formulating nursing diagnoses that are amenable to intervention. Establishing realistic goals and outcome criteria and planning interventions follow in logical order, as Box 11-6 illustrates.

Conclusions

The health history is the first component of health assessment. The history constitutes the subjective data that guide the examiner to assess more fully specific client concerns or areas identified through health risk appraisal.

Box 11-6. Applying the Nursing Process to Health Assessment

Introduction

Mrs. L. is a 58-year-old, healthy-looking woman who visits a glaucoma screening booth at a health fair. The nurse integrates health assessment data and nursing process while talking to Mrs. L. and testing her visual acuity.

Biographical Data

Married. Works full time as a legal secretary. Has one married child who lives out of state.

Physical Health History

History negative for significant health problems. Postmenopausal. Reports seeing rings around lights and decreased side vision most noticeable when reading.

Health Risk Appraisal

Mother had cataracts. Family history positive for hypertension. Nearsighted since age 10 and wears corrective lenses. Last eye examination 5 years ago. Has smoked one pack of cigarettes per day for 40 years.

Physical Examination

Snellen chart results (with corrective lenses) are O.D. = 20/40, O.S. = 20/30, O.U. = 20/30. Visual fields to confrontation reveal superior fields less than those of the examiner. Pupils react sluggishly to accommodation. Further physical examination limited because of setting.

Nursing Diagnosis

High risk for altered health maintenance related to visual changes (decreased visual acuity and peripheral vision), family history of hypertension, and smoking history.

Expected Outcomes

Long Term

Mrs. L. will maintain present visual acuity and prevent further loss of vision.

Short Term

1. Mrs. L. will verbalize understanding of the need for an immediate, complete ophthalmologic examination.
2. Mrs. L. will identify an ophthalmologist whom she will contact no later than tomorrow for an appointment.

Intervention

1. Discuss results of visual screening with Mrs. L. and their significance.
2. Explain risk factors for glaucoma and Mrs. L.'s risk profile.
3. Assist Mrs. L. to choose an ophthalmologist.
4. Provide Mrs. L. with pamphlets about glaucoma from the National Society to Prevent Blindness.
5. Give Mrs. L. a self-addressed, stamped postcard that is to be returned by the ophthalmologist after the first visit.

Evaluation

Long Term

Ask Mrs. L. to restate her understanding of the need to have regular visual check-ups by an ophthalmologist and to follow the recommended medical regimen for eye care.

Short Term

Ask Mrs. L. whom she plans to contact for an eye appointment and when she intends to do this.

The history can be recorded in many ways, such as through computerized database assessments or on paper. Although a thorough history may seem time consuming, the data provided are crucial to fully understanding the client and his or her special needs.

Bibliography

1. Alfaro, R. (1994). *Applying nursing process: A step-by-step guide* (3rd ed.). Philadelphia: J. B. Lippincott.
2. Allen, P. T. (1986). Screening. In C. Edelman & C. L. Mandel (Eds.), *Health promotion throughout the lifespan* (pp. 142–158). St. Louis: C. V. Mosby.
3. American Academy of Pediatrics. (1988). *Guidelines for health supervision II* (2nd ed.). Elk Grove Village, IL: Author.
4. American Medical Association. (1983). Medical evaluations of healthy persons (Report of the Council on Scientific Affairs). *JAMA, 249,* 1626–1633.
5. American Nurses Association. (1994). *Clinician's handbook of preventive services: Put prevention into practice.* Waldorf, MD: Author.
6. Andresen, G. P. (1992). How to assess the older mind. *RN, 55*(6), 34.
7. Bamberg, R., et al. (1989). The effect of risk assessment in conjunction with health promotion education on compliance with preventive behaviors. *Journal of Allied Health, 18*(3), 271–280.
8. Barkauskas, V. H., et al. (1994). *Health and physical assessment.* St. Louis: Mosby–Year Book.
9. Barry, P. D. (1989). *Psychosocial nursing assessment and intervention: Care of the physically ill person* (2nd ed.). Philadelphia: J. B. Lippincott.
10. Bernstein, L., & Bernstein, R. S. (1985). *Interviewing—A guide for health professionals* (4th ed.). Norwalk, CT: Appleton-Century-Crofts.
11. Bonheur, B., & Young, S. (1991). Exercise as a health-promoting lifestyle choice. *Applied Nursing Research, 4,* 2.
12. Braverman, B. G. (1990). Eliciting assessment data from the patient who is difficult to interview. *Nursing Clinics of North America, 25,* 743–750.
13. Brennan, P. F., & Romano, C. A. (1987). Computers and nursing diagnoses: Issues in implementation. *Nursing Clinics of North America, 22,* 935–941.
14. Breslow, L., & Somers, A. (1977). The lifetime health monitoring program. *New England Journal of Medicine, 296,* 601–608.
15. Brink, P. (1984). Value orientations as an assessment tool in cultural diversity. *Nursing Research, 35,* 198.
16. Brink, P. J. (1987). Cultural aspects of sexuality. *Holistic Nursing Practice, 1,* 12–20.
17. Burnard, P. (1988). Discussing spiritual issues with clients. *Health Vision, 61*(12), 371–372.
18. Cameron, C. T., & McNeil, E. L. (1976). The importance of history. *Journal of Emergency Nursing, 2*(3), 21–22.
19. Carpenito, L. J. (1995). *Nursing diagnosis: Application to clinical practice* (6th ed.). Philadelphia: J. B. Lippincott.
20. Carson, V. B. (1989). *Spiritual dimensions of nursing practice.* Philadelphia: W. B. Saunders.
21. Clark, C. C. (1986). *Wellness nursing: Concepts, theory, research, and practice.* New York: Springer-Verlag Publishing.
22. Cox, H. C., et al. (1993). *Clinical applications of nursing diagnosis: Adult, child, women's, psychiatric, gerontic, and home health considerations.* (2nd ed.). Philadelphia: F. A. Davis.
23. Diaz-Duque, O. F. (1982). Advice from an interpreter. *American Journal of Nursing, 82*(9), 1380–1382.
24. Dirckx, J. H. (1985). Talking with patients, the art of history taking. *Clinical Nurse Practitioner, 3,* 13–14.
25. Dudek, S. G. (1993). *Nutrition handbook for nursing practice* (2nd ed.). Philadelphia: J. B. Lippincott.
26. Fuller, J., & Schaller-Ayers, J. (1994). *Health assessment: A nursing approach* (2nd ed.) Philadelphia: J. B. Lippincott.
27. Geissler, E. M. (1994). *Pocket guide to cultural assessment.* St. Louis: C. V. Mosby.
28. Giger, J., & Davidhizar, R. (1995). *Transcultural nursing: Assessment and intervention* (2nd ed.). St. Louis: Mosby–Year Book.
29. Gordon, M. (1994). *Nursing diagnosis: Process and application* (3rd ed.). New York: McGraw-Hill.
30. Grasska, M. A., & McFarland, T. (1982). Overcoming the language barrier: Problems and solutions. *American Journal of Nursing, 82*(9), 1376–1379.
31. Grossman, D. (1994). Enhancing your "cultural competence." *American Journal of Nursing, 94*(7), 58–62.
32. Halloran, E. J. (1988). Computerized nurse assessments. *Nursing and Health Care, 9,* 497–499.
33. Hays, A. (1984). The set test to screen mental status quickly. *Geriatric Nursing, 5,* 96–97.
34. Helman, C. (1990). *Culture, health and illness.* Boston: Wright.
35. Hill, L. H., & Smith, N. (1990). *Self-care nursing: Promotion of health* (2nd ed.). Norwalk, CT: Appleton & Lange.
36. Holmberg, S. (1988). Physical health problems of the psychiatric client. *Journal of Psychosocial Nursing, 26*(5), 35–39.
37. Jarvis, C. (1996). *Physical examination and health assessment.* (2nd ed.). Philadelphia: W. B. Saunders.
38. Lipson, J., & Melies, A. (1985). Culturally appropriate care: The case of immigrants. *Topics in Clinical Nursing, 7*(3), 48–56.
39. Longo, D. C., & Williams, R. A. (1986). *Clinical practice in psychosocial nursing: Assessment and intervention* (2nd ed.). Norwalk, CT: Appleton-Century-Crofts.
40. McConnell, S. D., Inderbitzin, L. B., & Pollard, W. E. (1992). Primary health care in the CMHC: A role for the nurse practitioner. *Hospital and Community Psychiatry, 43,* 724–727.
41. Morton, P. G. (1993). *Health assessment in nursing* (2nd ed.). Springhouse, PA: Springhouse.
42. Murray, R. B., & Zentner, J. P. (1993). *Nursing assessment and health promotion: Strategies through the life span* (5th ed.). Norwalk, CT: Appleton & Lange.
43. North American Nursing Diagnosis Association (NANDA). (1994). *Classification of nursing diagnoses: Proceedings of the 10th conference.* St. Louis: Author.
44. Overfield, T. (1985). *Biologic variation in health and illness: Race, age, and sex differences.* Menlo Park, CA: Addison-Wesley.
45. Pender, N. J. (1987). *Health promotion in nursing practice* (2nd ed.). Norwalk, CT: Appleton & Lange.
46. Pulsch, R. W. (1985). Cross-cultural interpreters in health care. *JAMA, 254*(23), 3344–3348.
47. *Quick reference to cultural assessment.* (1994). St. Louis: Mosby–Year Book.
48. Rahe, R. H. (1975). Life changes and near-future illness reports. In L. Levi (Ed.), *Emotions: Their parameters and measurement.* New York: Raven Press.
49. Saba, V. K. (1988). Taming the computer jungle of NISs. *Nursing and Health Care, 9,* 487–491.
50. Schneiderman, H. (1982, June). The review of systems, an important part of comprehensive examination. *Postgraduate Medicine, 71,* 151–158.
51. Selleck, K. J. (1991). Nurses' interpersonal behavior and the development of helping skills. *International Journal of Nursing Studies, 28*(1), 3–11.
52. Sparks, S. M., & Taylor, C. M. (1991). *Nursing diagnosis reference manual.* Springhouse, PA: Springhouse.
53. Spillane, R. K. (1987). Getting the patient's point of view—Early. *Nursing Manager, 18*(5), 20–28.
54. Spradley, B. W. (1990). *Community health nursing: Concepts and practice.* Glenview, IL: Scott, Foresman.
55. Tom, C. K. (1976). Nursing assessment of biological rhythms. *Nursing Clinics of North America, 11,* 621–630.
56. Topf, M. (1988). Verbal interpersonal responsiveness. *Journal of Psychosocial Nursing, 26*(7), 8–16.
57. U. S. Preventive Services Task Force. (1989). *Guide to clinical preventive services: An assessment of the effectiveness of 169 interventions.* Baltimore: Williams & Wilkins.
58. Utz, S. (1990). Motivating self-care: A nursing approach. *Holistic Nursing Practice, 4*(2), 13–21.
59. Wenger, A. F. Z. (1993). Cultural meaning of symptoms. *Holistic Nursing Practice, 7*(2), 22–35.
60. Werner, J. S., & O'Neill, S. E. (1992). Nursing assessment and role in stress management. In S. M. Lewis & I. C. Collier (Eds.), *Medical-surgical nursing: Assessment and management of clinical problems* (3rd ed.). St. Louis: Mosby–Year Book.

Physical Examination

Annabelle M. Keene

The physical examination follows the health history interview. Physical examination skills require use of the ears, eyes, and senses of touch and smell. Repeated practice is necessary to learn how to integrate these skills into the nursing repertoire. The nurse learns the techniques and correct use of the equipment, as well as to discriminate normal from abnormal findings.

Objective data are collected systematically during the physical examination to supplement and validate the client's subjective data. The nurse's ability to perceive the client as a whole person is enhanced when both subjective and objective data are evaluated together. It is customary for the nurse to ask the client questions about abnormal physical findings. For example, if a mass is found during palpation, the nurse asks the client if the area is tender to the touch. The client's reply is recorded in the physical examination portion of the database (e.g., "nontender") even though it is an item of subjective data. If the nurse is palpating a lump or mass that the client did not report initially during the history interview, the nurse asks if the client is aware of the mass's existence. If the client knows the mass is present or admits to related symptoms, the nurse proceeds with a complete symptom analysis (see Chapter 11). These subjective data are recorded as part of the health history.

Physical examination is a skill used by nurses in all types of settings. Health fairs, screening clinics, physicians' offices, independent practice clinics, home healthcare, and hospitals are just some of the areas where nurses use physical examination skills to assess clients' health. The extent and depth of the physical examination are determined by the client's needs. For example, a home health nurse visits a client who has had total hip replacement surgery. During the first home visit, the nurse assesses the client to obtain baseline data. During subsequent visits, the nurse will use the initial assessment findings to guide the evaluation of the client's progress, for example, increased mobility and strength in the operative leg. Likewise, a coronary care unit nurse conducts periodic physical examinations of a client after a

myocardial infarction to assess for life-threatening complications.

The Purpose of Physical Examination

The purpose of physical examination is to differentiate normal from abnormal physical findings. The nurse must have a thorough understanding of basic anatomy (structure) and physiology (function) as a foundation. From this foundation, skill and expertise develop, which enable the nurse to appreciate the wide range of findings that are considered "normal."

In addition to collecting baseline data, physical assessment skills are used to make clinical judgments about a client's health status and evaluate the effectiveness of healthcare interventions. The examples of the home healthcare and coronary care clients illustrate this point.

Types of Physical Examination

Several types, or levels, of physical examination are performed, depending on the client's needs. A *screening physical examination* is an organized, superficial check of the major body systems for detecting abnormalities or possible problems. If the nurse detects a problem, the focus of the examination is directed to a *regional or branching examination,* which is an in-depth assessment of a specific body system. This chapter presents information that allows the nurse to perform a screening adult physical examination. Table 12–1 directs the reader to the assessments that are performed during regional examinations. Regional examinations are discussed further in

Text continued on page 225

Table 12–1. Assessments Performed During Regional Examinations

Assessment Area	Client Position or Activity*	Technique†	Equipment	What to Observe
1. General survey	▲ Standing and walking during entrance (a, c) ▲ Sitting during health history interview (a, c) ▲ Changing into examining gown (a, c, f) ▲ Walking to examining table (a, b, c, d, f) ▲ Sitting on edge of examining table (a, c, e, f)	▲ Inspection (a, b, c, d, e, f) ▲ Olfaction (a)		a. General appearance and behavior; apparent age; sex; race; general state of health; signs of distress; body build; posture; gait; obvious deformity; movements and gross ROM; skin color and texture of exposed areas; dress, hygiene, and grooming; body or breath odor; mental status (expression, affect, speech, memory, eye contact); level of consciousness; level of cooperation
			b. Balance scale with height measure	b. Height and weight measurements
				c. Balance, coordination (Romberg's test, arm drift)
			d. Snellen chart	d. Visual acuity (CN II)
			e. Thermometer; watch with second hand; sphygmomanometer; stethoscope	e. Vital signs: temperature; pulse; respirations; blood pressure, including check for auscultatory gap
			f. Tape measure; skinfold calipers	f. Nutritional status: body frame (wrist circumference); MAC; TSF; MAMC; IBW
2. Head and neck	▲ Sitting on edge of examining table (a, b, c, d, e, f, g)	▲ Inspection (a, b, c, d, e, f, g) ▲ Palpation (a, b, c, d, e, f, g) ▲ Percussion (e) ▲ Auscultation (a, f, g) ▲ Olfaction (a, f)		a. Head
			(1) Tape measure	(1) Inspect and palpate: skull size, shape, symmetry, contour, tenderness, lesions; measure circumference if abnormal size
				(2) Inspect hair and scalp: color, integrity; hair distribution and texture; presence of nits or lice; hygiene
			(3) Stethoscope	(3) Palpate temporal arteries: thickening, tenderness; auscultate for bruits if abnormality noted; rate amplitude
				b. Face
				(1) Inspect symmetry, skin color, hair distribution; facial movements (CN V and VII): clenched jaws, puffed cheeks, raised eyebrows, frown, eyelid strength
				(2) Palpate TMJ; temporal and masseter muscles (CN V); nodules
			(3) Cotton wisp; sterile safety pin	(3) Test facial sensation for light touch, pressure and pain (CN V) over forehead, cheeks, and jaw

214

c. *Eyes*

(1) Visual acuity, if not performed earlier (CN II)

(2) Visual fields (peripheral vision) by confrontation method (CN II)

(3) EOMs through six cardinal positions of gaze (CN III, IV, VI, VIII)

(4) Convergence and accommodation (CN III, IV, VI)

(5) Cover/uncover test (CN III, IV, VI) for movement

(6) Corneal light reflex (CN III, IV, VI) for alignment (Hirschberg's test)

(7) Inspect and palpate external eye structures:

  (a) Eyebrows' symmetry, alignment

  (b) Eyelashes' symmetry, hair distribution, direction of growth

  (c) Eyelids' position, skin characteristics, blinking

  (d) Lacrimal apparatus function

  (e) Eyeballs' symmetry, firmness

  (f) Conjunctivae and sclerae color, texture, lesions, foreign bodies

  (g) Corneas' texture, transparency; corneal reflex (CN V); omit corneal reflex testing if blinking intact

  (h) Anterior chambers' transparency, depth

  (i) Irises' and pupils' symmetry, color, size, reaction to light and accommodation (CN III, IV, VI)

(8) Inspect internal eye structures: red reflex, retina, retinal vessels, optic disc, macula, fovea

d. *Ears*

(1) Inspect and palpate external ear structures:

  (a) Auricles' symmetry, placement, skin integrity, color, mobility, tenderness over tragus

  (b) Ear canals' skin integrity, cerumen, obstruction, foreign body, discharge

  (c) Tympanic membranes' symmetry, color, light reflection, landmarks, scars, fluid

(2) Hearing acuity: response to normal conversation, whisper test, Weber's test for sound lateralization, Rinne's test for air and bone conduction of sound (CN VIII)

---

(1) Snellen chart; eye cover

(2) Eye cover; penlight or pen

(3) Penlight or pen

(4) Penlight or pen

(5) Eye cover

(6) Penlight

(7) Penlight; cotton wisp; cotton applicator

(8) Ophthalmoscope

(1) Otoscope

(2) Tuning fork (512 Hz)

Table continued on following page

Table 12–1. Assessments Performed During Regional Examinations (Continued)

Assessment Area	Client Position or Activity*	Technique†	Equipment	What to Observe
				e. *Nose and sinuses*
				(1) Inspect and palpate external nose alignment, symmetry; skin color, lesions, tenderness, discharge, nasal flaring, patency
			(2) Penlight	(2) Inspect vestibules' color, mucous membrane, septum alignment
			(3) Nasal speculum and penlight; or otoscope head with nasal speculum	(3) Inspect nares' mucosa for color, moisture; septum for alignment, masses, perforation; turbinates for color, exudate, inflammation
				(4) Palpate and percuss frontal and maxillary sinuses for swelling and tenderness
			(5) Penlight or transilluminator	(5) Transilluminate frontal and maxillary sinuses if client reports a problem
			(6) Various substances to smell (coffee grounds, cinnamon, cloves, peppermint)	(6) Sense of smell (CN I) not usually tested, but if done, test with coffee grounds, cinnamon, cloves, peppermint
			f. Gloves; tongue blade; penlight	f. *Mouth and pharynx*
				(1) Inspect and palpate lips and oral mucosa for color, symmetry, texture, hydration, lesions, Stensen's ducts
				(2) Inspect teeth and gums and palpate gums for state of repair, hygiene, teeth alignment, missing teeth, gum bleeding, gum integrity
				(3) Inspect and palpate tongue and floor of mouth for symmetry, color, tongue position and size, texture, mobility, lesions, presence of papillae
				(4) Tongue mobility and strength (CN IX, XII)
				(5) Inspect Wharton's duct under tongue, floor of mouth, and base of tongue for lesions
				(6) Inspect roof of mouth, palates, and uvula for color, symmetry, texture, bone deformity
				(7) Test rise of uvula and soft palate with phonation (CN X)
				(8) Inspect tonsils and pillars for color, size, shape
				(9) Inspect pharynx for color, discharge on posterior wall

Body region	Techniques	Equipment	Position	Procedure
				(10) Test gag reflex (CN IX, X) if swallowing impairment reported or noted
				(11) Note characteristics of voice, ability to swallow (CN IX, X)
				(12) Note presence of breath odor
		(13) Various substances to taste (sugar, salt, lemon juice, bitters)		(13) Test sense of taste (CN VII, IX) only if abnormality reported with sugar, salt, lemon juice, bitters
				g. Neck
				(1) Inspect neck muscles' symmetry, ROM, strength (CN XI); shoulder shrug
				(2) Palpate and inspect over parotid and submandibular salivary glands for swelling, tenderness
				(3) Palpate all cervical lymph nodes
				(4) Inspect and palpate trachea for symmetry and alignment
		(5) Stethoscope		(5) Inspect and palpate thyroid gland for symmetry, masses; auscultate for bruits if enlarged
		(6) Stethoscope		(6) Inspect and palpate carotid arteries; rate amplitude; auscultate for bruits
				(7) Inspect jugular venous distention
3. Upper extremities and spine	▲ Inspection (a, b) ▲ Palpation (a) ▲ Percussion (b)		▲ Sitting on edge of examining table (a, b)	**a. Upper extremities**
				(1) Inspect skin for lesions and palpate turgor
				(2) Inspect limbs for alignment and symmetry
				(3) Inspect fingernails and blanch to test capillary refill; inspect for clubbing
				(4) Palpate peripheral pulses: brachial, radial, ulnar; rate amplitude
				(5) Palpate epitrochlear lymph nodes
		(6) Tape measure		(6) Inspect and palpate muscle groups for size, symmetry, tone; measure if they appear unequal
				(7) Evaluate and rate muscle strength: upper arms, forearms, wrists, fingers
				(8) Inspect and palpate joints for swelling and tenderness, crepitus
		(9) Goniometer		(9) Assess ROM: shoulders, elbows, wrists, fingers; measure ROM if limitation noted
				b. Spine
		(1) Reflex hammer		(1) Test DTRs and rate response: biceps, triceps, brachioradialis; test lower extremity DTRs: patellar, Achilles, and plantar cutaneous reflexes
				(2) Assess cerebellar functions: finger-to-finger; hand supination and pronation; finger-to-thumb opposition

Table continued on following page

Table 12–1. Assessments Performed During Regional Examinations *(Continued)*

Assessment Area	Client Position or Activity*	Technique†	Equipment	What to Observe
4. Posterior thorax	▲ Sitting on edge of examining table; nurse stands behind client (a, b, c)	▲ Inspection (a, b) ▲ Palpation (a, b) ▲ Percussion (a, b, c) ▲ Auscultation (b)		a. *Spine, ribs, muscles* (1) Inspect spine for alignment; palpate spine processes for tenderness; inspect skin integrity (2) Inspect rib cage for symmetry, shape, movement with respiration (3) Measure anteroposterior-to-lateral diameter (4) Inspect and lightly palpate paravertebral muscles for tenderness, spasm (5) Assess thoracic expansion (respiratory excursion) b. *Lungs* (1) Observe respiratory pattern (2) Palpate tactile fremitus and respiratory excursion (3) Percuss posterior and lateral thorax and diaphragmatic excursion (4) Measure diaphragmatic excursion (5) Auscultate breath sounds, posterior and lateral thorax (6) Auscultate voice sounds if fremitus abnormal (bronchophony, egophony, whispered pectoriloquy) c. *Kidneys* Percuss over CVAs for kidney tenderness
			(4) Ruler and pen (5) Stethoscope (6) Stethoscope	
5. Anterior thorax	▲ Sitting on edge of examining table; nurse stands on right side of client (a, b, c, d, e) ▲ Sitting up and leaning forward (b, e) ▲ Sitting with arms at sides; with hands on hips; with arms raised over head (e) ▲ Supine, arm behind head (e) ▲ Supine, head elevated 30 degrees (f, g) ▲ Left lateral recumbent (f)	▲ Inspection (a, b, c, d, e, f, g) ▲ Palpation (a, b, e, f) ▲ Percussion (a) ▲ Auscultation (a, b, c, f)		a. *Lungs and thorax* (1) Inspect skin integrity (2) Observe respiratory pattern (3) Inspect rib cage for symmetry, movement with respiration, shape, use of accessory muscles (4) Palpate respiratory excursion (5) Palpate tactile fremitus (6) Percuss anterior thorax (7) Auscultate breath sounds and voice sounds (if fremitus abnormal) b. *Heart* (1) Inspect precordium for lifts, heaves, apical impulse (2) Inspect epigastrium for aortic pulsations (3) Palpate precordium for thrills, apical impulse, lift, heaves
			(7) Stethoscope	

(4) Auscultate heart sounds with client sitting up, then leaning forward

(5) Assess heart rate and rhythm

c. *Carotid vessels*

(1) Auscultate for bruits

(2) Rate amplitude if not done during neck examination

d. *Jugular veins*

Inspect for distention

e. *Breasts and axillae*

(1) Inspect breasts in 3 positions for size, shape, symmetry, contour, skin characteristics, lesions

(2) Inspect areolae and nipples for size, shape, color, contour, symmetry, lesions

(3) Inspect axillae for rashes, masses, lesions, pigmentation

(4) Palpate axillae for lymph nodes

(5) Palpate breasts for lumps, masses, consistency

▲ **Assist client to supine position**

(6) Palpate breasts, areolae, and nipples with client supine and arm behind head

f. *Heart*

(1) Inspect precordium for lifts, heaves, apical impulse

(2) Inspect epigastrium for aortic pulsations

(3) Palpate precordium for thrills, lifts, heaves, apical impulse

(4) Auscultate heart sounds with client supine, then in left lateral recumbent position

g. *Jugular veins*

(1) Inspect for level of venous distention with client's head elevated 30 to 45 degrees; measure level of distention between angle of Louis and angle of jaw

(2) Assess for hepatojugular reflux if right ventricular failure suspected

a. *Abdomen (general)*

(1) Inspect skin integrity and characteristics: striae, venous pattern, hair distribution

(2) Inspect contour, symmetry, umbilicus, pulsations, peristalsis, rectus muscles with straining; measure girth if distention noted

(3) Auscultate all quadrants for bowel sounds

(4) Stethoscope

(5) Stethoscope

(1) Stethoscope

(4) Stethoscope

(2) Tape measure

(3) Stethoscope

▲ Inspection (a, i, j)
▲ Auscultation (a)
▲ Percussion (a, b, c, h, j)
▲ Palpation (a, b, d, e, f, g, h)

▲ Supine with arms relaxed at sides or crossed over chest; may have knees flexed slightly (a, b, c, d, e, f, i)
▲ Turned to right lateral recumbent (g, h)

6. Abdomen

Table continued on following page

Table 12–1. Assessments Performed During Regional Examinations *(Continued)*

Assessment Area	Client Position or Activity*	Technique†	Equipment	What to Observe
			(4) Stethoscope	(4) Auscultate major vessels for bruits: abdominal aorta; renal, iliac, and femoral arteries
			(5) Stethoscope	(5) Auscultate over epigastrium for venous hum
			(6) Stethoscope	(6) Auscultate over liver and spleen for peritoneal friction rub
				(7) Percuss all quadrants for masses, tenderness, gastric bubble; over bladder and spleen
				(8) Blunt percussion over anterior right (liver) and left (spleen) lower rib margins for tenderness
				(9) Lightly palpate all quadrants for masses, tenderness
				(10) Deep palpation for masses and tenderness, all quadrants
				(11) Assess rebound tenderness over RLQ and LLQ
				b. *Liver*
			(1) Pen	(1) Percuss liver size at RMCL and MSL and mark borders
			(2) Ruler	(2) Measure liver span at RMCL and MSL
				c. *Spleen*
				(1) Percuss spleen size
				(2) Percuss for splenic enlargement if indicated
				d. *Aorta*
				Palpate for area of pulsation in epigastrium
				e. *Inguinal areas*
				(1) Palpate femoral arteries and rate amplitude
				(2) Palpate inguinal lymph nodes; note characteristics
				f. *Liver*
				Palpate for size, masses, nodules
				g. *Spleen*
				Palpate for size if enlargement suspected
				h. *Kidneys*
				(1) Palpate right and left kidneys for enlargement
				(2) Blunt percussion over CVAs (posterior thorax) for tenderness if not done earlier

Assessment	Position	Technique	Equipment
7. Lower extremities and spine	▲ Supine with arms relaxed (a, b) ▲ Prone if needed to assess popliteal lymph nodes (a)	▲ Inspection (a, b) ▲ Palpation (a) ▲ Percussion (b)	i. Tongue blade
8. General neurologic and spine	▲ Supine with arms at sides, eyes closed (a) ▲ Walking heel to toe (b) ▲ Walking on toes, then heels (b) ▲ Hopping on each foot (b) ▲ Knee bends (b) ▲ Standing with arms relaxed at sides (c)	▲ Inspection (a, b, c)	

Detailed procedures:

i. *Abdominal reflexes*
Assess each quadrant for presence of reflex
j. Test for ascites if indicated
a. *Lower extremities*
(1) Inspect skin for lesions, hair distribution
(2) Inspect limbs for alignment and symmetry
(3) Inspect toenails and blanch to test capillary refill
(4) Palpate peripheral pulses: popliteal, posterior tibial, dorsalis pedis; rate amplitude
(5) Palpate popliteal lymph nodes
(6) Inspect for edema and palpate for pitting if present
(7) Palpate for phlebitis, varicosities; measure circumference of calves or thighs if phlebitis present — Tape measure
(8) Assess for presence of Homan's sign
(9) Inspect and palpate muscle groups for size, symmetry, tone; measure if appear unequal — Tape measure
(10) Evaluate and rate muscle strength: hips, hamstrings, quadriceps, ankles, toes, feet
(11) Inspect and palpate joints for swelling, tenderness, crepitus
(12) Assess ROM: hips, knees, ankles, feet, toes; measure ROM if limitation noted — Goniometer
b. *Spine*
(1) Test DTRs if not done before at time of upper extremity evaluation; test patellar, Achilles, and plantar cutaneous reflexes
(2) Assess cerebellar functions; ability to slide heel down opposite shin; foot tapping
a. *Sensory function*
(1) Test perception of light touch over symmetric dermatomes distally, then proximally; trunk, face, neck — Cotton wisp
(2) Test perception of pain vs. pressure over symmetric dermatomes distally, then proximally; trunk, face, neck — Sterile safety pin or needle
(3) Test perception of vibration distally on toes and fingers; progress proximally if abnormal — Tuning fork (128 Hz)
(4) Test position sense, fingers and toes
(5) Test object identification, both hands (stereognosis) — Key, coins, safety pin, paper clip
(6) Test graphism, both hands — Closed pen

Table continued on following page

Table 12–1. Assessments Performed During Regional Examinations (Continued)

Assessment Area	Client Position or Activity*	Technique†	Equipment	What to Observe
			(7) Two sterile safety pins	(7) Test two-point discrimination, both index fingers
			(8) Test tubes filled with hot water and cold water	(8) Test temperature perception only if pain perception is impaired: distally, then proximally; trunk, face, neck
			(9) Finger touch	(9) Test point localization and tactile localization (double simultaneous stimulation) only if light touch perception is impaired
				▶ Assist client to standing position
				b. *Gross motor and balance*
				(1) Inspect gait and balance while client walks heel to toe, then on toes, then on heels
				(2) Observe balance while client stands on one foot, then the other
				(3) Observe balance and lower extremity strength while client hops on one foot, then the other
				(4) Observe balance and strength while client performs shallow knee bends
				c. *Spine*
				(1) Inspect spine from anterior, lateral, and posterior views for kyphosis, lordosis, or scoliosis
				(2) Assess spine ROM
9A. Genitalia (male)	▶ Standing facing nurse (a, b, c, d, e, f, g, h, i) ▶ Standing and performing Valsalva's maneuver (g, h, i)	▶ Inspection (a, b, d, f, g) ▶ Palpation (c, e, h, i)	A. Gloves worn throughout	A. *Male genitalia* a. Inspect pubic hair and skin, hair distribution, rashes, lesions, parasites
			b. Culture medium	b. Inspect penis: shaft, prepuce, glans, urethral meatus; culture discharge if present
				c. Palpate penile shaft for nodules, tenderness
				d. Inspect scrotum for size, symmetry, shape, swelling
				e. Palpate scrotum for presence of testes, epididymis, vas deferens
			f. Transilluminator or flashlight	f. Transilluminate scrotum if swelling or mass palpated
				g. Inspect inguinal areas for hernia, first with client standing quietly, then during Valsalva's maneuver
				h. Palpate for direct inguinal hernia with client at rest and performing Valsalva's maneuver

Examination area	Position	Technique	Equipment	Procedure
				i. Palpate for indirect inguinal hernia with client at rest and performing Valsalva's maneuver
9B. Anus and rectum (male)	▲ Standing and bending over examining table (a, c, f, g) ▲ Standing and bending over examining table, performing Valsalva's maneuver (b, d, e)	▲ Inspection (a, b, g) ▲ Palpation (c, d, e, f)	B. Gloves worn throughout	B. *Anus and rectum (male)* a. Inspect perianal skin integrity, color, excoriation, rash, lesions, fissures, ulcers, hemorrhoids b. Inspect anal area for rectal prolapse, fissures, fistulas, inflammation, hemorrhoids, polyps with client performing Valsalva's maneuver
			c. Lubricant	c. Palpate anus, anal canal, sphincter tone, anorectal junction, rectal walls, coccyx with client at rest d. Palpate anal sphincter tone during Valsalva's maneuver e. Palpate for a descending rectal mass with client performing Valsalva's maneuver f. Palpate prostate gland: median sulcus, two lateral lobes
			g. Hemoccult test; culture medium	g. Inspect gloved finger as it is withdrawn for stool and test stool for occult blood; obtain rectal culture if indicated **▲ Female client is assisted to lithotomy or dorsal recumbent position**
10A. Genitalia (female)	▲ Lithotomy position if both external and internal genitalia examined (a, b, c, d, e, f, g, h, i, j, k, l, m, n) ▲ Dorsal recumbent if only external genitalia examined (a, b, c, d, e, f, g, h, i)	▲ Inspection (a, b, c, d, e, g, j, k) ▲ Palpation (f, h, i, l, m, n)	A. Gloves worn throughout	A. *Female genitalia* a. Inspect mons pubis; pubic hair distribution and texture; perineal skin for color, lesions, irritation, parasites b. Inspect labia majora edema, symmetry c. Inspect labia minora symmetry d. Inspect clitoris color, presence of lesions e. Inspect introitus and hymen f. Palpate Bartholin's glands if inflamed or enlarged for size, tenderness g. Inspect urethral meatus for discharge, inflammation, swelling
			h. Culture medium; change gloves if discharge present	h. Palpate Skene's glands for discharge and obtain specimen for culture if present i. Assess integrity of pelvic floor muscles: strength, presence of cystocele or rectocele, discharge of urine
			j. Vaginal speculum; light source; wooden spatula; cotton-tipped applicator; glass slides; fixative; culture medium	j. Insert vaginal speculum and inspect cervix; adjust light as needed; note shape, position, color, lesions, discharge; obtain cervical specimens if indicated: cervical scraping, endocervical swab, vaginal pool scraping

Table continued on following page

Table 12–1. Assessments Performed During Regional Examinations *(Continued)*

Assessment Area	Client Position or Activity*	Technique†	Equipment	What to Observe
				k. Inspect vagina as speculum is removed: color, rugae, mucosa
			l. Lubricant	l. Palpate vagina and cervix for nodules, masses; cervix position, mobility, consistency, tenderness
				m. Bimanually palpate pelvic structures (1) Uterus (anterior wall and fundus) for masses, tenderness, position (2) Ovary and adnexa for ovary size, masses, tenderness
			n. Change gloves if vaginal examination performed; lubricant	n. Rectovaginal palpation of uterus for masses, position, tenderness
10B. Anus and rectum (female)	▲ Lithotomy position if done at same time as internal genitalia examination (a, b, c, d, e, g) ▲ Dorsal recumbent if done after external genitalia examination (a, b, c, d, e, f, g) ▲ Performing Valsalva's maneuver (b, d, e)	▲ Inspection (a, b, g) ▲ Palpation (c, d, e, f)	B. Gloves worn throughout	B. *Anus and rectum (female)* a. Inspect perianal skin integrity, color, excoriation, rash, lesions, fissures, ulcers, hemorrhoids
				b. Inspect anal area for rectal prolapse, fissures, fistulas, inflammation, hemorrhoids, polyps with client performing Valsalva's maneuver
			c. Lubricant	c. Palpate anus, anal canal, sphincter tone, anorectal junction, rectal walls, coccyx with client at rest
				d. Palpate anal sphincter tone during Valsalva's maneuver
				e. Palpate for a descending rectal mass with client performing Valsalva's maneuver
				f. Palpate cervix through anterior rectal wall for shape, position, mobility, tenderness
			g. Hemoccult; culture medium	g. Inspect gloved finger as it is withdrawn for stool and test stool for occult blood; obtain rectal culture if indicated
11. Examination complete	▲ Sitting			After removal of finger, assist client to clean perineum and to sit comfortably before leaving to allow client to dress

*Letters in parentheses after the client position or activity denote what the nurse observes.

†Letters in parentheses after technique denote when the nurse uses these skills to assist observations.

CN, cranial nerve; CVAs, costovertebral angles; DTRs, deep tendon reflexes; EOMs, extraocular movements; IBW, ideal body weight; LLQ, left lower quadrant; MAC, midarm circumference; MAMC, midarm muscle circumference; MSL, midsternal line; RLQ, right lower quadrant; RMCL, right midclavicular line; ROM, range of motion; TMJ, temporomandibular joint; TSF, triceps skinfold thickness.

the assessment chapters in each of the following units covering specific body systems. A *complete physical examination* includes ancillary examinations and procedures such as x-ray studies and clinical laboratory tests and is beyond the scope of this text.

In the clinical setting, *periodic head-to-toe assessment* is done to update baseline data and to assess for changes in the client's health status. The nurse individualizes the extent of examination for each major body system according to the client's needs. For example, a client with a CNS problem may be assessed using the Glasgow Coma Scale in addition to the rest of the head-to-toe evaluation (see Chapter 30 for discussion of this neurologic assessment tool). A client with intact neurologic function would not require this depth of assessment. An example of a head-to-toe periodic assessment guide is found in Box 12–1.

The Accuracy of Physical Examination

The physical examination helps to validate data collected during the health history interview. As with the health history, the nurse strives to collect accurate, thorough physical data. If difficulty is encountered while a physical assessment technique is performed or if the accuracy of a finding is questionable, the nurse consults with colleagues. A second opinion or evaluation of the client may be needed to obtain accurate data.

Physical Examination and the Nursing Process

An accurate database is essential to the formulation of individualized nursing diagnoses. It may be misleading for the nurse to diagnose a problem on the basis of one assessment finding. Significant findings (i.e., data that are either abnormal or indicate a potential risk) cue the nurse to collect additional information. A complete assessment is necessary before data are grouped into patterns and the etiologic basis is determined. The initial physical assessment is the baseline for the client's functional ability. Physical assessment is also used as intervention (e.g., monitoring lung sounds) and to evaluate changes in the client's physical condition and determine whether expected outcomes have been achieved.

Techniques of Physical Examination

Four primary techniques are used in physical assessment: inspection, palpation, percussion, and auscultation. These techniques enhance the data collected by the ears, eyes, and senses of touch and smell and are employed as indicated when each body region is examined (Fig. 12–1).

Box 12–1. Head-to-Toe Periodic Assessment Guide

1. Vital signs: Temperature, pulse, respirations, blood pressure
2. Pain: Location, type, quality, intensity
3. Neurologic: Orientation (person, place, time, situation,), level of consciousness, gait, extremity color, movement, sensation (CMS); pupillary responses to light
4. Pulmonary: Respiratory pattern and effort; breath sounds; cough quality; sputum production, color, and quantity
5. Cardiovascular: Heart sounds and rhythm, pulses (radial, dorsalis pedis, and right and left posterior tibial), capillary refill, edema (location and amount), skin color and temperature
6. Gastrointestinal: Oral assessment, abdominal appearance, bowel sounds, bowel elimination pattern
7. Genitourinary: Bladder distention, voiding pattern
8. Integument: Skin integrity, wounds, dressings, drainage
9. Psychosocial: Sociability, affect, anxiety, attitude

NOTE: Perform additional assessments according to the client's specific health status and needs.

Inspection

Inspection is the systematic, deliberate visual examination of the entire client or a region. Inspection yields information about size, shape, color, texture, symmetry, position, and deformities. It is the first technique of examination and begins at the outset of the client-nurse interaction. For example, the nurse inspects the facial skin while collecting the history. Inspection is important and is completed before progressing to the hands-on techniques of palpation, percussion, or auscultation.

Inspection is conducted in a well-lighted setting. The body region or part being inspected is uncovered sufficiently to permit complete visualization while the rest of the client's body is draped to preserve standards of modesty and client comfort. During inspection, the nurse compares what is observed with the known parameters of normal findings in clients of similar age, sex, race, and ethnicity.

Inspection is enhanced by the use of special instruments such as a penlight, oto-ophthalmoscope, and various specula (e.g., nasal and vaginal) that permit visual access to body cavities and orifices (Fig. 12–2). Other equipment used during inspection includes tongue blades, marking pen, ruler, tape measure, skinfold calipers, goniometer, and eye charts.

Palpation

Palpation, generally the second technique of physical assessment, is the use of touch. During palpation, varying

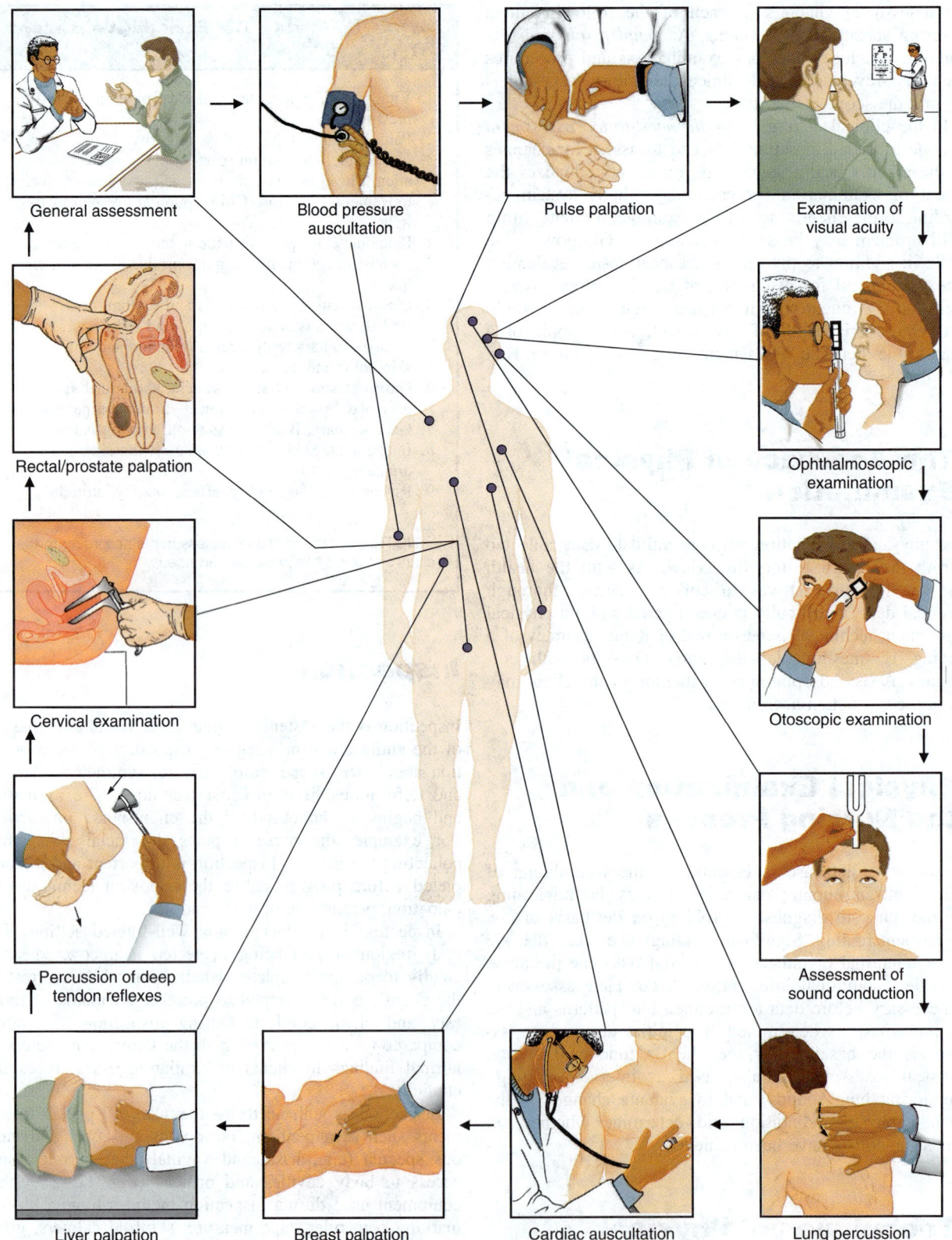

General assessment

Blood pressure auscultation

Pulse palpation

Examination of visual acuity

Rectal/prostate palpation

Ophthalmoscopic examination

Cervical examination

Otoscopic examination

Percussion of deep tendon reflexes

Assessment of sound conduction

Liver palpation

Breast palpation

Cardiac auscultation

Lung percussion

Figure 12–1. Common techniques of physical assessment used in a head-to-toe screening examination. Note that the examiner wears gloves for the pelvic, rectal, and prostate examinations.

amounts of pressure are exerted to determine information about masses, pulsation, organ size, tenderness or pain, swelling, tissue firmness and elasticity, vibration, crepitation, temperature, variation in texture, and moisture. In

addition, palpation is used to assess masses for position, size, shape, consistency, and mobility.

The nurse uses the most sensitive parts of the hands and fingers to palpate specific characteristics. For exam-

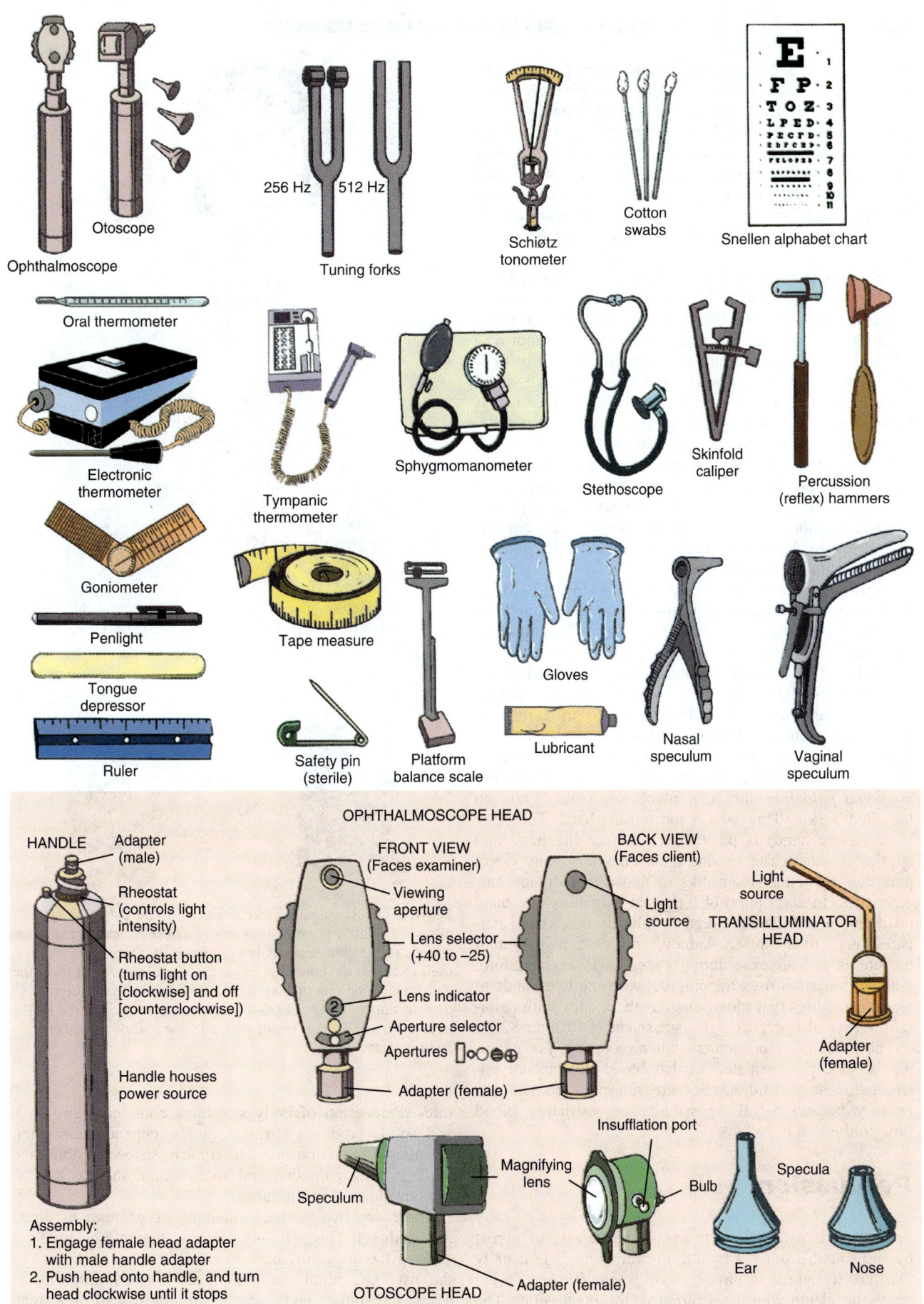

Figure 12–2. Special instruments used in physical examination.

ple, the *fingertips or pads* are the most sensitive for fine touch and are used to palpate pulses, lymph nodes, and breast tissue. The *dorsum,* or back of the hand and fingers, is used to discriminate skin temperature. The *palmar surface* of the hand over the metacarpophalangeal joints and *ulnar aspect* are used to assess vibration of the lung with vocalization (tactile fremitus). Position, consistency, mobility, size, shape, and skin turgor are assessed by lightly grasping tissue between the *thumb and index finger.*

Palpation is facilitated when the client is relaxed and comfortably positioned. Muscle tension is minimized, which lessens the possibility of the nurse's mistaking such tension for muscle rigidity. Relaxation is improved by having warm hands and short fingernails and using a gentle approach. Encouraging the client to take slow, deep breaths also assists relaxation. Tactile pressure is applied and increased gradually. Prolonged pressure decreases sensitivity in the palpating hand.

The client is asked to indicate tender areas before the nurse palpates. Tender areas are palpated last while the nurse observes the client for nonverbal signs of discomfort or pain. The nurse examines these areas, but this may result in discomfort for the client and reluctance to continue with examination.

Palpation proceeds from light to deep (Fig. 12–3). In *light palpation,* the underlying tissue is depressed approximately 1 to 2 cm (½ to ¾ inch). After light palpation, the nurse uses deep palpation to determine the size and condition of underlying structures such as abdominal organs. For *deep palpation,* the nurse depresses the underlying tissue approximately 4 to 5 cm (1½ to 2 inches), proceeding cautiously because prolonged pressure can potentially injure internal organs. Deep palpation is accomplished with either one or both hands (i.e., bimanual). For *bimanual palpation,* the nurse places one hand lightly on the client's skin. This hand is the sensing hand. The other hand (active hand) is placed over the sensing hand and applies pressure. The sensing hand does not apply direct pressure and remains sensitive to underlying organ characteristics. In a variation of bimanual palpation, one hand positions or stabilizes an organ while the other hand palpates (e.g., liver, spleen, kidney, or breast; palpation of the uterus and adnexae during gynecologic examination). Another variation uses trapping between the two hands to assess structures that move, such as the kidney with respiration. (See also gynecologic assessment in Chapter 82.)

The nurse takes precautions when palpating. For example, an artery is palpated so that blood flow is not obstructed. The carotid arteries are not palpated simultaneously because of the possibility of restricting blood flow to the brain.

Percussion

Percussion is a technique to assess the density of a part by the sound produced by striking the skin. It is usually the third technique in physical assessment. Three to 5 cm of tissue depth can be examined by percussion. The sounds and tissue vibrations that result from percussion are evaluated in relation to the underlying body struc-

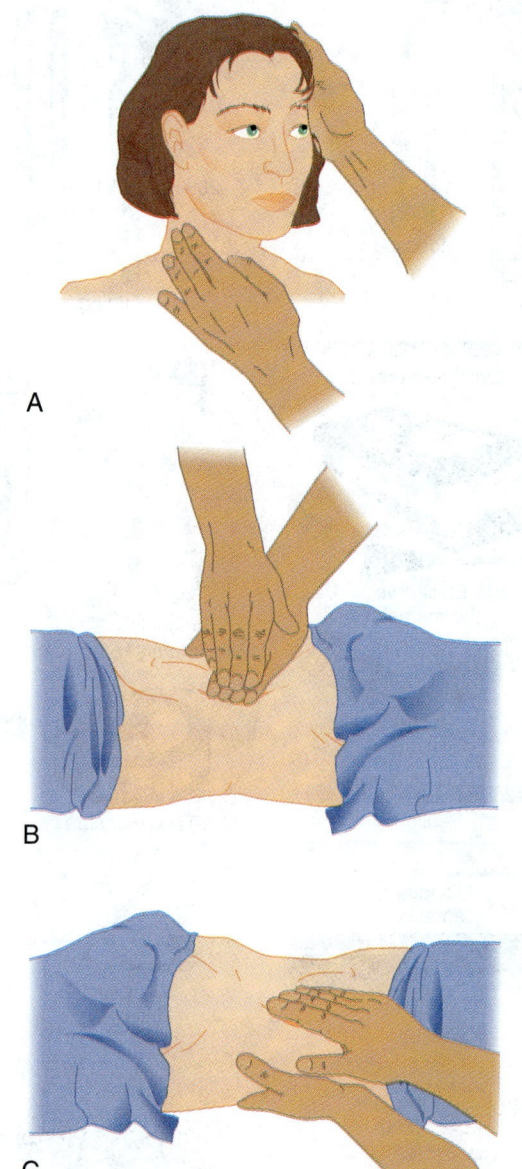

Figure 12–3. Palpation techniques. *A,* Light palpation employs the lightest possible pressure to assess structures under the surface of the skin, such as lymph nodes. *B,* Deep palpation is used to assess the condition of underlying organs, such as in the abdomen, using one or both hands. *C,* Bimanual palpation is used to trap and assess hard-to-palpate organs such as the kidneys or to stabilize an organ with one hand while the other hand palpates, as in liver palpation.

tures. Percussion of body structures containing air, fluid, and solids produces various sounds, depending on their densities. Percussion helps to confirm suspected abnormal findings from palpation and auscultation, such as a mass or consolidation in the lungs.

There are two primary methods of percussion: direct and indirect (Fig. 12–4). *Direct percussion* involves striking the body surface with either one or two fingers or the fist (i.e., blunt percussion). It is used primarily to assess the sinuses and over the thin chest wall of a small adult or a child. *Blunt percussion* is performed to elicit tenderness from an underlying structure such as the liver

DIRECT PERCUSSION

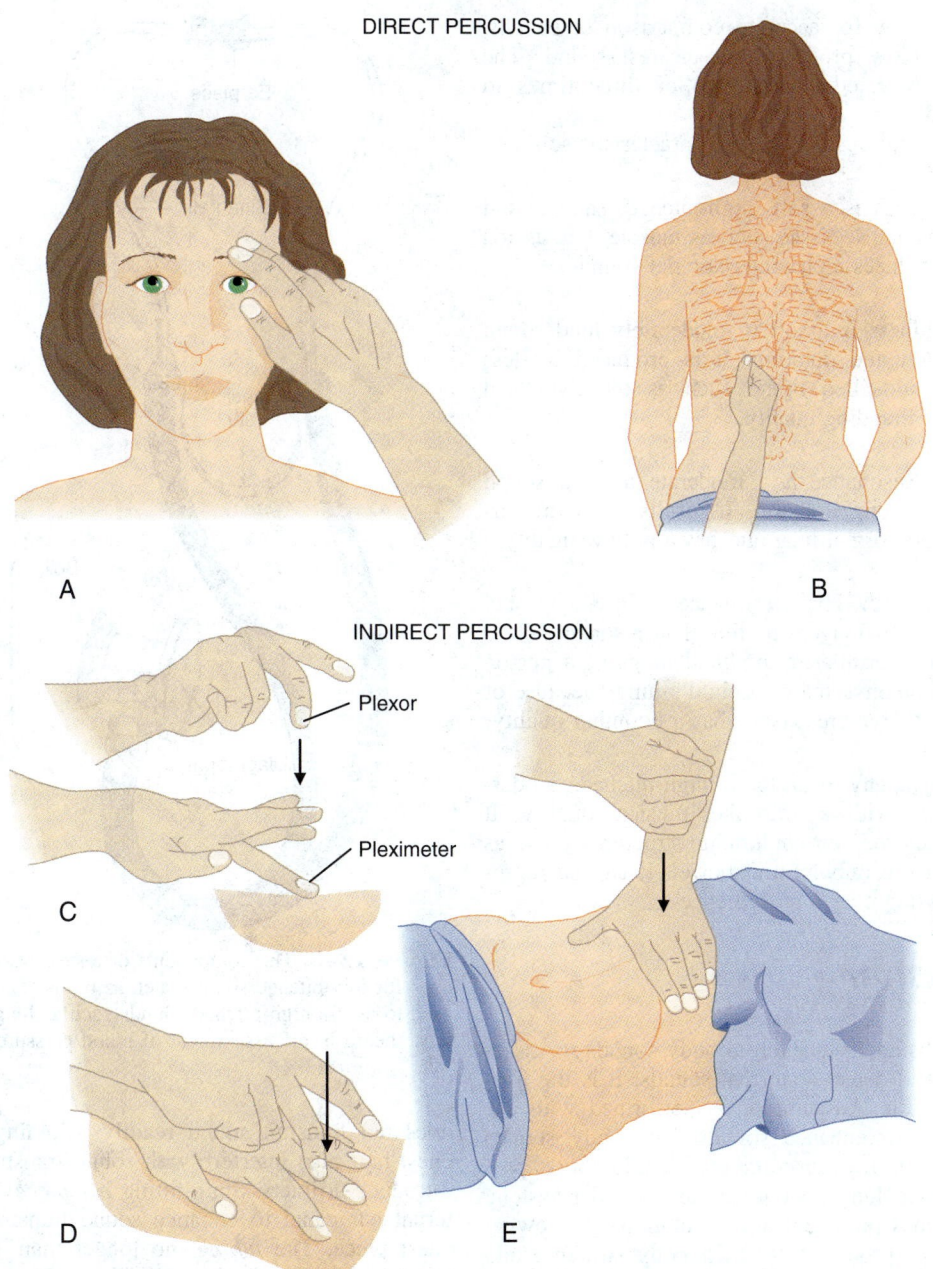

INDIRECT PERCUSSION

Plexor

Pleximeter

A

B

C

D

E

Figure 12–4. Techniques for the two primary types of percussion, direct and indirect. *Direct percussion. A,* Use one or two fingers to percuss directly against a body surface, such as over the sinuses to elicit tenderness. *B,* Use the ulnar surface of your fist to gently strike the surface of the client's body over an underlying organ, such as at the costovertebral junction to assess for kidney tenderness. *Indirect percussion. C,* Place the distal phalanx of the middle finger of your nondominant hand (the pleximeter) on the client's skin over soft tissue. Bend the middle finger of your dominant hand at its distal interphalangeal joint to create a "hammer" (or plexor). *D,* Pivot the plexor down quickly in an arc to strike the pleximeter. *E,* Place the palm of your left hand over the area to be percussed. Gently strike the left hand with the ulnar surface of your right fist.

or kidney and not to produce a sound. Use of a reflex hammer is another example of blunt percussion.

Indirect percussion involves striking an intermediary finger or hand that is placed firmly on the body's surface. Indirect percussion requires dexterity and practice to attain proficiency. In indirect finger percussion, the distal phalanx of the middle finger *(pleximeter)* (see Fig. 12–4) is placed firmly on the skin surface over soft tissue. The remaining fingers of the hand are hyperextended so that only the single digit is in contact with the skin. The

plexor must strike the pleximeter sharply and quickly, which is accomplished by relaxing the wrist, keeping the forearm stationary, and striking with the fingertip (not pad). Errors in technique dampen (or diminish) the sound produced. Common errors include placing the pleximeter over bone, resting the palm or other fingers of the nondominant hand on the body surface, losing contact of the pleximeter with the skin surface, delivering a weak blow with the plexor, or striking the pleximeter at a point other than the distal joint. The same amount of force is delivered with each blow for accurate comparison of sounds. A light, quick blow produces the clearest sound. The blows may be repeated rapidly two or three times to assess the sound.

Indirect percussion results in five characteristic sounds.

Flatness. Flatness is a soft, high-pitched, short sound produced by very dense tissue such as muscle. Percussion of the thigh reproduces a characteristic flat sound.

Dullness. Dullness is a soft to moderately loud sound of moderate pitch and duration. It is produced by less dense, mostly fluid-filled tissue such as the liver and spleen and has a thudding quality.

Resonance. Resonance is a moderate to loud sound of low pitch and long duration. It results from the air-filled tissue of the normal lung and has a hollow quality.

Hyperresonance. Hyperresonance is a very loud, low-pitched sound of longer duration than resonance. It is produced by the overinflated, air-filled lungs of a person with pulmonary emphysema or a child's lung (because of a thin chest wall). Hyperresonance has a booming quality.

Tympany. Tympany is a loud, high-pitched, moderately long sound with a drumlike, musical quality. It results from enclosed, air-containing structures such as the stomach (gastric bubble) and bowel. It can be reproduced by percussing over a puffed cheek.

Auscultation

Auscultation is listening to internal body sounds to assess normal sounds and detect abnormal sounds. It is the final step in examination. Auscultation is performed with use of a stethoscope to enhance sounds. The body sounds commonly assessed by auscultation include those produced by the heart, lungs, abdomen, and vascular system. The nurse becomes proficient at auscultation by knowing which sounds are produced by each body structure and the location at which they are most readily heard. Recognizing abnormal sounds is learned once the normal sounds have been mastered.

Acute hearing ability, a reliable stethoscope, and knowledge of how to use the stethoscope are essential to auscultation. Stethoscopes that amplify sounds are available for those who have difficulty hearing. The basic stethoscope (Fig. 12–5) has a chest piece with a bell and diaphragm and single or double tubing connected to double ear tubes (i.e., binaurals). A tension bar between the binaurals holds the ear pieces firmly in place and reduces kinking of the tubing.

The *diaphragm* is held between the index and middle fingers firmly against the skin surface. It is used to hear high-pitched sounds such as lung sounds, heart sounds, and blood pressure. The *bell* is placed lightly in contact with the skin to hear low-pitched sounds such as murmurs and bruits. The *chest piece* is placed on the skin so that it is between bones and not over them, because bone

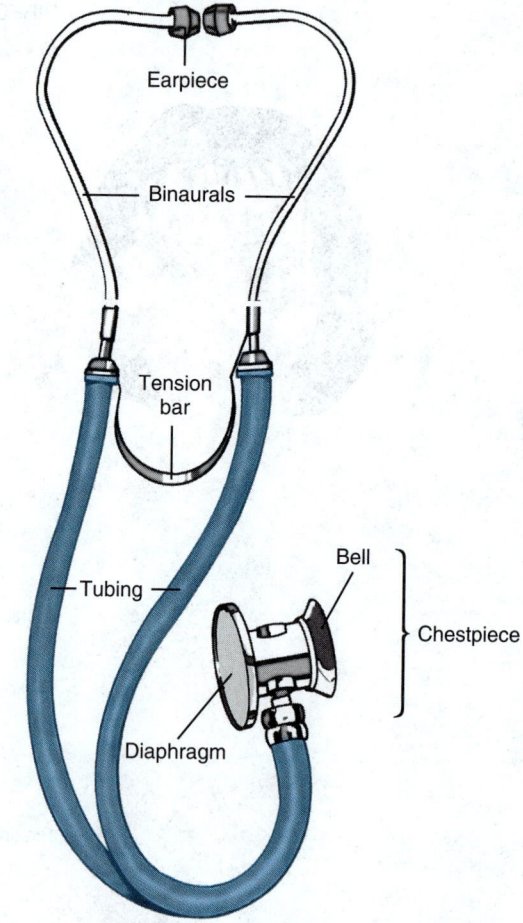

Figure 12–5. The components of a stethoscope. The *bell* is used for low-pitched sounds such as bruits. The *diaphragm* is used to assess high-pitched sounds such as lung sounds and those heard in the assessment of blood pressure.

does not transmit sound readily. Clothing and excessive chest hair also interfere with sound transmission and may introduce artifacts. Snug-fitting *ear pieces* occlude the external ear canal to enhance sound transmission from the chest piece. The *tubing,* no longer than 12 to 15 inches for the best sound transmission, is kept free of contact with all surfaces to prevent extraneous noises.

A quiet environment is essential for accurate auscultation. The nurse closes the door and draws the client's cubicle curtains for privacy. If necessary, the television or radio volume is turned down after informing the client about the importance of decreasing external sounds. The nurse concentrates on the body part being auscultated to determine what is causing the sounds that are heard. Once the nurse understands the source and characteristics of normal body sounds, recognition of abnormal sounds and their origin becomes easier.

There are four sound characteristics the nurse notes when auscultating.

Pitch. *Pitch* is the number or frequency of sound wave cycles per second. By varying the frequency, the pitch may be altered. For example, a high frequency results in a high-pitched sound, whereas a low frequency produces a low-pitched sound. Heart murmurs can be either high-pitched or low-pitched, depending on the structural cause. Pitch is a diagnostic clue.

Intensity. Intensity is the amplitude of a sound wave. The greater the amplitude, the louder the sound; the lower the amplitude, the softer the sound.

Duration. Duration is the length of time a sound endures. It may be long, medium, or short.

Quality. Quality is a description of a sound's character, such as "gurgling," "blowing," "whistling," or "snapping."

Olfaction

Olfaction is the use of the sense of smell to detect body odors. The sense of smell helps the nurse detect abnormalities not readily recognized by other means, such as inspection. For example, the smell of ammonia in urine suggests a urinary tract infection; a strong, musty odor from a casted body part suggests a wound infection under the cast; a strong fruity breath odor indicates enhanced production of ketone by-products. Findings from olfaction are considered with other assessments to determine the nature of the client's health problem.

Guidelines for Physical Examination

Physical examination proceeds in a logical, orderly fashion. The approach commonly used by examiners follows a head-to-toe system of organization so that findings are complete. This, however, is not an absolute rule, and the nurse who is beginning to use physical assessment skills practices and develops a system that is comfortable to use. Once a system is developed, the nurse uses it routinely to avoid inadvertently omitting portions of the examination. Successful physical assessment requires knowledge of both the techniques and the parameters of normal findings. The following guidelines are provided for planning and conducting a physical examination.

Preparation of the Environment

To prepare for physical examination, ensure that the environment is private, quiet, comfortable, and well-lighted. An examination may be conducted in a special examination room in an office or clinic; in a client's bedroom in the home; or in the area enclosed by drawn curtains around a client's bed in a hospital room. Eliminate or control extraneous noises to allow yourself to concentrate on the examination and to encourage the client to feel free to discuss problems or concerns. Make sure that the area is neither too warm nor too cool.

Preparation of Equipment

All necessary equipment is assembled and available before the examination is begun. Arranging equipment in order of use facilitates the examination. The nurse practices picking up equipment, holding it in the position of use, making adjustments, and assembling and disassembling. Equipment is also checked before use for adequate functioning. It is embarrassing as well as time-consuming to hunt for a replacement bulb for the oto-ophthalmoscope or to discover that the battery needs recharging in the middle of an examination.

Equipment commonly used in physical examination is shown in Figure 12–2. Additional equipment that may be used includes cotton balls, gauze sponges, a watch with a second hand, supplies for specimens, and substances to test taste and smell.

Preparation of the Client

The client is prepared physically and psychologically for the physical examination. Before beginning the examination, the nurse instructs the client to empty the bladder. If a urine specimen is needed the client is instructed in the technique for collection at this time. An empty bladder facilitates examination of the abdomen, genitalia, and rectum.

Draping

Physical preparation also includes instructing the client to dress according to the type and extent of examination to be conducted. A hospital or paper gown and drapes provide privacy (Fig. 12–6).

Positioning

During the examination, the client is assisted in assuming different positions to facilitate assessment. Figure 12–6 illustrates common positions for examination and the areas of the body that are assessed. The nurse considers limitations the client has that prevent optimal positioning, such as arthritis, back injury, joint deformities, or weakness. Alternative positions may have to be assumed for the examination to be completed. Several positions may be uncomfortable and embarrassing. The client is kept in these positions only as long as required and is draped to prevent unnecessary exposure. A sequence that minimizes the number of position changes during the examination appears in Table 12–1.

Psychological Preparation

The nurse approaches the client in a professional, calm manner. An organized, efficient approach and a relaxed tone of voice and facial expression put the client at ease

POSITION	AREAS EXAMINED	RATIONALE	CONTRAINDICATIONS
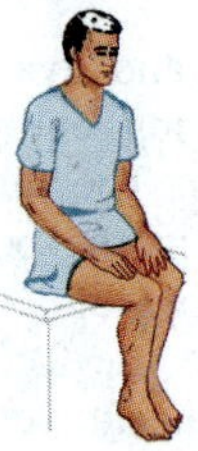 Sitting	Vital signs, head and neck, back, posterior and anterior thorax and lungs, breasts, axillae, heart, upper and lower extremities, reflexes	Sitting upright allows for full lung expansion and better visualization of upper body symmetry.	Elderly and weak clients may be unable to sit without support. An alternate position is supine with the head of the bed elevated.
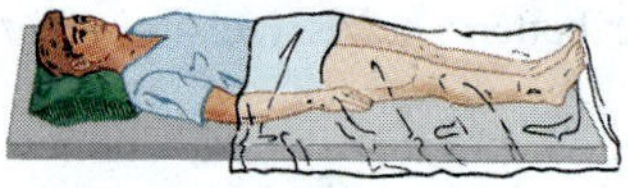 Supine	Vital signs, head and neck, anterior thorax and lungs, breasts, axillae, heart, abdomen, extremities, peripheral pulses	This is a relaxed position for most clients. It provides access to pulse sites and prevents contracture of abdominal muscles, especially if a small pillow is placed under the knees.	Clients with cardiovascular and respiratory problems may be unable to lie flat without becoming short of breath. An alternate position is to raise the head of the bed. Clients with lower back pain may be unable to lie flat without flexing the knees.
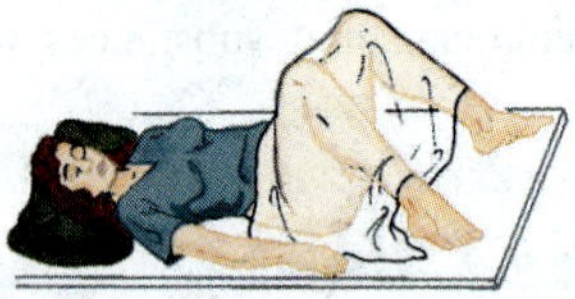 Dorsal recumbent	Abdomen and external genitalia	Flexed knees reduce tension on lower back and abdominal muscles and increase client comfort.	Same as for supine. The client should not raise the arms over the head or clasp the hands behind the head because this increases contraction of the abdominal muscles.
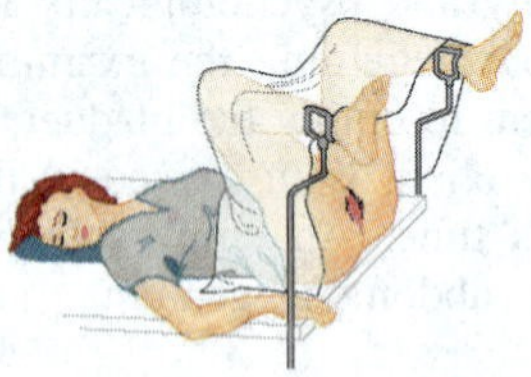 Lithotomy	Female genitalia, reproductive tract, and rectum	This position maximally exposes the genitalia and facilitates the insertion of a vaginal speculum.	This position is assumed immediately before it is needed because it is embarrassing and uncomfortable. The client is kept draped. Clients with arthritis or joint deformity may be unable to assume this position. Alternate positions are dorsal recumbent or Sims'.
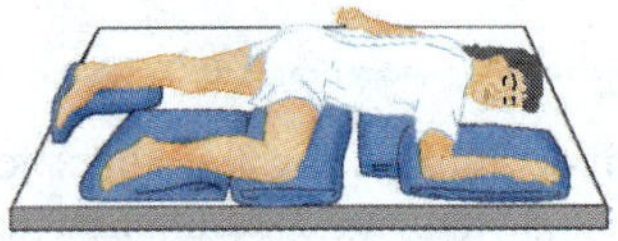 Sims' (posterior view)	Rectum, vagina	Flexion of the upper hip and knee improves exposure of the rectal area.	Clients with deformities of the hip or knee may be unable to assume this position. Elderly and obese clients may be uncomfortable.
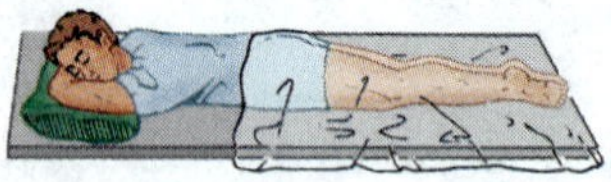 Prone	Posterior thorax, hip movement, popliteal pulses	This position is used to assess hip extension. Sometimes popliteal pulse palpation is facilitated in this position.	This position is not well tolerated by the elderly or clients with cardiovascular or respiratory problems.
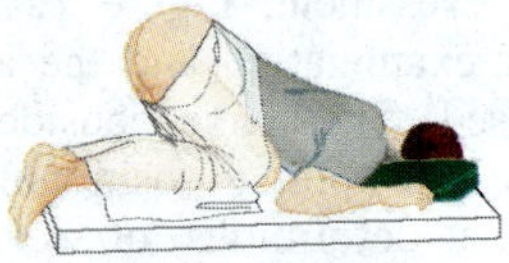 Knee-chest	Rectum, prostate	This position provides maximal exposure of the anal and rectal areas and facilitates insertion of instruments into the rectum.	Poorly tolerated by clients with cardiovascular or respiratory problems. Clients with difficulty flexing hips or knees may be unable to assume this position.
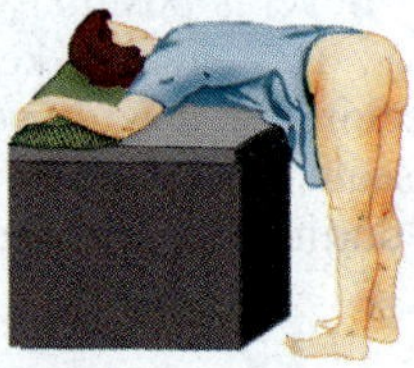 Standing, bent over examining table	Rectum, prostate	This is a more comfortable position than knee-chest and allows for palpation of the prostate gland.	This position is assumed immediately before it is needed because it is embarrassing. Clients with back problems may need assistance.

Figure 12–6. Draping and positioning the client to facilitate assessment and protect privacy.

and promote a relationship of trust. The client may feel anxious about the examination process and the possibility of the nurse's finding something abnormal. Some agencies require that a second staff person of the same sex as the client be present for examination of breasts and genitalia when the examiner is of the opposite sex. The nurse explains what will be done before proceeding so that the client knows what to expect and cooperates to the fullest extent possible.

The nurse first explains the physical examination in general terms and then provides a detailed explanation as each body system is examined. Simple terms are less confusing for clients to understand and are less threatening than complicated explanations. The nurse encourages the client to verbalize discomfort as the examination proceeds.

The nurse is sensitive to the client who is uncomfortable with exposing body parts to anyone other than those who are culturally sanctioned. For example, in some cultures, a woman is restricted from revealing most of her body to a male other than her husband or immediate family. In other cultures, women are restricted from touching men other than their immediate male relatives.

The nurse watches the client's facial expressions and body language throughout the examination. These nonverbal forms of communication may convey anxiety, fear, or concern. For example, the client may pull the drape closely around the body, or muscles may feel tight and tense. In extreme instances, the client may wish to stop the examination and the nurse should comply. The client is never coerced to continue. The nurse does, however, attempt to explain the purpose of the examination and to clarify any client misconceptions.

Preparation of the Examiner

The nurse begins the physical examination on meeting the client by focusing on the client's appearance, movements, position, and reaction to the assessment process. A mental plan (assisted by a general outline or checklist) is helpful so that the major portions of the examination are included. The outline may include the general sequence of the examination and the methods, equipment, and techniques needed to examine each body system.

Organization

Organization and efficiency provide a framework for a thorough physical assessment without wasting the time or energy of the nurse or client. Position changes are kept to a minimum so that the client is not fatigued. The nurse uses a specific piece of equipment to examine an entire region or body system. For example, the reflex hammer is used to test deep tendon reflexes in quick succession, proceeding from upper to lower extremities, while the client is either seated or supine.

Sequence of Examination

The importance of organizing the physical examination systematically has already been discussed. A suggested

format for sequencing the adult general screening physical examination is presented in Table 12–1. This format integrates a head-to-toe approach incorporating regional assessments of the head and neck, upper extremities and spine, posterior and anterior thorax, abdomen, lower extremities and spine, and genitalia and rectum, as well as each body system. Each examiner develops an individual style and approach to physical assessment. The examination is sufficiently complete to obtain the data necessary to diagnose the client's responses to physical problems, yet flexible enough to accommodate the client's individual needs.

Knowledge of Structure and Function

Anatomic landmarks are reference points for locating areas to examine and in recording findings. Reference to an anatomy book is recommended for the nurse who is a beginning practitioner in physical examination. Descriptive terms and anatomic reference points are discussed further with the examination of the respective body systems.

The Adult General Screening Physical Examination

General Survey

The general survey begins the physical examination and includes observing the client's general appearance and behavior, taking vital signs, and measuring height and weight. Additional assessments include the anthropometric parameters of triceps skinfold thickness and midarm muscle circumference.

General Appearance and Behavior

The nurse evaluates observations regarding general appearance and behavior in relationship to the client's background, that is, culture, educational level, socioeconomic status, and current health and illness status. Signs of problems or abnormalities direct the nurse to examine specific body areas thoroughly as the examination proceeds. For example, the client who is unkempt and has obvious body odor will need thorough examination of the hair, skin, and nails for assessment of hygiene. General appearance and behavior assessments include the following.

Apparent Age, Sex, and Race. The client's appearance may or may not be congruent with chronologic age, directing the nurse to assess each body system for potential problems related to aging. Other assessments are

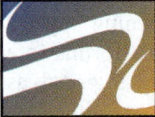

MANAGEMENT AND DELEGATION

Measuring and Recording Vital Signs and Other Client Data

The measurement and recording of routine vital signs may be delegated to unlicensed assistive personnel. The collection of data should only be delegated when caring for a stable client. Remember to emphasize the following when delegating these tasks to assistive personnel.

- Blood pressure: The proper placement of the blood pressure cuff is 1 to 2 inches above the antecubital fossa, with the cuff bladder overlying the brachial artery. The proper placement of the blood pressure cuff on the leg is 1 to 2 inches above the popliteal space, with the cuff bladder overlying the popliteal artery. The size of the cuff should properly accommodate the circumference of the client's arm or leg. Some clients may have contraindications to blood pressure measurement on the arm or leg. This must be communicated to the assistive personnel.
- Pulse: The radial pulse is counted for 30 seconds and multiplied by 2. If the pulse seems irregular, the pulse should be counted for a full minute.
- Respiratory rate: The rate of respiration should be counted with the client unaware that it is being done. This prevents the client from consciously controlling the respiratory rate. If the respiratory rate is regular, the rate is counted for 30 seconds and multiplied by 2. If the respiratory rate is irregular, the rate should be counted for a full minute.
- Temperature: Designate the route by which the temperature should be taken. Oral temperatures should not be taken for 15 minutes if the patient has just eaten, smoked, or consumed a hot or cold liquid. Dry mucous membranes and inability to hold the thermometer under the tongue with the lips closed are indications for measuring by the axillary, rectal, or tympanic routes. Some clients

may have contraindications to rectal temperature measurement. This must be communicated to the assistive personnel.
- Oxygen saturation: Designate the type of pulse oximeter sensor to be used. If a finger or toe sensor is used, nail polish or artificial nails may need to be removed. The skin at the sensor site should be clean, dry, and intact.

Findings that are immediately reportable to you, the RN, should be described for the assistive personnel. These may include a blood pressure outside the range of 95/60 to 140/90 mm Hg, or may be defined by the client's baseline blood pressure. For example, in a known controlled hypertensive client, a systolic reading of 140 to 170 mm Hg may be acceptable. Pulse rates less than 60 or greater than 110 beats per minute should be reported, as should any irregular pulse or inability to locate a pulse. Adult respiratory rates less than 10 or greater than 20 should be reported to you, as should any irregular respiratory rate. Temperatures outside the normal range of 97.6° to 99.4° F should be reported. An oxygen saturation level below 96% should be brought to your attention.

Remember, even though you have delegated the collection of this information, you remain responsible for the review and interpretation of the data, as well as for the full health assessment of the client. Assess the client's cardiovascular and respiratory status daily, and more frequently as his or her clinical condition warrants.

The competency of the assistive personnel in performing each of these tasks should be verified during orientation and annually thereafter. The competency verification should include the proper recording of the vital signs and any other client data delegated for collection.

---

sex-specific and affect the type of procedures performed. Data are interpreted and recommendations are made for health teaching and further screening on the basis of the client's health risk profile (Chapter 11).

Apparent State of Health. The nurse assesses whether the client looks "healthy," frail, or ill. Deformities or absent body parts are noted.

Signs of Distress or Discomfort. The client may display obvious signs of pain (wincing), anxiety (eyes darting around room), difficulty breathing (gasping), or other problems. The nurse adapts the examination to the client's needs by including only the necessary assessments. The ideal situation is that in which the client is comfortable and in no acute distress.

Body Build, Height, and Weight. The client's body build is assessed for proportionate distribution of weight for height. Body build may be thin, obese, trim, or muscular and reflect the client's level of wellness, age, and life-style.

Posture. Posture may reflect the client's mood or the presence of a physical problem. The nurse observes the client's posture throughout the health assessment process. Normal findings are an erect posture while standing, with the shoulders and hips aligned over the knees and ankles. Sitting posture is with a straight back and slight rounding of the shoulders. Deviations from normal include stooping, slouching, or a curved posture. An ethnic variation may include an increased forward lumbar spine curvature (i.e., lordosis) accompanied by a forward tilt of the pelvis and abdominal protrusion.

Gait. Gait is observed as the client enters the examination room or ambulates. It is smooth and coordinated with arms swinging freely at the sides, opposite to leg movement. Head and face orient in the direction the client is moving. Shuffling steps and hesitancy are abnormal findings. Devices to assist ambulation are noted.

Movements. The nurse observes the client's body movements as the examination proceeds. They are usually purposeful and controlled without tremors, tics, muscle fasciculations, signs of spasticity, or decreased muscle tone. Immobile body parts are noted.

Dress. The client's manner of dress is appropriate to the time of year, temperature, age, socioeconomic status, and current circumstances. A depressed client may wear clothing that is dull, unkempt, or mismatched. A client with a thyroid disorder may be dressed more warmly than others (hypothyroid) or may wear lightweight clothing despite a cool or cold environment (hyperthyroid).

Hygiene and Grooming. The nurse notes the client's cleanliness of hair, nails, skin, and clothes. Does the client present a pleasant image? The nurse considers what activity the client engaged in before the examination and if it affects the client's appearance.

Body and Breath Odor. These are noted in relationship to the client's activity level, such as strenuous exercise. Deficient hygiene may result in body and breath odors that are considered unpleasant or offensive. Odors include cigarette smoke, perfume, perspiration, alcohol, acetone, blood, decaying tissue, or odors associated with a disease process.

Mental Status. Mental status includes the client's level of consciousness, orientation, affect, speech, and thought processes. If abnormalities are noted in these areas, the nurse proceeds with a full mental status assessment. See Chapters 11 and 30 for discussion.

Level of Cooperation. The nurse assesses the client's cooperation with the examination. Is the client interested, concerned, and willing to discuss information? Or is the client silent, withdrawn, hostile, angry, or suspicious? Is the client relaxed and willing to engage in eye contact? Or is the client tense and avoiding eye contact? The nurse also considers the client's cultural influences when assessing eye contact and body language. In some cultures, direct eye contact is perceived as being hostile or as dominant behavior and averted eyes are the norm when talking to another person. Similarly, some cultures

Table 12–2. Metropolitan Life's Table of Adult Weight Standards

Weights* for men (according to frame, ages 25–59) for greatest longevity†

Height‡ Feet	Inches	Small Frame	Medium Frame	Large Frame
5	2	128–134	131–141	138–150
5	3	130–136	133–143	140–153
5	4	132–138	135–145	152–156
5	5	134–140	137–148	144–160
5	6	136–142	139–151	146–164
5	7	138–145	142–154	149–168
5	8	140–148	145–157	152–172
5	9	142–151	148–160	155–176
5	10	144–154	151–163	158–180
5	11	146–157	154–166	161–184
6	0	149–160	157–170	164–188
6	1	152–164	160–174	168–192
6	2	155–168	164–178	172–197
6	3	158–172	167–182	176–202
6	4	162–176	171–187	181–207

Weights* for women (according to frame, ages 25–59) for greatest longevity†

Height‡ Feet	Inches	Small Frame	Medium Frame	Large Frame
4	10	102–111	109–121	118–131
4	11	103–113	111–123	120–134
5	0	104–115	113–126	122–137
5	1	106–118	115–129	125–140
5	2	108–121	118–132	128–143
5	3	111–124	121–135	131–147
5	4	114–127	124–138	134–151
5	5	117–130	127–141	137–155
5	6	120–133	130–144	140–159
5	7	123–136	133–147	143–163
5	8	126–139	136–150	146–167
5	9	129–142	139–153	149–170
5	10	132–145	142–156	152–173
5	11	135–148	145–159	155–176
6	0	138–151	148–162	158–179

*Weight in pounds (in indoor clothing weighing 5 lb for men, 3 lb for women).
†Metropolitan no longer labels these weights "ideal" or "desirable," because these adjectives mean different things to different people.
‡In shoes with 1-inch heels.
Courtesy of Metropolitan Life Insurance Company, copyright 1983.

do not directly face a person while talking if that person is perceived as being an authority figure.

Height and Weight

The nurse measures height and weight while the client is standing. This often is done immediately after the health history interview, before the client sits on the examination table. A balance scale (see Fig. 12–2) is preferable because of its greater accuracy. (Alternatives to the standing platform scale include bed and chair scales.) The standing scale has a telescoping ruler to measure height.

Height and weight are compared with tables such as that developed by the Metropolitan Life Insurance Company (Table 12–2). Weight should fall within the range for the client's sex, height, and body frame. (Determining body frame is discussed later.) Weight that is more than 20% above or 10% below the *ideal body weight (IBW)* indicates that the client may be at increased risk for nutritional problems. To calculate IBW, the nurse uses a formula specific to the client's sex and body frame Box 12–2.

Box 12–2. Calculating Ideal Body Weight

Adult Male*

Take 106 lb for the first 5 ft of height; add 6 lb/inch for each additional inch over 5 ft

Adult Female*

Take 100 lb for the first 5 ft of height; add 5 lb/inch for each additional inch over 5 ft

Small Frame — Calculate 10% of the amount for medium frame and subtract it from the first amount (i.e., IBW is 10% *less* for persons with small frames)

Large Frame — Calculate 10% of the amount for medium frame and add it to the first amount (i.e., IBW is 10% *more* for persons with large frames)

Example — An adult male is 6'1" tall with a large body frame. His IBW is calculated as follows:

6'1" = 5 ft plus 13 inches
First 5 ft of height = 106 lb
Additional height over 5 ft = (13) × (6)
= 78 lb
Medium frame IBW = 106 + 78
= 184 lb
Allowance for large frame = (10%) × 184 = 18.4 lb
Large frame IBW = 184 + 18.4
= 202.4 lb

---

*These formulas are for adults with a medium body frame. Adjust formulas for clients with small or large frames (adjustment is the same formula for both sexes).
Data from The American Dietetic Association. (1981). *Handbook of clinical dietetics.* New Haven: Yale University Press.

Clients who are missing all or part of an extremity (e.g., amputation) should have their weight adjusted to account for the absent body mass. This may be done by using a chart or table for segmental weights.

Balance (Romberg's Test)

Balance is assessed after measurement of height and weight and before the client sits down. Romberg's test and the test for pronation assess cerebellar function. They may be done later during the neurologic examination. The nurse instructs the client to stand quietly with hands at the sides and feet together. Once equilibrium is attained, the nurse instructs the client to close the eyes. The client should be able to stand upright with minimal swaying and no loss of balance. The nurse is close by and intervenes should the client begin to lose balance and fall. While standing, the client is instructed to raise and extend the arms to shoulder height, then close the eyes. The client should be able to maintain the arms in extension with no downward drifting or pronation (pronation sign). (See other cerebellar assessments in Chapter 30.)

Once this portion of the examination is completed, the nurse may elect to test the client's visual acuity if the eye chart is located at the correct distance from the examination table. Otherwise, visual acuity is tested when the eyes are examined.

The nurse instructs the client to sit on the edge of the examination table for assessment of vital signs and anthropometric measurements (see Table 12–1).

Vital Signs

Once the client is comfortably seated, the nurse measures vital signs after a brief stabilization period. Body temperature and blood pressure are measured during the general survey. The nurse may measure specific vital signs during examination of the upper extremities or heart (peripheral pulse) and thorax (respirations). See a nursing fundamentals textbook for discussion of the techniques of vital signs measurement and equipment selection.

Temperature. Oral body temperature ranges from 96.8° to 99.5° F (36° to 37.5° C) with an average of 98.6° F (37° C). Temperatures above the normal range are *hyperthermic;* those below are *hypothermic.*

Pulse. Resting pulse rate ranges from 60 to 100 beats per minute (BPM). A rate above 100 BPM is *tachycardia;* below 60 BPM is *bradycardia.* The nurse notes general characteristics of the pulse, such as rhythm (regular or irregular), amplitude (weak or bounding), and pattern. Rhythm is regular with pulsations occurring at equal intervals and being of similar amplitude. Slight variation in rhythm occurs with respiration and is normal. *Pulse amplitude* is rated on a scale ranging from 0 to 3+ (Box 12–3). Irregular patterns are described. Further discussion of pulse assessment is found in Chapter 49.

Box 12-3. Rating and Recording Pulse Amplitude

The following scale is commonly used to rate and record pulse amplitude. Note that the rating 2+ is considered "normal." When the nurse records a pulse amplitude, it may be expressed in relationship to the rating scale norm, for example, 3+/2+ (i.e., the pulse is rated 3+ on a rating scale in which 2+ is normal).

0   *Absent.* The pulse is indiscernible to palpation.
1+   *Weak, thready.* The pulse is difficult to palpate and easily obliterated by slight pressure.
2+   *Normal.* The pulse is easily palpable and can be obliterated only with strong pressure.
3+   *Bounding.* The pulse is easily palpable, forceful, and not easily obliterated by pressure.

Respiration. Respirations range from 12 to 20 per minute; have a regular, smooth pattern; and are of consistent depth. They are quiet and effortless, without abnormal sounds such as wheezing. Respiratory depth reflects tidal volume (i.e., the amount of air taken in with each breath). The rise and fall of the client's chest is used to estimate whether respirations are shallow, moderate, or deep. The nurse notes the respiratory pattern and records its characteristics (Fig. 12-7). Further discussion of respiration assessment is found in Chapters 30 and 39.

Blood Pressure. Blood pressure varies greatly among individuals. Normal systolic pressure ranges from 100 to 140 mm Hg, and diastolic pressure ranges from 60 to 90 mm Hg. It is more accurate to evaluate consecutive blood pressure readings over time rather than make an isolated measurement for determining blood pressure abnormalities. *Hypotension* is a systolic pressure below 95 mm Hg or diastolic pressure below 60 mm Hg. *Hypertension* is a systolic pressure above 140 mm Hg or diastolic pressure above 90 mm Hg. The difference between the systolic and diastolic pressure readings (i.e., *pulse pressure*) is noted. A difference of more than 40 mm Hg is abnormal and is reported. A slightly elevated blood pressure may be considered a normal finding in the elderly.

The nurse assesses the client's blood pressure by using the bell of the stethoscope initially. Assess both arms and compare the two readings. A pressure difference of 5 to 10 mm Hg between the two arms is normal. Larger differences are reported. The nurse assesses for an *auscultatory gap* the first time a client's blood pressure is measured. This phenomenon occurs as a period of silence between two levels of systolic pressures that may range as much as 40 mm Hg. Further discussion of blood pressure is found in Chapter 49.

Body Frame

The nurse assesses the client's body frame by measuring the wrist circumference and dividing it into the height. The resulting *r*-value is compared with a chart to determine whether the client's body frame is small, medium, or large (Box 12-4). This information is necessary for calculating the IBW. An alternative method to calculate body frame is to measure the elbow breadth (Box 12-4).

Adipose Tissue Measurement

The nurse measures the triceps skinfold (TSF) thickness and midarm circumference (MAC) to estimate the client's nutritional status. The TSF and MAC are used to calculate the midarm muscle circumference (MAMC), which is an indication of protein and calorie reserves. All measurements are compared with published norms for age and sex. The techniques for measuring TSF, MAC, and MAMC and their norms are shown in Figure 12-8.

Skin Color

Overall skin color is assessed as the nurse interviews the client. A more thorough assessment is conducted as the nurse proceeds with the remainder of the physical examination. The nurse observes the client's face and visible skin surfaces for color tones that should be congruent with the client's stated race. Abnormal findings include pallor (paleness), flushing or a ruddy complexion, cyanosis (blue cast), jaundice (yellow cast), and areas of irregular pigmentation. (See skin assessment in Chapter 77.)

Processing the Data
Comparison of Findings

The client is used as a "control" or self-standard for comparison during the physical examination. Findings from one side of the body are compared with those of the opposite side, or *bilaterally*. Even though both sides of the human body are not exactly identical (i.e., symmetrical), similarities in structure and appearance are individualized and unique. Comparisons are useful and valid when the nurse assesses findings such as a joint deformity or extremity swelling. If a client is missing part of a limb (such as from an amputation), bilateral comparison is impractical. The nurse must then compare findings with a known standard.

Comparison with Known Standards

The nurse compares physical examination findings with known parameters of "normal" for the client's age, sex, and racial background. For example, decreased skin elasticity and loss of subcutaneous adipose tissue are expected findings for an elderly client but not for a 30-year-old.

RESPIRATORY PATTERN	DESCRIPTION

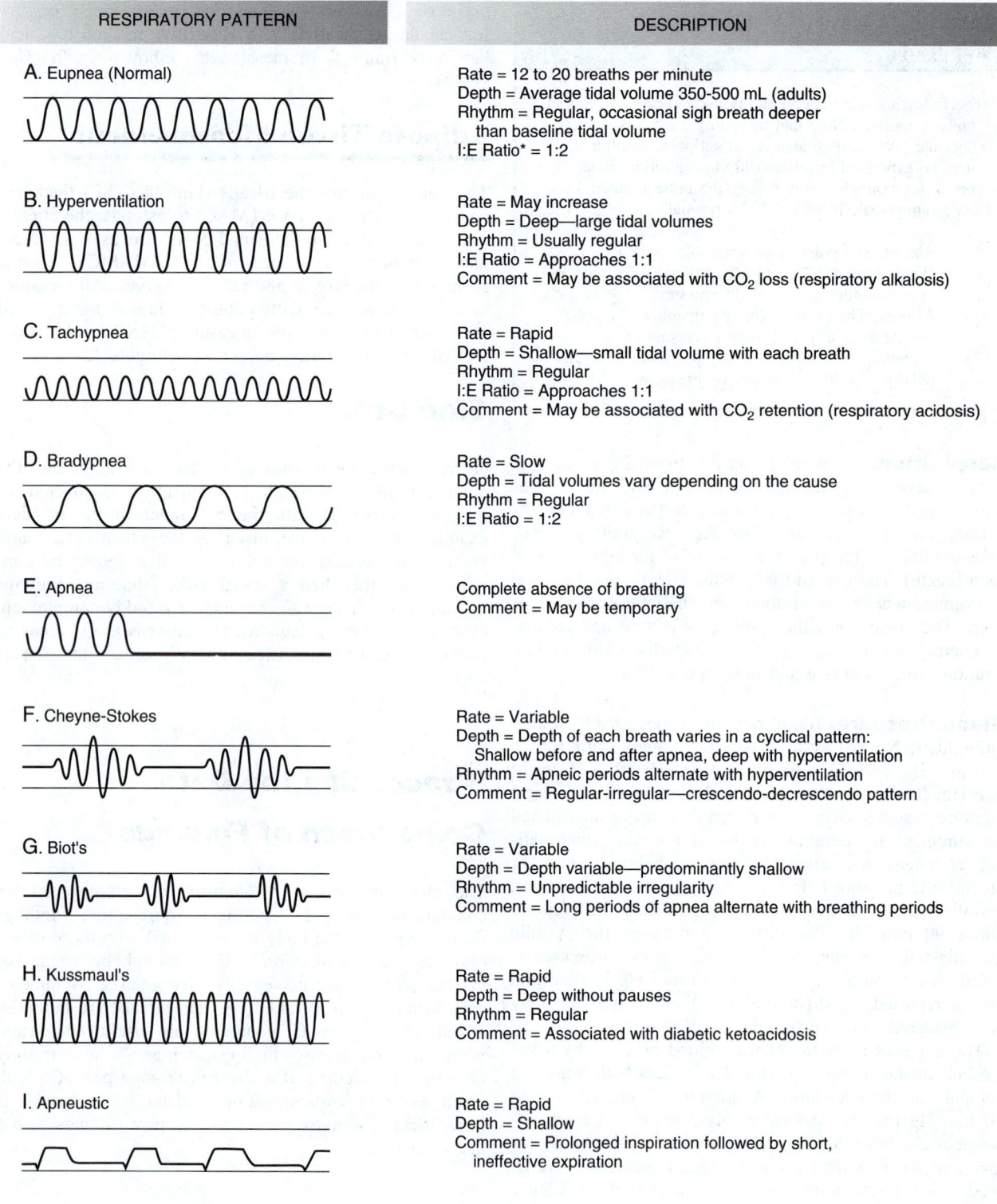

A. Eupnea (Normal)

Rate = 12 to 20 breaths per minute
Depth = Average tidal volume 350-500 mL (adults)
Rhythm = Regular, occasional sigh breath deeper
    than baseline tidal volume
I:E Ratio* = 1:2

B. Hyperventilation

Rate = May increase
Depth = Deep—large tidal volumes
Rhythm = Usually regular
I:E Ratio = Approaches 1:1
Comment = May be associated with CO_2 loss (respiratory alkalosis)

C. Tachypnea

Rate = Rapid
Depth = Shallow—small tidal volume with each breath
Rhythm = Regular
I:E Ratio = Approaches 1:1
Comment = May be associated with CO_2 retention (respiratory acidosis)

D. Bradypnea

Rate = Slow
Depth = Tidal volumes vary depending on the cause
Rhythm = Regular
I:E Ratio = 1:2

E. Apnea

Complete absence of breathing
Comment = May be temporary

F. Cheyne-Stokes

Rate = Variable
Depth = Depth of each breath varies in a cyclical pattern:
    Shallow before and after apnea, deep with hyperventilation
Rhythm = Apneic periods alternate with hyperventilation
Comment = Regular-irregular—crescendo-decrescendo pattern

G. Biot's

Rate = Variable
Depth = Depth variable—predominantly shallow
Rhythm = Unpredictable irregularity
Comment = Long periods of apnea alternate with breathing periods

H. Kussmaul's

Rate = Rapid
Depth = Deep without pauses
Rhythm = Regular
Comment = Associated with diabetic ketoacidosis

I. Apneustic

Rate = Rapid
Depth = Shallow
Comment = Prolonged inspiration followed by short,
    ineffective expiration

* Inspiration to Expiration (I:E) ratio

Figure 12–7. Assessing respiratory patterns.

Suspected Problem Areas

The nurse examines known or suspected problem areas or regions carefully. Areas to include are those identified by the client during the health history interview, as well as those the nurse predicts to be at risk based on the client's history and reactions to the physical examination. For example, the client who reports difficulty swallowing receives a thorough assessment of mouth and neck structures (see Chapter 59). To allay anxiety, the nurse ex-

Box 12–4. Calculating Body Frame Size

Wrist Circumference Method

1. Measure the client's right wrist (in centimeters) at the point of the smallest circumference, just distal to the styloid process of the radius and ulna.

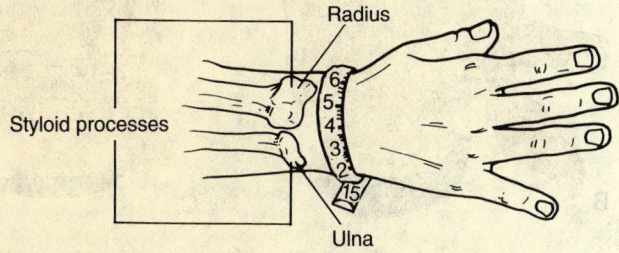

2. Obtain the client's height (in centimeters) without shoes.
3. Divide the client's wrist circumference into the client's height to obtain the *r*-value:

$$r = \frac{\text{height (in cm)}}{\text{wrist circumference (in cm)}}$$

4. Use the chart below to determine the client's body frame size based on the calculated r = value and sex:

	Men	*Women*
Small frame	$r > 10.4$	$r > 10.9$
Medium frame	$r = 9.6{-}10.4$	$r = 9.9{-}10.9$
Large frame	$r < 9.6$	$r < 9.9$

Elbow Breadth Method

1. Instruct the client to extend his or her right arm, then bend the forearm up to a 90-degree angle with the fingers pointing straight up.
2. Measure the width of the client's right elbow (in inches) across the greatest breadth of the joint between the bony prominences of the lateral and medial epicondyles of the humerus. To measure, either use calipers or place your thumb and index finger on the epicondyles and measure the distance between the thumb and finger.
3. Use the chart below to determine the client's body frame size based on the client's elbow breadth, sex, and height in 1-inch heels. The values shown are for a medium body frame. Measurements less than the values shown indicate a small frame; greater values indicate a large frame.

Height	Elbow Breadth
Men	
5'2"–5'3"	2½"–2⅞"
5'4"–5'7"	2⅝"–2⅞"
5'8"–5'11"	2¾"–3"
6'0"–6'3"	2¾"–3⅛"
6'4"	2⅞"–3¼"
Women	
4'10"–4'11"	2¼"–2½"
5'0"–5'3"	2¼"–2½"
5'4"–5'7"	2⅜"–2⅝"
5'8"–5'11"	2⅜"–2⅝"
6'0"	2½"–2¾"

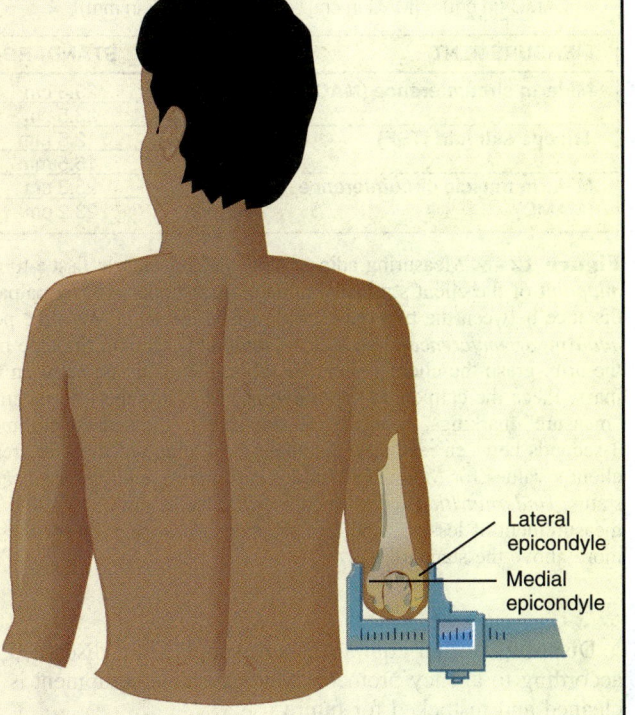

plains to the client why a particular portion of the examination is more thorough than is customary.

Health Teaching

The physical examination process lends itself to health teaching. There are opportunities for providing the client with accurate health information and correcting misconceptions. Examples include reinforcing the techniques for BSE and TSE and having the client perform a return demonstration.

Terminating the Health Assessment

After completion of the physical examination, the nurse closes the gown or allows the client to dress (assisting if needed) and assume a comfortable position. The nurse summarizes the examination findings in understandable terms for the client. If a serious abnormality is found, the nurse consults with the client's healthcare provider or refers the client to another healthcare professional for further assessment after explaining the general nature of the abnormality and the need for further examination.

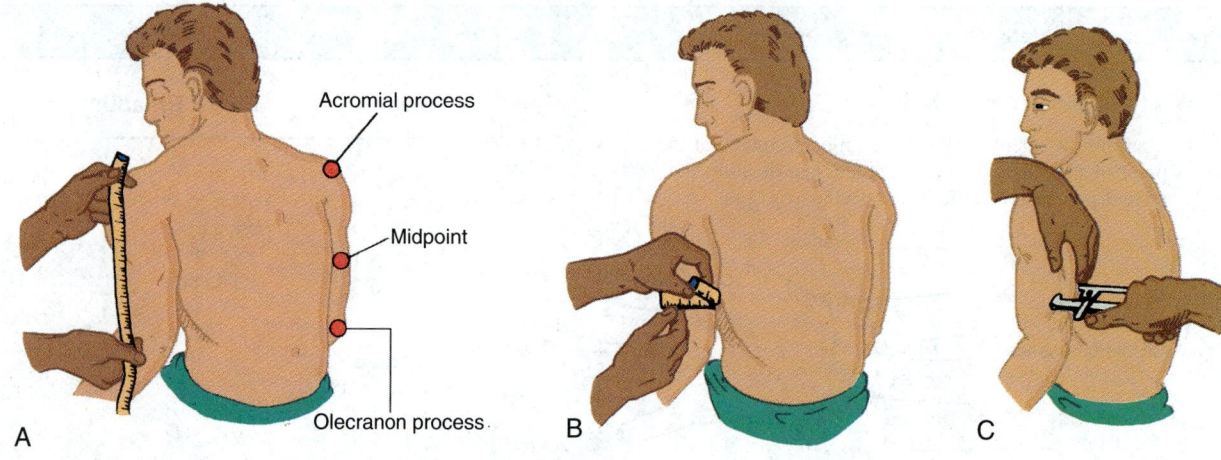

D   Calculate the midarm muscle circumference (MAMC) using the following formula:
MAMC (in cm) = [MAC in cm] − [(0.314) × (TSF in mm)]

MEASUREMENT		STANDARD	90%	60%
Midarm circumference (MAC)	Men	29.3 cm	26.4 cm	17.6 cm
	Women	28.5 cm	25.7 cm	17.1 cm
Triceps skinfold (TSF)	Men	12.5 mm	11.3 mm	7.5 mm
	Women	16.5 mm	14.9 mm	9.9 mm
Midarm muscle circumference (MAMC)	Men	25.3 cm	22.8 cm	15.2 cm
	Women	23.2 cm	20.9 cm	13.9 cm

Figure 12–8. Measuring adipose and skeletal muscle tissue to estimate the client's reserves of protein and calories. *A,* Locate the *midpoint* of the client's relaxed, nondominant upper arm by palpating the acromial and olecranon processes and measuring the distance between the two points with a tape measure. Mark the posterior aspect of the arm at the midpoint with a pen. *B,* Measure *midarm circumference (MAC)* at the midpoint, keeping the tape measure level. *C,* Just above the midpoint at the posterior aspect of the arm, grasp the client's skin and subcutaneous tissue between thumb and index finger, freeing it from the underlying muscle mass. Place the calipers at the midpoint just below the fold of grasped tissue. Squeeze the calipers until they are equilibrated at the "measure" markings. Read the measurement to the nearest millimeter. Repeat the readings two more times, allowing a rest period of 3 seconds between readings. Calculate the average of the three readings for the *triceps skinfold thickness (TSF). D,* Compare the client's values for MAC, TSF, and *midarm muscle circumference (MAMC)* to the following standards to determine nutritional risk status. *Undernutrition* is indicated by a measurement below 90% of the standard. *Protein-calorie malnutrition* is indicated by a measurement of less than 60% of the standard, especially for the MAMC. *Obesity* is indicated by a TSF measurement of 120% or more above the standard.

Disposable, used equipment and supplies are discarded according to agency protocol. Nondisposable equipment is cleaned and restocked for future use.

Recording Physical Examination Findings

The nurse documents physical examination findings using accurate, descriptive terms. Vague, subjective terminology, such as "normal," "slight," "moderate," "healthy," or "poor," is avoided because it is easily misinterpreted by others. The nurse strives to be objective, concise, clear, and thorough in the recording. However, it is better to err on the side of verbosity than to describe a significant finding vaguely or inadequately. A detailed recording is helpful as a baseline for comparison with future physical findings.

During the examination, the nurse may briefly note abnormal assessment findings on a notepad for later retrieval and detailed documentation. This avoids interrupting the flow of the examination to record detailed observations. After the examination, the nurse combines normal and abnormal findings in the final document.

Health Assessment, Nursing Diagnosis, and Nursing Process

After the collection of baseline data, which include both the health history and the physical examination results, the nurse summarizes the client's health problems. The client's areas of strength and health risk profile are assessed. Nursing diagnoses are formalized and prioritized. Tentative diagnoses formulated after the health history interview are re-examined and validated in light of the physical examination findings.

The nurse determines which health problems are nursing diagnoses and which are collaborative problems. Referrals are made when indicated so that the client receives continuity of care and either resolution or effective management of the health problems.

Conclusions

The physical examination is the second portion of physical assessment following the health history. The physical examination is the collection of objective data through inspection, palpation, percussion, and auscultation. Once all data are collected, the nurse compares the findings to known standards and makes appropriate referrals, intervenes, or provides health teaching.

Bibliography

1. American Dietetic Association. (1981). *Handbook of clinical dietetics.* New Haven: Yale University Press.
2. Andres, R., Muller, D. C. & Sarkin, J. D. (1993). Long term effects of change in body weight on all-cause mortality: A review. *Annals of Internal Medicine, 119,* 737–743.
3. Barkauskas, V. H., Stoltenberg-Allen, K., Bauman, L. C., & Darling-Fisher, C. (1994). *Health and physical assessment.* St. Louis: Mosby–Year Book.
4. Bates, B. (1995). *A guide to physical examination* (6th ed.). Philadelphia: J. B. Lippincott.
5. Blackburn, G. L., et al. (1977). Nutritional and metabolic assessment of the hospitalized patient. *Journal of Parenteral and Enteral Nutrition, 1*(1), 11–22.
6. Bowers, A. C., & Thompson, J. M. (1992). *Clinical manual of health assessment* (4th ed.). St. Louis: Mosby–Year Book.
7. Braunwald, E. (1992). *Heart disease* (4th ed.). Philadelphia: W. B. Saunders.
8. Colwell, C. B., & Smith, J. (1985). Determining the use of physical assessment skills in the clinical setting. *Journal of Nursing Education, 24*(8), 333–337.
9. Curtas, S., Chapman, G., & Meguid, M. M. (1989). Evaluation of nutritional status. *Nursing Clinics of North America, 24,* 301–313.
10. Doenges, M. E., & Moorhouse, M. F. (1992). *Application of nursing process and nursing diagnosis: An interactive text.* Philadelphia: F. A. Davis.
11. Erickson, R. S., & Yount, S. T. (1991). Comparison of tympanic and oral temperature in surgical patients. *Nursing Research, 40*(2), 90–93.
12. Fraden, J., & Lackey, R. P. (1991). Estimation of body sites temperature from tympanic measurements. *Clinical Pediatrics, Supplement,* 65–70.
13. Fuller, J., & Schaller-Ayers, J. (1990). *Health assessment: A nursing approach.* Philadelphia: J. B. Lippincott.
14. Geissler, E. M. (1994). *Pocket guide to cultural assessment.* St. Louis: Mosby–Year Book.
15. Giger, J. N., & Davidhizar, R. E. (1991). *Transcultural nursing: Assessment and intervention.* St. Louis: Mosby–Year Book.
16. Grant, J. P., Custer, P. B., & Thurlow, J. (1981). Current techniques of nutritional assessment. *Surgical Clinics of North America, 61,* 437–463.
17. Henneman, E. A., & Henneman, P. L. (1989). Intricacies of blood pressure measurement: Reexamining the rituals. *Heart Lung, 18,* 263–273.
18. Hogstel, M. O., & Keen-Payne, R. (1993). *Practical guide to health assessment through the lifespan.* Philadelphia: F. A. Davis.
19. Hurst, J. W. (1990). *The heart* (7th ed.). New York: McGraw-Hill.
20. Jacobson, N., Gift, A., & Jacox, A. (1990). Advances in physical assessment. *Nursing Clinics of North America, 25*(4), 743–833.
21. Jarvis, C. (1996). *Physical examination and health assessment.* (2nd ed.) Philadelphia: W. B. Saunders.
22. Morton, P. (1993). *Health assessment in nursing* (2nd ed.). Springhouse, PA: Springhouse.
23. Morton, P. (1994). *Quick reference to cultural assessment.* St. Louis: Mosby–Year Book.
24. Rice, E. M. (1989, May-June). Geriatric assessment. *Advancing Clinical Care,* 8–15.
25. Ross Laboratories. (1986). *Guidelines for anthropometric measurements* (Brochure G623). Columbus, OH: Author.
26. Seidel, H. M. et al. (1995). *Mosby's guide to physical examination* (3rd ed.). St. Louis: Mosby–Year Book.
27. Shinozaki, T., et al. (1988). Infrared tympanic thermometer: Evaluation of a new clinical thermometer. *Critical Care Medicine, 16*(2), 148–150.
28. Society of Actuaries and Association of Life Insurance Medical Directors of America. (1983). *Metropolitan Life Insurance Co. build study.* New York: Author.
29. Solomon, E. P., Schmidt, R. R., & Adragna, P. J. (1990). *Human anatomy and physiology* (2nd ed.). Philadelphia: Saunders College Publishing.
30. Swartz, M. H. (1994). *Textbook of physical diagnosis* (2nd Ed.). Philadelphia: W. B. Saunders.
31. Thomas, C. L. (1989). *Tabor's cyclopedic medical dictionary* (16th ed.). Philadelphia: F. A. Davis.
32. U.S. Department of Health and Human Services. (1988). The 1988 report of the Joint National Committee on detection, and treatment of high blood pressure. *Archives of Internal Medicine, 148*(5), 1023–1038.
33. Weber, J. (1993). *Nurses' handbook of health assessment* (2nd ed.). Philadelphia: J. B. Lippincott.

13

Diagnostic Testing

Cynthia Hromek

Diagnostic testing refers to the various methods used to assess body structures and functions to determine the presence or absence of a definite disease and the nature of the disease, if present. Diagnostic testing has many nursing implications. Nursing responsibilities extend from preparation of clients for diagnostic testing to interpretation of diagnostic test results to determine whether a client requires immediate medical intervention. This chapter discusses the general nursing management of clients undergoing laboratory, imaging, and endoscopic diagnostic testing. The specific uses of diagnostic tests for a given disorder are found throughout the book.

General Nursing Management of the Client Undergoing Diagnostic Testing

Assessment

When diagnostic testing is planned, the nurse should assess the client's ability to participate in testing. Consideration of the client's physical condition, sensory limitations, psychological status, and functional ability provides a baseline for selecting interventions that would enhance the client's ability to participate in diagnostic testing. Physical conditions involving disorders of cardiovascular or pulmonary systems may severely limit the client's tolerance of position changes required in diagnostic imaging. Sensory limitations such as impaired hearing or speech may interfere with communication regarding expectations or responses required during diagnostic testing. Psychological assessment should determine the client's mental ability to follow instructions and to remain motionless or remain calm in an enclosed space, and the need for family support during diagnostic testing. Assessment findings about patterns of self-care, mobility, and nutrition inform

the nurse about the client's functional ability to participate in diagnostic testing. The client with impaired mobility, restricted ability to provide self-care, or nutritional deficits may require interventions to prepare for testing and assistance during testing. For most imaging studies the client must be able to maintain a motionless position for at least 30 minutes. Those clients who are agitated or unable to maintain a motionless position need to be sedated prior to imaging studies. Clients who require imaging studies of the abdomen need to withhold food and fluids for 6 to 8 hours before examination (if the stomach is not empty, the study is postponed).

Nursing Intervention

Common independent nursing interventions related to diagnostic testing include client preparation, data collection, collection and transportation of clients and specimens, monitoring clients during diagnostic testing, and supportive teaching. It is important to obtain adequate specimens; see Box 13–1 for guidelines.

Common interdependent nursing interventions include transcribing orders, consultation with laboratory and radiology technicians, sedation, and interpretation of test results to determine if immediate action is required by the physician. Consider the underlying pathophysiology, current medical treatment, and whether the laboratory results indicate that immediate action is required by a physician. For example, if a client's serum potassium level has risen from 2.5 to 2.8 mEq/L, the client has no arrhythmias, and the client is receiving 80 mEq of potassium in a liter of intravenous fluid, the nurse may notify the physician about the potassium level during usual rounds. In contrast, if the potassium level has dropped from 2.5 to 2.0 mEq/L and the client is experiencing a flattened T wave and ventricular arrhythmia, the nurse should immediately notify the physician regarding the change in the client's status.

Box 13–1. Obtaining Adequate Specimens

- Ensure confidentiality and privacy for the client.
- If a culture is required, obtain it prior to initiating antibiotics, if possible.
- Avoid contamination of the specimen with secretions or excretions from uninvolved areas.
- Collect the correct amount of fluid or tissue for the sample.
- Use the proper instruments and collection tubes or bottles.
- To avoid contamination, do not open the collection bottle until you have the specimen.
- Label all containers accurately. Include the name of the client, source of the specimen, and date and time collected.
- Deliver the specimen to the laboratory immediately or keep it at the recommended temperature.

Specificity and Sensitivity of Diagnostic Tests

It would be nice to be able to say that all diagnostic tests are 100% accurate, but they are not. False-positives and false-negatives occur. No test is 100% specific and 100% sensitive, because there are interfering factors that can affect all tests.

Specificity is the ability of a diagnostic (or screening) test to correctly identify a person who is disease-free. Specificity equals the number of true-negatives divided by the sum of true-negatives and false-positives. For example, the presence of bacteria in a clean-catch urine sample does not always mean that the client has a urinary tract infection. This is because many other factors can account for the presence of bacteria, such as failing to clean the perineum.

Sensitivity is the ability of the test to correctly identify a disease. Sensitivity equals the number of true-positives divided by the sum of true-positives and false-negatives. For example, the antinuclear antibody (ANA) test is highly sensitive for detecting systemic lupus erythematosus, but it is not specific because clients with rheumatoid arthritis may also have positive ANA results.

Measurements Used to Report Laboratory Test Results

Reference Values

The term *reference value* rather than normal value is used for reporting laboratory studies, because the values change from laboratory to laboratory. In addition, some tests (e.g., serum calcium) have more than one accepted reference value.

Laboratory results may be influenced by several things. For example, the time of day, temperature, altitude, stress felt by the client, medications, and, of course, the underlying disorder may all influence the test. When analyzing your clients' laboratory test results, be certain to take all of these influencing variables into account.

The International System of Units (SI System)

A comprehensive modern form of the metric system is the SI system of units. The immediate rationale for the SI system is to provide a common international language for units of measurement. Adoption of the SI system in the United States has been very slow. The familiar meter and kilogram are used for length and weight. The most radical change is in reporting the amount per volume of a substance. Instead of using mass concentration units (e.g., mg), the SI system uses moles. A mole is the quantity of a substance in grams equal to its molecular weight.

The basic reason for a change to SI units is that biologic components react in vivo on a molar basis. When data are expressed in moles, a better understanding of the relative amounts of constituents of body fluids and of biologic processes and their interrelationships is obtained.

Laboratory Diagnostic Testing

Many nurses are responsible for peripheral testing and venous punctures in clinics or hospital units in order to obtain faster results and reduce costs (see Management and Delegation feature). The accurate outcome of any laboratory test depends on collecting the right kind of specimen in the proper manner, in the right container, at the right time. Examples include blood glucose needlesticks, pregnancy tests, slide tests for occult blood, and urine for specific gravity or culture. It is important for nurses to follow instructions on diagnostic test kits and maintain the integrity of test materials, that is, protect test materials from light and moisture, and check for expiration dates. Reliability of test results depends on the accuracy of procedures and the integrity of test materials.

Microbiologic Studies

There are many microorganisms that lead to infection, including bacteria, viruses, fungi, and protozoa. Many microbiologic studies can be used to identify the specific organism and guide treatment. Microbiologic studies are performed to determine whether bacteria are present in a sample of body fluid or tissue. The specific bacteria are identified (called a culture), and the type of antibiotics that will inhibit growth of the bacteria are also identified (sensitivity). Commonly, both tests are performed and they are abbreviated *C&S*.

To determine the specific microorganism, several tests can be performed:

A *smear* is a specimen that has been spread across a glass slide. It is examined under a microscope and usually stained.

A *stain* is the application of a dye or combination of dyes to aid in the identification of microorganisms. The Gram stain is commonly used and allows bacteria to be identified by their color. Gram-positive organisms stain

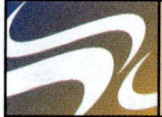

purple-black. Gram-negative organisms stain pink. Gram stain procedures can be done quickly, and many times knowing the Gram stain assists in empirical treatment of the client.

A *culture* is the placement of microorganisms on culture plates to facilitate the growth of the organism. After the microorganisms grow, they are isolated and identified. The culture process may take a few hours to several weeks, depending on the organism.

Sensitivity studies determine the type of antibiotic that will impede the growth of the organism. Small discs saturated with antibiotics are placed on the culture plate. In time, the culture is examined again. If the antibiotic stopped the growth of the microorganism, the microorganism is said to be *sensitive* to the antibiotic. In contrast, if the antibiotic does not halt growth of the microorganism, the organism is said to be *resistant.* Sensitivity reports list several antibiotics. The choice of antibiotics allows the proper prescription of antibiotics of reasonable cost.

Specimen collection and specimen handling is a common but risky procedure. There is risk of transmission of infection if specimens are mishandled. Hand washing and the use of latex gloves are important. Properly label and wrap specimens in plastic containers to reduce the risk of transmission to personnel.

Blood Cultures

Normally blood is sterile, but bacteria can enter the bloodstream and cause severe infections. *Bacteremia* is the term used to describe bacteria in the bloodstream. *Septicemia* is systemic disease caused by bacteria and their toxins in the blood. Blood cultures are commonly performed on clients with unexplained fever, clients at high risk of sepsis, and clients who appear to be in septic shock.

To collect blood cultures, the skin is thoroughly cleaned at the puncture site. Samples are drawn at specific intervals (e.g., 30 minutes apart) or from opposite arms. Blood samples may be examined for anaerobic or aerobic microorganisms. Ideally, blood cultures should be collected prior to beginning antibiotics. If clients have already received antibiotics, certain enzymes can be added to the growth medium to eliminate the activity of the antibiotic.

Nurses should note on the request slip for the laboratory that the client is receiving antibiotics. Once the specimen is drawn the client should receive any prescribed antibiotics and antipyretics.

Wound Cultures

Healing is delayed in wounds that are infected. Therefore, wound cultures may be used to identify specific microorganisms. Ideally, wound cultures should be collected prior to beginning antibiotics. Wound cultures should be collected using aseptic technique. Additional precautions, such as mask and gown, may be needed to culture wounds with drainage.

Culturettes, sterile cotton-tipped applicators in special containers, are commonly used for collecting wound cultures. The cotton tip should be placed deep into the wound without touching the skin around the wound. Swab the wound where the purulent drainage is most profuse. Return the applicator to the holder and break the bottom of it to release the culture medium. A syringe and needle can also be used to aspirate infectious material from the wound.

Be certain that the request slip indicates any antibiotics and the specific site from which the culture was obtained. Administer the antibiotics prescribed.

Urine Cultures

Normally, urine is sterile, but urinary tract infection (UTI) is a common disorder. Women are prone to UTI because of their short urethra. In addition, nosocomial UTI is a common sequela of indwelling catheterization. The goal of a clean-catch or midstream collection is to minimize contamination of the specimen by external organisms on the perineal skin. This type of specimen is usually collected if the urine is to be cultured. It is important to teach the client to begin voiding, stop voiding, resume voiding, then catch the specimen in the sterile container.

A catheterized specimen may be requested for culture. This technique for collecting a culture is not used often because of the risk of introducing organisms into the urinary tract during catheterization. When this procedure is needed, use a straight catheter of the smallest size to insert into the bladder under aseptic conditions, either through the urethra or as a suprapubic tap, allowing urine to flow directly from the end of the catheter into the sterile specimen container. Some hospitals provide special kits that include a catheter attached to a test tube.

A specimen also may be collected from an indwelling catheter. Urine standing in the collection bag undergoes chemical changes, may be contaminated with bacteria, and does not reflect the client's current urinary status. For these reasons, it should never be used for urine speci-

mens. Instead, obtain the specimen from the catheter or drainage tubing. Avoid opening the drainage system to air because this can introduce microorganisms. Most urinary drainage systems have a specimen collection port built into the top of the drainage tubing. This self-sealing rubber-covered area is cleaned, and the urine is aspirated with a sterile needle and syringe. The tubing may need to be clamped below the port for 15 to 20 minutes to allow enough urine to build up. If there is no collection port and the catheter is not Silastic, use a small 25-gauge needle and syringe to aspirate urine from the catheter itself. Using aseptic technique, insert the needle into the catheter distal to the sleeve leading to the balloon, slant the needle toward the drainage tubing, and avoid entering the balloon lumen. Puncture the catheter at an angle to allow resealing after the needle is withdrawn. This cannot be performed with a Silastic catheter because it will not reseal after being punctured.

Blood Studies

The nurse should check the facility's laboratory procedure manual to review collection procedures, available equipment, biohazard disposal procedures, and universal precautions. The types of blood collection methods include venipuncture, microcapillary collection, and serial port sampling.

Box 13–2. Procedure for Venipuncture

Step 1. Check physician's request to verify test and time requested, client's name, and client's identification number.

Step 2. Select materials needed—alcohol swabs, cotton or gauze swab, adhesive bandage, gloves, labels, needle, sharps container, tube holders, tourniquets, and Vacutainer or syringe.

Step 3. Label Vacutainer with client's name and identification number, collection date and time, specimen source, and test.

Step 4. Greet client; check test and client's name and identification number; and determine client's preparation for test. Wash your hands.

Step 5. Position the client's arm in such a way that it is comfortable for the client and for you to have clear access. The arm should be supported by a firm surface. The client should be sitting or lying down.

Step 6. Assemble the needle, needle holder, Vacutainer tube, alcohol swabs, cotton or gauze swab, and bandage. Take care not to engage the Vacutainer tube. Place any additional Vacutainer tubes in a convenient location. Use a 20- or 21-gauge 1- to 1½-inch needle for antecubital veins.

Step 6. Apply the tourniquet tightly enough to distend the veins but not so tightly that it cuts off circulation. Instruct the client to open and close the fist several times and to keep the fist closed while the vein is being located. If it is difficult to locate a vein, wrap the arm in a warm compress to promote venous distention. Another technique is to use a blood pressure cuff instead of a tourniquet to distend the veins; obtain a pressure between the systolic and diastolic

readings. Remember that a tourniquet or blood pressure cuff should never remain on the client's arm for more than 1 to 2 minutes.

Step 7. Choose the site. Try to locate the median cubital vein. Other acceptable veins are the cephalic and basilic veins. If hand veins are selected, use a 23- or 25-gauge needle.

Step 8. Clean the venipuncture site with 70% isopropyl alcohol by making outward concentric circles. Allow the site to air-dry or wipe with sterile gauze.

Step 9. Anchor the vein by stretching the skin below the site with your thumb. Reassure the client that any discomfort will be short-lasting. Insert the needle bevel-up into the vein and engage the Vacutainer tube. The needle should be at approximately a 15-degree angle to the client's arm and directly in line with the vein. If multiple samples are needed, remove the tube as soon as the blood flow stops and insert the next tube into the needle holder. Once good blood flow is established and before the final tube is filled, release the tourniquet.

Step 10. Remove the last Vacutainer tube from the needle holder. Remove the needle with a swift motion and quickly apply clean cotton or gauze over the puncture site. Apply pressure or direct the client to apply pressure to the puncture site. Properly dispose of the needle in the sharps container. (Do not lay down or recap the needle.) Immediately label the specimen. Remove gloves and wash your hands. Record the client's name, the test performed, disposition of the specimen, and any condition not meeting specimen collection criteria.

Table 13–1. Tubes Used for Venipuncture

Stopper Color	Principal Anticoagulant/Additive	Mode of Action	Commonly Used for
Red	None	NA	Cell/blood typing
	Clot activator and gel separator	Enhances clot formation	Serum blood group antibody testing
			Alkaline phosphatase
			Amylase
			Blood urea nitrogen (BUN)
			Creatine phosphokinase (CPK)
			Calcium
			Cholesterol
Speckled			Compatibility testing
			Drug monitoring
			Glucose
			High-density lipoprotein (HDL)
			Human immunodeficiency virus (HIV)
			Iron profile
			Low-density lipoprotein (LDL)
Gold (Hemoguard)			Liver enzymes
			Potassium
			Protein
			Rapid plasma reagin (RPR)
			Sodium
			Triglycerides
Lavender	Ethylenediaminetetraacetic acid (EDTA)	Binds calcium	Complete blood count (CBC)
			Erythrocyte sedimentation rate (ESR)
			Hemoglobin electrophoresis
			Platelet count
			Reticulocyte count
			Sickle cell screen
			White blood cell differential

From Flynn, J. C., Jr. (1994). *Procedures in phlebotomy*. Philadelphia: W. B. Saunders.

Venipuncture

The procedure for venipuncture is described in Box 13–2. Table 13–1 shows the various tubes, called Vacutainers. The tubes are vacuums and fill automatically with blood. Note that there are several types of tubes. Caution must be taken before drawing blood to ensure that the proper tube is being used. Remember that when cells are damaged, potassium leaks and platelets migrate. Therefore, if multiple blood tests are requested, it is important to draw a platelet test tube before the other test tubes. Another concern is that multiple venipuncture attempts may distort serum potassium results. Therefore, draw potassium early and, if needed, consider that abnormal results may be due to multiple punctures.

When it is preferable to obtain blood from a superficial

hand vein, use a butterfly needle. Insert the butterfly needle (Fig. 13–1). After flashback is noted, use a syringe or Vacutainer tube to withdraw blood from the vein.

Microcapillary Collection

Microcapillary blood collections may be used for a variety of purposes, including peripheral testing in clinics, for very young or very old clients, or for clients with skin disorders. The procedure for microcapillary collection is similar to the procedure for venipuncture. The site of the skin puncture is usually the finger tip. The ear lobe is used for edematous clients. No tourniquet is used. Hold the finger or ear lobe firmly. Clean the area with povidone-iodine (Betadine) or 70% alcohol. A microlance is used instead of a needle and Vacutainer. Make the punc-

Stopper Color	Principal Anticoagulant/Additive	Mode of Action	Commonly Used for
Blue	Sodium citrate	Binds calcium	Activated partial thromboplastin time (aPTT) Individual coagulation factor studies Fibrin degradation products (FDPs) Fibrinogen Prothrombin time (PT)
Green	Heparin	Inactivates thrombin and thromboplastin	Ammonia Chromosome screening Lupus erythematosus cell, preparation HLA typing
Gray	Potassium oxalate/sodium fluoride	Binds calcium Inhibits glycolysis	Glucose
Dark or royal blue	Heparin	Inactivates thrombin and thromboplastin	Trace metals, e.g., lead

ture perpendicular to the fingerprint lines and off the center of the finger. It is important to wipe away the first drop of blood with sterile gauze because it contains plasma. Place the hand in a dependent position and allow the next drops to flow without squeezing. A microtube or pipette may also be used to collect the blood specimen. Following completion of the blood collection, either you or the client must maintain pressure on the puncture site until bleeding has stopped.

Serial Port Sampling

Serial port sampling refers to collection of blood specimens from an indwelling venous catheter. The advantage of this method is that it reduces client discomfort from multiple venipunctures. The procedure for serial port sam-

pling is similar in preparation to the venipuncture procedure. Stop the intravenous fluid flow. After opening the stopcock or choosing the lumen, a 10-ml syringe is used to aspirate 10 ml of blood from the indwelling catheter. The first sample is discarded. Another 10-ml syringe (or 20-ml depending on the number of tests) is used to aspirate the blood specimen needed for the study. The indwelling line is flushed with saline and heparin according to agency procedure. Return the stopcock to the original position. Adjust the intravenous fluid rate as needed.

Arterial Blood Sampling

A sample of blood is collected from an artery for blood gas analysis and, rarely, for other studies. There are risks of bleeding and nerve injury, so arterial sampling is done

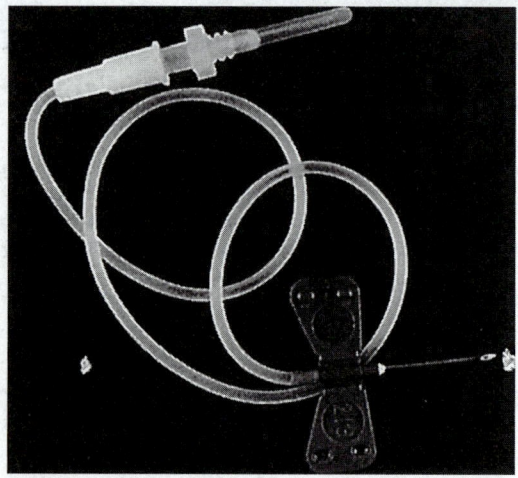

Figure 13–1. A butterfly needle used for venipuncture. (From Flynn, J. C., Jr. [1994]. *Procedures in phlebotomy.* Philadelphia: W. B. Saunders.)

only by trained personnel. The technique and how to analyze blood gases are discussed in Chapter 39.

Analyzing the Results of Blood Studies

The analysis of the results of blood studies should consider whether the findings are normal, expected abnormal, or unexpected abnormal. A laboratory manual can be used to guide your analysis.

Urine Studies

Urinalysis

Urinalysis is one of the oldest and most common laboratory tests. It yields a large amount of information about possible disorders of the kidney and lower urinary tract as well as about systemic disorders that alter the composition of urine. Urinalysis is also valuable because normal results can be used to exclude a number of alternative diagnoses. The advantages of urinalysis are that the test is noninvasive, the specimen is easily obtained, the results are obtained rapidly, and it is economical.

Information from a urinalysis includes color, specific gravity, pH, and the presence of protein, red (RBCs) and white (WBCs) blood cells, bacteria, leukocyte esterase, bilirubin, urobilirubin, glucose, ketones, casts, and crystals. A normal urinalysis does not show protein, bilirubin, urobilirubin, glucose, ketones, bacteria, or leukocyte esterase. A few RBCs, WBCs, casts, and crystals are normal findings.

A random-specimen urinalysis can be collected at any time. In general, an early-morning specimen gives more definitive results because the urine is concentrated and not influenced by the diet. Generally, no specific client preparation is needed. The urine should be collected in a clean container. This type of specimen cannot be used for

C&S tests because the container is not sterile, nor is the technique.

Twelve- or 24-Hour Urinalysis

A timed collection of urine allows for quantitative analysis of specific substances. A specimen collected over time is more accurate than a random specimen. A 12- or 24-hour specimen is usually collected in one large container. Some of the specimens may need a chemical preservative in the container and refrigeration during the collection process. If appropriate refrigeration is not available, the specimen container may be placed in ice or in insulated ice packs. In this case, make sure the cooling agent is replaced frequently so as to maintain the specimen at the necessary temperature. Likewise, if the client has an indwelling catheter, the bag can be placed on ice to collect a 24-hour specimen.

When the specimen collection begins, the client voids and this specimen is discarded. All urine voided in the next 12 or 24 hours, as appropriate, is placed in the container. Twelve or 24 hours from the time of the first voiding, instruct the client to void again and add this urine to the specimen. One of the major needs during this collection process is careful communication among all persons involved. If any single urine specimen is inadvertently discarded, the entire procedure must begin anew. The client should also be taught to limit moderately the amount of fluids consumed and to avoid alcohol. Other specific instructions may be needed, such as avoiding certain foods or medications.

Analyzing the Results of Urine Studies

The urinalysis should consider whether the findings are normal, expected abnormal, or unexpected abnormal. Table 13–2 can guide your analysis.

Diagnostic Imaging

Imaging refers to representations produced by x-rays, nuclear magnetic resonance, tomograms, ultrasound, radioisotopes, and so forth. Methods range from a simple x-ray to very complex and expensive magnetic resonance imaging (MRI) using magnetic fields and radiowaves. It is important to review the protocol to be followed at the particular facility, especially the guidelines for preparation and follow-up care. Nurses may need to consult with the imaging (radiology) department to obtain written guidelines for preparation and postimaging care, or to coordinate studies. For example, barium studies may make visualization of other abdominal tests impossible for up to 2 days.

Explain the procedure to the client and family and answer their questions. Many procedures may take up to an hour (follow-up x-rays are sometimes taken 30 minutes after an injection). Suggest that the client void before the procedure to be comfortable. (Note: There are some procedures for which the bladder must be full.)

Table 13-2. Normal Findings in a Routine Urinalysis	
Component	**Normal Values**
Color	Pale yellow to deep amber
Opacity	Clear
Specific gravity	1.002–1.035
Osmolality	275–295 mOsm/L
pH	4.5–8.0
Glucose	Negative
Ketones	Negative
Protein	Negative
Bilirubin	Negative
Red blood cells	None to 3
White blood cells	None to 4
Bacteria	None
Casts	None
Crystals	None

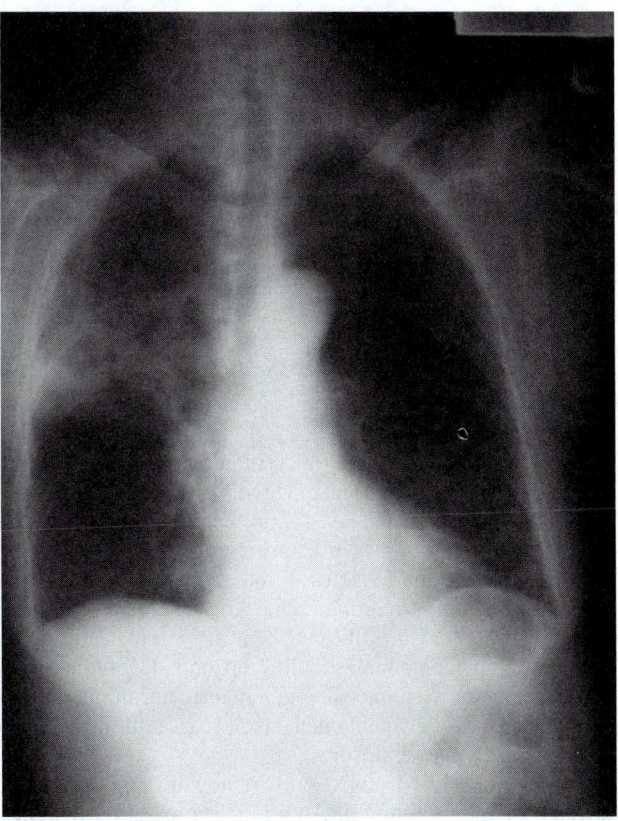

Figure 13–2. A chest x-ray showing right middle lobe pneumonia. The consolidation of lung tissue makes the area appear radiopaque.

X-Ray Studies

Procedure. Radiography is the most widely used diagnostic procedure for the study of soft tissues and bones. Radiographs are commonly called x-rays. Radiographs are negative images on photographic film made by exposure to x-rays that have passed through the body. The energy of the x-ray is adjusted by varying the voltage in the x-ray tube. Because each part of the body absorbs some of the x-rays, variable amounts of exposure are needed for optimal results depending on the body part being examined. Tissue is called *radiopaque* when transmission of x-rays is partially blocked, such as by bone. Bone appears white on an x-ray film. Tissues are said to be *radiolucent* when they allow x-rays to penetrate. Lung is translucent and therefore appears dark on x-ray film. X-rays are two-dimensional, so multiple views are often needed, such as anteroposterior (AP, front to back), posteroanterior (PA, back to front), lateral (from the side), or oblique (at an angle). It is important to note the position of the x-ray for proper interpretation; this is usually recorded by the x-ray technician.

X-ray examinations are important to (1) establish the presence of a mobility or structure problem, (2) follow its progress, and (3) evaluate the effectiveness of treatment. The following are some types of conditions that can be assessed by x-ray:

- A radiopaque (rather than radiolucent) area in the lung could mean pulmonary edema, pneumonia, or a tumor (Fig. 13–2).
- Alterations in normal contour or density of bones, such as develop with fractures or osteoporosis (Fig. 13–3).
- Changes in fat lines around soft tissues. When tumor or

inflammation is present, fat tissue is replaced by soft tissues.
- Enlargement in shadows produced by organs. For example, an enlarged heart shadow could mean an enlarged heart from congestive heart failure or athletic activity.

Preprocedure Care. Two potential risks from repeated exposure to radiation are genetic and somatic. The

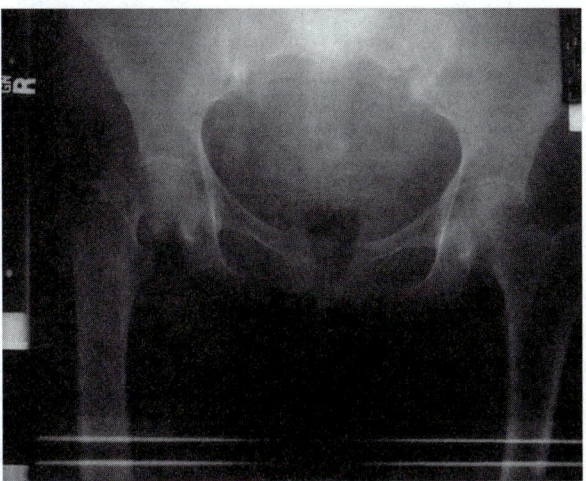

Figure 13–3. An x-ray showing a fracture of the hip.

genetic risk involves changes in the chromosomes. If a developing fetus (first trimester) is exposed to radiation, the chromosomes can mutate and the baby will be born with deformities. Likewise, eggs and sperm can be damaged, which may lead to similar problems with future pregnancies.

Somatic changes occur in body tissues receiving excessive doses of repeated exposure to radiation. The risks from radiation exposure are cumulative, and therefore potentially more dangerous to healthcare personnel than to clients. Side effects of the use of radiation for cancer treatment may be found in Chapter 24.

Several safety measures are used to avoid exposure to x-rays. The walls in rooms in which x-ray machines are located are lined with lead. Lead-lined protection, such as aprons, eyeglasses, and thyroid shields, are used by x-ray personnel. Maintaining adequate distance is also important and x-ray rooms have a protective divider for the technician. When x-rays are taken outside of the radiology department there is less protection available. If the nurse is assisting the client and must remain with the client during exposure, the nurse must wear a lead apron. Other nursing personnel should step outside of the room during exposure. Clients are given lead aprons to shield their gonads. X-ray personnel also wear a film badge to monitor accidental exposure.

Ask the client to remove any radiopaque objects (e.g., jewelry or metal buttons). Additional preparation depends on the type of study. If his or her condition makes it possible, the client may be asked to move into various positions so that x-ray films can be taken from the most useful angles.

Because various positions may be difficult or painful and x-ray tables are hard, analgesia and other pain-relieving interventions may be needed before and after the x-ray study. The focus of nursing care for the client having diagnostic imaging studies is on client preparation and follow-up care. Occasionally the nurse is asked to monitor the unstable client during an imaging procedure. The nurse needs an oximetry monitor, sphygmomanometer (an instrument for measuring blood pressure), stethoscope, extra intravenous fluids, and an emergency cart. Any pertinent findings, such as the presence of a pacemaker or an artificial joint, should be noted on the x-ray request.

Postprocedure Care. Although generally no specific care is needed after x-ray procedures, certain types of x-ray procedures do require specific postprocedure care. That care is discussed under the headings corresponding to the specific x-ray procedures.

Chest X-Rays

Chest x-ray studies may be taken to detect pulmonary disease and the status of respiratory problems or trauma, and to confirm endotracheal or tracheostomy tube placement. Instruct the client to remove all clothing and metal objects above the waist. The PA chest x-ray is taken with the client standing or sitting facing the x-ray film, with the chest and shoulders in direct contact with the film cassette. The shoulders are rotated forward to pull the scapulae away from the lung field. The radiograph is usually taken at full inspiration, which causes the diaphragm to move downward. Radiographs taken on expiration are sometimes requested to demonstrate the extent of diaphragm movement or to assist in the assessment and diagnosis of pneumothorax. For clients unable to be transported to the imaging department, a portable chest x-ray may be taken. Portable radiographs are usually taken with the film placed behind the client, and the x-ray beam penetrates from the front of the chest—the AP position. There is no follow-up care for a chest x-ray. A normal chest x-ray is shown in Chapter 39.

Plain Abdominal Films

A plain abdominal film ("flat plate") can reveal abnormalities such as tumors, obstructions, abnormal gas collections, and strictures. For this procedure the client wears a hospital gown without belts or jewelry. There is no follow-up care needed for this study.

Skeletal X-Rays

When fractures are suspected, x-rays are ordered for the bones in question. Generally, the procedure is not painful unless the extremity has to be moved for positioning. Some projections:

Waters' projection: A PA view of the skull to show the orbits and maxillary sinuses (be certain there is no risk of cervical spine fracture or do a negative lateral cervical spine x-ray)
Towne's projection: An AP view to demonstrate the occipital bone and facial structures, such as the zygomatic arch
Panorex: A 180-degree view of the teeth and jaw

Contrast X-Rays

■ Upper Gastrointestinal Series (Barium Swallow)

Procedure. An upper gastrointestinal (GI) series permits radiologic visualization of the esophagus, stomach, and duodenum. It can aid in the detection of strictures, ulcers, tumors, polyps, hiatal hernias, and motility problems.

Preprocedure Care. Instruct the client to abstain from food and fluids for 6 to 8 hours before the test. The client drinks a radiopaque contrast medium (barium) while standing in front of the fluoroscopy tube. The upper GI series takes about 45 minutes. The client is asked to move to other positions, such as lying on the x-ray table. Barium sulfate is a chalky-white radiopaque contrast agent that is not absorbed by the GI system. Defects such as tumors, strictures, and motility problems are detected in the radiograph patterns.

Postprocedure Care. Because barium may cause constipation, it is important to teach the client to drink extra fluids and eat adequate fiber. A laxative may be ordered to help expel the barium and prevent a fecal impaction. Assess the abdomen for distention and bowel sounds. Observe, or instruct the client to observe, the stool to determine whether the barium has been completely eliminated. Initially, the client's stool is white but it should return to its normal brown color within 72 hours. Constipation with a distended abdomen may indicate a barium impaction.

■ Lower Gastrointestinal Series (Barium Enema)

Procedure. A lower GI series is performed to visualize the position, movements, and filling of the colon. In a lower GI series, a radiopaque contrast medium (barium) is instilled rectally and x-rays are taken with or without fluoroscopy. The procedure is uncomfortable and may last 60 to 90 minutes. This test can aid in detection of tumors, diverticula, stenoses, obstructions, inflammation, ulcerative colitis, and polyps.

Preprocedure Care. Adequate bowel preparation is essential and varies among institutions. A typical preparation for most adults includes placing the client on a low-residue or clear liquid diet for 2 days prior to the test to reduce feces volume. The client usually receives a potent laxative and an oral liquid preparation for cleaning the bowel the day before the test. The client receives nothing by mouth (NPO) after midnight. The morning of the examination, a suppository or a cleaning enema may be administered. Note that if the client has active bleeding or an ileostomy, different bowel preparations may be needed. *If ultrasound, an abdominal scan, or colonoscopy is also indicated, it should be performed first because the barium will interfere with these tests.*

Postprocedure Care. A laxative or cleansing enema is often given after the test to empty the large bowel and prevent barium impaction. Stools are white for 24 to 72 hours following the examination. The client should increase intake of liquids to prevent fecal impaction. The client should report any pain, bloating, absence of stool, or bleeding.

Computed Tomography

Procedure. Computed tomography (CT) scans image differences in bone and soft tissue. The images are generated by computer synthesis of x-ray data obtained in many different directions in a cross-sectional plane. The computed data are assembled as three-dimensional images. CT is used to identify space-occupying lesions (masses) and shifts of structures caused by neoplasms, cysts, focal inflammatory lesions, and abscesses of the head, chest, abdomen, pelvis, and extremities (Fig. 13–4). To distinguish normal tissue from abnormal masses, contrast media may be administered. The CT scan can be performed quickly—within 20 minutes, not including analysis.

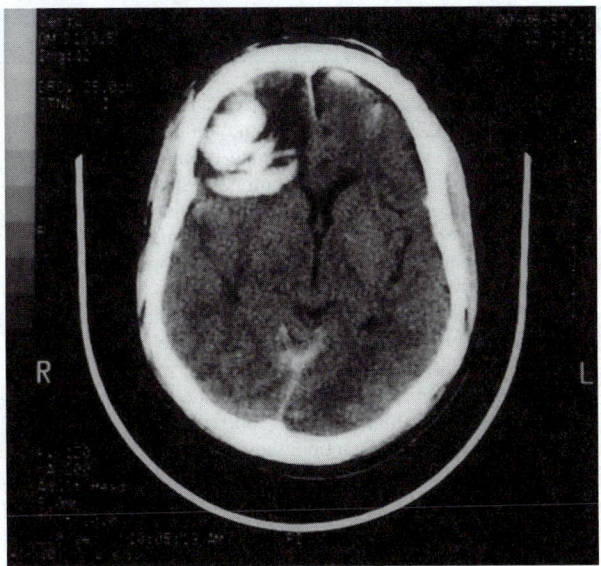

Figure 13–4. A computed tomography scan of the head. The brain tissue is gray and the skull is white. The mass in the left frontal lobe is blood from a head injury.

Preprocedure Care. Prior to the test, ascertain that informed consent has been obtained, and answer any questions the client and family may have about the CT scan. Explain that fasting usually is not required for CT of the head, but ask whether or not the client becomes nauseated easily and adjust food and fluid intake accordingly. For example, some clients prefer a light breakfast to reduce nausea while others prefer an empty stomach. Fasting is usually required for CT of the abdomen. Explain that a contrast agent is often given. Because the contrast (also called dye) is iodine-based, ask whether the client has allergies to iodine, contrast dyes, or shellfish. (See Box 13–3 on the use of contrast.)

If the CT is going to be of the head, remove any objects from the hair before the examination (wigs, barrettes, earrings, hair pins). The client's hair should be combed smoothly.

Explain the client's role in the scan. The client is positioned supine and the body part to be scanned is placed into the doughnut-shaped ring of the scanner. The table is moved by the technician from a control room during the scan to direct the study toward different levels. The client should expect to hear mechanical noises coming from the scanner. Some clients will feel claustrophobic during the test but should be assured that it is possible to communicate with the technician during the scan. Finally, the client is asked to remain still during the scan. If the client is unable to comply, sedation or even general anesthesia may be required. Clients who are agitated or unable to maintain a motionless position may require sedation prior to the scan. Instruct adults requiring sedation to (1) avoid alcohol and caffeine on the day of the scan, (2) not eat for 2 hours prior to scan time, and (3) arrange for a driver for escort home after the scan.

Postprocedure Care. Following the test, the client is assessed for reactions to the contrast agent, as well as

Box 13–3. Use of Contrast

Certain disorders are better visualized with the use of a contrast agent. For example, tumors are better visualized with contrast, whereas bleeding and edema can be seen better without it. The use of contrast agents is potentially dangerous. Contrast agents may irritate blood vessels. Clients who are sensitive to contrast agents may have allergic reactions, and if untreated they may develop anaphylactic shock.

Ask the client about a known allergy to contrast dye or possible allergy to iodine or shellfish (which has a high iodine content). Note the type of allergic response on the record: for example, "client states she develops hives from eating shellfish." Some clients report allergies but when asked to explain the reaction, they state that they "feel warm" when given the dye. This is a normal reaction, not an allergic one. Some clients are given contrast dye even though they report contrast allergy. To reduce the severity of the reaction, these clients are pretreated with an antihistamine or corticosteroids. Therefore, do not assure the client with a reported allergy to dye that contrast dye will not be given. Even if the client states that he or she has no history of allergy, observe the client for symptoms of an allergic reaction following the injection of contrast dye. Some anaphylactic reactions have occurred with the first dose of dye. Instruct the client that it is normal to feel a hot, flushed sensation and metallic taste in the mouth when the dye is

injected. The client should report any difficulty breathing or pruritus (itching) to personnel in the radiology department. After the procedure has been completed, the client can usually resume normal activities. Diuresis will occur shortly after the use of contrast agents. If the client is able to do so, encourage him or her to drink at least one glass of water or other liquid an hour following the procedure. Replacement fluid may be needed, and the client should be assessed for fluid balance. The fluid balance in clients with renal or cardiac disease should be assessed carefully after a series of tests requiring intravenous contrast agents.

Complications rarely occur but may include local and systemic allergic reactions, spasm, occlusion of the vessel by a clot, or bleeding at the injection site. Assess the affected extremity for color, warmth, pulses distal to the injection site, bleeding or hematoma formation, and ability to move the site.

In addition, assess the client for clinical manifestations of an allergic reaction, which include pallor, tachycardia, restlessness, sneezing, coughing, erythema, tachypnea, respiratory distress, facial flushing, urticaria, pruritus, hypotension, nausea, and vomiting. Assess the client for these reactions after the dye is injected, because clients have had respiratory and cardiac arrests while undergoing x-ray study. Emergency equipment should always be available.

---

for the presence of hematoma at the injection site and the quality of pulses in the extremity used for injection of the contrast. The client may resume normal activities, unless other diagnostic tests are planned. Diuresis from the dye should be expected. Following the test, encourage the client to drink liquids to excrete the contrast and to prevent nephrotoxic injury.

Magnetic Resonance Imaging

Procedure. MRI is a diagnostic tool similar to CT. The advantage of MRI is that it is noninvasive. MRI uses powerful magnetic fields and radiofrequency pulses to produce an image; therefore, the client is not exposed to ionizing radiation. The magnet in the scanner is 30,000 times more powerful than the earth's magnetic field. A contrast agent is often used to augment the images. MRI images are the opposite of CT images. Bone appears black on MRI and white on CT scan (Fig. 13–5). MRI is not used for pregnant clients and cannot be used in clients with pacemakers, implants, some types of ventilators, or metal fragments (e.g., shrapnel). The powerful magnet in the MRI can interfere with functioning and position of metallic devices and fragments.

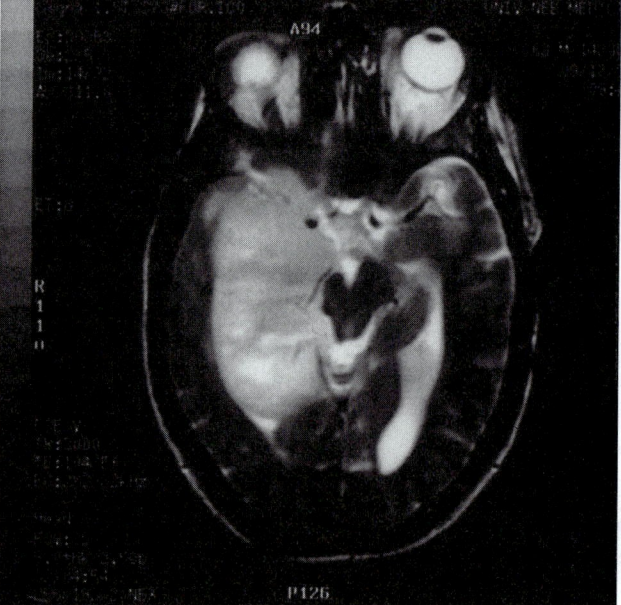

Figure 13–5. Magnetic resonance imaging of the head. The eyes are evident at the top of the image. This client has a brain tumor.

Preprocedure Care. The client and family should be told the purpose of the test, the sounds and sensations that the client will hear and feel during the examination, and the client's role during the test.

Prior to the test, the client should remove all metal-

containing objects (e.g., brassiere, jewelry, watch). Any internal metal objects, such as a prosthesis or pacemaker, should be noted for the physician. Intravenous fluid pumps need to be removed during the test. Special precautions are needed for clients with pulse oximeters. The cord from the sensor to the finger cannot be coiled around the body or any body part because it may cause a burn.[10]

The client can eat and take any prescribed medication prior to examination of the head. When an MRI is required for the GI system, the client must be NPO for 6 hours before the procedure. Instruct the client that the test requires that he or she lie still during the procedure, which can take from 60 to 90 minutes. Clients who are agitated or not able to maintain a motionless position may require sedation prior to the scan. If the use of contrast is planned, ask whether the client tends to become nauseated easily and adjust the intake of food and fluids accordingly.

The client lies supine on a narrow padded table. The client may be asked to lie still while the test is in progress. There will be loud clanging noises from the scanner while the images are being taken and the client should wear earplugs. Some clients will feel claustrophobic during the test, but should be assured it is possible to communicate with the technician during the scan. The examination takes about an hour.

Postprocedure Care. Following the test, the client may resume previous activities and diet. Expect diuresis if contrast was used.

Positron Emission Tomography

Procedure. Positron emission tomography (PET) allows imaging of metabolic and physiologic function. The function of diseased tissue often differs from that of normal tissues. The client is given doses of strong radioactive tracers (radionuclides), and the tracers emit signals showing the uptake and distribution of the substance. The images are formed by computer analysis of photons detected by annihilation of positrons emitted by the radionuclides (Fig. 13–6). PET has three primary uses:

1. To determine the amount of blood flow into specific body tissues
2. To reveal how adequately tissues use blood receptors, such as medications or neurotransmitters
3. To measure blood flow, glucose metabolism, and oxygen extraction

PET is used in the diagnosis of stroke, brain tumors, and epilepsy and to chart the progress of Alzheimer's disease, Parkinson's disease, head injury, schizophrenia, manic-depressive illness, and cardiac hypoxemia.

Preprocedure Care. Explain to the client and family the purpose of the test, the sounds and sensations that the client will hear and feel during the examination, and the client's role during the test. In contrast to CT and MRI, the PET scanner is absolutely quiet. Clients need to fast for 4 hours prior to the scan. If the client is diabetic, it is preferred that the blood sugar be below 150 g/dl. Clients who are agitated may require sedation prior to the scan. The client needs to remain motionless for approximately 45 minutes.

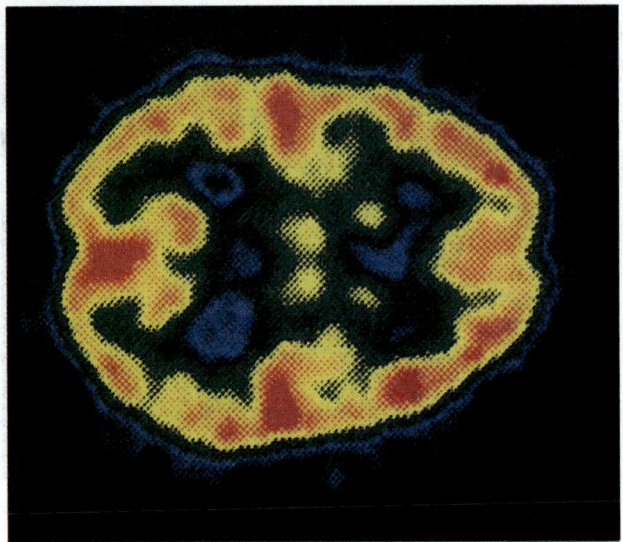

Figure 13–6. A positron emission tomographic scan showing decreased metabolic activity after a seizure (noted as green areas on the scan).

Postprocedure Care. No special care is required after the procedure.

Ultrasonography

Procedure. Ultrasonography (also called ultrasound or echography) is the use of high-frequency sound waves to visualize soft tissues by recording the reflection of sound waves off the tissues. It works on the same principle as sonar and radar. When the ultrasound waves are directed into the body, they spread through the tissues. Because tissues differ in structure, the sound waves are reflected in various ways. The reflected waves are processed and shown as an image and then recorded. There is no exposure to ionizing radiation during this test.

Ultrasound can be used to assess many structures in the body, including the heart, great vessels, liver, gallbladder, uterus and ovaries, kidney, and thyroid gland (Fig. 13–7). It is commonly used in obstetrics to determine gestational age.

Preprocedure Care. No special care is required prior to ultrasound. The client should be told the reason for the test and what to expect. Sometimes a bowel preparation with laxatives is used for viewing the abdominal organs. The bladder must be very full to view the uterus.

A gel is applied to the skin and the transducer is moved over the organ. The transducer is a device that changes reflected high-frequency sound to electrical energy. The procedure is painless and fairly quick. Sometimes the room must be darkened to see the scope.

Postprocedure Care. No special care is required after ultrasound.

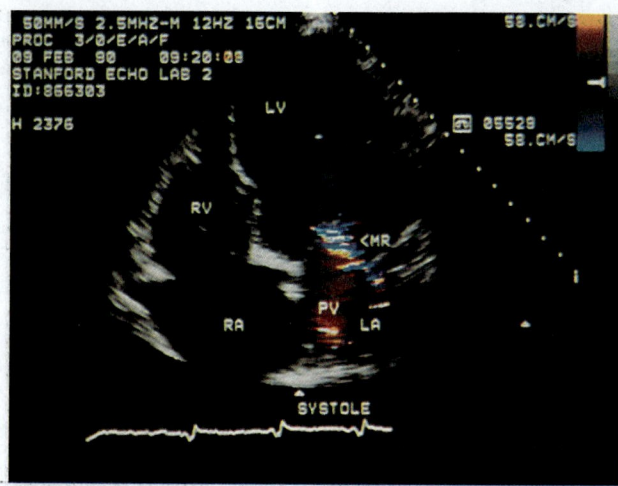

Figure 13–7. An ultrasound of the heart (an echocardiogram). (From Bennett, J. C., & Plum, F. [1996]. *Cecil textbook of medicine* [20th ed.]. Philadelphia: W. B. Saunders.)

Angiography

Procedure. Angiography is radiography of vessels after injection of contrast material to assess their patency or to determine if blood flow is normal. A common form of angiography is coronary angiography to determine the degree of obstruction of the myocardial circulation (Fig. 13–8). Angiography can also be used to outline veins (venography) or lymphatic vessels (lymphography). The terms *angiogram* and *arteriogram* are used interchangeably in practice.

Preprocedure Care. Prior to angiography see that the client understands the planned procedure. An in-

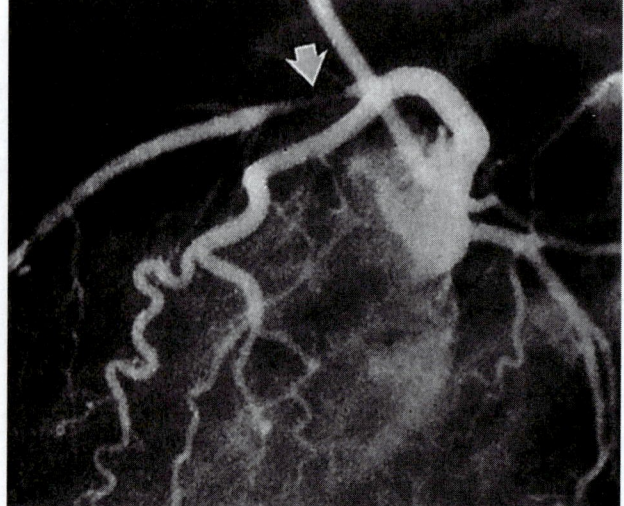

Figure 13–8. Coronary angiography shows stenosis (narrowing; *arrow*) of the left anterior descending coronary artery. (From Braunwald, E. [1992]. *Heart disease: A textbook of cardiovascular medicine* [4th ed.]. Philadelphia: W. B. Saunders.)

formed consent is signed after all questions are answered. Any known allergies to contrast, shellfish, or iodine must be noted. Baseline data should be collected on vital signs, quality and symmetry of pulses in the extremities, level of consciousness, speech patterns, and estimates of limb strength. These same assessments are made after the procedure. *A detailed baseline is critical to accurate assessment of postprocedure changes.*

The client is NPO for 6 to 8 hours in most institutions. Some centers do allow fluids to reduce the risk of dehydration and clotting. Be sure to follow your facility's protocol. The planned puncture site may be shaved.

Postprocedure Care. Hemorrhage or hematoma at the puncture site, with decreased perfusion of the distal extremity and allergic reaction to the contrast agent, are the two major complications that can develop after angiography. The nurse's assessment is critical to their early detection. The usual plan of care is given here, but be certain to follow your facility's protocol. Commonly, care includes the following:

- If the femoral approach was used, keep the leg immobile. Instruct the client not to flex the hip or leg for 12 hours. If the brachial approach was used, release the pressure dressing and apply an elastic bandage to the arm. The arm must remain straight. Movement of the extremity can dislodge the clots at the puncture site and result in bleeding.
- Monitor vital signs every 15 minutes for 2 hours, then hourly until stable. Review the manifestations of an allergic reaction (see Box 13–3).
- Keep a sandbag on the femoral puncture site to maintain pressure on the site. Check the puncture site every 15 minutes for 2 hours, then hourly.
- Monitor distal pulses every 15 minutes for 2 hours, then hourly until stable. Assess the quality of the pulses and note capillary filling time. Notify the physician if the quality of the pulse changes.
- Expect diuresis, provide ample fluids, and keep a urinal or bedpan nearby.
- If prescribed, resume medications and diet.

Radionuclide Scanning

Procedure. Radionuclides are radioisotopes or tracers that are used to visualize organs or regions that cannot be seen on plain films. Radioactive isotopes are treated by living cells in the same way as are the normal elements. Their radiation can be detected by suitable counters. Radionuclide studies may be used to diagnose disorders of the heart, thyroid, liver, brain, bone, kidney, spleen, pancreas, lung, and gallbladder. Various isotopes are used because they concentrate in one organ or body fluid. For example, thallium concentrates in the heart, whereas iodine concentrates in the thyroid. Used extensively in this area is an artificial radioactive element called technetium. Technetium emits gamma radiation only, and therefore is safer to use than other isotopes that emit more damaging radiation. When combined with pyrophosphate given intravenously, technetium is taken up by bone and the entire skeleton can be surveyed. This is helpful in detecting bone tumors (Fig. 13–9). When combined with albumin, technetium concentrates in the lung and can be used to estimate pulmonary blood flow. It can also be used to investigate lesions in other organs and has largely replaced the use of radioactive iodine for thyroid assessment.

If radioactive iodine is to be used for thyroid assessment, a blocking agent may be administered prior to the radionuclide to prevent uptake by other tissues. The blocking agent is not radioactive. For example, iodine is normally concentrated in the thyroid gland. When iodine-tagged radionuclides are used for other than thyroid studies, Lugol's solution is given to block the uptake of the iodine-tagged radionuclides by the thyroid.

The radionuclide is administered orally or intravenously about 1 to 3 hours prior to the test to allow sufficient time for distribution. During the waiting period the client is advised to drink extra fluids to clear the portion not taken up by the tissues. After the waiting period the client is placed on a table and an imaging device records the activity of the emitted radiation.

Radioactivity may be increased or decreased in comparison with normal activity in the organ. Areas of decreased activity, called *cold-spot imaging,* usually indicate tissues that are not functioning. This is common when normal tissues have been replaced by tumor. Increased activity, called *hot-spot imaging,* may occur in tissues that are metabolically more active. For example, a diseased thyroid gland or infection in bone can be detected by hot-spot imaging.

Preprocedure Care. The client should be told that only a very small amount of radioactivity is present in the radionuclide. Enemas may be required prior to scans of the abdomen. Radionuclide tests should be scheduled before other tests that use iodinated contrast or barium. These substances block the exit of protons from the radionuclides. This is especially important with radioactive iodine thyroid scans. The use of contrast for other studies can block uptake of radioactive iodine for months.

In addition, the following information is needed from the client:

- Age, weight, and height to calculate the amount of radioactive substance to be used
- Menstrual history to rule out pregnancy (pregnancy is a contraindication to many radionuclide studies)
- Whether the client is breast-feeding (breast-feeding is a contraindication to many radionuclide studies)
- A history of allergy
- Recent exposure to radionuclides
- Presence of internal prostheses that could block the view of the organ
- Current treatments, such as the need for oxygen, telemetry, or timed specimen collections

Postprocedure Care. The client is advised to drink extra fluids; otherwise, no special care is required.

Endoscopy

Endoscopy is direct visualization of a body system or part by means of a lighted, flexible tube. It is more accurate than radiologic examination because the physician can directly observe sources of bleeding and surface lesions and determine the status of healing tissues.

Arthroscopy

Procedure. Arthroscopy is an endoscopic examination for diagnosis and treatment of joints. An arthroscope is a thin fiberoptic instrument that allows examination of various joints, including hip, knee, shoulder, elbow, and wrists, without making a large incision into the joint. Biopsies can be taken, articular cartilage abnormalities

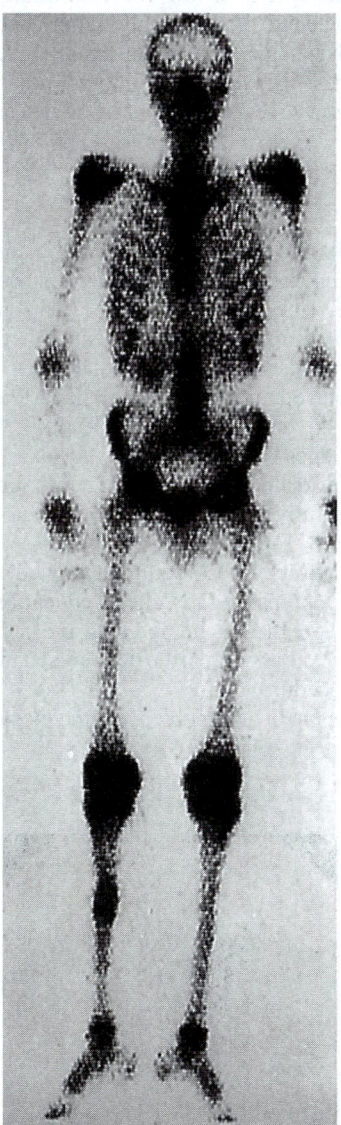

Figure 13–9. A technetium scan of the skeleton shows an area of increased radionuclide density on the right tibia that is a bone tumor. (From Walter, J. B. [1992]. *An introduction to the principles of disease* [3rd ed.]. Philadelphia: W. B. Saunders.)

can be assessed, loose bodies can be removed, and cartilage trimmed. Arthroscopy is usually an outpatient procedure performed under local anesthesia. The client is usually home and back to work sooner than if an arthrotomy (opening the joint) had been performed. Arthroscopy is contraindicated in clients whose joint flexion is less than 50% or if a skin or wound infection is present at the site. Complications are rare but include infection, hemarthrosis (blood in the joint), swelling, synovial rupture, joint injury, or thrombophlebitis.

Preprocedure Care. Instruct the client to fast from midnight the night before. Be sure the client and family know where the procedure will be performed and by whom and that appropriate consent forms are obtained. If a local anesthetic will be used, tell the client that there may be mild discomfort as it is administered and inserted.

Postprocedure Care. Instruct the client to watch for indications of postprocedure infection, such as temperature elevation or local inflammation at the incision site, and to report this promptly. Ensure necessary pain relief after the procedure. Tell the client that a normal diet may be resumed as soon as desired. Advise him or her that unless a surgical incision is performed and the surgeon gives specific instructions to the contrary, walking is usually permitted after sensation has returned, but excessive exercises should be avoided for a few days.

Bronchoscopy

Procedure. Bronchoscopy is the passage of a lighted bronchoscope into the bronchial tree (see Fig. 39–17). Bronchoscopy may be performed with rigid steel or flexible fiberoptic instruments. Bronchoscopy may be performed for diagnostic or therapeutic purposes. The diagnostic purposes include (1) examination of tissue, (2) further evaluation of a tumor for potential surgical resection, (3) collection of tissue specimens for diagnosis, and (4) evaluation of bleeding sites.

Therapeutic bronchoscopy is used to (1) remove foreign bodies, (2) remove thick, viscous secretions, (3) treat postoperative atelectasis, and (4) destroy and remove lesions.

Preprocedure Care. Explain the procedure to the client and family and obtain an informed consent. Instruct the client not to eat or drink anything 6 hours before the test. Tell the client that his or her throat may be sore after the bronchoscopy, and some initial difficulty swallowing will be present. Before sedation, dentures, contact lenses, and other prostheses are removed. Sedation is given to suppress cough, sedate the patient, and relieve anxiety. A topical anesthetic is also sprayed in the back of the throat.

During the procedure, the client lies supine with the head hyperextended. The nurse monitors vital signs, talks to and reassures the client, and assists the physician as necessary.

Postprocedure Care. After the procedure, vital signs are monitored per hospital protocol. The client is observed for signs of respiratory distress, including dyspnea, changes in respiratory rate, use of accessory muscles, and changes in, or absent, lung sounds. Pneumothorax is a possible complication. Sputum is inspected for evidence of hemoptysis. Nothing is given by mouth until the cough and swallow reflexes have returned, which is usually in 1 to 2 hours. Once the client can swallow, feeding may begin with ice chips and small sips of water. Lung sounds are monitored for 24 hours. Development of an adventitious sound should be reported to the physician.

Gastrointestinal Endoscopy

Procedure. Endoscopy of the upper GI tract includes esophagoscopy and esophagogastroduodenscopy (EGD). These procedures are useful for examining clients with acute or chronic GI bleeding, pernicious anemia, esophageal injury, dysphagia, substernal pain, and epigastric discomfort. Upper GI endoscopy should not be performed on clients with severe cardiovascular disease (Fig. 13–10).

Preprocedure Care. To prevent aspiration of the stomach contents, the client is NPO for 8 hours before the procedure. The client may receive an anticholinergic medication to decrease oropharyngeal secretions and prevent reflex bradycardia. Sedatives, narcotics, or tranquilizers such as diazepam (Valium) or meperidine (Demerol) also may be given before the procedure. Dentures and removable bridges should be removed prior to the procedure to prevent dislodgement. The client's oral cavity also should be carefully assessed for the presence of infection or any lesions.

Endoscopic procedures require a signed consent. Provide complete preprocedure client education to enhance cooperation. Tell the client not to drive a motor vehicle for at least 12 hours after the test if sedation was used during the procedure.

A local anesthetic is sprayed on the posterior pharynx

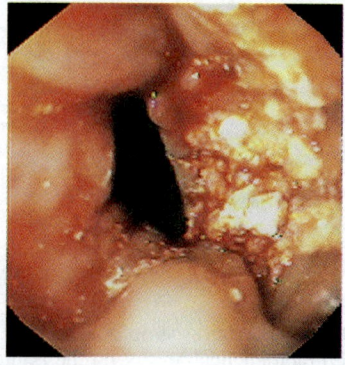

Figure 13–10. An endoscopic view of the esophagus shows an esophageal ulcer.

to ease discomfort and prevent gagging when the tube is inserted. This anesthetic often tastes unpleasant and makes the tongue feel swollen. The client should not swallow saliva after the throat has been anesthetized. Saliva can drain from the side of the mouth. The musculature of the GI tract tends to react with spasms and gagging if premedication is not used.

Postprocedure Care. Following the procedure check vital signs frequently. The client is placed on his or her side to prevent aspiration while the sedation and local anesthetic wear off. The client is NPO until the gag reflex returns (2–4 hours). Many endoscopic procedures are performed on an outpatient basis. The physician may order anesthetic throat lozenges or normal saline gargles for throat irritation or hoarseness.

Assess the client after endoscopy for signs of GI perforation, which include bleeding, fever, and dysphagia. The client with cervical perforation has crepitus (crackling) in the neck from the leakage. Neck and throat pain, aggravated by swallowing or moving, may also occur. Midesophageal perforation can result in referred substernal or epigastric pain. Also, assess for cyanosis, pleural effusion, and back pain. Distal esophageal perforation may result in shoulder pain, dyspnea, or clinical manifestations similar to those of perforated ulcer.

Cytologic Studies

Cytology is the study of the anatomy, physiology, pathology, and chemistry of the cell. A staining technique developed by George Papanicolaou is useful for determining the presence of malignant cells. This technique, called the *Pap smear*, is commonly used to study vaginal or cervical cells. Some tissue specimens can be obtained easily by smearing or by scraping the tissue. Smears are taken from the mouth, genital tract, and anus. Biopsies are used to obtain other tissue samples.

Biopsy is removal of tissue for diagnostic study. The tissue removed must be representative of the suspicious tissue, of adequate size to be examined, and kept intact until studied. Many times a fixative or refrigeration is used to prevent tissue decomposition. Not all tissues are placed in fixative. Breast tissue to be analyzed for hormones is not placed in a fixative. There are several types of biopsy procedures:

- *Needle aspiration biopsy* is performed by inserting a trocar or needle into the tissue. The aspirated cells are then examined. This technique is common for the biopsy of breast masses.
- *Stereotactic needle aspiration biopsy* is a relatively new procedure that creates a three-dimensional view of the abnormal tissue. Based on the imaging, a needle is inserted into the mass. The client must be able to remain motionless for 20 to 60 minutes while the coordinates are determined.
- *Core needle biopsy* is performed by using a special needle that can cut a specimen from tissues not in view. This technique is common for biopsy of kidney, prostate, liver, lung, and thyroid gland.

- *Punch biopsy* removes a small specimen by means of a special instrument that pierces the organ directly or through the skin. This technique is commonly used for biopsy of skin or cervix.
- *Excision biopsy* is the removal of the entire suspicious lesion and a margin of surrounding normal tissue. This is the procedure of choice for most lesions.
- *Incision biopsy* is the removal of a part of the suspicious lesion. This form of biopsy is commonly completed during endoscopic examination.
- *Shave biopsy* is the removal of skin lesions by shaving them from the skin surface with a surgical blade or razor blade.

Two methods are used to assess for malignant cells from tissue samples: *frozen sections* and *permanent* or *fixed sections*. Frozen sections are used for rapid microscopic diagnosis. A thin slice of tissue is cut from the frozen specimen and examined. The procedure requires about 10 to 15 minutes. The pathologist can determine if malignancy is present and if all of the tumor has been removed by looking for a margin of tumor-free tissue.

Permanent sections require about 48 hours. The tissue is placed in a fixative and then examined. It can be stained to facilitate pathologic study.

Prior to biopsy, the client should be told about the purpose of the procedure and a consent form obtained. The client may express concern or anxiety about the possible results of the biopsy and the nurse should be empathic with the client and family. Some clients will sign a permit that allows surgical excision of the mass if it is found to be malignant on frozen section. In these situations, the nurse should perform a complete baseline assessment for postoperative comparison. Certain types of biopsy require the client's cooperation. For example, to reduce the risk of liver laceration during biopsy of the liver, the client is instructed to hold the breath.

Postprocedural care varies with the type of biopsy. If organs such as the liver, lung, or kidney are biopsied, a risk of bleeding, peritonitis, and pneumothorax exists. Tailor the specific interventions to match the client's needs. Guidelines for care are offered in each chapter on assessment in this book.

Conclusions

Diagnostic testing is common in both hospital and ambulatory care settings. The nurse should be familiar with the various tests on urine, blood, and other body fluids. Many settings now require nurses to be "cross-trained" to collect these specimens. Knowledge of how to collect the specimen and the care needed by the client before and after the procedure are important aspects of nursing management. Diagnostic assessment of organs mandates that the nurse understand the test and the proper scheduling of multiple tests to avoid losing time. In addition, most laboratories call or fax results to the nurses. The nurse is responsible for determining whether the results warrant notification of the physician.

Bibliography

1. Caffery, L., & Claussen, D. (1991). Inpatient education for fiberoptic/videoptic diagnostic and therapeutic procedures for gastroenterology. *Gastroenterology Nursing, 14*(2), 106–109.
2. Corbett, J. (1992). *Laboratory tests and diagnostic procedures with nursing diagnosis.* Norwalk, CT: Appleton & Lange.
3. Flynn, J. C., Jr. (1994). *Procedures in phlebotomy.* Philadelphia: W. B. Saunders.
4. McFarland, M. (1994). *Nursing implications of laboratory tests.* Albany, NY: Delmar.
5. Monroe, D. (1991). Patient teaching for X-ray and other diagnostics. *RN, 54*(2), 44–46.
6. Pinner, J. (1991). Patient teaching for X-ray and other diagnostics. *RN, 54*(3), 32–36.
7. Putnam, C., & Ravin, C. (1994). *Textbook of diagnostic imaging.* Philadelphia: W. B. Saunders.
8. Zubay, R. (1988). Understanding magnetic resonance imaging from a nursing perspective. *Orthopaedic Nursing, 7*(6), 17–22.

UNIT 3

Foundations for Medical-Surgical Nursing Practice

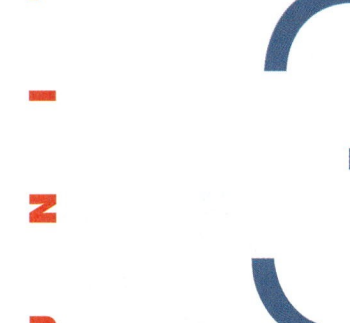

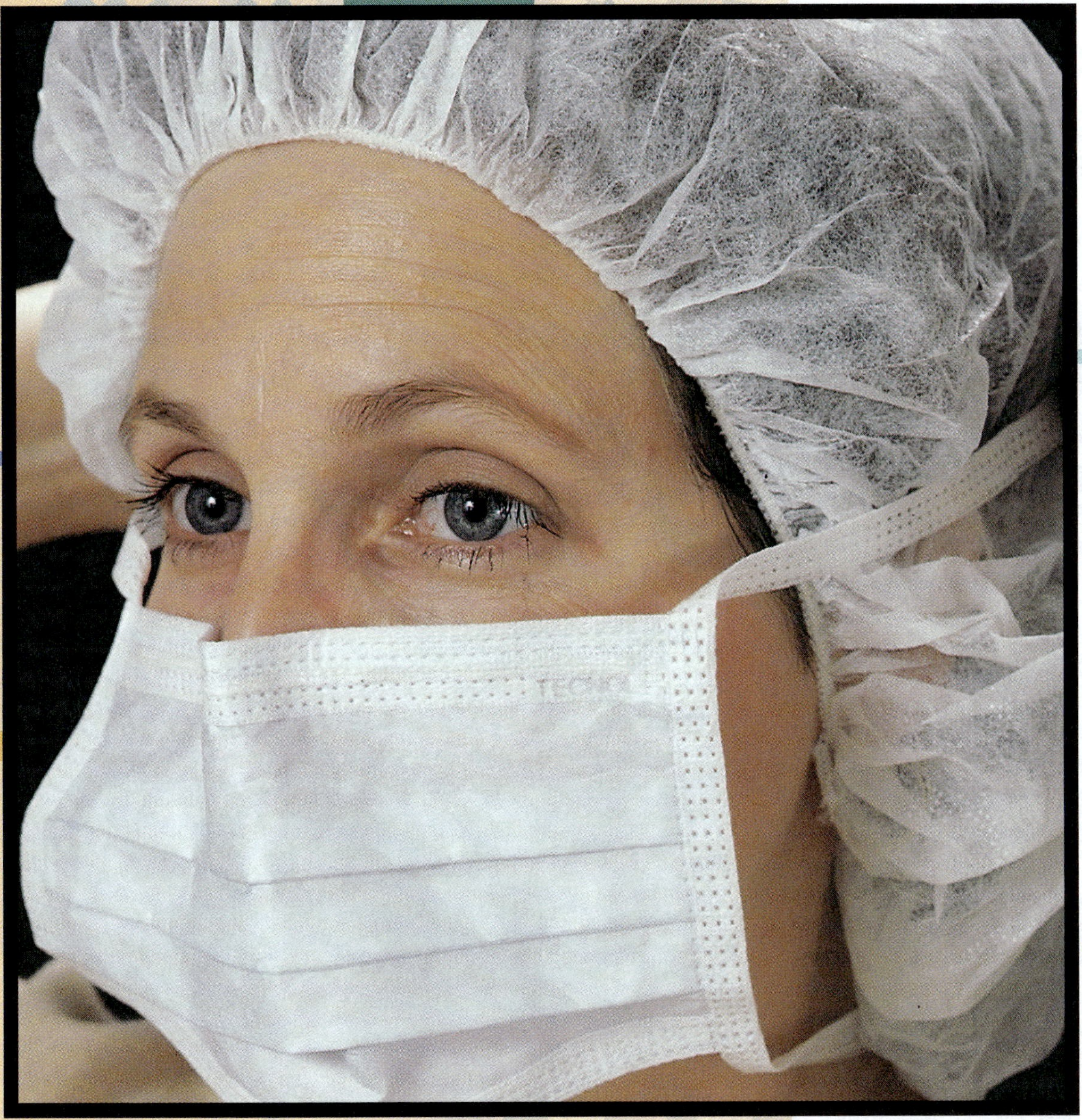

The Cell

R. B. Boley
Arlene L. Polaski

CHAPTER 14

The cell is the basic unit of structure and function in biologic systems. Two fundamental types of cells are recognized based on compositional and organizational patterns: prokaryotic and eukaryotic. An example of a prokaryotic cell is bacteria and examples of eukaryotic cells are human body cells and cells of higher plants and animals. All life systems utilize one or the other of these two patterns except for viruses, which have an acellular configuration and are taxonomically placed in a separate kingdom: the Akaryotae.

Structure and Function of the Cell

All cells, regardless of type, have the same basic structural pattern: a cytoplasmic matrix surrounded by a plasma membrane (Fig. 14–1). Scattered within the cytoplasm of eukaryotic cells are numerous membrane-bounded structures called organelles. Each organelle is a membrane-limited structure, many having a complex infrastructure, and each having a unique set of functions. This type of compartmentalization allows multistage metabolic pathways and other physiologic events to occur simultaneously while keeping one intercellular function separate from another. In marked contrast, the outstanding characteristic of prokaryotic cells is an absence of cytoplasmic organelles and a minimal degree of infrastructural organization. The differences between these two cell types allow clinicians to selectively attack a prokaryotic pathogen in vivo by using drugs that have no effect on eukaryotic cells. It is worth noting, however, that despite some marked differences in structure and composition, both cell types are able to perform the same basic functions. All cells must produce energy, take up and assimilate materials from outside the cell, synthesize macromolecules, maintain a homeostatic environment, and reproduce themselves as required.

Most of the substance of a cell is water (60%–95%) which serves as a solute for electrolytes and small and large organic molecules. Water is also a vehicle for intracellular chemical reactions and serves an important role in thermal regulation of the cell. The intracellular pool of molecules consists mostly of sugars, fatty acids, amino acids, and nucleotides which are used metabolically to produce energy and to synthesize macromolecules such as lipids, proteins, nucleic acids, and conjugates thereof. The electrolytes within the cytoplasm assist with various metabolic and physiologic activities and help maintain stable electrical and pH environments inside the cell. The most common intracellular electrolytes are calcium, potassium, magnesium, phosphate, and bicarbonate. Potassium is the most abundant intracellular cation.

Cell Replication

Human life begins as an undifferentiated single cell, derived from the fusion of a male gamete with a female gamete. On about the seventh day after fertilization, the original cell has undergone several cycles of proliferation. The progeny cells, under the influence of poorly understood microenvironments, begin to develop into distinctive tissues with specific functions. These fully differentiated cells in the embryo and fetus can be distinguished on the basis of both form and function. When tissues in the developing organism reach genetically programmed size limits, the rate of cell reproduction begins to slow and finally stops or attains a steady-state replacement level. This form of growth regulation, called contact or density-dependent inhibition, is initiated by physical (contact) and chemical (nutrient and cytokine) levels. When normal cells undergo transformation into cancerous cells, the latter fail to respond to these normal regulatory forces and show unrestrained growth. These unregulated replicating cells may then invade contiguous healthy tissues or become detached from the primary tumor and spread to other parts of the body where they continue to divide.

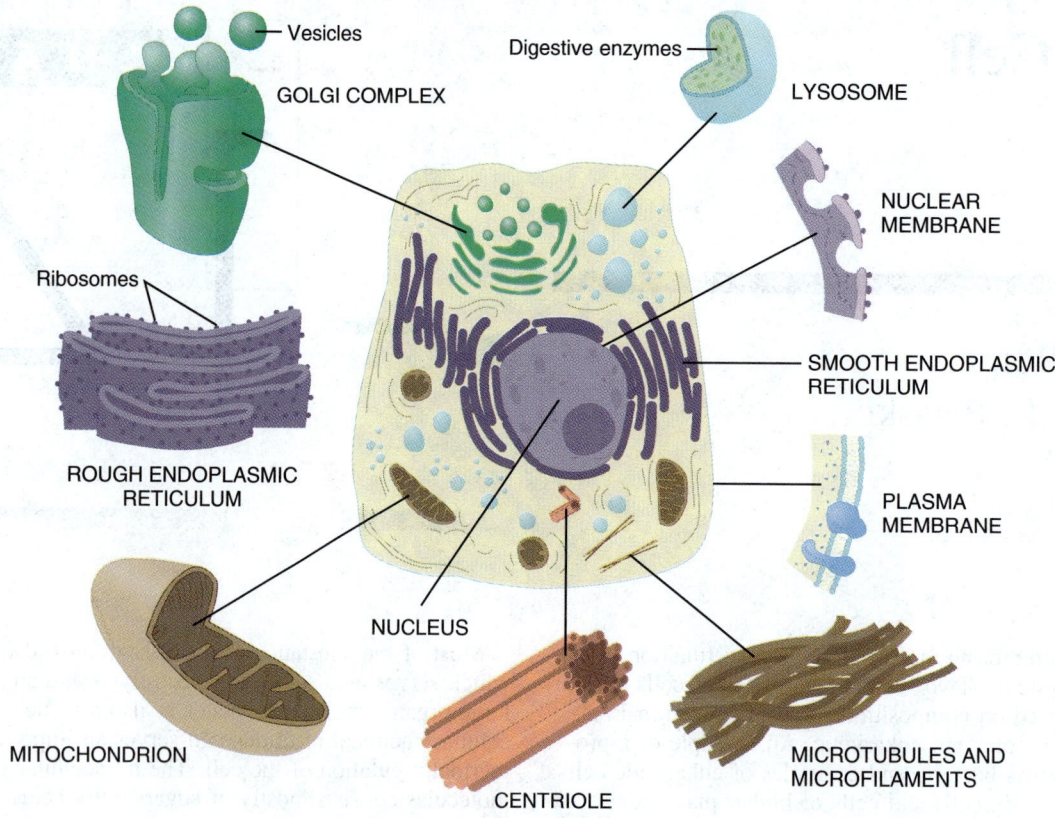

Figure 14–1. The components of a cell as seen through an electron microscope.

In the healthy adult body, somatic cells are replicated at varying rates. The cells of the skin and mucous membranes, the blood-forming cells in the bone marrow, and some cells in the reproductive system are replaced at a high constant rate. A second group of cells, such as hepatocytes and differentiated lymphocytes, undergo replication only in response to a stimulus. A third group of cells have very limited or no replicative capabilities. Individual smooth muscle cells may reproduce only once or twice in a lifetime. Striated muscle cells (heart and skeletal) and neurons are nonreplicating and any loss is permanent. For example, the person who is a paraplegic due to spinal cord injury will be permanently paralyzed because the spinal nerve cells (gray matter) cannot reproduce.

Replicating cells in eukaryotes may divide by mitosis or by meiosis. Somatic cells divide exclusively by mitosis, whereas the process producing gametes utilizes both mitosis and meiosis. Mitosis produces two daughter cells that have a gene content identical to the parent cell (unless altered by mutational events). The process of gametogenesis produces four progeny cells each having one-half the genetic content of the starting cell. A cell undergoing mitosis follows a cyclic sequence that is driven by a combination of signals that arise from both within and without the cell. The cycle of cellular reproduction is shown in Figure 14–2.

Cell Organelles

Cell Membrane

The cell membrane, or plasma membrane, is the outermost living boundary of the cell and provides many vital functions. The membrane consists of a lipid bilayer with a variety of proteins and conjugated proteins attached to or embedded within the membrane in a mosaic pattern (Fig. 14–3). Proteins that are weakly bound to the surface are called peripheral proteins. Those that span the lipid bilayer are called integral proteins. Individual integral protein molecules may cross the membrane once, four times, or seven times, thereby forming channels for the selective transport of ions and other water-soluble molecules.

Two of the most important activities of the cell membrane are the capacity to select which molecular species is to be transported, and the ability to transport substances into the cell (accumulation) or out of the cell (excretion, secretion) against both chemical and electrical potential gradients. The cell regulates entry and exit of materials across the membrane and into and out of the inner cell matrix by the following mechanisms.

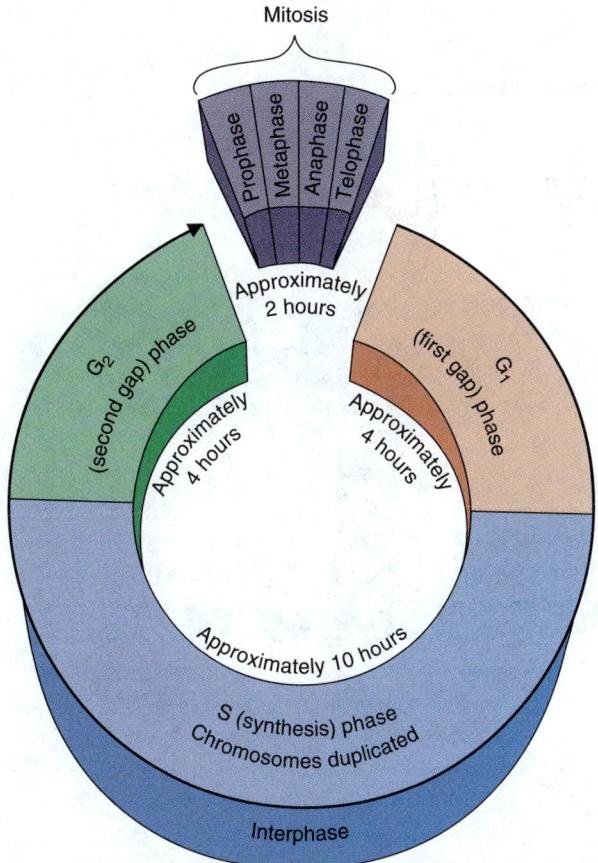

Figure 14–2. Phases in the life cycle of a cell. (Actual times vary, depending on the type of cell.)

Diffusion

Diffusion is the mode for entry of gases (oxygen and carbon dioxide) and small, relatively hydrophilic molecules (e.g., glycerol). The movement of water across a cell membrane is called osmosis. This process does not consume energy and can only occur with or along a concentration gradient (i.e., from higher to lower concentration).

Facilitated Diffusion

Small diffusible molecules having electrical charges such as cations, anions, and protons require special arrangements in order to cross a cell membrane. Transport is achieved by means of carrier proteins which show specificity for the molecule transported. In the case of ions, charge potential across the membrane as well as concentration of the given ion will regulate transfer. This process, like simple diffusion, can only occur with a concentration gradient. It is bidirectional and does not require energy. Sodium, potassium, and calcium ions, glucose, and amino acids are transported in this manner.

Active Transport

In active transport, ions or molecules are transported across the membrane against an electrochemical gradient. This mode, like facilitated diffusion, requires the presence of specific protein carriers in the cell membrane and is sensitive to metabolic toxins. The process for a given molecular species is unidirectional and requires the expenditure of energy (ATP). Protons, sodium ions, six-carbon sugars, and amino acids are accumulated by the cell using this process.

Bulk Transport

Many animal cells can take up substances from their external environment by trapping the material within an enclosing vesicle derived from the cell membrane. This type of transport is accomplished by endocytosis. Endocytosis includes pinocytosis, receptor-mediated transport, and phagocytosis.

Pinocytosis. This is the random, spontaneous, and nonspecific uptake of small amounts of extracellular fluid, including any solutes present. This mechanism is a part of the recurring process whereby a cell recycles membrane proteins.

Receptor-Mediated Transport. A specific receptor on the membrane binds to its ligand (a molecule needed for a chemical reaction) and initiates uptake. Unlike pinocytosis, this process permits ligand concentrations inside the cell to exceed those outside the cell. This type of transport is important in the uptake of a variety of molecules: such as transferrin (iron transport), antigens in solute form, and bacterial toxins.

Phagocytosis. This is similar to receptor-mediated endocytosis except that the material taken up is particulate (usually a cell) and the enclosing vesicle is much larger. This process is mainly observed with neutrophils, macrophages, lymphocytes, fibroblasts, and some endothelial cells. These cells function in defense against infectious agents, processing of antigen, tissue repair, and may contribute to the internal spread of contact sensitivity (e.g., poison ivy).

The intracellular fate of material after uptake in vesicles is controlled by the presence of signal sequences on enclosed molecules and by other, as yet undetermined, factors. Some substances taken up are enzymatically degraded and the fragments are metabolically assimilated. Viruses may be uncoated and the nucleic acid component released into the cytoplasm. Bacterial toxin molecules may be split and the active portion released into the cytoplasm to combine with a cytoplasmic or nuclear receptor. Other materials may be moved across the cell interior and exocytosed on the other side (e.g., transcytosis of substances across mucosal epithelia in the gut).

EXTERIOR OF CELL

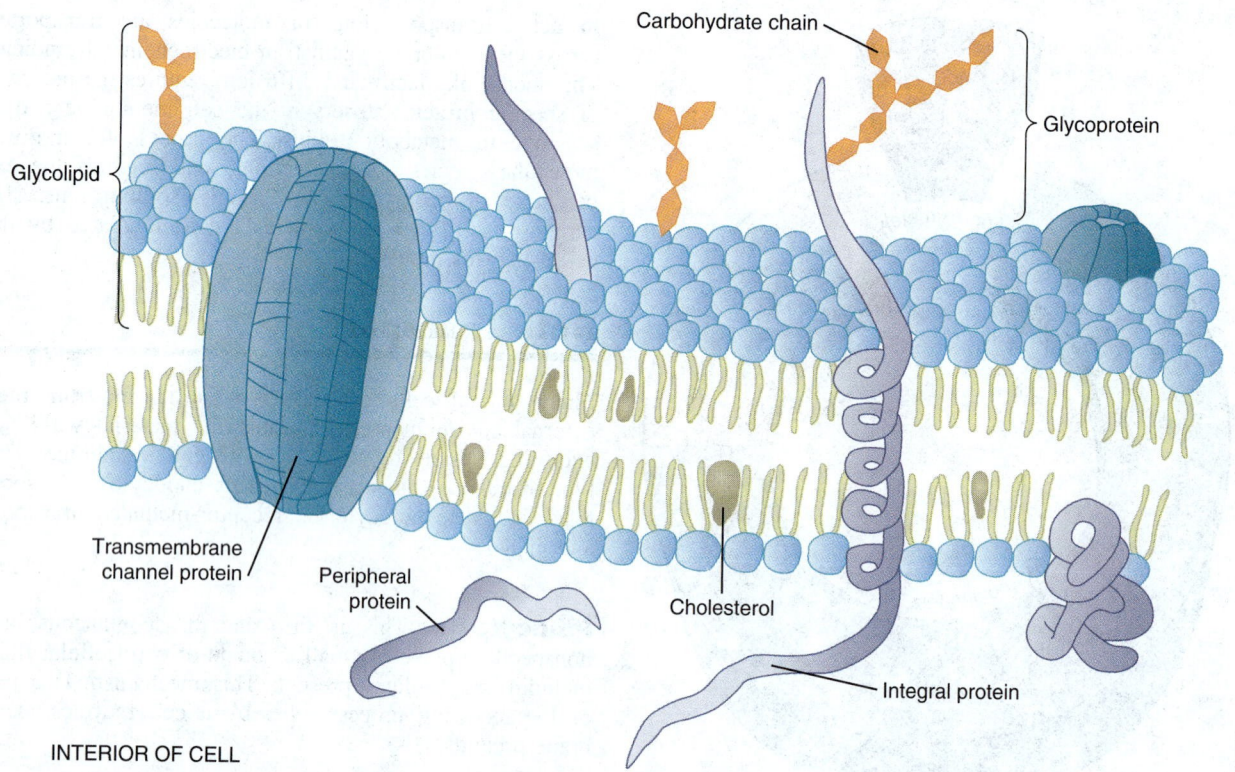

INTERIOR OF CELL

Figure 14–3. The cell membrane is composed of a bimolecular layer of lipids, primarily phospholipid and cholesterol. Proteins can be attached or embedded in the membrane. Peripheral proteins are attached to the surface; integral proteins are embedded in the cell membrane.

Intercellular Communication

Sites on cell membranes also play a role in communication and interaction between cells, both nearby and at distant sites. These mechanisms are mediated by membrane proteins serving as ligand-binding receptors and as signal transducers to initiate enzymatic function in inner membrane elements. Molecules involved in intercellular signaling include hormones and an extensive group of molecules called *cytokines.* The cytokines have many different functions, including cell activation, intercellular cooperation, and cell secretion.

Some of the cell surface molecules serve as mammalian blood group isoantigens (e.g., ABO, Rh) and others act as histocompatibility antigens which are the basis for self–non-self discrimination in immune function and in tissue and organ transplants. Membrane proteins also function as receptors for hormones, therapeutic agents, and many other ligands originating outside of the cell.

Contiguous cells within a tissue may interact with one another via tight junctions, desmosomes, and gap junctions. Cells that are transported throughout the body (in blood or lymph) can be induced to bind to other cells by interaction between surface ligands and receptors. These cellular adhesion molecules (CAMs) have important roles in organ development, inflammatory responses, in immune function, and in the spread of cancer cells.

Nucleus

The nucleus is the most prominent organelle in the eukaryotic cell. It is surrounded by a porous double membrane envelope. Prominent within the nucleus are one or more nucleoli visible among a mass of chromosomes. The nucleus is the site of deoxyribonucleic acid (DNA) replication (a prelude to cell reproduction) during interphase before the cycle of mitosis. Transcription products produced here provide the means for controlling all metabolic and physiologic activities of the cell.

The nuclear DNA molecules in cells that can divide are formed into chromosomes, each of which includes a centromere, a telomere, and a replication region. These elements are necessary for chromosomal replication and for movement of chromosomes during mitosis. Humans have 46 chromosomes with the inclusive DNA divided into coding sequences called exons interspersed with noncoding sequences called introns. The sequence of an RNA is specified by the base sequence of the section of DNA that is used as a template for RNA synthesis. The information in the transcribed RNA molecules is translated into protein molecules. While the amount of DNA present in the human genome is enormous (more than 3×10^9 base pairs), it is difficult to determine the productivity of the genome in terms of RNA and protein. Some geneticists have proposed that only about 10% of the human genome is needed to provide all necessary functions. It has been estimated that there are about 100,000 genes producing a maximum number of 60,000 essential proteins in a human. An upper limit for a single cell is the ability to synthesize about 20,000 different proteins (an awesome achievement nonetheless).

DNA replication is a crucial part of cell division. A new copy of an original strand of DNA must be made accurately and quickly. The mechanism of duplication requires DNA polymerase which catalyzes the stepwise incorporation of deoxynucleoside triphosphates onto a single-stranded DNA template. During the replication process, each chain of the original molecule serves as a template that provides two new DNA double-helix molecules each within one old and one new strand, a process called semiconservative replication.

RNA is synthesized from a DNA template using RNA polymerase enzymes. There are three types of RNA polymerases, each producing a different type of RNA. The three RNA products are (1) messenger RNA (mRNA), which carries the sequence information for building a peptide molecule and binds to ribosomal RNA; (2) ribosomal RNA (rRNA), which combines with protein to form ribosomes; and (3) transfer RNA (tRNA), which transfers amino acids to the ribosome. The synthesis of protein on the ribosome proceeds in several stages: initiation, elongation, termination and release, and polypeptide folding. Terminal signal sequences on the newly synthesized peptides direct their movement through routes that end with vesicular storage or lead to secretion across the cell membrane. Some antibiotics and bacterial cytotoxins interfere with or block one or more of these stages in protein synthesis (e.g., interferons, interleukin-2).

A major genetic problem is maintaining the integrity of the message contained in the nuclear DNA. Errors that occur in the replication process are called mutations. Mutational changes may be beneficial or harmful and possibly lethal. If such a change occurs in a somatic cell it may be inconsequential at one extreme, or, at the other, may result in cell death or a transformed cell that becomes malignant. If the mutation occurs during gametogenesis it will be passed on to the offspring. Thousands of abnormal changes are likely to occur on a daily basis during replication of human DNA due to thermal effects and inappropriate metabolic events, but in nearly all cases, the DNA is restored to normal configurations by a variety of repair mechanisms. Those abnormal genes that escape repair cause structural and functional problems leading to the development of diseases such as phenylketonuria (PKU) and sickle cell anemia.

Biotechnologists are applying recent advances in genetic engineering to the prevention and therapy of diseases. Using restriction endonuclease, which hydrolyses (cuts) DNA at specific sequences, and DNA ligase, which recombines the cut ends of DNA fragments, selected genes are cut out of sections of human DNA molecules. The human genes are then inserted into bacterial plasmids (extrachromosomal genetic elements in bacteria able to incorporate segments of human DNA). The bacteria can then, under controlled nutritional conditions, produce large quantities of the gene product.

Many benefits are being realized and anticipated from the use of this technology. Manipulation of gene systems in producing organisms are increasing yields and improving the antimicrobial action of antibiotics. The preparation of component virus vaccines increases both effectiveness and safety. A variety of mammalian proteins have been made, including clotting factors, insulin, human growth hormone, and interferons. Precise modification of reactive sites in antibodies makes possible the development of truly "magic bullets" for treating many conditions, including tumors. A peripheral benefit from this technology is the development of transgenic plants and animals for increasing and improving nutritional sources for humans.

Mitochondria

Mitochondria are self-replicating organelles present in almost all cells and are easily seen in electron microscopy. DNA and RNA are contained in the mitochondria. Each mitochondrion has an outer membrane, an inner membrane, and an internal matrix space. Transport proteins (porins) in the outer membrane form aqueous channels through the lipid layer. The inner membrane is selectively permeable to small molecules, especially ions, that are required by enzymes in the matrix. The matrix is the site of pyruvate metabolism, producing acetyl coenzyme A (acetyl CoA), and the enzymes for the citric acid cycle. The cell volume occupied by these organelles is proportional to the biochemical activity taking place in the cell. The main function of mitochondria is to provide large quantities of energy (in the form of adenosine triphosphate [ATP]) through oxidative processes involving the electron transport chain.

Endoplasmic Reticulum

The endoplasmic reticulum (ER) is an extensive membrane network that may represent up to half of the total membrane surface in the cell. In electron micrographs, it appears as tubules or compressed sacs. The ER membrane is thought to enclose a single interconnected space called the lumen or cisternal space. The major function of the ER is the synthesis of protein from RNA, and sex hormones. Ribosomes coat some of the ER membrane creating areas called rough ER. The regions of the membrane lacking ribosomes are called smooth ER, the quantity of which seems to be greatest in cells synthesizing lipoprotein (e.g., hepatocytes). Detoxification of some drugs (phenobarbital) increases the amount of smooth ER. After the drug is metabolized, the amount of smooth ER quickly returns to normal.

Ribosomes of the rough ER have a major role in synthesis of cell surface proteins such as hormone receptors, and secreted proteins, such as albumin and peptide hormones (insulin and follicle-stimulating hormone). Cell surface and secreted proteins synthesized by the ER-bound ribosomes are routed through the Golgi apparatus via membrane vesicles and glycosylated with carbohydrates on their way to the cell surface. Ribosomes that are not attached to the ER surface secrete their protein directly into the cytoplasm (glycolytic enzymes).

The sections of smooth ER that have no ribosomes bind enzymes to its surface that are involved in the synthesis of certain nonprotein substances, such as steroids and lipids (including cholesterol and phospholipids). Smooth ER also (1) contributes to the detoxification and metabolism of drugs, toxins, and other foreign substances; (2) releases enzymes that control glycogen breakdown; and (3) in muscle cells, sequesters and releases calcium ions, which are necessary for muscular contraction.

Golgi Apparatus

The Golgi apparatus consists of a stack of flattened membranes enclosing cisternae and vesicles. It connects the ER in the interior and the cell membrane of the exterior. Vesicle-enclosed proteins and lipids from the ER fuse with the *cis* face of the Golgi apparatus to expose the molecules to matrix enzymes. Enzymes may glycosylate; add sulfate, acetyl, and phosphate groups; or remove amino acid segments. In leaving the *trans* face of the Golgi apparatus, products may be routed into storage vesicles (lysosomes, reserved secretory vesicles) or transmitted directly to the outer cell membrane where the molecules are excreted or incorporated into the membrane.

Lysosomes

Lysosomes are cytoplasmic vesicles that contain digestive enzymes that break down lipids, proteins, certain carbohydrates, and nucleic acids into small molecules so that they can be oxidized by the mitochondria. The source of the substrates is material taken up via receptor-mediated endocytosis or phagocytosis. The products of enzyme action are transferred to the cytoplasm and assimilated into metabolic pathways. In the normal cell the membranes of the lysosome keep its potentially dangerous digestive enzymes separate from the cell contents. In the case of severe cell injury, however, lysosomal enzymes are released and the cell is destroyed, a process called autolysis. Lysosomes are abundant in white blood cells whose principal activity is phagocytosis of foreign material (e.g., bacteria) in the body.

Lysosomes are also responsible for tissue regression, as in the uterus following pregnancy, in muscles during long periods of inactivity, and in mammary glands after lactation. The mechanism controlling release of lysosomal enzymes in these circumstances is unknown. The programmed release of lysosomal enzymes also aids in the removal of injured cells or cell parts from damaged tissues as a prelude to the repair process.

Microtubules and Microfilaments (Cytoskeleton)

Most cells have what is referred to as a cytoskeleton that is based on the presence of three types of structures: (1) microfilaments, (2) microtubules, and (3) intermediate filaments. The cytoskeleton is related to cell movement,

determination of cell shape, and providing the basis for a structural network within the cytoplasmic matrix.

Microfilaments are present in many cell types and are involved in contractile processes. Intermediate filaments differ in composition and size from microfilaments but are also widely distributed in various cells. Data indicate the main function of intermediate filaments is to provide a framework for the cytoskeleton. Microtubules differ from the other types of filaments in both size, structure, and function. The two main functions are (1) attachment to spindles and centrioles to assist in movement and separation of chromosomes during mitosis, and (2) incorporation into eukaryotic cilia and flagella.

Tissues and Organs

Cells bond together according to their special functions to form definite units or structures called tissues. In turn, tissues unite to form individual organs. The four major specialized types of cells that unite into larger tissue units are the following:

1. *Epithelial cells,* which are arranged in sheets. They cover the outside of the body (epidermis) and form the absorptive covering that lines the inside of the body's cavities and tubular structures (mucosa).
2. *Nerve cells,* which form the highly specialized, irritable, and conductive nerve tissue. Injured or destroyed nerve cells cannot be replaced.
3. *Muscle cells,* which allow mobility by contracting and relaxing.
4. *Connective tissue cells,* which bind together and support other cells and tissues. They include blood cells and structural cells such as bones, tendons, and ligaments. Blood cells carry oxygen to the tissues and carbon dioxide and wastes from the tissues. Also, they defend the body against foreign substances. Structural cells build the bony scaffolding and form the critical intercellular proteins that bind together the cells of the body. Collagen is an important extracellular connective tissue protein.

Alterations in Structure and Function of the Cell

The major causes of cellular alterations are (1) changes in gene structure and function, (2) degeneration of normal tissue or infiltration by foreign substances, and (3) disorders of cell growth, including malignant growth, atrophy, and hypertrophy.

Genetic Disturbances

If a cell has a genetic abnormality, either newly acquired or hereditary, it may be exhibited in the cell as a disturbance of normal function. Cellular disorders of genetic causation are not apparent until the mutated gene is needed and is either nonfunctional or only partially functional.

Infiltrations

Injured cells have observable changes in their cytoplasm and nucleus. Infiltration describes a process whereby a substance that is external to the cell enters into the cell and damages its ability to function. For example, when large amounts of fat globules are deposited within the cell as the result of a metabolic systemic illness, the process is called fatty infiltration. Other infiltrates include water, glucogen, protein, and macropolysaccharides.

Disturbances of Cell Growth

Some major disturbances of cellular growth involve the problems of atrophy, hypertrophy, and precancerous changes (Fig. 14–4).

Atrophy

Atrophy is the wasting of a tissue or organ and a decrease in its size following normal development of the structure. This condition is due to a decrease in either the number of cells or the size of the cells composing a tissue or organ. Atrophy may follow disuse of an organ. For example, muscular atrophy may develop following denervation or prolonged immobilization. Atrophy due to aging can be greatly reduced by physical activity and isometric exercises. Because the adrenal glands normally secrete corticosteroids, atrophy of these glands can occur when large doses of corticosteroids are administered over a prolonged period. Atrophy accompanies the normal physiologic aging process. The thymus gland increases in size during childhood and very gradually starts to atrophy during adolescence. The ovaries atrophy after menopause.

Hypertrophy

Hypertrophy is an increase in the size of an organ or tissue resulting from an increase in the size of the cells. Hypertrophy sometimes represents the response of an organ to a greater workload. For example, when the heart is subjected to great strain, the left ventricle of the heart enlarges, or hypertrophies, in order to handle the additional stress. A second example of hypertrophy is the increase in size of the biceps muscle in persons engaged in strenuous physical activity.

Precancerous Changes

Dysplasia is deranged cellular growth or a form of hyperplasia. It occurs from persistent severe injury or irritation. *Hyperplasia* is an increase in the number of cells. Hyperplasia can be an expected cellular response, such as increased cell regeneration and the formation of calluses. Pathologic hyperplasia is usually a response to excessive hormone secretion. If the process continues, the cells can

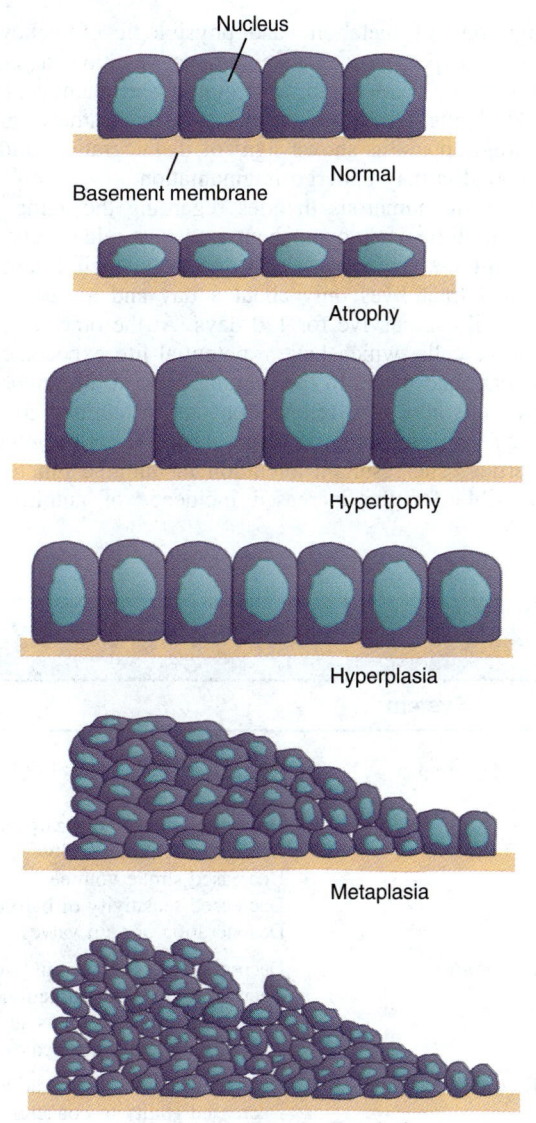

Figure 14–4. Adaptive alterations in simple cuboidal epithelial cells.

become cancerous. *Metaplasia* is the transformation of one mature cell type or tissue into another. Usually, the new cell does not perform the functions of the cell it replaced. Metaplastic cells can transform into malignant cancer cells.

Neoplastic Growth

Neoplastic growth is characterized by disturbances in cell differentiation and growth. Neoplasms fail to follow the rules of normal cellular proliferation. This alteration in normal cell reproduction is discussed in greater detail in Chapter 23.

The Aging Cell

In a young healthy person, cells are biochemically active, have a high turnover rate (in some tissues), and have a high rate of metabolic and physiologic efficiency. In the elderly person, cells are less active, have a slower turnover rate, and begin to decline in efficiency (Table 14–1). Aging cells shrink in size, protein synthesis slows, the Golgi apparatus shows signs of disintegration, and the mitochondria may undergo fragmentation.

There are numerous theories regarding the aging process, but little is known about how age-related changes occur. In the mature adult, an epithelial cell lining the intestinal tract lives only about a day and a half; a red blood cell can survive for 120 days. At the other extreme are nerve cells, which have a potential life expectancy of 100 years and more. In the immune system, immunocompetent cells appear to remain constant in numbers as people age but lose some of their interactive and regulatory properties. The resultant alteration in immune function is responsible for the increased incidence of autoimmune disease, the appearance of tumors, and the greater susceptibility to infection seen in this population.

Another theory of aging is that unrepaired mutations accumulate on DNA, causing changes that lead to aging. Highly specialized cells such as nerve cells do not reproduce. When these cells die from injury or disease, they are not replaced and the remaining cells must assume their functions. The greater workload may stress the remaining cells and cause them to age faster or hasten their dying. Other cells retain an ability to reproduce and replace injured or dead cells. This occurs in the liver and pancreas. One hypothesis is that each person is born with a genetic clock that governs that person's life span. This theory is based on the observation that each cell type has a finite number of divisions. This concept is supported in part by similarities in life spans seen in various family groups.

System	Physiologic Changes
Cardiovascular	Decreased vessel elasticity due to calcification and connective tissue (increased pulmonary vascular resistance)
	Decreased number of heart muscle fibers, with increased size of individual fibers (hypertrophy)
	Decreased filling capacity
	Decreased stroke volume
	Decreased sensitivity of baroreceptors
	Degeneration of vein valves
Respiratory	Decreased chest wall compliance due to calcification of the costal cartilage
	Decreased alveolar ventilation
	Decreased respiratory muscle strength
	Air trapping and decreased ventilation due to degeneration of lung tissue (decreased elasticity)
Renal and urinary	Decreased glomerular filtration rate due to nephron degeneration (decreased 33%–50% by age 70)
	Decreased ability to concentrate urine
	Decreased ability to regulate H^+
Gastrointestinal	Decreased muscular contraction
	Decreased esophageal emptying
	Decreased bowel motility
	Decreased production of HCl, enzymes, and intrinsic factor
	Decreased hepatic enzyme production and metabolic capacity
	Thinning of stomach mucosa
Neurologic and sensory	Degeneration and atrophy of nerve cells
	Decrease of 25%–45% in neurons
	Decrease in neurotransmitters
	Decreased rate of conduction of nerve impulses
	Loss of taste buds
	Loss of auditory hair cells and sclerosis of the eardrum
Musculoskeletal	Decreased muscle mass
	Bone demineralization
	Joint degeneration, erosion, and calcification
Immune	Decreased inflammatory response
	Decrease in T-cell function due to involution of the thymus gland
Integumentary	Decreased subcutaneous fat
	Decreased elastin
	Atrophy of the sweat glands
	Atrophy of the epidermal arterioles, causing altered temperature regulation

From Copstead, L. C. (1995). *Perspectives on pathophysiology*. Philadelphia: W. B. Saunders.

Mechanisms of Cell Damage

When cells are injured, the extent of the damage depends on the nature, intensity, and duration of the stressor, whether the blood supply to the cells is affected, and the state of differentiation or metabolic activity of the cells. Injured organelles are no longer capable of carrying out their specific functions (i.e., mitochondria stop producing ATP). Exposure of hepatocytes to noxious chemicals and some drugs places these cells at great risk of toxic injury. Nerve cells innervating cardiac muscle are extremely vulnerable to hypoxia due to a high rate of metabolism. Healthcare providers are reminded that when two clients are exposed to the same injurious substance both may not sustain the same degree of injury because of the influence of modifying factors. For example, the nutritional and emotional state of an individual can have a profound impact on the extent and consequences of a slight-to-moderate level of injury. There is, however, a point after which cell death inevitably occurs. The mechanisms responsible for the transition from reversible to irreversible cellular damage are not clearly understood.

Hypoxia

Hypoxia (inadequate tissue oxygenation) is a leading cause of cell injury and death. Hypoxia can arise secondary to (1) vascular disease or injury, which impedes blood flow to tissues, or (2) insufficient oxygenation of blood caused by conditions such as carbon monoxide poisoning. Depending on the severity of the hypoxic state, cells will compensate and recover or be killed. For example, if the femoral artery becomes stenotic, the skeletal muscles of the legs will eventually atrophy as a result of the inadequate blood flow and the consequent reduced oxygen supply. Severe or chronic hypoxia will result in cell injury or death. The most common cause of hypoxia is ischemia, or reduced blood supply. When ischemic injury is caused by gradual narrowing of arteries (atherosclerosis) the progressive hypoxia is better tolerated than sudden anoxia caused by an obstruction in the blood supply.

Temperature Extremes

Extreme heat will damage cells by coagulating cytoplasmic protein. Even mild heat results in permanent cellular damage if it is applied over a prolonged period to individuals with impaired circulation, as seen in peripheral vascular disease. Heat in these cases increases the metabolic needs of cells and tissues and leads to insufficient oxygen levels which, coupled with a reduced capacity to dispose of greater-than-normal amounts of waste products, will accelerate the damage to the affected tissue.

Cold will constrict the smaller blood vessels, thereby decreasing the circulation of blood and oxygen to tissues. Freezing temperatures may cause the intracellular water to crystallize, which destroys the cell's structure. Cold injury can result in frostbite, which permanently injures the tissues involved. Very low temperatures cause stasis of blood, leading to clot formation, which will occlude arteries, resulting in ischemia and, ultimately, in cell death and necrosis.

Ionizing Radiation

Exposure to radiation causes mutations, inactivates enzymes, and interrupts cell division. The fact that radiation stops mitosis makes radiation therapy important in the treatment of cancer—a disease involving pathologic cell reproduction. Radiation affects virtually all cells, but certain cells are more susceptible than others. Reproductive cells, cells in the lymph nodes and gastrointestinal tract, and bone marrow are highly sensitive to damage by radiation exposure, whereas cells of cartilage, muscle, brain, and endocrine glands are relatively insensitive. Individuals who work with radioactive materials or nuclear fission reactors, or who are giving or receiving radiotherapy, are most susceptible to cellular trauma from radiation.

Electrical Injury

Electrical energy generates heat when it passes through the body and may thus produce burns. It also interferes with neural conduction pathways and often causes death from cardiac dysrhythmias. The extent of damage from electrical energy depends on its voltage and amperage, tissue resistance, and the pathway of the current as it passes through the body. Users of electrical equipment should be aware that exposure to 100 mA can be lethal to humans. Electrical burns are discussed in Chapter 79.

Chemical Injury

Chemicals harm cells by destroying or altering their structure and by disrupting their metabolism. The capacity of a chemical to injure a cell depends on the strength and toxicity of the chemical, as well as the susceptibility of the cell. There are numerous chemicals that can cause cellular injury. Highly toxic substances are called poisons. Minute amounts of poisonous substances such as cyanide and arsenic cause death. Some of the most toxic substances known are bacterial exotoxins, such as diphtheria toxin and botulinus toxin. Environmental chemicals, such as herbicides, pesticides, and air pollutants, are potential causes of cellular injury. Lead-based paint, which tastes sweet, is often eaten by children. Lead-based paint on walls and window blinds comes off in dust particles and is inhaled. Dangerous amounts of lead are also found in water pipes in older homes and is present in the drinking water. The ingested or inhaled lead destroys cells in the nervous system (which may lead to mental retardation in young children), affects blood cell production, and damages the kidneys. Workers around machinery and home owners with gas appliances must guard against carbon monoxide poisoning. Carbon monoxide binds tightly and 210 times more rapidly than oxygen to hemoglobin and prevents normal exchange of oxygen and carbon dioxide.

Bacterial Injury

Microorganisms such as bacteria injure host cells by direct attack or by means of the toxins they produce. Bacterial toxins are classified as being either endotoxins or exotoxins. An endotoxin is a structural component of the outer envelope of gram-negative bacteria and consists of lipopolysaccharide. The toxic moiety is released only when the bacterium dies and the cell undergoes lysis. Endotoxins may act directly with macrophages and T lymphocytes causing the release of cytokines. Endotoxins acting on macrophages stimulate the production of interleukin-1 (IL-1) and tumor necrosis factor (TNF) (two cytokines) which in large quantities cause bacterial septic shock, a condition that is often fatal. Endotoxins may also activate the complement cascade, producing disseminated intravascular coagulation (DIC), another potentially fatal condition. Intervention in endotoxemia is difficult and often impossible to achieve.

An exotoxin is excreted by a bacterium into the surrounding medium. Exotoxins are proteins and have very specific toxic effects. *Clostridium tetani,* the organism that causes tetanus, produces a neurotoxin that blocks processes that inhibit neural transmission in the central nervous system (CNS). The disease is marked by painful spasms of the airway, generalized muscle tentanic contractions, and depression of the respiratory center. Preventive immunization is possible with a few exotoxins (such as *Clostridium tetani*), and in some cases an exotoxemia can be successfully treated with antitoxins (e.g., diphtheria).

Viral Injury

Viruses have been described as consisting of mobile genetic elements protected by outer layers of protein and lipoprotein. Viruses attach to specific receptors on host cell surfaces and are taken up by endocytosis. The nucleic acid core of the virus then passes through the vesicular membrane into the interior of the host cell. The viral genome then subverts the host cell metabolic machinery and begins to make viral components. While inside the host cell, the virus is protected from reactive cells and solutes of the host. The assembled virions may then exit the cell by either lysing the cell remnant or permitting the host cell to remain viable while continuously secreting virions across the cell membrane. Viruses damage host cells by killing, nutrient deprivation, or causing the cell to transform into a tumor state.

Mechanical Injury

Cells can be damaged by physical impact or irritation. Examples of this type of injury include blisters from tight shoes, abrasions, lacerations, and contusions (bruises). The cell can be injured in other ways as well. Light can damage cells of the cornea. Noise can damage the eardrum (tympanic membrane), the ossicle in the middle ear, and the organ of Corti in the inner ear. Prolonged contact with vibrating objects can alter muscle and bone struc-

ture, as well as nerve conduction. Clients at risk of these injuries are those who work with hand tools and pneumatic drills.

Nutritional Imbalance

Inadequate protein intake decreases the function of the intestinal mucosa and pancreas, which in turn reduces nutrient absorption. Plasma proteins, especially albumin, help retain fluid in blood vessels. When levels of plasma proteins decline, fluid tends to move into interstitial spaces, causing edema. Antibodies or immunoglobulins are protein; therefore, the lack of proteins adversely affects immune system function and will increase the risk of infection.

Inadequate carbohydrate intake forces the body to use fats for energy. The liver becomes overwhelmed and ketone bodies are formed that accumulate in the blood, a condition known as *ketosis*. Ketosis develops because of the rapid breakdown of fatty acids stored in adipose tissue. Fatty acids are used for energy when the intake of carbohydrates is less than 50 g. Clients at high risk for ketosis include diabetics, persons on starvation diets, and persons on low-carbohydrate diets.

Increased fat intake often causes fat deposition in heart, liver, and muscle and may lead to obesity, coronary heart disease, stroke, or breast and colon cancer.

Growth factors include amino acids, purines and pyrimidines, and vitamins. These nutrients are required but cannot be synthesized. Insufficient quantities of these substances will seriously impair the ability of the cell to take up and metabolize nutrients, or to synthesis macromolecules for structural building and reproduction.

Cell Death and Necrosis

Cells die as a result of being traumatized, through alteration by disease, from failure due to genetic alterations, or through a programmed process called apoptosis. Necrotic processes in tissues following the death of injured or altered cells have three patterns. (1) Coagulative necrosis results from the slowing or blocking of normal blood supplies to tissues. In this form of necrosis, the membrane of the cell is preserved but the nucleus is lost. The necrotic cell is removed by phagocytosis. (2) Caseous necrosis is usually associated with tuberculosis, but may be seen in other disorders. The cell membrane is destroyed, and the body walls off the damaged area. The central portion of the walled-off area looks cheesy and crumbly. (3) Liquifactive necrosis is seen in brain tissues. Death of the neuron releases lysosomes into the surrounding area. The lysosomes liquify the area and leave pockets of liquid and cellular debris. Cells undergoing death by apoptosis usually will not disturb the steady-state nature of the tissue and thus give no sign of its occurrence.

Somatic or body death occurs when respiration and cardiac function cease. Within minutes of death, noticeable changes occur that assist in determining that death has occurred. In addition to cessation of respiration and circulation, the skin becomes pale and yellow, body tem-

Box 14-1. The Value of Autopsy

Autopsy, or examination of the body after death, is invaluable for providing knowledge to clarify the cause of death. Autopsy can also serve as a monitor of clinical care and the quality of society's health. Autopsy can assist with recognition and identification of new diseases.

The purpose of autopsy goes beyond providing data on the effectiveness of medical therapy. The family of the deceased may be reassured that everything necessary and possible was done for the client. In addition, contagious illness and genetic illness can be identified and made known to the family. Autopsy also helps clarify the circumstances of violent and unexplained death.

Each state in the United States has its own laws on the need for permission for autopsy. Even though specific laws differ, there are some general similarities. Autopsy for the purpose of resolving medicolegal issues is ordered by an appropriate authority, such as a medical examiner. Death that is unexpected, occurring while in surgery, or in a client who is not under a physician's care, falls into this category. When there is no medicolegal reason for ordering an autopsy, permission can be given only by the next of kin. Usually, a client cannot order his own autopsy before death. Once death has occurred, the body becomes the property of the next of kin, or if there is no next of kin, of a legal entity such as the coroner or sheriff.

An autopsy is performed in privacy and in a professional manner. An incision is made from the axilla to groin to expose internal organs. Organs are examined and weighed. In addition, microscopic study and chemical, toxicologic, and microbiologic analyses are performed. The ideal time to perform an autopsy is within 24 hours of death. Autopsy can be performed after embalming.

The family may be concerned about the final appearance of the client at burial. Autopsy is customarily performed with great care so as not to disfigure the body. The family may meet with the pathologist and receive a copy of the findings. The cost of autopsy is usually built into the hospital costs; therefore, charges for autopsy do not appear on the bill.

---

currently a hotly debated subject. Advances in medical care options, such as ventilators and organ transplantation, have led to the development of specific criteria to document that brain death has occurred. These criteria are (1) coma with unresponsiveness, including the absence of brain stem reflexes (blinking, eye movement, pupil response to light, and swallowing); (2) cessation of automatic breathing when the patient is removed from ventilator support; and (3) an isoelectric electroencephalogram for 30 minutes in the absence of hypothermia and poisoning by CNS depressants. Once the patient is declared dead, undamaged organs can be taken from the body and used in transplantation. An autopsy is performed to determine the cause of death or for pathologic study, or if the family would benefit from knowing the cause of death (Box 14-1).

Conclusions

Cells are the basic units of life. They serve many functions. The integrity and existence of the organism is dependent on the individual and collective ability of body cells to digest and assimilate substances, protect themselves by reacting to stimuli, replicate, metabolize, and produce energy. When cells lose their ability to function normally because of injury or attack by pathogens, the organism will show signs of distress and develop disease.

Recent advances in molecular biology are providing the means for great improvements in the diagnosis and treatment of many human diseases. Only those persons who keep current in the field will be able to comprehend the nature and consequences of the pathologic changes associated with disease processes and have the knowledge to make and evaluate therapeutic decisions.

Bibliography

1. Alberts, B. D., et al. (1994). *Molecular biology of the cell* (3rd ed.). New York: Garland.
2. Barnes, D. E., Lindahl, T., & Sedgwick, B. (1993). DNA repair. *Current Opinion in Cell Biology, 5,* 424.
3. Becker, W. M., Reece, J. B., & Poenie, M. F. (1995). *The world of the cell* (3rd ed.). New York: Benjamin/Cummings.
4. Berridge, M. J. (1985). The molecular basis of communication within the cell. *Scientific American, 253,* 142.
5. Berridge, M. J. (1994). The biology and medicine of calcium signalling. *Molecular and Cellular Endocrinology, 98,* 119.
6. Dautry-Varsat, A., & Lodish, H. F. (1984). How receptors bring proteins and particles into cells. *Scientific American, 250,* 52.
7. Gierasch, L. (1989). Signal sequences. *Biochemistry, 28,* 923–930.
8. Jain, M., & Wagner, R. (1988). *Introduction to biological membranes* (2nd ed.). New York: John Wiley & Sons.
9. Hartwell, L. H., & Kastan, M. B. (1994). Cell cycle control and cancer. *Science, 266,* 1821.
10. Koshland, D. E. Jr. (1984). Control of enzyme activity and metabolic pathways. *Trends in Biochemical Sciences, 9,* 155–159.
11. Kraut, J. (1988). How do enzymes work? *Science, 242,* 533.
12. McPherson, M. A., & Dormer, R. (1991). Molecular and cell biology of cystic fibrosis. *Molecular Aspects of Medicine, 12,* 1–81.
13. Mulligan, R. C. (1993). The basic science of gene therapy. *Science, 260,* 926.

---

perature falls until it reaches the ambient temperature after 24 hours, blood pressure is absent, pupils become fixed and dilated, and limbs become rigid. The processes noted at death have been given specific names: *algor mortis* is loss of body temperature, *livor mortis* is a purple discoloration developing in body tissues following blood stasis, and *rigor mortis* is muscle stiffening. Rigor mortis affects the entire body within 12 to 24 hours and diminishes after 24 hours.

The legal and ethical issues surrounding death of the individual raise issues that require careful consideration on the part of all parties involved. People who have suffered for a long time may ask that no extraordinary measures be used to prolong their life. At other times, the family of a patient who has sustained an irreversible traumatic injury may view any evidence of life in the patient as a positive sign of possible recovery. The issue of promoting or facilitating death in the chronically ill is

14. Murray, A. W., & Kirschner, M. W. (1991). What controls the cell cycle? *Scientific American, 264,* 56.

15. Neufeld, E. F. (1991). Lysosomal storage diseases. *Annual Review of Biochemistry, 60,* 257.

16. Umbarger, H. E. (1992). The origin of a useful concept: Feedback inhibition. *Protein Science, 1,* 1392–1395.

17. Varmus, H. (1987). Reverse transcription. *Scientific American, 30,* 56.

18. Watts, A. (1989). Membrane structure and dynamics. *Current Opinion in Cell Biology, 1,* 691–700.

19. Weinberg, R. A. (1985). The molecules of life. *Scientific American, 253,* 48.

20. Welch, W. J. (1993). How cells respond to stress. *Scientific American, 268,* 56.

Fluid and Electrolyte Disorders

CHAPTER 15

Bernadette White

Physiologic homeostasis, and life itself, depends on normal fluid and electrolyte balance. Promoting balance in either a wellness or an illness state can prevent fluid and electrolyte imbalances that may be life-threatening. Nurses are the primary professional contact for most clients, whether the setting is in the hospital, an extended care facility, or the home. Therefore, it is natural for nurses to play an active role in the prevention, early detection, and treatment of fluid and electrolyte imbalances. Nurses not only have the opportunity, but they have a broad base of knowledge of normal physiology and pathology, to assist in the identification of clients at risk and in recognizing early clinical manifestations of *imbalance*. Nurses perform thorough assessments, assist in diagnosing the imbalance, set client goals with measurable outcomes, and implement independent and dependent nursing interventions to achieve these outcomes. Nurses also engage in an ongoing evaluation of a client's responses to the care plan and revise the care plan as necessary. This chapter assists the nurse in reviewing and updating practice recommendations for the primary, secondary, and tertiary care of a client who has or is at risk of having fluid and electrolyte imbalances.

Fluids

Fluid Balance

Fluid Compartments

Water is found everywhere on earth, including within the human body. In the adult, approximately 60% of the total body weight is water.

Two thirds of the body's water is found in the cell.

This is called the *intracellular fluid* (ICF). The remaining third of the water is found in the extracellular spaces and is known as *extracellular fluid* (ECF). The word "fluid" is used because more than water is found in these compartments. Substances such as glucose, sodium, and potassium are also found. The *ECF compartment* refers to the spaces outside the cell. ECF is further divided into *interstitial space* and *intravascular space*. CSF, lymphatic fluid, synovial fluid, and fluids in the eye are also part of the ECF.[72] The ECF transports nutrients, electrolytes, and oxygen to cells; carries waste products for excretion; regulates heat; lubricates and cushions joints and membranes; hydrolyzes food for digestive processes; and maintains vascular volume by passing easily through the capillary walls.

Interstitial fluid lies outside the vascular fluid and cells, and it constitutes 28% of the total body water. Interstitial space is also known as *tissue spaces* or the *third space*. Interstitial fluid is collected and transported by the lymphatic system. It provides the cells with the external medium necessary for cellular metabolism.

Plasma is the fluid found in the intravascular spaces. Plasma is similar to interstitial fluid, except that it contains more protein.

ICF provides the cell with the internal aqueous medium necessary for its chemical functions. Normally, the fluid volume inside and outside of the cells maintains a steady state due to compensatory responses. For example, in minor fluid losses, the compensatory responses maintain homeostasis, thereby minimizing the clinical manifestations that you might see with a major imbalance. For example, if a person has a mild case of the flu accompanied by vomiting and diarrhea, the body is able to shift fluids to restore balance until the person is able to drink and eat again. Fluid shifting is usually limited to the exchange between the interstitial and vascular compartments. When severe fluid changes occur, shifting in the intracellular compartment occurs. This shifting can cause irreversible changes in the structure and function of vital organs, such as the brain.

Clearly, water is not only responsible for the body's

This chapter incorporates material written for the fourth edition by Joyce Kee.

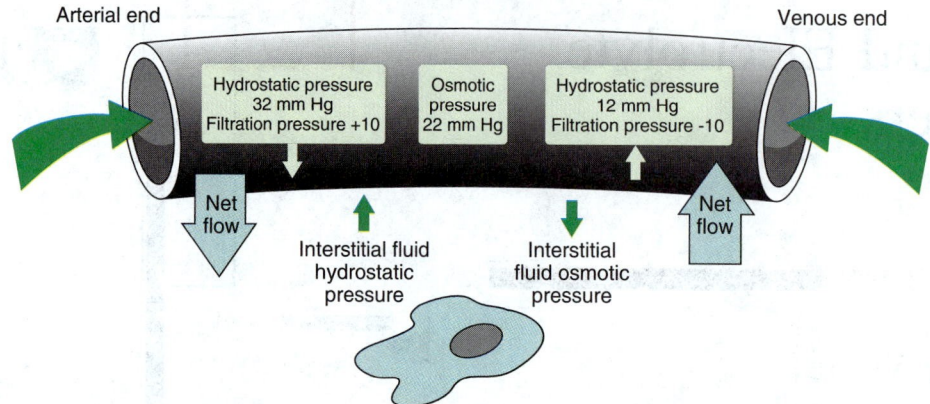

Figure 15–1. Pressure differences within the capillary are responsible for the movement of fluids. Fluid moves out of the capillary at the arterial end as a result of hydrostatic pressure in the vessel that exceeds the pressure in the tissues. Fluids return to the vessel at the venous end because the proteins (colloids) that remain in the vessel exert a pulling pressure on them. Under normal conditions, the movement of fluids is almost equal, and neither dehydration nor edema results. The remaining fluid in the interstitium is transported via the lymphatics to the vascular system. Abnormal conditions occur with the presence of too much fluid, too few proteins, changes in the capillary wall, or lymphatic obstruction.

structure and function, but it is also necessary for the maintenance of equilibrium and of life itself.

Fluid Pressures

As a result of pressure, body fluids shift between the interstitial space and the vascular space within the capillary. The pressures in the body fluids are either *hydrostatic* or *oncotic*. The pressure of the blood volume in the vessels creates hydrostatic pressure. When solutes in the capillary are too large to move outside of it, osmotic pressure is created.[35] The solutes are mostly proteins, such as albumin, that are more abundant in plasma than in interstitial fluids. The osmotic pressure resulting from protein solutes is called *oncotic pressure*. Oncotic pressure creates a "pulling" force for water movement. That is, water is pulled toward higher oncotic pressure.

Figure 15–1 demonstrates the movement of fluid through a capillary via the two pressures. The movement of fluid is called *filtration*. As blood enters the arterial end of the capillary, water and other particles pass through the thin-walled capillary, because the hydrostatic pressure (which would favor movement out) is greater than the oncotic pressure (which would favor pulling fluid in). Therefore, a great deal of filtered fluid leaves the arterial end of the capillary. At the venous end of the capillary, the hydrostatic pressure is low and the oncotic pressure (pulling) is great enough to pull fluid back into the capillary. This process is known as *reabsorption*. The system is not perfect, and some fluid is left behind in the interstitial spaces. The remaining fluid moves into the lymphatic capillaries due to the increase in tissue fluid pressure and movement, which causes the one-way valves in the terminal lymphatic capillaries to open. Contraction of the smooth muscles in the lymphatic vessels and pressure or movement from outside of the lymphatics propel the fluid forward into larger lymphatic vessels to the thoracic duct or the right lymph duct, and then into the venous systems. Valves within the lymphatic vessels pre-

vent backflow of fluid. Beside removing fluid, the lymphatics return small proteins that have leaked into the tissues to the venous system.

In some conditions, this system does not work smoothly, and excess fluid remains in the tissue spaces. When the level of plasma/serum protein is low, oncotic pressure in the vascular fluid is decreased and less water is reabsorbed back into the vascular space at the venous end. Normal albumin levels are critical, because albumin makes up 50% of the plasma proteins, but it is responsible for 80% of the oncotic pressure. Likewise, when the hydrostatic pressure is high because of fluid overload, the pressure gradient opposes fluid reabsorption into the venous end of the capillary. These conditions lead to edema. Concepts such as absorption, reabsorption, and resorption are often confusing. See Box 15–1 for an overview of these processes.

> ### Box 15–1. Concepts: Absorption, Reabsorption, and Resorption
>
> In addition to many other concepts, three often-confusing concepts are discussed often in this chapter: resorption, reabsorption, and absorption.
>
> **Absorption** usually refers to the initial movement of substances, such as end products of digestion or medications, from an organ such as the GI tract or tissues, such as the muscle, subcutaneous or dermal tissue, buccal or pharyngeal tissues, into the vascular spaces.
>
> **Reabsorption** refers to movement of water, electrolytes, vitamins, amino acids, glucose, lactate, or other essential substances from one compartment, such as the interstitium or renal tubules, back into vascular capillaries.
>
> **Resorption** refers to the process of calcium salts leaving the bone and moving to the blood in an ionized form.

Regulators of Fluid Balance

Thirst, many hormones, the lymphatic system, the nervous system, and the kidneys assist in the regulation of body fluids. These regulators may respond inappropriately to various stimuli and cause a fluid imbalance. Thirst is a primary factor in the maintenance of fluid intake. Figure 15–2 illustrates how the kidneys interact with hormones and the thirst mechanism to maintain fluid balance.

Osmolality

In the next sections, the role of osmolality in fluid balance is addressed. *Osmolality* and a related concept, *osmolarity*, refer to the amount of solutes (e.g., sugar, sodium, protein) in a liter of solution. The more solute present, the higher the osmolality. For example, distilled water is low in osmolality, sugar water is higher, and corn syrup is still higher. Fluids of high osmolarity tend to pull water across a membrane to reduce the ratio of solute to solvent.

Osmolarity is the concentration of all solutes or dissolved particles per liter of solution. Osmolality is measured by the number of dissolved particles per kilogram of water. Because 1 L of water is equal to 1 kg of weight, the terms osmolality and osmolarity are frequently used interchangeably. Sodium is the easiest solute to measure because it is abundant and readily accessible in the plasma. Electrolytes, especially sodium and protein, contribute the largest number of particles to the osmolality. Urea and glucose also contribute to osmolality. The role of osmolality in the human body is to control water movement and distribution among and within body fluid compartments by regulating the concentration of fluid in each compartment.

The hypothalamus is a regulatory center for osmolality. It manufactures antidiuretic hormone (ADH), which is released into the vascular system of the posterior pituitary gland. The hypothalamus also contains osmoreceptors that signal the posterior pituitary gland to release ADH as needed. Increased ECF osmolality causes the osmoreceptors to stimulate ADH release. Conversely, when ECF osmolality decreases, the osmoreceptors inhibit ADH secretion.

The kidney juxtaglomerular complex is also an important regulator of osmolality through its ability to sense and to regulate sodium concentrations via the renin-angiotensin-aldosterone hormonal system. Other hormones that affect osmolality because of their effect on sodium include prostaglandins, kallikrein, and natriuretic hormone.

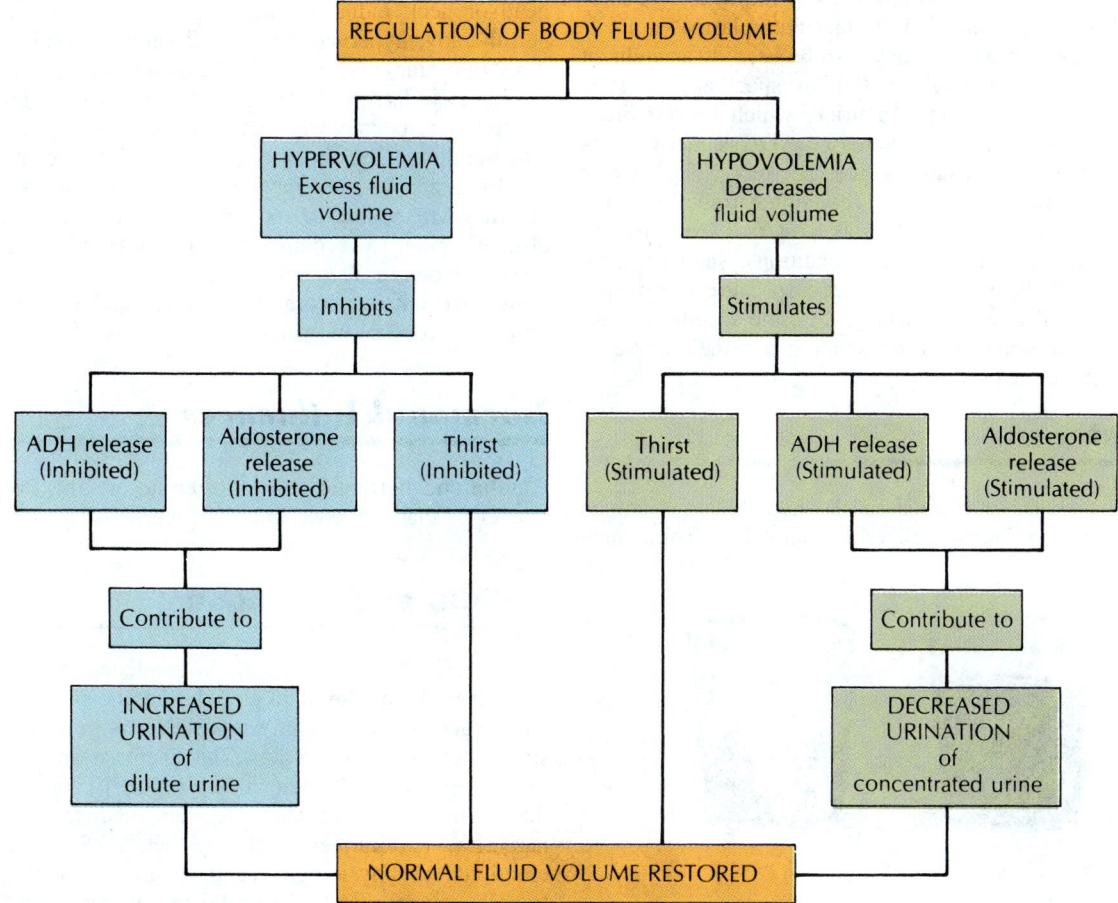

Figure 15–2. Regulation of body fluid volume depends on ADH, aldosterone, and thirst and fluid dynamics. (From White, B. [1994]. Maintaining fluid and electrolyte balance. In Bolander, V. B. [Ed.]. *Sorensen and Luckmann's basic nursing: A psychophysiologic approach* [3rd ed.]. Philadelphia: W. B. Saunders.)

(These are discussed under Sodium Homeostatic Mechanisms.)

One of the most powerful minute-to-minute controls of fluid and sodium concentrations in the body, however, is through the vascular changes secondary to the baroreceptor responses. (See the discussion under Nervous System.)

The plasma sodium value does not signify the total amount of sodium in the extracellular fluid, but rather it indicates the *relationship* of the amount of water to the amount of dissolved sodium.[11, 41] To illustrate this point, consider two glasses of water, one full and the other half full (Fig. 15–3). To each, add 1 tsp of salt. The half full glass on the right would taste saltier, yet it contains the same amount of salt as the glass on the left. The solution in the glass on the right is more concentrated (hyperosmolality) or, in other words, a lesser amount of water contains the same amount of salt.

The range of plasma osmolality (concentration of solutes in body fluid) is 275 to 295 mOsm/kg of water. When there are more than 295 mOsm/kg of water, a hyperosmolar state results. Isosmolar fluid contains particles and water in approximately equal proportions. Hyposmolar fluid has fewer particles than water. Solutions are considered hypertonic if they contain more than 375 mEq/L and hypotonic if they contain less than 250 mEq/L. Elevated plasma sodium levels (hypernatremia) usually indicate a state of hyperosmolality, and decreased plasma sodium levels (hyponatremia) usually indicate hyposmolality. Box 15–2 shows how to calculate plasma osmolality. Urine specific gravity may also be used as an indirect measurement of osmolality. A high specific gravity is found with very concentrated urine, which may indicate dehydration or result from increased ADH. Glucose, protein, and dyes will falsely elevate specific gravity. A low specific gravity is found with very dilute urine and may be normal with large fluid intake or as a response to diuretic therapy. More serious conditions, such as renal disease and diabetes insipidus, can also cause a low specific gravity. The nurse can measure urine specific gravity by using a urinometer or by sending a urine sample to the laboratory for testing.

Thirst

The thirst center is located in the hypothalamus and is activated by an increase in ECF osmolality. Thirst may

Box 15–2. How to Calculate Plasma Osmolality

To calculate plasma osmolality, the plasma sodium (Na) level should be known. Additionally, the glucose and blood urea nitrogen (BUN) should be known. The first formula may be used as a rough estimate of the plasma osmolality; the second formula gives a more exact plasma osmolality value.

$2 \times$ plasma Na = plasma osmolality
$2 \times$ plasma Na + (BUN/3) + (glucose/18) = plasma osmolality

result from hypotension, polyuria, fluid volume depletion as small as 0.5%, excess sodium intake, hypertonic feedings, and hypertonic intravenous (IV) fluids.

Although thirst can be reported and is an important clinical manifestation of fluid imbalances, it is not a true indicator of fluid balance in all persons. The thirst mechanism is depressed in the elderly, even those who are healthy, and in persons with debilitating illnesses.[82] Studies have identified inappropriate thirst mechanisms in persons with congestive heart failure due to an increase renin-angiotensin-aldosterone response. People may experience dry mouth from salivary gland dysfunction, head or neck radiation, smoking, mouth breathing, oxygen therapy, hyperventilation, and anticholinergic medications (atropine). Persons who have interstitial edema and an intracellular fluid deficit also experience thirst; the exception is people who are in a state of hyposmolality, which inhibits the thirst response.[83] Also, comatose and confused people may have very high serum osmolality, but they are unable to recognize the urge to drink. It is also important to recognize the cultural variations in fluid consumption. In Western society, offering a guest something to drink is a common practice and may influence total fluid consumption.

Hormonal Influences

Antidiuretic hormone and aldosterone are the two major hormones that influence fluid balance.

Antidiuretic Hormone

Antidiuretic hormone (ADH), is produced by the hypothalamus and is stored in vesicles in the posterior pituitary gland (neurohypophysis). ADH is released in response to many conditions: an increase in plasma or serum osmolality (hyperosmolality), ECF volume depletion, pain, stress, and use of certain medications such as narcotics, barbiturates, and anesthetics. Stress may be emotional or physiologic, such as the stress of surgery, trauma, severe anxiety, or prolonged exercise. As is obvious in the word *antidiuretic,* ADH prevents urine production. It promotes water reabsorption from the renal tubules. Stimulation of the thirst mechanism and ADH

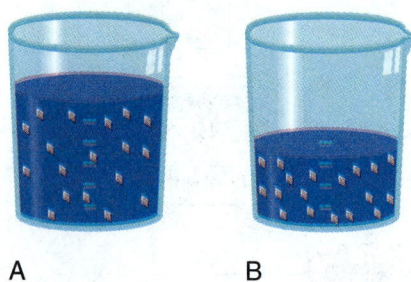

Figure 15–3. Although the actual salt content in both glasses is the same, glass B has a higher osmolality (concentration of salt to water) because it contains less water. Therefore, osmolality can be influenced by both water and sodium.

A   B

release usually occur concurrently in response to a body fluid deficit.

Factors suppressing ADH include hyposmolality of the ECF, increased blood volume, exposure to cold, acute alcohol ingestion, carbon dioxide inhalation, administration of some diuretics, lithium, and some antipsychotic medications. You could expect these situations to lead to increased urine output (diuresis). Sometimes diuresis is desirable. Can you see potential problems with unwanted diuresis or with diuresis in clients who cannot respond to thirst?

Aldosterone

Aldosterone is secreted by the adrenal cortex and promotes sodium reabsorption and potassium excretion from the kidneys. Aldosterone secretion is produced in a four-step process primarily by the renin-angiotensin system. Renin, secreted by the juxtaglomerular apparatus of the kidney (step 1) converts angiotensinogen in the blood to angiotensin I (step 2). Angiotensin I is further converted to angiotensin II in the capillary beds of the lungs (step 3). The presence of angiotensin II in the vascular system stimulates aldosterone secretion from the adrenal cortex (step 4). The two most powerful stimulants for aldosterone release are the increase in plasma potassium and the renin-angiotensin system. An increase in plasma sodium slightly decreases aldosterone secretion. The adrenocorticotropic hormone (ACTH) from the anterior pituitary is necessary for aldosterone secretion, but it has little effect on the rate of secretion.[35]

Hypovolemia is a common clinical condition in which aldosterone is secreted to maintain homeostasis. When arterial blood pressure falls, renal blood flow falls. Hypotension is sensed by the afferent arteriole of the nephron, which stimulates renin release from the juxtaglomerular cells. Following the four steps just outlined, aldosterone is produced, which increases sodium and fluid retention to raise the blood pressure.

Atrial Natriuretic Peptides, Prostaglandins, and Kinins

Atrial natriuretic peptides, prostaglandins, and *kinins* also contribute to the regulation of sodium balance. Atrial natriuretic peptides (ANP) are released from the atria in response to atrial distention, vasoconstriction, or direct cardiac damage. These factors increase the excretion of sodium and water and result in vasodilation.[9] Renal prostaglandins and the renal renin-kinin system also increase sodium excretion.

Lymphatic Influences

Plasma protein and fluid escaping from the tissue spaces cannot be directly reabsorbed into the blood vessels. The lymphatic system assists in returning any excess fluid and protein from the interstitial spaces to the blood. It is important to emphasize that this is a life-sustaining process.

Neurologic Influences

Neural mechanisms also contribute to the balance of water and sodium. Mechanoreceptors are sensory neurons that are found in the left atrium. When the ECF volume increases, these mechanoreceptors respond to stretching in the wall of the left atrium. This results in increased cardiac stroke volume. Also, the osmolality of the ECF stimulates osmoreceptors in the hypothalamus, which results in a decrease or an increase in ADH (depending on the fluid volume).

The baroreceptors, also known as pressoreceptors, which are located primarily in the carotid sinus and the wall of the aortic arch, are powerful nervous sensors that respond rapidly to changes in blood pressure. As the blood pressure rises, the baroreceptors send impulses to the medulla that result in inhibition of the vasoconstrictor center in the medulla and excitation of the vagal center. Vagal stimulation (parasympathetic) results in vasodilation, decreased heart rate, and decreased myocardial contraction to cause a decrease in blood pressure. The reverse process occurs when the blood pressure falls.

Renal Influences

The kidneys maintain fluid volume and the concentration of urine by filtering the ECF through the glomeruli. Reabsorption and excretion of ECF occurs in the renal tubules in response to ADH, aldosterone, and ANP.

Fluid Imbalances

The five types of fluid imbalances that may occur are as follows:

1. Extracellular fluid volume deficit (ECFVD)
2. Extracellular fluid volume excess (ECFVE)
3. Extracellular fluid volume shift
4. Intracellular fluid volume excess (ICFVE)
5. Intracellular fluid volume deficit (ICFVD)

Sodium is the major ion that influences fluid balance and imbalances. Water imbalances and sodium imbalances often occur concurrently, but they also may be seen separately. Therefore, they are discussed separately in this chapter.

Extracellular Fluid Volume Deficit

An ECFVD, commonly called *dehydration,* is a decrease in intravascular and interstitial fluids. ECFVD is a common and serious fluid imbalance that results in vascular fluid volume loss (hypovolemia). If the ECFVD is sudden or severe, it can lead to cellular fluid loss as well. This loss results because fluid shifts from the cells to the vascular spaces in an attempt to restore balance.

The three types of extracellular fluid volume deficits are as follows:

1. *Hyperosmolar fluid volume deficit*, in which the water loss is greater than the electrolyte loss
2. *Isosmolar fluid volume deficit*, in which there is equal proportion of both water and electrolyte (sodium) loss
3. Although it is less common, the third type of ECFVD, known as *hypotonic fluid volume deficit*, also occurs. In this type of deficit, the loss of electrolytes is greater than the fluid loss.

Etiology and Risk Factors

Several conditions leading to fluid losses can cause ECFVD. Common etiologies include severe vomiting, diarrhea, and diaphoresis, as well as traumatic injuries with excessive blood loss and insufficient water or fluid intake. Third-space fluid shifts, shifting of fluid from the vascular space to another body space where fluid cannot be easily exchanged, can result in ECFVD. (Conditions that cause third-space fluid shifting are discussed later in the chapter.) Spaces that are prone to third-spacing include the pericardial, pleural, peritoneal, and joint cavities. Other factors that increase the risk for ECFVD include fever, gastrointestinal (GI) suction, ileostomy, fistulas, burns, hyperventilation, hyperthyroidism, decreased ADH secretion, diabetes insipidus (nephrogenic and neurogenic), Addison's disease or adrenal crisis,[24] the diuretic phase of acute renal failure, and the use of diuretics.[31]

The elderly are at high risk for ECFVD for numerous reasons, including a decreased thirst mechanism, a decreased renal concentration of urine, and an altered ADH response.[27, 55] They also have increased drug-drug interactions and multiple chronic diseases.[40] Decreased access to fluids because of financial or transportation barriers, debilitation, chemical or physical restraint, and changes in mental status are significant risk factors for the elderly.[74]

Suggestions for primary, secondary, and tertiary prevention of ECFVD are presented in Risk Factors and Levels of Prevention.

Pathophysiology

The pathophysiologic changes in ECFVD are usually related to changes in *fluid balance* and *sodium levels*. Sodium has a major influence on water retention and water loss. Plasma sodium concentration is increased (hypernatremia) with an ECFVD from insufficient water intake or massive water loss. The seriousness of the manifestations and aggressiveness of the treatment are related to both the *amount* and *acuteness* of the fluid loss and the client's state of health at the time of loss. Sudden fluid loss does not give the compensatory mechanisms time to adapt; severe loss is often beyond the potential of compensatory mechanisms. Failure of compensation results in vascular collapse, shock, and intracellular fluid shifts. The fluid shift from the cells to the vascular spaces is an attempt to dilute the hypernatremic state. The resultant intracellular

cerebral dehydration may lead to vasospasm, intracerebral hemorrhage, and stroke. See Table 15–1 for the pathophysiologic basis of the clinical manifestations of ECFVD.

Clinical Manifestations and Diagnostic Findings

With mild ECFVD, 1 to 2 L of water or 2% of the body weight is lost. Moderate ECFVD is evidenced by 3 to 5 L of water loss or 5% weight loss. In severe ECFVD, the water loss is increased to 5 to 10 L and the weight loss is increased to 8%; the systolic blood pressure becomes alarmingly low ($\leq$70 mm Hg systolic pressure). Cells with high metabolic demands, such as cerebral, cardiac, and kidney tissues, experience signs of altered tissue perfusion. Immediate medical management is necessary. With fluid volume deficit, many laboratory findings are altered (see Table 15–1)

Acute and Subacute Care

■ Medical Management

Medical treatment of fluid volume deficit depends on the acuteness and severity of the fluid deficit. If the fluid loss is mild, the fluid intake should be increased in accordance with the client's physical condition. If the thirst mechanism is intact and the client can drink fluid, medical intervention may not be necessary.

Intravenous Therapy

When a hyperosmolar fluid volume deficit is present, a hypotonic IV solution, such as 5% dextrose in 0.2% saline (D_5/0.2% NaCl), may be prescribed. If the deficit has existed for more than 24 hours, it is dangerous to correct this deficit too rapidly. Sodium solutions should be infused at a rate of from 0.5 to 1.0 mEq/L/hr. If fluid is given too rapidly, cerebral edema may result.[11, 119]

If hemorrhage is the cause of the ECFVD and a client is symptomatic, packed red blood cells followed by hypotonic IV solutions may be necessary.[32] Acute blood loss resulting in even small volume losses can result in clinical manifestations such as hypotension, tachycardia, oliguria, thirst, pallor, cold and clammy skin, and anxiety. In contrast, chronic losses may result in hemoglobin levels of 7 or 8 g/100 ml without clinical manifestations. In situations in which the blood losses are less than 1 L, normal saline or lactated Ringer's solution may be used to restore fluid volume.[104]

The fluid needs of the client must be assessed within the context of the client's overall condition. A client with severe ECFVD accompanied by severe heart, liver, or kidney disease cannot tolerate large volumes of fluid or sodium. The client or family of a client suffering from terminal illness may have varied wishes as to fluid maintenance, as shown in Ethical Issues in Nursing.

Oral Rehydration

Mild fluid volume loss can usually be corrected with oral fluid replacement. Encourage consumption of clear liquids such as cola, broth, gelatin, or Gatorade. If the client tolerates, progress to full liquids. For a person who is able to eat solid foods, encourage 1200 to 1500 ml of oral fluids per day. If fluid intake is solely from oral liquids or parenteral fluids, increase the total intake to 2500 ml in 24 hours to compensate for the lack of fluids in foods.

It is important to remember that viral infections com-

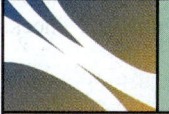

RISK FACTORS AND LEVELS OF PREVENTION

Extracellular Fluid Volume Deficit

Risk Factors

Clients with decreased intake, which often includes the elderly, confused, debilitated, restrained, or those with dysphagia.

Clients with increased loss from severe diaphoresis, use of diuretics, increased vomiting, fever, diarrhea, wounds, GI suction, burns, hyperglycemia, blood loss, diuresis, diabetes insipidus, or Addison's disease.

Levels of Prevention

Primary Prevention

- Teach clients to replace fluid (30 to 60 ml or more) hourly, as tolerated, with clear liquids, such as cola, to decrease nausea and to replace electrolytes.
- Teach the importance of consulting the physician if illness lasts longer than 24 hours or if chronic disease, such as diabetes or liver, kidney, or heart disease, is present. Elderly clients should also consult the physician, as should those who are experiencing severe weakness, cardiac palpitations, or acute weight loss.
- Teach people who exercise (1) to understand the importance of exercise and heat acclimatization, (2) to avoid exercise during high heat and humidity, (3) to wear appropriate clothing (excess clothing decreases evaporation), (4) to use more caution if obese, because obesity impairs the sweating mechanism, (5) to drink cool water before, during, and after finishing exercise, and to add carbohydrates (for energy and sodium), if exercise is prolonged, (6) to avoid rapid fluid replacement, as this fluid only overflows to kidney, and (7) to use caution when taking medications that interfere with thermoregulation, such as thyroid replacement, amphetamines, haloperidol, antihistamines, anticholinergic drugs, and phenothiazines.[67]
- Encourage diabetics who exercise to wear Medic-Alert identification jewelry and to increase protein intake, to decrease refined sugar intake, and to reduce insulin to half the usual dosage or to an amount recommended by the physician.[53]
- Teach persons taking cortisone the importance of not missing doses, of wearing Medic-Alert identification jewelry, and of consulting a physician about increased dosage during physical or emotional stress to prevent Addison's crisis.

Secondary Prevention

- Monitor intake and output and weights *accurately* in high-risk clients. Remember to record all sources of intake, including liquids with meals and between meals, with medications, IVs, tube feedings, and flushes. Record all sources of output including urine, diarrhea, diaphoresis, and hyperventilation.
- Give *hourly* fluids to elderly, confused, debilitated clients and to those who require restraints.
- Give thickened liquids to clients with dysphagia.
- Give water boluses with hypertonic tube feedings. Recommended dilution is 1 ml of water per 1 kcal of feeding formula. For example, if a can of formula has 380 kcal in 240 ml of feeding formula, give an additional 140 ml of water for a total of 380 ml of fluid.[10]
- Give antiemetics for nausea, antipyretics for fever, and antibiotics for infection.
- Consult the physician for IV maintenance/replacement needs, such as IV replacement for GI loss, and extra steroids before surgery if a client is taking cortisone.

Tertiary Prevention

- Give fluids "of choice" hourly.
- Place fluids within reach; use straws.
- Provide fresh, cool water.
- Give thickened fluids if client has dysphagia.
- Give fluid boluses if client is receiving hypertonic feedings.
- Examine elixirs for sorbitol content if diarrhea is a problem. If sorbitol is present, consult the physician for prescription change.[23]
- Encourage the family to participate in feeding.

monly result in lactose intolerance. To prevent the associated diarrhea, encourage avoidance of milk-based products. Also, persons who experience fluid loss from diarrhea should avoid fatty or fried foods.[102] Hypertonic tube feedings also place a person at risk for dehydration due to fluid shifting into the small bowel in response to the increased osmolality of the feeding. It is important to give water boluses between tube feedings to prevent this problem.[10]

■ Nursing Management of the Medical Client

Assessment

Current assessment recommendations for ECFVD are as follows. Assess the oral cavity for dryness of the mucous membranes. The most accurate site to assess mucous membranes is at the point at which the gums and cheeks

Table 15–1. Clinical Manifestations and Laboratory/Diagnostic Findings: Extracellular Fluid Volume Deficit

Clinical Manifestation	Pathophysiologic Basis
Thirst	Cells shrink, stimulating "thirst" osmoreceptors in the hypothalamus; with isosmolar fluid loss, thirst usually does not occur
Muscle weakness	Fluid imbalance alters electrolytes, especially Na
Decreased skin turgor	Decreased interstitial fluid causes skin tissue to "stick together" (not accurate in elderly)
Dry mucous membranes; dry, cracked lips or furrowed tongue	Cells of mucous membranes and tongue "dry out"
Eyeballs soft and sunken (severe deficit)	Water tension in eyeballs decreased
Apprehension, restlessness, headache, confusion; coma in severe deficit	Cerebral dehydration
Elevated temperature	Less fluid available for evaporation
Tachycardia, weak pulse	Pulse greater than 100 bpm may be due to circulatory compensation by the heart, decreased volume
Peripheral vein filling > 5 seconds	Decreased volume
Postural systolic blood pressure fall > 25 mm Hg and diastolic fall > 20 mm Hg, with pulse increase ≥30	Plasma volume is inadequate owing to hypovolemia; systolic pressure begins to fall
Narrowed pulse pressure, decreased CVP and PCWP	Decreased venous return
Flattened neck veins in supine position	Decreased venous return
Weight loss unless masked by third-spacing	A lack of the water component of body weight
Oliguria (<30 ml per hour)	Renal response to hypovolemia (compensatory)
Decreased number and moisture in stools	Decreased volume of fluid (compensatory)

Laboratory/Diagnostic Findings	
Increased osmolality (>295 mOsm/kg)	Due to hyposmolar fluid loss (more fluid than solutes lost)
Increased or normal serum sodium level (>145 mEq/L)	Hyposmolar fluid volume loss: water is lost in greater amounts than sodium Isosmolar fluid volume loss: serum sodium level within normal range
Increased BUN (>25 mg/dl)	The blood urea nitrogen (BUN) slightly elevated because of hemoconcentration
Hyperglycemia (>120 mg/dl)	Sugar increases serum osmolality, causing diuresis and water loss; glucose levels may also be elevated owing to hemoconcentration
Elevated hematocrit (>55%)	With hyposmolar fluid loss, hematocrit will be increased owing to hemoconcentration; with isosmolar fluid loss (e.g., hemorrhage), hematocrit may be within normal range
Increased specific gravity (>1.030)	Increased solute to solvent ratio (may be altered by renal function)

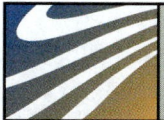

ETHICAL ISSUES IN NURSING

Should Hydration Measures Be Used on All Clients?

The electrolytes found in the body work together with amazing precision. Slight alterations in the electrolyte balance may cause physical symptoms as simple as muscle cramps or as grave as cardiac dysrhythmias. These imbalances may be corrected in many cases by the reintroduction, or the removal, of the electrolyte that is out of balance. This issue appears simple.

Scenario:

But, what if a person refuses to have his or her electrolyte imbalance corrected, for instance, through hydration measures? Or, in the case of a client in a persistent vegetative state, what if the family wishes to cease hydration measures, which will ultimately hasten the client's death?

The issue of hydration may be separated into two categories: life-sustaining and death-delaying. Life-sustaining measures of any kind mean to do just that—to sustain life. The ultimate goal may be to correct whatever is threatening life, which may be as simple as correcting an electrolyte imbalance. However, death-delaying measures are those that prolong the inevitable. Perhaps the disease process has passed beyond a controllable level, or a traumatic experience has rendered a person in a persistent vegetative state with no hope of recovery. In such cases, hydration may be considered a futile treatment, used only to prolong the process of death. Should hydration measures be used on all persons regardless of whether such measures are life-sustaining or death-delaying? Is hydration a basic measure of care that should never be denied to anyone for any reason? The following are questions to consider: Do clients experience pain if they are not hydrated, even if they are in a persistent vegetative state? Do nurses have the right to refuse to carry out orders not to hydrate clients if they believe this is a basic comfort never to be denied?[36] By hydrating clients who no longer may benefit from its treatment effects, are we really just comforting ourselves as caregivers? Should comfort be viewed from the beneficial effects of dehydration, such as less incontinence, less energy expenditure, less vomiting, fewer pulmonary secretions, less edema to exert pressure on nerve endings (and thus less pain), increased production of ketones and metabolites that reduce awareness of discomfort or from the perspective of negative effects of dehydration, such as thirst and dryness of mucous membranes?[77, 108]

Does it help to know that research studies have found only two major effects of terminal dehydration: drying of mucous membranes/lips and thirst?[4, 108] Each of these can be alleviated with frequent, thorough oral care and frequent small amounts of fluids. Does it help to know that pivotal court cases have decided in favor of the person's right to choose and have determined the cause of death to be the underlying illness instead of dehydration?

It is likely that nurses in all areas of healthcare will experience this type of dilemma sometime in their professional career. How a nurse reacts in a specific situation depends on many variables particular to that situation and to his or her ethical feelings at the time. All cases involving these issues should be evaluated individually so as not to trivialize the end results of taking such actions.

---

meet. At the same time, assess for tongue dryness and longitudinal furrows. Note speech difficulty.

Check skin turgor by gently pinching and lifting the skin (Fig. 15–4). Usually skin returns to a normal position within 1 or 2 seconds. A slower response may indicate loss of interstitial fluids. Recall that a return to normal is often slower in elderly people due to loss of subcutaneous fat and elastin.

Assess vital signs every 2 to 4 hours, depending on the severity of the fluid loss; compare with baseline vital signs and report marked differences. Assess for postural (orthostatic) blood pressure and pulse changes by taking a lying blood pressure and pulse; have the client stand up, then repeat the blood pressure and pulse. Report falls in standing systolic blood pressure of 25 mm Hg or more from the supine blood pressure with pulse increases of more than 30 beats/minute.[115] Assess peripheral vein filling time daily. Veins should fill within 3 to 5 seconds when the arm is lowered below the level of the heart.

If the ECFVD is mild, assess urinary output every 8

hours and compare daily outputs. Absence of adequate renal perfusion for several hours may result in permanent renal damage. Whenever the output drops to below 30 ml/hr for 2 consecutive hours, urinary output must be assessed hourly. Nurses must teach unlicensed assistive personnel to report urinary outputs of less than 30 ml/hr for 2 consecutive hours or less than 240 ml for an 8-hour period (see Management and Delegation).

Monitor and compare daily weights using a consistent approach. A loss of 2.2 lb is equivalent to 1 L of fluid. Therefore, an 8-lb weight loss equals approximately 3.5 L of fluid, or a moderate fluid volume deficit. Also, monitor plasma sodium, BUN, glucose, and hematocrit levels to determine the plasma osmolality. Monitor for confusion and upper body weakness, which are manifestations of ECFVD.

Research has suggested that some of the standard indicators of fluid balance may not be appropriate for all clients.[34] In some people, subjective sensations of thirst are not always reliable indicators of dehydration.[120] For

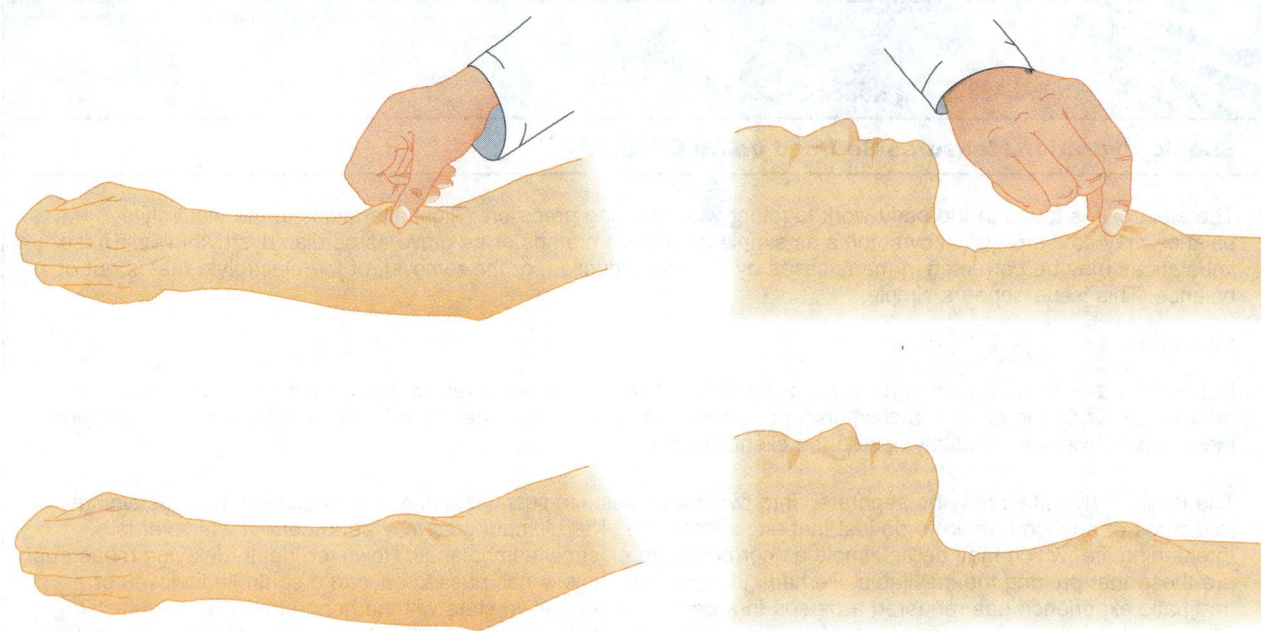

A Assessment of skin turgor on the forearm   B Assessment of skin turgor on the sternum

Figure 15–4. Skin turgor assessment. This can be done on the forearm of a young to middle-aged adult. However, testing skin turgor on the forearm of an elderly person yields inaccurate results; skin turgor should be assessed on the sternal area of elderly clients.

example, clients with hyposmolar dehydration do not experience thirst. Elderly clients have a decreased thirst mechanism.[72] Also, postural hypotension is not always a result of ECFVD. Autonomic neuropathy, dysrhythmias, and some medications, such as antihypertensives, can cause postural hypotension.[115] See Table 15–1 for the specific parameters for postural hypotension related to ECFVD.

Diagnosis, Planning, Implementation

Fluid Volume Deficit. Fluid volume deficit is the nursing diagnosis of choice. State the diagnosis as *Fluid Volume Deficit related to insufficient fluid intake, vomiting, diarrhea, hemorrhage, or third-space fluid loss (ascites, burns).* Be certain to specify the cause in your client's case.

Planning: Expected Outcomes. The client will have restored fluid balance, as evidenced by absence of postural vital sign changes; stabilization of body weight; absence of causative factor(s) of ECFVD; urine output greater than 720 ml/day; pink, moist mucous membranes and tongue, absence of tongue furrows; improvement in upper body strength; less confusion; and improvement in clarity of speech.

Implementation. In addition to assessment, numerous interventions are available to correct ECFVD. When fluid balance is present, the fluid not only provides some degree of cushioning against pressure but it also provides the vehicle for transportation of nutrients and removal of wastes to maintain cell function and growth. Therefore, when fluid balance is compromised, a person is at risk for tissue breakdown. It is also important to apply a moisturizer or skin barrier to the skin to protect the skin from the irritants, enzymes, and microorganisms found in urine

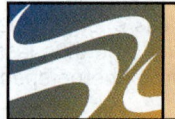

MANAGEMENT AND DELEGATION

Care of Clients with Fluid Volume Deficit

When working with unlicensed assistive personnel in the care of clients with fluid volume deficit, help them keep the following points in mind:

- Keep fresh water or other fluids in an easily accessible location. Remind elderly clients to drink fluids hourly, because their thirst mechanism is diminished.
- Try to provide fluids of choice every 1 to 2 hours.
- Encourage family members to assist with fluid intake.
- Provide oral care every 2 hours to help decrease the discomfort from dry mucous membranes.
- Record intake accurately. Remember that ice chips equal ½ of the container (e.g., 1 cup of ice chips = ½ cup of water).
- Assist clients as necessary to the bathroom/commode/bedpan every 2 hours. If the client is wearing disposable briefs, assess for incontinence and the need for perineal care at least every 2 hours.
- Record all output accurately. Include the amount of urine, the number of episodes of incontinence, and include the amount of any diarrhea (measure it).
- Report diarrhea, excessive sweating, or rapid breathing to the nurse.
- Report urine that is dark or is less than 30 mL per hour over 2 consecutive hours to the nurse.
- Report weight changes of 2 lb. or more from the previous day.

and feces. To prevent altered skin integrity, change the client's position every 2 hours. Give oral care, using a lip moisturizer, every 2 hours; avoid mouthwashes with an alcohol base. The frequency of positioning and oral care may need to be increased to hourly if reevaluation of the skin and oral assessment findings indicate lack of improvement.

If orthostatic hypotension is present, provide safety through step-progression position changes. Step-progression gives the client's body time to adapt to changes in position. First, raise the head of the bed. Next, sit the client at the edge of the bed (called dangling) until he or she is no longer dizzy. Then, have the client stand and, finally, assist the client to a chair. Do not progress to the next position until the client tolerates the preceding one (i.e., without dizziness or marked hypotension).

If the fluid loss is moderate or severe, administer IV fluids as prescribed. Monitor IV solutions, IV sites, and client responses hourly. Overhydration may occur from excessive and rapidly infused IV fluids or with pre-existing renal or cardiac disorders. Use minidrop IV tubing and/or infusion pumps to decrease the risk of overload. Notify the physician if the client shows no improvement or if the condition worsens. Manifestations of intracellular shifting (e.g., confusion) or of extracellular fluid overload (e.g., shortness of breath, auscultation of crackles in the lungs, and jugular vein engorgement) should be reported.

Evaluation

Fluid deficit should be correctable in 8 to 24 hours depending on the severity of fluid loss, whether the source of loss has been corrected (e.g., bleeding), and the age of the client.

■ Modifications for Elderly Clients

Research has suggested that some of the usual indicators of fluid balance are not appropriate for the elderly population[34] as shown in Nursing Research.

It is a common myth that reducing fluid intake decreases urinary incontinence. On the contrary, limited fluid intake increases bladder irritability, leading to uninhibited contractions, and alters the neurologic stimulus that controls normal bladder emptying. Emphasizing the importance of drinking even in the absence of thirst,[92] teaching pelvic muscle exercises, and instituting a toilet schedule may help an elderly person overcome the problem of incontinence.[74]

If satiety is the barrier, offer fluids of choice and in frequent, small amounts (30 to 60 ml/hr), and feed slowly. Involve the person and/or family in goal setting. When rehydrating an elderly person, it is important to rehydrate slowly because of frequent problems with renal and cardiac disease. Rapid replacement often results in overflow diuresis without cellular replacement. This only compounds the present dehydration and may result in hypernatremia.

If dysphagia is present, consult the physician for swallowing studies. Once the problem has been diagnosed, a speech pathologist can provide exercises to help the client with swallowing difficulties. The nurse reinforces the speech therapist's prescription during each feeding. Many of the prescriptions include such interventions as providing thickened fluids, elevating the headrest to 90 degrees

NURSING RESEARCH

Which Indicators of Dehydration Are Reliable in the Elderly?

Gross, C.R., et al. (1992). Clinical indicators of dehydration severity in elderly patients. *Journal of Emergency Medicine, 10*(3), 267–274.

Many studies have identified dehydration as the most common fluid and electrolyte problem in the elderly population. Some of the well accepted indicators of fluid and electrolyte balance have been found to be inadequate indicators of dehydration in the elderly.

Gross and colleagues conducted a prospective, correlational study on 55 clients older than 60 who came to two different university hospital emergency rooms. The clients presented with possible dehydration. The clients had a thorough history and physical examination in which 38 variables that have commonly been accepted as signs of dehydration were evaluated.

Of these, only seven variables were strongly correlated to dehydration. The most reliable indicators of the severity of dehydration in this population were tongue dryness, longitudinal tongue furrows, dryness of the oral mucous membranes, upper body weakness, confusion, speech difficulty, and sunken eyes. Thirst, skin turgor, orthostatic blood pressure changes, and lack of axillary moisture were found to be unreliable indicators of dehydration in the elderly.

Implications for Practice

A routine assessment of the mouth should be done on all clients 60 and older. If the client is a mouth breather, it may not be enough to assess for tongue dryness and furrows and dry mucous membranes. The nurse should also assess for other supporting data, such as upper body weakness, confusion, speech difficulty, and sunken eyes. Essential interventions include frequent oral care, fluid replacement, and diagnostic testing to validate the diagnosis.

before meals and for 1 hour after feeding, and flexing the head slightly forward when starting to swallow. In addition, the nurse can decrease the risk of aspiration by placing small amounts of food on the side of the mouth with the best sensation and muscle strength. Teaching the client to chew slowly and to swallow two or three times with each mouthful and inspecting the mouth for food pocketing can also decrease the risk of aspiration. Assessing fit of dentures is also important.

Community and Self-Care

Follow-up care is based on the original problem. If the client was fluid deficient because of inadequate fluid intake, teach the client or family member how to promote adequate fluid intake. Teach about medication risk factors, especially if the client is taking any that increase risk for fluid and/or electrolyte imbalance, such as diuretics and cortisone (see Risk Factors and Levels of Prevention). If the client is fluid deficient as the result of a traumatic injury, the problem may be resolved before dismissal.

Nurses working in extended care settings frequently care for clients receiving hypertonic tube feedings or elixir medications that contain a sorbitol base. Research has shown that these can cause abdominal distention, cramping, and osmotic diarrhea.[23] (For tertiary prevention measures, see Risk Factors and Levels of Prevention.) For addititonal information on managing IV therapy at home, see the Bridge to Home Healthcare.

Extracellular Fluid Volume Excess

ECFVE is increased fluid retention in the intravascular and interstitial spaces. Sodium and water retention in the same proportion is referred to as *isosmolar fluid volume excess.* Or the plasma sodium level may appear to be within the normal range, because of excess water retention, even though the actual sodium level is increased. In

---

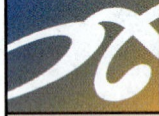

BRIDGE TO HOME HEALTHCARE

Managing IV Therapy at Home

Lisa Gorski, M.S., R.N.C.,
Franciscan Home Care,
Milwaukee, Wisconsin

Intravenous (IV) therapy is commonly administered in the home setting and is advantageous to many clients. Some recognized advantages include the comfort of being treated in one's own home, increased participation in care, and a reduced risk of infection in the home setting compared with the hospital. However, home therapy has associated risks. The presence of an invasive device (i.e., the IV catheter) and potential adverse reactions to specific home IV therapies certainly exist. Thus, it is important to provide home IV therapy with a primary goal of ensuring client safety. It is important that the nurse who is providing home IV therapy be educated and experienced in this area of practice. Clearly delineated policies and procedures and careful client selection are essential. Client selection criteria to consider when planning home IV therapy include client willingness and motivation, ability to learn and remember procedures, visual acuity, and manual dexterity. Some degree of self-care is usually the goal of home IV therapy. Depending on the type of therapy, clients or their caregivers may assume all or part of the responsibility for administering IVs. This may include taking care of the IV catheter site, flushing the catheter with heparin or normal saline to maintain patency, and administering IV medications. Home IV therapies that are usually taught to a patient or caregiver include antibiotic therapy and parenteral nutrition. However, in some cases, only the home care nurse administers the therapy, such as in home blood transfusions and complicated chemotherapy drug regimens.

Various methods are used to administer IV therapy in the home setting. The simple gravity drip method is cost effective and appropriate for administration of most antibiotics.

Infusion pumps are used when rate control is necessary. Pumps used in home care are usually computer programmable and are small, about the size of a portable radio. The pump is placed in a small nylon pouch with the IV fluid; IV tubing is threaded through the client's clothing to the IV catheter. The client can then ambulate while the pump is infusing the IV fluid; the pouch is often worn with an over-the-shoulder strap or sometimes as a fanny pack. Most home infusion pumps are fully alarmed; the alarm sounds if a battery is low or if IV tubing is occluded. Most home infusion pumps also have "lock-out" abilities to reduce the risk of tampering or of accidentally changing the program. Specific client education to be addressed when an infusion pump is used includes teaching the client how to safely maneuver while the pump is in use. Client education should also address dressing, bathing, checking pump function, and troubleshooting alarms.

The Intravenous Nursing Society (617–441–3008) is a national nursing organization devoted to the education of nurses practicing the specialty of IV nursing. This professional group is an excellent resource for home IV therapy; specific benefits include a professional journal, ongoing educational conferences, and local chapter meetings.

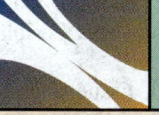

RISK FACTORS AND LEVELS OF PREVENTION

Extracellular Fluid Volume Excess

Risk Factors

Clients with heart, kidney, and/or liver disease, hyperaldosteronism, Cushing's syndrome, or those taking glucocorticoids. Clients with an increased ADH, such as after transurethral resection (TUR) or after general anesthesia, those taking barbiturates, or those receiving morphine drips.[7]
 Clients with nasogastric tubes.

Levels of Prevention

Primary Prevention

- Teach the client to weigh weekly and to call the physician if weight gain is greater than 3 lb.
- Teach the importance of limiting salt intake based on the physician's recommendation. This includes how to read labels to help avoid products containing sodium.
- Teach client to consult the physician for increase in shortness of breath, edema, or rapid weight gain.
- Encourage the client with edema to sit with the legs elevated and to avoid long periods of standing.

Secondary Prevention

- Monitor weight daily.
- Monitor for overload if receiving hypotonic irrigation during and/or after surgery. Consult the physician about changing the solution to normal saline.[5]
- Avoid overloading with IV fluids. Observe for pulmonary congestion.
- Use *only* normal saline for bladder and nasogastric tube irrigations.
- Report changes in respiratory difficulty: increased dyspnea, cough, or crackles.
- Report signs of increased systemic fluid, such as a weight gain greater than 3 lb in a week. Refer to Table 15–2.

Tertiary Prevention

- Assess lung sounds for increased respiratory difficulty.
- Compare weekly weights.
- Limit sodium intake.
- Provide rest periods between activities.
- Elevate edematous limbs.
- Keep heels off bed to prevent decreased tissue perfusion.
- Report a weight increase greater than 3 lb in a week.

---

this event, the sodium is diluted by the extra water. The discussion of the four types of volume changes as related to sodium can be found in the section Hyponatremia.

Etiology and Risk Factors

ECFVE usually results from an increase in the total body sodium content. Causes of ECFVE include heart failure, renal disorders, cirrhosis of the liver, increased ingestion of high-sodium foods (e.g., processed foods), excessive tap water enemas, excessive amounts of IV fluids containing sodium, electrolyte-free IV fluids, syndrome of inappropriate secretion of antidiuretic hormone (SIADH), sepsis, decreased colloid osmotic pressure, lymphatic or venous obstruction, stasis, or orthostatic edema.[120] SIADH has been associated with many central nervous system (CNS) and carcinogenic disorders.[7] Likewise, clients with hyperaldosteronism, Cushing's syndrome, and those taking glucocorticoids are at increased risk for ECFVE. Other risk factors include the use of hypotonic fluids to

irrigate nasogastric tubes and use of hypotonic bladder irrigations during or after transurethral resections.[75] General anesthesia also may cause ECFVE by promoting increased ADH secretion (stress response).[7]

Suggestions for primary, secondary, and tertiary prevention of ECFVE are presented in Risk Factors and Levels of Prevention.

Pathophysiology

With a fluid volume excess (fluid overload), the fluid pressure is even greater than usual at the arterial end of the capillary. Peripheral and pulmonary edema may result as fluid is pushed into the tissue spaces with greater force, as illustrated in Figure 15–5A. The fluid is not reabsorbed at the venous end because venous pressure also exceeds oncotic pressure. As the fluid pressure increases in the tissues, it creates a resistance to forward flow of blood and increases pressure throughout the circulatory system. A resistance to arterial flow occurs, which leads to increased pressure in the left ventricle and then in the left atrium. From the atrium, fluid is forced backward across the alveolar-capillary membrane of the lungs, resulting in pulmonary edema. Pulmonary edema is commonly seen when the left side of the heart is distended and fails to pump adequately. Also, because the lungs are low-pressure organs, they offer little resistance to fluid accumulation.[98] If the right side of the heart fails, peripheral edema occurs through the same retrograde process. Left-sided heart failure leads to right-sided failure and vice versa, so both pulmonary and peripheral edema may exist simultaneously.

When fluid overload results from renal disorders, sodium and water excretion are decreased. As fluid volume rises, the heart compensates through tachycardia and hypertrophy. When compensatory mechanisms fail, heart failure results. Uncontrolled heart failure can lead to multiple organ failure and death due to massive body water retention, also known as *anasarca*.

In cirrhosis of the liver,[52] renal disease, burns, or protein malnutrition, the plasma protein and albumin levels are decreased. Therefore, the oncotic pressure is decreased in the vascular fluids, resulting in less fluid reabsorption from the tissue spaces at the venous end. Peripheral edema and ascites result (see Fig. 15–5B).

When lymphatic channels are obstructed, tissue oncotic pressure rises and leads to edema, as illustrated in Figure 15–5C. See Chapters 75 and 79 for discussion of edema due to increased capillary permeability.

Clinical Manifestations and Diagnostic Findings

Some obvious indicators of severe fluid volume excess include dyspnea, engorged neck and hand veins, a bounding pulse, moist crackles in the lungs, rapid weight gain, and edema of the extremities. Table 15–2 lists the clinical manifestations and laboratory/diagnostic findings associated with fluid volume excess. With fluid volume excess or fluid overload, concentration of solutes is altered as reflected in laboratory values.

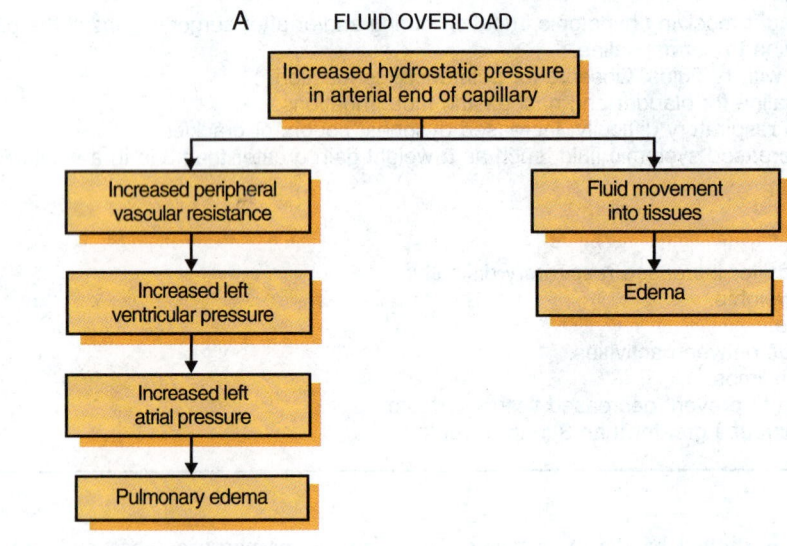

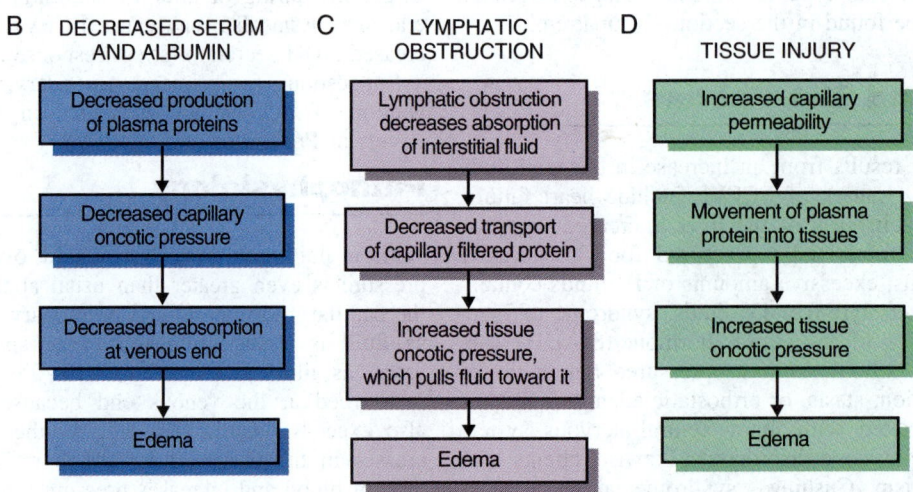

Figure 15–5. Mechanisms of edema formation. *A*, Fluid overload. *B*, Decreased plasma and albumin. *C*, Lymphatic obstruction. *D*, Tissue injury.

Table 15-2. Clinical Manifestations and Laboratory/Diagnostic Findings: Extracellular Fluid Volume Excess

Clinical Manifestation	Pathophysiologic Basis
Respiratory Manifestations	
Constant, irritating cough	Fluid accumulation in the alveolar sacs due to hypervolemia
Dyspnea	Fluid congestion in lungs
Crackles in lungs	Alveoli are congested with fluid owing to increased hydrostatic pressure
Cyanosis	Impaired oxygen transport due to the capillaries being filled with fluid
Pleural effusion	Increased hydrostatic pressure in pulmonary cells, causes fluid shifting
Cardiovascular Manifestations	
Neck vein engorgement in semi-Fowler position	Fluid overload and delayed right-sided heart emptying/filling
Peripheral vein emptying, >5 seconds	Peripheral vascular fluid overload
Bounding pulse, elevated blood pressure	Peripheral vascular fluid overload
S_3 gallop	Delayed ventricular filling and overdistention of ventricles from rapid filling during early diastole
Pitting edema of dependent tissues (lower extremities, sacrum)	Osmotic pressure in the venous end of the capillary exceeds oncotic pressure and fluid cannot return to the bloodstream
Sacral edema	Dependent edema in the supine client occurs in the sacral hollow rather than in the feet and legs, because the sacrum is the lowest place on the body
Weight gain (rapid)	Fluid retention; for every 2.2 lb gained, 1 L of body fluid is retained, greater weight gain if ICFVE
Increased CVP and PCWP	Fluid retention
Neurologic Manifestations	
Change in level of consciousness (malaise, confusion, headache, lethargy, and convulsion ICFVE)	Cerebral edema, early signs of ICFVE
Laboratory/Diagnostic Findings	
Serum osmolality <275 mOsm/kg	Indicates a diluted body fluid in which there are fewer solutes in proportion to the water volume
Serum sodium <135 mEq/L to >145 mEq/L (low, normal, or high value)	Depending on the amount of sodium retention or water retention, the serum sodium level may be normal, decreased, or elevated
Decreased hematocrit (<45%)	Hemodilution
Specific gravity below 1.010	Solvent in the urine exceeds solute
Decreased BUN (<8 mg/dl)	Hemodilution

Acute and Subacute Care

■ Medical Management

Diagnosis is determined by a clinical history of contributing and causative factors, drug history, manifestations of fluid overload, and laboratory findings. The presence of pulmonary edema is a medical emergency requiring im-

mediate interventions to prevent further respiratory distress and death.

Pharmacologic Management

To improve myocardial function, diuretics and a digitalis preparation are frequently prescribed for the treatment of ECFVE. Many diuretics cause potassium and magnesium to be excreted along with the sodium and water. To preserve potassium, a combination of potassium-wasting and potassium-sparing diuretics may be prescribed.

In people with congestive heart failure (CHF), angiotensin-converting enzyme (ACE) inhibitors and low-dose beta-blockers are being prescribed to improve myocardial contractility by decreasing cardiac oxygen demand and increasing cardiac oxygen supply. Improved cardiac function has led to a decreased morbidity and mortality in ECFVE secondary to CHF. It is important to remember that since most ACE inhibitors have a potassium-sparing effect, potassium supplements are usually not necessary and may produce a risk of hyperkalemia when given with potassium-wasting diuretics.[80] Research has shown that in persons in whom myocardial function is improved with ACE inhibitors, inotropic agents, and low-dose beta-blockers, the use of diuretics (and the sometimes lethal electrolyte imbalances that result) can be avoided completely.[56]

Dietary Management

A low-sodium diet is often prescribed to reduce fluid retention. Box 15–3 lists high- and low-sodium foods.

■ Nursing Management of the Medical Client

Assessment

Monitor vital signs for a bounding pulse and/or elevated blood pressure every 4 to 8 hours. Assess the apical pulse if the radial pulse is irregular or if the client is taking cardiac medication. Assess breath sounds every 4 to 8 hours for crackles, rhonchi, or wheezes, noting changes in location or severity. Assess for changes in respiratory effort with activity or rest. Observe for changes in level of consciousness, which may indicate intracellular fluid shifting.

Each morning, palpate the sacrum and lower extremities for pitting edema and observe the client for hand and bilateral neck vein engorgement. Jugular vein distention at or above a 45 degree headrest is indicative of ECFVE. Also assess for weight gain. Edema does not usually occur until 3 L or more of excess fluid has accumulated. Hand veins that do not flatten within 3 to 5 seconds when the hand is raised above the heart level suggest fluid overload. Compare intake and output every 4 to 8 hours. Monitor plasma osmolality, sodium level, hematocrit, and urine specific gravity. If the client is taking diuretics and digitalis, monitor plasma electrolytes and anticipate digitalis toxic effects secondary to hypokalemia.

Diagnosis, Planning, Implementation

Fluid Volume Excess. The nursing diagnosis of choice for clients with overhydration is Fluid Volume Excess. State this diagnosis as *Fluid Volume Excess related to congestive heart failure, renal or liver failure, or hypervolemia.* Be certain to specify the cause in your client's case. If your client has congestive heart failure, also consider using the diagnosis of altered cardiac output.

Box 15–3. High- and Low-Sodium Foods

High-Sodium Foods (~250 mg per Serving)

Breads/cereals

Cold cereal, 1 oz
Corn chips, 14 chips
Instant hot cereal, ½ cup
Potato chips, 14 chips

Cheeses

Natural cheese, 1 oz
Processed cheese, 1 oz
Creamed cheese, ½ cup

Meats

Sausage, 1 oz
Luncheon meats, 1 oz
Frankfurters, 1 oz
Cooked bacon, 2 slices
Ham, 1 oz

Convenience foods

Pizza, 2 to 3 slices
Pot pies, 8 oz
Ravioli, canned, 8 oz
Soups (canned/dehydrated), 1 cup

Low-Sodium Foods (<50 mg per Serving)

Fruits/vegetables

Fresh or canned, ½ cup
Fresh, frozen, ½ cup

Breads/Cereals

Unsalted pastas, ½ cup
Oatmeal, cooked, 1 cup
Popcorn (unsalted), 1 oz
Puffed rice, 1 cup
Shredded wheat, 1 biscuit

Meats

Fresh meat, 1 oz
Fresh chicken, 1 oz
Fresh fish, 1 oz

Data from Laquarta, I., & Gerlach, M. (1990). *Nutrition in clinical nursing.* Albany, NY: Delmar; and Burtis, G., et al. (1988). *Applied nutrition and diet therapy.* Philadelphia; W. B. Saunders.

Planning: Expected Outcomes. The client's fluid balance will be improved, as evidenced by absence of dyspnea, clear chest sounds, absence of dependent edema, presence of flat neck veins in semi-Fowler's position, peripheral vein emptying in 3 to 5 seconds, decreased body weight, and urine output exceeding intake.

Implementation. In addition to assessment, numerous interventions are available that are related to ECFVE. Notify the physician if there is an increase in pulmonary crackles, rapid weight gain, significant change in vital signs, or change in level of consciousness. Report low levels of plasma electrolytes (especially potassium). If clinical manifestations of cardiac or cerebral dysfunction are present, elevate the headrest from 30 to 45 degrees to decrease venous return from the lower body to the heart, which will decrease cardiac workload. Elevating the headrest also promotes jugular venous return, which decreases cerebral edema. Cardiac and cerebral function are also indirectly enhanced by the improved oxygen intake secondary to the improved breathing. Breathing improves with headrest elevation due to better diaphragmatic movement secondary to gravity and the decrease in abdominal pressure against the diaphragm.

Instruct the client and family about the rationale for fluid and sodium restrictions. Include fluids on meal trays and those given with medications as part of the total fluid intake. Collaborate with the dietitian in planning fluid restrictions. Schedule oral medications at meal times, if possible, to limit fluid intake. Use minimal amounts of water (5–10 ml) to dissolve crushed medications that need to be given per feeding tube. Flushing the tube with cola may decrease the need for large amounts of water and keep the tube patent. Cold fluids have been found to decrease the sensation of thirst more than warm or hot fluids.[87] Give ice chips, if allowed, and provide frequent oral care to decrease the thirst sensation. Remember that 1 cup of ice equals ½ cup of water. Use IV pumps and/or minidrop tubing to control IV fluid intake.

When peripheral tissue perfusion is altered because of edema and/or vascular disease, provide frequent skin care and turn the client often, control moisture, and prevent friction and shear. Heels are especially at risk for decreased capillary blood flow. Therefore, it is important to keep the heels elevated off the mattress and to remove elastic stockings when redness is noted. See Chapter 78 for more information on special mattresses and pressure ulcer prevention and treatment.

Evaluation

The client's improvement should be assessed at the end of every shift. Revisions in the plan of care may be required. Some forms of fluid volume excess are chronic, and it is unrealistic to expect complete resolution of all clinical manifestations. For example, clients with congestive heart failure may continue to develop dependent edema despite administration of diuretics and fluid restrictions.

■ Modifications for Elderly Clients

The elderly client commonly develops ECFVE secondary to many chronic diseases, such as congestive heart failure. In general, the interventions are the same, except that the elderly client responds more slowly to and is at higher risk for side effects related to the prescribed therapy. Assess renal and liver function and the potential for drug-drug interactions[74] before any therapy is begun. Monitor closely for signs of digitalis toxic effects.

Community and Self-Care

For a client who is dismissed on a low-sodium diet, review the allowed and restricted foods with the client and, if appropriate, the person who prepares the client's meals. Canned foods should be avoided; fresh and frozen foods are permissible. Buying these items in season and freezing them for later use will save money and provide more nutrients. Encourage the food purchaser to read food labels and to avoid products with high levels of sodium or salt or to avoid food whose labels contain the word "sodium" or the symbol "Na" as a prefix. Ask if she or he drinks softened water, which is high in sodium. Water may need to be obtained from another source, or a water distiller may be needed. Suggest alternatives for seasoning to enhance taste of foods and increase dietary compliance. Adding fresh lemon to vegetables and main dishes, condiments that come in powder form (e.g., garlic), or other low-sodium seasonings that can be found at a local health food store have been found to increase satiety. Remember that people taking ACE inhibitors cannot use potassium salt substitutes.[80]

Extracellular Fluid Volume Shift: Third-Spacing

A fluid volume shift is basically a change in the location of extracellular fluid between the intravascular and the interstitial spaces. Fluid shifts are of two types: (1) vascular fluid shifts to interstitial spaces and (2) interstitial fluid shifts to vascular spaces. Fluid that shifts into the interstitial spaces and remains there is referred to as *third-space fluid*. This abnormal fluid accumulation is not only due to a pathologic condition, but it also reflects an inability of the lymphatic system to compensate. Common sites for third-spacing include the abdomen, pleural cavity, peritoneal cavity, and pericardial sac. Abdominal third-spacing is commonly called *ascites*. Third-space fluid is physiologically useless because it does *not* circulate to provide nutrients for cells.

Etiology and Risk Factors

Fluid shifting may be minimal, as is seen with a simple sprain or blister, or it may be much more serious, as is common after major surgery. Clinical causes of third-spacing are varied. Increased capillary permeability causes massive fluid shifts from the vascular to the interstitial spaces, as is seen in crushing injuries, major tissue trauma, major surgery, extensive burns, acid-base imbalance, and sepsis. Increased fluid pressures also cause third-spacing, as is seen in perforated peptic ulcers, intestinal obstruction, lymphatic obstruction, and large venous thrombosis. Inflammatory responses to infectious, noninfectious, and autoimmune disorders cause pleural and pericardial fluid shifts. Conditions that promote hypoalbuminemia increase the risk for fluid shifting. These conditions include those that are characterized by decreased protein intake, such as malnutrition or alcoholism; decreased protein intake is also seen in elderly clients. Hypoalbuminemia also occurs with increased protein loss, which occurs with kidney or liver disease or large draining wounds or burns. Protein anabolism and catabolism both increase the risk of hypoalbuminemia. Increased protein anabolism can occur in the healing phase of fractures or wounds; increased protein catabolism can occur with fever, infection or sepsis, and malignancy. GI tract malabsorption also contributes to third-spacing by decreasing vascular oncotic pressure.

Suggestions for primary, secondary, and tertiary prevention of third-spacing are presented in Risk Factors and Level of Prevention.

Pathophysiology

Tissue injury causes the release of histamine and bradykinin, which increase capillary permeability, allowing fluid, protein, and other solutes to move into the interstitial spaces. Two phases of fluid shift are associated with tissue injury. The first phase is the fluid shift from vascular to interstitial spaces, which leads to a fluid volume deficit (hypovolemia, see Fig. 15–5D). Severe hypovolemia may lead to vascular collapse and death. If cellular damage is severe, toxic response may occur from intracellular ions, such as potassium, which leak into the vascular spaces. The second phase is the shift back from the inter-

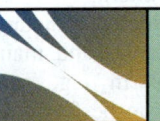

RISK FACTORS AND LEVELS OF PREVENTION

Third-Spacing

Risk Factors

Clients with liver or kidney disease, major trauma, burns, sepsis, wound healing or major surgery, malignancy, GI malabsorption, or malnutrition, or alcoholic or elderly clients.

Levels of Prevention

Primary Prevention

- Teach the importance of maintaining prescribed levels of protein as well as the importance of eating three well-balanced meals per day.
- Teach ways to decrease the cost of groceries and still provide protein needs (e.g., tofu instead of meat, cottage cheese, skim milk vs whole milk, eggs, combining incomplete protein sources, such as beans and rice, buying meat on sale and freezing it).
- Increase public awareness of homeless shelters that provide meals.
- Encourage the use of free dietary advice provided by many grocery stores.
- Refer alcoholics to support groups. Increase awareness of Meals-on-Wheels.

Secondary Prevention

- Monitor and compare daily weights.
- Anticipate side effects of medications.
- Monitor for lung congestion, fever, hypotension, tachycardia, and increased edema.
- Monitor intake and output of fluids and solids. Give high-carbohydrate diet to spare protein, vitamins, and minerals.
- Measure abdomen daily if ascites.
- Maintain universal precautions because less protein leads to decreased immunoglobulins.
- Prevent breakdown of edematous areas by turning, shifting weight, or using special mattresses.
- Maintain safety/seizure precautions, if cerebral signs are present.
- Consult physician for a dietary referral if the client's intake is inadequate to meet metabolic needs or if manifestations of protein deficit are seen.
- Report marked changes or lack of response to therapy.

Tertiary Prevention

- Assess vital signs if client is symptomatic. Consult physician if signs of infection or other marked changes are noted.
- Provide *balanced* nutrition via 3 to 6 small meals or food supplements.
- Use tube feedings as a last resort.
- Weigh weekly; report marked changes.
- Turn the client at least every 2 hours.
- Use special mattresses to prevent pressure.[43]
- Refer family to support groups.

stitial to the vascular space, which leads to a fluid volume excess (hypervolemia). If the hypervolemia is severe, it may lead to heart failure. Intracellular potassium ions shift back into the cell during this phase, which increases the risk for hypokalemia.

In burn trauma, for example, the fluid shifts out of the vessels into the injured tissue spaces as well as into normal unburned tissue. After 24 to 72 hours, the capillary permeability is restored, and fluid leaves the tissue spaces and returns to the vascular space. If renal function is inadequate, a fluid overload may result. If renal function is normal in the second phase, the urine output may be as high as 3000 ml/day. See Chapter 79 for further discussion of burns. The complex mechanism behind third-spacing with liver disease is discussed in Chapter 65.

Clinical Manifestations and Diagnostic Findings

Clinical manifestations of a fluid shift from the vascular to the interstitial spaces are similar to the manifestations of shock. Typical clinical manifestations include skin pallor, cold extremities, weak and rapid pulse, hypotension, oliguria, and decreased levels of consciousness. If the fluid collects and obstructs an organ, nerve, or vessel, other clinical manifestations may be noted. For example, bowel sounds may change in character throughout the abdomen. Extremities may become pale, cool, and pulseless. Laboratory results may indicate an elevated hematocrit and an elevated BUN level.

When the fluid returns to the blood vessels, the clinical manifestations are similar to those of fluid overload. Signs may include a bounding pulse, crackles, engorgement of peripheral and jugular veins, and an increase in blood pressure. Laboratory results may indicate a decrease in hematocrit and BUN level. Other abnormal findings depend on the area of the body affected.

Acute and Subacute Care

■ Medical Management

Medical treatment begins with the determination of the cause of the fluid volume shift. When hypovolemia results from tissue injury, such as burns or crush injuries, a large volume of isosmolar IV fluid administration is required. Albumin may be given if protein deficit is present. Because third-spacing is a common occurrence after major surgery, maintaining IV fluid intake is essential to maintaining kidney perfusion. The amount of fluid infusion may be three times greater than the urinary output. Generally, fluids are titrated for maintenance of an adequate blood pressure, pulmonary capillary wedge pressure or pulmonary artery wedge pressure (see Chapter 45), and urinary output. However, if replacement is too aggressive, a fluid overload can occur, due in part to the increase in antidiuretic hormone.

When the capillary regains integrity, fluid shifts from the tissue spaces back into the vessels. Therefore, if fluid replacement is too aggressive, a fluid overload can also occur in this phase.

■ Nursing Management of the Medical Client

If shock-like symptoms are present, assess vital signs every hour for at least 8 hours. If fluid loss is a result of ascites or peripheral edema, the fluid shift is slower, and changes in the vital signs are usually subtle.

Monitor IV fluid replacement needs. If fluids are administered too rapidly, fluid overload or hypervolemia may occur. Assess for and report pulmonary crackles, difficulty in breathing, and neck vein engorgement. As the fluid shifts back with the repair of tissue damage, IV fluid replacement volume is decreased.

In clients with ascites, measure the abdominal girth every 8 hours. If the extremities are involved, measure the circumference of the extremity and peripheral pulses every 8 hours. If the level of consciousness has changed, provide seizure precautions. Employ preventive measures to prevent skin breakdown of edematous areas.

Monitor urine output every hour and report an output of less than 30 ml/hr if it persists for more than 2 hours. Urine output is usually reduced after tissue injury because of decreased renal circulation and fluid shift into the injured tissue spaces. One to 3 days after tissue injury, fluid returns to the circulation and excess fluid is excreted by the kidneys unless renal function is impaired. Monitor plasma levels of BUN and creatinine.

■ Surgical Management

If the third-spacing of fluid has occurred as a result of pericarditis, pericardiocentesis may have to be done to preserve organ function. If third-spacing is due to a bowel obstruction, paracentesis is the procedure of choice. See Chapters 47 or 64 for nursing care of a client having either of these surgeries.

Intracellular Fluid Volume Excess: Water Intoxication

Although the cells are usually quite resistant to fluid shifts, certain conditions can lead to this imbalance. Hyposmolar disorders result from either water excess or solute deficit and are primarily due to sodium loss. In water excess, the number of solutes is normal, but they are diluted by excessive water. In solute deficit, the amount of water is normal, but there are too few particles per liter of water. In both cases, hyposmolality of vascular fluids exists and cellular swelling occurs.

Although intracellular fluid volume excess (ICFVE) is not as common a type of fluid imbalance as ECFVD and ECFVE, it presents a serious health problem if it is unrecognized and untreated. The most common cause of ICFVE is the administration of excessive amounts of hyposmolar IV fluids, such as 0.45% saline or 5% dextrose in water (D_5W). ICFVE may occur in clients who receive continuous D_5W IV fluid or in those who are elderly and consume excessive amounts of tap water without adequate nutrient intake. SIADH also leads to ICFVE, regardless of whether the SIADH is caused by CNS trauma, stress of surgery, pain, or narcotic use. People suffering from certain psychiatric disorders, such as schizophrenia, often have compulsive water consumption behaviors. Studies have found that as many as 80% of people admitted to a hospital with a diagnosis of schizophrenia suffer water intoxication. Nurses must monitor for compulsive water consumption in persons with a history or current manifestations of an organic psychiatric illness.[15, 17, 91, 103]

Hyposmolar fluids in the vessels move by osmosis to the region of higher concentration in the cells in an attempt to maintain equilibrium. Unfortunately, too much fluid accumulates in the cells, causing cellular edema. The brain cells are usually involved first, resulting in cerebral edema.

Early and common neurologic manifestations of ICFVE include headaches, behavioral changes, apprehension, irritability, disorientation, and confusion. Later signs of increased intracranial pressure include pupillary changes and decreased motor and sensory function. Vital sign changes signify late stages of increased intracranial pressure. These include bradycardia, elevated blood pressure, widened pulse pressure, and altered respiratory patterns.[75]

The urine output may be normal or decreased with water intoxication. Table 15–3 lists the clinical manifestations and laboratory/diagnostic findings associated with ICFVE.

The nurse should anticipate water intoxication in clients who have received excessive amounts of D_5W or tap water or who have had a recent operation, experienced pain or stress, undergone CNS trauma or other trauma, or who are taking depressant drugs.

Early administration of IV fluids containing some sodium chloride can prevent SIADH. Saline solutions, such as $D_5/0.45\%$ NaCl, increase the osmolality of vascular fluid and prevent or help correct hyposmolality. Also, give oral fluids, such as juices or soft drinks, hourly.[94]

Perform neurologic checks including level of consciousness (LOC), vital signs, reflexes, and pupillary responses every hour if cranial changes are present. Cerebral perfusion is altered if the systolic blood pressure drops too low or rises too high. Notify the physician if the client's sensorium changes from baseline assessment, if systolic blood pressure is less than 100 mm Hg or greater than 150 mm Hg, or if other signs persist or worsen.

Monitor IV fluids, fluid intake, and fluid output hourly, and monitor weight daily. Polyuria is a good sign and indicates that fluid has shifted to the vascular space and to the renal tubules, where it can be excreted. Administer antiemetics prophylactically as appropriate to promote food and fluid ingestion and retention.

Provide safety measures when the client displays behavioral changes, such as confusion or disorientation. Keep the bed in a low position with bedside rails raised. Keep suction equipment at the bedside in the event of seizures. If a client has a seizure, turn him or her to one

Table 15–3. Clinical Manifestations and Laboratory/Diagnostic Findings: Intracellular Fluid Volume Excess

Clinical Manifestation	Pathophysiologic Basis
Headaches, nausea, vomiting	CNS changes due to ICFVE cause increased intracranial pressure; cerebral cells absorb hyposmolar fluid more quickly than other cells do
Pupillary changes	Pressure on the second and third cranial nerves from increased cranial pressure
Behavioral changes: progressive apprehension, irritability, disorientation, confusion, drowsiness, decreased coordination	Swollen cerebral cells cause behavioral changes
Decreased muscle strength, unequal grasp, pronation drift	Frontal lobe swelling; if decreased coordination, cerebellar or basal ganglia swelling
Weight gain	Increased weight results from excess water retention
Severe CNS manifestations	Severe CNS changes occur when water excess progressively increases intracranial pressure, interferes with cell function
Vital signs: bradycardia with an increased systolic blood pressure (widened pulse pressure); altered respiratory patterns; neuroexcitability (muscle twitching); Babinski's response; decorticate-decerebrate posturing; flaccidity; projectile vomiting; papilledema; delirium; convulsions, coma	Vital sign changes are an *ominous* indicator of increased intracranial pressure and herniation of the brain stem (*late signs*)
Laboratory/Diagnostic Findings	
Serum sodium level <125 mEq/L	Low serum sodium level associated with hemodilution
Decreased hematocrit	Hemodilution; ECF excess often accompanies ICF excess

side to displace the tongue. Remain at the bedside until the client is safe and document all phases of the seizure. See Chapter 33 for care of the client during a seizure.

Intracellular Fluid Volume Deficit

Hypernatremia and dehydration can become so severe that the cells become dehydrated. This condition is relatively rare in the healthy adult, but it occurs quite often in the elderly client and in those with conditions that result in acute water loss. Symptoms include thirst, fever, oliguria, and CNS changes, such as confusion, coma, and cerebral hemorrhage.[84]

Electrolytes

Electrolytes are substances found in extracellular and intracellular fluid that dissociate into electrically charged particles known as *ions*. *Cations* are ions that carry a positive charge, and *anions* are ions that carry a negative charge. Sodium, potassium, calcium, magnesium, and hydrogen are the major cations, and chloride, phosphate, bicarbonate, and protein are the major anions that have been identified in the body. The electrolytes that are most plentiful inside the cells are potassium, magnesium, phosphate, and protein. The most plentiful ions in the ECF are sodium, calcium, chloride, and bicarbonate. The principal cation in the ICF is potassium and the principal cation in the ECF is sodium (Table 15–4). See Chapter 16 for the discussion of hydrogen and bicarbonate.

Electrolytes have major influences on the following:

1. Body water regulation and osmolality
2. Acid-base regulation
3. Enzyme reactions
4. Neuromuscular activity

Although all electrolytes affect osmolality, the sodium concentration in the extracellular fluid has a major effect on fluid balance due to its abundance. Sodium, potassium, chloride, hydrogen, bicarbonate, phosphate, and protein ions all play a role in acid-base balance within the body. See Chapter 16 for an in-depth discussion of acid-base homeostasis. Transmission of nerve impulses and stimulation of muscle activity would not be possible without the continual fluctuation of the anions and cations.[54] The concentration of electrolytes in various body fluids is shown in Table 15–5 and Figure 15–6.

Action Potentials

To understand the significance of the role of electrolytes in cell function, an understanding of the action potential system is necessary. All living cells in the body are electrically polarized, which means a difference exists in the electrical charge across the cell membrane. This potential difference in the electrical charge is known as the *resting membrane potential;* it is due to differences in the ion

Table 15–4. Distribution of Electrolytes in Body Compartments

Electrolyte	Extracellular Fluid (mEq/L)	Intracellular Fluid (mEq/L)
Cations		
Sodium	142	10
Potassium	5	156
Calcium	5	4
Magnesium	2	26
Total	154	196
Anions		
Bicarbonate	24	12
Chloride	104	4
Phosphate	2	40–95
Proteins	16	54
Other anions	8	31–86
Total	154	196*

From McCance, K., & Huether, S. (1994). *Pathophysiology. The biologic basis for disease in adults and children* (2nd ed.). St. Louis: Mosby–Year Book.
*Average value

composition between the ECF and ICF compartments. It is the high concentration of sodium cations on the outside of the membrane compared to a decrease in potassium cations and an increase in cations on the inside of the membrane that results in a negative resting membrane potential. A negative resting membrane is essential for cells to respond to electrochemical stimuli. For example, when a nerve or muscle cell receives a stimulus at a set level (threshold potential), a rapid change in the membrane potential occurs. This is known as the *action potential.* Figure 15–7 illustrates five phases of the action potential in a myocardial cell. First, a stimulus causes the membrane to become more permeable to sodium. As sodium moves across the membrane and the action potential is propagated along the entire length of the cell, the membrane potential becomes less negative. The steep upstroke of the action potential (phase 0) correlates with the opening of the fast sodium channels. A state of zero membrane potential is finally reached. This process is known as *depolarization.*[6]

As the membrane becomes less permeable to sodium, sodium channels begin to close. At the same time, the membrane becomes more permeable to potassium and potassium channels begin to open. The movement of potassium out of the cell causes the membrane potential to become more negative again. Slight repolarization occurs due to the closure of the fast sodium channels and the opening of the potassium channels (phase 1). This is followed by the plateau phase (phase 2), in which calcium channels open and close slowly, allowing a slow influx of calcium, which is offset by an efflux of potas-

Table 15–5. Concentration of Electrolytes in Various Body Fluids (in mEq/L)*					
Fluid	**Na⁺**	**K⁺**	**Cl⁻**	**HCO₃⁻**	**H⁺**
Plasma	135–145	3.5–5.0	98–106	25–29	7.35–7.45
Gastric juices	55–100	10–15	120	5–10	90
Pancreatic juices	145–160	5	65–90	50–80	—
Bile	130–145	5–9	75–100	10–45	—
Ileum	125	10–80	55	60	—
Sweat					
Insensible	8	10	15	—	—
Sensible	10–80	6	5–85	—	—

Na⁺, sodium; K⁺, potassium; Cl⁻, chloride; HCO₃⁻, bicarbonate; H⁺, hydrogen.
*Levels may vary depending on the physiologic state of the body.
From White, B. (1994). Maintaining fluid and electrolyte balance. In Bolander, V. B. (Ed.). *Sorenson and Luckmann's basic nursing: A psychophysiologic approach* (3rd ed.). Philadelphia: W. B. Saunders.

sium. Thus, little change in the membrane potential occurs. During phase 3, rapid repolarization occurs due to the closure of the slow calcium channels and continued potassium efflux. The active transport mechanism of the sodium-potassium pump continues to promote the rapid return of the membrane to its resting potential state (phase 4). The process of returning sodium ions to the outside of the cell and potassium ions back into the cell, to a resting potential, by the sodium-potassium pump is known as *repolarization*.[6]

A change in this fragile electrolyte balance can alter cell function dramatically. When the membrane potential is more negative than normal, the threshold rises. Thus, the cell is less excitable, or *hyperpolarized*, and requires a stronger than normal stimulus to reach threshold potential

and to generate an action potential. The opposite can also be true. When the membrane potential is more positive than normal, the threshold decreases and the cell is more excitable than normal, or *hypopolarized*, and responds to a weaker stimulus. See Figure 15–8 for an example of how low and high potassium levels affect the membrane potential.

Measuring Electrolytes

Because intracellular levels of electrolytes cannot be measured clinically, all values for electrolytes are reflected in plasma values. Plasma values for electrolytes can be expressed as milliequivalents per liter (mEq/L) or milli-

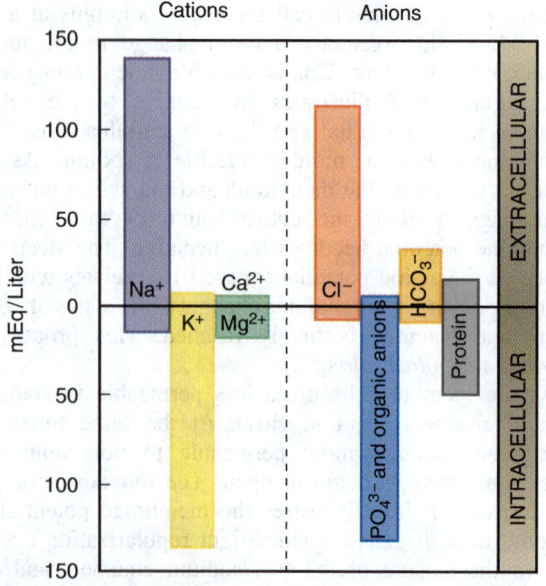

Figure 15–6. A comparison of electrolyte composition of the extracellular and intracellular fluid compartments. (From Guyton, A. C., & Hall, J. E. [1996]. *Textbook of medical physiology* [9th ed.] [p. 300]. Philadelphia, W. B. Saunders.)

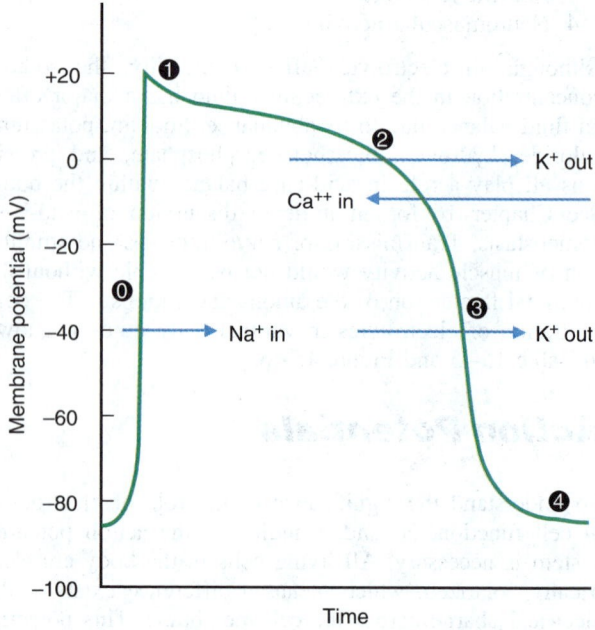

Figure 15–7. The five phases of the action potential in a myocardial cell.

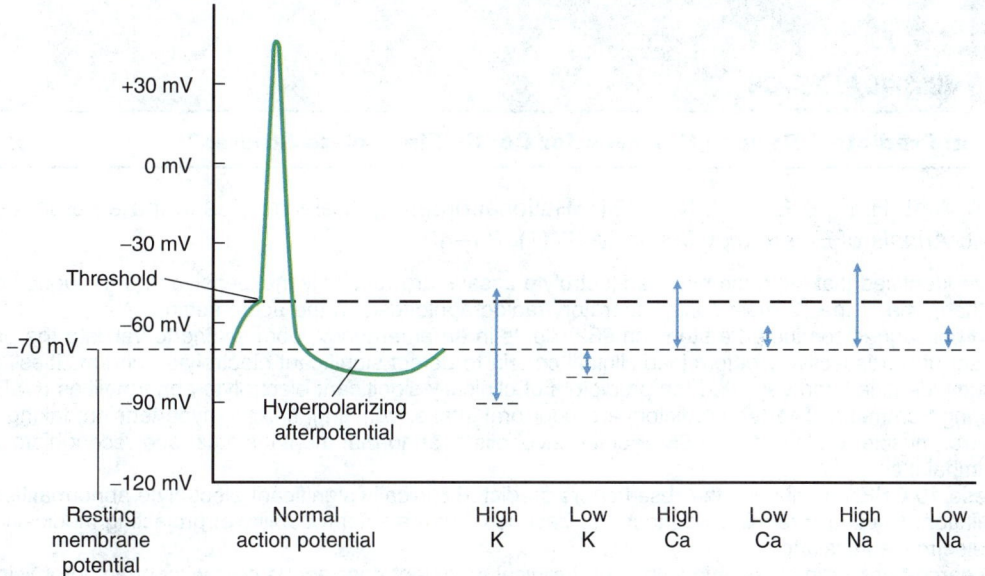

Figure 15–8. Effects of electrolyte imbalances on the membrane potential. Conductile tissue rests at negative millivolts, called a *resting membrane potential.* When the nerve is stimulated, ion channels for sodium, potassium, and calcium open to change the firing potential. Potassium tends to lower the potential by decreasing the millivolts to more negative levels. Sodium does the opposite: it raises the action potential to more positive values (above zero). Calcium also raises the resting membrane potential to a more positive value. The closer the resting membrane potential to threshold, the more rapid the nerve firing.

grams per deciliter (mg/dl). Both values are given in this text. Values reported as milliequivalents per liter can be converted to milligrams per deciliter by multiplying by 1.2.

Using Collaborative Problems

Currently, no NANDA diagnoses exist for electrolyte imbalances. The Iowa Interventions Project approached this problem from its collaborative foundation and developed a research-based list of critical and supporting activities for 15 fluid and electrolyte disorders. Because the nursing role primarily involves collaborating with the physician, the goal statements are also phrased differently. The reader will note that each expected outcome is preceded by the phrase: "The nurse will monitor the client for . . . ."[16] Nursing diagnoses that might apply to clients with electrolyte imbalances include *Risk for Injury, Risk for Activity Intolerance, Risk for Decreased Cardiac Output,* and *Risk for Impaired Skin Integrity.*

Besides identifying nursing interventions for electrolyte abnormalities, research has also identified risk factors to assist in predicting clinically significant electrolyte abnormalities as well as in promoting cost-effective care, as shown in Nursing Research.[61, 69] The rest of this chapter provides information about electrolytes that are monitored in current practice.

Electrolyte Imbalances

Sodium Imbalances

A sodium imbalance occurs when sodium concentration in plasma either decreases or increases. A sodium deficit

is known as *hyponatremia.* A sodium excess is known as *hypernatremia.*

Chloride is the anion that usually accompanies sodium imbalances; therefore, levels of chloride fall or rise along with levels of sodium. The manifestations of chloride imbalances are usually associated with the cation imbalance. Box 15–4 provides the normal plasma ranges for electrolytes, including sodium and chloride.

Sodium balance is regulated by the interaction between neural, hormonal, and vascular mechanisms. Sensing mechanisms in nerve endings in the atria, aorta, carotid sinus, liver, pulmonary tissue, and juxtaglomerular apparatus (JGA) in the kidneys detect changes in sodium intake and extracellular fluid volume by sensing an increase or decrease in pressure. CNS receptors also respond to changes in the sodium concentration in the cerebrospinal fluid (CSF). One example of a neural-hormonal interaction is the JGA sensory mechanism, which promotes a stimulation response of the renin-angiotensin-aldosterone hormonal system. Renin, excreted in response to hypotension, results in increased aldosterone secretion, which stimulates sodium reabsorption across the renal tubule. Other hormonal factors, including prostaglandins, kallikrein, and atrial natriuretic peptide, also control sodium homeostasis. Prostaglandins secreted by the kidney stimulate the production of renin. These hormones also maintain renal blood flow during periods of reduced blood volume. Kallikreins are high-molecular-weight proteins produced by the distal convoluted tubule that secrete kinin. Kinin is a potent renal vasodilator that increases renal excretion of sodium. Atrial natriuretic peptide (ANP) balances the effects of ADH by promoting sodium excretion (natriuresis), vasodilatation, and increased urinary output.[1, 35] See the section Nervous System for a review of the role of the baroreceptors.

The glomerular capillary filtration rate is an example of

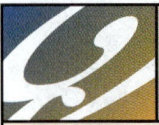

NURSING RESEARCH

Can Clinical Predictors Reduce the Need for Costly Electrolyte Studies?

Lowe, R. A, Arst, H. F., & Ellis, B. K. (1991). Rational ordering of electrolytes in the emergency department. *Annals of Emergency Medicine, 20*(1), 35–40.

Studies have identified that although plasma electrolyte assays are relatively inexpensive, the frequency of testing has made them one of the 12 most costly laboratory/radiographic tests in the acute setting.

   Lowe and colleagues conducted a study on 982 clients in an emergency room setting to validate the predictive ability of a set of retrospectively determined clinical criteria to detect significant electrolyte abnormalities. The previous study identified and validated ten predictors of clinically significant electrolyte abnormalities (CSEA) (i.e., those requiring treatment). The ten predictors are poor oral intake, vomiting, chronic hypertension, taking diuretics, recent seizure, muscle weakness, age 65 or older, alcoholism, abnormal mental status, and recent history of electrolyte imbalance.

   Using these 10 CSEA predictors, the researchers predicted clinically significant electrolyte abnormalities in 94% of the population. Routine screening was found to have less than a 2% probability of projecting medically significant electrolyte imbalances.

   Using research-based clinical criteria with sound clinical judgment can reduce cost without compromising client outcomes. Although the CSEA predictors had a 94% sensitivity, the researchers emphasized the importance of using the CSEA predictors with skilled clinical judgment. Nurses should have a high level of suspicion for electrolyte imbalance in clients presenting with any of the ten clinically significant risk factors. The physician should be consulted if the client presents with any manifestations of electrolyte imbalance.

how vascular dynamics influence sodium homeostasis. The glomerulus filters 1000 mEq of sodium every hour, and about 99% of this is reabsorbed. This process is greatly influenced by the pressure of the blood entering the glomeruli. Blood pressure promotes filtration, which promotes capillary oncotic pressure due to protein in the blood after the initial fluid movement promotes reabsorption.

Hyponatremia

Hyponatremia is defined as a plasma sodium level below 135 mEq/L. It is one of the most common electrolyte disorders in adults, especially the elderly.[75, 101] Hyponatremia is usually associated with fluid volume status. The four types of hyponatremic states include the following:

1. Hypovolemic hyponatremia
2. Euvolemic hyponatremia
3. Hypervolemic hyponatremia
4. Redistributive hyponatremia[75]

When sodium loss is greater than water loss, hypovolemic hyponatremia occurs. Euvolemic hyponatremia results when the total body water (TBW) is moderately increased and the total body sodium remains at a normal level. Hypervolemic hyponatremia results when a greater increase occurs in TBW than in total body sodium. In redistributive hyponatremia, no change occurs in TBW or total body sodium; water merely shifts between the intracellular and extracellular compartments relative to the sodium concentration. Table 15–6 shows the relationship of total body water to body sodium in various types of hyponatremia.

Etiology and Risk Factors

Hyponatremia can result from numerous causes. Hyponatremia secondary to SIADH may follow many forms of drug therapy, including oral hypoglycemics, cancer chemotherapy, phenothiazines, opiates, barbiturates, and spinal or general anesthetics.[49]

Hyponatremia may result from the kidney's inability to excrete sufficiently dilute urine.[85, 97] Normally, when hyponatremia and hyposmolality occur, diuresis follows to promote sodium and water balance. Table 15–7 lists clinical conditions and disorders that may cause hyponatremia.

Risk factors leading to hyponatremia are more prominent in the elderly,[85] infants, and small children, because of the variations in total body water. Conditions such as vomiting, diarrhea, wounds, fistulas, GI suction, hyperglycemia, cardiac disease,[60] renal disease, and Addison's disease increase the risk of hyponatremia. Clients who are in

---

Box 15–4. Plasma Ranges for Electrolytes*

Sodium: 135–145 mEq/L
Chloride: 98–106 mEq/L
Potassium: 3.5–5.0 mEq/L
Calcium: 4.5–5.5 mEq/L
Ionized calcium: 1.18–1.30 mEq/L
Phosphorus: 1.2–3.0 mEq/L
Magnesium: 1.5–2.5 mEq/L

---

*Ranges may vary somewhat between laboratories.

Table 15-6. Relationship of Total Body Water to Body Sodium in Various Types of Hyponatremia (Serum Sodium < 135 mEq/L)		
Etiology	**Total Body Water**	**Body Sodium**
Hypovolemic hyponatremia	↓	↓↓
Euvolemic hyponatremia	↑	Normal
Hypervolemic hyponatremia	↑↑	↑ or normal
Redistributive hyponatremia	Normal	Normal

a postoperative phase,[40] those who are NPO and receiving IV solutions, and those who are receiving potent diuretics without sodium replacement are also at risk.[71, 105] Many persons with chronic psychosis suffer from dilutional hyponatremia secondary to compulsive water intake.[114]

Hyponatremia can also occur in persons who are considered healthy. For example, athletes[67, 87] and outdoor laborers are at risk for hyponatremia due to excessive perspiration. Any person with an altered thirst mechanism, an inability to access fluids, or who attempts to rehydrate too rapidly after excessive fluid loss is at risk for hyponatremia. Persons with high-volume-output ileostomies can also experience hyponatremia.

Suggestions for primary, secondary, and tertiary prevention of hyponatremia are presented in Risk Factors and Level of Prevention.

Pathophysiology

Recall that the majority of sodium is outside of the cell. As the ECF concentration of sodium decreases, the sodium concentration difference in gradient between the ECF and ICF also decreases. Water concentration is also changed when sodium content changes. When the extracellular sodium level falls, the ECF becomes hyposmolar. Water moves into the cell to the area of greater concentration to rebalance the water concentration. This osmotic shift can lead to intracellular edema. These changes also mean that less sodium is available to move across the excitable membrane, which usually results in a delayed membrane depolarization. Excitable tissues vary in their response to decreased sodium. The cells most sensitive to change are the CNS cells. An increase in brain cell volume as small as 5% can cause brain herniation.[95] The brain cells attempt to compensate by reducing cerebral blood flow, shifting CSF, and decreasing the brain's intracellular osmolality. Intracellular osmolality is reduced through decreasing the amount of intracellular ions, such as sodium, potassium, and amino acids.[75, 95] Clinical manifestations develop due to a failure of these compensatory mechanisms to overcome the increasing edema; this results in increased intracranial pressure. The decreased excitability of the membranes from hyponatremia is also responsible for many of the clinical manifestations. The total body sodium and the ECF volume measures are used to categorize the hyponatremic state.

If the hyponatremic state and body fluid volume disorders are not corrected, potassium, calcium, chloride, and bicarbonate electrolyte imbalances may occur. Uncorrected hypovolemic hyponatremia may result in shock from continued ECF volume loss. This severe hyponatremic state leads to neurologic changes varying from confusion to convulsion and coma.[75, 95] A hypervolemic hyponatremic state, if not corrected, results in ECFVE.

Table 15-7. Clinical Conditions and Disorders That May Cause Hyponatremia	
Type of Hyponatremia	**Clinical Conditions and Disorders**
Hypovolemic hyponatremia	Renal loss of sodium from diuretic use, diabetic glycosuria, aldosterone deficiency, intrinsic renal disease Extrarenal loss of sodium from vomiting, diarrhea, increased sweating, burns, high-volume ileostomy
Euvolemic hyponatremia	Sodium deficit resulting from syndrome of inappropriate secretion of antidiuretic hormone (SIADH) or the continuous secretion of ADH due to pain, emotion, medications, many cancers, CNS disorders
Hypervolemic hyponatremia	Edematous disorders resulting in sodium deficits: congestive heart failure, cirrhosis of the liver, nephrotic syndrome, acute and chronic renal failure
Redistributive hyponatremia	Pseudohyponatremia, hyperglycemia, hyperlipidemia

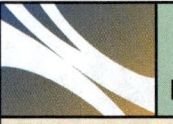

RISK FACTORS AND LEVELS OF PREVENTION

Hyponatremia

Risk Factors

Clients with conditions of increased loss: vomiting, diarrhea, severe diaphoresis (as with fever), GI or wound drainage, bulimia nervosa,[81] high-output ileostomy, Addison's disease, or chronic renal disease, clients taking diuretics, or diuretics plus a low-sodium diet.

Clients with decreased intake: NPO, NPO with dextrose IVs, or those with anorexia nervosa[81] and the elderly.

Clients with excess fluid retention: SIADH, excess tap water enemas.

Levels of Prevention

Primary Prevention

- Teach the client the importance of taking 30 to 60 ml of clear liquids or more per hour as tolerated. If client is on a low-sodium diet, do *not* be concerned about sodium restriction until the vomiting and/or diarrhea subside and the client is taking whole foods.
- Teach the client to consult the physician if vomiting and/or diarrhea persist for more than 48 hours, or sooner if extreme weakness, dizziness, palpitations, new onset of an irregular pulse, cough or dyspnea, or CNS changes, such as headache, confusion, or seizures, develop. Also consult physician if symptoms persist for more than 24 hours when the client has a chronic disease such as renal, liver, or heart disease or diabetes mellitus.
- Teach people to consult with the physician before taking over-the-counter medications.
- Review exercise precautions as listed in Risk Factors and Levels of Prevention for ECFVD.
- Refer persons with eating disorders to counseling and community support groups.

Secondary Prevention

- Monitor closely for manifestations of hyponatremia.
- Monitor intake and output and peripheral vein filling every 8 hours.
- Weigh daily.
- Irrigate nasogastric tubes and wounds only with isotonic saline.
- Give only *minimal* ice chips as ordered if a nasogastric tube is connected to suction.
- Consult with the dietitian to restrict total intake if the hyponatremia is due to hypervolemia.
- Give no more than 3 tap water enemas in a row without consulting the physician.
- Give antiemetics prophylactically with antineoplastics that have a high risk for producing vomiting.
- Monitor plasma electrolytes. Call the physician if sodium level is less than 125 mEq/L or sooner if client is symptomatic.
- Consult physician about IVs with electrolytes if the client is NPO or has an increased loss of electrolytes.
- Notify the physician of change in the level of consciousness; provide safety precautions.

Tertiary Prevention

- Monitor for manifestations of hyponatremia.
- Offer snacks between meals.
- Try clear liquids hourly if vomiting persists.
- Encourage the family to assist in feeding.
- Report vomiting and/or diarrhea that persists longer than 24 hours.
- Consult the physician for supplements if the client's intake is consistently less than half of meals.

Clinical Manifestations and Diagnostic Findings

Clinical manifestations of hyponatremia vary with the cause, type, and rate of fluid imbalance. A person may have a plasma sodium of 120 mEq/L that developed slowly and be asymptomatic. Another client with the same plasma sodium from an acute loss may have life-threatening clinical manifestations.[21] A sodium deficit may occur in the presence of decreased, normal, or increased total body sodium and water. An assessment of the body fluid volume is helpful in the determination of

treatment. With cardiac, renal, and liver disease, the total body sodium is usually high, although the plasma sodium level may appear normal or low due to dilution from water retention. In such instances, the increase in TBW is generally greater than the sodium indicates.[33]

A plasma sodium level of less than 115 mEq/L causes severe neurologic changes, such as confusion and behavioral changes, which lead to convulsions and death due to excessive water shift to the intracellular compartment, increased intracranial pressure, and brain herniation.[101] When the plasma sodium is greater than 125 mEq/L, signs and symptoms may not be apparent.[21, 101]

With a loss of body fluids and sodium, the heart rate

Table 15–8. Clinical Manifestations and Laboratory/Diagnostic Findings: Hyponatremia	
Clinical Manifestation	**Pathophysiologic Basis**
Gastrointestinal Manifestations	
Nausea, vomiting, diarrhea, hyperactive bowel sounds, abdominal cramps	Sodium is abundant in the gastrointestinal tract Altered neuromuscular irritability
Cardiovascular Manifestations	
Decrease in diastolic blood pressure, orthostatic hypotension, weak, thready pulse, tachycardia	Losses of sodium and water decrease circulating fluid volume, may result in shocklike symptoms, tachycardia compensatory response
Elevated blood pressure; full, rapid pulse	Dilutional hyponatremia with excessive fluid volume increases circulating fluids
Pulmonary Manifestations	
Changes in rate or rhythm of respirations	Changes in CNS, pulmonary overload
Adventitious lung sounds	Fluid overload, left ventricular failure
Neurologic Manifestations	
Headache, apprehension, lethargy, confusion, slowed problem solving, flat affect, diminished muscle tone in the extremities, decreased deep tendon reflexes, weakness and tremor, convulsions	Diluted body fluids move into the brain cells, affecting both cognition and reflexes; excitable membranes are less responsive to stimuli
Integumentary Manifestations	
Dry skin; dry tongue and mucous membranes	Decreased interstitial fluids
Laboratory/Diagnostic Findings	
Serum sodium <135 mEq/L Serum chloride <98 mEq/L	Symptoms become apparent when the serum sodium is <125 mEq/L, chloride main anion associated with Na
Urine sodium <40 mEq/L	Body sodium losses result in compensatory decrease in urinary excretion of sodium
Serum osmolality <275 mOsm/kg	Decreased concentration of sodium in body fluids

increases as a compensatory mechanism to overcome fluid and sodium losses. Clinical manifestations and diagnostic findings[46] and their pathologic bases are presented in Table 15–8.

Acute and Subacute Care

■ Medical Management

Medical management begins by attempting to determine the cause of the hyponatremia and correcting it. The goal of treatment is to correct the body water osmolality and, therefore, to restore cell volume by raising the ratio of sodium to water in the ECF. The increased ECF osmolality draws water from the cells and, therefore, decreases cellular edema. If the client has hyponatremia due to fluid volume excess, fluids will be restricted to allow the sodium to regain balance. If the plasma sodium level declines below 125 mEq/L, sodium replacement is needed.

Intravenous Therapy

With moderate hyponatremia, 125 mEq/L, IV normal saline solution (0.9% NaCl) or lactated Ringer's solution may be ordered if the client is symptomatic. When the plasma sodium level is 115 mEq/L or less, a concentrated saline solution such as 3% NaCl may be indicated until the plasma sodium reaches 125 mEq/L. A diuretic such as furosemide (Lasix) is often given intravenously to prevent fluid overload.[21, 94, 106]

Rapid elevation of plasma sodium concentrations to levels greater than 125 mEq/L increases intravascular fluid volume levels and may result in hypernatremia and CNS damage (demyelination). Other complications include pulmonary edema, pleural effusion, or cardiac tamponade. Recommendations for replacement include increasing plasma sodium 0.5 mEq/L/hr if the loss is chronic, not to exceed 12 mEq in 48 hours; and 1.0 mEq/L/hr if the loss is acute, not to exceed 25 mEq in 48 hours.[11, 110, 119] To prevent fluid shifts and exacerbation of vasospasm in persons with subarachnoid hemorrhage, normal saline is usually the IV solution of choice.[21, 75, 114]

Normal saline is the preferred treatment for hyponatremia unless the cause is SIADH. Demeclocycline (tetracycline), an agent that antagonizes ADH, is the preferred treatment for SIADH.

Dietary Management

A balanced diet is usually adequate therapy for mild hyponatremia (126 to 135 mEq/L). Foods high in sodium are listed in Box 15–3. If the client has hyponatremia due to excess fluids, a fluid-restricted diet may be prescribed. Fluids may be restricted to a range of 1000 to 1500 ml/day.[25]

■ Nursing Management of the Medical Client

Assessment

Nursing assessment focuses on data collection related to history of risk factors and manifestations in the client. Special emphasis should be placed on diet and medication history, including over-the-counter medications. The elderly are especially prone to drug-drug interactions that may alter sodium balance. The client and family should be asked about behavioral changes, headaches, increased weakness or sleepiness, dizziness, and palpitations.

Calculate ideal body weight by using height and weight and body frame and compare trends. Assess intake and output, peripheral vein filling time, and vital signs every 4 to 8 hours. Also, monitor plasma sodium levels and estimate the plasma osmolality. It is important to remember that in hyponatremic conditions, such as hypervolemic hyponatremia, plasma sodium levels may appear to be normal to low. Observe for signs of hypernatremia and pulmonary congestion (crackles) when IV 3% saline is being given.

Diagnosis, Planning, Implementation

Hyponatremia. The collaborative problem is stated as Hyponatremia. It may be related to vomiting, diarrhea, gastric suctioning, burns, SIADH, surgery, or fluid overload. You will need to specify the cause.

Planning: Expected Outcomes. The nurse will monitor the client for sodium levels to return to 135 mEq/L or above, reduction of factors contributing to the hyponatremia, fluid and electrolyte losses and replacement, and clinical manifestations of fluid and sodium imbalance.

Implementation. In addition to assessment, numerous interventions related to hyponatremia are available. For plasma sodium levels greater than 125 mEq/L, encourage the intake of a well-rounded diet. If the client is receiving nutrition only through tube feedings, it is sometimes necessary to add extra salt to the feeding to achieve the desired sodium level.[99] If the hyponatremia is secondary to hypervolemia, consult with the physician and dietitian to coordinate therapeutic fluid restriction. Strict behavioral modification or a psychiatric consultation may be necessary for a client with compulsive water drinking behavior. Offer ice chips and cold fluids, which increase satiety, to decrease thirst. However, if a person is suffering from a subarachnoid hemorrhage, it is not recommended to restrict fluids; restricting fluids in this situation may cause cerebral vasospasm and cell death.[21]

A plasma sodium level of less than 125 mEq/L indicates the need for prompt medical care if the client is symptomatic. *Caution:* Hypertonic saline must be given very slowly by IV piggyback infusion. Monitor the client *continuously* for signs of complications. Give the hypertonic saline in large veins to decrease the risk of phlebitis. Initiate safety and/or seizure precautions if the client is confused or agitated.

Evaluation

The client's plasma sodium levels should return to normal within 48 hours, depending on the severity of the deficit. If the client remains hyponatremic, the care plan may require revision while causes are being reassessed.

■ Modifications for Elderly Clients

Research outcomes have identified electrolyte imbalance, age greater than 79, and noninfectious postoperative complications as the major risk factors for death in the elderly in the postoperative phase. Hyponatremia and hypokalemia were the two most common imbalances. Most of these clients had received spinal anesthesia. The strongest predictors of electrolyte imbalances were intraoperative complications, use of cathartics preoperatively, and multiple pathologic conditions.[42] Clearly, the nursing implications are for more astute observations for manifestations of hyponatremia and hypokalemia, anticipation of imbalances, and early but cautious therapy, with ongoing monitoring.

Community and Self-Care

Instruct the client and family about the risk factors associated with prescribed medications and of the importance of not taking any over-the-counter medications without physician approval; reinforce dietary prescriptions. To enhance health promotion, suggest risk prevention activities such as those found in Risk Factors and Levels of Prevention.

Hypernatremia

Hypernatremia is defined as a plasma sodium level greater than 145 mEq/L. It occurs in approximately 1% of hospitalized clients and carries a high mortality rate, whether it has an acute or a chronic onset. Hypernatremia is usually associated with water loss or sodium gain. It can occur with increased, decreased, or normal total body sodium levels and decreased or increased water levels. The underlying cause of hypernatremia is a TBW deficit

Table 15–9. Clinical Conditions and Disorders That May Contribute to Hypernatremia	
Type of Hypernatremia	**Clinical Conditions and Disorders**
Hypovolemic hypernatremia	Renal losses; osmotic diuresis, diuretics, severe hyperglycemia Extrarenal losses: profuse diaphoresis, decreased thirst, diarrhea occurring with inadequate volume replacement or fluid replacement with hyperosmolar solutions, burns
Euvolemic hypernatremia	Excess fluid losses from the skin and lungs Hypodipsia in the elderly and infants Diabetes insipidus
Hypervolemic hypernatremia	Administration of concentrated saline solutions; hypertonic feedings, excess mineralocorticoids Accidental or intentional salt ingestion; commercially prepared soups and canned vegetables

relative to the total body sodium content, which results in hyperosmolality.

Etiology and Risk Factors

Body fluid loss resulting in hypernatremia may be due to renal or extrarenal causes such as gastrointestinal or skin problems. Hypernatremia can be classified into three types:

● Hypovolemic hypernatremia, in which TBW is greatly decreased relative to sodium (loss of hypotonic fluid)
● Euvolemic hypernatremia, in which TBW is decreased relative to the normal total body sodium
● Hypervolemic hypernatremia, in which TBW is increased but the sodium gain is in excess of the water gain

Hypervolemic hypernatremia is the least common type of hypernatremia.[41, 72] Table 15–9 presents clinical conditions and disorders that may contribute to the development of hypernatremia.

Clients with untreated diabetes insipidus do not secrete ADH; however, they tend to be only mildly hypernatremic. This is because the thirst mechanism is intact and stimulates the client to drink water and fluids, which helps to balance water losses and hypernatremia. See Chapter 71 for a more in-depth discussion of diabetes insipidus.

Populations at risk for developing hypernatremia are infants, the elderly, and debilitated persons. Major risk factors include inadequate water intake in conjunction with decreased thirst (hypodipsia) and excessive water loss or insufficient fluid replacement associated with febrile illness, vomiting, or diarrhea. Uncontrolled diabetes mellitus and renal disease are also major risk factors. Suggestions for primary, secondary, and tertiary prevention of hypernatremia are presented in Risk Factors and Levels of Prevention.

Pathophysiology

As with other imbalances, it is the water that moves in an attempt to create balance. However, the osmotic shift of water from the cells to the ECF in an attempt to dilute the hyperosmolar ECF only creates another problem: cellular dehydration. The higher level of sodium gradient between the ECF and the ICF creates a change in the membrane potential. With mild hypernatremia, almost all excitable (*irritable*) tissues are excited more easily. The CNS is most affected by hypernatremia, followed by skeletal, cardiac, and smooth muscles. If the hypernatremia occurs slowly or chronically, the brain develops its own osmotic particles, called *idiogenic osmoles*, to prevent fluid shifts in and out of the brain cells.[101] The pathophysiologic changes that relate to the clinical manifestations of and laboratory and/or diagnostic findings associated with hypernatremia are summarized in Table 15–10.

The cardiac system is sensitive to the increasing sodium levels. Calcium must move into the channel for cardiac muscle contraction. The sodium competes with calcium in the slow calcium channels of the heart, resulting in depression of myocardial contractility. Myocardial depolarization, however, occurs more easily with the increased sodium levels.

Generally, the body responds to increased sodium levels by suppressing the effects of aldosterone and ADH. These two mechanisms normally increase the renal blood flow and cause excretion of sodium and water. In hypernatremia, the problem is greater than the potential of these adaptive mechanisms to compensate.

Clinical Manifestations and Diagnostic Findings

Mild hypernatremia is usually asymptomatic. Early nonspecific manifestations such as polyuria followed by oliguria, nausea, vomiting, weakness, and restlessness, may be overlooked. Clinical manifestations are nonspecific because two thirds of the body water is intracellular, and primary water losses tend to cause only modest effects on circulating blood volume. If the vascular volume does decrease, orthostatic hypotension with compensatory tachycardia occurs. As hypernatremia progresses to sodium levels greater than 155 mEq/L, cells (especially brain cells) shrink due the increased ECF osmolality.

RISK FACTORS AND LEVELS OF PREVENTION

Hypernatremia

Risk Factors

Clients with decreased intake due to hypodipsia, lack of access, debilitation, restraint, mental confusion, or NPO status.

Clients with increased sodium intake, as with hypertonic saline IVs or hypertonic feedings or increased sodium retention, such as in heart, renal, or liver disease, Cushing's syndrome, increased aldosterone, or with cortisone therapy. Clients with decreased fluid intake or increased fluid loss, as in fever, vomiting, diarrhea, drainage, polyuria, or hyperventilation.

Levels of Prevention

Primary Prevention

- Teach client importance of taking hourly fluids (clear liquids), 30 to 60 ml or more if tolerated, and of keeping appropriate fluids on hand for replacement when symptoms appear.
- Teach client to avoid large amounts of caffeinated beverages or other fluids within a few hours of bedtime.
- Instruct client to consult physician if fever, vomiting, or diarrhea persists longer than 24 hours or if client is symptomatic. Manifestations that should be reported include extreme weakness, palpitations, change in mental state, new onset of cough, or increased restlessness. Consulting with the physician is especially important for a person with chronic disease of the heart, kidney, or liver or diabetes mellitus.
- Impress on family members the importance of providing fresh foods and variety of fluids for a loved one who lives alone.
- Encourage use of community resources such as Meals-on-Wheels.

Secondary Prevention

- Monitor daily weight, vital signs every 4 to 8 hours, input and output every 8 hours.
- Monitor plasma electrolytes.
- Monitor lung sounds every 2 to 4 hours. Notify physician if change in lung sounds. The client may need an IV diuretic to prevent or treat pulmonary overload.
- Provide 30 to 60 ml or more of clear liquids per hour; progress to medical liquids and increase amount as tolerated. Hypovolemic or euvolemic hypernatremia can usually be prevented by oral fluid replacement.
- Anticipate hypervolemic hypernatremia when giving hypertonic saline.
- Give IV fluids per IV pump at slow, prescribed rate.
- Restrict fluid and sodium intake.
- Teach client and family rationale for restrictions.
- Give 1 ml of fluid per 1 kcal of hypertonic feeding formula to prevent cellular dehydration.
- Teach clients taking cortisone the importance of limiting sodium, reading labels for "Na" content, and reporting weight gains greater than 3 lb/week.
- Encourage the family to assist in giving fluids.
- Consult the physician for IV to meet maintenance or replacement fluid and electrolyte needs, especially if the client is NPO.
- Consult the physician for hypotonic IV fluid replacement if the client develops symptoms or if fluid loss persists.

Tertiary Prevention

- Compare daily or weekly weights. Report gains greater than 3 lb/week.
- Restrict sodium intake if excretion decreased or retention of sodium increased.
- Give 1 ml of fluid per 1 kcal of hypertonic tube feeding.
- Notify physician if fever, vomiting, or diarrhea persists more than 24 hours.

Neurologic changes, including confusion, convulsions, coma, and irreversible brain damage, can occur. Hypernatremia is determined by elevated plasma sodium levels and increased osmolality. See Table 15–10 for other clinical manifestations of hypernatremia. Because chloride is the major ECF ion that balances sodium, the plasma chloride level is also higher.

Acute and Subacute Care

■ Medical Management

The goal of medical intervention is to identify the type of hypernatremia. The primary treatment for a client experi-

Table 15–10. Clinical Manifestations and Laboratory/Diagnostic Findings: Hypernatremia	
Clinical Manifestation	**Pathophysiologic Basis**
Gastrointestinal Manifestations	
Anorexia, nausea, and vomiting	Fluid retention in gastric cells
Integumentary Manifestations	
Skin dry and flushed; mucous membranes dry and sticky	Decrease of interstitial fluid in tissues
Thirst; tongue dry and rough; body temperature elevated	Less interstitial fluid to cool body by evaporation
Neurologic Manifestations	
Restlessness, agitation, irritability, confusion, lethargy, stupor, coma, fever	Neurologic symptoms are the result of cerebral cellular dehydration
Muscle weakness and twitching, tremor, hyperreflexia, seizures; rigid paralysis in late stages	Altered neuromuscular contractility and irritability
Cardiovascular Manifestations	
Tachycardia, hypotension or hypertension	Blood pressure relative to the type of hypernatremia. If hypovolemic, pressure will be decreased. If hypervolemic, pressure will be increased
Peripheral vein emptying >5 seconds S$_3$ gallop, NVD	Fluid overload, hypervolemic hypernatremia
Erratic heart rate and blood pressure dependent on fluid status	Myocardial depression as sodium ions compete with calcium ions in slow channels of heart
Weight gain, edema	If hypervolemic hypernatremia
Pulmonary Manifestations	
Crackles, dyspnea, pleural effusion	Increases hydrostatic pressure, seen in hypernatremic hypervolemia
Renal Manifestations	
Oliguria, dark and concentrated	Compensatory mechanism
Laboratory/Diagnostic Findings	
Serum sodium >145 mEq/L	Sodium retention and/or fluid loss
Serum osmolality >295 mOsm/kg	Sodium is the major solute of fluid concentration; hypernatremia increases serum osmolality

encing hypovolemia or euvolemic hypernatremia is correction of the presenting etiology and oral fluid replacement if manifestations are minor. However, clients with severe hypernatremia usually require hospitalization and the more aggressive approach of IV hypotonic saline.

Intravenous Therapy

To decrease total body sodium and replace fluid loss, either a hyposmolar electrolyte solution (0.2% or 0.45% NaCl) or D$_5$W is administered. These solutions do not cause a considerable dilution of body sodium; instead, the plasma sodium level gradually decreases as excess sodium is excreted. When administered continuously, D$_5$W is considered to be a hyposmolar solution because the dextrose is metabolized quickly and only water remains. If the plasma sodium level is lowered too rapidly, fluid shifts from the vascular fluid into the cerebral cells, causing cerebral edema. Slow administration of IV fluids with a goal of reducing plasma sodium levels not more than 2 mEq/L/hr for the first 48 hours decreases this risk.[11, 21]

Hypernatremia due to sodium excess may be treated with D$_5$W and a diuretic, such as furosemide (Lasix). When hypernatremia is due to diabetes insipidus, desmopressin acetate, in the form of a nasal spray, is commonly ordered to slow the rate of diuresis. It has a 20-hour duration compared to the 4- to 6-hour duration of vasopressin oil nasal spray.[21]

Sodium Restriction

Dietary sodium restriction is useful in preventing hypernatremia in high-risk clients. However, it will not bring a high sodium level down to normal. Persons with renal disease may need sodium intake restricted to 500 to 2000 mg/day (see Box 15–3). In hypervolemic hypernatremia, fluids must also be restricted. Persons with diabetes insipidus who are receiving antidiuretic medications must be taught to avoid excessive water intake. Drinking excess water defeats the purpose of the medication.

■ Nursing Management of the Medical Client

Assessment

Assess for the usual clinical manifestations, especially in high-risk clients such as head-injured clients. Obtain a thorough diet and medication history including corticosteroids and over-the-counter medications, such as cough medicine, and food flavorings and spices.

Depending on the client's condition, assess vital signs and peripheral vein filling time every 4 to 8 hours, measure intake and output every 8 hours, and compare daily weights. Use oral membrane and skin assessment tools to guide your interventions. Monitor for changes in plasma sodium and plasma osmolality (estimate). Report early signs of altered mental status, such as agitation, irritability, or confusion, to prevent the progression of hypernatremia and to detect lack of response to therapy or signs of overcorrection (hyponatremia).

Diagnosis, Planning, Implementation

Hypernatremia. The collaborative problem is simply stated as Hypernatremia. It can be related to decreased thirst or excessive administration of salt solutions or impaired excretion of sodium and water. Be sure to specify the cause.

Planning: Expected Outcomes. The nurse will monitor the client for response to IV fluid replacement of hyposmolar electrolyte solutions, absent clinical manifestations of hypernatremia, and return to normal sodium levels.

Implementation. Offer water and fluids frequently to the elderly and to people with debilitating diseases to prevent body fluid loss and hypernatremia. Exception, increasing fluid intake in persons with congestive heart failure or severe renal or liver disease is usually contraindicated. Caffeinated fluids and alcohol are avoided because they increase fluid loss and thereby increase the risk of hypernatremia. Initiate safety/seizure precautions if the client manifests weakness and/or cerebral changes. Involve the client and family in goal setting and preventive teaching (see Risk Factors and Levels of Prevention: Hypernatremia).

Monitor IV fluid/sodium replacements and IV sites hourly. Prevent osmotic diuresis from D_5W by maintaining the prescribed rate. Consult the physician if signs persist or worsen.

Altered Oral Mucous Membranes. Use the nursing diagnosis Altered Oral Mucous Membranes for clients with hypernatremia. State the diagnosis as *Altered Oral Mucous Membranes related to inadequate volume of oral secretions secondary to hypernatremia.*

Planning: Expected Outcomes. The client will have improved condition of oral mucous membranes, as evidenced by oral mucous membranes that are pink, moist, and intact; have an increased oral mucous membrane score on assessment tool; report no oral discomfort; and be able to consume fluids without pain.

Implementation. Give oral care every 2 hours with a nonalcoholic mouthwash. Avoid lemon-glycerin swabs because they dry the membranes and may cause pain. Saline and hydrogen peroxide (1:1) has been found to be an effective mouthwash for many clients. Use a soft toothbrush to prevent injury to the mucosa. Moisten lips every 1 to 2 hours. Offer cool, nonacidic fluids, such as apple juice. Low-acid juices provide fluid while decreasing pain and irritation. Limited ice chips may also decrease the discomfort from dry mucous membranes.

Evaluation

The nurse evaluates whether or not the goals of preventing and correcting fluid imbalance and hypernatremia have been met. If the client is elderly, 48 to 72 hours may be required to correct hypernatremia. The client's oral mucous membranes should be evaluated at every shift to detect a lack of improvement. Expect to see improvement in just a few hours with frequent oral care.

Community and Self-Care

The client and family may require dietary education to reinforce the need for fluid and sodium restriction. Teach avoidance of over-the-counter medications without physician approval and how to recognize the manifestations of hyponatremia and hypernatremia that warrant calling a physician.

Potassium Imbalances

Potassium is plentiful within the cell. Approximately 96% (150 mEq/L) of potassium is in intracellular fluid, and 4% (5 mEq/L) is in the intravascular fluid. Potassium is also plentiful in the gastrointestinal tract. Although the greatest amount of potassium is intracellular, it is valuable to measure plasma levels. However, because little potassium is extracellular, the range is very narrow. (See Box 15–4 for normal plasma ranges.) A plasma potassium level less than 2.5 mEq/L or greater than 7.0 mEq/L can result in cardiac arrest.

Potassium has many functions within the body. It assists in the regulation of intracellular osmolality and promotes the transmission and conduction of nerve impulses and the contraction of skeletal, cardiac, and smooth muscles. It promotes enzyme action for cellular metabolism and glycogen storage in the liver. Potassium also assists with the maintenance of acid-base balance through cellular exchange with hydrogen.

Requirements for a person with no active loss of potassium are 40 to 60 mEq/day. Potassium is poorly stored in the body, so *daily* potassium intake is necessary. A standard diet contains 50 to 100 mEq/day. Foods rich in potassium include vegetables, fruits (especially if dried), nuts, and meats.

Eighty percent to 90% of potassium is excreted through the kidneys and the remainder is excreted in feces. Renal excretion of potassium is influenced by plasma potassium concentration, blood flow into the kidney, acid-base status, and various hormones. An increased sodium intake promotes potassium loss.

The plasma and cellular levels of potassium are affected by acid-base imbalances. Alkalosis can cause hypokalemia. In an alkalotic state, hydrogen moves out of the cells to correct the alkalosis, and potassium shifts into the cells, thus lowering the plasma potassium level. In acidosis, the reverse is true; therefore, potassium leaves the cell and extracellular levels rise.

Insulin promotes potassium uptake by the cells. Therefore, insulin-deficient clients often manifest hyperkalemia. This is thought to be secondary to direct stimulation by insulin of the sodium-potassium pump, which moves potassium into the cell.

Glucagon increases plasma levels of potassium. It is thought that this is because glucagon stimulates potassium release from the liver and may promote potassium movement from muscle cells.

Adrenocortical hormones, such as cortisol and aldosterone, promote potassium excretion and sodium retention via the kidneys. During stress, cortisol and aldosterone levels are increased. Thus, hypokalemia is a risk factor in stress. Catecholamines and beta-adrenergic agonists promote cellular uptake of potassium.

In contrast with beta-adrenergic stimulation, alpha-adrenergic agonists increase plasma potassium concentration. Hepatic stores of potassium are released and muscle storage is altered.

Epinephrine, which has both alpha- and beta-adrenergic properties, causes an initial transient rise in potassium. The beta-adrenergic properties subsequently become dominant, and the major effect is a lowering of plasma potassium levels.

Hypokalemia

Hypokalemia is defined as a plasma potassium level of less than 3.5 mEq/L. It is a common electrolyte disorder, especially in the elderly. The many causes of hypokalemia are listed in Table 15–11.

Etiology and Risk Factors

The elderly and the young are at a higher risk for development of hypokalemia. The body does *not* preserve potassium. Thus, potassium deficit frequently occurs when there is an inadequate nutrient intake. People who take potassium-wasting diuretics or cathartics, or who have an ileostomy have a greater loss of potassium. Those who are in the healing phase after a severe tissue injury or who have cancer are also prone to develop hypokalemia.[63] Surgical clients often develop hypokalemia second-

Table 15–11. Clinical Conditions and Disorders That May Cause Hypokalemia
Gastrointestinal losses: Vomiting, diarrhea, nasogastric suctioning, intestinal fistula, laxative abuse, excessive tap water enemas, ileostomy
Dietary changes: Malnutrition, starvation, potassium-free diet, some weight reduction diets, potassium-free intravenous solutions when there is no dietary intake
Medications: Potassium-wasting diuretics (thiazide, loop of Henle, and osmotic), steroids (cortisone preparations), ingestion of large amounts of licorice (aldosterone-like effect), aminoglycosides, amphotericin B, digitalis preparations, and beta-adrenergics promote potassium loss, cisplatin, bicarbonate
Redistribution of potassium: Insulin moves glucose and potassium back into cells; potassium loss from osmotic diuresis in diabetic acidosis; alkalosis causes potassium to shift into cells in exchange for the hydrogen ion
Disorders: Cushing's syndrome, diuretic phase of acute renal failure, alcoholism, hyperaldosteronism, liver disease, cancer wounds; healing phase of severe stress, trauma, burns

ary to the increased cortisol levels during the stress adaptation period and to the wasting effects of general or spinal anesthesia. Recent studies have suggested that hypokalemia in alcoholics, as well as hypocalcemia, hypophosphatemia, and hypomagnesemia, is secondary to alcohol-induced nephrotoxicity. After several weeks of alcohol abstinence, these subjects experienced electrolyte normalization.[19, 64] Suggestions for primary, secondary, and tertiary prevention of hypokalemia are presented in Risk Factors and Levels of Prevention.

Pathophysiology

When plasma potassium levels decrease, a decrease in potassium gradient occurs between the cell and the plasma. The decreased gradient causes the resting membrane potential to increase, thus increasing excitability. Therefore, cell membranes are more responsive to stimuli (see Fig. 15–8).

Clinical Manifestations and Diagnostic Findings

The clinical manifestations of hypokalemia include abnormal electrocardiography, and manifestations related to GI, cardiac, renal, respiratory, and neurologic disturbances. Observable manifestations may not be apparent with mild hypokalemia (3.3 to 3.4 mEq/L), especially if the decrease is gradual. In such instances, the potassium imbalance may go undetected until the plasma potassium level continues to fall. With severe hypokalemia, ECG changes,

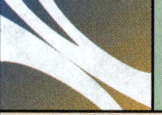

RISK FACTORS AND LEVELS OF PREVENTION

Hypokalemia

Risk Factors

Clients with decreased intake: debilitated, confused, those requiring restraint, those with poor access or finances, including many elderly and homeless; those with anorexia or bulimia nervosa, alcoholic, or NPO with potassium-free IVs or no IV.

Clients with increased loss from vomiting, diarrhea,[8] excess drainage, potassium-wasting diuretics, high-volume ileostomy, fistulas, wound drainage, osmotic diuresis with hyperglycemia, healing phase of major burns, trauma, stress, high carbohydrate intake, cathartics, GI suction, or conditions such as diuretic phase of renal failure, Cushing's syndrome, hyperaldosteronism, metabolic or respiratory alkalosis, or Bartter's syndrome, which is a chronic electrolyte-losing syndrome.[100]

Levels of Prevention

Primary Prevention

- Teach the client the importance of a well-rounded diet.
- Teach the client the importance of fluid replacement, 30 to 60 ml of clear liquids hourly. Cola contains potassium and assists in decreasing nausea.
- Increase awareness of the importance of not taking over-the-counter medications without consulting the physician, especially laxatives.
- Teach the importance of contacting the physician if vomiting and/or diarrhea persist longer than 24 hours, especially if chronic disease of the heart, liver, renal system, or diabetes mellitus is present.
- Teach the client to also consult the physician if he or she becomes symptomatic. This includes reporting severe weakness, irregular heartbeat, or change in mental status.
- Teach the client to take potassium with food and to avoid milk products if he or she is lactose intolerant.
- Encourage families of high-risk members to seek support for maintaining nutrient access, such as Meals-on-Wheels, food stamps, or respite care support services.
- Encourage family members to share responsibilities of care for the elderly or to seek assistance from friends or church support services.
- Refer client to Alcoholics Anonymous or other support services as appropriate.

Secondary Prevention

- Monitor apical pulses in clients receiving IV potassium chloride.
- Monitor renal function closely by calculating input and output every 8 hours. Report urine outputs less than 30 ml/hr if consistent for 2 hours or more.

---

such as are illustrated in Figure 15–9, may occur. Cardiac arrest may follow. Table 15–12 summarizes the pathophysiologic basis for the clinical manifestations and laboratory/diagnostic findings associated with hypokalemia. Although plasma levels are valuable, the ECG is the most reliable tool for determining intracellular potassium levels.

Acute and Subacute Care

■ Medical Management

Medical management is focused on determining and correcting the cause of the imbalance. The aggressiveness of the therapy is determined by the potassium level and the clinical manifestations. Extreme hypokalemia requires cardiac monitoring.

Potassium Replacement

Oral potassium replacement therapy is usually prescribed for mild hypokalemia (plasma potassium, 3.3 to 3.5 mEq/L) or for preventive purposes. Oral potassium (chloride or gluconate) is extremely irritating to the gastric mucosa. Therefore, it must be taken with a glass of water or juice or with meals.

Potassium chloride can be administered IV for moderate or severe hypokalemia. Potassium given intravenously *MUST ALWAYS BE DILUTED IN IV FLUIDS*. The usual concentration of IV potassium is 20 to 40 mEq/L. Potassium is *NOT* given intramuscularly and is *NEVER* given as a bolus (IV push) injection. Giving potassium by IV push may result in cardiac arrest. For severe potassium deficits, 10 to 20 mEq of potassium can be given per hour if *diluted* in IV fluids and if a heart monitor is being used. Saline dilution is recommended; avoid dextrose because it increases intracellular potassium shifting.

- Monitor plasma electrolytes and ECG. Report low normal levels and levels less than 3.5 mEq/L especially if not receiving potassium supplements.
- Monitor for digitalis toxic effects in clients at risk for hypokalemia, if on digitalis derivatives.
- Give antiemetics prophylactically.
- Wean TPN or consult physician for IV with dextrose to prevent rebound hypoglycemia; plasma insulin, which was released to transport glucose, is still active and will not only cause hypoglycemia, but will also cause potassium shifting into the cell. Anticipate need for increased potassium in TPN to replace the potassium that goes into cell as insulin is released to compensate for high glucose levels or sliding scale insulin.[63]
- Assist the client with intake of a well-rounded diet.
- Encourage the family to assist in feeding.
- Consult with the physician for supplements, such as IVs with potassium, or use of tube feedings or TPN if the client is NPO for more than 2 or 3 days.
- Consult the physician for a plasma electrolyte baseline for preoperative clients. Report any borderline or normal findings *before* surgery. Perioperative clients at *high risk* for cardiac dysrhythmias if hypokalemic.[28, 113]
- Consult the physician for oral potassium supplements if any conditions causing potassium wasting are present. Give the oral potassium supplements with food.

Tertiary Prevention

- Monitor for digitalis toxic effects. Manifestations include anorexia, nausea, vomiting, diarrhea; headache, weakness, visual changes such as blurring, yellow or green vision, a halo effect; mental changes; and almost any change in cardiac rate or rhythm. *Hypokalemia increases sensitivity of the myocardium to digitalis-induced dysrhythmia.*[79]
- Encourage intake of a well-rounded diet.
- Offer small, frequent feedings.
- Give oral potassium with food.
- Encourage family to assist in feeding.
- Consult the physician for supplements if client is eating less than half of meals or if loss of potassium is increased.
- Consult the physician for tube feedings if unable to meet the client's nutritional needs by a conservative approach.

Because potassium is irritating to the veins, higher concentrations increase the risk of phlebitis. Clients with plasma potassium levels between 3.0 and 3.4 mEq/L need approximately 100 to 200 mEq of IV potassium for the potassium level to rise 1 mEq/L. If the client's plasma potassium level is less than 3.0 mEq/L, it takes approximately 200 to 400 mEq of IV potassium to raise the level 1 mEq/L. High concentrations of potassium are extremely irritating to the heart muscle. Thus, correcting a potassium deficit may take several days.[63, 72]

Maintenance doses for clients not taking any source of potassium are 40 to 60 mEq/day in the IV solution. Larger amounts are needed with coexisting potassium losses.

Dietary Management

Administering foods high in potassium will help correct the problem and prevent further potassium losses. The adult recommended allowance for potassium is 1875 to 5625 mg/day. See Box 15–5 on page 313 for high- and low-potassium foods.

■ Nursing Management of the Medical Client

Assessment

Nursing assessments focus on collecting data related to the health problem and the clinical manifestations and laboratory findings associated with hypokalemia. Nurses need to anticipate hypokalemia in high-risk clients. Obtaining a diet history that focuses on intake, conditions promoting loss, and drugs such as diuretics, cortisone, and over-the-counter medications, is very important. Plasma potassium levels and the client's response to therapy need to be monitored.

In addition, monitor IV sites hourly for phlebitis, infil-

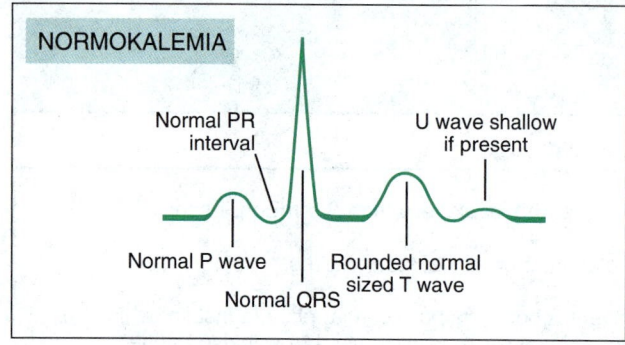

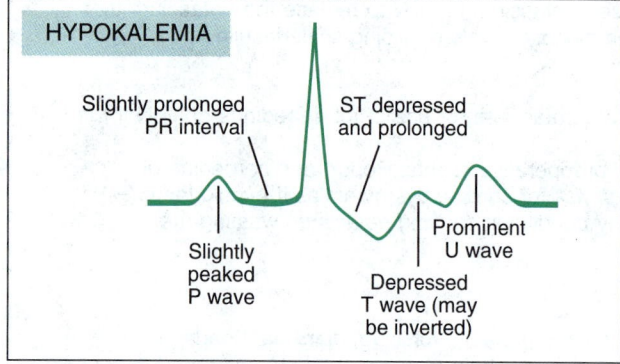

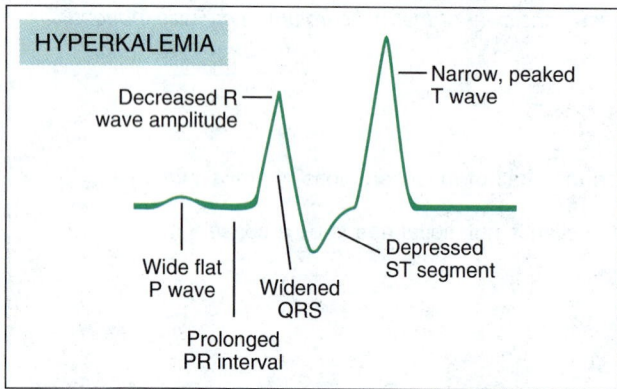

Figure 15–9. ECG changes seen in potassium imbalances. (From McCance, K. L., & Huether, S. E. [1994]. *Pathophysiology: The biologic basis for disease in adults and children* [2nd ed.]. St. Louis: Mosby–Year Book.)

tration, and rate of infusion. Assess neuromuscular and bowel function every 4 to 8 hours. Assess cardiac function, including apical pulses, and renal function every hour for severe hypokalemia and progress to every 8 hours as the client's condition improves. A urine output of 30 ml/hour is necessary to prevent rebound hyperkalemia. If the client receives digitalis, monitor for digitalis toxic effects. If the apical pulse is irregular, assess for pulse deficits. If hypokalemia is present or refractory to treatment, assess for manifestations of hypomagnesemia. Many persons who are hypokalemic are also hypomagnesemic. Hypokalemia that does not respond to treatment has frequently been associated with hypomagnesemia. Magnesium is necessary for the kidney to conserve potassium.[2, 65, 116]

Diagnosis, Planning, Implementation

Hypokalemia. Use the collaborative problem of Hypokalemia. It can be related to vomiting, diarrhea, Cushing's disease, prolonged or intensive diuretic use, cortisone therapy, decreased intake, or NPO status. Be sure to specify the cause.

Planning: Expected Outcomes. The nurse will monitor the client for plasma potassium level returning to normal range, absence of complications related to IV administration of potassium, and absence of the manifestations of hypokalemia.

Implementation. Give oral or IV potassium as prescribed, ensuring that it is *DILUTED IN IV FLUIDS; IT CANNOT BE GIVEN AS AN IV PUSH.* Always *agitate* IV bags before hanging them up to prevent giving a loading dose, which can cause cardiac arrest.[63, 109] Change IV sites every 72 hours or sooner if the vein becomes tender to palpation. Tenderness indicates damage to the intima of the vein; this is an early sign of phlebitis. Use the smallest IV catheter possible to allow a greater plasma flow around the site at which the potassium enters the vein. This dilutes the potassium and decreases the risk of phlebitis. If an IV with potassium infiltrates, consult the physician for advice. Potassium can cause tissue sloughing. Give IV fluids with potassium chloride by a controlled infusion pump to ensure the correct flow rate.

Consult the physician if the client's urinary output is less than 30 ml/hr while IV potassium is being given, if the pulse deficit is greater than 20 beats/minute, or if signs of impaired peripheral tissue perfusion are present. Also, notify the physician if signs of hypokalemia persist or worsen, such as increased dysrhythmia, or if signs of overcorrection occur, such as hyperkalemia.

Risk for Injury. Because potassium is needed for normal nerve conduction and muscle function, low serum potassium levels often lead to weakness and can lead to seizures. The nursing diagnosis is stated as *Risk for Injury related to muscle weakness and hypotension or seizures secondary to hypokalemia.*

Planning: Expected Outcomes. The client will remain free of injury, as evidenced by no falls or near falls and no seizures.

Implementation. Employ safety and/or seizure precautions to reduce the risk of injury. Keep the bed in a low position with side rails up. Before the client walks, clear the path of obstacles and place nonslippery shoes and an ambulation belt on the client. Use restraints only after all other alternatives to prevent inadvertent harm to self or others have been tried. In 1987, the Omnibus Budget Reconciliation Act (OBRA) included statements about nursing home residents' rights to be free from physical and/or chemical restraints that were used for the purpose of discipline or convenience. In 1992, the Health Care Financing Administration adopted these standards for clients in acute care facilities. It is imperative that the nurse comply with the client's rights and follow the defined protocol as required by these mandates. Refer to your agency's policy/procedural manuals for explicit guidelines for action and documentation.

Table 15–12. Clinical Manifestations and Laboratory/Diagnostic Findings: Hypokalemia

Clinical Manifestation	Pathophysiologic Basis
Gastrointestinal Manifestations	
Anorexia, vomiting, constipation, ileus, distention	Slowed smooth muscle contraction
Musculoskeletal Manifestations	
Muscle weakness, paralysis, leg cramps, muscle flabbiness	Slowed smooth and skeletal muscle contraction
Cardiovascular Manifestations	
Dysrhythmias, hypotension, slow, weak pulse	Increase in cell excitability; decreased myocardial contraction Dysrhythmias are more pronounced when the client is taking a digitalis preparation
Respiratory Manifestations	
Shallow respirations, shortness of breath, apnea, respiratory arrest	Weakness of the respiratory muscles due to a decrease in muscle contractions
Neurologic Manifestations	
Fatigue, lethargy, paresthesias, decreased tendon reflexes, dysphasia, irritability, confusion, depression, convulsions	Increased transmission and conduction of nerve impulses, alkalosis-compensatory cell buffer system
Renal Manifestations	
Polyuria, decreased serum osmolality, nocturia	Inhibition of the kidney's ability to concentrate urine
Laboratory/Diagnostic Findings	
Serum potassium <3.5 mEq/L	Hypokalemia is present when serum potassium level is <3.5 mEq/L
ECG: depressed, prolonged ST segment; depressed, inverted T, U wave	Prolongation of myocardial repolarization

Altered Nutrition: Less Than Body Requirements. If your client is not consuming adequate amounts of foods with potassium use the nursing diagnosis *Altered Nutrition: Less than Body Requirements related to insufficient intake of foods rich in potassium.* Use this diagnosis *only* if your client can eat and drink.

Planning: Expected Outcomes. Client will increase dietary potassium intake to correct hypokalemia, as evidenced by selecting a diet consisting of potassium-rich foods, consuming 1875 to 5625 mg of potassium each day, and consuming oral potassium supplements with food to prevent GI irritation.

Implementation. Instruct the client to choose and consume foods rich in potassium, such as fruits, fruit juices, dried fruits, and vegetables, including potatoes. Potato skins are very rich in potassium. Fish (but not shellfish), whole grains, and nuts, such as peanuts, almonds, or walnuts, are also good sources of potassium. Some fruits have more potassium than do others; bananas, cantaloupe, and honeydew melons have twice as much potassium as do oranges. Meat and milk have a moderate amount of potassium. Instruct the client to take liquid or tablet potassium supplements with a glass or more of water or juice and food.

Evaluation

The nurse evaluates whether the expected outcomes have been met: the plasma potassium level is within normal range; the client is free of the manifestations of hypokalemia; and the client did not suffer from any preventable adverse effects of potassium therapy. Evaluate the client's responses hourly if severe hypokalemia is present, and every 8 hours if mild hypokalemia exists. A revision of the plan of care may be required.

■ Modifications for Elderly Clients

The elderly have frequent problems with hypokalemia, mostly owing to a decreased intake and use of diuretics and cathartics. To promote an increased intake, provide puréed or finely chopped foods and small, frequent meals or fluids between meals. Offer cola if nausea is present; cola is also fairly high in potassium.

Elderly persons are more susceptible to impaired myocardial blood supply and alterations in cardiac rhythm or rate secondary to digitalis toxic effects. Therefore, it is a critical nursing intervention to teach clients and family members the skill of pulse-taking, the importance of calling the physician if signs and symptoms of digitalis toxic effects occur, or if the pulse drops below 60 beats/minute. Reinforce the importance of not taking any over-the-counter medication without physician approval. All teaching should be reinforced through a written handout.

Remember that the OBRA guidelines apply to all persons in nursing home settings and acute care facilities. The elderly make up the largest percentage of this group. You will be challenged to be creative and to find new alternatives to physical and chemical restraints. Review the videotape produced as an outcome of the OBRA act, to provide insight into alternatives to restraint.

Community and Self-Care

Review high-potassium foods with the client and, if appropriate, the person who prepares the client's meals. Provide a copy of the list of food groups and emphasize the importance of eating a well-rounded diet. Review alternative cooking methods, reinforcing that prolonged cooking of vegetables may result in potassium and vitamin loss. Suggest steaming, microwaving, or, if possible, eating raw vegetables, as methods to increase nutrient retention.

Teach clients and/or family the manifestations of potassium deficiency, and excess, if they are going home with potassium supplements. For clients taking digitalis, teach the signs and symptoms of digitalis toxic effects. Teach the client to take his or her pulse. Encourage the client to call the physician if any of these signs occur or if the pulse rate drops below 60 beats/minute. You may want to review the information on digitalis toxicity in Chapter 45. Provide written reinforcement of all of the teaching and a telephone number to call for further explanation. Reinforce the importance of not taking any over-the-counter medication without physician approval.

Hyperkalemia

Hyperkalemia is defined as an elevation of the potassium level above 5.0 mEq/L. Hyperkalemia is rare in clients with normal kidney function, but it occurs in more than 50% of persons with acute renal failure.

Etiology and Risk Factors

The three major causes of hyperkalemia are as follows:

1. Retention of potassium by the body as a result of decreased or inadequate urine output
2. Excessive release of potassium from the cells due to traumatic injury, burns, cell lysis, or acidosis
3. Excessive infusion of IV solutions containing potassium

All three potential causes of hyperkalemia limit the ability of the kidneys to excrete the excess potassium.

Table 15–13. Clinical Conditions and Disorders That May Cause Hyperkalemia
Retention of potassium: Renal insufficiency, renal failure, decreased urine output after surgery, adrenal insufficiency, Addison's disease, hypoaldosteronism, potassium-sparing diuretics, blood for transfusion that is 2 weeks old or more (as blood ages, hemolysis of the red blood cells occurs, which releases the intracellular potassium into the surrounding fluids)
Excessive release of cellular potassium: Severe traumatic injuries, crushing injuries, severe burns (first 24–72 hours), severe infection, metabolic acidosis (except diabetic acidosis), after open-heart surgery or surgery that requires a perfusion pump
Excessive intravenous infusions or oral administration of potassium: Excessive and rapid intravenous administration of potassium; excessive administration of large doses of oral potassium

Because the kidneys are responsible for 80% to 90% of potassium excretion, the underlying cause of hyperkalemia is often related to decreased kidney function. Persons with as little as 5% glomerular function can maintain normal plasma potassium if the urine output is at least 1 L/day. However, any illness can upset this delicate balance. The GI tract and skin cannot excrete enough potassium to compensate for an acute state of hyperkalemia. Shock compounds the problem because of low circulating vascular fluids and diminished kidney function.[88–90] People with high–growth rate cancers, such as non-Hodgkins lymphoma, acute leukemia, small cell tumors, and some metastatic cancers, are at risk for *tumor lysis syndrome* (TLS). TLS is the rapid destruction of tumor cells secondary to chemotherapy and/or radiation, which results in a state of hyperkalemia, hyperphosphatemia, hypocalcemia, and hyperuricemia.[37, 107] Disorders that decrease or inhibit secretion of aldosterone may also cause hyperkalemia. Hyperkalemia does not usually occur from increasing dietary potassium intake unless the potassium is administered in large doses, either orally or IV, or renal insufficiency is also present. Table 15–13 lists the clinical conditions and disorders that may cause hyperkalemia. Suggestions for primary, secondary, and tertiary prevention of hyperkalemia are presented in Risk Factors and Levels of Prevention.

Pathophysiology

Hyperkalemia increases the cell membrane's excitation threshold, causing the cell to become less excitable. This results in decreased nerve and muscle irritability. As hyperkalemia becomes more severe, muscles become weak and paralyzed. See Table 15–14 for the clinical manifestations and laboratory/diagnostic findings associated with hyperkalemia and their pathophysiologic bases.

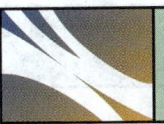

RISK FACTORS AND LEVELS OF PREVENTION

Hyperkalemia

Risk Factors

Clients with increased intake: excessive oral or IV potassium intake in presence of renal insufficiency, transfusion of stored blood with RBC release of potassium.

Clients who experience cellular shifting of potassium as in the early stages (usually the first 24 to 72 hours) of massive cell destruction, such as in trauma, burns, or sepsis, tumor lysis syndrome (TLS), or with metabolic or respiratory acidosis (exception: diabetic acidosis).

Clients with decreased output: chronic renal insufficiency or the onset of acute renal insufficiency, especially if taking potassium supplements.

Levels of Prevention

Primary Prevention

- Teach the importance of maintaining dietary potassium restrictions, reading labels, avoiding salt substitutes that contain potassium, avoiding over-the-counter medication without consulting a physician.
- Teach client to consult the physician if renal function worsens or if acute illness lasts more than 24 hours.

Secondary Prevention

- Monitor intake and output and vital signs every 1 to 8 hours, depending on severity of renal dysfunction and rate of IV potassium chloride administration.
- Monitor plasma electrolytes.
- Assess vital signs, especially apical pulses, for early detection of rate or rhythm change, every 1 to 8 hours.
- Assess for early changes in bowel sounds.
- Use cardiac monitoring for IV potassium chloride concentrations greater than 40 mEq/L, especially in presence of altered renal output. If early ECG changes indicative of hyperkalemia are present, notify physician. Maintain cardiac monitoring with narrow alarm limits.
- Keep in floor stock: 50% dextrose ampules, regular insulin, IV dextrose solutions, sodium polystyrene sulfonate (Kayexalate), oral and rectal form.
- Hydrate the client with 3000 ml of IV fluid 24 hours prior to, during, and 48 hours after rapid tumor lysis chemotherapy, and give diuretics and allopurinol to prevent TLS.[107]
- See Chapter 16 for the care of the client who has hyperkalemia secondary to respiratory acidosis.

Tertiary Prevention

- Monitor for manifestations of hyperkalemia.
- Monitor urinary output if client is taking potassium or if renal output is less than 240 ml/8 hours.
- Consult the physician for marked change in renal output or manifestations of hyperkalemia.

Clinical Manifestations and Diagnostic Findings

Clinical manifestations are related to the plasma potassium level and the suddenness of the imbalance. Acute hyperkalemia may cause manifestations when the plasma level is 6.0 mEq/L. However, if it has developed slowly, manifestations may not be present until the plasma level reaches 7.0 mEq/L. Clinical manifestations involve many body systems, including GI, cardiac, renal, and neurologic systems. Mild to moderate hyperkalemia (a plasma level near 6.0 mEq/L) causes muscle irritability, paresthesia (numbness, tingling), tachycardia, and intestinal colic. As the plasma potassium level approaches 7.0 mEq/L, disturbances in cardiac conduction, ventricular contraction, cardiac arrest, and severe neuromuscular weakness progressing to paralysis of the respiratory muscles can result.[44] Again, the key to the level of severity is the amount of

time the body has had to adapt to the imbalance. See Figure 15–9 and Table 15–14 for a summary of manifestations, including the laboratory and ECG changes. The ECG is the most reliable tool for identifying intracellular potassium levels. *Caution: Pseudohyperkalemia can result from hemolyzed blood specimens, when tourniquets are applied too tightly, when multiple attempts are made to obtain a sample from the same site, or when excess force is used to transfer blood into tubes or to aspirate blood into a syringe.*[44]

Other useful laboratory studies include BUN, creatinine, and carbon dioxide levels. Elevated BUN and plasma creatinine levels, which reflect decreased renal function, are important laboratory indicators for determining risk of hyperkalemia. If the venous total carbon dioxide levels are low, an arterial blood gas study should be done to rule out a metabolic or respiratory acidosis as a possible cause of hyperkalemia.

Table 15–14. Clinical Manifestations and Laboratory/Diagnostic Findings: Hyperkalemia

Clinical Manifestation	Pathophysiologic Basis
Cardiovascular Manifestations	
First tachycardia, and then bradycardia	Disturbances in cardiac conduction, especially through the Purkinje fibers and atrioventricular node, which may lead to ectopic beats; prolonged diastole
Dysrhythmia	Increase in pacemaker, ectopic foci excitability
Hypotension, decreased myocardial contraction	
Weaker cardiac contraction, cardiac arrest	Severe potassium elevation, inactivation of Na channels
Gastrointestinal Manifestations	
Nausea, explosive diarrhea, intestinal colic, hyperactive bowel sounds	Increased smooth muscle contraction, increased peristalsis
Neuromuscular Manifestations	
Paresthesia (tingling sensation), muscle weakness and later flaccid muscle paralysis, restlessness, muscle cramps, convulsions	Increased neuromuscular irritability of the skeletal muscles; muscle becomes weak secondary to depolarization block in the muscle and acidosis compensatory cell buffer system
Renal Manifestations	
Oliguria and later anuria	Usually due to preexisting renal dysfunction; limits potassium excretion in the urine
Laboratory/Diagnostic Findings	
Serum potassium >5.0 mEq/L	Hyperkalemia is present when serum potassium level >5.0 mEq/L
ECG changes: peaked, narrow T waves; wide QRS complex; depressed ST segment; widened PR interval, depressed P	Increased membrane excitability threshold

Acute and Subacute Care

■ Medical Management

Potassium elevation must be corrected before levels become severe. If the plasma potassium level is less than 5.5 mEq/L, dietary restriction of potassium may be all that is needed. If the level is greater, or if the client is symptomatic, then pharmacologic intervention is usually necessary. The onset of symptoms and the need for aggressive intervention are usually related to the acuteness of the development of hyperkalemia.

Reducing Potassium Levels

Improving urine output by forcing fluids, giving IV saline, or giving potassium-wasting diuretics usually corrects mild hyperkalemia.

When hyperkalemia is severe, immediate action is needed to avoid lethal cardiac disturbances. These measures may include the following:

● Infusion of IV calcium gluconate to decrease the antagonistic effect of the potassium excess on the myocardium
● Infusion of insulin and glucose or sodium bicarbonate to promote potassium uptake into the cells (useful in metabolic acidosis)
● Use of the beta-agonist albuterol (0.5 mg IV), which results in a decrease of plasma potassium level within 30 minutes that lasts for 6 hours[101]

These methods for decreasing potassium excess usually provide only temporary relief. Repeating these methods may not be effective.[20, 44]

As hyperkalemia persists or increases, a cation exchange resin, such as sodium polystyrene sulfonate (Kayexalate), may be given orally or rectally as a retention enema. When this medication is given, the potassium ion is exchanged for the sodium ion in the intestinal tract; the potassium ion is then excreted in the stool. To prevent the constipating effect of Kayexalate, sorbitol is usually combined with Kayexalate, and diarrhea often results. In marked renal failure, peritoneal dialysis or hemodialysis may be needed.[20, 44, 117] Prevention is the key to the treatment of tumor lysis syndrome;[107] see Risk Factors and Levels of Prevention for Hyperkalemia. Adequate hydration (3000 ml in 24 hours before therapy, during, and for 48 hours afterward) is key.

Dietary Management

When the plasma potassium level is 5.0 to 5.5 mEq/L, a low-potassium, high-carbohydrate diet may be all that is necessary. See Box 15–5 for a list of foods to teach clients with hyperkalemia to avoid.

■ Nursing Management of the Medical Client

Assessment

Nursing assessment focuses on the clinical manifestations and laboratory and ECG findings associated with hyperkalemia. The nurse should anticipate hyperkalemia in high-risk conditions.

In mild hyperkalemia, assess vital signs, bowel function, urine output, and monitor for pulmonary overload (crackles) and peripheral edema every 4 to 8 hours. Monitor plasma levels of potassium, BUN, and creatinine.

In severe hyperkalemia, assess vital signs, including apical pulses, hourly. ECG changes should be monitored continuously. In the absence of an ECG, apical pulses are the next most valuable assessment of intracellular potassium levels. Monitor urine output hourly if severe hyperkalemia or a history of renal insufficiency exists or if the urine output drops to less than 30 ml/hour for 2 consecutive hours.

Monitor not only for a therapeutic response (improvement) to treatment but also for signs of overcorrection. Rapid correction places a client at risk for hypokalemia and metabolic alkalosis. If a client is taking digitalis, the risk for digitalis toxic response is present if hypokalemia occurs.

Diagnosis, Planning, Implementation

Hyperkalemia. Use the collaborative problem of Hyperkalemia. State it as *Hyperkalemia related to renal dysfunction, shock from traumatic injuries, or burns (tissue destruction).* Again, be certain to specify the cause.

Planning: Expected Outcomes. The nurse will monitor the client for return of the plasma potassium level to normal, presence of adequate (30 ml/hr) urinary output, absence of manifestations of neuromuscular changes, and an apical pulse rate within a normal range and without dysrhythmia.

Implementation. In addition to the ongoing assessments, there are important interventions related to hyperkalemia. Report manifestations indicating the development of hypokalemia immediately: urine output of less than 30 ml/hr for 2 consecutive hours or less than 720 ml/day.

If the client is to receive a blood transfusion and is at risk for hyperkalemia, notify the blood bank so that "old" blood (more than 2 weeks old) is not given. Use a 19-gauge needle or 20-gauge catheter for the delivery of the packed cells to prevent RBC rupture and release of intracellular potassium. Use vacuum tubes when possible to

---

Box 15–5. High- and Low-Potassium Foods

High-Potassium Foods (Average: 7 mEq per Serving)

Vegetables (½ cup cooked or 1 cup raw)

Artichokes
Broccoli
Brussels sprouts
Cabbage
Carrots
Celery
Collards
Cucumber
Mushrooms
Spinach
Tomatoes

Fruits

Apricots, fresh, 4 medium
Apricots, canned, 4 halves
Apricots, dried, 7 halves
Banana, 7 inches
Cantaloupe, ¼ small
Guava, 1 medium
Honeydew melon, ⅛ medium
Nectarine, ½
Orange, 1 small
Prunes, 3 medium
Strawberries, 1¼ cups
Tangerine, 2 medium
Watermelon, 1¼ cups

Beverages

Brewed coffee
Tomato juice
Vegetable juice cocktail, unsalted

Low-Potassium Foods (Average: 3 mEq per Serving)

Vegetables

Corn, ⅓ cup
Sweet potato, yams, ¼ cup
Lima beans, ⅓ cup
French fried potatoes, 10 pieces

Fruit

Apple, 1 small
Apple juice, ½ cup
Applesauce, ½ cup
Blueberries, ¾ cup
Cranberries, 1¼ cups

Beverages

Coffee, instant
Cola
Cranberry juice cocktail, ⅓ cup
Ginger ale
Noncarbonated soft drinks
Root beer
Lemon-lime soda

Data from Mahan, K. L., & Arlin, M. (1992). *Food, nutrition and diet therapy* (8th ed.). Philadelphia: W. B. Saunders.

avoid pseudohyperkalemia when obtaining blood specimens.

Risk for Dysrhythmias. High potassium levels have the potential to induce life-threatening dysrhythmias. The collaborative problem is stated *Risk for Dysrhythmias related to hyperkalemia.*

Planning: Expected Outcomes. The nurse will monitor for dysrhythmias, assess ECG recordings, and intervene according to protocols or notify the physician.

Implementation. Report ECG changes that are related to hyperkalemia or hypokalemia secondary to treatment for hyperkalemia.[20] Set cardiac monitor alarms with narrow limits to ensure early detection of lethal dysrhythmias. *Remember, a machine DOES NOT replace the bedside assessment by the registered nurse.* Cardiopulmonary resuscitation may be required, but it is seldom successful in cases of severe hyperkalemia because the heart muscle will not respond to medications or countershock. Consult the physician if signs of decreased cardiac output, such as decreased tissue perfusion, crackles, oliguria, or peripheral edema, are present secondary to decreased stroke volume or to alterations in cardiac rate or rhythm.

Evaluation

Evaluate the client's responses to therapy every hour if severe hyperkalemia is present or every 8 hours if mild hyperkalemia exists. Hyperkalemia is usually corrected quickly because of the risk of dysrhythmia.

■ Modifications for Elderly Clients

The elderly are at high risk due to the increased incidence of chronic diseases that lead to multiple system (especially renal) dysfunction. Therefore, the frequency of assessments to monitor response to treatment may need to be increased during the acute stage of hyperkalemia. Nurses must focus more on prevention to decrease mortality or morbidity in this population (see Risk Factors and Levels of Prevention: Hyperkalemia).

 ## Community and Self-Care

If hyperkalemia is a chronic problem (e.g., with renal failure), the client needs to closely adhere to a diet that is low in potassium. Knowledge of food preparation is important, because cooking styles can affect potassium levels. Also, encourage clients not to take any over-the-counter medications or potassium salt substitutes without physician approval.

Calcium and Phosphorus Imbalances

Calcium, an extracellular and intracellular cation, has a normal plasma range of 4.5 to 5.5 mEq/L or 9 to 11 mg/dl. Approximately 99% of the body's calcium is in the bones and teeth. The other 1% is in the tissue and intravascular fluid. Approximately half of the 1% is bound to protein, mostly albumin, and the remaining half is free (*ionized calcium*). Therefore, the total plasma calcium level does not indicate the exact amount of free, active calcium in the body. Also, abnormal plasma albumin and pH levels influence the interpretation of plasma calcium levels. For example, when albumin is low, a falsely normal plasma calcium level can be present. Conversely, when plasma albumin is high, the functional ionized calcium is actually lower than the plasma laboratory level reveals. When albumin levels are abnormal, the total plasma calcium can be adjusted by adding or subtracting 0.8 mg/dl for every 1 g/dl decrease or increase, respectively, in plasma albumin. A basic pH causes an increase in calcium binding. The plasma level may appear normal, but the ionized, functional calcium level is actually lower. The opposite is true with an acid pH. Therefore, a plasma ionized calcium (iCa) assay should be done in clients that are critically ill, those with marginal calcium imbalances, or those with an albumin or acid-base imbalance. See Box 15–4 for normal ranges.

The normal plasma phosphorus level is 1.2 to 3.0 mEq/L. Less than 1% of phosphorus is contained in the vascular spaces; 85% is contained in the bones and 14% is contained in the soft tissues. However, rapid shifting between cell and blood can occur, which can create a risk for severe hypophosphatemia or hyperphosphatemia.

Calcium has many functions in the body. It acts as a catalyst in the transmission and conduction of nerve impulses and stimulates the contraction of skeletal, smooth, and cardiac muscle. Calcium maintains normal cellular permeability. Increased plasma calcium levels decrease cellular permeability, and decreased plasma calcium levels increase cellular permeability. Calcium also promotes coagulation of blood in all phases, but mostly in the prothrombin to thrombin phase. Calcium promotes absorption and utilization of vitamin B_{12}. Finally, calcium and phosphorus promote strong and durable bones and teeth. Phosphorus is also an integral part of the energy systems in the body (adenosine diphosphate [ADP] and adenosine triphosphate [ATP]) and in the phosphate acid-base buffer system.

Vitamin D promotes calcium absorption from the GI tract, whereas phosphorus (phosphate) inhibits its absorption. Therefore, calcium and phosphorus counterbalance each other.

The parathyroid hormone (PTH) regulates plasma levels of calcium and phosphorus in the following three ways:

1. By increasing resorption of calcium and phosphate from the bone
2. By increasing calcium reabsorption through inhibiting phosphate reabsorption from the renal tubule
3. By increasing calcium and phosphate absorption from the GI tract

Thus, increased PTH increases plasma ionized calcium levels and decreases plasma phosphorus levels. Calcitonin from the thyroid gland also promotes calcium balance by opposing the action of PTH; it inhibits bone resorption.

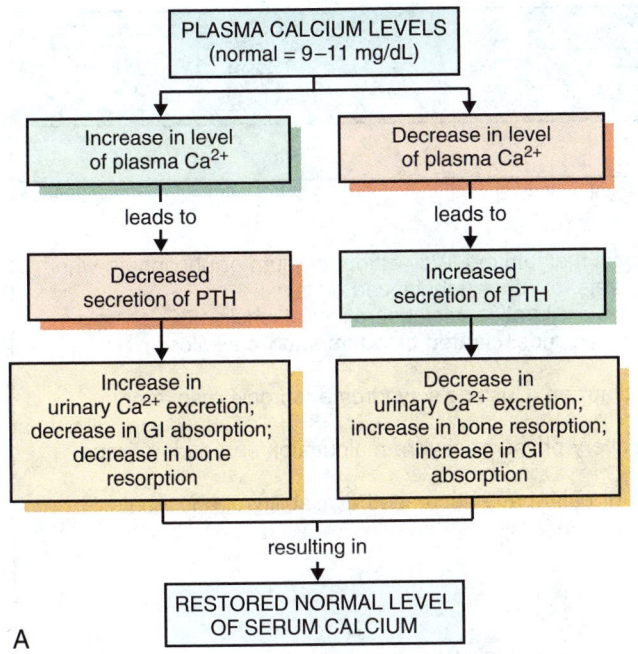

A

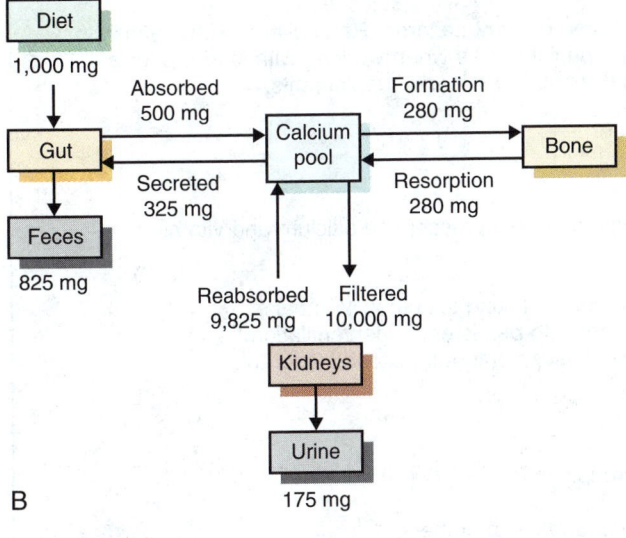

B

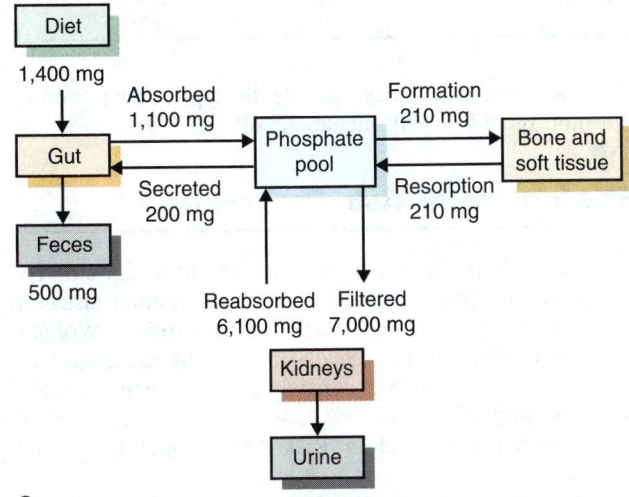

C

When the level of plasma calcium falls even slightly, PTH secretion increases. Within minutes, calcium is reabsorbed from the kidney tubules; bone resorption occurs within hours, and increased absorption from the gastrointestinal tract occurs within days (Fig. 15–10). Notice in Figures 15–10*B* and *C* how calcium and phosphate intake and output remain in balance.

Hypocalcemia and Hypophosphatemia

Although the overview of hypocalcemia and hypophosphatemia is presented together, it is important that the counterbalancing relationship of these ions is kept in mind. Depending on the cause, the client often presents with hypocalcemia and hyperphosphatemia.

Hypocalcemia is a plasma calcium level below 4.5 mEq/L (or 8.5 mg/dl). Hypocalcemia is a common and potentially serious electrolyte disorder that occurs more frequently in children, the elderly, and in postoperative clients. Overcorrection of acidosis may also lead to hypo-

Table 15–15. Clinical Conditions and Disorders That May Cause Hypocalcemia

Dietary changes: Inadequate dietary calcium intake, vitamin D deficiency, or both; excess intake of phosphorus combines with calcium, so neither electrolyte is absorbed

Gastrointestinal changes: Malabsorption of fat in the intestine, diarrhea

Calcium binding: Metabolic alkalosis (because there is less ionized calcium), multiple transfusion of stored blood (which is combined with citrate for storage)

Disorders: Renal failure with hyperphosphatemia, acute pancreatitis (which causes release of lipases into soft tissue spaces, so that free fatty acids that are formed bind with calcium), burns, Cushing's disease, hypoparathyroidism, inadvertent removal of the parathyroid gland with thyroidectomy, liver disease (decreased bile and vitamin D), wounds, alcoholism, tumor lysis syndrome

Medications: Magnesium sulfate, colchicine, neomycin inhibit PTH secretion; aspirin, anticonvulsants, estrogen alter vitamin D metabolism; phosphate preparations decrease serum calcium level; steroids decrease calcium mobilization; loop diuretics reduce calcium absorption from the renal tubules; antacids and laxatives decrease calcium absorption

Figure 15–10. *A,* PTH regulation of plasma calcium level. *B,* Calcium homeostasis. A pool of calcium exists in the body and remains in balance by dietary intake, bowel and kidney excretion, and bone formation and resorption. *C,* Phosphate homeostasis. A pool of phosphate exists in the body and remains in balance by dietary intake, urine and bowel excretion, and bone and soft tissue formation and resorption.

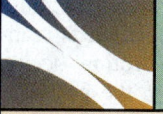

RISK FACTORS AND LEVELS OF PREVENTION

Hypocalcemia and Hypophosphatemia

Risk Factors

Clients with decreased intake of calcium or phosphate: chronic malnutrition, IVs without calcium or phosphate when NPO several days, lactose intolerant, high-protein reducing diets, or other unbalanced diets.

Clients with increased loss of calcium: from diarrhea,[8] diuresis, diuretics, malabsorption, alcoholism, Cushing's syndrome, renal failure, high protein diets, pancreatitis, burns, wounds, citrated blood, metabolic alkalosis, hypoparathyroidism.

Clients with increased loss of phosphate: malabsorption, diarrhea, Cushing's syndrome, chronic respiratory alkalosis, or hyperparathyroidism.

Clients with increased need for phosphate: during the recovery phase of severe malnutrition and during tissue growth or repair.

Also, persons who are exposed to lead through plumbing or paint have decreased availability of phosphate.

Levels of Prevention

Primary Prevention

● Teach importance of well-rounded diet.[14, 48]
● Teach clients about risk factors of nonprescribed high-protein diets for weight loss, importance of consulting nutritional resource for nutrient balance.
● Encourage exercise to prevent bone demineralization.
● Increase awareness of self or fetal injury through existing home or work hazards. Refer clients with this risk to the county health department for safety guidelines such as special masks when working with lead products.
● Consult physician, local pharmacist, or dietitian, regarding vitamin and mineral supplements.

Secondary Prevention

● Monitor appetite. Document I & O accurately.
● Encourage exercise.
● Teach client to avoid high-phosphate and high-protein foods, and take prescription calcium and vitamin D supplements, if low calcium is due to hypoparathyroidism.
● Ensure that IV TPN contains calcium and phosphorus.
● Consult physician for vitamin and mineral or feeding supplement if taking less than ½ meals.
● Consult the physician for plasma phosphate level in any client with persistent hyperventilation.
● Consult physician for lactase product or calcium and vitamin D supplement if lactose intolerant.
● Report manifestations of calcium overcorrection.

Tertiary Prevention

● Encourage person to consume nutrients from each food group.
● Encourage exercise.
● Encourage family to assist with feeding debilitated or confused family members.
● Consult the physician for food, vitamin and mineral supplements.

---

calcemia, because alkalosis causes decreased calcium ionization, leading to more calcium-protein binding. The many causes of hypocalcemia are shown in Table 15–15.

Like calcium, most phosphorus in the body resides in the skeleton. A deficiency (or less than 1.2 mEq/L) is rare. Phosphorus depletion can occur as a result of prolonged and excessive intake of antacids. Administration of high levels of glucose via tube feeding or IV causes phosphorus to enter the cell for glucose phosphorylation.[66] The increased sodium found in Cushing's syndrome, the increased calcium found in hyperparathyroidism, and the decreased $PaCO_2$ in chronic respiratory alkalosis also cause phosphorus to move into the cell. Long-term malnutrition, such as occurs with alcoholism; IV therapy without phosphorus; and malabsorption syndromes can also result in hypophosphatemia. Other causes

of phosphorus deficiency include lead poisoning, burns, and mild renal loss with metabolic alkalosis.

Etiology and Risk Factors

Those at risk for hypocalcemia are children, the elderly, and people on reducing diets or with debilitating diseases that limit dietary calcium intake or absorption. Women are at risk after menopause due to the slight increase in phosphate secondary to a deficiency of estrogen. Suggestions for primary, secondary, and tertiary prevention of hypocalcemia are listed in Risk Factors and Levels of Prevention.

Risk factors for hypophosphatemia primarily consist of long-term lack of intake or loss. However, risk factors that are often forgotten include periods of increased growth or tissue repair and recovery from malnourished states. Each of these increases the demand for phosphorus.[121] Failure to meet these increased needs results in a state of phosphorus depletion.

Pathophysiology

A deficiency of PTH results in a fall in plasma calcium levels secondary to decreased bone resorption and GI absorption and increased urinary excretion of calcium (see Fig. 15–10). Decreased calcium causes a partial depolarization of nerves and muscles because of a decrease in threshold potential. Therefore, a smaller stimulus initiates the action potential (see Fig. 15–8). Pathophysiologic changes as they relate to clinical manifestations and laboratory/diagnostic findings associated with hypocalcemia are summarized in Table 15–16.

Pathophysiologic changes that occur with hypophosphatemia can affect every organ system because of the effect of hypophosphatemia on optimal ATP and oxygen supply. Phosphate depletion impairs the conversion of glucose and many other intermediate substances to ATP. The ultimate result is a disruption in the sole mechanism responsible for regeneration of the ATP.

Clinical Manifestations and Diagnostic Findings

Hypocalcemia is suspected in persons with a history that indicates a risk (see Tables 15–15 and 15–16). As you can see, most of the clinical manifestations of hypocalcemia are related to neuromuscular hyperexcitability. Numbness and tingling of the hands, toes, and lips; irritability; and anxiety are seen in mild hypocalcemia. Early signs of hypocalcemia in the person with hypoparathyroidism secondary to an overingestion of phosphate products and/or protein are cardiac palpitations and restlessness. Both phosphate and protein increase calcium binding. Findings in severe hypocalcemia are cardiac insufficiency and dysrhythmias, a prolonged QT interval, carpopedal spasm, facial twitching, seizures, laryngeal stridor, and prolonged bleeding times.[122]

Table 15–16. Clinical Manifestations and Laboratory/Diagnostic Findings: Hypocalcemia

Clinical Manifestation	Pathophysiologic Basis
Neuromuscular Manifestations	
Tetany symptoms: twitching around mouth, tingling and numbness of fingers, carpopedal spasms, facial spasm, laryngospasm, and later convulsions, tetany-death Presence of Trousseau's and Chvostek's signs	Hypocalcemia causes increased neuromuscular excitability/irritability, producing hyperactivity of the motor and sensory nerves
Respiratory Manifestations	
Dyspnea, laryngeal spasm, stridor, death	Increased nerve excitability leading to tetany
Gastrointestinal Manifestations	
Increased peristalsis, diarrhea	Calcium absorption from the intestine is decreased; decreased calcium increases smooth muscle contraction
Cardiovascular Manifestations	
Dysrhythmias, palpitations, weak pulse, hypotension	Increase in cell excitability, decreased contraction of myocardium leads to decreased cardiac output
Musculoskeletal Manifestations	
Pathologic fractures	Calcium loss from bone, trying to compensate, causes bone to be brittle
Hematologic Manifestations	
Prolonged bleeding time, hemorrhage	Intrinsic pathway for blood coagulation is inhibited
Laboratory/Diagnostic Findings	
Serum calcium <4.5 mEq/L (<9 mg/dl) iCa <2.2 mEq/L (<4.4 mg/dl) ECG: prolonged QT	Hypocalcemia is present when serum level is <4.5 mEq/L (9 mg/dl) Conduction delay

With prolonged hypocalcemia, cataracts may develop because of increased uptake of sodium and water by the lens. In addition, pathologic fractures and trophic changes, such as dry, sparse hair and rough skin, may be seen.

The primary manifestations of hypophosphatemia include decreased cardiac and respiratory function, muscle weakness, fatigue, brittle bones, bone pain, confusion, and seizures.

Recognition of phosphate deficits is challenging, as the plasma level, whether normal or low, is not always reflective of the total body phosphate content. Careful review of a client's history, laboratory data, medications, and clinical manifestations, with emphasis on nutritional health in high-risk persons, increases the likelihood of identifying total body phosphate deficiencies.

Acute and Subacute Care

■ Medical Management

Medical management is focused on determining and correcting the cause of the hypocalcemia or hypophosphatemia. Other medical management is primarily focused on dietary and/or pharmacologic interventions.

Calcium Replacement

Asymptomatic hypocalcemia is usually corrected with oral calcium gluconate, calcium lactate, or calcium chloride. For increased absorption, the calcium supplement should be given with a glass of milk 30 minutes before meals. The vitamin D in the milk promotes calcium absorption. *Exception:* Vitamin D is given in pill form to a person with hypocalcemia secondary to hypoparathyroidism. Milk products are high in phosphate, and milk consumption causes impaired calcium absorption in a person with hypoparathyroidism.

Tetany from acute hypocalcemia needs *immediate* attention. Give IV calcium chloride or calcium gluconate slowly to avoid hypotension, bradycardia, and other dysrhythmias. Use D_5W solutions when dilution is necessary; saline promotes calcium loss.

Hypophosphatemia, if associated with signs of total body phosphate deficit, is usually treated with IV replacement. This is most commonly given in the form of total parenteral nutrition (TPN) if the client suffers from other electrolyte imbalances.

Increasing Dietary Calcium

Chronic or mild hypocalcemia can be treated in part by having the client consume a diet high in calcium. Foods high in calcium are listed in Box 15–6. If hypocalcemia is secondary to parathyroid deficiency, the client must avoid high-phosphate foods, such as milk products and carbonated beverages, and excess protein. Maintenance needs are met through calcium and vitamin D supplements.

Box 15–6. High- and Low-Calcium Foods

High-Calcium Foods (>100 mg per Serving)

Dairy Products

Cheese, all types
Ice cream, 1 cup
Milk, 1 cup
Yogurt, low-fat with fruit, 1 cup

Other Foods

Oatmeal, instant, ¾ cup
Rhubarb, cooked, 1 cup
Spinach, frozen, ½ cup
Tofu, regular, ½ cup

Low-Calcium Foods (<25 mg per Serving)

Apple, 1 medium
Banana, 1 medium
Chicken breast, baked, 3 oz
Ground beef, lean, 3 oz
Oatmeal, cooked, 1 cup
Pasta, cooked, 1 cup
Vegetable juices

Data from Laquarta, I., & Gerlach, M. (1990). *Nutrition in clinical nursing.* Albany, NY: Delmar; and Burtis, G., et al. (1988). *Applied nutrition and diet therapy.* Philadelphia: W. B. Saunders.

Good sources of phosphorus include milk products, eggs, fish, whole grains, vegetables, and carbonated beverages.

■ Nursing Management of the Medical Client

The nurse should obtain a thorough history of the client's current and chronic illnesses, diet intake, and medications, including over-the-counter medications. Be sure to ask if a digitalis preparation is being taken with calcium. This combination increases the risk for digitalis potentiation.

Check for Trousseau's and Chvostek's signs in high-risk clients. The Trousseau's sign is carpopedal spasm or contraction of the fingers and hand when a blood pressure cuff is kept inflated on the upper arm for 5 minutes at diastolic pressure. A positive test result is carpopedal spasm. The Chvostek's sign is spasm of the muscles innervated by the facial nerve. It is best elicited by tapping the client's face lightly below the temple. Spasm of the face, lip, or nose would also indicate a positive test for tetany. Figure 15–11 illustrates Chvostek's and Trousseau's signs. Also assess for paresthesias.

Assess the client's cardiac status by noting changes in the ECG and vital signs, especially the apical heart rate and rhythm. Frequency varies from 1 to 4 hours, depending on the client's condition. Assess color, motion, and sensation (CMS) and pulses of peripheral tissues to provide data for evaluation of the peripheral cardiac output.

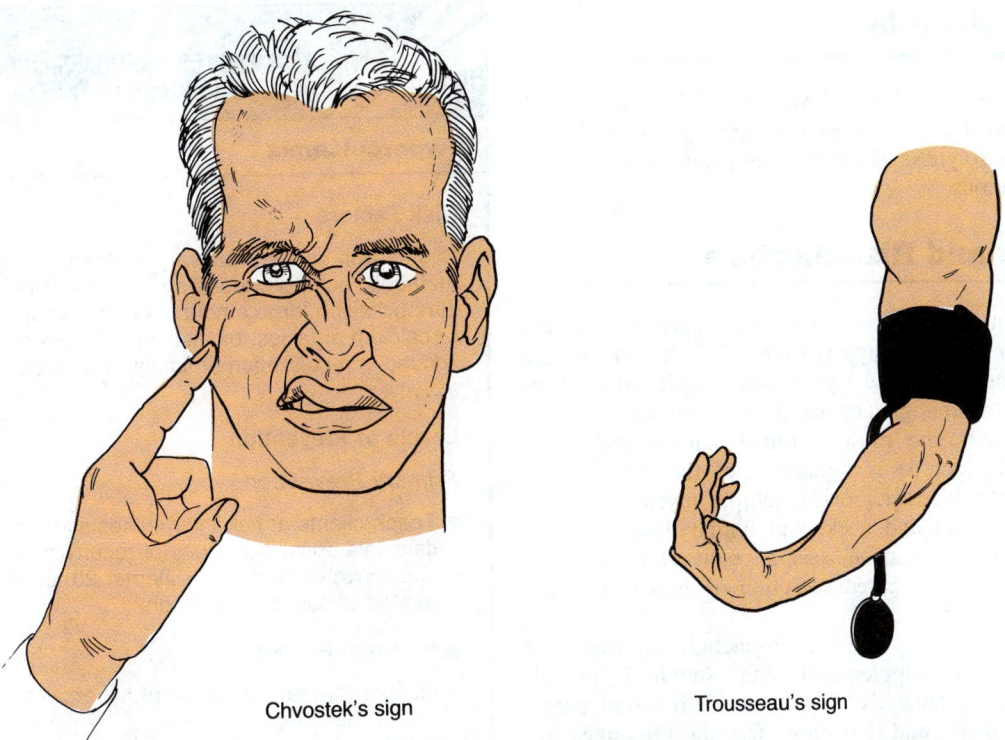

Chvostek's sign

Trousseau's sign

Figure 15–11. Chvostek's and Trousseau's signs. A calcium deficit (hypocalcemia) or magnesium deficit (hypomagnesemia) raises the resting potential of nerves. This rise allows nerve stimulation and firing with less stimulus. Touching the facial nerve adjacent to the ear produces twitching of the client's upper lip (Chvostek's sign). The hand and fingers can also spasm (Trousseau's sign or carpal pedal spasm). These spasms can occur spontaneously or when blood flow is decreased (e.g., during blood pressure cuff inflation).

Monitor also for signs of bleeding in the gums and petechiae or ecchymosis in the skin. Assess for changes in the clarity of urine, as microscopic bleeding causes clear urine to become cloudy before frank bleeding is apparent. Also, note occult, black or blood-streaked stool. Be suspicious of an intracerebral hemorrhage when a client reports new onset of headaches. Monitor plasma calcium levels for improvement or worsening.

Plasma levels of phosphate are rarely determined. Thus, the nurse's role in assisting the physician to identify hypophosphatemia is crucial in making a correct diagnosis. The nurse takes an in-depth history, emphasizing nutritional health and medication, and monitors for signs and symptoms. Monitoring a client's response to IV TPN is also essential. See Chapter 62 for more information on TPN.

In addition to an ongoing assessment, interventions include hourly monitoring of the IV site for infiltration or phlebitis when IV calcium is being infused. Calcium chloride is extremely irritating to the subcutaneous tissue. If infiltration occurs, notify the physician immediately, as tissue sloughing may occur. In either situation, change the IV site. Also notify the physician if the client's manifestations do not improve or if signs of overcorrection (hypercalcemia) occur. When possible, use fresh blood for transfusions. Avoid giving calcium and bicarbonate in the same IV, as a precipitate will form. Use filters with TPN solutions.

To prevent pathologic fractures, use caution by obtaining adequate help to turn or move the client. Use ambulation belts and/or extra personnel to walk or transfer the client to and from bed.

Instruct the client about foods that are rich in calcium, such as milk, cheese, yogurt, and green, leafy vegetables. Encourage taking of calcium supplements before meals and with vitamin D milk for better absorption. Exception: For persons with hypocalcemia secondary to hypoparathyroidism, phosphorus intake should be decreased by *omitting* milk, milk products, and other high-phosphorus foods. Calcium and vitamin D supplements are prescribed for this population as well. Several types of vitamin D are available. Therefore, the person must be advised not to take over-the-counter forms without first consulting with a physician to ensure that the right supplement is taken.

For clients with osteoporosis, see the dietary recommendations in Chapter 74.

■ Modifications for Elderly Clients

Elderly clients may have difficulty incorporating large amounts of food and fluids containing calcium into the diet. Part of the difficulty is in changing long-established eating habits. Many of today's elderly drink very little milk because of habits formed in childhood. Suggest other forms of calcium that may be more appealing, such as yogurt, cheese, milkshakes made with ice milk, or green, leafy vegetables.[14]

Hypercalcemia

Hypercalcemia is a plasma level over 5.5 mEq/L or 11 mg/dl. Hypercalcemia can occur in any age group. It is a common electrolyte disorder that can create serious physical complications.

Etiology and Risk Factors

The three most common causes of hypercalcemia are metastatic malignancy, hyperparathyroidism, and thiazide diuretic therapy. Severely high levels of calcium are usually due to the malignancy itself or to the treatment of the malignancy. The most common cancers that cause hypercalcemia include malignancies of the lung, breast, ovary, prostate, bladder, bone (multiple myeloma, leukemia), kidney, head and neck, and lymph tissues. Malignancy-induced hypercalcemia is a result of either bone destruction or an increased secretion of ectopic parathyroid hormone (PTH).

Other causes of hypercalcemia include an excessive intake of calcium supplements with vitamin D or calcium-containing antacids,[78] prolonged immobilization, metabolic acidosis, and hypophosphatemia. Prolonged immobilization causes resorption of calcium from the bone.[73] Metabolic acidosis causes displacement of bound calcium, thus increasing the plasma ionized calcium levels. The kidneys are unable to excrete the excess calcium that occurs secondary to hypophosphatemia. Suggestions for primary, secondary, and tertiary prevention of hypercalcemia are listed in Risk Factors and Levels of Prevention.

Pathophysiology

Destruction of bone tissue results in an increased release of calcium into the vascular spaces. See Chapter 23 for more information related to malignancies. Excessive PTH production promotes calcium retention, which leads to hypophosphatemia. Hypophosphatemia compounds the problem by promoting more calcium retention.

When excess calcium is present, the threshold potential becomes more positive, which results in cell membranes that are refractory to depolarization. This decreased cell membrane excitability requires a stronger stimulus for a response to occur (see Figure 15–8). As a result, cardiac and smooth muscle activity is decreased. Excess calcium in the bloodstream also impairs renal function and precipitates as a salt, which often forms renal stones. Pathophysiologic changes as they relate to the clinical manifestations and laboratory/diagnostic findings associated with hypercalcemia are summarized in Table 15–17.

Clinical Manifestations and Diagnostic Findings

The clinical manifestations of hypercalcemia, which are generally nonspecific, are determined by the plasma calcium level. Mild hypercalcemia, near 5.5 mEq/L or 11.5

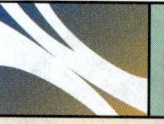

RISK FACTORS AND LEVELS OF PREVENTION

Hypercalcemia

Risk Factors

Clients with cancer, recovery or dormant state, or metabolic acidosis; those on thiazide diuretics or lithium; or taking large amounts of calcium medication or calcium antacids, or Vitamin D; those on prescribed immobilization or limited weight bearing activity.

Levels of Prevention

Primary Prevention

● Teach clients at risk the manifestations of hypercalcemia as well as signs of recurrent or metastatic involvement. See Chapter 23 for teaching related to cancer risk factors.

Secondary Prevention

● Monitor for manifestations of hypercalcemia in high risk clients.
● Monitor plasma levels.
● Perform resistive range-of-motion and increase weight bearing activities within limits of prescription.
● Consult physician for physical therapy referral.
● Consult the physician for change in diuretics if hypercalcemia secondary to thiazide therapy.

Tertiary Prevention

● Initiate resistive ROM and increase weight bearing activities within prescription guidelines as soon as possible on all clients in rehab or extended care.
● Consult the physician for a PT referral.

mg/dl, is usually asymptomatic. In mild cases, the plasma calcium level may increase momentarily when the client consumes calcium-containing antacids or a large dose of an oral calcium supplement, and the kidneys are initially unable to eliminate the excess. In moderate hypercalcemia, 6.2 mEq/L or 13 mg/dl, manifestations usually include anorexia, nausea, vomiting, polyuria, muscle weakness, fatigue, lethargy, dehydration, and constipation. Flank pain to severe renal or ureteral colic can occur if stones are present. As the hypercalcemic state becomes severe, the client becomes more lethargic and confused, and coma may result. In some instances, clients may complain of deep bone pain. Hypercalcemia is determined by the clinical manifestations and laboratory/diagnostic findings presented in Table 15–17.

Severe hypercalcemia may result in hypercalcemic crisis, which carries a 30% to 50% mortality rate. A hypercalcemic crisis occurs when calcium levels reach 7.1 mEq/L or 15 mg/dl. This level of plasma calcium can cause cardiac dysrhythmias, ECG changes (e.g., widened T wave and shortened QT interval), and cardiac arrest. Hypokalemia may occur as the body wastes potassium

Table 15–17. Clinical Manifestations and Laboratory/Diagnostic Findings: Hypercalcemia	
Clinical Manifestation	**Pathophysiologic Basis**
Gastrointestinal Manifestations	
Anorexia, nausea, vomiting, decreased peristalsis, distention, constipation	Increased calcium enhances hydrochloric acid, gastrin, and pancreatic enzyme release Slowed gastrointestinal transit time
Neuromuscular Manifestations	
Mild to moderate hypercalcemic state: weakness, fatigue, depression, difficulty in concentrating Severe hypercalcemic state: extreme lethargy, depressed sensorium, confusion, and coma	Neurologic depression
Cardiovascular Manifestations	
Dysrhythmias, heart block, cardiac arrest Digitalis toxicity	Increased transmission due to shortened repolarization, severe cardiac depression
Renal Manifestations	
Polyuria	Osmotic diuresis and volume depletion; reduces the kidney's ability to concentrate urine and results in polyuria
Kidney stones	Calcium precipitates
Renal failure	Decreased glomerular filtration due to contraction of renal vessels (decreased blood flow) from high calcium
Musculoskeletal Manifestations	
Bone pain, fracture	Cancer of the bone causes pressure on nerve endings and bone pain, which can be severe; decalcification of bones may cause osteoporosis and spontaneous fractures
Laboratory/Diagnostic Findings	
Serum calcium >5.5 mEq/L (>11.5 mg/dl)	Hypercalcemia is present when serum calcium level is > 5.5 mEq/L (11.5 mg/dl)

ABGs
  ph < 7.40
  HCO_3^- > 26 mEq/L
	Acidotic state inhibits calcium excretion from the kidneys

ECG changes: shortened ST segment, prolonged QT	Delayed transmission due to prolonged repolarization

rather than calcium. The usual treatment includes hydration with 6 to 10 L of IV normal saline in 24 hours and etidronate disodium (Didronel) therapy. If the client is not nauseated, encourage oral liquids. These actions are designed to lower the calcium level in 36 to 48 hours.[18]

Acute and Subacute Care

■ Medical Management

Immediate correction of moderate and severe hypercalcemia is essential. IV normal saline, given rapidly with furosemide to prevent fluid overload, promotes urinary calcium excretion. Antitumor antibiotics, such as plicamycin, inhibit the action of PTH on osteoclasts in bone tissue and result in a reduction of decalcification and a decrease in the plasma calcium level. However, plicamycin has many dangerous side effects. Calcitonin decreases the plasma calcium level by inhibiting the effects of PTH on the osteoclasts and increasing urinary calcium excretion. Corticosteroid drugs decrease calcium levels by competing with vitamin D, resulting in a decreased intestinal absorption of calcium, and by inhibiting prostaglandins, resulting in decreased bone resorption. IV phosphate decreases the plasma calcium level; however, it should be used cautiously because it may result in severe calcification of various tissues. Thiazide diuretics should be changed to furosemide or to another diuretic that does not cause retention of calcium. If the cause is excessive use of calcium or vitamin D supplements or calcium-containing antacids, these agents should be either avoided or used in a reduced dosage. Etidronate disodium (Didronel), a newer therapy, reduces plasma calcium by inhibiting precursors to calcium mineralization and secondarily by reducing bone formation. The client needs to be hydrated with normal saline before etidronate administration and given loop diuretics to enhance urine output and calcium excretion following drug administration. Gallium nitrate, also a new approach, has been effective in inhibiting bone resorption and decreasing osteoclastic activity. The drug should be stopped if the urinary output is less than 2 L/day or plasma creatinine is greater than 2.5 mg/dl.[47, 50, 76]

Review Box 15–6 for a list of high-calcium foods that should be restricted. Forcing fluids assists in lowering plasma levels by flushing excess calcium through the kidney. If manifestations of renal calculi are present, consumption of foods and fluids that increase urine acidity will help decrease stone formation. These include meat, cheese, eggs, whole grains, cranberry juice, and prune juice.

■ Nursing Management of the Medical Client

Since plasma calcium levels are not routinely assessed, it is essential that the nurse identify high-risk clients. This includes obtaining a thorough history, focusing on risk factors, medications (including over-the-counter calcium supplements or antacids), and diet history. Other nursing assessments include vital signs, apical pulses, and ECG every 1 to 8 hours depending on the severity of the client's manifestations. Bowel sounds, renal function, and hydration status should be assessed every 8 hours. Also, recall that it is important to monitor for fluid volume depletion secondary to hypercalcemia.

Early treatment may prevent a hypercalcemic crisis. Unless contraindicated (e.g., in clients with congestive heart failure), increase fluid intake. If flank pain or renal colic is present, strain all urine to capture renal calculi (stones). Report urinary output of less than 30 ml/hour for 2 consecutive hours. Report any manifestations that indicate worsening of the clinical status, such as an increase in dysrhythmias, a decrease in sensorium, or an overcorrection (hypocalcemia).

Instruct the client to avoid use of calcium supplements. Sodium intake is increased, unless contraindicated, to promote calcium loss through the kidneys. High-fiber foods and fluids may be suggested to prevent the constipation associated with hypercalcemia.

Provide safety precautions, including a low bed position with side rails elevated, if signs of confusion, lethargy, or coma are present. To prevent injury, turn and move the client with extreme caution and with adequate assistance. Ambulation belts, back braces, tripod canes, and walkers may be used to facilitate safer ambulation. Assist with resistive range of motion and weight-bearing activities to decrease calcium loss from bone. Report clinical manifestations of fractures immediately, such as bone pain or ecchymosis.

The client and family should be taught to continue an acid-ash diet, force fluids, and avoid calcium-containing medications. The client should also be taught to report clinical manifestations of renal calculi, such as flank pain, hematuria, or cardiac dysfunction (e.g., an irregular pulse or palpitations).

■ Surgical Management

Surgery may be used to remove an ectopic PTH-secreting tumor. Noninvasive or invasive lithotripsy or endoscopic removal of renal or ureteral calculi may be necessary. See Chapters 56 and 57 for more information related to these surgical procedures.

Hyperphosphatemia

Hyperphosphatemia is a rare but serious disorder. It is defined as a plasma phosphate level greater than 3.0 mEq/L. However, it is the total body phosphate level that determines the seriousness of the imbalance. The most common causes include excessive intake of high-phosphate foods, excess vitamin D (especially with renal insufficiency due to decreased excretion), impaired colonic motility due to increased absorption, hypoparathyroidism, and Addison's disease. Clinical manifestations are related to hyperphosphatemia or secondary hypocalcemia. Tachycardia, palpitations, and restlessness are among the earliest manifestations. Anorexia, nausea, vomiting, hyperreflexia, tetany, and more serious dysrhythmias may follow if the imbalance worsens.

In mild or asymptomatic hyperphosphatemia, the treatment focuses on limiting high-phosphate foods, especially milk products and carbonated beverages, and/or giving calcium or aluminum products to promote the binding and excretion of phosphate. Dialysis is the primary treatment for renal failure that is refractory to conservative approaches (either peritoneal dialysis or hemodialysis).[122] Nursing care focuses on assisting the physician in early detection of clinical manifestations, prevention through teaching of high-risk clients, and initiation of the nursing interventions associated with the secondary hypocalcemia. Review nursing implementation for hypocalcemia. Follow manufacturer recommendations when giving Fleet Phospho-Soda enemas. Hyperphosphatemia leading to death has been associated with Fleet Phospho-Soda enemas in the presence of altered renal or bowel function.[26]

Magnesium Imbalances

Magnesium is the second most abundant intracellular cation. The actions of magnesium in the body and the clinical manifestations of imbalance are similar to those of potassium imbalance. Fifty percent of the body's magnesium is stored in bone, 49% is contained in intracellular fluid, and 1% is contained in the extracellular fluid. Of the 1% in the plasma, 30% of the magnesium is bound to protein, 15% is combined with anions, and 55% is in a free, ionized form. Magnesium is absorbed from the small intestine at the same site at which calcium is absorbed. Thus, malabsorption affects both electrolytes. Magnesium is excreted in the urine and in small amounts in feces. See Box 15–4 for normal plasma levels. Figure 15–12 shows how magnesium balance is maintained.

The functions of magnesium include the transmission and conduction of nerve impulses and the contraction of skeletal, smooth, and cardiac muscle. Magnesium accomplishes this through its effect on more than 300 enzyme

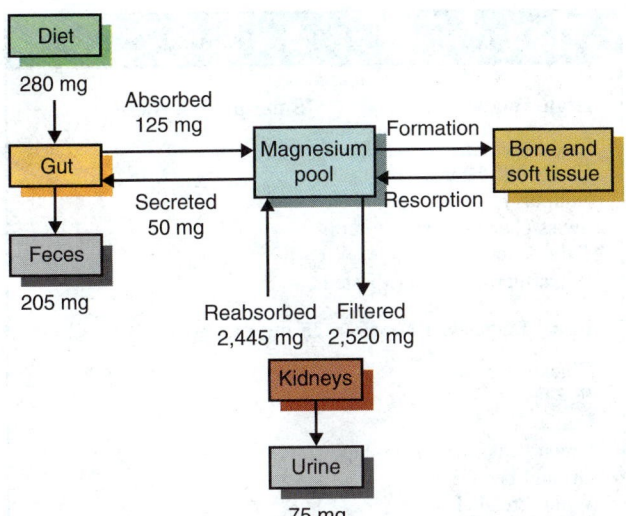

Figure 15–12. Magnesium homeostasis. A pool of magnesium exists in the body and is kept in balance by dietary intake, bowel and kidney excretion, and bone and soft tissue formation and resorption.

systems. It is responsible for the transportation of sodium and potassium across the cell membrane (sodium-potassium pump) and the synthesis and release of parathormone. Therefore, a deficit can lead to hypokalemia and hypocalcemia. Magnesium is necessary for the conversion of ATP to ADP and, thus, the release of energy. It influences the utilization of potassium, sodium, calcium, and phosphate, and it activates enzymes that are necessary for the metabolism of carbohydrates, proteins, lipids, and vitamin B_{12}. Finally, magnesium promotes vasodilation of peripheral arteries and arterioles.

Increased calcium or phosphorus intake can decrease magnesium absorption from the intestines. Conversely, a low calcium level increases magnesium absorption from the intestines.

Hypomagnesemia

Hypomagnesemia is defined as a plasma magnesium level below 1.5 mEq/L or 1.8 mg/dl. Magnesium deficits are being identified more often as a result of increased knowledge about this ion. Twenty-two percent to 42% of clients with calcium, phosphate, sodium, and potassium imbalances have been found to have a co-existing magnesium imbalance.[2] As with other intracellular ions, plasma levels may be normal in the presence of intracellular depletion. Also, hypomagnesemia is often overlooked because tests for plasma magnesium levels are not routinely ordered until a severe deficit has occurred. Plasma levels may be helpful in severe or acute changes, but a 24 hour urinalysis after an IV magnesium challenge, ion selective imaging, or nuclear MRI (to determine soft tissue levels) is more predictive of total body magnesium levels.[2] It is a rare imbalance in people who consume a well-balanced diet. However, it is becoming recognized as a common cause of refractory hypokalemia and hypocalcemia.[2, 65, 116] (*Refractory* means not responsive to treatment.) The hy-

pomagnesemic state inhibits potassium reabsorption; hypomagnesemia therefore needs to be normalized before potassium and calcium imbalances respond to treatment.

Magnesium deficits are often seen in the critically ill[39, 96] and in alcoholics. Alcoholism decreases intestinal absorption secondary to a decrease in enzymes that are normally produced by the liver. Alcoholism also promotes magnesium wasting due to nephrotoxicity and leads to malnutrition. Other causes of hypomagnesemia include severe or chronic malnutrition; malabsorption syndromes, such as Crohn's or celiac disease or pancreatitis; and gastrointestinal losses secondary to vomiting, GI suction, diarrhea, high-volume ileostomies, fistulas, laxative abuse, or radiation enteritis. Renal losses include the diuretic phase of acute renal failure and hyperphosphatemia. Prolonged IV or TPN therapy without magnesium replacement also increases the risk for hypomagnesemia. Excess calcium (e.g., in hyperparathyroidism) and excess sodium (e.g., in Cushing's syndrome or hyperaldosteronism) inhibit magnesium. The hyperglycemia seen in diabetic acidosis causes osmotic diuresis and loss of magnesium. Alkalosis is also associated with hypomagnesemia. Pregnancy and/or lactation increase the demand for magnesium. Low plasma magnesium levels are also associated with toxemia of pregnancy.[2, 65]

Many medications increase the risk of hypomagnesemia. Excessive amounts of phosphorus in the intestine (e.g., from overuse of antacids) inhibit the uptake of magnesium from the intestinal villi. Some medications interfere with renal handling of magnesium as either a primary action or a side effect. The primary drugs are diuretics and antibiotics. Loop, osmotic, and thiazide diuretics; aminoglycoside antibiotics (gentamicin, tobramycin); carbenicillin; amphotericin B; cisplatin; corticosteroids; and digitalis are the usual offenders. The neurologic trauma associated with cocaine abuse is also being linked to hypomagnesemia.[2]

The mechanism behind the myocardial irritability seen with hypomagnesemia seems to be a result of changes in the resting membrane potential associated with the altered relationship between the potassium and the magnesium ions. It is thought to be secondary to the stimulation of beta-2 adrenergic cells or, more commonly, associated with digitalis intake. Magnesium depletion and digitalis both promote potassium loss from myocardial cells. Digitalis uptake also seems to be increased in hypomagnesemia.[116] GI changes from decreased contractility, such as anorexia, nausea, and abdominal distention, can occur. Psychological disorders, such as depression, psychosis, and confusion, may also develop.[30, 111]

Severe hypomagnesemia causes neuromuscular manifestations such as Chvostek's and Trousseau's signs, tetany, convulsions, and vasospasm leading to stroke. Cardiac dysrhythmias include premature ventricular contractions, atrial or ventricular fibrillation, and ECG changes (e.g., prolonged QT intervals, widened QRS complexes, and broadening of T waves). Other ECG changes are related to the accompanying low levels of potassium. Low magnesium levels have been linked with increased ventricular dysrhythmias and decreased 1-year survival rates in persons with CHF as well as with lethal dysrhythmias in clients with myocardial infarctions.[3, 116]

Studies are also suggesting a link between estrogen therapy in postmenopausal women and increased coagulation risk; estrogen promotes tissue uptake of magnesium and, thus, hypomagnesemia. IV magnesium reduces bronchoreactivity and has been found useful in the treatment of acute asthma that has been refractory to other therapy. The positive inotropic, negative chronotropic, and vasodilatory effects of magnesium have also been found to increase cardiac output and decrease oxygen consumption in persons with shock and sepsis. Magnesium has also been successfully used as a mood stabilizer in persons suffering from bipolar disease.[2]

Treatment of hypomagnesemia includes oral magnesium replacement in the form of magnesium-containing antacids or parenteral magnesium sulfate. Increasing dietary intake of magnesium also helps ensure balance and stability.

Nursing management includes monitoring vital signs every 4 to 8 hours and reviewing ECG readings hourly, depending on the client's condition. Safety and seizure precautions should be initiated for persons who are extremely confused or at risk for seizure. Plasma magnesium, potassium, and calcium levels should be monitored. Also, many experts recommend assessing the client's deep tendon reflexes. The presence of normal reflexes is indicative of normal body magnesium levels.[65]

Nurses should consult the physician for magnesium maintenance/replacement if severe malnutrition exists, if the client is NPO for more than 3 days (especially in the presence of coexisting losses), or if manifestations of hypokalemia or hypocalcemia persist even after treatment. TPN may be necessary for the coexistence of other nutrient imbalances, which is common. Studies suggest that 25% to 40% of diabetics who have hyperglycemia also have hypomagnesemia.[65, 70] Therefore, maintaining glucose control in persons with diabetes mellitus will decrease the risk for hypomagnesemia.

When administering magnesium intravenously, dilute it according to pharmacy recommendations. Rapid infusion of magnesium sulfate can cause a hot or flushed feeling and phlebitis. Avoid giving magnesium in saline solutions.

Instructing clients and family about foods rich in magnesium may prevent a magnesium deficiency or correct a mild deficit. See Box 15–7 for a list of high- and low-magnesium foods. Caution clients about taking mineral supplements without the advice of a dietitian or pharmacist. The calcium-to-magnesium ratio should be maintained at 4:1; a greater ratio can cause deposition of calcium in the soft tissues and vessels.[2] Taking magnesium without potassium causes potassium shifting into the cell. In the alcoholic, magnesium should be taken with thiamine to promote nerve regeneration.[2]

Hypermagnesemia

Hypermagnesemia is defined as a plasma magnesium level greater than 2.5 mEq/L or 3.0 mg/dl. It is a rare disorder. Hypermagnesemia may occur with renal insufficiency, excessive use of magnesium-containing antacids or laxatives, or administration of potassium-sparing diuretics. Many potassium-sparing diuretics conserve magnesium. Hypermagnesemia is also seen with severe dehydration from ketoacidosis, in conditions that decrease the synthesis of aldosterone (e.g., Addison's disease or adrenalectomy), and from overuse of IV magnesium sulfate for controlling premature labor or pregnancy-induced hypertension.

Clinical manifestations are related to the blockage of the release of acetylcholine from the myoneural junction, which results in a decrease in muscle cell activity. With mild hypermagnesemia, peripheral vessels dilate, causing hypotension. ECG changes include prolonged PR and QT intervals. Extreme hypermagnesemia has a more profound sedative effect on the neuromuscular system, leading to severe muscle weakness, lethargy, drowsiness, loss of deep tendon reflexes, respiratory paralysis, and loss of consciousness. Cardiac signs include delayed myocardial conduction as seen in ECG changes, such as wide QRS complexes, elevated T wave, heart block, and premature ventricular contractions.

Treatment of hypermagnesemia includes decreasing the use of magnesium sulfate and enhancing its elimination. A saline infusion with a diuretic increases renal elimination of magnesium. However, a side effect of the treatment is a loss of calcium. Hypocalcemia may intensify the hypermagnesemic state. Calcium antagonizes magnesium. Thus, IV calcium salts in solution have been used for extreme hypermagnesemia. Albuterol is a drug being used to reduce magnesium levels. The presence of severe respiratory distress requires ventilatory assistance. If renal failure is present, hemodialysis may be necessary.[112]

Nurses should monitor for early signs of hypermagnesemia in high-risk clients. Assessments include vital signs, respiratory function, ECG recordings, urinary output, and the level of sensorium; these should be performed every 1 to 4 hours, depending on the client's condition. Safety/seizure precautions should be initiated if

Box 15–7. High- and Low-Magnesium Foods

High-Magnesium Foods (>75 mg per Serving)

Cashews, roasted, ¼ cup
Chili, with beans, 1 cup
Halibut, baked, 3 oz
Swiss chard, cooked, ½ cup
Tofu, ½ cup
Wheat germ, ¼ cup, toasted

Low-Magnesium Foods (<25 mg per Serving)

Chicken breast, 3 oz
Egg, 1
Fruits
Green peas, frozen, ½ cup
Ground beef, 3 oz
White bread, 1 slice

Data from Mahan, K. L., & Arlin, M. (1992). *Food, nutrition and diet therapy* (8th ed.). Philadelphia: W. B. Saunders.)

confusion or seizure risk is present. Changes in deep tendon reflexes should be reported. Remember, if the person has normal reflexes, body levels of magnesium are normal. Keep IV calcium salts in the code cart for emergency reversal of severe hypermagnesemia.

Fifty-five percent of diabetics who have hypoglycemia have also been found to have hypermagnesemia. Therefore, maintaining glucose control in persons with diabetes mellitus may decrease the risk of hypermagnesemia. Also teach clients to avoid constant use of laxatives and antacids containing magnesium, especially if urinary output is decreased. Encourage eating foods that contain fiber and drinking adequate fluids to promote fecal elimination.

Conclusions

Fluid and electrolyte disorders are fairly common problems. A fluid or electrolyte imbalance rarely occurs in isolation. The nurse must anticipate multiple imbalances in high-risk persons regardless of the setting (e.g., community, acute, or long-term). Nurses play a key role in primary, secondary, and tertiary prevention of fluid and electrolyte imbalances. This role includes the following:

Teaching clients and their families about positive health behaviors, about the importance of nutrient intake (even during non-acute illnesses), and about manifestations of fluid and electrolyte imbalance that necessitate physician consultation

Promoting nutritional maintenance and replacement in clients who are at high risk or who are experiencing fluid and/or electrolyte imbalance

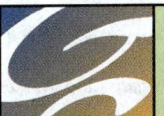

CRITICAL MONITORING

Fluid and Electrolyte Imbalance Secondary To Any Etiology

- New onset of dysrhythmia
- Worsening of dysrhythmia, such as premature ventricular contractions greater than 6 per minute, bradycardia less than 50, tachycardia greater than 120
- Sudden change in level of consciousness, including sudden restlessness, lethargy, convulsions
- Tetany, laryngeal spasm or stridor
- Postural systolic blood pressure drop greater than 25 mm Hg with a pulse increase of 30 or more
- Rapid weight loss
- Severe dryness of oral mucous membranes with tongue furrowing
- Hemorrhage
- Urinary output less than 30 ml/hour for two consecutive hours
- Rapid weight gain, especially with sudden pulmonary signs such as crackles, dyspnea, S$_3$ gallop

Assisting the physician in early detection of imbalances and of poor response to treatment or signs of overcorrection

Promoting balanced nutrition in rehabilitation or extended care settings through family support, early physician referrals for supplements, dietary consults, or management of imbalances

During this era of health cost explosion, the nurse plays a pivotal role in cost containment through primary, secondary, and tertiary prevention.

Thinking Critically

1. The admitting receptionist just called your floor to secure a room for a 69-year-old woman with a history of 2 days of vomiting and diarrhea and a fever of 103° F secondary to suspected influenza virus. The client has a history of hypertension and congestive heart failure. Home prescriptions include digoxin, 0.125 mg/day; furosemide (Lasix), 40 mg bid; and potassium chloride, 40 mEq/day. The client has also been advised to consume a low-sodium diet. An IV of 5% dextrose/normal saline, with 30 mEq of potassium chloride was started.

Factors to Consider. Will you place the patient in a private or a semi-private room? What assessments are a priority? What interventions should you anticipate?

2. A middle-aged client is admitted to your unit with shock-like symptoms. He has pale skin, cold extremities, a weak, rapid pulse, and hypotension. There is a decrease in the output of urine via the indwelling catheter. His level of consciousness varies from adequate response to little or no response to external stimuli. What are the implications for care of the client who has a fluid shift associated with third spacing? How does management differ when the fluid shifts from the vascular space to the interstitial space? From the interstitial space to the vascular space?

Factors to Consider. What assessments are important? What occurs to the body when the fluid shifts from one space to the other and back?

Bibliography

1. Abraham, W., & Schrier, R. (1994). Body fluid volume regulation in health and disease. *Advances in Internal Medicine, 39,* 23–43.
2. Altura, B., et al. (1994). Magnesium: Growing in clinical importance. *Patient Care, 28*(1), 130–150.
3. Altura, B., et al. (1994). Magnesium therapy: Coming of age. *Patient Care, 28*(2), 79–94.
4. Andrews, M., et al. (1993). Dehydration in terminally ill patients. *Postgraduate Medicine, 93*(1), 201–208.
5. Attah, C. (1993). Effect of continuous irrigation with normal saline

after prostatectomy. *International Urology Nephrology, 25*(5), 461–467.

6. Banasik, J. (1995). Alterations in cardiac function. In L. Copstead (Ed.), *Perspectives on pathophysiology* (pp. 346–374). Philadelphia: W. B. Saunders

7. Batcheller, J. (1994). Syndrome of inappropriate antidiuretic hormone secretion. *Critical Care Nursing Clinics of North America, 6*(4), 687–692.

8. Binder, H. (1990). Pathophysiology of acute diarrhea. *American Journal of Medicine, 88*(S6A), 2S–4S.

9. Birney, M., & Penny, D. (1990). Atrial natriuretic peptide: A hormone with implications for clinical practice. *Heart and Lung, 19*(2), 174–183.

10. Bowman, M., et al. (1989). Effect of tube-feeding osmolality serum sodium levels. *Critical Care Nurse, 9*(1), 22–28.

11. Brown, R. (1993). Disorders of water and sodium balance. *Postgraduate Medicine, 93*(4), 227–246.

12. Burge, F. (1993). Dehydration symptoms of palliative care cancer patients. *Journal of Pain and Symptom Management, 8*(7), 454–464.

13. Carpenito, L. (1993). *Nursing diagnosis: Application to clinical practice* (5th ed.). Philadelphia: J. B. Lippincott.

14. Constans, T., et al. (1994). Effects of nutrition education on calcium intake in the elderly. *Journal of the American Dietetic Association, 94*(4), 447–448.

15. Cosgray, R., et al. (1993). A program for water-intoxicated patients at a state hospital. *Clinical Nurse Specialist, 7*(2), 55–61.

16. Cullin, L. (1992). Interventions related to fluid and electrolyte balance. *Nursing Clinics of North America, 27*(2), 569–597.

17. Davidhizar, R., & Kriesl, R. (1993). Water intoxication: One nursing staff's response and intervention. *Journal of Advanced Nursing, 18*, 1975–1980.

18. Davis, K., Attie, M. (1991). Management of severe hypercalcemia. *Critical Care Clinics, 7*(1), 175–189.

19. DeAngelis, R. (1992). Hypokalemia. *Critical Care Nurse, 12*(7), 71–75.

20. DeAngelis, R., & Lessig, M. (1992). Hyperkalemia. *Critical Care Nurse, 12*(3), 55–59.

21. Diringer, M. (1992). Management of sodium abnormalities in patients with CNS disease. *Clinical Neuropharmacology, 15*(6), 427–444.

22. Dwyer, K., et al. (1992). Severe hypophosphatemia in postoperative patients. *Nutrition in Clinical Practice, 7*, 279–283.

23. Edes, T., et al. (1990). Diarrhea in tube-fed patients: Feeding formula not necessarily the cause. *American Journal of Medicine, 88*, 91–93.

24. Epstein, C. (1991). Fluid volume deficit for the adrenal crisis patient. *Dimensions of Critical Care Nursing, 10*(4), 210–218.

25. Escott-Stump, S. (1992). *Nutrition and diagnosis related care* (3rd ed.). Philadelphia: Lea & Febiger, 1992.

26. Fass, R., Son, D., & Hixson, L. (1993). Fatal hyperphosphatemia following Fleet Phospho-Soda in a patient with colonic ileus. *The American Journal of Gastroenterology, 88*(6), 929–932.

27. Faull, C., Holmes, C., & Baylis, P. (1993). Water balance in elderly people: Is there a deficiency of vasopressin? *Age and Ageing, 22*, 114–120.

28. Felver, L., & Pendarvis, J. (1989). Electrolyte imbalances: Intraoperative risk factors. *AORN, 49*(4), 992–1008.

29. Fischbach, F. (1992). *A manual of laboratory and diagnostic tests* (4th ed.). Philadelphia: J. B. Lippincott.

30. Friday, B., & Reinhart, R. (1991). Magnesium metabolism: A case report and literature review. *Critical Care Nurse, 11*(5), 62–71.

31. Gershan, J., et al. (1990). Fluid volume deficit: Validating the indicators. *Heart and Lung, 19*(2), 152–156.

32. Giesecke, A., et al. (1990). Fluid therapy and the resuscitation of traumatic shock. *Critical Care Clinics, 6*(1), 61–71.

33. Graber, M., & Corish, D. (1991).The electrolytes in hyponatremia. *American Journal of Kidney Diseases, 18*(5), 527–545.

34. Gross, C., et al. (1992). Clinical indicators of dehydration severity in elderly patients. *Journal of Emergency Medicine, 10*(3), 267–274.

35. Guyton, A., & Hall, J. (1996). *Textbook of medical physiology* (9th ed.). Philadelphia: W. B. Saunders.

36. Hall, J. (1994). Caring for corpses or killing patients? *Nursing Management, 25*(10), 81–89.

37. Hawthorne, J., et al. (1992). Common electrolyte imbalances associated with malignancy. *AACN, 3*(3), 714–722.

38. Henkelman, W., et al. (1991). Fluid volume dynamics. *Critical Care Nurse, 11*(4), 74–76.

39. Holtzman, G. (1990). Magnesium. *Critical Care Nurse, 10*(7), 81–83.

40. Hoot-Martin, J., & Larsen, P. (1994). Dehydration in the elderly surgical patient. *AORN, 60*(4), 666–671.

41. Howard, R., & Schrier, R. (1990). A unifying hypothesis of sodium and water regulation in health and disease. *Hormone Research, 34*, 118–123.

42. Incalzi, R., et al. (1992). Post-operative electrolyte imbalance: Its incidence and prognostic implications for elderly orthopaedic patients. *Age and Ageing, 22*, 325–331.

43. Inman, K., et al. (1993). Clinical utility and cost-effectiveness of an air suspension bed in the prevention of pressure ulcers. *JAMA, 269*(9), 1139–1143.

44. Innerarity, S. (1992). Hyperkalemic emergencies. *Critical Care Nursing Quarterly, 14*(4), 32–39.

45. Jones, A., et al. (1991). Fluid volume dynamics. *Critical Care Nurse, 11*(4), 74–75.

46. Kamel, K., et al. (1990). Urine electrolytes and osmolality: When and how to use them. *American Journal of Nephrology, 10*(2), 89–102.

47. Kaplan, M. (1994). Hypercalcemia of malignancy: A review of advances in pathophysiology. *Oncology Nursing Forum, 21*(6), 1039–1046.

48. Karanja, N., et al. (1994). Impact of increasing calcium in the diet on nutrient consumption, plasma lipids, and lipoproteins in humans. *American Journal of Clinical Nutrition, 59*(4), 900–907.

49. Karb, V. (1989). Electrolyte abnormalities and drugs which commonly cause them. *Journal of Neuroscience Nursing, 21*(2), 125–128.

50. Kaye, T. (1994). Hypercalcemia. *Postgraduate Medicine, 97*(1), 153–160.

51. Kee, J. (1991). *Laboratory and diagnostic tests with nursing implications* (3rd ed.). Norwalk, CT: Appleton & Lange.

52. Kelso, L. (1992). Fluid and electrolyte disturbances in liver failure. *AACN, 3*(3), 681–685.

53. Koivisto, V., et al. (1992). Fuel and fluid homeostasis during long-term exercise in healthy subjects and type I diabetic patients. *Diabetes Care, 15*(4), 1736–1742.

54. Kokko, J., & Tannen, R. (1990). *Fluids and electrolytes* (2nd ed.). Philadelphia: W. B. Saunders.

55. Kositzke, J. (1990). A question of balance: Dehydration in the elderly. *Journal of Gerontological Nursing, 16*(5), 4–11.

56. Krueger, S., et al. (1994). Treatment of heart failure: Update 1994. *Nebraska Medical Journal, 8*, 292–297.

57. Kuhn, M. (1991). Colloids vs. crystalloids. *Critical Care Nurse, 11*(5), 37–51.

58. Lacy, J. (1991). Albumin overview: Use as a nutritional marker and as a therapeutic intervention. *Critical Care Nurse, 11*(1), 46–49.

59. Laquarta, I., & Gerlach, M. (1990). *Nutrition in clinical nursing.* Albany, NY: Delmar.

60. Leier, C., Livio, D., & Metra, M. (1994). Clinical relevance and management of the major electrolyte abnormalities in congestive heart failure: Hyponatremia, hypokalemia, and hypomagnesemia. *American Heart Journal, 128*(3), 564–574.

61. Lowe, R., Arst, H., & Ellis, B. (1991). Rational ordering of electrolytes in the emergency department. *Annals of Emergency Medicine, 20*(1), 35–40.

62. Mahan, K., & Arlin, M. (1992). *Food, nutrition and diet therapy* (8th ed.). Philadelphia: W. B. Saunders.

63. Mahon, S., & Casperson, D. (1993). Pathophysiology of hypokalemia in patients with cancer: Implications for nurses. *Oncology Nursing Forum, 20*(6), 937–948.

64. Marchi, S., et al. (1993). Renal tubular dysfunction in chronic alcohol abuse: Effects of abstinence. *New England Journal of Medicine, 329*(26), 1927–1934.

65. Matz, R. (1993). Magnesium: Deficiencies and therapeutic uses. *Hospital Practice, 28*(4A), 79–92.

66. Matz, R. (1994). Parallels between treated uncontrolled diabetes and the refeeding syndrome with emphasis on fluid and electrolyte abnormalities. *Diabetes Care, 17*(10), 1209–1213.

67. Maughan, R. (1992). Fluid balance and exercise. *International Journal of Sports Medicine, 13*, S132–S135.
68. McCance, K., & Huether, S. (1994). *Pathophysiology: The biologic basis for disease in adults and children* (2nd ed.). St. Louis: Mosby–Year Book.
69. McCullough, M., et al. (1991). Feasibility of outpatient electrolyte balance studies. *Journal of the American College of Nutrition, 10*(2), 140–148.
70. McDermott, K., Almadrones, L., & Bajorunas, D. (1991). The diagnosis and management of hypomagnesemia: A unique treatment approach and case report. *Oncology Nursing Forum, 18*(7), 1145–1152.
71. Mendyka, B. (1992). Fluid and electrolyte disorders caused by diuretic therapy. *AACN, 3*(3), 672–680.
72. Metheny, N. (1992). *Fluid and electrolyte balance: Nursing considerations* (2nd ed.). Philadelphia: J. B. Lippincott.
73. Meythaler, J., Tuel, S., & Cross, L. (1993). Successful treatment of immobilization hypercalcemia using calcitonin and etidronate. *Archives of Physical Medicine Rehabilitation, 74*, 316–319.
74. Miller, C. (1995). *Nursing care of older adults: Theory and practice* (pp. 133–537, 2nd ed.). Philadelphia, J. B. Lippincott.
75. Mulloy, A., & Caruana, R. (1995). Hyponatremic emergencies. *Medical Clinics of North America, 79*(1), 155–169.
76. Mundy, G. (1994). Evaluation and treatment of hypercalcemia. *Hospital Practice, 6*, 79–86.
77. Musgrave, C. (1990). Terminal dehydration: To give or not give intravenous fluids? *Cancer Nursing, 13*(1), 62–66.
78. Newmark, K., & Nugent, P. (1993). Milk-alkali syndrome. *Postgraduate Medicine, 93*(6), 149–156.
79. Olin, B., et al. (1994). *Drug facts and comparisons.* St. Louis: Wolters Kluwer.
80. Oster, J., & Materson, B. (1992). Renal and electrolyte complications of congestive heart failure and effects of therapy with angiotensin-converting enzyme inhibitors. *Archives of Internal Medicine, 152*, 704–710.
81. Palmer, T. (1990). Anorexia nervosa, bulimia nervosa: Causal theories and treatment. *Nurse Practitioner, 15*(4), 12–21.
82. Phillips, P., Johnston, C., & Gray, L. (1992). Disturbed fluid and electrolyte homeostasis following dehydration in elderly people. *Age and Ageing, 22*, 26–33.
83. Porth, C., & Erickson, M. (1992). Physiology of thirst and drinking: Implication for nursing practice. *Heart and Lung 21*(3), 273–282.
84. Puterbaugh, S. (1991). Fluid volume deficit related to active loss. *Today's OR Nurse, 13*(9), 35–36.
85. Radke, K. (1994). The aging kidney: Structure, function, and nursing practice implications. *ANNA, 21*(4), 181–190.
86. Reber, P., & Heath, H. (1995). Hypocalcemic emergencies. *Medical Clinics of North America, 79*(1), 93–107.
87. Rehrer, N. (1994). The maintenance of fluid balance during exercise. *International Journal of Sports Medicine, 15*, 122–125.
88. Rice, V. (1991). Shock, a clinical syndrome: An update. Part 1. *Critical Care Nurse, 11*(4), 20–27.
89. Rice, V. (1991). Shock, a clinical syndrome: An update. Part 3. *Critical Care Nurse, 11*(6), 34–39.
90. Rice, V. (1991). Shock, a clinical syndrome: An update. Part 4. *Critical Care Nurse,* 11(7), 28–38.
91. Ribbe, D., & Thelander, B. (1994). Patients with disordered water balance. *Journal of Psychosocial Nursing, 32*(10), 35–42.
92. Rolls, B., & Phillips, P. (1990). Aging and disturbances of thirst and fluid balance. *Nutritional Reviews, 48*(3), 137–144.
93. Rousseau, P. (1992). Why give IV fluids to the dying? *Patient Care, 26*(12), 71–74.
94. Rutecki, G. W., & Whittier, F. C. (1994). Hyponatremia: Cause of hypotonicity directs management. *Consultant, 34*(5), 705–707, 711–712.
95. Rutecki, G., & Whittier, F. (1994). Hyponatremia: Physiologic clues to a state of disordered tonicity. *Consultant, 34*(5), 688–690, 700–702.
96. Salem, M., et al. (1991). Hypomagnesemia in critical illness. *Critical Care Clinics, 7*(1), 225–247.
97. Sands, J., & Kokko, J. (1990). Countercurrent mechanism. *Kidney International, 38*: 695–699.
98. Schuller, D., Calandrino, F., & Schuster, D. (1991). Fluid balance during pulmonary edema. *Chest, 100*(4), 1068–1075.
99. Seshadri, V., & Meyer-Tettambel, O. (1993). Electrolyte and drug management in nutritional support. *Critical Care Nursing Clinics of North America, 5*(1), 31–36.
100. Shipway, K. (1992). Bartter's syndrome: A chronic electrolyte losing syndrome. *ANNA, 19*(6), 559–565.
101. Sica, D. (1994). Renal disease, electrolyte abnormalities, and acid-base imbalance in the elderly. *Clinics in Geriatric Medicine, 10*(1), 197–211.
102. Simmons, B., et al. (1990). Infection control for home health. *Infection Control Hospital Epidemiology, 11*(7), 362–370.
103. Snider, K., & Boyd, M. (1991). When they drink too much: Nursing interventions for patients with disordered water balance. *Journal of Psychosocial Nursing, 29*(7), 10–16.
104. Sommers, M. (1990). Fluid resuscitation following multiple trauma. *Critical Care Nurse, 10*(10), 74–81.
105. Sonnenblick, M., Friedlander, Y., & Rosin, A. (1993). Diuretic-induced severe hyponatremia. *Chest, 103*(2), 601–606.
106. Sterns, R. (1991). The management of hyponatremic emergencies. *Critical Care Clinics, 7*(1), 127–141.
107. Stucky, L. (1993). Acute tumor lysis syndrome: Assessment and nursing implications. *Oncology Nursing Forum, 20*(1), 49–59.
108. Sutcliffe, J., & Holmes, S. (1994). Dehydration: Burden or benefit to the dying patient? *Journal of Advanced Nursing, 19*, 71–76.
109. Terry, J. (1994). The major electrolytes: Sodium, potassium, and chloride. *Journal of Intravenous Nursing, 17*(5), 240–247.
110. Toto, K. (1994). Regulation of plasma osmolality. *Critical Care Nursing Clinics of North America, 6*(4), 661–674.
111. Toto, K., & Yucha, C. (1994). Magnesium. *Critical Care Nursing Clinics of North America, 6*(4), 767–783.
112. Van Hook, J. (1991). Hypermagnesemia. *Critical Care Clinics, 7*(1), 215–223.
113. Vaska, P. (1992). Fluid and electrolyte imbalances after cardiac surgery. *AACN, 3*(3), 664–670.
114. Vieweg, W. (1994). Treatment strategies in the polydipsia-hyponatremia syndrome. *Journal of Clinical Psychiatry, 55*(4), 154–160.
115. Wandel, J. (1990). The use of postural vital signs in the assessment of fluid volume status. *Journal of Professional Nursing, 6*(1), 46–54.
116. Wester, P. (1992). Electrolyte balance in heart failure and the role of magnesium ions. *The American Journal of Cardiology, 70*(44C–49C), 93.
117. Williams, M. (1991). Hyperkalemia. *Critical Care Clinics, 7*(1), 155–173.
118. Wood, N. (1992). Reader offers strategies of identification and treatment of dilutional hyponatremia. *Nurse Practitioner, 17*(10), 9–10, 16.
119. Woodtli, A. (1990). Thirst: A critical care nursing challenge. *Dimensions of Critical Care Nursing, 9*(1), 6–15.
120. Yucha, C., & McKay, S. (1992). Idiopathic edema. *ANNA, 19*(1), 29–32.
121. Yucha, C., & Toto, K. (1994). Calcium and phosphorus derangements. *Critical Care Nursing Clinics of North America, 6*(4), 747–766.
122. Zaloga, G. (1991). Hypocalcemic crisis. *Critical Care Clinics, 7*(1), 191–199.

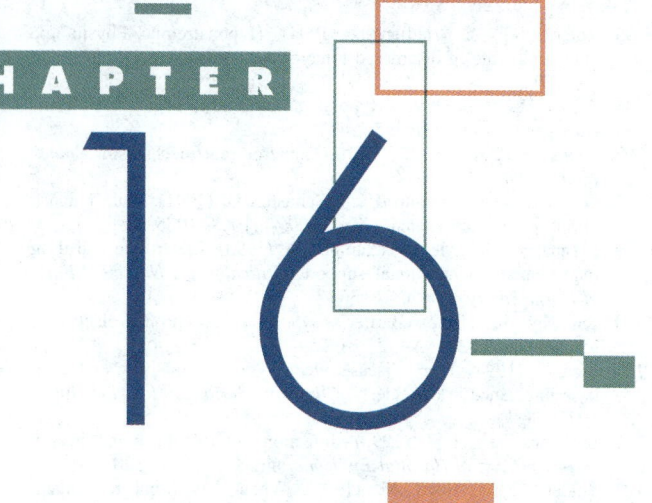

Acid-Base Disorders

Margie J. Hansen

Normal function of body cells depends on regulation of hydrogen ion concentration [H⁺] within very narrow limits. Acid-base imbalances occur when these limits are exceeded and are recognized clinically as abnormalities of serum pH. Because acid-base imbalances may result from disorders of virtually any body system, their incidence in clinical settings is very high. The nurse is responsible, along with other healthcare professionals, for prevention, detection, and intervention in acid-base imbalances.

Regulation of Acid-Base Balance

The symbol pH stands for the negative log of the hydrogen ion concentration. It is used to express the degree of acidity or alkalinity of a solution. A pH of 7.0 is neutral, having an equal number of acids and bases. An acidic solution has a pH below 7.0; an alkaline solution has a pH above 7.0. Because pH is the *negative* log, a rise in pH reflects a fall in H⁺. Conversely, a decline in pH indicates an increase in H⁺.

Normal serum pH is 7.35 to 7.45. Cell function is seriously impaired when pH falls to 7.2 or lower or rises to 7.55 or higher. Rapid *rates* of change in pH are especially detrimental. Serum pH below 6.8 or above 7.8 may be incompatible with life.

Three physiologic systems act interdependently to maintain normal serum pH: excretion of acid by the *lungs,* excretion of acid or reclamation of base by the *kidneys,* and buffering of excess acid or base by *chemical buffer systems.*

Regulation of Volatile Acid by the Lungs

Volatile acids are acids that can be converted to gases. As a consequence of normal ventilation, the lungs exhale large quantities of "potential" acid in the form of carbon dioxide gas (CO_2). CO_2 is continuously produced by body cells as an end product of complete oxidative metabolism of nutrients for energy. CO_2 diffuses from body cells into venous blood, where it may combine with water to form carbonic acid. Carbonic acid then dissociates, or separates into its component ions, H⁺ and HCO_3^-. This *hydrolysis reaction,* which is reversible, is shown below:

$$H_2O + CO_2 \rightleftarrows H_2CO_3 \rightleftarrows HCO_3^- + H^+$$

It is apparent from this equation that CO_2 and H_2CO_3 are directly related. As CO_2 levels in the blood rise, acid [H⁺] levels also rise, and pH declines. The reverse is also true. The hydrolysis reaction also demonstrates that some of the CO_2 entering the blood forms the base, bicarbonate (HCO_3^-). While some hydrolysis occurs in the plasma, most takes place within the cytoplasm of the red blood cell (RBC), where the enzyme *carbonic anhydrase* (CA) catalyzes the reaction at much more rapid rates than in the plasma. Presence of CA in other cells, notably the renal tubular cells, is also important to acid-base homeostasis, as discussed later.

Figure 16–1 demonstrates the hydrolysis reaction at the tissue level. Consistent with the *law of mass action,* the rate and direction of this reaction are determined by addition of substrate or removal of end product. In the tissues, addition of CO_2 to the blood by metabolizing cells drives hydrolysis in the forward direction, forming H⁺ and HCO_3^-, with most of this activity occurring within the RBC. The H⁺ formed would cause the pH of the blood and RBC cytoplasm to fall (i.e., become more acidic) if it were to remain free in solution. As discussed later, most of this H⁺ combines with hemoglobin and other *buffers* so that pH changes are minimized. The HCO_3^- formed within RBCs diffuses out into the plasma, while another anion, chloride (Cl⁻), moves in to maintain electroneutrality. This anion countertransport is known as the *chloride shift.* The HCO_3^- formed in this way accounts for the major portion (80%) of CO_2 transported in the blood. Small amounts are transported dissolved in

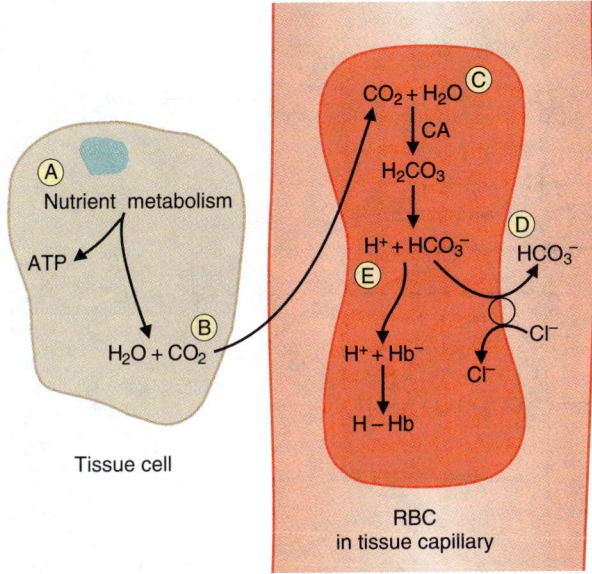

Figure 16–1. Tissue level hydrolysis. *A,* CO_2 is formed during cellular energy metabolism. *B,* CO_2 diffuses into plasma, then into red blood cells. *C,* CO_2 enters hydrolysis catalyzed by carbonic anhydrase, yielding H^+ and HCO_3^-. *D,* HCO_3^- diffuses into plasma in exchange for Cl^- (chloride shift). *E,* H^+ is buffered by hemoglobin *(Hb)* and other intracellular buffers.

plasma (8%) or combined with hemoglobin (as *carbaminohemoglobin*) or other proteins (12%). The amount of carbonic acid in the blood at any time is negligible (0.0006%).

In the lungs, CO_2 diffuses along its concentration gradient from the plasma to the alveoli, from which it is exhaled. Removal of CO_2 drives the hydrolysis reaction in reverse, as shown in Figure 16–2. In a reversal of the chloride shift, HCO_3^- reenters RBCs while Cl^- exits. HCO_3^- combines with H^+, which has been released from its buffers, regenerating CO_2 and H_2O.

Regulation of Fixed Acids and Bicarbonate by the Kidneys

Acids that cannot be converted to gases must be eliminated in the urine. These fixed acids include the sulfuric, phosphoric, and other acids produced during protein metabolism; ketones produced during accelerated lipid metabolism (as in diabetic ketoacidosis); lactic acid produced during anaerobic glycolysis (as in shock and hypoxemia); and, occasionally, acid metabolites of exogenous toxins such as salicylate drugs or methanol.

The kidneys regulate serum pH by secreting H^+ into the urine and by regenerating HCO_3^- for reabsorption into the blood. HCO_3^- is filtered from the blood into the tubules at the glomerulus, and as a large, charged particle it is poorly reabsorbed in that form. Any HCO_3^- filtered in excess of H^+ is excreted in the urine. H^+ is actively secreted into the renal tubules, primarily by proximal tubular cells, but also in the distal tubule and collecting duct. Secretion of large amounts of H^+ into the renal tubules would result in a rapid fall in tubular pH and inhibit further H^+ secretion if not for the presence of

urinary buffer systems. These allow the tubular fluid to accept large quantities of H^+ while limiting the degree to which urinary pH falls.

■ Urinary Buffer Systems

Buffer systems consist of a weak acid (one that does not readily release H^+) and a salt of its conjugate base. For example, carbonic acid, a weak acid, and sodium bicarbonate ($NaHCO_3$) constitute the *bicarbonate buffer* found not only in the renal tubules but also inside cells and in the plasma. The fixed organic acids formed during metabolism are strong acids, that is, they readily contribute free H^+ to solution, potentially producing marked alterations in pH. The pH of buffered solutions tends to remain fairly stable in spite of the addition of strong acids or bases because the buffer system combines with the added acid or base to convert it to a weaker form. Since only free H^+ contributes to pH, changes in pH are minimized.

The three principal buffer systems in renal tubules are the bicarbonate, ammonia, and phosphate (titratable acid) systems. In the *bicarbonate system* (Fig. 16–3), H^+ is secreted into the tubular lumen by tubular cells in countertransport with sodium (Na^+). The combination of H^+ with filtered bicarbonate regenerates CO_2 in a reversal of the hydrolysis reaction. The CO_2 formed is reabsorbed into the tubular cell, where hydrolysis proceeds efficiently due to the presence of CA. The HCO_3^- formed is then reabsorbed with sodium into the blood. Thus, for every molecule of H^+ secreted, a molecule of HCO_3^- is returned to the blood to restore components of the plasma bicarbonate buffer system (see later discussion of blood buffers).

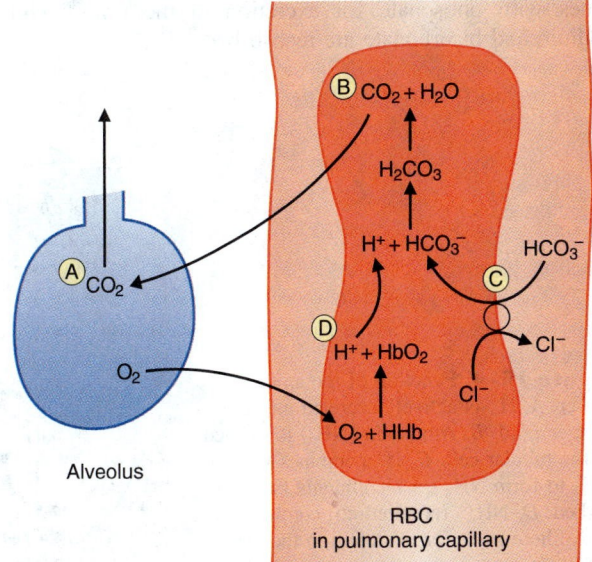

Figure 16–2. Reversal of hydrolysis in the lung. *A,* CO_2 is exhaled, creating a gradient for diffusion of CO_2 from the blood to the alveolus. *B,* Removal of CO_2 drives reverse hydrolysis in the red blood cell. *C,* HCO_3^- reenters the red blood cell in exchange for chloride (reverse chloride shift). *D,* Oxygen binding to hemoglobin *(Hb)* promotes H^+ release (reverse Haldane effect).

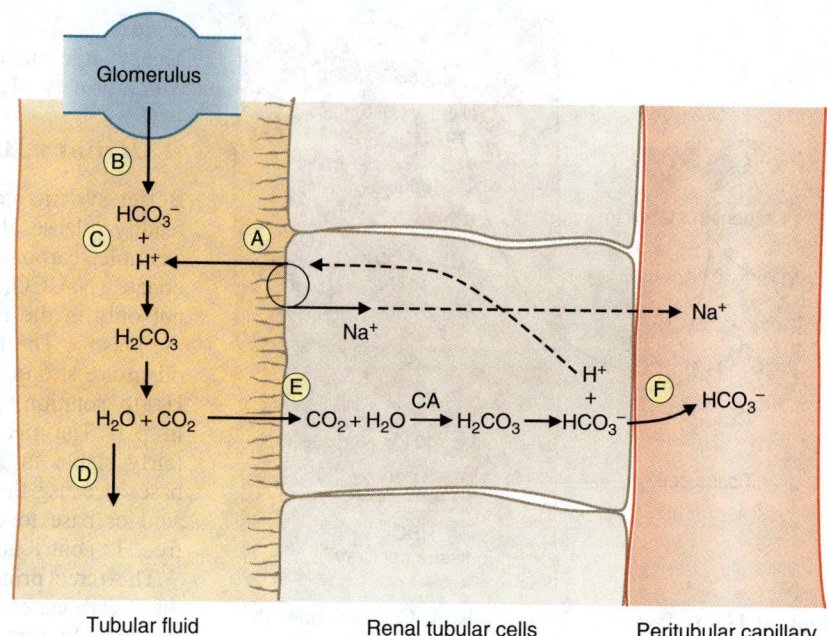

Figure 16–3. Function of the urinary bicarbonate buffer. *A,* H⁺ is actively secreted into the tubule in exchange for Na⁺. *B,* HCO_3^- is filtered into the tubule at the glomerulus. *C,* H⁺ and $H_2CO_3^-$ enter reverse hydrolysis, yielding H_2O and CO_2. *D,* H_2O remains in the tubule as urine unless reabsorbed. *E,* CO_2 diffuses into tubular cells and enters hydrolysis, catalyzed by carbonic anhydrase *(CA),* yielding H⁺ and HCO_3^-. *F,* HCO_3^- is reabsorbed, with Na⁺, into the blood.

The *ammonia system* depends on the generation of ammonia (NH_3) from the amino acid glutamine in renal tubular cells (Fig. 16–4). NH_3 diffuses into the tubular lumen, where it may combine with secreted H⁺ to form ammonium (NH_4^+), a large, charged particle which cannot be reabsorbed into the tubular cell. H⁺ in this form is thus "trapped" in the tubule. NH_4^+ combines with Cl⁻ from NaCl, and is excreted in the urine. Na⁺ is actively reabsorbed, along with tubular HCO_3^-. The *phosphate system* operates similarly (Fig. 16–5). Secreted H⁺ combines with phosphate for excretion in the urine, while sodium and bicarbonate are reabsorbed.

■ The Role of Other Electrolytes

While H⁺ and HCO_3^- are critical determinants of acid-base balance, they are also electrolytes, subject to the *principle of electroneutrality,* which holds that total cations must equal total anions in any fluid compartment. Renal regulation of serum pH is greatly influenced by the concentrations of other electrolytes, particularly potassium (K⁺), sodium (Na⁺), calcium (Ca²⁺), chloride (Cl⁻), and protein (Pr⁻).

When serum potassium is elevated (hyperkalemia), renal tubular cells secrete more K⁺, while retaining H⁺ for

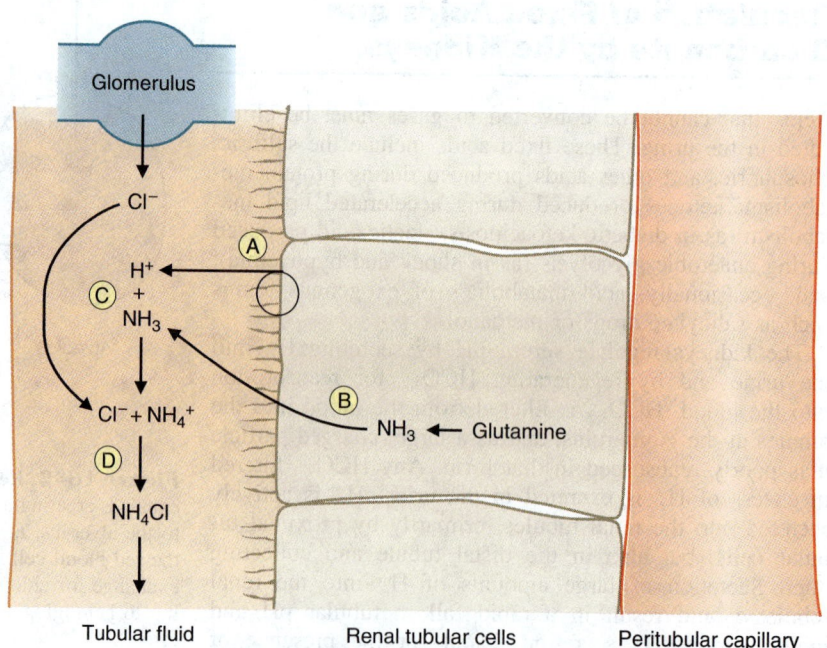

Figure 16–4. Function of the ammonia buffer. *A,* H⁺ is actively secreted into the tubular fluid. *B,* Ammonia (NH_3) is formed in the tubular cell. *C,* H⁺ combines with NH_3 to form NH_4^+, which cannot be reabsorbed. *D,* NH_4^+ (ammonium) combines with filtered Cl⁻ for excretion in the urine.

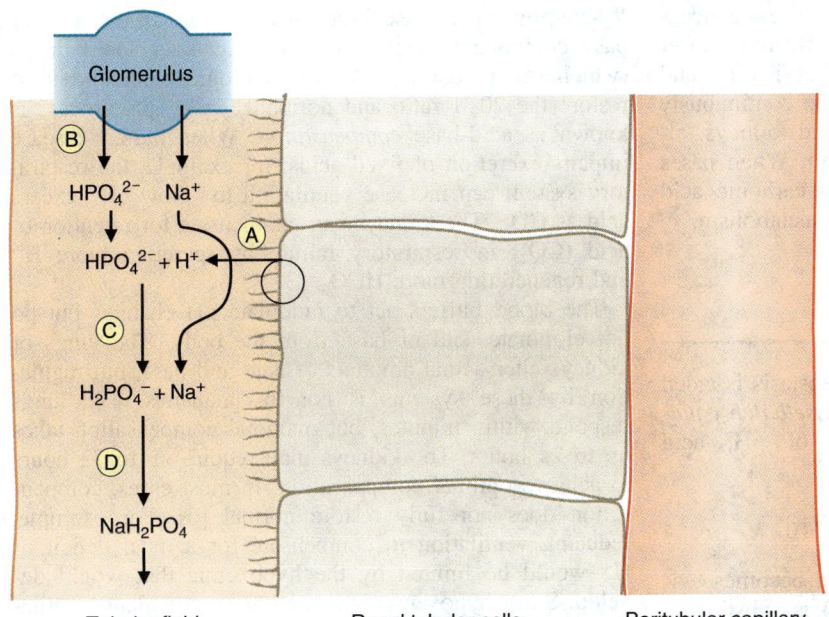

Tubular fluid   Renal tubular cells   Peritubular capillary

Figure 16–5. Function of the phosphate buffer. *A*, H^+ is actively secreted into the tubule. *B*, HPO_4^{2-} and Na^+ are filtered into the tubule at the glomerulus. *C*, H^+ and HPO_4^{2-} combine to form dihydrogen phosphate ($H_2PO_4^-$). *D*, $H_2PO_4^-$ combines with filtered Na^+ for excretion in the urine.

electroneutrality. The opposite occurs in hypokalemia, which promotes renal secretion of H^+. Similarly, H^+ imbalance influences both renal regulation and cellular shifts in potassium. In cases of serum H^+ excess, more H^+ is secreted by renal tubular cells, while K^+ is retained, promoting hyperkalemia. At the tissue level, H^+ moves into cells to be buffered by intracellular proteins, while K^+ moves out into the blood to maintain electroneutrality. This shift does not represent a true K^+ excess, but does contribute to clinical manifestations of hyperkalemia, which include potentially lethal cardiac dysrhythmias. Treatment of the H^+ excess causes a shift in the opposite direction, promoting hypokalemia. In cases where there is a deficit in serum H^+, renal cells retain H^+ while secreting more K^+, and cellular proteins release H^+ to the extracellular fluid while K^+ shifts intracellularly. The degree of hypokalemia associated with H^+ deficit is usually mild, however.

Sodium and chloride are of particular importance in maintenance of fluid balance, and the kidney is the principal site of their regulation. Active reabsorption of sodium from the renal tubules creates gradients which drive the reabsorption of anions such as Cl^- and HCO_3^-. Low extracellular volume is sensed by juxtaglomerular cells of the renal glomeruli, triggering the renin-angiotensin-aldosterone system (RAAS). Release of the mineralocorticoid hormone aldosterone from the adrenal cortex results in stimulation of renal reabsorption of sodium from the distal tubule and proximal collecting duct. A concurrent increase in (1) secretion of H^+ and K^+ or (2) HCO_3^- reabsorption is required for maintenance of electroneutrality. The kidney's priority in such cases is to restore *volume* balance, but this happens at the cost of worsening pH status. Clinical conditions that result in low serum Na^+ (hyponatremia) almost invariably result in low Cl^- (hypochloremia) as well. In Cl^- deficit, the kidney reabsorbs more HCO_3^- to maintain electroneutrality. Con-

versely, in conditions in which excess HCO_3^- is lost in the urine, Cl^- will be retained.

While intracellular proteins are the most important buffers in whole-body acid-base homeostasis, serum proteins, particularly albumin, also play a significant role. In H^+ excess, for example, serum proteins bind circulating H^+, displacing other cations such as calcium. The level of ionized Ca^{2+} thus rises, promoting clinical manifestations of hypercalcemia. In H^+ deficit, a greater fraction of serum calcium is bound, decreasing ionized levels. The clinical effects of this interaction are usually mild, however. Because H^+ excess creates a need for more urinary buffers, including ammonia, which is derived from protein, increased buffering of acid promotes depletion of protein. Similarly, deficiency of serum albumin caused by renal disease or other disorders may promote H^+ excess.

Modulation of Serum pH by Blood Buffer Systems

Several buffer systems are present in the blood, both within RBCs (e.g., hemoglobin, phosphate, bicarbonate) and in the plasma (e.g., bicarbonate, plasma proteins, phosphate). These systems act instantaneously to minimize the impact of the addition of strong acid or base to the blood by converting these to weaker forms. Blood buffers thus constitute the body's first line of defense against acid-base imbalance. Examples of *buffering reactions* are shown.

Strong acid buffered:

$$HCl + (H_2CO_3/NaHCO_3) \rightarrow NaCl + H_2CO_3$$

Strong base buffered:

$$NaOH + H_2CO_3 \rightarrow NaHCO_3 + H_2O$$

Whereas hemoglobin is present in the greatest concentration, *plasma bicarbonate* is the most effective buffer because it is an *open* buffer system. That is, the end products of acid buffering reactions can be continuously eliminated from the body by the lungs and kidneys, allowing the reaction to continue unimpeded. When bases must be buffered, the CO_2 consumed by carbonic acid formation is readily replenished by normal metabolism.

Interaction of Acid-Base Regulatory Systems

Clinical evaluation of total acid-base homeostasis is aided by an understanding of the *Henderson-Hasselbalch equation,* which describes the relationship of pH, acid (H_2CO_3), and base (HCO_3^-).

$$pH = pK_a + \log [HCO_3^-]/[H_2CO_3]$$

The clinical importance of this equation becomes evident when the normal value for pH (7.4) is substituted. Because pK_a is a constant (6.1), the equation reveals that a ratio of 20 parts base to 1 part acid must be present to yield a normal pH. An increase in the numerator (base) tends to increase blood pH; a decrease tends to decrease pH. An increase in the denominator (acid) lowers pH; a decrease causes a rise in pH (Fig. 16–6).

■ Acid-Base Compensation

In terms of commonly reported laboratory tests, normal acid-base balance translates the 20:1 ratio to 24:40 (24 mEq/L HCO_3^- to 40 mm Hg $PaCO_2$) (Fig. 16–7). $PaCO_2$ is the partial pressure of carbon dioxide in arterial blood.

When primary disease processes alter either the acid or base component of the ratio, the lungs or the kidneys (whichever is unaffected by pathologic change) act to restore the 20:1 ratio and normalize pH. This process is known as acid-base *compensation.* When kidney disease impairs excretion of fixed acids, for example, the respiratory system can increase ventilation to "blow off" excess acid as CO_2. The kidneys can compensate for retention of acid (CO_2) in respiratory failure by secreting more H^+ and regenerating more HCO_3^-.

The blood buffers act to modulate pH changes but do not eliminate acid or base from the body. The lungs or kidneys alter actual amounts of acid and base, but regulation by these systems is not instantaneous. The lungs respond within minutes, but maximal compensation takes up to 24 hours. The kidneys may require up to 72 hours to achieve optimal compensation. In most cases, compensation does not fully restore normal pH. For example, reducing ventilation to compensate for a renal deficit of H^+ would be limited by the hypoxemia that would develop. Since hypoxemia is a respiratory stimulant, ventilation would again increase. Likewise, renal compensation for ventilatory disorders is potentially limited by many factors, including renal perfusion, tubular flow rates, and saturability of tubular transport processes.

■ Acid-Base Correction

Although compensatory responses for primary acid-base disorders may nearly restore the 20:1 ratio of base to acid, the actual amounts of acid and base remain abnormal. Thus, compensation must be differentiated from *correction,* in which not only is the ratio restored but absolute quantities of $PaCO_2$ and HCO_3^- are returned to the

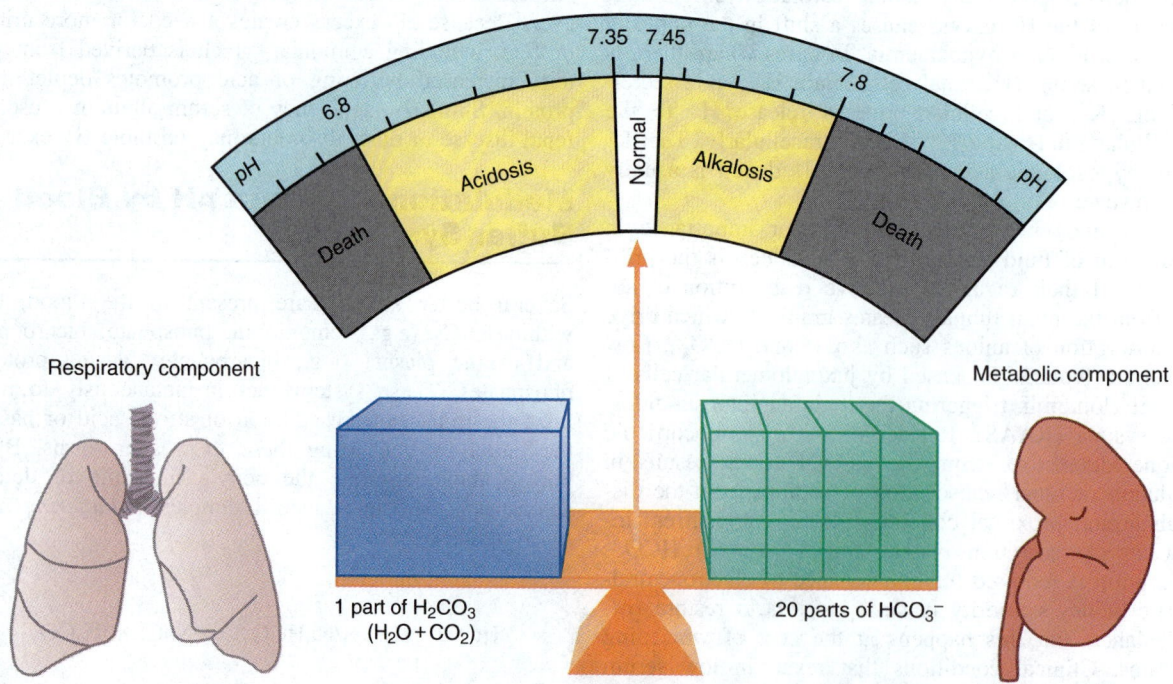

HENDERSON–HASSELBALCH RELATIONSHIP

Figure 16–6. Regulation of acid-base balance.

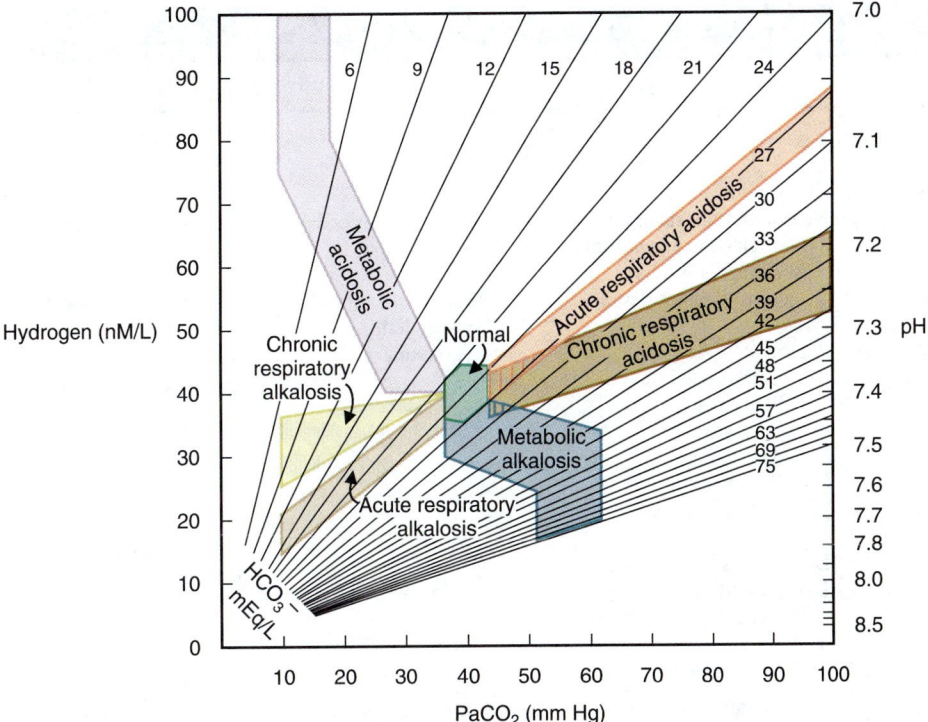

Figure 16–7. An acid-base map. To use the acid-base map, plot the pH on the vertical axis and the partial pressure of arterial carbon dioxide (PaCO₂) on the horizontal axis. Note the point at which the values intersect. If the result falls outside the *normal* area or the 95% confidence bands for the major primary disorders, the client most likely has a complex acid-base imbalance. However, a point falling *within* one of the bands does not rule out a complex disorder.

normal range. Correction occurs only with resolution of the underlying disorder.

Disorders of Acid-Base Balance

The four general classes of acid-base imbalance are respiratory acidosis, respiratory alkalosis, metabolic acidosis, and metabolic alkalosis. *Acidosis* refers to any pathologic process causing a relative excess of acid (volatile or fixed) in the body. *Acidemia* is excess acid in the blood. The presence of acidemia does not necessarily confirm an underlying pathologic process; technically it is merely a laboratory finding. The same distinction may be made between the terms *alkalosis* and *alkalemia;* alkalosis indicates a primary condition resulting in excess base in the body. Care must be taken not to confuse these terms conceptually, and they must not be used interchangeably in clinical practice.

The incidence of acid-base imbalances in clinical settings is high. A study of 110 consecutive admissions to a general hospital revealed an overall incidence of acid-base imbalances of 56%. The most common disorder was respiratory alkalosis (26 cases), followed in order by respiratory acidosis (16), metabolic alkalosis (10), and metabolic acidosis (6). Eleven persons had more than one acid-base imbalance concurrently.[11]

Overview of Acid-Base Disorders

Table 16–1 summarizes pathophysiologic mechanisms, common etiologic factors, clinical manifestations, and medical management of the four imbalances.

■ Respiratory Acidosis and Alkalosis

Respiratory acidosis is nearly always due to hypoventilation. Chronic respiratory acidosis is most commonly caused by chronic obstructive pulmonary disease (COPD). In endstage disease, pathologic changes lead to airway collapse, air trapping, and disturbance of ventilation-perfusion (V/Q) relationships. Acute respiratory acidosis also occurs in these clients when superimposed respiratory infection or concurrent cardiac disease increases the work of breathing. Hypoventilation with resultant respiratory acidosis is also seen in diseases of the neuromuscular junction in which diaphragmatic movement is impaired (such as Guillain-Barré syndrome) and in depression of the medullary respiratory center by drugs or lesions of the central nervous system (CNS).

Respiratory acidosis may be caused iatrogenically by inadequate mechanical ventilation or by excessive oxygen administration to clients with COPD. In the latter case, hypoventilation results from (1) depression of the medullary respiratory center with removal of the hypoxemic

Table 16–1. Overview of Acid-Base Imbalances

Mechanism	Etiology	Clinical Manifestations	Treatment
Respiratory Acidosis			

Hypoventilation	COPD
	Neuromuscular disease
	  Guillain-Barré syndrome
	  Myasthenia gravis
	  Respiratory center depression
	    Drugs
	      Barbiturates
	      Sedatives
	      Narcotics
	      Anesthetics
	    CNS lesions
	      Tumor
	      Stroke
	Late ARDS
	Iatrogenic disorders
	  Inadequate mechanical ventilation
	  CO_2 narcosis
		Dyspnea
		Disorientation or coma
		Dysrhythmias
		pH <7.35
		$PaCO_2$ >45 mm Hg
		Hyperkalemia
		Hypoxemia
			Treat underlying cause
			Support ventilation
			Correct electrolyte imbalance
			Intravenous $NaHCO_3$*

Excess CO_2 production	Hypermetabolism
	  Sepsis
	  Burns
	Excess carbohydrate intake
	  Total parenteral nutrition
	  Enteral feeding		

Respiratory Alkalosis			

Hyperventilation	Hypoxemia
	  Emphysema
	  Pneumonia
	  ARDS
	Impaired lung expansion
	  Pulmonary fibrosis
	  Ascites
	  Scoliosis
	  Pregnancy†
	Thickened alveolar-capillary membrane
	  Congestive heart failure
	  Early ARDS
	  Pneumonia
	  Pulmonary embolism
	Chemical stimulation of respiratory center
	  Bacterial toxins (sepsis)
	  Ammonia (hepatic failure)
	  Salicylates (aspirin overdose)
	Traumatic stimulation of respiratory center
	  CNS trauma
	  CNS tumor
	  Increased intracranial pressure
	  Excessive exercise
	  Extreme stress
	  Severe pain
		Tachypnea
		Hyperpnea‡
		Giddiness, dizziness, syncope, convulsions, or coma
		Weakness, paresthesias, tetany
		pH >7.35
		$PaCO_2$ <35 mm Hg
		Hypokalemia
		Hypocalcemia
			Treat underlying cause
			Increase CO_2 retention
			  Mechanical hypoventilation
			  CO_2 rebreathing§
			  Sedation

Table 16–1. Overview of Acid-Base Imbalances (Continued)

Mechanism	Etiology	Clinical Manifestations	Treatment
Metabolic Acidosis			

Fixed acid excess	Renal failure
	Diabetic ketoacidosis
	Lactic acidosis
	Ingested toxins
	  Aspirin
	  Antifreeze
		Hyperventilation (compensatory)
		Drowsiness, confusion, or coma
		Headache
		pH <7.35
		HCO_3^- <22 mEq/L
		Anion gap greater than 16 mEq/L
		  if excess acid
			Treat underlying cause
			Correct electrolyte imbalance
			Intravenous $NaHCO_3$*

Base deficit	Renal tubular acidosis
	Carbonic anhydrase inhibitors
	  Acetazolamide (Diamox)
	  Mafenide acetate (Sulfamylon cream)
		Hyperchloremia if base deficit
		$PaCO_2$ normal or slightly decreased	

Metabolic Alkalosis			

Fixed acid loss (with resultant base excess)	Hypokalemia
	  Diuresis
	  Steroids
	Gastric fluid loss
	  Vomiting
	  Nasogastric aspiration
		Hypoventilation (compensatory)
		Dysrhythmias
		pH >7.45
		Hypokalemia
		Hypocalcemia
		$PaCO_2$ normal or slightly increased
			Treat underlying cause
			Administer acetazolamide
			Administer KCl
			Intravenous acidifying salts* (e.g., NH_4Cl) in extreme cases

Excessive HCO_3^- intake	Milk-alkali syndrome Overcorrection of acidosis with $NaHCO_3$ Massive transfusion of whole blood		
Excessive HCO_3^- reabsorption	Hyperaldosteronism Licorice intoxication		

ARDS, adult respiratory distress syndrome; CNS, central nervous system; COPD, chronic obstructive pulmonary disease; $PaCO_2$, partial pressure of arterial carbon dioxide.
* Use of therapeutic compensation, e.g., intravenous acid or base administration, is controversial. (See text.)
† In the third trimester of pregnancy, the hormone progesterone also stimulates respiration.
‡ Restrictive lung disorders may preclude increased tidal volume.
§ Specific measures include breathing into a paper bag or increasing tubing dead space with mechanical ventilation.

stimulus and (2) worsening of V/Q relationships secondary to nitrogen washout. Normally, the most important stimulus for ventilation is the increase in acidity of the cerebrospinal fluid (CSF) resulting from CO_2 diffusing in from the blood. However, the increased HCO_3^- resulting from renal compensation for chronic respiratory acidosis minimizes the effect of increasing $PaCO_2$ in these patients. Oxygen therapy may worsen V/Q relationships since it displaced nitrogen, a much less soluble gas, in alveoli. As oxygen is absorbed, alveoli may collapse, contributing to hypoventilation. The second, much less common mechanism of respiratory acidosis is excessive CO_2 production due to excessive metabolic rate or excessive metabolism of carbohydrate.

Respiratory alkalosis is caused by alveolar hyperventilation, in which excess CO_2 is eliminated. The most common cause of respiratory alkalosis is hypoxemia. Low levels of oxygen partial pressure in arterial blood (PaO_2) are sensed by the peripheral chemoreceptors in the carotid bodies and aortic arch. These receptors then increase their rate of firing to the respiratory center in the medulla, and rate and depth of ventilation increase. The peripheral chemoreceptors are also stimulated in low blood flow states such as shock.

Conditions that physically impede expansion of the lungs (such as pulmonary fibrosis) stimulate activation of the respiratory center via the Hering-Breuer or stretch reflex. The J receptors, located in the alveolar-capillary membrane, are thought to stimulate increased ventilation in disorders such as adult respiratory distress syndrome (ARDS), which causes thickening of this membrane.

The central chemoreceptors and respiratory center may be stimulated excessively by chemicals or toxins. In the case of salicylate (aspirin) overdose, it is interesting that adults usually exhibit respiratory alkalosis, whereas children more often have metabolic acidosis due to the acid ingestion. The reason for this is unknown. Other conditions that may overstimulate the respiratory center include CNS lesions or trauma, fever, exercise, extreme emotional stress, or severe pain.

■ Metabolic Acidosis and Alkalosis

Metabolic acidosis may be caused by two different mechanisms: accumulation of fixed acid or loss of base. These mechanisms may be differentiated clinically by the presence or absence of a high *anion gap* (A^-). Normally, the anion gap is 12 to 14 mEg/L. A^- is calculated by subtracting the sum of the major anions, bicarbonate and chloride, from the sodium concentration. The "gap" represents anions in the serum other than HCO_3^- or Cl^-, often referred to as unmeasured anions. When acidosis is the result of the addition of acid (as in lactic acidosis), bicarbonate is consumed in buffering, and unmeasured anions increase to maintain electroneutrality.

Common causes of high anion gap acidosis include azotemic renal failure, in which acid end products of protein metabolism cannot be effectively excreted because of impaired glomerular filtration; diabetic ketoacidosis, in which ketoacids accumulate because of accelerated lipid metabolism in the absence of insulin; and lactic acidosis, a consequence of anaerobic carbohydrate metabolism. Less commonly, ingestion of toxins with acid metabolites is the cause.

Normal anion gap acidosis, due to loss of base, is also called *hyperchloremic metabolic acidosis.* Chloride is retained by the kidney when excess bicarbonate is lost in order to maintain electroneutrality. Excess bicarbonate may be lost through either the kidneys or the intestinal tract. In renal tubular acidosis, the renal tubular cells are unable to reabsorb bicarbonate; thus it is lost in the urine.

Intestinal secretions, high in bicarbonate, may be lost through enteric drainage tubes (e.g., ileostomy) or with diarrhea. Drugs such as acetazolamide (Diamox), which inhibit carbonic anhydrase, interfere with bicarbonate reclamation during urinary buffering.

Metabolic alkalosis develops through a two-phase mechanism. In the *generation phase,* the imbalance is first created by loss of acid (as with HCl loss during vomiting) or gain of base (as with administration of $NaHCO_3$), or with loss of intestinal fluids containing more Cl^- than HCO_3^-. The latter form is very common, and is referred to as *contraction alkalosis.* Another common type, *posthypercapneic metabolic alkalosis,* results from too-rapid correction of chronic respiratory acidosis. The compensatory increase in HCO_3^- then persists as a primary disorder. In the *maintenance phase,* alkalosis is perpetuated by impairment of renal HCO_3^- excretion, which would otherwise correct the disorder. This impairment may be due to hypovolemia or, much less commonly, aldosterone excess. In hypovolemia, increased Na^+ reabsorption by the distal tubule results in increased H^+ secretion and HCO_3^- regeneration. In aldosterone excess (or with prolonged corticosteroid administration in which mineralocorticoid effects are also seen), the hormone stimulates increased Na^+ reabsorption by the same distal tubular pump. Metabolic alkalosis due to fluid loss is referred to as "saline-sensitive," because restoration of volume with NaCl permits the kidneys to restore acid-base homeostasis. Alkalosis in cases of aldosterone excess is not correctable with saline administration, and is termed "saline-resistant."

Loss of gastric fluid via nasogastric suction or vomiting causes metabolic alkalosis due to loss of hydrochloric acid (HCl). When HCl is lost, new HCl must be produced by gastric cells via the hydrolysis reaction. H^+ is secreted into the stomach with Cl^-; the HCO_3^- produced in the reaction is reabsorbed into the blood in exchange for chloride.

Hyperaldosteronism leads to metabolic alkalosis via increased renal tubular reabsorption of sodium and subsequent loss of hydrogen ions. Rarely, excessive licorice ingestion (e.g., 20–40 g) causes metabolic alkalosis owing to its structural similarity to aldosterone. Overcorrection of acidosis with $NaHCO_3$ administration may cause alkalosis, as can massive transfusion of whole blood. The citrate anticoagulant used for storage of blood is metabolized to bicarbonate. Packed RBCs contain much less citrate; thus, their use in multiple transfusion is preferred. Treatment of hypovolemia with Ringer's lactate may also contribute, since lactate is metabolized to bicarbonate.

■ Complex Acid-Base Disorders

Complex acid-base disorders, in which two primary acid-base imbalances coexist, are frequently seen in clinical situations. In cardiac arrest, for example, lactic acid quickly accumulates as a result of anaerobic metabolism; carbonic acid is elevated because of respiratory arrest. In COPD, underlying respiratory acidosis may be complicated by metabolic alkalosis secondary to diuretic or steroid therapy.

A *triple* acid-base disorder is present when metabolic acidosis and metabolic alkalosis coexist with either respiratory acidosis or respiratory alkalosis. (The two respiratory imbalances cannot coexist because they have opposite effects on ventilation.) As an example of a triple disorder, ingestion of methanol (an exogenous toxin producing metabolic acidosis), vomiting (producing metabolic alkalosis), and respiratory arrest due to aspiration (producing respiratory acidosis) could be present simultaneously.

Prevention

The nurse must maintain a high index of suspicion in *clients at risk* for acid-base imbalance. These include (1) clients with known disease of the pulmonary, cardiovascular, or renal systems; (2) clients who manifest hypermetabolic states, as in fever, sepsis, or burns; (3) clients receiving total parenteral nutrition or enteral tube feedings high in carbohydrate; (4) mechanically ventilated clients; (5) clients with insulin-dependent diabetes; (6) clients with vomiting, diarrhea, or enteric drainage; and (7) the elderly, whose age-related decreases in respiratory and renal function may limit their ability to compensate for acid-base disturbances.

The *normal aging process* results in decreased ventilatory capacity as well as loss of alveolar surface area for gas exchange; thus, the elderly are prone to respiratory acidosis due to hypoventilation and to respiratory alkalosis due to hypoxemia. Elderly persons are frequently taking multiple medications for hypertension or cardiovascular disease; these drugs may contribute to hypokalemia and metabolic alkalosis. Respiratory compensation in this condition is compromised because of the structural and functional changes mentioned. Decreased cardiac output in the aging person diminishes renal perfusion and glomerular filtration. Aldosterone is less effective in the elderly, as is ammonia buffering. These changes limit renal compensation for respiratory imbalances and place the individual at higher risk of metabolic imbalance.

Clinical Manifestations and Diagnostic Findings

Ventilatory disturbance is present in all imbalances, either as a contributing cause in respiratory imbalances or as a compensatory response in metabolic imbalances. Cellular enzyme systems must operate outside their optimal pH ranges, resulting in manifestations which vary within dif-

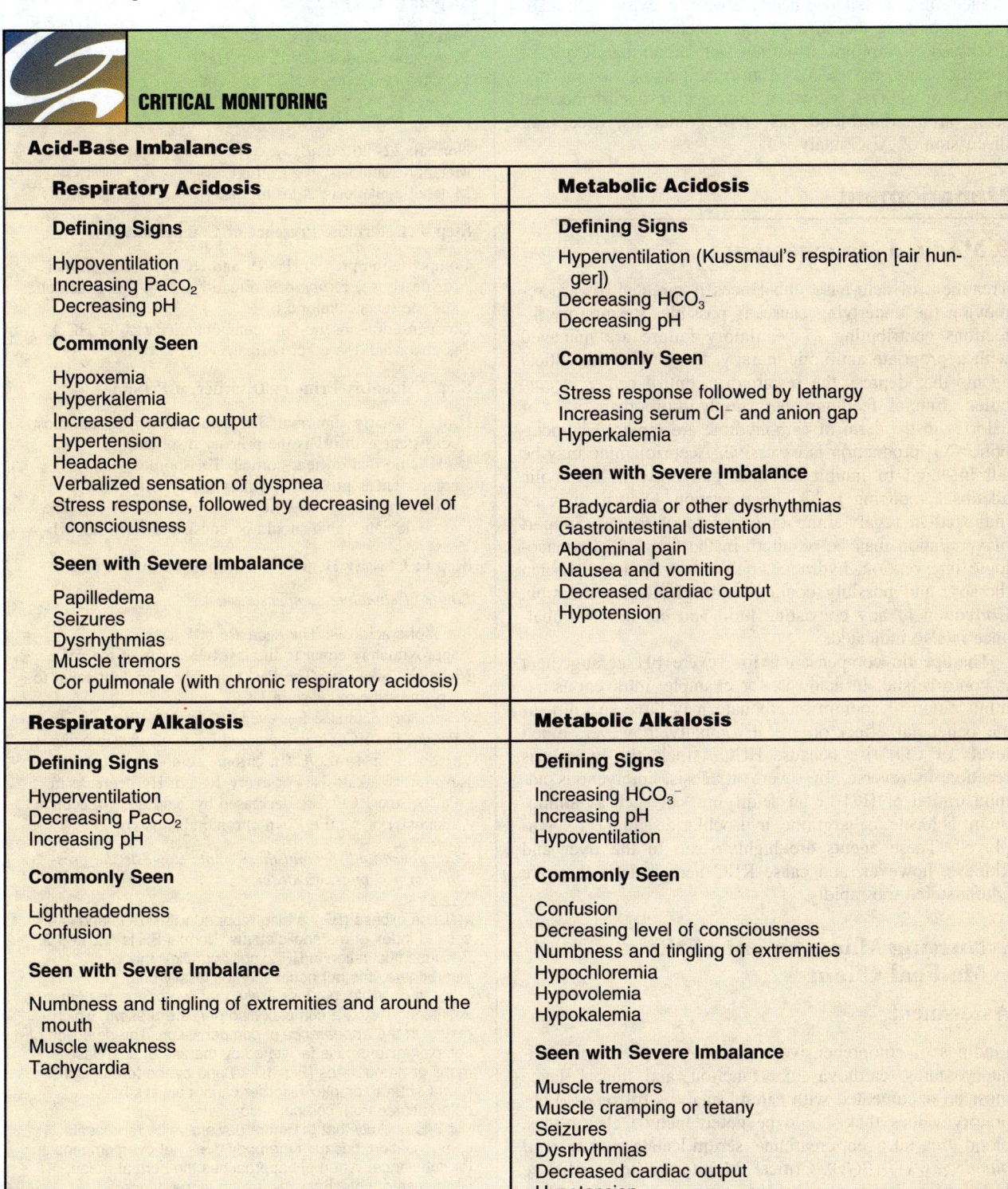

CRITICAL MONITORING

Acid-Base Imbalances

Respiratory Acidosis

Defining Signs

Hypoventilation
Increasing $PaCO_2$
Decreasing pH

Commonly Seen

Hypoxemia
Hyperkalemia
Increased cardiac output
Hypertension
Headache
Verbalized sensation of dyspnea
Stress response, followed by decreasing level of
  consciousness

Seen with Severe Imbalance

Papilledema
Seizures
Dysrhythmias
Muscle tremors
Cor pulmonale (with chronic respiratory acidosis)

Metabolic Acidosis

Defining Signs

Hyperventilation (Kussmaul's respiration [air hunger])
Decreasing HCO_3^-
Decreasing pH

Commonly Seen

Stress response followed by lethargy
Increasing serum Cl^- and anion gap
Hyperkalemia

Seen with Severe Imbalance

Bradycardia or other dysrhythmias
Gastrointestinal distention
Abdominal pain
Nausea and vomiting
Decreased cardiac output
Hypotension

Respiratory Alkalosis

Defining Signs

Hyperventilation
Decreasing $PaCO_2$
Increasing pH

Commonly Seen

Lightheadedness
Confusion

Seen with Severe Imbalance

Numbness and tingling of extremities and around the
  mouth
Muscle weakness
Tachycardia

Metabolic Alkalosis

Defining Signs

Increasing HCO_3^-
Increasing pH
Hypoventilation

Commonly Seen

Confusion
Decreasing level of consciousness
Numbness and tingling of extremities
Hypochloremia
Hypovolemia
Hypokalemia

Seen with Severe Imbalance

Muscle tremors
Muscle cramping or tetany
Seizures
Dysrhythmias
Decreased cardiac output
Hypotension

ferent organ systems (see Table 16–1). Excitable tissues (nervous tissue, cardiac muscle, smooth muscle, and skeletal muscle) demonstrate effects of altered ion conductance. Particularly notable are the effects of varying $PaCO_2$ on cerebral blood flow. Increased $PaCO_2$ (hypercapnea) increases cerebral blood flow, whereas hypocapnea decreases cerebral flow. Acidosis depresses the CNS; alkalosis stimulates it. Ultimately, severe, untreated acidosis and alkalosis both lead to coma.

Electrolyte imbalance nearly always coexists with acid-base imbalance because of the mechanisms previously discussed. Symptoms resulting from abnormal levels of specific ions are seen. Abnormalities of serum pH, $PaCO_2$, or HCO_3^- typical of the specific disturbance are seen on arterial blood gas (ABG) analysis. (See later discussion of ABG analysis.)

Management

■ Medical Management

Treatment of acid-base imbalances is directed toward removing the underlying cause, if possible. Respiratory infections contributing to ventilatory failure are managed with appropriate antibiotic therapy. Use of pharmaceutical agents that depress the respiratory control center is curtailed. Enteral feedings that supply more than 50% of calories in the form of carbohydrate are replaced if metabolic CO_2 production is excessive. Acetazolamide may be administered to inhibit carbonic anhydrase in metabolic alkalosis, reducing HCO_3^- regeneration. Dialysis may be indicated in renal failure or overdose of toxins. Support of ventilation may be required, in the form of pharmacologic intervention, hydration, pulmonary hygiene, oxygen therapy, and possibly continuous mechanical ventilation. Correction of any coexisting fluid and electrolyte imbalance is also indicated.

Therapeutic compensation for severe pH derangement is controversial. In acidosis, for example, intravenous administration of sodium bicarbonate may have an immediate beneficial effect on pH. Eventually, however, blood levels of CO_2 rise because HCO_3^- fuels the hydrolysis reaction in reverse. In severe alkalosis, intravenous administration of HCl or an acidifying salt such as ammonium chloride or arginine hydrochloride might be employed. These agents are highly toxic to the liver and kidneys, however, and cause RBC hemolysis if they are administered too rapidly.

■ Nursing Management of the Medical Client

Assessment

Findings of comprehensive *physical assessment* of ventilatory status, cardiovascular function, and fluid balance must be documented with careful analysis of trends. Laboratory values that should be noted include electrolytes, blood urea nitrogen, creatinine, serum lactate, and *arterial blood gases (ABGs)*. Critical Monitoring in Acid-Base Imbalances details the important clinical manifestations and laboratory values which should be monitored.

Box 16–1. Analysis of Arterial Blood Gases (ABGs)

Step 1: Classify the pH

Normal: 7.35–7.45
Acidemia: <7.35
Alkalemia: >7.45

Step 2: Assess $PaCO_2$

Normal: 35–45 mm Hg
Respiratory acidosis: >45 mm Hg
Respiratory alkalosis: <35 mm Hg

Step 3: Assess HCO_3^-*

Normal: 22–26 mEq/L
Metabolic acidosis: <22 mEq/L
Metabolic alkalosis: >26 mEq/L

Step 4: Determine Presence of Compensation

Compensation present: $PaCO_2$ and HCO_3^- are abnormal (or nearly so) in *opposite* directions, e.g., one is acidotic and the other alkalotic.†
Compensation absent: One component ($PaCO_2$ or HCO_3^-) is abnormal, the other normal.

Step 5: Identify Primary Disorder, if Possible

If pH is clearly abnormal: The acid-base component most consistent with pH is the primary disorder.
If pH is normal or near-normal: The more deviant component is probably primary.‡ To verify, note whether pH is on acidotic or alkalotic side of 7.4. The more deviant value should be consistent with this pH.

Step 6: Classify Degree of Compensation, if Present

Limits of complete compensation:

Metabolic acidosis: The decrease in $PaCO_2$ is approximately equal to the last two digits of the pH.
Metabolic alkalosis: The $PaCO_2$ is approximately equal to 0.6 times the increase in HCO_3^-.
Respiratory acidosis: For every 10-mm Hg increase in $PaCO_2$, the HCO_3^- is increased by 1 mEq/L (in acute acidosis) or 4 mEq/L (in chronic acidosis).
Respiratory alkalosis: For every 10-mm Hg decrease in $PaCO_2$, the HCO_3^- is decreased by 2 mEq/L (in acute alkalosis) or 5 mEq/L (in chronic alkalosis).

"Compensation" beyond these limits suggests the presence of a complex disorder.

---

*Base excess (BE) is also reported with ABGs and is a second index of metabolic status. Normal BE is −2 to +2. Because fluctuation in BE exactly parallels that of bicarbonate, it is not necessary to classify both.

† It is possible, but less likely, that two opposing primary imbalances (e.g., a complex disorder) are present, which results in the *appearance* of compensation. The detection of complex disorders is facilitated by the use of acid-base maps or nomograms (Fig. 16–7) and by the formulas in Step 6, but a complex disorder cannot always be differentiated from compensation.

‡ It is unlikely that the more deviant value represents compensation, because the body does not overcompensate for imbalance. When pH approaches the normal range, compensatory mechanisms are no longer triggered.

The nurse's knowledgeable interpretation of ABGs is critical for timely, appropriate intervention in acid-base disturbances. Often, ABG results are first reported to the nurse, who is the communication link between respiratory therapists and physicians regarding potential changes in client status or treatment. In critical care units, many nurses are using bedside ABG analyzers to obtain these results. Clinical trials of systems for continuous in vivo monitoring of blood gases are now ongoing. Whereas ABG interpretation is essential to diagnosis and treatment of acid-base imbalance, it must be emphasized that ABG findings are of value only when they are considered in the context of the total clinical picture. The recommended procedure for evaluation of ABGs is detailed in Box 16–1. The data from ABGs can also be interpreted by using the acid-base map (see Fig. 16–7).

Diagnosis, Planning, Implementation

Nursing Diagnoses. Several *nursing diagnoses* may apply to the management of underlying causes and clinical manifestations of acid-base disturbances. For example, *Ineffective Breathing Pattern, Altered Tissue Perfusion,* or *Risk of Injury* may be appropriate. Acid-base imbalances per se are perhaps best conceptualized as *collaborative problems,* however, in that the interventions of several healthcare professionals, including nurses, respiratory therapists, and physicians, are required for effective treatment.

Planning: Expected Outcomes. When acid-base imbalances are approached as collaborative problems, the expected outcomes for the client entail monitoring for clinical manifestations of the imbalances. Likewise, the nurse monitors clinical manifestations of the imbalances following treatment. Expected outcomes for nursing diagnoses are shown in the Care Plan for the Client with Acid-Base Imbalance.

Implementation. *Protection of the client* from injury during diagnostic procedures is a priority nursing responsibility. Before radial puncture for obtaining an arterial specimen for ABGs, Allen's test should be performed to ascertain adequate ulnar circulation (see Chapter 39). Allen's test is done by first having the client tightly close the hand into a fist. Both the radial and ulnar arteries are then occluded by applying pressure over the pulse points. The client's hand is then opened; it will have a blanched appearance due to lack of blood. The ulnar pressure is then released. If ulnar circulation is adequate, color will return to the hand within 10 to 15 seconds. Failure to assess collateral circulation could result in severe ischemic injury to the hand if damage to the radial artery occurs with arterial puncture.

Critically ill clients commonly have femoral or radial arterial catheter systems from which blood specimens are drawn. Frequent sampling can result in significant blood loss if an open system is used. Nursing research has demonstrated that a minimum discard specimen of 2 ml is sufficient to clear the arterial line of heparinized solution before aspiration of blood for ABG testing.[12] Closed systems (e.g., the VAMP system) allow reinstillation of initially aspirated heparinized solution and blood. Nursing responsibilities for clients with arterial lines are discussed in Chapter 44.

The nurse is also responsible for minimizing errors in ABG analysis due to faulty specimen collection and handling. Potential sampling errors, their consequences, and nursing implications are summarized in Table 16–2.

Despite quality-control procedures, erroneous blood gas data are sometimes reported. The nurse should suspect sampling error or transcription error when the reported values lack internal consistency or external congruity. Internal consistency means that the values make sense when considered as a whole. An alkalotic pH, for example, is inconsistent with excess $PaCO_2$ *and* a deficit of HCO_3^-. External congruity means that the ABG findings are consistent with other laboratory data as well as with clinical assessment findings. The client with a pH of 7.10 should appear profoundly ill.

Providing supportive care involves preserving an *acceptable* (not necessarily normal) pH and preventing life-threatening deviations in pH. The nurse optimizes respiratory and renal function through positioning, pulmonary hygiene, and hydration. The nurse intervenes in helping clients cope with the anxiety that often accompanies— and may contribute to—acid-base imbalance. The nurse collaborates in the administration of drug therapy, oxygen therapy, and mechanical ventilation when indicated. In extreme circumstances in which therapeutic compensation (intravenous administration of acid or base) is required, the nurse is knowledgeable about potential risks of this therapy and carefully monitors administration rates and therapeutic response.

Corrective interventions address the underlying causes of *primary* acid-base imbalances and are the mainstay of treatment in such disorders. Compensatory imbalances are not treated but instead resolve spontaneously as the primary disorder is reversed. Chapters on the specific diseases responsible for acid-base imbalances should be consulted for detailed discussion of appropriate nursing intervention.

Evaluation

The client's status should be evaluated frequently, because many acid-base imbalances are life-threatening. Revisions in the care plan may be required.

Conclusions

Normal function of all body cells depends on the regulation of acid-base balance. The kidneys, lungs, and blood buffers can usually balance acids and bases. Disorders of the lungs, kidneys, and metabolism can impair the balance, leading to respiratory or metabolic acidosis or alkalosis. Nurses play an instrumental role in early detection of high-risk clients.

Thinking Critically

1. The client is a 65-year-old widow with a long history of type II diabetes mellitus. She was a heavy

Table 16–2. Sources of Error in Sampling of Arterial Blood Gases

Sampling Error	Effect	Nursing Implications
Air bubbles in syringe	$\uparrow$ PaO_2 $\downarrow$ $PaCO_2$ $\uparrow$ pH	Expel all air bubbles immediately Do not agitate syringe Do not use any sample that appears frothy
Inadvertent venous sample or venous contamination of arterial sample	$\downarrow$ PaO_2 $\uparrow$ $PaCO_2$ $\downarrow$ pH	Avoid use of femoral artery Use short-beveled needle Do not overshoot artery and then withdraw to "catch" it Watch for autofilling of syringe with arterial puncture Verify questionable results with new sample
Anticoagulant effects: alteration of pH	$\downarrow$ pH	Use lithium heparin, if possible Use 1:1000 units/ml concentration Use minimum 2-ml discard sample with arterial line aspiration
Anticoagulant effects: dilution of sample	$\uparrow$ pH $\downarrow$ in all other values	Use syringe with minimal dead space Use dried heparin if available
Effects of metabolism of white blood cells in sample	$\downarrow$ PaO_2 $\uparrow$ $PaCO_2$ $\downarrow$ pH	Place sample in ice water immediately Have sample analyzed within 20 min Have sample analyzed immediately if client has leukocytosis

$PaCO_2$ and PaO_2, partial pressure of carbon dioxide and oxygen, respectively.
Data from Malley, W. J. (1990). *Clinical blood gases: Application and noninvasive alternatives.* Philadelphia: W. B. Saunders.

smoker for 40 years, but has not smoked in the last 5 years. She is admitted to the general medical unit because of a 1-week history of profuse diarrhea, attributed to food poisoning. She appears to be in respiratory distress. Her admission ABG values are as follows: pH, 7.26; $PaCO_2$, 13 mm Hg; HCO_3^-, 5 mEq/L. What acid-base imbalance is present? Should the nurse encourage the client to breathe more slowly? Other than ABGs, what laboratory values should be closely monitored by the nurse in this case? Why?

Factors to Consider. What acids or bases are lost through diarrhea? Why might the client have developed a respiratory change when the primary problem is gastrointestinal (e.g., metabolic)?

2. A 19-year-old college student is brought to the emergency room (ER) at 4:30 AM by his friends. While studying for final examinations, he had grown increasingly anxious during his "cram session," frequently voicing doubts about passing a particularly difficult course. His breathing became increasingly labored, and he seemed dazed and confused. He said his "face felt numb." His pulse was rapid (165 bpm) and he was diaphoretic. The client was diagnosed with bleeding duodenal ulcers 2 years ago. ABG analysis of samples drawn in the ER revealed the following: pH, 7.58; $PaCO_2$, 21 mm Hg; HCO_3^-, 20 mEq/L. What acid-base imbalance is represented? What caused it? What bedside assessments should the nurse perform and why? What interventions should the nurse consider which might prevent future episodes?

Factors to Consider. Can rapid breathing alone alter excretion of components needed for acid-base balance?

3. A 72-year-old retired college professor has a 55-pack-year history of cigarette smoking and advanced emphysema. He had an acute myocardial infarction 5 years ago, from which he recovered uneventfully. He sees his physician in the clinic, complaining of a "cold" that he "just can't get rid of" and "soreness" in his chest. His blood pressure is 165/90 mm Hg and he has inspiratory crackles in both lung bases. His ankles are edematous. ABGs drawn during the visit revealed: pH, 7.34; PCO_2, 65 mm Hg; HCO_3^-, 34 mEq/L. What acid-base imbalance is represented? What is the probable cause? What additional information would be helpful in planning his care? What variables should the nurse consider in determining priorities of care?

Factors to Consider. Consider that the client has developed heart failure. When the lungs fill with fluid, what happens to O_2/CO_2 exchange and, thereby, acid-base balance?

Bibliography

1. Anderson, S. (1990). ABGs: Six easy steps to interpreting blood gases. *American Journal of Nursing, 90*(8), 42–45.
2. Carpenito, L. (1995). *Nursing diagnosis: Application to clinical practice* (6th ed.). Philadelphia: J. B. Lippincott.
3. D'Addesio, J. (1992). Metabolic and respiratory acidosis. *Topics in Emergency Medicine, 14*(1), 51–55.
4. Dirks, J. (1995). Innovations in technology: Continuous intra-arterial blood gas monitoring. *Critical Care Nurse, 15*(4), 19–20, 22, 24–27.

5. Feeney-Stewart, F. (1990). The sodium bicarbonate controversy. *Dimensions of Critical Care Nursing, 9*(1), 22–28.

6. Horne, M., Heitz, U., & Swearingen, P. (1991). *Fluid, electrolyte, and acid-base balance: A Case study approach.* St. Louis: Mosby–Year Book.

7. Malley, W. (1990). *Clinical blood gases: Application and noninvasive alternatives.* Philadelphia: W. B. Saunders Co.

8. Marik, P., et al. (1991). Acetazolamide in the treatment of metabolic alkalosis in critically ill patients. *Heart and Lung, 20*(5), 455–459.

9. Metheny, N. (1992). *Fluid and electrolyte balance: Nursing considerations* (2nd ed.). Philadelphia: J. B. Lippincott.

10. Narins, R. (Ed.). (1994). *Maxwell & Kleeman's clinical disorders of fluid and electrolyte metabolism* (5th ed.). New York: McGraw-Hill.

11. Palange, P., et al. (1990). Incidence of acid-base and electrolyte disturbances in a general hospital: A study of 110 consecutive admissions. *Recenti Progressi in Medicina (Roma), 81*(12), 788–791.

12. Preusser, B., et al. (1989). Quantifying the minimum discard sample required for accurate blood gases. *Nursing Research, 38*(5), 276–279.

13. Rose, B. (1994). *Clinical physiology of acid-base and electrolyte disorders* (4th ed.). New York: McGraw-Hill.

14. Russell, J. (1991). Successful methods for arterial blood gas interpretation. *Critical Care Nurse, 11*(4), 14, 16–19.

15. Rutecki, G., & Whittier, F. (1991). Acid-base interpretation: Five rules, and how they help in everyday cases. *Consultant, 31*(11), 44–46, 55, 59.

16. Rutecki, G., & Whittier, F. (1991). Acid-base interpretation: Five rules, and how they simplify complex cases. *Consultant, 31*(12), 19–22, 24, 26.

17. Sica, D. (1994). Renal disease, electrolyte abnormalities, and acid-base imbalance in the elderly. *Clinics in Geriatric Medicine, 10*(1), 197–211.

18. Toto, R. (1991). Acid-base balance in the CCU patient. *Hospital Medicine, 27*(8), 103–105, 108, 111.

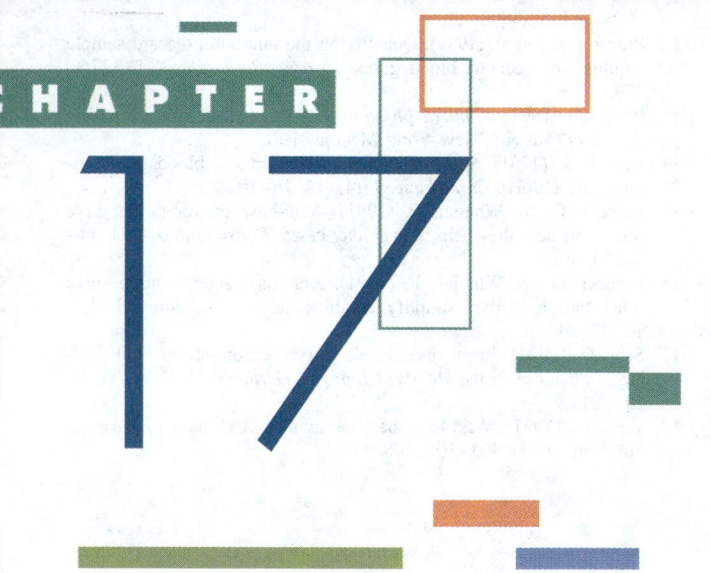

Pain

Esther Matassarin-Jacobs

Pain prompts people to seek healthcare more often than any other problem. Pain is very costly to the person experiencing it, to those around the person, and to society. Persons in pain are often not able to function to capacity or maintain their quality of life.

How would you define *pain?* Does your definition include ideas, such as a feeling of agony, distress, or suffering? Or do you define it in a structural or physiologic manner and say that pain results from stimulation of nerve endings? Your definition probably includes some personal words reflecting your own painful experiences. The pain you have experienced is the only pain you know.

We all know that others experience pain. Ultimately, however, each of us defines pain based on his or her own personal experience. Perhaps pain is simply whatever a person says "hurts."

In this chapter, a variety of definitions of pain are discussed, along with many ways in which pain can be treated. Nurses are in an excellent position to work with the client in pain and to help that client overcome the pain. This is an important but not an easy task. This chapter assists nurses to provide pain management care.

Definition of Pain

Pain is a multidimensional phenomenon; therefore, it is difficult to define. It is a personal and subjective experience with no objective measurements. Pain has been defined in many different ways by healthcare practitioners. Some of the definitions enhance the nurse's ability to assess the client who is in pain by focusing on specific aspects of the pain experience. The nurse may find pain control a difficult problem when caring for individual clients. It is, however, one of the most important areas of care, because people cannot function fully when they are in pain. Pain is best viewed as an experience, not merely as a manifestation.

Mountcastle[119] defined pain as "that sensory experience evoked by stimuli that injure or threaten to destroy tissue, defined introspectively by every man as that which hurts." The International Association for the Study of Pain offers the accepted medical definition of pain as "an unpleasant sensory and emotional experience associated with actual or potential tissue damage, or described in terms of such damage."[74]

Sternbach[150] defines pain as "an abstract concept which refers to (1) a personal, private sensation of hurt; (2) a harmful stimulus that signals current or impending tissue damage; and (3) a pattern of responses to protect the organism from harm." This definition helps the nurse's understanding of the client's pain. It focuses on pain as something that belongs to the client, because pain is both personal and private. Sternbach's definition also reminds the nurse that pain can and often does have a protective function.

McCaffery defined pain as "whatever the experiencing person says it is and existing whenever the person says it does."[95] This definition makes the client the expert about his or her own pain. Because clinical pain is subjective and no objective measures of it exist, the only people who can accurately define their own pain are the people experiencing that pain. In spite of its subjective nature, the nurse is charged with accurately assessing and helping to relieve the client's pain and McCaffery's definition helps nurses achieve this goal.

The Process of Pain

Pain is a complex phenomenon. It is elicited by threatened or actual tissue damage that stimulates nociceptive (pain-sensitive) neural receptors. Pain also may be caused by damage to the pain transmission system itself. However, these stark statements do not actually help nurses understand a client's actual pain experience. It is like describing the experience of a sunset as the physical stimulation of the retina! We need to know about pain recep-

CHAPTER 17

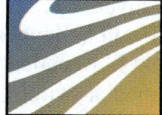

ETHICAL ISSUES IN NURSING

Pain: Who Is the Expert?

Pain is a relative term. People experience pain in many different ways. What might be considered painful to one person may not be considered so by another. Even so, healthcare providers tend to conceptualize what type and intensity of pain a certain person should experience for a certain type of illness, trauma, medical-surgical procedure, and postoperative course. If clients do not conform to the nurse's expectations, the client may be labeled by the nurse as a "weakling" or as having a "dependent" personality. The client may be requesting pain medication more frequently than the nurse expects and therefore is seen as "demanding" or "irritable."

It is useful for healthcare providers to anticipate the type and degree of pain a client may experience for a given condition in order to better care for him or her. What would happen, however, if a certain client did not fit into the anticipated pain experience and pain medication schedule? Perhaps pain medication of a certain type was ordered every 4 hours, but the client began to complain of severe pain 2 hours after administration. Should the nurse assess the client's complaint of pain? Certainly, there are physical signs that should be assessed in these clients, such as blood pressure, heart rate, wound appearance, and the inspection of the area in which the pain is located. After having assessed the client's complaint, what should the nurse do? Should the nurse tell the client no matter what, he or she must wait 2 more hours until the next dose of medication is due? (After all, a client should not have that much pain after a simple procedure such as hernia repair.) Should the nurse try diversional activities to help the client forget his or her pain? Should the nurse call the doctor and report the client's complaint and physical assessment?

Unfortunately, some clients may indeed become dependent on certain pain medications. This would cause them to ask for frequent doses. However, it is wrong to assume that all clients have such dependencies if given pain medications frequently. Do not prejudge a client's pain by whatever personal standards they may have. The obligation exists to assess clients' complaints of pain and address such complaints on an individual basis without preconceived notions about what type of pain they "should" or "should not" be experiencing.

tors and their pathways to the brain, but we also need a broader understanding of what may happen when pain is perceived, reacted to, and acted on. One way to gain this understanding is to conceptualize pain as a process made up of the *transduction, transmission,* and *modulation* of pain; *perception* of pain; and *reaction* to pain. Examining each of the parts of the process helps the nurse better understand the pain experience and better treat the client in pain.

Transduction, Transmission, and Modulation of Pain

Pain transduction, transmission, and modulation are physiologic processes dependent on an intact peripheral and central nervous system (CNS).

Pain Transduction

The train of events that leads to pain begins when pain fibers are excited by a variety of types of stimuli. The stimuli consist of mechanical events (such as stretching of organs or pressure), extremes of temperature (heat or cold), and chemical changes (such as ischemia). Specific fibers that react to these stimuli are classified as mechanical, thermal, or chemical nociceptors. Fast pain is usually elicited by the mechanical and thermal type receptors (A delta fibers), whereas slow pain can be elicited by all receptors (C fibers). Together these fibers are referred to as primary afferent fibers.

Fast pain is the pain that occurs in about 0.1 second when painful stimuli are applied. It is often referred to as sharp, pricking, acute, or electric pain. It is transmitted through A delta pain fibers. It is the pain felt when the skin is cut, burned, or an electric shock is felt. Fast pain is caused by a more superficial stimulus, so it is rare in deep tissues.[66]

Slow pain is pain that begins 1 second or more after stimulation and increases slowly over seconds or minutes. This pain is also known as burning, aching, throbbing, or chronic pain. It is often associated with tissue destruction and is felt in both superficial and deep tissues. It is transmitted through the more primitive type C fibers.

A wide variety of chemical substances, including bradykinin, serotonin, histamine, substance P, potassium ions, acids, proteolytic enzymes, prostaglandins, and acetylcholine, are significant in stimulating the slow pain that often follows tissue injury. These substances are released when tissue is damaged by injury, disease, or inflammation and enhance the nociceptive input and, therefore, increase pain. Since a variety of chemical mediators of pain are released, a variety of pharmacologic and non-pharmacologic interventions can be used successfully to treat this pain (discussed later in this chapter).

Nociceptors differ from the complex receptors for vision and other senses. Nociceptors are simply free nerve endings occurring in almost all types of tissue. Nociceptors react only to changes very close to them, and they require a relatively high level of stimulation to be activated. The chemical mediators mentioned previously increase the pain input into the nociceptors. However, once the threshold of the nociceptors is exceeded, they actively continue to communicate the presence of a painful stimulus (slow adaptation). Nociceptors also can become sensitized so they continue to discharge long after the stimulus is removed. Most is known about pain originating from receptors in the skin. It is assumed that pain receptors in deeper tissues are similar, but they may operate differently. ■

Pain Transmission

Once nociceptors are stimulated, the impulse they discharge travels as electric activity to the spinal cord and on to the brain. This electric activity becomes the experience of pain when it reaches the brain. There are no pain impulses as such, that is, impulses from nociception are not actually "pain" because pain is a perception mediated by multiple factors. However, if the neural pathway for these impulses is blocked, pain is also blocked because the impulses do not reach the brain. Pain pathways can be blocked by (1) surgical cutting, (2) medications that inhibit the activity of the pathway's fibers, and (3) natural (endogenous) methods that block portions of the pain pathway.

Nerve fibers that carry somatosensory information from the body periphery to the spinal cord include A beta, A delta, and C fibers. A-type fibers have a myelin sheath that speeds up information transmission. A delta fibers transmit pain stimuli. A beta fibers are larger and carry other sensory information such as touch. C fibers transmit pain stimuli more slowly because they have no myelin sheath. C fibers also conduct thermal, chemical, and strong mechanical impulses.

Pain sensation following stimulation of A delta fibers differs from that following C fiber stimulation. A delta activity is felt as a sharp, easily localized pain. C fiber activity is felt more slowly after painful stimulation, but the sensation is more constant and continuous. It is persistent, dull, and aching and is difficult to localize. Recall when you hit your elbow. A sharp, well-localized sensation occurred first (A delta activation), followed by a persistent, dull, aching sensation (C fiber activation).

These afferent fibers enter the dorsal root of the spinal cord, which transmits the pain impulses. The fibers separate as they enter the cord and then re-form in the dorsal horn. This area receives, transmits, and processes sensory impulses. The afferent nociceptors end at the level of the first, second, and fifth laminae. The substantia gelatinosa (SG), found in the second laminae, is hypothesized to be the gating mechanism described in the gate-control theory.

Different transmission pathways in the spinal cord contribute to the experience of various qualities of pain, such as slow pain versus fast pain. The major spinal tract carrying information to the brain is the spinothalamic tract. These ascending tracts transmit impulses through the spinal cord. Some fibers in this tract lead directly to the thalamus. From there, they pass to the somatosensory cortex, which is involved in discriminating the quality and localization of the pain.

Other fibers branch diffusely out to the many areas of the brain associated with emotion and motivation. The direct path of pain from the spinal cord to the thalamus to the somatosensory cortex is called the neospinothalamic tract, a tract that occupies the more lateral portion of the cord. This pathway contains few synapses, allowing for more rapid conduction of impulses. It projects into the posterior nucleus of the thalamus and is important in providing discriminative functions, such as the location, intensity, and duration of the painful stimulus.

The diffuse path of pain leads to more diverse brain centers, such as the reticular formation, medulla, hypothalamus, and limbic structures of the brain. It is called the paleospinothalamic tract and is more medial within the cord. This multisynaptic tract provides for slower conduction. It is associated with the unpleasant emotional component of pain and with the autonomic responses to pain.

Other ascending pathways include the spinoreticular, spinomesencephalic, spinocervical, spinohypothalamic, and second-order dorsal column tracts.

Pain Modulation

There is a great deal of variation in the way clients perceive similarly painful stimuli. The pain modulation system is one reason this variance occurs. There are a variety of mechanisms that contribute to this modulation (Fig. 17–1).

Modulation via the Dorsal Horn. The dorsal horn was once considered a simple relay for impulses, but is now known to contain extremely complex circuitry and multiple biochemical agents that both transmit and modulate nociceptive input. The dorsal horn is now thought to modulate the nociceptive impulses rather than simply receive and transmit these impulses. A high degree of processing of the sensory impulses occurs at this level.

Modulation via Descending Pathways. The descending serotoninergic inhibitory fibers originate in the periaqueductal gray matter (PAG) of the midbrain and descend downward into the nucleus raphe magnus. Neurons from the PAG project downward into the dorsal horn at the first and fifth lamina levels. The neurotransmitters serotonin and substance P are released into these areas, contributing to the modulation of pain.

Modulation via Endogenous Chemicals. Some chemical compounds released by injury or inflammation stimulate nociceptors, for example, histamine, bradykinin, serotonin, substance P, and prostaglandin E. Pain may be reduced by medications that block these agents, such as steroids, aspirin, and other nonsteroidal anti-inflammatory drugs (NSAIDs) that reduce inflammation and block prostaglandins. There is also a naturally occurring system within the nervous system called the analgesia system.

This analgesia system, described in Guyton and Hall,[65] has three major parts: (1) Neurons from the *periaqueductal gray area* of the mesencephalon and upper pons surrounding the aqueduct of Sylvius send their signals to (2) the *raphe magnus nucleus,* a thin midline nucleus located in the lower pons and upper medulla. Whence the signals are sent down the dorsolateral columns in the spinal cord to (3) a *pain inhibitory complex located in the dorsal horns of the spinal cord.* At this point in the system, pain can be blocked.

Other compounds are associated with pain transmission. Their action occurs at various points in the pain

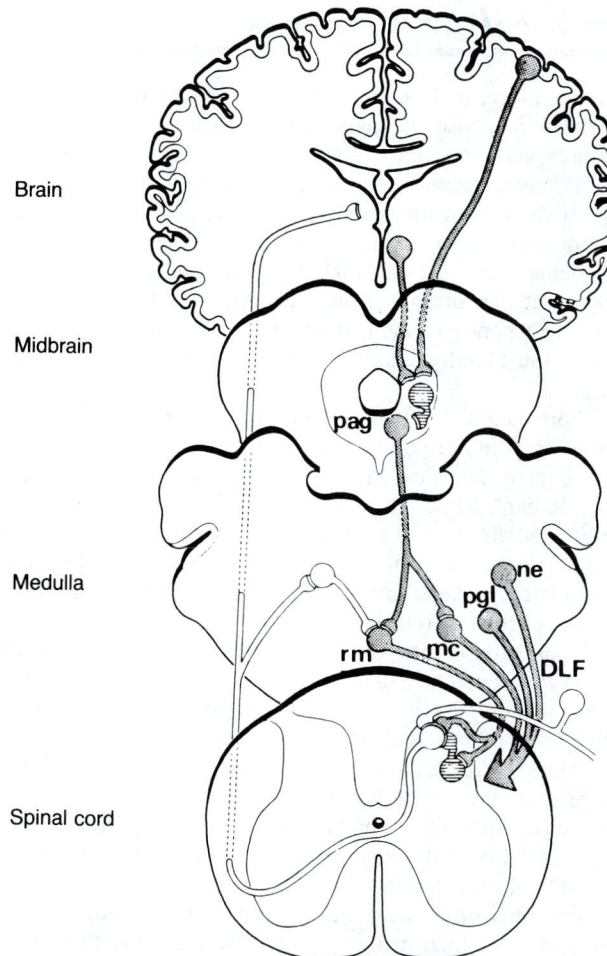

Brain

Midbrain

Medulla

Spinal cord

Figure 17–1. Pain-modulating network. Diagram of critical structures that contribute to control of pain-transmission neurons. The network includes connections from midbrain periaqueductal gray (*pag*) to medullary nucleus raphe magnus (*rm*), recticularis magnocellularis (*mc*), and, via the dorsolateral funiculus (*DLF*), to the spinal cord dorsal horn. Additional bulbospinal pathways potentially relevant to analgesia arise from the nucleus paragigantocellularis (*pgl*), which also receives input from pag and the noradrenergic medullary cell groups (*ne*) lateral to pgl. In addition to this brain stem-to-spinal cord network, connections from neocortex and hypothalamus to pag have been documented. Hypothalamic stimulation produces analgesia. The role of the cortex in pain modulation is unknown. At the spinal level, descending pathways inhibit nociceptive projection neurons through direct connections, as well as through interneurons in superficial layers of the dorsal horn. There is evidence that endorphin-containing interneurons (*crosshatched*) in pag and dorsal horn play an active role in pain modulation. (From Wall, P. D., & Melzack, R. [Eds.]. [1989]. *Textbook of pain* [2nd ed., p. 208]. New York: Churchill Livingstone.)

pathways described earlier. Substance P, a neuropeptide, appears to be a pain-specific neurotransmitter that is present in the spinal cord's horn (at the gate in the gate-control model), among other places. Other neuropeptides undoubtedly facilitate pain transmission.

Other peptides are associated with inhibiting pain. A group of naturally occurring (endogenous) peptides have properties similar to those of morphine and other opioid analgesics. The CNS has specific neuroreceptors that bind morphine. The body also manufactures opium-like compounds called endogenous opioids, or endorphins, that bind to these sites and have analgesic properties. The term *endorphins* actually refers to a group of peptides with similar properties, including the alpha- and beta-endorphins and enkephalin. The effect of the endorphins is long-lasting whereas that of enkephalin is much shorter. Electric and other stimulation of brain stem centers provides a profound analgesic effect, which can block pain in the analgesia system and appears related to endorphin release.

Enkephalins are also neurotransmitters that modulate pain. Enkephalins are smaller peptides found throughout the brain and dorsal horn of the spinal cord. Enkephalins inhibit the release of substance P, thereby modulating pain.

Other neurotransmitters are involved in the downward inhibition of pain. Serotonin, which facilitates pain in peripheral nociceptors, also acts as one of the transmitters in the descending pain inhibition system. The background level of many of these neurotransmitters varies throughout the day. Pain sensitivity is higher (lower pain threshold) in the afternoon than in the morning. Also, an individual's analgesic requirement may differ at different times of the day. There is increasing evidence that people who experience chronic pain may be deficient in some neurotransmitter.

Perception of Pain

Pain perception or interpretation is the next phase of the pain process. Once the nociceptive input has been received and transmitted, it must be perceived or interpreted. Because every individual perceives and interprets pain based on his or her individual experience, this is one point at which pain becomes different for each person. Pain modulation also occurs as it is being transmitted. For example, other sensory input will help reduce the amount of nociceptive information that is transmitted supraspinally.

Pain perception does not depend solely on the degree of physical damage. It is generally agreed that both physical stimuli and psychosocial factors influence a person's experience of pain. Although there is little consensus on the specific effects of these factors, it is known that anxiety, experience, attention, expectation, and the meaning of the situation in which injury occurs affect pain perception. Brain activities, such as distraction or anxiety, may also affect the severity and quality of the pain experience.

In the past, pain was viewed as a primary sensation, and motivational and cognitive processes were believed to influence only our reaction to pain. However, it now seems apparent that there are mechanisms within the body that can modify pain-related neural impulses even before they are transmitted to the brain. Thus, pain is likely to be determined by a relative balance between the sensory peripheral input and mechanisms of central control (brain) input to gating mechanisms in the spinal cord.

The first point the nurse needs to consider is the client's *pain threshold*. This is defined as the lowest intensity of a painful stimulus that is perceived by the client as pain. The pain threshold may vary based on physiologic factors such as inflammation or injury near pain receptors, but essentially it is similar for all people if the central and peripheral nervous systems are intact.

The second part of pain perception is the individual's tolerance for pain. Tolerance is different for each person who experiences pain. This may vary within each person based on many subjective factors, such as the meaning of the pain and the setting. It really refers to the amount of pain the client is willing to endure. Some individuals have a high tolerance, that is, they can tolerate a lot of pain without distress, whereas others have a very low tolerance. This tolerance will also vary for a given individual depending on a variety of factors that influence pain such as nausea, fatigue, and other sensory input. Only the client, not the healthcare team, can tell what the client's tolerance level is. The nurse must remember this and remember that pain tolerance can vary from situation to situation.

Another aspect that will alter a person's perception of pain is his or her experience with pain. This may be the reason that people incorrectly assume infants do not have pain. When the infant feels pain, it is simply that the infant has no experience with pain and, therefore, is unable to interpret it, and cannot communicate what is being felt. The reverse is also true. When a person has a bad experience with pain, the anticipation that future pain may be as bad can make any pain worse. There is also a physiologic reason if the pain is in the same area, that is, persons with recurrent low back pain actually have a lower pain threshold in that area than persons who have not had low back pain.

Response to Pain

The individual's reaction to pain adds even more variation to the pain process. There are many variables in this part of the process, including situation, culture, age, sex, cause of pain, tolerance, value and meaning of pain, and various psychological factors such as fear, anxiety, and depression. Each of these factors is discussed so the nurse will be better able to understand the client's experience.

Situational Factors

The situation associated with the pain will influence the person's response to it. A person's response to pain experienced in a formal or crowded situation may differ greatly from the response were he or she alone or in a hospital. Another example might be the woman who has a hysterectomy for cancer versus a woman who has a cesarean section. Although both may feel pain, it may seem worse to the woman with a diagnosis of cancer. In order not to underestimate the amount of pain, the nurse must decide whether the client's expression of pain is being influenced by the situational factors and how these may be altering that expression.

Sociocultural Factors

Race, culture, and ethnicity are critical factors in an individual's response to pain. These factors influence responses and, especially, responses to pain. The individual learns much about how to respond to pain and other experiences from his or her family and ethnic peer group. Although numerous studies have been done on a variety of sociocultural factors, including race and ethnicity, it is important that the nurse not stereotype individuals. Every person responds to pain in an individual manner, and the nurse must individualize assessment and treatment of pain.

Zborowski's[178, 179] studies on cultural and ethnic influences on pain are considered the classic studies conducted in this area. He identified four major groups, Old American, Italian, Irish, and Jewish, and looked at how each responded to pain. These studies have been disputed in recent years, especially as many cultures have become assimilated. There are also many important cultural groups excluded from his works.

Racial groups may differ in the way they react to pain according to some studies. Blacks may react differently from whites. Davitz and Davitz[34] report that southern blacks are more vocal in their reports of pain than northern blacks. Problems also may arise because of the views these groups have of healthcare team members. They often have difficulty communicating what they are feeling to physicians and nurses who are from different backgrounds or ethnic groups.[34, 68]

Hispanics often view health as the absence of illness. Stoicism is valued in this culture. They believe that difficulties and illness should be borne with dignity. There may be many folk beliefs associated with illness in this group, so any treatment has to fit into their patterns of belief. If the client is not convinced that the pain is related to an illness, he or she might refuse treatment for it.[110]

There are characteristics of many other groups, such as stoicism among Asians. One of the most important things for the nurse to remember is that clients of any culture may deal with pain in a wide variety of ways. The problem arises when the nurse does not recognize the client's way of dealing with pain or does not accept it. More study on the cultural influences of pain is needed, including research to clarify the effect that culture has on pain assessment, pain expression, and pain treatment.

Age

Age may release a client from culturally imposed norms in relation to pain expression. A young girl in a stoic culture may be allowed to cry because of pain. Children are usually given greater freedom of action, but boys may have more constraints on their behavior than girls.

There is controversy about pain in the elderly. There is no reason to assume that pain reception is altered in the elderly unless some damage has occurred in the CNS. The transmission and perception might be slowed with aging, but this does not diminish the pain that is felt.

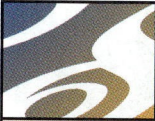

DIVERSITY IN HEALTHCARE

Cultural Perspectives on Pain

Expressions, meanings, and care associated with pain are learned in early childhood within the cultural context of the family. An individual's perception and reaction to pain is culturally influenced. The conceptualization of pain as a health-related problem is culturally determined. Culture also influences a nurse's perception, meaning, and decision-making in the care of persons who are experiencing pain. If the cultural meaning of pain is markedly different for the nurse, client, family, and others significant to the client, then the assessment, care, and evaluation of specific actions to alleviate pain may be problematic. There is the potential for cross-cultural miscommunication and provision of culturally inappropriate care.

Much can be understood about the cultural meaning of pain by the language used to communicate experiences with pain. For example, consider a 45-year-old Chinese-American man who complains of "chest pain" following the death of his wife. The client continues to complain of pain even though a complete cardiac work-up reveals no significant cardiac findings. Within the Chinese belief system the heart is the center of emotions. All emotions, good and bad, originate there. In Chinese culture the symptom is viewed as the primary illness problem. Therefore, care of this client will need to focus on the symptom (chest pain) rather than the cause of the symptom (loss or sadness). This scenario presents Western biomedical healthcare providers with the challenge of intervening in culturally congruent ways.

Perhaps the most cited study on culture and pain is the work of Zborowski. In this classic study, interviews were conducted with men hospitalized for chronic pain. Zborowski identified four groups, Old American, Italian, Irish, and Jewish, and examined how each responded to pain. Although more recent studies reflecting the influences of assimilation have been conducted, findings from this research support the premise that differences exist between cultural group members in

the reactions and meanings associated with pain.

Much of the research since this study has focused on identifying differences in pain responses among cultural groups. Both differences and similarities have been found in relation to pain anxiety, pain attitudes, tolerance, responses, perception, and coping behaviors used by members of cultural groups in response to pain.

The research of Davitz and Davitz in the 1970s and 1980s demonstrated racial differences in responses to pain. Southern blacks are more vocal in their reports of pain than northern blacks or whites. Cross-cultural communication issues also may influence the black client's openness in communicating pain to physicians and nurses who are from different cultures.

In a study of men experiencing the symptoms of myocardial infarction, Perkoff and Strand report that white men are more likely to report chest pain, whereas black men are more likely to report dyspnea. Research by Neill, however, found no statistically significant differences in sensory, affective, evaluative, or pain intensity measures among white, Irish, Italian, Jewish, and black men. However, black men in the study were more likely to report shortness of breath than were men from the other groups.

Abu-Saad studied Arab-American, Asian-American, and Latin-American children. Descriptors of pain varied by cultural group. Arab-American children use such words as "sore," "uncomfortable," and "tingling" to describe the pain. Asian-American children describe pain as "scary," "paralyzing," and "cold." Latin-American children use such words as "hitting," "terrible," and "sickening" to describe pain. Arab-American and Asian-American children often report feeling nervous, embarrassed, or angry when in pain, whereas Latin-American children say that they are feeling "bad" when in pain.

Several studies have examined single cultural groups. Calatrella found that Mexican-Americans rarely acknowledge signs and symptoms

of pain because they consider lack of stamina a sign of weakness. These persons, however, may moan while in pain because this is seen as an acceptable expression of pain and may be used in an attempt to relieve the pain. In many Hispanic groups, stoicism is valued. Difficulties and illness should be borne with dignity. Religious beliefs about suffering held by some Hispanics may contribute to the stoic response, especially if the pain is perceived as God's will or divine punishment for sinful transgressions.

In a study by Meleis, Arab-Americans were found to view pain as unwelcome and unpleasant. Accordingly, responses to pain are directed at avoiding painful situations, controlling existing ones, and attending to pain immediately. Expressions of pain are influenced by the environmental context and the presence of family members. For example, responses in the presence of family members were characterized by loud moans, screams, and gasps for air, but were considerably more subdued in the presence of non-family members. In contrast, the pain associated with childbirth requires a public expression of pain. Descriptions of pain by Arab-Americans tend to be more encompassing than one would infer from the primary site of injury or pain, involving references to the entire body, life, and overall functioning. Metaphors such as "fire" and "flame" frequently are used when describing a burning sensation of pain.

Kagawa-Sincer studied the expressions and behaviors of Japanese-Americans (Nisei) experiencing cancer pain. The researcher noted that, although Nisei appear stoic in situations that are likely to be painful, this stoic behavior does not mean that within the culture there is a high tolerance to pain. Rather, there are cultural norms which determine how pain should be expressed. For example, within the culture the belief exists that one should be able to withstand discomfort. Expression of pain indicates a weakness of character. Stoicism

Feature continued on following page

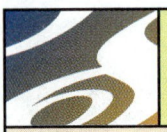

DIVERSITY IN HEALTHCARE

Cultural Perspectives on Pain (*Continued*)

may be related to Buddhist beliefs about pain and suffering.

The majority of nurses in the United States are white, middle-class women who have been socialized to believe that self-control is better than open displays of strong feelings. In a study of 52 white nurses, Acheson found that the nurses reported their own behavior while experiencing pain as "stoic" and "nonverbal." They also indicated a minimal use of analgesics when personally experiencing pain. Using vignettes that described Native-American, Southeast Asian, white American, and Mexican-American clients, nurses were asked to infer physical pain, psychological distress, and intervention choices. Nurses tended to infer the greatest physical pain for Southeast Asian clients, followed closely by Mexican-American clients. Inferences of pain were identical for Native-American and white American clients. A statistically significant relationship was found between the level of pain inferred and the choice of intervention.

Nurses may deny the pain that they observe in others. In a study of the biases of healthcare professionals, Baer and colleagues found that social workers tend to infer the greatest degree of pain, while physicians and nurses infer less pain. The researcher speculated that individuals who are in frequent contact with people in pain may protect themselves from becoming overwhelmed by denying the pain.

In a 1981 study by Davitz and Davitz, it was found that the client's ethnic background is an important determinant for inference by American nurses of suffering caused by physical and psychological distress. Nurses viewed Jewish and Spanish clients as suffering most and Asian, Anglo-Saxon, and Germanic clients as suffering least. In addition, nurses who inferred relatively greater client pain tended to report their own experiences as more painful than nurses who inferred less client pain. In general, nurses with eastern European, southern European, or African backgrounds tended to infer greater suffer than did nurses with northern European backgrounds. Years of experience, current position, and area of practice were unrelated to inferences of suffering.

The undertreatment of pain by nurses has been a significant problem for many years. Several studies suggest that nurses' perceptions of pain do not coincide with those of patients and that the undertreatment has resulted in unnecessary suffering for patients. Rankin and Snider found that 58% of nurses have the goal of reducing rather than eliminating pain. Sixty-seven percent of the patients in the study continued to have moderate pain despite interventions. Dudley and Holme found that nurses tend to infer a greater degree of psychological distress than physical distress from pain. This may lead to inappropriate interventions such as psychological support without other pain interventions. Streltzer and Wade studied postcholecystectomy pain in whites, indigenous Hawaiians, and Asians. They found that nurses limited the amount of analgesia given to all groups, with significantly less analgesia given to Japanese, Filipino, and Chinese patients, the least vocal group in this study.

Treatment of Pain

Although a large number of practices have been used for centuries in the management of pain, the predominant biomedical system has adopted or adapted very few of them. Most interventions for pain are limited to medication and biostimulation techniques. Research suggests that approximately one third of the 260 million people in the United States currently use alternative or complementary healing treatments. These are sometimes ridiculed and labeled pejoratively with terms such as "unconventional" or "unscientific." Fortunately, the National Institutes of Health has created the Office of Alternative Medicine for the purpose of testing the effectiveness of efficacy of these nontraditional treatments.

The following alternative or complementary methods of pain management may be used either alone or in combination by clients from varied cultural backgrounds. Pharmacologic, surgical, and other biomedical interventions may be used concurrently. Some of the methods have gained increasing acceptance in the professional healthcare arena, whereas others are viewed with skepticism. This overview is intended to familiarize the nurse with the many options available to clients. Success is highly variable and depends on the underlying cause and severity of the pain, the knowledge and skill of the healer(s), and the client's belief in the method's power to relieve pain and restore health.

Just as the symptoms and causes of pain are culturally defined, so is the treatment. Treatment may include single or multiple interventions. Folk, indigenous, and spiritual healing methods may be used either by themselves or in conjunction with Western biomedical interventions. Clients from some cultural groups may seek the help of

Physical factors such as paralysis or aphasia may change the response to pain, but it does not mean that pain is not occurring, only that the older person might be having difficulty reporting that pain. This is a very important point for the nurse to remember: lack of response does not mean lack of pain in older adults. Even confused clients need to be closely assessed because their expression of pain may be altered. It is vital that the nurse

Alternative or Complementary Methods of Pain Control

Method	Potential Benefit
Acupuncture, Acupressure	Target peripheral nerves (acupoints) to achieve analgesia. Pain relief is achieved through needle insertion at acupoints with *acupuncture* and through application of pressure at acupoints with *acupressure*
Biofeedback	Provides client with information about body function and muscle tension to overcome pain
Cutaneous stimulation	Reduces intensity of pain
Distraction	Protects client from awareness of pain by diverting attention with singing, dancing, conversation, or play
Guided imagery	Decreases awareness of intensity of pain by focusing thoughts on a place or activity that is pleasant to the client
Herbal remedies	Nourishes the body with natural ingredients that are believed to reduce or eliminate pain
Massage	Promotes muscle relaxation. Decreases anxiety. Manipulation of musculoskeletal system may reestablish normal alignment of bones and muscles, thus reducing or eliminating pain. (*Note:* Chiropractors are certified and licensed to practice chiropractic care. Chiropractic is a system of healthcare based on the premise that the relationship between the spinal column and nervous system is essential to the restoration and maintenance of health. Folk healers, such as Hispanic *sabadors,* are unlicensed persons who use massage and manipulation of muscles and bones.)
Music therapy	Decreases anxiety, promotes relaxation, and distracts client from awareness of painful stimuli (*Note:* Licensed music therapists base treatment on research and clinical expertise gained in formal academic programs at universities and colleges.)

Relaxation techniques
  Autogenic training
  Benson's relaxation response
  Hypnosis
  Meditation
  Progressive relaxation
  Yoga
	Reduce stress. Promote a sense of well-being by reducing muscle tension. Enhance client's feeling that he she is participating actively in the therapeutic regimen aimed at relieving pain

Religious rituals	Promote holistic healing. Decrease anxiety. Some rituals use distraction, guided imagery, herbal remedies, and therapeutic use of music, individually and severally
Therapeutic touch	Promotes client's self-healing potential. Moves healing energy field from therapist to client
Topical salves and balms	Provide local relief of skin and joint pain

healers who represent various health-illness belief systems.

A nurse's knowledge of cultures can assist in the creative discovery and use of means of care for clients experiencing pain. The comfort of clients is dependent on the nurse's ability to understand and respect the diversity of meanings and expressions of pain.

1. Ludwig-Beymer, P. A. (1995). Transcultural aspects of pain. In M. M. Andrews and J. S. Boyle (Eds.), *Transcultural concepts in nursing care* (pp. 301–322). Philadelphia: J. B. Lippincott.
2. Villarruel, A. (1995). Cultural perspectives of pain. In M. M. Leininger (Ed.), *Transcultural nursing: Concepts, theories, research and practice* (pp. 263–296). New York: McGraw-Hill.

remember that altered expression does not mean absence of pain.

Older people may assign different meanings to their pain. Pain is often thought of by the elderly as a natural manifestation of aging. This may be interpreted in two ways. First, older people may think pain is simply something to be endured as a normal part of the aging process. Second, it may be seen as a sign of aging, and therefore something to be denied because it means they are getting old. Many older people are hesitant to express pain for fear of being labeled as a complaining elder. Again, careful assessment of the older person's pain is important.

Gender

Gender may be an important influence in response to pain. In most cultures in the United States, little boys are expected to show less expression of pain than little girls. As they grow older, men are also expected to express pain less than women. This does not mean that men feel pain less, only that they are assumed to show it less. In most cultures, men will be less expressive in their reports of pain. As men age, they may be allowed more freedom to express their pain.

Meaning of Pain

The meaning of a person's pain is a factor that influences his or her response to pain. Again, pain caused by childbirth may be responded to differently from pain caused by surgery. If the cause of pain is known, it may help the client respond to it. If the cause is unknown, more negative psychological factors such as fear and anxiety come into play and the pain can be misinterpreted, resulting in an inappropriate response.

Pain that is associated with a threat to body image may be much worse than pain that is not. Think of the client who has a devastating alteration in his or her body image such as a radical neck dissection or an amputation. If the client's psychological response to the pain is not considered, the nurse may not understand the client's suffering.

Anxiety

The degree of anxiety the client is experiencing also may influence the client's response to pain. It is not possible to separate the mind from the body, so pain always has both physiologic components and psychological components. When anxiety is high, pain is felt as greater. Anxiety is often related to the meaning of the pain. If the cause is unknown, anxiety is likely to be higher and the pain worse.

Other Factors

Other factors that also may alter pain reaction are (1) fatigue and insomnia, (2) stress, (3) experience with pain, and (4) depression and the associated isolation.

Therapeutic Implications of the Pain Process

Therapeutic implications of our current knowledge of pain include the following:

● Pain control might be achieved by selectively influencing pain transduction and transmission. Also, any procedure that reduces sensory input lessens the opportunity for pain to occur.
● A better understanding of the physiology and pharmacology of the peripheral central control mechanisms may lead to new ways of controlling pain with medications that excite or inhibit activity.
● Experience, attention, emotion, and other psychological factors influence pain perception and pain response by acting on the spinal cord's pain transmission system. Pain management includes motivational and cognitive aspects of an individual's pain experience.
● Stimulation or blocking the production of various endogenous CNS substances may prove useful in controlling transmission of pain in the CNS, blocking its transmission to the central cortex, or influencing descending modulation.

Theories of Pain

Specificity Theory

The specificity theory was described by Descartes in the seventeenth century. This theory is based on a belief that specialized pathways for pain transmission exist. It was thought that free nerve endings existed in the periphery that acted as pain receptors. These nerves were believed to be capable of receiving painful stimuli and transmitting the impulses via highly specific nerve fibers. The sensation would then be transmitted through the spinal cord to the thalamus and finally to the higher cortical areas. Pain would be interpreted in these higher areas, and a response would occur.

This theory did not address the multidimensional characteristics of pain, viewing it simply as a sense like all the other senses. It is mainly a biologic explanation of a highly complex process. It has been refuted and is given here only for historical purposes.

Gate-Control Theory

The physiology of pain transmission and perception is less well understood than the underlying physical structure (anatomy). There are various theoretical models that attempt to explain how neural units interact during the experience of pain. One such model is the gate-control theory, described more than 30 years ago and revised periodically. It explains many aspects of pain and how pain may be controlled by thoughts, emotions, and action.

In 1965, Melzack and Wall[112] presented the first version of the gate-control theory. They suggested the existence of a gate that could either facilitate or inhibit the transmission of pain signals. The gate is controlled by the dynamic function of certain cells in the spinal cord's dorsal horn. Afferent fibers bringing information about pain synapse for the first time in the laminae of the dorsal horns. Melzack and Wall proposed that the substantia gelatinosa (SG) within the dorsal horn is the anatomic location of the gate. Both A delta and C fibers converge in the SG. Also, descending fibers from the brain send pain-inhibitory information and act here. These fibers come from areas such as the PAG, hypothalamus, nucleus raphe magnus, and locus ceruleus.

Melzack and Wall[112] proposed that a spinal cord transmission cell (T cell) exists in the SG. Depending on its input from other cells, the T cell either facilitates (opens the gate) or inhibits pain transmission (closes the gate). The gate can be influenced (opened or closed) by information from various sources. Activity from large-diameter fibers (carrying information, such as touch) can inhibit pain transmission (close the gate); for example, one rubs one's elbow after banging it to ease the pain, thereby closing the gate.

Whether the gate is open or closed, it can be influenced by fibers carrying information from many different brain centers down to the T cells. According to this theory, information from non-pain fibers or information from the brain can reduce or totally block pain information before it is experienced. When the gate is open, pain information influences multiple centers in the brain. When working together, these centers produce the complex but integrated responses that occur in a person experiencing pain. The model suggests, however, that the brain also can influence whether or not the gate is open. Thus, factors such as attention, memory, thinking, and emotion may either inhibit or enhance the transmission of pain signals.

A recent version of the gate-control theory (called Mark II by Melzack and Wall[113]) is presented in Figure 17–2. The newer model emphasizes the probability that there is an inhibitory system within the brain stem that also acts as a gate inhibiting pain transmission. This brain stem inhibitory circuit has been described in detail by Basbaum and Fields[11] who believe that the system involves structures in the midbrain, medulla, and spinal

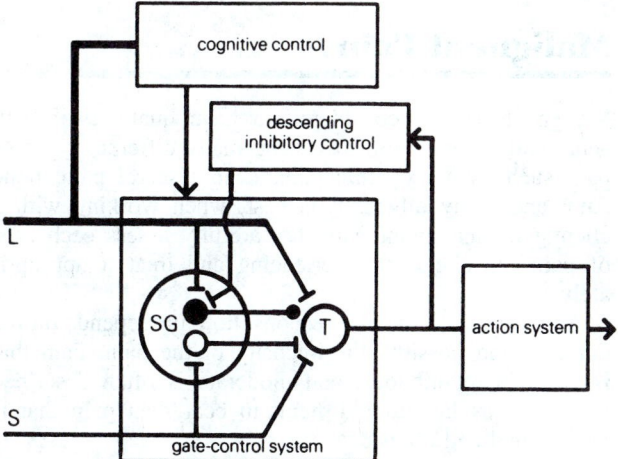

Figure 17–2. The gate-control theory: Mark II. The new model includes excitatory (*white circle*) and inhibitory (*black circle*) links from the substantia gelatinosa (*SG*) to the transmission (*T*) cells as well as descending inhibitory control from brain stem systems. The round knob at the end of the inhibitory link implies that its action may be presynaptic, postsynaptic, or both. All connections are excitatory, except the inhibitory link from SG to T cell. *L*, large-diameter fibers; *S*, small-diameter fibers. (From Melzack, R., & Wall, P. D. [1988]. *The challenge of pain* [2nd ed.]. New York: Penguin Books.)

cord. Activation of cells in the midbrain's PAG (by electric stimulation, opiate analgesic medications, or possible psychological factors), in turn, stimulates structures in the medulla. These medullary structures then project to and inhibit spinal pain transmission fibers. Pain itself might activate this system. Under some circumstances, it acts as a natural control mechanism that limits the severity of the pain experience, such the soldier severely injured in battle who is unaware of pain.

We now know that there is a pain inhibitory complex located in the dorsal horns of the spinal cord. Pain can be blocked at this point by signals from the brain. Nerve fibers terminating in the dorsal horns secrete serotonin, which causes local cord neurons to secrete enkephalin. Enkephalin then causes presynaptic and postsynaptic inhibition of incoming transmission from both type C and A delta pain fibers at the synapses in the dorsal horn. This natural analgesic system can block pain signals as they enter the spinal cord.

Types of Pain

It is important for nurses to realize that there are many different types of pain. There are various ways to define types of pain, including the following:

- Onset or time of occurrence, such as postoperative pain (see Chapter 21)
- Duration, such as chronic or acute pain
- Severity or intensity, such as severe or mild, or scored 0 to 10 on a scale
- Mode of transmission, such as through the usual pain pathways or referred pain
- Location or source, such as superficial, deep, or central pain
- Causation, such as pain due to receptor stimulation or nerve damage, or psychophysiologic pain
- Causative force or agent, such as spontaneous, self-inflicted, or other pain

Acute Pain

Acute pain is usually of short duration (less than 6 months) and has an identifiable, immediate onset, such as incisional pain after surgery. It is also seen as having a limited and often predictable duration, such as postoperative pain, which usually disappears as the wound heals. It is often described in sensory terms, such as "sharp," "stabbing," and "shooting."

Acute pain is seen as a useful and limiting pain in that it indicates injury and motivates the person to get relief by treatment of the pain and usually the cause. Acute pain is usually reversible or controllable with adequate treatment.

Figure 17–3 illustrates that as pain increases, so does a person's anxiety, until a certain point is reached. It demonstrates that the fear of pain can actually raise it above the level of tolerance.

Clients suffering from acute pain often come to terms with that pain because of the meaning or the limited nature of the pain, such as the pain of childbirth. When

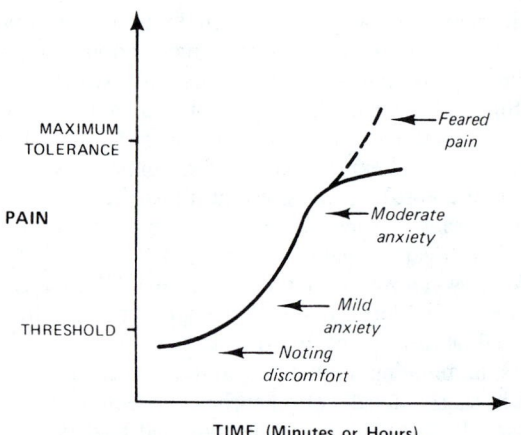

Figure 17–3. Sequence of reactions to acute pain. (From Sternbach, R. A. [1974]. *Pain patients—traits and treatment* [p. 6]. New York: Academic Press.)

the pain is relieved, the client again appears perfectly normal.

The physiologic response to acute pain is due to stimulation of the sympathetic nervous system. The client may exhibit the following manifestations: (1) increased or decreased blood pressure, (2) tachycardia, (3) diaphoresis, (4) tachypnea, (5) focusing on the pain, and (6) guarding the painful part.

In 1992, the Agency for Health Care Policy and Research (AHCPR)[2] released its first set of clinical practice guidelines. The topic was acute pain management. The purpose of the guidelines was to address problems of critical interest to both health professionals and the public. The guidelines had four major goals: "1) Reduce the incidence and severity of patients' acute postoperative or posttraumatic pain, 2) Educate patients about the need to communicate unrelieved pain so they can receive prompt evaluation and effective treatment, 3) Enhance patient comfort and satisfaction, and 4) Contribute to fewer postoperative complications and, in some cases, shorter stays after surgical procedures" (p. 3).

These guidelines were set up to help the client, family, and healthcare professionals work together to promote better relief of acute pain. Nurses can obtain valuable information from these guidelines including using them to help with both pain assessment and management. The nurse should use these guidelines to improve pain control for all clients. The guidelines emphasize the following.

> A collaborative, interdisciplinary approach to pain control, including all members of the health care team and input from the patient and patient's family, when appropriate;
>
> An individualized proactive pain control plan developed preoperatively by patients and practitioners (since pain is easier to prevent than to bring under control, once it has begun);
>
> Assessment and frequent reassessment of the patient's pain;
>
> Use of both drug and nondrug therapies to control and/or prevent pain;
>
> A formal, institutional approach to management of acute pain, with clear lines of responsibility. (p. 2)

Chronic Nonmalignant Pain

Chronic pain is usually considered pain that lasts more than 6 months (or 1 month beyond the normal end of the condition causing the pain) and has no foreseeable end except very slow healing, as with burns, or death. It is continuous or persistent and recurrent. There is some disagreement as to whether or not acute recurrent pain, as in migraines and sickle cell crisis, should be classified as chronic pain, but they usually are. The acute nature of this pain means that the nurse should be very careful when treating these clients.

Other characteristics of chronic pain are that it may have an identifiable cause (although the cause may be difficult to determine); is often described using affective terms, such as "hateful" or "sickening"; and is often much more difficult to treat than acute pain. It is considered a useless pain because it is not usually a manifestation of impending damage. For example, a client immobilized with the pain of severe rheumatoid arthritis may be further crippled by immobility.

Chronic pain is often frustrating and difficult for a person to live with. It gives no clues about how to lessen it. Healthcare providers may feel frustrated and incompetent when their attempts to relieve chronic pain are ineffective. However, if nurses understand the anatomy, physiology, and psychosocial aspects of chronic pain, they can be very helpful to the client. Professionals can intervene before extreme suffering occurs.

Clients experiencing continuous or continually recurring chronic pain often become increasingly engrossed by their illness. They may seem fearful, tense, fatigued, and depressed. Many persons with an unending chronic pain become withdrawn and isolated. Their pain often exhausts them and their families, physically and emotionally.

Malignant Pain

Malignant pain is considered to have qualities of both acute and chronic pain. It can be many different types of pain such as neuropathic pain, deep visceral pain, bone pain, and many others. It is best, when working with a client with malignant pain, to carefully assess each type of pain the client is experiencing and treat it appropriately.

An individual's mental response to pain depends on the duration and possibly the intensity of the pain. Pain that is constant, continuous, and moderate is often described by clients as far more difficult to bear than pain that is paroxysmal and intense.

The course of chronic pain includes months and years of pain, not minutes or hours. Chronic pain is associated with withdrawal and despair. Anxiety may give way to depression. Some chronic pain clients learn to adapt and cope with the pain, adjusting their lives.

The sympathetic arousal that may be associated with acute pain diminishes over weeks or months even though the pain itself persists. Sympathetic adaptation occurs over time. The nurse must remember, however, that absence of the expected expression of severe pain does not mean that the pain is gone. The nurse must depend on the client's description of pain, not the manifestations one expects to see. An example of severe chronic pain is causalgia. With causalgia, the nerve trunk itself is damaged, and prolonged, intense pain is experienced. Causalgia is often the cause of many types of chronic pain.

Intractable, chronic pain states, producing prolonged and intense bombardment of the CNS, are very difficult to bear. The client may become suicidal or at least take no steps to prolong life. Two days before her death, Alice James (sister of Henry James) wrote in her journal, "I am being ground slowly on the grim grindstone of physical pain, and on two nights I had almost asked for K's lethal dose; but one steps hesitantly along such unaccustomed ways, and endures from second to second."

Most clients have major affective and behavioral changes when experiencing pain for prolonged periods. Such changes may be compounded, and chronic pain syndrome can develop. Characteristics of clients experiencing chronic pain syndrome include the following:

● Depressed mood
● Increased or decreased appetite and weight
● Drastically restricted activity level, leading to reduced work capacity, poor physical tone, and increased depression
● Social withdrawal
● Preoccupation with physical manifestations
● Poor sleep and chronic fatigue, which may result from inactivity, analgesics, and depression, as well as pain

Some clients with chronic pain may not exhibit any of the above-mentioned manifestations, or they may exhibit only a few. However, once these changes take place, they may become more significant to treatment than the pain's original physical source.

Unfortunately, psychosocial implications about pain sometimes reinforce the idea that clients may "make too much fuss" over their pain. Clients with significant pain are rightfully resentful and angry if told this (either verbally or nonverbally), such as "your pain is all in your head." Such statements are not helpful and are based on (1) inadequate knowledge of the physical basis of pain, (2) behavioral consequences of having to endure persistent pain, (3) inadequate understanding of various therapies, and (4) the subjective nature of the pain experience (it is felt by the client, and if the client feels it, it is real).

Cutaneous or Superficial Pain

Two types of cutaneous pain are (1) pain with an abrupt onset and a sharp or stinging quality, and (2) pain with a slower onset and a burning quality. Cutaneous pain may be delineated by having the client point to the painful area. It may occur along each segment representing a portion of the body surface innervated by one dorsal root. A dermatome or skin segment is an area of skin supplied by one dorsal root. Each spinal nerve has a dorsal or sensory root. The boundaries of dermatomes may appear to be distinct in anatomic drawings, but nerve distribution actually overlaps. Irritation of one posterior root produces pain in adjacent dermatomes. A spinal nerve attaches to

the spinal cord with two roots—anterior and posterior. The anterior root contains efferent nerve fibers that carry impulses from the CNS to the periphery of the body. The posterior root contains afferent nerve fibers that carry impulses from the body's periphery toward the CNS. Cutaneous pain is relatively uncomplicated because it is readily localized, that is, the client can indicate exactly where it hurts.

Deep Somatic Pain

Pain in the somatic structures is a complicated phenomenon. Somatic structures are those of the body wall, such as muscles and bone. Table 17–1 compares deep pain with cutaneous pain. The main difference between cutaneous and deep sensibility (i.e., the capacity to receive stimuli and respond to them) is the different nature of the pain evoked by noxious (harmful) stimuli. For example, unlike cutaneous pain, deep pain (1) is poorly localized, (2) may produce nausea, and (3) is frequently associated with sweating and blood pressure changes.

Deep somatic pain is generally diffuse, less localizable than cutaneous pain. This is because the area supplied by one posterior nerve root (sclerotome) is less well defined than a dermatome and does not correspond with a dermal segment. Also, pain from deep structures frequently radiates (spreads) from the primary site (e.g., pain from a lumbar disc is felt along the sciatic nerve).

Somatic structures vary in their sensitivity to pain. Highly sensitive structures include tendons, deep fascia, ligaments, joints, bone periosteum, blood vessels, and nerves. Skeletal muscle is sensitive only to stretching and ischemia. Bone and cartilage respond to extreme pressure and chemical stimulation (e.g., rheumatoid arthritis, osteomyelitis).

Visceral Pain

Usually, the term *viscera* refers to abdominal viscera. Actually, however, a viscus (plural, *viscera*) is any of the large interior body organs occupying any body cavity, such as the cranial, thoracic, abdominal, or pelvic cavities. Visceral pain tends to be a diffuse, poorly localized, vague, dull pain. Nerve fibers innervating body organs follow the sympathetic nerves to the spinal cord. This may be the reason why autonomic manifestations (e.g., diarrhea, cramps, sweating, hypertension) frequently accompany visceral pain. Typical visceral pain includes acute appendicitis, cholecystitis, inflammation of the biliary and pancreatic tract, gastroduodenal disease, cardiovascular disease, pleurisy, and renal and ureteral colic.

Most viscera are not sensitive to stimuli that cause pain in somatic structures (such as cutting, burning, or pressure). This is understandable. Because viscera are not normally exposed to such traumas, the body does not "need" a response system. Although these types of stimuli do not produce pain in most viscera, other stimuli may cause severe pain, for example, violent or abnormal contractions of hollow viscera such as the ureters and alimentary tract.

Table 17–1. Comparison of Cutaneous and Deep Pain		
Characteristic	**Cutaneous Pain**	**Deep Pain**
Quality	Sharp, bright sensation or burning; felt superficially	Primarily dull and aching May be described as boring, crushing, throbbing, or cramping, or (if less intense) as a soreness or hurting
Duration	Typically short	Often fairly long
Localization	Tends to be precise Pain is often experienced as a point, surface, or line	Often diffuse and inaccurate; seems to originate in a fairly broad area Pain frequently is felt as if it were of three dimensions and occupied space
Hyperalgesia	May occur; of a primary nature	May exist; secondary in nature; occurring at a distance from the original noxious stimulus In referred pain, a superficial hyperalgesia may be associated with deep pain
Nausea	Never occurs	Sickening pain found only when deep structures are involved, as in renal and intestinal colic, gallstones, and angina
Associated symptoms	May be hyperalgesia, paresthesia, tickling, burning, or itching Also associated with brisk movements, a quick pulse, and a sense of invigoration	Due to autonomic responses including pallor, sweating, nausea, vomiting, and (at times) bradycardia, fall in blood pressure, syncope, faintness, and perhaps even death in shock Muscle contraction and tenderness often occur Segmental spread of pain frequently noted Pain may not remain confined to original spinal segment but may spread into one or more adjacent segments

Visceral pain differs from cutaneous pain in that highly localized damage to the viscera rarely causes severe pain, whereas such damage to the body surface would cause pain. For example, a surgical cut in the gut does not cause pain, whereas a cut on the skin would cause severe pain. If the stimulus to the viscera causes diffuse stimulation of nerve endings, then the resulting pain is severe, as in ischemia of the gut.

Visceral pain is transmitted through the sympathetic and parasympathetic fibers of the autonomic nervous system, with the pain being referred to the body surface, often in sites at a distance. Visceral pain also may be sent through the nerve fibers in the parietal pleura, pericardium, or peritoneum and is called parietal pain.

Parietal pain is transmitted directly to the spinal nerves, with the pain being felt directly over the painful area. Referred pain due to visceral disease follows dermatome patterns that somatic referred pain does not. Parietal tissue is well supplied with spinal nerves instead of sympathetic nerves. Pain starting in the parietal tissue is often very sharp.

Referred Pain

Deep pain may arise from disease of the viscera or from a lesion of a deep somatic structure (e.g., vertebra, muscle, interspinous ligament). However, both visceral and somatic pain are usually referred to a segment of skin because visceral fibers synapse at the level of the spinal cord close to fibers innervating some subcutaneous tissues.

Referred pain is peculiar because it is sometimes intense, although there is little or no pain at the point of noxious stimuli. For example, myocardial ischemia is not felt as pain in the heart; rather, it is felt as left arm, shoulder, or jaw pain. The fibers innervating these areas are close to those innervating the myocardium, resulting in the referred pain.

Identification of the segment of the spinal cord that is involved in transmitting referred pain is diagnostically helpful. Pain arising from a deep structure, whether a viscus or a deep somatic structure, has a referred segmental distribution, or a pattern of pain, determined according to the spinal cord segment supplying the structure.

Referred pain is often baffling and requires careful assessment. Examples of common patterns include pleural pain from the diaphragm referred to the shoulder, and the pain of cholecystitis referred to the back and in the angle of the scapula. Figure 17–4 illustrates common sites of referred pain.

Pathologic Pain Syndromes

Deafferentation or Neuropathic Pain

The types of pain discussed so far involve the stimulation of nociceptors by chemical, mechanical, or noxious ther-

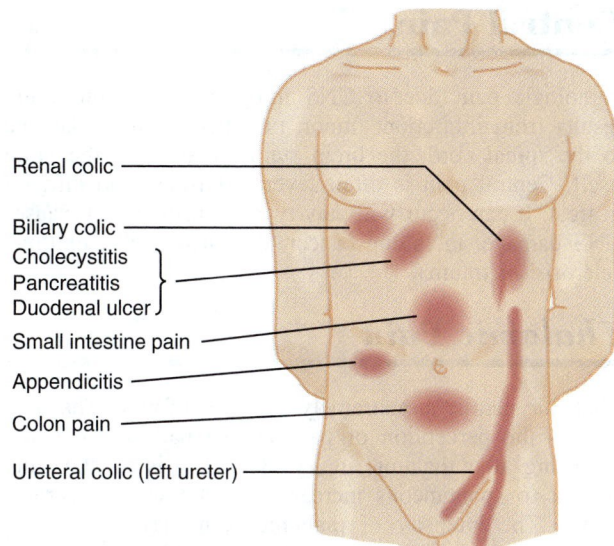

Renal colic

Biliary colic

Cholecystitis
Pancreatitis
Duodenal ulcer

Small intestine pain

Appendicitis

Colon pain

Ureteral colic (left ureter)

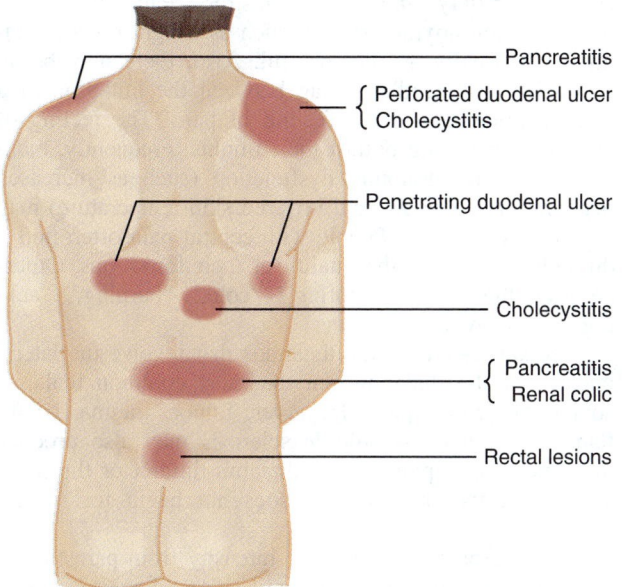

Pancreatitis

Perforated duodenal ulcer
Cholecystitis

Penetrating duodenal ulcer

Cholecystitis

Pancreatitis
Renal colic

Rectal lesions

Figure 17–4. Areas of referred pain.

mal (heat or cold) stimuli. Because they involve nociceptors, they are sometimes referred to as nociceptive pain. Severe pain also can be caused by nervous system damage, when the flow of afferent nerve impulses has been partially or completely interrupted. This type of pain is called neuropathic pain or deafferentation. (Other names include hyperpathia, causalgia, or spontaneous pain.) Most neuropathic pain syndromes have similar features, including the following:

● Pain is often present in the absence of stimulation or an obvious pathologic process to account for the pain, such as nonvascular peripheral neuropathies.

● Pain may be present in the absence of stimulation, with damage to small-caliber nerves, such as burning feet in a diabetic client.

● When nonpainful stimulation is applied to the area where pain is felt, as with a cotton wisp, the pain

sensation often increases, such as the sensitivity of postherpetic neuralgia.

● Although change in other somatosensory sensations, such as touch or position sense, may occur, the common finding is change in pain sensation due to damage of the normal pathways for pain transmissions, as with thalamic pain.

● Pain may appear to arise from a body part that has its pain pathway to the brain destroyed, as with an amputation. This seeming paradox (pain in the absence of a pathway) has given rise to such terms as *phantom* or *phantomlike pain.*

The lesions that cause neuropathic pain can occur at any location in the pain pathway. There may be damage to peripheral nerves as well as lesions of the spinal cord, brain stem, and thalamus and other subcortical and even cortical areas.

Pain of Muscular and Bony Origin

Ligaments, joint capsules, fascia, tendons, and muscle all vary in the density of their innervation. The periosteum is most sensitive. Spontaneous pain may occur from spasm, rupture, ischemia, inflammation, or other disturbances of the ligaments, tendons, muscles, and periosteum of bones and joints. The muscular ischemia of intermittent claudication and occlusive vascular disease induces pain in the extremities. Also, it is the basis of the pain of coronary occlusion. Although chemical irritants injected into muscles may give rise to considerable pain, muscular pain usually occurs in association with stretching, ischemia, or forceful or sustained contractile activity. An injury to muscle causes the release of lactic acid and other substances that increase pain.

The sustained clenching of muscles or their continued overuse may produce muscular pain. The primary cause of muscle pain does not appear to be muscle tension but rather the compression or constriction of blood vessels within the muscle or traction on periosteum.

When muscle pain causes a sustained reflex contraction of the muscle, a vicious circle may occur. The contraction successively increases muscular pain, and the pain gradually radiates into adjacent areas. A large proportion of headaches, especially those accompanied by stiffness or tenderness in the neck and occipital region, originate from the sustained contraction of underlying neck and scalp muscles (see the discussion of headache).

Vascular Pain

The precise mechanism of vascular pain is not understood but is believed to originate from some pathologic condition of the vessels or perivascular tissues. Some pain-producing substances also seem to be significant.

The blood vessels are often involved in various pain syndromes. Blood vessels are believed to be associated with pain induced by cold. Also, distortion of the cranial vessels by pulling, displacement, or distention is the source of a large proportion of headaches. These include migraine headaches and headaches associated with arterial hypertension, brain tumors, and variations in the hydrodynamics of the cerebrospinal fluid (CSF) (e.g., increased intracranial pressure).

Pain Caused by Inflammation

Inflammation is one of the most common pathologic conditions influencing pain sensitivity. Inflammation can be caused by numerous harmful agents, such as bacterial or chemical agents, or stressors, such as heat, cold, or trauma. Gross assessment findings associated with the inflammatory process are redness, swelling, heat, and pain. Inflammatory pain is secondary to the distention of stretch-sensitive tissue (i.e., periosteum, pleura) and the direct effect of released neuroregulators on afferent nerve endings. Principal chemical mediators of the inflammatory response are histamine, substance P, bradykinin, prostaglandins, and leukokinins. All of these mediators are highly acidic. Increased acidity at the site of the injured tissue seems to heighten sensitivity in pain fibers. This allows less stimulation to cause a sensation of pain and makes pain more intense (e.g., if one has a paper cut then the mildest touch, usually nonpainful, can cause pain). These acidic mediators are also capable of provoking pain directly.

In the chest, the parietal pleura is richly supplied with pain endings through the intercostal nerves and through the phrenic nerve, on the surface of the diaphragm. The visceral pleura in the chest, however, is insensitive to pain. The bronchi, on the other hand, are sensitive to pain. Elsewhere and throughout its serous surfaces, the visceral pericardium is insensitive to pain, with the exception of the lower portion of the fibrous pericardium, which appears to have pain fibers from the phrenic nerve.

Pain in the gastrointestinal tract is common. It appears to arise mainly from the tract's muscular and serous coats. Gastrointestinal pain seems to occur when intestinal mucosa is inflamed, ulcerated, or otherwise abnormal, or when the visceral muscles contract strongly or pass into spasm. Thus, while the wall of the intestine is not sensitive to cutting, burning, or crushing, it does produce pain under other conditions, such as widespread ischemia.

Abdominal pain may also occur when body organs are perforated and their contents drain into the peritoneal cavity. Intraperitoneal fluids that may accumulate are listed below, from the most irritating to the least irritating:

- Pancreatic enzyme fluid
- Gastric or duodenal fluid
- Fecal fluid from the colon, appendix, or small bowel
- Bile
- Urine
- Blood
- Lymph

The parietal peritoneum, the mesentery, and many blood vessels are sensitive to injuries such as cutting, stretching, and handling. Also, the mucosal linings of the urethra, bladder, ureter, and pelves of the kidneys are sensitive to nociceptive pain and stretching.

Central Pain

Pathologic pain due to CNS injury (central pain) often results from infarction, tumor, or other localized damage to the spinal cord, the brain stem, or areas of the brain itself. Central pain is often severe, constant, and difficult to treat. It can occur with any type of disorder that causes CNS damage, including cancer, diabetes, stroke, multiple sclerosis, or trauma.

Thalamic Pain

Thalamic pain is an extremely rare type of pain. Thalamic pain is the perception of pain in one half of the body, occurring after thalamic injury. It usually is constant and subject to spontaneous increases in pain without serious injury. The intensity of thalamic pain may also be increased by specific stimuli, such as sudden temperature changes, anxiety, and emotional stress. Pain may be induced by non-noxious stimuli such as a light touch, stimuli that normally are not painful. Also, there may be an unusually prolonged time lag between the initiation of a painful stimulus and the feeling of pain. The feeling of pain may then long outlast the stimulus. Frequently, manifestations of autonomic dysfunction (such as increased perspiration, cyanosis, and lowered skin temperature) may accompany the pain. People with central pain often find it difficult to describe the quality of their sensations. Others describe the pain as "boring," "cold," "burning," "aching," or "gnawing."

Vascular lesions of the thalamus that involve the lateral nucleus of the thalamus are the most common thalamic source of central pain. However, tumor, trauma, or inflammation such as multiple sclerosis may also produce thalamic central pain. When thalamic infarct or thrombosis occurs, the pain usually does not begin for several weeks.

Thalamic pain may range in intensity from paresthesias (sensations of numbness, tingling, or prickling) to agonizing, boring, burning pains that are often associated with a feeling that the hand or foot is being twisted. Following a thalamic infarct (cerebrovascular accident [CVA], i.e., stroke), these often excruciating thalamic pains may involve the entire half of the body. Thalamic pain may be intensified by emotional disturbances. Increased emotional lability (e.g., unmotivated crying or laughing) is often associated with this syndrome.

Back Pain

Back pain is one of the most common pain complaints, second only to headache. This pain usually occurs as either cervical or lumbosacral (low back) pain. Back pain results from herniation of the nucleus pulposus in the intervertebral disc, degeneration of the vertebra, or disc injury from hyperreflexia. Herniation, degeneration, or injury results in spinal root compression, leading to subsequent motor and sensory manifestations.

Low back pain is often difficult to diagnose. This leads to questioning the pain in clients with low back pain. It is important for the nurse to objectively assess, without preconceived notions, any client reporting pain. For more information on back pain, see Chapter 75.

Pain from Lesions of the Cerebral Cortex

These lesions (e.g., brain tumors and other mass lesions), as well as cortical ischemic lesions resulting from cerebrovascular occlusive disease, may involve the cerebral cortex and not the thalamus. They may produce central pain in the opposite (i.e., contralateral) side of the body.

Peripheral or Mixed Central and Peripheral Pathologic Pain

Postherpetic Neuralgia

One type of mixed central and peripheral pathologic pain presenting histologic changes in nerve structure is postherpetic neuralgia. After the extremely painful vesicles of herpes zoster (shingles) have subsided and disappeared, some people experience persistent, severe, intractable pain in the area of the original skin eruption. This is postherpetic neuralgia or postherpetic pain. This syndrome is very annoying and tormenting. Its unrelenting pain may cause sleepless nights and unbearable days. Some people are willing to undergo anything in hope of relief. However, the results of therapy may be poor and the postherpetic pain may continue. Neurologic pain is often treated with anticonvulsants or tricyclic antidepressants, such as phenytoin or amitriptyline (see discussion of adjuvant medications for more information).

The cause of postherpetic neuralgia is not fully understood. However, scarring and degenerative changes involving the spinal cord, ganglia, nerve trunks, and skin may be important factors.

Causalgia

The pain syndrome of causalgia typically has a history of peripheral nerve injury. The brachial plexus and the median and sciatic nerves are involved most frequently. Although peripheral nerve damage is the usual cause, other conditions may rarely precipitate the problem. Examples of these are sprains, bruises, fractures, amputations, and arterial and venous occlusions.

Assessment findings in causalgia include burning pain that is often severe, persistent, diffuse, spontaneous, and aggravated by motion, touch, or emotional stimuli. A client with causalgia may appear apathetic and haggard. The pain may cause emotional disturbance if it is prolonged. If the suffering increases in intensity and the area of involvement spreads, intractable pain may lead to severe depression and even suicide.

As with many types of deafferentation pain, virtually any stimulus may set off paroxysms of excruciating pain (e.g., drafts of air, eating, temperature changes, contact with clothing). Consequently, a person may try to prevent pain by keeping the affected joints rigid or by wrapping the part in a moist cloth. Because of a realistic fear of severe pain, a person experiencing causalgia may adopt elaborate precautions to prevent the paroxysms of pain from being triggered. Those who do not understand the reasons for these actions may view them as absurd and unreasonable. Such judgments only further hurt the person and cause additional suffering.

Generally, causalgia is associated with dystrophic and vasomotor changes. Reflex sympathetic dystrophy is a disorder of the sympathetic nervous system that may follow not only injuries to nerves but also those to blood vessels, or it may follow fractures or sprains. Assessment findings of reflex sympathetic dystrophy include rubor or pallor, sweating or dryness, edema, pain, or skin atrophy.

Trigeminal Neuralgia (Tic Douloureux)

This severe lancinating pain occurs along the sensory area of the fifth or ninth cranial nerve. The paroxysmal attacks of pain may be triggered by minimal stimuli, such as drafts of cold air, temperature changes, brushing teeth, clothing pressed against the area, eating, or talking, or even without any stimulus. This pain occurs as a result of a mild mechanoreceptive stimulus rather than a painful stimulus. The pain is described as feeling like a sudden electric shock. The severity of the attacks may lead to attempts to avoid all triggering by not talking or even eating, and the person becomes weak and often depressed.

Often, this condition can be treated with drug therapy. Carbamazepine (Tegretol), used to treat epilepsy, is usually effective in the treatment of this painful condition. Surgery, with the severing of the sensory portion of the fifth cranial nerve, also relieves the pain. This procedure leaves the motor function intact but causes anesthesia of the affected side of the face.

Phantom Pain

Following amputation of a body part (e.g., limb, breast), a client may feel phantom sensations in the area of the amputation, as if that part were still present. These abnormal sensations (paresthesias) commonly include feelings of itching, pressure sensations, tingling, or "pins and needles."

Although phantom sensations are relatively common, phantom pain is less common. Most phantom paresthesias are tolerable, but some types of phantom pain are severe. A formerly painless phantom area may gradually become painful. More typically, however, phantom areas that pose severe problems tend to be painful immediately after amputation.

When phantom pain does occur, throbbing, burning, stabbing, boring, or viselike sensations are experienced in the amputated area. Pain quality varies widely. Phantom pain also may be experienced as cramped, twisted, and abnormal posturing of a phantom limb.

With abnormal posturing sensations, the phantom limb feels as if it were being held immovably rigid in spite of the person's desire to change its position. The fist of an amputated hand may feel clenched so tightly that the nails are tearing into the palm. Clients with amputated legs or feet may experience their missing toes as cramped and curled. This type of pain does not occur in persons who maintain the feeling they can move the phantom limb voluntarily. The condition may be exacerbated by fatigue, excitement, sickness, weather changes, emotional stress, and other stimuli.

Stump pain (pain in the tissues adjacent to the amputation) is often associated with phantom pain. However, it is not necessarily related to it since it may be caused by a neuroma, which can be removed surgically. Clients who have phantom pain usually experience some stump discomfort with their phantom pain, but some clients have phantom pain without stump pain.

Headache

Headache is the most common type of pain. There are many causes of headache, involving both intracranial and extracranial structures. The brain itself is almost insensitive to pain, although the venous sinuses, tentorium, dura, some of the cranial nerves, and associated vasculature are pain-sensitive. One of the most sensitive areas in the brain is the middle meningeal artery. Changes in intracranial pressure, either increases or decreases, may lead to headache because the pressure changes cause the pain-sensitive structures in the head to shift. For example, when a person undergoes a lumbar puncture, the loss of CSF leads to a decreased cushioning of the brain and a downward displacement of the pain-sensitive structures.

There are many types of headache of intracranial origin. Vascular headache is a common type of intracranial headache. This headache can be caused by a variety of problems, such as hypertension, sepsis, hypoxia, and various medications. Other causes of intracranial headache include infection, hemorrhage, and, as mentioned, changes in intracranial pressure.

Probably the best-known headache of intracranial origin is the migraine. Although the cause of migraine is unknown, it seems to involve some abnormality of the vasculature. People suffering from migraine often experience prodromal manifestations, ranging from nausea to visual and auditory changes. One theory is that something triggers extreme vasospasm in some of the arteries in the cranium, leading to ischemia, which would explain the prodromal manifestations. The combination of vasospasm and ischemia leads to a decrease in vascular tone, causing vasodilation for 24 to 48 hours, with intense pulsating of these vessels. This process may cause stretching of intracranial and extracranial arteries, including the temporal artery, causing the pain. Shifting of pain-sensitive structures in the head also may lead to pain.

Headaches of extracranial origin also are common and have many causes. Many extracranial structures are sensitive to nociceptive stimuli. These structures include the skin, subcutaneous tissues, muscles, arteries, and periosteum of the skull. Problems in the eyes, sinuses, ears, teeth, nose, and jaws also may lead to headaches. The mechanisms of these headaches are similar to those causing headaches of intracranial origin. Stimuli such as traction, distention, dilation and spasms of vessels, irritation of nerves, and inflammation of various structures can cause them. The common types of extracranial headaches are muscle tension, temporomandibular joint syndrome, ocular, sinus, dental, and otic.

Headaches of both intracranial and extracranial origin are best treated by first identifying the cause and, if possible, treating it. Medications such as aspirin, acetaminophen, muscle relaxants, sumatriptan, ergotamine, and dexamethasone are used to treat a variety of headaches. The nurse should carefully assess the client to identify the cause so that correct treatment can be started.

Pain of Malignancy

Cancer pain is a common pain syndrome because one in three people in the United States develops cancer. Cancer pain is uncommon in some cancers such as leukemia. However, pain occurs in 60% to 80% of people with solid tumors.[7] The Oncology Nursing Society issued a three-part position paper on cancer pain in 1990.[147-149] This paper addresses issues such as the scope of nursing practice regarding cancer pain, ethical issues, practice issues, education of staff and clients, research recommendations, and sections on nursing administration, social policy, and pediatric cancer pain. The paper also contains a list of cancer and pain management resources. It is an excellent reference for the nurse working with cancer clients.

Cancer pain has multiple causes. Some pain is caused by pressure on or displacement of nerves. Pain also may result from interference with blood supply or blockage within hollow organs. A common cause of cancer pain is metastasis to the bone. This type of pain can occur as a result of pathologic fracture with resultant muscle spasms, as the spine is involved and nerves are affected. Another cause of pain is iatrogenic, such as surgery, radiation therapy, and chemotherapy. Immobility and inflammation also can lead to pain.

Treatment of this pain syndrome is also difficult because it has a variety of causes. Bone pain usually responds to a combination of radiation therapy and NSAIDs, whereas other pain may require opioid analgesics such as morphine. The client and the nurse must know and believe that cancer pain is controllable if adequate and correct medications are used in adequate amounts.

In 1994, the AHCPR developed clinical practice guidelines for the management of cancer pain.[91] These guidelines put forth 10 goals to improve the management of cancer pain:

1) To inform clinicians and patients and their families that most cancer pain can be relieved by available methods; 2) To dispel unfounded fears that addiction results from the appropriate use of medications to control cancer pain; 3) To inform clinicians that cancer pain: a) accompanies both disease and treatment, b) changes over time, c) may have multiple simultaneous causes, d) if unrelieved, can affect

the physical, psychological, social, and spiritual well-being of the patient; 4) To promote prompt and effective assessment, diagnosis, and treatment of pain in patients with cancer, 5) To strengthen the ability of patients with cancer and their families to communicate new or unrelieved pain in order to secure prompt evaluation and effective treatment; 6) To provide clinicians with a synthesis of the literature and expert opinion for application to the management of cancer pain; 7) To familiarize patients and their families with options available for pain relief and to promote their active participation in selecting among these; 8) To provide a model for cancer pain management to guide therapy in selected painful, life-threatening conditions such as AIDS; 9) To provide information and guidelines on the use of controlled substances for the treatment of cancer pain that distinguishes the use of these drugs for legitimate medical purposes from their abuse as illegitimate drugs; 10) To identify health policy and research issues that affect cancer pain management.[91(p2)]

These guidelines provide the nurse with a valuable tool in the understanding, assessment, and management of cancer pain. The nurse should become familiar with these guidelines and use them appropriately. The client guide includes excellent assessment tools for client use and client education information. These guidelines emphasize

> A collaborative, interdisciplinary approach to pain control, including all members of the health care team, with participation of the patient and the patient's family;
> An individualized pain control plan developed and agreed on by the patients, their families, and practitioners;
> Ongoing assessment of the patient's pain;
> Both drug and nondrug therapies to prevent and/or control pain;
> A formalized, institutional approach to the management of cancer pain, with clear lines of responsibility for pain management and for monitoring the quality of pain management. (p. 2)

Pain Associated with HIV

Pain is common in persons with active human immunodeficiency virus (HIV) infection. The major recommendation from the AHCPR is that pain in clients with HIV be treated using cancer pain as a model. Reports on the prevalence of pain in this population range from 25% to 40% in early and ambulatory clients to 60% to almost 100% in endstage disease.[91] The sources of pain in this population include gastrointestinal or abdominal pain from colitis, esophagitis, gastritis, herpes, and cytomegalovirus (CMV); peripheral neuropathy; headache; pleuritic pain from pneumonia; oropharyngeal pain from oral candidiasis or herpes; and pain from Kaposi's sarcoma lesions causing lymphatic obstruction.

As with most types of pain, pain associated with HIV is usually undertreated, even late in the disease. It is often complicated by a previous history of drug abuse or addiction. This prior addiction should not alter the way clients are treated. It simply means that higher doses of analgesics may be needed since the client may have a high tolerance to opioids. It is important that this pain be treated vigorously, using the model of cancer pain treatment. This is particularly true in clients with endstage disease when clients must receive humane pain relief.

Pain of Psychological Origin

Malingering

Rarely, a nurse may meet a client who says that pain is being experienced, who is seeking treatment for pain, but who actually has no pain. This is called malingering. Such clients are aware that they are not experiencing pain. They may make this pretense to achieve the following:

● Avoid a task
● Obtain possible economic gain, for example, money to compensate for an injury
● Obtain opioid analgesics or other psychoactive medications to which they have become physically or psychologically dependent
● Obtain attention or sympathy from others (such clients usually lack more effective social coping techniques)

Never assume that pain is pretended. An accurate diagnosis of pretended pain is difficult to make and is rarely made correctly. Much suffering has resulted when clients actually experiencing pain were treated as if they were just pretending. Pretended pain should not be confused with psychogenic pain, which is very real to the client.

Psychogenic Pain

The term *psychogenic pain* is often used, but is difficult to define. Psychogenic pain refers to pain believed to be due primarily to emotional factors rather than to physiologic dysfunction. Clients experiencing psychogenic pain have a real pain experience. This is sometimes referred to as somatiform disorder.

Psychogenic pain is different from pretended pain. Although psychogenic pain starts without a physical basis, repeated severe stress probably alters the complex physiology of pain transmission, modulation, and perception. The pain the client feels is real to that client, and the tension or stress the client is feeling may lead to pronounced physiologic changes. Unfortunately, this diagnosis is often assigned prematurely to a client's pain, when careful assessment would uncover a treatable physiologic dysfunction (such as either the cause of the pain or a result of the stress). Obtaining pain relief from a placebo does not mean the client is not experiencing pain (see Placebos). Psychogenic pain requires that the cause be found and treated.

When the psychogenic effect of stress, anxiety, fear, and anger produces painful alterations in physiology, this can be called psychophysiologic pain. For example, stress can produce chronic excessive muscle contraction, as though the client were continually prepared to meet danger. In turn, this chronic muscle contraction can produce pain. Most often, this occurs in the scalp muscles (muscle contraction or tension headache; see Headache) and postural muscles leading to low back pain. Stress also can produce visceral changes that can result in painful structural damage over a long period.

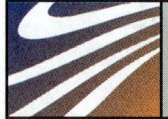

ETHICAL ISSUES IN NURSING

Is It Ethical to Give a Client a Placebo?

Consider the following case. You are caring for Mr. Adams who was in an automobile accident a month ago. His child was killed in the crash while not wearing a seat belt. Mr. Adams suffered abdominal injuries, fractures of both knees, the right ankle, and the right hip. He has undergone several surgeries. His postoperative course has been fraught with difficulties: an unexpected allergy to an intravenous antibiotic, infection, and much pain. Mr. Adams has been receiving narcotic injections for his entire hospitalization. He sleeps a great deal. He requests pain medication at frequent intervals. When the physician tries to replace the narcotic with another medication, Mr. Adams cries and complains. The physician asks you to give Mr. Adams an injection of saline (a placebo) for every other narcotic injection. He tells you not to tell the client what medication you are giving. What should you do?

A placebo is a substance (like saline or sterile water) that is of no pharmacologic use for the client's condition. Research studies have suggested that clients with selected conditions experience some symptomatic relief approximately 35% of the time with the use of placebos. The effectiveness of the placebo requires that the client believe that he or she is receiving a pharmacologically active medication.

The use of placebos in this case involves an act of deception. If you give Mr. Adams an injection of sterile saline for pain but give the impression that it is morphine or some other narcotic medication, you are deceiving the client. If you tell Mr. Adams it is a narcotic, you are lying.

The use of placebos is not recommended. It deceives the client and can ruin the trusting relationship between the nurse and the client. It is not good for the nurse either. The deceptive behavior gives the nurse the impression that it is all right to deceive a client. If the use of a placebo is being considered, it may be beneficial to all concerned to present the case to the institutional ethics committee.

In rare cases, placebo medication may be deemed necessary. In these cases, the client should be informed after the fact that placebos were used.

Assessment

Because pain is a subjective experience, one of the priorities for adequate treatment of pain is an accurate assessment. Assessment, however, is highly influenced by the client's ability to delineate aspects of the pain experience accurately. If the client cannot communicate clearly (e.g., is a child, unconscious, aphasic), then this aspect of the pain assessment is altered. Without the subjective information, it is difficult to intervene effectively, except by trial and error.

Blocks to Accurate Pain Assessment

Myths and Misconceptions About Pain

Many myths and misconceptions exist about pain (Table 17–2). These may influence the nurse's assessment of the client's pain. If nurses continue to believe these myths, then adequate pain assessment and relief are hampered.

Because pain is a subjective phenomenon, that does not mean it is not real. All pain is real to the individual who is experiencing it. This does not mean that a physical cause can always be found. Sometimes, the cause is obscure, as with many nerve pains, and it is difficult to diagnose. The inability to identify a cause does not negate that the pain exists.

Pain of psychological origin is also very real. Think of the last time you had a tension headache. The cause is purely psychological—tension. Knowing that fact does not make the pain any less; in fact, a tension headache is usually very painful and can be difficult to treat. Psychological stimuli lead to physiologic responses, and one such response can be pain. The nurse must remember that pain is always a combination of physiologic and psychological stimuli.

There are both physiologic and psychological responses to acute pain. These responses, however, vary over time as adaptation occurs. Initial physiologic responses are due to sympathetic stimulation that causes increased blood pressure and pulse and respiratory rates; dilated pupils; and diaphoresis. The initial psychological responses are usually a focusing on the pain, with a report of pain, crying or moaning, increased muscle tension, and guarding of the painful part. With time, the client with even extremely severe pain develops an adaptive response. The adaptive physiologic response is a return to normal vital signs and other physiologic parameters.

The adaptive psychological responses include a shifting away from the pain, reporting pain only if asked directly, sleepiness (which may also be due to insomnia secondary to the pain), decreased physical activity, and often a blank facial expression. These do not in any way mean that the client is not experiencing pain, simply that the client has adapted some responses to pain.

Although some of the responses to pain are predictable, how much pain any given stimulus causes in an individual is not. It is impossible to predict how much pain something will cause. When the members of the healthcare team make this sort of assumption, they are usually wrong. You may hear comments like, "A third-day postoperative hysterectomy client should not be having that much pain." No one except the client can tell how much pain is occurring.

The only way the nurse can overcome these myths, misconceptions, and prejudices is through education. By knowing the facts about pain, pain assessment, and pain treatment, the nurse can provide more complete care for the client.

Table 17–2. Common Pain Myths, Misconceptions, and Facts	
Myth/Misconception	**Fact**
Pain that is real has an identifiable cause	There is always a cause of pain, but it may be very obscure and must be assessed carefully. Also pain that has a psychological origin is just as real as pain of physiologic origin
There are predictable signs that a client in pain will exhibit	Pain is unpredictable in the physiologic changes that are produced. Even severe pain may not produce the typical pain symptoms. Lack of pain expression does not mean lack of pain
Very young or very old people do not experience as much pain	All clients with an intact CNS experience pain. Age is not a determinant of pain, although it may influence expression
Pain is predictable. Certain stimuli produce predictable amounts of pain for all people	Pain is individualized. There is no standard pain produced by a particular stimulus. An identical surgical incision in different people produces different amounts of pain
The healthcare team is the expert about the client's pain. They know how much pain the client should be feeling and how it should be treated	The client experiencing the pain is the only expert on that pain. The client is the only one who knows whether any given treatment works
Nurses can best assess pain using their own definitions of pain and cultural beliefs and values about pain	Using your own values and beliefs to assess another's pain is a mistake. People define pain for themselves, in terms of their own values and beliefs. The only way to understand the client's pain is to have the client tell you about it
A person can learn to increase tolerance to pain and that is good. With prolonged pain, a person's tolerance increases	High pain tolerance has no value in and of itself. There is no reason for a client to suffer unnecessarily. Prolonged pain actually lowers the client's tolerance of pain
If people can sleep, then they are not in pain	Pain is exhausting. People will sleep, however poorly, in spite of pain. People with severe or prolonged pain often sleep because of exhaustion. Sleep may also be how the client escapes from pain
Clients with chronic pain often have psychological problems	Clients with any unrelieved pain may experience depression or anxiety. If pain continues, then these other symptoms may increase, but they are caused by the pain, not the reverse
If distraction or other noninvasive pain relief methods work for the client, then the pain is not real	Noninvasive pain relief methods can be very effective in relieving both acute and chronic pain. You must believe the client's pain and the method of relief he or she chooses, as long as it does not hurt anyone

Data from McCaffery, M., & Beebe, A. (1989). *Pain: Clinical manual for nursing practice.* St. Louis: Mosby–Year Book.

Client Misinformation About Pain

One of the major blocks to accurate assessment of the client's pain is the client. If the healthcare team members still have myths and misconceptions about pain, then it is likely the client also has been misinformed about pain and pain control. Clients pick up on the expectations of the healthcare team about their own pain. Clients have learned that they are expected to tolerate certain levels of pain and not to complain excessively. They have also learned to be afraid of pain medications, especially opioids.

A major nursing responsibility, therefore, is to educate the client about pain and pain control. The nurse needs to help clients see that it is the clients who are the experts on their pain, not the healthcare team. The nurse is also responsible for helping the client provide an accurate pain history and assessment.

When discussing or documenting pain, avoid saying that a client "complains" of pain. This term tends to invalidate or minimize the client's experience, as if the client is fussing unnecessarily. It is more accurate and helpful simply to use the word "states" or "reports."

When discussing pain (e.g., with those experiencing it) or when documenting pain, avoid using the word "attack." Feeling that one is under attack may produce a greater feeling of powerlessness, such as feeling like a victim. "Victim" is another word best avoided in these situations, for similar reasons. Use the term "episode" rather than attack to promote self-control and a sense of being able to do something to manage the episode.

Basic Principles of Pain Assessment

Ongoing assessment of pain is vital. This ongoing assessment should include subjective and objective assessment, that is, the individual's verbal descriptions of the pain and observations of a person's behavior.

Each person has a basic human need to be free of pain and discomfort. Humans are motivated to avoid pain. Pain can occur as a result of inadequate satisfaction of other basic human needs. For example, if the need to eliminate urine is not met because urinary stones block the bladder outlet, pain occurs. Similarly, if a person does not experience affection and caring from someone else (i.e., to satisfy the need for love and belonging), some form of psychogenic pain may occur. Part of the nursing assessment is to identify any unmet needs that may contribute to a person's pain.

Pain assessment is difficult because there are no objective tests for pain. Also, psychic and somatic factors interact indivisibly. Each person experiences and expresses pain uniquely, and attaches personal meanings or explanations to pain experiences. The personal meanings nurses attach to pain may interfere with their assessments. For example, nurses may interpret a person's pain according to their own personal experiences rather than from the person's point of view. The frequent exposure nurses have to others experiencing pain may lead them to underestimate the significance of this person's pain.

Personal meanings attached to pain result from personal pain experiences throughout life and may arise from a person's (1) individual experiences and (2) sociocultural experiences. The cultural and familial role modeling a person is exposed to as a child teaches the following:

- What pains are appropriate or inappropriate to talk about
- Behavior that is appropriate or inappropriate when one experiences pain
- Circumstances likely to produce pain, which should therefore be avoided
- Various methods to avoid or relieve pain
- "Reasons" why one may experience pain, such as punishment, testing by supernatural or divine powers, or bad thoughts
- Possible consequences of pain, such as attention or lack of attention from others, imminent death

A pain experience is also affected by personal factors:

- Pain expectancy (the anticipation of pain)
- Pain acceptance (willingness to experience pain)
- Pain apprehension (generalized desire to avoid pain)
- Pain anxiety (the anxiety pain provokes because of its associated mystery, loneliness, helplessness, threat)

Pain evokes emotional responses that may have behavioral expressions. Observations of behavior provide a nurse with some understanding of a person's feelings and of what pain means to a particular person. By accepting behaviors and trying to understand their origins, nurses can help individuals experiencing pain. To do this well, nurses must (1) accurately observe clients' behavior, (2)

listen to all that clients say, and (3) never judge clients or jump to conclusions.

Perception of pain is influenced by these factors:

- Integrity of the nervous system
- State of consciousness
- Age
- Physical state (fatigue, debility, lack of sleep, and prolonged suffering all reduce a client's ability to tolerate pain) (Fig. 17–5)
- Emotional state (worry, fear, and anxiety reduce a person's ability to tolerate pain)

History

An accurate history is essential to assess a client's experience of pain. A detailed symptom analysis (see also Chapter 11) is performed using the following guidelines.

Location

To determine the location of the client's pain, ask the following questions:

- Where in the body is the pain? (Use a figure of a person and have the client point to or mark painful areas.)
- Is the pain inside (internal) or on the surface (external)?
- Is the pain always in these areas?
- If the pain is in more than one spot, are the pains equal, or does one trigger the others?
- Is the pain on both sides of your body? If so, is it the same on each side?

Extension or Radiation

To determine the extension and radiation of the client's pain, ask the following questions:

- Does the pain extend from where it started? Does it cover a wide area, or can you point to where it is?
- Is there a pattern in which the pain spreads?
- Is the pain on the surface or deep inside?

Onset and Pattern

To determine the onset and pattern of the client's pain, ask the following questions:

- When did the pain begin? Is it a regular pain, or does it vary? Does it occur in cycles, for example, at the same time every day, every month, or every spring?
- What triggers the pain? Are there specific things that always trigger it? Can you identify any particular patterns?
- Does the pain begin suddenly or gradually over time? Is it continuous, or does it vary? Are there separate episodes of pain? If so, does the pain go away completely between episodes, or does it just get better?

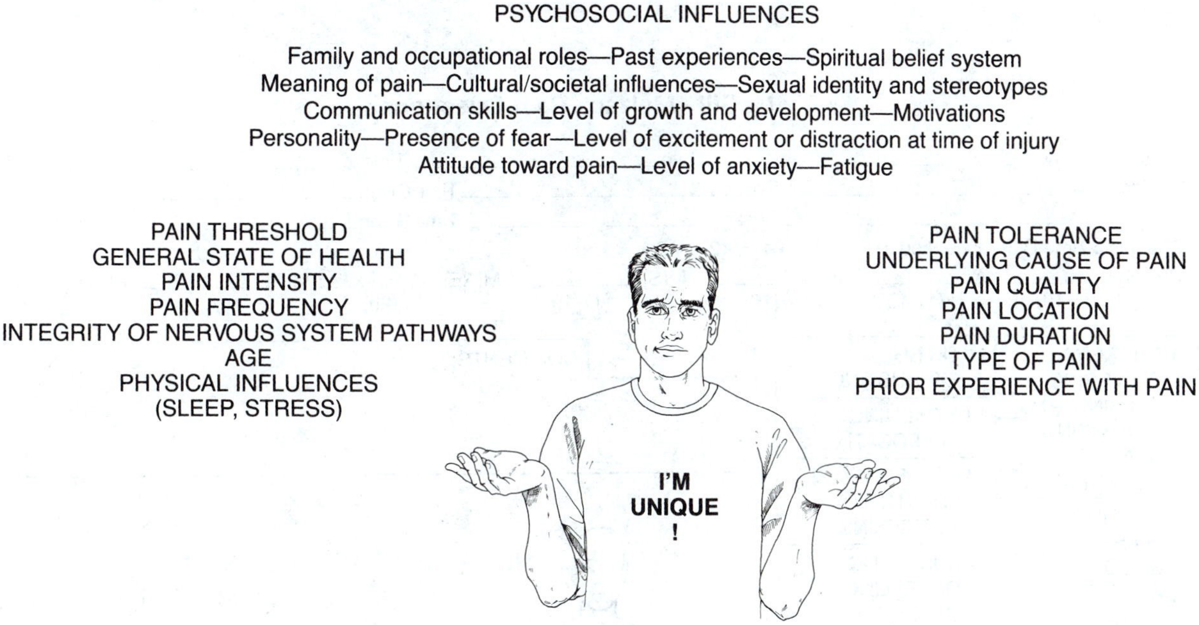

PSYCHOSOCIAL INFLUENCES

Family and occupational roles—Past experiences—Spiritual belief system
Meaning of pain—Cultural/societal influences—Sexual identity and stereotypes
Communication skills—Level of growth and development—Motivations
Personality—Presence of fear—Level of excitement or distraction at time of injury
Attitude toward pain—Level of anxiety—Fatigue

PAIN THRESHOLD
GENERAL STATE OF HEALTH
PAIN INTENSITY
PAIN FREQUENCY
INTEGRITY OF NERVOUS SYSTEM PATHWAYS
AGE
PHYSICAL INFLUENCES
(SLEEP, STRESS)

PAIN TOLERANCE
UNDERLYING CAUSE OF PAIN
PAIN QUALITY
PAIN LOCATION
PAIN DURATION
TYPE OF PAIN
PRIOR EXPERIENCE WITH PAIN

I'M UNIQUE !

Figure 17–5. Factors influencing responses to pain.

- Has the pain pattern changed at all since it began?
- Has your life-style changed since the pain began?

Duration

To determine the duration of the client's pain, ask the following questions:

- How long does the pain last? Are you free of pain between episodes?
- Is the pain constant, intermittent, or rhythmic?

Character or Quality

To determine the character or quality of the client's pain, ask the client to describe it:

- Is the pain dull, sharp, throbbing, burning, "electric," or shooting? (If the client cannot describe the pain, offer terms like those on the McGill-Melzack Pain Questionnaire[113] (Fig. 17–6). When recording the history, record the client's exact terms.)

Precipitating, Aggravating, and Alleviating Factors

To determine the factors that precipitate, aggravate, and alleviate the client's pain, ask the following questions:

- What seems to trigger the pain? Can you identify a specific cause or event that always or sometimes precedes the pain?
- Does anything alter the pain? Does anything make it worse, such as smoking, drinking alcohol, eating, heat, or tension? Is there anything that makes the pain better, such as rest, activity, heat or cold, or medications?

Intensity

To determine the intensity of the client's pain:

- Ask: On a scale of 0 to 10, with 0 being no pain and 10 being the worst pain you can imagine, how would you rate your pain now? How would you rate it at its worst? How would you rate it at its best? How would you rate it at rest? How would you rate it with activity? (When treatment starts, always have the client rate the pain before and after treatment.)
- Note what nonverbal manifestations of pain the client exhibits, such as grimacing, crying, moaning, sleeping, appearing exhausted, or remaining immobile.

Associated Manifestations

To determine whether there are any manifestations associated with the client's pain ask:

- Are there any other problems caused by your pain?
- Do you have any nausea, restlessness, insomnia, excessive sleeping, or loss of appetite?

Effect on Activities of Daily Living

To determine how the client's pain affects activities of daily living, ask:

- Does the pain interfere with work, sleep, driving, eating, schoolwork, sexual relations, housework, social activity, or other activity? (Box 17–1)
- Has the pain caused any changes in your life-style?
- When did you last have a good night's sleep?

McGill - Melzack Pain Questionnaire

Person's Name_____ Date_____ Time_____ am/pm

Analgesic(s)_____ Dosage_____ Time Given_____ am/pm

_____ Dosage_____ Time Given_____ am/pm

Analgesic Time Difference (hours):   +4   +1   +2   +3

PRI: S_____ A_____ E_____ M(S)_____ M(AE)_____ M(T)_____ PRI(T)_____
       (1-10)   (11-15)   (16)   (17-19)   (20)   (17-20)   (1-20)

1 FLICKERING QUIVERING PULSING THROBBING BEATING POUNDING	11 TIRING EXHAUSTING

1 FLICKERING
  QUIVERING
  PULSING
  THROBBING
  BEATING
  POUNDING

2 JUMPING
  FLASHING
  SHOOTING

3 PRICKING
  BORING
  DRILLING
  STABBING
  LANCINATING

4 SHARP
  CUTTING
  LACERATING

5 PINCHING
  PRESSING
  GNAWING
  CRAMPING
  CRUSHING

6 TUGGING
  PULLING
  WRENCHING

7 HOT
  BURNING
  SCALDING
  SEARING

8 TINGLING
  ITCHY
  SMARTING
  STINGING

9 DULL
  SORE
  HURTING
  ACHING
  HEAVY

10 TENDER
   TAUT
   RASPING
   SPLITTING

11 TIRING
   EXHAUSTING

12 SICKENING
   SUFFOCATING

13 FEARFUL
   FRIGHTFUL
   TERRIFYING

14 PUNISHING
   GRUELLING
   CRUEL
   VICIOUS
   KILLING

15 WRETCHED
   BLINDING

16 ANNOYING
   TROUBLESOME
   MISERABLE
   INTENSE
   UNBEARABLE

17 SPREADING
   RADIATING
   PENETRATING
   PIERCING

18 TIGHT
   NUMB
   DRAWING
   SQUEEZING
   TEARING

19 COOL
   COLD
   FREEZING

20 NAGGING
   NAUSEATING
   AGONIZING
   DREADFUL
   TORTURING

PPI
0 NO PAIN
1 MILD
2 DISCOMFORTING
3 DISTRESSING
4 HORRIBLE
5 EXCRUCIATING

PPI_____

COMMENTS:

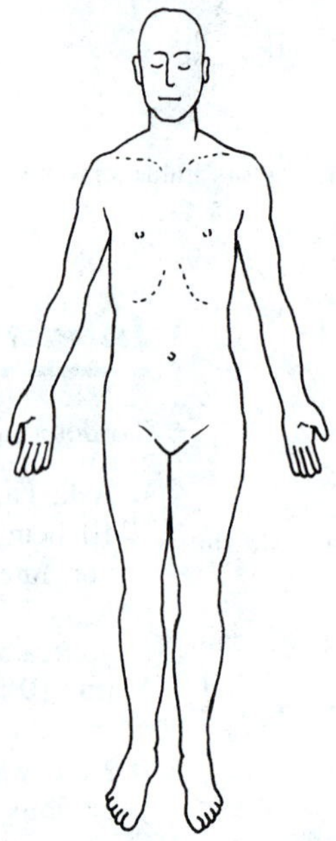

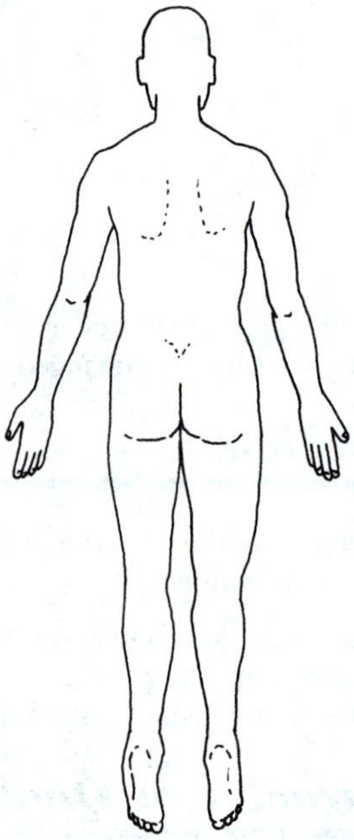

CONSTANT____
PERIODIC____
BRIEF____

ACCOMPANYING SYMPTOMS:
NAUSEA
HEADACHE
DIZZINESS
DROWSINESS
CONSTIPATION
DIARRHEA

COMMENTS:

SLEEP:
GOOD____
FITFUL____
CAN'T SLEEP____

COMMENTS:

FOOD INTAKE:
GOOD____
SOME____
LITTLE____
NONE____

COMMENTS:

ACTIVITY:
GOOD____
SOME____
LITTLE____
NONE____

COMMENTS:

Figure 17–6. The McGill-Melzack Pain Questionnaire, adapted for the study of narcotic drugs. The descriptors listed at left comprise four groups: 1 to 10, sensory; 11 to 15, affective; 16, evaluative; 17 to 20, miscellaneous. The rank value for each descriptor is based on its position in the word set. Total rank values comprise the pain-rating index (PRI). The present pain intensity (PPI) is based on a scale from 0 to 5. The drawings are used to designate the site of pain. (From Bonica, J. J. [1980]. *Pain* [p. 145]. New York: Raven Press.)

Box 17–1. Effects-of-Pain-on-Daily-Living Scale

Instructions

On a scale of 0 (no pain) to 5 (maximum pain), the client should indicate the areas of life currently affected and the severity of the interference. If the client's current level of pain is less than that usually felt, the client also should be asked to rate the most pain (effects) ever experienced in these areas.

Sleep
Appetite
Concentration
Work
School
Interpersonal relationships
Marital relations, sex
Home activities
Driving
Walking
Leisure activities
Emotional status (mood, irritability, depression, anxiety)

From Matassarin-Jacobs, E. (1981). *Pain assessment* (unpublished data). Presented in Chicago, May 1981.

Methods of Pain Relief

To determine how the client obtains pain relief, ask:

- What do you do to relieve the pain? (Ask about both invasive and noninvasive pain relief methods.)
- What has *not* worked to relieve your pain?

Physical Examination

Begin the examination by having the client show where the pain is and describe how it feels. Remember that the client is the expert on the pain and is the one who can best describe and pinpoint it.

Objective manifestations of pain can be divided into three categories: (1) sympathetic responses, (2) parasympathetic responses, and (3) behavioral responses. These responses are not diagnostic of pain, but they may give clues to its cause.

Sympathetic Responses

Sympathetic responses are often associated with minimal to moderate pain intensity or superficial pain. They signify that body defenses are mobilized and that the fight-or-flight response has begun. Objective manifestations include pallor, increased blood pressure, increased pulse, increased respirations, skeletal muscle tension, dilated pupils, and diaphoresis.

Parasympathetic Responses

Parasympathetic responses are often associated with pain of severe intensity, or with deep pain. In parasympathetic responses, body defenses may collapse in an attempt to lessen the effects of an external threat. Manifestations of a parasympathetic response include decreased blood pressure, decreased pulse, nausea and vomiting, weakness, prostration, pallor, and loss of consciousness.

Behavioral Responses in Acute Pain

The client may exhibit the following:

- Assume a posture that minimizes pain, such as lying rigidly, guarding, drawing up the legs, or assuming the fetal position
- Moan, sigh, grimace, clench the jaws or fist, become quiet, or withdraw from others
- Blink rapidly
- Cry, appear frightened, exhibit restlessness
- Have a drawn facial expression
- Have twitching muscles
- Withdraw when touched
- Hold or protect the painful area, or remain motionless

Although it is unreasonable to think that the nurse would be performing this detailed an assessment constantly with a client, portions of it are important and should be done at regular intervals.

Tools Used to Assess Pain

Simple pain assessment tools to use for both nurse and client are the visual analog and visual descriptor scales (Fig. 17–7). These scales can be combined with numbers and verbal anchors. These tools are easy to use and provide the client and nurse with a way to quantify pain. Some clients, especially the visually impaired and confused, may have difficulty with the scale. Another assessment tool used to assess pain is the McGill-Melzack Pain Questionnaire (see Fig. 17–6), used mainly with chronic pain clients. Although this tool is complex, it can be very useful in helping to initially diagnose the cause of the pain.

Nursing Intervention

Basic Principles of Pain Intervention

When caring for a client in pain, identify and remove the cause whenever possible. Work with the client in seeking ways to reduce or remove the pain. Listen to what the client thinks will help, and decide with the client and other healthcare team members what should be done. Allow the client a sense of control over the pain experience, rather than promote a feeling that the client is helpless in the grip of an episode of pain.

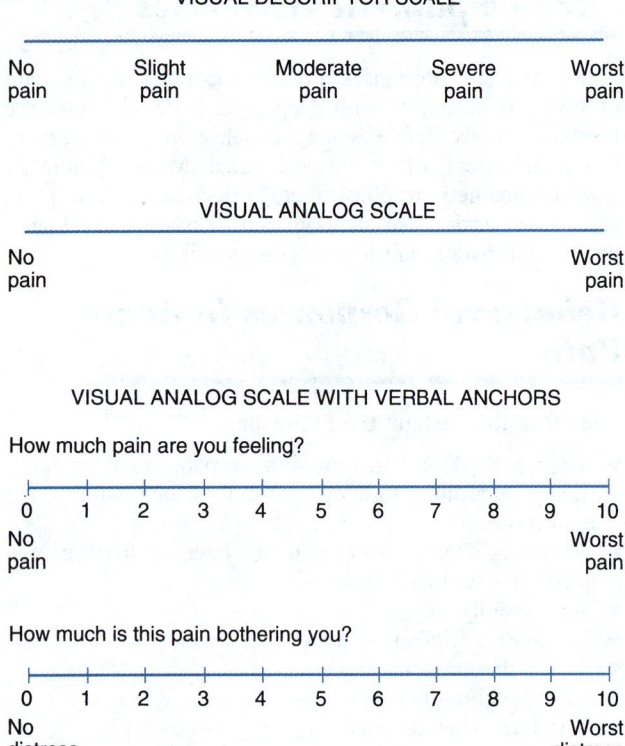

Figure 17–7. Visual analog and visual descriptor scales.

It is important to make frequent reassessments and evaluations and adjust nursing interventions accordingly. Reassessment should be done routinely after treatment and when anything changes in relation to the pain. Realize that an intervention that is helpful at one time for one client is not necessarily helpful at another time for another client—or even for the same client.

Also remember that the quality of your relationship with the client in pain may be as important as the pain-relieving skills you use. Create a relationship characterized by genuineness, warmth, empathy, and respect.

The client's basic human needs, such as those for food and elimination, should also be met. If they are, pain or discomfort (physical and psychological) may be reduced significantly.

Although specific therapy is, whenever possible, directed at removing the cause of the client's pain, you must also intervene for other problems that aggravate pain. Such problems include coughing, anorexia, diarrhea, and constipation. Management of these ancillary problems may also be used for palliation when the primary cause of pain cannot be treated or removed, or while a search for the primary cause of pain is in progress.

Alleviating Anxiety

Another nursing role is to help relieve anxiety. The greater a client's anxiety, the greater the suffering associated with pain.

To help alleviate anxiety, stay with the client for a while. Allow the client to talk and express feelings and fears. Communicate empathy and a willingness to listen. Give the client some sense of control by encouraging input into the nursing care plan and by encouraging the client to practice self-directed pain prevention or pain reduction techniques, such as meditation. Use therapeutic touch or other measures, such as giving a back rub and applying a cool cloth to relieve physical tension, promote comfort, and help the client relax. Do what you can to relieve the pain, and be sure that the client understands that everything possible is being done. Always seek help if the client's pain is not being controlled and anxiety is increasing. Finally, inform the client whenever a procedure is likely to be painful, and encourage the client to express the pain.

Distraction or Diversion

Another nursing measure used for clients in pain is distraction or diversion. Generally, the intensity of a client's suffering depends on the extent to which the pain dominates his or her consciousness. Pain perception, therefore, can be reduced by reducing the client's conscious awareness of pain. Distraction, which reduces this conscious awareness of pain, usually works better with mild pain than with severe pain.

Distraction may take many forms. Occupational therapy, conversation, reading, watching television, listening to the radio, meditation, self-hypnosis, biofeedback, and autosuggestion are a few forms of distraction that may be helpful. It is important to remember, however, to check with the client to determine what works best for him or her. To some clients, for example, small talk, idle chatter, and excessive noise are tiring rather than helpful. Likewise, some clients find that a low background noise such as a radio playing softly is relaxing, whereas others find this same stimulus irritating and tension-producing. When seeking to use distraction to relieve pain, encourage clients to use any methods that they have found helpful in the past to relieve pain, provided that these methods are not harmful or bothersome to others.

Another means of distraction is to involve the client in self-care, such as deep breathing, turning, and moving the legs. Be sure to give specific, clear instructions such as, "Concentrate on slow, deep breathing, in through the nose and out through the mouth for about 10 breaths" or, "Hold onto the side rail of the bed and turn to your right side."

Distraction is also useful during painful procedures. However, you must be careful to maintain a delicate balance between keeping the client informed and focusing his or her attention on other things. Be sure to use appropriate timing and a sincere manner, or the client may feel that you are discounting his or her pain.

Combatting Anticipatory Fears

Anticipatory fears are those fears that occur prior to an experience of pain-producing stimuli. Help prepare clients to meet pain realistically by talking with them about the pain they fear.

Before painful procedures, talk with the client about what to expect. This method may encourage relaxation and reduce muscle resistance, which, in itself, produces pain. Discuss the kind of pain or discomfort that the client may expect. For example, "You will feel a sharp prick." "You will probably feel some pressure, which may be uncomfortable but should not be painful." Clients who are given information about the sensation they can expect have less anticipatory distress and are more relaxed throughout the procedure than are those who are not prepared in this way. Also, before painful procedures, help clients assume body alignment and positions that will help them tolerate painful procedures more comfortably. For example, place a pillow between the client's legs if a side-lying position is required.

For preoperative clients, assure the client that he or she will be given adequate medication to control postoperative pain. If a postoperative client's analgesics are prescribed on a prn (as needed) basis, give the medication at prescribed intervals for the first 24 to 72 hours after surgery. Analgesics given around the clock provide better pain control and less sedation than analgesics provided intermittently. Make sure that the client knows that if the medication is not offered, he or she should ask for it at regular intervals. Patient-controlled analgesia (PCA) helps reduce anticipatory fears since the client controls the administration of the pain medication.

If a client who receives prescribed, scheduled analgesics is worried about pain, review with the client the times when the medication may be given. The routine of giving analgesics on a scheduled basis should be used to treat chronic pain, especially the pain of malignancy. Reassure clients who will require pain-relieving medications that you will supply them promptly as necessary. Clients who know this in advance are less likely to request medication unnecessarily or too early in anticipation of pain.

In addition to the measures outlined earlier for reducing anticipatory fear, teach the client techniques for reducing stress and help the client to communicate pain to healthcare providers.

Providing Physical Care

Effective physical nursing care for clients experiencing pain is directed at reducing mechanical, chemical, and thermal stressors that lower pain tolerance. This includes protecting clients from local irritations or inflammations such as infection or thrombosis, muscle spasm or muscle strain, interference with local blood supply and venous and lymphatic drainage, distention of hollow visceral organs such as the bowel and bladder, and further damage to traumatized tissue.

There are several important principles of physical nursing care. Identify the source of pain, and eliminate or reduce the pain. Handle sensitive or injured tissue carefully. Always perform painful procedures when pain-relieving medications are producing their maximal effect. Check drainage tubes frequently to ensure that they are not caught, stretched, pulled, kinked, or looped, and that

BRIDGE TO HOME HEALTHCARE

Controlling Pain

Joanie Kush, R.N., B.S.N., *Immanuel Visiting Nurse Association, Omaha, Nebraska*

In order to control pain in the home healthcare client it is important to be aware of many things that contribute to the pain. It is necessary to evaluate physical, social, emotional, and spiritual pain because each of these adds to the total pain experience. The plan of care should include a multidisciplinary approach to pain to be effective.

Assessment of the client with pain should include the type of pain, acute or chronic or malignant; its intensity and definitive location; and a description of the pain. Treatment modalities differ according to the type of pain experienced. It is often difficult to obtain this information from the home care client. The introduction of a pain inventory or pain assessment tool can help the client describe the pain in detail.

Many times in the treatment of malignant pain (as seen with cancer), medication is given on a regular schedule to prevent exacerbations in pain. This is in contrast to medication being taken at the time of pain or the prn (as needed) schedule used in acute care settings. This prophylactic scheduling is very effective, but requires client education to ensure compliance. Scheduling may well be the single most important instruction in the use of analgesics for malignant pain. Use of adjuvant therapy, such as for pain control, should also be considered because this often increases the effectiveness of the analgesic. It is also important to consider various methods of analgesia such as continuous, patient-controlled analgesia pumps, time-released skin patches, sustained-released oral medications, and suppositories.

Fear of addiction is a major problem. It is essential to explain that medication taken as directed will not cause addiction. The client should be assured that pain can and will be relieved.

Individualizing care is essential, and the various options available should be recognized. Providing the medical team with an assessment of the client's condition and home situation will help the team arrive at the safest, most effective pain management possible.

they are positioned correctly. Additional important principles of physical care include protecting the client from fatigue and helping the client get a good night's sleep, because overtiredness lowers pain tolerance.

It is also important to be alert to inflammation and ischemia caused by immobilization. If pain is caused by swollen body parts, elevating these parts may help. Likewise, a position of semiflexion may reduce the pain of joint disorders. Consult with a physical therapist about mobilization, positioning, and supportive devices that might be used to relieve pain.

If the client is experiencing pain from muscle spasms, a position change may help. Frequent position changes with good body alignment may also prevent painful muscle contractures. Know exactly what you are going to do before moving clients who are experiencing pain. Listen to the client's advice about the move. Whenever possible, allow the client to control the movement.

Additional physical care measures include gentle massage and applications of heat and cold. Gentle massage may help relieve muscle pain and prevent clot formation. However, never vigorously massage the client's calf, and instruct the client never to do this. Blood clots may form in that area, and massage could dislodge the clots and possibly cause a fatal embolism! Application of heat and cold may block pain, as explained by the gate-control theory.

Administration of Pain-Relieving Medication

Too often nurses view the administration of pain-relieving medications as all they need to do for pain management. The nurse must remember that medication can be more effective when combined with other pain relief techniques. When the nurse administers medication plus repositions the client, gives a back rub, or simply interacts with the client, the effectiveness of the drug may be increased. Simply giving an injection or a pill does not replace thoughtful, comprehensive pain management.

Therapeutic interaction with someone experiencing pain may include (1) facilitating the client's expression of feelings, which gives the client a sense of being cared for; (2) providing support, assurance, and understanding that

may relieve present pain or prevent future pain; and (3) teaching the client self-management of pain.

Numerous medications are used in pain relief. They are administered in a variety of ways—by mouth, rectum, topically, sublingually, by inhalation, or by injection. Medications may be injected by subcutaneous, intramuscular, and intravenous routes. Also, certain medications are sometimes injected spinally, paravertebrally, or into selected nerves to produce nerve blocks. The latter types of injections are performed by physicians, and nurses often assist with the procedures.

Managing Chronic Intractable Pain

Chronic intractable pain (pain that cannot be satisfactorily relieved) causes additional difficulties for people experiencing it. Clients experiencing chronic intractable pain may be helped by applying the psychological and physical nursing interventions discussed earlier. Nursing and medical therapeutic regimens must be coordinated and consistent to ensure a unified approach. The client must not be promised complete pain relief, however, because this may be unrealistic. These measures may help the client to better cope with the pain and may provide some relief.

Managing Progressive Pain

Clients experiencing progressive pain may be helped by the methods described in this chapter (Fig. 17–8). One important difference is that these individuals may require

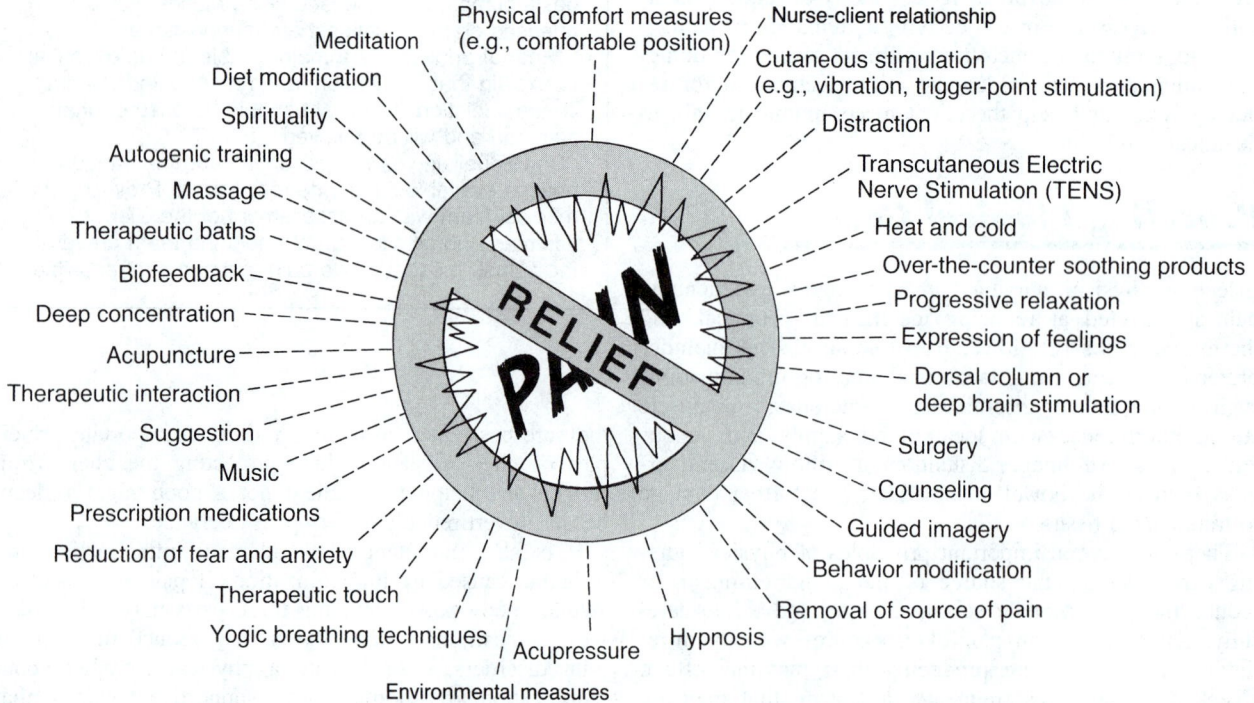

Figure 17–8. Pain relief measures.

pain-relieving medications routinely as a preventive measure (in the same way that vasodilators are routinely taken by people with ischemic heart disease). Some clients hesitate to take pain-relieving medications routinely for fear of addiction. However, clients experiencing pain because of widespread cancer have a disorder that requires pain-relieving medications. Thus, they are no more addicted to opioids than clients with heart disease are addicted to vasodilators. Help clients and their significant others understand this important point. The incidence of actual addiction to pain medications following their legitimate use is less than 1%.[95]

Noninvasive Interventions

Behavioral Techniques

It was not until the end of the nineteenth century that scientific attention was given to physiologic phenomena that accompany various yogic disciplines, hypnotism, and spiritual practices. It is now well known that activities such as meditation, relaxation, and hypnosis cause various physiologic changes. For example, peripheral blood vessels may dilate, blood sugar levels may change, and muscle tension is reduced. Thus, techniques such as these can be used to manage pain and promote healthy living.

A variety of behavioral techniques can reduce pain in many clients. It is important for the nurse to remember, however, that most of these techniques require a great deal of client participation. Some clients may be emotionally or developmentally unable to participate in these activities or may have religious convictions against using some of these techniques. Assess the client carefully before encouraging these methods. The client's response to the use of behavioral techniques should also be carefully assessed. If they are inappropriate or unsuccessful, the client will require other interventions.

It may be possible to teach clients a combination of these techniques to maximize their opportunities for self-control over manifestations. When a client is able to use these techniques successfully to control pain, this in no way indicates that the pain is primarily psychological in origin. Such techniques may activate inhibitory fibers in the spinal cord or activate the descending analgesic system.

Many of the noninvasive techniques require the cooperation and even active participation of the client. It is difficult, however, to teach people who are already in severe pain. We must teach clients before a painful procedure or a painful period occurs, if possible. Clients with chronic pain may require longer times for the teaching so they do not become overstressed with this new information.

Learning plays an important role in chronic pain. Unfortunately, healthcare providers often react to an indication of pain in ways that promote and strengthen pain behaviors. For example, many healthcare professionals are accustomed to working with clients experiencing acute pain and to responding to their reports of pain. However, when using behavior control methods, health professionals attend to a client when the client is not reporting pain

or demonstrating pain behavior. When pain behaviors are reinforced, increases in pain severity and related functional impairment may occur without a worsening of the underlying disease. For example, when a client's pain behavior is reinforced, that client may inhibit his or her range of motion or activities of daily living.

Clients experiencing chronic pain over long periods often learn (or become conditioned) to display a complex set of pain behaviors. Then, by using these pain behaviors, they actually reinforce their feelings of pain. For example, grimacing, guarding, and vocalizations can have a reinforcing effect by making other people respond to the client's pain.

When clients have learned pain behaviors, modification of these behaviors can be helpful. There are several behavioral modification techniques in which the person controls what is happening, including meditation, hypnosis (see Hypnosis), operant conditioning, biofeedback, autogenic training, and progressive relaxation training. The nurse must continue to be sensitive to the client's cultural and religious background when teaching any of these techniques.

Meditation. Meditation focuses the attention of people experiencing pain away from their pain. It also provides energy and peace to the meditator. Meditation involves simply sitting comfortably and quietly with oneself and focusing attention. Focuses vary. Examples include flow of the breath, a mantra, and a picture or mental image of a great spiritual being or peaceful place. Sometimes the meditator communicates with a great spiritual being. There are many meditation techniques, some with a spiritual base, such as Siddha meditation. Meditation is easily practiced anywhere and involves no special equipment. The positive experiences available through meditation are available to anyone, including individuals experiencing pain.

Autogenic Training. The purpose of autogenic training is to help individuals become self-motivated. The technique teaches relaxation and physiologic control by a system of self-suggestion in which people repeat phrases to themselves suggesting changes toward relaxation and self-control. This may help clients who are unable to participate in more directive forms of hypnosis.

Progressive Relaxation Training. Progressive relaxation training (PRT) is used to treat various physical and psychosocial problems, including pain. The client is taught to gradually tighten, then deeply relax, various muscle groups, proceeding systematically from one area of the body to the next. The deep relaxation produced by this method can decrease anxiety and excessive muscle contraction, and promote the onset of sleep. Audiotape cassettes are available to guide clients through PRT.

Guided Imagery. Imagery is a way to relieve pain through several mechanisms. First, using imagery is a way to help clients distract themselves from their pain, which may increase their pain tolerance. Second, imagery may produce a relaxation response that helps produce muscle relaxation and relieve pain. Last, the image can be a healing one, designed not only to relieve the pain but possibly to diminish the source of the pain.[145] Imagery is often combined with relaxation and biofeedback to produce a multifocal pain relief technique.

The image the client uses in this technique could be a complex scene that requires the client to think of each detail. This image would increase distraction. The image might be a relaxing scene such as a beach or meadow, which would help with the relaxation response, or the image could be one that visualizes the pain being worn away until it is so small it can be blown away. This is an example of a more healing image. When introducing an image setting, it is always wise to ask the client what setting is relaxing. Be sure not to use an image that may provoke anxiety in a client such as using a beach for someone who is afraid of water or a meadow for a client with severe allergies to pollen.

Rhythmic Breathing. Rhythmic breathing is a method of both relaxation and distraction. This method can be combined with rhythms such as music, a ticking clock, or a metronome. The technique does not require a lot of concentration because once the client begins the process, it takes on an automatic quality. This method focuses the client's attention away from the pain and on the breathing and the rhythm. The Lamaze method of childbirth is a good example of this method of pain control.

Operant Conditioning. An operant conditioning program does not cure pain. However, it can help reduce associated functional impairment. Operant conditioning is a program designed for clients whose high levels of chronic pain behavior interfere with their ability to function. It is useful for clients whose pain is caused by chronic, stable, organic disease, not progressive disease.

A successful operant conditioning program fully informs the client and significant others of every element before proceeding. The purposes of an operant conditioning program are (1) to reduce pain behaviors by withdrawing positive reinforcement for such behavior, (2) to increase the client's well behaviors by programming positive reinforcement when the client increases well behaviors, (3) to teach significant others to reinforce well behaviors and not to reinforce the pain behaviors, and (4) to refer clients having pain to other health professionals who can help with other functional impairments once the limitation of pain is successfully removed. An example of (1) is not attending to a client's verbal or nonverbal demonstrations of pain, such as saying that washing dishes is too painful. An example of (2) is attending a client when the person is not demonstrating pain behavior: for example, by praising the client for performing a task that previously was not done because of pain.

Biofeedback. Biofeedback refers to a wide variety of techniques that provide a client with information about changes in bodily functions of which the client is usually unaware, such as blood pressure. Biofeedback equipment provides a client with immediate, continuous information.

Some clients learn to use this information to control previously involuntary functions. The purpose of biofeedback in pain management is to teach the client self-control over physiologic variables that relate to the pain, such as muscle contraction and blood flow.

Information used to reduce muscle contraction is obtained by an electromyogram (EMG) recorded from body surface electrodes. (Needle EMG electrodes are not used.) Changes in blood flow are produced by monitoring skin temperature, which increases with increased blood flow. Depending on the equipment used, individuals can self-monitor their changes through (1) auditory displays (decreases in muscle contractions are heard as decreases in the pitch of a tone) or (2) visual displays (increases in skin temperature are seen as increases on a dial). A client using biofeedback tries to change the display of information in the desired direction, such as to reduce muscle contraction (relax muscle tension) and reduce blood flow. The continuous, precise information received shows the effectiveness of the effort and often helps a client learn physiologic control of these functions.

Biofeedback can be performed at home with purchased or rented biofeedback equipment under the guidance of a suitably prepared healthcare worker. Alternatively, it may be performed in an office or clinic setting with a biofeedback therapist or other specialist, such as a nurse trained in biofeedback. The equipment is expensive.

Establishing a Therapeutic Relationship

The client must be able to establish a therapeutic relationship with the nurse or someone else on the healthcare team. Pain is a lonely state. Clients suffering from pain often find their world shrinking until sometimes the pain becomes the only focus. When the healthcare team cannot relieve the client's pain, the impulse is to stay away, thereby increasing the client's sense of isolation and loneliness. When the nurse is unable to help in any other way, the nurse can stay with the client. By setting up a therapeutic relationship with the client, the nurse can decrease the client's sense of isolation and can actually be a distraction for the client.

Therapeutic Touch

Therapeutic touch is a type of holistic pain management. It is a derivative of the laying on of hands. If the human body is thought of as having energy fields, therapeutic touch is a way to realign these fields. Unlike some of the behavioral techniques, this technique requires learning and practice on the part of the nurse.

Because of the nature of therapeutic touch, make sure that your client is receptive to this type of pain relief. This type of treatment may not be accepted by all clients and consent should be obtained before beginning treatment.

Briefly, therapeutic touch involves three steps. First, the nurse must be centered, or focused in a meditative state. This helps the nurse become aware of the vibrations in the surrounding energy fields. In the second step, the nurse assesses the client's energy field. The hands are passed over the client's body at a distance of 2 to 6 inches to sense changes in the field. The last step is treatment. During this step, the nurse helps to rearrange the client's energy field and return it to normal.

Cutaneous Stimulation

Cutaneous stimulation is stimulation of the skin to relieve pain. This technique draws its rationale from the gate-control theory of pain transmission. Cutaneous stimulation activates the large- and small-diameter fibers, which close the gate to painful stimuli. A wide variety of stimuli include cold, heat, massage, vibration, menthol application, and transcutaneous electrical nerve stimulation (TENS). The nurse should remember that a back rub is a good method of providing cutaneous stimulation. It is particularly relaxing at bedtime and may block pain so the client can sleep more comfortably.

Cutaneous stimulation can decrease the intensity of pain the client feels and, in some instances, eliminate it. It also can help change the sensation in a painful or noxious area to a more pleasant sensation, such as warmth. This process may also be seen as a form of distraction, because the client usually focuses on the sensation being created rather than the pain.

Cutaneous stimulation can be applied to the unaffected side and still elicit positive benefits. This is because the stimulated fibers cross within the spinal cord. This method is particularly useful when an area is too painful to be directly stimulated, as with burns.

This method of pain relief also may produce prolonged pain relief. It has been theorized that cutaneous stimulation may cause the body to secrete the natural pain killers—endorphins and enkephalin.

Hypnosis

An individual's reaction to pain can be significantly altered by hypnosis. Hypnosis is based on suggestion and the process of focusing attention. Not all clients can or want to be hypnotized, so always be sure the client has consented to this procedure.

Various procedures may be used to relieve pain following induction of a trance state including (1) suggestion to alter the character of the pain or the individual's attitude toward it, (2) body disorientation and dissociations, and (3) anesthesia and analgesia for superficial and deep sensation.

In situations of chronic pain, posthypnotic suggestion may be used in combination with autohypnosis (self-hypnosis) to provide prolonged relief. Many hypnotic subjects successfully learn to use deliberate spontaneous trance induction or autohypnosis.

Hypnosis cannot change organic lesions that are producing pain. However, it can often reduce discomfort. It is not without hazards. The procedure itself is fairly simple and innocuous compared with the administration of many anesthetic and analgesic medications.

Hypnosis may be used as an adjunct to other pain-relieving therapies. Alteration of pain by hypnosis should be performed by those who are aware of the possible diagnostic implications of pain in the medical management of a person's disease. A hypnotherapist must be skilled and informed, and the client carefully selected to avoid untoward effects.

Music

Music is another way to relieve pain. It is believed to work in several ways. Music can be the background to relaxation tapes that help the client relax. The use of music can be more specific, such as having the client sing. It can be used as a specific distraction. Some clients find the use of a radio and headphones a quiet way to listen to distracting music without bothering others with the noise. These radios also allow the client to turn the music up or play it softly. When using this method, make sure to let clients choose the kind of music most suited to them.

There are other types of tapes available to promote relaxation. These include nature sounds, such as birds, water, and rainstorms. These tapes also can help the client form images to use to reduce the pain.

Acupressure

Acupressure is a noninvasive pain relief method based on the principles of acupuncture. In this case, pressure, massage, or other cutaneous stimulation such as heat or cold is applied over acupuncture points. Charts are available that pinpoint each of the pressure points. Stimulation is accomplished in a variety of ways, such as a circular massage, pressure with the thumbs, or cold applied to the pressure point.

Ice Massage

Massaging an area with ice is another way to reduce pain. Ice is believed to invoke local anesthesia by reducing the nerve conduction velocity of the nociceptors. This may provide temporary pain relief.

Invasive Interventions

An analgesic is a pharmacologic substance that diminishes or eliminates pain without producing unconsciousness. An anesthetic is a pharmacologic substance that, in addition to abolishing pain, generally causes loss of feeling and sensation. Many analgesics, depending on their mode of action and route of administration, act as anesthetics when given in larger doses. There are many different types of anesthesia. General anesthesia is usually accompanied by loss of consciousness and amnesia. Local anesthetics produce anesthesia in a restricted area of the body without loss of consciousness. (Anesthetics are also discussed in Chapter 21.)

A technique frequently used in minor surgery and other

procedures is infiltration of a local anesthetic into the skin and subcutaneous tissue to produce loss of sensation or local anesthesia. The same agent injected near a sensory nerve causes anesthesia in the distribution of the nerve, that is, regional anesthesia. Often, nerves are mixed in function; that is, they carry both sensory and motor fibers. Hence, a nerve block may cause motor weakness or paralysis, in addition to loss of sensation, in the innervated area. A nerve block is the application of a pharmacologic substance that inhibits nerve conduction (e.g., to numb the mouth).

Local anesthetic agents may be applied topically (on the skin or mucous membranes), infiltrated locally, used for specific nerve blocks (e.g., spinal anesthetic for surgery), or administered intravenously, depending on the reason for their use. An example of a local anesthetic given intravenously is one below a tourniquet for extremity surgery, such as a Bier block. Local anesthetic agents act by temporarily blocking nerve impulses between the peripheral structures and higher centers. Such blocks are reversible because the nerves regain their function over a period of minutes to hours.

Prolonged nerve blocks are produced by neurolytic agents, such as phenol and alcohol, which destroy the nerves. Neurolytic blocks may not be truly permanent because nerve fibers regrow after several months. However, the growth is often disorganized. Hence, the sensation from these nerve fibers is often abnormal or painful. Consequently, neurolytic blocks are generally used only in terminally ill persons with a short life expectancy, such as those with cancer-related pain.

Local Anesthesia

Local anesthetics are chemically divided into two classes: the esters and the amides. The esters, of which procaine (Novocain) is an example, are metabolized in the plasma, are less heat-stable than the amides, and account for most of the rarely occurring allergic reactions to local anesthetics. The amides lidocaine (Xylocaine) and bupivacaine (Marcaine, Sensorcaine) are metabolized in the liver.

Procaine produces analgesia in 3 to 10 minutes and lasts less than 1 hour. It is one of the least toxic of the local anesthetics, although allergies occur rarely. Procaine is not effective for topical use.

Lidocaine is one of the most commonly used local anesthetics. It acts within 5 to 10 minutes and lasts about 2 hours. It has a wide range of applications, including topical and intravascular block. Allergy to lidocaine is rare. A Bier block (see discussion of nerve blocks) is an example of an intravascular block.

Bupivacaine is long-acting (4–8 hours) but has a slow onset. It is four times more potent than lidocaine and four to six times more toxic. Therefore, a lower concentration is used. Bupivacaine appears to block sensory nerves in preference to motor nerves when used in low concentration. Thus, good analgesia may result without accompanying motor weakness.

Local anesthetics are usually vasodilators, increasing blood flow into the area in which they are injected. Thus, they shorten the duration of their own action by enhancing their own vascular absorption. Adding epinephrine, a vasoconstrictor, to local anesthetic solutions prolongs the anesthetic effect by decreasing the vascular uptake of the anesthetic, allowing it to stay in contact with the nerve tissue for a longer period. The client may sense an increase in heart rate from the epinephrine.

Caution: Epinephrine-containing solutions are not used for nerve blocks of the penis, fingers, or toes where vasoconstriction could cause inadequate blood flow and necrosis of the distal extremity.

In addition to prolonging anesthesia, epinephrine-containing local anesthetic solutions offer other advantages. The supplementary use of a vasoconstrictor reduces the possibility of the anesthetic's reaching a toxic blood level. The toxicity of local analgesic medications depends on their concentration in the blood. This, in turn, depends on the speed of absorption. Vasoconstricting medications delay absorption of a local analgesic solution and thus prevent a suddenly high blood concentration. This gives the body more time to metabolize and detoxify the medication. Vasoconstrictors also inhibit bleeding in the area of the injection. Larger doses of epinephrine containing local anesthetic should be used cautiously in persons with coronary artery disease.

Topical Local Anesthesia

Dilute solutions of local anesthetics may be applied topically in the form of pastes, sprays, or other preparations. They may reduce the severe pain of burns, abrasions, and necrosis of the mucous membranes and skin. Remember, once an area is anesthetized, it does not transmit painful sensation, so the area is at greater risk of injury.

A new agent, Emla cream, is a mixture of lidocaine and prilocaine. It is useful in preventing pain from venipuncture and also from minor plastic surgery. It must be applied in advance to the area and covered with an occlusive dressing.

Caution: Cocaine, a highly toxic agent, is sometimes used for topical anesthesia (as in an atomizer for a topical spray). Cocaine should never be used for infiltration anesthesia (i.e., injected) because it is highly toxic.

Toxic reactions to overdoses of topical medications can easily occur. Therefore, use dilute solutions of these medications and take care not to exceed the recommended total dose.

If topical anesthetic agents are applied to burned or abraded skin or mucous membranes, absorption of the medication is almost as rapid as that following intravenous administration!

Analgesia

Various factors are considered in selecting the most effective analgesic for a specific client. These include the cause, quality, intensity, duration, and distribution of the client's pain. The World Health Organization[175] has formulated a tool called a pain ladder (Figure 17–9), which is used to aid in the decision of what pain medications to use for cancer pain. The first step is to use non-opioids (such as acetaminophen) with or without adjuvants (such

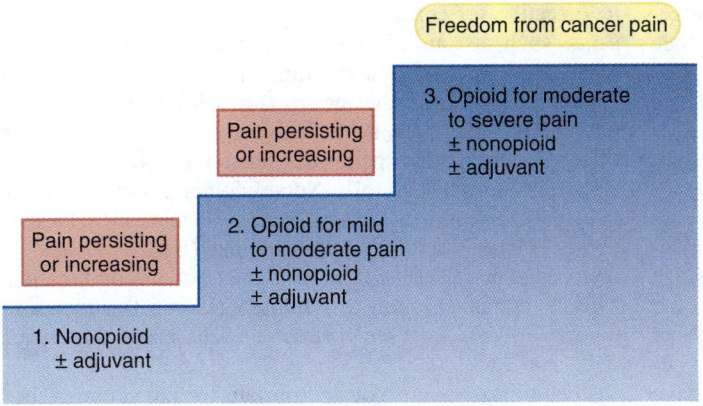

Freedom from cancer pain

3. Opioid for moderate
to severe pain
± nonopioid
± adjuvant

Pain persisting
or increasing

2. Opioid for mild
to moderate pain
± nonopioid
± adjuvant

Pain persisting
or increasing

1. Nonopioid
± adjuvant

Figure 17–9. World Health Organization (WHO) Three-Step Pain Ladder, which describes the steps in treating cancer pain.

as hydroxyzine). If the pain persists or increases, step 2 uses opioids (such as codeine) plus non-opioids with or without adjuvants. If the pain persists or increases, step 3 uses opioids (such as morphine) with or without non-opioids with or without adjuvants.

Systemic analgesic medications are the 9 most frequently used means of pain control. Analgesics are the most commonly prescribed medications and, therefore, the most widely used of all medications. They are also purchased extensively over the counter. This is not unexpected, because pain is usually the first manifestation of injury, and most diseases begin with or include pain at some time during their course.

Mechanisms of Analgesia

Analgesics do not all act in the same way. For example, aspirin and other NSAIDs act peripherally and do not seem to alter CNS processing. They also decrease inflammation and, therefore, the source of pain. Opioids, on the other hand, control the response to pain as well as raise the pain perception threshold.

Opioids produce analgesia by mimicking the natural opioid peptides (endorphins), mainly at the mu receptors (Table 17–3). These receptors are found in regions of the brain and spinal cord associated with pain perception. Opioid analgesics, therefore, modulate the perception of pain. Opioid analgesics, including local anesthetics, can raise or obliterate the pain threshold. The pain threshold is the stimulus intensity at which a person perceives pain.

Some analgesics, such as morphine, besides affecting the perception of pain, also affect the response to pain. Thus, clients receiving these medications may report that some pain is still felt but that the pain no longer bothers them. It is important to remember that these medications do nothing to decrease the source of pain, only the response to it.

Opioid analgesics have long been thought to produce their effects in the brain. In addition to their activity in the brain, special opioid receptors have now been identified. Multiple receptor sites exist within and outside the CNS. The three major opioid receptors are the mu, kappa, and sigma receptors (see Table 17–3). Delta receptors produce analgesia in response to endogenous endorphins. The mu receptors mediate analgesia, respiratory depres-

Table 17–3. Drug Actions at Specific Receptor Sites*

Drug Classification	Specific Drugs	Type of Opioid Receptor		
		Mu	Kappa	Sigma
Pure opioid agonists	Morphine, codeine, and all other opioids	Agonist	Agonist	No action
Pure opioid antagonist	Naloxone (Narcan) or naltrexone (Trexan)	Antagonist	Antagonist	Partial antagonist
Mixed, opioid agonist-antagonists	Pentazocine (Fortral, Talwin) or nalbuphine (Nubain)	Antagonist Antagonist	Agonist Partial agonist	Agonist Agonist
	Buprenorphine (Buprenex) or butorphanol (Stadol)	No action Partial agonist	Agonist Unknown action	Agonist No action

*Agonist means it enhances the action of that receptor. Partial agonist means it acts as a weak stimulant of the receptor when given alone, but can block the action of a pure agonist. Antagonist means it blocks the action of that receptor.
Adapted from Lehne, R. A., et al. (1990). *Pharmacology for nursing care.* Philadelphia: W. B. Saunders.

sion, and euphoria. Kappa receptors also mediate analgesia and respiratory depression, and in addition, mediate sedation and miosis (pupil constriction). Sigma receptors cause psychotropic reactions (e.g., hallucinations, euphoria).

NSAIDs act in several ways. As mentioned earlier, they are anti-inflammatory and because the swelling associated with inflammation is a cause of pain, these medications help relieve this pain. NSAIDs are also prostaglandin inhibitors. Remember that prostaglandins sensitize pain receptors to mechanical and chemical stimulation. By blocking prostaglandin synthesis, NSAIDs prevent stimulation of nociceptors. These medications work peripherally, not centrally, although some types may have some as yet undefined central action.

Because analgesics work at a variety of sites by differing mechanisms, a combination of analgesics is sometimes prescribed. Giving an NSAID plus an opioid can relieve severe visceral pain while also relieving the peripheral muscle aches and pains.

Types of Analgesics

Analgesics are usually divided into two classes on the basis of their clinical effectiveness: (1) strong opioids (agonists) and agonist-antagonist analgesics, and (2) weak non-opioid, antipyretic analgesics and NSAIDs.

Each class is distinguished by what type of pain it relieves and where in the nervous system it seems to work, rather than on its analgesic potency. Generally, opioid analgesics are given to relieve severe central pain; non-opioid analgesics are given for peripheral pains, such as muscle aches, headaches, and pains of inflammatory origin.

■ Weak Non-Opioid Analgesics

Nonsteroidal Anti-inflammatory Drugs. The NSAIDs were originally developed to treat arthritis. They are effective, however, in treating a number of mild to moderate pains of nonarthritic origin. NSAIDs act to decrease inflammation, but it is their ability to block prostaglandin synthesis that is thought to be responsible for most of their pain-relieving properties. As described earlier, prostaglandins are mediators of painful stimuli. Aspirin is one of the oldest NSAID pain relievers and one of the most widely used. Many others, however, exist today, and if one is ineffective for the client, another can be tried. A comparison of the analgesic quality of NSAIDs and aspirin is given in Table 17–4.

The most common problem associated with NSAIDs is gastrointestinal upset and possible bleeding. These agents also inhibit platelet aggregation, increasing the risk of hemorrhage. Clients taking NSAIDs must be monitored closely for the development of peptic ulcers. In clients who are taking high doses of NSAIDs for long periods of time, mainly those clients with arthritis, histamine H_2-receptor antagonists such as ranitidine (Zantac) or misoprostol (Cytotec) may be used.

Nonanalgesic Pain Relievers. A number of other medications not typically associated with analgesics may be effective for certain types of pain. Tricyclic antidepressants such as amitriptyline (Elavil) are very effective when used for neuropathic pain. They can be given daily at bedtime so the drowsiness associated with them helps the client sleep. Other medications that are effective in treating neuropathic pain are phenytoin (Dilantin) and carbamazepine (Tegretol). Nerve compression and bone pain may respond to dexamethasone (Decadron). Hydroxyzine (Vistaril) and diphenhydramine (Benadryl) are effective against a variety of pains alone or in combination. Muscle relaxants, such as baclofen (Lioresal) and diazepam (Valium), are used to treat muscle spasm associated with pain.

Phenothiazines are not appropriate for pain relief. They are good antiemetics. When given for pain, phenothiazines simply increase sedation, hypotension, and respiratory depression. A phenothiazine, such as promethazine (Phenergan), should never be used for pain relief. Promethazine actually increases the perception of pain, even in doses as low as 12 mg.[105]

■ Strong Opioid (Narcotic) Analgesics

Opioids are generally used when other methods of pain relief are not feasible, have failed, or the pain is moderate to severe. Although physical dependence and tolerance can occur when potent analgesics are given, this does not mean that these medications should be withheld. Tolerance and physical dependence are unlikely to occur in short-term pain therapy.

Examples of opioid analgesics are morphine and various morphine-like agents, such as opioid agonists. Agonists are opioids that stimulate the activities of selected pain receptor sites. Antagonists are medications that counteract both the CNS and the analgesic effects of opioids. Some medications are combinations of agonists and antagonists, such as butorphanol (Stadol) and pentazocine (Talwin). The morphine-like medications differ from morphine only in individual characteristics such as rate of onset, duration of action, route of administration, adverse side effects, and chemical configuration.

Opioid Agonists. The pharmacologic action of opioid agonists is similar to those of their parent compound, morphine. They all share certain desirable and undesirable characteristics (Box 17–2).

Opioid Antagonists. A pure antagonist, naloxone, reverses the effects of opioids, both side effects and analgesia. It has no agonist effects, that is, it produces no analgesia or CNS depression. This medication is used only to counteract against an overdose of an opioid.

Opioid Agonist-Antagonists. The combined agonist-antagonist medications act in two ways. When they are given following long-term use of opioids, they reverse the opioid and can precipitate acute withdrawal. When the combination agents are given alone, they produce analgesia and the positive effects of opioids without as many side effects. They are less likely to produce respiratory

Table 17–4. Oral Analgesic Equianalgesic Chart

Medication	Oral Dosage (mg)	Comments
Aspirin (ASA)	650	Aspirin 650 mg PO is the analgesic dose all other drugs in this table are compared to Aspirin is the best NSAID if the client tolerates it, and is much less expensive Major side effect is GI irritation and bleeding Contraindicated in client with a history of ulcers or with active bleeding or on anticoagulants Available in enteric-coated form Maximum dosage 4–6 g/day
Acetaminophen (Tylenol)	650	Acetaminophen has little or no anti-inflammatory effect; however, it is still an effective weak analgesic with few side effects May be given in combination with NSAIDs Use with care in clients with renal or hepatic disease Maximum dosage 4–6 g/day in healthy clients
Sodium salicylate	1000	Same as aspirin, but fewer GI side effects and less bleeding tendency
Ibuprofen (Motrin)	200	Available in 200-mg doses as nonprescription forms; 400 mg is prescription dose Effective, with similar but fewer side effects than aspirin Rapid onset, but shorter duration than aspirin
Naproxen (Naprosyn)	250	Relatively long action: 8–12 hr; side effects similar to aspirin
Indomethacin (Indocin)	25	Very effective NSAID, but with high incidence of GI side effects; cannot be given to clients with aspirin sensitivity
Codeine	32	Weak opioid Often combined with Tylenol as Tylenol No. 3 (30 mg codeine + 325 mg acetaminophen) or with Codeine with aspirin as Empirin No. 3 (30 mg codeine + 325 mg aspirin) Can cause severe constipation in high or prolonged doses Effectiveness is increased by giving Tylenol No. 3 + 700 mg acetaminophen; however, watch daily maximal dose of 4–6 g
Meperidine (Demerol)	50	Opioid with usual side effects (see Table 17–8) Not recommended because of buildup of metabolite normeperidine
Oxycodone	5	Opioid, available as a single agent or in combination with aspirin or acetaminophen; also as suppository Good analgesic potential, especially during first 2 hr after administration Side effects similar to other opioids
Hydrocodone	5	Opioid, available in combination with 500 mg of acetaminophen as Vicodin; similar to oxycodone
Pentazocine (Talwin)	30	Agonist-antagonist Available in 50-mg scored tablets High incidence of psychomimetic effects Do not give to clients who have been on pure agonists; may lead to acute withdrawal
Propoxyphene hydrochloride (Darvon)	65	Used for mild to moderate pain May cause GI symptoms Considered mild narcotic
Propoxyphene napsylate (Darvon-N)	100	Similar to propoxyphene hydrochloride

ASA, acetylsalicylic acid; GI, gastrointestinal; NSAID, nonsteroidal anti-inflammatory drug.

Box 17–2. Effects of Morphine and Opioid Agonists as Analgesics

Desirable Effects

Effective analgesia
Relief of anxiety
Euphoria*
Sedation*

Undesirable Effects

Psychological dependence
Tolerance
Physical dependence
Mental clouding
Dysphoria
Nausea, vomiting
Spasmogenic effects
Euphoria*
Sedation*
Constipation*
Respiratory depression*
Suppression of cough reflex*

---

*May be either desirable or undesirable depending on circumstances.
Data from Houde, R. W. (1974). The use and misuse of narcotics in the treatment of chronic pain. *Advances in Neurology, 4,* 527.

---

depression, although many of them are more likely to produce psychomimetic effects.

Methadone. Methadone is a potent, long-acting opioid analgesic that gained popularity in the management of cancer pain before the development of the long-acting forms of morphine. Unlike most morphine preparations, methadone has a long plasma half-life. This long plasma half-life, when repeated doses are given, may account for methadone's longer duration of analgesic action. The long plasma half-life of methadone also poses certain problems. This medication is not recommended for elderly people and persons with compromised hepatic and renal function. The long plasma half-life necessitates close monitoring of any client receiving repeated doses of this medication because cumulative effects develop over 1 to 2 weeks. If the client becomes oversedated, the dosage should be reduced or the intervals between administration lengthened.

Meperidine. A note of caution about the opioid meperidine (Demerol): This is a popular analgesic medication with limited potential. It should not be used on a prolonged basis, more than a few days, because of the potentially toxic breakdown product that is produced during its biotransformation, normeperidine. This by-product is a CNS stimulant and can build up in the client leading to seizure activity. It should not be used in clients with altered renal function. The AHCPR guidelines for chronic pain recommend against its use in pain management.

Side Effects and Adverse Effects of Opioid Analgesics

Some side effects of opioid analgesics, constipation in particular, last as long as the medication is administered. Others, such as nausea and vomiting and drowsiness, decrease as the administration is continued. Other side effects, such as respiratory depression, are extremely rare and the incidence decreases even more with longer administration of the opioid.

Constipation, another expected side effect of morphine and other opioids, results from increased smooth muscle tone and decreased motility of the gastrointestinal tract. Opioids diminish the propulsive peristaltic contractions in the small and large intestine and delay the passage of gastric contents through the duodenum. Tolerance does not develop to constipation as it does to the other side effects of opioids. Clients taking opioid analgesics need to follow some type of bowel regimen to prevent constipation. A diet high in fiber with plenty of fluids and stool-softening medications, such as docusate sodium (Colace) or docusate sodium–casanthranol (Peri-Colace), is common prophylactic treatment. It is better to prevent constipation than to begin treatment after it develops.

Opioids may precipitate *nausea and vomiting* because of their action on the brain stem centers. Morphine-like medications also affect the vestibular system, which can produce these manifestations. Changing the type of opioid used may stop the side effect, or the addition of an antiemetic agent may help. This is particularly true with the newer antiemetic agents. It is important to remember that this side effect decreases with analgesic use. No one should be denied pain relief because of this effect. Instead, they should simply receive treatment for the nausea and vomiting until it subsides.

Respiratory depression, one adverse effect of opioid analgesic therapy, is caused by diminished sensitivity of the respiratory center to carbon dioxide. All opioids can potentially produce respiratory depression, but this does not have to be a life-threatening problem, because this effect can be rapidly reversed with an opioid antagonist. This potential problem should not interfere in any way with the proper use of opioids to relieve pain in clients of all ages. The development of respiratory depression is not necessarily dose-related because even lesser amounts of an opioid may produce respiratory depression. The problem is related more to individual differences and the type of pain being experienced rather than to the medication being used. Opioid agonist-antagonists cause respiratory depression to a lesser degree than do opioids. Opioid antagonists also cause respiratory depression, although the extent of respiratory depression is limited. Rather than limit the use of opioid analgesics, carefully assess each client after giving the pain medication for the occurrence of side effects.

Deaths that occur secondary to opioid overdose are usually due to respiratory depression and usually occur in clients who have not received opioids in the past. With morphine, maximal respiratory depression usually occurs within 15 minutes of intravenous administration, within 30 minutes of intramuscular administration, within 90 minutes of subcutaneous administration, and within 4 to

12 hours of epidural administration.[151] It is very important to remember these time ranges when assessing the client's respiratory status following administration of opioids. For overdose to occur, however, doses well above the therapeutic level would have to be given. Accumulated doses, especially in clients with liver or renal failure and the elderly, can cause overdose.

Treatment of respiratory depression includes arousing the client, establishing a patent airway, administering an opioid antagonist such as naloxone, and providing artificial ventilation as necessary.

Circulatory depression is a second adverse effect of opioid analgesics. In a supine client, therapeutic dosages of morphine or synthetic opioids have very little effect on blood pressure and cardiac rate or rhythm. However, some clients experience orthostatic hypotension when moving from a supine position to a head-up or standing position. This hypotension is secondary to a direct dilating action on the peripheral blood vessels caused by the opioids, which reduces the capacity of the cardiovascular system to respond to gravitational shifts. Avoid abrupt body position changes in clients who have received opioids. For this reason, opioids are used very cautiously in clients with reduced blood volume since the effect is more pronounced. Increasing fluid volume will decrease the orthostatic changes.

Paresthesias may complicate the use of intramuscular opioid analgesics. The intramuscular injection of analgesic agents is generally not irritating to the local tissues. However, two exceptions are meperidine and methadone. Subcutaneous methadone may cause local tissue irritation. Both subcutaneous and intramuscular meperidine cause local painful tissue irritation and induration, and frequent administration can lead to severe fibrosis of muscle tissue and should be avoided whenever possible.

If any analgesic is deposited in the region of a nerve when it is injected intramuscularly, paresthesia and paresis may result along the course of the nerve. Proper injection techniques prevent nerve injury.

Physical dependence, a side effect of opioid analgesics, is defined as the altered physiologic state produced by repeated administration of a medication. When the medication is stopped abruptly, physiologic manifestations of withdrawal occur. Continued administration of the medication is necessary to prevent withdrawal syndrome. Physical dependence on opioids can develop as well as dependence on other substances such as alcohol, barbiturates, and nicotine.

Physical dependence is not the same as addiction, but it is an involuntary physiologic response that is an expected effect of the medication when it is taken for a time and then stopped. The nurse must observe the client for these physiologic manifestations. Gradual withdrawal of the medication can usually prevent this response.

Clients who receive a therapeutic dose of morphine several times a day develop some physical dependency in approximately 2 weeks. This means that if morphine were suddenly discontinued, a withdrawal syndrome would occur. Assessment findings that indicate a withdrawal syndrome include diarrhea, lacrimation, sweating, dilated pupils, restlessness, tremor, drug craving, and anorexia. Most manifestations, if untreated, subside in 5 to 10 days.

Withdrawal manifestations can be avoided by gradually (over 1–2 weeks) reducing and, finally, discontinuing a client's opioid intake as the pain decreases.

Tolerance to opioid analgesics, another expected side effect, is characterized by a shortened duration of pain relief, a decrease in peak analgesic effect, and an increase in the amount of opioid needed to relieve the pain. An example of tolerance is when stable pain has been adequately controlled by a particular dosage of opioid, but it begins to be less effective for the same length of time. In cancer clients, extension of disease is always a possible cause of the need for an increased dosage. A higher dose is needed to obtain the desired effect. The usual treatment for tolerance when pain relief is necessary is to increase the analgesic dose or decrease the interval between doses.

Addiction, an adverse effect of opioid analgesics, is a behavioral pattern of drug use characterized by (1) overwhelming involvement with the use of a drug (compulsive use) and securing a supply of it, and (2) a high tendency to relapse after withdrawal from the drug, that is, to begin taking it again. This behavior is sometimes described as the "three Cs"—compulsive, craving for the drug, and seeking and using the drug despite the consequences. The vast majority of clients who take opioid analgesic medication for pain do not become addicted. The nurse should never use the term *addict* unless a medical diagnosis has been established since many clients exhibiting "drug-seeking behavior" are simply seeking better pain relief, not the medication itself.

■ Adjuvant Analgesics

Adjuvant analgesics are medications whose primary use is not pain control, but act as analgesics for particular types of pain. Adjuvant analgesics may be used in combination with analgesics or may be used alone in specific instances. A wide variety of medications can be classified as adjuvant analgesics.

Antidepressants. Antidepressants are an effective treatment of pain of neuropathic origin. Tricyclic antidepressants are particularly effective, enhancing the descending pain inhibitory system by blocking cellular uptake of serotonin and epinephrine. The analgesia is above any antidepressant effect that may occur, although the relief of depression is usually a positive step in pain relief. When amitriptyline is used with morphine, it has been shown to increase the serum concentration of the morphine.[107] Tricyclics can be given as a single daily dose at bedtime or in divided doses. Analgesic effect usually begins within a week of starting the medication.

Anticonvulsants. Some of the anticonvulsants are effective against lancinating neuropathic pain. Medications such as carbamazepine and phenytoin are the most frequently used agents. The mechanism of action is unknown.

Steroids. Steroids can be used as pain relievers for a number of different types of pain. An example is pain

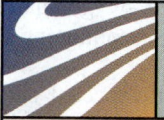

ETHICAL ISSUES IN NURSING

What Should the Nurse Do About an Incompetent Colleague?

You have been working on a general surgical unit for several years. Sandy, a new registered nurse, began working on your unit 4 months ago and you have become friends. About 2 months ago you noticed that Sandy was not very good at answering her clients' call lights. You would answer them as you continued with your own work. You began to notice that when you answered the call lights, clients would complain very bitterly that they had requested pain medication over an hour ago and had not received any medication from Sandy.

At first you do not think too much about it. But over the next several weeks you notice that Sandy's clients are frequently complaining that they had requested pain medication and had not received it. You decide to talk to Sandy about it. Sandy tells you that she does not want to "get her clients addicted." You tell her that they have just had major surgery, and that research has shown that they will not become addicted. Sandy tells you that she does not believe you. She has an aunt that became addicted in the hospital. You tell her that you will bring in books and journal articles that give detailed information about the current understanding of pain and its treatment.

Several weeks pass. You have given Sandy numerous resources that discuss pain therapy. Sandy is still not medicating the majority of her clients for pain. You are outraged. What should you do?

There are rare instances in which a nurse may discover that another nurse's practice is not up to accepted standards. The incompetent nurse puts clients at risk of harm. This situation is uncomfortable to both nurses and must be addressed.

The Code for Nurses of the American Nurses Association clearly states that a "nurse maintains competence in nursing." The code also requires that the "nurse must act to safeguard the client when health care and safety are affected." There seems little doubt that the nurse has an obligation to act to prevent harm to clients caused by another nurse's incompetence.

The American Nurses Association requires action on the part of the nurse to help maintain the public's trust in nurses and the nursing profession. This trust is supported by the professional's duty to be knowledgeable and proficient and to practice within accepted standards of care. The institution's responsibility to protect clients and to enhance the trust of the public is to encourage nursing administration and staff to develop and approve standards of care. These institutional standards of care should be clearly written and communicated to all those delivering nursing care to clients.

The peer review system used at various institutions for evaluating nurses helps to ensure that high standards are maintained. Nurses are evaluated by their peers by written, published criteria. This system improves healthcare delivery by holding each practitioner accountable to appropriate nursing care.

When instances of nursing malpractice exist, they should be communicated to nursing administrators. You may feel a bond of professional loyalty to Sandy that may make reporting the incident(s) to nursing administrators difficult. However, loyalty to Sandy does not excuse you from the duty to report the incident(s). Silence about an incident is not ethically acceptable. Clients will continue to suffer serious harm if Sandy persists in practicing in this manner.

---

related to inflammation or autoimmune causes such as rheumatoid arthritis. Its antiedema effect may reduce the compression caused by swelling and its anti-inflammatory action may reduce tissue levels of chemical mediators of nociception. Steroids are also used to treat malignant bone pain, neuropathic pain due to infiltration or tumor compression, lymphedema, and pain due to hepatic capsular distention.

Membrane-Stabilizing Agents. Some local anesthetic agents produce analgesia by suppressing aberrant electrical activity in central neurons or peripheral axons. Membrane-stabilizing agents include mexiletine (Mexetil) or tocainide (Tonocard). These agents appear to be effective against lancinating and continuous neuropathic pain. Membrane-stabilizing agents are used primarily for their antiarrhythmic effect and clients with heart disease must be carefully assessed before these medications are started.

Miscellaneous Agents. *Baclofen* is a gamma-aminobutyric acid (GABA) antagonist used as an analgesic for lancinating or paroxysmal neuropathic pain. *Capsaicin* is a topical medication that depletes peptides (such as substance P) in small primary afferent neurons that mediate nociceptive transmission. It has been found to be useful in clients with postherpetic neuralgia. It has also been shown to be effective for postmastectomy pain in some clients.

Factors Influencing the Effectiveness of Analgesics

■ Relative Analgesic Potency

Relative analgesic potency refers to the ratio of the doses of two analgesics required to produce the same effect. Estimates of relative analgesic potency provide a basis for prescribing the dose when changing from one analgesic to another, or from one route of administration to another. The equianalgesic table (Table 17–5) gives examples of the common analgesics and their relative analgesic potential compared with morphine. The nurse will find this information useful when assessing analgesic effectiveness.

■ Time Action

The time action of an analgesic agent is the result of factors such as pain intensity, the size of the dose, and the person's ability to absorb, biotransform, and eliminate the medication. The duration of action for the analgesics listed in Table 17–5 is based on a dose that produces a peak effect equivalent to that of morphine. The time of peak effect and the duration of action of a particular opioid vary with the route of administration. For instance, the peak analgesic effect of intramuscular morphine occurs between 30 minutes and 1 hour after administration. The peak analgesic effect of orally administered morphine occurs from 1½ to 2 hours after administration. The duration of analgesic action of orally administered opioids is usually somewhat longer than that of those given intramuscularly. Duration of analgesia may not be the same as the effect of analgesia. The nurse should be aware of information about peak and duration of analgesic effect so painful activities can be planned to coincide with these periods.

Several new forms of morphine have been developed. An oral liquid can be given for more rapid but short-acting effects. A controlled-release form also exists. With the long-acting morphine, the onset is somewhat slower, but the duration ranges from 8 to 12 hours. Fentanyl is available as a patch, effective for 48 to 72 hours, and as a shorter-acting lozenge.

■ Oral Potency

Opioids differ in the degree to which they are active as they are absorbed from the intestine and pass through the liver and into the systemic circulation. This difference in absorption accounts for the different oral doses listed in Table 17–5 for oral morphine. The older tablets had a low bioavailability and therefore required higher doses. The newer forms of morphine, such as Roxanol, have greater bioavailability and therefore the dosages of these are lower than those of the older oral form. Also, the different oral equianalgesic doses were based on a single dose. Dose requirements decrease after the client has received a loading dose.

Failure of healthcare providers to recognize differences in the oral and intramuscular potencies of opioids and the concept of equianalgesic doses can lead to undertreatment of a client's pain.

Principles of Administration of Analgesics

The goal of analgesic administration is to provide pain relief while maintaining the ability of the client to be in control of the environment and participate in care. As-sessment of a client before and after administering an analgesic is necessary to ensure safe and adequate pain relief. Factors to be assessed prior to analgesic administration include the following:

- Medication allergies or sensitivities
- Previous response to analgesics
- Other medications the client is taking
- Body weight
- Individual pain experience
- Other characteristics, such as age, general state of health, mental status, probable duration of pain, and probable life expectancy
- Cardiac, respiratory, renal, hepatic, and nervous system status

Medication Allergies or Sensitivities. Before administering an analgesic such as morphine, ensure that the client does not have a history of untoward reactions to the medication. When possible, ask the client or significant others, and review the chart or other documentation for such information.

Other Medications Being Taken. Clients on monoamine oxidase (MAO) antidepressants should not receive meperidine. Many other medications that may cause sedation, constipation, or orthostatic hypotension must also be considered when the client is on opioids.

Body Weight. Morphine 10 mg/70 kg body weight is considered standard. This produces satisfactory analgesia in about 70% of clients with moderate-to-severe postoperative pain. Some clients require higher or lower doses. The analgesic effect is dose-related. Review documentation concerning the client's body weight, or ask the client or significant others as necessary.

Individual Pain Experience. As we have seen, variation exists in pain experiences. There is no way to tell for certain how much, if any, pain a person is experiencing from a particular health problem or intervention (e.g., surgery). Likewise, one cannot know what dosage of analgesics is needed to control a client's pain. One method of treating postoperative pain is to administer a standard medication and dosage following a particular surgical procedure, and then to increase or decrease the potency of subsequent doses on the basis of an evaluation of the response to the initial dose. This is referred to as titrating the amount and kind of analgesic needed in accordance with the client's statements about pain and pain relief (see Ethical Issues in Nursing).

Other Individual Characteristics. A client's age determines, to a great extent, the length of time an analgesic will be effective. Clients older than 70 years of age respond to a standard dose of morphine as though they had received three to four times the dosage given to clients aged 18 to 49 years. In other words, 3 hours after the medication is administered, about 20% of 70-year-old people are no longer receiving pain relief from a standard

Drug	IM Route (mg)	PO Route (mg)	IM/PO Peak (hr)	IM/PO Duration (hr)	Comments
Table 17–5. Opioid Equianalgesic Chart					
Morphine	10	20–60	½–1 IM ½–2 PO	3–5 IM 4–5 PO	Morphine 10 mg IM is the analgesic dose all other drugs in this table are compared to PO dose varies from 3–6 times the IM dose depending on form used Also comes in rectal suppositories, timed release, and for spinal injection
Buprenorphine (Buprenex)	0.3–0.4	NA	½–1 IM	5–6 IM	Agonist-antagonist Can produce withdrawal from opioids More likely to produce nausea and vomiting Respiratory depression rare but severe and not easily reversed by naloxone
Butorphanol (Stadol)	2	NA	½–1 IM	4–5 IM	Agonist-antagonist Can produce withdrawal from opioids May produce psychomimetic effects, but less than pentazocine Contraindicated in clients with cardiac abnormalities Also available in nasal inhalation form
Codeine	130	200	½–1 IM 2 PO	4–5 IM 3–4 PO	More toxic in higher doses than morphine Causes more nausea and vomiting and is extremely constipating Adding 650 mg of acetaminophen or aspirin will significantly increase analgesic effect
Fentanyl (Sublimaze)	0.05	NA	7–8 min IM	1–2 IM	Commonly used for anesthetic, IV Substituted for high-dose morphine in terminally ill
Hydromorphone (Dilaudid)	1.5	7.5	½–1 IM ½–2 PO	3 IM 3–4 PO	Shorter-acting than morphine Also available as rectal suppository or high-potency injection 10 mg/ml May be used in PCA or as epidural anesthesia
Levorphanol (Levo-Dromoran)	2	4	½–1 SC ½–2 PO	6–8 SC 6–8 PO	Longer-acting than morphine when given in repeated, regular doses Good alternative to methadone Drug accumulates, so analgesic effect may increase with repeated doses Subcutaneous route better than IM

CNS, central nervous system; IM, intramuscular; IV, intravenous; NA, not available; PCA, patient-controlled analgesia; PO, oral; SC, subcutaneous.

dose of morphine. However, 50% of clients aged 18 to 49 years are no longer receiving pain relief under the same circumstances.

An older person tends to receive pain relief from an opioid for a longer time than a younger person. This difference in duration of action may relate to the speed with which an opioid is cleared from the body. A younger person clears a narcotic (opioid) faster than an elderly person. Also, people with debilitating diseases, whether old or young, have a heightened sensitivity to the effects of opioids.

Assess a client's general mental status, the probable duration of the pain, and the client's probable life expectancy in planning medication therapy for pain relief. A mentally anxious client may benefit from a mild tranquilizer or antihistamine in addition to an analgesic. A client whose life expectancy is relatively short may be given opioids more readily than a client with a chronic pain problem that will probably continue for a long time. When it appears that a client will require prolonged therapy for relief of acute or chronic pain, the side effects of analgesics must be considered.

Drug	IM Route (mg)	PO Route (mg)	IM/PO Peak (hr)	IM/PO Duration (hr)	Comments
Meperidine (Demerol)	75	300	½–1 IM ½–2 PO	2–4 IM 2–4 PO	*Oral dose of 300 mg not recommended* Shorter-acting than morphine Biotransformed to normeperidine, a toxic metabolite that stimulates the CNS and causes seizures Effects of normeperidine not reversed by naloxone Normeperidine has a long half-life so it is even more dangerous with repeated doses
Methadone (Dolophine)	10	20	10–20 min IM ½–1 PO	4–6 IM 4–12 PO	Long plasma half-life, so regular doses lead to accumulation of drug and increased analgesia; dosage must be carefully titrated over days to weeks Use with caution in elderly or in clients with liver or kidney failure
Nalbuphine (Nubain)	10	NA	½–1 PO	4–5 PO	Agonist-antagonist Similar to butorphanol May cause withdrawal if used in clients receiving opioids Longer-acting and less likely to cause hypotension than morphine Less respiratory depression
Oxycodone	NA	30	1 PO	3–4 PO	Faster onset and higher peak effect than most oral opioids Available as single agent and in combination with acetaminophen
Oxymorphone (Numorphan)	1.0–1.5	NA	½–1 IM	3–4 IM	Also available as rectal suppository; 10 mg by suppository equivalent to 10 mg IM morphine
Pentazocine (Talwin)	60	180	½–1 IM ½–2 PO	3–4 IM 3–4 PO	Agonist-antagonist Similar to butorphanol but much higher incidence of psychomimetic effects May cause withdrawal if used in clients receiving opioids
Propoxyphene (Darvon)	NA	500	½–2 PO	4–5 PO	*Never given in 500-mg dose* May be used for mild to moderate pain Doses of 65–130 mg are usual

Body System Assessment. Because all analgesics have the potential to produce mild-to-severe side effects, it is important to assess a client's cardiac, respiratory, renal, and nervous system status before administering analgesics. Hepatic function is also assessed since the role of the liver in detoxifying analgesics is important. The presence of increased intracranial pressure is cause for concern.

Potent opioid analgesics are used with caution in the presence of increased intracranial pressure. This is because opioids can potentially increase CSF pressure. This increase is secondary to increased arterial carbon dioxide tension, which may follow opioid-induced respiratory depression (see Side Effects and Complications of Opioid Analgesics). Clients who are being artificially ventilated do not experience respiratory depression and carbon dioxide retention after receiving morphine. Hence, they can receive opioids in spite of an elevated CSF pressure.

As a general rule, opioids are used cautiously in clients who have internal abdominal injuries, respiratory distress, or head injuries. Small, frequent doses of fast-acting opioids such as fentanyl may be used since they are of short duration and wear off quickly if they cause vomiting or interfere with neurologic status. Morphine may actually help relieve respiratory distress in some cases.

With head injuries (in addition to the danger of increasing CSF pressure, discussed earlier), internal cerebral hemorrhage may be present. Cerebral hemorrhage depresses the respiratory center, and morphine could worsen the condition. Also, the fact that opioids affect pupil size[76] makes assessments of pupil size inaccurate and misleading. These assessments are important following head injuries.

Previous Response to Analgesics. A number of instruments have been developed to assess and document pain location, pain severity, pain character, and the client's response to analgesic medications. Any of the instruments may be used as long as they help to accurately assess the client's response to the analgesic. Question the client carefully regarding allergies to medications. The client may be referring to side effects that can be prevented or controlled.

Methods of Administration of Analgesics

■ Nurse-Administered (Demand) Analgesia

The traditional method of treating pain is by nurse-administered pain medication on a schedule, or on a prn basis. This system has advantages. For example, it allows the nurse to assess the pain, helps the nurse detect or avoid untoward reactions or side effects due to the analgesic, and permits dose adjustment as necessary. It is also the best for clients who are unable to use PCA for a variety of physical or psychological reasons. In spite of these advantages, it is unfortunate that pain is often significantly undertreated with this system.[103] Undertreatment may occur because (1) it is difficult to assess the severity of another person's pain (unless the client is asked directly), (2) overconcern about possible opioid side effects and fear of inducing opioid addiction are often present in both the client (and significant others) and healthcare providers, (3) too low a dose of medication is ordered,[94] and (4) the interval between doses is too long. Also, with this system, the client experiencing the pain becomes dependent on others for pain relief. The client's pain may be worsened by anxiety about whether the nurse will give the next dose in time to prevent the return of severe pain.

Intermittent dosing causes wide swings in blood levels of the analgesic, resulting in sedation following one dose and unacceptable pain levels preceding the next dose. This problem is lessened if the nurse administers prn medications on a regular basis for clients with acute pain. If the medication is administered regularly rather than intermittently, the peaks and valleys of pain management are avoided.

■ Patient-Controlled Analgesia

One way to avoid some of the problems concerning nurse-administered pain medication is to use PCA instead. This method entails using an intravenous infusion pump, which contains the analgesic and is controlled by the client. The client can self-administer a dose of analgesic by pressing a button that releases a preset dose. The pumps are programmed to deliver preset demand doses of analgesic until a maximum dose is reached. There is then a minimal interval when no further analgesic can be administered (i.e., a lock-out period). With this system, clients control the administration of their own pain medication, within the limits prescribed by the physician.

There are many advantages to this system. First, the client usually reports that pain control is much better. This system also seems to relieve the client's anxiety about waiting for the nurse to administer the medication, thereby lowering the dose needed to relieve pain. This system also increases the client's independence. Another benefit is improved pulmonary function and fewer postoperative complications, probably because of the decreased sedation produced by this form of administration.[62]

Studies have shown that clients using these devices adjust their analgesic doses to a near-constant blood concentration. This method provides the best analgesia with minimal side effects. As the pain lessens, clients adjust themselves to lower doses, and finally stop taking the analgesic. Clients using PCA report superior analgesia with a lower incidence of side effects compared with the traditional nurse-administered method.

There are some problems associated with PCA. Some clients complain of inadequate analgesia at night requiring frequent wakening to redose themselves. Some institutions add a basal rate at night to prevent this. The success of this method depends on the nurse's understanding of the system and on how well the client is taught to use this system. If the client is taught properly, this method is usually successful. Failures can often be traced to a poor understanding on the part of the client or the nurse, or both.

■ Transdermal Analgesia

The primary opioid administered transdermally is fentanyl, a potent opioid. It is available in a variable-dosing transdermal application system that the client or significant other is able to apply independently. The patch is designed to deliver specified amounts of medication over a 72-hour period. This system provides the client with an easy way to maintain independence in medication administration.

In teaching the client about the system, it is important to stress that analgesia from the first application may take up to 24 hours to reach an adequate blood level. During this period, the client will need to be maintained on supplemental analgesia. It should also be remembered that the analgesic effect will continue for about 24 hours after the patch is removed. Teach the client to apply the patch to clean, dry skin on the chest or upper back. Excessive hair should be carefully clipped before application. The patch should not be applied over irritated or broken skin.

The patch is then left in place for up to 72 hours when it is removed and a new patch applied at a different site (to prevent irritation).

■ Continuous Subcutaneous Analgesia

Opioid analgesia can also be administered through continuous subcutaneous infusion. This can be done through a continuous infusion setup or continuous infusion with a PCA setup so the client can receive a bolus of medication on demand. A 25- or 27-gauge needle is used in this procedure or a special subcutaneous needle device can be implanted in the subcutaneous tissues. The site is rotated every 3 to 7 days depending on the type and volume of medication administered.

Observe the site for redness, excessive swelling, leakage of fluid around the infusion site, or edema in the area. If an extremity is used, you must carefully assess it for the presence of edema which will interfere with absorption of the medication. Also, closely monitor the client for the adequacy of analgesic effect. If the medication is ineffective, a higher concentration may be required.

■ Intraspinal Analgesia

A new advance in the treatment of severe pain, such as postoperative pain or chronic malignant pain, is a method of injecting opioids intrathecally or epidurally (Fig. 17–10).

The epidural space is outside the dura mater of the spinal cord and brain. The intrathecal space is inside the dura mater and contains the spinal fluid. The dorsal horns of the spinal cord contain receptors for endogenous opioid substances. These receptors also bind opioids and provide excellent pain relief of long duration (8–24 hours) without also causing sympathetic and motor nerve blockade. Relatively small doses provide high concentrations of the opioid in the spinal fluid that bathes the dorsal columns of the spinal cord. These concentrations are far higher than those that occur in the spinal fluid following similar doses given by standard parenteral routes.

Repeated bolus doses, PCA, or a constant infusion via an implanted refillable infusion pump of the opioid may be given through a small catheter placed in the epidural or intrathecal space. These catheters have been left in place for days to months without adverse effects. All the precautions observed for epidural and intrathecal nerve blocks (see Nerve Blocks) also apply to the placement of intraspinal catheters. Possible side effects of administering opioids by this route include pruritus, urinary retention, and delayed respiratory depression occurring 6 to 12 hours after a dose of medication. Low doses of naloxone may reverse these side effects without reducing analgesia.

Caution: Before giving a dose of opioid through an epidural catheter, carefully aspirate the catheter to ensure that there is no return of CSF. If CSF is aspirated, it is assumed that the catheter has migrated from the epidural space to the intrathecal space. Because an intra-

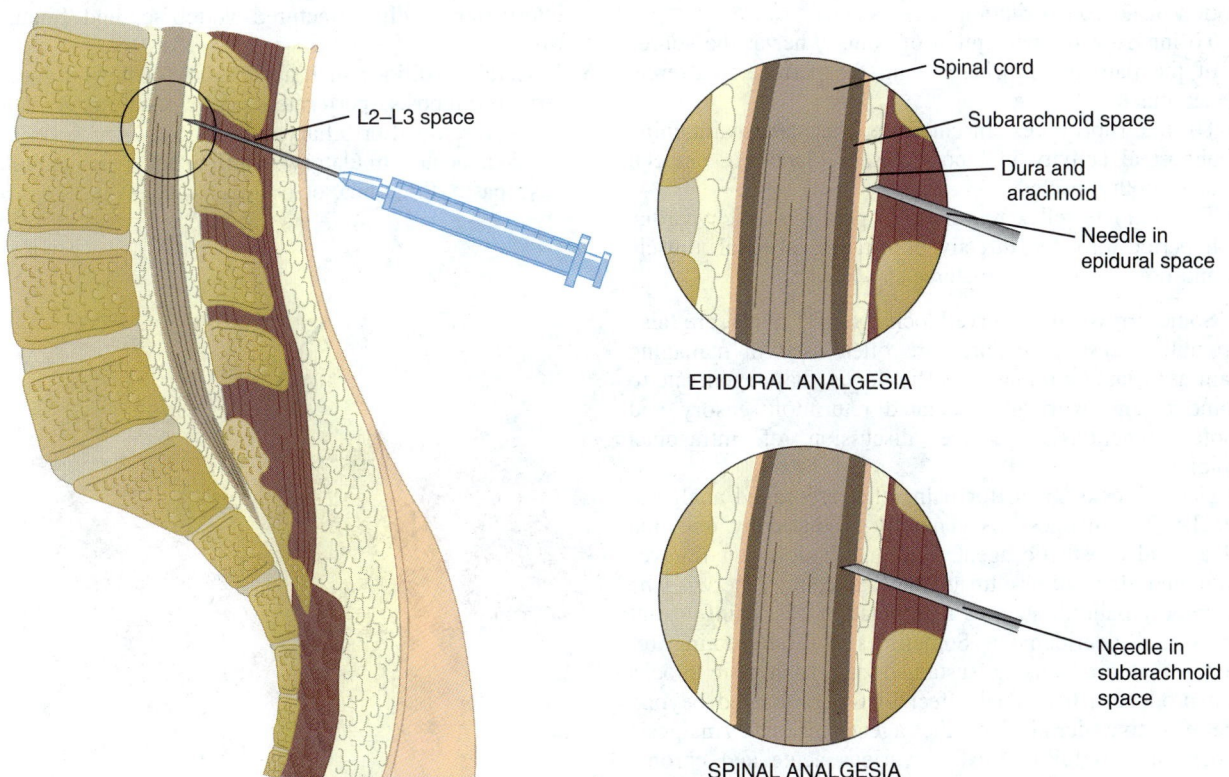

Figure 17–10. Epidural and spinal analgesia. *Top circle,* A small amount of analgesic medication, such as preservative-free morphine sulfate, is injected into the L2–3 space just outside the dura mater, that is, into the epidural space. *Bottom circle,* Analgesic medication is injected intrathecally into the subarachnoid space, which contains the cerebrospinal fluid.

thecal dose of opioid is about one-tenth that of an epidural dose, marked and potentially severe side effects (e.g., respiratory depression) occur rapidly.

Daily or every other day inspect the catheter insertion site for indications of infection (e.g., redness or swelling) and change the dressings. If they become moist or otherwise soiled, change the dressings.

Clients may experience exceptional analgesia from epidural or intrathecal opioids. It may then be possible to reduce or stop the previous regimen of parenteral or oral opioids.

Ommaya Reservoir. Another method of administering analgesic medications is via an Ommaya reservoir (see Chapter 24, Fig. 24–3). This reservoir is inserted into the anterior horn of the lateral ventricle. It consists of a catheter and a reservoir. In order to inject the medication, the physician or nurse first aspirates a small amount of CSF and then injects the analgesic. This route provides direct access to CSF. The same precautions must be used as with any intraspinal analgesia administration.

■ Nerve Blocks

Nerve blocks are commonly used for operative procedures as well as in pain clinics. Nerve blocks are performed by injecting various substances (e.g., local anesthetics) close to nerves, thereby blocking their conductivity. They may be used to produce a complete, reversible interruption of nervous pathways for the following purposes:

- To eliminate a local focus of pain-producing stimulation or nervous irritation
- To interrupt the perception of pain, either at the source of the pain or anywhere along the peripheral afferent neurons
- To interrupt reflex mechanisms that are maintaining abnormal activity in blood vessels, glands, or skeletal or smooth muscle
- To eliminate reflex responses to pain (e.g., tachycardia, hypertension) by directly infiltrating skeletal muscle and other involved structures

Some irreversible nerve-blocking procedures are also possible. These procedures are often used in managing pain associated with cancer. The nerves may regenerate to some extent, with an associated return of sensory and motor functions (see the discussion of intraspinal opioids).

Nerve blocks given for pain relief are called analgesic blocks. The analgesia is generally produced by injection of a local anesthetic agent. The anesthetic agent relieves pain and thus allows treatment that could otherwise be extremely painful, such as manipulation of a painful joint or wound debridement. Sometimes, by interrupting reflexes that are causing sustained pain, analgesic blocks can produce a beneficial effect that is prolonged beyond the effective duration of the agent injected. Analgesic blocks are useful in treating various acute and chronic disorders. They often reduce the amounts of analgesic medication that might otherwise be needed.

Injecting local anesthetics into tender points of muscle or skin (called trigger point injection) causes a type of analgesic block that may modify pain and break the pain cycle, allowing manipulation and stretching of a joint. However, the pain may not be permanently eliminated unless the primary afferent impulses are either chemically or surgically terminated, or until the underlying pathologic condition causing the pain is corrected.

Major types of nerve blocks include the following:

1. Local block by infiltration into skin or topical application to mucous membranes
2. Intravenous (Bier) block by injection distal to a tourniquet in an extremity
3. Peripheral nerve block (e.g., radial, median, and ulnar nerve blocks to anesthetize the hand)
4. Plexus block for analgesia of an extremity (brachial plexus, lumbosacral plexus; Fig. 17–11)
5. Somatic nerve block of spinal nerves by a paravertebral or intercostal approach
6. Prevertebral sympathetic (autonomic) block
7. Epidural block (caudal and segmental spinal epidural block)
8. Subarachnoid spinal block
9. Blocks of the cranial nerves

Examples of some acute painful situations that may be relieved with nerve blocks include the following:

1. Childbirth
2. Herpes zoster
3. Some neuralgias
4. Thrombophlebitis
5. Musculoskeletal problems such as acute, severe post-traumatic pain following ligamentous tears, a herniated intervertebral disc, fractured vertebrae, and fractured ribs
6. Visceral conditions such as coronary occlusion, mesenteric thrombosis, perforated peptic ulcer, pancreatitis, and severe renal or biliary colic
7. Sudden, acute circulatory insufficiency from embolus, vasospasm, thrombus, or trauma

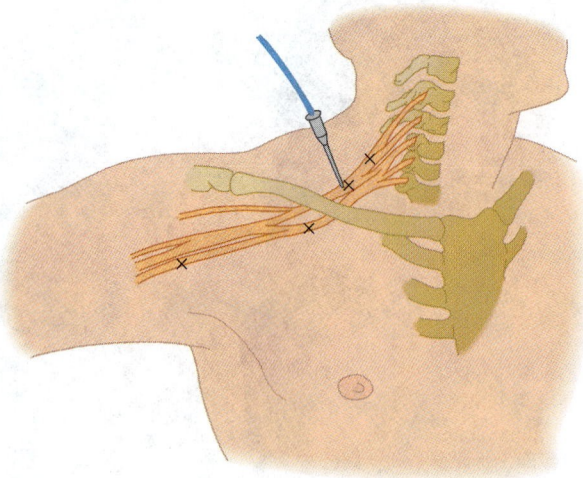

Figure 17–11. Nerve block of the brachial plexus may be performed at one of several levels. The X marks indicate (from distal to proximal) the axillary, infraclavicular, supraclavicular, and interscalene approaches.

Nerve blocks are useful as one modality in managing chronic pain (Table 17–6). The block breaks the pain cycle or provides temporary relief, allowing the person to use the painful part and regain more normal function. For example, reflex sympathetic dystrophy (overactivity of sympathetic nerves causing a cold, discolored, sweaty, swollen, painful extremity), if treated early (e.g., within 6 months of onset), often responds to a series of sympathetic blocks.

Cancer pain also can often be treated successfully by nerve block, particularly in the terminal stages with neurolytic block. Pancreatic cancer pain or other visceral abdominal pain responds to a celiac plexus neurolytic block. Low pelvic pain can be treated with lumbar sympathetic block. These procedures carry significant risks, including hypotension, loss of bowel and bladder function, paralysis, and loss of the useful warning signs that pain provides. However, freedom from pain and absence of the side effects of analgesic medication may outweigh the risks in this group of clients with terminal disease.

Nerve blocks may be unsuccessful owing to (1) difficulties in identifying the pain pathways or in locating the correct nerve for injection and (2) the complexity of pain. Some additional problems occur because only small amounts of solution can be injected at one time.

Nerve blocks are contraindicated in clients who (1) are receiving anticoagulant medication, (2) have an infection at the site of injection, or (3) are in shock, especially if extensive vasomotor paralysis will be produced or if large amounts of local anesthetic are required. They should be used cautiously in clients who are psychoneurotic, psychotic, or cachectic.

Caution: Because of potential complications, have re- *suscitative equipment and necessary medications readily available to combat untoward reactions when nerve block procedures are performed.*

Complications of nerve blocks include systemic toxic reactions related to peak blood concentrations of local anesthetics. These reactions are likely to involve the heart and CNS. Early assessment findings indicating the onset of these complications include lightheadedness, numbness of the tongue and lips, nausea, tinnitus, and hypertension or hypotension. The complications may culminate in loss of consciousness, seizures, and cardiac arrest. These complications may be prevented or minimized by (1) individualizing the dose, (2) using a test dose, (3) administering appropriate premedication, and (4) having readily available resuscitative medications and equipment (including oxygen, suction, adequate intravenous access, and appropriate monitoring). If a systemic toxic reaction occurs, treatment should immediately be directed to establishing a clear airway, providing oxygen and adequate ventilation, and ensuring a good pulse and blood pressure. Convulsions are treated effectively with diazepam. Complications such as pneumothorax, inadvertent subarachnoid (spinal) block, postinjection neuropathy (a late complication), respiratory dysfunction and paralysis, and hematoma relate to needle misplacement. Other complications relate to vasoconstrictor overdose or to idiosyncratic or allergic medication reaction.

Following a nerve block procedure, make the following assessments, and document the findings:

1. Indications of complications or untoward effects
2. The client's descriptions of manifestations and pain relief or continued presence of pain
3. The apparent amount, type, and duration of pain relief

Table 17–6. Indications for Therapeutic Nerve Blocks for Chronic Pain	
Indications	**Types of Nerve Block**
Causalgia and other reflex sympathetic dystrophies Acute herpes zoster and postherpetic syndrome	Blockade of appropriate sympathetic pathways Occasionally, epidural or subarachnoid injection of opioids or local anesthetics to interrupt preganglionic pathways
Chronic pancreatitis Upper abdominal cancer	Blockade of celiac plexus (injection of neurolytic agents)
Chronic myofascial pain dysfunction syndromes	Infiltration of trigger areas with anesthetic agents
Chronic back pain with nerve root irritation (no myelographic evidence of acute herniated intervertebral disc)	Injection of steroids and a local anesthetic into subarachnoid or epidural space Continuous epidural techniques (to provide profound muscle relaxation as an adjunct to bedrest and traction)
Post-traumatic, post-thoracotomy, and postinfectious neuralgia in upper torso	Intercostal nerve blocks
Terminal stage of metastatic cancer in clients with clearly unilateral and well-circumscribed pain	Celiac plexus block Lumbar sympathetic block
Painful spasticity	Fanwise injections of 45% alcohol into clonic and stretched muscle belly (to decrease muscle tone and clonus)

Adapted from Ghia, J. N., et al. (1979). Therapeutic nerve blocks for chronic pain. *American Family Physician, 20,* 74.

4. Instructions to the client about reporting changes in pain
5. Analgesics administered

Such assessment may continue for several weeks to help evaluate the effectiveness of the nerve block. If alcohol is used for the block, the maximal effects do not occur for several days. If epidural steroids are used, pain may actually increase for several days before pain relief occurs.

Neurosurgery for Pain Relief

For a client suffering from long-standing pain, the problem can become totally absorbing, completely dominating the person's life. The lives of significant others are also affected by the client's prolonged pain and his or her responses to it. When such pain is alleviated by surgical interruption of pain pathways and pain perception is abolished, the problem is not entirely solved. Because of the complicated nature of chronically painful conditions, such clients frequently require long-term counseling and rehabilitative measures after surgery. Once pain relief is obtained by surgery, function must be restored and new goals found. Occupational therapy may be necessary. The client's significant others should be included in the therapeutic approaches used.

When a client is experiencing persistent, intractable pain of high intensity, and less invasive modalities of treatment fail, neurosurgical procedures may be considered. Such procedures attempt to relieve pain by interrupting parts of nervous system tracts that relay sensations to the brain from their point of origin.

The goal of neurosurgical procedures for pain relief is to provide pain relief without causing the loss of other sensations, such as the loss of all feeling in an area or loss of movement following some procedures. Many procedures are used only in terminally ill clients because relief may be short-lived. In some clients, the same pain returns, and in others, the pain becomes even worse. Neurosurgical approaches should be used cautiously in clients with chronic pain.

These operations may be performed peripherally or centrally (on the spinal cord or brain). In addition, surgery on the autonomic nervous system (sympathectomy) may be performed alone or in combination with other procedures for the pain of causalgia or vascular disease.

Summarized next are some of the neurosurgical procedures performed for pain management (Fig. 17–12).

Neurectomy interrupts cranial or peripheral nerves by an incision. This procedure is used when pain is localized to a small part of the body. Neurectomies are performed infrequently because it is difficult to isolate sensory and motor fibers. Also, regeneration of the cut peripheral nerve fibers may occur, causing pain to return. There has been some success in treating localized pain, such as trigeminal neuralgia (tic douloureux). When a cranial neurectomy is performed, a craniotomy is necessary.

Rhizotomy is the interruption of the anterior or posterior nerve root area close to the spinal cord. Either a surgical procedure takes place or a radiofrequency electrode needle is used. Rhizotomy is performed when pain

is distributed beyond a small area. This technique is not generally useful for diffuse cancer pain because the extent of denervation and laminectomy is too extensive. Unpleasant dysesthesias may result from this procedure, such as "pins and needles" or crawling skin sensations (formication).

Chordotomy or *spinothalamic tractotomy* is the surgical interruption of pain-conducting pathways within the spinal cord. An incision a few millimeters in length is made in the anterolateral pathway opposite the side on which the pain is located. When pain is midline, a bilateral chordotomy must be performed. A laminectomy is necessary for this surgery.

Percutaneous cervical chordotomy is a preferred procedure for the relief of intractable pain in persons who are poor surgical risks or who have terminal cancer. It is used for lateral pain below T4. The operation is relatively simple, it is well tolerated, and there is a short convalescence period and a low morbidity rate. However, persons with preexisting respiratory disease are at a greater risk. By means of this procedure, a surgical incision is avoided and stereotactic destruction of the anterolateral spinothalamic tracts is possible. Percutaneous chordotomy is a simplified form of surgical chordotomy that interrupts or destroys the conduction of pain in the pain pathways of the spinal cord. The procedure is performed under local anesthesia by inserting a radiofrequency electrode needle into the neck, below and behind the mastoid process. X-ray control is used to guide the needle into the spinal cord. There, a thermal lesion is produced by passing radiofrequency current through the needle and heating the tip. This process coagulates a small area of nerve tissue at the tip of the needle. Some physicians believe that percutaneous chordotomy is simpler, more accurate, and safer than surgical chordotomy. A lateral cervical approach and an anterior approach have been used.

Tractotomy is the surgical division of the anterolateral pathway in the brain stem. Morbidity and mortality rates are high and limit the usefulness of this procedure in pain management. A craniotomy is necessary to accomplish this procedure.

Gyrectomy involves removal of the postcentral gyrus (part of the sensory cortex of the brain) corresponding to the painful part. This procedure is performed in an attempt to remove the registration of pain within the cortex of the brain.

Hypophysectomy is accomplished by destroying the pituitary gland, usually by injecting it with absolute alcohol. This technique may bring relief of pain associated with advanced cancer.

Prefrontal leukotomy, medial frontal leukotomy, cingulotomy, and *frontal lobectomy* are all procedures that interrupt the connections of the frontal lobe to the rest of the brain. To varying degrees, these procedures permanently change the client's personality. Hence, these interventions are reserved for only those clients most seriously affected by intractable pain and whose pain has not responded to other therapies.

Remember: When sensory nerves are cut, the tissues that no longer receive sensory innervation become highly susceptible to injury. With sensory innervation gone, feelings of pain, pressure, and temperature are no longer

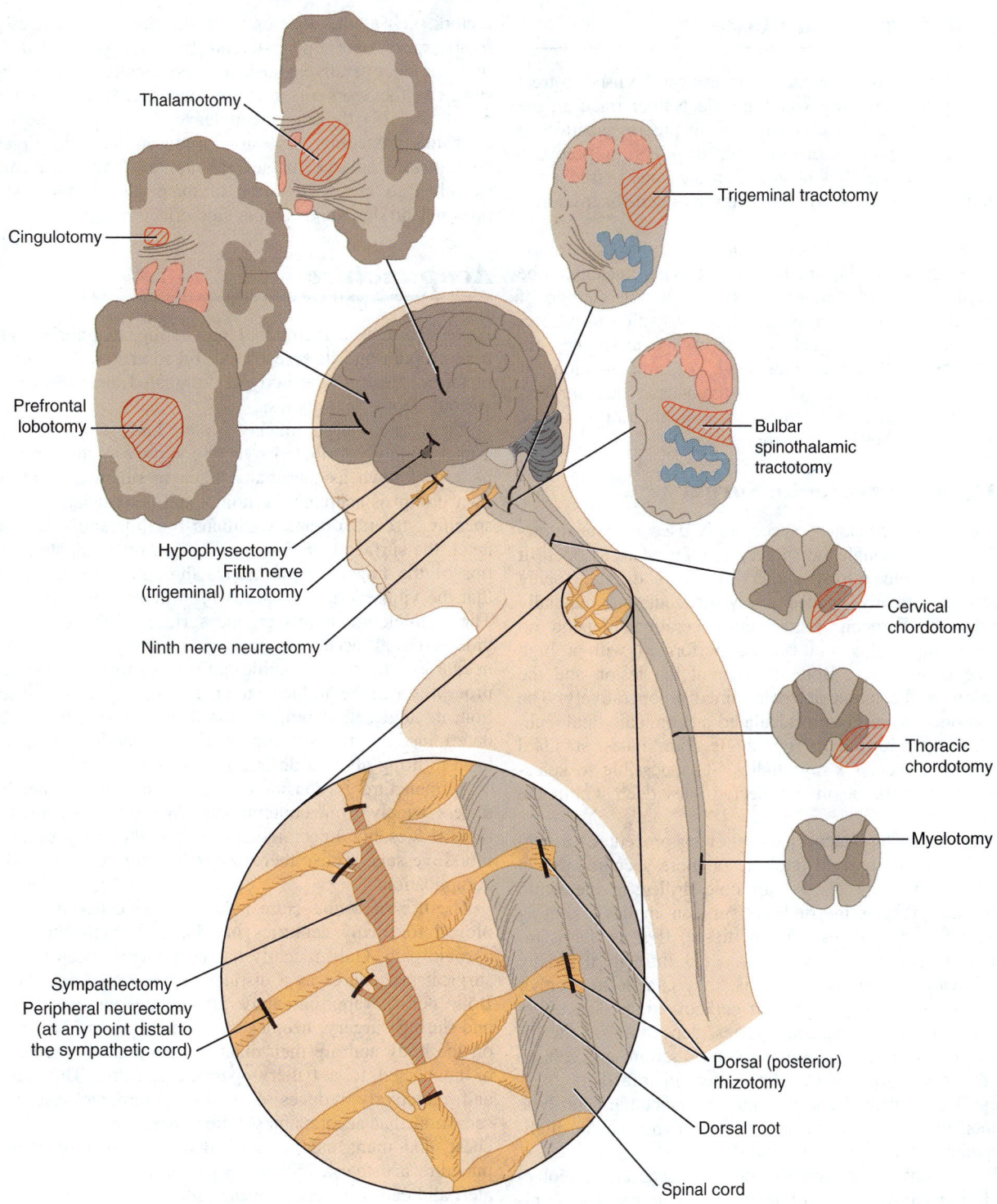

Figure 17–12. Diagram of various surgical procedures designed to alleviate pain.

present. Therefore, injury can occur without the client's being aware that it has happened. Because the interruption of sensory nerve pathways deprives body tissues of these protective mechanisms, this procedure is usually not carried out unless other less radical treatment measures have failed.

Once such procedures are performed, the individual (and significant others as appropriate) must be taught how to protect the affected area from damage. Frequent inspection of the area for indications of tissue damage is essential because the client cannot feel when tissue damage has occurred.

Stereotactic Pain Surgery

The techniques of stereotactic surgery can be used to treat some types of pain by sectioning deep fiber tracts in the brain. The word *stereotactic* refers to precise positioning in space. In relation to surgery, it refers to precisely locating operative sites deep within the body—frequently within the cranium—by use of three-dimensional coordinates.

Stereotactic brain surgery, aimed at modifying cerebral function by sectioning tracts and destroying nuclei, can be divided into two categories according to the method of approach: (1) open stereotactic surgery, which uses electrodes or other techniques such as cryogenic surgery, radiofrequency heating, ultrasound, or implantation of radioisotopes; and (2) closed stereotactic radiosurgery, which uses ionizing radiation, that is, gamma rays, x-rays, protons, and other heavy particles.

■ Open Stereotactic Surgery

These techniques can be successfully used to treat intractable pain. Although the surgery is referred to as open, it is not like conventional surgery in which the area being treated is actually opened up, visualized, and manually felt by the surgeon. Stereotactic operations depend on technical apparatus and can be performed with a high degree of accuracy. Both the size of the lesion and the position of the target are determined preoperatively. The operation is precisely precalculated anatomically and technically. By referring to right-angle coordinates, standard charts, and special x-ray studies, it is possible to selectively destroy tissue in preselected sites deep within the brain.

With open stereotactic pain-relieving procedures a needle or probe is inserted into one or more specific sites in the brain, by way of a small hole drilled in the skull. When the probe is inserted, the surgeon applies a heating current that coagulates adjacent tissue. If a needle is inserted, a neurolytic agent is injected through it. Many agents can be neurolytic, that is, they can destroy either nerve fibers themselves or their cells of origin. The effectiveness of injectable agents varies, depending on the location of the injection and the concentration and volume of the neurolytic agent. Hot water, disinfectants (e.g., phenol), and alcohol are examples of injectable neurolytic agents. Other agents that can be neurolytic include high-frequency sound, radiation, and dry ice.

It is technically possible to place an accurate stereotactic lesion anywhere in the depth of the brain with minimal risk and with little discomfort for the client. However, this type of surgery is not without problems. For example, there is often a tendency for pain to recur in time, as with more conventional pain surgery. However, it is also possible for these minute lesions to produce permanent pain relief. The clinical result often cannot be judged until several months after the operation.

■ Closed Stereotactic Radiosurgery

With radiosurgery, also, the operative effect does not appear immediately, but after a latent period that varies with factors such as the dose of radiation. Some advantages of radiosurgery over open stereotactic surgery are that (1) there is no operative shock and practically no mortality risk, (2) the risks of infection and bleeding are eliminated, and (3) the client can leave the hospital the day after the procedure. A lesion produced by radiosurgery continues to enlarge for several months. Thus, care must be taken to ensure that the ultimate size of the lesion does not produce undesirable side effects.

Acupuncture

Acupuncture is a method of preventing, diagnosing, and treating pain and disease by skillful insertion of very thin metal needles into the body at designated locations and at various depths and angles.

There are approximately 1000 known acupuncture points widely distributed over the surface of the body in patterns known as meridians. Each meridian contains its own group of acupuncture points and is associated with a specific visceral organ. Meridians run bilaterally just beneath the surface of the skin and begin or terminate at the tips of the fingers or toes. It is through these meridians that the vital energy (or *Qi*, as the Chinese term it) flows. The acupuncture points on the surface of the body provide external access to this vital energy, and through needle insertion at specific points, various physiologic processes can be influenced or controlled. Needle insertion, its angle, its depth, and the degree of stimulation are determined by the specific pathologic condition and are used to bring about a desired physiologic effect.

Acupuncture is considered an invasive technique, but differs widely from contemporary Western procedures in that it does not inject medicines into the body or enter blood vessels. Thus, there are relatively few iatrogenic complications.

The use of acupuncture as an analgesic has been employed for many centuries in China for both acute and chronic pain. Only recently has acupuncture been used in surgical procedures as a distinctive method of anesthesia. Both before (approximately 20 minutes preoperatively) and during surgery, needles are inserted at various points on the body and are then manually stimulated by rotation or connected to a battery-operated pulsator. This safely and effectively reduces or entirely eliminates the pain sensation that accompanies major operations on the head, chest, abdomen, and limbs. A distinctive feature of acupuncture anesthesia is that the person remains awake and alert and can often assist in the procedure.

Acupuncture has advantages over other types of anesthesia, because it does not lower blood pressure or create respiratory tract complications. Because side effects are reduced or eliminated, postoperative recovery is often accelerated.

There are no simple explanations for the mechanisms that underlie the analgesic effects of acupuncture. The gate theory of pain proposed by Wall and Melzack (see Fig. 17–2) may be a partial explanation. Evidence that needle stimulation elicits biochemical changes because of the release of endogenous morphine-like substances is another theory. In Western society, it does not seem as effective, perhaps due to lack of familiarity with the procedure and its effectiveness.

Stimulation Therapy

The relief of chronic pain by electric stimulation became a new clinical management technique after Melzack and Wall proposed the gate-control theory of pain transmission. The gate-control theory describes a spinal cord–modulating mechanism in which one type of sensation, such as vibration or light touch, can impede the transmission of another sensation, such as pain. The former sensations are transmitted by larger, more rapidly conducting fibers in the peripheral nerves. These sensations reach the spinal cord sooner than sensations traveling in the small fibers that conduct painful impulses. Because sensations such as vibration or light touch reach the spinal cord before the painful impulses, they can activate a pool of modulating neurons and block the incoming pain signal. Another explanation is that the electric stimulation causes release of the body's own pain-relieving substances—endorphins or the pain-modulating substance enkephalins. Electric nerve stimulators can activate the large fibers and produce a tingling or vibratory sensation that blocks painful stimuli.

It is known that the dorsal columns carry most light touch and vibratory sensations to higher centers. The idea developed that stimulating the dorsal columns directly could achieve a wider area of stimulation and pain relief. Other techniques involve the thalamus, including implanting electrodes and the use of continuous stimulation for pain relief.

Transcutaneous Electrical Nerve Stimulation

Transcutaneous electrical nerve stimulation developed from the need to screen clients prior to dorsal column stimulator implants (see later). The screening apparatus was then found to relieve pain effectively in many clients. Success with TENS depends on the client's understanding of, interest in, and motivation to use the apparatus, as well as the skillfulness of application of the device by the clinician (Table 17–7, p. 390). Thoroughly familiarize the client with the TENS equipment, such as how to operate the machine and adjust electrical settings. Involve significant others as appropriate in learning and teaching sessions, as shown in the Client Education Guide. The client may need their help in applying the machine to areas that are difficult to reach, such as below the shoulder blades.

Usually, a superficial nerve close to the pain is selected for stimulation. Electrode placement depends on the site of the pain. Positive and negative poles are usually placed within several inches of each other. Voltage and pulsation are controlled by the client wearing the device. Before application, the electrodes are moistened with electrode jelly to ensure proper conduction. The skin and the electrodes are cleaned every 8 hours, and fresh jelly is ap-

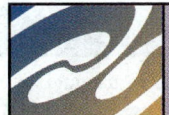

CLIENT EDUCATION GUIDE

Transcutaneous Electrical Nerve Stimulation (TENS) Units

Teaching and learning are very important to a client using a TENS unit. Teaching clients using a TENS unit includes the following items:

- A shock will not occur, and you do not need to fear electrocution.
- Wash the electrode sites and apply skin cream.
- Apply the electrodes properly; if they are not lying flat and making full surface contact, a burn may occur.
- You may conceal the unit's wires so that they are not visible to others.
- Use the TENS unit for as long as directed. [Regimens for the use of TENS units are highly individualized.]

plied. When stimulation is not effective, the entire painful area is explored for subsequent electrode placement.

The overall efficacy of TENS in clients with chronic pain is about 25%. TENS has been reported to be less effective for cancer pain than for other types of pain.

Percutaneous Epidural Dorsal Column Stimulation

A single (unipolar) electrode or two (bipolar) insulated-wire electrodes are placed through the skin (i.e., percutaneously) into the spinal epidural space. The dorsal column may then be temporarily stimulated to evaluate the mechanism's effectiveness in obtaining pain relief before permanent implantation of a stimulator. It is a necessary part of the assessment of a client to evaluate whether or not a permanent stimulator would be beneficial.

Local anesthesia is injected into the tissue overlying the interspinous space. A curved needle is inserted and the wire electrode is gently passed through the needle into the epidural space. After the electrode has been manipulated into proper position under fluoroscopy, the needle is withdrawn and the electrode left in place. This procedure is then repeated at the same site or at a different interspace to place the second electrode. The electrodes are then attached to an external power source, by which the person can control the amount of dorsal column stimulation received.

Dorsal Column Spinal Cord Stimulation

Success with this type of pain therapy requires careful assessment and selection of the client experiencing pain. The pain must have a definitively diagnosed organic

Table 17–7. Troubleshooting TENS Units

Following are some common problems of TENS use and some simple solutions. But remember, *always* turn the TENS unit off before checking it.

Problem	Solution
No stimulation	Change batteries Make sure batteries are inserted correctly Check that lead wires are plugged in securely at both ends Make sure electrodes are in total contact with the skin Look for corrosion on battery contacts Replace electrodes Check for defective wires
Cuts in and out	Check that both ends of the lead wire are plugged in securely Replace defective leads Check that batteries are securely in place Make sure electrodes are in total contact with the skin Check that amplitude is turned up enough
Skin irritation	Remove preoperative skin antiseptic Discontinue use temporarily, if necessary Treat rash (leave open to air; use skin cream) Reposition electrodes so they are not on irritated area Replace electrodes, if necessary Change type of electrode, if desired Make sure electrodes are in total contact with the skin Try a protective film (e.g., Skin-Prep), cream (e.g., Uniderm), or non-prescription cortisone cream Try a different adhesive tape Wash electrode (if made of reusable carbon rubber) Discontinue using TENS if problem does not resolve
Unpleasant sensation (itching, burning, pricking—without rash)	Use a different type of electrode Lower pulse-width dial Increase distance between electrodes Check electrode adhesion Try another brand of TENS
Unpleasant sensation (too intense, feels obnoxious, too distracting)	Turn down amplitude dial Turn down pulse-width dial Adjust rate Try another style of electrode Turn unit on less frequently Change electrode location Try another brand of TENS
Nausea	Reposition electrodes Vary rate, pulse width, amplitude Try another brand of TENS Discontinue using TENS if problem does not resolve
Headache	Turn down pulse-width dial Turn down amplitude dial Use shorter stimulation period (turn off more often) Use fewer electrodes and place them farther apart Reposition electrodes Vary the rate Try different brand of TENS Discontinue using TENS if problem does not resolve

From Meyer, T. H. (1982). TENS: Relieving pain through electricity. *Nursing 82, 12,* 57.

cause. Individuals selected should previously have tried many other types of pain management techniques and therapies in attempts to relieve their pain. Initial screening is performed with a percutaneous epidural dorsal column stimulator (see earlier). If the person experiences pain relief from this temporary technique, a dorsal column stimulation implant is surgically placed.

The implant stimulation device is a transistorized receiver that is surgically implanted. Electrode wires run into the epidural space and to an external transmitter. In a surgical procedure, a subcutaneous pocket is formed for the receiver. This pocket is usually in the infraclavicular region of the abdomen. Electrodes are passed subcutaneously from the receiver to a laminectomy incision. Electrode leads are threaded into the epidural space. Usually, the laminectomy is performed in the thoracic or lumbar region.

Relief of chronic pain from the dorsal column stimulator may diminish with time, and results have not been as encouraging as was hoped. Implantation of peripheral nerve stimulators is safer and easier than implanting dorsal column stimulators.

Intracranial Stimulation

Use of intracranial stimulation is becoming more common. It is considered for clients whose pain is diffuse and unresponsive to other treatments. This therapy is an alternative to destructive intracranial procedures. Under local anesthesia, a stimulating electrode is inserted into the posterior end of the third ventricle. The proximal end of the electrode is connected to a battery-driven stimulator, which is operated by the client. There is some evidence that the enkephalin levels in the CSF may be increased by this technique.[11]

Relief of chronic pain from the intracranial stimulator may diminish with time, and results have not been as encouraging as was hoped. Implantation of peripheral nerve stimulators is safer and easier than implanting intracranial stimulators.

Radiation Therapy

Because it may cause multiple complications, radiation therapy is not usually used to treat benign pain states if the condition can be managed by more conservative measures. Radiation therapy, however, is used extensively in treating pain caused by malignant conditions, such as bone pain. It is also very useful in reducing the size of tumors pressing on nerves and other organs.

Placebos

A placebo is thought of as a harmless, but useless, treatment designed to make the client feel better. It has been defined as any treatment that produces an effect in the client because of suggestion, not because of anything specific in its nature or in the therapeutic properties of the treatment.[99] If the client responds to a placebo, the client is said to be placebo-positive.

Unfortunately, placebos given instead of pain medications are not harmless. If nothing else, they usually require the nurse to lie to the client about what is being given. When the client discovers what has been done, all faith and trust in the healthcare team is lost. The nurse must question why the placebo is being ordered. If the client is placebo-positive, this only proves that the client is one of the one third of the population who respond positively to placebos. The problem arises when the client's response is considered to mean that the client's pain is not real.

There are many myths associated with response to placebos. These seem to have as a basis a disbelief of the client's report of pain. Any client who reports pain must be believed, because that pain is real for that client. Always closely question the use of placebos in the place of adequate pain medication. It is unethical to lie to a client, and placebos are a lie. You, the nurse, can be a positive influence (i.e., a placebo) by taking a positive approach to the usefulness of the treatment being done. This does not mean lying to the client, it simply means approaching each intervention with a very positive attitude.

Modification of Plan of Care for the Elderly

It is important for the nurse to be aware of problems associated with pain assessment and treatment in the elderly. There are many myths associated with both pain and treatment in this age group (Table 17–8). Some of these points were discussed previously in the section on response to pain.

When administering analgesics to the elderly, the nurse should be aware of the physiologic changes in these clients. The distribution of medications is altered by aging. There is usually a higher percentage of body fat in the elderly, which could increase the accumulation of fat-soluble medications, such as the lower muscle mass, resulting in the need for a lower dosage. Serum proteins are also lower, which affects the dosage of any medication that is bound to plasma proteins. This is important because NSAIDs are plasma protein–bound medications and are commonly used to treat some chronic pains, such as arthritis.

The liver is the major site of medication biotransformation. Aging alters the liver and therefore the biotransformation of medications may change in an unpredictable way. Medications such as acetaminophen are biotransformed more slowly, but other medications may not be affected. The interval between doses may have to be lengthened to avoid this problem. The maximum dose of a medication such as acetaminophen must be carefully checked to avoid liver toxicity. This includes acetaminophen used in combination medications such as Vicodin as well as the over-the-counter use of acetaminophen in non-aspirin combinations. The maximum 24-hour dose of 3 to 4 g of acetaminophen should not be exceeded in the elderly.

Excretion of medications is also affected by changes in renal mass, blood flow, glomerular filtration rate, and tubular secretion. Again, the length of time medications remain in the body is longer, so lower doses and longer intervals are needed. The clearance of morphine from the plasma is also reduced. This means that morphine remains in the body longer at higher concentrations. Giving lower doses at longer intervals will compensate for this problem.

Table 17–8. Misconceptions and Facts About Pain in the Elderly

Misconceptions	Facts
Pain is a natural part of the aging process	Pain does not accompany aging unless there is some specific disease process present. Older people are more likely to suffer from chronic diseases such as arthritis, but without disease there should not be pain
Pain perception decreases with aging	If the CNS is intact, then there is no alteration in pain perception. Pain response may be affected by a variety of factors, such as aphasia or paralysis. Lack of pain response, however, does not mean lack of pain
Elderly who appear occupied or are easily distracted from pain must not have significant pain	Many clients with chronic pain use distraction as a way of coping with their pain. What seems to be an easily distracted client may be one who could benefit from distraction techniques as a way of assisting with pain control. Lack of pain expression does not mean lack of pain
Opioids should never be used in the elderly. They are too dangerous	Opioids are appropriate to treat severe pain in the elderly as long as changes in sensitivity are accounted for. The elderly may have more problems biotransforming or excreting these medications, so lower doses and longer intervals between doses are safer
If the older person is confused, pain medications should not be given because they will increase the confusion	Pain itself can cause confusion in the elderly. It may interfere with sleep and rest, leading to confusion. Confusion will often resolve once the client has been adequately treated for pain
If an older person is showing signs of depression and chronic pain, the pain is caused by the depression. If the depression is treated, the pain will disappear	Depression is a normal response to, not a cause of, pain. Depression may influence the client's ability to cope with the pain, but is not the cause of it. When the pain is relieved, the depression will probably disappear

There are other factors that may alter medication therapy in the elderly. Intramuscular injections may be poorly absorbed because of loss of muscle mass. The possible alterations in circulation also may affect distribution of injected medications.

To treat pain adequately in the elderly, the nurse must rely on careful observation of the effectiveness of the treatment. If oversedation or other problems occur, the dose of medication should be reduced. Problems associated with pain medication and the elderly, however, should never mean that they are not being adequately treated for their pain.

Conclusions

Pain is a complex phenomenon, and it is one of the most common problems nurses face. Pain is an almost universal experience (except for the few clients who feel no pain), but, at the same time, it is a unique experience for each client. The nurse is in a good position to help the client with pain. The nurse can help the client communicate with the physician when pain relief is not sufficient. The nurse can establish a relationship with the client to help the client learn new ways of controlling pain.

The subject of pain control is changing constantly. New information about the physiology of pain transmission and control serves to broaden the options available to help the client in pain. Nurses are becoming more knowledgeable about pain and its control. Nurses have an ever-expanding role to play in the treatment of clients' pain.

Box 17–3. Internet Resources on Pain

Roxane Laboratories has a pain group on the World Wide Web at http://www.Roxane.com. Other sites of interest include:

http://www.painnet.com—a pain network
http://weber.u.washington.edu/~crc/OASP.html—the International Association for the Study of Pain

These sites often lead to other Web sites of interest to nurses interested in pain. The AHCPR guidelines are also available through the Roxane site.

Thinking Critically

1. A 33-year-old client arrives in the emergency department with a severe headache and a history of vomiting twice. She states, "This is the worst headache I have ever had." The headache has lasted for about 6 hours, and two doses of acetaminophen have given no relief. The client is unable to lift her head off of the pillow or to position herself for comfort. Her pupils are equal and there is no diaphoresis. What further nursing history and assessments should be done? How soon can medication to alleviate the headache be administered?

Factors to Consider. How crucial is a thorough pain assessment? How can a migraine headache mimic signs and symptoms of a cerebral disorder? Would it be advisable to delay giving analgesia? Why? Why not?

2. An elderly client, terminally ill with cancer, is prescribed an opiate analgesic for her pain. She is being cared for at home by a family that is concerned about pain control for their loved one. What should the client and family be taught regarding complications associated with use of opiate analgesia? Who would be the ideal person to assess and coordinate the client's response to dosing of a particular opiate and/ or combination of opiate and non-opiate medications?

Factors to Consider. What complications are associated with use of opiate analgesia? What factors contribute to the dosing schedule of a client with cancer-related pain? How much control over analgesia is given to the client? How should the caregiver and family monitor the response of the client to the prescribed medication regimen?

Bibliography

1. Abram, S. E. (Ed.) (1990). *The pain clinic manual.* Philadelphia: J. B. Lippincott.
2. Acute Pain Management Guideline Panel. (1992). *Acute pain management: Operative or medical procedures and trauma. Clinical practice guidelines.* AHCPR Publications No. 92-0032. Rockville, MD: Agency for Health Care Policy and Research, Public Health Service, U. S. Department of Health and Human Services.
3. Acute Pain Management Guideline Panel. (1992). *Acute pain management in adults: Operative procedures. Quick reference guide for clinicians.* AHCPR Publications No. 92-0019. Rockville, MD: Agency for Health Care Policy and Research, Public Health Service, U. S. Department of Health and Human Services.
4. Acute Pain Management Guideline Panel. (1992). *Pain control after surgery: A patient's guide.* AHCPR Publications No. 92-0021. Rockville, MD: Agency for Health Care Policy and Research, Public Health Service, U. S. Department of Health and Human Services.
5. Alpen, M. A., & Titler, M. G. (1994). Pain management in the critically ill: What do we know and how can we improve? *AACN Clinical Issues in Critical Care Nursing, 5*(2), 159–168.
6. Alspach, G. (1994). Pain management: Dispelling some myths. *Critical Care Nursing, 14*(5), 13–15.
7. American Pain Society. (1992). *Principles of analgesic use in the treatment of acute and cancer pain* (3rd ed.). Skokie, IL: Author.
8. Applying a sedation algorithm to ICU patients in pain . . . DCCN STATpack. (1995). *Dimensions of Critical Care Nursing, 14*(2), 67–68.
9. Arathuzik, D. (1994). Preliminary assessment: The Pain Inventory and the Pain Coping Tool. *American Journal of Hospice and Palliative Care, 11*(5), 25–29.
10. Atsberger, D. B. (1995). Relaxation therapy: Its potential as an intervention for acute postoperative pain. *Journal of Post Anesthesia Nursing, 10*(1), 2–8.
11. Basbaum, A. I., & Fields, H. L. (1978). Endogenous pain control mechanisms: Review and hypothesis. *Annals of Neurology, 4,* 451.
12. Bates, M. S., Edwards, W. T., & Anderson, K. O. (1993). Ethnocultural influences on variation in chronic pain perception. *Pain, 52,* 101–112.
13. Bates, M. S., & Rankin-Hill, L. (1994). Control, culture, and chronic pain. *Social Science and Medicine, 39*(5), 629–245.
14. Bombardier, C., et al. (1994). A guide to interpreting epidemiologic studies on the etiology of back pain. *Spine, 19*(Suppl. 18S), 2047S–2056S.
15. Bondville, J. (1994). Pain-free harvesting of skin grafts with Emla. *Plastic Surgical Nursing, 14*(4), 231–234.
16. Bonica, J. J., et al. (Eds.) (1990). *The management of pain* (vols 1 and 2, 2nd ed.). Philadelphia: Lea & Febiger.
17. Borneman, T. (1995). Controlling pain. Using nondrug interventions to relieve pain. *Nursing, 25*(2), 21.
18. Bostrom, J., & Batina, M. (1994). Managing pain in a diverse medical-surgical patient population. *MEDSURG Nursing, 3*(6), 469–474, 486.
19. Bowman, J. M. (1994). Perceptions of surgical pain by nurses and patients. *Clinical Nursing Research, 3*(1), 69–76.
20. Briggs, M. (1995). Principles of acute pain assessment. *Nursing Standards, 9*(19), 23–27.
21. Buck, M. M., & Paice, J. A. (1994). Pharmacologic management of acute pain in the orthopedic patient. *Orthopedic Nursing, 13*(6), 14–23.
22. Cain, J. M., & Hammes, B. J. (1994). Ethics and pain management: Respecting patient wishes. *Journal of Pain and Symptom Management, 8*(7), 474–482.
23. Cassetta, R. A. (1995). Waging a battle against cancer pain and fatigue. *American Nurse, 27*(1), 16.
24. Calcillo, E. F. & Flaskerud, J. H. (1991). Review of literature on culture and pain of adults with focus on Mexican-Americans. *Journal of Transcultural Nursing, 2*(2), 16–23.
25. Chapman, C. E. (1991). Can the use of physical modalities for pain control be rationalized by the research evidence? *Canadian Journal of Physiological Pharmacology, 69*(5), 704–712.
26. Chibnall, J. T., & Tait, R. C. (1994). The Pain Disability Index: Factor structure and normative data. *Archives of Physical Medicine and Rehabilitation, 75*(10), 1082–1086.
27. Choiniere, M., et al. (1990). Comparison between patients' and nurses' assessments of pain and medication efficacy in severe burn injuries. *Pain, 40*(2), 143–152.
28. Closs, S. J. (1994). Pain in elderly patients: A neglected phenomenon? *Journal of Advanced Nursing, 19*(6), 1072–1081.
29. Cooper, A. D. (1994). Pain assessment in accident and emergency. *Accident and Emergency Nursing, 2*(2), 103–107.
30. Copp, L. A. (1990). Treatment, torture, suffering, and compassion. *Journal of Professional Nursing, 6*(1), 1–2.
31. Cross, R. L., & Urbanski, B. A. (1994). Providing pain control for the critically ill substance-abuse patient. *Dimensions of Critical Care Nursing, 13*(6), 282–283.
32. Dahlberg, N., & Pendle, S. (1994). Developing an acute pain service in a multicultural setting. *Journal of Post Anesthesia Nursing, 9*(2), 96–100.
33. Dalton, J. A., et al. (1994). Behavioral pain profile: Development and psychometric properties. *Pain, 57*(1), 95–107.
34. Davitz, L. L., & Davitz, J. R. (1980). *Nurses response to patients' suffering.* New York: Springer Publishing.
35. Dietrick-Gallagher, M., Polomano, R., & Carrick, L. (1994). Pain as a quality management initiative. *Journal of Nursing Care Quality, 9*(1), 30–42.
36. Dowman, R. (1991). Spinal and supraspinal correlates of nociception in man. *Pain, 45*(3), 269–281.
37. Dudgeon, D., Raubertas, R. F., & Rosenthal, S. N. (1993). The

short-form McGill Pain Questionnaire in chronic cancer pain. *Journal of Pain and Symptom Management, 8*(4), 191–195.

38. Duggleby, W., & Lander, J. (1994). Cognitive status and postoperative pain: Older adults. *Journal of Pain and Symptom Management, 9*(1), 19–27.

39. Duncan, D. J., & Driscoll, D. M. (1991). Burn management. *Critical Care Nursing Clinics of North America, 2*(3), 165–267.

40. Eldridge, A. D., et al. (1994). Prevalence and characteristics of pain in persons with terminal-stage AIDS. *Journal of Advanced Nursing, 20*(2), 260–268.

41. Everett, J. J., et al. (1994). Pain assessment from patients with burns and their nurses. *Journal of Burn Care and Rehabilitation, 15*(2), 194–198.

42. Faucett, J. (1994). Depression in painful chronic disorders: The role of pain and conflict about pain. *Journal of Pain and Symptom Management, 9*(8), 320–326.

43. Faucett, J. (1995). Cumulative trauma disorder—Pain at work. *Healthline, 14*(2), 9.

44. Faucett, J., Gordon, N., & Levine, J. (1994). Differences in postoperative pain severity among four ethnic groups. *Journal of Pain and Symptom Management, 9*(6), 383–389.

45. Ferrell, B. R. (1994). Controlling pain: Switching to a longer-acting opioid. *Nursing, 24*(2), 22.

46. Ferrell, B. R. (1994). Using placebos ethically: Controlling pain. *Nursing, 24*(3), 28.

47. Ferrell, B. R., & Dean, G. (1995). The meaning of cancer pain. *Seminars in Oncology Nursing, 11*(1), 17–22.

48. Ferrell, B. R., & Griffith, H. (1994). Cost issues related to pain management: Report from the Cancer Pain Panel of the Agency for Health Care Policy and Research. *Journal of Pain and Symptom Management, 9*(4), 221–234.

49. Ferrell, B. R., et al. (1994). Cancer pain guidelines: Now that we have them, what do we do? *Oncology Nursing Forum, 21*(7), 1229–1231.

50. Ferrell, B. R., McCaffery, M., & Rhiner, M. (1992). Pain and addiction: An urgent need for change in nursing education. *Journal of Pain and Symptom Management, 7*, 117–124.

51. Ferrell, B. R., McGuire, D. B., & Donovan, M. I. (1993). Knowledge and beliefs regarding pain in a sample of nursing faculty. *Journal of Professional Nursing, 9*, 79–88.

52. Ferrell, B. R., Wendon, M., & Rollins, B. (1995). Pain and quality assessment/improvement. *Journal of Nursing Care Quality, 9*(3), 69–85.

53. Ferrer-Brechner, T. (Ed.) (1990). *Common problems in pain management.* St. Louis: Mosby–Year Book.

54. Fields, H. L. (Ed.) (1990). *Pain syndromes in neurology.* Boston: Butterworths.

55. Fields, H. L., et al. (1991). Neurotransmitters in nociceptive modulatory circuits. *Annual Review of Neuroscience, 14*, 219–245.

56. Finley, R. S. (1994). Clinical practice guidelines for the management of cancer pain. *Cancer Practice, 2*(3), 236–238.

57. Fox, A. E. (1994). Ethical issues: Confronting the use of placebos for pain. *American Journal of Nursing, 94*(9), 42–46.

58. Funk, B. (1995). Controlling pain. Using cognitive interventions. *Nursing, 25*(3), 30.

59. Gaukroger, P. B. (1991). Paediatric analgesia: Which drug? Which dose? *Drugs, 1*(41), 52–59.

60. Gilbert, M., et al. (1994). Spinal cord stimulation for chronic intractable pain: Nursing implications. *Journal of Neuroscience Nursing, 26*(6), 347–351.

61. Glover, J., et al. (1995). Mood states of oncology outpatients: Does pain make a difference? *Journal of Pain and Symptom Management, 10*(2), 120–128.

62. Graves, D. A., et al. (1983). Patient-controlled analgesia. *Annals of Internal Medicine, 99*, 360.

63. Greenwald, H. P. (1991). Interethnic differences in pain perception. *Pain, 44*, 157–163.

64. Gujol, M. C. (1994). A survey of pain assessment and management practices among critical care nurses. *American Journal of Critical Care, 3*(2), 123–128.

65. Guyton, A. C., & Hall, J. E. (1996). *Textbook of medical physiology* (9th ed.). Philadelphia: W. B. Saunders.

66. Hall, G. R., et al. (1995). Managing constipation using a research-based protocol. *MEDSURG Nursing, 4*(1), 11–20.

67. Hammes, B. J., & Cain, J. M. (1994). The ethics of pain management for cancer patients: Case studies and analysis. *Journal of Pain and Symptom Management, 9*(3), 166–170.

68. Harwood, A. (Ed.) (1981). *Ethnicity and medical care.* Cambridge, MA: Harvard University Press.

69. Henkelman, W. J. (1994). Inadequate pain management: Ethical considerations. *Nursing Management, 25*(1), 48A–B, 48D.

70. Herr, K. A., & Mobily, P. R. (1993). Comparison of selected pain assessment tools for use with the elderly. *Applied Nursing Research, 6*(1), 39–46.

71. Hitchcock, L. S., Ferrell, B. R., & McCaffery, M. (1994). The experience of chronic nonmalignant pain. *Journal of Pain and Symptom Management, 9*(5), 312–318.

72. Howell, S. L. (1994). A theoretical model for caring for women with chronic nonmalignant pain. *Qualitative Health Research, 4*(1), 94–122.

73. Hoyt, M. J., et al. (1994). The effect of chemical dependency on pain perceptions in persons with AIDS. *Journal of the Association of Nurses in AIDS Care, 5*(3), 33–38.

74. International Association for the Study of Pain (1986). Pain terms: A current list with definitions and notes on usage. *Pain, 3,* S216–S221.

75. Inturrisi, C. E. (1984). Pharmacology of narcotic analgesics. In *The management of cancer pain.* Nutley, NJ: Roche Laboratories.

76. Jaffe, J. H., & Martin, W. R. (1980). Opioid analgesics and antagonists. In A. G. Gilman, et al. (Eds.), *The pharmacological basis of therapeutics* (6th ed.). New York: Macmillan.

77. Johnson, A., et al. (1991). Inhibition of burn pain by intravenous lignocaine. *Lancet, 2*(338), 151–152.

78. Jurisson, M. L. (1995). Managing pain in rheumatic disease. *Physical Medicine and Rehabilitation Clinics of North America, 6*(1), 207–217.

79. Kenner, D. J. (1994). Pain forum: Part 3. Other types of pain. *Australian Family Physician, 23*(7), 1285–1289, 1292.

80. Kohr, J. (1995). Measuring your patient's pain. *RN, 58*(4), 39–40.

81. Kurz, J. M. (1994). Therapeutic touch for postop pain? *American Journal of Nursing, 94*(9), 48D.

82. Lawrence, S., et al. (1995). Epidural analgesia for effective pain control. *Critical Care Nurse, 15*(1), 20–21.

83. Lehne, R. A., et al. (1994). *Pharmacology for nursing care* (second edition). Philadelphia: W. B. Saunders.

84. Liebeskind, J. C. (1991). Pain can kill. *Pain, 44,* 3–4.

85. Lindaman, C. (1995). Talking to physicians about pain control. *American Journal of Nursing, 95*(1), 36–37.

86. Lloyd, G., & McLauchlan, A. (1994). Nurses' attitudes towards pain management. *Nursing Times, 90*(43), 40–43.

87. Lowdermilk, D. L. (1995). Home care of the patient with gynecologic cancer. *Journal of Obstetric, Gynecologic, and Neonatal Nursing, 24*(2), 157–163.

88. Lytle, S. A., et al. (1991). Postoperative analgesia with epidural fentanyl. *Journal of the American Osteopathic Association, 91*(6), 547–550.

89. Mackersie, R. C., & Karagianes, T. G. (1990). Pain management following trauma and burns. *Critical Care Clinics, 6*(2), 433–449.

90. Mahon, S. M. (1994). Concept analysis of pain: Implications related to nursing diagnosis. *Nursing Diagnosis, 5*(1), 14–25.

91. Management of Cancer Pain Guideline Panel. (1994). *Management of cancer pain: Clinical practice guideline.* AHCPR Publications No. 94-0592. Rockville, MD: Agency for Health Care Policy and Research, Public Health Service, U. S. Department of Health and Human Services.

92. Management of Cancer Pain Guideline Panel. (1994). *Management of cancer pain: Patient guide.* AHCPR Publications No. 94-0595. Rockville, MD: Agency for Health Care Policy and Research, Public Health Service, U. S. Department of Health and Human Services.

93. Management of Cancer Pain Guideline Panel. (1994). *Management of cancer pain: Quick reference guide for clinicians.* AHCPR Publications No. 94-0593. Rockville, MD: Agency for Health Care Policy and Research, Public Health Service, U. S. Department of Health and Human Services.

94. Marks, R. M., & Sachar, E. J. (1973). Undertreatment of medical inpatients with narcotic analgesics. *Annals of Internal Medicine, 78,* 173–181.

95. McCaffery, M. (1981). *Nursing management of the patient with pain* (2nd ed.). Philadelphia: J. B. Lippincott.

96. McCaffery, M. (1994). Ensuring pain relief. *Nursing, 24*(9), 81–82.

97. McCaffery, M. (1994). How reliable is your patient's pain assessment? *Nursing, 24*(1), 19.

98. McCaffery, M. (1994). How to use the new AHCPR cancer pain guidelines. *American Journal of Nursing, 94*(7), 42–47.

99. McCaffery, M., & Beebe, A. (1989). *Pain: Clinical manual for nursing practice.* St. Louis: Mosby–Year Book.

100. McCaffery, M., & Ferrell, B. R. (1991). How would you respond to these patients in pain? *Nursing, 21*(6), 34–37.

101. McCaffery, M., & Ferrell, B. R. (1991). Patient age: Does it affect your pain-control decisions? *Nursing, 21*(9), 44–48.

102. McCaffery, M., & Ferrell, B. R. (1994). Nurses' assessment of pain intensity and choice of analgesic dose. *Contemporary Nurse, 3*(2), 68–74.

103. McCaffery, M., & Hart, L. L. (1976). Undertreatment of acute pain with narcotics. *Nursing 76, 10,* 1586–1591.

104. McCorquodale, A., DeFaye, B., & Bruera, E. (1993). Pain control in an alcoholic cancer patient. *Journal of Pain and Symptom Management, 8*(3), 177–180.

105. McGee, J. L., & Alexander, M. R. (1979). Phenothiazine analgesia: Fact or fantasy. *American Journal of Hospital Pharmacy, 36,* 633–640.

106. McGuire, D. B. (1992). Comprehensive and multidimensional assessment and measurement of pain. *Journal of Pain and Symptom Management, 7*(5), 312–219.

107. McGuire, D. B., Yarbro, C. H., & Ferrell, B. R. (1995). *Cancer pain management* (2nd ed.). Boston: Jones & Bartlett.

108. McGuire, L. (1994). The nurse's role in pain relief. *MEDSURG Nursing, 3*(2), 94–98.

109. McGuire, L. (1995). Controlling phantom limb pain. *Nursing, 25*(2), 6.

110. Meinhart, N. T., & McCaffery, M. (1983). *Pain: A nursing approach to assessment and analysis.* Norwalk, CT: Appleton-Century-Crofts.

111. Melzack, R. (1987). The short form McGill pain questionnaire. *Pain, 30,* 191–197.

112. Melzack, R., & Wall, P. (1982). *The puzzle of pain.* New York: Basic Books.

113. Melzack, R., & Wall, P. (1983). *The challenge of pain.* New York: Basic Books.

114. Miakowski, C. (1993). Current concepts in the assessment and management of acute pain. *MEDSURG Nursing, 2*(1), 28–32, 40.

115. Miakowski, C., et al. (1994). Assessment of patient satisfaction utilizing the American Pain Society's Quality Assurance Standards on acute and cancer related pain. *Journal of Pain and Symptom Management, 9*(1), 5–11.

116. Mobily, P. R., Herr, K. A., & Nicholson, A. C. (1994). Validation of cutaneous stimulation interventions for pain management. *International Journal of Nursing Studies, 31*(6), 533–544.

117. Moret, V., et al. (1991). Mechanisms of analgesia-induced hypnosis and acupuncture: Is there a difference? *Pain, 45*(2), 135–140.

118. Morgan, A. E., Lindley, C. M., & Berry, J. I. (1994). Assessment of pain and patterns of analgesic use in hospice patients. *American Journal of Hospice and Palliative Care, 11*(1), 13–19.

119. Mountcastle, V. B. (1980). *Medical physiology* (p. 391). St. Louis: Mosby–Year Book.

120. Naber, L., Jones, G., & Halm, M. (1994). Epidural analgesia for effective pain control. *Critical Care Nurse, 14*(5), 69–72, 77–85.

121. Nash, R., Edwards, H., & Nebauer, M. (1993). Effect of attitudes, subjective norms and perceived control on nurses' intention to assess patients' pain. *Journal of Advanced Nursing, 18*(6), 941–947.

122. Nielsen, L. B., Svantesson-Martinsson, E. I., & Enberg, I. L. (1994). An interview study of nurses' assessment and priority of post surgical pain experience. *Intensive and Critical Care Nursing, 10*(2), 107–114.

123. Olesinski, N. (1994). Commentary on *Caveat emptor:* A critical analysis of the costs of drugs used to pain management. *AACN Nursing Scan in Critical Care, 4*(2), 24.

124. Patt, R. B. (Ed.). (1993). *Cancer pain.* Philadelphia: J. B. Lippincott.

125. Paice, J. A., & Buck, M. M. (1993). Intraspinal devices for pain management. *Nursing Clinics of North America, 28*(4), 921–935.

126. Paice, J. A., Penn, R. D., & Ryan, W. G. (1994). Altered sexual function and decreased testosterone in patients receiving intraspinal opioids. *Journal of Pain and Symptom Management, 9*(2), 126–131.

127. Pasero, C. L. (1994). Help for chronic pain sufferers. *American Journal of Nursing, 94*(10), 17.

128. Pasero, C. L., et al. (1995). Pain control. Antidepressants for pain relief. *American Journal of Nursing, 95*(2), 22, 24.

129. Patterson, J. (1994). The nurse's role in pain management. *Today's OR Nurse, 16*(6), 57–58.

130. Portenoy, R. K. (1995). Pharmacologic management of cancer pain. *Seminars in Oncology, 22*(2 Suppl. 3), 112–120.

131. Puntillo, K., & Weiss, S. J. (1994). Pain: Its mediators and associated morbidity in critically ill cardiovascular surgical patients. *Nursing Research, 43*(1), 31–36.

132. Puntillo, K. A. (1994). Dimensions of procedural pain and its analgesic management in critically ill surgical patients. *American Journal of Critical Care, 3*(2), 116–122.

133. Reilly, R. L. (1994). 12 steps to managing chronic pain: Chronic Pain Anonymous. *Patient Care, 28*(12), 117–121.

134. Rook, J. L. (1994). Managing chronic pain: The evolution of geriatric pain management will require a team approach . . . Part 1. *Rehab Management: The Interdisciplinary Journal of Rehabilitation, 75*(10), 1082–1086.

135. Rose, K. E. (1994). Patient isolation in chronic benign pain. *Nursing Standards, 8*(51), 25–27.

136. Ruta, D. A., et al. (1994). Developing a valid and reliable measure of health outcome for patients with low back pain. *Spine, 19*(17), 1887–1896.

137. Ryan, P., Vortherms, R., & Ward, S. (1994). Cancer pain: Knowledge, attitudes of pharmacologic management. *Journal of Gerontological Nursing, 20*(1), 7–16.

138. Scholz, M. J. (1995). Pain clinic: Assessing safety of opioids for chronic pain. *RN, 58*(4), 71.

139. Scott, I. E. (1994). Effectiveness of documented assessment of postoperative pain. *British Journal of Nursing, 3*(10), 494–501.

140. Seale, C., & Addington-Hall, H. (1994). Euthanasia: Why people want to die earlier. *Social Science and Medicine, 39*(5), 647–654.

141. Selbst, S. M. & Clark, M. (1990). Analgesic use in the emergency department. *Annals of Emergency Medicine, 19*(9), 1010–1013.

142. Simonton, O. C., et al. (1978). *Getting well again.* New York: Bantam Books.

143. Sorkin, L. S. (1991). Nociceptive transmission within the spinal cord. *Mount Sinai Journal of Medicine, 58*(3), 208–216.

144. Spross, J. A., McGuire, D. B., & Schmitt, R. M. (1990). Oncology Nursing Society position paper on pain: Part 1. *Oncology Nursing Forum, 17*(4), 595–614.

145. Spross, J. A., McGuire, D. B., & Schmitt, R. M. (1990). Oncology Nursing Society position paper on pain: Part 2. *Oncology Nursing Forum, 17*(5), 751–760.

146. Spross, J. A., McGuire, D. B., & Schmitt, R. M. (1990). Oncology Nursing Society position paper on pain: Part 3. *Oncology Nursing Forum, 17*(6), 943–947.

147. Stark, P. C. (1995). Problem solving in pain management by expert intensive care nurses. *Critical Care Nurse, 15*(1), 21.

148. Stein, W. M., & Miech, R. P. (1993). Cancer pain in the elderly hospice patient. *Journal of Pain and Symptom Management, 8*(7), 474–482.

149. Stephenson, N. L. N. (1994). A comparison of nurse and patient: Perceptions of postsurgical pain. *Journal of Intravenous Nursing, 17*(5), 235–239.

150. Sternbach, R. (1968). *Pain: A psychophysiological analysis* (p. 12). New York: Academic Press.

151. Stimmel, B. (1983). *Pain, analgesics, addiction: The pharmacologic treatment.* New York: Raven Press.

152. Sullivan, L. M. (1994). Factors influencing pain management: A nursing perspective. *Journal of Post Anesthesia Nursing, 9*(2), 83–90.

153. Tittle, M., & McMillan, S. C. (1994). Pain and pain-related side effects in an ICU and on a surgical unit: Nurses' management. *American Journal of Critical Care. 3*(1), 25–30.

154. Turk, D. C., & Feldman, C. S. (Eds.). (1992). *Noninvasive approaches in pain management in the terminally ill.* New York: Haworth.

155. Turk, D. C., & Marcus, D. A. (1994). Assessment of chronic pain patients. *Seminars in Neurology, 14*(3), 206–212.

156. Ufema, J. (1994). Placebos: Sugarcoated pain. *Nursing, 24*(9), 31.

157. Vallerand, A. H. (1991). The use of narcotic analgesics in chronic nonmalignant pain. *Holistic Nursing Practice, 6*(1), 17–23.

158. Vallerand, A. H. (1994). Street addicts and patients with pain: Similarities and differences. *Clinical Nurse Specialists, 8*(1), 11–14.

159. Villaruel, A. M., & de Montellano, B. O. (1992). Culture and pain: A Mesoamerican perspective. *Advances in Nursing Science, 15*(1), 21–32.

160. Walker, A. C., Tan, L., & George, S. (1995). Impact of culture on pain management: An Australian nursing perspective. *Holistic Nursing Practice, 9*(2), 48–57.

161. Wall, P. D., & Melzack, R. J. (Eds.). (1994). *Textbook of pain* (3rd ed.). New York: Churchill Livingstone.

162. Wallace, M. (1994). Assessment and management of pain in the elderly. *MEDSURG Nursing, 3*(4), 293–298.

163. Walsh, S. A., et al. (1995). A place for placebos? *American Journal of Nursing, 95*(2), 18.

164. Ward, S., & Gatwood, J. (1994). Concerns about reporting pain and using analgesics: A comparison of persons with and without cancer. *Cancer Nursing, 17*(3), 200–206.

165. Warfield, C. A. (Ed.) (1991). *Manual of pain management.* Philadelphia: J. B. Lippincott.

166. Waters, J., & Thomas, V. (1995). Pain from sickle-cell crisis. *Nursing Times, 91*(16), 29–31.

167. Watson, C. P. N. (1994). Antidepressant drugs as adjuvant analgesics. *Journal of Pain and Symptom Management, 9*(6), 392–405.

168. Webb, M. R., & Kennedy, M. G. (1994). Behavioral responses and self-reported pain in postoperative patients. *Journal of Post Anesthesia Nursing, 9*(2), 91–95.

169. Wenger, A. F. (1993). Cultural meaning of symptoms. *Holistic Nursing Practice, 7*(22), 22–35.

170. Wells, N. (1994). Perceived control over pain: Relation to distress and disability. *Research in Nursing and Health, 17*(4), 295–302.

171. Wild, L. (1990). Pain management. *Critical Care Nursing Clinics of North America, 2*(4), 537–547.

172. Wilke, K. J., Olsson, G. L., & Metclaf, C. L. (1993). *Essentials of pain management: A nursing handbook.* Seattle: Optioncare.

173. Williams, D. A., Robinson, M. E., & Geisser, M. E. (1994). Pain beliefs: Assessment and utility. *Pain, 59*(1), 71–78.

174. Woodward, S. (1995). Nurse and patient perceptions of pain. *Professional Nurse, 10*(7), 415–416.

175. World Health Organization. (1986). *Cancer pain relief.* Geneva: Author.

176. World Health Organization. (1990). *Cancer pain relief.* Geneva: Author.

177. Wotring, R. A. (1993). Cancer pain management. *Home Healthcare Nurse, 11*(5), 40–44.

178. Zborowski, M. (1952). Cultural components in responses to pain. *Journal of Sociological Issues, 8,* 16–30.

179. Zborowski, M. (1969). *People in pain.* San Francisco: Jossey-Bass.

Sleep and Sensory Disorders

Marlene Reimer

Most of us experience occasional problems of disturbed sleep, unwanted drowsiness, overstimulation, or understimulation. As a nurse you will frequently be involved with clients in whom these disturbances interfere with health and daily activities. Contributing factors may include personal life-style habits, environmental features, internal rhythms, or changes associated with episodic illness.

Sleep and Sleep Pattern Disturbances

Sleep can be defined as a normal state of altered consciousness during which the body rests and from which a person can be aroused by external stimuli.

Almost a third of the general population has some problems with sleep during any given year.[46] More than half of the 9000 participants in a study on sleep in elderly persons (65 years or older) reported the following as sleep pattern disturbances that they experience most of the time:

Trouble falling asleep
Frequent wakening
Waking too early
Needing to nap
Not feeling rested[18]

These disturbances may be secondary to situational, environmental, or developmental stressors, or they may be associated with illness or with pre-existing disorders. The relationship is often reciprocal in that the disorder decreases sleep and the decreased sleep affects the disorder. Sleep pattern disturbance also contributes to sensory disorders, such as intensive care unit psychosis.[58]

Sleep pattern disturbance is a nursing diagnosis that is defined as a disruption of sleep time that causes discomfort or interferes with a desired life-style.[7, 11, 47] The sleep pattern disturbance may relate to one of more than 70 sleep disorders identified in the International Classification of Sleep Disorders, a partial list of which is presented in Box 18–1. Intermittent sleep-related problems are also of concern for nursing diagnosis and intervention.

Chronobiology

Chronobiology refers to the study of biologic changes as they occur in relation to time. A knowledge of chronobiology is important to nurses in planning client care and teaching.

The menstrual cycle is an example of a complex, recurrent pattern extending over approximately 28 days. Sleep quality varies by stage of the menstrual cycle.[15]

The sleep-wake cycle is one of the circadian rhythms of the body. It follows an approximate 24-hour cycle through a complex process linked to light and dark. Illness and hospitalization may disrupt these rhythms. Elderly persons are particularly vulnerable to such changes. Nurses can minimize this impact by encouraging a regular schedule with appropriate environmental cues.

Ultradian cycles are biorhythms of less than 24 hours. The recurrent pattern of sleep stages, repeating approximately every 90 minutes in adults, is an example of an ultradian cycle. Recognizing this cycle, nurses can arrange care so as to avoid wakening patients more frequently unless absolutely necessary.

Chronopharmacology refers to the study of how biorhythms affect the absorption, metabolism, and excretion of drugs. For example, liver enzyme activity changes in relation to a circadian cycle. Thus, for example, the blood level achieved by a continuous infusion of heparin will vary. The risk of clotting is greater in the morning and the risk of bleeding is greater in the evening. Effectiveness of anticancer drugs varies according to the time of administration. Likewise, steroid medications should be administered in the morning to most closely approximate the natural variation in cortisol levels.

Box 18–1. International Classification of Sleep Disorders*

I. Dyssomnias
  A. Intrinsic sleep disorders
    1. Psychophysiologic insomnia
    2. Narcolepsy
    3. Obstructive sleep apnea syndrome
    4. Central sleep apnea syndrome
    5. Periodic limb movement disorder
    6. Restless legs syndrome
  B. Extrinsic sleep disorders
    1. Inadequate sleep hygiene
    2. Environmental sleep disorder
  C. Circadian rhythm sleep disorders
II. Parasomnias
  A. Arousal disorders
    1. Sleepwalking
    2. Sleep terrors
  B. Sleep-wake transition disorders
  C. Parasomnias usually associated with REM sleep
    1. Nightmares
    2. Sleep paralysis
  D. Other parasomnias
    1. Sleep bruxism
    2. Sleep enuresis
    3. Primary snoring
III. Sleep disorders associated with medical/psychiatric disorders
  A. Associated with mental disorders
  B. Associated with neurologic disorders
  C. Associated with other medical disorders
IV. Proposed sleep disorders

 * This is a partial listing of common sleep disorders. From the Diagnostic Classification Steering Committee, Thorpy, MJ, Chairman (1990). *International classification of sleep disorders: Diagnostic and coding manual.* Rochester, MN: American Sleep Disorders Association. Used with permission.

chemical messengers.[45] The onset of sleep and each subsequent sleep stage is an active process involving delicate shifts in the balance of several of these neurotransmitters.

The transition from the awake state to non-rapid eye movement (NREM) sleep is marked by decreases in the concentration of serotonin, norepinephrine, and acetylcholine. The later transition to rapid eye movement (REM) sleep is marked by a dramatic increase in acetylcholine and further drops in serotonin and norepinephrine.[26, 45] As REM sleep continues, the concentrations of serotonin and norepinephrine increase, eventually stopping REM sleep. Cholinergic activation with the release of acetylcholine seems to reestablish REM sleep.[26] The continuous interaction of these two systems is thought to produce the normal alterations between NREM and REM sleep.[26] Other neurotransmitters, such as gamma-aminobutyric acid (GABA) and dopamine, are also believed to have a part in the reciprocal processes involved in shifts in sleep state.

All of these neurotransmitters are actively involved in waking processes as well. For example, neurons that produce serotonin and norepinephrine play a role in the modulation of sensory input, mood, energy, and information processing, including attention, learning, and memory.[26] Thus, it can be seen that imbalances in these neurotransmitters induced through sleep pattern disturbances, medications, or diseases may reciprocally affect not only sleep but also aspects of sensory processing, mood, and cognition.

The Need for Sleep

Much is known about the architecture of the sleep cycle, but much less is known about the need for sleep. It is commonly held that sleep has a restorative and protective function.[29] Sympathetic activity decreases, whereas parasympathetic activity may increase. Hormonal shifts facilitate anabolic processes. Selective deprivation of slow-wave sleep is associated with vague physical complaints.[49]

REM sleep may be especially important for maintaining mental activities, such as learning, reasoning, and emotional adjustment. Sleep also appears to serve as an energy-conserving measure for most of the body except the brain.[30]

Sleep Stages

Sleep can be defined behaviorally, functionally, and electrophysiologically. Electrophysiologic monitoring of sleep, which is called *polysomnography,* includes at least three parameters: (1) brain wave activity, (2) eye movements, and (3) muscle tone. By using polysomnography, sleep can be divided into REM and NREM sleep. NREM can be further divided into stages 1 through 4. The stages vary in depth but are characterized by lack of eye movement, low and fragmented cognitive activity, maintenance of moderate muscle tone, and slower but generally rhythmic respirations and pulse rate. As individuals progress from stage 1 to stage 4 sleep, the waveforms recorded by

Physiology of Sleep and Arousal

The timing of the sleep-wake cycle and other circadian rhythms, such as body temperature, is controlled, at least in part, by the superchiasmatic nucleus in the anterior hypothalamus. Located above the optic chiasm, this area receives input from the retina, which provides information about darkness and light. The superchiasmatic nucleus controls the production of melatonin, which is believed to be a potent sleep inducer.[60]

Sleep is a naturally occurring, readily reversible altered state of arousal, characterized by a decreased responsiveness to the environment. The mediator of arousal and of sensory stimulation is the reticular activating system (RAS). The RAS is located in the brain stem and contains projections to the thalamus and cortex. The diffuse network of neurons in the RAS is in a strategic position to monitor ascending and descending stimuli through feedback loops.[45]

Although the RAS provides the anatomic framework for arousal, it is the neurotransmitters that serve as the

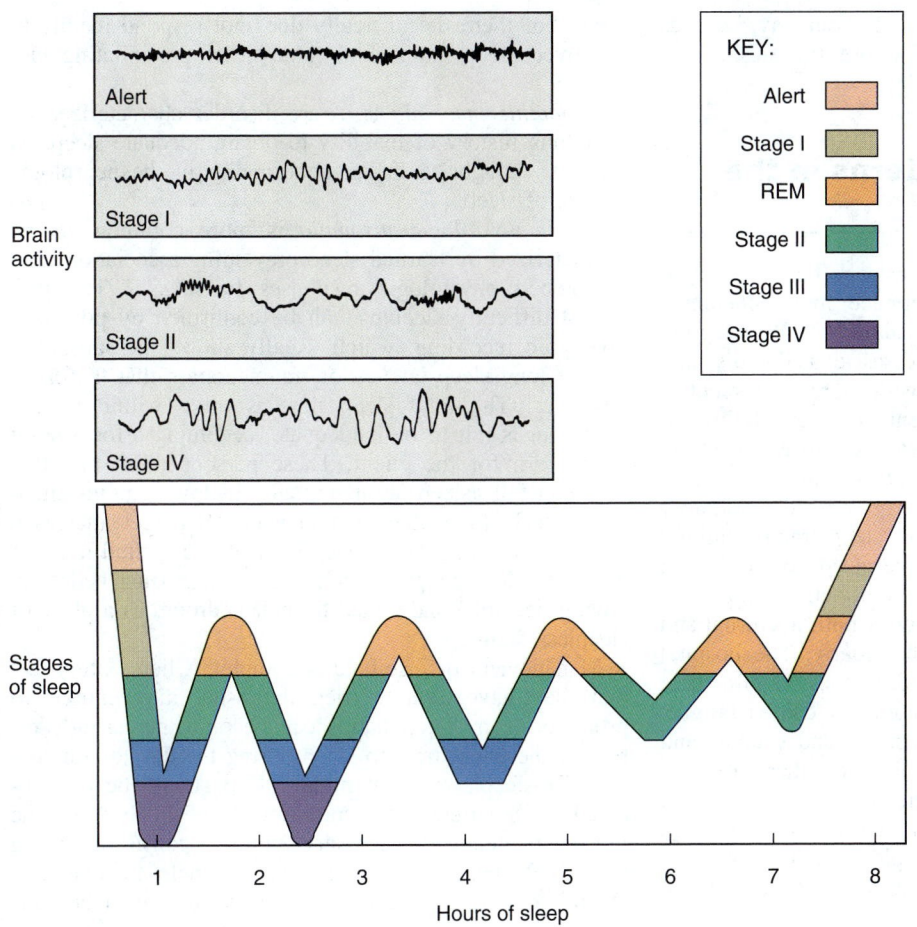

Figure 18–1. The electrical activity of the brain during various stages of sleep can be shown on electroencephalograms (EEGs). During the night, a person goes through three to five cycles. Each cycle includes a sequence of sleep stages. (From Solomon, E. P., Schmidt, R. R., & Adranga, P. J. [1990]. *Human anatomy and physiology* [2nd ed.]. Philadelphia: W.B. Saunders.)

electroencephalography (EEG) become more synchronized, slower, and of greater amplitude (Fig. 18–1).[63]

Stage 1 NREM sleep is very light. Respirations begin to slow, and muscles relax. At sleep onset, some erratic breathing may occur as well as sudden myoclonic jerks (sleep starts) as the body shifts from an awake to a sleep state. Stage 1 is such a light stage of sleep that persons wakened from it will often claim that they were not asleep at all.

Stage 2 NREM is still light sleep. The brain waves are frequently mixed and low voltage in pattern, with bursts of activity called *sleep spindles* and large-amplitude waves called *K complexes*.[60] More than 50% of sleep occurs as stage 2 sleep.

Stages 3 and 4 NREM are known as *slow-wave sleep*, named for the characteristic high-voltage, low-frequency delta waves. Respirations become slow and even. The pulse and blood pressure fall. Oxygen consumption by muscle tissues and urine formation are decreased.

Dreams that occur during the NREM stages of sleep are generally thought-like ruminations of recent events and current concerns, with little story line.[26]

REM sleep is characterized by low-voltage, random fast waves, as in stage 1 NREM. Clients in REM sleep have the characteristic rapid eye movements, erratic respirations, changes in heart rate, and very low muscle tone (see Fig. 18–1). During REM sleep, ventilation primarily depends on the movement of the diaphragm, because in-tercostal and accessory muscle tone is markedly diminished, and all postural and nonrespiratory muscles are essentially paralyzed.[56] The ventilatory response to hypoxia and hypercapnia is decreased. Thermoregulation is significantly reduced. Dreams in REM sleep are vivid, story-like, emotional, and bizarre.

Most persons move through an orderly progression of NREM sleep stages from 1 to 4 and back through 3 to 2 before initiating a period of REM (see Fig. 18–1). Although this is the typical progression, it is not essential or always seen. Atypical progressions are characteristic of some sleep disorders, such as narcolepsy, in which REM is entered almost immediately after sleep onset.

In adults, each sleep cycle through the various stages lasts about 90 minutes. During the first few cycles, more time is spent in slow-wave sleep, whereas the percentage of REM sleep increases later in the sleep period.[63]

Wide variations exist among individuals in relation to sleep patterns.[63] By explaining the range of these variations, the nurse can help clients to seek a pattern that leaves them feeling reasonably refreshed and alert. Eight hours of undisturbed sleep at night with no daytime naps has become the assumed ideal pattern in North American society. However, some adults do well on 6 hours or less; other healthy adults require 10 hours or more of nighttime sleep. Even young adults often waken once or twice a night, and with aging, such wakenings are more frequent. Humans may be physiologically inclined to have a long and a short sleep period each 24-hour day, such as is common in warmer climates, where the *siesta* is a normal part of the day's schedule.[14]

Changes in Sleep Patterns in the Elderly

The elderly take longer to fall asleep, have increased nocturnal wakefulness, and experience more sleepiness during the day than do younger adults.[6, 16] With aging, the percentage of stage 4 decreases considerably and REM sleep decreases somewhat, with more time spent in stage 1. REM sleep is more evenly distributed through the night. Sleep latency, the time it takes to get to sleep, increases, as does the average length of time it takes to get back to sleep after arousal.[63] Age-related respiratory dysfunction may be responsible for sleep fragmentation.[3] Other problems, such as pain, the need to void, and nocturnal dyspnea, may also decrease effective sleep.

Hospitalization affects the quality of both nocturnal and other sleep time, especially for the elderly. The hospital environment often lacks light and dark cues. Confinement curtails activity or exercise that normally causes fatigue. Additionally, there are unfamiliar sights and sounds, and frequent awakenings for vital signs and other interventions that disturb sleep. Finally, the elderly client is often in a poorer state of health and has more worry, anxiety, tension, and fatigue than does an older adult who is not hospitalized. These factors also decrease the quality of sleep.

Sleep Disorders

Dyssomnias

The dyssomnias include sleep disorders characterized by difficulty initiating or maintaining sleep (insomnia) or by excessive sleepiness. These disorders may arise predominantly from within the body (intrinsic), from external sources (extrinsic), or from disruptions of circadian rhythm.[13] The intrinsic sleep disorders are discussed first.

Intrinsic Sleep Disorders

Insomnia

Many persons experience transitory periods during which they have difficulty initiating or maintaining sleep. The onset or exacerbation of illness, with or without hospitalization, may precipitate such difficulty. These sleep pattern disturbances are most often associated with disrupted or inconsistent sleep habits (*inadequate sleep hygiene*) or environmental disruptions. These disorders do not constitute insomnia, but they do predispose individuals to insomnia.

A much smaller proportion of the population has developed persistent difficulty in initiating or maintaining

sleep. For them the difficulty does not respond readily to improved sleep habits and removal of precipitating factors.[13]

Idiopathic insomnia is a rare disorder characterized by a lifelong history of inability to obtain adequate sleep. Its cause is thought to be an abnormality in the neurologic control of sleep.

Psychophysiologic insomnia is more common and is characterized by learned sleep-preventing associations and heightened physiologic responses to stress.[13] The perceived difficulty sleeping can be confirmed by polysomnographic recording, which usually shows the same pattern of long sleep latency or fragmentation that the client describes. The total sleep time is often within normal range but is felt to be inadequate, becoming a focal point of concern for the client. These persons often find that they can fall asleep unintentionally in low-stimulus situations, such as watching television, but feel increased arousal when they go to bed. They also may find it easier to get to sleep in places other than their usual bedroom, having become conditioned to their bedroom as a place of sleepless nights.

Management of insomnia is complex. Clients often feel that they have already tried the usual interventions to promote sleep. Sleep habits can become increasingly erratic if the client tries to sleep during the day to compensate for sleeplessness at night. Sleep should be consolidated or restricted by curtailing time in bed to the minimum believed necessary with a consistent rising time.[25] Relaxation exercises can be helpful, but they should initially be practiced at times other than bedtime so that by the time they are introduced at bedtime, they are effective. Referral to a sleep specialist or mental health professional who can work with the client over a period of time should be considered.

Narcolepsy

Narcolepsy is one of the disorders characterized by excessive daytime sleepiness.[5, 61] The client also experiences disturbed nocturnal sleep and repeated episodes of almost irresistible daytime drowsiness followed by brief periods of sleep, especially when engaged in monotonous activities.[8] Many narcoleptic clients also experience *cataplexy*, a sudden loss of muscle tone at times of unexpected emotion (e.g., fright). Several other sleep-related abnormalities are commonly experienced by clients with narcolepsy. On initial wakening, they may experience *sleep paralysis* for 1 to several minutes, during which time they cannot move. This condition, like the other manifestations of narcolepsy, is thought to be linked to a malfunctioning of the mechanism controlling REM sleep. The REM sleep that is experienced is normal, but it occurs at different times. Another REM-like manifestation is *hypnagogic hallucinations*, hallucinatory experiences that occur at sleep onset or awakening. Some persons experience sleep paralysis or one of the other associated manifestations without narcolepsy, but when seen together with excessive sleepiness, they constitute the narcolepsy tetrad.[13] Automatic behaviors are also frequent during which there is a lapse of awareness.

On polysomnography, the most characteristic finding is sleep-onset REM periods. A multiple sleep latency test, to measure how long it takes to fall asleep during normal waking hours, shows a sleep latency of less than 5 minutes over four to five testing periods. Occurrence of REM periods at sleep onset at least twice during the test periods is another criterion for the diagnosis.[1, 8, 13, 20]

Narcolepsy is a genetically heterogeneous condition with autosomal dominance in some cases. Evidence suggests that genetic transmission of narcolepsy is multifactorial and involves a human leukocyte antigen (HLA) and another gene that is not HLA related.[8, 20] Environmental factors may also have a role. The prevalence is about 1 in 1000 persons in the United States.[46]

The effects of the disease on life-style are significant, with 60% to 80% of clients reporting episodes of having fallen asleep at work, while driving, or both.[1] The associated disruption of social and occupational roles and self-esteem is a major contributing factor to the depression and personality disorders frequently seen in clients who have narcolepsy.[19] Impaired release of neurotransmitters, such as dopamine, may be a factor in both the narcolepsy and the associated depression.[1]

Medical management for narcolepsy usually consists of low doses of stimulants to improve alertness and tricyclic antidepressants to control cataplexy.[1, 59]

Good sleep hygiene should be emphasized in counseling clients who experience narcolepsy. It is important that they maintain a regular schedule with adequate nocturnal sleep. Regular naps at times when they are prone to increased sleepiness can be recommended.[61] Safety is a major issue. Clients may need assistance in coping with the disruptive potential of their condition on family, work, and social roles.

Sleep Apnea Syndrome

Sleep apnea is characterized by recurrent periods of cessation of breathing for 10 seconds or longer occurring at least five times per hour. Sleep apnea can be differentiated as obstructive and central nervous system apnea. A mixture of the two may be seen.

■ Obstructive Sleep Apnea Syndrome

In obstructive sleep apnea syndrome, respiratory efforts of the diaphragm and intercostal muscles are apparent but ineffective against a collapsed or obstructed upper airway.[67] Snoring indicates partial obstruction. Escalating snoring followed by a silent pause, which ends with a gasp or snort, probably indicates complete airway obstruction. As hypoxia ensues, the client eventually awakens to breathe. The frequent awakenings impair the normal sleep cycle. With sleep, the muscles of the upper airway relax and may occlude an airway that is already narrowed by enlarged soft tissue structures, jaw structure, or obesity. Partial obstruction may result in upper airway resistance syndrome, with or without snoring. Repeated microarousals lead to excessive daytime sleepiness in most patients. A few, particularly the elderly, may present with insomnia.

Obstructive sleep apnea syndrome affects over 1% of the adult population.[52] Prevalence may be as high as 5% in middle-aged men and much higher in certain occupational groups, such as truck drivers.[46] Women are less likely than men to develop obstructive sleep apnea syndrome, particularly before menopause.[52] A much smaller percentage progresses to the classic pickwickian syndrome, characterized by obesity, severe sleep apnea, daytime hypercapnia, and cor pulmonale.[33]

Referral to a sleep disorders center should be considered for clients observed to have repeated periods of apnea (one a minute or more than 15 to 20 periods an hour) lasting longer than 10 seconds, whether or not these periods are associated with snoring. Because obstructive sleep apnea syndrome is particularly common among males who are obese with short, thick necks and who are heavy snorers, these clients should be observed during sleep for apneic periods. Question clients regarding the degree of daytime sleepiness, with particular concern for safety in relation to driving and occupational activities.

Milder cases of obstructive sleep apnea syndrome, in which excessive daytime sleepiness is not yet a concern, may respond to weight reduction, measures to promote sleeping in positions other than supine, and avoidance of alcohol. However, once the apneas are observed to occur most nights and in all body positions, more definitive treatment is usually required.

The application of continuous positive airway pressure (CPAP) by means of a face mask covering the nose is recognized as the treatment of choice for clients with moderate to severe obstructive sleep apnea syndrome. The CPAP device provides room air under increased pressure, essentially providing a pressure splint to keep the upper airway open. Bi-level positive airway pressure (BIPAP) operates by the same principle but offers a lower pressure during expiration.

The CPAP mask should be applied securely over the nose and held in place by the headgear. It should be turned on whenever the client is ready to go to sleep and be maintained at the preset pressure throughout the sleep period. Additional humidification may be necessary, especially in dry environments. Units are portable and contain features such as battery operation and voltage conversion to accommodate travel requirements.

Clients may experience nasal congestion, air leaks, pressure marks on the face, or pressure intolerance. Such problems are not uncommon and may lead to discontinuation of the therapy if they are not effectively managed. It is therefore important that nurses have a working knowledge of the therapy, the importance of regularity in its use, and sources available for technical assistance (e.g., sleep disorders center, respiratory equipment supplier).

Clients who regularly use CPAP should bring their units into the hospital with them. These clients need to be closely monitored when recovering from anesthetic and when receiving narcotics, because they are at risk for ineffective breathing patterns.[35]

A note should be made on the health record at the time of admission that the client has obstructive sleep apnea syndrome. It is imperative that the anesthetist and recovery room staff are alerted. It may be requested that the CPAP unit accompany the client to the recovery room.

Question any order for benzodiazepines or other hypnotic drugs for clients with obstructive sleep apnea syndrome, chronic obstructive pulmonary disease (COPD), or loud snoring, because of possible respiratory depression.[19, 35] Teach clients with such conditions that alcohol also may worsen their symptoms because of its selective effect in relaxing the muscles of the upper airway and depression of arousal (see the Client Education Guide).

Uvulopalatopharyngoplasty (UPPP) is a common surgical procedure for snoring. By resecting the uvula, posterior portion of the soft palate, tonsils, and any excessive pharyngeal tissue, the propensity to obstruction can be reduced in some patients.[65] However, concern has arisen that the reduction or elimination of snoring may place patients at unknown risk for obstructive sleep apnea syndrome. Therefore, preoperative assessment, including respiratory pattern during sleep, is recommended prior to UPPP or to the newer laser-assisted UPPP procedure,

which is done in stages in a doctor's office.[65] Tracheostomy may be required in severe obstructive sleep apnea syndrome.

Oral or dental appliances are being used increasingly as another treatment for sleep apnea. Essentially they act by keeping the jaw forward and the upper airway open.

■ Central Sleep Apnea Syndrome

Central sleep apnea is characterized by apneic periods during which no apparent respiratory effort occurs. It may be seen with central nervous system (CNS) lesions, such as in stroke or brain stem involvement, but it is most commonly mixed with obstructive sleep apnea. Cheyne-Stokes respirations are common. CPAP is the usual treatment. As with obstructive sleep apnea, sedative and hypnotic drugs should be avoided. In severe cases with CNS involvement, use of diaphragmatic pacemakers or mechanical ventilation may be required.

Periodic Limb Movement Disorder

Another disorder that may contribute to daytime sleepiness and frequent nocturnal wakenings is periodic limb movement disorder. Originally described as nocturnal myoclonus, it is characterized by periodic episodes of repetitive, stereotypic leg (or arm) movements that occur during sleep, causing partial arousals.[13, 34] The diagnosis can be confirmed during polysomnography with surface electromyography (EMG) of the anterior tibial muscles. Periodic limb movement disorder is common in the elderly. Clonazepam, a benzodiazepine, or baclofen, a skeletal muscle relaxant, may be ordered to diminish the magnitude of the movement and arousals. The anti-parkinsonian drug carbidopa-levodopa (Sinemet) and the tricyclic antidepressant imipramine seem to act more directly and almost eliminate the movements. However, most of the other tricyclic antidepressants aggravate the condition. For some clients, the use of transcutaneous electrical nerve stimulation (TENS) before sleep has been found to be helpful.[34]

Restless Legs Syndrome

Restless legs syndrome involves annoying crawling, itching, or tingling sensations of the legs while at rest, which cause an almost irresistible urge to move.[13, 34] The syndrome is often most severe prior to sleep onset. Clients with restless legs syndrome almost always have periodic limb movements during sleep. Treatment is similar to that used for periodic limb movements.

Extrinsic Sleep Disorders

All of the preceding dyssomnias are classified as intrinsic. The extrinsic sleep disorders encompass a range of factors, from environmentally to chemically induced. Some environmental factors temporarily present during hospital-

---

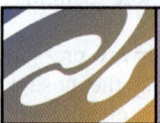

CLIENT EDUCATION GUIDE

Living with Obstructive Sleep Apnea Syndrome (OSAS)

1. Avoid sleeping on your back, because that is the position in which OSAS tends to be worse. Try sleeping with pillows at your back, wearing a small backpack, or sewing a tennis ball into the back of pajamas or nightgown.
2. Aim to reduce or stabilize your weight such that body mass index (weight in kilograms divided by height in square meters) is ≤27. Even a small weight loss may decrease the number of episodes of apnea or upper airway resistance. Increasing the amount of aerobic exercise is the most effective strategy.
3. Avoid alcohol, hypnotics, and other central nervous system depressants because of their relaxing effect on the upper airway.
4. Get adequate sleep. Chronic sleep deprivation can potentiate the effects of OSAS.
5. Have your blood pressure checked regularly. Hypertension is often associated with OSAS.
6. Try to limit driving to times when you feel well rested. If feeling drowsy, get someone else to drive or stop to have a nap. Snacks and caffeine drinks may provide temporary stimulation but they cannot overcome physiologic sleepiness.
7. Carry an identification card or bracelet that would alert emergency personnel to your OSAS.
8. If CPAP or an oral appliance is prescribed, use it regularly.

ization are discussed in the section on Hospital-Acquired Sleep Disturbances. Other predisposing factors are discussed in relation to Health Promotion and Sleep Hygiene.

Circadian Rhythm Sleep Disorders

In the general population, the circadian rhythm sleep disorders, such as *time zone change syndrome* and *shift work sleep disorder,* are not uncommon. In taking a nursing history, be alert to a history of long-time shift work.

Elderly and chronically ill clients who live alone may be vulnerable to *irregular sleep-wake pattern.* In this disorder, the prolonged ignoring or absence of external cues to time, such as regular mealtimes, work periods, and daylight, leads to erratic periods of sleeping and wakefulness. Internal circadian cues may also be dampened as a result of aging or diffuse brain disease.[13, 16]

Management strategies for circadian rhythm disorders include maintenance of a regular schedule (e.g., persons who regularly work night shift are encouraged to maintain their same sleep schedule on nights off) and exposure to natural sunlight. Light therapy is being used to facilitate adjustments in circadian rhythms as well as in the treatment of seasonal affective disorder (SAD).[36]

Some seasonal variation in mood, activity level, and appetite is common in latitudes where climate and length of daylight change markedly. SAD refers to a regular relationship between onset of a major depressive episode corresponding to a particular 60-day period of the year, usually late fall and early winter.

Administration of bright light in the early morning is most effective in treating SAD or for resetting habitual wakening to an earlier hour.[12, 71] Exposure to bright sunlight at those times can also be effective, but indoor lighting is inadequate. Dosage of light is measured in units of illuminance (lux).[38] Usual dosage is about 5000 lux-hours, which may be taken as 2500 lux for 2 hours, 5000 lux for 1 hour, or 10,000 lux for 30 minutes. This level of illumination requires special light boxes, a variety of which are now available.

It is important for clients to realize that light therapy should be commenced only under the guidance of a clinician experienced in its use. Teaching should include appropriate positioning of the head in relation to the light source. The most common side-effects are eyestrain and headache. Too much light may contribute to irritability and insomnia.[38, 71] The long-term risk of bright light therapy to the eyes is under investigation. Until more is known, the presence of retinopathy, glaucoma, or cataract is generally considered a contraindication.[38, 71]

Parasomnias

The parasomnias are disorders that occur during sleep but that usually do not produce insomnia or excessive sleepiness.[13] The underlying pathologic mechanism may involve partial arousal or abnormalities in sleep-wake transition.

Arousal Disorders

Partial arousals typically occur during slow-wave sleep.[13] *Sleepwalking*, also known as somnambulism, may include semipurposeful behavior, such as dressing. However, the behavior may be lacking in coordination and appropriateness, such as voiding in the closet. The occurrence of sleepwalking in adults is often associated with anxiety. *Sleep terrors* are sudden arousals from slow-wave sleep accompanied by screaming, tachycardia, tachypnea, diaphoresis, and other manifestations of intense fear.[13] If awakened, the person is often disoriented and has little recall of the nature of the dream image. Sleep terrors typically occur in young children but may develop in adults.

Sleep-Wake Transition Disorders

Sleep-wake transition disorders are common in the general population, rarely causing enough disruption to be legitimately called disorders. As mentioned earlier, *sleep starts* is the technical name for the sudden jerking movement of the legs that often occurs just as a person is falling asleep. Nocturnal leg cramps are also common. The frequency and intensity may be greater with high caffeine intake, stress, or intense physical activity prior to going to bed. *Sleeptalking* may also be more frequent during times of stress.

Parasomnias Associated with REM Sleep

As with the other parasomnias, those associated with REM sleep may be distressing but are seldom serious. *Nightmares* are frightening dreams arising in REM sleep for which the person often has vivid and detailed recall on wakening. These dreams are in contrast to night terrors, which occur in slow-wave sleep and about which there is little recall. *Sleep paralysis* is one of the classic signs of narcolepsy but can occur in isolation. At sleep onset or wakening, persons experience episodes of one to several minutes during which they are unable to move. This may be an extension of the normal state of low muscle tone during REM sleep.

Other Parasomnias

Other parasomnias are not specifically associated with a particular sleep stage. *Sleep bruxism* refers to grinding of the teeth during sleep and may lead to dental damage. *Sleep enuresis*, or bed-wetting, may occur in adults in association with other disorders, such as obstructive sleep apnea syndrome.[13] *Primary snoring* is distinguished from obstructive sleep apnea syndrome by its rhythmic nature without episodes of apnea or hypoventilation.

Sleep Disorders Associated with Medical and Psychological Disorders

Secondary sleep disorders are of particular relevance in considering problems common to medical-surgical clients. Whereas some clients have a pre-existing sleep disorder of the dyssomnia or parasomnia type, other clients develop a sleep disorder secondary to disease or its manifestations.[24] By remaining aware of the physiology of normal sleep, the nurse can anticipate the risk of sleep pattern disturbances in medical-surgical clients.

Neurotransmitter Imbalances

Neurotransmitter imbalances predispose to sleep pattern disturbances.[57] These imbalances may be disease related or drug induced.

Parkinson's disease is an example of a condition in which neurotransmitter imbalances may be related to sleep disorders. More than 70% of persons being treated for Parkinson's disease, which results from a deficiency of the neurotransmitter dopamine, report sleep pattern disturbances.[13] Insomnia is the most frequent initial concern, followed by sleep fragmentation, disturbances in the sleep-wake schedule, and visual hallucinations.

Depression is accompanied by sleep disturbance in at least 90% of people who suffer from it.[13] Milder forms of depression and those that occur in young persons are often associated with sleep-onset insomnia; more major depressions are characterized by broken sleep and early morning wakening. Some relationship appears to exist between the pathogenesis of depression and REM sleep mechanisms, in that depressed people who are deprived of REM sleep often show improved mood.[33] The action of tricyclic antidepressants in suppressing REM sleep has been proposed as the primary mechanism underlying their effectiveness in treating depression.[57]

Neurotransmitter imbalances may also contribute to the sleep disturbances frequently seen in people with Alzheimer's disease and other dementias. The most typical pattern with dementias is frequent wakenings, with agitation progressing to a loss of sleep-wake consolidation.[57] Assessment of sleep patterns, minimization of caregiver-initiated wakenings (e.g., for toileting), and ensuring a regular bedtime may help to reduce nocturnal and daytime agitation.[10, 28] The sleep-wake cycle may be completely reversed in the client with Alzheimer's disease. The client may nap during the day and be awake all night, restless, agitated, and wandering. The incidence of sleep apnea is higher in persons with Alzheimer's disease, possibly as a result of associated neuronal degeneration in the brain stem. Therefore, the nocturnal respiratory patterns of these clients should be carefully assessed, with referral to a sleep disorders center if apnea is suspected.[27]

Head Injury

Head injury of all degrees of severity affects sleep patterns. The appearance of differentiated sleep stages on EEG in comatose patients with severe head injuries is a favorable prognostic indicator. Sleep stages indicate that connections between the brain stem, diencephalon, and telencephalon are intact and allow shifts to occur between NREM and REM sleep.[2] However, even in mild head injury, some degree of sleep disturbance may persist for several months after the injury.[51] Teaching clients and their families that this unsettled sleep is a typical part of *postconcussion syndrome* can allay anxiety and hasten functional recovery. For clients in the confused-agitated stage of recovery that results from more severe head injury, use of environmental cues (e.g., light and darkness), regularity of daily schedule, and appropriate daytime exercise and activity can help to restore the sleep-wake cycle. Haloperidol (Haldol), which is often given to confused, agitated patients, blocks the activity of dopamine. This disruption in the delicate neurotransmitter balance may lead to insomnia. Thus, the healthcare team must balance the option of controlling agitated behavior—and its associated high consumption of energy—with the undesirable side effect of increasing sleep fragmentation through medication.[55]

Hormonal Imbalances

Hormonal imbalances also contribute to sleep pattern disturbance. *Hyperthyroid* clients tend to have fragmented, short sleep periods with an excess of slow-wave sleep. *Hypothyroidism* is characterized by excessive sleepiness, and polysomnographic recordings show a reduction in the proportion of slow-wave sleep.

Clients with *diabetes mellitus*, particularly type I, may experience hypoglycemic attacks during the night. Besides the usual clinical manifestations of sweating, palpitations, hunger, and anxiety that the client may recognize as a hypoglycemic reaction, the nurse should be alert to complaints of nightmares and early morning headaches.[43] If these manifestations are present, blood glucose levels should be checked at regular intervals during the night. Insulin dosage or timing may need to be changed. Diabetic clients who have developed autonomic neuropathy have a higher prevalence of breathing abnormalities during sleep because of the associated dysfunction of autonomic respiratory control; thus, nocturnal breathing patterns should be assessed in these clients.[41]

Sleep patterns normally vary across the menstrual cycle in response to estrogen and progesterone levels.[15] During the latter part of the cycle, when progesterone levels are higher, the first REM sleep period occurs earlier, and some studies have shown sleep disturbances to be more frequent.[37, 75] Women with *premenstrual syndrome* tend to have less slow-wave sleep throughout the menstrual cycle than their asymptomatic peers. With *menopause,* many women experience poorer sleep quality. Estrogen replacement therapy may help to reduce these symptoms. *Post-*

menopausal women are at higher risk for snoring and obstructive sleep apnea.

Respiratory Disorders

Nocturnal asthma attacks are common in cases of poorly managed asthma, contributing to frequent wakenings in up to 70% of people with asthma.[13, 75] Bronchial resistance increases during the early morning hours, even in healthy persons, as does sensitivity to histamine.

Chronic airway limitations, such as asthma and emphysema, contribute to difficulty initiating sleep, frequent arousals with shortness of breath or cough, and chronic fatigue. Oxygen saturation may fall, particularly during REM sleep, when ventilation depends on the diaphragm, which is often flattened and inefficient in clients with advanced chronic airway limitations.[31, 50] Additionally, ventilation and perfusion are altered. Dysrhythmias are common during sleep in clients with advanced respiratory disease, especially when oxygen saturation falls below 60%.[13] Pulmonary artery pressure increases secondary to the pulmonary vascular constriction induced by the low oxygen desaturation and the destructive processes of the underlying disease.

Ventilatory responses to hypoxia and hypercapnia are decreased during sleep, even in normal persons.[3] Clients with advanced respiratory disease are even more vulnerable; therefore, hypnotics and other CNS depressants that dampen arousal should be given with greater caution.

Some of the medications used in the treatment of chronic airway limitations, such as theophylline preparations, may contribute to insomnia. Anxiety and depression associated with effects of the disease may further exacerbate the tendency toward fragmented sleep. The nurse aims to provide a calm, secure, and relaxed environment for clients. Stimulants such as caffeine may need to be avoided.

The recumbent posture for sleeping is problematic for many people with respiratory disorders. They can be encouraged to use several pillows or to have the head of the bed elevated; during acute episodes, they may find it more comfortable to sleep in a reclining chair.

Cardiovascular Disorders

Up to 25% of people with hypertension have been found to have obstructive sleep apnea.[75] An association between snoring and hypertension has also been documented.[52] Thus, it is important that nurses assess clients who have hypertension or who snore while having repeated apneic periods during sleep.

In clients with severe congestive heart failure, periodic breathing of the Cheyne-Stokes type occurs. This pattern may result in significant hypoxemia, frequent arousals, increased stage 1 sleep, and reduced total sleep time.[22]

The variability of heart and respiratory rates during REM sleep may be a factor in nocturnal angina.[75] Clients recovering from myocardial infarction are often deprived of sleep during their stay in a critical care unit and may experience REM rebound on transfer to a step-down or standard unit. The greater cardiac demands during REM sleep may put some additional strain on the recovering heart, making continued nursing surveillance during this period particularly important.[40]

Gastrointestinal Disorders

Gastric acid secretion normally decreases during sleep, but people with duodenal ulcers have higher than average levels of secretion.[75] Recurrent wakenings with epigastric pain are common, especially in the first 4 hours after sleep onset,[13] and antacids or histamine antagonists may need to be administered.

Gastroesophageal reflux (heartburn) can be more serious when it occurs during sleep because the longer exposure of the esophagus to gastric acid can lead to esophagitis. Hypnotics should be used cautiously with such clients because the suppression of arousal makes them more vulnerable to esophagitis and pulmonary aspiration. In addition, the nurse may suggest that these clients avoid eating within 3 hours of bedtime, consider use of antacids or histamine antagonists, and raise the head of the bed on blocks to decrease the likelihood of reflux and subsequent aspiration.[48]

Other Disorders

Numerous other disorders seem to have some impact on or association with sleep. Any condition that results in pain, discomfort, or impaired mobility has the potential to disrupt sleep.[33] Various skin conditions, such as atopic eczema, are associated with decreased REM sleep.[75] Unrefreshing sleep and chronic fatigue along with diffuse musculoskeletal pain are among the diagnostic criteria for fibromyalgia. On EEG, clients with this condition often show a unique pattern of intrusion of alpha waves into slow-wave sleep, producing what is called *alpha-delta activity*.[13] Because the clinical manifestations tend to be vague, clients are often discouraged with the inability of healthcare professionals to diagnose and treat this condition. The nurse may be in a position to encourage referral to a sleep disorders center.

The effect of sleep or sleep deprivation on some disorders can be useful for diagnostic purposes. For example, the typical occurrence of erections in healthy males during REM sleep is being used as a diagnostic measure in differentiating sources of impotence.[73] REM-associated erections are also the reason that the nurse needs to be careful when securing an indwelling catheter in a male client and to allow a sufficient amount of loop to accommodate an erection.

Sleep deprivation and erratic sleep patterns reduce the seizure threshold, which is an important point for the nurse to consider in assessment and teaching of clients with seizure disorders. Seizure activity may also be a cause of sleep disturbance. Partial and focal seizures can arise in all phases of sleep, including REM; generalized tonic-clonic seizures are more likely to occur during slow-wave sleep than REM.[64] The tendency of sleep deprivation to trigger seizure activity is used diagnostically, in that clients may be required to stay awake all night prior to a sleep-deprived EEG. Some treatment regimens for clients susceptible to nocturnal seizures involve selective suppression by medication of sleep stages in which the client's seizures most frequently occur.

Hospital-Acquired Sleep Disturbances

Persons in the hospital may report difficulty getting to sleep, wakening frequently with difficulty getting back to sleep, or early morning wakening. The etiology and interventions are somewhat different.

Sleep Onset Difficulty

Sleep-onset difficulty is a common problem in hospitals because of the strange environment and the anxieties associated with illness and hospitalization. A sleep latency time of 20 to 30 minutes is within the normal range for most adults. Environmental control, such as reduction of noise and interruptions, and conservative relaxation measures, such as a back rub, should be tried before resorting to a hypnotic agent. The rapid-acting hypnotics, such as zolpidem (Ambien), are most effective with this type of insomnia.

If a hypnotic is given, monitor the client's safety in getting up at night. Most hypnotics cause some degree of antegrade amnesia, meaning that otherwise cognitively intact clients may become somewhat disoriented and forget where they are. The longer-acting hypnotics also result in some hangover effect. An increased risk of hip fractures from falls has been documented in persons who are taking long-acting benzodiazepines.[54]

Sleep Maintenance Disturbance

Sleep maintenance disturbance may be associated with sustained use of or withdrawal from a variety of medications and related substances. Alcohol hastens sleep onset but leads to wakening later in the night. In acute intoxication, REM sleep is suppressed. Abrupt withdrawal, as occurs with hospitalization, may trigger massive REM rebound. In chronic alcoholics, sleep architecture remains disturbed even several years after abstinence. Sustained use of or withdrawal from antidepressants, monoamine oxidase inhibitors, propranolol, and phenytoin can also contribute to insomnia.[60]

Other factors that contribute to sleep fragmentation include a variety of stimuli that tend to waken persons in the middle of the night. Internal stimuli, such as pain, discomfort, and the urge to void, are frequent disturbers of sleep. Sleep disorders, such as sleep apnea and periodic limb movement, are more frequently exhibited as excessive somnolence, but they do trigger wakenings from which some persons have difficulty getting back to sleep. Hospitalization provides an opportunity for nursing surveillance, which may be instrumental in detecting these disorders as distinct from those disturbances triggered by natural or transitory stimuli.

External stimuli include environmental factors, such as noise, light, and temperature, as well as disruptions from other persons. The nurse can reduce nocturnal stimuli by darkening the client's room. This can be accomplished by turning lights off (except for a small night light for safety purposes) and closing curtains. To reduce nocturnal stimuli, the nurse may also reduce as many sources of noise as possible, such as avoiding unnecessary conversation, minimizing equipment noise, and closing the client's door, if possible. Also, the nurse may adjust the temperature by providing bed coverings according to client preference and by modifying room temperature (either directly, by adjusting the thermostat or air conditioner when possible, or indirectly, through closing curtains and adjusting ventilation). The nurse may also remove disturbing objects to create a pleasant, tidy environment. An example is removing equipment associated with painful procedures. Other means of reducing nocturnal stimuli include spacing necessary caregiving activities (e.g., turning, taking vital signs) to allow periods of 90 minutes or more of undisturbed sleep and, when possible, synchronizing these activities with periods during which the client is already awake. Finally, the nurse may coordinate the nature and timing of interruptions by other caregivers (e.g., for laboratory testing or chest physiotherapy) to preserve periods of undisturbed sleep.

Early-Morning Wakening

Early-morning wakening is frequently seen among the elderly. Sensitivity to environmental disturbances increases toward morning for all age groups but even more so for the elderly. Clients who are disturbed by early morning wakening should be screened for indications of depression.

Sleeplessness and agitation may be associated with an acute confusional state (i.e., delirium). This transient cognitive disorder may be manifest, especially among elderly people, in association with acute illness and admission to hospital. Unlike dementia, the onset is rapid and is associated with a fluctuating level of consciousness. Thinking is disorganized and fragmented; memory is impaired; delusions and hallucinations are common. Sleep is grossly disturbed with frightening dreams, disorientation, and restlessness. Delirium is usually precipitated by treatable systemic illness such as dehydration, infection, drug toxicity, or renal failure. It is important for nurses to identify delirium and to pursue treatment possibilities. Once the cause is removed, recovery is rapid.

Sleep Deprivation

Sleep deprivation is of particular concern for clients in critical care units (see Nursing Research). The noise level, 24-hour lighting, and frequency of caregiver interruptions create a situation of sensory overload and sleep deprivation, which is thought to be a major contributing factor to postoperative psychosis.[58, 63]

Clients who have had surgery are also at risk for sleep pattern disturbance due to disruptions in circadian

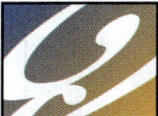

NURSING RESEARCH

How Well Do Clients Sleep in Critical Care Units?

Richards, K. C., & Bairnsfather, L. (1988). A description of night sleep patterns in the critical care unit. *Heart & Lung, 17*(1), 35–42.

Sleep deprivation has been identified as a research priority by critical care nurses. It is thought to be a major factor in the development of intensive care unit psychosis, a state of delirium observed in 10% to 20% of clients who have had open heart surgery. In this descriptive study, the investigators obtained polysomnographic recordings of the sleep patterns of 10 subjects during one or more of the first three nights in a critical care unit and compared them with 12 age- and sex-matched healthy subjects who slept in a sleep laboratory. The results indicated a wide variability among the critical care unit subjects but no significant differences among the three nights. The critical care subjects had significantly less total nocturnal sleep time, spent significantly more time awake and in stage 1 sleep, and had a significantly greater number of sleep stage shifts than did the healthy subjects. The sample size for this study was small, but the results are comparable to those of similar studies.

Implications for Practice

The authors suggest implications for critical care nurses based on the study results and their personal observations during data collection regarding noise and light control, postponement of routine laboratory work and nursing care until clients waken, and spacing of monitoring to allow sustained periods of uninterrupted sleep.

Their findings have implications for medical-surgical nurses as well. Clients transferred from critical care units can anticipate experiencing some degree of sleep deprivation. Besides planning interventions to promote sleep for these clients, nurses working with all types of hospitalized clients should monitor caregiver wakenings and noise and light levels in client sleeping areas.

rhythms. The cause is unclear, but it may be related to the length and type of anesthesia, postoperative analgesia, or mechanisms associated with the procedure itself.[4, 75] REM and slow-wave sleep are suppressed. It may take 4 to 6 weeks for the client's sleep patterns to return to normal after open heart surgery with cardiopulmonary bypass. Specific assessment of sleep quality and quantity should be incorporated into the care of all surgical patients.

Diagnostic Assessment

The primary diagnostic test for sleep disorders is polysomnography (Fig. 18–2). Clients may be referred to a sleep disorders center for an overnight recording of EEG, electro-oculography (EOG), and submental electromyography (EMG) from surface electrodes. Depending on the purpose of the investigation, other types of monitoring may include continuous recording of arterial oxygen saturation by ear or finger oximeter, airflow as detected by monitoring expired CO_2, respiratory movements by means of transducers placed around the chest and abdomen, and electrocardiogram (ECG) and heart rate from standard limb leads. Ambulatory monitoring systems are also available to facilitate studies in the natural home environment.

A multiple sleep latency test may also be performed to assess impairment of daytime alertness. The multiple sleep latency test is performed the day following a standard overnight polysomnogram. The time required for clients to fall asleep when in a relaxed state is evaluated at 2-hour intervals, with each nap limited to 20 minutes. The type of sleep is also assessed, making the test particularly useful in diagnosing narcolepsy, a condition in which clients typically have sleep-onset REM periods.[72]

Nursing Management

Assessment

A brief assessment of the client's usual sleep habits and recent sleep quality should be included as part of the initial nursing history. Notation should be made on the care plan of usual bedtime and rising time as well as preferences or rituals that may enhance sleep quality. For example, clients with ineffective breathing patterns secondary to conditions such as chronic obstructive pulmonary disease (COPD) and hiatal hernia may be accustomed to sleeping with several pillows or with the head of the bed elevated.

If sleep quality is reported to be poor, explore the nature of the disturbance by noting the following:

- Usual activities in the hour prior to retiring
- Sleep latency
- Number and perceived cause of wakenings
- Regularity of sleep pattern, shift work
- Consistency of rising time
- Frequency and duration of naps
- Events associated with initial onset of sleep disturbance
- Ease of falling asleep in places other than the usual bedroom
- Situations in which client fights sleepiness

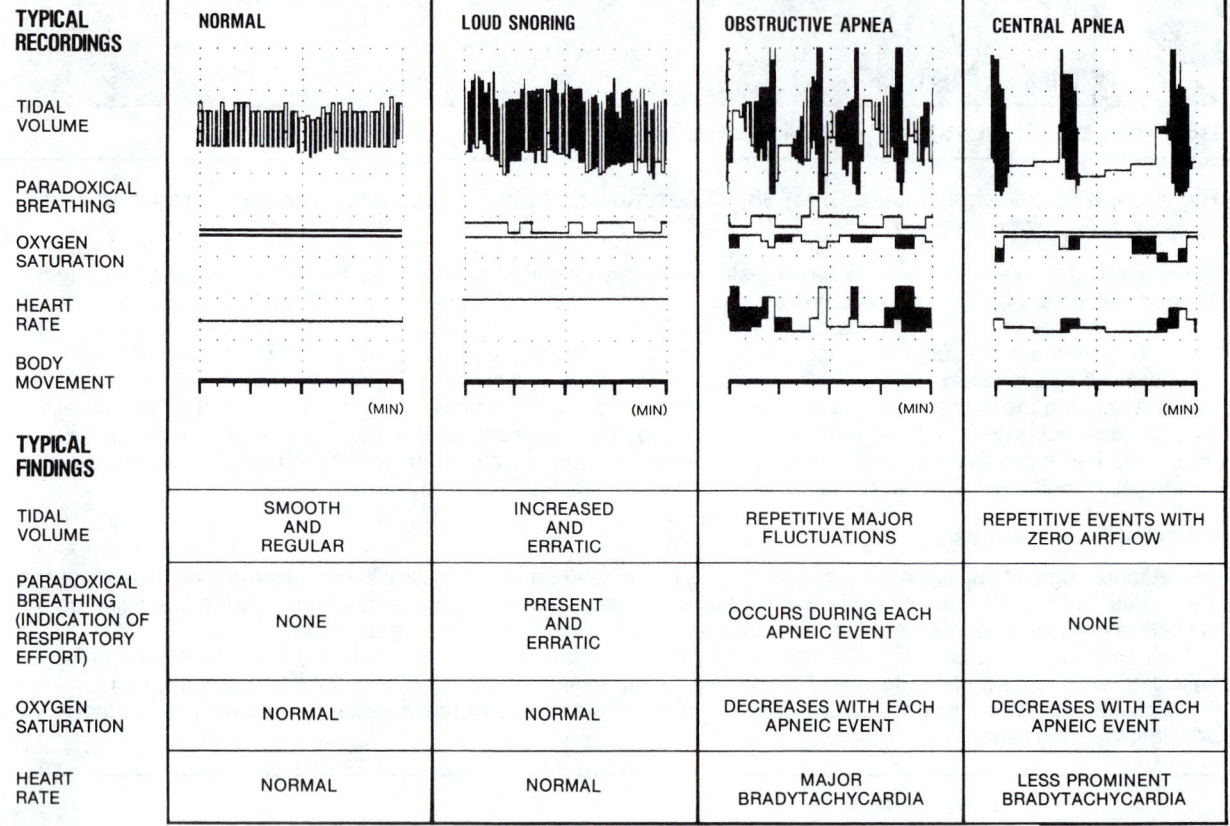

TYPICAL RECORDINGS	NORMAL	LOUD SNORING	OBSTRUCTIVE APNEA	CENTRAL APNEA
TIDAL VOLUME				
PARADOXICAL BREATHING				
OXYGEN SATURATION				
HEART RATE				
BODY MOVEMENT	(MIN)	(MIN)	(MIN)	(MIN)

TYPICAL FINDINGS	NORMAL	LOUD SNORING	OBSTRUCTIVE APNEA	CENTRAL APNEA
TIDAL VOLUME	SMOOTH AND REGULAR	INCREASED AND ERRATIC	REPETITIVE MAJOR FLUCTUATIONS	REPETITIVE EVENTS WITH ZERO AIRFLOW
PARADOXICAL BREATHING (INDICATION OF RESPIRATORY EFFORT)	NONE	PRESENT AND ERRATIC	OCCURS DURING EACH APNEIC EVENT	NONE
OXYGEN SATURATION	NORMAL	NORMAL	DECREASES WITH EACH APNEIC EVENT	DECREASES WITH EACH APNEIC EVENT
HEART RATE	NORMAL	NORMAL	MAJOR BRADYTACHYCARDIA	LESS PROMINENT BRADYTACHYCARDIA

Figure 18–2. Polysomnography used to determine the presence of sleep disorders. These examples are taken from a screening system that may be used in a person's home (as opposed to a laboratory), where sleep patterns are more typical. Screening studies can differentiate between obstructive (i.e., peripheral) sleep apnea and central sleep apnea, as well as loud snoring and normal sleep patterns. When a sleep disorder is identified, further assessment is needed, including EEG and ECG readings to further define the cause of the problem. (Courtesy of Vitalog, Mountain View, CA.)

- Daily caffeine intake
- Use of alcohol, sleeping pills, and other medications
- Incidence of morning headache
- Frequency of snoring, apparent pauses in breathing (apneas), and kicking movements. The latter information is best obtained from the sleeping partner or observed by a nurse while the client is in the hospital

Objective data may include visible signs of fatigue and lack of sleep, such as induration of the eyes, lack of coordination, drowsiness, and irritability.

Diagnosis, Planning, and Implementation

Sleep Pattern Disturbance. Sleep pattern disturbance is a common nursing diagnosis. Write the nursing diagnosis as *Sleep Pattern Disturbance related to changes in routine due to hospitalization and pain.* It may be related to change in sleeping environment, shift-work schedule, recurrent pain, or many other possibilities. Other nursing diagnoses may also be applicable (e.g., *Risk for Injury related to excessive daytime sleepiness*).

Planning: Expected Outcomes. The client will have improved sleep patterns within 3 nights as evidenced by sleeping for 6 to 8 hours at one time, stated feeling of lessened fatigue, and decreased irritability.

Implementation. The client's usual bedtime routine should be followed as closely as possible. For example, if the client usually watches television before sleeping, attempt to make this possible. Nursing assessments and interventions should be scheduled into blocks of time to allow 90 to 120 minutes of uninterrupted sleep. The environment should mimic nighttime, with lights dimmed and quiet maintained. External warmth with extra blankets should be offered. Milk has some tryptophan, which promotes sleep, and should be offered if the client's condition allows its use. Other techniques used to promote sleep include back massage, relaxing music, and progressive relaxation techniques (see Nursing Research).

Medications to promote sleep should be used judiciously because they can alter the architecture of sleep, often reducing the REM sleep and eventually leading to REM rebound. If the client is in pain, analgesics should be given rather than sleeping medications. Clients in pain do not sleep restfully.

At times, sleep medications are prescribed. They are commonly given before surgery to promote sleep and to make the client somewhat drowsy. A common method of prescribing these medications is to give them at bedtime and to repeat administration once if they are not effective. The nurse should consider the drug's half-life and the time of night before repeating it. Commonly, sleeping

NURSING RESEARCH

How Does Progressive Relaxation Affect the Sleep of Older Men and Women?

Johnson, J. E. (1993). Progressive relaxation and the sleep of older men and women. *Journal of Community Health Nursing, 10*(1), 31–38.

Older men and women commonly report problems initiating sleep, frequent wakening during the night, and early morning wakening. These changes are of concern to nurses working with the elderly because the lack of refreshing sleep may interfere with self-care ability, impair judgment and cognition, and alter behavior.

The purpose of this study was to determine the effect of progressive relaxation on the self-reported sleep patterns of healthy noninstitutionalized men and women older than 65 years. In this pre-test/post-test design, 99 men and women between 65 and 84 years old and 77 men and women over 85 years old completed a sleep pattern questionnaire for 3 nights before and after 5 days of instruction and practice with progressive relaxation. The same nurse instructed all of the subjects in a whole-body form of relaxation using controlled breathing and alternating contraction and relaxation of muscle groups.

The results indicated significant improvement in self-reported bedtime state of mind, time to sleep onset, soundness of sleep, number of nighttime arousals from sleep, and satisfaction with sleep. No significant differences were noted in perceived movement during sleep, time of morning wakening, feelings of freshness in the morning, or total sleep time. The younger group was more responsive to the intervention than the older group. Reasons for this response difference by age were not clear. Some differences by gender were also observed.

Implications for Practice

These findings suggest that teaching and reinforcing skills in progressive relaxation is an effective, nonpharmacologic intervention that nurses can use to improve the sleep quality of elderly persons living in the community.

medications are not repeated after 3 AM to avoid prolonged drowsiness. In this case, other measures to promote sleep should be tried, such as offering milk, analgesia, music, and back massage.

The client should be awakened with the least obtrusive stimulus possible, such as a soft touch or a soft voice. Startling the client may make it difficult for the client to go back to sleep. Many assessments and interventions can be performed without having the client completely awake.

Evaluation

The degree of expected outcome attainment should be determined and revisions made in the intervention or outcomes. Some sleep disturbances are due to the effects of aging and cannot be corrected at all; others are temporary and are due to the stress of hospitalization. It is possible that temporary stress problems will be corrected only by the client's return home.

Clients with sleep disturbances may need follow-up care with repeated assessments to determine whether or not the problem was corrected. The elderly client should be taught about the effects of aging on sleep and how to make the most of the new sleep patterns. Clients with long-term sleep disorders may need ongoing support to maintain the effectiveness of treatment.

Sensory Disturbances

Each person has an optimal level of sensory input that facilitates a sense of well-being and optimal cognitive and motor performance.[39] Sensory input comes from environmental and internal sources. Sensory input is received through peripheral receptors, transmitted via afferent neurons up the spinal cord, and channeled through the hypothalamus to the cerebral cortex, where it is interpreted in relation to previous patterns of experience.

Persons at risk for sensory overload or deprivation include those who are experiencing a new or unfamiliar environment, altered sensory input, altered cognitive processing, or impaired mobility.

It has been suggested that persons with dementia have a progressively lowered stress threshold because of declining cognitive and functional abilities.[69] Other situations, such as acute illness or losses, may also lower the ability to cope with a new or challenging environment.

Classification

Sensory Overload

Sensory overload is a state in which the degree and nature of sensory input exceeds the tolerance level of the individual, resulting in feelings of distress and hyperarousal with impaired thinking and problem-solving ability.

Sensory Deprivation

Sensory deprivation is a state in which the overall quantity or diversity of sensory input is decreased. People often compensate for an overall reduction in stimuli by increasing internal stimuli, such as by daydreaming or reminiscing.[70]

Prevention

The nurse can minimize the risk of sensory disturbances by modifying the environment to prevent overstimulation and by enhancing orientation, meaning, and pattern. Practical interventions include reducing noise and glare and explaining not only procedures but also sights and sounds in the environment (e.g., the intercom).

Clients who have had limited prior experience with hospitalization or with health technology are at particular risk for sensory overload because they lack memories and knowledge to make sense out of much of their changed environment.

Likewise, clients whose sensory input is restricted or distorted are at risk for sensory deprivation in the sense that the stimuli are inappropriate to their needs. For example, a client with a spinal cord injury may be kept in a supine position for several weeks during which time the field of vision is limited to the ceiling and the portions of the room that can be seen from each side.

Another major high-risk group of clients are those experiencing alterations in thought processes like those that occur with stroke, head injury, schizophrenia, or delirium of Alzheimer's type (DAT). Explanations to these clients should be kept simple and concrete. The environment should be structured and simplified, with the incorporation of normalizing cues (e.g., drapes open to sunlight, familiar pictures and objects). Agitation can be decreased through choice of colors, reducing television or visitor noise, and creating stability and predictability in the immediate environment.[42, 44, 69]

Associated factors that can increase the risk of sensory overload include confinement, lack of ability to control the environment, and pressures relating to time, decision making, and complex task performance.[39]

Consider the risks for an elderly, slightly deaf woman recovering from a fractured hip. She is confined to bed for much of the day except during physiotherapy sessions and short walks with the nurses. Learning to use the walker is a complex task. The faces surrounding her are strange. It is difficult to hear what the nurses are saying, so she just nods. She does hear a hissing, gurgling sound coming from above her head. She does not know that the sound comes from oxygen bubbling through water for humidification. She also hears a name that sounds like hers come booming out of the wall occasionally. She does not understand about intercom systems. The nights are the worst because then everything looks strange and unfamiliar.

This inability to integrate incoming stimuli may be exhibited as confusion.[53] Sensory overload from an excess of poorly understood environmental stimuli may be superimposed on disturbed cerebral metabolism from electrolyte disturbance, drugs, organic brain disease, and cardiopulmonary problems.[53, 66] The nurse should monitor the client for abnormal laboratory values and possible drug toxic response or interactions, with particular attention to implications of slower metabolic processes in elderly persons.[69] (For more information on assessing the confused client, see Chapter 31.)

Modification of the environment also has the potential to enhance psychological well-being for clients. The intervention has been called *environmental structuring*, which is defined as "an assortment of nurses' actions that directly or indirectly affect environmental features or conditions."[44(p.254)] As more has been learned about psychoneuroimmunology increasing evidence suggests that environmental conditions can be modified in ways that actually facilitate healing. Music therapy is an example of one such intervention that nurses can use to reduce psychophysiologic stress[21] and improve breathing patterns for the ability to communicate.[74]

Conclusions

The adequacy of sleep and rest and the appropriateness of sensory stimulation are important factors to consider in caring for clients with acute or chronic illness. In this chapter, disorders of sleep and sensory stimulation have been discussed with consideration of the reciprocity among these processes, illness, and hospitalization. The nurse can play a pivotal role in environmental modification and client teaching to minimize the impact of sleep and sensory disturbances.

Thinking Critically

1. The client has just been given a prescription for zolpidem (Ambien) to treat her insomnia. She confides in you that she has been using a product from a health food store, recommended by a friend. Now she is asking you if it is safe to continue taking that herbal remedy as well as her new prescription.

Factors to Consider. What is zolpidem? Can it interact with other medications? How could you find more information about the herbal medication the client is taking?

2. A late middle-aged client who is post-cerebrovascular accident and unable to move or speak is placed in a room at the end of the hall, away from the nurses' station. This client was assigned a window bed. He has few visitors. His roommate is a young man recovering from a mild head injury. The roommate has many visitors and uses the radio and television for loud and frequent entertainment. Which client would most likely develop sensory deprivation? Sensory overload? What nursing assessments and interventions would help prevent sensory disturbances?

Factors to Consider. What factors (age, environmental, physical, psychological) affect sensory functioning? How do clients receive and interpret incoming stimuli? Does the room assignment contribute to the development of sensory disturbance in either client?

3. A young adult comes to the neighborhood health clinic. She is unkempt, has circles under her eyes, and yawns frequently. She gives a history of being unable to sleep for any length of time as she recently gave birth to a set of twin sons. She took a variety of prescription "sleeping pills" before she became pregnant and wants a new prescription to help her sleep. What might be causing her sleeplessness? What sleep assessments should be completed? What effect will lack of sleep have on her life-style?

Factors to Consider. What information might help this young mother sleep naturally? How would her lack of sleep affect the health of her children? How normal is it for a young adult to experience difficulty with sleep and to take medications to assist with sleep?

Bibliography

1. Aldrich, M. S. (1990). Narcolepsy. *The New England Journal of Medicine, 323*(6), 389–394.
2. Alexandre, A., et al. (1983). Cognitive outcome and early indices of severity of head injury. *Journal of Neurosurgery, 59,* 751–761.
3. Ancoli-Israel, S., et al. (1991). Sleep disordered breathing in community dwelling elderly. *Sleep, 14,* 486–495.
4. Aurell, J., & Elmquist, D. (1985). Sleep in the surgical intensive care unit: Continuous polygraphic recording of sleep in nine patients receiving postoperative care. *British Medical Journal, 290,* 1029–1032.
5. Bergstrom, D. L., & Keller, C. (1992). Narcolepsy: Pathogenesis and nursing care. *Journal of Neuroscience Nursing, 24*(3), 153–157.
6. Bliwise, D. L. (1994). Normal aging. In M. H. Kryger, T. Roth, & W. C. Dement (Eds.), *Principles and practice of sleep medicine* (2nd ed.). Philadelphia: W. B. Saunders.
7. Carroll-Johnson, R. M., & Paquette, M. (1994). *Classification of nursing diagnoses: Proceedings of the tenth conference.* Philadelphia: J. B. Lippincott.
8. Cohen, F. L. (1988). Narcolepsy: A review of a common, life-long disorder. *Journal of Advanced Nursing, 13,* 546–556.
9. Cohen, F. L., & Merritt, S. L. (1992). Sleep promotion. In G. M. Bulechek & J. C. McCloskey (Eds.), *Nursing interventions: Essential nursing treatments* (2nd ed.; pp. 109–119). Philadelphia: W. B. Saunders.
10. Cohen-Mansfield, J., & Marx, M. S. (1990). The relationship between sleep disturbances and agitation in a nursing home. *Journal of Aging Health, 2*(1), 42–57.
11. Cox, H. C., et al. (1993). *Clinical applications of nursing diagnosis* (2nd ed.). Baltimore: Williams & Wilkins.
12. Czeisler, C. A., & Shapiro, C. M. (1995). Circadian rhythm disorders. In C. M. Shapiro (Ed.), *Sleep solutions manual* (pp. 190–207). Pointe Claire, Quebec: Kommunicom Publications.
13. Diagnostic Classification Steering Committee, Thorpy, M. J., Chairman. (1990). *International classification of sleep disorders: Diagnostic and coding manual.* Rochester, MN: American Sleep Disorders Association.
14. Dinges, D. F., & Broughton, R. J. (1989). *Sleep and alertness: Chronobiological, behavioral and medical aspects of napping.* New York: Raven Press.
15. Driver, H. S., & Taylor, S. R. (1993). Dealing with sleep disorders: Sleep patterns in women with regard to the menstrual cycle, pregnancy, and menopause. *Journal of the Society of Obstetricians and Gynecologists of Canada. 15*(7), S17–S19.
16. Evans, B. D., & Rogers, A. E. (1994). 24-hour sleep-wake patterns in healthy elderly persons. *Applied Nursing Research, 7*(2), 75–83.
17. Fleming, J. A., & Shapiro, C. M. (1995). Insomnia management. In C. Shapiro (Ed.), *Sleep solutions manual* (pp. 34–49). Pointe Claire, Quebec: Kommunicom Publications.
18. Foley, D. J., et al. (1995). Sleep complaints among elderly persons: An epidemiologic study of three communities. *Sleep, 18*(6), 425–432.
19. Fredrickson, P. A., et al. (1990). Sleep disorders in psychiatric practice. *Mayo Clinic Proceedings, 65,* 861–868.
20. Guilleminault, C. (1994). Narcolepsy syndrome. In M. H. Kryger, T. Roth, & W. C. Dement (Eds.), *Principles and practice of sleep medicine* (2nd ed.; pp. 549–561). Philadelphia: W. B. Saunders.
21. Guzzetta, C. E. (1989). Effects of relaxation and music therapy on patients in a coronary care unit with presumptive acute myocardial infarction. *Heart and Lung, 18,* 609–616.
22. Hanly, P. J., et al. (1989). Respiration and abnormal sleep in patients with congestive heart failure. *Chest, 96*(3), 480–488.
23. Hauri, P. J. (1994). Primary insomnia. In M. H. Kryger, T. Roth, & W. C. Dement (Eds.), *Principles and practice of sleep medicine* (2nd ed.; pp. 494–499). Philadelphia: W. B. Saunders.
24. Hauri, P. J., & Exther, M. S. (1990). Insomnia. *Mayo Clinic Proceedings, 65,* 869–882.
25. Hauri, P. J., & Linde, S. (1991). *No more sleepless nights.* New York: John Wiley & Sons.
26. Hobson, J. A. (1988). *The dreaming brain.* New York: Basic Books.
27. Hoch, C. C., Reynolds, C. F. III, & Houck, P. R. (1987). Sleep apnea in Alzheimer's patients and the healthy elderly. *Scholarly Inquiry for Nursing Practice, 1*(3), 221–235.
28. Hoch, C. C., Reynolds, C. F. III, & Houck, P. R. (1988). Sleep patterns in Alzheimer, depressed and healthy elderly. *Western Journal of Nursing Research, 10*(3), 239–256.
29. Hodgson, L. A. (1991). Why do we need sleep? Relating theory to nursing practice. *Journal of Advances in Nursing, 16,* 1503–1510.
30. Horne, J. A. (1988). *Why we sleep.* New York: Oxford University Press.
31. Johnson, M. W., & Remmers, J. E. (1984). Accessory muscle activity during sleep in chronic obstructive pulmonary disease. *Journal of Applied Physiology, 57*(4), 1011–1017.
32. Kaplan, H. I., Sadock, B. J., & Grebb, J. A. (1994). *Kaplan and Sadock's synopsis of psychiatry* (7th ed.). Baltimore: Williams & Wilkins.
33. Kaplan, J., & Staats, B. A. (1990). Obstructive sleep apnea syndrome. *Mayo Clinic Proceedings, 65,* 1087–1094.
34. Krueger, B. R. (1990). Restless legs syndrome and periodic movements of sleep. *Mayo Clinic Proceedings, 65,* 999–1006.
35. Kryger, M. H. (1994). Management of obstructive sleep apnea: An overview. In M. H. Kryger, T. Roth, & W. C. Dement (Eds.), *Principles and practice of sleep medicine* (2nd ed.; pp. 736–747). Philadelphia: W. B. Saunders.
36. Lahaie, U. (1991). Shift-workers and seasonal affective disorder. *Canadian Nurse, 87*(5), 33–34.
37. Lee, K. A., et al. (1990). Sleep patterns related to menstrual cycle phase and premenstrual affective symptoms. *Sleep, 13*(5), 403–409.
38. Levitt, A., & Shapiro, C. M. (1995). Seasonal affective disorder. In C. M. Shapiro (Ed.), *Sleep solutions manual* (pp. 126–146). Pointe Claire, Quebec: Kommunicom Publications.
39. Lipowski, Z. J. (1975). Sensory and information inputs overload: Behavioral effects. *Comprehensive Psychiatry, 16*(3), 199–221.
40. Littrell, K. D., & Schumann, L. L. (1989). Promoting sleep for the patient with a myocardial infarction. *Critical Care Nurse, 9*(3), 44, 46–49.
41. Lugaresi, E., et al. (1988). Sleep in clinical neurology. In R. L. Williams, I. Karacan, & C. A. Moore (Eds.), *Sleep disorders: Diagnosis and treatment* (2nd ed.; pp. 245–263). New York: John Wiley & Sons.
42. Maas, M. (1988). Management of patients with Alzheimer's disease in long-term care facilities. *Nursing Clinics of North America, 23,* 57–68.
43. McCance, K. L., & Huether, S. E. (1994). *Pathophysiology: The biologic basis for disease in adults and children* (2nd ed.). St. Louis: Mosby–Year Book.
44. Mion, L. C. (1992). Environmental structuring. In G. M. Bulechek & J. C. McCloskey (Eds.), *Nursing interventions* (2nd ed.; pp. 254–264). Philadelphia: W. B. Saunders.
45. Mitchell, P. H. (1988). Consciousness: An overview. In P. H. Mitchell, et al. (Eds.), *AANN's neuroscience nursing* (pp. 57–66). Norwalk, CT: Appleton & Lange.
46. *National Commission on Sleep Disorders Research: Wake up Amer-*

ica: A national sleep alert, Vol. 1. (Executive summary and executive report, Report of the National Commission on Sleep Disorders Research. National Institutes of Health. January 1993, pp 1–76. DHHS Publication, Washington, DC, Supervisor of Documents, US Government Printing Office). Philadelphia: W. B. Saunders.

47. North American Nursing Diagnosis Association (NANDA). (1994). *Nursing diagnoses: Definitions and classification 1995–1996.* Philadelphia: Author.

48. Orr, W. C. (1994). Gastrointestinal disorders. In M. H. Kryger, T. Roth, & W. C. Dement (Eds.), *Principles and practice of sleep medicine* (2nd ed.; pp. 861–869). Philadelphia: W. B. Saunders.

49. Oswald, I. (1987). The benefit of sleep. *Holistic Medicine, 2,* 137–139.

50. Parkosewich, J. A. (1986). Sleep-disordered breathing: A common problem in chronic obstructive pulmonary disease. *Critical Care Nurse 6*(6), 60–64.

51. Parsons, L. C., & Ver Beek, D. (1982). Sleep-awake patterns following cerebral concussion. *Nursing Research 31*(5), 260–264.

52. Partinen, M. (1994). Epidemiology of sleep disorders. In M. H. Kryger, T. Roth, & W. C. Dement (Eds.), *Principles and practice of sleep medicine* (2nd ed.; pp. 437–452). Philadelphia: W. B. Saunders.

53. Rasin, J. H. (1990). Confusion. *Nursing Clinics of North America, 25*(4), 909–918.

54. Ray, W., Griffen, M., & Downey, W. (1989). Benzodiazepines of long and short elimination half-life and the risk of hip fracture. *JAMA, 262*(23), 3303–3307.

55. Reimer, M. (1989). Sleep pattern disturbances related to neurological dysfunction. *Axon, 10*(3), 65–68.

56. Remmers, J. E. (1990). Sleeping and breathing. *Chest 97,* 77S–80S.

57. Reynolds, C. F. III, & Kuppfer, D. J. (1987). Sleep research in affective illness: State of the art circa 1987. *Sleep 10*(3), 199–215.

58. Richards, K. C., & Bairnsfather, L. (1988). A description of night sleep patterns in the critical care unit. *Heart & Lung, 17*(1), 35–42.

59. Richardson, J. W., Fredrickson, P. A., & Siong-Chi, L. (1990). Narcolepsy update. *Mayo Clinic Proceedings, 65,* 991–998.

60. Robinson, C. (1993). Impaired sleep. In V. K. Carrieri, A. M. Lindsey, & C. M. West (Eds.), *Pathophysiological phenomena in nursing* (pp. 390–417). Philadelphia: W. B. Saunders.

61. Rogers, A. E., & Aldrich, M. S. (1993). The effect of regularly scheduled naps on sleep attack and excessive daytime sleepiness associated with narcolepsy. *Nursing Research, 42*(2), 111–117.

62. Schmidt-Nowara, W., et al. (1995). Oral appliances for the treatment of snoring and obstructive sleep apnea: A review. *Sleep, 18*(6), 501–510.

63. Shaver, J. L., & Giblin, E. C. (1989). Sleep. *Annual Review of Nursing Research, 7,* 71–93.

64. Shouse, M. N. (1994). Epileptic seizure manifestations during sleep. In M. H. Kryger, T. Roth, & W. C. Dement (Eds.), *Principles and practice of sleep medicine* (2nd ed.; pp. 801–814). Philadelphia: W. B. Saunders.

65. Shepard, J. W., & Olsen, K. D. (1990). Uvulopalatopharyngoplasty for treatment of obstructive sleep apnea. *Mayo Clinic Proceedings, 65,* 1260–1267.

66. Sloane, P. D., & Mathew, L. J. (1990). The therapeutic environment screening scale. *The American Journal of Alzheimer's Care and Related Disorders & Research, 5*(6), 22–26.

67. Standards of Practice Committee of the American Sleep Disorders Association. (1994). Practice parameters for the use of laser-assisted uvulopalatoplasty. *Sleep, 17*(8), 744–748.

68. Steriade, M. (1994). Brain electrical activity and sensory processing during waking and sleeping states. *Principles and practice of sleep medicine* (2nd ed.; pp. 105–124). Philadelphia: W. B. Saunders.

69. Stolley, J. M., & Buckwalter, K. C. (1992). Confusion management. In G. M. Bulechek & J. C. McCloskey (Eds.), *Nursing interventions* (2nd ed.; pp. 120–134). Philadelphia: W. B. Saunders.

70. Suedfeld, P. (1985). Stressful levels of environmental stimulation. *Issues in Mental Health Nursing, 7,* 83–104.

71. Terman, M. (1994). Light treatment. In M. H. Kryger, T. Roth, & W. C. Dement (Eds.), *Principles and practice of sleep medicine* (2nd ed.; pp. 1012–1029). Philadelphia: W. B. Saunders.

72. Thorpy, M. (1988). Diagnosis, evaluation, and classification of sleep disorders. In R. L. Williams, I. Karacan, & C. A. Moore (Eds.), *Sleep disorders: Diagnosis and treatment* (2nd ed.; pp. 9–25). New York: John Wiley & Sons.

73. Ware, J. C., & Hirshkowitz, M. (1994). Monitoring penile erections during sleep. In M. H. Kryger, T. Roth, & W. C. Dement (Eds.), *Principles and practice of sleep medicine* (2nd ed.; pp. 967–977). Philadelphia: W. B. Saunders.

74. Wiens, M., Reimer, M., & Lemieux, L. (1994). Evaluation of music therapy as a treatment method to improve respiratory function and speech in multiple sclerosis. Unpublished data.

75. Williams, R. L. (1988). Sleep disturbances in various medical and surgical conditions. In R. L. Williams, I. Karacan, & C. A. Moore (Eds.), *Sleep disorders: Diagnosis and treatment* (2nd ed.). New York: John Wiley & Sons.

76. Zarcone, V. P. (1994). Sleep hygiene. In M. H. Kryger, T. Roth, & W. C. Dement (Eds.), *Principles and practice of sleep medicine* (2nd ed.; pp. 542–546). Philadelphia: W. B. Saunders.

Infectious Disorders

CHAPTER 19

Carol Sharkey

For one brief moment in human history (circa 1950–1980), management of infectious disease did not dominate healthcare practice. By the close of that era, morbidity and death from infectious diseases had plummeted as a result of multifaceted efforts in social, public health, and medical control. Environmental sanitation had curbed such killers as yellow fever, cholera, typhus, malaria, typhoid fever, and plague. International immunization programs had eradicated smallpox. Organized efforts to immunize all children lowered the occurrence of vaccine-preventable diseases, particularly measles, mumps, rubella, diphtheria, tetanus, and poliomyelitis. Improved living conditions and personal hygiene had diminished the occurrence of parasitic diseases and gastrointestinal infections. The widespread availability of sulfa and antibiotics quelled the fear of deadly tuberculosis, syphilis, gonorrhea, bacterial meningitis, scarlet fever, and rheumatic fever. Nosocomial (hospital-acquired) infections, which had earlier succumbed to medical asepsis, responded to further control with antibiotics; and medical technology continued to produce anti-infective agents to match the newly developing antibiotic-resistant organisms. Life for many was no longer clouded by fear of infectious disease. Health professionals were allowed to turn their attention to preventing and managing chronic disease.

This brief moment in history did not last. The 1980s and 1990s brought new infectious agents, such as *Legionella,* the human immunodeficiency virus (HIV), and the Ebola virus (which actually first appeared in 1976), reminders of human vulnerability to infectious disease. Hepatitis, tuberculosis, sexually transmitted diseases, and many vaccine-preventable diseases, such as pneumonia, persist, spread, and continue to kill. Antibiotic-resistant organisms flourish, particularly in hospitals. Normally nonpathogenic organisms create devastating disease in the immunocompromised and those with chronic diseases or malnutrition. Antibiotic-resistant organisms have developed as a result of chronic misuse and improper prescription of antibiotics. In addition, many of the major killers of the past, such as cholera and yellow fever, continue to cause death and destruction in many parts of the world where poor sanitation, hygiene, and poverty are endemic.

All persons, particularly healthcare professionals, must maintain vigilance. Such an attitude centers on preventing infectious disease rather than simply treating it. Prevention requires an understanding of the infectious process and the control measures that are needed. This chapter describes the process of infection and selected aspects of prevention and control. Other chapters address the nursing care of clients with specific infectious diseases.

The Process of Infection

Infection is a process by which an organism establishes a parasitic relationship with its host. The process begins with transmission of an infectious organism. Infection may end in infectious disease, a condition that depends on the response of the host to the invader. The entire process and its outcome hinges on a complex interaction of the infectious agent, an environment conducive to transmission of the organism, and a susceptible human host. This agent, host, and environment interaction is a prerequisite to infectious disease. All infectious diseases must be viewed in their unique multicausal context.

Agent

Humans coexist with many microorganisms in complex, mutually beneficial relationships. Many organisms establish residence on or in the host and usually cause no harm. Other organisms are parasitic, maintaining themselves at the expense of their host. Some parasites arouse a pathologic response in the host and are called *pathogens* or *pathogenic agents.* In one sense, pathogens are ineffective parasites because they stimulate an inflammatory response, leading to a disease that may harm the host and eventually kill the pathogen.

All microorganisms can be distinguished by certain intrinsic properties. These properties provide the basis for

This chapter incorporates material written for the fourth edition by Deanna E. Grimes.

identifying and classifying bacteria, viruses, fungi, and helminths. An organism's properties include the following:

- Shape
- Size
- Structure
- Chemical composition
- Antigenic make-up
- Growth requirements
- Viability under adverse environmental conditions
- Ability to produce toxins

Viability is a particularly important property to health-care professionals because it determines the pathogen's ability to survive outside its host. Organisms that can survive drying, sunlight, heat, or other adverse environmental conditions require more aggressive tactics to prevent their indirect transmission.

In addition to offering diagnostic clues, an organism's distinguishing properties also allow you to predict and understand its relationship with its host. Host interactions are influenced by the organism's

- Mode of action
- Infectivity
- Pathogenicity
- Virulence
- Toxigenicity
- Antigenicity

A pathogen's *mode of action* refers to how it produces a pathologic process. There is great variation here. Some intracellular pathogens, like viruses, invade cells and interfere with cellular metabolism, growth, and replication. Others invade and cause hyperplasia, necrosis, and cell death. Some pathogens, such as the tetanus bacillus, produce a toxin that interferes with intercellular responses. Others, such as group A beta-hemolytic streptococcus, stimulate a pathologic immune response in the host. Larger parasites, such as roundworms, interfere with the function of the gastrointestinal system. Some viruses, like cytomegalovirus and the herpes viruses, create a persistent latent infection. The deadly HIV virus causes immunosuppression by destroying helper T cells.

Infectivity refers to the pathogen's ability to invade and replicate in the host. The invasiveness of some pathogens is facilitated by enzymes produced by the organism. These enzymes dissolve host connective tissue or protect the pathogen from host defenses. Infectivity is high in measles because it takes very few viruses to establish infection. Infectivity is low in tuberculosis.

Pathogenicity is the ability of the organism to induce disease. This depends on the organism's speed of reproduction in the host, the extent of tissue damage, and the strength of the toxin that is released. The rabies virus is highly pathogenic; infection with it always results in disease. Poliomyelitis virus and *Mycobacterium tuberculosis* have low pathogenicity.

Virulence refers to the pathogen's potency in producing severe disease. It is measured by the *case fatality rate,* the proportion of people contracting a disease who die of that disease. Some pathogens, such as the rabies virus and HIV, are highly virulent. In contrast, herpes simplex and herpes zoster are much less virulent. Some pathogens change their virulence over time. Syphilis, for example, was frequently a fatal disease.

Toxigenicity, the amount and destructive potential of released toxin, is closely related to virulence. Some bacteria secrete water-soluble antigenic exotoxins that are quickly disseminated in the blood, causing potentially severe systemic and neurologic manifestations. Diphtheria and tetanus are examples of such pathogens. The cell walls of certain bacteria release endotoxins which may cause a state of shock and severe diarrhea. This is the case with *Shigella,* whose habitat is the intestinal tract.

Antigenicity, the ability of a pathogen to stimulate an immune response in the host, varies greatly among organisms. Generally, organisms that invade and localize in tissue initially stimulate a cellular (T cell) response. Organisms that disseminate quickly stimulate a humoral or antibody response. Some organisms, such as the influenza virus, have a high propensity for antigenic change.

One additional characteristic of pathogens and their interaction with their host is worth noting. Many parasites have the ability to adapt to new hosts over time. An example is the plague bacterium, *Yersinia pestis.* Before 1900, this species lived in domestic rats and fleas. As domestic rat populations have declined, the organism has been found in wild rodents and their parasites.

Environment

Transmission of infectious agents from a source to a susceptible host occurs within an environment. Organisms live and multiply in a *reservoir.* This can be a person, animal, plant, soil, food, or other organic substance or combination of substances. The reservoir provides what the organism needs for survival at specific stages in its life cycle. Some parasites have more than one reservoir but require only one. An example is the yellow fever virus, which can live either in humans or mosquitoes. A few parasites require more than one reservoir. Such is the case with *Schistosoma,* which is parasitic in snails and humans at different growth stages. Other parasites, such as most sexually transmitted organisms, require only a human reservoir. Infected people are the reservoirs for most bacteria and viruses that affect humans.

Both human and animal reservoirs may be infected and, therefore, also be hosts. An infected host may be asymptomatic, and a *carrier* of the pathogen. A carrier maintains an environment that promotes growth, multiplication, and shedding of the parasite without exhibiting signs of disease.

Organisms can have one or more than one *route of transmission* from the reservoir to a new host. There are three mechanisms through which transmission occurs: direct contact, airborne transmission, and indirect contact. Direct contact refers to immediate transfer from an infected person to a noninfected person, as in sexual contact, biting, touching, kissing, or droplet spray. Droplets from sneezing, coughing, spitting, or speaking are diminutive drops that travel a few feet at most. Droplets may contaminate the mucous membranes of the eye, nose, or mouth. Droplets either settle onto a surface or dry out while airborne. Relatively few organisms remain viable as airborne nuclei, but those that do have the potential for being transmitted in the air, and subsequently breathed into the lungs. Dust particles containing microorganisms can also become airborne. Airborne transmission requires that the pathogen survive in dried form in the air until it is inhaled.

Transmission by indirect contact implies a vehicle of transmission: a living vector, a common vehicle, or fomites (inanimate objects). Living vectors are usually animals that carry the pathogen internally as a biologic vector or externally by mechanical means. For example, a mosquito carries the malaria parasite in its body fluids and transmits the microorganisms through its bite; a fly picks up organisms on its feet and transmits them to food or water. Common vehicles are substances that have become contaminated with infectious organisms, such as water, soil, food, other biologic products, and air. Fomites are objects that may harbor a disease agent (e.g., clothing, bedding, eating utensils, needles, urinary catheters).

The *portal of exit* is the place whence the parasite escapes the reservoir. Generally, this site corresponds to the *portal of entry* into the next host. For example, the portal of exit for gastrointestinal parasites is generally the feces, and the portal of entry into a new host is the mouth. As is the case with other links in the transmission chain, there is variability here. Hookworm eggs, for example, are shed in the feces, but hookworm larvae enter through the skin of a person walking barefoot in soil containing hatched eggs. Common portals of exit include secretions and fluids (respiratory secretions, blood, tears, vaginal secretions, semen, breast milk), excretions (urine and feces), open lesions, and exudates. Some organisms, such as HIV, have more than one portal of exit. Knowledge of the portal of exit is essential for preventing transmission of a pathogen.

A pathogen may enter a new host by ingestion, inhalation, contact with mucous membranes, percutaneously, or transplacentally. Infectious diseases vary as to the number of organisms and the duration of the exposure required to start the infectious process in a new host.

Host

When it comes to infectious diseases, not all humans are created equal; some are more susceptible than others. A susceptible host has personal characteristics and behaviors that increase the probability of an infectious disease developing. Factors such as age, sex, ethnicity, heredity, altitude, and temperature influence the likelihood of a person's becoming infected. For example, the ethnic custom of eating raw fish may increase the risk of exposure to pathogens. General health and nutritional status, hormonal balance, and the presence of concurrent disease also play a role. Likewise, living conditions and personal behaviors such as drug use, diet, hygiene, and sexual practices all influence the risk of exposure to pathogens and resistance once exposed. Susceptibility is also influenced by the presence of anatomic and physiologic defenses, sometimes called lines of defense.

The first-line defenses are external and act to bar invasion by pathogens. These defenses are nonspecific in that they act against any invading pathogen. First-line defenses include physical and chemical barriers and the body's own natural flora. Physical barriers include intact skin and mucous membranes; oil and perspiration on skin; cilia in respiratory passages; gag and cough reflexes; peristalsis in the gastrointestinal tract; and the flushing action of tears, saliva, and mucus. All act to remove organisms before they have an opportunity to infect. The chemical composition of body secretions such as tears and sweat, together with the pH of saliva, vaginal secretions, urine, and digestive juices, further prevents or inhibits growth of organisms. Compromise in any of these natural defenses increases host susceptibility to pathogen invasion. Physical status is an important variable.

Another important first-line defense is the *normal flora* of microorganisms that inhabit the skin and mucous membranes of the oral cavity, gastrointestinal tract, and vagina. These microorganisms are indigenous to specific tissue. They generally coexist with their host in a mutually beneficial relationship as long as they do not migrate from the specific site. Through a mechanism called microbial antagonism, they control the replication of potential pathogens. The importance of this mechanism is evident when it is disturbed. An example of disturbance is the overgrowth of *Candida albicans* (thrush) that results from extensive antibiotic therapy that destroys normal flora in the gastrointestinal tract or vagina.

Some normal flora can become pathogenic under specific conditions, such as immunosuppression or displacement of the pathogen to another area of the body. The opportunistic infections experienced by clients with symptomatic HIV infection (see Chapters 26 and 86) are an example of the former. The latter is seen when *Escherichia coli,* normal flora in the gastrointestinal tract, become pathogenic when the organism invades the urogenital tract (see Chapter 55). Displacement of normal flora is a common cause of nosocomial infections. Invasive procedures increase the risk of displacing these organisms. For this reason, it is essential to maintain meticulous hand washing and asepsis.

The second line of defense, the inflammatory process, and the third line, the immune response, share several physiologic components. These include the lymphatic system, leukocytes, and a multitude of proteins and enzymes. (For discussion of inflammation and wound healing, see Chapter 20. See Chapter 25 for a description of the structure and function of the immune system.)

Even after successful transmission of a pathogen, the host may experience more than one possible outcome. The pathogen may merely contaminate the body surface. The process ends there if the host's first-line defenses, such as intact skin or mucous membranes, block the pathogen from further invasion. Successful invasion and replication of a pathogen that does not lead to clinical manifestations or a detectable immune response is referred to as *colonization.*

When microorganisms in or on the host cause an immune response, an infection is said to be present. The period of time when the pathogen is replicating but before it sheds from the host is called the *latent period.*

Table 19–1. Agents and Sites of Selected Infectious Diseases

	Infectious Agent	Site of Infection	Reservoir	Mode of Transmission
Viruses				
Influenza A	Influenza A virus	Respiratory tract	Humans	Direct contact by aerosol droplets; airborne spread
Measles (rubeola)	Paramyxoviridae	Skin, respiratory tract, systemic	Humans	Direct contact with nasal or throat secretions; airborne spread
Hepatitis B	Hepatitis B virus	Liver	Humans	Contaminated needles, blood transfusions, sexual contact, perinatal
AIDS	Human immunodeficiency virus	Helper T lymphocyte	Humans	Contaminated needles, blood transfusions, sexual contact, transplacental
Rabies	*Lyssavirus*	Systemic	Dogs, wild animals	Animal bite
Bacteria				
Cholera	*Vibrio cholerae*	Gastrointestinal tract	Humans	Ingestion of water contaminated with feces
Diarrhea	*Escherichia coli*	Gastrointestinal tract	Humans	Ingestion of contaminated food or water
Wound infection	*Staphylococcus aureus*	Connective tissue	Humans	Contaminated hands, surgical instruments
Pneumonia	*Streptococcus pyogenes*	Lung	Humans	Inhalation; aspiration of gastric content
	Pneumocystis carinii	Lung	Humans	Respiratory droplets
Pneumonia	*Mycoplasma pneumoniae*	Lung	Humans	Unknown
Meningitis	*Neisseria meningitidis*	Meninges	Humans	Direct contact with droplets from respiratory passages
Gonorrhea	*Neisseria gonorrhoeae*	Genitourinary tract	Humans	Sexual contact
Influenza	*Haemophilus influenzae*	Lung	Humans	Respiratory droplets
Tuberculosis	*Mycobacterium tuberculosis*	Lung	Humans	Inhalation of droplet nuclei
Lyme disease	*Borrelia burgdorferi*	Skin, joints, systemic	Wild rodents and deer	Tick bite
Rocky Mountain spotted fever	*Rickettsia rickettsii*	Vascular endothelium	Ticks	Tick bite
Malaria	*Plasmodium* spp.	Red blood cells, liver	Mosquito	Bite from infected mosquito
Toxoplasmosis	*Toxoplasma gondii*	Eye, lung, brain	Cats	Ingestion of cysts on fecally contaminated fingers or in food; transplacental
Giardiasis	*Giardia lamblia*	Gastrointestinal tract	Water, humans, wild animals	Ingestion of cysts in fecally contaminated water and food
Typhus	*Rickettsia prowazekii*	Vascular endothelium	Louse-human-louse cycle	Louse feces inoculated into skin by scratching

Table 19–1. Agents and Sites of Selected Infectious Diseases *(Continued)*				
	Infectious Agent	**Site of Infection**	**Reservoir**	**Mode of Transmission**
Trachoma	*Chlamydia trachomatis*	Conjunctiva and cornea	Humans, flies	Rubbing eyes with contaminated fingers, infected washcloths, bed linens
Genital chlamydia	*Chlamydia trachomatis*	Genital tract	Humans	Sexual contact
Fungi				
Candidiasis	*Candida albicans*	Skin, mucous membranes, genital tract	Humans	Overgrowth associated with damaged skin or mucosa or use of antibiotics
Histoplasmosis	*Histoplasma capsulatum*	Lung	Bat or bird feces	Inhalation of spores
Helminths				
Trichinosis	*Trichinella spiralis*	Gastrointestinal tract, muscle	Animals	Ingestion of raw or undercooked meat

Data from Institute of Medicine. (1992). *Emerging infections: Microbial threats to health in the United States.* Washington, DC.: National Academy Press; Hoeprich, P. D., Jordan, M. C., & Ronald, A. R. (1994). *Infectious diseases: A treatise of infectious processes* (5th ed.). Philadelphia: J. B. Lippincott.

During latency, host inflammatory and immune responses may ward off the organism or its products, thus preventing tissue damage; or the pathogen or its products may begin destroying undefended or poorly defended tissue, producing infectious disease. Disease manifestations herald the end of the *incubation period,* which is defined as the time from invasion of the disease to the time manifestations appear. By definition, infectious disease is the pathophysiologic response of a host to the destructive action of the pathogen, to its toxic products, or to the host immune responses to fight the pathogen. This pathophysiologic response is generally symptomatic. An asymptomatic pathologic response is called a *subclinical infection.*

An important point to note is that an asymptomatic host can still transmit a pathogen. The host may harbor a pathogen in sufficient quantities to be shed at any time after latency and toward the end of the incubation period. The time period when an organism can be shed is called the *period of communicability.* It usually precedes manifestations and coincides with part or all of the clinical disease, sometimes extending to convalescence. The communicable period, like the incubation period, varies with different pathogens and different diseases.

Table 19–1 gives examples of agents and sites of selected infectious diseases. At one time, infectious agents were considered the only causative factor in infectious disease. We now understand that the host's condition and physical and social environment are important elements in whether infection and clinical disease result. One must remember that pathogens can produce disease only when the host is susceptible. Non-pathogens, normal flora, also can produce disease when the host is immunocompro-

mised and defenseless. So, even though the term "etiologic agent" may be used to describe a pathogen, infection results from interactions among a variety of factors related to agent, host, and environment.

The Risks of Hospitalization

Nosocomial infections are a leading cause of death in the United States and are associated with significant morbidity.[10, 17] Nosocomial infections are infections that arise in a hospital or other healthcare facility. Infections present or incubating at the time of admission are referred to as community-acquired infections. From 5% to 10% of hospitalized clients acquire a nosocomial infection.[10] Occupationally acquired infections among the staff of a hospital are also considered nosocomial.

The source of nosocomial pathogens within healthcare facilities varies, but both healthcare workers and clients are reservoirs for most nosocomial pathogens. For example, *Staphylococcus aureus* is often carried on the skin and in the nasopharynx. Respiratory secretions, feces, urine, and blood are reservoirs for some nosocomial organisms. Liquids commonly found in the healthcare environment may become reservoirs for pathogens, and the inanimate hospital environment may also serve as a source of nosocomial infections. The most important means of transmission of nosocomial infections are the hands of healthcare workers. Hand washing, combined with principles of asepsis and proper use of gloves, is the best method of preventing nosocomial infections.

The most common sites of nosocomial infections in clients are the urinary tract, lower respiratory tract, surgi-

Table 19–2. Common Pathogens Causing Nosocomial Infections*

Site of Infection	Pathogen
Urinary Tract	*Escherichia coli* Enterococci *Pseudomonas aeruginosa*
Wound	*Staphylococcus aureus* Enterococci Coagulase-negative staphylococci *Escherichia coli*
Pneumonia	*Pseudomonas aeruginosa* *Staphylococcus aureus* *Enterobacter* spp.
Bloodstream	Coagulase-negative staphylococci *Staphylococcus aureus*

* Organisms are listed by major site and order of importance.
Data from Hoeprich, P. D., Jordan, M. C., Ronald, A. R. (1994). *Infectious diseases: A treatise of infectious processes* (5th ed.). Philadelphia: J. B. Lippincott.

cal wounds, and the bloodstream.[10] Various pathogens can cause nosocomial infections in multiple sites. For example, *E. coli* is the most common organism causing urinary tract infection, but it also causes wound infection, pneumonia, and bacteremia. *Staphylococcus aureus* is the most common cause of wound infection, and the second most common cause of both pneumonia and bacteremia; it occurs less frequently in urinary tract infection. Table 19–2 lists common nosocomial pathogens.

Urinary Tract Infections

Urinary tract infections (UTIs) remain the most common of all nosocomial infections, and about 80% are associated with urethral catheterization.[10] Major risk factors for catheter-associated UTIs include female sex, increased duration of catheterization, breaks in the closed catheter system, and lack of administration of systemic antimicrobials.[17] Chapter 55 provides a discussion of catheters and UTIs, including levels of prevention.

In the majority of catheter-associated infections in women, bacteria enter the bladder by the periurethral route. Organisms originating primarily from the fecal flora and found at the meatal and perineal areas may be introduced into the bladder during insertion of the catheter or may migrate along the external surface of the catheter into the bladder. In men, catheter-associated infections are usually a result of cross-infection (infection transmitted between clients), with bacteria introduced into the collection system at the catheter–drainage tube junction or at the outflow spigot. Bacteria that enter the catheter drainage bag migrate to the bladder in 24 to 48 hours. Once organisms are in the bladder, they multiply rapidly. Most nosocomial UTIs are easily managed, but bacteremia develops in 1% to 4% of clients with UTIs. Of these, 13% to 30% die.[10] It is important, therefore, that infections be prevented, recognized promptly, and treated appropriately.

Surgical Wound Infections

Nosocomial surgical wound infections are a major source of morbidity and account for nearly 60% of extra hospital days.[10] These infections usually result from endogenous or exogenous microorganisms that enter the wound at the time of the operation. Endogenous microorganisms normally reside within the host; exogenous microorganisms originate outside the host. The most common source of infecting bacteria is the client's own flora. Bacteria present in the client's nasopharynx and on the skin next to the operative site may serve as a source of infection. Although the physical environment of the operating room is an uncommon source of infection, operating personnel have been implicated in outbreaks of wound infections. Operating room personnel may shed bacteria-laden skin particles that travel through the air to the open wound.

Factors that influence the development of surgical wound infections include the number and types of organisms present in the wound, the type of operation, and the surgeon's technique. The duration of the operation is a major determinant of postoperative wound infection. Surgical wound infection rates almost double for each hour of surgery.[10] Client-related factors also influence the development of surgical site infections. Old age, obesity, malnutrition, and an underlying immunocompromised condition are associated with increased risk of postoperative wound infection.

Risk of surgical wound infection increases with the length of the client's preoperative hospital stay.[10] Limiting the length of the preoperative hospital stay tends to minimize the risk of infection by decreasing the opportunity for colonization with nosocomial bacteria. Proper preparation of the surgical site is also important. Shaving the operative site damages the epithelium, impairing the skin's defense mechanism.

Pneumonia

Nosocomial pneumonia is common and causes 15% of all in-hospital deaths.[10] While the most common cause of community-acquired pneumonia is *Streptococcus pneumoniae,* most nosocomial pneumonias are caused by gram-negative bacteria. *Pseudomonas aeruginosa* is the most common cause of nosocomial pneumonia, followed by *Staphylococcus aureus.* Aspiration of oropharyngeal or stomach organisms is the predominant mechanism by which nosocomial pneumonia develops. Stasis of respiratory secretions associated with immobility and decreased cough also contribute. Postoperative clients, particularly those undergoing thoracic and upper abdominal surgical procedures, and clients who require ventilatory support are at high risk of aspiration. Clients with diminished consciousness, impaired gag reflex, intubation, or tracheostomy are also at increased risk of aspirating oral secretions. Other risk factors include old age, decreased mobility, and severe disease conditions such as chronic lung disease, cardiovascular disease, renal insufficiency, and malignancies.

Nosocomial pneumonia is difficult to prevent because in most cases the microorganisms are derived from the client's own flora. Soon after hospitalization, the oropharynx of many clients becomes colonized with gram-negative bacteria that may be aspirated into the lungs. The use of histamine H_2-blockers, antimicrobial therapy, and enteral nutritional therapy have been found to promote colonization of the oropharynx with gram-negative bacteria.

Airborne transmission is usually not a major cause of nosocomial pneumonia. However, contaminated respiratory therapy equipment can serve as a source of pathogens. Contaminated nebulizers produce aerosols that can be inhaled into the terminal bronchioles. Mechanical ventilator tubing may become colonized from the client's secretions or from environmental contaminants, increasing the risk of pneumonia.

Device-Associated Infections and Bacteremias

The placement and use of intravascular devices, such as intravenous and intra-arterial infusion lines, is associated with increased risk of nosocomial infection. Other intravascular devices include diagnostic, therapeutic, and hemodynamic monitoring equipment. The risk of infection is influenced by factors related to the device itself, the site of insertion, and the technique used to place the device. Stiff catheters are associated with higher rates of infection than flexible catheters, and partially implantable catheters and totally implanted injection ports are associated with even lower infection rates.[10] Device-associated infections and bacteremias are usually caused by staphylococci found on the client's skin. Microorganisms invade disrupted tissue and migrate around the site of insertion and along the device into the intravascular space. The use of semipermeable membrane dressings over the site of insertion facilitates the growth of skin flora. Dressing changes following institution-specific protocols must be done at regularly scheduled intervals under aseptic conditions. Colonization of skin flora can also occur around the hub of the device, the tubing-device junction, or other connectors attached to the system. Although liquids given through the device may become contaminated, infusion-associated infection is relatively uncommon.

Client-related factors that contribute to the risk of device-associated infections include age, nutritional status, type and severity of underlying illness, skin condition, and immunosuppressive therapy. Bacteremia is especially common in clients with chronic diseases, malnutrition, and cancer.

Other Nosocomial Infections

Effective screening and processing of donated blood and blood products have greatly reduced the risk of transmission of HIV to clients in the healthcare setting. The risk of provider-to-client transmission of HIV is remote,[10] although the matter has created much anxiety in our society. The risk of occupational exposure to HIV in the healthcare setting has been primarily associated with parenteral exposures to blood from clients infected with HIV. Infection after exposure of mucous membranes to infected blood is much less common.

Nosocomial infection with hepatitis B virus is another concern in hospitals because the source clients of most nosocomial hepatitis B infections are never identified. While provider-to-client transmission of hepatitis B does not occur with routine client contact, client-to-provider transmission is a much larger problem. This is why healthcare workers must be vaccinated against hepatitis B.

The resurgence of tuberculosis is a major concern in healthcare facilities. Two factors responsible for this resurgence are poor compliance with therapeutic drug regimens and the emergence of drug-resistant strains of *Mycobacterium tuberculosis*. If clients infected with susceptible strains of the pathogen receive appropriate therapy, sputum smears begin to clear by the third week of treatment. Clients with resistant strains, however, continue to cough up large numbers of viable organisms, exposing many healthcare workers to the aerosols containing the organisms. Respiratory isolation must be closely followed with high-risk clients until adequate treatment has been given.

Methicillin-resistant strains of *Staphylococcus aureus* (MRSA) became important nosocomial pathogens in the 1980s. Epidemics MRSA have forced operating rooms and intensive care units to close. These organisms are resistant not only to methicillin but to all penicillins and cephalosporins. MRSA spreads through nasopharyngeal secretions and the hands of healthcare workers and clients. Infections may cluster in one area of the hospital, but spread is aided by transfer of clients or healthcare workers to other areas and even from facility to facility. One of the simplest methods of controlling the spread of MRSA is simple hand washing. Hand washing breaks the chain of transmission and prevents spread of the organism.

Nosocomial infections tend to occur more frequently and with more severity in debilitated, malnourished, and immunocompromised clients (Box 19–1). Susceptibility to infection increases when a host has an underlying illness, and when invasive procedures and indwelling devices are used. With the expanding use of invasive devices, more exposure to antimicrobial therapy, and more severely ill hospitalized clients, the risk of nosocomial infections will probably increase. Furthermore, the emergence of resistant organisms is likely to continue, resulting in infections that will be more difficult to treat. While resistance to infection may be enhanced by vaccines and immune globulin, it must be supplemented by manipulation of the physical environment to reduce the risk. This means that nurses must be more vigilant in administering care and in supervising those providing care.

Preventing and Controlling Infection

To be effective, strategies to prevent and control infection must be based on knowledge of agent-host-environment interactions. The goal in developing and implementing

---

Box 19–1. Infectious Disease in the Elderly

More than any other population, elderly clients are at risk of infection. In fact, studies show that elderly clients contract about three times as many nosocomial infections as younger clients. Infection frequently leads to hospitalization for nursing home residents, and it is one of the top 10 causes of death in the elderly. Many common infectious diseases, such as pneumonia, urinary tract infection (UTI), sepsis, skin and soft tissue infection, tuberculosis, and herpes zoster become more common with advancing age.

Elderly clients face an increased risk of infection partly from the normal consequences of growing older. With aging, mechanical barriers—such as skin and mucosa—undergo structural and functional decline. The physiologic reserve capacity of organ systems dwindles, and the immune system falters. When these defense mechanisms are compromised, infection can progress locally and even spread systemically.

Many older adults have chronic diseases that further jeopardize their host defenses. Conditions associated with aging, such as diabetes mellitus and malnutrition, probably exert more influence on immunity than age itself.

Not only do elderly people contract more infections, they tend to experience more complications from those infections. For example, an older client with pneumonia or a UTI is more likely to develop bacteremia than a younger client with the same infection.

To make matters worse, infection can be more difficult to detect and diagnose in the older client. Elderly people often do not manifest typical signs and symptoms of infectious diseases. Instead, they may exhibit worsening cognition or abnormal mental status, lethargy or agitation, loss of appetite, incontinence, and an increased tendency to fall.

Fever—the cardinal sign of infection—may be vague or absent in infected elderly clients, even those who have bacteremia or pneumonia. Remember that many other people have a low baseline temperature. Suspect infection in any elderly client with an oral temperature of 100° F or higher, or an increase in baseline temperature of 1.4° F or more. Coexisting diseases may mask the signs of infection even further.

Even the drugs used to treat infections are less successful when given to elderly clients. They produce a weaker response from the older person's body, while producing even more adverse reactions. Age-related changes in gastrointestinal, cardiac, and renal function alter the way antimicrobial agents are absorbed, distributed, and excreted.

Researchers are looking for better ways to detect and better drugs to treat infections in the elderly. While these agents are being investigated in the elderly population, nurses can help already-infected clients by encouraging individualized dosage regimens and monitoring these clients carefully.

Data from Yoshikawa, T. T., & Normal, D. C. (Eds.) (1994). *Antimicrobial therapy in the elderly patients.* New York: Marcel Dekker.

---

interventions is to prevent the spread of the infectious agent from its reservoir or source to susceptible hosts.

Methods for controlling transmission of infectious disease vary with the characteristics of the organism, its reservoirs, the type of pathologic response it produces, and available technology for control. In general, the aim is to intervene at the point where the greatest number of people can be protected, using the least amount of resources.

The simplest and most effective way to prevent transmission is meticulous hand washing. Hand washing is an absolute necessity, even when using gloves. Wash your hands before donning gloves and after removing them. Teach this procedure to all personnel and continually monitor for compliance. This simple, inexpensive technique, used appropriately, is one of the most potent weapons against the spread of infection.

Another method to prevent and control infectious disease involves environmental measures. Some pathogens can be controlled by disinfection, sterilization, or anti-infective drugs. Such is the case with *Staphylococcus aureus.* Other pathogens can be controlled best by eradicating their non-human reservoirs. This is accomplished through environmental sanitation, particularly water treatment; food safety programs; and control of animals, vectors, sewage, and solid wastes.

Transmission from the portal of exit can often be prevented by detecting and treating clients shedding a pathogen, such as gonococcus. Antimicrobials are among the most frequently prescribed drugs in the United States to treat infections. The use of antibiotics is not without problems, as shown in Box 19–2. Another example of prevention is the use of prophylactic antitubercular medications in clients exposed to tuberculosis who have positive skin tests.

Immunization Programs

Several infectious diseases have been dramatically reduced by maximizing host defenses through active and passive immunizations that stimulate the immune system to counteract the infectious agent. *Active* immunization refers to the deliberate administration of a modified infecting agent, called a *vaccine,* or a modified toxin, called a *toxoid,* to stimulate an immune response. Protection is not immediate because a period of time is needed to achieve protective antibody levels. However, induced active immunity usually results in long-lived protection against disease. In contrast, *passive* immunization refers to the administration of antibodies to a nonimmune person to provide temporary protection against a pathogenic agent or toxin. Passive immunity provides immediate but short-lived protection, lasting a few weeks.

Immunization programs in the United States have resulted in a significant reduction in the incidence of childhood infectious diseases. However, a major resurgence of measles occurred during 1989 to 1991, signaling a major

Box 19–2. The Problem of Resistance to Antibiotics

Among researchers and healthcare professionals, there is growing concern over the frequent, widespread use of antimicrobial drugs in hospitals and long-term care facilities. Nursing home studies have revealed frequent orders for antibiotics, often without adequate evidence of underlying infection. Worse, many of these drugs were prescribed for infections not responsive to antibiotic therapy, such as viral respiratory tract infections.

Studies in hospitals have found antimicrobial drugs used routinely as prophylaxis for invasive and even noninvasive surgical procedures.[19] While prophylaxis may be helpful when applied wisely, more than half the drugs studied were used inappropriately. Sometimes the wrong drug was ordered. Some were prescribed for unjustifiable reasons. Others were administered in the wrong dose or duration of therapy.

Misuse of antimicrobial drugs may alter a client's normal flora and encourage resistance to pathogenic organisms. To help avoid growing resistance to antimicrobial drugs, obtain appropriate cultures before starting antibiotic therapy. Also check sensitivity reports to be sure the client receives an appropriate antibiotic.

Controlling the spread of antimicrobial resistance is difficult and requires the appropriate selection and administration of antimicrobials, use of antibiotic combinations, and strict asepsis and infection control efforts.[17] While infection control practices—such as hand washing, aseptic techniques, and barrier precautions—do not directly limit the emergence of resistant strains, they do prevent transmission of resistant organisms from one client to another.

problem with childhood vaccination programs.[8] Baseline data from 1989 indicated that the immunization level of preschool children was approximately 70% to 80%, with some segments of the population having levels below 50%.[18] Urban minority populations, particularly black and Hispanic children, had much lower immunization levels than the general population.[8, 18] The goal of the Department of Health and Human Services is to immunize at least 90% of all children in the United States by 2 years of age.[18]

An entire population does not have to be immune to prevent an epidemic of a disease. When a large proportion of individual members of a community become immune to a disease, the chances of contact between susceptible persons and infected persons decrease. This phenomenon is called *herd immunity*. For example, epidemics of measles are less likely to occur when herd immunity increases and the number of susceptible persons in the community decreases.

Immunization schedules and recommendations are established by the Committee on Infectious Diseases of the American Academy of Pediatrics (AAP) and by the Advisory Committee on Immunization Practices (ACIP) of the Centers for Disease Control and Prevention (CDC). As of January 1996, the AAP and ACIP recommend that all children be immunized against measles, mumps, rubella, diphtheria, pertussis, tetanus, poliomyelitis, *Haemophilus*

influenzae type b (Hib), hepatitis B, and varicella zoster (Var).[7] The Hib, hepatitis B, and Var are recent additions to the routine childhood vaccination schedule. More than 85% of invasive Hib cases occur in children less than 5 years of age.[3] Since the introduction and widespread use of Hib vaccine in infants, the incidence of all Hib disease in children less than 5 years of age has decreased dramatically.[6] Hepatitis B is a worldwide problem; universal vaccination of children against the hepatitis B virus (HBV) has been recommended by the CDC, AAP, and World Health Organization (WHO).[10] In the United States, previous prevention strategies focused on vaccinating high-risk groups. Most vaccine doses have been administered to healthcare workers, who make up less than 5% of the cases of HBV infection.[18] The present strategy for HBV prevention is to include hepatitis B vaccine in the routine childhood immunization schedule. The routine use of varicella (chickenpox) vaccine in children is a 1996 addition to the immunization schedule.

Immunizations are as important for adults as they are for children. Infections seen primarily in children are being seen in older adolescents and adults who never developed active immunity. Adults who escaped natural infection or who were not adequately immunized as children are at risk of childhood diseases and their complications. All adults age 18 through 64 should complete a primary series of diphtheria and tetanus toxoids, and of measles, mumps, and rubella vaccines if they did not receive them during childhood. Adults 65 years and older should complete a primary series of diphtheria and tetanus, but are generally considered immune to measles, mumps, and rubella. Most persons born before 1957 are likely to have been infected naturally with these diseases.

The elderly and persons with chronic diseases are particularly at risk of infectious diseases because of a decline in their immune system. Approximately 80% to 90% of all deaths associated with influenza A and B viruses occur in people age 65 and older.[18] The most effective measure for reducing the impact of influenza is to vaccinate persons at high risk each year before the influenza season. The ACIP recommends that influenza vaccine be administered annually to people 65 years and older. For persons living in nursing homes and other chronic-care facilities, annual vaccination can reduce the risk of influenza outbreaks by inducing herd immunity. Annual vaccination with the current vaccine is necessary because new variants of influenza continue to occur and vaccination against one strain may not confer immunity to another.

Pneumococcal pneumonia, caused by *Streptococcus pneumoniae,* is an important cause of morbidity and mortality in the very young, the elderly, and others with certain high-risk or chronic conditions. The ACIP recommends that these persons receive a single dose of pneumococcal vaccine.

Nurses can be instrumental in ensuring that all children, adolescents, and adults are properly immunized. Every visit to a healthcare provider should be an opportunity to obtain a history of immunization status and provide vaccinations as needed. In addition, nurses and other healthcare professionals should be concerned about improving their own resistance to infectious diseases. One important approach is to maintain your immunization

Table 19–3. CDC Recommendations for Immunization of Adults in the United States

Disease	Recommendation
Polio	Primary series of oral poliovirus vaccine in childhood is sufficient. If no childhood series, vaccine need not be given except to adults at risk because of health occupation or foreign travel.
Tetanus, diphtheria	Booster dose of tetanus and diphtheria toxoids (Td) every 10 years after primary series of Td; tetanus toxoid may be repeated in 5 years if a dirty wound is sustained. If no childhood series, initiate series of 3 doses within 1 year.
Pertussis	Primary series of pertussis vaccine in childhood is sufficient
Measles	Documented immunity or 2 doses of vaccine at least 1 month apart. Adults who have received only 1 dose of vaccine since their first birthday should receive a second dose, particularly on enrolling in college, traveling to a foreign country, or entering a healthcare field.
Mumps	Documented immunity or 2 doses of vaccine at least 1 month apart.
Rubella	Documented immunity or 2 doses of vaccine at least 1 month apart. Vaccine particularly recommended for previously unimmunized women of childbearing age and susceptible healthcare professionals.
Hepatitis B	Complete series of 3 doses within 6 months for high-risk individuals including healthcare professionals, susceptible dialysis clients, persons with hemophilia, intravenous drug abusers, sexual and household contacts of hepatitis B virus carriers.
Influenza A and B	Annually for people over age 65; residents of nursing homes and other chronic-care facilities; adults with chronic cardiac or pulmonary disease, diabetes or other metabolic disorders, renal disease, severe anemia, or immunosuppression; healthcare professionals and others in close contact with persons in high-risk groups.
Pneumococcal	Single dose of vaccine for people over age 65; adults with chronic cardiac or pulmonary disease, cirrhosis, alcoholism, diabetes, Hodgkin's disease, nephrosis, renal failure, cerebrovascular fluid leaks, immunosuppression, sickle cell anemia, and asplenism. Revaccination should be considered after 6 years for persons at highest risk.

Data from Centers for Disease Control and Prevention. (1991). Updata on adult immunization. Recommendations of the Immunization Practices Advisory Committee (AICP). *Morbidity and Mortality Weekly Report, 40*(RR-12), 1–72; Centers for Disease Control and Prevention. (1994). Prevention and control of influenza: Part I. Vaccines. Recommendations of the Advisory Committee on Immunization Practices (ACIP). *Morbidity and Mortality Weekly Report, 43*(RR-9), 1–11.

status. This means being adequately immunized against hepatitis B, measles, mumps, rubella, polio, tetanus, and diphtheria. HBV infection is a major occupational hazard for healthcare providers because of their contact with blood and blood-contaminated body fluids from infected clients. The Occupational Safety and Health Administration (OSHA) has developed regulations that require employers to offer at-risk employees hepatitis B vaccine at the employer's expense. Influenza vaccination is recommended yearly for healthcare providers in hospital, chronic-care, and outpatient-care settings to reduce their risk of illness and to reduce the possibility of transmitting the virus to clients. Proper immunization not only protects the healthcare provider but also safeguards client health. An infected healthcare provider may spread the disease to clients, with life-threatening consequences. Current CDC recommendations for immunization of adults in the United States are shown in Table 19–3.

Infection Control Programs in Hospitals

Many nosocomial infections are preventable if healthcare personnel adhere to infection control practices. The CDC and the Joint Commission on Accreditation of Healthcare Organizations (JCAHO) issue guidelines and establish standards for control of hospital infection. The CDC continually develops and updates guidelines relating to the control and prevention of nosocomial infections, and JCAHO requires hospitals to establish infection control programs that meet accreditation standards. The 1995 JCAHO standards require hospital infection control committees to establish surveillance programs, implement infection control policies and procedures, and conduct continuing education for all hospital employees regarding infection control.

Infection control programs in hospitals address two major areas related to nosocomial infection: surveillance and reporting, and control and prevention. The purpose of surveillance is to establish and maintain a database that tracks the rates of nosocomial infections. Surveillance activities include early detection of infections in clients and personnel, and reporting relevant data to designated individuals for appropriate action. Surveillance systems to detect both agents and diseases are necessary components of prevention and control strategies. National data on nosocomial infections is obtained from selected hospitals in the United States by the CDC and used to estimate rates and trends.

The late 1960s saw the emergence of infection control practice as a specialty area for nurses. Most hospitals employ an infection control nurse or practitioner (ICP) who is responsible for the coordination of a hospital-wide infection control program. The ICP is recognized as the hospital's expert on infection control matters, and plays a major role in the collection of surveillance data. Other activities include developing infection control policies, conducting educational programs, and consulting with personnel regarding infection control practice. The ICP may also institute special studies when a problem is detected or when a new procedure or product requires evaluation.

The current focus of infection control strategies is on barrier precautions to reduce infection risk for all clients and personnel, and occupational health practices to protect healthcare staff from infection.

Barrier Precautions

Barriers are intended to prevent transfer of an infective organism to a susceptible site. By placing a clean layer of plastic or fabric between a susceptible site and a potential source of pathogenic organisms, the likelihood of transmitting an infection is reduced. The prevented transmission can be from client to caregiver or caregiver to client. The risk for clients increases when caregivers have contact with the client's mucous membranes and nonintact skin. The risk for caregivers increases whenever they are in contact with a client's moist body substances. Protective barriers include gloves, gowns, masks, and protective eyewear.

None of the protective barriers are intended to replace hand washing. *The most important means of preventing the spread of microorganisms is hand washing.* Hands become soiled during client care, particularly after contact with moist body sites and substances. Soiled hands have played a major role in transferring organisms to new client hosts. Unfortunately, gloves provide a false sense of security because hands can become contaminated even when gloves are used. The use of gloves is not a substitute for hand washing.

Historical Barrier Precautions

In the past, most barrier precautions were instituted after a client's infection was diagnosed. Once an infection was suspected or recognized, a system of barrier precautions, referred to as isolation procedures, were instituted to prevent transmission of pathogens among hospitalized clients, healthcare personnel, and visitors. Most hospitals used either a category-specific or disease-specific set of isolation procedures developed by the CDC. Depending on the diagnosis, one of several category-specific isolation strategies was used: strict, contact, respiratory, tuberculosis, enteric, blood and body fluid, or drainage and secretion precautions. Instructions for each category were printed on color-coded cards and placed on the doors and beds of clients. In the disease-specific isolation precautions, only those precautions (e.g., private room, mask, gown, and gloves) that interrupted transmission of the

infection were used. For these two isolation systems to be effective, the diagnosis of infection had to be made or suspected early. However, most infections are communicable for some period when manifestations are absent and the infection is undetected.

Universal and Other Precautions

In the early 1980s, unrecognized cases of HBV and HIV infection were identified as important sources of disease. Healthcare workers could potentially become infected through needle-sticks and body fluids contaminated with clients' blood. In response to this problem, the CDC revised a previous category of blood and body fluid precautions from the category-specific isolation system, and in 1985 recommended "universal precautions" as a means of preventing transmission of HIV, HBV, and other blood-borne pathogens. Universal precautions focuses on preventing transmission of bloodborne pathogens from infected or potentially infected clients to susceptible caregivers. Universal precautions requires the use of protective barriers with all clients regardless of their presumed infection status. Universal precautions emphasizes the use of gloves and gowns to reduce contamination of skin and clothing, and of masks and goggles to reduce contamination of the mucous membranes of the mouth, nose, and eyes. Prevention of needle-stick injuries is also emphasized. Used needles should not be recapped by hand, and puncture-resistant containers are to be used for disposal of sharps.

In 1987, body substance isolation (BSI) was proposed as an isolation system for all moist and potentially infectious body substances from all clients, regardless of their presumed infection status.[12] Personnel are to use clean gloves during contact with nonintact skin and mucous membranes, and when anticipating contact with blood, feces, urine, sputum, saliva, wound drainage, and other body fluids. BSI is based on the assumption that the blood and body substances of all clients may contain potentially infectious, transmissible organisms.

There has been considerable confusion surrounding the four isolation systems.[8,12] There is inconsistency in terminology and practice among hospitals, and uncertainty as to why and when a particular set of precautions should be implemented. Multidrug-resistant microorganisms are emerging, and appropriate precautions to contain them are not being implemented by some hospitals. In response to these problems, the Hospital Infection Control Practices Advisory Committee (HICPAC) of the CDC recently revised isolation guidelines. Rather than adjusting any of the existing isolation systems, HICPAC synthesized the various systems into one new set of guidelines.

The revised guidelines, published in 1996, propose two tiers of isolation strategies: Standard Precautions and Transmission-Based Precautions. Standard Precautions are the most important tier and are designed for the care of all clients in hospitals regardless of their diagnosis or presumed infection status. Standard Precautions synthesize the major components of Universal Precautions and body substance isolation. Standard Precautions apply to nonintact skin, mucous membranes, blood, and all body fluids, secretions, and excretions, except sweat. Recommended precautions include using gloves and washing hands immediately after gloves are removed, between client contacts, and after contact with blood, body fluids, secretions, excretions, and contaminated equipment or articles. Gowns, masks, and eye protectors are used during procedures that are likely to generate splashes or sprays of blood, body fluids, secretions, and excretions. Other precautions address the recapping of needles and the disposal of needles, scalpels and other sharps.

Transmission-Based Precautions form the second tier and are designed only for the care of clients with known or suspected infections, or who have been colonized with transmissible pathogens. Transmission-Based Precautions are *additional* precautions needed to interrupt transmission of a nosocomial infection and for use with Standard Precautions. There are three types of Transmission-Based Precautions: Contact Precautions, Droplet Precautions, and Airborne Precautions. They may be combined for infections that have more than one route of transmission.

Contact Precautions are designed to reduce direct and indirect contact transmission of microorganisms. Contact transmission is the most frequent mode of transmission of nosocomial infections. Direct-contact transmission involves skin-to-skin contact and transfer of organisms to a susceptible host from an infected person. Direct contact occurs when a caregiver turns a client, gives a client a bath, and performs other client-care activities that require direct, personal contact. Indirect-contact transmission involves contact of a host with a contaminated object such as an instrument, dressing, or gloves. Precautions emphasize hand washing and the use of gloves. Gowns are worn if contact with infected material is anticipated. Client-care equipment should not be shared, but if necessary, shared equipment should be cleaned and disinfected between clients.

Droplet Precautions are for infections transmitted on large-particle droplets such as those generated during coughing, sneezing, speaking, or suctioning. Droplets do not remain suspended in the air and transmission requires close contact (usually 3 ft or less) between source and host. Transmission occurs when droplets are propelled a short distance through the air and deposited on the host's conjunctivae, nasal mucosa, or mouth. Recommended precautions include wearing a mask and placing the client in a private room.

Airborne Precautions are designed to reduce the risk of transmission of pathogens on airborne droplet nuclei. Airborne droplet nuclei include evaporated droplets containing microorganisms that remain suspended in the air for long periods of time or dust particles containing the infectious agent. Airborne microorganisms can be inhaled by a host and be widely dispersed by air currents. Precautions include placing clients in a negative pressure isolation room with at least six air exchanges per hour, and the wearing of masks. Additional precautions for preventing the transmission of tuberculosis have been published under other CDC guidelines.[4]

Control of the nosocomial spread of infections depends on meticulous attention to good infection control practices. The CDC has provided excellent institutional infection control guidelines which can be tailored to meet the needs of specific situations or environments.

Occupational Health Practices

The second major component of an infection prevention and control program is to protect healthcare workers from infection. Occupational health practices include evaluating personnel for existing infections, administering immunizations, keeping records, managing exposures, educating employees, and developing and enforcing infection control procedures.

When it became recognized that healthcare workers who had contact with clients' blood were at increased risk for infection by bloodborne pathogens, infection control efforts focused on preventing employee exposure to blood. By 1989, most hospitals had implemented the universal precautions guidelines to protect employees at risk of transmission of HIV and HBV. In addition, efforts focused on delivery of hepatitis B immunization to employees at risk of blood exposure. New employees are screened for susceptibility to tuberculosis, hepatitis B, measles, rubella, and chickenpox: and periodic tuberculin skin testing is recommended for employees at risk of exposure to tuberculosis.

In 1989, OSHA published guidelines to protect employees exposed to blood and other potentially infectious materials. One of the most important components of the bloodborne pathogens standard is the requirement that all healthcare employees with the potential for blood and body fluid exposure be offered hepatitis B vaccine free of charge. In addition, OSHA requires all care providers to wear protective attire when they are likely to have contact with blood and other moist body substances that may contain pathogens. Since a third of occupational exposures to HIV are associated with recapping needles after use, OSHA standards urge the use of alternative needleless or recessed needle systems. Most elements of universal precautions have been incorporated into the OSHA bloodborne pathogens standard plus barrier precautions and needle disposal systems that must be available at the point of use.

Another major area of concern has been the role and selection of respiratory protection equipment to prevent transmission of tuberculosis in hospitals. OSHA has also proposed standards for respiratory protection programs to protect hospital personnel from pathogens spread by the airborne route. In particular, surgical masks have not been effective in preventing inhalation of droplet nuclei, and the use of disposable particulate respirators has been recommended. Regulations and recommendations are continually being updated by OSHA as changes in healthcare methodology and technology occur.

Conclusions

Infectious diseases have been killers of humans throughout recorded history. For most of this time, conquering infection has been the focus of healthcare. The nurse's role in preventing, detecting, and treating infectious disease is a vital one. You must be aware of agent-host-environment interactions, and take appropriate steps to prevent accidental transmission. Besides directly limiting the spread of disease, you also play an important role in teaching others how to avoid transmission. Clients are being discharged from healthcare facilities earlier than in the past, and it is important for them and their significant others to understand infection control. Teach clients and significant others how to prevent infection in the home. Important points to cover include hand washing; potential sources of infection in the home, such as plants and pets; food preparation precautions, such as careful washing of fresh fruits and vegetables and the importance of avoiding food pathogens; and sanitation issues, such as safe disposal of wastes and cleaning of contaminated objects. The nurse makes the difference in the prevention of infection.

Bibliography

1. Centers for Disease Control and Prevention. (1988). Update: Universal precautions for prevention of transmission of human immunodeficiency virus, hepatitis B virus, and other bloodborne pathogens in health-care settings. *Morbidity and Mortality Weekly Report, 37*(24), 377–387.
2. Centers for Disease Control and Prevention. (1990). Protection against viral hepatitis: Recommendations of the Immunization Practices Advisory Committee. *Morbidity and Mortality Weekly Report, 39*(S-2), 1–26.
3. Centers for Disease Control and Prevention. (1991). Update on adult immunization: Recommendations of the Immunization Practices Advisory Committee (ACIP). *Morbidity and Mortality Weekly Report, 40*(RR-12), 1–72.
4. Centers for Disease Control and Prevention. (1994). Guidelines for preventing the transmission of tuberculosis in health-care facilities. *Morbidity and Mortality Weekly Report, 43*(RR-13), 1–132.
5. Centers for Disease Control and Prevention. (1994). Prevention and control of influenza: Part 1. Vaccines. Recommendations of the Advisory Committee on Immunization Practices (ACIP). *Morbidity and Mortality Weekly Report, 43*(RR-9), 1–11.
6. Centers for Disease Control and Prevention. (1996). Recommended childhood immunization schedule—United States, January–June 1996. *Morbidity and Mortality Weekly Report, 44*(51,52), 940–943.
7. Cochi, S. L., et al. (1994). Meeting the challenges of vaccine-preventable diseases in child day care. *Pediatrics, 94*(6, Part 2), 1021–1023.
8. Garner, J. S., & Hospital Infection Control Practices Advisory Committee. (1996). Guideline for isolation precautions in hospitals. *Infection Control and Hospital Epidemiology, 17,* 54–80.
9. Harkness, G. A. (1995). *Epidemiology in nursing practice.* St. Louis: Mosby–Year Book.
10. Heoprich, P. D., Jordan, M. C., & Ronald, A. R. (1994). *Infectious diseases: A treatise of infectious processes* (5th ed.). Philadelphia: J. B. Lippincott.
11. Institute of Medicine. (1992). *Emerging infections:Microbial threats to health in the United States.* Washington, DC: National Academy Press.
12. Jackson, M. M., & Lynch, P. (1991). An attempt to make an issue less murky: A comparison of four systems for infection precautions. *Infection Control and Hospital Epidemiology, 12,* 448–450.
13. Joint Commission on Accreditation of Healthcare Organizations. (1995). *Accreditation manual for hospitals.* Chicago: Author.
14. McDonald, L. L. (1993). The influence of the Occupational Safety and Health Administration on infection control practice. *Infection Control, 28*(3), 613–623.
15. Occupational Safety and Health Administration. (1994). Respiratory protection. *Federal Register, 59*(219), 58884–58956.
16. Shulman, S. T., Phair, J. P., & Sommers, H. M. (Eds.). (1992). *The biologic and clinical basis of infectious diseases* (4th ed.). Philadelphia: W. B. Saunders.
17. Soule, B. M., Larson, E. L., & Preston, G. A. (1995). *Infections and nursing practice: Prevention and control.* St. Louis: Mosby–Year Book.
18. U.S. Department of Health and Human Services. (1990). *Healthy people 2000.* Washington, DC: U.S. Government Printing Office.
19. Yoshikawa, T. T., & Normal, D. C. (Eds.) (1994). *Antimicrobial therapy in the elderly patients.* New York: Marcel Dekker.

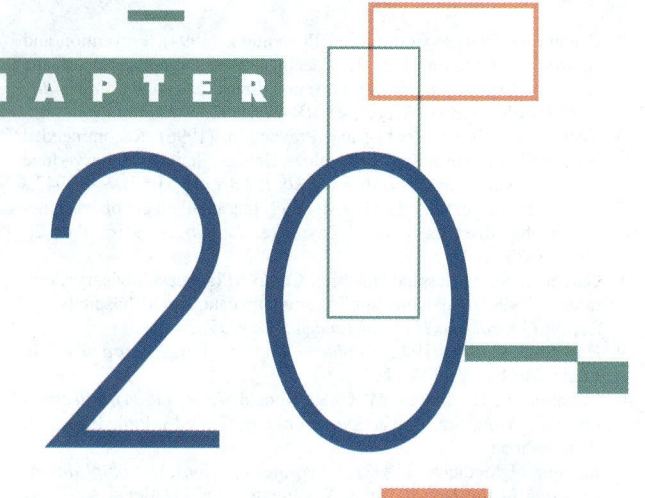

20

Wound Healing

Joyce M. Black

Healing is a fundamental property of living tissue, and if healing did not occur, all species would eventually become extinct. Unfortunately, many wound care practices seem to lack respect for this critical attribute of healing and accept the process as passive, inevitable, and unimprovable. Popular literature assumes that if people survived, they healed, and if people are healthy, they will heal.

Healing activities have always formed the basis of nursing practice. Florence Nightingale defined the nursing role as preparing the patient for the most favorable conditions for healing. Nurses today still serve as a crucial link in the process of wound healing. Nurses educate clients about disease management and wound care and support the client through the physical and psychological processes of healing.

This chapter focuses on tissue injury and repair. Tissue injury is common and is seen in clients who sustain trauma as well as those who have undergone surgery. Because tissue injury is common, the body is well equipped with mechanisms of defense and healing. Defense mechanisms include intact skin and mucous membranes, phagocytes, and the immune and inflammatory responses. They are discussed elsewhere in this book. In this chapter we limit our discussion to wound healing in general. Specific information on types of wounds can be found in other chapters: venous stasis ulcers are described in Chapter 50, diabetic foot ulcers are addressed in Chapter 69, and pressure ulcers are discussed in Chapter 78.

The Body's Defense Mechanisms

The first line of defense includes the skin, other organs, and secretions to reduce the risk of injury. When these systems function normally, little tissue injury occurs. Of

This chapter incorporates material written for the fourth edition by Susan Hockenberger.

course, many agents are able to overcome the structural, chemical, and biologic defenses. When invasion or trauma occurs, the second line of defense is set into action.

The white blood cells (WBCs) provide the major second line of defense. These defense mechanisms are called general or nonspecific responses because they occur in response to any form of injury. In addition to the WBCs, the immune system provides antibodies. Important to our discussion, the WBCs initiate the healing processes by removing cellular debris and microorganisms. They also stimulate many growth factors to promote healing.

Normal Wound Healing

Wound healing has been defined by the Wound Healing Society (WHS) as "a complex and dynamic process that results in the restoration of anatomic continuity and function." Wound healing is a continuous sequence of signals and responses in which several cells come together outside of their usual domains, interact, perform their tasks, and having done so, resume their normal functions. Healing, and specifically wound healing, is a process.

Healed wounds constitute a spectrum of repair. According to the WHS, an ideally healed wound is one that has returned to normal anatomic structure, function, and appearance. In humans, this degree of healing would only occur in epidermal tissue or mucous membrane, because once there is injury to the dermis, normal appearance cannot occur because scar tissue replaces missing tissue. The WHS defines a minimally healed wound as one that has restoration of anatomic continuity, but without a sustained functional result. Hence the wound may recur. Between these two extremes of healing, an acceptably healed wound is characterized by restoration of sustained function and anatomic continuity. The timeliness of wound healing is determined by the type of wound, and the intrinsic and extrinsic environments. The degree to

426

which wound healing can and does occur is based on several subconcepts of the healing process.

The type of injury itself has considerable influence on the form of repair. Clean approximated incisions heal with minimal synthesis of new tissue and barely test clients' resources. In sharp contrast, major burn wounds require complete regeneration of tissue and stimulate massive responses from all body systems to sustain life. The location of the wound also influences healing. Perineal wounds are likely to become infected, wounds over joints are subject to motion and therefore increased scarring, and wounds in peripheral areas or under pressure have limited perfusion and heal slowly.

Wound healing is most apparent on the skin, but occurs in all areas of the body. Bones, tendons, organs, and tissues can regenerate cells and restore function. The most favorable outcome of healing is the complete return to normal structure and function. This outcome is possible if tissue damage is minor, no complications occur, and the destroyed tissues are capable of regeneration. Body tissues have varying capabilities for regeneration. For example, mucous membrane is completely regenerated. Deep skin injury regenerates with a scar, which restores only a barrier. The central nervous system (CNS) cannot regenerate damaged cells. Therefore, damaged tissues in the CNS may be repaired with scar tissue, but they cannot be regenerated to regain their original function.

Phases of Wound Healing

Regardless of the cause of the wound, wound healing follows a predictable course. Events can be described in four phases: (1) vascular response, (2) inflammation, (3) proliferation, or resolution, and (4) maturation, or reconstruction. At the time of injury, many actions occur simultaneously. You may want to follow along on Figure 20–1 through this discussion.

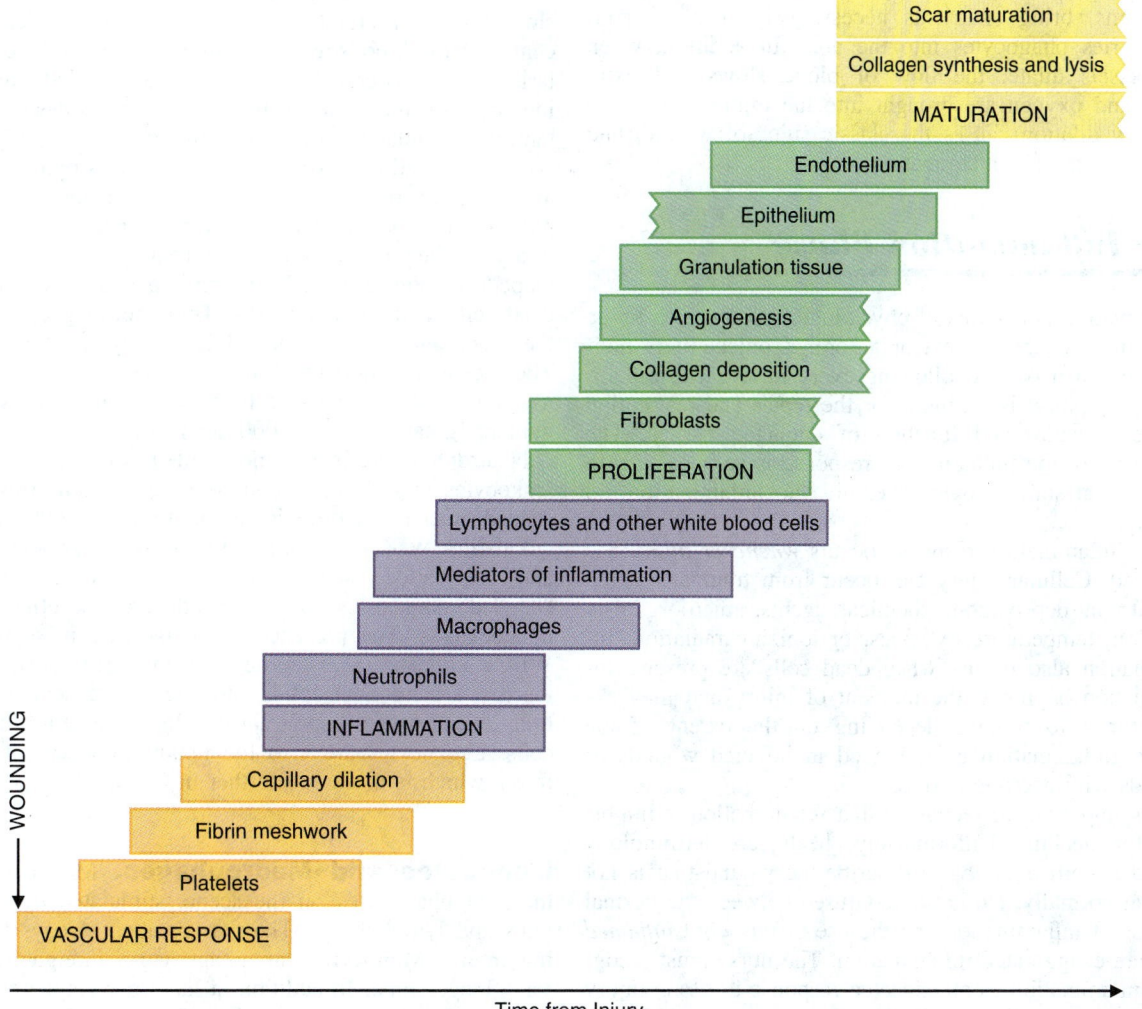

Figure 20–1. Normal wound healing. Wound healing proceeds through four phases: (1) the vascular response, (2) inflammation, (3) proliferation of cells to heal the wound, and (4) maturation of the wound. There are many components of each step. The jagged edge depicts an ongoing process. (Adapted from Cohen, I., et al. (Eds.). [1992]. *Wound healing.* Philadelphia: W. B. Saunders.)

The Vascular Response Phase

Within seconds after an injury, regardless of the source, blood vessels constrict to stop bleeding and reduce exposure to bacteria. Smooth muscle in the arterial walls contracts to reduce blood flow. The clotting process begins. Platelets, activated by the injury, aggregate to form a clot and stop bleeding. At the same time, the plasma protein system begins to form a fibrinous meshwork. When the platelets come in contact with the fibrin meshwork across the open vessel wall, they become sticky and adhere (aggregate) to the fibers, forming a plug. This meshwork of clotted blood and serum covers the wound while it heals and prevents further loss of blood and plasma. Platelets also release chemicals that promote clotting, such as adenosine diphosphate (ADP), to attract other platelets and a type of prostaglandin that activates other platelets. Platelets also release growth factors to stimulate healing; they are discussed later.

Capillaries dilate 10 to 30 minutes after injury and remain dilated for some time because of serotonin released by the platelets. Capillary dilation allows the ingress of plasma. Plasma dilutes toxins secreted by the organisms, brings nutrients necessary for tissue repair, and carries phagocytes into the area. In addition, when the vessels dilate, the flow of blood slows and extra blood and oxygen are brought into the injured area. The capillary dilation causes the classic signs of warmth and redness seen with inflammation.

The Inflammation Phase

Inflammation is a series of physiologic responses to tissue injury induced by trauma or a foreign object. It is nonspecific and it occurs following every injury. The inflammatory response is essential for the repair and restoration of the structure and function of damaged tissues. The mustering of the inflammatory response is so necessary to healing that some people have said "no inflammation, no healing."

The inflammatory response occurs *whenever injury* has occurred. Cellular injury can occur from trauma, oxygen or nutrient deprivation, chemical agents, microorganism invasion, temperature extremes, or ionizing radiation. Inflammation also occurs when dead cells are present. Inflammation begins at the moment of injury and may extend for 4 to 6 days depending on the extent of the injury. Inflammation is prolonged in infected wounds or wounds with necrotic tissues.

It is important to recognize that inflammation is important for healing. Unfortunately, healthcare terminology uses the word *inflamed* to describe the wound that is not healing normally. Do not be confused between the normal process of inflammation and the use of the word *inflamed* to mean exaggerated inflammation. The nurse must recognize inflammation as an expected response to tissue injury and not necessarily a pathophysiologic process. Although inflammation can cause additional tissue injury, it is an adaptation to injury. The purpose of inflammation is to limit the effects of harmful bacteria or injury by destroy-

ing or neutralizing the organism, and by limiting its spread throughout the body. The inflammatory response thereby sets up proper conditions to promote tissue repair. Unlike the immune response, which is slow and deliberate, using a system of specific antibodies, the effects of inflammation are immediate.

Inflammation is the second phase of wound healing. During this phase the WBCs become active to clean up the wound and initiate further healing processes. We need to look closely at these WBCs and the process of phagocytosis.

The Role of White Blood Cells

Neutrophils. Neutrophils are vital defense mechanisms because they are both the first and most numerous cell type to arrive at any area of disease or injury. Within 6 hours after release from bone marrow, neutrophils migrate into tissues where they survive for 4 to 5 days. Their role, along with tissue macrophages, is to phagocytose (ingest) injurious agents, thereby protecting against bacterial invasion.

They are attracted to the injury site by chemotaxis. The slowed flow of blood allows the neutrophil to leave the center of the bloodstream and line the walls of the capillaries, a process called pavementing (also called marginating) because they line up like bricks on a sidewalk. Histamine stimulates the cells lining the capillary to constrict, creating spaces in the wall. Neutrophils, which are normally too large to squeeze through the lining, can pass through the capillary wall and enter the site of tissue injury to begin phagocytosis, through a process called diapedesis (Fig. 20–2). Neutrophils phagocytose bacteria, dead cells, and cellular debris. They are phagocytosed by the macrophage and removed by the lymphatic system. These cells are short-lived, but they are effective in clearing a wound of debris if bacteria are not excessive in number (greater than 100,000 per gram of tissue).

Neutrophils are sometimes called polymorphonuclear leukocytes (PMNs or polys) because of their irregularly shaped nuclei. Neutrophils compose about 60% of the circulating WBCs. Mature neutrophils appear segmented, and are called "segs" for short. Immature cells are "banded" and called bands. Bands are not effective in phagocytosis. The presence of an increase in segmented WBCs indicates a bacterial invasion. The presence of increased band neutrophils indicates more severe infection, because the bone marrow has released immature cells. Leukocytes are also the major producers of interferon, which is discussed further in Chapter 25.

Monocytes and Macrophages. Monocytes are the next phagocytes on the scene, stimulated by neutrophils and lymphokines. They arrive about 4 days following injury. Monocytes can phagocytose foreign material for a longer time. In addition, a large percentage of monocytes enter the tissues and become macrophages. In the tissue, these cells continue to phagocytose large numbers of bacteria. If the need arises, these cells can reenter the circulation and become mobile macrophages. Macrophages have a greater role in chronic inflammation, and the process is discussed later. The macrophage is a critical cell in wound healing because it secretes angiogenesis factor (AGF). AGF stimulates the formation of new blood vessels at the end of injured vessels and stimulates fibroblasts to spew forth collagen. The macrophage also secretes other cytokines such as platelet-derived growth factor, transforming growth factor, interleukin-1, and basic fibroblast growth factor. This cell has a major role in wound healing. Wounds can heal without leukocytes, but wound healing is significantly impaired without macrophages.

The amount of oxygen in the wound influences the effectiveness of phagocytic cells. Both macrophages and neutrophils can function in an anaerobic environment, but their ability to effectively digest bacteria is slowed. Macrophages are inactivated when tissue levels of oxygen are below 30 mm Hg. (Normal tissue oxygen levels are not the same as levels of oxygen bound to hemoglobin or dissolved oxygen. Tissue oxygen levels are normal at 30 mm Hg.)

Lymphocytes and Other White Blood Cells.

Two other forms of WBCs exist and they have much less importance in wound healing, so they will be addressed only briefly. The lymphocytes are formed in the lymphoid tissues of the tonsils, intestines, and bone marrow, and they mature in the lymph nodes, thymus, and spleen. Lymphokines are sensitized lymphocytes. Lymphokines assist the macrophages to be more effective at the site of local injury through a number of processes. Lymphocytes are controlled by the adrenocortical hormones. Therefore, clients on steroid therapy have decreased numbers of lymphocytes. This change places the steroid-dependent client at increased risk of infection and delayed healing.

Eosinophils and basophils may also migrate to the injured area. Eosinophils will help control the inflammatory response by secreting antihistamine. Basophils secrete histamine.

The "Walling-Off" Effect.

The "walling-off" effect occurs in the damaged area to prevent the spread of injurious agents to other body tissues. The lymphatics and spaces in the tissues are blocked by fibrinogen clots so that fluid barely flows through the area. The process of walling off the area is partly dependent on the invading agent. For example, staphylococci invade and destroy nearby tissues quickly and, therefore, the process of walling off also develops quickly to control the spread. In contrast, streptococci do not cause an intense reaction in the tissues and can digest the walls. This allows the streptococci to multiply and spread. As a result, streptococcal infections have a much greater tendency to invade other organs (such as the heart valves) and are associated with a higher mortality rate.

Mediators of the Inflammation Phase

The specific mediators of inflammation are not shown in Figure 20–1. They are important, and their activity oc-

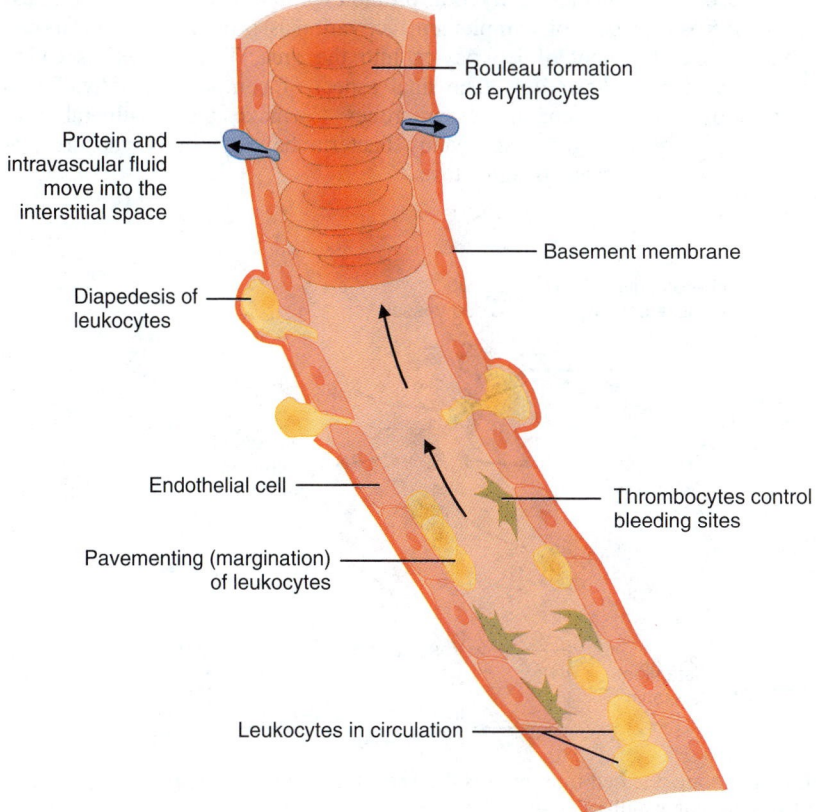

Protein and intravascular fluid move into the interstitial space

Rouleau formation of erythrocytes

Basement membrane

Diapedesis of leukocytes

Endothelial cell

Thrombocytes control bleeding sites

Pavementing (margination) of leukocytes

Leukocytes in circulation

Figure 20–2. Several changes occur in a capillary after injury. Neutrophils are attracted to the site of injury by chemotactic factors at the site. The neutrophil leaves the blood vessel by sliding through holes in the vessel wall (diapedesis). The leukocytes also line the vessel wall, and the erythrocytes stack like coins (rouleau formation) to slow blood flow.

curs throughout the healing phases. The chemicals that guide inflammation are shown in Understanding Inflammation and Its Treatment.

Mast Cells. There are several substances that mediate (control) inflammation. Mast cells are found in the tissue. Mast cells are filled with histamine and neutrophil chemotactic factors, substances called vasoactive amines. Histamine and serotonin cause capillary dilation (Fig. 20–3). The mast cell is stimulated by many factors, such as physical injury (wounds, burns, x-ray exposure), chemical injury (toxins, snake and bee venom), or immunologic means (the trigger of hypersensitivity reactions seen in allergies).

Mast cells also synthesize leukotrienes and prostaglandins. These two chemicals cause the same responses as histamine, except that the response they generate lasts longer. Prostaglandins also cause pain. They tend to appear in the later stages of inflammation. Leukotrienes and prostaglandins are produced from arachidonic acid released from the mast cell membrane. Aspirin and other nonsteroidal anti-inflammatory agents (NSAIDs) block the production of prostaglandins and can assist in reducing inflammation and pain (see Understanding Inflammation and Its Treatment). Leukotrienes and prostaglandins increase vascular permeability, and enhance the action of neutrophils. The increase in blood flow brings in more nutrients and WBCs. Bradykinin also causes vasodilation, induces pain, and facilitates the action of the leukocyte.

Kinin System. Kinins are plasma proteins involved in inflammation. Early in injury, kinins increase vascular permeability and allow the leukocytes to enter the tissue. Later in the inflammatory process, kinin acts with prostaglandin to cause pain and smooth muscle contraction, and to increase leukocyte chemotaxis. Kinin increases vascular permeability, fluid in the wound, and the number of leukocytes available to assist with phagocytosis. The primary kinin is bradykinin.

Free Radicals. Free radicals are commonly discussed as the cause of some diseases. During metabolism, an unstable form of oxygen is produced. This is a single oxygen atom, derived from molecular oxygen (O_2), having an unpaired electron. This form of oxygen is called an oxygen free radical or a superoxide radical. The molecule tries to become stable again by attaching to hydrogen, lipids, or vitamin E. If it attaches to hydrogen, hydrogen peroxide is produced which is toxic to the cell. If it attaches to lipids it can enter the cell or organelles and produce damage. When attached to vitamin E, it is stabilized and does not produce damage. Other vitamins support vitamin E: vitamin C restores vitamin E to the cell membrane. Vitamin A (beta-carotene) is present in high-density lipoproteins and is assumed to serve some role as an antioxidant, but that role is not fully understood. (A diagram of how free radicals injure cells and how they can be antioxidized is shown in Chapter 2.)

Unrestrained free radicals are known for being able to injure tissues and to induce breaks in both single- and double-stranded DNA, leading to mutations. In wound healing, free radicals serve as mediators of both acute and chronic inflammation, being stimulated by the PMN and the mast cell. They damage vascular endothelium (the inside lining of blood vessels). The exact role of free radicals in wound healing is being researched. The use of vitamin E as an antioxidant is becoming popular.

The Complement System. The complement system is composed of a group of plasma proteins that normally lie dormant in the blood, interstitial fluid, and mucosal surfaces. The complement system is activated by microorganisms (or antigen-antibody complexes). Complement activation promotes inflammation. The second aspect of complement activation is promotion of the movement of leukocytes into the area. This process is called *chemotaxis*. The final aspect of complement activation is the coating of microbes to make them vulnerable to phagocytosis. Many bacteria have an outer capsule that resists phagocytosis.

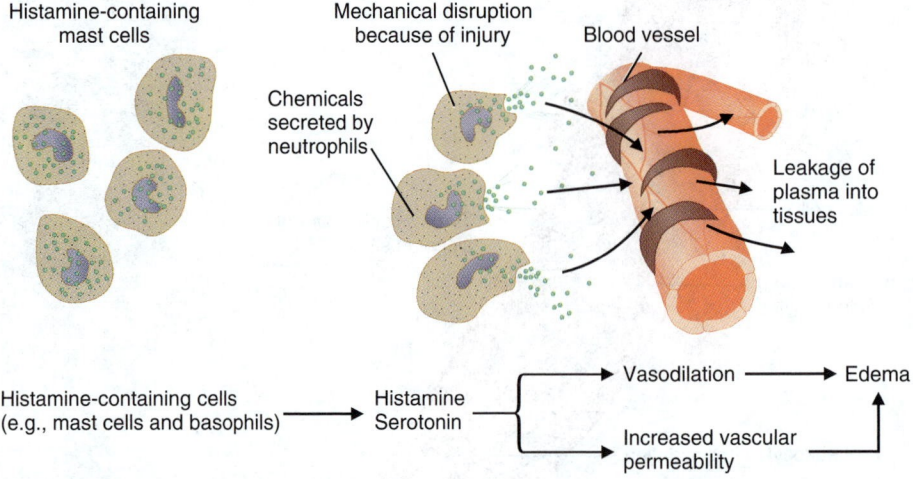

Figure 20–3. Histamine and serotonin are released from mast cells. These chemical mediators of inflammation lead to edema by increasing capillary permeability.

Understanding Inflammation and Its Treatment

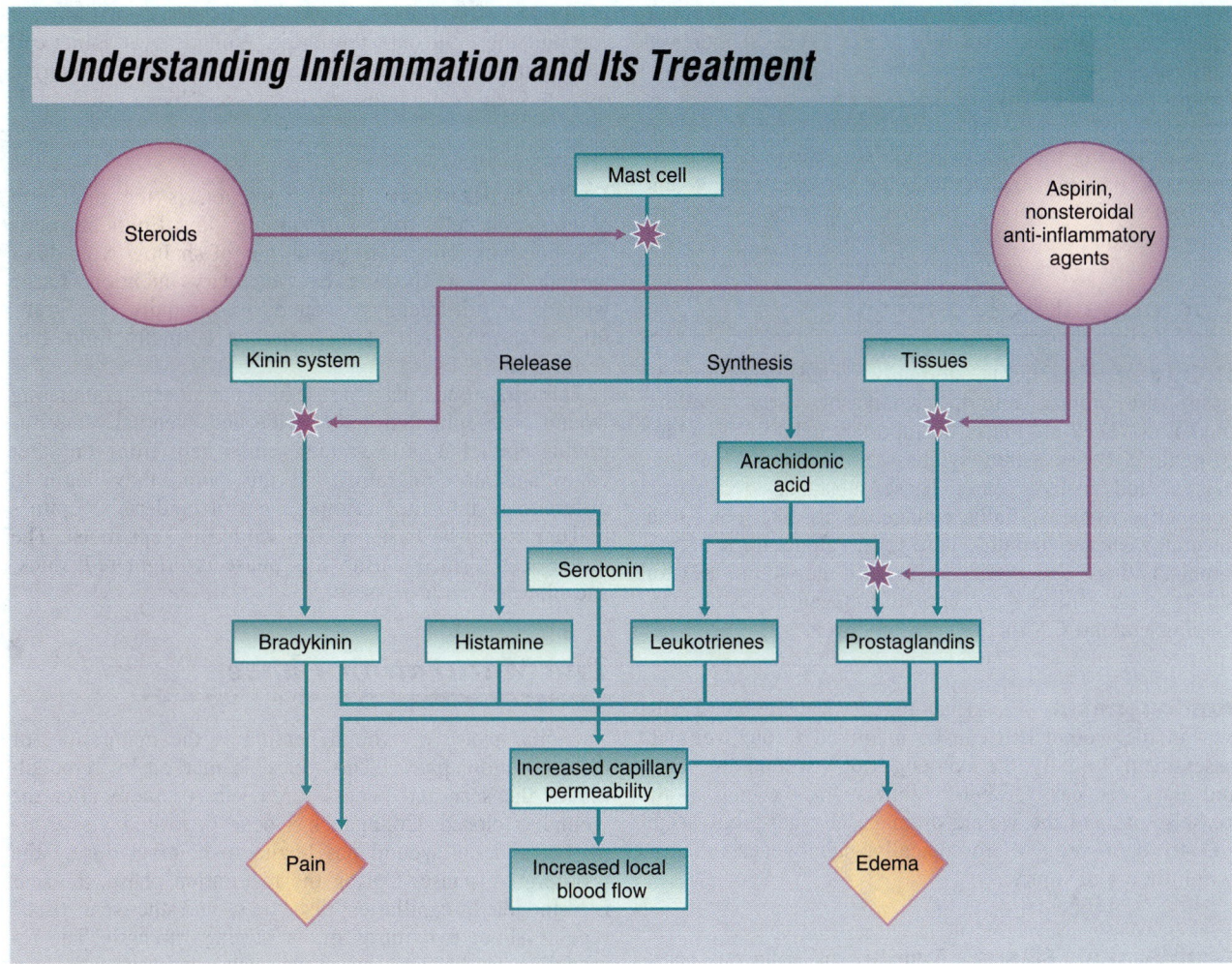

The Need for Phagocytosis

Phagocytosis, which is the engulfment and destruction of microorganisms, dead cells, and foreign material, is critical to wound healing. Two WBCs serve as phagocytes for wound healing: the leukocyte and macrophage. These cells are able to recognize foreign protein or damaged tissue, bind to it, engulf it, and destroy it. Disorders that lead to reduced numbers of phagocytic cells slow this process and make the person more prone to infection.

The Proliferative Phase

The third phase of wound healing is the proliferative or resolution phase. This phase contains overlapping processes of collagen deposition, angiogenesis, granulation tissue development, and wound contraction. This phase ends about 2 weeks after injury, but the processes of healing are not complete and continue for 1 to 2 years.

Mediators of the Proliferative Phase

Cytokines. Various substances act as mediators of wound healing. One group is called cytokines. They regu-

late the mobility, differentiation, and growth of leukocytes. Among the best-understood cytokines are interleukins and interferon. Interleukins promote the growth and function of several cells. Interleukin can account for many of the clinical manifestations of both acute and chronic inflammation, such as fever, anorexia, cachexia, and movement of leukocytes (PMNs) to the site of injury. Interferons augment immunity through several processes, especially the promotion of B cell maturation and moderating of suppressor T cell function.

Growth Factors. Catalysts for wound healing are growth factors released by platelets and macrophages. They can prime other cells to enter a growth phase or they can move a cell from a growth phase to a DNA production phase. Several types of growth factors have been identified. Only major families of wound healing growth factors will be described. Platelet-derived growth factor (PDGF) is named for the cell from which it originated. PDGF regulates the synthesis of fibronectin and fibroblasts in the matrix of the wound healing bed. Epidermal growth factor (EGF), named for the target cell, stimulates fibroblasts and endothelial cells. Fibroblast growth factor stimulates collagen synthesis and angiogenesis. Transforming growth factor alpha (TGF-α) stimulates epithelial cells and macrophages. It also controls cell growth and synthesis of the components of the matrix. Transforming growth factor beta (TGF-β) increases synthesis of the matrix components. Colony-stimulating factors are secreted by the bone marrow, monocytes, fibroblasts, and keratinocytes. Their major function appears to be enhancing the function of WBCs. Research in many centers is ongoing to determine the biologic activity and the potential benefits of topical application of these growth factors.

Components of Healing

Collagen. Fibroblasts, normally found in connective tissue, are brought into the wound by various cellular mediators. They are the most important cells in this phase of healing, because they synthesize and secrete collagen, elastin, and proteoglycans. These substances reconstruct connective tissue. Initially, collagen is gel-like, but within several weeks to months, it re-forms along lines of mechanical stress, which adds strength to the wound. Several substances are needed for normal collagen deposition, including vitamin C, zinc, oxygen, and iron.

Angiogenesis. The development of new blood vessels in the wound bed can be identified through clinical assessment. Initially, the skin edges of a wound are bright red and bleed easily. Then, within hours, the ends of the vessels seal and the wound drainage changes from bright red to dark red. Microscopically, angiogenesis begins within hours of injury.

Granulation Tissue. A matrix of collagen, capillaries, and cells begin to fill the wound space with new connective tissue, forming a scar. This tissue grows from the wound edges and the base of the wound. Granulation tissue is filled with new capillary buds, which gives it a red, bumpy, or granular appearance. It is also surrounded by fibroblasts and macrophages. The fibroblasts secrete collagen. The macrophages continue to debride the wound and stimulate fibroblasts and the process of angiogenesis. As granulation tissue is being formed, the process of epithelialization begins.

Wound Contraction. Wound contraction is the mechanism by which the edges of a wound are drawn together as a result of forces within that wound. Contraction is due to the action of myofibroblasts. Myofibroblasts bridge across a wound and then contract to pull the wound closed. The process of wound contraction is critical to survival. If a wound from an acute injury did not contract, infections would be lethal complications in all acute injuries. Contraction is undesirable in some wounds because of the cosmetic deformities that result from contracture.

Contracture. In large open wounds, like burns, wound contraction can go on to develop the more severe form of contracture. Contracture of the scar can produce profound deformities. Contracture of the scar at the neck can pull the chin onto the chest. Wounds over joints can also contract severely. Contracture also occurs in internal organs, such as the intestine, breast, and liver.

Epithelialization. Epithelialization is the migration of epithelial cells from surrounding skin. Epithelial buds also line hair follicles in the dermis of shallow wounds or wounds that are healing by secondary intention. Large wounds or full-thickness wounds may require skin grafting, because epidermal migration is normally limited to about 3 cm.

Epithelial buds can be seen in a clean granulating wound. The epithelial cells divide and eventually the migrating epithelial cells contact similar cells from the other edges and stop migrating. At this point, they begin to differentiate into the various layers of epidermis. Epithelialization can be hastened if a wound is kept moist. The initial scar formed during this phase is bright red, thick, and blanches with pressure.

The Maturation Phase

The final phase of wound healing is the maturation, or reconstruction, phase. This phase is marked by remodeling of the scar and occurs for a year or more after the wound is closed. Collagen has been deposited, tissue repaired, and the wound has begun to contract during the proliferative phase. During the maturation phase, the scar is remodeled, capillaries disappear, and the scar tissue regains about two thirds of its original strength. The remodeling is the process of collagen synthesis and lysis. Remodeling provides tensile strength to the wound. It is important to recognize that scar tissue is never as strong or durable as normal tissue. Tensile strength never reaches over 80% in scar tissue. The scar becomes mature, and appears thin and white instead of red and raised. Scarring is a normal part of wound healing. Some scars will become barely visible, whereas others will remain very visible throughout the client's lifetime. Factors that affect scarring are discussed in Chapter 80.

Wound Healing Intention

Wound healing intention is the term used to describe the probable process of healing for any wound. There are three types.

Primary Intention

Primary intention is the use of suture or other wound closures to approximate (place close together) the edges of an incision or clean laceration. Healing is primarily through collagen synthesis and very little scarring or contraction is needed (Fig. 20–4). The risk of infection and tissue defects is minimal. The eventual scar is usually thin and flat.

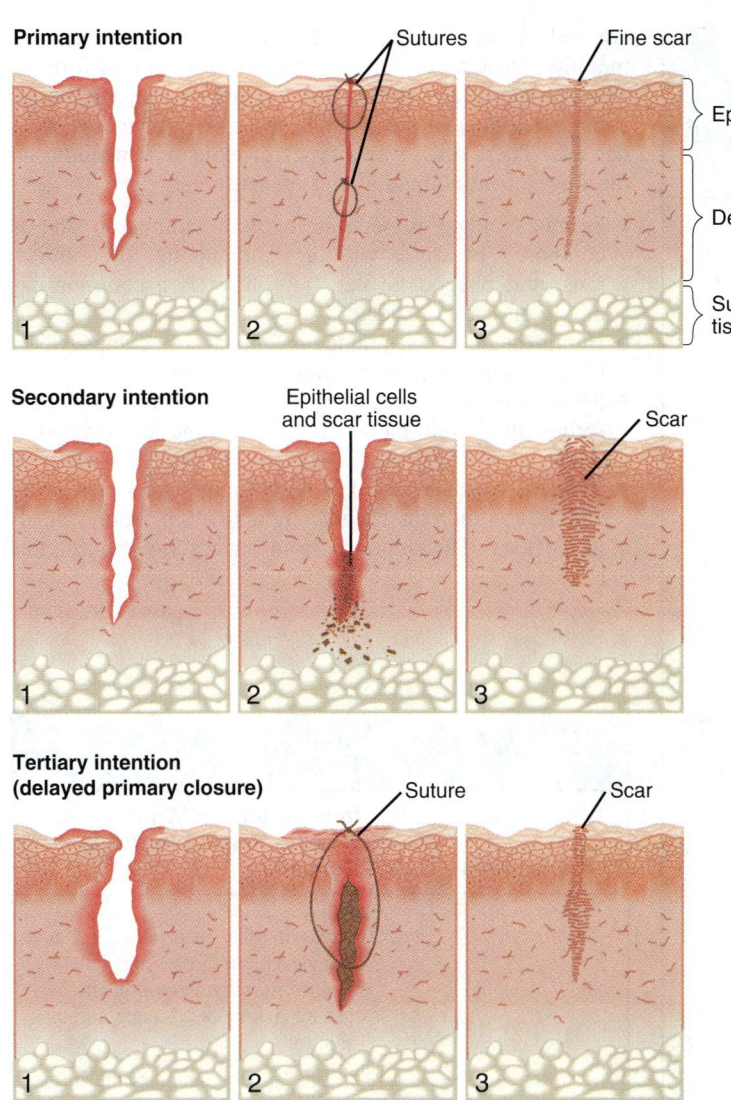

Figure 20–4. Wound healing by primary, secondary, and tertiary intention (delayed primary closure).

Secondary Intention

Wounds healing by secondary intention are left open rather than closed with sutures (stitches) and heal by the generation of connective tissue. Consider open wounds like pressure ulcers or abrasions. These open wounds require the regeneration of much more tissue than does the healing of an incision. There is also increased risk of infection with an open wound. Wounds healing by secondary intention have a prolonged phase of inflammation because there is more time required for phagocytosis of necrotic tissue. This chronic inflammation has macrophages and lymphocytes as the predominant cells. The ability of epithelial cells to migrate is limited, and epithelialization may not heal the wound. Therefore the wound has longer phases of proliferation and maturation leading to healing by contraction and the formation of scar tissue. Sometimes, the healing of these wounds is hastened by the application of skin grafts or musculocutaneous (also called myocutaneous) flaps (see Chapter 80).

Tertiary Intention

Certain wounds may be contaminated and although they could be closed by primary intention (e.g., sutured closed), they are not. Because of the increased risk of infection, these wounds are closed later when they are free of debris. This type of wound closure is called healing by *tertiary intention,* or *delayed primary closure.*

Risk factors and risk reduction for wound healing are shown in Risk Factors and Levels of Prevention.

Nutrition and Wound Healing

Protein and calories are needed for wound healing. Several vitamins and minerals are also needed for wound healing. Table 20–1 lists the various vitamins and minerals needed for healing. Malnutrition leads to impaired collagen synthesis and an increased risk of infection. Pro-

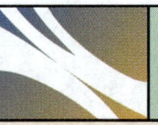

tein-calorie malnutrition is an all-too-common problem in the elderly, especially those in institutions.

Management of the Client with Inflammation

We have just reviewed the processes of wound healing. Now we discuss the management of clients during inflammation, with incisions, with open wounds, and with non-healing wounds. We begin with inflammation. Inflammation occurs in all clients that have any form of tissue trauma. The trauma can be from surgery, injury, changes in oxygen delivery to various tissues, and so on. Therefore, the information in this section can be applied to many clinical settings.

There are both local and systemic manifestations of inflammation. Because the response to inflammation is the same regardless of the cause, the manifestations of inflammation are relatively consistent.

The clinical manifestations of inflammation include redness, swelling, heat, pain, and loss of function. Tissues are red, warm, painful, and swollen and have limited mobility. In addition, an inflammatory exudate is formed. The exudate dilutes the toxins released by bacteria, brings certain nutrients to the wound, and carries phagocytes for defense. There are various types of exudate depending on the stage of inflammation and its cause.

- Serous exudate is seen in early inflammation and is composed of water with a small amount of colloids, ions, and phagocytic cells. A blister is a common example of serous exudate.
- Hemorrhagic or sanguineous exudate is composed of blood. Drainage is bright red or dark red.
- Serosanguineous exudate is drainage composed of both serous fluid and blood. It is pink and usually fairly thin.
- Purulent exudate is filled with more leukocytes (pus) and is common in chronic inflammation from walled-off lesions. The drainage from an abscess typifies this exudate.

Table 20–1. Nutrition and Wound Healing

Nutrient	Impairments in Wound Healing Related to Nutrient Deficiency
Protein	Decreased collagen production, angiogenesis, neutrophil and lymphocyte immune response; increased risk of dehiscence and infection
Calories	Too little glucose impairs the immune response because energy needs of white blood cells cannot be met
Fats	Impaired inflammation
Vitamin A	Impaired monocyte and macrophage activity; delayed inflammatory response including macrophage activity; increased risk of infection
Vitamin B complex	Not well understood; lack of vitamins interferes with enzyme production
Vitamin C	Decreased collagen production, angiogenesis, contraction; weakness in healed wound; increased risk of infection
Vitamin E	Delayed healing when given in excess
Zinc	Possibly impaired action of vitamin A, phagocytosis; increased risk of infection; decreased protein synthesis
Iron	Impaired oxygenation and secondary healing at very low levels

Initially, a surgical wound has sanguineous drainage, which then progresses to serosanguineous and finally to serous drainage (Table 20–2).

There are three systemic reactions to inflammation: (1) fever, (2) leukocytosis (a rise in the number of WBCs), and (3) an increase in the number of plasma proteins. *Fever* is caused by a pyrogen (fever-causing chemical) released from leukocytes, macrophages, and tumor necrosis factor (TNF). Prostaglandins also act on the hypothalamus to reset the internal thermostat. Fever is usually adaptive because bacterial reproduction is sensitive to even slight increases in temperature. Therefore, low-grade fevers should not be treated with antipyretics (e.g., acetaminophen). However, fever can be detrimental if it is extreme or prolonged. Therefore, the temperature is monitored closely to avoid harm to the client. The client may also experience malaise, nausea, anorexia, weight loss, tachypnea, and tachycardia.

Leukocytosis is due to the increase in the number of leukocytes in circulation to combat infection. Sometimes, in an effort to combat infection the bone marrow releases immature leukocytes, called banded neutrophils or bands. When the number of immature neutrophils is high, the client is said to have a "left shift." At times, the release of immature cells means that the body is having difficulty combating the infection with mature cells. (Interpretation of the WBC differential is shown in Table 20–3.)

The *sedimentation rate* also rises with inflammation. The sedimentation rate (or "sed rate") is the rate at which cells settle to the bottom of a glass test tube. Increased levels of fibrinogen cause the red blood cells to stack (like coins) and, therefore, settle more quickly. Additionally, plasma proteins rise during inflammation (e.g., fibrinogen, C-reactive protein). Most are released by the liver, and they are collectively called acute-phase reactants. They provide components of coagulation, transportation, and complement production.

Acute and Subacute Care

Since the inflammatory response is a desired response to promote wound healing, sometimes the client with inflammation requires only supportive care. The degree of inflammation is monitored to determine whether it is leading to healing. The area of inflammation is often elevated or wrapped to reduce edema. Analgesics may be required for pain control. Temperature is monitored and treated with antipyretics when it reaches levels that are detrimental to the client (e.g., more than 38.3° C [101° F]). If the inflammation is in response to a probable invasion by organisms, antibiotics may be prescribed.

Interpreting the Differential Count

The nurse should monitor the level of WBCs, differential counts, and temperature as indicators of infection. Unfortunately, as mentioned earlier, healthcare providers use the phase "inflamed" to describe wounds with increased inflammation and infection. This term can be confusing because the inflammatory process is normal, but the inflammation is not. Since the inflammatory process is normal, usually when the word "inflamed" is used it means an exaggerated response and that there are concerns about infection.

Managing the Client's Diet

The diet of the client with inflammation should be high in (1) vitamin C, to support the WBC function, production of collagen, and angiogenesis; (2) protein, to aid in the formation of blood cells and tissue; and (3) fluids, to remove metabolic waste and rehydrate the client, especially if the client has been febrile.

Table 20–2. Inflammatory Exudates		
Type	**Appearance**	**Significance**
Hemorrhagic, sanguineous	Bright red or bloody	Small amounts expected after surgery or trauma; large amounts may indicate hemorrhage; sudden large amounts of dark-red blood may indicate a draining hematoma
Serosanguineous	Blood-tinged yellow or pink	Expected for 48–72 hours after injury or trauma; a sudden increase may precede wound dehiscence
Serous	Thin, clear, yellow	Expected for up to 1 week after trauma or surgery; a sudden increase may indicate a draining seroma
Purulent	Thin, cloudy, foul-smelling; may be thick if filled with dead cells	Usually indicates infection; may drain suddenly from an abscess (boil)
Catarrhal	Thin, clear mucus	Seen with upper respiratory infection

Table 20-3. Interpretation of Differential Counts Within a Complete Blood Count

Cell Type	Function	Normal Value	Significance of Change
Segmented neutrophils (segs)*	Mature neutrophils act as phagocytes	50%–60%	Elevated with infection; a "left shift" means that many bands (immature) cells are present as the body fights infection; "right stuff" is the presence of more mature cells, seen with liver disease and pernicious anemia
Band neutrophils	Immature neutrophils	3%–8%	Elevated in acute stages of infection
Lymphocytes	Produced by lymphoid tissue, participate in humoral response	25%–40%	Elevated in infectious mononucleosis, cytomegalovirus infection, infectious hepatitis; decreased in AIDS, Cushing's syndrome, chronic uremia, and following trauma (e.g., burn injury)
Monocytes	A second line of defense, increasing in chronic infections	2%–8%	Elevated in chronic bacterial infection, viral disease, Hodgkin's disease, multiple myeloma, and some forms of leukemia
Eosinophils	Phagocytic, destroy antigen-antibody complexes before they can harm the body	1%–4%	Elevated in allergic disorders and parasitic infections; decreased in infectious mononucleosis, congestive heart failure, pernicious anemia, and during the use of steroids, epinephrine, and thyroxine

*To calculate the absolute neutrophil count (also called an absolute granulocyte count):

$$\text{Absolute neutrophil count} = \frac{\text{Total \% of neutrophils (segs + bands)} \times \text{WBC count (cells/mm}^3)}{100}$$

When the absolute neutrophil count falls below 1000/mm^3, the client is said to be 'neutropenic' and precautions must be taken to prevent infection.

Controlling the Effects of Edema

If the edema is causing a detrimental alteration of tissue perfusion, anti-inflammatory agents may be required. In certain areas of the body, such as the brain and extremities, the edema that accompanies inflammation can be detrimental to tissue perfusion. These clients may require surgery to release pressure in the area and restore blood flow. Burr holes and fasciotomy are examples of these operations, and are discussed in Chapters 32 and 75, respectively. If an extremity is edematous it should be elevated. Factors that impede venous flow should be controlled. For example, tight bandages that constrict venous return should not be worn.

Assessing the Client for Compartment Syndrome

Edema from the inflammatory response may restrict blood vessels and entrap nerves in the traumatized area. Dressings or casts over the affected area can also form a constriction. This response can be called *compartment syndrome*. Clients with visible injury causing inflammation should be assessed for the resolution of bleeding in the area, adequate blood flow, and nerve conduction distal to the area. Frequent assessment (every 2 hours) of the circumference of the area will provide data to indicate whether the area is becoming markedly edematous. To measure the same site, mark the area on the client with a pen. In addition to assessing the circumference, assess pulses, skin temperature, capillary refill, sensation, and movement in areas distal to the inflammation. Clients who have been injured or are having orthopedic surgery are at highest risk of developing compartment syndrome. See also Chapter 75 for further discussion.

Objects that may become entrapped in edematous tissues, such as rings, should be removed. The inflamed area should be elevated. Application of cold compresses will cause vasoconstriction and decrease the amount of edema. However, prolonged use of cold compresses may lead to rebound vasodilation and increase the risk of tissue injury. Vasoconstriction can also decrease the inflow of new blood and thereby slow the removal of toxins and waste from the site of injury.

Applying Heat and Cold

Most practitioners advocate using ice to control the inflammatory response in the extremities, especially edema and pain. Some physicians order ice for 24 to 72 hours to control inflammation, and then apply heat to remove the accumulated waste products. When ice is ordered be certain that it can touch the extremity and is not rendered ineffective by bulky dressings. Also assess for signs of skin damage if ice is applied directly to unprotected skin.

Community and Self-Care

If the client is capable of caring for a wound or area that is likely to become inflamed, he or she needs instructions on how to elevate the extremity, how to use heat or ice, how to follow the medication regimen, how to change dressings, what clinical manifestations of edema and infection must be reported, such as changes in color, pulse, or pain.

Management of the Client with Chronic Inflammation

Chronic inflammation is differentiated from acute inflammation by its duration and the cells that mediate the response. In acute inflammation there is altered capillary permeability, release of chemical mediators, and infiltration of leukocytes to engulf and destroy injured tissue and pathogens. If these elements are successful in cleaning the wound, it begins to heal. If the area is not cleaned, monocytes continue to perpetuate the inflammatory response, but this time the accumulation of inflammatory mediators may actually cause tissue destruction. The lymphocyte and tissue macrophage are the major phagocytes in chronic inflammation.

When the body is unable to kill the invading organisms during the acute stage of inflammation, it attempts to protect surrounding tissues from further invasion by building a wall around the infected site. The wall is called a granuloma. Some forms of infection, such as fungi, parasites, and, perhaps, antibody-antigen reactions (autoimmune disease), result in granuloma formation. Tuberculosis is a good example of granuloma formation. When a person develops tuberculosis, a thick wall forms around the mycobacteria. The bacteria continue to live in the walled-off area, and it is soon filled with dead tissue. As the tissue dies, the cellular enzymes are released and the fluid leaves the granuloma. The empty sac remains.

The chronically inflamed wound has purulent drainage (suppuration) and does not heal completely. A common example of chronic inflammation is seen when foreign objects are not removed from tissues (e.g., splinter, glass, dirt). Chronic inflammation can also occur when certain forms of bacteria cannot be killed by phagocytes. For example, the organisms that cause tuberculosis, syphilis, and leprosy have cell walls with a very high lipid and wax content, which makes them impermeable to the phagocyte.

Management of the Client with Incisions

Incisions are the most common example of wounds healing by primary intention. Wounds can be closed with suture, staples, or strips of tape.

The client's wound should be assessed every 8 hours. If the incision is not visible, check the dressings or assess for increased girth. The incision normally appears somewhat pink and swollen, but the erythema should not extend beyond a half-inch from the incision. If the wound was sutured in surgery, you should be able to palpate the presence of newly synthesized collagen by what is known as a "healing ridge" just under an intact suture line. When this ridge is not present 5 to 7 days after suturing, suspect slowed collagen synthesis.

The wound that is healing by primary intention should be protected from further trauma: kept free of pulling forces that stretch the sutured skin, kept clean (but not washed because water carries microorganisms into the wound along the sutures), protected from the external environment and drainage with dressings, and kept free from pressure. Dressings are applied using a sterile technique, but sterile gloves are usually not required. Hold the side of the dressing that will not touch the client's incision by the clean gloved hands and tape it in place. The type of dressing used will change as the wound responds to treatment. Use dressings that best suit the wound. Gauze dressings are the most common dressing used on a wound healing by primary intention. Dressings for open wounds are discussed in the following section.

Wound drainage tubes can be placed in the dead space created during surgery. Drainage of a wound is indicated when actual or potential fluid accumulation threatens the healing process. The drain facilitates removal of blood and bacteria from the wound. Assess the volume and type of fluid hourly immediately after surgery. If a reservoir is attached to the drain, measure the volume of drainage by markings on the reservoir. If the drainage is emptied from the reservoir, universal precautions must be followed for its disposal. In addition, if the drainage is caustic (e.g., bile) the skin around the site must be protected with skin barriers.

Teach the client how to care for the incision, the indications of wound infection, how to care for and empty the drain reservoir, and when to return for suture removal. Sutures in areas where scarring must be controlled (e.g., the face) are usually removed in 4 to 7 days; in other areas, sutures are usually removed in 7 to 10 days. Sutures in the hand and foot are removed in 1 to 2 weeks or more.

Management of the Client with Open Wounds

Acute and Subacute Care

■ Medical Management

The goal of management is to prepare the wound from the quickest and most durable form of healing. Clients with open wounds often have other problems, such as venous insufficiency and diabetes. These disorders decrease blood flow (and thereby oxygen) into the wound and delay healing. Medical management may include the use of oxygen and vasodilators to restore arterial flow, elevation to promote venous drainage, and antibiotics to reduce infection, based on the client's needs. The client's diet should be high in carbohydrates, protein, iron, and vitamins because all of these nutrients are required for wound healing. In addition, the client may remain at risk of further skin breakdown, such as pressure ulcers. Institute frequent assessment of pressure ulcer risk (see Chapter 80).

Some basic guidelines can be applied to all wound care.

Removing Devitalized Tissue from the Wound

Wound healing is optimized and the risk of infection is reduced when all necrotic tissue, exudate, and metabolic wastes are removed from the wound. Moist, devitalized tissue supports bacterial growth. Various forms of debridement are used to remove these tissues and are discussed later.

Keeping the Wound Moist

Wound healing is optimized in a moist environment. When the environment is moist, collagen synthesis and granulation tissue formation are enhanced, cell migration and epithelial resurfacing occur more rapidly, and scab, crust, and eschars cannot form. This moist environment, however, does create a medium conducive to infection. Heat lamps or dressings that dry the wound must be avoided.

Applying Safe Topical Agents in the Wound Bed

Avoid applying solutions on and in the wound that impair wound healing. For example, iodine, hydrogen peroxide, and Dakin's solution were once commonly used for wound care. It is now known that these solutions damage the wound. These solutions are toxic to the fibroblast and therefore delay healing. In addition, use of large volumes of iodine in wounds can lead to toxicity from excess iodine absorption.

Normal saline is the only solution recommended by the American Health Care Policy and Research (AHCPR) for wound care such as packing and cleaning. It is physiologic, will not harm tissues, and adequately cleans most wounds. Pressure may be applied to the irrigant for enhanced cleaning. If the wound is covered with adherent material, some solutions have surfactants in them to help clean the wound. Some of these chemicals can harm wound healing cells. If used, it is important to limit their use to as short a time as possible.

Protecting the Surrounding Skin

Moisture on normal, intact skin makes the skin more prone to breakdown. *The cardinal rule is to keep the wound bed moist and surrounding skin dry.* See Figure 20–5 for wound healing in a dry and moist environment. You will note that there is faster migration of epithelial cells on a moist wound bed.

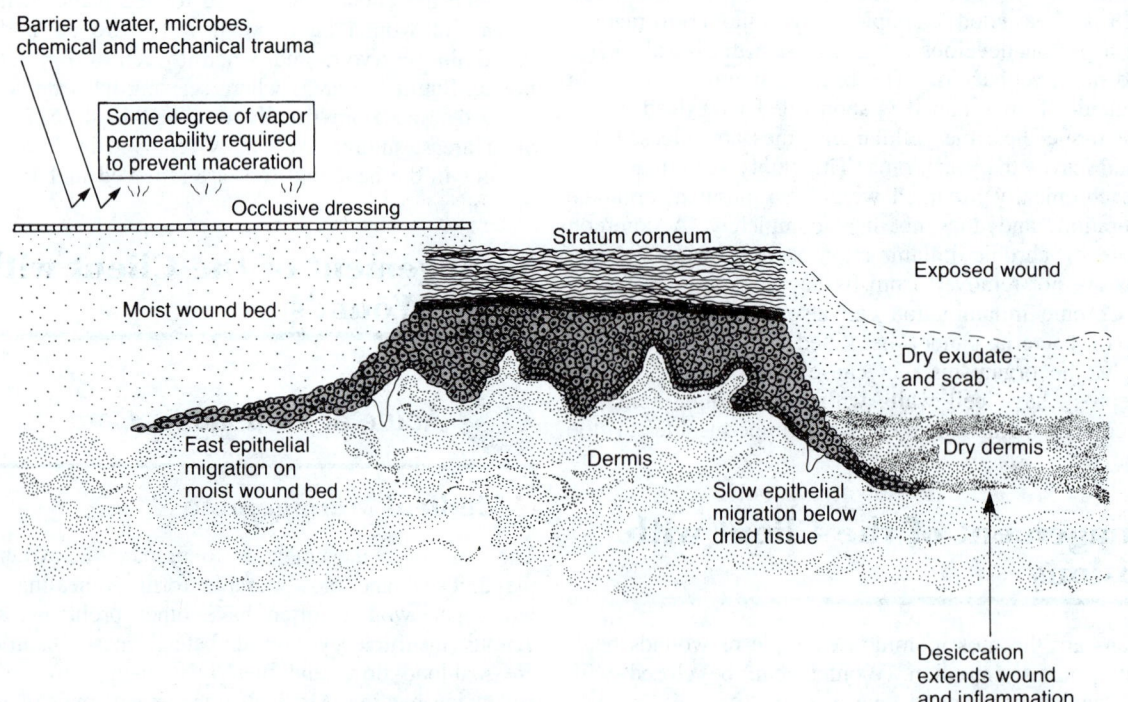

Figure 20–5. Wound healing under an occlusive dressing. (Adapted from Winter, G. D., & Scales, J. T. [1963]. Effect of air drying and dressings on the surface of a wound. *Nature, 197,* 91–92. Copyright 1963 Macmillan Magazines Limited.)

Filling Dead Space

Dead space is potential space within a wound. Dead space in an ulcer is the space between the base of the ulcer and the underside of the dressing around its perimeter. Since the space is closed, anaerobic infection is of concern. Long-acting normal saline gel is a good alternative to fill a clean wound before applying a topical dressing.

Matching the Wound to Its Care

Some wound care specialists advise using a color system as a guide in planning wound care. The colors are black, yellow, and red (Fig. 20–6). The use of colors is a good place to start, but wound care is more complex and many other factors need to be considered, such as nutrition. Many agencies have wound care nurses who should be contacted for up-to-date information and for assistance with complex wounds.

Black Wounds: Sharp Debridement. Black wounds have necrotic tissue and most often need debridement (see Fig. 20–6A). Sometimes this tissue is called an eschar, a term that is used to describe a burn wound. The tissue can also be called *devitalized tissue*. The risk of infection rises in proportion to the amount of necrotic tissue present. Systemic antibiotics seldom stop infection because they cannot penetrate avascular tissues. Topical antibiotics do not penetrate the avascular eschar either. Timely debridement is necessary to remove the eschar and reduce the risk of infection and the physical obstacle to granulation. In addition, the true size of the wound cannot be known until the necrotic tissue is removed.

There is one exception to debridement that should be considered. A black, dry eschar on heels should not be removed. The eschar provides a natural protective cover. If it is removed, there is no subcutaneous tissue to cover the heel and the ulcer usually worsens. Only if the wound becomes edematous, red, fluctuant, or develops drainage should the eschar be removed.

Sharp debridement is the fastest form of debridement and permits immediate treatment of the wound bed after the devitalized tissue is removed. The eschar is removed to the level of red, bleeding tissues. The wound then requires protection to begin healing. The wound size, depth of the wound, contamination, and the client's status influence whether the client is in satisfactory condition to tolerate sharp debridement that may require general anesthesia or sedation. Pain medications should be used for clients who are not taken to the operating room.

Sharp debridement is carried out under sterile conditions, usually in the operating room, treatment room, or an outpatient surgical setting. Risks associated with general anesthesia, blood loss, and infection are of major concern. This procedure is used for a larger wound or a wound that involves a thick eschar that could not be permeated by any topical agent, and for wounds that are acutely infected.

Following sharp debridement, the client is monitored for signs of bleeding and bacteremia (or sepsis). Sepsis is

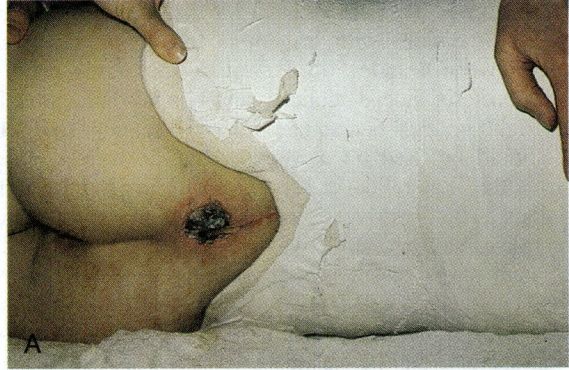
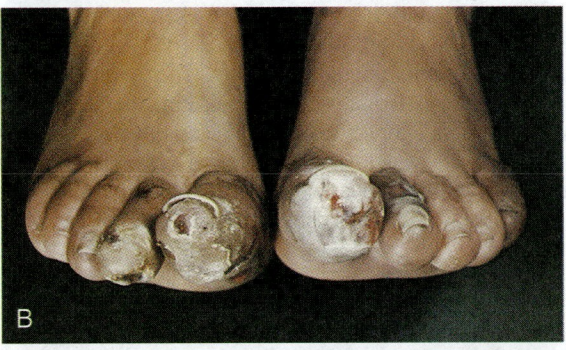
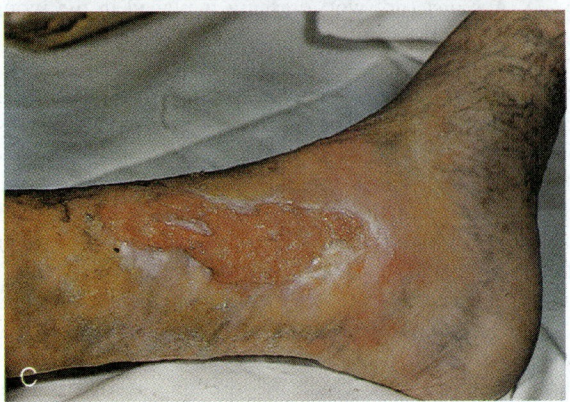

Figure 20–6. *A,* A "black wound" on the sacrum that needs debridement. *B,* Diabetic foot ulcers are an example of a yellow wound covered with soft slough that needs cleaning. *C,* Healing venous stasis ulcers have a red wound filled with granulation tissue that needs protection.

suspected if the client develops unexplained fever, tachycardia, hypotension, or deterioration in mental status. The physician should be notified of these changes. Usually blood cultures are taken and the client is started on a broad-spectrum antibiotic. Sepsis can be fatal if not recognized early and treated aggressively (see the discussion of septic shock in Chapter 22).

Yellow Wounds. Wounds that are yellow require cleaning (see Fig. 20–6B). Yellow wounds are covered with sloughy, necrotic material. Before a wound can heal, necrotic (devitalized) tissue must be removed. Debridement can be accomplished by using a variety of techniques: mechanical, enzymatic, and autolytic. This is in addition to sharp debridement.

Mechanical Debridement. Mechanical debridement includes treatments with irrigations and dressings. Irrigations, between 4 and 15 lb per square inch (psi), remove debris, bacteria, and necrotic tissue without damaging tissue. Eight pounds per square inch is the most pressure that should be used on a wound. High-pressure devices, such as the Water Pik, create too much force and trauma and may actually drive bacteria into the wound. Wound irrigation is safe and effective with a 35-ml syringe and a 19F angiocatheter (outer plastic tubing from an intravenous [IV] needle). This device provides 8 psi of force and removes most devitalized tissue. Hydrotherapy is also an option for wound cleaning.

Barrier precautions need to be taken with masks or goggles, gowns, and gloves because the nurse may be sprayed by contaminated solutions. The client may also need protection. Irrigation with pulsating devices is contraindicated in clients with wounds of the neck, eyes, or dura and in those with exposed blood vessels. To prevent further contamination of adjacent tissues, pressure should not be increased beyond the prescribed level.

Wet-to-Dry Dressings. Mechanical debridement can also be accomplished by using wet-to-dry dressings (Fig. 20–7). A moist (not wet) dressing is placed in the wound and held in place by an outer dressing or gauze wrap. The inner dressing is allowed to dry and then removed. As the dressing dries, debris, necrotic tissue, exudate, and drainage adhere to it. The wound is debrided as the dressing is gently removed. The wet dressing is obtained by saturating an all-gauze dressing with the prescribed solution and wringing the dressing out until it is just moist. The moist dressing should be placed in the wound and left long enough to begin to dry (usually 4–6 hours). Caution is needed so that normal (or high-risk) tissue on the edges of the wound are not made moist by the dressing. Topical skin protectants can be used to protect surrounding intact skin. Once the dressing is dry it is removed along with adherent tissues. The dressings are not remoistened to make removal easier because this practice defeats the purpose of the dressing, which is to debride the wound. The process is often painful and clients

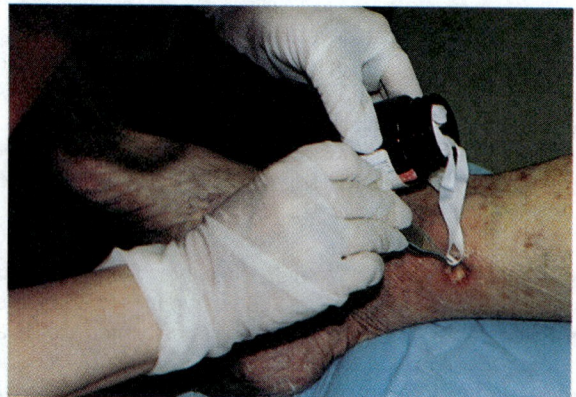

Figure 20–7. Wet-to-dry dressings being placed onto a wound using strip gauze.

should have adequate analgesia before changing the dressing. Wet-to-dry dressings are a nonselective form of debridement and can remove new granulation tissues as well as necrotic tissue, creating an environment that retards healing. Therefore, they are used only until the wound is clean and granulating.

Wet-to-Moist Dressings. Wet-to-moist or continuously moist dressings are used in clean and granulating wounds. Insert dressings into or place onto the wound while moist, again making certain to protect normal intact skin. Remove the dressings while still moist to avoid disrupting the granular bed. Bleeding should not occur when the dressing is removed. If the dressing is too dry to pull off, moisten it with sterile normal saline before attempting to remove it.

Wound Packing. Deep wounds with channels are at high risk of infection. These wounds can also heal with "false floors," which trap bacteria and lead to further infection. It is important that an open wound heal from the inside out.

Deep wounds are often packed with saline or gauze strips soaked in an antibiotic solution to debride the wound or prevent abnormal healing. Strips of gauze must be used to avoid having soiled dressings lost in the wound. The gauze is packed into the wound with enough force to hold the edges of the wound open but not so much force that the wound is under tension. Wounds packed too tightly compromise blood flow and delay healing. The outer edge of the dressing is covered with dry dressings. Packing is changed every 4 to 6 hours in most clients. Some gel packing strips are changed less often. Skin surrounding the wound should be assessed for breakdown from frequent tape removal, and dressings should be secured with other methods if needed (e.g., Montgomery straps).

Enzymatic Debridement. To avoid the risk of damaging new tissue growth, which is often experienced with wet-to-dry dressings, chemical agents such as enzymes offer nonsurgical options. Enzymatic agents are expensive and require diligent care. There are three available today: collagenase (Santyl), sutilains (Travase), and fibrinolysin-desoxyribonuclease (Elase). Collagenase and Travase convert denatured proteins to peptides and amino acids. Elase causes fibrin lysis. These agents cannot be used on wounds communicating with major body cavities, wounds with exposed nerves, or neoplastic ulcers. They must be used with caution around the eyes. The AHCPR recommends the use of collagenase. It was the only agent studied for wound care.

A dry eschar should be scored (have small cuts made into it) before the enzymatic ointment is applied. Scoring enhances penetration. The wound surface must be kept moist for the agent to work. The ointment is used until the eschar separates from the wound surface. These agents require frequent dressing changes and must be used only on necrotic tissue. They are usually only applied to about 2 to 4 square inches of necrotic tissue at one time. Medicate clients prior to the use of enzymatic agents; they cause burning.

Autolytic Debridement. Autolytic debridement uses the client's WBCs to destroy necrotic tissues. This form of debridement is the slowest but is well suited to clients who cannot tolerate other forms of debridement. Moisture-retentive dressings are a common method of autolytic debridement. The dressing is placed over the wound and allowed to remain in place for about 4 days. Several types of dressings can be used. The occlusion created by the dressing hastens the separation of the necrotic tissue by keeping enzymes normally present in wound fluid in intimate contact with the wound surface to lyse dead tissue. Autolytic debridement is contraindicated if the ulcer is infected, has tunneling, or is undermining, because the occlusive dressing can promote the growth of anaerobes.

It is important to inform caregivers that it is normal for a creamy fluid to develop beneath the dressing, and that this sign does not mean the ulcer is infected.

Red Wounds. Wounds that are red require protection (see Fig. 20–6C). Red wounds are filled with granulation tissue and are beginning to heal. These wounds should not be treated with lotions, ointments, or soaps because they may irritate or infect the area. Topical vasodilators can be used to stimulate capillary flow to the wound but require a physician's order. If the wound is shallow, a thin layer of antibiotic ointment and a nonadhering dressing (or synthetic dressing) is used to cover it. If the wound is deep, saline-moistened gauze can be used to pack the wound, but the dressing should not be allowed to dry out before changing it. A dried dressing removes the granulation tissue and new epithelium. If a wound is healing, the wound should be kept moist to facilitate healing.

Closing the Wound

Once the wound is clean, surgery may be used to speed healing and reduce the risk of infection and contracture. Skin grafts are commonly used to replace the epidermis. The partial-thickness burn wound is the best example of a wound that could heal by secondary intention but is often grafted to speed healing and reduce infection and scarring. Cutaneous or musculocutaneous flaps can also be used to close a large wound (see Chapter 80).

■ Nursing Management of the Medical Client

Assessment

The history of the present illness should include how long the client has had the wound, the client's beliefs about the causes and contributing factors of the wound, previous methods used in treatment, and degree of success. Sometimes wound treatments are used that actually impair healing, such as hydrogen peroxide or Dakin's solution, or that do not match the type of wound.

The nursing history should include information about the client's medical history, previous surgery, current and past medications (especially steroids), nutritional state (What type of diet has the client been eating? Any supplements?), serum glucose if diabetic, smoking, degree of immobility, level of continence, circulatory status, and presence of infection. It is important to recognize that many factors can lead to impaired wound healing. Assessments should be thorough and focus on the whole client, not just the wound.

Psychosocial assessment should include the client's age, occupation, living situation, financial status, healthcare benefits, roles and responsibilities, cultural and spiritual beliefs, body image and self-esteem, and the ability of the client to learn self-care and comply with the treatment plan. Compliance with underlying disorders, such as diabetes or collagen diseases, should also be noted.

A complete physical assessment should be performed. Focus data collection on height and weight; degree of range of motion; muscle wasting and level of activity; circulation, such as peripheral pulses, color, edema, and the temperature of extremities; lung sounds; and level of pain. The wound requires complete assessment (Box 20–1). Data about the wound should be documented clearly to allow for objective evaluation at a later date. It is

---

Box 20–1. Wound Assessment

When assessing an open wound, be certain to obtain the following information:

1. What is the size of the wound? Use objective measures to indicate the length and width (such as centimeters or millimeters). Avoid terms such as "the size of a grape." Use a sterile gloved finger or cotton swab to measure depth. Consider using photographs to provide a baseline and serial evaluations.
2. Where is the wound located anatomically?
3. What is the color of the wound? Give an estimate of the percentage of each color when more than one color is noted.
4. Is there granulation tissue or epithelial tissue? Granulation tissue is red, shiny, and bumpy; epithelial tissue looks like pale skin.
5. Are there sinus tracts or are the edges undermined? Use a gloved hand or swab to measure the extent. Indicate the location and direction of tunneling.
6. Are there signs of infection in the wound? Look for erythema extending beyond the edges of the wound, as well as warmth, edema, odor, and purulent exudate. (Consider systemic signs also.)
7. Is there any drainage? Note the color, odor, consistency, and approximate amount by the number of dressings saturated.
8. What is the condition of the surrounding skin? Is it intact, red, indurated, or macerated?
9. Is the wound painful?

Data from Faller, N., & Lawrence, K. (1991). Nursing to promote healing. *Ostomy/Wound Management, 32*(1), 43–46, 48; and Cuzzell, J. (1988). The new RYB color code. *American Journal of Nursing, 88*(10), 1342–1346.

helpful to describe the actual size of the ulcer by measuring the longest and widest areas, its depth, color, type of drainage, presence of undermining, and condition of periwound skin in the assessment data for later comparison. A photograph is an excellent means of documentation and determination of progress in healing. Consent must be obtained before photographs are taken.

The nurse should also examine the laboratory values for hemoglobin, hematocrit, albumin, and WBCs, specifically lymphocytes. These values indicate the degree of nutritional impairment that may be contributing to the wound's lack of healing. Generally, the risk of delayed healing correlates with low serum albumin levels. However, albumin levels are a slow-to-change indicator of nutritional state.

Diagnosis, Planning, Implementation

Impaired Skin Integrity. The nursing diagnosis of impaired skin integrity should be used to indicate an actual loss of skin. The actual statement might be phrased *Impaired Skin Integrity related to delayed wound healing secondary to impaired circulation, or to infection, or to malnutrition.*

Planning: Expected Outcomes. The client will have improvement in skin integrity, as evidenced by a cleaner wound within 1 week and no signs of infection in the wound. A long-term goal might be that the client will have a smaller wound in 3 weeks.

Implementation. The treatment of a wound includes the removal of its cause(s), the correction of underlying problems that are delaying healing, and the initiation of topical (or systemic) treatments to facilitate healing. If the client is immobile or incontinent, adequate prevention must be given to reduce the incidence of new areas of skin breakdown. If wound healing is delayed because of lack of venous return, the leg will require elevation. If the cause of the wound is lack of arterial flow, it should be positioned flat. Disorders such as diabetes mellitus and cardiovascular disease should be controlled as well as possible. The wound's appearance should be used as a guide in planning interventions (see earlier discussion).

Choosing Dressings. Gauze dressings still remain the most cost-effective dressing. Gauze is used as a dry cover for surgical wounds or wounds that heal by primary intention (Table 20–4). Wet-to-dry gauze dressings can be used for nonselective debridement of wounds. More absorbent dressings should be used with exudative wounds. Only mesh gauze dressings should be used in a wound. Use cotton-filled gauze as an outer dressing.

If the wound edges are friable or if the wound will be disrupted when the dressing is removed, a nonadherent dressing can be used. The nonadherent dressing can be impregnated or nonimpregnated. The intent of this dressing choice is that when it is removed, the disruption of the wound bed will be minimal.

Excessive exudate can delay healing. If the wound produces exudate, several absorption dressing products can be used. Absorptive dressings, calcium alginates, and hypertonic saline dressings can be used. Foams can also be used for absorption and autolytic debridement. Table 20–

4 describes the actions, indications, and nursing implications for various categories of wound dressings.

The selection of dressing type will change as the wound responds to treatment. Careful assessment and reassessment will indicate progress, or lack of progress, in wound healing. As the wound changes, variations in the dressing materials are made so that healing is maximized. There is no single dressing that provides the optimal atmosphere required during all healing stages of the wound.

Providing Nutritional Support. In addition to local wound care, the client must be provided with a diet that is high in protein, fat, carbohydrates, vitamins, and minerals to facilitate healing. Regardless of the client's actual body weight (e.g., obese), this is not the time to begin a weight loss diet. The wound must be healed first. If the client cannot or will not eat, the use of tube feeding or hyperalimentation should be considered.

Providing Pressure Control. If the client has pressure ulcers, pressure reduction is key to management and prevention. If the client has venous stasis ulcers or lymphadema, use graded pressure wraps. The specifics on the management of these ulcers may be found in Chapter 50.

Evaluation

Wound healing should be assessed every 24 hours, especially if the risk of infection remains high. If the wound shows no signs of healing after 2 weeks, AHCPR suggests a 2-week trial of topical antibiotics. If no healing occurs after another 2 weeks, AHCPR advises quantitative bacterial cultures to evaluate for infection and a bone scan to assess for osteomyelitis.

Community and Self-Care

The client with open wounds requires long-term care or community resources for safe self-care. Planning for discharge should begin several days before discharge so that the home situation can be appraised and necessary supplies and equipment obtained. Appropriate referral to the home health agency or wound healing clinic should be made. Social services, home healthcare, or a discharge planner should be involved in the plan of care. Financial status, home environment, and support systems must be evaluated. Third-party reimbursement may cover supplies, equipment, and nursing care.

Several areas of client education are needed. The client or family should demonstrate dressing removal, wound cleaning, and dressing application before discharge. Detailed written instructions should be provided to the client, family, and home healthcare nurse on wound care. The client also needs to understand what changes should be expected and what changes should be reported to the healthcare provider. Fever, change in drainage, or development of odorous drainage should be seen as reportable. If the client has a pressure ulcer, obtain a copy of *Treating Pressure Sores,* AHCPR publication number 95–0654 from the AHCPR, at 1–800–358–9295.

Table 20–4. Indications and Implications of Wound Dressings

Type of Dressing	Product	Indications for Use	Nursing Implications
Nonadhering Nonimpregnated	Telfa	Shallow open wounds	Require a second dressing or tape because they are nonadhesive
Impregnated	Adaptic gauze, Vaseline gauze, Xeroform	Moist wounds	Nonabsorbent, occlusive, not traumatic to remove
Gauze	Adaptic gauze, Kling gauze, Nu-Gauze, Primapore	Wet-to-dry debridement, wound packing	Moderately absorbent; can be used as wound packing for shallow wounds; use long strips of gauze to pack deep wounds. Gauze does not provide a bacterial barrier; if allowed to dry on a wound, it may remove viable tissue when removed
Transparent films	Bio-occlusive, Op-Site, Tegaderm	Coverage of shallow wounds (skin tears), intravenous sites, blisters, abrasions	Adhesive; therefore, no secondary dressing is needed; retain moisture, semipermeable, water-resistant; facilitate autolytic debridement
Hydrocolloids	Comfeel, Duoderm, Intrasite, Restore, Tegasorb, Intact, ulcer dressing	Shallow ulcers, as will provide autolytic debridement; donor sites; second-degree partial-thickness burns	Retain moisture, occlusive or semipermeable, water-resistant, adhesive; require replacement because the dressing melts; reduce pain
Hydrogels	Elastogel, wound gel, Spenco, Vigilon	Pressure ulcers, dermal ulcers, partial-thickness burns, abrasions, blisters	Hydrogels having cooling effect: maintain moist environment, relieve pain, permit autolytic debridement; easily removed unless they dry out
Exudate absorbers	Bard absorption dressing, Envisan	Deep wounds with eschar	Retain moisture, absorbent, promote autolytic debridement
Calcium alginates	Sorbsan, Kaltistat, Algiderm	Clean wounds with profuse drainage	Retain moisture, absorbent, left intact for several days

The average cost of skilled nursing services for treating wounds in the home was found to be $1600 per healed wound. Some cost-cutting measures for saline and gloves have been designed: It is possible to make normal saline for home use on wounds. Use this recipe: to 1 gal of distilled water or 1 gal of tap water boiled for 5 minutes (do not use well water or sea water), add 8 tsp of table salt. Mix the solution well before use. Cool to room temperature before use. This solution can be stored for up to 1 week.

In the home, rather than purchasing gloves for dressing changes, soiled dressings can be removed with a plastic sandwich bag (Fig. 20–8). The inside of the bag is used as a "glove" to remove the dressing, and the dressing is disposed of in the same bag. Methods of obtaining needed wound care supplies should also be discussed with the client and family.

The client should be alerted to signs of complications, such as infection, and given directions on when and how to contact the healthcare provider. A balanced diet with frequent high protein snacks should continue. A vitamin and mineral supplement should be taken as directed. The client may need to incorporate life-style changes into activities of daily living in an effort to promote healing.

Disorders of Wound Healing

Delayed Wound Healing

Nonhealing wounds result from the impairment of one or more of the normal processes of wound healing. These processes have been classified as intrinsic (factors within the wound) or extrinsic (factors outside of the wound).

Intrinsic Factors. When a wound is infected, the inflammatory response is prolonged and healing is delayed. Wounds will not heal while infection is present.

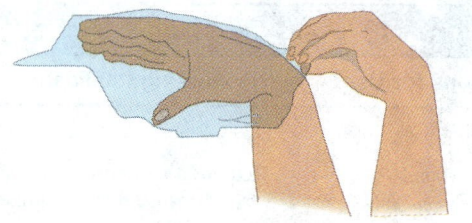

Place a small, clean bag over your hand like a mitten.

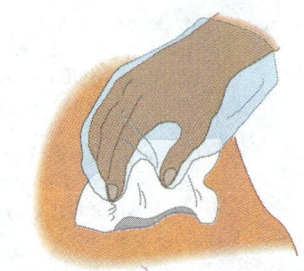

Carefully lift the dressing off the sore.

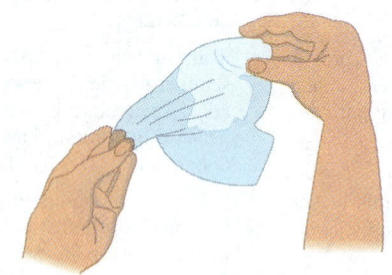

Turn the bag inside out to enclose the dressing.

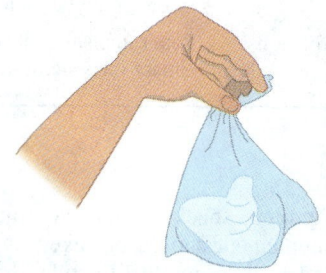

Seal the bag before throwing it away.

Figure 20–8. Plastic bags used as gloves to remove a dressing in the home. (Adapted from *Treating pressure sores.* Copyright 1994. U. S. Department of Health and Human Services, AHCPR Publication No. 95–0654.)

Infection can develop when the defense mechanisms are weakened, thus allowing a normal bacterial load to become overwhelming. Alternatively, the bacterial load can be greater than the body's defenses can handle. In healthy clients, the critical number is 100,000 bacteria per gram of tissue. This number is expressed as 10^5 on laboratory cultures of wounds (and other body fluids or tissues). This threshold number for bacteria holds true for all kinds

of bacteria except for group B streptococcus, which can cause infection in lesser quantities. Above that number, the body loses control over bacterial proliferation and invasion. Infection is present. The diagnosis of infection is through quantitative wound biopsy cultures. This requires 24 to 48 hours and the client is given a broad-spectrum antibiotic while awaiting results. Sometimes, foreign bodies within the wound are a source of infection. Examples include soil, hematomas (accumulations of blood) and bone fragments.

An adequate blood supply is essential for all aspects of wound healing. The blood supply can be restricted through disorders of the heart, vessels, or lungs. Hypoxia impairs delivery of oxygen and nutrients to the wound, and the action of the various defensive cells. Neutrophils require oxygen to generate hydrogen peroxide to kill the pathogens. Likewise, fibroblast and collagen proliferation are slowed. The only aspect of wound healing that can proceed in hypoxic states is angiogenesis.

Extrinsic Factors. Extrinsic factors that delay wound healing include malnutrition, changes associated with aging, and disorders like diabetes. Malnutrition can have an impact on several areas of the healing process. Protein malnutrition decreases synthesis of collagen and leukocytes. Fat and carbohydrate malnutrition slows all phases of healing because protein is broken down for energy during malnutrition. Vitamin deficiency leads to slowed production of collagen, immune responses, and coagulation responses.

The elderly client has decreased initial inflammatory responses, which slows the process of healing. The aged client may have decreased circulation, which delays WBC migration to the site and phagocytosis. In addition, the client may be malnourished and have concurrent disorders that retard healing, such as diabetes mellitus.

Diabetes is a disorder that predisposes many clients to difficulty in wound healing because of impaired collagen synthesis, angiogenesis, and phagocytosis. Elevated glucose levels interfere with cellular transport of ascorbic acid into various cells, including fibroblasts and leukocytes. Hyperglycemia also decreases leukocyte chemotaxis. Atherosclerosis, especially of small vessels, is also common in diabetes and impairs tissue oxygen delivery. Diabetic neuropathy further impairs healing by interrupting the neurologic components of healing (e.g., reducing vasodilation and the protective sensation of pain). Control of glucose levels after surgery facilitates normal wound healing.

Smoking causes vasoconstriction and hypoxia because of the carbon monoxide in the smoke. In addition to limiting oxygen supply, smoking increases atherosclerosis and platelet aggregation. These conditions further restrict the amount of oxygen in the wound.

The use of steroids slows healing by inhibiting collagen synthesis. Clients who are taking steroids have decreased wound strength, inhibited contraction, and impeded epithelialization. Fortunately, vitamin A has been shown to reverse the healing impairments caused by steroids.

Wound Infection

Wound infection is a serious consequence and delays wound healing. Topical antimicrobials can be used as the primary treatment. In addition, it is important to be certain that infected tissues are adequately perfused and oxygenated. This assists with delivery of WBCs to the area. Clinical manifestations of wound infection include increased drainage, erythema around the entire wound (not just the edges), development of purulent drainage, pain, fever, leukocytosis, and general malaise. The infected wound is slow to heal and may open (such as evisceration or dehiscence). Cultures can be used to diagnose wound infection. A swab culture can be obtained of wound drainage. A quantitative culture (an actual sample of tissue) is usually needed to study open wounds. All open wounds are colonized and using a swab culture on these wounds will not reveal the true offending organisms, only organisms growing harmlessly on the wound's surface.

The ideal antimicrobial would be broad-spectrum and preserve the regenerating tissues. But all of the antimicrobials compromise wound healing to some degree by being low in effectiveness against a particular organism or by interfering with healing. A variety of topical agents can be used to either clean or disinfect the wound. Table 20–5 describes some cleaning, antiseptic, and antibacterial agents that may be used. A word of caution on the use of disinfectants: they may retard healing and destroy tissue growth.

Hydrogen peroxide breaks down into water and oxygen. When it is used in a wound, it must be rinsed thoroughly with normal saline to remove any trapped oxygen before it can be absorbed by the tissues. Providone-iodine, acetic acid, and sodium hypochlorite are used only in debris-contaminated, infected, and malodorous wounds. These agents are cytotoxic and inhibit granular tissue growth and damage endothelial cells and fibroblasts.

■ Medical Management

Most chronic nonhealing wounds are managed by a team of healthcare providers that may include a wound care physician, vascular or orthopedic surgeons, wound care nurse, nutritionist, physical therapist, hyperbaric medicine specialists, and social workers and psychologists. Even for these teams, chronic nonhealing wounds are a challenge.

Table 20–5. Topical Agents Used in Treatment of Open Wounds		
Agent	**Indications**	**Impact on Wound Healing**
Antiseptic Solutions		
Normal saline	Used to moisten dry eschar; keep a clean wound healing by secondary intention	Speeds healing because solution is iso-osmolar, and it keeps the wound bed moist
Hydrogen peroxide	Used to dissolve clotted blood in a wound	Retards healing; do not use as a dressing on an open wound
Providone-iodine (Betadine)	Used for preparation of intact skin; may be used to clean very contaminated wounds	Retards healing; does not penetrate eschar
Dakin's solution	Used ¼ to ½ strength to clean contaminated wounds	Retards wound healing
Acetic acid	Used to treat wounds contaminated with *Pseudomonas*	Retards wound healing slightly
Antibiotic Solutions and Ointments		
Neomycin-bacitracin-polymyxin B (Neosporin)	Used to clean wounds contaminated with gram-negative and gram-positive bacteria	Increases epidermal healing but may sensitize tissues; high incidence of allergy
Polysporin	Treatment of gram-negative organisms	None known
Silver sulfadiazine	Used in wounds with eschar (e.g., burns); effective against gram-negative and gram-positive organisms	Enhances epidermal healing; penetrates eschar
Gentamicin	Most effective against gram-negative organisms, but its use may promote resistance in hospital flora	None known
Bacitracin	Effective against gram-positive and gram-negative organisms	May enhance epidermal healing

The focus of care is to fully examine the extrinsic and intrinsic factors that led to nonhealing. Not all of these factors can be eliminated, however. Clients cannot be made younger, and some clients refuse to stop smoking, even though their nonhealing is due to inadequate circulation. At times, bypass surgery may be required to restore adequate blood flow. Cultured epithelial grafts and hyperbaric oxygen are relatively new treatments in the care of nonhealing wounds. Wound healing accelerators, such as topically applied growth factors and electric currents, are being studied.

Chronic wounds are common in several groups of clients. Clients with diabetes, venous or arterial disease of the legs, and collagen diseases (such as scleroderma) commonly do not heal quickly or completely. There are several forms of adjunctive treatment for these wounds. They are discussed only briefly here.

Electric Stimulation

Pulsed galvanic stimulation (Diapulse) is a form of electricity applied to the skin's surface. The electric currents have been shown to stimulate DNA synthesis, increase blood flow, enhance fibroblast proliferation, and promote cell migration across the wound. It appears to be effective in promoting healing in wounds that have been refractory to other forms of treatment. Clients who are considering the use of electrotherapy should seek centers that have proper equipment and trained personnel.

Hyperbaric Oxygen Therapy

Hyperbaric oxygen (HBO) is the administration of oxygen at greater than atmospheric pressure. Oxygen is greatly increased in tissues, which promotes the growth of new vessels, fibroblast activity, collagen synthesis, and phagocytic action. HBO has been effective in managing complex wounds, especially those with osteomyelitis and other types of infection. HBO is available at only a few centers in the United States. Like electric stimulation, a properly trained staff is critical. Clients who are claustrophobic or have inner ear problems are usually not able to undergo HBO treatments.

Topical Application of Growth Factors

The same growth factors that are found in the wound bed naturally can be grown in a laboratory and applied to the wound bed. The efficacy of these treatments is still being studied.

■ Nursing Management of the Medical Client

The nurse's role in the care of the client with a nonhealing wound is to provide ample information for self-care. This includes a full understanding of how to change dressings, information on the disease process underlying the wound, and how to return to work or activities without increasing the risk of nonhealing. For example, a woman with venous stasis ulcers may need to return to

work, but can return to work safely only when the ulcer is healed. She also needs to know how to apply bandages, the time for elevating her legs while at work, and how to move her legs while working (such as walking rather than standing). The nurse serves a vital role in determining if these requirements are feasible for the client and employer.

Wound Disruption

Dehiscence is the interruption of a previously intact suture line (see Chapter 21). It is frequently preceded by the client experiencing a sharp pain in the suture line, or a cough and increased serosanguineous drainage from the wound. *Evisceration* is the opening of a wound with exposure of internal organs. It is obviously more serious than dehiscence. If a client experiences evisceration, the nurse should cover the exposed organs with sterile wet dressings, notify the physician, and prepare the client for surgery. The physician should also be notified about dehiscence, but it is not an emergency.

Altered Collagen Synthesis

Hypertrophic scars are scars that are raised above the suture line. They may be painful and itch. In general, hypertrophic scars tend to regress over time. Keloids are scars that extend well beyond the suture line (Fig. 20–9). These scars tend to occur in black clients and clients from the Mediterranean region. They can be excised from a wound but unfortunately tend to recur.

Conclusions

Wound healing is a complex process but often goes on with little effort on the part of the client. It is only when the wound does not heal or pressure ulcers develop, that the many steps in wound healing are evident. Wound care follows some basic principles: debride the wound of nonviable tissues, keep the wound bed moist, protect the surrounding skin, apply the proper dressings, use safe topical agents, and fill dead space.

Thinking Critically

1. You are caring for a man with large venous stasis ulcers on his lower legs. When he was admitted the ulcers were covered with soft yellow devitalized tissue. He has been treated with wet-to-dry dressings for the past 7 days. Today you notice that the ulcers are red and wet with a lumpy appearance. What should be done?

Factors to Consider. Is the appearance of red and lumpy tissue in a wound good or bad? What might be happening? What type of dressing is best used on this red and lumpy tissue?

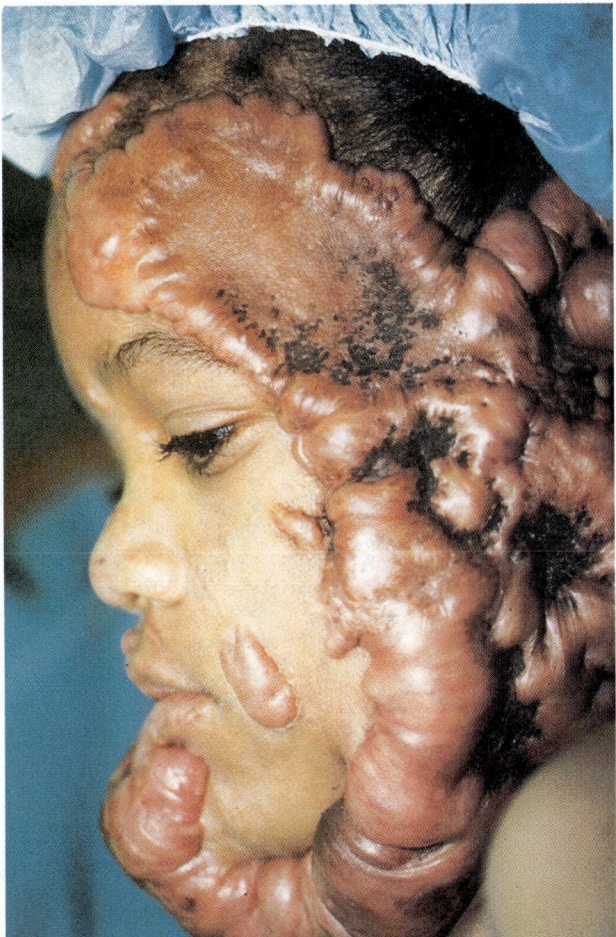

Figure 20–9. Keloid formation. Keloids are overgrowth of scar tissue above and beyond the normal boundaries of the scar. They are fairly resistant to treatment.

2. You are caring for an elderly homeless man after emergency abdominal surgery. He has had a nasogastric tube in place for 3 days for ileus and is receiving 1 L of intravenous fluids of 5% dextrose with 0.45 normal saline with 20 mEq of potassium every 8 hours. Prior to surgery his serum albumin was 3.2 g/dL, hemoglobin 9.6 g/dL, and WBCs 17,000/mm³. His weight was 104 lbs and height 5′5″. What are this client's chances of recovery? What interventions should be considered?

Factors to Consider. Does this client have evidence of malnutrition? If so, what effect does malnutrition have on wound healing? What short- and long-term interventions may need to be initiated? Does this client have a risk of fluid or electrolyte imbalance? If so, which ones and what can be done (or is being done) to reduce the risk?

Bibliography

1. Alvarez, O., Mertz, P., & Eaglestein, W. (1983). The effect of occlusive dressings on collagen synthesis and reepithelialization in superficial wounds. *Journal of Surgical Research, 35,* 142.
2. Alvarez, O., Rozint, J., & Wiseman, D. (1989). Moist environment for healing: Matching the dressing to the wound. *Wounds: A Compendium of Clinical Research and Practice 1*(1), 35–51.
3. Alper, J. C., et al. (1983). Moist wound healing under a vapor permeable membrane. *Journal of the Academy of Dermatology, 8*(3), 347–353.
4. Arnold, N. (1992). A study of wound healing in home care. *Ostomy/Wound Management, 38*(7), 38–44.
5. Bergstrom, N., et al. (1994). *Treatment of Pressure Ulcers.* Clinical Practice Guideline, No. 15. Rockville, MD, U.S. Department of Health and Human Services. Public Health Service, Agency for Health Care Policy and Research. AHCPR Publication No. 95–0652.
6. Black, S. (1995). Venous stasis ulcers. *Ostomy/Wound Management, 41*(8), 20–32.
7. Brown, S. (1990). Behind the numbers on the CBC. *RN, 53*(2), 46–51.
8. Bryant, R. A. (1992). *Acute and chronic wounds: Nursing management.* St. Louis: Mosby–Year Book.
9. Cooper, D. (1995). Indicies to include in wound assessment. *Advances in Wound Care, 8*(4), 18–25.
10. Cooper, D. (1990). Optimizing wound healing. *Nursing Clinics of North America, 25*(1), 165–180.
11. Curtis, A., et al. (1990). Hyperbaric oxygen therapy—an overview. *Plastic Surgical Nursing, 10*(2), 63–68.
12. Cuzzell, J. (1988). The new RYB color code. *American Journal of Nursing, 88*(10), 1342–1346.
13. Falanga, V., et. al. (1995). Experimental approaches to chronic wounds. *Wound Repair and Regeneration, 3*(2), 132–140.
14. Faller, N., & Lawrence, K. (1991). Nursing to promote healing. *Ostomy/Wound Management, 32*(1), 43–46, 48.
15. Gentzkow, G. D. (1992). Electrical stimulation for dermal wound healing. *Wounds: A Compendium of Clinical Research and Practice, 4*(6), 227–235.
16. Goss, R. (1992). Regeneration versus repair. In I. Cohen, et al. (Eds.), *Wound healing.* Philadelphia: W. B. Saunders.
17. Hotter, A. (1990). Wound healing and immunocompromise. *Nursing Clinics of North America, 25*(1), 193–203.
18. Jones, P., & Milliman, A. (1990). Wound healing and the aged patient. *Nursing Clinics of North America, 25*(1), 263–277.
19. Kerstein, M., & Polsky, S. (1995). Wounds associated with decreased sensibility. *Wounds: A Compendium of Clinical Research and Practice, 7*(1), 30–34.
20. Krasner, D. (1991). Resolving the dressing dilemma: Selecting wound dressings by category. *Ostomy/Wound Management, 35*(4), 62, 64–70.
21. Lawrence, W. (1992). Clinical management of nonhealing wounds. In I. Cohen, et al. (Eds.). *Wound healing.* Philadelphia: W. B. Saunders.
22. Lee, R. C., Canaday, D. J., & Doong, H. (1993). A review of the biophysical basis for the clinical application of electric fields in soft-tissue repair. *Journal of Burn Care and Rehabilitation, 14*(3), 319–335.
23. Netscher, D., & Clamon, J. (1994). Smoking: Adverse effects on outcomes for plastic surgical patients. *Plastic Surgical Nursing, 14*(4), 205–210.
24. Utley, R. (1992). Nutritional factors associated with wound healing in the elderly. *Ostomy/Wound Management, 38*(3), 22–27.
25. Walter, M. J., et al. (1994). Wound healing and nutritional state in patients undergoing reconstruction. *Wounds: A Compendium of Clinical Research and Practice, 6*(4), 128–131.

Perioperative Nursing

21

Ruth Plotkin Shumaker

Caring for perioperative clients is a challenging and gratifying specialty. Since the mid-1970s, dedicated researchers and practitioners have made tremendous advances in surgical intervention and postoperative care. Surgical procedures and other invasive procedures that were once considered last-resort measures are now routine. Clients no longer spend weeks in bed following surgery, a common practice in the past. Advances in anesthesia and surgical techniques allow clients to recover quickly from surgery and return home to productive lives.

A major change in the past decade has been the emergence of outpatient surgery centers and ambulatory surgery. Estimates vary, but according to some market analysts, more than 60% of all surgical care is now being provided on an ambulatory basis,[166] a development that is changing the focus of nursing care. Knowledge of the nursing process, technical skills, and responsibility for all phases of the client's perioperative experience has become essential to nursing care of the surgical client.

The Philosophy and Practice of Perioperative Nursing

What is perioperative nursing? A *perioperative nurse* is defined as the registered nurse who, using the nursing process, designs, coordinates, and delivers care to meet the identified needs of clients whose protective reflexes or self-care abilities are potentially compromised because they are under the influence of anesthesia during operative or other invasive procedures. Perioperative nurses possess and apply knowledge of the procedure and the client's intraoperative experience throughout the client's care continuum. The perioperative nurse assesses, diagnoses, plans, intervenes, and evaluates the outcome of interventions based on criteria and support of a standard of

care targeted toward this population. The perioperative nurse addresses the changing physiologic, pathophysiologic, psychological, sociocultural, and spiritual responses of the client that have been initiated by the prospect or performance of the invasive procedure.[14]

As with most areas of specialized nursing practice, perioperative nursing has adopted a distinctive set of standards of practice. The Association of Operating Room Nurses (AORN) has developed standards of nursing care that provide a basic model by which the quality of nursing practice can be measured for the operative client. The American Nurses Association (ANA) has developed standards of medical-surgical practice that outline standards for the nursing care of the preoperative and postoperative client. The American Association of Nurse Anesthetists (AANA) has developed standards of practice for the nurse-anesthetist. The American Society for Post Anesthesia Nursing (ASPAN) has also developed perioperative standards.

The scope of perioperative nursing practice consists of three phases: (1) preoperative, (2) intraoperative, and (3) postoperative.

Preoperative Phase

The preoperative phase begins when the decision for surgical intervention is made and ends with the transference of the client to the operative suite. Nursing activities range from a baseline assessment of the client during the preoperative interview at the clinic, physician's office, or even over the telephone, and continues with assessment in the preadmission unit, client room, holding area, or induction room on the day of surgery.

Intraoperative Phase

The intraoperative phase begins when the client is transferred to the operating room bed and ends when the client is transferred to an area for recovery from anesthesia. In this phase, nursing interventions range from com-

This chapter incorporates material written for the fourth edition by Maureen B. Barrett.

municating the client's plan of care, identifying nursing activities necessary for expected outcomes, and establishing priorities for nursing actions. Nursing activities are organized in a logical sequence. The perioperative nurse coordinates client needs with team members and personnel from other disciplines, coordinates the use of supplies and equipment, controls the environment, prepares for potential emergencies, and communicates and documents the client's plan of care.

Postoperative Phase

The postoperative phase begins with the client's transfer to an area for recovery and ends with the client's recovery, which usually extends to areas outside of healthcare facilities. Nursing activities range from communicating pertinent information about the client's surgery, to postanesthesia nursing staff, to a postoperative evaluation in the clinic or client's home. The nursing process is applied throughout the entire perioperative period to ensure that the client's physical and emotional needs are met.

Perioperative nurses interact with both the client and the client's significant others throughout the continuum of client care. Perioperative nursing practice takes place in the client's environment and includes, but is not limited to, surgical suites, ambulatory care settings, clinics, physicians' offices, community settings, and homes.

The management of clients' needs, both unique and predictable, may be through direct or indirect interventions. These interventions are planned to assist the client in meeting the projected outcome in an efficient and appropriate manner. Perioperative nursing care is implemented by registered nurses who strive to assist the client to meet projected outcomes by functioning in various roles—clinician, manager, client educator, and researcher.

Perioperative nursing varies and can include the following:

- Staff education and client and family teaching
- Support and reassurance
- Advocacy
- Control of the environment
- Efficient provision of resources
- Maintenance of asepsis
- Monitoring physiologic and psychological status
- Management of aggregate client needs
- Supervision of ancillary personnel
- Perioperative exploration and validation of current and future practices
- Integration and coordination of care across settings and among disciplines through collaboration and consultation

These activities are based on using the problem-solving approach in practice, management, education, and research.

The purpose of perioperative nursing practice is to care for persons undergoing operative and other invasive procedures. Perioperative nursing services are extended to a variety of other groups to enhance the care ultimately provided to the client. These groups include hospitals, clinics, schools and colleges of nursing, physicians, other nurses, insurers, and medical device and pharmaceutical manufacturers.[14]

Experienced perioperative nurses are alert to the emotional turmoil many clients and their significant others experience preoperatively. These nurses recognize that surgery involves expense, discomfort, emotional and physiologic stress, physical alterations, and disruption of the client's life. Nursing assessment and interventions are planned accordingly.

Basic Concepts of Perioperative Nursing

Of old, *surgeons* bored holes in skulls to provide a means "for disease to escape." Modern technology and advances in surgical technique and anesthesia have made procedures such as organ transplants and open heart surgery commonplace.

For many types of surgery, the client is admitted, surgery is performed, and the client is discharged the same day. To decrease the cost of care, infection rate, and client recovery time, many types of surgery are performed in ambulatory care settings (also known as surgicenters, same-day surgery centers, or outpatient surgery centers).

The Goal of Perioperative Nursing Practice

The goal of perioperative nursing practice is to assist clients and their significant others to achieve a level of wellness equal to or greater than that which they had prior to the procedure.

The Role of Perioperative Nurses

The perioperative nurse implements teaching according to measurable criteria.[156] Clients and family teaching should not be delegated or assigned to assistive personnel. Accountability and responsibility for client and family teaching rest with the perioperative nurse. The perioperative nurse is also the advocate for clients under the influence of anesthesia, a time of extreme vulnerability. The perioperative nurse also has specific roles that depend on the phase of care, for example, close physiologic monitoring in the postanesthesia care unit.

Services are extended to a variety of other groups to enhance the care ultimately provided to the client. These groups include but are not limited to hospitals, clinics, schools and colleges of nursing, physicians, other nurses, insurers, and medical device and pharmaceutical manufacturers.

The Recipients of Perioperative Care

The recipients of care are clients and their significant others who vary in age, degree of wellness, cultural background, and socioeconomic and educational status. Clients are those whose protective reflexes or self-care abilities are potentially diminished by the prospect or performance of an operative or other invasive procedure.

Recipients have widely diverse levels of knowledge and capabilities for self-care. They have both predictable and unique needs caused by these procedures. Some needs can be predicted based on the nurse's knowledge of the procedure and the technology to be used; others are unique to the individual.

Stress and the Perioperative Client

Stress must be considered in the care of the perioperative client. Surgery increases stress on all body systems, and stress can be exhibited psychologically or physically. *Stress* is a collective term used to describe the many psychological and physiologic factors that cause neurochemical changes within the body.

Stressors in the perioperative client include pain, tissue damage, blood loss, anesthesia, fever, and immobilization. The stressful stimuli imposed by surgery promote the stress response by combining both psychological (anxiety, fear of unknown) and physiologic (blood loss, anesthesia, pain, immobility) factors.

In response to the stress of surgery, the body mobilizes its defenses to maintain homeostasis. The systemic responses to surgical stress are outlined in Table 21–1. The success of the stress response in maintaining homeostatic balance is determined by a person's age, physical condition, and the duration of the stress. The ability to tolerate the stress of surgery and anesthesia is decreased significantly in neonates, infants, the aged, and debilitated persons. All body systems are affected by the response. In the perioperative period, the nurse must be able to assess stress in the client to plan interventions to reduce complications and to treat them effectively.

Invasive Procedures

Invasive procedures are those in which the body is entered by an instrument or device (e.g., a scalpel, tube) or by ionizing or non-ionizing radiation, and in which protective reflexes or self-care abilities are potentially compromised.[14]

Table 21–1. Responses to Surgical Stress

Response to Surgical Stress	Adaptive Responses	Maladaptive Responses
Vasoconstriction peripherally with increased coagulability	Blood increased to vital organs, away from periphery; increased clotting to decrease blood loss	Decrease in renal profusion possible; clotting and thrombus formation increase
Tachycardia with increased cardiac output, blood pressure, and coronary artery dilation	Increased perfusion of myocardium; increased oxygen perfusion to vital organs	Increased demand on heart possibly leading to heart failure; hypertension
Sodium and water retention secondary to increased ADH and aldosterone secretion	Increased volume to prevent hypovolemia, maintenance of blood pressure and cardiac output	Hypervolemia, circulatory overload, hypertension, and heart failure
Increased gastric acidity and decreased peristalsis	Blood shifted from large intestine to more vital areas	Paralytic ileus and stress ulcers
Bronchial dilation	Increased oxygen exchange, improved ventilation	No maladaptive change
Protein catabolism	Increased amino acids for wound healing	Negative nitrogen balance; eventual lack of tissue repair unless reversed
Proliferation of granulation and connective tissue	Increased wound healing	Development of excessive scar tissue and adhesions
Increased blood sugar and mobilization of fat stores	Increased energy available	Increased blood sugar detrimental to diabetics
Increased cortisol with increased anti-inflammatory response	Increased blood sugar	Possible infection if anti-inflammatory effect is prolonged
Increased metabolic rate	Increased energy available for adaptation	Increased heat loss may lead to hypothermia and shivering, with increasing oxygen demand

ADH, antidiuretic hormone.

Surgical Procedures

Common prefixes and suffixes can explain the type of procedure the client will undergo. Table 21–2 defines some common combining forms used in medicine and surgery.

Surgical procedures are categorized by their purpose, extent, and urgency. Knowledge of these categories may aid nurses in planning care for all phases of the client's surgery. Table 21–3 defines the main categories of surgical procedures.

Table 21–2. Common Medical Prefixes and Suffixes

Term	Definition
Prefixes	
supra-	Above; beyond
artho-	Joint
chole-	Bile or gall
cysto-	Bladder
encephalo-	Brain
entero-	Intestine
hystero-	Uterus
mast-	Breast
meningo-	Membrane
myo-	Muscle
nephro-	Kidney
neuro-	Nerve
oophor-	Ovary
pneumo-	Lung
pyelo-	Pelvis; kidney pelvis
salpingo-	Fallopian tubes
thoraco-	Chest
viscero-	Organ; especially abdominal
Suffixes	
-oma	Tumor, swelling
-ectomy	Removal of organ or gland
-rrhaphy	The suturing or stitching of a part or an organ
-scopy	Looking into
-ostomy	Making an opening or stoma
-otomy	Cutting into
-plasty	To repair or restore
-cele	Tumor, hernia, swelling
-itis	Inflammation of

Table 21–3. Categories of Surgical Procedures

Procedure	Definition
Purpose	
Diagnostic	To confirm a diagnosis
Exploratory	To estimate the extent of disease or confirm a diagnosis
Curative	To remove or repair damaged or diseased tissue or organs
Ablative	Involves removal of diseased organ
Reconstructive	Partial or complete restoration of a damaged organ or tissue to its original appearance and function
Constructive	Repair of a congenitally defective organ by improving its function or appearance
Palliative	Relieves symptoms but does not cure underlying disease
Extent	
Major	Extensive; involves significant, serious risk; may involve significant loss of blood, serious complications
Minor	Minimal, few serious complications; involves minimal loss of blood
Urgency	
Emergency	Must be performed immediately to (1) maintain life; (2) maintain organ or limb function; (3) remove a damaged organ; or (4) stop hemorrhage
Imperative	Requires surgical intervention within 24–48 hours
Planned or required	Surgical intervention is important, but it can be scheduled several weeks or months in advance
Elective	Performed for the client's well-being but is not absolutely necessary
Optional	Surgery performed simply for client's preference; is not needed

Preoperative Nursing

Careful preparation of clients undergoing surgery during the preoperative period reduces the operative risk and promotes postoperative recovery. In the case of emergency surgery, time may not permit complete preoperative assessment, care planning, and teaching. Nevertheless, essential preparation must be thorough.

Generally, preoperative preparation can take place in any of four places: (1) in the physician's office before admission to the healthcare facility, (2) on admission and during the days before the operation, (3) the night before surgery if the client is in the hospital, and (4) on admission on the morning of surgery.

The preoperative period begins once the client is scheduled for surgery and ends at the time of transfer to the surgical suite. During this phase, the nurse begins a complete assessment and establishes a plan of care based on the client's physical and psychosocial needs. Preoperative care focuses on preoperative teaching of the client and family to reduce anxiety and reduce the chance of postoperative complications.

General Preoperative Preparation

General Preoperative Assessment

Each client responds differently to surgery. Many variables influence a person's physiologic and psychological responses to the surgical experience. These include (1) physical and mental status, (2) extent of the disease, (3) magnitude of the surgery, (4) social and financial resources, and (5) psychological and physiologic preparation for surgery. When considered collectively, these variables reveal the degree of risk for a client undergoing surgery. Therefore, nursing assessment includes all these factors.

Physiologic nursing assessment before surgery elicits information about age, presence of pain, and nutritional status; fluid and electrolyte balance; presence of infection; physical mobility; skin integrity; cardiovascular, pulmonary, renal, gastrointestinal, liver, endocrine, neurologic, and hematologic function; sensory impairment; medication history; abnormalities, injuries, and previous surgeries; health habits; and social history. Table 21–4 lists common preoperative diagnostic tests, their reference range values, and their purpose.

Age. Infants, young children, and older adults have the lowest tolerance to the stressful effects of surgery. Consequently, their perioperative needs differ from those of older children, adolescents, and adults.

Infants. Immature organ development makes the infant less resistant to surgical stress. The infant's vital signs must be monitored closely. Also, the fluid and electrolyte balance of infants and young children is easily disrupted. It is important, therefore, to measure fluid intake, urine volume, and body weight accurately before and after surgery. Infants have decreased resistance to infection; therefore, assess postoperative wound status every 4 hours. Infants also exhibit ineffective thermoregulation requiring constant attention to body temperature and interventions to prevent excessive heat loss.

Table 21–4. Preoperative Diagnostic Tests

Test	Normal Ranges*	Purpose
Serum potassium	3.5–5.0 mEq/L	To identify hyperkalemia or hypokalemia
Serum sodium	136–145 mEq/L	To identify hypernatremia, hyponatremia, dehydration, or overhydration
Serum chloride	96–106 mEq/L	To identify hyperchloremia, hypochloremia, or metabolic alkalosis
Glucose	60–100 mg/dl	To identify hypoglycemia or hyperglycemia
Creatinine	0.7–1.4 mg/dl	To identify acute or chronic renal disease
Blood urea nitrogen (BUN)	10–20 mg/dl	To identify impaired liver or kidney function or excessive protein or tissue catabolism
Hemoglobin (Hgb)	Female: 12.0–15.0 g/dl Male: 13.0–17.0 g/dl	To identify the presence and extent of anemia
Hematocrit (Hct)	Female: 36%–45% Male: 39%–51%	To identify the presence and extent of anemia
Prothrombin time (PT)	11–18 seconds	To identify dysfunction of blood clotting (prothrombin level)
Partial thromboplastin time (PTT)	35–45 seconds	To identify deficiencies of coagulation factors
Chest x-ray study	No abnormal heart or lung lesions	To determine size and contour of heart, lungs, and major vessels
Electrocardiogram (ECG)	Normal rate and rhythm	To determine the electrical activity of the heart

*May vary for different laboratories.

Older Adults. Like extreme youth, old age produces physiologic changes that increase surgical risk. Physiologic changes and the presence of disease in the older adult's cardiovascular, pulmonary, musculoskeletal, gastrointestinal, hepatic, or renal system may affect surgical outcomes. Chronic conditions also increase the risk for older adults undergoing surgery. Table 21–5 outlines major physiologic changes that occur in older adults as a result of surgery and the appropriate nursing interventions.

Conditions that increase the risk include malnutrition, anemia, dehydration, atherosclerosis, chronic obstructive pulmonary disease (COPD), diabetes mellitus, cerebrovascular changes, and peripheral vascular disease, among many others. These are examples of common problems in older adults that should be corrected or controlled before surgery, if possible. A nutritious diet and adequate fluids help to counteract these problems, thus reducing the client's operative risk. Attention should also be paid to any altered visual or auditory impairments and the effects these would have on client understanding.

Pain. Pain is an important physiologic indicator that must be carefully monitored (see also Chapter 17). During the preoperative nursing assessment, ask the client to describe the pain and how it began. Find out if the pain developed rapidly, gradually, or in one explosive burst. Determine the regularity of the pain—whether it is constant or intermittent—and if anything has helped relieve it.

Judging the client's reaction to pain is as important as assessing the nature of the pain. Reactions vary from panic to apparent indifference, making it difficult to observe exactly what an individual is experiencing.

Nutritional Status. Nutritional status correlates directly with intraoperative success and postoperative recovery. The client who is well nourished preoperatively is better prepared to handle surgical stress and to return to optimal health after surgery.

Two major problems are nutritional deficiencies and excess. Nutritional deficiencies primarily affect clients with chronic illnesses, cancer, gastrointestinal conditions (e.g., ulcerative colitis, pyloric stenosis, bulimia), and advanced age. Nursing intervention for clients who are malnourished preoperatively includes encouraging a high intake of *carbohydrates* (for energy), *protein* (for wound healing), and *vitamins* (for healing), especially *vitamin C* (for wound healing) and *vitamin K* (for proper blood coagulation).

Total parenteral nutrition (TPN) or enteral nutrition may be administered for several days to a week before surgery. TPN plus lipids consists of total nutritional replacement with vitamin and mineral supplements. Enteral nutrition involves feeding directly through a tube placed into the stomach or small intestine. Enteral nutrition is also called tube feeding. Both methods help improve a client's nutritional status before surgery and are often continued postoperatively until satisfactory gastrointestinal function returns. See Chapter 60 for more information on enteral and parenteral feeding.

Table 21–5. Interventions for Physical Changes in Older Adults Undergoing Surgery

Physical Change	Nursing Interventions
Cardiovascular	
Decreased cardiac output Moderate increase in blood pressure Decreased peripheral circulation Arrhythmias	Know what anesthesia is used Monitor vital signs carefully Encourage early ambulation and leg exercises Assess for hypo- or hypertension or hypothermia Baseline ECG; note any changes
Respiratory	
Decreased vital capacity Reduced oxygenation of blood	Assess for pulmonary aspiration Monitor respirations carefully Vigorous pulmonary hygiene Postoperatively, auscultate lung sounds Oxygen saturation monitor
Renal	
Decreased renal blood flow and glomerular filtration rate Decreased ability to excrete waste products	Monitor urine output q 1–2 h during immediate postoperative period Evaluate intake and output Monitor fluid and electrolyte status
Musculoskeletal	
Decrease in lean body mass Increase in spinal compression Increased incidence of osteoporosis and arthritis	Assess level of mobility Position on operating table with padding to reduce trauma to bones and joints Spine, limbs, and pressure points may be padded to prevent fractures Early ambulation or exercises to client's ability Provide adequate nutrition Provide effective pain management
Sensorimotor	
Decreased reaction time Decreased visual acuity Decreased auditory acuity Thermoregulation	Orient client to environment Plan individual teaching, allow time to reinforce teaching Provide a safe environment Maintain warmth of client by use of warm blankets

ECG, electrocardiogram.

If possible, obesity should be corrected before elective surgery. A severely obese client faces a greater surgical risk than a client of normal weight because of the following problems:

● Obese clients frequently suffer from hypertension, congestive heart failure, and metabolic problems such as diabetes mellitus. These complicate the operative and postoperative course.
● Adipose tissue increases the technical difficulty of surgery. Incisions are usually deeper than normal, and the tissue is weaker. This increases the risk of postoperative infection, incisional hernias, and wound dehiscence and evisceration.
● An obese client is more susceptible to postoperative pulmonary complications. Obesity decreases the efficiency of coughing and deep breathing. The pressure of the abdominal contents on the diaphragm and lungs decreases expansion, leading to hypotension.
● An obese client is more prone to postoperative immobility, increasing the risk of venous stasis leading to deep vein thromboses and pulmonary emboli.

Treating obesity before surgery requires a reducing diet; mild exercise, if possible; and assessing and controlling conditions such as hypertension and diabetes mellitus, often with medications.

Fluid and Electrolyte Balance. Dehydration and hypovolemia (fluid volume deficit) predispose a client to complications during and after surgery. Dehydration results from prolonged vomiting, diarrhea, and bleeding, coupled with inadequate fluid intake. To correct dehydration, fluids are usually administered intravenously (IV) during the preoperative period.

Electrolyte imbalances also increase operative risk. It is particularly important to correct sodium, potassium, calcium, and magnesium deficiencies, as well as acid-base disturbances, before surgery through diet and IV infusions. Assessment and management of fluid and electrolyte imbalances is discussed in detail in Chapter 15.

Infection. Any infection, even a minor cold, can adversely affect surgical outcome. When the surgical site is near the lymph node or channel draining an infection, the likelihood of postoperative wound infection increases. During preoperative assessment, document such manifestations as sneezing, coughing, sore throat, elevated temperature, recent exposure to a communicable disease, and the presence of skin lesions, boils, or rashes. Also, note an elevated white blood cell (WBC) count. Communicate these findings to the surgeon or anesthesiologist, because these factors increase surgical risk. It may be necessary to reschedule surgery.

A low WBC count also can be dangerous for a client. A low WBC count may mean that the client is more susceptible to infection. A client who is immunosuppressed is at great risk of postoperative infections. Clients who test positive for human immunodeficiency virus (HIV) are at increased risk for postoperative infections.

Physical Mobility. The perioperative nurse should identify the client's level of mobility or impairment to determine the type of assistance needed to move the client. The nurse ensures that sufficient personnel and equipment are available to transfer the client. The perioperative nurse ensures that safety and comfort measures are used during client transportation. The client should be positioned using correct body alignment, padding, and positioning equipment to prevent the occurrence of, or an increase in, impaired physical mobility.

Skin Integrity. The perioperative nurse identifies all alterations in skin integrity preoperatively to establish a baseline for comparison postoperatively. Lesions, pressure ulcers, necrotic skin tissue, skin turgor, erythema or discoloration of the skin, and the presence of external devices should be reported and documented. The approximate size, color, and location of the skin breakdown is noted to determine if impaired skin integrity remained at perioperative levels or increased during surgery. The nurse should provide sufficient padding and positioning equipment for the client to prevent the occurrence of or an increase in, impaired skin integrity.

Cardiovascular Function. Cardiac conditions that increase operative risk include angina pectoris, a myocardial infarction within the last 6 months, uncontrolled hypertension, congestive heart failure, and peripheral vascular disease. All cardiac conditions could lead to decreased tissue perfusion, and peripheral vascular disease could impair wound healing in an extremity.

Assess all clients for elevated blood pressure; slow, rapid, or irregular pulse; edema; cold, cyanotic extremities; weakness; and shortness of breath. Laboratory and diagnostic studies, which are often ordered before surgery to determine cardiovascular function, include electrocardiogram (ECG), hemoglobin, hematocrit, and serum electrolytes (see Table 21–4).

Preoperative treatment of clients with cardiovascular disease includes rest, a low sodium or low cholesterol diet, heart medications such as digoxin, and the judicious administration of fluids. An attempt is made to improve the client's cardiovascular system to the best condition possible before surgery.

Pulmonary Function. Pulmonary conditions such as COPD, emphysema, asthma, and bronchitis increase operative risk because they impair gas exchange in the alveoli and predispose the client to postoperative pulmonary complications.

To evaluate pulmonary conditions, assess the client for shortness of breath, wheezing, clubbed fingers, chest pain, cyanosis, and coughing with expectoration of copious or purulent mucus. Question the client carefully about smoking habits. Obtain a history of respiratory allergies and infections. A chest x-ray is usually ordered for diagnostic purposes on appropriate clients, such as those with cardiorespiratory problems.

Often a baseline arterial blood gas study is obtained to evaluate pulmonary function in a client with known respiratory disease, as are pulmonary function studies (see Chapter 39). Clients with severe respiratory disease are usually treated preoperatively with aerosol therapy, postural drainage, and antibiotics. Clients who smoke are strongly encouraged to stop before surgery. To help prevent postoperative respiratory complications, these clients need careful preoperative instruction and practice in deep breathing and coughing exercises.

Renal Function. The surgical client needs adequate renal function to eliminate protein wastes, preserve fluid and electrolyte balance, and clear anesthetic agents. Emergency surgery must be performed, however, regardless of the client's renal function. Conditions that increase operative risk by affecting urine elimination include advanced renal insufficiency, acute nephritis, and benign prostatic hypertrophy (BPH). In older men, BPH may obstruct the normal flow of urine and predispose them to urinary tract infection.

To assess renal status, observe for manifestations of frequency, dysuria, and anuria. Also observe the appearance of the urine. Document and report urine that is cloudy or bloody.

The most commonly ordered preoperative tests to assess renal function are urinalysis, blood urea nitrogen (BUN), and creatinine.

Urinalysis, performed on either a clean voided specimen or a catheterized specimen, checks urine for the presence of the following:

- Red or white blood cells, which may indicate an infection or tumor
- Casts, which may indicate renal disease
- Protein, which may indicate renal disease
- Glucose, which usually indicates diabetes
- Specific gravity (if below 1.010, the kidney may be unable to concentrate urine; if over 1.025, the client may be dehydrated)

BUN and serum creatinine are studies that test the ability of the kidney to excrete urea and protein wastes. Elevated levels may simply reflect dehydration, although they may indicate more serious problems. Serious renal disease and urinary infections must be treated, if possible, before surgery.

Gastrointestinal Function. The client's gastrointestinal system should be functioning well before surgery to prevent postoperative complications. Impaired nutrition may be related to altered gastrointestinal function. The client should be questioned about normal bowel functioning, so postoperative expectations for return of function are appropriate. Clients with a long history of constipation may have more difficulty postoperatively than those with regular bowel function.

Liver Function. Liver disease, such as cirrhosis, increases risk because an impaired liver is unable to detoxify medications and anesthetic agents or to metabolize carbohydrates, fats, and amino acids. Liver disease may also be evidenced by decreased albumin levels leading to a decrease in immunoglobulins and fibrinogen. Low albu-

min levels predispose the client to fluid shifts, infection, and coagulopathy. In addition, inadequate liver function is associated with poor wound healing and a higher risk of infection. Clients with a history of alcoholism or ascites require a careful examination of liver function before surgery. Because these clients are usually malnourished and debilitated, the surgeon generally orders a high calorie diet, IV solutions, and vitamins during the preoperative period.

Endocrine Function. Endocrine function, particularly that of the thyroid, must be monitored carefully preoperatively to minimize operative risk. Hyperthyroidism can lead to thyroid storm or thyroid crisis, with manifestations of hypertension, tachycardia, and hyperthermia and, therefore, should be treated medically preoperatively (see Chapter 70). Likewise, hypothyroidism increases the risk of hypotension and cardiac arrest during anesthesia, and it should be recognized and treated before surgery.

Diabetes mellitus predisposes a client to infection and poor tissue healing and swings of blood sugar greater than usual. Cardiovascular, peripheral vascular, neurologic, and renal complications also increase surgical risk for a client with diabetes. The client with well-controlled diabetes is more likely to respond well to surgery. Chapter 69 discusses in detail the care of clients with diabetes mellitus.

Neurologic Function. When appropriate, the nurse should conduct a thorough neurologic physical assessment before surgery to determine the client's baseline function. Testing generally includes cranial nerves, reflex response of the upper and lower extremities, sensory reflexes, and cerebellar response (see Chapter 30).

Serious neurologic conditions, such as uncontrolled epilepsy or severe Parkinson's disease, increase surgical risk. Important neurologic preoperative findings include severe headache, frequent dizziness, lightheadedness, ringing in the ears, unsteady gait, unequal pupils, and a history of convulsions.

Sensory and Perceptual Alteration. The perioperative nurse identifies characteristics that indicate sensory and perceptual alterations and reviews the possible causative factors to assist the client in managing the environmental stimuli associated with the surgical experience (e.g., bright overhead lights and speaking clearly).[156]

Decreased sensory input is related to aging, excessive stimuli, a physiologic imbalance, or disorientation.[112]

The nurse assesses the client's orientation to time, place, and person, and then performs a neurologic check. The client may be instructed to leave hearing aids, glasses, and other health aids on the unit or at home, to avoid losing them. This may increase the client's anxiety and decrease his or her level of comprehension. The nurse should speak in a clear, low-pitched voice to clients with a hearing deficit or use appropriate visual aids.

Hematologic Function. Clients with blood coagulation disorders are at risk of hemorrhage and hypovolemic shock during and following surgery. Five factors pointing to abnormal hematologic factors are:

1. A history of bleeding
2. Manifestations such as easy bruising, excessive bleeding following dental extractions and razor nicks, and severe nosebleeds
3. The presence of hepatic or renal disease
4. Use of anticoagulants, aspirin, or other nonsteroidal anti-inflammatory drugs (NSAIDs)
5. Abnormal bleeding time, prothrombin time, or platelet count (see Chapter 53)

For a variety of reasons, including improved surgical hemostasis, blood transfusions are used less frequently than in past years. Many clients also fear the transmission of HIV and hepatitis B. If possible, clients are encouraged to donate their own blood before surgery (autologous blood transfusion) for use during or after surgery. Blood transfusions are discussed in Chapter 53.

Use of Medications. Many clients take prescribed and nonprescribed medications that may increase operative risk by (1) increasing coagulation time or (2) interacting unfavorably with the anesthetic. Some medications that may result in complications include the following:

● Anticoagulants, including aspirin and other NSAIDs, which cause clotting abnormalities
● Antibiotics, which combine with some muscle relaxants to increase postoperative respiratory depression
● Tranquilizers, which lower blood pressure and thus increase the risk of shock; they also potentiate the effects of narcotics and barbiturates
● Thiazide diuretics, which can create potassium depletion
● Steroids, which cause hypofunction of the adrenal cortex and thus impair physiologic response to the stress of anesthesia and surgery; their anti-inflammatory effects also delay wound healing and increase the risk of infection; steroid replacement also needs to be increased before, during, and after surgery
● Monoamine oxidase (MAO) inhibitors, which can cause hypertensive crisis when combined with anesthetic agents
● Anti-parkinsonian drugs, which cause hypotension or hypertension when combined with anesthetics
● Street drugs and alcohol abuse, which increase tolerance to narcotics
● Hypoglycemic agents, which require dosage alteration and close monitoring of blood sugar

When performing a nursing preoperative assessment, document whether the client has any drug allergies or reactions or is currently taking any prescribed or over-the-counter medications. Surgical risk is increased if (1) the client is allergic to the anesthetic or (2) the medications the client is taking interact adversely with the anesthesia. Clients often forget to list some medications they are taking. They also sometimes fail to recognize that nonprescription medications may pose a threat and, consequently, do not mention them. Therefore, question clients very carefully and obtain as complete a list of medications as possible. The physician's decision to discontinue, reduce, or continue preoperative medications is based on the client's surgical risk (Table 21–6).

Abnormalities, Injuries, and Previous Surgeries. When surgery must be performed following a traumatic event (e.g., gunshot wound, stab wound, serious accident, severe fall), document the details of the event as precisely as possible. If the client was injured in a fall or accident, ask questions such as, "What was your position when the accident occurred?" and, "Did you lose consciousness?" The answers may help to determine whether or not there is an underlying, undetected condition that may increase surgical risk (e.g., epilepsy, coronary artery disease, uncontrolled diabetes mellitus). Be especially alert to manifestations of severe trauma warranting surgery in children. Young children are often unable to talk about what happened to them. Some children are victims of child abuse, and the trauma may have been inflicted on them by an adult in their environment. If abuse is suspected, report the findings to your immediate supervisor, the surgical team, and the proper authorities. Also, remember that adults can be abused, often by a spouse.

Life-Style Habits. It is generally agreed that the client who smokes or abuses drugs has an increased surgical risk. The client who smokes has reduced hemoglobin levels and, therefore, less oxygen available for tissue repair. Smokers may be more susceptible to thrombus formation because of the hypercoagulability of their blood and their increased rate of arteriosclerosis. Smokers are also more likely to have damage to their lung tissue, including COPD and chronic bronchitis. Smokers should stop smoking at least a week before elective surgery.

Clients who use alcohol or drugs may experience withdrawal manifestations during hospitalization. Their surgical course may be complicated by poor nutrition, as well as unpredictable reactions to anesthetic agents. Remember, even two drinks a day can lead to withdrawal manifestations and the need for increased analgesia and anesthesia.

Clients who lead a sedentary life-style may have a complicated postoperative course because of poor muscle tone, limited cardiac and respiratory reserve, and decreased stress response to the physical demands of surgery.

Clients who are HIV-positive have several areas of increased surgical risk. If their immune systems are affected, they are at a much higher risk of developing a postoperative infection and of being unable to fight infection. If they have developed *Pneumocystis carinii* pneumonia, they are at increased risk of anesthetic and postoperative pulmonary complications.

Social History. The client's marital status, significant others, and support systems should be explored. The client's occupation should also be identified because it may be a source of difficulty after surgery if the client is unable to return to work. It is also important to determine whether the client has insurance or whether this surgery will cause severe financial hardship.

Table 21–6. Examples of Medications and Possible Effects on the Surgical Client

Medications	Possible Effects
Antibiotics	
Gentamicin (Garamycin) Penicillin	Produces mild respiratory depression, may mask infection, and affects metabolism of muscle relaxants
Antiarrhythmics	
Propranolol hydrochloride (Inderal)	Affects client's tolerance of anesthesia; interacts with epinephrine used in local anesthesia
Quinidine gluconate (Quinatime)	Depresses cardiac function
Procainamide hydrochloride (Pronestyl)	Potentiates anesthetics that are neuromuscular blockers
Antihypertensives	
Methyldopa (Aldomet) Captopril (Capoten)	May alter response to muscle relaxants and narcotics; may cause intraoperative or postoperative hypotensive crisis
Corticosteroids	
Dexamethasone (Decadron) Hydrocortisone sodium succinate (Solu-Cortef) Prednisone (Deltasone)	Delays wound healing; masks infection; increases risk of hemorrhage; increases serum glucose; decreases stress response (needs replacement during surgery)
Anticoagulants	
Heparin sodium Warfarin sodium (Coumadin) Aspirin	Increases risk of hemorrhage intraoperatively and postoperatively
Glaucoma Medications	
Pilocarpine hydrochloride	May cause respiratory or cardiovascular collapse during surgery
Antidiabetic Agents	
Chlorpropamide Glipizide Glyburide Insulin	Insulin needs decrease when client is to receive nothing by mouth; insulin levels may fluctuate during healing because of dietary and activity restrictions.

Because all of these factors can increase the client's stress and interfere with healing, the nurse should be aware of the potential risk factors that may jeopardize a successful surgical intervention. Significant or important conditions detected should be communicated to other members of the healthcare team.

Psychosocial Aspects of Preoperative Preparation

Most clients are somewhat fearful of surgery. The extent to which a client fears surgery depends on his or her personality, general responses to stress, mental health, past experiences with surgery, and preconceptions about surgery and anesthesia.

Fear of the unknown is one of the most important causes of preoperative anxiety. During the preoperative phase, clients also may fear postoperative pain, the discovery of cancer, the loss of an organ or limb, anesthesia, vulnerability while unconscious, the threat of loss of job or financial security, loss of social and familial roles, disruption of life-style, separation from significant others, and death.

Clients respond differently to fear. Some respond by becoming silent and withdrawn, childish, belligerent, evasive, tearful, or clinging. Most clients feel helpless when admitted to a healthcare facility. We need to remember that although surgery may be commonplace for the healthcare professional, it is a frightening experience for the client.

Based on the nursing assessment, a number of interventions may be appropriate for the preoperative client. First, provide explanations and printed information about the healthcare facility routines, visiting hours, mealtimes, the location of the chapel and waiting room, and so forth. Explain the procedures involved in the planned surgery to allay the client's anxiety. The client should have a complete idea of what the preoperative, intraoperative, and postoperative course entails. Consult with the physician before speaking to the client about specific or technical details. Explain all nursing care and any possible discomfort that may result as a consequence of nursing interventions. Also, tell the client what you will do to minimize any discomfort. If the client is scheduled to go to the intensive care unit (ICU) after surgery, ask what the client already knows or has heard about intensive care. At this point, take time to clarify any misconceptions or incorrect information.

Allow the client to take the lead in asking questions concerning surgery and the postoperative period. Provide the client with essential information, such as nothing-by-mouth (NPO) status and preoperative procedures, but then provide only as much additional information as the client wants to know. If the client is withdrawn, depressed, or apprehensive, use your communication skills to encourage expression of fears and concerns. For example, tell the client that preoperative fear is normal and that it is not unusual to experience anxiety. Invite the client to share his or her concerns. Find out if the client knows someone who had similar surgery and what the outcome was. Often clients' fears may be rooted in their own past experiences or stories of unpleasant experiences that happened to others.

Whenever possible, introduce the client and family to others who have successfully undergone similar surgery. If this is not possible preoperatively, it may be done after surgery. You may want to contact support groups, such as the local laryngectomy or colostomy organization, for instance, and ask for a volunteer to visit the client.

Find out the client's religious preference and arrange for a visit from clergy, if the client so desires. Finally, include the client's significant others in preoperative discussions whenever possible. Provide them with information they can use to assist in reducing the client's preoperative anxiety.

Handling fears in these ways can smooth the preoperative experience. Studies show that clients who are calm and emotionally prepared for surgery withstand anesthesia better and experience fewer postoperative complications.

Discharge Planning as Part of Preoperative Preparation

Identify the discharge needs of the client based on the planned surgical procedure and current health status. Referrals for assistance could include the following:

- Local visiting nurse or home healthcare services
- Local chapters of organizations offering help (e.g., the American Cancer Society, American Heart Association, American Diabetes Association, etc.)
- Local mastectomy, laryngectomy, colostomy support groups
- Medic Alert Foundation
- Malignant Hyperthermia Hotline
- Local senior citizens' assistance program
- Substance abuse treatment programs or groups
- Emergency social services
- Local sexual assault center (law requires that suspected sexual abuse of minors be reported)
- Child protection services
- Emergency legal assistance

Preoperative Assessment

History

Data gathered during the history help detect problems that may arise preoperatively or postoperatively. The manner is which the history is conducted plays a large part in determining the degree of preoperative and postoperative anxiety the client experiences.

The history allows clients to explain their understanding of the impending surgery. This information can be used to determine clients' learning needs. The preoperative history also allows the nurse to:

- Establish rapport with the client and significant others
- Begin a psychosocial assessment of the client: this information is valuable in developing the preoperative and postoperative teaching care plan (e.g., a client who is apprehensive preoperatively may need more frequent or repetitive instruction and more reinforcement than a less anxious client)
- Reassure the client and significant others, and answer general questions about the surgery, healthcare facility, etc.

Specific information to obtain during the preoperative history concerns:

- Previous surgery and experience with anesthesia
- Responses of family members to previous surgery and anesthesia
- Whether the client has had any serious illnesses
- Previous and current medications (prescription or over-the-counter)
- Allergies and reactions; dietary restrictions
- Alcohol, nicotine, or recreational drug use
- Current manifestations or discomforts
- Occupation
- Religious affiliation
- Significant others (Is the client single or married? How many dependents does the client have?)
- Whether the client has any questions about the surgery
- Chronic illnesses (e.g., arthritis, migraines, back pain)

In addition to helping the nurse establish valuable preoperative baseline data, this information uncovers the need for supportive services. If a client will need assistance after returning home, the nurse can initiate discharge plans.

Physical Examination

A physical examination is performed on all clients undergoing surgery to obtain baseline data and identify conditions that may interfere with the administration of anesthesia or produce problems postoperatively.

A complete physical examination should be performed, paying special attention to cardiac and respiratory systems. Baseline vital signs are obtained as one determination of the client's risk for postoperative complications. Any abnormal vital sign is significant and may cause a postponement of surgery until the problem is treated. Abnormal breath sounds may indicate the need for respiratory therapy both before and after surgery, or the need for bronchodilators. Clients with abnormal cardiac findings will need further evaluation to determine whether they can withstand the stress of surgery and anesthesia. Physical examination also should reveal any problems with joint mobility or deformities that may interfere with operative positioning, as well as the postoperative course. Special consideration of the elderly should include cardiac, respiratory, renal, and musculoskeletal assessment.

Preoperative Diagnostic Tests

Routine diagnostic tests are ordered less often than in past years. Now clients have specific tests ordered based on their health status to identify potential problems that would interfere with the surgery. Table 21–4 identifies commonly requested preoperative laboratory tests.

Informed Consent

Anyone undergoing any invasive procedure must give informed consent for that procedure. A consent form is the legal document that signifies the client's informed consent for the procedure. The consent form is the legal document that signifies the client's informed consent for the procedure. The consent form guards the client against unwanted invasive procedures. It also protects the healthcare facility and healthcare professionals.

A signed or oral consent is necessary for each invasive procedure. The client or client's surrogate must receive a full explanation of the operation before giving consent. Pictures and diagrams may be necessary for complete understanding of the surgical procedure. Moreover, the client or surrogate must be told about potential risks, complications, and disfigurement that may result from the surgery; about anesthesia; who will perform the surgery; and whether or not organs or body parts may be removed. The client or surrogate should be informed about alternative treatments. The surgeon should explain the procedure in terms the client or surrogate readily understands. Ensure that the client or surrogate receives an honest, accurate, and fair statement of what to expect during and after surgery, and understands it before informed consent is given.

The procedure for obtaining a signed consent varies from state to state and according to the policy of the healthcare facility. Generally, the surgeon explains the surgical procedure, the possible risks and complications, and the alternatives. The nurse, however, may obtain and witness the client's signature on the consent form (dependent on healthcare facility policy).

Adults sign their own operative permit unless they are unconscious or mentally incompetent. In such cases, a surrogate, such as a relative or guardian, is responsible for consent (see Ethical Issues in Nursing). If the relative or guardian is out of state, the physician can secure consent over the telephone in the presence of one or two witnesses on the same line. If no relative or guardian can be found, the court can appoint one.

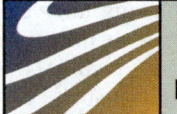

ETHICAL ISSUES IN NURSING

Should Clients Who Have a "Do Not Resuscitate" Order Undergo Surgery?

Surgical procedures are performed to enhance the lives of those receiving them. Such procedures may be elective (such as a cosmetic procedure), scheduled, but not emergent (such as a thyroidectomy), or emergent (such as emergency trauma procedures). In most instances, the clients undergoing surgery hope to have whatever problem they are experiencing corrected so they can go on living a normal life. There are times, however, when problems cannot be surgically corrected and such surgical procedures result in a poor outcome or possibly death.

No surgery is without risk, even for the most healthy of clients. There are cases when very unhealthy clients may require surgical procedures. The risks of surgery are, of course, far greater for these clients than for more healthy clients. If any of these clients need resuscitative measures during surgery, there should be no question that the operating room staff would administer such measures. There is really no dilemma present for such cases.

However, what if a seriously ill client has a "Do Not Resuscitate" (DNR) order prior to surgery? What should be done if this client should experience a cardiac or respiratory arrest on the operating table? Should the surgical staff honor the DNR order? Is a DNR order valid in the operating room where, routinely, patients are maintained with ventilator support, vasoactive drugs, and even electric shock to the heart?

In most hospitals and surgicenters, DNR orders are not honored in the operating room. The client may have a DNR order preoperatively and postoperatively, but during surgery, if there is a need for resuscitative measures, such measures would be administered. Nurses in operating room settings, as well as those caring for clients pre- and postoperatively, should know the institution's policies regarding DNR orders in the operating room.

The client should also be informed of the institution's DNR policies and understand the implications. The client's physician or anesthesiologist should have a long discussion with the client explaining the policies and setting goals with the client that would direct treatment decisions in the operating room. All persons involved in the client's care need to be working toward the same client-directed goals.

Children under legal age (18 in most states) who are not emancipated minors must have consent given by the child's parent or legal guardian. Emancipated minors are considered, in most states, to be those who are under legal age but because of marriage or other circumstances are independent of the family. If the child's family cannot be present to sign the permit, consent can be obtained from a parent by telephone, wire, or letter. When a minor's relatives cannot be located, a court order may be needed to permit surgery, depending on the state law.

Once the operative permit is signed, it becomes a permanent part of the client's record. Make sure it accompanies the record to the operating room. If oral consent was obtained, be sure that this is completely documented in the appropriate place in the client's record.

Preoperative Teaching

Preoperative teaching is an important component in the client's operative experience. Numerous research studies have supported the value of preoperative instruction in both reducing the incidence of postoperative complications and the length of stay. The client's teaching needs, anxieties, and fears about the surgery must be assessed individually.

The timing of preoperative teaching is highly individualized. Ideally, there will be enough time for the client to be given instructions and time to answer questions. If teaching is done too far in advance, the client may forget. On the other hand, clients who are taught immediately before the surgery may be too anxious to comprehend what is being taught. In many cases, the client is admitted on the day of surgery. Hopefully, they will have received written or oral instructions prior to this time and the nurse will be able to reinforce instructions and answer questions. A telephone interview is conducted in many ambulatory surgery units.

Preoperative teaching allays anxiety and encourages clients to participate actively in their own care. The basic areas that must be covered in preoperative teaching are the following:

- Deep breathing and coughing exercises
- Turning, extremity exercises, and ambulation
- Pain control methods
- Postoperative equipment

Deep Breathing Exercises

Breathing and coughing exercises help expand collapsed lungs and prevent postoperative pneumonia and atelectasis. Demonstrate correct deep breathing by inhaling slowly through the nose, distending the abdomen, and exhaling slowly through pursed lips. After you have demonstrated the method, ask the client to demonstrate the procedure (Fig. 21–1). Ask the client to do the following:

1. Sit on the edge of the bed or lie supine, with knees flexed to relax the abdominal musculature (the client may lie on either side if lying on the back is impossible)
2. Place hands on the abdomen
3. Inhale through the nose until the abdomen balloons outward
4. Exhale through pursed lips while contracting the abdominal muscles

Instruct the client to use this breathing method as often as possible, preferably 5 to 10 times every hour during the postoperative period of immobilization.

Coughing Exercises

For these exercises, the client may be in a sitting or lying position. Show the client how to splint an incision. Splinting minimizes pressure and helps to control pain when the client is coughing. Instruct the client to lace the fingers and hold them tightly across the incision before coughing. A small pillow or folded towel held over the incision also facilitates splinting. Have the client take a deep breath, exhaling through the mouth, before coughing from deep in the lungs. Encourage the client to perform deep breathing exercises *before* coughing, to stimulate the cough reflex.

Incentive spirometers are used to promote lung expansion. They promote alveolar inflation and strengthen respiratory muscles. They also help to prevent atelectasis in the postoperative client. They should be used about 10 times an hour after surgery.

Turning Exercises

The client also needs to practice turning from side to side, using the side rails to assist movements. Turning helps to prevent venous stasis, thrombophlebitis, decubitus ulcer formation, and respiratory complications. Teach the client to turn every 1 to 2 hours during the postoperative period.

Extremity Exercises

The client should practice extremity exercises. Ask the client to flex and extend each joint, particularly the hip, knee, and ankle joints, keeping the lower back flat as the leg is lowered and straightened. Have the client move each foot in a circular motion. These exercises help prevent circulatory problems, such as thrombophlebitis, by facilitating venous return to the heart.

Antiembolism stockings may be used on the lower extremities preoperatively, intraoperatively, and postoperatively, combined with turning and leg exercises to prevent thrombophlebitis or thromboembolism. Sequential compression stockings are now being used to massage legs rhythmically for even more effective prevention of clots.

Ambulation

Encourage ambulation after surgery when appropriate. Ambulation helps prevent postoperative complications. Include a projected schedule for postoperative ambulation in your preoperative teaching program. Teach the client proper methods of arising to decrease pain and the risk of hypotension. Always have the client sit up slowly and pause before attempting to stand. Show the client how to support the incision to decrease pain on arising.

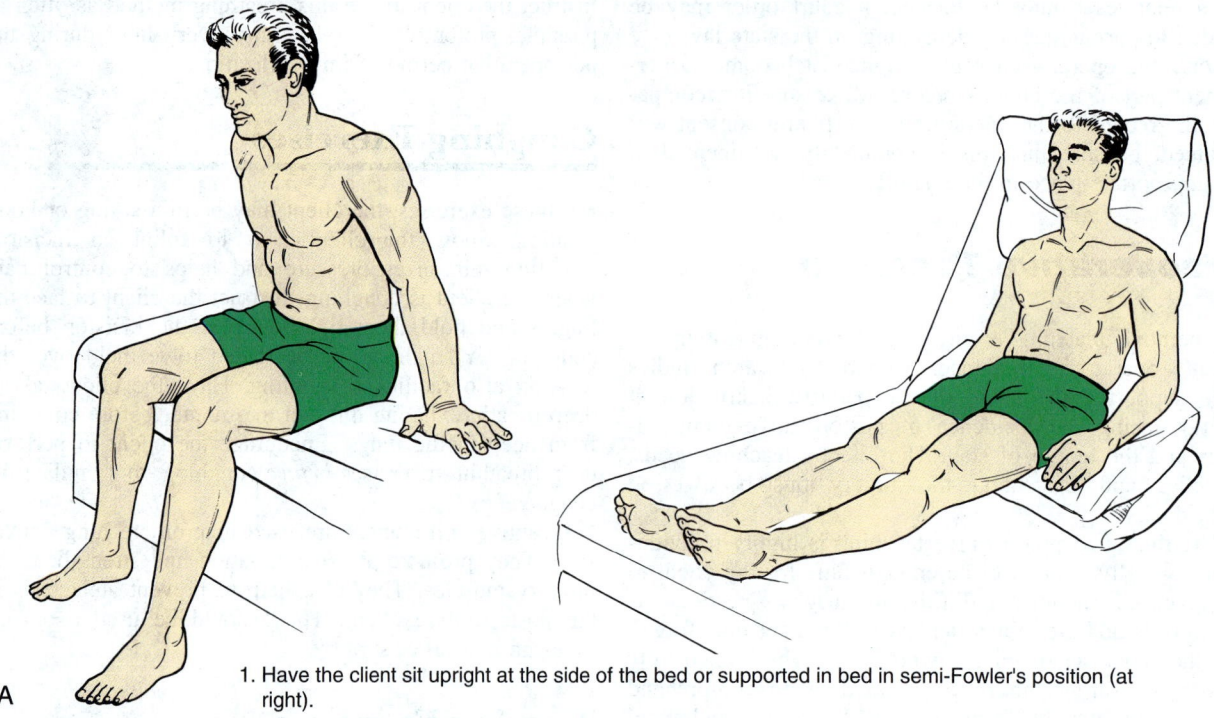

A

1. Have the client sit upright at the side of the bed or supported in bed in semi-Fowler's position (at right).

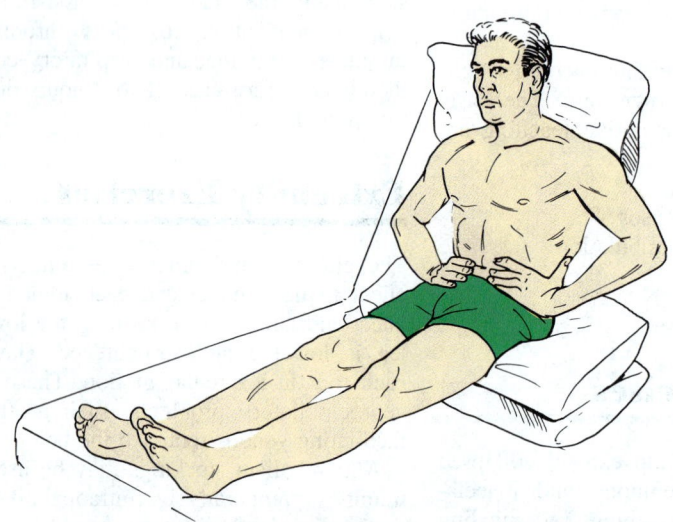

2. Instruct the client to place his or her hands on the abdomen to feel whether the chest rises to indicate that the lungs are expanding.
3. Have the client inhale through the nose until the abdomen distends.
4. Instruct the client to exhale through pursed lips while contracting the abdominal muscles.
5. Have the client repeat this exercise every hour during the first postoperative day.

B

Figure 21–1. Deep (diaphragmatic) breathing after surgery.

Pain Control

A common concern among preoperative clients is the pain they will experience in the postoperative period. It is important to assure clients they will be kept as comfort-able as possible while regaining their strength and mobility.

During the immediate postoperative period, clients will receive medication by IV, intramuscular, or epidural routes. If the pain medication is given IV or epidurally, it may be given by an infusion pump. Patient-controlled analgesia (PCA) allows clients to administer their own pain medication. If it is anticipated the client will use PCA postoperatively, the nurse should explain the operating instructions and allow the client time to practice operating it. Chapter 17 contains further information on current pain control methods.

Postoperative Equipment

Clients should be instructed about equipment that may be used postoperatively. Depending on the surgery, various tubes, drains, and IV lines will be used. Discussion should focus on the purpose of specific pieces of equipment and how they relate to the surgery.

Tubes. The most common type of tube is an indwelling catheter for the purpose of bladder drainage. Another common tube is the nasogastric tube. The purpose of the latter is to decompress the stomach and upper bowel and to drain stomach contents.

Drains. Drains are usually inserted during surgery to promote evacuation of fluid from the operative site. They act either by wick action, as with a Penrose drain, or with a mild amount of suction, as with a Hemovac or Jackson-Pratt drain.

Intravenous Infusion Devices. Intravenous infusions are usually started prior to surgery. The purpose of the infusion is to administer medications and fluids before, during, and after surgery.

Physical Preparation

Preparing the Skin

Usually the operative area is treated the night before surgery with an antiseptic such as povidone-iodine (Betadine) to clean and disinfect the skin.

Opinions differ as to preoperative skin preparation. Recent research studies show that not removing hair at all, clipping hair, or using an electric razor is associated with a lower rate of infection than traditional shaving.[5] The Centers for Disease Control (CDC) recommends that if shaving is necessary, it be performed in the operating suite prior to surgery. The nurse responsible for skin preparation should conduct a preoperative assessment for any skin abrasions, lacerations, or signs of infection at the operative area.

Preparing the Gastrointestinal Tract

The gastrointestinal tract needs special preparation on the evening before surgery to (1) reduce the possibility of vomiting and aspiration during anesthesia, (2) reduce the possibility of a bowel obstruction, and (3) prevent contamination from fecal material during intestinal tract or bowel surgery.

Preparation involves restricting food and fluid, administering enemas as needed, and inserting a gastric or intestinal tube when appropriate.

If a client undergoing surgery is to receive a general anesthetic, foods and fluids are restricted for 8 to 10 hours before the operation. This restriction significantly reduces the possibility of aspiration of gastric contents, which can cause aspiration pneumonia. Because solid food must be withheld 8 to 10 hours before surgery, most clients have an NPO status after midnight. When surgery is not scheduled until late afternoon, the client may eat a liquid breakfast in the morning if the surgeon permits.

When a client is NPO:

● Explain the reasons for the restriction
● Remove food and water from the bedside stand
● Place an NPO sign on the door and on the bed
● Mark the Kardex or nursing care plan NPO
● Inform the dietitian that the client is awaiting surgery
● Inform other caretakers that the client is NPO

If the client who is NPO consumes food or fluids, notify the surgeon and anesthesia provider, because the surgery may have to be canceled or delayed. The client is sometimes instructed to take important medications (such as digoxin) with a small sip of water at the usual time. Be sure that this fact is noted on the client care record.

Clients who are extremely debilitated or malnourished may receive IV infusions of glucose, amino acids, or plasma prior to surgery.

Enemas are not routinely ordered during the preoperative period except for surgical procedures involving the gastrointestinal tract, perianal or perineal areas, and pelvic cavity. Preoperative enemas help (1) prevent contamination of the peritoneal cavity by feces, (2) prevent colon injury, and (3) provide adequate visualization of the surgical site. Enemas are usually administered the evening before surgery. Clients who are admitted on the day of the surgery may be instructed to take one or more enemas at home the night before surgery. This requires teaching to ensure the client knows how to administer the enemas correctly and what results are to be expected. Some clients may require further bowel cleaning on the morning of surgery after admission to the facility.

Gastrointestinal tubes are usually inserted during surgery, if they are used at all. This procedure is usually performed for clients undergoing major abdominal or intestinal tract surgery.

Many types of surgery require special preparations. The specific protocol for each surgical procedure is usually available at the healthcare facility.

Preparing for Anesthesia

The anesthesia care provider visits the client before surgery to perform a complete respiratory, cardiovascular, and neurologic examination. Generally, the topics discussed with the client during the examination include the type of anesthesia planned and the sensations the client will experience when undergoing anesthesia. Fears the client has concerning anesthesia also are addressed. The client's risk of side effects and complications is also assessed. The American Society of Anesthesiology has developed a classification system rating clients from class 1 (no disturbances that would cause anesthesia problems) to class 5 (a client with little chance of survival). There is also a classification of emergency surgery.

Promoting Rest and Sleep

The preoperative client will rest more completely on the night before surgery if he or she is physically comfortable, mentally at ease, and adequately sedated. Measures to reduce preoperative sleeplessness and restlessness include a well-ventilated room, a comfortable clean bed, a back rub, and a warm beverage (if fluids are not contraindicated). With same-day surgery, the client may be at home the night before surgery and may have to get up early to get to the hospital for surgery. The client still needs to be encouraged to get as much sleep as possible before surgery. Encourage apprehensive clients to take ordered sleep medication the night before surgery to help them to sleep.

Always remember to talk in a positive manner with the client as you give preoperative care, and listen to any doubts or fears the client may have concerning surgery.

Preparing the Client on the Day of Surgery

Early-Morning Care

Immediate preoperative preparation begins at least 1 to 2 hours before surgery for clients in the hospital and as soon as same-day admission clients enter the hospital. At this time, the nurse asks whether the client has any questions or concerns. Continue to assess for manifestations of anxiety. Communicate any surgical delays to the client and significant others.

The following preoperative interventions help promote safety during surgery:

- Be sure that all allergies are recorded. In many institutions, a special allergy wristband is given to the client.
- Take and record the vital signs. Some increase in blood pressure or pulse is common because of anxiety. However, if marked differences from baseline information appear, report them to the surgeon. They might signify, for example, a respiratory infection and may require delay of surgery.
- Check the identification band to make sure it is legible, accurate, and securely fastened to the client.
- Be sure that informed consent has been obtained and is clearly documented.
- If a skin preparation has been ordered, check that it has been completed accurately and thoroughly.
- Check for and carry out any special orders such as administering enemas or starting an IV line.
- Verify that the client has not eaten for the last 8 hours. Check that fluids have been restricted, although sometimes the physician will order clients to take their usual

oral medications (e.g., digoxin) with a small sip of water.

- Ask the client to void; measure and record the amount of urine (if indicated).
- Assist the client with oral hygiene, if necessary.
- Remove dentures or bridgework that could obstruct the airway if left in place. Store these and other valuables according to healthcare facility policy or give them to family members.
- Have the client remove jewelry. Many facilities allow the client to keep wedding bands on as long as they are taped securely. If jewelry is removed, it should be stored according to policy or given to the family. Assist with the removal of hairpins, wigs, or prostheses.
- If the client is wearing a hearing aid, notify the operating room nurse. Leave it in place so that operating room personnel know it is there and can communicate with the client.
- Assist the client in donning a hospital gown, protective cap, Ace bandage, or antiembolic hose, if these items are being used.
- Remove colored nail polish from at least one nail for the pulse oximeter (although the device can accurately read oxygen saturation levels through light-colored polish).
- Remove make-up so skin color can be observed.

To prevent omissions in preoperative nursing interventions, most facilities supply nurses with a preoperative checklist. As each intervention on the list is completed, the nurse initials it.

Preoperative Medications

Prior to administering preoperative medications, check to be sure that the operative permit and transfusion permit (if required) are correctly signed and attached to the client record. These must be signed and witnessed before the client receives any medication that will alter his or her consciousness (such as a narcotic or tranquilizer).

The purposes of various preoperative medications are to allay anxiety, decrease pharyngeal secretions, reduce side effects of anesthetic agents, and induce amnesia.

The pharmacologic preparation for anesthesia is based on many variables, including the client's age and physical and psychological condition, the type of surgery, and the specific anesthesia to be administered.

Table 21–7 presents an overview of common preoperative medications. Specific drug choices are based on individual client variables, the goals for sedation, and the potential for undesirable side effects. Preoperative medications may be given in the preoperative area or on the nursing unit prior to the client leaving for surgery. If the preoperative medication is given on the unit, the nurse is responsible for raising the bed side rails. Lower the window shades, and turn off bright lights. *Instruct the client not to get up without assistance, because medications may cause drowsiness or dizziness.* Once the client is calm and drowsy, disturb the client only when necessary and then briefly and quietly. Observe the client for side effects from medication such as hypotension or respiratory depression.

Table 21–7. Commonly Used Preoperative Medications		
Medication	**Desired Effects**	**Undesired Effects**
Tranquilizers		
Diazepam (Valium)	Decrease anxiety	May cause dizziness, clumsiness, or confusion
Droperidol (Inapsine)	Decrease anxiety Produce an antiemetic effect	Anxiety Hypotension during and after surgery
Sedatives		
Midazolam hydrochloride (Versed)	Induce desired sleepiness and decrease anxiety	Hypotension, undesired respiratory depression
Promethazine hydrochloride (Phenergan)	Same as for droperidol	Hypotension during and after surgery
Secobarbital sodium (Seconal Sodium)	Decrease anxiety Promote sedation	Disorientation, especially in elderly patients
Pentobarbital sodium (Nembutal Sodium)	Same as for secobarbital sodium	Same as for secobarbital sodium
Analgesics		
Morphine sulfate	Relieve pain Decrease anxiety Sedation	Respiratory depression Hypotension Circulatory depression Decreased gastric motility causing potential for vomiting
Fentanyl citrate (Sublimaze)	Short-acting analgesic for minor or outpatient surgery; adjunct to general anesthesia	Same as for morphine sulfate
Meperidine hydrochloride (Demerol)	Same as for morphine sulfate	Same as for morphine sulfate
Anticholinergics		
Atropine sulfate	Control secretions	Excessive dryness of mouth, tachycardia
Glycopyrrolate (Robinul)	Same as for atropine sulfate	Same as for atropine sulfate
Histamine H_2-Receptor Antagonists		
Cimetidine (Tagamet) (See Table 61–3 for other H_2 antagonists)	Inhibit gastric acid production	Some mild dizziness, diarrhea, somnolence, and rash

Transporting the Client to Surgery

When surgical personnel call for the client, gently transfer the client to a stretcher (making sure you have enough help to transfer the client safely). Cover the client with blankets for protection from drafts, place side rails up, and secure with a restraining belt 2 inches above the knee. Make sure the client record accompanies the client to the operating room. Make the trip to surgery as smooth as possible so the sedated client does not develop nausea and dizziness. Avoid rapid walking and swinging the cart around corners.

The nursing unit should prepare the client's room for postoperative care as follows:

1. Arrange furniture so the stretcher can easily be brought to the bedside
2. Make a surgical bed
3. Set out an emesis basin
4. Bring in additional equipment, such as the blood pressure cuff, intravenous setup (if ordered), suction, and oxygen equipment as anticipated
5. Ensure that all equipment is in working order

Caring for Significant Others

During surgery, the significant others usually wait in a designated surgical waiting area. If they must leave the facility for any reason, ask them for a telephone number where they can be reached. Provide the telephone number of the client's unit and the client's room if appropriate.

When discussing surgery with significant others, be aware of information previously given by the surgeon regarding the immediate surgical outcome and eventual prognosis. You can then answer questions confident that the information you give agrees with previous statements.

Prepare significant others for any nasogastric tubes, chest tubes, suction equipment, respiratory equipment, IV infusions, dressings, or monitoring equipment the client might require. Inform significant others when the surgery is completed (this may be done by waiting room personnel). Make certain the surgeon knows who is waiting for information on the client and where they can be found.

Reassure significant others that the length of time the client is gone may not reflect the actual length of surgery. There are often unpredictable delays that might cause the client to wait before surgery. Reassure the family if this has happened so they will not worry unnecessarily.

Intraoperative Nursing

The intraoperative phase of the perioperative experience begins when the client enters the surgical suite and ends with admission to the recovery area. Nursing care during this phase focuses on the client's emotional well-being, as well as on physical factors such as safety, positioning, maintaining asepsis, and controlling the surgical environment. The nurses are the client's advocates upon induction of anesthesia.

In the surgical holding area, the nurse is responsible for reviewing the record for completeness, ensuring proper identification of the client, client safety, and providing emotional support. It is important to deal with the fears and concerns of a frightened or agitated client. A relaxed client undergoes anesthetic induction easier than one who is anxious. If the client still seems anxious despite sedation and reassurance, notify the surgeon or anesthesia personnel.

While in the holding area, the client is usually seen by the anesthesiologist. The IV fluids, if ordered, are usually started at this time. The anesthesiologist or nurse-anesthetist may also administer sedatives or other preoperative medications, especially if the client has not yet received such medications. The client usually remains in a holding area until the operating room is ready.

Procedures vary among institutions, but after admission to the operating room, the client is identified by the surgeon and then moved to the operating room bed. At this time, the client is anesthetized; positioned; has the skin prepared; has any other procedures done, such as catheterization; and is draped for surgery.

Members of the Surgical Team

The surgical team is a group of highly trained and educated individuals who must work together as a coordinated team for the welfare and safety of the client undergoing operative and other invasive procedures. The team is composed of a surgeon, anesthesiologist or certified registered nurse-anesthetist (CRNA), circulating person, scrub person or surgical technologist, and assistants.[147]

The surgeon heads the surgical team and makes the major decisions concerning the course of surgery, such as whether to remove an organ, amputate a limb, or make radical or extensive repairs. The surgeon must be alert at all times to reports from the anesthesia provider concerning the changing physiologic needs of the client undergoing the stress of surgery.

The anesthesiologist (a physician) or nurse-anesthetist (a registered nurse, or RN, with special education) alleviates pain and promotes relaxation with medications. These specialists must (1) maintain the client's airway; (2) ensure that the client has an adequate gas exchange; (3) infuse blood, fluids, and medications to maintain hemodynamic stability; (4) monitor circulation and respiration, including estimation of blood and fluid loss; and (5) alert the surgeon immediately to any complications.

The circulating registered nurse (1) checks that all equipment is working properly before surgery; (2) ensures sterility of the instruments for surgery; (3) assists with positioning the client; (4) performs a skin preparation on the client; (5) alerts team members to any break in sterile technique; (6) assists the anesthesiologist or anesthetist with monitoring vital functions, such as urine output and blood loss; (7) labels specimens; (8) coordinates activities with other departments such as x-ray and pathology; and (9) documents the care provided. The circulating nurse ensures that staff conversation and traffic are kept to a minimum (see Ethical Issues in Nursing feature).

The circulating nurse promotes smooth and safe function in the operating suite by bringing needed supplies and medications to the operating table; assisting with the sponge, sharps, and instrument counts; and removing unneeded items or specimens. The Joint Commission on Accreditation of Healthcare Organizations (JCAHO) recommends that an RN be in close proximity to each operating room.

The scrub person, who may be an RN or a surgical technologist, assists the surgeon during the procedure by handing instruments, sutures, and other supplies. During surgery, the scrub person maintains an accurate count of sponges, sharps, and instruments on the sterile field.

Scrubbing and circulating may become obsolete terms; these define functions that are only part of the perioperative nurse's responsibility. Many believe that the future may bring new titles and functions but will not erase the critical function every perioperative nurse fulfills.[131]

The direct assistants to the surgeon may be other surgeons, surgical residents, an RN first assistant (RNFA), and experienced paraprofessionals. RNFAs and paraprofessionals act under the surgeon's direction.

The surgical team may include other members of the healthcare team if the surgical procedure so dictates. For example, a pathologist may be requested to identify a pathologic finding. An x-ray technician may be needed to perform various radiologic procedures while the client is on the operating table. A cardiopulmonary perfusionist

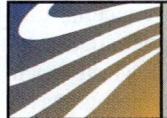

ETHICAL ISSUES IN NURSING

Is It Your Job to Protect the Client's Dignity?

Ms. Hall is having an appendectomy. You are the nurse caring for her in the operating room. During the surgery, one of the resident physicians begins to talk about Ms. Hall, making rude remarks about her. Ms. Hall is a prostitute and the police brought her to the hospital from jail. The statements by the physician are very unprofessional. You are uncomfortable and do not think this is appropriate behavior, even if the client is anesthetized and unable to hear what the resident is saying.

You have thought carefully about the scene in the operating room. You decide to contact the resident after surgery. You meet him in the hall and quietly tell him of the inappropriateness of his actions. The resident tells you that his actions in surgery are none of your business. You are very angry and upset about his disregard of the client and his disregard of your concerns.

After giving yourself some time to be certain that you were not reacting from anger, you decide to write a letter to the medical chief of staff explaining what happened. You have determined that the situation needs further attention. It is imperative that the nurse carefully analyze his or her own motives and biases. Client issues such as confidentiality and respect must define the problem, not old anger or bad feelings toward the resident physician.

Even if nurses are frequently in positions of less power than physicians, client safety, confidentiality, and dignity must be maintained.

---

may be required to assist during cardiothoracic surgery when cardiopulmonary bypass is necessary.

The RN First Assistant

Perioperative nursing practice has historically included the role of the RN as assistant at surgery. As early as 1980, documents issued by the American College of Surgeons supported the appropriateness of qualified RNs to first-assist. In 1983 the Association of Operating Room Nurses (AORN) officially recognized the role as a component of perioperative nursing and adopted the first official statement on RN first assistants (RNFAs) in 1984.

> The RN first assistant at surgery collaborates with the surgeon in performing a safe operation with optimal outcomes for the client. The RN first assistant practices perioperative nursing and must have acquired the necessary specific knowledge, skills, and judgment. The RN first assistant practices under the supervision of the surgeon during the intraoperative phase of the perioperative experience. The RN first assistant does not concurrently function as a scrub nurse.[14]

Scope of Practice

The scope of practice of the nurse performing as first assistant is a part of perioperative nursing practice. The activities include first assisting and are further refinements of perioperative nursing practice *executed within the context of the nursing process. Their observable nursing behaviors* are based on an extensive body of scientific knowledge.

These intraoperative nursing behaviors may include the following:

● Handling tissue
● Providing exposure of the surgical area
● Using instruments
● Suturing
● Providing homeostasis

These functions may vary depending on client populations, practice environments, services provided, accessibility of human and fiscal resources, institutional policy, and state nurse practice acts.[14]

Training for the RN First Assistant

The complexity of knowledge and skill required to care effectively for recipients of operating room nursing services requires nurses to be well-educated and to continue their education beyond generic nursing programs. Perioperative nurses who wish to practice as RNFAs, must develop a set of cognitive, psychomotor, and affective behaviors and demonstrate accountability and responsibility for identifying and meeting the needs of their nursing clients. Further preparation for the RNFA includes perioperative nursing practice with diversified experience in scrubbing and circulating. This should culminate in the nurse achieving certification as a certified registered nurse operating room (CNOR) and certified registered nurse first assistant (CRNFA). Additional preparation is then acquired through completion of formal education programs including instruction and supervised clinical learning activities. These programs should consist of the curricula and address all of the content area of the modules in the core curriculum for the RNFA, take place in institutions approved by the Association of Higher Education (or its equivalent), and award a degree of certification upon successful program completion.[147]

Anesthesia Providers

In the United States, anesthesia care is usually provided by (1) an anesthesiologist; (2) a CRNA working under the direction of the anesthesiologist or a physician; or (3) an anesthesiologist's assistant (i.e., physician's assistant in anesthesia) working under the direction of an anesthesiologist. An anesthesiologist is a physician with 4 or more years of specialty training in anesthesiology after medical school.

Nurse anesthesia programs are now a minimum of 2 years in length. They require a bachelor of science degree in nursing or other appropriate field plus 1 year of acute or intensive care nursing experience before acceptance. Many nurse anesthesia programs are master's degree level in a school of nursing or allied health, although a number of programs are based in community hospitals. In recent years, anesthesiologist's assistants (AAs) have also been trained. These are physician's assistants to the anesthesiologist. Acceptance into an AA program requires a BS degree, including a college-level premedical education and a satisfactory score on the medical college admission test (MCAT) or graduate record examination (GRE). These AA programs are offered only in medical schools with an approved residency program in anesthesiology. The 2-year training program is based upon the classified premedical education.

In this section, the term *anesthesia provider* denotes the person providing continuous anesthesia care of the client. Depending on the practice in a given hospital, this may be an anesthesiologist, nurse-anesthetist, or an AA.[147]

Anesthesia in Surgery

Anesthesia means the absence of pain (Greek *an-*, without + *aisthesis,* feeling). Anesthesia is an artificially induced state of partial or total loss of sensation, with or without loss of consciousness. Anesthesia produces muscle relaxation, blocks transmission of nerve impulses, and suppresses reflexes.

Clients are generally anxious about receiving anesthesia. Some are concerned about the adequacy of the analgesic effects. Others are concerned about being "put to sleep" with a drug. Some clients wonder if they will talk during anesthesia or experience nausea and vomiting after surgery. Reviewing the client's preoperative nursing assessment reveals some of these fears and concerns and allows the surgical nursing staff to offer continued support. A smile, a cordial introduction, and a warm touch help allay clients' fears in a threatening and strange environment.

The decision as to the type of anesthesia to be used is made largely by the anesthesia provider in consultation with the surgeon and client. The anesthetic agents chosen for a surgical procedure depend on many variables. These include (1) age and physical condition of the client; (2) type, location, and duration of the surgery; (3) degree of technical intricacy of the surgery; (4) previous anesthetic history; and (5) the personal preference, expertise, and judgment of the anesthesiologist or nurse-anesthetist. Also, the client undergoing surgery may prefer one type of anesthesia over another (e.g., spinal anesthesia rather than general anesthesia). A client's preference should be considered as part of the total profile when the type of anesthesia is selected.

There are two major classifications of anesthesia: (1) general and (2) regional. General anesthetics block pain stimulus at the cerebral cortex. General anesthesia is a drug-induced depression of the central nervous system (CNS) that is reversed either by metabolic elimination in the body or by pharmacologic means. General anesthetic agents produce analgesia, amnesia, and unconsciousness, characterized by loss of reflexes and muscle tone.

Regional anesthetics block the pain stimulus (1) at its origin, (2) along afferent neurons, or (3) along the spinal cord. Unlike general anesthesia, regional anesthesia produces a loss of painful sensation in only one region of the body and does not result in unconsciousness. The client also may receive sedative agents that produce drowsiness. The client might receive epidural narcotics, which have a systemic effect and produce some drowsiness. Table 21–8 illustrates the goal, method of administration, and assessment of these two major types of anesthesia.

Table 21–8. Types of Anesthesia			
Type	**Goal**	**Administration**	**Assessment**
General	Total loss of consciousness and sensation; produces amnesia by blocking awareness centers in brain	Intravenous Inhalation Rectal	Loss of reflexes and muscle tone
Regional	Reduces all painful sensations in one region of the body without inducing unconsciousness		
	Blocks transmission of nerve impulses at their origin	Topical Local infiltration	Produces analgesia over specific tissue area
	Blocks transmission of nerve impulses along afferent neurons	Field block Nerve block Intravenous regional	Produces analgesia over specific area of body
	Blocks transmission of nerve impulses along spinal cord	Spinal Epidural block	Produces analgesia over specific region of body

The Physical Status Classification of the American Society of Anesthesiology

One tool developed to determine the client's risk for side effects while undergoing anesthesia is the American Society of Anesthesiology's physical status classification:

Class 1: A client with no organic, physiologic, biochemical, or psychiatric disturbances.

Class 2: Mild to moderate systemic disturbances caused by a condition to be treated surgically or by a pathophysiologic process. Example: hypertension or diabetes.

Class 3: Severe systemic disease with more than one system involved. Example: hypertension and cardiac disease and pulmonary problems.

Class 4: Severe systemic disease or disturbances that are life threatening. Examples: heart disease with cardiac insufficiency; persistent angina; advanced degrees of pulmonary, hepatic, renal, or endocrine insufficiency.

Class 5: A client who has little chance of survival. Surgery may be a resuscitative measure with little anesthesia. Example: a ruptured abdominal aneurysm or major cerebral trauma with rapidly increasing intracranial pressure.

Emergency surgery: Any client in one of the classes listed who undergoes surgery in an emergency situation.[156]

General Anesthesia

Effects of General Anesthesia. The body systems affected by general anesthetics are the neurologic, respiratory, and cardiovascular systems. General anesthesia is best suited for surgery of the head, neck, upper torso, and back; for prolonged surgical procedures; or for clients who are unable to lie quietly for a prolonged period of time. General anesthetic agents affect all tissues in the body to some degree.

The anesthesia provider continually monitors body systems and tissues during induction of anesthesia, maintenance of the anesthetized state, and emergence of the client from anesthesia. These specialists understand when body systems are functioning adequately, and they recognize and intervene when systems are unstable. The depth of anesthesia is monitored by observing changes in respiration, oxygen saturation and end-tidal CO_2, heart rate, urine output, and blood pressure.

Stages of General Anesthesia. The four stages of anesthesia are described in Table 21–9. Surgery is performed in stage III. Although not apparent with all anesthetics, all three stages may be seen if the drug is given slowly. Clients emerge through all three stages after the anesthetic agents are discontinued.

Administration of General Anesthesia. General anesthesia can be administered by inhalation, IV,

Table 21–9. The Four Stages of Anesthesia

Stage	From	To	Assessment	Nursing Interventions
1: Onset	Anesthetic administration	Loss of consciousness	Client may be drowsy or dizzy May experience auditory or visual hallucinations	Close operating room doors; keep room quiet; stand by to assist client
II: Excitement	Loss of consciousness	Loss of eyelid reflexes	Increase in autonomic activity Irregular breathing Client may struggle	Remain quietly at client's side; assist anesthetist, if needed
III: Surgical anesthesia	Loss of eyelid reflexes	Loss of most reflexes Depression of vital functions	Client is unconscious Muscles are relaxed No blink or gag reflex	Begin preparation (if indicated) only when anesthetist indicates stage III has been reached and client is under good control
IV: Danger (death)	Vital functions too depressed	Respiratory and circulatory failure	Client is not breathing May or may not have a heartbeat	If arrest occurs, respond immediately to assist in establishing airway; provide cardiac arrest tray, drugs, syringes, long needles; assist surgeon with closed or open cardiac massage

Table 21–10. General Anesthetic Agents

Drug	Action	Side Effects	Nursing Implications
Inhalation Agents			
Nitrous oxide	Gas with very low anesthetic potency, so it must be used with other agents; highest analgesic effect of all agents; little or no effect on BP or P; no muscle relaxant properties	Minimal side effects; little or no hypotension or respiratory depression; low incidence of malignant hypothermia	Monitor vital signs, especially BP and P; monitor effects of CNS depressants for 24 hours after administration
Halothane (Fluothane)	Volatile liquid with high anesthetic potency, so it could be used alone; has weak analgesic effect; causes a moderate decrease in BP and a large decrease in respirations, and is only a mild muscle relaxant	Hypotension, depression of myocardium with decreased cardiac output, bradycardia, respiratory depression, sensitizes heart to catecholamines, malignant hyperthermia, hepatitis, postoperative mild nausea and vomiting, decreased urine output	Monitor all vital signs closely; monitor temperature for signs of malignant hyperthermia; keep client warm during recovery, and watch for severe shivering; avoid use of catecholamines (epinephrine or norepinephrine); monitor liver function after surgery; monitor urine output closely
Enflurane (Ethrane)	Volatile liquid with fairly high anesthetic potential; has weak analgesic effect; causes moderate decrease in BP, a large decrease in respirations, and is moderate muscle relaxant	Hypotension, respiratory depression, blocks labor, minimal sensitization of heart to catecholamines, and seizures with high doses	Do not give to clients with history of seizures; monitor vital signs, especially BP, P, and respirations; not for use during labor
Isoflurane (Forane)	Volatile liquid with high anesthetic potential; has weak analgesic effect; causes moderate decrease in BP, a large decrease in respirations, and is a moderate muscle relaxant; produces profound vasodilation	Hypotension related to vasodilating effect; respiratory depression; suppresses uterine contractions	Does not sensitize heart to catecholamines, so it can be used with epinephrine and norepinephrine; monitor vital signs; and avoid rapid position changes, because it may lead to hypotension due to vasodilation
Intravenous Drugs			
Thiopental sodium (Pentothal)	Short-acting barbiturate that produces rapid unconsciousness; a weak analgesic and muscle relaxant	Respiratory depression with momentary apnea after injection, retrograde amnesia, myocardial depression, hypotension, headache, and shivering	Monitor for allergic reactions; monitor respiratory function closely, especially during induction; monitor vital signs; cannot be mixed with solutions containing atropine, tubocurarine, or succinylcholine; avoid extravasation
Fentanyl citrate–droperidol (Innovar)	A potent opioid (fentanyl) combined with a neuroleptic (droperidol); produces indifference to surroundings and insensitivity to pain; CNS depressant, which produces calming, analgesia, and reduced motor activity	Emergence delirium with hallucinations, hypotension, vasodilation, nausea and vomiting, laryngospasm, respiratory depression, shivering, and apnea	Use with caution in clients with head injuries, increased intracranial pressure, COPD, hepatic or renal dysfunction, bradyarrhythmias, or with elderly; monitor vital signs; maintain patent airway; reduce narcotic doses to one fourth or one third for the first 24 hours postoperatively; when Innovar is used for induction, fentanyl citrate (Sublimaze) alone is used for maintenance of anesthesia

	Table 21–10. General Anesthetic Agents (*Continued*)		
Drug	**Action**	**Side Effects**	**Nursing Implications**
Ketamine hydrochloride (Ketalar)	Produces state of dissociative anesthesia. Causes sedation, immobility, analgesia, amnesia, and unresponsiveness to pain; short-acting (no antagonist)	Delirium, hallucinations, disturbing dreams, tonic and clonic movements, respiratory depression, hypotension or hypertension, decreased or increased pulse, nystagmus, increased salivation, laryngospasms, and mild nausea and vomiting	Contraindicated in clients with history of CVA and severe hypertension; use with caution in clients with alcoholism, or elevated CSF; maintain airway; do not give in same syringe as barbiturates; keep all stimulation to a minimum as client emerges from anesthesia; use diazepam if hallucinations occur or delusions are severe; excellent for anesthesia in young and elderly; pad side rails of gurney; place client in a quiet dark area; do not stimulate client inadvertently; any sudden moves will elicit hallucinations

BP, blood pressure; CNS, central nervous system; COPD, chronic obstructive pulmonary disease; CVA, cardiovascular accident; CSF, cerebrospinal fluid; P, pulse.

rectal, or oral routes. Inhalation and IV methods are the most common routes of administration. Table 21–10 describes the most common general anesthetic agents in use and their implications for nursing.

Neuroleptic (Balanced) Anesthesia. Balanced anesthesia is the practice of selecting drug combinations based on the individual client's need with consideration of the type of surgery. Balanced anesthesia is typically achieved with a combination of inhalation agent, oxygen, narcotic, and neuromuscular blocking agents.

Types of General Anesthesia

Intravenous Anesthesia. When general anesthesia is administered IV, the client experiences an extremely rapid induction. Unconsciousness generally occurs about 30 seconds after the initial IV administration. Intravenous anesthesia is most commonly used as an induction agent before inhalation anesthetics are given. However, IV anesthesia is sufficiently potent to be used alone in such minor procedures as dental extractions or pelvic examinations. Examples of IV anesthetics include thiopental sodium and ketamine. Ketamine has no antagonist but does metabolize quickly. The postanesthesia care unit (PACU) must be alerted to the use of ketamine because of its hallucinogenic properties. Sudden stimulation, loud noises, or bright lights can trigger hallucinatory episodes. The side rails should be padded, lights kept low, and noise kept to a minimum around these clients.

Inhalation Anesthesia. Inhalation anesthesia is a mixture of volatile liquids or gas and oxygen. The mixture is given through a mask or through an endotracheal tube (Fig. 21–2). These anesthetics are advantageous because of their ease of administration and elimination through the respiratory system.

When inhalation anesthesia is administered by mask, the gases generally flow into the mask via a finely calibrated vaporizer controlled by a machine. When an endotracheal tube is used to give anesthetic, the gases flow directly into the client's tracheobronchial tree.

Many different liquids and gases are used in inhalation anesthesia. Two commonly employed volatile liquid anesthetics are halothane and isoflurane. A commonly used gas anesthetic is nitrous oxide.

As mentioned earlier, an IV anesthetic is often administered before the use of inhalation anesthetic. This process promotes a rapid transition from the conscious stage to the surgical anesthesia stage (from stage I to stage III).

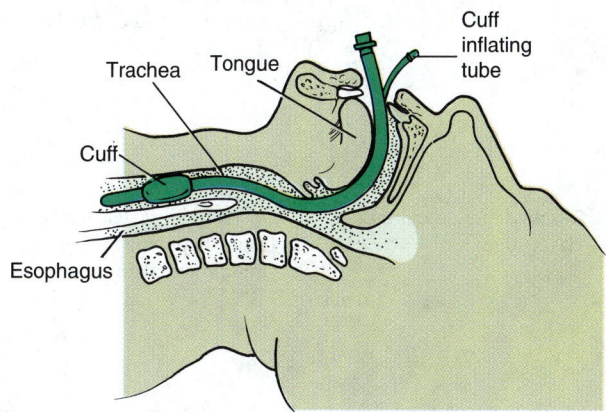

Figure 21–2. Correct placement of the endotracheal tube for anesthesia administration.

In this case, the early stages of anesthesia typically are not seen.

Although ether rarely is used today, it is important historically as one of the oldest known anesthetics. It produces a deep and prolonged anesthesia that rarely results in cardiovascular complications. It was, however, the leading medical cause of perioperative mortality in adults. Ether is sometimes used for high-risk clients, but its highly explosive properties make it a dangerous and less desirable choice.

Rectal Anesthesia. Rectal anesthesia is administered via a rectal tube. This form is rarely used today, although it is useful in children or when facial surgery makes it difficult to maintain an airway. Intravenous or liquid inhalation agents are instilled into the rectum. Methohexital sodium is one anesthetic agent that may be administered rectally. It is absorbed by the rectal mucosa and delivered to the CNS via the circulatory system. Because rectal anesthesia is used only during induction, it must always be supplemented with other types of anesthetic agents.

Neuromuscular Blocking Agents. Neuromuscular blocking agents are administered IV and are given mainly to facilitate intubation, relax the muscles within the surgical field, ease laryngospasms, and relax muscles for controlled ventilation. When given with neuromuscu-

lar blocking agents, potent general anesthetics can be administered in smaller, and thus safer, doses.

Neuromuscular blocking agents are classified as depolarizing and nondepolarizing agents that block the transmission of nervous impulses to the muscle fibers (Table 21–11). This block produces temporary paralysis of voluntary muscles, including the muscles that control respiration. Hence, respiration must be supported mechanically when muscle relaxants are used. Respiration in clients who have received muscle relaxants must be closely monitored for at least 1 hour after the relaxants appear to have worn off because paralysis may recur.

Common muscle relaxants are succinylcholine (Anectine), tubocurarine, pancuronium (Pavulon), and vecuronium (Norcuron).

Regional Anesthesia

Regional anesthetics are useful in many clinical situations. Local anesthetic agents can be used for local effects and also can be administered to function as central, peripheral, intravenous, regional, retrobulbar, or transbronchial nerve blocks. These anesthetic agents block the conduction of impulses in nerve fibers without depolarizing the cell membrane (Table 21–12).

Table 21–11. Muscle Relaxants

Drug	Action	Side Effects	Nursing Implications
Pancuronium bromide (Pavulon)	Nondepolarizing agent; prevents acetylcholine from binding to receptors on muscle endplate, blocking depolarization	Tachycardia, hypertension, prolonged dose-related apnea, allergic reaction, and excessive sweating and salivation	Use carefully in older or debilitated clients or in clients with renal, hepatic, or pulmonary disease, myasthenia gravis, or thyroid disease; measure intake and output carefully; have resuscitation equipment available; do not mix in syringe or solution with barbiturates; neostigmine reverses effect
Vecuronium bromide (Norcuron)	Nondepolarizing agent; prevents acetylcholine from binding to receptors on muscle endplate, blocking depolarization	Transient tachycardia; prolonged dose-related apnea, redness, itching, and induration	Has no effect on cardiovascular system; use with caution in clients with hepatic disease, obesity, or neuromuscular disease; tolerated well in renal disease; reversed with anticholinesterase and neostigmine; have emergency resuscitation equipment available
Succinylcholine chloride (Anectine)	Depolarizing agent that prolongs depolarization of muscle endplate	Increased or decreased pulse rate and blood pressure, dysrhythmias, increased intraocular pressure, prolonged respiratory depression, malignant hyperthermia, postoperative muscle pain, excessive salivation, and hypersensitivity	Monitor vital signs; maintain patent airway; postoperative stiffness is normal; drug of choice for short procedures; keep emergency resuscitation equipment on hand; repeat infusions can prolong apnea; reversible with neostigmine

Table 21–12. Local and Topical Anesthetic Agents

Drug	Action	Side Effects	Nursing Implications
Local Agents			
Bupivacaine hydrochloride (Marcaine HCl)	Amide-type local anesthetic that blocks depolarization, preventing generation and conduction of nerve impulses; combined with epinephrine, it has prolonged action	Edema, anaphylaxis; rarely, anxiety, convulsions, respiratory arrest, cardiac arrest, blurred vision, and shivering	Contraindicated for children under 12, for spinal or paracervical block or topical anesthesia; use with caution in older clients, or clients with hepatic disease or allergies; onset 4–15 minutes, duration 3–6 hours; keep resuscitative equipment available
Chloroprocaine hydrochloride (Nesacaine)	Ester-type local anesthetic that blocks depolarization, preventing generation and conduction of nerve impulses	Anaphylaxis, edema; rarely, anxiety, convulsions, respiratory arrest, cardiac arrest, blurred vision, and shivering	Contraindicated for clients with allergies to "caines," CNS disease; use cautiously with older adults; check solution for particles or discoloration; keep resuscitative equipment available; do not use solution with preservative for caudal or epidural blocks
Lidocaine hydrochloride (Xylocaine)	Amide-type local anesthetic that blocks depolarization, preventing generation and conduction of nerve impulses; combined with epinephrine, it has prolonged action	Edema, anaphylaxis, arrhythmias; rarely, anxiety, respiratory arrest, cardiac arrest, and tinnitus	Contraindicated in clients with hypersensitivity, severe hypertension, septicemia, spinal deformities, or neurologic disorders; use cautiously with older clients and clients with heart block, general drug allergies, or in severe shock; use solutions with epinephrine only in body areas with good blood supply; use preservative-free solution for spinal, epidural, and caudal blocks
Topical Agents			
Benzocaine (Americaine)	Blocks conduction of impulses at sensory nerve endings	Sensitization rash, possible tolerance	Contraindicated in clients with history of hypersensitivity to "caines"; discontinue if rash develops; avoid contact with eyes; avoid inhalation when using spray; has short duration of action; do not use over infected area; if used rectally, clean area well first
Ethyl chloride spray	Produces local anesthesia by producing sensation of cold	Frostbite, tissue necrosis from prolonged use, muscle spasms, and increased pain	Do not apply over broken skin; protect adjacent skin; avoid contact with eyes; avoid inhalation; highly flammable, do not use near open flame; very short duration
Tetracaine hydrochloride (Pontocaine HCl)	Blocks conduction of impulses at sensory nerve endings	Local sensitization and rash	Do not use in hypersensitive clients; clean rectal area well before applying; do not use if rash develops

Table continued on following page

	Table 21–12. Local and Topical Anesthetic Agents *(Continued)*		
Drug	**Action**	**Side Effects**	**Nursing Implications**
Cocaine	Ester-type topical anesthetic, blocks uptake of norepinephrine by adrenergic neurons	CNS stimulation, euphoria, decreased fatigue, tachycardia, vasoconstriction, and hypertension	For topical use only; produces psychological dependence with prolonged or repeated use; schedule II narcotic; use cautiously with clients with history of severe hypertension or heart disease; combined with epinephrine, it can lead to cardiovascular toxicity; monitor vital signs closely

CNS, central nervous system.

Sometimes, epinephrine is added to the local anesthetic agent to provide a more prolonged effect. Epinephrine causes local blood vessels to constrict, thus delaying absorption of the anesthetic agent. Epinephrine should be used with caution in elderly clients with cardiovascular or liver disease.

Types of Regional Anesthesia. There are several anesthetic techniques using regional anesthesia: (1) topical, (2) local infiltration, (3) field block, (4) peripheral nerve block, (5) spinal, (6) epidural, (7) caudal, and (8) IV regional block.

Topical Anesthesia. Topical anesthesia may be directly applied onto the area to be desensitized. The anesthetic may be a solution, ointment, gel, cream, or powder. This short-acting form of anesthesia can block peripheral nerve endings in the mucous membranes of the vagina, rectum, nasopharynx, and mouth. Topical anesthesia is used in minor procedures such as a rectal examination when painful hemorrhoids are present, or before a bronchoscopic examination to desensitize the bronchi.

One drug commonly used for topical anesthesia is cocaine, in a 4% to 10% solution. This agent is for topical use only, and is primarily used to anesthetize the eye and the mucous membranes of the nose, mouth, and urethra. Cocaine is highly toxic. If accidentally injected, it may cause severe excitement and seizures, followed by shock, respiratory failure, and cardiac arrest. Emergency resuscitation equipment must be available.

Other agents used for topical anesthesia include tetracaine, procaine, mepivacaine, bupivacaine, and lidocaine. To avoid an anaphylactic reaction from previous sensitization to anesthetic agents, check the client's drug allergies before topical anesthesia is applied (see Table 21–12).

Local Infiltration Anesthesia. Local infiltration anesthesia involves injection of an anesthetic agent, such as lidocaine (Xylocaine), into the skin and subcutaneous tissue of the area to be incised. Local anesthesia blocks only the peripheral nerves around the area of the incision.

When a local anesthetic is administered, the physician must not allow the needle to slip into one of the veins. If a local anesthetic agent becomes systemic by IV injection, cardiovascular collapse or convulsions may result. For this reason, the physician must always aspirate before injection to ensure the needle is not in a vein.

Field Block Anesthesia. In a field block, the area proximal to the incision is injected and infiltrated with local anesthetics, thereby forming a barrier between the incision and the nervous system. This procedure contrasts with local anesthesia, in which only the area of the incision is injected. Thus, a field block actually walls in the area around the incision and thereby prevents transmssion of sensory impulses to the brain from that area. Precautions to avoid IV administration must be taken in performing field blocks.

Peripheral Nerve Block Anesthesia. A nerve block anesthetizes individual nerves or nerve plexuses rather than all the local nerves anesthetized by a field block. Nerve blocks may be used to anesthetize, for example, a finger (digital nerve block), the entire upper arm (brachial plexus nerve block), or the chest or abdominal wall (intercostal nerve block). Nerves most commonly blocked are those within the brachial plexus and the intercostal, sciatic, and femoral nerves. Drugs commonly used as nerve blocks are lidocaine, bupivacaine, and mepivacaine. The anesthetist attempts to inject the anesthetic along the nerve, rather than into the nerve, to decrease the risk of nerve damage. Once the drug has been injected, it takes several minutes to anesthetize the area.

Nerve blocks, like local infiltration blocks, can produce severe systemic responses if the drug is accidentally injected into a blood vessel. Because epinephrine causes vasoconstriction, particularly of the extremities, surgery

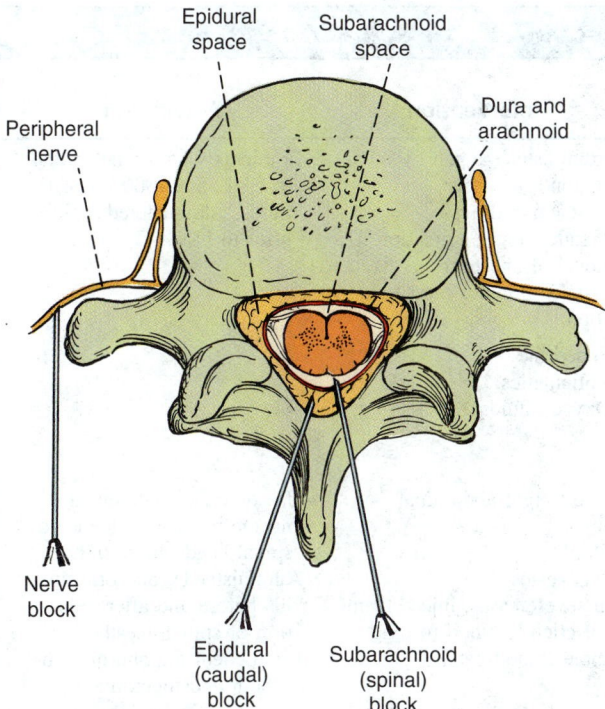

Figure 21–3. Cross section of the spinal cord, showing injection sites for anesthesia.

performed below the wrist or ankle typically uses anesthetics that do not contain epinephrine.

Spinal Anesthesia. Spinal anesthesia is achieved by injecting certain local anesthetics into the subarachnoid space (Fig. 21–3). Autonomic nerve fibers are the first to be affected by spinal anesthesia and the last to recover. Following autonomic blockage, spinal anesthesia blocks the following fibers in this order: touch, pain, motor, pressure, and proprioceptive fibers. Recovery is in reverse order.

Spinal anesthesia can be used for almost any type of major procedure performed below the level of the diaphragm, such as a hysterectomy or appendectomy. Figure 21–4 illustrates the proper positioning for spinal anesthesia. Within minutes after induction of spinal anesthesia, the client experiences a loss of sensation and paralysis of first the toes, then the feet and legs, and finally the abdomen. Most clients exhibit slight hypotension initially due to the vasodilation.

Spinal anesthesia offers many advantages for clients undergoing surgical procedures involving the lower half of the body. It has these major benefits:

- Is relatively safe
- Provides excellent muscle relaxation
- Does not cloud the client's consciousness or alertness (anxious clients, however, can be given a small dose of barbiturate or sedative to enable them to rest or even sleep throughout the operation)
- Can be used for clients with a full stomach, because they will be awake to maintain their airway if they vomit

The complications of spinal anesthesia are listed in Table 21–13 with their causes, prevention, and intervention. Remember that a client who has undergone spinal anesthesia is a candidate for serious neurologic, respiratory, or cardiovascular problems.

As the anesthetic agent wears off, monitor the client carefully. Return of motion to the extremities is checked by asking clients to move their toes. However, clients who can wiggle their toes have not necessarily recovered completely from the spinal anesthetic. An ability to move the toes simply means that the motor blockade is wearing off, although autonomic blockade may still be present. Clients who are still experiencing autonomic blockade are prone to hypotension despite having the ability to move their toes and extremities. Continue to monitor vital signs and for return of sensation.

Epidural Anesthesia. Epidural block is achieved by introducing an anesthetic agent into the epidural space (see Fig. 21–3). The epidural space is generally entered by a needle at the thoracic, lumbar, sacral, or caudal interspaces. The needle is carefully positioned in the epidural space, without penetrating the dura and entering the subarachnoid space. When the needle is properly positioned, the cerebrospinal fluid (CSF) cannot be aspirated.

Epidural block, like spinal anesthesia, produces autonomic blockade. Hypotension can result. Respiratory depression or paralysis also may occur if the level of the block is too high and affects respiratory muscles.

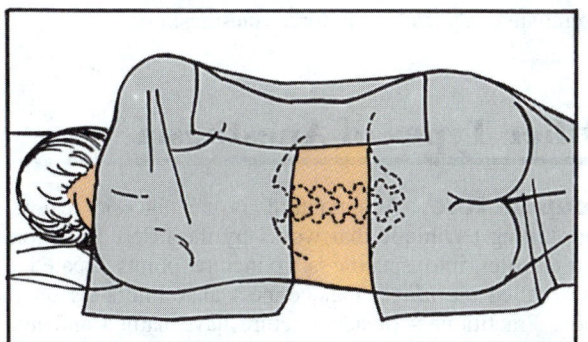
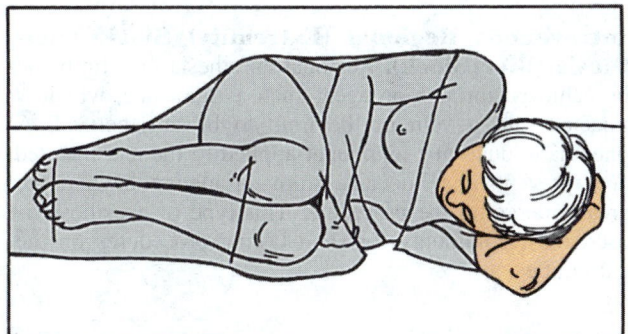

Figure 21–4. Proper positioning for spinal anesthesia administration.

Table 21–13. Complications and Discomforts of Spinal Anesthesia

Complications and Discomforts	Causes	Intervention	Prevention
Hypotension	Paralysis of vasomotor nerves; usually occurs shortly after induction of anesthesia	Administer oxygen by inhalation Vasoactive drugs Trendelenburg's position if level of anesthesia is fixed, 10–20 minutes after induction	In clients who are not prone to CHF, 500–800 ml of IV fluids, administered rapidly prior to block
Nausea and vomiting	Occurs mainly during abdominal surgery, because of traction placed on various structures within abdomen, or hypotension	Ephedrine Antiemetics Oxygen fluids	
Headache (can be extremely painful and may last a week)	Cerebrospinal fluid (which cushions the brain) is lost through dural hole; leakage of fluid and loss of cushioning effect increased by (1) use of a large spinal needle, (2) poor hydration	Apply tight abdominal binder Fluids Analgesics In severe cases, inject 10 ml of client's blood to plug hole (blood patch)	Use of very small spinal needle reduces incidence of spinal headache to 0.9% Administer IV and oral fluids before and after induction of spinal anesthesia Keep client flat and quiet 6–8 hours postoperatively
Respiratory paralysis	Occurs if drug reaches upper thoracic and cervical cord in large amounts or in heavy concentrations	Artificial respiration	Avoid extreme Trendelenburg's position before level of spinal anesthesia set, i.e., 10–20 minutes following induction
Neurologic complications (e.g., paraplegia, severe muscle weakness in legs)	Paralysis postoperatively may be due to (1) unsterile needles, syringes, and anesthetic medications; (2) preexisting diseases of CNS (e.g., multiple sclerosis and spinal cord tumors), which cause paralysis, rather than spinal anesthesia itself	See Unit 5	Strict sterile technique Heat-sterilized medications and instruments Careful preoperative neurologic examination to ascertain presence of neurologic disease

CHF, congestive heart failure; CNS, central nervous system.

Caudal Anesthesia. This type of anesthesia is produced by injecting the local anesthetic into the caudal or sacral canal. Caudal anesthesia is a variation of epidural anesthesia. This method of regional anesthesia is commonly used in obstetric clients.

Intravenous Regional (Extremity) Block Anesthesia (Bier Block). Regional anesthesia of a limb can be achieved through an agent such as lidocaine, which is injected into a vein of the limb to be anesthetized. A pneumatic dual cuff tourniquet applied to the anesthetized area prevents the lidocaine from circulating beyond the area undergoing the procedure. This type of anesthesia is used most commonly for short-lasting procedures on the extremities.

Monitored Anesthesia. Monitored anesthesia is provided when infiltration of the surgical site with a local anesthetic is performed by the surgeon and the anesthesia provider supplements the local anesthetic with IV drugs and provides sedation and systemic analgesia. The anesthesia care provider monitors the client's blood pressure, heart rate, and respiration. *Local standby* and *anesthesia standby* are older, less accurate terms frequently used interchangeably with monitored anesthesia care.[131]

Other Types of Anesthesia

Acupuncture. Acupuncture is an age-old Chinese pain-killing technique that works by the insertion of long, thin needles into specific acupuncture points located on lines called *meridians* that connect anatomic sites on the body. Practitioners of acupuncture have named and numbered around 1000 acupuncture points, each about 0.25 cm (⅛ inch) in diameter.

There are several Western theories to explain why acupuncture works. One, based on the gate theory of pain, holds that the technique stimulates the larger sensory nerve fibers that carry non-pain impulses. Another theory hypothesizes that acupuncture triggers the release of endorphins, endogenous polypeptides with analgesic properties.

Some advantages of acupuncture as an anesthetic include (1) no anesthesia-related side effects during or after surgery, (2) less blood loss during surgery, and (3) reduced need for postoperative analgesia, because acupuncture's pain-killing effects persist for several hours.

When performing major surgery, Chinese doctors use acupuncture as a form of anesthesia. Some Western physicians remain skeptical about the technique's pain-killing capabilities.

Cryothermia. Cryothermia is the use of cold to induce anesthesia. Because a very low surface temperature reduces pain, the surgical site is treated with ice before operating. Although there are many acceptable alternatives to cryothermia, this technique can be used in extreme conditions that threaten life and when the client cannot tolerate a conventional form of anesthesia.

Hypnoanesthesia. Hypnosis is an altered state of consciousness in which the person experiences a heightened state of concentration. As an anesthetic, hypnosis alleviates pain through relaxation, suggestion, and intense concentration on a particular object or sound to the exclusion of other distractions, including pain. Exactly how hypnosis relieves pain is unknown.

Some therapeutic hypnoanesthesia techniques currently used are the following:

● Manifestation suppression in which the client blocks awareness of pain through concentration
● Manifestation substitution in which the client substitutes warmth, pressure, or tingling for the sensation of pain
● Time distortion in which the therapist suggests to the client that the period of pain is very brief when in reality it may last for hours

Hypnoanesthesia has been used successfully in obstetrics and in certain dental procedures, but not everyone is susceptible to hypnotic suggestion. Moreover, it must be performed by a specially trained practitioner. Like cryothermia, there are better alternatives to hypnoanesthesia, especially for major surgery.

Nursing Care During Surgery

Providing Emotional Care

The client's emotional well-being is paramount during the operative phase. Before anesthesia, the nurse is responsible for ensuring that the client feels secure and that anxieties have been addressed.

If the client is awake during the procedure, the nurse should explain the procedure and support and reassure the client. When the client is recovering from the anesthesia, explanations and reinforcement of teaching should be given.

Assisting with Positioning

The perioperative nurse understands the various operative positions as well as the physiologic changes that occur when a client is placed in a specific position. Essential factors to consider when positioning a client on the operating room bed include (1) site of operation, (2) age and size of client, (3) type of anesthetic used, and (4) pain normally experienced by the client on movement, such as from arthritis. The position must not hinder respiration or circulation, apply excessive pressure to skin surfaces, or limit surgical exposure. The following surgical positions are shown in Figure 21–5:

● The *dorsal recumbent (supine)* position is commonly used for hernia repair, mastectomy, or bowel resection
● *Trendelenburg's* position permits displacement of the intestines into the upper abdomen and is often used during surgery of the lower abdomen or pelvis
● The *lithotomy* position exposes the perineal and rectal areas, and is ideal for vaginal repairs, dilatation and curettage, and most rectal surgeries
● The *laminectomy (prone)* position is used during surgical procedures involving the spine
● The *lateral* position is used for clients undergoing kidney, chest, or hip surgery

Whatever the client's position on the operating room bed, there are certain general considerations and rules of safety to observe:

● Explain to the client in simple, understandable terms, why the positions and restraints are necessary.
● Always place a safety strap 2 inches above the knees.
● Preserve the client's dignity and avoid undue exposure.
● Secure the client to the table with well-padded straps, usually placed above the knees. Nerves, muscles, and bony prominences are padded to prevent nerve and tissue damage.
● Maintain adequate respiratory exchange and vascular circulation to permit the exchange of gases. Avoid pressure on the chest and on body parts such as the female breast and male genitalia, especially in the prone position, because pressure can impair or slow circulation, resulting in the pooling of blood. Slow blood flow predisposes to thrombus formation.
● Do not allow the client's extremities to dangle over the sides of the table, because this may impair circulation or cause nerve and muscle damage.
● When using an armboard, do not abduct the upper extremity more than 90 degrees since this could crush the brachial plexus between the first rib and scapula.
● Avoid excessive strain on the client's muscles.
● Be certain the client's body does not rest on hands or fingers; circulation may be occluded.
● Always move both lower extremities at the same time when putting them up in the stirrups and when lowering them so that the hips are not dislocated or the muscles strained.

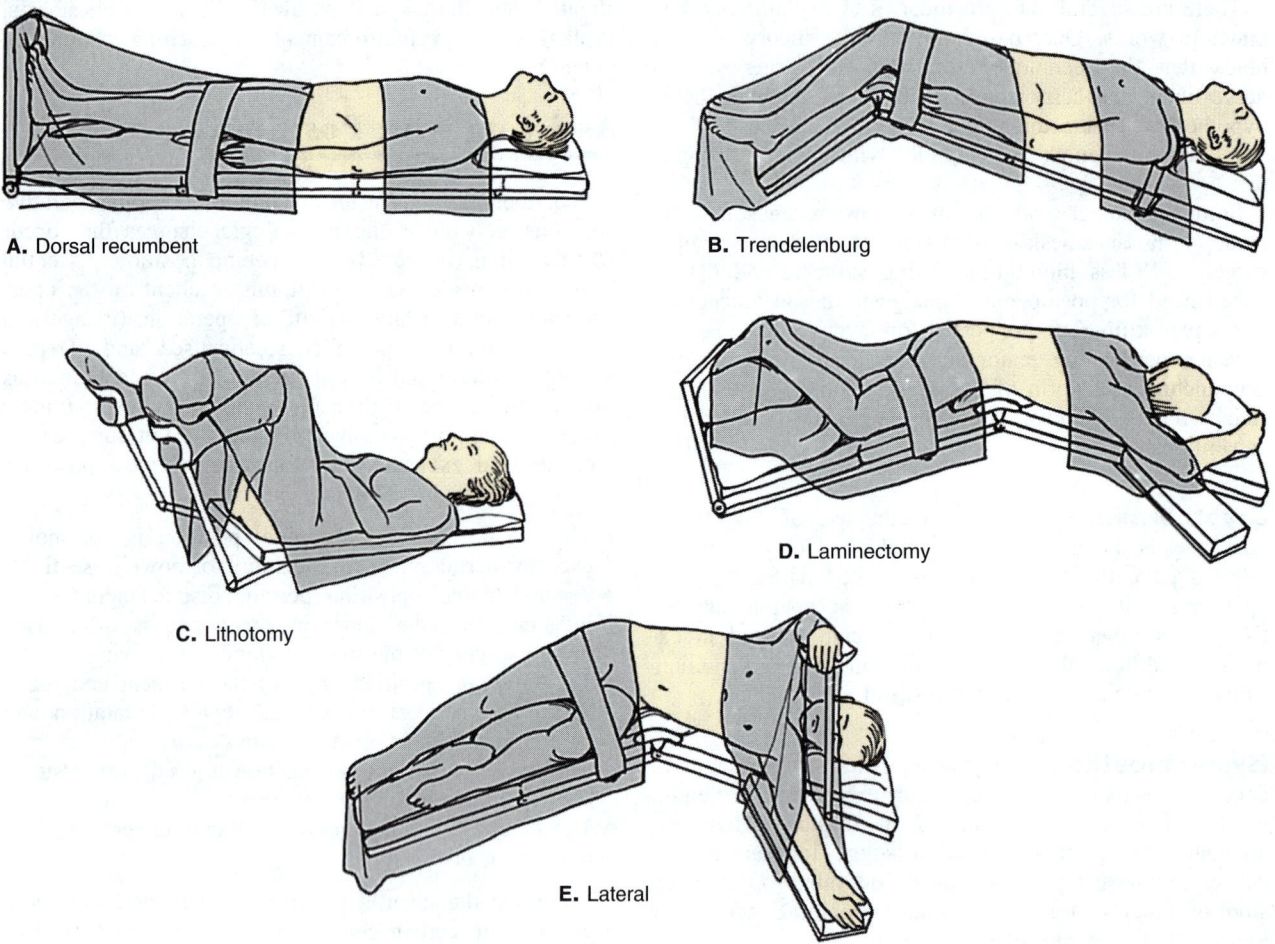

A. Dorsal recumbent

B. Trendelenburg

C. Lithotomy

D. Laminectomy

E. Lateral

Figure 21–5. Five surgical positions.

Remember that the client may remain in one position for hours. Even with careful positioning, most clients feel stiff and sore after a long surgical procedure. Therefore, observe the client throughout surgery, protect any unprotected bony prominence or pressure points, and readjust the client's position as needed.

Maintaining Safety

Other safety precautions include the need to count needles, sponges, and instruments before the incision is closed. When electrocautery is used, the client must be safely grounded. A ground pad is usually applied to the thigh or back so that electric shocks are prevented.

Maintaining Surgical Asepsis

The nurse is responsible for maintaining surgical asepsis during the procedure. The perioperative nurse is responsible for ensuring the sterility of supplies and equipment, and also for ensuring that all members of the health team use sterile technique. If a suspected or actual break in the sterile field occurs, the contaminated instruments or clothing are replaced with sterile items.

Preventing Client Heat Loss

The temperature in the operating room is maintained at a standard cool level (60°–75° F) and humidity (50%–60%) is regulated to inhibit bacterial growth. The client usually feels cold in the operating room if he or she is not well covered. The client loses heat from the skin and from the area open for surgery. When tissues that are not covered with skin are exposed to the air, heat loss is greater. The client should be kept as warm as possible to minimize heat loss without causing vasodilation that could cause more bleeding.

Monitoring for Malignant Hyperthermia

Malignant hyperthermia is a genetic disorder characterized by uncontrolled skeletal muscle contraction, leading to potentially fatal hyperthermia. It occurs in clients with this genetic disorder who receive a combination of succinylcholine and inhalation agents (especially halothanes). This condition can occur within 30 minutes of anesthesia induction or several hours after surgery. The initial manifestation is increased end-tidal CO_2, masseter muscle rigidity, cardiac arrhythmias, and a hypermetabolic state. The client's fever can rise as high as 109° F (43° C). Unless the triggering event is stopped and attempts are made to cool the body, death can result. Dantrolene, a skeletal muscle relaxant, can be used to decrease the skeletal muscle rigidity. There is a screening test for this disorder. A muscle biopsy must be taken from the vastus lateralis or abdominal rectus muscle and sent to a malignant hyperthermia laboratory for testing. This test is very expensive. A family history of general anesthetic problems may reveal the possibility of malignant hyperthermia.

Assisting with Wound Closure

The last step in the surgical procedure is closure of the surgical wound. Prior to closure, sponge, instrument, and needle counts must be done. Sutures are used to approximate the wound edges until wound healing is complete or to occlude the lumen of a blood vessel. A contaminated wound may be left open or partially open to drain and then to heal by secondary or tertiary intention.

The surgeon selects the method and type of closure to be used on the basis of surgical site, the size and depth of the surgical wound, and the age and condition of the client. The surgical wound is closed in layers with sutures, staples, skin closure strips, retention sutures, or zipperlike devices. In the process of closing the incision, the surgeon approximates the wound edges as closely as possible, with as little manipulation to the tissues as possible.

After the incision is closed, a dressing is applied to prevent wound contamination, absorb drainage, and provide support for the incision. If healing progresses without major complications, the sutures, clips, and staples are usually removed after 7 to 10 days. Common skin closures are illustrated in Figure 21–6.

Assessing Drainage

A drain is placed in a separate stab wound parallel to the incision to drain blood, serum, and debris from the operative site. If this material is allowed to collect, it may delay wound healing and promote infection. There are several types of surgical drains. The type of drain chosen

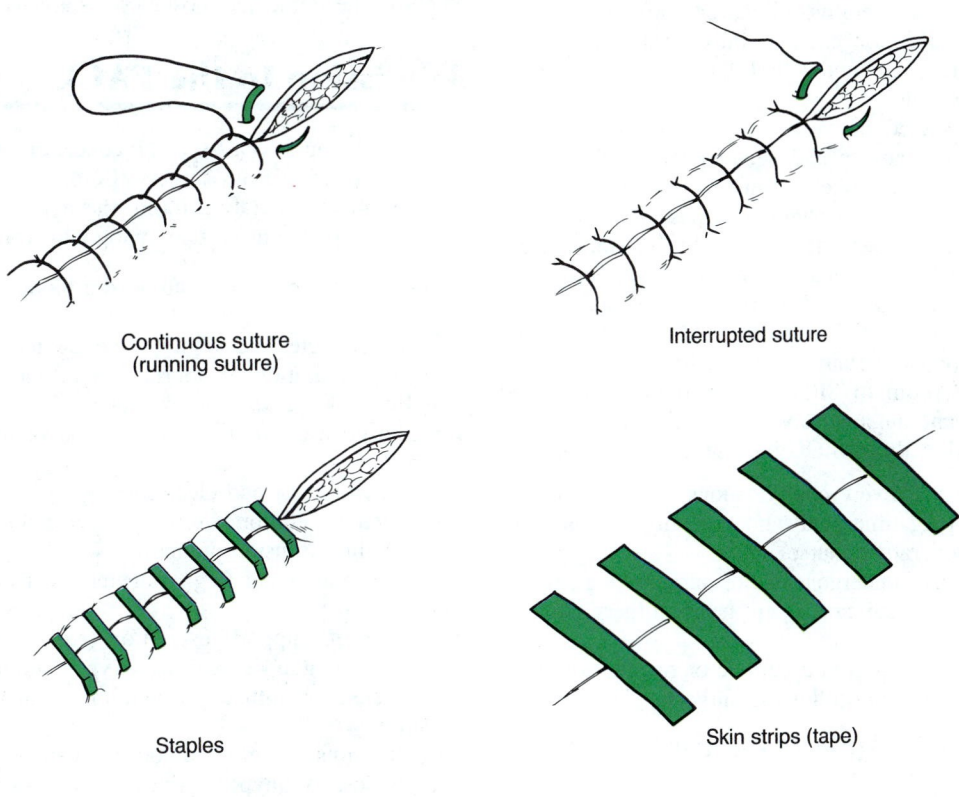

Continuous suture
(running suture)

Interrupted suture

Staples

Skin strips (tape)

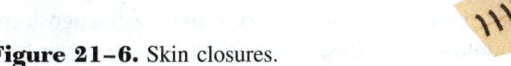

Retention suture

Figure 21–6. Skin closures.

is based on the size of the wound and type of drainage expected. Drains may be free-draining, attached to a suction apparatus, or self-contained with suction.

The nurse is responsible for assessing that the drainage is flowing freely through the system. Drains are usually removed when the drainage is reduced to an insignificant amount.

Transporting the Client

Following the operation, generally a member of the surgical team, wipes off any drainage, dresses the client in a clean gown, then assists with transfer of the client to a stretcher. During this transfer, the operating room personnel avoid exposure, which may be embarrassing and predispose the client to heat loss, respiratory infections, and shock. Also, avoid rough handling, which may strain the client's sutures and conveys lack of concern for the client's comfort and feelings. Finally, avoid hurried movements and rapid changes in position that predispose the client to hypotension. In particular, the client must be moved gradually from the lithotomy to the horizontal position and from the prone to the supine position, and the client must be moved carefully after receiving spinal or epidural anesthesia. When moving or transferring a client after surgery, always have adequate help to prevent injuries to the postoperative client or staff. Very large clients, some orthopedic clients, and clients going to the surgical intensive care unit (SICU) are often placed directly into their beds.

After being placed on the stretcher, the client is covered with warm blankets and secured with safety belts. The side rails of the stretcher must be up to ensure the client's safety in case the client becomes agitated during transport from the operating room. The anesthesia care provider, as well as another member of the operating room professional staff, and sometimes the surgeon or assistant accompany the client to the PACU.

In some hospitals, certain clients are transferred directly from operating room to SICU for continued specialized care and constant nursing supervision. Clients who may be transferred directly to SICU include the following.

- Those at risk of severe complications, who remain unstable for a long time, and who probably have a complicated postoperative course
- Those who have undergone major surgery (e.g., resection of aortic aneurysm, open heart surgery, kidney transplant)
- Those who have suffered a cardiac or respiratory arrest during or immediately following surgery

The client has now begun the postoperative phase.

Postoperative Nursing

The postoperative phase of surgery is the third and final phase of the surgical experience. Nursing plays a critical role in returning the client to an optimal level of functioning. The postoperative period can be divided into two

phases. The first phase, the immediate postanesthesia and postoperative period, is the first few hours after surgery when the client is recovering from the effects of anesthesia. The second phase, or later postoperative phase, is a time for healing and preventing complications. This period may last for weeks, months, or even years after surgery. There is certainly an overlap of these two phases, but for purposes of discussion they will be dealt with separately.

The Postanesthesia Care Unit

The immediate postanesthesia period is a critical time for the client. Close observation is important. The client's vital physiologic functions must be supported until the effects of the anesthesia abate. Until then, the client is dependent, drowsy, and may be unable to call for assistance. In the PACU, nurses assess the client during recovery from the immediate effects of surgery and intervene as appropriate.

ASPAN has described the goal of postanesthesia nursing as assisting the client to return to a safe physiologic level after anesthesia by providing safe, knowledgeable, individualized nursing care to clients and their significant others in the immediate postanesthesia phase.[9]

Admission to the PACU

The PACU nurse has special education in the care of clients recovering from surgery. Before the arrival of each client from the operating room, the nurse checks that the following equipment is functioning and ready for use:

- Sphygmomanometer or automatic blood pressure monitor
- Pulse oximeter—a noninvasive device that measures oxygen saturation of arterial blood, and the pulse rate, and provides a warning of hypoxemia
- Stethoscope to auscultate breath sounds and blood pressure
- Cardiac monitor and electrodes
- Intravenous equipment (e.g., insertion equipment, fluids, tubing, infusion pumps)
- Suction equipment (e.g., catheters, sterile saline, sterile gloves)
- Supplies to support respiration (e.g., artificial airways, oxygen, tongue depressors, oxygen tubing with masks and cannulas, intubation equipment, an anesthesia machine)
- Medications (e.g., narcotics, narcotic antagonists, hypnotics, antihypertensives, neuromuscular blocking agents)
- Emesis basins, mouth wipes, urinals, and bedpans
- Thermometers for oral, rectal, and tympanic membrane
- Warmed blankets or electric warming units to maintain body temperature
- Emergency cart containing emergency medications (cardiotonics, vasotonics, respiratory drugs), a tracheostomy tray, endotracheal tubes, a defibrillator, a cutdown tray,

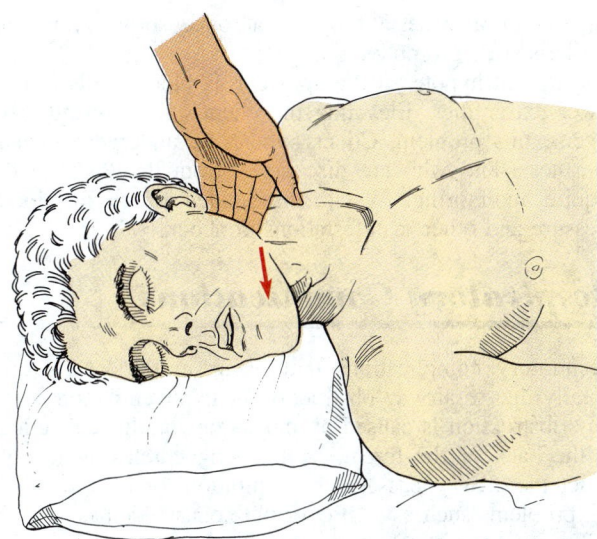

Figure 21–7. Position of the hand to move the jaw forward after anesthesia. The fingers are placed behind the angle of the jaw. As the jaw is moved, the tongue comes forward, opening the airway.

a ventilator, gastric suction equipment, and chest tube insertion equipment

The client is left on the stretcher while in the PACU. Proper positioning of an unconscious or semiconscious client ensures airway patency. Keep the adult client's head to the side and the chin extended forward; you may need to extend the neck and thrust the jaw forward (Fig. 21–7). The lateral Sims position allows the client's tongue to fall forward and mucus or vomitus to drain. There may be specific surgical or anatomic reasons to keep a client lying flat on the back while in the PACU. When this is the case, carefully monitor the client's respiratory status. Have suction equipment ready to suction vomit or oral secretions.

Immediate Baseline Assessment

On admission, the PACU nurse performs the following:

● Assesses airway patency and support as needed, and assesses for the presence of hoarseness, croup, stridor, wheezes, or decreased breath sounds
● Applies humidified oxygen via nasal cannula or face mask (unless otherwise ordered)
● Records vital signs (blood pressure; heart rate, strength, and regularity; respiratory rate and depth; oxygen saturation; skin color; and temperature
● Assesses the client's level of consciousness, muscle strength, and ability to follow commands
● Observes the client's IV infusions, dressings, drains, and special equipment
● Remains at the client's bedside, continuing close observation of the client's condition

After the client has been positioned safely and the baseline vital signs status has been ascertained, the nurse receives a verbal report from members of the operating room team and a detailed report of events from the anesthesia provider.

The following information is provided during the report:

● What operative procedure was performed?
● What was the incision time?
● What were the client's vital signs in the operating room?
● What were the client's blood loss, fluids or blood infused, and urine output?
● Was the procedure eventful or uneventful?
● What are the client's medical diagnosis, pertinent medical history, and daily medications?
● What anesthetic agents, narcotics, neuromuscular blocking agents, or antibiotics has the client received?
● Did the client suffer any complications during surgery? What interventions were instituted? Were drains inserted? What were the outcomes?
● What pathologic disorders were encountered during surgery? Was cancer or some other unexpected problem discovered?
● Are there any specific manifestations or complications to observe? What manifestations should be reported immediately?
● Are there physician orders to be carried out immediately?

With the anesthesia provider present, the PACU nurse then reviews the client's record, noting specifically (1) the anesthesia record for IV medications and blood received during surgery, and (2) the length of time the client was in surgery. Ideally, a preoperative nursing assessment and nursing history are available in the record for comparison with the postoperative assessment.

Following the baseline nursing assessments, review of the client's record, and the postoperative verbal report, the PACU nurse assesses and documents routine observations. Observations to document include the following:

● Time of admission to the PACU.
● The absence of reflexes, such as the pharyngeal reflex. Clients admitted to the PACU without a pharyngeal reflex are positioned on their side if their condition allows. *The nurse stays at the bedside until the client's gag reflex returns.*
● Level of consciousness. What is the response to stimuli such as light or touch? Does saying the client's name or giving simple commands bring a response? Is the client moving voluntarily or making audible or intelligible sounds?
● Temperature and vital signs. Monitor the vital signs every 15 minutes until they are stable, or more often as necessary. In some hospitals this assessment continues until the client leaves the PACU (usually a minimum of 1 hour). Monitor the temperature on admission and at intervals until the client is discharged as established by PACU policy. Usually, clients must achieve a minimum temperature of greater than 36° C (96.8° F) before they are discharged from the PACU.
● Skin color and dryness. Dusky, pale, cold, moist skin is an important manifestation of shock and should be considered with blood pressure. Also, observe the lips and

nail beds for pallor and cyanosis. Consider this information in relationship to oxygen saturation and hemoglobin.

- Skin condition and color. Pink color, free from inflammation, free from hematoma or serum collection, intact and dry.
- Condition of the dressing. (Dry or soiled? Intact?) If soiled, note the color, type, and amount of drainage.
- Drainage tubes, such as T tube, gastric tube, urinary catheter, or wound drains. Is the T tube unclamped and attached to a gravity drainage system? Are gastric, chest, and intestinal tubes attached to suction as ordered? Ensure that tubes are patent and drain freely, that there are no kinks in the tubes, and that the client is not lying upon them. Note the volume of drainage and color. Note any abnormalities in the appearance of the urine.
- Intravenous infusion. Note the type of IV solutions that are running. Also, check the amount of IV solution left in the bottle and the rate of infusion. Redness, soreness, and swelling at the insertion site may indicate that the solution has infiltrated. Note medications added to the IV solution or orders.
- Infusion of blood products or colloid infusion, if one is ordered. Check the rate of drip, and watch carefully for manifestations of a reaction.
- Maintenance of the client's comfort and safety. Side rails always must be up. Maintain proper body alignment, and turn the client from side to side. Offer psychological support.
- Pain. Observe and interview client about pain. Initiate analgesia in consultation with anesthesia personnel or PACU policy.

After completing the assessment, the nurse performs an assessment that relates to the specific surgical procedure. In most healthcare facilities, the nurse and other PACU staff record their observations on a postanesthesia recovery assessment form. The nurse reviews the physician's order sheet for further instructions and medication orders.

Assessment and Interventions for Immediate Postoperative Complications

Nursing intervention during the immediate postoperative period centers on performing interventions to prevent or treat complications. The most common immediate postoperative complications that occur are those related to spinal anesthesia and those affecting the respiratory, cardiovascular, and renal systems and fluid and electrolyte balance.

Complications of Spinal Anesthesia

An important nursing intervention for the client who has received spinal anesthesia is to check the blood pressure, heart rate, and depth of breathing every 10 to 15 minutes during the recovery period. If the blood pressure begins to fall rapidly or if breathing becomes labored, notify the

surgeon or anesthesia provider at once so interventions can be started promptly.

Transient hypotension may occur as blood pools in the lower extremities. Elevating the client's feet can quickly reverse this problem. Clients who have undergone spinal anesthesia and who are discharged from the PACU still require monitoring. Watch for sudden drops in blood pressure and other manifestations of shock.

Respiratory Complications

Respiratory complications that occur in the PACU are usually due to airway obstruction or hypoventilation. Airway obstruction is caused by mucus or vomitus collecting in the back of the throat, by the tongue relaxing to obstruct the airway passage, by aspiration, or by pre-existing problems such as COPD or pulmonary edema.

The primary intervention to prevent respiratory complications is ensuring that the airway is patent. All clients receive oxygen, usually at the rate of 60%/6 L, although clients with COPD will receive no more than 20%/2 L. In the immediate postoperative period, the head of a minimally responsive client may be turned to the side and the chin extended forward to prevent respiratory obstruction. An oral or nasal airway may be placed to help maintain airway patency and tongue control. The airway is a hollow rubber or plastic tube inserted through the nose or mouth that passes over the base of the tongue to keep the tongue from falling back and obstructing the anatomic airway (Fig. 21–8). Airways should not be taped in place. When clients awaken and the gag reflex returns, they may spit it out. When the gag reflex has returned, the PACU nurse may remove the airway for the responsive client who is unable to remove it unaided. Its continued presence could irritate or stimulate vomiting or laryngospasm. The client who is unable to clear mucus or vomitus from the throat requires suctioning immediately.

Some clients are intubated and ventilated. They require close monitoring and suctioning as needed. When the client is extubated, observe for the development of laryngospasms. If the client develops crowing respirations after extubation and is not moving air, the client is probably experiencing a laryngospasm. If this problem develops, the client could progress to respiratory arrest. The nurse

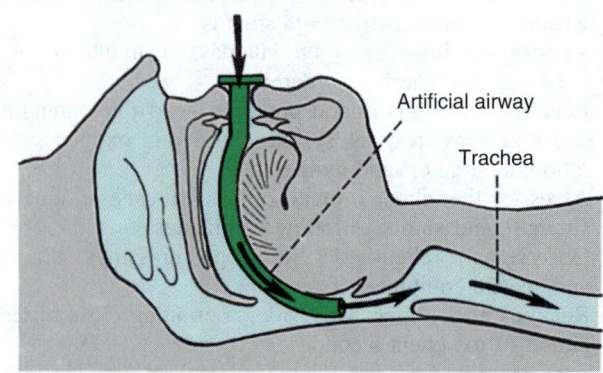

Figure 21–8. Artificial airway. The flattened, hollow tube prevents the tongue from falling back and occluding the natural airway.

should immediately attempt to ventilate the client using an Ambu bag with a tight fit. Positive pressure will sometimes alleviate the laryngospasm. If the spasm cannot be broken, a bolus of succinylcholine is given.

Other major respiratory problems include respiratory distress or depression, wheezing, and aspiration. Interventions may include the continued administration of oxygen, positive pressure airway support, or narcotic antagonists. Reversal agents, such as naloxone hydrochloride (Narcan), are administered to reverse the narcotic effect, or neostigmine with glycopyrrolate (Robinul) is given to reverse some neuromuscular blocking agents.

Cardiovascular Complications

Common cardiovascular complications include arrhythmias, hypertension, and hypotension resulting in shock. When assessing a client for postoperative cardiovascular complications, remember that a slight increase in a client's heart rate after surgery may be normal. However, a significant increase or decrease from baseline or the development of new dysrhythmias requires observation. ASPAN standards recommend that clients in the PACU be connected to a cardiac monitor.[9] In this way, diagnosis and treatment can be started immediately.

Causes of postoperative cardiac dysrhythmias include hypovolemia, pain, electrolyte imbalances, hypoxemia, and acidosis. When dysrhythmias develop, the PACU nurse monitors the client's blood pressure, oxygen saturation, and ventilation. When the ventilatory status is inadequate, the nurse institutes airway management. The nurse also consults with the surgeon and anesthesia provider, and intervenes with prescribed medications.

Postoperative hypotension can have numerous causes, including inadequate ventilation; side effects of anesthetic agents or preoperative medications; rapid position change; pain; fluid or blood loss; and peripheral pooling of blood after regional anesthesia. A drop in blood pressure slightly below a client's preoperative baseline reading is common after surgery. However, a significant drop in blood pressure, accompanied by an increase or decrease in heart rate, may indicate hemorrhage, circulatory failure, or fluid shifts. In addition to hypotension, manifestations of shock include tachycardia; cold, moist, pale, or cyanotic skin; and increased restlessness and apprehension.

When a client appears to be going into shock, the PACU nurse (1) applies oxygen or increases the rate of delivery; (2) raises the client's legs above the level of the heart; (3) increases the rate of IV fluids unless contraindicated; (4) notifies the anesthesia provider and surgeon; (5) administers medication or additional fluid volume as ordered; and (6) continues assessment on a one-to-one basis.

Clients in PACU also may develop hypertension. Older clients with a history of hypertension may exhibit hypertensive episodes after the stress of surgery. If the blood pressure rises above the baseline, the PACU nurse should consult with the anesthesia provider or surgeon and administer antihypertensive medications as ordered.

Complications Involving Renal Function and Fluid and Electrolyte Balance

Changes in renal function and fluid and electrolyte balance also may develop soon after surgery. Surgery and anesthesia stimulate the secretion of antidiuretic hormone (ADH) and aldosterone, which cause fluid retention. Urine volume decreases regardless of fluid intake. Avoid fluid overload while maintaining blood pressure, cardiac output, and adequate urinary output. Nursing interventions must include assessment of intake and output, blood pressure, pulse, and serum electrolytes. Any significant changes should be reported to the anesthesia provider or surgeon.

Temperature Changes

Malignant hyperthermia, as stated, can develop in the operating room or in the PACU. The PACU nurse must assess for severe muscle contractions and increased temperature (see Monitoring for Malignant Hyperthermia).

Hypothermia is another potential problem in the PACU. The heat loss from the operating room can continue in the PACU if the client is not warmed sufficiently. Warming requires maintaining the client's temperature without overwarming and causing excessive vasodilation (which could cause fluid shifts and a decrease in blood pressure). Warm blankets are applied to maintain the client's body temperature.

Pain

Clients must be assessed carefully in the PACU for postoperative pain. If clients become restless and state they are in pain, they should be medicated. The nurse consults with the anesthesia provider to determine the appropriate medication and dosage. After the client receives a pain medication, many PACUs have a policy requiring them to be closely monitored for another hour or until stable.

Other Complications

Diabetic clients require extra monitoring and care in the PACU. The stress of surgery can cause fluctuations in blood sugar. Blood glucose monitoring is conducted in the PACU and, based on the results, IV regular insulin may be ordered (see Chapter 69).

Clients who are on steroids also require special care in the PACU. The client should be assessed for the development of addisonian crisis. If the blood pressure drops, the pulse rate increases, and the client appears to be in shock, a low level of cortisol may be the problem. Intervention is immediate replacement with IV hydrocortisone after careful assessment of other possibilities (see Chapter 71).

Discharge from the PACU

Common criteria for evaluating the client's readiness for discharge from the PACU are the following:

- The client has recovered (many institutions use some variation of the Aldrete scoring system) and is ready for transfer. The criteria scored are activity, respiration, circulation, consciousness, and skin color. Each scale ranges from 0 to 3. A score of 9 or 10 usually indicates the client is ready for transfer to the postoperative unit. This requires a stay of about 1 hour in the PACU.
- The vital signs are stable at the preoperative level.
- There is only moderate or light drainage from any site.
- Essential postoperative care has been completed by PACU personnel.
- Urine output is maintained at a minimum of at least 30 ml/hour for an adult. The amount must be monitored and recorded. A urine output of less than 30 ml/2 hours is reported to the physician.
- Staff on the clinical unit to which the client is to be transferred have been alerted, a report has been given on the client's condition, and the unit is prepared to receive the client.
- Thorough documentation of the client's progress in the PACU is included in the client's permanent medical record.
- Notify significant others if the client required a prolonged PACU stay.

A client who has undergone ambulatory surgery in an inpatient or outpatient facility requires the same level of monitoring and support as if general or regional anesthesia were used. After surgery, the client may remain in the PACU until fully awake. The client is then transferred to the phase II care unit. In this area, clients are allowed to rest until they are able to tolerate fluids, ambulate, and void.

To prepare for discharge following ambulatory surgery, the client (1) receives complete postoperative written and oral instructions (which may have been given to and discussed with the client preoperatively), (2) knows when and how to seek help for any problems that may arise, and (3) has transportation home with assistance by a competent person. The next day there will be a follow-up telephone call from the staff.

Transfer to the Clinical Unit

After meeting the PACU discharge criteria, the client can be returned to the appropriate clinical unit to complete recovery. Clients who have experienced complications in the PACU generally may be transferred to the ICU for continued close observation.

The Clinical Unit

To carry out postoperative care, certain preparations need to be made on the clinical unit. These preparations include the following:

- A clear passageway to the client's bed to ensure easy transfer
- Clean bed linen, with pads if excessive drainage is anticipated; keep additional blankets available
- Necessary equipment that is contingent on the type of surgery, such as an emesis basin, IV pole, tissues, suction apparatus, and oxygen administration equipment

The PACU nurse calls the clinical unit to notify the staff that the client is ready for transfer. The client is transferred to the unit, accompanied by a PACU nurse. The nursing staff helps move the client into bed, making sure the client's body is in correct alignment and a comfortable position. All tubes and equipment are identified and adjusted appropriately. The PACU nurse gives a verbal report that includes the client's history, condition, the operative and PACU course, and any special orders that were initiated or need to be initiated.

The significant others should be notified of the client's status. The surgeon usually discusses the surgical procedure and outcome with the client and significant others. Thus, the nurse needs to be aware of the client's condition and of the information given to the client, family, and significant others by the surgeon.

Assessment. The nurse on the unit makes an initial assessment of the client after the transfer. The assessment includes the status of respiratory, cardiovascular, and neurologic systems, and of the surgical wound, IV lines, tubes, client position, and level of pain.

Respiratory Status. Assess for a patent airway. Listen for breath sounds and assess their character. Check the quality, depth, and rate of respirations. Remember that skin color and temperature also indicate the degree of oxygen exchange. Restlessness is an early sign of hypoxia, although it may have other causes, such as pain. Pale or dusky skin may signal poor oxygen exchange and the possible recurrence of narcotic effects. Cyanosis is a very late manifestation of hypoxia.

Cardiovascular Status. Assess vital signs, skin color, temperature, and degree of moistness. Assess for any abnormal pulses.

Neurologic Status. Assess the client's level of consciousness or ability to move extremities, and assess the lingering effects of regional anesthesia.

Status of the Surgical Wound. Assess the dressing and any drainage present. The nurse should measure and record the area of drainage to compare later assessments for changes.

Status of Intravenous Line. Assess the IV line for patency, type of fluid infusing, and rate.

Status of Tubes. Assesses drainage tube (e.g., nasogastric or chest tube) as to whether to attach it to suction or to use gravity drainage. Note the amount, color, and consistency of drainage and document.

Position. Assess the client for proper positioning to promote ventilation and decrease pain.

Pain. Assess the client for pain. Comfort measures are initiated. Assess the need for pain control through the use of narcotic analgesics. It is vital that pain be managed if the client is to comply with instructions for coughing, deep breathing, and ambulation.

Establishment of Postoperative Goals. The client has now entered the next phase of the postoperative course. At this point, a postoperative care plan is developed. This plan should include an assessment of the client's needs and goals as well as nursing interventions. Nursing diagnoses are used to specify and define postoperative problems and guide the plan of nursing care.

Goal 1: Restore Homeostasis and Prevent Complications

Surgery upsets the body's homeostatic balance, disrupting fluid and electrolyte balance, vital signs, and body temperature. Therefore, nursing care is directed toward reestablishing the client's normal balance, which, in turn, helps prevent complications.

One of the nurse's primary goals in caring for the postoperative client is to prevent complications after surgery. No matter how minor the surgery, the danger of postoperative complications is always present. Complications have caused death following relatively simple surgeries such as tonsillectomies and hernia repairs.

Postoperative complications can develop (1) directly in the wound, (2) in organs adjacent to or far from the operative site, (3) in body cavities, or (4) as a result of the client's medical condition. Complications may arise immediately after surgery or may develop later. Some authorities arbitrarily define a postoperative complication as any untoward event arising within 30 days after surgery. Complications may result directly from the surgical procedure, or may be a consequence of the condition being treated. For example, abdominal surgery may lead to an abdominal-peritoneal abscess, which, in turn, causes intra-abdominal infection. In this instance, the surgery itself resulted in a postoperative complication.

Complications are particularly common after a devastating illness or difficult surgery. These include disorders such as stress ulcer, renal failure, and hepatic failure. Most cardiovascular complications (e.g., cerebrovascular accident, myocardial infarction, pulmonary embolism) and virtually all life-threatening infections (e.g., peritonitis) follow some critical event such as postoperative shock or hemorrhage or preoperative rupture of an organ.

Preventing postoperative complications promotes rapid convalescence and saves time, expense, worry, pain, and even life. Know the manifestations of postoperative complications, and be able to recognize them quickly. Once postoperative problems develop, they are difficult to treat. One complication often leads to others, thereby prolonging morbidity and dependence. For example, the client who develops pneumonia following surgery has limited mobility, which may lead to thrombophlebitis, constipation, and further respiratory stasis. With pneumonia, appetite decreases and the client may develop a negative nitrogen balance, which slows wound healing. Fever and diaphoresis can result in fluid and electrolyte imbalance. Intravenous fluids probably will be ordered, but then this intervention causes additional discomfort and prolongs immobility. Additionally, these problems cause psychological reactions in the client and significant others.

One of the most common complications following surgery is postoperative shock. Causes include bleeding and hemorrhage (hypovolemic shock), sepsis (septic shock), cardiac arrest and myocardial infarction (cardiogenic shock), drug sensitivity (anaphylactic shock), transfusion reactions, pulmonary embolism, and adrenal failure.

Table 21–14 discusses, in brief, each type of shock, its causes, assessments, and interventions. See Chapter 22 for further information on shock.

Goal 2: Maintain and Promote Adequate Airway and Respiratory Function

Respiratory complications are among the more common complications that may occur in the postoperative period. Early assessment of respiratory problems can lead to immediate treatment.

Manifestations of pulmonary complications include increased temperature, restlessness, dyspnea, tachycardia, hemoptysis, pulmonary edema, altered breath sounds, and thick viscous sputum (with chest pain, if the client has pneumonia).

Pulmonary problems typically develop in the first 48 hours after surgery. Postoperative respiratory complications may be caused by one or several of the following factors:

- Pre-existing respiratory infections (colds, influenza, and sore throats) that were not resolved during the preoperative period
- Respiratory infection following surgery
- Use of anesthetics, endotracheal tubes, and oxygen— all of which irritate the tracheobronchial tree and cause increased mucous secretions
- Aspiration of vomitus
- Prolonged immobility of the client on the operating table during prolonged surgery
- A history of smoking
- Respiratory disease prior to surgery (e.g., asthma, chronic bronchitis, COPD)
- Depressive effects of many narcotics (especially codeine) on the cough reflex
- Collapse of the lung during surgery or inadequate reexpansion of lung tissue following surgery
- Severe postoperative pain, which makes the client reluctant or unable to turn, cough, or breathe deeply
- Surgery with a high abdominal or chest incision, which causes the client to neglect deep breathing exercises because of pain

Table 21–14. Types of Shock

Cause	Assessment	Intervention
Bleeding (hypovolemic shock)	Check wounds, drain sites, open wounds; central venous pressure low; bleeding usually in peritoneal or pleural cavities or retroperitoneal areas	Blood administration and immediate ligation of bleeding vessel by surgeon; measure arterial blood gases
Sepsis (septic shock)	Culture of blood or suspicion of gram-negative bacterial source of septicemia; tachycardia, hypotension, oliguria, fluid retention, respiratory failure	Massive IV antibiotics, fluids, corticosteroids may be ordered
Cardiac arrest, myocardial infarction, or arrhythmias (cardiogenic shock)	Check for pulse irregularities, ECG; absence of pulse and cyanosis suggest cardiac arrest; AST aids diagnosis of infarction; central venous pressure is high	Dependent on specific cause; general measures: oxygen; sedation; and cardiopulmonary resuscitation, if needed
Drug sensitivity (anaphylactic shock)	Obscure clinical picture; history of drug sensitivities is vitally important; urticaria and edema may aid diagnosis	Epinephrine, antihistamines, corticosteroids may be ordered; maintain airway, O_2 by mask or prongs, IV line, cardiac monitor, reassurance, arrange for ICU bed
Transfusion reaction (contaminated or incompatible blood)	Smears of blood show gram-negative organisms; shock rapidly follows blood administration	Discontinue blood; corticosteroids, massive doses of antibiotics IV may be ordered
Pulmonary embolism, respiratory distress, nasal flaring	No specific signs; chest pain, hemoptysis suggest diagnosis; angiography can make diagnosis; obesity, previous cardiac difficulties, cancer, pelvic operations, immobility, and increased age are associated factors	Embolectomy, fibrinolytic agents to dissolve clots are promising and may be ordered; O_2 by mask or prongs, arterial blood gases, ECG, cardiac monitor, pain relief, chest film; heparin therapy
Adrenal failure	Must be diagnosed by suspicion or history of steroid therapy, lack of other causes	IV corticosteroids (hydrocortisone) may be ordered

AST, aspartate aminotransferase; ECG, electrocardiogram; ICU, intensive care unit; IV, intravenous.
Adapted from Liechty, R. D. (1985). Postoperative care. In R. D. Liechty & R. T. Soper (Eds.), *Synopsis of surgery* (5th ed.). St. Louis: Mosby–Year Book.

● Extreme debilitation and old age, which lower the client's resistance to pulmonary infections
● Prolonged postoperative immobility, which leads to decreased chest expansion, pooling of mucus in the bronchi, and hypostatic pneumonia

The most common postoperative respiratory problems are atelectasis, pneumonia, and pulmonary emboli.

Atelectasis is the most common of these problems. Atelectasis is defined as collapse of the alveoli. Signs are increased pulse, increased temperature, and decreased breath sounds on auscultation. The chest x-ray verifies areas of consolidation.

Pneumonia is an acute infection causing inflammation of lung tissue. Typical findings include elevated temperature, tachycardia, tachypnea, productive cough, dyspnea, crackles, and a dullness over area of consolidation.

Pulmonary emboli, either a blood clot or a fat embolus, can occur after any major surgery, especially surgery involving the abdomen or long bones. It is a potentially fatal complication. It occurs when there is a passage of thrombi into the pulmonary vasculature, thus decreasing blood flow to the lungs. Manifestations are severe dysp-

nea, intense pleural pain, apprehension, fever, and hemoptysis.

Although the cause of each respiratory complication is different, some basic nursing interventions may prevent these and other pulmonary complications. Rigorous attention to these interventions is essential. First, provide preoperative instruction regarding moving, coughing, and deep breathing exercises. After surgery, coach the client during the performance of these exercises. Encourage the client to do deep breathing exercises every 1 to 2 hours, as described earlier. Encourage the client to cough every 1 to 2 hours. Splint the client's incision so coughing will be less painful and less likely to cause the incision to rupture. Check the color and consistency of the mucus expectorated with coughing. If a respiratory infection is present, the mucus may be thick, tinted, and odorous. Hydrate the client adequately because fluids thin mucous secretions. If the client is receiving IV infusions, check the drip rate and timeliness of administration. If the client can tolerate oral fluids, encourage fluid intake.

Assess the client for respiratory depression and suppression of cough, especially if the client is receiving narcotics (e.g., morphine) for pain. If respirations are de-

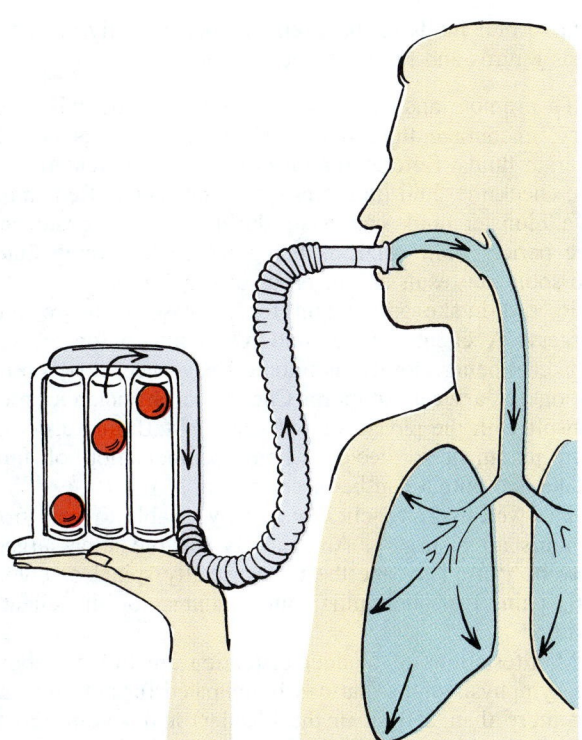

Figure 21–9. Using an incentive deep breathing exerciser to promote alveolar inflation, restore and maintain lung capacity, and strengthen the respiratory muscles.

pressed, notify the surgeon so a different narcotic can be prescribed. Assess and report manifestations of respiratory infection. If pneumonia develops, nasotracheal suctioning may be necessary to stimulate a cough. Also, antibiotics and antipyretics may be prescribed.

Encourage the client to stop smoking. Encourage the use of an incentive spirometer every 1 to 2 hours after surgery. This device provides physiologically correct exercise that encourages deep, prolonged, and voluntary inspiration. It also promotes maximal alveolar inflation, helps restore and maintain lung capacity, and strengthens respiratory muscles (Fig. 21–9). Encourage the client to ambulate as soon as possible because this will also improve respiratory functions. Finally, perform respiratory assessment and chest auscultation as part of routine postoperative care.

Goal 3: Maintain Adequate Cardiac Function and Promote Tissue Perfusion

Any surgical client is at risk of developing cardiac or perfusion problems, but clients at most risk are the elderly and clients with a history of cardiac or peripheral vascular disease. Two common problems that may occur in the postoperative client are thrombophlebitis (and possibly embolism) and myocardial infarction.

Thrombophlebitis (inflammation of the vessel lining) usually involves the peripheral veins, most commonly the calf veins. It develops because of direct pressure on the walls of veins during surgery or from venous stasis.

Postoperative thrombophlebitis generally occurs 7 to 14 days after surgery. Dehydration, prolonged bedrest, and inadequate circulation resulting from hemorrhage can result in circulatory stasis and increased blood coagulability, both of which can cause thrombophlebitis. The great danger of thrombophlebitis is that a clot will break loose from the vein wall and travel as an embolus to the client's lungs, heart, or brain.

Manifestations of phlebitis include redness, warmth, swelling, and tenderness of the extremity, and the presence of Homans' sign—pain in the calf when the foot is dorsiflexed (if the clot is in the calf). Preventive measures for thrombophlebitis include postoperative leg exercises, early ambulation, antiembolic support stockings, adequate hydration, and low-dose heparin.

Myocardial infarction occurs during the first 72 hours after surgery. The nurse must assess high-risk clients—those with a history of dysrhythmias or heart disease—or any client over 70 years of age. Because anesthesia might mask chest pain, the nurse should observe the client for dyspnea, tachycardia, cyanosis, and dysrhythmias. Interventions and nursing care for the client with a myocardial infarct are discussed in depth in Chapter 45.

Another postoperative condition related to tissue perfusion is blood loss. In the postoperative client, this can be the result of a pre-existing condition, blood loss during the surgery, or a postoperative complication.

Clients who are at high risk of experiencing blood loss postoperatively are those with pre-existing medical conditions, a history of aspirin use, a history of anemia or clotting disorders, and the elderly.

Manifestations of blood loss in the postoperative client include postural hypotension, tachycardia, tachypnea, decreased urine output, cool clammy skin, and decreased level of consciousness. Laboratory data should include hemoglobin, hematocrit, and clotting studies (prothrombin time, partial thromboplastin time, and platelet count).

Blood loss is treated with plasma expanders, albumin, large volumes of fluid, salvage of blood with the cell saver or other autotransfusion device, and, if necessary, transfusion. Whole blood may be used, but, more commonly, packed red blood cells are administered. Fresh frozen plasma or coagulation factors are used if the client has a coagulation problem. Blood transfusions are covered in detail in Chapter 53. It is important that the client needing transfusion maintain adequate tissue perfusion.

Goal 4: Maintain Adequate Fluid and Electrolyte Balance and Adequate Renal Function

After surgery, it is crucial to promote adequate fluid and electrolyte intake and output. Postoperative imbalances can lead to retention of metabolic wastes, neurologic and cardiac problems, and problems of overhydration or underhydration.

The goals of postoperative fluid and electrolyte therapy are twofold: (1) to give sufficient fluids to maintain extracellular fluid and blood volume (proper fluid volume ensures adequate blood pressure, cardiac output, and urinary flow); and (2) to prevent fluid overload with resultant congestive heart failure and pulmonary edema.

Normal fluid and electrolyte adjustments during the first 3 to 4 days following surgery include the following:

● Renal retention of water and sodium
● Expansion of extracellular fluid (ECF) in excess of sodium (Na^+) and chloride (Cl^-)
● A transient decrease in ECF Na^+ and Cl^-
● An increase in potassium excretion
● A decrease in hematocrit as a result of expansion of ECF

Normal fluid and electrolyte adjustments during the fifth through seventh days following surgery include the following:

● Diuresis
● Return of ECF volume to normal
● Return of serum Na^+ to normal
● Reduction of potassium (K^+) concentration in urine

Further information on fluid and electrolyte alterations may be found in Chapter 15.

Principal causes of postoperative dehydration and electrolyte deficits are (1) failure to replace deficits existing before surgery, (2) inadequate replacement of normal postoperative losses, and (3) excessive postoperative losses as a result of sweating, hyperventilation, wound drainage, gastrointestinal tract drainage, diarrhea, diuresis, or vomiting.

Principal causes of fluid overload are the administration of excessive amounts of IV fluids and inadequate renal function with low urine output.

Principal causes of respiratory acidosis (many of which cause hypoventilation) are the following:

● Narcotics, some of which reduce respiratory efficiency, especially in the elderly
● Postoperative pain and bulky, uncomfortable dressings that make clients reluctant to cough and breathe deeply
● Abdominal distention, a common postoperative problem that inhibits movement of the diaphragm, making deep breathing difficult
● Surgery with a high subcostal incision, such as hiatal hernia repair and gallbladder surgery, which causes painful postoperative ventilation
● Postoperative complications, such as atelectasis, pneumonia, and bronchitis, which cause respiratory obstruction and poor ventilation

To prevent fluid and electrolyte imbalance perform the following:

● Record intake and output accurately
● Assess serum electrolyte values and report abnormal findings to the surgeon immediately
● Obtain an order for an antiemetic (e.g., prochlorperazine maleate [Compazine]) if the client develops nausea and vomiting
● Irrigate nasogastric suction tubes properly (see Chapter 60)
● Instruct the client to cough and breathe deeply to prevent respiratory acidosis

● Give oral fluids to the client as soon as active peristalsis returns and fluids can be tolerated

To promote and maintain renal function following surgery, encourage fluid intake when the client is able to tolerate fluids. Before administering oral or parenteral fluids, check the fluid limits set by the physician. Remember to administer fluids cautiously during the early postoperative period while ADH is being released. Forcing fluids too soon can result in dangerous overhydration.

Record intake and output for at least 48 hours after surgery. A client with a fluid restriction, or one whose intake is being closely monitored, may need close observation for a week or more. Check the physician's order, consult with the physician and nursing staff, and use your own judgment to decide when documentation of fluid intake and output can be discontinued.

The well-hydrated client generally is able to void 6 to 8 hours after surgery. An inability to void after surgery may be caused by anesthesia (especially spinal or epidural), pain, fear, unfamiliar surroundings, or the client's position.

Manifestations of bladder distention are fullness above the symphysis pubis that can be palpated (usually indicating more than 250 ml in the bladder) and voiding 30 to 60 ml of urine every 20 to 30 minutes (indicating retention with overflow).

Possible nursing interventions to aid the client in voiding include the following:

● Running tap water so the client hears it
● Pouring warm water over the female perineum
● Assisting the male to sit or stand at the bedside (if not contraindicated)
● Administering prescribed pain medication
● Inserting a straight or indwelling catheter, as ordered

Catheterization is the most common cause of postoperative urinary tract infection. Manifestations of urinary tract infection generally occur between the third and fifth day after catheterization and include dysuria, frequency, and fever.

Intervention for urinary tract infections involves first sending a specimen of the urine to the laboratory for culture and sensitivity testing. The culture results indicate the organism causing the infection. The results of the sensitivity test indicate which antibiotic will be most effective in treating the infection. Appropriate antibiotics are prescribed on the basis of laboratory results. To prevent bladder infections, avoid catheterization, if at all possible.

Goal 5: Promote Comfort and Rest

Being comfortable and free from pain enables a client to progress more quickly and more easily through the postoperative period. Factors related to a high incidence and intensity of postoperative pain include the type of anesthesia used, high levels of anxiety, extensive and prolonged surgical procedures, and poor state of mental health. An example of pain related to type of anesthesia used is early pain following administration of nitrous oxide, a soluble agent that is rapidly eliminated from the body. Clients who have been given nitrous oxide during surgery may experience pain earlier in the postoperative period. Soluble inhalation agents cause CNS depression. However, because they are not excreted as rapidly as nitrous oxide, their anesthetizing effects continue for hours following surgery.

Nursing assessment of pain, especially prior to the administration of narcotics, involves carefully checking for the following:

● Hypotension or hypertension: Pain can cause an increase or decrease in blood pressure.
● Pressure points beneath a cast or splint: Relieving pressure by splitting the cast or cutting a window (usually done by a physician) may alleviate pain.
● Distended bladder: Obtain an order for catheterization if the client is unable to void.
● Abdominal distention and flatulence: A rectal suppository or tube may alleviate gas pain. Flatus is a common postoperative problem that is often alleviated by ambulation.

Nursing measures that help alleviate pain include the following:

● Comfort measures, such as changing the client's position, straightening bed linen, giving a back rub with lotion, and applying a cool cloth to the hands and face
● Administration of narcotics, such as morphine, meperidine, and codeine; narcotics are used primarily during the first 24 to 72 hours after surgery

A newer option is the use of patient-controlled analgesia (PCA), which allows the client to self-administer postoperative analgesia (often morphine, meperidine, or fentanyl). Note in Figure 21–10 that the PCA system is basically a pump that can be programmed to deliver a predetermined dose of analgesic when the client pushes the control button. A system also can be set up to deliver a continuous dose with the client able to trigger an increase in the dose as needed. An indwelling IV line delivers the analgesic.

The PCA system has the following advantages:

● Clients, who are the experts on their own pain, can monitor and meet their own analgesia needs
● PCA allows a constant blood level of analgesic, in contrast to an intramuscular injection, which delivers a bolus of pain medication that tapers off over hours
● Clients can self-administer small amounts of analgesia, sparing them the difficult cycles of escalating pain and heavy sedation

The pump is provided with safety features to prevent overdosing. An average setting for a PCA device is 1 mg morphine administered every 6 minutes; however, the setting for each client is based on the client's pain, body size, surgery, and anesthesiologist's choice. In one setup, the client must push the button to receive medication; there is no automatic administration. In another, the client receives a steady dose that can be augmented as needed. After receiving a dose of medication, there is a preset time (e.g., 6 minutes) during which the machine will not

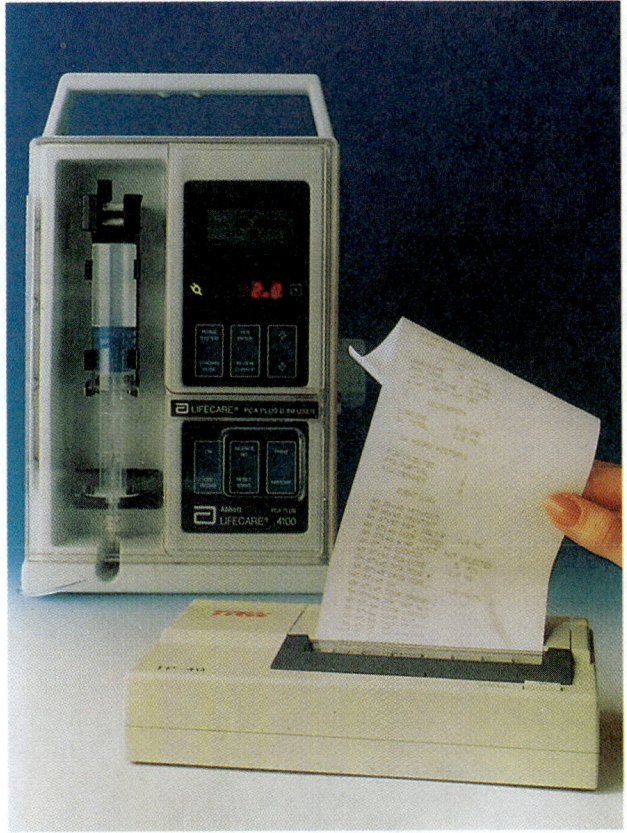

Figure 21–10. A patient-controlled anesthesia (PCA) device allows clients to control their own pain relief postoperatively. (Courtesy of Abbott Laboratories, Hospital Products Division, North Chicago, IL.)

deliver more medication. Contrary to what some healthcare providers expected, studies have shown that clients do not overmedicate. Most clients achieve a balance between pain relief and sedation. Studies have shown that clients using PCA (1) use less medication, (2) are able to ambulate earlier, and (3) recover pulmonary function sooner, as a result of increased activity levels.

On most PCA devices, the following settings can be programmed: (1) flow rate (dosage), (2) flow type (continuous or intermittent), (3) number of milligrams per dose, and (4) time required between injections. In addition, the device records (1) the number of injection attempts, (2) the number of injections actually given, (3) a low battery, (4) an error in the system setup, (5) little or no remaining infusion, (6) an unauthorized entry to the system, and (7) an occlusion or excessive pressure in the line.

Assessing IV catheter patency during PCA is the nurse's responsibility. Ensure that the IV line remains patent (so the analgesic is not deposited subcutaneously) and that the IV tubing is not occluded.

Narcotics should be given routinely during the first 24 hours after surgery and as needed for up to 72 hours. There is no real danger of overmedication as long as careful assessment is performed. The client will recover faster if comfortable and able to comply with postoperative breathing exercises and ambulation.

As convalescence progresses, pain medications are administered in decreasing dosages and strengths. Comforting and reassuring can help relieve any anxiety that might cause tension and increase pain. Most clients require less medication as the pain associated with the surgical procedure decreases. Drug dependence or tolerance is not a common problem for most surgical clients, and medication should never be withheld from a client who is in pain. For further information on pain, see Chapter 17.

If the client is having difficulty resting during the postoperative period or if restlessness is severe, a thorough assessment should be made of possible causes. Restlessness may be caused by pain, bladder or abdominal distention, fear, anxiety, hypoxia, wet or tight dressings, or hemorrhage.

Nursing interventions to promote rest include the following:

● Changing the client's position when necessary
● Keeping the bed linen clean, dry, and free of wrinkles
● Giving a back rub with lotion
● Administering pain medication as ordered and as needed
● Specific interventions for other potential causes of restlessness (e.g., administering oxygen, loosening the dressings, assisting with voiding, ambulating to decrease abdominal distention)

Goal 6: Promote Adequate Nutrition and Elimination

It is beneficial for the client to resume a normal diet as soon as possible after surgery. A normal diet promotes an early return of gastrointestinal function, aids in wound healing, and is psychologically healthy.

Nursing assessments to be made prior to feeding a client postoperatively are the presence of bowel sounds and ensuring that the abdomen is soft and palpable.

Certain surgical procedures (e.g., abdominal exploration and cholecystectomy) may require that the client abstain from oral fluids and food until bowel sounds return, usually within about 24 to 48 hours after surgery. Clients who are unable to eat for longer periods (after gastric or bowel resection) may have a nasogastric tube in place, which, because of its decompressive properties, removes flatus and stomach secretions. Clients who are NPO for a prolonged period after surgery usually receive nutritional support with hyperalimentation.

For the first 24 to 36 hours following surgery, many clients are nauseated and have episodes of vomiting. Antiemetics may be ordered for the nausea. If nausea persists, the surgeon should be notified. The initial postoperative diet is usually clear liquids. These liquids may include broth, tea with lemon and sugar, fruit juices, and Jell-O. Early solid foods may include toast, light cornstarch puddings, and easily digested meats and vegetables. As the client regains appetite and begins to eat well, a full diet is ordered to promote vitamin, mineral, and nitrogen balance. Muscle substance and strength return, and the client may regain some weight.

Normal peristalsis returns during the first 48 to 72 hours after surgery. It is important for the nurse to record any bowel movements in the postoperative period. Bowel function can be impaired by immobility, anesthesia, manipulation of abdominal organs, and the use of pain medications.

A common postoperative discomfort related to a decrease in peristalsis is abdominal distention. This causes a feeling of fullness and discomfort. Nursing measures to prevent and treat abdominal discomfort are early ambulation, adequate fluid intake, and an increase in dietary fiber. A rectal tube may be inserted if none of these interventions work.

Paralytic ileus is a postoperative complication that may occur when a portion of the bowel stops normal peristalsis. Nursing assessment includes diminished or absent bowel sounds, abdominal distention, and feelings of fullness. X-rays often reveal a distended bowel. A nasogastric tube may be inserted to prevent distention and vomiting until bowel function resumes.

Goal 7: Promote Wound Healing

Factors affecting wound healing are the location of the incision, type of surgical closure, nutritional status, presence of disease, presence of infection, and the presence of drains and dressings.

Nursing assessments to promote wound healing include the following:

● Assess the wound for manifestations of infection, such as redness, drainage, odor, pain, and induration
● Observe the wound for edema, bleeding, and color
● Observe the wound for approximation of the suture line
● Monitor drains, and assess the color, consistency, and amount of drainage

Maintaining strict asepsis during surgery and the postoperative period is the single most important factor in promoting wound healing.

Wound infections are often evident within 36 to 48 hours postoperatively, although most manifestations appear about 5 to 7 days after surgery. Important factors that predispose a client to develop wound infections are the following:

● *Obesity.* Adipose tissue is difficult for the surgeon to approximate and suture, and it does not heal readily.
● *Debilitation.* Clients debilitated by cancer, malnutrition, or ulcerative colitis have a lowered resistance to infections.
● *Advanced age.* Elderly clients, particularly those with atherosclerosis and poor circulation, have lowered defenses against infection.
● *Lengthy, complicated operations.* Complex operations are stressful and lower resistance. The longer the client is in surgery, the longer the tissues are exposed, making them more susceptible to infection.
● *Therapy with steroids, irradiation, and anticancer medications.* Certain medications and treatments affect the immune system and reduce the body's WBC count dramatically.

- *The presence of other diseases.* Hypogammaglobine-mia, diabetes mellitus, obstructive jaundice, ulcerative colitis, uremia, leukemia, aplastic anemia, and malignant neoplasms, in particular, lower resistance to wound infection.
- *Failure to maintain asepsis* in the operating room or during wound dressing changes.
- *Preoperative organ rupture or sepsis,* such as occurs with a ruptured appendix, perforated ulcer, or abscess drainage. When the organ is infected prior to surgery, the wound is usually considered contaminated and infected.

Studies show that the general attitude of the staff toward controlling infection is important in maintaining infection control. Healthcare personnel are sometimes careless in aseptic technique because they fail to recognize the importance of asepsis. In-service education that concentrates on the principles of asepsis is one important way to prevent wound infections.

The organism most commonly responsible for wound infections is methicillin-resistant *Staphylococcus aureus* (MRSA), a gram-positive, nonmotile organism. Staphylococci produce a golden-yellow pus. These organisms can be transmitted to the surgical wound from contaminated wound-dressing equipment or from staff who harbor the organism in their noses and throats as resident flora.

Clients with infected surgical wounds must be isolated from clients with clean wounds in order to stem the transmission of infections. Other organisms frequently responsible for wound infections are *Escherichia coli, Proteus vulgaris, Aerobacter aerogenes,* and *Pseudomonas aeruginosa.* Infectious diseases are covered in detail in Chapter 19.

Wound dehiscence and evisceration are possible complications of improper wound healing. *Wound dehiscence* is an opening of the wound edges (Fig. 21–11). *Wound evisceration* is the protrusion of internal organs (such as loops of bowel) through the incision (see Fig. 21–11). Malnourished, chronically ill, and obese clients are most prone to wound dehiscence and evisceration. Related causal factors are wound infection, faulty closure of the wound in surgery, and severe stretching of the abdominal wall as a result of coughing and vomiting.

Although wound dehiscence and evisceration can occur at any time, they generally develop on the sixth to seventh day after surgery. At this time, the client's incision is weakest because the sutures may have been removed, wound infection is likely to be present, and pulmonary complications may cause excessive pressure when the client coughs. Preventing wound dehiscence and evisceration includes splinting the wound during vigorous coughing or movement, preventing wound infection, and providing adequate nutrition and hydration. Obese or debilitated clients can wear a binder to increase support of the suture line. Any wound can rupture. However, midline abdominal incisions are most prone to dehiscence and evisceration.

When an abdominal wound ruptures suddenly, evisceration may occur because of the presence of intestine. When the wound edges part slowly, a gush of pinkish serous drainage is usually the major manifestation of dehiscence. The client feels something give way and may or may not complain of pain, tachycardia, and restlessness. In any postoperative client, sudden, profuse, pink, serous drainage from the wound is an ominous manifestation and must be investigated immediately!

Intervention for wound dehiscence and evisceration involves immediate closure of the wound under general or local anesthesia. The nurse's role in the event of wound dehiscence and evisceration includes the following:

- Remain calm
- Place the client in bed in a semi-Fowler position with the knees slightly elevated (William's position); if the wound has not completely opened or has not become eviscerated, this position may prevent further tear
- Ring the emergency bell, pull on the call light, or use the telephone to tell the hospital operator to notify the nurse's station on your floor to send help immediately
- Have another nurse notify the surgeon while you remain with the client
- Cover any protruding coils of intestine with sterile dressings moistened with sterile normal saline; if sterile supplies are not available, use clean towels or dressings
- Moisten the towels and dressings frequently with sterile normal saline
- Monitor the client's vital signs because shock may ensue
- Reassure the client that the physician is on the way
- Do not medicate the client with narcotics until after the client has signed an operative permit to reclose the wound
- Set up IV equipment, and prepare the client for surgery
- Notify the surgery department that the client will be returning to the operating room upon the surgeon's order

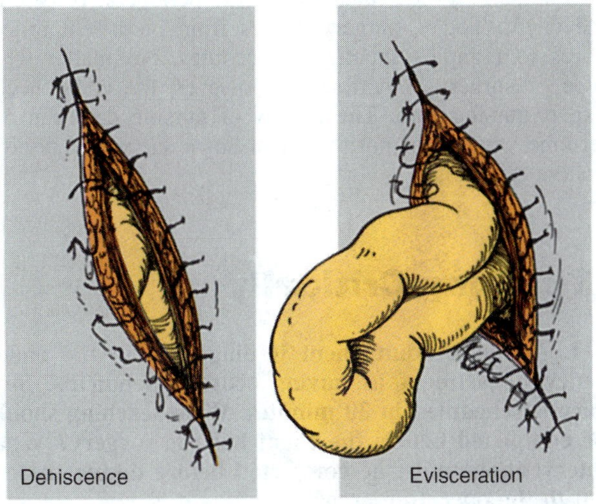

Dehiscence   Evisceration

Figure 21–11. Wound dehiscence and evisceration require immediate attention. Have someone notify the surgeon and return the client to bed. Using sterile technique, cover the wound site with gauze or a sterile towel moistened in sterile saline. Take measures to prevent shock (see text). Do not leave the client's side.

Goal 8: Promote and Maintain Activity and Mobility

Clients who are immobilized for long periods often become weak and develop respiratory diseases (e.g., pneumonia, atelectasis), circulatory problems (e.g., thrombophlebitis), osteoporosis, urinary retention and bladder stones, and a negative nitrogen balance. These same problems occur in clients who are immobilized after surgery.

After surgery, complications from immobility may be prevented by encouraging the client to (1) move around in bed, (2) cough and do deep breathing exercises, and (3) flex the ankles and legs. Allow the client to assume personal care as soon as possible to promote early movement. Encourage and assist with ambulation, if not contraindicated by the physician. Remember that clients vary. Some clients are ready to move or walk about sooner than others. Allowing the client to return to physical activity as soon as possible after surgery can hasten recovery, shorten the hospital stay, and reduce the client's expenses.

Goal 9: Provide Adequate Emotional Support and Foster a Positive Body Image

Surgery has different meanings and implications for each client. Recognize these differences and individualize your psychological approach to the client and significant others as he or she progresses through the surgical experience. The degree of psychological support the client needs depends on the client's social support as well as the type of surgery performed. A client whose postoperative course is complicated needs much more psychological support than the client who recovers quickly.

Maladaptive coping behavior may occur in response to a loss or change associated with surgery. Surgical incisions can alter a client's body image. Surgeries that are most likely to cause a change in body image are surgeries of the face, head, neck, breast, or gynecologic or genitourinary system. The onset of problems with coping with these changes may occur in the immediate or extended postoperative stage.

Assessment may reveal passivity, depression, reduced involvement in self-care, sleep disturbance, increased pain and use of analgesics, and hyperactivity. The client also may experience the onset of stress-related manifestations, such as gastrointestinal dysfunction and cardiovascular problems.

Nursing intervention primarily involves providing psychological support. Draw the client and significant others into discussions of anticipated changes and about how they feel these postoperative changes will affect their lives. Encourage the expression of feelings. Provide empathic listening. Reassure these clients that the grieving process they are going through is normal and that it will pass with time. Arrange support groups and community referrals for the client and significant others.

Goal 10: Plan for Discharge

Discharge planning and teaching should begin at the time of the client's admission to the hospital. Most clients are discharged within 5 days after major surgery and sometimes even sooner. Early discharge planning is a necessity.

Specific instructions that the client needs to receive prior to discharge should include the following:

● Wound care (manifestations of infection)
● Activity restrictions after abdominal and many other surgeries: driving, lifting heavy objects, and coitus are restricted for up to 6 weeks
● Dietary instructions
● Postoperative medication instruction
● Personal hygiene instruction
● Follow-up appointment with surgeon or clinic

Because of the anxiety associated with discharge, written instructions should be given to the client and significant others for reference. The type of planning and instruction required varies with the individual and type of surgery. Discharge teaching instructions need to be clear, and they must reinforce the material the client learned during the preoperative period and during recovery. Teaching plans and the client's understanding of them need to be included in the care plan and documented in the chart (see Bridge to Home Healthcare).

Finally, ascertain the quality of the client's support systems, because you may need to involve community resources for follow-up care. Community resources such as mental health facilities and home healthcare agencies help to ensure continuity of care.

Conclusions

The nurse plays a critical role in the perioperative care of the client. Today, surgery ranges from outpatient procedures to complex inpatient procedures. No matter what type of surgery is performed, however, the client needs expert nursing care. The quality of nursing care can determine whether or not the client has a successful perioperative experience.

Thinking Critically

1. **A young adult client is diagnosed in the emergency department as having acute appendicitis. Surgery is scheduled in 30 minutes. What teaching should be completed before the client has the surgery? What interventions must be completed before taking the client to the operating area?**

Factors to Consider. What important client teaching is completed before any surgery in which general anesthesia is used? Does discussion of possible complications occur at this time? What measures usually appear on a preoperative checklist?

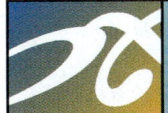

BRIDGE TO HOME HEALTHCARE

Recovery from Surgery

Deborah Bayliss, M.S., R.N., *Poudre Valley Hospital, Fort Collins, Colorado*

An 80-year-old man is discharged from 1-day surgery in stable condition following an inguinal hernia repair. Before discharge he is given postoperative instructions. Because he is elderly and lives alone, his physician orders a home care consult. On your initial visit to the patient's home, you perform an assessment that includes physical, environmental, and psychosocial status. As you review the patient's discharge instructions you realize that his vision is impaired. He cannot read the instructions without help. He was instructed to take his temperature twice daily but cannot read the thermometer. The patient is on a regular diet but has little food in his house. He tells you that he recently stopped driving because of poor vision and depends on neighbors for transportation, including trips to the grocery store. He was instructed to see his physician in 1 week but is not sure how he will get to the office. The patient says the doctor told him to call if there was drainage from his surgical incision but he is not sure what that means.

Before you leave, you review all of the postoperative instructions with the patient to be sure he understands them. You change his dressing and note serosanguineous drainage at the surgical site. You show him the drainage and explain that he should call you if it increases or changes color. You contact one of the patient's neighbors who agrees to take his temperature every morning and record it. You also call Meals-on-Wheels to have meals delivered to the patient's home. Most important, you tell the patient that you will be back to see him tomorrow and leave a phone number for him to call if he needs a nurse.

The above case study illustrates the issues that can arise for patients recovering from surgery at home and the value of a home care consult. To qualify for home care, certain guidelines must be followed. Under Medicare guidelines, the patient must be homebound, requiring skilled, intermittent care. All payor sources require a physician's order for home care and most third-party payors require preauthorization for services. The primary goals for the home care nurse are to monitor and prevent postoperative complications, instruct the patient or caregiver, and assist the patient in achieving an optimal level of wellness and functioning. In assessing the postoperative patient, some questions that should be asked include:

1. Does the patient understand the postoperative instructions?
2. Does the patient need specific equipment such as a walker or dressings?
3. Does the patient have adequate medication for pain control and know how to use it?
4. If a special diet is ordered, can the patient get the food needed for the diet?
5. What skilled needs does the patient have such as wound care or intravenous administration? Can the patient or caregiver be taught to perform this care?
6. Does the patient understand his or her level of activity?

You can assist the patient in learning and coping in the postoperative recovery period.

---

2. An elderly client has major abdominal surgery performed under general anesthetic. At age 80 years, she is in relatively good health following a cerebrovascular accident about 8 years ago. Her only medication is a 325-mg aspirin tablet taken once a day. What complications are most likely in an 80-year-old client? How can these complications be prevented? How is pain tolerated by the older client?

Factors to Consider. What complications are associated with general anesthesia? How does a thorough nursing history and assessment help you in your plan to prevent complications following surgery? What age-related considerations must be made?

Bibliography

1. Accreditation Association for Ambulatory Health Care. (1992). *Accreditation handbook for ambulatory health care.* Skokie, IL: Author.

2. Acute Pain Management Guideline Panel. (1992). *Acute pain management in adults: Operative procedures.* AHCPR Publications No. 92–0019. Rockville, MD: Agency for Health Care Policy and Research, Public Health Service, U.S. Department of Health and Human Services.

3. Acute Pain Management Guideline Panel. (1992). *Acute pain management: Operative or medical procedures and trauma.* AHCPR Publications No. 92–0032. Rockville, MD: Agency for Health Care Policy and Research, Public Health Service, U.S. Department of Health and Human Services.

4. Acute Pain Management Guideline Panel. (1992). *Pain control after surgery: A patient's guide.* AHCPR Publications No. 92–0021. Rockville, MD: Agency for Health Care Policy and Research, Public Health Service, U.S. Department of Health and Human Services.

5. Alexander, J. W. (1983). The influence of hair-removal methods on wound infection. *Archives of Surgery, 118,* 347.

6. Allen, A. (Ed.). (1991). *ASPAN's core curriculum for post anesthesia nursing practice.* Philadelphia: W. B. Saunders.

7. Alves, S. L., & Deisering, L. F. (1996). Cardiovascular changes associated with aging: The anesthetic implications. *CRNA: The Clinical Forum for Nurse Anesthetists, 7*(1), 2–8.

8. American Society of Anesthesiologists. (1992). *Relative value guide: Physical status classification.* Chicago: Author.

9. American Society of Postanesthesia Nurses. (1992). *Standards of nursing practice.* Richmond, VA: Author.

10. Anderson, K., & Harris, A. (1992). Is there a statistically significant difference in two post-surgical rewarming methods: Convection versus radiation. *Journal of Post Anesthesia Nursing, 7*(3), 219.

11. Aquavella, J. (1990). Ambulatory surgery in the 1990s. *Journal of Ambulatory Care Management, 13*(1), 21–24.

12. Arnovitch, S. (1995). Selecting the best dressing sponge. *Nursing, 25*(7), 52–54.

13. Association of Operating Room Nurses. (1995). *Perioperative core curriculum.* Philadelphia: W. B. Saunders.

14. Association of Operating Room Nurses. (1995). *Standards and recommended practices.* Denver: Author.

15. Association of Operating Room Nurses: Nursing Practices Committee. (1994). Proposed perioperative nurse translation of the federal clinical practice guidelines. *AORN Journal, 60*(5), 828, 832–833, 835–836.

16. Atkinson, L. J. (1992). *Berry and Kohn's introduction to operating room technique* (7th ed). New York: McGraw-Hill.

17. Augustin, P., & Hains, A. A. (1996). Effect of music on ambulatory surgery patients' preoperative anxiety. *AORN Journal, 63*(4), 750, 753–756, 758.

18. Augustine, S. (1990). Hypothermia therapy in the postanesthesia care unit: A review. *Journal of Post Anesthesia Nursing, 5*(4), 254–263.

19. Avoiding dehydration: How you can protect elderly patients. (1995). *Nursing, 25*(2), 52.

20. Badgwell, J. M. (1996). The postanesthesia care unit: A high-risk environment for bloodborne and infectious respiratory pathogens. *Journal of Post Anesthesia Nursing, 11*(2), 66–70.

21. Balcom, C. (1994). The new code of ethics: Implications for perioperative nurses. *Canadian Operating Room Nursing Journal, 12*(1), 6–8.

22. Ball, K. (1995). *Lasers: The perioperative challange* (2nd ed.). St. Louis: Mosby–Year Book.

23. Barash, P., Cullen, B., & Stoelting, R. (1992). *Clinical anesthesia* (2nd ed.). Philadelphia: J. B. Lippincott.

24. Barrett, J. B., & Deehan, R. M. (1992). Preoperative patient teaching: A video guide. *Nursing, 22*(2), 32F, 32H.

25. Batson, V. D. (1993). Conscious sedation: Implications for perioperative nursing practice. *Seminars in Perioperative Nursing, 2*(1), 45–57.

26. Bean, M. (1990). Preparation for surgery in an ambulatory surgery unit. *Journal of Post Anesthesia Nursing, 5,* 42–47.

27. Benumof, J., & Saidman, L. (1992). *Anesthesia and perioperative complications.* St. Louis: Mosby–Year Book.

28. Bosek, V., & Miguel, R. (1994). Comparison of morphine and ketorolac for intravenous patient-controlled analgesia in postoperative cancer patients. *Clinical Journal of Pain, 10*(4), 314–318.

29. Bowman, A. M. (1992). The relationship of anxiety to development of postoperative delirium. *Journal of Gerontological Nursing, 18*(1), 24–30.

30. Bryant, R. (1992). *Acute and chronic wounds: Nursing management.* St. Louis: Mosby–Year Book.

31. Burchiel, R. N. (1995). Does perioperative nursing include caring? *AORN Journal, 62*(2), 57–59.

32. Burden, N. (1993). *Ambulatory surgical nursing.* Philadelphia: W. B. Saunders.

33. Butterworth, J. (1992). *Atlas of procedures in anesthesia and critical care.* Philadelphia: W. B. Saunders.

34. Caldwell, L. (1991). Surgical outpatient concerns: What every perioperative nurse should know. *AORN Journal, 53,* 761–767.

35. Caldwell, L. M. (1991). The influence of preference for information on preoperative stress and coping in surgical outpatients. *Applied Nursing Research, 4*(4), 177–183.

36. Carmody, S., Hickey, P., & Bookbinder, M. (1991). Perioperative needs of families: Results of a survey. *AORN Journal, 54*(7), 561–567.

37. Carpenito, L. J. (1995). *Handbook of nursing diagnosis* (6th ed.). Philadelphia: J. B. Lippincott.

38. Chana, C. H. (1992). Documenting the nursing process: A perioperative nursing care plan. *AORN Journal, 55*(5), 1231–1235.

39. Chiarella, M. (1991). The role of the nurse in today's operating room. *AORN Journal, 4*(4), 15–16.

40. Christoph, S. B. (1991). Pain assessment. *Critical Care Clinics of North America, 3*(1), 11–16.

41. Clark, K. L. (1994). Nursing patient care rounds in the postanesthesia care unit setting. *Journal of Post Anesthesia Nursing, 9*(1), 20–25.

42. Controlling pain in the elderly. (1995). *Nursing, 95*(7), 73.

43. Corey-Plett, P. (1995). Special considerations of the elderly patient requiring anesthesia. *Canadian Operating Room Nursing Journal, 13*(1), 20–21, 24–25, 27–28.

44. Curtin, L. (1984). Ambulatory surgery: Organization, finance, and regulation. *Nursing Management, 15,* 22–24.

45. Cushing, M. (1992). Back to (PACU) basics . . . the legal side. *American Journal of Nursing, 92*(7), 21–22.

46. Davidhizar, R. (1992). When patients die in the operating room. *Today's OR Nurse, 14*(1), 4.

47. Davidhizar, T., & Bowen, M. (1992). Managing stress in the OR. *Today's OR Nurse, 14*(5), 24–29.

48. Davis, L. A., & O'Rourke, N. C. (1993). Pulmonary embolism: Early recognition and management in the postanesthesia care unit. *Journal of Post Anesthesia Nursing, 8*(5), 338–345.

49. Davis, J., & Sherer, K. (1994). *Applied nutrition and diet therapy for nurses* (2nd ed.). Philadelphia: W. B. Saunders.

50. Definition of perioperative nursing patient needs. (1993). *AORN Journal, 57*(2), 377–380.

51. Dellasega, C., & Burgrunder, C. (1991). Perioperative nursing care for the elderly surgical patient. *Today's OR Nurse, 13*(6), 12–17.

52. Dent, T. L., Ponsky, J. L., & Berci, G. (1991). Minimal access general surgery: The dawn of a new era. *American Journal of Surgery, 161,* 323.

53. Devine, E. C., & Cook, T. D. (1986). Clinical and cost-saving effects of psychoeducational interventions with surgical clients: A meta-analysis. *Research in Nursing and Health, 9*(2), 89–96.

54. DiBenedetto, R. J., et al. (1994). Pulse oximetry monitoring can change routine oxygen supplementation practices in the postanesthesia care unit. *Anesthesia and Analgesia, 78*(2), 365–368.

55. Dove-Bright, L., & Georgi, S. (1994). How to protect your patient from DVT. *American Journal of Nursing, 94*(12), 28–32.

56. Drago, S. S. (1992). Banking your own blood. *American Journal of Nursing, 92*(3), 62–64.

57. Drain, C. B. (1994). *The recovery room: A critical care approach to post anesthesia nursing* (3rd ed.). Philadelphia: W. B. Saunders.

58. Duggar, B. (1990). Ambulatory surgery facilities: Definition and identification. *Journal of Ambulatory Care Management, 13*(1), 1–9.

59. Eccelston, S. B. (1992). Gloving: Clinical question demands further research. *AORN Journal, 56*(2), 265–269.

60. Ehrlichman, R. J., et al. (1991). Common complications of wound healing. *Surgical Clinics of North America, 71*(6), 1323–1351.

61. Einhorn, G. W., & Chant, P. (1994). Postanesthesia care unit dilemmas: Prompt assessment and treatment. *Journal of Post Anesthesia Nursing, 9*(1), 28–33.

62. Elmquist, L. (1992). Decision making for extubation of the post-anesthetic patient. *Critical Care Nursing Quarterly, 15*(1), 82–86.

63. Entrup, M. H. (1991). Perioperative complications of anesthesia. *Surgical Clinics of North America, 71*(6), 1151–1176.

64. Erwin-Toth, P., & Hocevar, B. J. (1995). Wound care: Selecting the right dressing. *American Journal of Nursing, 95*(2), 46–51.

65. Fairchild, S. S. (1996). *Perioperative nursing: Principles and practice* (2nd ed.). Boston: Little, Brown.

66. Fallo, P. (1991). Developing a program to monitor patient satisfaction and outcome in the ambulatory surgery setting. *Journal of Post Anesthesia Nursing, 6,* 176–180.

67. Fawcett, D. L., & Lainof, C. A. (1996). A pilot study appraising the climate for perioperative nursing research. *AORN Journal, 63*(1), 205–208.

68. Fernsebner, M. E. (1992). *Core curriculum for perioperative nursing or manager publication.* Denver: The National Certification Board.

69. Ferrell, B. A. (1991). Pain management in elderly people. *Journal of American Geriatric Society, 39,* 64–73.

70. Fetzer-Fowler, S., & Huot, S. (1992). The use of temperature as a discharge criterion for ambulatory surgery patients. *Journal of Post Anesthesia Nursing, 7,* 398–403.

71. Figley, E., & Burden, N. (1991). Preparing for the unexpected in the ambulatory surgery unit. *Journal of Post Anesthesia Nursing, 6,* 117–120.

72. Gaberson, K. B. (1995). The effect of humorous and muscial distraction of preoperative anxiety. *AORN Journal, 62*(5), 784, 786–787, 788.

73. Garber, N. (1993). OSHA regulations for the OR nurse. *Today's OR Nurse, 15*(1), 27–30.

74. Gerber, D. E., & Workman, D. P. (1995). Death in the operating room and postanesthesia care unit: Helping nurses to cope. *Journal of Post Anesthesia Nursing, 10*(2), 84–88.

75. Gilbert, H. (1990). Pain relief methods in the postanesthesia care unit. *Journal of Post Anesthesia Nursing, 5,* 6–15.

76. Girard, N. (1994). Anesthesia and learning: The mind-body connection. *Seminars in Perioperative Nursing, 3*(3), 121–132.

77. Girard, N. (1993). Nursing care delivery models: The perioperative environment. *AORN Journal, 57*(2), 481–488.

78. Gliniecki, A. M. (1992). Postanesthesia shaking: A review. *Journal of Post Anesthesia Nursing, 7*(2), 89–93.

79. Golanowski, M. (1995). Do not resuscitate: Informed consent in the operating room and postanesthesia care unit. *Journal of Post Anesthesia Nursing, 10*(1), 9–11.

80. Goldman, D. R., Brown, F. H., & Guarnieri, D. M. (Eds.). (1994). *Perioperative medicine: The medical care of the surgical patient.* New York: McGraw-Hill.

81. Goldman, L. (1994). Assessment of perioperative cardiac risk. *New England Journal of Medicine, 330*(10), 707–709.

82. Groah, L. K. (1996). *Perioperative nursing* (3rd ed.). Norwalk, CT: Appleton & Lange.

83. Hagen, K. S., & Treston-Aurand, J. (1995). A comparison of two skin preps used in cardiac surgical procedures. *AORN Journal, 62*(3), 393–402.

84. Heffline, M. (1990). Exploring nursing interventions for acute pain in the postanesthesia unit. *Journal of Post Anesthesia Nursing, 5,* 321–328.

85. Heinen, C., & Paul, M. (1992). "Operation information" for ambulatory surgical patients. *Nurse Manager [OR/Ambulatory Surgery Edition], 23*(8), 64Q, T.

86. Hershey-Hannan, J., et al. (1992). A comparison study of three interventions to warm patients and reduce the duration of hypothermia. *Journal of Post Anesthesia Nursing, 7*(3), 223–224.

87. Hinohosa, R. J. (1992). Nursing interventions to prevent or relieve postoperative nausea and vomiting. *Journal of Post Anesthesia, 7*(1), 3–14.

88. Hodgson, B. B., Kizior, R. J., & Kingdon, R. T. (1995). *Nurse's drug handbook, 1995.* Philadelphia: W. B. Saunders.

89. Hogenson, K. D. (1992). Acute postoperative hypertension in the hypertensive patient. *Journal of Post Anesthesia Nursing, 7*(1), 38–44.

90. Holland, M. S., Gammill, B. G., & Mackey, D. C. (1990). New techniques in anesthesia: Update for nurse anesthetists—alternatives for postoperative pain management. *American Association of Nurse Anesthetists Journal, 58*(3), 201–210.

91. Holtzclaw, B. J. (1990). Shivering: A clinical nursing problem. *Nursing Clinics of North America, 25*(4), 977–986.

92. Horner, J. (1993). The aging client: A perioperative approach. *Seminars in Perioperative Nursing, 2*(4), 226–230.

93. Horstman, P., Helmick, L., & Sions, J. A. (1994). Perioperative nursing model redesign. *Nursing Management, 25*(4), 80A, 80D–80E, 80H.

94. Jacobson, B. S. (1994). Ethical dilemmas of do-not-resuscitate orders in surgery. *AORN Journal, 60*(3), 449–452.

95. Jespen, O. B., & Bruttomesso, K. A. (1993). The effectiveness of preoperative skin preparations. *AORN Journal, 58*(3), 477–479, 482–484.

96. Joint Commission on Accreditation of Health Care Organizations. (1990). *Ambulatory health care manual.* Chicago: Author.

97. Kang, S. B., et al. (1994). Postanesthesia nursing care for ambulatory surgery patients post-spinal anesthesia. *Journal of Post Anesthesia Nursing, 9*(2), 101–106.

98. Keene, A. (1991). Perioperative assessment and nursing implications for the elderly. *Plastic Surgery Nursing, 11*(4), 143–150, 163–137.

99. Khalil, S. N., et al. (1994). Ondansetron prevents postoperative nausea and vomiting in women outpatients. *Anesthesia and Analgesia, 79*(5), 845–851.

100. Kim, M. J., McFarland, G. K., & McLane, A. M. (1995). *Guide to nursing diagnoses* (3rd ed.). St. Louis: Mosby–Year Book.

101. Kjervik, D. K., & Weisensee, M. G. (1992). Empowering older people is a perioperative nursing challenge. *AORN Journal, 55*(4), 1086–1089.

102. Kleinbeck, S. V. (1993). What future will perioperative nurses choose by 2010? *AORN Journal, 58*(5), 902–908.

103. Kneedler, J. A., & Dodge, G. H. (1990). *Perioperative patient care* (3rd ed.). Boston: Jones & Bartlett.

104. Kneedler, J. A., & Purcell, S. K. (1989). Perioperative nursing research: II. Intraoperative chemical and physical hazards to personnel. *AORN Journal, 49,* 829–854.

105. Kneedler, J. A., & Purcell, S. K. (1989). Perioperative nursing research: III. Potential intraoperative biological hazards to personnel. *AORN Journal, 49,* 1066–1079.

106. Kuhn, M. (1990). *Pharmacotherapeutics: A nursing process approach.* Philadelphia: F. A. Davis.

107. Kurz, A., et al. (1995). Postoperative hemodynamic and thermoregulatory consequences of intraoperative core hypothermia. *Journal of Clinical Anesthesia, 7*(5), 359–366.

108. Lafountain, J. (1992). The RN first assistant in surgery. *Nursing Management, 23*(12), 51–53.

109. Lake, C. L., & Moore, R. A. (Eds.). (1995). *Blood: Hemostasis, transfusion, and alternatives in the perioperative period.* New York: Raven Press.

110. Lambert, D. H. (1992). Continuous spinal anesthesia. *Anesthesiology Clinics of North America, 10*(1), 87–102.

111. Lansen, K., Epstein-Stiles, M., & Olsson, G. L. (1992). Ketorolac: A new parental nonsteroidal anti-inflammatory drug for postoperative pain management. *Journal of Post Anesthesia Nursing, 7*(4), 238–242.

112. Lederer, J. R., et al. (1993). *Care planning pocket guide: A nursing diagnosis approach* (5th ed.). Menlo Park, CA: Addison-Wesley.

113. Lehne, R. A., et al. (1994). *Pharmacology for nursing care* (2nd ed.). Philadelphia: W. B. Saunders.

114. Leino-Kilpi, H., & Vuorenheimo, J. (1993). Perioperative nursing care quality: Patients' opinions. *AORN Journal, 57*(5), 1061–1063, 1066–1071.

115. Leske, J. S. (1992). Practice-based perioperative research. *AORN Journal, 55*(2), 581–590.

116. Litwak, K. (1994). *Core curriculum for post anesthesia nursing practice* (3rd ed.). Philadelphia: W. B. Saunders.

117. Litwak, K. (1995). *Post anesthesia care nursing* (2nd ed). St. Louis: Mosby–Year Book.

118. Longinow, L. T., & Rzeszewski, L. B. (1993). The holding room: A perioperative advantage. *AORN Journal, 57*(4), 914–924.

119. Longnecker, D., & Murphy, F. (Eds.). (1992). *Dripps/Eckenhoff/Vandam Introduction to anesthesia* (8th ed.). Philadelphia: W. B. Saunders.

120. Lord, E. V. (1993). General anesthesia: What the perioperative nurse needs to know. *Seminars in Perioperative Nursing, 2*(1), 4–7.

121. Malignant Hyperthermia Association of the United States. (1991). *Preventing malignant hyperthermia: An anesthesia protocol.* Westport, CT: Author.

122. Mamaril, M. (1993). Standard of care: Legal implications in the postanesthesia care unit. *Journal of Post Anesthesia Nursing, 8*(1), 13–20.

123. Marshall, M. (1993). Postoperative confusion: Helping your patient emerge from the shadows. *Nursing, 23*(2), 44–47.

124. Matassarin-Jacobs, E. (Ed.). (1994). *Saunders review for NCLEX-RN* (2nd ed.). Philadelphia: W. B. Saunders.

125. Mathis, J. M. (1992). Collaborative practices eases OR problems. *OR Manager, 8*(3), 8–9.

126. McConnell, E. A. (1992). Assessing postoperative chills and tremors. *Nursing, 22*(4), 110–114.

127. McConnell, E. A. (1992). Assessing wound drainage. *Nursing, 22*(7), 66.

128. McConnell, E. A. (1992). Diagnosing postoperative fatigue. *Nursing, 22*(3), 70–74.

129. McNamara, S. A. (1995). Perioperative nurses' perceptions of caring practices. *AORN Journal, 61*(2), 377, 380–385, 387–388.

130. Meeker, B. J., Todriguez, L. S., & Johnson, J. M. (1992). A comprehensive analysis of preoperative patient education. *Today's OR Nurse, 14*(3), 11–18, 33–34.

131. Meeker, M. H., & Rothrock, J. C. (1995). *Alexander's care of the patient in surgery.* St. Louis: Mosby–Year Book.

132. Metzler, D. J., & Fromm, C. G. (1993). Laying out a care plan for the elderly postoperative patient. *Nursing, 23*(4), 67–74.

133. Miller, K. M., & Taylor, B. T. (1991). Standard care plans for the post anesthesia care unit. *Journal of Post Anesthesia Nursing, 1*(1), 26–32.

134. Miner, D. G. (1990). Anesthesia: The perioperative nurse's role. *Today's OR Nurse, 12*(8), 24–25.

135. Mock, E. (1991). Electrosurgical unit safety: The role of the perioperative nurse. *AORN Journal, 53*(3), 744–752.

136. Moddeman, G. (1991). The elderly surgical patient: A high risk for hypothermia. *AORN Journal, 53*(5), 1270–1272.

137. Moore, J. L., & Rice, E. L. (1992). Malignant hyperthermia. *American Family Physician, 45*(5), 2245–2251.

138. Moss, M. T. (1995). Managed care 'marriage' benefits perioperative nursing. *Nursing Economics, 13*(3), 183–185.

139. Moss, M. T. (1994). The rebirth of quality: Managed care and managed cost in perioperative nursing. *Nursing Economics, 13*(1), 54–55, 57.

140. Moss, V. A. (1994). Assessing learning abilities, readiness for education. *Seminars in Perioperative Nursing, 3*(3), 113–120.

141. Mullen, C. (1992). Hypoxemia during transfer to the PACU. *Journal of Post Anesthesia Nursing, 7*(3), 220.

142. Murphy, E. K. (1993). Monitoring IV conscious sedation: The legal scope of practice. *AORN Journal, 57*(2), 512–514.

143. Murphy, E. K. (1991). OR nursing law: Counts, documentation revisited. *AORN Journal, 54*(4), 878.

144. Nash, C. A., & Jensen, P. L. (1994). When your surgical patient has hypertension. *American Journal of Nursing, 94*(12), 39–44.

145. Nathan, M. A. (1993). Malignant hyperthermia: Perioperative considerations. *Seminars in Perioperative Nursing, 2*(1), 38–44.

146. North American Nursing Diagnosis Association. (1994). *Nursing diagnoses: Definitions and classification, 1995–1996*. Philadelphia: Author.

147. Neuberger, G. B. (1987). Wound care: What's clear, what's not. *Nursing 17*(2), 34–37.

148. Nora, P. F. (1991). *Operative surgery: Principles and techniques* (3rd ed.). Philadelphia: W. B. Saunders.

149. Null, S., Richter-Abt, D., & Kovac, J. (1995). Development of a perioperative nursing diagnoses flow sheet. *AORN Journal, 61*(3), 547–554, 557.

150. Nussbaum, W., deCastro, N., & Campbell, F. W. (1994). Perioperative challenges in the care of the Jehovah's Witness: A case report. *AANA Journal, 62*(2), 160–164.

151. Omogui, S. (1995). *The anesthesia drug handbook* (2nd ed.). St. Louis: Mosby–Year Book.

152. Oetker-Black, S. L. (1992). Preoperative self-efficacy and postoperative behaviors. *Applied Nursing Research, 4*(4), 177–183.

153. On-site preregistration: An idea whose time has gone? (1993). *Same Day Surgery, 17*(1), 8–10.

154. Operating room nurses: On the "cutting edge" of change. (1993). *Nursing, 23*(2), 73–83.

155. Parsons, E. C., Kee, C. C., & Gray, D. P. (1993). Perioperative nurse caring behaviors: Perceptions of surgical patients. *AORN Journal, 57*(5), 1106–1107, 1110–1114.

156. Phippen, M. L. Y., & Wells, M. P. (1994). *Perioperative nursing practice*. Philadelphia: W. B. Saunders.

157. Pobojewski, B. J., et al. (1992). Documenting nursing process in the perioperative setting: Continuity of care, patient evaluation. *AORN Journal, 56*(1), 98–112.

158. Ponte, J., & Green, D. W. (1994). *Handbook of anesthetics and perioperative care*. Philadelphia: W. B. Saunders.

159. Poole, E. L. (1993). The effects of postanesthesia care unit visits on anxiety in surgical patients. *Journal of Post Anesthesia Nursing, 8*(6), 386–394.

160. Ratner, L. E., & Smith, G. W. (1993). Intraoperative fluid management. *Surgical Clinics of North America, 73*(2), 229–241.

161. Rhodes, V. (1990). Nausea, vomiting, and retching. *Nursing Clinics of North America, 25*, 885–900.

162. Rothrock, J. C. (1993). *The RN first assistant: An expanded perioperative nursing role* (2nd ed.). Philadelphia: J. B. Lippincott.

163. Rothrock, J. C. (1996). *Perioperative nursing care planning* (2nd ed.). St. Louis: Mosby–Year Book.

164. Sabiston, D. C. Jr. (1996). *Textbook of surgery: The biological basis of modern surgical practice* (15th ed.). Philadelphia: W. B. Saunders.

165. Saleh, K. (1992). Practical points in understanding local anesthetics. *Journal of Post Anesthesia Nursing, 7*(1), 45–47.

166. Same-day surgeries surpass inpatient rate. (1992). *Hospital Purchasing News, 16*(6), 1, 16.

167. Seifert, P. C., et al. (1993). ANA Code for Nurses with interpretive statements: Explications for perioperative nursing. *AORN Journal, 58*(2), 369–388.

168. Shepard, S. (1990). Helping ambulatory surgery patients cope with emotions. *Journal of Post Anesthesia Nursing, 5*, 103–105.

169. Smith, R. N., et al. (1995). Instilling the facts about autotransfusion. *Nursing, 25*(3), 52–55.

170. Steelman, V. M., Bulechek, G. M., & McCloskey, J. C. (1994). Toward a standardized language to describe perioperative nursing. *AORN Journal, 60*(5), 786–790, 793–795.

171. Stuttard, D. (1994). The effects of minimally invasive surgery on the future of perioperative nursing. *Canadian Operating Room Nursing Journal, 12*(3), 5–12.

172. Summers, S., & Ebbert, D. W. (1992). *Ambulatory surgical nursing: A nursing diagnosis approach*. Philadelphia: J. B. Lippincott.

173. Terranova, A. (1991). The effects of diabetes mellitus on wound healing. *Plastic Surgery Nursing, 11*(1), 20–25.

174. Thomas, B. L. (1991). Pain management for the elderly: Alternative interventions. *AORN Journal, 51*(1), 126–132.

175. Thornhill, A. M. (1994). Perioperative nursing in a national health care system. *AORN Journal, 60*(2), 302–309.

176. Valdrighi, J. B., et al. (1994). Effect of intraoperative ketorolac on postanesthesia care unit comfort. *Journal of Pain and Symptom Management, 9*(3), 171–174.

177. Vance, A., & Davidhizar, R. (1992). The element of care in the operating room. *Today's OR Nurse, 14*(11), 24–27.

178. Vidor, K. (1990). Anxiety related to impending surgery. *Today's OR Nurse, 12*(9), 36.

179. Vogelsang, J. (1992). Research in PACU. *Journal of Post Anesthesia Nursing, 7*(3), 218.

180. Vogelsang, J. (1992). The Bair Hugger system does not stop shaking. *Journal of Post Anesthesia Nursing, 7*(3), 222.

181. Vogelsang, J., & Fetzer, S. J. (1995). An integrative review of postanesthesia care unit: Phase I. Patient outcome research: 1982 to 1993. *Journal of Post Anesthesia Nursing, 10*(4), 197–207.

182. Walhout, M. F. (1992). Treat for hypothermia. *RN, 55*(4), 50–55.

183. Walsh, J. (1993). Postop effects of OR positioning. *RN, 56*(2), 50–57.

184. Walsh, K. (1990). Communication: The heart of patient education. *Plastic Surgery Nursing, 10*, 171–172.

185. Watson, D. (1990). *Monitoring the patient receiving local anesthesia*. Denver: Association of Operating Room Nurses.

186. Watt-Watson, J. H., & Donovan, M. I. (1992). *Pain management: Nursing perspective*. St. Louis: Mosby–Year Book.

187. Waugaman, W., Foster, S., & Rigor, B. (1992). *Principles and practice of nurse anesthesia* (2nd ed.). Norwalk, CT: Appleton & Lange.

188. White, P. (Ed.). (1990). *Outpatient anesthesia*. New York: Churchill Livingstone.

189. Who has the responsibility to monitor OR blood loss? (1992). *Regan Report on Nursing Law, 33*(4), 2.

190. Whitman, G. R. (1991). Hypertension and hypothermia in the acute postoperative period. *Critical Care Nursing Clinics of North America, 3*(4), 661–673.

191. Wild, L., & Coyne, C. (1992). The basics and beyond: Epidural analgesia. *American Journal of Nursing, 92*(4), 26–35.

192. Woodin, L. M. (1993). Cutting postop pain. *RN, 56*(8), 26–34.

193. *Wound closure manual* (publication No. EPB010). (1994). Somerville, NJ: Ethicon, Inc.

194. Zeller, J. (1995). Developing a quality indicator logbook for the postanesthesia care unit setting. *Journal of Post Anesthesia Nursing, 10*(5), 259–264.

Shock

CHAPTER 22

Louise Nelson LaFramboise

Shock is a complex clinical syndrome that may occur at any time and in any place. It is a life-threatening condition often requiring team action by many healthcare providers, including nurses, physicians, laboratory technicians, pharmacists, and respiratory therapists. Shock causes thousands of deaths and unknown numbers of permanent injuries each year. Because shock is potentially lethal, it is essential that you be able to identify clients at risk of developing shock, recognize the early assessment findings indicating shock, and initiate appropriate interventions before shock ensues. In order to recognize the development of shock, it is important for you to understand the processes taking place in the body.

Shock is defined as failure of the circulatory system to maintain adequate perfusion of vital organs. Various disorders leading to inadequate tissue perfusion result in decreased oxygenation at the cellular level. This inadequate oxygenation results in anaerobic cellular metabolism and accumulated waste products in cells. If the condition is untreated, cell and organ death occur.

This chapter discusses three major classifications of shock: (1) hypovolemic, (2) cardiogenic, and (3) distributive. Various etiologic factors related to each classification are also addressed. Included in the discussion are the pathophysiologic mechanisms of shock, its complications, and its medical and nursing management. Knowledge of the pathophysiology of shock will enable you to identify accurate, individualized interventions paramount to the effective care of the client in shock.

Hypovolemic shock is due to inadequate circulating blood volume resulting from hemorrhage with actual blood loss, burns with a loss of plasma proteins and fluid shifts, or dehydration with a loss of fluid volume. Hypovolemic shock is the most common type of shock and develops when the intravascular volume decreases to the point where compensatory mechanisms are unable to maintain organ and tissue perfusion.

Cardiogenic shock is due to inadequate pumping action of the heart because of primary cardiac muscle dysfunction or mechanical obstruction of blood flow caused by myocardial infarction (MI), valvular insufficiency due to disease or trauma, cardiac dysrhythmias, or an obstructive condition, such as pericardial tamponade or pulmonary embolus. Cardiogenic shock occurs in 15% to 20% of all clients following MI and has at least an 80% mortality rate. Cardiogenic shock after an MI usually occurs when 40% or more of the myocardium has been damaged.

Sometimes, the term *obstructive shock* is used as another category of shock to include those conditions that lead to a sudden obstruction of blood flow. These problems include cardiac tamponade, tension pneumothorax, and pulmonary embolism. We will incorporate a discussion of obstructive etiologies within cardiogenic shock because the ability of the heart to pump effectively is the primary problem.

Distributive shock is due to changes in blood vessel tone that increase the size of the vascular space without an increase in the circulating blood volume. This results in a relative hypovolemia (total fluid volume remains the same but is redistributed). Distributive shock is further divided into three types: (1) anaphylactic shock, a severe hypersensitivity reaction resulting in massive systemic vasodilation; (2) neurogenic shock, interference with nervous system control of the blood vessels, such as with spinal cord injury (especially cervical spine injury), spinal anesthesia, or severe vasovagal reactions due to pain or psychic trauma; and (3) septic shock, due to a release of vasoactive substances.

Some amount of neurogenic shock is seen with all spinal cord injuries. The more dramatic cases of neurogenic shock are seen with cervical spine injuries. The duration of neurogenic shock is usually 1 to 6 weeks, provided there has been no irreparable cord injury. The incidence of septic and anaphylactic shock is variable. Persons who are at risk for either type of shock should be monitored closely.

Etiology and Risk Factors

Since shock is a disorder of perfusion, all the causes of shock focus on some component of the distribution of blood throughout the body. There can be an insufficient quantity of blood (hypovolemic shock), an incompetent pump (cardiogenic shock), or ineffective delivery of blood (distributive shock).

Hypovolemic Shock

The primary event precipitating hypovolemic shock is a large reduction in the circulating blood volume so that the body's metabolic needs cannot be met. Hypovolemic shock may be due to loss of plasma or blood. Conditions that may cause a reduction in the circulating volume include hemorrhage, burns, and dehydration.

■ Hemorrhage

Hemorrhage is the loss of blood. Clinical manifestations indicative of hypovolemic shock may begin to appear with a blood volume deficit of 15% to 25%, or about 500 to 1500 ml in an adult with a normal circulating volume. Shock fully develops if a previously healthy client loses about one third of the normal circulating blood volume of 5 L.

The loss of smaller amounts of blood may cause shock in persons less able to compensate rapidly (e.g., the elderly with decreased vascular tone and impaired cardiac function). The extent to which a person develops shock after blood loss also depends on the length of time over

which the blood loss occurs. Clients with slow blood loss over a period of days or weeks tolerate their blood loss better than do those whose blood loss occurs rapidly over minutes or hours. Hypovolemic shock following trauma is typically the result of hemorrhage. The classes of hemorrhage and the associated assessment findings are listed in Table 22–1.

■ Burns

Hypovolemic shock produced by burns occurs most often in persons with large partial-thickness or full-thickness burns. It is caused primarily by a shift of plasma from the vascular space into the interstitial space. In addition to these fluid losses or shifts, the client may have cardiac dysfunction due to the presence of *myocardial depressant factor (MDF)*. MDF affects the contractility of cardiac muscle by depressing myocardial muscle function. The result is impaired cardiac output, even in the presence of a normal circulating volume. Shock related to burns is discussed in Chapter 79.

Other causes of hypovolemic shock which may produce fluid shifts similar to those in burns include nephrotic syndrome, severe crush injuries, starvation, surgery, and conditions causing plasma fluids to accumulate in the abdominal cavity (e.g., cirrhosis of the liver, pancreatitis, and bowel obstruction).

■ Dehydration

Shock may also occur from either reduced oral fluid intake or significant losses of fluid. Examples of situations in which inadequate oral fluid intake may occur are (1) rigorous exercise causing fluid loss from sweating and insensible fluid loss through the respiratory tract and (2)

Table 22–1. Assessment Findings and Classifications of Acute Hemorrhage

Assessment Finding	Class I	Class II	Class III	Class IV
Blood loss (%)	15	15–30	30–40	>40
Blood loss (ml)	<750	1000–1250	1500–1800	2000–2500
Pulse rate/min	<100	>100	>120	>140
Respiratory rate/min	Normal (14–20)	20–30	30–40	>35
Blood pressure	Normal	Normal or slightly increased	Decreased	Not obtained
Pulse pressure	Normal	Narrowed	Narrowed	Narrowed
Capillary refill	Normal	Prolonged	Prolonged	Prolonged
Skin circulation	Pale, pink, cool	Slightly pale, cool	Pale, cold, moist	Cyanotic, cold, clammy
Level of consciousness	Slightly anxious	Mildly anxious	Anxious/confused	Confused, lethargic, or obtunded
Urinary output (ml/hr)*	≥30	25–30	5–15	Negligible
Intravenous fluid replacement	Crystalloid at 3 ml/1 ml of blood loss	Crystalloid at 3 ml/1 ml of blood loss	Crystalloid plus blood	Crystalloid plus blood

*Assumes a normal 70-kg man.
Data from American College of Surgeons Committee on Trauma guidelines.

hot environments. Loss of fluid, leading to dehydration-induced hypovolemic shock, may occur in persons with excessive urine output or prolonged vomiting or diarrhea. People with chronic illnesses, especially the elderly, may be at increased risk because of impaired recognition of thirst or inability to obtain fluids, inadequate maintenance of chronic conditions (i.e., increased blood sugar with diabetes), or inadequate monitoring of therapeutic regimens (i.e., diuretic-induced dehydration). With a prolonged fluid deficit, all compartments—intravascular, interstitial, and intracellular—are depleted.

Cardiogenic Shock

Cardiogenic shock results primarily from an inability of heart muscle to function adequately or mechanical obstructions of blood flow to or from the heart. Similar to the other causes of shock, the lack of blood flow decreases tissue and organ perfusion. Clients with hypovolemic shock may develop cardiogenic shock. The myocardium normally receives its blood supply during diastole. If the heart rate is increased to compensate for the decreased circulating volume and decreased cardiac output, diastole will be shortened and the myocardium's oxygen needs will rise. This predisposes the myocardium to injury because of decreased blood flow and decreased oxy-gen. In addition, the decreased venous return associated with hypovolemia results in decreased coronary artery perfusion and inadequate oxygenation of the myocardium. Finally, shock results in the release of MDF and lactic acid, which depress myocardial function.

■ Myocardial Infarction

Impaired heart muscle action is most often caused by MI (see Chapter 45). The area of dead or dying tissue that occurs with infarction impairs contractility of the myocardium, and the cardiac output decreases. Impaired myocardial contractility may also occur with blunt cardiac trauma, cardiomyopathy, and congestive heart failure.

Clients with cardiogenic shock may also develop some degree of hypovolemic shock. This is most often due to therapeutic use of diuretics or edema in the extremities or other dependent areas (due to inadequate cardiac pumping activity and venous congestion).

■ Obstructive Conditions

Mechanical obstructions to blood flow causing cardiogenic shock include a large pulmonary embolism, pericardial tamponade, and tension pneumothorax. An embolus is usually the result of a blood clot that breaks loose in a person with deep vein thrombosis. This embolus travels through the venous system to the right side of the heart and into the pulmonary artery. The size of the embolus determines at what point it lodges in the pulmonary ar-

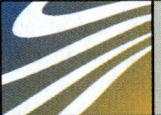

ETHICAL ISSUES IN NURSING

Are Healthcare Workers Required to Continue Life-Supporting Interventions Until the Client's Body No Longer Responds?

Interventions directed at sustaining life become more progressive, capable, and invasive on a daily basis. Medical science has advanced to the point where we can sustain life for extended periods of time in some clients. Healthcare professionals often find themselves asking, Have we gone too far?

Consider the client in cardiogenic shock. Mary is a 61-year-old woman with a past history of hypertension, palpitations, and angina. She has suffered a massive anterior myocardial infarction. Mary is being sustained by a ventilator to support respiratory status and vasoactive drugs to support cardiovascular status. Without these interventions, Mary would die.

Mary's only living relatives are her two daughters. One daughter says that Mary would not want all of these life-sustaining interventions if there were "no hope," whereas the other daughter indicates that Mary would want every possible chance at life. Mary does not have a living will.

Unless Mary has specified who has the right to make healthcare decisions for her when she is unable to do so, the eldest daughter is the one who can legally make Mary's healthcare decisions. However, when a client's relatives have such differing opinions on care, legal considerations are only a part of the decision-making process. Ethically, healthcare providers attempt to have all involved family members agree on decisions that are made. To accommodate this, healthcare institutions often have ethics committees to help work through these dilemmas.

An ethics committee comprises representatives from multiple areas of the hospital, including medicine, nursing, social work, and pastoral care. This committee can help the family work through the decision-making process for care.

Be aware of your feelings about client care and when you believe it is appropriate to stop interventions, but your beliefs should not affect your care. The nursing role is as facilitator for the family: helping to arrange conferences, serving as advocate, and ensuring the family clearly understands what is being said by other healthcare providers. It is your responsibility to assess families to determine disparities in their ideas about treatment. If differences of opinion are identified, help families access resources that will assist in the decision-making process.

tery. A large embolus can inhibit perfusion of a major portion of the lung field, resulting in an increased workload for the right ventricle. Pericardial tamponade is an accumulation of blood or fluid in the pericardial space that compresses the myocardium and interferes with the myocardium's ability to expand. Tension pneumothorax is a significant amount of air in the pleural space compressing the heart and great vessels and thus interfering with venous return to the heart.

■ Other Causes

Other causes of cardiogenic shock include cardiac valvular insufficiency from trauma or disease, myocardial aneurysms (usually due to previous MI or congenital abnormalities), rupture of a valvular papillary muscle, rupture of a ventricle, aortic stenosis, mitral regurgitation, and cardiac dysrhythmias.

Clients with hypovolemic shock may also develop cardiogenic shock. This happens when the rapid heart rate initiated to compensate for decreased volume and to increase cardiac output does not allow time for the coronary arteries to fill with blood. Because these arteries supply blood to the myocardium, the myocardial oxygen supply is impaired. Also, the increased heart rate increases the myocardium's need for oxygen. In addition, the decreased venous return associated with hypovolemia results in decreased coronary artery perfusion and inadequate oxygenation of the myocardium. Finally, shock results in the release of MDF and lactic acid, which depresses myocardial function.

Distributive Shock

Distributive shock (also sometimes called vasogenic shock) results from inadequate vascular tone. With distributive shock, the blood volume remains normal. However, the size of the vascular space increases dramatically because of massive vasodilation. The result is maldistribution of the blood due to decreased blood pressure and lack of blood returning to the heart. This maldistribution of the blood is often referred to as "relative" hypovolemia. The volume of blood remains constant, but the blood has pooled due to increase capacity of the vascular system.

After extensive vasodilation, blood pressure (BP), return of venous blood to the heart, and cardiac output are decreased. As with other forms of shock, tissue anoxia and cell destruction result. The massive vasodilation present with distributive shock has several major causes.

■ Acute Allergic Reaction (Anaphylactic Shock)

Anaphylactic shock occurs as a result of an acute allergic reaction from exposure to a substance to which the client has been sensitized. Common sensitizing agents are peni-

cillin, penicillin derivatives, bee stings, chocolate, strawberries, peanuts, snake venom, iodine-based contrast for x-rays, foods, and nonsteroidal anti-inflammatory agents (NSAIDs).

Reexposure to the foreign substance results in the offending antigen binding to previously made immunoglobulins (IgE) located on the mast cell. This binding causes the release of several chemical mediators from the cell, such as histamine, kallikrein, platelet-activating factor, leukotrienes, and prostaglandins. Reactions depend on the route and dose of exposure. The more systemic the exposure, the more rapid is the onset. Manifestations include massive vasodilation, urticaria (hives), laryngeal edema, and bronchial constriction. Without prompt treatment, a person suffering from anaphylactic shock will die from cardiovascular collapse and respiratory failure.

■ Spinal Cord Injury (Neurogenic Shock)

With injury to the cervical spine, the autonomic nervous system is affected. Below the level of injury, there is blocking of sympathetic nervous stimulation and the parasympathetic system goes unopposed. This unopposed stimulation causes vasodilation, decreased venous return, decreased cardiac output, and decreased tissue perfusion.

■ Infection (Septic Shock)

Before discussing septic shock, it is important to understand sepsis. Sepsis is the systemic response to infection. The process begins with the growth of various microorganisms at the site of infection. The organisms may invade the bloodstream directly (leading to positive blood cultures) or may remain in one area. The organisms release various substances into the bloodstream. These substances include structural parts of the organism such as endotoxins and elements synthesized by them called exotoxins. Once these substances are released into the body, they activate the complement cascade (see Chapter 25). The client develops a complex shock picture, which is discussed later. Septic shock is very lethal, having a mortality rate of up to 50%!

Since shock is such a serious and often lethal development, it is important for nurses to identify high-risk clients and prevent shock whenever possible. The risk factors for shock are shown in Risk Factors and Levels of Prevention. It is evident that there is little primary prevention except for the person with allergies and maintenance of nutrition in high-risk immunocompromised persons.

Pathophysiology

Before we begin to discuss the pathophysiology behind shock, it is important to review the physiologic basis of blood flow through the body. Adequate circulating volume is dependent on three interrelated components of the cardiovascular system: (1) the heart, (2) vascular tone, and (3) blood volume. A minor impairment in one component will be compensated for by the other two. Pro-

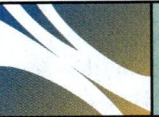

RISK FACTORS AND LEVELS OF PREVENTION

Shock

Risk Factors

- Trauma, heart muscle injury or valve incompetence, cardiac output obstruction, allergen exposure, compromise of body's natural defenses (immunosuppression, impaired skin integrity, invasive procedures), exposure to pathogens

Levels of Prevention

Hypovolemic Shock

Primary Prevention

- Teach clients safety measures to avoid injury

Secondary Prevention

- Provide support oxygenation
- Help clients to maintain fluid and electrolyte balance

Tertiary Prevention

- Provide cardiac rhythm monitoring
- Provide hemodynamic monitoring
- Provide vasoactive medications
- Provide for blood and fluid replacement

Cardiogenic Shock

Primary Prevention

- Teach clients to reduce risk factors with diet and exercise

Secondary Prevention

- Provide support oxygenation
- Administer inotropic agents and vasodilators

Tertiary Prevention

- Provide an intra-aortic balloon pump
- Administer inotropic agents and vasodilators

Distributive Shock

Anaphylactic Shock

Primary Prevention

- Teach clients to avoid precipitators
- Teach clients to wear medical alert bracelets for known allergens
- Provide for allergy desensitization.

Secondary Prevention

- Teach clients to wear medical alert bracelets for known allergens
- Encourage clients to discontinue or remove the allergen
- Provide an EpiPen (for injection of epinephrine)

Tertiary Prevention

- Provide respiratory support
- Provide cardiovascular support
- Administer glucocorticoids

Neurogenic Shock

Primary Prevention

- Teach clients safety measures to avoid injury

Secondary Prevention

- Maintain the client's airway and breathing
- Provide circulatory support
- Protect the client's spine (especially the cervical spine)
- Provide for thermoregulation

Tertiary Prevention

- Maintain the client's airway and breathing
- Provide circulatory support
- Protect the client's spine (especially the cervical spine)
- Provide for thermoregulation
- Begin the client's rehabilitation when he or she is stable

Septic Shock

Primary Prevention

- Teach clients to maintain adequate nutrition for maximal immune system functioning
- Teach immunosuppressed clients to take precautions

Secondary Prevention

- Take body fluid cultures
- Administer antibiotics

Tertiary Prevention

- Provide respiratory support
- Provide cardiovascular support
- Administer naloxone
- Administer vasoactive agents

---

longed or severe impairments will lead to shock. You will see in the following paragraphs that some of the problems with decreased organ and tissue perfusion in shock are due to failure of the normal mechanisms.

Blood flows throughout the body because of the driving pressure it carries with it as it leaves the left ventricle (LV). Nowhere else in the cardiovascular system is blood under as high a pressure as it is in the LV; hence it "is all downhill from there." We will follow it briefly.

About 100 ml of blood (called stroke volume) leaves the LV at systolic blood pressure about 80 times a minute. Since the metabolic demands are continuous rather than intermittent, blood is delivered into muscular walled arterioles where it can be stored and released more consistently into the capillaries. From here the blood flows slowly through the capillaries that have greatest demand. When you run, more blood flows to your legs and lungs and less to your gastrointestinal tract. After you eat, the opposite is true. The microcirculation has the potential capacity to hold a great volume of blood. Nonetheless, the capillaries normally are relatively ischemic, containing only about 5% of the body's volume of blood. Typically, blood flow through the capillary bed is influenced by the varying needs of the cells located near the vessel. The capillaries open on demand of the cells adjacent to them. The size of the body's larger blood vessels is regulated by the autonomic nervous system. However, this is not so for the microcirculation. Arteriole and capillary sphincters are separate mechanisms governed by different controls.

The microcirculation is relatively autonomous as a functional entity. Its patterns of behavior (in both normal and abnormal situations) are highly independent of the vasomotor influences affecting the systemic circulation lying next to it. The systemic circulatory bed and the microcirculatory bed apparently do not have sensing devices that would allow a unified, coordinated response throughout the entire circulation. Thus, events occurring within one bed do not influence events in the other. As shall be seen, the relative autonomy of the microcirculation and the lack of coordination between it and the systemic circulation are important in determining the course of events in shock.

In the capillaries, nutrients in the blood are delivered to interstitial spaces to be picked up by the cells, and wastes are transported to the capillary. The microcirculation is governed locally by vasoactive substances (i.e., affecting blood vessels) released into the area by the actions of various types of cells. This local regulation is a sensitive mechanism that can adjust blood flow from moment to moment according to tissue needs. The capillaries eventually join and meet veins that deliver blood to the heart. Veins have no muscle and are very low-pressure systems in which blood returns to the heart by using one-way valves. Veins can also store very large amounts of blood.

Now that normal flow has been discussed, how does the body make needed adjustments? There are two major receptors that sense blood flow and volume. The arterial baroreceptor located in the aortic arch senses how "full the system is." If pressure in the muscular arterioles is low because of increased demand, the baroreceptor stimulates the sympathetic nervous system. This stimulation results in increased cardiac output, both by increasing rate and increasing stroke volume and increased muscle tension on the arteriole walls (called systemic or peripheral vascular resistance). If blood pressure was low to begin with, there will be insufficient pressure for perfusion at the capillary end. On the right side of the heart is another receptor, the atrial baroreceptor. This receptor measures the fluid volume returning to the heart. It also stimulates the sympathetic nervous system and constricts vessels storing blood in areas that are not considered vital to survival. The heart and brain are the organs considered most vital to survival. All other areas, most notably the

gastrointestinal tract, skin, muscle, and kidneys, are not considered by the body to be vital to survival.

There are also chemoreceptors located in the aortic arch and carotid bodies. These receptors sense decreased pH and increased partial pressure of arterial carbon dioxide ($PaCO_2$). When tissues do not receive adequate blood, they maintain their metabolism using an anaerobic pathway. A product of this pathway is lactic acid. When there is inadequate perfusion, CO_2 accumulates in the tissues. If breathing is also impaired, CO_2 is not exhaled. When these changes are sensed by chemoreceptors, respiratory rate and depth increase and cardiac output increases to correct the imbalance.

There is a juxtaglomerular receptor in the kidney which measures blood flow to the kidney. When blood volume falls, the cells in the receptor release renin. Renin begins a cascade of response (angiotensin I, angiotensin II) that eventually produces very potent peripheral vasoconstriction. In addition, antidiuretic hormone (ADH) is released when osmoreceptors in the hypothalamus are triggered. Osmoreceptors sense the osmolality, that is, how "concentrated" the blood is. When osmolality is increased, ADH release prevents diuresis, increases water returned to the body from the kidney, and thus increases total blood volume.

All of these receptors and hormones work minute by minute to maintain volume and thus arterial pressure. When the circulatory system is functioning properly, mean arterial pressure (MAP) is maintained at normal levels (70–105 mm Hg).

$$MAP = (systolic + [2 \times diastolic])/3$$

MAP is the average effective pressure that drives blood through the systemic organs.[23] If MAP is not maintained at normal or near-normal levels, tissues are inadequately perfused. Let us explore the problems seen when shock is induced by problems of inadequate blood volume, a failing pump, or changes in vasoconstriction.

If one of the three components of circulation fails, other parts of the system initiate compensatory mechanisms. For example, vasoconstriction and increased cardiac output may be used to compensate for decreased volume. Thus, as long as two of these factors can maintain a satisfactory compensatory action, adequate blood circulation can be maintained even though the third factor is not functioning normally. However, if compensatory mechanisms fail or if more than one of the three factors necessary for adequate circulation malfunction, circulatory failure results, and shock develops.

Stages of Shock

■ Early Compensation Stage

During the initial or compensated stage of shock (Fig. 22–1), cardiac output is slightly decreased because of loss of actual or relative blood volume. During this stage, the body's compensatory mechanisms are able to maintain

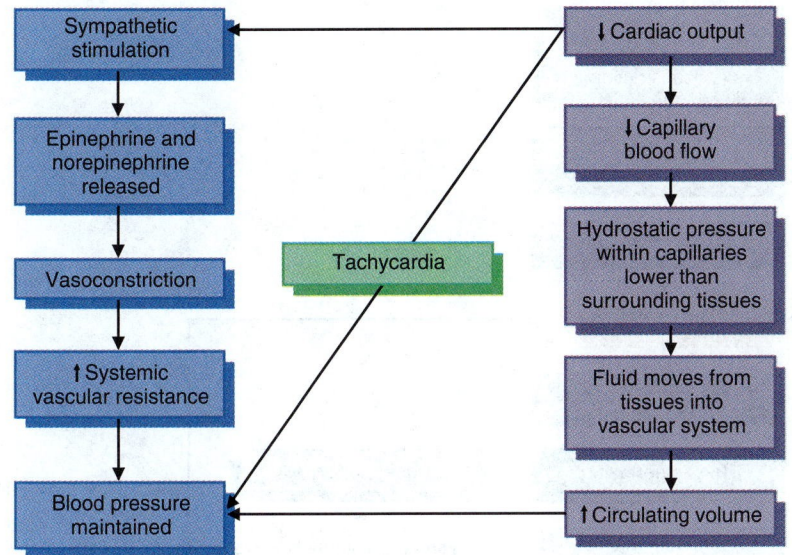

Figure 22–1. Compensated stage of shock. Regardless of the cause, a decreased cardiac output is generally the stimulus that precipitates the body's response to compensate for the hypovolemia (relative or actual) to maintain blood pressure.

BP within a normal to low-normal range and are able to maintain tissue perfusion to the vital organs. During the compensatory phase, the systemic circulation and microcirculation work together. Both undergo a major readjustment in which their activities are coordinated to preserve the entire system.

Decreased cardiac output causes a reduction in blood flow through the capillaries, which results in a fall in hydrostatic pressure within the capillaries. As the hydrostatic pressure decreases to a level below that of the surrounding tissues, fluid moves from the higher-pressure tissues into the lower-pressure vascular system, thereby increasing circulating volume. The decreased cardiac output also stimulates the sympathetic nervous system. The vasoconstriction caused by this stimulation and the accompanying tachycardia further maintain BP.

■ Decompensation Stage

If shock and the compensatory vasoconstriction persist, the body begins to decompensate and the systemic circulation and microcirculation no longer work in unison. As vasoconstriction continues, there is a decreased supply of oxygenated blood to the tissues. This results in anaerobic metabolism and lactic acidosis. Acidosis and the increasing $PaCO_2$ cause the microcirculation to dilate. This dilation causes decreased venous return and decreased circulation of reoxygenated blood.

Lactic acidosis also causes increased capillary permeability and relaxation of the capillary sphincters. Relaxation of the sphincters allows increased blood in the capillaries and increased capillary pressure. This increased pressure, along with the increased capillary permeability, allows fluid to move out of the vascular space and back into the tissues. In doing so, the microcirculation has reversed its pattern and is trying to secure for itself (and the tissue it supplies) more of the limited supply of available blood. Thus, the blood supply is progressively retained in the capillary bed. In other words, blood pools in the microcirculation. Because the cells demand greater perfusion time, many or most of the capillaries remain open at any one time. This increases the vascular space in the microcirculation.

Increased vascular capacity, decreased blood volume, or decreased heart action reduces the MAP. In turn, the pressure gradient for the venous return of blood decreases. This also contributes to venous pooling of blood, decreased venous return to the heart, and decreased cardiac output.

Because there are no feedback systems within the body to change this pattern, the cycle of events becomes progressively more severe. Eventually, the circulation is totally disrupted. Once the vascular space enlarges (owing to vasodilation of the microcirculation), even a normal blood volume cannot fill all these small vessels and the larger ones as well. The result is a low central venous pressure (CVP) (except in cardiogenic shock) and inadequate venous return to the right side of the heart, with a further decrease in cardiac output.

This resultant decrease in circulating volume and capillary flow does not allow adequate perfusion and oxygenation of the vital organs. With the prolonged decrease in capillary blood flow, the tissues become hypoxic. This process is described in Figure 22–2.

■ Progressive Stage

The progressive stage of shock occurs if the cycle of inadequate tissue perfusion is not interrupted. The shock state becomes progressively more severe, even though the initial cause of the shock is not itself becoming more severe. Cellular ischemia and necrosis lead to organ failure and death.

Systemic Effects of Shock

Shock affects every system within the body. Equally important to understanding the cellular level of shock is

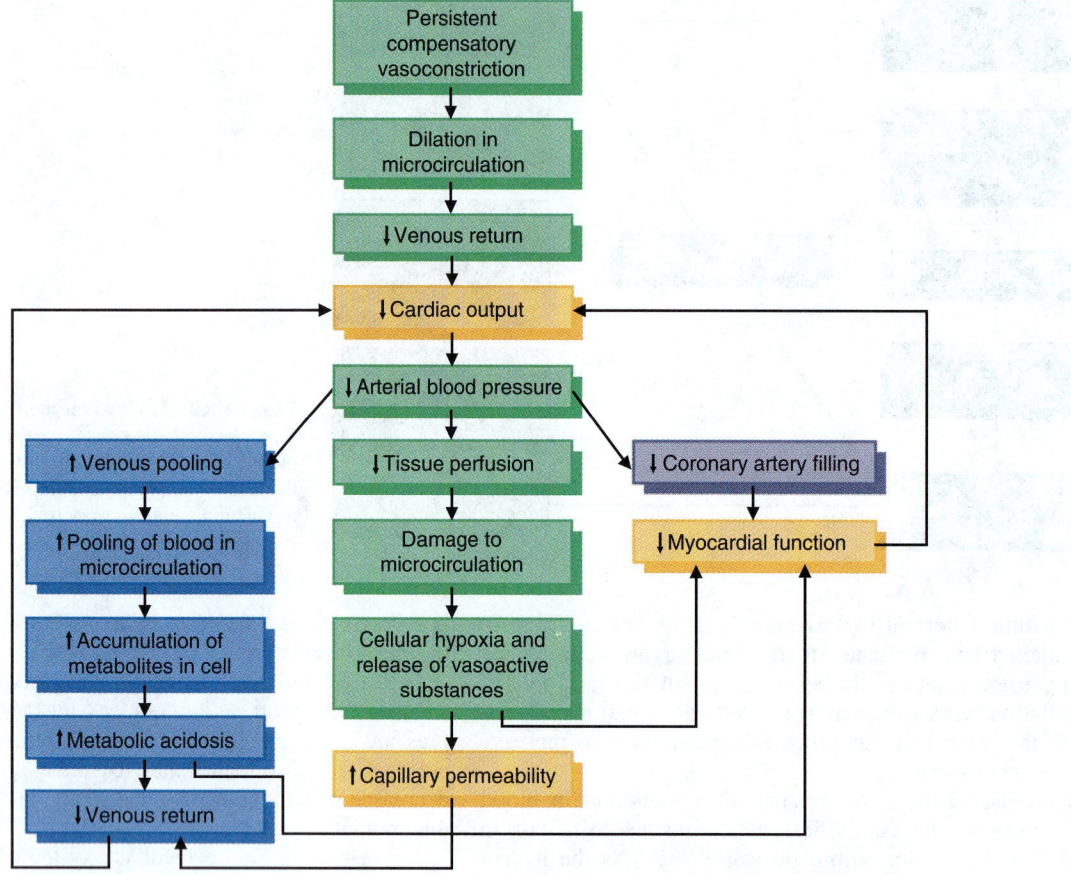

Figure 22–2. Vicious circle of events occurring in shock. The shock syndrome can be initiated anywhere in the circle, depending on the precipitating cause, for example, impaired myocardial function due to myocardial infarction, blood loss due to trauma, or the release of vasoactive toxins due to sepsis. Hypovolemic shock resulting from blood loss, for example, results in decreased arterial blood pressure, setting in motion a cascade of events that worsen the shock state.

understanding what happens to the various organs. Figure 22–3 presents the systemic effects of shock in a flow chart.

■ Effects on the Respiratory System

Getting oxygen in (ventilation) and delivering oxygenated blood to the tissues (perfusion) are critical for survival. As previously emphasized, shock produces prolonged circulatory insufficiency. This leads to variable and inadequate perfusion of certain organs and tissues, particularly at the microcirculation level. Such circulatory deprivation results in tissue hypoxia and anoxia. Hypoxia and anoxia can be tolerated for a short time. However, as the time lengthens, the chances of recovery diminish. A lack of oxygen appears to stimulate development of the progressive stage of shock. The greater the difference between the amount of oxygen available and the amount needed, the more rapidly progressive shock develops. If sufficient oxygen is available to the cells to meet the body's needs, progressive shock is less likely to occur.

Despite many advances in shock prevention, early recognition, and management, respiratory failure continues to be a major cause of death in shock. The magnitude of this problem surfaced during the Vietnam War when sol-diers sustaining massive injuries and profound blood loss were successfully resuscitated only to die several days later from acute respiratory distress syndrome (ARDS) (see Chapter 42). While ARDS remains the greatest contributor to respiratory failure, other causes of respiratory failure during shock include aspiration and loss of neurologic control of breathing.

Effects on Acid-Base Balance

To function properly, cells depend on adequate circulation to receive nutrients, electrolytes, and oxygen and to remove waste products. Oxygen and nutrients are essential to life because they make possible complex chemical transformations resulting in the synthesis of adenosine triphosphate (ATP). ATP is the ultimate source of energy for life processes.

When oxygen is not present, ATP is produced through a different set of reactions called anaerobic metabolism. Production of ATP in this manner is a useful emergency measure. However, it is inefficient, compared with the normal process of aerobic (oxidative) metabolism. Anaerobic metabolism produces anaerobic metabolites, such as lactic acid (which causes intracellular acidity with consequent cellular damage) and substrates of the adenylic acid system (which depress the heart) (Fig. 22–4).

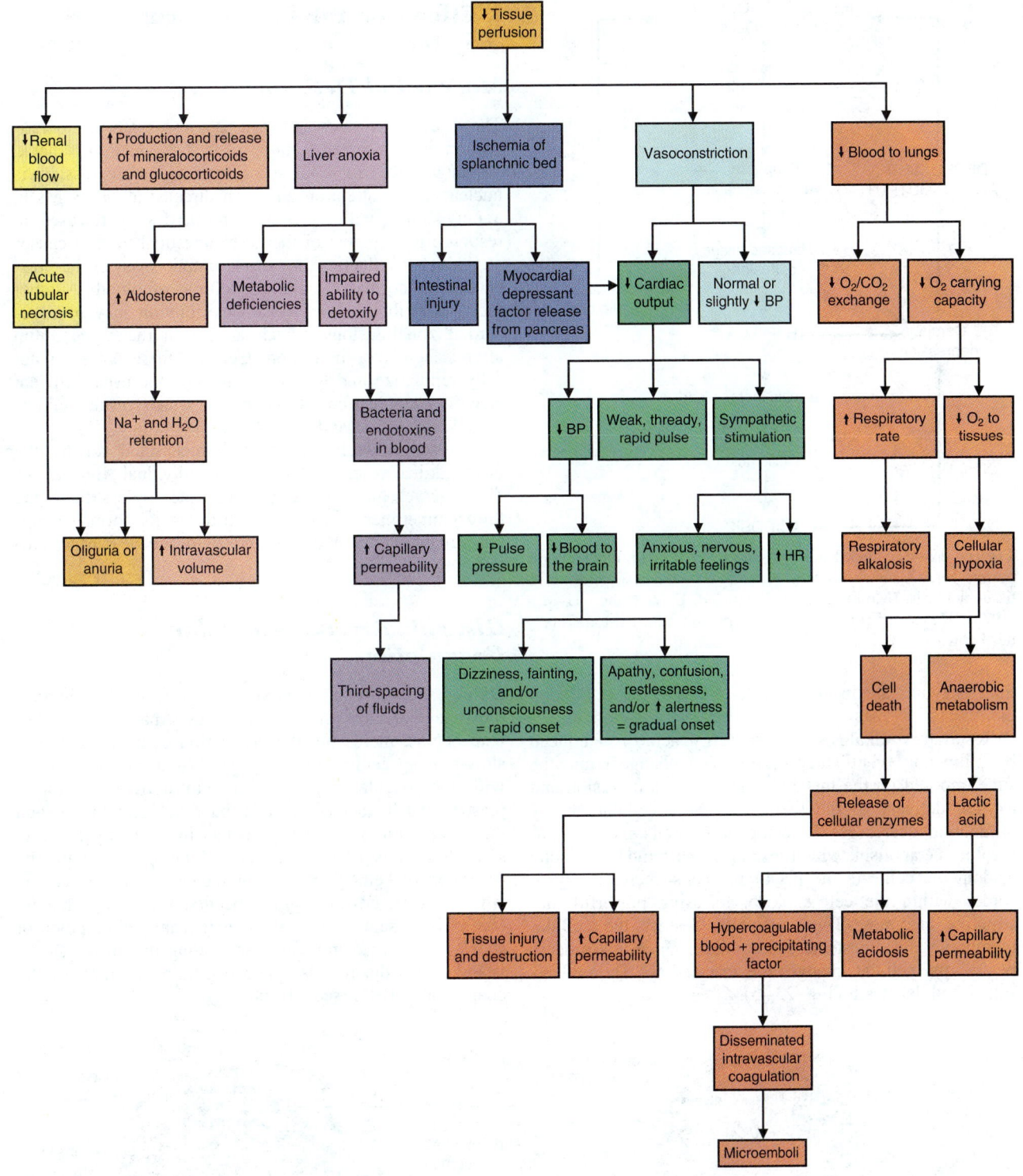

Figure 22–3. The systemic effects of shock.

In response to the chemoreceptors sensing decreased pH, the rate and depth of respirations are increased to blow off CO_2 in an attempt to compensate for the metabolic acidosis. This results in respiratory alkalosis. However, the cellular hypoxia is not caused by inadequate ventilation but by inadequate tissue perfusion. Therefore, the increased respiratory effort does little to correct the problem.

Because lactic acid is not exhaled, it accumulates in tissue fluids. This causes them to become increasingly acidic. Eventually, metabolic acidosis is produced. During metabolic acidosis, blood pH and bicarbonate fall. Pyruvate, lactate, phosphate, and sulfate rise. Unless circulation is restored, the acidotic reaction resulting from metabolic acidosis ultimately kills the cells. The buildup of lactic acid causes such a severe local acidosis that cel-

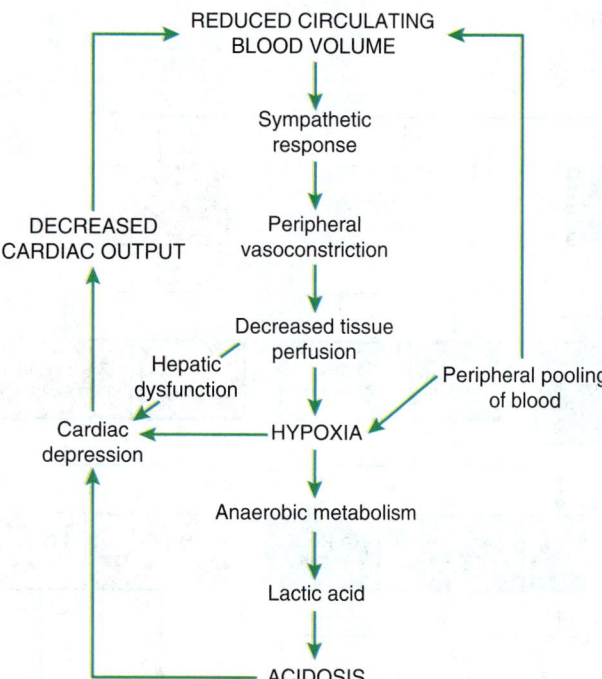

Figure 22–4. Shock leads to tissue hypoxia, with blockage of normal aerobic metabolism. Lactic acid accumulates, resulting in tissue acidosis. (Modified from Condon, R. E., & Nyhus, L. M. [1978]. *Manual of surgical therapeutics* (4th ed.). Boston: Little, Brown.)

lular enzymes are inactivated. As a result, the cells soon die.

Respiratory alkalosis or respiratory acidosis (induced by pulmonary ventilatory or diffusion changes) may be superimposed on the metabolic acidosis. As perfusion and oxygen delivery to the tissues decrease, cellular energy production decreases. To compensate, cells increase anaerobic metabolism, which results in the buildup of lactic acid in the cell. As the pH of the cells decreases, lysosomes within the cell explode, releasing powerful, destructive enzymes. These enzymes destroy the cellular membrane and digest the cell contents. Once this process begins, the cellular changes are irreversible. The end result is cellular death (Fig. 22–5).

■ Effects on the Cardiovascular System

Myocardial Deterioration

The heart deteriorates as shock progresses. Cardiac deterioration is one of the major causes of death in shock. Although the exact cause of myocardial depression is unclear, much attention has been directed at MDF. MDF, a polypeptide with vasoactive properties, is released in response to ischemia of the gastrointestinal tract. It causes a significant reduction in cardiac output, even in the presence of a normal circulating volume of blood. Another factor contributing to cardiac deterioration may be myocardial zonal lesions, which appear in the myocardium after ischemia or infarction. Cells in these areas do not fully repolarize and thus interfere with the usual efficient electrical conduction in the heart, which results in impaired contraction and possibly cardiac failure.

Cardiac depression is often compensated for by the large cardiac reserve of a normal individual. Because of this reserve, the heart can deteriorate to less than one third (sometimes less than one fifth) of its normal pumping strength without measurable evidence of cardiac failure.

Disseminated Intravascular Coagulation

During shock, tissue hypoxia results from the sluggish movement of blood in the capillaries. Anaerobic metabolism begins, increasing the production of lactic acid. The slow-moving acidic blood is hypercoagulable; however, it will not coagulate unless some clot-initiating factor is present. Such factors include bacterial endotoxins and thromboplastin of red blood cells (liberated by hemolysis). Hemolysis (destruction of red blood cells with the liberation of hemoglobin) accompanies trauma, especially when massive crushing injury occurs. When any of these factors is present, along with the stagnant, acidic blood of shock, widespread intravascular clotting may occur in the vessels. This disorder is called disseminated intravascular coagulation (DIC) (see Chapter 53).

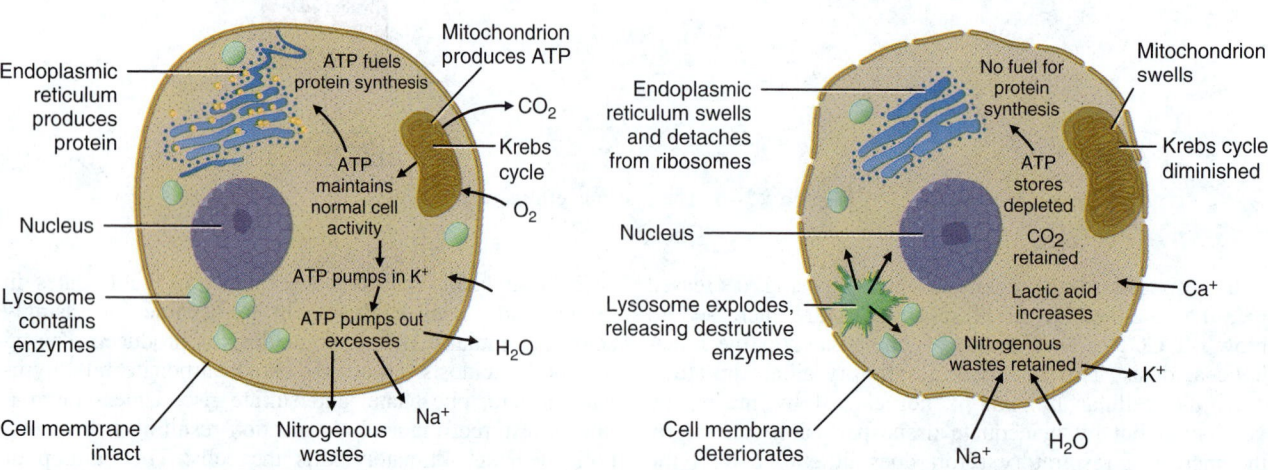

Figure 22–5. *Left,* Normal cell. *Right,* Alterations in cell function during late shock.

DIC is associated with multiple thrombi or emboli that are deposited in the microvascular circulation, with resultant organ obstruction and increased tissue ischemia. As blood attempts to flow through partially obstructed vessels, widespread hemolysis may occur. When red blood cells are destroyed, again hemoglobin is liberated. Anemia occurs because the liberated hemoglobin is excreted by the kidneys.

Because of the inappropriate clotting that occurs with DIC, the body attempts to reverse the process by breaking down clots. However, clots are destroyed throughout the body, not just the inappropriately formed clots. This results in bleeding in areas previously sealed by clots (i.e., venipuncture sites, vascular leaks in the brain).

As DIC progresses, clotting factors are depleted, causing an inability for normal clot formation in the presence of bleeding. Treatment of the precipitating cause, anticoagulant therapy, and replacement of clotting factors need to be started as soon as possible for maximal effectiveness. DIC is a serious complication and often is fatal.

Vasoconstriction

Sluggish circulation also results in decreased removal of CO_2 from the tissues. Increased CO_2 dilates arterioles located in active tissues and constricts those in nonactive tissues. Because of the heart's increased activity, excessive CO_2 is produced in the myocardium. This directly dilates the coronary arteries leading to the myocardium, which allows the myocardium to receive more arterial blood (with its oxygen and nutrients). CO_2 is also a powerful stimulant of the vasoconstrictor center in the sympathetic nervous system. With vasoconstriction of nonactive tissues, blood is shunted to the more active tissues, which have a greater immediate need.

Release of Lysosomal Enzymes

Lysosomal enzymes are released from dead cells undergoing autolysis. They are also released just before cell death produced by cellular anoxia or some other form of injury. For example, these enzymes may be liberated as a result of trauma and endotoxins. During shock, the disruption of lysosomes and the release of their enzymes seem to occur in the liver. This is one mechanism of cell destruction resulting from prolonged shock. The presence of hepatic lysosomal active enzymes in the bloodstream, along with blocking of the reticuloendothelial system (RES), may contribute to death from shock. Blockade of the RES drastically reduces its capacity to clear bacteria from the bloodstream.

Lysosomal enzymes become most active in an acid pH range. Thus, as long as normal acid-base balance is maintained within the body, these enzymes are repressed within normal cells. During shock, however, the accompanying metabolic acidosis accelerates the activation of these enzymes in hypoxic tissues.

The activation of lysosomal hydrolases within the cells and their release into the circulation markedly exacerbate the tissue injury that occurs during shock. The release of active lysosomal proteases and other enzymes from damaged tissue into the bloodstream and their action on extra-cellular and intracellular structures probably contribute to the progression of injury from cell to cell.

Vasoactive Substances. Vasoactive substances are highly variable in promoting vasoconstriction or vasodilation in a person experiencing shock. The influence they exert may be altered by factors such as pH, the specific tissue (e.g., heart, lung), the presence of drugs or other substances, serum electrolyte levels, and the sensitivity of the end organ.

Catecholamines. Catecholamines, such as epinephrine and norepinephrine, are present early in shock and are related to the fight-or-flight response. Their general effects are to increase blood flow to the brain, heart, and striated (skeletal) muscle and to decrease blood flow to the skin, kidneys, and splanchnic bed. Although the initial effect of vasoconstriction in the skin, kidneys, and splanchnic bed (GI tract) serves to increase the intravascular volume, sustained vasoconstriction contributes to stagnant hypoxia and cellular death.

Histamine. Histamine causes vasodilation, increased capillary permeability, bronchoconstriction, coronary vasodilation, and cutaneous reactions (flares, wheals). The effects of histamine are especially obvious in anaphylactic and septic shock.

Vasoactive Polypeptides. Bradykinin, angiotensin, and MDF are among the more important vasoactive polypeptides that appear to play significant roles in shock.

● Bradykinin (a kinin peptide) is known to produce vasodilation, increased capillary permeability, smooth muscle relaxation, pain, and infiltration of an area with leukocytes. Kinins appear to be most active in late shock. They may be a factor in the development of pulmonary insufficiency associated with shock.

● Angiotensin results from the action of renal renin on angiotensinogen. This potent substance causes vasoconstriction and increased vascular resistance. Although similar to norepinephrine in effect, angiotensin may have fewer negative effects. The role of angiotensin in sodium and water retention (through the stimulation of aldosterone secretion) is discussed under the sympathoadrenal response.

● MDF is a vasoactive polypeptide that contributes to cardiac failure in clients in shock by depressing cardiac muscle contraction.

■ Effects on the Neuroendocrine System

GAS Response

Neuroendocrine responses during shock are defensive reactions that occur during the body's stage of resistance in the general adaptation syndrome (GAS), discussed in Chapter 2. Recall that the length of the stage of resistance varies among persons and is determined by a body's ability to compensate for its deficiencies. Hence, one person may be able to combat shock longer than another. For example, a previously healthy person may have a longer stage of resistance against shock than will a client who is debilitated before shock develops.

Adrenal Response

Some basic features of the neuroendocrine responses are (1) the release of epinephrine and norepinephrine from the adrenal medulla, which results in increased respiratory and heart rates, increased BP, increased blood flow to organs, and decreased blood flow to peripheral tissues; and (2) the release of mineralocorticoids (which control fluid and electrolyte balance) and glucocorticoids (which affect energy and tissue resistance) from the adrenal cortex.

Increased production of adrenocortical mineralocorticoid hormones occurs. The main mineralocorticoids, aldosterone and desoxycorticosterone, help to increase intravascular fluid volume by stimulating the kidneys to retain sodium and hence water. The renal tubular conservation of sodium occurs with any type of fluid loss or blood volume depletion. Aldosterone is essential to conservation of sodium. Because water is retained in the body along with sodium, urine excretion is diminished during shock. This fluid is retained in the bloodstream in an effort to increase blood volume. Increasing the volume of blood in this way is aimed at increasing venous return, cardiac output, and BP.

Pituitary Response

Of major importance in regulating water and sodium balance are aldosterone and ADH, also called vasopressin. ADH is produced by the posterior pituitary gland. The blood's osmolality (osmotic concentration) increases with dehydration. This stimulates osmoreceptors in the hypothalamus to release ADH from the posterior pituitary gland. Via the blood, the ADH is carried to the kidneys. There it causes the body to retain water.

Various components of the sympathoadrenal (sympathetic part of the autonomic nervous system and adrenal medulla) response to a major stressor are shown in Figure 22–6.

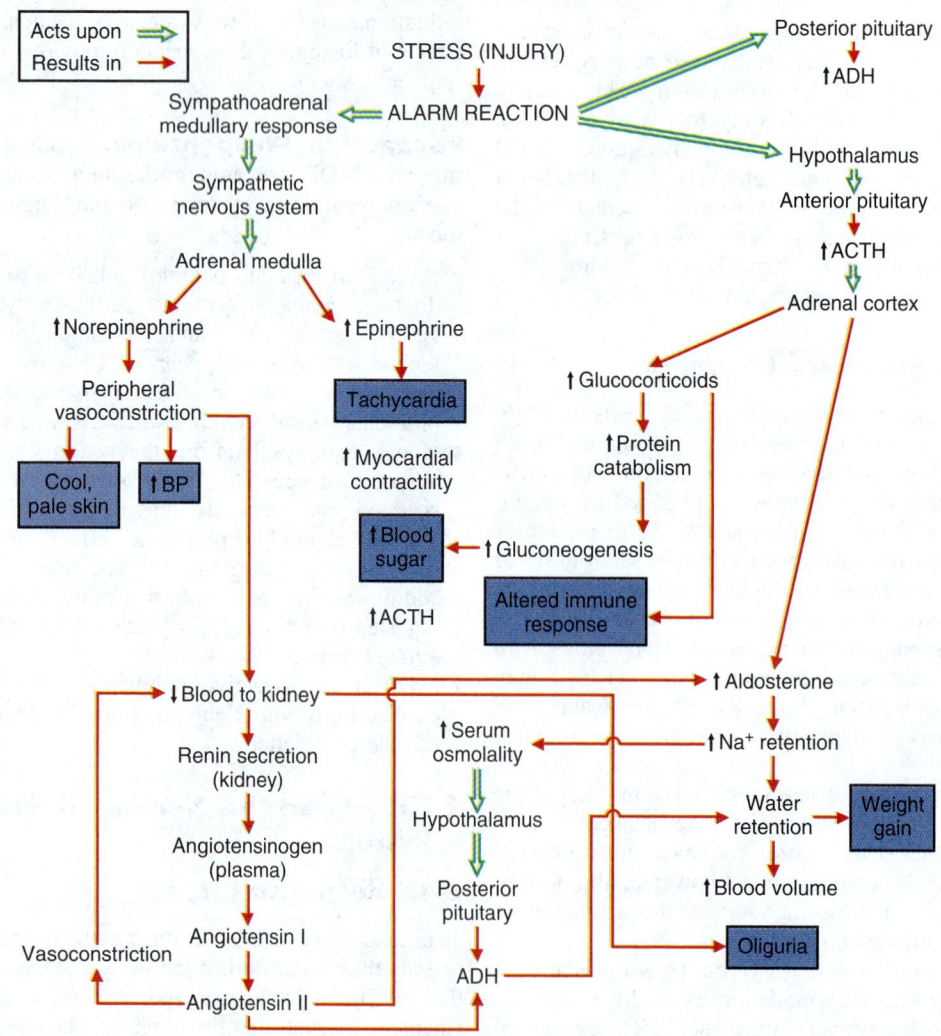

Figure 22–6. Components of the neuroendocrine response to a major stressor. Readily observed clinical signs as well as laboratory values are indicated by the boxes.

Metabolic Response

Generally, the hormonal response to stress rapidly provides fuel for the body's various tissues, organs, and systems. These fuels (e.g., amino acids, fatty acids and glucose) are produced by the breakdown of food. These substances are then chemically converted into energy, resulting in the formation of ATP. ATP is the main source of energy produced and used inside the body's cells.

The glucocorticoids, particularly hydrocortisone, mobilize energy stores. During the initial phase of shock, the body's small stores of available carbohydrate are rapidly depleted. It then becomes necessary to mobilize protein and fat stores to meet the body's energy requirements. Protein catabolism and negative nitrogen balance occur as part of the metabolic response, because of gluconeogenesis (resulting from glucocorticoid action) and starvation.

Neurologic Response

With shock, cerebral blood flow and, thereby, cerebral metabolism may become insufficient to maintain normal mental functioning and level of consciousness. Brain cells are highly sensitive to a shortage of oxygen and glucose and to fluid imbalances. When the brain becomes hypoxic, the cerebral vessels dilate to restore blood flow. Likewise, blood is diverted to the brain from the other, less vital organs.

■ Effects on the Immune System

All forms of shock severely depress macrophages, which are located in both the blood and tissues. (Macrophages used to be called the reticuloendothelial system [RES] because of their ability to exist in both blood and tissues.) The capacity of macrophages to remove bacteria and the constantly formed endotoxins from the bloodstream is greatly reduced. Alterations in the blood itself are partially due to tissue hypoxia and impairment of monitoring activities of the macrophage. The stasis, sludging, tendency for venular thrombosis, impaired capillary permeability, and subnormal vascular reactivity that occur during shock can all be traced to macrophage dysfunction.

The impaired ability of macrophages to ward off toxic agents is critical. Reduced blood flow through the intestines during shock extensively impairs the integrity of intestinal tissue. This results in the movement of normal gastrointestinal flora across the impaired intestinal tissue into the bloodstream, leading to a possible bacteremic state. The person in a state of shock is more susceptible than normal to bacterial products, particularly bacterial endotoxins, because of alterations in macrophage function.

■ Effects on the Gastrointestinal System

Under sympathetic stimulation, vagal stimulation to the GI tract slows or stops. This results in no peristalsis, a condition called ileus. A lack of nutrient blood supply to the intestines increases the risk of tissue necrosis and sepsis.

Gastrointestinal changes now appear to have a more important role in the progression of shock than was previously thought. The submucosa of the intestine becomes ischemic early in shock. If prolonged, actual tissue necrosis of intestinal mucosa occur. The intestinal arterioles and venules seem highly susceptible to the extensive vasoconstriction that occurs during shock. The massive amount of tissue destruction within the intestines that results from vasoconstriction and tissue anoxia is sufficient to cause death even if bacteria are not present. Bacteria and their toxins contribute to shock by escaping into the systemic circulation following destruction of the intestinal mucosa barrier.

As seen in the intestines, shock causes serious changes in the functions of the liver. The liver also suffers from this impaired circulation and appears to be a source of toxic materials.

The liver is the major detoxifying organ. Normally, the liver protectively traps and disposes of toxic materials (released from the bowel contents) that are products of bacterial enzyme actions. During shock, the anoxic liver develops metabolic deficiencies, an impaired ability to detoxify, and may release vasoactive substances. In addition, enhanced bacterial invasion of the liver from the intestine apparently occurs.

Finally, during shock, pooling of blood occurs in the viscera. Pooling of blood in the liver and portal bed may result from masses of agglutinated (clotted) blood plugging numerous small hepatic vessels, sinusoids, and intrahepatic radicles of the portal vein and hepatic artery.

■ Effects on the Renal System

The rate of urinary production reflects visceral blood flow and body fluid balance. Thus, urinary output indicates the status of circulation through the vital organs. Adequate urinary output indicates adequate circulation even if the arterial blood pressure is below normal.

Changes in Capillary Blood Pressure and Glomerular Filtration

Glomerular filtration within the kidneys depends on the pressure at which the blood is circulating through the glomerular capillaries. Usually, the average capillary pressure of blood is much higher in the kidneys' glomeruli than in other capillaries. Interestingly, under usual circumstances, the kidneys can maintain this heightened capillary pressure in the glomeruli in spite of changes in systemic BP. Afferent arterioles supplying the glomeruli dilate as the BP falls and constrict as it rises. However, eventually this adaptive mechanism cannot protect the kidneys against damage from a falling systemic BP.

During shock, when the blood volume and BP decline steadily, glomerular filtration is progressively reduced. This reduction in filtration leads to inability of the kidneys to excrete sodium and water. To compensate, the body excretes some sodium and water through the sweat glands. Damaged kidneys also lose their crucial ability to regulate electrolyte and acid-base balance.

Inadequate perfusion of renal capillaries is believed to be the cause of early renal failure in shock. The afferent and efferent arterioles constrict, shunting blood away from the glomeruli. Later, if shock persists, actual renal shutdown occurs from focal tubular necrosis. Unfortunately, vasoconstriction in the kidneys may continue for a prolonged period of time after the systemic BP is restored to normal levels.

Renal Ischemia

The kidneys may suffer from renal ischemia during shock because microcirculatory failure commonly develops in the abdominal organs. Because the kidneys have a high rate of metabolism, they are highly susceptible to injury of the tubule cells when the blood supply is deficient. When injury to the kidneys is extensive and renal failure ensues, acute tubular necrosis (ATN) occurs. With appropriate intervention, including careful fluid administration, the kidneys can heal. Normal kidney function returns after 10 to 14 days.

Clinical Manifestations and Diagnostic Findings

General Clinical Manifestations of Shock

Because the body is made up of many cells, which may function or malfunction at different stages of metabolic impairment, shock causes many diverse clinical manifestations. Subjective complaints are usually nonspecific and may not be particularly helpful to the clinician attempting to diagnose and treat the client in shock. The client may report feeling sick, weak, cold, hot, nauseated, dizzy, confused, frightened, thirsty, or short of breath. Observable and measurable manifestations (Fig. 22–7) are often con-

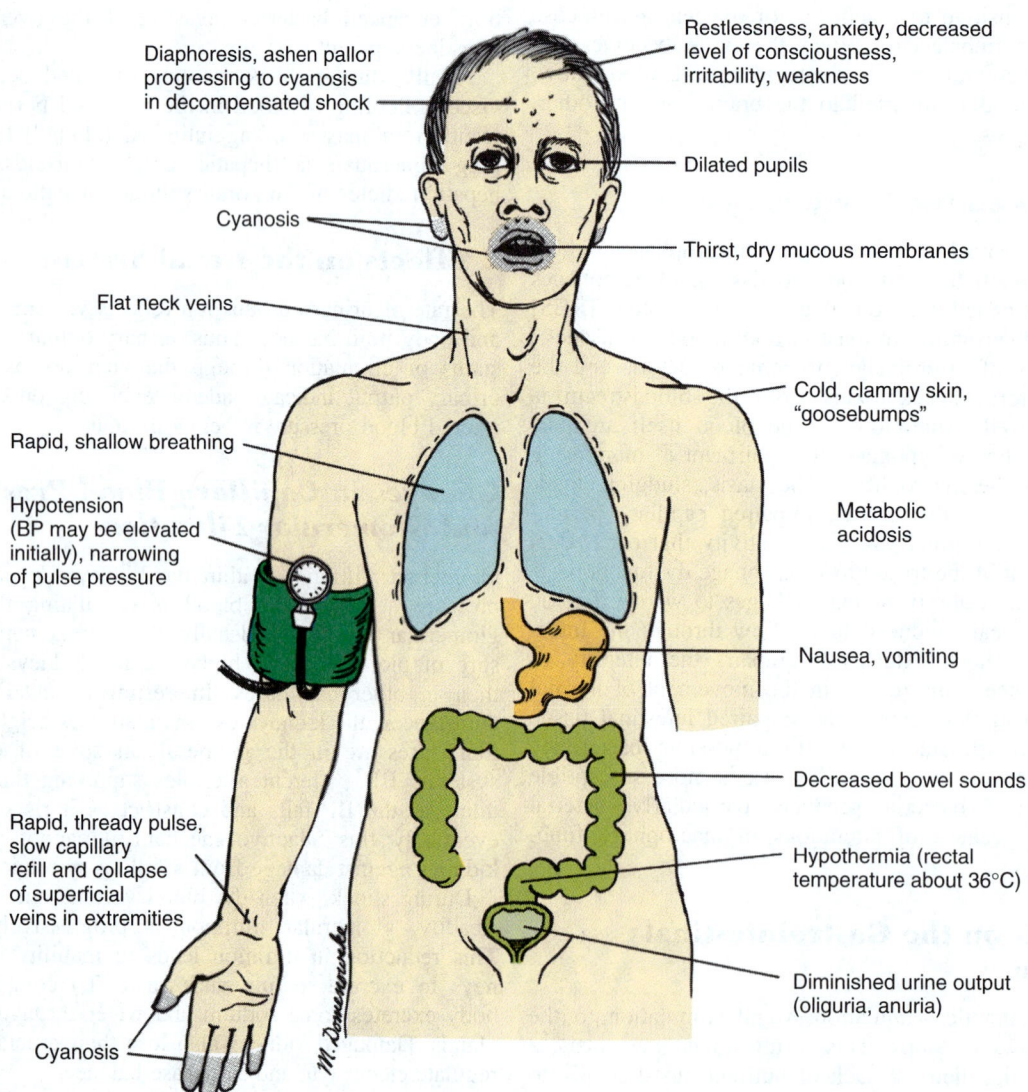

Diaphoresis, ashen pallor progressing to cyanosis in decompensated shock

Cyanosis

Flat neck veins

Rapid, shallow breathing

Hypotension (BP may be elevated initially), narrowing of pulse pressure

Rapid, thready pulse, slow capillary refill and collapse of superficial veins in extremities

Cyanosis

Restlessness, anxiety, decreased level of consciousness, irritability, weakness

Dilated pupils

Thirst, dry mucous membranes

Cold, clammy skin, "goosebumps"

Metabolic acidosis

Nausea, vomiting

Decreased bowel sounds

Hypothermia (rectal temperature about 36°C)

Diminished urine output (oliguria, anuria)

Figure 22–7. Clinical manifestations of the client with hypovolemic shock.

flicting. BP, cardiac output, and urinary output are usually—but not always—decreased. Respiratory rate is usually increased. Variable indicators of shock include alterations in heart rate, core body temperature, skin temperature, systemic vascular resistance, and skin color. Dyspnea, diaphoresis, and altered sensorium may be present. The following manifestations are usually present in persons with shock of any type.

■ Tachypnea

Rapid, shallow respirations (tachypnea) typically occur during shock because of decreased tissue perfusion. The respiratory rate increases as the blood's oxygen-carrying capacity decreases. These changes may signal the development of hypoxemia and respiratory alkalosis.

■ Tachycardia

Generally, the pulse rate increases (tachycardia) in shock from increased sympathetic stimulation. This occurs in an attempt to maintain adequate cardiac output when the blood's circulating volume is declining.

With increased rate, the pulse becomes typically weak and thready. At the onset of shock, the pulse rate does not relate as directly to the severity of shock as does BP. This is because in the early stage of shock, worry, excitement, and fear may influence the heart rate out of proportion to the underlying conditions. However, when emotional factors are no longer significant, serial observations of the pulse rate over a period of time are highly useful to (1) assess the client's condition and the direction of the shock state and (2) evaluate the effectiveness of intervention. Elderly clients (with and without various degrees of heart block) and clients taking beta blockers are exceptions to this. Their heart rates may show little change in spite of the presence of conditions causing circulatory failure (e.g., hemorrhage). The pulse rate may become extremely slow in the terminal stages of shock and is usually slow in neurogenic shock.

■ Hypotension

The systolic BP indicates the integrity of the heart, arteries, and arterioles. The diastolic BP indicates the peripheral resistance (peripheral vascular resistance [PVR] or vasoconstriction) of blood vessels. For example, an increasing diastolic BP indicates increasing peripheral blood vessel resistance. Conversely, a declining diastolic BP indicates decreasing peripheral resistance. When the diastolic BP falls significantly, vasoconstriction is being lost as a compensatory mechanism. When vasoconstriction is replaced by marked vasodilation, there is no resistance to blood flow, and an adequate BP is difficult to maintain.

Usually, the BP begins to fall when total blood volume is decreased by about 15% to 20%. However, some people lose as much as 25% of their total blood volume without having a fall in BP. This is especially true in young adults; therefore, in young adults, falling BP is a *very* late sign of shock.

Typically, as shock progresses, both the systolic and diastolic BPs drop—the systolic pressure dropping more

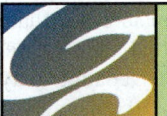

CRITICAL MONITORING

Worsening Shock

Systolic blood pressure decreased more than 20 mm Hg with heart rate increased more than 20 beats indicates actual or relative hypovolemia requiring immediate assessment of need for fluid replacement and support of cardiovascular status.
Decreased oxygen saturation or any signs and symptoms of respiratory distress require immediate intervention.

than the diastolic. The pulse pressure narrows because it is equal to the difference between the systolic and diastolic blood pressures.

During shock, the pulse pressure is actually more significant than the BP, because it tends to parallel cardiac stroke volume. The pulse pressure is affected by stroke volume (amount of blood ejected by the LV during contraction) and peripheral resistance. If stroke volume is decreased from a decreased circulating blood volume, pulse pressure decreases. In shock, pulse pressure may decrease even in the presence of an acceptable systolic BP. This may provide a clue to worsening of shock. In shock, pulse pressure is often less than 20 mm Hg. See Critical Monitoring.

In order to supply the myocardium with blood (i.e., maintain coronary circulation), a minimal systolic BP of 60 to 70 mm Hg is necessary. In interpreting BP readings, you need to know what the client's BP was previously. A systolic BP of 100 mm Hg or less is significant for clients whose systolic BP usually ranges from 110 to 140 mm Hg. When a client is in a supine position, a decline in BP may be a late finding. It is important to note that hypotension by itself (without other abnormal assessment findings) is not shock. Healthy clients often have BP readings lower than textbook normals.

Additional problems need to be considered in assessing BP and make it (particularly the systolic BP) an unreliable criterion for assessing the presence and severity of shock. In the early, compensated stages of shock, BP changes are generally unreliable because the arterial pressure may actually be normal or slightly elevated even though shock is present. In fact, blood volume deficits of a liter or more may occur even though arterial and venous pressures are normal or elevated.

When severe vasoconstriction is present, the BP may be normal even though the circulation is actually highly inadequate. Also, conversely, the blood flow may be adequate even though the BP is decreased (e.g., because of mechanisms such as vasodilation).

Valuable information about the level of arterial pressure in vasoconstricted clients can be gained by assessing the strength of the femoral pulses. It may also be appropriate to do a Doppler study (Chapter 49) to obtain an accurate peripheral blood pressure. With displaced or depleted blood volume, it is important to consider adequate venous filling. Hypovolemia, whether actual or relative, will cause superficial veins to flatten. This change may hamper attempts to insert intravenous (IV) catheters for fluid replacement.

■ Changes in Level of Consciousness

Early in shock, hyperactivity of the sympathetic nervous system with increased secretion of epinephrine usually causes the client to feel anxious, nervous, and irritable. Anxiety and worry are seen in the client's facial expressions.

Assessment findings associated with lack of blood to the brain are determined by the suddenness with which the shock develops and by its severity. With sudden, severe shock, the body may not have time to initiate its compensatory adjustment mechanisms. Consequently, the brain is deprived of its blood supply. The client may feel dizzy and faint on sitting up from a horizontal position because of postural hypotension. Fainting and unconsciousness may occur. If shock develops gradually over a period of hours, early assessment findings may include apathy and confusion or the opposite, restlessness and unusual alertness.

The systolic BP is important in maintaining blood flow to the brain. A cerebral perfusion pressure (CPP) of at least 50 mm Hg is required to deliver blood to the brain (CPP = MAP−ICP [intracranial pressure]). Usually, a decrease in systolic BP is accompanied by a reduced flow of blood to the brain. However, the brain's vessels, like those of the heart, are not constricted by the vasoconstrictor center in the medulla oblongata. Thus, blood from the peripheral vessels can be shifted to the brain as an emergency compensatory measure.

A client's level of consciousness decreases as circulation to brain tissue becomes increasingly impaired. Confusion, agitation, and restlessness may occur. In trauma situations, restlessness can be mistaken for pain. If narcotics are given, the client's situation may be worsened or it may be difficult to detect worsening hypoxia.

Drowsiness and stupor are more likely to occur in shock related to severe infection than in shock caused by trauma and hemorrhage. As compensatory mechanisms fail, apathy may ensue. Ultimately, a comatose condition may be reached.

■ Oliguria

A fall in urinary volume is often the earliest sign of developing shock. Recall that the kidneys are not organs of primary perfusion. A fall in urine volume may occur even while arterial BP and pulse remain stable. Urinary output is one of the most sensitive indices in shock. However, it should be kept in mind that any form of shock that develops very rapidly (e.g., due to trauma) shows other symptoms before decreased urinary output is noticed.

Urinary output should be kept above 0.5 ml/kg/hour (approximately 35 ml in an average 70-kg adult male). If the hourly output diminishes significantly, treatment must be instituted to prevent renal failure. Urinary flow of less than 20 ml/hour can cause ATN from inadequate renal circulation.

Clinical Manifestations of Specific Types of Shock

■ Clinical Manifestations of Hypovolemic Shock

Initially, urine osmolality and specific gravity increase because of sodium and water reabsorption, which attempts to support circulating volume. As altered tissue perfusion and the hypovolemic shock progress, urine osmolality and specific gravity decrease because of the kidneys' inability to reabsorb sodium and water.

Sympathetic nervous system stimulation of the skin leads to marked diaphoresis. Clients sweat profusely, increasing insensible fluid loss leading to further hypovolemia and temperature instability. Sympathetic stimulation also results in decreased tissue perfusion to the skin, causing the skin to feel cool and clammy and to appear pale; increased heart rate; and increased respiratory rate.

Cyanosis may indicate either decreased tissue perfusion or decreased oxygenation or both. Cyanosis is a late sign of decreased oxygenation.

■ Clinical Manifestations of Cardiogenic Shock

Because of the impaired muscle action or mechanical obstruction that caused the cardiogenic shock, blood is inadequately pumped through the heart. This results in a back-up of blood. When the shock is due to right-sided heart failure, this back-up will be evidenced as jugular venous distention and increased CVP. (See Chapters 42 and 45 for discussions of cardiac tamponade and tension pneumothorax.) When the shock is due to left-sided failure, blood backs up into the pulmonary circulation, resulting in pulmonary edema, crackles in the lungs, and increased pulmonary capillary wedge pressure (PCWP). As in hypovolemic shock, there is stimulation of the sympathetic nervous system due to decreased cardiac output and decreased BP. The sympathetic nervous system causes decreased tissue perfusion to the skin and all of its resultant clinical manifestations.

■ Clinical Manifestations of Distributive Shock

Clinical Manifestations of Anaphylactic Shock

Initially, the client may complain of a vague feeling of uneasiness or a feeling of impending doom. The massive vasodilation that occurs with anaphylaxis may cause complaints of headache as well. This may be followed by severe anxiety, dizziness, disorientation, and loss of consciousness.

Respiratory involvement may be manifested through a variety of symptoms. The initial complaint may be a feeling as though there were a lump in the throat. This is due to laryngeal edema and is followed by hoarseness, coughing, dyspnea, and stridor. Diffuse wheezes and prolonged expiratory phase are heard on auscultation. If a pulse oximeter is in use, there may be a rapid decline in oxygen saturation.

Additional complaints may include pruritus and urticaria. Direct observation may also demonstrate edema of the eyelids, lips, or tongue (angioedema).

Clinical Manifestations of Neurogenic Shock

In neurogenic shock, abnormal distribution of fluid volume occurs from interruption or loss of innervation. Exceptions to the usual clinical manifestations are bradycardia and hypotension (which cannot be corrected because of loss of ability of vasoconstriction). Below the level of injury, skin temperature takes on the same temperature as the room (poikilothermia). There is also an inability to sweat, so skin feels dry to the touch.

Clinical Manifestations of Septic Shock

In the early stages of septic shock, the body experiences massive vasodilation. Warm, dry, flushed skin is apparent during this hyperdynamic stage of septic shock. It is the compensatory increase in cardiac output and resultant increased perfusion of the skin that gives this stage the name "warm shock."

During later stages, when compensatory mechanisms fail, the release of MDF and decreased venous return result in decreased perfusion and "cold shock," or the hypodynamic stage. At this point, the skin becomes pale, cold, clammy, and mottled. Body temperature drops to subnormal levels. Auscultation of the lungs reveals crackles and wheezes, which develop secondary to pulmonary congestion as ARDS ensues. In addition to the clinical manifestations seen with shock in general, changes in the level of consciousness may include drowsiness and stupor progressing to coma.

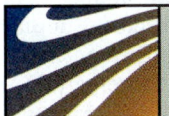

ETHICAL ISSUES IN NURSING

Is There a Moral Difference Between Withholding and Withdrawing Treatments?

Your patient Mr. Charles was in a severe automobile accident during the night. He sustained third-degree burns over 55% of his body and severe internal injuries including a ruptured spleen, torn colon, and lacerated liver. He has returned to your burn unit from surgery. He is intubated and on a ventilator, requires dopamine for blood pressure support, and even with the anesthesia out of his system, his Glasgow Coma Scale is category 5. Without ventilator assistance, he breathes on his own, but not as effectively.

Several weeks pass. Mr. Charles continues with a Glasgow Coma Scale of 5, remains on a ventilator, experiences multisystem organ failure, and continues on vasoactive drugs for blood pressure support. Since his wife has been named as a decision-maker for Mr. Charles on his durable power of attorney for healthcare, she has helped to direct his care. Mrs. Charles has been told by the physicians that Mr. Charles is dying from septic shock. Mrs. Charles wants to discontinue the ventilator and vasoactive drugs. You are concerned that this is unethical.

When caring for very sick clients, nurses sometimes feel very uncomfortable when treatments are withdrawn. If the treatments are life-sustaining, nurses may feel better about withholding treatments that were never started, but not about withdrawing treatments that have already been started.

Nurses may be more uncomfortable when life-sustaining treatments are withdrawn because they somehow feel responsible for a client's death. But they feel less responsible if the treatment is never started. While these feelings are important, they can sometimes lead to misunderstandings of proper treatment.

A treatment that can be withheld because it is of no benefit to the patient can also be withdrawn. This includes life-sustaining treatment. There is a need to balance benefits and burdens to the client to determine the appropriateness of a treatment. Whether the treatment has already been started or not is of no moral consequence. Sometimes it is necessary to start a life-sustaining treatment to give physicians enough time to make a sound medical diagnosis and prognosis so that the benefits and burdens to the client can be properly analyzed.

It is not uncommon to give a client a "trial run" of a specific treatment. Maybe it will help the client improve. If it does not, it can be withdrawn. The beginning of a new treatment should include periodic reevaluation of the diagnosis, prognosis, and the benefits and burdens of treatments to the client.

In this case, Mr. Charles is dying of septic shock. His infections have not responded to many courses of antimicrobial drugs. It is ethically permissible to withdraw the ventilator and the vasoactive drugs because they are prolonging the dying process. They are not going to cure the underlying disease processes.

Staying in touch with your feelings is essential to nursing. Feeling uncomfortable about withholding and withdrawing treatment is understandable. However, there is no moral difference between withdrawing and withholding treatment.

It is exceedingly important to remember that although treatments may be withdrawn, care for Mr. Charles is never withdrawn. And, in fact, when life-sustaining treatments are withdrawn, the nursing care needs of the client frequently increase.

▪ Diagnostic Assessment

Diagnostic assessments of clients in shock should include oxygenation, organ perfusion, and fluid balance. Assessment of respiratory status can be accomplished to some degree by noninvasive procedures. Spirometry measures tidal volume and minute volume. A pulse oximeter assesses arterial oxygen saturation through a fiberoptic probe placed on the client's skin (either on the pinna of the ear or on a finger). Oxygen saturation of arterial blood (SaO_2) is determined by the amount of light transmitted through the skin. Corneal oxygen sensors may also be used to assess arterial oxygen saturation. The pulse oximeter does not replace arterial blood gas (ABG) analysis, which provides information about partial pressure of arterial oxygen (PaO_2), $PaCO_2$, and pH. However, it may be valuable in determining when ABGs are needed.

The $PaCO_2$ is measured by ABG analysis to determine whether the metabolic acidosis that occurs with shock is being effectively combated by hyperventilation. A low $PaCO_2$, along with low pH and bicarbonate levels (metabolic acidosis), indicates that hyperventilation is trying to compensate. However, a rising $PaCO_2$ in the presence of a persistently low pH indicates that respiratory assistance is needed. It will also be important to monitor PaO_2 levels to determine whether the client is being adequately oxygenated. (See Critical Monitoring and Chapter 40 for discussion of therapeutic respiratory interventions.)

CVP measurement is one of the first invasive assessments made in the presence of shock. CVP is an important means of estimating fluid loss. A pulmonary artery or Swan-Ganz catheter may also be inserted to assist with assessments of fluid status, cardiac function, and tissue oxygen consumption.

Other noninvasive assessment and monitoring tools are the cardiac monitor and the 12-lead electrocardiogram (ECG). Laboratory studies include a complete blood count and blood chemistry. Other specific studies, such as blood and body fluid cultures, may be indicated for certain clients.

Emergency Care

▪ Medical Management

It is difficult to know when shock actually exists and when therapy should begin. Treatment should generally be instituted for shock whenever at least two of the following three conditions occur: (1) systolic BP of 80 mm Hg or less, (2) pulse pressure of 20 mm Hg or less, and (3) pulse rate of 120 or more. Pulse pressure is calculated by subtracting diastolic BP from systolic BP. Normally pulse pressure is between 30 and 50 mm Hg.

Methods for treating inadequate tissue perfusion vary according to the specific cause of a client's shock state. Thus, assessment and an accurate differential medical diagnosis, which establish the specific cause of the shock state, form the basis for treatment. The differential medical diagnosis is usually readily made unless the shock is in an advanced stage, in which several specific forms of shock may exist at the same time. Some forms of shock more easily recognized are hypovolemic shock due to extensive burns or trauma and cardiogenic shock with severe chest pain and acute MI. Septic shock is probably the most difficult shock state to diagnose because of its insidious onset and complex symptoms. The emphasis here is on maintaining adequate circulating volume with reference to additional treatments for shock. Remember that the overall goal in treating all forms of shock is to achieve optimal tissue perfusion and oxygenation. Therefore, many aspects of care are similar for all types of shock.

The therapeutic management of shock has changed markedly over recent years. Lowering the head, raising the feet, and administering potent vasoconstrictor drugs were once the foundation of treatment for a client in shock. Now, emphasis is placed on maintaining adequate circulating volume, positions that do not interfere with pulmonary ventilation, and the use of medications having both vasoconstrictor and vasodilator effects.

Interventions in the treatment of shock are being continuously updated. See, for example, the Nursing Research feature concerning fingerstick measurements of blood glucose. The informed nurse must keep up to date with changes. As with any care, recognize that intervention for shock is individualized and follow specific physician prescriptions or agency guidelines.

Maintaining Adequate Perfusion

The primary aim in treating shock is to increase tissue perfusion. Unless this is accomplished early, subsequent therapeutic measures are of no avail, and death can be anticipated. Of central importance in current shock intervention is establishing and maintaining an adequate circulating blood volume. In addition, other treatment adjuncts are necessary and are discussed in the following paragraphs. The adjuncts facilitate the distribution of blood to the body and enhance perfusion and oxygenation of the tissues with the circulating blood. Table 22-2 lists vasoactive medications commonly used to treat shock.

Vasoconstrictors. Vasoconstrictors elevate the systemic BP by constricting peripheral arterioles. Vasoconstrictor agents may be used briefly in shock if compensatory vasoconstriction is unable to maintain blood flow to vital organs. They may also be used to correct hypotension secondary to vasoconstrictor nerve paralysis, as in spinal anesthesia or conditions associated with massive vasodilation. However, vasoconstrictors should not be used exclusively but should be given concomitantly with IV fluids in an attempt to restore adequate circulation and perfusion.

Perfusion of vital organs with blood is impossible when systolic BP is below 50 mm Hg. Usually, the goal of using vasoconstrictors is to achieve and maintain a mean BP of 70 to 80 mm Hg. This maintains a BP level sufficient to perfuse tissues. Generally, attempts to increase the BP beyond this level are not advisable because vasoconstrictors increase the heart's oxygen demand and

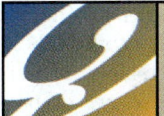

NURSING RESEARCH

Are Fingerstick Measurements of Blood Glucose Accurate in Clients with Decreased Peripheral Tissue Perfusion?

Sylvain, H.F., et al. (1995). Accuracy of finger-stick glucose values in shock patients. *American Journal of Critical Care, 4*(1), 44–48.

Clients in shock have decreased peripheral tissue perfusion due to the effects of norepinephrine. Because blood flow is reduced there is a concern that the accuracy of blood glucose assessment may be altered. Furthermore, if blood glucose assessment is not accurate, improper treatment could follow. The purpose of this study was to determine the accuracy of fingerstick blood glucose samples for clients in shock.

The sample consisted of 38 emergency room and intensive care clients determined to have inadequate tissue perfusion. Venous blood samples were drawn from clients. One drop of the venous sample was tested with the One Touch II glucose meter; the rest of the sample was sent to the hospital's chemistry laboratory for glucose analysis. Within 4 minutes of drawing the venous sample, a fingerstick sample was obtained and tested on the same One Touch II glucose meter. All three glucose values were recorded for statistical analysis.

Findings indicate that there was no difference in the mean values of the venous sample, whether tested on the One Touch or by the laboratory. However, there was a significant difference between the laboratory value and the fingerstick One Touch value, with the mean laboratory value significantly higher than the fingerstick One Touch value.

Implications for Practice

All clients were on sliding-scale insulin. In this study, all clients would have received less insulin based on the fingerstick glucose result than if doses had been based on laboratory values. These results indicate that patients in shock who require careful blood sugar control are inappropriate candidates for fingerstick blood glucose determinations.

may cause fatal dysrhythmias. Vasoconstrictors would be used with extreme caution in cardiogenic shock.

Major adverse effects of vasoconstrictors include the following:

● Increase myocardial oxygen consumption.
● Ventricular dysrhythmias.
● Decreased renal and splanchnic blood flow.
● Excessive or sudden rise in arterial BP, which may precipitate heart failure.
● Pulmonary edema or LV decompensation.
● Gangrene of the fingers and toes from prolonged vasoconstriction.

Although the use of vasoconstrictors during shock is being critically evaluated, they do favorably increase blood flow to the brain and heart in severely hypotensive clients. Reduced tissue perfusion when systolic pressures are below 60 to 70 mm Hg may precipitate MI or a cerebrovascular accident.

Vasodilators. Agents that induce vasodilation or inhibit vasoconstriction may promote recovery from shock in which intensive vasoconstriction is contributing to the problem. These include adrenergic blocking agents, ganglionic blocking agents, and direct-acting peripheral vasodilators.

Adrenergic blockade prevents harmful effects of prolonged vasoconstriction such as increased pressure in capillaries, promoting fluid loss from the vascular to the interstitial compartment, and altered blood flow, especially in the splanchnic area. Prolonged vasoconstriction also impairs cellular nutrition and allows accumulation of waste products. Not only does adrenergic blockade prevent these changes in circulation, it may also induce opposite beneficial changes.

Vasodilators may be helpful during shock when vasoconstriction is severe and persists even though fluids have been infused in what should be adequate amounts for fluid replacement. As discussed, during shock, peripheral blood vessels are fully constricted as a result of the large output of norepinephrine from sympathetic stimulation. Vasodilators may be administered to try to inhibit vasoconstriction so that blood can be redistributed. That is, blood trapped peripherally would become available to enhance tissue perfusion, and the vascular volume would increase.

When shock is caused by hypovolemia, rapid and adequate fluid replacement is essential before vasodilators are used. Vasodilators are dangerous because they lower arte-

Table 22–2. Vasoactive Medications Used in Shock Management	
Medication	**Action**
High-dosage dopamine (Intropin); norepinephrine (Levophed); phenylephrine (Neo-Synephrine)	Systemic vasoconstruction, especially in the gastrointestinal tract, skin, and kidney
Amrinone (Inocor); epinephrine (Adrenalin); dobutamine (Dobutrex); isoproterenol (Isuprel)	Increased heart rate, increased contractility
Amrinone; dobutamine; epinephrine; isoproterenol; nitroprusside (Nipride)	Vasodilation of blood vessels in heart and skeletal muscle
Low-dosage dopamine	Vasodilation of renal and mesenteric blood vessels
Amrinone; nitroglycerin (Tridil); nitroprusside	Relaxation of vascular smooth muscle

rial blood pressure if they are given while circulating blood volume is deficient. When the circulating blood volume is inadequate, the body depends on vasoconstriction to try to maintain arterial pressure. However, when the vascular space is full and cardiac venous return is adequate, vasodilation should open arterioles in the lungs and elsewhere. This lets blood circulate, increasing cardiac output and capillary perfusion without lowering systemic BP. In fact, a vasodilator may produce a dramatic, sustained rise in the systemic arterial pressure.

Keep clients who are receiving vasodilators lying relatively flat. Elevation of the head can produce dangerous orthostatic hypotension. Older clients may have sclerotic blood vessels and may not tolerate the hypotension that may accompany administration of vasodilators. In this situation, a cardiotonic drug (such as dobutamine) may be given with the vasodilator to increase cardiac output.

Vasoconstrictor medications are sometimes given in combination with vasodilator medications. This may be done to offset the profound effects that may occur with some vasoconstrictors. This may also be done to provide the benefits both types of drugs have to offer.

Characteristically, impaired tissue perfusion is correctable during early shock. However, it may be fatal if treatment is not received or is inadequate. In the later stages of shock, impaired tissue perfusion apparently becomes "irreversible," leading to death in spite of treatment. However, treatment for "irreversible" shock is never abandoned while the client remains alive. Before a client's shock state is viewed as probably irreversible, the following therapies must have been attempted:

- Restoration of circulating volume
- Identification and treatment of occult bleeding
- Identification and treatment of any factors interfering with cardiopulmonary functioning
- Identification and treatment of overwhelming infection

During shock intervention, all of the basic pathophysiologic changes associated with the development of shock must be corrected. Some problems that must often be treated are the vascular problem of vasoconstriction, with the diminished tissue perfusion it causes; the intravascular problem of coagulation and sludging of blood cells; and the extravascular problem of extravasation of fluid into the extravascular space.

Treatment modalities discussed in the following pages can be divided into two major categories: (1) those used to treat the shock state itself and (2) those used to prevent or treat complications of shock through early symptom intervention. Interventions discussed in the following sections and in Critical Monitoring include respiratory support, positioning, circulatory assist devices, IV fluid therapy, vasoactive and other medications, renal support, and gastrointestinal tract support.

Improving Oxygenation

Maintaining the client's airway is vital to the treatment of shock. In all types of shock, supplemental oxygen is administered to protect against hypoxemia. Oxygen can be delivered via nasal cannula, mask, high-flow nonrebreathing mask, endotracheal tube, or tracheostomy tube.

Endotracheal intubation, or tracheostomy, may be performed to rest an exhausted client during severe or prolonged shock and to correct respiratory failure. By increasing the rate of pulmonary ventilation (through spontaneous or mechanical hyperventilation), it is possible to compensate for minor degrees of metabolic acidosis. This increased "blowing off" of carbon with hyperventilation begins to compensate for acid-base imbalance. Positive end-expiratory pressure (PEEP) may be added when the client is being mechanically ventilated. This assists in preventing atelectasis and may provide a higher PaO_2 for the client at a lower oxygen concentration setting. The goal of therapy is to maintain a PaO_2 greater than 50 mm Hg and SaO_2 greater than 90% to avoid anaerobic metabolism. If the chest is congested, chest physical therapy, including vibration, percussion, and postural drainage, may be required.

Sometimes the interventions discussed cannot establish optimal tissue oxygenation. In these instances, hyperbaric oxygenation (HBO) or extracorporeal membrane oxygenation may be used. HBO involves the administration of 100% oxygen under 2 to 3 atm of pressure. This raises tissue oxygen tension to normal or above-normal levels. HBO requires the use of special chambers, which usually are available only in highly specialized institutions (see Chapter 20).

Extracorporeal membrane oxygenation is most commonly used in adults as a temporary intervention for refractory ARDS. Arterial and venous catheters are inserted, and some of the client's blood is diverted through them into a machine that artificially oxygenates the blood. This is a relatively expensive form of therapy and is usually done only in large medical centers.

Assisting Circulation

Mechanical devices that assist circulation or decrease the heart's workload may be used as temporary measures in managing clients in shock. Examples of these include the military or medical antishock trousers (MAST), intra-aortic balloon pump, and external counterpulsation device. (See Chapter 45 for more information.)

MAST Garment. MAST, also called pneumatic antishock garment (Fig. 22–8), encases the lower part of the body in a one-piece, three-chambered (two leg chambers and one abdominal chamber) suit from the lower costal margin to the ankles. The external pressure provided by the MAST garment causes increased vascular resistance and reduces the diameter of the blood vessels in the abdomen and legs. This results in impedance of blood flow and may decrease leakage into the tissues, resulting in increased perfusion of vital organs. Cardiac output increases, and arterial BP improves.

MAST garments are most often used in trauma situations occurring outside the hospital setting for management of massive blood loss with no obtainable BP, fluid loss other than hemorrhage, and cardiac arrest due to severe fluid or blood loss. Also, they help further reduce bleeding in areas being compressed, immobilize fractures

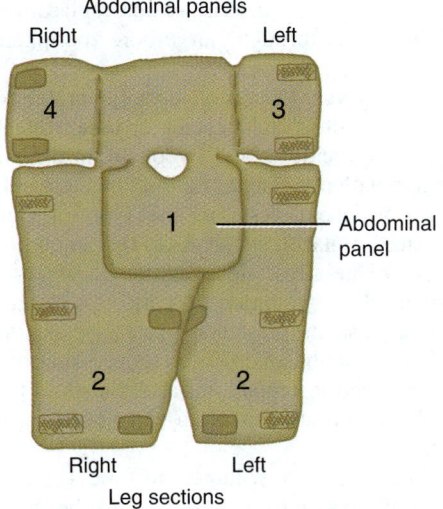

Abdominal panels
Right   Left

Abdominal panel

Right   Left
Leg sections

A MAST suit

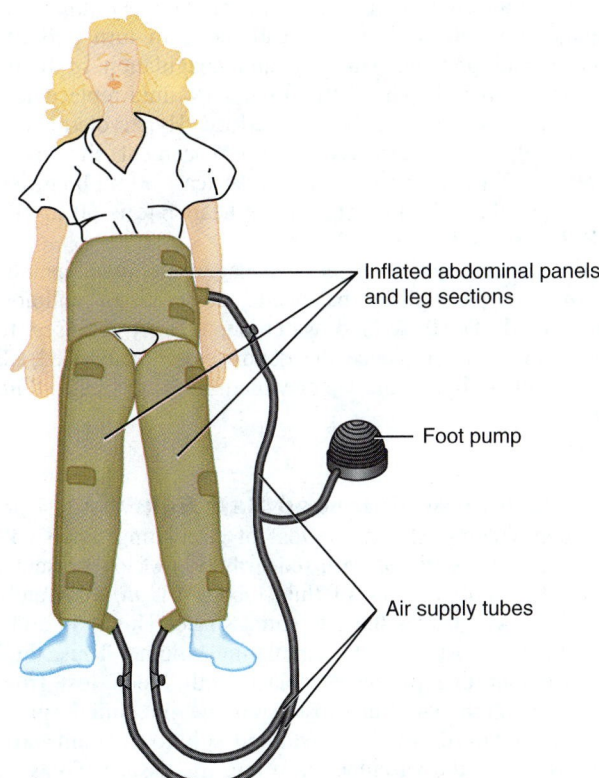

Inflated abdominal panels and leg sections

Foot pump

Air supply tubes

B MAST suit applied to client

Figure 22–8. MAST suit, or pneumatic antishock garment. *A,* The suit is composed of two leg compartments and an abdominal compartment. *B,* The MAST suit in place. Abdominal and leg compartments are attached to air tubes and a foot pump for inflation.

of the femur and pelvis, and facilitate insertion of the IV line by increasing upper extremity cardiac output and vein filling. The use of MAST garments continues to be controversial because the decreased perfusion in the lower extremities leads to acidosis in the compressed tissues. MAST garments may be contraindicated in cardiogenic shock.

Intra-aortic Balloon Pump. An intra-aortic balloon pump (IABP) is used primarily in clients with cardiogenic shock and after open heart surgery. The heart's ability to pump blood adequately is augmented by a balloon-tipped catheter placed in the descending thoracic aorta. The catheter is attached to a unit that inflates during diastole and deflates just before systole. This counterpulsation displaces blood back into the aorta and improves coronary artery circulation. In cardiogenic shock, use of the IABP reduces preload, allowing the heart to more efficiently empty, thereby increasing cardiac output. Details of the IABP are found in the Bridge to Critical Care feature on IABP in Chapter 45.

External Counterpulsation Device. This device uses the same general principles as an IABP but is applied externally to the legs. The legs are encased in air- or water-filled tubular bags connected to a pumping unit. Pressure is applied to the legs during diastole and is released in systole.

Modified Trendelenburg's Position. A client in shock is usually positioned in a modified Trendelenburg's position with the lower extremities elevated 30 to 45 degrees, knees straight, trunk horizontal or very slightly raised, and the neck comfortably positioned with the head level with the chest or slightly higher (Fig. 22–9). This position promotes increased venous return from the lower extremities without compressing the abdominal organs against the diaphragm.

Elevating the legs mobilizes blood that has pooled in the lower extremities. As a result of gravity, the additional circulating blood increases venous return to the heart, thus improving cardiac output. The position is of temporary value in moderate hypovolemia. However, it does not help in severe hypovolemia, because the extremities have very little blood in them in such a state. Generally, the modified shock position is not used with cardiogenic shock, when there is already circulatory overload.

As discussed in Nursing Research, Trendelenburg's position (head down, with legs elevated at least 30 degrees

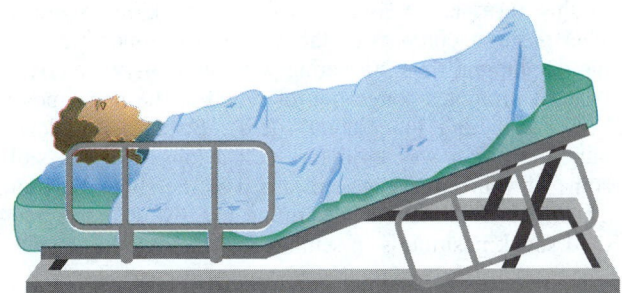

Figure 22–9. Positioning of the person in shock. This position is a modification of Trendelenburg's position and includes elevating the legs, leaving the trunk flat, and elevating the head and shoulders slightly.

NURSING RESEARCH

Does the Modified Trendelenburg's Position Improve Cardiac Output and Blood Pressure?

Ostrow, C. L., Hupp, E., & Topjian, D. (1994). The effect of Trendelenburg and modified Trendelenburg positions on cardiac output, blood pressure, and oxygenation: A preliminary study. *American Journal of Critical Care, 3*(5), 382–386.

Trendelenburg's position was used for many years to raise blood pressure by increasing venous return. A problem with placing clients in Trendelenburg's position was decreased lung capacity because of the shift of gastrointestinal contents by gravity toward the chest. The modified Trendelenburg's position was introduced to provide ample venous return and not reduce lung capacity. But did this modified position cause the desired changes in cardiac output and blood pressure?

The purpose of this research was to study the effects of the Trendelenburg's and modified Trendelenburg's positions on five dependent variables, cardiac output, cardiac index, mean arterial pressure, systemic vascular resistance, and oxygenation, in critically ill normovolemic and normotensive clients following cardiac surgery. Baseline measurements were taken in the supine position. Clients were then randomly assigned to one of the experimental positions.

In the 18 clients who completed the study, no statistically significant differences were found in the five dependent variables.

Implications for Practice

This research indicates that, in normovolemic and normotensive clients, the modified Trendelenburg's position (legs raised 30 degrees) is as effective as Trendelenburg's position for increasing cardiac output and blood pressure.

above the head) was once the classic shock position, but in this form is no longer used for shock management. This position compresses the abdominal contents against the diaphragm, thus interfering with pulmonary excursion. Also, it promotes congestion of blood in the brain, possibly contributing to cerebral edema. Because Trendelenburg's position was used for such a long time, possibly some of your colleagues still use it as the shock position. Thus, it is important to determine exactly what the standard shock position is in settings in which you practice.

Replacing Fluid Volume

The mainstay of hypovolemic shock therapy is expansion of circulating blood volume by IV administration of blood or other appropriate fluids. Fluid replacement should be administered through large-bore peripheral lines, central venous lines, or both.

Various fluids are given to correct specific problems, such as electrolyte or protein deficiencies or other defects of the blood, including acidosis and hyponatremia. However, in treating hypovolemic shock, the immediate results of therapy seem to depend less on the type of fluid administered for fluid replacement than on the amount of fluid administered. Generally, enough fluid is given to exceed the normal blood volume. In part, this "extra" fluid is required because the vascular space is expanded as a result of dilation of the microcirculation. Additional fluid is also administered to replace intracellular fluid that was mobilized into the circulation as an early response to the hypovolemia.

In replacing fluids, enough volume must be administered to fill the capillaries and run through into the veins. Such fluid replacement maintains CVP and provides an adequate venous return to the heart. This promotes additional cardiac output. In addition, adequate fluid replacement decreases the blood catecholamine level and thus produces a vasodilation that promotes capillary flow. Adequate flow of fluids in the capillaries in turn perfuses tissues and prevents sludging and coagulation of blood within the vessels. Carefully monitor IV fluid replacement therapy to prevent circulatory overload. Hypervolemia can be lethal, thus aggressive fluid replacement should be tapered off when urinary output is at least 60 ml/hour, BP is greater than 100 mm Hg, or the heart rate is 60 to 100 BPM.

IV fluids used in shock management may include warmed crystalloids or balanced salt solutions, colloids, and blood. Dextrose and water should not be used to resuscitate a client; once the dextrose is metabolized, all that is left is hypotonic water which leads to greater fluid shifts.

Crystalloid or Balanced Salt Solutions. During hypovolemic shock, the loss of circulating blood volume is also associated with redistribution of extravascular fluid. A sizable amount of fluid (about 4 L in moderately severe shock) leaves the interstitial space. This is in addition to fluid lost from the circulating volume. Thus, fluid replacement therapy must replace both blood lost from the circulation and fluid lost from the interstitial space. About two thirds of the crystalloid solution administered moves out of the vascular space into the tissues. To assist with fluid administration, a 3 : 1 rule has been developed. For a client's estimated blood loss, three times as much crystalloid solution must be administered for adequate volume resuscitation. Crystalloid solutions that may be administered include normal saline, Ringer's lactate, or half-normal saline.

Electrolyte solutions such as Ringer's lactate or saline buffered with bicarbonate help expand extracellular volume, reduce viscosity, and prevent sludging. In a client with impaired liver function, a solution containing lactate could further compound the problem of lactic acidosis since lactate is converted to bicarbonate by the liver. If the liver is functioning normally, lactate does not accumulate. Since the liver is not an organ of primary perfusion during times of stress for the body, other solutions should be considered before Ringer's lactate.

Abnormalities of electrolyte and acid-base balance are corrected with the specific substance needed rather than with a solution that administers multiple electrolytes and acid-base components. Therapy is gauged by serial ABG and electrolyte determinations.

Colloid Solutions. Colloid solutions contain proteins too large to exit normally at the capillary, thus they remain in the vascular compartment and increase osmotic pressure of the capillaries. This increased osmotic pressure helps retain fluid in the vascular compartment and maintain circulating volume. These solutions may be used in conjunction with crystalloid solutions in treating hypovolemic shock in an attempt to maintain an adequate circulating volume. The most commonly used colloid solutions include plasma and its components, plasma substitutes (e.g., dextran), oxygen-carrying solutions other than blood (e.g., perfluorochemicals), and hetastarch. (See discussions of blood and blood transfusions, Chapter 53.) Colloid solutions are often not used in initial fluid resuscitation after major burn injury. The capillary leakage is large enough that even the proteins escape.

Plasma is sometimes used in treating clients with low serum protein levels in an effort to control fluid escape from the vascular system. Fresh frozen plasma (FFP) is the form commonly used to improve serum protein levels. FFP may be administered after massive transfusions to restore some clotting factors deficient in "banked" blood. FFP requires 15 to 30 minutes to thaw. Hence, it is not used in initial fluid resuscitation with shock.

Albumin may also be used to achieve adequate osmotic pressure. Occasionally, it is administered when sufficient amounts of other fluids fail to restore an adequate circulating volume. Use of albumin is controversial because it may move into the pulmonary interstitial space, drawing water along with it. Thus, albumin may contribute to the development of ARDS.

Dextran may be used in both high- and low-molecular-weight forms. By initiating therapy with low-molecular-weight dextran and then progressing to high-molecular-weight forms, the incidence of hypersensitivity reactions to dextran can be lowered. The advantage in using dextran is that it contains large-sized molecules that should effectively and rapidly expand the intravascular volume. Dextran can interfere with blood type and crossmatch procedures and with clotting factors. It should therefore be used only after type and crossmatch have been done and until blood is available for transfusion.

Although the administration of crystalloids, albumin, and blood has been the standard treatment of hypovolemic shock for many years, several new substances have recently been introduced for shock management. Perfluorochemicals such as Fluosol are non-blood, oxygen-carrying solutions that remain in the circulation for about 12 to 24 hours. Major limitations associated with the use of perfluorochemicals relate to limited immediate availability (the product must be stored frozen), administration of 80% to 100% O_2 for the solution to be effective, and accumulation of the chemicals in the body. Advantages include the high solubility of Fluosol, making it readily available to the tissues, and its acceptability to clients whose religious beliefs prohibit the use of blood products. Perfluorochemicals have been researched since the 1970s and are still considered experimental at this time. Hetastarch is a glycogen-like synthetic colloid that has been used to treat hypovolemic shock and also may provide alternatives to blood administration.

Blood. When hemorrhage is the primary cause of shock, the rapid administration of large volumes of packed cells or whole blood may be necessary. Type-specific, crossmatched blood is the most desirable form of blood replacement. However, if the client is hemorrhaging, it may be necessary to administer type-specific, uncrossmatched blood: O-negative blood or O-positive, low–antibody titer blood. Women should receive Rh-negative blood.

When shock resulting from hemorrhage is treated, crystalloid is usually given as an initial emergency treatment to sustain blood pressure. Later, the acute anemia resulting from the hemorrhage must be corrected by administration of packed cells for prevention of hypoxemia.

During fluid replacement, a normal red blood cell mass should be maintained. Fluids given in excess of normal volume should be fluids other than blood so that they can be easily removed from the circulation by the kidneys once the shock is corrected. If the normal red blood cell mass is exceeded, it is difficult for the body to get rid of the excess red blood cells after the vascular volume contracts to normal (after adequate perfusion of tissues with blood is achieved). Also, because dangers are involved in blood transfusions, blood should not be used if another fluid can satisfactorily maintain an adequate oxygen-carrying capacity and can sufficiently increase blood volume. Clients can become so dilute that there are relatively few blood cells as the result of up to 8 to 12 L of fluid being administered in only a few hours.

Providing Autotransfusion

Autotransfusion involves collecting and retransfusing blood into the same client. Autotransfusion is used in the prevention or treatment of existing hypovolemic shock caused by hemorrhage. It is common in the treatment of chest injuries.

Evaluating Fluid Replacement

Often, fluid replacement is the only treatment required for shock. However, it is difficult to evaluate whether fluid replacement is adequate. Internal losses of circulating fluid volume, including whole blood, into areas of traumatized tissue, infection, and so forth are difficult to estimate. If a vasoconstrictor drug has been administered or if prolonged vasoconstriction occurs, an additional considerable loss of circulating volume may also occur because of vasoconstriction. Large volumes of IV fluid may be administered either until systemic BP, urinary volume, and lactate levels become relatively normal or until central venous or pulmonary artery pressures, or both, become elevated.

Infusion of blood or other fluids usually continues only as long as the CVP is low, that is, below 4 cm H_2O or 2 mm Hg. When the CVP is higher than normal (e.g., above 15 cm H_2O or 11 mm Hg), benefit cannot be expected from the continued infusion of fluids or blood beyond maintenance amounts. When the CVP is low and the lungs are clear, with no indications of congestive heart failure, fluids are administered to improve the return of blood to the heart. However, some clients have a normal or low CVP in spite of faulty LV function. They readily develop congestive failure or pulmonary edema. Thus, a low or normal CVP does not always mean that fluid administration is advisable.

IV fluid administration should be stopped before extremely high elevations of pulmonary artery pressure occur if there is an adequate systemic response. Adequate volume of circulating fluid causes an ample venous return to the right side of the heart and increases the right-sided output. Pulmonary artery hypertension may develop if continued pulmonary obstruction is present because of coagulation in the microcirculation or vasoconstriction. This appears as increased pulmonary artery pressure. In the presence of right-sided heart failure, this increased pressure may back up through the right side of the heart, causing an abnormal elevation in CVP. Vasodilators may help open this partially blocked pulmonary microcirculation.

Providing Pharmacologic Management

Antibiotics. Antibiotics are essential when shock is due to infection. If septic shock is suspected, a blood specimen for culture and sensitivity is taken at once, and broad-spectrum antibiotics are started even though the specific infectious organism has not yet been identified. When the blood sample is drawn, samples of urine, sputum, and fluid from draining wounds, sinuses, and so forth are also taken for culture. The antibiotic selected depends on the cause of the infection and should not be initiated until after all cultures have been taken. However, once cultures have been obtained, treatment with empiric broad-spectrum antibiotics should be initiated. Cephalosporins, gentamicin, and aminoglycosides may be used in combination until specific culture and sensitivity information is available.

Antibiotics may be administered along with appropriate surgical management to clients with open or potentially contaminated wounds who are experiencing hypovolemic shock. Common antibiotics include third-generation cephalosporins and aminoglycosides.

Monoclonal Antibodies. A new treatment for gram-negative septic shock is the use of monoclonal antibodies. These agents neutralize the endotoxin or toxicity of the offending pathogen or the immune response itself. Two antiendotoxins being researched are HA-1A and E5.

Heparin. The anticoagulant effect of heparin may help prevent complications or treat DIC. The dosage is usually adjusted according to clotting studies. Heparin is also used because of the prolonged immobility often associated with shock. Immobility predisposes to venous thrombosis and pulmonary emboli. The treatment of DIC may include heparin administration to minimize consumption of clotting factors. Also, heparin may be appropriate for clients with ARDS if the primary cause of the respiratory insufficiency is believed to be from DIC or massive microembolism.

Steroids. Steroids have several effects that may assist the client in neurogenic shock after spinal cord injury. They are given to reduce edema in the cord and have been shown to improve recovery. They assist in treatment by stabilizing lysosomal membrane and preventing intracellular release of enzymes. Complications from high-dose steroid therapy include acute gastrointestinal bleeding; aggravation of diabetes; and immunosuppression. Steroids used to be given for treatment of septic shock, but this practice was not shown to reduce mortality and therefore was abandoned.

Naloxone. Naloxone (Narcan), an opiate antagonist, is commonly used to treat narcotic and synthetic narcotic overdosages. During stress, opiate-like substances known as enkephalins and endorphins are released from the brain. Although the mechanisms of action are not clear, endorphins may play a role in capillary bed vasodilation found in all forms of shock. Studies indicate that when naloxone is administered to animals not in shock, no significant cardiovascular effects are noted. However, when administered during shock, naloxone reverses the hypotension and decreases cardiac contractility. It is believed that naloxone blocks the effects of endorphins and enkephalins.

Epinephrine. Epinephrine is the drug of choice for emergency treatment of allergic reactions (anaphylaxis). Epinephrine inhibits histamine release and antagonizes its effects on end organs, resulting in reversal of the bronchial constriction, increased capillary permeability, and vasodilation, which occur with acute anaphylactic reactions. The overall effect is improved respiratory status and cardiovascular stability.

Diphenhydramine Hydrochloride. Anaphylaxis can also be treated with antihistamines, like diphenhydramine hydrochloride (Benadryl). This medication acts primarily to relieve clinical manifestations associated with anaphylaxis rather than to stop the release of histamine. Therefore, epinephrine is always administered first in treating anaphylaxis.

Histamine H_2-Receptor Antagonists. Cimetidine, famotidine, and ranitidine are histamine H_2-receptor antagonists, which inhibit gastric acid secretion. Any of them may be administered to a client experiencing shock to prevent stress ulcers, which are often lethal complications of severe illness or injury produced by continuous shunting of blood from the gastrointestinal tract from extended sympathetic nervous system stimulation. They are commonly given IV to the client in shock and may be prescribed in combination with oral antacids.

Narcotics. The need for pain relief may be obvious in clients experiencing different types of shock. However, the use of narcotics for pain management may, unfortunately, be dangerous. Narcotics interfere with vasoconstriction, and vasoconstriction may be the mechanism by which the client's BP is maintained. Morphine sulfate, however, causes pooling of blood in the extremities and contributes to a decrease in anxiety. These effects may prove useful for the client in cardiogenic shock.

Cardiotonic Medications. Medications that improve myocardial contraction are basic in treating those forms of shock that decrease cardiac output (e.g., hypovolemic shock and cardiogenic shock).

- Digitalis is often used if there is evidence of cardiac failure. By strengthening and slowing the heart beat, digitalis supports a weakened heart and may reduce the heart rate to a more normal level.
- Lidocaine, bretyllium, quinidine, and procainamide may treat dysrhythmias that tend to reduce cardiac efficiency. However, these medications reduce myocardial contractility.
- Atropine may treat bradycardia, which predisposes clients to cardiogenic shock.

Calcium. Calcium is needed for normal functioning of the nervous and cardiovascular systems and for blood clotting. The value and dosages of calcium in treating shock are not clear. However, calcium may be administered if impaired cardiac function is evident. Calcium may precipitate toxic effects in a person who has received digitalis. It is given only with extreme caution to such a person. Monitor for evidence of digitalis toxicity (e.g., bradyarrhythmias or tachyarrhythmias, ST segment depression).

Calcium chloride should be given IV only. Calcium gluconate may be given intramuscularly, but is very irritating to tissues. Whereas calcium chloride and calcium gluconate are both available as 10% solutions, they are not identical in concentration. Do not substitute one for the other. Indications of hypocalcemia may be subtle. Careful assessment is essential. (See discussions of calcium in Chapter 15.)

Monitoring Urinary Output

Impaired kidney function and ATN may result from inadequate renal tissue perfusion, as discussed earlier. In an attempt to prevent acute renal damage, the urinary output is monitored with an indwelling catheter, and diuretics (e.g., furosemide) may be given. Correcting metabolic acidosis (see Chapter 15) and using other measures to increase blood volume and improve cardiac output also benefit the kidney as well as other tissues. If tubular necrosis is present, peritoneal dialysis or hemodialysis

may be needed until regeneration of functioning renal tubular epithelium occurs. (See also Chapter 57.)

During shock, urinary output should be measured and compared with normal urinary production. The normal rate of urinary excretion from the kidneys is 1 ml/minute or 60 ml/hour. A client who becomes acutely hypovolemic or is experiencing a redistribution of circulating volume cannot maintain an hourly output of 40 to 60 ml of urine. Decreased urinary output (oliguria) typically occurs in shock. Often during shock, the urinary output may stop completely (anuria). When this occurs, the client is said to be in renal shutdown or renal failure.

Oliguria does not contraindicate the administration of large volumes of fluid in the treatment of shock. In fact, restoring renal capillary perfusion along with that of other vital capillaries restores urine volume production as long as tubular necrosis is not already present. Fluid administration may, in fact, prevent ATN in the kidneys.

A large amount of tissue damage (e.g., crush injuries) may cause a release of myoglobin from muscle tissue. Because the myoglobin molecule is large, a type of mechanical renal failure may result from attempts to excrete large amounts of myoglobin. Fluid administration is again important to decrease damage to the tubules.

Preventing Gastrointestinal Bleeding

Recall that an early physiologic response to shock is a decrease in splanchnic circulation. This reduces the blood supply to the stomach and bowel, causing inadequate gastrointestinal tissue perfusion and delayed gastric emptying; thus, vomiting with aspiration of gastric contents into the lung may occur. For this reason and for diagnostic purposes, nasogastric suction is often used during treatment of shock. A double-lumen, 16F nasogastric tube (Salem sump tube) is usually used in adults.

Assess gastric aspirate periodically for blood. Guaiac solution or Hemoccult tablets and reagent can be used to check for blood; litmus paper checks the pH to determine the acidity of the stomach. Promptly report new findings of blood or increases in the amount of blood. Histamine blockers and proton pump inhibitors are used to reduce gastric acid in the stomach. Antacids may also be instilled through the tube when the pH is acidic.

When shock is caused by gastrointestinal bleeding, other nasogastric tubes may be used. For example, if the suspected cause of bleeding is a gastric ulcer, a 36F Ewald tube may be used. This tube's many large holes facilitate saline lavage and removal of blood clots. If esophageal varices are suspected or present, a Sengstaken-Blakemore tube is often used. This triple-lumen tube exerts pressure on the lower portion of the esophagus and the upper portion of the stomach, where varices are most prominent. Pressure is created by esophageal and gastric balloons inflated with air. Gentle traction is applied to keep the balloons in proper position (see Chapter 61).

The medical management of shock has been discussed in general. Tables 22–3, 22–4, and 22–5 give some of the specific interventions for hypovolemic, cardiogenic, and distributive shock, respectively.

Table 22–3. Summary of the Management of Hypovolemic Shock

Etiology	Clinical Situation	Intervention*
Blood loss	Massive trauma Gastrointestinal bleeding Ruptured aortic aneurysm Surgery Erosion of vessel from lesion, tubes, or other devices DIC	Stop external bleeding with direct pressure, pressure dressing, tourniquet (as last resort) Reduce intra-abdominal or retroperitoneal bleeding by applying MAST garment or prepare for emergency surgery Administer lactated Ringers solution or normal saline Transfuse with fresh whole blood, packed cells fresh frozen plasma, platelets, or other clotting factors, if significant improvement does not occur with crystalloid administration; administer crystalloids as well Use non-blood plasma expanders (albumin, hetastarch, dextran) until blood is available Autotransfusion if appropriate
Plasma loss	Burns Accumulation of intra-abdominal fluid Malnutrition Severe dermatitis DIC	Administer low-dose cardiotonics (dopamine, dobutamine) Administer lactated Ringer's solution or normal saline Administer albumin, fresh frozen plasma, hetastarch, or dextran if cardiac output still low
Crystalloid loss	Dehydration (e.g., diabetic ketoacidosis, heat exhaustion) Protracted vomiting, diarrhea Nasogastric suction	Isotonic or hypotonic saline with electrolytes as needed to maintain normal circulating volume and electrolyte balance

DIC, disseminated intravascular coagulation; MAST, *military or medical anti-shock trousers*.
*Assumes that airway management and cardiac monitoring are ongoing.

▪ Nursing Management of the Medical Client

Assessment

Because a client's condition can change rapidly in shock, frequent nursing assessment is essential. Documentation of progress and response to intervention needs to be concise, yet convey the client's status minute by minute.

Initiate a flow sheet containing all pertinent data in an easily read format. This flow sheet must accompany the client at all times. At the bedside, immediate laboratory assessments are essential in treating shock. Blood chemistries, blood gases, oxygen saturations, and electrolytes need to be determined frequently and reported promptly so therapy can be adjusted to the client's rapidly changing physiologic status.

Do not administer narcotics to a client suffering from acute, multiple trauma without first knowing if the blood volume is adequate. Narcotic administration causes vasodilation, which results in severe hypotension or shock. Also, if a narcotic is administered intramuscularly to a client in shock, it may not be completely absorbed because of the vasoconstriction that is present. Then, because the client experiences little or no pain relief, a second injection may be given. Once fluid resuscitation is complete and the circulating volume is restored, the client may absorb both doses of the narcotic. No one in shock should be given intramuscular medications.

When narcotics are appropriate for a client in shock, they are most effective if administered IV in small doses.

When caring for trauma victims, especially those with massive injury, remember that the extent of the injury does not necessarily coincide with the amount of pain being experienced. Careful assessment is necessary once narcotic administration seems safe (in terms of the client's hemodynamic status). Assess the client's blood pressure more closely after IV administration of narcotics to watch for hypotension.

When caring for clients experiencing shock, carefully make nursing diagnoses concerning pain and impaired gas exchange. Restlessness is an assessment finding common to both and can thus be easily misinterpreted. Too often, clients who are restless, especially trauma victims, are given narcotics because their behavior is incorrectly interpreted as resulting from pain. However, the restlessness frequently is actually due to hypoxia, and narcotics worsen the problem. The decision to administer narcotics is often a nursing decision. It is important to assess the need for these medications carefully. Attention to positioning, splinting of injured areas, breathing techniques, and comfort measures may provide safer and more effective pain relief than narcotics. (Pain is discussed in detail in Chapter 17.)

Even though a person in shock may feel cold and may be hypothermic, do not apply heat to the skin. Heat application dilates peripheral blood vessels and draws blood away from the vital organs (where it is life-sustaining) into the vessels of the skin. This interferes with the body's initial compensatory mechanism of peripheral vasoconstriction. Also, heat increases the body's metabolism. In turn, this increases the need for oxygen and puts an added strain on the heart.

Table 22–4. Summary of the Management of Cardiogenic Shock		
Etiology	**Clinical Situation**	**Intervention***
Myocardial disease or injury	Acute myocardial infarction Myocardial contusion Cardiomyopathies	Fluid-challenge with up to 300 ml of normal saline solution or Ringer's lactate to rule out hypovolemia, unless congestive failure or pulmonary edema is present Insert CVP or pulmonary artery catheter; monitor cardiac output, pulmonary artery pressure, and PCWP; administer IV fluids to maintain left ventricular filling pressure of 15–20 mm Hg Administer inotropics (e.g., dopamine or dobutamine) Vasodilators (e.g., sodium nitroprusside, nitroglycerin, calcium channel blockers, morphine) Diuretics (e.g., mannitol or furosemide) Cardiotonics (e.g., digitalis) Beta blockers (propranolol) Glucocorticosteroids† Intra-aortic balloon pump or external counterpulsation device if unresponsive to other therapies
Valvular disease or injury	Ruptured aortic cusp Ruptured papillary muscle Ball thrombus	Same as above: if rapid response does not occur, prepare for prompt cardiac surgery
External pressure on the heart interferes with heart filling or emptying	Pericardial tamponade due to trauma, aneurysm, cardiac surgery, pericarditis Massive pulmonary embolus Tension pneumothorax Ascites Hemoperitoneum Mechanical ventilation	Relieve tamponade with ECG-assisted pericardiocentesis; repair surgically if it recurs Thrombolytic (streptokinase) or anticoagulant (heparin) therapy; surgery for removal of clot Relieve air accumulation with needle thoracostomy or chest tube insertion Relieve fluid accumulation with paracentesis Reduce inspiratory pressure
Cardiac dysrhythmias	Tachyarrhythmias Bradyarrhythmias Pulseless electrical activity	Treat dysrhythmias; be prepared to initiate CPR, cardiac pacing

CPR, cardiopulmonary resuscitation; CVP, central venous pressure; ECG, electrocardiogram; IV, intravenous; PCWP, pulmonary capillary wedge pressure.
*Assumes that airway management and cardiac monitoring are ongoing.
†Controversial.

This does not mean that the person is kept in a cold environment. The environment is kept warm because it is important that the person not become chilled. Chilling and shivering require energy expenditure needed to maintain vital functions. Also, chilling contributes to sludging of blood in the microcirculation. Hypothermia slows the heart, increases the likelihood of ventricular fibrillation, and inhibits the body's reparative processes.

Various invasive and noninvasive techniques are used to assess a client's status during shock and to evaluate the effectiveness of interventions.

Noninvasive Techniques. Because nurses often provide healthcare in settings other than hospitals, it helps to know about assessment and monitoring techniques that do not require sophisticated machinery or invade body tissues or cavities. These noninvasive techniques can be performed rapidly and relatively easily, they require little equipment, and are readily observable.

The first step in assessing a person in shock is a general overview, giving attention as necessary to the ABCs—Airway, Breathing, and Circulation. Once the airway is patent, air exchange is adequate, a pulse is present, and the cervical spine is immobilized (if it is a trauma situation), perform a rapid, cursory initial head-to-toe physical assessment. The initial assessment goal is to identify major problems and gross abnormalities. Give further detailed attention to specific injuries or problems after shock is stabilized.

Table 22–5. Summary of the Management of Distributive Shock

Etiology	Clinical Situation	Intervention*
Anaphylactic shock	Allergy to food, medicines, dyes, insect bites, or stings	Prepare for surgical management of the airway Decrease further absorption of antigen (e.g., stop IV fluid, place tourniquet between injection or sting site and heart if feasible) Epinephrine (1:100) 2 inhalations every 3 hours, *or* Epinephrine (1:1000) 0.2–0.5 ml every 5–15 min given subcutaneously, *or* Epinephrine (1:10,000) 0.5–1.0 ml every 5–15 min given at a rate of 1 mg/min IV fluid resuscitation with isotonic solution Diphenhydramine hydrochloride or H_1-receptor antagonist IV Theophylline IV drip for bronchospasm Steroids IV Vasopressors (e.g., norepinephrine, metaraminol bitartrate, high-dosage dopamine) Gastric lavage for ingested antigen Ice pack to injection or sting site Meat tenderizer paste to sting site
Septic shock	Often gram-negative septicemia but also caused by other organisms in debilitated, immunodeficient, or chronically ill clients	Identify origin of sepsis; culture all suspicious sources Vigorous IV fluid resuscitation with normal saline Empirical antibiotic therapy: until sensitivities are reported. If suspected organism is gram-positive, vancomycin is used; if suspected organism is gram-negative, give expanded-spectrum penicillin or cephalosporin and aminoglycoside Administer cardiotonic agents (e.g., dopamine or dobutamine, norepinephrine, isoproterenol, digitalis, calcium) Naloxone (narcotic anatagonist) Prostaglandins Monoclonal antibodies Temperature control (both hypothermia and hyperthermia are noted) Heparin, clotting factors, blood products if DIC develops
Neurogenic (spinal) shock	Spinal anesthesia Spinal cord injury	Normal saline to restore volume Treat bradycardia with atropine Vasopressors (e.g., norepinephrine, metaraminol bitartrate, high-dosage dopamine, and phenylephrine) may be given Place client in modified Trendelenburg's position
Vasovagal reaction	Severe pain Severe emotional stress	Place client in a head-down or recumbent position Give atropine if bradycardia and profound hypotension; eliminate pain

DIC, disseminated intravascular coagulation; IV, intravenous.
*Assumes airway management and cardiac monitoring are ongoing.

With the use of physical assessment skills, the following observations should be made:

- Airway patency: presence of noisy respirations, obstructions
- Breathing: respiratory rate and effort
- Respiratory pattern: chest wall expansion; chest wall bulges or defects
- Circulation: pulse, blood pressure, skin color, and temperature
- Level of consciousness: orientation ×3 (i.e., person, place, time); ability to move extremities; sensation in all extremities; hand grasps; response to verbal and painful stimuli; pupil size and reaction to light; presence of abnormal posturing; and so on to evaluate neurologic function

- State of hydration and perfusion of the skin (e.g., capillary refill time <3 seconds); condition of mucous membranes, sclera, and conjunctivae; presence of pallor or cyanosis
- Fullness of neck veins (jugular venous distention, JVD): JVD may suggest right heart failure cardiogenic shock
- Position of trachea: tracheal deviation may indicate tension pneumothorax
- Heart sounds
- Presence, location, intensity, duration of pain; what relieves the pain
- Abdominal distention: rigidity; bowel sounds
- Circumference of abdomen or extremities
- Peripheral pulses
- Presence of lacerations, contusions, ecchymoses, petechiae, purpura (also check for bruising over flank area)
- Bone deformities
- Presence of medical alert tags or bracelets

After potentially life-threatening problems are treated, take complete vital signs with BP taken in both arms to rule out other causes of hypovolemic shock (i.e., thoracic dissection, aneurysm). It is important to take postural vital signs if applicable and if it is safe to do so. Do not take postural vital signs if the client has multiple traumatic injuries; if there is evidence of vertebral, pelvic, or femoral fracture; or if hypotension already exists. Clients with postural hypotension should not be sent to the x-ray department for upright films until they are adequately volume-resuscitated. If x-rays must be taken, clients require constant attendance by a nurse who monitors vital signs, administers IV fluids if necessary, and provides guidance to x-ray department personnel regarding movement, positioning, and timing of studies.

Measurement of postural vital signs is indicated under the following circumstances:

- History or presence of significant blood loss
- Unexplained tachycardia
- History of fluid loss (e.g., diarrhea, vomiting, diuretic therapy, or third-space loss)
- Unexplained syncope
- Blunt chest or abdominal trauma
- Abdominal pain

Alternative Methods of Blood Pressure Monitoring. Often when a client is in shock it is difficult to hear the BP with a standard stethoscope. Two commonly used techniques to obtain BP measurements are palpation of the radial or brachial pulse during deflation of the BP cuff and use of a Doppler instrument. When palpation is used, the first palpable pulse noted during deflation of the cuff is the systolic BP. Document the BP as such (e.g., 90/palp). A Doppler amplifies arterial and venous pulsations by ultrasonography. Various Doppler probes are available and are used instead of a stethoscope to measure BP. Systolic BP is easily heard by placing the probe over the brachial artery after applying transmission gel. The diastolic BP is not obtainable when the Doppler is used.

For clarity and accuracy, document the method by which BP readings are taken (in addition to the readings themselves) and if palpation or a Doppler monitor is used. This is important because these readings may be higher or lower than those obtained in the standard way with a cuff and stethoscope. Likewise, document whether readings are obtained by automatic BP machines even though readings from these machines may not differ from those taken in the standard way.

Direct measurement of arterial BP by use of an arterial line often is done during shock. Discussion of arterial lines is found in Chapter 47.

Temperature Monitoring. An accurate core temperature measurement is important in assessing a client in shock. Sometimes an indwelling flexible rectal probe connected to a continuous display monitor is more accurate and less traumatic than intermittent rectal temperature measurements with a standard thermometer. Core temperature can also be measured with a thermometer inserted by the manufacturer into an indwelling urinary catheter. Tympanic temperatures are commonly used in critical care settings and also provide core temperature measurements. Core temperature can also be obtained if the client has a thermodilution (Swan-Ganz) catheter in place.

Oral temperature measurement is neither accurate nor safe. During shock, the buccal mucosa is poorly perfused, and the client should be receiving oxygen by mask or nasal prongs. (Because clients in shock are hypoxemic, the procedure of removing the oxygen long enough to obtain an oral temperature is not routinely recommended.)

Cardiac Monitoring. For assessment and evaluation purposes, the electrical activity of the heart needs to be continuously monitored in all clients in shock, regardless of age. Nurses caring for clients experiencing shock need to be able to initiate cardiac monitoring, recognize cardiac dysrhythmias, and initiate treatment for any potentially lethal dysrhythmias that occur (see Chapter 46).

During the initial resuscitation period, it may be more appropriate to place the ECG monitor electrodes on the client's shoulders rather than on the chest. This placement does not interfere with chest film findings. Also, it allows better access to the chest for thoracic procedures such as insertion of chest tubes, pericardiocentesis, and CVP line placement. Once the client is stabilized, the electrodes may be moved to the chest.

Invasive Techniques
Hemodynamic Monitoring. Measurement of CVP is one hemodynamic technique that may be used in initial shock management, especially with hypovolemic shock. However, because CVP only provides information regarding preload, peripheral intra-arterial lines or a pulmonary artery catheter is inserted as soon as possible. Blood volume needs to be expanded as the vascular space enlarges, and CVP measurements are used to determine the amount of fluid needed to fill the enlarging vascular space. The rate of fluid replacement is adjusted to maintain the desired CVP. It is serious if the CVP continues to fall in spite of fluid replacement. This means that the rate and volume of fluid replacement are not sufficient to meet the client's physiologic needs.

Peripheral arterial catheters are commonly used in shock to measure arterial BP and MAP and to obtain blood samples for chemical and blood gas analysis. These catheters are usually placed in the radial artery, but may also be placed in the femoral or brachial arteries. Pulmonary artery and PCWP measurements are monitored to assess left-sided heart function and to guide fluid administration. These pressures are measured through a Swan-Ganz catheter. The PCWP corresponds to the LV end-diastolic pressure. This is the pressure in the LV just before contraction. A rise in this pressure in a client with cardiogenic shock may indicate left-sided heart failure. A low value in a client with hypovolemic shock may indicate that volume replacement is needed. In a client with septic shock, lower values would be expected during the warm phase and higher values during the cold phase.

Depending on the type of Swan-Ganz catheter used, additional measurements may be obtained. Some catheters have a fiberoptic tip that allows measurement of oxygen saturation of hemoglobin in the venous blood (SvO_2). SvO_2 is measured in the pulmonary artery, just before the blood's reoxygenation in the lungs. This reading gives an average of the tissue's uptake or use of oxygen in the body. The normal range for SvO_2 is 60% to 80%. When the SvO_2 falls below 60%, it may indicate either decreased arterial oxygenation or increased tissue oxygen demand. If the SvO_2 is greater than 80%, the indication, in relation to shock, is that the oxygen is unable to either reach the tissues or to be extracted by the tissues.

Most Swan-Ganz catheters also have a thermistor bead just proximal to the balloon. This may be used to determine cardiac output by a thermodilution technique. A fourth lumen opens at the level of the right atrium, and CVP measurements (preload) can be obtained through this lumen.

Monitoring Cardiac Output. Cardiac output, measured in liters per minute, is the amount of blood pumped by the LV into the aorta each minute. During shock, cardiac output may be decreased because of myocardial damage resulting from an MI or, in hypovolemic shock, from inadequate volume replacement.

Because of the widespread use of Swan-Ganz catheters and the ease of performing measurements, cardiac output monitoring is used in managing all types of shock. These measurements assess overall cardiac function and the function of the LV. Factors that may alter cardiac output include heart rate, PVR, age, body size, exercise, and (in persons with cardiac problems) decreased filling or emptying of the LV.

Cardiac index is the cardiac output divided by the body surface area. Cardiac output as a separate reading does not take into account the amount of tissue that needs to be perfused. By figuring body size into the calculation, a more accurate assessment is obtained.

Using the cardiac output and the MAP, PVR can be determined. PVR measures afterload and provides information regarding vasoconstriction or vasodilation. Decreased PVR indicates systemic vasodilation and may indicate the need for administration of vasoconstrictors. Increased PVR indicates systemic vasoconstriction, and the potential need for vasodilators. Arterial BP and cardiac function should always be taken into consideration before administering vasoconstrictors or vasodilators.

Monitoring Urinary Output. An indwelling urinary catheter is a simple means of monitoring a client during shock. Continuously measuring urinary flow provides important information about peripheral blood flow and kidney function. Because the amount of urine excreted during shock is often very small, it is important to have an accurate, calibrated urine collector. In some settings, the catheter may be attached to a urimeter collector or to a more complex electric urimeter.

Urinary volume changes can be highly important as an index of the success or failure of therapy. Minimal (< 30 ml/hour or 240 ml/8 hours) or absent urinary output indicates treatment is not successful. Increasing urinary output is a favorable sign. Assess the client's urinary output routinely and record it at least every hour.

Diagnosis, Planning, Implementation

Nursing Diagnosis. Some potential nursing diagnoses for the client in shock are listed in Box 22–1.

Planning: Expected Outcomes. Nursing care of the client with shock is complex. Frequent reassessment of the client and nursing activities is essential because the client's status often changes rapidly. Specific nursing and medical interventions vary according to individual needs and the setting in which care is delivered (e.g., emer-

---

Box 22–1. Potential Nursing Diagnoses for Client in Shock

Ineffective airway clearance
Ineffective breathing pattern
Impaired gas exchange
Altered tissue perfusion: cerebral, cardiopulmonary, renal, gastrointestinal, peripheral
Decreased cardiac output
Fluid volume deficit
Altered nutrition: less than body requirements
Constipation
Activity intolerance
Impaired physical mobility
Sensory/perceptual alterations: visual, auditory, kinesthetic, gustatory, tactile
Sleep pattern disturbance
Impaired or risk for impaired skin integrity
Self care deficit: feeding, bathing/hygiene, dressing/grooming, toileting
Body image disturbance
Self esteem disturbance
Altered role performance
Personal identity disturbance
Anxiety
Fear
Pain
Impaired verbal communication
Spiritual distress
Altered thought processes
Ineffective family coping: compromised
Altered family processes
Anticipatory grieving

gency room versus intensive care unit). However, four major outcomes of care are desired:

1. Return of tissue perfusion and cellular function to normal
2. Meeting metabolic demands
3. Preventing further injury
4. Effective coping by the client and significant others

Implementation. Other nursing considerations in caring for clients in shock include the following:

- Continuous assessment of the client. Cardiovascular and respiratory changes can occur rapidly, and intervention must promptly be adjusted accordingly. Document observations clearly and concisely.
- Help the client (and family) to feel physically and emotionally comfortable.
- Facilitate expression of concerns and questions by the client and family. For example, try to reduce the client's fears and anxieties about what is happening and about the equipment being used.
- Keep equipment and supplies (e.g., suction, emergency drugs) available and in working order.
- Implement appropriate, planned nursing interventions to prevent complications that can develop from enforced immobilization.
- Provide adequate pain relief, because pain intensifies shock. Base this intervention on careful assessment.
- Provide care to the family also.

A client in shock is extremely ill and may die. In addition, the stress of the situation is compounded by emergency medical treatment with all the people, equipment, and movement this entails. During shock management, nurses have numerous delegated medical care activities to attend to. However, there must be sufficient nursing resources to provide psychosocial care (e.g., reassurance, emotional support) to the client and family. All of these people involved may be frightened, anxious, perhaps confused, and certainly very dependent.

Keep the client's family informed of what is happening. They need information on which to base decisions. Because of their anxiety, the nurse may need to calmly repeat information several times. See the Client Education Guide for information to be conveyed. Remember that the client and significant others may be experiencing "psychological shock." Often they need (and greatly appreciate) opportunities to discuss with care providers their important concerns.

Do not keep loved ones away from the client unnecessarily. There may be times when, because of limited space, they will have to wait in another room for a period of time. However, they should not be kept away long. They should not be asked to leave their loved one without being given a reasonable explanation of why it is necessary.

A client experiencing shock requires emotional support. When caught up in the sudden drama of an emergency or of critical care, health professionals sometimes forget that the experience and setting are often new and very frightening for the client. Unfortunately, "dehumanization" of the client may occasionally occur during the rush of

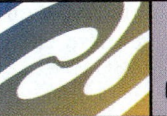

CLIENT EDUCATION GUIDE

Shock

It is difficult to prevent the occurrence of shock because the causes are often unpredictable. If your family member is in shock, obtain precise, consistent information about his or her current status and prognosis.
 Learn about the monitoring equipment in use
 Learn how to communicate with the client who is intubated or unconscious
 Learn how to demonstrate love and caring to someone surrounded by equipment
 Participate in your family member's care during the hospital stay; this will increase your ability to provide care at home.
 Learn how to prevent recurrence if the cause was avoidable.

emergency treatment. Whether a client appears to be conscious or not, always explain what is happening. Keep the atmosphere as quiet and orderly as possible. Eliminate unnecessary chatter. Commonly, recovered clients remember hearing what was said and were aware of what happened to them even though they appeared to be unconscious.

Among nurses' greatest responsibilities are those of providing support, comfort, and advocacy to clients receiving care and to their significant others. In nursing clients who are critically ill and experiencing shock, this is very important.

Evaluation

The expected outcomes should be evaluated frequently; revisions in the plan of care may be required hourly to maintain tissue perfusion.

Continually monitor BP and CVP when vasodilator drugs are being used. Usually, a mean BP of 70 mm Hg is acceptable. However, if abrupt severe hypotension occurs, administration of the vasodilator is generally stopped and fluid administration increased.

Carefully monitor arterial BP during vasoconstrictor administration as well. Watch for undesirable BP elevations. Carefully adjust IV flow to establish and maintain the desired BP. Inspect IV sites frequently for evidence of infiltration. However, the excessive vasoconstriction they cause may actually impede rather than enhance tissue perfusion.

■ Surgical Management

Surgical interventions that can help in shock states are limited; however, they may be very useful in trauma situations. In hypovolemic shock due to trauma, surgery can be performed in an attempt to control sources of bleeding. Once bleeding has been controlled, interventions aimed at restoring adequate fluid volume are more effective.

Community and Self-Care

Shock must be fully resolved before a client is transferred or discharged (unless the client is being transported for the treatment of shock). Clients who have survived shock find that recovery of the precipitating problem is delayed. They may also experience some feelings of confusion, depression, or grief when they realize that they lived through a very critical illness.

Multiple Organ System Failure/ Systemic Inflammatory Response Syndrome

Single organ failure (e.g., heart failure, renal failure) has long been recognized as a cause of mortality and morbidity in critically ill clients. In trauma centers in the late 1960s a new form of organ failure was recognized, that of sequential failure of lung, liver, and kidney usually followed by death. By the 1970s, the syndrome of sequential organ failure was well described. Today this problem is named multiple organ system failure (MOSF), multiple organ dysfunction syndrome, or multiorgan system failure. More recently the precursor to MOSF has been labeled as systemic inflammatory response syndrome.

Etiology and Risk Factors

There are several etiologies of MOSF. They include dead tissue, injured tissue, infection, perfusion deficits, and persistent sources of inflammation such as pancreatitis or pneumonitis. Acute lung injury is usually present in some form. Persons known to be at high risk for developing MOSF include clients with impaired immune responses. These clients include the elderly, clients with chronic illnesses, clients with malnutrition, and clients with cancer. In addition, clients with prolonged or exaggerated inflammatory responses are at risk. These clients include victims of severe trauma and clients with sepsis.

Prevention is a major direction of current therapy for MOSF. Source control is a major emphasis. Whenever possible, the potential source of sepsis or inflammation is excised or removed (e.g., full-thickness burn wound). Unfortunately, the source cannot be removed in many cases, such as pneumonia, pancreatitis, soft tissue injury, and hematoma. When the source cannot be removed, empirical antimicrobial agents are used to reduce risk.

It would be helpful to clinicians to be able to predict which clients are at the highest risk, but accurate prediction remains illusive. The variables that appear to be the most predictive are: the ratio of arterial oxygen tension (PaO$_2$) to the fraction of inspired oxygen (FiO$_2$) on day 1; the plasma lactate on day 2; the serum bilirubin on day 6;

and the serum creatinine of day 12 postinjury.[15] When nurses note these predictors, increased surveillance should begin.

Pathophysiology

In the healthy person, the normal integrated inflammatory immune response (IIR) functions to protect tissue from microbial invasion and rid the body of cellular debris and foreign material. The IIR is a continual process of responses until the insult slows and the client's condition stabilizes. The IIR stops once it is no longer needed. SIRS is a case of unchecked inflammatory responses. MOSF is the end result of the prolonged response.

Most inciting events start with a local injury from trauma, infection, or lack of perfusion. Bacteria introduced into the wound or allowed to grow in necrotic tissues due to decreased immune activate the systemic inflammatory responses. Bacteria release toxins that activate systemic mediators of inflammation. Activation of the systemic response is an effort to "recruit help" to battle the invasion of microorganisms.

Once the inflammatory response becomes systemic, it is controlled by chemical mediators of inflammation. Mediators include bradykinin, complement, histamine, interleukin-1, prekallikrien, prostaglandins, and tumor necrosis factor. These powerful mediators of inflammation induce a systemic response. Endothelial cells are a common target for some mediators. The endothelium is destroyed, and blood flow is reduced to the tissues. Endothelial damage is produced by endotoxins from bacteria, tumor necrosis factor, interleukin-1, platelet activating factors, and many others. When this inflammatory response is unchecked, it produces damage to organs and tissues by altering perfusion, disturbing oxygen supply or demand, or changing metabolic dysfunctions. Metabolism increases under the direction of mediators such as cortisol and the catecholamines.

Many organs "respond" to MOSF. The lungs are usually the first to malfunction, owing to the large surface area of pulmonary epithelium combined with the presence of bacterial contamination from systemic blood return. The gastrointestinal (GI) tract is the second system to malfunction, and it propagates conditions for further deterioration of other organs. Once malfunctioning, bacteria quickly relocate from the GI tract to other organs. Additionally, the hypermetabolic state increases gastric acid production increasing the risk of ulceration and bleeding. The most serious metabolic problem is hypermetabolism. The hypermetabolic state is continued by cell to cell communication and the sympathetic nervous system responding in its usual "fight or flight" response.

Types of MOSF

There are two types of MOSF: Type I and Type II. In Type I, MOSF is the terminal event, and MOSF becomes evident only a few days before death. Type I is most commonly seen after a primary pulmonary injury, such as aspiration. Only a small percentage of clients develop Type I MOSF. Type II MOSF does not become progressive for 7 to 14 days after the initial event. The form occurs with septic shock and ARDS.

Clinical Manifestations and Diagnostic Findings

There is usually a precipitating event to MOSF, including aspiration, ruptured aneurysm, or septic shock, which is associated with hypotension. The client is resuscitated; the cause is treated; and the client appears to do well for a few days. A possible sequence of events develop, and we will present a prototype of this pattern.

Before MOSF develops, the client experiences SIRS. Within a few days, there is an insidious onset of a low-grade fever, tachycardia, increased numbers of banded and segmented neutrophils on the differential count (called a left shift), and dyspnea develop with the appearance of diffuse patchy infiltrates on the chest x-ray. The client often has some deterioration in mental status with reasonably normal renal and hepatic laboratory results. Dyspnea progresses, and intubation and mechanical ventilation are required. Some evidence of consumptive coagulopathy (DIC) is usually present. The client is usually stable hemodynamically, has relative polyuria, has an increased cardiac index (over 4.5 L/min), and systemic vascular resistance of under 600 dynes cm^{-5}.[15] Clients often have increased serum glucose levels in the absence of diabetes. Before MOSF is diagnosed, some physicians use the criteria presented in Table 22–6 to make the diagnosis.

Between 7 and 10 days, the bilirubin level rises and continues to rise, followed by an increase in serum creatinine. Blood glucose and lactate levels continue to rise because of the hypermetabolic state. Other progressive changes include excretion of urinary nitrogen and protein combined with decreased levels of serum albumin, prealbumin, and retinol-binding protein. Bacteremia with enteric organisms is also common. In addition, infections

---

Table 22–6. Modified Apache II Criteria for Diagnosing Multiple Organ System Failure

Cardiovascular Failure (presence of one or more of the following)

Heart rate <54 beats/min
Mean arterial pressure ≤49 mm Hg (systolic pressure ≤60 mm Hg)
Occurrence of ventricular tachycardia or ventricular fibrillation
Serum pH ≤7.24 with a $PaCO_2$ of ≤40 mm Hg

Respiratory Failure (presence of one or more of the following)

Respiratory rate ≤5 breaths/min or ≥49 breaths/min $PaCO_2$ ≥50 mm Hg
Alveolar-arterial oxygen difference ≥350 mm Hg (calculate as follows, at sea level): (713 × % oxygen in inspired gas) − $PaCO_2$ − PaO_2
Dependent on ventilator or CPAP on the second day

Renal Failure (presence of one or more of the following)

Urine output ≤479 ml/24 hr or ≤159 ml/8 hr
Serum BUN ≥100 mg/dl (35.7 mmol/L)
Serum creatinine ≥3.5 mg/dl (309 μmol/L)

Hematologic Failure (presence of one or more of the following)

WBC count ≤1000/μl (1 × 10^9/L)
Platelets ≤20,000/μl (20 × 10^9/L)
Hematocrit ≤20%

Neurologic Failure

Glasgow Coma Score ≤6 (in absence of sedation)

Hepatic Failure (presence of both of the following)

Serum bilirubin ≥6 mg%
Prothrombin time ≥4 sec over control in the absence of systemic anticoagulation

CPAP, Continuous positive airway pressure; BUN, blood urea nitrogen; WBC, white blood cell.
From Knaus, W. A., & Wagner, D. P. (1989). Multiple systems organ failure epidemiology and prognosis, *Critical Care Clinics* 5:221.

from *Candida* and viruses such as herpes and cytomegalovirus are common. Surgical wounds display delayed healing, and pressure ulcers may develop. During this time, the client needs increasing amounts of fluids and inotropic medications to keep blood volume and cardiac preload near normal and to replace fluids lost through polyuria.

Between day 14 and day 21, the client is unstable and appears close to death. The client may lose consciousness. Renal failure worsens to the point of considering dialysis. Anasarca or edema may be present due to low serum protein levels. Mixed venous oxygen levels may rise because of problems with tissue uptake of oxygen due to mitochrondial dysfunction. Liver enzymes continue to rise. Lactic acidosis worsens. Coagulation disorders become impossible to correct.

By day 21, it is usually evident that the client will die. Death usually occurs between days 21 and 28 after the injury or precipitating event. Not all persons with MOSF die; however, MOSF remains the leading cause of death in the intensive care unit (ICU) despite the development of better antibiotics, better resuscitation, and more sophisticated means of organ support.

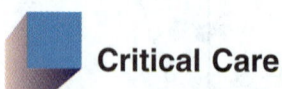

Critical Care

The management of the client with MOSF is directed at restraining the activators of the process, controlling the mediators of inflammation, and protecting the various organs affected by the process.

■ Restraining the Activators

Signs of potential infection must be quickly treated to restrain the activators of MOSF. If the agent is known, antibiotics to which the organisms is sensitive should be administered. If the organism is not known, broad-spectrum antibiotics are given. Antibiotics are sometimes directed at the probable organism (an empirical treatment). Early aggressive management of sources of infection should be carried out. For example, the client may need to have a large infected wound incised and drained or necrotic tissue excised. Extreme caution must be taken to avoid infecting the client. These clients have many invasive monitors and may have open wounds. Unfortunately, clients in critical care units exist in a paradox. The ICU is the only environment with sophisticated equipment and healthcare professionals to provide safe care, yet it is an environment where the risk of infection is higher. In addition, there is a high prevalence of multiresistant organisms, such as vancomycin-resistant *Enterococcus* (VRE) and methicillin-resistant *Staphylococcus aureus* (MRSA).

Because the lungs are common first organs to fail, they require special attention. Aggressive pulmonary care is needed in all clients who are at risk of MOSF. Interventions may be as simple as coughing and deep breathing to ambulation. The client's oxygen saturation should be monitored.

Likewise, because malnutrition develops from the hypermetabolism and the GI tract often seeds other areas with bacteria, some clinicians require the client to be fed enterally. They believe that feeding will enhance perfusion and decrease the bacterial load and the effects of endotoxins. Nutrient intake is usually 30 to 35 kCal/kg/day of carbohydrates. Fats are restricted to 0.5 to 1 g/kg/day. Proteins are given to the client via modified amino acids. Some practitioners administer protein until a rise in plasma transferrin or prealbumin is noted. Increases in these values indicate hepatic protein synthesis rather than a breakdown of body stores. Decontamination of the GI tract and pharynx have been found to decrease infection but have shown no effect on the death rate from MOSF.[46]

■ Controlling the Mediators

Controlling the mediators of inflammation is both directed at general levels of care and specific treatments targeted at the problem cells. Maintenance of a positive nitrogen balance via nutrition, promotion of sleep and rest, and management of pain are important general care areas. Specific treatments include monoclonal antibodies to control mediators such as endotoxins, interleukin-1, and tumor necrosis factors. These therapies are shown in Table 22–7. Outcomes from the research in these treatments are conflicting, and it appears that there is no "magic bullet" to cure the problem. Research and development of more specific monoclonal antibodies are ongoing.

■ Protecting the Organs Affected

While remembering the organs that fail with MOSF, you can direct care to maintain their function for the client. The client is intubated and mechanically ventilated in order to maintain adequate oxygenation. Oxygen is given to the client until blood levels of lactate decrease toward normal. Elevated serum lactate levels indicate the use of anaerobic metabolism. Nurses must recognize that certain clinical problems further increase the need for oxygen. Problems such as fever, seizures, and shivering increase oxygen demands. These problems should be controlled with medications or environmental changes (e.g., warming).

Fluids and inotropic drugs are used to support hemodynamic parameters. The client often becomes more and more unstable and needs more continuous monitoring. Nutritional support is also critical to reduce the catabolism that accompanies hypermetabolism. Dialysis is often used to reduce azotemia from renal failure.

This complex disorder taxes the client and family. Nurses must remain sensitive to the needs of the family. Caring for the family of critically ill clients is a challenge in that understanding, predicting, and intervening with families in crisis is less exact than the calculation of

Table 22–7. Summary of Potentially Useful Therapies for MOSF	
Rationale	**Therapy**
Treatment of infection	Monoclonal antibodies Passive antibody protection Gut decontamination regimens
Support of gut function	Mucosal trophic agents: e.g., glutamine, bombesin, ketone bodies Early enteral feeding Regulation of gut microbial flora
Improved resuscitation	Hypertonic saline In-line sensors Tissue-specific sensors Noninvasive monitoring
Endothelial cell protection	PAF inhibitors WBC adherence inhibition Antioxidant therapy Eicosanoid modulation
Modulation of macrophage function	n3 polyunsaturated fatty acids Signal transduction modulation
Stimulation of lymphocyte function	Arginine w3 polyunsaturated fatty acids

PAF, platelet activating factor; WBC, whie blood cell.
From Lekander, B. J., & Cerra, F. B. (1990). The syndrome of multiple organ failure. *Critical Care Clinics of North America* 2(2), 338.

oxygen needs. There are no easy formulas to use to provide hope, courage, coping, and caring. Nurses must remain alert to the needs of the family as well as the client during this stressful time.

■ Outcomes

Current intensive care technology has allowed prolonged support of the client with MOSF. The patient's average duration of ICU stay is about 21 days, and the rehabilitation is about 10 months. Rehabilitation is directed at recovery of muscle mass and neuromuscular function.

Conclusions

This chapter has discussed shock under three major classifications: hypovolemic, cardiogenic, and distributive. The pathophysiology, complications, and medical and nursing management have been presented. Shock is a critical condition with a high mortality rate. Early diagnosis and intervention are necessary for the best possible outcomes. Multiple organ system failure is a syndrome of multiple organs progressively falling due to prolonged inflammatory responses.

Thinking Critically

1. The client is a 20-year-old man with a gunshot wound to the right chest and massive hemorrhage. His BP is 60 (palpated), heart rate 130, respiratory rate 36. **The skin is pale, cold, and clammy; capillary refill is less than 3 seconds; pulses are weak and thready. What priority assessments should be done? What interventions might be performed?**

Factors to Consider. What do his vital signs tell you? What injuries might have occurred with a major chest trauma? How can his need for fluid and blood replacement best be met?

2. **A 69-year-old man was brought to the emergency room by a rescue squad. He had a colon resection 2 weeks ago. His wife said that he was having increased difficulty breathing and he could feel his heart beating in his chest. He also has seemed "slower" to her. He is not moving as fast as usual and he gets very dizzy when he stands up; he almost passed out, which is why she called the rescue squad. What priority assessments should be done? What interventions might be performed?**

Factors to Consider. What might be happening that could lead to all of the problems with breathing, dizziness, and confusion? What risk might be present as a result of the surgery?

3. **A 65-year-old man in the coronary care unit was diagnosed 3 days ago with an acute myocardial infarction (MI). The monitor alarms and assessments reveal his BP is 76/50, respiratory rate is 20. His pulse is rapid (128) and thready; skin is cool and diaphoretic with a slight ashen color; capillary refill is less than 3 seconds. David is restless and confused. What priority assessments should be done? What interventions might be performed?**

Factors to Consider. What form of shock can quickly develop in a client after an MI? Does he need fluid resuscitation to increase his blood pressure? Why or why not? What medications are commonly used to support a heart in distress? Are special forms of monitoring needed while these medications are used?

Bibliography

1. Adomat, R. (1992). Understanding shock. *British Journal of Nursing, 1*(3), 124–128.
2. Aguilar, M. M., & Hartley-Winkler, M. (1990). CAVHD during extracorporeal membrane oxygenation. *Dialysis and Transplantation, 19*(8), 436–439.
3. Barone, J. E., & Snyder, A. B. (1991). Treatment strategies in shock: Use of oxygen transport measurement. *Heart and Lung, 20*(1), 81–85.
4. Barron, R. L. (1993). Clinical frontiers: Pathophysiology of septic shock and implications for therapy. *Clinical Pharmacy, 12,* 829–845.
5. Bell, T. N. (1990). Disseminated intravascular coagulation and shock: Multisystem crisis in the critically ill. *Critical Care Nursing Clinics of North America, 2*(2), 255–268.
6. Blansfield, J. (1990). Emergency autotransfusion in hypovolemia. *Critical Care Nursing Clinics of North America, 2*(2), 195–199.
7. Brass, N. J. (1994). Predisposition to multiple organ dysfunction. *Critical Care Nursing Quarterly, 16*(4), 1–7.
8. Bone, R. C., Balk, R. A., Fein, A. M., et al. (1995). A second large controlled clinical study of E5, a monoclonal antibody to endotoxin: Results of a prospective, multicenter, randomized, controlled trial. *Critical Care Medicine, 23*(6), 994–1005.
9. Burns, K. M. (1990). Vasoactive drug therapy in shock. *Critical Care Nursing Clinics of North America, 2*(2), 167–178.
10. Coffland, F. I., & Shelton, D. M. (1993). Blood component replacement therapy. *Critical Care Nursing Clinics of North America, 5*(3), 541–556.
11. Colletti, R. C., Dew, R. B., & Goulart, A. E. (1993). Antiendotoxin therapy in sepsis. *Critical Care Nursing Clinics of North America, 5*(2), 345–354.
12. Collins, A. S. (1990). Gastrointestinal complication in shock. *Critical Care Nursing Clinics of North America, 2*(2), 269–277.
13. Dofferhoff, A. S. M., et al. (1992). Patterns of cytokines, plasma endotoxin, plasminogen activator inhibitor, and acute-phase proteins during the treatment of severe sepsis in humans. *Critical Care Medicine, 20*(2), 185–192.
14. Glauser, M. P., et al. (1994). Pathogenesis and potential strategies for prevention and treatment of septic shock: An update. *Clinical Infectious Diseases, 18*(2), S205–S216.
15. Graham, P., & Brass, N. J. (1994). Multiple organ dysfunction: Pathophysiology and therapeutic modalities. *Critical Care Nursing Quarterly, 16*(4), 8–15.
16. Goldenberg, I. F. (1992). Nonpharmacologic management of cardiac arrest and cardiogenic shock. *Chest, 102*(5), 596S–616S.
17. Houston, M. C. (1990). Pathophysiology of shock. *Critical Care Nursing Clinics of North America, 2*(2), 143–149.
18. Hoyt, N. J. (1990). Preventing septic shock: Infection control in the intensive care unit. *Critical Care Nursing Clinics of North America, 2*(2), 287–297.
19. Jillings, C. R. (1990). Shock: Psychosocial needs of the patients and family. *Critical Care Nursing Clinics of North America, 2*(2), 325–330.
20. Lancaster, L. E. (1990). Renal response to shock. *Critical Care Nursing Clinics of North America, 2*(2), 221–233.
21. Lancaster, L. E., & Rice, V. (1990). Nurse care planning: overview and application to the patient in shock. *Critical Care Nursing Clinics of North America, 2*(2), 279–286.
22. Lekander, B. J., & Cerra, F. B. (1990). The syndrome of multiple organ failure. *Critical Care Nursing Clinics of North America, 2*(2), 331–342.
23. Lekander, B. J., & Cerra, F. B. (1990). The syndrome of multiple organ failure. *Critical Care Nursing Clinics of North America, 2*(2), 331–342.
24. Livingston, D. H., Mosenthal, A. C., & Deitch, E. A. (1995). Sepsis and multiple organ dysfunction syndrome: A clinical-mechanistic overview. *New Horizons, 3*(2), 257–266.
25. Lorenz, A. (1989). Lactic acidosis: A nursing challenge. *Critical Care Nurse, 9*(4), 64–73.
26. Marelli, T. R. (1994). Use of a hemoglobin substitute in the anemic Jehovah's Witness patient. *Critical Care Nurse, 14*(1), 31–38.
27. Martin, E., et al. (1989). Autotransfusion systems. *Critical Care Nurse, 9*(7), 65–73.
28. McCloskey, R. V., et al. (1994). Treatment of septic shock with human monoclonal antibody HA–1A. *Annals of Internal Medicine, 121*(1), 1–5.
29. Mims, B. C. (1989). Physiologic rationale of SvO₂ monitoring. *Critical Care Nursing Clinics of North America, 1*(3), 619–628.
30. Mohrman, D. E., & Heller, L. J. (1991). *Cardiovascular physiology.* New York: McGraw-Hill.
31. Ostrow, C. L., Hupp, E., & Topjian, D. (1994). The effect of Trendelenburg and modified Trendelenburg positions on cardiac output, blood pressure, and oxygenation: A preliminary study. *American Journal of Critical Care, 3*(5), 382–386.
32. Phoenix, J. (1990). Low blood pressure: How to investigate this ominous sign. *Nursing, 20*(11), 34–39.
33. Rice, V. (1991). Shock, a clinical syndrome: An update. Part 1. *Critical Care Nurse, 11*(4), 20–27.
34. Rice, V. (1991). Shock, a clinical syndrome: An update. Part 2. The stages of shock. *Critical Care Nurse, 11*(5), 74–82.
35. Rice, V. (1991). Shock, a clinical syndrome: An update. Part 3. Therapeutic management. *Critical Care Nurse, 11*(6), 34–39.
36. Rice, V. (1991). Shock, a clinical syndrome: An update. Part 4. Nursing care of the shock patient. *Critical Care Nurse, 11*(7), 28–40.
37. Roach, A. C. (1990). Antibiotic therapy in septic shock. *Critical Care Nursing Clinics of North America, 2*(2), 179–186.
38. Robins, E. V. (1990). Burn shock. *Critical Care Nursing Clinics of North America, 2*(2), 299–307.
39. Robinson, N. (1993). Cardiogenic shock. *Nursing Standard, 8*(8), 48–49.
40. Rodney, P. A. (1991). Dealing with ethical problems. An ethical decision-making model for critical care nursing. *Canadian Critical Care Nursing Journal, 8*(1), 8–10.
41. Sable, C. A., & Wispelwey, B. (1991). Pharmacologic interventions aimed at preventing the biologic effects of endotoxin. *Infectious Disease Clinics of North America, 5*(4), 883–898.
42. St. John, R. C., & Dorinsky, P. M. (1993). An overview of multiple organ dysfunction syndrome. *Journal of Laboratory and Clinical Medicine, 124,* 478–488.
43. Schott, K. E. (1990). Intra-aortic balloon counterpulsation as a therapy for shock. *Critical Care Nursing Clinics of North America, 2*(2), 187–193.
44. Schumann, L. L., & Remington, M. A. (1990). The use of naloxone in treating endotoxic shock. *Critical Care Nurse, 10*(2), 63–71.
45. Siskind, J. (1990). Handling hemorrhage wisely. *Nursing, 20*(3), 137–143.
46. Stoutenbeek, C. P., & Van Saene, H. K. (1992). Prevention of pneumonia by selective decontamination of the digestive tract. *Intensive Care Medicine 18(suppl),* S18–S24.
47. Stroud, M., et al. (1990). Cellular and humoral mediators of sepsis syndrome. *Critical Care Nursing Clinics of North America, 2*(2), 151–160.
48. Summers, G. (1990). The clinical and hemodynamic presentation of the shock patient. *Critical Care Nursing Clinics of North America, 2*(2), 161–166.
49. Sylvain, H. F., et al. (1995). Accuracy of fingerstick glucose values in shock patients. *American Journal of Critical Care, 4*(1), 44–48.
50. Vaughan, P., & Brooks, C. (1990). Adult respiratory distress syndrome: A complication of shock. *Critical Care Nursing Clinics of North America, 2*(2), 235–253.
51. Waters, L. M., Christensen, M. A., & Sato, R. M. (1990). Hetastarch: An alternative colloid in burn shock management. *Journal of Emergency Nursing, 16*(4), 279–285.
52. Young, L. M. (1990). DIC: The insidious killer. *Critical Care Nurse, 10*(10), 26–33.

Basic Concepts of Neoplastic Disorders

CHAPTER 23

Joann Petty

Overview

Caring for clients with cancer is one of the most significant tasks facing healthcare professionals today. Currently, cancer is the second leading cause of death in the United States, exceeded only by cardiovascular disease. Cancer claims over 500,000 lives per year and affects many thousands more. It will strike at least 4 out of 10 people in this country and about half will survive.[6] Within the United States and throughout the world, cancer has a tremendous economic and sociologic impact. It influences people in every realm of their lives: physical, emotional, spiritual, cognitive, social, and economic.

Since 1985, cancer research has made significant strides toward solving the mysteries of cancer causation and the many problems of cancer treatment. The National Cancer Institute (NCI) has set a target for the year 2000 to reduce the nation's cancer mortality to 50% or less.

Nurses in all areas of practice are likely to come into contact with people who are ill with cancer, and, therefore, must be familiar with its diagnosis and treatment. More important, the nurse is often the professional in closest contact with clients and is in a unique position to teach prevention and to practice early detection.

The Terminology of Cancer

The first task in understanding cancer is to define some commonly used terms associated with the disease. It is vital that both the client and the healthcare provider have a mutual understanding of the terms associated with cancer so the disease and its treatment can be discussed without confusion.

The word *cancer,* often abbreviated Ca, is a term that frightens most people. Cancer is synonymous with the term *malignant neoplasm.* Other terms that suggest malignant neoplasm include *tumor, malignancy, carcinoma,*

and *aberrant cell growth.* Strictly speaking, these words are not interchangeable.

Cancer is a collective term describing a large group of diseases characterized by uncontrolled growth and spread of abnormal cells. This group of diseases (1) arise from any tissue or organ, (2) differ greatly from one another in appearance and growth, (3) may follow very different courses of development in their hosts, and (4) respond differently to the variety of therapies applied to them.

The word *neoplasm* is derived from the Greek word *neos,* new, and *plasis,* molding. Thus *neoplasm* is defined as an abnormal new growth, or formation, of tissue that serves no useful purpose and may harm the host organism.

A neoplasm can be either benign or malignant. *Benign* is defined as a usually harmless growth that does not spread or invade other tissue. *Malignant* is defined as a harmful tumor, capable of spread and invasion of other tissues far removed from the site of origin. Table 23–1 lists other important terms.

The Challenge of Cancer Nursing

For too many people, the word cancer means death. As recently as *20 years ago,* cancer was usually incurable. Today, because of advances in early diagnosis and treatment, more and more people are living longer after the diagnosis has been made. In fact, more than 8 million Americans with a history of cancer are alive today. According to American Cancer Society estimates, more than 1.35 million Americans will be diagnosed with cancer during 1996, and during the same year more than 550,000 Americans will die from their disease.

Nurses are involved in all phases of the cancer experience: prevention, detection, diagnosis, treatment, rehabilitation, survivorship, and palliative and terminal care. Many malignancies can be prevented or be greatly decreased in incidence by life-style changes and minimizing exposure to carcinogens. The nurse plays a major role in helping clients identify risks and make needed changes.

This chapter incorporates material written for the fourth edition by Esther Matassarin-Jacobs and Lynn Allchin Petardi.

Table 23–1. Cancer Terminology

Terms	Definition
Anaplastic	Tumor cells that are completely undifferentiated and bear no resemblance to cells of tissues of their origin
Hyperplasia	An increase in the number of normal cells in a normal arrangement in a tissue or organ; usually leads to an increase in the size or part and an increase in functional activity
Metaplasia	The replacement of one type of fully differentiated cell by another fully differentiated cell in another part of the body where the second cell type does not normally occur
Dysplasia	An alteration in the size, shape, and organization of differentiated cells; cells lose their regularity and show variability in size and shape, usually in response to an irritant; cells may revert to normal when the irritant is removed but may transform to a neoplasia
Metastasis	The ability of neoplastic cells to spread from the original site of the tumor to distant organs, spreading as the same cell type as the original neoplastic tissue
Carcinoma	A form of cancer that is composed of epithelial cells that tend to infiltrate surrounding tissues and may eventually spread to distant sites
Oncogenes	Cancer genes that are altered versions of normal genes
Proto-oncogenes	Repressed oncogenes existing in normal cells which can be activated by many different factors and cause the host cell to become malignant
Tumor	Usually synonymous with neoplasm

Cancer nursing skills are vital in all healthcare settings because clients are seen in the home, office, clinic, acute care setting, rehabilitation setting, and hospice.

Perhaps the greatest role a nurse can play is assisting in the prevention and early detection of cancer. Nurses meet a variety of people daily (family, friends, co-workers), and there is always an opportunity to teach and encourage good health habits. Nurses can and must take advantage of time spent with the general public to engage in health promotion teaching and encourage people to follow cancer prevention guidelines.

The nurse, whether a generalist or a specialist, assists in caring for clients in all phases of the cancer experience. Through teaching, using clinical expertise, research,

and supporting the client, the nurse delivers the highest quality of care possible to a group of clients requiring intensive nursing services.

Cancer occurs in all strata of our society. It strikes people of all ages, socioeconomic and cultural backgrounds, and of both sexes. It is the second leading cause of death in the United States, affecting one in three to four persons. Nurses are in the unique position to influence and care for clients in all phases of the cancer experience. Rather than being seen as a uniformly terminal illness, many cancers are now seen as more of a chronic illness, or at least one with a long course.

Epidemiology

Epidemiology is the study of the distribution and determinants of diseases and health problems in specified populations. The goal of an epidemiologic study is the control or prevention of the health problem. An epidemiologic approach to cancer evaluates patterns of the disease, identifies possible causes, and infers relationships between patterns of disease and determining factors. Although the causes of many cancers remain unknown, some epidemiologic studies have helped to identify those factors that underlie theories of causation. The knowledge gained from epidemiologic findings gives the nurse greater insight into the magnitude of cancer risk or complications.

The NCI established the Surveillance, Epidemiology, and End Results (SEER) Program in 1973 as a way to report population-based data in site-specific incidences of cancer, mortality, and survival rates. This report is based on a sample of 12% of the U.S. population and includes six large cities (San Francisco, Oakland, Detroit, New Orleans, Atlanta, and Seattle). It also contains data from six states (New Jersey, Utah, Connecticut, New Mexico, Hawaii, and Iowa) and the Commonwealth of Puerto Rico. This is an ongoing project and provides a great deal of information about different geographic areas and ethnic groups.

Incidence

The *incidence rate* for cancer reflects the number of new cases occurring in a given population at risk during a specified time (Fig. 23–1). The incidence gives a perspective on the current magnitude of the problem and provides a source for establishing future priorities in cancer control programs. Factors that influence cancer incidence and deaths include gender, age, geographic location, socioeconomic status, ethnic background, personal habits (including diet), occupation, and personal and family histories of cancer or precancerous conditions.

The incidence of reported cases of cancer has been increasing steadily since 1900. There are at least three reasons for this apparent increase. First, diagnostic methods are more precise today than in the past. Thus, people who would have died from what were believed to be unknown causes or pulmonary hemorrhage in the past are now correctly diagnosed with cancer. Second, the gathering, analysis, and publication of cancer statistics have become more sophisticated over the years. Formerly,

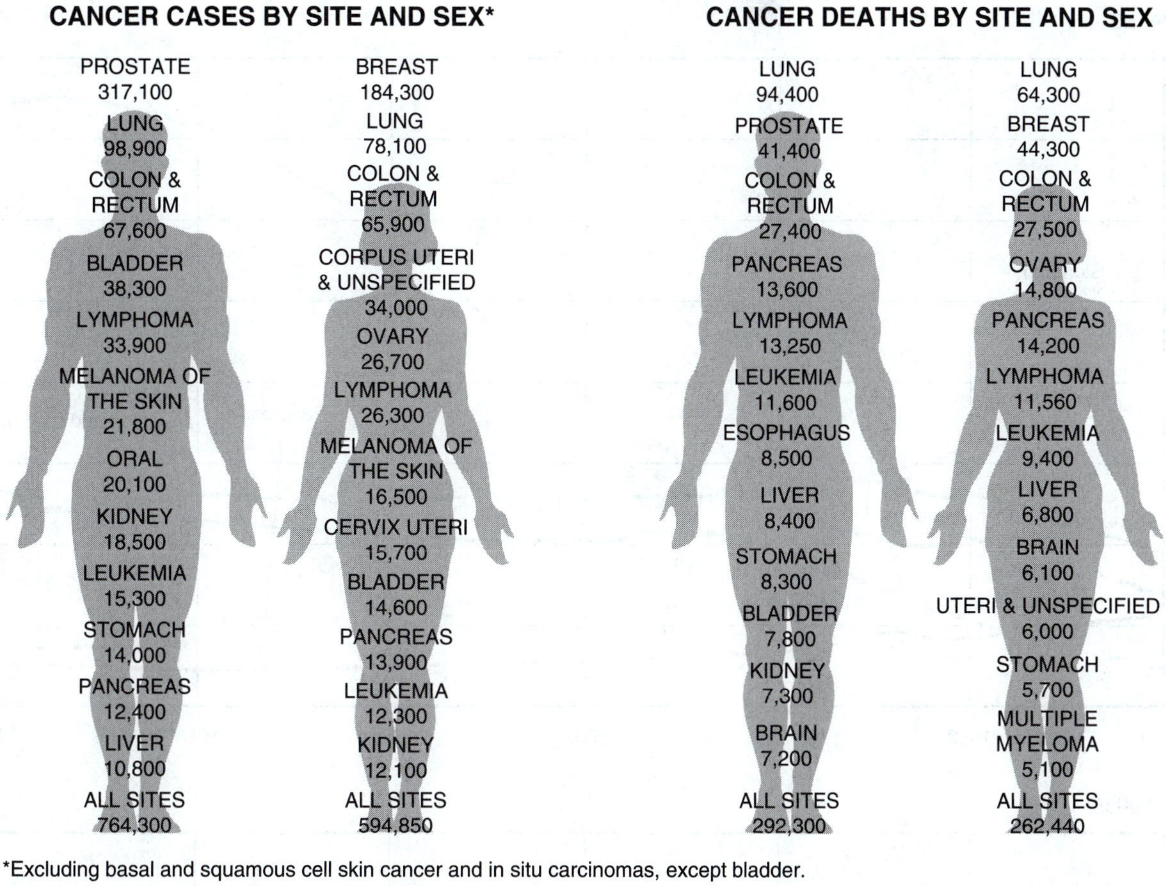

CANCER CASES BY SITE AND SEX*

PROSTATE
317,100

LUNG
98,900

COLON & RECTUM
67,600

BLADDER
38,300

LYMPHOMA
33,900

MELANOMA OF THE SKIN
21,800

ORAL
20,100

KIDNEY
18,500

LEUKEMIA
15,300

STOMACH
14,000

PANCREAS
12,400

LIVER
10,800

ALL SITES
764,300

BREAST
184,300

LUNG
78,100

COLON & RECTUM
65,900

CORPUS UTERI & UNSPECIFIED
34,000

OVARY
26,700

LYMPHOMA
26,300

MELANOMA OF THE SKIN
16,500

CERVIX UTERI
15,700

BLADDER
14,600

PANCREAS
13,900

LEUKEMIA
12,300

KIDNEY
12,100

ALL SITES
594,850

CANCER DEATHS BY SITE AND SEX

LUNG
94,400

PROSTATE
41,400

COLON & RECTUM
27,400

PANCREAS
13,600

LYMPHOMA
13,250

LEUKEMIA
11,600

ESOPHAGUS
8,500

LIVER
8,400

STOMACH
8,300

BLADDER
7,800

KIDNEY
7,300

BRAIN
7,200

ALL SITES
292,300

LUNG
64,300

BREAST
44,300

COLON & RECTUM
27,500

OVARY
14,800

PANCREAS
14,200

LYMPHOMA
11,560

LEUKEMIA
9,400

LIVER
6,800

BRAIN
6,100

UTERI & UNSPECIFIED
6,000

STOMACH
5,700

MULTIPLE MYELOMA
5,100

ALL SITES
262,440

*Excluding basal and squamous cell skin cancer and in situ carcinomas, except bladder.

Figure 23–1. Cancer incidence by site and sex, and cancer deaths by site and sex—1996 estimates. (Data from American Cancer Society [1996]. *Cancer facts and figures—1996.* Atlanta: Author.)

many cases of cancer were not included in the yearly reports on cancer morbidity and mortality. Finally, people are living longer than even a few decades ago. Older adults are at greater risk for many cancers; therefore, the incidence of cancer is higher now than when people died younger. Therefore, the apparent rise in the incidence of cancer may be somewhat misleading. It may simply reflect more precise diagnostic and statistical methods combined with the trend toward a longer lifespan. It is also true, however, that many life-style behaviors, such as smoking, alcohol intake, and multiple sex partners, are linked to an increased risk of cancer.

Mortality

The *mortality rate* is the number of deaths that occur in the population at risk in a specific period (Fig. 23–2). The data used to determine mortality rates are from death certificates. Although some of that information may be inaccurate or incomplete, it is a solid beginning in helping describe and determine the number of deaths attributed to cancer.

Survival

Generally, clinicians consider that the person who has no evidence of disease and has the same life expectancy as a person who has never had cancer is said to be cured of the cancer. The old 5-year survival marker is referred to as the relative survival rate. Although the 5-year determination is arbitrary, in many cancers this waiting period decreases the probability that the condition will recur or spread.

Survival data for the most common cancer sites are displayed in Figure 23–3. A 5-year relative survival rate of 50% is expected in many of the cancers listed. The lower survival in blacks for most cancer classifications is striking. This difference may be due to a variety of factors, including limited access to healthcare, no or little medical insurance, no primary healthcare provider, homelessness, poverty, lack of knowledge regarding early diagnosis and treatment, attitude toward primary and secondary prevention, and greater exposure to carcinogens.

Survival analysis is used to evaluate the effectiveness of cancer therapies, determine whether or not the interval between disease onset and treatment initiation could be modified to reduce cancer morbidity or mortality, and develop hypotheses regarding cancer risk factors.

Trends

The change in 5-year relative survival rates is shown in Table 23–2. Although the 5-year survival rate has increased from 1960 to 1990 when races are combined, not all cancers have seen significant increases in survival. In

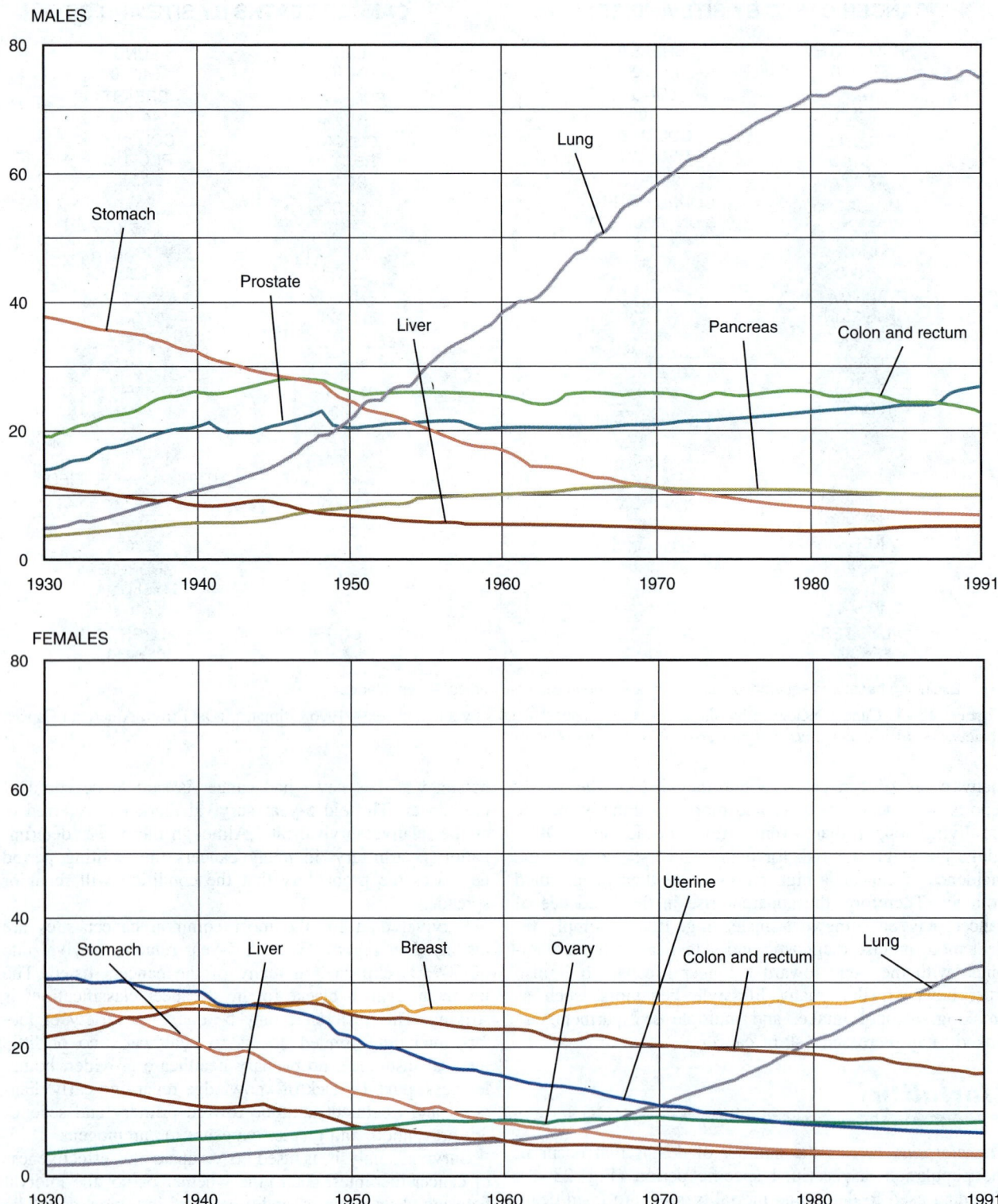

Figure 23–2. Cancer death rates by site in males and females in the United States from 1930–1991. Rates are per 100,000 and are age-adjusted to the 1970 U.S. census population. (From American Cancer Society [1995]. *Cancer facts and figures—1995.* Atlanta: Author.)

fact, cancer of the oral cavity and pharynx, liver, pancreas, esophagus, and colon have decreased or increased less than 10%. At the same time, the survival rate for Hodgkin's disease and prostate, testicular, and bladder cancers has increased by at least 25%.

Despite significant advances in detection, diagnosis, and treatment, cancer continues to be a significant health problem. It is believed that 75% of all cancers could be prevented if primary prevention (such as smoking cessation) was initiated against known causative factors by the

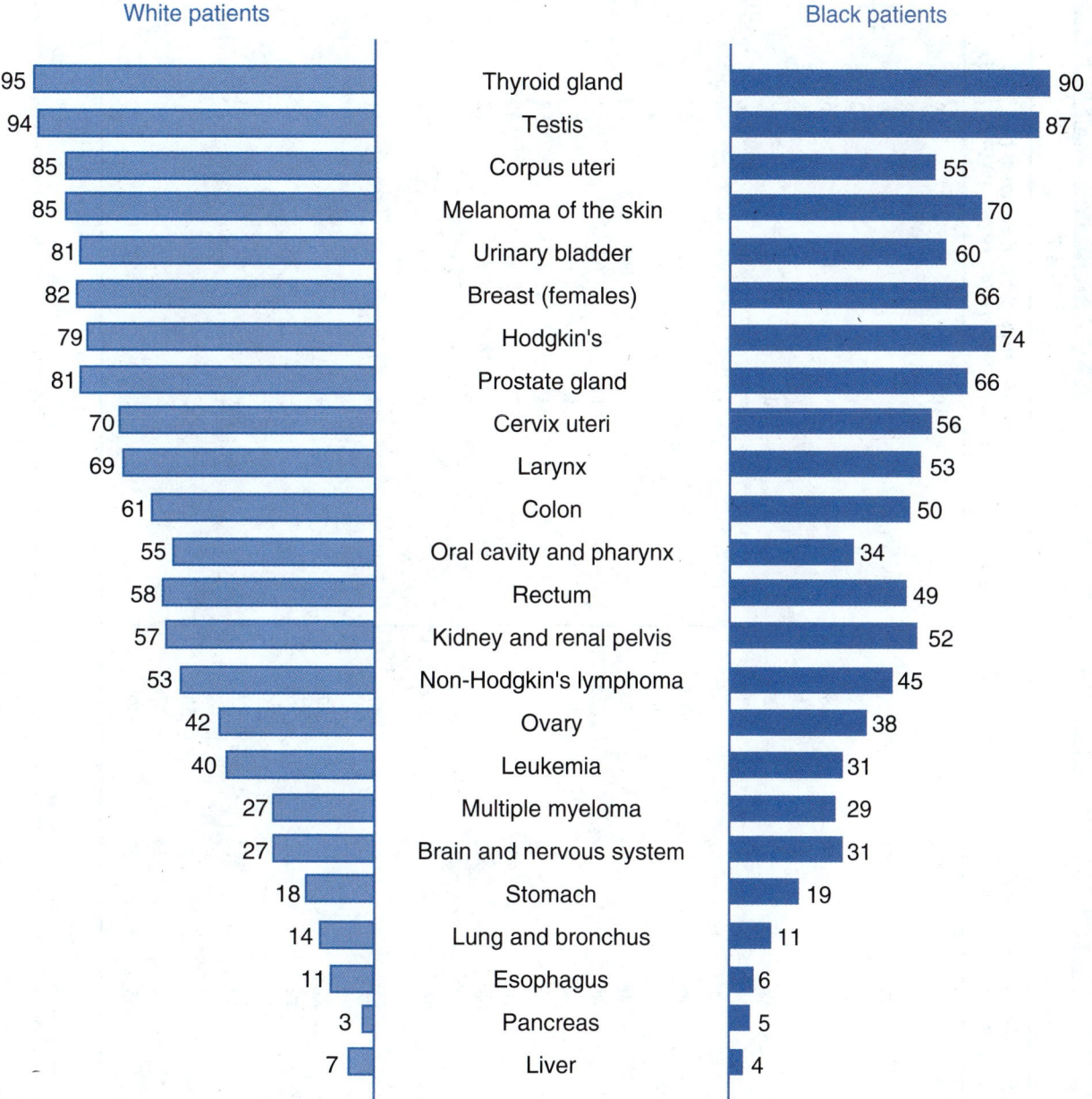

Figure 23–3. Five-year relative cancer survival rates from the Surveillance, Epidemiology, and End Results (SEER) program from 1983–1990. (From American Cancer Society [1995]. *Cancer facts and figures—1995*. Atlanta: Author. Data from Cancer Statistics Branch, National Cancer Institute, based on data from population-based registries in Connecticut, New Mexico, Utah, Iowa, Hawaii, Atlanta, Detroit, Seattle-Puget Sound, New Orleans, and San Francisco-Oakland. Rates are based on follow-up of patients through 1991.)

government, industry, and the public. Prevention and early detection of cancer must be a high priority to further decrease cancer morbidity and mortality rates.

Pathogenesis

The exact causes and methods of the development of cancer are unknown. The theories of cellular transforma-

tion and derangement and failure of the immune response are common explanations for the development of cancer.

Cellular Transformation and Derangement

Although scientists have learned a great deal about the causes of cancer, the exact mechanism by which these

Table 23-2. Trends in Survival by Site of Cancer, by Race

Site/Tumor	White Relative 5-Year Survival (%)					Black Relative 5-Year Survival (%)				
	1960–1963*	1970–1973*	1974–1976†	1977–1979†	1983–1990†	1960–1963*	1970–1973*	1974–1976†	1977–1979†	1983–1990†
All sites	39	43	50	51	56‡	27	31	39	39	40‡
Oral cavity and pharynx	45	43	55	54	55	—	—	36	36	34
Esophagus	4	4	5	6	11‡	1	4	4	3	6‡
Stomach	11	13	14	16	18‡	8	13	16	15	19
Colon	43	49	50	53	61‡	34	37	46	48	50‡
Rectum	38	45	49	51	58‡	27	30	42	38	49
Liver	—	2	4	3	7‡	1	—	1	6	4
Pancreas	1	2	3	2	3‡	1	2	2	4	5‡
Larynx	53	62	66	68	69§	—	—	59	55	53
Lung and bronchus	8	10	12	14	14‡	5	7	11	11	11
Melanoma of skin	60	68	80	82	85‡	—	—	66§	51¶	70§
Female breast	63	68	75	75	82‡	46	51	63	63	66‡
Cervix uteri	58	64	69	69	70	47	61	64	62	56‡
Corpus uteri	73	81	89	86	85‡	31	44	60	58	55
Ovary	32	36	36	38	42‡	32	32	40	40	38
Prostate	50	63	68	72	81‡	35	55	58	62	66‡
Testis	63	72	79	88	94‡	—	—	76§	—	87
Urinary bladder	53	61	74	76	81‡	24	36	48	55	60‡
Kidney and renal pelvis	37	46	51	51	57‡	38	44	49	51	52
Brain and nervous system	18	20	22	24	27‡	19	19	27	28	31
Thyroid gland	83	86	92	92	95‡	—	—	88	91	90
Hodgkin's disease	40	67	72	73	79‡	—	—	68	73	74
Non-Hodgkin's lymphoma	31	41	48	48	53‡	—	—	48	50	45
Multiple myeloma	12	19	24	25	27‡	—	—	27	34	29
Leukemia	14	22	35	38	40‡	—	—	32	30	31

Modified from American Cancer Society (1995). *Cancer facts and figures—1995.* Atlanta: Author.

* Rates are based on end results group data from a series of hospital registries and one population-based registry.

† Rates are from the Surveillance, Epidemiology, and End Results program. They are based on data from population-based registries in Connecticut, New Mexico, Utah, Iowa, Hawaii, Atlanta, Detroit, Seattle–Puget Sound, and San Francisco-Oakland. Rates are based on follow-up of patients through 1991.

‡ The difference in rates between 1974–1976 and 1983–1990 is statistically significant (*p* > .05).

§ The standard error of the survival rate is between 5 and 10 percentage points.

¶ The standard error of the survival rate is greater than 10 percentage points.

agents transform healthy cells into neoplastic cells remains obscure. One accepted premise is that cancer develops as a result of genetic alteration from one or more causes, resulting in uncontrolled cellular reproduction and growth. When a defective cell divides, the new cells contain the defective genetic code within the DNA. Over time, defective cells divide and multiply, and the malignancy grows.

Carcinogens are substances that, when introduced into the cell, cause changes in the structure and function of the cell that lead to cancer. It is not a simple cause-and-effect mechanism, however. There are three identified stages of carcinogenesis: (1) initiation, (2) promotion, and (3) progression.

Initiation occurs when a chemical, physical, or biologic agent damages DNA. This damage may be reversible or may lead to genetic mutation if not repaired; however, the mutation may not lead immediately to cancer. After this damage, cells are more susceptible to progression into malignancies. Irreversibly initiated cells do not display their changes and are not detectable until exposed to a promoting agent.

Promotion is usually the result of a second factor acting on the initiated cell. Some agents are called complete carcinogens because they produce both initiation and promotion. However, promotion may occur after very long periods of latency, which varies with the type of agent, dose, and characteristics of the target cell. Promoting agents work by changing the expression of genetic information within the cell, increasing DNA synthesis, increasing the number of copies of a particular gene, and altering cellular communications. Often exposure to the promoting agent is under the control of the client, as with tobacco, alcohol, and dietary fat.

Progression involves the morphologic and phenotypic changes in cells, which are associated with increasingly malignant behavior, leading to invasion of surrounding tissue and metastasis to distant body parts.

Failure of the Immune Response

Researchers are actively pursuing the role of immunity in preventing, controlling, and treating cancer. According to the immune theory of cancer control, cancer cells continually form within the body. The immune system perceives these cancer cells as foreign and destroys them. However, certain conditions either cause a breakdown or overwhelm the immune system. Thus, the malignant cells reproduce more rapidly than the immune system can destroy them.

Data from postoperative heart and kidney transplant clients support this theory. These clients are intentionally immunosuppressed to prevent the rejection of their transplanted organs. The risk of developing cancer is at least 80 times greater among persons who have undergone transplantation surgery than among the population as a whole. Further support for this theory comes from data on people with acquired immunodeficiency syndrome (AIDS). These persons have a much higher incidence of a number of cancers such as non-Hodgkin's lymphoma and

Kaposi's sarcoma. The immunodeficiency of AIDS makes them more susceptible to cancers.

Investigators are trying to determine whether the immune system controls the spontaneous regression of tumors, a mysterious phenomenon. Spontaneous regression of cancers occurs in about 1 in 100,000 cases. The role of the immune system in bringing about this seemingly miraculous change remains a provocative and unanswered question.

Etiology

There are approximately 150 types of cancers found in humans, and there are probably at least 500 different cancer-causing agents. Researchers suspect that cancer results from multiple agents working together.

Viruses

The study of viruses as carcinogens is one of the most rapidly advancing areas in cancer research today. Researchers now have proof that some viruses cause certain cancers in animals.

The study of viruses in tumors has led researchers to discover oncogenes. Oncogenes are small segments of genetic DNA that can transform normal cells into malignant cells, independently or incorporated into a virus.

Viruses probably do not, as single agents, cause cancer. However, viruses may be one of multiple agents acting to initiate carcinogenesis. Viruses have been associated with hepatocellular carcinoma, T-cell lymphoma, T-cell leukemia, Burkitt's lymphoma, nasopharyngeal carcinoma, and cervical cancer.

Chemical Agents

Some of the most common chemical carcinogens include tar, soot, asphalt, aniline dyes, hydrocarbons, crude paraffin oil, fuel oils, nickel, and arsenicals. Most of these agents cause cancer only after close and prolonged contact, and persons affected are usually workers in industries where these chemicals are used or occur as by-products such as in tanning, die making, refineries, and in battery-making factories.

Because organisms have different metabolic systems, potential carcinogens are metabolized one way in some organisms and in other ways in other organisms. Some organisms, humans included, may be more sensitive than others to certain carcinogens because of their metabolic differences.

Physical Agents

Physical carcinogens cause cellular damage just as chemical carcinogens do. Radiation and asbestos are physical carcinogens.

Two forms of radiation can lead to cancer: ultraviolet radiation and ionizing radiation. Ultraviolet radiation from the sun can cause changes in DNA structure that can lead to malignant transformation if it is not repaired. Basal and squamous cell carcinomas of the skin, as well as melanoma, are linked to ultraviolet exposure.

Excessive exposure to ionizing radiation can cause permanent DNA mutation and transformation into a malignant growth. Most radiation exposure is from natural sources (radon, cosmic, terrestrial, and internal radiation). Preventive measures are usually focused on minimizing exposure to manufactured sources of radiation such as x-rays and isotopes, which are used in medical diagnosis and treatment.

In the United States, asbestos, a carcinogenic fiber, contributes significantly to the occurrence of bronchogenic cancer and mesothelioma. There is a strong synergistic relation between tobacco smoke and asbestos. The mechanism of action of asbestos is unknown. Another example of a synergistic effect is that of alcohol and tobacco. The combination of agents is a much stronger carcinogen.

Drugs and Hormones

Scientists have demonstrated that a relationship exists between hormonal secretion, action, tumor development, and growth. Exactly what the relationship is remains obscure. Do hormones actually cause normal cells to change into cancer cells? Do hormones act only to promote the growth of tumors caused by other factors? The answers to these questions lie in future research.

One of the most controversial topics in carcinogenesis is the role of estrogen. Animal studies have shown that estrogen is involved in the development of breast cancer. Human studies indicate that estrogen is related to human breast cancer but the relationship is poorly defined.

Cancer chemotherapeutic agents are carcinogenic, and cancer clients are at risk for future development of leukemia and other cancers (see Chapter 53 for further discussion on this topic).

Predisposing Factors

In addition to the carcinogens described, there are also predisposing factors that influence the host's susceptibility to various etiologic agents.

Age

While cancer affects people of all ages, it is generally considered a disease of older age, with 67% of cancer deaths occurring after the age of 65.[6] Many cancers, such as prostate and colon cancer and some chronic leukemias, have increased incidence in older people. Older people may be more susceptible to cancer simply because they have been exposed to carcinogens longer than younger people. Also, as people age, their immune system becomes impaired. The immune response failure theory suggests that this problem alone could make people more susceptible to cancers.

Also, there are cancers that occur within very narrow age ranges. Testicular cancer is found in men from about 20 to 40 years of age. Ovarian cancer is more common in women over 55 years of age. Many cancers occur mainly in childhood, such as Ewing's sarcoma, certain acute leukemias, Wilms' tumor, and retinoblastoma.

Sex

Women are more susceptible to certain types of cancer than men are, and vice versa. Since 1949, more men than women have died from all types of cancer. The increased incidence of cancer deaths among men apparently relates to the higher incidence and mortality of lung cancer, which is currently almost twice that of women. More women, however, are smoking, leading to an increase in lung cancer in women. Lung cancer is now the leading killer of both men and women. Oral cancer death rates are almost twice as high for men as for women.

Geographic Location

The incidence of different types of cancer varies on a geographic basis. For example, the incidence of stomach cancer is higher in Japan than in the United States. On the other hand, breast cancer is rare in Japan but has a high incidence in the United States, Europe, and Israel. These differences may reflect the influence of environmental factors (diet, customs, pollutants in the environment) rather than genetic differences between races and nationalities. This explanation seems likely because when Japanese women live in the United States, their rate of breast cancer is the same as that of other women in the United States.

Geographic differences exist in this country also. In highly urbanized areas, colon cancer is more prevalent than in rural areas. The industrialized areas have higher amounts of polluted air, so rates of lung cancer are higher. In rural areas, particularly among farmers, skin cancer is more common. Colon cancer is more common in the industrialized Northeast and Great Lakes region. The greater susceptibility in certain geographic areas is probably related to exposure to different carcinogens, especially substances in the environment. There is also an increase in skin cancer in the Sun Belt of the United States.

Occupation

People in certain occupations are more susceptible to certain cancers because of their greater contact with specific carcinogens. For example, workers in asbestos factories have a higher incidence of lung cancer because of their chronic exposure to asbestos. People who work around hydrocarbons, especially benzene, have a higher rate of bladder cancer. Radium miners have a higher incidence of leukemia from the exposure to radioactivity. Radiologists also have a higher rate of leukemia.

Heredity

There are a number of cancers that provide evidence of a heritable predisposition to cancer. Fanconi anemia, ataxia-telangiectasia, and xeroderma pigmentosum are examples of autosomal recessive conditions that predispose persons to a variety of malignancies. Familial polyposis coli, retinoblastoma, Wilms' tumor, and neurofibromatosis are examples of autosomal dominant disorders that follow classic mendelian patterns of inheritance.[38] Breast, ovarian, and colon cancers may also show a familial pattern.

Diet

Links between diet and nutrition have been detected. People 40% or more overweight have an increased risk of colon, breast, prostate, gallbladder, ovary, and uterine cancer. Studies have shown that daily consumption of vegetables and fresh fruits is associated with a decreased risk of lung, prostate, bladder, esophagus, colorectal, and stomach cancers. High fiber diets may reduce the risk of colon cancer. A diet high in fat may be a factor in the development of breast, colon, and prostate cancers. Excessive alcohol, especially when accompanied by cigarette smoking, increases the risk of cancers of the mouth, larynx, throat, esophagus, and liver. A higher incidence of cancer of the esophagus and stomach has been noted in areas of the world where salt-cured, smoked, and nitrite-cured foods are eaten frequently.

The American Cancer Society Guidelines on Diet, Nutrition, and Cancers[2] were developed with the above considerations in mind. Although the potential for substantial reduction in cancer incidence by dietary modification alone appears remote, a diet rich in fruits and fiber and low in animal fats is desirable for many health reasons.

Fad anticancer diets and drugs prey on the ignorance and fear of many people. Before a specific diet is recommended as helpful in the fight against cancer, it is important to evaluate its overall nutritional content and be aware of any harmful effects it may generate.

Stress

Recent research suggests that stress may increase the risk of cancer. Chronic physical or emotional stress preys on the hypothalamus, the portion of the pituitary gland that regulates hormone and immune systems. Increased stress causes hormonal or immunologic changes, or both, which in turn may spur the growth and proliferation of cancer cells. The field of study that explores these relationships is called *psychoneuroimmunology.*

Precancerous Lesions

Precancerous lesions and some benign tumors may undergo transformation later into cancerous lesions and tumors. Common precancerous lesions include pigmented moles, burn scars, senile keratoses, leukoplakia, and benign adenomas or polyps of the colon or stomach. These lesions need to be periodically assessed for malignant changes.

Impact

Physical Impact

Physical changes can occur in the client throughout the cancer experience. The malignant tumor itself may cause obvious disfigurement or internal organ changes even prior to diagnosis. For example, some skin cancers are potentially disfiguring and colon cancer can cause internal change, including obstruction, before diagnosis.

Treatment for a malignant tumor also may cause the client to experience physical changes. Surgery may be mutilative, as in the amputation of a breast or an extremity. Radiation therapy may cause changes in body functions and skin integrity. Chemotherapy may lead to hair loss, weight gain or loss, and skin pigmentation changes.

Clients, therefore, live not only with the physical indicators of the disease but with the sequelae of its treatment as well. Although some of the physical changes of cancer are a result of treatment, the changes affect a client's self-concept, self-esteem, and general feelings of worth and acceptance (see Chapter 24 for further discussion).

Psychosocial Impact

Historically, studies of persons with cancer were used to identify unique psychosocial responses to cancer, describe types of coping behaviors, and guide healthcare professionals in assisting the client with cancer to adjust to the diagnosis, the demands of treatment, and the requirements of living with cancer. The variability of psychosocial responses is increased by the fact that people bring their own sets of values, beliefs, attitudes, resources, and coping mechanisms to the cancer experience.

Anxiety and depression are the most common psychosocial reactions in people with cancer.[15] Each person reacts to the diagnosis differently and has unique concerns and problems regarding the diagnosis and treatment.

Health professionals can guide and facilitate open communication between the client, significant others, and healthcare providers to reduce anxiety and depression and foster optimism. These discussions with the client and significant others must be honest and open regarding the disease, treatment options, and prognosis so that false hope or unrealistic fears can be lessened. The nurse can help the client in many ways. First, the nurse can help the client recognize the manifestations of anxiety. Often, simply helping the client identify these behaviors can help him or her to cope more effectively. If the client is suffering from severe depression, the nurse should spend time with the client and possibly suggest counseling. It is also helpful for the client to know that these feelings are normal. There are many support groups (such as I Can Cope, Make Today Count, New Voice Club) available for these clients to help them establish effective support systems.

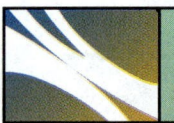

RISK FACTORS AND LEVELS OF PREVENTION

Common Cancers

Risk Factors

Bladder Cancer: Exposure to aniline dye, print, coal, tar, or asbestos; occupations in the apparel, textile, leather, and painting industries; white race

Colon and Rectal Cancer: History of ulcerative colitis, colorectal adenomas, or bladder, breast, colon, or female genital cancer; increasing age; sedentary life-style; familial predisposition

Gastric Cancer: Family history of gastric cancer; history of gastric resection; blood group A; atrophic gastric mucosa; gastric ulcers; pernicious anemia; stomach polyps; low socioeconomic level; nonwhite race

Leukemia: Age (childhood for acute and old age for chronic); Down or Klinefelter's syndrome; an identical twin with leukemia; viruses; immunologic factors; genetic factors; exposure to ionizing radiation or benzene; occupation as poultry farmer, explosives or rubber cement worker, radiologist, distiller, dye user, painter, radium miner, or chemist

Lung Cancer: Family history of lung cancer; exposure to environmental pollution; cigarette smoking

Skin Cancer: Family history of melanoma; fair skin or hair; increasing age; history of organ transplant, dysplastic nevi, burns, topical ulcers, or scars from squamous or basal cell carcinoma

Special Risk Factors in Men: Increased risk of bladder cancer and leukemia. *Prostate cancer:* black race; increasing age; exposure to cadmium; history of venereal disease; possibly sexual activity. *Testicular cancer:* white race; cryptorchidism; age between 20 and 40 years; family history of testicular cancer, diethylstilbestrol (DES) exposure in utero; atrophic testicles

Special Risk Factors in Women: **Breast cancer:** Family history of breast cancer, especially on the maternal side and occurring before menopause; history of previous breast cancer or other gynecologic cancer or benign breast disease; early menarche or late menopause; birth of first child after age 30; nulliparity; Jewish; white; single; high socioeconomic level; increasing age. **Cervical cancer:** black race; intercourse with uncircumcised males; early frequent intercourse with multiple sex partners, multiparity; chronic cervicitis; history of genital herpes or human papilloma virus (HPV) infection. **Ovarian cancer:** history of breast cancer or pelvic radiation; nulliparity or first pregnancy after age 30; white; high income level. **Uterine and endometrial cancer:** history of hypertension, diabetes mellitus, menstrual disorders; high socioeconomic level; nulliparity; infertility related to anovulation; long-term use of conjugated estrogens; Stein-Leventhal syndrome

Levels of Prevention

Primary Prevention

Encourage clients to stop smoking cigarettes and pipes and to avoid smokeless tobacco and snuff to prevent bladder, lung, laryngeal, throat, and oral cancer; educate clients about the risk of secondary smoke to nonsmokers

  Advise clients, especially those who work outdoors, to limit sun exposure to prevent basal and squamous cell skin cancer, melanoma, and oral (lip) cancer; excessive sunbathing or sunburn before age 20 may predispose to skin cancer

  Educate clients to the risks of radon exposure in their homes; this exposure may increase their risk of lung cancer, especially if they are smokers

Financial Impact

■ Impact on the Client and Family

The diagnosis and treatment of cancer are expensive. Medical intervention is intricate and drawn out. Not surprisingly, the financial consequences of the illness are a major concern to the cancer client. Sometimes, even if the client has health insurance, the cost can be astronomical. The client without private insurance may be unable to afford needed care. Medicaid, in some states, will not pay for expensive treatments such as bone marrow transplants (BMTs). A BMT can cost from $60,000 to $250,000, more than most people can afford. Moving cancer care to outpatient, ambulatory care centers or the home helps reduce the cost. This move, however, means that the client must have adequate support at home, potentially leading to an increasing caregiver burden.

  Unfortunately, not all procedures can be administered outside the hospital. Primary and secondary prevention

Encourage overweight clients to lose weight to lower the risk of colorectal, breast, uterine, and endometrial cancers

Teach clients that high-fat diets may contribute to development of breast, colon, or prostate cancer; diets that are high in sugar also may be a risk factor for prostate cancer; saccharin use may contribute to bladder cancer

Encourage clients to eat high fiber foods to reduce risk of colon cancer; emphasize the importance of a varied diet including vegetables and fruits rich in vitamins A and C to reduce the risk of a wide range of cancers; salt-cured, smoked (especially fish and mutton), nitrite-cured foods, and rice treated with talc have been linked to esophagus and stomach cancer

Encourage clients to avoid high alcohol intake, especially if they smoke cigarettes or chew tobacco, to lower the risk of oral cancer and cancers of the bladder, larynx, throat, esophagus, and liver

Advise women to consult with a physician to assess the personal risks and benefits of estrogen treatment, which increases the risk of endometrial cancer (including progesterone in estrogen replacement therapy helps to minimize the risk)

Teach clients that exposure to various industrial agents (e.g., benzene, nickel, chromate, asbestos, vinyl chloride) increases the risk of various cancers; risk from asbestos is greatly increased when combined with cigarette smoking

Encourage clients to maintain good oral hygiene, dental care, and well-fitting dentures to prevent oral cancers

Secondary Prevention

Teach women to begin mammography screening by age 40 to detect breast cancer; women age 40 to 49 should have mammography every 1 to 2 years, depending on physical and mammographic findings; women age 50 and older should have mammograms yearly

Encourage women 20 years and older to practice breast self-examination monthly

Encourage women age 20 to 40 to get clinical breast examinations every 3 years; women older than 40 should get clinical breast examinations yearly

Advise patients older than 40 to get a digital rectal examination by a physician every year to detect colorectal and prostate cancer; patients older than 50 should have a stool blood test done every year. Ensure that patients have a sigmoidoscopy every 3 to 5 years, based on the advice of the physician

Teach women who are 18 and older, or who are or have been sexually active, to have an annual Pap test and pelvic examination to detect cervical cancer; after a woman has had three or more normal annual examinations, the Pap test may be performed less frequently at the discretion of her physician

Encourage men age 50 and older to have annual prostate-specific antigen blood testing to detect prostate cancer

Monitor clients who take drugs such as melphalan, cyclophosphamide (Cytoxan), or chloramphenicol; they have an increased risk of leukemia

Monitor clients with schistosomiasis or who are being treated with cyclophosphamide for evidence of bladder cancer

Monitor clients with vitamin B complex and iron deficiencies for oral cancers

Monitor clients being treated with PUVA for psoriasis for development of skin cancer

---

Adapted from Groenwald, S., et al. (1993). *Cancer nursing: Principles and practice* (3rd ed.). Boston: Jones and Bartlett; and American Cancer Society (1995). *Cancer facts and figures*—1995. Atlanta: Author.

methods, described in the Risk Factors and Levels of Prevention feature, also can help lower the cost either by preventing the cancer or by treating it sooner.

Although up to 80% of clients with cancer return to work after diagnosis and treatment of cancer,[17] depending on the type and stage of cancer, a client may find it necessary to work fewer hours, find a different line of work, or in extreme cases, stop working altogether. If the client is the main source of income and insurance benefits, a reduction in work hours or loss of work may have catastrophic consequences.

Because a social stigma is still associated with the diagnosis of cancer, clients may be denied their former jobs or job benefits (insurance included) when their cancer becomes known to those in the workplace. It is, however, illegal to terminate someone based on the diagnosis of cancer. The Federal Rehabilitation Act of 1973 and the Americans with Disabilities Act prohibit discrimination against an employee based on a real or perceived handicap. The Americans with Disabilities Act applies to any private employer with 15 or more employees and prohibits discrimination in hiring, promotions, firing, pay, job training, and job benefits (including insurance). Many states also protect cancer clients against job discrimination.

Unfortunately, there is no federal protection against the loss of insurance that occurs. An estimated 25% to 30% of persons with cancer face some form of insurance discrimination.[18] The COBRA federal law requires employers with 20 employees or more to offer a continuation of group medical coverage to those whose circumstances warrant reducing or changing work hours or to those who must leave a job.[16] To help the client and family deal with the overall cancer experience, the nurse must discuss personal financial obligations and responsibilities and the changes diagnosis and treatment may bring.

■ Impact on the Economy

Costs may be direct or indirect. Direct costs involve cancer prevention, diagnosis, and treatment. They also include payment for chronic and acute care facilities, nursing and medical services, research, and professional education. Indirect costs include loss of national productivity due to the absence of clients with cancer and caregivers of clients who opt for many more ambulatory treatments, especially that of bone marrow transplant, from the workforce.

Cancer also affects the economy of the society. In this time of limited access to healthcare, questions are being raised about the cost of cancer care. Cancer care costs an estimated $104 billion annually. As technology advances and medical costs increase, the cost of cancer care will become even greater in the future. It is unlikely that this nation can afford the ever-increasing cost of healthcare.

Research

Both physicians and nurses contribute to cancer research. Medical research focuses on the natural history of the disease, new treatment approaches, and single versus multimodal approaches to medical treatment. Nursing research focuses on the client with cancer and the client's family rather than on the cancer, and may include biologic, psychological, and social aspects.[29] The Oncology Nursing Society (ONS) has fostered a great deal of nursing research. The *ONS Standards of Nursing Practice* includes a statement about the importance of research and the need for the oncology nurse to be actively involved. Research priorities within oncology include symptoms and symptom management, such as care of clients with fatigue, pain, and nausea.

Clinical Trials

The NCI has developed a method of testing new cancer treatments, especially chemotherapy. There are several stages in this method, commonly known as phase I, II, III, and IV clinical trials. Information is available on these trials from the Physician's Data Query, a computer program accessible by modem, through a medical library, or by calling 1-800-4-CANCER. Each phase has well-defined guidelines. Phase I studies determine the maximum tolerated dose of a new agent and access its toxicity. Phase II trials determine the efficacy of the agent in different types of cancer. Phase III trials compare the new agent with the standard treatment, and in phase IV trials, the agent is given to large numbers of people with the same tumor type to confirm its efficacy. If an agent successfully meets the criteria of the clinical trials, Food and Drug Association (FDA) approval is granted and the agent is approved to treat specific cancers.

Ethical Issues

Ethical issues related to cancer research include informed consent, which encompasses client competence; disclosure and understanding of information; voluntariness; and confidentiality. Although in any given institution it may be the physician's responsibility to obtain informed consent prior to the client's inclusion in a research protocol, it is always the nurse's responsibility to ascertain a client's competence, and his or her understanding of the given information, and to obtain voluntary participation prior to the initiation of any treatment or therapy. Clients need to know that they can withdraw from the trial at any time without jeopardizing their access to medical care. The nurse must also oversee that protocols are followed and extra tests are not performed without the client's knowledge.

Prevention and Assessment

Characteristics of Normal Cells

Chapter 14 explores general characteristics of normal cells. Specific characteristics of normal cells that help us understand changes that occur in neoplastic cells are (1) the cell cycle, (2) differentiation, and (3) contact inhibition.

The Cell Cycle. The concept of the cell cycle has increased researchers' understanding of how both normal and neoplastic cells replicate (Fig. 23–4). The cell's replication cycle is divided into the following intervals, or steps, with the letter G standing for "gap"—the interval separating mitosis (M) and synthesis (S).

G_0 Phase. This phase is the interval in which the cell is at rest (until a trigger in the immediate environment signals the beginning of the G_1 phase). Some cells do not replicate, or they replicate so infrequently that they are always said to be in G_0 state.

G_1 Phase. This phase is the interval in which RNA and protein are synthesized. The period of time the cell is in G_1 varies, depending on the type of cell and the proliferative activity of the tissue. With high activity, the G_1 interval is short. The interval lengthens when activity is low. The acquisition of the ability to begin DNA synthesis marks the termination of G_1.

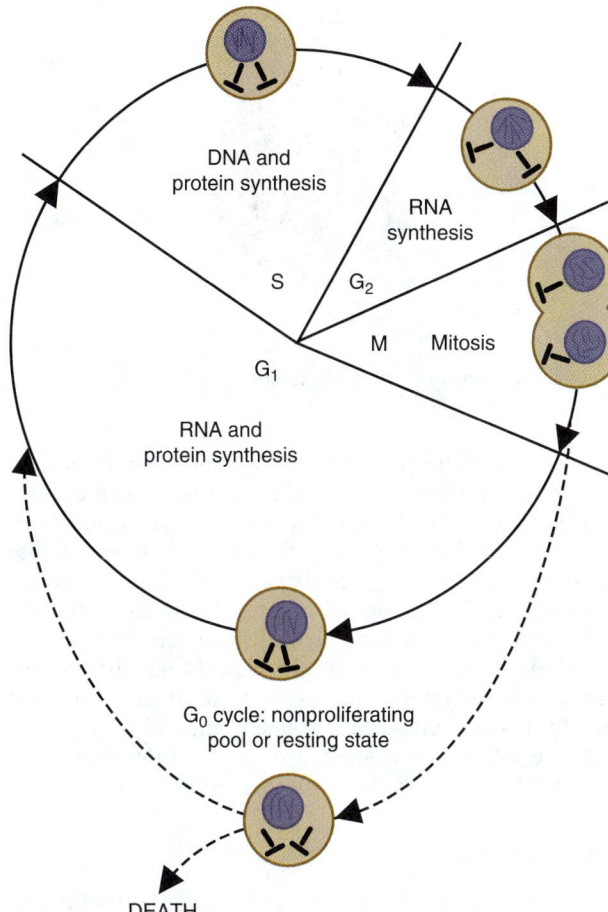

Figure 23–4. The cell cycle. Periods of DNA synthesis *(S)* and mitosis *(M)* are divided by gaps *(G)* in which the cell is in a resting state *(G₀)*, producing substances in preparation for DNA synthesis *(G₁)*, or producing proteins and some RNA in preparation for mitosis *(G₂)*.

S Phase. Synthesis of both DNA and proteins of new chromosomes occurs. The interval of time is probably 6 to 8 hours. It varies in certain cell populations and under different circumstances.

G₂ Phase. Biochemical processes, including synthesis of some RNA, occur in preparation for mitosis. Little is known about this phase, which may last only a few hours.

M Phase. Actual division of the cell—mitosis—occurs, producing two daughter cells. The duration of this phase usually ranges from less than an hour to a few hours.

In the normal mature organ, cell cycling is carefully controlled so that the organ maintains its function. Cells that die are replaced, but no extra cells are produced. Researchers are investigating the mechanisms of this control, which are not fully understood.

Differentiation. In the embryo, genetically identical cells assume various structures and functions. One muscle cell looks like all the other muscle cells but not much like a kidney or liver cell. The process is called differentiation.

Contact Inhibition. When normal cells are grown outside the body on culture plates, they exhibit an interesting characteristic called contact inhibition. Normal cells spread freely about the culture medium until they contact another cell. Then they adhere to one another and align themselves in parallel. The cells grow until they reach the edges of the container, covering the surface in a single layer. At this point active growth stops.

Growth of Cancer Cells

Tumor growth is actually an increase in the number of cells. Cells may increase in number by (1) shortening the length of the cell cycle, (2) increasing the fraction of cells going through the cell cycle, or (3) decreasing cell loss. At one time, researchers believed that neoplastic cells divided much more rapidly than other cells in the body. This rapid division was thought to account for the mass of cells that developed. Later, investigators discovered that some normal cells proceed through the cell cycle faster than neoplastic cells. The current belief is that the fraction of proliferating cells in a tumor is higher, thus accounting for the tumor mass. There is also a decrease in cell death, with the ratio of cell birth exceeding cell death.

The concept of doubling time is central to the study of tumor growth. Theoretically, cancer could start as a single abnormal cell that divides to form two cells, then four cells, and so on. Provided that the amount of time for the cell cycle remains constant, the tumor mass would double with each cell cycle (Fig. 23–5). Cancer cells are capable of having more than two daughter cells at one time.

Although some tumors steadily enlarge, this factor does not entirely account for their growth. Also, cycling times vary with the type of tumor. Cell losses are considerable in all tumors, and may counterbalance new cell output in some. Approximately 20 doublings will occur before a 1 mm³ tumor is produced. This is the smallest mass that can be detected clinically. At 30 doublings, the mass would be about 1 cm³, weighing 1 g, still a small lesion by any standards. Ten more doublings bring the mass to 1 kg, but only five more doublings bring the mass to 32 kg, or half the body weight! Another five doublings and the tumor would weigh about 1000 kg.

Clearly, the cell cycle of a tumor is of great clinical significance. First, the slower the cell cycle of the tumor, the longer it is before the tumor can be identified. Second, Figure 23–5 shows that the preclinical period of growth is approximately two thirds of the total growth period. This fact helps us to understand how metastasis or spread of a tumor occurs, even when the original tumor is small. It also explains why the physician requires a long period of time following removal of the tumor before being assured that the person is cancer-free. Also, malignant cells with a short cell cycle are typically more sensitive to chemotherapy.

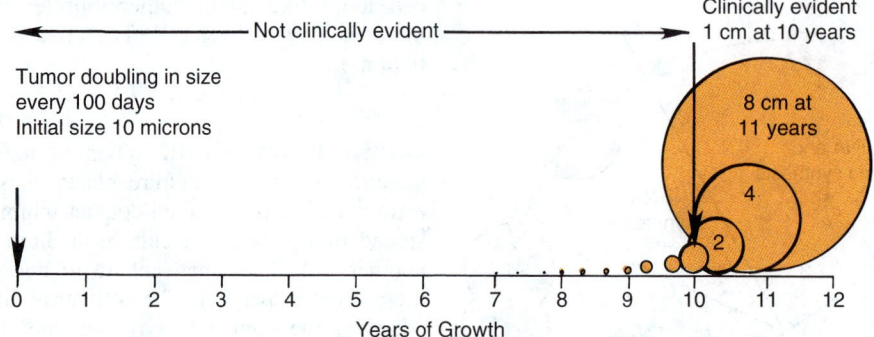

Figure 23–5. A depiction of tumor growth, showing doubling time related to tumor size.

Neoplastic Cell Division and Differentiation

Despite research advances, investigators still have unanswered questions about cancer. What is a cancer cell? How does it differ from a normal cell, and what are the factors that cause cancer cells to develop? To better define abnormal cells and explain why they develop, researchers are learning more about normal cells and their regulation at the genetic level.

Characteristics of Neoplastic Cells

■ Appearance

Neoplastic cells differ from normal cells in appearance, pattern of growth, and physiologic function. The cells themselves are larger than normal and grow more rapidly. The nuclei of these cells are larger and more prominent than normal. The neoplastic cells exhibit pleomorphism (variability or heterogeneity in size and shape). The neoplastic cells bear little resemblance to the normal cells in the afflicted tissue and lack the characteristic organization of the host cells. Neoplastic tissue that differs radically from the host tissue is referred to as anaplastic. Anaplastic cells lack the differentiated cell characteristics, specific functions, and organization of normal cells (Table 23–3). Differentiated cells are functionally and structurally specialized, and are often nondividing.

■ Growth

The growth patterns of neoplastic cells also differ from those of normal cells. These cells flourish in antagonistic physical, chemical, hormonal, and viral environments. Neoplastic cells invade adjacent tissue. Malignant cells grow well under adverse conditions that would keep other cells from growing. The growth rate is also very erratic.

There is a loss of cellular control in neoplastic cells as a consequence of changes in the cell membrane. They exhibit increase mitosis, with multiple mitotic spindles, leading to the development of more than the normal two daughter cells at the end of mitosis. The normal limits of replication do not exist in neoplastic cells, which leads to

uncontrolled replication. Also, neoplastic cells do not exhibit contact inhibition, and cell birth exceeds cell death.

Neoplastic cells also exhibit other growth characteristics that normal cells do not. Neoplastic cells are able to break off proliferative cells that enter the circulation and migrate from their tissue of origin. These cells form emboli that lodge in distant areas, where they are able to extravasate (leak out) from the vessels and begin new proliferation in foreign tissues. Neoplastic cells are also able to invade lymphatic channels and move with the lymph to other nodes. They also can seed throughout the body cavities, such as the peritoneal cavity.

■ Function

Malignant cells, unlike normal cells, serve no useful purpose. The result of neoplastic growth is an abnormal tissue mass that does not contribute in any way to the well-being of the host. The mass occupies space and draws nutrition and sustenance from the host. If the malignant cells function at all, they do not function normally and may even act in a way that causes damage to the host. For example, a functional tumor of the thyroid gland produces excess amounts of thyroid hormone, leading to a hypermetabolic state.

■ Other Differences

Malignant cells exhibit other differences. First, they develop antigens that are completely different from those associated with normal cells. Chromosomal aberrations also occur as the malignant cell matures. There is a return to a more primitive and simplified metabolic and enzyme pattern, and these cells can invade, erode, and spread.

Neoplastic cells grow in adverse conditions, such as in the presence of necrosis and inflammatory cells, lymphocytes, and macrophages. Malignant cells also exhibit varying periods of latency. When the cells group to form tumors, they develop their own blood supply and supporting stroma (structure).

Growth of Malignant Tumors

Neoplastic cells mass together to form neoplastic tissue growths, or tumors. What accounts for the growth and spread of these tumors?

Table 23–3. A Comparison of the Characteristics of Normal and Malignant Cells

Characteristic	Normal Cells	Malignant Cells
Mitotic cell division	Mitotic division leads to two daughter cells	Mitosis leads to multiple daughter cells that may or may not resemble the parent. Multiple mitotic spindles
Appearance	1. Cells of same type homogeneous in size, shape, and growth 2. Cells cohesive, form regular pattern of expansion 3. Uniform size to nucleus 4. Have characteristic pattern of organization 5. Mixture of stem cells (precursors) and well-differentiated cells	1. Cells larger and grow more rapidly than normal. Pleomorphic, i.e., heterogeneous in size and shape 2. Cells not as cohesive, irregular patterns of expansion 3. Larger, more prominent nucleus 4. Lack characteristic pattern of organization of host cell 5. Anaplastic, lack of differentiated cell characteristics, specific functions
Growth pattern	1. Do not invade adjacent tissue 2. Proliferate in response to specific stimuli 3. Grow in ideal conditions (e.g., nutrients, oxygen, space, correct biochemical environment) 4. Exhibit contact inhibition 5. Cell birth equals or is less than cell death 6. Stable cell membrane 7. Constant or predictable growth rate 8. Cannot grow outside specific environment (e.g., breast cells grow only in breast)	1. Invade adjacent tissues 2. Proliferation in response to abnormal stimuli 3. Grow in adverse conditions such as lack of nutrients 4. Do not exhibit contact inhibition 5. Cell birth exceeds cell death 6. Loss of cell control a result of cell membrane changes 7. Growth rate erratic 8. Able to break off cells that migrate through bloodstream or lymphatics, or seed to distant sites and grow in other sites
Function	1. Have specific, designated purpose 2. Contribute to the overall well-being of the host 3. Cells function in specific predetermined manners (e.g., cells in the thyroid secrete thyroid hormone)	1. Serve no useful purpose 2. Do not contribute to the well-being of the host; parasitic, actually feed off host without contributing anything 3. If cells function at all, they do not function normally, or they may actually cause damage (e.g., malignant lung cancer cells secrete ACTH and cause excessive stimulation of adrenal cortex)
Other	1. Develop specific antigens, characteristic of the particular cell formed 2. Chromosomes remain constant throughout cell division 3. Complex metabolic and enzyme pattern 4. Cannot invade, erode, or spread 5. Cannot grow in presence of necrosis or inflammation	1. Develop antigens completely different from a normal cell 2. Chromosomal aberrations occur as cell matures 3. Have more primitive and simplified metabolic and enzyme pattern 4. Invade, erode, and spread 5. Grow in presence of necrosis and inflammatory cells such as lymphocytes and macrophages 6. Exhibit periods of latency that vary from tumor to tumor 7. Have own blood supply and supporting stroma

ACTH, adrenocorticotropic hormone.

Some neoplastic cells have the ability to spread from the original site of the tumor to distant organs of the body. This characteristic is called metastasis. The word is derived from the Greek words *meta,* beyond, and *stasis,* standing. The capacity of a neoplastic tumor to metastasize to other sites is a major characteristic of malignancy, and it distinguishes malignant from benign growths.

Researchers do not fully understand the mechanisms of tumor spread. Studies have revealed that the walls of tumor cells are different from those of their normal counterparts. Furthermore, the "contact inhibition" noted in normal cells is extremely variable in tumor cells.

For the purposes of study, the metastatic process may be divided into three stages (Fig. 23–6).

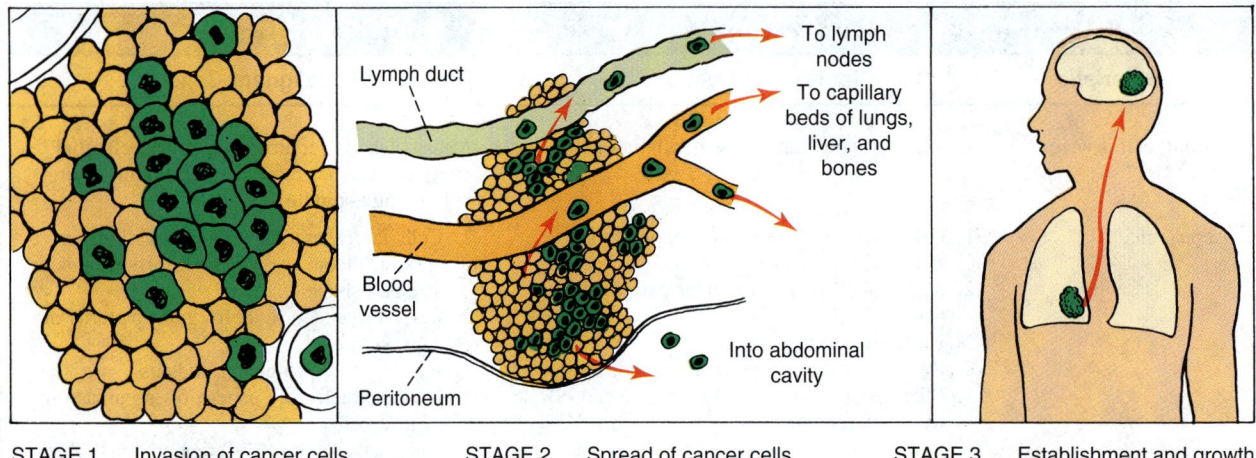

STAGE 1.   Invasion of cancer cells into adjacent tissue   STAGE 2.   Spread of cancer cells   STAGE 3.   Establishment and growth at secondary site

Figure 23–6. The three stages of the metastatic process.

Stage 1

Stage 1 involves invasion of neoplastic cells from the primary tumor into surrounding tissue, and penetration of blood or lymph vessels. Tumor invasion may be caused by any of the following:

- Increasing tumor size, leading to tissue pressure and mechanical expansion
- Loss of tumor cell cohesiveness, with increasing motility
- Destruction of the host stroma (the supporting tissues of an organ)
- Factors in the host response to tumor cell invasion

Stage 2

Stage 2 involves spread of tumor cells via the lymph or blood circulation or by direct expansion. The lymphatic system provides the most common pathway for initial spread of cancer cells. The spread may be to the lymph nodes draining the region of the primary site. Distant lymph nodes may be affected later in the disease or if the regional lymph nodes are obstructed by inflammation or other processes. Lymph node involvement is seen in about one half of all fatal cancers. The blood vessels (including both veins and arteries) carry cancer cells from the primary tumor to the capillary beds of the lungs, liver, and bones. Metastatic spread to distant organs and tissues is almost always the result of cells moving through the bloodstream. Direct expansion of tumors in body cavities occurs as cells travel throughout the cavity to develop new growth on other serosal surfaces. Cancers of the ovary are often said to seed the entire peritoneal cavity. Primary tumors of the CNS appear to spread by direct extension, or via gravity, in the cerebral fluid. Direct extension of tumors to directly adjacent tissues also occurs. For example, some breast cancers spread directly to the chest wall.

Stage 3

Stage 3 involves establishment and growth of tumor cells at the secondary site. The tumor develops its own vascularization in the new site and has the ability to infiltrate adjacent tissue. Researchers have observed that certain tumor cells have, for unknown reasons, an affinity for certain sites.

As previously mentioned, the cell cycle time and host factors determine the length of time necessary to detect metastatic growth. If the cells replicate quickly, a tumor may attain a size of 1 cm within months. If the cells proliferate slowly, it may be many years before the metastatic lesion is large enough to be detected.

The growth of metastatic tumors puts severe stress on the person both physiologically and psychologically. As the tumor burden (the amount of tumor in the body) increases, fewer metabolic resources are available for normal cells.

Although there is no clear explanation about the exact mechanism of metastasis, the metastatic sites of many tumors are fairly predictable. The predilection of certain tumors for particular sites may be due to the ability of the tumor to live within only certain tissues, or it may be due to some other, unknown factor. The most common site of metastasis is to lymphatic tissues. The next most common sites of metastasis are liver, lung, bone, and brain.

Classification of Neoplasms

Classification as Benign Versus Malignant

Neoplastic tumors are classified as either benign or malignant. Deciding whether a tumor is benign or malignant is probably the most important decision a physician must make when treating a person with a neoplastic growth.

The word "benign" comes from the Latin *benignus,* meaning "kind." A benign tumor, however, does occupy

Table 23–4. A Comparison of the Characteristics of Benign and Malignant Neoplasms

Characteristic	Benign Neoplasm	Malignant Neoplasm
Speed of growth	Grows slowly, usually continues to grow throughout life unless surgically removed; may have periods of remission	Usually grows rapidly, tends to grow relentlessly throughout life; rarely, neoplasm may regress spontaneously
Mode of growth	Grows by enlarging and expanding; always remains localized; never infiltrates surrounding tissues	Grows by infiltrating surrounding tissues; may remain localized (in situ) but usually infiltrates other tissues
Capsule	Almost always contained within a fibrous capsule; capsule does not prevent expansion of neoplasm but does prevent growth by infiltration; capsule advantageous because encapsulated tumor can be removed surgically	Never contained within a capsule; absence of capsule allows neoplastic cells to invade surrounding tissues; surgical removal of tumor difficult
Cell characteristics	Usually well differentiated; mitotic figures absent or scanty; mature cells; anaplastic cells absent; cells function poorly in comparison with normal cells from which they arise; if neoplasm arises in glandular tissue, cells may secrete hormones	Usually poorly differentiated; large numbers of normal and abnormal mitotic figures present; cells tend to be anaplastic, i.e., young, embryonic type; cells too abnormal to perform any physiologic functions; occasionally a malignant tumor arising in glandular tissue secretes hormones.
Recurrence	Recurrence extremely unusual when surgically removed	Recurrence common following surgery because tumor cells spread into surrounding tissues
Metastasis	Metastases never occur	Metastases very common
Effect of neoplasm	Not harmful to host unless located in area where it causes compression of tissues or obstruction of vital organs; does not produce cachexia (weight loss, debilitation, anemia, weakness, wasting)	Always harmful to host; results in death unless removed surgically or destroyed by radiation or chemotherapy; causes disfigurement, disrupted organ function, nutritional imbalances; may result in ulcerations, sepsis, perforations, hemorrhage, tissue slough; almost always produces cachexia, which leaves person prone to pneumonia, anemia, etc.
Prognosis	Very good; tumor generally removed surgically	Depends on cell type and speed of diagnosis; poor prognosis indicated if cells are poorly differentiated and evidence of metastic spread exists; good prognosis indicated if cells still resemble normal cells and there is no evidence of metastasis

space. Consequently, if it is located near a vital tube or organ, it could be fatal, as with a brain tumor. As a rule, though, the person with a benign tumor has a good prognosis because the tumor can be readily excised.

Malignant tumors, on the other hand, represent a serious threat to the life and well-being of the host. Table 23–4 compares the characteristics of benign and malignant neoplasms.

Classification by Tissue of Origin

Neoplasms are classified not only as benign or malignant but also according to the tissue from which they arise. Almost all names for tumors end in the suffix *oma,* meaning tumor (Table 23–5). This suffix is usually attached to a term for the parent tissue of the tumor. Thus, adenoma comes from the Greek *aden,* or gland, plus *oma.* When more than one parent tissue enters into the formation of a neoplasm, the names of the tumors are even more descriptive. For example, an adenomyoma is a benign neoplasm that contains both glandular and muscle (Greek genitive *myos*) cells.

Because epithelial tissues vary greatly, benign tumors of epithelial origin are classified according to either their microscopic appearance (e.g., adenoma) or their macroscopic appearance (e.g., polyp, from the Greek *polys* [many] + *pous* [foot]).

Three of the most common benign tumors listed in Table 23–5 are the fibroma, lipoma, and leiomyoma.

The *fibroma* may grow anywhere in the body, but it very frequently makes its home in the uterus. Fibromas are generally small, but occasionally they grow to great size. These encapsulated, relatively harmless tumors do not cause manifestations unless, because of their location,

Table 23–5. Classification of Neoplasms by Tissue of Origin

Tissue of Origin	Benign	Malignant
Connective tissue		Sarcoma
Embryonic fibrous tissue	Myxoma	Myxosarcoma
Fibrous tissue	Fibroma	Fibrosarcoma
Adipose tissue	Lipoma	Liposarcoma
Cartilage	Chondroma	Chondrosarcoma
Bone	Osteoma	Osteogenic sarcoma
Epithelium		Carcinoma
Skin and mucous membrane	Papilloma	Squamous cell carcinoma
Glands		Basal cell carcinoma
		Transitional cell carcinoma
	Adenoma	Adenocarcinoma
	Cystadenoma	Cystadenocarcinoma
Pigmented cells (melanocytes)	Nevus	Malignant melanoma
Endothelium		Endothelioma
Blood vessels	Hemangioma	Hemangioendothelioma
		Hemangiosarcoma
		Kaposi's sarcoma
Lymph vessels	Lymphangioma	Lymphangiosarcoma
		Lymphangioendothelioma
Bone marrow		Multiple myeloma
		Ewing's sarcoma
		Leukemia
Lymphoid tissue		Malignant lymphoma
		Lymphosarcoma
		Reticulum cell sarcoma
Muscle tissue		
Smooth muscle	Leiomyoma	Leiomyosarcoma
Striated muscle	Rhabdomyoma	Rhabdomyosarcoma
Nerve tissue		
Nerve fibers and sheaths	Neuroma	Neurogenic sarcoma
	Neurinoma	
	(Neurilemoma)	
	Neurofibroma	(Neurofibrosarcoma)
Ganglion cells	Ganglioneuroma	Neuroblastoma
Glial cells	Glioma	Glioblastoma
Meninges	Meningioma	Malignant meningioma
Gonads	Dermoid cyst	Embryonal carcinoma
		Embryonal sarcoma
		Teratocarcinoma

they press on a bone or nerve. Fibromas are easily removed surgically.

The *lipoma,* a very common benign tumor, arises in adipose tissue. Lipomas rarely cause manifestations, but they are poorly encapsulated and may put pressure on surrounding tissues as they expand.

The *leiomyoma,* a benign neoplasm of smooth muscle origin, is the most common benign tumor in women. Leiomyomas may develop anywhere in the body, but they most commonly grow in the uterus. Rarely (in approximately 1% of cases), these tumors become malignant.

Let us now consider the classification of malignant tumors. A malignant tumor that arises from epithelial tissue is called a carcinoma, whereas a malignant neoplasm that arises from mesenchymal origins (i.e., blood

vessels, lymphatic, nerve tissue) is called a sarcoma (Greek *sarx,* flesh).

Three representative examples of malignant neoplasms are carcinoma in situ, fibrosarcoma, and bronchogenic carcinoma.

Carcinoma in situ is a neoplasm of epithelial tissue that remains confined to the site of origin. In situ carcinoma typically affects the cervix, and it may occur in squamous epithelium in other parts of the body. This form of cancer is, by definition, localized, and thus can be removed surgically. However, in situ carcinoma can become invasive, eroding into surrounding tissues.

Malignant fibrosarcomas are similar to benign fibromas. Fibrosarcomas tend to grow in the same sites and may originate as benign fibromas, later becoming malignant. These bulky, well-differentiated tumor masses are usually responsive to surgery. Fortunately, fibrosarcomas rarely metastasize.

Bronchogenic carcinomas account for 90% of all cases of lung cancer. Bronchogenic carcinomas usually develop in the lower trachea and lower bronchi. Surgical excision of the tumor is the intervention of choice. However, this type of cancer readily gives rise to metastases, and if this occurs, surgery is contraindicated.

Prevention

Risk Analysis and Modification

Although cancer is the second most common cause of death in this country, many forms of cancer have identifiable risk factors and are preventable (see the Risk Factors and Levels of Prevention feature). Some cancers can be avoided through primary prevention. However, some cancers cannot be prevented from occurring. For these cancers, there is secondary prevention, or early detection. Dietary modifications are among the important ways to reduce the occurrence of cancer in general (Fig. 23–7).

The nurse needs to know the risk factors for each client and the common factors for each type of cancer. The Risk Factors and Levels of Prevention feature identifies specifics of primary and secondary preventions.

Genetic Testing

The Human Genome Project, a federally funded, multibillion dollar international initiative, was begun in 1990, with the goal of locating, mapping, and sequencing the more than 100,000 genes of a human's genetic composition. Approximately 60 genes have been linked to cancer. Many are used as molecular biologic markers of tumor prognosis while others are useful markers for the screening and early detection of common cancers, including those of the breast, ovary, and colon.[38] Of recent interest is the BRCA1 gene, isolated in 1994, the mutation of which has been linked to susceptibility to breast and probably ovarian cancers in a small percentage of women.

Engelking,[21] in a comprehensive review of the topic, predicts a profound impact of genetic discoveries on oncology nursing in several areas. Genetic discoveries will change the traditional perspective on screening, diagnosing, preventing, and treating cancer. Precise identification of cancer-causing genetic abnormalities will significantly improve the accuracy of cancer prediction and thus the capacity to target preventive interventions to at-risk populations. As a result, the perspective of nursing care will shift from symptomatic individuals diagnosed with cancer to counseling asymptomatic at-risk individuals. Issues of confidentiality and discrimination as well as the dilemma of predicting as yet incurable illnesses may have an enormous negative impact on the individual's and family's quality of life and psychological state. The first Ethical

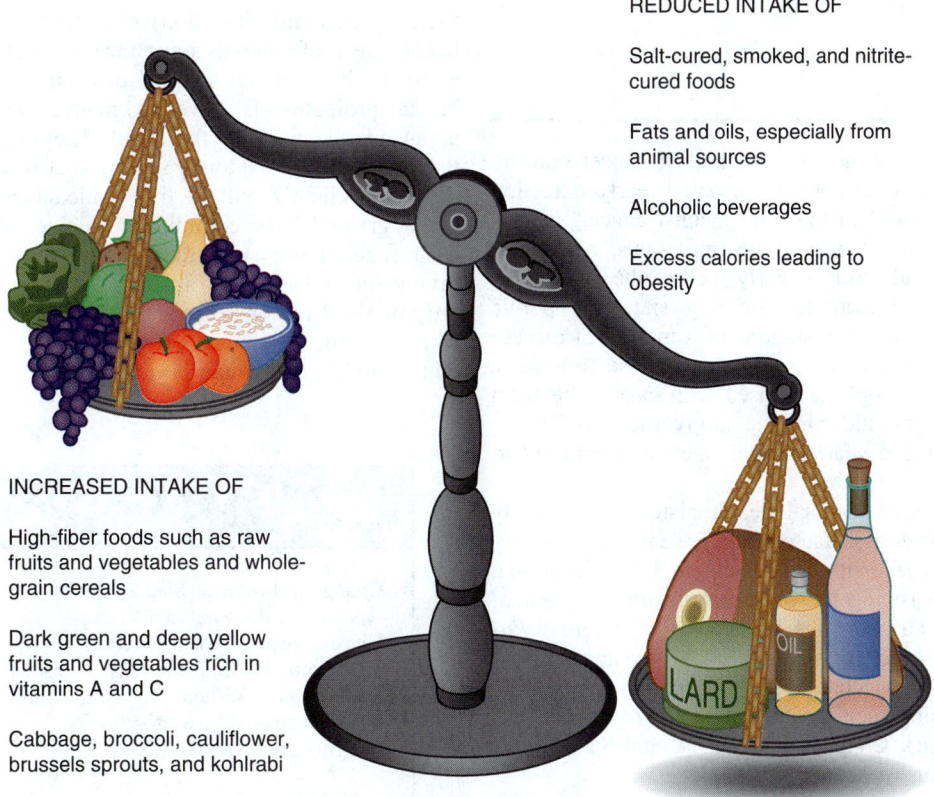

REDUCED INTAKE OF

Salt-cured, smoked, and nitrite-cured foods

Fats and oils, especially from animal sources

Alcoholic beverages

Excess calories leading to obesity

INCREASED INTAKE OF

High-fiber foods such as raw fruits and vegetables and whole-grain cereals

Dark green and deep yellow fruits and vegetables rich in vitamins A and C

Cabbage, broccoli, cauliflower, brussels sprouts, and kohlrabi

Figure 23–7. Dietary changes to reduce cancer risks.

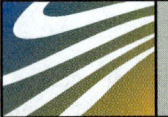

ETHICAL ISSUES IN NURSING

Bioethical Questions Generated by Genetic Advances

- Should the ability to predict presymptomatic risk precede the ability to treat or cure cancer?
- Can the revelation of family secrets be avoided when conducting genetic testing?
- What strategies should be used to obtain family consensus for testing when conflicts exist among family members?
- Should the genome be the "private property" of the individual or a component of the public domain?
- How can individual ownership of the genome be protected while simultaneously ensuring the rights of insurers and employers?
- How can employment and work discrimination based on cancer risk alone be prevented?
- How can one prevent prenatal diagnosis of genetic abnormalities from becoming a "search and destroy" mission?
- Who will bear the liability for and costs of aborting a defective fetus?

Adapted from Engelking, C. (1995). Genetics in cancer care: Confronting a Pandora's box of dilemmas. *Oncology Nursing Forum, 22* (Supplement), 27–34.

Issues in Nursing feature highlights several bioethical issues concerning genetic testing.

Screening

Primary prevention is the ideal method of cancer control. Because all cancers cannot be prevented, early detection is the next major tool in the fight against cancer. Nurses must emphasize to the public the importance of finding the cancer and eradicating it early, before the cancer begins to metastasize from the primary site. The public needs to realize that manifestations of a malignant disease can mimic those of other, less serious disease processes. Currently 6 of 10 people diagnosed with cancer die from it.[6] Early detection could raise the survival rate to 50% or more. The relative 5-year survival rate has increased to about 54%.[6]

The person's age, personal health history, and family history may indicate risk factors and are vital to the early detection of cancer. Nurses can help in this educational process by emphasizing the need for an *annual physical examination,* by stressing the importance of a *yearly Papanicolaou (Pap) test* for sexually active women, and by teaching women the technique for *breast self-examination (BSE)* and teaching men the technique for *testicular self-examination (TSE).* Chapters 82, 83, 84, and 85 describe these examinations in detail.

The public should be aware of cancer's seven warning signals (Box 23–1). Table 23–6 summarizes the Ameri-

can Cancer Society's (ACS) *most recent* guidelines for screening asymptomatic populations.

It is a normal human response to procrastinate in scheduling an examination when cancer is suspected. People are frightened by the thought of cancer. They do not always realize that cancer is curable when found early. Early detection improves survival. Part of the process of screening clients is educating them as well. The Ethical Issues in Nursing feature on p. 554 lists screening priorities.

Diagnosis

What specifically is involved in cancer detection? The primary healthcare provider employs both general and special techniques in a complete cancer diagnostic examination. General techniques include obtaining the client's history, including familial and environmental histories (see Chapter 11), performing a thorough physical examination, and ordering and evaluating laboratory examinations of blood, tissue, sputum, urine, and other specimens.

Psychosocial Issues During Diagnosis

When people undergo the diagnostic process associated with suspicious lumps or other cancer manifestations, they are usually somewhat afraid and anxious. They are experiencing unfamiliar and possibly painful tests.

In the past, if the diagnosis was cancer, there was often a debate about whether or not to tell the client. Today, nurses and physicians respect the client's right to know the diagnosis and all options for treatment. Consequently, healthcare professionals must face the difficulty of telling a client the bad news. One problem, however, is that health professionals have as many feelings and fears about this diagnosis as the client. They do not want to be the bearers of bad tidings, fearing that this diagnosis may destroy a client's will to live, which could result in the client giving up or committing suicide. Most clients exhibit much more strength than might be expected, and giving up or suicide is a rare response. Therefore, these are not valid reasons or excuses for avoiding our responsibility to the client. To provide support through a difficult period, nurses must be able to discuss the diagnosis,

---

Box 23–1. Cancer's Seven Warning Signals

Change in bowel or bladder habits
A sore that does not heal
Unusual bleeding or discharge
Thickening or lump in breast or elsewhere
Indigestion or difficulty in swallowing
Obvious change in wart or mole
Nagging cough or hoarseness

If YOU have a warning signal, see your doctor!

Table 23-6. American Cancer Society Guidelines (1995) for Early Detection of Cancer in Asymptomatic Populations

Test	Age (yr)	Sex	Frequency
Chest x-ray study			No longer recommended for smokers to screen for lung cancer
Sputum cytology			No longer recommended for smokers to screen for lung cancer
Physical examination	40+	M,F	Yearly for all people over 40, including examination of skin, lymph nodes, mouth, thyroid, breast, testes, rectum, and prostate
Health teaching	20	M,F	Every 3 years, teach proper diet, exercise, health habits, breast and testicular self-examination, avoidance of sunlight, and smoking cessation
Breast self-examination	20+	F	Every month after menses before menopause; after menopause, monthly, on any specified day such as the first or last of the month
Mammography	35–40	F	Baseline mammogram between 35 and 40; between 40 and 49, a mammogram should be done every 1–2 years and yearly after 50; high-risk women should check with their physician
Pap smear	18+	F	Sexually active women should have Pap smears regardless of age; should be performed yearly until there are three negative examinations in a row; at this point, they can be performed yearly or as physician advises
Pelvic examination	20–40, 40+	F	Every 3 years, earlier if sexually active; yearly after 40
Endometrial tissue sample	At menopause	F	High-risk women (obese, abnormal uterine bleeding, estrogen therapy, history of infertility, diabetes, hypertension, failure to ovulate) should have this test performed at menopause
Testicular self-examination	20–40	M	Monthly, on a set date such as the first of the month, following a shower
Digital rectal examination	40+	M,F	Annually for rectal cancer in men and women and prostate in men
Fecal occult blood	20–40, 40–49, 50+	M,F	Done per physician's recommendation; women at higher risk Done per physician's recommendation, yearly
Proctoscopy, flexible sigmoidoscopy	50+	M,F	Every 3–5 years
Oral examination	20+	M,F	Annually
Breast physical examination	20–39 40+	F	Every 3 years Annually

treatment, care, and expected outcomes with the client and significant others.

When working with clients whose cancer is being diagnosed, it is usually helpful to give the client the information over time. If the client knows the alternatives that are being ruled out during the diagnostic process, the confirmation of one alternative, even if unpleasant, will not be as much of a shock. Having time to prepare for an event is part of successful coping. Second, gear expectations to the client's level of understanding. Listen to the clients and the terms they are choosing. Sometimes they avoid the word "cancer" and use "tumor" or "growth" instead.

If the diagnosis of cancer is made, make sure that the client understands the terms the physician is using. Third, clients will need to hear the information several times and often from several people they trust. Often, clients repeat the same questions several times. Sometimes, clients are reluctant to take up the time of the busy nurse or physician with their repeated questions. Clients need to feel that people are willing to take the time to talk to them. The client's needs should be communicated to other members of the healthcare team as well.

Finally, at the time the diagnosis is confirmed, the client needs to know that alternatives are available. There should be time for the client to assimilate the information before being asked to make choices about interventions. The nurse needs to be informed about the diagnosis and plan of care, about the disease and interventions in general, and about what the client actually knows.

If the diagnosis of cancer is made, expect a wide variety of reactions. This is a period of crisis for the client. This time is marked by fear, denial, withdrawal, anger, and other reactions to a crisis situation. A few clients will

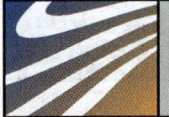

ETHICAL ISSUES IN NURSING

Who Should Be Screened for Cancer, and What Tests Should Be Used?

There are several ethical dilemmas associated with screening tests for cancer. First, not all screening tests are as effective as others. Screening tests can be very expensive. Also, should everyone be screened, or should only those at highest risk (e.g., because of age or race) be screened routinely?

To be most effective, tests should be (1) specific for one type of cancer in one anatomic site, (2) reliable, (3) acceptable to the client, and (4) economical in terms of the cost-benefit ratio. The question then becomes: Should only those tests that meet these standards be used?

There are no easy answers; however, those at highest risk for a disease are a priority for screening.

---

say that they do not want to hear anything about the disease or treatment. They cope by saying, "Don't tell me anything. Just do what you have to do." Because this is probably a temporary coping strategy, remain sensitive to clients' requests for no information now, knowing that later they will probably want to know more.

The goal of care during this time is to help the client cope with the diagnosis, recommended treatment, and prognosis. People cope in different ways during a crisis situation. Nevertheless, the client can be helped to explore new and more effective coping strategies. The foundation for successful coping is receiving accurate information about the situation and possible solutions.

It is also important for the client to be both physiologically and psychologically intact enough to understand and use the information. The client should not be physically suffering, and he or she must have a sense of control over the situation. The nurse must be especially aware of the client's feelings. Hospitalization makes most people feel helpless and out of control, all of which interferes with coping.

If the client can cope successfully during the period of diagnosis and the beginning of treatment, he or she may cope better during the entire course of the disease. People with cancer and their significant others often demonstrate great strength as they learn to deal with their fears and with the difficulties of being treated for cancer.

History and Physical Assessment

The first step in the diagnostic process is obtaining a complete history and physical examination. Some cancers are linked with certain genetic and environmental factors. Therefore, learn about the health of the client's family members, the work history of the client, and the environ-

ment in which the client lives. (See Chapters 11 and 12 for health history and physical assessment.)

When a malignant tumor is in its early stages, there are often few manifestations. Clinical manifestations usually appear once the tumor has grown to a sufficiently large size to cause one or more of the following problems:

- Pressure on surrounding organs or nerves
- Distortion of surrounding tissue
- Obstruction of lumen of tubes
- Interference with the blood supply of surrounding tissues
- Interference with organ function
- Disturbance of body metabolism
- Parasitic use of the body's nutritional supplies
- Mobilization of the body's defensive responses, resulting in inflammatory changes

Common clinical manifestations that may arise secondary to cancer include weight loss, weakness or fatigue, CNS alterations, pain, and hematologic and metabolic alterations. Close assessment of such manifestations may reveal that they are directly or indirectly related to the tumor growth.

Anorexia, weight loss, weakness, and fatigue are related to the body's inability to consume and use nutrients appropriately. Mechanical interference by tumors, malabsorption, paraneoplastic endocrine secretions (such as excessive secretion of thyroid hormones), and tumor use of nutrients may all contribute to a cycle that must be interrupted to avoid general physical debilitation.

The client who has difficulty with vision, speech, coordination, or memory may be experiencing primary or metastatic CNS disease. Increased intracranial pressure caused by tumor growth may cause headache, lethargy, nausea, and vomiting.

Although pain is not a common early manifestation of cancer, it may occur as a result of obstruction or destruction of a vital organ, pressure on sensitive tissues or bone, or involvement of nerves. If it occurs and is not adequately treated, it may become constant and progressively severe. Bone cancer is particularly painful because the rigidity of bone allows for little or no expansion as the tumor cells proliferate. It also becomes more painful because pathologic fractures produce instability and muscle spasms. In spite of the fact that pain is usually a late manifestation, it may be the manifestation that brings the client to healthcare.

Unexplained anemia often indicates a malignancy. Hematologic changes also include leukopenia, leukocytosis, and bleeding disorders, which in some diseases may occur before local manifestations. Metabolic manifestations such as Cushing's syndrome, hypercalcemia, inappropriate antidiuretic hormone (ADH) secretion, and carcinoid syndrome also signify the possibility of malignant disease.

A localized tumor usually produces manifestations related to increased pressure or obstruction in a single region. Metastatic disease and extensive tumors of major organs may display a variety of local and systemic manifestations.

Cancer-Specific Diagnostic Examinations

The ideal diagnostic test would find cancer at an early stage, when it is composed of only a few cells. It would be specific for one type of cancer, and a positive test would provide a definitive diagnosis. It should also be inexpensive, easy to perform, and noninvasive. Unfortunately, no such test exists. Some laboratory tests can detect cancer when there are 10^4 cells, whereas the more routine laboratory and x-ray examinations detect cancer when 10^7 cells are present. A general physical assessment does not detect most tumors until there are 10^8 cells, and cancer is symptomatic at about 10^{10} cells.

■ Radiographic Procedures

Basic X-ray Studies

X-ray studies are particularly useful in diagnosing obstructive tumors of the gastrointestinal, respiratory, and renal tracts. They are also valuable in identifying bone malignancies and, aided by computers, help pinpoint the location of brain tumors and the degree to which the tumors are compressing surrounding tissues.

Radioisotope Studies (Scans)

Radioisotopes are capable of entering into the same chemical reactions and the same metabolic processes in the body as stable elements. When a radioactive isotope enters a person's body, the fate of the element can be followed, or traced, by scanning machines. Abnormal tissue appears different on the scan because the isotope is metabolized differently by this tissue. Thyroid, bone, brain, liver, lung, and spleen are areas of the body most frequently scanned for diagnostic purposes.

When employed diagnostically, radioisotopes are used as tracers. A tracer is administered either orally or by injection. The isotope is then identified, located, and traced by a radiosensitive apparatus as the radioactive material circulates through the body and concentrates in particular organs and tissues.

The scintillation scanner is a device for locating and pinpointing malignant growths by measuring the uptake of a radioisotope. This scanner is passed back and forth over the area of the body that is being studied.

Radioisotopes are useful in the diagnosis of cancer and other diseases for several reasons. First, radioisotopes can be administered in extremely small doses, for example, one billionth of a gram of a radioisotope can be used for administration as a tracer dose. With such small doses, the body absorbs a minimal amount of radiation, and consequently, the cells suffer no damage. Thus, radioisotopes can be employed diagnostically without the danger of cellular destruction.

Second, radioisotopes can be used to study the functions of specific organs and tissues. A classic example of this type of study is the ^{131}I uptake test that is used to evaluate thyroid function. If the examiner suspects the presence of thyroid disease, the client receives a tracer dose of radioactive iodine (^{131}I). The radioactive iodine circulates to the thyroid gland and there converts into thyroxine in precisely the same manner as regular (nonradioactive) iodine. The scintillation counter or scanner can then trace, locate, and measure tagged atoms to determine the presence of disease.

Radioisotopes are also employed to measure blood volume, blood circulation rate, red blood cell turnover, cardiac output, and lung blood flow, using the same types of procedures.

Finally, radioisotopes are used to locate tumors and lesions within the brain, kidneys, liver, lungs, pericardium, and bones. Certain radioisotopes have an affinity for particular organs or tissues; for example, ^{131}I has an affinity for thyroid tissue, ^{198}Au has an affinity for the liver, and so forth. In some cases, if the organ harbors a malignant tumor, the tagged atoms will tend to concentrate in the area of tumor growth. Consequently, a scan of the organ will reveal a high uptake of the radioisotope at the site of the tumor. For example, ^{131}I is used to locate cancerous tissues that have metastasized from the thyroid gland to other parts of the body. An area in which the concentration of a radioisotope is unusually high is called a hot spot. In other cases, the tagged atoms tend to concentrate less densely in the diseased portion of the organ than in the normal portion. The area of less concentration of a radioactive isotope is called a cold spot.

An organ scan is a simple and completely painless procedure. There are three steps involved.

1. *Administration of the radioisotope.* The client receives a tracer dose of the appropriate radioisotope either orally or by injection.
2. *Waiting period.* Before the scanning procedure can be performed, the radioisotope must be assimilated by the organ under study. The length of time required for assimilation varies. A brain scan should be performed 1 1/2 hours after an injection of radioactive mercury, and 18 to 48 hours after an injection of radioiodinated human serum albumin (RIHSA).
3. *The scanning procedure.* The client is asked to lie still and breathe normally while the scintillation scanner measures the radioactive atoms concentrated in the organ under study and records its findings. Sedation before this procedure may help the restless, agitated, or anxious client.

Positron-Emission Tomography

Position emission tomography (PET) is an imaging technique that provides information about physiologic and biochemical processes. Functional images of the distribution of radioactively labeled compounds are obtained using the PET scanner, which produces 35 simultaneous cross-sectional images of the organs of interest. It is particularly useful in differentiating low-grade tumors from high-grade tumors and in distinguishing treatment-induced tissue necrosis from recurrent tumor. This unique imaging technology has shown promise for improving client outcomes in several somatic cancers (lung, colon, breast, soft tissue and bone, brain) by aiding in the staging, treatment planning, and monitoring of disease.[33]

Computed Tomography

The computed axial tomogram, or computed tomographic (CT) scan, is an x-ray technique that produces sequential cross-sectional body images at progressive depths. CT scans can help differentiate malignant and nonmalignant masses, and accurately identify their size and location. Occasionally, an oral or intravenous contrast agent is administered to increase the sensitivity of the CT scan. Always check for an allergy to the dye.

Depending on the area to be scanned, the client may be placed on a restricted diet. Clients should be taught that they will lie on a table and the x-ray machine will move around them. This is a painless test unless an intravenous contrast dye, which may cause a burning sensation on injection, is given. The dye also may cause nausea, vomiting, flushing, itching, and a bitter taste. The x-ray machine is very noisy and could frighten the client if he or she is not warned.

Mammography

A mammogram is a radiologic examination using a minimal and safe amount of radiation to allow visualization of breast masses, differentiating tumors from fibrocysts. The breast is compressed between two plates. The use of compression decreases the amount of radiation that must be used to visualize the tumors. Some women, particularly those with multiple fibrocysts in the breast, will find the compression uncomfortable; otherwise, the examination is painless. Two views are taken of the breast: a craniocaudal and a lateral view.

Angiography

Angiography is used infrequently to check the resectability of tumors. This examination involves the injection of a radiopaque dye that circulates to the tumor, and then a radiographic study is performed. This procedure clearly outlines the blood supply of the tumor and surrounding structures.

Depending on the site of the angiography, the client may be placed on a restricted diet. Clients may be sedated before the examination to help them relax and lie still during the test. The skin over the injection site is cleaned, shaved if necessary, and anesthetized. The radiopaque dye injected may cause some feelings of nausea, vomiting, flushing, itching, or a bitter or salty taste. Check whether or not the client has an allergy to the dye before it is administered.

After the test, a pressure bandage is applied to the site of the cannulation. This site is then immobilized for up to 24 hours. If a cutdown (an incision to locate the vein) is used, then the site is sutured and wound care should be done.

Lymphangiography

The lymphangiogram is a very useful diagnostic test because it examines the lymphatic system, the primary site of metastasis for tumors with good lymphatic drainage.

Although the test cannot rule out metastasis, it is an excellent marker when there is known disease because it can show tumor growth or remission.

The lymphangiogram cannot be performed for 48 hours after another contrast study. There is no preparation before this examination except client education. Explain to the client that the test is fairly long and uncomfortable. The test is performed by injecting blue dye into the interdigital webs of the feet. This dye is picked up by the lymphatic system so it can be cannulated. The skin on each foot over the lymphatics is anesthetized and cutdown performed so cannulas can be inserted to infuse the dye. The dye may take several hours to infuse into the lymphatics of the abdomen. X-ray studies are then obtained.

After the test, the client should drink plenty of fluids. The dye may continue to discolor the urine for several days. The feet also will remain tinted blue for a long time after the test. The client must return the following day for follow-up x-ray studies.

■ Blood Studies

A variety of blood tests can be performed to help diagnose cancer (Table 23–7). Some of the more routine tests, such as the complete blood count (CBC) and differential, do not test for specific types of cancer but indicate the presence of any number of problems. Other blood tests, such as tumor markers and biochemical tests, including acid phosphatase, identify the extent of a particular type of cancer. These tests, however, are not used to make the diagnosis of cancer but only to check its progression.

■ Cytologic Examination

The *Pap smear* is a valuable diagnostic test that was developed by George N. Papanicolaou in 1943. Its original purpose was to discover cancer of the cervix during the early, noninvasive, asymptomatic stage. Today, the test is also used to detect early cancers of the digestive, respiratory, and renal tracts, and occasionally, those of the breast. The Pap smear is also used to evaluate responses to chemotherapy and radiation therapy, as well as to detect malignant disease when it recurs postoperatively.

Materials that can be examined by Pap smears include: (1) cervical scrapings, (2) bronchial secretions and washings obtained by bronchoscopy, (3) urine sediment, (4) coughed-up sputum, (5) aspirated gastric secretions, and (6) mammary gland discharge fluid.

The method of obtaining a Pap smear is fairly simple. First, the examiner either scrapes cells from a tissue (e.g., the cervix) or obtains cells by aspirating fluid or sediment from an organ (e.g., the stomach or bronchi). Next, the examiner fixes the smear by immersing it in a chemical solution of equal parts of ether and 95% ethyl alcohol. Finally, the fixed slide is allowed to dry. It is then stained and evaluated.

The laboratory technique used to analyze the Pap smear is called *exfoliative cytology,* which means the ex-

Table 23–7. Laboratory Blood Tests for Cancer

Test	Reference Values	Conditions in Which Levels May Be Altered
Hematologic Tests (CBC)		
Hemoglobin	M: 14–18 g/dl F: 12–16 g/dl	↓ Anemia, nonspecific, may indicate malignancy
Hematocrit	M: 40–54 ml/dl F: 37–47 ml/dl	↓ Anemia, nonspecific, may indicate malignancy
Leukocytes (WBC)	4500–11,000 mm³	↑ Leukemia and lymphomas ↓ Leukemia and metastatic disease to bone marrow
Percent neutrophils	54%–62%	↑ AML, CML, and lymphoma ↓ Leukemia, carcinoma, myeloma, sarcoma, bone marrow depression
Percent lymphocytes	25%–33%	↑ ALL and CLL, multiple myeloma, lymphoma, carcinoma ↓ Hodgkin's disease, nonlymphocytic leukemias, lymphosarcoma, bone marrow depression
Percent monocytes	3%–7%	↑ Hodgkin's disease, lymphoma, monocytic leukemia, CML, multiple myeloma ↓ Hairy cell leukemia
Percent eosinophils	1%–3%	↑ CML ↓ Hodgkin's disease, bone marrow depression
Percent basophils	0%–1%	↑ CML, Hodgkin's disease
Platelets	150,000–300,000 mm³	↑ Myeloproliferative disorders, CML, Hodgkin's disease ↓ ALL, AML, multiple myeloma, bone marrow depression
Blood/Serum Tests		
Acid phosphatase	0.11–0.60 milliunits/ml	↑ Metastatic prostate cancer
ACTH	10–80 pg/ml (in AM)	↑ Lung cancer
Alkaline phosphatase	20–90 milliunits/ml	↑ Cancer of bone or bone metastasis, liver cancer, lymphoma, leukemia
Calcitonin	Undetectable	↑ Medullary thyroid cancer >100 pg/ml
Calcium	9.0–11.0 mg/dl	↑ Bone metastasis, breast cancer, leukemia, lymphoma, multiple myeloma, lung, kidney, bladder, liver, parathyroid cancers
Gastrin	<200 pg/ml	↑ Gastric and pancreatic cancer
IgG	500–1900 mg/dl	↑ IgG myeloma
IgA	60–333 mg/dl	↑ IgA myeloma
IgM	45–145 mg/dl	↑ IgM Waldenström's macroglobulinemia
IgD	0.5–3.0 mg/dl	↑ IgD myeloma
IgE	500 ng/ml	↑ IgE myeloma
LDH	100–190 milliunits/dl	↑ Liver cancer and liver metastasis, lymphoma, acute leukemia
Lysozyme	4–13 mg/L	↑ AML and CML
Parathyroid hormone	430–1860 ng/L	↑ Squamous cell lung, kidney, pancreatic, ovarian cancers
Serotonin	50–200 ng/ml	↑ Carcinoid syndrome
SGPT (AST)	5–35 milliunits/ml	↑ Metastatic cancer to the liver
SGOT (ALT)	7–40 milliunits/ml	↑ Metastatic cancer to the liver
Testosterone	M: 275–875 ng/dl F: 23–75 ng/dl	↑ Adrenal and ovarian cancers

Table continued on following page

Table 23–7. Laboratory Blood Tests for Cancer *Continued*		
Test	**Reference Values**	**Conditions in Which Levels May Be Altered**
Uric acid	M: 2.5–8.0 mg/dl F: 1.4–7.0 mg/dl	↑ Leukemia and multiple myeloma ↓ Hodgkin's disease, multiple myeloma, and lung cancer
Tests for Tumor Markers		
AFP	<10 ng/ml	↑ Lung, nonseminomatous testicular, pancreatic, colon, stomach cancers, choriocacinoma
CA–125	<35 units	↑ Ovarian, pancreatic cancers
Calcitonin	<100 pg/ml	↑ Medullary thyroid, small cell lung, breast cancers; carcinoid
CEA	0–2.5 ng/ml nonsmokers <3.0 ng/ml smokers	↑ Colorectal, breast, lung, stomach, pancreatic, prostate cancers
Estrogen receptors (ER)	Positive >10 femtomoles/mg	↑ ER + breast cancer
HCG	0–5 IU/L	↑ Choriocarcinoma and germ cell testicular cancer; ectopic production in lung, liver, stomach, pancreatic, colon cancers
Progesterone (PR) receptor assay	Positive >10 femtomoles/mg	↑ PR + breast cancer
Prostatic acid phosphatase	0.26–0.83 u/L	↑ Metastatic prostate cancer
PSA	0–4 ng/ml	↑ Prostate cancer
CA–19–9		↑ Pancreatic, colon, gastric cancers
CA–15–3		↑ Breast cancer

ACTH, adrenocorticotropic hormone; AFP, alpha-fetoprotein; ALL, acute lymphocytic leukemia; AML, acute myelogenous leukemia; CBC, complete blood count; CEA, carcinoembryonic antigen; CLL, chronic lymphocytic leukemia; CML, chronic myelogenous leukemia; HCG, human chorionic gonadotropin; LDH, lactic dehydrogenase; PSA, prostate-specific antigen; SGOT, serum aspartate aminotransferase; SPGT, serum alanine aminotransferase.

amination of desquamated or sloughed-off cells. Under the microscope, the cells may have either a normal or an anaplastic appearance. Cells are graded on the following 5-point scale:

Class I: Normal
Class II: Inflammation
Class III: Mild to moderate dysplasia
    CIN (cervical intraepithelial neoplasia) I: Mild dysplasia
    CIN II: Moderate dysplasia
Class IV: Possibly malignant
    CIN III: Severe dysplasia and carcinoma in situ
Class V: Probably malignant

If the Pap smear indicates a class II finding, the smear is simply repeated in 3 months. If the test reveals a class III, CIN I, or CIN II finding, the Pap smear will be repeated in 6 weeks to 3 months, and if it is class IV, CIN III, or class V, a biopsy is performed immediately.

■ Biopsy

A biopsy is the surgical excision of a small piece of tissue for microscopic examination. Physicians most commonly use this method to either rule out or confirm a diagnosis of malignancy.

The client is usually scheduled for minor surgery. If the site for biopsy is easily accessible (e.g., cervix, breast), the person is draped appropriately and adminis-

tered a local anesthetic. Then the surgeon removes a piece of the suspicious tissue. Additional procedures (e.g., bronchoscopy, cystoscopy, and sigmoidoscopy) are necessary for an internal tumor.

There are two types of biopsy procedures. The type used depends on the size of the tumor and the purpose of the biopsy. If the suspicious tumor is small, the entire tumor is excised for examination. This is called a total or excisional type of biopsy. If the tumor is large, only a part of the neoplasm is excised. This procedure is termed a subtotal or incisional type of biopsy. There is some question as to the safety of the subtotal biopsy. Some surgeons believe that this procedure opens vascular channels and releases tumor cells that may then metastasize to other sites during the time the excised tissue is being examined. However, there are no studies to date that confirm this fear.

Following the excision, the pathologist prepares a frozen section or permanent paraffin section to examine the specimen. To prepare a frozen (or rapid) section, the tissue is immediately frozen. Then the pathologist cuts the tissue into thin sections and examines the tissue slices under the microscope. The main advantage of the frozen section is the speed with which the section can be prepared and the diagnosis made. Only minutes are required. In contrast, the slower, more classic method of embedding the tissue in paraffin takes about 24 hours. However, the paraffin section provides the pathologist with clearer detail than does the frozen section.

Needle or aspiration biopsy is used mainly to obtain tissue samples for identification from liver, kidney, spleen, lung, or breast. The physician aspirates a core of tissue from a suspicious nodule or mass rather than excising it. Stereotactic breast biopsy is an x-ray-guided method for localizing and sampling small, nonpalpable breast lesions discovered on mammography and considered to be suspicious for malignancy.

■ Ultrasound

Ultrasound uses high-frequency sound waves to visualize the interfaces around organs and within pathologic masses. Special equipment is used to detect and map echoes of varying densities from various organs and tumors. This technique is used to detect lesions in the female pelvis, abdominal lymph nodes, the prostate through a transrectal approach, and other areas of the body. One advantage of this procedure is that it is a noninvasive way to demonstrate and follow the growth or neoplasms without radiation exposure.

Preparation for the test includes cleaning the bowel with enemas if the abdominal area is to be tested and having the client drink six to eight glasses of water without voiding before the test. The water distends the bladder, used as a landmark for a pelvic ultrasound, and the client is not allowed to void until after the test. The test is painless, with only a slight pressure being felt. A lubricant gel is applied, but is easily wiped off after the test. The client is allowed to void after the test is completed.

■ Direct Visualization

An endoscopy involves direct visualization of the gastrointestinal tract, bronchoscopy of the lungs, laryngoscopy of the larynx, colposcopy of the cervix and vagina, cystoscopy of the bladder, laparoscopy of the pelvic or abdominal cavities, and so on. These tests use a rigid or flexible scope, which allows the physician to view the internal anatomy directly, without major surgery. During these tests, suspicious areas can be examined, tissue samples and aspirates taken for biopsies, the extent of the disease staged, and pathologic processes excised. These tests are discussed in detail in later chapters.

■ Magnetic Resonance Imaging

Magnetic resonance imaging (MRI) identifies abnormalities by creating sectional (tomographic) images of the body without the use of ionizing radiation. The client's nuclei are aligned in a magnetic field, absorb energy from radio frequency pulses, and emit signals as their excitation decays. These signals are converted into tomographic images. MRI provides clear images of the CNS, spine, head and neck, and musculoskeletal system.

All materials that might be affected by a magnet should be removed before the test. This test cannot be performed if any material affected by a magnet cannot be removed, such as a pacemaker or surgical clips. The test is painless, although some clients may feel somewhat claustrophobic because of the narrow tunnel in the machine in which they must lie. Inform clients that the machine makes a loud hammering sound during the test, so that they will not be frightened. If an intravenous contrast dye is used to enhance the image, the client may experience some nausea, vomiting, and itching. There is no specific nursing care required after the test. As with all diagnostic tests, the client must be supported while awaiting the results.

■ Antigen Skin Testing

Recall that the immune system apparently plays a vital role in preventing tumor growth and in destroying tumors that do develop. The immune response can be repressed by (1) immunosuppressive drugs, (2) physical or emotional stress (which stimulates the release of plasma cortisol), (3) smoking, (4) alcohol, and (5) blocking agents released by the tumor. A repressed immune response usually indicates a poor prognosis. The dinitrobenzene (DNCB) skin test is one method currently used to assess whether the person has a properly functioning immune system. Approximately 90% to 95% of healthy persons can be sensitized to the chemical DNCB when it is placed on a small area of the skin. The healthy person develops a positive response (redness, itching, perhaps blistering) within 24 to 48 hours. When given a second (challenge) dose of DNCB 14 days later, a delayed cutaneous hypersensitivity response (a raised red site) appears on the skin.

Other common antigens used for intradermal testing include tetanus toxoid, *Streptococcus*, tuberculin, *Candida*, *Trichophyton*, and *Proteus*. The application of multiple antigens is referred to as an anergy battery. Response is assessed by measuring the induration in millimeters at 24 and 48 hours.

Skin testing is useful for several reasons. First, it acts as a diagnostic aid. For example, clients who have a negative reaction or who cannot be sensitized are said to be anergic (i.e., have diminished ability to react to specific antigens). This signals inadequacy of the immune response. Second, skin testing can assess the client's immunocompetence before and during radiotherapy and chemotherapy. Both of these treatments can suppress the immune system. A candidate for immunotherapy (see Chapter 27) is tested prior to therapy to determine the immune function. Clients in immunotherapy (biotherapy) programs are monitored throughout their therapeutic regimen to determine their response to therapy.

Staging and Grading

When a neoplastic growth is definitely diagnosed, it must be further defined in terms of its extent. This diagnostic process, called *staging*, involves a systematic search for (1) the characteristics of the primary tumor, (2) involvement of lymph nodes, and (3) evidence of metastasis, based on knowledge of the natural history of the disease.

The TNM system is the accepted system for staging today. In this system, T stands for tumor, N refers to the regional lymph nodes, and M refers to metastasis. Table 23–8 summarizes the TNM staging system.

Based on the TNM classification, cancers may also be

Table 23–8. The TNM Staging System	
Tumor	
T_0	No evidence of primary tumor
T_{IS}	Carcinoma in situ
$T_1\ T_2\ T_3\ T_4$	Progressive increase in tumor size and involvement
T_X	Tumor cannot be assessed
Nodes	
N_0	No regional lymph node metastasis
$N_1\ N_2\ N_3$	Increasing involvement of regional lymph nodes
N_X	Regional lymph nodes cannot be assessed clinically
Metastasis	
M_0	No evidence of distant metastasis
M_1	Distant metastasis
M_X	Presence of distant metastasis cannot be assessed

Modified from Beahrs, O. H., et al. (1992). American Joint Committee on Cancer: *Manual for staging of cancer* (4th ed.). Philadelphia: J. B. Lippincott.

grouped into one of four stages (I–IV), or stage 0 for carcinoma in situ. Higher stages signify more extensive disease, with stage IV consistently representing distant metastases and the worst prognosis. Other established classifications may be used for particular malignancies, such as Clark's classification for malignant melanomas and Duke's classification for colorectal cancer. Clark's classification considers the level of invasion of melanomas, and Duke's system refers to the depth of invasion of colorectal cancer. Hodgkin's disease uses the Ann Arbor classification which refers to both the distribution of the tumor and the associated manifestations.

The *tumor grade* is an evaluation of the extent to which tumor cells differ from their normal precursors. Low numerical grades, grades I and II, mean the cells are well differentiated and deviate minimally from normal cells. High grades, grades III and IV, refer to cells that are poorly differentiated and the most aberrant compared with normal cells.

The histologic grade is determined by a pathologist. Tumor grading involves a histologic and anatomic description of the malignant neoplasm. Staging and grading information guides the physician in the choice of intervention and in estimating the client's prognosis. It is therefore very important that this procedure be done consistently.

Assessment of the Client's Physical Performance

The Karnofsky Performance Status Scale, the Eastern Cooperative Oncology Group (ECOG) scale, and the American Joint Committee on Cancer (AJCC) scale help assess the client's ability to continue activity. The last two are compared in Table 23–9.

Since 1985, multidisciplinary research has begun to focus on measuring the impact of cancer and its treatment on the quality of a person's life. Prior to this, length of survival was considered to be the primary outcome in oncology treatment research. Because of its abstract, multidimensional, and elusive nature, many different definitions of "quality of life" are found in the literature, along with equally diverse measurement tools. Most instruments encompass such subconcepts as satisfaction and successful adjustment to illness and treatment in the physical, social, psychological, and spiritual domains. A comprehensive review of this topic is provided by Mast.[39]

Table 23–9. Performance Status Scales			
Eastern Cooperative Oncology Group (ECOG) Scale		**American Joint Committee on Cancer (AJCC) Scale**	
Score	*Status*	*Score*	*Status*
0	Asymptomatic	HO	Normal activity
1	Symptomatic; fully ambulatory	H1	Symptomatic and ambulatory; cares for self
2	Symptomatic; in bed <50% of day	H2	Ambulatory >50% of time; occasionally needs assistance
3	Symptomatic; in bed >50% of day, but not bedridden	H3	Ambulatory <50% of time; nursing care needed
4	Bedridden	H4	Bedridden; may need hospitalization

Adapted from Groenwald, S., et al. (1993). *Cancer nursing: Principles and practice* (3rd ed.). Boston: Jones and Bartlett.

Conclusions

Cancer is a disease that strikes two of five people in the United States. It is a condition most nurses will work with at some point during their careers. An understanding of the basic principles concerning its development, prevention, and early detection is essential.

Bibliography

1. American Cancer Society. (1995). *The case for screening mammography for women ages 40–49* (ACS PUBL NO 6129PE). American Cancer Society Illinois Division.
2. American Cancer Society. (1992). *American Cancer Society guidelines on diet, nutrition, and cancer.* Atlanta: Author.
3. American Cancer Society. (1992). Update January 1992: The American Cancer Society guidelines for the cancer-related checkup. *CA: A Cancer Journal for Clinicians, 42,* 44–45.
4. American Cancer Society. (1993). *American with Disabilities Act: Legal protection for cancer patients against employment discrimination* (ACS PUBL NO 93-100M-No. 4571). Atlanta: Author.
5. American Cancer Society. (1993). *Cancer, employment rights and you* (ACS PUBL NO 6099PS). American Cancer Society Illinois Division.
6. American Cancer Society (1995). *Cancer facts and figures.* Atlanta: Author.
7. American Nurses' Association & Oncology Nursing Society (1987). *Standards of oncology nursing practice.* Kansas City: American Nurses' Association.
8. Americans with Disabilities Act, 42 USC 12101, et seq.
9. Baird, S. B., et al. (1991). *Cancer nursing: A comprehensive textbook.* Philadelphia: W. B. Saunders.
10. Beahrs, O. H., et al. (1992). *American Joint Committee on Cancer: Manual for staging of cancer* (4th ed.). Philadelphia: J. B. Lippincott.
11. Benedict, W. (1987). Hereditary factors: Human cancer susceptibility genes. *Proceedings of the Second National Conference on Cancer Prevention and Detection.* New York: American Cancer Society.
12. Black, B. L., Schweitzer, R., & Dezelsky, T. (1993). Report on the American Cancer Society workshop on community cancer detection, education, and prevention demonstration projects for underserved populations. *CA: A Cancer Journal for Clinicians, 43,* 226–233.
13. Boring, C. C., Squires, T. S., & Heath, C. W. (1992) Cancer statistics for African Americans. *CA: A Cancer Journal for Clinicians, 42,* 7–18.
14. Brawer, M. K. (1995). How to use prostate-specific antigen in early detection for screening for prostate carcinoma. *CA: A Cancer Journal for Clinicians, 45,* 148–164.
15. Clark, J. (1993). Psychosocial responses of the patient. In S. L. Groenwald, et al. (Eds.), *Cancer nursing: Principles and practice* (3rd ed., pp. 449–467). Boston: Jones and Bartlett.
16. Consolidated Omnibus Budget Reconciliation Act (COBRA) (1986). 42 U.S.C. 300 bb et seq.
17. Crothers, H. M. (1986). Employment problems of cancer survivors: Local problems and local solutions. In American Cancer Society, *Proceedings of the workshop on employment, insurance, and the patient with cancer* (pp. 51–57). New Orleans: Author.
18. Crothers, H. M. (1987). Health insurance: Problems and solutions for people with cancer histories. In American Cancer Society *Proceedings of the 5th National Conference on Human Values and Cancer* (pp. 100–109). San Francisco: Author.
19. DeVita, V. T., Hellman, S., & Rosenberg, S. A. (1993). *Cancer: Principles and practice of oncology* (4th ed.). Philadelphia: J. B. Lippincott.
20. Eddy, D. M. (1986). Secondary prevention in cancer: An overview. *Bulletin of the World Health Organization, 64,* 421–429.
21. Engelking, C. (1995). Genetics in cancer care: Confronting a Pandora's box of dilemmas. *Oncology Nursing Forum, 22 (Supplement),* 27–34.
22. Engelking, C. (1995). The human genome exposed: A glimpse of promise, predicament, and impact on practice. *Oncology Nursing Forum, 22 (Supplement),* 3–9.
23. Frank-Stromborg, M. (1986). The role of the nurse in early detection of cancer: Population 66 years of age and older. *Oncology Nursing Forum, 13,* 107–115.
24. Frank-Stromborg, M. (1988). Nursing's role in cancer prevention and early detection: Vital contributions to attainment of the Planning, goals/expected outcomes year 2000 goals, *Cancer, 62,* 1833–1838.
25. Frank-Stromborg, M. (1989). Reaction to the diagnosis of cancer questionnaire (RDCQ): Development and psychometric evaluation. *Nursing Research, 38,* 364–369.
26. Frost, P., & Fidler, I. J. (1986). Biology of metastasis. *Cancer, 58,* 550–553.
27. Garfinkel, L. (1991). Nutrition and cancer: Current status. *CA: A Cancer Journal for Clinicians, 41,* 325–327.
28. Garfinkel, L. (1995). Perspectives on cancer prevention. *CA: A Cancer Journal for Clinicians, 45,* 5–7.
29. Grant, M. M., Padilla, G. V., & Ferrell, B. R. (1993). Cancer nursing research. In S. L. Groenwald, et al. (Eds.), *Cancer nursing: Principles and practice* (3rd ed., pp. 1599–1613). Boston: Jones and Bartlett.
30. Greenwald, P., et al. (1995). Chemoprevention. *CA: A Cancer Journal for Clinicians, 45,* 31–49.
31. Greenwald, P., & Sondik, E. (Eds.) (1986). Cancer control objectives for the nation. *National Cancer Institute Monograph, 1985–2000.* (NIH Publication No. 86—2880). Washington, DC: United States Government Printing Office.
32. Groenwald, S., et al. (1993). *Cancer nursing: Principles and practice* (4th ed.). Boston: Jones and Bartlett.
33. Groenwald, S. L., et al. (1996). *Cancer symptom management.* Boston: Jones and Bartlett.
34. Gupta, N. C., & Frick, M. P. (1993). Clinical applications of positron-emission tomography in cancer. *CA: A Cancer Journal for Clinicians, 43,* 235–254.
35. Holleb, A. I., Fink, D. J., & Murphy, G. P. (1991). *American Cancer Society textbook of clinical oncology.* Atlanta: Author.
36. Kritchevsky, D. (1991). Diet and cancer. *CA: A Cancer Journal for Clinicians, 41,* 328–333.
37. Levine, E. G., et al. (1989). The role of heredity in cancer. *Journal of Clinical Oncology, 7,* 527–540.
38. Littrup, P. J. (1993). The benefit and cost of prostate cancer early detection. *CA: A Cancer Journal for Clinicians, 43,* 134–150.
39. Loescher, L. J. (1995). Genetics in cancer prediction, screening, and counseling. *Oncology Nursing Forum, 22 (Supplement),* 10–19.
40. Mast, M. E. (1995). Definition and measurement of quality of life in oncology nursing research: Review and theoretical implications. *Oncology Nursing Forum, 22,* 957–964.
41. Sandberg, A. (1994). Cancer cytogenetics for clinicians. *CA: A Cancer Journal for Clinicians, 44,* 136–159.
42. Schmidt, R. A. (1994). Stereotactic breast biopsy. *CA: A Cancer Journal for Clinicians, 44,* 172–191.
43. Slawin, K. M., et al. (1995). Screening for prostate cancer: An analysis of the early experience. *CA: A Cancer Journal for Clinicians, 45,* 134–147.
44. Steele, G. D., et al. (1995). Clinical highlights from the National Cancer Data Base: 1995. *CA: A Cancer Journal for Clinicians, 45,* 102–111.
45. Stromborg, M., et al. (1986). Carcinogens: Are some risks acceptable? *American Journal of Nursing, 86,* 814–817.
46. Teneriello, M. G., & Park, R. C. (1995). Early detection of ovarian cancer. *CA: A Cancer Journal for Clinicians, 45,* 71–87.
47. Weinberg, R. A. (1994). Oncogenes and tumor suppressor genes. *CA: A Cancer Journal for Clinicians, 44,* 160–170.
48. Wynder, E., et al. (1986). Diet and breast cancer in causation and therapy. *Cancer, 58,* 1804–1813.
49. Yasko, J. M., & Greene, P. (1987). Coping with problems related to cancer and cancer treatment. *CA: A Cancer Journal for Clinicians, 37*(2), 106–125.

Treatment Modalities for Neoplastic Disorders

Joann Petty

Psychosocial Aspects of Cancer

Cancer is a feared and dreaded disease for several reasons. It may present in an advanced stage with no manifestations. Compliance with vigorous and sometimes disfiguring treatment does not guarantee a cure. In addition, cancer may recur after many years of remission. A healthy life-style does not ensure that a person will escape from the disease.[46]

Great variability exists in the distress, changes, and effects of cancer on the lives of clients and their families. Responses to cancer depend on (1) the client and the client's psychological make-up, (2) the client's family and social community, and (3) the disease, disabilities, and disfigurement it may cause. Responses also depend on preexisting medical conditions that may limit treatment options.

Cancer can affect the client at all levels of functioning. Intellectual function can be clouded by physical and psychological distress, medication, or the disease itself. The client's self-concept is affected by the physical changes and changes in role or function. The client who was the breadwinner in the family may become dependent on others and become a consumer of family savings and resources. The young adult, striving for independence, may need to revert to an earlier level of dependency. Changes in body image occur in most clients. Weight loss, loss of hair (alopecia), and skin changes can result from treatment. Radical surgical procedures can produce devastating and permanent changes in appearance and function. Procedures such as laryngectomy, glossectomy, quadrant resection, hemicorpectomy, or pelvic exenteration produce changes that may humiliate and overwhelm the client.

The diagnosis of cancer has an impact on the entire family. The daily life of the family is changed. If the

client is the breadwinner, other family members will need to assume this role. If the family functioned poorly before the illness, the additional stress may increase the dysfunction.

Imposed on the intrinsic complexity of individuals, families, and cultures is the variability of cancer as a disease. Some cancers are relatively easy to treat and have a reliable potential for cure, whereas others require extensive, rigorous treatment without a guarantee of cure. Manifestations of cancer vary among clients as well. Some may have considerable physical distress, whereas others have none.

Although each cancer experience is unique, people with cancer have some common problems. All persons undergo a period of diagnosis and initial treatment. If the cancer is considered curable and the client completes definitive treatment for the cancer, a period of survivorship ensues. This is characterized by watchful waiting for disease recurrence.[49] Those clients who have metastatic disease at the time of treatment or who have a cancer recurrence must deal with the chronicity of the disease.

Specific psychosocial problems, assessment, and intervention strategies are addressed for each of the distinct phases of the cancer continuum: (1) diagnosis and treatment, (2) survivorship, (3) recurrent disease, chronicity or palliation, and (4) terminal illness.

Phases of the Cancer Continuum

Diagnosis and Treatment

Cancer clients reach the point of diagnosis in many ways. They may have had vague manifestations, such as weight loss and fatigue, that have been ignored or a cause of some anxiety for weeks or months. They may have manifestations such as pain or abdominal bloating that evaded diagnosis. Many times, cancer is found incidentally dur-

This chapter incorporates material written for the fourth edition by Patricia F. Jassak and Mary Ann Krol.

ing a routine examination. Often, the person suspects cancer, but many people are shocked when the diagnosis is made. The diagnostic period may be long and extremely stressful. This period is filled with anxiety over each test result, especially when staging procedures are done. More than 70% of clients consider the time of diagnosis and treatment as the most stressful in the cancer experience.[74]

Most clients fear death during the first few months of the cancer experience. Weisman[74] called this stage "the existential plight." Whether clients can express their fears or not, it is an underlying cause of distress. During diagnosis, the magnitude of the client's problems becomes apparent. Is my disease curable? Will my disabilities be temporary or permanent? What types of physical impairment will occur? What will be the side effects of treatment? Will my symptoms be relieved? Will I be able to return to work? What adjustments have to be made in family life or work? Will finances be adequate? What plans need to be abandoned? Which changes in life-style will be temporary and which permanent?

Clients must not only deal with specific problems but also the emotional distress experienced throughout this time. They may feel angry and frustrated because their lives have been changed; they may feel isolated or may worry about being abandoned by family and friends. They may be shocked and unbelieving that they are the ones with cancer. They may also feel guilty if they feel they contributed to their disease (i.e., by smoking, drinking, or putting themselves at risk for sexually transmitted diseases).

There is great variability in clients' reactions. Some have minimal distress, whereas others may be overwhelmed and devastated. The magnitude and intensity of

---

Box 24–2. Enabling and Hindering Factors in Coping with Cancer

Enabling Factors

Social support systems
Perception of control
Hardiness
Humor
Positive appraisal
Hopefulness
Positive comparisons
Religiosity
Self-esteem
Information-seeking
Open communication
Social skills
Problem-solving ability

Hindering Factors

Denial
Avoidance
Helplessness
Powerlessness
Hopelessness or despair
Depression
Guilt
Erosion of autonomy
Isolation or withdrawal
Wishful thinking
Anger or hostility
Blaming others
Noncompliance

From Jalowiec, A., & Dudas, S. (1991). Alterations in patient coping. In S. Baird, R. McCorkle, & M. Grant (Eds.), *Cancer nursing: A comprehensive text* (pp. 806–820). Philadelphia: W. B. Saunders.

Box 24–1. General Coping Strategies

- Seek more information (rational inquiry)
- Share concern and talk with others (mutuality)
- Laugh it off; make light of the situation (affect reversal)
- Try to forget; put it out of your mind (suppression)
- Do other things for distraction (displacement, redirection)
- Take firm action based on present understanding (confrontation)
- Accept but find something favorable (redefinition, revision)
- Submit to the inevitable (fatalism, passive acceptance)
- Do something, anything, however reckless or impractical (impulsivity)
- Consider or negotiate a feasible alternative (if x, then y)
- Reduce tension with excessive drink, drugs, danger (life threats)
- Withdraw into isolation; get away (disengagement)
- Blame someone or something (externalization, projection)
- Seek direction; do what you are told (cooperative compliance)
- Blame yourself; sacrifice or atone (moral masochism)

Modified from Weisman, A. (1979). *Coping with cancer* (p. 23). New York: McGraw-Hill.

---

emotions and problems depend on the client's psychological make-up; their social support; their emotional, social, and financial resources; and the disease itself. Many nurses think clients respond inappropriately (i.e., too little or too much). It is very important to acknowledge the client's mode of response as acceptable and unique for that client.

Coping is the dynamic process by which a client responds to a problem to bring about relief or equilibrium. Weisman identified coping styles used by many cancer clients (Box 24–1). Denial, which is a part of coping, allows a client to "repudiate what cannot be avoided, by substituting a more favorable or agreeable idea.[49] Denial can be useful in the diagnostic phase when the number of problems may be overwhelming. Denial is harmful when it prevents the client from seeking appropriate treatment. Awareness and denial can exist at the same time.

Clients who are good problem solvers or who cope well confront reality, avoid excessive denial, remain flexible, accept support, and remain hopeful and optimistic. Clients who cope poorly use avoidance and excessive denial; they are pessimistic and feel hopeless.[49] Box 24–2 lists factors that enable or hinder the client's ability to cope. The client will use a variety of strategies to cope with cancer.

Families also should be assessed for their coping ability. Use of a specific family assessment tool often is not possible, but high-risk families should be identified. Families have a lot of baggage and unresolved past problems that may affect their ability to cope with cancer in the present. Families who use excessive denial, exhibit strong anger and guilt, or are unreasonably demanding may be at increased risk of dysfunction. When the client is the pivotal person in the family or when the family has had a previous experience of cancer with a negative outcome, family needs may be increased.[45]

To assess the psychosocial needs of the client, learn about the general types of emotions and problems of clients with cancer and be sensitive to their expression by the client. Asking tactful questions will determine the accuracy of your perception. The complexity and uniqueness of each client requires validation of that client's individual problems.

Expressing emotions may be difficult for many clients. Help clients by listening actively and maintaining a non-critical relationship with the client that allows expression of negative feelings. Referrals to counseling or more formal methods of emotional expression such as music or art therapy may be appropriate, if available. Providing social support and improving the client's sense of control help reduce anxiety. Stress reduction or relaxation techniques can be taught. Many clients are encouraged by speaking with former clients. Programs such as Reach to Recovery and CanSurmount (American Cancer Society) provide this opportunity.

Informational needs are very high during the diagnostic and treatment periods. Tests, procedures, and treatments, which are often very technical and complicated, need to be explained. Present consistent, accurate information in as much detail as the client wants. Be sure all healthcare providers are telling the client the same thing. When

---

Box 24–4. Cancer Resources

Many organizations provide information on request. The following are a few key resources for the nurse caring for the client and family with cancer to contact for further information:

Oncology Nursing Society (ONS)
501 Holiday Dr.
Pittsburgh, PA 15220–2749
(412) 921–7373

Office of Cancer Communications
National Cancer Institute
Building 31, Room 11A52
Bethesda, MD 20892–4200
1–800–4–CANCER

American Cancer Society (ACS)
1599 Clifton Rd. NE
Atlanta, GA 30329
1–800–ACS–2345

National Coalition for Cancer Survivorship
1010 Wayne Ave., 5th Floor
Silver Spring, MD 20910
(301) 650–8868

Oncolink
University of Pennsylvania
http://www.oncolink.upenn.edu

Roxane Pain Institute
Roxane Laboratories
http://www.Roxane.com

---

clients from a cancer clinic were surveyed, the need for information and support from family, friends, and caregivers were identified as high-priority items[23] (Box 24–3).

During this time of anxiety and stress, the simplest explanation is usually the most appropriate and all that the client can assimilate. Identify and correct misconceptions. Clients need to feel they have your undivided attention, and that enough time is allowed to ask questions. If the client feels information is provided too fast or in too little detail, he or she may get the impression that information is being withheld.

Address specific problems by helping the client to identify the problem, providing information when necessary, and referring the client to appropriate resources (Box 24–4). Common problem areas in oncology are identified in Box 24–5. If these areas are thoroughly assessed and evaluated for each client during each phase of the cancer experience, the physical and emotional distress of cancer may be minimized.

Survivorship

Clients who have completed curative treatment enter an indeterminate period of survivorship. With increasing numbers of clients being cured of cancer, more attention

---

Box 24–3. Needs of Clinic Patients with Cancer

The following needs were identified and rank-ordered by a sample of clinic patients. The last three items were ranked of equal importance.

- Information about operating special equipment
- Information about radiation
- Information provided in a way that is understandable
- Ways to be active in decision-making
- Adequate preparation before discharge from hospital
- Support from family
- Support from friends
- Information about chemotherapy
- Time off from work to recuperate
- Information about what to expect in the future
- A patient caregiver
- Time off work for treatment

Modified from Gates, M. F., Lackey, N. R., & White, M. R. (1995). Needs of hospice and clinic patients with cancer. *Cancer Practice, 3*(4), 226–232.

Box 24–5. Common Problem Areas in Oncology

Prevention and early detection
Coping
Nutrition
Mobility
Sexuality
Circulation
Information
Comfort
Protective mechanisms
Elimination
Ventilation

From American Nurses' Association & Oncology Nursing Society. (1987). *Standards of oncology nursing practice.* Kansas City, MO: American Nurses' Association.

The time of survivorship has been divided into a time of extended survival followed by a period of so-called permanent survival.[49] The transition between these periods is not precise but evolves as time passes and cancer does not recur.

The period of extended survival may be one of physical fatigue and limitation, depending on the extent of treatment. Physical rehabilitation to improve functioning may dominate the client's energy in this early period. Efforts must focus on returning the client to his or her previous level of functioning. The long-term physical effects of cancer treatment are now becoming apparent as data accumulate, especially from pediatric cancer clients. The physical effects may range from minimal restriction to life-threatening complications. The effects can be organ-specific, such as cardiomyopathy or pulmonary fibrosis, or general, such as fatigue. The potential for developing a second malignancy as a result of primary treatment exists, although it rarely occurs. Establish routine follow-up and long-term healthcare with the client and significant others at this time.[41]

Psychologically, the period of extended survival is one in which clients must take up previous roles or adjust and reorganize their lives. The possibility of recurrence may dominate their lives. Plans may be suspended. Decisions

is being focused on the physiologic and psychological needs of this group. Clients have organized into advocate groups to provide mutual support and to lobby for legislation to address some of their specific needs in employment and insurance coverage.

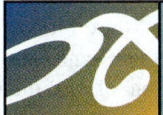

BRIDGE TO HOME HEALTHCARE

Helping Clients Cope with Cancer Treatment After Returning Home
Susan Haibeck, R.N., M.S., *Oncology Nurse Specialist, Elmhurst, Illinois*

Now that clients are being discharged earlier from hospitals, home nursing care of clients with cancer may be more intense and more frequent than ever before. The effects of cancer treatment may not develop until the client returns home after hospitalization, and they may be overwhelming to clients, caregivers, and others. When you visit clients with cancer at their home, you will frequently be the first healthcare professional to assess and report the significant side effects of cancer treatment. Depending on the client's condition and insurance coverage, you may also be the one to administer chemotherapeutic agents and blood products as part of home care. Coordination of such complex care requires excellent communication and a good working relationship with the client, the oncologist, and the oncologist's office staff. Knowledge of the expected side effects of cancer treatment and of appropriate nursing interventions increases the probability of prompt, effective treatment, allays anxiety, and reduces the number of unnecessary telephone calls or visits to the physician.

Using community resources can help the client adjust to physical changes resulting from the disease or its treatment. For example, specialty clothing stores geared toward the special needs of the woman who has undergone a mastectomy are invaluable for obtaining properly fitted breast forms and clothing. Wig suppliers that work exclusively with people who have cancer will often make home visits and are sensitive to the special needs of people with cancer. As the client learns about the resources available and develops trust in you, he or she will be better prepared to get on with the activities of daily living.

Virtually every hospital maintains or provides referrals to support groups and educational classes for people learning to cope with cancer. Some of these groups are site-specific; others are more general and are open not only to clients but to their families as well. These groups, usually led by an oncology nurse or social worker, are not therapy groups, but they do provide the opportunity for clients with cancer to learn how others have coped under similar circumstances. Some clients and their families also benefit from referrals to other support groups, the local chapter of the American Cancer Society, and mental health and counseling services.

Returning to the work place during cancer treatment is an individual decision based on the client's physical condition, the client's occupation, the recommendations of the client's physician, and treatment schedules. Many clients can return to their previous work, while others may require lighter duty or schedule adjustments to accommodate therapy. Some clients, however, are unable to return to their previous employment. If clients are able to work, most will want to and need to maintain their income and their insurance coverage, and most will want to return to work just to keep busy and know that they are contributing to the welfare of their families.

concerning changing jobs, buying a house, starting a family, or retirement may be difficult in the face of the uncertainty of recurrence. Referral to support groups may be helpful.

Employment discrimination has been a problem for cancer survivors. Although clients with a cancer history have proved themselves to be dependable and productive, studies show that as many as 84% of blue-collar workers and 38% of white-collar workers with cancer experience some type of discrimination in employment.[57] Over the years, these issues have been partially rectified by state laws protecting the rights of the disabled.

Like employment, obtaining insurance coverage for a client with a history of cancer has been difficult, ruinously expensive, and sometimes impossible. Legislative efforts have rectified some of these problems. Insurance discrimination can be legally appealed. Federal programs such as COBRA (*C*onsolidated *O*mnibus *B*udget *R*econciliation *A*ct) protect the insurance coverage of an employee for 18 months following employment termination, but at an increased monthly premium. Many states have passed comprehensive health insurance plans to provide coverage for clients who are unable to obtain commercial insurance. Direct clients who have difficulty with insurance coverage to the American Cancer Society, their state department of human rights, or their state insurance department. The booklet *Facing Forward* from the National Institutes of Health provides detailed information resources.

With time, problems usually recede and clients may become "permanent survivors." The experience of cancer is nonetheless indelibly printed on their lives. Amazingly, most clients cope very well and face the difficulties in their lives with courage. For many, the experience brings about a reappraisal of goals and values, making life richer and more meaningful.

Recurrent Disease and Palliation

The recurrence of cancer provides the basis for a chronic phase of the cancer experience. Most clients with cancer live with the threat or reality or recurrent disease. Weisman[74] describes the impact that this phase has on the client as "the hope for a cure" becoming the "struggle for existence."

With recurrent disease, therapy may once again be used to eradicate or stabilize the disease process. Yet, although subsequent recurrent disease may occur, it is usually the first recurrence that involves surprise, shock, and disbelief. Assess the client's coping skills and provide assistance in helping to mobilize resources and support. Many cancers have a propensity for recurrence, including adult acute leukemias, non-Hodgkin's lymphoma, breast, and lung cancers.

Physical impairment may be increased and quality of life may be limited because of disease or treatment. The client who previously projected an optimistic outlook may now express a more guarded attitude. Maintain open communication and be sensitive to the informational and support needs of the client and family with cancer.

Palliative treatment and palliative care are two distinct options for the client whose cancer persists. Surgery, radiation therapy, or chemotherapy may be used to palliate complications caused by persistent tumor growth. For example, surgery may be used to manage a malignant obstruction, or radiation therapy to reduce or prevent paralysis from spinal cord compression.

Palliative care is not curative, but rather aimed at improving the quality of the remainder of the client's life for a long as possible. Palliative care is the provision of symptom management and psychosocial support, best provided by a multidisciplinary healthcare team. Communicate to the client that disease manifestations can be managed successfully and that resources are available to assist in providing supplies and support. Palliative care is effective in decreasing the stress and discomfort related to advanced cancer and provides the client and family with options to assist them as the disease enters the terminal phase.

Terminal Illness

More than 50% of clients with cancer die from their disease.[2] The time from diagnosis to death ranges from weeks to years. Not all clients with cancer become terminally ill. Some clients die during the initial treatment; others die from complications of treatment. Many clients, however, reach an endpoint, at which time their cancer no longer responds to treatment and progression of the disease cannot be controlled. Now the goal of treatment is directed toward supportive care and minimizing distress until death occurs.

During the past 25 years, hospice care has become the standard of care for terminally ill cancer clients in the United States. This philosophy of care emphasizes symptom control and pain management, providing comfort and dignity for the client during the dying process.

Hospices date back to medieval times when they were way stations for travelers and pilgrims. Most were run by Christian religious orders. The Irish Sisters of Charity opened the first hospice specifically for the dying in the mid-19th century in London. However, it was not until 1967 when Dr. Cicely Saunders opened the St. Christopher's hospice in London and pioneered techniques for adequate pain control that the modern concept of hospice care emerged.[44]

The first hospice in the United States was established in 1974 in New Haven, Connecticut. Since that time, more than 1600 hospice facilities have been established in the United States. The hospice can be affiliated with a hospital, community, home care agency, or skilled nursing facility and care can be provided in an inpatient hospital, a separate facility, or in the home. The basic characteristics of a hospice program include the following:

● Control of client manifestations and pain relief
● Treatment of client and family as a unit
● Provision of care by a physician-directed interdisciplinary team
● Twenty-four-hour, 7-day coverage

- An autonomous hospice administration providing coordinated home care with back-up inpatient services
- Use of trained volunteers to augment staff services
- Structured systems of staff support
- Spiritual support
- Bereavement follow-up
- Services given based on need and not ability to pay

Community-based hospices also include services such as family respite care, running errands or shopping, light housework, transportation, provision of medical equipment, basic care, nutritional support, and assistance to allow the client to die at home.

To qualify for hospice services, clients must have a life expectancy of less than 6 months and be on supportive treatment only.

When clients reach the point at which treatment is no longer effective, they are considered terminally ill. The Ethical Issues in Nursing feature explores ways to care for clients who can accept or resign themselves to the approaching end of their life, as well as those who cannot and continue to seek treatment despite the futility of further treatment.

Hospice programs have been innovators in encouraging clients to identify their wishes related to cardiopulmonary resuscitation, invasive procedures, and identification of family and friends to assist in decision-making if the client becomes incapacitated.[43] The Patient Self-Determination Act of 1991 seeks to promote client decision-making regarding medical interventions at the end of life through the use of legal, written documents known as advance directives. An advanced directive is a statement made by a competent individual directing his or her medical care in the event he or she is unable to make healthcare decisions.[15] The law does not specifically require that

persons execute advanced directives, rather that they know they have the opportunity to do so.

The two most commonly used advanced directives are the living will and durable power of attorney for healthcare. A living will focuses on limiting the use of life-sustaining treatment for a person who has a documented terminal illness.[15] The durable power of attorney for healthcare identifies a proxy appointed by the person to make healthcare decisions in the event he or she becomes incapacitated. It is not limited to persons in a terminal state.[15]

Clients approach death in as many ways as they approach life. Some try to remain active despite tremendous physical limitations. Others may withdraw into depression. This period is a time of suffering for both client and family as the physical loss of function and the psychological pain of anticipated and real losses in relationships and roles are intensified.

Nursing care of the terminally ill addresses pain and symptom management while maintaining the dignity of the client and promoting the maximum quality of life. As family members become caretakers, they must be taught simple nursing skills and pain management. Open communication and continued revalidation of the concerns and needs of client and family need to be maintained.

Family members need constant reassurance that they are providing good care. Although it is often a new and unfamiliar experience, most families are able to focus their energies and strengthen their family bonds through the experience of caring for a dying family member with the continued support of an interdisciplinary healthcare team. When death occurs, families are usually physically exhausted but psychologically strengthened.

Clients without families or friends to function as primary caretakers have few options for their care. A few freestanding hospices exist to provide them with care.

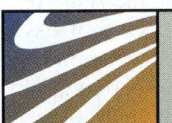

ETHICAL ISSUES IN NURSING

Who Should Decide to Continue or End Cancer Treatment?

Great strides have been made in the treatment of neoplastic disorders. The word *cancer* no longer synonymous with death. There is much hope in the treatment of many cancerous conditions. Nevertheless, disease processes remain that cannot be cured, and patients with these diseases must rely on care.

Are there times when a client should accept the fact that nothing more can be done—that treatment options are futile? Are physicians obligated to treat clients with therapies that are hopeless even if the client might want such therapies? Are there times when clients can say they wish no more treatment—no more chemotherapy, radiation therapy, or even surgery—even if there is a chance that such treatments might be helpful? Perhaps they believe the end stages of their life would be better lived without the side effects of such treatments.

Nursing care for clients with cancer presents many challenges. Be sensitive to the emotional aspect of the client's illness, use your skills with the technical aspects of care (such as chemotherapy), be available to teach both client and significant others about the disease process and treatments, and be a healthcare advocate for the client. If a client decides that he or she no longer wants treatment, put all of your skills to work to help meet the client's current and anticipated needs. If treatment is no longer an option for the client, be there to provide care for the client and significant others.

To cure should not always be seen as success and not to cure as failure. Caring can be just as successful as curing when curing is not an option. Nurses have an important role in the caring process of a client's illness, especially when such care is exercised during the final stages of life.

Many nursing homes have hospice programs. Clients without insurance or financial means are less fortunate, although some home care may be available.

Masterful use of basic nursing skills, combined with creative symptom management and compassion for the client and family, is the essence of hospice nursing care. Nursing care remains the mainstay of the client and significant others.

Beyond what machines and medicines and procedures can do for the client, the act of caring remains a powerful weapon in the fight against disease. It is the one thing that technology can never replace. When everything is done that can be done, compassion is the only thing that brings beauty and meaning to our lives. It is "the irreplaceable gift."[68]

Treatment and Nursing Care of Clients with Cancer

Goals of Intervention

The major objective of cancer therapy is to treat the client effectively with appropriate therapy for a sufficient duration so a cure results with minimal functional and structural impairment.[10] If a cure is not possible, important alternative goals are to (1) prevent further metastasis, (2) relieve manifestations, and (3) maintain a high quality of life for as long as possible. Decisions made at the time of first diagnosis are crucial, because early aggressive intervention usually offers the best hope of cure.

Methods of treating clients with cancer include surgery, radiation therapy, chemotherapy, bone marrow transplantation, and biologic response modifiers. The choice of method depends on the type of tumor, extent of disease, the client's physical status, and the client's wishes. In most cases, a client is treated with a combination of methods rather than a single therapy. This approach is called combined modality, or multimodal therapy. Combined modality therapy is used in most cancer treatment regimens because it is more effective in destroying cancerous cells.

Surgery

Surgery plays a major role in the diagnosis, staging, and treatment of cancer. It is also an integral part of the rehabilitation and palliation of clients with cancer. It is used with less frequency as a method of cancer prevention.

Although many aspects of surgical care of the client with cancer are similar to all surgical clients (see Chapter 21 and those chapters that address surgery of a specific part of the body), some differences exist.

Preoperatively, clients with cancer may be nutritionally compromised and require hospitalization or home nutritional therapy before surgery. Those who have had adjuvant or palliative chemotherapy or radiotherapy may have low red or white blood cell counts, which need correction

before surgery. Clients undergoing a palliative surgical procedure must have their pain assessed from the perspective of normal postoperative pain in addition to pain secondary to tumor invasion.

The current insurance-driven practice of shortened hospital stays leaves little time for preoperative assessment of the client's psychological state. Is is important that you evaluate the client's understanding of the proposed procedure and the changes it involves preoperatively. Some clients anticipate surgery with relief because it represents a physical removal of the tumor and the endpoint of what may have been a protracted diagnostic interval. On the other hand, the client may suffer from great anxiety if the extent of the tumor is unknown preoperatively and the procedure will determine the curability or noncurability of the disease. Support from the client's clergyman or clergywoman may be helpful.

Diagnostic Surgery

The diagnosis of cancer is established by microscopic identification of malignant cells from tumor tissue. A variety of methods are used to obtain tissue for diagnostic purposes. The biology of the tumor, its size and location, and the proposed method of treatment determine which biopsy method should be used.

Cytology Specimens. Cytology specimens can be obtained from tumors that tend to shed cells from their surface. Tumor cells can often be obtained from cytologic examination of fluids aspirated from effusions, ascitic fluid, or endoscopic brushings.

Needle Biopsy. Needle biopsy is a simple method of obtaining tissue samples. In a fine-needle aspiration, tumor cells are withdrawn from the tumor by a needle and syringe. A core-needle biopsy is essentially the same procedure; however, the needle is larger and a core of tissue is obtained. This allows the pathologist to examine the cells with their spatial relationships intact, whereas aspiration biopsy provides individual cells or clumps of cells for review. Needle biopsies are useful in obtaining samples from tumors in subcutaneous tissue, muscle, breast, pancreas, liver, and lung.

Cytology and needle biopsies are relatively simple procedures. Care must be taken to obtain needle biopsies from areas that will be surgically removed if the tumor is malignant, because malignant cells can be deposited in the needle tract. A negative biopsy does not prove the absence of cancer but rather may be an indication of inadequate or misplaced tissue sampling. Negative needle biopsies must be followed by additional biopsies to obtain an accurate diagnosis.

Incisional Biopsy. An incisional biopsy removes a small sample of tissue for examination. It is performed during endoscopic examinations of the bronchus, stomach, bladder, and colon and in removal of samples of large tumor masses in which a diagnosis must be made before definitive surgical treatment. Surgical techniques are used to prevent seeding of tumor cells in the biopsy site. As with needle biopsy, cancer can be proved with a positive result but not ruled out with a negative one. When negative results are obtained, additional biopsies may be done.

Excisional Biopsy. An excisional biopsy removes all of the tumor mass and provides the pathologist with an entire sample. It is used for small tumors (2–3 cm) in which the biopsy also may serve as the treatment if the tissue margins contain no tumor cells. If tumor cells remain, a wider excision is required. Excisional biopsies are useful in skin cancers, melanomas, and in breast cancer. It is important that these biopsies have clean margins if this is to be the only surgery.

Staging Exploratory Surgery

Cancer staging is the process of determining the extent of disease as the basis for treatment decisions. Clinical staging is based on evidence acquired before treatment and obtained from physical examination, imaging, endoscopy, biopsy, and surgical exploration. It is based on all information prior to the first definitive treatment used.[4] Pathologic staging is based on the evidence acquired before treatment, supplemented or modified by information from surgery and the pathologic examination of resected specimens, including the primary tumor, regional lymph nodes, and metastatic nodules.[4] For example, the true stage of colon cancer is usually determined after surgery, when the regional lymph nodes are examined for the presence of tumor cells. Staging of ovarian cancer is based on the extent and location of disease found at surgical exploration.[80]

In lymphomas, although radiation therapy and chemotherapy are the primary treatment modalities, a surgical laparotomy is sometimes necessary to determine the precise extent of the disease. When indicated for lymphoma staging, the laparotomy includes liver biopsy, splenectomy, and multiple nodal biopsies.

Curative Surgery

Surgery for Primary Lesions

Surgery is performed in 55% of clients with cancer. Forty percent of clients are treated with surgery alone. Cancers that are localized to the organ of origin and the regional lymph nodes are potentially curable by surgery, although multimodal treatment is more likely to be used.[58]

Historically, the generally accepted concept of tumor growth was an orderly sequence of growth from the organ of origin to adjacent tissue, regional lymph nodes, and eventually, systemically to distant sites. The logical surgical approach to this type of growth was the widest excision possible of the tumor, surrounding tissue, and regional lymph nodes. Thus, radical surgery became the standard for cancer treatment. Analysis of treatment results, however, demonstrated that despite radical excisions, tumors recurred.[72] Current concepts in tumor biol-

ogy hold that tumors probably shed cells into the systemic circulation throughout their growth and, therefore, local therapies, surgery, and radiation must be combined with systemic therapies, chemotherapy, and biotherapy to improve client survival.

When surgery is performed with curative intent, the extent of the excision is determined by the type of tumor. For slow-growing tumors, such as those of the skin, a wide local excision may be sufficient. Tumors of the colon and breast that spread to the regional lymph nodes are removed with an en bloc excision of the tumor and regional lymph nodes. Large tumors, such as sarcomas, which tend to spread locally without metastasizing, are removed with radical excisions, such as amputations. In all surgical procedures, various operative techniques, such as glove changing, instrument cleaning, and wound irrigation with cytotoxic agents, are used to prevent dissemination of tumor cells into and beyond the operative field.

Surgery for Recurrent Lesions

Cancer that recurs locally can be resected, resulting in occasional cure, remission, or both. Local recurrences of sarcomas, colon, breast, and skin cancers have been successfully excised, resulting in cures.

Surgery for Metastatic Lesions

Solitary metastatic lesions that appear in the lungs, liver, or brain can be removed to effect a surgical cure. Excision of metastatic lesions is considered if no other evidence of disease exists and the metastatic lesion appeared after a relatively long disease-free interval. The metastatic lesion must exhibit some degree of stability and be refractory to chemotherapy and radiotherapy. Metastatic renal cell carcinomas, sarcomas, melanomas, and colon carcinomas have been removed in selected clients, resulting in cures or prolonged survival times.

Palliative Surgery

Because surgical procedures carry an inherent potential for morbidity, use of surgery in palliative care is carefully considered and used only if the risk-benefit ratio is favorable. Examples of palliative surgery that can benefit the client with cancer and improve quality of life include procedures that (1) reduce pain, (2) relieve airway obstructions, (3) relieve obstructions in the gastrointestinal and urinary tracts, (4) relieve pressure on the brain or spinal cord, (5) prevent hemorrhage, (6) remove infected and ulcerating tumors, and (7) drain abscesses.

Reconstructive Surgery

Advances in reconstructive surgery offer a different perspective on rehabilitation to the client who has experienced curative surgery. Restoration of form and function is possible in varying degrees, depending on the site and extent of surgery. Reconstructive surgery may be performed concurrently with the radical procedure or delayed for optimal outcome. The major goal of reconstructive surgery is to improve the client's quality of life by restoring maximal function and appearance.

Preventive Surgery

The client at unusually high risk of cancer may elect to have preventive surgical intervention. Certain conditions or diseases increase the risk of cancer occurrence so significantly that removal of the target organ is justified to prevent cancer development. Clients with familial polyposis have a 50% risk of developing colon cancer by the age of 40. By the age of 70, all clients with this inherited trait have developed colon cancer. Clients with ulcerative colitis also have an increased risk for colon cancer. Prophylactic subtotal colectomies may be indicated for this group.[58] Clients with multiple high-risk factors (see Chapter 23) may consider prophylactic surgery. Prophylactic mastectomy or oophorectomy, although infrequently indicated, are forms of preventive therapy in certain high-risk clients.

Radiation Therapy

More than 60% of all clients with cancer receive radiation therapy (RT) at some point during the course of their disease. RT may be used as a primary, adjuvant, or palliative treatment modality. As a primary modality, RT is the only treatment used and aims to achieve local cure of the cancer (e.g., early-stage Hodgkin's disease, skin cancer, carcinoma of the cervix). As an adjuvant, RT can be used either preoperatively or postoperatively to aid in the destruction of cancer cells (e.g., colorectal cancer, early breast cancer). In addition, it can be used in conjunction with chemotherapy to treat disease in sites not readily accessible to systemic chemotherapy, such as the brain. Chemotherapy also can be combined with RT and is administered before the RT dose in an attempt to potentiate the effects of RT. RT also can be used as a palliative treatment modality to relieve pain caused by obstruction, pathologic fractures, spinal cord compression, and metastasis.

How Radiation Therapy Works

RT is the use of high-energy ionizing rays to treat a variety of cancers. Ionizing radiation destroys the cell's ability to reproduce by damaging the cell's DNA. Rapidly dividing cells, such as some cancer cells, are more vulnerable to radiation than more slowly dividing cells. Furthermore, normal cells have a greater ability than cancer cells to repair the DNA damage from radiation.

In addition to the DNA effects, a complex chain of chemical reactions occurs in the extracellular fluid resulting in the formation of free radicals. Well-oxygenated tumors show a much greater response to radiation than poorly oxygenated tumors. Oxygen free radicals formed during ionization interact readily with nearby molecules, causing cellular damage (including genetic material).

Radiosensitivity, the relative susceptibility of tissues to radiation, depends on the individual cells and the characteristics of the tissue itself. A highly radiosensitive tumor is greatly affected by radiation because it divides rapidly, is well vascularized, and has a high oxygen content.

Types of Radiation Therapy

RT can be administered from a variety of sources. Sources can be divided into those used outside the body (external RT) and those used close to the surface of the body or inside the body (internal RT).

External Radiation Therapy

External beam radiotherapy, or teletherapy, refers to radiation delivered from a source placed at some distance from the target site. It is usually administered by high-energy x-ray machines (e.g., the betatron and linear accelerator) or machines containing a radioisotope (cobalt 60).

The major advantage of high-energy radiation is its skin-sparing effect. This means that the maximum effect of radiation occurs within the tumor deep in the body and not on the skin surface.

Neutron beam therapy delivered from a cyclotron particle accelerator is currently used to treat many types of cancers, including salivary gland tumors, sarcomas, and tumors of the prostate and lung.

Internal Radiation Therapy

Internal RT involves the placement of specially prepared radioisotopes directly into or near the tumor itself (brachytherapy) or into the systemic circulation. The two major types of internal RT are the sealed source, in which the radioactive material is enclosed in a sealed container, and the unsealed source, in which the radioactive material is administered systemically, such as by injection or orally.

Sealed-Source Radiation Therapy. Sealed-source RT includes intracavity and interstitial therapy. In intracavity therapy, the radioisotope, usually cesium 137 or radium 226, is placed into an applicator, then placed in the body cavity for a carefully calculated time, usually 24 to 72 hours. Intracavity radiation therapy is used to treat cancers of the uterus and cervix.

In interstitial therapy the radioisotope of choice (e.g., iridium 192, iodine 125, cesium 137, gold 198, or radon 222) is placed in needles, beads, seeds, ribbons, or catheters and then implanted directly into the tumor. For example, clients with prostate cancer may receive implanted seeds as therapy. Implants may be left in the tumor either temporarily (e.g., when ribbons, needles, or catheters are used) or permanently (prostatic seeds), depending on the half-life of the isotope being used.

Unsealed-Source Radiation Therapy. Unsealed sources are used in systemic therapy. Radioisotopes may be administered intravenously, into a body cavity, or orally. For example, sodium phosphate P32 is administered intravenously to treat polycythemia vera. Iodine 131 is given orally in very low doses to treat Graves' disease (see Chapter 70) or in high doses to treat thyroid cancer. Strontium chloride 89 (Metastron) is administered intravenously for relief of painful bony metastases.

Side Effects of Radiation Therapy

Several factors determine the side effects of RT. The size of the treatment field is important. If a small area is treated, the client will tolerate a higher dose of radiation than if a larger area is treated. Different areas of the body are affected differently by radiation. Certain tissues are more sensitive to radiation and may incur permanent damage as a result of radiation. In general, only the area in the treatment field is affected by the radiation. For example, hair loss occurs only in the area being treated with radiation.

The total dose of radiation is also related to the side effects a client may experience. Radiation dose is prescribed in units called grays (Gy). This term has replaced the unit of dose known as the rad (radiation absorbed dose). One Gy equals 100 rad. One cGy (centigray) equals 1 rad. A client receiving 5000 cGy for cure probably will experience more side effects than someone receiving 2000 cGy for palliation. The side effects are minimized by administering the radiation in divided rather than single doses.

Combined modality therapy with chemotherapy and radiation has the potential for enhanced tumor destruction as well as enhanced side effects. The gastrointestinal, integumentary, and myeloproliferative systems are at greatest risk of damage.

The goal of RT is to destroy the malignant tumor without harming surrounding tissues. Several factors help achieve this goal. Fractionation refers to dividing the total radiation dose into small, frequent doses. A common dosage schedule for external radiation therapy is 150 to 200 cGy, 5 days per week, for a total of 4 to 5 weeks. Fractionation increases the probability that tumor cells will be in a vulnerable phase of the cell cycle when treated. Fractionation also allows normal cells time to repair themselves.

Another way in which normal cells are spared is to alternate the sites of entry (ports) of radiation. For example, radiation for cervical cancer can be directed at the cervix through the front, back, and sides of the body. The maximum effect of the radiation beam is on the cervix, with the normal tissues receiving only a portion of the total dose. Additionally, customized shielding "blocks" may be created to protect normal tissues from ionizing rays.

Radiation therapy can be a source of fear and misunderstanding for clients and their families (Box 24–6). Education can dispel common fears and misconceptions.

In general, skin reactions, fatigue, nausea, and anorexia may occur with RT to any site, whereas other side effects occur only when specific areas are involved in the treatment field. Many manifestations do not develop until ap-

proximately 10 to 14 days into treatment, and some do not subside until 2 or more weeks after treatment.

The response of normal skin to radiation treatment varies from mild erythema to moist desquamation, similar in appearance to a second-degree burn. However, the term "burn" should not be used to describe these skin reactions because this may unnecessarily frighten the client. Because megavoltage and cobalt deliver the maximum dose beneath the skin, skin reactions have become less significant. Provide clients with explicit oral and written instructions for skin care (see the Client Education Guide for skin care within the treatment field).

Site-specific manifestations include mucositis, xerostomia, radiation caries, esophagitis, dysphagia, nausea and vomiting, tenesmus, cystitis, urethritis, alopecia, and bone marrow suppression. During radiation therapy a complete blood count is usually done weekly. The degree of mye-

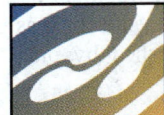

CLIENT EDUCATION GUIDE

Skin Care Within the Treatment Field

- Keep your skin dry.
- Do not wash the treatment area until you are instructed to do so. When permitted, wash the treated skin gently with mild soap, rinse well, and pat dry. Use warm or cool water, *not* hot water.
- Do not remove the lines or ink marks placed on your skin.
- Avoid using powders, lotions, creams, alcohol, or deodorants on the treated skin.
- Wear loose-fitting clothing to avoid friction over the treatment field.
- Do not apply tape to the treatment site if dressings are applied.
- Shave with an electric razor; do not use pre-shave or after-shave.
- Protect your skin from exposure to direct sunlight, chlorinated swimming pools, and temperature extremes (e.g., hot water bottles, heating pads).
- Consult your radiation therapist or nurse about specific measures for individual skin reactions.

losuppression varies with the amount of bone marrow in the treatment field. Areas at greatest risk are the pelvic region, sacrum, skull, lumbar and thoracic spine, ribs, shoulder region, and sternum. In the client of childbearing age, radiation therapy may cause prolonged or permanent infertility.

Many of the symptom management strategies are similar to those for chemotherapy side effects described in this chapter. Strohl[64] provides a comprehensive review of symptom management of acute and chronic RT reactions.

The Role of Radiation in Cancer Research

Radiation is a vital area in medical research. Radioactive isotopes are being attached to monoclonal and polyclonal antibodies to treat certain tumors on an investigational basis.[8] Several centers in the United States are using intraoperative radiation to deliver a high dose of radiation directly to the tumor, with little damage to normal structures in the beam pathway.[62] Hyperfractionation (increased total dose delivered in two to three treatments per day) for particularly resistant tumors is being tested.

Another area of research involves the use of hyperthermia with RT. Hyperthermia and radiation therapy work together in three ways: (1) hypoxic tumor cells are radioresistant but heat-sensitive, (2) tumor cells in the S phase of replication tend to be radioresistant but heat-sensitive, and (3) heat directly impairs the repair process of irradiated cells.

Hyperthermia can be provided locally, regionally, or to the entire body. Local hyperthermia is usually generated with electromagnetic coupling or ultrasound. Regional hyperthermia may involve perfusion with heated solutions. Whole-body hyperthermia can be accomplished by placing the client in a heated enclosure, such as a heated water tank or a water-heated space unit. Studies involving hyperthermia continue and may prove to significantly potentiate the efficacy of radiation therapy.[71]

In addition, the use of radiosensitizers and radioprotectors is being explored. Radiosensitizers and radioprotectors are chemical compounds that may be used to change the effect of radiation on cells and tissues. Radiosensitizers are compounds that enhance the damaging effect of ionizing radiation. Because hypoxic cells are resistant to radiation, research is being directed toward increasing the oxygen supply to the tumor. Hypoxic cell sensitizers are chemical agents that take the place of oxygen in hypoxic cells and, thus, promote radiation effectiveness. Agents under current investigation include metronidazole and etanidazole. Radioprotectors are compounds that can protect normal healthy tissue while having a limited effect on tumor cells.

Radiation Safety

Three key principles to follow to protect nurses and others from excessive radiation exposure are distance, time, and shielding.

Distance

The greater the distance from the radiation source, the less the exposure dose of ionizing rays. Distance and radiation exposure are inversely related. The intensity of radiation decreases inversely to the square of the distance from the source. For example, if a person stands 4 ft from a source of radiation, the person is exposed to approximately one-fourth the amount of radiation the person would receive at 2 ft (Fig. 24–1).

Figure 24–1. Radiation safety. (From Sedhom, L. N., & Yann, M. I. Y. [1985]. Radiation therapy and nurses' fears of radiation exposure. *Cancer Nursing, 8,* 129–134.)

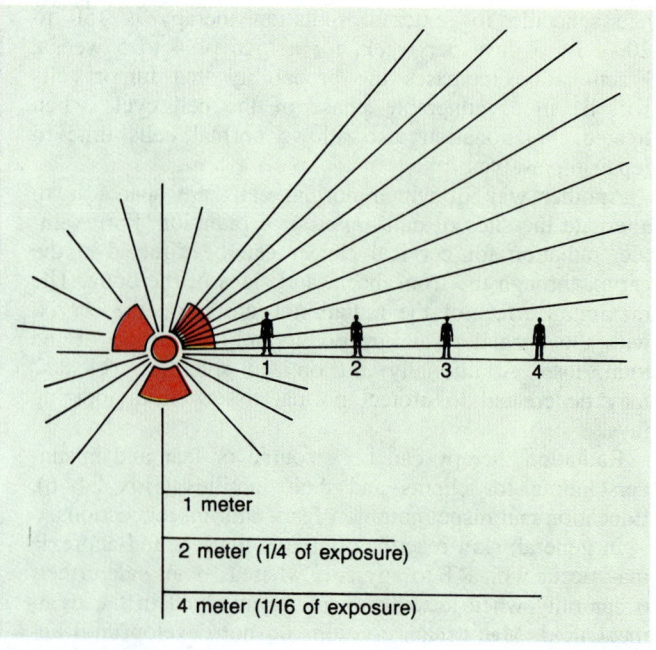

Time

Minimal exposure time should be promoted, although client care needs must still be met. A nurse's exposure time is generally limited to 30 minutes of direct care per 8-hour shift.[16]

Shielding

The choice of whether or not to use shielding devices to reduce exposure depends on the source of radiation. The dose of x-rays and gamma rays is reduced as the thickness of the lead shield is increased. In practice, nurses have found that lead shielding can be cumbersome to work with. By maintaining maximum distance from the radioactive source and limiting duration of exposure, nurses can safely protect themselves with or without shielding.[16]

Safety Standards

The U.S. Nuclear Regulatory Commission requires that radiation exposure be kept as low as reasonably achievable.[70] All institutions using radioactive materials must have written policies concerning radiation protection. In addition, a radiation safety officer licensed by the U.S. Atomic Energy Commission to work with radioactive material must be available at all institutions using radioactive materials.

Monitoring devices such as a film badge are required by law for healthcare workers exposed to radiation and to provide a record of an individual's exposure. Film badges should not be shared. The film badge provides a measure of whole-body exposure. The general precautions listed earlier apply to all forms of internal RT, both sealed and unsealed sources. However, because sealed and unsealed sources differ from each other in certain respects, each type requires additional precautionary measures for safe use.

Sealed Sources

Sealed sources of internal radiation differ from unsealed sources in that the radioisotope is completely enclosed by nonradioactive material. Thus, the radioisotope cannot circulate through the client's body, nor can it contaminate urine, sweat, blood, or vomitus. Consequently, the client's excretions are not radioactive. However, radiation exposure can result from direct contact with the sealed radioisotope, such as touching the container with bare hands or from lengthy exposure.

Afterloading devices have been developed in which an empty applicator (the product that holds the radiation source) is placed during an operative procedure, and the radioactive source is not loaded until the client returns to the hospital room. The technique of remote afterloading may be used to deliver frequent, short-term high doses of radiation directly to a selected tumor. Generally, hollow applications are surgically inserted. The radioactive source is inserted into the applicator and left in place for a specific time afterward. The source is removed while the applicator is left in place and the client returns to the hospital room until the next treatment. Thus, the use of afterloading devices has helped to decrease exposure.

Clients with radioactive implants require a private room and bath because of the risk of dislodgement. Client rooms at the ends of halls or stairwells may be designated for use because their location provides less chance of exposure to others. Institutions with a high volume of radiation implants may have specially designed rooms with lead-shielded walls. Address the feelings of isolation these clients may experience. Stay in verbal contact with the client from the doorway, keeping your distance from radiation exposure.

A lead container and a pair of long-handled forceps should always be present in the client's room. If the source becomes dislodged, forceps are used to pick up the source, which is then placed immediately in the lead container. Generally, the radiation therapist and the radiation safety officer are notified immediately of the situation.[16] They in turn retrieve and secure the radiation source.

Table 24–1 summarizes radiation safety precautions. Use these guidelines for your own protection as well as for the protection of other staff and visitors. Teach clients receiving internal radiation therapy about the precautions that must be followed and why they are necessary.

Unsealed Sources

Unsealed sources used for internal radiation therapy are colloid suspensions and come into direct contact with body tissues. Unsealed sources are given intravenously, orally, or by instillation directly into a body cavity. Because the source is not encased in a protective container, a potential contamination hazard exists. The isotope may be excreted in any body fluid. Instruct clients to flush the toilet several times after each use for several days, depending on the radiation source used. Additional precautions may be necessary depending on the radioisotope used and individual practice setting policies and procedures.

Foods are served on disposable plates along with disposable utensils. Trash is kept in the client's room and not removed until the client is ready for discharge. Bed linens are generally not changed unless they are grossly soiled to further decrease the risk of radiation exposure to caregivers. Prior to discharge, the client should be scanned by the radiation safety officer to be certain that the level of radiation has decreased to a safe level.

Chemotherapy

Drug Development and Clinical Trials

The era of modern chemotherapy can be considered to have begun in 1948 with the introduction of nitrogen

Table 24–1. Safety Precautions and Rationales for Clients Receiving Internal Radiation Therapy

Safety Precaution	Rationale
Place the client in a private room.	Prevents undue exposure to other clients and to nurses caring for these clients.
Plan care well so minimal time is spent in direct contact with the client. Do not spend more than 30 minutes per shift with the client.	To limit the amount of radiation exposure, plan care well in advance, change linens less frequently, prepare meal trays outside the room, and work as quickly as possible. If the client can get up, have him or her sit as far as possible from the bed while you change the linen.
Stand at the client's shoulder (for cervical implants) or at the foot of the bed (for head and neck implants), avoiding close contact with unshielded areas.	The client's body will help to shield you.
If you must have prolonged contact with the client or if you will be exposed to an unshielded area, use a lead shield.	Lead will decrease your exposure to radiation.
Do not care for more than one client with a radiation implant at one time.	Caring for more than one client with an implant could expose you to unnecessarily high amounts of radiation.
All healthcare personnel should wear appropriate monitoring devices.	Keep records to monitor the exact amount of radiation exposure of each person in contact with the client. If any employee is receiving too much exposure, this person should not be assigned to radiation care for a while.
The room should be marked with appropriate signs stating the presence of radiation; do not allow children under 18 or pregnant women to visit; limit visitors' time to 30 minutes at a distance of at least 6 ft from the radioactive source; do not care for these patients if you are pregnant.	Warn all personnel (and visitors) of the presence of radiation so that undue exposure does not occur.
Carefully check all linens or other materials removed from the bed for the presence of implants.	If the client has excessive drainage requiring frequent linen changes, the linen may be examined with a Geiger counter to be certain no portion of the implant is lost. Careless discarding of linens could lead to unnecessary exposure of personnel to radiation.
Keep long-handled forceps and a lead-lined container available on the nursing unit or in the client's room while the implant is in place.	In case of accidental dislodgement of the implant, use long-handled forceps to pick up the implant and place it in the lead-lined container. Notify the radiation therapy department immediately.

mustard. Since that time, scientists have continued to search for medications to treat neoplasms.

The National Cancer Institute methodically screens 50,000 compounds each year, of which only a few become commercially available. First, pharmacologic studies are carried out in the laboratory. If these experiments demonstrate antitumor activity and the absence of prohibitive toxicity, the drug advances to supervised clinical trials in humans. Clinical trials are carried out on a nationwide basis, and the pooled results of these investigations are used to determine and validate the effectiveness of treatment regimens. Nurses have a major role to play in these research trials.

Phase I trials determine the maximum tolerated dose with acceptable toxicity, define drug side effects, and provide information on bioavailability and pharmacologic data. During this phase, the investigational drug is given to a small number of human subjects with cancer. Although the drug has been tested in the laboratory and in animals, it is not known how humans will respond. No direct benefit in terms of disease remission can be guar-

anteed. Because these trials may involve significant risks for the subject and only minimal, if any, benefit, they are offered only to those whose cancer has spread and would not be helped by other known treatments. Safety, comfort, and ethical considerations are primary nursing concerns during this phase of clinical trials. Give clients as much information as possible, including the fact that the drug may have no benefit.

The information obtained in phase I trials is then used to conduct phase II trials, which determine the effect of the drug on various types of cancer. After tumor specificity has been determined in phase II, a phase III trial then compares the investigational therapy against an established form of treatment for a particular type of cancer. This phase often involves randomization (random selection of who is treated with the usual therapy and who will receive the new treatment).

Nursing responsibilities associated with caring for a client participating in a clinical trial include documentation of treatment benefits and side effects, anticipation of adverse reactions and early recognition of toxicity, management of side effects, preparation for diagnostic procedures, and client education. A client education pamphlet prepared by the National Cancer Institute, *What Are Clinical Trials All About?*,[50] describes important questions a client should ask when considering participation in a clinical trial.

Objective of Chemotherapy

The objective of chemotherapy is to destroy all malignant tumor cells without excessive destruction of normal cells. Chemotherapy is a systemic intervention and is appropriate when disease is widespread or when the risk of undetectable disease is high.

Chemotherapy leads to a cure for many clients with cancer. Guidelines for treating curable cancers stress early aggressive therapy. Another important use of chemotherapy is to control tumor growth when a cure is not possible. Chemotherapy may also be given for palliation without curing the underlying disease. Many clients with cancer have benefited from an extended life span and an improved quality of life as a result of chemotherapy.

In recent years, chemotherapeutic agents have come into use as adjuvant therapy. This means that after initial treatment with either surgery or radiotherapy, medications are used to eliminate any remaining cancer cells. The client at high risk of recurrence but with no evidence of current disease may be a candidate for adjuvant therapy. Adjuvant therapy is now well established in the treatment of breast cancer. Neoadjuvant chemotherapy refers to the initial use of chemotherapy to reduce the bulk and lower the stage of a tumor, making it amenable to cure with subsequent local therapy.[40]

Significant advances in the field of chemotherapy have been made in the last 30 years. Twelve types of cancer are now considered curable with chemotherapy, even in advanced stages.[40] Unfortunately, these 12 tumors account for only about 10% of all cancers. The most common cancers have not yet shown a significant response to systemic therapy, and in the intermediate and less favorable groups of cancer, the responses to chemotherapy are mainly temporary.[39, 40] The response of specific neoplasms to chemotherapy is summarized in Box 24–7.

How Chemotherapy Works

The phases of the cell cycle are common to all cells (see Chapter 24). Normally, cells respond to the body's need for growth, repair, or regeneration in an orderly manner and cease production by entering a resting phase or slowing growth when the need is met. At any given time, normal cells may be found in all phases of growth. Cancer cells reproduce in the same manner as normal cells. However, growth occurs in an uncontrollable manner. In general, cells that are actively dividing are the most sensitive to chemotherapy.

Chemotherapy directly or indirectly disrupts reproduction of cells by altering essential biochemical processes. The desired outcome is control or eradication of all malignant cells.

Box 24–7. Response of Selected Tumors to Chemotherapy

Cures in Advanced Cancers

Gestational trophoblastic tumors
Acute lymphoblastic leukemia (children)
Acute lymphoblastic leukemia (adults)
Acute myeloblastic leukemia
Non-Hodgkin's lymphoma (children)
Diffuse large cell lymphoma
Hodgkin's disease
Burkitt's lymphoma
Testicular tumors

Cures with Adjuvant Chemotherapy

Wilms' tumor
Osteogenic sarcoma
Rhabdomyosarcoma

Minor Responses with Chemotherapy and Adjuvant Chemotherapy, but with No Demonstrable Prolongation of Life

Non–small cell lung cancer
Head and neck cancer
Large bowel cancer
Cancer of the adrenal cortex
Soft tissue sarcoma
Stomach cancer
Pancreatic cancer
Liver cancer
Cervical cancer
Melanoma

Complete and Partial Remissions with Uncertain Prolongation of Survival with Chemotherapy and Adjuvant Chemotherapy

Multiple myeloma
Ovarian cancer
Endometrial cancer
Neuroblastoma

Complete Remissions with Increased Survival with Chemotherapy and Adjuvant Chemotherapy

Small cell carcinoma of the lung
Acute myeloblastic leukemia
Non-Hodgkin's lymphoma, indolent
Chronic granulocytic leukemia
Breast cancer
Prostate cancer
Hairy cell leukemia

From Krakoff, I. H. (1991). Cancer chemotherapeutic and biologic agents. *CA: A Journal for Clinicians, 41*, 265–266.

Experiments and clinical experience suggest that most types of chemotherapy do not kill all cancer cells during one exposure. According to the cell kill hypothesis, only a percentage of cancer cells will be killed with each course of chemotherapy. Repeated doses of chemotherapy therefore must be used.

The use of medications in combination, known as combination chemotherapy, has consistently been far superior

Table 24–2. MOPP Regimen for Hodgkin's Disease

Component	Dosage
M = Nitrogen *M*ustard	6.0 mg/m² IV on days 1 and 8
O = *O*ncovin (vincristine)	1.4 mg/m² IV on days 1 and 8
P = *P*rocarbazine	100 mg/m² PO on days 1–14
P = *P*rednisone	40 mg/m² PO on days 1–14
Repeat cycle every 28 days for a minimum of 6 cycles	

to single-agent therapy. When combined, medications destroy malignant cells more effectively and produce fewer side effects because they strike the cancer cells at different points in the cell cycle. Combination chemotherapy is now the standard, and the regimens are complex, cyclic, and individualized based on the client and type of cancer. An example of chemotherapy regimen for Hodgkin's disease is shown in Table 24–2.

Classification of Chemotherapy

Chemotherapeutic agents generally are classified according to their pharmacologic action and effect on the cell generation cycle. However, the method by which cancer cells are inhibited or destroyed is not always known. A classification of common chemotherapeutic agents is shown in Box 24–8.

Administration of Chemotherapy

Depending on the clinical setting, chemotherapy may be administered by the physician, staff nurse, or specialized team member, such as the oncology clinical nurse-specialist or intravenous therapist. Only adequately prepared registered professional nurses who are skilled in administering chemotherapy should assume responsibility for its administration to ensure quality of client care and maintain the highest standards of client and personnel safety.[53] Recommendations for course content, clinical practicum, and nursing practice can be found in the Oncology Nursing Society's *Cancer Chemotherapy Guidelines.*[53]

Safe Preparation, Handling, and Disposal

The safe administration and disposal of chemotherapeutic agents is controversial. Although evidence suggests that these agents may be carcinogenic, no valid and reliable studies have determined the risks of exposure to the healthcare provider.

Undue exposure to antineoplastic drugs can occur from three major routes: (1) inhalation of aerosols, (2) absorption through the skin, and (3) ingestion of contaminated materials.[26] Several organizations, including the Occupational Safety and Health Administration, the National Study Commission on Cytotoxic Exposure, and the Oncology Nursing Society, have prepared guidelines for the safe preparation, handling, and disposal of antineoplastics.[51, 52, 53] These guidelines call for the use of gloves and gowns during preparation and administration and the use of a biologic safety cabinet for drug preparation.

Antineoplastic agents and their metabolites are found in the excreta and body fluids of clients undergoing chemotherapy. For this reason, gloves and disposable gowns should be worn when handling body secretions such as blood, vomitus, or excreta of clients who have received chemotherapy within the previous 48 hours.[26, 53]

Extravasation Management

Careful assessment of the intravenous site is required during and after the infusion of antineoplastic agents because some agents may cause tissue damage if extravasated (infiltrated). Nonvesicant agents have no significant soft tissue toxicities. Vesicant chemotherapeutic agents can cause or form a blister and cause tissue destruction (Box 24–9). Irritant drugs can produce venous pain at the site and along the vein, with or without an inflammatory reaction. Pain, erythema, swelling, and lack of a blood return indicate an extravasation.

Procedures for management of extravasation are controversial and unique to each clinical setting. Institutionally approved guidelines for the management of extravasation should be readily available. Guidelines for the management of extravasation are included in the Oncology Nursing Society's *Cancer Chemotherapy Guidelines.*[55] General recommendations include the following:

- Stop drug administration
- Leave the needle in place and attempt to aspirate any residual drug from the tubing, needle, and site
- Administer an antidote if appropriate
- Remove the needle and do not apply direct manual pressure to the site
- Apply warm (for vinca alkaloid) or cold compresses as indicated
- Observe the site regularly for pain, erythema, swelling, induration, and necrosis

The appearance of the site before and after chemotherapy should be carefully documented in the client's record.

Box 24–8. Classification of Chemotherapeutic Agents

Alkylating Agents

Busulfan (Myleran)
Carboplatin (CBDCA, Paraplatin)
Chlorambucil (Leukeran)
Cisplatin (Platinol)
Cyclophosphamide (Cytoxan)
Dacarbazine (DTIC)
Ifosfamide (Ifex)
Mechorethamine hydrochloride (Mustargen, nitrogen mustard)
Melphalan (Alkeran, L-PAM)
Thiotepa

Antimetabolites

Cladribine (Leustatin)
Cytarabine (ara-C, Cytosar-U)
Floxuridine (FUDR)
Fludarabine (Fludara)
5-Fluorouracil (Adrucil, 5-FU)
5-Fluorouracil topical (Efudex, Fluoroplex)
Mercaptopurine (Purinethol, 6-MP)
6-Thioguanine (6-TG)
Methotrexate sodium (Folex, Mexate)
Pentostatin (Nipent, 2-DCA)

Antitumor Antibiotics

Bleomycin sulfate (Blenoxane)
Dactinomycin (Actinomycin D, Cosmegen)
Daunorubicin (Cerubidine, Daunomycin)
Doxorubicin (Adriamycin, Rubex)
Epirubicin (Pharmorubicin)
Idarubicin (Idamycin)
Mitomycin (Mitomycin C, Mutamycin)
Mitoxantrone (Novantrone)
Plicamycin (Mithramycin)

Nitrosoureas

Carmustine (BiCNU)
Lomustine (CCNU)
Semustine (methyl-CCNU)
Streptozocin (Zanosar)

Plant Derivatives

Docetaxel (Taxotere, investigational)
Etoposide (Vepesid, VP-16-213)
Paclitaxel (Taxol)
Teniposide (Vumon, VM-26)
Vinblastine sulfate (Velban)
Vincristine sulfate (Oncovin)
Vindesine sulfate (Eldisine)
Vinorelbine tartrate (Navelbine)

Hormones and Steroids

Androgen

Dromostanolone proprionate (Drolban)
Fluoxymesterone (Halotestin)
Methyltestosterone (Android)
Testolactone (Teslac)
Testosterone (Android-5,-10,-25)
Testosterone cypionate (DEPO-testosterone)
Testosterone enanthate (Delatestryl)
Testosterone proprionate (Malogen, Testex)

Antiandrogen

Flutamide (Eulexin, Euflex)

Estrogens

Chlorotrianisene (Tace)
Conjugated estrogens (Premarin)
Diethylstilbestrol (DES)
Estradiol (Estrace)

Antiestrogen

Tamoxifen (Nolvadex)

Luteinizing Hormone–Releasing Hormone Agonists

Goserelin acetate (Zoladex)
Leuprolide acetate (Lupron)

Progestational Agents

Megestrol (Megace)
Medroxyprogesterone (Depo-Provera, Provera)

Adrenal Cortical Compounds

Cortisone acetate (Cortone Acetate)
Dexamethasone (Decadron)
Hydrocortisone sodium succinate (Solu-Cortef)
Prednisone (Deltasone)
Prednisolone (Cortalone, Delta-Cortef)
Methylprednisolone sodium succinate (Solu-Medrol)

Adrenal Cortical Steroid Inhibitor

Aminoglutethimide (Cytadren)

Miscellaneous Agents

Altretamine (Hexalen)
Amsacrine (*m*-AMSA)
Asparaginase (Elspar, L-ASP)
Estramustine (Emcyt)
Hydroxyurea (Hydrea)
Levamisole (Ergamisol)
Mesna (Mesnex)
Mitotane (Lysodren)
Procarbazine (Matulane)

Note: Category headings and drug groupings may differ depending on the source consulted.
Data from Chabner, B. A. (1993). Anticancer drugs. In V. T. DeVita, S. Hellman, & S. A. Rosenberg (Eds.): *Cancer: Principles and practice of oncology* (4th ed., pp. 325–328). Philadelphia: J. B. Lippincott; Tenenbaum, L. (Ed.) (1994). *Cancer chemotherapy and biotherapy: A reference guide* (2nd ed., pp. 70–72). Philadelphia: W.B. Saunders.

Box 24–9. Vesicant and Irritant Chemotherapeutic Agents

Common Vesicants

Amsacrine
Dactinomycin
Daunorubicin
Doxorubicin
Epirubicin
Idarubicin
Mechorethamine
Menogaril
Mitomycin C
Vinblastine
Vincristine
Vindesine
Vinorelbine

Rare Vesicants

Cisplatin
Mitoxantrone
Paclitaxel

Common Irritants

Carmustine
Cisplatin
Dacarbazine
Etoposide
Fluorouracil
Plicamycin

Rare Irritants

Bleomycin
Paclitaxel
Streptozotocin
Teniposide

Data from Boyle, D., & Engelking, C. (1995). Vesicant extravasation: Myths and realities. *Oncology Nursing Forum, 22*(1), 57–67; Oncology Nursing Society. (1992). *Cancer chemotherapy guidelines: Recommendations for the management of vesicant extravasation, hypersensitivity, and anaphylaxis.* Pittsburgh, PA: Author.

Hypersensitivity Reactions

Hypersensitivity reactions to chemotherapy, although rare, can be serious and life-threatening. The antineoplastic agents most commonly implicated in the development of hypersensitivity reactions are L-asparaginase, carboplatin, cisplatin, paclitaxel, bleomycin, and teniposide.[66]

When administering a drug with anaphylactic potential, take the following precautions to ensure client safety:

- Obtain an allergy history from the client
- Administer a test dose when ordered by the physician
- Stay with the client the entire time the drug is being administered
- Have emergency equipment and drugs readily available
- Obtain baseline vital signs

- Establish a free-flowing intravenous line for the administration of fluids and emergency drugs should the need arise

The manifestations of an immediate hypersensitivity reaction include dyspnea, chest tightness or pain, pruritus, urticaria, tachycardia, dizziness, anxiety, agitation, inability to speak, abdominal pain, nausea, hypotension, cloudy sensorium, flushed appearance, and cyanosis.

If an anaphylactic reaction is suspected, immediately stop drug administration, maintain intravenous access with 0.9% saline, and notify the physician. Maintain the airway, and place the client in a supine position with the feet elevated, unless contraindicated. Monitor the client's vital signs every 2 minutes until he or she is stable. Administer epinephrine, aminophylline, diphenhydramine, and corticosteroids based on the physician's orders.

Routes of Administration

Appropriate routes of medication administration are determined by the properties of the medication and the purpose of the therapy. Some agents may be safely administered by a variety of routes. Therapy may be systemic or local.

Intravenous Routes

■ Peripheral Access

Large veins in the fleshy part of the forearm are the preferred peripheral access sites. Avoid areas of impaired lymphatic drainage, phlebitis, invading neoplasm, hematoma, inflamed or sclerosing areas, areas of impaired venous circulation, the lower extremities, and sites distal to a recent venipuncture site. Also avoid veins that are on the dorsal aspect of the hand or over an area of flexion such as the wrist or elbow.

■ Vascular Access

In the past, vascular access devices (VADs) were placed as a last resort in clients with poor venous access. Today, because chemotherapy regimens are complex and supportive care is extensive, they are being used during the initial treatment of clients requiring continuous chemotherapy, total parenteral nutrition (TPN), multiple access, parenteral fluids and antibiotics, and frequent blood testing.

These catheters are usually inserted into one of the major veins of the upper chest. The brachial or cephalic vein in the forearm is used for peripherally inserted central catheters (PICCs). The distal catheter tip is advanced to the level of the superior vena cava at or above the junction of the right atrium. Proper catheter tip placement is confirmed by fluoroscopy or radiography.

A variety of VADs are currently available, including (1) catheters that are subcutaneously tunneled for several inches from the catheter exit site to the venous insertion site, (2) catheters that enter the vein 1 inch from the exit site, (3) totally implanted venous access ports that lie completely beneath the skin, and (4) peripherally inserted

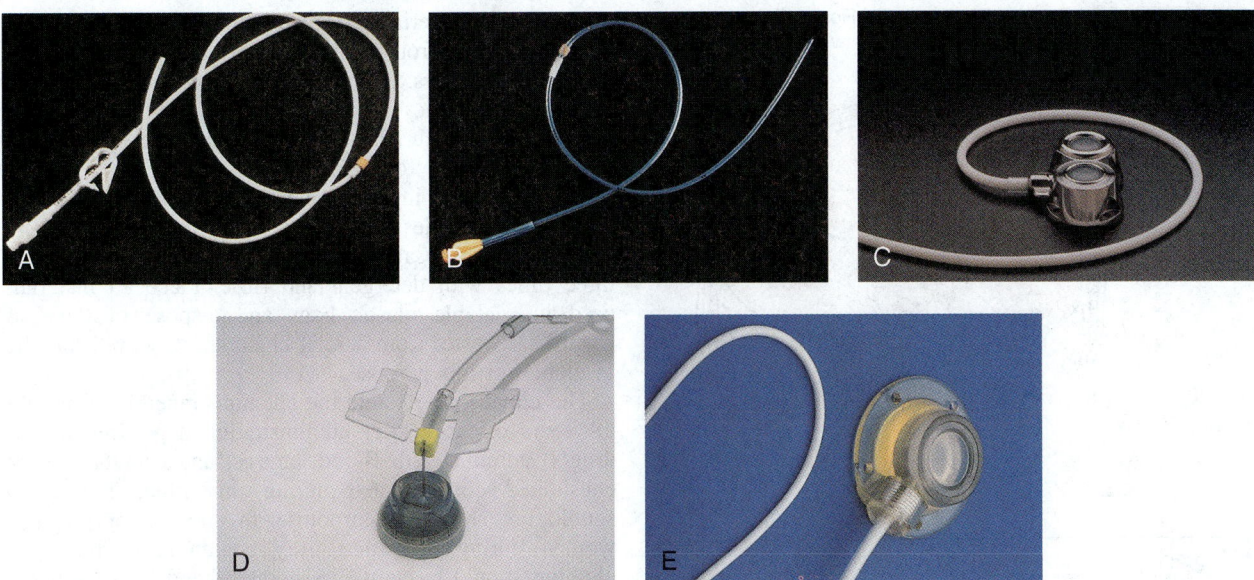

Figure 24–2. Venous access devices. *A,* Hickman single-lumen catheter. *B,* Groshong single-lumen catheter. *C,* Port-A-Cath Dual-Lumen Venous Access System. *D,* OmegaPort, a port designed to protect against accumulation of infectious sludge. *E,* Infusaid Microport. (*A* and *B,* courtesy of Bard Access Systems, Inc., Salt Lake City, UT; *C,* courtesy of SIMS Deltec, Inc., St. Paul, MN; *D,* courtesy of Norfolk Medical Products, Inc., Skokie, IL; *E,* courtesy of Strato/Infusaid, Inc., Norwood, MA.)

central catheters. Examples of various types are shown in Figure 24–2A to E. There are advantages and disadvantages to each type of device, including factors such as maintenance requirements, ease of use, cost, ease of insertion, longevity, and effect on body image.

The most frequently reported complications are infection and catheter occlusion. The prevention of VAD infections centers on catheter care, daily assessment for manifestations of infection, and client education. Intraluminal occlusion may occur secondary to a blood clot or precipitate. Prevention strategies include proper flushing, vigilance for drug incompatibilities, and adherence to proper drug dilutions. Procedures for the care and maintenance of VADs vary with each clinical setting and type of device. Nursing management strategies for VADs are extensively described elsewhere.[7, 42, 54, 67, 77]

Alternative Routes

Regional chemotherapy allows high concentrations of chemotherapy to be directed to localized tumors. Methods of regional administration include topical, intrathecal, intracavitary, and intra-arterial chemotherapy. Although intra-arterial infusions involve some risk, major organs or tumor sites do receive maximal exposure with limited serum levels of medications. As a result, systemic side effects are minimal.

Most medications given systemically are not effective against central nervous system (CNS) tumors because they cannot cross the blood-brain barrier. The physician may instill chemotherapeutic agents into the CNS through a reservoir placed in the ventricle (Fig. 24–3) or via a lumbar puncture.

Intracavitary therapy instills the medication directly into areas such as the abdomen, bladder, or pleural space.

Intraperitoneal chemotherapy is an option for cancer involving the intra-abdominal area, such as ovarian cancer. With this method, a high concentration of a chemotherapeutic agent is delivered to the actual tumor site with minimal exposure of healthy tissues, thereby decreasing toxic side effects.

Outpatient Chemotherapy Delivery

Aggressive, complex, and sophisticated cancer therapies are currently being delivered in ambulatory, office, and home care settings. This shift in provision of services from the hospital setting is a result of cost-containment efforts, advanced techology, competition, and increased competence of nurses.[79]

Cost containment is a major consideration in today's healthcare environment. Outpatient care is less expensive and allows for the maintenance of a more normal lifestyle. Technical developments such as VADs and implantable and external infusion pumps make it possible to deliver chemotherapy, hyperalimentation, antibiotics, blood components, and parenteral and epidural analgesics outside the hospital. Increasingly sophisticated support is available from home healthcare agencies as well.

Different nursing challenges exist in outpatient settings. First, a high level of commitment is required from the client and caregivers. Both require education regarding complex treatment regimens; identification, prevention, and treatment of disease manifestations experienced at home; the operation of medical equipment; and the care of a variety of VADs. Second, a mechanism for immediate access to healthcare personnel is required. Finally, when chemotherapy is administered in the home setting, provisions must be made for the safe handling and dis-

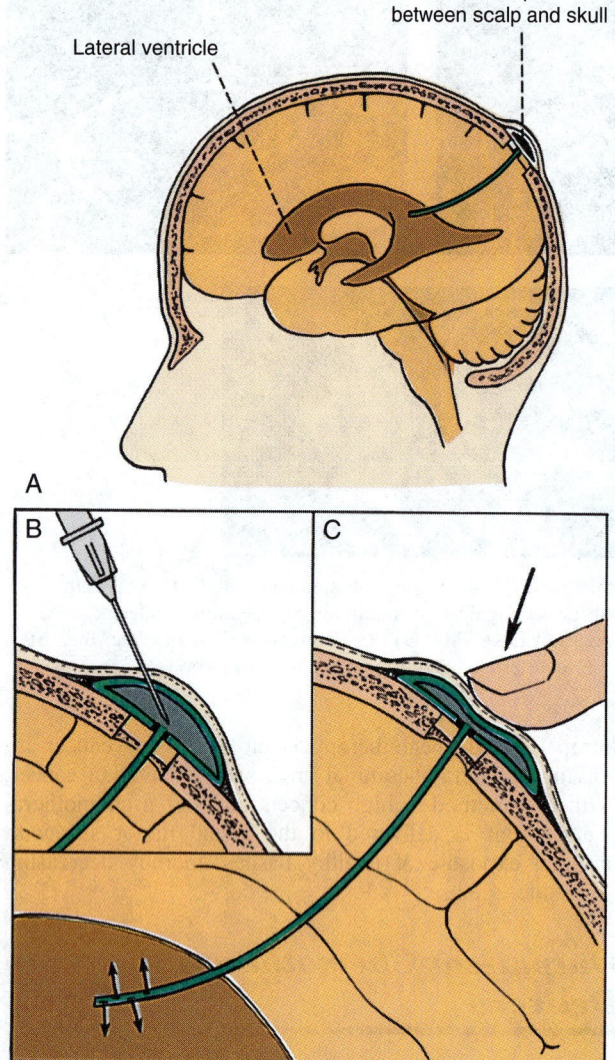

Figure 24–3. Ommaya reservoir. *A,* Placement of Ommaya reservoir in the ventricle. *B,* Injection of chemotherapeutic agent into the reservoir. *C,* Delivery of chemotherapeutic agent into the ventricle and into the cerebrospinal fluid. (Adapted from Ratcheson, R. A., & Ommaya, A. [1968]. Experience with the subcutaneous cerebrospinal fluid reservoir. *New England Journal of Medicine, 279,* 1026. Reprinted by permission of *The New England Journal of Medicine.*)

posal of cytotoxic drugs to minimize client, family, and nurse exposure.

When the chemotherapeutic medication is obtained from the healthcare facility, it should be labeled as cytotoxic, securely sealed, and packed in an impervious material for transportation.

Whenever possible, prepare chemotherapy outside of the home setting. If you must prepare the medication in the home for administration, be sure to work in an area away from food and anywhere the family, particularly children, congregate. Clean the area and cover it with a plastic-backed absorbent pad. Then assemble all needed materials for the chemotherapy administration on this surface. Use the same precautions for administering the chemotherapy as are used in the hospital setting.[3]

The waste materials are disposed of in biohazard containers obtained from medical supply companies or pharmaceutical vendors. Place all empty containers and tubing in sealable plastic bags with appropriate labels. These items are then returned to the healthcare facility or pharmaceutical vendor for proper disposal.

If spills occur in the home, wear a protective gown, gloves, and goggles to clean it up. Wiped the area completely with disposable absorbent towels and then wash it three times with detergent and rinse. Place all materials used in sealable plastic bags and dispose of them as hazardous waste. Commercial chemotherapy spill kits are available for this purpose.

The client may excrete the chemotherapeutic agents for 48 hours or more after administration depending on the drug(s) administered. Blood, emesis, and excreta may be considered contaminated during this time. The client should not share a bathroom with children or pregnant women during this time. Any contaminated linens or clothing should be washed separately, and then washed a second time with the rest of the laundry. All contaminated disposable items should be sealed in plastic bags and disposed of as hazardous waste.[52] The contaminated items should be double-bagged in waterproof bags and returned to the healthcare facility for disposal in a biohazards container.

Toxic Effects of Chemotherapy

Antineoplastic medications can damage and destroy not only malignant cells but also certain normal cells. Normal cells most vulnerable to antineoplastic medications are those that divide and proliferate rapidly, specifically cells of the bone marrow, hair, and mucosa. Damage to these cells can result in myelosuppression, alopecia, oral mucositis, gastrointestinal irritation, and diarrhea. In addition to these effects on proliferative cells, drugs may exert organ-specific toxicities resulting in cardiac, renal, pulmonary, hepatic, reproductive, and neurologic dysfunction. Box 24–10 summarizes the side effects of antineoplastic agents.

Side effects are evaluated or graded according to degree of severity. Mild-to-moderate side effects generally do not warrant discontinuing the drug or decreasing the dose. More severe or unexpected toxicities require careful evaluation and dose reduction. Box 24–11 lists risk factors for the development of toxicities.

The onset of side effects of chemotherapy may be acute or delayed. Acute toxicities tend to occur in tissues composed of rapidly dividing cells, are frequently intermittent, and generally resolve with complete recovery; in contrast, late effects tend to occur in different tissues and may produce lifelong problems.[59] The client and all healthcare providers must be aware of, monitor for, and report side effects.

Myelosuppression

Myelosuppression is one of the most common and lethal side effects of chemotherapeutic drugs. Infection and

---

Box 24–10. Side Effects of Antineoplastic Agents

Gastrointestinal

Nausea and vomiting
Constipation
Anorexia
Stomatitis
Esophagitis
Taste alterations
Diarrhea
Weight loss
Pharyngitis

Integumentary

Dermatitis
Alopecia
Perianal ulcers
Vulvar ulcers
Hyperpigmentation
Photosensitivity
Nail changes

Hematopoietic

Anemia
Thrombocytopenia
Neutropenia

Genitourinary

Nephrotoxicity
Urine color change
Hemorrhagic cystitis
Hyperuricemic nephropathy

Hepatic

Hepatotoxicity
Cirrhosis
Hepatic fibrosis
Portal hypertension

Reproductive

Amenorrhea
Sterility
Loss of libido
Impotence
Azoospermia
Gonadal dysfunction
Menopausal manifestations
Irregular menses
Gynecomastia
Oligospermia

Cardiac

Electrocardiogram changes
Arrhythmias
Cardiomyopathy, chronic heart failure
Tachycardia

Pulmonary

Pneumonitis
Pulmonary fibrosis

Metabolic

Tumor lysis syndrome

Neurologic, Sensory-Perceptual

Ototoxicity
Subacute meningeal irritation
Peripheral neuropathy
Cranial nerve neuropathy
Autonomic neuropathy
Cerebellar toxicity

Data from Hydzik, C. A. (1990). Late effects of chemotherapy: Implications for patient management and rehabilitation. *Nursing Clinics of North America, 25,* 423; Ruccione, K., & Weinberg, K. (1989). Late effects in multiple body systems. *Seminars in Oncology Nursing, 5,* 4.

Box 24–11. Risk Factors for Chemotherapy Toxicity

- Drug dose, route, and method of administration
- Extent of cancer and client's overall physical condition
- Prior chemotherapy or radiation therapy
- Concomitant organ dysfunction or illness
- Age
- Nutritional status
- Self-care behavior
- Combination versus single-agent therapy

Adapted from Goodman, M.S. (1989). Managing the side effects of chemotherapy. *Seminars in Oncology Nursing,* 5(2)(Suppl. 1), 29.

---

bleeding as a result of diminished white blood cell and platelet production are two common causes of death in cancer clients. For this reason, complete blood counts must be checked before administration of myelosuppressive drugs and monitored periodically after drug administration.

The time after chemotherapy administration when the white blood cell or platelet count is at the lowest point is referred to as the *nadir.* For most myelosuppressive agents, the nadir occurs within 7 to 14 days after drug administration. Knowledge of blood count nadirs helps you predict when the client is at greatest risk for infection and bleeding.

Granulocytopenia, also known as neutropenia, predisposes the client to infection, especially by opportunistic endogenous organisms. Neutrophils are the first and most numerous type of cell to arrive at any area of disease or tissue injury. When the number of neutrophils is substantially reduced, one of the body's prime defenses against infection is impaired.

The absolute neutrophil count (ANC) is calculated by multiplying the white blood cell count (WBC) by the percentage of granulocytes (neutrophils) in the differential: ANC = WBC × % granulocytes. For example, if the WBC is 1200/mm³, and the percentage of neutrophils, including the percentage of segmented and band neutrophils, is 34%, the ANC is 408 (1200 × 34% = 408). *Neutropenia* is commonly defined as an ANC of less than 1000/mm³.[56] The frequency of infection increases as the ANC decreases below 500/mm³, and the longer the client remains neutropenic.[56] Granulocyte colony-stimulating factor (G-CSF) or granulocyte-macrophage colony-stimulating factor (GM-CSF) may be prescribed to reduce the duration and severity of neutropenia (see Biologic Response Modifiers).

Teach clients measures to protect against infection:

- Maintain adequate nutrition and fluid intake
- Avoid raw or uncooked foods
- Avoid crowds, people with infections, and children who have been recently vaccinated with live or attenuated vaccines
- Avoid contact with animal excrement (e.g., bird, cat, and dog feces)
- Immediately report any manifestations of infection, such as fever over 38° C (100° F), cough, sore throat, chills or sweating, or frequent or painful urination
- Maintain personal hygiene, especially hand washing
- Get adequate rest and exercise
- Avoid indiscriminate use of antipyretics (e.g., acetaminophen, aspirin) because they can mask fever

Because infections are associated with increased morbidity and mortality, infection must be treated promptly and aggressively in the neutropenic client. The typical manifestations of infection are often absent because these clients are not able to produce an adequate inflammatory response to infection. Fever is the single most important and often the only manifestation of infection in the neutropenic client.[56] The development of fever in a neutropenic client should be treated as a medical emergency and mandates prompt assessment, diagnosis, and initiation of antibiotic therapy. Management includes culturing all suspected infection sites and administration of broad-spectrum antibiotics.

Thrombocytopenia increases the client's risk of bleeding. A high risk of hemorrhage exists when the platelet count is less than 20,000/mm³. Fatal CNS hemorrhage or massive gastrointestinal hemorrhage can occur when the platelet count is less than 10,000/mm³. Assess for changes in level of consciousness, which may be an early indication of an intracranial hemorrhage. Instruct clients to report any of the following:

- Bleeding gums
- Increased bruising, petechiae, or purpura, especially on the lower extremities
- Hypermenorrhea
- Tarry stools, blood in urine, coffee-ground vomitus
- Headaches
- Blurred vision
- Visual changes (thrombocytopenic clients may have retinal bleeding)
- Hemoptysis
- Nosebleed

Some controversy exists as to whether clients should receive prophylactic transfusions when platelet counts reach a certain level, or emergent transfusions when bleeding is noted.[22] Most oncologists will transfuse to keep the platelet count above 20,000/mm³ unless the client is known to have a platelet antibody. Platelet products for transfusion include multiple- or random-donor, single-donor, and human leukocyte antigen (HLA)–matched.

Anemia may cause fatigue, headache, dizziness, fainting, pallor, dyspnea, palpitations, and tachycardia. Packed red blood cell transfusions may be required to relieve anemia that is producing manifestations. Erythropoietin may be prescribed to elevate or maintain the erythrocyte level and decrease the need for transfusions (see Biologic Response Modifiers).

Additional precautions are necessary when administering blood components to selected groups of oncology clients. Cytomegalovirus-negative products are required for cytomegalovirus-negative clients undergoing bone marrow transplant. Irradiated products are transfused to severely immunocompromised clients to prevent graft-versus-host disease secondary to the transfusion of immunocompetent lymphocytes present in donor platelet and packed cell products. Leukocyte-poor products, administered through a leukocyte filter, are indicated for clients with a history of repeated nonhemolytic febrile transfusion reactions. They are also used as a prophylactic measure to prevent alloimmunization to leukocytes. McGuire and Braine[47] provide a comprehensive discussion of transfusion practices in the oncology setting.

Gastrointestinal Effects

Gastrointestinal effects of chemotherapy include nausea and vomiting, anorexia, taste alteration, weight loss, oral mucositis, diarrhea, and constipation. The emetic potential of a particular chemotherapeutic regimen depends on the drugs given, the dose and route of administration, and the client's susceptibility to emesis.

Adequate control of nausea and vomiting is an essential factor in compliance with chemotherapy. Uncontrolled nausea and vomiting can result in anorexia, malnutrition, dehydration, metabolic imbalances, psychological depression, and decreased immunity.[48]

Management of nausea and vomiting has greatly improved during the last decade because of heightened interest and research. Successful management depends on an understanding of the pathophysiology of the manifestations, recognition of patterns of nausea and vomiting, and an appreciation of pharmacologic and nonpharmacologic interventions.[30]

Research indicates that the vomiting center, located in the medulla oblongata, is responsible for coordinating the act of vomiting.[25] It is postulated that stimulation of the vomiting center occur via a variety of pathways and is mediated by a variety of neurotransmitters.[48] Pharmacologic blockade of these potential neurotransmitters is the hypothesized mechanism of action of drugs used as antiemetics.

Three common patterns of nausea and vomiting have been described. After the client has experienced nausea and vomiting, anticipatory nausea and vomiting may occur before the administration of further therapy. Acute, post-therapy nausea and vomiting occur within the first 24 hours following therapy. Delayed nausea and vomiting refers to manifestations that persist or develop 24 hours after chemotherapy.

Antiemetics are usually prescribed 6 to 12 hours prior to the administration of chemotherapy and are continued every 4 to 6 hours for at least 12 to 24 hours, or for as long as the manifestations persist. Specific drug combinations, doses, and schedules are described elsewhere.[30, 48] Ongoing evaluation is essential to find the most effective dose, schedule, and combination of drugs for each client. Nonpharmacologic interventions include adjusting oral and fluid intake, relaxation, exercise, hypnosis, biofeedback, guided imagery, and systemic desensitization.[25, 30]

Anorexia and weight loss occur as a result of the disease process as well as the treatment. The client with cancer is at risk for protein-calorie malnutrition. Many variables, in addition to the effects of chemotherapy, may alter the client's ability to ingest food via the oral route. Common problems that may interfere with oral intake include anorexia, nausea and vomiting, early satiety, taste alterations, dry mouth, stomatitis, esophagitis, viscous saliva, lactose intolerance, pain, diarrhea, and constipation.

Assessment of nutritional status includes the following:

● Current and normal weight and height
● Caloric intake
● Anthropometric measurements
● Laboratory values (albumin, transferrin, creatinine, lymphocyte count, nitrogen balance)
● Diet history
● Physiologic factors (difficulty in swallowing, malabsorption, taste alterations)

When medically appropriate, oral nutrition can be enhanced by relaxing dietary restrictions and emphasizing the need for a high-protein, high-calorie diet with fortification from natural food sources or commercial supplements. Monitor the client's nutritional status by daily calorie counts and assessment. If the nutritional requirements cannot be met orally, another method must be considered. Enteral and intravenous feedings are two possibilities (see Chapters 60 and 61 for a detailed discussion of these methods).

Stomatitis, or *oral mucositis,* is the term used to describe inflammation and ulceration of the mucosal lining of the mouth. What is seen in the mouth is present throughout the gastrointestinal tract. Consequences of stomatitis include pain, decreased nutritional and fluid intake, oral infections, malabsorption, and diarrhea.

An oral hygiene program should start before therapy and continue throughout treatment. A plan for oral care includes a dental examination prior to and during therapy, thorough and gentle cleaning to avoid further trauma, moisturization if saliva is scanty or absent, avoidance of alcohol and smoking, culture and antimicrobial therapy for infections, and topical anesthetics and analgesics for pain or discomfort. Dietary modifications include avoiding extremely hot or cold foods, spices, and citrus fruits and juices; eating soft foods; and taking nutritional supplements.

Diarrhea is most often the result of antimetabolite drugs. A low residue or liquid diet is usually advised. Electrolytes and intake and output should be carefully monitored. Scrupulous perineal hygiene is encouraged, especially in the neutropenic client. Antidiarrheals may be prescribed.

Constipation is frequently the effect of vinca alkaloids (vinblastine, vincristine) on bowel peristalsis. Other causes of constipation include narcotic use, immobility, decreased fluid and bulk intake, tumor invasion of the gastrointestinal tract, and depression. Preventive measures include increasing fluid and bulk intake, administering stool softeners prophylactically, increasing activity, and administering laxatives when necessary.

Integumentary Effects

Alopecia is a common side effect of many antineoplastic agents. The extent of hair loss depends on the specific drug, dosage, and method of administration. Alopecia is temporary, with regrowth often occurring before chemotherapy ends, although hair color and texture may change. Approaches to lessen or prevent chemotherapy-induced alopecia remain controversial. One method is the use of scalp hypothermia to decrease blood flow to the hair follicle and thereby reduce contact between the drug and epithelial cells. This is contraindicated in clients with metastatic disease in this area and in clients with brain tumors.

The type of skin reactions that may occur in the client receiving chemotherapy depend on the drug(s) administered:

● Red patches (erythema) or hives (urticaria) at the drug injection site or on other body parts: These reactions generally disappear within several hours.
● Darkening of the skin (hyperpigmentation) in the nail beds, mouth, on gums or teeth, and along the veins used for intravenous chemotherapy, or generalized: Hyperpigmentation usually occurs 2 to 3 weeks after administration of chemotherapy and continues for 10 to 12 weeks after the end of therapy.
● Sensitivity to sunlight (photosensitivity): This may result in an acute sunburn after just a short exposure to the sun. The sensitivity disappears once treatment stops. Clients must be taught to use sunscreen or protective clothing before sun exposure.
● Radiation recall: This skin reaction may occur in clients who received radiation therapy prior to the administration of chemotherapy. When chemotherapy is given several weeks or months later, a recall reaction occurs in the previously irradiated skin area. Skin effects range from redness, shedding, or peeling, to blisters and oozing. After the skin heals, it is permanently darkened.[29]

It is important to maintain meticulous hygiene to avoid a superimposed infection. Antibiotic therapy should be initiated at the first manifestation of infection.

Effects on the Reproductive System

The effects of chemotherapy on gonadal function and reproductive capacity may be temporary or permanent. Azoospermia, oligospermia, and sterility have been documented in males. Amenorrhea, menopausal manifestations, and sterility have been noted in females.

Not all clients experience these effects to the same degree, however. Preliminary studies suggest that the effects of chemotherapy on gonadal function vary with respect to the client's age at the time of therapy, the drugs administered, and the total drug dosage.[2] Surgery and radiation therapy may likewise produce temporary or permanent sterility. Therefore, in clients who had received combined modality therapy, the effect of any one modality on reproductive function is less well defined.

Administration of antineoplastic agents during the first trimester of pregnancy increases the risk of spontaneous abortion and fetal malformations.[38] Second- and third-trimester chemotherapy exposure may result in low birth weight or prematurity.[38] For these reasons, many physicians advise the use of birth control during cancer treatment and for up to 2 years following completion of treatment.

Pregnancy conceived after cytotoxic chemotherapy has about the same chance of a successful outcome as a normal pregnancy.[2] However, the genetic effects of chemotherapy may not be evident for several generations of offspring. Therefore, discuss the unpredictability of occurrence, degree, or duration of genetic damage with the client and spouse or significant other.

Pretreatment sperm banking offers the possibility of retaining reproductive capacity for some clients. Kaempfer et al.[38] provide an in-depth discussion of fertility considerations, procreative alternatives, and sexuality with respect to the cancer client.

Nursing Management of the Client Undergoing Chemotherapy

Assessment

A thorough client evaluation is necessary before cytotoxic drugs can be administered. Review the client's medical history to identify potential risk factors for chemotherapy toxicity, such as a history of impaired cardiac, pulmonary, or renal function. Carefully assess the severity and duration of side effects experienced since the previous course of therapy. Abnormal laboratory values may indicate organ-specific toxicities. Drug doses may have to be modified or delayed based on these results.

The client's chart should have either a copy of the formal drug protocol or a written summary of the planned chemotherapy regimen. Chemotherapy doses are usually based on body surface area in square meters (m^2), which is determined by the client's height and weight. Clear and complete chemotherapy prescriptions include the name of the drug, dose/m^2 and total dose, route of administration, administration rate of intravenous infusions, and frequency of administration. Plans for antiemetic therapy, hydration, diuresis, and electrolyte supplementation are frequently included as well.

Before administering antineoplastic agents, consult with the pharmacologist and review chemotherapy drug handbooks and investigational drug protocols for detailed information regarding drug actions, dosages, administration guidelines, and potential side effects.

Client and Family Education

Client and family education about chemotherapy and the identification, prevention, and management of side effects are primarily nursing functions. Box 24–12 identifies educational objectives for clients who are receiving chemotherapy.

Bone Marrow Transplantation

Early efforts to cure leukemia with supralethal radiation and bone marrow transplantation (BMT) began in the 1950s.[35] Current advances in cell typing, prevention and treatment of graft-versus-host disease, antimicrobial therapy, and management of marrow aplasia have broadened the application of BMT to a variety of cancers, as well as aplastic anemia and immunodeficiency diseases.[21, 78]

Box 24–12. Educational Objectives for Clients Receiving Chemotherapy

Client demonstrates knowledge of rationale for treatment with chemotherapy

■ Talks about the need for chemotherapy
■ Understands the use of chemotherapy in conjunction with other treatment modalities, if applicable
■ States expected response to treatment

Client demonstrates knowledge of treatment plan and schedule

■ Identifies drugs to be given and frequency and duration of administration
■ Identifies studies and procedures that will be performed before administration of chemotherapy
■ Identifies follow-up studies and procedures to be performed

Client demonstrates knowledge of potential side effects of drugs

■ Identifies side effects that may occur
■ Knows self-management strategies to control side effects
■ Identifies manifestations to report to healthcare persons
■ Knows procedures for reporting manifestations

Adapted from Somerville, E. T. (1991). Knowledge deficit related to chemotherapy. In J. C. McNally, et al. (Eds.), *Guidelines for cancer nursing practice* (2nd ed., pp. 36–39). Philadelphia: W.B. Saunders.

BMT is a unique treatment modality with the single goal of cure. It is a complex therapy with a high potential for complications. BMT allows the client to receive lethal and potentially more effective doses of chemotherapy and radiation therapy without regard to hematopoietic toxicity. The damaged bone marrow is replaced by healthy donor marrow.

Types of Bone Marrow Transplantation.

There are three types of donor bone marrow: autologous, allogeneic, and syngeneic. The autologous BMT is the most common type of transplant performed and is often referred to as a rescue. The marrow donor is also the recipient. The bone marrow is generally harvested during disease remission, it may or may not be chemically treated, and is stored (frozen) to be reinfused later. Autologous BMTs (ABMTs) are now common for solid tumor diseases that are chemotherapy-sensitive or radiosensitive.[75] These tumors include breast, ovarian, testicular, neuroblastoma, and lung (small cell and non-small cell) cancers. In addition, ABMTs are being performed for hematologic malignancies such as Hodgkin's and non-Hodgkin's lymphoma, myeloma, and acute and chronic leukemias when an HLA match is unavailable from an allogeneic donor. In these cases, once the bone marrow is harvested, the marrow may be purged (treated) with the use of a biophysical, pharmacologic, or immunologic agent to kill any cancer cells present while sparing normal cells.[61]

One type of autologous BMT is the peripheral blood stem cell (PBSC) transplant. In this type of transplant, the client's peripheral blood stem cells are harvested by leukapheresis. During leukapheresis, the client's blood is circulated through a high-speed cell separator, the peripheral stem cells are retained and stored, and the plasma and erythrocytes are reinfused in the client. The procedure takes approximately 2 to 4 hours and may require three to seven harvests to achieve an adequate number of stem cells.[36] The client then receives lethal doses of chemotherapy, RT, or both, and the PBSCs are reinfused.

Allogeneic PBSC transplant can also be performed either from a donor or using cord blood from a newborn. In an allogeneic BMT, the marrow donor is usually a sibling or parent with a similar HLA tissue type. In rare instances, an unrelated donor, found through the National Bone Marrow Registry or through a local tissue typing drive, may be the donor.[73] A syngeneic BMT uses bone marrow from an identical twin (see also Chapter 27).

The Process of Bone Marrow Transplantation.

The transplant process consists of several phases: conditioning, harvest, marrow infusion, pre-engraftment, and engraftment. Conditioning refers to the immunosuppression treatment regimen (chemotherapy, RT, or both) used to eradicate malignant cells, provide a state of immunosuppression, and create space in the bone marrow for the engraftment of new marrow.

The harvest procedure consists of multiple bone marrow aspirations from the posterior and anterior iliac crests and sternum. The procedure is performed in the operating room with the donor under general or spinal anesthesia.

The time of the bone marrow harvest depends on the type of transplant being performed. In ABMT and PBSC transplants, the cells are harvested before the initiation of the conditioning regimen. Instruct clients undergoing a bone marrow harvest about the procedure and requirements after the procedure.

Marrow is usually infused 48 to 72 hours after the last dose of chemotherapy or RT. Potential side effects include fluid overload, development of micropulmonary emboli, and hypersensitivity reactions to the white blood cells present in the marrow.

Once the marrow has been infused, the client starts an arduous upward climb. In allogeneic or syngeneic transplants, the pre-engraftment period lasts for 2 to 4 weeks, during which time the marrow cannot produce any cells. In autologous transplants, there is a period of 1 to 2 weeks of limited marrow development. Before engraftment occurs, the client is at high risk of bleeding and infection. Be vigilant in assessing and monitoring the client for the development of complications during this time. When successful, engraftment follows, indicated by a rise in the client's granulocyte and platelet counts. Because of the severe immunosuppression that occurs with the conditioning regimen, BMT clients will have a deficient immune system for up to a year after the transplant.[35]

Complications of Bone Marrow Transplantation.

In addition to infection and bleeding, potential complications of the conditioning regimen include renal insufficiency; gastrointestinal effects; veno-occlusive disease (VOD), a condition in which the small veins of the liver become obstructed; and graft-versus-host disease. Management of these transplant complications is beyond the scope of this chapter.[9, 19, 76] See Chapter 27 for more information on transplantation.

Biologic Response Modifiers

The search to understand and manipulate the human immune system has engaged scientists for decades. Under the proper circumstances, malignant tumors are susceptible to immunosurveillance and subsequent destruction. Thus, the quest to isolate and identify effective biologic agents continues.

In the last decade, four major technological advances have assisted scientists in their search. These advances include an increased understanding of the complex cellular nature of the immune system; advances in genetic engineering that have led to recombinant biologic agents; advances in molecular biology; and refined and advanced laboratory equipment and computer systems.[31, 34]

Biologic response modifiers aim to boost immune system function or to attack tumor cells directly. Clark and Longo[12] identified three major categories of biologic response modifiers according to their mechanism of action: (1) agents that restore, augment, or modulate the host's normal immune function; (2) agents that have direct antitumor effects; and (3) agents that demonstrate other biologic effects, such as interference with a tumor cell's ability to metastasize, promotion of cell differentiation, and tumor cell transformation.

Biologic response modifiers currently in use include interleukins; interferons (IFNs); monoclonal antibodies (MoAbs); tumor necrosis factor (TNF); colony-stimulating factors (CSFs) including granulocyte-macrophage (GM-CSF) and granulocyte (G-CSF) colony-stimulating factors; and erythropoietin (EPO). G-CSF, GM-CSF, and EPO have received Food and Drug Administration (FDA) approval and are available on the market.

Interleukins. Interleukins are substances produced by mononuclear phagocytes and function to promote normal hematopoiesis. Interleukin-2 (IL-2) is derived from T cells, augments various T cell activities, and enhances natural killer cell function. Clients with tumors previously unresponsive to standard therapy, such as renal cell carcinoma, melanoma, and non-Hodgkin's lymphoma, have responded to therapy with IL-2. Phase I and II clinical trials continue in an attempt to document the efficacy and therapeutic use of IL-2.

Major toxic responses reported with IL-2 therapy include increased capillary permeability, which may produce hypotension, ascites, pulmonary edema, and generalized weight gain.[37] Additionally, integumentary changes occur and may include generalized redness, rash, pruritus, and occasionally skin desquamation. Toxicities with IL-2 vary greatly with the dose of drug administered. Higher doses produce greater toxicities and require astute clinical management.

Interleukin-3 (IL-3), or multi-CSF, targets bone marrow progenitor cells.

Interferons. IFNs are small proteins that have cellular activity in three areas: antiviral, immunomodulatory, and antiproliferative. IFN received FDA approval for use in hairy cell leukemia in 1986, and in 1989 the drug's clinical indications were broadened to include AIDS-associated Kaposi's sarcoma. Currently, clinical trials are being conducted to investigate its use in other hematologic (particularly chronic leukemias) disease and solid tumors.

Toxicities appear to be dose-related, with lower doses of IFN exhibiting few side effects, whereas high doses may require therapy to be interrupted or stopped.[28] A flulike syndrome is a common side effect of IFN therapy and may include the following manifestations: fever, chills, tachycardia, muscle aches, malaise, fatigue, and headaches. Continued use of IFN produces a tachyphylactic response such that these manifestations decrease in intensity over time. Premedication with acetaminophen and diphenhydramine are helpful in reducing the client's discomfort.

Monoclonal Antibodies. MoAbs are specific antibodies directed against a single antigenic determinant on the cell surface.[60] MoAbs provide high specificity lacking in other types of treatment modalities. They can be used either diagnostically or therapeutically. Diagnostic uses include the early detection of cancer by identification of surface markers on tumor cells and as a delivery agent of radioisotopes to the tumor site to aid in tumor visualiza-

tion. Therapeutically, MoAbs may be used to deliver immunotoxins, such as ricin; chemotherapeutic agents; and radioactive isotopes directly to the tumor site.[14] To date, MoAbs have demonstrated limited success as a therapeutic option, and clinical trials continue for a variety of cancers.

Colony-Stimulating Factors. CSFs are naturally occurring growth factors that mediate hematopoiesis.[27] Generally, CSFs are named for the major cell lineage they mediate: GM-CSF affects both the granulocyte and macrophage lineage; G-CSF affects only granulocytes. GM-CSF is approved for myeloid reconstitution after autologous bone marrow transplantation and for use in clients experiencing BMT failure or engraftment delay. G-CSF is approved for the treatment of chemotherapy-associated neutropenia.

G-CSF is administered by subcutaneous injection, intravenous short infusion, or intravenous continuous infusion daily, starting at least 24 hours after chemotherapy is completed. The recommended dose of G-CSF is 5 μg/kg/day.[5] Filgrastim (Neupogen), a G-CSF, is not compatible with saline. The drug is continued for 10 to 14 days, or until the client's absolute neutrophil count is greater than or equal to 10,000/mm³. When G-CSF is discontinued, a 50% decrease in circulating neutrophils will occur within 1 to 2 days, and a return to pretreatment values occurs within 1 to 7 days. Thus, for optimal benefit, the drug should be continued beyond the expected nadir period. G-CSF is well tolerated, with minimal toxicities reported. The most commonly reported side effect is bone pain, and the problem appears to occur more frequently in high doses administered intravenously. The bone pain may be the result of the marrow expansion that occurs from the rapid increase in the neutrophil pool. Clients report pain in bone areas that have large marrow reserves, such as the pelvis, sternum, and long bones.

GM-CSF can be administered by continuous intravenous infusion (over 2 hours) or by subcutaneous injection daily. The recommended dose of GM-CSF is 250 μg/m²/day for 21 days starting 2 to 4 hours after reinfusion of autologous bone marrow, at least 24 hours after chemotherapy, and at least 12 hours after radiotherapy is completed.[5] Sargramostim (Leukine), a GM-CSF, is not compatible with dextrose. GM-CSF should be discontinued if the absolute neutrophil count exceeds 20,000/mm³ or the platelet count exceeds 500,000/mm³. For clients receiving either G-CSF or GM-CSF, monitoring of the complete blood count with a differential is recommended twice weekly during therapy to avoid potential complications of excessive leukocytosis. GM-CSF is generally well tolerated. Side effects include mild-to-moderate flulike manifestations such as fever, myalgias, bone pain, fatigue, and headache; cutaneous rash; a transient increase in liver enzymes; and thrombocytopenia.

Erythropoietin. Erythropoietin was approved by the FDA in 1989 for use in treating anemia secondary to end-stage renal failure and was approved in 1993 to treat anemia associated with cancer chemotherapy. EPO can be administered either as an intravenous or subcutaneous injection. The recommended dose for clients with cancer and anemia receiving concomitant chemotherapy is 150 units/kg body weight subcutaneously; three times weekly.[5] Minimum response time is 2 weeks, but it can take as long as 4 to 6 weeks to see an effect. The client's clinical response will determine if dose adjustments up to 300 units/kg three times weekly are required. Clients with serum erythropoietin levels greater than 200 mU/mL are unlikely to respond to therapy. Hematocrit levels should be monitored twice a week until a stabilized target range (30%–33%) is achieved and the maintenance dose is established.[5] It is important to maintain adequate levels of iron, folic acid, and vitamin B_{12} because these are essential for the development of red blood cells. The most commonly reported side effect is transient flulike manifestations, such as arthralgias and myalgias. Hypertension is a potential side effect more commonly seen in persons with chronic renal failure.

Most biologic agents are still investigational, so it is important to understand the potential side effects of the agent to be administered and to be prepared for, and continually assess and document, the client's response to therapy. Client and family teaching is of the utmost importance because many clients will seek alternative therapies if standard therapy fails to achieve a tumor response.

Second Malignancies

The term *second malignancy* refers to the occurrence of a new, unrelated neoplasm following initial cancer therapy. The risk of carcinogenesis associated with RT and chemotherapy is under intense investigation. Determination of treatment-related risks is complicated by the interaction of additional risk factors such as the natural history of the disease, genetic predisposition, age, immune status, and environmental factors.[32]

An increased risk of leukemia and solid tumors has been noted following treatment of childhood malignan-

---

BRIDGE TO HOME HEALTHCARE

Helping Clients Cope with the Reality of a New Diagnosis of Cancer

Barbara Michaud, R.N., B.S.N., *The Visiting Nurse Association of Omaha, Omaha, Nebraska*

Stunned by the reality of a new diagnosis of cancer, a person requires considerable emotional support, as well as support in the management of symptoms. Ideally, symptom management will result in a renewed sense of well-being for the client, and a determination to continue as an active participant in life despite the illness. Providing emotional support simply means showing, through active touch and listening, that you care. When all else is forgotten, that touch and those kind words will provide comfort.

During home visits with the client newly diagnosed with cancer, teaching quickly becomes the focus as the client begins to relax in his or her own home and actually begins to *hear* information that will help him or her to feel better.

Be familiar with the rationales behind your suggestions, and present these rationales when appropriate. Start with simple information about nutrition and fluid intake. Teach the client to eat a large breakfast, because appetite normally wanes as evening draws on. The client should eat small, frequent meals, eat foods at room temperature, and avoid fatty, fried, or spicy foods. Advise the client to use a dietary supplement, such as powdered instant-breakfast products, between meals to boost caloric intake and provide energy. If nausea is a problem, advise the client to take antiemetic medication regularly, as ordered. Drinking plenty of water supports the client's blood pressure, flushes out the bladder, and replaces fluids that might be lost through vomiting and diarrhea.

Remind the client to pay attention to mouth care. The client should watch for the development of mouth sores and report them immediately. Also, advise the client to use a soft toothbrush, keep lips moist, and rinse the mouth before and after meals.

Bowel elimination is a major concern of clients with cancer. If diarrhea is a problem, advise the client to decrease fluid intake, and to include nutmeg, cooked apples, or bananas in meals to slow peristalsis. Advise the client to use vitamin A and D ointment on the anus after washing, and to use prescribed medications. If constipation is a problem, suggest that the client increase fluid intake, fiber intake, and activity. A concoction of prune juice, milk of magnesia, and a buffered saline laxative (Fleet Phospho-Soda) is one of a number of remedies that may also be helpful for the client with constipation.

Fatigue remains a troublesome symptom for many clients with cancer. Remind the client that it is OK to take the time needed for recovery, and that a longer recovery period is likely with each succeeding cancer treatment. Clients in treatment are likely to have low blood cell counts. Therefore, stress the necessity of avoiding people with contagious illnesses. Have the client take his or her temperature twice a day. Teach good hand-washing technique. Advise the client to avoid bumping or cutting the skin. Suggest that the client use an electric shaver rather than a razor.

Pain, whether real or anticipated, frightens everyone with cancer. Two simple suggestions go a long way to promote comfort: Take medication when scheduled, rather than as needed, and reorder medication 1 week before the supply is gone.

cies, Hodgkin's disease, multiple myeloma, non-Hodgkin's lymphomas, gastrointestinal cancers, lung cancer, and ovarian cancer.[20] Acute nonlymphocytic leukemia following treatment with alkylating agents and solid tumors following RT account for most second cancers.

Most treatment-related leukemias occur within 10 years of treatment. Acute nonlymphocytic leukemia that occurs following cancer therapy is refractory to therapy and almost always fatal within 6 months of diagnosis.

In contrast to leukemia, most radiation-related cancers appear after 10 years. The majority of these cancers occur either within the direct field of radiation or in contiguous organs. The relationship of chemotherapy alone to subsequent solid tumor development is not clear.

When instructing clients and families about treatment-related risks, reassure them that the risk of second malignancy is small and must be balanced against the benefits of therapy for a life-threatening disease. Once therapy is completed, emphasize the importance of lifelong surveillance.

Ethical Issues

Ethical considerations have long been a central concern of nurses caring for clients with cancer. A recent survey of oncology nurses identified those issues thought to be the most important[18] (Box 24–13).

Conclusions

Cancer therapy has progressed over time. Many cancers once considered incurable are now controlled with a variety of combination therapies. The care of clients undergo-ing these therapies mandates that you keep abreast of new developments in this rapidly expanding field.

Thinking Critically

1. You are a nurse working in a health clinic that focuses on prevention of disease. This month the targeted goal is cancer prevention. How will you assess each client for cancer risk factors?

Factors to Consider. How would you develop an assessment tool for the clinic nurses to use? What teaching can help clients to avoid factors that increase their risk for cancer?

2. The client is a 22-year-old man who comes to the neighborhood health clinic with fears of testicular cancer. His companion has pain and a lump in the right testicle. What teaching should be completed during this visit? What psychosocial concerns would the companion have?

Factors to Consider. What diagnostic studies should you anticipate? What care should be given to the client awaiting diagnosis after cancer testing?

Bibliography

1. American Nurses' Association & Oncology Nursing Society (1987). *Standards of oncology nursing practice.* Kansas City, MO: American Nurses' Association.
2. Averette, H. D., et al. (1990). Effects of cancer chemotherapy on gonadal and reproductive capacity. *Ca-A Cancer Journal for Clinicians, 40,* 199–209.
3. Barry, L. K., & Booher, R. N. (1985). Promoting the responsible handling of antineoplastic agents in the community. *Oncology Nursing Forum, 12*(5), 41–46.
4. Beahrs, O. H., et al. (Eds.). (1992). *American Joint Committee on Cancer: Manual for staging of cancer* (4th ed.). Philadelphia: J.B. Lippincott.
5. Bockheim, C. M., & Jassak, P. F. (1993). The expanding world of colony stimulating factors. *Cancer Practice, 1*(3), 205–216.
6. Boyle, D., & Engelking, C. (1995). Vesicant extravasation: Myths and realities. *Oncology Nursing Forum, 22*(1), 57–67.
7. Brown, J., & Scelci, D. B. (1994). Management of complications associated with the use of venous access devices. In L. Tenenbaum (Ed.), *Cancer chemotherapy and biotherapy: A reference guide* (2nd ed., pp. 481–498). Philadelphia: W. B. Saunders.
8. Bucholtz, J. (1992). Radiolabeled antibody therapy. In K. H. Dow & L. J. Hilderley (Eds.), *Nursing care in radiation oncology* (pp. 275–284). Philadelphia: W.B. Saunders.
9. Buchsel, P. C., & Whedon, M. B. (Eds.). (1995). *Bone marrow transplantation: Administration and clinical strategies.* Boston: Jones & Bartlett.
10. Carbone, P. P. (1990). Progress in the systemic treatment of cancer: Concepts, trials, drugs, and biologics. *Cancer, 65,* 625–633.
11. Chabner, B. A. (1993). Anticancer drugs. In V. T. DeVita, S. Hellman, & S. A. Rosenberg (Eds.), *Cancer: Principles and practice of oncology* (4th ed., pp. 325–417). Philadelphia: J.B. Lippincott.
12. Clark, J. W., & Longo, D. L. (1986). Biological response modifiers. *Mediguide Oncology, 6,* 1–10.
13. DeVita, V. T., Hellman, S., & Rosenberg, S. A. (Eds.). (1993). *Cancer: Principles and practice of oncology* (4th ed.). Philadelphia: J.B. Lippincott.

Box 24–13. Ethical Issues for Oncology Nurses

Ranked in order of importance:

- Undertreatment of pain
- Truth-telling
- Right to refuse treatment
- Do-not-resuscitate orders
- Informed consent for procedures or treatments
- Withdrawal of life support
- Withdrawal of food or fluid
- Use of high-tech interventions for pain management
- Euthanasia
- Use of investigational procedures
- Allocation of scarce resources
- Rights of pediatric patients
- Care of patients with AIDS

Modified from Ersek, M., et al. (1995). Priority ethical issues in oncology nursing: Current approaches and future directions. *Oncology Nursing Forum, 22*(5), 803–807.

14. Dillman, J. B. (1988). Toxicity of monoclonal antibodies in the treatment of cancer. *Seminars in Oncology Nursing, 4,* 107–116.

15. Dimond, E. P. (1994). Two years of the patient self-determination act. *Oncology Nursing: Patient Treatment and Support, 1*(2), 1–14.

16. Dow, K. H. (1992). Principles of brachytherapy. In K. H. Dow & L. J. Hilderley (Eds.), *Nursing care in radiation oncology* (pp. 16–29). Philadelphia: W.B. Saunders.

17. Dunne-Daly, C. F. (1994). Nursing care and adverse reactions of external radiation therapy: A self-learning module. *Cancer Nursing, 17*(3), 236–256.

18. Ersek, M., et al. (1995). Priority ethical issues in oncology nursing: Current approaches and future directions. *Oncology Nursing Forum, 22*(5), 803–807.

19. Ford, R., & Ballard, B. (1988). Acute complications after bone marrow transplantation. *Seminars in Oncology Nursing, 4*(1), 15–24.

20. Fraser, M. C., & Tucker, M. A. (1989). Second malignancies following cancer therapy. *Seminars in Oncology Nursing, 5*(1), 43–55.

21. Freedman, S. E. (1988). An overview of bone marrow transplantation. *Seminars in Oncology Nursing, 4*(1), 3–8.

22. Fuller, A. K. (1990). Platelet transfusion therapy for thrombocytopenia. *Seminars in Oncology Nursing, 6*(2), 123–128.

23. Gates, M. F., Lackey, N. R., & White, M. R. (1995). Needs of hospice and clinic patients with cancer. *Cancer Practice, 3*(4), 226–232.

24. Goodman, M. (1989). Managing the side effects of chemotherapy. *Seminars in Oncology Nursing, 5*(2, Suppl. 1), 29–52.

25. Grant, M. (1988). Nausea and vomiting. In *Nursing management of common problems* (pp. 16–24) (A.C.S. No. 3480.06-PE). New York: American Cancer Society.

26. Gullo, S. M. (1990). Safe handling of chemotherapy. *Oncology Nursing Forum, 17*(11), 113–116.

27. Haeuber, D., & DiJulio, J. E. (1989). Hemopoietic colony stimulating factors: An overview. *Oncology Nursing Forum, 16*(2), 247–255.

28. Hahn, M.B., & Jassak, P. F. (1988). Nursing management of patients receiving interferon. *Seminars in Oncology Nursing, 4*(2), 95–101.

29. Hilderley, L. (1993). Radiotherapy. In S. L. Groenwald, et al. (Eds.), *Cancer nursing: Principles and practice* (3rd ed., pp. 235–269). Boston: Jones & Bartlett.

30. Hogan, C. M. (1990). Advances in the management of nausea and vomiting. *Nursing Clinics of North America, 25,* 475–497.

31. Hood, L. A., & Abernathy, E. (1996). Biological response modifiers. In R. McCorkle, et al. (Eds.), *Cancer nursing: A comprehensive text* (2nd ed.; pp. 434–457). Philadelphia: W. B. Saunders.

32. Hydzik, C. A., & Miaskowski, C. (1994). Chemotherapy-induced second malignancies. In L. Tenenbaum (Ed.), *Cancer chemotherapy and biotherapy: A reference guide* (2nd ed., pp. 319–370). Philadelphia: W.B. Saunders.

33. Jalowiec, A., & Dudas, S. (1991). Alterations in patient coping. In S. Baird, R. McCorkle, & M. Grant (Eds.), *Cancer nursing: A comprehensive text* (pp. 806–820). Philadelphia: W.B. Saunders.

34. Jassak, P. F. (1993). Biotherapy. In S. L. Groenwald, et al. (Eds.), *Cancer nursing: Principles and practice* (3rd ed., pp. 366–392). Boston: Jones & Bartlett.

35. Jassak, P. F., & Porter, N. A. (1990). Bone marrow transplantation. In K. M. Sigardson-Poor & L. M. Haggerty (Eds.), *Nursing care of the transplant recipient* (pp. 280–306). Philadelphia: W.B. Saunders.

36. Jassak, P. F., & Riley, M. B. (1994. Autologous stem cell transplant. *Cancer Practice, 2*(2), 141–145.

37. Jassak, P. F., & Sticklin, L. A. (1986). Interleukin-2: An overview. *Oncology Nursing Forum, 13*(6), 17–22.

38. Kaempfer, S. H., et al. (1985). Fertility considerations and procreative alternatives in cancer care. *Seminars in Oncology Nursing, 1*(1), 25–34.

39. Krakoff, I. H. (1987). Cancer chemotherapeutic agents. *CA: A Cancer Journal for Clinicians, 37,* 93–105.

40. Krakoff, I. H. (1991). Cancer chemotherapeutic and biologic agents. *CA: A Cancer Journal for Clinicians, 41,* 264–277.

41. Loescher, L. J., et al. (1989). Surviving adult cancers: I. Physiologic effects. *Annals of Internal Medicine, 111*(5), 411–432.

42. Lucas, A. B. (1992). A critical review of venous access devices: The nursing perspective. *Current Issues in Cancer Nursing Practice, 1*(7), 1–10.

43. Martinez, J., & Wagner, S. (1993). Hospice care. In S. L. Groenwald, et al. (Eds.), *Cancer nursing: Principles and practice* (3rd ed., pp. 1432–1450). Boston: Jones & Bartlett.

44. McCabe, S. V. (1982). An overview of hospice care. *Cancer Nursing, 5,* 103–108.

45. McCaffery, D. (1989). Family issues in cancer care: current dilemmas and future directions. *Journal of Psychosocial Oncology, 6*(1/2), 199–211.

46. McGee, R. F. (1993). Overview: Psychosocial aspects of cancer. In S. L. Groenwald, et al. (Eds.), *Cancer nursing: Principles and practice* (3rd ed.,pp. 437–448). Boston: Jones & Bartlett.

47. McGuire, D. B., & Braine, H. G. (Guest Eds.) (1990). Blood component therapy. *Seminars in Oncology Nursing, 6*(2), 89–177.

48. Morrow, G. R. (1989). Chemotherapy-related nausea and vomiting: Etiology and management. *CA: A Cancer Journal for Clinicians, 39,* 89–104.

49. Mullan, F. (1985). Seasons of survival: Reflections of a physician with cancer. *New England Journal of Medicine, 313,* 270–273.

50. National Cancer Institute. (1986). *What are clinical trials all about?* (NIH Publication No. 86-2706). Washington, DC: U.S. Government Printing Office.

51. National Study Commission on Cytotoxic Exposure (1984). *Recommendations for handling cytotoxic agents.* Providence, RI: Rhode Island Hospital.

52. Occupational Safety and Health Administration (Jan. 29, 1986). *Work practice guidelines for personnel dealing with cytotoxic (antineoplastic) drugs.* (OSHA Instruction Publication No. 8-11). Washington, DC: Office of Occupational Medicine.

53. Oncology Nursing Society. (1996). *Cancer chemotherapy guidelines.* Pittsburgh, PA: Author.

54. Oncology Nursing Society. (1989). *Access device guidelines: Recommendations for nursing education and practice: Module I, II, III.* Pittsburgh, PA: Author.

55. Oncology Nursing Society. (1992). *Cancer chemotherapy guidelines: Recommendations for the management of vesicant extravasation, hypersensitivity, and anaphylaxis.* Pittsburgh, PA: Author.

56. Oniboni, A. C. (1990). Infection in the neutropenic patient. *Seminars in Oncology Nursing, 6*(1), 50–60.

57. Quigley, K. M. (1989). The adult cancer survivor: Psychosocial consequences of cure. *Seminars in Oncology Nursing, 5*(1), 63–69.

58. Rosenberg, S. A. (1993). Principles of surgical oncology. In J. T. DeVita, S. Hellman, & S. A. Rosenberg (Eds.), *Cancer: Principles and practice of oncology* (4th ed., pp. 238–247). Philadelphia: J.B. Lippincott.

59. Ruccione, K. & Weinberg, K. (1989). Late effects in multiple body systems. *Seminars in Oncology Nursing, 5*(1), 4–13.

60. Rumsey, K. A., & Rieger, P. T. (Eds.). (1992). *Biological response modifiers: A self-instruction manual for health professionals.* Chicago: Precept Press.

61. Schryber, S., et al. (1987). Autologous bone marrow transplantation. *Oncology Nursing Forum, 14*(4), 74–80.

62. Smith, R. (1992). Intraoperative radiation therapy. In K. H. Dow & L. J. Hilderley (Eds.), *Nursing care in radiation oncology* (pp. 295–306). Philadelphia: W.B. Saunders.

63. Somerville, E. T. (1991). Knowledge deficit related to chemotherapy. In J. C. McNally, J. Campbell Stair & E. T. Somerville (Eds.), *Guidelines for cancer nursing practice* (2nd ed., pp. 36–39). Philadelphia: W.B. Saunders.

64. Strohl, R. (1988). The nursing role in radiation oncology: Symptom management of acute and chronic reactions. *Oncology Nursing Forum, 15*(4), 429–434.

65. Tenenbaum, L. (1994). *Cancer chemotherapy and biotherapy: A reference guide* (2nd ed.). Philadelphia: W.B. Saunders.

66. Tenenbaum, L., Leshin, D., & Hydzik, C. (1994). Other systems affected by chemotherapy and biotherapy. In L. Tenenbaum (Ed.), *Cancer chemotherapy and biotherapy: A reference guide* (2nd ed., pp. 371–408). Philadelphia: W.B. Saunders.

67. Tenenbaum, L., & Scelsi, D. (1994). Central venous access devices. In L. Tenenbaum (Ed.), *Cancer chemotherapy and biotherapy: A reference guide* (2nd ed., pp. 411–428). Philadelphia: W.B. Saunders.

68. Theisen, A. (1991). The irreplaceable gift. *Journal of the American Medical Association, 266*(9), 1283.

69. U.S. Department of Health and Human Services. (1990). *Facing Forward: A Guide for Cancer Survivors* (National Institutes of Health Publication No. 90-2424). Washington, DC: National Cancer Institute.

70. U.S. Nuclear Regulatory Commission. (1981). *Instruction concerning risks from occupational radiation exposure.* Regulatory Guide 8:29, Washington, DC.: Office of Nuclear Regulatory Research.

71. Valdagni, R., et al. (1988). Important prognostic factors influencing outcome of combined radiation and hyperthermia. *International Journal of Radiation Oncology, Biology, Physics, 15,* 959–972.

72. Veronisi, U. (1987). Rationale and indications for limited surgery in breast cancer. *World Journal of Surgery, 11,* 493–498.

73. Weinberg, P. A. (1991). The human leukocyte antigen (HLA) system, the search for a matching donor, national marrow donor program development, and marrow donor issues. In M. Whedon (Ed.), *Bone marrow transplantation: Principles, practice, and nursing insights* (pp. 3–19). Boston: Jones & Bartlett.

74. Weisman, A. (1979). *Coping with cancer.* New York: McGraw-Hill.

75. Whedon, M. (1991). Autologous bone marrow transplantation: Clinical indications, transplant process and outcomes. In M. Whedon (Ed.), *Bone marrow transplantation: Principles, practice, and nursing insights* (pp. 49–69). Boston: Jones & Bartlett.

76. Whedon, M. (Ed.) (1991). *Bone marrow transplantation: Principles, practice, and nursing insights.* Boston: Jones & Bartlett.

77. Wickham, R. S. (1990). Advances in venous access devices and nursing management strategies. *Nursing Clinics of North America, 25,* 345–364.

78. Wingard, J. R. (1991). Historical perspective and future directions. In M. Whedon (Ed.), *Bone marrow transplantation: Principles, practice, and nursing insights* (pp. 3–19). Boston: Jones & Bartlett.

79. Yasko, J. M., & Rust, D. (1989). Trends in chemotherapy administration. *Seminars in Oncology Nursing, 5*(2, Suppl. 1), 3–7.

80. Young, R. C., Perez, C. A., & Hoskins, W. J. (1993). Cancer of the ovary. In V. T. DeVita, S. Hellman, & S. A. Rosenberg (Eds.), *Cancer: Principles and practice of oncology* (4th ed., pp. 1226–1263). Philadelphia: J. B. Lippincott.

Immunologic Disorders

MODIFIED-PROTECTIVE ISOLATION
VISITORS – REPORT TO NURSES' STATION BEFORE ENTERING ROOM
Do not enter room if you have a cold or flu-like symptoms.

HANDWASHING – on entering room

Masks – for close face contact over an extended length of time or if you have a cold and must enter the room.

Gowns

Door closed

No live plants, flowers, dried plants, fresh fruits or vegetables.

Check with nursing staff before taking other articles in the room.

Structure and Function of the Immune System

CHAPTER 25

R. B. Boley

Arlene L. Polaski

The human body defends itself against attack by viruses, bacteria, and other parasites by using two sets of separate but interrelated functions: (1) resistance (called by some innate immunity) and (2) immunity. Both of these systems must be present and operating properly in order to block establishment of infectious agents, minimize damage caused by disease in progress, and, finally, expel, destroy, or isolate infectious agents that gain access to inner tissues.

The immune system is an intricate network of specialized cells, tissues, and organs that evolved early in vertebrate development. The added functions were needed to supplement primitive defenses that were being overwhelmed by continually evolving pathogens and parasites. Some of the newly acquired mechanisms provided assistance in recognizing and killing body cells that develop into malignant growths. Through time, the old and new defenses merged together to form a sort of three-layered approach providing both surveillance (inside threats) and defense (outside threats) functions. This combination improved resistance to surface attachment of parasites, created an ability to mobilize phagocytic cells and reactive solutes to sites where surface tissues were breached, and made possible the production of special molecules and cells that were able to specifically recognize and combine with parasites and their products within the tissues and thus accelerate their removal. Some of the newly acquired cells were also able to detect self cells that were infected or transformed and selectively kill them.

The importance of these mechanisms to the health and well-being of an individual becomes apparent when the defenses of a healthy body are compromised by infection or suppressed by medication or chemotherapy. An individual thus affected will, if the condition persists, develop overwhelming infections, malignant disease, or both. The presence of such powerful means of defending ourselves against environmental and autogenous threats is, however, accompanied by some penalties. Parts of the defense system in a healthy body may function inappropriately to reject organ and tissue transplants and produce autoimmune disease or hypersensitivity states that cause pathologic changes and, sometimes, death.

Within the past decade or so, immunologists have come to realize that the pervasive nature and fundamental function of the immune system justifies including the system of immune functions as a core control mechanism of equal importance to the neural and endocrine systems. It is becoming increasingly clear that these three control systems serve together as a homeostatic continuum acting in concert to assist the body when it is threatened by stress, attacked by pathogens and parasites, or by other circumstances that threaten the integrity of the body.

Resistance

Resistance components are usually the first to encounter infectious agents or parasites. Many of these functions operate independently of the immune system but, as will be seen later, some of the components and features participate in or amplify acquired immune responses. A survey of resistance functions discloses the following types of functions:

Surface Defenses

Barriers. Intact skin and mucous membranes are sufficient to prevent penetration to underlying tissues by many pathogens.

Biochemical Defenses. Lysozyme in tears and bile in the gut inhibits gram positive bacteria; hydrochloric acid in the stomach is lethal to all pathogens; and fatty acids help protect the skin from infectious agents.

Surface-Clearing Mechanisms. These include washing of oral surfaces by saliva, tear-washing, urine-flushing, the mucociliary escalator in the trachea, and mucoperistaltic propulsion in the small intestine. The cough reflex is very important in protecting the lower recesses of the respiratory tract from infectious agents.

Autochthonous (Natural) Flora. Autochthonous flora interfere with colonization of pathogens by both niche (function) and habitat (location) competition.

Reticuloendothelial System (RES). The RES includes mononuclear phagocytic cells (macrophages). Fixed (attached) macrophages in the sinusoids of the liver, spleen, and bone marrow monitor the circulating blood and remove all foreign particulates and any moribund self cells. Resident mobile macrophages in lymph nodes remove foreign particulate matter. Macrophages in the alveolar spaces are the most active of the RES cells and act to remove inspired particulates (1 μm or less in diameter) that reach the lower recesses of the lung.

Inflammation

Inflammation is a combined fluid and cellular response to tissue injury, septic or sterile, that acts to clear debris, remove or neutralize septic agents, and set the stage for repair of damage. There are two types of inflammation: (1) acute and (2) chronic. *Acute inflammation* follows sublethal tissue injury. The chief cell is the neutrophil. It is usually quickly resolved. *Chronic inflammation* occurs when injury is prolonged, as in persistent bacterial, fungal, or parasitic infections. The chief cell is the macrophage. Resolution is slow and may persist for years.

Inflammation is a complex response to sublethal injury to a tissue and has both local and systemic consequences. The process can be initiated by products released from damaged cells, components from microbial cells, and from the interaction of effector units and antigen. Visible external signs are erythema, edema, warmth, pain, and decrease or loss of function of the affected part. Within the injured tissue site, the first indication is a transient constriction followed by a sustained dilation of small blood vessels (Fig. 25–1). Swelling at the site is caused by the escape of plasma (with its solutes: complement, fibrinogen, immunoglobulins). At about the same time the

vessels are responding, white blood cells begin to stick to the vascular endothelium, a process called margination. Neutrophils are the first to escape from the vessels (diapedesis) and, in response to a chemotactic gradient, accumulate at the site of injury. After a few hours, monocytes from the local circulation and macrophages present in local connective tissues begin to infiltrate the site of injury and soon replace the neutrophils as the dominant cell type (Fig. 25–2). In a limited type of injury, the healing and resolution process begins shortly afterward. Some cytokines produced by stimulated macrophages act locally to stimulate vascular changes and to activate fibroblasts and other cells. The same or other cytokines are distributed systemically and serve to initiate the acute phase response.

The Acute Phase Response

This is a systemic response that attends a strong local inflammatory response. Many aspects of the acute phase response are initiated by the action of cytokines produced by stimulated macrophages. These stimulatory molecules include interleukin-1 (IL-1), tumor necrosis factor (TNF), and interleukin-6 (IL-6). The systemic responses of the host include elevation of serum cortisol; induction of fever; leukocytosis; de novo appearance of a protein called C-reactive protein, an opsonizing protein that aids in phagocytosis; increased production of complement components, and increased production of siderophores (iron-binding proteins).

The Natural Killer Cell System

Natural killer (NK) cells are a poorly understood group of lymphoid cells that make up about 5% to 10% of the circulating lymphocytes. NK cells are not immunocompetent and have no well-defined ligand binding sites. They are involved in killing some tumor cells and some virally infected cells. Their cytotoxicity can be enhanced by exposure to cytokines, which convert a naive NK cell into a lymphokine-activated cell. After binding to a target cell,

Figure 25–1. Movement of white blood cells by the process of chemotaxis toward an area of tissue damage. (From Miller, M. J. [1983]. *Pathophysiology* [p. 149]. Philadelphia: W. B. Saunders.)

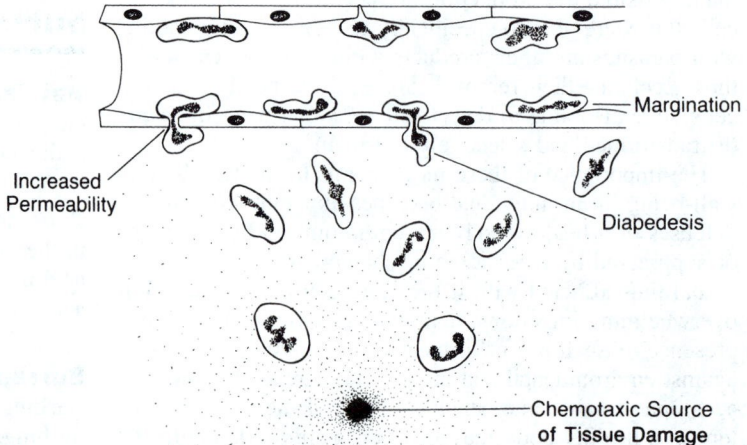

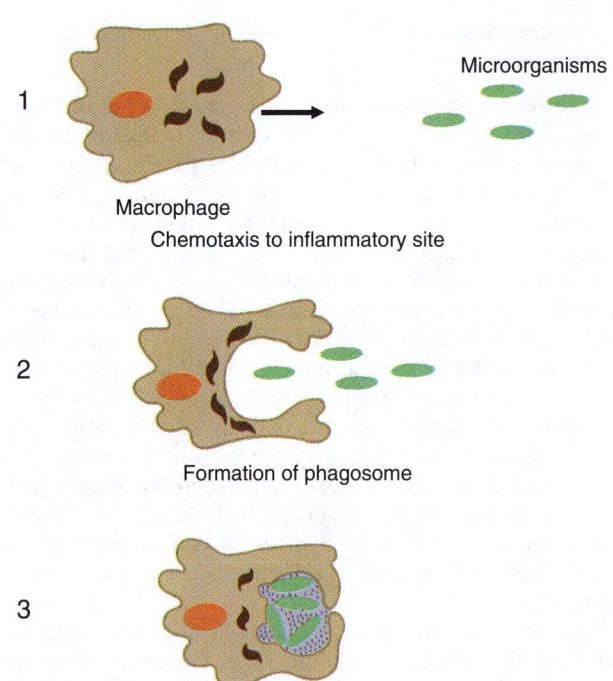

Figure 25–2. *1*, Macrophages migrate to an inflammatory site by chemotaxis. *2*, Macrophages engulf the microorganisms by extending pseudopodia around them. A phagosome or phagocytic vacuole forms around the microorganisms. *3*, Lysosomes attach to the phagosome and release their enzymes, which destroy the microorganisms.

the NK cell, like the cytotoxic T cell, secretes special protein molecules called perforins into the intercellular space. The perforins are then inserted into the target cell membrane in a manner analogous to the membrane attack complex of complement which causes holes to form in the membrane. An interesting observation is that individuals who have normal T and B cell populations but who are deficient in, or have reduced numbers of, NK cells experience repetitive life-threatening infections by viruses such as varicella and cytomegalovirus.

These diverse resistance functions, acting singly or in concert, are highly effective in preventing many types of microbial agents from initiating or maintaining an infectious process. Failure or even a slight reduction in normal function of one or more of these processes can have serious consequences for the individual involved.

Immunity

An individual can become immunized by direct (active) or indirect (passive) means:

- Active immunity. The individual produces effector units following stimulation by antigen. Natural immunity is produced by disease and environmentally acquired allergies. Artificial immunity is produced via vaccinations and allergies from therapeutic drugs.
- Passive immunity. The individual receives effector units that are produced by an animal, another human,

or by gene-engineering procedures. Natural immunity is produced via colostrum (topological protection in humans) and across the placenta (systemic protection in humans). Artificial immunity is produced through pooled γ (immune)-globulin, $Rh_0(D)$ immune globulin (RhoGAM), and genetically engineered human antibody.

Categories of Acquired Immunity

Four types (or compartments) of active immunity are identified based on the type and body location of the effector units:

1. Humoral immunity. The effector units are immuno-globulins (IgM, IgG, and IgA) present in the peripheral blood.
2. Mucosal immunity. The effector unit is an immuno-globulin (secretory IgA) present in mucous secretions of the respiratory tract, intestinal tract, and urogenital tract.
3. Cell-mediated immunity. The effector units are cytotoxic T cells that circulate in peripheral blood and are present in peripheral lymphoid tissues.
4. Atopic hypersensitivity (type I hypersensitivity). The effector unit is IgE, which is attached via the Fc portion to surface receptors on mast cells found in connective tissues and subsurface tissues of the respiratory and gastrointestinal tract.

Anatomy of the Immune System

The organs of the immune system are presented in Figure 25–3.

Central Lymphoid Organs

■ Bone Marrow

The bone marrow in an adult human is a major organ. Its combined weight can attain about 3000 g. In mammals, the bone marrow has several functions (Fig. 25–4). These include the following:

1. Maintenance of an undifferentiated stem cell population that is the source of all blood cells, including those active in immune functions
2. A significant storage site for erythrocytes and neutrophils
3. Sinusoids bearing fixed macrophages which serve an RES function in blood clearing
4. A site of antibody production in a secondary immune response to thymic-dependent antigens administered intravenously
5. The site in mammals for converting noncommitted or null lymphocytes into immunocompetent B cells.

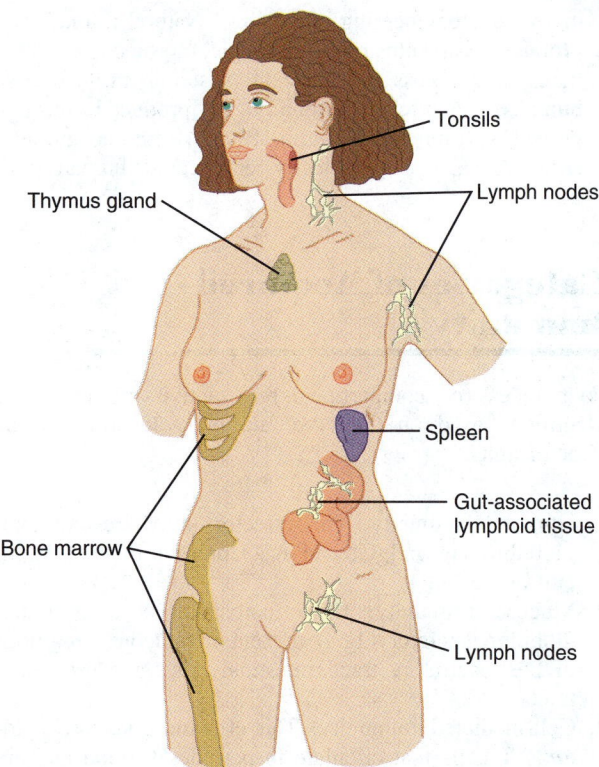

Figure 25–3. Organs of the immune system. The bone marrow, spleen, lymph nodes, tonsils, and gut-associated lymphoid tissue function in both specific and nonspecific immunity, whereas the thymus functions primarily in specific immunity.

■ Thymus

The thymus is a lymphoepithelial organ located in the mediastinum (thoracic cavity between the lungs and above the heart) which reaches peak development during childhood. After puberty it begins to atrophy (involute) and the cortex becomes less cellular and infiltrated with fatty tissue. Remnants of the thymus, however, persist into old age. The thymus is an endocrine organ and secretes several hormones that contribute to the maintenance and function of peripheral T cell populations. The interior of the early thymus is heavily populated with thymocytes derived from incoming null lymphocytes from the bone marrow and from a high rate of cell replication within the organ. During the course of converting null lymphocytes into T cells, the following major events take place within the thymus:

1. Conversion of null lymphocytes from the bone marrow into immunocompetent T cells
2. Rearrangement of gene sets to produce specific antigen recognition molecules (T cell antigen receptor [TCR])
3. Selection of those T cells that are able to bind self-recognition molecules of the major histocompatibility complex (MHC) (positive selection)
4. Destruction of those T cells that respond to self antigens (negative selection)
5. Synthesis of thymic hormones (several peptides that are ill-defined but are proposed to have a role in the

development and maintenance of peripheral T cell function)

The rearrangement of germ line genes during differentiation of lymphocytes in the central lymphoid tissues leading to the production of molecules for the recognition of antigen is the basis of the clonal selection hypothesis, a fundamental paradigm in immunology. In both cell types, the antigen recognition unit is inserted into the membrane with the antigen-reactive ends extending out into the extracellular environment. The T cell uses the T cell antigen receptor, and the B cell has a tetrapeptide monomer called a surface immunoglobulin (SIg). The individual cells each have a unique receptor capable of reacting only with a single antigenic determinant (Fig. 25–5). Each of these specifically reacting cells is called a clonotype, and when properly stimulated by antigen will produce effector units (either antibody molecules or specially reactive cells) and a memory cell clone, both of which have the identical specificity of the original clonotype.

The positive and negative selection processes acting on cells in the thymus make possible the mechanism for discrimination between self and nonself in immune function. This distinction is effected by making antigen recognition absolutely dependent on the variable but individually unique composition of the transcription products of gene loci located in the major histocompatibility region of the genome:

● Class I MHC molecules are found on nearly all nucleated cells in the body and represent a major antigenic distinction between individuals of a given species with different genotypes. This molecule is necessary for antigen recognition by T cells with CD8 surface markers.
● Class II MHC molecules are found on some antigen-presenting cells, on all B cells, and on antigen-activated T cells. This molecule is necessary for antigen recognition by T cells with CD4 surface markers. MHC antigens in humans were initially discovered on leukocyte membranes and are thus called human leukocyte antigens (HLAs).

The genes coding for these products are located on chromosome 6. Each of these genes is thought to have 25 or more alleles, making possible a large degree of diversity in the gene pool for MHC antigens and reducing the probability of duplication between two or more members of a species. It is this recognition system that forms the basis for the rejection of foreign or transplanted tissue. The cells in the recipient's immune system recognize the surface HLA proteins of the donor's tissue as being nonself.

It has been observed that persons possessing certain HLA proteins may develop a pattern of certain diseases at a higher rate than individuals who do not possess the proteins. Such diseases include several that affect the joints, endocrine glands, and skin. Examples are rheumatoid arthritis, Graves' disease, and psoriasis. The suspected association between the individual HLA patterns and the related disease is of a statistical nature that shows

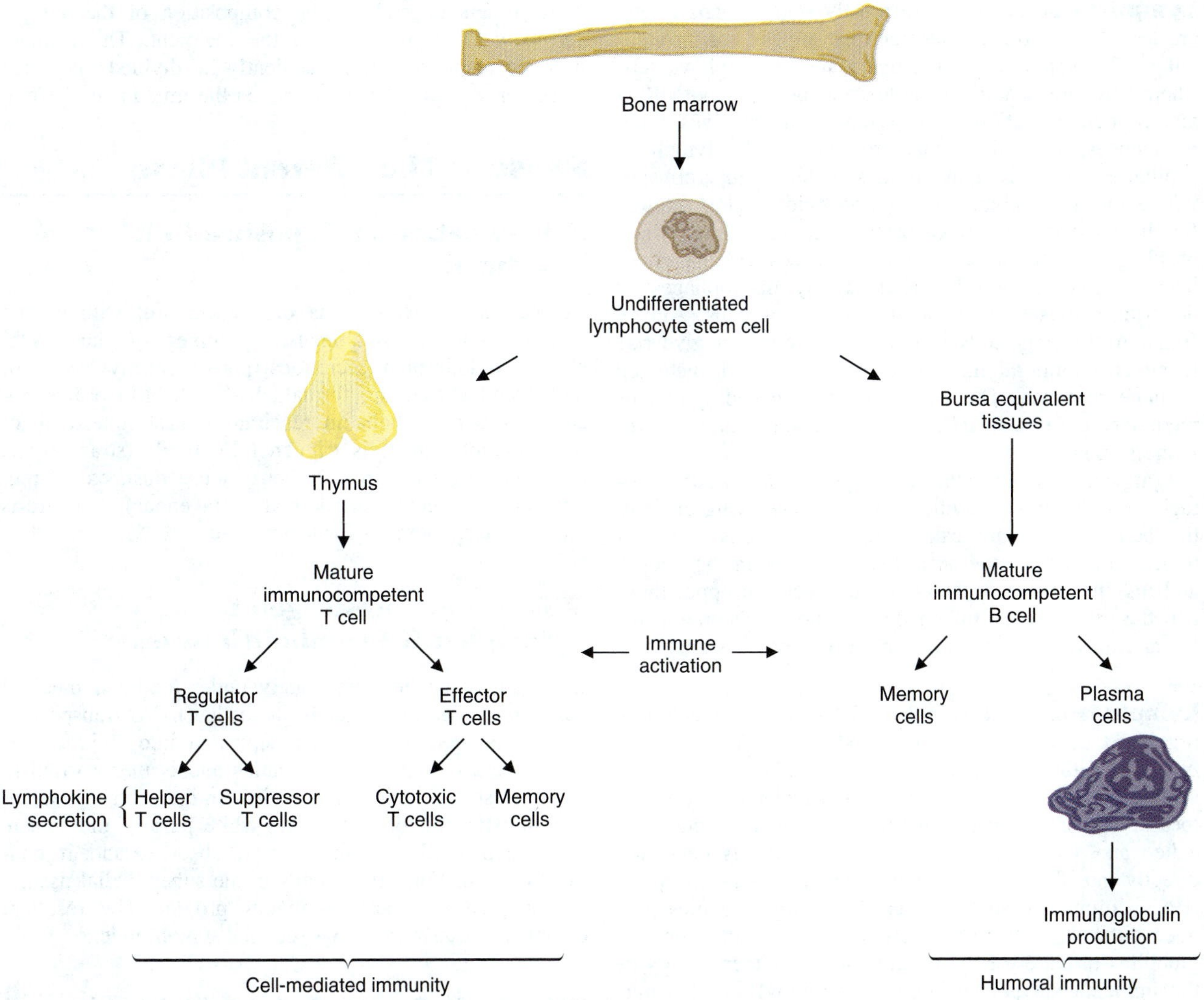

Bone marrow

Undifferentiated
lymphocyte stem cell

Thymus

Bursa equivalent
tissues

Mature
immunocompetent
T cell

Mature
immunocompetent
B cell

Immune
activation

Regulator
T cells

Effector
T cells

Memory
cells

Plasma
cells

Lymphokine { Helper
secretion { T cells

Suppressor
T cells

Cytotoxic
T cells

Memory
cells

Immunoglobulin
production

Cell-mediated immunity

Humoral immunity

Figure 25–4. The pathway of lymphocyte maturation. Undifferentiated lymphocyte stem cells are derived from the bone marrow. Those stem cells that are processed in the thymus differentiate into mature immunocompetent T cells, whereas those that are "processed" in bursa-equivalent tissues (most likely in the bone marrow) become mature immunocompetent B cells. Activation of either T or B cells by antigens leads to proliferation of immune cells that mediate either cell-mediated immunity or humoral immunity.

strong relationships in some cases and weak connections in others. Analysis of the indicated relationships is complicated by the fact that all persons with a given HLA phenotype do not develop the associated disease (half or more fail to do so in some cases). This suggests that the cause-effect relationship is multifactorial. None of the proposed hypotheses have been validated.

Peripheral Lymphoid Tissue

Peripheral lymphoid tissues are sites for antigen processing and presentation, and for T cell and B cell activation. These are the only locales for the production of the molecules and cells that serve as effector units of the immune response.

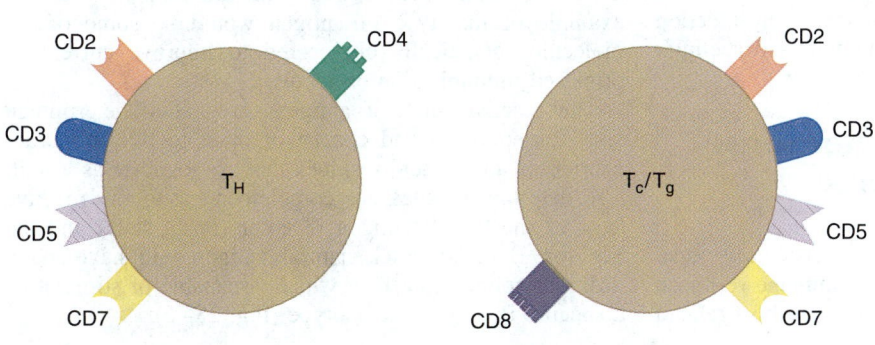

CD2   CD4

CD3

CD5

CD7

T_H

CD2

CD3

CD5

CD8   CD7

T_c/T_g

Figure 25–5. T cells can be distinguished by distinctive molecules located on their cell surfaces. They are called cluster designations (CDs). All mature T cells carry markers known as T2 (or CD2), T3 (or CD3), T5 (or CD5), and T7 (or CD7). T helper cells carry a T4 (CD4) and suppressor and cytotoxic T cells carry a T8 (CD8) marker.

Lymph Nodes. These are mostly small organs (many are less than 5 μm in diameter) that are present throughout the body interconnected by means of lymph vessels. Their structure is fairly complex and provides both RES and immune functions. The lymph node receives fluid, particulates, and solutes that are taken up by lymphatic capillaries from distal tissue sites. Resident macrophages within the node monitor the lymph fluid passing through for the presence of foreign particulates and remove them by phagocytic action. Antigenic substances, either particulates or solutes, will be taken up by macrophages or dendritic cells serving as antigen-presenting cells (APCs). Immunocompetent cells in the lymph node can give rise to either a humoral immune response or a cell-mediated immune response. The masses of cells called lymph or medullary cords also is a site of secondary humoral immune responses.

Lymph nodes are found in large numbers in the thoracic and abdominal cavities. Lymph nodes lying close to the body surface are called superficial nodes. Cervical nodes lie alongside the neck, axillary nodes in the armpit, and inguinal nodes in the crease between the upper thigh and the trunk. When inflamed, these nodes become swollen and may be palpated, serving as diagnostic signs.

Lymph Nodules. Lymph nodules have a much less organized structure than lymph nodes. They occur in the mucosal epithelium lining the respiratory, the gastrointestinal, and urogenital tracts. Antigenic materials are translocated across a dome epithelium through a special cell, called an M cell. The translocated material is deposited directly into the nodule structure where it is taken up by APCs. Immunocompetent B cells in lymph nodules produce either IgE or IgA. These two classes of immunoglobulins provide for the development of either allergy of the immediate hypersensitivity type (atopy), or of a mucosal immune response.

Lymph nodules exist either singly or in clusters. Examples of the latter are the tonsils, appendix, and Peyer's patches. These structures do not have a defined outer boundary, and are not connected with the lymph drainage system that connects the lymph nodes.

Spleen. The spleen is the largest lymphoid organ in the body. Its defensive functions include participation in the blood-clearing process via fixed macrophages in sinusoids as well as being a major site for humoral immune responses to bloodborne antigens. The splenic pulp is divided into red zones and white zones. The white zones are accumulations of lymphocytes and APCs. Loss of the spleen or diminished function due to injury or infection greatly increases the risk of infection with extracellular bacteria.

The Primary Immune Response and the Immune Cascade

A primary immune response arguably occurs only once. The quality and quantity of the primary immune response depends on many factors, some of which are host-related while others depend on the composition of the antigen and how it is presented to the recipient. The primary immune response can conveniently be divided into three stages or phases collectively called the immune cascade.

Phase 1: The Afferent Phase

■ Application or Exposure to the Antigen

Topical (skin) exposure is only successful with certain materials called proantigens. Examples of these substances include plant secretions (poison oak, ivy), salts of nickel and chromium, formaldehyde, etc. Mucosal exposure, through epithelia in respiratory, gastrointestinal, or the urogenital tract, is triggered by foods (strawberries, peanuts), drugs (aspirin), pollens, house dust, etc. Parenteral (subcutaneous, intradermal, intravenous) exposure is via vaccines, allergens for testing, etc.

■ Transport of Antigen to Peripheral Lymphoid Tissues

Lymph nodules lie immediately under modified mucosal epithelium (bearing M cells in the gut). No transport of antigen is required. Antigen deposited into solid tissues gain access to draining lymphatics and is then carried to the nearest regional lymph node. Antigen introduced intravenously will localize in the white pulp of the spleen. Proantigens applied to the skin are absorbed and, in conjunction with Langerhans cells in the subepithelial tissues, are coupled with an autogenous protein. The resultant complex is transported to a regional lymph node.

■ Arrival of Antigen in Peripheral Lymphoid Tissue

Arrival of antigen in peripheral lymphoid tissue is followed by its uptake by APCs.

Any exogenous molecule or any cell that does not have the self-markers of the recipient can serve as an antigen. Antigens may be natural, artificial, or synthetic. Natural antigens include unmodified bacteria, fungi, viruses, parasites, foreign tissue cells, and large individual molecules such as proteins. Artificial antigens are natural antigens that have been altered, usually to produce a vaccine: killed or attenuated bacteria, inactivated viruses, and toxoids. Artificial antigens are substances that are not found in nature, but are synthesized in the laboratory. A modern example of this type of antigen would be some of the molecules genetically engineered to improve current or proposed immunization protocols.

The reactive sites of antigens are called determinant sites (or epitopes) and consist of three to five monosaccharide or amino acid residues that act together as a unit. The determinant sites are complementary to the reactive sites of the T cell antigen receptor (on T cells) and the SIg (on B cells). Each natural antigen will have many different epitopes, each of which is capable of stimulating a specific B or T cell clonotype (Fig. 25–6).

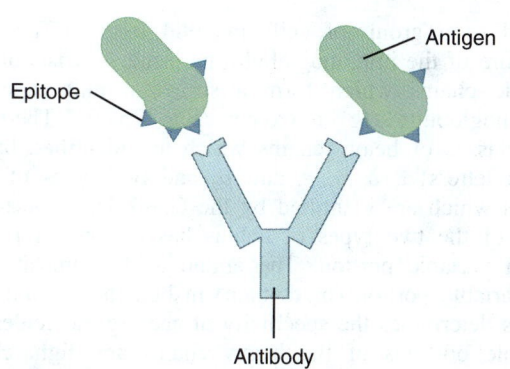

Figure 25–6. Epitopes protrude from the surface of an antigen and combine with the appropriate receptor of an antibody, much as a key fits into a lock.

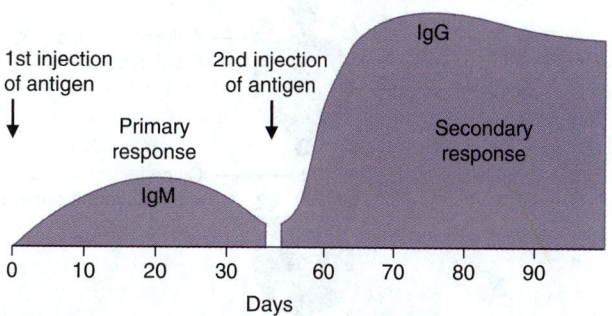

Figure 25–7. Primary and secondary antibody response. The second exposure of an antigen to the host causes a more rapid, stronger, and longer-acting response than the first exposure, owing to the presence of memory cells. IgM is most often produced in the primary response, whereas IgG is more likely to be produced predominantly in the secondary response.

Phase 2: The Central Phase

In phase 2, the central phase, antigen is taken up by or becomes affiliated with processing and presenting cells. Protein antigens are processed intracellularly by the APCs into peptide fragments and the fragments, in association with the major histocompatibility molecules, are placed on the surface of APCs for presentation to T cells, B cells that react to antigen in solute form, or adsorbed to the surfaces of follicular dendritic cells. T and B lymphocytes become activated and produce effector units and memory clonotypes.

Phase 3: The Efferent Phase

Effector units and memory clonotypes are exported to all body sites. If residual antigen remains in the tissues, effector units may combine with it causing signs and symptoms until the antigen is neutralized or removed. Residual antigen is most often seen with obligate or facultative intracellular parasites or pathogens. This condition is not likely to occur with an extracellular pathogen.

The Secondary Immune Response

The secondary immune response occurs when an individual who has been previously immunized with an antigen is rechallenged later with the same substance. This second (and any subsequent) response is characterized by several features that distinguish it from the primary immune response. Effector units are generally produced in greater quantity for a longer period of time, and antibody molecules may exhibit a higher affinity for antigen (Fig. 25–7).

Antigen Processing and Presentation

T cell recognition of antigen is limited to peptide fragments presented by an APC in conjunction with an MHC molecule. The recognition process is assisted by CD4 or CD8 molecules on the T cell surface. Class I MHC molecules are used to present peptides to CD8 cells and class II molecules present peptides to CD4 cells. This recognition process is said to be self-MHC–restricted which means that the APCs and the T cell both must have the same MHC molecules (i.e., each must recognize the other as self). The cells that can function as APCs in peripheral lymphoid tissue sites are B cells, dendritic cells, and some macrophages. Other locations include endothelial cells in peripheral vasculature (in humans), and Langerhans cells in the skin.

B Cells and the Antibody Response

B cells recognize antigen in one of two forms. (1) When free, unprocessed antigen, characteristically carbohydrate is encountered, the response is limited in that only IgM is produced and there are no memory B clonotypes developed (Fig. 25–8). (2) When proteins or protein conjugates are used as antigens, the APCs must first process the molecules to produce peptide fragments which are combined with MHC molecules and then presented to T helper cells. The activated T cells secrete cytokines which assist the B cell in responding to its own set of determinant sites present on the protein antigen. The cytokines stimulate growth and maturation in B cells, induce isotype switching, and make possible the development of memory clonotypes in both T and B cell lines. After being activated by antigen, and stimulated by cytokines, the B cell is transformed morphologically and physiologically into a distinct cell type: the plasma cell. Plasma cells are highly differentiated and specialized cells that are capable of producing large quantities of secreted immunoglobulin.

Immunoglobulins

Antibodies, or immunoglobulins, are a family of glycoprotein molecules that are present in the body as solutes in body fluids (plasma and mucous secretions) and at-

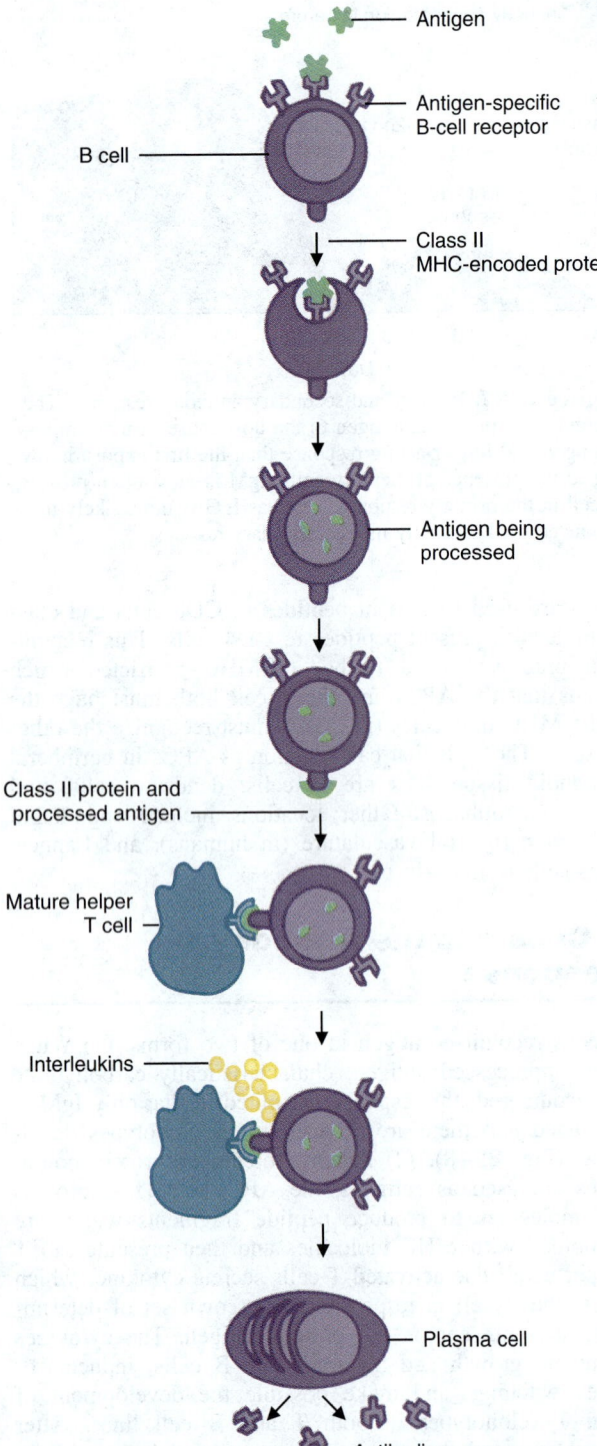

B cell
Antigen
Antigen-specific
B-cell receptor
Class II
MHC-encoded protein
Antigen being
processed
Class II protein and
processed antigen
Mature helper
T cell
Interleukins
Plasma cell
Antibodies

Figure 25–8. Activation of B cells to make antibody. The B cell uses its receptor to bind matching antigen, which it engulfs and processes. The B cell then presents a piece of antigen, bound to class II protein, on its surface. The complex binds to the mature T helper cell, which releases interleukins that transform the B cell into an antibody-secreting plasma cell. (Redrawn from Schindler, L. W. [1991]. *Understanding the immune system*. Washington, DC: National Institutes of Health.)

tached to a group of cells in solid tissues. The basic structure of the immunoglobulin molecule consists of four peptide chains which form a structural unit called an immunoglobulin (Ig) monomer (Fig. 25–9). There are five classes of heavy chains which are identified by the Greek letters α, δ, γ, ϵ, and μ, and two types of light chains which are identified by the Greek letters κ and λ. Each of the two types of chains has a constant portion and a variable portion. The amino acid composition of the variable portion (or domain) in both heavy and light chains determines the specificity of each Ig molecule. The variable portions of the heavy chains and light chains combine to form two identical antigen-combining sites called paratopes. The bottom part or tail of the Ig molecule, consisting of constant domains of two heavy chains, is called the Fc region. The terminal amino acid residues of this segment are reactive with receptors on the surface of macrophages, neutrophils, B cells, and mast cells.

■ IgG

IgG makes up about 75% of the total immunoglobulins in plasma (Table 25–1). It is available to react with any antigen that gains access to the circulating blood, either opsonizing it for accelerated uptake by RES cells or by activating complement via the classic pathway. When inflammation occurs in extravascular tissues, IgG is carried out of the vascular compartment to the septic site. IgG is the immunoglobulin that crosses the placenta and protects the newborn during the first few months of life. There are four subclasses of IgG based on variation in amino acid composition in the heavy chain. The properties of the subclasses differ from one another but the significance of these differences is not known.

■ IgA

IgA makes up approximately 15% of the immunoglobulin pool. It is present in small quantities in the circulation, but is the predominant immunoglobulin in saliva, tears, colostrum, breast milk, and in intestinal and bronchial secretions. The secretory (or mucosal) form of IgA serves to prevent the adherence of microorganisms to mucosal epithelium and thus supplements resistance mechanisms against local infections in the respiratory, gastrointestinal, and urogenital tracts.

■ IgM

IgM represents about 10% of the total plasma immunoglobulin and is normally present as a pentamer stabilized by a peptide J chain. It is the largest of the immunoglobulin molecules and is the class identified by the designation "natural." It is produced in response to challenge by bacteria in the normal gut flora and acts not only against these and similar bacteria that may infect tissue sites but is the main immunoglobulin composing the isoagglutinins reacting with blood group antigens. IgM is more effective than IgG in activating complement since only a single pentameric molecule bound to a cell is sufficient to initiate the cascade sequence (IgG requires the presence of

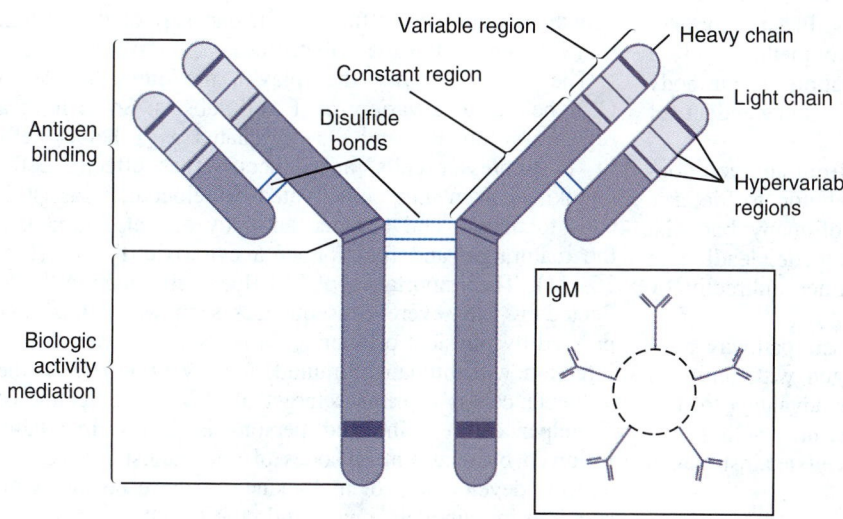

Figure 25–9. The immunoglobin G molecule (IgG) consists of two heavy chains joined by disulfide bonds to two light chains. Both chains have regions of constant and variable amino acid sequences. All five major immunoglobulin classes are composed of variations of this structure; combinations from pentamers of the IgM molecule, for example (*see inset*). The antigen-binding portion of the Y is responsible for the immunologic specificity of the IgG molecule; the biologic activity mediation portion is responsible for facilitating complement, phagocytosis, cell specificity, and IgG transport across the placenta.

two adjacent molecules bound to the cell surface). IgM is the early antibody seen in response to a thymic-dependent antigen, and the sole antibody produced against a thymic-independent antigen.

■ IgE

IgE is normally present only in trace amounts within the blood of most people. Exceptions are individuals who have active atopic allergies or who are infected with parasitic worms. In humans IgE is normally found bound to a surface Fc receptor on mast cells, where, following antigen binding, it triggers the release of chemical mediators such as histamine, which helps initiate the cascade of events leading to the expression of atopic allergy.

■ IgD

IgD contributes less than 1% of the total circulating immunoglobulins. The physiologic function of this immunoglobulin is unknown. It is present in large numbers on the cell membrane of naive B lymphocytes and its only role is thought to be for antigen recognition.

Monoclonal Antibodies

Monoclonal antibodies were first discovered as products of plasma cell tumors arising from a single B cell clonotype. These immunoglobulins can be synthesized by a hybridized cell produced by fusing a normal plasma cell (for antibody) with a myeloma cell (for longevity). The products of such a hybrid cell consist of a population of immunoglobulins with an identical specificity. Current technology enables large quantities of immunoglobulins with almost any specificity to be produced at reasonable cost. Because they have a single specificity, they are widely used in research and for diagnostic and therapeutic regimens. Some of the applications include leukocyte identification, parasite and pathogen identification, quantitative estimation of peptide hormones, antitumor therapy, immunosuppression, and fertility control.

Complement and Amplification of Antibody Function

Complement is the name given to a group of proteins that exist as solutes in plasma. When activated, the various components react in a cascade fashion whose most recog-

Table 25–1. Classes and Characteristics of Immunoglobulins (Ig)		
Class	% of Total	Characteristics
IgG	75	Present in the circulation and tissue spaces Opsonizes antigen Activates complement Transferred transplacentally First Ig synthesized in secondary immune response
IgA	15	Present in the circulation and seromucous secretions Prevents adherence of microorganisms to mucosal surface
IgM	10	Present primarily in the circulation Powerful agglutinating antibody First Ig of the primary immune response Activates complement
IgE	<1.0	Mediates hypersensitivity reactions Binds to mast cells and triggers mediator release
IgD	<1.0	Lymphocyte differentiation Full function unknown

nized function is the destruction of cells. Plasma complement can be activated by either of two methods: (1) a classic pathway requiring the participation of antibody and (2) an alternative pathway that is independent of antibody (Fig. 25–10).

The alternative pathway is the older from an evolutionary standpoint and is a major contributor to defense against pathogens. Surface molecules of many bacterial species can initiate the complement cascade, leading to the destruction of the bacterial cell either indirectly by opsonization or by direct cell lysis.

Activation of complement by the classic pathway must be preceded by the interaction of antigen with antibody (which must be either IgG or IgM). The advantage of this pathway is that complement can be recruited to assist in the removal of any solute or of any cell against which antibody can be produced.

T Lymphocytes and Cell-Mediated Immunity

Cell-mediated immunity (CMI) includes immune responses in which antibodies are not involved. CMI is vital in protecting the body against infection by viruses, slow-growing bacteria, and fungal infections. It also has a major role in immunosurveillance, reacting to abnormal clones of self cells, some of which are malignant. Such altered self cells can be destroyed in early stages by cytotoxic T cells or by NK cells, preventing them from becoming established tumors. Other CMI functions include primary rejection of allografts and development of delayed hypersensitivity reactions such as contact dermatitis (poison oak) and hypersensitivity to products of the tubercle bacillus. Many, if not all, of the biologic actions of T lymphocytes are mediated through the secretion of factors called lymphokines (cytokines). Although humoral and cell-mediated responses are often discussed separately, it is important to realize that these two arms of the immune system work together, sometimes inseparably,

and that failure or malfunction in one part of the system will frequently alter the effectiveness of the other.

The T lymphocytes that play a predominant role in CMI belong to a variety of T cell subsets. Some have a regulatory function and are designated as T helper cells or T suppressor cells, and others act as effector cells. Cytokines from antigen-activated T helper cells assist B cells to mature and produce antibody and also modulate the maturation and function of a cytotoxic T cells (Fig. 25–11). The importance of T helper cell function is reflected by the severe consequences seen when it is suppressed by physical or chemical means or depleted during infection with human immunodeficiency virus (HIV) (the T helper cell is a primary target of HIV). The decline of T helper cells in infected persons is almost inevitably followed by recurrent episodes of opportunistic infections and the development of malignancy in those persons with acquired immunodeficiency syndrome (AIDS).

The homeostatic reduction or suppression of B and T cell responses to antigen is no longer considered to be restricted to a single suppressor cell population (once thought to be a subset of T cells bearing the CD8 marker). A current hypothesis suggests that this type of negative regulation may be a function of essentially all T cells. Whether a given cell will act to produce a positive immune response (produce effector units) or mediate a negative response (tolerance) may be a function of the mechanism by which an individual T cell is activated by antigen.

The cytotoxic T lymphocyte reacts individually with target cells to establish a contact boundary that is required for target cell destruction. The intimate contact between the target cell and the cytotoxic T lymphocyte is mediated by an antigen-specific process and allows the cytotoxic T lymphocyte to release lytic molecules called porins directly into the membrane of the target cell. Cytokines produced and released by the cytotoxic T lymphocyte during the cell contact phase enhances the action of the porins. The cytotoxic T lymphocyte function is to kill viral-infected host cells, malignant cells, and cells in allograft transplants.

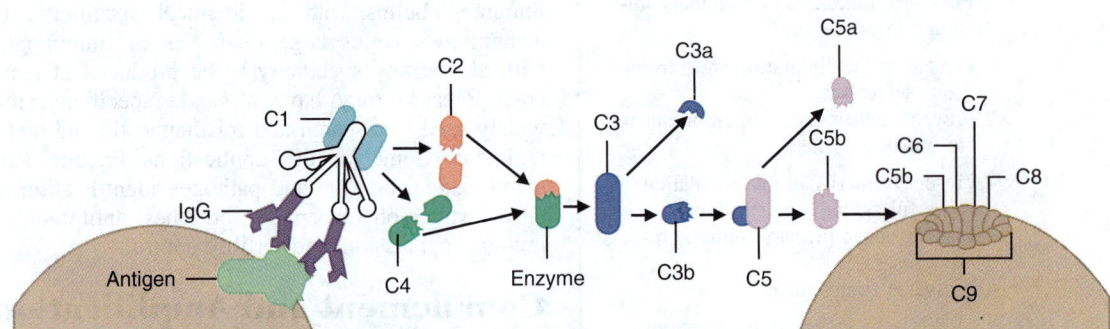

Figure 25–10. The classic complement pathway becomes activated when the first complement molecule, C1, recognizes antigen-antibody complex. Each of the remaining complement proteins, in turn, performs its specialized job, cleaving or binding the complement molecule next in line. The end product is the cylindrical membrane attack complex. (Redrawn from Schindler, L. W. [1990]. *Understanding the immune system.* Washington, DC: National Institutes of Health.)

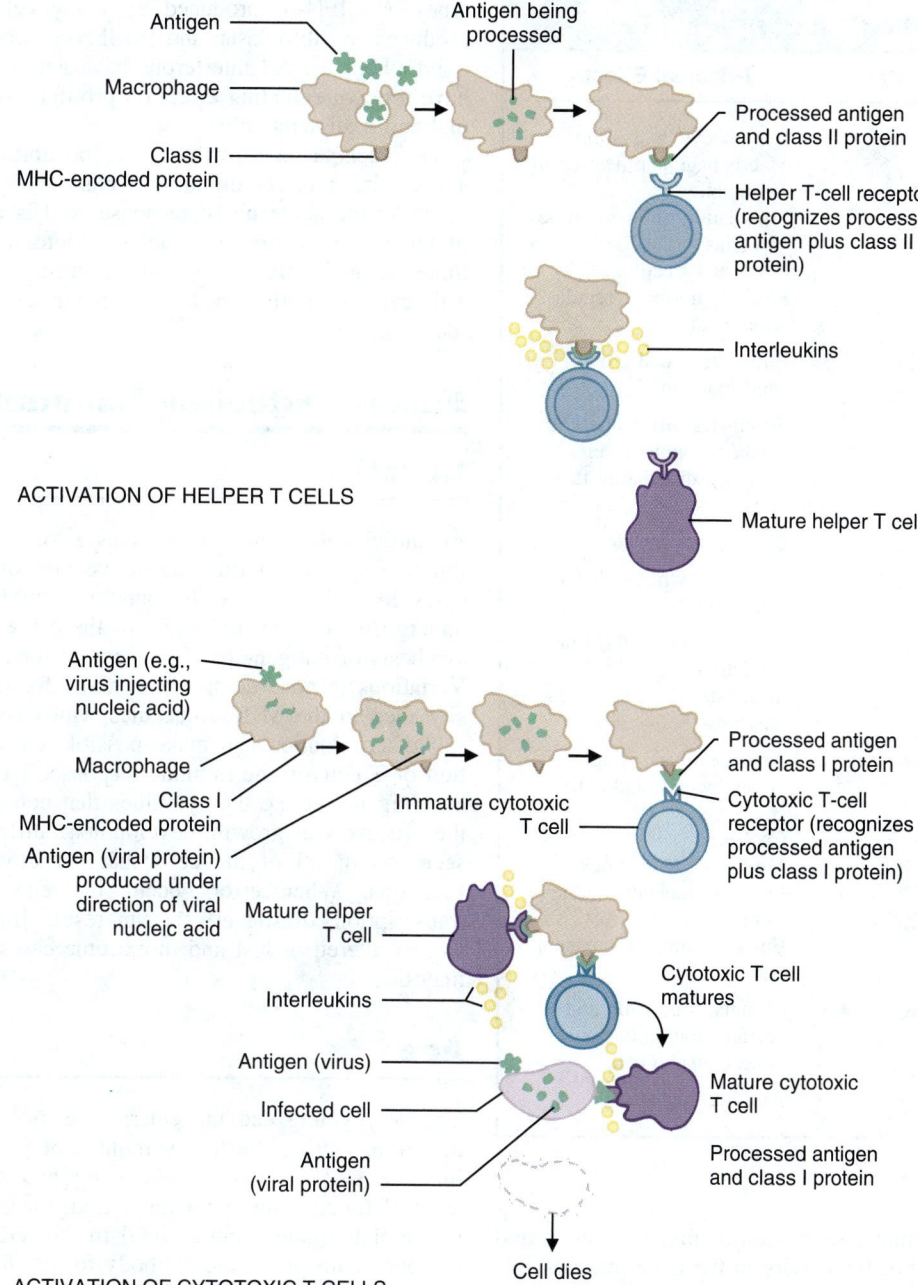

ACTIVATION OF HELPER T CELLS

ACTIVATION OF CYTOTOXIC T CELLS

Figure 25–11. Activation of cytotoxic T cells. After the macrophage internalizes and processes antigen, it presents antigen fragments on its surface. Antigen combined with class II protein attracts the T helper cell; interleukins help the T cell mature. Antigen plus the class I protein binds to the cytotoxic T cell; aided by the T helper cell, the cytotoxic T cell matures. (Redrawn from Schindler, L. W. [1990]. *Understanding the immune system.* Washington, DC: National Institutes of Health.)

The Role of Cytokines

Cytokine is a general term for cell-derived factors that mediate interactions between cells. Those produced by lymphocytes are called lymphokines and those produced by the monocyte-macrophage cells are called monokines.

Some of these factors are called interleukins, indicating service as regulatory signals between various leukocytes (Table 25–2).

Cytokines are a diverse group of proteins with four areas of function: (1) enhancement of mononuclear phagocytes; (2) regulation of lymphocyte growth, differentiation, maturation, and secretory activities; (3) inflamma-

Table 25–2. Major Cytokines

Cytokine	Principal Effects
Interleukin-1 (IL-1)	Lymphocyte activation Macrophage and neutrophil stimulation Stimulation of acute phase proteins Fever and sleep Pituitary hormone regulation
Interleukin-2 (IL-2)	Enhances T cell growth and function
Interleukin-3 (IL-3)	Stimulates differentiation of hematopoietic cells (colony-stimulating factor)
Interleukin-4 (IL-4)	B cell growth factor
Interleukin-5 (IL-5)	B cell growth and differentiation
Interleukin-6 (IL-6)	B cell growth and differentiation Stimulates the acute phase response
Tumor necrosis factor (TNF)	Activates macrophages, granuloctyes, and cytotoxic cells Cachexia Mediates septic shock Increases leukocyte adhesion Enhances antigen presentation
Colony-stimulating factor (CSF)	Stimulates division and differentiation of bone marrow stem cells
Interferon	Antiviral factor

tion; and (4) systemic effects such as fever induction and induction of hemopoietic activity in the bone marrow.

One of the best known cytokines is interleukin-1 (IL-1) which was originally described in the early 1960s. Produced by macrophages, its functions include induction of fever, as a coactivator of T cells, assisting in activation of B cells and NK cells, and induction of the acute phase response. Interleukin-2 (IL-2) is also well known from its first identification as a T-cell growth factor. The growth-enhancing function was crucial in the original studies of some of the retroviruses. Current research efforts are directed toward finding an application for IL-2 for treatment of malignant conditions. Interleukin-3 and -4 (IL-3, IL-4) are necessary for inducing antigen-stimulated B cells to undergo isotype switching to change from synthesis and secretion of IgM to IgG (or IgA or IgE). IL-3 also stimulates bone marrow stem cells to differentiate into monocytic and granulocytic precursors.

Interferons (IFNs) are another group of molecules that serve as intercellular messengers. There are three major

types: (1) IFN-α, produced by many cells; (2) IFN-β, produced by fibroblasts; and (3) IFN-γ, produced only by T lymphocytes. All interferons have antiviral activity and have a downregulating effect on proliferation of both normal and malignant cells.

TNF acts as a growth factor for fibroblasts and has a necrotizing effect on tumor cells. TNF participates in inducing the acute phase response, and is apparently one of the major factors in inducing endotoxic shock (sometimes seen in infections with gram-negative bacteria). This cytokine is thought to be a major cause of infection-related cachexia.

Factors Affecting Immunity

Genetics

An individual's genotype provides a foundation for one's immune system. During the conversion of null lymphocytes into T and B cells, gene sets in both cell lines undergo rearrangement as part of the process that leads to synthesis of antigen-specific receptors for each clonotype. Variations in gene composition allow for the great diversity seen in the MHC molecules which control self-non-self discrimination and make possible the specific activation of T cells in the immune response. T cells stimulated by antigens secrete the cytokines that control or fine-tune the processes of growth, development, differentiation, and secretion of all of the cells that participate in immune functions. When errors occur in gene replication or transcription, drastic effects can result. Immune function can be altered or lost and in extreme cases the individual may die.

Age

The very young and the elderly are most susceptible to infection. During the first 9 months of postnatal life, the immune system is still developing and exhibits a low level of function and poor regulation. Placental transfer of maternal immunoglobulin (IgG) to the fetus provides the newborn with protective antibody for the first few months of life. The breast-fed infant also is bolstered by receiving secretory IgA and immune cells from breast milk which protect the mucosal surfaces of the respiratory and gastrointestinal tracts. Artificial active immunization of an infant typically is not started until approximately 3 months of age when the infant is able to start producing antibody and memory cells in response to the antigens used in the vaccines. By about 1 year of age, the infant is able to produce about 60% of the adult level of IgG, 75% of the adult level of IgM, and 20% of the adult level of IgA.

After puberty the thymus begins a slow process of atrophy. As the individual ages, immune function becomes progressively weaker and there are emerging signs of loss of regulation. Consequences of these changes in elderly people include lower titers of humoral antibody, an increase in the frequency of autoimmunity, and an increase in the occurrence of malignancies. Other signs of altered immune function in this group are greater numbers of infections caused by direct pathogens and by opportunistic agents that normally do not cause disease in younger people.

The decline in immune function with age may be exacerbated by the presence of chronic illness. Certain diseases, such as diabetes mellitus, chronic renal failure, and liver disease, are characterized by impaired immune function. The elderly also have impaired physical barriers to infectious agents, associated with breakdown of skin and mucous membranes and decreased muscle mass. Changes in the endocrine system leading to alterations in hormone levels that occur with aging further contribute to impaired immunity. Finally, poor nutrition, which is common in this age group, will also adversely affect immune function.

Nutrition

The immune system is ordinarily robust. It requires extreme changes in nutrition or frank malnutrition before it is affected. A normal diet is usually adequate in proteins, vitamins, and minerals, but significant nutritional deficiencies can occur in the critically ill client with impaired gastrointestinal function, renal failure, and in catabolic states, such as burns and sepsis, as well as in chronic illness marked by cachexia, as seen with cancer.

Nutritional deficiencies are more likely to affect T cell function than B cell responses. Starvation will cause the thymus to undergo atrophy with a subsequent decline in thymic hormones. The number of circulating T cells declines and CMI responses are diminished. Other observations in starving animals include impairment of the inflammatory response, less than normal complement levels, and loss of resistance to invasive bacteria.

Zinc deficiency leads to thymus involution with a consequent decrease in T cell number and function. Low levels of this metal can also depress NK cell activity. Individuals with a vitamin A deficiency exhibit increased susceptibility to infection, which suggests a role for the vitamin in a humoral immune response. On the other hand, diets high in calories, especially from fats, appear to be involved in the development of autoimmunity.

Medications

A large number of medications can depress the immune system. Some medications are taken specifically for their anti-inflammatory or immunosuppressive properties. Some drugs produce bone marrow depression as a side effect that reduces the number of peripheral blood cells, for example, antibiotics (cephalosporins and penicillin) and antipsychotic drugs (phenothiazines). Glucocorticoids, commonly prescribed for a large number of conditions, have many anti-inflammatory and immunosuppressive effects, including a decrease in phagocytic cell activity and a lowered production of immunoregulatory cytokines. The administration of high doses of glucocorticoids is associated with increased susceptibility to infection and delayed wound healing.

Stress

For decades, stress has been suspected as being a cause of immunosuppression. Acute physical stressors, such as trauma and burns, are always accompanied by depressed immune cell function. If the affected individual survives the initial insult, he or she remains at great risk of infection. Emotional stress, such as grieving the loss of a loved one, is also marked by immunosuppression. Recent advances in cell biology, endocrinology, and neurology are beginning to clarify some of the mechanisms relating to the connections between stress and immunity. Stress due to both emotional and physical causes will trigger responses from the autonomic nervous system and the endocrine system. Both of these systems contribute to normal function of organs and tissues of the immune system. Untimely or excessive secretion of hormones and neurosecretory products can downregulate immune function or alter its normal course of activity.

A number of so-called stress hormones secreted by glands of the endocrine system modulate immune activity. The best-known stress hormone is cortisol, secreted by the adrenal cortex, which has multiple anti-inflammatory and immunosuppressive effects. However, other hormones released during stress, such as pituitary endorphins, growth hormone, prolactin, thyroid hormones, and reproductive hormones, also influence immune cell function. Furthermore, the link between the immune and endocrine systems appears to be a two-way street because secretory products from the immune system, such as IL-1, can also affect endocrine gland secretion. The relationship between the immune, endocrine, and nervous systems and the client's psychological make-up has evolved into an area of study called psychoneuroimmunoendocrinology.

Data from studies involving persons participating in a moderate exercise program indicate that they become more resistant to disease (and possibly to tumor development and growth). Persons engaged in forms of very strenuous physical activity may show signs of immunosuppression related to the physiologic stresses induced by the high level of activity.

Conclusions

The immune system is an extremely complex system. It has evolved through the years to become a pervasive and highly structured group of complex functions that defend the body against pathogens and parasites from the outside and are able to detect and attack altered self cells that pose threats to organismal homeostasis. At least three distinct cell lines are able to work cooperatively to produce a variety of effector units that carry out the defense and surveillance responsibilities. The remarkable advances made by molecular biologists during the past two decades have enabled immunologists to describe in increasing detail the molecular mechanisms that underlie immune function. Knowledge about cell adhesion molecules, signal transduction, recombination processes in genes, and positive and negative selection processes that act on differentiating cells will give the clinician enormous latitude in designing and using therapeutic protocols for all forms of disease regardless of cause.

Bibliography

1. Ada, G. L., & Nossal, G. (1987). The clonal selection theory. *Scientific American, 257*(2), 62.
2. Ader, R., & Cohen, N. (1993). Psychoneuroimmunology: Conditioning and stress. *Annual Review of Psychology, 44,* 53.
3. Ahmed, R. A., & Blose, D. A. (1983). Delayed hypersensitivity skin testing: A review. *Archives of Dermatology, 119,* 934.
4. Arai, K., et al. (1990). Cytokines: Coordinators of immunity and inflammatory responses. *Annual Review of Biochemistry, 59,* 783.
5. Balkwill, F. R., & Burke, F. (1989). The cytokine network. *Immunology Today, 10,* 299.
6. Bloom, B. (1989). Vaccines for the third world. *Nature, 342,* 115.
7. Bohnsak, J. F., & Brown, E. J. (1986). *Annual Review of Medicine, 37,* 49. The role of the spleen in resistance to infection.
8. Bos, J. D., & Kapsenberg, M. L. (1986). The skin immune system: Its cellular constituents and their interactions. *Immunology Today, 7,* 235.
9. Grey, H. M., Sette, A., & Buus, S. (1989). How T cells see antigen. *Scientific American, 261*(5), 56.
10. Hedrick, S. M. (1992). Dawn of the hunt for nonclassical MHC function. *Cell 70,* 177.
11. Knight, S. C., & Stagg, A. J. (1993). Antigen-presenting cell types. *Current Opinion in Immunology, 5,* 374.
12. Lanzavecchia, A. (1993). Identifying strategies for immune intervention. *Science, 260,* 937.
13. Rose, N. R., et al. (1992). *Manual of clinical immunology* (4th ed.). Washington, DC: American Society for Microbiology.
14. Slater, J. (1992). Latex allergy—What do we know? *Journal of Allergy and Clinical Immunology, 90,* 3.
15. Springer, T. A. (1990). Adhesion receptors in the immune system. *Nature, 346,* 425.
16. Tomlinson, S. (1993). Complement defense mechanisms. *Current Opinion in Immunology, 5,* 83.
17. Trowsdale, J., Ragoussis, J., & Campbell, R. D. (1991). Map of the human MHC. *Immunology Today, 12,* 443.
18. Virella, G., Patrick, C. C., & Goust, J. M. (1993). Diagnostic evaluation of lymphocyte functions of cell-mediated immunity. *Immunology Series, 58,* 291.
19. von Boehmer, H., & Kisielow, P. (1991). How the immune system learns about self. *Scientific American, 265*(4), 74.
20. Young, J. D. E., & Cohn, Z. A. (1988). How killer T cells kill. *Scientific American, 258*(1), 38.

Assessment of Clients with Immune Disorders

CHAPTER 26

Esther Matassarin-Jacobs

History

Biographical and Demographic Data

The client's age should be noted because immune function becomes less competent with age. The client's environment should also be assessed by asking questions about where he or she lives and works because environmental agents often trigger allergic responses.

Current Symptoms

The client may report a range of manifestations depending on the part of the structure or function of the immune system affected.

Chief Complaint

Manifestations can result from allergic responses, altered immune system function, or disorders of the lymphatic system.

Symptom Analysis

Timing. Ask the client when the manifestations began. Many times allergic manifestations begin in childhood, whereas other clients develop allergies later in life. Ask what allergens trigger allergic responses. Ask also about the development of frequent infections since this could indicate an immune disorder.

Ask the client how long allergic manifestations last. Are they relieved once the allergen is removed or do they continue?

Quality and Quantity. What manifestations is the client exhibiting? The client may report allergic manifestations such as rhinitis, sneezing, nasal stuffiness, postnasal drip, sore throat, voice changes, hoarseness, wheezing, persistent cough, dyspnea, malaise, fatigue, rashes, pruritus, vomiting, diarrhea, intestinal colic, excessive tearing, or altered hearing acuity. Manifestations vary depending on the nature of the allergen and the client's individual sensitivity pattern. Complete a symptom analysis (see Chapter 11) for each reported manifestation to assist in the identification of the allergen.

The client may report localized swelling over an underlying lymph node (or nodes) or generalized swelling and edema of an extremity. Other manifestations include increased redness or streaks (indicating cellulitis), pain, tenderness, fever, anorexia, headache, and irritability.

Severity and Location. How severe are the allergic manifestations? Are they simply skin rashes, nasal stuffiness, and cough, or are they more severe manifestations such as wheezing and respiratory distress? Do different allergens trigger different responses? Ask if the client has ever experienced an anaphylactic reaction to an allergen.

Precipitating Factors. Ask the client what allergens trigger an allergic reaction. The major types of allergens include inhalants (e.g., pollens, molds, spores, dust, mites, trees, grasses, and animal dander); contact agents (e.g., dyes in clothing, fibers, cosmetics, metals in jewelry, plant oils and secretions, topical drugs, and numerous chemicals); ingested agents (e.g., foods, food additives, drugs); and injectable agents (e.g., drugs, vaccines, and insect venom).

The nurse asks the client about infections, both systemic and local. These infections may be associated with breaks in the skin, ingrown nails, fungal infections, or puncture wounds. Lymphedema can result from congenital deformity of the lymph vessels or as a result of altered structure and function. Therefore, ask the client about surgery or trauma to extremities, radiation therapy, and the presence of a malignancy or neoplasm, which may

---

This chapter incorporates material written for the fourth edition by Linda Janusek.

have obstructed lymphatic vessels or nodes and drainage from an area.

If the client is experiencing frequent infections, ask what exposure the client has had that might be causing them. Ask if the client has a history of taking steroids or immunosuppressant agents.

Aggravating and Relieving Factors. Ask the client what he or she takes to relieve the allergic manifestations. Does the client take antihistamines or antipruritics? If the problem is a rash, what does the client use to relieve this? Is the client using an inhaler for a respiratory manifestations?

Ask whether elevation relieves swelling of an affected extremity and whether a dependent position leads to increased swelling. Does the client use a compression wrap (e.g., an elastic bandage) on an extremity to relieve or prevent swelling?

Associated Manifestations. If the client has swelling in the lymph nodes, is there associated pain, tenderness, redness, or drainage? Is there an accompanying fever?

Past Health History

Childhood and Infectious Diseases

Ask if the client has always had allergic manifestations. Did the client have frequent infections as a child? What childhood diseases did the client have? Has the client recently been exposed to a known infectious disease?

Immunizations

Ask if the client has ever received any desensitization injections for allergies. If so, ask the client what allergens were given, when they were given, and how effective they were in preventing allergic reactions. Is the client current with recommended immunizations?

Major Illnesses and Hospitalizations

Ask the client about any history of hospitalizations associated with allergic manifestations. Also ask the client about the occurrence of any major illness such as cancer, human immunodeficiency virus (HIV) infection, or autoimmune disease that might affect the immune system.

Inquire about previous problems with swelling, injury, or trauma to extremities, including surgery. Has the client had a systemic infection, immunologic reaction, or neoplastic disorder? If so, ask the client to describe the disorder and its treatment. For example, a client who has had axillary node dissection accompanying a mastectomy often has upper extremity edema of the ipsilateral side. Also ask about disorders affecting the vascular system such as congestive heart failure, renal disease, and periph-

eral vascular problems. These disorders are often accompanied by edema of the extremities.

Allergies

Ask the client about past episodes of allergic reactions. Ask the client if there is a seasonal pattern associated with these episodes, what manifestations developed, what treatment was given for these allergies and its effectiveness. Inquire about drug and food allergies or sensitivities. Has the client ever suffered an anaphylactic reaction? Has the client ever been hospitalized for an allergic reaction? Has the client had previous series of treatment for desensitization with allergy injections? If so, were the treatments effective? Ask about allergies to iodine or seafood. Diagnostic studies of the lymphatic system use an iodine-based contrast medium.

Family Health History

Ask the client to identify allergies and sensitivities in family members, particularly atopic reactions. Hay fever also tends to occur among family members. Ask if family members have immune system problems such as frequent infections, delayed healing responses to injury, or an autoimmune response.

Psychosocial History

Occupation

Ask about the client's occupation. If the client is exposed to allergens at work, this could trigger allergic reactions. What possible occupational exposure might the client have that would predispose to the development of cancer (see Chapter 23)? Does the client work around agents that might predispose to the development of immune disorders such as asthma?

Geographical Location

Where does the client live? Allergic responses to inhalants and contact agents are more severe in certain areas of the country. Some parts of the country have a higher level of air pollution, which might increase the client's respiratory problems. Does the client live in parts of the country that have a higher incidence of immune diseases such as multiple sclerosis or thyroiditis?

Environment

Information about the client's physical environment and psychosocial patterns is important in obtaining a complete allergy history. Ask about the home and work (or school) environments. Are there pets in the home? Are there houseplants or fresh-cut flowers in the home? What type of vegetation is in the immediate vicinity of the home or workplace? Ask the client to describe the type of heating and cooling systems both in the home and at work. If food-related allergies are suspected, ask the client to keep a food diary, including descriptions of any reactions to ingested foods. Encourage the client to discuss current levels of stress and whether there is a relationship to the appearance of allergic manifestations. Also ask how the client reacts to outbreaks of allergic manifestations. For example, some clients break out in hives when they are under psychological or emotional stress. Their appearance triggers more emotional stress, which, in turn, leads to further outbreaks of hives. A cycle develops that is difficult to interrupt.

Nutrition

Does the client have any allergies to food or food additives? Have the allergies limited the client's intake of any particular nutrients such as citrus fruits or grains? Is the client allergic to eggs and other protein sources that may lower immunoglobulin levels? Does the client ingest sufficient protein to sustain immunocompetence?

Habits

Ask if the client smokes or has smoked in the past. Does anyone around the client smoke? Smoking may make inhalant allergies worse and tobacco smoke is a known carcinogen. What is the client's alcohol intake? Excessive alcohol ingestion may lead to poor nutrition and decreased immunity.

Review of Systems

Prior to the physical examination, ask the client about the following problems associated with allergies:

- General: fatigue, malaise, unusual reactions to insect bites or medications, including over-the-counter drugs
- Integumentary: rashes, urticaria, itching, scratching, dryness, scaling
- Eyes: dark circles around the eyes, excessive tearing, rubbing or blinking, conjunctivitis, styes
- Ears: altered hearing acuity, feeling of fullness in the ears, ear pain, ruptured tympanic membranes
- Nose: sneezing, sniffling, rhinitis, nasal polyps, nasal voice quality, nose twitching or rubbing, nasal stuffiness, recurrent epistaxis, postnasal drip
- Throat: swollen lips or tongue, frequent clearing of the throat, sore throat, itching of the throat or neck, hoarseness
- Respiratory: wheezing, dyspnea, frequent cough, ineffective cough, respiratory distress
- Gastrointestinal: diarrhea, vomiting, cramping, food intolerances

Ask the client to describe problems in the following areas for information about the lymphatic system:

- General: malaise, fatigue, fever, lassitude, chills, sweating, pruritus
- Head and neck: localized swelling, pain or tenderness, swollen nodes, headache, irritability

- Cardiovascular: hypertension; congestive heart failure; peripheral vascular disorders such as varicose veins; edema of the hands, feet, or legs
- Gastrointestinal: anorexia, hepatomegaly, splenomegaly
- Renal: kidney disease, including renal failure
- Immunologic: recent infections such as influenza, measles, mononucleosis, viral infections; neoplasms, including lymphoma; injury or trauma resulting in a break in the skin barrier; date of last tetanus toxoid injection

Physical Examination

The client with allergies should receive a head-to-toe physical examination. Focus on the area that is the target for the allergen. Disorders of the lymphatic system (lymphadenopathy) include inflammation (lymphangitis), an increased amount of lymph (lymphedema), or enlargement of lymph nodes. A complete history and physical examination help determine the cause of the problem and direct treatment.

The portions of the lymphatic system accessible to physical examination are the superficial lymph nodes, liver, and spleen. Examination of the liver and spleen is discussed in Chapter 64. The techniques used to examine superficial lymph nodes are inspection and palpation. Use a methodical approach when examining lymph nodes so as not to overlook single nodes or chains of nodes. The nodes of the head and neck, supraclavicular areas, axillae, and epitrochlear areas are most easily palpated while the client is sitting. Inguinal and popliteal nodes are more accessible when the client is lying down.

Inspection

Inspect the surfaces overlying nodes for masses or scars and look for symmetry. If masses are seen, palpate the area and compare it with the contralateral side.

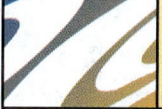

NORMAL PHYSICAL ASSESSMENT FINDINGS
Immune System
Inspection
Areas overlying the superficial lymph nodes of the head, neck, axillae, epitrochlear chains, inguinal chains, and popliteal fossae without masses or drainage.
Palpation
All nodes nontender. Several round, small (less than 0.5 cm), discrete, soft, mobile nodes palpable in submandibular area.

Palpation

Palpation is used to assess lymph nodes for size, shape, consistency, discreteness, mobility, and tenderness. To palpate the nodes, use the finger pads of the middle three fingers in a gentle, circular motion. Keep the fingertips in contact with the skin and slide them over the underlying nodes. Avoid excessive pressure so as not to miss small, yet palpable nodes. Lymph nodes are not normally palpable, yet it is common to find small (diameter 1 cm or less), round, soft, single, mobile, nontender nodes, particularly in the cervical and inguinal areas. Nodes that are large (diameter greater than 1 cm), hard, that feel matted together or fixed to underlying structures, or tender are abnormal findings. Describe their characteristics thoroughly.

Specific guidelines for palpating the *head and neck lymph nodes* are given in Table 26–1. The techniques for palpating these nodes are shown in Figure 12–3. Use a methodical approach when examining head and neck nodes. These nodes are normally not palpable, but small, mobile, nontender nodes are common because they enlarge with repeated local and systemic infections. The lymph nodes accessible to examination in the arms are the *epitrochlear chains*. These nodes are located in the groove between the biceps and triceps muscles, proximal to the medial epicondyle of the humerus. They are not usually palpable. *Axillary nodes* are usually examined during assessment of the anterior thorax, as part of the

Table 26–1. Sequence and Palpation Technique for Lymph Nodes in the Head and Neck

Nodes	Location	Palpation Technique
Occipital	Posterior at base of skull and lateral to cervical spine	Flex the client's neck forward slightly to relax the trapezius. Palpate right and left node centers simultaneously
Posterior auricular (mastoid)	Behind auricle of ear, over outer surface of mastoid process	Palpate over both mastoid processes simultaneously
Posterior cervical chain	Along anterior edge of trapezius, in the posterior triangle	Flex the client's neck to relax the trapezius muscles. Palpate slowly against the trapezius muscles, progressing from the mastoid processes toward the clavicles
Supraclavicular (scalene)	Above the clavicle, in the angle formed by the clavicle and the sternocleidomastoid	Flex client's neck sharply with one hand and encourage the client to relax the shoulders so that clavicles drop. Palpate one side at a time with fingers over the client's right clavicle lateral to the sternocleidomastoid. Ask the client to inhale deeply while pressing in and behind the clavicle. Repeat using the right hand to palpate the client's left node centers
Superficial (anterior) cervical chain	Along and over (anterior to) the sternocleidomastoid, in the anterior triangle	Flex the client's neck forward to relax the sternocleidomastoid. Palpate one side at a time. Palpate slowly against the sternocleidomastoid, progressing from the clavicle toward the jaw
Deep cervical chain	Under the sternocleidomastoid	Flex the client's neck laterally toward the side being examined to relax muscles and soft tissue. Palpate one side at a time. Hook thumb (on one side) and fingers (on the other side) around the sternocleidomastoid muscle to feel deep to the muscle. Progress from the jaw toward the sternum
	Along the anterior edge of the sternocleidomastoid, in the anterior triangle	With the client's neck still flexed laterally, palpate along the anterior edge of the sternocleidomastoid from the sternum to the jaw angle. Repeat on the opposite side of the neck
Tonsillar	Near the angle of the jaw at the jaw margin	Flex the client's neck slightly in the midline. Palpate behind both jaw angles simultaneously
Submandibular (submaxillary)	Along the medial border of the mandible, between the angle of the jaw and the chin	Palpate along the medial borders of the mandible from the angle of the jaw toward the chin. Palpate right and left node centers simultaneously
Submental	At the midline, posterior to the tip of the mandibles under the chin	Palpate with one hand under the client's chin just behind the tip of the mandible. Steady the client's head with the free hand if necessary
Anterior auricular	In front of the tragus of the ear	Palpate right and left sides simultaneously, anterior to the tragus and posterior to the temporomandibular joint

breast examination. See Chapter 85 for a discussion of axillary lymph node palpation. The superior (horizontal) and inferior (vertical) chains of the *inguinal lymph nodes* are not palpable, although small, soft, mobile, nontender nodes are common. The inguinal area is normally free of bulges or masses. The lymph nodes examined in the lower extremities are the *popliteal nodes*. The popliteal nodes are located in the popliteal fossae on the lateral aspects and are not normally palpable.

If an extremity appears edematous, measure its circumference and compare it with the contralateral extremity. Differences of less than 1 cm (about ½ inch) are considered within normal limits.

The techniques of percussion and auscultation are not done in association with the lymphatic system.

Diagnostic Tests

Acquired Immunodeficiency Syndrome (AIDS) Tests

Enzyme-Linked Immunosorbent Assay

The enzyme-linked immunosorbent assay (ELISA) is the first test performed when HIV infection is suspected. Although this is a relatively inexpensive, quick, and easy test, there is a high rate of false-positive results. In other words, ELISA is highly sensitive, but not as specific.

Western Blot

The Western blot is a more specific test for the presence of the HIV antibody. It is also more expensive and labor-intensive compared with ELISA. The usual course of events when a client requests testing for HIV is as follows:

1. Pretest counseling is provided, and informed consent is signed.
2. Serum is drawn and tested by ELISA for the presence of the HIV antibody. If this test is negative, the tests stop here.
3. If the test is positive twice by ELISA, then a Western blot is performed. If this is also positive, the client is considered HIV-positive and, therefore, infected with HIV.
4. If the Western blot is negative, a confirmatory test is often run, and if this is still negative, the client is considered HIV-negative. Most laboratories will confirm positive results by running the Western blot a second time on a new specimen.

Radioimmunoprecipitation Assay

The radioimmunoprecipitation assay (RIPA) is another serum test performed on clients with suspected AIDS. This test is more time-consuming and labor-intensive than the Western blot; however, it is considered to be more sensitive and more specific. It also requires the use of radioactive materials, making it a poor choice for routine screening.

Tests of Immunologic Status

Hematologic Studies

See Chapter 52 for standard hematologic studies.

CD4 Cell Count

The hallmark of HIV infection is depletion of T-helper lymphocytes. Clients with HIV infection have CD4 counts done. This is a simple blood serum test.

T- and B-Lymphocyte Assays

T- and B-lymphocyte assays require a peripheral blood sample. There is no pre- or postprocedure care required. Increased levels of T lymphocytes are associated with acute lymphocytic leukemia, infectious mononucleosis, and multiple myeloma, while reduced levels may indicate AIDS, chronic lymphocytic leukemia, severe combined immunodeficiency disease (SCID), and long-term immunosuppressive therapy. Increased levels may indicate chronic lymphocytic leukemia, multiple myeloma, and lupus erythematosus. Reduced levels are associated with acute lymphocytic leukemia and SCID.

Immunoglobulin Assays

This is another simple blood serum test requiring no pre- or postprocedure care. The examination measures the levels of the various immunoglobulins: IgG, IgA, IgM, IgD, and IgE. Clients with autoimmune and allergic disorders may show increased levels of IgA and IgE. Clients with lymphocytic leukemia may exhibit reduced levels of IgG, IgA, and IgM.

Tests of Bone Marrow and Lymphatics

Chapter 52 discusses bone marrow aspiration. Diagnostic assessment of the lymphatic system may be found in Chapters 52, 53, 64, and 85.

Lymphangiography

Procedure. A lymphangiogram is a test that allows visualization of the lymphatic system to assess the presence of primary malignancy (lymphoma) or metastatic disease (e.g., testicular cancer) in tumors involving the lymphatic system or with typical lymphatic spread. The test involves injection of an oil-based dye into the lymphatic system. The tops of the feet are first numbed using local anesthesia, and a blue dye is injected that is taken up by the lymphatics. A surgical cutdown is done, a catheter is inserted into the lymphatic channel, and an oil-based dye is injected. The feet are elevated to aid in distribution of the dye throughout the lymphatic system. X-ray studies are done to visualize the lymphatic system.

Preprocedure Care. Tell the client that the test takes several hours on the first day, and that follow-up x-ray studies will be performed the next day. The dye itself is excreted very slowly, taking months to more than a year for it to be completely excreted. The dye is excreted through both the urine and respiratory system. Food and fluids are not restricted prior to the test.

Postprocedure Care. Monitor the extremities for changes in pulse or sensation. Possible adverse reactions associated with the test include fever, allergic reaction to the dye, infection at the incision site, and possible pulmonary oil embolism. The client should monitor the site of the incision closely for infection. Tell the client that the urine will have a bluish discoloration for a while after the test and the tops of the feet may remain blue for months. Also tell the client to report any fever, signs of redness or swelling at the incision, or respiratory distress to the physician. Warm compresses can be applied to the site if there is discomfort.

Tests for Allergies and Autoimmune Disorders

Skin Testing

Procedure. In addition to blood tests, skin testing confirms sensitivity to a specific allergen. These tests involve placing a known antigen on or directly below the skin (intradermal) to check for the presence of antibodies. The antigen is applied using one of three methods: (1) scratch test, (2) patch test, or (3) intradermal test. In the first test (also known as a tine or prick test), the allergen is applied to a superficial scratch that cuts the outer layer of skin. For a patch test, the antigen is applied directly to the skin, and then covered with a gauze dressing. Intradermal testing involves injecting a small amount of the antigen into the intradermal layer of the skin. Intradermal testing is the most accurate method, but carries a higher risk of severe allergic reactions.

Often, nurses administer skin tests and interpret test results. To interpret results, observe for the following reactions. An immediate reaction (i.e., appearing within 10–20 minutes after injection), marked by erythema and wheal formation, denotes a positive reaction. Positive reactions indicate an antibody response to previous exposure to this antigen, and suggest the client is allergic to the substance causing the reaction (see Chapter 27, Fig. 27–1). Negative reactions may be inconclusive, indicating the need for further assessment. Negative results may indicate that (1) antibodies have not formed to this antigen, (2) the antigen was deposited too deeply into the skin (e.g., subcutaneously), or (3) the client is immunosuppressed as a result of disease or therapy (e.g., chemotherapy, steroids, radiation therapy).

Preprocedure Care. There is no specific preprocedure care for the client other than a thorough history.

Postprocedure Care. Problems arising from skin testing range from minor itching to anaphylaxis. Itching and discomfort at the injection site, for example, are common and are relieved by the application of cool compresses and topical steroids. Ulceration of the injection site is best treated by keeping the area clean and dry. Anaphylactic shock is a rare but potentially lethal complication of skin testing. A client with a history of an anaphylactic reaction to a substance should never be skin-tested for an allergy to that substance. This is especially true of allergens such as penicillin, which can produce lethal anaphylaxis in susceptible persons. Anaphylaxis is treated with emergency oxygen administration, epinephrine administered subcutaneously, intravenous aminophylline, and intravenous antihistamines, as necessary.

Food Allergy Testing

Food allergies are tested by skin testing, or by either the challenge or elimination diet. In the challenge diet, the suspect food(s) is given to the client in progressively larger doses until a reaction is evoked. Manifestations of a reaction range from the typical erythema, itching, and rash to vomiting or diarrhea. Manifestations such as fatigue, depression, or restlessness are not conclusive.

In the elimination diet, foods are eliminated from the diet one by one until the manifestations are relieved. This may indicate allergies to food additives or to the food(s) itself.

Conclusions

The immune system is extremely complex. Understanding the structure, function, and assessment of the immune system helps the nurse provide more consistent and appropriate care for the client with inflammatory, infectious, or immune disorders.

Bibliography

1. Araki, S., et al. (1993). Decrease of CD4-positive T lymphocytes in workers exposed to benzidine and beta-naphthylamine. *Archives of Environmental Health, 48*(4), 205–208.
2. Bancroft, B. (1994). Immunology simplified. *Seminars in Perioperative Nursing, 3*(2), 70–78.
3. Bates, B. (1991). *A guide to physical examination* (5th ed.). Philadelphia: J. B. Lippincott.
4. Beeson, P. B. (1994). Age and sex associations of 40 autoimmune diseases. *American Journal of Medicine, 96*(5), 457–462.
5. Bennett, J. C., & Plum, F. (Eds.). (1996). *Cecil textbook of medicine* (20th ed.). Philadelphia: W. B. Saunders.
6. Blaylock, B. (1993). The aging immune system and common infections in elderly patients. *Journal of ET Nursing, 20*(2), 63–67.
7. Bower, A., & Thompson, J. (1992). *Clinical manual of health assessment* (3rd ed.). St. Louis: Mosby–Year Book.

8. Chang, B. L., Vredevoe, D., & Hirsch M. (1995). Allergy as a risk factor for nursing care problems in the elderly cancer patient. *Cancer Nursing, 18*(2), 83–88.
9. Chernecky, C. C., Krech, R. L., & Berger, B. J. (1993). *Laboratory tests and diagnostic procedures*. Philadelphia: W. B. Saunders.
10. Christiansen, J. L., & Grzbouski, J. M. (1993). *Biology of aging*. St. Louis: Mosby–Year Book.
11. Colosio, C., et al. (1993). Toxicological and immune findings in workers exposed to pentachlorophenol (PCP). *Archives of Environmental Health, 48*(2), 81–88.
12. Colvin, R. B., Bhan, A. K., & McCluskey, R. T. (Eds.). (1995). *Diagnostic immunopathology*. New York: Raven Press.
13. Corbett, J. (1991). *Laboratory tests and diagnostic procedures with nursing diagnoses* (3rd ed.). Norwalk, CT: Appleton & Lange.
14. Cotran, R. S., Kumar, V., & Robbins, S. L. (1994). *Robbins pathologic basis of disease* (5th ed.). Philadelphia: W. B. Saunders.
15. Ershler, W. B. (1993). The influence of an aging immune system on cancer incidence and progression. *Journal of Gerontology, 48*(1), B3–7.
16. Fuller, J., & Schaller-Ayers, J. (1994). *Health assessment: A nursing approach* (2nd ed.). Philadelphia: J. B. Lippincott.
17. Golde, D. W. (1991). The stem cell. *Scientific American, 261*, 86–93.
18. Grammer, L. C., et al. (1993). Evaluation of a worker with possible formaldehyde-induced asthma. *Journal of Allergy and Clinical Immunology, 92*(1, Pt. 1), 29–33.
19. Gurevich, I. (1985). The competent internal immune system. *Nursing Clinics of North America, 20*, 151–161.
20. Guyton, A. C. (1992). *Human physiology and mechanisms of disease* (5th ed.). Philadelphia: W. B. Saunders.
21. Guyton, A. C., & Hall, J. E. (1996). *Textbook of medical physiology* (9th ed.). Philadelphia: W. B. Saunders.
22. Hyde, R. M. (1995). *Immunology* (3rd ed). Baltimore: Williams & Wilkins.
23. Jarvis, C. (1996). *Physical examination and health assessment* (2nd ed.). Philadelphia: W. B. Saunders.
24. Kee, J. L. (1995). *Laboratory and diagnostic tests with nursing implications* (4th ed.). Norwalk, CT: Appleton & Lange.
25. Kenny, R. A. (1992). *Physiology of aging: A synopsis*. St. Louis: Mosby–Year Book.
26. Klein, D. M., & Witek-Janusek, L. (1992). Advances in immunotherapy for sepsis. *Dimensions in Critical Care Nursing, 11*, 75–89.
27. Klein, J. (1990). *Immunology*. Boston: Blackwell Scientific.
28. McCance, K., & Huether, S. (1990). *Pathophysiology*. St. Louis: Mosby–Year Book.
29. Meliska, C. J., et al. (1995). Immune function in cigarette smokers who quit smoking for 31 days. *Journal of Allergy and Clinical Immunology, 95*(4), 901–910.
30. Porth, C. M. (1994). *Pathophysiologic concepts of altered health states* (4th ed.). Philadelphia: J. B. Lippincott.
31. Powers, D. C., Morley, J. E., & Coe, R. M. (Eds.). (1994). *Aging, immunity, and infection*. New York: Springer-Verlag.
32. Price, S., & Wilson, L. (1992). *Pathophysiology* (4th ed.). St. Louis: Mosby–Year Book.
33. Rennie, J. (1990). The body against itself. *Scientific American, 260*, 106–115.
34. Roit, I. M., Brostoff, J., & Male, D. K. (1996). *Immunology* (4th ed). St. Louis: Mosby–Year Book.
35. Seeley, R., Stephens, T., & Tate, P. (1995). *Anatomy and physiology* (3rd ed.). St. Louis: Mosby–Year Book.
36. Sheehan, C. (1990). *Clinical immunology*. Philadelphia: J. B. Lippincott.
37. Shils, M. E., Olson, H. A., Shike, M. (Eds.). (1993). *Modern nutrition in health and disease* (8th ed.). Philadelphia: Lea & Febiger.
38. Strauss, J. F. III. (1991). Steroid hormones: Synthesis, metabolism, and action in health and disease. *Endocrinology and Metabolism Clinics of North America, 20*(4), 681–924.
39. Thibodeau, G. A., & Patton, K. T. (1992). *Anatomy and physiology* (2nd ed.). St. Louis: Mosby–Year Book.
40. Thibodeau, G. A., & Patton, K. T. (1992). *The human body in health and disease*. St. Louis: Mosby–Year Book.
41. Thrasher, J. D., Madison, R., & Broughton, A. (1993). Immunologic abnormalities in humans exposed to chlorpyrifos: Preliminary observations. *Archives of Environmental Health, 48*(2), 89–93.
42. Toto, K. H. (1994). Endocrine physiology: A comprehensive review. *Critical Care Nursing Clinics of North America, 6*(4), 637–659.
43. Tribett, D. (1989). Immune system function. Implications for critical care nursing practice. *Critical Care Nursing Clinics of America, 1*, 725–740.
44. Virella, G., Goust, J. M., & Fudenberg, H. H. (Eds.) (1990). *Medical Immunology*. New York: Marcel Dekker.
45. Watson, J., & Jaffee, M. S. (1995). *Nurse's manual of laboratory and diagnostic tests* (2nd ed.). Philadelphia: F. A. Davis.
46. Workman, M. L. (1995). Essential concepts of inflammation and immunity. *Critical Care Nursing Clinics of North America, 7*(4), 601–615.

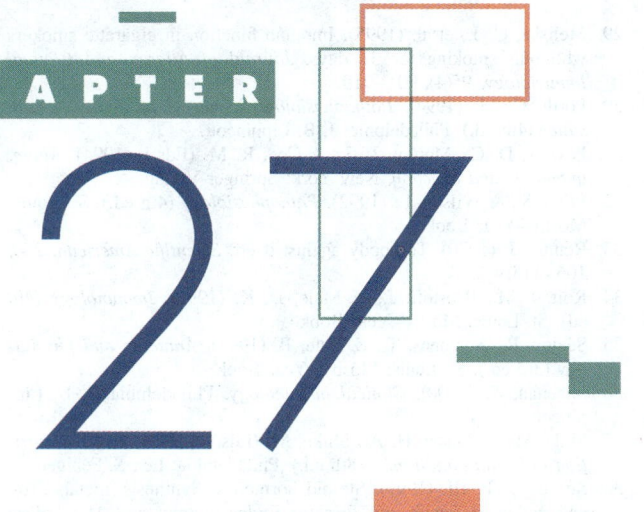

CHAPTER 27

Nursing Care of Clients with Altered Immune Systems

Peter J. Ungvarski
Esther Matassarin-Jacobs

The immune system controls the body's response to invading foreign substances. A functioning immune system protects the body from a wide variety of pathogens. On the other hand, an immune system that is malfunctioning predisposes the client to the development of a wide variety of disorders ranging from severe infection to autoimmune disease. Chapter 25 describes the normally functioning immune system; this chapter looks at alterations in the immune system and how these changes affect the individual.

Human Immunodeficiency Virus Infection

Etiology and Risk Factors

■ Etiology

The etiologic agent associated with AIDS was first isolated by French scientists in 1983 and originally named the *lymphadenopathy-associated virus* (LAV). One year later, an American scientist claimed the discovery of the etiologic agent and named it the *human T-cell lymphotropic virus type III* (HTLV-III). Although it was discovered that both scientists had identified the same virus, much confusion and arguing took place. In 1986, the International Society on the Taxonomy of Viruses renamed the virus, calling it the human immunodeficiency virus. In that same year, much to the surprise of everyone, a second and distinctly different strain of the virus was discovered in Africa. Therefore, since 1986, the scientific names to distinguish between the two viruses are HIV-1 and HIV-2. This was a major discovery that alarmed everyone, because it was the first clue that the HIV virus had the ability to change its appearance, or mutate, very rapidly. The capability of HIV to mutate

rapidly is often referred to as *genetic promiscuity,* and it has become the hallmark of this virus, creating a monumental challenge for scientists and researchers alike. HIV-1 is distributed worldwide, but it is most prevalent in Europe and the United States. HIV-2 is predominantly found in west African nations, but it has been isolated in other parts of the world. The majority of infections worldwide are due to HIV-1.

By 1996, scientists had discovered that HIV-1 had also mutated several times. HIV-1 has two major subtypes or clades, and they have been designated HIV-1 group "M" viruses or HIV-1 group "O" virus. Group "M" viruses have been assigned to ten genetic subtypes and are designated HIV-1, group "M," subtype A, B, C, D, E, F, G, H, I, and J, according to the phylogenetic analysis of their genes. The distribution of the subtypes varies worldwide. For example, whereas subtype B predominates in North America and Europe, subtypes A, B, C, and E have been identified in India. There is concern that subtypes other than B will be found in the United States, because U.S. servicemen assigned to overseas duty who have become infected with HIV-1 have been found to be infected with subtypes A, D, and E. Although all of this detail may sound confusing, it is important to mention it to illustrate the rapidly changing nature of this virus. It poses a considerable challenge to researchers investigating new drugs to treat the disease or developing vaccines to prevent the disease, as their work is usually limited to one specific subtype of HIV-1. Vaccine trials have demonstrated that a vaccine for one subtype may not work for other subtypes.

The other major strain of HIV-1 is classified as HIV-1 group "O". The designation "O" was deliberate, because this mutation was an outlier and was very different from the others in that it cannot be detected with the routine HIV antibody tests that are used in the United States. Group "O" was primarily identified in west and central Africa, with a few isolated cases identified through special tests in France and the United States. The CDC is currently working with the manufacturers of HIV-1 anti-

---

This chapter incorporates material written for the fourth edition by Carol Bova.

body test kits to ensure that the testing methods are reconfigured to detect HIV-1 group "O" as well as group "M."

■ Risk Factors

The modes of transmission have remained constant throughout the course of the HIV pandemic. HIV is spread through certain sexual practices, exposure to blood, and/or through perinatal transmission. The patterns in the spread of HIV have changed considerably during the first 15 years of the epidemic in the United States. Comparing the early 1980s with the early 1990s, significant increases have been noted in IV drug users, women, and heterosexuals. Overall, the number of new HIV infections among men who have sex with men has decreased considerably. This decline, however, has been limited to white men, and the number of new cases among racial and ethnic minority men who have sex with men continues to increase (see Diversity in Healthcare). In young adults (ages 19 to 29 years), the number of new infections has been increasing, especially in the South and Midwest. Death due to HIV in youths aged 15 to 24 years increased by 38% between 1987 and 1993.

Perhaps the most overlooked population in the HIV epidemic is adults older than 50 years. In 1996, 11% of the nation's total number of reported AIDS cases occurred in this age group. Women older than 50 years are primarily acquiring HIV infection through heterosexual contact. Although the largest cumulative total number of AIDS and HIV infections have been reported in large cities such as New York and San Francisco, there has been a shift of newly diagnosed cases to small cities and rural areas, especially in the South and Midwest.

The principal mode of transmission of HIV throughout the world has been through sexual exposure. With the exception of Australia, Europe, and the United States, most of the transmission of HIV has been through heterosexual activities. One important lesson that healthcare professionals have learned from the HIV epidemic is that sexual practices, not sexual preferences, place people at risk for sexually transmitted diseases. Gay men who do not engage in unprotected anopenile sex or expose themselves to another person's body fluids are no more at risk for acquiring HIV infection than anyone else. Likewise any couple, heterosexual or homosexual, in a long-term monogamous relationship are not at risk for acquiring HIV. The problem of unsafe sexual encounters outside of these relationships does, however, pose an actual risk.

Sexual practices that are absolutely safe include autosexual activities (e.g., masturbation), mutually monogamous relationships between noninfected partners, and, of course, abstinence. Very safe sexual practices include non-insertive sexual practices. Insertive practices with a condom are considered probably safe as long as the condom doesn't break and no contact with body fluids occurs. Everything else is considered risky. Other co-factors, such as engaging in sexual activities while under the influence of drugs or alcohol, having multiple sex partners, and the presence of sores in the genital area, have been identified as increasing the risk of acquiring HIV. Although the number of reported cases is small, oral sexual practices, whether performed on a man or a woman, have been implicated as a possible transmission activity.

Transmission by exposure to blood is a very broad category that encompasses numerous possible routes. The most obvious is through the administration of blood or blood products, transplantation of donated tissue or organs, or implantation of semen contaminated with HIV. Prevention of HIV infection by any of these means is possible by donor exclusion (excluding persons from high-risk groups), routine serologic testing of donated tissues or fluids for HIV antibodies, and heat inactivation of certain blood products, such as factor VIII concentrate. Other means of preventing HIV infection related to blood products are autologous blood programs and limiting the administration of any blood product to situations in which it is absolutely necessary.

Injection drug use accounts for the largest number of HIV infections due to exposure to contaminated blood. The only absolutely safe injection drug use behavior is not to inject. Very safe practice for injecting drug use is only using sterilized injection paraphernalia and never sharing needles and syringes. Probably safe practice is to clean injection paraphernalia with full-strength bleach before injecting, although disposable needles and syringes are difficult to clean. Anything else is considered risky. Other co-factors that increase the chances of acquiring HIV by drug injection include the seroprevalence of HIV in the geographic location of the drug user, the social setting of injection drug use (e.g., "shooting galleries," where injection paraphernalia is shared), and the frequency of the injections.

Needle exchange programs (NEPs) provide sterile injection equipment, latex condoms, counseling, and access to social and health programs, including drug detoxification treatment. Numerous studies have shown that needle exchange programs not only decrease the spread of HIV as well as hepatitis B and C, but do not increase or promote injection drug use. Despite the proven success of this approach to disease prevention, legislators both at the state and federal level have been reluctant to appropriate funds to support this model of care. In the United States, because of existing attitudes to IV drug use, NEPs operate as either legal, illegal-but-tolerated, or illegal/underground programs. In Europe, where the approach to preventing disease has received more favorable support, governments providing national healthcare services for their citizens have found that NEPs not only have reduced the incidence of disease, but also have significantly reduced healthcare spending for diseases associated with intravenous drug injecting.

Occupational exposure to blood is not only a potential problem for healthcare workers (HCWs), but for members of other occupations, such as police and corrections officers. The state of Connecticut legalized the sale of sterile needles and syringes in certain drug stores and found that they not only reduced the incidence of needle sharing in IV drug users, they also resulted in a significant decrease in the number of occupationally acquired needle-stick injuries in police officers.

Concern over HCWs becoming infected with HIV (patient-to-HCW) is an ongoing concern of workers, employ-

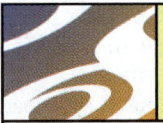

DIVERSITY IN HEALTHCARE

HIV and AIDS in Minority Populations

Although acquired immunodeficiency syndrome (AIDS) has been called an "equal opportunity disease," the human immunodeficiency virus (HIV) that causes the disease is more prevalent among blacks and Hispanics than other groups. AIDS incidence rates are six times higher among blacks than whites, and three times higher among Hispanics than whites. Men who have sex with men continue to be the population most affected by AIDS, but there is growing concern over heterosexual transmission.[1]

As indicated in the table, blacks account for one third of the AIDS cases in adults (age 13+ years) whereas 17% of cases occur in Hispanics. For the first time, in 1994, blacks and Hispanics combined accounted for the majority of all AIDS cases (53% when adults and children are considered). Seventy-five percent of all women with AIDS are black or Hispanic. Seventy-nine percent of the 6611 children (<13 years) diagnosed with AIDS are black or Hispanic. The AIDS epidemic in communities of color is cause for alarm because the number of minorities afflicted with HIV and AIDS is projected to continue its steady growth.[1,2]

Reported Cases of AIDS by Ethnicity in Adults (Age 13+ Years): June 30, 1994–June 30, 1995

	Men (%)	Women (%)	Total (%)
White	211,856 (52)	15,570 (24)	227,426 (48)
Black	121,017 (30)	35,372 (55)	156,389 (33)
Hispanic	68,051 (17)	13,293 (20)	81,344 (17)
Asian, Pacific Islander	2902 (0.7)	325 (0.5)	3227 (0.7)
Native American	1010 (0.2)	173 (0.3)	1183 (0.2)
Unknown ethnicity	626 (0.1)	89 (0.2)	715 (0.1)
Totals	405,462	64,822	470,284

From: Centers for Disease Control, National Center of Infectious Diseases, Division of HIV/AIDS. (1995). *HIV/AIDS surveillance information report. US HIV and AIDS cases reported through December 1994.* Atlanta: Author.

Sexual preferences and practices govern sexual behavior between and within racial groups. This premise is central to the epidemic spread of HIV and to the risks of contracting AIDS.[3] Given the absence of a cure, changes in individual behaviors provide the major weapon against the transmission of HIV. These behavioral changes should be based on knowledge of risky sexual practices, modes of HIV transmission, and the potential harm to self and others. Efforts to change sexual behavior, and thereby slow the spread of transmission of HIV, have been limited and often misdirected. Educational messages often lack detailed information about an individual's behavior, gender differences, and considerations of the social, cultural, and economic realities of people's lives. In addition to the information contained in this chapter, the following culture-specific considerations may be helpful in reducing the spread of HIV and AIDS.

Blacks

While only 14% of the young adults in this country are black, they constitute more than 30% of the AIDS cases in their age group.[2] It is projected that more than 1 million blacks will be affected with AIDS unless there are changes in their risk behavior patterns or there is major scientific breakthrough. Condom use by black males remains low despite educational efforts in schools and in the mass media. In the development of educational programs aimed at such culturally informed experiences as sexual behavior, ignoring the unique social and cultural experiences of the black population has frequently resulted in ineffective programs and has alienated some blacks.[3] Conversely, programs that incorporate culture tend to be successful. For example, the "Be Proud, Be Responsible" program was developed by an African-American husband-

and-wife team who understood the culture of black youths. The program consists of a 6-hour intervention for black males between the ages of 12 and 19. Follow-up 3 months after the program revealed that participants had sexual intercourse on fewer occasions and with fewer women. Those who had intercourse used condoms more consistently and a smaller percentage reported engaging in anal intercourse. Representatives from 20 states have attended a training session that will enable them to train others to deliver the curriculum.[4]

Most blacks with AIDS contracted the disease from intravenous (IV) drug use.[1] The complex interrelationships among addiction, poverty, absent or inadequate health insurance, poor nutrition, and other socioeconomic factors must be considered when addressing the difficult problem of AIDS in this population. Some black drug abusers may be afraid that legal authorities will be contacted when they seek healthcare. Mistrust of the police and other officials tends to be high, especially in low-income black neighborhoods. This mistrust and suspicion of authority figures may extend to nurses and other healthcare providers. Although needle exchange programs in many urban areas have been successful, their early history was marked by poor participation resulting from fear of arrest. Needle exchange programs for IV drug users continue to be controversial and reflect the diverse social, political, religious, and cultural views of society. Some blacks have expressed disbelief that the government could be interested in helping them. The history of discrimination against blacks in this country has fueled skepticism about current programs aimed at the prevention of HIV and AIDS.[5]

Black women account for 55% of all adult cases (age 13+ years) with AIDS, compared with 24% for their white counterparts. The reason for this discrepancy is blamed, in part, on the dynamics occurring in black women's relationships. Some experts believe that black women need to develop both the skills to communicate with their partners about sexual behaviors and the technical skills to prevent spread of the disease.[3]

Hispanics

For Hispanics with HIV and AIDS, cultural differences, migratory patterns, seasonal influences, and language barriers interfere with receiving adequate healthcare. Among Puerto Ricans, IV drug use is a common cause of infection. In Mexican-American and Cuban-American populations, heterosexual transmission is more common, but IV drug use is still a factor.[1, 2]

For many Hispanics, there is a cultural norm that discourages open discussion of sexual practices, even in the presence of immediate family members. Importance is placed on the patriarch whose sexual behaviors seldom are questioned because of his position in the family hierarchy. Women are expected to comply with the sexual requests of their husbands. Unfortunately, the patriarch frequently transmits HIV to his unsuspecting wife who in turn passes the disease to her children. A combination of machismo and guilt over marital infidelity may keep some Hispanic men from seeking early care for HIV. Until symptoms become severe enough to interfere with functioning, some Hispanic men may avoid seeking healthcare. By the time care is sought, transmission of the virus already has occurred.

For migrant workers, such as those who assist farmers with seasonal needs, access to healthcare is often difficult or impossible. Seasonal migration, long work days, and separation from family and social support networks create obstacles to healthcare-seeking behaviors. The location of health facilities, hours of operation, perceived lack of cultural respect by care providers, lack of transportation, and language barriers may prevent Hispanic migrant workers from receiving preventive education about HIV and AIDS. These factors also prevent them from receiving treatment after the diagnosis has been made.

Although Spanish-language materials about HIV and AIDS have been developed, nurses and other healthcare providers need to make them more readily available to Hispanic clients. The nurse must assess the client's ability to read and comprehend information in Spanish and in English. Contained in the list at the end of this diversity feature are sources of Spanish-language information about HIV and AIDS. Ideally, written and audiovisual materials should be accompanied by a verbal explanation from the healthcare provider, preferably in Spanish. It should be noted that the stress accompanying a diagnosis of HIV or AIDS may result in language regression. Clients whose English communication had been very good may find it easier to understand Spanish in times of stress, especially when terms concerning sexual behaviors and reproduction are used. As with other groups, the Hispanic client should be given the opportunity to ask questions in a private and confidential setting. If an interpreter is needed, he or she should be the same sex as the client to foster communication and avoid embarrassment.

Asians and Pacific Islanders

Although the incidence of HIV and AIDS is relatively low in the Asian and Pacific Islander population compared with other groups, AIDS case management and educational programs with preventive goals have been implemented. The San Francisco Asian AIDS Project, for example, targets limited-English-speaking Asians and Pacific Islanders. Through outreach and the distribution of educational materials, the project targets four groups: men who have sex with men, women working in massage parlors, youth in detention centers, and transgenders.[6]

In general, many people with Asian and Pacific Islander backgrounds consider it inappropriate to discuss openly subjects related to sexual behavior. Discussing sexual matters with strangers—a group that includes nurses and other members of the healthcare team—is inconsistent with their cultural values and practices. For these reasons, peer education has been particularly successful with the Asian and Pacific Islander population. This approach relies on friends talking with friends about the cause and transmission of HIV and AIDS, Peer education enables cultural issues to be explored frankly, in a language familiar to the client. The Asian AIDS Project primarily serves recent immigrants and provides opportunities for interaction between people who know how it feels to deal with AIDS, while also dealing with assimilation.

Many Asians and Pacific Islanders encounter barriers when they seek information and healthcare re-

Continued on following page

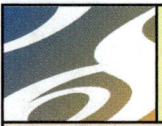

DIVERSITY IN HEALTHCARE *(Continued)*

HIV and AIDS in Minority Populations

lated to HIV and AIDS. Some feel self-conscious about their English-language skills and avoid situations in which there is no interpreter. It should be noted that there are dozens of different languages represented by the heterogeneous group labeled Asian and Pacific Islander. The nurse must identify the client's primary language and arrange for an interpreter who is fluent in it. If an interpreter is unavailable, explore whether there is a third language that is known by both client and interpreter. For example, many Vietnamese immigrants are fluent in French. The interpreter should be the same sex and approximate age as the client. In some Asian cultures, the use of an interpreter who is younger than the client is unacceptable. Age is believed to afford the client a certain level of status. When topics of such a personal nature as sexual behavior are discussed, it is expected that information will be conveyed by someone of the same sex who has the equivalent age-related status.

If no interpreter is used, nurses and other healthcare providers should be attentive to both verbal and nonverbal communication. Some Asians and Pacific Islanders speak softly as a sign of respect. Many find it disconcerting when nurses raise their voices and ask them to speak up. Chinese-American clients may be perplexed when nurses ask them to relate their chief complaint or reason for seeking healthcare. It is expected that the healthcare provider will provide answers, not ask questions. Some persons of Asian descent will avoid direct eye contact to avoid staring, behavior they perceive to be rude

and aggressive. The degree of acculturation will determine the extent to which cross-cultural communication issues emerge in the nurse-client interaction. More recent immigrants are likely to have more traditional beliefs and practices. The plan of care for clients from Asian and Pacific Islander backgrounds who have HIV or AIDS should be developed only after a comprehensive cultural assessment has been completed. Whenever possible, the nurse and client should develop mutual goals. The plan of care should include all parties whom the client has identified as significant. This may include a domestic partner of the same sex, folk or indigenous healers, and extended family members.

Native Americans

With more than 500 Native American tribes in the United States, cultural attitudes, beliefs, and practices about sexual behavior and HIV and AIDS vary widely. Many tribes, however, have ceremonies in which the skin is broken with a razor blade. The purpose of breaking the flesh may be to obtain a skin offering, symbolically show one's stoicism in the face of pain, or convey other cultural meanings. Sometimes the same instrument slices the skin of more than one person, a dangerous practice that allows HIV to be transmitted through the exchange of body fluids.[7]

The appropriate response to such risky behavior is not to criticize tribal ceremonies, but rather to support AIDS prevention activities based on Native-American practices. The In-

dian Health Service works with tribal health boards to distribute, at no cost, disposable razors and scalpels to discourage reuse. In this way, Native Americans can preserve and maintain their cultural traditions while promoting health and preventing disease.[7]

The Minneapolis Indian Health Board has implemented a successful AIDS education program by including the traditional value of self-realization. The four parts of self—mind, body, spirit, and feeling—must be an integral component of the HIV-AIDS program for Native Americans. In addition to discussing how to protect the mind and body from disease, educational programs generally include loss issues specific to native communities such as how loss of land and loss of culture affect attitudes about health.[7]

The key to successful AIDS prevention on reservations lies in training local tribal health educators. Under the auspices of the Native Americans Against AIDS Project, local tribal educators in North Dakota have been prepared to lead training sessions, provide advice for fellow tribe members, and make appropriate healthcare referrals. Federal and private foundation funds have been provided for several demonstration projects aimed at implementing culturally appropriate Indian AIDS prevention programs.[7]

The National Native American AIDS Prevention Center (NNAAPC) is an organization established by and for American Indians, Alaskan Natives, and Native Hawaiians. NNAAPC operates a hotline and clearinghouse, maintains statistics compiled by the Centers for Disease Control and Prevention, and con-

ers, and public health officials. In the United States, by 1996, the cumulative total of number of HCWs with documented occupationally acquired HIV/AIDS was 49, and the number with possible (less clear evidence) transmission was 102. Although the majority of occupationally HIV-infected HCWs acquired disease after percutaneous exposure, other modes of transmission included mucocu-

taneous exposure and direct exposure to HIV in the laboratory setting. The actual average risk to an HCW for exposure is extremely low (0.3%). The risk, when an exposure occurs, is increased in situations in which a deep injury is sustained by the HCW, there is visible blood on the device causing the injury, the device involved was previously placed in an artery or vein of the

ducts training for AIDS trainers. Traditional healing treatments for HIV and AIDS are among the topics explored in training sessions. The center publishes and distributes several publications for patients and health and human services workers. For more information about NNAAPC, call (800) 283-2437 or (510) 444-2051.

For further information about HIV and AIDS and members of minority groups, contact the following organizations:

Office of Minority Health
P.O. Box 37337
Washington, DC 20013–7337
(800) 444–6472

CDC National AIDS Clearinghouse
P.O. Box 6003, Rockville, MD
  20849–6003
Publications: (800) 458–5231
National AIDS Hotline: (800) 342–2437
Spanish Hotline: (800) 344–7432

National Council of La Raza AIDS
  Center
111 19th St. N.W., Suite 1000
Washington, DC 20036
(202) 785–1670

National Native American AIDS Prevention Center
2100 Lake Shore Ave., Suite A
Oakland, CA 94606
(800) 283–AIDS

National AIDS Office
Indian Health Service
U.S. Public Health Service
Rockville, MD 20857
(505) 837–4116

American Indian Health Care Association
1550 Larimer St., Suite 225
Denver, CO
(303) 607–1048

Gay and Lesbian Medical Association
273 Church St.
San Francisco, CA 94114
(415) 255–4547

Minority AIDS Project
5149 W. Jefferson Blvd.
Los Angeles, CA 90016
(213) 936–4949

Office on HIV/AIDS Policy
Hubert H. Humphrey Building,
  Room 733E
Independence Avenue S.W.
Washington, DC 20201
(202) 690–6248

People of Color Against AIDS Network
4900 Rainer Ave. S.
Seattle, WA 98118
(206) 721–0852

National Black Women's Health
  Project
1237 Abernathy Blvd. S.W.
Atlanta, GA 30310
(404) 758–9590

National Association of People with
  AIDS
1413 K St. N.W., 7th Floor
Washington, DC 20005
(202) 898–0414

AIDS Action Council
1875 Connecticut Ave. N.W., Suite
  700
Washington, DC 20009
(202) 986–1300

[1] Fleming, P. S. (1995). Minority health perspective: No time to retreat. In *Closing the gap* (p.3). Office of Minority Health, Public Health Service, U.S. Department of Health and Human Services.

[2] Centers for Disease Control, National Center on Infectious Diseases, Division of HIV/AIDS. (1995). *HIV/AIDS surveillance information report.* Atlanta: Author.

[3] Odulana, J. A., et al. (1995). Knowledge and beliefs of HIV modes of transmission among African-American and Caucasian college students. *Journal of Multicultural Nursing and Health, 2*(1), 10–15.

[4] Casetta, R. A. (1993). The new faces of the epidemic. *American Nurse, 16* (March).

[5] Office of Minority Health. (1995). Be proud! Be responsible! Strategies to empower youth to reduce their risk for AIDS. In *Closing the gap* (p. 8). Office of Minority Health, Public Health Service, U. S. Department of Health and Human Services.

[6] Office of Minority Health. (1995). Asian AIDS project hits the streets. In *Closing the gap* (p. 7). Office of Minority Health, Public Health Service, U. S. Department of Health and Human Services.

[7] Office of Minority Health. (1995). Recognizing the link between Indian culture and health. In *Closing the gap* (p. 4). Office of Minority Health, Public Health Service, U. S. Department of Health and Human Services.

patient, and the source patient has recently died of AIDS (since it is known that at end-stage disease the concentrations of HIV in the blood are very high). Accidental needle-stick exposure poses the greatest hazard to HCWs. All HCWs are taught and encouraged to follow universal precautions (Box 27–1) when handling blood and body fluids and performing procedures that may potentially expose them to blood and body fluids. When any incident that reflects potential exposure to bloodborne pathogens occurs, the HCW should seek medical treatment immediately. The U.S. Public Health Service has issued guidelines for evaluating and treating exposures to HIV, and in

Box 27–1. Universal Precautions

Universal precautions are intended to prevent parenteral, mucous membrane, and nonintact skin exposures of healthcare workers to bloodborne pathogens. Universal precautions apply to blood and to other body fluids containing visible blood, semen, vaginal secretions, cerebrospinal fluid, synovial fluid, pleural fluid, peritoneal fluid, pericardial fluid, and amniotic fluid. Most institutions now include feces, urine, vomitus, and sputum even if blood is not visible. Universal precautions do not apply to feces, nasal secretions, sputum, sweat, tears, urine, and vomitus unless they contain visible blood.

Barrier Guidelines

1. Disposable gloves (vinyl, latex) should be worn when in contact, or when there is potential for contact, with blood, body fluids, or other fluids that may contain human immunodeficiency virus (HIV). Gloves should be removed after each client contact. Rubber gloves can be used for cleaning equipment.
2. Hands should be washed between clients, after any exposure, and after removal of gloves.
3. Protective eyewear, face shields, or masks, or a combination of these, should be worn during procedures that may aerosolize blood.
4. Impervious gowns should be worn when there is potential for exposure to large quantities of blood, as in the labor and delivery area or emergency room.

Needle Precautions

1. Needles should never be recapped after use; keep in mind that most needle-sticks are the result of missed needle recapping.
2. Needles should not be cut, broken, or bent after use; this may release aerosolized blood from the needle shaft.
3. Needles should not be left lying around.
4. Needles should not be disposed of in ordinary receptacles; instead, use appropriately labeled, impermeable needle containers.

the case of high-risk exposures, they have recommended that combination antiretroviral therapy be given for at least 4 weeks for post-exposure prophylaxis.

There has only been one documented case of HIV transmission from an HIV-infected HCW to clients. Six clients of a Florida dentist reportedly became HIV-infected as a result of dental care. The circumstances surrounding this case all implied that adequate precautions for disinfection and sterilization of instruments were not followed in the dental office.

Perinatal HIV exposure can occur in utero during pregnancy, during the birth process in vaginal deliveries, and postpartum through breast feeding. Of all babies born to HIV-infected women, approximately 25% are actually infected. The risk of mother-to-child (vertical) transmission is increased if the amount of viral activity is high and the CD4+ titer is low, which is usually the case in later stages of HIV disease, when the woman is diagnosed with AIDS. Therefore, clinical trials were conducted to

see if giving pregnant women antiretroviral therapy for HIV could reverse this (control the HIV activity and raise the CD4+ cell count). The results of clinical trials, in which zidovudine was given to pregnant women, demonstrated that there was a 68% reduction in the incidence of vertical transmission. The CDC has published guidelines for the use of zidovudine therapy for pregnant women and their newborn infants. There has been no increase in birth defects noted in babies born to mothers who have taken zidovudine during pregnancy.

The only absolute method of preventing perinatal exposure is to avoid pregnancy. All HCWs should discuss HIV infection as part of routine prenatal care with all patients, because many mothers may be unaware that they are infected with HIV. For HIV-infected women who do carry to term, they should be advised against breast-feeding, as this has been implicated as a mode of HIV transmission.

Pathophysiology

HIV-1 is a member of the lentivirus subfamily of human retroviruses. Diseases caused by lentiviruses are characterized by an insidious onset with progressive involvement of the central nervous system and may result in disorders of the immune system. HIV-1 is one of five viruses in the lentivirus family. The others are HIV-2 and human T-lymphotropic viruses types I, II, and IV. A retrovirus belongs to the family Retroviridae and possesses RNA-dependent DNA polymerase (reverse transcriptase). HIV infects T helper cells (T4 lymphocytes), macrophages, B cells, and certain cells in the brain and central nervous system. T helper cells are infected more readily than are other cells. This depletion of the T helper cell occurs in the following steps:

1. Once inside the host, HIV attaches to the target cell membrane by way of its receptor molecule, CD4+.
2. The virus is uncoated, and the RNA enters the cell.
3. The enzyme known as reverse transcriptase is released; thereby, the viral RNA is transcribed into DNA.
4. This newly created DNA moves into the nucleus and the DNA of the cell.
5. A provirus is created when the viral DNA integrates itself into the cellular DNA or genome of the cell.
6. Once the provirus is in place, its genetic material is no longer pure cell but part virus.
7. The cell may function abnormally.
8. The host cell dies, and viral budding occurs; the new virus proceeds to infect other cells.

The main target for HIV is the T4 helper cell. However the "glue" to which HIV is attracted is the CD4+ molecule, which acts as the receptor for HIV on the T4 helper cell. Despite the fact that the CD4+ molecule is also found on other cells, such as macrophages, monocytes, and glial cells, clinicians usually refer to T4 helper cells as CD4+ cells. Therefore, when reading articles about HIV disease, research papers, or laboratory reports, the labels *T4, T4 helper, CD4+,* and *CD4+ T-helper cell* are used synonymously.

The CD4+ T-helper cells are the regulating cells within the immune system; they interact with monocytes, macrophages, cytotoxic T cells, natural killer cells, and B cells. Using the analogy of an orchestra and a conductor, the T cells are the conductor within the immune system, directing all of the activity (music) produced by the other immune cells (orchestra). Therefore, it becomes quite apparent that the loss of the CD4+ T-helper cells results in total chaos, and the body loses its basic ability to maintain a constant state of health. With significant losses of these regulatory cells, not only does the HIV-infected person become readily susceptible to acquiring infection, but pathogens that have previously caused disease in the individual may reactivate and also cause infection. A prime example is the varicella zoster virus, which may have caused chickenpox in the HIV-infected person as a child and may reactivate when the CD4+ T-cell count drops to low levels, causing shingles.

The average laboratory range for the CD4+ T cell count is approximately 500 to 1600/mm³. It should be noted that a gradual physiologic decline occurs in these cells over the life of an individual. In fact, CD4+ T cell counts in newborns are almost double those of an adult. In the adult, CD4+ cell counts below 200/mm³ are considered seriously low, and infection is likely to develop. Other laboratory changes that indicate immune dysfunction include (1) an overall decline in the total numbers of white blood cells (WBCs), (2) decreases in both the total number and percentage of lymphocytes, (3) significant changes in the CD4+/CD8+ ratio, (4) decreased CD4+ T cell test findings, (5) absent or decreased skin test reactivity (anergy), and (6) increased immunoglobulin levels.

The cause of all this damage to the immune system is the extensive amount of HIV activity that takes place in the body of an infected person from the time of infection. HIV replicates at a very rapid rate. In fact, it has been estimated that HIV produces 10 million new virions daily. Although a person with HIV may be asymptomatic, and the CD4+ cell counts may be within the normal range, insidious destruction of the immune system is taking place.

The course of HIV illness often varies from individual to individual. Several co-factors that may accelerate the immunodeficiency seen in HIV disease include malnutrition, continued use of injection drugs and recreational substances, allergic conditions, genetics, age, pregnancy, gender, and presence of infections. In some instances, research has clearly implicated some of these co-factors as contributing to a more rapid decline in CD4+ cell levels; for some, the evidence is less clear. Factors that have been linked to increased mortality and morbidity include lower socioeconomic status, lack of access to adequate care, receiving care in a hospital with limited AIDS experience, and being treated by a physician with little experience in AIDS care. Overall, comparing the 1980s with the 1990s, survival with the diagnosis of AIDS has doubled. Most authors attribute increases in survival to the introduction of prophylactic drugs to prevent opportunistic infections when the CD4+ count falls below 200/mm³ and to the introduction of antiretroviral agents to treat HIV disease.

To illustrate further the differences observed in HIV-infected individuals, scientists have reported that approximately 5% of all HIV-infected individuals are perfectly healthy after many years and show no signs of disease progression. These persons, referred to as *long-term non-progressors* (LTNPs), possess the following features: (1) they have had documented evidence of HIV infection for more than 10 years, (2) they are asymptomatic, (3) they have both normal and stable immune profiles, and (4) they have never required any treatment for HIV disease. LTNPs appear to produce vigorous amounts of serum antibodies, which keep the HIV activity at extremely low levels, thus preventing immune system damage. LTNPs should not be confused with long-term survivors who are defined as individuals who have survived for more than 8 years after an AIDS diagnosis, show all clinical and laboratory signs of disease, and continuously require treatment.

Although the principal target of HIV is the immune system, considerable damage occurs to other parts of the body as a direct result of HIV in body tissues. A few examples of clinical conditions that can be directly attributed to HIV include (1) cranial and peripheral neuropathies, (2) uveitis, (3) cardiomyopathy, (4) pneumonitis, (5) malabsorption in the small intestines, (6) nephritis, (7) cervicitis, (8) arthritis, (9) psoriasis, and (10) gonad dysfunction and adrenalitis. Additionally, the hematologic system damage, due in part to impaired blood cell production, often results in anemia, granulocytopenia, and thrombocytopenia, which are common abnormalities seen in patients throughout the course of disease.

In addition to managing HIV disease, clinicians will also be challenged with addressing those illnesses that existed before the individual acquired HIV infection. These will not only require continuing treatment and attention, but also may complicate the course of illness. Frequently encountered preexisting and co-morbid conditions seen in HIV-infected clients include, but are not limited to, alcoholism, drug dependence, liver and/or kidney disease, psychiatric illness, and a history of sexually transmitted diseases.

Clinical Manifestations and Diagnostic Findings

As knowledge has evolved regarding the HIV disease process, the CDC has developed and revised numerous classification systems. The most recent classification system for HIV disease in adults and adolescents is based on two monitoring parameters used to follow a patient: laboratory data (CD4+ cell counts) and the clinical presentation of an individual (the signs and symptoms or diseases that develop) (Box 27–2). The period in which a person gets infected has a distinct name and is referred to as *primary infection.* If HIV is detected in a client at the time of initial infection, the client is considered to be in category "A."

Primary infection is the initial period after an individual has acquired HIV, usually through a high-risk behavior such as certain sexual practices or IV drug use. The length of time that primary infection lasts varies from

Box 27–2. Human Immunodeficiency Virus (HIV) Classification System for Adolescents and Adults

The Centers for Disease Control and Prevention (CDC) classification system for HIV-infected adolescents and adults emphasizes the importance of CD4+ lymphocyte testing in clinical management. The classification system is divided into laboratory and clinical categories as follows.

Laboratory Categories

Category 1: Greater than or equal to 500 CD4+ cells
Category 2: 200 to 499 CD4+ cells
Category 3: Less than 200 CD4+ cells

Clinical Categories

Category A: One or more of the following conditions occurring in an adolescent or adult with documented HIV infection. Conditions listed in categories B and C must not have occurred.

- Asymptomatic HIV infection
- Persistent generalized lymphadenopathy (PGL)
- Acute (primary) HIV infection with accompanying illness or history of acute HIV infection

Category B: Symptomatic conditions occurring in an HIV-infected adolescent or adult that are not included among conditions listed in clinical category C and that meet at least one of the following criteria:

- The conditions are attributed to HIV infection or are indicative of a defect in cell-mediated immunity.
- The conditions are considered by physicians to have a clinical course or management that is complicated by HIV infection.

Examples of conditions in clinical category B include, but are not limited to, the following:

- Bacterial endocarditis, meningitis, pneumonia, or sepsis
- Candidiasis, vulvovaginal; persistent for more than 1 month, or poorly responsive to therapy
- Candidiasis, oropharyngeal (thrush)
- Cervical dysplasia, severe; or carcinoma
- Constitutional symptoms, such as fever (>38.5° C) or diarrhea lasting more than 1 month
- Hairy leukoplakia, oral
- Herpes zoster (shingles), involving at least two distinct episodes or more than one dermatome
- Idiopathic thrombocytopenic purpura
- Listeriosis
- *Mycobacterium tuberculosis* infection, pulmonary
- Nocardiosis
- Pelvic inflammatory disease
- Peripheral neuropathy

Category C: Any condition listed in the 1987 surveillance case definition of acquired immunodeficiency syndrome (AIDS) and affecting an adolescent or an adult.

- The conditions in clinical category C are strongly associated with severe immunodeficiency, occur frequently in HIV-infected clients, and cause serious morbidity or mortality.
- According to the proposed classification system, HIV-infected clients would be classified on the basis of both (1) the lowest accurate (not necessarily the most recent) CD4+ lymphocyte determination, and (2) the most severe clinical condition diagnosed regardless of the client's current clinical condition.

Adapted from (1993). Revised classification system for HIV infection for adolescents and adults, November 15, 1993. U.S. Department of Health and Human Services, Public Health Service, CDC.

several weeks to a few months. During primary infection, 50% to 70% of people get sick. Many clinicians are unaware of this fact; they tend to think that primary infection is "silent." In addition to constitutional symptoms (fever, fatigue, lymphadenopathy, nausea, vomiting), people may experience headache, truncal (torso and upper extremities) rash, ulcers of the mouth and/or genitalia, "thrush," pharyngitis, diarrhea, hepatomegaly, myalgia, arthralgia, anemia, thrombocytopenia, and leukopenia. Although in some individuals the symptoms may be mild, often comparable to those of mononucleosis, they can be quite severe in others, and even require hospitalization.

During primary infection, a sudden and intense burst of HIV activity results in a high viral load and a dramatic drop in the CD4+ cell count. In fact, there have been reports of the CD4+ cell count dropping at the time of primary infection to below 100/mm^3, with the concomitant development of an AIDS-defining illness. This is also the period in which most newly infected individuals develop antibodies to HIV, which can then be detected through enzyme immunoassay (EIA) testing.

Unfortunately, most individuals are not diagnosed at

the time of primary infection, either because they do not seek medical care when the symptoms occur or because clinicians caring for them do not take adequate histories that would lead to suspicion of HIV infection. This is quite a serious situation, because preliminary studies have shown that initiating therapy at the time of initial infection may prevent HIV from inflicting damage to both the immune system and other body systems.

Except in certain instances, such as seeking a federal job or in infant umbilical cord blood testing, the decision to seek the EIA test for HIV antibodies is left up to the individual. Going for testing involves pretest and posttest counseling. Laws governing the reporting of HIV antibody test results vary from state to state, and testing may be performed either anonymously or confidentially. If the EIA test is positive, a second test, the Western blot test, is performed to confirm that the test is in fact a positive HIV test. Serum antibodies to HIV usually develop in about 3 months from the date of initial HIV infection. If testing is performed too early in this period, a false-negative result may occur. False-positive results can also occur, and have been reported in blood donors after influenza vaccination.

In general, test results are reported as either positive, negative, or indeterminate. A positive test results means that the person is HIV-infected, but it does not predict the future course of disease. A negative test result means that HIV antibodies were not detected. Indeterminate results usually mean that the EIA test was positive, but the Western blot test failed to confirm those findings. Repeat testing on indeterminate results often shows an HIV-negative antibody test. Repeat testing at a later date is commonly recommended as a means of validating initial test results.

The period following primary infection is one in which the person usually remains asymptomatic for many years. Therefore, clients with HIV disease are frequently categorized in group "A" for extended periods. Although the individual remains without any obvious major symptoms, he or she may start to notice recurrent infections of the sinuses or respiratory tract or increasing fatigue. Although no significant disease is apparent, viral destruction takes place throughout the body. A major portion of this destructive activity takes place in lymph tissue and results in a slowly declining CD4 cell count. The damage to lymphatic structures also has a negative effect on the quality of CD4 cells that are continuously produced within the body. After a while, although the numbers may be adequate, CD4 cells lose their ability to contain the destructive nature of HIV.

Since the beginning of the HIV epidemic, the focus of clinical monitoring has been on evaluating the quantity of CD4 cells. In essence, CD4 cell counts are an indirect measurement of the clinical course of HIV disease, showing the end result of HIV activity. In 1996, viral load testing became available to directly measure how much viral activity was occurring in a person with the disease. Viral load tests measure the amount of HIV RNA in plasma, quantify HIV activity, determine prognosis, indicate the need for treatment, evaluate the biologic response to treatment, and detect treatment failure. CD4 cell counts should not be a substitute for viral load testing, because the correlation between the results of the two tests is weak. High viral loads may not always correlate with clinical symptoms and a low CD4 cell count, and vice versa. Viral load results are reported in copies per milliliter (e.g., 10,000 copies/ml). The actual numbers may be reported as decimal numbers (10,000 copies), or exponents (10^4 [the exponent 4 just indicates the number of zeros after the 1]), or they may be reported as a logarithm (in this case 4 [or $10^4 = 10,000$]). Reading a report indicating viral activity at 5 logs is interpreted as 10^5, or 100,000 copies/ml.

As the disease progresses, symptoms such as "thrush" or vulvovaginal candidiasis usually appear, which are distinct signs of an underlying immunodeficiency. It is at this time that many individuals seek HIV antibody testing and discover that they are infected. Persons with symptomatic illness are then classified into group "B" (see Box 27–2). Eventually the client with HIV infection develops one or more of the diseases listed as AIDS-defining diseases and is finally classified into group "C." Once again, this may be the first time that HIV infection is discovered.

Community and Self-Care

■ Medical Management of HIV Disease

The goals for medical management of the HIV-infected person are to monitor the clinical status of the individual and to provide appropriate therapy to treat HIV disease and prevent the development of opportunistic diseases. This requires medical follow-up at specified intervals.

Laboratory Evaluation

Initial and follow-up laboratory testing provides invaluable information on disease progression, serves as guide for treatment decisions, and determines the efficacy of treatment prescribed. The complete blood count is necessary to identify anemia, thrombocytopenia, leukopenia, and developing infections. Multichannel chemistry panels and urinalysis reveal renal, liver, metabolic, or nutritional disease. A tuberculin skin test detects mycobacterial disease and a chest x-ray identifies pulmonary problems. For women, a pregnancy test and Papanicolaou test are usually performed. Screening for venereal diseases includes testing for syphilis, gonorrhea, and *Chlamydia.* Hepatitis B panel testing is performed to identify acute or prior infection. The only serologic testing for potential pathogens that may be of use is testing for antibodies to toxoplasmosis.

Finally, CD4+ cell counts, ratios, and percentages are performed to determine the degree of immunodeficiency, and viral load testing is ordered to calculate the amount of viral activity. Viral load test result interpretations are as follows: (1) <10,000 copies/ml is a low risk for AIDS; (2) at 10,000 to 100,000 copies/ml, the risk doubles; (3) >100,000 copies/ml is a high risk for developing AIDS. The initial test, without any treatment, may reveal viral loads of 80,000 to 1,000,000 copies/ml. These same tests will be repeated at intervals determined by the presence or absence of symptoms or disease in the HIV-infected person, through the course of illness. Because several viral load tests have been approved for use, clinicians are advised to use the same viral load test when performing serial measurements to control variations in test results. Diseases such as influenza, herpes, or pneumonia, as well as testing immediately after the influenza vaccine is administered, can cause a temporary rise in test results. Therefore, testing should be deferred in the presence of any of these situations.

Antiretroviral Therapy

The decision to treat HIV disease is a joint decision between the primary care provider and the client. Many individuals, because of personal experience or preference, may choose to refuse antiretroviral therapy that is recommended. Clinicians should, in a non-coercive manner, provide as much objective information as possible, so that the person with HIV can make an informed choice about taking these drugs. Because viral load testing is new, there is no consensus on when to initiate therapy. However many primary care providers recommend that when the viral load is >5,000 to 10,000 copies/ml and signs and symptoms of clinical or immunological deterioration are present, or when the viral load is >30,000 to 50,000 copies/ml, regardless of signs and symptoms, therapy should be started. Trials are also under way to determine if antiretroviral therapy should in fact be initiated close to primary HIV infection, as soon as HIV infection is identified. The hypothesis behind these trials is that less damage will be done to the immune system the sooner therapy is started.

Three classes of antiretroviral agents have been approved in the United States for therapy and include nucleoside analogs, protease inhibitors, and non-nucleoside reverse transcriptase inhibitors (NNRTIs). Nucleoside analogs block HIV replication by protecting non-infected cells. Protease inhibitors render HIV particles noninfectious in cells already infected with HIV. NNRTIs work similarly to nucleoside analogs.

The first nucleoside analog, approved in March 1987, was zidovudine (Retrovir, AZT). The original dosage was 1200 mg/day taken at specified intervals. The most profound side effect was myelosuppression, resulting in anemia and leukopenia, which often required repeated transfusions. Many individuals currently diagnosed with HIV infection remember a friend's or loved one's experiences, and this has influenced their reluctance to try antiretroviral therapy. By 1990, research demonstrated that half of the original dose or 600 mg/day of zidovudine was sufficient to achieve the desired effects. Other nucleoside analogs include didanosine (Videx, ddI, approved in 1990), zalcitabine (Hivid, ddC, approved in 1992), stavudine (Zerit, d4T, approved in 1994), and lamivudine (Epivir, 3TC, approved in 1995).

Eager anticipation preceded the approval of new classes of drugs, because large numbers of patients had developed resistance to nucleoside analogs. Protease inhibitors currently approved include saquinavir (Invirase, approved in 1995), indinavir (Crixivan, approved in 1996), and ritonavir (Norvir, approved in 1996). Finally the first of the newest class of drugs (i.e., the NNRTIs), nevirapine (Viramune), was approved in 1996.

Perhaps the greatest challenge to treating HIV disease has been the genetic promiscuity of this virus. As stated earlier, HIV mutates rapidly, and in the presence of antiretroviral agents it can develop resistance to the drug and continue to grow in the presence of the drug. Three types of drug resistance are of concern: (1) genotype resistance, in which the virus mutates; (2) phenotype resistance, in which a decrease occurs in the sensitivity of the virus to the drug; and (3) cross-resistance, in which the virus, having developed resistance to one drug, becomes resistant to other drugs within that class of agents. Monotherapy, prescribing one antiretroviral agent at a time, is more likely to result in drug resistance than is combination therapy. Subtherapeutic levels of a drug will also lead to drug resistance. Subtherapeutic levels can occur when the patient does not take the prescribed dosage and/or does not take the dosages at specified intervals, and when other drugs are prescribed that interact with the

antiretroviral agent by lowering serum plasma levels of the drug.

In an attempt to prevent the development of drug resistance, combination therapy is currently ordered. The hypothesis is that combinations of drugs will "confuse" the virus, thus interfering with its ability to develop resistance. Unfortunately, preliminary data are showing that even in combinations of three drugs at one time, resistance develops to one or more of the agents being taken. Combination therapy includes two or more drugs given simultaneously from either the nucleoside analog group exclusively or in combination with a protease inhibitor or an NNRTI. The goal is to find combinations that are the least toxic and that produce the largest and most long-lasting viral response (lowest viral load) and the best immune response (highest CD4+ cell counts). Because this is a new approach to treating HIV disease, the best combinations of drugs have not as yet been identified.

Evaluating the efficacy of antiretroviral therapy is based on the clinical presentation of the client (the presence of signs and symptoms) and laboratory data (viral load tests and CD4+ cell counts). The most reliable objective determinant is viral load testing, which is performed 3 to 4 weeks after initiating or changing therapy. If the decrease in viral load is not at least three times the original laboratory reports, or decreased by at least 0.5 log, the therapy is usually changed. Repeat testing to make sure that the drugs are working is usually performed at 3- to 4-month intervals.

Vaccines

Since 1987, approximately 15 HIV experimental vaccines have been tested on more than 2,000 healthy people. Vaccines are being developed to prevent HIV disease (preventive vaccine) and as therapy for HIV-infected individuals (therapeutic vaccine). To date, vaccine development has focused on recombinant vaccines structured from envelope glycoproteins gp120 and gp160 of HIV. Preparation has begun to test approximately 5,000 volunteers to determine the effectiveness of these vaccines.

Immunomodulator Therapy

Research continues to investigate the development of immunomodulators, drugs designed to modulate or reconstitute the immune system. Agents being studied include tumor necrosis factor alpha, interleukin-12, and interferon alpha. Although no single agent has been identified as a safe and beneficial adjunct to antiretroviral therapy, research continues.

Prophylaxis for Opportunistic Infection

By 1986, surveillance data indicated that more than 80% of individuals with HIV disease developed *Pneumocystis carinii* pneumonia (PCP) at least once before they died. Research studies eventually demonstrated that morbidity and mortality could be significantly reduced by administering a drug prophylactically for PCP. Since 1989, the U.S. Public Health Service has recommended that PCP prophylaxis be provided for all HIV-infected individuals with a CD4+ cell count <200/mm³. Therapies that may be prescribed include trimethoprim-sulfamethoxazole (TMP-SMX), dapsone, dapsone plus pyrimethamine plus leucovorin, or aerosolized pentamidine. Alternatives include intermittent parenteral pentamidine, pyrimethamine-sulfadoxine, clindamycin plus primaquine, atovaquone, or intravenous trimetrexate. It is interesting to note that TMP-SMX and dapsone also provide protection against the development of toxoplasmosis.

Although surveillance data alone do not reflect the true incidence of infection due to *Mycobacterium avium-intracellulare* complex (MAC), postmortem examinations revealed that more than 60% of all HIV-infected persons had active infection due to MAC. Since 1993, the U.S. Public Health Service has recommended that MAC infection prophylaxis be provided to all HIV-infected persons with a CD4+ cell count <75/mm³. The recommended drugs include rifabutin or clarithromycin. There may be a problem with ordering either of these drugs, because both may interact with the currently available protease inhibitors.

All HIV-infected patients who test positive to a tuberculin skin test and have no evidence of active tuberculosis should receive 12 months of preventive therapy with isoniazid. Pyridoxine should be added to reduce the potential for peripheral neuropathy. Other recommended prophylactic measures include prevention of respiratory infections using pneumococcal vaccine and influenza vaccine, and prevention of "traveler's diarrhea" when traveling to countries where diarrhea is common, using antimicrobials such as ciprofloxacin. Finally, cytomegalovirus prophylaxis using oral ganciclovir is under study.

■ Nursing Management of HIV Disease

The goals of nursing management of the HIV-infected person are (1) to collect baseline information for planning to manage the client throughout the course of illness, (2) to provide health teaching to prevent complications associated with HIV disease, and (3) to provide accurate information to the client so that informed choices can be made.

Assessment

In most instances, HIV disease is viewed as a chronic illness. Therefore, assessment should not be restricted to the immediate clinical status of the individual, but it should focus on potential problems that may be encountered during the illness trajectory. For example, federal legislation passed in 1996 barred states from providing Medicaid to legal immigrants to the United States. It is of no value to hand someone a prescription if they have no insurance and no money to pay for it. Social work intervention will be needed to find an alternative source of obtaining the medication, such as applying directly to the drug company to get free medicine or asking a community-based AIDS service organization for assistance. Likewise, if the client lives alone and has absolutely no one willing to assist when needed, when the illness progresses, institutional placement may be necessary. As a coordinator of care, the nurse should have information available to identify problems and plan ahead.

Assessment should also include the preexisting level of knowledge of HIV disease. Some clients may be very knowledgeable about HIV disease and may even have suspected that they were infected but avoided testing. The nurse should attempt to assess exactly what the client does or does not know about HIV disease before assuming that there is a complete lack of knowledge regarding transmission and health-promoting behaviors.

The psychological burden of HIV disease can frequently be overwhelming. Crisis points at which the nurse can anticipate anxiety, fear, or depression include the following: (1) the time of initial diagnosis of HIV infection, (2) the time of the initial AIDS diagnosis, (3) changes in treatment, (4) the development of new symptoms, (5) recurrence of problems or relapse, and (6) terminal illness. Psychological conflicts that clients often experience include (1) fear of transmitting HIV to others, (2) constant worry about getting an infection, (3) guilt over previous life-style, and (4) changes in personal relationships. Social stressors may include (1) disclosure of HIV status, (2) stigma, (3) insecurity with employment and insurance, and (4) loneliness and social isolation.

Diagnosis, Planning, Implementation

Knowledge Deficit. The primary nursing diagnosis encountered with newly diagnosed HIV-infected individuals is *Knowledge deficit related to behaviors that will improve the level of health and prevent complications.* Although some patients may have knowledge of HIV disease, it is highly improbable that they know all that can be done to improve their health.

Planning and Implementation. Health teaching should be ongoing and repeated at frequent intervals. An HIV-infected person can adopt several behaviors that will not only improve their immune function but also increase their sense of well-being. A high-protein, high-calorie diet; learning to control stress through relaxation and attending support groups; and exercising regularly will all have a positive effect on the immune system. Smoking cessation will reduce the risk of pneumonia and other infections. Learning and following food and water safety guidelines will reduce the potential for infections of the gastrointestinal system.

Support groups are an excellent means of coping with HIV and to express fears and concerns and process large amounts of information received from both healthcare providers and the media. Local support groups are available, even in rural areas of the United States. The nurse should encourage the client to seek out assistance from community-based AIDS service organizations.

Evaluation

Evaluation includes whether or not the client understands the teaching that has been provided and the choices that

BRIDGE TO HOME HEALTHCARE

Following Universal Precautions at Home

Gina Miranda, R.N., B.S.N. *Mount Sinai Medical Center Home Health Agency, Bronx, New York*

Infection control in the home presents a unique challenge to the nurse, patient, and caregiver. Unlike the hospital, the home is an unstable environment and, as such, requires special measures to assure that the patient and caregiver adhere to infection control measures referred to as universal precautions.

You are required to investigate the potential or existing sources of infection in the home, and teach the patient and caregiver about areas in the home that may harbor bacteria. Surfaces and cutting boards in the kitchen and bathroom are prime areas for bacteria to live and grow and require extra care and cleaning measures to prevent the spread of bacteria to the susceptible patient. A 1:10 solution of bleach and water is the best method for cleaning these surfaces.

In the kitchen, for example, raw meats placed on the countertop may leave behind bacteria such as salmonella, while the bathroom may be a haven for bacteria from the hands, mouth, and skin. Usually, these bacteria are encountered on an everyday basis. However, when someone is susceptible to infection, these common bacteria can be very harmful.

Following universal precautions in the home requires a great deal of creativity on the part of the nurse working with the patient and caregiver. The following tips provide a guide for teaching the patient and caregiver about following universal precautions in the home:

- Hand washing is the first defense in preventing the spread of infectious diseases. Instructing patients and caregivers about good hand-washing techniques is extremely important. Using a "pump" liquid soap device is preferred over bar soap sitting in a dish filled with soap scum, which may support the growth of bacteria.
- Wear gloves, gowns, masks, and aprons when you handle blood or body fluids.
- Wash bathroom and kitchen surfaces with a 1:10 bleach-and-water solution (as recommended by universal precautions) should they become contaminated with blood or body fluids. Do not share toothbrushes and razors. Dispose of razors, which may be contaminated with blood, in the same manner as needles (described below).
- Maintain adequate ventilation and lighting to reduce the growth of bacteria.
- Wash dishes and utensils as usual. If a dishwasher is used, include the heat drying cycle.
- Wash laundry contaminated with blood or body fluids (urine, blood, sputum, or feces) separately with a 1:10 bleach-and-water solution.
- Pets should not be cared for by someone who is at risk of infection.
- Dispose of sharps (needles, syringes, razor blades) in a can or detergent bottle and decontaminate with a 1:10 solution of bleach and water. Remind the patient and caregiver not to recycle this container and to never recap a needle.
- Have double bag at the bedside for disposal of tissues or other waste contaminated with blood or body fluids. Do not discard these items with the household waste.
- The nursing bag should be waterproof to prevent contamination of the contents and have an outside pocket for soap and paper towels. Clean all items that are not disposable with alcohol before returning them to the nursing bag. Never place the bag on a unclean surface. Use a paper towel or the inside of a newspaper as a clean surface.

Be sensitive as you follow universal precautions and help patients and caregivers follow the precautions.

---

each person may make. If a client chooses not to adopt a recommended behavior, it does not mean that he or she is noncompliant. The HIV-infected person who smokes may find that his or her stress level rises to high levels during attempts to quit, and even when offered a nicotine patch or gum, such a client may choose to continue to smoke. Healthcare providers have a difficult time with evaluating outcomes of teaching, and weighing them against the free choice of the individual. It is important to remember that the ultimate decision as to whether to follow the advice of healthcare providers is up to the client, and this in no way reflects failure on the part of the healthcare professional.

A totally different situation exists when minimal learning has taken place because of cognitive impairment. It is well documented in the literature that problems with thinking or memory may exist and go undiagnosed if they are not obvious. This is more likely to occur in HIV-infected individuals with less than a 12th grade education and in persons older than 50 years. In this type of situation, a designated care-partner should be identified, to whom all information is provided when it is provided to the patient. Whenever the care-partner can't make a clinic or office visit, the nurse should provide telephone teaching and document that this was provided.

Persons with HIV should be encouraged to inform their healthcare providers of any self-prescribed therapies they may be taking, because this may have either a positive or negative impact on the outcomes of care. Keeping track of over-the-counter medications is important, as they may interact with prescribed therapies. Some patients may also obtain medications through buyers' clubs or "underground" pharmacies. This can not only be detrimental to the effectiveness of treatments prescribed, but it can also have an adverse effect on observations made in experimental drug trials in which some patients may be enrolled.

Alternative or complementary therapies may be chosen by some individuals and include (1) spiritual or psychological interventions, such as guided imagery, meditation, or faith healing; (2) nutritional alternatives, such as macrobiotics; (3) drug and biologic therapies, such as homeopathy, oxygen, or ozone therapy; and (4) physical forces, such as acupuncture, acupressure, or massage therapy. In most instances, these choices have a positive effect on the emotional well-being of the individual. However, in some cases they can also have a negative effect on health, such as a macrobiotic diet that can lead to vitamin and mineral deficiencies as well as weight loss, or herbal remedies that may cause nausea, vomiting, diarrhea, or central nervous system depression. Despite these effects, some clients may continue to use them. Documenting this information will help in evaluating the overall effectiveness of the plan of care.

Acute and Subacute Care

■ Medical Management of AIDS

As both the quantity and quality of CD4+ cells diminish, the client develops AIDS-indicator diseases. The categories of AIDS-defining illnesses include opportunistic infections (OIs), neoplasms, and/or other conditions specific to HIV disease. The four major categories of OIs include bacterial, fungal, protozoal, and viral infections. The list is presented in rank order of ease of treatment, as bacterial infections are the easiest to treat and viruses are the most difficult. Neoplasms associated with AIDS include Kaposi's sarcoma, non-Hodgkin's lymphoma, and invasive cervical cancer. Two other conditions that are unique to AIDS are HIV encephalopathy and HIV wasting syndrome.

Opportunistic Infections

Most of the pathogens responsible for OIs are ubiquitous in nature, that is, they are all around us. *Pneumocystis carinii* is an organism that is in the air we breathe. The reason most people do not get sick from this organism is that their immune systems are intact. However once the regulators of the immune system, the CD4+ cells, are destroyed by HIV, infection occurs. Most OIs are infections due to previously acquired pathogens. They are secondary reactivation of organisms that caused an infection in the person previously, as opposed to a new or primary infection. For example, most individuals have been infected with *Pneumocystis carinii* in early preschool years, when it presented with respiratory symptoms and was probably dismissed as a common cold. Because of an intact immune system, the infection was brought under

control. However, the organism remained dormant within the body of the person. The potential then exists that if an immunodeficiency does occur, the organism will reactivate, causing disease again. This concept applies to any person who develops an immunodeficiency, regardless of the cause. To illustrate further, clients with cancer who receive chemotherapy and become immunodeficient may also develop infection due to *Pneumocystis carinii*.

Many of the OIs that occur in persons with HIV are not curable. Because the immune system no longer has the strength to contain the infection, it becomes chronic in nature and requires lifetime suppressive therapy. Assisting the client in complying with taking antibiotics to keep the OI under control becomes an essential part of the care planning process. Because the client has to take antibiotics for extended periods, drug resistance may develop, and both doctors and nurses must constantly observe the client for recurrence of symptoms that may indicate the infection is reactivating and the drugs no longer work. Finally, single OIs are rare, and clients may have multiple infections.

Bacterial Infections

Mycobacterium tuberculosis. Co-infection with *Mycobacterium tuberculosis* (TB) and HIV is common, especially in large metropolitan areas. Because TB is airborne, the presence of an immunodeficiency makes the person with HIV very susceptible. All HIV-infected persons should be tested annually to detect new or active infection. Nosocomial spread of TB among clients hospitalized and placed on AIDS units has been a problem. Signs and symptoms of active infection are categorized as constitutional, pulmonary, or extrapulmonary. Constitutional manifestations include fever, chills, weight loss, night sweats, lymphadenopathy, and fatigue. Pulmonary symptoms may include cough, dyspnea, chest pain, and hemoptysis. Extrapulmonary presentation may involve lymph nodes, bones, joints, liver, spleen, central nervous system, skin, gastrointestinal tract, mass lesions, urine, and blood.

The recommended therapy includes four drugs: isoniazid, rifampin, pyrazinamide, and either ethambutol or streptomycin, administered for at least 9 months. Multiple drug–resistant tuberculosis (MDR-TB) was identified as an emerging problem in the United States around 1987. By 1990, significant numbers of cases were identified, especially among persons with HIV infection. Studies attributed the development of MDR-TB to doctors prescribing insufficient numbers of drugs to treat new cases of TB and, once again, the development of strains of TB that were resistant to the most widely prescribed agents, isoniazid and rifampin. Based on drug-sensitivity reports, second-line therapy for MDR-TB includes ciprofloxacin, ofloxacin, kanamycin, amikacin, capreomycin, ethinomide, cycloserine, aminosalicylic acid, and/or clofazimine. In institutional settings, the client is placed in respiratory isolation until sputum tests reveal that the client is no longer infectious. In many cases of MDR-TB, despite therapy, sputum results indicate the presence of organisms, and it is not uncommon to have the client remain in respiratory isolation until discharge. TB is a reportable communicable disease, and healthcare professionals are required to report new cases to local health authorities.

Follow-up care focuses on symptom management. Monitoring drug compliance is essential to ensure effective treatment and to prevent recurrent active disease. In cities where MDR-TB has become a significant problem, local health departments have established monitoring programs (Directly Observed Therapy, DOT) and workers go to the client and watch them take their medications. Psychological stressors for the client include coping with the stigmata attached to both HIV and TB.

Mycobacterium avium Complex.
Mycobacterium avium complex (MAC) is also sometimes referred to *Mycobacterium avium-intracellulare* (MAI). The organism is ubiquitous in nature and exists in the soil, water, animals, eggs, and unpasteurized dairy products. It is important to realize that not all members of the *Mycobacterium* family of bacteria are communicable. MAC is referred to as atypical, noncommunicable mycobacterial disease. Because it is well known that the majority of HIV-infected individuals will develop active disease, and the risk of infection increases with CD4+ cell counts $< 75/mm^3$, prophylaxis to prevent infection is recommended. Additionally, MAC infection is much easier to prevent than to treat.

The clinical presentation of MAC infection includes fever, night sweats, fatigue, anorexia, weight loss, abdominal pain, and diarrhea. Because the disease is difficult to treat and the side effects of the medications are numerous, the decision whether to treat MAC infection depends on the severity of symptoms and the presence of renal or hepatic disease. Anywhere from two to six drugs may be used at one time, including azithromycin, amikacin, clarithromycin, clofazimine, ethambutol, ciprofloxacin, rifampin, rifabutin, cycloserine, ethionamide, and/or streptomycin.

Follow-up care focuses on managing symptoms, as they may persist despite drug therapy. Evaluating the client's ability to comply with the prescribed therapy is important, because some clients may decrease the dosage of prescribed pills on their own to minimize side effects. Both clients and their care providers need to be taught that this is not a communicable disease.

Salmonellosis.
Salmonella infection is a disease that can be prevented by teaching the client food and water safety and proper food handling. Infection occurs with ingestion of contaminated food, including beef, pork, poultry, and eggs; drinking contaminated water; ingesting contaminated medications or diagnostic agents; directly handling contaminated feces; or through sexual activity involving oral-anal contact. Food handlers may be asymptomatic carriers, and pets, especially turtles, may be a source of exposure. Presenting signs and symptoms include fever, night sweats, fatigue, anorexia, weight loss, abdominal pain, and diarrhea. Treatment includes ampicillin, chloramphenicol, trimethoprim-sulfamethoxazole, cephalosporins, amoxicilin, ciprofloxacin, or norfloxacin. Follow-up care is focused on symptom management, including preventing or managing skin breakdown in the perianal region.

Bacterial Pneumonia.
Recurrent bacterial pneumonia is common among IV drug users. Predisposing factors include needle sharing, environmental exposure, heavy alcohol use, smoking, and inadequate nutrition. Pathogens most often associated with bacterial pneumonia, seen in HIV-infected persons, are *Streptococcus pneumoniae,* and *Haemophilus influenzae*. The risk of bacterial pneumonia increases when the CD4+ cell count is $< 200/mm^3$. Treatment with antibiotics is based on culture and sensitivity reports. Follow-up care includes focusing on behavioral changes that would decrease the possibility of recurrence (e.g., smoking cessation, adequate nutrition, using clean needles to inject drugs).

Fungal Infections

Candidiasis.
Candida albicans is not only ubiquitous (in soil and food, on fomites), but it is also a commensal organism normally found in the mouth, vagina, large intestine, and on the skin. The majority of infections that occur are endogenous (the person's own organism is the source of the infection). Nosocomial spread in institutions such as hospitals and nursing homes can also occur. Human-to-human transmission can occur from mother to infant during vaginal delivery and between sexual partners. Clinical presentation is related to the site of infection: (1) dysphagia with esophagitis, (2) oral lesions with "thrush," (3) cutaneous lesions with intertrigo, (4) vulvovaginal irritation and discharge with vaginitis, and (5) constitutional symptoms with disseminated disease. Treatment is also site dependent: (1) for oral/esophageal candidiasis, clotrimazole troches, nystatin suspension, ketoconazole, fluconazole, and amphotericin B oral suspension (for esophagitis only) is given; (2) for intertrigo and vaginitis, clotrimazole, miconazole, ketoconazole, fluconazole, imidazole, and itraconazole (for nail infection) is given; and (3) for disseminated disease, amphotericin B, with or without flucytosine, is given. Follow-up care includes teaching routine skin and mouth care. Encouraging the patient to eat 8 oz of yogurt made from live cultures (*Lactobacillus acidophilus*) may be of benefit in controlling recurrent infection due to *Candida*.

Cryptococcosis.
Cryptococcus neoformans is ubiquitous and is found in pigeon droppings, nesting places, soil, fruit, and unpasteurized fruit juices. The organism is aerosolized and inhaled, and as an AIDS-indicator disease it causes both lung and brain infection. HIV-infected smokers are more prone to developing cryptococcosis. The clinical manifestations primarily involve the central nervous system but can also include the lungs, skin, and mouth. Central nervous system signs and symptoms include low-grade fever, fatigue, headaches, nausea and/or vomiting, and altered mental status. Pulmonary symptoms include cough, dyspnea, and pleuritic chest pain. Cutaneous and oral manifestations include painless lesions that may mimic Kaposi's sarcoma or molluscum contagiosum. Treatment includes amphotericin B, with or without flucytosine, fluconazole, or itraconazole. Maintenance lifetime suppressive therapy is required, and follow-up care focuses on assisting with medication compliance and moni-

toring for recurrence of symptoms that indicate resistance to maintenance drug therapy.

Histoplasmosis. *Histoplasma capsulatum* is a fungus that is endemic to certain regions of the United States. It is most prevalent in the middle, central, and south central states and Puerto Rico. Therefore, persons with HIV disease living in these areas are prone to the disease. When diagnosed in other parts of the country (e.g., New York and California), the disease is usually limited to those individuals who either grew up in or traveled to the endemic regions. The signs and symptoms include fever; weight loss; enlarged lymph nodes, liver, and spleen; abdominal pain; oral and skin lesions; anemia; leukopenia; and thrombocytopenia. Treatment includes amphotericin B, itraconazole, or fluconazole. Maintenance lifetime suppressive therapy is required, and follow-up care focuses on assisting with medication compliance and monitoring for recurrence of symptoms that indicate resistance to maintenance drug therapy.

Coccidioidomycosis. *Coccidioides immitis* is a fungus that is endemic to the southwestern part of the United States. It was originally discovered in the San Joaquin Valley in southern California, and it is also referred to as *valley fever*. As an AIDS-defining diagnosis, it is frequently seen in HIV-infected persons residing in Arizona, California, Nevada, New Mexico, Texas, and Utah. When diagnosed in other parts of the country, the disease is usually limited to those individuals who either grew up in or traveled to the endemic regions. Clinical presentation includes fever, dyspnea, fatigue, weight loss, and cough. Treatment includes amphotericin B, ketoconazole, itraconazole, or fluconazole. Maintenance lifetime suppressive therapy is required, and follow-up care focuses on assisting with medication compliance and monitoring for recurrence of symptoms that indicate resistance to maintenance drug therapy.

Protozoal Infections

Pneumocystosis. *Pneumocystis carinii* is a ubiquitous organism that is airborne and can be found in the lungs of humans and animals. Most healthy individuals have had primary infection by the age of 4 years. Although most of the literature supports the theory that *Pneumocystis* infection in HIV-infected individuals is a secondary appearance of a previously acquired pathogen (reactivation), recent information has revealed that some patients have different strains of the organism, which may indicate the reinfection is possible through airborne transmission. Clinical presentation can be elusive, and approximately 7% of patients developing infection are asymptomatic. With *P. carinii* pneumonia (PCP) coughing is a frequent first symptom, which begins as nonproductive progressing to a productive cough. Eventually the client develops fever and dyspnea on exertion, and then dyspnea at rest. Extrapulmonary *Pneumocystis* infection can occur in the eyes, ears, lymph nodes, heart, spleen, liver, pleural space, and on the skin. Clients who are receiving PCP prophylaxis sometimes also develop infection be-

cause of poor compliance, unusual or erratic pharmacokinetics, or the development of drug resistance. Treatment includes trimethoprim-sulfamethoxazole, pentamidine, atovaquone, trimethoprim-dapsone, clindamycin-primaquine, or trimetrexate. Maintenance lifetime suppressive therapy is required, and follow-up care focuses on assisting with medication compliance and monitoring for recurrence of symptoms that indicate resistance to maintenance drug therapy.

Toxoplasmosis. *Toxoplasma gondii* is ubiquitous in nature and is acquired through ingestion of contaminated meat (lamb and pork), vegetables, eggs, and unpasteurized dairy products. The only documented human-to-human transmission noted is mother-to-fetus, if the mother acquires primary infection during pregnancy. Toxoplasmosis can also be acquired through direct handling of contaminated cat feces. However, it is important to note that not all cats are infected with *Toxoplasma gondii*. In fact, fewer than 1% of domestic cats are infected, and a veterinarian can perform a simple blood test to determine the presence of infection. Studies of HIV-infected cat owners have not shown any increased risk for development of toxoplasmosis.

The potential for the development of toxoplasmosis increases when the CD4+ cell count is < 100/mm.[3] If trimethoprim-sulfamethoxazole or dapsone is prescribed for PCP prophylaxis, these agents will provide prophylaxis against toxoplasmosis.

Signs and symptoms of central nervous system infection include headache, impaired cognition, hemiparesis, aphasia, ataxia, vision loss, cranial nerve palsies, motor problems, and seizures. Infection can also involve the heart, lungs, skin, stomach, abdomen, and testes. Treatment includes pyrimethamine plus sulfadiazine, dexamethasone, phenytoin, leucovorin, clindamycin plus pyrimethamine, or azithromycin. Maintenance lifetime suppressive therapy is required, and follow-up care focuses on assisting with medication compliance and monitoring for recurrence of symptoms that indicate resistance to maintenance drug therapy.

Cryptosporidiosis. *Cryptosporidium* is a pathogen that is found in mammals, birds, reptiles, and fish. The primary mode of transmission in HIV-infected persons is through the ingestion of contaminated food or water. Waterborne transmission can occur when water supplies used for drinking become contaminated, including municipal water supplies, as chlorine does not destroy the organism. The disease can also be acquired from contaminated swimming pools, from handling infected animals, and through anal-oral sexual contact with an infected person. When cryptosporidiosis occurs in immunocompetent individuals, the disease is self-limiting. In the HIV-infected, immunodeficient person, the disease is chronic, causing malabsorption, dehydration, and malnutrition, and it can lead to death. Clinical presentation includes profuse diarrhea, steatorrhea (1 to 25 L/day), flatulence, abdominal cramping and pain, anorexia, nausea, vomiting, profound weight loss, fever, fatigue, myalgia, and electrolyte imbalance. There is no effective treatment for cryptosporidiosis.

Drugs that may be tried include paromomycin, letrazuril, azithromycin, clarithromycin, nitazoxanide, and symptomatic therapy to decrease peristalsis and control pain. Special attention is also needed to manage skin breakdown in the perianal region. Clients with cryptosporidiosis are prone to depression and social isolation.

Isosporiasis. *Isospora belli* is a parasite that is transmitted through contact with infected animals, humans, or contaminated water. The disease is often seen in immigrants from Mexico, Haiti, and Central America. The signs and symptoms of disease include diarrhea, anorexia, nausea/vomiting, weight loss, abdominal pain, and fever. Drug therapy includes trimethoprim-sulfamethoxazole, sulfadoxine-pyrimethamine, or pyrimethamine alone. Treatment is usually successful, and lifetime suppressive therapy is not usually required.

Viral Infections

Cytomegalovirus Disease. Cytomegalovirus (CMV) is ubiquitous in humans throughout the world. Almost everyone eventually becomes infected with CMV, which is transmitted through direct contact with infected secretions including saliva, cervical secretions, urine, semen, breast milk, feces, or blood. In HIV-infected persons CMV infection can be asymptomatic or can result in chorioretinitis, pneumonitis, encephalitis, adrenalitis, colitis, esophagitis, hepatitis, or cholangitis. Drugs used to treat CMV infection include ganciclovir, foscarnet, or cidofovir. Treatment of CMV retinitis may also involve intraocular ganciclovir implants or intravitreal injection of ganciclovir, foscarnet, or cidofovir. Maintenance lifetime suppressive therapy is required, and follow-up care focuses on assisting with medication compliance and monitoring for recurrence of symptoms that indicate resistance to maintenance drug therapy.

Herpes Simplex Virus Disease. Herpes simplex virus (HSV) is ubiquitous throughout the world and is spread by direct contact with infected secretion; HSV-1 is present in oral secretions and HSV-2 is present in genital secretions. Transmission also takes place with symptom-free excretors (persons previously infected with HSV and with no apparent lesions). Clinical presentation includes painful vesicular lesions that coalesce and rupture. Lesions usually occur in the mouth or genital or perianal region. HSV can also cause encephalitis, esophagitis, bronchitis, keratitis, pericarditis, and hand infection. Treatment includes acyclovir, foscarnet, or famciclovir. Topical acyclovir will also relieve pain and itching associated with skin lesions. Follow-up care focuses on monitoring the client for recurrent disease. If it is chronic in nature, lifetime suppressive therapy is prescribed.

Progressive Multifocal Leukoencephalopathy Disease. Progressive multifocal leukoencephalopathy (PML) is caused by the J.C. virus (the virus was named by using the initials of the first client in whom it was discovered). The J.C. virus is ubiquitous in nature and appears to infect most individuals by middle adulthood. Active disease in HIV-infected persons results in extremity weakness, ataxia, cognitive impairment, vision loss, speech impairment, and headache. In the latter stages of illness it progresses to dementia, blindness, paralysis, and death. There is no effective therapy, but drugs that may be used include prednisone, acyclovir, adenine arabinoside, cytosine arabinoside, and human leukocyte antigen. Follow-up care focuses on palliative therapy, safety measures, and preventing complications due to immobility.

Neoplasms

Kaposi's Sarcoma

There are four types of Kaposi's sarcoma (KS) that may be encountered in clinical practice. Three are not associated in any way with HIV infection: (1) classic KS, which tends to occur in older men who are black, of Mediterranean descent, or from certain Jewish populations; (2) African KS, seen in Africa; and (3) transplant KS, seen in persons who receive transplanted organs. The fourth type is HIV-related KS, which differs from the others in that it runs a fulminant course, is disseminated throughout the body, and results in shorter survival. In HIV disease, KS has been predominantly diagnosed in men who have sex with men, and it is thought to be associated with a sexually transmitted pathogen that then predisposes the individual to the development of KS. A new type of herpes virus is suspected. KS differs from most AIDS-defining diseases in that it is not related to low CD4+ cell counts and can occur early in HIV infection.

Clinical presentation generally starts with an initial "patch," which is flat, pink, looks like a bruise, and is symmetrical on both sides of the body, later turning into dark violet or black plaques (see Fig. 78–19). Clinical presentation of the lesions can include the mouth, skin, mucous membranes, head, neck, torso, extremities (soles of feet), genitals, lung, brain, intestines, and lymph nodes, and they can be painful. Treatment depends on the extent of tumors (tumor burden), CD4+ cell count, associated symptoms and diseases, and functional ability of the patient. Local therapy includes radiation, localized chemotherapy, and cryotherapy. Systemic therapy includes vincristine, vinblastine, etoposide, doxorubicin, daunorubicin, bleomycin, and alpha-interferon, with or without an HIV-specific antiretroviral agent. Experimental therapies currently under investigation include the possible treatment of the underlying viral cause of KS with foscarnet. Initially several therapies may be tried, which may be effective in suppressing the course of KS; however, eventually the clinical decline in the client's condition makes continued treatment impossible.

Non-Hodgkin's Lymphoma

Non-Hodgkin's lymphoma (NHL) tends to occur late in the course of HIV disease and is related to low CD4+ cell counts. The primary sites of occurrence are the brain, gastrointestinal tract, bone marrow, and liver. The initial clinical presentation may be nonspecific and include fever, night sweats, and weight loss, all of which are associated with MAC infection, TB, and CMV infection. Treatment includes methotrexate, bleomycin, doxorubicin, cyclophosphamide, vincristine, and dexamethasone. Despite aggressive treatment, the prognosis is poor.

Invasive Cervical Cancer

Cervical intraepithelial neoplasia (CIN), the precursor to cervical cancer, occurs at a high rate in HIV-infected women. In HIV-infected women, CIN progresses more rapidly, is less responsive to therapy, and is related to low CD4+ cell counts. In early stages of disease, the client is asymptomatic and cervical dysplasia is usually detected by Pap smear. Early symptoms include postcoital bleeding, metrorrhagia, and a blood-tinged vaginal discharge. Symptoms of more extensive disease include back, pelvic, and leg pain; weight loss; vaginal bleeding; anemia; lymphadenopathy; and edema of the lower extremities. Treatment of CIN can include conization, laser therapy, cryosurgery, electrocautery, or hysterectomy. For invasive cancer, treatment may involve surgery, radiation, and chemotherapy using cisplatin, vincristine, bleomycin, or mitomycin. Follow-up care focuses on recurrent disease and/or metastasis and symptom control.

Conditions Specific to HIV Disease

HIV Encephalopathy

HIV encephalopathy is also referred to as AIDS dementia complex (ADC). The very young and the older person with HIV is more likely to develop ADC as are clients with anemia and weight loss. There is also some evidence that HIV-infected persons with less than a 12th grade education may be more likely to show signs and symptoms of ADC. ADC is a triad of symptoms that includes cognitive dysfunction, motor problems, and behavioral changes. Cognitive symptoms include inability to concentrate, decreased memory, impaired judgment, and slowness in thinking. Motor impairment may be manifested as leg weakness, ataxia, and clumsiness. Behavioral changes can range from apathy, reduced spontaneity, and social withdrawal to irritability, hyperactivity, anxiety, mania, or delirium. The staging system for ADC is as follows: (1) stage 0: normal; (2) stage 0.5: minimal; (3) stage 1: mild; (4) stage 2: moderate; (5) stage 3: severe; and (6) stage 4: end stage. While some studies have shown a favorable response to treatment with zidovudine, no specific therapy has been identified that will ameliorate this condition. Follow-up monitoring is directed at detecting progression of ADC and evaluating the client's ability to safely maintain independent living and comply with prescribed therapies.

HIV Wasting Syndrome

Weight loss occurs at some point in HIV disease in more than 90% of HIV-infected individuals. HIV wasting is defined as profound involuntary weight loss >10% of total body baseline weight plus either chronic diarrhea or chronic weakness and fever. The primary causes are reduced food intake, malabsorption of nutrients, and altered metabolism of nutrients. The clinical work-up of the client with HIV wasting includes attempting to determine the cause. For example, if it is due to gastrointestinal infection (e.g., salmonellosis), then treating the underlying infection will usually alleviate the progressive weight loss. Once wasting has begun, treatment usually only results in partial recovery. The goal of drug therapy to treat wasting is to stimulate appetite, produce weight gain, and increase lean muscle mass. Weight gain that results in increased fat in the body is of little benefit. Agents used to treat HIV wasting include oxandrolone, megestrol acetate, and dronabinol. The latter two agents usually result in weight gain that is primarily fat. Follow-up therapy includes constant assessment for factors that may interfere with the plan of care (e.g., the client develops cognitive impairment, or has severe fatigue, or lacks resources to buy or prepare food).

■ Nursing Management of AIDS

In advanced HIV disease, the goal of nursing care is to diagnose and treat human responses to actual or potential health problems related to symptom development and the diagnosis of AIDS. All efforts are directed at symptom control. Actual or potential problems seen in people living with HIV/AIDS include fever, fatigue, weight loss, nausea, diarrhea, dry painful mouth, dry skin, skin lesions, pain, dyspnea, cough, impaired cognition, impaired vision, insomnia, and sexual dysfunction. Common nursing diagnoses that have been identified through nursing research associated with the diagnosis of AIDS are contained in Box 27–3. Three of the most common problems, seen in the majority of AIDS clients, are discussed in detail.*

Fever

Etiology

A. Chronic HIV infection
B. Secondary opportunistic infection(s)
C. Malignancy
D. Autoimmune disorders
E. Diarrhea
F. Dehydration
G. Allergic response to medications (drug fever)
H. Infections of intravenous lines, catheters, drains, and incisions

Nursing Assessment

A. Subjective data
 1. History of clinical manifestations
 2. Associated clinical manifestations
 3. Twenty-four hour dietary history, including fluid intake

---

*The following sections of this chapter, dealing with fever, fatigue, and weight loss, are adapted from Flaskerud, J. H., & Ungvarski, P. J. (1995). *HIV/AIDS: A guide to nursing care* (3rd ed.). Philadelphia: W. B. Saunders.

Box 27–3. Common Nursing Diagnoses for Patients with HIV/AIDS

Risk for Ineffective Individual Coping
Impaired Physical Mobility
Altered Nutrition: Less than Body Requirements
Fatigue
Altered Health Maintenance
Body Image Disturbance
Pain
Altered Thought Processes
Impaired Skin Integrity
Altered Oral Mucous Membranes
Knowledge Deficit
Ineffective Breathing Pattern
Diarrhea
Risk for Altered Body Temperature
Sensory/Perceptual Alterations
Powerlessness
Impaired Tissue Integrity
Ineffective Management of Therapeutic Regimen
Sleep Pattern Disturbance
Risk for Injury

4. Medical and surgical history
5. Current drug therapy

B. Objective data
  1. Vital signs
  2. Mental status, including alertness, cognition, and orientation
  3. Skin assessment, including integrity, temperature, turgor, appearance, and signs of injury or infection
  4. Assessment for dehydration, including the preceding, plus fluid intake and output estimates, and assessment of urine color, quantity, and consistency

NOTE WELL: It is important for clinicians to remember that because of the underlying immunodeficiency resulting in an impaired inflammatory response, clinical manifestations of infection, including fever, may be greatly muted.

Nursing Diagnoses

Risk for Altered Body Temperature
Risk for Fluid Volume Deficit

Goals

After discussing the finding of assessment and the nursing diagnosis, the client and/or care partner and the nurse will select interventions to control fever and replace fluid loss.

Considerations for Nursing Care and Health Teaching

A. Nonpharmacologic interventions
  1. Promote heat loss by
    a. Allowing heat to escape from trunk by applying a sheet and a loosely woven blanket

    b. If no skin lesions are present and client is ambulatory, immerse in a tub bath with water temperature at 39° C (102.2° F); avoid chilling when emerging from bath
  2. Avoid counterproductive treatments such as
    a. Tepid water sponge bathing, which causes defensive vasoconstriction (this has not been shown to be an effective coolant in fever, it can cause shivering, and it is also distressing)
    b. Alcohol sponging causes vasoconstriction, shivering, and toxic fumes, and may be absorbed cutaneously, causing hypoglycemia
  3. Holtzclaw (1992) recommended that the use of cooling blankets and ice packs be reserved for conditions in which core temperature is rising uncontrollably to potentially damaging levels (others suggested that hypothermia blankets and similar devices not be used in interleukin-1–mediated temperature elevations [pyrogenic fever], because the associated shivering is counterproductive to core temperature reduction)
  4. Prevent febrile shivering
    a. Keep client in a warm room to avert shivering
    b. Avoid fanning bedcovers, skin exposure, or rapid removal of clothing that might cause chilling
  5. Control febrile shivering by wrapping the arms from fingertips to axillae and the legs from toes to groin with three layers of terrycloth toweling

B. Increase caloric and fluid intake
  1. Provide a plan for six feedings distributed over a 24-hour period
  2. Provide high-protein, high-calorie nutritional supplements, especially in the presence of anorexia
  3. Provide at least 2 to 2.5 L of fluid to drink daily
  4. Record intake and output

C. Maintain comfort and safety
  1. Provide dry clothes and bed linens; use cotton materials rather than synthetics
  2. Use emollient creams for dry skin
  3. Monitor mental status frequently, especially when client is febrile
  4. Evaluate client's need for assistance with all activities of daily living

D. For chronic recurrent night fever and night sweats
  1. Suggest that client take the antipyretic agent of choice before going to sleep
  2. Have a change of bedclothes nearby in case a change is necessary
  3. Keep a plastic cover on the pillow
  4. Place a towel over the pillow in case of profuse diaphoresis
  5. Keep liquid at bedside to drink

E. Pharmacologic treatment should include consideration of the following:
  1. Clinicians should assess the client's patterns of use of aspirin, nonsteroidal antiinflammatory agents, and acetaminophen
  2. Follow-up should include comparing patterns of use of these agents with laboratory evaluation of hepatic and hematologic abnormalities, as well as interactions with other agents

Evaluation

The client will:

A. Identify appropriate measures to be taken in the presence of fever
B. Demonstrate the ability to initiate and maintain adequate hydration and nutrition
C. Demonstrate the ability to take and record the temperature accurately

Fatigue
Etiology

A. Chronic HIV infection
B. Secondary opportunistic infection(s) or malignancies
C. Anemia
D. Malnutrition
E. Diarrhea
F. Prolonged immobility
G. Psychological factors
H. Situational factors

Nursing Assessment

A. Subjective data
   1. History of symptoms
   2. Associated symptoms (e.g., anxiety, depression, dyspnea)
   3. Current ability to perform activities of daily living safely and to exercise
   4. Factors that increase fatigue (e.g., weather, alcohol consumption, bathing)
   5. Medical and surgical history
   6. Current drug therapy
   7. Nutrition history
B. Objective data
   1. Assess activity tolerance by taking vital signs before and immediately after the performance of an activity such as bathing, dressing, or ambulating
   2. Assess client for associated signs and symptoms such as pallor, diaphoresis, or complaints of dyspnea or dizziness

Nursing Diagnosis

Fatigue

Goals

After discussing and validating the findings of assessment and nursing diagnosis, the client and/or care partner and nurse will select interventions to

A. Increase self-awareness of fatigue, associated symptoms, environmental factors affecting fatigue, and activity tolerance
B. Identify the importance of resting when needed
C. Develop a plan for activity and rest
D. Accept assistance when needed

E. Develop a life-style that keeps client involved in activities of daily living (ADL), independent, and socially active

Considerations for Nursing Care and Health Teaching

A. Promote self-care and self-awareness
   1. Have client keep a daily fatigue diary for at least 1 week to identify sources of fatigue and appropriate interventions, as well as patterns of peak fitness
   2. Use an assessment tool to evaluate fatigue
B. Promote adequate sleep
   1. Increase the amount of sleep
   2. Reduce the amount of sleep cycle interruptions by
      a. Preparing for sleep
      b. Keeping needed items at bedside (e.g., ice water, urinal, towel to absorb perspiration)
C. Encourage adequate nutrition
   1. Substances such as coffee, tobacco, or alcohol may, in some individuals, increase fatigue
   2. Abstain from or curtail foods that the client may be sensitive to
D. Promote rest and activity
   1. Assist the patient in pacing of activities
      a. Plan a written 24-hour schedule for ADL that alternates short activities with rest periods
      b. Assist in identifying activity priorities such as eating breakfast and then resting before bathing in the morning, as opposed to the reverse
      c. Evaluate the individual's needs and point out ways to conserve energy, such as
         (1) Sitting down while dressing, shaving, or preparing food
         (2) Sitting in a shower chair while bathing
         (3) Using disposable items for eating so that no cleanup is needed
   2. Write up a plan, progressing from daily to weekly, for rest and activities
   3. Always plan activities ahead of time
   4. Several short periods of rest may be more effective than fewer long rest periods
   5. Plan an exercise schedule (physiologic immobilization may lead to increased fatigue as a result of decreased endurance)
      a. Plan exercise at peak energy times (after a rest period)
      b. Follow exercise with rest
      c. Have physical therapist assess the client and plan an exercise program
      d. Aerobic exercise, which increases endurance, has been shown to reduce fatigue
E. Additional natural techniques that may be of benefit include
   1. Progressive muscle relaxation
   2. Acupressure
   3. Massage
   4. Reflexology
   5. Imagery and visualization
   6. Autogenic relaxation
   7. Reframing and positive affirmations

8. Therapeutic touch
9. Social support and support groups

Evaluation

The client will

A. Identify causative factors that increase fatigue
B. Demonstrate the ability to plan a schedule of paced activity for a 24-hour period
C. Demonstrate the ability to participate in a program of exercise
D. Verbalize a decrease in the fatigue experienced for a 24-hour period

Weight Loss

Etiology

A. Increased nutrient requirements resulting from primary systemic infection with HIV or secondary systemic (opportunistic) infection, causing
   1. Hypermetabolism
   2. Fever
   3. Catabolism
B. Decreased food intake resulting from side effects of medication or systemic infection, causing
   1. Anorexia
   2. Nausea
   3. Vomiting
   4. Alterations in taste
C. Oral or esophageal infection, causing
   1. Impaired chewing
   2. Difficulty in swallowing
D. Decreased assimilation of food because of primary intestinal infection with HIV or secondary (opportunistic) gastrointestinal infection, causing
   1. Malabsorption
   2. Diarrhea
E. Inability to obtain food because of
   1. Fatigue
   2. Lack of money
   3. Distance from shopping
   4. Lack of utilities to store and prepare food
F. Lack of knowledge of the importance of nutrition in HIV infection and its impact on survival
G. Neuropsychiatric problems such as
   1. Depression
   2. Impaired cognition
   3. Paralysis

Nursing Assessment

A. Subjective data
   1. Medical and surgical history, including clinical manifestations, stage of HIV infection, opportunistic infections and/or neoplasms, and related therapy
   2. Medication profile, including prescribed medications, over-the-counter medications, alternative therapies, and recreational drugs
   3. Diet history, including food patterns, tolerances and allergies, cultural preferences, and knowledge of nutrition
   4. Mental status, including cognitive impairment, anxiety, and depression
   5. Resources to buy, store, and prepare food
   6. Related signs and symptoms such as dyspnea and/or fatigue
   7. Social supports
B. Objective data
   1. Height and weight
   2. Anthropometric measurements
   3. Examination of skin, hair, nails, and oral cavity
   4. Examination of cranial nerves I (olfactory), V (trigeminal), IX (glossopharyngeal), and X (vagus)
   5. Evaluation of ability to feed self
   6. Laboratory data including blood cell count and serum albumin level

Nursing Diagnosis

Altered Nutrition: Less than Body Requirements

Goals

After discussing and validating the findings of assessment and the nursing diagnosis, the client and/or care partner and the nurse will select interventions to

A. Preserve lean body mass
B. Provide adequate levels of all nutrients

Considerations for Nursing Care and Health Teaching

A. Minimize factors contributing to anorexia
   1. For alterations in the sense of smell
      a. Hyperosmia (increased sense of smell): avoid cooking odors by keeping windows open and the home well aerated; encourage meals that include cold foods
      b. Hyposmia (decreased sense of smell): use spices such as basil, oregano, rosemary, thyme, cloves, mint, cinnamon, or lemon juice to enhance smell
   2. For alterations in sense of taste (especially related to distaste for red meat)
      a. Marinate meat before cooking in commercial marinade, wine, or vinegar
      b. As substitutes for red meat, use other protein sources such as eggs, peanut butter, tofu, cheeses, poultry, or fish
   3. For persons living alone or experiencing fatigue or depression:
      a. Eat small meals frequently throughout the day; try to eat "by the clock"
      b. Include high-calorie snacks and/or commercially prepared supplements (liquids or bars)
      c. Indulge desires for favorite foods
      d. Consume more nutrient-dense foods and bever-

ages, rather than filling up on low-calorie items
   e. Drink liquids a half hour before eating instead of with meals
   f. Prepare meals (such as soups or casseroles) ahead of time so that they can be divided into individual servings and frozen until ready to use
   g. Keep easy-to-prepare foods on hand, such as frozen dinners, canned foods, and eggs
   h. Make food presentation and service appealing
   i. Encourage dining with friends or family in pleasant surroundings
   j. Get family members and friends involved in meal preparation; the warm atmosphere that they can provide may stimulate the patient's appetite
   k. Utilize home food delivery service (e.g., Meals on Wheels programs)
   l. Direct the patient to support services in the community; sources of information on available food programs may include outpatient dietitians at local hospitals or public health department nutritionists
   m. Carry powdered forms of liquid dietary supplements because they may be easier to carry than ready-to-use forms in cans
B. Minimize factors related to difficulty in chewing, dysphagia (difficulty in swallowing), or odynophagia (painful swallowing)
   1. Avoid
      a. Rough foods such as raw fruits and vegetables
      b. Spicy, acidic, or salty foods
      c. Alcohol or tobacco
      d. Excessively hot or cold foods
      e. Sticky foods such as peanut butter and slippery foods such as gelatin, bologna, and elbow macaroni
   2. Encourage
      a. Eating foods at room temperature
      b. Choosing mild foods and drinks (e.g., apple juice rather than orange juice)
      c. Eating dry-grain foods such as breads, crackers, and cookies after softening in milk, tea, or other mild beverage
      d. Eating nonabrasive, easy-to-swallow foods such as ice cream, pudding, well-cooked eggs, noodle dishes, baked fish, and soft cheese
      e. Eating Popsicles to numb pain
      f. Using straw when drinking
      g. Tilting head back or moving it forward to make swallowing easier
C. Minimize factors related to inability to obtain food:
   1. Evaluate financial resources and the need for referral for Medicaid, food stamps, and other services
   2. Evaluate the home and the client's ability to prepare and obtain food, looking for such factors as
      a. Absence of cooking facilities (e.g., living in a shelter or hotel for homeless persons)
      b. Need for alternative housing arrangements

   3. Explore community resources that provide free meals
D. Discuss nutritional requirements for persons with HIV disease, including
   1. High-protein sources and ways to increase protein intake by
      a. Adding skim milk powder to regulate whole milk
      b. Preparing canned creamed soups with heavy cream instead of water or milk
      c. Increasing intake of peanut butter and eating it on whole-wheat bread
      d. Adding pasteurized processed cheeses to soups and vegetables
      e. Eating hard-boiled eggs for snacks
   2. Increasing caloric intake by
      a. Using extra peanut butter, cream cheese, sugar, honey, sour cream, and mayonnaise
      b. Substituting heavy creams for milk in coffee, tea, soups, and other foods
      c. Eating sweets for snacks
      d. Drinking commercially prepared liquid dietary supplements
      e. Making a liquid nutritional supplement at home by mixing:
         (1) A 1-quart packet of powdered milk with
         (2) One quart of whole milk and
         (3) Four packets of a flavored instant breakfast mix
            Note: This powdered package recipe is significantly easier to travel with than ready-to-use canned preparations.
      f. Eating small, frequent meals instead of a few large meals
   3. Reviewing a balanced diet selection for a 24-hour menu plan
E. Review essential elements of a low-microbial diet and food safety and preparation

NOTE WELL: The nutritional teaching should, as much as possible, follow the client's usual pattern of food intake rather than expect the client to follow a totally new, unfamiliar prescription for meal planning.

Evaluation

The client will

A. Demonstrate weight maintenance or gain
B. Identify factors related to anorexia, difficulty in chewing, dysphagia, or odynophagia
C. Identify sufficient resources to obtain and prepare food—or social work intervention has been established to obtain food stamps or public assistance
D. Identify means of increasing protein and calorie intake
E. Identify key concepts in planning a low-microbial diet
F. Select a balanced 24-hour menu

■ Modifications for Elderly Clients

People older than 50 years account for 11% of the AIDS cases reported in the United States. Providing nursing care to this specific population of HIV-infected individuals poses numerous unique challenges. They are from generations in which open discussion of sex was taboo. Gay men and lesbians born in the 1930s and 1940s grew up during a period when they could be arrested by police just for gathering in a public place. Having experienced such a repressive societal attitude, they are often reluctant to discuss sexual matters, which makes HIV prevention efforts more difficult. Likewise, older heterosexual men and women are also often reluctant to discuss the fact that they may be sexually active, because society tends to think that sexual desires and feelings disappear after age 50 years. Therefore, many older people with HIV/AIDS are guilt ridden, and when they are diagnosed with the disease they find a need to tell healthcare providers that they were infected through a transfusion, viewing this a more socially acceptable explanation.

The literature has cited numerous instances in which older adults are misdiagnosed as having simple pneumonia and Alzheimer's disease, when in fact they had PCP and ADC. HIV risk assessment, including sexual history taking, should be collected on all patients regardless of their age.

Understanding these barriers to communication will assist the nurse in establishing an environment in which all matters related to health can be discussed openly and nonjudgmentally. Older persons may also have difficulty speaking openly with younger nurses, who may be the same age as their children, grandchildren, nieces, or nephews.

The co-morbid conditions encountered in the older person with HIV/AIDS will include commonly diagnosed conditions of the elderly such as cardiac disease, diabetes, cancer, and arthritis. The presence of these conditions along with the fact that older people with HIV/AIDS have a shorter survival, means that the care management is more complex. They may also be more sensitive to prescribed medications and will require more frequent monitoring than younger patients.

■ Surgical Management of HIV/AIDS

The most frequent surgical procedures performed on people with HIV/AIDS are the insertion of venous access devices and diagnostic biopsies for neoplasms and infections. Additional surgery may be necessary for AIDS-related conditions such as a cholecystectomy for a gallbladder with active CMV infection that is causing intractable pain, or removal of obstructing tumors of the bowel. Likewise, during the course of HIV illness, patients may sustain trauma or experience other common problems, such as appendicitis, and require surgery.

Hypersensitivity Disorders

Although the immune system protects the body from harmful invaders, an overactive or overzealous response is detrimental. Overreaction to a substance, or hypersensitivity, is often referred to as an allergic response. Although "allergy" is widely used, the word "hypersensitiv-

ity" is more appropriate; this term designates an increased immune response to the presence of an antigen (in this case referred to as an allergen) that results in tissue destruction.

Factors Influencing Hypersensitivity

The occurrence and intensity of hypersensitivity responses depend on several factors: host defenses, the nature of the allergen, the concentration of the allergen, the route of allergen entrance into the body, and the exposure to the allergen.

Host Defenses. Some people are more prone to hypersensitivity than others for reasons that are unclear. About 1 in 4 Americans have serious allergies. The term *atopy* is used for a genetically determined state of hypersensitivity to allergens. Persons with atopy produce IgE antibodies to allergens.

Nature of the Allergen. Like all antigens, allergens are usually high molecular weight proteins. However, some haptens (e.g., penicillin) are highly allergic. A hapten is a low molecular weight substance that binds with an antigenic substance to elicit an allergic response.

Concentration of the Allergen. Higher concentrations usually result in hypersensitivity responses of greater intensity.

Route of Allergen Entrance into the Body. Routes include inhalation, injection, ingestion, or direct contact. Most allergens are inhaled.

Exposure to the Allergen. Hypersensitivity responses occur after initial exposure. The first contact with the substance causes a primary immune response, slower and less severe than the secondary immune response, which occurs with subsequent exposure to the allergen. Also, if much time elapses between each contact with the allergen (i.e., several years), the immune response diminishes.

Diagnostic Findings

Laboratory tests also provide valuable data, especially when they are evaluated with consideration of a history of allergic responses. Common tests include assays of IgE levels: the radioallergosorbent test, radioimmunosorbent test, and paper radioimmunosorbent test. These tests reveal elevated levels of IgE, but a normal or even decreased level may occur in IgE-mediated sensitivities. The last two tests are more sensitive. Elevated serum eosinophil levels also suggest hypersensitivities.

Pulmonary function studies may also be done to evaluate the status of the respiratory system in asthma. Ventilatory capacity and lung volume are both abnormal in asthma. This test can also indicate the presence of complications such as pneumothorax.

In addition to blood tests, skin testing confirms sensitivity to a specific allergen. These tests involve placing a known antigen on or directly below the skin (intradermal) to check for the presence of antibodies. The antigen can be applied in one of three methods: scratch test, patch test, or intradermal test. In the first (also known as a tine or prick test), the allergen is applied to a superficial scratch that cuts the outer layer of skin. For a patch test, the antigen is applied directly to the skin and then covered with a gauze dressing. Intradermal testing involves injecting a small amount of the antigen into the intradermal layer of the skin. Intradermal testing is the most accurate method, but carries a higher risk of severe allergic reactions.

Nurses often administer skin tests and interpret test results. To interpret results, observe for the following reactions. An immediate reaction (i.e., appearing within 10–20 minutes after the injection) marked by erythema and wheal formation denotes a positive reaction. Positive reactions indicate antibody response to previous exposure to this antigen and suggest the person is allergic to the particular substance causing the reaction (Fig. 27–1). Negative reactions may be inconclusive, indicating the need for further assessment. Negative results may indicate that (1) antibodies have not formed to this antigen, (2) the antigen was deposited too deeply into the skin (e.g., subcutaneously), or (3) the client is immunosuppressed from disease or therapies (e.g., chemotherapy, steroids, radiation therapy).

Problems arising from skin testing range from minor itching to anaphylaxis. Itching and discomfort at the injection site, for example, are common and can be relieved by the application of cool compresses and topical steroids. Ulceration of the injection site is best treated by keeping the area clean and dry.

Anaphylactic shock is a rare but potentially lethal complication of skin testing. A client with a history of an anaphylactic reaction to a substance should never be skin-tested for an allergy to that substance. This is especially true of allergens such as penicillin which can produce lethal anaphylaxis in susceptible clients. Anaphylaxis is treated with emergency oxygen administration, epinephrine subcutaneously, intravenous aminophylline, and antihistamines intravenously, as necessary.

Food allergies can be tested by skin testing or by either food challenges or an elimination diet. In the challenge test, suspected foods are given to the client in progressively larger doses until a reaction occurs. Manifestations of a reaction range from the typical erythema, itching, and rash to vomiting or diarrhea. Manifestations such as fatigue, depression, or restlessness are not conclusive of an allergy. In the elimination diet, foods are eliminated from the diet one by one until the manifestations are relieved. This may indicate allergies to food additives or the foods themselves.

Pathophysiology

There are two general categories of hypersensitivity reaction: immediate and delayed. These designations are based on the rapidity of the immune response. Recent research, however, suggests there is a biochemical and a cellular component in both types of reaction. Immunoglobulins mediate immediate reactions, whereas T cells govern delayed hypersensitivity responses. Humoral responses occur more rapidly than cell-mediated responses.

In addition to the delayed and immediate categories, hypersensitivity reactions are divided into four main types (Table 27–1): (I) immediate or anaphylactic, (II) cy-

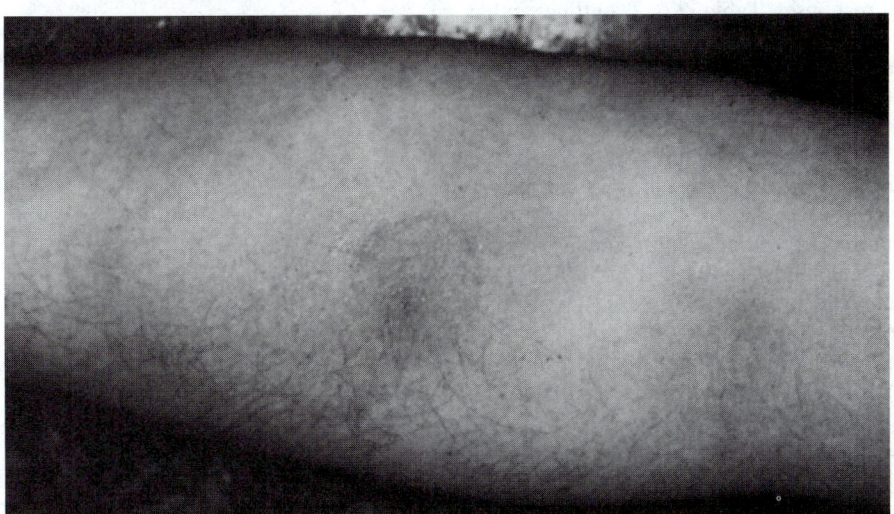

Figure 27–1. Delayed hypersensitivity reaction. This positive reaction to intradermal challenge with tuberculin supplies a convenient window through which to observe the cell-mediated inflammatory processes at work. (From Dwyer, J. M. [1983]. The cell-mediated immune system. In Dwyer, J. M., et al. (Eds.), *Management of the immune-compromised patient.* Berkeley, CA: Pharmaceutical Division of Miles Laboratories.)

Table 27–1. Types of Hypersensitivity Reactions

Type		Causative Component	Pathologic Process	Reaction
I	Immediate/anaphylactic	IgE	Mast cell degranulation ↓ Histamine and leukotriene release	Anaphylaxis Atopic diseases Skin reactions
II	Cytolytic/cytotoxic	IgG IgM Complement	Complement fixation ↓ Cell lysis	ABO incompatibility Drug-induced hemolytic anemia
III	Immune complex	Antigen-antibody complexes	Deposition in vessels and tissue walls ↓ Inflammation	Arthus reaction Serum sickness Systemic lupus erythematosus Acute glomerulonephritis
IV	Cell-mediated delayed	Sensitized T cells	Lymphokine release	Tuberculosis Contact dermatitis Transplant rejection

tolytic or cytotoxic, (III) immune complex, and (IV) cell-mediated delayed.

■ Type I (Anaphylactic) Hypersensitivity

This response is a rapidly occurring reaction mediated by IgE antibodies. The allergen stimulates IgE production, which in turn causes mast cell degranulation. Mast cells release histamine and leukotrienes (formerly slow-reacting substances of anaphylaxis [SRS-A]). Mast cells cause vasodilation and increased capillary permeability, which promotes fluid loss into the interstitial space. Leukotrienes cause spasm of the bronchial smooth muscles, which elicits an asthmalike response. Table 27–2 outlines other chemical mediators of these reactions.

Anaphylactic shock represents the most severe form of type I hypersensitivity. Initial manifestations of anaphylaxis may include localized itching, edema, and sneezing. These seemingly innocuous problems are followed in minutes by wheezing, dyspnea, cyanosis, and circulatory shock.

Anaphylaxis requires immediate emergency treatment. Common causes of anaphylaxis are listed in Table 27–3. See Chapter 88 for a discussion of emergency care of clients with anaphylaxis.

Prevention is the key in anaphylaxis. A careful nursing history reveals individual susceptibility to such reactions. Always mark known allergies clearly on the permanent health record, nursing Kardexes, and nursing care plans.

Special identification bracelets worn by the client at all times or signs placed on the client's bed also help. If the physician suspects a client might be allergic to a certain medication or substance, the physician will order an intradermal skin test. A localized reaction to such a test may be an indication that a more severe reaction will occur if the full dose is given.

Atopic allergies are less severe forms of type I response. These reactions are common: 15% to 25% of people in developed countries suffer from atopic allergies. Atopic allergies include hay fever (allergic rhinitis), some types of bronchial asthma, atopic dermatitis, some food

Table 27–2. Chemical Mediators of the Allergic Reaction

Mediator	Function
Histamine	Increased vascular permeability → erythema Increased respiratory airway resistance → increased cAMP
Leukotrienes (formerly SRS-A)	Increased vascular permeability Increased smooth muscle contraction
Eosinophil chemotactic factor of anaphylaxis (ECF-A)	Increased eosinophils to site
Neutrophil chemotactic factor	Increased neutrophils to site
Heparin	Anticomplement action Anticoagulation
Bradykinin	Slowed smooth muscle contraction Increased vascular permeability Increased mucous secretions Stimulation of pain fibers
Platelet-activating factor	Secretion and aggregation of platelets

cAMP, cyclic adenosine monophosphate; SRS-A, slow-reacting substance of anaphylaxis.

and drug allergies, and urticaria. Urticaria is an area of localized edema and itching resulting from exposure to an allergen, most commonly a food or drug. Table 27–4 lists some clinical manifestations of allergic reactions to selected medications.

■ Type II (Cytolytic or Cytotoxic) Hypersensitivity

These reactions are complement-dependent and thus involve IgG or IgM antibodies. The antigen-antibody complex and complement attach to a cell, usually a circulating blood cell, with resultant cell lysis. During blood transfusion, blood group incompatibility causes cell lysis, which results in a transfusion reaction. The antigen responsible for initiating the reaction is a part of the donor red blood cell membrane.

Manifestations of a transfusion reaction result from intravascular hemolysis of red blood cells. They include:

● Headache and back pain (flank)
● Chest pain similar to angina
● Nausea and vomiting
● Tachycardia and hypotension
● Hematuria
● Urticaria

Transfusions of more than 100 ml of incompatible blood can result in severe, permanent renal damage, circulatory shock, and death. Therefore, stop the transfusion immediately, maintain an open intravenous line, check the client's vital signs, and notify the physician immediately when these problems develop. For detailed nursing interventions related to transfusion reactions, see Chapter 53.

■ Type III (Immune Complex) Hypersensitivity

Immune complex disease results from the formation or deposition of antigen-antibody complexes in tissues. The molecular size of the antigen-antibody complexes is an important feature in eliciting immune complex disease. Larger complexes are rapidly cleared by phagocytic cells. The smaller complexes formed in antigen excess persist longer in the circulation because they are not as easily captured by phagocytic cells in the spleen and liver. Inflammation results and leads to acute or chronic disease of the organ system in which the immune complexes were deposited.

Immune complex–mediated inflammation is produced by IgG or IgM antibodies, antigen, and complement. The mediators of inflammatory injury include the complement cleavage peptides, which can degranulate mast cells and basophils. Also, release of lysosomal granules from white blood cells and macrophages causes further tissue injury.

The antigen may be tissue-fixed or released locally, as in Goodpasture's syndrome, in which circulating antibodies react with autologous antigens in the glomerular basement membranes of the kidneys causing inflammation of the glomerulus. Alternatively, antigen-antibody complexes may form in the joint space, with resultant synovitis, as in rheumatoid arthritis. The antigen may also be circulating, as in serum sickness. Antigen-antibody complexes are formed in the bloodstream and get trapped in capillaries or deposited in vessel walls, causing urticaria, arthritis, arteritis, or glomerulonephritis. The Arthus reaction is a localized area of tissue necrosis that results from immune complex hypersensitivity.

Serum sickness is another type III hypersensitivity response, which develops 6 to 14 days after injection with foreign serum. Deposition of complexes on vessel walls causes complement activation with resultant edema, fever,

Table 27–3. Common Agents Causing Anaphylaxis	
Drugs	
Penicillins (most common)	Vancomycin
Cephalosporins	Amphotericin B
Tetracyclines	Polymyxin
Streptomycin	Bacitracin
Kanamycin	Aspirin, other
Neomycin	anti-inflammatory agents
Heparin	Colchicine
Protamine	Tranquilizers
Foods	
Seafoods	Citrus fruits
Eggs	Strawberries
Nuts	Legumes
Insect Venoms	
Hymenoptera (honeybees, wasps, yellow jackets, hornets, fire ants)	
Biologicals	
Heterologous antisera (especially equine)	
Enzymes	
Hormones	
Vaccines (especially egg-cultured types)	
Blood Products	
Plasma	
Cryoprecipitate	
Whole blood	
Gamma globulin	
Allergen Extracts	
Skin-testing agents	
Desensitization	
Diagnostic Agents	
Sulfobromophthalein	
Iodinated contrast media	

Table 27–4. Clinical Manifestations of Allergic Reactions to Selected Medications

Drug	Systemic Manifestations	Cutaneous Manifestations
Penicillin	Anaphylaxis Serum sickness syndrome Pulmonary alterations (e.g., bronchial asthma) Vasculitis	Contact dermatitis Urticaria Rash Pruritus
Sulfonamides	Hepatic alterations Vasculitis Polyarteritis Renal disturbances Hematologic alterations	Rash Pruritus Exfoliative dermatitis Erythema multiforme Purpuric eruptions Photosensitivity
Salicylates	Bronchial asthma	Angioneurotic edema Urticaria Pruritis
Para-aminosalicylic acid	Fever Löffler's syndrome (pulmonary infiltrate with eosinophilia) Hepatic alterations Hematologic alterations	—
Phenytoin sodium (Dilantin)	Eosinophilia Lymphadenopathy Hepatic alterations	Erythema multiforme
Barbiturates	—	Rash Exfoliative dermatitis Fixed eruptions

inflammation of blood vessels and joints, and urticaria. Today, classic serum sickness is rare because large doses of heterologous sera (e.g., horse antisera to human lymphocytes) are seldom used.

However, the serum sickness–like reaction may occur after administration of such medications as penicillin, sulfonamides, streptomycin, thiouracils, and hydantoin compounds. Rather than being dominated by cutaneous vasculitis, these reactions more often manifest with fever, arthralgias, lymphadenopathy, and urticaria. This illness is usually benign and self-limiting. It resolves after the offending medication is discontinued.

Nursing care of the client with serum sickness depends on the severity of the reaction. For a mild reaction, care includes control of fever and pain with aspirin and antihistamines. A severe reaction may require steroids for control of the problem.

Serum sickness can be prevented by avoiding allergen exposure. Nursing assessment includes obtaining an allergy history and information about previous reactions to drugs or vaccines. Document findings in the client's chart, care plan, Kardex, and medication record so that risk of subsequent exposure is minimized.

■ Type IV (Cell-Mediated or Delayed) Hypersensitivity

In cell-mediated hypersensitivity, sensitized T cells respond to antigens by releasing lymphokines, which direct phagocytic cell activity. This reaction occurs 24 to 72 hours after exposure to an allergen. Delayed hypersensitivity is induced by chronic infection (e.g., tuberculosis) or by contact sensitivities, as in contact dermatitis.

Type IV reactions occur after the intradermal injection of tuberculosis antigen or purified protein derivative. If the client has been sensitized to tuberculosis, sensitized T cells react with the antigen at the injection site. The reaction leads to edema and fibrin deposits, which result in the induration characteristic of a positive tuberculosis reaction.

Graft-versus-host disease (GVHD) and transplant rejection are also type IV reactions. In GVHD, immunocompetent donor bone marrow cells (the graft) react against various antigens in the bone marrow recipient (the host), which results in a variety of clinical manifestations including skin, gastrointestinal, and hepatic lesions. Transplant rejection and GVHD are discussed later.

Contact dermatitis is another type IV reaction which occurs after sensitization to an allergen, commonly a cosmetic, adhesive, topical medication, drug additive (such as lanolin added to lotions), or plant toxin (such as poison ivy). With the first exposure, no reaction occurs; however, antigens are formed. On subsequent exposures, hypersensitivity reactions are triggered, which leads to itching, erythema, and vesicular lesions.

Community and Self-Care

Allergies are chronic problems that require prolonged and often multiple treatments. The client often requires a combination of treatments ranging from avoidance of known allergens to environmental control and immunotherapy.

Avoidance of the allergen is often the easiest, cheapest, and safest way of dealing with allergies. However, identification of the specific allergen is sometimes difficult, especially if the client refuses or cannot afford or locate allergen-testing services. Sometimes, even if the allergen can be identified, complete avoidance may not be possible, as with pollens, dust, and some food additives.

Environmental control sometimes helps eliminate airborne allergens. Figure 27–2 illustrates ways to desensitize a room. These environmental controls, combined with air filters that remove small particles from the air, can help eliminate many allergens.

Clients with atopic allergies can have their manifestations alleviated or controlled by many prescription and over-the-counter medications. Usually, clients will self-administer these agents, although in some settings the nurse or a family member administers them. Instructing clients about these medications, however, is always an important nursing responsibility.

Antihistamines

Antihistamines are the major group of prescription and over-the-counter drugs used to alleviate allergic manifestations. These medications relieve sneezing, rhinorrhea, itching, and other manifestations of allergic rhinitis. Newer agents (such as terfenadine, Seldane) do not cause the drowsiness that limited the use of older medications.

Decongestants

Decongestants (oral sympathomimetics) help relieve nasal congestion. These drugs can be combined with antihistamines to treat multiple manifestations of the allergy. The nasal sprays of these agents can be used for several days to treat nasal congestion; however, overuse of these agents can lead to recurrence of congestion and exacerbation of the nasal manifestations secondary to chemical rhinitis.

Steroids

Corticosteroids, anti-inflammatory agents, and immunosuppressants can be used to treat a variety of manifestations associated with allergies. Topical steroids can be used to treat dermatitis and other skin manifestations (e.g., urticaria). Beclomethasone dipropionate (Beconase) is a steroidal aerosol useful in treating allergic rhinitis. It has fewer side effects than dexamethasone. This drug is also available via inhalation for asthma.

Aerosols

Cromolyn sodium is a topical or aerosol medication used to treat allergic rhinitis and asthma. It helps prevent the release of chemical mediators, such as histamine and leukotrienes, from mast cells.

Desensitization

Immunotherapy (sometimes called desensitization therapy) is designed for type I, IgE-mediated hypersensitivity reactions. Precise doses of allergens are injected at intervals over a prolonged period. The doses are increased gradually over time. Immunotherapy increases IgG antibody levels and may increase suppressor T-cell function. It also decreases IgE binding to allergens. The decrease in IgE binding occurs because allergens bind more readily to IgG. Therefore, immunotherapy mitigates the hypersensitivity response. Although there is some controversy regarding the efficacy of this treatment, it is widely used. The greatest success has been achieved with allergic rhinitis (hay fever) and Hymenoptera sensitivity (bee, yellow jacket, wasp, and hornet stings).

Nurses often administer these injections and assess and treat side effects. Clients are asked to wait at least 20 minutes after receiving the injections so immediate reactions can be treated. Side effects are similar to those seen in skin testing. Some clients are taught to administer the desensitization injections themselves. In this case, teach clients the proper injection technique and the signs of any untoward reactions to the medication.

Organ Transplantation

Histocompatibility

With recent advances in technology and immunology, organ and tissue transplantation is becoming commonplace. Thus, nurses need to (1) gain a clear understanding of the immunology on which this intervention is based and (2) learn how to assess and provide intervention for clients with transplants. See the specific chapters (e.g., Chapter 57 for renal transplants) for specific information on each type of transplant.

There are several different types of transplants. *Syngeneic* transplants are between genetically identical members of the same species (identical twins); they are also

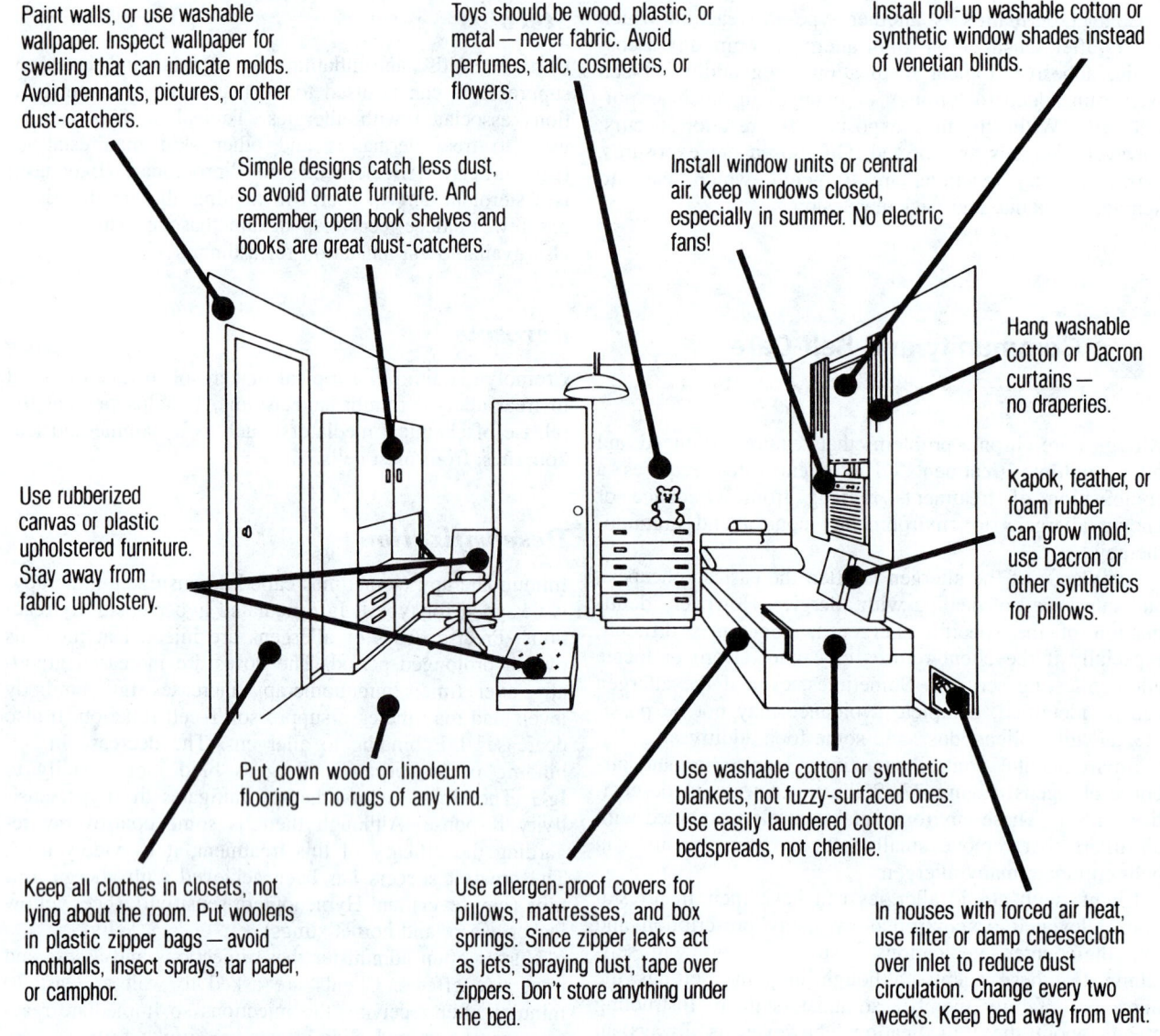

Paint walls, or use washable wallpaper. Inspect wallpaper for swelling that can indicate molds. Avoid pennants, pictures, or other dust-catchers.

Toys should be wood, plastic, or metal — never fabric. Avoid perfumes, talc, cosmetics, or flowers.

Install roll-up washable cotton or synthetic window shades instead of venetian blinds.

Simple designs catch less dust, so avoid ornate furniture. And remember, open book shelves and books are great dust-catchers.

Install window units or central air. Keep windows closed, especially in summer. No electric fans!

Hang washable cotton or Dacron curtains — no draperies.

Use rubberized canvas or plastic upholstered furniture. Stay away from fabric upholstery.

Kapok, feather, or foam rubber can grow mold; use Dacron or other synthetics for pillows.

Put down wood or linoleum flooring — no rugs of any kind.

Use washable cotton or synthetic blankets, not fuzzy-surfaced ones. Use easily laundered cotton bedspreads, not chenille.

Keep all clothes in closets, not lying about the room. Put woolens in plastic zipper bags — avoid mothballs, insect sprays, tar paper, or camphor.

Use allergen-proof covers for pillows, mattresses, and box springs. Since zipper leaks act as jets, spraying dust, tape over zippers. Don't store anything under the bed.

In houses with forced air heat, use filter or damp cheesecloth over inlet to reduce dust circulation. Change every two weeks. Keep bed away from vent.

Figure 27–2. Controlling the environment of a room. (Courtesy of A. H. Robins Company, Richmond, VA.)

called *isografts*. *Allogeneic* transplants are between individuals of the same species (e.g., human to human). *Autologous* transplants are grafts in the body of the same individual (e.g., a skin graft from leg to hand). *Xenogeneic* transplants are between individuals of different species (e.g., pigskin grafts).

In all cases of graft rejection, the cause is incompatibility of cell-surface antigens. As expected, there is a better chance of graft acceptance with autologous or syngeneic transplants, because the cell-surface antigens are identical.

A major role of the immune system is to distinguish between self and nonself. This fact is the major problem facing the candidate for transplantation: the immunologic response of the client to the donor's tissues. This ability to distinguish between self and nonself is central to proper immune function.

The identification process causes problems, however, when a tissue or organ from one client or animal (donor)

is transplanted to another client or animal (recipient). In the immunocomponent recipient, the client's immune system recognizes the transplanted tissue or organ as "foreign" (nonself) and produces antibodies and sensitized lymphocytes against it. The cell-mediated delayed hypersensitivity response causes damage to or destruction of the donated tissue. *Graft rejection* is the term describing the immune responses leading to graft destruction by the recipient's immune system.

The closer the match between the donor's and recipient's antigens, the less chance rejection will occur. Although many hundreds of antigens may differ between donor and recipient, certain antigens are critical to a successful transplant. These are (1) ABO and Rh antigens present on red blood cells and (2) histocompatibility antigens. Most important in this latter group is the human leukocyte antigen (HLA). To increase compatibility and reduce the chance of graft rejection, physicians and scientists attempt to match donors and recipients who have similar immune characteristics, especially those involving the ABO, Rh, and HLA systems.

Genes in the area known as the major histocompatibility complex (MHC) on the sixth chromosome contain the human histocompatibility antigens. All people inherit one MHC zone from each parent. Histocompatibility antigens reside on the surface of most body cells. There are five specific HLAs within the MHC: HLA-A, HLA-B, HLA-C, HLA-D, and HLA-DR. HLA-A, HLA-B, and HLA-C are referred to as class I antigens and the others as class II antigens. Class I antigens are those recognized by the host during the rejection process. Class II antigens are found mainly on B cells, activated T cells, and macrophages. These antigens act to stimulate the proliferation of T helper cells, activating T killer cells, and antibody-producing B cells.

The process of finding compatible donors and recipients is called tissue typing. After tissue typing of the donor and recipient, the laboratory performs a matching procedure called mixed lymphocyte culture. Various lymphocyte antibodies form after blood transfusions, pregnancy, (prior) exposure to foreign bodies, or infections. In the mixed lymphocyte culture, lymphocytes from the donor are mixed with serum from the recipient and then observed for immune responses. This test can determine whether antibodies incompatible with the donor have been formed by the recipient (a positive crossmatch). If the crossmatch is positive, the transplant will fail; therefore, a negative test is necessary for a successful transplant.

Graft Rejection

Rejection is the body's normal immune response to invasion of foreign tissue (the transplanted tissue or organ). Although this response is normal, it is not the desired response after a transplant. The physiologic mechanisms in rejection (the normal immune response) involve B lymphocytes forming antibodies and T lymphocytes producing cell-mediated immunity. Acute rejection is caused by the T-lymphocyte activity and chronic rejection by that of B lymphocytes.

There are three basic kinds of rejection: hyperacute, acute, and chronic.

▪ Hyperacute Rejection

Allografts transplanted into presensitized recipients may be rejected very quickly. This rejection may occur from the time of the transplant up to 48 hours after the transplant. These recipients have performed cytotoxic antibodies to donor antigens as well as sensitized lymphocytes, which reject the graft immediately. Rejection occurs before vascularization takes place.

The manifestations of hyperacute rejection include general malaise and high fever. In renal transplants, the kidney becomes infiltrated with leukocytes, which results in thrombosis of arterioles and glomerular capillaries. In car-

diac transplants, the heart becomes hard and a mottled purple.

Hyperacute rejection is not treatable; removal of the rejected tissue or organ is the only way to stop the reaction. The client must then be maintained until another transplant can be arranged.

▪ Acute Rejection

This occurs usually within 3 months but may occur as late as 2 years after the transplant. The graft becomes vascularized in 2 to 3 days. In acute rejection, the response is primarily cell-mediated. The reaction begins when the recipient becomes sensitized to the donor antigens. Memory cells are formed that can trigger rapid rejection of a subsequent transplant of the same histocompatibility type.

In 6 to 10 days, the first signs of rejection may be observed. Sensitized lymphocytes and macrophages appear at the graft site. Later, the vascular bed itself begins to deteriorate, and the graft becomes necrotic.

Acute rejection is treatable with immunosuppressant medications including corticosteroids, azathioprine, cyclophosphamide, antithymocyte globulin (ATG) and antilymphocyte globulin (ALG), cyclosporine, OKT3, and tacrolimus (FK506, Prograf) (Table 27–5). Intravenous methylprednisolone sodium succinate (Solu-Medrol) is usually given first with good response (i.e., rejection reversed). Repeated episodes of acute rejection can lead to permanent damage of the organ.

▪ Chronic Rejection

Months or even years after the transplant, function of the transplanted tissue or organ may deteriorate gradually. The problem is a recurring and continuing one. Antibodies and complement play a role in this type of rejection, causing arteriolar narrowing due to deposition of fibrin, platelets, and complement along vessel walls. The body tries to repair the endothelial damage that leads to intimal proliferation, necrosis, and collagen deposits, which further blocks circulation.

The manifestations of chronic rejection are related to deterioration of organ function. In renal transplants, there is a gradual increase in serum creatinine and blood urea nitrogen, electrolyte imbalance, weight gain, hypertension, decreasing urine output, and peripheral edema. In cardiac transplants, there is myocardial fibrosis and increasing blockage of the coronary arteries, which leads to myocardial ischemia and infarction. In liver transplants, there is progressive thickening of the hepatic arteries and narrowing of the bile ducts, which leads to progressive liver failure. In pancreatic rejections, the vessels begin to thicken, which leads to fibrosis and a decrease in insulin secretion and hyperglycemia.

Clients with chronic rejection may be asymptomatic. Others will demonstrate manifestations directly related to failure of the transplanted organ.

Treatment of chronic rejection is not usually successful. Deterioration is gradual and progressive. Antirejection

Table 27–5. Medications Used in Transplants

Medication	Action	Side Effects	Nursing Implications
Azathioprine (Imuran)	Inhibits DNA and RNA; blocks antibody production	Leukopenia, bone marrow depression, pancreatitis, liver dysfunction, immunosuppression	Monitor for manifestations of liver dysfunction; monitor CBC; warn client to avoid people with known infections; teach client to report signs of even mild infection; avoid IM injections if client is thrombocytopenic
Cyclosporine (Sandimmune)	Inhibits action of T lymphocytes and cell-mediated immunity	Hypertension, tremor, infection, gum hyperplasia, hirsutism, nephrotoxicity, hepatotoxicity, flushing	Monitor BUN and creatinine, liver function studies; always give in conjunction with corticosteroids; monitor levels of drug because oral absorption is erratic; give dose daily, at same time of day; give with meal to decrease nausea; comes suspended in olive oil, so administer in juice or milk, in glass so container does not absorb drug; emphasize to client importance of never varying or stopping medication without physician's approval
Antithymocyte globulin (ATG) Antilymphocyte globulin (ALG)	Either alters T-cell function or eliminates antigen-reactive T cells to inhibit cell-mediated immunity	Leukopenia, hemolysis, hypotension, chest pain, dyspnea, laryngospasms, nausea, vomiting, serum sickness (horse serum), anaphylaxis	Client should be skin-tested before first dose; do not use in clients allergic to horse serum; solution very heat-sensitive, keep refrigerated; monitor client for signs of infection; use filter when administering drug

BUN, blood urea nitrogen; CBC, complete blood count; IM, intramuscular.

medications may slow the process, so it is years before the organ fails completely and retransplantation is required.

Graft-Versus-Host Disease

A different type of rejection occurs when the transplanted material is an allogeneic bone marrow transplant. GVHD is a variation of the traditional graft rejection, but involves the same immunologic principles. GVHD occurs with bone marrow transplantation in which immunocompetent donor cells are infused into an immunosuppressed recipient. Thus, if rejection occurs, it is the immunocompetent T lymphocytes from the graft (i.e., the donated marrow) rather than the host cells that cause the problem.

GVHD has acute and chronic forms. Acute GVHD manifests itself as early as 1 to 100 days after transplant, with a peak time of onset in 30 to 50 days. Chronic GVHD usually occurs or persists later than 100 days. The major organs affected by GVHD are the skin, liver, and gastrointestinal tract. Skin involvement often begins with an erythematous rash, which may progress to a severe, sloughing stage. Figure 27–3 shows erythroderma of the trunk and extremities.

Abnormalities in liver function tests (as evidenced by increased liver enzymes and bilirubin), right upper quadrant pain, hepatomegaly, and jaundice signal liver involvement. Gastrointestinal tract manifestations of GVHD include nausea and vomiting, mild to severe diarrhea, malabsorption, ileus, and sloughing of intestinal mucosa.

Chronic GVHD resembles autoimmune collagen-vascular disease, such as lupus erythematosus. Skin changes resemble scleroderma-like fibrosis. The same organs are affected in chronic and acute forms; however, in chronic GVHD, the changes are less than in the acute form.

Prevention of GVHD is similar to that of transplant rejection and involves immunosuppression of the recipi-

Medication	Action	Side Effects	Nursing Implications
Muromonab-CD3 (OKT3)	IgG antibody, reacts in T-lymphocyte membrane to block T-cell function and proliferation; may reverse rejection, but carcinogenic and used with caution	Chest pain, fever, nausea, vomiting, severe pulmonary edema, dyspnea, increased incidence of malignant lymphomas	Used only in cases of acute rejection not responding to other agents; monitor cardiopulmonary system closely during administration; assess for signs of fluid overload; administer antipyretic before drug to decrease chills and fever
Methylprednisolone sodium succinate (Solu-Medrol)	Anti-inflammatory, prevents leukocyte infiltration during rejection, decreases antibody production and inhibits antigen-antibody reaction	Infection, delayed wound healing, peptic ulcers, hypertension, congestive heart failure, hypokalemia, weight gain, hyperglycemia; withdrawal symptoms if stopped suddenly	Monitor client for infection; teach client to prevent infection; tell client not to decrease or stop dose suddenly because of possibly life-threatening reaction; treat side effects symptomatically; give with food or antacids to prevent ulcers.
Cyclophosphamide (Cytoxan)	Action similar to azathioprine, used mainly when cyclosporine or azathioprine not tolerated	Bone marrow depression, leukopenia, nausea, vomiting, hemorrhagic cystitis, alopecia	Monitor for infection; teach client to avoid infections and notify physician at first sign of infection; increase fluid intake and encourage client to void every 2 hr; monitor CBC regularly
Tacrolimus (FK506, Prograf)	Inhibits T-lymphocyte activation	Tremors, headache, hepatotoxicity, constipation, diarrhea, nausea and vomiting, renal dysfunction	Monitor renal and liver function studies; teach client ways to avoid infection; tell client not to alter dosage without physician's consent; teach client to report any unusual bleeding or bruising, sore throat, mouth sores, or fatigue

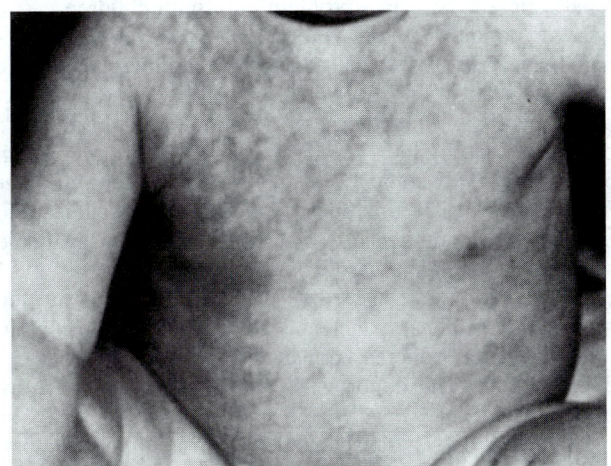

Figure 27–3. Erythroderma of trunk and extremities in a child with graft-versus-host disease.

ent. For further information on bone marrow transplants, see Chapters 24 and 53.

Criteria for Transplantation

The basic criteria for transplantation include the following:

1. The presence of endstage disease in a transplantable organ
2. Failure of conventional therapy to treat the condition successfully
3. Progression of problems associated with the organ failure which in themselves may be fatal
4. The absence of untreatable malignancy or irreversible infection
5. The absence of disease that would attack the transplanted tissue

6. Ability of the client to survive the surgical procedure

The first, fourth, fifth, and sixth criteria apply to all transplants, whereas the second is mainly for liver and heart, and the third for pancreas and kidney. Different institutions apply other criteria, such as age limits and the absence of drug or alcohol abuse.

For kidney transplants, the most common organ transplant procedure, the candidates have endstage renal disease without systemic infection or major uncontrollable complication, with diabetes being the most common cause of the endstage disease. For heart transplants, candidates have irreversible endstage cardiac disease. Cardiomyopathy and left ventricular disease are the most common causes. The client should not have severe renal, pulmonary, or liver complications. Heart-lung transplant candidates have terminal cardiopulmonary disease or endstage cardiac disease associated with severe pulmonary disease. The client should not have severe pulmonary hypertension or other serious organ failure.

Candidates for liver transplants suffer from endstage liver disease, congenital biliary abnormalities, inborn errors of metabolism, chronic active hepatitis, sclerosing cholangitis, vascular disorders, fulminant disease such as hepatitis B, and cirrhosis. Clients with continuing alcoholism are evaluated carefully before transplant. If the clients are willing to enter substance abuse recovery programs, they are considered for transplant. Candidates for pancreatic transplants are usually clients with diabetes who have progressive disease of other organs (kidney, heart) and are often also scheduled for kidney transplant.

Corneal transplants are done on clients with corneal opacity or ulceration. Skin transplants are typically done on clients with severe burns, which make autografts impossible. Bone marrow transplants are done for clients with leukemia, aplastic anemia, genetic hematopoietic disorder, or experimentally on others with late-stage malignant disease (these are usually autologous transplants). Criteria for selection of bone marrow transplant candidates are mainly based on the stage of disease and the potential for improvement.

Donor Procurement and Preparation

Organ procurement is a subject that makes many healthcare professionals uncomfortable. They hesitate to approach the family of a potential donor when the family is suffering the potential loss of their loved one. There is, however, a federal requirement that hospitals have request protocols for organ donation; otherwise they risk losing Medicare and Medicaid reimbursement. Most states now have laws requiring that families be given the opportunity for organ donation.

Families often have been very receptive to possible donation as a living memorial to their loved one. The approach must be sensitive, sincere, and stated in a positive way. Many institutions have set up organ procurement nurses or teams to handle this process. The request for organ donation occurs only after the family has been completely informed about the hopelessness of the situation. The discussion can be initiated by asking the family if their loved one ever thought about organ donation and how they feel about this option.

Organ donors typically have been either living relatives or cadavers. More recently, however, living unrelated donors have been used for bone marrow transplants (see Chapters 24 and 53). The ideal living donor is an identical twin, who will have the same genetic make-up. Close relatives with similar genetic make-up are the most common living donors.

Cadaver donors are usually people who have died suddenly, often in accidents that spare the vital organs, and who have signed organ donor cards or whose family gives permission for the donation. The organs are removed when the donor is declared brain-dead. The organs must remain viable until they can be used for transplant. The primary concern, at this point, is adequate perfusion of the organs. Once the family has agreed to the transplant, all costs are assumed by the organ procurement organization. There are many ethical considerations associated with donor procurement (see Ethical Issues in Nursing).

The potential donor, living or cadaver, must undergo thorough assessment for eligibility for donation to be determined. The donor must be free of communicable diseases, especially hepatitis B and HIV infection. The involved organ cannot be diseased; therefore, clients with diabetes are often unable to donate most organs. The presence of a malignancy is also usually a contraindication, except the cornea and skin if they are not involved. Of course, the donor must be histocompatible with potential recipients.

Not all organs from a cadaver donor are suitable for transplant. Heart donors should be less than 40 years old without cardiac disease or chest trauma. The heart has the shortest hypothermic preservation time (about 4 hours). Heart-lung donors are even harder to find because size is an additional criterion. The donor must also have good pulmonary function without history of any pulmonary disorder.

Kidney donors may be 1 to 65 years old, with normal renal function. Size is a problem only with children.

Liver donors can be live donors or cadavers. Live donors have been used for adult-to-child donations in the last few years. Liver donors must have well-perfused organs; therefore, only those on a ventilator with adequate perfusion are eligible. The donor should be younger than 55 years. MHC compatibility is not a concern in liver transplants because this does not seem to affect rejection. Size is important because the liver bed limits available space for transplantation.

Pancreas donors can be live or cadavers; therefore, the islet cells or distal pancreas can be taken from living relatives. Total pancreas transplants must come from cadaver donors. The donor must be younger than 55 years of age.

Bone marrow is transplanted only from living donors. For autologous transplants, the marrow is donated by the client, frozen, and then returned to the client after treatment.

All living donors must be in good health without se-

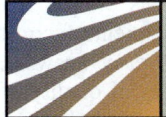

ETHICAL ISSUES IN NURSING

Do Transplant Clients Have an Obligation to Comply with Their Post-transplant Self-Care?

The transplantation of human organs from one client to another is a major miracle of modern medicine. These transplants give life to clients who would surely die without such procedures. Although certain organ transplant operations are common these days, the postoperative course that transplant clients go through may be very complicated. Organ transplant clients must take medications for help in preventing rejection of the "foreign" part. These medications alter one's immune system, causing immunosuppression. The postoperative transplant regimen can be quite rigorous, and clients must be counseled regarding this before surgery.

All transplant clients are grateful for being given a second chance at life. Most usually follow their postoperative course of treatment rigidly. There will be times, however, when organ rejection will take place, even though everything was done by the clients as ordered. The dilemma faced by the healthcare providers of transplant clients has to do with clients who do *not* follow their postoperative treatment regimens or who abuse their bodies in ways that may cause organ rejection. Examples of this include the liver transplant client who continues to drink alcohol or any transplant client who does not follow dietary and medication protocols. With limited availability of organs for transplant, should clients be strictly screened and those showing potential lack of postoperative treatment compliance be placed on a longer waiting list than those who show more promise in complying with treatment orders? Do transplant clients, by accepting organs, have an obligation to take care of themselves as prescribed by their physicians in order not to "waste" their transplanted organ?

Nurses who care for post-transplant clients have a duty to reinforce their clients' treatment protocols. Those clients who choose not to comply with such protocols pose many challenges to the nurses caring for them. When clients do not comply with their treatments, seek out reasons in order to identify problems. Perhaps a client's reason for noncompliance might be misunderstanding of the treatment, or perhaps there is a financial constraint that might need social work intervention. Be aware of potential problems due to possible lack of compliance in your clients in order that maximal benefit might come to these clients.

potential cadaver donor so that the organs are maintained in prime condition. Continued evaluation requires that specimens be collected and that vital signs be assessed continually. A great deal of physical care is required to ensure that the organs are adequately perfused, which includes managing parenteral fluids to maintain adequate blood pressure, medications, and ventilatory support. These potential donors are usually in critical care areas where they can receive continuous monitoring and care.

Many donors have suffered head injuries and require strict control of fluids for control of cerebral edema. The restriction of fluids often leads to a decreased perfusion of the kidneys and other organs. Once brain death has been established, the donor is rehydrated to improve perfusion. Antibiotics may also be initiated.

Living donors and the families of cadaver donors must be given a great deal of psychological support. The living donor often seems to be forgotten in the joy of a successful transplant. This client has undergone major surgery and requires expert physical and psychosocial nursing care. The families of cadaver donors often find that the usefulness of their loved one's organs is of help in their grief. These families should not be forgotten in the rush to transplant the organs successfully.

The organ for transplantation is removed under sterile conditions for both live and cadaver donors. With live donors, the organ is transplanted immediately. With cadaver donors, once the organs are removed, they must be transplanted immediately or preserved at 4° C in a special electrolyte solution. The organs are then transported to the recipient's hospital as soon as possible for transplantation. The kidney can last about 48 hours with hypothermic preservation; the liver lasts 18 to 24 hours; the pancreas about 18 hours; and the heart-lung about 4 hours. Corneas and skin can be preserved for longer periods.

Nursing Management

▪ Pretransplantation

Before the transplant, the priority nursing intervention is to maintain the health of the recipient. The client's disease as well as any other problems that develop during the pretransplant period must continue to be vigorously treated. The client must be monitored closely for the development of any new problems and must be protected as much as possible from developing an infection or other problem that might delay the transplant. Clients should have careful dental screening and receive any needed treatment before the transplant. Also, any chronic condition, such as ulcers or gastritis, should be adequately treated before the stress of a transplant. Any condition that can be resolved before the transplant should be, because the immunosuppressed client will be at much greater risk of disease after the transplant. The client should be in the best health possible for the transplant.

Administration of immunosuppressants may begin before the transplant in some cases. In the case of clients undergoing bone marrow transplant, the recipient's marrow must be destroyed before the transplant (see Chapters 24 and 53 for further information).

vere disease. Kidney donors must have normally functioning kidneys. Kidney disease is often genetic, so with living donors assessment must be made for the presence of the same genetic disorder. The donor's ability to withstand the transplant must be a prime consideration.

The nurse is responsible for continuing care of the

The psychological care of the transplant recipient is very important. These clients are often very ill and may have unrealistic expectations about the outcome. Listen closely to what the client is saying and what the client's expectations are. Many transplant programs include psychological evaluation and follow-up, but expert nursing care is of vital importance. All concerns are usually addressed in multidisciplinary conferences. The family or significant others should also be assessed for their coping abilities and strategies.

Once the decision is made to undergo transplantation, the client is placed on a transplant list with others awaiting the availability of the same organ. This wait can be almost unbearable for the client and significant others. The client, however, must continue with treatment of the underlying disease and maintain a high level of wellness.

One issue that is often discussed before the transplant is the client's ability to comply with therapy after the transplant. Often, it is the client's failure to comply with therapy that has led to the organ failure and the need for transplant. The question is raised whether the client is capable of compliance and, therefore, whether the client is an acceptable candidate. Organs are rare, and there are many needy candidates. An ethical question arises whether clients "responsible" for their own illness are appropriate transplant candidates. There is no one answer to this question. Clients are screened, and the reasons for past noncompliance are explored. If there is strong evidence that clients will not be able to comply with the complex post-transplant regimen, they will probably not be placed on the transplant list.

Nutrition is important before the transplant. Many clients are malnourished and need extra vitamins and protein before the procedure. Liver transplant clients need to have ascites reduced and may need total parenteral nutrition to reach a better physical condition for the transplant.

There is a great deal of teaching that must be done before the transplant. The client must be instructed in pulmonary exercises for preventing postoperative respiratory problems. Education about the post-transplant medication and treatment regimen is also begun preoperatively. The client should also be taught what to expect throughout the transplant process, from the uncertainty of the waiting period to the intensive care required postoperatively. Some of the appropriate nursing diagnoses for transplant clients are listed in Box 27–4. Specific care for each type of transplant can be found in the appropriate chapter.

The financial impact of the transplant on the family and on society must also be considered. Transplant surgery is extremely expensive. Many clients are not employed at the time of the transplant, having left their jobs as their disease progressed. Post-transplant medications alone may cost between $5000 and $10,000 a year. Many of these clients have only Medicare, and perhaps Medicaid, to provide insurance coverage. Those with coverage often find they have reached their policy limit.

In the United States, without national health insurance, many clients simply cannot afford transplants. Financial costs also affect the nation. In this time of increasingly scarce healthcare resources, the cost of a transplant and client maintenance must be considered. Many policymakers argue that the cost of transplantation is simply not worth the quality of life post-transplant recipients face. It is not an easy question, and there are no easy answers. Nursing research is being conducted in areas of quality of life after transplants to address some of these issues.

■ Post-transplantation

In many ways, care after a transplant is the same as care after any major abdominal or cardiothoracic surgery (see Chapter 21). Infection control, however, is even more important for these clients because of the immunosuppression required by the transplant. Nosocomial (hospital acquired) infections can be fatal in these clients, so the nurse must be meticulous about preventing them. Use strict aseptic technique in caring for these clients, especially those with indwelling urinary catheters and intravenous lines.

A variety of complications, other than organ rejection, are possible after transplant (Table 27–6). These must be anticipated and, if possible, prevented. Postoperative nursing care of clients receiving specific transplants is discussed in the appropriate chapters.

Fluid and electrolyte balance is vital postoperatively. The client's intake and output must be measured carefully so signs of fluid imbalance can be diagnosed early and treated before complications occur. Fluid balance is monitored hourly in most clients and determined by subtracting output plus 500 ml for insensible fluid loss from intake for a 24-hour period. Wound care and care of all tubes are also vitally important. Tubes in transplant cli-

---

Box 27–4. Common Nursing Diagnoses and Collaborative Problems for the Client Undergoing a Transplant

■ Knowledge Deficit related to transplant procedure, postoperative course, post-transplant self-care requirements, and medication regimen
■ Anxiety related to endstage organ disease and pending transplant
■ Risk for Ineffective Breathing Pattern related to surgical procedure and need for ventilator
■ Risk for Fluid Volume Excess related to postoperative fluid management
■ Pain related to surgical procedure
■ Risk for Infection related to immunosuppressant medications
■ Risk for Ineffective Individual and Family Coping related to possible rejection phenomena
■ Risk for Altered Tissue Perfusion related to leakage or thrombosis at graft anastomosis sites
■ Risk for Injury related to side effects of immunosuppressant medications
■ Activity Intolerance related to post-transplant weakness and fatigue
■ Risk for Altered Home Maintenance Management related to post-transplant activity intolerance
■ Risk for Ineffective Management of Therapeutic Regimen (Individuals) related to complexity of medication and immunosuppressed condition

Table 27–6. Potential Post-transplant Complications

Organ	Potential Complications
Kidney	Rejection, fluid and electrolyte imbalances, acute tubular necrosis, post-transplant diabetes, problems related to immunosuppression (e.g., infections), renal artery thrombosis or leakage at anastomosis sites, decreased renal function, hypertension, renal abscess
Liver	Rejection, fluid and electrolyte imbalance, clotting disorders, post-transplant diabetes, problems related to immunosuppression (e.g., infections), hepatic artery or vein thrombosis or leakage at anastomosis sites, liver failure, subphrenic abscess, atelectasis and pneumonia secondary to ascites, peritonitis
Heart (lung)	Rejection, post-transplant diabetes, problems related to immunosuppression (e.g., infections), thrombosis or leakage at anastomosis sites, heart (lung) failure, pulmonary hypertension, mental status changes, effusion
Pancreas	Rejection, problems related to immunosuppression (e.g., infections), thrombosis or leakage at anastomosis sites for total replacement, decreased pancreatic function, peritonitis, pancreatic abscess
Bone marrow	Graft-versus-host disease, clotting disorders, problems related to immunosuppression (e.g., infections), agranulocytosis, failure of engraftment

ents range from nasogastric to chest and other drainage tubes.

Client education about these potential problems is an important nursing function. The educational program for a transplant client is complex and often must be taught and mastered in a short time under less than ideal conditions. Do everything possible to facilitate client learning.

The focus of nursing care after transplant, in addition to the prevention of infection, is on prevention of rejection. Early recognition of rejection leads to early treatment, which improves the chances that rejection can be reversed. The pathophysiology of rejection has been covered earlier in this chapter. The actual manifestations of rejection vary with the affected organ (see the appropriate chapter for the specific organ).

All clients receive immunosuppressant therapy, but when rejection actually occurs, the doses of the immunosuppressants must be increased. The nurse must then watch the client closely for the side effects and potentially toxic effects of these medications.

Each medication administered has its own side effects (see Table 27–5). These drugs produce immunosuppression and, therefore, possible infection. Clients and significant others must understand their medications, the side effects, and complications. Often clients with transplants are also taught to keep track of their own laboratory values as well as to understand them.

Clients on cyclosporine must be closely monitored for signs of nephrotoxicity. In renal transplant clients, this must be carefully differentiated from rejection. If the cyclosporine level is not elevated, then rejection is the possible cause of fever and graft tenderness.

When the immunosuppressant antithymocyte globulin (ATG) or antilymphocyte globulin (ALG) is begun, closely assess the client for anaphylaxis. Skin testing is usually done first to assess for possible allergy. Have diphenhydramine hydrochloride (Benadryl) and epinephrine on hand in case of an adverse reaction.

Psychosocial care is also extremely important at this point. The client often plummets from the joy of survival to the dark depression of possible rejection. The client needs a great deal of emotional support at this point and needs to focus on the reality of the situation. Clients often assume the worst once rejection begins, even if the rejection is minor and expected. If the rejection is serious, the client still needs to understand the reality of the situation and help in understanding it. Significant amounts of research have been done in this area.

Long-Term Follow-up Care

The post-transplant client requires follow-up care for a prolonged period. The client will continue immunosuppressant therapy, which can usually be gradually decreased over time.

Infection is one of the most serious prolonged problems after transplant. The client must be continually vigilant to avoid obvious potential sources of infection. This includes precautions such as avoiding crowds, wearing a mask when out in public, and immediately seeking treatment for even a minor infection. Prevention of infection, however, remains the priority.

Immunosuppressant medications have major side effects, and much of the post-transplant client's long-term care needs revolve around controlling these side effects. Clients must learn what to do to control these problems. The common side effects are given in Table 27–5. It is important to help the client understand that although the side effects from these medications can be severe and even fatal, these medications are necessary to maintain the viability of the transplant. The client must decide between the often distressing side effects of the immunosuppressants and survival of the transplant. Although this is discussed thoroughly before the transplant, clients often seem dismayed when reality sets in.

Future Considerations

The use of organ transplantation continues to grow. The use of living donors who share their liver, kidney, pancreas, or bone marrow with the recipient exemplifies this. As improvements in antirejection medications continue, transplants are increasingly successful and survival is prolonged.

Renal grafts have a success rate of 85% for the first year and about 60% thereafter. Heart transplant survival has similar rates, with about 80% success in the first year and 60% thereafter. Pancreatic transplants successfully produce insulin, which eliminates diabetes. Bone marrow transplants are very successful in good matches. Remember that GVHD and recurrence of the cancer in bone marrow transplants are the problems, rather than rejection. At present, there have not been enough heart-lung transplants to assess long-term survival and benefits accurately.

Liver transplants have previously not had good success in many clients because of the severity of illness before the transplant is performed. As these transplants have become more frequent, clients are receiving transplants earlier. This has helped increase the survival rate.

The nurse has a major role to play in the future of transplantation. Nurses are becoming increasingly involved in procurement. Nurses also provide care to potential donors in intensive care units. The nurse must provide increasingly complex care to keep the organs viable and then provide the complex care required by the recipient. Organ transplantation will continue to grow in this country, and the nurse's involvement should grow with it. The role of the nurse in helping clients learn self-care is vital.

Conclusions

The immune system is a complex, interrelated system that affects the whole body. The nurse must understand this system in order to provide clients with complete and individualized care. This chapter covers a wide variety of disorders ranging from AIDS, to allergies, to transplantation. The care of these clients requires complex interventions for meeting the wide variety of problems. The nurse must be able to plan and implement complex care to meet the needs of these clients.

Thinking Critically

1. A 35-year-old client is diagnosed with acquired immunodeficiency syndrome (AIDS). His most recent CD4+ cell count was 145. He has candidiasis of the esophagus and trachea and his physician suspects *Pneumocystis carinii* pneumonia (PCP). How will the client be diagnosed and treated? Which body systems should you focus on during assessment?

Factors to Consider. What tests confirm the diagnosis of acquired immunodeficiency syndrome? How is the CD4+ cell count used? How do opportunistic infections occur?

2. A client has been on dialysis for several years awaiting a kidney transplantation. She is notified during dialysis that a kidney match is available and that she should proceed to the hospital immediately. What

teaching will be completed before she undergoes surgery? What psychological care should be offered?

Factors to Consider. What criteria are used to select candidates for transplantation?

3. You are working in a homeless shelter and are scheduled to present a 20-minute program on AIDS prevention. A small class of four men and three women have gathered. They are all known to you and you suspect that one couple may be infected with human immunodeficiency virus (HIV). What should you plan to teach?

Factors to Consider. What main areas of HIV education should be addressed? What is an effective method of communicating this information?

Bibliography

1. Agency for Health Care Policy and Research. (1994). *Evaluation and management of early HIV infection.* Rockville, MD: U. S. Department of Health and Human Services, Publication no. 94-0572.
2. Aiken, L. H., et al. (1993). Nurse practitioner managed care for persons with HIV infection. *IMAGE: Journal of Nursing Scholarship, 25*(3), 172–177.
3. Arnold, R. M. (Ed.). (1995). *Procuring organs for transplant: The debate over non-heart-beating cadaver protocols.* Baltimore: Johns Hopkins University Press.
4. Bach, F. H., & Auchincloss, H., Jr. (1995). *Transplantation immunology.* New York: Wiley-Liss.
5. Barre-Sinousi, F. (1996). HIV-1 as the cause of AIDS. *Lancet, 348*(9019), 31–35.
6. Bancroft, B. (1994). Immunology simplified. *Seminars in Perioperative Nursing, 3*(2), 70–78.
7. Bayer, R., Dubler, N. N., & Landesman, S. (1993). The dual epidemics of tuberculosis and AIDS: Ethical and policy issues in screening and treatment. *American Journal of Public Health, 78*(4), 649–654.
8. Bauer, C. L. (1993). Commentary on differences in immunosuppressant agents. *AACN Nursing Scan in Critical Care, 3*(4), 14.
9. Bechtel-Boenning, C. (1996). State of the art: Antiviral treatment of HIV infection. *Nursing Clinics of North America, 31*(1), 1–13.
10. Blaylock, B. (1993). The aging immune system and common infections in elderly patients. *Journal of Enterostomal Therapy Nursing, 20*(2), 63–67.
11. Breault, A. J., & Polifroni, E. C. (1992). Caring for people with AIDS: Nurses' attitudes and feelings. *Journal of Advanced Nursing, 17,* 21–27.
12. Brodine, S. K., Mascola, J. R., Weiss, P. J. et al. (1995). Detection of diverse HIV-1 genetic subtypes in the USA. *Lancet, 346*(8984), 1198–1199.
13. Centers for Disease Control. (1987). Revision of the CDC surveillance case definition for acquired immunodeficiency syndrome. *Morbidity and Mortality Weekly Report, 36*(suppl. 1), 3–15.
14. Centers for Disease Control. (1988). Update: AIDS worldwide. *Morbidity and Mortality Weekly Report, 37,* 286–295.
15. Centers for Disease Control and Prevention. (1991). Recommendations for preventing transmission of human immunodeficiency virus and hepatitis B virus to patients during exposure-prone invasive procedures. *Morbidity and Mortality Weekly Report, 40*(RR–8), 1–9.
16. Centers for Disease Control. (1991). Women and AIDS: The growing crisis. *HIV/AIDS Prevention Newsletter, 2*(1), 1–19.
17. Centers for Disease Control and Prevention. (1992). Recommendations and reports: 1993 revised classification system for HIV infection and expanded surveillance case definition for AIDS among adolescents and adults. *Morbidity and Mortality Weekly, 41*(RR-17), 1–19.

18. Centers for Disease Control and Prevention. (1993). *HIV/AIDS prevention fact sheet: Facts about the human immunodeficiency virus and its transmission.* Atlanta: Author.

19. Centers for Disease Control and Prevention. (1994). Birth outcomes following zidovudine therapy in pregnant women. *Morbidity and Mortality Weekly Report, 43*(22), 409, 415–416.

20. Centers for Disease Control and Prevention. (1994). Recommendations of the U.S. Public Health Service Task Force on the use of zidovudine to reduce the perinatal transmission of human immunodeficiency virus. *Morbidity and Mortality Weekly Report, 43*(RR–11), 1–19.

21. Centers for Disease Control and Prevention. (1995). First 500,000 AIDS cases—United States, 1995. *Morbidity and Mortality Weekly Report, 44*(46), 850–853.

22. Centers for Disease Control and Prevention. (1995). *HIV/AIDS surveillance report: US HIV and AIDS cases reported through December 1994.* Atlanta: Author.

23. Centers for Disease Control and Prevention. (1995). Syringe exchange programs—United States, 1994–1995. *Morbidity and Mortality Weekly Report, 44*(37), 684–685, 691.

24. Centers for Disease Control and Prevention. (1995). Update: HIV–2 infection among blood and plasma donors—United States, June 1992—June 1995. *Morbidity and Mortality Weekly Report, 44*(32), 603–606.

25. Centers for Disease Control and Prevention. (1996). Update: Provisional Public Health Service recommendations for chemoprophylaxis after occupational exposure to HIV. *Morbidity and Mortality Weekly Report, 45*(22), 468–472.

26. Chang, B. L., Vredevoe, D., & Hirsch, M. (1995). Allergy as a risk factor for nursing care problems in the elderly cancer patient. *Cancer Nursing, 18*(2), 83–88.

27. Corley, M. C., et al. (1995). Patient and nurse criteria for heart transplant candidacy. *MEDSURG Nursing, 4*(3), 211–215.

28. Corley, M. C., & Sneed, G. (1994). Criteria in the selections of organ transplant recipients. *Heart and Lung, 23*(6), 446–457.

29. Currier, J., Fliesler, N. (1995). Demographics of HIV survival revisited. *AIDS Clinical Care, 7*(11), 94.

30. Duffy, M. M., & Uber, L. (1994). Immunosuppressive medications. *Dialysis and Transplantation, 23,* 571.

31. Enger, C., Graham, N., Peng, Y., et al. (1996). Survival from early, intermediate, and late stages of HIV infection. *Journal of the American Medical Association, 275*(17), 1329–1334.

32. Eichner, E. R., & Calabrese, L. H. (1994). Immunology and exercise: Physiology, pathophysiology, and implications for HIV infection. *Medical Clinics of North America, 78*(2), 377–388.

33. Evans, D. L., et al. (1995). Stress-associated reductions of cytotoxic T lymphocytes and natural killer cells in asymptomatic HIV infection. *American Journal of Psychiatry, 152*(4), 543–550.

34. Fegan, C. (1996). Cryptosporidial disease in the adult HIV-infected patient. *Journal of the Association of Nurses in AIDS Care, 3,* 17.

35. First, M. R. (1993). Long-term complications after transplantation. *American Journal of Kidney Disease, 22,* 477.

36. Flaskerud, J. H., & Ungvarski, P. J. (1995). *HIV/AIDS: A guide to nursing care* (3rd ed.). Philadelphia: W. B. Saunders.

37. Flye, M. W. (Ed.). (1995). *Atlas of organ transplantation.* Philadelphia: W. B. Saunders.

38. Gift, A. G., & Pugh, L. C. (1993). Dyspnea and fatigue. *Nursing Clinics of North America, 28*(2), 373–384.

39. Grayce-Barnes, K. B. (1995). Nutrition, immunity, and HIV disease. *Physician Assistant, 19*(8), 57–58, 60, 62–65.

40. Helderman, J. H., & Frist, W. H. (Eds.). (1995). *Grand rounds in transplantation.* New York: Chapman & Hall.

41. Henry, K., Sullivan, C., & Campbell, S. (1993). Deficits in AIDS/HIV knowledge among physicians and nurses at a Minnesota public teaching hospital. *Minnesota Medicine, 76*(2), 23–27.

42. Hurley, P. M., & Ungvarski, P. J. (1994). Home health care needs of adults living with HIV disease/AIDS in New York City. *Journal of the Association of Nurses in AIDS Care, 5*(2), 33–40.

43. Hussar, D. A. (1994). Immunosuppressant: Tacrolimus. *Nursing, 24*(12), 54.

44. Jewitt, J. F., & Hecht, F. M. (1993). Preventive health care for adults with HIV infection. *JAMA, 269*(9), 1144–1153.

45. Johnson, C. C. S. (1994). Knowledge of immunology is essential to plan effective nursing for immunocompromised patients. *Intensive and Critical Care Nursing, 10*(2), 121–126.

46. Kelly, P. J., & Holman, S. (1993). The new face of AIDS. *American Journal of Nursing, 93*(3), 26–34.

47. Kleinpell, R. M. (1993). Commentary on transplantation immunology. *AACN Nursing Scan in Critical Care, 3*(4), 15.

48. Larson, E., & Ropka, M. E. (1991). An update on nursing research and HIV infection. *Image: Journal of Nursing Scholarship, 23*(1), 4–12.

49. Mann, J., Tarantola, D. J., & Netter, T. W. (1992). *A global report: AIDS in the world.* Cambridge, MA: Harvard University Press.

50. Mellors, J. W., Rinaldo, C. R., Gupta, P., et al. (1996). Prognosis in HIV–1 infection predicted by the quantity of virus in plasma. *Science, 272*(5265), 1167–1170.

51. Merrill A. (1995). AIDS and malnutrition: Dual assaults on the body. *Home Healthcare Nurse, 13*(1), 56–63.

52. Newshan, G. T. (1993). Pain characteristics and their management in persons with AIDS. *Journal of the Association of Nurses in AIDS Care, 4*(2), 53–59.

53. Nichols, L. (1992). Future trends in transplantation. *Seminars in Perioperative Nursing, 1*(1), 55–57.

54. Nolan, M. T., & Augustine, S. M. (Eds.). (1995). *Transplantation nursing: Acute and long-term management.* Norwalk, CT: Appleton & Lange.

55. Olbrisch, M. E., & Levenson, J. L. (1995). Psychosocial assessment of organ transplant candidates: Current status of methodological and philosophical issues. *Psychosomatics, 36*(3), 236–243.

56. Peterson, R. (1993). An emerging cancer risk: Organ transplantation. *Cancer Nursing, 16*(6), 468–472.

57. Quinn, T. C. (1996). Global burden of the HIV pandemic. *Lancet, 348*(9020), 99–106.

58. Rose, M. (1993). Concerns of women with HIV/AIDS. *Journal of the Association of Nurses in AIDS Care, 4*(3), 40, 44.

59. Sande, M. A., & Volberding, R. A. (1995). *The medical management of AIDS* (4th ed.). Philadelphia: W. B. Saunders.

60. Santangelo, J., & Schnack, J. (1991). Primary care intervention and management for adults with early HIV infection. *Nurse Practitioner, 16*(6), 9–15.

61. Sax, P. (1996). Viral load testing. *AIDS Clinical Care, 8*(4), 31–32.

62. Shaefer, M. S., & Collier, D. S. (1993). Immunosuppression for solid organ transplantation. *Dialysis and Transplant, 22,* 541.

63. Shronts, E. P. (1993). Basic concepts of immunology and its application to clinical nutrition. *Nutrition in Clinical Practice, 8*(4), 177–183.

64. Sinclair, B. P. (1991). Epidemiology and transmission of infection by human immunodeficiency virus. *NAACOG's Clinical Issues in Perinatal Women's Health Nursing, 1*(1), 1–9.

65. Smith, S. L. (Ed.). (1990). *Tissue and organ transplantation.* St. Louis: Mosby–Year Book.

66. Suthanthran, M., & Strom, T. B. (1995). Immunobiology and immunopharmacology of organ allograft rejection. *Journal of Clinical Immunology, 15*(4), 161–171.

67. Thompson, G., Ruane-Morris, M., & Lawton, S. (1994). Lines of defence . . . hypersensitivity. *Nursing Times, 90*(41), 48–51.

68. Ungvarski, P. J. (1994). Comorbidities of HIV–1/AIDS in adults. *Journal of the Association of Nurses in AIDS Care, 5*(6), 20–29.

69. Ungvarski, P. J. (1995). Meeting the challenge of HIV/AIDS. *Imprint, 42*(4), 51–54.

70. Ungvarski, P. J. (1995). Adults and HIV/AIDS: Clinical considerations for care management. *The Journal of Care Management, 1*(3), 40–42, 45–46, 49, 51–63.

71. Ungvarski, P. J. (1996). Waging war on HIV wasting. *RN, 15*(20), 26–33.

72. Whipple, B., Scura, K. W. (1996). The overlooked epidemic: HIV in older adults. *American Journal of Nursing, 96*(2), 22–28.

73. World Health Organization. (1992). *Global programme on AIDS: Current and future dimensions of HIV/AIDS pandemic. A capsule summary.* Geneva: Author.

74. Workman, M. L. (1993). The immune system: Your defensive partner and offensive foe. *AACN Clinical Issues in Critical Care Nursing, 4*(3), 453–470.

75. Workman, M. L. (1995). Essential concepts of inflammation and immunity. *Critical Care Nursing Clinics of North America, 7*(4), 601–615.

76. Zeller, J. M., Swanson, B., & Cohen, F. L. (1993). Suggestions for clinical nursing research: Symptom management in AIDS patients. *Journal of the Association of Nurses in AIDS Care, 4*(3), 13–17.

Nursing Care of Clients with Connective Tissue Disorders

Cleda L. Meyer

Imagine trying to wear an antique suit of armor 24 hours a day. Consider how it would limit your movements. Think about how painful it would be if some of the joint hinges were rusty. Walking or even moving would cause you to feel tired and worn out. For many people living with rheumatoid arthritis or one of the other connective tissue disorders referred to as "rheumatic disorders," life is like living in a painful suit of armor.

Over 100 different connective tissue disorders, or collagen disorders, have been identified and classified by the American College of Rheumatology (ACR).[40] According to the Arthritis Foundation, 1 in every 7 persons, over 37 million people, annually have evidence of some form of arthritis. The term *rheuma,* meaning "flux," was used in the 1st century A.D. Early physicians believed these diseases originated in the brain as viscous fluid, "a bad humor" which flowed down into the body and attacked joints. We use a more common term, *arthritis,* which means inflammation of a joint.

Connective tissue, the most abundant tissue in the body, is found as loose connective tissue, dense connective tissue, elastic connective tissue, hematopoietic tissue, and strong connective tissue (Box 28–1). The primary functions of connective tissue are to bind cells, organs, and tissues; provide warmth; and permit ease of mechanical movement. Collagen and elastin are the major components of connective tissue. The underlying problem in connective tissue disorders is alteration or disruption of the protein component in the collagen.

The most common disorders are osteoarthritis, osteoporosis, gout, rheumatoid arthritis, systemic lupus erythematosus, scleroderma, and ankylosing spondylitis. Less common disorders include rheumatic syndromes associated with infectious agents, metabolic and endocrine diseases associated with rheumatic states, connective tissue neoplasms, extra-articular disorders, and miscellaneous disorders associated with joint symptoms. Disorders with an autoimmune etiology are discussed here. Other orthopedic disorders are discussed in Chapter 74. Although the conditions have different clinical patterns, pain and impaired mobility are common problems with these disorders. Many connective tissue diseases are autoimmune disorders without a known cause or cure. Most of these disorders are chronic and follow a course of progressive deterioration. Before discussing the specific disorders, an understanding of autoimmunity is important.

Autoimmunity

Overview

Connective tissue disorders are due to problems with the immune system. You will remember that the immune system provides antibodies that recognize and destroy invaders, called antigens. Antigens can include bacteria, fungi, parasites, viruses, our own damaged tissues, or foreign bodies (e.g., wood splinters). Antibodies have the ability to recognize "self" and "nonself" markers. All cells with a nucleus have protein markers on their cell membranes known as *major histocompatibility complexes (MHCs).* Foreign cells also have cell markers called *antigenic determinants* or *epitopes.* Properly functioning antibodies recognize both types of markers and either attack them or leave them alone as appropriate.

Crucial to the process of immunity is the ability to recognize normal tissue and *not* invade or destroy it. When the immune system loses its ability to distinguish normal from abnormal tissue, normal tissue is destroyed. We call this process *autoimmunity* and the disorder arising therefrom, *autoimmune disease.* A growing number of disorders have compelling evidence that they are due to autoimmune responses.

Autoimmune disorders form a spectrum. At one end are conditions in which autoantibodies are directed at a single organ or tissue, resulting in local tissue damage. A classic example is Hashimoto's thyroiditis, in which autoantibodies have absolute specificity for the thyroid tissues (see Chapter 70). At the other end of the spectrum is systemic lupus erythematosus (SLE), which is discussed

This chapter incorporates material written for the fourth edition by Esther Matassarin-Jacobs.

in this chapter. In SLE autoantibodies react with virtually every cell. The result is widespread lesions throughout the body. In the middle of the spectrum falls Goodpasture's syndrome, in which autoantibodies destroy the basement membrane of the lungs and kidneys, leading to disease in these organs. Goodpasture's syndrome is discussed in Chapter 57.

Although it would be appealing to explain all autoimmune disorders by a single mechanism, it is clear that there are a number of ways in which normal tolerance of self is bypassed. More than one defect might be present in a disorder, and the defects may vary from one disorder to the next. Furthermore, the development of autoimmune disorders is through the interaction of immunologic, genetic, and environmental components. Not everyone with the same genetic susceptibility develops autoimmune disorders. Therefore we can conclude that other factors, such as the environment, play a role. Here we can only scratch the surface of a rapidly evolving area of healthcare.

Bypass of T Helper Cell Tolerance

Normal T helper cell tolerance is critical to the prevention of autoimmunity. Developing T cells that have the ability to recognize normal tissues are normally deleted in the peripheral T cell pools and therefore never reach the tissues. In autoimmune disorders this tolerance is bypassed. Four general mechanisms for the loss of self-tolerance have been postulated.

Modification of the Molecule

If a potentially damaging molecule, called an autoantigenic determinant, is attached to a new carrier, part of the new complex may be recognized as foreign. This process can happen with drugs or microorganisms. Some drugs, like the antihypertensive agent methyldopa, alter the surface of the red blood cell (RBC). This change makes the damaged RBC look foreign and it is attacked (Fig. 28–1A).

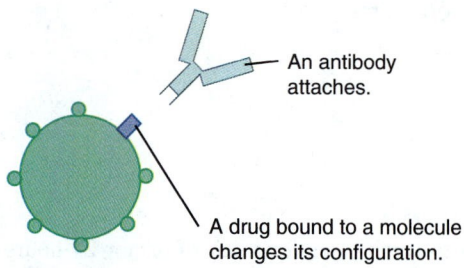

An antibody attaches.

A drug bound to a molecule changes its configuration.

A Modification of the molecule

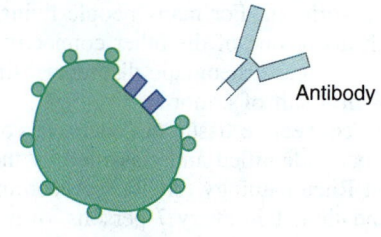

Antibody

B Release of sequestered antigens

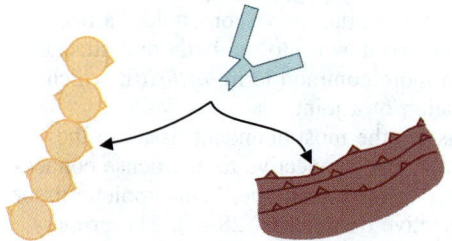

Streptococcus viridans bacteria are attacked.

A sarcolemma with a similar configuration is also attacked.

C Molecular mimicry

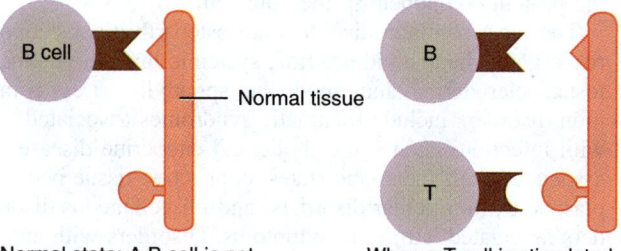

B cell

Normal tissue

Normal state: A B cell is not stimulated without a T cell.

When a T cell is stimulated, a B cell is also triggered.

D Interaction of B cells and T cells

Figure 28–1. Theories of autoimmunity.

Release of Sequestered Antigens

This theory proposes that the self-antigens are isolated from the immune system within an organ during the neonatal period. When the organ is damaged later in life, these antigens are exposed to the immune system, which does not recognize them as self and therefore destroys the damaged cells. Bacteria, viruses, and parasites can degrade collagen and γ-globulin. There are specific autoantibodies developed for γ-globulin called rheumatoid factors, which we will look at more closely later (Fig. 28–1B).

Molecular Mimicry

Several infectious agents cross-react with human tissues because of similarities between the molecular segments or epitopes of the foreign antigens and the person's own cells. There is evidence that rheumatic heart disease sometimes follows streptococcal infection because an antibody to the streptococcal M protein cross-reacts with the M protein in the sarcolemma of the cardiac muscle. Once the infectious agent provokes tissue damage, the process continues because tissue injury releases more self-antigens (Fig. 28–1C).

Interaction of T Cells and B Cells

One of the tolerance mechanisms is inactivation of T lymphocytes when fully competent B lymphocytes are present. This normal process is called clonal anergy. Several microorganisms are capable of producing polyclonal (antigen-nonspecific) B cells. Failure of this process leads to the production of nonspecific B lymphocytes. The Epstein-Barr virus is often cited as a cause of autoimmune disorders (Fig. 28–1D).

Any loss of T suppressor cell function will contribute to autoimmunity. Conversely, excessive T cell help may drive B cells to extremely high levels of autoantibody production. Enhanced T helper cell function is seen in persons with SLE.

Rheumatoid Arthritis

Rheumatoid arthritis (RA) is an autoimmune connective tissue disease that most commonly causes inflammation of the joints and subsequent joint deformity. According to the American Rheumatism Association, the incidence of RA is about 1% of the worldwide population.[40] More than 3 million people in the United States alone have been diagnosed with RA. A higher incidence of RA is found in blacks and whites, a lower incidence in Asians and Hispanics. The onset of RA may occur at any age; however, it is found in only 0.3% of the population under age 35 years. In those age 65 or older, 10% have been diagnosed with RA. The incidence is two to three times higher in women until age 65, when men are affected equally. Women are most likely to develop clinical manifestations during the menopausal years (ages 48–52). The life expectancy of people with established RA is less than that of control populations. A 35-year review of research studies showed that median life expectancy for people with RA was shortened by 7 to 10 years in males and 3 to 7 years in females.[42]

Etiology and Risk Factors

A combination of factors, rather than a single cause, seems to be responsible for the onset of RA. It seems that RA occurs in genetically predisposed persons, and it appears to be triggered by some unknown infectious agent or endogenous antigens (antigens occurring naturally within the person). Seventy percent of persons with RA have the HLA-D4 and HLA-DR4 genes supporting a possible genetic predisposition. These genes tend to bind to antigens. Persons with more of these genes have more severe clinical manifestations and a shorter life expectancy. Despite continued research, however, a specific bacterium triggering RA has eluded investigators. There is some evidence to associate the Epstein-Barr virus, parvo-

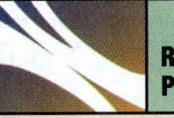

RISK FACTORS AND LEVELS OF PREVENTION

Rheumatoid Arthritis

Risk Factors

The cause of RA and factors that trigger the onset of the disease remain unknown, so there are no known risk factors. Factors that are found in RA include genetic association; increased incidence with age; and predilection for women, who are affected two to three times more often than men.

Levels of Prevention

Primary Prevention

● None

Secondary Prevention

● Assess reports of joint pain and swelling for RA
● Consider RA as an explanation for morning stiffness

Tertiary Prevention

● Administer analgesics and other medications as ordered
● Teach clients to use joint protection devices as ordered
● Teach need for compliance with prescribed therapies
● Monitor clients for side effects of medications
● Promote exercises developed for arthritis
● Teach clients to avoid unproven remedies
● Provide psychosocial support for coping with chronic illness
● Encourage participation in self-help classes
● Provide contacts for obtaining assistive devices

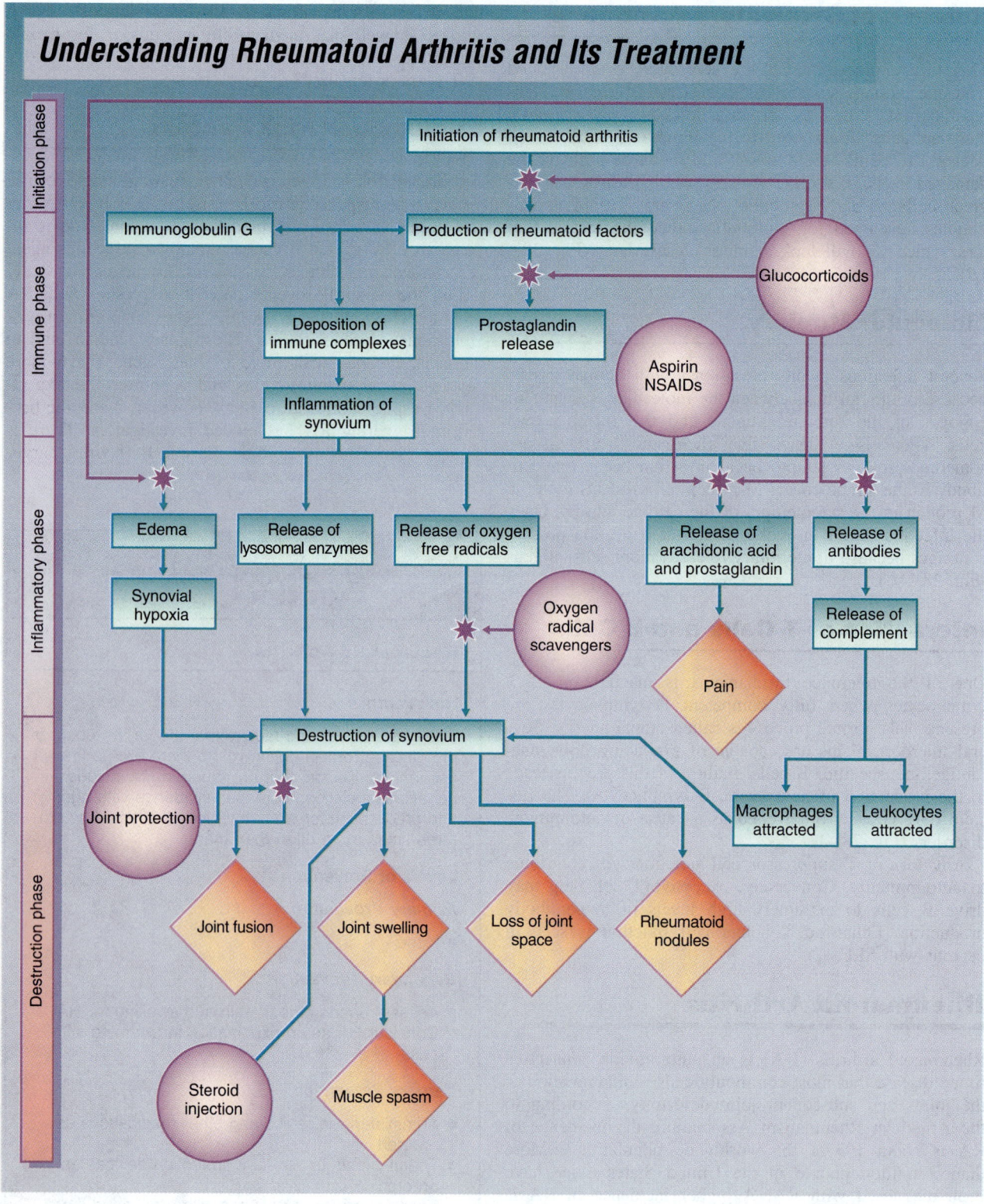

Understanding Rheumatoid Arthritis and Its Treatment

virus, and other viruses[15] with RA. Stressful events have been linked to increased clinical manifestations. Also, hormonal factors appear to influence the course of the disease, since clinical manifestations tend to be less severe during pregnancy. In some cases the disease goes into remission during pregnancy.

Pathophysiology

Regardless of the initial stimulus, altered B cell regulation leads to nonspecific polyclonal immunoglobulin G (IgG) response. This response leads to lymphocyte production of antibodies that recognize the host (the client's tissues) as foreign and attack them. The altered antibodies are called *rheumatoid factors* (RFs). RF forms immune complexes with IgG that are deposited in the synovial membranes, where they stimulate inflammation.

Joint deformity in RA occurs from repeated episodes of inflammation. The damage to the joint occurs in four distinct phases: the initiation phase, the immune response phase, the inflammatory phase, and the destruction phase (Fig. 28–2). The mechanism of the first phase, *initiation,* is not understood. Some changes in the synovial lining are present.

During the *immune response* phase, large numbers of infiltrating lymphocytes (T cells, most of them CD4 cells) and RF are present in the synovial fluid. These antibodies trigger the release of complement, which attracts leukocytes and macrophages to the area. RF also stimulates the release of prostaglandins, which attract more leukocytes to the synovial fluid. Cytokines normally stimulate re-

modeling and rebuilding of cartilage; however, in RA this process is disrupted and cartilage is destroyed.

As the disease process continues during the *inflammatory* phase, the resultant swelling damages tiny blood vessels in the synovial membrane that contains the synovial fluid. In response to this damage, the body releases arachidonic acid and lysosomal enzymes. Oxygen radicals are also present. These substances create fissures in the surface of the synovium. They intensify the inflammation, eventually causing cells to enlarge and change into hyperactive stromal cells that thicken the membrane. Although the stromal cells are similar to malignant cells, they are considered to be nonmalignant.

The *destruction* phase occurs over time. If the inflammatory process is not arrested, a thickened fibrous scar tissue called "pannus" is formed. Pannus adheres to the articular surface of the cartilage and eventually invades the bone, causing bony erosions which can be seen on x-ray. In this phase, fibrous tissue may become calcified,

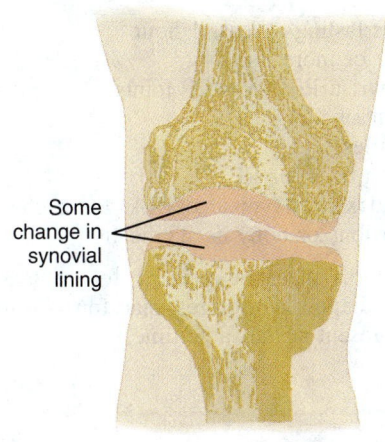

Some change in synovial lining

INITIATION PHASE

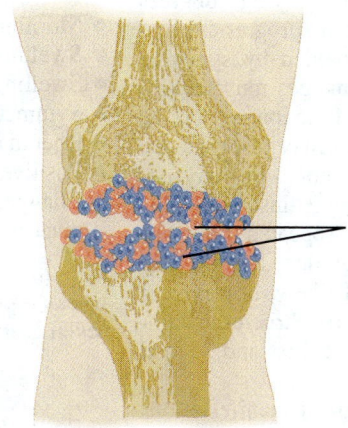

Influx of immune cells: B cells, T cells, macrophages, Ag–Ab complexes

IMMUNE RESPONSE PHASE
Hyperplasia of synovium

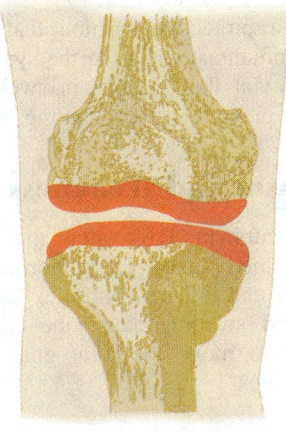

INFLAMMATORY PHASE
Oxygen radicals, arachidonic acid radicals, and lysosomes destroy synovial tissue

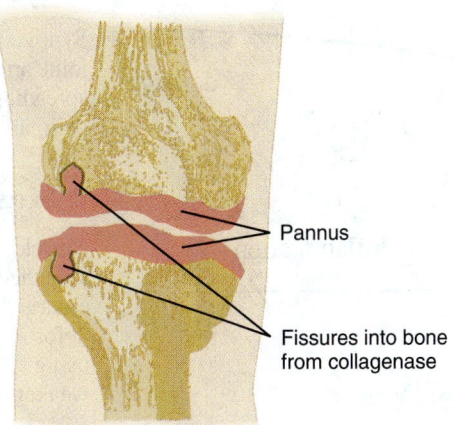

Pannus

Fissures into bone from collagenase

DESTRUCTION PHASE

Figure 28–2. The four phases of joint damage in rheumatoid arthritis.

leading to joint fusion with permanent deformity. Vasculitis occurs when inflammation of the tiny blood vessels with platelets, leukocytes, and fibrin occludes the vessels. When vessels are occluded, infarction results from lack of oxygen to the tissue, causing further tissue damage.

Clinical Manifestations and Diagnostic Findings

For most clients, the manifestations of RA begin as increasing fatigue, accompanied by diffuse musculoskeletal pain. Stiffness occurs after inactivity, such as sleep or prolonged sitting. In fact, the duration of stiffness in the morning (morning stiffness) is one measure of the severity of RA.

In about 20% of clients, the onset of RA is acute.[40] During this acute phase, the manifestations are intermittent. With the passage of time, however, the manifestations become more sustained. Some people will have no more than a few months of discomfort, but others quickly become disabled. The more common course includes repeated periods of inflammation of varying degrees throughout the course of RA, leading to progressive debilitation. The inflammation is accompanied by synovitis and the formation of pannus, which damages muscles and tendons and leads to decreased joint function. After the initial flare of the disease, inflammation may resolve even without treatment, and a spontaneous remission may occur for months or 1 to 2 years. In some instances, this remission may last up to 25 years. Repeated bouts of inflammation and remission lead to a gradual loss of joint function (Fig. 28–3). Remission is not likely, however, if RA has persisted for more than 2 years. Structural damage of joints tends to occur between the first and second year of the disease.

Since RA is a systemic disease, clinical manifestations may occur in various parts of the body. However, the joints are generally affected first. In RA, joints also tend to be affected symmetrically. For example, if one wrist is affected, the other is likely to be affected also. The wrist, proximal interphalangeal (PIP), and metacarpophalangeal (MCP) joints are usually involved first. Joint swelling is more apparent in the morning after an accumulation of fluid during the night.

Since RA is a systemic disorder, manifestations of RA may occur in other organs. They include skin changes, pulmonary disease, cardiac disease, ocular disease, neurologic disease, Felty's syndrome, vasculitis, Sjögren's syndrome, and Caplan's syndrome. Felty's syndrome, vasculitis, Sjögren's syndrome, and Caplan's syndrome can also occur alone.

Other conditions that may produce clinical manifestations similar to those found in RA include Crohn's disease, ulcerative colitis, tuberculosis, hyperthyroidism, hyperparathyroidism, sickle cell crisis, and psoriasis. Treatment of these primary conditions usually leads to a decrease in the severity of the arthritis.

Clients presenting with manifestations suggestive of RA are diagnosed with RA only if they meet the following criteria:

- Morning stiffness lasting at least 1 hour
- Swelling of three or more joints
- Swelling of the wrist, PIP, or MCP joints
- Symmetrical joint swelling
- Rheumatoid nodules
- Positive results on tests for RF
- Changes on hand x-rays typical of RA; these changes must include erosions or bony decalcification

The first four criteria must be present for at least 6 weeks. A definite diagnosis requires that four of these seven features be present at the same time.

Articular Manifestations

■ Synovitis

Synovial fluid is a protective cushion that permits free joint articulation. Inflammation inside the synovial capsule, spreading into synovial fluid, results in swelling, warmth, pain, and increased pressure on surrounding tissue.

■ Muscle Spasm and Weakness

Muscle spasm occurs in RA when the muscles are stretched over inflamed joints. The abnormal position of enlarged bone ends and inflamed muscles leads to further deformity. Pain and swelling cause the client to avoid using the joint or to move the joint guardedly, further weakening the muscles.

■ Hand Deformity

The inflammatory process of synovitis causes the tendons and ligaments to become shortened and less flexible, leading to deformity. The wrist, PIP, and MCP joints are

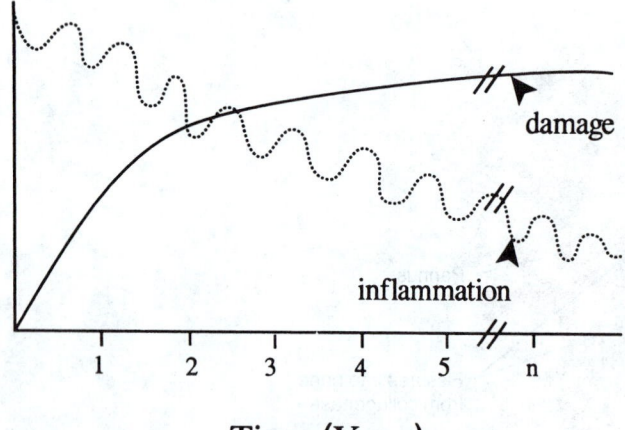

Time (Years)

Figure 28–3. Joint damage in rheumatoid arthritis is both irreversible and cumulative. Inflammation gradually subsides over time but is never completely absent. (From McCarty, D. J. [1993]. Treatment of rheumatoid arthritis. In D. J. McCarty, & W. J. Koopman [Eds.], *Arthritis and allied conditions* [12th ed., Vol. 1, p. 1146]. Philadelphia: Lea & Febiger.)

most commonly involved. The result of this involvement is three types of hand deformity; ulnar drift, boutonnière deformity, and swan-neck deformity (Fig. 28–4).

Ulnar drift occurs when synovitis stretches and damages the tendons. Eventually, the tendons become shortened and fixed. An imbalance of damaged extensor tendons and intact flexor tendons causes the subluxation (drift) of the MCP joint. *Boutonnière deformity* results from flexion of the PIP joint and hyperextension of the distal interphalangeal (DIP) joint extensor tendon, causing it to shift. *Swan-neck deformity* is due to flexion contracture of the MCP joint, hyperextension of the PIP, and flexion of the DIP.

■ Rheumatoid Nodules

Rheumatoid nodules are composed of granulation tissue surrounding a central core of fibrous debris. These firm, nontender nodules are usually found in subcutaneous tissue, although they have been found in visceral organs, including the lungs and the heart. They tend to develop during exacerbations of the disease. The most common sites are the wrist, carpal, knee, and elbow joints, and MCP and PIP joints of the fingers (Fig. 28–5). Rheumatoid nodules behind the knee may be tender, and this tenderness may be mistaken for a positive Homans' sign.

Extra-articular Manifestations

Extra-articular manifestations of RA—manifestations outside the joints—may occur at any time in the course of the disorder and may, at times, overshadow the articular manifestations. These systemic manifestations must be treated quickly, because they are major predictors of morbidity and even mortality.

■ Skin Changes

Rheumatoid vasculitis occurs when small blood vessels outside the joints become inflamed. Vasculitis leads to skin ulceration, lesions of the finger pads and nail beds, and peripheral neuropathy. Generalized vasculitis may also occur. Biopsy of involved tissue may be needed to determine the extent. Treatment is symptomatic and includes smoking cessation, low-dose prednisone, antiplatelet agents, and local wound care.

■ Pulmonary Disease

Pulmonary fibrosis is a common problem with RA. It is caused in part by smoking. Up to 28% of persons with RA develop pulmonary fibrosis. Treatment is usually with glucocorticoids. Caplan's syndrome is pneumoconiosis with RA. Persons with Caplan's syndrome have multiple, large nodules throughout the lungs. This syndrome most commonly occurs in people with RA who have been exposed to silica, usually through occupational exposure, such as granite workers. Treatment options vary.

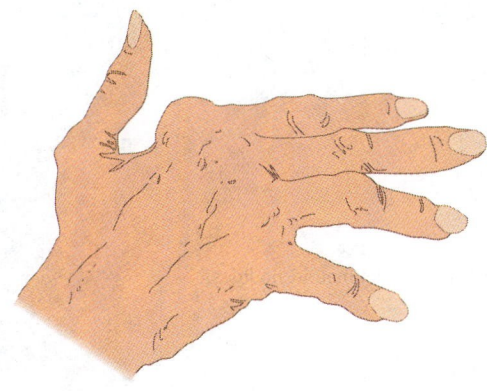

Ulnar drift

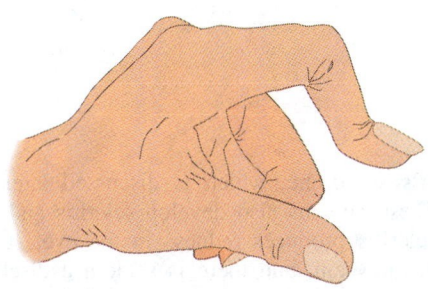

Boutonnière deformity

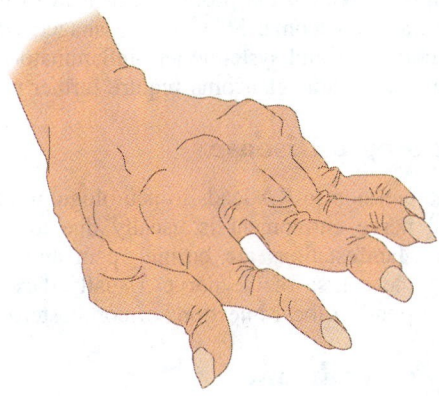

Swan-neck deformity

Figure 28–4. Three types of hand deformity characteristic of clients with rheumatoid arthritis.

■ Cardiac Disease

Pericarditis is the most common cardiac disorder to appear in people with RA. It develops in about 50% of those with RA. Like pulmonary fibrosis, pericarditis related to RA also responds to glucocorticoid therapy. Mitral and aortic valve disease have been noted. The valves develop nodules and thickening of the cusps.

■ Ocular Manifestations

Ocular problems are commonly associated with connective tissue disorders. Many of the problems are potentially blinding. The most common ocular problem seen in RA

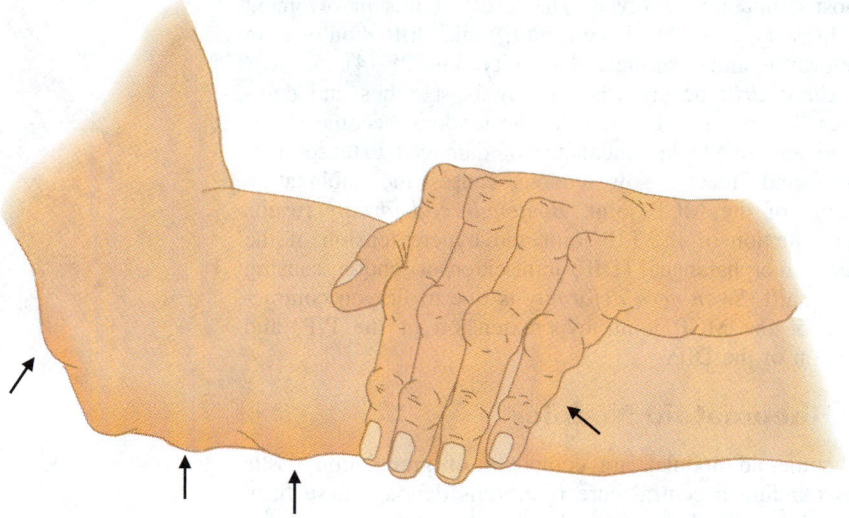

Figure 28–5. Rheumatoid nodules.

is Sjögren's syndrome, which is discussed later in this chapter. These persons also develop scleritis and episcleritis. Episcleritis produces redness in the eye, some discomfort but no pain, and there is seldom a discharge. It rarely if ever causes loss of vision. Episcleritis is a benign self-limiting problem that seldom requires treatment.

In contrast, scleritis can lead to blindness and severe ocular pain. Untreated, the problem can lead to ulcers of the cornea and glaucoma. Scleritis is managed with topical glucocorticoids and systemic anti-inflammatory agents. Complications such as glaucoma require further treatment.

■ Neurologic Disease

Nerve compression in RA leads to neurologic impairment. Peripheral nerve entrapment is usually due to extensive synovitis. Manifestations are burning pain and paresthesias along the course of the nerve. Usually these inflammations respond to local injections of corticosteroids.

■ Felty's Syndrome

Felty's syndrome is defined as the presence of leukopenia with splenomegaly. It is not common overall in RA. However, it tends to develop in people with long-standing RA (more than 10 years' duration), seropositive RA (RA with positive tests for RF), nodular RA (RA with rheumatoid nodules), and destructive RA. Persons with Felty's syndrome usually have high levels of RF, antinuclear antibodies (ANAs), cryoglobulins, and diminished levels of serum complement. The neutropenia predisposes to infections, and 60% to 90% of persons with Felty's syndrome develop pneumonia or joint infections. Some studies indicate that the best treatment for Felty's syndrome is with what are called "disease-modifying antirheumatic drugs" for RA, such as gold salts or methotrexate.

■ Vasculitis

Vasculitis is actually a group of disorders, including polyarteritis nodosa, systemic necrotizing vasculitis, and aller-

gic agranulomatosis angiitis. All of these disorders result in necrotizing inflammation of the blood vessels. Circulating immune complexes deposit in the blood vessels, causing inflammation and damage to large and small vessels.

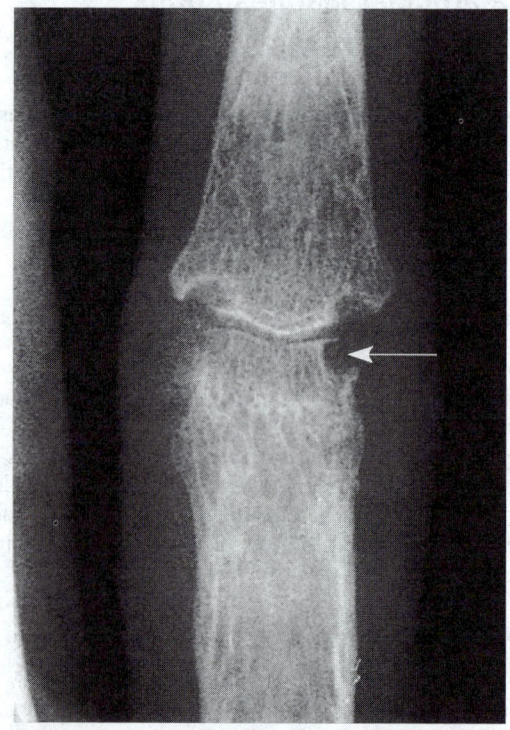

Figure 28–6. X-ray of an interphalangeal joint affected by rheumatoid arthritis. Marginal erosions *(arrow)* are present on both sides of the joint. There is also joint space narrowing and soft tissue swelling. (From Resnick, D., Berthiaume, M. J., & Sartoris, D.: Imaging. In W. N. Kelley, et al. [Eds.] [1993], *Textbook of rheumatology* [4th ed., p. 600]. Philadelphia: W. B. Saunders.)

The result is end-stage organ damage. The specific symptoms vary depending on the organs affected, but corticosteroids are the treatment of choice regardless.

■ Other Manifestations

During the initial onset of RA, people may complain of fatigue, weakness, low-grade fever, anorexia, weight loss, and generalized aching.

Additional manifestations are visible only on x-rays, which are of value in diagnosis and in the evaluation of treatment. High-resolution films, as used in mammography, aid in the early detection of bony erosions. X-rays are also helpful for identifying narrowing of the joint spaces and loss of cartilage (Fig. 28–6). On x-rays, invasion of the bone by the disease can be seen as "pocket" erosions (Fig. 28–7). These erosions may first be detected at the edges of the bone that have direct contact with the inflamed synovium. The formation of pannus and osteoporotic changes may also be detected on x-rays.

Laboratory tests for the presence of RF aid in definitive diagnosis. However, elevations in RF take a while to appear. Within the first 3 months after the onset of clinical manifestations, tests for RF are positive in only 25% of people with RA. After 1 year, however, RF is found in 80% of people with RA. Nevertheless, RF is not specific for RA and may be found in 3% of the population without any clinical manifestations of RA. Other laboratory findings in RA include an accelerated ESR (erythrocyte sedimentation rate), elevated serum globulins, and a positive test for C-reactive protein. A secondary finding is normochromic, normocytic anemia, which is often found in chronic disease. Synovial fluid may be aspirated for examination. Abnormal findings in the synovial fluid of clients with RA include reduced viscosity and WBC (white blood cell) counts as high as 50,000/mm³.

Community and Self-Care

■ Medical Management

Most clients with RA are diagnosed and treated in a community setting. Part of the initial and ongoing assessment of people with RA involves determining their degree of functional impairment. The American College of Rheumatology identifies four categories for rating functional ability in people with arthritis. The ratings are as follows:

1 = normal function
2 = adequate function for normal activities
3 = limited function for activities of daily living (ADL)
4 = inability to function independently

With current therapies, most people with RA are able to remain at functional level 2 without progressing to level 3. Management of RA is interdisciplinary and involves the client, physician, nurse, physical therapist, occupational therapist, and social worker.

The physician's goals in clients with RA are to arrest the inflammatory process before serious bony erosion and joint destruction occur, and to provide relief from pain. In recent years, the philosophy of management toward those goals has changed; Figure 28–8 illustrates both the older, "pyramid," philosophy, and the new philosophy that now guides the management of RA. The foundation of this new philosophy is a balanced program of pharmacologic therapy with nonsteroidal anti-inflammatory drugs (NSAIDs), education, physical therapy, occupational therapy, and psychosocial therapy. With this balanced program, many clients with RA are able to maintain function and continue active, productive life-styles. If these measures are unsuccessful, pharmacologic therapy with dis-

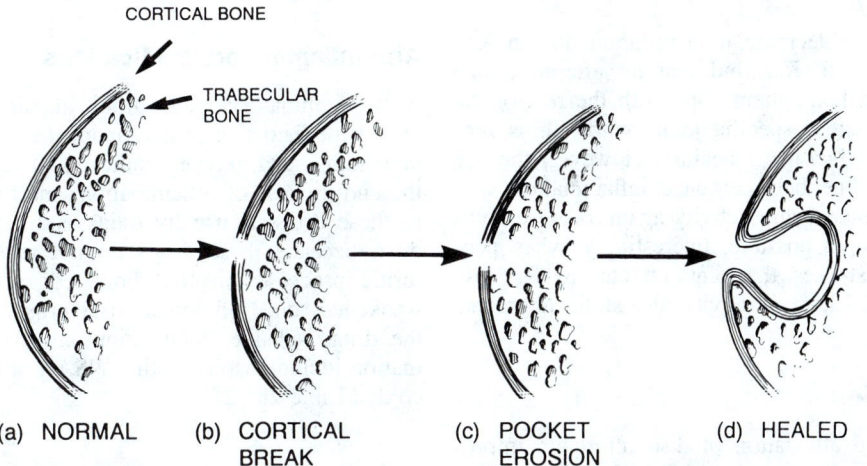

Figure 28–7. Formation of pocket erosions. Inflammation of synovial fluid may spread to the cortex of a bone. When the erosion breaks through the cortex of the bone, a cortical break is said to occur. The erosion then spreads into the trabecular bone, forming a pocket erosion. If the inflammatory process is arrested at this stage, cortical bone may re-form in this pocket, but the total bone surface remains weakened because of the presence of the pocket erosion. Pocket erosions may be seen on high-resolution x-rays. (From McCarty, D. J. [1993]. Treatment of rheumatoid arthritis. In D. J. McCarty, & W. J. Koopman [Eds.], *Arthritis and allied conditions* [12th ed., Vol. 1.]. Philadelphia: Lea & Febiger.)

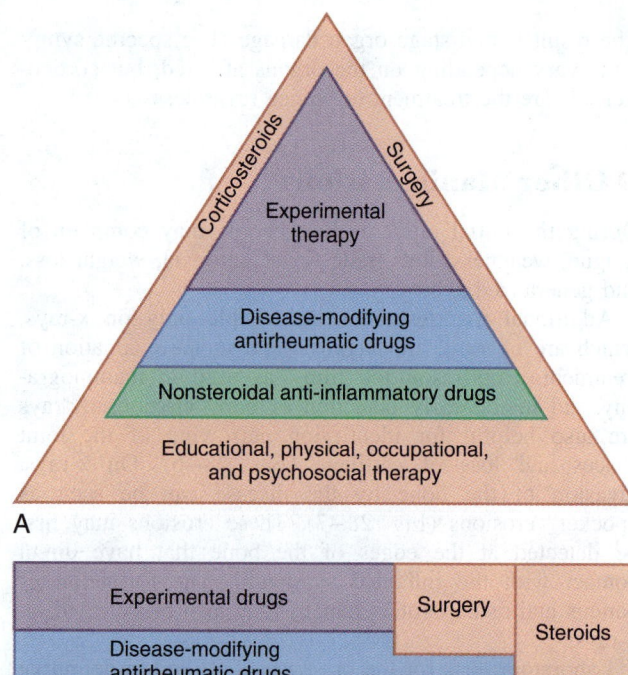

Figure 28–8. The old treatment pyramid for rheumatoid arthritis *(A)* and today's "overlapping" approach *(B)*. Clients with rheumatoid arthritis now have multidisciplinary care early in the course of their disease to help maintain function. (*A* adapted from *Primer on the Rheumatic Diseases* [ed. 10], copyright 1993. Used by permission of the Arthritis Foundation. For more information, please call the Arthritis Foundation's information line 1–800–283–7800. *B* from Starz, T. W., & Miller, E. B. [1993]. Diagnosis and treatment of rheumatoid arthritis. *Primary Care, 20*[4], 832.)

ease-modifying antirheumatic drugs may be used. Corticosteroid therapy, surgery, and therapy with experimental drugs are reserved for RA resistant to less aggressive approaches. In managing clients with RA, many physicians attempt to limit the number of inflamed joints to four, using this number as a benchmark of progress or lack of progress.

Rest

Whole-body rest can decrease joint inflammation in RA, and many clients with RA find that an afternoon nap reduces fatigue and helps them cope with the rest of the day. In addition, rest of specific joints with splints protects the joints and facilitates healing. However, the use of rest requires a fine balance; once inflammation subsides, the client should begin activity again to preserve as much joint function as possible. Interestingly, when people with RA have strokes, the joints affected by RA lose their inflammation. Clearly, activity and strain aggravate the inflammation.

Joint Protection

Joint protection and alleviation of discomfort are important aspects of the management of RA. Joint protection techniques and techniques for carrying out tasks without pain are typically taught by an occupational therapist and reinforced by nurses. Table 28–1 lists the principles of joint protection and strategies for lessening discomfort.

Pharmacologic Management

A combination of medications forms the first line of pharmacologic management. The goal is to decrease inflammation and to modify the course of the disease. NSAIDs are used to decrease pain and swelling from inflammation. Disease-modifying antirheumatic drugs (DMARDs) are used to slow the course of the disease.

Anti-inflammatory Medications

Anti-inflammatory medications impair the natural action of the mediators of inflammation (arachidonic acid, prostaglandins, and oxygen radicals). These drugs work on the end process of inflammation, and the client's response to these drugs is usually quick and easily noticed. However, because these drugs do not reverse the initial arthritic processes in RA, bone edges remain rough and weakened, and inflammation returns once the effects of the drugs subside. Medications used to decrease inflammation include aspirin, other NSAIDs, and the glucocorticoids (Table 28–2).

Aspirin. Aspirin (acetylsalicylic acid, ASA) is a prostaglandin inhibitor used to decrease inflammation. Aspirin has historically been one of the first drugs used to treat RA. However, it is used less often today because the high

Table 28–1. Principles of Joint Protection and Strategies for Lessening Discomfort	
Principles of Joint Protection	**Strategies for Lessening Discomfort**
Respect pain (Fear of pain can lead to inactivity; ignoring pain can lead to joint damage)	Carry out activities and exercise only to the point of fatigue or discomfort Reduce the time spent in doing painful activities Avoid doing activities (other than gentle ROM) when joints are inflamed
Balance work and rest	Rest 5–10 min periodically when doing tasks that take more time Get sufficient sleep Take a 30-min rest during the afternoon
Reduce effort by joints	Slide objects rather than lift them Store items at convenient heights Avoid stooping, bending, or overreaching Sit to work whenever possible
Avoid positions of stress on joints	Avoid tight pinch or grip: use built-up handles and holders for objects such as toothbrushes and pens Avoid turning fingers toward the little finger: turn fingers toward the thumb Avoid wrist flexion and rotation during stirring (e.g., use spoon like a dagger) Use two hands to lift or carry objects Always consider adaptive devices (jar opener, reachers, built-up keys)
Use larger, stronger joints	Lift with palm and forearm instead of fingers Use a backpack, waist pack, or shoulder bag instead of a handbag
Use joints in most stable positions	Avoid or minimize excessive stretch of joint ligaments (e.g., rise from chair symmetrically and avoid leaning to either side) Maintain good posture
Avoid remaining in one position	Change position (or stretch) every 20 min Balance sitting tasks with those that require moving around
Avoid activities that cannot be stopped	Break activities into defined parts

From A. Maher, S. Salmond, & T. Pellino (Eds.) (1994). *Orthopedic nursing.* Philadelphia: W. B. Saunders.

doses required in RA leave the client susceptible to troublesome side effects, such as gastrointestinal (GI) irritation and bleeding, impaired platelet function, and ototoxicity. To achieve anti-inflammatory effects, the therapeutic dose of aspirin is 1000 to 1600 mg/day. At these high doses, aspirin is frequently toxic. In addition, to sustain therapeutic blood levels, aspirin must be taken four times a day, and such frequent dosing often leads to problems with compliance with the medication regimen. As with the other NSAIDs, clients should be instructed to take aspirin with food and watch for clinical manifestations of GI bleeding, easy bruising, and tinnitus. Few patients tolerate the doses needed to achieve therapeutic benefit.

Other Nonsteroidal Anti-inflammatory Drugs.
NSAIDs are used extensively to decrease inflammation and provide pain relief in clients with RA. Many NSAIDs are available over the counter at low doses. The most common NSAIDs are ibuprofen (Motrin, Advil), naproxen (Naprosyn), tolmetin (Tolectin), sulindac (Clinoril), piroxicam (Feldene), diclofenac (Voltaren), and ketoprofen (Orudis). The therapeutic effect of these drugs is to inhibit prostaglandin synthesis, thus decreasing the pain and swelling that accompany the inflammatory response. Unfortunately, because NSAIDs suppress prosta-

glandin production, they also decrease production of gastric mucus and intestinal bicarbonate. These unwanted changes in the GI mucosa greatly increase the risk of bleeding and ulceration. These drugs are therefore usually taken with food, and a histamine receptor antagonist such as ranitidine (Zantac) is usually prescribed concurrently to reduce secretion of stomach acids. NSAIDs also decrease platelet adherence ("stickiness") and therefore increase the risk of bleeding. Clients therefore need to be taught to watch for bruising and clinical manifestations of gastrointestinal bleeding. When about to undergo surgery or dental work, clients should also inform the surgeon or dentist of their current medications.

Most NSAIDs permit simpler dosing schedules and have fewer side effects than aspirin. Nevertheless, clients need to be taught the importance of using the prescribed dosage and the need for continued medical monitoring during therapy.

Glucocorticoids. Glucocorticoids, such as prednisone and cortisone, have both anti-inflammatory and immunosuppressive effects; however, they do not directly modify RA. Long-term use of these drugs is accompanied by serious side effects, such as adrenal suppression, osteoporosis, paper-thin skin, delayed healing, and cataracts. The

Table 28–2. Medications Used in the Treatment of Rheumatoid Arthritis

Medication	Action(s)	Nursing Considerations
Aspirin; choline salicylate (Arthropan)	Analgesic, anti-inflammatory, antipyretic, anticoagulant	Take with food, milk, or antacid: prolong clotting time; may cause occult bleeding; toxic levels cause tinnitus
Other Nonsteroidal Anti-inflammatory Drugs (NSAIDs)		
Diclofenac (Voltaren)	Analgesic; inhibits prostglandin synthesis, anti-inflammatory	Enteric-coated, do not crush; may cause dizziness, GI upset; take with food or milk
Fenoprofen (Nalfon)	Analgesic, anti-inflammatory	Absorption is delayed if taken with food; may cause headache, somnolence, drowsiness, dyspepsia
Ibuprofen (Motrin, Advil)	Analgesic, anti-inflammatory, antipyretic	Absorption is delayed if taken with food; may cause dyspepsia, dizziness, rash
Indomethacin (Indocin)	Analgesic, anti-inflammatory	Take with food or antacid; may cause headache, GI upset, CNS symptoms
Ketoprofen (Orudis)	Analgesic, anti-inflammatory	Causes frequent heartburn
Ketorolac (Toradol)	Analgesic, anti-inflammatory	Most commonly given by IM injection; may cause diarrhea/constipation, rash
Naproxen (Anaprox, Naprosyn)	Analgesic, anti-inflammatory	Side effects include: headache, dyspepsia, nausea, dizziness, pruritus, rash, ecchymoses, tinnitus
Piroxicam (Feldene)	Analgesic, anti-inflammatory	Take with food or antacid (do not crush or break capsule)
Sulindac (Clinoril)	Analgesic, anti-inflammatory	Age increases risk of side effects: GI distress, rash, dizziness, headaches
Tolmetin	Analgesic, anti-inflammatory	GI side effects most common especially in elderly
Glucocorticoids		
Dexamethasone, hydrocortisone, methylprednisolone, prednisolone, prednisone	Potent anti-inflammatories	With high doses/prolonged use may lead to immune suppression, cushingoid changes
Slow-Acting Antirheumatic Drugs (SAARDs)		
Safe		
Auranofin (Ridaura)	Anti-inflammatory gold salt	Monitor closely with CBC and urinalysis to check renal function
Hydroxychloroquine (Plaquenil)	Anti-inflammatory, action unknown	May cause GI disturbances; retinal edema may cause blindness
Sulfasalazine (Azulfidine)	Anti-inflammatory	May cause anorexia, GI symptoms, headache
Toxic		
Azathioprine (Imuran)	Purine antagonist	May cause occasional nausea, vomiting, diarrhea
Cyclosporine (Sandimmune)	Immunosuppressant	In high doses may cause hypertension, hirsutism, tremor, acne, gum hyperplasia
Gold salts (Solganal, Myochrysine)	Anti-inflammatory	Monitor closely with CBC and urinalysis to check renal function
Methotrexate	Mild immunosuppressant	Anorexia, nausea, vomiting, diarrhea
Penicillamine (Cuprimine)	Anti-inflammatory	May cause rash, altered sense of taste, GI disturbances, glossitis
Very toxic		
Chlorambucil (Leukeran)	Immunosuppressant	GI effects are less at low doses (<20 mg): mild nausea, vomiting, anorexia
Cyclophosphamide (Cytoxan)	Immunosuppressant	Monitor laboratory values for leukopenia

healthcare provider, therefore, usually tries to control manifestations with other medications first. The lowest possible dose to establish control of pain and inflammation is used. The dose is reduced as soon as possible to keep the client on the smallest dose that keeps the symptoms under control. The dosage must be increased during periods of major physiologic stress, such as illness or surgery, because the suppressed adrenal glands cannot respond with the usual cortisol boost during stress. Careful monitoring of the client taking glucocorticoids is essential because of the serious complications that result from their long-term use.

When inflammation and tenderness are localized to particular joints, intra-articular injections of corticosteroids may be helpful. Reduced pain and improved function may last for weeks or months after these injections. Corticosteroid injections have been useful in delaying surgery for carpal tunnel syndrome, and they can decrease the need for larger oral doses of corticosteroids. Intra-articular injection of corticosteroids is a sterile procedure requiring careful skin preparation. The physician first aspirates excess fluid, then injects the corticosteroids. The client should keep the needle insertion area clean, dry, and covered with a sterile dressing for the first 24 hours after the procedure.

Slow-Acting Antirheumatic Drugs

Slow-acting antirheumatic drugs (SAARDs), also called disease-modifying antirheumatic drugs (DMARDs), are gaining acceptance for primary therapy. These medications—gold salts, antimalarials, immunosuppressive agents, and D-penicillamine—seem to slow progression of RA by blocking the immunologic aspects of inflammation. However, like other drugs used in the treatment of RA, they do not correct the underlying cause of the disease. Previously used for clients who did not respond adequately to symptomatic therapy, these drugs are being used more aggressively to arrest clinical manifestations and thus decrease joint destruction. They may be used alone or in combination with NSAIDs. Because the DMARDs are generally slow-acting, they must be taken for several months before an effective response becomes noticeable. Some of these agents are also used in cancer treatment. Because the doses in RA are much lower than those used in cancer treatment, the side effects are therefore decreased, but careful monitoring for toxicity is still important. These drugs are summarized in Table 28–2.

Experimental Drugs

Experimental drugs are also used in the treatment of RA. Such drugs include biologic response modifiers, immunomodifiers, antioxidants, and inhibitors of cartilage metabolism. Of course, when these drugs are used, clients are monitored closely so that therapy can be adjusted to avoid or decrease side effects.

Physical Therapy

Physical therapists have an important role in helping the client with arthritis. Physical therapists are trained to evaluate joints, conduct endurance testing, and develop an exercise plan. Safe and effective exercises strengthen weakened muscles and improve function. Exercises may be carried out in group activities or independently. Daily range-of-motion (ROM) exercises are an important component of this program and can actually relieve pain (see the Nursing Research feature). Isometric exercises are important in maintaining muscle function, even when the client wears splints. Physical therapists also measure clients for orthoses, splints, and assistive devices that may be necessary in advanced disease. A correct fit of such devices is important to preserve a functional joint and maintain skin integrity. Physical therapists also help clients learn the correct methods of using walkers and wheelchairs when the lower extremities are severely impaired by RA.

Occupational Therapy

Occupational therapists teach clients ways to avoid placing strain on weak joints. For example, to protect joints during ADL, occupational therapists may teach clients to use both hands to carry items, or they may teach clients with weak grips how to use jar openers, levers attached to doorknobs, and other adaptive devices (Fig. 28–9). Occupational therapists can also recommend workplace modifications and modifications in clothing to assist in dressing. For example, they might recommend wearing clothing with Velcro closures rather than zippers. Occupational therapy promotes independence and enhances self-esteem.

Complications

Complications of RA may be the result of disease progression or the side effects of treatment. The use of any medication has potential risk. Side effects of anti-inflammatory medications include bleeding, gastrointestinal distress and ulceration, and delayed healing. NSAIDs can cause some liver and renal dysfunction; they also lead to gastric ulceration. Aspirin toxicity is usually dose-dependent but can include hypersensitivity reactions, tinnitus, and hearing loss. Adverse reactions to therapy with gold injections or oral gold preparations include allergy, kidney disorders, and anemia. There also are several drug-drug interactions.

The stress of living with a chronic disease such as RA with pain and loss of independent function can lead to depression. Altered body image, sexual problems, and decreased ability to work outside the home also contribute to depressed mood. Depressed clients report more pain, fatigue, and decreased activity with further loss of independence and function.

Outcomes

Living with a progressive painful chronic debilitating condition like RA presents many problems. Current therapeutic regimens enable many people to preserve function and lead productive lives with less pain. However, as with other autoimmune diseases, the person's immune

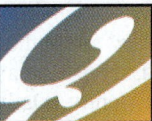

NURSING RESEARCH

What Can Healthcare Workers Do to Encourage People to Develop an "Exercise" Habit?

Minor, M. A., & Brown, J. D. (1993). Exercise maintenance of persons with arthritis after participation in a class experience. *Health Education Quarterly, 20*(1), 83–95.

What are the different types of exercise people with arthritis use? What encourages people with arthritis to continue to exercise? The purpose of this study was to examine the effects of different types of exercise and the reasons people continue to exercise.

The study included 120 subjects, 40 with rheumatoid arthritis (RA) and 80 with osteoarthritis (OA). Physical fitness, arthritis-related disability, pain, duration of arthritis, anxiety, depression, social support, age, sex, and exercise participation were recorded. Subjects were encouraged to choose a preferred exercise: aerobic walking, aerobic aquatics, or nonaerobic range of motion (ROM). All groups met with the same instructors for 60 minutes, three times a week for 12 weeks.

After 12 weeks the walking and aquatic groups showed the greatest improvement with decreased pain and morning stiffness and greater aerobic capacity. All of the groups demonstrated improved flexibility and muscle strength. By 1 year after beginning to exercise, even the ROM groups' aerobic capacity improved significantly, nearly to the level of the other groups.

After the 12-week formal program ended, 75% of the subjects continued to exercise. They selected different types of exercise, including walking, aquatic exercise, stationary bicycle, calisthenics, or flexibility exercise, singly or severally. The average number of

minutes per week devoted to exercise at 9 months was 109.8 (SD 167.8 minutes). By 18 months the subjects exercised 110.4 min/week (SD 132.6 minutes).

When subjects were evaluated again at 3 months, 9 months, and 18 months after starting an exercise program, different reasons were listed for continuing to exercise. At 3 months less depression and the benefits of social activity were rated as important reasons to exercise. At 9 months, decreased anxiety, improved physical activity, and support of friends were indicated as major factors. By 18 months, improvement over initial aerobic capacity and less pain were the reasons people continued to exercise.

Implications for Practice

The implications for practice are that even low-intensity exercise continued over a period of time can improve the client's chronic pain levels, flexibility, muscle strength, and aerobic capacity. A variety of exercise methods can be used to permit exercise throughout the year. Patients need extra encouragement to exercise when they feel depressed. It is important to include family and friends in the activity to support the exercise habit.

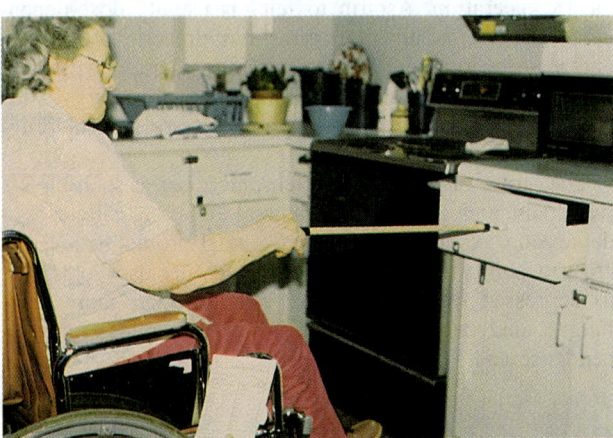

Figure 28–9. There are various devices for a client with rheumatoid arthritis to protect affected joints during activities of daily living. (From *Guide to Independent Living for People with Arthritis,* copyright 1988. Used by permission of the Arthritis Foundation. For more information, please call the Arthritis Foundation's information line at 1–800–283–7800.)

system is compromised, which increases the risk of infection. The presence of higher levels of RF and genetic markers is an indicator of more serious disease and more rapid deterioration. In addition, many of the medications have serious side effects. The psychosocial problems associated with this disease present additional challenges for nursing management.

■ Nursing Management of the Medical Client

The primary nursing goal in the management of a client with RA is to promote the healthiest possible life for the client. As case manager, the nurse's role is to assess, educate, coordinate treatments, facilitate adaptations in the home, reevaluate periodically, and serve as client advocate. Providing information to help the client deal with chronic pain, comply with treatment, and cope with a chronic disease are some of the challenges faced in managing clients with RA. The nurse provides information and encourages the client's self-management by allowing choices about when to exercise, which adaptive equipment to use, and what other self-care techniques to employ.

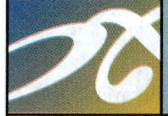

BRIDGE TO HOME HEALTHCARE

Promoting Independence in Clients with Rheumatoid Arthritis

By Beverly Sheehan, M.B.A., O.T.R., V.N.A. *Health Services, San Diego, Carlsbad, California*

Rheumatoid arthritis can affect every aspect of a person's life. For example, people with rheumatoid arthritis may not be able to remove food from the refrigerator, or heavy pots and pans from the cupboards. They may experience pain and lingering discomfort every time they open heavy, sliding closet doors to take out clothing. Changes in fine motor skills and decreased strength can cause routine functional tasks to result in frustration, loss of self-esteem, and feelings of incompetence and lack of control. The disease makes independent self-care and homemaking difficult—if not impossible—without the use of assistive devices and techniques to protect joints from continued injury. For people with rheumatoid arthritis who live alone, routine tasks may pose special challenges that require special approaches.

By using simple assistive devices and techniques, people with rheumatoid arthritis can often remain in their homes independently and can lead productive, satisfying lives. Special stores and catalogues are full of adaptive aids and gadgets that can help clients with the tasks of self-care and homemaking. However, every device and new technique causes subtle life-style changes, and too much change can be overwhelming.

It is important that you problem-solve together with the client, so that he or she can decide which of the many available devices and techniques would be most helpful for managing the tasks of self-care and homemaking. Listen closely and be sensitive to any reluctance to try new approaches. Clients may feel more comfortable, emotionally, using a cumbersome

can opener that was a gift from one of their children than they would with a lightweight, battery-operated one that would be easier on their finger joints. Always offer *suggestions* or *recommendations* for assistive aids and techniques rather than *tell* clients what they should do. For example, you could say, "I've seen this used, and it seems to work really well."

Be familiar with the devices yourself. *Use* a battery-operated can opener, a long-handled reacher, and the adaptive techniques for dressing, so that you can anticipate problems and be ready with solutions for clients. For example, be ready to offer suggestions such as, "The shorter reacher may be better for you. I've noticed that the longer one is top-heavy and is hard to hold."

If a technique, rather than a device, can be used to solve a problem, recommend the technique. Techniques are versatile and can often be applied in multiple ways. Equipment is situation-specific. For instance, instead of a long-handled reacher, recommend that the person organize an area in such a way that commonly used articles are within easy reach, and items that are used once a year for special occasions are placed higher up, lower down, or farther back. This strategy works anywhere—in the kitchen, bedroom, bathroom, office, or garage—and it even saves the client the energy that he or she would spend in searching for the assistive device.

Living with rheumatoid arthritis is a creative challenge to both the client and the healthcare professional. Assistive aids and techniques can solve functional problems and make the difference between painful limitations and optimal independence.

Assessment

Nursing assessment begins by identifying the client's concerns and needs. The history should include information about the duration of clinical manifestations and ways the client has been managing those manifestations, particularly pain. It is important to identify other conditions that the client may have. The patient's current understanding of RA and the coping strategies used for dealing with pain and fatigue are important. Determine the methods that the client is now using to obtain pain relief (and the amount of pain that the client considers tolerable). Find out what methods the client is using for joint protection.

Evaluate the amount of swelling and pain in each joint, and the number of affected joints (to obtain a "joint count"). Recall that disease severity is based on the joint count, laboratory findings, and radiographic changes. In

addition, physiologic measures of function such as a timed walk, measures of grip strength, and results of self-report instruments that evaluate flexion and extension enable further evaluation of functional impairment and the impact of the disease on the client's life. Assess for current clinical manifestations in the client's eyes, heart, lungs, and peripheral nerves. It is important to note new manifestations and marked changes in previous clinical manifestations.

RA can be a crippling disorder. After 10 to 15 years with the disorder, less than one half of clients can still perform their own ADL. These physical limitations can greatly alter the usual role of the client in the family, the ability to work gainfully, the ability to participate in family events, and the ability to be an active sexual partner. Extreme fatigue and pain usually lead to early bedtimes and a reluctance to socialize. In addition, physical changes in the body can lead to lowered self-esteem. Western society values beauty and youth. Clients may find it psychologically difficult to be seen in public and deal with stares brought on by a hand deformity and other changes. As the client grieves the loss of a healthy, youthful body, thoughts of suicide can occur. Be sensitive to these issues and bring them into the discussion if the client or family hints at suicidal thoughts. Despite these changes, however, RA does not have to be a crippling disorder; with good medical and nursing care, many clients can maintain a healthy, productive, active life-style.

In caring for clients with RA, the nurse also acts as a liaison to obtain orders and arrange appointments with physical therapists, occupational therapists, and other providers. In rural settings, where these "extra" services are limited, you may need to provide supplemental information that these specialists would otherwise provide, and you may need to use printed resources to help clients.

Diagnosis, Planning, Implementation

Chronic Pain. The primary diagnosis of clients with RA is *Chronic Pain related to inflammation and swelling from pressure on surrounding tissues, joint deformity, and joint destruction.* The amount of pain that these clients experience permeates all aspects of their life. Recall the earlier analogy of living in a rusty armored suit.

Planning: Expected Outcomes. The client's pain will be controlled at a level that permits the client to perform his or her ADL.

Implementation. Chronic pain must be managed to allow the client to perform daily activities and function normally, to increase mobility, and to reduce fatigue. Teach the client the purpose and expected action of prescribed analgesics. You can use a handout to describe which side effects the client should report. Other pain relief interventions that may be used include the use of heat or cold, exercise, and massage. Paraffin baths have been used for arthritis of the hands; however, the greatest benefit from this intervention occurs when the client exercises immediately after the treatment. Cold therapy is applied by cold packs, ice massage, immersion, or vapocoolant sprays. While heat or cold may reduce pain, they may not be effective in decreasing inflammation. Transcutaneous electrical nerve stimulation (TENS) units have been used to reduce pain and local joint inflammation if only one or two joints are involved. Caution should be used when applying topical creams, rubs, or sprays, as shown in the Client Education Guide.

Relaxation techniques such as guided imagery help some people cope with pain. Classes to teach coping techniques have also been effective in decreasing pain and anxiety. When correctly performed, massage may also help relieve muscular aches and pain. However, it is important to massage only the surrounding muscles.

CLIENT EDUCATION GUIDE

Using Topical Pain Relievers

Topical pain relievers work in several ways, depending on their ingredients. Some, which contain salicylates, the substance found in aspirin, may penetrate through the skin to the joint and reduce pain. Other pain relievers contain ingredients such as menthol or camphor that irritate the skin and distract attention from the actual pain. Still others contain capsaicin, a substance found in hot peppers, which reduces the pain signal to the brain. Regardless of the mechanism of action of the pain reliever, the Arthritis Foundation recommends that topical pain relievers be only one part of a comprehensive treatment program that includes medication, exercise, rest, joint protection, and, in severe cases, surgery. Additional instructions to convey to the client are as follows:

Client Instructions in English *(Instrucciones para el cliente en inglés)*	**Client Instructions in Spanish** *(Instrucciones para el cliente en español)*
Read and follow the directions on the package.	Lea y siga las instrucciones en el paquete.
Wash your hands after every application.	Lávese las manos después de cada aplicación.
Keep topical pain relievers away from your eyes, mucous membranes, cuts, or irritated skin.	No aplique analgésicos tópicos cerca de los ojos, membranas mucosas, heridas, o piel que esté irritada.
If you are allergic to aspirin or are taking an anticoagulant ("blood thinner"), talk with your doctor before using any rubs, creams, or sprays that contain salicylates.	Si tiene alergias a la aspirina o si está tomando anticoagulantes (para adelgazar la sangre), consulte a su doctor antes de frotarse cremas o usar espray (atomizadores) que contengan salicilatos.
Keep all topical pain relievers out of the reach of children.	Guarde todos los analgésicos tópicos fuera del alcance de los niños.

Never massage acutely inflamed joints because doing so may aggravate inflammation.

Many clients with RA are perceived as demanding and manipulative. This misconception has stemmed from clients' attempts to control what little of their world they can. Chronic pain and fatigue often push coping skills to the limit. With what little energy is left, these clients attempt to control other parts of their lives. Approach these clients with compassion and appreciation for their problems. Many of their idiosyncrasies, such as statements like "Don't put the covers over my toes," are attempts to reduce pain. There is no such thing as a rheumatoid personality.

Impaired Physical Mobility. Another common nursing diagnosis is *Impaired Physical Mobility related to pain, stiffness, and joint deformity.* Using the armored suit analogy once again, you can see how movement of any kind is hampered when most or all of the articular joints are inflamed.

Planning: Expected Outcomes. The client will maintain mobility at the highest possible level to carry out desired activities.

Implementation. Encourage the client to stay active. In cooperation with a physical therapist or trained exercise physiologist, help the client to develop an exercise program to preserve ROM while protecting joints. Maintaining function and mobility are necessary for the client to manage self-care activities.

Exercise can decrease morning stiffness, pain, and fatigue and enhance the client's self-esteem. Participating in group exercise programs, such as community water exercise programs (Fig. 28–10), provides social support and strengthens coping. Seek programs led by arthritis-certified instructors who monitor movement for adequate joint protection. Each session should include a warm-up period, full ROM exercises, endurance exercises, muscle-strengthening exercises, and cool-down exercises. Clients may use analgesics prior to exercise to permit increased freedom of movement. However, if a joint becomes painful during the exercise and the pain persists for 2 hours or more after the exercise, the activity should be modified.

Fatigue. Fatigue is a complex physiologic process involving the muscles, heart, lungs, and immune system. Clients with RA often experience fatigue, in part because of their chronic inflammatory process, pain, and depression. The diagnosis you may be working with is *Fatigue related to chronic inflammation, pain, or depression.*

Planning: Expected Outcomes. The client will develop methods to balance rest and activity and will express satisfaction with his or her current level of activity and energy.

Implementation. Help the client to explore reasonable options for gaining enough sleep and finding time during the day to rest or nap. This may require changes in job performance or work relationships (if others need to do the client's work while he or she rests). Be sensitive to these concerns and ask if your suggestions are reasonable in the client's personal setting. Practitioners can find it easy to say "be sure to rest now" without determining the feasibility of this protocol. For example, if the client is a young mother, she may need to send her young children to a neighbor for an hour or two each afternoon or nap while the children nap.

Altered Role Performance, Body Image Disturbance, Self-Esteem Disturbance. Several psychosocial nursing diagnoses may apply to the client with RA. You will want to choose the one that best fits the client. All of these diagnoses may be related to chronic pain, the need for others to perform previous

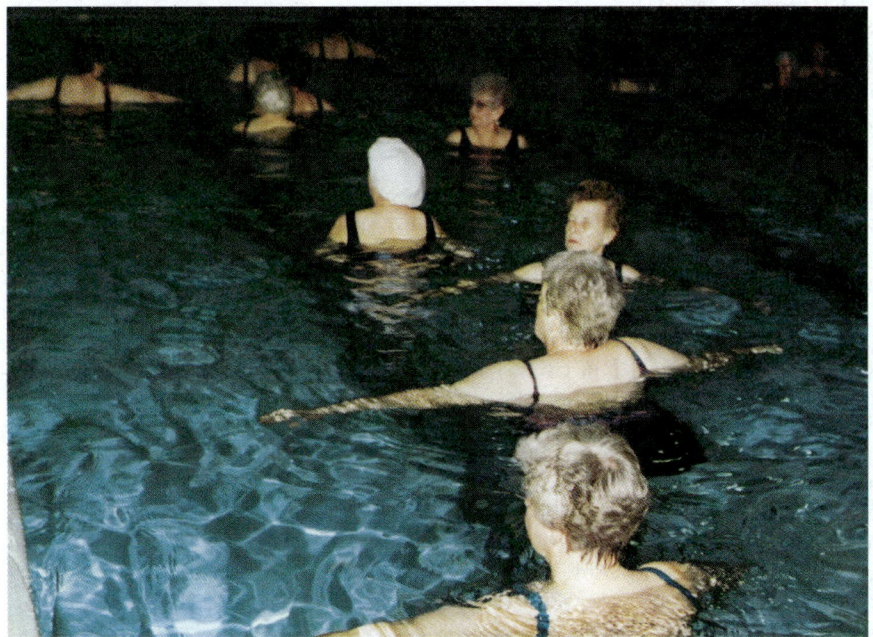

Figure 28–10. A community water exercise program. Many clients with rheumatoid arthritis find that water exercise helps to control pain and disability and improves exercise tolerance. The people in this class demonstrate the importance of keeping the shoulders submerged to allow the buoyancy of the water to protect their joints.

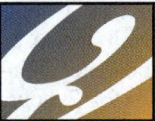

NURSING RESEARCH

Are Community Water Exercise Programs Effective?

Meyer, C. L., & Hawley, D. J. (1994). Characteristics of participants in water exercise programs compared to patients seen in a rheumatic disease clinic. *Arthritis Care and Research, 7* (2), 85–89.

A benefit of water exercise is the buoyancy of the water, which supports the joints, decreasing stress and pain during movement. This study was designed to ascertain if people with arthritis participating in a community water exercise program report less pain and better function than people not known to exercise regularly.

This question was investigated using 87 participants in water exercise programs and comparing them with 164 people coming to an outpatient arthritis clinic. The subjects were matched by type of arthritis, age, and sex. For this study, 82% of the subjects were female with an average age of 68 years, (range 44–83). The exercise group contained more retired subjects (63%) than the clinic group (49%). To compare the two groups, grip strength was measured and subjects were asked to complete a questionnaire designed to measure their arthritis-related disability, pain, anxiety, and depression. The exercise sessions were led by an Arthritis Foundation–certified instructor. Each session included a warm-up period and full range-of-motion, endurance, muscle strengthening, and cool-down exercises. Most people attend the 45- to 50-minute sessions two to three times a week.

Water exercise participants demonstrated a stronger grip, reported better function, less pain, decreased anxiety, and less depression than the outpatient group. Nearly 50% of those attending water exercise attended for 3 or more years. They reported "feeling better" and "social interaction" as other benefits of the water exercise program.

Implications for Practice

Nurses working with clients with arthritis should encourage participation in water exercise programs. Collaboration with an exercise physiologist may be required.

Implementation. Not only does the disease itself alter appearance, but if the client is being treated with corticosteroids, there are several side effects from these medications that can alter self-esteem. Corticosteroids cause abnormal deposition of fat in the face (giving the client a "moon face" appearance) and shoulders (causing a "buffalo hump"); other side effects include acne, paper-thin skin that bruises easily, striae, and weight gain. Because of these and other side effects, the prescriber must always consider the risk-benefit ratio when initiating corticosteroid therapy. Also, the client may question their use because the physical changes caused by corticosteroids can be humiliating, even though the medications slow the inflammation. Most of these changes are permanent, and the client needs time to work through a new body image. Body image changes take months to accept. Be sensitive to negative self-talk by the client, and express acceptance of the client's appearance; suggest clothing options to minimize visible changes.

The client and family will need time to plan for and accept the changes in the client's ability to perform previous tasks. Initially, it may seem easy to fill the role of two people in the home, and clients and their families may seem wary of efforts to encourage them to think about this change over the years that follow. Clients may also think initially that they will be able to go back to work full-time and that joint inflammation is only temporary. Be sensitive to this type of denial and work with the client and family "where they are." Gradually, as the disease progresses, clients and families may need additional help as they try to come to terms with the long-term implications of the disease.

Risk of Ineffective Management of Therapeutic Regimen (Individuals).

A final nursing diagnosis for the medically managed client with RA is *Risk for Ineffective Management of Therapeutic Regimen related to complex medications, schedules, high risk of side effects from medications, health maintenance, and self-care.* The management of any chronic disorder is complex, and the management of RA is no exception. Clients often have to take several types of medications with many undesirable side effects. They must plan for exercise and rest, and cope with daily pain and stiffness.

Planning: Expected Outcomes. The client will make informed decisions about the management of the disease that will lead to a satisfactory quality of life despite the disease.

Implementation. Education focuses on coping skills, alternative methods of managing pain, joint protection, exercise, and adaptations for retaining functional independence. Inadequate knowledge may contribute to noncompliance with treatment regimens. Also, because of the pattern of remissions and exacerbations characteristic of RA, people tend to become discouraged with their prescribed treatments. Likewise, the medications used in the treatment of RA may provide only moderate pain relief, and many are slow-acting. Clients with RA therefore often fall prey to "quack" cures and unproven remedies (Box 28–2).

roles, feelings of helplessness, and feelings of embarrassment. In this section we present several avenues of care; select those that apply best to the particular client.

Planning: Expected Outcomes. Although the actual outcome statement will depend on the client's particular diagnosis, most outcomes focus on the client's being able to express improved satisfaction with the problem. The problems identified by the three psychosocial diagnoses are usually very closely related, and improvement in one area will lead to improvement in others.

Box 28–2. Unproven Remedies for Arthritis

Harmless	Harmful	Unknown
■ Copper bracelets	■ DMSO (dimethyl sulfoxide)	■ Biofeedback
■ Mineral springs		■ Diets
■ Uranium mines	■ Large doses of vitamins	■ Fish oil
■ Vibrators		■ Lasers
■ Vinegar and honey	■ Drugs with hidden ingredients such as steroids	■ Yucca
	■ Snake venom	

The Arthritis Foundation estimates that most people with arthritis have tried an unproven arthritis remedy at some point.

One in 10 people who have tried unproven arthritis remedies report harmful side effects, according to a Health and Human Services survey.

An estimated $1 billion is spent yearly on unproven arthritis remedies.

Any unproven remedy, no matter how harmless, can become harmful if it stops or delays someone from seeking a prescribed treatment program from a physician.

How Can People Determine if a Remedy Is Unproven?

It may be hard to spot an unproven remedy at first glance. The only source of information about a remedy may be what is given out by its promoters. People with arthritis should be cautious if the proposed remedy falls into one or more of the following categories:

Works for all types of arthritis

There are over 100 types of arthritis and treatments vary for each kind.

Uses case histories and testimonials

Claims of individuals helped by a treatment need to be backed up by repeated studies on large numbers of people.

Cites only one study

A single study may get results which other studies cannot repeat. A number of scientists must repeat the same study and get similar results for a treatment to be considered proven. A single study may, however, suggest a treatment that may have promise and should be studied further.

Cites a study without a control group

The use of a control group helps show that the results are due to the new treatment and not to some other factor.

Does not list contents

Some ads for a miracle drug for arthritis actually are just aspirin at a high price. Other treatments have been found to contain corticosteroids and other powerful drugs. These drugs may have severe side effects and should not be taken without a doctor's supervision.

Has no warnings about side effects

There should be warnings on the label or instructions stating who should not use the treatment.

Claims to be based on a secret formula

Scientists share their discoveries so that other experts in arthritis can review and question their findings.

Courtesy of the Arthritis Foundation, Atlanta, GA.

Unproven arthritis remedies are treatments that in scientific studies have not been shown to work and to be safe. Proven treatments for arthritis must show in repeated, controlled scientific tests that they work by meeting one or more of the following goals:

● Pain reduction
● Reduction of inflammation
● Safe joint mobility
● Avoidance of stress damage to joints

Proven treatments also must show how safe they are. The benefits of a treatment in controlling arthritis should be greater than the risk of unwanted or harmful effects. Some unproven remedies are harmless. Others are harmful. Still others have health effects that are unknown. Even if an unproven remedy is in itself harmless, it can still have a detrimental effect if it causes a person to stop or slow down proven treatments to control arthritis. Nevertheless, despite the many problems that people with RA face daily, many of these people courageously overcome these problems to maintain active, productive lives. There are news groups on America On-Line for arthritis that

clients or healthcare providers can access and Web browsers can go to http://www.arthritis.org/.

Evaluation

The process of RA is slow to improve. It will take several weeks to months for the expected outcomes for most of these diagnoses to be met. When joints are already severely damaged and pain is uncontrollable, joint replacement becomes an option. These and other surgical therapies are discussed under the heading Surgical Management.

Modifications for Elderly Clients

Elderly people can slowly succumb to the pain and immobility associated with the disease, becoming complacent and sedentary. Some of these elderly people with RA virtually *never* leave home for fear of pain and embarrassment about being slow to walk and move. Help these elderly clients to find ways of improving mobility by having them work among other clients of their own age and abilities. In addition, elderly clients are often being treated for several other problems, such as lung or heart disease, each with its own treatment regimen. The proper integration of all of these medications and other treatments is important.

 Acute and Subacute Care

■ Surgical Management

Surgical procedures may be helpful for clients with arthritis. Surgery may be used to relieve pain, improve function, and correct deformities. Previously, surgery was considered only late in the course of arthritis, often after severe joint destruction or deformity had developed. Now, however, preventive surgery is used to prevent deformities during the early phases or active stages of the disease.

Tendon Transfer and Osteotomy

Tendon transfers can prevent progressive deformity caused by muscle spasm. During these procedures, nodules or benign bony tumors (called exostoses) may be surgically removed, and flexion contractures may be surgically relieved. Osteotomies (excising or cutting through bone) may improve the function of deformed joints or limbs. For example, a femoral head osteotomy may give symptomatic relief by changing the position of the head of the femur when it is being subjected to the stress of impact against the acetabulum. Postoperative care varies depending on the joint treated. In general, joints operated on are immobilized for a short time and then remobilized with physical therapy.

Synovectomy

Synovectomy (surgical removal of synovia, as in the elbows, wrists, fingers, or knees) may be used in RA to help maintain joint function. With RA, joint destruction begins in the synovial tissue and then proceeds to involve bone, cartilage, and other structures. Early synovectomy helps prevent recurrent inflammation. Short-term immobilization is needed after surgery.

Arthrodesis

Arthrodesis is an operation to produce bony fusion of a joint. Most often arthrodesis is used for clients with bone loss after joint infection, with tumors, with musculoskeletal trauma, and with paralysis, Arthrodesis can also help certain clients with RA or degenerative arthritis to regain some mobility. The surgeon usually uses metal screws and plates to fuse the joint. Although arthrodesis immobilizes the joint, the procedure eliminates much of the pain of the arthritic process and improves the client's functional mobility. The ankle is the joint most commonly treated with arthrodesis, usually to relieve post-traumatic arthritis. However, the hip and knee can also be fused.

Despite its limited benefits, arthrodesis also has its drawbacks. It often results in stiffness in adjacent joints and increases the energy required for ambulation. It is possible, at times, to convert some fused joints to arthroplasties later in life. Bone grafts can also be used to stabilize the joint when desired union fails to occur after arthrodesis or when the use of screws or other devices is inadvisable. Following surgery, the limb is casted, and nursing care is the same as for clients with casts (see Chapter 75).

Joint Replacement

Joint replacement (arthroplasty) is surgical replacement of natural diseased joints or joint components with artificial joints or joint components. The operation restores motion to a joint and function to the muscles, ligaments, and other soft tissue structures that control a joint. The concept of joint replacement surgery is actually several hundred years old, but the modern ideas of joint replacement began in the 1960s, with the development of replacement components for the hip joint made of stainless steel and polyethylene (a lightweight plastic). Soon after, replacement joints were designed for the knee, shoulder, elbow, and fingers. Today, joint prostheses are still a combination of a metal surface articulating with a polyethylene surface (Fig. 28–11). The metal surfaces are made of strong, lightweight alloys such as cobalt-chromium, and titanium-aluminum-vanadium. Both surfaces of an arthritic joint are replaced. If only one surface were replaced, the prosthesis would rub against the remaining tissue and not relieve pain or improve function. Arthritic joints can be replaced. This chapter discusses arthroplasty of the shoulder, elbow, and fingers. Discussion of hip and knee replacement is found in Chapter 74 following discussion of osteoarthritis.

Shoulder Arthroplasty

Disorders of the shoulder that require arthroplasty are much less common that those problems in weightbearing joints. Although the shoulder is classified as a ball-and-socket joint, the shoulder permits more mobility than any other joint in the body. The large head of the humerus articulates against, and not inside, the small glenoid cavity. This freedom of movement comes at the expense of stability. No inherent stability exists in the shoulder joint. The shoulder relies on soft tissue and ligaments for stability, particularly the rotator cuff muscle-tendon unit. Four muscles and their tendons compose the rotator cuff, which allows the normal shoulder to move through three planes: flexion and extension, abduction and adduction, and internal rotation and external rotation. Shoulder pain can have several causes. Therefore it is important to determine the true cause of the problem before treatment begins. Common manifestations of glenohumeral disorders include difficulty in flexion and extension and increased pain with attempted movement. An increase in joint stiffness may occur after sleeping. Local injections of steroids and physical therapy can usually delay surgery.

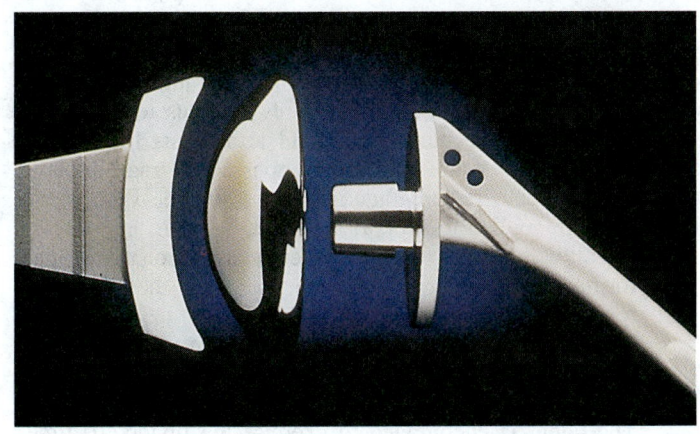

Figure 28–11. This shoulder joint prosthesis is a typical joint prosthesis consisting of a metal surface articulating with a polyethylene surface. (Courtesy of Zimmer, Inc., Warsaw, IN.)

Shoulder arthroplasty is replacement of the humeral head and glenoid articulating surface with a metal and polyethylene prosthesis (Fig. 28–12). The primary indication for total shoulder replacement is pain caused by incongruity of the glenoid and humeral head. Improvement in function and ROM is a secondary objective of the operation. Usual problems that are treated with total shoulder arthroplasty are RA, osteoarthritis, fractures, and dislocations. There are no specific age limitations, but the client must be well motivated and be a reasonable surgical risk. In many clients with RA, the rotator cuff is thin and diseased. This is a disadvantage for full recovery of shoulder function. Contraindications include infection and inability to comply with rehabilitation, such as clients with physiologic problems (e.g., neuropathy) or psychological problems. Complications include brachial nerve palsy, prosthetic loosening, joint dislocation or subluxation, and impingement syndrome.

Nursing assessment includes neurovascular assessment of the operative arm at least every 4 hours, as summarized in the Critical Monitoring feature. A possible complication is development of impingement syndrome because of the proximity of the brachial plexus. Hemovac

drainage should be less than 100 ml during the first 12 hours. Elevate the head of the bed 30 degrees to reduce swelling and improve comfort. Aggressive pain management is needed; the shoulder arthroplasty usually causes more pain during the first 24 hours than the other joint replacements. Patient-controlled analgesia (PCA) works well when supplemented with non-narcotic anti-inflammatory agents (e.g., ketorolac tromethamine [Toradol]). Ice is applied to the shoulder. It may be difficult for the client to find a comfortable position to lie in; the nurse should position the shoulder to comfort without forcing it into motion. Personal items should be placed within easy reach of the nonoperative arm.

After surgery, the client's arm is placed in a sling or Velpeau bandage. Clients with rotator cuff repair wear a light brace to prevent abduction and external rotation. A

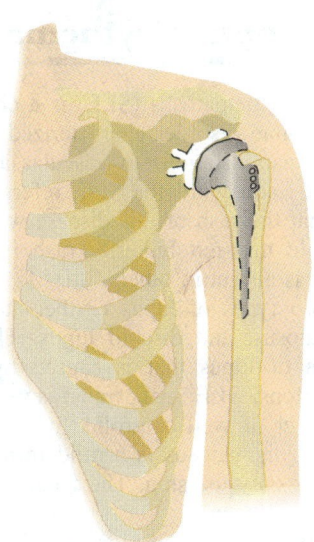

Figure 28–12. Total shoulder arthroplasty.

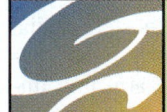

CRITICAL MONITORING

Postoperative Brachial Plexus Compromise

- To assess median nerve status, have the client grasp your hand. Note the strength of the first and second fingers. A weak grip may indicate compromise of the median nerve.
- To assess radial nerve status, note the movement of the client's thumb toward the palm, and back to neutral. Problems with this motion may indicate compromise of the radial nerve.
- To assess ulnar nerve status, have the client spread all the fingers wide and resist pressure. Weakness against pressure may indicate compromise of the ulnar nerve.
- To assess cutaneous nerve status, assess for flexion of the biceps by having the client raise the forearm. Poor biceps flexion may indicate compromise of the cutaneous nerve.
- To assess axillary nerve status, have the client push the elbow outward against pressure. Hold the arm still while you palpate the deltoid for contraction. Weak contraction may indicate compromise of the axillary nerve.

shoulder CPM (continuous passive motion) can be used for all three planes of motion. Initially, the shoulder is placed in forward flexion and external rotation. Shoulder rehabilitation begins quickly after surgery and continues for about 6 weeks. For no other joint is rehabilitation as important as for the shoulder. The shoulder is placed through progressive external and internal ROM, hyperextension, and finally exercises with resistance once the rotator cuff has healed (at about 6 weeks). Usually the client can be taught how to use the nonoperative arm to move the operative arm through ROM.

Elbow Arthroplasty

Early forms of elbow arthroplasty were metal-to-metal hinges, replacing the hinge structure of the elbow joint. Few of these prostheses are used today because they loosen after 2 to 3 years. Later, hinge joints were made that contained metal and polyethylene. This metal and plastic joint allows for some medial-to-lateral and rotational movements. There is also a nonhinged elbow joint that contains a metal and polyethylene component. Indications for elbow arthroplasty are pain, mechanical instability, and bilateral elbow arthrodesis (fusion of the elbow). It is also possible to correct pain in the elbow by resecting the olecranon; this is called a resection arthroplasty. Clients with severe RA are the most common clients having total elbow arthroplasty. After surgery the arm is dressed in compressive dressings or splinted, and wound drains are placed.

Postoperative care includes elevating the arm above the shoulder for 4 to 5 days. Assess the client every 4 hours for ulnar nerve entrapment. Check the client's hand strength; especially assess thumb and index finger's ability to pinch and ability to adduct the fourth and fifth fingers. The ulnar nerve lies close to the posteromedial surface of the elbow. It is called the "funny bone" because of the uncomfortable sensation in the arm and fingers when it is hit. Also assess for radial and ulnar pulses and capillary refill. Some institutions use pulse oximetry to continuously assess tissue perfusion. Pain is managed with PCA narcotics. Elbow flexion and extension are allowed as tolerated. Personal items should be placed within easy reach of the nonoperative arm. An occupational therapist should guide the client on how to modify ADL. Clients should not lift more than 5 lb or begin triceps and biceps strengthening exercises for 3 months. The client will never be able to lift heavy items or play sports with the operative arm.

Hand Arthroplasty

Various hand deformities develop from the synovitis of RA (see Figure 28–4). Synovitis stretches the central portion of the extensor tendon, causing it to shift. Eventually the tendons become shortened and fixed. Ulnar drift occurs when the imbalance of damaged extensor tendons and intact flexor tendons cause subluxation of the metacarpophalangeal (MCP) joint. Other hand deformities develop from synovitis of the proximal interphalangeal joint (PIP) joint: boutonnière deformity and swan-neck deformity. A boutonnière deformity is flexion of the PIP and hyperextension of the distal interphalangeal joint (DIP). There is no loss of MCP joint mobility. In the swan-neck deformity, the DIP is flexed and the PIP joint is hyperextended. Surgery for arthritic hands includes tendon transfers to improve pinch grasp and arthrodesis for strength and position of the thumb for opposition. Hinge implants are placed to restore function to the fingers. Fluff dressings are applied to support the hand.

Following surgery, neurovascular assessments are performed every hour for several hours. If the client has regional block anesthesia, the hand may be numb. The hand is elevated off of the bed to prevent ulnar pressure. Usually the hand is placed in a stockinette and suspended from the bed. An opening is made to assess the fingers. The client is encouraged to exercise the fingers 10 times every hour, attempting full extension and flexion. Finger exercises will reduce edema and pain. Personal items should be placed within easy reach of the nonoperative arm. If the opposite hand is equally deformed from RA, the client is quite helpless and will require assistance with most components of ADL. Encourage the client to use the nonoperative arm as much as possible. Some clients may express great concern about being dependent. The nurse should promote independence and praise actions that foster self-care.

Rehabilitation is very long. Most clients are fitted with outrigger splints with rubber bands that allow exercise with resistance after 1 week. Therapy continues for several weeks to assist the client to regain strength and control.

Modifications for Elderly Clients

Older clients may have adapted to the RA very well but often find any further dependency needed after surgery difficult to handle. They tend to be slower in their recovery from total joint replacement. They may require prolonged hospitalization in an extended care facility or subacute care setting until they regain adequate mobility to function independently or with some assistance and safety.

Systemic Lupus Erythematosus

Systemic lupus erythematosus (SLE) is a chronic, inflammatory, autoimmune disorder characterized by a wide array of clinical manifestations in vascular and connective tissue. *Lupus* is Latin word for wolf, referring to a belief in the 1800s that the rash of this disease was caused by a wolf bite. While this red butterfly rash is distinctive is some clients, it is absent in others.

There are two types of lupus erythematosus: systemic lupus erythematosus, and discoid lupus. There is also a reversible form of lupus that is caused by reactions to various medications. SLE is the most severe form of the disorder. However, if well controlled it can also be mild. Discoid lupus erythematosus is a mild form of the disorder that involves only the skin. The face, neck, and upper chest are usually affected.

SLE is relatively rare, occurring in 1 in 2000 persons. It most commonly develops in younger women between the ages of 15 and 40. It is also more common in blacks, followed by Asians and then whites. It is almost 10 times more common in women than in men. This suggests a hormonal influence.[11]

Etiology and Risk Factors

There is a theory that the genetic predisposition for the disease is present in some clients and a virus or some other agent triggers it and the disease occurs. This theory is as yet unsupported. SLE also has a familial tendency, and when one twin has the disease, the other twin has a 25% to 50% greater incidence of the disorder. Although the exact cause of SLE is unknown, sources of disease exacerbation have been identified. These include sunlight and other forms of ultraviolet light, physical and emotional stress, and pregnancy.

Several medications have been implicated in the development of a reversible form of lupus. They are listed in Box 28–3. These drugs bind to and alter DNA, possibly enhancing the response. There may also be a correlation between the client's ability to metabolize the medication and a predisposition to SLE.

Pathophysiology

Persons with SLE produce several autoantibodies. The primary autoantibodies produced are directed at the cell nuclei and are called antinuclear antibodies, or ANAs. SLE produces autoantibodies against double-stranded DNA, and the presence of these antibodies in the serum are considered typical of SLE. Normally, the T suppressor cells prevent autoantibody formation. In SLE a defect in the T suppressor cell prevents this protective process. Natural killer cell function is also suppressed; they cannot kill abnormal cells as readily. There are inherited defects in complement factors and cell surface receptors that normally assist with clearing immune complexes.

ANA does not cause a lot of cellular destruction alone, primarily because ANA does not come in contact with intact cell nuclei. However, when cells die, the nuclei are released and then bind to the ANA. The immune complex that is formed triggers the inflammatory response, which is the primary cause of tissue damage. In addition, the immune complex is large and is often deposited in tissues. The deposit of this complex causes even more tissue damage by initiating the complement cascade and further increasing inflammation. A common site for deposit is the basement membrane of the kidney, which leads to glomerulonephritis. The complexes can also cause vasculitis, or inflammation of the vessels, leading to a decrease of oxygen in organs and tissues. The immune complexes can also be deposited in the heart and brain.

Clinical Manifestations and Diagnostic Findings

SLE is not a single specific disorder, and therefore the manifestations of SLE can vary greatly among people. The course of SLE also has exacerbations or flares and

---

Box 28–3. Lupus-Inducing Drugs

Definite	Possible	Unlikely
Hydralazine	Phenytoin	Griseofulvin
Procainamide	Penicillamine	Phenylbutazone
Isoniazid	Quinidine	Oral
Chlorpromazine	Sulfonamide	contraceptives
Methyldopa	Propylthiouracil	Gold salts
	Practolol	Penicillin
	Acebutolol	Hydrazine
	Lithium carbonate	L-Canaverine
	p-Aminosalicylate	
	Nitrofurantoin	
	Tartrazine	
	Atenolol	
	Metoprolol	
	Oxprenolol	
	Mephenytoin	
	Trimethadione	
	Ethosuximide	
	Methimazole	
	Captopril	

From Schur, P. (1993). Clinical Features of SLE. In W. Kelley, et al. (Eds.), *Textbook of rheumatology* (4th ed.). Philadelphia: W. B. Saunders.

---

controlled periods called remissions. Persons with SLE often present with nonspecific symptoms, such as weight loss, fever, malaise, and lethargy. In some persons, the manifestations are insidious and resemble other conditions such as arthritis because of the joint involvement. Many of the manifestations of SLE are due to the deposition of immune complexes in the tissues.

■ Acute Forms

Manifestations of acute SLE may include fever, musculoskeletal aches and pains, butterfly rash on the face, pleural effusion, basilar pneumonia, generalized lymphadenopathy, pericarditis, tachycardia, hepatosplenomegaly, nephritis, delirium, convulsions, psychosis, and coma.

■ Chronic Forms

Manifestations of chronic SLE depend on the organs involved but may include fever, malaise, weight loss, cutaneous discoid LE lesions, erythema of exposed skin, generalized lymphadenopathy, severe hemolytic anemia, thrombocytopenic purpura, hypersplenism, pericarditis, pleural effusion, tachycardia, peripheral vascular syndromes (e.g., Raynaud's phenomenon, gangrene), ulcerative mucous membrane lesions, abdominal pains, nausea, vomiting, anorexia, bloody stools, hepatic dysfunction, hepatomegaly, focal glomerulitis progressing to glomerulonephritis, myalgia, arthralgia, neuritis, hemiplegia, psychosis, convulsions, and coma.

Laboratory tests reveal

● Presence of LE cells (autoantibodies); the severity of SLE usually correlates with the degree of LE cell formation
● Decreased complement levels
● Presence of immune complexes in the serum
● Presence of immune antibodies to DNA anti-samarium (Sm) and ANA
● Decreased levels of red blood cells, white blood cells, and platelets
● Increased γ-globulin fraction due to increased antibody production
● An elevated ESR

At some point, abnormalities in the kidneys can be noted on an intravenous pyelogram (IVP); a barium enema would reveal colonic ulceration; a magnetic resonance imaging (MRI) study might reveal CNS involvement; and an ECG or echocardiogram might show cardiac changes.

Community and Self-Care

■ Medical Management

The goals of care for the client with SLE focus on (1) maintenance of skin integrity, (2) promotion of a healthy life-style and reduction of stress, (3) maintenance of proper nutrition, (4) promotion of comfort, (5) increase in the client's independence, and (5) maintenance of emotional well-being.

The client is examined every 3 months with a CBC, determination of creatinine and cholesterol levels, urinalysis, and sometimes serum C3, C4, and anti-dsDNA (double-stranded DNA).

Management of SLE is based on the organ systems involved. For example, if the client has cardiac involvement with either pericarditis or pleural effusion, intravenous pulse methylprednisolone may be used for 3 days, followed by oral prednisone. Cutaneous manifestations are managed with antimalarial agents. Most treatments are with medications; an algorithm has been developed to guide care (Figure 28–13). Plasmapheresis may also be used to remove circulating autoantibodies and immune complexes from the blood before organ and tissue damage occur. The efficacy of this treatment has not been determined.

SLE requires more than medications for proper management. The client is advised of life-style changes needed to reduce the risk of coronary artery disease, including management of hypertension, smoking cessation, and prevention of obesity and hyperlipidemia. Hypertension is aggressively managed with medications because it commonly leads to renal failure and death. The client is also advised to reduce salt, fat, and cholesterol intake.

People in the United States have been called sun worshipers because they strive for a "healthy tan." Of course,

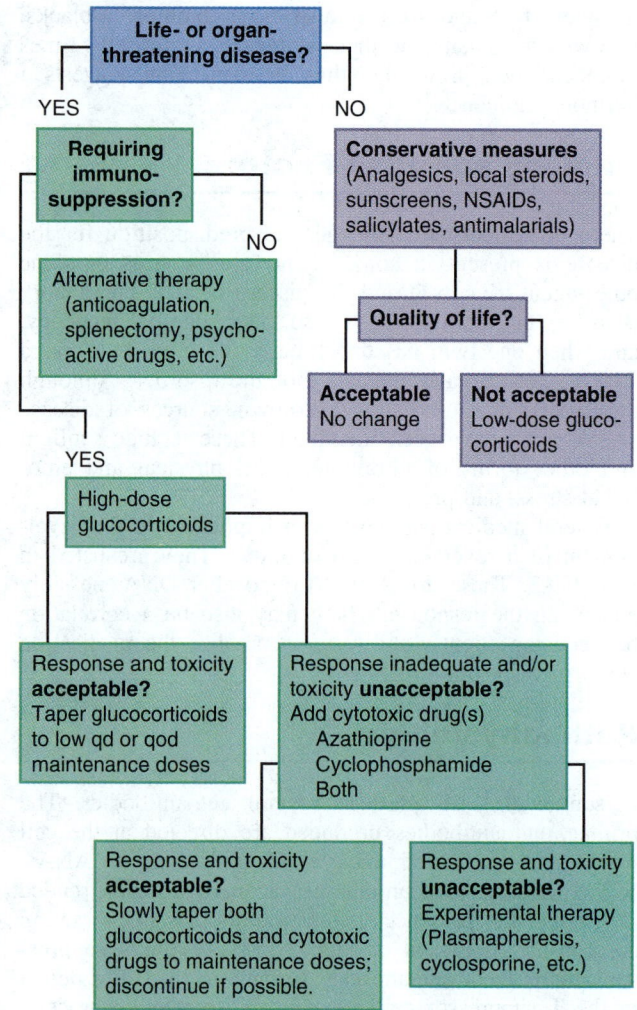

Figure 28–13. An algorithm for the management of clients with systemic lupus erythematosus. (From Hahn, B. H. [1993]. Management of systemic lupus erythematosus. In W. N. Kelley, et al. [Eds.]. *Textbook of rheumatology* [4th ed.]. Philadelphia: W. B. Saunders.)

tanning is dangerous to everyone, but the client with SLE must consider the sun an enemy. Photosensitivity is common; many develop a rash after sun exposure as a result of stimulation of inflammatory processes.

All SLE clients receiving corticosteroids or immunosuppressants should receive the pneumococcal pneumonia vaccine and yearly influenza vaccine. Clients should be taught to report any signs of infection quickly. If possible, sulfa antibiotics should be avoided because of their tendency to cause allergy and flares of SLE. Ongoing dental care is important to avoid a potential source of systemic infection. Yearly ophthalmologic examinations are also important to monitor for side effects of antimalarial therapy and to detect and treat cataracts secondary to long-term corticosteroid use.

Renal disease, such as nephritis leading to renal failure, is a common outcome. Again, high-dose corticosteroids are given initially. If the creatinine level rises above 3 mg/dl, dialysis is considered.

■ Nursing Management of the Medical Client

Nursing intervention for clients with SLE depends on how they respond to the condition and on the severity and specific types of clinical manifestations. In a newly diagnosed client, the nurse can expect knowledge deficits with respect to the diagnosis itself, prescribed drug therapies, and the prognosis. Provide the client and significant others with instructions on relieving anxiety and avoiding misunderstandings. This is particularly important in terms of the prescribed medications. Advise the client and significant others of the actions, side effects, and potential interactions of prescribed medications, especially corticosteroids.

During follow-up visits, review changes in all body systems. A physical examination is needed with attention given to skin, muscles, and joints. Central nervous system involvement is common, and a complete psychosocial assessment is important to detect changes in cognition and emotional stability.

During exacerbations, provide physiologic support to prevent skin breakdown, maintain nutritional and metabolic status, and minimize the risk of opportunistic infection. Also, provide emotional support to the client facing a chronic, potentially fatal disease. Clients may experience grief reaction following diagnosis, with exacerbations, or both. It is important to allow for verbalization of these feelings. In such situations, be supportive and understanding, and when necessary, refer the client or significant others for counseling.

■ Outcomes

In general, the clinical pattern and prognosis of SLE are variable. The illness may develop rapidly and have an acute fulminant course. More commonly, it develops insidiously and becomes chronic, with remissions and exacerbations. The course of the disorder is more severe when onset occurs at a young age. The survival rate has improved dramatically in recent years, although the disease is still potentially fatal. More than 95% of clients are alive 5 years after diagnosis. Improvements in treatments mean that clients can now live for many years.

The leading cause of death in clients with SLE is renal failure. There is some degree of kidney involvement causing progressive changes within the glomeruli in most clients with SLE. With progression of SLE nephritis, the glomeruli become increasingly abnormal and accumulate immune complex deposits. Once 75% of the glomeruli have been affected, the client will show signs of renal failure. The heart is the other major organ involved in SLE. The immune complexes deposit in the coronary vessels, myocardium, and pericardium. CNS involvement, usually leading to cerebral infarction, can also occur.

Progressive Systemic Sclerosis

Progressive systemic sclerosis (PSS) is a disorder caused by excessive collagen deposition, microvascular injury, and changes in humoral and cellular immunity. PSS is commonly known as scleroderma, although the skin is not the only organ system affected by the progressive sclerosis. Actually, this is a connective tissue disease characterized by fibrosis and degenerative changes of the skin, synovium, digital arteries, and parenchymal and small arteries of the internal organs.

The exact mechanisms that cause PSS are not fully understood. Excess deposition of collagen is the characteristic feature of PSS but the cause of excess collagen production is not known. However, the collagen that is produced is normal in other aspects. Vascular changes include fibrosis of the endothelium of small arterioles. Endothelial damage and cell death activate platelets and cause more inflammation. The activated platelets also lead to vasoconstriction and increased capillary permeability and recruit other inflammatory cells (e.g., fibroblasts) into the area. Alterations in humoral immunity are seen in the development of antibodies to type IV collagen found in the basement membranes of tissues. Persons with PSS have hypergammaglobulinemia, with the greatest increase in IgG. Cellular immunity is also altered. In PSS, T lymphocytes accumulate in involved tissues; therefore circulating T lymphocytes may be slightly decreased.

Scleroderma is classified into two categories: localized and generalized. *Localized scleroderma* is the less severe form and affects primarily the skin. It may involve muscles and bones but does not affect the internal organs. Localized scleroderma is further divided into morphea and linear scleroderma. Morphea is the development of skin lesions that are hard, oval, and white with a purple ring around them. Morphea often improves in time. Linear scleroderma is seen as a skin lesion that looks like a thick line of skin. It often begins in childhood and develops on the arms, legs, or forehead. The lesion can extend into the muscle and bone beneath it and alter growth.

Generalized scleroderma, or what is truly called PSS, involves the skin and many other internal organs such as the kidneys, lungs, joints, muscles, cardiovascular system, and digestive system. Generalized PSS can also be further divided into limited subcutaneous scleroderma or diffuse subcutaneous scleroderma, often called CREST (Box 28–4).

Calcinosis is the development of small white calcium deposits beneath the skin. The lumps may break open and drain a chalky fluid. Most clients have Raynaud's syndrome. Raynaud's syndrome is spasms of the arteries and arterioles. Spasms can occur spontaneously but most often are brought on by exposure to cold or emotional stress. Esophageal motility is decreased from excessive deposits of collagen and muscle atrophy. Sclerodactyly is scleroderma of the fingers and toes. Telangiectasia is permanent dilation of the capillaries, arterioles and venules.

Box 28–4. CREST

C = calcinosis
R = Raynaud's phenomenon
E = esophageal motility changes
S = sclerodactyly
T = telangiectasia

Limited subcutaneous scleroderma usually has a slow onset and may take 10 to 20 years before manifestations appear. Manifestations are usually one of the CREST constellation. Prognosis is favorable. Diffuse subcutaneous scleroderma affects the entire body and most of the manifestations of CREST appear.

Progressively fatal PSS is associated with a generalized skin thickening and invasion into internal organs. Common clinical manifestations include subcutaneous edema, fever, and malaise. The skin becomes thickened and hidelike and loses normal skinfolds (Fig. 28–14). Ulcerations around the fingertips and subcutaneous calcification occur. Polyarthritis and polyarthralgias are also present. Dysphagia due to esophageal dysfunction, from abnormalities in motility, and later from fibrosis, occurs in about 90% of clients. Fibrosis and atrophy of the GI tract cause hypermotility and malabsorption. Diffuse pulmonary fibrosis and pulmonary vascular disease are reflected by low oxygen-diffusing capacity and decreased lung compliance. Hypertensive uremic syndrome, resulting from obstruction in small renal vessels, is serious. RF may be present in a small number of clients. Mild anemia is often present. An elevated ESR and hypergammaglobulinemia are also common. PSS typically progresses slowly. When death occurs, it is usually from infection or renal or cardiac failure.

Treatment of PSS is supportive and symptomatic. The primary goal of medical treatment is to trigger a remission of the disease. Steroids and immunosuppressants are used to treat the disease, often in high doses.

Nursing interventions are directed at control of clinical manifestations. One of the major areas of concern is skin care to prevent breakdown and ulceration. The skin should be carefully inspected daily so any injury or breakdown is noted and treatment begun immediately. The client should be taught to use gentle soaps and nonalcohol astringent lotions to maintain skin integrity. Helping the client control acute pain, which is sometimes associated with Raynaud's phenomenon, polyarthralgia, and polyarthritis, is another important nursing function. The client must learn to avoid activities that might trigger pain. This includes actions such as joint protection behaviors, avoiding extreme cold, wearing gloves when hands are exposed to cold (even when removing food from the

freezer), eliminating smoking, and resting the painful part when pain is acute.

If the client is experiencing esophageal dysfunction, modification of the diet may be necessary. Clients usually tolerate small, frequent, bland feedings better than three regular meals a day. The client also should learn to sit up for at least 1 hour after meals to promote digestion and food motility. Histamine receptor antagonists and antacids may be prescribed to decrease the acidity some clients feel.

The client will need continued follow-up care and monitoring. As with SLE, the client also needs psychosocial support to cope with this chronic debilitating disease. Encourage the client to continue to receive psychological support as needed after hospitalization.

Ankylosing Spondylitis

Ankylosing spondylitis (AS), or Marie-Strümpell disease, is a chronic, progressive inflammation of the spine and sacroiliac joints. It affects 1% of the population, mostly males. The exact cause of AS is not known, but it does have a genetic transmission. The joints of the sacroiliac begin to inflame and then ossify (fuse) as the joints and disc spaces are replaced by bone. The process moves up the spinal column until the spine is stiff and rigid, and then the disorder extends into the hips, knees, and shoulders. AS begins insidiously in adolescence or young adulthood, usually with morning backache and stiffness in the lumbar area. The pain and stiffness subside with movement but return with inactivity. Other manifestations associated with AS include iritis, arthritis or arthralgia, weight loss, and malaise. In advanced stages of AS, the client is rigid and stooped forward (Figure 28–15). The spine is rigid and looks like bamboo shoots on x-ray. Laboratory tests reveal increased HLA-B27. ESR and RF are usually negative.

There is no management to prevent or slow the progress of AS. Since stiffening of the spine is inevitable, the goals of management are to relieve pain, maintain optimal posture, and prevent respiratory involvement from minimal chest movements. Pain is usually treated with NSAIDs and heat. The client is instructed to try to maintain an erect posture, and rest frequently throughout the day. Splints and back braces are helpful for support. Surgical management may include osteotomy for marked deformities of the hip or spine. Occasionally hip or knee arthroplasty is used.

Sjögren's Syndrome

Sjögren's syndrome is a chronic inflammatory disorder of the eyes. It can be a primary problem or secondary to RA. It involves a decrease in lacrimation and salivation due to obstruction of the secretory ducts by immune complexes. Persons with Sjögren's syndrome exhibit dry eyes (keratoconjunctivitis sicca) and a dry mouth (xerostomia). Common manifestations include swelling of the lacrimal ducts and parotid glands and fatigue. This disorder affects mainly women, who experience an additional manifesta-

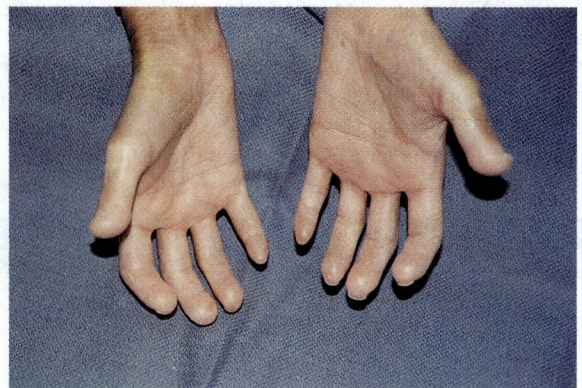

Figure 28–14. Appearance of the hands in a client with scleroderma.

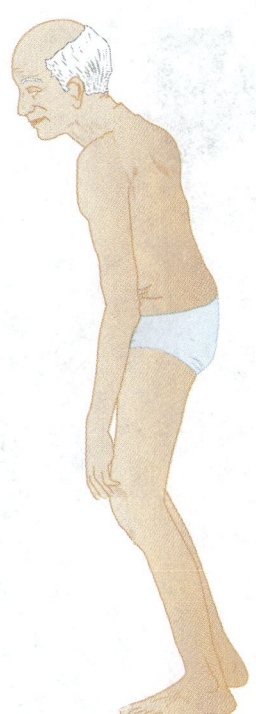

Figure 28–15. Posture of a client with advanced ankylosing spondylitis.

tion of vaginal dryness. Almost half of the persons with Sjögren's syndrome also exhibit another connective tissue disorder, especially RA. Diagnostic tests reveal hyper-gammaglobulinemia and the presence of RF, ANA, and anti-extractable nuclear antigen (anti-ENA). Autoantibodies against salivary duct antigens are also found. If the client also has RA, the treatment is directed at the underlying arthritis. Artificial tears are helpful for keeping the eyes moist and preventing corneal abrasions. Artificial saliva can be used for the xerostomia. If the syndrome is left untreated, the client can develop visual problems, oral ulcerations, dental caries, and dysphagia.

Clients with Sjögren's syndrome have difficulty when going to surgery. Placing these clients NPO (nothing by mouth) can cause great oral discomfort because they have decreased saliva. Artificial saliva should be used. In addition they are at risk of corneal abrasion in surgery because of the low humidity in the surgery suite. Ocular lubricants should be used before surgery.

Fibromyalgia Syndrome

Not all people complaining of musculoskeletal pain have arthritis. Fibromyalgia syndrome is an increasingly recognized chronic musculoskeletal pain disorder of unknown cause. It is estimated to occur in about 2% of the general population, predominately in girls and young women. Active research is being conducted to find the cause; at present some data indicate that there may be alterations in several hormones (e.g., adrenocorticotropin hormone [ACTH], growth hormone) and the hypothalamus-pituitary-adrenal axis.

Clinical manifestations include fatigue, morning stiffness, nonrefreshing sleep due to lack of stage 4 sleep, and postexertional muscle pain. About one third of clients have associated problems such as irritable bowel syndrome, tension headaches, premenstrual syndrome, numbness and tingling, and Raynaud's phenomenon. Fatigue is the most common clinical manifestation, and the most common cause of the fatigue is chronic depression. The physical examination is often unremarkable unless attention is paid to the tender points (Fig. 28–16).

These points should be palpated with moderate pressure with the pulp of the thumb or forefinger. It is important to intersperse examination of tender points with nontender points to avoid anticipation reactions if every point is associated with pain.

Management includes L-tryptophan to increase sleep, tricyclic antidepressants to inhibit serotonin uptake, benzodiazepines for the treatment of anxiety associated with depression, and corticosteroids and NSAIDs for pain control. Low-intensity exercise is also important and helps to decrease pain. Biofeedback, acupuncture, and hypnotherapy have also been used to help manage nonmuscular problems such as functional diarrhea, tension headache, and fatigue. The efficacy of these treatments is yet to be fully ascertained.

Many clients with fibromyalgia perceive themselves to be significantly disabled and have a reduced quality of life that rivals conditions such as RA and terminal emphysema. Clients with fibromyalgia have difficulty coping with "daily hassles" and this, in turn, increases the psychological stress. Cognitive behavioral therapy is often effective in providing these clients a sense of control over their lives.

Polymyositis and Dermatomyositis

Polymyositis is an acute or chronic inflammatory disorder of the striated muscles causing symmetrical weakness. When there is a rash associated with polymyositis, it is referred to as dermatomyositis. As with other connective tissue diseases, polymyositis and dermatomyositis are characterized by periods of remission and exacerbation, and are chronically progressive. This disorder is twice as common in women as in men and occurs equally among all races. People between the ages of 30 and 60 are most likely to get the disease. Polymyositis may be associated with a malignancy. Diagnostic tests reveal positive ANA and focal deposition of complement, IgG, and IgM in vessels of the involved muscles.

Clinical manifestations of the disease, besides the symmetrical muscle weakness and rash, include polyarthralgia, polyarthritis, and Raynaud's phenomenon. Clients with dermatomyositis have characteristic heliotrope B (lilac) rash and periorbital edema. The muscle weakness can lead to problems with speaking and swallowing. These disorders are treated with high-dose corticosteroids and immunosuppressants. Nursing care is mainly supportive. The client's ability to swallow should be monitored closely so that aspiration does not occur.

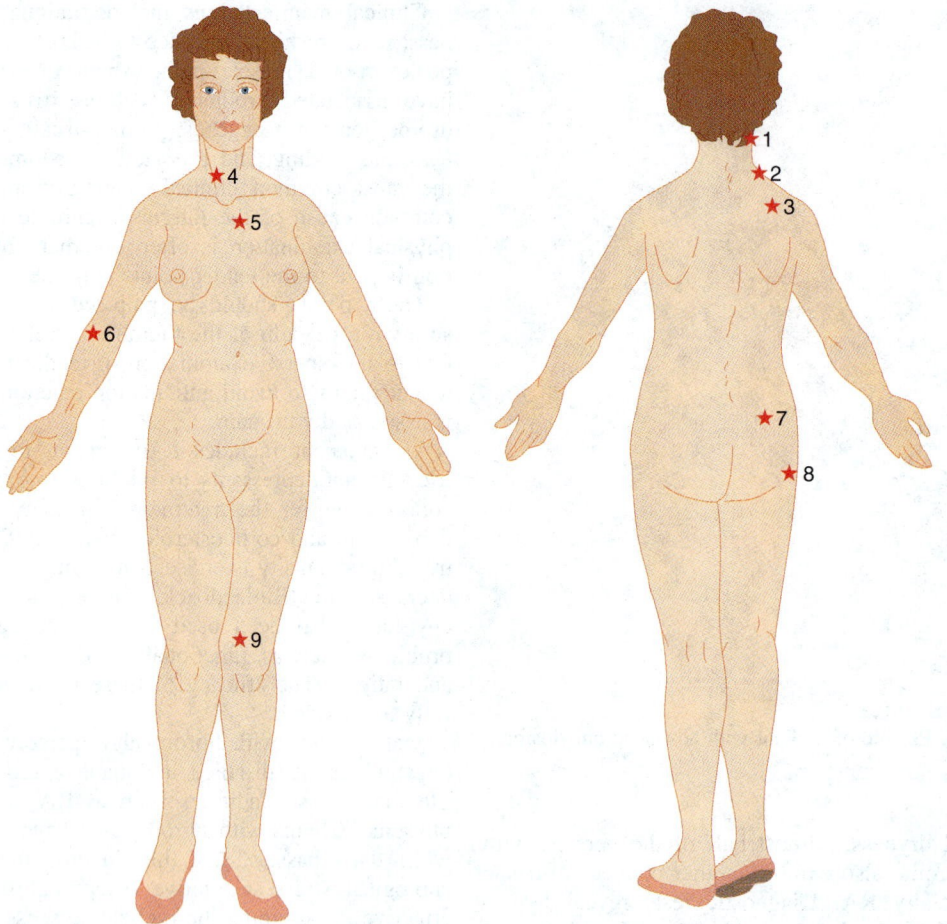

Figure 28–16. The nine paired tender points recommended by the 1990 American College of Rheumatology Criteria Committee for establishing a diagnosis of fibromyalgia: (1) insertion of the nuchal muscles into the occiput; (2) upper border of the trapezius—midportion; (3) muscle attachments to the upper medial border of the scapula; (4) anterior aspects of C5 and C7 intertransverse spaces; (5) second rib space, about 3 cm lateral to the sternal border; (6) muscle attachments to the lateral epicondyle—about 2 cm below the bony prominence; (7) upper outer quadrant of the gluteal muscles; (8) muscle attachments just posterior to the greater trochanter; (9) medial fat pad of the knee proximal to the joint line. Eleven or more tender points in conjunction with a history of widespread pain are characteristic of the fibromyalgia syndrome. (From Bennett, R.: The fibromyalagia syndrome. In W. N. Kelley, et al. [Eds.] [1993]. *Textbook of rheumatology* [4th ed., p. 472]. Philadelphia: W. B. Saunders.)

Vasculitis

Vasculitis is a group of disorders leading to inflammation and necrosis of blood vessel walls. Soluble immune complexes are deposited in blood vessel walls in areas where capillaries have increased permeability. Once deposited, the immune system is activated and the complex is destroyed but so is the blood vessel wall. These disorders include polyarteritis nodosa, systemic necrotizing vasculitis, and allergic agranulomatosis angiitis. With these disorders, there is inflammation and damage to large and small vessels, resulting in end-stage organ damage. The specific manifestations vary, depending on the organs affected. Steroids are the treatment of choice for these disorders.

Reiter's Syndrome

Reiter's syndrome is a triad of arthritis, urethritis, and conjunctivitis. The syndrome is triggered by genitourinary

or gastrointestinal infections. Other manifestations may include prostatitis, penile or vaginal lesions, and urethral discharge. HLA-27 is present in most clients and indicates an immunologic aspect. It is treated with steroid therapy and aggressive physical therapy. NSAIDs may be used to treat the joint pain. Antibiotics are not used, since no organism can be cultured. The major nursing concerns are with pain and stiffness. Most problems are similar to those seen in clients with RA.

Polymyalgia Rheumatica and Cranial Arteritis

Polymyalgia rheumatica is a clinical syndrome occurring more commonly in women than in men. It is a disease of aging, rarely occurring before the age of 60 years. It is characterized by pain and stiffness in the neck, shoulder, back, and pelvic girdle, especially in the morning. Headaches or painful areas on the head may be present. The client also may have a low-grade fever or temporal arteritis. Laboratory findings include an elevated ESR, mild anemia, and possible elevation of immunoglobulins. Steroids usually produce symptomatic relief within days.

Giant cell arteritis is also known as temporal or cranial arteritis. This is also a disease of older people. The client often has symptoms of polymyalgia rheumatica for months, then suddenly develops the severe headaches associated with temporal arteritis. The onset of this disorder is usually sudden, with severe pain often appearing in the temporal area. The pain also may be felt in the occipital area, face, jaw, or side of the neck. It is usually associated with hyperesthesia, which makes any touch exquisitely painful. The client may experience visual changes, including sudden onset of blindness in one or both eyes. It is very important to diagnose and treat this disorder before blindness occurs. Because older women are often affected, their complaints of decreased vision and headaches are sometimes ignored as normal aging. Treatment is with corticosteroids, which are highly effective in controlling this disorder.

Mixed Connective Tissue Disease

Mixed connective tissue disease (CTD) is a combination of several CTDs. Clients have manifestations that are not typical of any one disorder. This diagnosis is applied to about 10% of clients with CTD. Frequent combinations are SLE and PSS and RA. Mixed CTDs are managed according to their manifestations. Often clients are managed as if they had SLE. The term is used less frequently today.

Lyme Disease

Lyme disease is one form of rheumatic joint disease with a known cause. It is included as a connective tissue disorder because the skin, joints, nervous system, and heart are involved. This complex multisystem disease is caused by the tickborne spirochete *Borrelia burgdorferi*. Clinical manifestations found from 3 to 32 days after the bite may include a red flat rash that clears in the center, severe headache, stiff neck, fever, chills, myalgias, joint pain, severe malaise, and fatigue. The disease can be treated with a course of antibiotic therapy. Doxycycline is the most common antibiotic used. Neurologic abnormalities may occur if treatment is ineffective. Intra-articular steroids and NSAIDs may be used to relieve joint inflammation and pain.

Secondary Arthritis

Whipple's Disease

Whipple's disease is a secondary arthritis associated with a gastrointestinal disorder. The disease was first described in the early 1900s as a condition characterized by arthral-

gias, diarrhea, abdominal pain, and weight loss. Other manifestations include fever, lymphadenopathy, and increased skin pigmentation. The disease can affect almost every organ system in the body. Whipple's disease occurs most commonly in middle-aged white males. Although an organism was described as the cause, it was not isolated until 1992. Treatment of Whipple's disease consists of broad-spectrum antimicrobials.

Other Disorders Causing Arthritis

Other conditions that may produce arthritis-type symptoms include Crohn's disease, ulcerative colitis, tuberculosis, hyperthyroidism, hyperparathyroidism, sickle cell anemia crisis, and psoriasis. Treatment for the primary condition usually leads to a decrease in the severity of the arthritis.

Conclusions

Autoimmune disorders most often lead to problems of the joints, such as rheumatoid arthritis, and problems with other connective tissues, such as scleroderma. These chronic problems and resulting pain and deformity quickly test the resources of the client. Client education for self-care is critical. Most of these problems have no cure, so the nurse considers the effects of chronic pain, multiple treatments, and progressive deformity on self-concept, role performance, and family systems.

Thinking Critically

1. You are working in an outpatient clinic and receive a call from a 66-year-old woman who is experiencing a flare-up of rheumatoid arthritis. She was seen 2 days ago in the clinic and given a high dose of prednisone. Now, she reports epigastric abdominal pain. A symptom analysis reveals the following: her pain has a burning quality, is worse between meals, relieved by food, and aggravated by coffee. She has taken some over-the-counter ibuprofen for the pain but states, "It didn't help." What other information do you need to collect? What interventions would you advise?

Factors to Consider. Consider the side effects of corticosteroids and NSAIDs.

2. A 55-year-old woman with a history of joint pain is scheduled for a total hip replacement. She has experienced increasing pain while walking and hopes to be able to walk pain-free so she can resume her job as a waitress. What nursing assessments are pertinent to this type of condition and proposed surgery? How

realistic is the client's desire to return to work as a waitress?

Factors to Consider. How will assessments help in the prevention of postoperative complications? Are clients able to return to an improved level of functioning following joint replacement surgery?

Bibliography

1. Anderson, R. J. (1993). Clinical features and laboratory. In J. Schumacher (Ed.), *Primer on the rheumatic diseases* (10th ed., pp. 90–96). Atlanta: Arthritis Foundation.
2. Awerbach, M. (1995). Different concepts of chronic musculoskeletal pain. *Annals of Rheumatic Disease 54*(5), 331–332.
3. Belza, B. L., et al. (1993). Correlates of fatigue in older adults with rheumatoid arthritis. *Nursing Research, 42,* 93–99.
4. Bertsch, C. (1995). CREST syndrome: A variant of systemic sclerosis. *Orthopaedic Nursing, 14*(3), 53–60.
5. Bonafede, R. D., Downey, D. C., & Bennet, R. M. (1995). An association of fibromyalgia with primary Sjögren's syndrome. *Journal of Rheumatology, 22*(1), 133–136.
6. Carson, D. A., & Tan, E. M. (1995). Apoptosis in rheumatic disease. *Bulletin on the Rheumatic Diseases, 44*(1), 1–3.
7. Dale, K. G., Orr, P. M., & Harrell, P. B. (1992). Total elbow replacement. *Orthopaedic Nursing 11*(5), 23–29.
8. Dav, P. C., & Callahan, J. P. (1994). Immune modulation during treatment of systemic sclerosis with plasmapheresis and immunosuppressive drugs. *Clinical Immunology and Immunopathology, 76*(2), 159–165.
9. Eisenberb, R. A., & Cohen, P. L. (1993). The role of immunologic mechanisms in the pathogenesis of rheumatic disease. In J. Schumacher (Ed.), *Primer on the rheumatic diseases* (10th ed., pp. 27–35). Atlanta: Arthritis Foundation.
10. Ekdahl, C., et al. (1990). Dynamic training and circulating levels of corticotropin-releasing factors, β-lipoprotein, β-endorphin in rheumatoid arthritis. *Pain, 40,* 35–42.
11. Gladman, D. D., & Urowitz, M. B. (1993). Clinical features of SLE. In J. Schumacher, J. H. Klippel, & W. J. Koopman (Eds.), *Primer on the rheumatic diseases* (10th ed., pp. 106–112). Atlanta: Arthritis Foundation.
12. Golddenberg, D. (1995). Fatigue in rheumatic disease. *Bulletin on the Rheumatic Diseases, 44*(1), 4–7.
13. Gray, M. A. (1995). NSAIDs revisited. *Orthopaedic Nursing, 14*(1), 52–54.
14. Halverson, P. B. (1995). Extraarticular manifestations of rheumatoid arthritis. *Orthopaedic Nursing, 14*(4), 47–50.
15. Harris, E. (1993). Etiology and pathogenesis of rheumatoid arthritis. In W. N. Kelley et al. (Eds.), *Textbook of rheumatology.* Philadelphia: W. B. Saunders.
16. Hughes, R. A. (1994). The microbiology of chronic inflammatory arthritis: an historical review. *British Journal of Rheumatology, 33,* 361–369.
17. Johnson, R. L. (1993). Total shoulder arthroplasty. *Orthopaedic Nursing, 12*(1), 14–22.
18. Katz, P. P., & Yelin, E. H. (1994). Life activities of persons with rheumatoid arthritis with and without depressive symptoms. *Arthritis Care and Research, 7*(2), 69–77.
19. Laskin, R. S. (1990). Total condylar knee replacement in patients who have rheumatoid arthritis. *Journal of Bone and Joint Surgery, American Volume, 72,* 529–535.
20. Legerton, C. W. (1995). Systemic sclerosis, Clinical management of its major complications. *Rheumatic Disease Clinics of North America, 21*(11), 203–216.
21. McCarty, D. J. (1993). Treatment of rheumatoid arthritis. In D. J. McCarty & W. J. Koopman (Eds.), *Arthritis and Allied Conditions* (12th ed., Vol. 1, p. 1146). Philadelphia: Lea & Febiger.
22. Meyer, C. L. (1991). *Community arthritis water exercise programs: A controlled study.* Unpublished masters of nursing science thesis, Wichita State University, Wichita, KS.
23. Meyer, C. L., & Hawley, D. J. (1994). Characteristics of participants in water exercise programs compared to patients seen in a rheumatic disease clinic. *Arthritis Care and Research, 7*(2), 85–89.
24. Minor, M. A., & Brown, J. D. (1993). Exercise maintenance of persons with arthritis after participation in a class experience. *Health Education Quarterly, 20*(1), 83–95.
25. Morrow, A. K., Parker, J. C., & Russell, J. L. (1994). Clinical implications of depression in rheumatoid arthritis. *Arthritis Care and Research, 7*(2), 58–63.
26. Mudge-Grout, C. (Ed.). (1992). *Immunologic Disorders.* St. Louis: Mosby–Year Book.
27. Neuberger, G. B., et al. (1993). Promoting self-care in clients with arthritis. *Arthritis Care and Research, 6*(3), 141–148.
28. Osial, T. A., Jr., Cash, J. M., & Eisenbeis Jr., C. H. (1993). Arthritis-associated syndromes. *Primary Care, 20,* 857–879.
29. Parker, J. C., et al. (1992). Psychological factors, immunologic activation, and disease activity in rheumatoid arthritis. *Arthritis Care and Research, 5*(1), 196–201.
30. Pincus, T., & Callahan, L. F. (1992). Early mortality in RA predicted by poor clinical status. *Bulletin on the Rheumatic Diseases, 41*(4), 1–4.
31. Rankin, J. A. (1995). Pathophysiology of the rheumatoid joint. *Orthopaedic Nursing, 14*(4), 39–46.
32. Riott, I. M. (1994). Autoimmune disease. In *Essential immunology* (8th ed., pp. 412–418). Cambridge, MD: Blackwell Scientific Publications.
33. Sipos, D. A. (1993). MP implants for rheumatoid arthritis of the hand. *Orthopaedic Nursing, 12*(5), 7–15.
34. Sisk, T. D. & Wright, P. E. (1992). Arthroplasty of shoulder and elbow. In A. H. Crenshaw (Ed.), *Campbell's operative orthopaedics* (pp. 627–673). St. Louis: Mosby–Year Book.
35. Starz, T. W., & Miller, E. B. (1993). Diagnosis and treatment of rheumatoid arthritis. *Primary Care, 20,* 827–837.
36. Stillerman, C. B., Schneider, J. H., & Gruen, J. P. (1993). Evaluation and management of spondylolysis and spondylolisthesis. *Clinics in Neurosurgery, 40* 384–415.
37. Swezey, R. L. (1993). Rehabilitation medicine and arthritis. In D. H. McCarty & W. J. Koopman (Eds.), *Arthritis and allied conditions* (12th ed., Vol. 1, p. 1146). Philadelphia: Lea & Febiger.
38. Syle, D. A. (1991). Orthopedic complications. *Nursing Clinics of North America, 26*(1), 113–131.
39. Tooms, R. E. (1992). Arthroplasty of ankle and knee. In A. H. Crenshaw (Ed.), *Campbell's operative orthopaedics* (pp. 389–439). St. Louis: Mosby–Year Book.
40. Wilder, R. L. (1993). Rheumatoid arthritis: Epidemiology, pathology, and pathogenesis. In J. Schumacher, J. H. Klippel, & W. J. Koopman (Eds.), *Primer on the rheumatic diseases* (10th ed., p. 349). Atlanta: Arthritis Foundation.
41. Williams, H. J. (1993). Rheumatoid arthritis: Treatment. In J. Schumacher, J. H. Klippel, & W. J. Koopman (Eds.), *Primer on the rheumatic diseases* (10th ed.). Atlanta: Arthritis Foundation.
42. Wolfe, F., et al. (1994). The mortality of rheumatoid arthritis. *Arthritis & Rheumatism, 37,* 481–494.
43. Wolfe, F., & Cathey, M. A. (1991). The assessment and prediction of function disability in rheumatoid arthritis. *Journal of Rheumatology, 18,* 1298–1306.
44. Zuckerman, J. D., et al. (1991). The painful shoulder: Part II. Intrinsic disorders and impingement syndrome. *American Family Practitioner, 43* (February), 497–512.

UNIT 5

Neurologic Disorders

Unit Editor: **BERNADETTE WHITE**

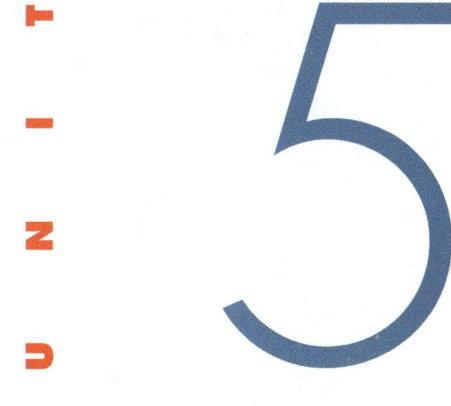

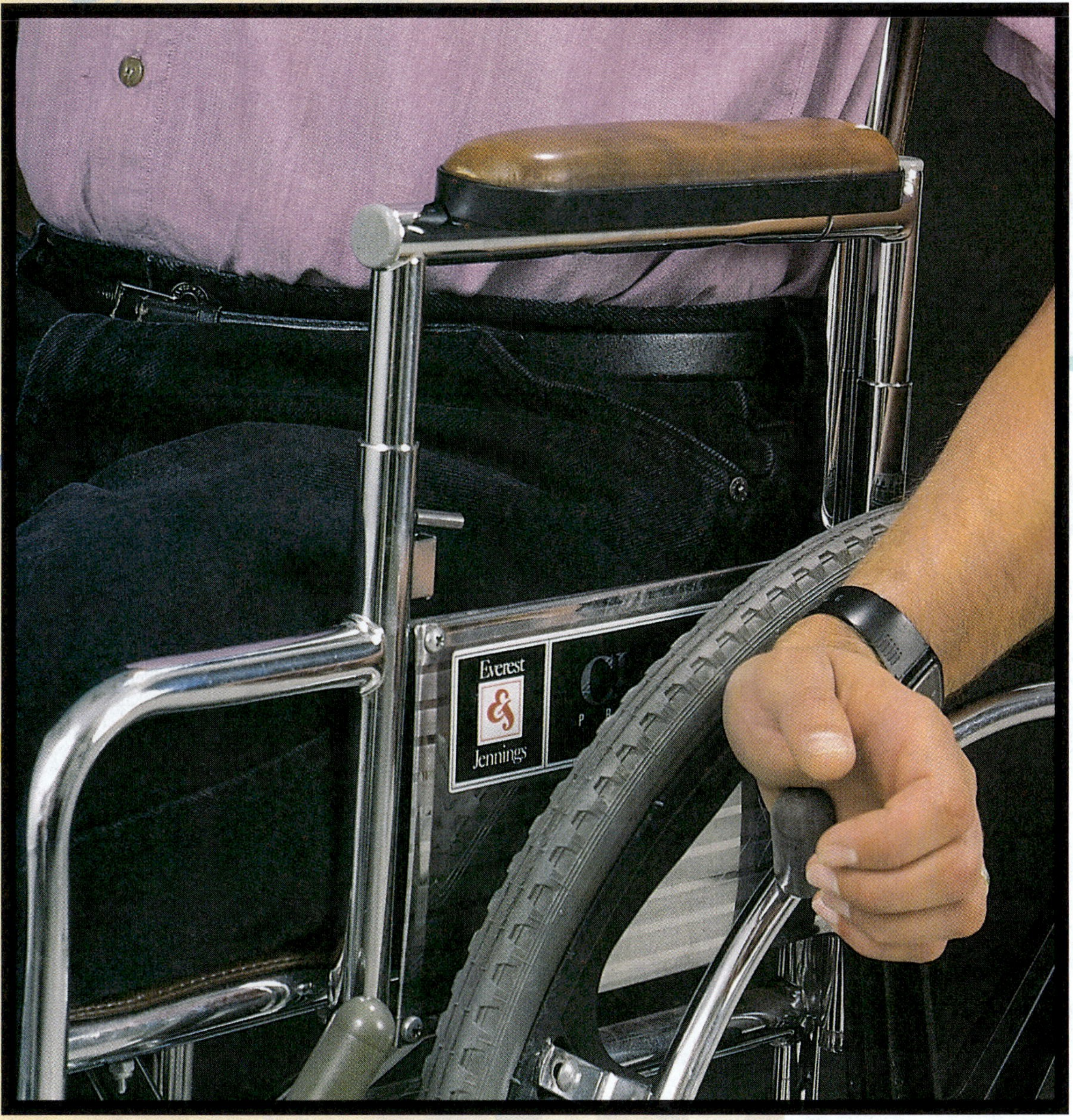

Structure and Function of the Nervous System

Bernadette White

The nervous system is the body's most organized and complex structural and functional system. It profoundly affects both psychological and physiologic function. This unit discusses the importance of the nervous system to human function and the major consequences of neurologic disorders. Providing quality nursing care for clients experiencing neurologic disorders is challenging and requires extensive knowledge of neurologic structure and function and neurologic disease processes.

The onset of neurologic problems may be sudden, as in traumatic spinal cord severance or ruptured cerebral aneurysm, or insidious, as in Parkinson's disease or multiple sclerosis. Neurologic problems can be frightening and even devastating to the client and significant others, especially if the process is irreversible. Many such problems produce varying degrees of physical or psychosocial dependency, or both. Memory loss and confusion may be slow and subtle, or sudden, with gross changes in consciousness. These changes may result in the client not being able to control his or her behavior or perform self-care. Whether the neurologic insult is temporary or permanent, a grief reaction is common and appropriate for both the client and his or her significant others. Their entire way of life may be altered.

This unit provides the information necessary to plan appropriate nursing care for clients experiencing neurologic problems in both acute and rehabilitative stages. Chapter 29 is an overview of neurologic structure and function. Chapter 30 describes the overall assessment of clients with neurologic problems. Of the disorders chapters, Chapter 31 discusses the care of clients who are confused or comatose, the nursing care of clients with cerebral disorders is explored in Chapters 32 and 33, Chapter 34 focuses on nursing care of clients with degenerative neurologic disorders. Disorders of the spinal cord, peripheral nerves, and cranial nerves and accompanying nursing care are discussed in Chapter 35.

Knowledge of the structure (anatomy) and function

(physiology) of the nervous system is essential to an understanding of alterations in neurologic function and disorders of the nervous system. The basic structural and functional units of the nervous system, the neurons and neuroglia, and their functions, including nerve impulse transmission, are discussed first. Next, the central nervous system and the protective and nutritional structures are described, followed by a description of the peripheral nervous system, which includes the spinal and cranial nerves and the autonomic nervous system. Finally, nervous system regeneration and normal changes in the nervous system seen with aging are presented.

Cells of the Nervous System

Structure

Nervous tissue consists mainly of neurons and neuroglia (as well as vascular and some connective tissues). Neurons are responsible for communications. Neuroglia cells provide support for the activity of the neurons. The nervous tissue that composes the brain and spinal cord is known as the *central nervous system (CNS)*. The neurons and neurilemma cells that are found outside the CNS compose the *peripheral nervous system (PNS)*.

Neurons

A neuronal cell body (soma) is much like other cells, in that it contains cytoplasm, mitochondria, lysosomes, Golgi apparatus, microtubules, and a nucleus. It also contains neurofibrils, or networks of threadlike structures that provide support to the other structures. Nissl bodies, membranous sacs containing endoplasmic reticulum, are also unique to the neuron.

Threadlike extensions called dendrites and one axon are part of the neuron (Fig. 29–1). Dendrites carry messages to the neuronal cell body, whereas the axon carries

This chapter incorporates material written for the fourth edition by Barbara J. Boss.

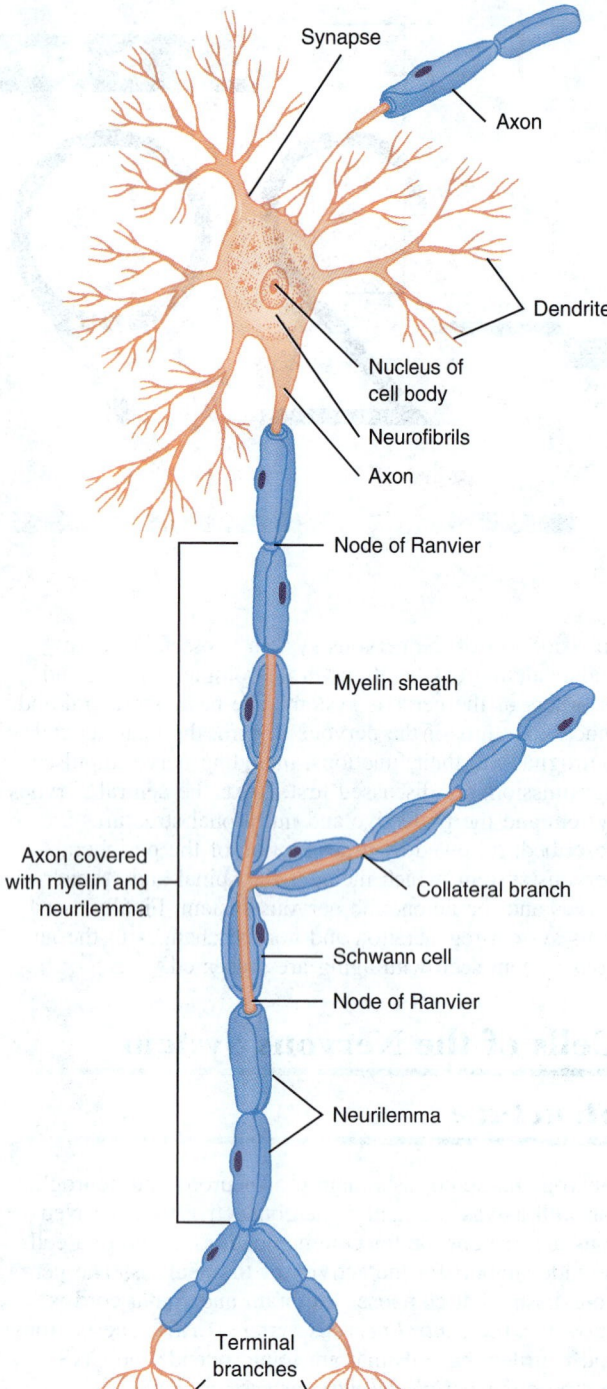

Figure 29–1. A neuron, the basic element of the nervous system.

which have only one dendrite and one axon, are found in the eyes, nose, and ears. Unipolar neurons have only one nerve fiber leaving the cell body, but branch to form a dendrite and axon. Some unipolar cell bodies aggregate into special masses of nerve tissue outside the brain and spinal cord and are called ganglia.

Synapses are a very important part of nerve function. They are small spaces between neurons, or between neurons and their target (also called effector) organs, such as muscles and glands. (These organs are known as *effectors* because they perform the function dictated by the nerve stimuli.) Of the two types of synapses, chemical and electrical synapses (which have gap junctions), chemical synapses dominate the CNS. In an electrical synapse, two cells' electrical nerve impulses cross directly through a very small separation (called gap junctions) from the presynaptic to the postsynaptic cell; this type of synapse is found in smooth and cardiac muscle cells.

As a message travels down the neuron, it reaches a synapse that it must cross in order to "jump" to the next neuron. Chemical substances called *neurotransmitters* exist in the space (called a cleft) between two neurons and propel the message onto the next neuron. Neurotransmitters are synthesized in the synaptic knobs, stored, and then secreted from the vesicles in the first neuron (presynaptic neuron) into the synaptic cleft (Fig. 29–2). The neurotransmitter either excites, inhibits, or modifies signals to the second neuron (postsynaptic neuron) by interacting with the receptors on its membrane. Within the CNS, each neuron may receive messages from thousands of presynaptic vesicles.

More than 50 neurotransmitters have been identified. There are two basic groups: the small-molecule, rapidly acting neurotransmitters, and the slow-acting neuropeptides. See Box 29–1 for a listing of the more common transmitters.

Each neuron synapses with many other neurons. Divergence occurs when one neuron synapses with several neurons. Convergence occurs when several neurons synapse to one neuron.

messages away from the cell body. Most of the neurons in the CNS are multipolar neurons, meaning they have many dendrites. Multipolar neurons called interneurons are responsible for sending messages received from the PNS to the appropriate sites for interpretation. They play a major role in memory, reasoning, communication, judgment, and emotions. The interneurons in the cerebral cortex are also known as association fibers. Bipolar neurons,

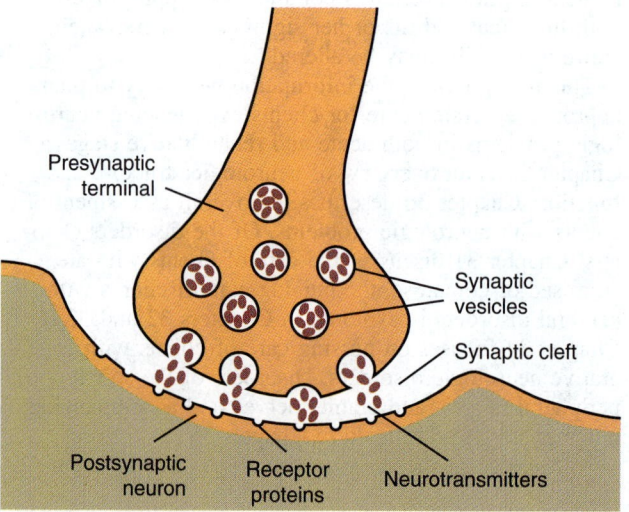

Figure 29–2. The chemical synapse.

Box 29-1. Common Neurotransmitters and Neuropeptides

Small-molecule, transmitters

Acetylcholine
Dopamine
Norepinephrine
Epinephrine
Histamine
Serotonin
Gamma-aminobutyric acid (GABA)
Glycine
Glutamate
Aspartate
Nitric oxide

Neuropeptides

Hypothalamic-releasing hormones (thyrotropin, luteinizing, growth)
Pituitary hormones
Beta-endorphin
Enkephalin
Substance P
Gastrin
Insulin
Glucagon
Cholecystokinin
Angiotensin II
Bradykinin
Calcitonin

Adapted from Guyton, A. C., & Hall, J. E. (1996). *Textbook of medical science* (9th ed., pp. 572–573). Philadelphia: W. B. Saunders.

Neuroglia

Neuroglia make up approximately half of the total brain and spinal cord and are 5 to 10 times more numerous than neurons. These cells play a role in the support and protection of other vital cells within the nervous system. They also control ion concentrations within the extracellular space, and contribute to the transport of nutrients, gases, and waste products between neurons and the vascular system and the cerebrospinal fluid (CSF). Four types of neuroglial cells exist (Fig. 29–3). In addition to the above functions, each type of neuroglia has specific functions. *Astrocytes* (Fig. 29–3, *A*) appear to be the cells of the CNS that respond to brain trauma by forming scar tissue. They also have specialized contacts with blood vessels in the pial-glial membrane, which is a critical part of the blood-brain barrier. These cells also contain calcium channels, which are essential to nerve transmission. *Oligodendrocytes* (Fig. 29–3, *B*), are comparable to the Schwann cells in the PNS, in that they produce myelin. *Microglia* (Fig. 29–3, *C*) are phagocytic scavenger cells related to macrophages. *Ependymal cells* (Fig. 29–3, *D*) form the lining of the ventricles, choroid plexuses, and the central canal that extends downward through the spinal cord. They create a one-cell-layered membrane that allows easy diffusion of substances between the interstitial fluid and the CSF.

Function and Impulse Conduction

Resting Potential

A neuron not conducting a nerve impulse is called a resting cell. Although it is called "resting" it remains charged and potentially ready to fire. The potential to fire is produced by a difference in electrical charge between the interstitial fluid outside the neuron and the intracellular fluid within (Fig. 29–4). The inside of the nerve cell is electrically negative, the interstitial fluid electrically positive. A resulting membrane potential measured in millivolts results from this difference in electrical potential between the two compartments. The resting membrane potential (RMP) of neurons is −70 mV (Fig. 29–4*A*). RMP varies with cell types. RMP in a neuron is −70 mV; in cardiac and skeletal cells it is −90 mV.

Interstitial fluid has a much higher concentration of sodium and chloride ions. Intracellular fluids have a much higher concentration of potassium and organic protein ions. The difference in the ion concentration is the result of three mechanisms:

1. The resting membrane (see Fig. 29–4*B*) is more permeable to potassium than sodium
2. There is a greater concentration of negative ions (phosphate, sulfate, and protein) that cannot diffuse out of the cell membrane
3. The sodium-potassium active transport pump maintains the differential concentrations of sodium, potassium, and chloride across the semipermeable membrane

Calcium is essential to membrane excitability and to the release of neurotransmitters. It is necessary for the closure of sodium channels in the nerve fiber. When calcium levels are low, more sodium leaks into the neuron and the resting potential is lowered. This makes the cell more excitable and results in the cell firing spontaneously. When calcium is high, sodium is less able to enter the neuron. The neuron is less excitable and harder to fire. Also, when the action potential reaches the membrane of the presynaptic knob, the membrane's permeability to calcium increases, allowing increased calcium influx. Calcium promotes fusing of the vesicles with the membrane and release of the neurotransmitters inside; this process is called *exocytosis*[8] (see Fig. 29–2). To maintain neurotransmitter balance, the vesicle returns to the cytoplasm to pick up more neurotransmitters. Some neurotransmitters are transported back into the vesicles (reuptake). Others are decomposed by an enzyme process. For example, acetylcholinesterase decomposes acetylcholine at the postsynaptic membrane. Monoamine oxidase inactivates epinephrine and norepinephrine after reuptake. Many other factors affect normal nerve impulse transmission, including other electrolytes (see Chapter 15), acid-base balance, oxygen, and glucose.

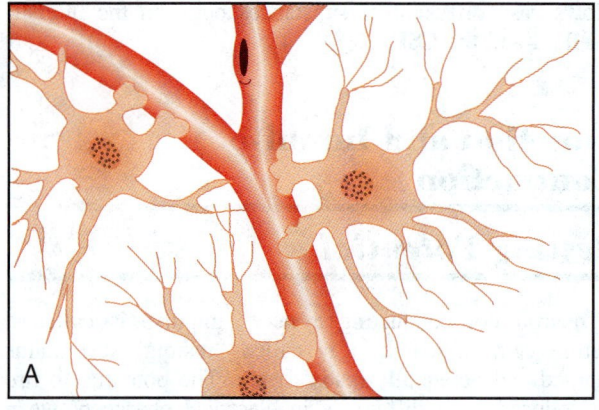
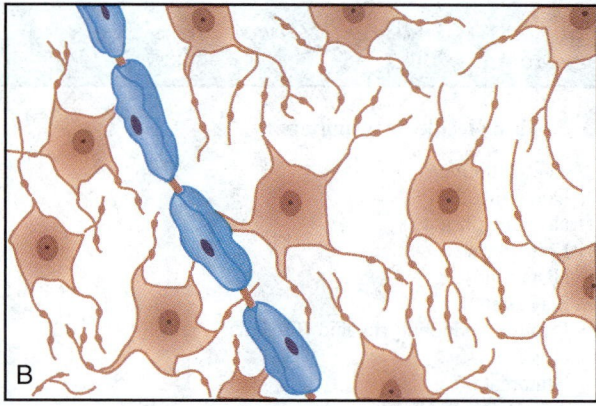
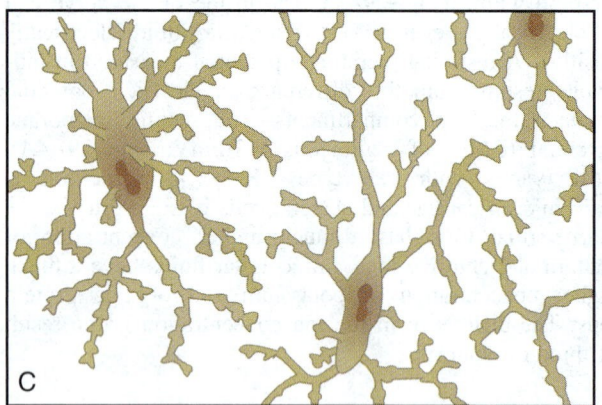
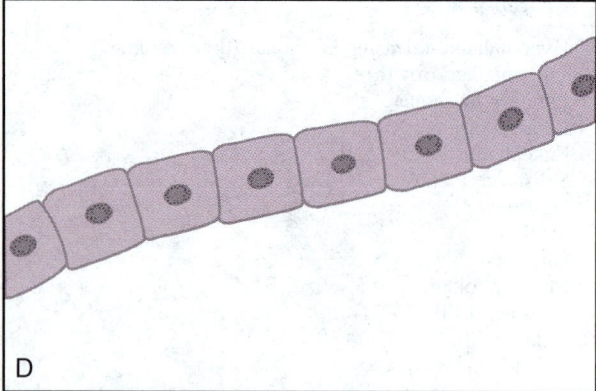

Figure 29–3. Neuroglial cells. *A*, Astrocytes. *B*, Oligodendrocytes. *C*, Microglia. *D*, Ependymal cells.

Nerve Impulse

A nerve impulse is an electrochemical phenomenon involving a sequence of ion exchanges (see Fig. 29–4). If the axon's membrane potential is lowered to a critical point, called the *threshold value,* an action potential (nerve impulse) is generated. More than one stimulus may be required to reach threshold potential if the stimuli are not strong. When the action potential has been achieved, it passes along the axon to all parts of the neuron. The axon responds with an all-or-none response; that is, the stimulus either generates an action potential or it does not. A strong stimulus will produce the same action potential as a weaker one because of the all-or-none response.

The generation of an action potential in the nerve cell has two phases that are related to permeability of the cell membrane. The first phase involves an opening of sodium channels which allows an influx of sodium into the cell. This influx of positive ions changes the electronegativity from -70 mV to $+30$ mV. This change is called *depolarization* (see Fig. 29–4C). Depolarization progresses along the nerve fiber. This progression of the action potential along a fiber is known as the *nerve impulse.*

The sodium influx is immediately followed by the second phase, an increased permeability of the plasma membrane to potassium. Potassium ions diffuse from the cell until the resting potential of the membrane is reestab-

lished (see Fig. 29–4D). This process, known as repolarization, occurs within a millisecond or so after the action potential. To restore the resting membrane potential, the sodium is pumped out of the cell by the sodium-potassium active transport pump.

The integrated sum of the excitatory and inhibitory potentials determine whether an action potential will result. In other words, the excitatory potential must outweigh the inhibitory stimuli for an action potential, or depolarization, to occur. If the level of excitation is subthreshold, the impulse is not triggered, but the neuron will be more excitable to the next stimulus; this is called *facilitation.* If the inhibitory potential is the stronger, *hyperpolarization* occurs.

Refractory Period

After an action potential is generated, no segment of the nerve fiber can conduct another action potential for a brief period of time (less than a millisecond). This is called the *absolute refractory period.* Sodium and potassium are returning to their original locations during this period, and sodium cannot enter the nerve cell. During the next period, called the *relative refractory period,* only a stimulus stronger than ordinary will produce an action potential. On average, a return to a resting potential takes approximately 10 to 30 ms.

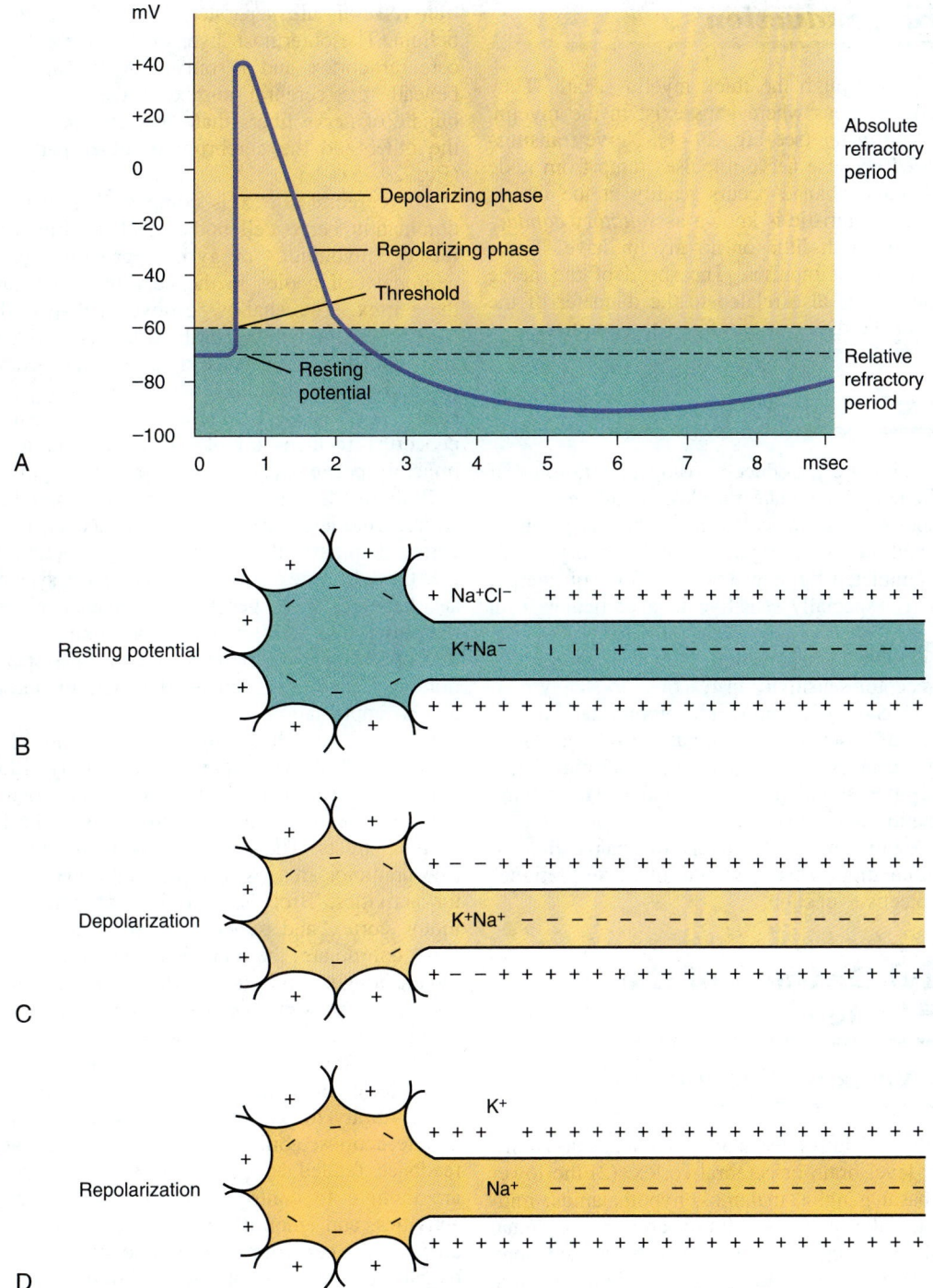

Figure 29–4. *A–D,* Generation of nerve impulses. The resting membrane potential is shown at −70 mV.

Myelin

Myelin, a lipid substance that insulates the nerve fiber, is deposited around the axon in many layers by Schwann cells. Neurons with their axons covered by myelin are called *myelinated nerve fibers.* Neurons with little or no myelin are called *unmyelinated nerve fibers.* The myelinated fibers in the CNS compose the *white matter* in the brain and spinal cord. The *gray matter* consists of nonmyelinated nerve fibers.

Schwann cells also form lipid layers of cellular membrane, the *myelin sheath,* which acts as an insulator to ion transfer. Parts of the Schwann cells also make up the neurilemma, a sheath that surrounds the myelin sheath (see Fig. 29–1). Neurilemma is essential to nerve regeneration and is discussed later under Regeneration.

In unmyelinated nerves the plasma membrane acts as insulation to nerve conduction. When myelin is present, the velocity of nerve impulses is increased because the myelin alters resistance.

Saltatory Conduction

Ions cannot flow through the thick myelin sheath. They can flow easily in areas where gaps exist in the myelin, called *nodes of Ranvier* (see Fig. 29–1). Nerve transmission is increased because nerve impulses jump from node to node, and ion exchange occurs readily at the nodes. This jumping characteristic is known as *saltatory conduction*. Nerve fibers with little or no myelin have slower transmission of nerve impulses. The speed of the nerve impulse conduction is also related to the diameter of the fiber; the greater the diameter, the faster the impulse.

Receptors

Receptors are biologic transducers, using the stimulus of one form of energy to initiate the "electrical" energy of the nerve impulse—mechanical energy, chemical energy, light energy, and thermal energy. Although sensory receptors may be stimulated by more than one form of energy, each receptor is especially sensitive to a particular form of energy.

Receptors exhibit a phenomenon known as *adaptation,* a decreased receptor sensitivity in response to steady continuous stimuli. Slowly adapting receptors can maintain the lower rate of discharge for minutes to even hours. Fast-adapting receptors' bursts of impulses terminate less than a second after initiation of the stimulus. The mechanism of adaptation is not known.

Receptors respond more effectively to change than to continuous stimulation. This syndrome of nerve "fatigue" provides a protective function.

Structural Divisions of the Nervous System

Central Nervous System

The CNS is divided into three major functional divisions: (1) the higher-level brain or cerebral cortex, (2) the lower brain level (basal ganglia, thalamus, hypothalamus, midbrain, pons, medulla, and cerebellum), and (3) the spinal cord level. These structures are protected by a rigid bony encasement, three layers of membranes, a fluid cushion, and a blood-brain or blood–spinal cord barrier.

Brain

■ Cerebrum

The brain is the largest and most complex part of the nervous system. It is composed of over 100 billion multipolar neurons and associated fibers. The brain tissues have a gelatin-like consistency. This semisolid organ weighs about 1400 g (approximately 3 lb) in the adult. The cerebrum is divided by a longitudinal fissure (deep groove) into two sections called *cerebral hemispheres.* A

transverse fissure separates the cerebrum from the cerebellum. The outermost layer of the cerebrum is called the cerebral cortex and is only 2 to 5 mm thick. Directly beneath the cerebral cortex is the *corpus callosum,* a bundle of nerve fibers that connects one hemisphere with the other and the cerebrum to other parts of the brain (Fig. 29–5).

The cerebral cortex is composed of gray matter (predominantly nerve cell bodies and dendrites) formed into raised convolutions or gyri. Approximately 75% of the neuronal cell bodies in the nervous system are found in the cortex. The shallow grooves between the gyri are called sulci. Each cerebral cortex is divided by major sulci into five lobes: the frontal, parietal, occipital, temporal, and central (insula) lobes (Fig. 29–6). The term *neocortex* is often used to refer to the cerebral cortex. The neocortex includes all of the cerebral cortex except the olfactory portions and the hippocampal regions.

Both the left and right cortex interpret sensory data, store memories, learn, and form concepts. However, each cortex dominates the other in many functions. For example, the left cortex has a dominance for systematic analysis, language and speech, mathematics, abstraction, and reasoning. The right cortex has a dominance for assimilation of sensory experiences such as visuospatial information and activities such as dancing, gymnastics, music, and art appreciation.

In the frontal lobes, the precentral gyrus (the motor cortex) controls voluntary motor activity. Most of these fibers cross to the opposite side of the brain at the medulla and descend via the spinal cord as the lateral corticospinal tracts. The area anterior to the precentral gyrus (the premotor area) is also associated with voluntary motor activities. Broca's area lies anterior to the primary motor cortex and superior to the lateral sulcus. These cells coordinate the complex muscular activity of the mouth, tongue, and larynx, which makes expressive (motor) speech possible. Damage to this area leaves the client unable to speak clearly, a disorder called *aphasia.*

The prefrontal areas control attention over time (concentration); motivation, ability to formulate or select goals; ability to plan; ability to initiate, maintain, or terminate actions; ability to self-monitor, and ability to use feedback (called executive functions). These same areas are thought to contribute to reasoning, problem-solving activities, and emotional stability by inhibiting the limbic areas of the cerebrum. The limbic system, which consists of parts of the upper and lower brain levels, is discussed later.

Each parietal lobe, located posterior to the central sulcus of Rolando, contains a primary somatic (tactile) receptive area and the somatic (tactile) association areas. The postcentral gyrus and the posterior portion of the paracentral lobule are the primary receptive (interpretation) areas for tactile sensations such as temperature, touch, and pressure. The association areas occupy the remainder of the parietal lobe. Concept formation and abstraction are carried out by the parietal association areas. The right parietal areas are also dominant for spatial orientation and awareness of size and shapes (stereognosis) and body position (proprioception). The left parietal areas assist with right-left orientation and mathematics.

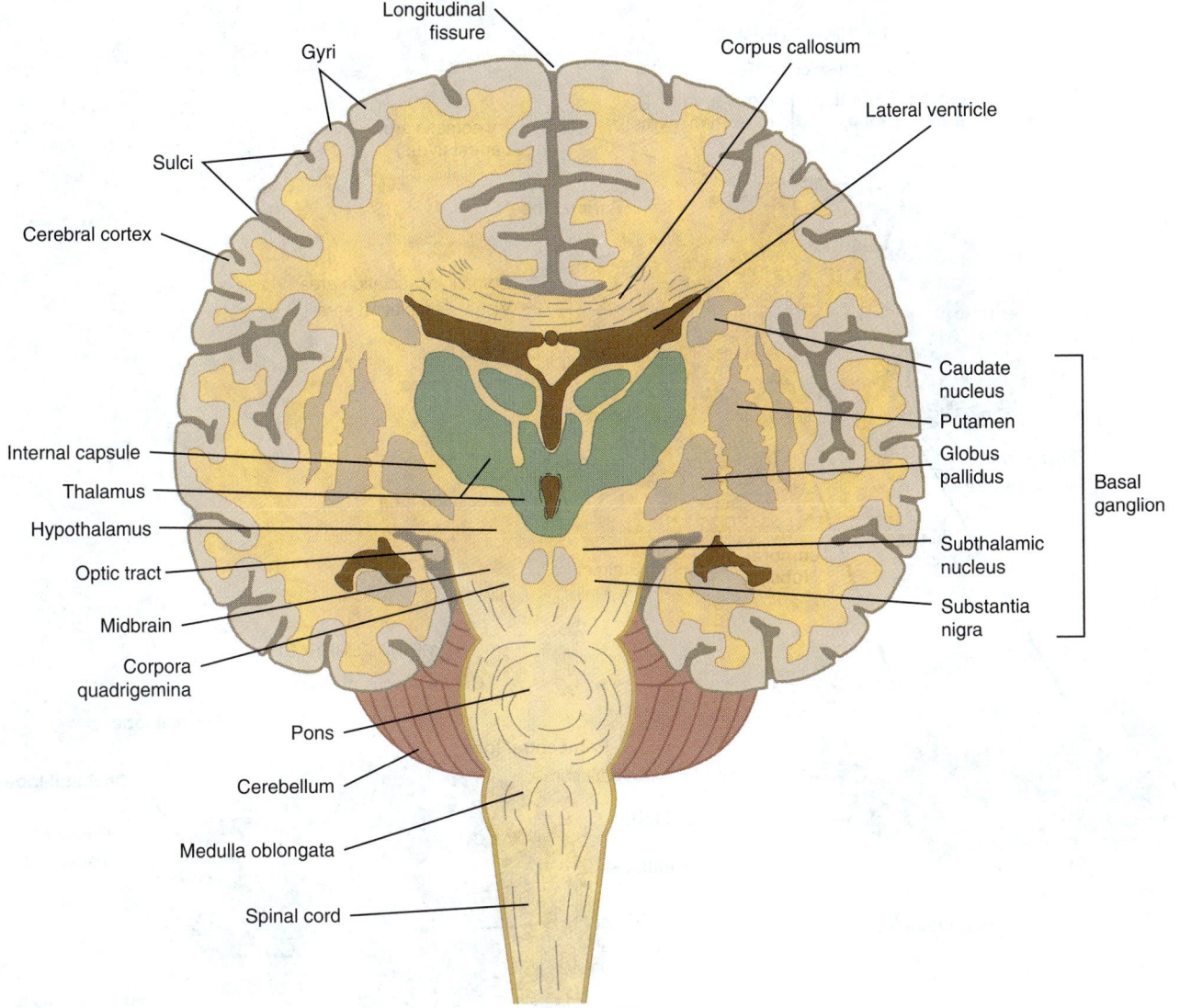

Figure 29–5. The structures of the brain (coronal section).

Each occipital lobe contains a primary visual receptive (interpretation) area and visual association areas. The primary visual cortex is on either side of the calcarine sulcus (see Fig. 29–6). The other areas of the occipital cortices are visual association areas. Visual memories are stored in these visual association areas, which contribute to a person's ability to visually recognize and understand his or her environment.

Each temporal lobe is located under (caudal to) the lateral sulcus. The temporal lobe contains a primary auditory receptive (interpretation) area and secondary auditory association areas. Spoken language memories are stored in the left temporal auditory association areas. All other sound memories that are not language, such as music, various animal sounds, and other noises, are stored in the right temporal auditory areas. Damage to these temporal lobe areas leaves the person unable to understand spoken or written language or to recognize music or other environmental sounds. The cells that function in understanding language are found in a group of cells called *Wernicke's area.*

The central (insula) lobe is located deep within the lateral sulcus and is surrounded by the frontal, parietal, and temporal lobes. Nerve fibers for taste pass through the parietal lobe to the insular lobe. Many association fibers leading to other parts of the cerebral cortex pass through this lobe.

■ Hippocampus

The hippocampus, which is a part of the medial section of the temporal lobe, plays an essential role in the process of memory. *Memory* is a very complex phenomenon. Three levels of memory, short-term (recent), intermediate, and long-term, have been identified. Short-term memory is lost after seconds or minutes. Intermediate memory lasts days to weeks and eventually is lost. Long-term memory (remote) is stored and lasts a lifetime. Theories about the physiologic basis behind memory posit reverberating neuronal messages that cause short-term memory and actual neuronal structural changes that lead to long-term memory. The hippocampus assists in the conversion

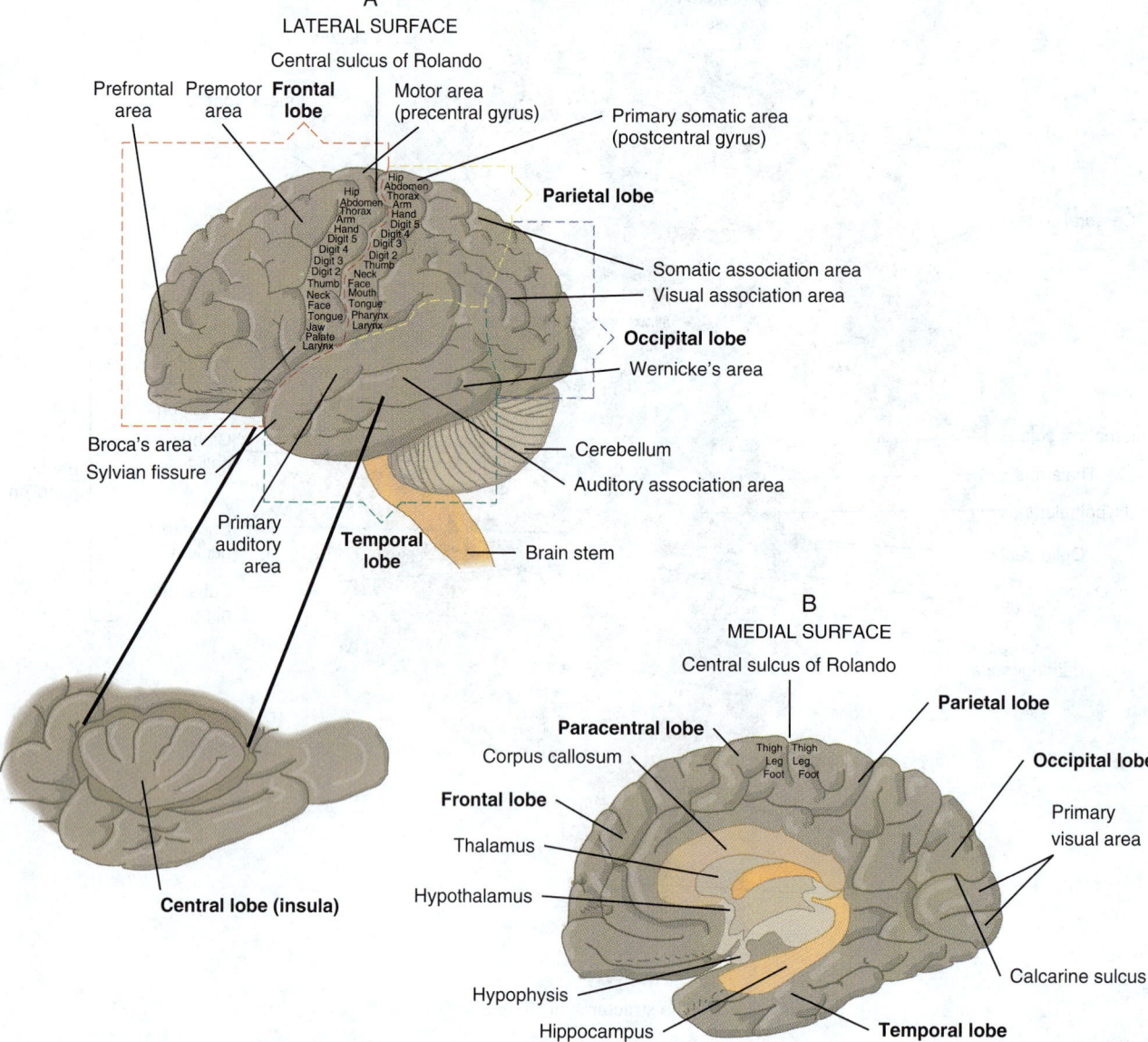

Figure 29–6. The lateral (*A*) and medial (*B*) surfaces of the cerebral cortex.

of short-term memory into intermediate and long-term memory in the thalamus. The association fibers of the frontal, parietal, temporal, and occipital lobes, as well as the diencephalon, also play an important role in long-term memory.[2]

■ Basal Ganglia

The basal ganglia consist of several structures of subcortical gray matter buried deep in the cerebral hemispheres. These structures include the caudate nucleus, putamen, globus pallidus, substantia nigra, and subthalamic nucleus (see Fig. 29–5). The basal ganglia serve as processing stations linking the cerebral cortices to thalamic nuclei. Almost all the motor and sensory fibers connecting the cerebral cortex and the spinal cord travel through the white matter pathways in the caudate nucleus and putamen ganglia. These pathways are known as the *internal capsule*. The basal ganglia play a significant role in asso-

ciation with the corticospinal tract in controlling complex motor activity.

■ Diencephalon

The diencephalon is comprised of the thalamus and the hypothalamus. The *thalamus* lies between the cerebral hemispheres and superior to the brain stem. Its gray matter surrounds the lateral edges of the third ventricle (see Fig. 29–5). The *hypothalamus* forms the floor of the third ventricle. Other important structural parts found in and near the diencephalon include the optic tracts and optic chiasm, the pituitary gland on the floor and the pineal gland on the roof of the diencephalon.

The thalamus channels all ascending (sensory) information except smell to the appropriate cortical cells and acts as a relay station for descending (motor) fibers. The hypothalamus regulates autonomic nervous system functions such as heart rate, blood pressure, water and electrolyte

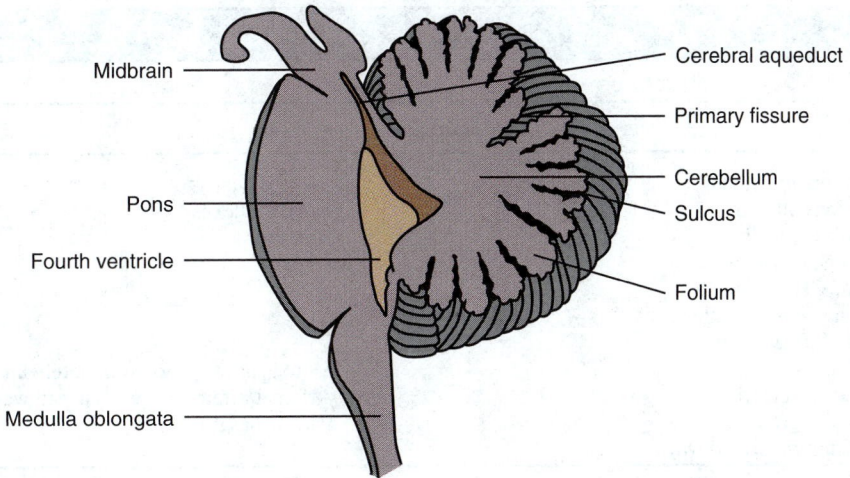

Figure 29-7. Sagittal view of the brain stem, fourth ventricle, and cerebellum.

balance, stomach and intestinal motility, glandular activity, body temperature, hunger, body weight, and sleep-wakefulness. It also serves as the master over the pituitary gland by releasing factors that stimulate or inhibit pituitary hormone output.

■ Limbic System

The limbic system is made up of many nuclei including parts of the medial portion of the frontal and temporal lobes (hippocampus), thalamus, hypothalamus, and the basal ganglia. It is considered the center for feelings and control of emotional expression (fear, anger, pleasure, sorrow). The limbic system (temporal lobe component) also receives nerve fibers from the olfactory bulbs and thus plays an essential role in the interpretation of smells.

■ Brain Stem

The brain stem is composed of the midbrain, pons, and medulla oblongata (see Figs. 29-5 and 29-7). These structures are continuous segments of the diencephalon nuclei. They are composed of ascending pathways, the reticular formation, cranial nerves and their nuclei, and descending autonomic and motor pathways. For a detailed listing of these important structures, see Table 29-1.

■ Reticular Formation

The reticular formation is composed of a complex network of gray matter (nuclei), ascending reticular pathways, and descending reticular pathways. Its nuclei extend from the superior part of the spinal cord to the diencephalon and communicate with the basal ganglia, cerebrum, and cerebellum.

The reticular formation assists in regulation of skeletal motor movement and spinal reflexes. It also filters incoming sensory information to the cerebral cortex. Approximately 99% of sensory information is disregarded as unessential. One component of the reticular formation, the reticular activating system, controls the sleep-wake cycle (see Chapter 18) and consciousness.

■ Cerebellum

The cerebellum is composed of gray and white matter. The cortex of the cerebellum is a thin layer of gray matter arranged in parallel long and deep gyri, called folia, and separated by cerebellar sulci (see Fig. 29-7). Deep fissures divide the cerebellum into three lobes, but the functional division of the cerebellum consists of a right and left hemisphere separated by a narrow band of white matter called the *vermis*. An extension of dura mater, the falx cerebelli, partially separates the hemispheres.

The cerebellum integrates sensory information related to position of body parts, coordinates skeletal muscle movement, and regulates muscle tension, which is necessary for balance and posture. Three pairs of nerve tracts (cerebellar peduncles) provide the communication pathways. The inferior peduncles are sensory (afferent) pathways from the spinal cord and medulla, which carry information related to the position of body parts to the cerebellum. The middle peduncles carry information from the cerebral cortex to effector cells that control voluntary (purposeful) motor activities. The cerebellum also receives sensory input from the receptors in the muscles, tendons, joints, eyes, and inner ear. After this information is integrated and analyzed, the cerebellum sends impulses via the superior peduncles (efferent pathways) to the brain stem and spinal cord and then to the appropriate body parts (effectors) to make corrections.

Most of the tracts in the cerebellum travel through various nuclei without crossing. Therefore, the right cerebellar hemisphere predominantly affects the right (ipsilateral) side of the body and vice versa.

Spinal Cord

The spinal cord, that portion of the CNS surrounded and protected by the vertebral column, is continuous with the medulla and lies within the upper two thirds of the vertebral canal (the cavity within the vertebral column). The lower spinal cord terminates caudally in a cone-shaped structure known as the *conus medullaris* at the level of

Table 29–1. Brain Stem Structures and Their Functions

Structures	Functions
Midbrain	
Corpora quadrigemina	
Superior colliculi	Visual reflexes
Inferior colliculi	Auditory reflexes
Cerebral aqueduct	
Origin of CN III and IV	
Ascending sensory pathways	
Reticular formation	
Red nuclei	Motor pathways to cord, cerebellum
Paired crura cerebri	Afferent/efferent cerebellar pathways
Substantia nigra	Part of basal ganglia
Descending motor pathways	
Pons	
Fourth ventricle	
Nuclei of inferior colliculus	Auditory processing
Nuclei of CN V, VI, VII	
Locus ceruleus	Secretes norepinephrine
Raphe nuclei	Secretes serotonin
Ascending sensory pathways	
Medial lemniscus, auditory pathway	Proprioceptive pathways
Descending motor pathways	
Medial longitudinal fasciculi	Efferent pathway to cord
Pyramids (corticospinal, corticobulbar, corticopontine)	Voluntary motor
Reticular formation	
Respiratory centers	
Pontine nuclei; pontocerebellar fibers	
Medulla Oblongata	
Fourth ventricle	
Central canal	
Raphe nuclei	Secretes serotonin
Ascending sensory pathways	
Medial lemniscal pathways	Proprioceptive pathways
Spinothalamic tracts	Pain pathways
Trigeminothalamic tracts	Tactile, temperature
Lateral lemnisci	Audition pathways
Nuclei of CN VIII, IX, X, XI, XII	
Olive and vestibular-cerebellar systems	
Reflex centers: respiratory, vasomotor, cardiac, coughing, swallowing, sneezing, vomiting	
Reticular formation	
Descending motor pathways (pyramids)	Voluntary motor

the first (L1) and second (L2) lumbar vertebrae. The spinal cord is subdivided into four areas: (1) the cervical cord, (2) the thoracic cord, (3) the lumbar cord, and (4) the sacral cord (the conus medullaris) (Fig. 29–8).

Within the spinal cord, butterfly-shaped gray matter (mostly unmyelinated) is surrounded by mostly myelinated white matter. The white matter consists of ascending and descending tracts that conduct nerve impulses between the brain and the cells outside the CNS. The cell bodies in the gray matter are grouped into clusters of nuclei and laminae (a defined group or column of cells). The tracts in the white matter are arranged into three paired columns: the posterior, lateral, and anterior columns (Fig. 29–9).

Ascending and Descending Pathways (Tracts)

The ascending (sensory) pathways eventually terminate in the cerebral and cerebellar cortex. Motor impulses from the brain, which travel through the descending pathways, terminate in the muscles and glands. For example, a spinothalamic tract, which is a sensory tract, begins in the spinal cord and ends in the parietal lobe. The corticospinal tract is a descending tract that originates in the frontal lobe of the cerebral cortex, travels through the spinal cord, and terminates in the muscle cells. This group of motor cells that originate in the frontal lobe and continue

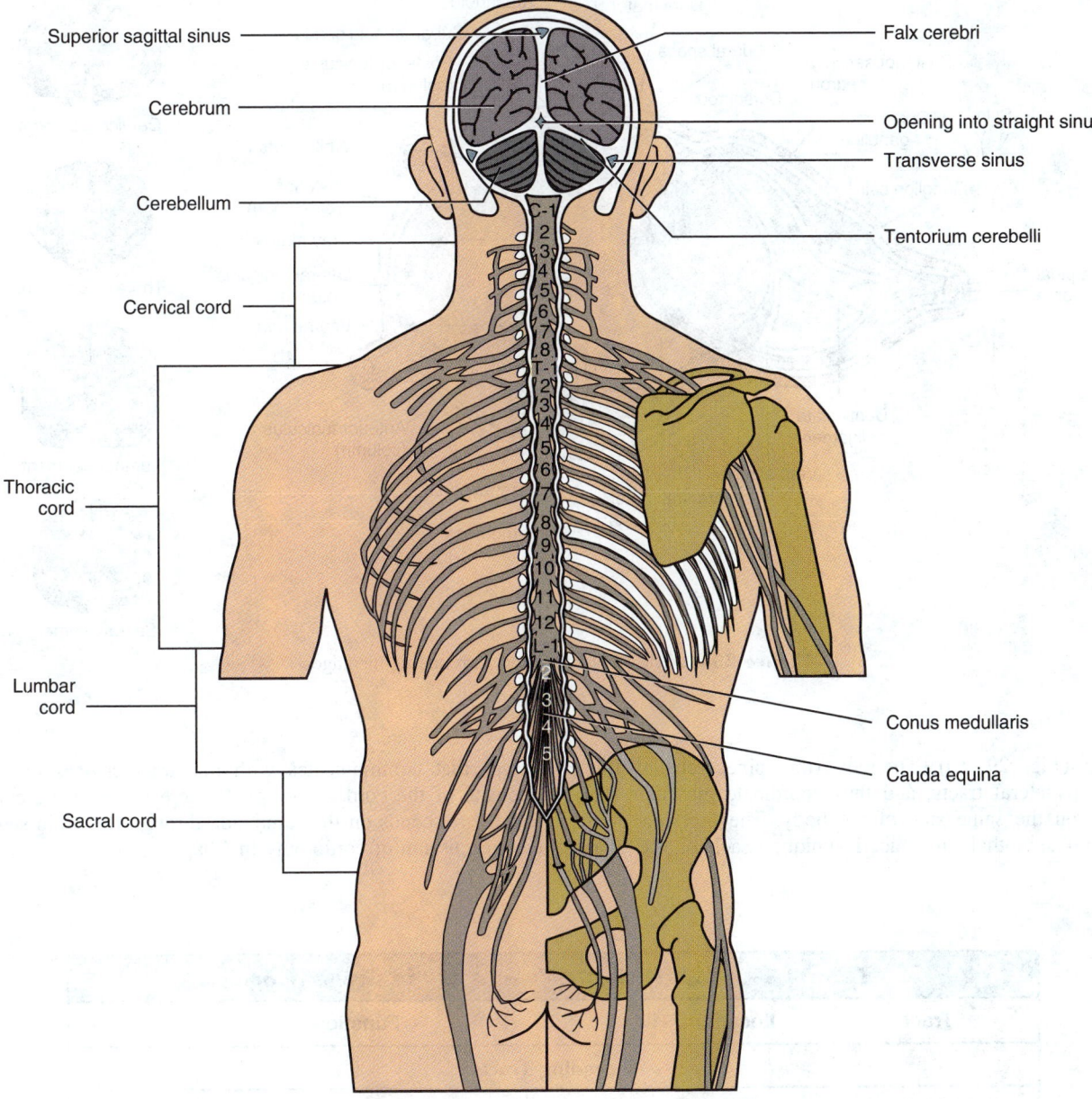

Figure 29–8. The cranial vault, vertebral column, and peripheral nerves.

through the corticospinal tract are also referred to as upper motor neuron cells. Lower motor neurons refer to those motor cells that begin in the anterior horn of the spinal cord and communicate with the spinal nerves. Impulses from the autonomic nervous system also descend from the hypothalamus, other brain levels, and cranial nerves to neurons within the spinal gray matter which synapse with preganglionic neurons of the sympathetic and parasympathetic nervous systems. Table 29–2 summarizes the specific functions of the major brain and spinal cord tracts.

Knowledge of spinal cord tract crossing is essential to primary, secondary, and tertiary prevention in clients with spinal cord injury. Many of the tracts communicating

with the cerebral cortex cross (decussate), but not all cross at the same place. The term *contralateral* is used to refer to those tracts that cross at the medulla and ascend or descend to the opposite side of the body. Tracts that do not cross are referred to as same-sided or *ipsilateral* tracts. For example, sensory tracts, including the anterior spinothalamic, the posterior, and anterior spinocerebellar tracts, cross in the medulla as they ascend to the cerebral cortex. Therefore, the sensory neurons in the cerebral cortex interpret sensory stimuli from the contralateral side of the body.

The lateral corticospinal spinal tract, also referred to as the pyramidal tract, crosses at the medulla as it descends from the frontal lobe of the cerebral cortex to the spinal

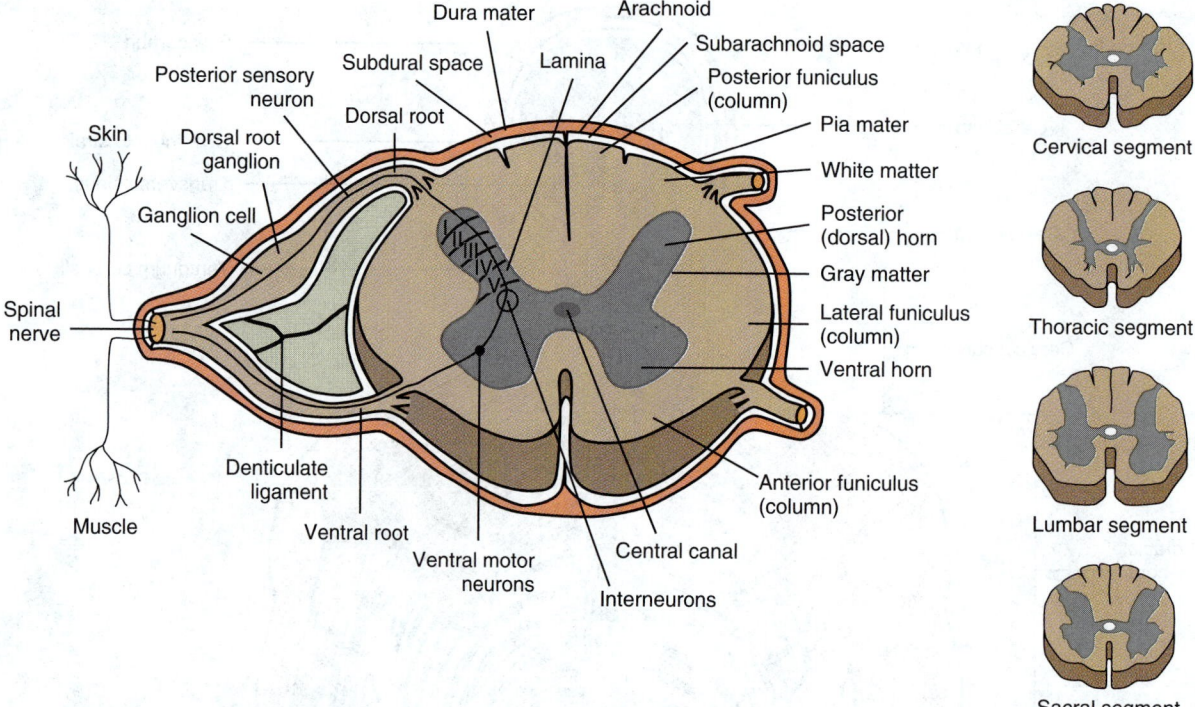

Figure 29-9. The spinal cord and surrounding meninges.

cord (Fig. 29–10). The posterior spinocerebellar tracts are ipsilateral tracts, and thus coordinate muscular function on the same side of the body. The crossing of the lateral spinothalamic tract is unique. Each of the spinal nerves that communicates with this tract crosses to the opposite of the cord at the level where it enters the cord and then ascends on the same side through the brain stem (see discussion of cordotomy in Chapter 35).

Tract	Location	Function
Table 29-2. Major Nerve Tracts of the Spinal Cord		
Ascending Tracts		
Fasciculus gracilis	Posterior column	Touch, pressure, body movement, position
Fasciculus cuneatus	Posterior column	
Spinothalamic		
Lateral	Lateral column	Pain, temperature
Anterior	Anterior column	Light (crude) touch
Spinocerebellar		
Posterior	Lateral column	Coordination of muscle movements
Anterior	Lateral column	
Descending Tracts		
Corticospinal		
Lateral	Lateral column	Voluntary motor
Ventral	Anterior column	Voluntary motor
Reticulospinal		
Lateral	Lateral column	Autonomic nervous system fibers, muscle tone, sweat glands
Anterior	Anterior column	
Medial	Anterior column	
Rubrospinal	Lateral column	Coordination of muscle movements

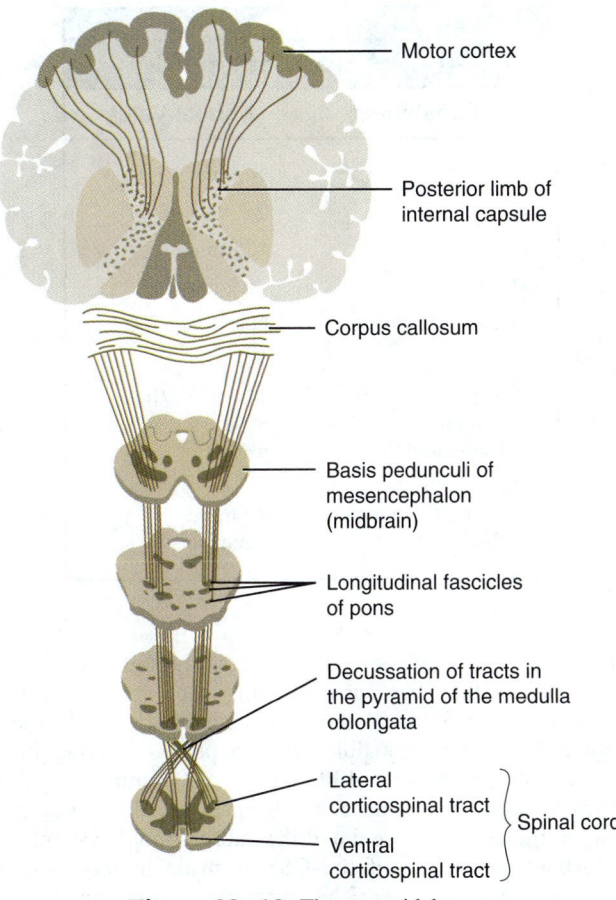

Figure 29–10. The pyramidal tract.

- Motor cortex
- Posterior limb of internal capsule
- Corpus callosum
- Basis pedunculi of mesencephalon (midbrain)
- Longitudinal fascicles of pons
- Decussation of tracts in the pyramid of the medulla oblongata
- Lateral corticospinal tract
- Ventral corticospinal tract
- Spinal cord

Protective and Nutritional Structures

■ Cranium and Vertebral Column

Eight bones that fuse early in childhood compose the cranium. The fused junctions are called *sutures*. The cra-nium predominantly encloses the brain structures and serves as a source of protection.

The floor, or basilar plate, of the cranial vault has three depressions, called *fossae*. The frontal lobes lie in the anterior fossa. The anterior temporal lobes and the base of the diencephalon lie in the middle fossa. The cerebel-lum rests in the posterior fossa. The floor, which supports the undersurface of the brain, is a very vulnerable part of the cranial vault because it contains many openings (*fo-ramina*) from which cranial nerves, blood vessels, and the spinal cord exit.

The vertebral column, a flexible series of vertebrae, surrounds and protects the spinal cord. The vertebral col-umn consists of 7 cervical vertebrae, 12 thoracic verte-brae, 5 lumbar vertebrae, 5 sacral vertebrae fused into a sacrum, and a coccyx. Ligaments hold the vertebrae to-gether, and discs between the vertebrae prevent the bones from rubbing together. In the adult, the vertebral column is much longer than the spinal cord; the spinal cord ends at L1−2.

■ Meninges

The meninges, three membranes enveloping the brain and spinal cord, are predominantly for protection (see Figs. 29–9 and 29–11). Each layer, the pia mater, arachnoid, and dura mater, is a separate but continuous membrane.

The *pia mater* is a vascular layer of connective tissue and is so closely connected to the brain and spinal cord that it follows every sulcus and fissure. This layer serves as a supporting structure for blood vessels passing through to the tissues of the brain and spinal cord. The pia mater and astrocytes together form the membrane part of the blood-brain barrier (see Blood-Brain Barrier).

The *arachnoid* is a thin layer of connective tissue. It extends from the top of each gyrus to the top of the adjacent gyrus. It does not extend into the sulci and fissures. The space between this layer and the pia mater is known as the subarachnoid space. The CSF flows through this space.

The cranial *dura mater* is a tough, nonstretchable vas-

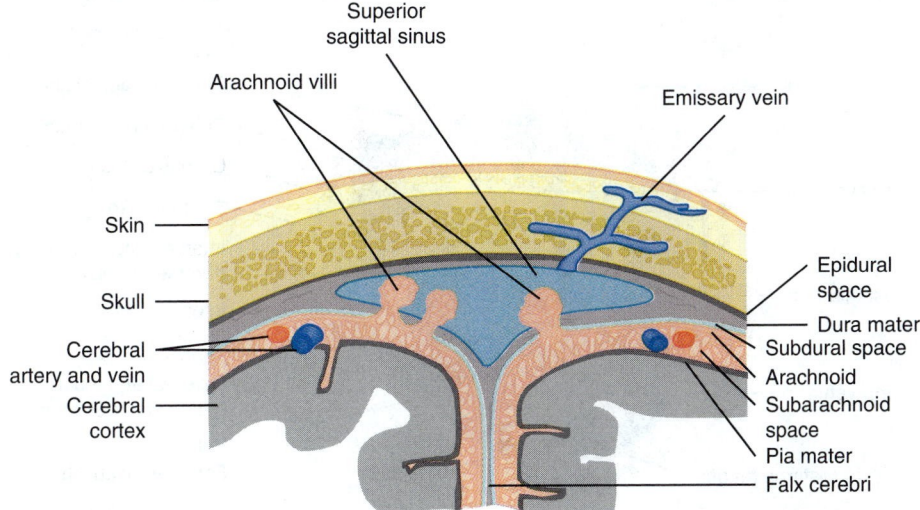

- Superior sagittal sinus
- Arachnoid villi
- Emissary vein
- Skin
- Skull
- Cerebral artery and vein
- Cerebral cortex
- Epidural space
- Dura mater
- Subdural space
- Arachnoid
- Subarachnoid space
- Pia mater
- Falx cerebri

Figure 29–11. The meninges (coronal section through the superior sagittal sinus).

cular membrane with two layers. The outer dura mater is actually the membrane (periosteum) of the cranial bones. The inner dura mater forms the plates that separate the two cerebral hemispheres (falx cerebri) (see Figs. 29–8 and 29–11), the cerebrum and the brain stem and cerebellum (tentorium cerebelli) (see Fig. 29–8), and the roof of the pituitary fossa (diaphragma sellae). The *tentorium cerebelli* is a landmark term that is often used by clinicians to separate parts of the brain; it is often referred to as "tentorium." The term *supratentorial* refers to the cerebrum and all the structures superior to the tentorium cerebelli. *Infratentorial* refers to those structures inferior to the tentorium cerebelli, the brain stem and the cerebellum.

Venous sinuses, which collect venous blood for return to the heart, are located between the dural layers. Note the superior sagittal sinus in Figure 29–11 as an example.

Brain spaces that often fill with blood after head trauma include the potential space called the subdural space between the inner dura and arachnoid and the epidural space between the dura mater and periosteum.

The meninges anchor the spinal cord. The pia mater, which closely surrounds the spinal cord, continues from the tip of the conus as a threadlike structure, called the filum terminale, to the end of the vertebral column, where it is anchored into the ligament on the posterior side of the coccyx. The denticulate ligaments, paired strips of epidural tissue, extend laterally from the pia mater to the dura mater to suspend the spinal cord from the dura. Two common spaces that are often accessed by physicians include the subarachnoid space, which extends below the level of the spinal cord to the second sacral (S2) vertebral level, and the epidural space, which lies between the dural sheath and the vertebral bones. The subarachnoid space is used for diagnostic studies and the epidural space is often used for medication delivery.

■ Cerebrospinal Fluid and Ventricular System

Cerebrospinal fluid is a clear, colorless fluid. Reference values for its constituents are listed in Table 29–3. Ap-

Table 29–3. Composition of Cerebrospinal Fluid	
Constituent	**Normal Value**
Na⁺	148 mmol/L
K⁺	2.9 mmol/L
Cl⁻	125 mmol/L
HCO₃⁻	22.9 mmol/L
Glucose (fasting)	50–75 mg/100 ml
pH	7.3
Protein	15–45 mg/100 ml
Albumin	80%
Gamma-globulin	6%–10%
Blood cells	
White (lymphocytes)	0–4/mm³
Red	0/mm³

proximately 135 ml of CSF circulates through the ventricles and within the subarachnoid space (80 ml in the ventricles and 55 ml in the subarachnoid space). The average pressure of the fluid when a person is lying in a horizontal position is 130 mm H₂O (10 mm Hg). The flow of CSF is produced by the pressure difference between the arterial system and the subarachnoid system.

About two thirds of the CSF is made in the choroid plexus of the four ventricles, primarily in the lateral ventricles. Small amounts are produced by ependymal, arachnoid, and other brain cells. The choroid plexus is a network of blood vessels within the pia mater that is in direct contact with the lining of the ventricle. The choroid plexuses together produce approximately 500 ml of CSF per day.

The ventricular system is a series of cavities within the brain. CSF flows from each of the lateral ventricles via the *foramen of Monro* into the third ventricle (Fig. 29–12). The third ventricle is midline just beneath the corpus callosum. CSF drains from the third ventricle through the *aqueduct of Sylvius* into the fourth ventricle. The fourth

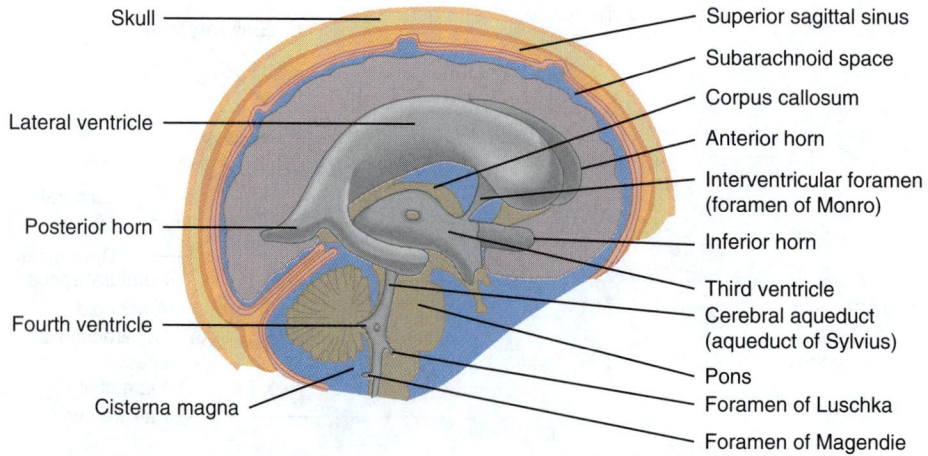

Figure 29–12. The ventricular system (lateral view).

ventricle is located in the brain stem just anterior to the cerebellum. From the fourth ventricle, CSF passes via one of three foramina (two *foramina of Luschka* and one *foramen of Magendie*) into a large subarachnoid space that lies behind the medulla and below the cerebellum, called the *cisterna magna*. The cisterna magna is continuous with the subarachnoid space, which surrounds the brain and spinal cord. Eventually, the CSF circulates upward into the region of the superior sagittal sinus (see Fig. 29–11), where it is absorbed across the arachnoid granulations, because of a pressure difference, into the venous system. The arachnoid granulations are extensive tufts of pia-arachnoid that along with the inner dura extend into the superior sagittal sinus and permit one-way flow of CSF into the sinus (see Fig. 29–11).

The brain and spinal cord float in the CSF, which absorbs shocks, thus cushioning the CNS. CSF also prevents the brain from tugging on meninges, nerve roots, and blood vessels.

■ Blood-Brain Barrier

Three barriers exist: (1) a blood-brain barrier, (2) a blood-CSF barrier, and (3) a brain-CSF barrier. The primary role of these brain barriers is to regulate and maintain an optimal and stable chemical environment for neurons. Brain barriers are either physical barriers or physiologic processes (transport systems) that slow movement of certain substances from one CNS compartment to another by regulating ion movement between the compartments. Tight junctions of the endothelial cells lining the capillaries, pores of the capillaries of the choroid plexuses, the basement membrane (ependymal cells) next to the choroid plexuses, and the pial-glial membrane serve as the physical barriers. An intact blood-brain barrier may prevent some drugs from crossing into the brain. This must be taken into consideration when medications are prescribed for nervous system disorders. Certain events, including dilutional hyponatremia, acute hypertension, high doses of some anesthetics, vasodilation, and hypercarbia, can increase the permeability of the blood-brain barrier; hypothermia stabilizes the blood-brain barrier.[6]

■ Blood Supply

The brain requires one third of the cardiac output and uses 20% of the body's oxygen. It makes energy almost exclusively from glucose. The gray matter has higher metabolic needs than white matter. The brain receives 800 ml of blood flow per minute. This blood flow can be affected by metabolic end products such as carbon dioxide, which alters the vascular tone of cerebral vessels. By this means, the brain ensures that its blood flow is adequate.

The vertebral arteries and the internal carotid arteries (Fig. 29–13) provide the arterial supply to the brain. The vertebral arteries branch from the subclavian arteries, travel through the transverse foramina in the cervical vertebrae, and enter the cranial vault through the foramen magnum. The vertebral arteries are located on the antero-lateral surface of the medulla. At the junction of the medulla and pons, the vertebral arteries join to form the basilar artery. The basilar artery bifurcates at the midbrain level to form two posterior cerebral arteries. The vertebral artery system supplies the brain stem, cerebellum, lower portion of the diencephalon, and the medial and inferior regions of the temporal and occipital lobes.

The internal carotid arteries branch from the common carotid arteries and enter the cranial vault at the base of the skull. The internal carotid arteries pass through the cavernous sinus and bifurcate into the anterior and middle cerebral arteries. Near this bifurcation, the circle of Willis, a ring of blood vessels at the base of the brain, is formed by the posterior cerebral arteries, posterior communicating arteries, internal carotid arteries, anterior cerebral arteries, and anterior communicating branches. The internal carotid arteries supply the upper diencephalon, basal ganglia, lateral temporal and occipital lobes, and parietal and frontal lobes. The middle cerebral arteries supply large portions of the frontal, parietal, temporal, occipital, and insular lobes; and the basal ganglia, internal capsule, and thalamus. The anterior cerebral arteries supply the medial portions of the frontal and parietal lobes and the upper basal ganglia and internal capsule (see Fig. 29–13).

The cerebral veins are grouped into superficial (external, surface) veins and deep veins. Blood from the upper lateral and medial cortices drains into the superior sagittal sinus flowing occipitally through other sinuses until it reaches the right jugular vein. The deep veins drain into the internal cerebral vein through venous sinuses and into the left internal jugular vein.

The spinal cord derives its arterial blood supply from small spinal arteries that branch off larger arteries, including the vertebrals, ascending cervical, deep cervical, intercostal, lumbar, and sacral arteries. These arteries and their branches form the three main arteries of the spinal cord, the anterior spinal artery and a pair of posterior spinal arteries, which extend the length of the cord. The anterior and posterior spinal arteries arise from the intracranial portion of the vertebral arteries.

The venous distribution is similar to the arterial distribution of the spinal cord. The venous system drains into the venous sinuses located between the dura mater and the periosteum of the vertebral column.

■ Reflex Mechanisms

Our subconscious automatic responses to internal and external stimuli, known as reflex responses, provide many homeostatic functions. Although the spinal cord is often thought of as the reflex center (Fig. 29–14), it is not the only site for reflex regulation. Many of the complex reflexes controlling heart rate, breathing, blood pressure, swallowing, sneezing, coughing, and vomiting are found in the brain stem.

Some intrinsic reflex circuits in the spinal cord create patterns of movement (flexion and extension) that are the basis for posture and forward progression. Other reflex circuits are the bases for spinal cord reflexes, which include the myotatic (deep tendon, stretch) reflex, the flexor

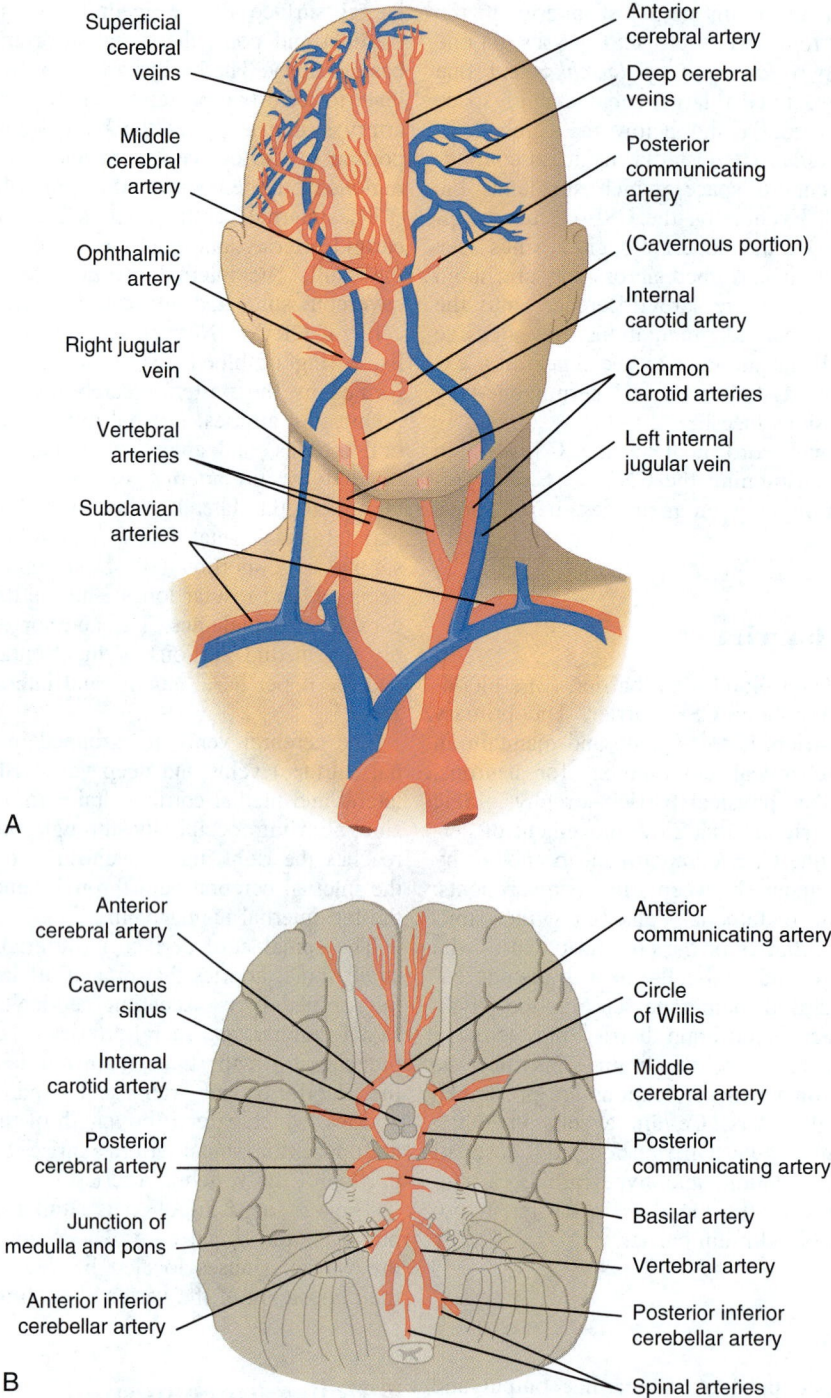

Figure 29–13. Cerebral circulation. *A,* Anterior circulation. *B,* Posterior circulation.

withdrawal reflex, the crossed extension reflex, and the extensor thrust reflex. Viscerosomatic reflexes can also excite or inhibit the motor neurons, producing changes in muscle tone and even movement.

Neuromuscular spindles monitor muscle length. As a muscle contracts, the neuromuscular spindle within the muscle becomes shorter, which reduces the rate of spindle firing to the motor neuron in the ventral horn, making continued contraction of the muscle impossible. Tone, residual tautness of the muscle, exists because some mus-

cle fibers in a muscle are always contracted. This is primarily a function of the muscle spindle.

The Golgi tendon organs are sensory nerve endings that respond to increased tendon tension. As the tension within the tendon increases, these endings increase their rate of firing, which increases the inhibitory stimulation to the motor neurons. The Golgi tendon organs protect against excessive stretch of tendons and muscles.

Simple reflexes require only two or three neurons. For example, the knee jerk reflex that helps maintain upright

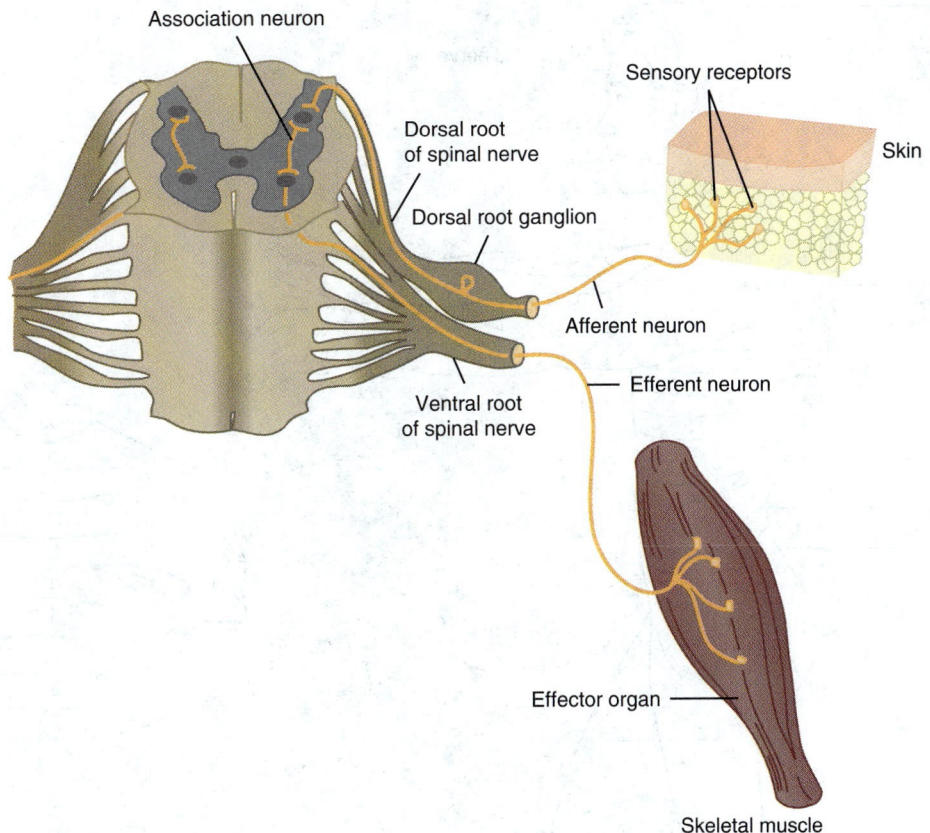

Figure 29–14. A simple reflex arc.

posture requires only a sensory and a motor neuron. The withdrawal reflex helps prevent or decrease tissue injury when a body part touches a potentially harmful object. The harmful stimuli are sent via the sensory neuron to the interneuron in the spinal cord for interpretation and the response message is sent via the motor neuron which results in the withdrawal response (see Figs. 29–9 and 29–14).

Reflexes are often used to evaluate the health of the nervous system because they are very sensitive to alterations in tissue perfusion and acid-base and electrolyte balance.

Peripheral Nervous System

In addition to dividing the peripheral nervous system into the spinal and cranial nerves and the autonomic nervous system (ANS), many authorities divide it into functional systems: the somatic nervous system and the ANS. The somatic nervous system refers to the nerve pathways that regulate voluntary motor control (skeletal muscles). The ANS refers to those nerve pathways that govern involuntary control in the internal environment (viscera).

The cranial and spinal nerves connect the brain and spinal cord to the skin, skeletal muscles, and special sensory organs. These nerves mostly affect voluntary activities. Those nerves that conduct impulses to the brain and spinal cord are called sensory (afferent) nerves. Those that conduct impulses away from the brain and spinal cord are called motor (efferent) nerves. Most nerves are

mixed, having both sensory and motor components. Each cranial and spinal nerve is composed of an axon and neurilemma cells with their neurilemma sheaths. They also have connective tissue coverings that provide structural support, a network of blood vessels, and the interstitial spaces essential for nerve impulse conduction.

Spinal Nerves

The spinal nerves develop from a series of nerve rootlets that collect laterally as spinal roots. Each spinal nerve consists of a dorsal (sensory) root and a ventral (motor) root which unite to form a spinal nerve. The dorsal root emerges from the posterolateral cord. The ventral root emerges from the anterolateral spinal cord. There are 31 pairs of spinal nerves: 8 pairs of cervical nerves, 12 pairs of thoracic nerves, 5 pairs of lumbar nerves, 5 pairs of sacral nerves, and usually 1 pair of coccygeal nerves (see Fig. 29–8). The specific area of sensory reception for each dorsal root is called a dermatome (Fig. 29–15). Cervical and thoracic nerves have a horizontal dermatome, whereas the lumbar, sacral, and coccygeal nerve roots extend beyond the spinal cord in the adult. This is because the growth phase of the vertebrae is faster than the cord growth. This collection of nerve fibers gives the appearance of a "horse's tail" *(cauda equina)*, at the end of the cord (see Fig. 29–8). Spinal nerves exit through an intervertebral foramen and they divide into four major branches. The meningeal branch reenters the vertebral canal and supplies the meninges, the blood vessels of the

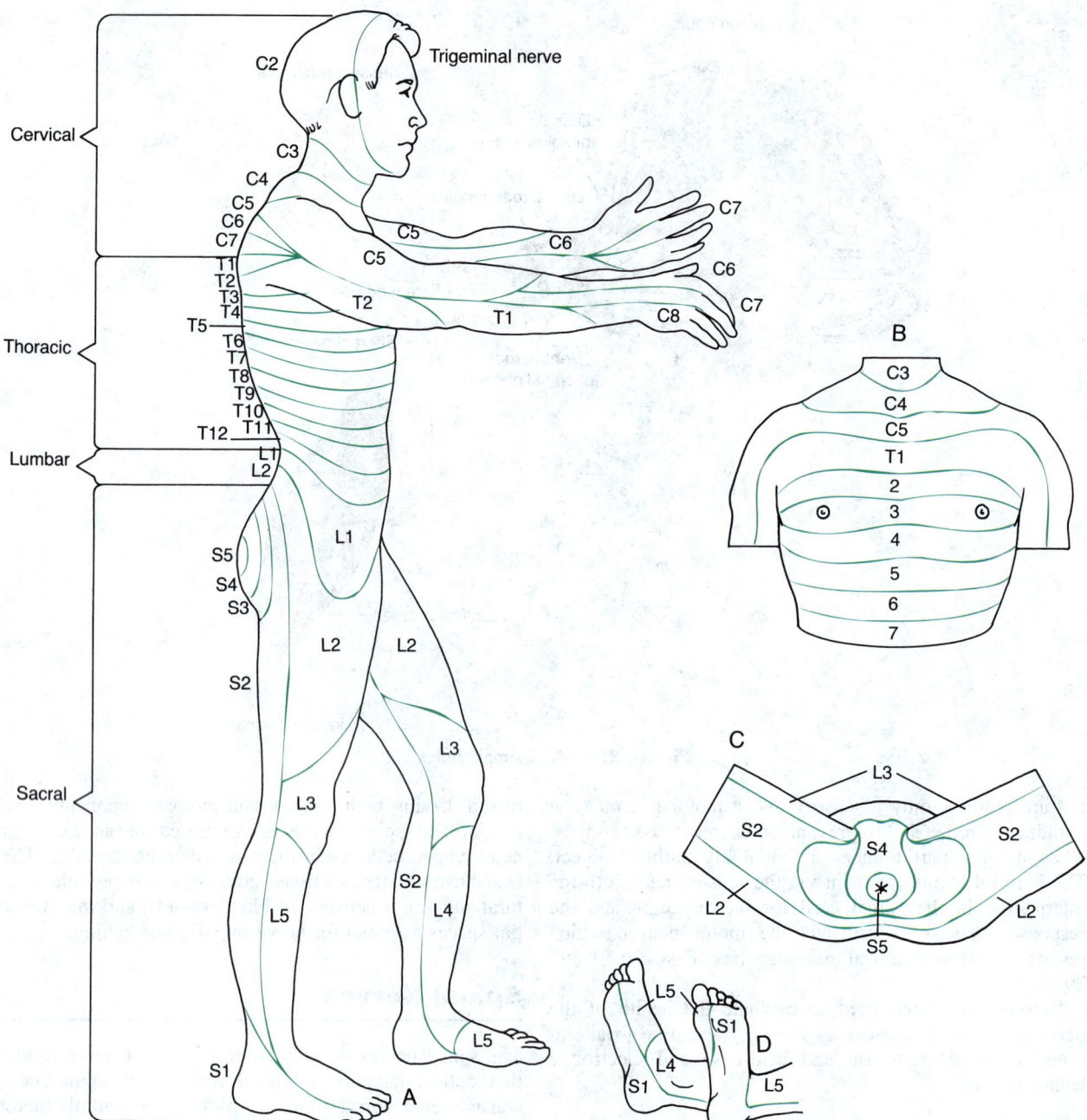

Figure 29–15. Dermatomes indicate distribution of spinal nerves. *Solid lines* divide the regions of the spinal cord (i.e., cervical, thoracic, lumbar, sacral). *Dotted lines* indicate segments of the spinal cord, or dermatomes. *A*, Torso and limbs. *B*, Anterior chest. *C*, Perineum. *D*, Feet. Dermatomes are used during assessment to identify specific areas of sensory impairment (e.g., touch, pain, temperature).

cord, the intervertebral ligaments, and the vertebrae. The posterior branch supplies the muscles and skin of the back. The anterior branch supplies the muscles and skin of the front and sides, trunk, and limbs. The visceral branch supplies the ANS fibers. Some of the anterior branches form complex nerve networks called *plexuses.* The three major plexuses are the cervical, brachial, and lumbosacral plexuses. The cervical plexus supplies the muscles and skin of the neck and branches to form the phrenic nerve, which innervates the diaphragm. The brachial plexus supplies the muscles and skin of the shoulders, axilla, arm, forearm, and hand. It branches to

form the ulnar, median, and radial nerves. The lumbosacral plexus supplies sensory and motor impulses to the muscles and skin of the perineum, gluteal region, thighs, legs, and feet. Its many branches include the pudendal, gluteal, femoral, sciatic, tibial, and common peroneal nerves.

Cranial Nerves

Cranial nerves arise in pairs and transmit nerve impulses from the special and general senses to the muscles of the

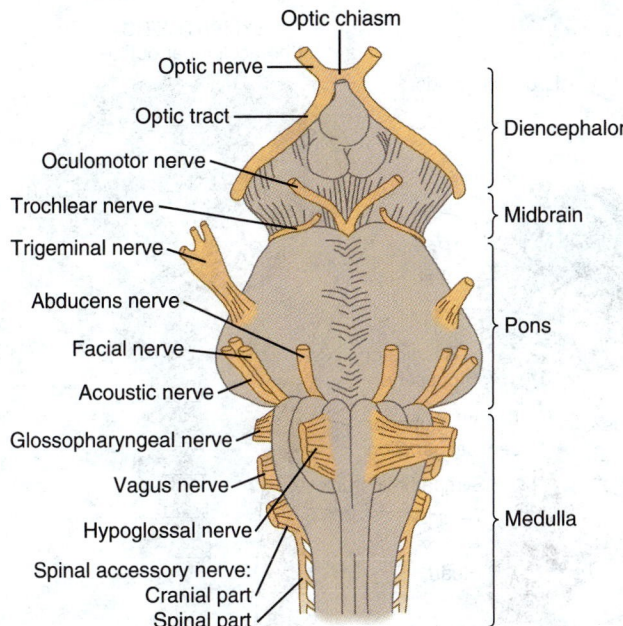

Optic chiasm
Optic nerve
Optic tract — Diencephalon
Oculomotor nerve
Trochlear nerve — Midbrain
Trigeminal nerve
Abducens nerve
Facial nerve — Pons
Acoustic nerve
Glossopharyngeal nerve
Vagus nerve
Hypoglossal nerve — Medulla
Spinal accessory nerve:
    Cranial part
    Spinal part

Figure 29–16. The brain stem (ventral view) and the cranial nerves that exit from it.

eyes, mouth, face, pharynx, larynx, and tongue to affector organs on their respective sides (Fig. 29–16). With the exceptions of the olfactory and optic nerves, whose nuclei lie just below the cerebrum, all the other cranial nerve nuclei lie within the brain stem.

Cranial nerves also carry the parasympathetic nervous system fibers to the head region (Fig. 29–17). The vagus nerve carries parasympathetic innervation to the thoracic and abdominal organs. Table 29–4 describes the functions and types of the 12 pairs of cranial nerves.

Peripheral Ganglia

Ganglia are groups of neuronal cell bodies that are usually located outside the CNS (see Fig. 29–9). They consist of proximal portions of axons and dendrites and the connective tissue of the ganglion. There are two types of ganglia: sensory ganglia, which are close to the CNS and have no synapses; and the motor ganglia of the ANS, which are at a distance from the CNS.

Autonomic Nervous System

The ANS is the part of the PNS that coordinates involuntary activities, such as visceral functions, smooth and cardiac muscle changes, and glandular responses. Although it can function independently, its primary control is from the brain and spinal cord. The ANS has two divisions, the sympathetic and parasympathetic nervous systems. The efferent ANS fibers travel within the cranial and spinal nerves. These two systems are highly integrated

and interact with each other to maintain a stable internal environment.

Unlike the somatic nerves, which usually are single neurons that link the CNS to a muscle or gland, the ANS has a two-neuron chain prior to the effector organ. The cell body of the first neuron is located in the CNS and synapses with nerve fibers whose cell bodies are within an autonomic ganglion. The axon of the second neuron (postganglionic fiber) carries impulses to the target viscera. An exception to this is the adrenal medulla, which is innervated directly by preganglionic fibers.

The sympathetic nervous system (SNS) coordinates activities that are used to handle stress. The SNS is geared for action as a whole for sustained periods. The preganglionic neurons of the sympathetic nervous system emerge from the spinal cord via the motor (ventral) roots of the thoracic and upper two lumbar spinal nerves (T1–L2) (see Fig. 29–17). The preganglionic axons are short, whereas the postganglionic axons are long.

The parasympathetic nervous system is associated with conservation and restoration of energy stores. The parasympathetic nervous system is geared to act locally and discretely and for a short duration. There is no mass discharge activity, as in the SNS. The preganglionic fibers emerge from the brain stem via the cranial nerves and from the spinal cord via the sacral spinal nerves at S1–4 (see Fig. 29–17). These preganglionic fibers have long axons that synapse with the postganglionic neurons in ganglia close to or located within the organs to be innervated. Each postganglionic neuron has a relatively short axon. Most organ systems, but not all, have both a parasympathetic and sympathetic nervous system. Approximately 75% of the parasympathetic fibers are in the vagus nerve.

Table 29–5 lists the effects of both the sympathetic and parasympathetic nervous systems on different organs. These functions and responses are related to the type of neurotransmitter released. The preganglionic fibers of the sympathetic and parasympathetic nerves and the postganglionic fibers of the parasympathetic nerves release acetylcholine. The postganglionic fibers of the sympathetic nerves release norepinephrine. Fibers secreting acetylcholine are called *cholinergic fibers;* those secreting norepinephrine are called *adrenergic fibers.* The complexity of the sympathetic and parasympathetic responses are also dependent on the type of receptor that combines with the neurotransmitter. The SNS has four types of receptors: $alpha_1$, $alpha_2$, $beta_1$, and $beta_2$. The parasympathetic nervous system has muscarinic and nicotinic receptors. Muscarinic receptors are found at the ends of all postganglionic parasympathetic and cholinergic SNS fibers. Responses are slow and excitatory. Nicotinic receptors are found between preganglionic and postganglionic synapses of the parasympathetic and sympathetic nervous systems. Responses are rapid and excitatory. Nicotinic receptors are found in the neuromuscular junction of the skeletal muscles.

Homeostasis is not only provided by the counterbalance between the SNS and the parasympathetic nervous system but also by enzyme decomposition. Acetylcholinesterase is the enzyme responsible for rapid decomposition of acetylcholine. Monoamine oxidase, found in the

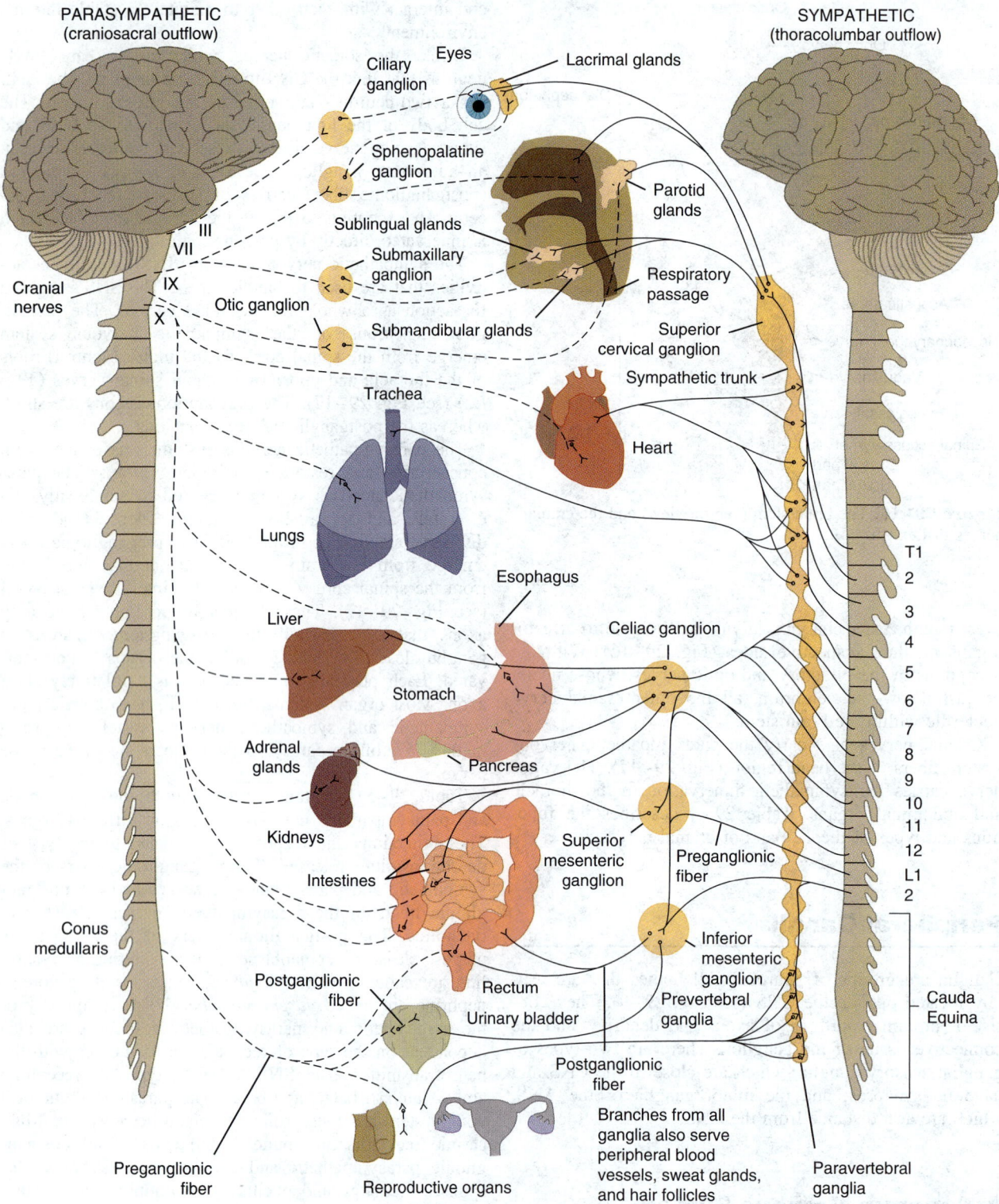

Figure 29–17. The autonomic nervous system.

mitochondria, is the enzyme that inactivates norepinephrine after it returns to the presynaptic vesicles. Some norepinephrine diffuses into the tissues and bloodstream, which results in a longer decomposition and a more last-

ing effect. Many drugs affect either the sympathetic or the parasympathetic nervous system. Many of the drug side effects occur because all innervated organs are affected, not just the one organ requiring treatment.

Table 29–4. Functions and Types of Cranial Nerves

	Name	Function	Type
I	Olfactory	Olfaction (smell)	Sensory
II	Optic	Vision	Sensory
III	Oculomotor	Extraocular eye movement	Motor
		Elevation of eyelid	
		Pupil constriction	Parasympathetic
IV	Trochlear	Extraocular eye movement	Motor
V	Trigeminal		
	Ophthalmic division	Somatic sensations of cornea, nasal mucous membranes, face	Sensory
	Maxillary division	Somatic sensations of face, oral cavity, anterior two thirds of tongue, teeth	Sensory
	Mandibular division	Somatic sensation of lower face	Sensory
		Mastication (chewing)	Motor
VI	Abducens	Lateral eye movement	Motor
VII	Facial	Facial expression	Motor
		Taste, anterior two thirds of tongue	Sensory
		Salivation	Parasympathetic
VIII	Vestibulocochlear		
	Vestibular	Equilibrium	Sensory
	Cochlear	Hearing	Sensory
IX	Glossopharyngeal	Taste, posterior third of tongue; pharyngeal sensation	Sensory
		Swallowing	Motor
X	Vagus	Sensation in pharynx, larynx, external ear	Sensory
		Swallowing	Motor
		Thoracic and abdominal visceral parasympathetic nervous system activities	Parasympathetic
XI	Spinal accessory	Neck and shoulder movement	Motor
XII	Hypoglossal	Tongue movement	Motor

Effects of Injury and Aging on the Nervous System

Regeneration

Nerve cell bodies are not able to regenerate. Regeneration is possible, however, if only the axon is injured. Initially, there is breakdown of the myelin sheath and axon. The axon swells and fragments while the myelin sheath disintegrates distal to the injury. The cell body takes up water. Macrophages phagocytose the breakdown products.

Neurilemma cells near the injury and in the entire segment distal to the injury undergo cell multiplication. These neurilemma cells form continuous cords (tubes) of cells that maintain the nerve fiber pattern. Neurilemma cells migrate into the emerging space.

The injured axon tip forms a new plasma membrane. Within a few days after injury, sprouts emerge from the tip. Peripheral nerve sprouts enter the distal stump and often come in contact with a neurilemma cord, which serves as a guide. The regenerating axon grows along the cord at a rate of 4 mm/day. Later, the neurilemma cells encapsulate the regenerating nerve fibers. With time, the axon and myelin sheath both thicken. Axons within the

CNS sprout and form growing tips but appear unable to sustain the metabolic responses necessary for extensive regeneration. It is believed that the axon tip is not able to penetrate the glial scar formed at the injury site, such as after spinal cord injury.[13]

An uninjured axon may sprout a collateral branch at a node of Ranvier that may enter into an adjacent denervated neurilemma cord. Collateral nerve regeneration occurs in both the peripheral and central nervous systems, for example, after peripheral nerve trauma or inflammation of a peripheral nerve, as in Bell's palsy.

Changes Related to Aging

Neurons undergo senescence. Intracellular, cellular, and biochemical changes occur. Lipofuscin accumulates in the cell. Neurofibrillary tangles and senile plaques develop. The neurons decrease in number after 30 years of age; the neuroglial cells increase in size and number. The number of dendrites decreases but the intrinsic dendritic changes have been found to be quite variable in hippocampal areas of the brain on postmortem examination in the normal aging population.[3] Variations in dendrite

Table 29–5. Effects of the Sympathetic and Parasympathetic Nervous Systems on Organs

Organ	Effect of Sympathetic Stimulation	Effect of Parasympathetic Stimulation
Eye		
Pupil	Dilation (alpha)*	Constriction
Ciliary muscle	Slight relaxation (far vision)	Constriction (near vision)
Glands	Vasoconstriction and slight secretion	Stimulation of copious secretion (containing many enzymes for enzyme-secreting glands)
Nasal		
Lacrimal		
Parotid		
Submandibular		
Gastric		
Pancreatic		
Sweat glands	Copious sweating (cholinergic)	Sweating on palms of hands
Apocrine glands	Thick, odoriferous secretion	None
Heart		
Muscle	Increased rate (beta$_1$)	Slowed rate
	Increased force of contraction (beta$_1$)	Decreased force of contraction (especially of atria)
Coronaries	Dilated (beta$_2$); constricted (alpha)	Dilation
Lungs		
Bronchi	Dilation (beta$_2$)	Constriction
Blood vessels	Mild constriction	? Dilation
Gut		
Lumen	Decreased peristalsis and tone (beta$_2$)	Increased peristalsis and tone
Sphincter	Increased tone (alpha)	Relaxation (most times)
Liver	Gluconeogenesis, glycogenolysis (beta$_2$)	Slight glycogen synthesis
Gallbladder and bile ducts	Relaxation	Contraction
Kidney	Decreased output and renin secretion	None
Bladder		
Detrusor	Relaxation (slight) (beta$_2$)	Contraction
Trigone	Contraction (alpha)	Relaxation
Penis	Ejaculation	Erection
Systemic arterioles		
Abdominal viscera	Constriction (alpha)	None
Muscle	Constriction (alpha)	None
	Dilation (beta$_2$)	
	Dilation (cholinergic)	
Skin	Constriction	None
Blood		
Coagulation	Increase	None
Glucose	Increase	None
Lipids	Increase	None
Basal metabolism	Increase up to 100%	None
Adrenal medullary secretion	Increase	None
Mental activity	Increase	None
Piloerector muscles	Contraction (alpha)	None
Skeletal muscle	Increased glycogenolysis (beta$_2$)	None
	Increased strength	
Fat cells	Lipolysis (beta$_1$)	None

*Sympathetic Nervous System comprised of alpha (α) and beta 1 (β_1) and beta 2 (β_2) receptors.

Adapted from Guyton, A. C., & Hall, J. E. (1996). *Textbook of medical science* (9th ed., pp. 774–775). Philadelphia: W. B. Saunders.

length, stability, and growth have been attributed to compensatory response to death of dendrites. Age has little effect on sensory and primary memory, but causes a decrease in working memory, including longer retrieval times for short-term memory, categorization, and episodic memory.[4] Dendritic changes are quite pronounced in pathologic conditions such as Alzheimer's disease (see Chapter 34). The axons also change in normal aging; their diameters thin, and the receptors decrease in number.

The amount of available neurotransmitters decreases by the age of 65 or 70 years. Oxygen consumption is decreased. Neuronal activity decreases, as evidenced by a decrease in the frequency and amplitude of brain waves on an electroencephalogram. Conduction velocity (speed of transmission) decreases by about 10%, thereby increasing response time.

Conclusions

The CNS is composed of the brain and spinal cord. These structures are protected by the skull and vertebrae, protective membranes, CSF, blood-brain barrier, and various cells. The PNS is comprised of the spinal and cranial nerves and the ANS.

The neuron is the structural and functional unit of the nervous system. The typical neuron is composed of a cell body, one axon, and several dendrites. The impulses along the nerve are carried through the action of several electrolytes and neurotransmitters. Unfortunately, only the axon (which is covered with myelin) can regenerate. Therefore, injury or disease and changes with aging create permanent losses of function within the central and peripheral nervous systems.

The nervous system is like a fine orchestra: as a whole it functions with a high level of harmony. But if one component of that system fails, the whole presentation is affected.

Bibliography

1. Bakey, L. (1991). Discovery of the arachnoid membrane. *Surgical Neurology, 36,* 63–68.
2. Bondy, K. N. (1994). Assessing cognitive function: A guide to neuropsychological testing. *Rehabilitation Nursing, 19*(1), 24–30.
3. Flood, D. G., & Coleman, P. D. (1990). Hippocampal plasticity in normal aging and decreased plasticity in Alzheimer's disease. In J. S. Mathisen, J. Zimmer & O. P. Ottersen (Eds.), *Progress in brain research* (Vol. 83, pp. 435–440). New York: Elsevier Science Publishers.
4. Green, P. M., & Gildemeister, J. E. (1994). Memory aging research and memory support in the elderly. *Journal of Neuroscience Nursing, 26*(4), 241–244.
5. Guyton, A. C., & Hall, J. E. (1996). *Textbook of medical science* (9th ed.). Philadelphia: W. B. Saunders.
6. Lewis, B. (1992). AANA journal course: Update for nurse anesthetists—Blood brain barrier function alteration during anesthesia. *Journal of the American Association of Nurse Anesthetists, 60*(6), 573–577.
7. Louis, E. D. (1993). The origins of the term "extrapyramidal" within the context of late nineteenth- and early twentieth-century neurology, neurophysiology and neuropathology. *Journal of the History of Medicine, 48,* 68–79.
8. McCance, K. L., & Huether, S. E. (1994). *Pathophysiology: The biologic basis of disease in adults and children* (2nd ed.), St. Louis: Mosby–Year Book.
9. Monti, E. J., Kerr, M. E., & Bender, C. (1995). Monitoring neuromuscular function. *Journal of Neuroscience Nursing, 27*(4), 252–256.
10. Pressman, E. K., Zeidman, S. M., & Summers, L. (1995). Primary care for women: Comprehensive assessment of the neurological system. *Journal of Nurse-Midwifery, 40*(2), 163–171.
11. Shier, D., Butler, J., & Lewis, R. (1996). *Hole's human anatomy and physiology* (7th ed.). Dubuque, IA: W. C. Brown Publishers.
12. Sur, M., & Cowey, A. (1995). Cerebral cortex: Function and development. *Neuron, 15,* 497–505.
13. Tower, D. B. (1992). A century of neuronal and neuroglial interactions, and their pathological implications: An overview. In A. C. H. Yu, et al. (Eds.), *Progress in brain research* (Vol. 94, pp. 3–17). New York: Elsevier Science Publishers.

Assessment of Clients with Neurologic Disorders

Mary Vorder Bruegge

The assessment of a client experiencing a neurologic disorder is a nursing challenge. Neurologic disorders range from simple to complex with widespread involvement of the central nervous system (CNS). Some neurologic disorders have profound consequences on activities of daily living (ADL) and even on survival. Neurologic assessment is used by physicians and nurses to establish a baseline of client data. This baseline is used to compare ongoing assessments, diagnose actual and potential health problems, plan the management of client care, and evaluate the client's outcome. Some of these functions are physician-oriented assessments, and others are assessments shared by nurses and physicians. Because of the complexity of the nervous system, the neurologic assessment is both multifaceted and lengthy. There are three main components to a neurologic assessment: (1) a comprehensive history, which includes symptom analysis; (2) a neurologic physical examination; and (3) general and specific neurodiagnostic studies.

The physician's assessment of the client with neurologic disorders is usually focused on the organic basis of the disorder. Physicians assess the client's clinical manifestations to pinpoint the anatomic location of the disorder, for example, the brain versus the spinal cord. The cause of the clinical manifestations is identified, for example, a tumor versus trauma. These data are combined with all other data and allow a medical diagnosis to be made from which a treatment plan is determined.

The focus of the nurse's assessment is both anatomic and functional. The nurse makes continuous observations of the client and compares them with baseline data. Astute observations are essential because most neurologic changes occur subtly. Nurses also collect data on the ability of the client to function physically (e.g., self-care deficit) and mentally (e.g., confusion and altered problem solving). Finally, because many neurologic disorders are very serious, the nurse provides skillful, crisis-oriented support for the client and significant others.

This chapter presents basic neurologic assessment procedures. Additional assessment techniques are discussed throughout this unit for other specific neurologic disorders.

Novice practitioners may want to follow the assessment sequence described in this chapter to avoid missing parts of a complex examination. More advanced clinicians may develop a preferred sequence based on personal experience. The sequence suggested in Table 30–1, "Neurologic Assessment Guidelines," integrates cranial nerve and reflex testing into motor and sensory examinations.

History

The purpose of the history is to determine past and present health status and to obtain a description of the onset of the current illness. It includes biographical data, the chief complaint and history of present illness, past health history, family health history, psychosocial history, and review of systems.

Biographical and Demographic Data

Biographical data include demographic, administrative, and insurance data. Often included are (1) a personal profile or brief description of the client, (2) the source of the history (e.g., client or significant other), and (3) the client's mental status (indicating the reliability of the data). Neurologic problems often affect mental status, sometimes making it difficult to get an accurate history directly from the client.

Chief Complaint

The nurse obtains a detailed description of the events that led the client to seek care. Avoid suggesting symptoms to the client and use open-ended questions.

This chapter incorporates material written for the fourth edition by Joyce M. Black and Ellen Barker.

Text continued on page 714

Table 30-1. Neurologic Assessment Guidelines

Functional Category	Specific Category	Area of Nervous System Involved	Assessment Technique	Examples of Disorders
1. Consciousness (awareness of self and environment)	Arousal response to verbal, tactile, and visual stimuli	Reticular activating system (mesencephalon, diencephalon) Both hemispheres	Is client alert? What is attention span? Is there normal response to visual and auditory stimuli?	Elevation: insomnia, agitation, mania, delirium
			Reaction to loud noises, shaking, deep pressure over eye orbits or sternum? Are vital signs, pupils, and reflexes normal?	Depression: somnolence, lethargy, semicoma, coma
2. Mentation	Thinking	Cerebral hemispheres plus specific regional functions	Is client oriented (time, place, person)?	Disorientation
	Insight, judgment, planning	Frontal lobe, with association fibers to other areas of cerebrum	Does client recognize implication of illness? Are goals congruent with abilities? How would client respond to given situation (e.g., house on fire)?	Lack of judgment, inattention to grooming, appearance, and personal habits
	Fund of information	Basic biologic intellect (frontal lobe) integrated into other areas	Calculation ability, knowledge of current events consistent with educational level. Who is U.S. president?	Impairment—functioning not congruent with level of education
	Memory	Temporal lobe and association to most other areas of cortex		
	Recent	Hippocampus	What was eaten for breakfast? What happened yesterday?	Organic brain disease
	Past	Frontal lobe	Recall past events during taking of history	Lapses of memory for past events may coincide with past CNS problems (e.g., trauma, infection, psychic trauma)
	Feeling (affect) (congruence of response to stimulus)	Limbic system (usually involves both hemispheres)	Compare observed with expected reactions. Are emotions labile? Appropriate?	Blunted affect: hysteria, schizophrenia, bilateral frontal lobe lesions
	Perceptual distortions (illusions, hallucinations)	General and specific cortical areas in hallucinations	Observations for behavior indicating perceptual problems. Ask client	Irritative lesions of cortex may → hallucinations (occipital cortex → visual, postcentral gyrus → somatic sensation, uncus → smell)
3. Language and speech	Dysarthria (defects in articulation, enunciation, and rhythm in speech)	Impairment of muscles of tongue, palate, pharynx, or lips (may be due to ↓ impulses or incoordination) Brain stem, cerebellum, or extraneural causes; CN V, VII, IX, X, XII	Have client repeat a difficult phrase (e.g., "Susie sells seashells by the seashore")	Slurring, slowness, indistinctness, nasality, break in normal speech rhythm (i.e., speech of intoxication), amytrophic lateral sclerosis; pseudobulbar palsy; myasthenia gravis)

Table 30–1. Neurologic Assessment Guidelines *(Continued)*

Functional Category	Specific Category	Area of Nervous System Involved	Assessment Technique	Examples of Disorders
3. Language and speech *Continued*	Dysphonia (abnormal production of sounds from larynx)	Many extraneural causes Recurrent laryngeal nerve problems (part of vagus); CN X Medulla (area of nucleus of CN X)	Is client hoarse? Whispered voice is intact Use indirect laryngoscopy findings	Compression of recurrent laryngeal nerve by bronchogenic carcinoma of left mainstem bronchus Left atrial hypertrophy Brain stem tumors, occlusion of posterior inferior cerebellar or vertebral artery
	Aphasia (inability to use and understand written and spoken words)	Fluent (receptive) left temporal and parietal lobes (Wernicke's area)	Observe vocal expression, written expression, comprehension of spoken and written language, and gesture communication	Cerebrovascular disease of middle cerebral artery Trauma, tumor, abscess, etc., in left temporal and parietal lobe areas
		Nonfluent (expressive) Broca's area (lateral) inferior portion of frontal lobe of dominant side Global (combined)		Damage to Broca's area or association fibers (stroke, tumor, etc.)
	Agnosia (inability to recognize objects or symbols by means of senses)	Primarily in parietal temporal and occipital areas	Sense organs intact? Can the client recognize objects by sight, touch, hearing, etc?	Cerebrovascular disease
4. Motor function	Expression (facial)	CN VII	Symmetry of smile, frown, raising eyebrows	Central facial weakness (upper motor neuron dysfunction); weakness of lower half of face Causes: cerebral vascular accident, corticobulbar tract Peripheral facial weakness (lower motor dysfunction); weakness of entire half of face Causes: Bell's palsy, brain stem tumor, fracture of temporal bone
	Eating (chewing, swallowing)	CN V, VII, IX, X, XII	Strength of masticator muscles, gag reflexes, ability to swallow	Tetanus, peripheral spasm of muscle; amyotrophic lateral sclerosis, medullary tumor; pseudobulbar palsy may be associated with dysarthria
	Eye movements	CN III, IV, VI	Extraocular movement, pupil size, reactivity, pupils react equally to accommodation, diplopia, nystagmus	Cerebral peduncle pressure → CN III dysfunction, cavernous sinus thrombus → CN III, IV, VI problem Muscular problems (e.g., myasthenia gravis, hyperthyroid)

Table continued on following page

Table 30–1. Neurologic Assessment Guidelines (Continued)

Functional Category	Specific Category	Area of Nervous System Involved	Assessment Technique	Examples of Disorders
4. Motor function *Continued*				Horner's syndrome (ptosis, constricted pupil), anisocoria
	Moving	Motor precentral gyrus (pyramidal) and cerebellar systems, basal ganglia, CN XI, spinal cord, upper motor neuron, (brain → spinal cord via corticospinal tract)	Gait, heel-to-toe walking, presence or absence of involuntary movements, coordination, muscle tone, mass, strength, Romberg's test, ability to shrug shoulders and to rise from chair	*Upper motor neuron* Brain and cord-sparing anterior horn cell
				Tone ↑ ↑ (spastic)
				Bulk ↓ due to atrophy of disuse
				Reflexes ↑ ↑ due to loss of central inhibition No fasciculations
				Frequent clonus
		Lower motor neuron (motor cells of cranial and spinal nerves and anterior horn cells → peripheral muscles)		*Lower motor neuron* Segment anterior horn cell peripheral nerve
				Tone ↓ ↓ (flaccid)
				Bulk ↓ due to tone loss
				Reflexes ↓ or absent due to loss of anterior horn cell
				Fasciculations
		Involves cerebellum		No clonus *Cerebellar problem* → loss of coordination and balance
5. Sensory function	Seeing	CN II Optic, occipital lobe	Acuity, visual fields, funduscopy	Field test: loss in retina or optic nerve → loss in eye involved, optic chiasm → bitemporal hemianopsia Optic tract → homonymous hemianopsia, parietal lobe → quadrant problems (inferior), temporal lobe → superior quadrant problems ↑ Intracranial pressure → papilledema (raised disc → hemorrhage)
	Smelling	CN I Temporal lobe (uncus)	Ability to detect familiar odors	Usually ↓ smell due to extraneural causes (e.g., upper respiratory infection, allergy, smoking), olfactory groove; meningioma, olfactory hallucinations

Table 30-1. Neurologic Assessment Guidelines (Continued)

Functional Category	Specific Category	Area of Nervous System Involved	Assessment Technique	Examples of Disorders
5. Sensory function *Continued*	Hearing	CN VIII Cochlear division, temporal lobe	Acuity of hearing, presence or absence of unusual sounds, Weber's and Rinne tests	May have conductive (nerve OK) or neural hearing loss; Méniere's syndrome (tinnitus, hearing loss, vertigo, and nystagmus), basilar skull fracture → otorrhea
				Brain stem vascular dysfunction or tumors → ↓ hearing
	Taste	CN VII, IX Insula lobe	Ability to differentiate sweet, salt, sour, and bitter	Brain stem or insula lesions → ↓ taste; extraneural causes, smoking, poor oral hygiene
	Feeling (sensory)	Peripheral nerves → Dermatomes → Spinal cord → Tracts (leading to) Pain-temperature-tactile, anterolateral system, proprioception, stereognosis, dorsal roots → thalamus leading to somasthetic area (postcentral gyrus, parietal lobe)	Pain: pinprick Touch: cotton touched to skin Proprioception: check where digit is in space Vibration: place vibrating tuning fork on bony prominence Temperature: test tubes of cold and warm water laid against skin; person identifies whether hot or cold	Polyneuropathy, (e.g., diabetes, anemia) Spinal cord lesions → dermatome alterations; upper pons → thalamus, contralateral loss; thalamus → contralateral loss + paresthesia; thalamus → cortex → cortical sensory loss
6. Bowel and bladder function	Bowel function	Afferent Spinal nerve S3–5 External sphincter (voluntary control) Internal sphincter Spinal nerve S3–5 Autonomic nervous system	Check for fecal impaction or incontinence Check muscle tone	Fecal incontinence with lesions S3–5 Anal anesthesia—conus medullaris and tabes dorsalis May be extraneural causes
		Cerebral cortex		Loss of inhibitory control (e.g., stroke)
	Bladder function	Autonomic nervous system Afferent Spinal nerve T9–L2, S2–4 Pudendal nerve	Feel when bladder is full, complete emptying. Does client have urgency, frequency	Urinary incontinence Flaccid bladder
		Efferent Spinal nerve T11–L2 External sphincter (voluntary) Spinal nerve S2–4 Cerebral cortex		Spastic bladder Loss of inhibitory control (e.g., stroke) May be extraneural causes

History of Present Illness

The onset and sequence of symptoms and their progress are important to determine. Neurologic disease processes should be described with great accuracy to facilitate the diagnostic process. Ask the client to describe symptoms in detail using his or her own words. Data regarding symptom characteristics and their progression are elicited using a symptom analysis (see Chapter 11).

The health history guides the nurse in the following physical examination. For example, a complaint of dizziness cues the nurse to focus on examination of the eyes, ears (vestibular), and cerebellar function instead of motor and sensory functions. A detailed neurologic examination is indicated in situations in which the client reports behavioral changes, altered level of consciousness, growth and development problems, pain, changes in motor or sensory function, infection, or trauma. The nurse is alerted to assess for neurologic problems that may be related to other problems such as alcohol and recreational drug use, metabolic imbalances, or metastatic lesions.

Past Health History

The past health history encompasses previous illnesses, hospitalizations, childhood and infectious diseases, medications, perinatal period, growth and development, family health history, and psychosocial history and life-style. Neurologic illnesses often subtly affect a client's ability to function in an integrated fashion. The nurse asks about changes in consciousness, vision, speech, motor or sensory functions, headaches, seizures, dizziness, vertigo, gait, and body posture.

Childhood and Infectious Diseases and Immunizations

Data are collected regarding common childhood diseases and immunizations. Diseases associated with neurologic sequelae include rubella, rubeola, cytomegalovirus infection, herpes simplex, influenza, and meningitis. Ask whether or not the client has been immunized for polio, tetanus, and measles.

Major Illnesses and Hospitalizations

There are a number of major illnesses associated with neurologic changes, such as diabetes mellitus, pernicious anemia, cancer, infections, and hypertension. Advanced liver disease and renal disease result in metabolic disturbances such as fluid and electrolyte imbalances and acid-base changes that affect mental function. Inquire about hospitalization, injury, or surgery for problems related to the neurologic system, such as head trauma, seizures, stroke, or crushing tissue injury. Has the client had any neurologic diagnostic studies performed, such as an electroencephalography (EEG), electromyography (EMG), or computed tomographic (CT) scan? Results of such diagnostic studies provide valuable data for future comparison.

Medications

The medication history includes all medications that the client is taking or has taken, both prescription and over-the-counter medications. Specifically, ask about aspirin, anticonvulsants, CNS stimulants and depressants, sedatives, anticoagulants, narcotics, tranquilizers, and antihypertensive medications. Many preparations for allergies and colds contain ingredients that cause drowsiness. Inquire about the current use of recreational drugs or past use, type of drug, and duration of use.

Growth and Development

The client's history of growth and development may help determine whether or not neurologic dysfunction was present at an early age. The perinatal history may include data about in utero exposure to viruses (rubella), maternal consumption of alcohol and tobacco or other drugs, and radiation. Ask the client whether gestation was full term or premature, because premature birth increases the risk of neurologic damage from inadequate oxygenation and intracranial bleeding if ventilator support was used. A difficult or prolonged labor and delivery can result in hypoxia or use of forceps for delivery, with consequent central and peripheral neurologic damage.

The nurse asks the client when major developmental tasks such as walking and talking occurred. Was the client able to participate in games, sports, and other childhood activities with peers? Were there any problems with coordination, balance, or agility?

Family Health History

Ask the client about the family history of neurologic disorders to determine whether genetic risk factors are present. Inquire about the familial occurrence of epilepsy, Huntington's disease, amyotrophic lateral sclerosis, muscular dystrophy, hypertension, stroke, mental retardation, and psychiatric disorders.

Psychosocial History

An understanding of personal psychosocial factors (e.g., educational background, level of performance, and personality changes) enhances accurate assessment. The nurse specifically inquires about changes that have occurred in the client's daily routines. Ask about changes in sleep patterns, exercise routines, hobbies and recreation, occupation, perceived stressors, and sexual interest and performance. Is the client at risk of exposure to neurotoxic fumes or chemicals, such as pesticides, paints, or bonding agents (glue), or is he or she in an inadequately ventilated living area or workspace?

Review of Systems

The client is asked to describe symptoms associated with the neurologic system, such as behavior changes, mood swings, loss of consciousness, seizures, memory deficits, motor function problems (e.g., unstable balance, tics, tremors), and sensory function problems (e.g., pain, paresthesia or tingling, paralysis). Significant data related to the neurologic assessment include those given in Box 30–1. Detailed questions for the review of systems are found in Box 11–2.

The client with a neurologic problem may be unaware of its presence. The nurse attempts to supplement and corroborate the client's history and review of systems with a family member or significant other who knows the client well. Ask specifically about mental or physical changes that have been noticed.

Physical Examination

The neurologic physical examination is intended to detect abnormalities in neurologic functioning. Variations in the client's age, physical condition, and level of consciousness determine how detailed the examination can be. The components of a comprehensive neurologic examination are described here. The nurse must adapt the comprehensive neurologic examination to the client's level of neurologic function. Box 30–2 is a guide to adapting the assessment in various situations.

The comprehensive neurologic examination consists of vital signs, mental status, language and communication, cranial nerve assessment, motor response, sensory response, and reflexes. A suggested sequence of the physical examination is as follows:

1. Vital signs
2. Mental status (including language and communication)
3. Head, neck, and back
4. Cranial nerves (including pupils)
5. Motor system
6. Sensory function
7. Reflexes
8. Autonomic nervous system

The normal physical assessment findings are summarized in the feature on page 717.

Vital Signs

Although cortical changes occur first (e.g., level of consciousness [LOC]), vital signs are assessed first because neurologic disorders can cause life-threatening changes in a client's vital signs. Clients with cervical spinal cord injuries exhibit a classic triad of hypotension, bradycardia, and hypothermia related to loss of sympathetic nervous system function. Inadequate perfusion of vital organs may result from hypotension if the blood pressure is not supported.

Changes in vital signs can also accompany the late stages of increased intracranial pressure (ICP). The body attempts to provide an adequate supply of oxygen and

---

Box 30–1. Manifestations Related to Neurologic Assessment

Eye

Visual loss
Diplopia
Ptosis
Proptosis

Ear, Nose, and Throat

Infections
Hearing loss
Tinnitus
Dizziness
Vertigo
Voice change
Dysphagia
Changes in taste or smell
Experiences of unusual smells

Cardiovascular

Syncope
Palpitations
Hypotension
Hypertension
Vertigo
Transient ischemic attacks
Stroke

Neurologic

Weakness
Numbness
Paresthesias

Headache
Pain
Altered thinking
Speech difficulty
Vomiting
Vertigo
Ataxia
Fainting
Seizures
Any loss of consciousness
Distortions of reality
Use of consciousness-altering drugs
Disorientation
Altered sleep patterns
Changes in ability to speak, read, or understand language
Changes in memory of recent or remote events
Changes in ability to concentrate

Skin

Hair and nail changes

Musculoskeletal

Tremor
Weakness
Altered coordination
Staggering
Difficulty climbing stairs

---

glucose to the brain by increasing the blood flow to the brain to compensate for increased ICP. Cushing's response consists of elevated systolic blood pressure, widened pulse pressure, and bradycardia. Respiratory rate and rhythm can be altered by increased ICP on the brain stem.

Mental Status

Document general data about the client's mental status (e.g., LOC, orientation, memory, mood and affect, intellectual performance, judgment and insight, and language and communication). The mental status examination is discussed in Chapter 11.

Level of Consciousness

The *level of consciousness (LOC)* is the most sensitive indicator of changes in the neurologic status of a client. Consciousness is maintained by the function of the cerebral hemispheres and the reticular activating system. LOC is tested using stimuli to determine arousability. Stimuli include verbal, visual, tactile, and noxious agents such as painful pressure.

Box 30–2. The Initial Neurologic Examination in the Clinical Setting

The sequence in which the neurologic examination is performed and the amount of time devoted to each section is dictated by the client's situation. For example, assessment of the head-injured client in the emergency room requires evaluation of vital signs, pupil reactivity, level of consciousness, and motor response. These clients may not be stable or cooperative enough to complete the cranial nerve and sensory response assessment. Spinal cord–injured clients, however, are usually coherent and able to participate in the sensory examination. This information is essential for documenting changes in the status of spinal cord–injured clients.

As clients become more stable and cooperative, the examination can be performed in more depth and with less frequency. Remember that neurologically impaired clients frequently experience fluctuations in status. Alter the assessment schedule and technique to detect and report these fluctuations.

The following are suggested modifications in the screening neurologic examination based on the client's initial presentation.

■ Initial examination for diagnosis and triage:
   Client history based on chief complaint
   Physical examination including vital signs
   LOC
   Pupil response
   Brain stem function (corneal reflex)
   Motor and sensory function in all four extremities
■ If the client is conscious and stable:
   Complete baseline neurologic examination
   Focused examination at prescribed levels

■ If the client is conscious and unstable:
   Quick baseline physical assessment
   Frequent focused examinations until stable
   Vital signs
   LOC
   Pupil response
   Brain stem function
   Motor and sensory function in extremities
   Spinal cord function
■ If the client is unconscious yet stable:
   Vital signs
   LOC and arousal
   Cranial nerve function
   Motor and sensory function
   Pathologic reflexes
■ If the client is unconscious and unstable:
   Vital signs
   LOC
   Cranial nerve function
   Motor and sensory function relative to the ability to test for these
   Pathologic reflexes
   Frequent focused examination on ongoing basis (hourly or more often)
■ If the client is suspected of having spinal cord involvement:
   Motor function in detail with testing of specific muscle groups
   Sensory function
   Reflexes
   Bowel and bladder function
   Vital signs

When assessing LOC, stimuli are provided and observations are made regarding the response. Start with visual cues, such as walking in front of the client, and note the response. If a response is not elicited, provide stimulation by use of the voice. Touch and painful (noxious) stimuli are used only if the client does not respond to the milder forms of stimulation. If the nurse must use a painful stimulus to elicit a response, it should be a central stimulus, such as a sternal rub, and not fingernail pressure, which is local. Document location and type of stimuli applied along with the client's response so that the examination can be accurately compared with future examinations. Noxious stimuli are also discussed in Chapter 31.

The Glasgow Coma Scale is an assessment tool designed to note trends in a client's response to stimuli (see Chapter 33). The original Glasgow Coma Scale was developed for use with head injury patients. Many variations of this scale now exist for use with other patient populations.

Terms such as "alert," "lethargic," "stuporous," "semicomatose," and "comatose" are vague and should be avoided, unless your facility has explicit definitions so that consistency is maintained.

Orientation

Establish *orientation* to time, place, person, and event (or situation). (What is your name? What year is this? What kind of place is this? Where are you? What brought you to the hospital today?)

Memory

Identify gross deficits in *long- and short-term memory* by using simple tests. For example, long-term memory is tested during history-taking when the client is asked to give a past health history. (Of course, there must be another source to validate such data.) Test short-term memory by giving the client three words to remember (e.g., red, Broadway, three), and asking the client to immediately repeat the words and repeat the same words in a few minutes.

Mood and Affect

Assess *mood and affect* both by the way the client appears (e.g., euphoric, depressed) and by the reports of

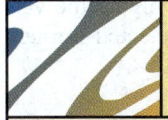

NORMAL PHYSICAL ASSESSMENT FINDINGS

Neurologic System

Inspection

Mental Status. Oriented to person, place, time, situation. No difficulty recalling recent and past events. Serial 7s deferred. Mood and affect congruent; cooperative, pleasant. Thought process clear, logical. Demonstrates effective problem solving. Speech articulate, clear, fluent.

Head, Neck, and Back. Normocephalic without obvious lesions. Maintains head position. Spine in straight alignment with normal cervical, thoracic, and lumbar curves. Neck and back have full range of motion.

Cranial Nerves. CN I: Discerns smell of coffee, cinnamon, alcohol. CN II: Visual acuity per Snellen's chart is OU = 20/20. Visual fields full to confrontation. Optic disc margins sharp, no cupping; cup-to-disc ratio is 1:3. Retina: Arteriovenous ratio is 2:3, without nicking. Fovea visualized. CN III, IV, VI: PERRLA, direct and consensual. Accommodation present. EOMs intact without nystagmus or strabismus. Cover-uncover test negative. Corneal light reflections symmetrical. CN V: Opens, closes mouth; chews, clenches teeth, moves jaw side to side voluntarily. Sensation intact to forehead, cheeks, chin. Corneal reflexes present. CN VII: Face movements symmetrical with smiling, frowning, eyebrows raising, lips pursing, cheeks puffing. Discerns sweet, salty, sour, and bitter tastes (also CN IX). CN VIII: Gross hearing intact. Whisper heard at 3 ft. Air conduction greater than bone conduction bilaterally. CN IX and X: Tongue and uvula midline. Uvula and soft palate rise in midline with phonation. Gag reflex present bilaterally. Swallows, coughs, speaks without difficulty. CN XI: Performs shoulder shrugs. Turns head against resistance. Maintains head position against resistance. CN XII: Tongue protrudes midline without deviation; pushes side to side with equal strength.

Motor Function. Muscle groups symmetrical. Gross and fine motor coordination intact. Moves all extremities through range of motion. Romberg's test negative. Pronator drift absent. Gait smooth, steady. Maintains balance walking on toes, heels. Rapid alternating movements and point-to-point maneuvers performed without difficulty.

Sensory Function. Sensation to light touch, pain, and vibration intact distally, over trunk, neck, and face. Position sense of fingers and toes intact. Stereognosis and graphesthesia present bilaterally. Two-point discrimination: 2 mm on index fingers. Discerns two-point simultaneous stimulation.

Palpation

Head, Neck, and Back. Skull without lesions or tenderness; smooth, firm. Neck and paravertebral muscles firm, relaxed, nontender. No pain or tenderness over spinous processes.

Motor Function. Muscle groups firm, elastic; strength rated as 5/5.

Percussion

Reflexes. Deep tendon reflexes rated 2+ (on scale of 0–4+) in triceps, biceps, wrists, knees, ankles. Plantar reflexes present. Abdominal reflexes present in all four quadrants.

Auscultation

Vascular Flow. Absence of bruit over carotid arteries bilaterally.

---

significant others. Is the client's affect appropriate to the situation?

Intellectual Performance

Intellectual performance includes the client's fund of knowledge and calculation ability. Ask the client to identify commonly known people, places, events, and the like. Assess calculation ability by asking the client to subtract 7 from 100, then 7 from the remainder and so on. If the client is unable to perform reversed serial 7s, have the client perform simple addition or subtraction (e.g., 3 + 4 = 7, 13 − 5 = 8).

Judgment and Insight

Judgment and insight include reasoning, abstract thinking, and problem solving, as well as the client's perception of the situation. Assess reasoning, abstract thinking, and problem solving for indications of major thought content problems related to the mental status examination discussed in Chapter 11. Listen to the way the client answers questions. Are the answers logical? Do they relate to the question? Can the client concentrate and remain focused on the examination, or is the client easily distracted? Abstract thinking is assessed by asking the client to explain a proverb such as "a rolling stone gathers no moss." Reasoning and problem solving are assessed by describing a problem situation and asking the client to give a solution. For example, "What would you do if you lost your house keys?" Assess insight and perception of the situation by asking the client to give an opinion of what may be the cause of the chief complaint.

Language and Communication

The *language and communication* assessment tests the client's ability to express and comprehend his or her environment. Expression and comprehension can be grossly evaluated during the initial interview. Does the client initiate speech? Is the speech fluent and appropriate? Does the client follow verbal commands? The content of speech is assessed as above (orientation, intellect, logic). Assess speech for articulation problems (usually motor disorders) or comprehension or expression problems (aphasic disorders). Assess the client's ability to communicate and understand verbally, in writing, mathematically, and nonverbally.

The quality of speech is assessed. Is speech clear and intelligible, or garbled due to facial droop or poor dentition?

■ Comprehension and Expression

Comprehension and expression are then assessed in more depth. Test the client's ability to comprehend spoken language by asking the patient to follow basic commands ("Show me your right thumb." "Stick out your tongue.") Ask the client to read several words or sentences and explain them to determine comprehension of written language. Or write a simple command ("Stick out your tongue") and have the client read and then perform the command.

Expression is evaluated as the client responds to questions. Ask questions that require more than a nod or a yes or no answer. Evaluate speech for flow, choice of words, and completion of phrases or sentences. If the client is expressively aphasic, comprehension can be tested by asking yes or no questions or having the client follow simple verbal commands as above. Written expression is assessed by having the client write answers to simple questions on paper (e.g., "Write your name and address").

■ Integrated Sensory Functions

Testing of *integrated sensory functions* involving language is often done with this portion of the neurologic examinations. Ask the client to perform simple addition or subtraction without writing. Ask the client to orally identify common objects, such as a pen, a key, and a watch. These skills require integration of cortical functioning (calculation) and visual recognition with expressive speech.

Head, Neck, and Back

Head, neck, and spine are examined by inspection, palpation, percussion, and auscultation. Tumors, vascular disorders, traumatic disorders, and problems involving the vertebrae and surrounding muscles may be detected through examination.

Inspection

The head is inspected for size, shape, contour, and symmetry. Note any ecchymosis around the eyes or behind the ears. Anterior basilar skull fractures often result in "raccoon eyes" with periorbital ecchymosis and occasionally cerebrospinal fluid (CSF) draining from the nares. Middle fossa basilar skull fractures often result in ecchymosis over the mastoid process behind the ears (Battle's sign) and drainage of blood or CSF, or both, from the ears.

Palpation

Palpate the skull lightly for nodules or masses and to supplement abnormal inspection findings. If there are open or draining areas, wear gloves. The skull normally feels smooth and firm. Areas of bogginess or depressions are abnormal. Palpation of neck muscles may identify masses or areas of tenderness. Ask the client to flex his or her neck with the chin touching the chest; look for nuchal rigidity, which is a sign of meningeal irritation.

Inspect the spine and palpate for alignment, noting any deviation from the normal curvatures. Palpate the paravertebral muscles for masses, tenderness, and spasm.

Percussion

Gentle percussion over the spinous processes may produce pain or tenderness.

Auscultation

Auscultation of major neck vessels and other vessels may reveal bruits or other abnormal sounds indicative of an abnormality.

Cranial Nerves

The cranial nerves (CN) are referred to by specific name or Roman numeral. Cranial nerve examination is important for two reasons.

First, CN III through XII arise in the brain stem. Testing their function provides information about the brain stem and related pathways.

Second, three reflexes involving cranial nerves are called protective reflexes (corneal, gag, and cough reflexes). The presence or absence of protective reflexes indicates the client's ability to protect the eye surfaces and airway. This is especially important for unconscious patients.

Normal cranial nerve function requires an appropriately received input stimulus that produces an appropriate response (output). When testing cranial nerves, failure to

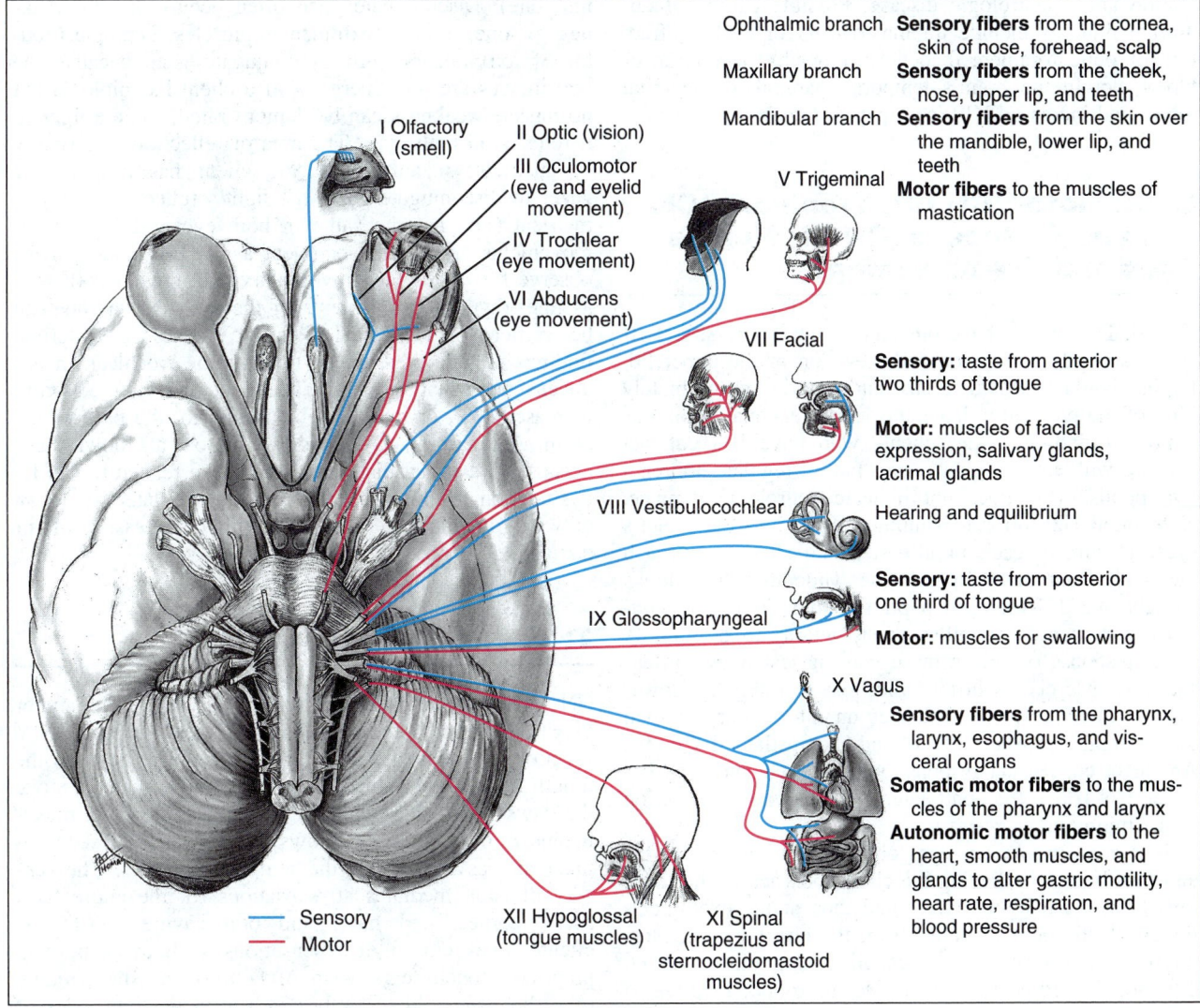

Figure 30–1. Distribution of the cranial nerves. Study this figure along with Table 30–1.

get a normal response may mean (1) failure to receive stimuli (input failure), (2) failure to respond appropriately (output failure), or (3) a combination of input and output failure. Determining which problems exist is often a challenge. For example, vision is a function of CN II, and pupillary light response is a function of both CN II and CN III (Fig. 30–1; see Table 30–1). The structure and function of the cranial nerves are discussed in Chapter 29.

Olfactory Nerve (CN I): Smell

CN I has a purely sensory function. Ask the client to smell and then identify an aromatic, nonirritating odor (e.g., coffee, isopropyl alcohol, toothpaste) with each nostril with the eyes closed. Test with several different odors. If the client can perceive any one smell, consider the nerve functional. Although inability to smell (called anosmia) may develop in elderly people, problems such as basal skin fracture or olfactory groove tumor also may be present. Other possible causes of anosmia include crib-

riform plate fracture, an olfactory bulb, or a tract tumor, or previous sinus disorders or surgery.

Optic Nerve (CN II): Vision

CN II has a purely sensory function. Assessing the optic nerve involves (1) inspecting the globe for foreign bodies, cataracts, inflammation, or other obvious abnormalities; (2) testing visual acuity; (3) testing visual fields; and (4) examining the eye fundus with an ophthalmoscope. (Details of eye assessment are in Chapter 36.) Test *visual acuity* generally by having the client read from a newspaper, a sign (from a distance), or Snellen's chart while wearing glasses (if usually worn). Refraction errors are not significant in neurologic assessment. Test *visual fields* to determine whether vision is absent in one or more directions or in a portion of the visual field, such as half of the visual field, the middle portion, or both sides. Such losses may indicate various problems and may correlate with the area of the brain involved. Gross inspection of the eyes and examination of the fundus can provide information about neurologic disease. Possible causes of abnormal findings include trauma to orbit or eyeball; fracture of optic foramen; diabetic retinopathy; laceration or blood clot in the brain's temporal, parietal, or occipital lobes; and increased ICP (e.g., papilledema).

Oculomotor (CN III), Trochlear (CN IV), and Abducens (CN VI) Nerves: Eyes and Eye Movement

CN III, IV, and VI have only motor components. CN III controls pupil constriction and elevation of the upper lid. Pupils should be equal in size and round. Approximately 20% of the population have anisocoria (unequal pupils) as a normal finding. Older clients who have had cataract surgery with lens implants may have irregular, nonreactive pupils. This does not indicate neurologic damage. Note pupil size prior to shining a light into the client's eyes. Document each pupil's size and shape. Approach the pupil from the temporal side while the client looks straight ahead. Test each pupil for both *direct* and *consensual responses* (pupillary constriction) to a light. A direct response occurs in the eye being tested. A consensual response occurs in the other eye at a slightly slower rate. A direct response indicates an intact connection in the midbrain between CN II and the ipsilateral CN III. An intact consensual response indicates a connection between CN II and the contralateral CN III via a connection in the midbrain.

Test *accommodation* (eyes able to focus on both near and far objects) by having the client look across the room (away from the light source) and then at the examiner's fingers, held about 6 inches from the client's nose. Normally, the lens shape changes and the pupils constrict. The notation PERRLA (*p*upils *e*qual, *r*ound, *r*eactive to *l*ight, and *a*ccomodation) indicates these functions are normal. When testing pupillary light reflex only (not accommodation) the abbreviation PERL is used (i.e., *p*upils *e*qual, *r*eactive to *l*ight).

CN III lies over the edge of the uncal portion of the temporal lobe. Increased ICP or edema causes that area of the brain to shift, and CN III is stretched or compressed. This disruption of the CN III pathway causes either a sluggish or absent response to light. This response can be unilateral or bilateral, depending on the site and severity of edema. Hippus is the rhythmic constriction and dilation of a pupil and is caused by early compromise of CN III with increased ICP; it is not seen in all clients.

Destruction of part of CN III can cause ptosis (drooping) of the eyelid. Disorders or pressure on a specific side of CN III can cause the ipsilateral pupil to dilate, the eyelid to droop, and the eye to deviate outward.

CN III, IV, and VI coordinate to control eye movements in all six cardinal directions of gaze (see Chapter 36). The function of these nerves is tested in various ways. Ask the client to move the eyes in the six directions. Alternatively, move an object in the six cardinal directions, and ask the client to follow it with the eyes. *Conjugate gaze* allows for the eyes to move in a coordinated effort for binocular vision (two images "merged" into one). Disconjugate gaze often occurs due to weakness of one or more extraocular muscles. Diplopia (double vision) occurs with dysconjugate gaze because the two images are not "merged." If a client has diplopia but no muscle weakness can be demonstrated, shine a light so it reflects on both eyes. The area of reflection is normally symmetrical, meaning that the client has a conjugate gaze. In disconjugate gaze, the light's reflection is asymmetrical (i.e., not the same in both eyes). If extraocular movements are intact, document as "EOMs intact." Also observe for *nystagmus* (involuntary eye movements), seen as fine, rhythmic movements of the eyes. Nystagmus can be vertical or horizontal. Possible causes of abnormal findings include pressure on oculomotor, trochlear, or abducens nerves at the brain stem due to fractured orbit, increased ICP, or tumor at, or trauma to, the base of the brain. An inability to look down or to walk down steps because of a visual disturbance could be related to CN IV dysfunction. Failure of an eye to move laterally in an outward direction is associated with compression of, or damage to, CN VI.

Trigeminal Nerve (CN V)

CN V has a motor and a sensory division. The motor division innervates the muscles of mastication. Test CN V function by asking the client to clamp the jaws, open the mouth against resistance, open the mouth widely, move the jaws from side to side, and make chewing movements. A normal CN V allows all these activities. Document any asymmetry in the temporal muscles. The sensory division mediates all sensations for the entire face, scalp, cornea, and nasal and oral cavities. With the client's eyes closed, test sensations such as pain (e.g., pinprick), touch (e.g., wisp of cotton), and temperature (e.g., hot and cold test tubes of water) on both sides of the face from the top of the head (vertex) to the chin. Test the *corneal reflexes* by gently touching the cornea with a sterile wisp of cotton or gently stroking the eyelash. (This test is omitted during the screening examination.) The normal response is brisk eyelid blinking. The corneal reflex involves CN V and CN VII. CN V is the afferent (sensory) arc while CN VII controls closure of the eye (motor). Possible causes of abnormal findings include a tumor at, or trauma to, the base of the brain, a fractured orbit, and trigeminal neuralgia.

Facial Nerve (CN VII)

CN VII has a motor and sensory division. The motor division innervates muscles controlling facial expression. Observe the face for symmetry and the ability to use facial muscles. Ask the client to smile, frown, raise the forehead and eyebrows, tightly close the eyes and resist attempts to open them, whistle, show the teeth, and puff out the cheeks. Test the anterior part of the tongue for taste by asking the client to close the eyes and protrude the tongue. Then place a taste substance on one side of the anterior tongue. Have the client keep the tongue protruded while identifying the taste. Ask the client to rinse the mouth or drink a small amount of water before testing the other side. Test taste on each side with sweet, salty, acidic or sour (e.g., vinegar or lemon), and bitter (e.g., coffee) substances. Common abnormalities noted include loss of the nasolabial fold, inability to close the eye and blink reflexively, facial asymmetry, drooling, difficulty swallowing secretions, loss of tearing, and loss of taste on the anterior two thirds of the tongue. Possible causes of abnormal findings include Bell's palsy, temporal bone fracture, and peripheral laceration or contusion to the parotid region.

The lower half of the facial muscles, especially around the mouth, also receive innervation from the voluntary motor area of the frontal lobes. Deficits of lower facial muscles can be related to a lesion in the contralateral frontal lobe (i.e., a stroke patient with a flattened nasolabial fold and facial droop on the opposite side who retains the ability to close the eyelid on the same side of the face). Deficits on the lower half of the face only are called central deficits because the lesion is in the CNS. A deficit involving both the upper and lower face is called a peripheral deficit because the lesion involves the CN VII, which is a peripheral nerve.

Vestibulocochlear or Acoustic Nerve (CN VIII)

CN VIII is a sensory nerve with two divisions, cochlear and vestibular. The cochlear nerve permits hearing. Test *auditory acuity* by having the client listen to and report on a whispered voice, rustling fingers, or a tuning fork at various distances from the ear. Test *bone and air conduction* with a tuning fork. Audiometry may be used for a precise assessment. The vestibular nerve helps maintain equilibrium by coordinating the muscles of the eye, neck, trunk, and extremities. Equilibrium tests include Romberg's and caloric tests (oculovestibular reflex) and electronystagmography. (For details on hearing and equilibrium assessment, see Chapter 37.) Possible causes of abnormal findings include Ménière's syndrome and acoustic neuroma.

Glossopharyngeal (CN IX) and Vagus (CN X) Nerves

CN IX and X have both motor and sensory components. Because of the overlapping innervation of the pharynx, assess CN IX and X together. Ask the client to open the mouth widely and say "Ah." Observe the position and movement of the uvula and palate. Do they rise midline? Test the gag reflex by gently touching the pharynx on each side with a tongue depressor. This normally elicits a brisk gag response. With a small amount of water, assess the client's ability to swallow. Test the posterior third of the tongue for taste, as with the seventh cranial nerve (may be performed when testing CN VII). Dysfunction of CN IX includes loss of taste and sensation of glossopha-

ryngeal pain. Ask the client to cough and to speak to test CN X. Damage to CN X causes an ineffective cough and a weak, hoarse voice. To differentiate areas of weakness, ask the client to vocalize different sounds: "kuh-kuh" (soft palate), "mi-mi" (lips), "la-la" (tongue). Possible causes of abnormal findings include brain stem trauma, neck trauma, brain stem tumors, and stroke.

Spinal Accessory Nerve (CN XI)

CN XI has only a motor component. CN XI innervates the sternocleidomastoid muscle and the upper portion of the trapezius muscle. To test, ask the client to (1) elevate the shoulders (with and without resistance), (2) turn (not tilt) the head to one side, and then the other, (3) resist attempts to pull the chin back toward midline, and (4) push the head forward against resistance. Disorders may produce drooping of a shoulder, muscle atrophy, weak shoulder shrug, or turn of the head. Possible causes of abnormal findings include neck trauma, radical neck surgery, and torticollis.

Hypoglossal Nerve (CN XII)

CN XII has only a motor component. CN XII innervates the tongue. Ask the client to open the mouth widely, stick out the tongue, and rapidly move the tongue from side to side and in and out. Document any deviation of the tongue to the side. Assess tongue strength by having the client push the tongue strongly against the inside of the cheek while pressure is applied to the area externally. Possible causes of abnormal findings include neck trauma associated with major blood vessel damage.

Motor System

Assessing the motor system thoroughly involves numerous procedures. The following discussion focuses on the screening examinations and common abnormalities.

Included in the motor examination are muscle size, muscle strength, tone, coordination, gait, station, and movement disorders.

Muscle Size

Inspect the major muscle groups bilaterally for symmetry. Inspect the trunk, intercostal, and abdominal muscles.

Muscle Strength

Assess muscle power in major muscle groups against resistance (see Chapter 73). Muscle strength is assessed and rated on a five-point scale in all four extremities, comparing one side to the other as follows:

5/5 = Normal full strength. Muscle is able to move actively through full range of motion against the effects of gravity and applied resistance.

4/5 = Muscle is able to move actively through full range of motion against the effect of gravity with weakness to applied resistance.

3/5 = Muscle is able to move actively against the effect of gravity alone.

2/5 = Muscle is able to move with support against the effect of gravity.

1/5 = Muscle contraction is palpable and visible; trace or flicker movement occurs.

0/5 = Muscle contraction or movement is undetectable.

Next, test for subtle weakness in upper and lower extremities. For upper extremities, have the client hold the arms straight out in front with palms up ("like holding a tray"). Ask the client to close the eyes and maintain the position. A *pronator drift* is said to be present if one arm pronates and falls lower than the other. For lower extremities, have the client walk on the heels, then on the toes. This tests dorsal and plantar flexion and balance.

Assessment of specific muscle groups can be completed to assess deficits in certain areas, such as spinal cord disorders. Disorders of muscle strength may be exhibited by weakness on one side of the body, in both lower extremities, or in both upper and lower extremities.

If an asymmetry is detected, the client or family is asked if this is a long-standing or new finding. The age and physical condition of the client should be considered when interpreting the results of muscle strength testing. One would not expect the same strength from a physically fit young client as from an elderly or debilitated client.

If abnormalities are found in muscle power, more detailed assessment may be conducted with procedures such as EMG, discussed later in this chapter.

Muscle Tone

Muscle tone is assessed while moving each extremity through passive range of motion. When tone is decreased (hypotonic), the muscles are soft, flabby, or flaccid. Increased muscle tone exists if the muscles are resistant to movement, rigid, or spastic. Note the presence of abnormal flexion or extension posture.

Muscle Coordination

Muscle coordination assessment includes testing rapid alternating movements, point-to-point maneuvers, and maintenance of truncal balance and head position. To test *rapid alternating movements,* ask the client to touch (approximate) each finger to the thumb quickly in succession. Alternatively, ask the client to pat the thighs first with palms, then with the back of the hands. In *point-to-point testing,* the examiner holds up an index finger approximately 18 inches away from the client. The client is asked to first touch his or her nose with a finger, then the examiner's index finger. This is repeated several times while the examiner moves the index finger to different points. The test is performed bilaterally for both the client's right and left hands. Lower extremity coordination is tested by asking the client to place the heel of the foot below the opposite knee and then to slide the heel down the shin toward the great toe. Repeat for the opposite leg.

Truncal balance is assessed with the client sitting. Can the client remain upright without support? Gently push the client to a leaning position. Can the client return to an upright position? *Head position* is assessed by observing the ability of the client to move the head while following movements of the examiner.

Disorders related to coordination are indicative of cerebellar or posterior column lesions. The defining characteristics of cerebellar dysfunction include ataxia, intention tremor (tremor upon nearing the object), nystagmus, ocular dysmetria (inability to gaze on an object), and dysdiadochokinesia (arresting one motor impulse and substituting an opposite one).

Gait and Station

Assess *gait and station* by having the client stand still, walk, and walk in tandem (i.e., one foot in front of the other in a straight line). Walking involves the functions of motor power, sensation, and coordination. The ability to stand quietly with the feet together requires coordination and intact proprioception. If the client has difficulty standing, further assessment is needed to determine whether the client is weak or unsteady. If the client is weak, the nurse needs to protect the client from falling. (See Box 30–3 for terms used to describe gait disorders.)

Movement

Examine the muscles for fine and gross abnormal movements. Examples of fine movements are fasciculations

---

Box 30–3. Terms Associated with Gait Disorders

- *Ataxic.* Staggering and unsteady
- *Double step.* Alternate steps differ in length or rate
- *Dystonic.* Irregular and nondirective
- *Dystrophic or broad-based.* Legs far apart, and weight shifting from side to side (waddling)
- *Equine.* High-stepping
- *Festinating.* Walking on toes at an accelerating pace
- *Helicopod.* Feet (or foot) makes a half-circle with each step
- *Hemiplegic.* Paralyzed on one side, paralyzed limb swings outward, foot drags, arm on affected side does not swing freely.
- *Parkinsonian.* Short, accelerating steps; shuffling; forward-leaning posture; head, hips, and knees flexed; difficult to start and stop
- *Scissors.* Legs cross while walking with short, slow steps
- *Spastic.* Stiff, short steps; toes catch and drag; legs held together; and hips and knees flexed
- *Steppage.* Foot and toes lifted high, heel comes down heavily
- *Tabetic.* High steps, foot slaps down

Box 30–4. Abnormal Movements Associated with Extrapyramidal Disease

- *Akinesia.* Reduced body movement in the absence of weakness or paralysis. Habitual movements (e.g., swinging arms) are limited or absent.
- *Athetosis.* Gross, writhing, wormlike movements of body, face, or extremities.
- *Ballismus.* A form of chorea. Involuntary dramatic movements of arms and legs. Hemiballismus involves only one side.
- *Bradykinesia.* Slow movement.
- *Chorea.* Discrete, jerky, purposeless movements in distal extremities and face.
- *Dystonia.* Prolonged twisting movements.
- *Myoclonus.* Sudden muscle contractions of varying intensity, which may involve a small part of one extremity or the entire body; may violently fling a client to the floor.
- *Tic.* Involuntary movement of groups of muscles in stereotypic patterns. May be physical or psychogenic in origin. Pathologic causes of tics include Tourette's syndrome and tic douloureux.
- *Tremors.* Involuntary trembling or quivering. May vary in direction, amplitude, rhythmicity, parts involved, speed, and timing in relation to rest or activity. Types include parkinsonian, familial, and senile.

(involuntary ripples or twitches occurring while relaxed), which may indicate lower motor neuron disease. Examples of more grossly abnormal movements, often representing extrapyramidal disease, are described in Box 30–4.

Move all joints through a full range of passive motions. Abnormal findings include pain, contractures, and muscle resistance.

Test for *apraxia* (inability to carry out a learned movement on command in the absence of weakness or paralysis). Ask the client to perform common activities, such as tying shoes or combing hair. True apraxia is present only if a client can do the activity spontaneously but cannot do it on request.

Motor Testing of Unconscious Patients

The term *patient* is used in this chapter to describe the client who is unconscious and who cannot be an active participant in care. The family is considered the client in these situations.

An unresponsive patient can be tested only for response to painful stimuli (e.g., reflex withdrawal of limbs, wincing, grimacing). Although a pain stimulus is used, the response is usually recorded as a motor system response. These responses are often incorporated into the motor scale of the Glasgow Coma Scale.

In an unconscious client, deep pain is used to elicit a sensory response when superficial pain does not produce such a response. The minimal amount of stimulus is used. Means of producing noxious stimuli include pressing on the nail beds to test a basic response. To assess for cerebral response to pain, use techniques such as rubbing the sternum, applying pressure to the orbital rim, squeezing the sternocleidomastoid muscle, or squeezing the clavicle. Document the site and type of stimulus used so the examination can be adequately reproduced at a later time. The client's response to the noxious stimuli is noted. The following responses are those most commonly seen when painful stimuli are applied:

- *Localization*—the client reaches for the source of the stimulus and attempts to push the examiner away.
- *Flexion withdrawal*—the client moves without purpose and may exhibit minimal movement, grimacing, or wincing.
- *Decorticate posturing* (abnormal flexion)—the client flexes, adducts, and internally rotates the wrists and arms to the chest and rigidly extends the legs. This posture indicates damage in the corticospinal tracts near the cerebral hemispheres.
- *Decerebrate posturing* (abnormal extension)—the client extends and pronates the arms while rigidly extending the legs. This indicates damage in the diencephalon or upper brain stem.
- *No response*—there is no visible movement to painful stimulus.

Sensory Function

The sensory function examination incorporates assessment of responses to superficial and mechanical sensations as well as cortical discrimination. Sensory assessment involves testing for touch, pain, vibration, position (proprioception), and discrimination. Assessing hearing, vision, smell, and taste is also sensory assessment. Sensory assessment may identify dermatomes (skin areas innervated by various nerves) having absent, reduced, exaggerated, or delayed sensation. Dermatomes are shown in Figure 27–14, and are discussed in Chapter 27.

A complete sensory examination is possible only on a conscious client because it requires cooperation. Always test sensation with the client's eyes closed. Help the client become as relaxed as possible.

Conduct sensory assessment systematically. Test a particular area of the body, and then test the corresponding area on the opposite side. Proceed in a systematic fashion. Begin testing a selection of dermatomes that represents cervical, thoracic, lumbar, and sacral segments of the spinal cord. If a sensory loss is noted, a more detailed testing of surrounding dermatomes can be done. Document any asymmetrical findings, that is, those varying from one side to the other. If the client has a sensory loss, document the area of loss and where normal sensation begins. Sensation assessment may be documented on a body chart of dermatomes.

Superficial Sensation

Superficial sensations are tested by stimulating the skin in symmetrical areas on each side of the body according to the dermatome distribution. Superficial pain is tested by alternating the sharp and dull ends of a sterile safety pin.

■ Touch and Pain

Ask the client to close the eyes and say that there will be a sharp and a dull stimulus. Demonstrate how sharp and dull feel. Touch the client with the dull end of the safety pin. Then apply a painful stimulus by using the pin's sharp end. Moving from the fingers to the shoulders, alternate the two stimuli inconsistently (so the client cannot predict which is being used) and ask the client to distinguish between which is sharp and which is dull. Then test the toes to the thigh. Finally, test the anterior and posterior trunk and buttock. Keep in mind the dermatomal pattern while testing. When there is a loss of the sense of pain, test for temperature awareness. Otherwise, it is not necessary to test for temperature, because pain and temperature travel on related pathways.

■ Other Modalities

Other modalities for testing superficial sensation in the conscious client include using a cotton wisp to assess *light touch*. Follow the same guidelines as for testing superficial pain sensation, stimulating symmetrical areas of the dermatomes.

Temperature sensation is not assessed routinely, and the test is performed only when pain and light touch responses are abnormal. If performed, use test tubes, one filled with warm water and one with cold water (test first to ensure that the warm water is not too hot). Assess each major dermatome symmetrically. Alternatively, the side of the tuning fork could be used to test temperature because it is always cold.

Mechanical Sensation

Mechanical sensations are assessed by vibration and proprioception.

■ Vibration

Use a tuning fork to test for vibration. Place the end of a vibrating tuning fork on a distal bony prominence such as a finger or great toe joint. Ask the client to indicate when and where vibration (not touch) is felt. If vibration is not felt, move proximally to the wrist or elbow or foot or ankle.

■ Proprioception

Test sense of body position by holding the side of the client's fingertips, then the great toes, between thumb and index finger. As each of the client's fingers and toes are gently flexed and extended, ask the client to state when movement is felt and in what direction. If impairment is detected, test more proximal joints.

Discrimination

Cortical discrimination depends on the ability to discriminate between superficial and deep sensations. Discrimination tests the integrative functions of sensation and memory in the brain's parietal lobe. Included are tests for stereognosis, graphism, extinction phenomenon, and two-point stimulation.

To test *astereognosis* (i.e., discernment of the form and configuration of objects felt, or three-dimensional discrimination), place three small, familiar objects one at a time in the client's hands, such as coins, keys, or a paper clip, and ask the client to identify each.

To test *agraphesthesia* (recognition of the form and configuration of written symbols), trace different separate letters and numbers on the client's palm with the blunt end of a pen, asking the client to identify each.

To test for the *extinction phenomenon* (simultaneous stimulation) simultaneously prick the client's skin at the same place on both sides of the body, and ask the client to say whether one or two pricks are felt.

To perform *two-point stimulation,* simultaneously prick the client's skin with two pins at varying distances apart to identify the smallest distance in which the client can perceive two pricks. Normal distances for loss of two-point stimulation discrimination are: upper arms, 75 mm; thighs, 75 mm; back, 40 to 70 mm; chest, 40 mm; forearms, 40 mm; palms, 8 to 12 mm; toes, 3 to 8 mm; fingertips, 2.8 mm; tongue, 1 mm.

Sensation abnormalities may include the following:

- *Dysesthesias* (well-localized irritating sensations such as warmth, cold, itching, tickling, crawling, prickling, and tingling)
- *Paresthesias* (distortions of sensory stimuli, e.g., light touch may be experienced as burning or painful sensation)
- *Anesthesia* (absent sense of touch)
- *Hypoesthesia* (reduced sense of touch)
- *Hyperesthesia* (pathologic overperception of touch)
- *Hypalgesia* (reduced sensation to pain)
- *Hyperalgesia* (increased sensation to pain)
- *Agraphesthesia* (inability to identify symbols traced on the palm with eyes closed)
- *Analgesia* (absence of pain sensation)
- *Astereognosis* (loss of sense of three-dimensional discrimination)

Figure 30–2 summarizes patterns of sensory loss. Sensory changes are part of the normal aging process. Careful assessment of such changes is the basis of nursing intervention for elderly clients. Table 30–1 is an assessment guide.

Reflex Activity

Reflexes test the integrity of specific sensory and motor pathways. Reflex arcs consist of the following:

- Receptor (sensory) organ
- Afferent (sensory) nerve

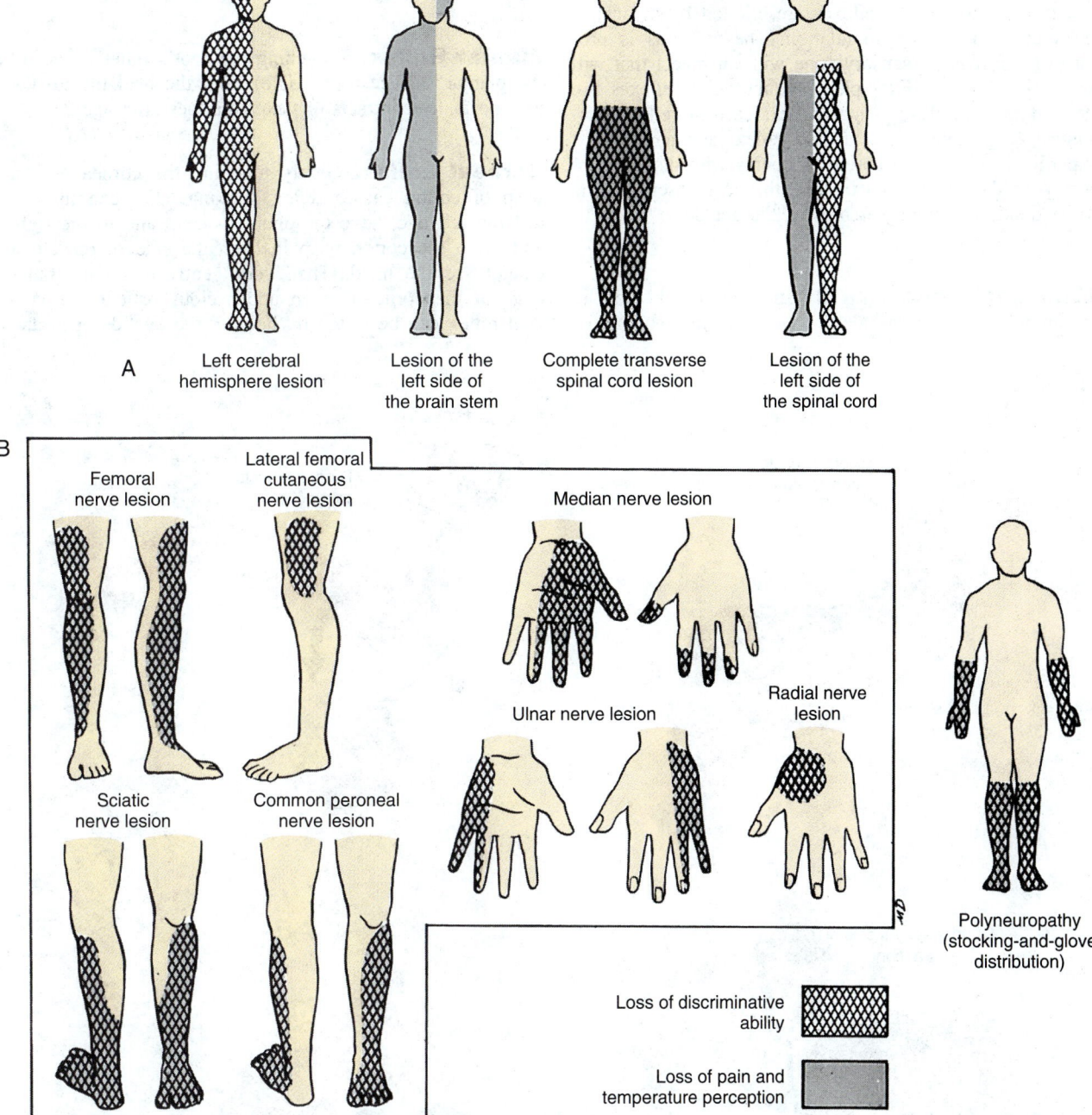

Figure 30–2. Patterns of sensory loss with *(A)* brain and spinal cord disorders and *(B)* peripheral nerve lesions.

- Connection in spinal cord or brain
- Efferent (motor) nerve
- Effector (motor) organ

Reflex activity assessment, always a part of neurologic assessment, provides information about the nature, location, and progression of neurologic disorders.

Normal Reflexes

Two types of reflexes are normally present: (1) superficial, or cutaneous, reflexes and (2) deep tendon, or muscle-stretch, reflexes (see Table 30–2).

■ Superficial (Cutaneous) Reflexes

Superficial (cutaneous) reflexes are elicited by cutaneous or mucous membrane stimulation. The stimulus is produced by stroking a sensory zone with an object that will not cause damage. Examples of superficial reflexes are the abdominal reflex, plantar reflex, corneal reflex, pharyngeal (gag) reflex, cremasteric reflex, and anal reflex. Superficial reflexes are absent in clients with disorders of the pyramidal tract. For example, they are absent on the affected side following cerebrovascular accident.

Abdominal Reflex. Lightly stroking the skin on an abdominal quadrant normally contracts the abdominal

muscle in that quadrant, and the umbilicus moves toward the stimulated side.

Plantar Reflex. Scratching the foot's outer aspect of the plantar surface (outer sole) from the heel toward the toes normally contracts or flexes the toes after age 2.

Corneal Reflex. Gently touching the cornea with a wisp of cotton causes reflex blinking. (For example, to test the left eye, have the client look up and to the right and bring the cotton wisp in from the side so the client cannot see the hand. Then very gently touch the outer edge of the cornea.) In an unconscious patient, the corneal reflex can be tested by holding the eyelids open and

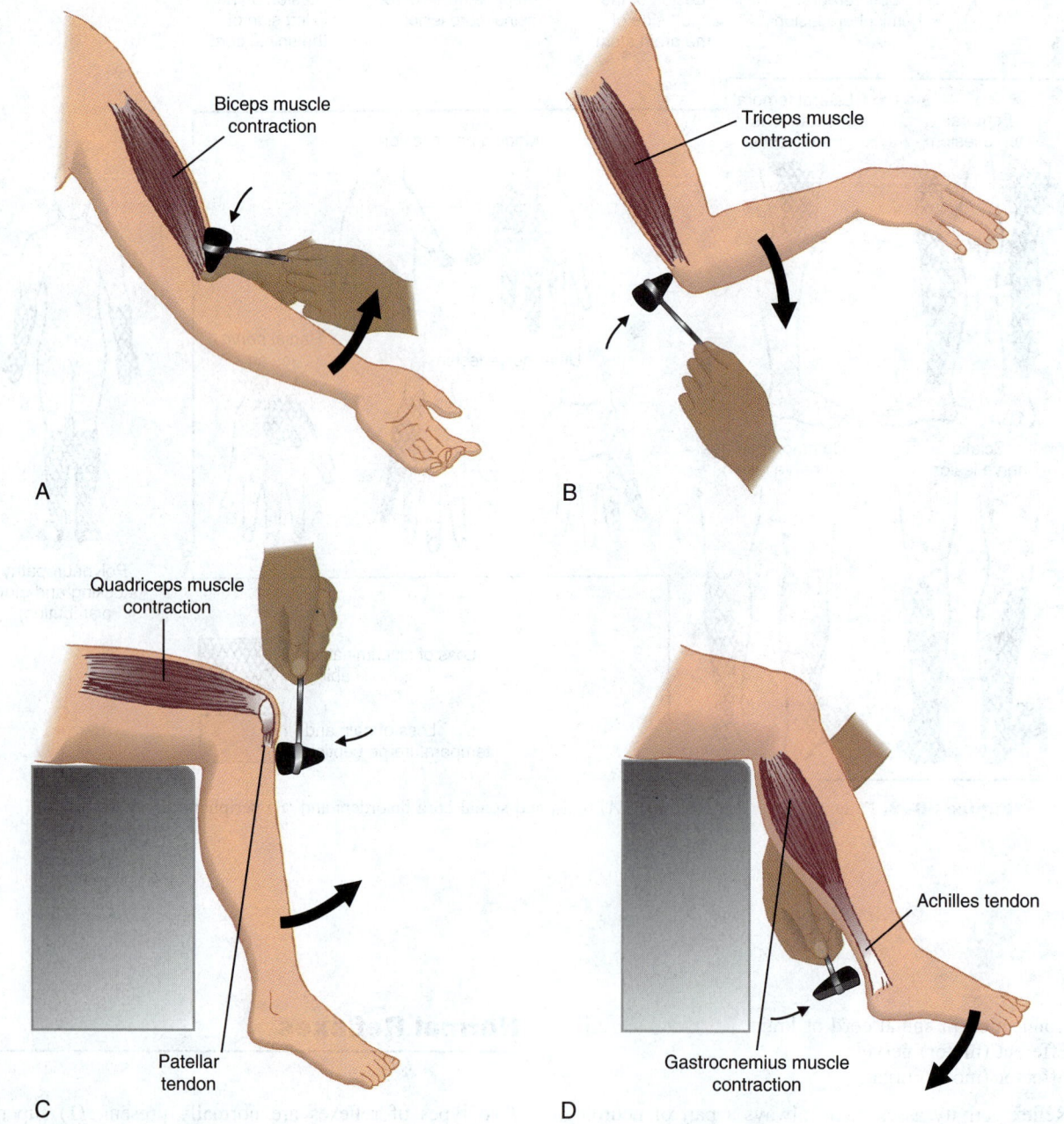

Figure 30–3. Deep tendon (muscle-stretch) reflexes. *A*, Biceps jerk (C5–6). *B*, Triceps jerk (C7–8). *C*, Patellar reflexes (L2–4). *D*, Ankle jerk (S1–2).

placing a drop of sterile saline on the cornea. This technique prevents inadvertent corneal abrasions.

Pharyngeal (Gag) Reflex. Gentle stimulation with a tongue blade at the back of the throat and pharynx normally produces gagging. The corneal and pharyngeal reflexes are usually assessed with the cranial nerves, discussed earlier in this chapter.

Cremasteric Reflex. Stroking the inner thigh of a male normally elevates the ipsilateral testicle.

Anal Reflex. Stimulate the perianal skin or gently insert a gloved finger into the rectum. Normal response is contraction of the rectal sphincter.

■ Deep Tendon (Muscle-Stretch) Reflexes

Deep tendon reflexes are also called muscle-stretch, or myotatic, reflexes because reflex muscle contraction normally results from rapidly stretching the muscle. This is produced by striking a muscle tendon's point of insertion sharply with a sudden, brief blow using a reflex hammer (Fig. 30–3 and Box 30–5).

Box 30–5. Guidelines for Assessment of Deep Tendon Reflexes

■ Test deep tendon reflexes with the client either sitting or supine.
■ Support the joint where the tendon is being tested so that the attached muscle is relaxed.
■ Use the pointed end of a triangular reflex hammer to strike over small areas, as the thumb is placed over the biceps tendon. Use the flat end of the hammer to strike over larger areas, such as the Achilles tendon.
■ Hold the reflex hammer loosely between thumb and fingers so it can swing in an arc.
■ Swing the reflex hammer using only wrist motion, not the arm or elbow.
■ Tap the tendon briskly.
■ Note the speed, force, and amplitude of reflex responses.
■ Compare reflex responses bilaterally.
■ Grade reflexes on a 0 to 4+ scale. Consider the strength of the reflex in relation to the bulk of the muscle mass.
■ Repeat testing of reflexes graded 0 or 1+ by using the technique of *reinforcement*. Note in the record that reinforcement was used. *Reinforcement* is a maneuver used to enhance deep tendon reflex responses when they are graded 0 or 1+:

Ask the client to perform isometric contraction of other muscles, which may increase the generalized reflex response, or
For the upper extremities, have the client either clench the teeth together or contract the quadriceps muscles (i.e., push the thighs against the table), or
For the lower extremities, have the client lock fingers together and try to pull them apart at the same time the tendon is tested.

Reflex sites commonly assessed include the Achilles tendon, patella, biceps, and triceps.

● An *ankle jerk* (plantar flexion of the foot) is produced by tapping the Achilles tendon.
● A *knee jerk, quadriceps jerk,* or *patellar reflex* (leg extension) is produced by tapping the quadriceps femoris tendon just below the patella.
● A *biceps jerk* (forearm flexion) is produced by tapping the biceps brachii tendon.
● A *triceps jerk* (forearm extension) is produced by tapping the triceps brachii tendon at the elbow.

■ Other Normal Reflexes

Some other normal reflexes involve structures other than skeletal muscles. For example, reflex mechanisms help maintain respiration and keep blood pressure within normal limits. Reflex salivation may follow taste (or smell) of food. Flashing a light in an eye causes the pupils of both eyes to constrict (*light reflex,* or *pupillary reflex;* see also the section on cranial nerve assessment).

Abnormal Reflexes

Pathologic (abnormal) reflexes are reflexes that do not normally occur. Their presence indicates neurologic disorders, often related to the spinal cord or higher centers.

These responses include Babinski's, jaw, palm-chin (palmomental), clonus, snout, rooting, sucking, glabella, grasp, and chewing reflexes.

Babinski's Reflex. Babinski's reflex is tested by gently scraping the sole of the foot with a blunt-pointed object. To elicit Babinski's reflex, start the stimulus at the midpoint of the heel and carry it upward and laterally along the outer border of the sole to the ball of the foot. Then direct the stimulus across the ball of the foot (without touching the toes) toward the medial side and off the foot. Alternatively, start the stimulus at the midlateral sole and carry it down toward the heel. A normal response (absent Babinski's reflex) is plantar flexion of the toes. An abnormal response (present Babinski's reflex) is dorsiflexion of the great toe and often fanning of the other toes (Fig. 30–4). In extreme circumstances, a present Babinski reflex may be accompanied by dorsiflexion of the foot at the ankle and flexion at the knee and hip. This flexion at the ankle, knee, and hip is called triple flexion.

When exaggerated deep reflexes are present, superficial reflexes are usually diminished or absent, and pathologic reflexes (e.g., Babinski's reflex) also exist.

Jaw Reflex. Jaw reflex (jaw contracts and closes the mouth as a result of downward tapping on the lower jaw, when the mouth is relaxed and passively hanging partially open) occurs rarely in healthy persons, but is noticeably present in some disorders, for example, sclerosis of the lateral columns of the spinal cord. Jaw reflex is also called mandibular reflex, or jaw jerk.

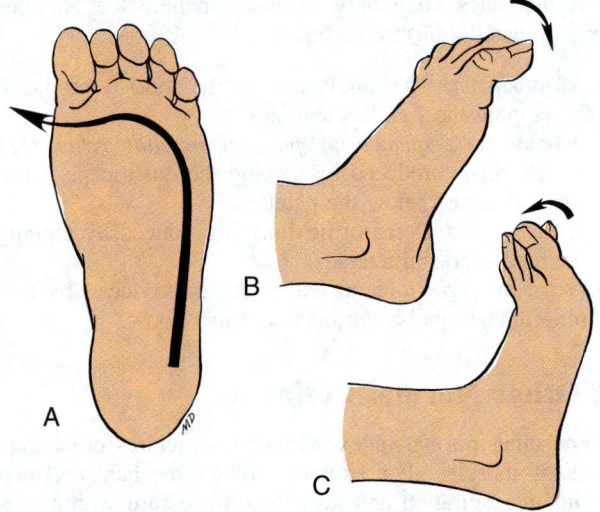

Figure 30–4. Babinski's reflex. *A,* Test maneuver: Scratch the sole of the foot as shown, using a blunt point. *B,* Normal response (absent Babinski's response) is plantar flexion of the toes. *C,* Abnormal response (present Babinski's response) is dorsiflexion of the big toe and often a fanning of the other toes.

Palm-Chin (Palmomental) Reflex. Palm-chin (palmomental) reflex is produced by vigorous, rapid irritation on the mound of the palm at the thumb's base with a blunt instrument causing the chin muscles to pull up on the same side.

Clonus. Clonus is rapidly alternating joint flexions and extensions, resulting from continuous rhythmic contractions of a stretched muscle. This is not like a normal stretch reflex, which typically produces one reflex action. With clonus, the action continues.

Snout Reflex. A brisk midline tap above or below the mouth results in pursing of the lips.

Rooting Reflex. Stroking the side of the face causes the mouth to open and the head to turn to the stimulated side.

Sucking Reflex. Touching the lips with a blunt object results in movement of the tongue, lips, and jaws.

Glabella Reflex. Tapping the forehead between the eyebrows results in sustained closure of the eyelids.

Grasp Reflex. Placing an object in the palm of the hand causes the fingers to curl around the object.

Chewing Reflex. A tongue blade placed between the teeth results in the jaws closing tightly.

Grading Reflex Activity

Superficial reflexes are graded 0 (absent), ± (slightly present), and + (normally active). Deep reflexes are graded from 0 through 4+; 2+ is normal. Although 1+ or 3+ responses are not considered normal, they may not be significant findings (Fig. 30–5). Asymmetrical responses are much more significant. Abnormal reflexes may be present in both neurologic and metabolic disorders. Table 30–2 summarizes important reflexes.

Autonomic Nervous System

Clinical manifestations of disorders of the autonomic nervous system occur in many body systems. This unit focuses on neurologic disorders (e.g., heatstroke, autonomic dysreflexia). Disorders of other portions of the autonomic system are discussed in the cardiac, urinary, digestive, reproductive, and endocrine chapters of this book.

Clinical manifestations of autonomic disorders include (1) altered perspiration patterns; (2) faulty body temperature regulation (hypothermia and hyperthermia); (3) abnormal pulse rate; (4) pilomotor responses; (5) skin, vasomotor, and pupillary changes; and (6) digestive changes.

When assessing for autonomic disturbances, ask about polyuria and abnormal motility of the gastrointestinal tract. Examine the abdomen for evidence of bowel and urinary bladder distention. Changes in thirst, energy, potency, libido, weight, and appetite may also be significant.

Examine the client's skin, mucous membranes, hair, and nails for trophic changes. Such changes occur in various diseases causing loss of innervation, including the autonomic nerve supply. Trophic changes may be indicated by (1) changes in the affected area's sweating, temperature, and color (e.g., pallor, cyanosis, and erythema); (2) nails that may become curved, brittle, broken, and thickened; (3) skin that may be painlessly ulcerated, thickened, atrophied, pigmented, oily, scaly, rough, tight, shiny, or dry; (4) oily, brittle, or dry hair with hair loss or abnormal hair growth; and (5) pressure sores in denervated regions of the skin, beginning in areas subjected to

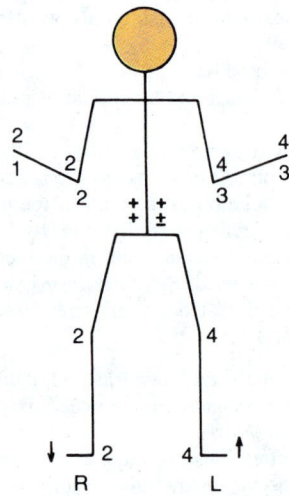

Figure 30–5. Documentation of muscle stretch and superficial reflexes in left hemiparesis. Muscle stretch reflex grades: 0, absent; 1, diminished; 2, normal; 3, brisker than normal; 4, hyperactive (clonus). Superficial reflex grades: 0, absent; ±, equivocal or barely present; +, normally active.

Table 30–2. Important Reflexes

Reflex	Assessment Technique	Expected Response	Pathway Involved
Tendon Reflexes			
Biceps reflex	A blow on the examiner's thumb placed over the biceps tendon	Flexion of elbow	C5–6
Brachioradialis reflex (supinator)	Styloid process of radius is tapped while forearm is in semiflexion and semipronation	Flexion of elbow, fingers, and hand with supination of forearm	C5–6
Triceps reflex	Strike on triceps tendon just above the olecranon	Extension of elbow	C6–8 (C7 primarily)
Patellar reflex (knee jerk)	Tap on patellar tendon	Leg extends	L2–4
Achilles reflex (ankle jerk)	Tap on Achilles tendon	Plantar flexion of foot	S1–2
Superficial Reflexes			
Corneal reflex	Light touch at the corneoscleral junction	Closure of eyelids	CN V, VII
Palatal and pharyngeal reflexes	Light touch to soft palate and pharynx	Elevation of palate; gagging	CN IX, X
Abdominal reflexes	Stroke skin of upper, middle, and lower abdomen toward umbilicus	Contraction of abdominal wall toward stimulus	Upper—T7–9 Middle—T9–11 Lower—T11–12
Cremasteric reflex	Stroke medial surface of upper thigh	Elevation of ipsilateral scrotum and testicle	T12–L2
Anal reflex	Stroke perianal region	Contraction of external anal sphincter	S3–5
Plantar reflex (normal)	Stroke sole of foot	Flexion of toes	L4–S2
Plantar reflex (pathologic; Babinski's sign)	Stroke sole of foot	Dorsiflexion of great toe and fanning of other toes	L4–S2

Adapted from Mitchell, P. A., et al. (1988). *AANN's neuroscience nursing: Phenomena and practice.* Norwalk, CT: Appleton & Lange.

prolonged pressure. Palpitation (i.e., a rapid heart rate felt by the client) may also indicate autonomic dysfunction.

Functional Assessment

A client with a neurologic disorder is usually experiencing problems that disrupt basic function either permanently or temporarily. The client's ability to cope effectively with ADL (ability to meet basic needs) is often altered. For example, a client may have problems seeing, hearing, breathing, walking, talking, or eating. Remember that a client with a neurologic disorder may be frustrated just trying to do the things most people take for granted.

Functional assessment can be incorporated into the neurologic examination as well as into daily care of the client. During the examination, note what deficits the client experiences and how they are managed. Ask the client or family what changes have been made in daily routines to accommodate deficits. Document not only the deficit but also the functional response. Examples:

- Motor strength of right arm 4/5—the client reports independence in ADL but notices difficulty in carrying books or groceries with the right arm.

- Diplopia present—the client uses an eye patch, alternating the side covered every few hours to reduce headache and nausea caused by diplopia.
- Right gaze preference—the client can overcome gaze preference and move the eyes past midline to the left when asked. The client turns head to the left to see visitors enter room.

Clinical Applications

The initial assessment for diagnosis and triage of the client with a possible neurologic deficit includes a history, *brief* physical examination, and a neurologic examination. The *initial* neurologic examination usually consists of assessment of the *level of consciousness* using the Glasgow Coma Scale, *pupillary response, focal motor and sensory abnormalities* in all four extremities, and *brain stem function* via assessment of *protective reflexes* consisting of gag, cough, and corneal reflexes (see Box 30–2).

The initial assessment provides the baseline for comparison when serial assessments are completed. When recorded on a time-oriented flow sheet, changes in the client's status can be quickly identified. The frequency of serial assessment is determined by the client's diagnosis and may be as frequent as every 15 minutes. The nurse has an important responsibility to monitor the client's progress and report any unexpected deviations. A complete neurologic assessment is done initially on all clients. Serial examinations may focus on deficits or functions that may indicate potential danger (i.e., pupil responses and LOC for suspected increased ICP).

Thorough assessment and reporting of changes in a client serve a major role in determining the plan of care. Often, the client's current condition, for example, a decreased level of responsiveness and a change in pupillary reaction, is compared with initial data.

Because nurses are with clients continually, it becomes the nurse's responsibility to develop sound assessment skills and recognize trends in the client's condition that warrant further care. *In no other area of practice are subtle changes as important to detect and act on than in the care of the client with neurologic disorders.*

Diagnostic Tests

The complexity of the CNS combined with the relative inaccessibility of the brain requires indirect techniques to study it. Early techniques such as lumbar puncture, plain x-ray study, pneumoencephalography, and EEG have provided the foundation for new techniques that allow direct visualization of the brain structure, blood supply, and metabolism. Air contrast studies, such as pneumoencephalogram and ventriculogram, were performed for client assessment prior to the development of CT and magnetic resonance imaging (MRI). The nurse may find the results of these tests recorded in the history of a client who has had neurologic disorders for many years. These tests used air to provide contrast so that various portions of the brain could be viewed by x-ray study. The tests were painful and had potentially serious side effects. Today's neurodiagnostic studies are much safer for the client. The tests begin with the least invasive and move to the more invasive forms.

The focus of nursing care for the client having diagnostic assessment is centered on physical and psychological preparation for the study. The nurse also plans for the specific assessments that will need to be made after the study is completed, such as continued neurologic assessment. Prior to the study, the nurse should perform a baseline neurologic examination and provide education to the client and family about the purpose of the study, the preparation needed, and the client's role during the test. The nurse may also have to assist the client in reducing anxiety about the test, and can usually do so by providing information and answering questions. Serial scans may be necessary when the client has an evolving disease (e.g., cerebral bleeding) that reveals more abnormalities in 2 or 3 days than within the first 24 hours.

After the diagnostic procedures have been performed, the nurse assesses the client for possible side effects and neurologic changes and assists the client in understanding the results of the studies, as needed. More information on diagnostic testing can be found in Chapter 13.

Noninvasive Tests of Structure

Skull and Spinal X-Ray Studies

Procedure. Skull x-ray studies reveal the size and shape of the skull bones, suture separation in infants, fractures or bony defects, erosion, calcification, sella turcica erosion, and pineal gland shift (after age 12). Spinal x-ray studies show fractures, dislocation, compressions, curvature, erosion, narrowed spinal cord, and degenerative processes.

Preprocedure Care. Some clients with neurologic disorders require nursing support throughout an x-ray study, especially clients who are confused, combative, or ventilator-dependent. Whenever a client is unable to act as a self-advocate, a nurse is required. If the client has a suspected spinal fracture, the neck is immobilized prior to moving the client to make the x-ray films. A lateral view of the cervical spine is taken first because the x-ray study can usually be taken with minimal movement to determine whether fractures have occurred. Metal items should be removed from body parts undergoing the x-ray procedure, for example, barrettes. Nurses should document thick or heavy hair, because hair may affect interpretation of the x-ray film.

Postprocedure Care. Until the results of the study are known, preprocedure precautions, such as spinal immobilization, are maintained.

Computed Tomography

Procedure. The CT scan is a highly informative diagnostic test based on the principle of tissue density using the computer to analyze data. The primary purpose of CT scans is to detect intracranial bleeding, space-occupying lesions, cerebral edema, and shifts of brain structures. Infarctions, hydrocephalus, and cerebral atrophy can also be identified. Aneurysms and arteriovenous malformations (AVMs) are best detected by angiogram. The basilar cisterns and posterior fossa are not as well visualized on the CT scan. These areas have a large density contrast between the bone and air-filled sinuses (see Fig. 30–6).

Preprocedure Care. Providing information about the CT scan is the major focus of nursing intervention. Prior to the test, ascertain that informed consent has been obtained, and answer any questions the client and family have about the CT scan and explain the following items.

Fasting usually is not required for CT of the head, but ask whether the client tends to become nauseated easily and adjust the intake of food and fluids accordingly. For example, some clients prefer a light breakfast to reduce nausea and others prefer an empty stomach.

Explain that a contrast agent often is given. Because the agent (also called dye) is iodine-based, ask whether the client has known allergies to iodine, contrast dyes, or shellfish. (See the section on the use of contrast.) If an

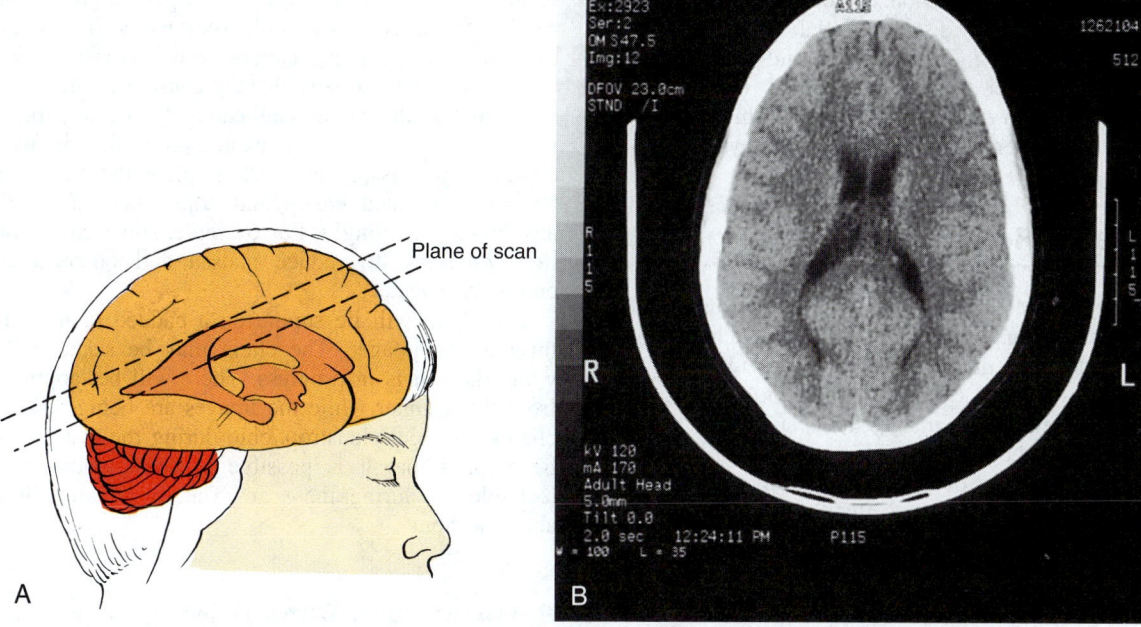

Figure 30–6. Computed tomography scans are taken at various cross-sections of the brain. *A* illustrates the cross-section used for the scan shown in *B.*

intravenous infusion has not been established, one will be before the study begins.

Remove any objects from the hair before the examination, including wigs, barrettes, earrings, and hairpins. The client's role in the scan should be explained. The client will be positioned supine and the head placed into the doughnut-shaped ring of the scanner. The table is moved by the technologist from a control room during the scan to direct the study toward different levels of the head. The client should expect to hear mechanical noises coming from the scanner as it scans. Some clients will feel claustrophobic during the test but should be assured that it is possible to communicate with the technologist during the scan. Finally, the client will be asked to remain still during the scan. If the client is unable to comply, sedation, or even general anesthesia, may be required.

Postprocedure Care. Following the test, the client should be assessed for reactions to contrast media, as well as other specific assessments, such as presence of hematoma at the injection site and manifestations of intravenous infiltration of contrast material or fluids. Report infiltrations of contrast medium to the radiologist. The client can resume normal activities, unless other diagnostic tests are planned. Diuresis from the dye should be expected.

Replacement fluids may be needed, and the client should be assessed for fluid balance. The fluid balance in clients with renal or cardiac disease should be assessed carefully after a series of tests requiring intravenous contrast agents.

Complications rarely occur but may include local and systemic allergic reactions, spasm or occlusion of the vessels by a clot, and bleeding at the injection site. The nurse should assess the affected extremity for color,

warmth, pulses distal to the injection site, bleeding or hematoma formation, and ability to move the site.

Use of Contrast Agents. Certain pathologic conditions are better visualized with the use of a contrast agent. For example, tumors are better visualized with contrast, whereas bleeding and edema are seen better without it. The use of contrast agents is potentially dangerous. They may irritate blood vessels. Clients who are sensitive to contrast agents may have allergic reactions, and, if untreated, these clients may develop anaphylactic shock.

The nurse should ask the client about a known allergy to contrast dye or possible allergy to iodine or shellfish. This type of allergic response should be noted on the record, for example, "client states she develops hives from eating shellfish." Some clients report allergies, but when asked to explain the reaction, they state they "feel warm" when given the dye. This is a normal reaction, not an allergic one. Some clients will be given contrast dye even though they report allergy to it. This is done to obtain a clear picture and assist with diagnosis. To reduce the severity of the reaction, these clients are pretreated with an antihistamine or corticosteroids. Therefore, the nurse should not assure the client with a reported allergy to dye that contrast dye will not be given. Even if the client states that he or she has no history of allergy, the client should be observed for symptoms of an allergic reaction following the injection of contrast dye. Some anaphylactic reactions have occurred with the first dose of dye.

The nurse should instruct the client that it is common to feel a hot, flushed sensation and a metallic taste in the mouth when the dye is injected.

The nurse should assess the client for clinical manifestations of an allergic reaction, which include restlessness, tachypnea, respiratory distress, facial flushing, urticaria, nausea, and vomiting. The client should be assessed for these reactions after the dye is injected, because clients have had respiratory and cardiac arrests while undergoing x-ray study. Emergency equipment always should be available.

Magnetic Resonance Imaging

Procedure. MRI is a diagnostic tool similar to CT. The advantages are that MRI provides much more anatomically detailed pictures than are provided by a CT scan, and it does not expose the client to ionizing radiation. In fact, the MRI images look strikingly like anatomic slices of the brain (see Fig. 30–7). MRI provides more detailed images of the optic chiasm, posterior fossa, brain stem, and spinal cord than does CT. MRI also detects disorders in white matter pathways caused by loss of myelin, as in multiple sclerosis.

Preprocedure Care. Teach the client and family about the purpose of the test, the sensations that the client will hear and feel during the examination, and the client's role during the test.

Prior to the test, the client should remove all metal-containing objects, such as a brassiere, jewelry, and a watch. Such objects may be drawn into the magnetic field by the powerful magnet and become harmful projectiles. Any internal metal objects should be assessed for, such as prostheses and pacemakers. Check procedural guidelines for contraindications to MRI testing. For example, an MRI is contraindicated in a client with a pacemaker or implanted defibrillator. Clients who have prostheses may be able to have MRI depending on the location of the

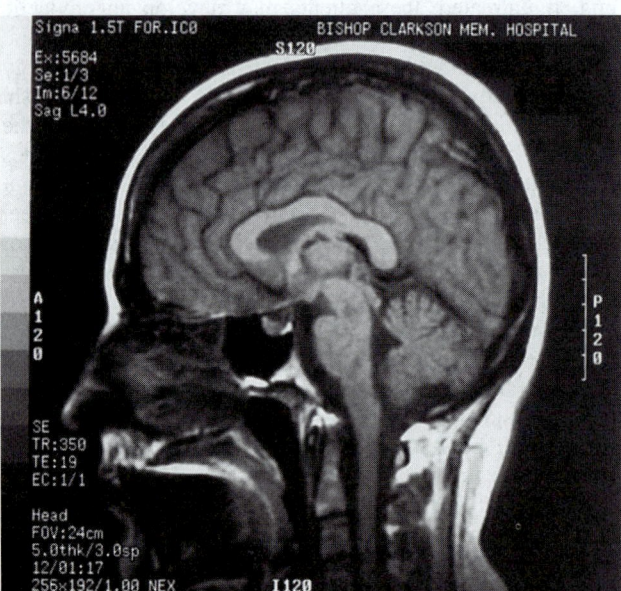

Figure 30–7. A normal magnetic resonance image. This sagittal section shows the cerebrum, ventricles, cerebellum, and medulla.

prostheses. Intravenous fluid pumps need to be removed from the client during the test. Special precautions are needed for clients with pulse oximeters. The cord from the sensor to the finger cannot be coiled around the body or any body part because it may cause a burn.

Normally, the client can eat and take any prescribed medications prior to the examination. If the use of a contrast agent is planned, ask whether the client tends to become nauseated easily and adjust the intake of food and fluids accordingly. For example, some clients prefer a light breakfast to reduce nausea and others prefer an empty stomach.

The client will lie supine on a padded table and move through the imager. The client may be asked to lie still while the test is in progress. There will be tapping noises from the scanner while the images are being taken. Some clients will feel claustrophobic during the test, but should be assured that it is possible to communicate with the technologist during the scan. The examination will take about an hour.

Postprocedure Care. Following the test, the client can resume previous activities. Expect diuresis if a contrast agent was used.

Positron Emission Tomography

Positron emission tomography (PET) allows the visualization of physiologic function in body areas. Often, the function of diseased tissue is different from normal tissues.

Procedure. The client is given doses of strong radioactive tracers, and the high concentration of tracers creates signals that are picked up by a scanner. The tracers, although potent, have a very short half-life, which makes their use safe. The tracers release positive particles, which emit a signal when they come in contact with electrons. PET has three primary uses: (1) to determine the amount of blood flow to specific body tissues; (2) to reveal how adequately tissues use blood or nutrients, such as oxygen; and (3) to map specific receptors, such as medications or neurotransmitters. PET can be used to measure cerebral blood flow, cerebral glucose metabolism, and oxygen extraction. PET is used in the diagnosis of stroke, brain tumors, and epilepsy, and to chart the progress of Alzheimer's disease, Parkinson's disease, head injury, schizophrenia, and manic-depressive illness.

One major disadvantage is that PET is expensive. PET requires its own positron to manufacture high-energy radioactive tracers; a PET system can cost $5 million initially. As a result of the cost, a modification of the test has been developed. It is called single photon emission computed tomography (SPECT). This test uses less precise but more stable and more readily available isotopes to measure cerebral blood flow rather than metabolic activity, as is measured with PET. The test appears to be an effective diagnostic tool. A PET scan is shown in Chapter 13.

Preprocedure Care. Educate the client and family about the purpose of the test, the sensations that the client will hear and feel during the examination, and the client's role during the test. In contrast to CT and MRI, the PET scanner is absolutely quiet. Clients need to fast for 4 hours prior to the scan. If the client is diabetic, it is preferred that the blood sugar be below 150 g/dl. Clients who are agitated may require sedation prior to the scan.

Postprocedural Care. Following the test, the client can resume usual activities.

Tests for Vascular Abnormalities

Noninvasive tests are useful in assessing cerebrovascular disease.

■ Ophthalmodynamometry

Ophthalmodynamometry compares the retinal artery pressures in both eyes. It may help diagnose extracranial vascular disease. While the retina is observed through an ophthalmoscope, pressure (or suction) is applied to the eyeball by a dynamometer, and readings are obtained.

■ Doppler Ultrasonography

Doppler ultrasonography may be used to measure blood flow (including direction and velocity) in the supraorbital region. In occlusion or stenosis of the internal carotid artery, the direction of blood flow is altered (reversed) in the supraorbital artery, which may be detected by ultrasonography. Transcranial Doppler studies evaluate arterial flow in the circle of Willis and its major branches.

■ Doppler Scanning

This is a test combining Doppler ultrasonography with pulse echo. Visual representation of moving blood is obtained. A mobile artery and vein imaging system is commonly used.

■ Quantitative Spectral Phonoangiography

This is a noninvasive method of assessing the extent of carotid stenosis by spectral analysis of bruits arising from the carotid bifurcation.

Invasive Tests of Structure

Lumbar Puncture

Procedure. A lumbar puncture (LP, or spinal tap) is the insertion of a needle into the subarachnoid space in the lumbar region of the spine below the level of the spinal cord. CSF can be withdrawn or substances can be injected into this space.

LP is performed for assessment and therapeutic purposes. LP enables assessment of CSF pressure and collection of CSF for evaluation. When meningitis or subarach-

noid hemorrhage is suspected, the CSF is examined for white blood cells and blood. *Myelogram* is an x-ray study in which contrast is injected into the subarachnoid space after CSF is removed in order to examine the spinal canal. Therapeutically, LP is used to administer spinal medications and anesthetics.

Even though LP is generally a safe procedure, it does have some potential hazards. The procedure can be uncomfortable for the client. The client will feel pressure in the lower back and may experience pain if a nerve root is touched with the needle during insertion. The potential complications of LP are CSF leakage, infection, intervertebral disc damage, and herniation of the brain. A space-occupying lesion within the cranium, such as a tumor or bleeding, increases ICP. Therefore, LP is not performed in clients with papilledema (a sign of increased ICP), suspected intracranial lesions, or increased ICP or infection of the skin at the puncture site. CT scans are used in these clients to rule out masses before an LP is performed. If an LP were performed in clients with increased ICP, there would be a rapid decrease in pressure within the CSF around the spinal cord. This change in pressure might allow the structures within the brain to drop (herniate) into the spinal canal. The process of herniation creates pressure on the vital centers in the medulla (cardiac and respiratory centers) and could cause sudden death.

Preprocedure Care. Educate the client and the family about the purpose of LP, the sensations that the client will feel during the examination, and the client's role during the examination. An informed consent form must be signed by the client prior to the test. The bladder and bowels should be emptied, if possible. The client will need to lie on one side with the legs pulled onto the abdomen and the head tucked into the chest in order to open the spaces between the vertebrae. It will be important for the client to lie still during the test. Sedation may be ordered before the procedure.

The necessary equipment should be assembled in the client's room. Spinal tap trays are available which contain all needed equipment. In addition, have laboratory request forms available and a marking pencil to label the samples of spinal fluid.

Care During the Procedure. LP to remove a sample of CSF is described here. The same general principles apply to any LP procedure, however.

Position the client on the side (lateral recumbency) with the client's back close to the edge of the bed. Place a pillow under the flank so that the spinous processes are horizontal. Use additional pillows between the client's knees and under the head to keep the spine horizontal. Ask the client to draw the knees up to the abdomen and the chin onto the chest (Fig. 30–8). Help the client maintain this curved position to separate and increase space between the vertebrae so that the needle can be inserted more easily. Stand in front of the client and place one hand behind the client's knees and the other around the neck. Keep the client's upper shoulder from falling forward, thus preventing rotation of the spine. (An alterna-

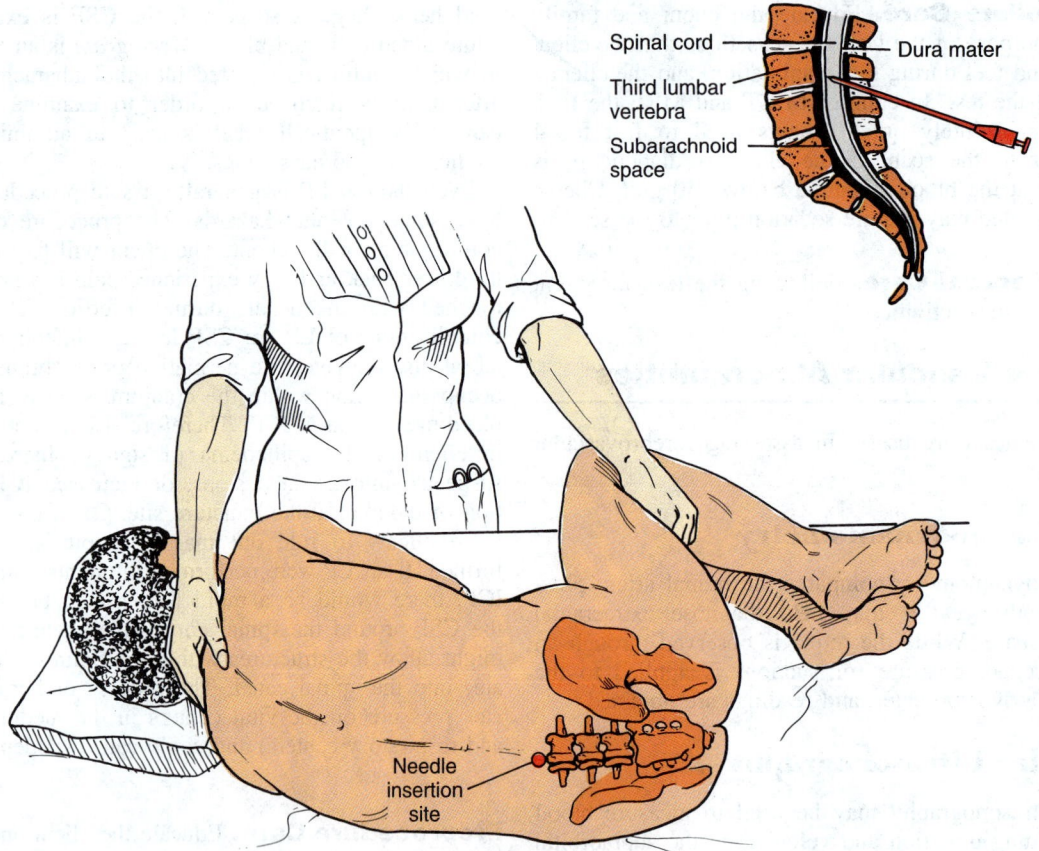

Figure 30–8. Lumbar puncture. Position the client laterally, with the knees drawn up to the abdomen and the chin brought down to the chest. This position increases the spaces between the vertebrae. The sterile lumbar puncture needle is inserted as shown, between the third and fourth (or fourth and fifth) vertebrae, and enters the subarachnoid space.

tive position is with the person sitting up with head and chest bent toward the knees.)

After a local anesthetic is given, a small needle will be placed into the space between the vertebrae in the lower back. In adults, the needle is inserted about level with the top of the iliac crests (hip bones) or at the next lower vertebral level (usually between the third and fourth or fourth and fifth lumbar vertebrae). In adults, the spinal cord normally ends at the lower border of the first lumbar vertebra. Thus, the puncture site is low enough to avoid spinal cord injury.

The needle bevel is usually held parallel to the longitudinal fibers of the dura. This position limits the size of the dural tear and reduces the risk of CSF leak. A little local pain may occur as the needle passes the dura mater. Ask the client to mention additional discomfort because it may indicate misplacement of the needle.

When the needle has entered the subarachnoid space, the physician removes the stylus and attaches a stopcock and manometer. A manometer measures CSF pressure. The first stabilized CSF pressure is the opening pressure. Normal opening CSF pressure with the person in a horizontal position is 6 to 13 mm Hg (80 to 180 mm H_2O). Pressures over 200 mm H_2O are abnormal. Normally, CSF oscillates (fluctuates) in the manometer, readily responding to coughing, straining, and changes in the person's breathing. If there is a blockage in the spinal canal, the CSF pressure may not oscillate.

CSF specimens are collected in a series of small sterile test tubes, numbered in sequence of collection (e.g., no. 1, no. 2). Two to 3 ml of CSF are collected in each tube; 8 to 10 ml may be removed. The needle is withdrawn, and a dry sterile dressing is placed over the puncture site.

In adults, CSF is assessed for cells, chloride, glucose, protein, pressure, and lactate dehydrogenase (LDH). Table 30–3 lists common abnormalities of CSF. When analyzing CSF, the first vial obtained is not assessed for blood because it may contain blood from the puncture.

Postprocedure Care. Vital signs should be recorded after an LP. Sometimes, lying flat for several hours is prescribed. The client can eat and drink as prior to the test. Forcing fluids will help restore CSF volume. If the CSF measurement indicated a high ICP, the client should be assessed for decreasing LOC, indicating increasing ICP.

Post-LP headache (spinal puncture headache, spinal headache) is typically throbbing, bifrontal, and suboccipital, developing a few hours to several days after an LP. The headache is probably due to continuing CSF leakage through the opening in the dura made by the needle. As a result of the leak, the CSF circulating around the cranium is depleted. The fluid loss allows abnormal movement of the brain in the skull. When the brain moves, tension is placed on the meninges and venous sinuses, which causes

Table 30–3. Normal Cerebrospinal Fluid (CSF) Values and Significance of Abnormal Values

Substance	Normal Value (Conventional Units)	Significance of Abnormal Values
Blood	None; CSF should be clear	Gross blood is seen in CNS hemorrhage. If the CSF is grossly bloody, other tests may not be able to be performed. Rarely, there are some blood cells in the first tube of CSF collected, because of trauma during the tap. The collection of specimens should be marked in sequence, so that it is possible to determine whether there is more blood in the first tube than in the last tube.
Cells	0–5 mononuclear	Increased neutrophils may be seen in bacterial infections such as bacterial meningitis. Lymphocytes may be increased in tuberculosis and some viral disorders. Aerobic pathogens can be cultured.
Glucose	50–75 mg/dl, should be 20 mg less than serum glucose level	Glucose level is lowered in neoplasm, inflammation, and bacterial infections. Be certain to compare CSF glucose with serum glucose. Ideally, a serum specimen should be drawn 30–60 minutes before lumbar puncture, because it takes glucose about 30–60 munutes to diffuse into the CSF.
Protein Albumin	15–45 mg/dl 10–30 mg/dl	Lesions that interrupt the blood-brain barrier increase proteins because there is increased diffusion. Decreased proteins can be seen when water reabsorption occurs, as with increased intracranial pressure.
IgG Oligoclonal bands	1–4 mg/dl Absent	IgG and oligoclonal bands (an abnormal type of protein band seen on immunoelectrophoresis) are often present in multiple sclerosis and neurosyphilis.
Pressure	70–180 mm H$_2$O	Elevated in bacterial meningitis, cerebral bleeding, and tumors. Decreased in conditions that obstruct CSF flow, such as tumors of the spinal canal.

pain. The headache is usually relieved when the client lies down and is made worse by sitting up or a sudden jolt of the head. Such headaches usually disappear within 24 hours but may last for several days.

To reduce the risk of post-LP headache, have the client remain in bed following the examination. Although physician's orders may differ on the length of time, an average time in bed is 3 hours. Fluids should be encouraged to replace the CSF withdrawn during the test. Once a headache begins, treatments may include bedrest in a dark, quiet room, and the administration of analgesics and fluids. If the headache continues, an epidural blood patch may be required. Blood is withdrawn from the client and injected into the epidural space, usually at the LP site. The blood acts as a fibrin patch to seal the hole in the dura and prevent further CSF leakage. Blood patches cannot be performed when the client has bleeding tendencies or infection at the puncture site.

Myelography

Procedure. Myelography is an x-ray examination of the spinal cord and vertebral canal following introduction of contrast media into the spinal subarachnoid space (Figure 30–9). It is used to study the spinal canal and subarachnoid space. This study is a particularly valuable assessment tool when the spinal cord is thought to be compressed (e.g., by a herniated intervertebral disc or a tumor encroaching on the spinal subarachnoid space). Myelography is also useful in diagnosing such spinal cord disorders as intramedullary tumors, syringomyelia, and AVMs. In the radiology department, an LP is performed, a small amount of CSF is withdrawn, and the contrast material is injected. With the needle in place, the client is turned on the abdomen and secured to the table by foot and shoulder supports. While the radiologist follows carefully with fluoroscopy, the table is slowly tilted. This procedure causes the column of dye to move up or down within the subarachnoid space, permitting visualization of the desired areas. Standard films are taken of these areas. If the contrast material used is water-soluble, it is not removed from the spinal column.

Preprocedure Care. Preparation for a myelogram includes hydration for at least 12 hours before the procedure. Phenothiazines lower the seizure threshold; hold prior to this procedure.

Postprocedure Care. Following the myelogram, the client may have to remain flat in bed (if the dye used is oil based) or with the head of the bed elevated 15 to 30 degrees if water based contrast is used. Usually, the client

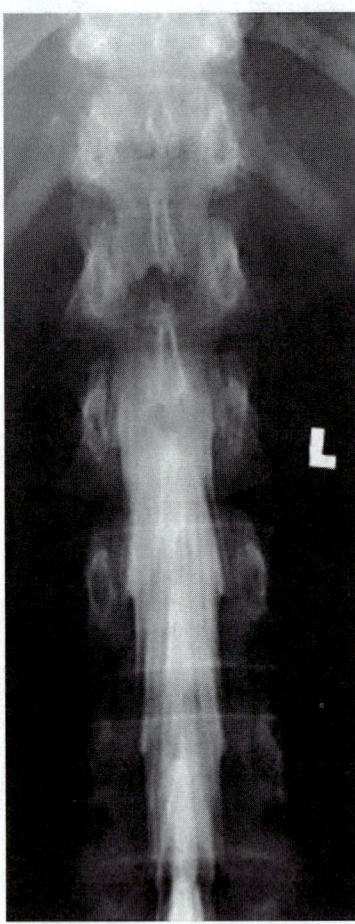

Figure 30–9. A myelogram of the lumbar spine shows contrast flowing throughout the subarachnoid space without obstruction.

remains in bed 6 to 8 hours and then resumes normal activity. Encourage the client to take extra fluids. Assess neurologic status frequently. Back pain (ranging from mild discomfort to severe pain) in the area of the needle insertion may develop and may last a few days. Also, the client may experience a stiff neck and headache for a few days, particularly if the contrast medium was allowed to rise to high cervical levels. The discomfort is usually relieved by lying flat and by administration of fluids and analgesics. (See also Lumbar Puncture.)

Cisternal Puncture

On rare occasions, access to the CSF cannot be made by LP and cisternal puncture may be used.

Procedure. Cisternal puncture is puncture of the cisterna magna (a small reservoir of CSF between the cerebellum and medulla). A physician introduces a short-beveled needle below the occipital bone, between the first cervical lamina and the rim of the foramen magnum. Cisternal puncture is performed either to drain CSF or to obtain a CSF specimen when there is a block in the spinal subarachnoid space or if LP is contraindicated. If the client has a lesion on the spinal cord, the top edge of the lesion can be determined by contrast injected via the cisternal puncture.

Preprocedure Care. Position the client at the edge of a treatment table or bed, lying on the side with a sandbag under the head to keep the cervical spine and head straight with the thoracic spine. Flex the client's head forward and hold it firmly in position. Following skin preparation, a local anesthetic may or may not be injected. A cisternal needle with stylet in place is inserted to a depth of about 5 cm.

Postprocedure Care. Subsequent assessments and interventions are essentially the same as with LP.

Cerebral Angiography

A cerebral angiogram is the injection of contrast into an artery to visualize intracranial circulation (Fig. 30–10). Angiography is the procedure used most often to visualize aneurysms, AVMs, major vessel displacement, vascular occlusion, and thrombi. Not only is cerebral angiography an invasive procedure, but it is a test in which small errors can result in permanent disability or death. Meticulous attention must be given to the client before, during, and following angiography.

Procedure. The procedure is performed by inserting a catheter (a soft needle) into the femoral artery and then guiding the catheter, with the aid of a fluoroscope, into the carotid or vertebral arteries. This approach has replaced previous approaches in which the carotid, vertebral, or brachial vessel was punctured directly. The use of the femoral artery is less traumatic, and local complications, such as infection or bleeding at the puncture site, occur away from the neck. Once the vessels are reached, the contrast agent is injected and a series of x-ray studies are taken from lateral, anteroposterior, and oblique approaches. Sequential views of the vessels show the movement of the dye in the vessels. After the catheter is removed, a sterile dressing is placed over the puncture site and firm pressure is applied to the site for 10 minutes to prevent hematoma formation. Sandbags and a pressure dressing may be used to provide firm pressure. Ice bags may also be used to provide pressure and relieve tenderness. The injection site may be tender.

Interventional Angiography. Interventional angiography is a recent advance in client care. This technique uses a polymer glue or Gelfoam (an absorbable gelatin sponge that stops bleeding) to occlude feeding vessels in tumors or AVMs. Blocking feeding vessels reduces the size and vascularity of the tumor or AVM, thus reducing the need for, or the complications of, surgical removal.

Interventional angiography also provides balloon angioplasty for cerebral vessels to expand athlerosclerotic narrowed vessels.

Digital Venous Angiography. Computerized digital video subtraction systems allow visualization of vascular

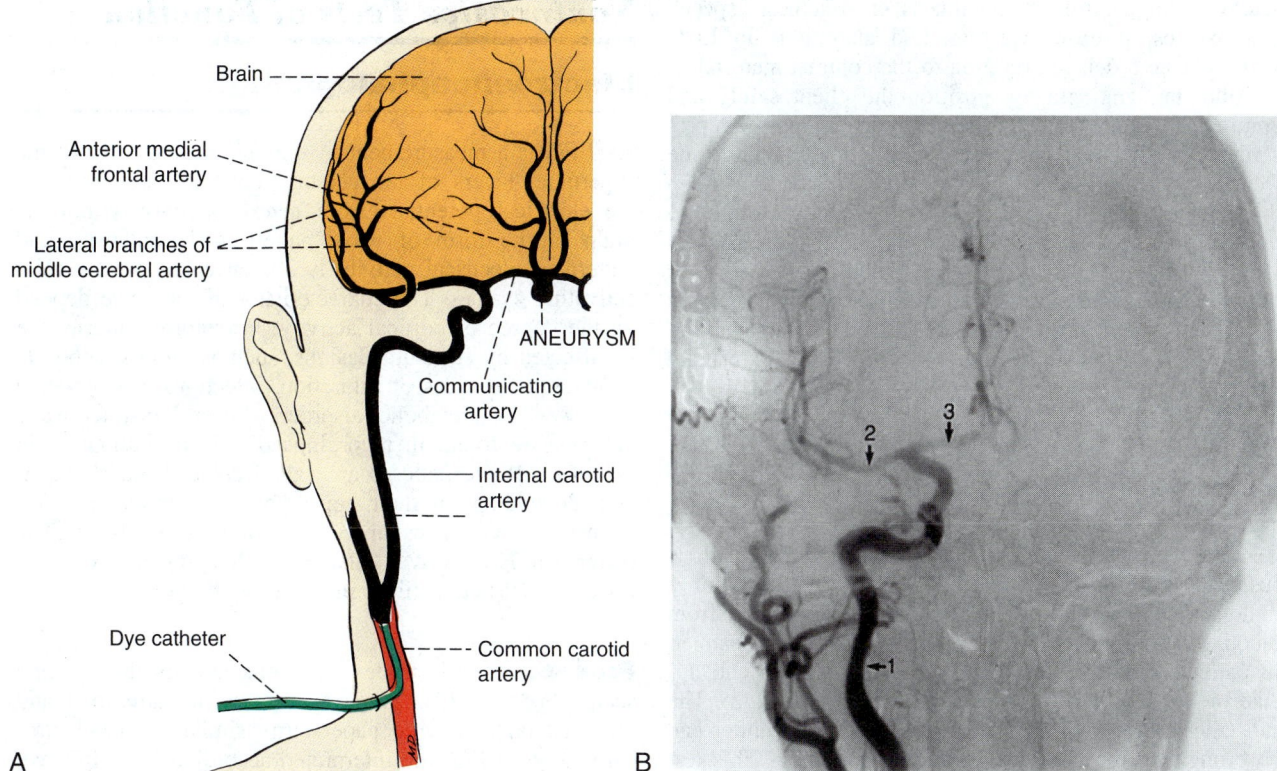

Figure 30–10. Cerebral angiography allows x-ray visualization of the brain's vascular system when a contrast dye is injected arterially. *A,* Insertion of dye through a catheter in the common carotid artery, subsequently outlining vessels of the brain. *B,* An angiogram using the subtraction technique. *1,* internal carotid artery; *2,* middle cerebral artery; *3,* middle meningeal artery.

structures. Much less contrast medium is required than that used in cerebral angiography. A central venous line is necessary to inject the contrast medium. Raw data are stored in digital form and can be retrieved at any time. Images with the best vascular visualization are selected and subjected to electronic manipulation to improve image detail.

Indications for digital video subtraction systems include assessment for (1) transient ischemic attacks, (2) serial follow-up for clients with known carotid stenoses, (3) intracranial tumors, (4) postoperative aneurysm, (5) extra-cranial-intracranial bypass procedure follow-up, and (6) dural venous sinuses. Three to four venous injections are usually required for a complete diagnostic craniocerebral study. The only potential complication is a reaction to the contrast material.

Preprocedure Care. Educate the client and family about the purpose of the test, the sensations that the client will experience during the test, and the client's role during the procedure. Prior to the test, the client may not take anything by mouth for 4 to 6 hours but should be well hydrated prior to that time. Intravenous fluids may be prescribed. The nurse should document the neurologic status of the client to serve as a baseline after the examination. The client should remove any metal items from the hair, such as barrettes and earrings. Allergies to io-

dine should be reported. During the test, the client will be given an injection of local anesthetic prior to placement of the catheter. There will also be a warm flushed feeling when the dye is injected. (See the discussion on use of contrast agents.) While the angiogram is being conducted, the client is continually assessed for neurologic deterioration.

Postprocedure Care. Following the test, assess the client closely for complications. Complications are rare but include (1) local and systemic allergic reactions to the contrast dye, (2) spasm or occlusion of the vessel by a clot, (3) hemorrhage, and (4) obstructive clot formation above a femoral injection site. Assess for reactions to the contrast. Spasm or occlusion of the target vessel(s) causes symptoms similar to those of a stroke. (Stroke, or cerebral vascular accident, is discussed in Chapter 33.) Clot formation at the injection site also causes ischemic reactions in the affected area. These adverse reactions are usually reversible and rarely cause permanent damage.

Potential complications vary, depending on their cause. For example, indications of centrally located reactions may include changes in LOC, aphasia, hemiplegia, hemiparesis, convulsive seizures, or increased focal symptoms. A hematoma in the neck may cause difficulty in breathing or swallowing. If it is large, it may compress the trachea and esophagus, requiring emergency tracheostomy. Nausea, vomiting, extremity numbness or weakness, speech disturbances, profuse sweating, and alterations in LOC may indicate a delayed reaction to the contrast material.

Following angiography, position the client safely and comfortably and maintain bedrest for as long as prescribed (often about 12 hours). Check the injection site frequently for bleeding and hematoma formation. Keep the affected extremity (arm or leg) or neck straight to prevent kinking the vessel and clot formation. Assess vital signs (every 15 minutes for 1 hour, then every 30 minutes for 1 hour, then every hour for 4 hours), pulses distal to the puncture site, color, temperature, and ability to move the distal extremity. A regular diet is usually resumed.

Cerebral Perfusion Studies

Cerebral perfusion can be assessed when brain death is suspected. The patient is injected with technetium 99m, a radioisotope. The ability of the substance to perfuse from blood vessels into brain tissue is assessed with a scanner. In patients who are clinically brain-dead, there is no uptake of the substance by the cerebrum or cerebellum. The substance is injected at the bedside, and the scanner can be brought to the bedside to evaluate perfusion. This test allows appropriate medical care to continue when brain death cannot be determined, and conversely, medical care can stop for those patients who are brain-dead. The nurse's role in this test is informing the patient's family of the significance of the test and its findings. Once the patient is declared brain-dead, it is the end of meaningful life. The family may need help accepting the results of this very final test. Organ donation should be considered for these clients. See discussion in Chapter 32.

Noninvasive Tests of Function

Electroencaphalogram

An EEG is a measurement of the electrical activity of the superficial layers of the cerebral cortex. It demonstrates the electrical potentials from neuron activity within the brain in the form of wave patterns. The intensity and pattern of electrical activity is influenced by the reticular activating system. The characteristics of the wave depend on the degree of cortical activity. Waveform patterns can be affected by structural lesions, such as tumors, subdural hematomas or areas of infarction, infections, degenerative processes, or metabolic disorders. Several distinct wave patterns are found in recordings of clients without brain disorders. Wave patterns are called delta, theta, alpha, or beta depending on their appearance (amplitude and frequency). EEG waves are shown in Figure 30–11. The pattern of EEG waves changes with aging and disease; for example, beta activity increases with age.

Procedure. Electrodes are attached to the client's scalp (Fig. 30–12). The wave forms are amplified and recorded on a moving paper strip, similar to an electrocardiogram. EEGs are interpreted according to brain wave characteristics, frequency, and amplitude.

If the patient is comatose or unable to be moved, EEG can be performed at the bedside. For routine diagnostic examination, the client is taken to an EEG laboratory for a more controlled environment. The client's scalp is cleaned, and electrodes are applied to the scalp and ear lobe (for reference) with collodion. Leads can also be placed in the nasopharynx to assess disorders in the temporal lobe. The first portion of the test is performed with

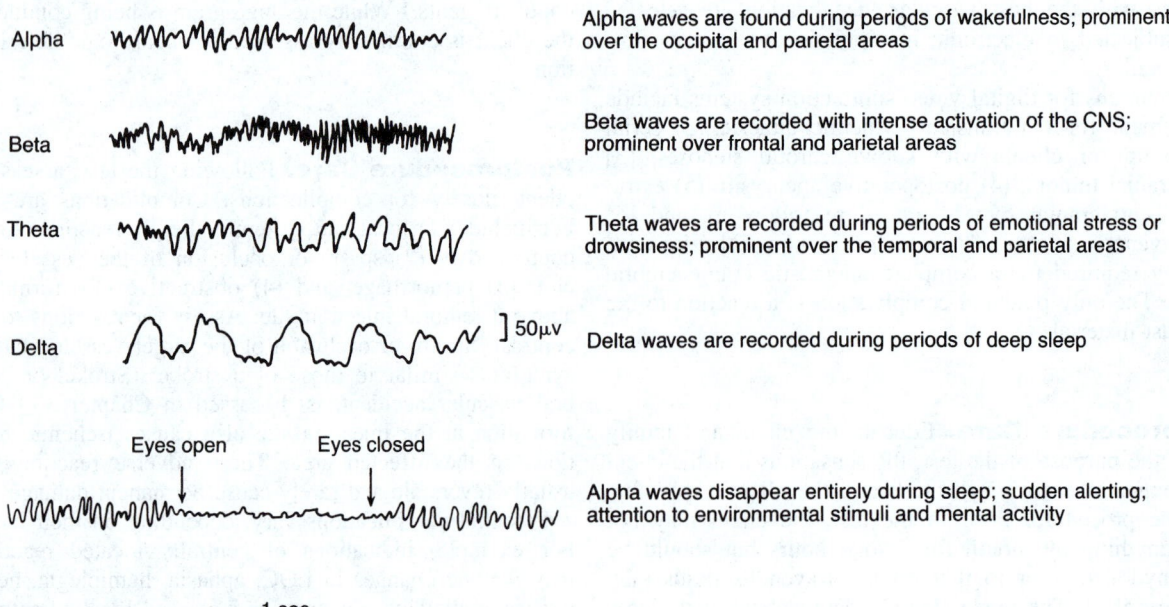

Figure 30–11. Electroencephalographic waves. (Modified from Guyton, A. C., & Hall, J. [Ed.]. [1996]. *Textbook of medical physiology* [9th ed]. Philadelphia: W. B. Saunders.)

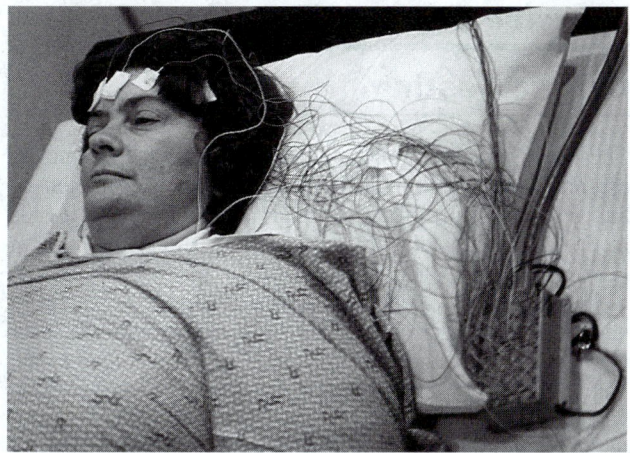

Figure 30–12. Client undergoing an electroencephalogram.

the client as relaxed as possible to obtain a baseline recording. Further readings are taken while the client is hyperventilating, sleeping, or viewing flickering lights. Hyperventilation alters acid-base balance (respiratory alkalosis) and decreases cerebral blood flow. Flickering lights may trigger seizures. Sleep may evoke abnormal EEG patterns not present while the client is awake. The client may be kept awake the night preceding the test or sedated to induce sleep.

An EEG is useful in assessing clients with any type of seizure disorder. An EEG is diffusely abnormal in various metabolic disturbances, toxic conditions (e.g., drug overdose), coma, organic brain syndrome, and infections such as meningitis and encephalitis. The EEG may be used in the operating room to monitor cerebral activity during surgery on the blood vessels in the head or neck. Sleep patterns in depressed clients may also be assessed with EEGs. Some clients are assessed for temporal lobe epilepsy by using a 24-hour EEG recording. An EEG is also used to assist in diagnosing narcolepsy and insomnia.

Absence of EEG waves (flat lines) on EEG may be one of the criteria for defining brain death. Studies on comatose patients show that findings of the EEG have a high correlation with the survival or death of the client in a coma.

Preprocedure Care. Explain the purpose of the test and the procedure to the client and family. Reassure the client and family that electricity does not enter the brain (shock is not given) and the machine is not able to read the mind. Before the EEG is performed, the client's hair must be shampooed. Stimulants, (e.g., coffee, alcohol, tea, cola, and cigarettes), antidepressants, tranquilizers, and anticonvulsants should be avoided for 24 to 48 hours prior to the test. Sometimes sleep is withheld for many hours. Normal meals should be consumed because a lowered serum glucose level will alter the test results. If the client will be asked to sleep for a portion of the test, sleep should be minimized the night before the test. The client will be asked to relax during the test, because anxiety can block alpha rhythms and produce artifacts from increased muscle tone in the head and neck. Be sure

to send adequate supplies (i.e., intravenous fluids or oxygen) to the laboratory.

If the EEG is being performed to evaluate the possibility of brain death, it is important to keep artifacts to a minimum. Artifacts can be caused by the manipulation of electrodes, electrical interference, cycling of respirators, and even walking in the room. Institutional guidelines should be followed for the avoidance of artifacts when EEG is performed at the client's bedside.

Postprocedure Care. Following the EEG, the client can resume previous activity, medications, and diet. If seizure activity is possible, seizure precautions need to be followed. The hair can be washed and acetone may be required to remove the collodion from the scalp and hair.

Evoked Potential Studies

Evoked potential (EP) studies are a form of EEG in which the client's brain waves are monitored as the client is given various stimuli. The test is used to assess the function of the cerebral hemispheres and the brain stem. A variety of types of stimuli are used, such as auditory, somatosensory, and visual. Typical stimuli include flashing lights, buzzing tones, and peripheral nerve stimulation. EP studies can be used to assess blindness, deafness, and brain stem injury. Specific brain signals can be accentuated and others filtered out, allowing assessment of brain waves from other areas. EP studies are carried out in the same fashion as EEGs. EP studies can detect abnormalities even if the client is sedated or paralyzed with neuromuscular blocking agents. Some clinicians believe that EP studies are more reliable than clinical assessments in predicting neurologic recovery in comatose, head-injured patients. Nursing interventions are the same as for the client having an EEG, except in the explanation of the variations between the tests.

Neuropsychological Testing

Neuropsychological testing involves a series of tests to evaluate the presence of cortical function and impairment by localizing the area and degree of impairment, and determining the rate of progression or recovery. The tests are sensitive to brain function and gauge many types of abilities (i.e., motor, perceptual, language, visuospatial, cognitive).

With careful interpretation, inferences can be made about the extent of brain function impairment and the effect it may have on the client's ability to function. Results from the neuropsychological evaluations, clinical manifestations, neurologic examinations, and neurodiagnostic studies are correlated and used to predict the client's potential functioning in 6 months, 12 months, and so on.

Results of neuropsychological testing assist in the diagnosis of specific cognitive dysfunctions and the development of an individualized rehabilitation program. Serial testing is valuable for monitoring rehabilitative progress and recovery in clients with problems such as head injury and epilepsy.

There is poor correlation between the degree of brain damage as revealed, for example, by CT scan and neuropsychological testing. A small lesion can create a large functional deficit, and, in contrast, a large lesion may cause only small changes. There are even instances in which testing clearly demonstrates brain dysfunction in the absence of a demonstrable lesion on CT scan.

A client may be referred for neuropsychological assessment in the acute phase or months after an injury. For example, after a head injury in which the physical neurologic assessment is normal and the EEG reveals only mild generalized abnormalities, the client may complain of being unable to work because of persistent headaches. Recommendations from testing may be made about treatment, including educational and vocational rehabilitation.

Neuropsychological tests measure deficits in coping skills by assessing the skills directly. They may be helpful when deficits in adaptive abilities are suspected. An individual test may be performed in the case of a disorder with only one specific symptom, or a complete series of tests with extended evaluation may require several hours or days of testing. The client's level of performance is compared with scores that represent normal levels of performance. General measures of intelligence (e.g., Wechsler Adult Intelligence Scale), as well as tests of emotional and personal adjustment, such as the Minnesota Multiphasic Personality Inventory, are used.

Testing may be nonspecific in implicating the presence of brain damage or very narrow in scope with sensitivity for certain areas of the brain. Results may indicate that something is wrong, but may not be able to identify the problem specifically.

Memory loss is common following head injury and in neurologic disorders. Skills such as reading, which have been stored in the brain over the years, may be retained in contrast to new learning or short-term memory, which may be impaired. The client's impaired memory may interfere with the nurse's ability to teach and the client's ability to learn. Knowing that a brain-injured client has damage to the limbic system, especially the hippocampus, amygdala, or areas of the temporal and prefrontal lobes is a good indicator for neuropsychological testing to determine memory loss.

Testing will identify problems in cognitive, psychomotor, and affective domains. Left hemisphere lesions impair factual information functions like problem solving, decision-making, and judgment. Client and family teaching must be modified to address these deficits.

Both the right and left hemispheres are involved with psychomotor learning, with the right hemisphere controlling visuospatial abilities and the left verbal instructions and sequencing of activities. Repetition and time are needed for the individual to perform activities automatically. Memory loss diagnosed from damage to the right or left hemisphere causing affective learning deficits can be improved with role modeling and one-to-one and group therapy.

Your documentation of client behavior and functional abilities assists the neuropsychologist in following the client's progress and recovery.

Invasive Tests of Function

Caloric Testing

The oculovestibular reflex, or caloric test, is a diagnostic examination providing information about the function of the vestibular portion of the eighth cranial nerve. It aids in the differential diagnosis of cerebellum and brain stem lesions (see also Chapter 31).

The test is performed only on an unconscious patient to determine if any brain stem function exists. Either cold or warm water is introduced into the external auditory canal. Patency of the external canal is confirmed first. Typically, when the vestibular eighth cranial nerve is normal, stimulation of the auditory canal with warm water produces a horizontal nystagmus toward the side of the irrigated ear. When cold water is used, the normal response is horizontal nystagmus away from the irrigated ear if the brain stem is intact. If brain stem death exists, nystagmus does not occur. Caloric tests are contraindicated in clients with perforated eardrums or with acute labyrinthine disease. As with pupil signs, abnormalities in eye movements help to localize the area of a disorder. They also help differentiate between structural and metabolic causes of coma.

Peripheral Nerve Studies

■ Electromyography

EMG measures and documents electrical currents produced by skeletal muscles, called muscle action potentials. Small needle electrodes are inserted into muscles. The electrical potentials of each muscle are amplified, transmitted to an oscilloscope, and displayed on a screen. The recording can be made audible and documented on paper (Fig. 30–13).

EMG can provide objective information that is helpful in diagnosing various neuromuscular diseases. EMG can differentiate between primary muscle disease and disease secondary to denervation. It helps identify specific primary muscle diseases. It may indicate a defect in transmission at the neuromuscular junction, such as myasthenia gravis. It can help to differentiate diseases of the anterior horn cells from those primarily of peripheral nerves. Peripheral nerve degeneration and regeneration can often be monitored with EMG before any clinical changes appear.

■ Nerve Conduction Velocity Study

A nerve conduction velocity study is often performed in conjunction with EMG, which studies the excitability and conduction velocities of motor and sensory nerves. It is helpful in diagnosing diseases of peripheral nerves. A stimulating electrode and a recording electrode are placed to test specific nerves (usually on a limb). The time required for the passage of a nerve impulse from the point of stimulation to the point of recording is measured pre-

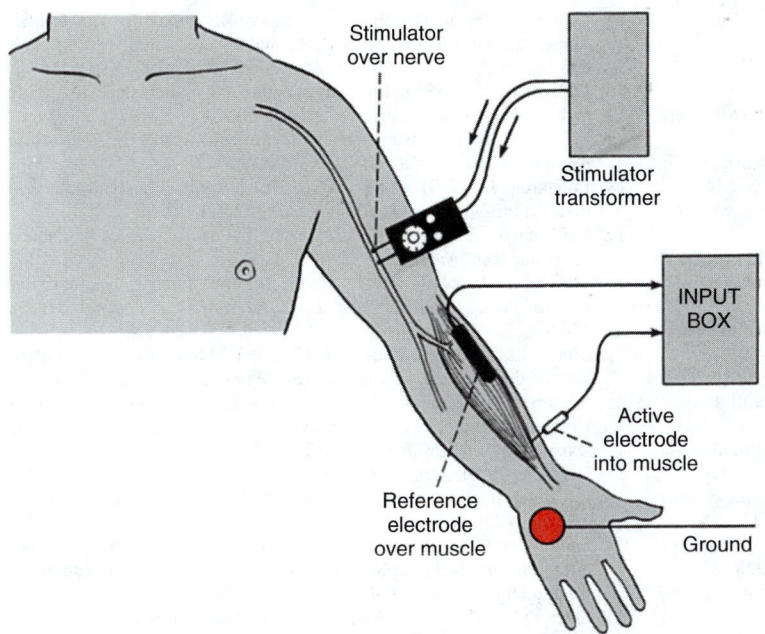

Figure 30–13. Electromyography measures and documents electrical currents produced by skeletal muscles. A stimulator is placed over the peripheral nerve being tested. A small pin is inserted into the muscle being assessed for nerve innervation, and a ground wire is placed on the client's skin.

cisely. Conduction velocity is calculated. Both motor and sensory modalities are altered in peripheral nervous system disorders (e.g., carpal tunnel syndrome), whereas only motor fibers are affected in chronic disease of the anterior horn cell or motor nerve roots.

Explain the procedure to the client and significant others. They are often concerned about the outcome of the test. They may be very anxious and stressed. The person should avoid all stimulants, depressants, and sedatives for 24 hours before the test. There may be some discomfort when the electrodes are inserted. If many muscles are tested, there may be some residual discomfort. The client may experience a mild electrical shock during the procedure. The client lies flat and may be asked to move various muscles at specific times during the test.

Clients with neuritis may have residual pain from testing. Mild analgesia may be needed.

Muscle Biopsy

Muscle biopsy is used in diagnosing neuropathies and myopathies. It is useful in distinguishing between neurogenic and myopathic processes. However, muscle histologic findings are nonspecific for any neurogenic atrophy. An EMG is helpful in locating those muscle areas that are most abnormal. It is important that areas that have been traumatized by needle electrodes be avoided when tissue is taken for biopsy. Biopsy site care is needed.

Cellular Assessment

Chromosome analysis is used to (1) assist diagnosis of some abnormal neurologic conditions and (2) provide the basis for genetic counseling in families with evidence of congenital neurologic malformations. Chromosomes can

be prepared for microscopic examination from tissue culture of cells obtained from peripheral blood, bone marrow, or skin.

Mental retardation and convulsive seizures may result from neurologic dysfunction associated with inborn errors of metabolism. Diagnosis of disorders of carbohydrate and lipid metabolism may require measurements of specific enzyme concentration in blood cells or tissue biopsied from brain, muscle, liver, or peripheral nerve cells. Usually, protein metabolism disorders are indicated by increased amounts of particular amino acids in the urine or blood. Postprocedural care is usually directed at anxiety control while the client awaits test results. Several days will be required before results are available.

Conclusions

The neurologic assessment of a client begins as all assessments do—with the history of the disorder—and then proceeds to the physical examination. The physical examination of the client can be lengthy because of the complexity of the CNS. The neurologic examination includes assessment of cognition, sensation, motor function, and reflexes. The complexity and length of time required to complete the assessment may tend to make the examiner want to omit sections to speed up the process. Before omitting any sections, it is important to realize that these assessments often provide the baseline for further evaluation and at times legal proof of a client's status.

Common diagnostic tests include LP, CT and MRI scans, and angiography. The nurse needs to understand how the test is performed so that the client can be adequately prepared and appropriate follow-up assessments can be conducted.

Bibliography

1. The American Association for Neuroscience Nurses. (1990). *Core curriculum for neuroscience nursing.* Chicago: Author.

2. Baker, D. (1993). Assessment and management of impairments in swallowing. *Nursing Clinics of North America, 28*(4), 793–805.

3. Barker, E., & Moore, K. (1992). Neurological assessment. *RN, 55*(4), 28–35.

4. Bell, T. A., et al. (1992). Transcranial Doppler: Correlation of blood velocity measurement with clinical status in subarachnoid hemorrhage. *Journal of Neuroscience Nursing, 24*(4), 215–219.

5. Bondy, K. (1994). Assessing cognitive function: A guide to neuropsychological testing. *Rehabilitation Nursing, 19*(1), 24–30.

6. Brocklehurst, R., Tallis, J., & Fillit, H. (1992). *Textbook of geriatric medicine and gerontology* (4th ed.). New York: Churchill Livingston.

7. Cason, C. L., & Sample, J. C. (1995). Preparatory information for myelogram. *Journal of Neuroscience Nursing, 27*(3), 182–187.

8. Chernecky, C., Krech, R., & Berger, B. (1993). *Laboratory tests and diagnostic procedures.* Philadelphia: W. B. Saunders.

9. DiDonato, O., & Schaffer, V. (1994). The importance of outcome data in brain injury. *Rehabilitation Nursing 19*(4), 219–228.

10. Gilman, S. (1992). Advances in neurology: Part 2. *New England Journal of Medicine, 326*(25), 1671–1676.

11. Gilroy, J. (1990). *Basic neurology* (2nd ed.) New York: Pergamon Press.

12. Guyton, A., & Hall, J. (1996). *Textbook of medical physiology* (9th ed.). Philadelphia, W. B. Saunders.

13. Hickey, J. V. (1991). *Clinical practice of neurological and neuroscience nursing.* J. B. Lippincott.

14. Jarvis, C. (1996). *Physical examination and health assessment* (2nd ed.). Philadelphia: W. B. Saunders.

15. Lauren, N., et al. (1989). Cerebral perfusion imaging with technetium-99m HM-PAO in brain death and severe central nervous system injury. *Journal of Nuclear Medicine, 30*(10), 1627–1635.

16. Lederman, R. (1996). Lumbar puncture: Essential steps to a safe and valid procedure. *Geriatrics, 51*(6), 51–58.

17. Lower, J. (1992). Rapid neuroassessment. *American Journal of Nursing, 92*(6), 38–48.

18. Lundgren, J. (1990). Computerized EEG: Applications and interventions. *Journal of Neuroscience Nursing, 22*(2), 108–112.

19. McDonagh, A. (1991). Getting your patient ready for a nuclear medicine scan. *Nursing 91, 21*(2), 53–57.

20. McGruder, J., et al. (1988). Headache after lumbar puncture: Review of the epidural blood patch. *Southern Medical Journal, 81*(10), 1249–1252.

21. Monti, E., Kerr, M., & Bender, C. (1995). Monitoring neuromuscular function. *Journal of Neuroscience Nursing, 27*(4), 252–256.

22. Pressman, E., Zeidman, S., & Summers, L. (1995). Primary care for women: Comprehensive assessment of the neurological system. *Journal of Nurse Midwifery, 40*(2), 163–171.

23. Reid, R., et al. (1989). Clinical use of technetium-99m HM-PAO for determination of brain death. *Journal of Nuclear Medicine, 30*(10), 1621–1626.

24. Sand, T. (1989). Which factors affect reported headache incidence after lumbar myelography? A statistical analysis of publications in the literature. *Neuroradiology, 31*(1), 55–59.

25. Shier D., et al. (1996). *Hole's human anatomy and physiology* (7th ed.). Dubuque, IA: Wm. C. Brown.

26. Solomon, E. P. (1992). *An introduction to human anatomy & physiology* (2nd ed.). Philadelphia: W. B. Saunders.

27. Sur, M., & Cowey, A. (1995). Cerebral cortex: Functional development. *Neuron, 15,* 497–505.

28. Swartz, M. H. (1989). *Textbook of physical diagnosis.* Philadelphia: W. B. Saunders.

Nursing Care of Comatose or Confused Clients

CHAPTER 31

Sally Strong Schnell

Clients who are comatose or confused, perhaps more than any other clients we encounter, need to be cared for in a holistic manner. All aspects of physiologic and psychological function need to be addressed. Even if the client cannot interact with the environment it is important to care for him or her in a respectful and dignified manner. It is important that family members see their loved one spoken to and cared for in a professional and caring way.

The brain serves many functions in the body. In contrast to other body systems that monitor and regulate a group of functions, such as the gastrointestinal tract regulating digestion, the nervous system monitors and regulates all other body systems. Some of these functions are self-protective and include the ability to think, be awake, respond appropriately to the environment, and move about. Other functions are automatic and include the regulation of body temperature and protective reflex responses. When these protective functions are lost, the clinical manifestations reflect the complexity of the nervous system. The term *patient* is used in this chapter to describe the client who is comatose. It is assumed that such a client cannot be an active participant in care, and the family serves as the client in these circumstances.

Disorders of Consciousness

Consciousness is a state of being that has two important aspects: (1) wakefulness and (2) awareness of self, environment, and time. Awareness of self means that the client can identify himself or herself. Awareness of environment indicates that the client can identify his or her present location and reason for being there. Awareness of time indicates that a client knows the date, month, and year and can identify common current phenomena such as the name of the president of the United States.

Unconsciousness can be brief, lasting for a few seconds, to an hour or so, or sustained, lasting for a few hours or longer. To produce unconsciousness, a disorder must (1) disrupt the ascending reticular activating system, which extends the length of the brain stem and up into the thalamus; (2) significantly disrupt the function of both cerebral hemispheres; or (3) metabolically depress overall brain function, such as drug overdose.

Coma is a state of sustained unconsciousness in which the patient does not respond to verbal stimuli, may have varying responses to painful stimuli, does not move voluntarily, may have altered respiratory patterns, may have altered pupillary responses to light, and does not blink. In general, the longer the state of unconsciousness lasts, the more likely it is irreversible and due to a permanent disorder in the structure of the brain. Higher mortality rates and poorer neurologic outcomes have been associated with the length of coma.[12]

Etiology and Risk Factors

Three kinds of disorders produce sustained unconsciousness (Fig. 31–1). They are:

1. Structural lesions in the brain that place pressure on the brain stem or the structures within the posterior cranial fossa, which include the cerebellum, the midbrain, pons, and medulla. These types of lesions destroy the reticular activating system.
2. Metabolic disorders and diffuse lesions that impair the cerebrum and arousal functions by reducing the supply of oxygen or allowing waste products to accumulate.
3. Psychogenic causes, in which case the patient looks comatose but his or her self-awareness is usually intact, as is in catatonia and hysteria. Only physiologic causes of coma are discussed here.

Structural causes of unconsciousness include brain tumors, head trauma, and cerebral hemorrhage. The cause of primary brain tumors is unknown. The brain can be a site of metastatic tumors from many organs such as breast and lung. Automobile and motorcycle accidents, physical assaults, gunshot wounds, and falls are common causes of

This chapter incorporates material written for the fourth edition by Joyce M. Black and Ellen Barker.

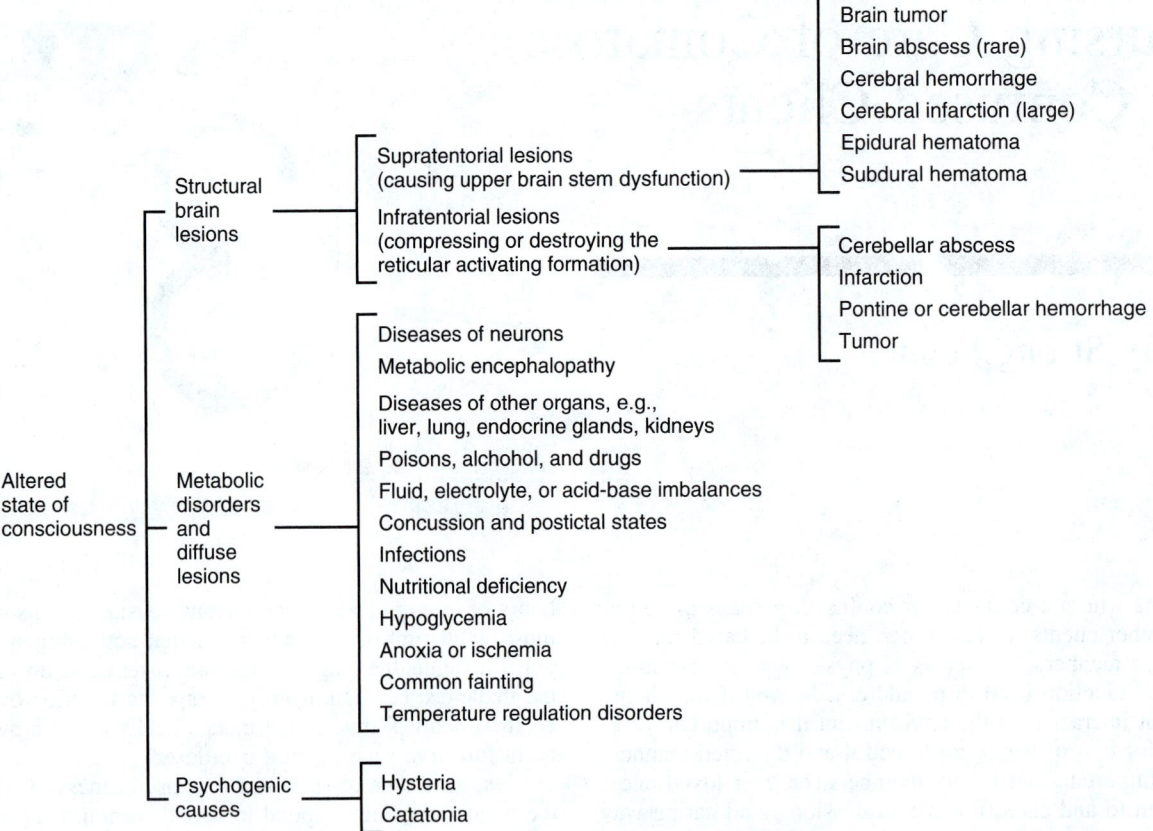

Figure 31–1. Some causes of altered states of consciousness. (Note: *Supratentorial* lesions are located *above* the dura roofing in the cerebellum, which separates the cerebellum from the cerebrum. *Infratentorial* lesions lie *beneath* the dura roofing in the cerebellum.)

head injury. A common problem after head injury is the accumulation of blood between the skull and dura (epidural hematoma) or beneath the dura (subdural hematoma). Epidural hematomas are common when an unprotected head is injured, as in assault victims, bicyclists, motorcyclists, and baseball players without helmets. Subdural hematomas are common in the elderly who fall and hit their heads, as well as in clients with decreased platelet aggregation because of alcohol abuse or other causes. In addition to direct injury to the brain tissue and the pressure caused by accumulating blood, clients with head injury may also have sustained injury to their chest or airways, which increases the risk of hypoxia. Trauma physically damages the brain, and the brain may be damaged as a result of the edema and hemorrhage that follow. Cerebral hemorrhage can cause unconsciousness by placing pressure on brain tissue.

There are many metabolic causes of coma. The term *metabolic* is used to describe problems that do not originate in the brain but begin in another system and eventually cause a disorder in the nervous system. *Hypoxia* is a common cause of metabolic brain disorders. Blood loss, high altitudes, or carbon monoxide poisoning may deprive the brain of oxygen. *Ischemia,* inadequate tissue levels of oxygen, may occur with cardiac disorders in which cardiac output is decreased, such as cardiac arrest or even fainting. Disorders of the liver, lungs, and kidney may produce coma because of the accumulation of metabolic waste products. Finally, there are many agents that

affect the metabolism of neurons. They include toxins; hypoglycemia; fever; infections, such as encephalitis; and fluid, electrolyte, or acid-base imbalance.

Pathophysiology

Masses within the brain alter the functioning of the brain in many ways. Masses or lesions, whether they are growing tumors, edema, or bleeding, place pressure on the brain. Because the brain is encased in the cranium, there is no space within the skull for the expanding brain. Pressure slows blood and CSF flow in and out of the brain and reduces cerebral function. The level of consciousness and ability to move purposefully are affected. When pressure reaches the diencephalon or brain stem, vital functions such as heart rhythm and respiration are affected. The patient's outcome depends on the location of the mass, the size and rate of enlargement, and the amount of edema and necrosis in brain tissues.

A blow to the head can cause brain lacerations or contusions because the brain is jarred and strikes the bony cranium. In addition, the brain can suffer diffuse injury as tissues are torn and sheared.

Metabolic disorders producing coma do so through various mechanisms. Infections of the brain, such as encephalitis, cause inflammation of the meninges and brain tissues. Hyperglycemia and hypoglycemia starve the cells of needed glucose for metabolism. Overdoses of sedative drugs suppress the central nervous system (CNS), especially the centers for breathing. Failure of the liver, kidney, and lungs allows metabolic waste to accumulate; this waste poisons the neurons.

Clinical Manifestations and Diagnostic Findings

Decreased levels of consciousness are most often caused by disorders in the reticular activating system of the brain stem and thalamus. Conditions such as confusion and decreased attention span can be caused by disorders of one of the cerebral hemispheres, such as stroke. Coma itself is due to extensive damage to both cerebral hemispheres or the reticular activating system.

Masses located in the supratentorial area (above the dura roofing the cerebellum) of the brain cause a fairly predictable set of clinical manifestations. Supratentorial lesions can involve the entire cortical or subcortical level of the brain tissue, as in hemorrhage. The disorder may also be located in one hemisphere, as with stroke. These masses first produce manifestations such as headache, sensorimotor deficits, aphasia, visual loss, or seizures. The specific manifestations are related to the specific area of the brain that is affected.

For example, if the client has a mass in the temporal lobe, early clinical manifestations may include headaches, memory deficits, or focal seizures. Focal seizures are located in one area of the body, such as the hand. As the mass expands, manifestations worsen because the mass places pressure on nearby areas as well as the diencephalon. The client may develop a unilateral sensorimotor deficit (cannot raise the right leg or has numbness in the right leg), aphasia, and a deficit in the visual field (blind in the left visual field). These clients usually have intact pupillary and oculovestibular reflexes. If the mass is not detected or cannot be treated and progresses, the client will eventually develop coma. Coma indicates that the mass has grown and compressed structures deep in the brain stem.

Infratentorial disorders (beneath the dura roofing the cerebellum) cause the client to lose consciousness in two ways: (1) by directly affecting the reticular activating system or its pathways or (2) by invading the brain stem or reducing its blood supply. Infratentorial lesions may produce unusual respiratory patterns. The medulla houses the center for rhythmic breathing. This center's function is lost as consciousness decreases, and the lower brain stem regulates breathing by responding to changes primarily in the carbon dioxide levels, as well as changes in acid-base balance and oxygen levels. The result is a very irregular breathing depth and pattern (Fig. 31–2). The cranial nerves are commonly compressed by the mass or edema in the brain, and various cranial nerve palsies can be seen. Specific patterns of pupil size and reactivity to light occur when pressure is exerted at various locations of the cranial nerves (see Fig. 31–2).

An important difference in coma caused by a metabolic disorder is the presence of bilateral or symmetric manifestations, because the disorder affects the entire brain rather than just one section. The client usually develops confusion and stupor before any physical signs are noticed. Physical signs include tremor, asterixis (flapping tremors of the hands), myoclonus (a single, sudden jerking movement), and seizures. Pupillary response is usually normal

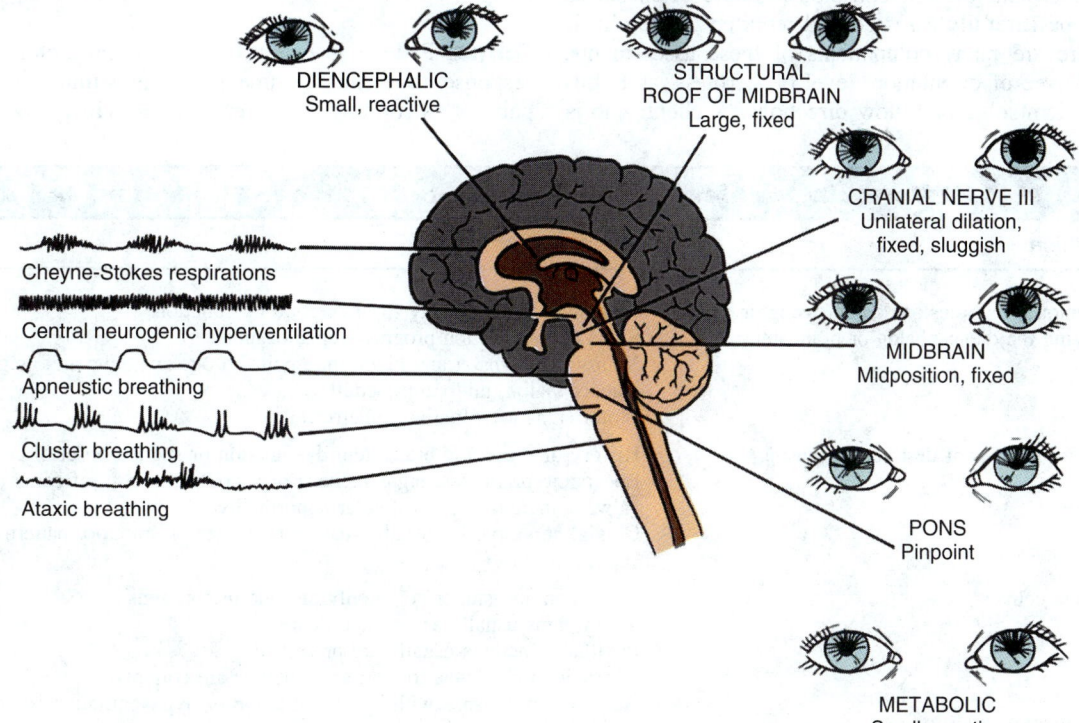

Figure 31–2. Respiratory patterns and pupil appearances associated with lesions of various neurologic structures. Cheyne-Stokes respiration may occur because of altered cerebral perfusion deep within the cerebral hemisphere or from within the diencephalon.

unless the condition is related to drug overdose. Depending on the underlying cause, acid-base imbalances may be noted. For example, metabolic acidosis would be present in a patient with diabetic coma.

Clients who are unresponsive because of a psychiatric disorder, rather than a true coma, do not have the same manifestations. These clients have intact eyelid muscles and their eyelids close tightly; the pupils are small but react normally; oculocephalic responses are unpredictable; and oculovestibular stimulation produces the normal nystagmus. Motor tone is inconsistent, no pathophysiologic reflexes are present, and the electroencephalogram (EEG) is normal.

Some patients in coma awaken slowly and begin to respond normally. They often require physical, occupational, and speech therapy for return to maximal levels of function. Irreversible coma is caused by damage to the cerebral hemispheres that destroys the patient's ability to respond to the environment. The brain stem and cerebellum remain intact and functional, however, so that vital functions, such as heart, lung, and gastrointestinal function, continue. Patients can remain in irreversible coma for years. Significant ethical and legal debates have arisen regarding the maintenance of nutritional intake for these patients, particularly when the family questions the rationale for artificial feeding.

Table 31–1 describes the clinical manifestations of structurally induced and metabolic coma.

■ Level of Consciousness

The level of consciousness is the most critical clinical piece of data assessed in the neurologically impaired patient. Changes in level of consciousness are often subtle and must be carefully assessed and reported to the physician. There are many components of these assessments, such as degree of orientation, level of alertness, and ability to problem-solve or follow directions. A client who is awake, alert, and fully oriented to self, others, place, and time is considered to be fully conscious. As changes in the level of consciousness occur, the client may either be improving or deteriorating. From the normal alert state, consciousness deteriorates in stages, with each stage having its own definition.

Confusion. *Confusion* is the loss of the ability to think rapidly and clearly; an impairment in judgment and decision-making.

Disorientation. *Disorientation* marks the beginning of loss of consciousness. Disorientation to time is followed by disorientation to place and inability to recognize others. The last step of disorientation is inability to know self. These manifestations are sometimes referred to as "disoriented times 3," meaning time, place, and person.

Lethargy. *Lethargy* is restriction in activity related to a decreased level of alertness. The patient is easily aroused by speech or touch but returns to lying quietly or sleeping when not stimulated.

Obtundation. *Obtundation* is reduced ability to be aroused and limited response to the environment. The patient sleeps unless stimulated by speech or touch. Verbal response to questions is minimal, perhaps a grunt or nod.

Stupor. *Stupor* is a condition of deep sleep or unresponsiveness from which a patient may be aroused only with vigorous, sometimes painful, stimulation. Patients respond by withdrawing from or grabbing at the source of pain.

Coma. Patients in *coma* demonstrate no motor or verbal response to the environment or any stimuli, even deep pain or suctioning or other noxious (irritating, hurtful)

Table 31–1. Differential Manifestations of Structurally Induced and Metabolic Coma

Mechanism	Manifestations
Supratentorial mass lesions compressing or displacing the diencephalon or brain stem	Initiating sign is usually focal cerebral dysfunction Signs of dysfunction progress cephalocaudad Neurologic signs at any given time point to one anatomic area (e.g., diencephalon, midbrain, medulla) Motor signs are often asymmetrical
Infratentorial mass of destruction causing coma	History of preceding brain stem dysfunction or sudden onset of coma Localizing brain stem signs precede or accompany onset of coma and always include oculovestibular abnormality Cranial nerve palsies usually manifest "bizarre" respiratory patterns that appear at onset
Metabolic coma	Confusion and stupor commonly precede motor signs Motor signs usually are symmetrical Pupillary reactions usually are preserved Asterixis, myoclonus, tremor, and seizures are common Acid-base imbalance with hyperventilation or hypoventilation is frequent

Adapted from McCarce, K. L., & Huether, S. E. (1994). *Pathophysiology: The biological basis for disease in adults and children* (2nd ed., p. 479). St. Louis: Mosby–Year Book.

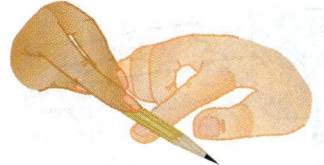

Placing a pencil or pen across the fingernail bed and applying firm pressure produces a constant noxious stimulus and a minimal amount of tissue trauma.

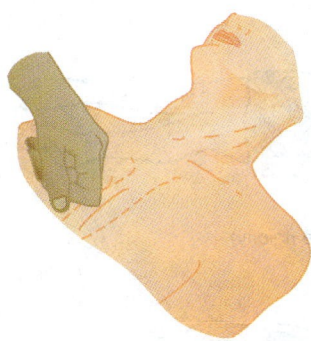

Sternal rub or compression is a common form of noxious stimulus but may, over time, cause severe tissue trauma. In the elderly, in whom bones may be very brittle, it can also cause fractured ribs and/or accompanying pulmonary complications.

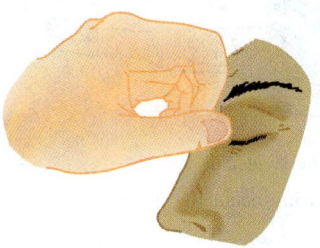

Supraorbital pressure is not recommended as a noxious stimulus when testing for the eye opening response. The grimacing associated with supraorbital pressure may actually cause eye closure.

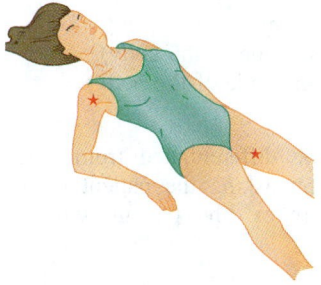

Pinching various parts of the extremity or trunk is the most appropriate stimulus when a response in each extremity is desired. Examples of where to apply the stimulus are shown.

Figure 31–3. Painful or noxious stimuli may need to be used to elicit a response from a patient in a coma or with decreased levels of consciousness. (From Marshall, S., et al. [1990]. *Neuroscience critical care: Pathophysiology and patient management.* Philadelphia: WB Saunders.)

stimuli.[8] See Figure 31–3 for other examples of noxious stimuli.

In the clinical setting, these terms can be confusing, and their true meaning is debatable. Document the behavior to validate the terminology chosen. For example, "does not respond to spoken words or light touch, will pull away from painful stimuli" is much more descriptive than just using the word "stuporous." Also, determine how these terms are defined at each healthcare facility.

Breathing Pattern

Respiration is a complex process controlled by the cerebrum, pons, and medulla. Disorders causing coma and decreased levels of consciousness also commonly cause respiratory abnormalities. Changes in respiratory rate and rhythm have many causes. Rapidly expanding lesions in the cerebrum, brain stem, or cerebellum may lead to compression of the pons and medulla, which leads to respiratory failure. Common abnormal respiratory patterns are shown in Figure 31–2.

Airway obstruction and aspiration are common complications in unconscious patients. An obstructed airway leads to inadequate gas exchange, which in turn causes one or both of the following: (1) carbon dioxide retention, contributing to vasodilation, cerebral edema, and increasing ICP; (2) reduced arterial oxygen levels, resulting in decreased oxygen delivery to the brain and increased ICP. These events can create a vicious cycle of deterioration if interventions are not successful. Respiratory failure will occur if a patient has insufficient lung ventilation and inadequate gas exchange. Respiratory failure may be prevented by oxygen administration and assisted ventilation.

Eye Movement

The cranial nerves (CN) responsible for eye movement exit through the brain stem; when the cranial nerves are compressed, eye movement is impaired. Eye movements in the comatose patient are uncoordinated, and pupillary response is abnormal. The eyes of an awake and alert client at rest normally gaze straight ahead. Eyes normally track together to look at something. When the eyes move in this way, gaze is said to be *conjugate*. *Dysconjugate* gaze or conjugate deviation of the eyes at rest indicates a disorder of one or more of the ocular muscles due to weak muscles or damage to the cranial nerves supplying the eye muscles (CN III, IV, and VI). Several types of abnormal involuntary eye movements may occur: ocular bobbing (i.e., the eyes appear to be slowly jumping up and down); or roving eye movements (i.e., the eyes slowly wander or move around); or nystagmus (involuntary oscillation, or vibration, of the eyeballs). Nystagmus may be horizontal, vertical, oblique, rotary, or mixed, with various rates of movement.

Pupillary Changes

The nuclei of CN II are located directly below the cerebrum and the nuclei of CN III are located in the midbrain. Therefore, one can readily understand why pupillary changes are used to assess brain stem function. Severe cerebral hypoxia and ischemia cause pupils to become fixed and dilated. Fixed and dilated pupils are also seen late in the herniation syndromes. Hypothermia may also result in the pupils being fixed but this is usually due to paralysis of the pupillary muscles caused by exposure to cold temperatures, not cerebral changes. There are also several medications that affect pupil size and reaction to light. These medications include large doses of atropine and scopolamine, which fix and fully dilate the pupil; miotics, which constrict the pupil; mydriatics, which dilate the pupil; narcotics (especially morphine), which cause the pupils to become pinpoint in size; and barbiturates, which produce fixed pupils (see Fig. 31–2). A mass lesion affecting only one hemisphere may result in only the ipsilateral (same-sided) pupil being less reactive or nonreactive to light. A lesion affecting both hemispheres affects both pupils.

■ Motor Response

Motor response is often used as a predictor of outcome in patients with severe neurologic impairment. The patient may respond appropriately to commands such as "raise your right arm." Other patients may not respond to verbal requests but have purposeful movement, such as pushing away a source of pain. For example, the patient may push away a suction catheter during suctioning. As consciousness decreases further, the patient may only draw up the knees and arms without directing any response to the stimuli.

The patient may also exhibit some abnormal motor movements and postures. *Posturing* is abnormal flexion and extension caused by hyperreflexia. Posturing can occur in patients with severe brain dysfunction, lesions pushing on the midbrain and pons from the posterior cranial fossa, herniation, or advanced metabolic coma. Both abnormal flexion and extension posturing usually appear in response to painful stimulation in patients in profound coma. The postures may also appear without stimulation. They may be so intense that the bed shakes as spasms of rigidity pass through the body. At times, shivering, hyperpnea, and teeth clenching may accompany the posturing.

When the ICP is increased at the cortical level, abnormal flexion (decorticate) posturing is seen as flexion of the arms, wrists, and fingers with the arms adducted at the shoulder. The legs are fully extended and internally rotated, with the feet in plantar flexion (see Fig. 31–4A). As the pressure increases to the level of the upper pons, abnormal extension (decerebrate) posturing occurs. In this posture, the legs are extended abnormally, similar to decorticate posturing. The arms are extended stiff and adducted and the hands are hyperpronated (see Fig. 31–4B).

Just as decerebrate posturing is a graver sign than decorticate posturing, *flaccidity* (Fig. 31–4C) is yet a graver sign. Flaccidity is extreme weakness. The body and extremities are limp and remain in whatever position they are placed. A patient in a flaccid posture offers no resistance to movement. Bilateral flaccidity is considered the most severe of motor impairment signs. True flaccidity, the absence of any movement or tone in response to deep painful stimuli, is one of the criteria for brain death. Therefore, great caution is used in determining whether flaccidity is present. Disorders such as stroke and spinal cord injury also may produce flaccidity.

Other motor signs in a patient with cerebral hemisphere damage may include the following:

- Primitive sucking or snout reflexes
- Strong reflexive hand grasps

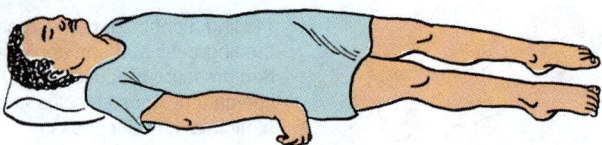

A. Extension posturing (decerebrate rigidity)

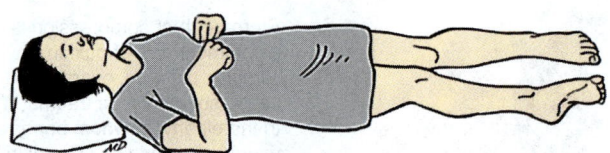

B. Abnormal flexion (decorticate rigidity)

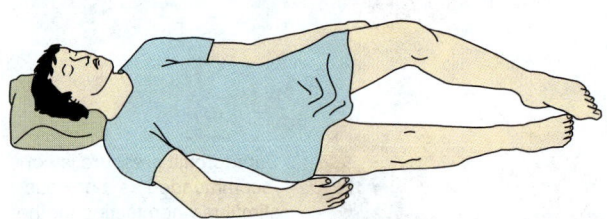

C. Unilateral flaccidity (right side is flaccid)

Figure 31–4. Pathologic posturing occurring in patients with severe brain injury.

- Restlessness
- Resistance to passive movement
- Hemiplegia (paralysis on one side of the body)
- Hemiparesis (weakness on one side of the body)
- Seizures

Reflexive hand grasps can be differentiated from a response to verbal command by asking the patient to release the grasp. If it is a reflex, the patient will not release on command.

■ Changes in Vital Signs

Wide variations in vital signs may occur in patients with various levels of consciousness. Some changes relate directly to the cause of the unconsciousness. Others relate to complications of the initial disorder, treatment, or immobility, such as shock, cardiac dysrhythmias, fluid and electrolyte imbalances, and hypertension. Some conditions causing coma produce autonomic nervous system instability because of impairment of the hypothalamus. These disorders may cause a wide variation in blood pressure, pulse, and body temperature.

■ Cushing's Triad

Cushing's response may develop with increased ICP. These changes include decreased pulse and increased systolic blood pressure with diastolic pressure remaining the same (or rising slightly) to create a widened pulse pressure and slowing of respirations. These physiologic responses are an attempt to restore adequate blood flow through compressed cerebral vessels. Cushing's response is not a reliable warning of increasing ICP because it does not always occur, and when it does occur, it is often *late* in the course of rising pressure. Cushing's response is sometimes difficult to differentiate from other causes of hypertension or slowing pulse rate. See Figure 31–5 for vital sign changes associated with Cushing's response.

▪ Diagnostic Tests

The goal of medical management of the patient in coma is to remove or correct the cause. Frequently, time is required to perform all the tests to find the specific cause. In the interim, the patient's brain must be protected from further injury.

Computed Tomography and Magnetic Resonance Imaging.
A computed tomographic (CT) scan or magnetic resonance imaging (MRI) usually provides data that indicate whether the cause of the coma is structural. Tumors or areas of bleeding will be evident on the scan. Sometimes the patient will require emergency surgery to remove the mass or drain the fluid and thereby relieve pressure.

Lumbar Puncture.
A lumbar puncture can be done when it is known from data provided by the CT or MRI scans that the patient has no expanding intracranial mass. Obtaining this information prior to lumbar puncture avoids the risk of herniation due to sudden changes in CSF pressures (low in the spinal column and high in the ventricles). A lumbar puncture can assist with the diagnosis of infection or bleeding as a cause of coma. CSF may be cloudy or bloody when the patient has an infection or bleeding into the ventricles or the subarachnoid space.

Electroencephalography.
EEG can be used to determine if the patient is comatose because of continuous seizures. EEG results are abnormal in many patients with structural and metabolic coma and do not serve as a clear diagnostic tool. A portion of the general population may have an abnormal EEG as well.

See Chapter 30 for more information related to care of a client undergoing specific diagnostic tests.

Tests for Abnormal Reflexes.
Test for Oculocephalic Reflex Response.
The *doll's eye reflex* is movement of the eyes in the opposite direction to that which the head is moved, for example, doll's eyes are considered present if the eyes move to the right when the head is rotated to the left and vice versa (Fig. 31–6). Assessment for the presence of doll's eye movement is a rapid method of detecting potential abnormalities of the brain stem. This test can be done only on unconscious patients because this is a normal response in unconscious patients and indicates some remaining brain stem function. The doll's eye reflex does not occur in awake clients or clients without brain stem problems. Do not perform the doll's eye test on comatose patients with suspected or known cervical spine injury. The head movement could produce permanent spinal cord damage.

Patients in metabolic coma, except for that caused by barbiturate or phenytoin (Dilantin) poisoning, retain ocular reflexes. The presence of a brisk doll's eye movement indicates a decrease in the level of consciousness with an intact brain stem (see Fig. 31–6A). The brain stem in a comatose patient may be functioning even with the absence of doll's eye movement (see Fig. 31–6B). Other agents and disorders can block the eye's response. Neuromuscular drugs, such as succinylcholine, and Menière's disease, which destroys the labyrinth in the ear, cause an absent oculocephalic response. However, negative oculo-

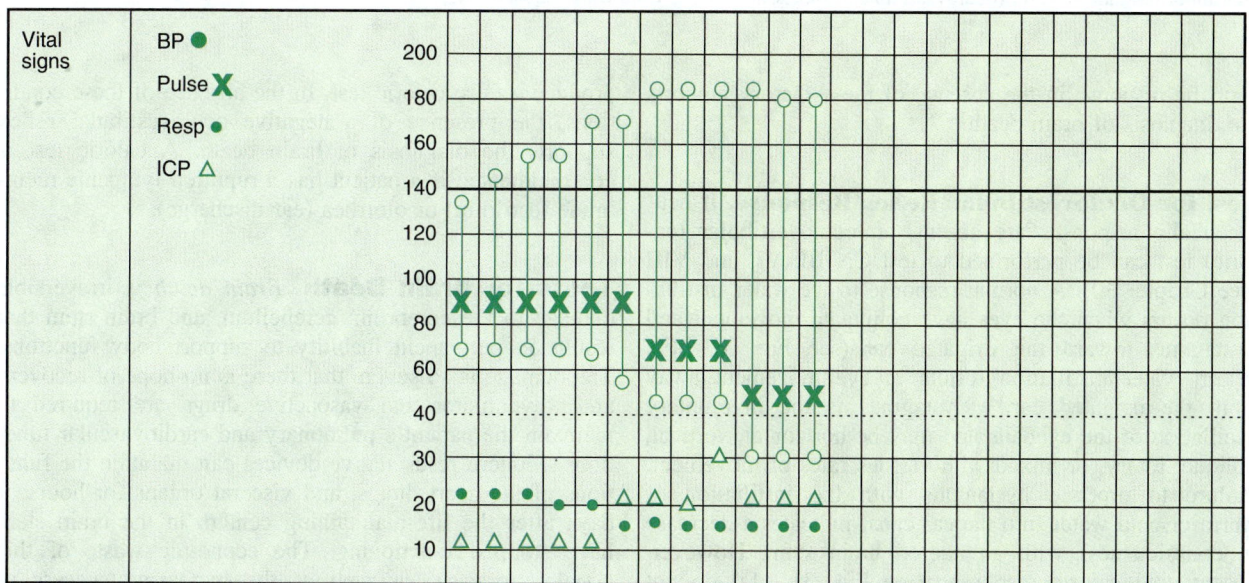

Figure 31–5. Cushing's response (Cushing's triad) includes bradycardia, systolic hypertension, and a wide pulse pressure that occur from pressure on the medulla. These signs often occur with intracranial hypertension or herniation syndrome. Alterations in respiratory patterns also accompany Cushing's triad.

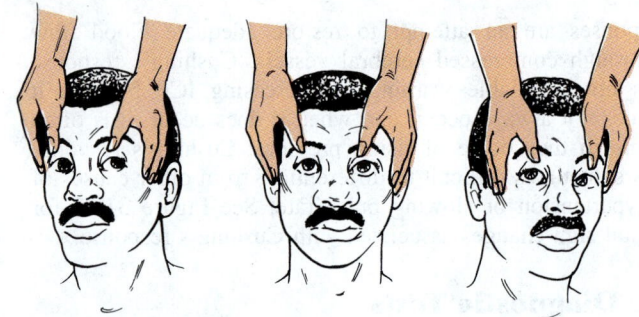

A. NORMAL REACTION:
Eyes move from side to side when head is turned

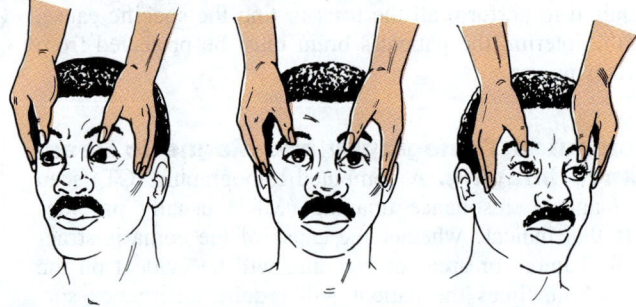

B. ABNORMAL REACTION:
Eyes remain in fixed position in skull when head is turned

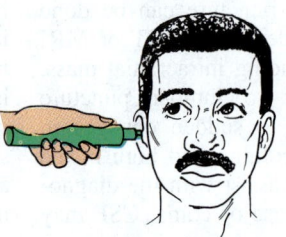

C. NORMAL CALORIC:
Eyes deviate to side of
ice water application

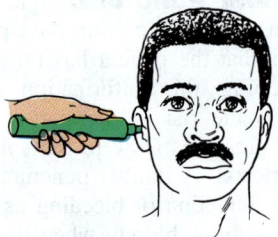

D. ABNORMAL CALORIC:
Eyes do not deviate

Figure 31–6. *A* and *B,* Normal and abnormal doll's eye reflexes (oculocephalic response). *C* and *D,* Normal and abnormal caloric tests (oculovestibular response).

cephalic response in the absence of these factors supports the diagnosis of brain death.[16]

Test for Oculovestibular Reflex Response. If oculocephalic responses are absent, an oculovestibular (caloric) test can be performed to test CN III, VI, and VIII (see Chapter 30). A normal response to ice water instillation occurs when the eyes have conjugate movement and nystagmus toward the irrigated ear (see Fig. 31–6C). Warm water instillation results in eye movement away from the irrigated ear.[16] Nystagmus is the involuntary oscillation of the eyeballs and may be horizontal, vertical, oblique, rotary, or mixed with various rates of movement. Failure to produce nystagmus with the instillation of warm or cold water into the ear canal indicates a decrease in consciousness with an altered brain stem. However, absent cold caloric responses (see Fig. 31–6D) do not always indicate a brain stem disorder. The use of ototoxic drugs, barbiturates, sedatives, phenytoin, or tricyclic antidepressants or the presence of Menière's disease may

produce a false caloric test. In the absence of these conditions, the presence of a negative oculovestibular reflex supports the diagnosis of brain death. A caloric test is contraindicated if a patient has a ruptured tympanic membrane (eardrum) or otorrhea (ear discharge).

Tests for Brain Death. *Brain death* is irreversible damage to the cerebrum, cerebellum, and brain stem that results in permanent inability to support body functions. The damage is so severe that there is no hope of recovery and a ventilator and vasoactive drugs are required to maintain the patient's pulmonary and cardiovascular functions. Modern resuscitative devices can maintain the functions of the heart, lungs, and visceral organs for hours or days after the life-maintaining centers in the brain stem have stopped functioning. The economic waste of this hopeless process, as well as the increasing success of organ transplant programs, has led countries worldwide to adopt the principle that death of a person occurs when either the brain or the heart irreversibly fails to function.

In the United States, the time of brain death has been accepted as the legal time of death. The Presidential Commission set the criterion for brain death as the "irreversible cessation of all functions of the entire brain, including the brain stem."

Certain points in diagnosing brain death need emphasis. Recoverable drug depressant poisoning can in all ways, except stopping cerebral circulation, resemble brain death and must be explicitly ruled out. If ever there is doubt that a person is brain dead, all life support must be maintained until a clear diagnosis can be made. EEG activity or brain stem reflexes means there is some brain activity. In contrast, purely spinal reflex activity can persist after brain death. Spinal reflexes can lead to some remarkably complex movements, such as flexion of the trunk and raising of outstretched arms.

Guidelines for establishing brain death are as follows:

1. Nature and duration of coma must be known
   a. Known structural disease or irreversible systemic metabolic cause
   b. No chance of drug intoxication or hypothermia; no paralyzing or potentially anesthetizing drugs recently given for treatment
   c. Body temperature must be greater than 34° C
   d. Observation of no brain function for 6 hours is sufficient in cases of known structural cause when no drug or alcohol is involved in causation or treatment; otherwise, 12 hours plus negative drug screen required
2. Absence of cerebral and brain stem function
   a. No behavioral or reflex responses can be elicited by noxious stimuli applied above foramen magnum level
   b. Fixed pupils
   c. No oculovestibular response to 50 ml ice water calories
   d. Apneic off ventilator with oxygenation for 10 minutes
   e. Systemic circulation may be intact
   f. Purely spinal reflexes may be retained
3. Supplementary (optional) criteria (any one is diagnostic)
   a. EEG must be largely isoelectric for 30 minutes at maximal gain
   b. Brain stem−evoked responses must reflect absent function in vital brain stem structures
   c. No cerebral circulation present on angiographic examination[11]

Emergency Care

Initial care of an unconscious patient includes clearing the airway immediately and loosening all tight clothing, especially around the neck. Never move a recently injured or unconscious patient without using a stiff collar to protect the neck if there is any possibility of spinal injury. Anyone with a head injury is treated as if he or she has sustained cervical spine injury until diagnostic tests have determined otherwise. Maintain a patent airway by the jaw-thrust method. Remove and store any dentures or bridgework. These could cause airway obstruction or could be broken and swallowed.

Noisy respirations or obvious efforts to breathe indicate partial airway obstruction. If it is possible to do so without moving the neck, remove the cause of obstruction. If spinal cord injury has been ruled out, place the patient in a lateral or semiprone position to facilitate drainage of pulmonary secretions and prevent the tongue from falling into the posterior pharynx and occluding the airway. Elevation of the headrest may be prescribed, particularly in patients experiencing increased ICP. Do not position the patient on his or her back, unless intubated, because this position can compromise respirations. In addition to the tongue occluding the airway, secretions may pool in the pharynx and be aspirated.

The patient's airway, ventilation, and circulation must be maintained. A nasal or oral airway may be inserted for a short time. If the patient is completely unresponsive, an endotracheal tube is carefully inserted, avoiding injury to the cervical spine. The head-injured patient may be hyperventilated while on a ventilator to reduce partial pressure of arterial carbon dioxide ($PaCO_2$) to between 30 and 35 mm Hg. Hyperventilation is an effective way to reduce cerebral blood flow. *Hypocapnia* (decreased arterial concentration of CO_2) causes desirable vasoconstriction. This results in reduced blood flow to the head and reduced ICP. Use caution, however, to avoid decreasing the blood supply to the point of causing ischemia, which may result in increased ICP and possibly infarction. Normal cerebral perfusion is promoted by monitoring blood pressure and maintaining the systolic pressure between 100 and 160 mm Hg. Blood pressures lower or higher than these levels may decrease cerebral perfusion pressure. This may require using vasoactive agents to keep the systolic pressure at 100 mm Hg or *mean* systolic blood pressure above 80 mm Hg or medications to lower the blood pressure. If the patient is breathing spontaneously, the airway and respirations need to be closely monitored because the airway may become obstructed and aspiration may occur as consciousness decreases. Respiratory patterns may become ineffective, requiring intubation.

Initial assessment of the comatose patient includes the following:

● Level of consciousness by observing responses to stimuli.
● Presence of localizing neurologic symptoms indicating focal intracranial disease.
● Pupil sizes and reactivity to light for indications of increased ICP or other causes of coma.
● Deep and superficial reflexes (see Chapter 30). Reflex assessment is particularly valuable in comatose patients because it provides objective information about the condition without requiring conscious participation. Assess the corneal reflex carefully to avoid corneal abrasion.
● Response to painful stimuli. Other aspects of sensory assessment are not possible or are unreliable in patients with decreased consciousness.

- Evidence of trauma. Trauma may be the result of coma rather than the cause of it (e.g., a tongue bite may result from a seizure). Examine ears for ruptured eardrums or otorrhea.
- Determination of serum oxygenation, blood alcohol, blood urea nitrogen, ammonia, and glucose levels if manifestations suggest a metabolic disorder.
- History from significant others (or observers of what has happened) when possible.

Immediate interventions include treatment of common causes of coma while assessment of neurologic status continues. For example, after blood is drawn, intravenous (IV) glucose is given to reverse potential insulin reactions. Many comatose patients are malnourished and subject to Wernicke's encephalopathy related to alcohol abuse. These patients are commonly given thiamine, especially if they are given glucose.

If the patient is having repetitive seizures, coma and brain damage can follow; give the patient IV diazepam or lorazepam to stop the seizures. If the patient is not intubated, closely monitor the airway because of the respiratory depressant effects of these medications.

Many metabolic causes of coma lead to acid-base and fluid-electrolyte imbalances. The patient's acid-base balance should be restored quickly. Fluid imbalances should be restored slowly to prevent rebound fluid shifts into the brain. Fluids may be given if the patient is dehydrated or withheld if the patient is fluid-overloaded. Fluids such as isotonic saline are usually given because these fluids will not passively diffuse into the brain and increase edema. Patients with increased ICP are frequently kept slightly dehydrated. If cerebral edema is present, osmotic diuretics may be used to promote shifting of the edematous fluid from the brain cells back into the plasma. Other medications that promote a decrease in ICP through more indirect means include steroids, barbiturate therapy, and neuromuscular blocking agents. Treatment of electrolyte imbalances is discussed in Chapter 15.

Take cultures of the blood, nose, throat, and wounds (if present). Once the cultures are taken, give antibiotics, as ordered, to combat infection. Body temperature should be normalized as much as possible by means of antipyretics, air circulation, and cooling mattresses. Care must be taken to ensure that the patient does not shiver, because this will increase ICP.

Drug overdose–induced coma may be reversed by specific antidotes if the ingested drug can be identified. Many times, however, the specific drug ingested is not known. Blood should be drawn for a toxicity screen. Narcotic overdose may be reversed with naloxone (Narcan). The duration of action of naloxone is 2 to 3 hours shorter than that of most narcotics, and naloxone may need to be readministered. Seizures resulting from cocaine overdose can be treated with diazepam. Patients with cocaine overdose often have cardiac arrhythmias and irregular respirations. Gastric lavage may be used to remove ingested agents, followed by activated charcoal instillation.

To stimulate your thought process, refer to the Thinking Critically section at the end of the chapter for a scenario involving a client with head trauma.

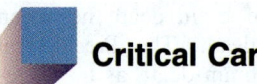

Critical Care

Once emergency care is given, medical management centers on trying to diagnose and treat the cause of the coma. Body functions are maintained, and complications that may slow recovery or cause residual problems are prevented. The Nursing Research feature on early intervention advocates early use of coma stimulation in the critical care phase.

NURSING RESEARCH

Does Coma Stimulation Affect Prognosis?

Sosnowski, C. (1994). Early intervention: Coma stimulation in the intensive care unit. *Journal of Neuroscience Nursing, 26*(6), 336–341.

Coma stimulation has been used more often for patients in a rehabilitation setting than in an intensive care setting. Such an intervention in the early stages of a person's recovery may play a vital role in patient outcome.

Sosnowski described the case of an 18-year-old girl who suffered a serious head and thoracic injury from a motor vehicle accident. She was received in the emergency department with a Glasgow Coma Scale score of 3 and with fixed and dilated pupils. One week after admission, she did not respond to verbal or tactile stimuli, but did withdraw from pain and her pupils were reactive. On day 14, she developed acute respiratory distress syndrome and had to be chemically paralyzed to maintain her oxygenation level on a ventilator.

Rehabilitation had been provided since day 3, but the family and rehabilitation team decided that the therapy needed to be more formalized. The team (nurses, family, speech pathologists, occupational therapists, and physical therapists) initiated a formalized coma stimulation program. This program included auditory, visual, olfactory, gustatory, tactile, and kinesthetic stimulation.

Coma stimulation continued after the patient was discharged to a head injury rehabilitation unit on day 67. The patient had a slow, continual improvement. Ten months after the trauma, she was able to speak, read, recognize people, complete simple mathematics problems, and use a wheelchair with minimal assistance for transfers.

Implications for Practice

It is important to work with the brain's inherent ability to reorganize after an acute brain injury. The rehabilitation team, with the family's help, provided a consistent and controlled stimulation program that resulted in a positive outcome for this patient.

Table 31–2. Clinical Signs of Good or Poor Outcome From Coma

Good Prognosis	Poor Prognosis
1 day: Awake. No neuro-ophthalmologic abnormalities; speaking at least words. Possibility of poor outcome = 30%	Not awake. Pupils and oculocephalic reflexes absent and flaccid motor system. Possibility of good outcome = 2%.
3 days: Corneal responses present, speaks words, moves. Possibility of poor outcome = 26%	No words; corneal responses and appropriate motor responses absent. Possibility of good outcome = 0%
1 week: Eyes open, says words, makes localized motor responses. Possibility of poor outcome = 1%	No wakefulness, motor system flaccid. Possibility of good outcome = 0%

Data derived from best outcome studies of 500 optimally treated patients in coma from nontraumatic, non-drug poisoning causes. From Levy, D. E., et al. (1981). Prognosis in non-traumatic coma. *Annals of Internal Medicine, 94,* 293. Used with permission.

If the coma is prolonged, initiate enteral feeding to promote nutrition and prevent muscle wasting. Parenteral nutrition may be used if paralytic ileus occurs. Provision of nutritional needs must be balanced against the possible increase in ICP related to glucose delivery. However, brain cells have a high glucose need compared with other cells; supplying the cell need without inducing osmotic shifts requires a delicate balance. Prevent the complications of immobility, such as pneumonia and pressure ulcers, with oscillating beds. Continually assess for these complications and treat them promptly if they occur.

In the past, little information was available on which to base a prediction about the outcome of a patient in coma. Most of the time, a "wait-and-see attitude" was used. The family and the healthcare team should have some idea of the probable eventual outcome for the patient. It is discouraging and inappropriate to vigorously treat a patient with no chance of recovery, but it is even more inappropriate to deny treatment to a patient with a reasonable chance of recovery.

Coma after head injury has a statistically better outcome than that associated with medical illness. About 50% of patients in coma from head injury die, many instantly. Acute treatment may somewhat improve the outcome of those who reach the hospital. Recovery in traumatic cases is closely linked to age: the younger, the better. As with medical coma, severely abnormal neuro-ophthalmologic signs reflecting brain stem dysfunction imply a poor prognosis; approximately 90% of such patients either die or remain in near-vegetative states.[11]

The absence of pupillary, corneal, or oculovestibular responses during early stages of coma is highly predictive of mortality or significant morbidity (e.g., persistent vegetative state). The recovery of these responses and a return to purposeful movement correlate with a better prognosis. Patients who lapse into coma from metabolic disorders have an extremely poor prognosis if the coma lasts more than 1 week. Clinical manifestations associated with good or poor outcomes are shown in Table 31–2.

■ Organ Donation

The passage of the Uniform Anatomical Gift Act in 1968 recognized the right of every person to determine the disposition of his or her organs after death. This act provided legal documentation of the intent of the deceased and prompted many states to place uniform donor cards on the state driver's license. As people became more aware of the right to donate organs and the benefit from donation, another law was passed that required hospitals to develop a procedure for identifying potential donors, a mechanism to approach family members in a sensitive manner, and a provision to notify appropriate procurement organizations about potential donors. This law does not state that all families must be approached; it only requires that mechanisms be in place within a hospital (see Ethical Issues in Nursing). Therefore, organ donation today is still in the process of overcoming many obstacles. Each year in the United States approximately 20,000 people die under circumstances in which organ donation could have been an option for the family. Unfortunately, from this pool of 20,000, only about 20% actually donate. The main cause of this shortfall is the failure of the healthcare team to present the option of organ donation to the family. These lost opportunities are underscored by the number of people who die while waiting for organ transplants.

It has been estimated that 95% of all organ donors originate in critical care units. As the primary caregiver, the nurse may be the first to recognize that a client's survival is unlikely. The fact that grieving families rarely have the presence of mind to initiate a request highlights the importance of the nurse's role in informing the family about the options. The nurse also serves a crucial function in meeting the psychological and emotional needs of the family during the donation process. Fundamental to meeting the family's needs is an understanding of the donor process.

Step 1. The potential donor is identified. Organ and tissue donation criteria are kept intentionally broad so as not to exclude a potential candidate. Some general rules that govern donor criteria are age (65 years for tissues and 70 years for organs), no unresolved sepsis, no metastatic cancer, no communicable diseases, and declaration of brain death.

The hospital's organ donation procurement coordinator should be notified. He or she will ascertain the current local and national transplant needs. In some cases organs from a marginal candidate can be used as a "bridge" until a more suitable organ is found. It is often wise to ask the procurement coordinator to see the patient before the family is approached. A thorough evaluation of the potential donor can prevent a situation in which the family is willing to donate and then finds out the option does not exist.

Step 2. The patient is declared brain dead (see earlier discussion).

Step 3. Determination of eligibility. Assessment includes medical history (e.g., surgery, illnesses, evidence of high-risk behaviors). Laboratory tests are performed to assess for the presence of transmissible diseases. There is no cost to the family for these tests, regardless of their decision about organ donation.

Step 4. The family is approached about the option of donation. A team approach is usually the best. The nurse is often the person who establishes a relationship of trust with the family. From this foundation, the option of do-

nation is presented. Approaching the family about organ donation is believed to be one of the most emotionally draining experiences in the practice of nursing. Many nurses believe that they are intruding or worsening the grieving process by offering organ donation. In fact, the opposite is often true; most families report that they welcome the opportunity to consider donation.

Nurses must realize that this is a very difficult decision, especially if no previous discussion has ever been held on organ donation. This difficulty is compounded by the fact that physicians and nurses have made the decisions about treatment for the patient in intensive care. Families need time to think and need to have an open environment in which to do so. Feelings of pressure or coercion will not lead to organ donation.

The nurse is in a pivotal role to clarify common misconceptions about brain death and organ donation. Many family members do not understand "brain death." Their loved one does not appear dead, and he or she is breathing and has a heartbeat. A clear explanation of brain death is imperative. It is also important to clarify that machines such as the ventilator maintain rudimentary functions and should not be misinterpreted as maintaining life.

Another common issue surrounds burial and cost of donation. All costs associated with the assessment, management, and recovery of donated organs are not charged to the family. There usually needs to be no change in funeral plans. The body will not look deformed in any way as a result of organ donation.

Invariably, issues surrounding the meaning of life ensue. It is not unusual for the family to make their spiritual needs known, and the nurse may provide the family with access to the hospital chaplain or personal clergy. An accurate assessment of the family's spiritual beliefs helps the nurse frame the discussion of organ donation in a manner that is consistent with their spiritual needs.

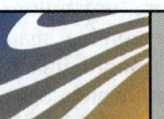

ETHICAL ISSUES IN NURSING

Should Organ Procurement and Donation Be Discussed with the Dying and Their Families?

When a client's condition is such that death appears imminent, family members need the support of the healthcare team. It is at this most uncomfortable time that nurses have the opportunity to speak to clients and their families about organ donation. Ideally, this issue should be addressed prior to ill health or trauma, but the reality is that organ donation is not something many people plan prior to ill health or trauma.

How does a nurse approach an upset or grieving family about organ donation? Should they be approached about organ donation at all? Is there an ethical responsibility to discuss the procurement of organs with the dying and their family? Thousands of living persons are on waiting lists for organ transplants. Should they have the opportunity to receive an organ from someone who no longer has need of it? Should we have to get consent to procure organs from the deceased? In some parts of the world, human organs are procured from the deceased automatically, without need for consent. In fact, consent is needed only in cases in which donation is not to occur.

Nurses need to be aware of their state laws and institution's policies regarding organ donation. It is not an easy task to discuss this matter with clients and their families, but nurses should assess their clients when the possibility of donation is present.

Step 5. Once the family has decided in favor of organ donation, steps are taken to ensure the viability of the organs. Hemodynamic stability, oxygenation, and temperature are maintained. These efforts might be more rigorous than before donation.

Step 6. Suitable recipients are identified. A national organ center matches donor organs to recipients. The search begins locally and then proceeds nationally until the organs are placed. Organs are allocated among recipients according to strict criteria, including tissue type, medical urgency, and logistic factors (e.g., distance, time). Recovery surgery is performed to remove the organs. The donor is treated like any other surgical patient except that no anesthesia is used.

Many families like to know how the recipient's new transplanted organs have fared and how the recipient is progressing. Some centers offer a service for a year. Some families actually meet each other if the desire is mutual.[17]

Acute and Subacute Care

■ Nursing Management of the Medical Client

Assessment

Frequent, systematic, and objective nursing assessment, including neurologic status, is essential. Serial observations are important for comparison and to facilitate prompt reporting of even subtle changes in status. Even if assessment findings seem insignificant for long periods, documentation provides an objective pattern and an important baseline for future observations. Assessment of orientation levels is most effective when the caregivers performing the assessments are consistent. The neurologic assessment is performed as often as every 15 minutes during the first few hours of unconsciousness. Depending on the patient's condition, assessments may need to be continued hourly for several days.

Periodically assess the entire body, observing for lacerations, bruises, ulcerations, fractures, dislocations, and contractures. Also note skin color, texture, and temperature. Inspect dressings frequently for purulent or bloody drainage and head dressings for CSF leakage.

The Critical Monitoring feature lists the neurologic manifestations of a person who is unconscious. Note that it is ordered according to the seriousness of the presenting manifestation. Remembering these subtle changes in assessment will help you in early identification of a patient's improvement or worsening. A decrease in the patient's Glasgow Coma Scale (GCS) score also indicates worsening. The GCS is the most common neurologic assessment tool used in clinical practice. See Chapter 30 for a copy of the GCS and further discussion.

Diagnosis, Planning, Implementation

This section describes interventions appropriate for all unconscious patients regardless of the cause of the coma. Interventions specific to particular etiologic factors are described in other sections of the book (e.g., hepatic coma in Chapter 65, and uremic coma in Chapter 57).

Unconscious patients are completely dependent on others because their protective reflexes are impaired. Nursing intervention provides the safety normally afforded by protective reflexes. Unconsciousness is often life-threatening and requires aggressive medical intervention. Physicians are concerned with establishing a medical diagnosis and prescribing appropriate treatment; nurses are responsible for meeting basic human needs and preventing complications associated with unconsciousness. Nurses are also responsible for assessing and intervening to reduce ICP.

Altered tissue perfusion is one of the highest risks for a patient with an altered level of consciousness. This outcome is often seen as a direct consequence of increasing ICP. The nursing management of this problem is described in Chapter 32.

Risk for Suff
cannot swallow
or coughing
Airway ob
to patien
nosis a

Pl
exhibit n.
by no sign.
equal lung exp
pallor.

Implementation.
oral airway can be inser.
Endotracheal intubation, with
required to maintain airway pat
tion.

For extended airway management, a
be required to (1) allow long-term continu.
ventilation, (2) facilitate removal of tracheob.
cretions, and (3) separate the upper and lower
(see Chapter 40).

Risk for Aspiration. The lack of effective airway clearance and gag reflex makes the comatose patient at very high risk of aspiration. Write the diagnosis as *Risk for Aspiration related to lack of effective airway clearance and loss of gag reflex.*

Planning: Expected Outcomes. The patient will exhibit no signs of aspiration, as evidenced by clear lung sounds, no stridor, no fever, minimal amounts of clear mucus upon suctioning, and a clear chest x-ray.

Implementation. Keep suctioning equipment available. Often, an open route (tracheostomy or endotracheal tube) for tracheal suction is lifesaving for a comatose patient. Assess breath sounds every hour or two in acutely ill patients. Monitor the results of arterial blood gas analysis and pulse oximetry to determine the degree of oxygenation provided by ventilators or oxygen. Perform frequent tracheobronchial suctioning to prevent or decrease the accumulation of secretions from immobility, the lack of a cough and sigh reflex, or pneumonia. While suctioning, observe the cardiac monitor for dysrhythmias (e.g., premature ventricular contractions) secondary to hypoxia. Hyperoxygenating the patient before, between, and after suctioning will decrease the risk of dysrhythmias. Suctioning should be gentle and the catheter should not remain in the airway for longer than 10 seconds. Hyperoxygenation and limiting the suctioning time to 10 seconds will minimize increased ICP associated with suctioning. Transient increases in ICP do not cause irreversible brain damage. However, not suctioning a person who cannot expectorate his or her own secretions can cause hypoxia and result in neurologic damage. Never suction the nasal passages in patients who have had brain surgery or head injuries. The suction catheter can cause further trauma, increase the risk of CSF leakage, and introduce bacteria leading to meningitis. Premedication with lidocaine may minimize the increase in ICP with suctioning. Lidocaine can be given intratracheally or IV.

A comatose patient may lack pharyngeal reflexes and is therefore unable to swallow. Pneumonia secondary to as-

CRITICAL MONITORING

Manifestations of Changes in Neurologic Status

Anticipation is the key word. Notify the physician whenever there is a change in the patient's neurologic status. The following manifestations are listed in the order that indicates a _worsening_ in the patient's condition. Remember that the patient may display a "transient" deterioration in neurologic responses that does not warrant calling a physician. For example, after you have just suctioned a patient, or turned him or her, you would anticipate a possible change in neurologic status. If you hyperoxygenate the patient and ensure proper positioning for venous return from the jugular veins and airway maintenance, however, any signs of increased deficit should last only a few seconds or no more than 4 or 5 minutes. Signs of increased deficit that last longer than this increase the risk for irreversible brain injury.

Normal

Alert, oriented to person, place, time
Responds appropriately to verbal commands
Eyes open spontaneously with any stimulus, unless in a deep sleep

Abnormal; Related to Altered Perfusion of Cerebral Cortex

Altered level of consciousness
Altered perception of time, then place, and lastly person
Motor deficits (e.g., hemiparesis, hemiplegia)
Speech deficits (e.g., expressive or receptive speech, or both)
Memory deficits (e.g., recent, intermediate, remote)
Hyperreflexia
Babinski's sign
Seizures
Decorticate rigidity
Emotional lability
Altered sensory interpretation
Cheyne-Stokes respiration
Headache, nausea, vomiting, papilledema

Abnormal; Related to Altered Perfusion Just Inferior to the Cortex

Pupillary changes: asymmetry of size, shape, or time-responsiveness
Loss of reaction to direct light
Visual field changes (e.g., homonymous hemianopsia; see Chapter 32)

Abnormal; Related to Altered Perfusion of the Diencephalon

Altered temperature; first high fevers, then hypothermia
Cheyne-Stokes respiration

---

piration is a common cause of death in unconscious patients. To decrease the risk of aspiration, never give a comatose patient fluids to swallow. Secretions also accumulate in the posterior pharynx and may be aspirated. Suction the upper trachea and posterior pharynx as often as necessary to remove secretions. After tracheal suctioning, the same suction catheter can be used for oral or pharyngeal suctioning, but not vice versa. Also, turn the patient from side to side every 2 hours to facilitate drainage of secretions and prevent pneumonia. Note, however, that a patient suffering from a stroke has altered perfusion on the affected side and may only be able to tolerate 30 minutes on that side.

While performing mouth care, place a comatose patient in a lateral position to prevent aspiration. If facial paralysis is present, keep the affected side uppermost. Keep the patient's mouth open by placing an oral airway or bite-block between the teeth. Pay close attention to the roof of the mouth in patients who breathe through their mouth for long periods. Crusts may form, break off, and be aspirated. Use of artificial moisturizers may help prevent crust formation.

As consciousness returns and the client begins to respond to verbal stimuli and has a gag reflex, test the client's ability to suck and swallow liquid. Before the test, position the client in high Fowler's position and have suction equipment nearby in case it is needed. Use a thick juice, nectar, or ice chips rather than water. A thick consistency is easier to swallow. Place about 1 tsp of liquid into the back of the mouth. Observe for swallowing. Suction as needed to prevent aspiration. If a client cannot suck through a straw or drink from a glass because of facial paralysis, place fluids into the unaffected side of the mouth with an Asepto syringe. Watch for

Abnormal; Related to Altered Perfusion of the Posterior Pituitary

Diabetes insipidus (decreased antidiuretic hormone, resulting in abnormally large urinary output)

Abnormal; Related to Altered Perfusion of the Midbrain

Dysfunction of CN III (loss of reaction to indirect or consensual light, dysconjugate eye movement)
Dysfunction of CN IV (dysconjugate eye movement)
Central neurogenic hyperventilation

Abnormal; Related to Altered Perfusion of the Upper Pons

Dysfunction of CN V (altered sensory function to cornea, nasal membranes, face, oral cavity, tongue, teeth, or altered mastication)
Dysfunction of CN VI (altered lateral eye movement)
Dysfunction of CN VII (altered facial expression, taste, and salivation)
Central neurogenic hyperventilation
Abnormal extension posture
Pinpoint pupils

Abnormal; Related to Altered Perfusion of the Lower Pons

Apneustic breathing
Flaccidity

Abnormal; Related to Altered Perfusion of the Medulla

Dysfunction of CN VIII (altered equilibrium and hearing)
Dysfunction of CN IX (altered taste, pharyngeal sensations, and cough and swallowing)
Dysfunction of CN X (altered sensations in pharynx, larynx, external ear, and altered cough and swallowing; altered parasympathetic nervous system functions in thoracic and abdominal viscera)
Dysfunction of CN XI (altered neck and shoulder movement)
Dysfunction of CN XII (altered tongue movement)
Projectile vomiting
Cushing's triad (increased systolic blood pressure, wide pulse pressure, bradycardia)
Ataxia (Biot's) breathing

difficulty in swallowing. Suction as needed. If there is any question as to a client's ability to swallow, a formal swallowing evaluation should be done by a speech therapist. Clients who cannot swallow for long periods of time may require placement of a gastrostomy tube. Many rehabilitation and extended care facilities require gastrostomy tubes rather than NG tubes because there is less risk of aspiration with gastrostomy feedings.

Swallowing can be stimulated by having the client lean the head forward and, after taking fluid, quickly tip the head backward. Stroking the anterior neck may also promote swallowing.

Once a client can safely swallow, begin small oral liquid feedings, progressing to a soft diet. Discontinue tube-feedings only when the client can take adequate nutrition orally. Many clients are fed orally during the daytime and tube-fed at night to maintain adequate nutrition.

When changing from tube-feeding to oral feeding, turn off the tube-feeding several hours before the meal. This will stimulate the appetite. When a client begins to eat independently, be reassuring and encouraging. Remind the client to eat slowly and to swallow after each bite. Position the client sitting up as tolerated.

Altered Oral Mucous Membrane. Several factors can lead to altered oral mucous membranes. The comatose patient is usually NPO (nothing by mouth), has an inability to swallow, and mouth-breathes. A possible nursing diagnosis might be *Altered Oral Mucous Membrane related to mouth breathing.*

Planning: Expected Outcomes. The patient will maintain intact oral mucous membranes, as evidenced by having oral and nasal mucous membranes that are pink, moist, and without lesions, crusts, or bloody drainage.

Implementation. Inspect the patient's mouth every 8 hours, using a flashlight and tongue depressor. Keep the patient's lips coated with a water-soluble lubricant to prevent encrustation, drying, and cracking. Carefully inspect a paralyzed cheek for crusts or other conditions requiring intervention. Provide oral hygiene to prevent excessive drying of oral mucous membranes and complications such as parotitis, aspiration, and respiratory tract infections.

Brush the patient's teeth with a small toothbrush at least twice a day. Then, rinse the mouth. Clean the oral mucous membranes (especially the roof of the mouth), tongue, and gums with toothettes. Avoid agents containing lemon or alcohol because these agents dry the membranes. While performing mouth care in an unconscious patient, suction excess secretions to prevent aspiration. Toothbrushes with suction attachments are now available at many agencies.

Nasal passages may become occluded because an unconscious patient is unable to sniff, blow, sneeze, or clear the nose. To clear the nasal passages of mucus and crust formations, gently swab the nose with an applicator moistened with water or normal saline. Then, apply a thin coat of water-soluble lubricant with a cotton-tipped applicator.

Do *not* clean the nasal passages or ears of patients who have had brain surgery or head injuries. If bleeding occurs from the ears or nose, or if CSF (a watery discharge) appears to be draining from these areas, notify the physician.

Risk for Impaired Skin Integrity. Normal reflexes reduce the risk of skin ischemia by signaling conscious (even sleeping) persons to shift their body weight. Comatose patients have lost these protective reflexes and are completely immobile. Sometimes the patients are agitated and can shear the skin with frequent nonpurposeful movements. This diagnosis also applies to these patients. Write the diagnosis as *Risk for Impaired Skin Integrity related to immobility.*

Planning: Expected Outcomes. The patient will have intact skin, as evidenced by no reddened areas over bony prominences and no areas or signs of skin irritation or dryness.

Implementation. Provide nursing intervention for all self-care needs, including bathing and care of the hair, skin, and nails. Patients often scratch themselves as the depth of unconsciousness lessens; therefore, keep the nails trimmed. Patients who are comatose for long periods may be lifted occasionally into a bathtub half-filled with warm water. It may be helpful to apply superfatty solutions (e.g., Castile soap, baby oil, or cold cream) daily and bathe the patient weekly to prevent loss of cutaneous oils and skin irritation and dryness. Perineal care should be performed at least every 8 hours and after every episode of incontinence. If perineal care is not effective for women with vaginal discharge or odor, consult the physician for cleaning douches.

When the patient cannot respond to local tissue hypoxia from being in one position for an extended period of time, the risk of pressure ulcers increases. Patients should be repositioned at least every 2 hours. If this is impossible because of the patient's medical condition, place the patient on a special mattress or bed (see Fig. 31–7). However, the use of a special bed does not eliminate the need to pad bony prominences and assess the skin every 4 hours. In addition, meet the nutritional needs of the patient to reduce the risk of pressure ulcers.

Risk for Contractures. Normal movement and stretch are needed to prevent tightening of one group of muscles. When muscle groups are not used during periods of immobility, contractures of joints can develop. Footdrop is of special concern. Write the diagnosis as *Risk for Contractures related to disuse.*

Planning: Expected Outcomes. Monitor the patient for risk of contractures, as evidenced by muscle resistance to full range of motion in any joint; presence of flexion positioning in wrists, elbows, and knees; and signs of footdrop.

Implementation. Prevent contractures by maintaining the patient's extremities in functional positions with proper support. Hand and forearm splints prevent flexion contracture of the fingers and wrist. Orthotic devices or high-top tennis shoes are used to support the feet. Remove the support devices every 4 hours for skin care and passive exercises.

Altered Nutrition: Less Than Body Requirements. Unconscious patients cannot eat and yet have normal or even increased metabolic needs, so they can quickly develop malnutrition. Write the diagnosis as *Altered Nutrition: Less than Body Requirements related to inability to eat or swallow.*

Planning: Expected Outcomes. The patient will demonstrate the following signs of adequate nutrition: stable weight; adequate calories for age, height, and weight; intake equaling output; incisions and wounds healing within 12 to 14 days; and hemoglobin, blood urea nitrogen, total lymphocyte count, total protein, and albumin levels within normal limits for age and sex.

Implementation. IV fluids are begun on admission for comatose patients. Initially the IV site provides access to the circulatory system for the administration of medications. Because fluid intake is restricted and limited glucose and few electrolytes are given by the IV route, an IV infusion cannot be considered nutritional support. Consider that a 1-L solution of 5% dextrose provides only 200 kilocalories!

Just because a patient is comatose, never assume that hunger is not present and caloric needs are reduced. In fact, the opposite is true; caloric needs are increased in patients with head injury. Nutritional and fluid needs of comatose patients are usually met through enteral feedings because of the risk of aspiration from the oral route. If the patient does not have paralytic ileus or delayed gastric emptying and if bowel sounds are audible, start enteral feedings (see Management and Delegation feature).

The nutritional requirements that follow brain injury

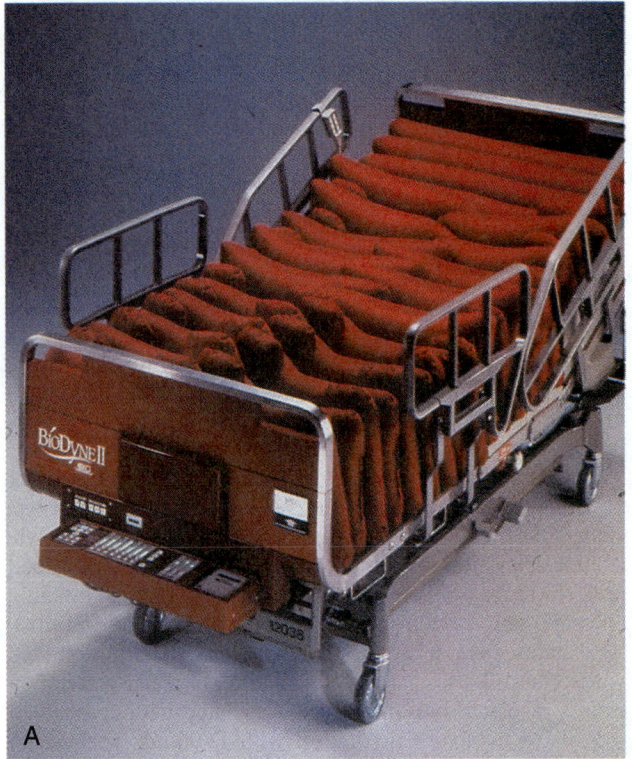

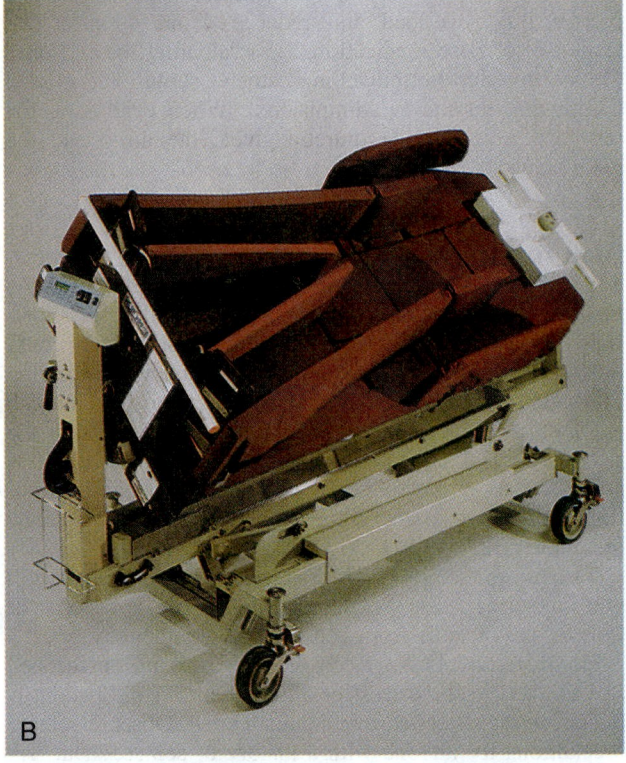

Figure 31–7. *A*, BIODYNE, an oscillating air support surface. *B*, ROTO REST, an oscillating bed. Both devices are used to treat hypoxemia and to reduce the incidence of nosocomial pneumonia. ROTO REST is also used for clients with spinal cord injury and skeletal traction. (Courtesy of Kinetic Concepts, Inc., San Antonio, TX.)

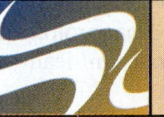

MANAGEMENT AND DELEGATION

Preparing Enteral Nutrition

Enteral nutrition may be delivered via oral, nasal, gastrostomy, or jejunostomy tubes. The delivery of enteral nutrition, including the verification of tube placement, is your responsibility. You may choose to delegate the reconstitution or preparation of enteral feedings to assistive personnel. Before delegating the preparation of tube feeding or refilling the nutrition reservoir bag, consider the following:

- Your abdominal assessment does not reveal abdominal distention, pain, discomfort, or complaints of nausea. Your examination includes verification of tube placement and the residual volume is less than 50% of the previous hour's intake. The presence of any of these findings would prompt you to hold the tube feeding and notify the physician of your examination findings.
- You have checked the physician's order for the type and rate of tube feeding to be delivered.
- The assistive personnel are instructed in the proper dilution and handling of enteral feeding. (*Hint:* When mixing powdered enteral feedings, always place the powder in the mixing container before the water; this will ensure the powder dissolves fully.)
- Assistive personnel are instructed to place a 4-hour supply of feeding in the reservoir bag and to store the remaining mixture in a refrigerator for future use. Label the storage container with the client's name, date on which mixture was prepared, and description of mixture.
- Assistive personnel may prime the pump. You must set the pump and ensure that the flow rate matches the ordered flow rate.
- You are responsible for performing any irrigation of the tube.
- Gastrostomy and jejunostomy tube site care may be delegated to assistive personnel.

Findings that are immediately reportable to you should be described for assistive personnel. This includes any difficulty in preparing the enteral feeding and client complaints of fullness, nausea, or vomiting.

The competence of the assistive personnel in performing these tasks should be verified during orientation and annually thereafter.

are complex; a complete nutritional assessment with comparison of height and weight charts, laboratory tests, and clinical examination is essential. There is a marked increase in metabolic needs with severe brain injury. Malnutrition increases the morbidity and mortality of neurologically ill patients. Diarrhea and delayed gastric emptying may result from malabsorption. Healing will not take place in the presence of a negative nitrogen state. Immunodeficiency with increased risk of infection, sepsis, stress ulcers, weight loss, skeletal muscle protein wasting, and lung tissue catabolism leading to diaphragmatic weakness with respiratory reduction result from prolonged calorie and protein deprivation. Starvation can lead to death.

Nursing responsibilities in tube-feeding unconscious patients are critical because these patients (1) cannot communicate and (2) may have lost protective cough and gag reflexes. The possible complications from enteral feeding include the following:

- Vomiting and aspiration if the stomach is overfilled.
- Tube dislocation into trachea or lungs, causing aspiration. Some facilities use food coloring to tint the tube feeding. Then, if suctioned secretions are the same color, aspiration is suspected. Unconscious patients are often restless. Watch that they do not pull out the tube. Aspiration may occur if a feeding tube is pulled out during a feeding session or whenever it is unclamped. During feeding sessions, cloth wristlets or wrist restraints may be needed. When tube-feeding a patient, elevate the head of the bed (HOB) at least 30 degrees to minimize possible aspiration. When possible, verify tube placement by aspirating for gastric contents. Some agency policies and some manufacturers of small-bore nasogastric (NG) tubes require checking placement by listening with a stethoscope for air "whooshing" when instilling air through the NG tube. Never tube-feed a patient in the supine position unless all other positions are impossible. Leave the HOB elevated 30 degrees for at least 30 minutes after bolus feedings.
- Ulcerated or crusted nares from local pressure from the feeding tube.
- Tracheoesophageal fistula, that is, breakdown of the anterior esophageal wall from prolonged contact between the NG tube and a tracheostomy tube. This complication is manifested by gastric contents in tracheal secretions. Notify the physician immediately.
- Trauma to the gastric mucosa if the tube's distal end hardens, as may happen over time.
- Delayed gastric emptying. Check residual volumes every 4 hours. If the residual volume is more than 100 ml, hold the feeding for 1 hour, then reassess. Also assess bowel sounds and check for gastric distention. If this complication persists after several hours, notify the physician. If there is a high suspicion that the patient has developed a bowel obstruction, do not return the gastric residue to the stomach.
- Fluid volume deficit if hypertonic tube feedings are given. To prevent this problem, ensure that the client receives approximately 1 ml of fluid for every kilocalorie of feeding. Depending on your agency's policy, this may require consulting with the dietitian or the physician.
- Constipation or diarrhea may develop from the osmolarity of the feeding, the use of liquid medications with a sorbitol base, or a too rapid infusion.

Risk for Fluid Volume Deficit. The comatose patient cannot drink fluids and respond to normal thirst mechanisms and is therefore at *Risk for Fluid Volume Deficit*. Recall that hypertonic tube feedings also increase this risk.

Planning: Expected Outcomes. The patient will demonstrate the following signs of fluid balance: as evidenced by intake and output that are equal for 24, 48, and 72 hours; stable body weight; no signs of excessive perspiration, diarrhea, or vomiting; serum glucose, hematocrit, and blood urea nitrogen, creatinine, sodium, potassium, and chloride within normal limits. Oral mucous membranes are moist and there are no tongue furrows.

Implementation. Important aspects in maintaining fluid-electrolyte balance in unconscious patients are (1) accurate intake and output documentation; (2) daily weighing with comparison of trends; and (3) assessing and documenting conditions that may increase fluid volume deficit (e.g., diaphoresis, polyuria, diarrhea, vomiting, or hypertonic tube feedings).

Before fluid and electrolyte intervention is planned for a comatose patient, carefully assess the fluid-electrolyte status. The coma itself may be due to fluid-electrolyte causes. Blood tests such as blood sugar, hematocrit, blood urea nitrogen or creatinine, serum sodium, potassium, chloride, and carbon dioxide help determine fluid-electrolyte status (see Chapters 13 and 15). Dehydration and water intoxication (true hyponatremia) are common causes of electrolyte imbalance associated with coma.

Always avoid overhydration with IV fluids because of the risk of cerebral edema. Diuretics may be prescribed to correct fluid overload and reduce edema. Monitor the response to these medications. In evaluating the response to any diuretic, the indwelling catheter should be emptied before the diuretic is administered. When evaluating the response, consider the diuretic given, the dose, and the renal status.

Risk for Injury. It may not be apparent that the comatose patient is at *Risk for Injury* because there is no movement. If the patient's coma starts to lighten, however, he or she can move and without protection could fall or be injured. In addition, use caution when moving the patient, since he or she cannot voice pain. Although the loss of the corneal blink reflex, which increases the risk of corneal abrasions, is also a type of injury, it is addressed as a collaborative problem. Nursing interventions for a loss of the corneal blink reflex are discussed in Chapter 32.

Planning: Expected Outcomes. The patient will not sustain injury, as evidenced by no abrasions or bruises and no falls from bed.

Implementation. Keep the side rails up on the bed and the bed in the lowest position whenever the patient is not receiving direct care or is unattended. Observe seizure precautions for anyone with a history of seizure or at risk of seizure. Protect the patient from injury during seizures or periods of agitation (e.g., use padded side rails, keep the patient's nails short and filed). It is of utmost importance to protect the patient's head. Give the prescribed seizure medication on time to maintain a high seizure threshold. If the client misses a dose of the medication for any reason (e.g., vomiting), notify the physician. Anticonvulsant medication should not be withheld without a physician order.

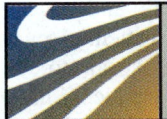

ETHICAL ISSUES IN NURSING

What Are the Ethical Concerns Surrounding the Use of Physical Restraints?

You are working in an acute care unit and are assigned to care for a 72-year-old man who tripped at home and sustained a mild subdural hematoma. The client is confused and is climbing over the bed rails. To safeguard him, you must either watch him at all times or apply physical restraint. Unfortunately, you are also caring for five other clients and have only one aide to help with all the patients on the unit. Is it appropriate to use physical restraints on this client?

Nurses use physical restraints in healthcare institutions to protect confused clients from injury. Unfortunately, nurses often fail to analyze carefully the ethical issues involved in the use of restraints before applying them. In the case of this 72-year-old client, as with every client, it is important to assess the person individually to determine the appropriateness of physical restraints. Be certain that the only reason for the use of restraints is to protect the client from harm. Restraints have often been used for other, inappropriate reasons such as to protect the institution from legal liability or for the convenience of the nursing staff.

To determine whether restraints are appropriate for this client, assess the client's risk of harm. Consider the magnitude of the risk and probability of injury to the client. This risk must be significant to justify the use of restraints.

Assess the client's capacity to make genuine autonomous decisions in light of any mental confusion or other mental disturbances. Restraints impair the client's autonomy, so you must determine that the client no longer has the capacity to make genuine autonomous decisions before applying restraints.

Also, assess the client's ability to deal with the psychological trauma of being restrained. Physical restraints can pose a significant psychological burden to a client, and some people are much more sensitive to the use of restraints than others.

The consideration of other clients is also important. If you do not use physical restraints for a client who is confused and trying to get out of bed, other clients may suffer. For example, you might be tempted to stay in the room with the confused client when you should be providing care for other clients. By not restraining the confused 72-year-old man, you might bring harm to other clients who need your attention.

If you determine that leaving your client alone and unrestrained poses a significant risk of injury and jeopardizes the care of your other clients, and if you must leave him alone, you can carefully apply restraints and monitor them according to the standards of the institution. The use of physical restraints requires prudent ethical analysis.

Give adequate support to the limbs and head when moving or turning an unconscious patient. Limbs without tone may dislocate if they are allowed to fall unsupported. Always turn an unconscious patient toward you or someone else to prevent falls. Protect an unconscious patient from external sources of heat (e.g., heating pads).

Do not restrain the patient unless it is absolutely necessary because restraint is likely to increase confused and combative behavior. The Ethical Issues in Nursing feature explores the ethical concerns surrounding the use of restraints. If used, restraints must be released at least every 2 hours for range-of-motion and skin checks. Do not leave unstable patients unattended. Sometimes agencies hire "sitters"; ask for volunteer services, or rely on family members or friends to assist in providing this need. Avoid oversedation because it may alter respirations, which increases ICP and masks changes in a patient's level of consciousness.

Fecal Incontinence. Once the patient's gastrointestinal tract is moving food, the client will produce feces. Most patients are incontinent because voluntary control is required for the function of the external anal sphincter. Write the diagnosis as *Bowel Incontinence related to inability to respond to normal cues about evacuation.* Also consider using the nursing diagnosis of *High Risk for Impaired Skin Integrity related to fecal incontinence.*

Planning: Expected Outcomes. The patient will have reduced fecal incontinence, as evidenced by a bowel movement every 2 to 3 days and no signs of fecal impaction.

Implementation. Plan interventions to (1) control bowel movements, (2) maintain the patient's normal schedule, and (3) prevent fecal impaction or constipation. As soon as the patient is able, begin a program of bowel retraining. Maintain a regular schedule of stool softeners, suppositories, and digital removal at approximately the same time each day. Examine the abdomen frequently for distention. Constipation and fecal impaction may occur. Small, frequent liquid stools may indicate impaction. If diarrhea or constipation persists, assess for possible causes such as medications, enteral feedings, or intestinal bacterial infections.

Caution: Consult with the physician prior to doing a digital removal on a patient with an altered level of consciousness. This intervention has been known to induce seizures. Use of an anesthetic jelly rectally prior to the stimulus decreases this risk.

Altered Family Processes. Having a family member in a coma is a significant stressor for the family. A lot of nursing care will be directed toward the family. A possible diagnosis is *Altered Family Processes related to uncertain future or impending death of a family member.* Individualize the etiology portion of the diagnosis to fit your specific patient and family.

Planning: Expected Outcomes. The family members will exhibit positive coping behaviors, as evidenced by showing an ability to solve problems, meet the needs of other family members, and ask questions about the patient that indicate that previous teaching has been understood.

Implementation. The significant others of a comatose patient are often very stressed. It is difficult for the family when they cannot communicate with the patient. The uncertainty of not knowing whether the patient will recover is a major stressor. Include family members in the patient's care to the extent that they can and want to be involved. It is important that the family see the patient receiving high-quality, professional, and caring nursing care. For example, talk to the patient as if he or she can understand. Initially, this behavior will seem awkward, but in time it will feel appropriate. Tell the patient that he or she will be turned to the side, bathed, and so on. Depending on the depth of the coma, the patient's sense of hearing may still be intact. Therefore, speak to the patient as if he or she can hear. Comatose patients have awakened and reported that they remember hearing specific voices.

The family is often in a state of shock, needing someone to recognize their needs and help them through this difficult situation. They may experience various conflicting feelings such as guilt and anger. The Client Education Guide suggests ways for the patient's family members to cope with these feelings.

Allow the significant others to stay with the patient

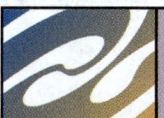

CLIENT EDUCATION GUIDE

When a Loved One Is in an Altered State of Consciousness

Family Instructions in English *(Instrucciones para la familia en inglés)*	**Family Instructions in Spanish** *(Instrucciones para la familia en español)*
Seeing a loved one in this state causes a roller coaster of feelings (e.g., denial, anger, depression, guilt, bargaining). There is no "correct" order for these feelings; they may recur even after one thinks they have been worked through. Feelings are normal. It is important to "give yourself permission" to feel, so that you can work through the grieving process.	El ver a una persona amada en un estado de coma causa una serie de sentimientos inexplicables (p. ej.: rechazo de la realidad, enojo, depresión, culpa, deseo de nacer tratos). No se sabe en qué orden van a surgir estos sentimientos; pueden ocurrir aún cuando se piense que se han resuelto. El sentir estas emociones es normal. Es importante "permitirse" experimentar estos sentimientos para dominarlos y poder resolver su pena.
Talk to and touch your loved one. Research supports the positive outcomes of coma stimulation, which includes talking to and touching the person.[14]	Acaricie y hable con su ser amado. Las investigaciones apoyan resultados positivos producidos por el estímulo durante el estado de coma, los cuales incluyen tocar y hablarle a la persona.[17]
Become involved in the care of your loved one, including care plan decisions.	Participe en el cuidado de su ser amado inclusive en las decisiones del planeamiento del cuidado.
Learn about the devices and equipment used to monitor and treat your loved one.	Aprenda como funcionan los aparatos y el equipo que se usan para controlar y tratar a su ser amado.
Stay informed of your loved one's condition. Ask a nurse to reinforce or explain information provided by the physician and to clarify any medical jargon that you do not understand.	Manténgase informado sobre el estado de salud de su ser amado. Pidale a la/al enfermera(o) que le explique la información que le da el/la médico(a) y le aclare cualquier término médico que no entienda.
If the physician has indicated that there is no chance for your loved one's recovery, refocus your energies into hoping for a peaceful death. Consider organ donation; this has helped other families with their healing.	Si el/la médico(a) ha indicado que su ser amado no podrá recuperarse, enfoque sus energías en esperar una muerte tranquila. Considere la donación de órganos; esto ha ayudado a otras familias a recuperarse de su pesar.
Join a support group, whether your loved one is expected to die or stay at this level of altered consciousness for an indeterminate time. Through reaching out, you may be able to find strength and meaning in this tragedy.	Unase a un grupo de apoyo, bien sea que se espere la muerte de su ser amado, o que se espere que quede en estado de coma por un tiempo indeterminado. El aceptar ayuda le podrá dar fuerza para sobrellevar y comprender esta tragedia.

when and where this is possible. At times, family members may become zealous in attending and stay at the patient's bedside continuously. Encourage family members to care for themselves also by encouraging adequate meals and sleep. Have them consider using external support systems (e.g., neighbors and church groups). Tell them that they will be called if any significant changes occur, and ask them to leave a phone number where they can be reached. Encourage family members to call if they have questions or concerns.

Some hospitals, especially tertiary care centers, have "family homes" that provide family members who travel a long distance to the hospital a place to stay and be close to the hospital and patient.

Evaluation

The patient may remain comatose for a few hours or even months. Some comatose patients (e.g., patients with diabetic coma) awaken and make a complete recovery while in the hospital. Therefore, some expected outcomes have brief time frames (e.g., airway obstruction), whereas others are prolonged, requiring frequent reevaluation (e.g., family coping). Your evaluation may identify a need for a care plan revision.

■ Modifications for Elderly Clients

The aged patient in a coma requires the same quality of care as other age groups. However, the aged patient is at higher risk of all complications of immobility, especially pressure ulcers and pneumonia. Urinary retention is common in male patients because of prostatic enlargement. Finally, fully assess the patient for the common disorders of aging (e.g., diabetic coma) that might be the cause of the coma.

Community and Self-Care

The site of discharge from an acute care setting is totally dependent on the condition of the patient, the cause of the coma, and the level of family support available. If the patient is still in a coma and recovery is expected, plan for placement in a rehabilitation center. In these centers, besides supportive care, the focus is often centered on coma stimulation.[6]

If the patient is in a coma and is not expected to awaken but may live for a time with nutritional support, placement in a skilled nursing center is common. In these centers, supportive care is given. Family members usually specify how aggressively they want the patient treated in case of deterioration in status. Your role in discharge of the comatose patient centers on communication with the receiving nurses and family. If the patient is ventilator-dependent or combative, special consideration is required for transport to the new facility. Provide a complete plan of care.

Confusional States

Confusion is a mental state marked by alterations in thought and attention deficit followed by problems in comprehension. Confusion is accompanied by a loss of short-term memory and often irritability alternating with drowsiness. Confusion is a common clinical manifestation in many neurologic and metabolic disorders. *Sundowning* is defined as agitation, confusion, and restlessness that occurs after the sun sets[13, 15]; however, diurnal variations may be responsible for these changes as well.[1]

The Nursing Research Feature describes the relationship between confusion and increased morbidity and increased length of hospital stay. This relationship has major implications in terms of cost containment, especially because people over age 85 are the fastest-growing U.S. age group.

Etiology and Risk Factors

There are many causes of confusion. Common causes of acute confusion are alcohol withdrawal and drug ingestion. Confusion can also follow fever, heart failure, head injury, or anesthetics. Other causes of confusion are hypoxia, hypoglycemia, severe fluid and electrolyte disorders, sepsis, liver and renal failure, poisons, and drug overdose. Delirium and dementia are classifications of types of confusion.

Three commonalities exist with all types of *delirium:*

1. A disturbance of consciousness with a reduced ability to focus, sustain, or shift attention
2. A change in cognition (memory, language, disorientation) or development of a perceptual disturbance that is not better accounted for by a preexisting, established, or evolving dementia
3. A change that develops over a short period of time (hours to days) and may fluctuate during the course of the day

There are several classifications that have each of the three commonalities but have specific causes. These include the delirium related to a general medical condition, to substance intoxication (prescribed, over-the-counter medications, or street drugs), to substance withdrawal, to multiple causes, and the delirium "not otherwise specified."[5]

Dementia is the chronic form of confusion. As with delirium, there are commonalities that exist among the many types of dementia. They include:

1. The development of multiple memory impairments
2. One or more of the following cognitive disturbances: aphasia, apraxia, agnosia, impaired executive functioning
3. Significant impairment and decline in social or occupational functioning
4. A gradual onset and continuing cognitive decline

The classifications of dementia include the four commonalities with variable causes and characteristics. There are many subtypes of dementia of the Alzheimer's type.

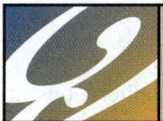

NURSING RESEARCH

How Does Client Confusion Affect Intervention and Discharge Choices?

Shedd, P. P., Kobokovich, L. J., and Slattery, M. J. (1995). Confused patients in the acute care setting: Prevalence, intervention, and outcomes. *Journal of Gerontological Nursing, 21*(4), 5–12.

Managing confused patients is a major problem for nurses. Confusion also has been associated with increased morbidity, length of stay in the hospital, and need for placement in extended care facilities.

Shedd and colleagues conducted a descriptive study of all clients on three medical-surgical units (N = 843 clients) over a 2-year period. The purpose of the study was threefold: (1) to determine nurses' assessment of the prevalence of confused clients at an institution before and after relocation to a new facility, (2) to determine whether environmental factors, such as noise and the surroundings, in the new facility were related to the incidence of confusion, and (3) to describe the characteristics of confused clients.

The authors found that out of the 843 clients, 82 were confused. Of the confused clients, 37 (45%) had neurologic alterations, 22 (26%) had hematologic or oncologic problems, and 23 (28%) had experienced general surgery. Confused clients were also significantly older: 64.5 years (SD=18) compared to 58 years (SD=17) for nonconfused clients.

Thirty-six clients (48%) were identified as having restlessness. Interventions for restlessness included restraints for 19 clients (53%), sitters for 8 clients (22%), and medications for 17 clients (47%).

The relationship between confusion and outcome at discharge was significant. Only 9% of the confused clients went home, whereas 60% of the nonconfused clients went home. Thirty-four percent of the confused clients went home with a visiting nurse referral; 24% of the nonconfused clients needed referral. Forty-four percent of the confused clients were institutionalized and 11% died; 10% of the nonconfused clients required institutionalization and 4% died.

Documentation of confusion was found in 63 (78%) of the nurses' notes but only 34 (42%) had a nursing care plan follow-up. None of the interventions for confusion were mentioned in either the nurses' notes or care plans.

Implications for Practice

Regardless of the cause of confusion, healthcare costs were high because of extended hospital stays and increased need for posthospital care. Cost is also a major concern because this population continues to increase. Using home health services and caregivers instead of extended care placement for the mildly confused, whenever possible, will help to decrease costs and keep the client at home. In addition, initiating discharge planning at the time of admission to include long-term placement will avoid transfer delays.

Care strategies also must address these environmental and long-term considerations. An accurate history is essential to gauge a client's change in level of confusion. Documentation in the nurses' notes and the care plan is essential to continuity of care.

Finally, methods for confusion intervention (such as use of restraints) must be evaluated using a team approach and data in current literature.

Essentially, all other causes such as CNS disorders, systemic conditions, substance-induced conditions, depression, and schizophrenia must be ruled out. The other types of dementia include vascular dementia (multi-infarct), the dementia secondary to other general medical conditions, the substance-induced persisting dementia, the dementia due to multiple causes, and the dementia "not otherwise specified."[5] An in-depth discussion of the care related to specific types of delirium and dementia, as well as the memory changes with amnestic disorders and other cognitive disorders not meeting the criteria for any of the above classifications, is beyond the scope of this book. The reader is referred to a psychiatric textbook for this information. This section focuses on the general care of a client with confusion. However, since dementia of the Alzheimer's type is an increasing problem, Chapter 34 presents an in-depth discussion of the pathology and care related to a client with this type of degenerative disease.

Risk factors leading to confusion vary with the specific etiologic factors. In general, the proper management of various diseases, such as diabetes mellitus, would reduce the incidence of confusion. Disorders such as Alzheimer's disease have no known prevention at this time. Primary, secondary and tertiary prevention are discussed in Risk Factors and Levels of Prevention.

Pathophysiology

Three mechanisms account for the development of acute confusion: (1) damage to the brain with swelling or loss of oxygen, blood, or both (functional disorder); (2) impairment of the action of the nervous system by chemicals or other substances (metabolic disorder); and (3) the rebound overactivity of a previously depressed center in the brain. Chemicals that cross the blood-brain barrier, such as alcohol, impair the metabolism of neuronal cells. When the drug action wears off or the client is withdrawn from the drug, the lower centers in the brain are overactive. This overactivity accounts for the development of acute confusion, combativeness, and other abnormal behaviors.

Chronic confusional states are disorders that cause brain tissue destruction, biochemical imbalances, or compression of the brain. For example, persons with Alzheimer's disease have a lack of acetylcholine, a neurotransmitter that is necessary for short-term memory. Other disorders causing chronic confusion may be inherited, be secondary to a transmissable agent as with Creutzfeldt-Jakob disease, or follow diseases such as encephalitis.

Clinical Manifestations and Diagnostic Findings

The earliest sign of a brain disorder is a *disorder of attention.* The client may report the loss of concentration or appear preoccupied. At the same time, restlessness, emotional lability, insomnia or drowsiness, and vivid nightmares may begin. Clients may appear anxious and fear that they are "going crazy." As the disorder progresses, stupor and coma develop. Behaviors seen in the client are reflective not of personality but of the cause of the disorder. For example, barbiturate or alcohol abuse and withdrawal and liver disorders cause agitated delirium. In contrast, anoxia and kidney and lung disorders are associated with a quieter response. Disorders that develop rapidly are more likely to cause an agitated response than are those that develop slowly.

Fluctuations in cognition (the ability to think and reason) are common in patients with metabolic brain disorders. Clients may be totally irrational one moment and lucid the next. Some of the fluctuations are caused by the environment. Delirious clients become more disoriented at night, in unfamiliar surroundings, when unfamiliar noises are heard, when unfamiliar people are seen, or when restraints are used. The lack of a window in the room has caused many clients to become disoriented.

Loss of memory for recent events is a hallmark of metabolic brain disorders. The client will commonly have difficulty with immediate recall and ability for abstract thought. Clients who are delirious quickly lose orientation to time. Normal persons can readily recall six or seven digits forward and five or six backward and identify the commonalities between an orange and an apple or a tree and a bush. Delirious clients cannot do this. However, the client's general intelligence level can have an impact on the data seen. If possible, the client's level of education should be known before the assessment.

Perceptual errors (e.g., mistaking the nurse for a daughter) as well as hallucinations, illusions, and delusions are common accompaniments of delirium.

Hallucinations are sensations occurring in the absence of external stimuli. A client may hear, see, feel, smell, or taste something that is not present. The client may or may not realize that the experience is "unreal."

Illusions differ from hallucinations in that illusions are the misinterpretation of something in the environment. For example, if a client sees a shadow on the drape and mistakes it for a real person, the client is experiencing an illusion.

Delusions are thoughts or beliefs that have no basis in fact. For example, a client may think that he or she has been robbed or poisoned, when there is no basis for this thought.

There are no specific diagnostic tests for confusion. The client may have a CT or MRI scan to determine whether there is a structural cause of the confusion, such as a tumor. In addition, a series of laboratory studies may be performed to determine whether there is a metabolic cause. Common studies include a complete blood count, electrolyte determinations, determination of vitamin B_{12} and folate levels, thyroid and liver function studies, drug toxicity screening tests, and an EEG. A lumbar puncture may be performed for the analysis of CSF.

 ## Acute and Subacute Care

In all care settings, the medical management of the confused client begins by determining the cause of the confusion and correcting it, if possible. When no specific cause is found, the medical management focuses on controlling manifestations. At times, haloperidol can be given to calm agitation. Nutritional needs also must be monitored.

■ Nursing Management of the Medical Client

Assessment

The confused client needs a thorough history. The history should include the onset of the confusion, past medical illnesses, work and occupational history, and past injuries. Disorders such as diabetes or liver failure may be out of control and the cause of the confusion. The client may have been exposed to heavy metals or toxic wastes at work. Record past injuries, especially head injury. Depending on the level of confusion, the client may not be able to answer each question, and you may need to rely on the family or others who have been with the client. Specific questions as to the client's ability to handle routine financial transactions or home safety with tasks such as cooking, dressing, and driving will help determine whether the client can be safely returned home or is in need of an alternative arrangement. At times the family may report a change in personality, such as apathy, social isolation, disinterest in current events, and irritability. Record these data because they may be clinical manifestations of Alzheimer's disease or frontal lobe lesions.

The confused client needs ongoing assessment with the Glasgow Coma Scale or the Mini-Mental State examination. The Mini-Mental State examination is much more sensitive for serial evaluations of confused clients.[3] Analyze the data collected to determine whether the confusion is improving, worsening, or unchanged.

The confused client is often combative and argumentative. Assess whether the client is able to refrain from self-injury or injury to others. If not bedfast, the client may

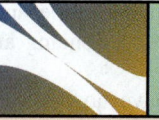

RISK FACTORS AND LEVELS OF PREVENTION

Injury Secondary to Confusion

Risk Factors

- Medical conditions that alter cognitive function directly (e.g., brain injury from a stroke or head trauma; lesions such as hematomas; tumors; inflammatory processes such as meningitis or encephalitis; degenerative diseases such as Alzheimer's dementia, AIDS encephalopathy, Parkinson's disease, Huntington's disease, Pick's disease, or Creutzfeldt-Jakob disease)
- Metabolic changes (e.g., liver, kidney, respiratory, or cardiac diseases; fluid, electrolyte, or acid-base disturbances)
- Side effects of administration or withdrawal of medication, including prescription, over-the-counter, and street drugs

Levels of Prevention

Primary Prevention

- Teach the client and family to monitor for periods of confusion.
- Teach the client to avoid high-risk activities during periods of confusion: operating heavy machinery, driving a vehicle, engaging in high-risk sports or recreational activities (e.g., bicycling, motorcycling, skateboarding).

Secondary Prevention

To minimize agitation, confusion, and psychological pain:

- Help the client to interpret his or her reality (avoid global issues and time-oriented responses if they increase agitation).
- Allow time for a slower response.
- Provide individual attention, reassurance, and support.
- Use a quiet, calm approach.
- Use familiar phrases.
- Redirect or distract if repetitive thoughts are increasing agitation or confusion.
- Minimize environmental stimuli, unless it has a calming effect.

To maintain normalcy and increase a feeling of security, self-esteem, and social adequacy:

- Encourage family members to visit and call on the telephone.
- Assign the same staff to care for the client.
- Provide environmental cues such as a name or picture on the client's door and a sign on the bathroom door.
- Provide familiar objects, music, and personal items.
- Manage behavioral disturbances.

---

wander about and get lost or injured if harmful items are not secured (e.g., knives).

Confusion can occur in clients of any age, culture, or from variable causes. The nurse's role as a client advocate supersedes personal bias related to any of these variables. See the Ethical Issues in Nursing feature for an example of this type of advocacy.

Diagnosis, Planning, Implementation

One of our roles as nurses is to teach unlicensed personnel how to care for a client with confusion. The Nursing Research feature describes the interventions and outcomes in a study in which nurses' aides were trained to care for residents with sundowning.

Altered Thought Processes. Use the nursing diagnosis *Altered Thought Processes related to failure in*

memory and lack of self-protective behavior to address needs for safety.

Planning: Expected Outcomes. The client will have improved thought processes, as evidenced by improving scores on the Mini-Mental State examination and decreased frequency of hallucinations, illusions, and delusions.

Implementation. The confused client will benefit from consistency in the environment and care routine. Keep objects in the same place, such as the tray table and bedside chair. If possible, the same staff should care for the client. When the routine is changed, give the client short explanations as events occur, such as "You need an x-ray" and "Please sit in the wheelchair." Telling the client that "in 2 hours an x-ray tech will be coming to take you for a CAT scan" will be neither understood nor remembered.

Reorient the client as often as necessary, but use caution as to the specific communication used. Clients with

To meet basic needs:

- Maintain a routine care schedule for eating, toileting, activity, and rest.

To manage behavior disturbances and to guide the client through the experience of disturbance as quickly as possible with minimal physical or chemical intervention:

- Identify the specific early signs, patterns, or triggers that initiate a behavioral disturbance. Communicate these signs to other staff when planning for the client's care.
- Intervene calmly and redirect the client away from the situation.
- Tolerate or ignore repetitive behavior or speech if the client cannot be redirected and is not harming himself or herself or others.
- Provide the client with space and remove other clients or dangerous objects if the behavior disturbance escalates and there is potential for harm.
- Give psychotropic medications in low doses that maintain the client's functional abilities but reduce behavioral disturbances that cannot be managed by other interventions.
- Use physical restraints as a last resort to protect the client from harm to himself or herself or others.

Tertiary Prevention

All the interventions for secondary prevention are appropriate for tertiary prevention. In addition:

- Encourage the family to bring in familiar items such as pictures for an album or a personal bulletin board.
- Try to schedule group activities (e.g., dining, music, games) in the same room, with the same residents, at the same time of day, and with the same group leaders.
- Involve the resident in pet therapy.
- Involve the resident in reminiscence therapy.
- Use "wandering bracelets" or other alarm-activated systems to reduce the risk of the resident wandering from designated boundaries.

Adapted from Rantz, M. J., & McShane, R. E. (1994). Nursing-home staff perception of behavior disturbance and management of confused residents. *Applied Nursing Research, 7*(3), 132–140.

chronic untreatable confusion do not benefit from reorientation and may become more agitated when you attempt to reorient them. For example, in one study when a 92-year-old client was told that her mother or father could not possibly be alive, the client reacted each time as if it was the first time she had been told and grieved deeply each time.[11] For these select clients, avoid reorienting and "go along" with the confusion. Of course, when the client is at risk of injury, safety precautions must be foremost. Clocks and calendars in the room also help with reorientation. The use of familiar objects is helpful when remote memory is intact. For example, the use of a quilt from home on the bed may help the confused client recognize the bed as his or her own.

Unfamiliar noise should be reduced because it adds to the confusion. The client's room should be quiet and softly lighted without producing shadows.

Consistency in care of a client with confusion requires communication between caregivers. This communication is not only through the oral reporting method but also in the care plan and documentation records.

Risk for Injury. Confusion greatly increases risk of harm. The client cannot interpret or may not be able to respond to environmental stimuli that precede danger. Write the nursing diagnosis as *Risk for Injury related to the unpredictable behavior and inability to interpret environmental stimuli.*

Planning: Expected Outcomes. The client will not sustain injury and will not injure others.

Implementation. The client must be protected from self-injury. The client should be in a room near the nursing station so that frequent assessments can be performed every 30 to 60 minutes. In addition, the bed should be in low position. The routine use of physical restraints (e.g., side rails, cloth restraints) or chemical restraints (e.g., medication) has been discouraged since the Omnibus Budget Reconciliation Act (OBRA) of 1987. The use of

ETHICAL ISSUES IN NURSING

How Can Nurses Serve as Advocates for Confused Clients?

States of consciousness can be altered by many different factors, including disease, emotional stress, fatigue, poor nutrition, alcohol abuse, age-related pathologic changes, and sedation by medication. Such altered states may be temporary, induced by alcohol or sedatives, or long-lasting, like Alzheimer's disease or another disease process affecting cerebral activity. When a client experiences a change in consciousness, he or she may or may not be able to make rational decisions, particularly decisions about healthcare.

There is little question reqarding the decision-making capabilities of someone who is in a more permanently altered state of mind or who is unconscious. A patient who is in a coma or has severe senile dementia would never be deemed competent to make personal health-related decisions. A surrogate would always need to be consulted to make such decisions on behalf of and in the best interest of the patient. The client who is experiencing a *transient* altered state of mind, however, may erroneously be deemed competent to make healthcare decisions on his or her own behalf. The following is a true case presentation that illustrates this dilemma.

A 23-year-old gang member came to the emergency room of a local hospital with a puncture wound to the left eye and surrounding facial tissue. He was alone and was not combative. The smell of alcohol was heavy on his breath, and the stat alcohol level confirmed that he was legally intoxicated. The ophthalmology surgeon examined him and decided that he must have surgery as soon as possible to prevent possible loss of vision. The surgeon had the client sign a consent-for-surgery form; however, she would have to wait to operate until a second alcohol level could be drawn, approximately 2 hours later, because the client could not go to surgery with an elevated blood alcohol level. The nurse caring for the young man noticed that the consent form was signed while his blood alcohol level was high. She approached the surgeon and explained that such an "informed" consent was not valid, because the client was temporarily incompetent to sign such a document, and that another consent must be obtained before surgery, when the client's blood alcohol level was within normal limits. The surgeon did not think that this was necessary but did obtain a second consent when the client was no longer incompetent because of alcohol intoxication.

This case is an excellent example of the nurse's role as a client advocate. However tragic the loss of vision might have been for this client, he had a right to informed consent. Informed consent can never be obtained from a client who is not capable, for whatever reason, of understanding what he or she is consenting to. Nurses have an obligation to speak out when they believe, on the basis of their knowledge of the client, that their client's competence to make healthcare decisions is in doubt. However, medical personnel must always compare the risk of waiting to treat a client until informed consent is obtained against the right to informed consent. If the risk of waiting is too great, the procedure may need to be performed as a medical emergency.

---

side rails and restraints does not guarantee that clients will not fall, and often they make them more agitated or they suffer worse injury when they do fall. If all other alternatives have been unsuccessful, and restraints are used, make frequent assessments and record the data. Cloth restraints must be removed every 2 hours to assess the skin beneath them and range-of-motion exercises need to be performed. The side effects of chemical restraint (e.g., tranquilizers) can result in increased confusion and tremors (extrapyramidal symptoms). The client with brain alteration is not in control of his or her behavior. Behaviors may be unpredictable, irrational, impulsive, or the patient may be frightened and suspicious. Never "punish" a client for inappropriate behavior or comments. Instead, remember that these personality changes are a result of brain lesions and adjust the care plan accordingly. The Risk Factors and Levels of Prevention feature shows how managing confusion will assist in reducing a person's risk of injury.

Sleep Pattern Disturbance. A common problem seen in confused clients is daytime napping and nighttime hallucinations. This problem is stated as *Sleep Pattern*

Disturbance related to alterations in usual sleep habits.

Planning: Expected Outcomes. The client will have improved sleep patterns, as evidenced by sleeping 4 to 6 hours continuously at night and will not sleep as often during the day.

Implementation. Plan nighttime interventions to allow 4 to 6 hours of uninterrupted sleep. Recall that a sleep cycle requires 2 to 3 hours and the loss of REM (rapid eye movement) sleep can increase confusion. When you enter the room at night, assess the client for REM. When REM is present, the client should be allowed to complete the REM portion of the sleep cycle and you should return later to care for the client.

Keep the client active during the day so that there is some fatigue by nighttime. Daytime sleeping is a difficult pattern to break, and the client may have to be kept awake for this pattern to be reversed. For the elderly client, the normal changes in sleep with aging need to be considered, such as the increased use of short naps and less sleep during the night. Sleeping medications are seldom given to confused clients because they often alter sleep cycles and deplete the client of REM sleep. See Chapter 18 on sleep disorders for a more in-depth discussion.

NURSING RESEARCH

Can Training Help in the Management of Sundown Syndrome Behaviors?

Wallace, M. (1994). The sundown syndrome: Will the specialized training of nurse's aides help elders with sundown syndrome? *Geriatric Nursing, 15*(3), 164–166.

For this study, the *sundown syndrome* was defined as behavioral disturbances that occur between 3 PM and 7 PM in individuals in whom these disturbances do not occur at other hours. These behaviors include wandering, verbal outbursts, upset behavior or agitation, resistance to or refusal of care, and acts of violence toward self, staff, or others. The sundown syndrome primarily affects elderly people with a history of dementia.

Wallace used a case study approach to determine if specialized training of nurses' aides would result in a decrease in the number of sundowning behaviors experienced by residents of a long-term care facility. Four elderly residents from a 60-bed long-term facility demonstrated sundowning. Five nurses' aides received half-hour training sessions that provided a basic overview of the sundown syndrome and introduced appropriate interventions to manage the behavioral disturbances. These interventions included maintaining continuity in staff assignments; ensuring consistency in timing for care delivery; maintaining specific times for residents to rest, sleep, and have quiet times; providing adequate nutrition; monitoring the residents' elimination patterns; introducing one's self at the beginning of the shift and every few hours; maintaining an awareness of the residents' whereabouts at all times; taking time to sit and talk to residents about their lives, pictures, or other topics of interest; gently redirecting wandering residents back to their units and staying with them until redirection is successful; encouraging residents to feed themselves and participate in other activities of daily living without forcing them; ensuring that residents use sensory deficit aids (e.g., eyeglasses, hearing aids); and reporting any behavior problems to the nurse, and documenting these behaviors on a preprinted flow sheet.

After the specialized nurse's aide training, most sundowning decreased. These behaviors included verbal outbursts; wandering; acts of violence toward self, staff, and others; and displays of upset behavior or agitation. Resistance to care or refusal of care increased.

Implications for Practice

Although the sample size was small, the outcomes were so positive that more research is indicated to further support for these interventions. Most long-term settings employ unlicensed professionals for the care of their residents. Half-hour training sessions are a small investment compared to the potential outcomes for residents with sundown syndrome.

Ineffective Family Coping. The unfamiliar behavior of the client or the stress of providing continual care for the client at home may increase stress in the family and alter their ability to cope. This diagnosis is stated as *Ineffective Family Coping related to caregiver stress.*

Planning: Expected Outcomes. The client's family will demonstrate improved coping strategies, as evidenced by improved use of support systems and appropriate analysis of the client's condition.

Implementation. When confusion is a new problem for the client, the family will be distressed by the behavior. Explain to the family that the client is not able to control behavior or speech at this time. Assess whether the client becomes calm or agitated when the family is present and advise visitations accordingly. If possible, the need for and use of restraints should be explained to the family before they see the client. The family may become very upset when they see the client "tied" to the bed. Advance explanations can avert some of this reaction. There have also been instances in which the client suffered an injury because the family did not understand the purpose for the restraints and untied them.

If the client's confusion is due to a chronic disease, such as Alzheimer's disease, the family may need to find support systems to provide continual supervision of the client in the home. Advise the family to have legal counsel determine the client's competence and determine the need for guardianship or durable power of attorney.

Evaluation

The degree of goal attainment should be assessed at regular intervals. If expected outcomes have not been met, the care plan may need revision. More commonly, the degree of confusion will require more time to abate and the expected outcome will need a new time frame. A diagnosis of a chronic, progressive condition such as Alzheimer's disease or dementia of the Alzheimer's type may require an entire change in care plan prioritization. These conditions are discussed in Chapter 34.

■ Modifications for Elderly Clients

It is common, but incorrect, to think that elderly people have a marked deterioration in mental function. In general, most elderly people have difficulty recalling new information, but remote memory is intact. In addition, depression occurs in 20% to 30% of the elderly. Depression may follow the loss of friends, spouse, health, and independence and may lead to manifestations such as memory loss and confusion.

Elderly people are particularly at risk of confusion during hospitalization. Not only are they dealing with the stress of being ill but they have the additional stress of an unfamiliar environment. Elderly clients may rely heavily on familiar landmarks and routines to help them maintain an independent life-style. These cues are often lost in the hospital or extended care setting. A large percentage of the population in hospital and extended care settings are elderly, who typically have other conditions that contribute to confusion. By using a team approach and teaching unlicensed personnel to utilize interventions such as those listed in the Nursing Research feature on the sundown syndrome, nurses can effectively manage elderly clients with confusion.[11]

Community and Self-Care

Choosing sites for discharge placement from the hospital for a confused client varies with the cause of confusion. If the confusion is acute and full recovery is expected, sometimes the patient can go home under the care of family members. If the confusion is chronic, the patient will need either care or supervision at home or placement in an extended care facility. Some communities offer adult day care and respite services that allow family members a relief from constant care of the confused person. See Chapter 34 for care of the client with Alzheimer's disease at home.

Conclusions

Clients who are confused or comatose are vulnerable to injury, aspiration, malnutrition, skin breakdown, and more. Nurses provide a lifeline for these clients, providing protection and promoting normal body functions. The families of these clients require therapeutic management as they face many difficult decisions.

Thinking Critically

1. The client is a 48-year-old man who was brought to the emergency department (ED) by his wife, who stated that he had been out shoveling the sidewalk when he fell and hit his head. She said that she noticed a small cut by his ear but did not think too much about it until he started complaining of a terrible headache and blurring of vision. She then decided to bring him to the hospital. Is this possibly a serious problem? What was his neurologic baseline when you received him in the ED? Were this headache and blurring of vision a change for this client?

Factors to Consider. What other signs or symptoms did the client display? Were there any other physical signs of injury to his head or other parts of his body? Does he have any other significant medical history or allergies?

2. You are caring for an 18-year-old high-school senior who was involved in a head-on motor vehicle accident on the previous day. He has not been conscious since the accident. He has no response to painful stimuli, and EEGs are ordered to assess brain function. His mother has been informed about his lack of neurologic response. When she is told that EEGs have been ordered, she says "He's not dead! He moves his eyes when I talk to him." How would you respond?

Factors to Consider. What abnormal eye movements can develop after head injury? What are the possible effects of medications on neurologic response? How will the mother's anxiety affect her ability to process information?

Bibliography

1. Bliwise, D. L. (1994). What is sundowning? *Journal of American Geriatrics Society, 42*(9), 1009–1011.
2. Cutchins, C. (1991). Blueprint for restraint free care. *American Journal of Nursing, 91*(7), 36–44.
3. Dellasega, C., & Morris, D. (1993). The MMSE to assess the cognitive state of elders. *Journal of Neuroscience Nursing, 25*(3), 147–152.
4. Foreman, M. (1990). Complexities of acute confusion. *Geriatric Nursing, 11*(3), 136–139.
5. Frances, A., et al. (1994). *Quick reference to the diagnostic criteria from DSM-IV.* Washington, DC: American Psychiatric Association.
6. Helwick, L. D. (1994). Stimulation programs for coma patients. *Critical Care Nurse, 8,* 47–51.
7. Keller, C., & Williams, A (1993). Cardiac dysrhythmias associated with central nervous system dysfunction. *Journal of Neuroscience Nursing, 25*(6), 349–355.
8. Maher, M. E., & Strong, S (1989). Organ donation: A nursing perspective. *Journal of Neuroscience Nursing, 21*(6), 257–361.
9. Marshall, S. (1990). *Neuroscience critical care.* Philadelphia: WB Saunders.
10. Newbern, V. (1991). Is it really Alzheimer's? *American Journal of Nursing, 91*(2), 50–54.
11. Plum, F. (1996). Brain death. In J. C. Bennett and F. Plum (Eds.). *Cecil textbook of medicine* (20th ed.). Philadelphia: W. B. Saunders.
12. Rantz, M. J., & McShane, R. E. (1994). Nursing-home staff perception of behavior disturbance and management of confused residents. *Applied Nursing Research, 7*(3), 132–140.
13. Ross, B. L., et al. (1994). Neuropsychological outcome in relation to head injury severity: Contributions of coma length and focal abnormalities. *American Journal of Physical Medicine Rehabilitation, 73*(5), 341–347.
14. Shedd, P. P., Kobokovich, L. J., & Slattery, M. J. (1995). Confused patients in the acute care setting: Prevalence, intervention, and outcomes. *Journal of Gerontological Nursing, 21*(4), 5–12.
15. Sosnowski, C. (1994). Early intervention: Coma stimulation in the intensive care unit. *Journal of Neuroscience Nursing, 26*(6), 336–341.
16. Wallace, M. (1994). The sundown syndrome. *Geriatric Nursing, 15*(3), 164–166.
17. Willis, R., & Skelley, L. (1992). Serving the needs of donor families: The role of the critical care nurse. *Critical Care Nursing Clinics of North America, 4*(1), 63–77.
18. Zegeer, L. (1989). Oculocephalic and vestibulo-ocular responses: Significance for nursing care. *Journal of Neuroscience Nursing, 21*(1), 46–55.

Nursing Care of Clients with Cerebrovascular Disorders

CHAPTER
32

Sally Strong Schnell

Cerebrovascular disorders comprise a large group of problems that affect blood supply to the brain. Blood supply can be altered by narrowing or clotting of an artery supplying the brain, abnormal blood vessels within the brain, or traumatic bleeding in brain tissue or brain linings. Cerebrovascular disorders include cerebrovascular accidents (commonly called *strokes*) and head injury. Most of us know someone who has suffered from a cerebrovascular disorder and have seen the devastating effects. Caring for these clients requires as much attention to psychosocial factors and family dynamics as it does to physiologic parameters.

Whatever the origin, increased intracranial pressure is a frequent consequence of cerebrovascular disorders. The skull is a rigid compartment and cannot stretch when the brain beneath it swells. As a result, the brain tissue becomes compressed, impairing consciousness and function. If the intracranial pressure is not controlled, the client will die. This chapter describes the care of clients with cerebrovascular accidents, transient ischemic attacks, arteriovenous malformations, headaches, traumatic brain injury, and hematomas. The pathogenesis and care related to the syndrome of intracranial pressure is essential to each of these conditions, so it is discussed first.

Increased Intracranial Pressure

Intracranial pressure (ICP) is the pressure exerted in the cranium by its contents: the brain, blood, and cerebrospinal fluid (CSF) (Fig. 32–1). Intracranial pressure is measured via monitors either in the ventricle brain parenchyma or in the subarachnoid space. The normal pressure of CSF is 5 to 15 mm Hg. Pressures over 20 mm Hg are called *increased ICP,* and they seriously affect cerebral perfusion. Recognition of increased ICP is one of the most important assessments made by nurses caring for clients with neurologic disorders.

Cerebral perfusion pressure (CPP) is the amount of blood flow from the systemic circulation that is required to provide adequate oxygen and glucose for brain metabolism. In cases of profoundly increased ICP, the MAP and ICP become the same, and brain perfusion ceases. The formula for calculating cerebral perfusion pressure is as follows:

$$CPP = MAP - ICP$$

Etiology and Risk Factors

The Risk Factors and Levels of Prevention feature notes that increased ICP is most often associated with a destructive expanding lesion (e.g., tumor or hemorrhage), cerebral infarction, hydrocephalus (an obstruction to the outflow of CSF), an abscess, or an ingested toxin.

Pathophysiology

The skull is a hard bony vault filled with brain tissue, blood, and CSF. The pressure within the cranium is maintained by a balance between these three components. The modified Monro-Kellie hypothesis, a theory for understanding ICP, states that since the bony skull cannot expand, when one of the three components expands, the other two must compensate by decreasing in volume in order for the total brain volume and pressure to remain constant.

As a mass enlarges, initial compensation occurs through displacement of CSF into the spinal canal. The ability of the brain to adapt to increasing pressure without increasing ICP is called *compliance*. The movement of CSF is the first and major compensatory mechanism, but it can accommodate increasing intracranial volume only to a point. When the ability of the brain to be compliant is exceeded, the ICP rises, clinical manifestations develop, and other compensation efforts to reduce pressure begin.

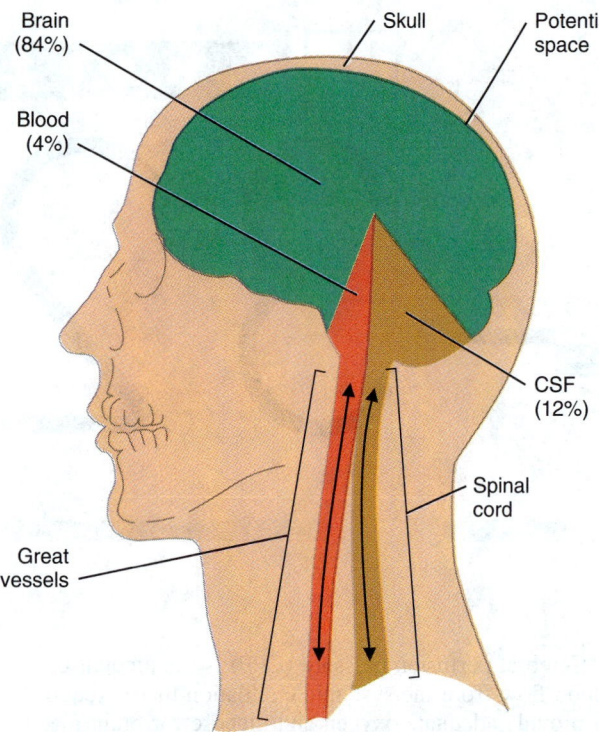

Brain (84%)
Skull
Potential space
Blood (4%)
CSF (12%)
Spinal cord
Great vessels

Figure 32–1. Components of the intracranial vault.

The second form of compensation is reduction of blood volume in the brain. When blood flow is reduced by 40%, cerebral tissue becomes acidotic. When 60% of blood flow is lost, the electroencephalogram (EEG) begins to change. This stage of compensation alters cerebral metabolism and eventually produces brain tissue hypoxia and areas of brain tissue necrosis.

The last stage of compensation and the most lethal is displacement of brain tissue across the tentorium, under the falx cerebri, or through the foramen magnum into the spinal canal. This process is called *herniation* and often results in death from brain stem compression. *Autoregulation,* which is the compensatory alteration in the diameter of the intracranial blood vessels designed to maintain a constant blood flow during changes in cerebral perfusion pressure, is lost with increasing intracranial pressure. When this happens, small increases in brain volume can cause dramatic increases in intracranial pressures with a longer time required to return to baseline. When intracranial pressure approaches systemic blood pressure, cerebral perfusion decreases and the brain suffers from severe hypoxia and acidosis.

The brain is supported within various intracranial compartments (Fig. 32–2). The supratentorial compartment contains all of the brain tissue from the top of the midbrain upward. This section is divided into right and left

---

RISK FACTORS AND LEVELS OF PREVENTION

Increased Intracranial Pressure

Risk Factors

Epidural, subdural, subarachnoid, or intracerebral bleeding; swelling of the brain; tumors or other lesions in the brain; inflammatory processes in the brain; increased cerebral blood flow or impairment of cerebral venous flow; increased production, decreased absorption, or blockage of CSF flow; vasodilation from increased CO_2 or decreased O_2; uncompensated hypertension; increased intrathoracic pressure.

Levels of Prevention

Primary Prevention

- Teach clients to reduce the risk of head injury by wearing seat belts and helmets.
- Encourage clients to avoid alcohol, drugs, and dangerous weapons.
- Instruct clients to use caution when diving.
- Position at-risk clients with their heads elevated and necks in neutral position.
- Ventilate clients to keep Pao_2 and $Paco_2$ normal.

Secondary Prevention

- Monitor high-risk clients with Glasgow Coma Scale and ICP monitors.
- Treat these clients with steroids and diuretics.
- Hyperventilate high-risk clients to reduce $Paco_2$.

Tertiary Prevention

- Initiate fall prevention protocols for clients at risk for falls.
- Use seizure precautions for clients at risk for seizures.
- Ensure that the client receives the prescribed dose of anticonvulsants; consult the physician for replacement if necessary.
- Suction as needed to remove secretions that impair O_2 and CO_2 exchange.

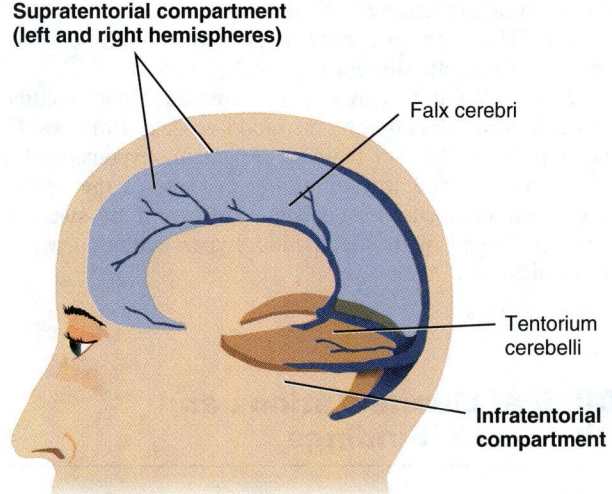

Figure 32–2. The intracranial compartments.

chambers by the tough, inelastic fibers of the falx cerebri. The supratentorial compartment is separated from the infratentorial compartment (containing the brain stem and cerebellum) by the tentorium cerebelli. The brain is capable of some movement within these compartments. Pressure increases in one compartment affect surrounding areas of lower pressure.

■ Herniation Syndromes

Herniation syndromes have been classified into five types (Fig. 32–3). These conditions occur late in the course of increased ICP and represent the body's last attempt to restore normal brain volume and pressure.

Supratentorial Herniation Syndromes

Transcalvarial Herniation

Transcalvarial herniation occurs with open head injuries when brain tissue is extruded through an unstable skull fracture.

Central Transtentorial Herniation

Central transtentorial herniation is the end result of the downward displacement of the diencephalon through the tentorial notch. It is caused by injuries or masses located in the cerebral cortex or on the outward perimeter of the cerebrum.[32] An early indication of central transtentorial herniation is a rapid change in the level of consciousness. As the pressure increases it causes changes in respiratory patterns: first, Cheyne-Stokes respirations, then central neurogenic hyperventilation; later, apneustic breathing and ataxic (Biot's) respirations; and, finally, apnea. Pupils become small, but they remain reactive, and they progress to a dilated and fixed state. Pathologic reflexes begin with a positive Babinski's sign (see Chapter 30) and then progress from abnormal flexion to abnormal extension posturing. Doll's eye reflex and a positive response to caloric testing are present when brain stem function is still intact, but absent if the brain stem dies. The Critical Monitoring feature in Chapter 31, lists the specific areas of brain involvement that are correlated with pathologic manifestation.

Lateral (Uncal) Transtentorial Herniation

Lateral transtentorial herniation occurs from masses in or along the temporal lobe. It is also called *uncal herniation,* because as the temporal lobe is compressed, the uncus

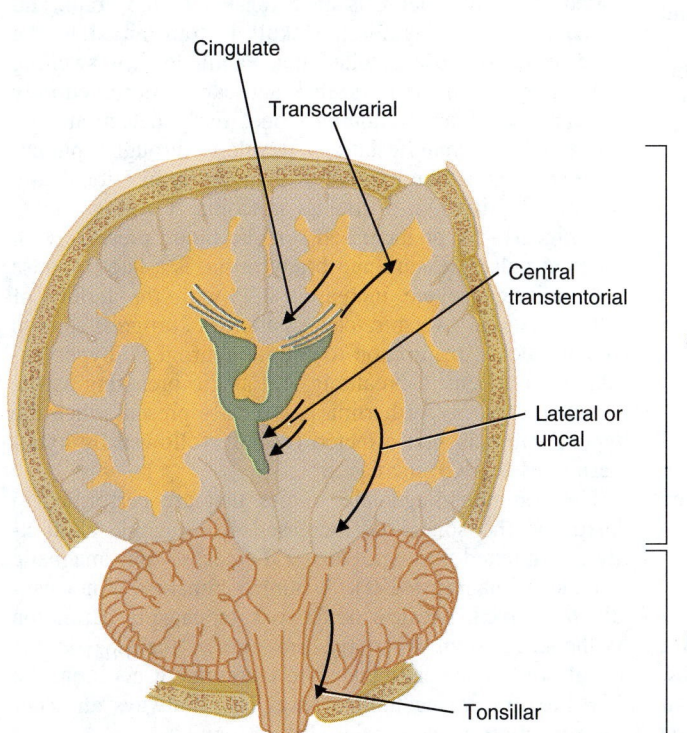

Figure 32–3. Types of herniation syndromes. In transcalvarial herniation, edematous brain tissue is extruded through the skull. In central transtentorial herniation syndrome, a lesion located centrally or superiorly in the cranium may compress central and midbrain structures. In lateral, or uncal, herniation syndrome, a lateral lesion within the cranium causes pressure on the midbrain. Cingulate herniation occurs between the two frontal lobes; the brain is pressed under the falx cerebri. Tonsillar herniation syndrome occurs when the cerebellar tonsils are driven between the posterior arch of the atlas and the medulla and compressed.

(the anteromedial portion of the hippocampus) and/or the hippocampal gyrus shift from the middle fossa through the tentorial notch into the posterior fossa.[32] As the herniation progresses, the pupils first become sluggish in response to light and then become unresponsive; lack of response is seen first in the ipsilateral pupil and then in the contralateral pupil, secondary to third nerve compression at the midbrain level. Other progressive clinical manifestations include a decreasing level of consciousness (stupor to coma), Cheyne-Stokes respirations followed by central neurogenic hyperventilation, and abnormal flexion posturing that progresses to abnormal extension posturing.

Cingulate Herniation

Cingulate herniation occurs when the frontal lobes of the cerebrum are compressed and results in the cingulate gyrus (an arch-shaped convolution situated just above the corpus callosum) being pressed under the falx cerebri.[32] Manifestations are related to cerebral artery compression, resulting in ischemia and congestion, edema, and increasing intracranial pressure.

Infratentorial Herniation Syndrome

Tonsillar Herniation

Tonsillar herniation, also known as cerebellar herniation, occurs when the cerebellar tonsil shifts through the foramen magnum, compressing the medulla and upper portion of the spinal cord. It is caused by increasing pressure in the posterior fossa, often secondary to cerebellar bleeding. Manifestations often progress rapidly and include erratic changes in blood pressure, pulse rate, and breathing; decreased level of consciousness; an arched stiff neck; and quadriparesis.

Herniation, regardless of the type, is always an emergency. *Notify the physician immediately of any manifestations that indicate a worsening of the client's condition due to increasing intracranial pressure.*

■ Brain Swelling and Brain Edema

The terms *cerebral edema, brain swelling,* and *increased ICP* are sometimes used interchangeably, but they are not the same. Cerebral edema and brain swelling are causes of increased ICP. An increase in brain bulk caused by an increase in cerebral blood volume is called *brain swelling.* *Brain edema,* in contrast, is an increase in the fluid content surrounding the tissues of the brain, such as in the extracellular spaces or the white matter, or within the cells themselves. The distinction between these two conditions is important because the interventions differ.

After head injury, edema develops as a result of a disruption of the blood-brain barrier. This type of edema is similar to other forms of edema, such as that seen in a sprained ankle. The fluid contains electrolytes, proteins, and even blood. Edema reaches its maximum within 48 to 72 hours after brain surgery or injury. The fluid returns to the systemic circulation via the CSF or the venous systems. This form of edema may be treated with corticosteroids or osmotic diuretics, or both.

Brain swelling is caused by increased blood volume resulting from dilated cerebral blood vessels. Brain swelling appears to be the major mechanism responsible for increasing ICP and for decreasing the size of the ventricles when compensation occurs. This form of swelling may be treated with therapeutic hyperventilation via a mechanical ventilator.

Clinical Manifestations and Diagnostic Findings

Manifestations of increased ICP are caused by traction on the cerebral blood vessels by swelling tissues and pressure on the pain-sensitive dura mater and various structures within the brain and eye. Increased ICP is actually composed of several entities that occur at the same time, rather than being one process. No single set of clinical manifestations occurs in all clients. Indications of increased ICP relate to the location and the cause of the raised pressure and the speed and extent of its development.

The manifestations of increased ICP are subtle, and you must be diligent in observing for changes in the client's condition. Clinical manifestations include any alteration in level of consciousness, restlessness, irritability, confusion, and a decrease in the Glasgow Coma Scale (GCS) score. In addition, the client may have changes in speech, pupillary reactions, motor or sensory changes, or cardiac rate and rhythm changes. Headache, nausea, vomiting, or blurred or double vision (diplopia) may be reported. The optic nerve is an extension of the brain, and increased tension within the skull is transmitted to the optic nerve to cause papilledema. Papilledema is swelling and hyperemia of the optic disk and can be observed only through use of an ophthalmoscope. Early detection (i.e., before clinical manifestations develop) through ophthalmic examinations and use of ICP monitors in critical care can greatly improve a client's outcome. *Cushing's triad* (see Fig. 31–5), or increased systolic blood pressure with widened pulse pressure and bradycardia, is a late response and indicates severe increased ICP with the failure of autoregulation. Respiratory patterns progress from Cheyne-Stokes respiration to central neurogenic hyperventilation to apneustic breathing and ataxic breathing as the ICP increases. Hyperthermia is typically present when the hypothalamus is first affected by ICP, followed by hypothermia as the ICP increases.

The common diagnostic studies that are performed to determine the source of increased ICP include skull x-rays, computed tomographic (CT) scans, and magnetic resonance imaging (MRI). A lumbar puncture is not usually performed, because of the risk of causing herniation of the brain stem when the pressure of the CSF in the spinal cord is lower than in the cranium. In addition, the CSF pressure at the lumbar level is not always an accurate reflection of the cranial CSF pressure.

Emergency Care

Emergency care of the client who is at high risk of developing increased ICP focuses on maintaining the airway, improving breathing, and promoting circulation. Immediate interventions may include intubation followed by hyperventilation, osmotic diuretics, steroids, and elevation of the head to promote venous drainage.

Critical Care

■ Medical Management

Hyperventilation

Carbon dioxide causes dilation of cerebral blood vessels. By increasing the ventilator settings to cause hyperventilation, a hypocarbic (low carbon dioxide) blood level is created. A $PaCO_2$ level between 30 and 35 mm Hg will result in vasoconstriction of the cerebral blood vessels, decreased blood flow, and thus, decreased ICP.

Increasing the respiratory rate and depth adjusts carbon dioxide. It is also important to maintain oxygenation. The swollen or bruised brain has an increased need for oxygen and glucose because of an increased metabolic rate. The PaO_2 must be kept between 90 and 100 mm Hg.

Medication

Mannitol, a hyperosmotic agent, is the preferred agent for treating increased ICP because it does not cross an intact blood-brain barrier and has fewer rebound effects.[15] It is given in doses of 0.25 to 1.0 g/kg by IV. Hyperosmotic agents increase intravascular pressure by drawing fluid from the interstitial spaces and from the brain cells. If the blood-brain barrier is damaged, the medication enters the brain and increases swelling. Renal function needs to be monitored when using Mannitol. Diuresis is expected.

Steroids, such as dexamethasone, are used by many practitioners to stabilize the cell membrane and reduce the leakiness in the blood-brain barrier. Clients must be withdrawn slowly from steroid therapy to decrease the risk of adrenal crisis.

Blood pressure medication, either to raise or lower blood pressure, may be required to maintain cerebral perfusion pressure at a normal level. Cerebral perfusion pressure is a result of the relationship between blood pressure and intracranial pressure. If the physician has not left orders to cover blood pressure changes, then you must notify him or her if the blood pressure range is below 100 or above 150 mm Hg systolic.

Antibiotics may be prescribed, especially in the case of an open head injury or an infection in another body system. Infections increase metabolism and, thus, ICP. Therefore, antipyretics are indicated.

Anti-seizure medication (e.g., phenytoin, phenobarbital, diazepam) may be given prophylactically because of the risk of seizures. Seizures increase metabolic requirements and cerebral blood flow and volume; thus an increase in ICP occurs. Chapter 33 describes the care of the client with seizures.

Intravenous (IV) fluids are given by IV pump to help minimize the amount of IV fluids given. Hypertonic IVs are avoided because of the risk of promoting more cerebral edema.

Temperature reduction decreases metabolism, cerebral blood flow, and, thus, ICP. Antipyretics may be used, but a hypothermic blanket is more commonly the intervention of choice. Muscle relaxants are given to prevent shivering.

Barbiturates

Some clients are given large doses of barbiturates to treat uncontrolled ICP. This therapy requires sophisticated monitoring and special training, but its use has shown increased survival outcomes. The client is intubated and placed on ventilatory support and has a pulmonary artery catheter inserted. Pentobarbital, 5 to 10 mg/kg by slow IV injection over 30 minutes, is often given in a loading dose, followed by a maintenance dose of 1 mg/kg/hour until the ICP is under control. Monitor the client's mean arterial blood pressure (MAP), because pentobarbital is a cardiac depressant. The MAP should not be allowed to fall below 80 mm Hg. The serum drug level should be monitored daily; the dose should be reduced if the serum levels exceed 5 mg/100 ml. Temperature should also be monitored because barbiturates reduce metabolism and have a concurrent cooling effect on the body. If the temperature falls below 91.4° F (33° C), the client should be warmed. Pupillary assessment should also continue. Even if a client is in a coma, the pupils dilate if the brain stem becomes compressed. Notify the physician of this change. Barbiturate therapy eliminates the client's normal protective functions. The client is completely dependent on you for all his or her basic needs. Clients should be weaned slowly from barbiturate therapy.

Neuromuscular Blocking Agents

Nondepolarizing neuromuscular blocking agents are sometimes used to induce skeletal muscle relaxation to help manage clients on mechanical ventilation. Decreasing muscle activity may be necessary to control ICP. Nurses are trained in the use of a peripheral nerve stimulator to monitor for adequacy of drug dosage as well as for the risk of overdosage.

Intracranial Pressure Monitoring

Continuous ICP monitoring is used for clients experiencing conditions associated with potentially elevated ICP (e.g., head trauma, preoperative and postoperative aneurysms, tumors, posterior fossa lesions). However, ICP monitoring devices never replace serial clinical observations of the client's condition.

Several methods of ICP monitoring are available. The most common types measure CSF pressure in the ventricles or subarachnoid space. Intraventricular and subarachnoid screws give more accurate results than the epidural

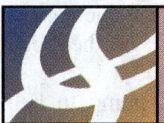

BRIDGE TO CRITICAL CARE

Intracranial Pressure (ICP) Monitoring

Guidelines for Management of ICP

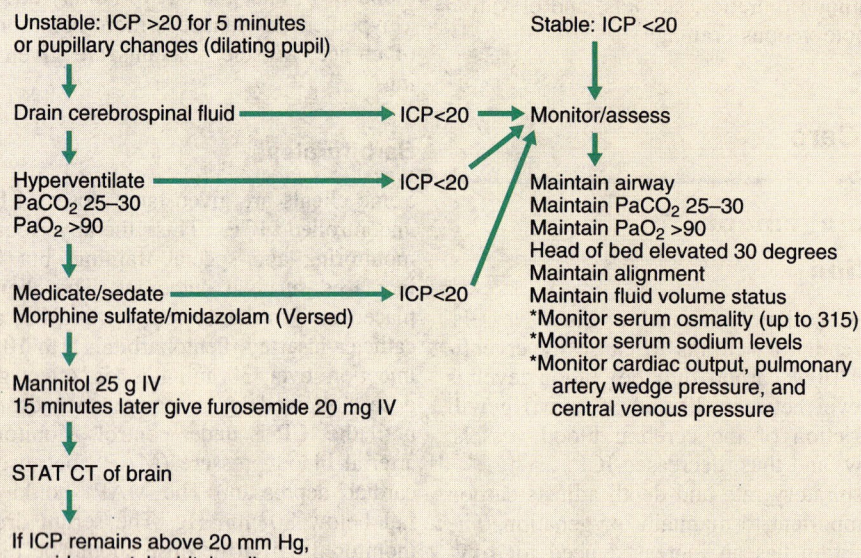

Unstable: ICP >20 for 5 minutes
or pupillary changes (dilating pupil)

Stable: ICP <20

Drain cerebrospinal fluid ⟶ ICP<20 ⟶ Monitor/assess

Hyperventilate ⟶ ICP<20
PaCO$_2$ 25–30
PaO$_2$ >90

Medicate/sedate ⟶ ICP<20
Morphine sulfate/midazolam (Versed)

Mannitol 25 g IV
15 minutes later give furosemide 20 mg IV

STAT CT of brain

If ICP remains above 20 mm Hg,
consider pentobarbitol sodium coma

Maintain airway
Maintain PaCO$_2$ 25–30
Maintain PaO$_2$ >90
Head of bed elevated 30 degrees
Maintain alignment
Maintain fluid volume status
*Monitor serum osmality (up to 315)
*Monitor serum sodium levels
*Monitor cardiac output, pulmonary
 artery wedge pressure, and
 central venous pressure

Intracranial Pressure Waveforms

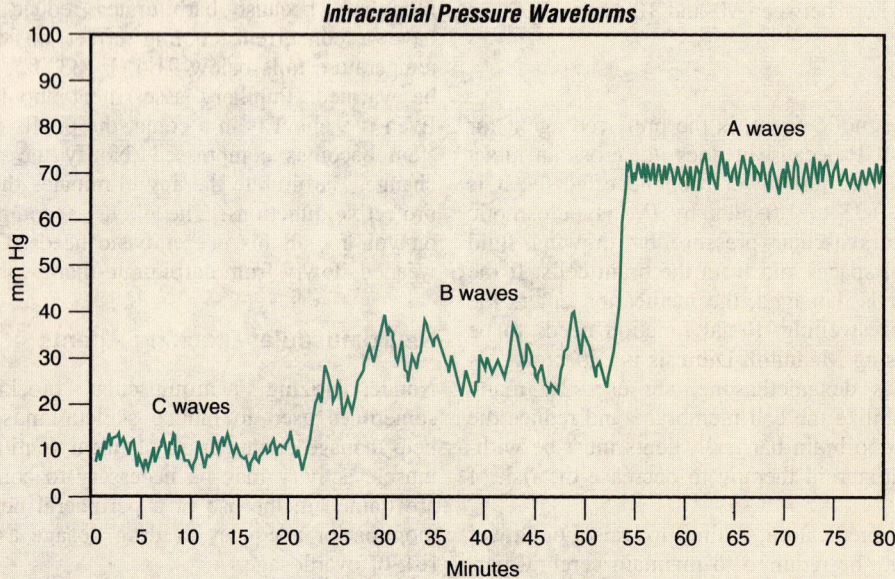

The shape of the waves is influenced by cardiac pulsations and respirations as well as by ICP. The waves have been named A, B, and C waves.

C waves occur four to eight times per minute and reflect fluctuations in arterial pressure. C waves are not
 considered significant.
B waves occur at intervals of 30 seconds to 2 minutes and represent increases in ICP to 50 mm Hg.
A waves are most pronounced when the cranial contents are increased. These waves, also called *plateau waves,*
 represent recurrent ICP elevations to 100 mm Hg. A waves may be caused by coughing or straining but, if

recurrent or sustained, may indicate a reduced ability of the brain to compensate. The client may also show other signs of increasing intracranial pressure.

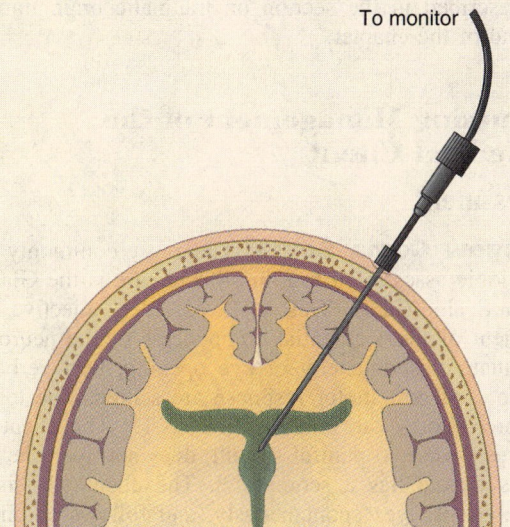

Ventricular catheter (ventriculostomy)

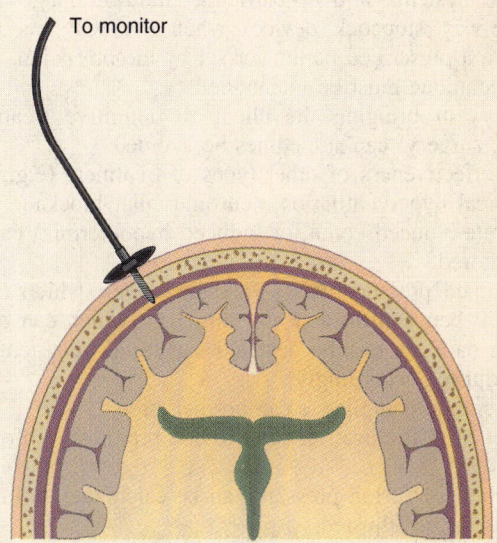

Subarachnoid screw (bolt)

General Interventions for Intracranial Pressure Monitoring

- Ensure that the tubing is long enough to allow the client to be moved in bed but not longer than 14 feet. Tubing longer than 14 feet may cause inaccurate readings.
- Be careful to prevent kinks in the tubing.
- Place the transducer and screw (or catheter) at the preset level of the transducer to take a reading.
- Use sterile technique when working with the device.
- Monitor for signs of infection.
- Flush the catheter if the readings dampen.
- Check for the following if inaccurate readings occur:
  Leaks in the system
  Differences in the height of the transducer and the device
  Kinks in the tubing
  Client performing the Valsalva maneuver
  Obstruction in the system

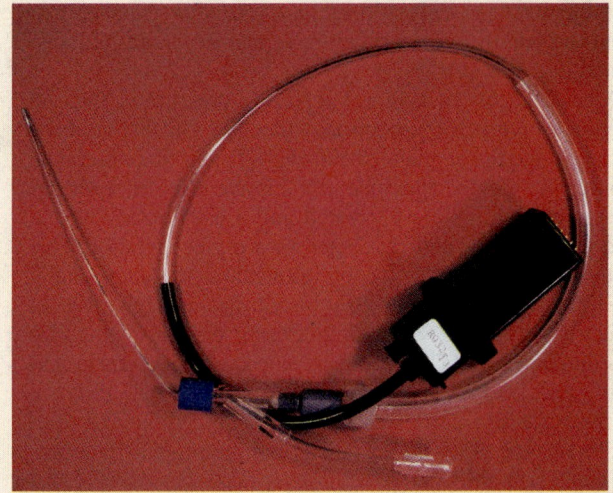

■ A ventricular catheter.

types, but their use carries a higher incidence of infection. Some institutions also use intraparenchymal monitors. (See the Bridge to Critical Care feature and the second Thinking Critically question for your role in ICP monitoring).

The following are advantages of ICP monitoring:

- Pressure increases may be recognized and treated before the onset of clinical manifestations.
- Some systems allow ventricular fluid drainage (e.g., three-way stopcock device) when the ICP has risen above a prescribed parameter set by the physician. Sterile technique must be maintained.
- Delays in bringing the client to definitive treatment (e.g., surgery) can sometimes be avoided.
- The effectiveness of other types of treatment (e.g., mechanical hyperventilation, neuromuscular blockade, barbiturate-induced coma, or induced hypothermia) can be monitored.
- Sustained pressure waves (plateau waves, which occur at ICP between 50 and 100 mm Hg), which can cause brain damage, can be detected early and treatment can be adjusted accordingly.
- Intracranial compliance can be measured.
- Level of ICP elevation can provide prognostic information.
- Cerebral perfusion pressure can be calculated and treatment can be adjusted.
- The effect of nursing interventions on ICP can be monitored. The timing of procedures that raise ICP (e.g., turning) can be altered to coincide with periods of "lower" pressure.

Monitoring ICP also allows the measurement of intracranial compliance. Compliance is tested by introducing a known volume of fluid into the ventricle and measuring its effect on ICP. Detecting a change in the critical relationship between volume and pressure allows early treatment before the onset of clinical manifestations or sustained elevated ICP.

Measurements of cerebral perfusion pressure (CPP) can be made with ICP monitors. Ideally, CPP should be maintained greater than 70 mm Hg. Types of intracranial monitoring devices include the intraventricular catheter, for which a burr hole is created and a catheter is inserted into the ventricle and connected to a digital monitor. This is the most accurate type of intracranial monitor, and it can be used to drain CSF, but it has a high risk of infection. Another type of monitoring device is the subarachnoid screw. The screw is placed into the subarachnoid space, which allows pressure readings and removal of fluid but also carries a high risk of infection. The third common type is an intraparenchymal monitor. It measures pressure in brain tissue.

Complications

Intracranial Hypertension

The development of intracranial hypertension is ICP of 20 to 25 mm Hg. It is usually managed by mannitol administration, hyperventilation, and barbiturate therapy, if needed.

The most serious complication of increased ICP is herniation of the brain. When the herniation is at the level of the medulla, death is imminent.

Other complications of increased ICP include Cushing's stress ulcer (which results from decreased mucosal blood flow and hypersecretion of acid from overstimulation of the vagal nuclei), neurogenic pulmonary edema, diabetes insipidus, and syndrome of inappropriate secretion antidiuretic hormone (SIADH). These complications are described in the section on traumatic brain injury at the end of the chapter.

■ Nursing Management of the Medical Client

Assessment

Glasgow Coma Scale. The most commonly used neurologic assessment tool in clinical care is the Glasgow Coma Scale (GCS). This scale provides objective measurement of three essential components of the neurologic examination: spontaneity of eye opening, best verbal response, and best motor response are scored. The total of the three scores can range from 3 to 15. The client who is unresponsive to painful stimuli, does not open the eyes, and is flaccid has a score of 3. The client who is oriented, opens eyes spontaneously, and follows commands scores 15. A score of 7 or less is equal to coma. Because the scoring of the GCS is based on the client's ability to respond and to communicate, always note whether the following characteristics apply to the client:

1. Is intubated and cannot speak
2. Eyes are swollen closed
3. Is unable to communicate in English
4. Has a hearing loss
5. Is blind
6. Is aphasic
7. Is paralyzed

The presence of these criteria may render the GCS invalid for that individual.

The first GCS score recorded on the client becomes the baseline score. Subsequent scores allow assessment of trends or changes in neurologic status. The scale also can be used to recognize disorders as well as to predict outcomes. Use consistent criteria for client assessment. Specific behaviors indicating a given score should be used. If variations occur in scoring criteria, the value of the scale is lost and serious changes in the client's condition can be overlooked or treated unnecessarily (Fig. 32–4).

Level of Consciousness. The first change in a client who presents with altered cerebral tissue perfusion is a change in the level of consciousness. When decreased levels of consciousness are present, serial and detailed assessments are required until the client has achieved maximum recovery.

To eliminate the subjectivity of using terms such as *lethargy, obtundation, semi-coma,* or *coma,* the GCS both objectifies the client's level of consciousness and assists in identifying very subtle changes. The Nursing Research feature explains the results of a study regarding the rela-

MISSION HOSPITAL
REGIONAL MEDICAL CENTER

ADULT NEURO FLOW SHEET

TIME

GLASGOW COMA SCALE		Eyes Open			
		Best Motor			
		Best Verbal			
		TOTAL			

VOLUNTARY MOTOR	Right	upper extremity			
		lower extremity			
	Left	upper extremity			
		lower extremity			

CRANIAL NERVES	PUPILS	Right	Size			
			Reaction			
		Left	Size			
			Reaction			
	EOMS	Conjugate				
		Dysconjugate				
		Tracking	Right			
			Left			
	Blink Reflex				
	Gag Reflex				
	Facial Symmetry				

KEY

MOTOR
5+ Normal Power
4+ Weakness
3+ Anti-gravity
2+ Not anti-gravity
1+ Trace
0 No movement

B = Brisk
Pupil S = Sluggish
Size   A = Absent

2mm 3mm 4mm 5mm

6mm 7mm 8mm

✔ = Present
O = Absent
S = Symmetrical
A = Asymmetrical

Date

TIME

Speech Patterns: _____

Comments: _____

GLASGOW COMA SCALE	Eyes Open	4 Spontaneously
		3 To verbal command
		2 To Pain
		1 No Response
	Best Motor Response	6 Obeys Commands
		5 Localize Pain
		4 Flexion to pain withdraw
		3 Flexion Decorticate
		2 Extension to pain (decerebrate)
		1 No Response to pain
	Best Verbal Response	5 Oriented
		4 Confused
		3 Inappropriate words
		2 Incomprehensible sounds
		1 No Response

Unit _____

R.N. Signature _____ Shift: _____

R.N. Signature _____ Shift: _____

R.N. Signature _____ Shift: _____

ADDRESSOGRAPH

#408 10:89

Adult Neuro Flow Sheet

Figure 32–4. A neurologic observation chart. (Courtesy of Mission Hospital Regional Medical Center, Mission Viejo, CA.)

Illustration continued on following page

NEUROLOGIC FLOW SHEET

1. Glasgow Coma Scale (GCS). Three areas are assessed: Best eye opening, Best motor response, and Best verbal response. Assign the appropriate numerical score for each category (1st box—best eye, 2nd box—best motor, and 3rd box—best verbal). Place the total score in the fourth box (total score 3-15).

2. Voluntary Motor is evaluated by assessing each extremity on both the right and left side. Note **symmetry vs. asymmetry.** In the cooperative patient, voluntary motor strength is assessed by asking the patient to close their eyes and hold their arms straight ahead with palms up for about 30 seconds. The leg strength is evaluated by asking the patient to push downward against the examiner's hands.

Scoring: Normal power (5+) is the score given if the patient's arms stay in the same position and/or if the legs have equal strong power.

Weakness (4+) is the score given if one of the pt.'s arm drifts downward (hands may pronate) or if the leg strength is diminished. Some resistance to force is noted.

Anti-gravity (3+) is the score given if the patient is able to move an extremity above the plane of gravity (ie flexing & extending a hand up/down against gravity).

Not anti-gravity (2+) is the score given to a patient who can move the extremity back and forth on the bed but not against the forces of gravity.

Trace movement (1+) is the score given to a patient who can move an extremity slightly.

No movement (0) is the score given if a patient cannot move the extremity.

3. **Cranial Nerve Exam:**

Pupillary response: Each pupil is assessed individually. Note the size of the pupil prior to shining the light into the eye. Place your hand at the bridge of the nose to block light to the opposite eye. Using the penlight, shine the light from outside the right eye to midpoint across the eye to assess the direct light reflex. Note the pupillary constriction (Brisk, sluggish, or non-reactive) in the right eye. Also, observe for constriction in the left pupil (consensual light reflex). Repeat the above steps for the left eye observing the direct light reflex in the left eye and the consensual reflex in the right eye. Document the pupil size (prior to light in the eye) and the reaction on the flow sheet.

Extra-ocular movements (EOMS's) are tested on patients who are awake enough to follow instructions. Ask the patient to follow your fingers with his eyes without moving the head. Move your fingers in a figure H and observe both eyes as they move across/up/down. **Conjugate eye movements** occur when both eyes move in parallel motion. **Dysconjugate eye movements** occur when the eyes do not move in a lateral direction together (one eye may move laterally while the other is fixed or moves in another direction). **Tracking** occurs when the patient is consciously following someone's or something's movement around the room. Place a check for present or a 0 for absent.

The Blink reflex is elicited by lightly stroking the patient's eyelashes. When the eyelids are closed, the eyelids will flutter slightly if the reflex is present. In the conscious alert patient, observe for blinking. Place a check for present or a 0 for absent.

The Gag reflex is evaluated by asking the alert, cooperative patient to cough or swallow. If the patient is unable to do so or is unconscious, take a long cotton tipped swab and stroke the back of the patient's throat. Note if the reflex is present (place a check) or absent (place a 0).

Muscles of the face: Note the muscle symmetry of the facial muscles. Note the ability of the eyelids to open spontaneously and equally. Ask the patient to close their eyes as tightly as possible. Note asymmetry. Ask the patient to smile—note the corners of the mouth to identify symmetrical patterns. Ask the patient to frown/wrinkle his forehead—note the symmetry of the muscles. Place a S for symmetrical and an A for asymmetrical.

Speech patterns: Note if speech is clear, slurred, rambling, or aphasic.

Comments: Utilize this section to elaborate on any abnormal findings or document other pertinent data.

Sign your name and document shift worked. Complete the date/unit and addressograph. The neurological flow sheet is for a 24 hour period. Each day at 7 am, obtain a new flow sheet. Document your findings in the appropriate time box.

Figure 32–4. *Continued*

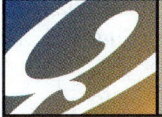

NURSING RESEARCH

Is Intracranial Pressure Influenced by the Comatose Client's Awareness of Bedside Conversation?

Johnson, S. M., Omery, A., & Nikas, D. (1989). Effects of conversation on intracranial pressure in comatose clients. *Heart and Lung, 18*(1), 56–63.

Many studies have validated the effect of various activities on intracranial pressure (ICP). These studies have found anecdotal information about the effects of emotionally laden conversations on ICP in comatose clients.

Johnson and co-workers studied the effects of conversation on ICP using a time series design. Two conversation types were used and continuous measurements of ICP were recorded. The type 1 conversation was emotionally laden and reflected an actual nursing report of the client's current condition. The type 2 conversation was a predetermined dialogue unrelated to the client. Clients served as their own controls. Student's *t*-test was used to analyze mean scores of the minimum, average, and maximum ICP measurements before, during, and after both conversations.

The data collected revealed a wide variation in client responses and that the effect of conversation on ICP was related to the client's level of consciousness, not specifically to the conversation. Clients with a Glasgow Coma Scale rating of less than 5 may not interpret verbal language, and the type of conversation may therefore be irrelevant. A significant decrease occurred in ICP when minimum ICP measurements taken before type 2 conversations were compared with measurements recorded during type 2 conversations.

Implications for Practice

A client may hear and misinterpret the conversation at the bedside. Direct conversation toward information that supports rehabilitative goals such as cognitive stimulation. Speak to the client about, for example, his or her identity, family, time and place orientation, hobbies, and favorite music.

---

tionship of level of consciousness to conversation at the bedside.

Eye Opening. Observe eye opening without speaking to the client. Does the client open the eyes and look around? If the eyes are closed, call the client's name. If no response is noted, raise your voice. If there is still no response, use a mildly painful stimulus, such as squeezing the trapezius muscle or pressing on a nail bed (see Fig. 31–3). Avoid supraorbital pressure, as it can cause damage to the eyes.

Motor Response. Motor responses are assessed by asking the client to follow specific commands, such as "raise your right arm" or "wiggle your toes." Do not ask the client to squeeze your hand because grasp is a reflexive response that occurs in clients with head injury. If agency protocol lists grasp as a neurologic assessment, ask the client to "let go" after grasping, to measure the cognitive ability to control movement. Assess clients who are unable to follow commands by observing their response to a painful stimulus. Responses may include the following: localizing (trying to remove the stimulus), withdrawing, or posturing. Or a response may not be elicited, and the client may remain motionless. Compare the right and left sides and upper and lower extremities. Record the best response while also recording any abnormality that indicates decreased movement in that extremity.

Posturing. Review the discussion on posturing in Chapter 31 (see Fig. 31–4). Recall that as the client's intracranial pressure increases at the cortical level, abnormal flexion posturing occurs. As it increases to the pons level, abnormal extension posturing occurs. When the pressure reaches the medullary level, flaccidity occurs or response is totally lacking, which is the gravest of all signs.

Motor Activity. Motor activity assessment is the measure of strength of voluntary movement of the arms and legs. If a client cannot cooperate with testing, paralysis may be difficult to detect. Observe the client carefully. If a client is restless, paralysis may become obvious because the paralyzed part does not move as other body parts move. Additional information may be obtained by the following means:

1. Compare the tone of one side of the body with that of the other
2. Lift the arms or legs on both sides, release them, and watch them drop to the bed
3. Observe the position of the limbs at rest

If a client can cooperate, assessing "drift" may show subtle tone alterations. To do this, have the client hold both arms up in front of the body with palms upward and eyes closed. Muscles are weak if one arm "drifts" (i.e., moves downward) or if the hand pronates. This is often referred to as the *pronator drift test.*

Verbal Response. Verbal responses assess the client's orientation to self, environment, and time. Ask appropriate questions, such as, "What is your name?" "Where are you?" "What is the month, year, season, nearest holiday?" Avoid asking questions about the date or day of the week. Being hospitalized can alter accuracy of that response even in a person with normal cognitive function. The conversation should include information that can be verified by family, such as home address or employer's name. Many times, slight degrees of confusion are not noticeable until you spend some time with a client. You may find the apparently oriented client asking the same question a few minutes after it was originally asked and answered. Likewise, the client may have "learned" the answers to common questions such as "What is your name?" and "What hospital are you in?" Therefore, it is helpful to reassess a client regularly to check memory or to challenge him or her with various questions.

After obtaining the data for all three parts of the GCS, total the score and compare it to the client's baseline score. If a decrease in the score of even one point occurs, complete a detailed neurologic assessment, including pupillary responses, and notify the physician. Documentation should contain specific descriptive terms. For example, instead of just indicating that the client is "stuporous," record "no response to verbal commands, responded only to tracheal suctioning with abnormal flexion posturing."

Pupil Response. A pupil check includes assessing pupil appearance and physiologic response. The affected pupil is usually on the same side (ipsilateral) as the brain lesion, whereas the motor and sensory deficits are usually on the opposite side (contralateral). Be careful not to mistake a prosthetic eye for a fixed pupil.

Pupil Equality. Document pupil equality, noting the relative size of each pupil.

Pupil Size. Estimate the size of each pupil in millimeters (mm) before and after light stimulation. A penlight provides more accurate data than a flashlight.

Pupil Position. Note whether the pupil is midline or deviated from midline.

Pupil Reaction to Light. Bring the penlight from the lateral side of the client's head toward the eye. Observe for constriction in that eye as well as in the opposite eye. Then test the opposite eye in the same way. The detection of subtle change may require four approaches with the penlight. Brisk and equal constriction of the pupil to direct and indirect light is a normal response. Sluggish or unequal direct or indirect (consensual) response is abnormal. Anisocoria, or unequal pupils, occurs normally in about 17% of the population, with one pupil being about 1 mm larger.

Pupil Shape. The pupillary shape is normally round. Describe abnormal shapes with a drawing.

Pupil Accommodation. Normally, the size of the pupil and the lens (which is not visible to the naked eye) adjust to accommodate to varying focal lengths. Accommodation is usually tested by having the client focus on a distant object and then quickly focus on a close object. Pupils should become smaller as the object is brought near the eye and dilate when the object is moved away from the eye.

The acronym PERRLA is often used in practice and indicates that the *p*upils are *e*qual, *r*ound, *r*eactive to *l*ight and *a*ccommodate. Notify the physician immediately if any change occurs in the pupillary response.

Eye Movement. Document eye movement changes. Observe the position of the eyes when assessing the pupils.

Vital Signs. Initially, vital signs should be assessed every 15 minutes until they are stable. Body temperature should be monitored every 2 hours. If hypothermia or hyperthermia occurs, continuous temperature monitoring should be used. Trends in vital signs and respiratory patterns should be analyzed. As ICP increases to the level of the medulla, the Cushing's response occurs (see Fig. 31–5).

Vital sign changes are *late* changes. See the following discussion of altered cerebral tissue perfusion for care of a client with increasing ICP.

Diagnosis, Planning, Implementation

Any changes in neurologic manifestations may be very significant and must be reported to the physician, no matter how minor they may seem.

Altered Cerebral Tissue Perfusion. If your patient is in a coma because of increased ICP, use this diagnosis to reflect the risk to cerebral tissue perfusion. Write the diagnosis as *Altered Cerebral Tissue Perfusion related to increased intracranial pressure.* The term *patient* is used to discuss persons in a coma. The *client* in this case is the patient's family, who serves as his or her advocate.

Planning: Expected Outcomes. The patient will maintain normal cerebral perfusion, as evidenced by stable or improving levels of consciousness; stable or improving GCS score; ICP of 15 mm Hg or less; no restlessness, irritability, or headache; and no pupillary changes, no seizures, no widening pulse pressure, no respiratory irregularity, and no hypertension or bradycardia.

Implementation. Administer the medications that are ordered to reduce cerebral edema (e.g., osmotic diuretics, corticosteroids) and to decrease risk for seizure (e.g., anticonvulsants), and monitor the patient's response to these medications. If the patient's baseline manifestations of increased ICP are not improving or if seizures develop, notify the physician. Also, consult the physician for medication to promote bowel evacuation without straining, as straining increases ICP.

Position the Client. Place the client supine with the head elevated 30 degrees unless contraindicated (e.g., some spinal injuries, some aneurysms). Keep the patient's head in a neutral position to facilitate venous drainage from the brain. Avoid extreme rotation and flexion of the neck because these positions compress the jugular veins and increase ICP. Also avoid extreme hip flexion because this position increases intra-abdominal and intrathoracic pressure, which increases ICP.[75] As coma lightens, the patient may become disoriented and combative, making it difficult to maintain proper positioning. Restraints must be used as a last resort, because they often increase agitation, which increases ICP.

Suction the Airway. Maintain a patent airway by suctioning to help prevent buildup of CO_2 and elevation of ICP. Adequately oxygenate intubated patients before initiating suctioning, between suctioning, and after suctioning. Try to limit suctioning to three passes and limit each pass to 10 seconds. Recall that nasal drainage may indicate a dural tear; therefore, suctioning of the nares is contraindicated because of the risk of meningitis.

Restrict Fluids. There is some controversy about the type of IV solution to use. Cerebral edema is a major concern, so maintain fluid restriction by use of IV pumps and precise intake and output comparisons (all sources). Never play "catch up" if fluid therapy has fallen behind; consult the physician. Mechanical ventilation causes a client to retain fluid.

Control the Client's Temperature. As noted earlier, hyperthermia increases ICP. Therefore, notify the physician immediately if hyperthermia occurs. If a client's intracranial pressure is being managed with a hypothermia blanket, notify the physician if the client's response is not within the prescribed parameters. Observe for shivering because it increases metabolism and ICP. Assess for skin breakdown if cooling blankets are used for extended periods or in patients who are thin.

Observe the Intracranial Monitor. An ICP monitor requires continuous observation. Nursing responsibilities include the following:

1. Observing for increased ICP
2. Intervening when increases occur
3. Preventing infection

The ICP reading should be less than 15 mm Hg, the MAP reading 80 mm Hg or above, and the CPP reading above 70 mm Hg.

Elevated (plateau) waves, ICP waves above 50 mm Hg, indicate a serious condition if sustained for over 5 minutes (see the Bridge to Critical Care feature). Whenever these sustained pressures are present, assess for contributing factors and intervene appropriately. For example, neck flexion, excessive hip flexion, airway secretions, excess water in the ventilator tubing, an endotracheal tube taped tightly over the jugular veins, discussing the client's condition at the bedside (see the Nursing Research feature) have all been known to increase ICP. Spacing and planning of nonessential nursing interventions (e.g., turning the client), when the client's ICP is not elevated help to prevent plateau waves.

Prevent infection or promote early intervention if infection occurs by assessing the ICP monitor site for signs of infection and leakage, using sterile technique for dressing and drainage bag changes, and by maintaining a closed system. If CSF drainage is required, most systems have a stopcock to attach the tubing and drainage bag. The system is opened only to change the drainage bag.

Evaluation

Evaluate the client's response to treatment as often as every 15 minutes, progressing to hourly, then every 2 to 4 hours, and every 8 hours as the client improves. Once the physician has determined that the client's condition has reached its maximum potential, the frequency and degree of evaluation will diminish even further. In the immediate and acute stages, anticipate ongoing modification in the care plan to help the client reach the maximum potential.

■ Surgical Management

Various surgical techniques are used to treat increased ICP. Optimally, the cause is located and removed. Other techniques include (1) surgical placement of a ventriculoperitoneal shunt to allow drainage if CSF circulation is blocked (Fig. 32–5) and (2) decompressive surgery. The latter is done by removing some brain tissue (e.g., part of the temporal lobe) to give the remaining structures room to expand. If compliance is low at surgery, the bone flap removed to gain access to the brain is not replaced or the dura may not be closed. Subsequent surgery is then required to repair the defect. Postoperative care is the same as that required after craniotomy.

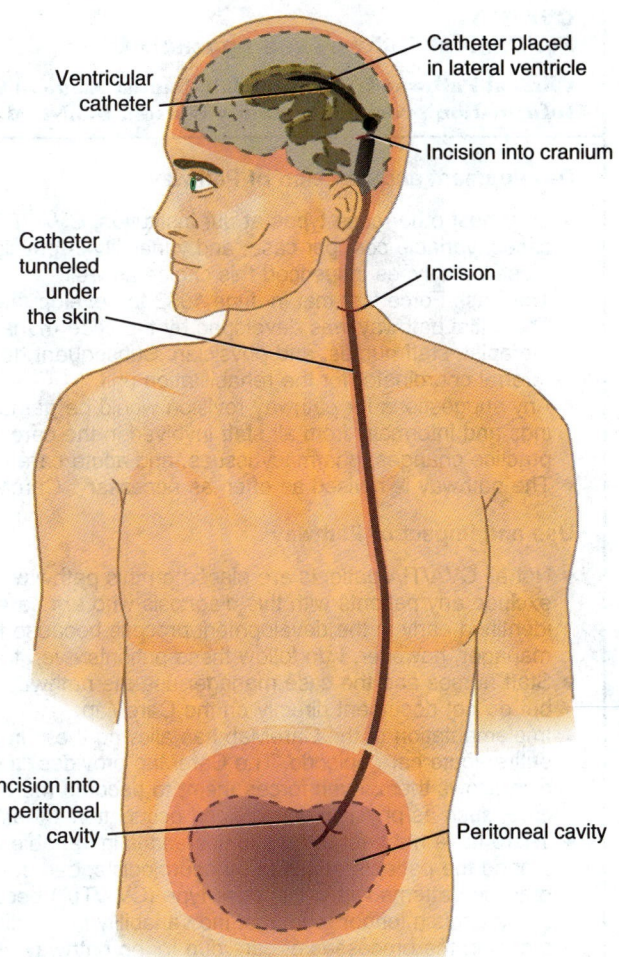

Figure 32–5. Ventriculoperitoneal shunt placed for chronic hydrocephalus.

Cerebrovascular Accident

A *cerebrovascular accident*, commonly known as a *stroke*, is a term used to describe neurologic changes brought on by an interruption in blood supply to the brain (ischemia). The two major causes of ischemia are occlusion and hemorrhage. The occlusion of a blood vessel can be brought about by either progressive thrombosis or emboli. Approximately 75% of strokes are from brain infarctions, 15% are from intracerebral or subarachnoid hemorrhages, and the remaining 10% are from other causes. Cerebrovascular disorders are the third most common cause of death in the United States, preceded only by heart disease and cancer. Approximately 3 million Americans are living with varying degrees of disability from stroke.[55] Along with a high mortality rate, strokes produce significant morbidity in people who survive them. In the large Framingham Study, a 20-year follow-up of stroke survivors in the 45- to 74-year age group found that 31% needed assistance with self-care, 20% required assistance with ambulation, 71% had some impairment in vocational ability up to 7 years following the stroke, and 16% were institutionalized.[25] Fortunately, the incidence of stroke has been declining since the mid-1960s, partly as a result of control of atherosclerosis through the improved control of hypertension, increased diet consciousness, and a reduction in smoking in some segments of the population. In 1996, a national campaign was begun to increase public awareness of stroke.

Etiology and Risk Factors

Narrowing or complete closure of one of the vessels supplying the brain by thrombosis or embolism is the most common cause of cerebrovascular accident (Fig. 32–6). Hemorrhage, vascular compression, and arterial spasm are less frequent causes. (See Risk Factors and Levels of Prevention.)

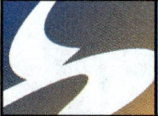

CASE MANAGEMENT

CVA/TIA
For Clinical Pathway see Appendix D

Clinical Pathway from Montclair Baptist Medical Center, Birmingham, Alabama
Information provided by Cindy Watson, B.S.N., M.Ed.

Development and Revision of Pathway

- Like most other case types at our institution, CVA (DRG 14) and TIA (DRG 15) were chosen based on volume of cases, variable cost per case, and variability in physician practice. The availability of a physician champion for these case types influenced this choice as well.
- The Task Force first met in June 1993 to develop the CareMap. It was implemented in February 1994.
- The initial pathway was developed by the case manager, discharge planner, physical therapist, occupational therapist, staff nurses, and physician. Subsequent development involved pharmacists, pastoral care, and the referral coordinator for the rehabilitation unit.
- Any suggestions for pathway revision would be gathered formally at Clinical Process Improvement Team meetings and informally from all staff involved in the care and treatment of these patients. This may include physician practice changes, pharmacy issues, and acute care or rehabilitation issues.
- The pathway is revised as often as necessary. CareMaps are reviewed frequently on rounds with the staff also.

Use and Impact of Pathway

- Not all CVA/TIA patients are placed on this pathway. There are exclusions for cerebral hemorrhage, and we also exclude any patients with this diagnosis who are cared for by a cardiovascular surgeon. These exclusions were identified early in the development process because the care of these types of patients is different. As case manager, however, I do follow these patients even though they are not placed on the CareMap.
- Staff nurses and the case manager use the pathway every day. Other disciplines review the plan of care daily, but do not document directly on the CareMap.
- Implementation of the CareMap has allowed the nursing staff to look at the "big-picture" plan for the patient's entire acute care episode. The CareMap provides "triggers" for the nurses to ensure that all goals are met. It also allows them, even forces them, to become more involved with other disciplines and with other aspects of care, such as physical therapy and occupational therapy.
- There have not been dramatic decreases in variable cost per case and length of stay for all patients; however, among the patients admitted by neurologists, decreases have been significant. It is more difficult to change practice patterns within this case type (CVA/TIA) because all medical physicians treat these patients. Therefore, it takes much longer to impact the variability in practice among physicians. There have been quality improvements in the processes of care due to the pathway. We inserted a mandatory "rehab team consult" on the pathway early in the patient's stay. Planning for discharge now takes place much earlier and is better coordinated. Improvements such as this have an indirect impact on cost over time.

■ Ischemia

Ischemia, lack of blood supply perfusing the brain tissue, occurs whenever blood supply is interrupted or totally obstructed. Ultimate survival of ischemic tissue is dependent on the length of time the brain is deprived plus the degree of brain metabolism. Ischemia is commonly due to thrombosis or embolism.

Thrombosis

Thrombosis starts with damage to the lining of the vessel walls. Most often, atherosclerosis is the primary culprit that causes endothelial damage. Atherosclerosis causes fatty material to cluster and form plaques on vessel walls. These plaques accumulate and alter the usual flow of blood. Blood swirls around the plaques and platelets adhere to the plaque. Eventually the vessel lumen becomes obstructed. Rarely, occlusion is due to inflammatory reactions in the vessel walls. Thrombosis may occur anywhere along a carotid artery or its branches. A common site is at the bifurcation of the common carotid into the internal and external carotid arteries. Thrombotic stroke is the most common stroke in diabetics.

Embolism

Cerebral embolism is the occlusion of a cerebral vessel by emboli. A common embolus is plaque. Atrial fibrillation, in particular, is associated with a high incidence of embolic stroke. Blood pools in the poorly emptying atria. Tiny clots form in the left atrium and move through the heart and into cerebral circulation. Artificial cardiac valve replacements, which have a rougher surface than the nor-

mal endocardium, also cause an increased risk of clots. Finally, bacterial vegetations produced in endocarditis can break off and travel through the circulation. Other sources of emboli include tumor, fat, bacteria, and air. The embolus most often lodges at the bifurcation of the middle cerebral artery. The incidence of cerebral embolism increases after age 40 years.

■ Hemorrhage

Intracerebral Hemorrhage

Intracerebral hemorrhage results from rupture of a cerebral vessel, which causes bleeding into brain tissue. Intracerebral hemorrhage is most often secondary to hypertension. Large hemorrhages usually come from arteries. Small hemorrhages may come from veins and capillaries. Intracerebral hemorrhage, caused by arteriosclerosis and hypertension, is most common after age 50 years. These hemorrhages usually produce extensive residual functional loss and have the slowest recovery of all types of stroke. Brain herniation causes death in more than 50% of clients within the first 3 days after intracerebral hemorrhage.

Aneurysm Rupture

Bleeding may also occur from rupture of an aneurysm or a vascular malformation. The effects of these hemorrhages depend on the site and the extent of the bleeding.

■ Other Causes

Cerebral arterial spasm, caused by irritation, reduces blood flow to the area of the brain supplied by the con-

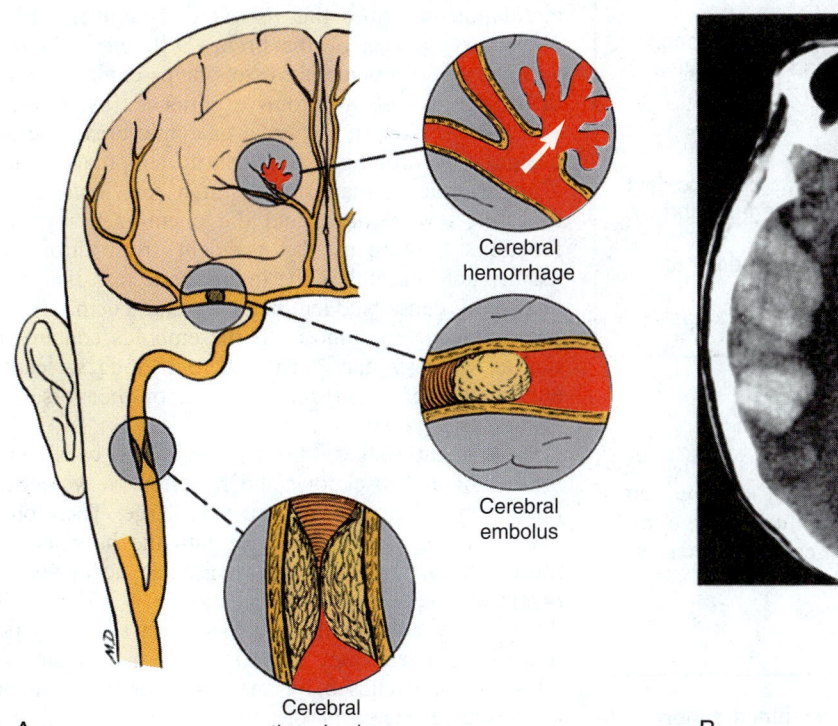

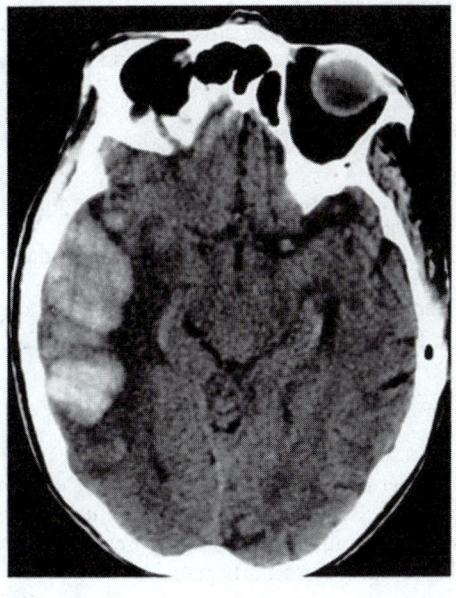

Figure 32–6. *A*, Events causing CVAs. *B*, An MRI showing a hemorrhagic CVA in the left cerebrum.

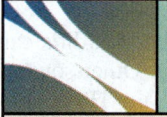

stricted vessel. Spasm of short duration does not necessarily cause permanent brain damage. Also, compression of cerebral vessels may result from a tumor, large blood clot, swollen brain tissue, brain abscess, or other disorders. These causes are fairly rare.

Pathophysiology

The brain is very sensitive to loss of blood supply. Unlike other body tissues, such as muscle, the brain cannot resort to anaerobic metabolism in the absence of oxygen and glucose. The brain is perfused at the expense of other less vital organs to preserve cerebral metabolism. Hypoxia (inadequate oxygen) can cause cerebral ischemia. Short-term ischemia leads to temporary or transient ischemic attacks (TIAs). Long-term ischemia leads to permanent infarction (death) of cerebral cells. The most common form of cerebral infarction is deprivation of blood supply to a localized area of the brain. The extent of infarction depends on factors such as the location and size of an occluded vessel and the adequacy of collateral circulation to the area supplied by the occluded vessel.

During periods of anoxia (no oxygen) cerebral metabolism is quickly altered. Cell death and permanent changes can occur within 3 to 10 minutes of anoxia. The client's baseline oxygen level and ability to compensate will determine how quickly irreversible changes occur. Regardless of whether blood flow is altered from localized perfusion problems, such as stroke or generalized problems (e.g., cardiac arrest), cerebral perfusion pressure must fall to two-thirds of normal (a mean arterial pressure of 50 mm Hg or below) before the brain does not receive adequate blood flow. These numbers are based on a normal baseline. A client who has lost compensatory autoregulation would have increasing signs of neurologic deficit sooner. Without blood flow, electrical dysfunctions occur, which impair neuronal function.

Most forms of decreased cerebral perfusion are caused by occlusion or hemorrhage. Thrombosis produces ischemia in the brain tissue supplied by the affected vessel and edema in the surrounding areas. An area of infarction occurs in brain tissue not being perfused by the affected artery (like the zone of infarction after myocardial infarction). A zone of hypoperfusion (ischemia) also exists around the infarcted area. The size of this zone depends on the amount of collateral circulation present. Collateral circulation describes the vessels that augment the major circulatory vessels of the brain. Differences in the size and number of collateral vessels helps explain differences in the severity of symptoms experienced by different clients with strokes in the same anatomic area. The area of edema after thrombosis may lead to temporary neurologic changes. Edema may subside in a few hours or sometimes in several days, and the client may regain some function. Cerebrovascular accident from thrombosis is usually not fatal unless the infarction is massive.

Emboli cause sudden necrosis and edema similar to that following thrombosis. If the embolus contains bacteria, an abscess may form where it lodges, leading to encephalitis or aneurysmal dilation of the vessel, called *mycotic aneurysm*.

Most hemorrhages into the brain are caused by the rupture of arteriosclerotic and hypertensive vessels. Most intracerebral hemorrhages are very large. Therefore, it is not surprising that hemorrhage into the brain causes the most fatalities of all cerebrovascular accidents. Aneurysms are weakened outpouchings in a vessel wall. Although they are usually quite small in the brain (2 to 6 mm in diameter), they can rupture. An estimated 6% of all strokes are caused by aneurysm rupture. (Aneurysms are discussed later in the Intracranial Hemorrhage section.) A stroke secondary to bleeding often produces spasm of cerebral vessels because the blood outside of the vessels acts as an irritant to the tissues.

Clinical Manifestations and Diagnostic Findings

■ Early Warning Signs

Although they are not often recognized, focal warning signs of impending stroke may occur. Such warning signs may precede an actual cerebrovascular accident by a few hours or days. Warning signs of thrombotic stroke include transient hemiparesis, loss of speech, and paresthesias involving one side of the body. These manifestations are called *transient ischemic attacks* (TIAs) and should not be ignored. Unfortunately, there are no warning signs of embolic stroke. (See the section on TIAs.)

Common manifestations that may precede cerebral hemorrhage in hypertensive clients include severe occipital or nuchal (back of neck) headaches, vertigo (dizziness) or syncope (fainting), paresthesias (abnormal sensations), transient paralysis, epistaxis (nosebleed), and retinal hemorrhages.

■ General Findings

Some general findings of cerebrovascular accident that are not related to specific vessel sites include headache, vomiting, seizures, mental changes (including coma), fever, and electrocardiographic (ECG) changes. ECG changes include T-wave changes, shortened P-R interval, prolonged Q-T interval, premature ventricular contractions, sinus bradycardia, and ventricular and supraventricular tachycardias.[37]

■ Specific Deficits after a Cerebrovascular Accident

Manifestations of deficit must persist longer than 24 hours to be diagnostic of a cerebrovascular accident. These manifestations can be correlated with the cause (Table 32–1) and with the area of the brain in which perfusion is impaired (Table 32–2). The client's deficit also varies according to whether the dominant or the nondominant side of the brain is affected. The degree of deficit can also vary from very little impairment to serious functional loss.

Hemiparesis and Hemiplegia

Hemiparesis (weakness) or hemiplegia (paralysis) of one side of the body may occur following a stroke. Complete hemiplegia involves half of the face and tongue as well as the arm and leg of the same (ipsilateral) side of the body. Hemiplegia results from damage to the motor area of the cortex or to pyramidal tract fibers. Infarction in the brain's right side causes left-sided hemiplegia, and vice versa, because nerve fibers cross over in the pyramidal tract as they pass from the brain to the spinal cord. Other cortical areas may be affected, producing localized manifestations (e.g., hemianesthesia, hemianopia, apraxia, agnosia, and aphasia). Muscles of the thorax and abdomen

Table 32–1. Clinical Manifestations of the Various Causes of Cerebrovascular Accident

Cause	Clinical Manifestations
Thrombosis	Tends to develop during sleep or within 1 hour of arising Ischemia is produced gradually; therefore, the clinical manifestations develop more slowly than those caused by hemorrhage or emboli Relative preservation of consciousness Hypertension
Embolism	No discernible time pattern, unrelated to activity Clinical manifestations occur rapidly, within 10–30 seconds and often without warning; no headache May have rapid improvement Relative preservation of consciousness Normotension
Hemorrhage	Typically occurs during active, waking hours Severe headache occurs (if client is able to report symptoms) Rapid onset of complete hemiplegia, occurs over minutes to 1 hour; form most likely to be fatal Usually results in extensive, permanent loss of function with slower, less complete recovery Rapid progression into coma Nuchal rigidity

are usually not paralyzed because they are innervated from both cerebral hemispheres.

When voluntary muscle control is destroyed, strong flexor muscles overbalance the extensors. This can cause serious deformities. For example, a hemiplegic client's affected arm tends to rotate internally and to adduct, because adductor muscles are stronger than abductors. Also, the elbow, wrist, and fingers tend to flex. The affected leg tends to rotate externally at the hip joint, flex at the knee, and plantar flex and supinate at the ankle joint (Fig. 32–7).

Apraxia

Apraxia is a condition in which a client can move the affected part but cannot use it for specific purposeful actions (e.g., walking, speaking, or dressing). The part is not paralyzed or uncoordinated. An apraxic client can conceive or conceptualize the content of messages to send to muscles (e.g., "stand"). However, the motor patterns or schema necessary to convey the impulse message cannot be reconstructed. Thus, accurate "instructions" do not reach the limb from the brain, and the desired action or movement does not happen. Apraxia ranges from relatively simple to highly complex disorders. For example, a

Table 32–2. Clinical Manifestions of Cerebrovascular Accidents Associated with Area of Brain Affected

Location	Middle Cerebral Artery	Anterior Cerebral Artery	Posterior Cerebral Artery	Internal Carotid Artery	Vertebrobasilar System	Anteroinferior Cerebellar (Lateral Pontine)	Posteroinferior Cerebellar
Motor changes	Contralateral hemiparesis or hemiplegia	Contralateral hemiparesis, foot and leg deficits greater than arm, footdrop gait disturbances	Mild contralateral hemiparesis (with thalamic or subthalamic involvement) Intention tremor	Contralateral hemiparesis with facial asymmetry	Alternating motor weaknesses Ataxic gait, dysmetria (uncoordinated actions)	Ipsilateral ataxia Facial paralysis	Ataxia Paralysis of larynx and soft palate
Sensory changes	Contralateral hemisensory alterations Neglect of involved extremities	Contralateral hemisensory alterations	Diffuse sensory loss (thalamic)	Contralateral sensory alterations	Numbness of the tongue	Ipsilateral loss of sensation in face, sensation changes on trunk and limbs	Ipsilateral loss of sensation in face, contralateral on body
Visual or ocular changes	Homonymous hemianopia Inability to turn eyes toward affected side	Deviation of eyes toward affected side	Pupillary dysfunction (brain stem) Loss of conjugate gaze, nystagmus Loss of depth perception Cortical blindness Homonymous hemianopia	Hemianopia Ipsilateral periods of blindness (amaurosis fugax)	Double vision Homonymous hemianopia Nystagmus, conjugate gaze paralysis	Nystagmus	Nystagmus
Speech changes	Dyslexia, dysgraphia, aphasia	Expressive aphasia	Perseveration Dyslexia	Dysphasia	Dysarthria, dysphasia		Dysarthria, dysphasia, dysphonia
Mental changes	Memory deficits	Confusion, amnesia Flat affect, apathy Shortened attention span Loss of mental acuity	Memory deficits		Memory loss Disorientation		
Other changes	Vomiting may occur	Apraxia (inability to carry out purposeful movements in nonaffected areas	Visual hallucinations	Mild Horner's syndrome Carotid bruits	Drop attacks Tinnitus, hearing loss	Horner's syndrome Tinnitus, hearing loss	Horner's syndrome Hiccoughs and coughing

client may have less difficulty writing than speaking or vice versa.

Aphasia

Aphasia is a defect in using and interpreting the symbols of language. Aphasia may involve any or all aspects of language use, such as speaking, reading, writing, and understanding spoken language. There are about 50 types of aphasia, only a few of the most common are described here. Aphasia may be categorized as follows:

1. Sensory (receptive aphasia), which affects speech comprehension
2. Motor (expressive aphasia or executive aphasia), which affects speech production
3. Global, which affects both

Receptive aphasia is also called *Wernicke's aphasia.* Expressive aphasia is also called *Broca's aphasia.* Other methods of classifying aphasia are by fluency or by the degree of difficulty in articulation. Clients with fluent aphasia (Wernicke's) have speech that is well articulated and grammatically correct but lacks content. Clients with nonfluent aphasia (Broca's) produce very little speech, and what words are spoken are uttered slowly, with great effort and poor articulation. Clients with global aphasia typically repeat the same sounds they hear and have poor comprehension.

Sensory or fluent aphasias involve loss of the ability to comprehend written, printed, or spoken words. For example, auditory or acoustic aphasia produces deafness in the hearing center of the brain, and clients have difficulty understanding what is being said. They are not deaf. They hear sound but they cannot make sense of it, because they cannot understand the symbolic communication associated with the sound. Visual aphasia ("word blindness") is similar. Affected clients cannot read words but can see them. They cannot understand the symbolic content of printed or written symbols.

Motor (expressive or nonfluent) aphasias include aphasias in which the ability to write, make signs, or speak is lost. For example, with motor aphasia, words may be recalled, but the client cannot combine speech sounds into words and syllables. Pure motor or pure sensory aphasias are rare. Most aphasias are mixed (expressive-receptive), affecting both expressive and receptive elements.

Most aphasias are partial rather than complete. The severity of aphasia varies with the area and the extent of cerebral damage. The Nursing Research feature describes how severe damage may deprive the client of any meaningful relationship with the environment and family. Global aphasia (total aphasia) is so extensive that neither expressive nor receptive language abilities are retained. Early determination of the client's yes-no reliability facilitates communication. Verbal skills are often the best. Reading and writing are usually more impaired. Use gestures to aid in communication.

Aphasia may occur if blood supply to a client's speech center is cut off. Aphasia is associated with hemiplegia involving the dominant hemisphere. The speech center for a right-handed client is usually located in the left cerebral hemisphere. The speech center for a left-handed client may be in the brain's right or left side. Thus, a right-handed client with right-sided hemiplegia usually has aphasia, because the speech center is in the damaged left hemisphere. Most people have left-sided speech dominance.

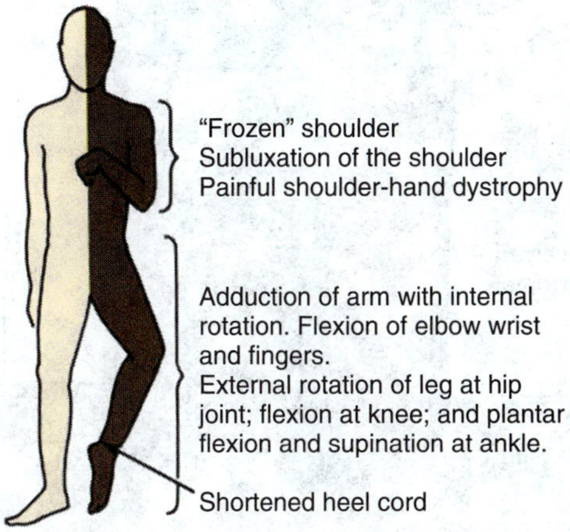

Dysarthria

Dysarthria is imperfect articulation that causes difficulty in speaking. It is important to differentiate between dysarthric and aphasic speech. With dysarthria, the client understands language but has difficulty pronouncing words and may slur them, enunciating poorly. No disturbance is evident in grammar or in phrase or sentence construction. A dysarthric client can understand verbal speech and can read and write (unless the dominant hand is paralyzed, absent, or injured).

Dysarthria is caused by cranial nerve dysfunction. It may result from weakness or paralysis of the muscles of lips, tongue, and larynx or from a loss of sensation. In addition to speaking problems, clients with dysarthria often have difficulty chewing and swallowing food (dysphagia) because of poor muscle control. Dysarthria is a problem for clients with bulbar disorders.

Dysphagia

Recall that swallowing is a complex process requiring the function of several cranial nerves. The mouth must open (cranial nerve V), the lips must close (cranial nerve VII), and the tongue must move (cranial nerve XII). The mouth must sense the quantity and quality of the food bolus (cranial nerves V and VII), and send messages to the swallowing center (cranial nerves V and IX). During swallowing, the tongue moves the food bolus toward the oropharynx. The pharynx elevates and the glottis closes. Contraction of the pharyngeal muscles transports food from pharynx to the esophagus. Peristalsis moves food to the stomach.

"Frozen" shoulder
Subluxation of the shoulder
Painful shoulder-hand dystrophy

Adduction of arm with internal rotation. Flexion of elbow wrist and fingers.
External rotation of leg at hip joint; flexion at knee; and plantar flexion and supination at ankle.

Shortened heel cord

Figure 32–7. Hemiplegic deformities. Note that the elbow is bent, the wrist is flexed, and the fingers are curled into palmar flexion; the knee is bent and the heel cord is shortened.

NURSING RESEARCH

How Does Stroke Affect Marriage?

Williams, S. E. (1993). The impact of aphasia on marital satisfaction. *Archives of Physical Medicine and Rehabilitation, 74*, 361–367.

The person who is most typically affected by stroke, other than the client, is the spouse, whose life is often permanently altered in innumerable ways. A stroke has an overwhelming effect on family dynamics, so the spouse's perception of the impact must be assessed.

Williams studied the affect of aphasia on marital satisfaction. Forty spouses were grouped according to the severity of the client's stroke. The spouses completed two questionnaires on marital satisfaction (Marital Satisfaction Scale and Marital Comparison Level Index) and one questionnaire on their knowledge of aphasia.

The severity of the aphasia was not found to independently alter marital satisfaction. Even spouses of persons with mild aphasia felt less satisfaction. Spouses felt that marriages were more confining, less pleasant, and more unhappy than before the stroke. They also reported that their own health had been affected and sexual desire had decreased. Favorable changes after stroke included having more time together, less arguing over petty issues, and less conflict over how to spend leisure time. The more knowledge the spouse had about aphasia, the less negative the effect on marital satisfaction.

Implications for Practice

The effect of aphasia on spouses is an important consideration in planning and implementing a rehabilitation program for clients who have had a stroke. Include spouses in any program, and provide adequate follow-up of family dynamics. Teach spouses about the characteristics of aphasia, methods of improving communication, and available community support services.

Visual Changes

Lesions in the parietal and temporal lobes may interrupt visual fibers of the optic tract (en route to the occipital cortex) and produce visual defects. Depth perception and visual perception of horizontal and vertical planes may also be impaired. In clients with hemiplegia, this causes motor performance problems in gait and posture (Fig. 32–8). Clients may or may not be aware of a perceptual difficulty, but it may cause them to be accident prone and their behavior to appear bizarre. Visual disorders may interfere with a client's ability to relearn motor skills.

Homonymous Hemianopia

Homonymous hemianopia (Fig. 32–9) is defective vision or visual loss in the same half of the visual field of each eye, so the client has only half of normal vision. For example, the client may see clearly on one side of the midline but see nothing on the other side. Clients with homonymous hemianopia cannot see past the midline without turning the head toward that side.

Horner's Syndrome

Horner's syndrome is the paralysis of sympathetic nerves to the eye, causing sinking of the eyeball, ptosis of the upper eyelid, slight elevation of the lower lid, constriction of the pupil, and lack of tearing in the eye.

Agnosia

Agnosia is a disturbance in interpreting visual, tactile, or other sensory information. The client is unable to recognize objects. Agnosia may be visual, auditory, or tactile,

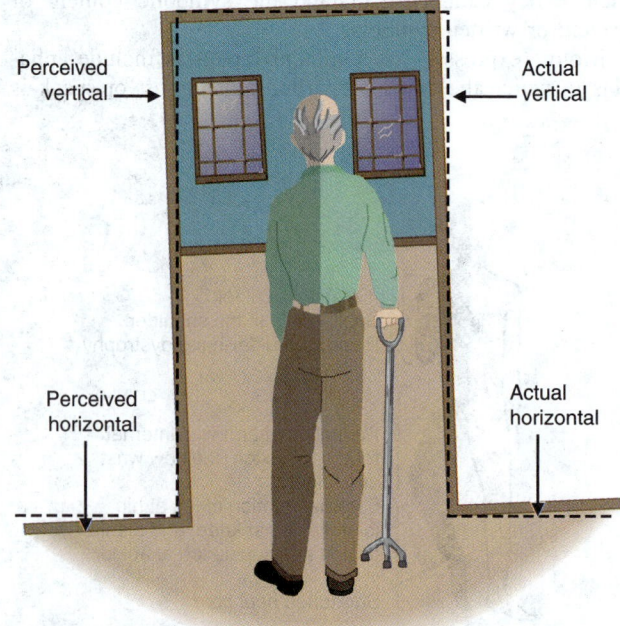

Figure 32–8. Perceptual disturbances in hemiplegia. Such disturbances can be both unpleasant and unsafe.

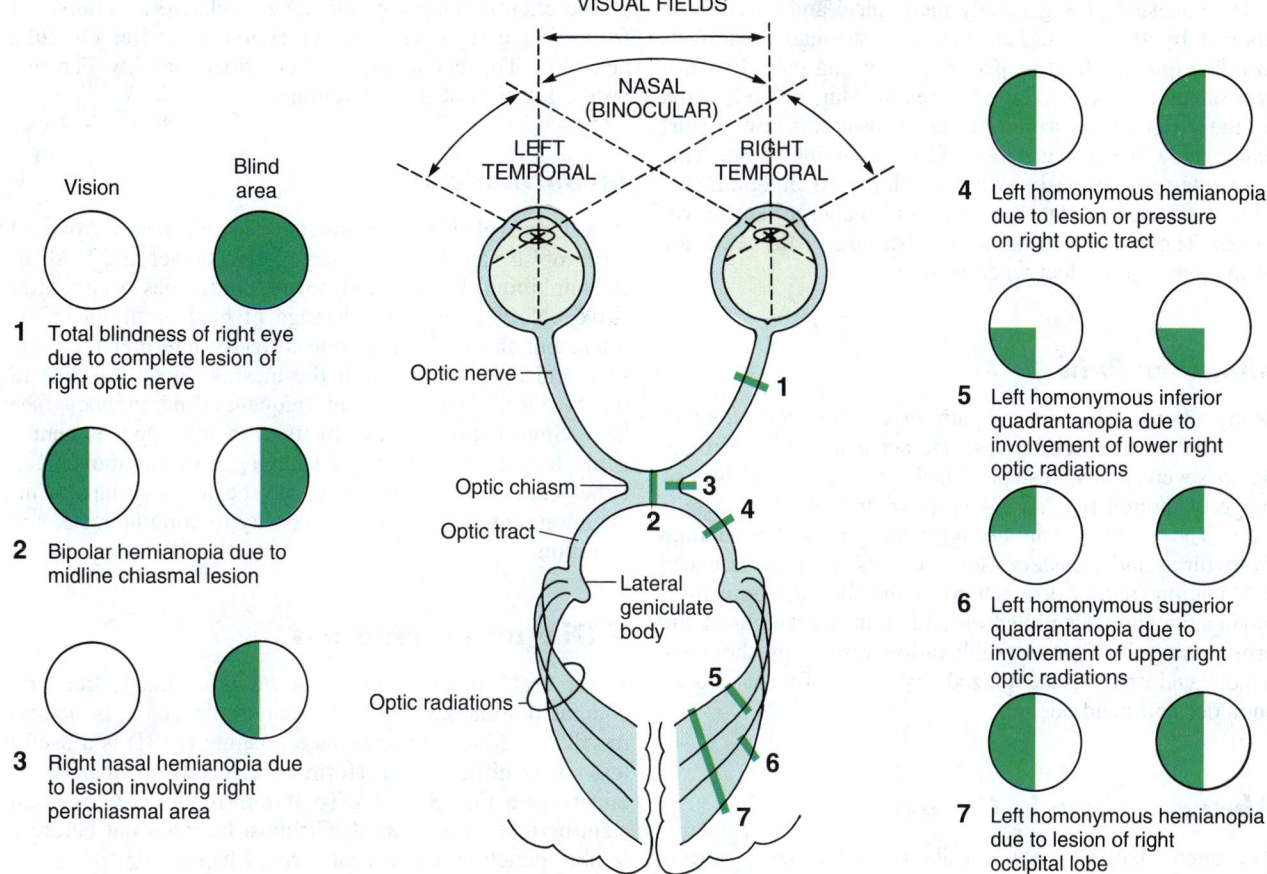

Figure 32–9. Visual field defects associated with optic nerve lesions.

but is not the same as blindness, deafness, or paralysis. Loss of muscle-joint sensation may be accompanied by inaccurate beliefs about the position of a limb in space or its existence or ownership. For example, a man with agnosia may not feel that his arm is part of his body, he may be unaware of his arm's position, or he may deny that a limb is paralyzed when it is.

This problem has been termed *unilateral neglect*. In nursing literature *Unilateral Neglect* is described as a deficit of looking, listening, touching, and searching as opposed to a deficit of seeing, hearing, feeling, or moving. Clients with neglect often have intact vision but will not look at or search for specific areas of the environment. Clients with injury to the temporoparietal lobe, inferior parietal lobe, lateral frontal lobe, cingulate gyrus, thalamus, and striatum most commonly develop neglect. Because of the dominance of the right hemisphere in directing attention, neglect is most commonly seen in clients with right hemisphere damage. Clinical manifestations of neglect appear on the side contralateral to the lesion and include failure to attend to one side of the body, failure to report or respond to stimuli on one side of the body, failure to use one extremity, and failure to orient the head and eyes to one side.[35]

Another type of agnosia affects only half of external space. Objects on one side are correctly interpreted, whereas those on the other side are not. For example, a client may be able to tell time only if it is between 12:00 and 6:00 and not between 6:00 and 12:00. A client with this condition (neglecting the left half of external space) usually has a right brain injury causing left hemiplegia and tends to avert the head and eyes to the right.

A client with visual agnosia sees objects but is unable to recognize or attach meaning to them. Disorientation occurs because of an inability to recognize environmental cues, familiar faces, or symbols. Such a client may examine objects curiously but be unable to know their function. This can cause considerable self-care deficit when common, necessary objects, such as silverware, clothing, or toilet articles, are unfamiliar. Visual agnosia greatly increases risk of injury because the client cannot recognize danger or symbols that warn of danger. Extensive visual agnosia can produce such extreme behavioral effects that the client may be inaccurately diagnosed as having diffuse dementia.

Kinesthesia

Kinesthesias are alterations in sensation. They occur on the affected side of the body and include the following:

1. Hemianesthesia (loss of sensation)
2. Paresthesia (feelings of heaviness, numbness, tingling, prickling, heightened sensitivity)
3. Loss of muscle-joint sense

Hemianesthesia is generally incomplete and may not be noticed by the client. Paresthesia occasionally manifests in a hemiplegic client as persistent, burning pain. Proprioception (ability to perceive the relationship of body parts to the external environment) and postural sense disturbance may occur with loss of muscle-joint sense. This may interfere seriously with the ability to ambulate because of lack of balance control and inappropriate movements. The risk of falling is high because of the tendency to malposition the feet when walking.

Shoulder Pain

Many clients have severe pain in the affected shoulder and hand after a cerebrovascular accident. This pain can be so severe that it results in lack of balance and loss of range of motion (ROM), which restricts mobility and self-care. The problem can be aggravated by overstretching from turns and transfers. Some clients have experienced subluxation (partial dislocation) of the shoulder both from having the shoulder pulled on and from the weight of the arm pulling it. Chronic subluxation results in shoulder-hand syndrome, characterized by a painful or frozen shoulder and hand edema.

Abstract Thought Changes

The client may also have difficulty in localizing objects within the environment and estimating their size or distance. The client may have difficulty finding routes or following directions to new places. This is caused in part by problems with memory, spatial perception, and loss of direction. Some clients lose their ability to recognize numbers; this prohibits them from using a telephone or telling time. The client may also have an inability to discriminate right from left.

Emotional Lability

Various portions of the brain assist with control of behavior and emotions. The cerebral cortex interprets various stimuli. The temporal and limbic areas modulate emotional responses to stimuli. The hypothalamus and pituitary coordinate the motor cortex and language areas. The brain can be seen as an inhibitor of emotions, and when the brain is not fully functional, emotional reactions and responses lack this inhibition.

After a cerebrovascular accident, clients are often emotionally labile, confused, forgetful, and frustrated. They tend to burst into tears, or, less commonly, laughter, without provocation. Clients may also use profanity, which is often termed *automatic language*. The client may often be distracted away from this behavior. Also, a client may appear highly distressed but not feel distressed. Depression, which has a negative effect on recovery, occurs in 23% to 63% of clients with strokes.[38] Other emotional or behavioral reactions may occur, including severe mood swings, social withdrawal (especially in aphasic and dys-

phasic clients), inappropriate sexual behavior, outbursts of frustration and anger, and regression to earlier childlike behavior. The actual type of emotional lability depends on the location of the infarction.

Incontinence

Bowel and bladder incontinence do not result from all types of stroke. A type of neurogenic bowel and bladder, an uninhibited bladder and bowel, sometimes occurs after stroke. Nerves send the message of bladder filling to the brain, but the brain does not correctly interpret the message and does not transmit the message not to urinate to the bladder. This results in frequency and urgency (see Case Study). Sometimes clients with this type of neurogenic bowel seem fixated on having a bowel movement. Other causes of incontinence may be memory lapses, inattention, emotional factors, inability to communicate, and infection.

■ Diagnostic Findings

A cerebral infarction may not be immediately seen on computed tomographic (CT) scan if its cause is nonhemorrhagic. Magnetic resonance imaging (MRI) is a useful test but is difficult to perform on critically ill or unstable clients (see Fig. 32–6b.) To minimize the risk of brain stem herniation, increased ICP must be ruled out before a lumbar puncture is performed. See Chapter 30.

Emergency Care

Most strokes occur at home or at work and are often confused with drunkenness, seizures, or diabetic coma. Emergency care includes maintaining a patent airway. Turn the client on the affected side if he or she is unconscious, to promote drainage of saliva from the airway. The collar of the shirt should be loosened to facilitate venous return. The head should be elevated but the neck should not be flexed. The person should be kept quiet and emergency help contacted.

Once in the emergency department (ED), airway patency is maintained and oxygen is supplied. The client is assessed for cardiac disorders, such as atrial fibrillation, that increase the risk of small emboli. Blood pressure is also evaluated and hypertension may be reduced with vasodilators. Thrombolytic treatments, such as administration of tissue plasminogen activator (tPA), may be undertaken once a hemorrhage has been ruled out. In a recent study, when tPA was given within 3 hours of ischemic stroke in a group of 291 clients, no significant effect was noted in neurologic improvement in the first 24 hours. However, in a second group of 333 clients, the clients were at least 30% more likely to have minimal or no disability at 3 months. Intracerebral hemorrhage incidence was increased in 6.4% of the treated clients versus 0.6% of the group not treated with tPA.[51]

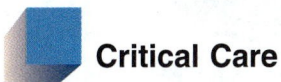

Critical Care

■ Medical Management

Medical management of the client after a cerebrovascular accident is directed toward to following:

1. Preserving life
2. Minimizing residual deficits
3. Reducing ICP
4. Preventing extension or recurrence

Because there are several causes of cerebrovascular accident, medical management differs based on the cause.

Clients who have received tPA in the ED will need critical monitoring for hemorrhage and reperfusion dysrhythmias for at least 24 hours. All clients are placed on bedrest. The head is elevated to 30 degrees to reduce ICP and to facilitate venous drainage in clients with hemorrhagic strokes. The head is kept flat for clients with ischemic strokes. External ventriculostomy drainage is sometimes used for a few days to reduce pressure from CSF accumulation. This involves placing a burr hole through the skull and passing a catheter into the lateral ventricle. This allows drainage of CSF. Blood pressure and level of consciousness (LOC) are closely monitored. The goal is to maintain blood pressure low enough to prevent another stroke or hemorrhage without decreasing cerebral perfusion. Fluids are administered carefully to avoid fluid volume excess and further cerebral ischemia. The client may require continuous mechanical ventilation.

Pharmacologic Management

Hypervolemic Hemodilution

Hypervolemic hemodilution is a relatively new approach in stroke management. The purpose is to dilute hematocrit to 30% to 35%, to raise cardiac output, and to thereby augment cerebral perfusion to reverse the ischemia. Hypervolemic hemodilution must begin within a few hours of the stroke to be effective, and it usually continues for 3 days. Albumin, low molecular weight dextran, and hetastarch have been used. Obviously, this procedure incurs risk of bleeding, cerebral edema, congestive heart failure, and pulmonary edema. Hypervolemic hemodilution requires constant monitoring in a critical care unit. Hemodynamic monitoring is used to assess the client's cardiovascular response. Short-term outcomes are better than in treatment with usual methods of stroke management.[28, 39]

Anticoagulation

For embolic or thrombotic stroke, anticoagulants and antiplatelet medications are commonly used to improve blood flow after hemorrhage has been ruled out. Initially these are administered IV, and then they are administered orally. Intravenous medications are delivered with an infusion pump to improve accurate delivery. Monitoring of clotting times is important to detect over-anticoagulation, which increases the risk of bleeding. Partial thromboplastin time (PTT) should be at 1.5 to 2 times normal for anticoagulation to be effective. After a therapeutic anticoagulant level has been achieved with heparin therapy, oral anticoagulants, such as warfarin, are begun. Because warfarin (Coumadin) has a long half-life, the physician initiates the warfarin therapy while the client is still receiving IV heparin. Once the client has a therapeutic response to warfarin, in about 24 to 48 hours, the physician discontinues the heparin and continues the warfarin therapy. Many agencies are now using the *international normalized ratio* (INR) instead of the prothrombin time (PT) for monitoring oral anticoagulation therapy; it provides a more consistent base for monitoring anticoagulant therapy responses. The therapeutic INR level for treatment and prophylaxis against venous thrombosis or systemic embolization is 2.0 to 3.0.[31]

Clients receiving anticoagulation should be assessed for bruising, hematuria, blood in feces, bleeding in mucous membranes, and new-onset or worsening headaches.

Antiplatelet Therapy

Antiplatelet aggregation medications work under the premise that inhibiting platelet function decreases the risk of thrombus formation. Aspirin prevents the synthesis of prostaglandins and thromboxane, which decrease platelet aggregation (clumping). However, larger doses of aspirin also inhibit prostacyclin, a substance that facilitates vessel dilation and inhibits platelet aggregation. Therefore lower doses of aspirin are more effective in reducing the risk of second stroke. Some studies have suggested that dipyridamole (Persantine) has not proved to provide additional stroke protection.[10] Ticlopidine (Ticlid), another antiplatelet therapy, demonstrated a 24% decreased stroke incidence over aspirin in 3069 clients. Ticlopidine also reduced risk in both men and women, unlike aspirin, which has been shown to affect only men.[6, 10]

Edema Control

Steroids or osmotic diuretics may be used to reduce ICP. Hypertension is commonly controlled with antihypertensives and diuretics. Headache and neck stiffness can usually be treated with mild analgesics, such as codeine and acetaminophen. Stronger narcotics are usually avoided; these agents sedate the client, depress respirations that result in increased ICP, and thus make the neurologic assessment inaccurate.

Seizure Control

If seizures develop, phenytoin (Dilantin) or phenobarbital may be used. Barbiturates and other sedative agents are avoided. If fever develops, antipyretics may be prescribed.

Meningioma, Fractured Hip, and Possible Cerebrovascular Accident

Mrs. Olsen is a 72-year-old white woman who resides at Shady Oaks Care Center. She fell today and could not get up again because of the pain. An x-ray obtained at the nursing home showed a proximal femoral fracture near the right hip joint. She has been transferred to your hospital for a preoperative medical evaluation in preparation for possible surgical repair of her right hip fracture later today.

Mrs. Olsen has a history of a meningioma, which she has had resected three times. Two days ago the client had an episode of apparent dysfunction of the left upper and lower extremities associated with a period of hypertension and agitation, all of

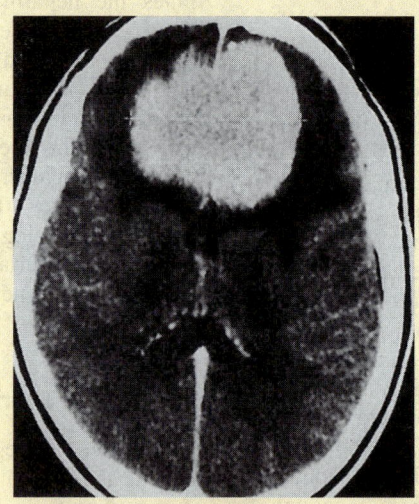

■ This contrast CT scan shows Mrs. Olsen's meningioma, prior to resection.

placed on phenytoin (Dilantin). The daughter states that her mother has had several falls during the past several days and seems imbalanced at times when she changes position. Mrs. Olsen is a World War II immigrant from Denmark, where her siblings continue to live. Since her last craniotomy, she has been lapsing into intervals where she uses her native language and believes that her daughter is her sister Ingrid. Consider the implications of this in your preoperative preparations. Mrs. Olsen denies discomfort at this time.

Mrs. Olsen taught high-school mathematics until the time of her first craniotomy 10 years ago. Her husband died last year of a myocardial infarction.

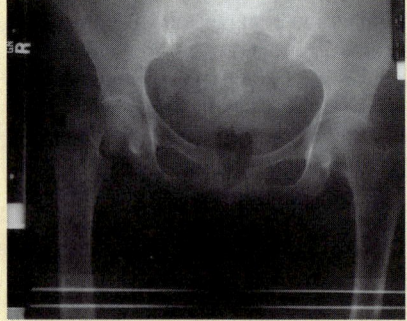

■ An x-ray of Mrs. Olsen's fracture of the proximal femur, near the right hip joint.

which resolved within 24 hours. Mrs. Olsen also has a history of deep vein thrombosis (DVT) following one of her surgeries, but is not on long-term anticoagulation therapy. What ramifications will this have for her current treatment?

Nursing Admission Assessment

Mrs. Olsen has lived at Shady Oaks since her last craniotomy, after which she developed seizures and was

Selected Admission Laboratory Values

RBC	3.76 million/mm³
Hgb	11.7 g/dl
Hct	34%
WBC	10,200/mm³
Sodium	141 mEq/L
Potassium	4.3 mEq/L
Chloride	101 mEq/L
CO_2	22 mEq/L
Glucose	157 mg/dl
ABO/Rh type	O⁺
Phenytoin level	7.6 μg/ml

Nursing Physical Examination

Height: 5′6″
Weight: 135 lb (61.4 kg)
Vital signs: BP = 170/90;
  TPR = 99.6, 102, 22
LOC: Awake, alert, slightly confused; daughter states that she is asking in Danish where she is and what happened
EENT: PERRLA, evidence of cranial surgical scars on right frontal region, slight left facial droop, hand grasps equal
Cardiac: Regular rate and rhythm without gallop or murmur
Pulmonary: Clear bilaterally
Abdominal: Soft, nontender, active bowel sounds
Genitourinary: Foley catheter inserted in ER draining clear yellow urine
Peripheral pulses: 3/4 without edema, some shortening of right lower extremity

Initial Treatment Plan

Meds: Phenytoin (Dilantin) 200 mg PO or IV bid
IV: D5LR TKO
Diet: NPO
Activity: Bedrest with mattress overlay and trapeze
Additional assessments: Vital signs, neurologic checks, and cerebrospinal meningitis (CSM) checks q 4 h
Treatments: Ice to right hip continuously
Diagnostic Tests: CT scan of head

Mrs. Olsen's CT scan revealed no further progression of her meningioma. She successfully underwent surgery for endoprosthetic replacement of the right proximal femur. Postoperatively, the surgeon orders:

advance diet as tolerated, soft wrist and Posey restraints as needed to protect self, physical therapy to initiate progressive ambulation with weightbearing as tolerated, incentive spirometer while awake, cefazolin (Ancef) 1 g IV q 8 h × 4, Lovenox 30 mg SQ q 12 h, docusate (Colace) 100 mg PO daily, and meperidine (Demerol) 75 mg with hydroxyzine (Vistaril) 25 mg IM q 3 h prn. Vicodin 500 mg q 4 h prn.

Mrs. Olsen pulls out her Foley catheter 36 hours postoperatively. The urine had become cloudy and odorous. Recordings of the time and amount of voiding and trimethoprim-sulfamethoxazole (Bactrim) 1 tablet PO bid are ordered. Consider the factors that precipitated the need for this drug. Mrs. Olsen continues to speak primarily in Danish and because she is incontinent, she requires disposable undergarments. She also refuses to eat, and the nurse is unable to determine why. The IV infusion was discontinued after Mrs. Olsen pulled it out during her bath. Attempts at ambulation have been unsuccessful because of communication difficulties. A Danish interpreter is not available, and although Mrs. Olsen's daughter speaks Danish, she has had to return to her job and family responsibilities. The physician is planning to release Mrs. Olsen to Shady Oaks tomorrow.

Discharge Criteria

Average LOS (insurance certification): 7.6 days with transfer to skilled care on day 4.
Complete transfer form.
Initiate social services referral to coordinate transfer.

Questions to Be Considered

1. Mrs. Olsen becomes increasingly agitated while in restraints. What alternative measures might the nurse consider to protect Mrs. Olsen? Discuss the ethical implications surrounding physical and chemical restraints.
2. Consider the implications that Mrs. Olsen's neurologic problems—the meningioma, seizures, and a possible CVA—may have had in relationship to her fall. What other factors may have contributed to the fall? What actions should the nurse take to protect her from future injury?
3. Based on her admission assessment data, calculate Mrs. Olsen's score on the Glasgow Coma Scale. What influence does Mrs. Olsen's use of the Danish language have on your calculation? How is her situation different from someone who is not bilingual?
4. How has Mrs. Olsen's recovery been compromised because of her lack of mobilization? Identify potential complications that may occur as a result of immobility. How may they be prevented? Discuss methods of communication you might use to facilitate Mrs. Olsen's recovery and rehabilitation.
5. Discuss the effects that Mrs. Olsen's refusal to eat will have on the processes of wound healing and immunity.
6. Review the nursing implications and related patient education for administration of phenytoin and trimethoprim-sulfamethoxazole.
7. Compare and contrast brain tumors in terms of treatment and prognosis.

Dietary Management

Because of the high risk of aspiration, choking, excessive coughing, and vomiting, oral food and fluids are generally withheld for 24 to 48 hours. If the client cannot eat or drink after 48 hours, alternate feeding routes are used, such as tube feeding or hyperalimentation.

When the swallowing mechanism has returned, the client can be fed orally. Progressive feeding programs for dysphagia are based on the degree of swallowing ability (Table 32–3).

Controlling blood pressure is key in management. A blood pressure that is too high or too low can decrease cerebral perfusion. Chronic hypertension is a risk factor for cerebrovascular accident and clients are often evaluated in ED with blood pressures well above normal limits. When blood pressure must be lowered, it is done so gradually. Clients are placed in a supine position to promote cerebral perfusion. Unlike most healthy people who are able to maintain cardiac output and cerebral perfusion with position changes, the client is unable to do so following a stroke. Stroke victims have difficult maintaining cerebral perfusion, especially when moving from a lying to a standing position.

Supportive Care

The general care of clients after stroke was discussed previously. Each type of stroke also requires specific care especially when the client has had a life-threatening infarction.

Thrombotic Stroke

Thrombotic stroke of a large portion of the brain is usually poorly tolerated, especially in the elderly. If the dominant hemisphere is involved, aggressive medical management may be withheld if rehabilitative potential is slim. The choice of whether to pursue aggressive treatment focuses on several factors, such as the client's age, his or her preference (if known), the presence and severity of other disorders, the size of the infarction, how much time has elapsed since the infarction, and the rehabilitation potential. At present, the treatment for most clients with large areas of infarction is supportive care. It is hoped that future research can improve the treatment outcomes for these clients.

Table 32–3. Progressive Feeding Program for Clients with Dysphagia

	Stage 1	Stage II	Stage III	Stage IV
Description	Severe swallowing difficulty	Swallowing difficulty with various textures and chewing	Less difficulty swallowing, beginning to control foods better in mouth, also able to tolerate various food textures and consistencies	Able to swallow most foods very well
Meats	Puréed meat with gravy, baby food, egg yolks	Junior baby food meats with gravy; scrambled, soft, or poached eggs; cottage cheese	Ground meat with gravy; soft meats (tuna) in casseroles; macaroni and cheese; fish without bones; chopped meats	Soft diet
Starch	Mashed potatoes with gravy	Muffins (no seeds); pancakes; French toast; cooked cereal (thick)	Toast (no seeds); rice; soft baked potato	Soft foods
Vegetables	Puréed	Junior vegetables	Peas, squash, carrots; avoid stringy foods (celery, spinach)	Soft foods
Fruits	Puréed, ripe watermelon, cantaloupe, or honeydew (no seeds)	Cooked fruit, ripe banana, soft canned fruit	Grapefruit and orange sections; peeled ripe peaches, pears, and nectarines	Soft foods
Dessert	Custard, pudding	Cakes (no seeds, nuts)	Pies, cakes, sherbet, ice cream	Soft foods
Liquids	None	None	Thick liquids, nectars, strained cream soups, eggnog, liquid caloric supplements, milk shakes	May be able to have thickened liquids

Embolic Stroke

In addition to the critical care management, treatment is directed at prevention of further emboli by resolution of the underlying problem. Clients may need treatment of cardiac dysrhythmias (see Chapter 46).

Hemorrhagic Stroke

Treatment of hemorrhagic stroke depends partly on the condition of the client when first seen and partly on the cause of the stroke. A client who presents with a severe headache but who is fully conscious will probably survive no matter what the therapy. The client who is in a coma is likely to do poorly despite intensive medical or surgical intervention.[45] Hypoxia often occurs in these clients because of inadequate ventilatory effort. Intubation and continuous mechanical ventilation may be required to prevent secondary injury to the brain from hypoxia.

Again, hypertension may have been the culprit that caused the aneurysm to leak. Therefore, rampant hypertension must be brought under control. The ideal range for systolic blood pressure is usually 100 to 150 mm Hg (which more closely matches the client's usual blood pressure). Clients have increased intracranial pressure and are positioned with the headrest at 30 degrees, without neck flexion, to promote venous drainage.

Intracranial hemorrhage is often accompanied by hyperthermia. This condition increases oxygen use by the brain at a time when the oxygen supply is compromised. Antipyretics may be prescribed. In addition, a hypothermia blanket or ice packs may be required to reduce body temperature. Causing the client to shiver should be avoided, however, because shivering increases oxygen consumption and ICP.

Stroke in Evolution

A *stroke in evolution* is a term used to describe a client in whom the cerebral infarction is still evolving. The client presents with increasing neurologic deficits over a period of hours to days. The client has the potential to become severely impaired and also has the potential to not develop further damage. Treatment focuses on improving cerebral blood flow by avoiding fluid volume deficits and hypotension. The goal is to maintain the systolic blood pressure between 100 and 150 mm Hg. In addition, hypoxia is also avoided by administration of oxygen and maintenance of a patent airway. Thrombolytic agents or IV heparin therapy may be used.

■ Nursing Management of the Medical Client

Assessment

The initial assessment of the client who is suspected of having a stroke is very important. Initial assessment includes the following: level of consciousness, pupillary response to light, movement to command or painful stimuli, changes in speech, sensory changes, reflexes, presence of headache, and vital signs. These data are often recorded and scored on the Glasgow Coma Scale (GCS). In addition, if intracranial pressure monitors are in place, baseline pressure values and waveforms should be noted. See the Bridge to Critical Care feature for intracranial pressure monitoring. The assessment must be complete and accurate to provide a baseline for ongoing assessments. Report abnormal neurologic assessments promptly to the physician. Refer to the earlier discussion of the GCS and the neurologic assessment in Chapter 30.

A complete history of the presenting problem as well as past medical and social history provide data about the etiology of the cerebrovascular accident. For example, a history of hypertension or cardiac valve disorders is commonly associated with a cerebrovascular accident.

Diagnosis, Planning, Implementation

Many acute care agencies have begun to use critical pathways for the management of clients with cerebrovascular accident. An example of one is shown in Appendix G.

Altered Cerebral Tissue Perfusion. Perfusion of the cerebrum is critical for survival. Therefore, it should be the first priority in care of clients with acute stroke. Decreased cerebral blood flow may be secondary to thrombus, embolus, hemorrhage, edema, or spasm. Data that indicate that the altered perfusion has become an actual problem include the following:

- Intracranial pressure greater than 15 mm Hg sustained for 15 to 30 seconds or longer
- Cerebral perfusion pressure less than 70 mm Hg
- Decrease in GCS score of two or more points from baseline
- Decreasing levels of consciousness
- Mean arterial pressure of less than 80 mm Hg or systolic blood pressure less than 100 mm Hg or greater than 150 mm Hg
- Bradycardia or altered pattern of breathing (e.g., central neurogenic hyperventilation, apneustic, ataxic)
- Loss of response to painful stimuli
- Change in pupil size or response to light
- Headache
- Vomiting
- Abnormal flexion or extension posturing

Planning: Expected Outcomes. The client will have improved cerebral tissue perfusion as evidenced by ICP less than 15 mm Hg, CPP greater than 65 mm Hg, no type A waves (when using intracranial monitors), no reports of headache, no decreases in LOC, and stable or improving GCS score.

Implementation. Serial assessments of these data may be required as often as hourly for unstable clients. Analyze data for trends, and if the client is deteriorating (decreasing LOC, changes in motor or sensory function, pupillary changes, respiratory difficulty, development of visual or perceptual defects or aphasia), notify the physician.

Administer medications to improve cerebral tissue perfusion as prescribed. The drugs prescribed to decrease risk of further thrombus formation include anticoagulants (e.g., heparin, warfarin) or antiplatelet drugs (e.g., aspirin, ticlopidine). Ticlopidine has been shown to be even more effective than aspirin in stroke prevention and had significant stroke reduction in both women and men. Research on aspirin has only been shown to be effective with men.[10] Nimodipine, a calcium-channel blocking agent, is also approved for treatment of vasospasm secondary to subarachnoid hemorrhage.[53]

Delirium and restlessness should be controlled, with sedatives if necessary. Be certain, however, that restlessness is not the result of treatable causes, such as a hypoxia, full bladder, bowel impaction, or pain. Restraints should be avoided, because they often increase agitation and cerebral pressure.

Straining at stool or with excessive coughing, vomiting, lifting, or use of the arms to change position should be avoided, because it increases intracerebral pressure. Mild laxatives and stool softeners are often prescribed.

The client who is awake and alert should be taught about the pathologic process and instructed to inform you about any changes in sensation, movement, or function, regardless of how minor a change may seem. Increasing neurologic deficit indicates either progression of the infarction or ischemia.

Other nursing diagnoses and collaborative problems that are used in planning care of the stroke client in critical care are listed in the following section. Common problems include impaired physical mobility, risk for impaired skin integrity, impaired verbal communication, risk for corneal abrasion, hyperthermia, risk for injury/aspiration, and ineffective individual coping.

Acute and Subacute Care

■ Medical Management

During the acute and subacute stages, residual deficits from a stroke are treated, and intervention is directed toward helping the client function at the maximum capacity. Clients with stroke and their families face difficult adjustments as the acute stages pass and residual disabilities become obvious. A multidisciplinary rehabilitative team may help to assist and support clients during this time. Assessing the functional abilities of the client and setting realistic goals are part of this approach. To optimize recovery, all clinicians should use the Clinical Practice Guidelines developed by the Agency for Health Care Policy and Research (AHCPR) on post-stroke rehabilitation to guide care of a client suffering from a stroke.[57]

- Treat the client with multidisciplinary services
- Document the client's condition and course fully, including deficits, status of other diseases, complications, changes in status, and functional status before stroke
- Begin physical activity as soon as the client's medical condition is stable; use caution with early mobilization in clients with coma, severe obtundation, progressing neurologic clinical manifestations, subarachnoid or intracerebral hemorrhage, severe orthostatic hypotension, acute myocardial infarction, or acute deep vein thrombosis.

- Assist in managing general health functions throughout all stages of treatment, such as managing dysphagia, nutrition, hydration, bladder and bowel function, sleep and rest, co-morbid conditions, and/or acute illnesses
- Prevent complications, including deep vein thrombosis and pulmonary embolism, dysphagia and aspiration, skin breakdown, urinary tract infections, falls, spasticity and contractures, shoulder injury, and seizures (anticonvulsants are not recommended in clients who have not had any seizures).
- Prevent recurrent strokes through control of modifiable risk factors, oral anticoagulation, antiplatelet therapy, and/or surgical intervention
- Assess throughout acute and rehabilitation stages
- Use reliable standardized instruments for evaluation
- Evaluate for formal rehabilitation during acute stage
- Choose individual or interdisciplinary program based on the individual's and the family's needs; success of the program requires full support and active participation of the client and family; families must be involved at the outset
- Choose the local rehabilitation program that best meets the client's and/or family's needs

Several other disciplines join to facilitate recovery of the client following a cerebrovascular accident. It is the coordinated effort of the entire team that best serves the client and family.

Physical Therapy

Physical therapists work with the client to build strength, preserve range of motion (ROM) and tone in non-involved muscles, and build ROM and tone and retrain muscles affected by the stroke. The client also works on balance and proprioception skills. This may enable the client, with continued improvement, to sit on the edge of the bed and to eventually ambulate. Exercise and bed mobility skills are taught at the client's bedside, as are wheelchair mobility and transfers. If the client is able to wear an orthosis (brace), he or she is instructed on how to apply and remove it. A hemiplegic client is usually able to ambulate using either a quad cane or a Lofstrand crutch, following gait training.

Occupational Therapy

Occupational therapists work with the client to relearn activities of daily living (ADLs) and to use assistive devices that promote independence. For example, a client with hemiplegia may be able to dress if the clothing can be closed with Velcro fasteners rather than buttons.

Speech Therapy

Speech therapists work with the client to foster the maximum amount of speech recovery possible through relearning, accentuation of speech sounds, or use of alternative communication devices.

Outcomes

It was previously thought that damage to the CNS was irreversible. Now it has been shown that even in adults with significant brain injury, relearning can take place. But it is extremely important that relearning take place as soon as possible after the injury. When healing takes place without demands, potential function will be lost. It has been reported that Pasteur did some of his best work after a small stroke.

Complications

Complications of stroke depend primarily on the location of the lesion or infarcted tissue. If the brain stem is affected, blood pressure fluctuations, altered respiratory patterns, and cardiac dysrhythmias are all possible. Aspiration, injury, and the complications secondary to immobility related to the client's inability to realize his or her physical limitations are also risk factors.

Coma can follow strokes of various causes. The blood supply to the brain stem or reticular activating system may have been directly occluded. Likewise, the deep structures of the thalamus that relay information to the cerebral cortex may be involved. Vascular occlusion of the internal carotid artery or one of its major branches may also decrease the level of consciousness. Sometimes, the cerebral edema that follows stroke may produce midline shifts, resulting in coma.

Strokes caused by occlusive disease (e.g., thrombus, embolus) rarely cause sudden death. When stroke is fatal, death may occur within 3 to 12 hours, but it more often occurs between 1 and 14 days after the original episode. Typically, with any type of fatal stroke, a rise in temperature, heart rate, and respiratory rate occurs along with deepening coma several hours or days before death. These are a result of damage to the vasomotor and heat-regulating centers.

The two primary causes of death with stroke are (1) respiratory infection and (2) brain stem failure. Impaired consciousness, altered attention, and feeding and swallowing problems all predispose the stroke victim to respiratory infections. These infections often lead to death from progressive hypoxia. Increasing ICP, central herniation, and brain stem hemorrhage lead to death from depression of the vital centers in the medulla, that is, brain stem failure.

■ Nursing Management of the Medical Client

Assessment

Ongoing assessments of all body systems are needed. Assess the client's LOC, heart sounds, heart rate and rhythm, respiratory rate and rhythm, temperature, ability to move, levels of nutrition, ability to swallow, bladder and bowel elimination, sensation and perception, communication, sexuality, and self-concept. The assessment of life-threatening problems should be continuous; the psychosocial aspects need assessment every day or so unless, of course, obvious abnormal data are noted.

Diagnosis, Planning, Implementation

Altered Cerebral Tissue Perfusion. This diagnosis was initiated in critical care if the client was admitted to critical care with an acute stroke. Management of cerebral perfusion does not end in critical care, though. Ongoing assessment and interventions are required.

Planning: Expected Outcomes. The client will have improved cerebral tissue perfusion as evidenced by no reports of headache, no decreases in LOC, and stable or improving GCS score.

Implementation. Ongoing assessments of these data may be required as often as every 2 to 4 hours for clients who have undergone recent cerebrovascular accidents. Analyze assessment data for trends, and if the client's condition is deteriorating, notify the physician. Such data include decreasing LOC, changes in motor or sensory function, pupillary changes, respiratory difficulty, development of visual or perceptual defects, or aphasia. See the Critical Monitoring feature in Chapter 31 for a more complete listing of the changes that indicate progressive deterioration.

Various medications to improve cerebral tissue perfusion are used. Anticoagulants (e.g., heparin, warfarin) or antiplatelet drugs (e.g., aspirin, ticlopidine) are used if a thrombus is present; calcium-channel blocking agents also are given to reduce cerebral vasospasm. Other interventions are directed at reducing intracranial pressure. Straining at stool or with excessive coughing, vomiting, lifting, or use of the arms to change position should be avoided. Mild laxatives and stool softeners are often prescribed. See the section on care of a client with increased ICP earlier in this chapter.

Teach the client who is awake and alert about the pathologic process and to inform you about any changes in sensation, movement, or function regardless of how minor a change may seem. Increasing neurologic deficit indicates either progression of the infarction or ischemia of the area from cerebral edema or bleeding.

Risk for Aspiration. An increased risk of aspiration is listed first here because of its importance in maintaining airway and oxygenation. Not all clients are at risk of aspiration after stroke, and their risk depends on time since injury and area of infarction. When considering this diagnosis, use the following etiologies of aspiration to guide your problem solving: impaired swallowing, depressed cough and gag reflexes, and decreased LOC.

Planning: Expected Outcomes. The client will develop no clinical manifestations of aspiration, as evidenced by easily managing own saliva, no choking while eating, no coughing while eating, no fever, and no crackles or rhonchi.

Implementation. Assess the client for clinical manifestations of aspiration, such as fever, dyspnea, crackles and rhonchi, confusion, and decreased PaO_2 in arterial blood gases. Use caution in feeding the client, either orally or enterally. See Table 32–3 for a list of foods for the client with dysphagia. If the client has enteral feedings, add food coloring to the tube feeding to assist with identifying aspiration via suctioned aspirate. Monitor chest x-ray results, and report findings of pulmonary infiltrate.

Impaired Physical Mobility.
Almost all clients have some degree of immobility after a stroke. In the early phases of stroke recovery, the client may be completely immobile and need assistance just to turn over in bed. Later in recovery, mobility may only be hampered in one extremity. Various causes can be used to individualize this diagnosis. They include loss of muscle tone secondary to flaccid paralysis or spasticity or reluctance to move associated with fear of self-injury or prolonged disuse.

Planning: Expected Outcomes. The client will achieve maximal physical mobility within the limitations imposed by cerebrovascular accident as evidenced by more normal movement of affected extremity, improved muscle strength, and effective use of adaptive devices.

Implementation. Assess the client's degree of muscle strength to use as a baseline and for setting expected outcomes. A comprehensive assessment by a physical therapist will help to determine appropriate activity levels.

Doing Exercises in Bed. Encouraging clients with hemiplegia to exercise while they are still in bed not only prepares for later activities but also offers hope and a sense of optimism about recovery. A hemiplegic client can learn to move the weak leg by sliding the unaffected leg under it to lift and move the weak leg. Be aware that clients may have difficulty crossing the midline.

Hourly gluteal muscle setting and quadriceps muscle setting exercises during the day help prepare for later ambulation. Begin with five repetitions and increase gradually to 20 repetitions each time. Instruct the client as follows:

- Gluteal setting: "Pinch" or contract the buttocks together and count to five. Then relax and count to five. Repeat.
- Quadriceps setting: Contract the quadriceps muscles, on the anterior portion of the thigh, while raising the heel and trying to squash a rolled towel placed under the popliteal fossa against the mattress. While keeping the muscle contracted, count to five; then relax and count to five. Repeat. Perform on each extremity if possible. Start quadriceps setting exercise as soon as the client is conscious. The quadriceps muscle is the most important in giving knee joint stability in walking.

Sitting Up. Help the client out of bed as soon as the client's condition is medically stable. Remember, however, that hemiplegia severely affects balance. Assistance is needed to provide security and safety. Raise the client's head slowly in bed to reduce orthostatic hypotension.

When the client first sits up, support the affected side, especially the back and the head. Gradually, the client learns to sit alone with the head of the bed elevated, and then to sit on the edge of the bed with the feet on a firm surface. Help the client maintain balance by extending the affected arm and placing the palm flat on the bed. Be patient and encouraging as the client regains balance. When the client is sitting in a chair, support the weak side with pillows.

Eventually, the client learns to raise the weak leg with the unaffected leg and to swing both legs laterally over the side of the bed onto the floor. It is safest to have the client pivot on the unaffected leg. Therefore, position the chair at a right angle to the unaffected side.

Using a Wheelchair. A hemiplegic client needs to learn safe transfers from bed to chair, commode, or wheelchair. The Client Education Guide shows one method. A hemiplegic client usually does better with a "hemi" wheelchair, which sits approximately 1 to 2 inches lower than a conventional wheelchair to make propulsion easier. The client with unilateral paralysis can propel a wheelchair with the unaffected arm and leg; also, one-arm-drive wheelchairs are available. Once in a wheelchair, a client's level of independence increases greatly. Deficits in spatial relations, decreased awareness, and neglect can result in problems such as falling and running into doors. A client must not be allowed to do wheelchair self-transfers until he or she has demonstrated competence.

Walking. A tilt table may be used in physical therapy to help the client assume a standing position if difficulty with balance is a problem. Begin standing as soon as the quadriceps muscles on the unaffected side have normal strength. Have the client seated on the edge of the bed. Encourage the client to rise, using the muscle power of the unaffected leg. The client may tend to swing around toward the affected side. Gradually, the client learns to take increasing amounts of weight onto the weaker side. Despite weakness in the affected limb, a hemiplegic client often develops an extensor reflex, which facilitates standing. Position yourself on the weaker side when helping the client to stand. A cane should be used on the unaffected side, to allow walking with a three-point gait.

Most hemiplegic clients can be taught to walk. Remind them to keep the body weight forward over the feet. Practice is important for learning to walk correctly. Incorrect habits, once developed, may be difficult to overcome later. Supervise clients carefully until they can safely walk alone without fear of falling. When walking, the client should not show circumduction or toe scraping or stoop forward. Heel-toe walking with a reciprocal gait pattern is the goal of ambulation.

Bracing. If bracing is used, teach the client and family how to apply and remove the brace, to observe skin for breakdown, to give proper skin care, and to care for the brace itself.

Hyperthermia.
Bleeding or edema of the hypothalamus leads to ischemia of the thermoregulatory center of the brain.

Planning: Expected Outcomes. The client will have decreasing temperature or normal temperature.

Implementation. Treat fever with antipyretics. Sometimes a hypothermia blanket is used to bring down a high temperature quickly. When hypothermia blankets are used, the skin must be frequently assessed for pressure points. Shivering must also be avoided as the muscle activity increases body temperature. Sometimes keeping the feet warm with blankets decreases shivering. Pheno-

CLIENT EDUCATION GUIDE

Transfer from Bed to Wheelchair by a Hemiplegic Client

(Shading on the right side of the client indicates the affected side.) Lock the wheelchair for safety and keep it beside the bed on your unaffected side. Use your unaffected arm and leg (*A* and *B*) to move your affected arm and leg. As your legs drop over the edge of the bed, swing your torso up to a sitting position (*C*). Push yourself up to a standing position (*D*) by using your unaffected arm and leg. Reach across the wheelchair (*E*) to grasp the far arm of the chair, and turn to seat yourself.

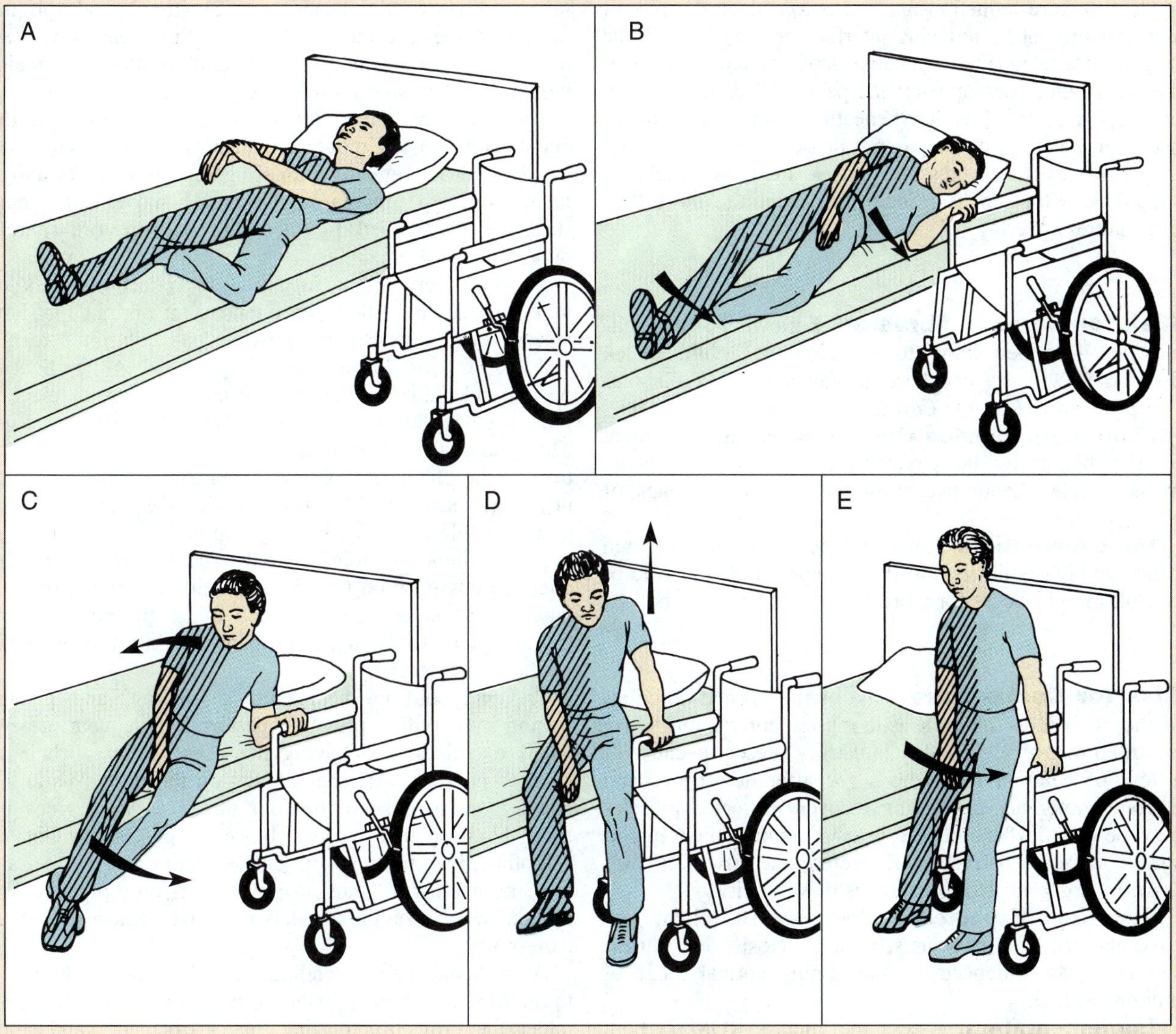

A

B

C

D

E

thiazines may be used to help stabilize neuronal membranes if the fever is related to damaged brain structures.

Risk for Impaired Skin Integrity. The loss of protective sensation and decreased ability to move increases the risk of injury to the skin. In addition, the client may develop skin damage from friction and shearing or increased skin fragility from inadequate nutritional status or edema.

Planning: Expected Outcomes. The client's skin will remain intact as evidenced by no stage I pressure ulcer development and no signs of redness from friction or shearing.

Implementation. Assess the skin often, such as every 2 to 4 hours. If stage I pressure ulcers are noted, turn the client more frequently.

Change a hemiplegic client's position every 2 hours. Develop a written turning schedule for other healthcare providers and family members to follow. When positioning the client on the affected side, make sure that body weight does not harm affected limbs. Support the affected leg when turning and positioning a hemiplegic client. Complete hip dislocation can occur if the flaccid leg falls forward and downward when the client is turned onto the unaffected side. Place a pillow between the client's legs to provide support. At night, apply a padded posterior splint to the affected leg to maintain correct positioning and to prevent leg flexion. Also, the client may only be able to tolerate lying for 30 minutes on the affected side because of the impaired circulation.

Use pressure reduction mattresses to reduce the risk of skin impairment by reducing interface pressure. Check the mattress for adequacy in padding depth by reaching under the client with your outstretched palm. If less than 1 inch of support material is felt beneath the hips, sacrum, or heels, the mattress overlay is not dense enough and is not reducing interface pressure. Ideal mattress thickness should be 3 to 4 inches. Some clients require more than one mattress overlay.

Risk for Corneal Abrasion. Following stroke, clients may lose their ability to blink. Without a blink reflex the cornea will dry and become abraded. The collaborative problem is *Risk for Corneal Abrasion.*

Planning: Expected Outcomes. Monitor the client for risk factors for the development of corneal abrasion, including absence of eye closure or blinking or lack of eye moisture.

Implementation. Protect the eye with an eye patch if no blinking is noted. Instill prescribed artificial tears or consult the physician for a prescription if none exists.

Risk for Contracture. One of the normal activities of the brain is to inhibit spastic muscle contraction. Early in stroke recovery, flaccidity is usually present because of a loss of cerebral connections for afferent sensory and efferent motor nerves. During recovery, affected muscles may be spastic because the injured brain cannot inhibit spastic muscle contraction. Therefore the *Risk for Contracture* is due to flaccid paralysis or spasticity.

Planning: Expected Outcomes. The client will have absence of contractures, joint ankylosis, and muscle shortening as evidenced by maintaining normal range of motion (ROM).

Implementation. Assess the client's ROM in both the involved and non-involved joints. These findings can be used as a baseline and also as an expected outcome.

Perform passive ROM exercises two times daily after the first 24 hours following a stroke unless otherwise prescribed. Motor impulses usually begin to return between 2 and 14 days after a stroke. The affected part (initially flaccid) becomes spastic as the spinal cord motor systems establish their autonomy and the potential for contractures increases. Passive exercises are more difficult to perform once affected muscles begin to tighten. Do not force extremities beyond the point of initiating pain or continuous spasm. Always support the joint you are exer-

cising and move the extremity smoothly, without jerking movements. Frequent passive ROM exercises prevent joint immobility, tendon contractures, and muscle atrophy. They also stimulate circulation and help reestablish neuromuscular pathways. By performing these exercises before dressing and undressing the client, you may facilitate self-care.

Teach the client to use the unaffected hand to lift the weak arm and put it through ROM exercises. Exercise each finger separately. Also, while the client is in bed, teach him or her to (1) exercise the affected arm by grasping it at the wrist with the unaffected hand and raising it above the head, and (2) stretch and rub the fingers of the affected hand several times each day. Active ROM to the unaffected extremities assists in maintaining or increasing muscle strength.

Once some voluntary movement returns, encourage the client with assisted movements. Support the affected arm during such movements with sling-suspensions. As movement strength increases, resisted movements may strengthen weakened muscles and help restore muscle bulk.

Several interventions are used to reduce the risk of joint contracture. Allow the client to sit upright for short periods only, because this position can contribute to hip and knee flexion deformities. Likewise, when the client is on one side, do not flex the hip acutely. Do not place a pillow under the affected knee when the client is supine. This encourages flexion deformity and impedes circulation. If the clients knees have a tendency to hyperextend, however, place a folded towel under the knee for short periods while the client is lying supine.

If the client can tolerate the prone position, place the client in this position for 15 to 30 minutes several times a day, with a small pillow placed under the pelvis (from the umbilicus to the upper third of the thigh) to hyperextend the hip joints.

Prevent footdrop, heel cord shortening, and plantar flexion by avoiding pressure, performing frequent passive ROM exercises, and having the client sit in a chair as soon as possible with the feet flat on the floor. While the client is in bed, keep the foot flexed at 90 degrees by using high-top tennis shoes, braces, a posterior splint, or a footboard. A footboard is only effective if both feet are pressing against it. Thus, a footboard is only practical for a client who is supine and has no movement in the lower extremities.

A trochanter roll, extending from the crest of the ilium to midthigh, prevents external hip rotation by wedging under the projection of the greater trochanter and stopping the femur from rolling. Trochanter rolls increase the risk of skin impairment; assess the skin beneath the roll often.

When the client is in bed, prevent adduction of the affected shoulder by placing a pillow in the axilla, between the upper arm and the chest wall, to keep the arm abducted about 60 degrees. Keep the arm slightly flexed in a neutral position. Place the forearm on another pillow with the elbow above the shoulder and the wrist above the elbow. This position stretches the shoulder's internal rotators. Elevating the arm also helps prevent edema and resultant fibrosis.

Place the affected hand in a position of function, that is, slightly supinated with fingers slightly flexed and thumb in opposition. Frequent passive ROM exercises are important. The use of splints to prevent flexion contractures is more effective if they are individually designed by occupational therapists and are scheduled for "on-and-off" periods to allow for skin assessment and ROM. Squeezing a rubber ball is no longer recommended because it promotes flexion when extension is desirable.

The weight of an immobile arm may cause (1) pain and movement limitation ("frozen shoulder") secondary to shoulder joint fibrositis or (2) subluxation, that is, incomplete dislocation of the shoulder joint. Prevent these by supporting a completely flaccid arm in a sling when the client is walking and with a pillow when the client is in bed or seated in a chair.

Self Care Deficit. Self care deficits may range from not being able to reach with a weak or paralyzed arm to full dependence on others. This diagnosis is applicable if an achievable outcome can be obtained. Clients with complete paralysis and cognitive deficits may not be able to perform self care. Other diagnoses may be more accurate in these cases, such as *Impaired Physical Mobility* and *Impaired Skin Integrity*. Several terms can be used to describe *Self Care Deficit*, including *Impaired Physical Mobility, Visual and Sensory-Perceptual Alterations, Unilateral Neglect*, or *Altered Thought Processes*.

Planning: Expected Outcomes. The client will perform as many ADLs as possible within limitations, as evidenced by use of adaptive devices and techniques.

Implementation. At first, a client who has had a stroke may need considerable help with all self-care activities (e.g., washing, eating, grooming). Help the client to use the affected arm as much as possible and to avoid the tendency to do everything with the unaffected limb. As soon as hemiplegic clients can sit up in bed, encourage the client to do all self-care activities possible with the unaffected hand (e.g., brushing teeth, eating, combing hair, shaving, bathing). This helps preserve independent self-care and prevents immobility complications. Be patient and allow the hemiplegic clients to do as much for themselves as possible. Because this is often difficult, a lot of encouragement is needed. This is also an excellent opportunity for family teaching. Family members find it very difficult to watch a loved one struggle with a task, and they often perform the task for the client. It is important to explain how it benefits the client to be as independent as possible.

In clients with diplopia, an eye patch over one eye removes the second image and promotes better vision. Alternating the patch daily will help maintain the function and strength of the extraocular muscles in both eyes. Provide mouth care at least three or four times a day, giving special attention to the affected side of the tongue and mouth. Focus rehabilitation plans on self-care deficits and ADLs.

Risk for Injury. The *Risk for Injury* and trauma continues throughout recovery from stroke. It may also extend into the home environment, where clients attempt to perform former activities, such as cooking or driving. Factors that increase risk for injury include decreased LOC, motor, visual and spatial-perceptual impairments, weakness, flaccidity, spasticity, impulsive behavior, and altered thought process.

Planning: Expected Outcomes. The client will not experience injury, as evidenced by no abrasions, burns, or falls. The client will also seek needed help to perform tasks that are beyond his or her capabilities.

Implementation. Keep the side rails of the bed raised for clients with recent hemiplegia to protect them from rolling out of bed. As recovery proceeds, the client may pull against side rails when sitting up or turning. Once the client can get out of bed unassisted, half side rails may be more useful. Full side rails hinder ambulation.

A client with impaired sensation is especially prone to injury. Frequent skin inspections for signs of injury are essential. Visual disturbances may also increase a hemiplegic client's potential for injury. (See the Agnosia section earlier in the chapter.) Weakness on one side makes clients prone to falls. Remind clients to walk slowly, rest adequately between intervals of walking, use effective lighting, and look where they are going. Be especially alert during toileting. Make sure that ancillary personnel know not to leave these clients alone in the bathroom.

Altered Nutrition: Less than Body Requirements. Use the nursing diagnosis *Altered Nutrition: Less than Body Requirements* if your client has an inability to swallow secondary to stroke. Support the diagnosis with data on intake and output, ability to swallow, caloric intake over past 3 days, hemoglobin, hematocrit, albumin, lymphocyte count, and weight change over the past 3 days.

Planning: Expected Outcomes. The client will demonstrate signs of adequate nutrition, as evidenced by stable weight; consumption of adequate calories for age, height, and weight; intake equaling output; hemoglobin and hematocrit levels within normal limits for age and sex; and lymphocyte count and albumin levels within normal limits; and incisions/wounds healing within 12 to 14 days (as applicable). (Make these outcomes more specific for your client by using the agency laboratory norms and your client's age and weight.)

Implementation. Carefully assess the client's diet to ensure adequate nutrition. Assess total intake. Feeding clients with partial paralysis of the tongue, mouth, and throat requires patience and care for prevention of choking and aspiration (see Bridge to Home Healthcare). Clients often fear choking and are embarrassed and frustrated by eating difficulties. Consequently, they may avoid eating and not get sufficient nutrition. Give supplemental meals as necessary. If the client is not able to swallow at all, tube feeding may be used. With help and encouragement, hemiplegic clients can usually learn to feed themselves. Many helpful orthotic devices are available through consultation with an occupational therapist. Make mealtimes pleasant and unhurried. Serve food attractively and at an appropriate temperature.

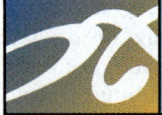

BRIDGE TO HOME HEALTHCARE

Managing Swallowing Difficulties

Bernice Christopher, R.N., B.S.N., *Keystone Home Health Services, Trevose, Pennsylvania*

Swallowing difficulty or "dysphagia" varies in severity and duration. It can be mild to severe, short term or long term. Initially, the services of a certified speech therapist may be needed to help clients reach their optimal rehabilitation potential. The home health nurse should try to schedule some shared visits with the speech therapist to promote continuity of care.

When you feed a client with dysphagia, use good observational skills and plenty of communication and patience. Observe the client's response to what you are doing. The client may turn his head away when food is not appealing or frown, spit, clamp the jaws together, or cough. Respect your client's opinion and try to adapt meals to his or her tastes. Another way to increase your effectiveness includes involving the client in food selection. For example, if a client enjoys bananas, they can be diced, mashed, or blended into a shake, depending on the consistency best tolerated.

The client with dysphagia often does not tolerate clear, thin liquids well. You may have to spoon thick liquids into the least affected side of the client's mouth. Be careful not to succumb to baby talk, cheek pinching, or "airplane landings" if you are not feeding a young child. If a bib or clothes protector must be worn, apply it in a casual, dignified manner. Remember to avoid all crackers, pretzels, and foods that make crumbs.

A high Fowler's position with 90 degree flexion of the hips is usually the best position for mealtime. Remember to position the client so that the shoulders are back and the torso is erect. It is usually best to keep the head erect. However, slightly flexing the neck forward facilitates swallowing for some clients, whereas others do best with very mild neck hyperextension. Placing a pillow at the lower back and a towel roll behind the neck can facilitate a smooth flow of food from the mouth into the stomach. Observe your client to see what position makes him most comfortable. Cushions, pillows, or bed rolls should be used to support any dependent limbs or "weak" sides. Increasing the client's comfort will reduce his stress and allow him to focus on eating.

Consider techniques to prompt the swallowing reflex if there is a delay after chewing. Use a very light-touch throat massage with instructions to "swallow," or touch a lemon to your client's tongue once food has entered the mouth. These same techniques can prompt a "dry" swallow between bites of food as well, clearing bothersome saliva. Maintain the high Fowler's position or at least a 75 to 80 degree flexion at the hips for at least 30 minutes after meals to help reduce reflux and aspiration.

Check the mouth carefully after all meals for lingering food pockets. Carefully swipe around the outer upper and lower gums with a toothette (sponge swab) or gloved finger. Check the back of the tongue, cheeks, inner lower gums, and between the teeth for food particles that could become dislodged and cause aspiration long after the meal. Remove and rinse dentures after meals. Also, have the client swish and spit with warm water or use a soft toothbrush or mouth swab. Never place your unprotected fingers inside the inner lower gums when checking for food. This will prevent involuntary (or voluntary!) movements that can cause a nasty bite! Your nursing knowledge will make the difference between a pleasurable and humiliating experience for your client at mealtime.

Feeding can be very frustrating for a dysphagic client, especially if you are not familiar with the client's specific disabilities. If unlicensed personnel are expected to feed hemiplegic clients they need to be taught basic techniques. These individuals also need to be informed of each client's individual needs and limitations. To facilitate feeding, assess the following and intervene as necessary.

- **Head Control.** If the client has limited or no voluntary head control, placing a hand on the forehead may help. Have the client face forward rather than to the side. Remind the client not to throw the head back to propel food, because this can lead to aspiration. The head should be midline and flexed slightly forward.
- **Position.** Have the client in an upright position, as close to 90 degrees as possible, either in bed or on a chair. Support the head to counteract hyperextension.
- **Mouth Opening.** If the client cannot open the mouth, lightly touch both lips with the tip of a spoon. If this

does not work, apply light pressure with a finger to the chin just below the lower lip. Ask the client to open at the same time. Stroking the muscle under the chin (digastric muscle), without crossing the midline, also stimulates mouth opening.
- **Mouth Closing.** If a client cannot close his or her lips, swallowing is more difficult. Stimulate lip closure by (1) stroking the lips with a finger or ice or (2) applying gentle pressure just above the upper lip with your thumb or forefinger.
- **Sucking.** If a client cannot remove food from a spoon, the sucking reflex needs strengthening. Place a small disk at the end of a short straw and have the client suck on it. Gradually lengthen the straw. Use thicker liquids as the sucking reflex strengthens.
- **Tongue Movement.** Tongue movement can be improved by
  1. Lightly touching various parts of the cheek with a tongue blade to encourage the tongue to move to that place

2. Icing weak tongue muscles
3. Applying pressure to soft tissue under the mandible to correct tongue protrusion
4. "Walking" a tongue blade from the tip of the tongue to the back (this inhibits tongue thrust and stifles the gag reflex).

- **Chewing.** Chewing each bite carefully decreases the risk of aspiration. Do not mix foods. Puréed foods lose their appeal when they are mixed.
- **Salivary Secretion.** Ice (plain ice or a Popsicle) stimulates saliva secretion.
- **Swallowing.** A dysphagic client must concentrate on swallowing. A quiet environment, free from distractions, is helpful. Feed the client slowly and offer small amounts. Alternate liquids with solids whenever possible to prevent food from being left in the mouth. Avoid nonthickened liquids. Place food in the unaffected side of the mouth. After clients have swallowed, teach them to check for food on the paralyzed side by turning the head to the unaffected side and checking with the tongue.

Impaired Verbal Communication. The inability to speak is very frustrating for clients. Early recognition of this problem decreases some of the frustration in meeting everyday needs. Loss of verbal communication is usually caused by loss of the function of muscles that produce speech or ischemia of the dominant cerebral hemisphere.

Planning: Expected Outcomes. The client will be able to effectively communicate. The client's needs will be understood and met, and the client will indicate understanding of the communication of others.

Implementation. Communication involves the dual processes of sending and receiving language. Although either can be affected, the expressive deficit is usually greater than the receptive deficit after initial recovery. Clients may understand more than they are able to respond to.

Most aphasic clients regain some speech through spontaneous recovery or speech therapy. Speech therapy should be started early. Occasionally, residual brain function is not adequate for an aphasic client to relearn the complicated processes of communication. Assessment of dysarthria usually includes examination of the peripheral speech mechanism, tests for specific speech skills, otolaryngologic consultation, and assessment of the client's functional ability based on the clarity of speech in conversation. Speech therapy is beneficial for many dysarthric clients. A picture board may be helpful.

Reinforce the lessons that a speech therapist has initiated. Remember that the client may have a short attention span. Use every encounter to encourage and support communication, yet be careful not to cause fatigue. In general, when working with an aphasic client, practice expanded speech (a slower rate) and self-pacing (give the client time to respond). Listen and watch carefully when an aphasic client attempts to communicate. Try hard to understand. This reduces the client's frustration. Anticipate an aphasic client's needs, to reduce feelings of communication helplessness.

When a client *cannot identify objects by name*, give practice in receiving word images. For example, point to an object and clearly state its name (e.g., *hand, glass*). Then have the client repeat the word.

When a client *cannot understand spoken words*, repeat simple directions until they are understood (e.g., *Drink this juice.*). Do not shout. The client can hear. Speak slowly and clearly. Talk without pressing for a response. Also use nonverbal methods of communication.

When a client has *difficulty with verbal expression*, give practice in repeating words after you. Begin with simple words and then progress to simple sentences (e.g., *Yes. No. Here is breakfast.*).

When talking to a client with *receptive difficulty*, stand within 6 feet and face the client directly. Gradually shift topics of conversation and say when you are going to change the topic.

Help the family to communicate with the aphasic client. Act as a model for such communication by being calm, patient, and gentle. Explain how damaging it can be to the client's self-image if others appear embarrassed or amused by attempts to communicate. Likewise, the family should not do all of the speaking for the client.

Always try to put aphasic clients at ease. Reduce the feelings of panic that may occur when they first realize that they cannot communicate as before. The fact that others understand the problem is helpful. Offer calm reassurance. Demonstrate use of the call light and allow the client to practice. Use gestures and one-step commands.

Altered Thought Processes. Sometimes it is difficult to make a diagnosis of *Altered Thought Processes* unless you spend some time with the client. Asking simple or common questions may get fixed, yet correct, answers. Often, after spending a morning with a client, you will note difficulty with thought processing that was not evident on first assessment. It can be caused by impaired cerebral blood flow, altered sensations, and faulty interpretation of environmental stimuli.

Planning: Expected Outcomes. The client will have reduced confusion, as evidenced by recall of information (recent/remote), improved Mini-Mental State Examination scores, decreased agitation, cooperation with interventions, and appropriate responses to questions about recent and past events.

Implementation. Prevent intellectual regression and disorientation. Reorient the client as consciousness returns. Continually reorient a confused and aphasic client. Position a calendar and a clock where the client can see them. Cerebrovascular diseases contribute to many behavioral deviations, including confusion, memory loss, language disorders, and emotional lability. To decrease agitation, explain all nursing activities before initiating them. Avoid sensory overload. Use alternate methods of communication.

Additional changes in behavior may be caused by alterations in body image, sensation, vision, mobility, and perception. Cerebral edema may also increase confusion. Imagine what it would be like to regain consciousness after a stroke and find that the right half of your body is numb and paralyzed and that you cannot talk. Perhaps you cannot even understand what is being said to you. This is the plight of many hemiplegic, aphasic clients. Empathic understanding is necessary as the client regains consciousness after a stroke. Personal conversations and joking may be misunderstood and should not be conducted around clients.

Visual Sensory/Perceptual Alterations. Ische-
mia of visual pathways can lead to some bizarre changes in vision. A thorough assessment of visual fields is usually needed for this diagnosis. Sometimes you will notice that the client fails to notice you on one side of the bed or the other or fails to eat food from one side of the food tray. Use that cue to do a complete visual field assessment.

Planning: Expected Outcomes. The client will successfully compensate for altered visual perceptions, as evidenced by safely performing ADLs and safely compensating for visual deficit through scanning or other techniques.

Implementation. Approach the client from the side that is not visually impaired. Position the call light and phone on that side. If possible, position the bed so that the side that is not visually impaired is toward the center of the room. Teach clients to position the head to increase the visual field. Warn hemiplegic clients to be very careful when crossing streets because they may not see traffic approaching from the affected side. An eye patch over one eye in clients with diplopia removes the second image and assists vision.

A client with perceptual defects benefits from simplicity. A busy or noisy environment is difficult to interpret and may increase confusion. Reduce complexity and the need for decision making. For example

1. Obtain clothing that is simply designed and easy to put on
2. Give brief, simple directions
3. Prepare food trays with a minimum number of utensils, dishes, and foods

Unilateral Neglect. *Unilateral Neglect* is a pattern
of lack of awareness of body parts, such as paralyzed arms or legs. The client behaves as if the part is simply not there. He or she does not look for the paralyzed limb when moving about. It is caused by damage to portions of the nondominant cerebral hemisphere (usually the right hemisphere). Obviously unilateral neglect creates increased risk of injury. It is possible to relearn to look for and to move the limb.

Planning: Expected Outcomes. The client will be free of unilateral neglect, as evidenced by being free from injury, demonstrating an awareness of the neglected body side, and compensating for neglect of the affected side.

Implementation. Initially, adapt the environment to the deficit by focusing on the client's unaffected side. Keep personal care items and a bedside chair and commode on the unaffected side. Position the client's extremities in correct alignment. Gradually begin to focus the client's attention to the affected side. Move the personal items, bedside chair, and commode to the affected side. Assist client from the affected side. Have the client groom the affected side first. Cue the client to scan the entire environment.[35]

Ineffective Individual Coping. Coping strategies
are quite varied among people. Any major illness or change in the body challenges a client's or family's coping skills. This is particularly true after a stroke because of the physiologic changes and frustrations associated with the deficits that occur after a cerebrovascular accident. The term *coping* refers to the use of all forms of coping strategies: emotional, cognitive, support systems, and risk appraisal.

Planning: Expected Outcomes. The client will develop effective coping strategies, as evidenced by appropriate life-style modifications, use of the assistance of others, and appropriate social interactions.

Implementation. After a cerebrovascular accident, the client may experience grief over lost mobility, inability to speak, alterations in sensation and vision, and loss of roles within society. These reactions can be understood when the extent of the change and dysfunction in a client's life is appreciated. Be understanding and kind. Supportive statements are often helpful, such as "I am sure it's hard for you not to be able to dress alone." Saying "I understand how you feel" is never an appropriate response, even if you have actually experienced a similar situation. Remember, that perception to illness is subjective and, therefore, individual.

Care for clients with hemiplegia in a way that their dependency is minimized. Arrange the environment and anticipate needs to reduce frustration. Praise all successes, however small. When necessary, point out disruptive or inappropriate behavior kindly and ask them to stop. Significant others often need help to understand these behaviors. It is often difficult for them to see their loved one behave in these ways. They may feel at a loss about what to do. Recall that these behaviors may be caused by the damage to the inhibitory centers or they may be a part of the normal grief response. Provide support by helping the client and family to understand this.

Aphasic clients often express their emotional state by irritability and "moodiness." These frustrated clients are often anxious, bewildered, and depressed. Emotional lability may also be present. Accept such behavior in a matter-of-fact but kind manner, without embarrassment. Help families by encouraging short visits by one or two people. If children are allowed to visit, ensure that they are adequately supervised.

Psychosocial Nursing Diagnoses. Various psy-
chosocial nursing diagnoses may be appropriate for clients experiencing stroke, depending on the client and the circumstances. These include *Altered Family Processes*, (see Chapter 4); *Diversional Activity Deficit; Anxiety; Fear; Powerlessness; Self Esteem Disturbance;* and *Social Isolation*. Include significant others in the plan of care. Let them help care for the client if they wish. Provide them with the information they need to under-

stand the client's condition. Many clients with strokes are in intensive care units (ICUs) during the acute phase. The complexity of equipment and activity within an ICU may be frightening to the client and to significant others. Provide opportunities for questions and discussion; explain carefully what is happening. Give frequent reassurance and support.

Evaluation

Evaluate the degree of outcome attainment on an ongoing basis. After a cerebrovascular accident, some outcomes are achieved early (e.g., cerebral perfusion); others may require rehabilitation (e.g., self-care deficit). Monitor progress toward outcomes, working with both the client and the family.

■ Surgical Management

Several criteria are used to determine candidates for rapid evacuation of the hematoma in hemorrhagic stroke. The clients most likely to benefit from surgery are those who are younger than 70 years, can open their eyes and follow commands, have elevated ICP (usually above 30 mm Hg), or are rapidly deteriorating neurologically. Clients who have large blood clots removed have been shown to recover a substantial portion of speech. Surgery is usually not performed on clients with bleeding in the basal ganglia or thalamus.

Surgery is also performed on some intracranial aneurysms and on the carotid arteries (e.g., carotid endarterectomy) to reduce the risk of cerebrovascular accident. These operations and the associated nursing care are discussed later in this chapter.

■ Modifications for Elderly Clients

Because cerebrovascular accident strikes the elderly population more than any other, the nursing care discussed here does not have to be significantly altered for the elderly client. Elderly clients often have multiple medical problems that must be monitored and treated simultaneously.

Community and Self-Care

Clients who have experienced a cerebrovascular accident often are transferred to a rehabilitation unit after they are medically stable. If this transfer moves the client a long distance from home, it may be stressful for the client and family, particularly an elderly spouse. In some cases, care by nurses and allied health professionals in the home may prevent placement in an extended care facility. If both partners are elderly or in poor health, placement in an extended care facility may be the only option. This can create feelings of guilt and abandonment. Emotional support must be provided to both the client and family members. Education in how to choose a facility and how to monitor care can be helpful.

Once transfer to an extended care facility has taken place, the client is evaluated for rehabilitation potential

and plans are made for ongoing therapy. The plan of care established during acute care can continue. The major nursing diagnoses and collaborative problems include: *Impaired Physical Mobility, Self Care Deficit, Impaired Verbal Communication, Risk for Contracture, Altered Nutrition: Less than Body Requirements,* and *Ineffective Individual Coping.*

Three adjuncts to discharge from rehabilitation settings to home include self-medication, use of therapeutic passes, and rehabilitation home visits. Self-medication means that the client is in charge of managing his or her own medications and of getting medications refilled as needed. The goals of self-medication are to help the client learn about the medications, including dosage, action, and side effects. Provide a supervised trial to evaluate the client's knowledge and compliance and to enable the client to develop increased responsibility for his or her own care. A clear and accurate medication chart is helpful.

Therapeutic passes are defined as the process of allowing the client to return to home or family for short stays. They facilitate discharge planning and improve the transition into the community. Passes help the stroke survivor adjust to the home environment and practice self-care activities at home. Passes also help the family adjust to living with the stroke survivor and to any alterations in physical, cognitive and emotional functioning. They can practice problem solving and perform some physical care skills that will be needed after discharge. Much effort goes into planning for the passes and preparing the client and family. Passes usually begin with an 8-hour pass and then increase to a weekend. When the client returns, the client and family discuss any difficulties they had during the pass interval, and team members intervene with information, retraining, or procuring needed supplies.

The rehabilitation home visit is another adjunct to facilitate discharge. Team members, commonly the nurse, social worker, and physical and/or occupational therapist, visit the client's home. The purpose of the visit is to evaluate the accessibility of the home and the safety of the home environment based on the client's level of functioning. Specific things to be evaluated include the client's probable ability to get in and out of the house; perform specific tasks in each room; transfer onto and off of the toilet, bed, and chair; and move about from room to room. The client's ability to safely use the telephone and various appliances is also evaluated. Based on findings from the visit, the team makes recommendations for home modifications, further teaching, or adaptive equipment.

The family needs a clear understanding of the client's residual deficits. If spatial or perceptual deficits or unilateral neglect are present, emphasize the need for assistance with daily activities and the need for adherence to safety precautions to prevent injury. Clients with impaired memory may be helped by writing lists of tasks or activities. It is important to reinforce measures to improve ability to perform ADL and be mobile. The client should have a plan for exercises. Of equal importance, the family and client need to have realistic expectations about the client's abilities, so they can encourage independence when and where the client is able.

The client and family need to be taught about reportable manifestations of another stroke (see Client Education Guide) and cautioned that seizures can develop as scar tissue forms. People often delay seeking treatment because they think the manifestations will pass. The average length of time between the onset of a stroke and treatment is 24 hours. A public education campaign is under way to promote awareness of the signs and symptoms of a stroke with the same intensity that those of a myocardial infarction have been promoted. Prompt recognition and treatment of a stroke in the early stages may lessen residual deficits. Finally, validate the ability of the family (especially an elderly spouse) to safely care for the client.

Written documentation of any anticoagulant schedule should be provided, as well as a list of warning signs of bleeding. The need for caution when using sharp instruments and tools should be reinforced. If appropriate, contact sports will also have to be curtailed while anticoagulation drugs are being taken. The INR is closely monitored and medications adjusted as needed. The client should be taught to carry Medic-Alert identification.

Provide information about community resources that can assist the client and family with home management and adjustments to residual deficits. These groups include Meals-on-Wheels, American Heart Association, stroke support groups, social services, local service groups to assist with the purchase of equipment, and individual and family counselors.

Transient Ischemic Attacks

Etiology and Risk Factors

Transient ischemic attacks (TIAs) are brief, reversible episodes of neurologic dysfunction caused by temporary, focal cerebral ischemia. By definition, a TIA lasts less than 24 hours. A TIA is analogous to angina pectoris. TIAs are also called *mini-strokes* because they often serve as warning signs of an impending stroke. A reversible ischemic neurologic deficit (RIND) is similar to a TIA, except that the manifestations can last from 24 to 48 hours. The client then returns to previous level of function.

During a TIA, a transient decrease in blood supply to a focal area of the cerebrum or brain stem occurs. Many factors can cause this ischemia. Occlusive disease of the extracranial cerebral vessels from progressive atherosclerosis is the most common cause of TIAs. The most frequent site of occlusion is the origin of the internal carotid artery. Occlusions may occur in the vertebrobasilar system. Emboli can also cause TIAs. Common sources of emboli include blood clots forming on diseased or replaced heart valves, atrial fibrillation, or breakdown of plaque. Refer to the Risk Factors and Levels of Prevention feature for stroke; the preventive measures are essentially the same for TIAs.

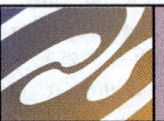

CLIENT EDUCATION GUIDE

Transient Ischemic Attacks

Client Instructions in English *(Instrucciones para el cliente en inglés)*	Client Instructions in Spanish *(Instrucciones para el cliente en español)*
See your doctor if any of the following occur:	Visite a su médico si le ocurre cualquiera de los síntomas siguientes:
● If you develop sudden weakness or paralysis on one side of your body	● Si se le debilita o paráliza repentinamente un lado del cuerpo
● If you experience sudden changes in speech, vision, or hearing	● Si le aparecen cambios inesperados en el lenguaje, la visión, o el oído
● If you suddenly develop abnormal sensations in one side of your body (e.g., face, arm, or leg)	● Si de repente se le presentan sensaciones anormales en un lado del cuerpo (p. ej., en la cara, un brazo, o en una pierna)
● If you suddenly develop a headache that increases in intensity	● Si de repente siente un dolor de cabeza que aumenta en intensidad
● If you experience a sudden change in your thought processes or personality	● Si experimento cambios súbitos en la actividad mental o en la personalidad
● If you develop seizures, or—if you already experience seizures—if you notice changes in the characteristics of your seizures	● Si usted tiene ataques repentinos o—si ya está sufriendo estos ataques—si nota cambìos en las características de los ataques

Pathophysiology

The pathophysiology of a TIA is similar to that of a cerebrovascular accident, or stroke. The major differences are the short duration of ischemia and the lack of permanent deficits.

Clinical Manifestations and Diagnostic Findings

Clinical manifestations of TIAs vary, depending on which area of the brain is affected. Common manifestations include a rapid onset of weakness or numbness in an arm or leg, seizures, alterations in speech patterns, and decreased vision in one eye.

Generally, TIAs last only minutes (often 2 to 15 minutes) to hours. The manifestations can persist for 24 hours. Although TIAs are often recurrent, some clients have only one or two episodes prior to having a complete stroke. TIAs may occur for as long as 2 years before cerebral infarction, or clusters of TIAs may first appear only a few hours or days before a cerebral infarction. Between episodes, neurologic assessment findings are usually normal.

TIAs are diagnosed by the client's reported symptoms. The causes of the TIA and potential risk of cerebrovascular accident are diagnosed by the following examinations:

1. Auscultation and palpation for a carotid bruit
2. Doppler and angiogram studies of the carotid arteries (Fig. 32–10)
3. CT to rule out cerebrovascular accident
4. Electrocardiogram to assess for atrial fibrillation
5. Echocardiogram to rule out mural thrombosis and valvular disorders

If the Doppler reveals 70% or greater narrowing of the carotid, the results are considered to be indicative of significant cerebrovascular disease. Atrial fibrillation, valve disorders and mural thrombosis are possible causes of cerebral ischemia.

Management

Preventing the progression of a TIA to a cerebrovascular accident is the goal of medical management. Antihypertensives or antiplatelet drugs (e.g., aspirin, ticlopidine) may be prescribed. In some instances, warfarin (Coumadin) may be administered to prevent clot development. Every effort is made to determine the cause of the TIAs.

Teach the client and family manifestations of cerebrovascular accident (see the Client Education Guide) and emergency care if a cerebrovascular accident occurs at home. See medical management of cerebrovascular accident. If the client is hospitalized, assess his or her neurologic status frequently for progressive ischemia. Refer to the pharmacologic management of cerebrovascular accident for further discussion.

Clients experiencing TIAs are often afraid that they are having a cerebrovascular accident. They need emotional support and education during this stressful time. The di-

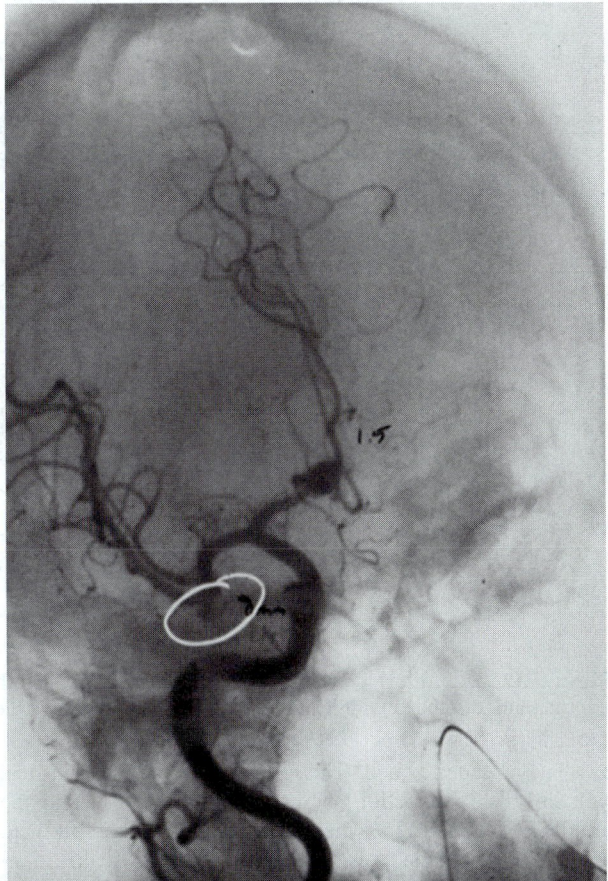

Figure 32–10. An angiogram revealing an aneurysm of the right middle cerebral artery and the right anterior communicating artery.

agnostic work-up as well as the symptoms themselves can produce anxiety. Thorough, simple explanations of upcoming events can help. Stress the importance of completing the work-up. Baseline neurologic status must be recorded for postoperative comparison.

■ Surgical Management

High-resolution ultrasound duplex real-time imaging with transcranial Doppler sonography assists in localizing the lesion. Ophthalmodynamometry and oculopneumoplethysmography may also be ordered. These tests are commonly performed on an outpatient basis. Prior to surgery, administration of oral anticoagulants and heparin is stopped. If the client was asymptomatic before surgery, inform the client of the manifestations that may develop because of the lesion. For example, if the client had asymptomatic stenosis of the left carotid artery, he or she should be taught to report right hand, arm, or leg numbness, tingling or weakness, speech changes, or any changes in vision.

Extracranial-Intracranial Bypass

If vascular insufficiency is detected in the distribution of the middle cerebral artery, an extracranial-intracranial by-

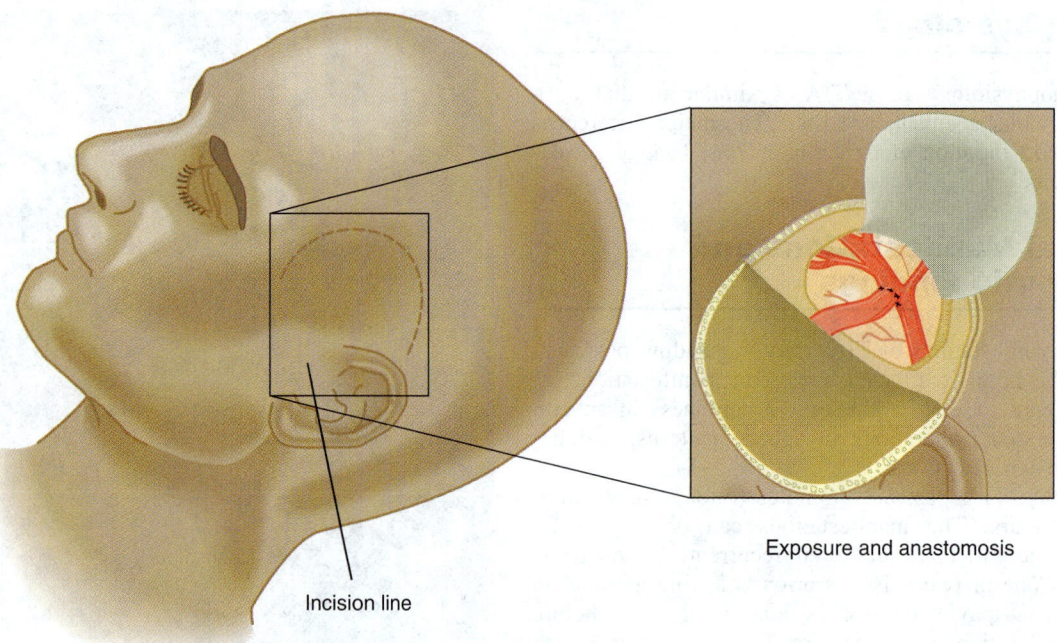

Incision line

Exposure and anastomosis

Figure 32–11. An extracranial-intracranial bypass, in which the superficial temporal artery and pedicle are dissected from the skin flap and distended with heparinized saline. This artery is then anastomosed to a cerebral artery.

pass may be performed. This procedure creates a surgical anastomosis (connection) between a scalp artery and the middle cerebral artery, thereby increasing blood flow to the brain. An incision is made alongside the scalp artery selected, usually the superficial temporal artery (Fig. 32–11). The artery is dissected away from the scalp and the dura is opened through a small burr hole. The superficial vessel is usually anastomosed to one of the branches of the middle cerebral artery. Occasionally, the superficial vessels are not available. In these cases, superficial veins from the arm or leg can be used.

Several outcomes have been reported for extracranial-intracranial bypass. The procedure has been found to be relatively safe, with a 30-day mortality rate of 2% to 4%. Specific complications include occlusion of the anastomosis site, infection, scalp necrosis, subdural hygroma, hematoma, and some systemic complications. Neurologic function and quality of life[65] may improve. Extracranial-intracranial bypass is designed to decrease the incidence of stroke, so stroke incidence is an important outcome measure. When other vessels have been used to perform extracranial-intracranial bypasses for highly selected clients with extensive extracranial disease, these clients have had a high survival rate and positive clinical outcomes.[5, 55]

atheroma) is dissected out. Because of extensive occlusion in each carotid artery, some clients are at increased risk of decreased cerebral perfusion during the operation; for them, a temporary blood supply can be created by shunting blood through other vessels to the brain. Clients commonly treated with shunts include those with bilateral stenosis of the carotid, neurologic deficits, known decreases in cerebral blood flow, a history of cerebrovascular accident, or a stroke in evolution. Once the plaque is removed, the carotid artery is sutured closed and the incision is closed with a drain in place. A pressure dressing is usually not applied because of the risk of impairment to carotid blood flow; pressure is provided to the site immediately postoperatively in the surgery room. Carotid endarterectomy is useful in preventing stroke.[52] It has also been used to improve functions such as vision, comprehension of language, fluency of speech, swallowing, lower and upper limb function, shopping and social visiting.[27] Surgery is usually performed only on stenotic arteries, not on those that are totally occluded. A client may require bilateral extracranial-intracranial bypass and endarterectomy. Interval between surgeries is determined by the client's tolerance of the procedure and the likelihood of symptom progression from the remaining stenotic vessel.

Carotid Endarterectomy

Carotid endarterectomy is the opening of the carotid artery to remove obstructing and embolizing plaque. After coronary artery bypass, carotid endarterectomy is the second most common vascular surgery. Carotid endarterectomy is performed through an incision on the anterior border of the sternocleidomastoid muscle (Fig. 32–12). The vessel is clamped and the plaque (sometimes called

Outcomes

The lowest morbidity and mortality rates are reported in clients who had stable TIAs or were asymptomatic before surgery. Clients who had progressive strokes, more than one stroke, or delayed operations had much higher mortality. Carotid endarterectomy reduces the risk of stroke in persons with recent symptomatic or asymptomatic TIAs.[27]

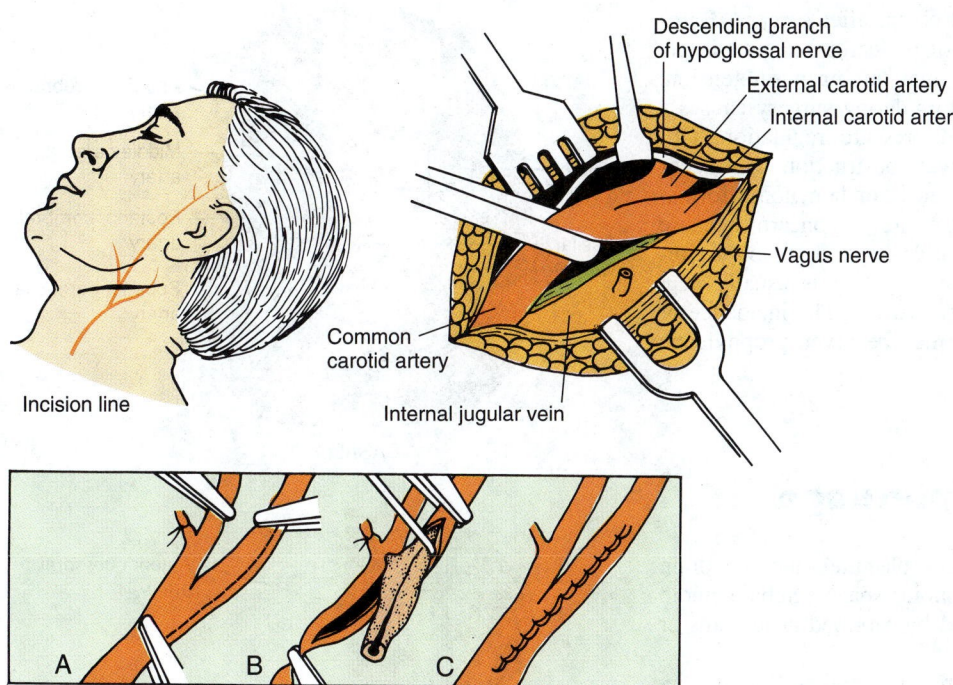

Descending branch
of hypoglossal nerve

External carotid artery

Internal carotid artery

Vagus nerve

Common
carotid artery

Internal jugular vein

Incision line

Figure 32–12. Carotid endarterectomy. *A*, The external carotid is clamped, and an incision is made along the carotid bifurcation. *B*, Plaque is removed. (Sometimes, portions of the artery are also removed and reconstructed with vein grafts or Dacron.) *C*, The artery is sutured closed, and the clamps are removed.

Complications

Neurologic complications of carotid endarterectomy include the following:

1. Embolization during surgery, causing cerebral occlusion and ischemia
2. Clotting (thrombosis) of the artery at the endarterectomy site, causing cerebral ischemia
3. Increased ICP due to intracranial hemorrhage
4. Inadequate cerebral perfusion from intolerance of the temporary artery clamping during surgery.

■ Nursing Management of the Surgical Client

Extracranial-Intracranial Bypass

The care of clients undergoing an extracranial-intracranial bypass is the same as that of clients having other types of cranial surgery. Careful, frequent (every 1 to 2 hours) assessment of vital signs and neurologic function is essential. Report immediately any changes in status compared to baseline. In addition, the surgical anastomosis creates a pulse that should be palpated or assessed with a Doppler ultrasound probe during vital sign assessments. This pulse is located just below the curve of the incision. If the pulse changes in character, notify the surgeon immediately. Keep the client's blood pressure within 20 mm Hg of the preoperative normal values. Hypertension or hypotension may lead to hemorrhage or occlusion of the anastomosis. Medicate the client to prevent seizures.

Length of hospital stay is about 5 days. Discharge instructions include no driving for 1 week. Any visual changes should be evaluated before the client drives. Activity is not limited, except that no heavy lifting (over 20 lb) is allowed. Sexual activity is permitted. An occasional mild headache is normal and usually can be treated with

acetaminophen (Tylenol). Persistent or severe headaches need to be reported. Once the scalp sutures or staples are removed, usual hair care can resume. There will be a small depression in the skull, where the bypass was performed. This area will close in time. Prolonged pressure from eyeglasses, wigs or hats over the site should be avoided. Sleeping on the bypass side is permissible. Any manifestations of TIAs should be reported.

Carotid Endarterectomy

Postoperative care after carotid endarterectomy is most important during the first 24 hours. Frequent neurologic assessments (at least every 2 hours) are essential. Immediately report indications of deterioration of neurologic impairment. In addition, because of the close proximity of several cranial nerves to the operative site, the function of the following cranial nerves are assessed: facial (VII), vagus (X), spinal accessory (XI), and hypoglossal (XII) (see Chapter 30). Cranial nerve damage is usually temporary, but it may last for months. The most common cranial nerve damage causes vocal cord paralysis or difficulty managing saliva and tongue deviation. Horner's syndrome may result from damaged sympathetic nerve fibers. This is usually temporary.

Keep the client's head in a straight position to help maintain airway patency and to minimize stress on the operative site. Medications to promote blood flow may include anticoagulants or antiplatelet aggregates. The client can lie supine or on the side, so long as the neck is not flexed. Elevate the head of the bed when vital signs are stable. Local applications of cold to the operative site may be prescribed. Frequently assess the client's breathing pattern, pulse, and blood pressure. Maintain the client's blood pressure within 20 mm Hg of the preoperative normal values. Hypertension or hypotension may lead to hemorrhage or occlusion of the anastomosis. Labile blood pressure is a common problem after surgery. Baroreceptors located in the lining of the carotid sinus are one of the primary mechanisms of maintaining normotension. Manipulation of the baroreceptors during surgery causes a short-term disruption in blood pressure regulation. Observe the operative site. Airway obstruction can occur from excessive swelling of the neck or hematoma formation. Bleeding and hemorrhage are a concern because anticoagulation from intraoperative heparin is not yet reversed. An emergency tracheostomy tray is usually kept at bedside for use in respiratory distress. The incidence of seizures is low, but the client may be given prophylactic anticonvulsants.

Intracranial Hemorrhage

Intracranial hemorrhage includes bleeding into the brain tissue itself or the subarachnoid space. Subarachnoid hemorrhages are usually caused by ruptured aneurysms or head trauma.

Intracranial aneurysms are congenital, traumatic, arteriosclerotic, or septic weakenings or outpouchings in vessel walls. Ninety percent of aneurysms are congenital. Eighty percent occur on the circle of Willis (Fig. 32–13).[61] Sometimes these aneurysms weaken, leak, or rupture and cause bleeding into the subarachnoid space. This is called *subarachnoid hemorrhage* (SAH). SAH from ruptured intracranial aneurysms occurs in about 18,000 clients annually in the United States. Women are more commonly affected. Ruptures occur most frequently between the ages of 30 and 60 years; the peak incidence is in the fifth decade.[45]

Etiology and Risk Factors

The most common cause of spontaneous SAH is leaking or rupture of an intracranial aneurysm. This is the cause of death in more than half of all fatal cerebrovascular lesions in clients younger than 45 years. It is not clear why some aneurysms bleed (rupture), but it is probably related to degenerative changes in the vessel wall at the site of the aneurysm, hypertension, and constant stress caused by the force of blood flow, particularly at a bifurcation.

Meningeal vessel rupture from head trauma is another cause of subarachnoid bleeding. Spontaneous hemorrhage that is not associated with trauma may be caused by blood dyscrasias, primary or metastatic intracranial tumors, vascular anomalies (e.g., angiomas or arteriovenous malformations), CNS infections, or intracerebral hemorrhages spreading to the subarachnoid space. (See the Risk Factors and Levels of Prevention feature for cerebral hemorrhage.)

Pathophysiology

Fusiform and saccular aneurysms are the two most common types of cerebral aneurysm (see Fig. 50–10). Both

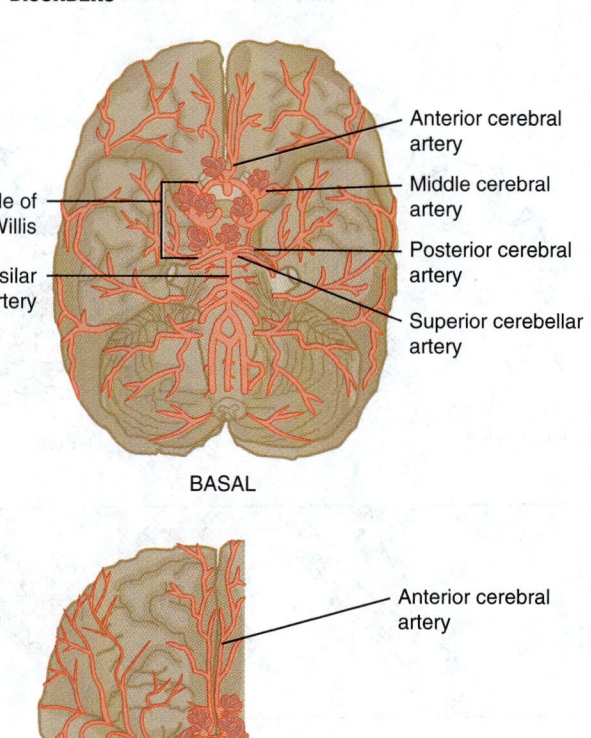

BASAL

ANTERIOR

LATERAL

Figure 32–13. Common aneurysm sites.

are caused by a congenital weakness in artery walls. Saccular (berry) aneurysms are the most common. More than one aneurysm may be present. Saccular aneurysms usually have a *neck*, or narrowed portion attached to the vessel. Most develop around the anterior portion of the circle of Willis at the junction of the posterior communicating and the internal carotid arteries. Fusiform aneurysms most often occur on the larger basilar and carotid arteries. These aneurysms do not usually rupture. They develop from atherosclerotic changes that impair vascular elasticity. Dissecting aneurysm occurs when the intima of the vessel wall is torn. Blood escapes the lumen of the

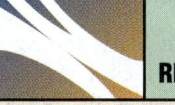

RISK FACTORS AND LEVELS OF PREVENTION

Cerebral Hemorrhage

Risk Factors

Head trauma, hypertension, cocaine use, and congenital aneurysms.

Levels of Prevention

Primary Prevention

- Promote the use of bicycle and motorcycle helmets.
- Prevent driving after alcohol consumption.
- Provide information regarding the ability of cocaine to elevate blood pressure and possibly trigger rupture of a blood vessel.

Secondary Prevention

- Treat hypertension. High blood pressure can increase the flow of blood against a weakened blood vessel wall and possibly increase the chance of aneurysm rupture.

Tertiary Prevention

- Prevent rebleeding and complications of the initial hemorrhage. Rebleeding is prevented by early clipping of the aneurysm if the client's condition allows it. In the case of traumatic or cocaine-induced SAH, hypertension is controlled as closely as possible.
- Minimize or prevent the complications associated with immobility, aspiration, or injury related to paralysis.

vessel through the tear. Eventually, the expanding mass occludes the vessel. Almost a third of clients who have a ruptured aneurysm die from the initial hemorrhage.[49]

The blood mixed in the CSF causes irritation of the meninges. It also clots in the subarachnoid space and can obstruct CSF flow, leading to hydrocephalus and increased ICP. After an aneurysm ruptures, a clot forms at the site of the hemorrhage. This reduces the risk of rebleeding for a few days. As the clot begins to dissolve, the possibility of rebleeding increases.

Clinical Manifestations and Diagnostic Findings

An aneurysm is usually asymptomatic until it ruptures. Occasionally, mild premonitory indications are present, such as mild headache, confusion, fainting, or vertigo. However, the onset of the hemorrhage is usually sudden. The client experiences a sudden, severe headache, often accompanied by vomiting. The client often says, "This is the worst headache I have ever had." The client may lose consciousness immediately, he or she may become confused and lethargic and gradually become comatose within hours, or the client may remain conscious and coherent. Generalized seizures may occur. Signs of meningeal irritation (e.g., stiff neck and leg and back pain) are often present, caused by blood in the subarachnoid space. Focal neurologic deficits include cranial nerve involvement (usually the third and sixth cranial nerves,

causing pupil dilation and dysconjugate gaze) and motor weakness (usually monoparesis or hemiparesis).

Clinical manifestations of SAH have been divided into five grades for classification of severity of the neurologic deficits associated with the bleeding (Table 32–4). The classifications help the surgeon to determine the timing of surgery.

Table 32–4. Classification of Subarachnoid Hemorrhages	
Grade	**Clinical Manifestations**
Grade I	Minimal bleeding, alert, no neurologic deficit, no symptoms, slight nuchal rigidity
Grade II	Mild bleeding, alert, headache, minimal neurologic deficit (e.g., compressed 3rd nerve, stiff neck)
Grade III	Moderate bleeding, drowsiness or confusion, headache, stiff neck, with or without neurologic deficit
Grade IV	Moderate to severe bleeding, semiconsciousness, moderate to severe hemiparesis, decerebrate posturing
Grade V	Severe bleeding, coma, decerebrate or decorticate posturing, moribund appearance

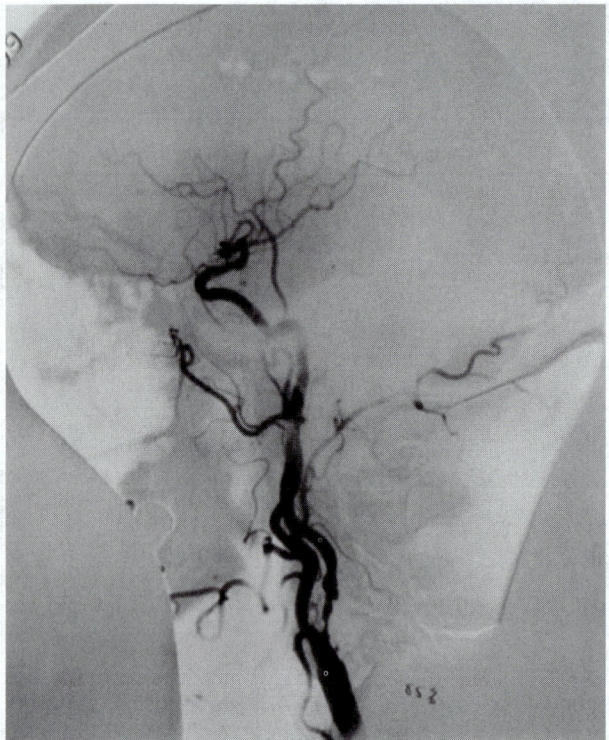

Figure 32–14. An angiogram taken before an endarterectomy reveals an 85% occlusion of the internal carotid artery.

Diagnosis of SAH is usually based on history and physical examination. CT scan may identify blood in the subarachnoid space, intracerebral clots, and large clots surrounding an aneurysm. Lumbar puncture usually confirms the presence of blood in the subarachnoid space. Variations occur in the pressure, color, and cell content of CSF, depending on the timing of the lumbar puncture in relation to the hemorrhage.

Angiography is the definitive diagnostic test. A four-vessel study provides adequate visualization of the carotid and vertebrobasilar circulation. An angiogram usually demonstrates the following:

1. Aneurysm structure and location
2. Vessels supplying the aneurysm
3. Presence or absence of an intracerebral clot or vasospasm of any vessels surrounding the aneurysm or distal to it (Fig. 32–14)

Depending on the client's condition, the angiogram may be done immediately or when the client's condition stabilizes. (See Chapter 13 regarding angiography.)

 Critical Care

■ Medical Management
Pharmacologic Management

Medical intervention focuses on management of vasospasm because untreated vasospasm leads to ischemia and infarction.

Hypertensive Hypervolemic Hemodilution

Although no definitive prevention or cure exists for cerebral vasospasm, there are treatment modalities. Hypertensive, hypervolemic hemodilution can minimize the impact of vasospasm. This is usually accomplished by infusion of serum albumin. Through osmosis, this colloid helps maintain a high intravascular volume, which results in hemodilution. A low hematocrit reflects decreased blood viscosity. The less viscous the blood, the more easily it flows through narrowed vessels. If the hypervolemia does not adequately elevate blood pressure, then vasopressors may be instituted. Systolic blood pressure is maintained between 100 and 150 mm Hg. The increase in volume and pressure helps force blood through narrowed vessels.

Antispasmodic Therapy

Nimodipine, a calcium-channel blocker that is selective to cerebral blood vessels, has been administered in an effort to inhibit this influx. Research is ongoing in the use of this and other drugs in the treatment of vasospasm.[14, 53]

Intracranial Pressure Reduction

Nonsurgical measures to decrease ICP often include the following:

1. Administration of dexamethasone (Decadron) and osmotic agents
2. Elevating the head of the bed 20 to 30 degrees
3. Maintaining a patent airway to prevent increased $PaCO_2$; mechanical hyperventilation may be used to decrease $PaCO_2$, thereby promoting vasoconstriction, decreasing cerebral blood flow, and decreasing ICP.

Some of the systemic effects of SAH include neurogenic pulmonary edema, cardiac arrhythmias, and stress ulcers. Clients are assessed for these problems routinely, and prophylactic treatment may be given.

Complications

Several complications of SAH may affect intervention.

Rebleeding is a major complication that may occur at any time with an unclipped aneurysm (i.e., one that has not been surgically obliterated by placement of a metal clip). Rebleeding commonly occurs within the first few days after hemorrhage, but may occur anytime over the first few months if the aneurysm is unclipped. Mortality is high following rebleeding. Clipping the aneurysm is definitive management of rebleeding.

Vasospasm is a spasm of the vessel that causes a narrowing of the vessel lumen. Vasospasm is a major concern because of its location. Aneurysms commonly occur in the circle of Willis; therefore, when vasospasm occurs, the major cerebral vessels are affected. Spasm usually occurs in the vessel adjacent to a ruptured aneurysm and may spread throughout all the major vessels at the base of the brain. Vasospasm produces symptoms of ischemia and, if extensive and prolonged, results in infarction and permanent neurologic deficit. The breakdown of blood after SAH may be the etiologic factor behind vasospasm.

Research has identified several breakdown products that affect the contractility of vessel walls. Another theory of the cause of vasospasm is the influx of calcium into the muscular layer of the blood vessel wall.

Hydrocephalus is caused by blood in the subarachnoid space that prevents adequate CSF circulation. It often occurs in the acute stage following SAH and contributes to increased ICP. Hydrocephalus often resolves spontaneously but may be treated by short-term external ventriculostomy drainage to help decrease ICP. Hydrocephalus may develop again after several weeks, this time more slowly, resulting in dementia and ataxia. Chronic hydrocephalus is usually treated with a ventriculoperitoneal (see Fig. 32–5) or a ventriculoatrial shunt.

■ Nursing Management of the Medical Client

Nursing care of the client with SAH is a complex task that takes place in an intensive care unit (ICU). The condition of the client may range from alert and oriented to comatose and ventilator dependent. This is a disorder of sudden onset, often striking young people in the prime of their lives. Helping the family to understand what has happened and what is being done can be time consuming. Repeat explanations frequently to help family members develop realistic expectations.

Assessing arterial blood pressure is especially important after SAH. Elevated arterial pressure may contribute to further bleeding from the ruptured aneurysm. At the same time, pressure sufficient to maintain cerebral perfusion pressure must be maintained. Administer vasoactive agents as prescribed and evaluate the effects carefully. The physician will write parameters for the ideal blood pressure range. If the blood pressure exceeds or falls below the parameters, contact the physician. If no parameters have been written, contact the physician if the systolic blood pressure goes below 100 mm Hg or above 150 mm Hg. Assess and document vital signs frequently, especially blood pressure. Observe carefully for changes in the client's status, particularly a decrease in LOC or progression of motor weakness, and notify the physician of significant changes.

Attempt to provide a quiet, calm environment for clients with SAH. This may be difficult to do in a busy ICU. Evaluate the client's response to visitors and adjust visiting schedules as needed (see the Nursing Research feature earlier in the chapter). Keeping a restless client quiet and in bed for an extended period of time is difficult, especially if visual problems or attention deficits preclude reading or watching television for diversion. Avoid sedation whenever possible.

Follow Aneurysm Precautions. Follow individualized aneurysm precautions during the acute stages of SAH to prevent rupture of the vascular abnormality. These precautions may also be used after surgery and in clients with AVMs. Typical aneurysm precautions include the following:

  Dim lights
  Limit visitation

  Decrease noise
  Place the client in a private room
  Elevate the head of the bed
  Ensure that the client avoids the Valsalva maneuver
  Administer analgesics and sedatives

Elevate the Head of the Bed. Elevate the head of the bed 15 to 30 degrees, as prescribed. Advise the client to avoid straining. Place necessary items, such as the call light, within easy reach. Assist with position changes and turning. During these activities, encourage the client to relax and not to tighten muscles. Advise the client to minimize turning the head and to neither rotate nor flex the neck. Isometric or active exercises are not permitted. Passive ROM exercises are acceptable.

Avoid the Valsalva Maneuver. A Valsalva response is an increase in intrathoracic pressure secondary to straining or vagal stimulation. This response should be avoided whenever possible because it causes a decrease in venous return and, thus, an increase in ICP.

Valsalva's maneuver occurs with activities such as straining to pass urine, sneezing, coughing, straining at stool, bending, and vomiting and during suctioning. Avoid rectal stimulation (e.g., rectal temperatures) or straining at stool (e.g., use of bedpan). Enemas are contraindicated, because a vagal effect may result from distention of the lower colon. Manage bowel elimination with prescribed stool softeners, mild laxatives, and use of a commode for clients whose condition allows (grades I and II), to help decrease the risk of a Valsalva response. When straining is unavoidable, teach clients to take a deep breath; this opens the epiglottis and decreases intrathoracic pressure, which may decrease the risk.

Administer Analgesics and Sedatives. Administer prescribed medications such as analgesics (e.g., codeine) for headache and sedatives to promote rest. Avoid oversedation, because the client must be easily aroused as necessary for neurologic assessment. Phenobarbital may be prescribed for sedation or to help prevent seizures.

■ Surgical Management

Aneurysm Clipping

Surgical obliteration of the aneurysm with a metal clip or suture eliminates the risk of rebleeding. A craniotomy is performed to expose the aneurysm. The aneurysm is isolated, and a clip is placed over the neck of the aneurysm. Many neurosurgeons advocate surgery as soon as possible after the rupture. Early surgery is not recommended for all clients. However, clients with SAH grades IV and V may not be operated on because early surgery may contribute to morbidity or mortality. Also, if vasospasm is present, most surgeons will delay surgery. Operating while vessels are in spasm increases morbidity and mortality. Unfortunately, medical instability, delay in transfer from one hospital to another, or client or family reluctance to consent to surgery may also delay prompt surgery.

Following surgery, carefully monitor neurologic status, hemodynamic parameters, and systemic functioning. (See Care of the Client after Craniotomy in Chapter 33.) Prompt identification of changes, notification of the physician, and intervention are keys to improving client outcome.

Ventriculoperitoneal/Ventriculoatrial Shunt

Chronic hydrocephalus can be treated with a shunt to redirect CSF into the peritoneum or atria (see Fig. 32–5). Avoid positioning the client so that pressure is placed on the incision. Monitor the client for increased ICP, wound infection, headache and seizures, shunt occlusion (which would cause hydrocephalus again), and overshunting (which could collapse the ventricles). Teach the family and client to report any signs of infection in the shunt such as fever, headache, irritability, and signs of increased ICP.

Other Cerebrovascular Disorders

Arteriovenous Malformations

Arteriovenous malformations (AVMs) are congenital malformations that consist of tangles of thin-walled blood vessels without intervening capillaries. Arterial and venous blood shunt together. Hence, perfusion of brain tissue cannot occur through them. The vessels may "leak" small amounts of blood or they may rupture, causing hemorrhage into the subarachnoid space or brain, depending on the location of the bleeding AVM. Whereas some AVMs are huge, others are microscopic. Most commonly, they occur in the posterior portions of the cerebral hemispheres. Over time, they may change in size. Large AVMs may decrease somewhat, whereas small ones may enlarge. Bleeding into brain tissues usually produces focal neurologic clinical manifestations. However, cerebral infarction or ischemia may occur without rupture. A ruptured AVM produces clinical manifestations and laboratory results similar to those of SAH. The smaller AVMs are most prone to rupture.

Aneurysm precautions (see the preceding section on SAH) may be prescribed. About half of AVMs can be completely removed surgically. Laser intervention may be used preoperatively to decrease the size of the AVM, or neuroradiologic procedures may be performed to reduce the blood supply to the AVMs. These procedures may also be used on inoperable AVMs. Other techniques that may be used to reduce the size of AVMs include the following:

1. Use of radiation energy from a proton beam
2. Detachable balloon procedures

3. Artificial embolization (clotting) of the AVM
4. Ligation of the feeding arteries to the AVM

These interventions are not without such hazards as provoking hemorrhage or infarction or enlarging the area of ischemia. Carefully assess clients for signs of neurologic deterioration.

Lesions of Cerebral Veins and Sinuses

Lesions do not often occur in the small cerebral veins. However, these vessels may be affected by extension of infectious or thrombotic processes from the large dural sinuses. Focal neurologic symptoms occur from occlusion of the cortical and subcortical veins. The large dural sinuses may become thrombosed from infection within or from the epidural or subdural spaces. In adults, the dural sinuses may be occluded by trauma, tumor masses, or effects of other conditions, such as the formation of clots in clients with polycythemia.

The superior sagittal, lateral, and cavernous dural sinuses are most often thrombosed. The superior sagittal sinus is less commonly affected by infective thrombosis than is the lateral or cavernous sinus. Thrombosis of the lateral sinus is usually secondary to otitis media and mastoiditis. This condition is rare because of effective antibiotic treatment.

Cavernous sinus thrombosis is typically secondary to suppurative processes in the orbit, nasal sinuses, or upper half of the face. The infection commonly first involves one sinus and then rapidly spreads to the opposite side. The client is acutely ill and has a septic febrile reaction and pain in the eye. Visual acuity may or may not be affected, and pupillary reactions may or may not be preserved. The pupils may be small or dilated, the cornea may be cloudy, and corneal ulcers may develop. Although it was formerly a fatal condition, cavernous sinus thrombosis can now be treated with antibiotics and possibly with anticoagulants.

Carotid–cavernous sinus fistula may develop after head trauma or occur spontaneously. In this condition, an abnormal communication exists between the carotid artery and the cavernous sinus. This abnormality allows rapid blood flow into vessels not accustomed to such rapid flow. Carotid–cavernous sinus fistula produces several characteristic signs.

Exophthalmos, a protrusion of the eyeball, is caused by blood flowing in a retrograde fashion into the ophthalmic veins from the cavernous sinus. These veins dilate and can displace the eyeball laterally and inferiorly. The displacement may be severe enough to prevent the eyelids from closing. Rapid flow through veins surrounding the orbit may result in palpable ocular pulsations.

Dilation and arterial blood flow through the small veins of the sclera and conjunctiva cause chemosis (edema of the conjunctiva). This edema surrounding the cornea may herniate beyond the eyelids. Vigilant eye care is required to prevent irreversible damage to the affected eye. The eye must be kept lubricated and protected from trauma. Traditional eye patches have limited usefulness in exophthalmos because pressure from the patch may actually cause tissue damage. Plastic bubbles, which allow protrusion of the eye and assist in maintaining a moist environment, are available.

Visual impairments and extraocular palsies can result from changes in blood vessels and cranial nerves. Changes in blood flow also cause headaches and bruits. The bruit may be the first sign actually exhibited. Sleeping may be difficult because the bruit tends to become louder when the client is lying down and little surrounding noise is present.

The treatment goal in carotid–cavernous sinus fistula is to eliminate the fistula while maintaining patency of the carotid artery. This may be accomplished by embolization of the fistula. In embolization, a catheter is introduced via the femoral artery. When the catheter is properly positioned, the fistula is occluded. In most cases, this is accomplished by inflating a balloon and detaching it from the catheter. Other materials have also been used for embolization.

Obliteration of the fistula usually results in reversal of the signs and symptoms. If the carotid artery is sacrificed or occluded, the client may develop manifestations of ischemia. If collateral circulation is inadequate, the client may experience a cerebrovascular accident. A baseline neurologic assessment should be obtained before the procedure and then repeated frequently after the procedure. Report any change from baseline to the physician immediately.

Headaches

Headaches, the most common of pains, may occur either in the absence of organic disease or as a manifestation of serious disease. Most headaches are transient and of only moderate or slight severity. However, a few are chronic, intense, and recurrent over a period of months or years.

Headache is a symptom of an underlying disorder, rather than a disease itself. The cause of headache must be identified so that appropriate treatment can be given.

Clients often self-treat headaches with over-the-counter medications (available without prescription). Most headaches do not indicate serious disease. However, encourage clients with persistent or recurrent headaches to seek neurologic assessment. Serious disorders that typically produce headache include the following:

1. Intracranial tumors and infections
2. Bacterial or viral meningitis
3. Acute systemic infections
4. Head injuries
5. Cerebral hypoxia
6. Severe hypertension
7. Acute or chronic diseases of the eye, ear, nose, or throat

There are many types of headaches. The following are the most common:

1. Migraine headaches
2. Cluster headaches
3. Tension headaches (muscle contraction headaches)
4. Head pain related to the eyes, ears, teeth, and paranasal structures (Fig. 32–15)

Some clients experience several types of headaches. For example, migraine and tension headaches are often associated.

Assessment of headaches includes detailed history, psychosocial assessment, and physical examination. Neurologic assessment is particularly important. Possible neuro-

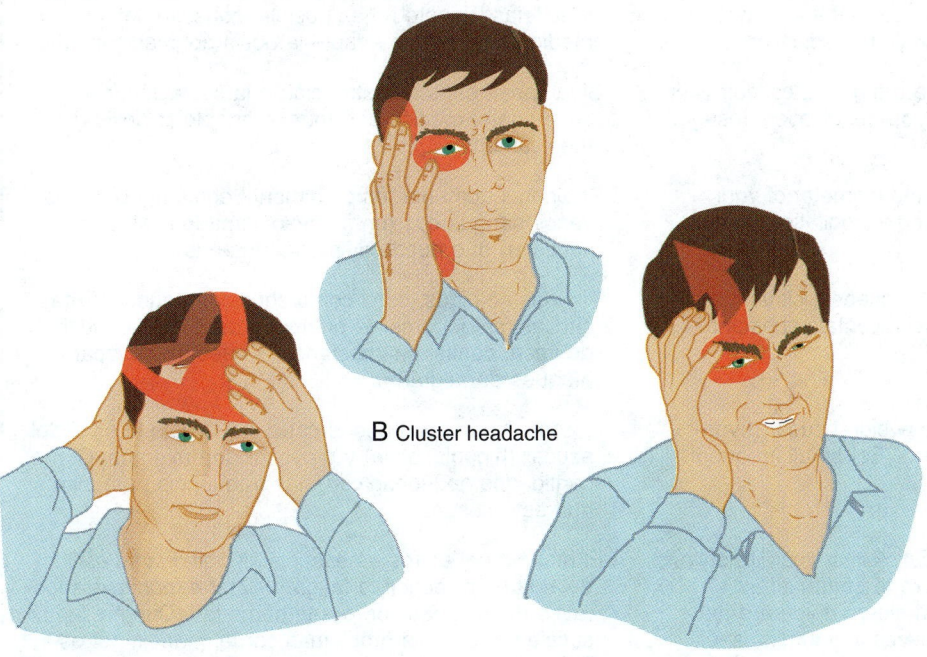

Figure 32–15. Types of headaches. The red areas show the regions of greatest pain. *A*, Muscle contraction headache. *B*, Cluster headache. *C*, Migraine headache.

B Cluster headache

A Muscle contraction headache

C Migraine headache

logic diagnostic tests include skull x-rays, computed tomography (CT), electroencephalography (EEG), and lumbar puncture with CSF examination.

History includes asking about the following:

1. Pain localization, intensity, and paths of radiation
2. Character of the headache (e.g., sharp, dull, throbbing)
3. Mode of headache onset, duration, and frequency
4. Way in which headaches stop
5. Presence of localized tenderness
6. Associated phenomena or precipitating factors
7. Familial incidence

Migraine Headaches

Migraine headaches are episodic headaches that are unilateral or bilateral, pulsating in quality, moderate to severe in intensity, and exacerbated by activity. Headache episodes begin during puberty or ages 20 to 40 years. Generally, they decrease in frequency and severity with advancing years. Migraines affect about 5% to 10% of the population. Women are more susceptible than men.

Migraine headaches usually occur at irregular intervals. Their frequency varies from several times a week to only several times a year.

The pathophysiology of migraine is complex. The vascular theory is currently accepted. It states that early neurologic symptoms are caused by constriction of intracranial vessels. The later intense, throbbing headaches are caused by dilation of extracranial and intracranial branches of the external carotid artery. The underlying mechanism causing this periodic spasm and dilation of vessels is not known.

Psychosical factors also influence migraine headaches. They tend to occur in clients who have perfectionistic tendencies. Migraine episodes may be precipitated by various, often repetitive conditions such as fatigue, excess sleep, hunger, refractive errors, bright light, surprises, mental and emotional excitement, excessive smoking, high altitudes, or drinking alcoholic beverages. As the Client Education Guide indicates, certain foods appear to precipitate migraine episodes. There appears to be a familial character to these headaches. Oral contraceptives may exacerbate migraines or induce their onset in women previously free of significant headaches. Headaches often

---

CLIENT EDUCATION GUIDE

Migraine Headache

Client Instructions in English *(Instrucciones para el cliente en inglés)*	**Client Instructions in Spanish** *(Instrucciones para el cliente en español)*
Many things can trigger a migraine headache. Find out what triggers your headaches and avoid those triggers. If this is not possible, consult your physician about adjusting the dosage of your medication.	Muchas cosas pueden desencodenar una migraña. Investige qué cosas le provocan los dolores de cabezc, y evítelas. Si esto no es posible, consulte con el médico para que le adapte la dósis del medicamento.
If menstruation and ovulation are triggers, consult your physician for adjustments to your medication dosage.	Si la causa es la menstruación o la ovulación, consulte con el médico para que le adapte la dosis del medicamento.
Alcohol temporarily increases the diameter of your blood vessels (a process called vasodilation) and may trigger migraines.	El alcohol aumenta temporalmente el diámetro de los vasos sanguíneos (un proceso llamado dilatación vascular) que puede disparar migrañas.
Some foods, such as chocolate, cheese, citrus fruits, coffee, pork, and dairy products, contain substances that may trigger migraines.	Algunas comidas, tales como chocolate, queso, frutas cítricas, café, carne de puerco, y productos de leche de vaca, contienen substancia y pueden provocar ataques de migraña.
Low food intake may lead to low blood sugar (hypoglycemia) and trigger migraines. Eat small, frequent meals to decrease this risk.	El comer muy poco puede causar que baje el nivel del azúcar (hipoglucemia) y provocar una migraña. Coma cantidades pequeñas con más frequencia para disminuir este riesgo.
Stress management is essential. Adjust your life-style to reduce fatigue and exposure to bright sunlight, heat, or humidity. Get enough sleep. If you are having trouble managing the stresses in your life, seek expert guidance.	El manejo del estrés es esencial. Modifiqua su estilo de vida para reducir la fatiga y evitar exponerse a los rayos del sol, al calor, o a la humedad. Duerma lo suficiente. Si tiene problemas con el manejo del estrés en su vida, busque ayuda profesional.

occur during menstruation and are rare during pregnancy. There are numerous variants of the migraine syndrome and many variations among clients.

Classic or Typical Migraines

The headache may be preceded by an aura or prodromal phase in which the client may feel depressed, irritable, restless, and perhaps anorexic. The client may also experience transient neurologic disturbances, including visual phenomena (flashes of lights, bright spots, distorted vision, diplopia, transitory impaired vision), vertigo, nausea, diarrhea, abdominal pain, paresthesias (numbness or tingling of lips, face, or extremities), or transient hemiparesis. Prodromal symptoms may last a few minutes or several hours.

A migraine headache has a crescendo quality. It gradually increases in severity until the pain becomes intense and all-encompassing. Pain varies in intensity from mild discomfort to a prostrating, throbbing pain that forces the client to seek seclusion and lie in bed in a darkened room. The pain may be described as viselike, dull and boring, pressing, throbbing, or hammering. Initially throbbing in nature, the pain may later become a steady ache. The pain is usually unilateral and may be localized to the front, back, or side of the head. It may begin at any part of the head, often the temple and the eye areas. Prodromal symptoms and head pain rarely occur in the same location in every episode.

During an acute migraine episode (often 4 to 6 hours), the client is acutely ill and may be extremely irritable. Various somatic signs and symptoms such as photophobia, nausea, vomiting, vertigo, tremor, diarrhea, and excessive sweating or chilliness accompany severe episodes. The common symptoms of nausea and vomiting explain why many clients call migraine headaches "sick headaches." There is usually a general hypersensitivity of all the sensory organs, and the client withdraws from light and sound. Arteries of the head may become prominent, and the amplitude of their pulsations increases. The client's scalp may be very tender. Swelling, redness, and excessive tearing of the eyes and swelling of the nasal mucosa, sometimes accompanied by epistaxis, may occur.

Atypical, or Common Migraines

The atypical, or common migraine headache begins suddenly, with or without prodromal symptoms; may be generalized or unilateral; and may or may not be accompanied by nausea and vomiting.

Treatment of migraine headaches involves prevention of episodes and treating of the two phases of migraine, that is, vasoconstriction and vasodilation. Treatment of an acute migraine episode varies with symptom intensity. The transient neurologic symptoms are not treated. Analgesics such as acetaminophen, acetylsalicylic acid, or codeine may relieve a mild headache. Combination drugs such as acetaminophen, isometheptene, and dichloralphenazone (Midrin) and aspirin with caffeine and butalbital (Fiorinal) have potential to lead to a dependency and a propensity to induce headache.[71]

More severe headaches respond to ergot preparations, but only if they are taken 30 to 60 minutes after headache onset. Ergot must be taken before the vessels become rigid from edema in the vessel walls. Ergot may be prescribed orally, intravenously, or rectally. Once a migraine headache becomes intense, ergot is of little value, and sumatriptan and dopamine agonists are more effective. Sumatriptan given orally has been shown to relieve migraine headaches in 65% to 78% of a group of clients with migraines (N = 187) as well as to relieve nausea and photophobia.[62] Lidocaine nasal drops have also been found to be an effective treatment of migraine.

Some sources recommend reducing the pain of migraine by applying pressure on the common carotid artery and the affected superficial artery. Lying in a dark, quiet room with ice on the back of the neck is often helpful during an acute episode.

Between migraine attacks, the client is usually in a normal state of health. If migraine episodes occur as often as once a week or more, preventive treatment may be possible. There are several types of medications used to prevent migraines. They include: beta-adrenergic blockers (propranolol), 5-hydroxytryptamine–influencing drugs (methysergide and amitriptyline), and calcium-channel blockers (nifedipine). Low-doses of caffeine are also effective to prevent headache. Some clients with migraine benefit from relaxation techniques, biofeedback, or counseling directed at preventing episodes by helping the client understand tensions and resolve major life conflicts. Another prophylactic measure is following a restrictive diet to avoid any beverages that contain tyramine and have vasoactive qualities that appear to predispose to migraine headaches.

Cluster Headaches

Cluster headaches are sometimes classified as a form of migraine. Most clients experiencing cluster headaches do not have a history of migraine headaches. Cluster headaches are excruciatingly painful, are unilateral, and tend to occur in clusters. There is usually no aura, as often occurs with migraines. Numerous episodes may occur within a few days, weeks, or, occasionally, months, followed by a remission with no symptoms for months or years. Then the headaches again recur in clusters. Men are affected five times more often than are women. Episodes usually begin in middle life and are often worsened by alcohol consumption. Recurrent episodes are dreaded by the client because of the intense suffering they cause.

A cluster of episodes subsides as suddenly and inexplicably as it began. Cluster headache may recur at irregular intervals for many years, often related to times of stress, anxiety, or emotional upset. The mechanism underlying cluster headaches is not well understood but is believed to be vascular in origin. These headaches were formerly believed to be caused by sensitivity to histamine.

Individual cluster headaches begin suddenly and may last only a few minutes or as long as 2 to 3 hours. Often they begin at night at approximately the same time. During an episode, the client experiences excruciating throbbing or steady pain arising high in the nostril and spreading to one side of the forehead, around and behind the eye on the affected side. The nose and affected eye water, and the skin reddens on the affected side. Nasal congestion and conjunctival injection are common.

Intervention for cluster headaches is ineffective because of the shortness of episodes. The client is acutely ill during the attack and desires to be alone and quiet. Applying cold relieves pain for some clients. Indomethacin (Indocin) or other nonsteroidal anti-inflammatory drugs are the medications of choice. Tricyclic antidepressants can also be used in treatment. Supportive care is important, because clients with cluster headaches often become depressed over their condition and fearful of recurrent episodes. Some feel they cannot survive another episode.

Tension Headaches (Muscle Contraction Headaches)

Tension headaches result from the long-sustained contraction of skeletal muscles around scalp, face, neck, and upper back. The muscles become tender, and as a result, the client tenses even more. This prolonged muscle contraction is the primary source of many headaches associated with excessive emotional tension, anxiety, and depression. Vasodilation of associated cranial arteries may also contribute to muscle irritability and head pain.

Tension headaches begin in adolescence but occur most often in middle age. They may increase significantly with menopause. Premenstrual headaches are usually of this type.

Sustained muscle contraction may also cause headaches secondary to painful stimuli from other cranial structures such as brain tumor; distended arteries; or eye, ear, nose, paranasal, or tooth inflammation.

Assessment of tension headaches typically reveals a steady, nonpulsatile ache (unilateral or bilateral) in any region of the head. Pain often occurs in the occipital and upper cervical regions and extends diffusely over the top of the head. The pain is frequently described as feeling of tightness, fullness, drawing sensations, or pressure. The pain of tension headache may be localized, or frequent changes may occur in location and intensity. Sometimes these headaches are fleeting but recurrent.

The onset of tension headaches is more gradual than with migraine headache. Nausea and vomiting may accompany tension headache but occur as a late reaction to pain. Also, the headache may be accompanied by dizziness, tinnitus, or lacrimation, or these symptoms may be elicited by pressing on the tender muscles. Palpation may demonstrate contracted muscles with localized painful areas or nodules. Pain may be precipitated or aggravated by combing the hair, wearing a hat, or exposure to cold. Tension headaches may be unrelieved for weeks, months, or years.

Tension headaches are treated when possible by removing the primary source of stimulation (e.g., treating diseased teeth). Clients with prolonged or recurrent muscle tension headaches of psychological origin may be helped by psychotherapy. Symptomatic treatment for the headaches themselves includes massaging affected muscles, applying local heat, rest, and various relaxation techniques. Sometimes, local injections of procaine are helpful. Tension headaches respond best to a medication that combines a non-narcotic analgesic with an anxiety-relieving drug. Occasionally, a stronger analgesic is needed (e.g., codeine sulfate).

Head Pain Related to Other Structures

Headaches may result from errors of refraction, glaucoma (with increased intraocular pressure), inflammation, and ocular muscle equilibrium disturbances (see Chapter 36).

Pain associated with sinus infection is usually caused by irritation and inflammation of sinus openings. Sinus walls are less sensitive. The pain of a sinus headache may be relieved or eliminated by decongestants and analgesics. Sometimes antibiotics are needed. Surgery to drain the sinuses may also be required (see Chapter 40).

Traumatic Brain Injury

Traumatic brain injury is a traumatic insult to the brain capable of producing physical, intellectual, emotional, social, and vocational changes. In the United States, a head injury is experienced approximately every 15 seconds. Head injuries occur in about 2 million Americans every year. Of these people, more than 750,000 are hospitalized, 50,000 experience chronic disability, and 100,000 die.[67]

Fatal head injuries occur in more than 30% of cases prior to arrival at the hospital due to the seriousness of the injury. An additional 20% of people die later because of secondary brain injury.[30] Secondary brain events include ischemia from hypoxia and hypotension, secondary hemorrhage, and cerebral edema.

Clients with traumatic head injuries often have other major injuries. These injuries include facial fractures, lung and heart injuries, cervical fractures, abdominal injuries, and musculoskeletal injuries. Facial fractures and lung injuries may contribute to respiratory insufficiency. Airway obstruction and decreased ability to breathe (e.g., from pulmonary contusion, flail chest, pneumothorax) contribute to respiratory insufficiency and poor oxygenation of the brain and other tissues. Brain death may result.

Hemorrhagic shock in clients with multiple trauma is rarely caused by head injury alone. Frequently it relates to (1) ruptured abdominal organs or (2) musculoskeletal injuries (e.g., fractured femur and pelvis). Circulation may be further compromised by cardiac contusion and associated arrhythmias.

Etiology and Risk Factors

Males aged 15 to 30 years are three times more likely to succumb to a traumatic head injury than are females. Peak occurrence is during evenings, nights, and weekends. Motor vehicle accidents are the foremost cause of head injuries. Other causes are assaults, falls, and accidents. Alcohol is a major contributor to this type of injury.

■ Mechanisms of Injury

Head injuries are caused by a sudden force to the head (Fig. 32–16). The results are complex. Three mechanisms contribute to head trauma: (1) acceleration, (2) deceleration, and (3) deformation. An acceleration injury occurs when the immobile head is struck by a moving object (see Fig. 32–16*A*). Deformation refers to injuries in which the force results in deformation and disruption of the integrity of the impacted body part (e.g., skull fracture, see Fig. 32–16*B*). If the head is moving and hits an immobile object, a deceleration injury occurs (see Fig. 32–16*C*). This injury can be seen in an auto accident when the head hits the steering wheel. In an acceleration-deceleration injury, a moving object hits the immobile head, and then the head hits an immobile object. Acceleration-deceleration injuries are also associated with rotation injury, where the brain is twisted within the skull.

Blunt Trauma

Head trauma is also categorized by describing the injury (e.g., blunt or penetrating trauma or a coup or contrecoup injury). Acceleration and deceleration injuries often result in blunt trauma. These are complex injuries involving several cranial structures, including brain parenchyma and vessels. Because the brain is able to move within the skull, movement of the brain can result in injuries at different locations. The brain is partially tethered (at its base) and is also suspended in CSF. Therefore, a blow to the skull can cause the hemispheres to twist on the fixed brain stem. As the brain moves, it scrapes over the skull's irregular inner prominences, which bruise and lacerate brain tissue. Disruption of the brain's small surface blood vessels may occur. Changes in vascular integrity may lead to fluid shifts and petechial hemorrhages. Cranial nerves, nerve tracts, larger blood vessels, and other tissues may be stretched, twisted, or rotated, and their functions disrupted.

Penetrating Trauma

Penetrating injuries include those made by foreign bodies (e.g., knives or bullets) or those made by bone fragments from a skull fracture. The damage caused by a penetrating injury often relates to the velocity with which a penetrating object pierces the skull and brain. Bone fragments from a skull fracture may cause local brain injury by lacerating brain tissue and damaging other structures (e.g., nerves and blood vessels). If a major blood vessel is severed or ruptured, a large clot (hematoma) may form, with damage to adjacent or even to remote structures (e.g., brain compression from one of the herniation syndromes). Thus, a secondary event, a hematoma, can also cause extensive brain tissue damage.

High-velocity objects (e.g., bullets) produce shock waves in the skull and brain. The shock waves may significantly damage brain structures beyond those in the

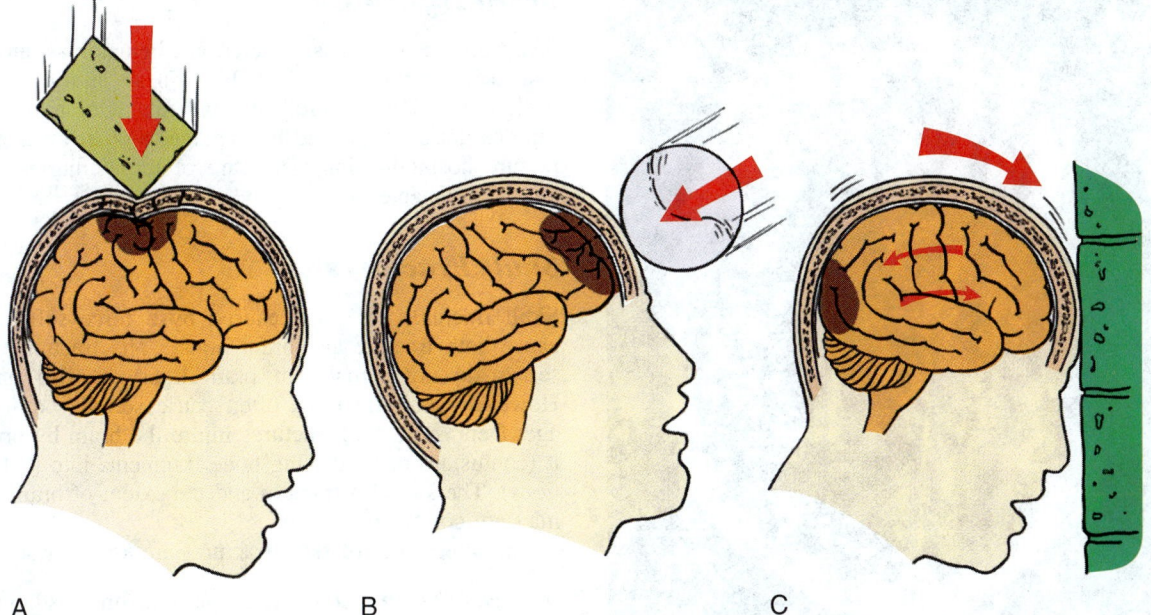

A   B   C

Figure 32–16. Some mechanisms of head injury. Head injury results from penetration or impact. *A*, Direct injury (a blow to the skull) may fracture the skull. Contusion and laceration of the brain may result from fractures. Depressed portions of the skull may compress or penetrate brain tissue. *B*, In the absence of a skull fracture, a blow to the skull may cause the brain to move enough to tear some of the veins going from the cortical surface to the dura. Subdural hematoma may then develop. Note the areas of cerebral contusion (dark brown). *C*, Rebound of the cranial contents may result in an area of injury opposite the point of impact. Such an injury is called a *contrecoup injury*. In addition to the three injuries depicted, additional brain dysfunction or damage may occur.

object's path. Frequently, penetrating wounds create an open communication between the external environment and the cranial cavity. Thus, infection is a possible complication.

Coup and Contrecoup Injuries

A *coup* (French for *blow*) injury occurs immediately at the point of impact. Because of movement within the skull, the same blow may cause injury on the opposite side of the brain, that is, a contrecoup injury (Fig 32–16C). *Contrecoup* is French for *counterblow*. In addition multiple areas of injury often occur along the line of the blow's force. Tissues around major injured areas often swell, which increases damage to the brain (Fig. 32–17).

The major factor contributing to the occurrence of head injury is alcohol consumption. Alcohol slows reflexes and alters cognitive processes and perception. These physiologic changes increase the chances of being involved in an accident or altercation. (See Risk Factors and Levels of Prevention.)

■ Types of Primary Injuries

Primary injury is an injury that results from the impact itself. It is contrasted to secondary injury, which is caused by hypoxia, hypercapnia, hypotension, and intracranial hypertension. The secondary problems occur hours to days after the initial impact.

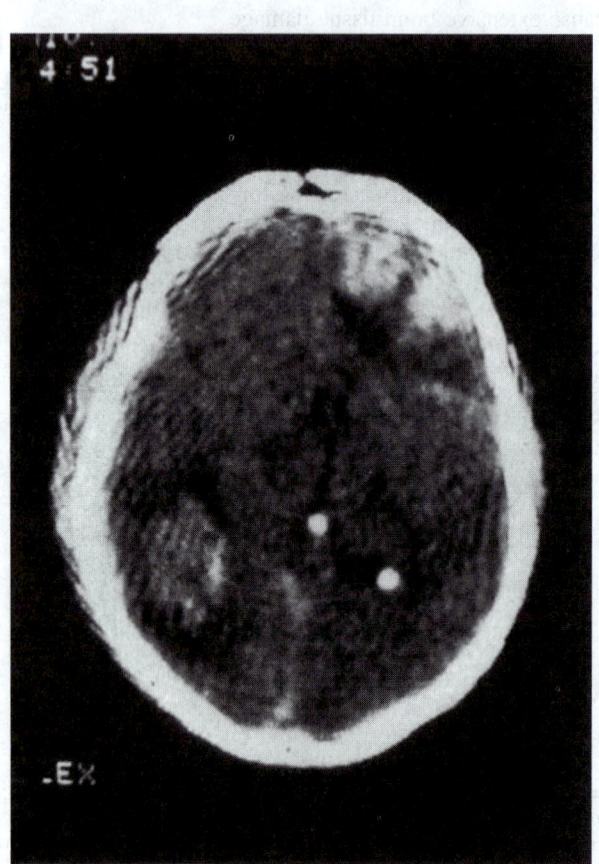

Figure 32–17. An MRI showing coup-contrecoup injury after head injury.

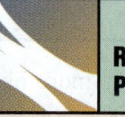

RISK FACTORS AND LEVELS OF PREVENTION

Head Injury

Risk Factors

Alcohol abuse, drug abuse, careless driving, failure to wear seat belts and protective gear, and improper use of weapons.

Levels of Prevention

Primary Prevention

- Teach clients to use safety restraints in cars and to wear bicycle helmets, motorcycle helmets, and roller blade helmets.
- Instruct clients not to drive after drug or alcohol ingestion and to use a designated driver when drinking

Secondary Prevention

- Help the client to control pre-existing conditions that may affect recovery from head injury.

Tertiary Prevention

- Stabilize and transport the client to a tertiary care center.
- Prevent falls in high-risk populations.

Scalp Injuries

Scalp injuries can cause lacerations, hematomas, and contusions or abrasions to the skin. These injuries may be unsightly and bleed profusely. Clients with minor scalp injuries not accompanied by damage to other areas do not require hospitalization. The care of these injuries is discussed in Chapter 89.

Skull Fractures

Skull fractures are often caused by a force sufficient to cause both fracture and brain injury. The fractures themselves do not signal that brain injury is also present. However, skull fractures often cause serious brain damage. Depressed skull fractures injure the brain by bruising it (contusion) or by driving bone fragments into it (lacerations). The site of a fracture and the extent of brain injury may not correlate.

The three types of skull fractures are as follows:

- *Linear skull fractures* appear as thin lines radiographically and do not require treatment; they are important only if there is significant underlying brain damage
- *Depressed skull fractures* may be palpated and are seen radiographically
- *Basilar skull fractures* occur in bones over the base of the frontal and temporal lobes

Brain Injuries

A single classification of brain injuries does not exist. However, the terms *open, closed, contusion,* and *concussion* are often applied to brain injuries. Open head injuries are those that penetrate the skull. Closed injuries are from blunt trauma.

Concussions. A concussion is head trauma that may result in loss of consciousness for 5 minutes or less and retrograde amnesia. There is no break in the skull or dura, and no visible damage on a CT or MRI scan.

Contusions. Contusions cause more extensive damage than do concussions. Contusions damage the brain itself, causing multiple areas of petechial and punctate hemorrhage and bruised areas. Diffuse axonal injury resulting in anatomic disruption of the white matter may result from serious contusions. Microscopic nerve fiber lesions also occur. Abnormalities may be mainly in one area of the brain, but other areas may also be injured. This is particularly true of brain stem contusions, which are a very serious type of lesion.

Diffuse Axonal Injury. Diffuse axonal injury is the most severe form of head injury. Diffuse axonal injury is classified into mild, moderate, and severe. Mild diffuse axonal injury consists of loss of consciousness lasting 6 to 24 hours. Moderate diffuse axonal injury is coma less than 24 hours with incomplete recovery on awakening. Severe diffuse axonal injury includes primary injury to the brain stem. Diffuse axonal injury begins with immediate loss of consciousness, prolonged coma, abnormal flexion or extension posturing, increased ICP, hypertension, and fever.

Pathophysiology

A concussion usually causes injury to the brain that is reversible. Some biochemical and ultrastructural damage, such as depletion in mitochondrial adenosine triphosphate and changes in vascular permeability, also can occur.[82]

Major head injuries cause direct damage to the parenchyma of the brain. Kinetic energy is transmitted to the brain and bruising occurs that is analogous to what is seen in soft tissue injuries. A blow to the surface of the brain leads to rapid brain tissue displacement, disruption of blood vessels and bleeding, tissue injury, and edema.

Clients with diffuse axonal damage have shearing injury with severe cerebral concussion, contusion of the cerebri, diffuse neuronal injury, and stretch injury to many other fibers. Widespread white matter injury, white matter degeneration, neuronal dysfunction, and global cerebral edema occur. Diffuse axonal injury is a microscopic lesion; therefore, CT scans may appear normal. Sometimes diffuse axonal injury appears on CT as small areas of bleeding.

Studies have noted a double mortality rate with hypotension because of the disruption of autoregulation. When autoregulation is disrupted, cerebral hypoperfusion leads to brain tissue ischemia. Hypoxia has a lesser effect on mortality as long as cerebral perfusion is adequate, because the brain can extract extra oxygen for short periods of time. Prolonged hypoxia, however, leads to brain tissue ischemia.[30]

Reperfusion injury occurs when ischemia is reversed and blood flow is re-established; it also leads to secondary injury. Reperfusion injury is probably caused by oxygen free radicals, which are normal byproducts of aerobic metabolism that usually break down into oxygen and water. In cell injury, breakdown of these radicals is impaired and they accumulate, causing destruction of nucleic acids, proteins, carbohydrates, lipids, and, eventually, cell membrane destruction in the brain tissue. Currently, research is targeted at developing neuroprotective agents that prevent delayed injury progression.[30]

Clinical Manifestations and Diagnostic Findings

■ Skull Fractures

Other than a history of head injury, clients with skull fractures may not have clear manifestations of their injury. Therefore, they need careful ongoing assessment. They may develop other clinical signs, including the following:

1. CSF or other fluid draining from the ear or nose
2. Various cranial nerve injuries
3. Blood behind the tympanic membrane
4. Periorbital ecchymoses (bruises around the eyes)
5. Later, a bruise over the mastoid (Battle's sign)

Basilar fractures are rarely seen radiographically.

Indications of cranial nerve and inner ear damage may occur at the time of the initial injury or may develop later. They include the following:

- Vision changes from optic nerve damage
- Hearing loss from auditory nerve damage
- Loss of the sense of smell from olfactory nerve damage
- Squint or fixed, dilated pupil and loss of some eye movements from oculomotor nerve damage
- Facial paresis or paralysis (unilateral) from facial nerve damage
- Vertigo from damage to otoliths in the inner ear
- Nystagmus from damage to the vestibular system

Basilar skull fractures, depressed fractures, and other open (compound) fractures allow communication between the external environment and the brain. Infection is therefore a possible complication. See Chapter 33 for a discussion of brain abscess and meningitis.

■ Concussions

Following concussion, observers report a loss of consciousness for 5 minutes or less. Retrograde amnesia, post-traumatic amnesia, or both may be present. The duration of amnesia may directly correlate with severity of the concussion. The client usually presents with headache and dizziness and may complain of nausea and vomiting. There is no break in the skull or dura, and no visible damage is seen on CT or MRI.

■ Contusions

The clinical manifestations of contusions are various. This is partly because any area of the brain can suffer contusion. Contusions are often associated with other serious injuries, including cervical fractures. Secondary effects (e.g., brain swelling and edema) accompany serious contusions. Increased ICP and herniation syndromes may result. Contusions may be divided into (1) cerebral contusions and (2) brain stem contusions.

Cerebral Contusions

Manifestations of cerebral contusions vary, depending on which areas of the cerebral hemispheres are damaged. An agitated, confused head-injured client who remains alert may have a temporal lobe contusion. Hemiparesis in an alert head-injured client may indicate a frontal contusion. An aphasic head-injured client may have a frontotemporal contusion. Other findings indicate contusions in other areas. Although these findings correlate with cerebral contusion, they do not rule out other abnormalities, such as a developing mass or lesion. Adverse changes in the client's condition require immediate medical attention. If treated early, these complications may be reversible.

Brain Stem Contusions

Brain stem contusions render a client immediately unresponsive or partially comatose because of significant brain stem disruption. Typically, an altered LOC continues for at least several hours and usually days or weeks. The client may regain partial consciousness within hours or remain in a coma.

Damage to the reticular activating system may render the client permanently comatose. Other neurologic abnormalities are present and are usually symmetrical (i.e., evenly distributed on both sides of the body). Some may be lateralized (asymmetrical, or on one side of the body only), indicating development of a secondary event, such as a hematoma.

In addition to the altered LOC that is always present with brain stem contusion, respiratory, pupillary, eye movement, and motor abnormalities may occur.

- Respirations may be normal, periodic, very rapid or ataxic.
- Pupils are usually small, equal, and reactive. Damage to the upper brain stem (third cranial nerve) may cause pupillary abnormalities.
- Loss of normal eye movements may occur because pathways controlling eye movements traverse the midbrain and pons.
- The client may respond to light or noxious stimuli by purposeful movements, such as pushing the stimulus away, or the client may have no response to stimuli (i.e., may be in a flaccid state). In the presence of profound LOC alterations, flexion and extension posturing may be elicited with or without noxious stimuli (see Chapter 31).

Brain stem contusions do not usually injure the brain stem alone. Swelling or direct injury to the hypothalamus

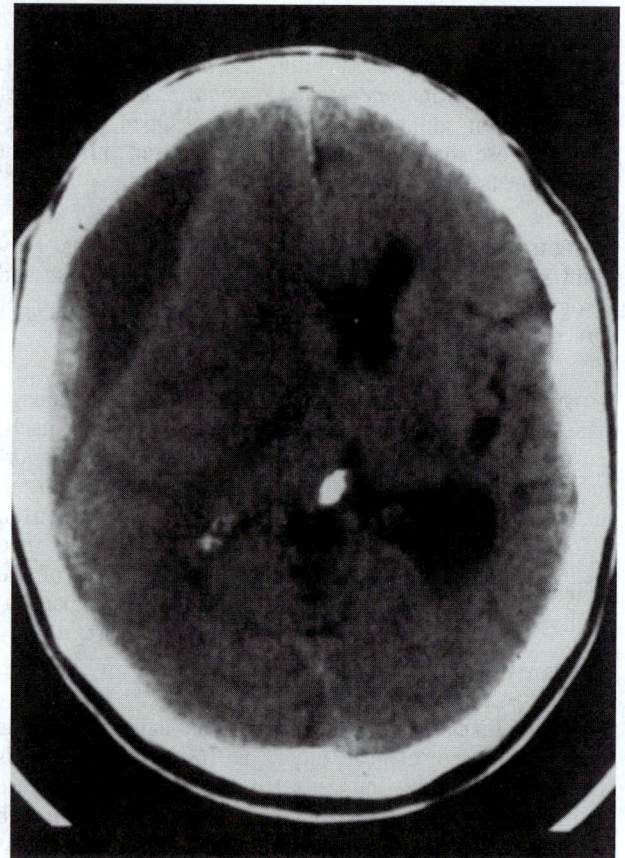

Figure 32–18. An MRI showing chronic subdural hematoma with an area of acute bleeding, causing a severe midline shift.

may produce autonomic nervous system effects. The client has a high temperature, a rapid pulse and respirations, and perspires profusely. These effects may wax and wane but, if sustained, can lead to serious complications.

These clinical manifestations often vary from one observation to another, whereas findings indicating a developing hematoma are more consistent. Carefully document assessment findings to identify patterns or trends in the client's condition.

Diagnostic assessments, such as a CT or MRI scan, may reveal fractures and areas of bleeding or brain shift (see Figs. 32–17 and 32–18). Lumbar puncture can also be used to assess for bleeding within the subarachnoid space.

Emergency Care

The initial management of clients with head injury is the same as for any other injured client: airway, breathing, and circulation. There is a high association of cervical fracture with head injury; therefore, the client must be immobilized at the scene of the injury. Lateral cervical spine x-rays are obtained before the client's head is moved or the immobilization is removed. Protect the client with head injury from possible complications of cord injury by immobilizing the head and neck immediately by using a cervical collar or sandbags until a collar can be obtained. Maintain cervical immobilization until an injury is ruled out by x-ray examination. If resuscitation is necessary, a jaw thrust maneuver must be used. Obtain a baseline of the client's motor and sensory function. Continue to monitor and document hourly. Notify the physician immediately if any progressive signs of deficit occur.

An IV line is started and fluids are given to stabilize the blood pressure. Head injury alone does not cause major loss of blood. If a large blood loss is suspected, look for other injuries (e.g., fractures, abdominal injury).

A complete history is taken of the mechanism of injury. These data allow the physician to determine the probable extent of injury. Diagnostic findings are reviewed.

Cover open head wounds and apply pressure to control bleeding unless there appears to be underlying depressed or compound skull fracture. Do not attempt to remove foreign objects or any penetrating objects from the wound. Uncomplicated scalp wounds (that do not lie over depressed or compound skull fractures) are anesthetized locally, cleansed, and sutured.

 ## Critical Care

Ongoing care to reduce intracranial pressure is the focus of critical care. Osmotic diuretics, hyperventilation, and adequate oxygenation continue. The cerebral metabolic rate is reduced by using sedatives, barbiturates, paralytic agents, antipyretics, and hypothermia. Codeine is a good narcotic for the head-injured client. It reduces pain without causing marked sedation or respiratory depression. Paralytic agents may be used to promote adequate ventilation. Always administer these agents in conjunction with a sedative because paralytic agents have no sedative effect.

■ Medical Management

The medical management of severely head-injured clients focuses on supporting all organ systems while recovery from the injuries takes place. This involves (1) ventilatory support, (2) management of fluid balance and elimination, and (3) management of nutrition and gastrointestinal function. Head trauma affects all systems of the body, and managing the effects requires a holistic perspective. Clinical manifestations may be the result of the initial head injury or may arise from a complicating process. Major goals in the care of severely head-injured clients are as follows:

1. Prompt recognition and treatment of hypoxia and acid-base disorders that can contribute to cerebral edema
2. Control of increasing ICP resulting from factors such as cerebral edema or expanding hematoma
3. Stabilization of other conditions

Complications

Complications of head injury develop after several hours or days. Histamine antagonists (e.g., cimetidine or raniti-

dine) are given to reduce the risk of stress ulcers. Antibiotics may also be prescribed. Osmotic diuretics may be required to reduce ICP. Initially, the client is given nothing by mouth until peristalsis returns, usually about 5 days. Enteral feedings are begun when peristalsis returns, because metabolic needs increase after head injury. The risk of aspiration with nasogastric feeding must be prevented by elevating the client's head during feedings and monitoring pulmonary changes. Total parenteral nutrition (TPN) can also be used, but some clients develop hyperglycemia from the solution. Hyperglycemia can increase ICP; therefore, monitor blood glucose levels carefully.

Cerebral Edema. Cerebral edema and brain swelling are almost always associated with serious head injuries. The skull is a closed compartment with little room to accommodate swelling. A mass effect occurs once the space is filled and ICP increases. Clinical manifestations of compromised brain function develop. Edema is one of the common causes of death in clients who survive the initial injury and who do not develop an intracranial mass lesion.

Infection. Infections such as meningitis and a brain abscess may occur after head injury. They are more common after open head injuries.

Acute Hydrocephalus. Acute hydrocephalus develops when increased CSF accumulates in the ventricles. This results from the defective reabsorption of CSF or blockage of the CSF flow. Traumatic or infectious blockage of CSF flow can occur with head injuries. As the CSF pressure rises, signs of increased ICP develop. Intervention includes surgical shunting or the placement of a ventriculostomy.

Diabetes Insipidus. Diabetes insipidus of the neurogenic type is often seen with closed head injuries. Lesions that affect the hypothalamus, the antidiuretic hormone (ADH) storage vesicles, or the posterior pituitary can also cause diabetes insipidus. The client experiences severe polyuria followed by polydipsia secondary to a deficiency of ADH. Clients who have a urine output of more than 9 L/day and a urine osmolality of less than 100 mOsm/kg after a dehydration or water restriction test usually require ADH replacement (desmopressin/DDAVP).

Syndrome of Inappropriate Secretion of Antidiuretic Hormone. The syndrome of inappropriate secretion of antidiuretic hormone (SIADH) is characterized by high levels of ADH that result in oliguria in the absence of normal physiologic stimuli for its release. Pituitary surgery may stimulate the release of ADH, but the most common cause of SIADH is ectopic tumors, as in many forms of cancer, that secrete ADH. Some psychiatric illnesses and some medications are also associated with SIADH.

Dysrhythmias. Head injuries can cause dysrhythmias that further complicate the client's recovery. Some clients survive initial head trauma only to develop intracranial mass lesions, such as expanding hematomas (e.g., epidural and subdural hemorrhages), which may be fatal unless promptly diagnosed and treated.

Neurogenic Pulmonary Edema. Clients with massive head injury may develop neurogenic pulmonary edema in about 24 to 48 hours. It is very similar to adult respiratory distress syndrome (ARDS), so some people think it is a variant of ARDS. Treatment is the same as for ARDS.

Arteriovenous Aneurysms. Arteriovenous aneurysms are often caused by traumatic laceration of the internal carotid artery (as it passes through the cavernous sinus). Typical injuries include penetration by missiles or a sphenoid bone fracture. Manifestations include exophthalmos, distended orbital and periorbital veins, and cranial nerve paralysis. These result from increased tension in the cavernous sinus caused by accumulated arterial blood. Surgery may be necessary to ligate the internal carotid artery in the neck and the internal carotid and ophthalmic arteries intracranially.

Altered Behavior. On regaining consciousness after several days of unconsciousness that follow head injury, a client's behavior may be noisy, generally disturbed, and confused. Such a client is usually experiencing traumatic delirium resulting from cerebral irritation. He or she is not deliberately being difficult. During this temporary phase, the client needs protection, reassurance, and care, as during other delirious states. This state of partial confusion may remain even after the client can speak clearly and is able to cooperate in some activities. The family needs complete explanations and reassurance. Family members are often upset with the client's behavior. After this phase comes a time during which the client appears to have fully regained mental faculties. The client may be up and about, may recognize others, and may cooperate, yet memory of these events is impaired. This is a state of automatic behavior during which the client has no memory of day-to-day events and yet is able to carry on activities in a seemingly normal manner.

Post-trauma Response. Post-trauma response is a set of complications emerging in the recovery phase after head injury; it may continue for months or years. This response generally occurs in clients who have sustained a minor head injury. Assessment findings include the following:

  Headache
  Poor concentration (especially in reading)
  Dizziness
  Unsteadiness related to sudden head movements
  Irritability
  Sensitivity to noise
  Insomnia
  Restlessness

  Hyperhidrosis (excessive perspiration)
  Depression
  Personality changes
  Nervousness
  Impaired memory
  Anxiety
  Alcohol intolerance
  Easy fatigability

Although as many as half of head-injured clients may experience these symptoms in a mild form for a short time, the manifestations are not appropriately referred to as *post-trauma response* unless they persist for weeks or even years and impair the client's employability.

Post-trauma response is seen in clients with the following characteristics:

1. Condition progressively worsens
2. Extent of injury does not correlate with the severity of the syndrome
3. Complex overlapping neurologic and psychogenic symptoms tend to coexist

Whether the manifestations arise from brain damage or are psychogenic in origin is not known and is the subject of much controversy. Sometimes an organic cause cannot be found by physical examination, but careful neuropsychological testing demonstrates abnormalities compatible with brain damage.

Intervention for post-traumatic response is usually supportive. The client and family may be relieved to know that this syndrome sometimes occurs after head injury. Explain that the problems usually diminish and eventually clear. Supporting the client and family usually alleviates the anxiety. If not, professional counseling may be helpful. Cognitive rehabilitation may help the client compensate for memory impairment and attention deficits.

Outcomes

Not many clients die instantly from head injury. However, many head-injured clients die within the first few minutes after injury from shock or impaired respiration. Early death may also result from brain stem damage. Sullivan and co-workers[67] reviewed several studies that concluded that coma duration is the best predictor of damage severity because it correlates highly with probability of death, intellectual deficit, and social skills impairment. The results of these studies classified a mild head injury as loss of consciousness for 20 minutes or less, a moderate head injury as 21 to 59 minutes of unconsciousness, and severe head injury as coma for 1 hour or more.

■ Nursing Management of the Medical Client

Assessment

A history of how a client was injured is helpful in understanding the nature of a head injury. When accident witnesses accompany a head-injured client to the care facility, obtain as much information as possible about the accident and about the client's neurologic responses at the scene of the accident. Try to find out if the client lost consciousness.

As soon as possible after head injury, assess and document the client's vital signs and neurologic status. This initial assessment and the data from the witnesses at the accident scene establishes a baseline for later observations. Carefully document all assessment findings.

In the healthcare facility, the frequency of assessing vital signs and neurologic status varies according to the client's condition. However, it is usually every 15 minutes until the client's condition is stable; consider age and other previous conditions. It may be necessary to wake up a head-injured client hourly for assessment during the first 24 to 48 hours after injury. Parameters assessed include the following:

1. LOC and responsiveness
2. Pupillary size, direct and consensual responses to light, extraocular movement
3. Vital signs: blood pressure, temperature, pulse rate and quality, respiratory rate and quality
4. Motor strength
5. Speech
6. Vision
7. Reaction to auditory and painful stimuli
8. Response to command
9. Spontaneous activity
10. General responsiveness to stimulation

The GCS is commonly used. Oxygen needs are also monitored by assessing tissue perfusion, oximetry readings, and arterial blood gas analysis (ABG) results. Fluid and electrolyte balance must also be monitored. Note bleeding; check the hemoglobin and hematocrit.

Promptly report to the physician any findings that indicate the possible development of complications. It is particularly difficult to assess the condition of a head-injured client who has ingested large amounts of alcohol or other drugs before injury, because these substances may obscure significant clinical assessment findings.

Diagnosis, Planning, Implementation

Many nursing and collaborative problems are present in the client with a head injury, such as risk for *Ineffective Airway Clearance, Altered Tissue Perfusion,* seizures, paralysis, infection, diabetes insipidus, and *Post-trauma Response.* Other problems that a client with a head injury may experience include the following:

Risk for contractures
Impaired Skin Integrity
Altered Oral Mucous Membranes
Altered Nutrition
Altered fluid volume
Risk for Injury
Risk for increased ICP
Altered Thought Processes
Altered Family Processes

These diagnoses are discussed in Chapters 31 and 32. The etiologies of these problems and the interventions for them must be individualized to your client.

Risk for Ineffective Airway Clearance. The client with traumatic brain injury may have an altered state of consciousness and may not be able to expectorate secretions. This client is also at increased risk for aspiration.

Planning: Expected Outcomes. The client will have effective airway clearance. He or she will have an upper airway free of secretions; a regular respiratory rate (16 to 22 respirations/minute), rhythm, and depth; clear breath sounds in both lungs; symmetrical chest movement; a midline position of the trachea; absence of dyspnea, agitation, confusion, or yawning; absence of aspiration; PaO_2 greater than 90 mm Hg and $PaCO_2$ between 35 and 45 mm Hg; and a clear chest film.

Implementation. Nursing actions aimed at maintaining adequate airway clearance include clearing the mouth and oral pharynx of foreign bodies (e.g., teeth) and suctioning the oropharynx and trachea every 1 to 2 hours and additionally as needed. Never suction the nasopharynx until after a basilar fracture and meningeal tear is ruled out. A semiprone, lateral position may facilitate drainage of secretions and prevent aspiration but is contraindicated with increased ICP or a cervical fracture. Humidified oxygen, endotracheal intubation, a tracheostomy, or a mechanical ventilator may be required to maintain the client's PaO_2.

Altered Cerebral Tissue Perfusion. Clients who suffer from traumatic brain injuries are at *Risk for Altered Cerebral Tissue Perfusion secondary to hypotension, hypertension, intracranial hemorrhage, hematoma, or other injuries.*

Planning: Expected Outcomes. The client will have adequate cerebral tissue perfusion. He or she will have; stable, improving LOC; a GCS of 9 or above; a temperature less than 38.5° C; equal, direct, and consensual pupil response to light; intact extraocular movements; stable or improving motor response or response to pain; ICP of 15 mm Hg or less; MAP of 80 mm Hg or above with systolic blood pressure between 100 and 150 mm Hg; normal sinus rhythm with minimal dysrhythmia; minimal urinary output of 30 ml/hour; normal hemoglobin/hematocrit with no bleeding; and a normal central venous pressure.

Implementation. Although anticipatory, prudent monitoring is key to early detection of altered cerebral tissue perfusion, nursing interventions can actually prevent, delay, or minimize altered cerebral perfusion. For example, treating hyperthermia early with antipyretics or lowering or maintaining temperature by using a temperature controlled blanket can prevent alterations in cerebral metabolism. Elevating the head of the bed to at least 30 degrees, keeping the head in neutral position, and avoiding extreme hip flexion can facilitate venous jugular drainage and decrease cerebral edema. Consulting the physician for early treatment of dysrhythmias and blood replacement as indicated may be necessary for maintenance of an adequate cardiac output. Control active bleeding by compression when possible, unless a skull fracture is present. Communicating a client's neurologic status accurately and completely through verbal reporting and documentation is essential to early identification of change and early intervention.

Intracranial monitoring may be required. It is discussed earlier in this chapter.

Risk for Diabetes Insipidus.

Almost any brain lesion, whether a tumor, aneurysm, thrombosis, infection, immunologic response, closed head injury, or a hypophysectomy, can place a client at risk for diabetes insipidus, which is caused by a deficiency of ADH secondary to damage to the hypothalamus, storage vesicles, or posterior pituitary.

Planning: Expected Outcomes. Monitor the client for risk of diabetes insipidus, as evidenced by polyuria, nocturia, polydipsia, and low urine specific gravity.

Implementation. Assess and record urinary output hourly. Compare output with intake. If the output exceeds the hourly intake by 200 ml for 2 consecutive hours, notify the physician. The physician may order assays of specific gravity, urine osmolality, or a plasma osmolality to be done after a period of water deprivation. A client with this syndrome will have low specific gravity, low urine osmolality, high plasma osmolality, and electrolyte imbalance. A client with normal ADH response will have a decrease in urinary output, but a person with diabetes insipidus will continue to have polyuria. This client is at risk for fluid volume deficit secondary to the loss of 9 L or more of fluid volume per day and is placed at further risk for circulatory collapse or hypertonic encephalopathy during the water deprivation test. Therefore, monitor cerebral function and blood pressure at least hourly during the water deprivation period (usually 8 hours). If the test result is positive, the physician will order replacement with a synthetic vasopressin (desmopressin DDAVP), commonly given intranasally.

Risk for Seizures.

Any disorder that causes a change in the neuronal environment of the brain can put a client at risk for seizures. A traumatic head injury is a common cause. See Chapter 33 for more discussion of seizures.

Planning: Expected Outcomes. Monitor the client for seizure development, protect the client from injury, and maintain a patent airway if a seizure should occur.

Implementation. Protect the client at risk, prophylactically, by placing padding on side rails, keeping the bed in a low position, giving the anticonvulsant medication on time, and reporting missed dosages or low or high plasma levels of medication to the physician. If a seizure does occur, call for help as you are protecting the client's head and turning the client to a lateral position to displace the tongue and to promote an open airway. Stay with the client; protect the client from harm; and observe the onset, progression, and duration of the seizure. Suction as necessary and monitor vital signs. Never attempt to insert a tongue blade or oral airway once the client is having convulsions; it will only increase the risk of damage to the teeth or oral cavity and cause more risk for airway obstruction. Seizures that become continuous are life threatening; notify the physician immediately, give

oxygen, and prepare for administration of an IV anticonvulsant (e.g., diazepam).

Risk for Infection.

Clients who have a head injury with meningeal tearing have a *Risk for Infection secondary to invasion of organisms to a damaged meningeal membrane*; this can lead to meningitis or encephalitis.

Planning: Expected Outcomes. The client will have no infection secondary to meningeal membrane tearing, no fever, and no signs of meningitis.

Implementation. Prevent risk for infection by not suctioning a client nasally if an anterior fossa or basilar fracture or CSF leakage from the ears (otorrhea) or nose (rhinorrhea) is present. If drainage is present, test it for the presence of glucose. CSF drainage is clear, tests positive for glucose, and dries in concentric rings: blood-tinged fluid that contains CSF will dry with a "halo sign." When drainage is present, use sterile dressings to absorb the fluid. Change them whenever they become wet to decrease the entry of microorganisms. If the client is conscious, discourage nose blowing, coughing, and inhibition of sneezing. Instruct the client to sneeze through an open mouth; suppressing a sneeze forces the bacteria backward. Administer prescribed antibiotics on time. Report any signs of meningitis: fever, severe headache, photophobia, neck pain and rigidity with flexion (nuchal rigidity), flexion of the legs and thighs with neck flexion (Brudzinski's sign), and inability to extend the leg with the hip flexed at a right angle (Kernig's sign). Also report any manifestations of increased ICP.

Post-trauma Response.

A client who has experienced a head injury often experiences a *Post-traumatic Response*. See earlier discussion.

Evaluation

Assess the degree of attainment of expected outcomes often in the early phases of care. Later in rehabilitation, expected outcomes may require weeks for full attainment. Because the care of the head-injured client goes on in many areas of a healthcare setting (e.g., the ICU, a general nursing unit, a rehabilitation unit), complete communication about the client, family, and goals should always be a part of care plan.

Modifications for Elderly Clients

Although most head injuries do not occur in the elderly population, diagnosis is often more difficult in the elderly because of an atypical presentation. These clients also experience more complications. An elderly client may be less able to tolerate respiratory problems or cardiac dysrhythmias. The presence of chronic diseases such as chronic obstructive pulmonary disease or congestive heart failure can make managing ventilation and fluid balance more difficult. If any type of mental impairment was present before the injury, recovery to full independence is less likely. Rehabilitation may be impeded by poor stamina and medical complications.

■ Surgical Management

Some conditions that may require surgery include subdural and epidural hematomas, depressed skull fractures, and penetrating foreign bodies. Intracranial pressure is reduced as much as possible before surgery. Baseline neurologic data are documented. Informed consent needs to be obtained from the family if the client is unconscious or confused.

Simple skull depressions are electively treated by surgically elevating the depressed bone tissue, removing fragments, and repairing lacerated dura. Compound depressed skull fractures are immediately treated surgically. The scalp, skull, and devitalized brain are debrided, and the wound is cleaned thoroughly. Unless all foreign material is removed, a brain abscess develops. Debridement of a penetrating wound or depressed skull fracture frequently leaves a cranial defect that is cosmetically unsightly. The defect may be surgically corrected by cranioplasty at a later time. Following surgery, care for the client following guidelines for craniotomy (see Chapter 33).

Community and Self-Care

Clients with possible head injury or mild head injury were previously hospitalized for observation for a minimum of 6 hours (ideally for 48 hours) because of the risk of extradural hemorrhage. If the client is sent home, give clear instructions to help the clients caregiver assess for complications (see the Client Education Guide).

Almost any client who is hospitalized for more than 48 hours because of a head injury will require some rehabilitation. This treatment may take place in an inpatient or outpatient setting, depending on the client's condition. Rehabilitation, which can include physical, occupational, speech, and cognitive therapy, is essential in returning the client to maximal function. Nurses play a major role in the rehabilitation of the head-injured client and significant others. (See the section on cerebrovascular accident earlier in this chapter for additional suggestions.)

Clients may be sent to rehabilitation facilities with feeding tubes or tracheostomy tubes in place. Clients and families need assistance in choosing a new healthcare facility that can deliver the level of care needed. If recovery is unlikely, the client may need to be transferred to an extended care facility. Because many head-injured clients are young, previously healthy people, placement in a nursing home may be a very difficult reality for family members to accept. Your teaching and support can greatly improve coping.

The rehabilitation of clients with brain injuries is challenging. Sometimes, community reintegration is unsuccessful. Some programs have found improvement in the client's ability to lead a productive life with interdisciplinary techniques that include rehabilitation in cognition, compensatory techniques, social skills, emotional adjust-

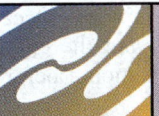

CLIENT EDUCATION GUIDE

Monitoring Family Members After Head Injury

Family Instructions in English *(Instrucciones para la familia en inglés)*	Family Instructions in Spanish *(Instrucciones para la familia en español)*
Observe your family member for 24 hours. Take him or her to the hospital immediately if any of the following occur:	Observe al miembro de su familia por 24 horas. Llévelo(a) al hospital inmediatamente si ocurre cualquiera de los síntomas siguientes:
● Increased drowsiness or confusion	● Aumento en el estado de confusión o somnolencia
● Inability to be awakened	● Incapacidad de despertarse
● Vomiting	● Vómito
● Convulsions	● Convulsiones
● Bleeding or drainage from the nose or ears	● Hemorragia o drenaje por la nariz o los oídos
● Weakness in either arm or leg	● Debilidad en un brazo o en una pierna
● Loss of feeling in either arm or either leg	● Pérdida de sensación en un brazo o en una pierna
● Blurring of vision	● Visión borrosa
● Slurring of speech	● Lenguaje indistinto
● Enlargement or shrinkage of one pupil	● Agrandamiento o empeanehñecimientu de una de las pupilas

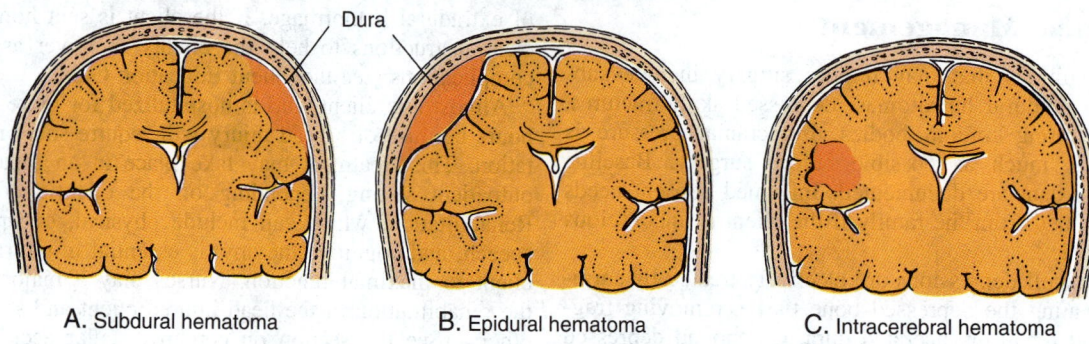

Figure 32–19. Formation of a hematoma after head injury.

ment, leisure skills, physical fitness, and health maintenance. Most clients require 6 months in such a program.[65]

Secondary Brain Injuries

Secondary injuries are complications of the initial injury. Several have been listed in the section on traumatic brain injury. Epidural and subdural hematomas (Fig. 32–19) require special consideration.

Epidural Hematoma

An epidural hematoma, also called an *extradural hematoma*, forms between the skull and the dura mater (see Fig. 32–19*B*). It occurs in about 10% of severe head injuries and is usually associated with skull fracture. An epidural hematoma occurs from injury to the extracerebral blood vessels, most often the middle meningeal artery and vein. Bleeding is almost always continuous, and a large clot forms, which separates the dura from the skull.

Manifestations are usually acute in onset because the bleeding is often arterial. With a classic epidural hematoma, the following sequence of events occurs:

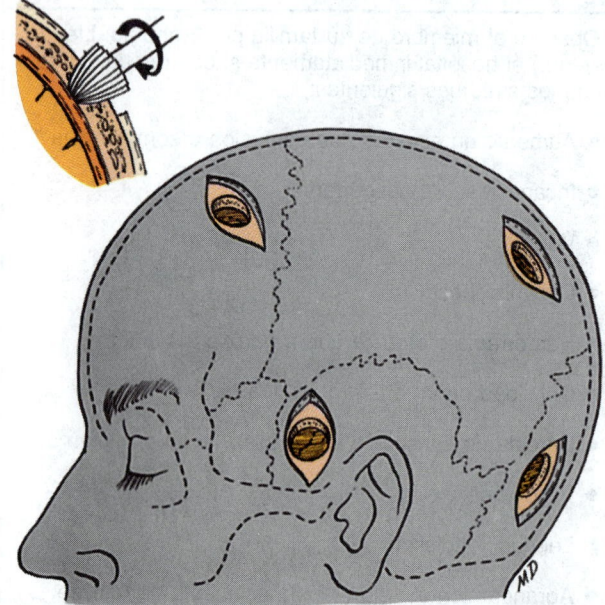

Figure 32–20. Placement of burr holes in the skull.

1. The client is unconscious immediately after head trauma
2. The client awakens and is quite lucid
3. Rapid deterioration takes place in LOC, pupil dilation, and eye movement paralysis on the same side as the hematoma
4. The client lapses into a coma

Hemiparesis on the opposite side or seizures may also occur. The client may deteriorate rapidly, showing signs of increasing ICP and tentorial herniation until death occurs from respiratory arrest. Bleeding ceases only with medical interventions or death.

No indications of extradural hemorrhage may be present immediately after the initial trauma. Within several hours, the hematoma may grow to a critical level, and the client deteriorates rapidly and may die. For this reason, head-injured clients are usually hospitalized for observation even after apparently minor injuries. Occasionally, an epidural clot develops slowly, and the client remains asymptomatic for a week or even a month before neurologic changes become evident.

Skull radiography and CT scan may confirm the diagnosis. Rapid diagnosis and prompt intervention are essential with an epidural hematoma. Careful, ongoing assessment of neurologic status is also necessary. Notify the physician of changes immediately.

Intervention includes lowering the ICP with hyperventilation by mechanical ventilation or by manually ventilating the client with an Ambu bag. An epidural clot may be surgically evacuated through burr holes (Fig. 32–20), twist drills, or a craniotomy. During surgery, the wound may be drained and bleeding vessels ligated. Following surgery, the client is cared for like any client recovering from a craniotomy.

Subdural Hematoma

Subdural hematoma is a collection of blood in the subdural space (i.e., between the dura mater and arachnoid mater) (see Fig. 32–19*A*). Blood escaping into the subdural space is not absorbed but becomes organized or encapsulated by the dura. As a blood clot forms, blood cells within the clot's membrane undergo lysis to form a fluid of high osmotic character. This draws fluid from the surrounding subarachnoid space into the clot, which produces a gradually increasing intracranial mass. Large clots may produce such high ICP that cerebral herniation occurs, and death may result.

Subdural hematomas may be classified as acute, subacute, or chronic, depending on how rapidly clinical manifestations develop. Another classification recognizes only acute and chronic, combining the acute and subacute categories.

Acute and Subacute Subdural Hematoma

Acute subdural hematoma usually results from brain laceration. Acute subdural hematomas are a serious complication requiring prompt treatment because they compress and distort an already damaged, edematous brain. Occasionally, acute subdural hematoma results from a ruptured saccular aneurysm or an intracerebral hemorrhage if there is tearing of the arachnoid mater. Acute subdural hematoma is symptomatic within 24 hours of injury. Acute subdural hematoma is seen in approximately 24% of clients with severe head injuries.

Clinical manifestations of acute subdural hematoma are similar to those of acute epidural hematoma. The onset and development of the clinical manifestations may be somewhat slower because the bleeding is more often venous, rather than arterial. Symptom recognition may be difficult because subdural hematoma is often associated with moderate or severe brain injury. A client developing an acute subdural hematoma may remain unconscious after injury or may have a variable LOC (depending on the extent of injury). A conscious client usually has a headache. The client may become irritable and confused and lapse into a coma or show a fluctuating LOC. Manifestations of increasing ICP occur. Subtle changes in LOC and development of lateralizing changes (i.e., on one side) such as hemiparesis, pupillary dilation, or extraocular eye movement paralysis may be the only findings.

Chronic Subdural Hematoma

Chronic subdural hematoma is most common in elderly and alcoholic clients. These clients experience atrophy of the brain, which results in stretching of the bridging veins. These stretched veins are easily ruptured in a fall, even if it does not result in other injuries. It develops several weeks or even months after injury. Elderly or alcoholic clients may not even recall the mechanism of injury. The initial injury may have been relatively minor, and the client may not associate current clinical manifestations with the past injury.

Gradually the blood clot causes pressure on the brain. There is an interval during which the client appears to be recovering or seems completely recovered. Later, manifestations of neurologic deterioration develop. The client may become drowsy, inattentive, and incoherent and display personality changes. Headaches are another prominent symptom. These indications of chronic subdural hematoma may be overlooked until focal or lateralizing signs appear (e.g., hemiparesis, pupil signs). Changes in LOC continue and may fluctuate widely. Educate the in-

jured client and significant others of the possible complications so that they can seek medical help promptly if necessary.

Clinical assessment of subdural hematoma is similar to that for epidural hematomas. Surgical intervention usually consists of placing several burr holes or performing a craniotomy to remove the hematoma. Treatment results depend on the client's condition before surgery and the degree of primary brain tissue damage.

A client who has had evacuation of a chronic subdural hematoma usually has a drain placed in the cavity to prevent reaccumulation of the fluid and blood. These clients are typically kept flat during the immediate postoperative period. This allows the brain to reexpand and fill the cavity, without the effects of gravity hindering the reexpansion.

Intracerebral Hematoma

Intracerebral hematomas occur less often than epidural or subdural hematomas. They are caused by bleeding directly into brain tissue and may occur at the area of injury, some distance away or deep within the brain. These hematomas cause problems with increased ICP. Surgical resection may cause as much damage as the clot itself and is usually not performed unless the clot is easily accessible. Clinical manifestations are similar to those that occur with epidural or subdural hematomas, although hemiplegia is more common than hemiparesis. Many assessment findings relate to the lesion's mass effect secondary to increased ICP. Various other clinical manifestations may also be present, depending on the location of the intracerebral hematoma. A diagnosis is established as with other types of hematomas. One form of hematoma, called *delayed traumatic intracerebral hematoma*, occurs after a few days. It is most common in persons with disseminated intravascular coagulation (DIC), hypotension, alcohol abuse, and hypoxia. It carries a poor prognosis.

Conclusions

Because of the complexity of brain disorders and the emotional reactions of the client and family to these problems, neurologic nursing is one of the most challenging areas of practice. Common nursing problems center on cerebral perfusion and cognition as well as on assisting the client to a maximal level of functional rehabilitation. Prevention and early intervention are key to client outcome.

Thinking Critically

1. A 70-year-old man had a left cerebral hemisphere cerebrovascular accident (CVA) 2 days ago. While obtaining his assessment, you note that his

blood pressure is elevated at 200 mm Hg systolic; his usual systolic blood pressure is 140 to 160 mm Hg. He is receiving oxygen at 5 L, but his oxygen saturation has dropped from 95% to 88% in the last hour. The client was oriented to person, place, and time an hour ago, but has become increasingly restless and slightly confused. The confusion has led him to pull out a nasogastric tube that had been placed for nutritional maintenance. What other neurologic assessments should you do? What is the first priority? Is the suddenness of this change significant?

Factors to Consider. How has the client's assessment changed from baseline? Is there any relationship between the increased blood pressure and the hypoxia? Is the removal of the nasogastric tube an immediate problem?

2. You are caring for a client who had a malignant brain tumor resected 72 hours ago. During prior assessments, she was alert and oriented, her pupils were equal, round, reactive to light, and accommodative, her eyes opened spontaneously, and she was moving all four extremities equally and on command. Her Glasgow Coma Scale (GCS) score was 15. Currently she is slow to respond, though still oriented to person, place, and time. Her right pupil is equal in size to the left but exhibits a sluggish reaction to direct light. Her left pupil responds normally. She still responds to verbal commands appropriately, has equal motor strength, and opens her eyes spontaneously. Thus, her score on the GCS is still 15. You decide to notify the physician. Why?

Factors to Consider. How sensitive is the Glasgow Coma Scale? What might the decreased response time and the change in pupil reaction indicate?

Bibliography

1. Adams, R. J. (1995). Management issues for patients with ischemic stroke. *Neurology, 45*(Suppl 1), S15–S18.
2. Andrus, C. (1991). Intracranial pressure: Dynamics and nursing management. *Journal of Neuroscience Nursing, 23*(2), 85.
3. Baggerly, J. (1991). Sensory perceptual problems following stroke: The "invisible" deficits. *Nursing Clinics of North America, 26*(4), 997–1005.
4. Baker, D. M. (1993). Assessment and management of impairments in swallowing. *Nursing Clinics of North America, 28*(4), 793–805.
5. Berguer, R., & Gonzalez, J. A. (1994). Revascularization by the retropharyngeal route for extensive disease of the extracranial arteries. *Journal of Vascular Surgery, 19*, 217–225.
6. Blisset, P. A. (1992). Ticlopidine hydrochloride. *Journal of Neuroscience Nursing, 24*(5), 296–300.
7. Boss, B. J. (1991). Managing communication disorders in stroke. *Nursing Clinics of North America, 26*(4): 985–996.
8. Breslau, N., et al. (1994). Migraine and major depression: A long-term study. *Headache, 34*(7), 387–393.
9. Bronstein, K. S. (1991). Psychosocial components in stroke: Implications for adaptation. *Nursing Clinics of North America, 26*(4), 1007–1015.
10. Bronstein, K. S., & Chadwick, L. R. (1994). Ticlopidine hydrochloride: Its current use in cerebrovascular disease. *Rehabilitation Nursing, 19*(1), 17–20.
11. Bronstein, K. S., et al. (1991). *Promoting stroke recovery: A re-search-based approach for nurses.* St Louis: Mosby–Year Book.
12. Brooke, M. M., et al. (1992). The treatment of agitation during initial hospitalization after traumatic brain injury. *Archives of Physical Medicine And Rehabilitation, 73,* 917.
13. Camp, Y. G., et al. (1995). Stop and look: Two approaches to manage stroke patients. *Journal of Neuroscience Nursing, 27*(1), 24–28.
14. Counsell, C., et al. (1995). Nimodipine: A drug therapy for treatment of vasospasm. *Journal of Neuroscience Nursing, 27*(1), 53–55.
15. Davis, M., & Lucatorto, M. (1994). Mannitol revisited. *Journal of Neuroscience Nursing, 26*(3), 170–174.
16. DiDonato, B. A., & Schaffer, V. L. (1994). The importance of outcome data in brain injury. *Rehabilitation Nursing, 19*(4), 219–228.
17. Dring, R. (1989). The informal caregiver responsible for home care of the individual with cognitive dysfunction following brain injury. *Journal of Neuroscience Nursing, 21*(1), 42.
18. Farzan, D. T. (1991). Reintegration for stroke survivors. *Nursing Clinics of North America, 26*(4), 1037–1047.
19. Fowler, S. B., et al. (1995). Pharmacological interventions for agitation in head-injured patients in the acute care setting. *Journal of Neuroscience Nursing, 27*(2), 119–123.
20. Gfeller, J. D., Chinball, J. T., & Duckro, P. M. (1994). Post-concussion symptoms and cognitive functioning in post-traumatic headache patients. *Headache, 34*(9), 503–507.
21. Gilman, S. (1992). Advances in neurology: Part 2. *New England Journal of Medicine, 326*(25), 1671–1676.
22. Godbole, K. B., et al. (1991). A head injured patient: Caloric needs, clinical progress and nursing care priorities. *Journal of Neuroscience Nursing, 23*(5), 290.
23. Goldstein, L. B., & Matcher, D. B. (1994). Clinical assessment of stroke. *JAMA, 271*(14), 1114–1120.
24. Gregory, R. J. (1995). Understanding and coping with neurological impairment. *Rehabilitation Nursing, 20*(2), 74–78.
25. Gresham, G. E. (1979). Epidemiologic profile of long-term stroke disabilty: The Framingham study. *Archives of Physical Medicine and Rehabilitation, 60,* 487–493.
26. Gwynn, M. (1993). tPA in Acute Stroke—Risk or Reprieve? *Journal of Neuroscience Nursing, 25*(3), 180–186.
27. Haynes, R. B., et al. (1994). Prevention of functional impairment by endarterectomy for symptomatic high-grade carotid stenosis. *JAMA, 271,* 1259.
28. Hemodilution in Stroke Study Group (1979). Hypervolemic chemo-dilution treatment of acute stroke: Results of a randomized multi-center trial using pentastarch. *Stroke, 20*(3), 317–323.
29. Hickey, J. V. (1992). *The clinical practice of neurological and neurosurgical nursing.* Philadelphia: J. B. Lippincott.
30. Hilton, G. (1994). Secondary brain injury and the role of neuro-protective agents. *Journal of Neuroscience Nursing, 26*(4), 251–255.
31. Hirsh, J., et al. (1992). Oral anticoagulants: Mechanism of action, clinical effectiveness, and optimal therapeutic range. *Chest, 102*(Suppl), 3125–3265.
32. Huether, S. E., & McCance, K. L. (1996). *Understanding pathophysiology.* St Louis: Mosby–Year Book.
33. Hydo, B. (1995). Designing an effective clinical pathway for stroke. *AJN, 95*(3), 44–51.
34. Johnson, S. M., et al. (1989). Effects of conversation on intracranial pressure in comatose patients. *Heart and Lung, 18,* 56–63.
35. Kalbach, L. R. (1991). Unilateral neglect: Mechanisms and nursing care. *Journal of Neuroscience Nursing, 23*(2), 125–129.
36. Keller, C., et al. (1989). Psychological responses in aphasia: Theoretical considerations and nursing implications. *Journal of Neuroscience Nursing, 21*(5), 290.
37. Keller, C., & Williams, A. (1993). Cardiac dysrhythmias associated with central nervous system dysfunction. *Journal of Neuroscience Nursing, 25*(6), 349–355.
38. Kelly-Hayes, M., & Paige, C. (1995). Assessment and psychologic factors in stroke rehabilitation. *Neurology, 45* (Suppl 1), S29–S32.
39. Koller, M., et al. (1990). Adjusted hypervolemic hemodilution in acute ischemic stroke. *Stroke, 21*(10), 1429–1434.
40. Leahy, N. M. (1991). Complications in the acute stages of stroke. *Nursing Clinics of North America, 26*(4), 971–983.
41. Lewis, T. A., & Solomon, G. D. (1995). Advances in migraine

management. *Cleveland Clinic Journal of Medicine, 62*(3), 148–154.

42. Little, N., et al. (1992). Think subarachnoid hemorrhage early. *Patient Care, 26*(5), 108–122.

43. Lugger, K. E. (1994). Dysphagia in the elderly stroke patient. *Journal of Neuroscience Nursing, 26*(2), 78–84.

44. Mackey, W. C., et al. (1989). Carotid endarterectomy in patients with intracranial vascular disease: Short-term risk and long-term outcome. *Journal of Vascular Surgery, 10*(4), 432–437.

45. Marshall, S. B., et al. (1990). *Neuroscience critical care: Pathophysiology and patient management.* Philadelphia: W. B. Saunders.

46. Mattson, A. J., & Levin, H. S. (1990). Frontal lobe dysfunction following closed head injury. *The Journal of Nervous and Mental Disease, 178*(5), 282.

47. McCrory, S., & Matchar, D. (1996). Stroke prevention: Emerging strategies. *Hospital Practice, 31*(3), 123–140.

48. Meyer, F. B. (1990). Calcium antagonists and vasospasm. *Neurosurgery Clinics of North America, 1*(2), 367–376.

49. Meyer, F. B., et al. (1995). Medical and surgical management of intracranial aneurysm. *Mayo Clinic Proceedings, 70,* 153–172.

50. Mitchell, M. (1989). *Neuroscience nursing: A nursing diagnosis approach.* Baltimore: Williams & Wilkins.

51. National Institute of Neurological Disorders and Stroke rt-PA Stroke Study Group. (1995). Tissue plasminogen activator for acute ischemic stroke. *New England Journal of Medicine, 333*(24), 1581–1587.

52. North American Symptomatic Carotid Endarterectomy Trial Collaborators. (1991). Beneficial effect of carotid endarterectomy in symptomatic patients with high-grade carotid stenosis. *New England Journal of Medicine, 325,* 445–453.

53. Olin, B. R., et al. (Eds.). *Drug facts and comparisons* (48th ed.). St. Louis: Facts and Comparisons, 1994.

54. Origitano, T. C., et al. (1990). Sustained increased cerebral blood flow with prophylactic hypertensive hypovolemic hemodilution ("triple-H" therapy) after subarachnoid hemorrhage. *Neurosurgery, 27*(5), 729.

55. Piepgras, A., et al (1994). STA-MCA bypass in bilateral carotid artery occlusion: Clinical results and long-term effect on cerebrovascular reserve capacity. *Neurological Research, 16*(2), 104–107.

56. Plylar, P. A. (1989). Management of the agitated and aggressive head injury patient in an acute hospital setting. *Journal of Neuroscience Nursing, 21*(6), 353.

57. Post-stroke Rehabilitation Guideline Panel. (1995). Post-stroke rehabilitation: Clinical Practice Guidelines, *American Family Physician, 52*(2), 461–470.

58. Pulsinelli, W. (1996). Cerebrovascular diseases: Principles. In Bennett, J., Plum, F. (Eds.), *Cecil textbook of medicine* (20th ed.). Philadelphia: W. B. Saunders.

59. Raps, E. C., & Galetta, S. L. (1995). Stroke prevention therapies and management of patient subgroups. *Neurology, 45*(Suppl 1), S19–S24.

60. Raskin, N. H. (1996). Approach to the patient with migraine. *Hospital Practice, 31*(2), 93–106.

61. Sacco, R. L. (1995). Risk factors and outcomes for ischemic stroke. *Neurology, 45*(Suppl 1), S10–S14.

62. Sargent, J., et al. (1995). Oral sumatriptan is effective and well tolerated for the acute treatment of migraine. *Neurology, 45*(Suppl 7), S10–S14.

63. Shepard, T. J., & Fox, S. W. (1996). Assessment and management of hypertension in acute ischemic stroke. *Journal of Neuroscience Nursing, 28*(1), 5–12.

64. Sisson, R. A. (1995). Cognitive status as a predictor of right hemisphere stroke outcomes. *Journal of Neuroscience Nursing, 27*(3), 152–156.

65. Smigielski, J., et al. (1992). Mayo Medical Center brain injury outpatient program: Treatment procedures and early outcome data. *Mayo Clinic Proceedings, 67*(8), 767–774.

66. Stewart-Amidei, C., & Penckofer, S.: Quality of life following cerebral bypass surgery. *Journal of Neuroscience Nursing, 20,* 50–55.

67. Sullivan, T. E., et al. (1994). Closed head injury assessment and research methodology. *Journal of Neuroscience Nursing, 26*(1), 24–29.

68. Toni, D., et al. (1995). Progressing neurological deficit secondary to acute ischemic stroke. *Archives of Neurology, 52,* 670–675.

69. Tosch, P. (1988). Patients' recollections of their posttraumatic coma. *Journal of Neuroscience Nursing, 20*(4), 223–228.

70. Veltman, R. H., et al. (1993). Cognitive screening in mild brain injury. *Journal of Neuroscience Nursing, 25*(6), 367–372.

71. Welch, K. M. (1993). Drug therapy of migraine. *The New England Journal of Medicine, 329*(20), 1476–1483.

72. Whitney, C. M., & Daroff, R. B. (1988). An approach to migraine. *Journal of Neuroscience Nursing, 20*(5), 284.

73. Whitney, F. (1994). Drug therapy for acute stroke. *Journal of Neuroscience Nursing, 26*(2), 111–117.

74. Williams, A. (1994). What bothers caregivers of stroke victims? *Journal of Neuroscience Nursing, 26*(3), 155–161.

75. Williams, A., & Coyne, S. M. (1993). Effects of neck position on intracranial pressure. *American Journal of Critical Care, 2*(1), 68–71.

76. Williams, S. E. (1993). The impact of aphasia on marital satisfaction. *Archives of Physical Medicine and Rehabilitation, 74,* 361–367.

77. Willis, D., & Harbit, M. D. (1989). A fatal attraction: Cocaine related subarachnoid hemorrhage. *Journal of Neuroscience Nursing, 21*(3), 171.

78. Wilson, L. D. (1993). Sensory perceptual alteration. *Nursing Clinics of North America, 28*(4), 747–765.

79. Wilson, S. F., et al. (1988). Determining interrater reliability of nurses' assessments of pupillary size and reaction. *Journal of Neuroscience Nursing, 20*(3), 189.

80. Youmans, J. R. (Ed.) (1990). *Neurological surgery: A comprehensive reference guide to the diagnosis and management of neurosurgical problems.* Philadelphia: W. B. Saunders.

81. Zasler, N. D. (1994). Mild traumatic brain injury and post-concussive disorders: Neuromedical and medicolegal caveats. *Network, 5*(3), 3–5.

(*Note:* CT scan of meningioma on p. 794 from Stimac, G. K. [1992]. *Introduction to diagnostic imaging.* Philadelphia: W. B. Saunders.)

33

Nursing Care of Clients with Cerebral Disorders

Sally Strong Schnell

Seizure Disorders

In this section, an important distinction is made between seizures and epilepsy. A *seizure* is a sudden, abnormal electrical discharge from the brain that results in changes in sensation, behavior, movements, perception, or consciousness. A seizure may occur in isolation or with some acute problem within the central nervous system (CNS), such as low blood sugar, drug or alcohol withdrawal, or head injury. *Epilepsy* is a chronic disorder of recurrent seizures. An isolated, single seizure does not constitute epilepsy.

Epilepsy

Epilepsy is derived from the Greek *epilepsia,* meaning "seizure." In early times, epilepsy was viewed as being of divine origin and was called "the sacred disease" because it was thought that someone with epilepsy was "seized" or "struck down" by the gods. Today, epilepsy is understood to be a syndrome of paroxysmal neurologic disorders causing recurrent episodes of one or more of the following manifestations: loss of consciousness, convulsive movements or other motor activity, sensory phenomena, and behavioral abnormalities. Approximately 0.5% to 1.0% of people in the United States experience epileptic seizures.[32]

The last two decades have brought significant advances in the understanding, diagnosis, and treatment of epilepsy. But despite improvements in electroencephalographic (EEG) monitoring, neuroimaging, and surgery, a cure has not been found. Some important terms used in the discussion of epilepsy are defined in Box 33–1.

Etiology and Risk Factors

Epilepsy can be caused by any process that disrupts the stability of the neuronal cell membrane. Some people have a lower threshold for seizures because of either genetic factors or an acquired condition such as brain injury. A tendency to have a lower threshold is inherited, but the actual seizure disorder itself is not. This form of epilepsy is called *idiopathic epilepsy,* because no specific cause can be found. A genetic predisposition to epilepsy exists in monozygotic twins.

Idiopathic epilepsy most often begins before age 20 and rarely begins after age 30. Seizures beginning in newborns and infants are often caused by congenital brain defects, birth injuries, or metabolic problems such as anoxia, hypoglycemia, or hypocalcemia. Although the underlying cause may be perinatal, seizures may not begin for many years, often during puberty. Other than children under age 5, the highest incidence of new-onset epilepsy is in persons over age 65.[26] The increased risk in this age group is attributed to the increase in conditions that cause neurologic changes in this group. These include cerebrovascular disease, tumor, delirium of Alzheimer's type (Alzheimer's disease), infection, accumulated trauma, and chronic alcoholism, as well as the aging process itself.[26]

When the cause of seizures is known, the disorder is called *secondary epilepsy.* After age 20, generalized seizures usually have an identifiable cause. These causes include traumatic brain injury, brain tumor, and infection. Approximately two-thirds of cases of epilepsy are idiopathic and one-third are secondary. The Risk Factors and Levels of Prevention feature outlines risk factors and preventive measures for epilepsy.

Pathophysiology

Seizures occur from a malfunction of hypersensitive neurons in the cerebral cortex and the limbic centers in the hippocampus. These cells are called the *epileptogenic focus.* The membrane of the cell is more permeable, which makes the cell more likely to become activated by hyperthermia, hypoxia, hypoglycemia, hyponatremia, sensory overload, and certain phases of sleep. These cells begin

Box 33–1. Terms Used in the Discussion of Epilepsy

Seizure: a paroxysmal, uncontrolled, abnormal discharge of electrical activity in the brain's gray matter. A seizure causes events that interfere with normal function. It is a symptom rather than a disease.

Prodromal phase: precedes some seizures and may last minutes or hours. A vague change occurs in emotional reactivity or affective responses (e.g., depression or anxiety).

Aura: generally, a brief sensory experience (e.g., a feeling of weakness, dizziness, strange sensations in an arm or leg, numbness, or odor) that occurs at the onset of some seizures. An aura may localize the area of the brain from which the seizure originates. For instance, a seizure arising from a focus in the motor strip could produce twitching in the client's thumb. A focus in the temporal lobe could cause a client to experience an unpleasant odor. Usually, an aura precedes other manifestations of the seizure by only a few seconds. Occasionally, an aura gives the client enough time to lie down before seizure activity occurs. It may or may not be followed by a complete seizure.

Epileptic cry: a cry, occurring in some seizures, caused by a thoracic and abdominal spasm, which expels air through the narrowed spastic glottis.

Ictus, postictal: ictus is synonymous with seizure; *postictal* refers to that time immediately after a seizure during which the client usually experiences some change in consciousness, behavior, or activity.

by firing in increasing frequency and amplitude. When the intensity of the discharges reaches a threshold, it spreads to adjacent normal neurons and then spreads over the entire cerebral cortex, the basal ganglia, thalamus, and brain stem. These discharges block normal inhibition and perpetuate a feedback loop (Fig. 33–1). Discharges in the brain stem cause muscle contraction and possibly loss of consciousness. The excitation of the cells can spread to the spinal cord.

Eventually, inhibitory neurons in the cortex, anterior thalamus, and basal ganglia slow the neuronal firing. This inhibition interrupts the seizure and produces an intermit-

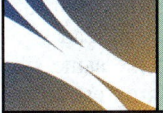

RISK FACTORS AND LEVELS OF PREVENTION

Seizures

Risk Factors

Any occupying lesion (e.g., brain tumor, hematoma, abscess); inflammatory problem (e.g., meningitis, encephalitis); metabolic disturbance that affects the brain secondary to metabolic waste buildup or toxin overdose (e.g., uremia, liver failure, lead poisoning, alcohol, illicit drug use or overdose of any drug affecting the CNS; any condition that leads to cerebral hypoxia or hypercapnia, or head trauma.

Levels of Prevention

Primary Prevention

- Advise clients to wear helmets when appropriate.
- Advise clients to avoid overuse of alcohol, illicit drug use, and taking over-the-counter medications, especially if they are also taking prescription medications. Encourage clients to consult with their physician about medications.
- Tell clients to avoid driving when drinking.

Secondary Prevention

- Control pre-existing conditions that have a high risk of seizure activity.
- Avoid unnecessary nursing care during periods of increased ICP.
- See that plasma levels of anticonvulsants are maintained; if any dose is missed, notify the physician.
- Monitor the client for signs of hypoxia; notify the physician if they are present.
- Prevent further brain injury to the client by using padded side rails.
- Hyperoxygenate the client with suctioning.

Tertiary Prevention

- Implement all the secondary prevention interventions.
- Ensure that the client gets the total dose of anticonvulsant, even when the route is via a gastrostomy tube.
- At least every 3 months, consult the physician to check the client's plasma levels of anticonvulsants.

tent contraction-relaxation phase. As the epileptogenic neurons are exhausted and inhibitory processes build, the seizure stops. These later events depress CNS action and impair consciousness. This period of impaired consciousness after a seizure may be manifested as sleep, confusion, or fatigue. It is called a *postictal state*.

Seizure activity increases the need for adenosine triphosphate by 250% and cerebral oxygen consumption by 60%. Supplies of oxygen and glucose are rapidly consumed. To meet these demands, the cerebral blood flow increases by 250% during a seizure. If the seizure is ongoing (as in status epilepticus), severe hypoxia and lactic acidosis occur. These conditions may result in brain tissue destruction.

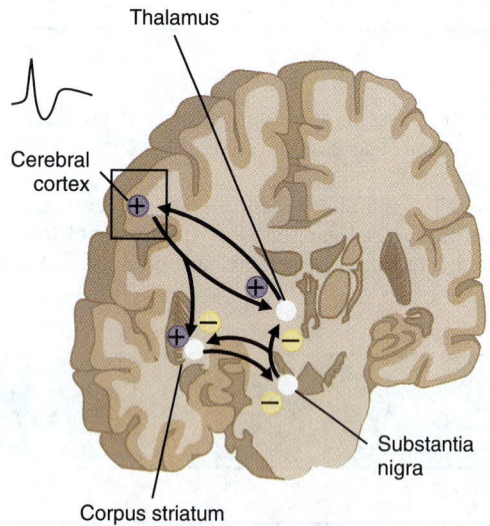

A

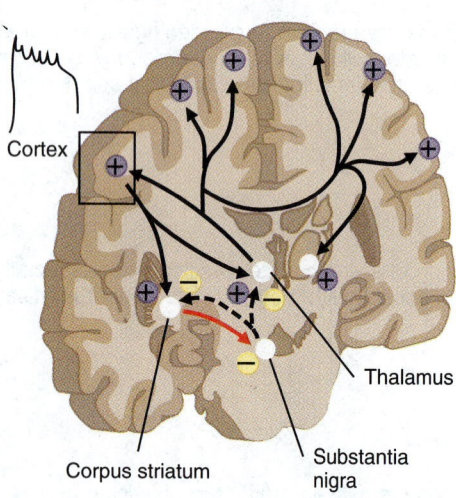

B

Figure 33–1. *A*, Normally, excitatory messages from the cerebral cortex are modulated by deeper structures. *B*, In epilepsy, there are bursts of activity from the cortex that are not modulated, and these bursts spread. (From Devinsky, O. (1994). Seizure disorders. *Clinical Symposia, 46*(1), 1–54. Adapted from an original illustration in the *Clinical Symposia,* illustrated by John Craig, M.D., copyright by Ciba-Geigy Corporation.)

Clinical Manifestations and Diagnostic Findings

Epilepsy has been classified according to the age of onset, cause, area of origin, EEG abnormalities, and clinical type of seizure. The International Classification of Epileptic Seizures, used here, is based on the clinical seizure type and on EEG findings during seizures (the *ictal* period) and between seizures (the *interictal* period).

■ Partial (Focal, Local) Seizures

Partial seizures are the most common type of epilepsy. The first clinical and EEG changes indicate initial activation of neurons in one part of the cerebral hemisphere. They are further classified according to whether or not consciousness is impaired. There are four types of simple partial seizures that do not impair consciousness. These include those with motor signs, sensory signs, autonomic signs, and subjective symptoms.

Motor Signs. Partial seizures with motor signs arise from a focus in the region of the brain's motor cortex. The resulting motor activity (seizure) occurs in the part of the body innervated by motor neurons originating in the affected region of the cortex. Because the hand and fingers have the largest cortical representation, most focal motor seizures begin with convulsive twitching in an upper extremity. Involuntary movements may spread centrally and involve the entire limb, and even the same side of the face and lower extremity. This progression or spread is known as the *jacksonian march*. The client also may exhibit changes in posture or spoken utterances.

Sensory Signs. If the epileptogenic focus is in the parietal region, the patient experiences sensory phenomena such as numbness and tingling in the affected area. If the focus is in the occipital region, the patient may experience bright, flashing lights in the field of vision opposite the side of the focus. Likewise, the patient can have changes in speech or taste. Involvement of the posterior temporal area of the dominant hemisphere (usually the left) causes difficulty with speaking, or aphasia.

Autonomic Signs. Stimulation of the autonomic system produces epigastric sensations, pallor, sweating, flushing, piloerection (erection of hair), and pupillary dilation.

Subjective Symptoms. These seizures usually arise in the anterior temporal lobe. There are two types: complex partial seizures and partial seizures evolving into generalized seizures. These seizures frequently begin with an *aura*, a subjective sensation that helps localize the focus. An aura may be a strange smell, noise, or sensation preceding a seizure, or a sense of "rising" or "welling up" in the epigastric region. Visual distortions and feelings such as déjà vu are common.

Complex Partial Seizures

The most characteristic part of a complex partial seizure is automatisms during the seizure. These include purposeless, repetitive activities such as lip-smacking, chewing, patting a part of the body, or picking at clothes while in a dreamy state. Inappropriate or antisocial behavior may also automatically occur during the seizure. This unusual behavior may cause the client to be viewed as psychotic or otherwise mentally disturbed. However, some abnormalities are very subtle and may not be detected by an untrained observer.

Temporal lobe seizures usually last 2 to 3 minutes but may last up to 15 minutes. The patient is usually unaware of any activity during the seizure and may be confused or drowsy postictally. Attempts to restrain the patient during a seizure may cause combative and uncooperative behavior.

Partial Seizures that Generalize

These seizures start from a particular focus, and then the electrical discharges spread throughout the brain. Clinically, the client first shows focal signs; for example, one side of the face moves, and then the whole body becomes involved. Consciousness is lost if the discharges spread through the brain.

▪ Generalized Seizures

Generalized seizures are those in which the first clinical manifestations involve both hemispheres. Consciousness may be impaired, and this impairment may be the first clinical manifestation. About one third of seizures are generalized. Types of generalized seizures include absence, myoclonic, tonic-clonic, and atonic seizures.

Absence Seizures

Formerly known as petit mal seizures, absence seizures consist of brief periods of altered consciousness lasting 5 to 30 seconds. These seizures may diminish or disappear after puberty. Clients with absence seizures may also have clonic or tonic components or automatisms. Absence seizures may be idiopathic (unknown cause) or may be secondary to identifiable disorders such as birth injuries or acute febrile childhood infections. These "little," or minor seizures usually begin during childhood and are primarily limited to childhood and early adolescence. Grand mal or partial seizures may develop at any time in patients who have had absence seizures.

Myoclonic Seizures

Myoclonic seizures involve sudden uncontrollable jerking movements of either a single muscle group or multiple groups, sometimes causing the client to fall. Usually the client loses consciousness for a moment and then is confused postictally. These seizures often occur in the morning, and clients often report that they spill their coffee with their fall.[13]

Tonic-Clonic Seizures

Formerly known as grand mal seizures, tonic-clonic seizures are the type of seizures most closely associated with epilepsy. Actually, however, this type makes up only about 10% of all seizures. A tonic-clonic seizure typically proceeds as follows:

1. Aura may or may not be present.
2. Sudden loss of consciousness may occur.
3. In the *tonic phase,* the entire body becomes rigid (Fig. 33–2A). If standing or sitting, the client falls stiffly to the floor. A cry may be uttered. Respirations are interrupted temporarily, and the client may become cyanotic. The jaw is fixed and the hands are clenched. The eyes may be opened widely; the pupils are dilated and fixed. The tonic phase lasts 30 to 60 seconds. At the end of this phase the client breathes deeply.
4. The *clonic phase* begins next, with rhythmic, jerky contraction and relaxation of all body muscles, especially the extremities (Fig. 33–2B). The client is usually incontinent and may bite the lips, tongue, or inside of the mouth. Excessive saliva is blown from the mouth, which creates a frothing at the lips.
5. An entire seizure may last from 2 to 5 minutes, after which the client enters the *postictal phase,* during which he or she relaxes and remains totally unresponsive for a time. The client may rouse briefly and then go into a postictal sleep lasting 30 minutes to several hours. This may be followed by general fatigue, depression, confusion, or headache, all of which gradually resolve. The client has complete amnesia for the seizure episode and may feel nauseated, stiff, and sore. Falling during the seizure may cause injury.

Tonic-clonic seizures vary in frequency from many times daily to once or twice a year. Tonic-only and clonic-only seizures may also occur.

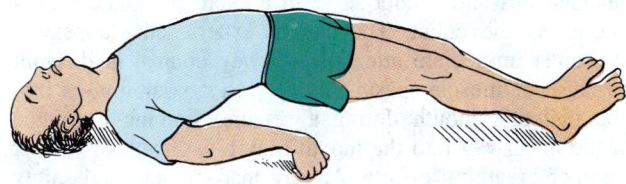

A Tonic phase

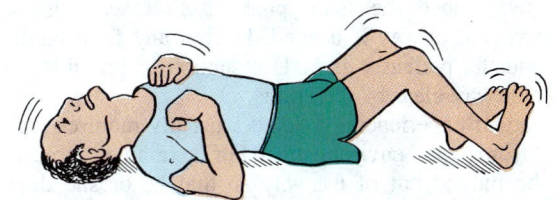

B Clonic phase

Figure 33–2. *A,* The tonic phase of a seizure is marked by loss of consciousness, falling, crying, and generalized stiffness. There may be incontinence. *B,* During the clonic phase, there is jerking of the limbs and salivary frothing.

Atonic Seizures

Atonic seizures cause a total loss of muscle tone. They may be mild with the client briefly nodding the head, or the client may fall to the floor. Consciousness is impaired only briefly. These seizures are often called "drop attacks."

■ Diagnostic Tests

The diagnostic assessment of clients suspected of having epilepsy includes an EEG. This test assists in (1) locating the focus of abnormal electrical discharges, if present; (2) establishing a diagnosis of epilepsy; and (3) identifying the specific type of seizures. However, a normal EEG does not always exclude a diagnosis of epilepsy, and EEG abnormalities do not always confirm the diagnosis. During a seizure, EEG abnormalities involve all parts of the cortex. Between seizures, clients with epilepsy may show EEG abnormalities not characteristic of seizure disorders. An ambulatory EEG can be used to clarify suspected seizures that are occurring frequently. The monitor used is similar to a Holter monitor. Long-term video EEG monitoring may also be used to rule out pseudoseizures.

Occasionally, diagnostic tests such as skull x-ray, computed tomography (CT), and magnetic resonance imaging (MRI) are used to rule out brain lesions that could trigger seizures. Positron emission tomography (PET) and single photon emission computed tomography (SPECT) may be helpful to measure cerebral blood flow in clients having surgery for epilepsy.

Emergency Care

The term *patient* is used here because this person is unconscious and cannot serve in a client role. The family serves as the client. The patient experiencing a seizure demands immediate attention. Airway control is difficult because of muscle spasms. Never insert your fingers into the patient's mouth during a seizure. Forcing a tongue blade or airway into the mouth may break teeth or further hamper breathing efforts. Airway management and safety are the top two priorities. Turning the patient to his or her side will displace the tongue and usually result in an open airway once the tonic phase has ceased. Use a nasopharyngeal airway if needed. Loosen any tight clothing around the patient's neck. Use suction, if possible, to keep the airway clear of secretions.

The patient experiencing a seizure usually requires protection from the environment. For example, objects should be moved out of the way so that he or she does not strike the head or extremities. Put a pillow or folded blanket under the patient's head.

Observers' comments about a patient's seizures can be very helpful in making a diagnosis, especially if they can describe them in detail, including the sequence in which phenomena occurred. Instruct the family and unlicensed assistive personnel to make the following observations:

- How long did the seizure last?
- Where in the body did the seizure begin and how did it progress?
- Did the client's eyes deviate?
- Were the respirations labored or frothy?
- Was the client incontinent?
- Did the client lose consciousness?
- What were the type of movements and what body parts moved?

Acute and Subacute Care

■ Medical Management

Intervention for epilepsy includes (1) elimination of factors that may cause or precipitate seizures, (2) measures to improve the client's physical and mental health, (3) specific medical treatment, and (4) possible surgical treatment. The main focus in intervention for epilepsy is preventing seizures from recurring.

The most effective method of controlling idiopathic seizures is with anticonvulsant drugs, also called antiepileptic drugs. Table 33–1 lists and describes the most common anticonvulsants. Large doses of a single anticonvulsant are often more helpful than smaller doses of several drugs. Ideally, initial treatment begins with a single drug (primary anticonvulsant) until either seizure control is attained or unacceptable side effects appear. If side effects become intolerable before seizures are controlled, another drug is added. Combining medications does carry the potential risk of drug-drug interactions, which decrease effectiveness.

Medical intervention focuses on prescribing anticonvulsants to arrest or prevent a client's seizures. Developing such a program requires weeks of medication trial and error and adjustment.

■ Nursing Management of the Medical Client

Epilepsy is not usually treated by hospitalization. However, a client may initially be hospitalized for assessment, diagnosis, and education and again later if seizures become uncontrolled or if status epilepticus develops. Nurses have a role in assessing for altered health maintenance related to knowledge deficit or other barriers, anticipating risk of injury, and providing support for clients and their families who experience life changes related to seizure disorders.

Assessment

Assessment of clients not actively experiencing seizures includes the following:

- History: prenatal, birth, and developmental history; family history; age of seizure onset; history of all illness and trauma; previous brain surgery or stroke; complete description of seizures, including precipitating factors; presence of an aura

Table 33–1. Anticonvulsant Agents

Classification of Seizure	Medication	Side Effects

Focal and major generalized seizures
    Tonic-clonic
	Primary
	    Phenytoin (Dilantin)
	    Carbamazepine (Tegretol)
	    Phenobarbital
	
	    Primidone (Mysoline)
	
	    Valproate (Depakene)
		Mental dullness, ataxia, diplopia, hypertrophy of gums
		Nystagmus, ataxia, rash, blood dyscrasias
		Mental changes, withdrawal seizures if drug is stopped abruptly
		Emotional and mental changes including depression, irritability, impotence; withdrawal seizures if drug is not discontinued slowly
		Transient nausea, potential bleeding problems, liver damage

	Secondary
	    Succinimides
	        Phensuximide (Milontin)
	        Methsuximide (Celontin)
	    Inhibits neurotransmitters
	        Vigabatrin (Sabril)
	        Lamotrigine
	        Gabapentin
	    Benzodiazepines
	        Diazepam (Valium)
	        Clonazepam (Klonopin)
	
	    Ancillary
	        Acetazolamide (Diamox)
		
		Drowsiness, headache
		Drowsiness, headache
		
		Drowsiness, blurred vision, headache, gastrointestinal problems
		
		Respiratory depression, lethargy, ataxia
		Drowsiness, exacerbation of childhood hyperactivity, withdrawal seizures, and status epilepticus if drug is removed too quickly
		
		Anorexia, numbness of extremities

Absence seizures	Primary
	    Ethosuximide (Zarontin)
	    Valproate (Depakene)
	    Clonazepam (Klonopin)
	Secondary
	    Trimethadione (Tridione)
		Gastric distress, nausea, dizziness, drowsiness
		See above
		See above
		
		Hemeralopia ("glare effect"), blood immune disorders

Minor generalized motor seizures
    Atonic (akinetic) seizures
    Myoclonic seizures
	Same drugs as for focal and major generalized seizures
	
	Phenytoin (Dilantin)
	Valproate (Depakene)
	Clonazepam (Klonopin)
		See above
		
		See above
		See above
		See above

- Medication use and postictal symptoms
- Psychosocial assessment, including mental status examination
- Complete physical examination, focusing on neurologic signs; usually the physical examination findings between seizures are normal

Diagnosis, Planning, Implementation

Altered Health Maintenance. This diagnosis is appropriate for clients who are having difficulty adjusting their life to their epileptic condition. Knowledge deficit of the significance of managing medication is a common problem. State the diagnosis as *Altered Health Maintenance related to chronic disorder management.*

Planning: Expected Outcomes. The client will have improved health maintenance related to knowledge deficit as evidenced by maintaining routine dosing, con-

sulting a physician whenever there is a problem, and wearing a medical alert identification.

Implementation. Provide the client with verbal information and written reinforcement about (1) how anticonvulsants prevent seizures, (2) the importance of taking prescribed medication regularly, and (3) care during seizures. Plan with the client ways to make taking medication part of daily activities (e.g., keeping medication by the toothbrush). Also, help the client identify factors that precipitate seizures and ways of avoiding these factors. Such factors include increased stress, lack of sleep, emotional upset, and alcohol use. See the Client Education Guide for other important teaching information.

Evaluation

The short-term outcomes for the client actively seizing are usually met within hours. An example is that the seizure stops and the client returns to the previous level

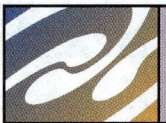

CLIENT EDUCATION GUIDE

Status Epilepticus

Client Instructions in English *(Instrucciones para el cliente en inglés)*	Client Instructions in Spanish *(Instrucciones para el cliente en español)*
Take prescribed dosages of medications to maintain your blood levels.	Tome las dosis del medicamento anticonvulsivo que se le recetó para mantener un nivel apropiado en la sangre.
Consult your physician if you are unable to take medication because of illness.	Llameal médico si no puede tomar el medicamento debido a una enfermedad.
Observe for side effects of anticonvulsant drugs. Do not stop taking them because of annoying side effects; this is very dangerous. Consult your physician first.	Observe los efectos adversos de las drogas anticonvulsivas. No deje de tomar el medicamento por los efectos adversos; esto es muy peligroso. Consulte primero con el médico
Notify the physician if your seizure activity is not being controlled. Provide specific descriptions of the seizure activity.	Llame al médico si no puede controlar la actividad de las convulsiones; dé descripciones específicas sobre la actividad de la convulsión.
Do not take any over-the-counter medications without consulting with your physician.	No tome medicamentos sin receta sin consultar primero con el médico.
Obtain a medication alert identification with the name of the drug, dosage, and frequency, and your physician's name and phone number. Carry this identification with you at all times.	Use siempre una forma de identificación con el nombre del medicamento, la dosis, la frequencia, y el nombre y número de teléfono del médico.

of functioning. Nursing care of clients with confirmed epilepsy should focus on the long-term outcomes of self-care.

■ Modifications for Elderly Clients

With the increasing frequency of epilepsy in the elderly, nurses need to be more aware of the changes in pharmacokinetics in this age group. Concurrent diseases, food, and other drug interactions affect absorption of anticonvulsant medication. A decrease in albumin, as is commonly seen in the elderly, can increase the free plasma level of these drugs. Decreased metabolism can increase the half-life of these drugs and decreased elimination can result in higher plasma levels. Enteral feedings inhibit the absorption of phenytoin (Dilantin). Therefore, the feeding should be turned off 2 hours before and after administration of phenytoin or the dose should be altered based on plasma levels. Altered vitamin D metabolism with phenytoin increases the risk of osteoporosis. Carbamazepine (Tegretol) has an increased risk of slowed conduction and congestive heart failure; hyponatremia secondary to increased antidiuretic hormone, especially if the client is on a low-sodium diet; and altered cholesterol metabolism in the elderly. Valproate (Depakene) carries an increased risk of causing hyperammonemia in elderly clients, leading to hepatic dysfunction, decrease in platelets, and toxicity because of a longer half-life in the elderly.[26]

■ Surgical Management

For approximately 75% of people with seizures, medical management with antiepileptic agents and follow-up suffice. The remaining 25% continue to have seizures. For about 5% of people with epilepsy, surgery is a last resort to control the disease.

When seizures do not respond to medication, surgical therapy may be considered. The safest and most effective surgical treatment is cortical resection of the anterior temporal lobe for complex partial seizures.[10,13] Criteria for resection include (1) failure of the medical approach and (2) localization and identification of a focus of abnormal discharge that is easily accessible surgically and is located in dispensable cortex. Cortical resection is a long procedure. The client must be awake during most of it. It is important that the client be highly motivated and psychologically well prepared.

Thorough assessment is necessary before surgery. This is usually done in three phases. Phase 1 involves using video EEG to locate the epileptogenic focus. This stage can also include SPECT and PET studies.[41] IQ testing and psychological assessments are usually performed.

Phase 2 is used when surface EEG electrodes are not sensitive enough to locate the seizure focus exactly. Electrodes are placed in the temporal and frontal lobes of the brain or in the subdural space. These techniques allow detailed maps of the brain for surgery.

Phase 3, the final stage, involves cerebral angiography with Wada's test to determine hemispheric dominance and location of the speech center. The functional supremacy of one cerebral hemisphere is critical to language function. Wada's test is a method of determining which side of the brain is dominant. An injection of sodium amytal is introduced into the left internal carotid artery. If the left hemisphere is dominant, speech is arrested for 1 or 2 minutes, followed by misnaming and misreading for 8 to 9 minutes altogether. After 30 minutes, the process is repeated in the right internal carotid artery. The physician looks for changes in sensation, abstract thought, and coordination. Postprocedural care is the same as for cerebral angiography.

Cortical Resection

Corpus callosal resection is considered a palliative surgery designed to make the seizures more tolerable. It involves the excision of one section of cortex to reduce the spread of epileptic discharges (Fig. 33–3*A*). One complication, called *disconnection syndrome,* results when the pathways responsible for communication from one hemisphere to another are severed. Clinical manifestations range from motor apraxias and mutism to minimal losses detected only with neuropsychological testing. Staged resections are now performed to reduce the risk of disconnection syndrome.

Temporal Lobectomy

This form of curative surgery for epilepsy removes the area where the seizures begin without causing neurologic or cognitive deficits (Fig. 33–3*B*). If the dominant hemisphere is removed, the client will experience some language defects for a few weeks. Visual defects from loss of visual projection fibers are compensated for quickly.

Hemispherectomy

The removal of most of the cortex of one hemisphere is done in children with intractable seizures to control those that are injurious, not to stop all seizures (Fig. 33–3*C*).

Implantation of a Vagal Nerve Stimulator

A new therapy in which an implanted vagal nerve stimulator which delivered programmed bursts via an electrode attached to the vagus nerve showed a 50% reduction in seizure activity in 6 of 15 clients over a 1-year period.[29] All clients were maintained on therapeutic levels of antiseizure medication. Research continues in this area.

Other Surgical Procedures

Some seizures are caused by brain lesions that can be surgically removed (e.g., operable brain tumors, cysts, or abscesses). Other options may include stereotactic laser therapy and implantation of a vagal nerve stimulator that the client can activate when he or she experiences an aura.

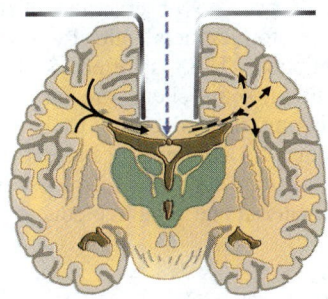

Corpus callosotomy

Division of the corpus callosum disrupts the interhemispheric pathway for secondary generalization of partial
A   seizures (unilateral seizure focus)

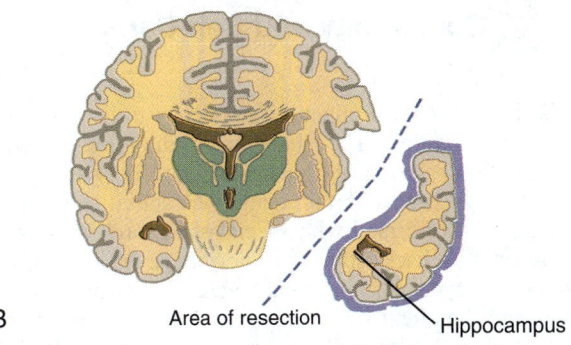

Temporal lobectomy

B   Area of resection — Hippocampus

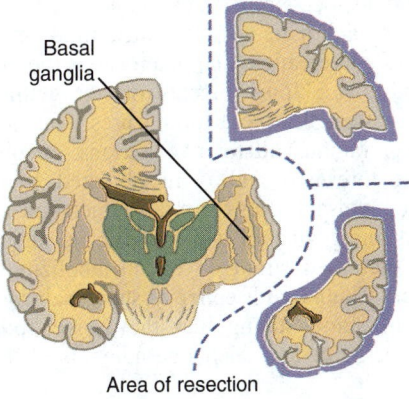

Hemispherectomy

Basal ganglia

C   Area of resection

Figure 33–3. Surgery for epilepsy can include corpus callosotomy (*A*), temporal lobectomy (*B*), or hemispherectomy (*C*). (From Devinsky, O. (1994). Seizure disorders. *Clinical Symposia, 46*(1), 1–54. Adapted from an original illustration in the *Clinical Symposia,* illustrated by John Craig, M.D., copyright by Ciba-Geigy Corporation.)

■ Nursing Management of the Surgical Client

Preoperative Care

The role of the nurse during the evaluation phase prior to surgery is to provide support and education. These clients have been trying to control their seizures for most of their lives. Now, as part of the preoperative assessment, the healthcare team will want to observe the client during seizure activity. Therefore, antiepileptic drugs will be tapered and discontinued. This is often confusing and frightening. In addition, some clients are far from family and may be rethinking their decision to have surgery. Memory impairments are common because of both the side effects of medications and postictal states. Be certain to provide written material and reinforce education often.

Postoperative Care

After surgery, the client is placed in critical care. Postoperative nursing care is the same as for any client undergoing a craniotomy.

Community and Self-Care

It is important for a client with epilepsy to live as normal a life as possible. The client and family must learn to accept the condition and not exaggerate it or overprotect the client. Whereas certain dangerous activities should be avoided or performed with special safeguards (e.g,. swimming or horseback riding), a wide range of activities can still be enjoyed. Driving motor vehicles depends on local laws and the client's medical control of seizures. In many states, clients with epilepsy may drive a car after they have been seizure-free for 1 year. This restriction can be emotionally and economically devastating for clients of all ages and socioeconomic backgrounds.

A regular pattern of adequate diet, fluid intake, sleep, and moderate recreation and exercise is helpful. Many clients find that skipping meals or not getting enough sleep lowers their threshold for seizures. Alcoholic beverages are contraindicated for two reasons. Alcohol lowers the seizure threshold and is metabolized by the liver. Most anticonvulsant drugs are also metabolized by the liver. Consuming alcohol while taking an anticonvulsant places an increased strain on the metabolizing functions of the liver. Clients with epilepsy should always wear or carry identification stating that they have epilepsy and providing the name and telephone numbers of their physician.

For some clients, the psychosocial impact of epilepsy is overwhelming. Because most seizures occur without warning, many clients spend their lives anticipating inappropriate behavior, embarrassment, and self-injury. Clients with epilepsy often have a poor self-image, feelings of inferiority, self-consciousness, guilt, anger, depression, and other emotional problems. Education and support can help clients deal with the emotional impact of epilepsy. Support groups can be very helpful.

The client and family should be taught that epilepsy is a chronic disorder that requires long-term management. Even though the client does not actively seize, it is important to take medication as prescribed. Phenytoin, a common anticonvulsant, leads to excessive gingival (gum tissue) growth. Brushing two to three times daily helps retard its growth. Some clients have excess gingival tissue

excised every 6 to 12 months. Medications may also cause diplopia, ataxia, sedation, and bone marrow depression. Most anticonvulsants require periodic monitoring of serum drug levels, liver function, and complete blood counts.

If the client is able to recognize that certain activities trigger the seizure, the activities can be avoided or the client can be desensitized in some cases. For example, flickering lights can trigger seizures. Fluorescent lights and flickering shadows from trees on the road while driving during the late afternoon are common precipitators of seizures. If the client has an aura, precautions should be taken immediately to prevent self-injury from the impending seizure; for example, lying down on the ground or floor, or if driving a vehicle, pulling over to the side of the road and lying on the seat. Instruct clients to carry a large pillow in the vehicle or to use their arms to protect their head.

Some clients with epilepsy cannot find work if they admit to having seizures. However, falsifying job applications can result in dismissal from employment. These factors contribute to a higher incidence of depression among clients with epilepsy. Nurses can educate the public regarding epilepsy and help dissipate prejudices. When discussing the long-term impact of epilepsy with the client, be empathic but realistic. It is hoped the client can accept the life-style limitations of the disorder and not be overwhelmed by them.[5]

The client's family needs to know what to do in the event of a seizure. The patient should be protected from self-injury. Clothing should be loosened, the head protected from impact, and sharp objects in the environment removed. The patient should not be forcibly restrained during a seizure but protected from self-injury. Hard objects or fingers should not be inserted into the mouth; patients do not swallow their tongues. After the head is protected, the patient should be positioned on the side to displace the tongue and allow oral secretions to drain from the airway. Someone should stay with the patient until full consciousness has returned. An ambulance should be called if the seizure lasts over 10 minutes, another seizure occurs before consciousness returns, there is respiratory difficulty, evidence of injury, or the patient is pregnant.

Various organizations are working at public education, introduction of appropriate legislation, and assisting people with epilepsy. In the United States, these include the Epilepsy Foundation of America, 4351 Garden City Dr., Landover, MD 20785 and Epilepsy Services, 22 W. Monroe, Chicago, IL 60601. Similar organizations exist in other countries.

Seizures

Recall that not all seizures are epilepsy. This section covers isolated seizures not associated with epilepsy.

The cause of seizures varies widely in adults. Brain tumors are the most common cause. Seizures are often the first manifestation of an intracranial mass. Head trauma is another common cause of seizures in young adults. With severe closed head injuries, seizures occur in a small percentage of clients. However, with open head injuries in which the skull and dura are penetrated, the incidence of seizures rises markedly.

Arteriosclerotic cerebrovascular disease is the most common cause of seizures in clients over age 50. These seizures usually accompany a stroke. In other vascular lesions, such as arteriovenous malformations, seizures may be the first manifestation.

CNS infections frequently produce seizures, either in their acute phase or chronically thereafter. Seizures can develop from viral infections, brain abscesses, and meningitis. Postinfectious encephalitis can cause persistent seizures.

Toxic substances that interfere with brain metabolism or with the supply of oxygen or glucose to the brain can cause seizures. Alcohol is one of the most frequently ingested toxins and can cause seizures either during ingestion or during withdrawal. Chronic substance abuse, especially of barbiturates, can lead to seizures when the drug is withdrawn (see Chapter 87).

Simulated convulsive episodes may occur in clients with psychiatric disorders. These are called pseudoseizures. One key to differentiating between pseudoseizures and actual seizures is to look for stereotypical movements and a paroxysmal nature to the episodes. Clients with recurrent seizures exhibit the same stereotypic movements with each seizure. Clients exhibiting pseudoseizure make different movements with each seizure.

The management of clients who have a single seizure focuses on protecting the client during the seizure and then identifying and correcting the underlying problem. Care of clients during a seizure is discussed under Emergency Care in the section on epilepsy.

There is controversy as to the best pharmacologic approach to seizure management. Many authorities are recommending a single antiepileptic drug therapy approach, which decreases the risk of drug interactions and adverse effects, makes monitoring easier, and increases client compliance.[13] However, about 30% of clients with epilepsy remain refractory to this approach. Two new anticonvulsants (gabapentin and lamotrigine) have been shown to have efficacy and safety as add-on therapy for clients with refractory simple or complex partial seizures with or without secondary generalized tonic-clonic seizures.[41]

Status Epilepticus

Status epilepticus, an emergency condition, is a state in which a patient has continuous seizures or seizures in rapid succession, without regaining consciousness, lasting at least 30 minutes. A patient experiencing status epilepticus may remain comatose, have repetitive seizures for hours, have irreversible brain damage, or die.

The most common cause of status epilepticus is the sudden withdrawal of anticonvulsant medication.

During a seizure, the brain's metabolic needs increase dramatically. If these heightened requirements continue without opportunity for the body to recover, the supply of glucose and oxygen to the brain becomes inadequate, and permanent brain damage may occur. The underlying

cause of the seizure is initially assessed through blood chemistry, liver function, and toxicology (for cocaine and heroin) studies.

Treatment of status epilepticus is best carried out in a setting with emergency equipment and skilled personnel. Intervention for status epilepticus includes the following:

● Maintaining a clear airway. Prevent aspiration by positioning and suctioning, and provide adequate oxygenation. Intubation may be necessary.
● Assessing the client constantly. Even when seizures are controlled, the client may be unconscious for a while. If a client does not awaken within 2 hours, careful reassessment is needed. Document and report recurrent seizures immediately.
● Protecting the client from injury (e.g., padded side rails).
● Administering prescribed emergency anticonvulsant therapy to terminate seizures and prevent exhaustion. Intravenous infusion is begun immediately and maintained during treatment. Status epilepticus is treated with diazepam in doses of 5 to 10 mg every 10 to 20 minutes up to 30 mg in an 8-hour period. Lorazepam can also be given in 4-mg doses over 2 to 5 minutes, repeated every 10 to 15 minutes to a maximum of 8 mg. In addition, phenytoin can be given to a total dose of 15 to 18 mg/kg by slow intravenous push (no more than 50 mg/min). Assess the client for bradycardia and heart block while the medication is given. If this agent is not effective, diazepam or lorazepam can be used. Because all of these medications can depress respirations, emergency ventilation equipment should be readily available.

If the diazepam or lorazepam is not effective, then pentobarbital can be used to bring on a barbiturate coma and suppress brain activity. This step is used only after all others have been tried and proved unsuccessful. The client in barbiturate coma is ventilator-dependent and requires care in an intensive care unit (ICU).

A last resort involves the use of general anesthesia. If general anesthesia or neuromuscular blockade agents such as vecuronium bromide (Norcuron) are required, there must be mechanical ventilation, continuous EEG monitoring, and hemodynamic monitoring. Absence of signs of seizure does not mean the seizure has stopped. After the seizures have been controlled, maintenance anticonvulsants are prescribed.

Clients experiencing status epilepticus are especially difficult for significant others to watch. They need support and assessment. Always explain to them the treatment being given.

Intracranial Tumors

Intracranial (or brain) tumors have profound implications for the client and family. Brain tumors are among the most destructive lesions of the CNS. Without treatment, brain tumors may be fatal, whether they are benign or malignant, located inside or outside of the brain, invasive or noninvasive, rapid- or slow-growing.

Intracranial tumors can be defined in several different

ways. *Primary tumors* develop from CNS tissue. *Secondary tumors* have metastasized from other locations in the body. *Intra-axial tumors* originate from glial cells within the cerebrum, cerebellum, or brain stem. These tumors infiltrate and invade brain tissue. *Extra-axial tumors* have their origin in the skull, meninges, cranial nerves, or pituitary gland. These tumors have a compressive effect on the brain.

Intracranial tumors are second only to cerebrovascular disease as the most common endogenous neurologic problem; 36,000 new cases of primary brain tumor develop yearly in the United States.[28] It is not known whether the incidence of brain tumors is actually increasing or whether it appears so because of increasingly sophisticated diagnostic tests. Tumors of this type occur equally in males and females of all ages. Nearly 20% of all cancers affect the brain, yet only 2% originate there.[40] There are about 18,000 secondary brain cancers yearly.[28]

Types of Intracranial Tumors

Intracranial tumors are classified by histologic origin. Tumors can be encapsulated, nonencapsulated, or invasive. In addition, the tumors are staged based on biopsy or excision.

■ Glial Tumors

Gliomas are tumors of the neuroglia. Astrocytomas are the most common type of glial tumor and the frontal lobe is the most common site. The first clinical manifestation is usually seizure followed by changes in mental status. Grades I and II are considered benign and usually occur in younger clients. Grades III and IV are considered malignant. The most aggressive form is called glioblastoma multiforme. This form is the most common and most lethal primary CNS cancer. Even with surgery, radiation, chemotherapy, or a combination of these, survival may be limited to months or a few years (Fig. 33–4).

■ Oligodendrogliomas

Oligodendrocytes are the cells that produce myelin. Oligodendrogliomas are tumors of the white matter of the brain. They tend to develop in the cortex of the frontal and parietal lobes. This tumor is fairly slow-growing and calcifies. The calcification makes it recognizable on x-ray. Oligodendrogliomas peak in clients between the ages of 30 and 50. Early manifestations are headache, seizures, personality changes, and papilledema. Papilledema is edema and hyperemia of the optic disc as noted on ophthalmic examination. Many clients are treated with chemotherapy or radiation therapy, or both.

■ Ependymomas

Ependymomas develop from cells that line the ventricles and central canal of the spinal cord. This tumor affects all ages. Manifestations are caused by ventricular obstruction and include headache, vomiting, diplopia, dizziness, ataxia, and vision changes. Radiation therapy is often used as an adjunct to surgery.

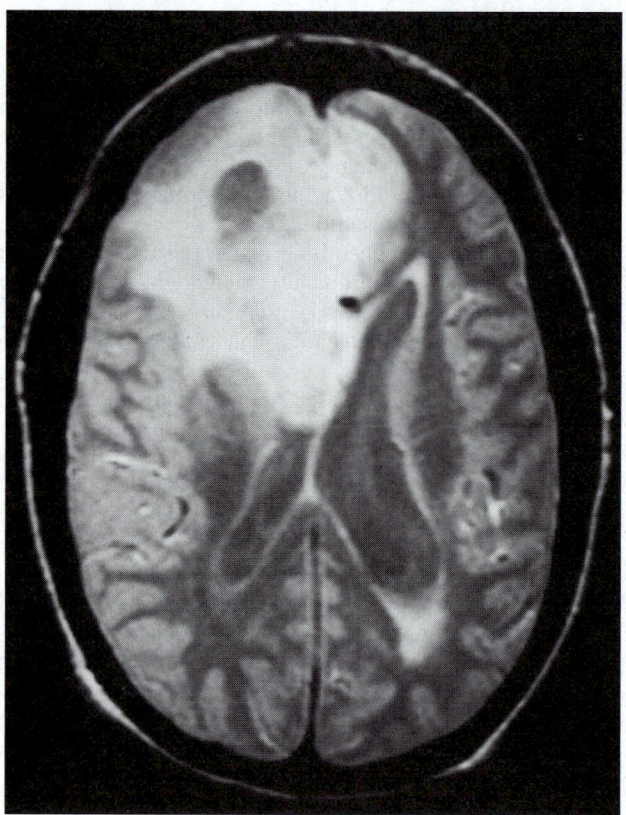

Figure 33–4. An MRI showing a mixed glioma in the right frontal lobe, with ventricular compression.

■ Pituitary Tumors

Pituitary tumors are usually slow-growing tumors that involve only the anterior lobe of the pituitary gland or extend into the floor of the third ventricle. Most of these are benign, small, and encapsulated. Manifestations of pituitary tumors are often overlooked for months because they are so diverse. Manifestations can be related to hypofunctioning of the gland and include visual field defects, irregular or absent menstrual cycles, infertility, decreased libido, impotence, decreased body hair, and decreased production of pituitary-stimulating hormones; this decrease results in decreased thyroid and adrenal function. Hypersecretion can also occur and is related to the hormones that are in excess. A combination of hypo- and hypersecretion can also be seen. Clients are usually diagnosed by testing blood for the presence of stimulating hormones.

A fairly common effect of pituitary surgery is the development of transient diabetes insipidus (DI) due to a decreased secretion of antidiuretic hormone (ADH). Clients with DI have large volumes (2–15 L/day) of dilute urine with a specific gravity of 1.005 or less. These clients require laboratory assessment of serum and urine levels of sodium and osmolality. Aside from the inconvenience of polyuria, the client often suffers no serious side effects from DI unless deprived of oral or intravenous fluids. When this happens, circulatory collapse (hypovolemic shock) and hypertonic encephalopathy occur as a result of fluid shifts in the brain. Usual treatment is with intravenous vasopressin (Pitressin) or inhalation desmopressin (DDAVP). Long-acting forms of these agents can be used for chronic DI.

■ Tumors of Supporting Structures

Meningiomas

Meningiomas are common benign tumors of arachnoid cells in the meninges (Fig. 33–5). A rare few are malignant. They are slow-growing and occur at any age, most commonly at midlife. Manifestations are based on site and can be quite diverse. Outcomes are based on the site of the tumor. Recurrence is a concern.

Acoustic Neuromas

Acoustic neuromas are tumors of the Schwann cells of the vestibular nerve. Manifestations are tinnitus, dizziness, and unilateral hearing loss. If the tumor is allowed to grow, it can displace the other cranial nerves (especially CN IV–X) and the brain stem. Excellent outcomes should be expected with surgical resection and preservation of the remaining cranial nerves. However, most clients experience at least temporary tinnitus, balance problems, and facial weakness after surgery.[11]

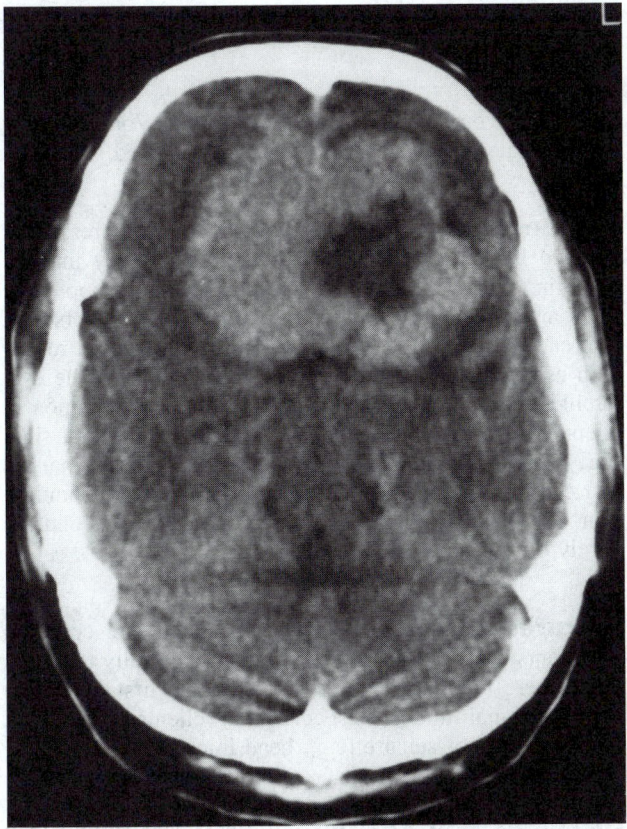

Figure 33–5. An MRI revealing a midline frontal meningioma.

■ Metastatic Brain Tumors

Metastatic brain tumors are those whose primary sites are outside of the brain. Cancers of the lung, breast, kidney, and malignant melanoma are the major sources of metastatic brain cancers. The sites may also be within the brain or on the arachnoid. The common locations of brain tumors are shown in Figure 33–6.

Etiology and Risk Factors

Heredity is not a significant risk factor in primary brain tumors, except for the rare tumors neurofibromatosis and tuberous sclerosis. A clear etiologic factor has not been established for any of the primary intracranial tumors. Although the type of cell that gave rise to the tumor can often be identified, the mechanism causing the cells to act abnormally remains unknown. Primary intracranial tumors do not metastasize to other sites in the body unless the protective barriers are damaged. Because the etiologic mechanism of primary intracranial tumors is uncertain, there are no specific risk factors or primary and secondary preventive measures. Aggressive treatment of the primary site of any cancer may prevent the development of metastatic tumors within the brain. Unfortunately, such treatment is not always successful, and not all clients can tolerate aggressive treatment. Experimental evidence suggests that some chemotherapeutic agents given for systemic cancer actually disrupt the blood-brain barrier. These clients may develop metastatic tumors because of the disruption of the protective barriers.

The cause of secondary tumors can be traced to the primary site from which they metastasized. Changes in the permeability of the blood-brain barrier may allow for seeding of these tumors into the brain.

Tertiary prevention addresses those clients who have an intracranial tumor. Depending on the location of the lesion and the type and extensiveness of medical intervention, the client may exhibit various neurologic deficits. Tertiary prevention focuses on preventing complications associated with these deficits.

Pathophysiology

Primary brain tumors are thought to originate from a cell or colony of single stem cells with abnormal deoxyribonucleic acid (DNA). Abnormal DNA leads to uncontrolled mitotic division of the cells. The immune system is unable to limit or stop the aberrant, self-renewing growth. As the tumor enlarges it causes death by infiltration and compression of brain tissue. Not only are the tumors space-occupying lesions but they often produce considerable cerebral edema. The skull is rigid and has little room for expansion of the contents. If not successfully treated, brain tumors progressively increase intracranial pressure (ICP), which causes displacement of brain stem structures (herniation). Pressure on the brain stem causes alteration in critical vital sign centers that control blood pressure, pulse, and respirations; this alteration may lead to death. See Chapter 32 for a more in-depth discussion of herniation syndromes.

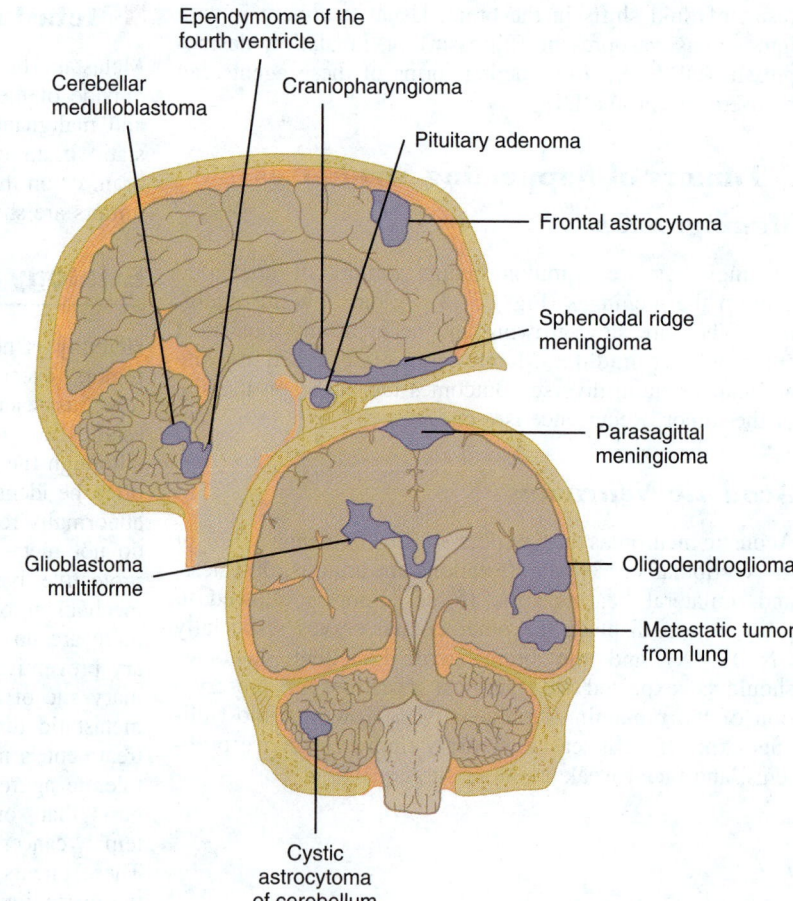

Figure 33–6. Common intracranial tumors and their usual locations. (From Snyder, M., & Jackle, M. [1981]. *Neurologic nursing: A critical care nursing focus.* Bowie, MD: Brady.)

Clinical Manifestations and Diagnostic Findings

Despite the extremely sensitive and sophisticated equipment available, brain tumor diagnosis is often delayed because of difficulty recognizing early manifestations. Older clients, especially, fail to report them during regular examinations because they forget or feel the manifestations "are just part of growing old."

General clinical manifestations are caused by changes in cerebral function resulting from edema and increased ICP. Headache, vomiting, and papilledema are considered the clinical triad of increased ICP and significant indicators of brain tumors.

Headaches. Headaches (localized or generalized) are often most severe in the frontal or occipital region. They are usually intermittent, are of increasing duration, and may be intensified by a change in posture or straining. Recurrent, severe headaches in a client previously free of them or recurrent headaches in the morning, increasing in frequency and severity, may indicate an intracranial tumor and require further assessment.

Nausea and Vomiting. Nausea and vomiting may occur late in the tumor progression because of the location of the vomiting center in the medulla. Vomiting may not be related to meals. Nausea may be marked.

Papilledema. Cranial nerves may be compressed or invaded by benign or malignant tumors, or they may be the primary site of tumors. The underlying pathophysiologic mechanism of papilledema is not clearly understood. The cause may be increased pressure in the central retinal vein as a result of obstructed venous return from the eye. Papilledema, also known as "choked disc," is common in clients with intracranial tumors and may be the first sign. Early papilledema does not cause visual acuity changes and can only be detected through an ophthalmic examination. Prolonged papilledema causes optic atrophy and severely diminished visual acuity.

Seizures. Seizures, focal or generalized, are common in clients with intracranial tumors, especially cerebral hemisphere tumors. Seizures are often the first indication of intracranial tumors, especially in clients without an obvious cause of seizure (e.g., head injury).

Dizziness and Vertigo. Dizziness and vertigo may develop from impairment of intracranial circulation or pressure on cranial nerves.

Mental Status Changes. Mental and emotional status changes such as lethargy and drowsiness, confusion, disorientation, and personality changes may accompany an intracranial tumor. As with other cranial disorders, the clinical manifestations associated with an intracranial tumor correlate with the area of the brain involved.

Localized Manifestations. Localized clinical manifestations are caused by destruction, irritation, or compression of the part of the brain in or near the tumor. Blood supply to the affected area is also impaired. Localized manifestations include the following:

- Focal weaknesses (e.g., hemiparesis)
- Sensory disturbances, including absence of feeling (anesthesia) or abnormal sensation (paresthesia)
- Language disturbances
- Coordination disturbances (e.g., staggering gait)
- Visual disturbances (e.g., diplopia [double vision] or visual field deficit [hemianopia])

As an intracranial tumor enlarges, it shifts intracranial structures and may produce brain stem herniation. Table 33–2 lists specific clinical manifestations based on tumor location.

A complete history from the client or family, followed by a thorough physical examination, is especially important. If an intracranial tumor is suspected, noninvasive studies such as CT, MRI, and x-ray are done first. Other disorders may be ruled out with EEG, radionuclide scans, angiogram, or a lumbar puncture. Three-dimensional thresholding techniques help visualize the tumor's projection in the brain, and can assist with plans for surgery. PET scans can also be used to study the biochemical and physiologic effects of the tumor. A stereotactic biopsy may confirm the diagnosis of a brain tumor and help in planning chemotherapy and radiation therapy.

Acute and Subacute Care

■ Medical Management

Intervention depends on the type and location of an intracranial tumor and the client's condition. Management is always interdisciplinary, with several members forming a clinical team to support the client through care. Medical knowledge and technology, to date, have been unable to provide a complete cure or design a technique for complete removal of malignant brain tumors. The clinical course of a client with an intracranial tumor varies with the specific type of tumor present. For example, a client with a low-grade glioma who has undergone partial surgical excision of the tumor followed by radiation may survive 5 to 15 years. Clients with malignant gliomas may

Table 33–2. Clinical Manifestations of Brain Tumors by Location	
Location	**Clinical Manifestations**
Frontal lobe	Disturbed mental state, apathy, inappropriate behavior, dementia, depression, emotional lability, inattentiveness, inability to concentrate, indifference, loss of self-restraint and social behavior, impaired long-term memory, difficulty with abstraction, quiet but flat affect, dominant hemisphere expressive speech disturbance, impaired sphincter control with bowel and bladder incontinence, motor disorders, gait disturbances, paralysis, "frontal release signs," seizures
Temporal lobe	Receptive aphasia, generalized psychomotor seizures, visual field changes, personality changes, ataxia, headache, signs and symptoms of increased ICP, tinnitus, recent memory impairment
Parietal lobe	Sensory deficits, motor and sensory focal seizures, agnosias, hypesthesias, paresthesias, dyslexia, visual field cut, diminished appreciation of the side opposite the tumor, headache, apraxia, tactile inattention, right and left disorientation
Occipital lobe	Headache, signs and symptoms of increased ICP, visual impairment (homonymous hemianopsia), visual agnosia, cortical blindness, hallucinations, seizures
Cerebellar	Unsteady gait, falling, ataxia, incoordination, tremors, head tilt, nystagmus, CSF obstruction/hydrocephalus, truncal ataxia if vermis is tumor site
Brain Stem	Vertigo, dizziness, vomiting, CN III–XII palsies/dysfunction, nystagmus, decreased corneal reflex, headache, vomiting, gait disturbance, motor and sensory deficits, deafness, intranuclear ophthalmoplegia, sudden death from cardiac and respiratory failure
Pituitary and hypothalamus	Visual deficits, headache, hormonal dysfunction, sleep disturbances, water imbalance, temperature fluctuations, imbalance in fat and carbohydrate metabolism, Cushing's syndrome
Ventricular	Obstruction of CSF circulation, hydrocephalus, rapid rise in ICP, postural headache

Adapted from Barker, E. (1994). *Neuroscience nursing.* St. Louis: Mosby–Year Book.

die within 1 to 2 years, despite aggressive treatment. Likewise, a glioblastoma multiforme grows rapidly and may cause death within 6 months to 1 year, even with radiation therapy.

Chemotherapy

Chemotherapy is used for selected types of brain tumors. Chemotherapy may be given to the client:

1. Immediately after surgical debulking (tumor reduction) in combination with radiation therapy
2. After the client completes a course of radiation
3. After tumor recurrence

Several factors are considered before using chemotherapy, such as the client's age, neurologic status, type and stage of the tumor, and predicted outcomes of each specific chemotherapy. There are no known curative combinations of chemotherapy. Not all chemotherapeutic agents cross the blood-brain barrier, which limits the usefulness of chemotherapy with many types of brain cancers. Some alkylating agents, antimetabolites, and natural products are currently being used (see Chapter 24). The better route of administration, systemic or intra-arterial, is under investigation. The Ommaya reservoir is another route of administration. It is an implanted device used to obtain repeated access to the CNS. The device has a dome-shaped reservoir and a ventricular catheter made of silicone. The advantage is that chemotherapeutic agents can be injected directly into the CNS. Corticosteroids are also used as an adjunct to other chemotherapeutic agents to reduce cerebral edema.

Stereotactic Radiation Therapy

Stereotactic refers to precise localization of target tissue by use of three-dimensional coordinates. Radiation therapy often uses this approach to slow tumor growth and improve the quality of life. Radiation may be administered in the conventional manner or via several innovative systems. The gamma knife uses multiple low-dosage radiation sources. These sources are arranged around the client's head in a helmet device to focus on the tumor. In radiosurgery, a linear accelerator is used to deliver the radiation. The single radiation source is moved in arcs around the client's head, again focusing on the tumor. The benefit of these systems is that the area being irradiated can be clearly identified. This minimizes the effect on healthy brain tissues and other body tissues. These techniques can also be used on tumors or arteriovenous malformations (AVMs) that are surgically inaccessible. In brachytherapy (internal radiation), radioactive seeds are inserted, through catheters, into the tumor. These seeds are left in place for approximately 2 days and then removed to minimize radiation to healthy brain tissue. These techniques can be used after traditional radiation treatments.

Complications of chemotherapy and radiation therapy in clients with brain tumors are similar to those in clients being treated for other types of cancer. See Chapter 24 for a complete discussion.

■ Nursing Management of the Medical Client

Assessment

Assess and document a baseline neurologic check when the client is admitted (see Chapter 30). Reassessment frequency varies with progression of clinical manifestations. Reassess whenever there is a change in the client's condition or in treatment intervention. Compare findings to baseline information.

Diagnosis, Planning, Implementation

Nursing management of the client having chemotherapy or radiation therapy for brain tumors follows the usual care of these clients, which is discussed in Chapter 24. The client remains at risk of increased ICP and seizures related to cerebral edema plus displacement of brain structures by the tumor. Common nursing diagnoses include the following:

- *Pain from stretching of the dura and cerebral edema*
- *Self Care Deficit related to decreased motor function secondary to tumor growth or pressure on the motor strip*
- *Altered Cerebral Tissue Perfusion related to increased ICP*
- *Anxiety related to brain tumor treatment and possible outcomes*
- *Risk for Injury related to seizures*
- *Fear of death*

Implementation for most of these diagnoses can be found in the sections on stroke and care of the client in a coma in Chapters 31 and 32.

Altered Cerebral Tissue Perfusion. The client with a brain tumor, whether benign or malignant, is at risk for altered cerebral tissue perfusion related to the mass. An increase in ICP is caused by the mass itself or by the damage to the surrounding brain tissues that results in edema. Write the nursing diagnosis as *Risk for Altered Cerebral Tissue Perfusion related to cerebral mass and edema*.

Planning: Expected Outcomes. The client will maintain normal tissue perfusion as evidenced by maintaining or improving the present level of Glasgow Coma Scale scores. The client will experience no worsening or improvement in pupillary responses, absence of seizures, absence of Cushing's response (widening pulse pressure, high systolic blood pressures, bradycardia), or absence of respiratory alterations.

Implementation. The care of a client with altered tissue perfusion related to an intracranial tumor focuses on management of the ICP. See Chapter 32 for an in-depth discussion.

■ Surgical Management

Stereotactic Radiosurgery

Stereotactic radiosurgery is the application of ionizing beams of radiation focused with the help of intracranial guiding devices. Three techniques are used: Bragg peak photon beam, linear accelerator radiosurgery, and gamma knife radiosurgery. Disorders treated with radiosurgery include AVMs, primary and metastatic tumors, and chronic pain syndromes.

Craniotomy

A craniotomy is a surgical opening into the skull (Fig. 33–7). A craniectomy (removal of a portion of the cranium) is sometimes performed for decompression, that is, to relieve pressure on brain structures by providing space for expansion. General anesthetics are used. The brain itself has no pain receptors, so a light anesthetic can be used except during opening and closure. During surgery, the client's head is supported in a special frame. The frame may cause pressure sores on the client's head, edema of the face, and muscle soreness, especially in the neck. Depending on the type of surgery being performed, the surgeon may use a laser or an ultrasonic aspirator. These devices can minimize the trauma suffered by normal brain tissue.[4] After some craniectomies (e.g., large), a protective prosthesis made of methyl methacrylate is later surgically inserted.

The surgeon may place a catheter in the brain to drain excess fluid or blood from a ventricle or other fluid-filled space. A Jackson-Pratt suction drain (Fig. 33–8) may be surgically inserted if a large cavity remains after removal of a tumor or large hematoma. During brain surgery, the brain may become edematous and expand so that the

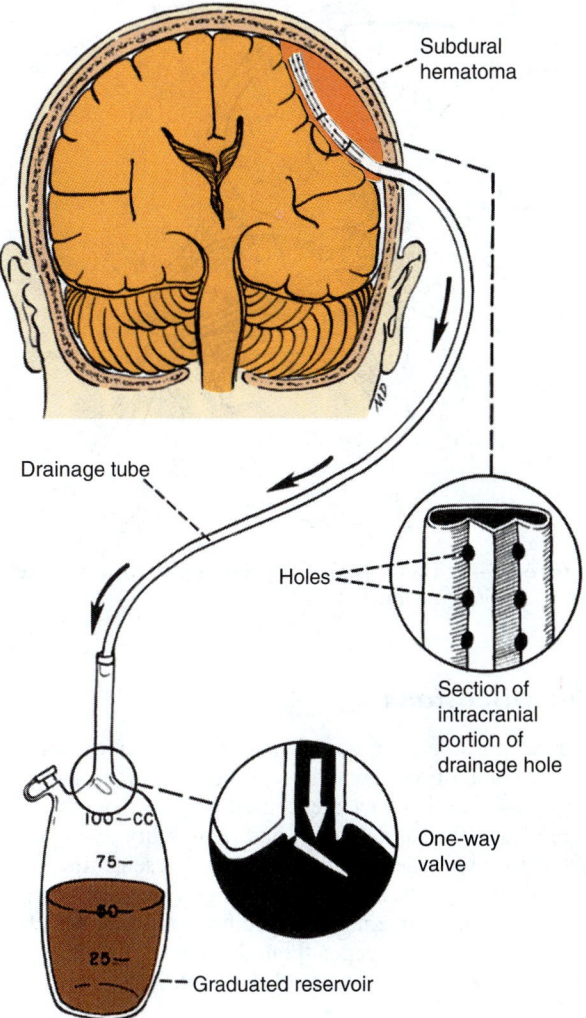

Figure 33–8. A Jackson-Pratt suction drain.

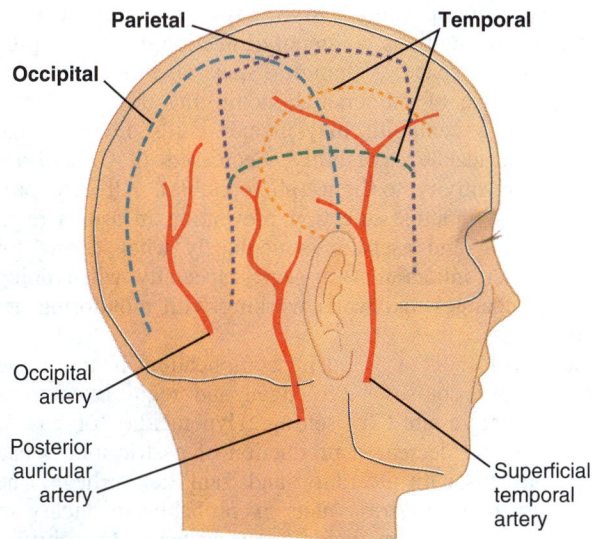

Figure 33–7. Basic craniotomy incisions. (From Wilkins, R. H., & Odom, G. L. [1982]. Anesthesia and operative technique. In J. R. Youmans [Ed.], *Neurological surgery* [2nd ed.]. Philadelphia: W. B. Saunders.)

surgeon cannot close the dura. Sometimes the bone flap is left out to permit expansion of such an edematous brain. Rarely, a client with an expanding brain tumor has a small craniectomy performed to provide for expansion when the tumor grows.

Transsphenoidal Hypophysectomy

Pituitary tumors can usually be removed successfully with surgery. The most common procedure is called transsphenoidal hypophysectomy. This operation is performed through the anterior upper gum or nose to avoid entering the cranium (Fig. 33–9). The nose is packed to control bleeding. After surgery, the client is positioned with the head elevated. Postoperative care is similar to that of other clients after craniotomy, with several additions. Mouth care is especially important for these clients because they cannot breathe through their noses. The client may require replacement pituitary hormones if the gland is nonfunctional.

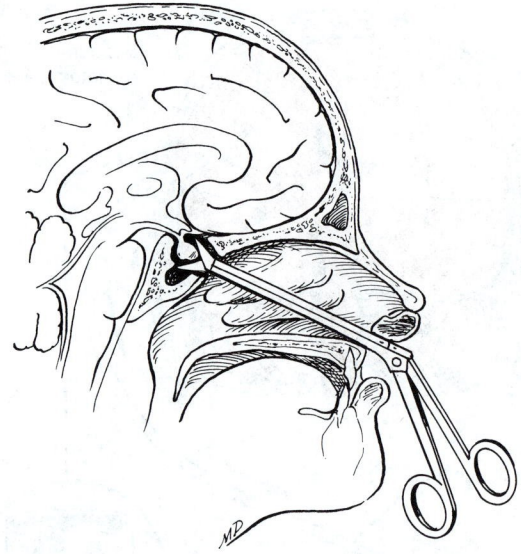

Figure 33–9. Transsphenoidal hypophysectomy for the excision of pituitary tumors.

Complications

General postoperative complications after intracranial surgery do not differ from those following other forms of surgery. Complications are caused by the depressive effects of anesthesia, narcotics, and immobility. Ecchymosis and periorbital edema are commonly present after intracranial surgery, but are transient. They can be very frightening to family members. Specific complications from intracranial surgery depend on the area of surgery and the procedure being performed. Examples include the following:

• Increased ICP
• Cerebrospinal fluid (CSF) leaks
• Memory loss
• Paralysis
• Loss of or impaired special senses (e.g., blindness)
• Loss of or impaired speech
• Mental confusion

Obviously, because of the loss of significant functions, these problems can be psychosocially and physically devastating. Some postoperative complications gradually improve, but others are permanent.

Increased ICP (caused by cerebral edema or bleeding) is the major complication of intracranial surgery. Clinical manifestations may include the following:

• Change in level of consciousness (LOC) with associated headaches
• Visual and speech disturbances
• Muscle weakness or paralysis
• Pupil changes
• Seizures
• Vomiting
• Respiratory changes

Conventional management of increased ICP includes osmotic diuretic therapy and steroid administration. Me-

chanical hyperventilation reduces the carbon dioxide in the bloodstream, which leads to vasoconstriction and thereby reduces ICP. Mechanical ventilation also prevents hypoxia. Elevation of the client's head (varies with the surgical site) and maintaining the head in a midline position facilitates venous drainage and reduces ICP. ICP monitoring (see Chapter 32) and CSF drainage are used to guide therapy and reduce ICP. Further surgical intervention may be necessary, depending on the suspected cause of the increased ICP.

CSF leak may be manifested postoperatively by saturation of the surgical head dressing or drainage from the ear (otorrhea) or nose (rhinorrhea) of clear, thin fluid that dries in concentric circles (halo sign). The fluid should be tested with enzymatic test tape for glucose or sent to the laboratory to determine if it is CSF. CSF leaks increase the risk of infection and therefore are managed with antibiotics and bedrest. In some instances a spinal drain is inserted to relieve pressure at the operative site and promote healing. If the site does not close spontaneously, a dural patch may be used to repair the site.

Body temperature regulation may be erratic after intracranial surgery. Hypothermia can result from excessive body dehydration because of the client's condition before surgery. Hyperthermia may be secondary to blood in the cranium or underlying infection. Postoperative respiratory complications are the most common cause of hyperthermia. When the hypothalamus has been operated on or manipulated, wide variations in temperature regulation may occur.

Seizures may occur in clients with intracranial surgery. There may be only one seizure or many, possibly progressing to status epilepticus. Seizure activity greatly increases the brain's metabolic needs and may cause further brain damage. Seizures are suppressed by prophylactic anticonvulsants. Phenytoin is the most commonly used drug for prophylactic management of seizures.

Meningitis (see Neurologic Infections), when it develops, typically appears 2 to 3 days after surgery. The cause of meningitis is commonly infection or blood in the subarachnoid space. Meningitis may also develop with prolonged use of intracranial monitoring devices. Manifestations of meningitis may include chills, fever, nuchal rigidity, headache, irritability, decreased LOC, and increased sensitivity to light (photophobia). All care providers must practice infection prevention measures (e.g., handwashing and asepsis) meticulously when caring for clients after intracranial surgery, especially when doing dressing changes and when working with monitoring devices.

Stress ulcer is a frequent complication if the acute postoperative course is prolonged and requires complex management in an ICU setting. Hyperacidity of gastric secretions and decreased production of gastric mucus can cause gastritis with ulceration and frank hemorrhage. The development of a stress ulcer is probably secondary to insult to one or more major organ systems. The physiologic stress stimulates the sympathetic nervous system, which reduces blood flow to the abdominal organs. Steroid administration and mechanical ventilation are also predisposing factors. Intervention includes monitoring gastric contents to keep the pH above 4.5 and administering prescribed antacids or histamine-blocking agents.

Clients undergoing surgery in the posterior fossa region are also at risk of development of postoperative complications. These complications are related to the potential manipulation of vital brain stem structures. Cardiac dysrhythmias and air embolism may relate to the client's sitting position during surgery. Other complications relate to dysfunction of CN VIII through XII (e.g., hearing loss, inability to swallow, aspiration, and impaired airway protection). Pressure on the pituitary gland from increased ICP can cause DI or syndrome of inappropriate antidiuretic hormone (SIADH). See Chapter 71 for more information on SIADH.

■ Nursing Management of the Surgical Client

Preoperative Care

Clients usually undergo blood tests and an anesthesia evaluation prior to surgery. Assess the client's physical condition for surgery and anesthesia. Address any disorders that require correction or improved management, such as atrial fibrillation or electrolyte imbalances. Provide client and family education at this evaluation regarding NPO (nothing by mouth) status, admitting procedures, and expected events on the day of surgery.

Assessment

Assess and document the following:

- Vital signs; LOC; orientation to person, place, time; ability to follow instructions; pupil size, equality, and reaction to light; extraocular movements (EOMs); skin color and palpable skin temperature (cool, warm); cranial nerve function.
- Limb movements; limited or exaggerated movements; pronator drift, strength in extremities (grip); any paresis or paralysis; sensory abnormalities; edema; indications of skin pressure, burns, irritations, abrasions, bruises, or hematomas.
- Manifestations of increasing ICP. Report these findings immediately.
- Manifestations of pulmonary congestion. Report these findings immediately.
- Any other abnormal findings (e.g., indications of dehydration, seizures, aphasia, visual or auditory problems).
- Fluid and electrolyte balance and renal function.

These assessment findings provide preoperative baseline data for comparison with postoperative assessment findings. It is thus possible to determine if a client's condition is improved, worsened, or remains unchanged after surgery.

Diagnosis, Planning, Implementation

Preoperative preparation for elective intracranial surgery generally differs slightly from that for general surgery. This is particularly true for nonemergency surgery when the client's general condition is stable. In addition to a thorough neurologic assessment, preparation for intracranial surgery should include psychosocial preparation.

A client requiring neurosurgery often has an altered ability to tolerate conventional premedications. Thus, for example, if narcotics are prescribed by the anesthesiologist, be sure to confirm these orders with the neurosurgeon before administering the narcotics. Narcotics may cause hypoventilation and circulatory depression and may be problematic for clients with increased ICP. Prophylactic steroids and antibiotics are commonly given.

Anxiety and Fear. Clients with suspected or known brain tumors are frightened and apprehensive. State this diagnosis as *Anxiety and Fear related to unknown outcome of surgery for brain tumor.*

Planning: Expected Outcomes. The client will report that the anxiety and fear are at an acceptable level. It is not realistic to expect that a client facing this much uncertainty with potential risk of death or major changes in quality of life will be free of anxiety and fear.

Implementation. The client and his or her significant others require your kindness, patience, and understanding. Encourage open communication between the client and significant others. Offer spiritual support through accessing resources in the hospital or community. Do not provide false hope. The Nursing Research feature suggests ways to support a client with a brain tumor.

The loss of hair can be very traumatic. Offer reassurance that the hair will grow back. The cut hair is typically saved for the client. Suggest colorful scarves or loose-fitting hats for use after surgery.

Knowledge Deficit. A client will often have questions about the nature of brain tumors and about brain surgery. Find out whether the client has been told about the tumor and what else has been discussed concerning diagnosis and treatment. State the diagnosis as *Knowledge Deficit of Craniotomy related to no previous experience.*

Planning: Expected Outcomes. The client will be able to explain the prescribed plan of treatment.

Implementation. Accompany the physician on rounds, so an accurate explanation of the proposed treatment can be reviewed with the client later if necessary. Provide a quiet and private environment when asking the client to explain his or her understanding of the treatment plan. Offer support and clarification as necessary. Involve significant others as appropriate. If the client is still uncertain about the treatment or has specific questions about morbidity or mortality risks, notify the physician of the client's need for further clarification.

Evaluation

The care plan must be evaluated in a short time frame. If the expected outcomes are not being achieved, a revision in the care plan is warranted.

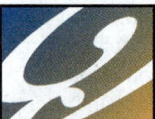

NURSING RESEARCH

How Can You Support a Client with a Brain Tumor?

Newton, C., & Mateo, M. A. (1994). Uncertainty: Strategies for patients with brain tumor and their families. *Cancer Nursing, 17*(2), 137–140.

The client with a brain tumor and his or her family have many uncertainties related to the tumor and the treatment. You can help them deal with these uncertainties.

Newton and Mateo used a case report to illustrate how the changing needs of a client and his family were met using different strategies.

The client was faced with inability to care for his wife, loss of control, and feelings of worthlessness. He also struggled with changes in his role and the desire for life to return to "normal." His wife was faced with guilt and the need to learn more about brain tumors. She was afraid of returning to work, of leaving her husband alone, and of the unknown. She became overprotective and worried about the change in her role and life-style. Client and family education, support groups, and counseling (pastoral and social service consults) helped this client and his family deal with the uncertainty of the brain tumor and treatment. These services also helped them make informed decisions, which restored their sense of control. Although some degree of uncertainty remained, the couple were able to share quality time together before the husband died. The wife continued to attend a support group to facilitate her grief work and help others who were going through the same type of experience.

Implications for Practice

Provide client and family education and referrals to other disciplines such as pastoral care and social services as appropriate. Help clients to get involved with structured support groups with other professionals or refer them to unstructured support groups in which the participants dictate the forum.

Postoperative Care

Assessment

The client is usually admitted to a critical care unit after surgery. Frequent and thorough neurologic assessment of the client after neurologic surgery is essential. These clients can deteriorate quickly. Assess vital signs and neurologic signs such as LOC, ability to move extremities, and speech every 15 minutes for 1 hour, every 30 minutes for the next 2 hours, every hour until stable, and then every 4 hours. This format may not be what your facility uses, so be certain to check the policy. It is important to keep the client's blood pressure within normal limits. Vasoactive medications may be required. Carefully document intake and output every hour. Monitor electrolytes, especially serum glucose, sodium, potassium, osmolality, and hematocrit. Take appropriate measures to keep electrolytes within normal range while avoiding extremes of hydration (see Chapter 15).

Inspect the dressing and the underlying linens for evidence of bleeding or CSF leak. Sometimes a small amount of bloody drainage occurs on the dressing if a catheter or drain is in place. CSF is clear fluid that dries in concentric circles. Assess (character, estimated amount) and document prolonged "oozing" bleeds or oozing wound drainage. Immediately report and document such evidence. Assess whether the dressing is comfortable. It should not be constrictive around the client's head or ears or over the eyes.

Evaluate the response of the client and significant others to the surgery. This is a very stressful experience,

particularly if the tumor was malignant or the client experiences neurologic deficits after surgery.

Diagnosis, Planning, Implementation

Nursing diagnoses and collaborative problems that may apply to the client after a craniotomy include the following:

- *Impaired Verbal Communication related to aphasia or dysarthria*
- *Risk for Contractures*
- *Self Care Deficit related to weakness and cognitive impairments*
- *Risk for Injury related to seizures*

These have already been discussed in the care of the client with stroke and brain injury (see Chapter 32).

Prophylactic anticonvulsant drugs are typically ordered postoperatively. Observe the client carefully for focal or generalized seizure activity. Such activity requires prompt, aggressive nursing and medical intervention. The client must be protected from harm and seizures stopped as quickly as possible, because continuous seizures damage the brain. Immediately report a seizure to the physician. Do not restrict the client's movement during the seizure, but provide physical protection. Administer prescribed medication promptly.

Prevention of meningitis or other infection is also of great concern. Most neurosurgeons usually prefer to perform the initial change of the head dressing after intracranial surgery. You may reinforce the original dressing if it becomes contaminated before the first dressing change (e.g., from serosanguineous drainage). Inform the physician if frequent reinforcement is necessary. Nurses usually perform subsequent dressing changes. Use sterile technique during dressing changes. Place a gauze dressing over the incisional site or around a drain or catheter insertion site to keep this area clean, dry, and free of abrasion by the overlying bulky dressings. During dressing changes, inspect the operative site and sites around drains or catheters for edema and signs of infection. Document and report these assessment findings.

As postoperative edema subsides and the client's wound heals and improves, replace bulky dressings with modified dressings to suit individual needs. For example, sutures or staples are usually kept covered with gauze pads, and a stockinette cap is placed over the client's head. To remove dried flaky skin and residue, soften the scalp with baby oil or glycerin and then gently wash the head with soap and water. Do not cause any tension on the suture line. While giving wound care, assess the suture line and wound healing. Document and report any sutures or staples inadvertently left in place, openings in the suture line, or other complications of wound healing.

There may also be a Jackson-Pratt drain to remove fluid buildup in the space. Maintain only "thumbprint" suction to the drain unless the physician prescribes otherwise. More suction pressure can cause tissue trauma.

Altered Cerebral Tissue Perfusion. The client remains at risk for altered cerebral tissue perfusion related to increased ICP, cerebral edema, and possible bleeding. State this common diagnosis as *Risk for Altered Cerebral Tissue Perfusion related to postoperative cerebral edema.*

Planning: Expected Outcomes. The client will maintain normal ICP and cerebral perfusion. He or she will experience a maintained or improved LOC; a maintained or improved Glasgow Coma Scale score; absence of restlessness, irritability, or headache; no worsening of pupillary changes; absence of seizures; and absence of widening pulse pressure, respiratory irregularity, hypertension, or bradycardia.

Implementation. Continuously assess the client's neurologic status, comparing postoperative findings with preoperative status. General interventions to reduce ICP are discussed in Chapter 32. The use of diuretics and CSF drainage devices are common interventions.

During the acute phase of care after intracranial surgery, correct postoperative positioning of the client is extremely important to prevent pressure on the operative site, prevent or minimize ICP increases, promote jugular venous outflow, facilitate tissue perfusion, and prevent pressure ulcers. If a client is neurologically unstable and the ICP elevation is within a critical range (greater than 20 mm Hg), avoid procedures that require a flat position (e.g., daily weight-taking). Lowering the client's head can dangerously elevate ICP.

When a client must remain in a head-elevated position on the side, remember to support his or her head. For example, prop the client's head on a small pillow or folded blanket or apply a soft cervical collar to prevent the head from turning and thus lowering venous outflow. Reduced venous outflow from the head elevates ICP. When the client is in the side-lying position, place a pillow between his or her legs to maintain correct body alignment, to make the client comfortable, and to protect the knees from pressure sores. However, avoid sharp hip flexion, which increases intra-abdominal pressure and consequently increases ICP.

Positions allowed vary with the type of surgery performed and specific postoperative orders. If in doubt, always double-check orders before repositioning the client. Incorrect positioning of a client after intracranial surgery may have serious, possibly fatal consequences. Know whether the client's head is to be elevated or kept flat. The client may not be positioned on the operative side if there is no bone flap. To help ensure proper positioning, post a sign clearly stating safe and unsafe positions for the client. Some guidelines for typical positions after intracranial surgery follow.

In *supratentorial surgery* (surgery above the brain's tentorium), the client's head is usually elevated 30 degrees to promote venous outflow through the jugular veins. Do not lower the client's head or the head of the bed in the acute phase of care after supratentorial surgery. An order should be obtained from the neurosurgeon before the head is lowered. If central venous lines are present for hemodynamic monitoring purposes, assess and document pulmonary artery or central venous pressure readings at least every 2 hours. If the client is to remain in this head-elevated position, be certain to take these readings consistently while the client is in this position and document the position.

An exception to typical positioning is the client who has undergone evacuation of a chronic subdural hematoma. The neurosurgeon may order the client's head to remain flat after supratentorial surgery to remove a chronic subdural hematoma. Clients with this problem are usually older and their brains are less expandable. When the hematoma is removed, a large space may remain between the dura and brain. To allow the brain to reexpand, the client lies flat. Increased ICP rarely occurs with chronic subdural hematomas.

An *infratentorial surgery* involves tissues below the brain's tentorium, which includes the brain stem and cerebellum. Postoperatively, the neurosurgeon may order the head of bed (HOB) at 30 to 45 degrees, or more commonly, a flat position without head elevation. Care should be taken not to place the neck at an angle, either laterally or anteriorly. The client is turned every 2 hours. If the client is unconscious, position him or her on the side to facilitate drainage of oral secretions.

Do not elevate the client's head (or the HOB) in the acute phase of care after infratentorial surgery for any procedure without permission from the neurosurgeon.

After *posterior fossa surgery,* the client is typically positioned on the side, with a pillow under the head for support, and not on the back. This protects the operative site from pressure and minimizes tension on the suture line.

If a bone flap was surgically removed for decompression (to allow further expansion of an already edematous brain), place the client on the side that was not operated on or the back. This facilitates brain expansion. The client should be turned from the back to the uninvolved side, but not to the side operated on if a bone flap is not present.

Ineffective Airway Clearance.
Cerebral edema, decreased LOC, or neck edema can all impair the ability of the client to clear the airway of secretions. State this diagnosis as *Risk for Ineffective Airway Clearance related to decreased level of consciousness.* Other etiologies may be used if appropriate.

Planning: Expected Outcomes. The client will show no signs of airway obstruction, as evidenced by clear lung sounds; full, equal lung expansion; and quiet respirations.

Implementation. Assess respiratory parameters frequently to avoid hypercapnia and to ensure maximal oxygenation of the brain (cerebral oxygenation). Arterial lines and pulse oximetry may be used. Maintain airway patency. However, do not suction through the nose. If the cribriform plate is damaged during suctioning, CSF will leak and meningitis may result. Preoxygenate the client and do not suction longer than 10 seconds at one time to avoid hypoxia, which increases ICP. Prolonged suctioning increases intrathoracic pressure.[7] This, in turn, increases ICP because of decreased venous return. Hyperventilate between each pass of the catheter. This may be done using an Ambu bag or the ventilator. Monitor arterial blood gases after intracranial surgery to ensure adequate oxygenation.

Risk for Fluid Volume Deficit.
DI from alterations in ADH can develop in clients undergoing pituitary resection. State this diagnosis as *Risk for Fluid Volume Deficit related to inappropriate secretion of ADH.*

Planning: Expected Outcomes. The client will maintain adequate fluid volume as evidenced by:

1. Urine output less than 250 ml/hr
2. Specific gravity greater than 1.005
3. No excessive thirst
4. Normal serum sodium levels
5. Plasma osmolarity greater than 295 mOsm/kg H_2O
6. Stable weight
7. Stable blood pressure

Implementation. For all clients after pituitary surgery, assess intake and output and urine specific gravity every 2 hours and assess for indications of fluid and electrolyte imbalance. If the client develops DI, explain the condition to the client and significant others. Emphasize the need for fluid balance and educate the client about the pharmacologic treatment. Some clients may need lifelong medication.

Altered Nutrition: Less than Body Requirements.
Clients who are unconscious, combative, or confused cannot eat. Those clients who are able to eat may choke or aspirate their food and fluids. This diagnosis may be stated as *Risk for Altered Nutrition: Less than Body Requirements, related to confusion.* Other etiologies should be used for clients who are not confused.

Planning: Expected Outcomes. The client will demonstrate signs of adequate nutrition, as evidenced by weight remaining stable; consuming adequate calories for age, height, and weight; intake equaling output; incisions or wounds healing within 12 to 14 days; hemoglobin level within normal limits for age and sex; and lymphocyte level within normal limits.

Implementation. A client with an uncomplicated postoperative course after intracranial surgery usually requires minimal intravenous maintenance and electrolyte therapy. As the level of wakefulness improves and the swallowing and gag reflexes return, the client usually begins a clear liquid diet and progresses to a diet as tolerated. Total fluid intake may be curtailed to minimize overhydration and cerebral edema.

Enteral feedings may be prescribed for clients who are unable to eat once peristalsis is present. Long-term tube feedings may be given via gastrostomy or percutaneous endoscopic gastrostomy (PEG) tubes to reduce nasal irritation and the risk of aspiration. To minimize the potential subsequent development of diarrhea from tube feedings, begin with dilute feedings, infuse the feedings at a continuous rate with an infusion pump, and if possible, avoid using elixir-based medications. The sorbitol base of elixirs can cause osmotic diarrhea.

If diarrhea becomes uncontrollable, reduce tube feedings in concentration and rate until it subsides. Typically, the intravenous fluid infusion rate is increased to replace fluid loss from diarrhea and to maintain adequate hydration. If it is still not possible to maintain adequate nutrition and there is only minimal decrease of the diarrhea, total parenteral nutrition (TPN) may be ordered. The main advantage of TPN is its high-calorie, high-protein content. This begins to maximize the client's nutritional state. Consult a fundamental nursing text for interventions for clients receiving intravenous therapy, tube feedings, and TPN.

Self Esteem Disturbance.
Changes in the appearance of the head or in bony contour may challenge the client's coping abilities. In addition, changes in functional ability can also alter role performance and personal identity. State the diagnosis as *Risk for Self Esteem Disturbance related to charges in appearance and identity.*

Planning: Expected Outcomes. The client will develop effective coping strategies, as evidenced by appropriate life-style modifications, use of the assistance of others, appropriate social interactions, and ability to integrate the changes into his or her new body image.

Implementation. Assist the client to talk about the way he or she feels. Help the client to look at the incision and the face when he or she expresses interest. Do not force the client to look at himself or herself. If a defect remains in the skull after surgery, it may be helpful for the surgeon to discuss possible cranioplasty before the client sees the defect. Cranioplasty is the surgical repair of the defect with a custom-made implant. Naturally, it may be depressing for the client to experience a disturbance in self-esteem because of a body image change, and the client may fear additional surgery. Assure the client that cranioplasty can not only improve his or her appearance but also protect the brain from further injury.

Problems with loss of function should be referred to the appropriate therapy discipline. A psychiatric clinical nurse-specialist may also be of help in discussing feelings and concerns with the client and family.

Altered Thought Processes.

Thought processing requires very complex neuronal connections. Even somewhat minor changes can limit a client's ability to think. After a craniotomy, changes can be brought about by numerous conditions, including the actual loss of brain tissue from surgical resection, damage to the brain tissue from the underlying problem (e.g., tumor, bleeding), cerebral edema, sleep deprivation, or electrolyte imbalances. State this commonly used nursing diagnosis as *Altered Thought Processes related to surgical resection*. Again, other etiologies may be better suited to your client.

Planning: Expected Outcomes. The client will recognize limitations and attempt to minimize them, as evidenced by participation in prescribed therapies, consideration of physical capabilities during activities, and verbalization of limitations and adaptations.

Implementation. Alteration in thought processes may be temporary (e.g., due to sleep deprivation or cerebral swelling) or permanent (e.g., due to surgical removal of brain tissue). If thought process disturbances continue to persist, make suggestions about how to live with this problem. For any brain function change (verbal thought, memory), neuropsychological testing helps establish parameters of dysfunction.

Pain.

The only pain sensors in the brain are the dura and scalp, so pain is usually relatively mild and incisional. Headaches may occur. *Pain related to surgical incision* is a clear statement of this nursing diagnosis.

Planning: Expected Outcomes. The client will experience adequate pain relief, as evidenced by verbalization of improvement in comfort level without excessive drowsiness or lethargy, the ability to rest without interruption by pain, and the ability to participate in therapies without hindrance by pain.

Implementation. Avoid abrupt movements such as bumping the bed. Keep the environment quiet, calm, and dimly lighted. Administer prescribed medications as indicated for pain relief. Acetaminophen or codeine may be prescribed for pain relief. Codeine, although a narcotic, does not alter respirations as do other narcotics. Thus, it is the exception to the "no narcotics" rule in clients with increased ICP. Evaluate the effectiveness of pain-relieving medications and make adjustments as needed.

Altered Family Processes.

The family's ability to cope with irreversible changes in the function or personality of the client after surgery may be severely stressed. Recovery of neurologic function may be very slow and it is difficult to predict outcomes. State this nursing diagnosis as *Risk for Altered Family Processes related to difficulty coping with changes in client*.

Planning: Expected Outcomes. The family members will exhibit positive behaviors, as evidenced by their ability to problem-solve, to support and care for one another, and to ask questions indicating concern toward the client as appropriate, showing that they have understood previous conversations.

Implementation. An assessment of the family's previous coping styles can help you individualize the interventions. Family members are also affected by the client's postoperative changes. Some are able and willing to help the client and themselves grow and meet postoperative challenges. Others are unable to adapt effectively in this way, finding it difficult to accept changes in the client. Emotional lability or memory loss may be particularly difficult for family members to deal with.

Facilitating the expression of concerns, providing support and understanding, careful listening, and an unhurried empathic manner may all help the client and significant others if postoperative problems occur (e.g., paralysis, infection, speech disorders, skull defects) or if the surgery is unsuccessful. The client and family may also experience spiritual distress, powerlessness, or anticipatory grieving if the surgery was not successful and the client is unimproved, has postoperative complications, or is dying. Social workers, the psychiatric clinical nurse-specialist, and pastoral care personnel are all excellent resources.

Evaluation

The client's progression toward expected outcomes should be evaluated on a regular basis. Some expected outcomes, such as normal ICP and adequate cerebral perfusion, will need to be met before discharge from the ICU. Other expected outcomes, such as improved cognition and speech, may require months to obtain. Setting appropriate and achievable goals with the client and family is important.

If the physician has determined that the client has succumbed to an irreversible state, consult the family or guardian regarding transfer from the ICU and eventual long-term placement.

Community and Self-Care

Many clients can be discharged home and return to a gratifying life after brain surgery. Others will require short-term or ongoing rehabilitation to achieve complete recovery. Still others will never regain complete competence because of the amount of brain tissue damaged as a result of the disorder or surgery, or both. For these clients, the greater burden rests on the family to provide ongoing care either at home or in an extended care facility.

Family support groups are available to families with brain-damaged members within most hospitals and communities. These groups help the significant others to know they are not alone. Clinical nurse-specialists in neuroscience are often the facilitators for these groups. Participation by both client and significant others should be encouraged. Care should be taken to include all persons whom the client perceives as supportive.

Appropriate referrals to rehabilitation specialists such as speech therapists, physical therapists, and vocational therapists facilitate recovery. They may help the client and significant others to experience hope, personal growth, and recovery and to build effective coping skills.

Neurologic Infections

Almost any pathogenic microorganism may invade the nervous system and related structures, including the neurologic parenchyma, coverings, and blood vessels. The term *parenchyma* refers to the essential or functional elements of an organ. Neurologic infectious syndromes may be categorized according to the main area of involvement (e.g., meningeal subdural and epidural infections) or by causative mechanism. This section discusses the following:

1. Bacterial and pyogenic infections
2. Viral infections
3. Fungal infections
4. Parasitic infections

Bacterial and Pyogenic Infections

In bacterial infections, the invading organisms reach the CNS by the vascular system after systemic or bloodstream infection or by direct extension from adjacent cranial structures such as infection entering through a cranial fracture or a fracture through mastoid or nasal sinuses. Infection may also be unintentionally introduced into the CNS during invasive procedures.

Bacterial Meningitis

Bacterial meningitis is an inflammation of the arachnoid or pia mater membranes. The infection spreads throughout the subarachnoid space via the CSF around the brain and spinal cord and usually involves the ventricles. Approximately 20,000 to 25,000 cases of meningitis occur yearly in the United States.[40]

Factors predisposing to bacterial meningitis include the following:

1. Head trauma
2. Systemic infection
3. Postsurgical infection
4. Meningeal infection
5. Anatomic defects
6. Other systemic illness

When pathogenic organisms enter the subarachnoid space, an inflammatory reaction occurs, with these results:

1. CSF clouding
2. Exudate formation
3. Changes in subarachnoid arteries, including engorgement with blood, rupture, and thrombosis
4. Congestion of adjacent tissues

The pia-arachnoid tissues become thickened, and adhesions form, especially in the area of the basal cisterns. Little change occurs in brain structure in the early stages of meningitis.

Almost any bacteria entering the body can cause meningitis. The most common are meningococcus *(Neisseria meningitidis)*, pneumococcus *(Streptococcus pneumoniae)*, and *Haemophilus influenzae*. These organisms are often present in the nasopharynx. It is not known how they enter the bloodstream and the subarachnoid space. *S. pneumoniae* and *N. meningitidis* occur most often in adults.

Initial clinical manifestations include headache, prostration, chills, fever, nausea, vomiting, back pain, stiff neck, and generalized seizures. The client may be irritable at first, but as the infection progresses, the sensorium often becomes clouded, and coma may develop. Clients experiencing meningitis appear acutely ill and confused, stuporous, or semicomatose. A petechial or hemorrhagic rash may develop. Temperature is moderately elevated, and pulse and respiratory rate are increased. Blood pressure is usually normal. The client usually shows signs of meningeal irritation. These include the following:

1. Nuchal rigidity (rigidity of the neck)
2. Positive finding of Brudzinski's sign
3. Positive finding of Kernig's sign

Kernig's and Brudzinski's signs are elicited as follows.

To assess for *Kernig's sign,* begin with the client recumbent and the thigh flexed at a right angle to the abdomen, and with the knee flexed at a 90-degree angle to the thigh. Then extend the client's lower leg. In meningeal irritation, extending the leg upward causes pain, spasm of the hamstring muscles, and resistance to further leg extension at the knee (Fig. 33–10*A*).

To assess for *Brudzinski's sign,* with the client supine lift the head rapidly up from the bed. If meningeal irritation is present, forward neck flexion produces flexion of both thighs at the hips and flexure movements of the ankles and knees (Fig. 33–10*B*).

Medical diagnosis is made by assessment of clinical manifestations and is confirmed by isolating the causative organism from the CSF. Gram stain of the CSF reveals organisms in 70% to 80% of cases.[40] When the organism cannot be identified, bacterial antigens can be determined. *H. influenzae* is frequently diagnosed with this technique. Clients with bacterial pneumomeningitis show the following:

1. Moderately elevated CSF pressures
2. Elevated CSF protein (over 100 mg/dl)
3. Decreased CSF glucose (40 mg/dl)
4. Elevated white blood count, usually an increased cell count (100–10,000/cm), with predominantly polymorphonuclear leukocytes

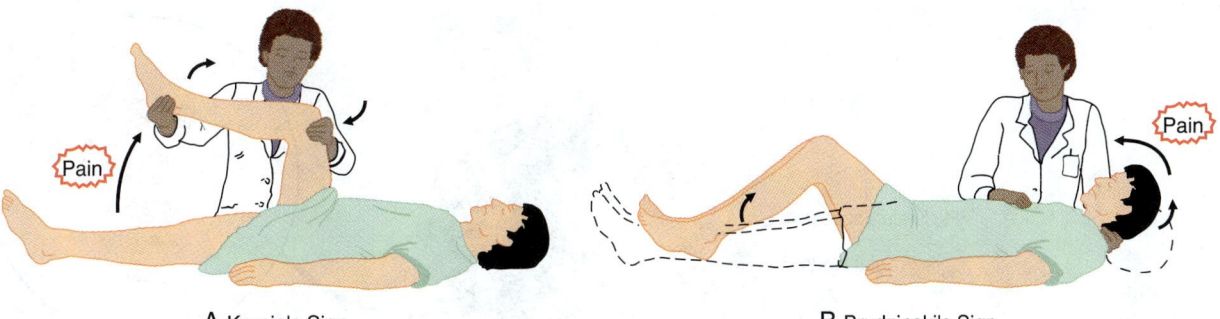

A Kernig's Sign   **B** Brudzinski's Sign

Figure 33–10. Assessment of meningeal irritation. *A,* Kernig's sign. *B,* Brudzinski's sign.

Bacterial meningitis is a medical emergency. If untreated, it can be fatal within hours to days. Intervention depends on the causative microorganism and the source of the infection. Large doses of the appropriate antibiotic are usually prescribed for at least 10 days. With the exception of chloramphenicol, common antibiotics do not readily penetrate the normal blood-brain barrier. Fortunately, meningeal inflammation improves passage. High doses of penicillins and third-generation cephalosporins are the preferred agents. Antibiotics are given intravenously; the blood-brain barrier recovers as inflammation subsides and high doses are required in order to reach the CSF. Adequate fluid and electrolyte balance needs to be maintained. Assess neurologic status frequently, hourly if appropriate, to detect early signs of increasing ICP and seizures. Anticonvulsants may be prescribed for seizures. If the primary focus of infection is located in specific parts, such as the parasinuses, or if mastoid or cranial osteomyelitis is present, surgery may be indicated after the acute phases of meningitis have subsided. Outbreaks of meningitis can be a major health problem in the community, especially when they occur in schools. Refer to your facility's isolation protocols.

The use of antibiotics has reduced the mortality rate of all types of bacterial meningitis. Prognosis varies according to the causative organism. Mortality is less than 5%.[40] Deaths most often occur in newborn infants and the elderly. Complications are rare but may include septic shock, vasomotor collapse, seizures, and increased ICP due to hydrocephalus, brain swelling, and fluid overload. Residual neurologic deficits are rare in adults.

Bacterial Toxins

Toxins produced by several pathogenic bacteria have a special affinity for the nervous system. They cause conditions such as tetanus, diphtheria, and botulism.

Tetanus is caused by the anaerobic spore-forming rod *Clostridium tetani.* The spores produce a toxin when introduced into a wound. The toxin suppresses spinal and brain stem inhibitory neurons and may act directly on skeletal muscle at the point of entry.

Clinical manifestations may be limited to painful mus-

cular spasms and contractions in the affected extremity. However, generalized tetanus is more common, with production of spasms beginning with the spasm of the masticatory muscles of the jaw (trismus) and progressing to spasms of the muscles of the neck, trunk, limbs, and the respiratory and pharyngeal muscles. Seizures and impaired respiration may occur. The affected muscles become constantly rigid, with painful paroxysms of tonic contractions in response to even the slightest external stimuli.

Interventions include the following:

● Surgery to debride any associated wounds
● Single dose of tetanus immune globulin (Hyper-Tet)
● Ten-day course of penicillin G (tetracycline, erythromycin, and chloramphenicol are alternative agents)
● Respiratory support, including possible mechanical ventilation
● Chlorpromazine, meprobamate, or diazepam to control muscle spasms
● Enteral feeding if the client has dysphagia
● Prophylactic anticoagulation to prevent thrombus

The overall mortality rate for tetanus is 25% to 50%, even in modern facilities with extensive resources. Tetanus is best prevented by immunization and regular booster doses of toxoid.

Brain Abscess

A brain abscess is a collection of either encapsulated or free pus within brain tissue arising from a primary focus elsewhere (e.g., ear, mastoid sinuses, nasal sinuses, heart, distal bones, lungs, or primary bacteremia [Fig. 33–11]). Brain abscess occasionally follows penetrating head trauma or intracranial surgery. *Staphylococcus* is the most common organism in trauma-related cases, whereas *Toxoplasma* is the usual agent found in clients with human immunodeficiency virus (HIV) infection. Brain abscesses vary in size. A large abscess may involve most of one cerebral hemisphere. Other abscesses are microscopic. Brain abscesses are relatively rare. They may occur at any age but more commonly occur in persons under age

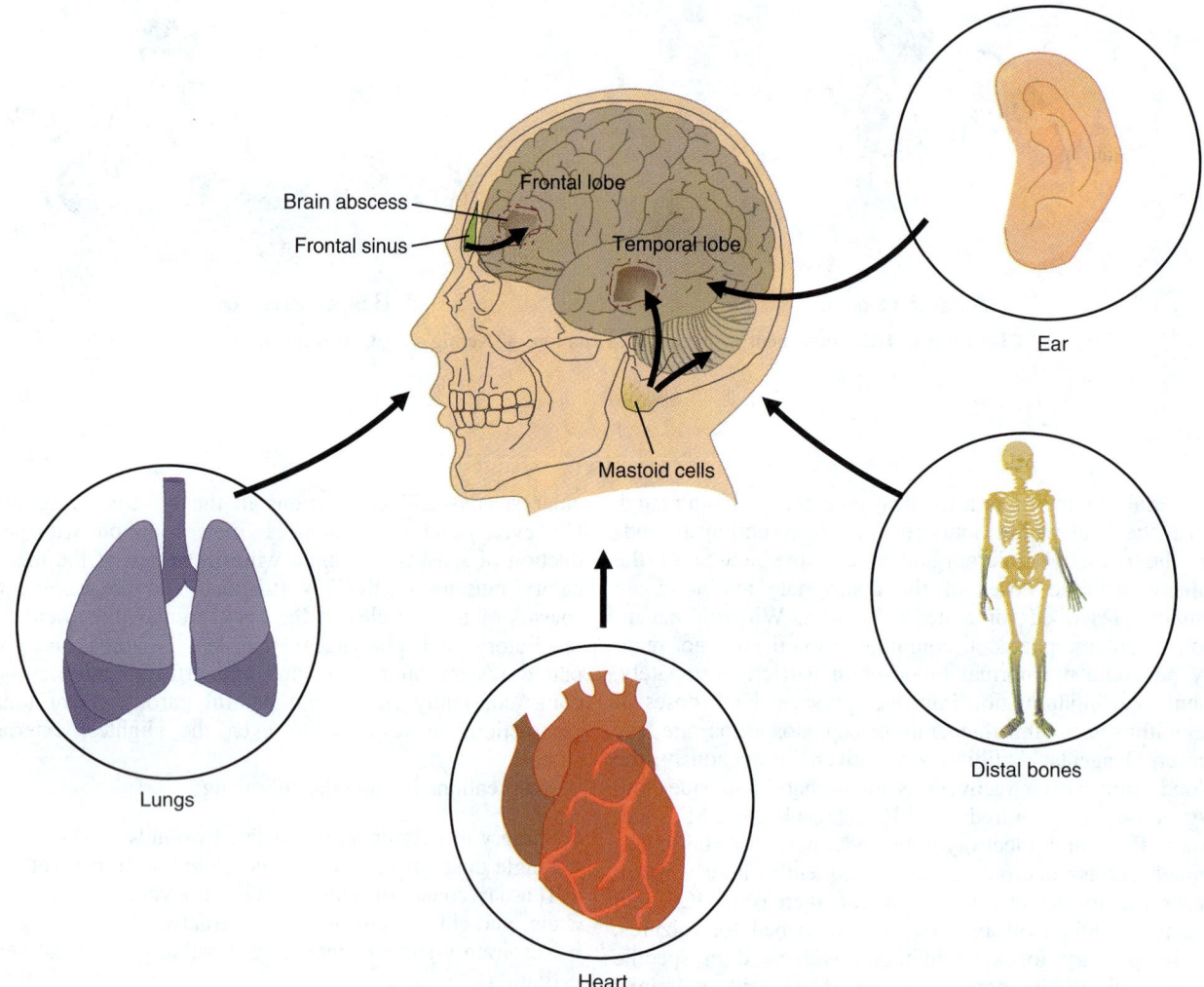

Figure 33–11. Origins and locations of cerebral abscesses. (After Bullock, B. L., & Rosendahl, P. P. [1992]. *Pathophysiology: Adaptations and alterations in function* [3rd ed., p. 1080]. Philadelphia: J. B. Lippincott.)

30. The current mortality rate is 5% to 15%, depending on the location of the abscess and the client's preexisting problems. Age, cause, number of abscesses, or use of corticosteroids does not affect outcome.[36]

In its early stages, the abscess produces inflammation, necrotic tissue, and surrounding edema. Within several days, the center of the abscess is purulent, and a wall of granulation tissue forms, encapsulating the abscess. Infection may spread through thin places in the wall of the capsule, resulting in development of additional abscesses.

Clinical manifestations of a brain abscess are essentially the same as with any space-occupying brain lesion. Headache and lethargy are the most common symptoms. Clinical indications of infection (e.g., fever, chills) are present about half the time. Other early findings include the following:

1. Drowsiness and confusion
2. Transient focal neurologic disorders (e.g., weakness on one side, loss of speech)
3. Depressed mental status

Early manifestations may improve or subside, and within

a few days or weeks, indications of increasing ICP may develop (e.g., recurrent headaches, changes in LOC, and focal or generalized seizures). Medical diagnosis of brain abscess is made through CT and MRI.

Pyogenic brain abscess may be treated with antibiotic therapy alone or antibiotics combined with surgical aspiration or excision. Needle aspiration may be performed stereotactically (guided by CT imaging) while the client is under local anesthesia. Corticosteroids may also be given to reduce cerebral edema. Penicillin is the antibiotic of choice for this type of infection. When antibiotics are used to treat the abscess, follow-up CT scans are used to monitor progress.

Viral Infections

Neurologic viral infections are usually associated with systemic viral infections and can be devastating. Viruses may enter the body via the respiratory system, mouth, or genitalia or from an insect or animal bite. The organism invades the CNS via the cerebral capillaries and choroid plexus or along peripheral nerves. Viruses multiply in the body and cause viremia (blood infected with viruses). Some viruses appear to have an affinity for specific cell types within the CNS.

There is no adequate treatment for most CNS viral infections. Immunizations are available for a few viral conditions (e.g., poliomyelitis and rabies). However, they are not available for most viral encephalitides. Currently, mass immunization is practical only for acute anterior poliomyelitis. The best control of other viral disorders is to identify and eliminate vectors responsible for their transmission.

Viral Meningitis

Acute viral meningitis ("aseptic" meningitis) is most often caused by the mumps virus or one of the picornaviruses. Aseptic meningitis infecting the subarachnoid space usually resolves within 2 weeks.

Clinical manifestations are mild. The client may be drowsy, photophobic, may have a headache and pain when moving the eyes, and may experience neck (nuchal rigidity) and spine stiffness on flexion. Other generalized manifestations include weakness, rash, and painful extremities. Fever and signs of meningeal irritation may be present. Physical examination reveals the presence of nuchal rigidity, and positive Brudzinski's and Kernig's signs. Acute and convalescent serologic testing and appropriate viral cultures may identify the specific virus.

Interventions for clients with aseptic meningitis are related to symptom management. Keep the client at bedrest during the acute phase. Plan intervention to relieve headache, control fever, and increase comfort. If seizures occur, anticonvulsants are prescribed.

Viral Encephalitis

Encephalitis is an inflammation of the brain parenchyma. Many viruses can cause encephalitis. The two most common are arthropod-borne (arbo)virus encephalitis and herpes simplex type 1 virus encephalitis. Also, the viruses that cause viral meningitis may cause severe viral encephalitis. They become very destructive when they invade brain parenchyma. The course of the illness is unpredictable. Death occurs in about 10% of cases. Herpes simplex encephalitis has a mortality rate of 10% to 40%. Of the clients who recover, about 20% have some disability, including mental deterioration, personality changes, and hemiparesis. Residual disability is even higher with eastern equine encephalitis.

Viral encephalitis is an acute febrile illness. Clinical manifestations include the following:

1. Meningeal irritation
2. Seizures
3. Confusion and delirium
4. Stupor or coma
5. Aphasia

6. Motor involvement (e.g., hemiparesis and asymmetrical reflexes)
7. Involuntary movements

■ Arbovirus Encephalitis

Arbovirus encephalitis is caused by arboviruses that multiply in a blood-sucking vector (e.g., mosquito or tick) and are transmitted to humans by the insect's bite. The incidence of diseases caused by arboviruses is characteristically seasonal and geographical. Become familiar with those in your area. In the United States, they occur in late summer and early fall. The most common types are the St. Louis and eastern and western equine encephalitides.

The infection sites are usually microscopic and scattered throughout the cerebral gray and white matter except for eastern equine encephalitis, which may destroy major parts of a lobe or hemisphere. Two-thirds of persons who develop eastern equine encephalitis either die or develop severe residual disabilities including mental retardation, seizures, blindness, deafness, speech disorders, and hemiplegia.

Clinical manifestations with all arbovirus encephalitides are similar. The onset is gradual in adults and older children, with headache, nausea, vomiting, listlessness, and fever. After a few days, seizures, nuchal rigidity, stupor, and coma develop. Photophobia, hemiparesis, and asymmetrical reflexes may be present. Fever and neurologic signs subside within 2 weeks if the client does not develop irreversible CNS changes or die.

■ Herpes Simplex Virus Encephalitis

Herpes simplex virus encephalitis occurs at any time of year and throughout the world. It affects particularly the middle-aged. The gradually evolving initial clinical manifestations are similar to those of other acute encephalitides. However, this virus has an affinity for the inferomedial portions of the frontal and temporal lobes. The client soon becomes acutely ill with headache, fever, vomiting, and, often, seizures. Signs of a localized lesion develop, including visual field deficits. If not aggressively treated, temporal lobe swelling leads to transtentorial herniation, coma, and brain death. A biopsy may be done in an attempt to identify the herpesvirus. Although biopsy is definitive for the disease, there are risks. MRI is an effective and safe diagnostic tool.

Intervention for herpes simplex encephalitis is a 10-day course of intravenous acyclovir, an antiviral agent. To be effective, it must be given early in the course of the disease. Despite treatment, the course of the disease may continue. The prognosis is grave but not hopeless. The mortality rate is above 30%, and the client may die within 2 weeks. Of those who survive, many are left with severe neurologic and mental disabilities such as global dementia, seizures, and aphasia.

Nursing intervention is a challenge. An acutely ill client is often restless and combative and exhibits bizarre behavior. Extensive rehabilitation is often needed. Such clients need careful protection from injury, and the family requires supportive care. If residual behavior changes and mental deterioration develop, help the family adjust to changes in the client. Refer the family to agency or community support groups.

Acute Anterior Poliomyelitis

The poliovirus, an RNA picornavirus, is the causative agent of acute poliomyelitis. Outbreaks are sporadic in areas where there are nonimmunized persons. It most commonly infects the victim in summer and early fall.

Since the 1950s, mass immunization programs have significantly reduced the worldwide incidence of acute anterior poliomyelitis. The goal of the World Health Organization is to have polio eradicated by the year 2000. Significant progress toward this goal has been made.[33] The best time for this immunization is in infancy. Trivalent oral poliomyelitis vaccine has almost completely replaced both the inactivated (Salk) and monovalent (Sabin) vaccines because it is easy to administer and supervise. A few infections secondary to other enteroviruses in unvaccinated clients occasionally occur.

Acute anterior poliomyelitis ("polio," infantile paralysis) is characterized by destruction of motor cells, particularly anterior horn cells in the spinal cord and brain stem (bulbar), especially the medulla, and flaccid paralysis of muscles innervated by affected neurons. Poliomyelitis is caused by one of three types of poliovirus and spreads from the gastrointestinal tract to the nervous system.

Spinal paralysis, restricted to spinal segments, is flaccid, asymmetrical, and scattered in distribution. It tends to be more severe in one extremity (most often a leg). Involvement of the diaphragm and intercostal muscles or damage to the respiratory center involving the reticular activating center in the medulla oblongata may produce respiratory paralysis. Occasionally, transient bladder paralysis occurs. Bulbar paralysis involves the muscles supplied by the cranial nerves because bulbar nuclei are also affected. These muscles may be paralyzed alone or in combination with spinal musculature. Bulbar paralysis is often unilateral. Protein and white blood cell levels in the CSF are elevated. It is difficult to distinguish polio from Guillain-Barré syndrome (see Chapter 34). However, for practical purposes, no other acute disorder produces headaches, stiff neck, fever, and asymmetrical flaccid paralysis without sensory loss coupled with an increase in white blood cells in the CSF.

Clients with respiratory muscle paralysis need intensive care. Mechanical ventilation at the first sign of respiratory compromise greatly increases the client's chances of recovery.

Postpolio syndrome is a recently recognized disorder affecting survivors of polio. This syndrome is characterized by new onset of progressive muscle weakness, fatigue, decreased endurance, pain in the joints and muscles, and respiratory problems beginning 30 or more years after the original attack. Clients may experience any or all of these manifestations. The cause and pathophysiology of this syndrome are not well understood, particularly because the interval between the original illness and the postpolio syndrome is so long.

Postpolio syndrome can be very discouraging to clients who have successfully adapted to a certain level of disability. Further restriction of physical capabilities is difficult for the client and significant others to accept. Emotional support is as vital as teaching the client to balance rest and activity and to utilize new adaptive techniques. Development of respiratory difficulty may be particularly frightening to those clients who required ventilatory support with an iron lung (a respirator that encompassed all of the body except the head) during their initial illness.

Fungal Infections

Fungi may cause meningitis, meningoencephalitis, intracranial thrombophlebitis, or brain abscess. CNS fungal infections are rare. When they do occur, these infections are usually complications of another condition. Conditions that increase the risk of fungal infections include those that interfere with the body's normal flora or suppress the immune response, such as acquired immunodeficiency syndrome (AIDS), leukemia, organ transplant, diabetes, and collagen-vascular disease.

● Coccidioidomycosis mainly involves the lungs; it occasionally spreads to the meninges.
● Cryptococcosis is the most frequent CNS fungal infection. The *Cryptococcus,* a common soil fungus, can cause granulomatous meningitis. Small granulomas and cysts are found within the cortex, and large granulomas and cystic nodules are found deep within the brain. This organism is an opportunist, and the incidence of cryptococcosis has risen since the onset of the AIDS epidemic. Assessment findings vary, and diagnosis is confirmed by finding *Cryptococcus neoformans* in the CSF. If untreated, this infection is fatal within a few weeks.
● Mucormycosis, a malignant infection of cerebral vessels, is a rare complication of diabetic acidosis. It begins in the nose and paranasal sinuses and spreads to the brain. It may be associated with fungal meningitis.

CNS fungal infections produce clinical manifestations similar to those of bacterial infections. The main interventions for these infections are intravenous amphotericin B combined with flucytosine for 4 to 6 weeks. With this treatment, recovery is almost certain, except for clients with advanced infections or other overwhelming, fatal diseases. Cryptococcal meningitis in clients with AIDS is highly refractory and has a 50% to 60% relapse rate.

The most common opportunistic infection to attack the CNS of the AIDS patient is toxoplasmosis. It is usually manifested as single or multiple brain abscesses.

Initial clinical manifestations are headache, confusion, lethargy, and low-grade fever. Greater than 65% of clients develop such focal signs as weakness, ataxia, speech disturbances, apraxia, seizures, and sensory disturbances.[35] Treatment consists of pyrimethamine (Daraprim), sulfadiazine or clindamycin (Cleocin), and leucovorin (folinic acid or Wellcovorin). If a therapeutic response is seen, the client is kept on maintenance dosages.

Parasitic Infestations

In South America and Mexico the parasite most commonly affecting the CNS is *Cysticercus*. The tapeworm, in larval form, causes a systemic infestation. Pork may contain tapeworms. If pork is eaten in a raw or undercooked state, the tapeworm is passed into the human gastrointestinal tract, where it grows. It enters the bloodstream and establishes a cyst within an organ. The cyst, which may be 3 to 15 mm in diameter, contains the larvae of the tapeworm. These larvae die approximately 18 months after infestation. Calcification of the cyst and inflammation follow. Clients may have more than one cyst.

CT scan or MRI identifies the cysts. Cysticercosis titers may be identified in the blood and CSF; however, surgical biopsy is often performed to confirm the diagnosis. Praziquantel is the drug used to treat cysticercosis. The mechanism of action is to eliminate the tapeworm from the gastrointestinal system. If pharmacologic treatment is ineffective, surgical excision of the cyst may be recommended.

Bulbar Disorders

Some neurologic disorders involve the lower brain stem, altering bulbar function and resulting in difficulties in respiration, talking, swallowing, and coughing. Such conditions include tetanus, myasthenia gravis, and bulbar poliomyelitis.

Bulbar involvement is evidenced by hoarseness, dysarthria, pooling of food and saliva in the pharynx, increased oropharyngeal secretions, inability or difficulty swallowing (dysphagia), hypoxia, and laryngeal stridor. Airway obstruction, pulmonary aspiration, and asphyxia may occur. Mortality is high with bulbar disorders.

When caring for clients with bulbar dysfunction, watch for early indications of hypoxia such as anxiety, restlessness, apprehension, sleeplessness, increasing respiratory effort, decreasing arterial oxygen saturation via pulse oximeter, and increasing pulse rate. Early indications of hypoxia may be very subtle.

Quickly assess for possible causes of airway obstruction if hypoxia is evident. A tracheostomy and possibly mechanical ventilation may be needed. Many clients with bulbar problems are conscious but immobile and have difficulty speaking. Their progressive loss of respiratory function is terrifying. Thorough, ongoing assessment and supportive communication help reduce distress. Intervene before the client becomes apneic.

Nursing intervention for clients with bulbar involvement is similar to that described for clients with altered states of consciousness. This is especially true for assessing vital signs, preventing deformities, and maintaining a patent airway and fluid and electrolyte balance.

Clients with bulbar disorders may benefit from having a formal swallowing evaluation done by a speech therapist. If the client has no manifestations of dysphagia, conduct a bedside evaluation. To test the client's ability to swallow, have him or her sit up with the head slightly flexed. Do not tilt the client's head backward because this opens the airway. Offer a small amount of nectar (e.g., thick, fruity juice such as apricot nectar) or firm gelatin or pudding. The consistency of these foods is easier to swallow than thin liquids. Watch to see if the client is able to swallow. If aspiration occurs, suction the fluid quickly from the back of the mouth and throat.

Before feeding, give mouth care to keep the mouth clean and induce salivation. Soft foods are easiest to swallow. Avoid milk products. Offer liquids in a small glass or cup. The client may not be able to suck or swallow when using a straw. Clients with progressive dysphagia may need enteral feedings to maintain adequate nutrition. Make sure they obtain enough calories.

The extent of bulbar paralysis and return of muscle function vary. A client with persisting partial bulbar paralysis is particularly disabled and may need a permanent tracheostomy tube. When suction equipment is needed in the client's home, someone must be taught to use it efficiently. Eating, drinking, and common colds are all potentially hazardous for clients with bulbar problems.

Conclusions

Neurologic nursing is one of the most challenging nursing specialties. Nurses play a pivotal role in early detection of manifestations related to an intracranial tumor or infection. Nurses also play an essential role in the prevention of further neurologic damage through management of seizures and ICP associated with cranial tumors and infections.

Thinking Critically

1. A client suffered a temporal lobe contusion from a motor vehicle accident 3 days ago. He is disoriented to time and place and has short-term memory deficits. During your assessment of the client, he stops answering questions and begins tonic movements of his extremities.

Factors to Consider. What are the highest priorities at this time? What are the interventions related to these priorities? What interventions come next? What significance does the site of injury have?

2. A 78-year-old woman with a history of hypertension has a cerebrovascular accident (CVA). Her family reports that she has felt good and has refused to take her anti-hypertension medication. She has hemiparesis and is able to respond verbally. She does not recognize people or objects who are in her line of vision on the left side. Three days post-CVA she is able to move her fingers and wiggle her toes on the affected side, and she is transferred to the rehabilitation unit. What are the most likely multidisciplinary plans for this client? How should you proceed with teaching about prevention of complications, motivation to comply

with the prescribed therapies, and the importance of anti-hypertension medications?

Factors to Consider. How soon will the client be transferred to a rehabilitation unit? How soon can teaching begin? How will you teach the client and family to best prepare them for care after discharge to the home for continuing care?

3. A client with a history of headaches, dizziness, and vertigo experienced a first-time seizure at age 27. Following this episode, he experienced blurred vision. Subsequent studies revealed the presence of a brain tumor, and cranial surgery was scheduled. Two days after surgery, the client is transferred to the regular unit. What are your responsibilities regarding monitoring for an increase in intracranial pressure? What are the general interventions for the client after craniotomy?

Factors to Consider. What is the major complication following intracranial surgery? How do the general interventions prevent complications associated with this type of surgery?

Bibliography

1. Adams, B. A., Clancey, J. K., & Eddy, M. S. (1991). Malignant glioma: Current treatment and perspectives. *Journal of Neuroscience Nursing, 23*(1), 15–20.
2. Adams, J. H., & Duchen, L. H. (1992). *Greenfield's Neuropathology.* New York: Oxford University Press.
3. Albrecht, H., et al. (1995). Disseminated toxoplasmosis in AIDS patients—Report of 16 cases. *Scandinavian Journal of Infectious Diseases, 27,* 71–74.
4. Arbour, R. (1994). Laser and ultrasound technology in aggressive management of central nervous system tumors. *Journal of Neuroscience Nursing, 26*(1), 30–35.
5. Barfield, H., & Mae, D. (1996). Recognizing post-polio syndrome. *Hospital Practice, 31*(5), 75–94.
6. Begley, C. E., et al. (1994). Cost of epilepsy in the United States: A model based on incidence and prognosis. *Epilepsia, 35*(16), 1230–1243.
7. Beyers, V. L. (1993). Novel antiepileptic drugs: Nursing implications. *Journal of Neuroscience Nursing, 25*(6), 375–379.
8. Brucia, J. J., Owen, D. C., & Rudy, E. B. (1992). The effects of lidocaine on intracranial hypertension. *Journal of Neuroscience Nursing, 24*(4), 205–214.
9. Dean, E. (1991). Clinical decision making in the management of the late sequelae of poliomyelitis. *Physical Therapy, 71*(10), 752–761.
10. Desmeules, M., Mikkelsen, T., & Mao, Y. (1992). Increasing incidence of primary malignant brain tumors: Influence of diagnostic methods. *Journal of the National Cancer Institute, 84*(6), 442–445.
11. Devinsky, O. (1994). Seizure disorders. *Clinical Symposia, 46*(1), 1–54.
12. Foote, A. W., Holcombe, J. (1994). Acoustic neuroma: Suggestions for helping the patient adapt after translabyrinthine surgery. *Journal of Neuroscience Nursing, 26*(3), 162–165.
13. Fowler, S. B., Wagner, B. K., & Hertzog, J. (1995). Pharmacologic interventions for agitation in head-injured patients in the acute care setting. *Journal of Neuroscience Nursing, 27*(2), 119–123.
14. French, J. (1994). The long-term therapeutic management of epilepsy. *Annals of Internal Medicine, 120,* 411–422.
15. Gilman, S. (1992). Advances in neurology. Pt. 2. *New England Journal of Medicine, 326*(25), 1671–1676.
16. Gregory, R. J. (1995). Understanding and coping with neurological impairment. *Rehabilitation Nursing, 20*(2), 74–78.
17. Guyton, A. C., & Hall, J. E. (1996). Textbook of medical science (9th ed.). Philadelphia: W. B. Saunders.
18. Habel, M., & Strong, P. (1996). The late effects of poliomyelitis: Nursing interventions for a unique patient population. *Medsurg Nursing, 5*(2), 77–86.
19. Hauser, W. A., & Hesdorffer, D. C. (Eds.). (1990). *Epilepsy: Frequency, causes and consequences.* New York: Demos Press.
20. Hickey, J. V. (1992). The clinical practice of neurological and neurosurgical nursing. Philadelphia: J. B. Lippincott.
21. Hodges, K., & Root, L. M. (1991). Surgical management of intractable seizure disorders. *Journal of Neuroscience Nursing, 23*(2), 93–98.
22. Howes, D. S. (1992). Bacterial meningitis: Closing in on the standards of care. *Emergency Medicine, 24*(5), 35–36, 41–42, 44, 47–48.
23. Johnson, R. T. (1996). Emerging viral infections. *Archives of Neurology, 53,* 18–22.
24. Kovalic, J. J., et al. (1993). Intracranial ependymoma: Long term outcome, patterns of failure. *Journal of Neuro-Oncology, 15,* 125–131.
25. Krause, E. A., et al. (1991). Radiosurgery: A nursing perspective. *Journal of Neuroscience Nursing, 23*(1), 24–28.
26. Lannon, S. L. (1993). Epilepsy in the elderly. *Journal of Neuroscience Nursing, 25*(5), 273–282.
27. Macabasco, A., & Hickman, J. (1995). Thrombolytic therapy for brain attack. *Journal of Neuroscience Nursing, 27*(3), 138–151.
28. Mahaley, M. S. (1989). National survey of patterns of care for brain-tumor patients. *Journal of Neurosurgery, 71*(6), 826–830.
29. Marshall, S. B., et al. (1990). *Neuroscience critical care: Pathophysiology and patient management.* Philadelphia: W. B. Saunders.
30. McCance, K. L., & Huether, S. E. (1994). Pathophysiology: The biologic basis for disease in adults and children (2nd ed.). St. Louis: Mosby–Year Book.
31. Michael, J. E., Wegener, K., & Barnes, D. W. (1993). Vagus nerve stimulation for intractable seizures: One year follow-up. *Journal of Neuroscience Nursing, 25*(6), 362–366.
32. Mitchell, M. (1989). *Neuroscience nursing: A nursing diagnosis approach.* Baltimore: Williams & Wilkins.
33. *Morbidity and Mortality Weekly Report.* (1995). Progress toward global poliomyelitis eradication, 1985–1994. *44*(14), 273–275.
34. Newton, C., & Mateo, M. A. (1994). Uncertainty: Strategies for patients with brain tumor and their families. *Cancer Nursing, 17*(2), 137–140.
35. Newton, H. B. (1995). Common neurologic complications of HIV-1 infection and AIDS. *American Family Physician, 51*(2), 387–398.
36. Quagliarello, V., & Scheld, M. W. (1992). Bacterial meningitis: Pathogenesis, pathophysiology and progress. *New England Journal of Medicine, 327*(12), 864–871.
37. Sabiston, D. (1991). *Textbook of surgery* (14th ed.). Philadelphia: W. B. Saunders.
38. Simon, R. (1992). Parameningeal infections. In J. Wyngaarden, L. Smith, & J. Bennett (Eds.), *Cecil Textbook of Medicine.* Philadelphia: W. B. Saunders.
39. Singer, J. M. (1995). Supratentorial low grade gliomas in adults: A retrospective analysis of 43 cases treated with surgery and radiotherapy. *European Journal of Surgical Oncology, 21,* 198–200.
40. Swartz, M. N. (1992). Bacterial meningitis. In J. Wyngaarden, L. Smith, & J. Bennett (Eds.), *Cecil textbook of medicine.* Philadelphia: W. B. Saunders.
41. Theodore, W. H., et al. (1992). Temporal lobectomy for uncontrolled seizures: The role of positron emission tomography. *Annals of Neurology, 32*(6), 789–793.
42. Vick, N. A. (1992). Intracranial tumors: General considerations. In J. Wyngaarden, L. Smith, & J. Bennett (Eds.), *Cecil textbook of medicine.* Philadelphia: W. B. Saunders.
43. Wilder, B. J. (1995). The treatment of epilepsy: An overview of clinical practices. *Neurology, 45*(Suppl. 2), S7–S11.
44. Willis, D. (1991). Intracranial astrocytoma: Pathology, diagnosis and clinical presentation. *Journal of Neuroscience Nursing, 23*(1), 7.
45. Wilson, L. D. (1993). Sensory perceptual alteration. *Nursing Clinics of North America, 28*(4), 747–765.
46. Wyngaarden, J., Smith, L., & Bennett, J. (1992). *Cecil textbook of medicine.* Philadelphia: W. B. Saunders.
47. Youmans, J. R. (Ed.). (1990). *Neurological surgery: A comprehensive reference guide to the diagnosis and management of neurosurgical problems* (3rd ed.). Philadelphia: W. B. Saunders.

Nursing Care of Clients with Degenerative Neurologic Disorders

Judith Ozuna

CHAPTER

34

Degenerative neurologic disorders pose a great challenge to the client, the family, and the caregiver, be it the nurse, a family member, or a significant other. By their very nature these disorders cause progressive decline in neurologic function. Some progress relatively quickly, that is, over months to 1 or 2 years, while others progress more gradually, sometimes over decades. Common nursing diagnoses for clients with these disorders are impaired thought processes, memory deficit, visual-perceptual alteration, impaired physical mobility, incontinence, self-care deficit, and impaired individual and family coping. A major goal of intervention is to help the client achieve an optimal level of functioning in light of chronic neurologic deficits.

Clients with degenerative neurologic disease will most often be diagnosed in an outpatient setting. However, they may require hospital admission when acute relapses or life-threatening events occur. Many clients return to their homes and have regular follow-up in outpatient clinics. However, some may require rehabilitation, in either inpatient or outpatient settings, for newly acquired deficits. Others may require transfer to long-term care facilities because of significant decline in ability to provide self-care. Still others may not survive their acute illness.

Alzheimer's Disease

Alzheimer's disease (AD) is a form of dementia. Dementia involves progressive decline in two or more areas of cognition, usually memory and one or more of the following: language, calculation, visuospatial perception, constructional praxis, judgment, abstraction, and personality. Dementia of the Alzheimer's type (DAT) constitutes at least half of all dementias (see Chapter 31 for a general discussion of dementia).

Recent studies have shown that the prevalence of DAT is higher than previously thought.[8, 19] DAT occurs in 10% to 15% of people over age 65, in 19% of people over age

75, and in 47% of people over age 85. Thus, the incidence of DAT increases greatly with increasing age.

Etiology and Risk Factors

The cause of DAT has not been found, although several risk factors have been identified. As can be seen by the statistics listed earlier, increasing age is a risk factor. Genetic factors can influence DAT. At least four chromosomes (1,14,19,21) are involved in some forms of familial DAT. However, the lack of 100% concordance in studies of identical twins implies that environmental, metabolic, and other factors also may play a role. Nearly all persons with Down syndrome develop dementia and the pathologic features of DAT. Female sex, head trauma, lack of education, and myocardial infarction have been linked to AD, but these associations are weak.[6] Some have postulated that aluminum intoxication, disordered immune function, and viral infection are causes of DAT; however, these factors have not been proved.[7]

Although the major risk factors for AD (age, family history) cannot be controlled, efforts to reduce the incidence of head trauma and cardiovascular disease may help reduce the incidence of Alzheimer's and other types of dementia.

Pathophysiology

Alois Alzheimer first described presenile dementia in 1907. He used a new staining technique of human brain tissue to demonstrate the pathologic changes. The changes he noted are now termed *neurofibrillary tangles* and *neuritic plaques* (Fig. 34–1). These are abnormal proteins that accumulate in the brain. The neuritic plaque is a cluster of degenerating nerve terminals, both dendritic and axonal, that contain amyloid protein. Neurofibrillary tangles are abnormal neurons in which the cytoplasm is filled with bundles of abnormal protein called *paired heli-*

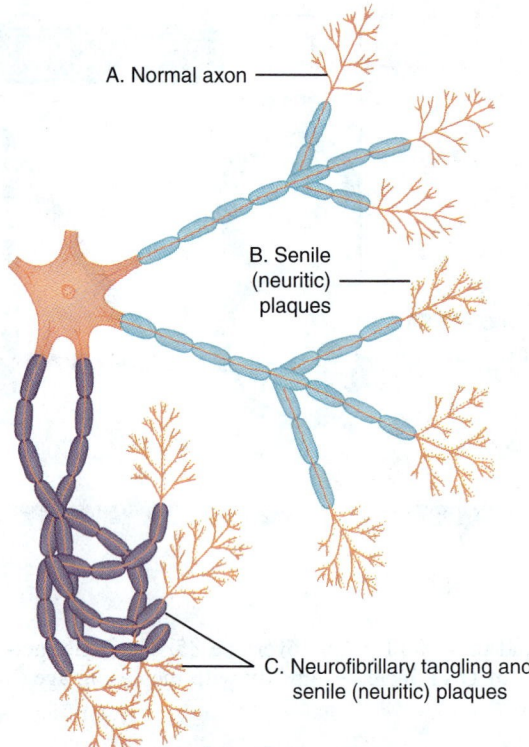

A. Normal axon

B. Senile (neuritic) plaques

C. Neurofibrillary tangling and senile (neuritic) plaques

Figure 34–1. Neurofibrillary tangles. Neurofibrillary tangles replace the normal neuronal cytoplasm in Alzheimer's disease and some other neurologic disorders. The tangles are often seen with senile plaques and appear throughout the cortex, hippocampus, and amygdala. The number of plaques and tangles correlates roughly with the severity of the dementia. *A,* Normal axon. *B,* Senile plaques on ends of axon. *C,* Neurofibrillary tangles and senile plaques replacing normal axon.

cal filaments. Neuritic plaques and neurofibrillary tangles are located in areas of cell loss in the brain of the person with DAT. These areas are the association areas of the neocortex and the hippocampus, which account for the cognitive decline. The term "association" is used to describe all the intellectual activities of the cerebral cortex. These functions include learning and reasoning, memory storage and recall, language abilities, and even consciousness.

In addition to structural changes, there are neurotransmitter changes in the brains of clients with DAT. A decline in cholinergic neurons in the basal nucleus leads to loss of choline acetyltransferase in the neocortex and hippocampus. Also affected are neuronal systems that project to the neocortex: the noradrenergic locus ceruleus and the serotonergic dorsal raphe nucleus in the brain stem. These two areas also contain neurofibrillary tangles. Involved neurons in the neocortex include those using corticotropin-releasing factor, somatostatin, and glutamate.[15]

Clinical Manifestations and Diagnostic Findings

Clinically, Alzheimer's disease is characterized by a relentless impairment of decision-making that generally be-

gins insidiously and can progress for a decade or so. The onset of DAT typically occurs in late middle age (age 65 and older), although some familial cases occur in the 40s and 50s.

First Stage. The sequence of loss of higher cognitive functions is a helpful clue in establishing the clinical diagnosis. The clinical progression of manifestations is usually divided into three stages (Box 34–1). Memory disturbance is usually the first feature of the disease. Family members or co-workers often notice the memory

---

Box 34–1. Common Clinical Manifestations in Each Stage of Dementia of the Alzheimer's Type

Stage I (duration of disease 1–3 years)

Memory—new learning defective, remote recall mildly impaired
Visuospatial skills—topographic disorientation, poor complex constructions
Language—poor wordlist generation, anomia
Personality—indifference, occasional irritability
Psychiatric features—sadness or delusions in some
Motor system—normal
EEG—normal
CT/MRI—normal
PET/SPECT—bilateral posterior parietal hypometabolism/hyperperfusion

Stage II (duration of disease 2–10 years)

Memory—recent and remote recall more severely impaired
Visuospatial skills—poor constructions, spatial disorientation
Language—fluent aphasia
Calculation—acalculia
Praxis—ideomotor apraxia
Personality—indifference or irritability
Psychiatric features—delusions in some
Motor system—restlessness, pacing
EEG—slowing of background rhythm
CT/MRI—normal or ventricular dilation and sulcal enlargement
PET/SPECT—bilateral parietal and frontal hypometabolism/hypoperfusion

Stage III (duration of disease 8–12 years)

Intellectual functions—severely deteriorated
Motor—limb rigidity and flexion posture
Sphincter control—urinary and fecal incontinence
EEG—diffusely slow
CT/MRI—ventricular dilation and sulcal enlargement
PET/SPECT—bilateral parietal and frontal hypometabolism/hypoperfusion

---

EEG, electroencephalogram; CT, computed tomography; MRI, magnetic resonance imaging; PET, positron emission tomography; SPECT, single photon emission computed tomography.

From Cummings, J. L., & Benson, D. F. (1992). *Dementia: A clinical approach.* Boston: Butterworth-Heinemann.

loss before the individual does. The individual may demonstrate poor judgment and problem-solving skills and become careless in work habits and household chores. He or she may do well in familiar surroundings and be able to follow well-established routines but lack the ability to adapt to new challenges. The person may become irritable, suspicious, or indifferent. Agitation, apathy, dysphoria, and aberrant motor behavior have been associated with cognitive impairments.[16a]

Second Stage. In the second stage of illness, the client may demonstrate language disturbance, characterized by impaired word-finding and circumlocution (talking around a subject rather than directly about it). Later, spontaneous speech becomes increasingly empty, and paraphasias (words used in the wrong context) are used. The person may repeat words and phrases just spoken by himself or herself (palilalia) or by others (echolalia). Motor disturbance (apraxia) is characterized by difficulty in using everyday objects such as a toothbrush, comb, razor, and utensils. Apraxia combined with forgetfulness can create serious safety problems. The person may leave a burner on in the kitchen or forget to extinguish a cigarette. Indifference worsens and restlessness with frequent pacing appears. Hyperorality (the desire to take everything into the mouth to suck, chew, or taste) may develop. Swallowing may become difficult. Depression and irritability may worsen, and delusions and psychosis may appear. The person fears personal harm, theft of property, or infidelity of the spouse. He or she may see bugs crawling on the bed or throughout the house. Wandering at night is common. Occasional incontinence may occur.

Third Stage. In the final stage, virtually all mental abilities are lost, including speech. Voluntary movement is minimal, and the limbs become rigid with flexor posturing. Urinary incontinence and fecal incontinence are frequent. The person has lost all ability for self-care.

Because there is no definitive test for DAT, the diagnosis is made by exclusion of known causes of dementia (e.g., toxic or metabolic alterations, drug side effects, cerebrovascular disease, neoplasm, and infection). The diagnosis of DAT requires the presence of dementia involving two or more areas of cognition, insidious onset, steady progression, and loss of normal alertness.[16] When these criteria are applied, 9 of 10 persons given this diagnosis have DAT confirmed at autopsy. Postmortem examination of the brain is the only way DAT can be definitively diagnosed. The brain is viewed under the microscope for the presence of neuritic plaques and neurofibrillary tangles.

Diagnostic assessments such as the electroencephalogram (EEG), computed tomography (CT), and magnetic resonance imaging (MRI) are sometimes used in the diagnosis of DAT. Recently, PET scans have also been used to diagnose DAT. In general, these studies rule out other causes of dementia, such as seizures and cerebral bleeding, but do not diagnose DAT. Changes on EEG, CT, and MRI do not appear until the later stages of DAT. Finally, laboratory studies are performed to rule out metabolic and drug-related causes of dementia. They include urinalysis, complete blood count, sedimentation rate, electrolytes, blood urea nitrogen (BUN) and creatinine values, thyroid and liver function tests, calcium, serum B_{12} levels, syphilis serology, and human immunodeficiency virus (HIV) testing.[5]

Community and Self-Care

■ Medical Management

There is no cure for DAT. Results of studies in which acetylcholine (ACh) precursors (choline, lecithin, and deanol) and anticholinesterase agents (physostigmine and tetrahydroaminoacridine) are used to enhance memory and cognitive function have been disappointing. Tacrine (Cognex) was recently approved for delaying cognitive decline in DAT. It inhibits breakdown of acetylcholinesterase in the brain, allowing more ACh to be available for nerve impulse transmission. Because of potential liver toxicity, liver function tests must be checked weekly for 18 weeks. Other pharmacologic therapy is primarily aimed at treating behavioral problems, although behavioral and environmental manipulations are often more effective (Table 34–1). Low-dose antipsychotic agents, like haloperidol (Haldol), can be effective for agitation and confusion. The lowest effective dose should be used and should be given just before bedtime. Sometimes twice-a-day dosing is required. Adverse side effects such as akathisia (motor restlessness), parkinsonian symptoms, tardive dyskinesia, orthostatic hypotension, anticholinergic symptoms (urinary retention and confusion), and sedation should be monitored. Antidepressants (e.g., nortriptyline and desipramine) that have few anticholinergic side effects, fluoxetine, and trazadone are helpful for depression. Table 34–1 lists drugs that can be used to treat behavioral problems in DAT.

■ Nursing Management of the Medical Client

Assessment

When DAT is suspected, a complete history should be taken to assess for other causes of dementia. Data should be obtained from the client, family, and co-workers (if possible). Secondary sources are used because the client is often unaware of a problem with thought processing and minimizes it. The nurse should ask specific questions about difficulties with activities of daily living (ADL), increasing forgetfulness, and changes in personality. Past medical history should be assessed for previous head injury or surgery, recent falls, headache, and a family history of DAT. A Mini-Mental State examination may provide objective data for ongoing evaluation of the client (see Chapter 30).

DAT has a profound impact on psychosocial behaviors. The nurse should ask about the client's reactions to

Table 34-1. Pharmacologic Treatment of Behavioral Problems in Dementia of the Alzheimer's Type

Problem	Treatment Options

Suspiciousness, paranoia, sundowning	Behavioral
	Environmental
	Correct sensory impairment
	Low-dose antipsychotics
	  Loxapine (5–25 mg/day)
	    Causes fewer EPS
	    More sedative
	    Low-potency antipsychotic
	  Risperidone (1–4 mg/day)
	    Observe for EPS
	  Haloperidol (0.25–1.0 mg/day)

Anxiety	Treat underlying physical problems (pain, dyspnea, urinary urgency, sensory impairment) If acute, offer reassurance If related to confusion, use antipsychotics If diffuse or chronic, use short-acting benzodiazepine (e.g., oxazepam) Avoid non-benzodiazepine sedative-hypnotics, especially barbiturates Role of buspirone unclear
Acute catastrophic reactions	Lorazepam 1–4 mg IM Haloperidol 2–5 mg IM

Insomnia	Environmental, behavioral
	If associated confusion, use low-dose antipsychotics
	If associated depression, use:
	  Nortriptyline
	  Doxepin
	If associated restlessness with antipsychotic treatments:
	  Lorazepam
	  Observe for disinhibition or increased confusion
	  Ambien

Angry or violent outbursts	Very difficult to control
	Behavior log is key to determine relationship to stimuli such as:
	  Pain from arthritis or other chronic illness
	  Urinary problems
	  Constipation
	Low-dose antipsychotic
	  Risperidone, loxapine, clozapine
	Carbamazepine
	Lithium

EPS, extrapyramidal symptoms such as restlessness, drooling, stiffness, shuffling, cogwheel rigidity (like Parkinson's disease); IM, intramuscularly.

changes in routine or in the environment. It is not uncommon for a client with DAT to become very agitated over small changes. Likewise, apathy, social isolation, and irritability may be noted. As the brain continues to atrophy and the limbic system becomes dysfunctional, the client becomes paranoid, uses abusive language, and becomes suspicious of others.

DAT has a profound impact on the family. The nurse needs to assess the family for strengths and weaknesses, their ability to provide care for the client, and their financial concerns. In large centers, the assessment of the client and family is performed through a team approach. The Client Education Guide provides instructions and resources for caregivers of people with AD.

Diagnosis, Planning, Implementation

Impaired Verbal Communication. Use the nursing diagnosis *Impaired Verbal Communication related to neuronal degeneration* to describe the client with DAT.

Planning: Expected Outcomes. The client's needs will be communicated effectively, as evidenced by making his or her needs known and interacting meaningfully with others.

Implementation. In the initial stage of DAT, the client's receptive and expressive language skills are relatively intact. The nurse must be prepared to adapt to the communication level of the client. If the client speaks only single words or short phrases, the nurse should do

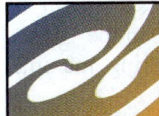

CLIENT EDUCATION GUIDE

Caring for Family Members with Alzheimer's Disease

Client Instructions in English (Instrucciones en Inglés)	Client Instructions in Spanish (Instrucciones en Español)
Be sure that you have verbal and written information about the disease, the results of diagnostic testing (including the results of neuropsychological testing), legal and financial resources, and social support resources such as support groups.	Asegurese de tener información oral y escrita sobre la enfermedad, los resultados de comprobación de examenes neuropsicológicos, recursos legales y financieros, y recursos de apoyo social tales como grupos del apoyo.
Meet regularly with your healthcare providers to discuss the demands of caring for people with Alzheimer's, strategies for reducing stress, and resources for support.	Reunase regularmente con su medico o enfermera/o para discutir las demandas del cuidado de personas con Alzheimer, estrategias para reducir tensión, y recursos de apoyo.
Contact the local branches of national and regional Alzheimer's groups, which can be found in Box 34–3. A good place to start for information is the National Alzheimer's Association, 919 Michigan Ave., Suite 1000, Chicago, IL 60661. Call 1–800–272–3900.	Mantenga contacto con las ramas locales de los grupos de Alzheimer nacionales y regionales, que se pueden encontrar en su guía telefónica. Una buena fuente de información es la Asociación de Alzheimer Nacional, que se localiza en 919 Michigan Avenue, Suite 1000, Chicago, IL 60661. Puede llamar a NAA al = 1 (800) 272-3900.
Many caregivers have also found it helpful to read the following publications:	Muchos proveedores de cuidado también han encontrado útil leer las publicaciones siguientes:

Alzheimer's Disease: A Guide for Patients and Families, by Lenore Powell and Katie Courtice, Reading, MA, Addison-Wesley, 1983.

The 36-Hour Day, by Nancy Mace and Peter Rabins, Baltimore, Johns Hopkins University Press, 1981.

Alzheimer's: A Caregiver's Guide and Sourcebook, by Howard Gruetzner, New York, John Wiley & Sons, 1988.

Understanding Difficult Behaviors, by A. Robinson, B. Spencer, and L. White, Ypsilanti, MI, Eastern Michigan University, 1991.

---

likewise. It is best to speak slowly and simply, with firm volume and low pitch. The tone of voice should always be calm and reassuring and project control of the situation. However, when language becomes impaired in the second stage of the illness, the nurse must be prepared to apply new techniques for communicating with the client.

Bartol,[4] in 1979, wrote a very useful guide for nurses that is still useful today. Nonverbal behavior can provide the nurse with clues. Clients with DAT often avert their eyes, look down, back away, and increase hand gesturing when they do not understand. If they are frustrated, angry, or hostile, they may increase motor activity by pacing, rattling doorknobs, waving their arms or shaking their fists, frowning, raising their voice volume and pitch, or tightening their facial muscles. These behaviors should signal staff to increase their alertness, search for the cause of the distress, and prepare to intervene. Interventions can include the following:

- Decreasing environmental stimuli
- Approaching the client calmly and with assurance

- Taking care not to place any more demands on the client
- Distracting the client
- Making sure that all verbal and nonverbal communication cues are concordant
- Using multiple sensory modalities (visual, auditory, and tactile) to send the message.

The client's memory loss can be an advantage in distracting him or her from the stressful situation. If removed from the situation and provided with a calm, nonthreatening environment, the client may forget why he or she was upset. Bartol suggested that nurses can elicit listening behavior from DAT clients by reaching out and touching, holding a hand, putting an arm around the waist, or in some way maintaining physical contact with the client. Dementia sufferers can perceive nonverbal behavior from others and can become agitated or upset if they sense negative nonverbal behavior from others.

The identification of pain or discomfort in clients with advanced DAT is also difficult. Hurley et al.[11] have developed a tool to facilitate assessment. Behavioral indicators of discomfort include noisy breathing, negative vocalization (constant muttering, making sounds with a negative quality), a sad or frightened facial expression, frowning, tense body language, and fidgeting.

Altered Thought Processes. Neuronal degeneration also affects thought processing. State this diagnosis as *Altered Thought Processes related to neuronal degeneration.*

Planning: Expected Outcomes. The client will have improved thought processing, as evidenced by exhibiting retention of information to maximal capacity, maintaining orientation to maximal capacity, and sharing meaningful life experiences.

Implementation. Because memory deficit occurs in all stages of DAT, the nurse must continually apply interventions to enhance memory. The nurse should reorient the client as necessary by placing a calendar and clock in obvious places. Since DAT clients' long-term memory is retained longer than their short-term memory, the nurse

should allow clients to reminisce. The nurse should be aware of a client's past so experiences can be shared meaningfully. Repetition is useful for ensuring maximal retention of information by the client.

Risk for Injury. Altered thought processes lead to impaired judgment and forgetfulness. These changes increase risk for injury. State this common diagnosis as *Risk for Injury related to impaired judgment, forgetfulness, and motor impairments (specify).*

Planning: Expected Outcomes. The client's physical and environmental safety will be maintained, as evidenced by the absence of physical injury and the existence of a safe living environment.

Implementation. Impaired judgment, forgetfulness, and motor impairment can make any environment unsafe for the client with DAT. In the home, electrical devices, toxic substances, loose rugs, hot tap water, inadequate lighting, and unlocked doors can be sources of injury. Family members should be educated on how to eliminate these safety hazards. In the inpatient setting, nurses

---

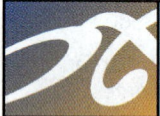 **BRIDGE TO HOME HEALTHCARE**

Safety Solutions for People with Alzheimer's Disease

Tammi Hardiman, R.N., B.S.N., Anacortes Convalescent Center, Anacortes, Washington

To live with damaged thinking and judgment is to live at risk. People with Alzheimer's disease have diminished ability to take responsibility for their own safety. They have diminished ability to evaluate the potential consequences of their actions. They are often forgetful. Accidents can easily happen.

When caring for a person with Alzheimer's disease, be sure that you know firsthand the limitations of the person's abilities. Do not take the person's word for it that he or she is able to cook supper or get into the tub alone.

A neat house is safer than a cluttered one. In a neat house there are fewer things to trip over or knock over, and hazards are more easily seen. Although it is helpful to keep the arrangement of furniture essentially the same for the person with Alzheimer's, it may be necessary to remove furniture with sharp corners, rockers that tip easily, coffee tables, and fragile possessions. Hot radiators can be blocked off by putting a sturdy chair in front of (but not against!) them. Eliminate hazards such as telephone cords, extension cords, and other wires.

Most accidents happen in the kitchen and bathroom. You may be able to take the knobs off the stove so that the person with Alzheimer's disease cannot operate it alone. If the stove is electric, you can have a switch installed behind it so that when the switch is off the burners will not operate. If the stove is controlled by its own fuse or circuit breaker, you can remove it when the stove is not in use.

Remove rugs and runners that tend to slide, especially from the bathroom. Grab bars can help people with Alzheimer's get into and out of the tub or shower and prevent falls. Make sure that the bars are firmly attached to studs behind the wall rather than just to plaster or drywall. Bath benches with nonskid feet are helpful, and handheld showers minimize the need for the person to move about in the shower or tub. Consider having a raised toilet seat installed if the person finds it difficult to rise from a standard toilet seat; obtain a bedside commode for nighttime use if the person finds urinary urgency to be a problem. These items are available at medical supply stores. Lower the temperature setting on the water heater if the water from the hot water faucet is hot enough to scald. If hot water pipes are exposed, make sure that they are covered with insulation.

Although walking is good exercise and can reduce stress, wandering can become an issue for the person with Alzheimer's. To deal with that problem, doors can be secured with locks placed high or low, where the person is less likely to notice them. Or, locks can be camouflaged by painting them the same color as the surrounding door and walls. When wandering starts to become a problem, it may also be good to sign up for the Alzheimer's Association's "Safe Return" program. When a family registers for this low-cost program, the Alzheimer's Association provides the family with information, an identification bracelet, and several identification labels. It also places identifying information, pictures of the person, and a list of contacts (family, neighbors, and local police) into a nationwide computer database. For applications, call the Alzheimer's Association at 1-800-272-3900.

should ensure that clients cannot leave the premises without being noticed, that they wear an identification badge in case they become lost, and that doors and windows are secured. Dangerous objects should be kept out of reach, and potentially dangerous activities, such as cooking, should be supervised. Driving skill should be evaluated at regular intervals.

Self Care Deficit. State the diagnosis of self-care problems as *Self Care Deficit related to loss of memory and motor impairments.*

Planning: Expected Outcomes. The client will have improved self-care ability, as evidenced by completing the tasks he or she is capable of performing and receiving assistance with ADL he or she is incapable of performing.

Implementation. The client with DAT should be encouraged to do as much as possible, as long as it is safe and appropriate. The nurse must carefully balance helping the client with maintaining his or her autonomy. This will boost the client's confidence and self-respect, which can be very fragile during the early and middle stages of the disease. The client should be given plenty of time to complete a task. Constant encouragement, urging, and reminding the client in a step-by-step approach is necessary.

Urge Incontinence. DAT clients develop urge incontinence as cortical neurons degenerate and no longer provide inhibition of the micturition and defecation responses. State this diagnosis as *urge incontinence related to neuronal degeneration and forgetfulness.*

Planning: Expected Outcomes. The client will have optimal continence of bladder and bowel, as evidenced by having clean, dry clothing and bedding as much as possible; having intact skin; and voiding appropriately in the bathroom.

Implementation. Anticipation of elimination needs and scheduled voiding and defecation times can help in the initial stages. The client may show nonverbal signs of needing to void or defecate, like restlessness, grasping the genital area, or picking at clothing. Sometimes the client forgets where the bathroom is located. Having clear, bright signs indicating where the bathroom is and frequently taking the client there may help control incontinence. Fluid intake after the dinner meal can be restricted to help maintain continence during the night. A bowel program can be arranged to coincide with the client's usual pattern. In the later stages of DAT, clients may need to wear incontinence pads during the day and external urinary drainage devices at night. Indwelling catheters should be avoided because of the risk of infection and injury.

Caregiver Role Strain. Family members and especially caregivers (usually a spouse or adult child) of clients with DAT face a great deal of emotional and physical burden. State this diagnosis as *Caregiver Role Strain*

related to grieving the loss of a family member to DAT, change in social role, and intense demands for time commitment and provision of care.

Planning: Expected Outcomes. The family will demonstrate decreased role strain, as evidenced by voicing their emotional concerns, seeking appropriate assistance, and providing adequate care for the client.

Implementation. Family members grieve the loss of the person they used to know. Each decline in cognitive function becomes another source of grief. Jones and Martinson[12] describe two stages of grief in the family. The process of grief begins during the caregiving stage and continues after the client's death. Normal family routines are lost, and the relationship between the family member and the dementia sufferer changes. Morris et al.[17] summarized studies of the factors that affect the emotional well-being of caregivers of dementia sufferers. The behavior problems most likely to be reported by caregivers are incontinence, overdemanding behavior, and the need for constant supervision. Wives tend to experience a higher degree of emotional burden as caregivers than do husbands. Paradoxically, the closer the emotional bond between caregiver and dementia sufferer, the less the strain for the caregiver. Conversely, a low past level of intimacy is associated with an increased level of both perceived strain and depression in the spouse caregiver. Caregivers are most likely to be depressed if they feel a loss of control over their spouse's behavior, if they feel unable to cope with the impact of caregiving, and if they perceive the situation to be stable and to affect everything. Studies have not determined that formal support of the caregiver (home visits by special practitioners, chore workers, and day-care workers) relieves the caregiver's burden more than informal support (family member visits and support groups). The Alzheimer's Disease and Related Disorders Association has local chapters that offer support groups in many major cities in the United States. The toll-free number is 1-800-272-3900 for information on nearby local chapters.

Family members should be interviewed to determine their understanding of the diagnosis and prognosis of DAT and to allow them to discuss their concerns about caring for the client. Do they know about community resources? Do they have someone to call when they can no longer cope with caregiving? The home environment should be evaluated for safety before the client is sent home from the hospital. Is the home on a busy street? Can doors be secured so that the client cannot get out without supervision? Are potentially dangerous appliances out of reach?

A variety of options are available to caregivers. Chore service workers can help with household chores and relieve the caregiver of these duties. Other paid help can provide in-home respite care by observing the dementia sufferer while the caregiver tends to business outside the home, seeks social interaction, or meets recreational needs. Adult day care provides time away from home for the dementia sufferer. Day care usually offers a lunchtime meal as well as several hours of scheduled activities that are tailored to the client's abilities. These activities may include games, crafts, music, and exercise. Respite care involves admission to an extended care facility for a few

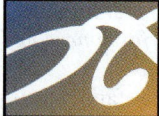

BRIDGE TO HOME HEALTHCARE

Respite Care for Caregivers of People with Alzheimer's Disease
Cyndy Hunt, M.S., R.N., *Poudre Valley Hospital, Fort Collins, Colorado*

When providing home care for people with Alzheimer's disease, be alert to how well the caregivers themselves are managing their own health. In order for people with Alzheimer's disease to remain at home for as long as possible, caregivers must remain healthy themselves. If *their* health fails as a result of the stress of caregiving, the person with Alzheimer's may need to be placed in a nursing home much sooner than expected.

You can help caregivers find physical and emotional respite by following these suggestions:

- Encourage caregivers to be realistic about what needs they can meet for their loved ones, and what needs they cannot meet.
- Suggest that caregivers make a list of all the tasks they perform for the person with Alzheimer's. Next to each task, have them write down who else could do the job. (Caregivers may find that they are performing some tasks that the person with Alzheimer's could still be doing on his or her own.) This exercise will help caregivers identify tasks that they could delegate to someone else.
- Help caregivers identify friends and neighbors who could offer them support. These friends might take the caregiver out for dinner or come to house-sit with the person with Alzheimer's, giving the caregiver some precious time alone. Often, friends of caregivers are more supportive than family members, because friends can maintain more objectivity.
- Know the community resources that provide in-home day care for people with Alzheimer's.
- Know the community centers that provide day care outside the home. Find out about the qualifications of the staff, the cost of services, eligibility criteria, availability of financial assistance, daily activities at the centers, and the environment of the centers. Having firsthand knowledge of the centers will help you guide families in making choices.
- Encourage caregivers to make use of support groups offered by the local chapter of the Alzheimer's Disease and Related Disorders Association. These support groups often provide physical respite care, but the emotional respite of knowing that the caregiver is not alone can be even more valuable.
- Validate the caregiver's feelings of anger, guilt, exhaustion, and frustration. Let caregivers know that you understand how bad things can get at home with a person with Alzheimer's, even though people with Alzheimer's may appear alert and pleasant when company visits.
- Caregivers may complain about "going crazy" as they watch their loved ones perform tedious, repetitive tasks; for example, picking up falling leaves one leaf at a time rather than raking up the leaves. Help caregivers analyze activities in terms of safety. Does the activity harm the person with Alzheimer's? If not, caregivers can reframe their perceptions of the activity and accept it as harmless.
- Laugh with caregivers. Help them realize that finding humor in the absurdities of life can make it possible to deal with a situation that might otherwise be unbearable.

Respite care for caregivers of people with Alzheimer's must include not only physical but also emotional respite. Anything that you can do to help caregivers find such respite may enhance the health of both the caregiver and the person with Alzheimer's.

---

days to a few weeks to allow the caregiver time to recover from the demands of providing 24-hour care. Nursing home care is usually the final, and most difficult and trying option for a caregiver. This decision creates guilt, self-doubt, and anxiety. However, it is often the only option when the caregiver suffers burnout and becomes unable to provide adequate care. Table 34–2 lists nursing guidelines for meeting family needs.

When the person with DAT reaches the terminal stage of illness, questions about end-of-life treatments arise. Should a feeding tube be used to provide nourishment? Should antibiotics be used to treat pneumonias or other infections? Should cardiopulmonary resuscitation be used? Ideally, decisions about these questions are raised and discussed with the client and family members before the individual loses the capacity to make decisions. Mezey

found that spousal decisions to forego life-sustaining treatments were more common when the client was comatose.[16b] Two forms of advance directives (means of expressing one's wishes about life-sustaining treatment after losing the mental capacity to make informed decisions) are available. One is the living will, a written document signed by the individual (while he or she is still mentally capable of making informed decisions) in the presence of a witness. The living will lists conditions under which the person wishes life-sustaining treatments to be withheld or withdrawn. The other advance directive is a durable power of attorney for healthcare. This is a legal document in which the individual (while still mentally capable) assigns a person to act on his or her behalf in matters of healthcare decisions if the individual loses decisional capacity (e.g., becomes demented).

Table 34–2. Nursing Guidelines for Meeting the Needs of the Family of the Client with Dementia of the Alzheimer's Type

Goals	Selected Interventions
Physical	
Monitor chronic health problems or physical limitations of family caregiver	Obtain health history of family caregiver to identify past and new health problems
Identify development of new health problems	Support family in following through with routine health examinations
	Refer family member(s) to physician when health problems are observed
	Assess family's understanding of medical management of own health problems
	Teach family members to preserve own health in order to continue caring for patient with Alzheimer's disease (AD)
Identify cues for stress	Emphasize family's need for adequate nutrition, hydration, exercise, and rest
Examine somatic health problems	Help family members to be alert to signs of caregiver stress
Psychosocial	
Assist family in coping positively with stress	Instruct family to get respite regularly for rest and relaxation
	Teach stress management techniques (i.e., relaxation, supportive relationships, goal setting, time management, diversion)
Identify destructive methods of coping (i.e., alcohol, drugs, tobacco, over- or undereating, physical abuse of patient)	Refer family to physician, therapist when stress remains unmanageable even with social or psychological resources
	Refer signs of physical abuse to adult protective services
Assess family dynamics	Recognize the family's role, discuss capacity to provide care, and give reinforcement for care provided
Assist family members in dealing with role change and conflict	Counsel family in dealing with role conflicts, unmet expectations, or interpersonal conflicts
	Teach family the need to maintain roles and social activities outside caregiving experience
	Administer burden interview
	Reinforce family's attempt to cope
	Acknowledge family fears of being unable to continue with caregiving
If need for support identified, direct family members to sources	Refer family to a support group to share with others in similar situations
	Refer family to nearest office on aging or Alzheimer's Disease and Related Disorders Association, Inc. (ADRDA) to identify benefits in community available to AD patients
Identify family's mixed emotions (i.e., depression, anger, resentment, pity, embarrassment, guilt)	Listen to family and facilitate sharing of emotions and feelings in supportive, empathic environment
Identify alternative plans for care if family members or social support systems become unable to provide care or are ineffective	Counsel and support family if patient placed in care of others (i.e., day care, respite service, home care, nursing home); allay feelings of guilt
	Facilitate family meeting to identify time for socialization
Identify financial limitations	Encourage family to be specific about financial limitations
	Offer family referrals (legal, financial, or social service) for information on eligibility for private, county, state, or federal financial support for home services, and advise and counsel regarding power of attorney or guardianship, trust or estate planning
Assess family's ability to make funeral plans	Help family anticipate and cope with grief process
	Assist family in making prefuneral arrangements
	Address family's fear regarding the possible role of heredity in development of AD and assist in making decision regarding autopsy

Table continued on following page

Table 34–2. Nursing Guidelines for Meeting the Needs of the Family of the Client with Dementia of the Alzheimer's Type *(Continued)*	
Goals	**Selected Interventions**
Environmental	
Identify compatibility of environment with family and patient	Conduct a family meeting to discuss relationship of family, patient, and environment
Assess learning needs regarding patient care tasks	Teach management of concurrent physical health problems of the AD patient
	Include family in development of patient care plan
	Teach family to encourage AD patient to continue daily habits to extent possible
	Complete behavior problems checklist
	Anticipate likely problems and teach how to manage them
	Teach environmental modification (consistent, simple, calm routines) to maximize family endurance and enhance safety
	Teach family to relate to patient with creative connectedness (touch, humor, flexibility, reminiscence, music, planned activities)
Assess family need and desire for information about AD and how it affects patient's behavior	Assist family in understanding symptoms related to memory loss, nature of the illness, symptoms, stages of disease progression, and behavior manifestations
	Provide written material to reinforce education and understanding (i.e., *The 36-Hour Day, Coping and Caring: Living with Alzheimer's Disease;* literature from local, state, or national ADRDA chapters)
	Supply ADRDA 24-hour hotline number: 1-800-621-0379

Adapted from Stevenson, J. P. (1990). Family stress to home care of Alzheimer's disease patients and implications for support. *Journal of Neuroscience Nursing,* 22(3), 185.

Evaluation

The nurse continually evaluates the degree of expected outcome attainment. The nurse should expect progress toward outcomes to be slow. If the client is transferred to a new center (e.g., hospital), some regression can be expected. Family evaluation should be completed on regular intervals.

Creutzfeldt-Jakob Disease

Creutzfeldt-Jakob disease (CJD) is a subacute CNS disorder that produces progressive dementia, myoclonus, and distinctive EEG changes. CJD is a unique disease that can apparently arise from two separate mechanisms, genetic and infectious. Persons with the genetic form have been shown to have a mutated gene present. The infectious form does not develop from a known virus or other pathogen, and therefore words like *virion, slow virus,* and *prion* are sometimes used to describe the etiologic agent. Several reports document human-to-human spread of CJD from cornea transplants, dural allografts, human pituitary growth hormone injections, and reuse of stereotactic EEG electrodes that had been previously implanted in a person with CJD. Apparently, there was a group of infected cadavers that were used for growth hormone replacement. Incubation periods have ranged from 4 to 21 years, which indicates the enormous difficulty of tracing the infection. Additional cases may still appear in persons who received

the hormone prior to its discontinuation in 1985. In 1996, CJD was associated with ingestion of infected beef.

The incidence of CJD peaks in the age group 40 to 70 years. It affects both sexes equally. A higher incidence has been noted in Libyan-born Jewish persons and in some groups from Chile and the former Czechoslovakia. Clinical manifestations include vague psychiatric or behavior changes suggesting a personality change. About one third of clients report weight loss, anorexia, insomnia, malaise, and dizziness for a period of weeks to months. In the early stages, there is progressive memory loss, visual impairment, and dysphagia. Within a few weeks or months a relentlessly progressive dementia develops, and notable deterioration is noted from week to week. Myoclonus (twitching) is usually present. Deterioration is rapid, with 90% of clients dying within 1 year. Diagnosis attempts to differentiate CJD from AD. AD has a more protracted course and no myoclonus or EEG changes. Lithium toxicity can mimic the manifestations, but they clear within about 2 weeks after discontinuing the drug. Brain biopsy during hospitalization or on autopsy is the usual method of establishing a definitive diagnosis. No effective treatment is available, and CJD appears to be uniformly fatal. Nursing care is directed at supportive care preventing skin breakdown, furnishing nutrition, providing emotional support to client and family. Families require much support, care, and concern as they try to cope with the sudden onset of this debilitating disease and with the problem of management of day-to-day care of the client.

Although CJD can be transmitted, the risk to healthcare workers and others having contact with the client is no more than that to the general population. Isolation of clients is not indicated, but personnel should wear gloves when handling tissues, blood, and spinal fluid. Accidental skin contact with possibly infected material should be followed by washing in 1N sodium hydroxide or a 1:10 solution of 5% household chlorine bleach. The agent can be inactivated on surfaces by using a 1:10 bleach solution for 1 hour. Surgical and pathologic instruments should be steam-autoclaved for 1 hour at 132° C. No organs, tissue, or tissue products from clients with CJD or any other ill-defined neurologic disorders should be used for transplantation or replacement therapy.

Multiple Sclerosis

Multiple sclerosis (MS) is a progressive degenerative disease that affects the myelin sheath of neurons in the CNS. The myelin sheath is essential for normal conduction of nerve impulses. Patches of myelin deteriorate at irregular intervals along the nerve axon, causing slowing of nerve conduction.

The onset of MS usually occurs between ages 20 and 40, and it affects women twice as often as men. Whites are affected more often than Hispanics, blacks, or Asians. The disease is most prevalent in the colder climates of North America and Europe. If someone is born in an area of high risk for MS and moves to an area of low risk after age 15, he or she carries the risk of the country of origin.

Etiology and Risk Factors

The exact cause of MS is unknown. Most theories suggest that MS is an immunogenetic-viral disease, that is, an immune-mediated demyelination triggered by a viral infection. A genetic susceptibility apparently alters the body's immune response to viral infection. Multiple genes are probably involved. However, the only consistently identified disease locus is on the HLA gene complex on chromosome 6.[23]

A variety of precipitating factors can precede the onset or an exacerbation of MS. They include infection, physical injury, emotional stress, pregnancy, and fatigue. Most pregnancy-related exacerbations occur 3 months post partum and may relate more to the stress of labor and fatigue during the puerperium than to the pregnancy itself.

MS has no known areas of primary prevention (see Risk Factors and Levels of Prevention).

Pathophysiology

Myelin is a highly conductive fatty material that surrounds the axon and speeds conduction of nerve impulses along the axon. In MS, plaques form along the myelin sheath, causing inflammation, edema, and eventually scarring and destruction (Fig. 34–2). Plaques are characterized by primary demyelination and death of oligodendro-

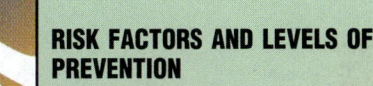

RISK FACTORS AND LEVELS OF PREVENTION

Multiple Sclerosis

Risk Factors

Viral infection leading to immune reactions
Living in cold environments
Genetic predisposition

Levels of Prevention

Primary Prevention

● None known

Secondary Prevention

● Advise clients to avoid infection by:
    Using good handwashing technique
    Avoiding being around people with infections
    Employing measures to keep the urinary tract free from infection
● Advise clients to use good stress management techniques
● Assist clients to make informed choices about pregnancy
● Advise clients to avoid hot environments

Tertiary Prevention

● Maintain fluid intake of 2000 ml each day
● Void every 3 hours while awake
● Eat a high fiber diet
● Balance activity and rest
● Maintain muscle flexibility by daily stretching and range-of-motion exercises
● Try to minimize stress response

cytes in the center of the lesion. Initially, perivascular inflammatory cells (autoreactive T cells) invade the myelin-covered axons in the CNS. This is followed by extensive gliosis or scarring by astrocytes and aberrant attempts at remyelination, with oligodendrocytes proliferating at the edges of the plaque. When edema and inflammation subside, some remyelination occurs but is often incomplete. Although plaques may occur anywhere in the white matter of the CNS, the areas most commonly involved are the optic nerves, cerebrum and cervical spinal cord.

Clinical Manifestations and Diagnostic Findings

MS has two major courses: exacerbating-remitting and chronic-progressive. In the former, the client has episodes of neurologic dysfunction (exacerbations) from which he or she recovers and is able to function normally (remission). In some cases, the recovery from each exacerbation is not complete, causing a stepwise decline in function with each exacerbation. In the second major course of

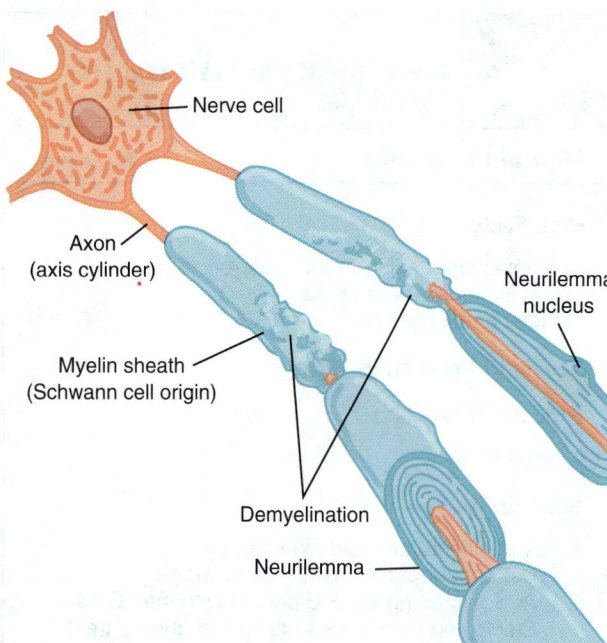

Nerve cell

Axon
(axis cylinder)

Myelin sheath
(Schwann cell origin)

Neurilemma
nucleus

Demyelination

Neurilemma

Figure 34–2. Changes in the nerve sheath with multiple sclerosis. Myelin is made by the oligodendrocyte and coats peripheral nerves, facilitating nervous impulse. In multiple sclerosis, the myelin degenerates in patches, making nerve transmission erratic.

MS, the client experiences a steady decline in neurologic function that can occur over several years. In acute, fulminant cases, the decline may occur rapidly within a year or two. Life expectancy is about 85% that of the general population. The usual cause of death is bacterial infection of the lungs or bladder, or pressure ulcers.

The random distribution of MS plaques leads to a variety of clinical manifestations: weakness or tingling sensations (paresthesias) of one or more extremities due to involvement of the cerebrum or spinal cord; vision loss from optic neuritis; incoordination due to cerebellar involvement; and bowel and bladder dysfunction as a result of spinal cord involvement. Seizures may develop in some clients.

Bladder dysfunction can have several forms, depending on which neural pathways are affected. Dysfunction may involve hesitancy, frequency, loss of sensation, incontinence, and retention. There may be increased or decreased detrusor, bladder neck, or external sphincter tone, or a combination of these problems. The ultimate bladder dysfunction, however, is usually a hyperreflexic bladder in association with sphincter dyssynergia (sphincter contraction during detrusor contraction).[3] Proper diagnosis of the type of bladder dysfunction requires a good history, laboratory assessment of kidney function, and a search for and identification of infection. If bladder emptying is defective, further investigation using urography, cystoscopy, and urodynamic studies should be performed.

Stool incontinence and constipation are commonly experienced by clients with MS. Dysfunction can result from one or more of the following factors: spinal cord lesion, immobility, dehydration, medications, and nutritional deficiencies.

Sexual dysfunction can also occur, as a result of lesions in the ascending or descending autonomic and sensory fibers in the spinal cord.

Fatigue is a common symptom in MS. It usually worsens as the day progresses. Spasticity can reduce energy; inhibit motor control; and interfere with self-care, sexuality, vocational responsibilities, and recreation.

Because MS strikes young adults during their years of establishing a family and occupation, the impact of the disease can be devastating. Depression often occurs in MS clients, but it is not clear whether depression is a reaction to disability or a function of the disease itself.[1] Others may experience euphoria, emotional instability, or apathy.

Because there is no definitive test for MS, clinicians rely on a detailed history, clinical findings, and a variety of diagnostic tests. The history should reveal at least two episodes of neurologic dysfunction, separated by time and by different locations in the CNS. Diagnostic tests include spinal fluid evaluation for the presence of oligoclonal banding, evoked potentials of the optic pathways and auditory system to assess the presence of slowed nerve conduction, and MRI of the brain and spinal cord to determine the presence of MS plaques.

Community and Self-Care

▪ Medical Management

Several treatments for MS have been tested, but because many clients experience spontaneous remission within days to weeks, the effects of treatment are difficult to evaluate. Corticosteroids, which have both anti-inflammatory and immunosuppressive properties, are often used to enhance recovery from an exacerbation. These include methylprednisolone and adrenocorticotropic hormone (ACTH), which are given intravenously, and prednisone, which is given orally. Azathioprine (Imuran), another immunosuppressive agent, may be used for progressive MS.

Interferon beta-1b (Betaseron) was approved in 1993 for ambulatory clients with exacerbating-remitting MS. Interferon beta-1b is a genetically engineered complex protein with both antiviral and immunoregulatory properties. It has been shown to reduce the number of MS exacerbations. The drug is injected subcutaneously every other day. Numerous other therapies are undergoing clinical trials.

Several strategies are available for the variety of complications that occur with MS. Pharmacologic interventions can be used for bladder dysfunction (oxybutinin, probanthelene); constipation (psyllium hydromuciloid, bisacodyl [Dulcolax] pills or suppositories); fatigue (amantadine); spasticity (baclofen, diazepam, dantrolene); tremor (propranolol, phenobarbital, clonazepam); and dysesthesias and trigeminal neuralgia (carbamazepine, phenytoin, amitriptyline). Transcutaneous electrical nerve stimulation (TENS) is also helpful for dysesthesias. Areas of numbness should be inspected regularly to prevent injury and development of pressure ulcers. Skin should be kept dry and free of urine and feces. A pressure-distributing seat cushion should be used for wheelchair-bound clients with insensate buttock skin. Blindness or severely impaired vision may occur. In this case, refer the client to Services for the Blind for rehabilitation. Cognitive and perceptual impairment necessitates psychometric and functional testing for accurate assessment and rehabilitation services.

■ Nursing Management of the Medical Client

Assessment

If the client is being assessed for possible MS, the nurse should assess the client for clinical manifestations of the disorder. Ocular symptoms are very common. Likewise, as a result of the fluctuations of clinical manifestations, the client may report a past history of similar findings that went away.

If the client is being hospitalized for an exacerbation of MS, the nurse should focus on the client's ability to perform ADL as well as other areas that require fine motor movements. Gross motor activities such as walking may also be impaired and lead to problems with bowel and bladder continence (see the Nursing Research feature).

Diagnosis, Planning, Implementation

Altered Urinary Elimination. Demyelination alters bladder function. This diagnosis is stated as *Altered urinary elimination related to bladder dysfunction.*

Planning: Expected Outcomes. The client will maintain urinary continence and normal bladder filling, as evidenced by residual volumes of less than 100 ml, application of appropriate bladder elimination procedures, and verbalization of personal satisfaction with urinary elimination status.

Implementation. The following interventions are for neurogenic bladder, the most common type of bladder dysfunction in MS. Fluid intake should be maintained at 2000 ml/24 hours, ideally, 400 to 500 ml with each meal and 200 ml at midmorning, midafternoon, and late afternoon. Avoiding fluid intake after the evening meal reduces the need for emptying the bladder during the night. Voiding should be attempted every 3 hours during waking hours. If voiding is not successful, a catheter should be inserted into the bladder and then removed once emptying is complete. This is called *intermittent catheterization.* If the volume of catheterized urine exceeds 500 ml, the catheterization schedule may need to be more frequent. The nurse instructs the client on how to do self-catheterization if he or she is capable. A clean red rubber catheter can be reused for up to 1 week, as long as it is washed thoroughly with soap and water and placed in a clean, tightly sealed plastic bag after every catheterization. Sterile equipment is not required for ongoing self-catheterization in the hospital or at home for these clients.

Constipation. Immobility and demyelination lead to constipation. State this common diagnosis as *Constipation related to immobility and demyelination.*

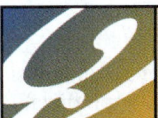

NURSING RESEARCH

How Do Clients with Multiple Sclerosis View Their Health?

Gulick, E., & Bugg, A. (1992). Holistic health patterning in multiple sclerosis. *Research in Nursing and Health, 15*(3),175–186.

Gulick and Bugg examined self-assessments of health patterns over a 5-year period in clients with multiple sclerosis (MS). Health patterns are composites of interrelationships between the client and the environment that have occurred in the past. Health patterns include way of life, functions, abilities, and social relationships and are influenced by heredity, culture, and values. Four areas were studied: (1) fine and gross motor movement, (2) socializing and recreation, (3) sensory and communication, and (4) intimacy.

Symptoms occurred in all clients in all four areas and validated that clients with MS must learn to cope with a wide array of clinical manifestations. Fine and gross motor movement and intimacy declined in all groups. There was little change in socializing, perhaps because the disease had already affected social interactions.

Implications for Practice

It is important that nurses have a full understanding of the clinical manifestations of MS and the impact it has on many body functions so that health teaching with the client and family can focus on anticipation of needs. The client will benefit from knowing the various symptoms that are part of MS and what resources are available, such as a motorized wheelchair.

Most reports about MS related to changes in neurologic function, such as changes in bowel and bladder function, sensation, cerebellar alterations, visual changes, and the like. Because the progression of MS alters a client's way of life, abilities, and social relations, a holistic-focused research study was seen as an important contribution to the nursing literature.

Planning: Expected Outcomes. The client will have bowel movements of normal consistency and frequency.

Implementation. A high fiber diet, bulk formers, and stool softeners are useful for maintaining stool consistency. Adequate fluid intake also assists bowel elimination; 2000 ml should be taken. Teach the client that laxatives and enemas should be avoided because they lead to dependence. A bowel program should be performed every other day, approximately 45 minutes after the largest meal, to take advantage of the gastrocolic reflex. Rectal evacuation may be augmented by the use of glycerin or bisacodyl suppositories or digital stimulation.

Activity Intolerance. State this common diagnosis as *Activity Intolerance related to fatigue and muscle weakness.*

Planning: Expected Outcomes. The client will demonstrate improved activity tolerance, as evidenced by maintaining a balance between work, rest, and exercise and recreation; performing ADL without excessive fatigue; using energy-saving devices and techniques; avoiding elevations in environmental and body temperatures; and consuming a diet adequate in calories and protein for body size, frame, and age.

Implementation. Because fatigue can be precipitated by warm temperatures, the environment should be kept cool. If air conditioning is unavailable, cool baths and ice packs may help lower body temperature.

Assist the client to plan activities at his or her peak energy level, which is usually in the morning. This schedule promotes optimal synchrony between circadian rhythms and the client's physical demands. The client should plan for periods of rest throughout the day. Collaboration with the physical and occupational therapist can reveal methods to reduce energy consumption with repeated tasks and apply adaptive devices for ambulation and toileting. The drug amantadine (Symmetrel) may alleviate fatigue in some clients.

Impaired Physical Mobility. Several problems lead to difficulties with mobility. State this diagnosis as *Impaired Physical Mobility related to weakness, contractures, spasticity, and ataxia.*

Planning: Expected Outcomes. The client will achieve optimal physical mobility, as evidenced by improved or maintained range of motion in all joints, optimal control of spasticity, and effective use of adaptive aids.

Implementation. Although some clients are bothered by painful muscle spasms, others may rely on spasticity to stabilize weak limbs during transfers and ambulation. Spastic muscles must be stretched at least twice daily through their full range of motion. The drug baclofen (Lioresal) provides synaptic inhibition of spinal reflexes, which can reduce spasticity, although it may increase weakness and fatigue in some clients. Diazepam (Valium) and dantrolene (Dantrium) are other antispasmotic drugs. Surgical intervention or nerve blocks may be necessary if contractures develop. The nurse monitors the effect of medications on spasticity, promotes activity to decrease spasms, and utilizes spasms for muscle strength when transferring.

Strengthening exercises for muscle weakness (paresis) must be done with caution because they can aggravate paresis by causing muscle fatigue. However, selective strengthening of nonaffected or less affected muscles can enhance physical function and well-being. Range-of-motion exercises should be performed at least twice daily. Active movement is preferable to passive movement. Correct body alignment should be maintained to reduce the risk of contractures. Splints may help maintain position and provide support for weak hands and ankles. Ataxia and tremor of the extremities can be lessened by the use of small weights applied to the distal extremities or the use of weighted utensils. Weakness and fatigue can aggravate ataxia. Ambulation aids such as a cane or a walker may be necessary.

Risk for Self Care Deficit. Clients with MS may experience a decline in self-care abilities. State this diagnosis as *Risk for Self Care Deficit related to muscle weakness.*

Planning: Expected Outcomes. The client will reduce the risk of self-care deficits by using ADL aids.

Implementation. Clients may require aids, such as wheelchairs or canes, to perform ADL and ambulate. The performance of ADL may be enhanced if counters and table tops are adjusted to a comfortable working height. The nurse works in combination with the physical therapist, occupational therapist, social worker, and home health nurse to identify, purchase, and teach the client how to use ADL aids.

Knowledge Deficit. The client with a new diagnosis of MS often lacks knowledge about MS, its unpredictable course, and the role of stress in MS. State this diagnosis as *Knowledge Deficit related to new diagnosis of MS.*

Planning: Expected Outcomes. The client will have more knowledge about MS as evidenced by stating facts about the course of MS, and the role of stress in MS.

Implementation. The client with MS needs to have a clear understanding of the unpredictability of this disorder. The client may be symptom-free for many weeks to months, even years, and then develop symptoms. If the client can identify stressors that exacerbate the symptoms, sometimes these stressors can then be avoided.

Self Esteem Disturbance. Because of the age of the client, loss of independence and fear of disability can be devastating. Psychosocial diagnosis is important in providing holistic care. State this diagnosis as *Self Esteem Disturbance related to loss of independence and fear of disability.*

Planning: Expected Outcomes. The client will achieve improved self-esteem, as evidenced by verbalizing awareness that personal goals and body image will need to be adjusted, willingness to maintain appropriate independence, and positive self-thoughts and statements about self.

Implementation. Regardless of the cause of disturbance in self-esteem, the nurse should carefully assess the individual and family history for presence and type of depressive episodes and the clinical manifestations. Previous treatment for depression should be identified, including psychotherapy and drug therapy. By assessing the client's problem-solving strategies, the nurse can identify coping behavior strengths and defense mechanisms such as denial, avoidance, or intellectualization that the client may use to mask depression. The client's social support system should also be evaluated because this contributes to his or her sense of well-being. Grieving the loss of function in MS can lead to a reactive depression and require provision of support group therapy for both the client and family. Some clients may not benefit from this kind of therapy, however, because they may see people whose condition is much worse than their own and may fear developing that level of disability. Online computer services for MS clients can provide a means of social support.

Evaluation

The degree of expected outcome attainment should be evaluated on an ongoing basis. Most outcomes are long-term and may require weeks to months to attain.

Guillain-Barré Syndrome

Guillain-Barré syndrome (GBS) is an inflammatory disease of unknown cause that involves degeneration of the myelin sheath of peripheral nerves. GBS is seen worldwide and affects people of all ages and races. Since the virtual elimination of poliomyelitis, GBS has become the most common cause of acute generalized paralysis, with an annual incidence of 0.75 to 2.0/100,000 population. In one half to two thirds of cases, an upper respiratory or gastrointestinal infection precedes the onset of the syndrome by 1 to 4 weeks. Cytomegalovirus and Epstein-Barr virus have been implicated in these antecedent illnesses, as have *Mycoplasma pneumoniae, Salmonella typhosa,* and *Campylobacter jejuni.* An association between human immunodeficiency virus (HIV) and GBS has also been reported, so clients with GBS should be tested for HIV.[19]

The characteristic feature of GBS is ascending weakness, usually beginning in the lower extremities and spreading, sometimes rapidly, to the trunk, upper extremities, and even the face. The weakness evolves over days to weeks, with maximal deficit by 4 weeks in 90% of cases. Deep tendon reflexes are lost. Paresthesias (tingling sensation) in the limbs may occur early in the course of the illness. Deep, aching muscle pain in the shoulder girdle and thighs is common. The two most dangerous features of the disease are respiratory muscle weakness and autonomic neuropathy involving both the sympathetic and parasympathetic systems. The latter feature can in-

volve orthostatic hypotension, hypertension, pupillary disturbances, sweating dysfunction, cardiac dysrhythmias, paralytic ileus, and urinary retention. Improvement and recovery occur with remyelination. However, if nerve axons are damaged, some residual deficits may remain. Recovery is usually maximal at 6 months, although severe cases may take up to 2 years for maximal recovery. Fortunately, 85% to 90% of clients with GBS recover completely.

Diagnosis of GBS is based on history and physical examination, cerebrospinal fluid (CSF) examination, and electrophysiologic studies. The CSF contains increased protein, with few or no white blood cells. Nerve conduction velocity is slowed, although it may be normal in the early stage of the illness. Conduction block, a diminution in amplitude or an absence of elicited muscle action potentials from stimulation of a peripheral nerve, also occurs.

The focus of therapy is supportive care. Respiratory or cardiovascular status must be monitored carefully. This includes vital signs, serial measurement of vital capacity, peripheral oxygen saturation, and electrocardiography. When vital capacity falls to 15 ml/kg of body weight, intubation and artificial ventilation are usually necessary. Early treatment with plasmapheresis accelerates recovery, although the exact mechanism for this effect is not known (hypotheses include the removal of circulating antibodies or other humoral myelinotoxic or immunopathogenic factors[6]). Intravenous IgG therapy may prove to be the treatment of choice because it can be administered easily and can be given with other drugs simultaneously (plasmapheresis removes comedication jointly with adverse disease factors).[24]

During the first 5 days after hospital admission, it is critical to assess respiratory, swallowing, and autonomic function (see the Critical Monitoring feature). Assess the following every 4 hours: vital signs, forced vital capacity, swallowing, strength in the extremities, and intake and output balance. If ascending weakness is noted, increase the frequency of assessment to every 2 hours or even more often. Cardiac monitoring and supplemental oxygen are often needed. Common complications include bladder infection, deep vein thrombosis, pulmonary emboli, pneumonia, and syndrome of inappropriate antidiuretic hormone (SIADH).

Interventions to control infection and prevent complications of immobility are important. Proper body alignment should be maintained to prevent deformities and injury to paralyzed limbs. Once the client's condition has stabilized, rehabilitative interventions can be implemented.

The nurse also assists the client to cope with the progressive nature of GBS. During the early stages, clients are frightened because each day their paralysis has climbed upward. They are often admitted to an acute care agency with progressive weakness and within days are completely paralyzed. Clients fear they will never recover. Nurses assist clients in verbalizing their fears and offer support and encouragement that although the disorder is progressive, most clients gain full recovery. Encouragement is not hollow, however. The client is not taught to expect immediate resolution but is assisted to realize the usual time frames for recovery.

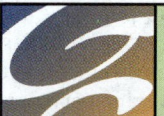

CRITICAL MONITORING

Respiratory Distress with Guillain-Barré Syndrome

- Monitor the client for:
  Complaints of headache
  Myoclonic jerks
  Drowsiness
  Confusion
  Restlessness
  Reduced cough
  Decreased ability to move pulmonary secretions
- Assess pulmonary function studies for:
  Decreased forced vital capacity (<15 ml/kg)
  Decreased tidal volume (<3–4 ml/kg)
  Decreased maximum inspiratory pressure (<10–20 H_2O)
  Decreased maximum expiratory pressure (<40 cm H_2O)
- Assess arterial blood gases for:
  Decreased Pao_2 (<80 mm Hg on 50% Fio_2 with normal Pco_2)
  Alveolar-arterial gradient >300 on 50% Fio_2
  $Paco_2$ >50 mm Hg
  Vd/Vt >0.6

Fio_2, fraction of inspired oxygen; $Paco_2$, partial pressure of arterial carbon dioxide; Pao_2, partial pressure of arterial oxygen; Vd/Vt, ratio of dead-space volume to tidal volume.

Parkinson's Disease

Parkinson's disease (PD) is an idiopathic syndrome characterized by disability from tremor and rigidity. There are various other forms of parkinsonism that cause similar symptoms but have known causes. They include the following:

- Postencephalitic parkinsonism, which occurred after the large epidemic of encephalitis in 1919
- Athereosclerotic parkinsonism, which results from ischemia in the basal ganglia
- Drug-induced parkinsonism, which occurs after long-term use of phenothiazines
- Toxin-induced parkinsonism, which can result from carbon monoxide, mercury, or manganese exposure
- Recently the role of agricultural herbicide and pesticide exposure as a cause of PD has been investigated.
- Trauma-induced parkinsonism, resulting from injury to the midbrain

PD is the focus of this section because it is the most common form of parkinsonism. PD involves degeneration of dopamine-producing cells in the substantia nigra, which leads to degeneration of dopaminergic neurons in the basal ganglia. Once cell loss in the substantia nigra reaches 80%, manifestations appear. The cause of nigral

cell degeneration is not known. The net result of the loss of dopaminergic neurons is an imbalance of dopamine in relation to ACh in the basal ganglia, which leads to the clinical characteristics of PD.

PD most often develops in people in their 60s. It occurs worldwide. About 1% of people over age 50 have PD. PD has three cardinal features: tremor, rigidity, and bradykinesia. Early in the disease, the client may notice a slight slowing in the ability to perform ADL. This is called *bradykinesia*. A general feeling of stiffness (rigidity) may be noticed, along with mild diffuse muscular pain. Tremor is a common early sign that usually occurs in one of the upper limbs. It occurs at rest and involves a coarse "pill-rolling" movement of the thumb against the fingers that can vary in intensity and distribution. Voluntary movement stops or reduces the tremor in some people; however, others may have tremor during voluntary movement (intention tremor as well).

Bradykinesia makes voluntary movements difficult to execute. When manifestations are severe, total lack of movement (akinesia) may occur and the client is literally frozen in one spot. Bradykinesia also affects gait. Initially there may be a slight stiffness of one leg while walking, and the ipsilateral arm may be held flexed at the elbow and abducted at the shoulder. The person may catch or drag one foot. Later, when both sides of the body are involved, the typical shuffling gait with short steps may develop. There is lack of associated swinging of the arms while walking. In advanced PD, the client stands with head, shoulders, and spine flexed forward, giving the appearance of a stooped posture (Fig. 34–3).

The face of someone with advanced PD appears stiff, masklike, and without expression. The speech is low in volume, monotonous in tone, and slow. Words are poorly articulated (dysarthria). Saliva may flow involuntarily from the mouth because of the lack of spontaneous swallowing.

Rare complications of PD are (1) oculogyric crisis, in which the eyes fix upward and to one side or downward, and (2) blepharospasm, which causes almost total closure of the eyelid. Various autonomic effects may accompany PD, including decreased lacrimation (tearing) and sexual capacity, constipation, incontinence, excessive perspiration, and heat intolerance.

PD does not usually affect intellectual ability; however, 15% to 20% of PD sufferers develop a dementia similar to that of Alzheimer's disease. Mood disturbance can occur, and emotional stress may intensify signs and symptoms.

The course of the disease is slowly progressive. The person becomes more rigid and more disabled, eventually requiring full assistance with ADL.

■ Medical Management

The manifestations of PD can be relieved by various medications, particularly levodopa and anticholinergic drugs. The purpose of levodopa is to provide dopamine to the basal ganglia. The purpose of anticholinergic drugs is to block release of acetylcholine, thereby creating a better balance between acetylcholine and dopamine. The most common levodopa drug is carbidopa-levodopa (Sinemet).

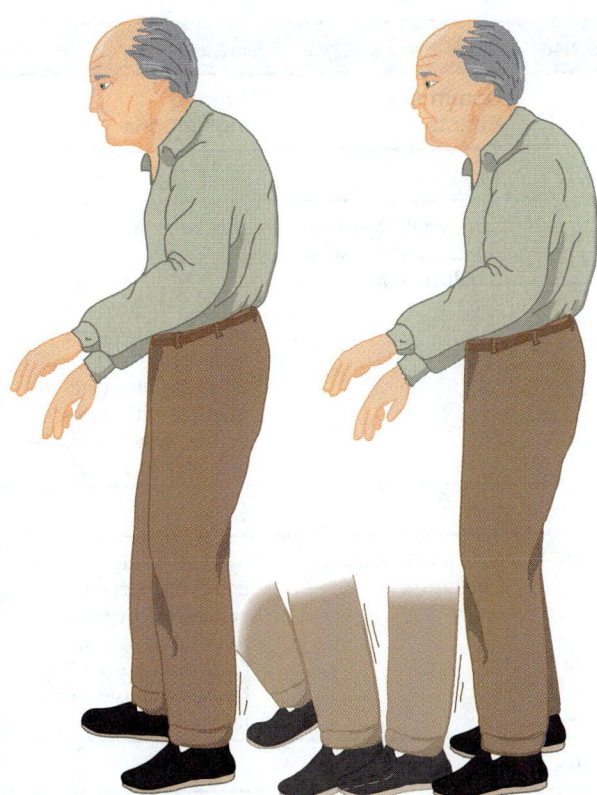

Figure 34–3. Gait changes seen in Parkinson's disease. Some of the clinical manifestations of Parkinson's disease are stooped posture, bradykinesia, and a festinant gait.

Levodopa is a synthetic metabolic precursor of dopamine. Dopamine itself cannot be used because it cannot cross the blood-brain barrier. Carbidopa must be given with levodopa because it prevents peripheral metabolism of levodopa, allowing levodopa to reach the brain. Initiation of carbidopa-levodopa therapy is usually delayed until manifestations affect ADL because the benefit of the drug seems to decline with prolonged use. The therapy is more effective in treating bradykinesia and rigidity than tremor. The dosage of levodopa is gradually increased until the optimal therapeutic response is achieved. This process may take several months. When the daily dose of levodopa approaches the desired level, the client often has involuntary dyskinesias (jerky, writhing movements), especially of the face, mouth, and tongue. Some clients prefer this stage to being severely bradykinetic, because at least they can be mobile and perform voluntary movements more easily. Table 34–3 lists drugs used in PD.

A former treatment of clients with PD was to taper their medications for a short period of time. This was called a "drug holiday." The premise behind the drug holiday was that it allowed neurotransmitter receptor sites to regain sensitivity to medications. Clients became very ill during the holiday. For the most part the treatment has been abandoned.

Managing the Parkinsonian Crisis

Occasionally, clients with PD experience a parkinsonian crisis as a result of emotional trauma or sudden or inad-vertent withdrawal of antiparkinson medication. Severe exacerbation of tremor, rigidity, and bradykinesia, accompanied by acute anxiety, sweating, tachycardia, and hyperpnea, occur. Intervention for parkinsonian crisis includes respiratory and cardiac support. The person should be placed in a quiet room with subdued lighting. Barbiturates may be prescribed, as well as antiparkinson drugs.

Managing the On/Off Response

An "on/off response" (rapid fluctuation of clinical manifestations) may occur in clients with PD. A person may be mobile and active ("on") one moment and akinetic and rigid ("off") the next. This transition may happen quickly, within 1 to 2 minutes. Initially, the off periods tend to occur 3 to 4 hours after a dose of antiparkinson medication. Later, the transition may happen at any time and be unrelated to medication ingestion. Apparently off periods are due to dopamine deficit, but this factor is not clear. A person experiencing on/off response may be temporarily helped by shortening the interval between medication doses or by gradually increasing the total dosage.

■ Nursing Management of the Medical Client

Nursing care of the PD client includes health assessment, medication instruction and monitoring, liaison with other members of the healthcare team, and client and family education.

Advise the client to maintain fluid intake of 2000 ml/24 hours and increase intake of dietary fiber. Stool softeners and mild laxatives can be used. A regular time for bowel movements should be established, usually a half-hour after the morning or evening meal.

Teach the client various techniques to enhance voluntary movement. Clients often need to try different things on their own to find what helps most. Some clients grasp coins in their pocket to reduce embarrassing hand tremor. Others grip the arms of a chair. Mental thoughts, such as walking over imaginary lines, can aid ambulation. One client found that tossing small scraps of paper in front of him aided his walking. Another found that rocking back and forth helped initiate movement. Daily range-of-motion exercises should be encouraged to avoid rigidity and contractures. Remind the client to maintain good posture and to avoid flexion of the neck and shoulders. The client should sleep on a firm mattress. When resting, the client should avoid using a pillow to prevent flexion of the spine. Periodically lying prone also helps.

Because self-care activities are performed more slowly by the client with PD, extra time should be allowed for completion of tasks such as dressing, bathing, and eating. Warming trays can keep food hot. Rest periods should be encouraged during meals to avoid aspiration.

As PD progresses, clients become rigid and unresponsive to verbal stimuli. During these stages, continue to treat the client with dignity, speaking to the client rather than ignoring him or her.

Teach the client about home safety. Loose carpeting should be removed. Grab bars should be placed in the

Table 34–3. Pharmacologic Management of Parkinson's Disease

Drug Classification and Example	Action	Indications	Common Side Effects	Nursing Implications
Anticholinergics				
Trihexyphenidyl (Artane) Benztropine (Cogentin) Procyclidine (Kemadrin) Ethopropazine (Parsidol)	Inhibit action of endogenous acetylcholine and muscarine agonists to block the excitatory effect of the cholinergic system	Tremor, rigidity, drooling	Dry mouth, constipation, blurred vision, confusion, hallucinations	Usually contraindicated in clients with acute-angle glaucoma and tachycardia; monitor pulse and blood pressure during periods of dosage adjustment; administer with meals; do not withdraw medication suddenly
Antihistamines				
Diphenhydramine (Benadryl)	Mild anticholinergic	Tremor, rigidity, insomnia	Dry mouth, lethargy, confusion	Use with caution in clients with seizures, hypertension, hyperthyroidism, heart and renal disease, and diabetes; administer with meals or antacids
Dopaminergics				
Amantadine (Symmetrel)	Cause the release of dopamine in the central nervous system	Rigidity, bradykinesia	Dizziness, ataxia, insomnia, leg edema	Monitor client for postural hypotension, do not administer at bedtime
Carbidopa-levadopa (Sinemet)		Tremor, rigidity, bradykinesia	Orthostatic hypotension, nausea, hallucinations, dystonia, dyskinesias	Monitor blood pressure; use elastic stockings to increase venous return; monitor client for urinary retention
Dopamine Agonists				
Bromocriptine (Parlodel)	Activate dopamine receptors in the central nervous system	Fluctuation of symptoms, dyskinesia, dystonia	Hallucinations, mental fogginess, orthostatic hypotension, confusion	Monitor blood pressure and mental status
Pergolide (Permax)			Orthostatic hypotension, nausea, insomnia	Monitor blood pressure; do not administer at bedtime
Monoamine Oxidase Inhibitors				
Selegiline (Deprenyl)*	Inhibit monoamine oxidase B, an enzyme that converts chemical by-products in the brain into neurotoxins that prevent substantia nigra cell death	Adjuvant treatment	Nausea, dizziness, confusion, hallucinations, dry mouth	Monitor for levodopa side effects as selegiline may increase effect of levodopa

* Note: A recent study showed that levodopa in combination with selegiline provided no clinical benefit over levodopa alone in treating early, mild Parkinson's disease. Moreover, mortality was significantly higher when these two drugs were used together.[14a]

bathroom. An elevated toilet seat should be installed. Clients with severe tremor should avoid carrying hot liquids. Walking aids such as a cane or walker can provide added stability. See the Client Education Guide.

The client and family need emotional support. Support groups are available in most major cities. Refer the client and family to the American Parkinson Disease Association and to referral centers by contacting the American

CLIENT EDUCATION GUIDE

Parkinson's Disease

Client Instructions in English *(Instrucciones para el cliente en inglés)*	**Client Instructions in Spanish** *(Instrucciones para el cliente en español)*

Make sure that you understand how to take your medications, the importance of following the correct diet, and what side effects you can expect from your medications.

Aprenda a tomar su medicamento, la importancia de seguir una dieta apropiada, y los efectos que le puedan causar los medicamentos.

To avoid rigidity and the development of contractures:

Para prevenir el desarroyo de contracciones:

- Exercise and stretch regularly.
- Perform the exercises recommended in your self-help booklets.
- Exercise first thing in the morning, when your energy levels are highest.
- Exercise in bed if getting to the floor is difficult

- Haga ejercicio y estirese con regularidad.
- Haga los ejercicios que le recomiendan en los libritos (foyetos) de auto-cuidado.
- Haga los ejercicios al levantarse, cuando el nivel de energía es mayor.
- Haga ejercicio en cama si se le hace difícil hacerlo en el piso.

- Get out of a chair by bending over slowly so that your head is over your toes; avoid soft, deep chairs.

- Levantese de la silla y doble la cabeza despacio hasta que vea los dedos de los pies; no se siente es sillas suaves o muy hondas.

If your healthcare provider has told you that you have bradykinesia (slow movements):

Si su proveedor de cuidados le ha dicho que tiene bradykinesia (movimientos muy lentos):

- Rock back and forth to get going.

- Imagine that you are stepping over an imaginary line when you walk.
- Throw small objects (e.g., small scraps of paper) in front of you to practice fine motor movements.
- Count to yourself while walking.
- Visualize your intended movement.

- Mesase hacia el frente y para atrás para poder empezar a caminar.
- Imagine que está pisando una linea imaginaria cuando camina.
- Tire objetos pequeños adelante de usted para practicar movimientos delicados.
- Cuente números cuando camine.
- Visualize (imaginese) que movimiento va a hacer.

If you have a tremor:

Si empieza a temblar:

- Hold change in your pocket or squeeze a small rubber ball.
- Use both hands to accomplish tasks.
- Lie face down on the floor and relax your entire body.
- Sleep on the side that has the tremor.

- Ponga monedas en el bolsillo del pantalón y detengalas o apriete una pelotita de hule.
- Use las dos (2) manos cuando haga quehaceres.
- Acuestese boca abajo en el piso y relaje todo el cuerpo.
- Duerma del labo donde tiene el temblor.

If you have trouble getting dressed:

Si tiene problemas al vestirse:

- Dress and undress in front of a mirror.
- Use adaptive devices like long-handled shoe-horns and button fasteners.

- Buy clothes with Velcro fasteners and slide-locking buckles.

- Vistase y desnudese delante de un espejo.
- Use aparatos adaptables como los cuernos de mango largos para ponerse los zapatos y el su-jeta-broches.
- Compre ropa con broches de Velcro y con hebillas que se cierran de un lado.

To ensure safety:

Para su seguridad:

- Wear good, sturdy shoes.
- Use a cane or walker.
- Concentrate on standing upright.

- Consciously pick up your feet to take steps.
- Remove all throw rugs, electrical cords, and clutter from the floor.

- Use buenos zapatos firmes.
- Use un bastón o un trípodo de sostén.
- Concentrece en levantarse lo más derecho posible.
- Levante los pies al dar pasos.
- Quite todas las alfombras, cordones electricos y otros artículos del suelo.

Chart continued on following page

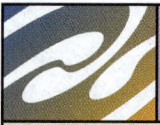

CLIENT EDUCATION GUIDE *(Continued)*

Parkinson's Disease

To ensure safety:	Para su seguridad:

To ensure safety:

• Make sure that you have adequate lighting.
• Arrange essential items so that they are within easy reach.
• Use a bath chair and a handheld shower nozzle.

• Have grab bars installed in the bathroom.
• Have a raised toilet seat installed

To ensure good communication:

• Pause between every few words.
• Exaggerate the pronunciation of words.
• Finish saying the final consonant of a word before starting to say the next word.

• Express ideas in short, concise phrases.
• Plan what to say.
• Face the listener.

To ensure adequate swallowing and prevent aspiration:

• Think through the steps of swallowing:
  1. Keep your lips closed.
  2. Keep your teeth together.
  3. Put food on your tongue.
  4. Lift your tongue up and back.
  5. Swallow.

• Eat slowly, taking small bites.
• Chew hard and move food around with your tongue.
• Finish one bite before taking another.

To keep saliva from building up in your mouth:

• Make a conscious effort to swallow saliva often.
• Keep your head in an upright position so saliva will collect in the back of your throat and stimulate automatic swallowing.
• Swallow excess saliva before attempting to speak.

Para su seguridad:

• Asegurese que tenga iluminación adecuada.
• Arregle artículos esenciales cerca de usted para tenerlos al alcance de su mano.
• Use una silla en el baño y una ducha (regadera) que pueda detener con la mano.
• Instale agarraderas en la pared del baño.
• Instale un asiento alto en el inodoro (excusado).

Para asegurar una buena comunicación:

• Haga pausas entre las palabras.
• Exagere la pronunciación de las palabras.
• Termine de decir la última consonante en una palabra antes de empezar a decir la próxima palabra.
• Exprese sus ideas en frases cortas y concisas.
• Planee lo que quiere decir.
• Pongase al frente de la persona con quien está hablando.

Para asegurar que puede tragar bien y para prevenir la aspiración:

• Piense en los pasos que debe tomar al tragar.
  1. Mantenga los labios cerrados.
  2. Mantenga los dientes juntos.
  3. Ponga la comida sobre su lengua.
  4. Levante la lengua y empuje hacia atras.
  5. Trague.

• Coma despacio y en bocadillos pequeños.
• Mastique duro y mueva la comida con la lengua.

• Termine un bocado antes de tomar otro.

Para evitar la acumulación de saliva en la boca:

• Haga el esfuerzo de tragar la saliva a menudo.
• Mantenga la cabeza erecta (derecha) para que la saliva se junte atrás de la garganta y para estimular el tragar automaticamente.
• Trague el exceso de saliva antes de tratar de hablar.

Parkinson Disease Association, 116 John St., New York, NY 10038, 1-800-223-APDA.

■ Surgical Management

Surgical intervention is not often used for PD. However, intractable tremor may be ameliorated by thalamotomy or pallidotomy. Autologous transplantation of adrenal medullary tissue into the brains of PD clients, in the hope that these cells will produce dopamine, has yielded disappointing results. Fetal tissue transplantation has produced better results, although no cases resulted in complete reversal of parkinsonian symptoms.[2] Transplantation of genetically engineered cell lines or vector-mediated gene transfection might ultimately prove to be the most effective strategy for the surgical treatment of PD.[2]

Huntington's Disease

Huntington's disease (HD), also known as Huntington's chorea, is a genetically transmitted degenerative neurologic disease. It is characterized by abnormal movements (chorea), intellectual decline, and emotional disturbance. Clinical manifestations usually begin in the 30s and 40s, although occasionally they begin in young adulthood or even in children. Women and men are equally affected. The disease is relentlessly progressive, leading to disability and death within 15 to 20 years. Death usually results from respiratory complications caused by aspiration.

The disease is autosomal dominant, meaning that offspring of an affected person have a 50% chance of inheriting the disease. Because HD does not skip generations, offspring who have not inherited the disease will not pass it on to their offspring. The abnormal gene has been isolated on chromosome 4.

The pathologic changes of HD involve degeneration of the striatum (caudate and putamen) in the basal ganglia. Other subtle changes occur in the cortex and cerebellum, namely, loss of neurons and an increased number of glial cells (gliosis). The degeneration of the caudate nucleus leads to a reduction in several neurotransmitters, including gamma-aminobutyric acid, ACh, substance P, and metenkephalin, and their synthetic enzymes. This leaves relatively higher concentrations of the other neurotransmitters, dopamine and norepinephrine. The relative excess of dopamine in HD, a disorder of excessive movement, can be contrasted to the lack of dopamine in PD, a disorder of lack of movement.

The abnormal movements in HD are subtle at first. The person may appear restless or fidgety. The person may be aware of these movements and try to mask them by making them seem to be parts of intentional movements, such as head scratching or leg crossing. As the disease progresses, the rapid, jerky choreiform movements become more pronounced and involve all muscles. The person is constantly in motion. Stress, emotional situations, and attempts to perform voluntary movement can aggravate the abnormal movements. During sleep, the movements diminish or disappear.

Emotional disturbances and mental deterioration may precede the abnormal movements. The person may become negative, suspicious, and irritable. This condition may progress to depression and psychosis. Temper outbursts and sexual promiscuity may also occur. Severe mood swings are common. Cognitive decline progresses, and eventually the person becomes demented, unkempt, incontinent, and completely helpless.

The diagnosis of HD is made on the basis of clinical signs and symptoms and family history, because there is no specific diagnostic test for the disease itself. CT or MRI imaging of the brain may show atrophy of the head of the caudate, but this factor alone is not diagnostic of HD.

There is no known treatment to cure or alter the course of HD. Haloperidol, a dopamine blocker, can control the abnormal movements and some behavioral manifestations.

Diazepam can be used to lower anxiety, aiding in control of movements. Antidepressants can help depression.

One of the most common and dangerous middle- to late-stage problems is dysphagia. Several interventions should be tried.[10] Medications need to be evaluated for their anticholinergic and sedative effects, which may impair swallowing. Mealtimes should be free of stress and clutter and have an unhurried atmosphere. Use of adaptive eating utensils can encourage and extend independence in eating. The diet should include foods that are easy to swallow, those that form a bolus in the mouth (e.g., canned peaches, chopped meat in gravy and mashed potatoes, custards). Because many clients with HD require high caloric intake because of excessive movements, they should try eating frequent, small meals containing high-calorie foods. Clients should sit bolt upright while eating. While swallowing they should keep the chin down toward the chest. They can be trained to hold their breath before swallowing and cough after each mouthful is swallowed to clear the throat of any residual food.

If the client continues to have difficulty eating and loses weight despite dietary and environmental modifications, a feeding tube may become necessary. However, artificial feeding methods often frighten families and they pose ethical dilemmas about prolonging life. Nurses can help clients and their families make these difficult decisions by clarifying the issues and providing information on the types, risks, benefits, and long-term effects of artificial feeding methods.[9]

Poor control of oral and respiratory muscles can make communication difficult. The nurse can assist the family to develop signals such as raising a hand or keeping the eyes open or closed for yes/no responses. If physical signals are not an option, cards with printed words may be helpful. Keep communication simple and unstrained. Repeat words that are understood to let the client know that communication has been successful.

Excessive movements and falls may cause physical injury and can restrict independence. Pads on wheelchairs and beds, shin guards, and walking belts can prevent injury. Aids for ambulation (e.g., walking behind a wheelchair) can extend independence. Clothing should be light, and simple to get on and off.

HD has a major impact on the family, not only because of the burden of caregiving but also because of the risk to offspring of inheriting the disease (see Ethical Issues in Nursing). Because a blood test is now available to check for the presence of the abnormal gene, family members face difficult choices about whether to find out if they have the Huntington's gene.

Myasthenia Gravis

Myasthenia gravis (MG) is an autoimmune disease that presents as muscular weakness and fatigue that worsens with exercise and improves with rest. It is caused by loss of ACh receptors in the postsynaptic neurons of the neuromuscular junction. The cause of MG is unknown, but 80% of people with the generalized form of the disease have elevated titers of antibodies to the ACh receptor in

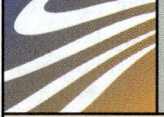

ETHICAL ISSUES IN NURSING

In Revealing Information About Huntington's Disease, Which Should Take Precedence: Client Confidentiality or Beneficence?

Huntington's disease is a degenerative neurologic disorder that is autosomal dominant and has a 50% chance of affecting offspring. The disease usually appears in a person's 30s or 40s, bringing on irreversible dementia that leads to death within approximately 10 years after onset. The disease, at present, is incurable. Often, parents have had children before they know that one of them has the possibility of passing on the disease. Currently, there are diagnostic tests that detect the disease long before symptoms are present. Because offspring of a parent with Huntington's disease have a 50% chance of developing the disease, early testing may assist them in their own decisions about having children.

Many ethical dilemmas surrounding the issue of privacy can surface in cases of Huntington's disease. Whether a person's test results are positive or negative, the results are of interest to the spouse, the other family members, employers, and insurers. Does the affected person have a special duty to inform the spouse? Is there a duty to inform other family members? What rights do employers or insurance companies have regarding the client's diagnosis?

There are several ethical principles that must be considered in this case. First, there is confidentiality. *A person has the right not to have medical information disclosed to anyone unless he or she consents to do so.* Is this right absolute, even if it means that others may be harmed by such confidentiality? The American Nurses' Association code states that there is a duty to tell the truth and not to deceive others. If a family member asks the nurse if another family member has a positive test for Huntington's chorea, what should the nurse do? Is there any duty of beneficence toward family members in disclosing information that could ultimately affect their lives?

The profession of nursing is one that assists others in maintaining or improving their health status. Information gathered from diagnostic tests can greatly influence the treatment decisions of healthcare providers. Information regarding a positive test for Huntington's disease may assist in the counseling of those family members at risk for developing the disease. However, if information is withheld from those family members, counseling may not be given. Nurses must be sensitive to their clients' desire for confidentiality, but should also use this opportunity to teach their client about the effect the disease may have on other family members.

---

their serum. MG may appear at any age, although there are two peaks of onset. In early-onset MG, at age 20 to 30 years, women are more often affected than men. In late-onset MG, after age 50, men are more often affected. The overall incidence of MG is 0.4/100,000 and the prevalence is 0.5 to 5.0/100,000.

The primary feature of MG is increasing weakness with sustained muscle contraction. For instance, if the person is asked to hold the arms up, the power of muscle contraction diminishes and the arms gradually drift downward. After a period of rest, the muscles regain their strength. Muscle weakness is greatest after exertion or at the end of the day. Ocular symptoms are most common, with ptosis (drooping of the upper eyelid) or diplopia (double vision) occurring in the majority of clients. Ptosis is due to weakness of the levator palpebrae muscles of the eye. If not present at the time of examination, ptosis can be elicited by prolonged upward gaze, which creates fatigue of the muscle. Diplopia is a result of weakness or fatigue of the extraocular muscles. Other symptoms are weakness of the orbicularis oculi muscles (which help close the eye), the facial muscles, the muscles of chewing and swallowing, and the limbs. Weakness of the facial and levator palpebrae muscles produces an expressionless face, with droopy eyelids, smoothed features, and a tendency for the mouth to hang open. An attempt to smile often turns into a snarl because of the weakness. A person may hold a hand under the jaw to keep it closed. Dysphagia and a nasal quality to speech occur when the muscles of chewing and swallowing are involved. In severe cases, respiratory muscle weakness may occur, which may necessitate intubation and mechanical ventilation (see discussion of myasthenic crisis).

The course of MG varies, and there may be remissions and exacerbations. Clinical manifestations may progress quickly or slowly and may fluctuate from day to day. The severity of the disease varies greatly from person to person.

The diagnosis of MG is based on the clinical presentation. It can be confirmed by testing the client's response to anticholinesterase drugs. These drugs inhibit cholinesterase, an enzyme that breaks down ACh in the neuromuscular junction, thereby allowing more ACh to bind to the remaining ACh receptors. Edrophonium (Tensilon) is a short-acting drug that is given intravenously. A test dose of 2 mg (for adults) is injected first. If no untoward reaction occurs (such as increased weakness, change in heart rate or rhythm, nausea, or abdominal cramps), the remaining 8 mg is injected. The client is then observed for objective signs of improvement in muscle strength. The effect is transitory, wearing off after 3 to 5 minutes. Another drug, neostigmine methylsulfate (Prostigmin), may be used because of its longer duration of effect on muscle strength (1–2 hours) which allows better analysis of its effect. When either drug is used, atropine sulfate should be available to inject intravenously as an antidote. This medication counteracts any severe cholinergic reactions (cardiac arrhythmias or abdominal cramping). Electromyography (EMG) helps confirm the diagnosis. Repetitive stimulation of the nerve with recording from the involved muscle shows a characteristic decrementing response of the muscle action potential.

■ Medical Management

There is no cure for MG. Pharmacologic intervention consists of two groups of medications: (1) short-acting anticholinesterase compounds and (2) corticosteroids. The most effective anticholinesterase drugs are pyridostigmine (Mestinon) and neostigmine (Prostigmin). Dosages are highly individualized, based on physiologic response to the medication. The goal is to achieve the maximum benefit (muscle strength and endurance) with the fewest side effects (excessive salivation, sweating, nausea, diarrhea, abdominal cramps, or tachycardia). Corticosteroids (usually prednisone) are directed toward reducing the levels of serum ACh receptor antibodies. Corticosteroids may temporarily worsen symptoms; however, this is followed by gradual improvement in muscle strength. After a peak of improvement is reached and maintained for several weeks, the dosage of both prednisone and anticholinesterase medication may be gradually decreased. A low maintenance dose of alternate-day prednisone may be effective for many months or years. The precautions of any steroid therapy are important, including potassium supplements if indicated and liberal use of antacids. Potential complications of steroid use are cataracts, hypertension, diabetes, fluid retention, delayed wound healing, insomnia, and osteoporosis. Other treatments include azathioprine (Imuran) and cyclosporine (Sandimmune), which reduce the level of circulating ACh receptor antibodies, and plasmapheresis and intravenous immunoglobulin G (IgG).

Plasmapheresis

Plasmapheresis is an adjunctive therapy for clients with refractory MG. It is a process by which plasma is separated from formed elements of blood. The plasma is discarded and the packed red blood cells are joined with albumin, normal saline, and electrolytes and returned to the client. The purpose is to remove plasma proteins containing antibodies that are believed to cause MG. Plasmapheresis produces transient improvement in clients who have actual or pending respiratory failure. Usually three to five treatments are required. Potential complications include myasthenic or cholinergic crisis and, rarely, hypovolemia. Muscle strength should be assessed before and after the procedure, with particular attention paid to vital

capacity, swallowing ability, diplopia, and ptosis to evaluate the effectiveness of the treatment.

Complications

Two major complications of MG may occur. One is *myasthenic crisis*. Clients with moderate or severe generalized MG, especially those who have difficulty swallowing or breathing, may experience a sudden worsening of their condition. This is usually precipitated by an intercurrent infection, but it may occur spontaneously. If an increase in the dosage of the anticholinesterase drug does not improve the weakness, endotracheal intubation and mechanical ventilation may be required. In many instances, drug responsiveness returns in 24 to 48 hours, and weaning from the respirator can proceed.

The other major complication of MG is *cholinergic crisis*. This occurs as a result of overmedication. The muscarinic effect of a toxic level of anticholinesterase medication causes abdominal cramps, diarrhea, and excessive pulmonary secretions. The nicotinic effect paradoxically worsens weakness and can cause bronchial spasm. If respiratory status is compromised, the client may need intubation and mechanical ventilation, and treatment is similar to that of the client in myasthenic crisis. Box 34–2 outlines the features and interventions of cholinergic and myasthenic crises.

■ Nursing Management of the Medical Client

Clients with MG are usually managed in an outpatient setting. Kernich and Kaminski[13] provide a detailed overview of nursing and collaborative care of clients with MG. When clients are hospitalized for diagnosis or during a crisis, the following nursing management procedure may be pertinent.

Because MG may involve the muscles of respiration, the client may experience dyspnea and ineffective cough and swallow mechanisms. This may lead to aspiration and pneumonia. Deep breathing and coughing should be encouraged. Suction equipment should be available at the bedside; instruct the client on how to use it. Instruct the client to sit bolt upright when eating, to swallow only when the chin is tipped downward toward the chest, and never to speak while food is in the mouth. Oxygen and, in severe cases, mechanical ventilation may be required.

In MG, weakness is usually greatest following exertion and at the end of the day. Activities should be carefully planned to include rest periods so that energy is conserved and the muscles have a chance to regain their strength. Rearrangement of the home environment may help prevent unnecessary energy expenditure. Vocational retraining may be indicated for those who can no longer meet the physical demands of their jobs. Clients with severe disease or an acute exacerbation will be totally dependent on nursing care for ADL. This level of care requires that complications of immobility be avoided.

Provide the client and family with information about MG and its treatment (see resources at end of chapter).

Box 34–2. Myasthenic and Cholinergic Crises in Clients with Myasthenia Gravis

Myasthenic Crisis Is Caused by Undermedication

Clinical Manifestations

Sudden marked rise in blood pressure due to hypoxia
Increased heart rate
Severe respiratory distress and cyanosis
Absent cough and swallow reflex
Increased secretions, increased diaphoresis, increased
  lacrimation
Restlessness, dysarthria
Bowel and bladder incontinence

Intervention

Increased doses of cholinergic drugs as long as the client
  responds positively to edrophonium treatment
Possible mechanical ventilation if respiratory muscle
  paralysis is acute

**Cholinergic Crisis Is Caused by Depolarization Block
Resulting from Excessive Medications**

Clinical Manifestations

Weakness with difficulty swallowing, chewing, speaking,
  and breathing
Apprehension, nausea and vomiting
Abdominal cramps, diarrhea
Increased secretions and saliva
Sweating, lacrimation, fasciculations, blurred vision

Intervention

Discontinue all cholinergic drugs until cholinergic effects
  decrease
Provide adequate ventilatory support
1 mg IV of atropine may be necessary to counteract
  severe cholinergic reactions

IV, intravenous.

They should be aware of adverse reactions of both anti-cholinesterase drugs and steroids. They also should know how to recognize myasthenic and cholinergic crises and have a plan to seek medical intervention, if necessary.

■ Surgical Management

Another intervention for MG is thymectomy. The thymus gland, located in the superior mediastinum, is important during fetal development for development of the immune system. It is usually atrophied and nonfunctioning in adulthood. The effect of thymectomy is not fully understood. It may alter some immunologic control mechanism that affects the production of antibodies to the ACh receptor, or it may eliminate a trigger to antibody production. Thymectomy is indicated for clients with thymoma, selected clients with generalized MG without thymoma, and selected clients with disabling ocular MG.[14] The procedure should be done early in the course of the disease. Nursing management is similar to care following thoracic surgery.

Eaton-Lambert Syndrome

Eaton-Lambert syndrome is a myasthenia-like condition in which weakness is noted in the limbs. It is also called myasthenic syndrome. This syndrome is characterized by defective release of ACh possibly caused by autoantibodies (IgG). Eaton-Lambert syndrome is found almost exclusively in persons with oat cell carcinoma of the lung, and has been noted less often in persons with cancers of the prostate, stomach, rectum, and breast. Eaton-Lambert syndrome has an insidious onset and the clinical manifestations are progressive. In comparison with MG, diplopia is less common and there is proximal weakness of the legs, arms, and pelvic girdle. There is reduced muscle action potential when muscle is stimulated, but repetitive stimulation augments muscle action. Weakness tends to develop with exertion, although some clients have a temporary increase in power when muscles are repeatedly stimulated. Autonomic dysfunction is common, presenting as dry mouth, impotence, and peripheral paresthesias. Treatment is directed at the primary cancer. Guanidine hydrochloride is a medication that may improve manifestations by increasing ACh release. Plasmapheresis and immunotherapy have also been used. Calcium channel blockers can worsen the transmission defect. Since MG can precede the development of cancer by many years, clients with Eaton-Lambert syndrome should be assessed yearly for the development of cancer.

Amyotrophic Lateral Sclerosis

Amyotrophic lateral sclerosis (ALS) is the most common of the motor neuron diseases. The onset of ALS usually occurs in middle age. Men are affected more often than women. The overall incidence of ALS is 0.4 to 1.8/100,000 and the prevalence is 4 to 6/100,000. ALS involves degeneration of both the anterior horn cells and the corticospinal tracts. Consequently, both upper and lower motor neuron clinical manifestations are seen. Lower motor neuron clinical manifestations include weakness, atrophy, cramps, and fasciculations (irregular twitchings of muscle fibers or bundles). Upper motor neuron signs include spasticity and hyperreflexia. Involvement of the corticobulbar tracts causes dysphagia (difficulty swallowing) and dysarthria (slurred speech). The sensory system is not involved nor is cognition affected. The client remains alert and mentally intact throughout the course of the disease.

The course of the disease is relentlessly progressive. Death usually results from pneumonia due to respiratory compromise within 2 to 5 years. Weakness typically begins in the upper extremities and progressively involves the upper arms and shoulders and then the muscles of the neck and throat. The trunk and lower extremities are usually not affected until late in the disease. When the intercostal muscles and diaphragm become involved, respirations become shallow and coughing is ineffective. Cognition, as well as bowel and bladder sphincters, remains intact, even when the client is totally debilitated. In some cases, weakness begins in the brain stem, causing problems with speech and swallowing. This is called *bulbar ALS.*

Diagnosis of ALS is made by the clinical presentation and electromyography (EMG). EMG criteria for the diagnosis of ALS include the presence of widespread anterior horn cell dysfunction with fibrillations, positive waves, fasciculations, and chronic neurogenic motor unit potential changes in multiple nerve root distribution in at least three limbs and the paraspinal muscles in the presence of normal sensory responses.

Supportive therapy was the only intervention for ALS until riluzole (Rilutek) was approved in 1996. Its mechanism of action is unknown, but it is thought to have a neuroprotective effect. The drug extends the life of ALS patients by a few months. Clients with ALS are usually admitted to healthcare facilities only twice in their illness, first for diagnosis and later in the final stage of debilitation.

Supportive nursing care is an important aspect of managing the ALS client. In the outpatient arena, the nurse can provide ongoing assessment of daily living needs and make suggestions for modifications in activity level, clothing, and diet. Often, just allowing the client or family to talk about problems reduces anxiety and helps them find solutions to problems.[21] Interventions should be aimed at conserving energy. Activities should be spaced during the day. Muscle stress, strenuous activity, and extremes of hot and cold should be avoided. Leg braces, canes, and walkers can prolong independence in ambulation. Hand braces, special utensils, and adaptive devices such as buttonhooks can help with dressing and self-feeding. Pressure ulcers are not usually a problem because the sensory system remains intact and the client can feel when pressure on a body part is too great.

In the acute care setting, the nurse gathers information from the client and family about communication needs and what positions are best for respiration, handling secretions, eating, and turning routines.

Fluid intake should be encouraged regularly, when the client is not fatigued. Proper positioning is imperative. Providing a cup with a spout may prevent liquid from running out of the corners of the mouth. Liquids may be given by using a large syringe with short tubing on the tip. The tube is placed on the anterior portion of the tongue, and gentle force is used to deliver small amounts of liquid.

Small, frequent, high nutrient feedings should be encouraged. The client should be told to sit bolt upright, with the head slightly flexed forward while eating. Papase tablets placed under the tongue 10 minutes before meals can make thick saliva less sticky. Plenty of time should be allowed for eating, and the client should not attempt to speak while food is in the mouth. Suction equipment should be available during meals to reduce the risk of aspiration of food and secretions that become lodged in the mouth and pharynx. The head may need to be stabilized with a soft cervical collar. The dietitian should be consulted for special diet recommendations.

Although speech remains intelligible, the client can be trained to slow the rate of speech and exaggerate articulation. As symptoms progress, the client may need to repeat words or have an interpreter (usually the spouse). At this

stage, it is important to eliminate extraneous noise, face the client when he or she is talking, and maintain eye contact. When speech contains only one-word phrases or is no longer possible, writing can be an effective means of communicating and should be encouraged. When writing is no longer possible, a speech pathologist can provide communication devices such as alphabet boards and portable memo writers.[9]

If the client is a smoker, encourage him or her to stop. Exposure to people with respiratory infections should be

Box 34–3. Resources for Clients Affected by a Degenerative Neurologic Disorder

Myasthenia Gravis Foundation
53 W. Jackson Blvd., Suite 660
Chicago, IL 60604
1/800/541–5454 or 312/427–6252

National Alzheimer's Association
919 Michigan Ave., Suite 1000
Chicago, IL 60661
1/800/272–3900

National Multiple Sclerosis Society
733 Third Ave.
New York, NY 10017
212/986–3240

The American Parkinson's Disease Association
60 Bay St.
Staten Island, NY 10301

National Parkinson's Foundation, Inc.
1501 NW 9th Ave.—Bob Hope Rd.
Miami, FL 33136

The Parkinson's Disease Foundation
William Black Medical Research Building
640 W. 168th St.
New York, NY 10032

United Parkinson's Foundation
360 W. Superior St.
Chicago, IL 60610

Parkinson's Support Group of America
13376 Cherry Hill Rd., Apt. 204
Beltsville, MD

Guillain-Barré Syndrome Foundation International
P.O. Box 262
Wynnewood, PA 19096
215/667–0131

ALS Society of America
15300 Ventura Blvd., Suite 315
Sherman Oaks, CA 91403
(818) 990–2151

Muscular Dystrophy Association (for ALS)
810 Seventh Ave.
New York, NY 10019
(212) 586–0808

avoided. Remind the client to use good posture. Pulmonary function tests should be performed regularly to assess ventilatory status. Clients generally experience respiratory fatigue when vital capacity is less than 1.5 L. Some clients can be taught to use their abdominal muscles to enhance respirations when the intercostal muscles and diaphragm become weak. A sign of pending respiratory insufficiency is shortness of breath while eating.

The client and family should be encouraged to talk about the losses they are experiencing and the feelings associated with them. Family members should be encouraged to take time for rest and activities away from the client. The client and family can be referred to an ALS support group.

Eventually, clients face the difficult choice of deciding whether or not they will accept artificial ventilation. Encourage them to discuss this with family and friends and to seek input from ALS support groups. Information about these groups can be obtained from the agencies listed in Box 34–3. Encourage clients to complete advance directives to indicate whether they desire life-sustaining treatments such as cardiopulmonary resuscitation, but this should be reassessed at regular intervals. Clients may change their minds on the basis of their experience with their illness, changes in their subjective appreciation of their quality of life, or changes in their evaluation of the benefits and burdens of life-sustaining measures as they come to terms with the imminence of death.[21]

Conclusions

Degenerative neurologic disorders have many causes, including viruses, autoimmune responses, and heredity. Some have no known cause. Because of the many causes, these disorders are feared by both the client and family. In general, they are relentlessly progressive, slowly taking away both physical and mental ability. The nurse needs to focus care on the management of clinical manifestations and prevention of complications. Family support throughout the process of care is essential.

Thinking Critically

1. A 52-year-old man with multiple sclerosis, who is wheelchair-bound and has a neurogenic bladder, complains of a sudden onset of generalized weakness, fever, and chills and is admitted to the hospital. What priorities should be set for his care?

Factors to Consider. What do generalized weakness, fever, and chills suggest in *any* client? If your client has not been following good bladder management, how can you intervene?

2. A 70-year-old man with Parkinson's disease is admitted to the hospital after experiencing severe nightmares and periods of confusion. During lucid periods, he is very disturbed by these symptoms. At other times, he believes that his wife is participating in a conspiracy to harm him. What assessments and interventions should you consider?

Factors to Consider. Are hallucinations and paranoia typical manifestations of Parkinson's disease? Could the client's manifestations be related to treatment, or to some cause other than his Parkinson's?

3. A 41-year-old woman with myasthenia gravis, who is taking pyridostigmine and prednisone, complains of increased fatigue and weakness, and difficulty breathing. What concerns should you have?

Factors to Consider. Might the client's difficult breathing be related to her fatigue and weakness? Could these symptoms be related to her myasthenia gravis or its treatment?

Bibliography

1. Acorn, S., & Andersen, S. (1990). Depression in multiple sclerosis: Critique of the research literature. *Journal of Neuroscience Nursing, 22*(4), 209–214.
2. Ahlskog, J. E. (1993). Cerebral transplantation for Parkinson's disease: Current progress and future prospects. *Mayo Clinic Proceedings, 68:* 578–591.
3. Bansil, S., Cook, S. D., & Rohowsky-Kochan, C. (1995). Multiple sclerosis: Immune mechanisms and update on current therapies. *Annals of Neurology, 37*(Suppl. 1), S87–101.
4. Bartol, M. (1979). Nonverbal communication in patients with Alzheimer's disease. *Journal of Gerontological Nursing, 5*(4), 21–31.
5. Corey-Bloom, J., et al. (1995). Diagnosis and evaluation of dementia. *Neurology, 45,* 211–218.
6. Corey-Bloom, J., Galaski, D., & Thal, L. J. (1994). Clinical features and natural history of Alzheimer's disease (pp. 631–645). In Calne, D. B. (Ed.), *Neurodegenerative diseases.* Philadelphia: W. B. Saunders.
7. Cummings, J. L., & Benson, D. F. (1992). *Dementia, a clinical approach.* Boston: Butterworth-Heinemann.
8. Evans, D. A., et al. (1989). Prevalence of Alzheimer's disease in a community population of older persons. *Journal of the American Medical Association, 262*(18), 2552–2556.
9. Hillel, A. D., & Miller, R. (1989). Bulbar amyotrophic lateral sclerosis: Patterns of progression and clinical management. *Head and Neck, 11*(1), 51–59.
10. Hunt, V. P., & Walker, F. O. (1989). Dysphagia in Huntington's disease. *Journal of Neuroscience Nursing, 21*(2), 92–95.
11. Hurley, A. C., et al. (1992). Assessment of discomfort in advanced Alzheimer patients. *Research in Nursing and Health, 15*(5), 369–378.
12. Jones, P. S., & Martinson, I. M. (1992). The experience of bereavement in care givers of family members with Alzheimer's disease. *Image: Journal of Nursing Scholarship, 24*(3), 172–176.
13. Kernich, A., & Kaminski, H. J. (1995). Myasthenia gravis: Pathophysiology, diagnosis, and collaborative care. *Journal of Neuroscience Nursing, 27,* 207–215.
14. Lanska, D. J. (1990). Indications for thymectomy in myasthenia gravis. *Neurology, 40*(12), 1828–1829.
14a. Lees, A. J. (1995). Comparison of therapeutic effects and mortality data of levodopa and levodopa combined with selegiline in patients with early, mild Parkinson's disease. *British Journal of Medicine, 311,* 1602–1607.
15. McKhann, G., et al. (1984). Clinical diagnosis of Alzheimer's disease: Report of the NINCDS-ADRDA Work Group under the auspices of Department of Health and Human Services Task Force on Alzheimer's Disease. *Neurology, 34*(7), 939–944.
16. Mayeux, R., & Chun, M. (1995). Dementias. In Rowland, L. P. (Ed.), *Merritt's textbook of neurology* (9th ed). Baltimore: Williams & Wilkins.

16a. Mega, M., Cummings, J., Fiorello, T., & Gornbein, J. (1996). The spectrum of behavioral changes in Alzheimer's disease. *Neurology, 46*(1), 130–135.

16b. Mezey, M., Kluger, M., Maislin, G., & Mittelman, M. (1996). Life-sustaining treatment decisions by spouses of patients with Alzheimer's disease. *Journal of the American Geriatric Society, 44*(2), 144–150.

17. Morris, R. G., Morris, L. W., & Britton, P. G. (1988). Factors affecting the emotional wellbeing of the caregivers of dementia sufferers. *British Journal of Psychiatry, 153,* 147–156.

18. Mocsny, N. (1991). Precautions to prevent the spread of Creutzfeldt-Jakob disease. *Journal of Neuroscience Nursing, 23*(2), 116–119.

19. Pfeffer, R. I., Afifi, A. A., & Chance, J. M. (1987). Prevalence of Alzheimer's disease in a retirement community. *American Journal of Epidemiology, 125*(3), 420–424.

20. Ropper, A. H. (1992). The Guillain-Barré syndrome. *New England Journal of Medicine, 326*(17), 1130–1136.

21. Silverstein, M. D., et al. (1991). Amyotrophic lateral sclerosis and life-sustaining therapy: Patients' desires for information, participation in decision making, and life-sustaining therapy. *Mayo Clinic Proceedings, 66*(9), 906–913.

22. Stone, N. (1987). Amyotrophic lateral sclerosis: A challenge for constant adaptation. *Journal of Neuroscience Nursing, 19*(3), 166–173.

23. Tienari, P. J. (1994). Multiple sclerosis: multiple etiologies, multiple genes? *Annals of Medicine, 26,* 259–269.

24. van der Meche, F. G. A. (1994). The Guillain-Barré syndrome: Plasma exchange or immunoglobulin intravenously? *Journal of Neurology, Neurosurgery, and Psychiatry, 57*(Suppl.), 33–34.

25. Vernon, G. M. (1989). Parkinson's disease. *Journal of Neuroscience Nursing, 21*(5), 273–282.

Paula Carson

Nursing Care of Clients with Disorders of the Spinal Cord, Peripheral Nerves, and Cranial Nerves

The intricacies and complexity of the nervous system permit the individual to collect, process, and interpret information about the surrounding world. Failure of these nerve pathways to accurately perform their tasks can significantly affect a person's interactions with others as well as his or her self-appraisal. This chapter examines disorders of the spinal cord and peripheral nerves, including the spinal and cranial nerves.

Disorders of the Spinal Cord

Spinal Cord Injury

Injury to the spinal cord can range in severity from mild flexion-extension "whiplash" injuries to complete transection of the cord with permanent quadriplegia. Trauma to the cord can occur at any level but most commonly occurs in the cervical and lower thoracic–upper lumbar vertebrae. This finding is due in part to the support given by the ribs to the thoracic spine.

Although this discussion focuses on nursing management of acute spinal cord injury (SCI), it should be remembered that there are approximately 200,000 spinal cord–injured people living in the United States.

Etiology and Risk Factors

Trauma is the most common cause of SCI. Each year approximately 10,000 people sustain an SCI. Most of these people are males under the age of 40. Traumatic spinal injuries are often caused by automobile or motorcycle accidents, gunshot or knife wounds, falls, or sporting mishaps.

The feeling of immortality often held by adolescents and young adults contributes strongly to their risk of SCI. Young people may believe they can engage in dangerous behavior without being injured. The use of alcohol and

This chapter incorporates material written for the fourth edition by Sally Strong Schnell.

illicit drugs can reinforce this belief in immortality. The Risk Factors and Levels of Prevention feature lists factors that contribute to SCI. The message of primary prevention may be best delivered by a young person who has experienced the devastation of SCI. There are several nationwide programs in which head and spinal cord–injured persons speak at school-sponsored educational programs. You can assist with these educational programs, as well as share your knowledge of SCI prevention on the basis of your experience.

Nontraumatic disorders may also result in SCI. These problems include the following:

- Cervical spondylosis with myelopathy (spinal canal narrowing with progressive injury to the cord and roots)
- Myelitis (infective or noninfective)
- Osteoporosis, causing vertebral compression fractures
- Syringomyelia (central cavitation of the cord)
- Tumors, both infiltrative and compressive
- Vascular diseases, usually infarction or hemorrhage

Whatever the cause, SCIs produce distinctive and debilitating damage. Nowhere else in the body can a local insult produce such devastation in proportion to the extent of tissue involved.

Flexion-Rotation, Dislocation, and Fracture-Dislocation Injuries. By far the most common spinal injuries are flexion injuries. For example, when a person strikes the head against the steering wheel or windshield, the spine is forced into acute hyperextension (Fig. 35–1). Rupture of the posterior ligaments results in forward dislocation of the vertebrae. Blood vessels may be damaged, leading to ischemia of the spinal cord. The cervical spine, usually at C5–6, is most commonly affected by a flexion injury. In the thoracic-lumbar spine, this type of injury is most frequently seen at T12–L1.

Hyperextension Injuries. Hyperextension injuries result after a fall in which the chin hits an object and the

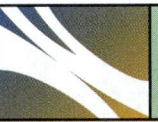

RISK FACTORS AND LEVELS OF PREVENTION

Spinal Cord Injury

Risk Factors

Alcohol consumption while operating a moving vehicle; diving; recreational activities such as bicycling, motorcycling, rollerblading, or horseback riding, especially without a helmet; occupations that require the use of ladders, climbing, or heights 5 ft or more above the ground

Levels of Prevention

Primary Prevention

- Educate the public on the hazards of drinking and driving and on the risk of diving into water of uncertain depth.
- Encourage clients to wear helmets when bicycling, motorcycling, rollerblading, and horseback riding.

Secondary Prevention

- Stabilize the client's spine to correct the already compromised spinal cord.
- Help clients to maintain the use of traction, specialized beds, halo braces, and lumbar braces.
- Prevent twisting of the client's spine during position changes or transfers.

Tertiary Prevention

- Encourage clients to maintain cardiovascular and pulmonary integrity.
- Educate the client and caregiver regarding:
  - Maintenance of skin integrity.
  - Achievement of adaptive activities of daily living.
  - Maintenance of bowel and bladder function.
  - Psychosocial adaptation to life-style changes.
  - Prevention and early recognition of autonomic dysreflexia.

head is thrown back (Fig. 35–1B). The anterior ligament is ruptured with fracture of the posterior elements of the vertebral body. Hyperextension of the spinal cord against the ligamenta flava can lead to dorsal column contusion and posterior dislocation of the vertebrae. Complete transection of the cord can follow a hyperextension injury. Complete lesions of the cord result in loss of all voluntary movement below the lesion and loss of reflex function in isolated segments of the cord.

Compression Injuries. Compression injuries are often caused by falls or jumps in which the person lands directly on the head, sacrum, or feet (Fig. 35–1C). The force of impact fractures the vertebrae and the fragments compress the cord. Disc and bone fragments may be propelled backward into the spinal cord upon impact. The lumbar and the lower thoracic vertebrae are the most commonly injured regions following a compression impact. About 50% of these injuries result in incomplete lesions. Incomplete lesions occur when some of the spinal tracts remain intact.

Unique Cervical Injuries. Two types of fractures are unique to the cervical spine: odontoid and hangman's fractures (Fig. 35–2). Fractures of the odontoid process (the odontoid process is the superior projection of the bone on C2) may be intact (no movement) or displaced with movement and entrapment of the spinal cord (Fig. 35–2A). A hangman's fracture is a break through the pedicles of C2, dividing the vertebrae (Fig. 35–2B). Clients with these two types of fractures either die from the injury immediately or are stable and actually walk into the emergency department reporting only neck pain.

Pathophysiology

SCIs most often occur as a result of injury to the vertebrae. The most common sites of injury are at the C1–2, C4–6, and T11–L2 vertebrae. These segments of the spine are the most mobile and thereby most easily injured.

The cord is injured as the result of acceleration, deceleration, or another force (e.g., impact) applied to the spine. The forces injure the spinal cord by compressing, pulling, or tearing the tissues. Microscopic bleeding occurs immediately after injury, primarily in the gray matter of the cord. Within the first hour, edema develops and often spreads along the length of the spinal cord. Edema is caused by arachidonic acid and its metabolites (prostaglandins, thromboxanes, and leukotrienes). Cord edema peaks within 2 to 3 days and subsides within the first 7 days after injury. Although the site of the initial injury has the most edema and bleeding, some edema and bleeding extend at least for two cord segments on either side of the injury. The edema of the cord leads to temporary loss of sensation and function. Therefore, immediately after injury, it is not easy to determine the degree of permanent impairment.

Further changes include fragmentation of the axonal covering and loss of myelin. Phagocytic cells can injure surviving axons as they scavenge cellular debris. Chemotactic and inflammatory mediators further extend tissue necrosis. Macrophages engulf so much spinal cord that a central cavity (called post-traumatic syringomyelia) develops as early as 9 days after injury.

In addition, the oligodendroglial cells that support the cord are lost. Injury to the cord produces rapid losses of axonal conduction due to ion changes, such as very rapid increases in extracellular potassium and influx of calcium into the cell. Finally, free radicals are produced. Free radicals are normally found in the body but are quickly controlled by antioxidant enzyme systems. When the antioxidant systems are overwhelmed, the free radicals damage tissues.

The physiologic response to SCI extends beyond changes within the spinal cord. For example, the sympathetic nervous system stress response results in reduced perfusion of the gastrointestinal tract and reduced produc-

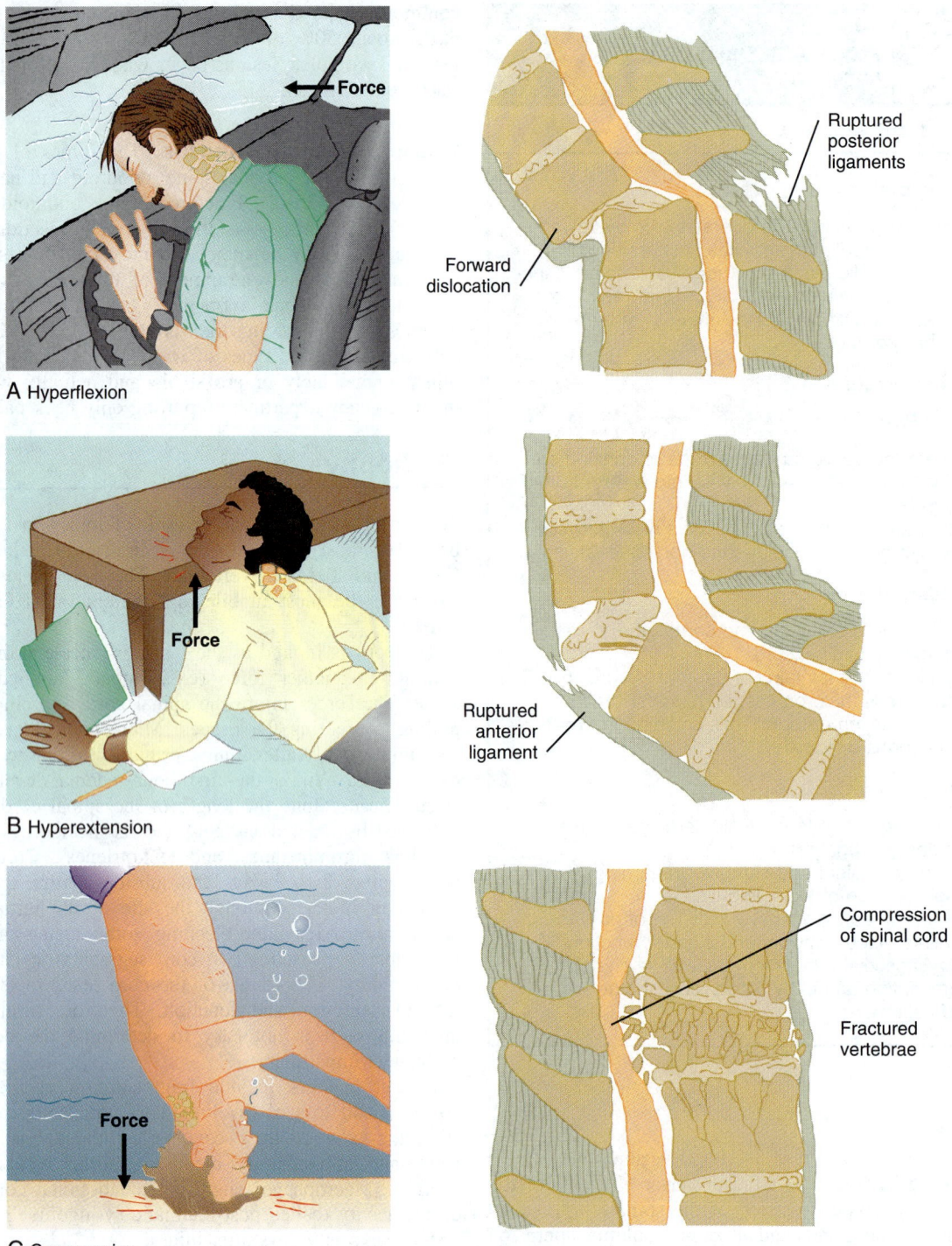

A Hyperflexion

Force

Forward dislocation

Ruptured posterior ligaments

B Hyperextension

Force

Ruptured anterior ligament

C Compression

Force

Compression of spinal cord

Fractured vertebrae

Figure 35–1. *A,* Flexion injury of the cervical spine ruptures the posterior ligaments. *B,* Hyperextension injury of the cervical spine ruptures the anterior ligaments. *C,* Compression fractures crush the vertebrae and force bony fragments into the spinal canal.

tion of gastric mucus to protect the lining. Ulceration and bleeding may develop.

Spasticity is the increased tone or contraction of muscles, producing stiff movements. Various central nervous system (CNS) injuries or diseases, such as SCIs, cerebrovascular accidents, and cerebral palsy may result in spasticity. Following spinal cord transection, the brain can no longer influence reflex movements built into the spinal cord. Eventually the lower part of the cord, using spinal reflexes, begins to work automatically. Spinal reflex activities occurring automatically after spinal cord severance include the flexor withdrawal reflex and reflex emptying of the bladder and bowel. These primitive spinal mechanisms, normally kept inactive by higher centers, are "re-

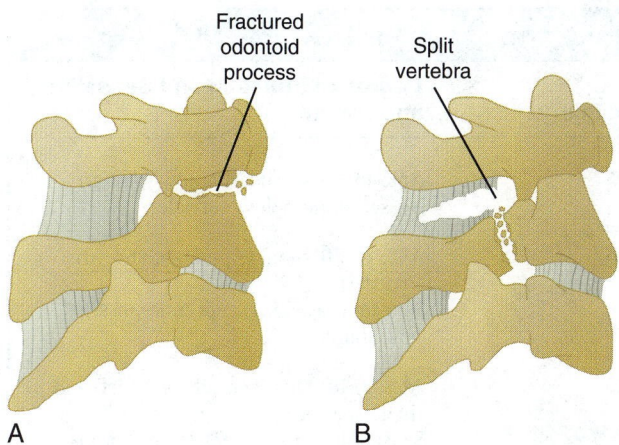

Figure 35–2. *A,* Odontoid fractures are fractures of the superior projection of C2 that normally projects into C1. Stabilization is required for healing. *B,* Hangman's fractures are of the pedicle of C2. The vertebra is split in half. These fractures are usually treated with a halo brace.

leased" when the normal inhibitions of the higher centers are destroyed. As recovery progresses after cord transection, flexor responses are interspersed with extensor spasms. These movements ultimately develop into predominantly extensor activity. The client's limbs spasm into extension with movement. Spasticity may remain indefinitely or gradually decrease over time.

Clinical Manifestations and Diagnostic Findings

■ Level of Injury

The initial clinical manifestations of acute SCI depend on the level and extent of injury to the cord. Below the level of injury or lesion, there is *loss of*

1. Voluntary movement
2. Sensation of pain, temperature, pressure, and proprioception
3. Bowel and bladder function
4. Spinal and autonomic reflexes

The level of injury may be described in terms of (1) skeletal injury and (2) neurologic level of injury. Skeletal injury refers to the vertebral damage demonstrated by x-ray. The criterion of the American Spinal Injury Association (ASIA) is useful in describing the level of spinal cord involvement: *The neurologic level of injury is the lowest segment of the spinal cord with bilateral intact sensory and motor function.* Sensory function is assessed by using dermatomes to identify the areas of skin with normal sensation. Motor function is measured by testing myotomes to identify muscles with active movement and full range of motion (ROM) against gravity. The ASIA Impairment Scale describes functioning in terms of normal and four degrees of impairment:

Normal with sensory and motor function preserved
Incomplete with the majority of motor function preserved
Incomplete with nonfunctional motor function preserved
Incomplete with only sensation preserved
Complete with loss of sensation and motor function

Injury to the cervical spine and cord produces quadriplegia. Injuries above C4 may be fatal because of loss of innervation to the diaphragm and intercostal muscles. Without immediate rescue breathing after the accident, the person will die of respiratory failure. Today, with the general public's knowledge of cardiopulmonary resuscitation, many people survive injury to the cervical spine. Injuries to the remainder of the cervical spine create specific patterns of motor loss (Table 35–1). Note that a person with a C7 injury is able to lift the shoulders, elbows, wrists, and have some hand function, but below C7 there remains no motor function or sensation.

Injuries to the thoracic or lumbar spine produce paraplegia. Persons with such injuries have function of their upper extremities and can be mobile in a wheelchair or with crutches and braces. Table 35–1 describes the extent of paralysis as it relates to the level of injury. Persons with L5 injury can extend their great toe and dorsiflex the ankle. They have no sensation in the perianal area, calf, heel, or small toe.

■ Changes in Reflexes

Reflexes, which normally cross the spinal cord and return to the stimulated limb, are absent in early SCI because of spinal cord edema. Blood pressure and temperature in denervated (without nervous function or innervation) areas fall markedly and respond poorly to reflex stimuli.

After cord edema subsides, some body functions may return by reflex (e.g., control of the urinary bladder), but they lack integration with other visceral activities. Visceral activities may be initiated by atypical stimuli. For example, scratching the skin may cause vasodilation, sweating, and urination. Nervous system lesions may produce defective urinary bladder function known as cord bladder. For example, stimulation of the skin on the lower abdomen or thighs may cause reflex urination. This form of cord bladder is called an automatic bladder. Such stimulation may also cause reflex ejaculation and priapism (persistent abnormal penile erection without sexual desire) in paralyzed men.

■ Muscle Spasms

Intense and painful muscular spasms of the lower extremities occur following a traumatic complete transverse spinal cord lesion. In assisting the client and his or her family to understand these movements, tell them that these muscle spasms are involuntary and do not mean that voluntary movement is returning. This information, although disappointing, is essential.

Muscle spasms vary from mild muscular twitching to vigorous mass reflexogenic states. Extreme, involuntary muscle spasms can actually throw a client out of bed. Bed side rails are kept up and restraining straps are comfortably secured over the client lying on a stretcher. Muscle spasms, often aggravated by cold weather, prolonged periods of sitting, or emotionally upsetting events, may

Table 35–1. Spinal Cord Injury and Impairment

	Level of Injury	Degree of Function and Sensation Impairment
	C5	Able to lift shoulder, elbow (partial) No sensation below clavicle
	C6	Able to lift shoulder, elbow, and wrist (partial) Sensation as C5, except more in arms and thumb
	C7	Able to lift shoulder, elbow, wrist, and hand (partial) Sensation as C6 except more in arms and middle finger
	C8	Able to lift shoulder, elbow, wrist, and hand (partial) Sensation as C7 except more in arms and little finger
	T4	Able to use arms and hands normally No sensation below nipple line
	T6	Able to use intercostal muscles No sensation below 6th intercostal space
	L2	Able to use abdominal muscles and flex hips No sensation below midanterior thigh or in perianal area
	L5	Able to extend great toe and dorsiflex ankle No sensation in perianal area or calf, heel, or little toe
	S1	Able to plantar-flex ankle No sensation in popliteal fossa, ischial tuberosity, or perianal area
	S2–5	No sensation in perianal area

Diagram labels: T4, T6, C5, C6, S3–5, C8, L2, C7, S2, L5, S1

become intolerable. Reflex spasms may be triggered by extrinsic or visceral stimuli, such as a distended bladder.

Spastic movements may be initiated by (1) emotion (e.g., anxiety, crying, anger, or laughing) or (2) cutaneous stimulation (e.g., tickling, stroking, or pinching). By learning to recognize events that trigger such reflex spasms, the client may use these potentially annoying movements to achieve functional activities such as urination.

■ Autonomic Dysreflexia

Autonomic dysreflexia, a life-threatening syndrome, is a cluster of clinical manifestations that results when multiple spinal cord autonomic responses discharge simultaneously. This syndrome, observed in as many as 85% of clients with injury above T7, can occur anytime after

spinal shock has resolved. Dysreflexia often resolves 3 years after injury, but it may reoccur. The manifestations of autonomic dysreflexia result from an exaggerated sympathetic response to a noxious stimulus below the level of the cord lesion. Stimuli commonly are bladder and bowel distention but can be pressure ulcers, spasms, pain, pressure on the penis, excessive rectal stimulation, bladder stones, ingrown toenails, abdominal abnormalities, or uterine contractions.

Exaggerated sympathetic responses cause the blood vessels below the level of injury to constrict. As a result, the client develops hypertension (possibly as high as 300 mm Hg), a pounding headache, flushing, nasal stuffiness, diaphoresis, piloerection ("gooseflesh"), dilated pupils with blurred vision, bradycardia (30–40 beats per minute), restlessness, and nausea. The manifestations are a result of the success and failure of compensatory efforts to overcome the severe hypertension. Initially, baroreceptors sense the hypertensive stimuli and stimulate the parasympathetic nervous system, which results in vasodilation above the level of cord injury (headache, flushing) and bradycardia. The problem is that the visceral and peripheral vessels do not dilate because the efferent impulses cannot pass through the damaged cord. Thus, the overall effect is one of extreme hypertension. Seizures and cerebral hemorrhage occur in approximately 10% to 15% of cases. See the discussion of Risk for Autonomic Dysreflexia for interventions.

■ Clinical Syndromes Causing Partial Paralysis

There are five spinal cord syndromes causing partial paralysis: (1) central cord syndrome, (2) anterior cord syndrome, (3) Brown-Séquard syndrome, (4) conus medullaris syndrome, and (5) cauda equina syndrome (Fig. 35–3). Each has distinctive neurologic findings.

Central Cord Syndrome. Central cord syndrome (most common with hyperextension-hyperflexion injuries) produces more weakness in the upper extremities than in the lower. The weakness is caused by edema and hemorrhage in the central area of the cord, which is predominantly occupied by nerve tracts to the hands and arms (Fig. 35–3A).

Anterior Cord Syndrome. A lesion in the anterior spinal cord causes anterior cord syndrome, with complete motor function loss and decreased pain sensation (Fig. 35–3B). Touch, position, and vibration sensations remain intact. Cervical cord concussion may produce varying degrees of motor and sensory deficit, which completely resolve within hours. Occasionally, cervical cord trauma produces only root injuries, which may paralyze isolated muscles or muscle groups in the arms and shoulders. These deficits are usually permanent.

Brown-Séquard Syndrome. Brown-Séquard syndrome (Fig. 35–3C) is caused by lateral hemisection of the cord (i.e., when a lesion cuts or affects half the cord) such as with a bullet wound or knife wound. This results in ipsilateral motor paralysis, loss of vibratory and position sense, and contralateral loss of pain and temperature sensation.

Conus Medullaris Syndrome. Conus medullaris syndrome follows damage to the lumbar nerve roots and the conus medullaris in the spinal cord (Fig. 35–3D). The client usually has bowel and bladder areflexia and flaccid lower extremities. The bulbospongiosis penile (erection) and micturition reflexes may be preserved when damage occurs to the upper sacral segments of the spinal cord.

Cauda Equina Syndrome. Injury to the lumbosacral nerve roots below the conus medullaris is called cauda equina syndrome (Fig. 35–3E). The client experiences areflexia of the bowel, bladder, and lower extremities.

■ Spinal Shock

The immediate response to cord transection is called spinal shock or post-traumatic areflexia. The spinal cord–injured person experiences complete loss of skeletal muscle function, bowel and bladder tone, sexual function, and autonomic reflexes. Loss of venous return and hypotension also occur. The hypothalamus cannot control temperature by vasoconstriction and increased metabolism; therefore, the client assumes the environmental temperature.

Spinal shock may last for 7 days to 3 months. Indications that spinal shock is resolving include return of reflexes, development of hyperreflexia rather than flaccidity, and return of reflex emptying of the bladder. The earliest reflexes recovered are the flexor reflexes evoked by noxious cutaneous stimulation. The return of the bulbospongiosis reflex in male patients is also an early indicator of recovery from spinal shock. Babinski's reflex (dorsiflexion of the great toe with fanning of the other toes when the sole of the foot is stroked) is an early-returning reflex.

■ Diagnostic Assessment

Initially, full spinal x-rays are obtained. If a high cervical lesion is suspected, films of the odontoid bone through the open mouth may be required. Computed tomographic (CT) scans or tomograms may be obtained after the client has achieved hemodynamic and pulmonary stabilization. They provide more information regarding the nature of fractures and the status of the spinal cord. They are also useful if a fracture is not seen on x-ray study, but neurologic deficit is present. Magnetic resonance imaging (MRI) may also be used to locate the level of the lesion. Although controversial, myelography may be used if SCI is suspected and the degree of deficit is increasing. Somatosensory evoked potentials (SEPs) are used to establish the extent of injury and are often performed within 48 hours of admission.

Emergency Care

Both the initial (especially during the first hour after injury) and long-term intervention provided for a client experiencing SCI significantly influence

1. The extent of the injury and associated deficits
2. How well the person survives the acute phase of injury
3. The success of recovery and rehabilitation

People with SCI can lead productive and, in some cases, independent lives.

At the scene of the accident, the injured person should be moved only when there are adequate numbers of people to accomplish this and immobilize the spine. The neck should be stabilized in a neutral position without

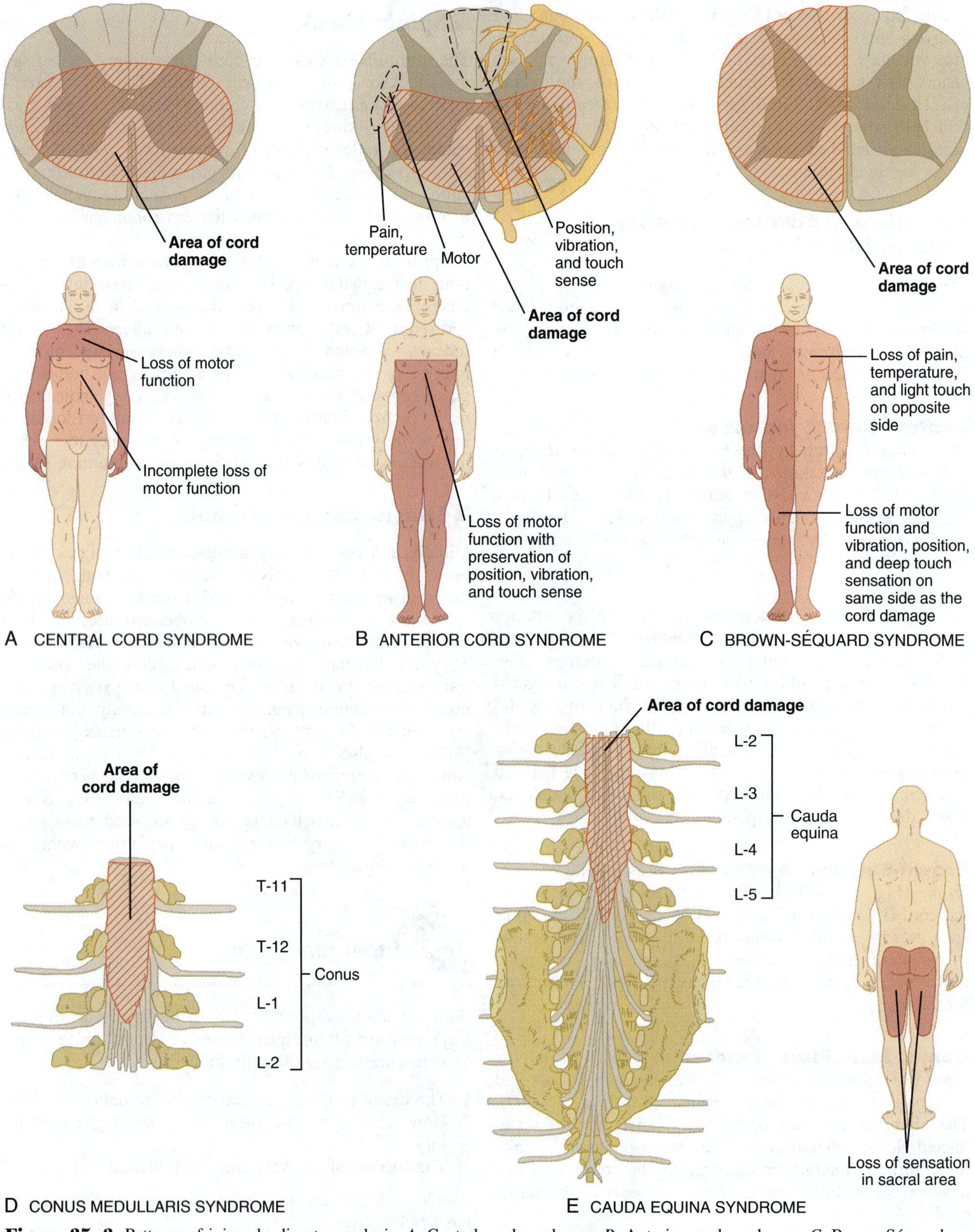

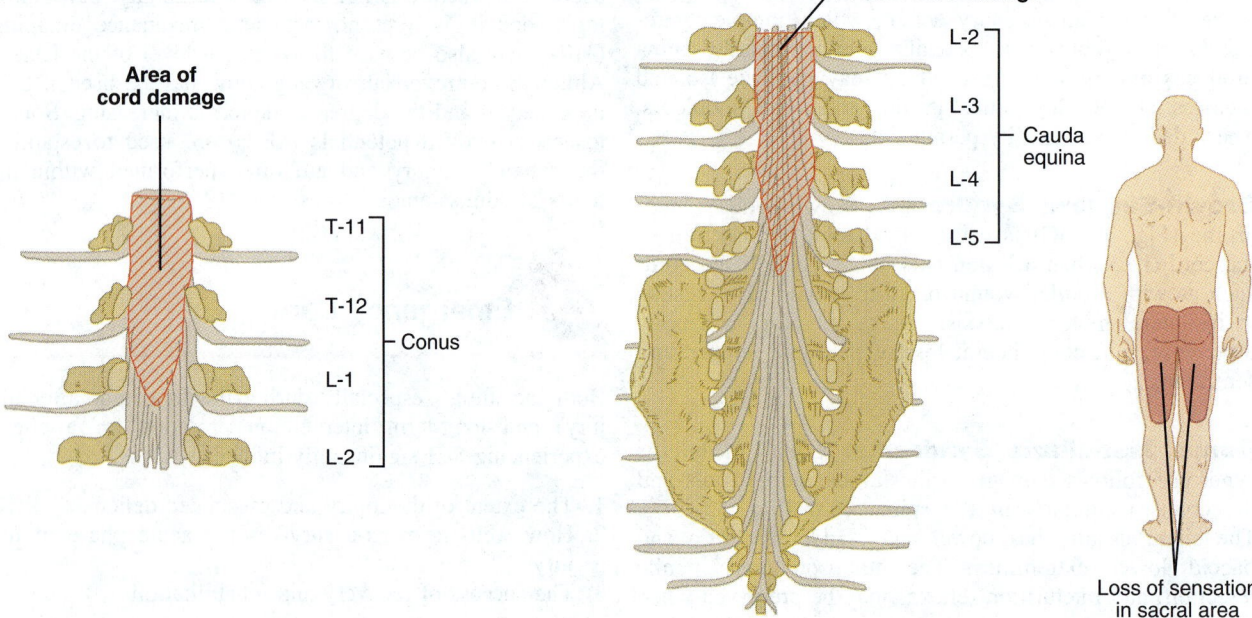

Area of cord damage

Loss of motor function

Incomplete loss of motor function

A CENTRAL CORD SYNDROME

Pain, temperature Motor

Position, vibration, and touch sense

Area of cord damage

Loss of motor function with preservation of position, vibration, and touch sense

B ANTERIOR CORD SYNDROME

Area of cord damage

Loss of pain, temperature, and light touch on opposite side

Loss of motor function and vibration, position, and deep touch sensation on same side as the cord damage

C BROWN-SÉQUARD SYNDROME

Area of cord damage

T-11
T-12 Conus
L-1
L-2

D CONUS MEDULLARIS SYNDROME

Area of cord damage

L-2
L-3 Cauda equina
L-4
L-5

Loss of sensation in sacral area

E CAUDA EQUINA SYNDROME

Figure 35–3. Patterns of injury leading to paralysis. *A*, Central cord syndrome. *B*, Anterior cord syndrome. *C*, Brown-Séquard syndrome. *D*, Conus medullaris syndrome. *E*, Cauda equina syndrome.

flexion or extension until a fixed immobilizing device can be applied. Cervical traction should not be applied. Without an x-ray to guide movements, the spinal cord can be injured. The simplest method of immobilizing the spine is to place the individual on a spine board and secure the spine with a hard collar around the neck and Velcro ties across the torso and legs. Transparent stiff collars have become popular because they allow visualization of the carotid arteries and trachea. Excellent on-the-scene care has increased the number of persons who are neurologically intact despite vertebral column fractures.[28] Also, accurate reporting of the person's baseline deficits is essential to help the physician plan the aggressiveness of treatment interventions.

Spinal trauma is often associated with other injuries such as head injury, chest trauma, extremity fractures, and abdominal injury. Anyone who has sustained multiple trauma should be handled as if spinal injuries are present until assessment proves otherwise. When handling a client suspected of having a cervical spine injury, the spine is kept in neutral alignment and flexion is prevented. If turning is required, a logrolling maneuver is used. The client is placed in a supine position on a firm surface. The head is supported in alignment with the body and is immobilized with a firm, padded, cervical collar. Some physicians use halter traction immediately to keep the cervical spine aligned and prevent movement. Clothing is cut off rather than removed. The client is transported on a flat, firm stretcher with the neck immobilized. SCI personnel should remain with the person while x-ray studies are taken to ensure that the cervical spine is not moved.

Cervical spine injury may produce respiratory distress. In this case, immediate action is taken to maintain a patent airway and provide adequate oxygenation. It is important that the client's neck not be hyperextended during intubation; therefore, the jaw thrust technique is used. Suction is performed as necessary to maintain a patent airway. Mechanically assisted respiration is required when definite loss or impairment of respiratory muscle function occurs. Respiratory parameters can be used to guide a decision to mechanically ventilate the client. Serial decreases in vital capacity, along with an increase in partial pressure of arterial carbon dioxide ($PaCO_2$) are good predictors of impending pulmonary failure. A vital capacity of less than 15 ml/kg is cause for serious concern.

In the emergency department, a person who has sustained a severe cervical injury should be placed immediately in skeletal traction to immobilize the cervical spine and reduce the fracture and dislocation. Various types of skull tongs may be used for this: Crutchfield or Gardner-Wells. The tongs are inserted through the outer table of the skull (Fig. 35–4). Traction is applied to the tongs via rope, pulleys, and weights. Weights begin with 10 to 20 lb (4.5–9.1 kg) and are gradually increased to accomplish bone reduction. When proper alignment is obtained and verified by x-ray examination, the traction weight may be lessened to maintain the reduction. Traction is not used to stabilize and immobilize thoracic or lumbar spinal fractures or fracture-dislocations because there is no effective way to provide it. Therefore, the spine is kept in alignment and logrolling is used as needed until surgical stabilization can be obtained.

A cross-table lateral x-ray film of the cervical spine is obtained prior to transport. Lateral and anteroposterior x-ray studies are not usually sufficient. To visualize lower cervical fractures, it is necessary to either apply downward traction to the arms or have the arms in the swimmer's position during x-ray examination. If a high cervical lesion is suspected, a view of the odontoid bone through the open mouth may be required. A brief but thorough neurologic examination is made to assess the

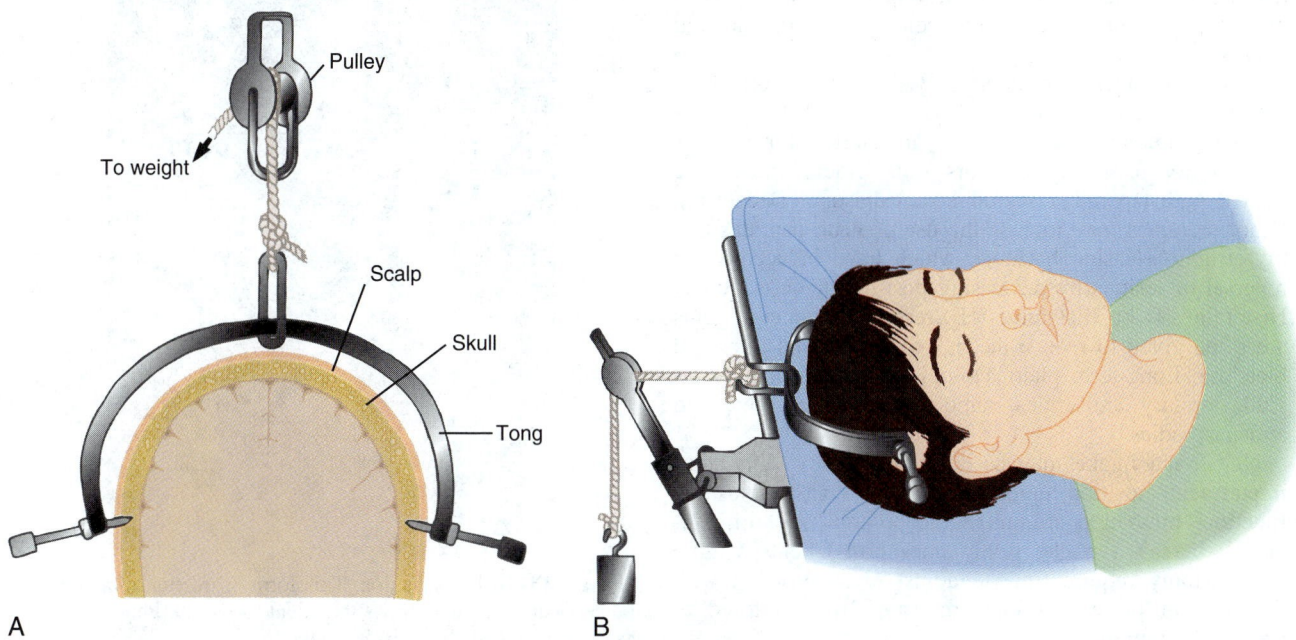

Figure 35–4. Skeletal traction for cervical injuries. *A,* Crutchfield tongs. *B,* Gardner-Wells tongs.

extent of injury and establish a baseline of function and involvement for later comparison.

Common emergent interventions include insertion of an intravenous (IV) line and infusion of normal saline, insertion of an indwelling catheter, administration of potent steroids, administration of vasoactive medications to maintain systolic blood pressure, insertion of a nasogastric tube, and provision of oxygen if oxygen saturation is low.

Once the client is stabilized, the client is transferred to an intensive care unit (ICU, hyperacute care area) or to an SCI center. It is important that the client be appropriately immobilized prior to transport.

Critical Care

■ Medical Management

Once the client's spine and emergent medical conditions have stabilized, a complete neurologic assessment is performed. Several complications commonly accompany SCI. These include orthopedic injury to the spine, head injury, chest injury, abdominal injury, and genitourinary injury. Some of these injuries may not be immediately evident in the emergency room, and ongoing assessments are made until the problem is ruled out.

The client is monitored for spinal shock and the effects of hypotension, bradycardia, and decreased cardiac output. Respiratory compromise may occur if the client develops diaphragmatic fatigue; mechanical ventilation may be needed. Arterial blood gases are monitored closely. The client may be transferred to a Stryker frame or Roto-Rest bed to reduce the risk of pressure ulcer development and other complications of immobility. These beds are shown in Figure 31–7.

Complications include atelectasis, pneumonia, bradycardia, hypotension, deep vein thrombosis, gastrointestinal bleeding, pressure ulcers, joint contractures, denial, and depression.

Vasoactive agents are commonly used to support blood pressure immediately after injury. Short-term high doses of methylprednisolone 30 mg/kg are started for persons with injury less than 8 hours old. Older injuries are treated with tapered doses of dexamethasone (Decadron). Other therapies may include the use of neuropeptides and thyrotropin-releasing hormone which have induced some reversal of lesions by decreasing post-traumatic ischemia. Histamine-H$_2$ or Histamine (H$_2$)-receptor blocking agents are often given to reduce the risk of gastric and intestinal bleeding. Long-term pharmacologic management may include urinary antiseptics, anticoagulants, laxatives, and antispasmodics.

Nutritional intake may be compromised by respiratory impairment, position, emotional status, or gastrointestinal function. Intubation eliminates the possibility of oral intake, whereas a tracheostomy does not. Clients with a tracheostomy require time to adjust to swallowing with the tube in place and must be carefully monitored to prevent aspiration.

Aspiration is also a risk for clients who must remain flat while in tongs and traction. Although these clients may be capable of swallowing, it is unlikely that they will be able to safely consume enough food to meet their metabolic needs. Clients in halo jackets (Fig. 35–5) often experience difficulty eating because their head is immobile. They should be encouraged to take small bites, eat slowly, and concentrate on swallowing.

Depression is a common reaction to SCI and may inhibit the appetite. Choosing when and what to eat may be one of the few areas of control left to the person with an SCI. As much free choice of dietary intake as is feasible should be encouraged.

Any of these conditions can severely limit a spinal cord–injured client's oral intake at a time when a high calorie, high protein diet is needed. Enteral feeding or total parenteral hyperalimentation is often prescribed until oral intake is sufficient to meet body needs.

■ Nursing Management of the Medical Client

Assessment

A holistic assessment is essential when caring for clients with SCI. Every system of the body is affected. A complete baseline assessment is obtained initially. The results of subsequent serial assessments are then compared with the baseline. Specific components in the assessment of the client with an SCI depend on the phase of treatment the

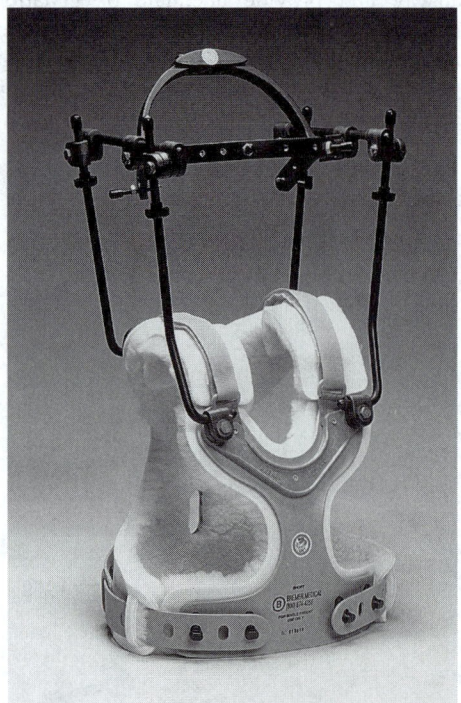

Figure 35–5. Halo traction. This form of traction immobilizes the cervical spine and allows the client to move. (Photo courtesy of Bremer Medical, Jacksonville, FL.)

client is in at that moment. Therefore assessment is addressed within each section of care.

Careful monitoring of hemodynamic parameters is essential. Heart rate, blood pressure, temperature, respirations, fluid balance, and pulse oximetry should be monitored continuously.

If the client is conscious, ask where any pain is occurring. Sensation is tested by determining whether the person can feel a touch or a pinprick in the feet, legs, trunk, hands, and arms. Levels of sensation are documented according to dermatomes. To assess motor function, ask the client to wiggle the toes, move the ankles, flex the knees, and move the hands and arms. The location, symmetry, and strength of muscle movement are documented (Table 35–2). The major reflexes, that is, the Achilles, patellar, biceps, and triceps, are briefly tested. Look for areas of sensory sparing, such as sacral sparing, in which the perineum retains sensation.

If the client is unresponsive, assessment is more limited. Assess respiratory status by observing for spontaneous movement and thorax expansion. Sensation and movement of extremities are assessed by watching the client for a few moments or by applying a painful stimulus (nail-bed pressure) and observing for withdrawal. Obtain details of the injury and the client's condition immediately after the injury from witnesses.

Usually the client is awake and may be concerned about obtaining pain relief, the chances of surviving, and

Table 35–2. Motor Assessment After Spinal Cord Injury

Spinal Nerve	Assessment Technique
C4–5	Shoulders are shrugged against downward pressure of examiner's hands
C5–6	Arm is pulled up from resting position against resistance
C7	From the flexed position, arm is straightened out against resistance
C7	Index finger is held firmly to thumb against resistance to pull apart
C8	Hand grasp strength is evaluated
L2–4	Leg is lifted from bed against resistance
L5–S1	Knee is flexed against resistance
L2–4	From flexed position, knee is extended against resistance
L5	Foot is pulled up toward nose against resistance
S1	Foot is pushed down (stepping on the gas) against resistance

Modified from Marshall, S. B., et al. (1990). *Neuroscience critical care: Pathophysiology and patient management* (p. 327). Philadelphia: W. B. Saunders.

the safety of other people in the accident. Once these issues are addressed, the client may begin to appraise the severity of his or her own injury.

Rehabilitation begins when the client is admitted to the healthcare facility. During the acute stage, nursing and medical attention is appropriately focused on immediate needs. However, it is also imperative to remember that the client probably has severe residual disabilities and must make major life-style changes. Care provided in the acute period can significantly affect the client's later life. Prevention of complications such as infection, pressure sores, and contractures facilitates rehabilitation and reduces suffering, disability, and expense.

Diagnosis, Planning, Implementation

Risk for Hypotension. Clients suffering from SCI are at *Risk for Hypotension.* This collaborative problem is related to vasodilation and the inability to vasoconstrict, not volume depletion.

Planning: Expected Outcomes. Expected outcomes for collaborative problems address actions of the nurse, rather than client outcomes. The problem is within the physician's domain; therefore, nurses monitor for it. The nurse will monitor for hypotension. The client will have no manifestations of pulmonary fluid overload.

Implementation. Hypotension associated with spinal shock is initially treated with IV fluid. It is important to remember that fluid depletion is not the cause of hypotension. Therefore, fluid resuscitation should be carefully monitored to avoid fluid overload, which can lead to pulmonary edema. Vasopressor agents are often given in the acute phase of SCI to maintain blood pressure.

Inability to Sustain Spontaneous Ventilation, Ineffective Airway Clearance, Impaired Gas Exchange. Cervical SCI carries a high risk of respiratory compromise. Any or all three of these nursing diagnoses may be appropriate.

Planning: Expected Outcomes. The client will show no signs of respiratory compromise, as evidenced by clear lung sounds; partial pressures of arterial oxygen (PaO_2), $PaCO_2$, pH, and oxygen saturation within normal limits; and unlabored respirations and normal vital capacity.

Implementation. Chest physical therapy can help mobilize secretions and prevent pneumonia, as can suctioning and assisted coughing. When spinal cord edema has temporarily impaired respiratory function, mechanical ventilation is used to support respiration. Intubation and ventilation can be frightening to a person who has been able to breathe independently. Provide reassurance that mechanical ventilation will probably not be permanent. Sedation is administered as needed after intubation.

For extended airway management, a tracheostomy may be required to (1) allow for long-term controlled ventilation, (2) facilitate the removal of tracheobronchial secretions, and (3) seal off the esophagus from the trachea to prevent aspiration. An abdominal binder is often used to provide abdominal support, facilitate diaphragmatic breathing, and increase venous return.

Risk for Aspiration. Clients with tracheostomies, ineffective airway clearance, or an absent gag reflex are at higher *Risk for Aspiration.* Aspiration is a common cause of morbidity in spinal cord–injured clients.

Planning: Expected Outcomes. The client will exhibit no signs of aspiration, as evidenced by clear lung sounds; absence of stridor and fever; minimal amounts of clear mucus upon suctioning; and PaO$_2$, PaCO$_2$, pH, and oxygen saturation within normal limits.

Implementation. Suctioning equipment should be kept available, and breath sounds assessed every 1 or 2 hours in acutely ill clients. The results of arterial blood gases and pulse oximetry are monitored to determine the degree of oxygenation provided by ventilators or supplemental oxygen. Tracheobronchial suctioning is performed frequently to prevent or reduce the accumulation of secretions from immobility, lack of a cough reflex, or pneumonia. Monitor the electrocardiogram for dysrhythmias (e.g., premature ventricular contractions [PVCs]) due to hypoxia during suctioning.

Ineffective Thermoregulation. Thermoregulation may be altered because of loss of hypothalamic control of the sympathetic nervous system in clients with SCI above the T6 level.

Planning: Expected Outcome. The client will maintain normothermia.

Implementation. Rectal or core temperature is monitored every 4 hours during the first 72 hours after injury. Skin surfaces are palpated for areas of warmth, coolness, and moisture. Control the environmental temperature by using bed linens as needed to warm the client, eliminating drafts in the room, and using hypothermia blankets cautiously.

Evaluation

The problems identified in the early period of SCI care should resolve within 72 hours, especially if there are no other serious injuries or medical problems. If the client remains in an ICU for a prolonged time, implement other aspects of SCI care as discussed below.

Acute and Subacute Care

■ Medical Management

In 1970, the United States Rehabilitation Service Administration adopted a model system for rehabilitation of spinal cord–injured persons. The key to the system is the use of multidisciplinary teams of physicians, nurses, and allied healthcare providers (physical therapists, occupational therapists) to reduce morbidity, maximize the extent of functional recovery, and promote independence.

Establishing Functional Goals

Prediction of functional ability after SCI can generally be guided by the degree of residual muscle function (Table 35–3). Clients with all levels of injury and of all ages benefit from rehabilitation. The client and family are involved in all phases. The client is taught skills that he or she cannot perform to pass on to those who will provide this skill at home. Likewise, skills learned in a rehabilitation setting must be adapted to the home environment and community setting prior to discharge. This process can be accomplished by use of therapeutic weekend passes and participation in community activities as a part of the rehabilitation process.

In all phases of rehabilitation, it is imperative that a motivated client be given the opportunity to perform any skill, even if it can be accomplished more quickly by the nurse or physician. Allowing the client to attempt a complex skill demonstrates support of the client's self-care abilities. A description of functional outcomes for rehabilitation is provided in Table 35–3. It is intended to be a guide and may not represent the ability of all clients with various levels of injury.

Promoting Mobility. Wheelchairs provide mobility, and having the proper wheelchair is critical. The wheelchair design must provide the client with the ability to propel the chair and prevent development of spinal deformities and pressure ulcers. A high back and head support are needed for clients without arm function (Fig. 35–6). Clients who can use their arms should have the back of the wheelchair at the level of the scapula and the wheelchair should be lower than normal to facilitate transfers. Cushions help reduce pressure and the risk of pressure ulcers. However, cushions do not prevent pressure ulcers, and the client still needs to shift weight every 10 to 15 minutes while in the chair. Physical therapists work with the client to teach how to transfer from bed to a wheelchair, from a wheelchair into and out of a car, and from the wheelchair onto a toilet.

Current emphasis is on strengthening muscles rather than using braces. However, back braces may be prescribed following lumbar spinal injury or intervertebral disc problems. A Taylor back brace (Fig. 35–7), splint, or heavy muslin corset with stays may be worn initially while the client is in bed. More frequently, a thoracolumbosacral orthosis (TLSO) is used. This is a custom-made plastic brace with front and back pieces that fasten together with Velcro straps. This brace provides stability for the healing spine. The nurse is responsible for supervising the unlicensed professional whenever he or she is assisting with positioning or mobility for a client with a spinal abnormality.

Reducing Spasticity. Spasticity often interferes with positioning and functional activities. Spasticity does maintain muscle bulk and venous return and serves to aid transfers. Treatment includes ROM exercises and pharmacologic agents such as baclofen, dantrolene sodium, and clonidine. Medications for the treatment of spasms are

Table 35-3. Functional Goals in Spinal Cord Injury		
Spinal Cord Level	**Muscle Function**	**Functional Goals**
C1-2	Has no phrenic nerve function	Respirations managed with phrenic pacemaker
C3-4	Neck control Scapular elevators Diaphragm function may be weak or absent	Manipulate electric wheelchair with breath control, chin control, or voice activation Limited self-feeding with ball-bearing feeders Operate environmental control units
C5	Fair-to-good shoulder control Functional deltoids/biceps Elbow flexion	Dress upper trunk Turn self in bed with or without arm slings Propel wheelchair with or without friction-surface hand-rims Self-feeding with hand splints or following tenodesis Assist getting to and from bed May learn to write or type
C6	Good shoulder control Wrist extension Supinators	Dress upper trunk, sometimes dress lower trunk Turn self in bed with arm slings Propel wheelchair with hand-rim projections Self-feeding with hand splints Transfer from wheelchair to bed with or without minimal assistance (e.g., sliding board) Assist getting to and from commode chair Self-catheterization
C7	May have weak shoulder depression Weak elbow extension Some hand function Triceps	Independent in transfer to bed, car, and toilet Total dressing independence Wheelchair without hand-rim projections Self-feeding with no assistive devices
T1-4	Good-to-normal upper extremity muscle function Intrinsic muscles of the hand No trunk control	Independent in transfer to bed, car, and toilet Total dressing independence Wheelchair with standard hand-rims Self-feeding with no assistive devices Transfer from wheelchair to floor and return Wheelchair up and down curb Transfer from wheelchair to tub and return
T5-L2	Partial-to-good trunk stability	Total wheelchair independence Limited ambulation with bilateral long leg braces and crutches (injury at T12 or below)
L3-4	All trunk-pelvic stabilizers intact Hip flexors Adductors Quadriceps	Ambulation with short leg braces with or without crutches, depending on level
L5-S3	Hip extensors Abductors, knee flexors, ankle control	No equipment needed if plantar flexion is strong enough for pushoff at end of stance

Modified from Physical Therapy Department, Rancho Los Amigos Hospital, Downey, CA.

given only when the spasms cause discomfort or safety concerns.

Improving Bladder and Bowel Control. The term "neurogenic bladder" is used to describe bladder control changes that occur with both upper and lower motor neuron disorders. Upper motor neuron disorders produce a spastic or reflex bladder. Lower motor neuron disorders produce a flaccid bladder. There are many ways to manage the bladder, and treatment options must be tailored to fit the client's preferences and life-style as well as his or her functional abilities.

Most clients with arm function are taught to empty their bladder using the Credé maneuver over the bladder to relax the sphincter and express urine (see Bladder Retraining under Nursing Management of the Medical Client). To ensure complete emptying, this method is often combined with other techniques such as catheterization and external catheters. Intermittent catheterization reduces the risk of infection and bladder stone formation caused by indwelling catheters. Clients with C6 and lower injuries can perform self-catheterization, although the technique requires adequate hand function and the ability to manage lower extremity clothing. External catheters

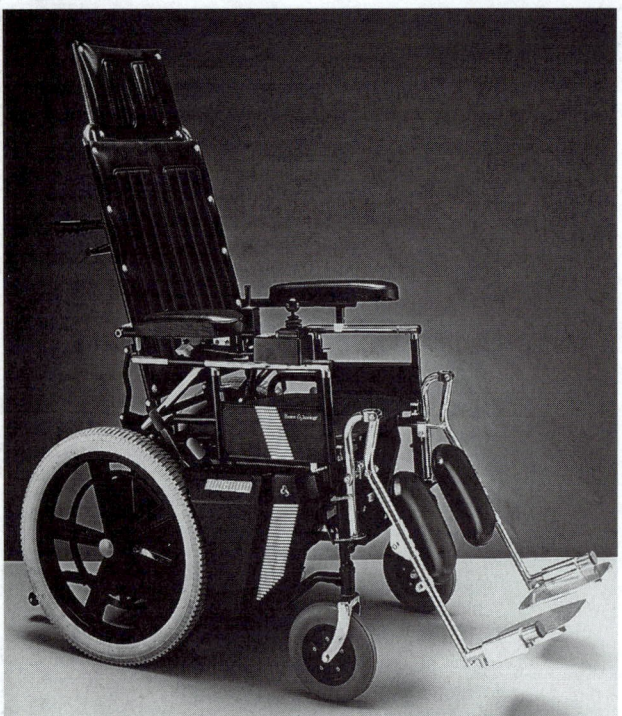

Figure 35–6. A C1–3 spine injury wheelchair with power hand controls for clients with cervical injury. A respirator can be attached to the wheelchair. (Courtesy of Everett and Jennings, St. Louis, MO.)

are used for men who can void between catheterizations or for those who leak urine during bladder spasms. Suprapubic catheters can also be inserted and seem to offer the advantages of less infection and urethral injury over indwelling catheters. Indwelling catheters are not ideal from a medical standpoint but are preferred by many clients because of the ease of management. Complications include infection, bladder stones, urethral damage, and a

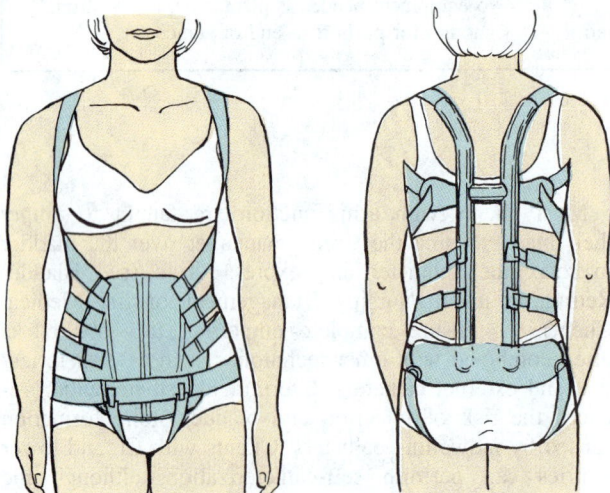

Figure 35–7. A Taylor back brace.

reported increased incidence of bladder cancer. A neurogenic bladder may also be treated with medications such as bethanechol (Urecholine) to stimulate bladder contraction. Urine acidifying agents may also be prescribed to reduce the risk of infection.

A neurogenic bowel is similar to a neurogenic bladder because the client cannot control defecation. The goal is to develop a bowel elimination method that is convenient, effective, and least expensive for the client. Sufficient fluid and fiber intake is essential. When fiber is added to or increased in the diet, it must be done slowly to avoid cramping and diarrhea. Stool softeners and bulk laxatives may also be used.

The bowel movements of clients with upper motor neuron damage are generally regulated with suppositories or digital stimulation every day or every other day to prevent autonomic dysreflexia. A lower motor neuron neurogenic bowel is more difficult to regulate, and often the client requires manual removal of an impaction.

Preventing Pressure Ulcers. Anesthetic skin increases the risk of pressure ulcers. During the acute care period, pressure ulcer development was associated with the level of injury, completeness of the injury, and length of time immobilized. As stated in the first Nursing Research feature on the facing page, 6 hours of immobilization significantly increases the risk of ulcers.[12] Although 6 hours was the time frame validated in the study cited, guidelines based on many other studies recommend that clients be turned or have their weight shifted at least every 2 hours. The Agency for Health Care Policy and Research (AHCPR) guidelines for prevention of skin injury include completing a daily systematic skin inspection, using proper positioning techniques (to minimize shearing and friction effects), maintaining adequate nutritional support, minimizing environmental exposure (i.e., excessive moisture or dryness), and avoiding massage over bony prominences. Prevention of pressure ulcers should include a pressure-relieving device. Wheelchair-bound clients are taught to relieve pressure every 15 minutes.

Reducing Respiratory Dysfunction. Respiratory dysfunction is a significant cause of morbidity and mortality after SCI. The diaphragm is often the only functional muscle because the intercostal and abdominal muscles are paralyzed. Vital capacity and inspiratory reserve volume are markedly diminished. The client should be taught to use incentive spirometry and diaphragmatic breathing to enhance vital capacity. Glossopharyngeal breathing uses the tongue and muscles of the pharynx to force air into the lungs. This technique enhances vital capacity and promotes chest expansion.

Providing Ongoing Care

SCI is permanent and affects all aspects of life. The second Nursing Research feature on the facing page identifies eight areas in which the client's quality of life can be enhanced. Ongoing care addresses the holistic needs of the client and the long-term complications seen with SCI.

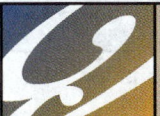

NURSING RESEARCH

How Is Immobility Related to Pressure Ulcer Formation in Clients with Spinal Cord Injuries?

Curry, K., & Casady, L. (1992). The relationships between extended periods of immobility and decubiti formation in the acutely spinal cord–injured individual. *Journal of Neurosurgical Nursing, 24*(4), 185–189.

Immobility has been associated with pressure ulcer formation. Loss of sensation and motor function places persons with spinal cord injury (SCI) at even higher risk.

Curry and Casady conducted a study involving 49 persons who sustained an SCI. The sample included individuals with complete or incomplete cord injuries. The questions asked were (1) what variables influence pressure ulcer formation in the immediate post-injury period and (2) when is the rate of pressure ulcer formation accelerated?

Curry and Casady found that immobilization for more than 6 hours resulted in an accelerated rate of pressure ulcer formation. Factors not found to be associated with the formation of pressure ulcers included level of injury and completeness of injury.

Implications for Practice

Development of pressure ulcers is an unwarranted drain on personal and financial resources. During the immediate care period following SCI, prolonged delay in clearing x-rays can result in the client being burdened with preventable injury. Early use of pressure-relieving methods is necessary. Six hours of immobility almost guarantees pressure sore development. Practice guidelines based on other studies recommend a minimum of 2-hour turning schedules.

Promoting Expression of Sexuality. Sexual function in spinal cord–injured males depends on the location of the lesion (Table 35–4). Reflex erection is possible in some clients with upper motor neuron lesions. Reflex erections occur with some lower motor neuron lesions. Ejaculation is possible with lower motor neuron lesions and if the lesion is more caudal. Unfortunately, fertility is about 5%, but it is hoped that this rate will improve with advances in technology. It is becoming a common practice for semen to be collected and frozen for later in vivo fertilization. Sexual dysfunction is approached from two avenues: (1) psychological counseling and (2) education about technological advances to facilitate sexual activity. Erection can be restored with external aids, an implantable penile prosthesis, and medications.

Female clients retain fertility after SCI. Problems with sexual function generally relate to positioning and the lack of vaginal lubrication. These problems can usually be addressed through client education.

Reducing Pain. Long-term pain occurs in almost all spinal cord–injured clients with intact sensation. Dysesthetic pain, which is distal to the site of injury, is extremely disabling. It is similar to the phantom pain seen after amputation. It is described as cutting, burning, piercing, radiating, or tightening. The usual treatment is with non-narcotic analgesics and transcutaneous nerve stimulators. Pain management prn (as needed) is not recommended as a primary treatment for chronic pain. How-

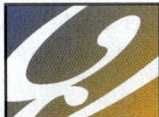

NURSING RESEARCH

How Can Quality of Life Be Improved for Quadriplegic Clients?

Bach, C. A., & McDaniel, R. W. (1993). Quality of life in quadriplegic adults: A focus group study. *Rehabilitation Nursing, 18*(6), 364–367.

Although advances in technology have resulted in more people with quadriplegia surviving and having a projected life span nearly equal to the general population, little is known about how these people view quality of life or life satisfaction.

Bach and McDaniel conducted a study involving 14 patients who had completed a rehabilitation course in a midwestern rehabilitation center. Data were collected using focus group sessions. The participants were asked to identify and discuss what they considered to constitute components of quality of life for them personally.

Bach and McDaniel found that quality of life was identified using eight categories: relationships, job and productivity, dependence versus independence, finances, health, inner strength and survival, assertiveness, and level of activity. Seven of the eight categories identified in this group have also been identified in quality-of-life studies in the general population. Assertiveness is the category not reported in the general population studies. This population described having to ask others for assistance in achieving daily activities. Assertiveness, which helped them claim opportunities for achieving independence, was an important characteristic in their quality of life.

Implications for Practice

The nature of quadriplegia can place the individual in a constant balancing act of independence and dependence. Usually quadriplegic clients are knowledgeable about their care and can direct others providing this care. Support these clients in becoming more assertive in directing others to help them achieve their daily activities.

Table 35-4. Sexual Function in Clients with Spinal Cord Injury

Sexuality	Reproductive Functioning	Special Considerations for Contraceptive Methods
Females 　Lesions at C1–3: Reflex lubrication is probable. Erogenous areas may develop above injury. Libido is intact 　Lesions at C4–6: Psychogenic lubrication is unlikely. Nongenital orgasm may be experienced 　Lesions at C7: Able to use hands for holding and caressing 　Lesions at T12–L5: Psychogenic stimulation of the clitoris, lubrication, labial swelling, and skin flush are possible but unlikely	Menstruation and fertility unaffected Pregnancy is not affected Incidence of bladder infection during pregnancy increases Risk of autonomic hyperreflexia during delivery and labor increases	Birth control pills are contraindicated when circulatory problems are present; thrombophlebitis could go undetected owing to lack of sensation in extremities Intrauterine device may be contraindicated because of pelvic inflammatory disease, and other problems could remain undetected owing to lack of sensation Client must be able to assess for vaginal bleeding
Males 　Lesions at C1–3: Reflex erection is caused by genital stimulation. Psychogenic erection is not possible. Erogenous areas above injury site may develop. Libido is intact 　Lesions at C4–6: Reflex erection is possible. Nongenital orgasm may be experienced; no ejaculation. Oral sex is possible. Libido is intact 　Lesions at C7: Holding and caressing with hands are possible 　Lesions at T12–L6: Psychogenic stimulation and erection are possible; no reflex erection 　Lesions at S2–4: Reflex erection is possible. Ejaculation is possible but may be retrograde	Semen can be obtained from the bladder of clients who have retrograde ejaculation For clients who cannot ejaculate, semen can be obtained through glandular vibratory stimulation In general, semen quality is impaired, with poor motility the most common abnormality Some clients are candidates for penile prosthesis	Client or partner may apply condom

ever, routine analgesics may need to be supplemented by analgesics prn during a client's pain peaks.

Reducing Abnormal Bone Growth. Heterotopic ossification is the formation of bone in abnormal locations, most often around the hips and knees after SCI. The client may develop swelling in the joint or loss of ROM. Heterotopic ossification is diagnosed by x-ray study or bone scan. Treatment includes the use of etidronate disodium (Didronel) and ROM exercises of the affected areas. Sometimes the bone is removed surgically.

Promoting Psychological Adjustment. Psychological counseling is ongoing. Commonly, spinal cord–injured clients participate in peer group sessions to share their experiences and help newly injured clients to cope better with their situation. Vocational rehabilitation may help clients reach their maximal rehabilitation potential.

■ Nursing Management of the Medical Client

Assessment

The client usually is transferred from a hyperacute nursing unit after becoming hemodynamically stable. Clients with high cervical injuries may remain on ventilators. The care of the ventilator-dependent client is discussed in Chapter 39. Some of the nursing diagnoses that applied in the critical care unit may still apply now. The client will remain at risk for skin impairment and may still have difficulty swallowing and therefore be at risk for aspiration. You will need to evaluate each client individually. A baseline assessment should be completed upon transfer.

Diagnosis, Planning, Implementation

Impaired Physical Mobility. SCI causing permanent impaired physical mobility produces problems with ambulation and potential complications arising from immobility. Write the diagnosis as *Impaired Physical Mobility related to inability to move upper and/or lower extremity secondary to paralysis.*

Planning: Expected Outcomes. The client will have maximal physical mobility, as evidenced by absence of tendon contractures, joint ankylosis, and muscle shortening, and effective use of adaptive devices.

Implementation. Throughout the acute and rehabilitative phases of nursing care, every effort should be made to maximize the client's functional abilities and independence by encouraging the client to perform independently any activities of daily living (ADLs) for which capability remains.

Positioning and Adaptive Equipment. Tendon contractures, joint ankylosis, and muscle shortening are caused by improper positioning of the client in the bed or chair and lack of joint movements (e.g., because of spasticity or immobility). Intervention to prevent such problems includes the following:

1. Frequent position changes
2. Proper positioning of joints
3. Use of splints and removable casts
4. Intermittent turning to a prone position
5. Positioning of upper extremities away from the body
6. Draping of bedding over frames to keep pressure off the feet
7. Keeping knee joints flexed 15 degrees when supine
8. Use of active and passive conditioning exercises (see Risk for Contractures).

Wristdrop and footdrop will develop in paralyzed extremities unless prevented. Footdrop may be prevented by keeping the client's feet firmly supported in dorsiflexion at right angles to the hips (high-topped athletic shoes are commonly used) to counteract the force of gravity on weakened muscles. Support a paralyzed arm in a sling when the client is out of bed, and in a cock-up splint while in bed. Usually, the hand end of the splint is elevated 2 inches to support the wrist, and the fingers are maintained in a position of function. Posterior molded casts may be used instead of splints to support a paralyzed wrist while in bed. For some clients, pillows and a hand roll are adequate.

Transfers and Ambulation. Rehabilitative programs often require strength and endurance. To prepare a client for ambulation, the unaffected parts of the body must be strengthened and suitable exercises started early. Tolerance for activity gradually increases. Take care not to fatigue the client. Periods of planned rest and recreation are important.

Physical therapy is essential for all clients with SCIs. Paraplegic clients need to learn various transfers to become self-sufficient. One transfer is illustrated in Figure 35–8. Learning to sit up precedes learning to transfer. Many paralyzed clients become mobile by using a wheelchair. Many types of wheelchairs are available, and selection needs to be made carefully, according to individual needs (Fig. 35–6). Prolonged, unrelieved periods of immobility can result in renal calculi and pressure ulcers. Pressure is relieved by position changes (see Nursing Research feature). When sitting up, a paralyzed client needs to shift body weight every 10 to 15 minutes and lift the

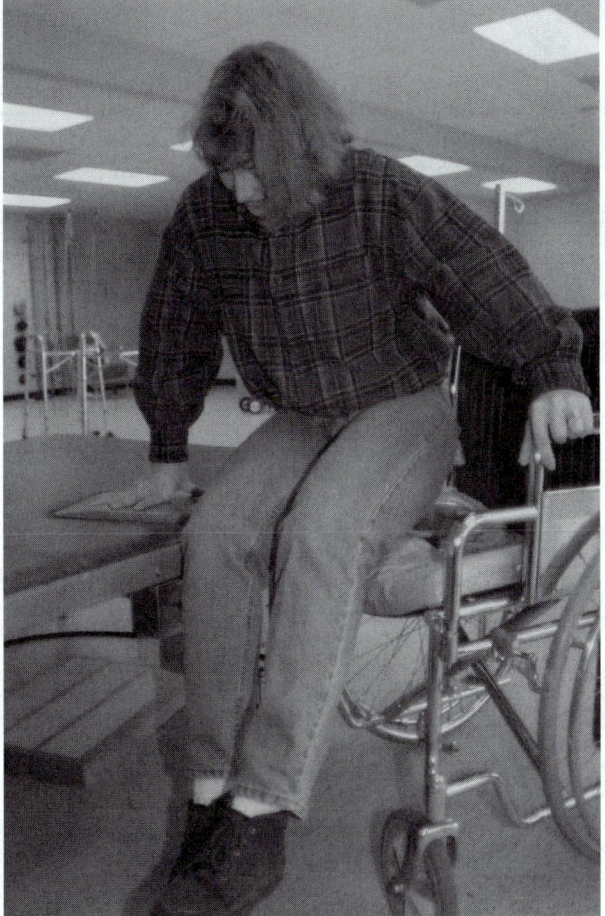

Figure 35–8. Bed-to-wheelchair lateral transfer using a sliding board.

body by pushing with the arms and hands against the chair arms or seat. Pressure reduction can also be performed by leaning forward. This relieves pressure on the buttocks and prevents skin breakdown. Apply the brace or corset before helping the client out of bed. A thin, knitted undershirt is worn under the brace or corset to protect the skin and keep the appliance clean. To apply the brace or corset, turn the client to one side, place the appliance against the back, and then roll the client back into it. The brace or corset is secured while the client lies supine. As recovery and rehabilitation progress, many clients learn to apply their own braces and corsets while in bed. Others continue to need help. The degree of arm and hand function determines the client's ability to apply a brace.

Weightbearing begins as early as possible after SCI. This stimulates osteoblastic activity and thus decreases demineralization of bone (osteoporosis) that develops with prolonged immobilization. Standing boards or tilt tables assist the person gradually to assume a standing position. Having the person assume a standing position periodically each day also helps prevent contractures (e.g., hip contractures from long periods of sitting). Care must be taken when helping clients to stand or sit in a chair for the first time. Because of the effects of loss of muscular activity on the peripheral venous system, these clients are

NURSING RESEARCH

Can Pressure Be Relieved by Position Changes in Seated Clients with Spinal Cord Injuries?

Henderson, J. L., et al. (1994). Efficacy of three measures to relieve pressure in seated persons with spinal cord injury. *Archives of Physical Medicine and Rehabilitation, 74,* 535–539.

Pressure ulcers are a major risk for persons with a spinal cord injury (SCI). More time and financial resources are being spent on treatment of pressure ulcers over the ischial tuberosities than other sites.

Henderson and colleagues conducted a study involving seated spinal cord–injured persons to determine whether pressure could be adequately relieved by position change. Using a new mapping system, the study compared dynamic pressure changes while tipping the wheelchair back to 35 degrees, tipping the wheelchair back 65 degrees, and leaning the person forward in a chest-to-thigh position. Ten adult volunteer subjects with either a cervical or thoracic SCI participated in the study. The participants used their personal cushion and either personal or hospital-loaned wheelchairs.

Henderson and colleagues found that the greatest relief of pressure was measured in the forward-leaning position. The 35-degree tip-back position was least useful in reducing pressure over the ischial tuberosities. Pressure was appreciably reduced in the 65-degree tip-back position.

Implications for Practice

Various methods to relieve pressure are currently practiced by SCI persons and taught by healthcare professionals. Present and discuss different pressure-relieving methods with the SCI client. The results of this study suggest that the forward-leaning position may prevent pressure ulcer formation. Evaluate SCI clients regarding their ability to use and tolerate the forward-leaning position. Caution SCI clients to not use the 35-degree tip-back position. Present the 65-degree tip-back position as an option for the individual who cannot tolerate the forward-leaning position but not as the sole relief used during periods of long, uninterrupted sitting.

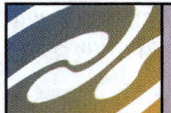

CLIENT EDUCATION GUIDE

Use of a Halo Vest

The vest or the halo ring bolts are only to be adjusted by the neurosurgeon or his or her designee.

If the bolts become loose, tell your physician.

Use fleece or foam inserts to relieve pressure points.

Keep the vest lining dry; if the fleece gets wet, dry it with a hair dryer (on a cool setting); do not allow the fleece to become matted.

Clean the pin at least once a day; cleaning agents include soap and water with cotton-tipped swabs, alcohol swabs, or shampoo soap if hair is being washed. Crusting can be removed using peroxide or alcohol. Ointments and antiseptics are not recommended for routine care. Use a separate sterile swab for each pin site.

Report redness, swelling, drainage, open areas around the pin (tracking), pain, tenderness, or a clicking noise from the pin site. Retightening is usually necessary during the first 24 to 48 hours for the first week.

Recheck the pin every 2 to 3 weeks.

Wash the skin under the vest. Use a bath towel wrung out in hot water (alcohol is permitted) and pull it back and forth. Do not use soap, lotion, or powder because it cannot be removed adequately. Assess daily for skin breakdown under the vest using a flashlight. Showering is prohibited. A sponge bath or tub bath with minimal water to prevent the vest liner from getting wet may be permitted. When shampooing the hair, the shoulders and neck of the vest must be protected with plastic. Do not use any products other than shampoo on your hair (no dyes, tints, sprays, or conditioners).

When getting out of bed, roll onto your side and push on the mattress with your arm; sitting straight up puts too much stress on the front pins. *Never use the metal frame for turning or lifting!*

A rolled towel or pillow case between the back of your neck and the bed or next to your cheek when lying on your side and raising the head of the bed will increase sleep comfort.

Adapt your clothing to fit over the halo or have button, Velcro, or zipper closures. The vest will be needed for about 3 months, followed by a hard collar.

Eat food products high in protein and calcium to promote bone healing.

Have the correct size of wrench with you in case of an emergency; the anterior portion of the vest including the anterior bolts will need to be loosened; the posterior portion of the vest should remain in place to provide stability for the spine during cardiopulmonary resuscitation.

Adapted from Reid, B., & Marr, J. (1990). *Health professional's guide to caring for the client with a halo vest* (pp. 1–12). Bremer Medical.

prone to orthostatic hypotension. Blood pressure should always be checked before and after transfers. Syncope during a wheelchair transfer may be avoided with the quadriplegic client by use of an abdominal binder, thigh-high support hose, and slowly elevating the head of the bed (HOB) to 90 degrees. Using a recliner or a wheelchair with an adjustable back will help achieve gradual elevations.

Clients easily lose their balance when wearing braces, particularly the halo brace, and must be very careful to avoid falling. The Client Education Guide describes the use of a halo vest. A brace feels surprisingly heavy at first, especially if the client is weak. Some braces are now made of plastic and are considerably lighter. For safety, shoes, rather than slippers or just stockings, should be worn during ambulation. Shoes should tie or have Velcro straps for firm support and have a low heel. High-top athletic shoes give added support. Slick soles, high or narrow heels, or stocking feet are hazardous. Wearing shoes also helps prevent footdrop when the client lies down.

The fit, comfort, and appearance of braces, corsets, and shoes are important to the client. Try to assist clients who want to be as stylish as possible as well as benefit from therapeutic garments. Disabled clients are helped by (1) being encouraged to express their feelings concerning their self-image and (2) having their feelings taken into consideration when being fitted for therapeutic garments. Some garments can be painful when first worn. The pain worsens if the garments do not fit properly. The client's skin should be inspected frequently, especially at first, because pressure sores can develop very quickly.

Ineffective Airway Clearance. Airway clearance may be impaired because of paralysis of the abdominal and intercostal muscles. Write this nursing diagnosis as *Ineffective Airway Clearance related to inability to cough.*

Planning: Expected Outcomes. The client will participate in "quad-assisted" coughing, remain afebrile, and have normal blood gas or oximetry values and clear sputum.

Implementation. Use the quad-assist cough to promote airway clearance. Like the Heimlich maneuver, place a fist or heel of the hand between the umbilicus and the xiphoid process. Press inward and upward during the client's cough. Other interventions, such as turning, hydration, and chest physical therapy may also be used.

Risk for Contractures. Active ROM is severely limited or nonexistent in the upper extremities and nonexistent in the lower extremities in a client with cervical cord damage; it is also nonexistent in the lower extremities in a client with thoracic or lumbar cord damage. This deficit increases the risk for contractures. Write the diagnosis as *Risk for Contractures related to inability to move purposefully.*

Planning: Expected Outcomes. Monitor the client for changes in ROM in all joints. The client will have no change in ROM compared with the level prior to injury.

Implementation. Passive exercises prevent contractures and painful reflex dystrophies of the hand and shoulder. Such exercises may be prescribed as soon as 48 to 72 hours after injury. Active exercises, massage, and electrical stimulation may also be prescribed. Begin shoulder and arm exercises early. Strength in these areas and in the chest and back is essential for effective self-transfers and ambulation when the lower spine is stable enough to permit mobilization.

Self Care Deficit. The client who has suffered an SCI is often unable to perform many self-care activities.

This can lead to a feeling of powerlessness. Assisting him or her to maximize independence can lessen this feeling.

Planning: Expected Outcomes. The client will independently perform as many ADLs as possible. If the client is unable to independently perform an activity, he or she will be able to direct a caregiver's performance. These goals will be evaluated by successful performance of ADLs by the client or under the client's direction.

Implementation. The client is assisted with muscle-strengthening exercises and the use of adaptive devices. Clients with high cervical injuries are able to perform very few activities independently. Allow them adequate time to accomplish whatever tasks they can. If the client needs help with ADLs, adapt nursing care to the client's routine. In collaborating to maintain intact oral mucous membranes, a schedule is established for brushing teeth at least twice daily and cleaning the tongue, roof of the mouth, and gums with agents not containing lemon or alcohol.

Once the client is able to be responsible for some ADLs, educate the client about the risk of pressure ulcers and teach techniques to reduce risk. The client should shift body weight every 10 to 15 minutes while sitting in a wheelchair. Shifting weight promotes reactive hyperemia and vasodilation to bring blood into hypoxic tissues. Finally, the client should use a mirror to inspect for signs of pressure ulcers each evening before bedtime.

Risk for Altered Nutrition: Less than Body Requirements. After traumatic injury there is increased metabolic demand because of the response to stress and to allow healing. This nursing diagnosis is written *Risk for Altered Nutrition: Less than Body Requirements related to increased metabolic demand and inability to access nutrients.* Anorexia related to depression may be another etiology.

Planning: Expected Outcomes. The client will not experience excessive weight loss (more than 10 lb) during hospitalization.

Implementation. The client should be weighed on admission to serve as a baseline measurement. Nutrient supplementation should begin by 72 hours after injury if the client is not eating. Enteral feeding can be used if the client has bowel sounds. If the client still has paralytic ileus, hyperalimentation is commonly used. Weigh the client at least once a week to monitor progress.

Total Incontinence. Observe the client carefully for indications of faulty bladder control and infection, including incontinence, retention, urgency, dribbling, frequency, enuresis, and precipitate micturition. Document such observations and inform the physician. This nursing diagnosis is written as *Total Incontinence related to paralysis.*

Planning: Expected Outcomes. The client will have improved bladder control, as evidenced by no infection and emptying of the bladder every 4 to 6 hours.

Implementation. Nursing intervention is planned to (1) prevent urinary tract infection, (2) preserve existing bladder capacity and muscle tone, and (3) establish and maintain a routine pattern of elimination requiring minimal artificial assistance.

Urinary bladder atony (absence of tone) may last several weeks or months after SCI. In clients with upper motor neuron lesions, when spinal shock subsides and the reflex arc returns, as evidenced by an increase in rectal tone, a reflex contraction will empty the bladder. During the period of atony, a retention catheter may be inserted to prevent bladder distention and keep the client dry and comfortable. Bladder overdistention causes stretching and fissure formation, a predisposition to infection, and may result in bladder rupture. When sensory pathways are damaged, the client does not feel the discomfort of bladder distention. However, prolonged catheter use also predisposes to infection. This is why catheterization every 6 hours is preferred over a retention catheter.

Urinary complications may be avoided by (1) periodically examining the client for bladder distention, (2) accurately documenting fluid intake and output, (3) using aseptic technique when handling urinary catheters, and (4) observing for signs of bladder infection. Encourage the client to drink water to keep the urine diluted and lessen the possibility of infection. Urine acidifiers may be prescribed. Urinary complications occur because of incomplete emptying of the bladder, necessitating catheterization. Catheterization may predispose the client to infection and vesicoureteral reflux, which may lead to kidney complications. Renal calculi, pyelonephritis, and hydronephrosis are major causes of death and of considerable disability in paralyzed clients.

To prevent development of renal calculi, encourage the client to drink about 3000 ml of fluid per day, unless contraindicated by other medical conditions. This is sufficient to maintain a minimal urinary output of 2000 ml/day. Drinking this much fluid may increase incontinence but is necessary to prevent renal calculi.

Bowel Incontinence or Constipation.
Bowel dysfunction is a common but manageable problem in a client with an SCI. This common nursing diagnosis is written as *Constipation related to paralysis.*

Planning: Expected Outcomes. The client will have reduced risk of bowel incontinence or constipation, as evidenced by a bowel movement every 1 to 2 days, no signs of fecal impaction, and no incontinence.

Implementation. Nursing intervention is planned to (1) prevent constipation, distention, and impaction; (2) detect and treat these conditions if they occur; and (3) reestablish habitual, controlled bowel movements by conditioned reflex activity. Paralytic ileus is a common sequela of SCI. By frequently assessing bowel sounds and documenting the passage of stool, you can determine when peristalsis has returned and the client is capable of digesting food. The client is observed carefully for indications of constipation, diarrhea, or tenesmus (straining at stool). If a client becomes impacted, a cleaning enema may be prescribed to initially empty the lower bowel. However, enemas should be avoided for long-term bowel management. A paraplegic or quadriplegic client cannot retain an enema solution nor can the degree of intestinal distention be felt. Therefore, enemas must be administered carefully to avoid overdistending the intestine with excessive fluid; 500 ml or less is usually given.

The client's intake of fluid and food and elimination pattern are documented. The routine daily pattern of bowel elimination is established, with the client using suppositories and other means of stimulating evacuation until reflex evacuation occurs.

A daily fluid intake of 3000 to 4000 ml/day is important for proper bowel function as well as bladder function. Also, the diet must be high in bulk and roughage such as bran, whole grains, fresh and dried fruits, and leafy green and raw vegetables. A stool softener such as docusate sodium (Colace) may be taken daily, but laxatives should be carefully administered. Bulk-forming medications (e.g., psyllium hydrophilic mucilloid [Metamucil]) are very effective for spinal cord–injured clients as long as adequate hydration is maintained.

Risk for Impaired Skin Integrity.
Clients with SCI are at higher *Risk for Impaired Skin Integrity* because of immobility and loss of protective functions.

Planning: Expected Outcomes. The client will have intact skin, as evidenced by no reddened areas over bony prominences and no areas or signs of skin irritation or dryness.

Implementation. The spinal cord–injured client cannot respond to local tissue hypoxia resulting from being in one position for an extended period of time. Impaired skin sensation occurring with quadriplegia and paraplegia predisposes the client to pressure ulcers and burns. Spinal cord–injured clients should be placed on pressure-reducing beds or mattresses. However, the use of these special beds does not eliminate the need to assess the skin every 2 to 4 hours. In addition, the client's nutritional needs must be met to reduce the risk of pressure ulcers.

A client with spinal fractures may be placed on a Roto-Rest bed. A Roto-Rest bed is currently popular for clients with SCIs or other disorders requiring prolonged immobilization (see Fig. 31–7). It is equipped with supportive packs and straps that keep the body in neutral alignment while it continuously oscillates from side to side. The continuous motion helps (1) prevent skin breakdown, (2) reduce urinary stasis, and (3) promote lung aeration. Unfortunately, the constant movement may also stimulate peristalsis, resulting in severe diarrhea. Some clients also experience disorientation from the constant movement. These clients also express fear of falling. Staff members should remain with the client initially to provide emotional support and reassurance. Also, it is important to pull window curtains at night, as a client in a Roto-Rest bed can see himself or herself "floating" in the window reflection and become disoriented or frightened.

Chronic Pain.
Clients with spinal injuries may experience pain at the level of the injury and radiating along spinal nerves originating in the area. Phantom pain may also be experienced. Pain usually occurs later than muscle spasms. Some paraplegic and quadriplegic clients experience both pain and spasm. Pain most often occurs in the lower extremities.

Planning: Expected Outcomes. The client will experience adequate pain relief, as evidenced by verbalization of improvement in comfort, ability to rest without interruption by pain, and ability to participate in therapies without hindrance by pain.

Implementation. Analgesics such as aspirin and nonsteroidal anti-inflammatory agents may be prescribed. Narcotics are seldom used after the initial injury and are contraindicated in clients with high cervical injuries because of the risk of respiratory depression.

Clients with thoracic injuries often tend to breathe more shallowly to avoid pain. This can lead to respiratory complications. Give prescribed pain medication and encourage deep breathing and coughing to aerate the lungs and remove secretions from the respiratory tract.

Antispasmodics, nonsteroidal anti-inflammatory agents, and non-narcotic analgesics are prescribed for pain associated with spasticity. Surgery (e.g., neurectomy or chordotomy) is sometimes required for pain relief.

Risk for Autonomic Dysreflexia. Autonomic dysreflexia is a serious complication of SCI when injury is above T7. Write this collaborative problem as *Risk for Autonomic Dysreflexia related to SCI.*

Planning: Expected Outcomes. The nurse will monitor for clinical manifestations of autonomic dysreflexia and respond to them quickly.

Implementation. Assess the client for sudden indications of severe hypertension, severe throbbing headache, profuse diaphoresis, flushing of the skin above the level of the lesion, nasal stuffiness, pilomotor spasm, blurred vision, nausea, and bradycardia. (See Critical Monitoring.)

Educate the client about the warning symptoms of autonomic dysreflexia and the importance of calling for a nurse immediately should any occur. Adaptive call lights are available to facilitate nurse calling. If autonomic dysreflexia does occur, do the following:

1. Elevate the HOB to a sitting position immediately.
2. Check the blood pressure.
3. Check for possible sources of irritation (e.g., kinked or clogged catheter or distended bladder or lower bowel).

4. Remove the stimulus if it can be done quickly. Once the source of irritation is removed, manifestations of autonomic dysreflexia usually subside.
5. If blood pressure remains elevated, antihypertensive medication (nitrates, nifedipine, hydralazine, guanethidine, or diazoxide) may be administered according to the physician's prescription or procedural policy (IV, intranasally, or sublingually).
6. If there is no order or policy or if the above measures do not correct the problem, notify the physician.

Once manifestations have subsided, observe the client's vital signs and neurologic status closely for 3 to 4 hours. If an antihypertensive medication has been given, the client may become hypotensive after the stimulus is removed. Autonomic dysreflexia may recur if the stimulus is not completely removed. If the identified source is bladder distention, use caution when emptying the bladder. Remove 500 ml every 5 to 15 minutes. If the identified source of irritation is bowel distention, be very careful when removing an impaction from the client. An anesthetic lubricant is used, and another nurse must monitor the client's blood pressure every few minutes. The stimulation of trying to remove the impaction can increase the severity of the autonomic response. Remember, when a quadriplegic client complains of a headache, do not automatically give analgesics prn without first checking the blood pressure.

Risk for Injury. Clients with SCI are at *Risk for Injury related to abnormal reflexes, spasms, and corneal drying,* which can lead to corneal abrasions.

Planning: Expected Outcomes. The client will sustain no injuries due to spasms, as evidenced by no abrasions or bruising. Corneal abrasions will not occur.

Implementation. Injections should be avoided whenever possible. Medications should be given orally. Use saline locks if necessary. When injections are unavoidable, give above the level of the cord lesion whenever possible. Absorption may be compromised in denervated areas of the body with impaired capillary and precapillary circulation. Moisten the cornea with natural tears every 4 hours for a client with altered blinking reflexes.

Clients can also be injured from involuntary spasms. Avoid unnecessary stimulation of areas that elicit reflex spinal automatisms. When such reactions do occur, an unembarrassed, accepting response helps relieve the client's anxiety and embarrassment. Gentle, slow hyperextension of a limb in spasm can often override the trigger points and interrupt the spasm. Abnormal spinal reflexes make people respond to stimuli in ways that may be puzzling to them and others unless the origin of such responses is explained. For example, stimulation of the limbs (perhaps toe flexion while the person's foot is being dried) may cause mass flexion of the upper and lower extremities. Mass flexion reactions may be accompanied by massive contractions of the abdominal wall, evacuation of the urinary bladder and bowel, and automatic response such as sweating, flushing, penile erection, or pilomotor reactions below the level of the lesion.

CRITICAL MONITORING

Autonomic Dysreflexia

Severe hypertension (>300 mm Hg)
Pounding headache
Flushing
Piloerection
Diaphoresis
Dilated pupils, blurred vision
Nasal stuffiness
Bradycardia (pulse <60 beats/min)
Restlessness
Nausea

Risk for Thrombophlebitis. Muscular activity is a major factor in venous circulation. A paralyzed client experiences slowed venous return and pooling of blood in dependent limbs. These phenomena increase the *Risk for Thrombophlebitis.*

Planning: Expected Outcomes. The nurse will monitor for thrombophlebitis, as evidenced by unilateral leg edema, erythema, and warmth.

Implementation. In the acute phase of SCI, antiembolism stockings, sequential compression devices, and subcutaneous heparin may be used prophylactically.

Education is vital to preventing vascular complications and minimizing their impact. When you apply stockings and perform ROM exercises, teach the client the importance of these activities. During assessment of the legs for signs of clot formation (i.e., redness and unilateral swelling and warmth), explain what is being done and why this activity needs to be incorporated into daily routines. Measuring calf diameter on both legs daily and noting changes is a more objective way of assessing swelling. Clients also learn not to cross their legs while sitting in a wheelchair.

Ineffective Individual Coping. When the reality of the injury and the permanence of deficit are understood, coping skills may need to be taught. The nursing diagnosis can be written as *Ineffective Individual Coping related to paralysis.*

Planning: Expected Outcomes. The client will use adaptive coping strategies and resources appropriately.

Implementation. Clients need to find appropriate methods to cope with new means of performing activities and managing bodily functions. The learning needs of spinal cord–injured clients and their family members are complex and ongoing. In the acute phase, education about spinal anatomy and physiology is needed. This teaching begins in the acute phase of hospitalization and should be incorporated into all aspects of care. Successful learning in this stage affects the client's entire life.

Anticipatory Grieving. Clients with SCI experience many changes (e.g., functional ability, role definition, body image, financial security). Grief is a normal response to these losses. Write the diagnosis as *Anticipatory Grieving related to multiple losses.*

Planning: Expected Outcomes. The client will progress through the grieving process and develop adaptive coping strategies, as evidenced by verbalizing his or her feelings about the injury and the future, participating in community activities, and expressing positive thoughts about the future.

Implementation. Adjusting to paralysis is difficult physically and psychosocially for the client and family. The family may experience the same reactions and need the same kind of help as the disabled client. Sudden paralysis in a previously healthy, active person can be devastating. Typically, the sudden life-style changes brought about by serious SCI cause a grief reaction. This may involve initial shock and denial, leading to depression and anger. Crying and talking about the injury may be helpful.

It takes time to adjust to disability and develop ways of coping. Psychological adjustment occurs when the client can function appropriately in the real world.

A client may use psychological defense mechanisms in adjusting to paralysis. When caring for such a client, assess the possible reasons for the behavior. Hostility, depression, anger, or withdrawal may be upsetting to the staff and family. These behaviors are coping mechanisms and should not be taken personally. Paralysis may cause complex changes in self-concept and body image. In the acute phase, immobilization can contribute to sensory deprivation (e.g., hallucinations). This may be minimized by providing visual, auditory, and tactile stimulation, as desired by the client.

Paralyzed clients are often helped initially by being with others who are experiencing similar problems. Clients should be allowed to wear their own clothing as soon as possible and encouraged to be out of bed and out of their rooms. Planned social activities may reduce feelings of social isolation and help clients regain self-confidence. Peer counseling, such as allowing newly disabled clients to talk with others who have adjusted to similar disabilities, may be helpful.

A sense of security is particularly important for a newly paralyzed client adjusting to enforced dependency. A paralyzed client should always have a means of summoning help, yet needs to learn that it is safe to be alone at times. Blow lights, minimal pressure call lights, pads, and voice-activated call lights are now available in many settings.

Gradually, the client develops trust in his or her abilities and resources, and relinquishes some reliance on others. These feelings and attitudes develop slowly as people experience truly trustworthy relationships.

To avoid unnecessary frustrations, try to keep each person's environment comfortable, with necessary items conveniently placed. It is difficult and depressing for the client to have to ask for help repeatedly. Although recent advances have been made in the rehabilitation prognosis of paraplegic and quadriplegic clients, it is important to be realistic as well as optimistic. The nurse needs to understand the tremendous life-style changes disabled clients must make. Some can be rehabilitated to a level of near independence: walking (perhaps with braces or other appliances), driving a car, and coping with full-time employment outside the home. Quadriplegic clients usually rely on a wheelchair and other devices and appliances.

Most paralyzed clients can become productive and happy. A recent SCI victim, the actor Christopher Reeve, is serving as a positive role model regarding *abilities* that remain after SCI. Even if some are unable to be "productive," all disabled clients have a right to a satisfying, happy life. Although many paralyzed clients achieve complete rehabilitation, others lead lives that are difficult, frustrating, and psychophysiologically complex. At times, severe mental depression develops. Depression is assessed and professional counseling is offered as indicated. Suicide is frequent.

Ineffective Family Coping: Compromised. A family is a unit. A trauma as devastating as SCI to one of the members of the family unit affects the entire family. The diagnosis can be written *Ineffective Family Coping: Compromised related to multiple changes in the family roles.*

Planning: Expected Outcomes. The client and family will identify areas of significant or potential loss and changes in family roles, work together to overcome obstacles, seek appropriate support services, and be able to restore a supportive family structure.

Implementation. The injury affects not only physical functioning but also the psychological, vocational, educational, and social aspects of life. An organized team approach is vital to helping the injured client and family cope with life-style changes. Nurses are often the first professionals to assess client and family coping. An open, empathic manner can allow these persons to express their grief and uncertainty and ask questions. Educate the family about the normal grief response. Also carefully probe into persistent denial of grief or lack of progression through grieving. Encouraging as much optimism as possible while remaining truthful and realistic may help SCI survivors to face the future.

Assess the previous roles of the client and other family members and how they handle stressful situations or losses. Identify the family's sources of strength. Assess patterns of interaction between family members as well as their spiritual, social, and economic status, their life-style, and cultural or ethnic influences. These variables often influence how the family responds to grief. Sometimes you play a valuable role simply by giving family members permission to have a day off from visiting.

Ineffective Management of Therapeutic Regimen (Individuals). Clients with SCI have bladder function changes. Bladder emptying has to be learned using a different approach. A common nursing diagnosis in this circumstance is *Ineffective Management of Therapeutic Regimen (Individuals).*

Planning: Expected Outcomes. The client will be able to manage his or her own bowels and bladder or instruct others how to do so.

Implementation. One of the most common stimuli for autonomic dysreflexia, a life-threatening complication in persons with SCI, is bladder distention. Therefore, intervention leading to bladder management is crucial.

Bladder Retraining. When the initial indwelling catheter is removed, a program of intermittent catheterization is commonly prescribed to empty the bladder regularly every 4 to 6 hours for several weeks. During this time, the client is taught methods of emptying the bladder without catheterization. Such methods promote urination by increasing intra-abdominal pressure on the bladder. For some clients with SCI, urinary flow may be initiated by using the Credé maneuver, Valsalva's maneuver, or the rectal stretch.

The *Credé maneuver* involves placing the fist or fingers directly over the bladder and pressing down toward the pubic bone with a kneading motion. This motion is continued until the bladder is empty.

Valsalva's maneuver involves inhaling deeply, holding one's breath, and bearing down as hard as possible, as if for a bowel movement.

The *rectal stretch* involves inserting a lubricated, gloved finger into the rectum. When the anal sphincter is relaxed, the client maintains the relaxation by gently pulling on the sphincter. This relaxes the perineal floor. Valsalva's maneuver is performed at the same time.

Urination may also be prompted by reflex stimulation. The following stimuli may be successful: tapping the suprapubic area; stroking the glans penis, thigh, or vulva; tugging pubic hairs; or flexing the toes. The stimulation may be applied by the client or caregiver. As training continues, less stimulation is needed to initiate urination.

Catheterization may be required at home. Teach the client and caregiver clean, rather than sterile, technique. This technique has the same infection rate as sterile insertion methods for home catheterization. Suprapubic catheters may be inserted for long-term bladder management. Occasionally, a surgical procedure such as sphincterotomy may be necessary. The bladder then empties continuously. An external, condom-type catheter connected to a straight closed drainage bag may be used to collect drainage in men. External appliances for females are not consistently effective.

Renal calculi, pyelonephritis, and hydronephrosis are major causes of death and disability in paralyzed clients. To prevent the development of renal calculi and bladder infections, encourage the client to drink 3000 ml of fluid per day, unless contraindicated by other medical conditions.

Bowel Retraining. Bowel retraining is possible for most paraplegic and quadriplegic clients. It involves developing controlled bowel movements by conditioned reflex activity. Begin bowel retraining as soon as feasible. Ensure privacy during the daily bowel routine, and if possible, have the client sitting upright. When possible, include appropriate family members in the bowel retraining program, as they may be involved in this aspect of long-term management. Always assess the family members' willingness to participate in such care. If the sexual partner is also responsible for hygiene and personal care, problems in role separation and intimacy may result. These issues should be openly discussed between partners.

With an effective bowel program, a client has a bowel movement once a day or every other day and is not incontinent at other times. Attaining continence may influence a paralyzed client's vocational future and positively affect his or her ability to have satisfying social relationships. It can also give the client the confidence to cope with other problems.

Sexual Dysfunction. Spinal cord–injured clients are often concerned about sexuality and their ability to achieve sexual fulfillment. They often worry about such concerns long before they express them to others. Nurses are often asked about sexuality issues before other professionals are approached, perhaps because nurses provide intimate care. Such care can promote a high degree of trust.

Planning: Expected Outcomes. The client will develop personally satisfying and socially acceptable means of expressing sexuality, as evidenced by interacting appropriately in social situations, verbalizing the effects of the injury on sexual function, discussing sexual issues with a team member, verbalizing methods of sexual expression, and verbalizing understanding of contraceptive implications.

Implementation. Some clients discuss their own sexual potential directly. Others refer to it subtly or appear crude in the way they introduce the topic, such as making inappropriate sexual comments or gestures. Such behaviors are attempts to acknowledge sexuality. Try to look beyond the behavior to the underlying emotional concerns. Acknowledge the client's concerns and offer to open a discussion, by saying, for example, "You seem concerned about your sexuality, James. This is a common concern that others with spinal cord injury have had. Sometimes talking about it helps. If you like, we can talk about how this has affected you, and when you are ready, I can share with you interventions that have helped others who have had similar problems."

To be helpful, nurses need to be able to talk about sexuality without embarrassment. They also need accurate information about "normal" sexuality and how physiologic changes that occur because of the injury affect sexual function.

The client can be referred to another person or an agency if appropriate. Referral should not be made too hastily, though. If someone talks with a nurse about this subject, it is probably because that person feels most comfortable speaking with that nurse at that time. Allow the client to lead the conversation, which may be difficult. Professionals often think they know what someone needs and wants, without listening to the client.

Generally, a physiologic sexual response requires an intact nervous system. For example, psychogenic erection requires an intact spinal cord, S2–4 nerve roots, and spinal reflexes; ejaculation is a function of skeletal muscle controlled by the somatic center in the pudendal nerve originating in the S2–4 roots; and orgasm involves contraction of both smooth and skeletal muscle. It should be remembered, however, that there is more involved in sexual expression than physiologic response.

To some extent, sexual function can be predicted by the level of the spinal cord lesion (see Table 35–4). For example, psychogenic erection is often difficult or impossible after most SCIs. However, although physical limitations certainly occur, every person is different. Many men do have reflex erections after SCI. Many disabled people enjoy paraorgasm (phantom orgasm) by developing alternative erogenous zones. The genitals are not the only body areas that can be sexually excited, and intercourse is not the only means of sexual expression.

Some persons find it disappointing, perhaps devastating, if they can no longer function sexually as they did before the injury. However, they can be helped to learn new ways of giving and receiving sexual pleasure. Sex and relationship counseling is sometimes helpful. Your role is to facilitate expression of feelings and convey hope that new and real sexual enjoyment can be experienced. Some form of sexual expression is possible for anyone, regardless of disability. Before making specific suggestions for alternative expressions of sexuality, you should interview the client regarding past sexual behavior and cultural taboos. Some clients may find some methods of giving and receiving sexual pleasure unacceptable. Lack of a sexual partner may be a deterrent, but should not preclude discussion of sexuality.

Society as a whole is becoming progressively more open about sexuality. Increasingly, the parenting potential of disabled people is receiving serious attention. Physical assessment is needed to determine a client's ability to reproduce. Male infertility is a frequent complication of SCI because of testicular atrophy, decreased sperm formation, and infrequent ejaculation. Most men are unable to ejaculate after SCI. Women usually remain fertile and can conceive and deliver a child. Adoption is a viable option, and conception by artificial insemination is possible.

Disabled people may have contraception concerns. Little is known about the effects of various kinds of contraceptives on disabled people. Oral contraceptives may be contraindicated. Paralyzed women often have slowed circulation, increasing the potential circulatory complications of oral contraceptives. To use an intrauterine device, a woman must have feeling in her pelvis to be able to recognize early manifestations of pelvic inflammatory disease. Many paralyzed women do not have such feeling. Barrier devices, such as a diaphragm, a condom, or foam, may be used if at least one partner has enough manual dexterity to insert the diaphragm or foam or put on the condom.

Risk for Injury. Sensory loss poses serious problems for paralyzed clients because they cannot feel the pain or pressure that normally warns of tissue damage.

Planning: Expected Outcomes. The client will be free of injury, as evidenced by no abrasions, reddened areas, ulcerations, or burns.

Implementation. SCI clients should not wear tight, restrictive clothing or ill-fitting shoes or braces. They need to develop the habit of preventive thinking to avoid potential danger. Dangerous situations include getting too close to heaters, radiators, and fireplaces and using heating pads or hot-water bottles. Burns can be a serious problem, because impaired circulation delays healing. External heat should not be applied if there is a loss of sensation, and the bath water should not be too hot.

Regular foot and nail care is required to prevent rubbing or cutting the skin and ingrown nails. Foot infections may be prevented by instructing the client not to cut corns or calluses. Cocoa butter or oils without alcohol may be used to soften calluses and reduce cracking.

Altered Health Maintenance. An SCI leaves a client with many alterations in physiologic functioning that place him or her at risk for maintaining a normal health status. A possible nursing diagnosis is *Altered Health Maintenance.*

Planning: Expected Outcomes. The client and family members will be able to meet the client's needs, as evidenced by intact skin, bowel and bladder continence, ability to transfer in and out of a wheelchair, absence of infection, maintenance of appropriate weight, and satisfying personal relationships.

Implementation. Teaching should be conducted in short sessions, using easily understood terms. For example, teach the caregiver the importance of providing good skin care on the hands and skinfolds to prevent *Candida* overgrowth. Complex tasks should be taught in steps with return demonstrations.

Most spinal cord–injured people are transferred from an acute care hospital to a rehabilitation facility. After functional capabilities have been maximized, the person is then discharged from the rehabilitation facility. The Bridge to Home Healthcare feature provides suggestions for helping caregivers support the client with an SCI who lives at home.

Evaluation

Spinal cord–injured clients are hospitalized for a long time. Therefore, some expected outcomes need to be evaluated frequently, such as respiratory and cardiac functions. Other expected outcomes will not be met for months, such as independence in ADLs. The plan of care for each client needs to reflect these individual problems.

■ Surgical Management

Intervention for progressive neurologic deficit is indicated when any of the following exist:

- Compound fractures and penetrating wounds of the spine
- Bone fragments in the spinal canal
- Syndrome of acute anterior spinal cord trauma[37]

Some neurosurgeons and orthopedic surgeons recommend decompressive laminectomy for complete SCIs. In this type of surgery, the lamina of the vertebrae are removed to minimize pressure on the spinal cord. Others believe that laminectomy should not be used routinely to treat SCI. Similarly, some surgeons recommend stabilization by surgical fusion within the first few days after

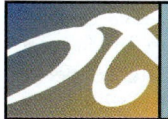

BRIDGE TO HOME HEALTHCARE

Managing the Immobile Client

Terrance Broadway, R.N., M.S.N., *Florida State Health Office, Tallahassee, Florida*

Assisting caretakers in the home as they provide supportive care and treatment to the client with spinal cord or other immobilizing injury is among the most challenging tasks in home healthcare. At one time or another, all members of the healthcare team will usually become participants in the care of these clients. Communication is one key to successful care. Maintain constant contact with the client, the caretakers, family members, and other members of the healthcare team to maximize client outcomes.

Prevention of the effects of immobility is the primary goal for clients and caregivers. Tissue anoxia and pressure sores develop over bony prominences when pressure is unrelieved. Therefore, total skin assessment should be done daily to evaluate potential areas of breakdown. Both active and passive preventive measures can be employed to preclude the effects of immobility.

Active measures include regular position changes in bed and while seated. Additionally, daily range-of-motion exercises promote circulation and help keep the skin well hydrated. Almost all physical activity improves air exchange, which helps to prevent upper respiratory infections and pneumonia. Adequate nutrition and hydration are important for healthy skin and for prevention of urinary tract infections. Use of universal precautions and avoiding cross-contamination can decrease the incidence of cellulitis.[13]

Passive prevention measures include waterbeds, alternating pressure mattresses, and specially designed cushions for wheelchairs. Skin should be as clean and dry as possible with folds, wrinkles, and debris removed from the areas beneath the patient. Pillows, foam supports, and blankets should be used to further protect immobilized limbs and bony prominences.

Contractures and spasticity are other complications of immobility. Preventive measures include passive range-of-motion exercises to maintain circulation and joint mobility. Passive range of motion should be accomplished daily and uninvolved limbs should be exercised to maintain strength. Slow, steady movement of limbs and joints is the best preventive measure for muscle spasms. Should a spasm occur during movement, the limb should be held firmly until the spasm subsides prior to finishing the movement. Forcing movement against a spastic response may cause fractures or other injury.

Immobile clients and their caretakers may need assistance with diversionary activities to assist in maintaining optimal mental health. Information on community resources, transportation, caregiver assistance, home adaptations, health services, financial assistance, and recreation should be provided.

Care can become complex when a home care client has a spinal cord or other immobilizing injury. Providers and caretakers must maintain constant contact to ensure that needs are being met and the effects of immobility are prevented.

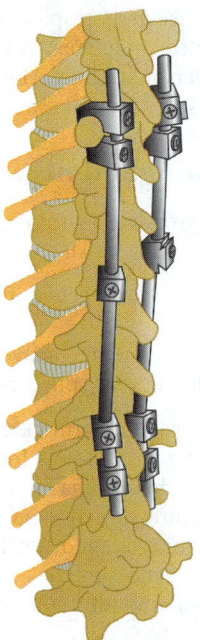

Figure 35–9. Fractures of the spine are often stabilized with internal fixation devices.

trauma, whereas others do not. Fusion is accomplished by insertion of metal plates and screws or the use of bone grafts, or a combination of these.

Cervical fractures can also be allowed to heal with bony stability by immobilization in a brace or halo jacket (see Fig. 35–5). The halo jacket has a ring that is fixed to the skull with pins. This ring is then attached to the jacket by rods. This system provides the traction required to maintain cervical alignment. A halo jacket allows early mobilization and rehabilitation. The wrench that comes with the brace should always be taped to the front of the jacket. This allows quick removal in case of emergency. Never grasp the rods to help in turning the client. If the client has some mobility remaining, always assist during the client's first attempt at any activity. The halo jacket changes the client's center of gravity and makes it easy for him or her to fall. Perform pin site care around the pin insertion sites daily. Refer to your agency's policy manual for guidelines.

Burst fractures of the thoracic and lumbar spine can be treated with body casts, Harrington rods, or other forms of spine stabilization. Spine stabilization devices are commonly inserted through a posterior incision (Fig. 35–9). Following the operation, the client has the usual postoperative assessments, including an assessment of the neurovascular status of the legs. Chest tubes and nasogastric tubes are inserted during surgery. The client is logrolled to facilitate respiration and skin perfusion. Pain is managed with continuous or injected narcotics. The client usually is fitted for a body brace and ambulates on the fourth day.

Complications of surgery include infection and poor wound healing, as well as the complications of anesthesia. Both infection and impaired wound healing are more likely to occur in a malnourished client.

■ Modifications for Elderly Clients

For elderly clients, the most important modification of the nursing care plan is increased vigilance. Elderly people are more prone to the complications of immobility. A person with congestive heart failure may have difficulty breathing when lying flat. When placing an elderly client in halo traction some neurosurgeons perform a temporary prophylactic tracheostomy because the elderly client has difficulty swallowing oral secretions and eating. Elderly people are also more susceptible to sensory deprivation. The nurse must make sure the client has his or her eyeglasses and hearing aid. If the person is not able to see a window or clock, he or she should be reoriented as needed. Discharge plans for elderly clients may be complicated if the caregiver is also elderly. The spouse of an elderly spinal cord–injured person may not have the physical strength to provide the needed care. Learning to provide home care may also be problematic.

Community and Self-Care

Paraplegic clients can usually live independently. Most quadriplegic people need some assistance with daily activities. Depending on the amount of assistance needed and the individual situation, this care may be provided by family members, a part-time paid attendant, or a full-time paid attendant. By using a wheelchair, clients may become completely independent in all ADLs, with minimal help of social services, a home health aide, or family. Many clients drive and hold outside jobs. Ventilator-dependent persons who cannot obtain in-home care and others who do not have the personal or financial resources for in-home care may have no option except institutional living. The Ethical Issues in Nursing feature addresses the problem of limited government resources for all clients requiring rehabilitative care. Group living situations, especially for young adults, are becoming more available.

Syringomyelia

Syringomyelia is often associated with the Arnold-Chiari malformation (an abnormal protrusion of the medulla into the spinal canal) or spina bifida. Syringomyelia consists of abnormal cavities filled with dense gluelike tissue in the spinal cord substance, especially the cervical cord. Scar tissue surrounds the cysts. Syringomyelia is characterized by (1) muscular weakness and wasting, (2) sensory defects, and (3) indications of injury to the long tracts of the spinal cord, such as hyperreflexia.

These disturbances may begin at any age but most often occur between ages 30 and 40. Syringomyelia often occurs with other developmental defects. Kyphosis (abnormal increased convexity in curvature of the thoracic spine when viewed from the side), scoliosis (lateral deviation in the normally straight vertical line of the spine), and clubfoot often occur with syringomyelia.

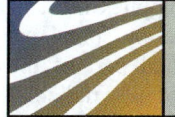

ETHICAL ISSUES IN NURSING

What Is the Government's Obligation to Put Care for Its Citizens Above Care for Non-Citizens, Given Scarce Resources?

Rehabilitative nursing has become more specialized to meet the various needs of clients who require physical rehabilitation. Clients who have spinal cord injuries often face long rehabilitative treatment regimens. Support is needed by these clients in several different areas of their lives. Emotional, technical, and financial support are the three major areas in which rehabilitation clients have great need. Financing a long rehabilitation course can be quite expensive. For many clients, this cost must be picked up by government-sponsored insurance programs (i.e., Medicare or Medicaid).

There is usually no opposition to such governmental reimbursement programs, because such programs benefit those members of society who are in need of specialized healthcare. But what happens when those who take advantage of governmental resources, such as an expensive rehabilitation course, are not citizens of the society where the treatment is being rendered, in particular, the United States? This dilemma is further complicated when resources are limited. For example, there may be two available openings for rehabilitative treatment and there are three persons in need of such treatment. Two of the persons are U.S. citizens and the third is not. Should the U.S. citizens receive first chance at the rehabilitation spots? What if the person who is not a U.S. citizen accepts treatment and then leaves the country halfway through the treatment course, thus wasting resources on an unfinished course and taking an opening that could have been given to someone who might have finished the course of treatment?

In large metropolitan areas, the number of clients who are not U.S. citizens may be fairly high. Nurses who work in these areas often care for such clients and probably are not even aware of their citizenship status. Nursing care should be the same for all clients, regardless of citizenship. The ethical dilemma remains, however, regarding the allocation of governmental financial assistance to those who are not U.S. citizens. Is there not an obligation by government to care for its own? Does this obligation include the exclusion of non-citizens? When resources become scarce, rationing takes place. No matter what governmental action takes place regarding financial reimbursement, strive for justice in nursing practice.

Early indications of cervical syringomyelia often include the following:

1. Atrophy, weakness, and fibrillations of the small muscles of the hands
2. Loss of pain sensation in the fingers or forearms
3. Weakness and atrophy of the shoulder girdle muscles
4. Horner's syndrome, which is characterized by ptosis of the upper eyelid, constriction of the pupil, anhidrosis (absence of sweating), and flushing of the affected side of the face
5. Nystagmus
6. Vasomotor and trophic disturbances of the upper extremities

Although there is segmental loss or impairment of pain and temperature sensation, sensation for light touch remains. Segments of sensory loss may be separated by zones of normal sensation. Spasticity, ataxia, or paralysis of the lower extremities may occur, as well as disturbed bladder control, if the lumbosacral region of the spinal cord is involved.

Cranial nerve involvement may produce additional problems such as impairment of facial pain and temperature sensation, loss of the corneal reflex (necessitating protection of the eye), dysphagia, dysarthria, laryngeal stridor (possibly necessitating tracheostomy), nystagmus, and atrophy and fibrillation of the tongue muscles.

Syringomyelia may progress rapidly at first and then become quiescent for many years. Some people live 40 years after onset. Others become incapacitated (from paralysis or sensory defects) or die within a few years.

Treatment includes relieving increased pressure on the cord from the fluid content of the cavities within the spinal canal. The fluid buildup can be removed and cerebrospinal fluid (CSF) outflow restored by direct surgical drainage or by shunt placement.

Spinal Tumors

Spinal tumors are similar in nature and origin to intracranial tumors but occur much less often. They are most common in young or middle-aged adults and most often involve the thoracic region. Spinal tumors may occur outside of the spinal cord such as in the meninges, nerve roots, or vertebrae (extramedullary) or within the substance of the spinal cord (intramedullary). Neurofibromas and meningiomas are the most common spinal cord tumors. Both are benign and operable and may not produce permanent damage if removed early.

Clinical manifestations of spinal tumors vary according to their location. Spinal cord compression is the common pathologic feature of all tumors within the spinal canal, because the cord has little room for expansion inside the bony vertebra. Compression of the spinal cord interrupts the function of peripheral nerves.

Extramedullary tumors cause manifestations by compressing the spinal cord or some of its nerve roots or by occluding blood vessels supplying the cord. Early characteristics of spinal cord compression include pain, sensory loss, muscle weakness, and muscle wasting. Progressive cord compression is manifested by spastic weakness below the level of the lesion, decreased sensation, and increased reflexes. Severe cord compression at the cervical level destroys cord function and produces quadriplegia; compression at the thoracic or lumbar level results in paraplegia.

Intramedullary tumors produce more variable clinical manifestations. High cervical cord involvement causes spastic quadriplegia and sensory changes. Tumors in descending areas of the spinal cord produce motor and sensory changes appropriate to functions at that level.

Medical diagnosis is made after a complete general neurologic examination. Diagnostic testing includes a spinal x-ray, CT scan, MRI, and a myelogram, individually or serially.

Intervention for spinal tumors is usually surgery, radiation therapy, or both. Immediate surgery is indicated if compression of the cord or nerve roots is evident. Often, surgery results in marked improvement or even complete restoration of function, especially if the tumor is benign and encapsulated (e.g., meningioma or lipoma). However, functional improvement is less common if cord necrosis has developed. Complete surgical removal of an intramedullary tumor is rare. However, partial resection followed by radiation may improve the client's condition. Usually, the course of the condition is gradually progressive.

Vascular Spinal Cord Lesions

The blood supply to the spinal cord is via the anterior and posterior spinal arteries and the radicular arteries (Fig. 35–10). The anterior spinal artery supplies most of the cord's cross-sectional area. The posterior spinal arteries supply the posterior white matter and part of the posterior gray matter. Various branches of the radicular arteries supply the superficial areas of white matter. A complex venous system drains the cord and empties into the anterior and posterior spinal veins and the two lateral veins.

As with stroke, spinal cord vascular lesions may be caused by rupture, thrombosis, or embolism. Trauma is the usual cause of hemorrhage into the spinal cord. Arteriosclerosis of spinal vessels is not a common cause of thrombosis. Thrombosis of the spinal vessels is usually secondary to meningitis or to compression of the vessels by tumors, granulomas, or abscesses in the epidural space.

Myelomalacia

Myelomalacia is softening or infarction of the spinal cord from spinal artery occlusion. This condition has a poor prognosis. There is little or no return of normal function to the involved areas. Myelomalacia is suspected when indications of transverse myelitis develop suddenly. Assessment findings in myelomalacia depend on the level of the lesion in the cord. There is always motor paralysis and dissociated sensory loss below the level of the lesion, accompanied by paralysis of bladder and bowel sphincters. Paralysis is usually bilateral but rarely complete. Initially, the limbs are flaccid and no deep tendon or superficial reflexes are elicited, as in spinal shock. After several weeks, spasticity, hyperreflexia, and clonus develop. Intervention focuses on maintaining body func-

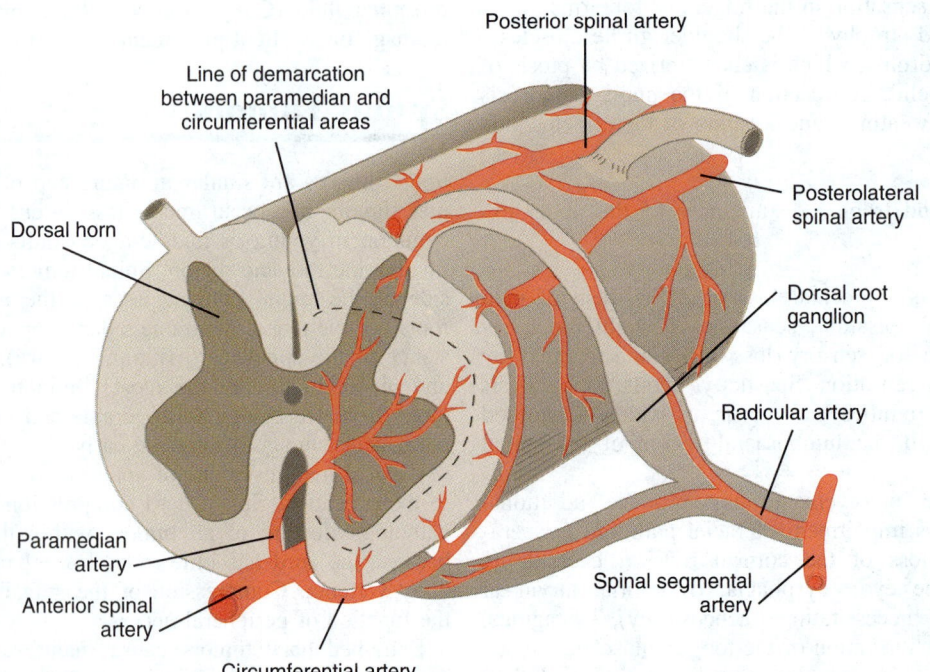

Figure 35–10. Arterial supply to the spinal cord.

tions, preventing complications of immobility, and providing pain relief. The person usually begins intensive rehabilitation 12 to 14 hours after onset of symptoms.

Hematomyelia

Hematomyelia is hemorrhage into the substance of the spinal cord. It almost always follows trauma but may be caused by vascular malformation or a bleeding disorder. Clinical manifestations of hematomyelia usually develop suddenly, immediately after spinal injury, and depend on the size of the hemorrhage. Following trauma, it is important to differentiate between hematomyelia and a vertebral fracture dislocation. Immediate surgery to relieve cord compression is indicated if fracture dislocation is evident on x-ray film. Spinal angiography, spinal CT scans, and MRI enable visualization of vascular lesions. Some of these lesions are treated by ligating their feeding vessels, others by excising the entire malformation. Management is the same as for myelomalacia. If surgery is needed, postoperative care is like that given to clients with other forms of spinal surgery.

Disc Herniation

An intervertebral disc is a pad that rests between the centers of two adjacent vertebrae. Discs provide cushions for spinal movement. The intervertebral disc is composed of three parts. (1) Cartilaginous plates act as the superior and inferior limits of the disc. These are composed of hyaline cartilage and cover the top and bottom of the vertebrae. (2) The annulus fibrosus is a ring of tissue that gives size and shape to the disc and holds the nucleus pulposus in place. (3) The nucleus pulposus is a semigelatinous material that forms the center of the disc and provides the cushioning effect.

Strenuous activity or degeneration of the disc or vertebrae can allow the disc to move from its normal location. Displacement of intervertebral disc material may be referred to as prolapse, herniation, rupture, or extrusion. Ruptured intervertebral discs may occur at any level of the spine. Lumbar discs are more likely to rupture than cervical discs, due to the force of gravity, continual movement in this region, and improper movements of the spine as with lifting or turning. As in SCI, thoracic disc disorders are the least common.

Etiology and Risk Factors

Several risk factors are associated with back pain. They include occupations that require strenuous or repetitive lifting in a stooped position, cigarette smoking, and jobs that require operating vibrating machinery. Genetic predispositions to back injury are found in persons with spondylolisthesis. Persons with postural problems from kyphosis and scoliosis do not appear to have a greatly increased risk.

Back Strain. More than half of the people with clinical manifestations of a herniated disc give a history of a previous back injury. Heavy physical labor, strenuous exercise, and weak abdominal and back muscles all increase the risk of herniated disc. Flexing the back without bending the knees and making rotating movements create significant stress on the intervertebral disc. Repeated stress progressively weakens the disc, resulting in bulging and herniation.

Lordosis. Lordosis is an excessive backward concavity in the lumbar spine. It is commonly associated with sagging shoulders, medial rotation of the legs, and an exaggerated pelvic angle. Excessive lordosis may result in swayback and kyphosis. Back pain is common.

Other causes of low back pain include spinal stenosis, spondylolisthesis, spondylolysis, and spinal tumors (see Spinal Tumors).

Spinal Stenosis. Spinal stenosis is narrowing of the vertebral foramen through which the spinal cord passes. It can develop at any level in the spine and usually occurs in older people. Severity can range from entrapment of one nerve root to compression of the entire cord.

Spondylolisthesis. Spondylolisthesis is the forward slipping of one vertebra. It commonly occurs at L5–S1, where L5 slips forward. Spondylolisthesis is graded from 1 to 4. Grades 1 and 2 are managed conservatively. Grades 3 and 4 usually require surgery for stabilization.

Spondylolysis. Spondylolysis is a structural defect in the lamina or neural arch of the spine. The vertebral arch slips forward. The lumbar spine is most commonly involved.

Approximately 80% of the population experience low back pain at some point in their lives. It is estimated that 10% of those who seek medical attention for back pain have herniated discs. Because of the frequency of herniated disc problems, health promotion is an essential activity for healthcare providers. The Client Education Guide provides suggestions for low back care.

Pathophysiology

The annulus fibrosus is weaker posteriorly than anteriorly, which explains why disc herniations are retrograde. When the disc only bulges, the annulus remains intact. With herniation, the annulus is usually torn, allowing extrusion of the nucleus pulposus (Fig. 35–11). Compression of spinal nerve roots may result from herniation of the disc. When the disc impinges on the sciatic nerve, the condition and resulting pain is called sciatica. Sciatica is a severe, usually constant pain in the leg that occurs along the course of the sciatic nerve and its branches.

The nucleus pulposus has no intrinsic nerves. However, when it extrudes, it irritates the dural membranes and creates pain that is referred to other body areas. The

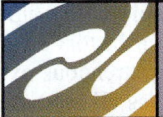

CLIENT EDUCATION GUIDE

Low Back Care

Get out of bed by rolling onto one side near the edge of the mattress. Push up to a straight position by pushing off the bed with your arms while keeping your spine straight and swing your legs over the edge. Avoid twisting while getting up.

Do not sleep while partially reclined or sitting in a chair. Sleep on a bed with a firm (not hard) mattress. Avoid riding in or driving a car for a long distance or time. Sit erect without slouching. Avoid low couches and chairs, and use your leg muscles when rising from a chair; a recliner chair is usually comfortable.

When you must stand for a long time, bend one knee to reduce stress on your low back.

Maintain a body weight that is close to ideal. Exercise and walk or swim to strengthen your back muscles. Wear low-heeled shoes.

Eat a diet high in fiber and fluids to soften bowel movements and reduce strain. (When adding fiber to your diet, add it slowly over days.)

Use proper body mechanics when lifting. Get adequate help if the object is heavy. Use the muscles of your legs, not your back, by bending at the knees to get close to the object being lifted. Never turn and lift at the same time.

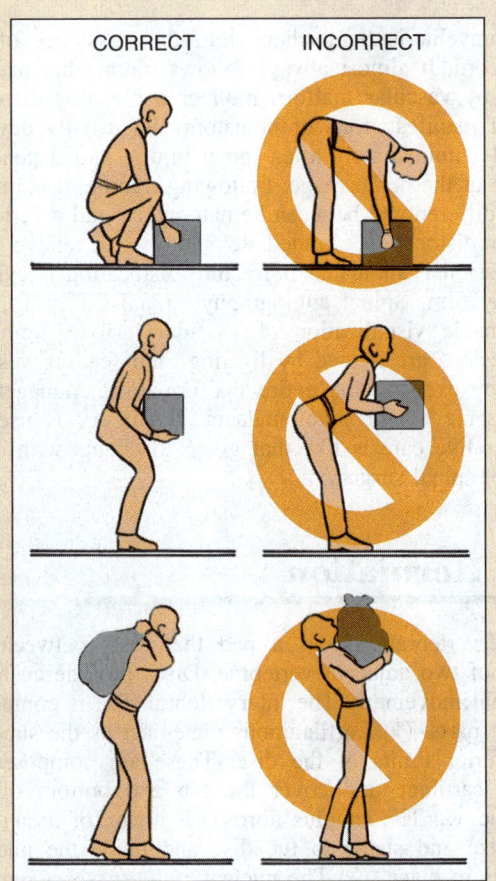

CORRECT　　INCORRECT

cause of the muscle spasms that develop with severe back pain is not fully understood. It is thought that a motor-reflex pathway is responsible for the pain.

Spinal stenosis (see Fig. 35–11) is due to ligamentous infolding and hypertrophy of the bone. It produces pressure on the entire spinal cord. If compression remains untreated, weakness or paralysis of the innervated muscle groups may result.

Clinical Manifestations and Diagnostic Findings

Rupture of a small, laterally placed cervical disc typically causes (1) a stiff neck, (2) shoulder pain that radiates down the arm into the hand, and (3) paresthesias and sensory disturbances in the hand.

Clinical manifestations seen in clients with a ruptured lumbar intervertebral disc include the following:

1. Low back pain that radiates down the sciatic nerve into the posterior thigh
2. Muscle spasm
3. Aggravation of pain by straining (coughing, sneezing, defecation, bending, lifting, and straight-leg raising)
4. Depression of deep tendon reflexes
5. Hyperesthesia in the area of distribution of affected nerve roots

Typically, the pain of sciatica begins in the buttocks and extends down the back of the thigh and leg to the ankle. Any movement of the lower extremities that stretches the nerve causes pain and involuntary resistance. Straight-leg raising on the affected side is limited. Complete extension of the leg is not possible when the thigh is flexed on the abdomen (Lasègue's sign).

Manifestations of spinal stenosis usually begin slowly and are due to pressure placed on nerve roots as they exit the vertebrae. The most common manifestations are pain with standing and walking, although bowel and bladder

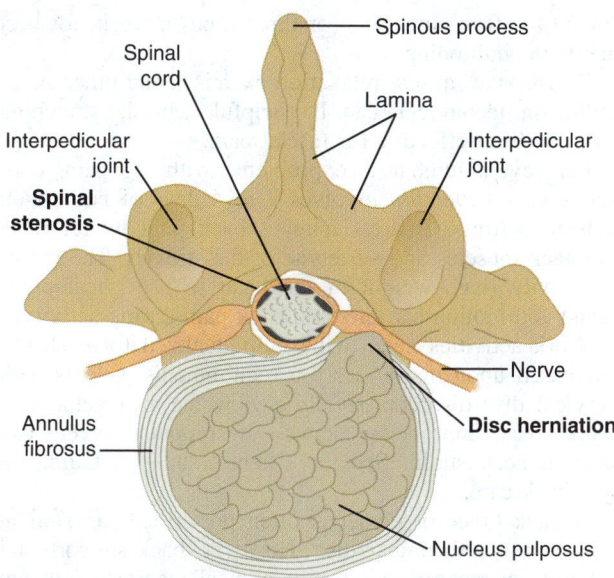

Figure 35–11. The usual causes of low back pain are disc herniation and spinal stenosis.

function can be altered with severe forms of the disorder.

X-ray studies may show spinal degenerative changes (at any level) that may indicate disc problems but usually do not show a ruptured disc. Osteophytes and narrowed disc interspaces are degenerative changes demonstrable on x-ray. Also, other spinal disorders (e.g., spinal tumors, vertebral fracture, rheumatoid arthritis, and osteoarthritis) can lead to the same manifestations.

MRI may demonstrate spinal stenosis (narrowing of the spinal canal), extrusion of disc material into the

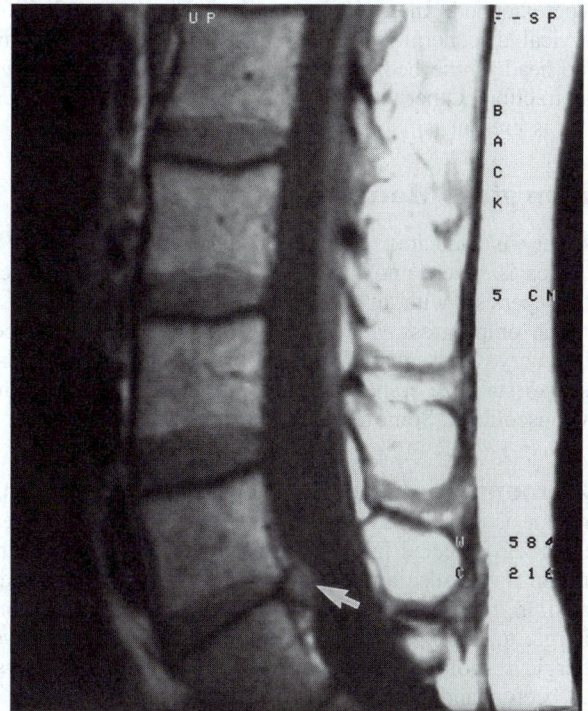

Figure 35–12. Magnetic resonance imaging of the lumbar spine showing herniation of the disc between L5 and S1.

spinal canal, and impingement of a spinal nerve root (Fig. 35–12).

Myelography may show narrowing of the disc space and impingement of a spinal nerve root. Myelography identifies the level of herniation and may rule out other spinal diseases. It is typically performed if the MRI is not conclusive. A CT scan is usually done following a myelogram. This sequence allows better imaging with only one administration of contrast material. CT scanning may demonstrate spinal stenosis or other changes associated with degenerative disc disease. CT scans are more useful at the thoracic or lumbar level than the cervical level.

Discography is the injection of a water-soluble imaging material into the nucleus pulposus. It is used to determine internal changes in the disc. During the injection, information is recorded about the amount of dye accepted and the pressure needed to inject the material. Clients can have allergic responses to the dye and develop disc space infections from the injection. Electromyography of the peripheral nerves may also be used to localize the site of the ruptured disc.

Acute and Subacute Care

■ Medical Management

Initial assessment of the client with low back pain is designed to help diagnose the cause. The client's medical history is obtained to help determine if a serious underlying condition is responsible for the pain, such as a fracture, tumor, infection, or cauda equina syndrome. The client's psychological and socioeconomic history is obtained, since these problems can complicate both assessment and management. The client is also asked to rate the pain. Physical examination is used to determine if lumbar nerve roots are involved by testing for reflexes, muscle strength, and the presence of neurologic deficits (Fig. 35–13). Once the clinician is certain that there is no serious condition, the client is assured that a rapid recovery may be expected.

Initial care is directed at managing the client's pain and directing activities. Pain is usually managed with nonsteroidal anti-inflammatory agents, muscle relaxants, and, at times, narcotics. Ice may be used to reduce pain with acute disc herniation for the first 48 hours. After that time heat is usually a better analgesic. A semi-sitting position (in a recliner chair) is usually comfortable and promotes forward lumbar spine flexion and thus reduces back strain. Other positions of comfort include (1) the supine position with pillows under the legs or (2) the lateral position, in which the client lies on the unaffected side with a thin pillow between the knees with the painful leg flexed to reduce tension on the sciatic nerve. Lying in a prone position and sleeping with thick pillows under the head should be avoided.

If the client has nonspecific low back pain, manipulation may be used by a physical therapist or chiropractor. *Spinal manipulation* may be defined as the use of the hands on the spine for therapeutic purposes. It is usually

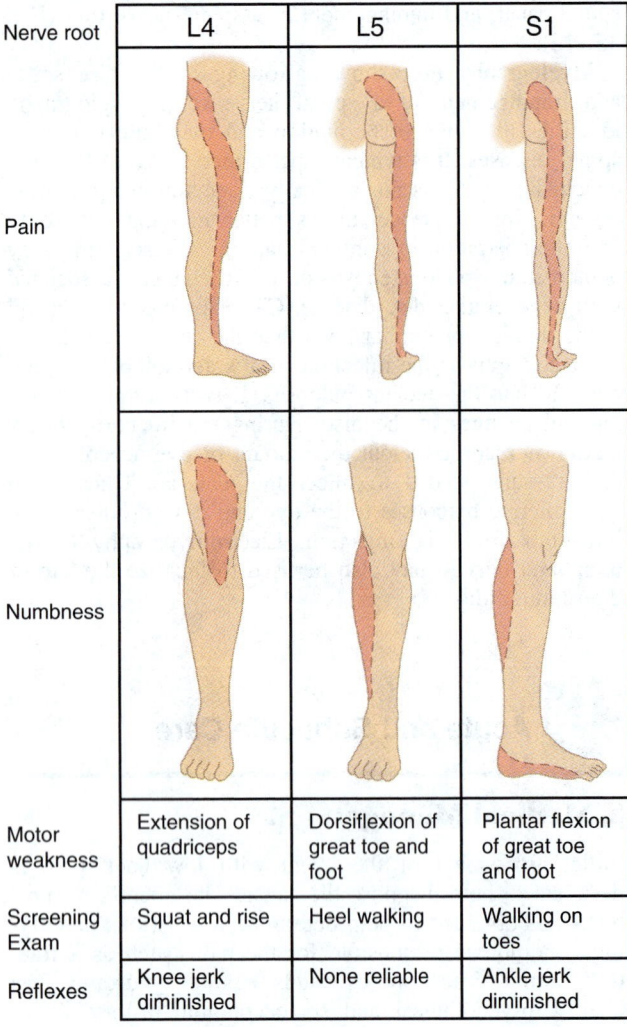

Nerve root	L4	L5	S1
Pain			
Numbness			
Motor weakness	Extension of quadriceps	Dorsiflexion of great toe and foot	Plantar flexion of great toe and foot
Screening Exam	Squat and rise	Heel walking	Walking on toes
Reflexes	Knee jerk diminished	None reliable	Ankle jerk diminished

Figure 35–13. Testing for lumbar nerve root compromise includes testing for motor weakness and reflexes, and to elicit pain (screening examination). (Redrawn from Agency for Health Care Policy and Research. [1994]. *Acute low back problems in adults: Assessment and treatment. Quick reference guide for clinicians,* No. 14. Rockville, MD: Author.)

performed for clients with manifestations that last more than 1 month. The AHCPR review panel found no evidence that spinal traction with weights was effective in reducing low back pain. Although yet unproven, deep ultrasonic heat treatment and moist local heat applications may help reduce pain.

Activity modifications are prescribed to reduce back irritation and prevent debilitation from inactivity. Most clients do not require bedrest. In fact, more than 4 days of bedrest can be debilitating and actually slow recovery. The client is taught to minimize the stress of lifting by keeping objects close to the body, and to avoid twisting when lifting. Sitting may aggravate leg pain and clients who sit at work should change positions often. Aerobic activities should be prescribed to help avoid debilitation. Walking, stationary bicycling, and even light jogging can be performed. Exercise should begin within the first 2 weeks after injury and each activity should be performed

for 20 to 30 minutes, two or three times a week, for best aerobic conditioning.

Progressive muscle relaxation exercises and other stress reduction techniques can be helpful. Muscle stretching has also been effective for fascial pain.

For severe lumbar disc problems with leg pain, conservative intervention involves 2 to 4 days of bedrest on a firm mattress. Bedrest relieves back pain by relieving the back muscles and vertebrae of the stresses. The forces of gravity (e.g., weight of the head with cervical problems) and motion can increase back pain during activity.

Work activities need to be individualized for each client based upon his or her job requirements. Clients with cervical disc disorders should review the arrangement of work areas. Improper placement of computer screens can lead to neck strain. See the Client Education Guide on low back care.

A back brace or corset is often prescribed for a client with a ruptured lumbar disc. However, back supports are usually not recommended once clinical manifestations are relieved, because restricted back motion progressively weakens muscles and causes further degeneration of spinal structures. Once the acute pain episode passes, progressive muscle-strengthening exercises may be prescribed. Strengthening the back and abdominal muscles helps prevent further problems if the exercises are done daily throughout life.

Opinions differ concerning the advisability of performing head and neck ROM exercises in the presence of significant cervical disease. Tell the client to avoid activities that increase cervical disc pain. To prevent neck extension when in bed, only one flat pillow (to prevent neck flexion) is recommended. A soft cervical collar may be prescribed for mild-to-moderate cervical disc problems to keep the head slightly flexed. The neck should not be hyperextended. Intermittent traction may be applied for cervical disc herniation (5–8 lb weight) to relieve pain. The head of the bed may be slightly elevated with cervical traction. Otherwise, it is best kept flat when cervical pain is present.

■ Surgical Management

Surgery is indicated with spinal disc problems when (1) sciatica is severe and disabling, (2) manifestations of sciatica persist without improvement for longer than 4 weeks, or progress, and (3) physiologic evidence of specific nerve root dysfunction is present. Surgery is also used to stabilize spinal fractures and correct scoliosis and kyphoscoliosis. Some surgeons use other criteria.

Chemonucleolysis. Chymopapain is a proteolytic enzyme isolated from papaya latex that is used as a meat tenderizer. Injected into the disc, chymopapain digests the protein in the disc and thereby shrinks it. It is contraindicated in persons with multiple allergies and in persons allergic to papaya. Immediate and delayed (after 15 days) allergic responses have been reported. Therefore, its use has been abandoned by most practitioners.

Discectomy. Discectomy is the use of microsurgical

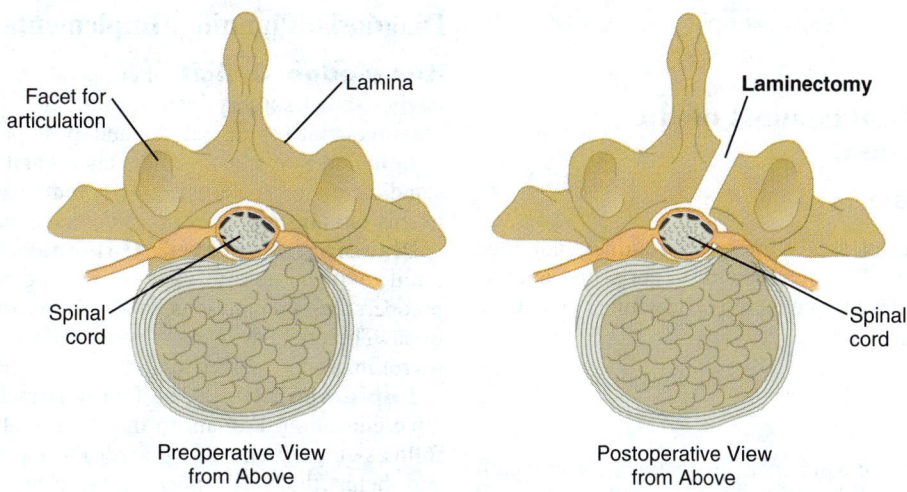

Figure 35–14. Laminectomy for the interlaminal removal of a herniated disc.

instruments to remove the herniated fragment of disc. This technique causes less trauma to the surgical site than standard surgery and preserves more tissue integrity. Advantages of microsurgery include minimal nerve root retraction, preservation of an intact joint capsule (no bone is removed), improved hemostasis, and minimal stripping of the muscle and fascia from the spine. Sometimes foraminotomy is performed to enlarge the intervertebral foramen if it is narrowed and osteophytic processes (overgrowth of bone) entrap the nerve root and impinge on neural structures.

Laminectomy. Laminectomy is surgical removal of the posterior arch of a vertebra, exposing the spinal cord

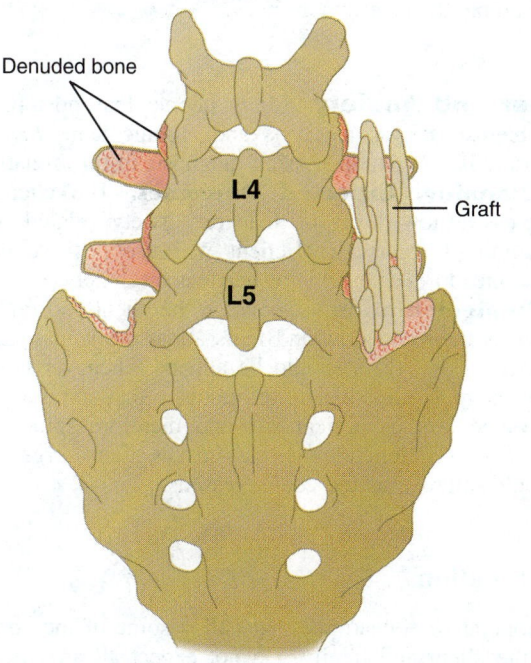

Figure 35–15. Lumbar interbody spinal fusion. Bone grafts are taken from the iliac crest and inserted between the vertebrae. In this illustration, the "bed" of raw bone is shown on the left, and the graft material is shown in place on the right.

(Fig. 35–14). This gives access to the spinal canal for (1) removing a spinal cord tumor, (2) removing the portion of the nucleus pulposus that is ruptured or protruding from a herniated disc, or (3) decompressing (relieving pressure on) the spinal cord.

Spinal Fusion. Spinal fusion is the placement of bone grafts (bone chips) between vertebrae (Fig. 35–15). The new bone that grows fuses the two vertebrae and immobilizes them. Usually no more than five vertebrae are fused; fusing more than five vertebrae causes considerable loss of movement in the spine. The bone graft may be obtained from a bone bank or the anterior superior iliac crest. During healing, the graft gradually grows onto the vertebrae and forms a bony union. This causes permanent stiffness in the area. After a while, the stiffness is hardly noticed in the lumbar area but is noticeable in the cervical area. Metal rods may be used to straighten and fuse the spine in disorders such as scoliosis or multiple vertebral fractures. An anterior or posterior surgical approach is taken to perform cervical and lumbar spinal fusions.

Complications. General potential complications following spinal disc surgery at any level include infection and inflammation, injury to nerve roots, dural tears, cauda equina syndrome, and hematoma. Nonunion of the surgical area is also a risk and is associated with smoking.

Complications after posterior cervical surgery include soft tissue hematoma, air embolism, and subcutaneous wound dehiscence. Complications following anterior cervical surgeries include laryngeal nerve damage and injury to neck structures such as the carotid arteries, trachea, esophagus, and soft tissue.

Outcomes. The AHCPR reviewed outcomes of surgery for low back problems.[1] In general, lumbar discectomy often relieved manifestations of pain faster than continued medical management in persons with severe and disabling leg pain. However, in other persons with no leg pain, there appeared to be little difference in outcome between discectomy and conservative care. Most clients who had chymopapain injections required eventual discectomy for permanent pain relief. Certainly, more study is needed to determine who is best served by the various techniques; client preference also plays a big role in the technique chosen.

■ Nursing Management of the Surgical Client

Preoperative Care

Clients undergoing elective surgery are routinely admitted the day of surgery. This significantly reduces the amount of time nurses have for preoperative teaching. (See Case Management feature.)

Assessment

A baseline neurologic assessment is obtained for comparison after surgery. Assessment should include motor and sensory function of extremities, and psychological readiness for surgery.

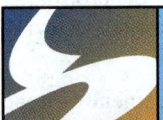

CASE MANAGEMENT

Lumbar Laminectomy
For Clinical Pathway, see Appendix D.

Clinical Pathway from Montclair Baptist Medical Center, Birmingham, Alabama
Information provided by Lee Ann Abernathy

Development and Revision of Pathway

- This diagnosis was selected for pathway development due to the high number of cases in our hospital.
- We have been using this pathway for approximately 2 years.
- Staff nurses and practical nurses were the initiators of this pathway.
- We have a task force meeting each quarter during which quality, financial, and clinical issues are discussed and reviewed. We solicit feedback from the staff as well, to help us keep current on the accuracy and usefulness of the CareMap.
- Initially we reviewed the pathway monthly. Now it is reviewed as needed.

Use and Impact of Pathway

- All patients who are admitted for lumbar laminectomy surgery are placed on this pathway.
- The nursing staff use the pathway daily.
- Standing orders, which complement the pathway, are available for the nurses to use when a patient is admitted for this procedure. Each day of the pathway has a set of standing orders which the physician can use or modify. Nurses know what to expect in caring for this type of patient.
- The pathway has helped cut length of stay by 2 days, and the cost of laboratory tests has also been reduced.

Diagnosis, Planning, Implementation

Knowledge Deficit. Perioperative care of a client having spinal surgery includes providing knowledge about the preoperative, operative, and postoperative phases. It also includes evaluating the client and family's understanding of the experience. A common nursing diagnosis in this circumstance is *Knowledge Deficit.*

Planning: Expected Outcomes. The client and family will be able to explain the surgical procedure, the preoperative preparations, and the postoperative precautions. The client will demonstrate safe mobility, including logrolling, and transfer to and from the bed.

Implementation. The family is included in preoperative education. Explain to the client that frequent turning follows surgery and that correct turning protects the back and helps the recovery process. Explain the logrolling method of turning, and the necessity for limitations on activity to prevent damage (flexion, extension, or twisting) to the surgical site, and the importance of not straining. Advise the client to ask for help rather than stretch to reach for objects. Stool softeners are given daily while the client is in the hospital to minimize straining with bowel movements. Clients with a recent injury may not be permitted to ambulate prior to surgery. For these clients, explain and demonstrate.

Clients who smoke are encouraged to stop smoking. Smoking increases cardiovascular complications and increases the risk of poor wound healing and nonunion if a fusion is performed.

If a fusion is to be done, clients need to be evaluated for autologous blood donations. Two or three units should be donated, the last one at least a week before the surgery. A fusion also necessitates informing the client of the bone graft site and the additional pain associated with the autograft bone donor site.

Fear and Anxiety. Many people fear postoperative problems such as paralysis and chronic pain. *Fear and Anxiety* is a common nursing diagnosis in this situation.

Planning: Expected Outcomes. The client will express a low level of fear or anxiety related to the upcoming surgery. The client will use positive coping strategies to decrease his or her fear or anxiety.

Implementation. Encourage the client and family to express their concerns and fears about the spinal surgery. Concerns and fears should be allayed whenever possible. For example, clients need to be aware that some edema is expected at the surgical site and therefore some of the preoperative deficit may still exist after surgery, but should improve as the edema lessens.

Evaluation

Preoperative education should allay some of the concerns of the client and family. Do not expect all anxiety to be relieved; in fact, some new areas of concern may arise. If questions come up about the operation, ask the surgeon to answer them. Do not attempt to provide information outside of your area of expertise.

Postoperative Care

Assessment

Following spinal surgery, assessment is similar to that performed for other surgical clients. A head-to-toe assessment is done. Dressings and drains are checked. The level of pain and the response to analgesia are evaluated. Neurologic function is assessed by asking the client to move his or her legs and comparing the results with those of the baseline evaluation. Question the client about the presence of numbness or tingling and changes in sensation or pain. These paresthesias are a consequence of the edema from the surgery, but should improve. If progressive weakness or paralysis of the lower extremities, loss of sphincter control, anal numbness, or urinary retention (called the cauda equina syndrome)[34] occur, notify the physician immediately. Emergency surgical decompression may be required. Clients who have had fusions are on bedrest longer, and thus have a higher risk of deep vein thrombosis (DVT). Observe for and report any manifestations of DVT: positive Homans' sign, redness or swelling in the leg, or sudden chest pain or dyspnea. Observe for signs of infection at the incision site. Take the client's temperature every 4 hours. A mild temperature elevation is expected after the prolonged surgery and hardware insertion. However, a temperature over 101° F may require removal of the hardware. Assess the wound for bulging or clear drainage which may indicate CSF leakage. Test the fluid for glucose. A positive test means CSF leakage. Notify the physician.

Disc problems often create fears and concerns related to pain, treatments, sexual activity, possible length of illness, and possible life-style changes. Provide psychosocial support to the client and family. Impaired mobility and altered urinary or bowel elimination are also common problems experienced after disc surgery. Considerations about employment and finances should be referred to a social worker.

Diagnosis, Planning, Implementation

Pain. Pain secondary to incisional trauma and edema is an expected response after spinal surgery. Write this common postoperative nursing diagnosis as *Pain related to incision.*

Planning: Expected Outcomes. The client will express an acceptable level of pain, for example, level 3 on a scale of 0 to 10.

Implementation. Although there will be pain from the incision, often the pain in an extremity will be significantly less after herniated disc surgery. In addition, many surgeons inject long-acting local anesthetics into disc spaces during surgery. This gives the client immediate relief from pain and promotes a positive attitude toward the outcome of surgery. Often the pain recurs on the second postoperative day. This is due to both the increase in swelling and the fact that the local anesthetic is wearing off.

Acute postoperative pain can be managed by using a basal dose of a narcotic per IV pump in combination with a patient-controlled analgesia (PCA) dose for pain peaks (breakthrough pain) not controlled by the continuous dose. Another method of providing basal (continuous) pain medication is by IV drip or epidural catheter. If the client is on prn pain management, teach him or her to keep pain levels tolerable by asking for narcotics before the pain is too great. Ice may also be applied to the incision using an abdominal wrap that holds sheets of ice along the lumbar area and reduces the risk of ice burns.

Impaired Physical Mobility. Clients who have spinal surgery will have varying degrees of mobility limitations. The diagnosis can be written as *Impaired Physical Mobility related to pain, leg weakness, prolonged immobility or fear of pain and spasms.* You may not need all of these etiologies; choose the one that best fits your client.

Planning: Expected Outcomes. The client will resume a maximal level of progressive activity, starting with logrolling on the day of surgery, progressing to independent movement from the bed to a standing position, followed by independent ambulation prior to discharge.

Implementation. Encourage the client to move the legs and feet while on bedrest to promote venous return. In addition, alternating compression stockings may be used to promote venous return. If the client requires assistance to turn, or when turning to place a bedpan, turn the client in the logrolling manner. A fracture bedpan is used to reduce back arching and strain.

When the client is being transferred to bed postoperatively, at least four people should assist. Transfer devices such as a sliding board may be used with adequate help. Transfer the client gently and smoothly, with the spine supported and properly aligned at all times.

Immediately following lumbar discectomy, the client typically is not turned for an hour or so but remains flat to aid hemostasis. Begin side-to-side logrolling and repeat every 2 hours. If a dural tear was repaired, the surgeon may order the client to remain flat longer to minimize the risk of CSF leak or a tear in the dural sutures.

Following lumbar fusion, the bed is generally kept flat. The client logrolls from side to side, usually beginning about 4 hours after surgery and then every 2 to 4 hours thereafter. Twisting the client's spine or twisting at the hips must be avoided. Ensure safety during turning to prevent straining of the spine or rolling off the bed. It is beneficial to have extra help in turning a client the first few times after spinal surgery. Spinal bone grafts are delicate and heal slowly. Eventually, turning is permitted without help, while keeping the spine rigid.

It is common for the client to have spasms and pain with turning, so administer pain medication prior to moving. Once turned, tilt the client back onto pillows to reduce pressure on the iliac crest. Once turned, back strain may be reduced by (1) keeping the spine straight, (2) flexing the upper leg and placing a pillow between the legs, and (3) placing a pillow to support the upper arm and prevent the upper shoulder from sagging. If the iliac crest was used as a donor site, the client may not be able to turn onto that side because of pain. Follow the surgeon's orders on how high the head can be elevated.

Use a pressure reduction mattress to reduce the risk of pressure ulcers if the client had spinal surgery for fracture stabilization or will be in bed for a long time. Use of a trapeze over the bed is contraindicated because it promotes twisting. The call light is placed so the client can touch it without straining. Once the client is allowed to reach for things, the objects needed should be convenient.

If a client is supine following spinal surgery (e.g., using a bedpan), the lower back muscles may be relaxed somewhat if pillows are placed under the entire length of the legs. This may also prevent thrombophlebitis in the femoral vessels. Do not flex the client's knees by placing anything under the popliteal space; this is hazardous because it increases the risk of DVT. A sign, which is discussed with the client, is placed on the bed describing the prescribed position for the bed. Also instruct the client clearly about contraindicated activities and positions.

To assist the client into a chair, teach the client to roll onto the side and push the torso from the bed with the arms to rise from the bed. This technique has often been used by clients with long-standing back pain and may be familiar to the client. In this case, review the client's technique for rising from the bed. Usually the client is assisted to a chair the morning following surgery. Be sure to follow the physician's activity prescriptions.

Following spinal surgery, a brace or corset may be required temporarily to support the spine. Persons who have lumbar or thoracic spinal fusions wear a fiberglass brace. Initially, back braces or corsets may be worn all the time, whether the client is in or out of bed. As the client's muscles strengthen, the use of braces or corsets is usually decreased. Casts may be used for a while following any thoracic spinal surgery for clients with unstable thoracic spines (e.g., thoracic spinal cord trauma).

Altered Urinary Elimination. Following spinal surgery, urinary retention may occur. Most commonly, it occurs due to pain and spasms when resting supine and as a side effect of narcotics. It also occurs when the cauda equina is affected. State the nursing diagnosis as *Risk for Altered Urinary Elimination related to pain and spasms with movement.*

Planning: Expected Outcomes. The client will resume normal bladder emptying by the time he or she is ambulating.

Implementation. Assess for bladder distention and pain 8 hours after surgery. If the client's bladder is distended and painful on palpation, noninvasive measures should be tried first. Commonly, the client is catheterized with an in-and-out catheter (straight catheterization) twice, after which an indwelling catheter is placed. It may be used for the first few days until the client is ambulating and using less pain medication. When the catheter is removed, generally clients can urinate when sitting or standing rather than lying supine. If the bladder is full or cannot be emptied completely, the physician may order straight catheterization to check for residual urine.

Risk for Paralytic Ileus. The most common bowel problem after laminectomy and spinal fusion is paralytic ileus. This loss of bowel sounds and abdominal distention is due to lack of peristalsis from a sudden loss of parasympathetic function innervating the bowels and manipulation of the intestines in anterior approaches to spinal surgery.

Planning: Expected Outcomes. The client will resume normal bowel function, including evacuation without straining, by the time he or she is ambulating.

Implementation. Assessment findings with paralytic ileus include nausea, vomiting, a hard abdomen, and absence of bowel sounds. The client is assessed every 4 hours postoperatively for bowel distention.

Intervention typically includes insertion of a nasogastric tube, which is connected to low intermittent suction, and initiation of a nothing-by-mouth status. When a client's gag reflex and bowel sounds have returned and the client passes gas or has a bowel movement, a clear liquid diet is usually prescribed and progresses to a regular diet.

Bowel dysfunction may occur for several days postoperatively. Inactivity often causes problems with bowel elimination. Bowel movements are documented. Fluids are forced as ordered; a regular time for bowel movements and bowel care is encouraged; fiber is provided in the diet (when allowed), and prescribed medications and enemas (e.g., stool softeners, mild bulk laxatives, or a suppository) are administered. Instruct the client not to strain for a bowel movement, because this increases pain and CSF pressure. Often clients find it difficult or impossible to defecate when lying flat. A bowel movement may not occur until sitting up is possible.

Evaluation

Expect pain to be controlled with mild to moderate narcotic analgesics, bowel and bladder function to be intact, the client to be able to walk steadily for several yards, and the client to be able to eat prior to discharge.

Cervical Disc Disorders

Discs may become entrapped in the cervical spine. The process is much like that with herniated lumbar discs. Manifestations include arm pain, neck pain and spasms, and loss of function (grip strength) and changes in sensation in the hands. Initial treatment is with nonsteroidal anti-inflammatory agents, muscle stretching, and teaching proper body mechanics. A review of posture at work is important for clients who work at computer terminals. Keyboards, screens, and written materials should be kept at a height that reduces strain on the neck and shoulders. Following fracture of a cervical vertebra, cervical disc rupture, or whiplash injury, the person may wear a neck brace (fitted so the chin rests on a cup and the neck is kept hyperextended), a hard collar (which extends up under the chin and prevents flexion of the neck), or a soft collar. Neck braces tend to limit vision, because people wearing them cannot look down at their feet. Safety awareness is important to prevent falls. Sometimes conservative treatment does not work and clients require surgery. Surgery to stabilize bone fragments is necessary if a neck injury involves a bone fracture. Cervical fusion (Fig.

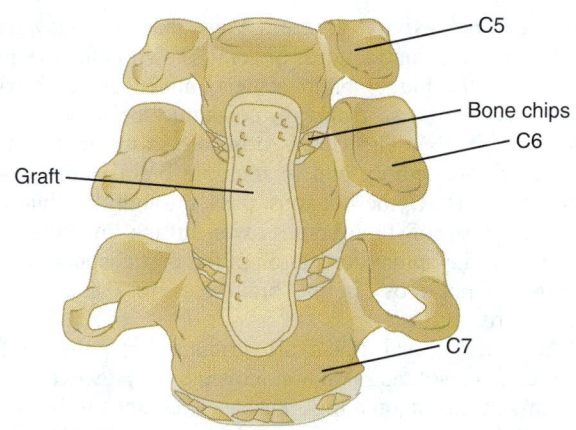

Figure 35–16. Anterior cervical fusion. A trough has been cut into the anterior cervical spine for insertion of an iliac graft as a splint. The intervertebral spaces have been filled with bone chips.

35–16) is most commonly performed through an anterior approach.

Following microdiscectomy, the client may have the head of the bed elevated to whatever position is comfortable. Following cervical spine surgery, the surgeon indicates the degree of head elevation for comfort and to reduce edema. A client who has had cervical surgery is positioned in essentially the same manner as are clients after lumbar surgery. Make sure the spine is in line at the cervical area. Immediately after a posterior cervical discectomy, a cervical collar is worn (Fig. 35–17). The client's head may be elevated and a folded small towel, bath blanket, or small pillow is placed under the head to maintain spinal alignment while the client lies supine or on the side.

Assess and document the client's neurologic status frequently. The development or worsening of a neurologic deficit must be promptly reported to the surgeon. During the first 24 hours following an anterior cervical discectomy, assess the client's ability to breathe, check the operative site for excessive swelling, and look for shifting of the trachea and changes in the client's voice. Laryngeal nerve damage during surgery may cause permanent vocal impairment, such as hoarseness. Difficulty swallowing and throat discomfort are usually present for several days and are usually due to local irritation from the endotracheal tube. A soft diet, throat lozenges, a viscous lidocaine (Xylocaine) solution, humidified air, minimal talking, and other comfort measures lessen the discomfort. If a spinal fusion was performed with the anterior cervical discectomy, the surgeon is notified if radicular pain suddenly recurs. This could mean that the bone graft has moved out of place and surgery needs to be repeated. Also assess the client for indications of postoperative improvement such as absence of paresthesias. Document these findings. Tell the client that it is not unusual for preoperative manifestations to persist for a few days secondary to edema at the operative site, although these manifestations are usually less uncomfortable.

Following surgery on the cervical spine, watch for indications of respiratory paralysis resulting from cord edema. Emergency tracheostomy equipment is kept at hand. Postoperatively, flexion of the neck is prevented by use of a collar.

A wound drain may be present and is usually removed by the surgeon on the second postoperative day, after drainage has decreased. Bladder and bowel management are the same as for clients after lumbar surgery. Cervical surgery may affect the parasympathetic chain, causing urinary retention. A hard cervical collar is usually prescribed following fusion. The Client Education Guide lists other suggestions for home care after a cervical laminectomy or fusion.

With shorter postoperative hospital stays, most clients are discharged prior to suture or staple removal. Instruction for care of the incision includes keeping the sutures or staples clean and dry and noting any increased redness or drainage from the wound. Clients need clear instructions on walking, lifting, driving, and returning to work. Most clients can resume activity 6 weeks after surgery. Specific physician instructions need to be followed.

Prolonged sitting or standing in one position strains the healing back. Contraindicated activities vary. The client is instructed to ask the surgeon when it will be safe to perform activities that could damage the back, for example, climbing stairs, lifting a weight greater than 5 lb, prolonged travel, sexual activity, sports, exercise, and driving a car. Clients must not smoke. Smoking reduces blood supply to the tissues and delays healing.

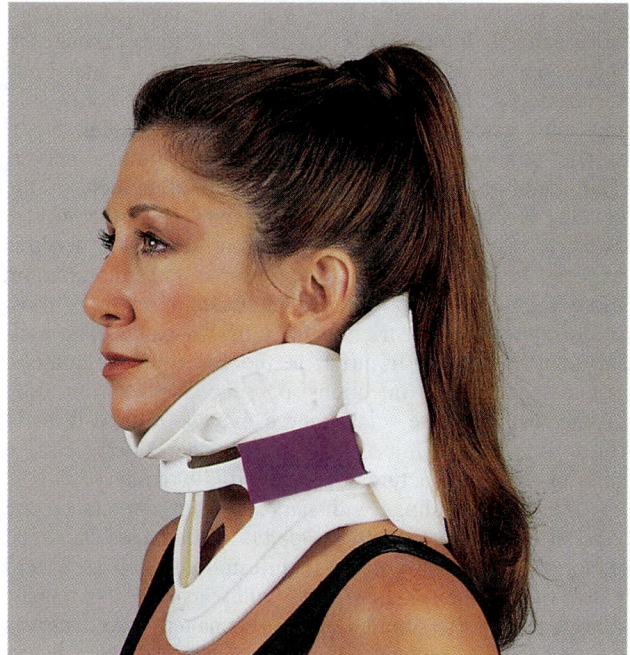

Figure 35–17. A cervical collar with a chin piece. This orthosis provides additional support for the head and some restriction of cervical spine motion. (Courtesy of Zimmer, Inc., Dover, Ohio.)

Lower Motor Neuron Lesions

Recall that lower motor neurons (LMNs) consist of the anterior horn cells located in the anterior gray matter of

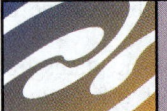

CLIENT EDUCATION GUIDE

Home Care After Cervical Laminectomy or Fusion

Wear the collar at all times for up to 6 weeks or until your physician gives you permission to stop.

You may wash under the collar with mild soap.

If the collar is hard and needs cleaning, you should lie flat, remove the front of the collar and wash the front first, using the back of the collar for neck support. Then replace the front of the collar and turn onto a pillow for support. Open one side of the collar and wash the back of your neck; then repeat on the other side.

If the collar itches, a small silk scarf between the neck and the collar may provide some comfort.

If a soft collar is prescribed, stockinettes made of soft fiber that fit over the collar can be purchased. Purchase two stockinettes, so when one is soiled, it can be removed, laundered, and replaced when dry.

Riding in a car is permissible, but driving is not allowed until your physician has given you permission.

---

the spinal cord. They are also located in the motor cranial nuclei of the brain stem. Each anterior horn cell has a long axon that leaves the cord via the anterior spinal root and extends out the peripheral nerve, eventually synapsing at the motor endplate of a neuromuscular junction. These structures form a motor unit that controls skeletal muscle activity, both voluntary and reflex activity. They are the last cells to carry information from the nervous system out to the muscles.

When a lesion develops in these structures, the client develops flaccid muscle weakness or paralysis, loss of reflexes, loss of muscle tone, and atrophy of the involved muscles. The degree to which these clinical manifestations develop depend on the extent of the lesion. Each anterior horn cell innervates several separate muscle fibers, and because several anterior horn cells exist at each spinal level, a lesion confined to one spinal segment may not damage all of the anterior horn cells innervating an entire muscle. This type of lesion would cause muscle weakness rather than paralysis. Paralysis occurs when a lesion involves the column or anterior horn cells in several spinal segments. If all the peripheral motor nerves are involved, the entire muscle becomes flaccid. The muscles atrophy early due to lack of innervation. LMN lesions are often associated with spinal cord injury or tumors and surgery on the aorta, which alters blood flow to the spinal cord.

Upper Motor Neuron Lesions

Because the LMNs send instructions for the muscles to contract, it follows that certain pathways in the CNS

influence the activity of the LMNs that facilitates and inhibits muscle contractions. Several known pathways that arise from the higher brain centers influence the activity of the LMNs. These pathways constitute the upper motor neurons (UMNs). The UMNs originate in the motor strip of the cerebral cortex and in multiple brain stem nuclei. From the cortex, these axons pass through the internal capsule; most of them cross over in the medulla and descend in the spinal cord through the corticospinal tracts. A few do not cross in the brain but cross later in the spinal cord.

The corticospinal tracts are primarily responsible for precise, fine, voluntary motor movements. However, they also assist in modulating muscle tone and reflexes to some degree. Any lesion that destroys the UMNs will result in contralateral paralysis, such as is seen with cerebrovascular accident (stroke). Initially, the involved area is flaccid and hyporeflexic. The flaccidity gradually recedes, and the reflex arc becomes hyperactive due to the lack of inhibition by the UMNs. Muscle tone is hypertonic and the extremity becomes spastic. Despite the spasms, the muscle becomes atrophied from disuse. The atrophy seen with UMN lesions occurs later than that seen with LMN problems. The Babinski reflex is present.

Disorders of the Peripheral Nerves

Peripheral nerves can be injured in many ways—from bone fractures, stretching of the nerves, infections, vascular or metabolic disturbances, constriction by fascial bands, pressure from tumors, trauma associated with perforating wounds, injection of drugs, and exposure to chemicals or toxins. Neuritis is nerve damage from any cause. Mononeuritis is injury to a single nerve as a result of localized injury. Polyneuritis is diffuse damage to many nerves as a result of toxic agents or metabolic disturbances. The peripheral nerves most commonly subjected to external pressure are the median, radial, ulnar, sciatic, common peroneal, tibial, and long thoracic nerves. The common peroneal nerve (a terminal branch of the sciatic) is injured more frequently than any other nerve. Because of its course and distribution, the sciatic nerve is exposed to internal and external trauma and inflammation more than any other nerve. The median nerve is most often injured by constriction from fascial bands. The axillary nerve may be injured as the result of an allergic reaction to serum injections or secondary to improper crutch walking. The sciatic nerve may be injured directly during medication injections. Any peripheral nerve can be injured by bone fractures or perforating wounds.

Assessment findings with nerve damage depend on the type of nerve injured and the extent of damage. Damaged motor nerves cause clinical manifestations such as flaccid paralysis, muscle wasting, and reflex loss in the muscle innervated by the injured nerve. Damaged mixed nerves or sensory nerves cause vasomotor and trophic disturbances following either partial or complete interruption of the nerve. Following partial injury or incomplete division of a nerve, the person may experience stabbing pains, paresthesias (pins-and-needles sensation), and occasionally the burning pains of causalgia. Damaged sensory nerves cause loss of sensation in the nerves' area of anatomic distribution.

Peripheral Neuropathies

Carpal Tunnel Syndrome

Carpal tunnel syndrome (CTS) is an entrapment neuropathy that occurs when the median nerve is compressed as it passes through the wrist along a pathway to the hand. The tunnel is called the carpal tunnel. The tunnel is bordered by the flexor retinaculum which is a band of fibrous tissue that prevents the wrist tendons from bowing when the wrist is flexed. Compression causes sensory and motor changes in the thumb, index and middle finger, and radial aspect of the ring finger (Fig. 35–18). CTS also leads to atrophy of the radial half of the thenar eminence. CTS may develop spontaneously without a known cause or may result from disease or injury. The most commonly reported cause of CTS is repetitive motion of the wrist, with the wrist in constant flexion. A higher incidence of CTS is reported among homemakers, factory workers, bricklayers, cashiers, musicians, secretaries, and computer operators. Pregnancy, hypothyroidism, gout, and rheumatoid arthritis are other conditions associated with CTS.

Initially, the person may be awakened at night by pain and paresthesia. Although these initial manifestations are temporary and relieved by shaking the hand, later stages may be accompanied by motor changes.

Assessment of the client begins with a thorough history, including occupational tasks. Diagnostic assessment for CTS includes assessing for Tinel's and Phalen's signs (Fig. 35–18A and B). Tinel's sign is the development of tingling in the hands and fingers when the wrist is tapped.

Phalen's test is assessing for the development of numbness and tingling following forceful flexion of the wrists for 20 to 30 seconds (see Fig. 35–18B). Finally, the wrist compression test is done. The wrist compression test is manual application of 30 seconds of pressure over the flexor retinaculum (Fig. 35–18C). If paresthesias develop after compression, the test is positive. The wrist compression test has been demonstrated to be 87% accurate in diagnosing CTS. Electromyography procedures may also be used in differential diagnosis to rule out other possible causes.

Initially the wrist is splinted in a neutral position to prevent mechanical irritation of the nerve. Injection of steroids into the flexor tendons is done less frequently now because of reported problems with scarring, median nerve damage, and infection. In addition to rest, pyridoxine hydrochloride (vitamin B_6) has been reported to be helpful.

Surgery is indicated with (1) severe manifestations of long duration, (2) muscle atrophy, or (3) progressive sensory loss in the fingers and hand. Regional anesthesia is used prior to carpal tunnel release (decompression of the median nerve by transecting the transverse carpal ligament).

Following surgery, blood flow is assessed hourly by checking the color, capillary refill, and warmth of the finger tips. When the anesthetic has worn off, assess the fingers for sensation.

Initially, postoperative care centers on wrist immobilization using bulky dressings and a wrist splint. The arm is elevated on pillows to reduce edema. Encourage the client to try to move the fingers, even though they are splinted.

The client and family are the care providers beyond the immediate postoperative period. Since this surgery is usually performed on an outpatient basis, provide detailed

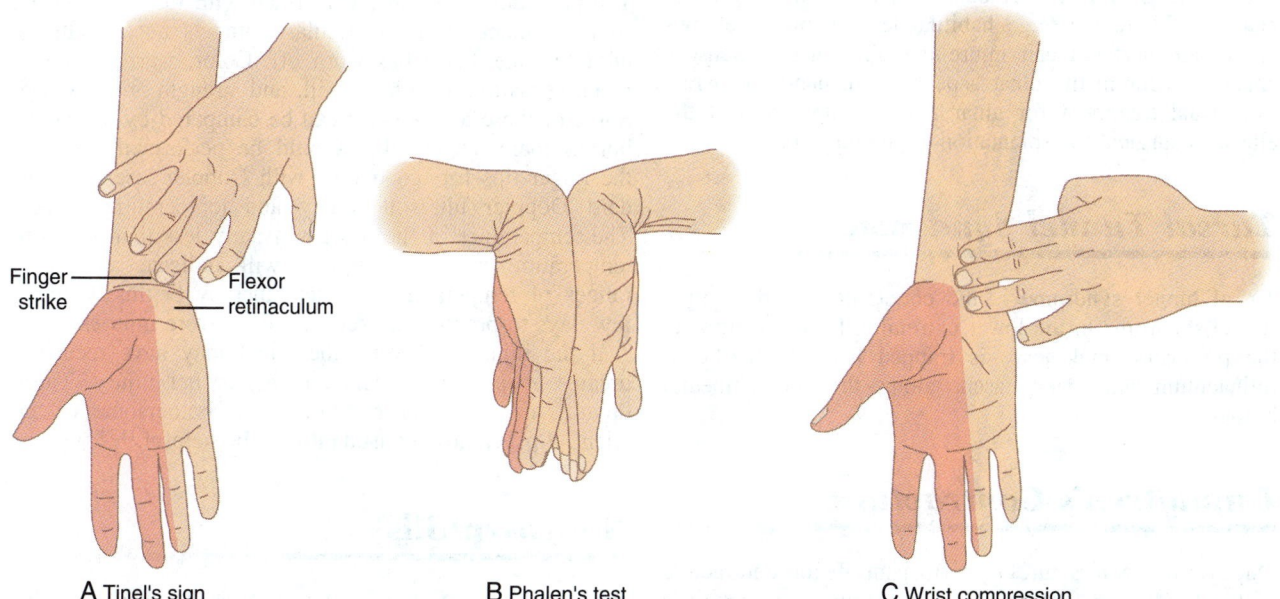

A Tinel's sign   B Phalen's test   C Wrist compression

Figure 35–18. Clinical examination for carpal tunnel syndrome includes tests for (A) Tinel's sign, (B) Phalen's sign, and (C) wrist compression. Each of these maneuvers will elicit numbness and pain in the thumb, index and middle fingers, and the radial aspect of the ring finger if carpal tunnel syndrome is present.

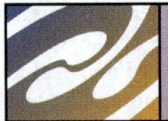

CLIENT EDUCATION GUIDE

Home Care After Carpal Tunnel Release

Check the circulation in your hand; notify the physician if any of the following occur: increased swelling that results in the hand or fingers becoming pale, tingly, or cold, or rings being too tight to remove, or if any of these symptoms or signs occur even without swelling.

Keep the affected wrist elevated as much as possible, using the splint to immobilize the wrist area.

Flex and extend your fingers hourly during waking hours.

Observe for signs of infection: odorous dressing, fever, or increased pain at the incisional site.

Use analgesia as directed for pain relief.

Restrict lifting for 2 months.

Wear a splint for 7 to 14 days after surgery or until the sutures are removed.

Avoid getting the incision site wet until after the sutures are removed.

---

instructions on home care. The Client Education Guide lists suggestions for home care after carpal tunnel release.

Ulnar Nerve Syndrome

Lying within a bony groove at the elbow, the ulnar nerve is susceptible to compression from direct trauma to the elbow (e.g., hitting the funny bone) or from changes within the groove that gradually squeeze the nerve. Repeated mild trauma (e.g., habitual leaning of the elbows on a hard surface) can injure the ulnar nerve. Sensory changes occur in the ulnar aspect of the hand and wrist. The usual treatment for ulnar nerve compression at the elbow is surgical transplantation of the ulnar nerve.

Tarsal Tunnel Syndrome

Tarsal tunnel syndrome is the counterpart of the carpal tunnel syndrome in the lower extremity. In this syndrome, the posterior tibial nerve is trapped beneath the flexor retinaculum and deep fascia along the foot's medial border.

Dupuytren's Contracture

Dupuytren's contracture is permanent flexor contracture of the fourth and fifth fingers. Dupuytren's contracture is inherited as an autosomal dominant trait and is common in people of Northern European descent. It is also more common in alcoholics and diabetics.

In severe forms of contracture, a longitudinal fibrous cord forms, which extends from the fingers to the palm and pulls the fingers into a locked position. Milder forms have less contracture and fewer nodules in the palmar fascia.

Ten years or more may pass before surgery is necessary. The decision to operate is usually made when the client can no longer lay the hand outstretched on a table. The operation consists of excision of part of the palmar fascia. After surgery the hand is dressed in a large compression dressing. ROM is encouraged. Frequent assessments of capillary refill and finger color are needed. Splints are often used at night to promote extension. Many months of physical therapy may be needed, and even then, full function may not be achievable.

Peripheral Nerve Injuries

Nerves can be injured in common household accidents (cut on glass) or in severe motor vehicle accidents. Assessment includes full examination of the hand, a discussion of the client's occupation, and documentation of the dominant hand.

Conservative management may include splinting, ice, elevation of the limb, or administration of anti-inflammatory and analgesic agents, or a combination of these. If a peripheral nerve is traumatically severed, the ends should be surgically anastomosed to enable healing. The nearer the site of injury occurs to the CNS, the less chance of regeneration. When nerves are only slightly damaged, mild edema occurs at the injury site. This may cause temporary manifestations that recede in a few days or possibly weeks.

Postoperative care of clients having nerve repair or grafting includes elevation of the extremity. Elevation is critical to reducing edema and improving venous return. The procedure is usually performed with local anesthesia, so assessment of neurovascular status is not conclusive until the anesthesia has worn off. Color, warmth, movement, sensation, capillary refill, and strength are assessed. Some of these assessments can be hampered by dressings, but as many as possible should be performed. Monitor the finger tips for blood flow with Doppler laser or standard Doppler ultrasonography and temperature probes. The temperature of the hand is usually less than the core temperature and the surgeon will indicate acceptable ranges of temperature. Physical therapy begins within a few days to promote movement after severe injuries.

If the injury is severe, the client may have recurring dreams about the accident and his or her injury. These dreams are generally normal, but if bothersome to the client, a psychiatric consultant may be helpful.[11,24]

Neurosyphilis

Neurosyphilis is a chronic or late stage of syphilis involving infection of the brain and/or spinal cord. The oculomotor nerves may be affected, leading to an inability of the pupil to react to light, called an Argyll Robertson pupil. The posterior columns and nerve roots of the spinal cord may be affected, which is called *tabes dorsalis*. Because these are sensory nerves, the most common manifestation is pain. The pain can occur almost anywhere in the body, although abdominal pain is most common. The pain is severe enough to be confused with gastric ulcers and gallbladder disease. In addition to pain, areas of paresthesias may be noted. A common finding in tabes dorsalis is the loss of position sense in the feet and legs. As a result, clients walk with a slapping step. They are at increased risk of falls when walking in the dark because they must rely on visual cues for placement of their feet with each step. In addition, since the gait is abnormal, bone alignment with walking is altered. Eventually the foot is abnormally shaped (called *Charcot's joint*). This alteration in foot structure can lead to foot ulcerations, because the client bears the body weight on abnormal areas. The brain can also be involved in later stages of syphilis. A general deterioration of mental status can develop.

With improved case finding and the use of penicillin to treat syphilis in its early stages, the management of syphilis is improving. However, with development of resistant strains of organisms and a recent rise in the incidence of sexually transmitted diseases, problems may recur in the future.

Peripheral Nerve Tumors

Although solitary tumors (generally neurofibromas) may develop on any peripheral nerve, multiple tumors most often occur and are part of a syndrome known as neurofibromatosis (von Recklinghausen's disease). This hereditary disorder is characterized by multiple tumors of the spinal and cranial nerves along with involvement of many other systems. The disease is usually not life-threatening, and lesions are excised only when they interfere with normal activity. Intracranial and intraspinal tumors are usually removed.

Surgery for peripheral nerve tumors is often done on an outpatient basis. In the recovery room, the dressings are checked for drainage; circulation, motion, and sensation in the extremity are also assessed. Clients are encouraged to perform ROM exercises. Clients and family members are taught the signs of circulatory compromise and infection, medication management, and care of the dressing and incision.

Disorders of the Cranial Nerves

Cranial nerves can be affected in many ways by various nervous system disorders. For example, they may be secondarily affected by compression resulting from increased intracranial pressure or they may be directly damaged as a result of head injuries. In this section, only the two most common disorders specific to the cranial nerves, not those associated with other disorders, are discussed. Regeneration of the first (olfactory) or second (optic) cranial nerve does not occur, because these nerves are actually part of the CNS.

Trigeminal Neuralgia

Chronic irritation of the fifth cranial nerve results in trigeminal neuralgia. Approximately 15,000 cases are diagnosed each year in the United States. Although most commonly occurring in 50- to 70-year-old persons, trigeminal neuralgia can occur in adults of any age. Approximately 60% of clients are female. The trigeminal nerve has three divisions: the ophthalmic, maxillary, and mandibular (Fig. 35–19). Trigeminal neuralgia may occur in any one or more of these divisions.

Causes of trigeminal neuralgia can be divided into intrinsic and extrinsic lesions within the nerve itself, such as gross abnormalities of the axon or myelin, as may occur with multiple sclerosis. Extrinsic lesions are outside the trigeminal root and include mechanical compression by tumors, vascular anomalies, dental abscesses, or jaw malformation.

Trigeminal neuralgia is characterized by intermittent episodes of intense pain of sudden onset. The pain is rarely relieved by analgesics. Tactile stimulation, such as touch and facial hygiene, and even talking, may trigger an attack. Trigeminal neuralgia is more prevalent in the maxillary and mandibular distributions and on the right side of the face. Bilateral trigeminal neuralgia is rare but does occur. The pain from trigeminal neuralgia can become so intense that the client ponders suicide.

None of the current diagnostic studies identify trigeminal neuralgia. A CT scan, MRI, and angiography can identify a causative lesion. The actual diagnosis is made on the basis of an in-depth history with attention paid to triggering stimuli and the nature and site of the pain.

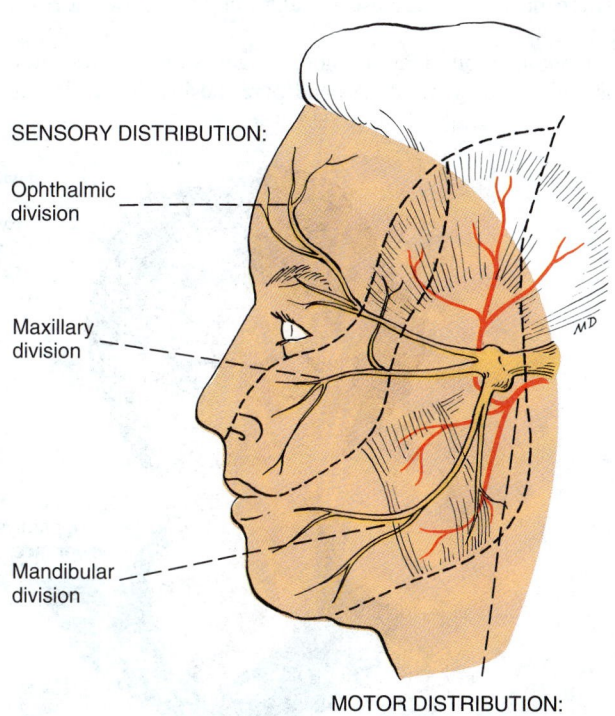

SENSORY DISTRIBUTION:

Ophthalmic division

Maxillary division

Mandibular division

MOTOR DISTRIBUTION:
to muscles of mastication

Figure 35–19. Distribution of the trigeminal nerve.

A careful history is obtained from the client regarding stimuli that trigger an attack. This information is used to plan care so as to minimize triggering events. The client's dental hygiene and nutritional intake are evaluated. These clients often do not eat enough to meet their daily nutritional needs and neglect their teeth because of the pain.

The nurse helps clients use and improve any pain control strategies they have developed. Clients with trigeminal neuralgia need emotional support to help them deal with pain that has often been present for a long time.

Anticonvulsants such as carbamazepine (Tegretol) and phenytoin (Dilantin) are often prescribed as the initial treatment of trigeminal neuralgia. These drugs may dampen the reactivity of the neurons within the trigeminal nerve. For some clients, these medications are all the treatment that is ever needed. Liver impairment may result from administration of both carbamazepine and phenytoin. Liver enzymes must be monitored before and during therapy. These medications should be used cautiously in clients with a history of alcohol abuse. Baclofen (Lioresal) is an antispasmodic that may be used alone or in conjunction with anticonvulsants. Narcotics are not particularly effective in relieving trigeminal neuralgia pain.

Surgery includes nerve blocks with alcohol and glycerol, peripheral neurectomy, and percutaneous radiofrequency wave forms which create lesions that alter pain transmission. The relief obtained with these procedures is not always permanent. Complications include development of facial paresthesias and muscular weakness. These procedures, being less invasive, are often better tolerated by elderly or debilitated clients.

The more invasive techniques involve major surgical procedures. Microvascular decompression involves removing the vessel from the posterior trigeminal root. A rhizotomy is the actual resection of the root of the nerve. These procedures require a craniotomy to allow access to the nerve.

Complications include those of any surgical procedure, as well as facial weakness and paresthesias. If facial anesthesia is present following surgery, clients must learn to test the temperature of food before putting it into their mouth. They should chew on the unaffected side and inspect mucous membranes for irritation. Assess for aspiration and advance the diet slowly. Teach clients to use a water jet device instead of a toothbrush for dental hygiene and advise them to visit the dentist as soon as possible after surgery.

If the corneal reflex has been impaired, the client will need to be taught eye care. During the acute postoperative period, apply eye drops and a protective shield. The client assumes these tasks with supervision and then independently.

Bell's Palsy

Bell's palsy affects the motor aspects of the facial nerve, the seventh cranial nerve (Fig. 35–20). Bell's palsy is the most common type of peripheral facial paralysis. It affects both women and men in all age groups. However, it is most common between ages 20 and 40.

Bell's palsy results in a unilateral paralysis of the facial muscles of expression. There is no evidence of a pathologic cause. Facial paralysis may be central or peripheral in origin. Central facial palsy is an upper motor neuron paralysis or paresis. Sometimes it produces dissociation of motor function. In this situation, the client cannot voluntarily show his or her teeth on the paralyzed side, but can show them with emotional stimulation such as that causing smiles or laughter. This phenomenon is called voluntary emotional dissociation.

Typical assessment findings on the affected side include (1) upward movement of the eyeball on closing the eye (Bell's phenomenon), (2) drooping of the mouth, (3) flattening of the nasolabial fold, (4) widening of the palpebral fissure, and (5) a slight lag in closing the eye. Eating may be difficult.

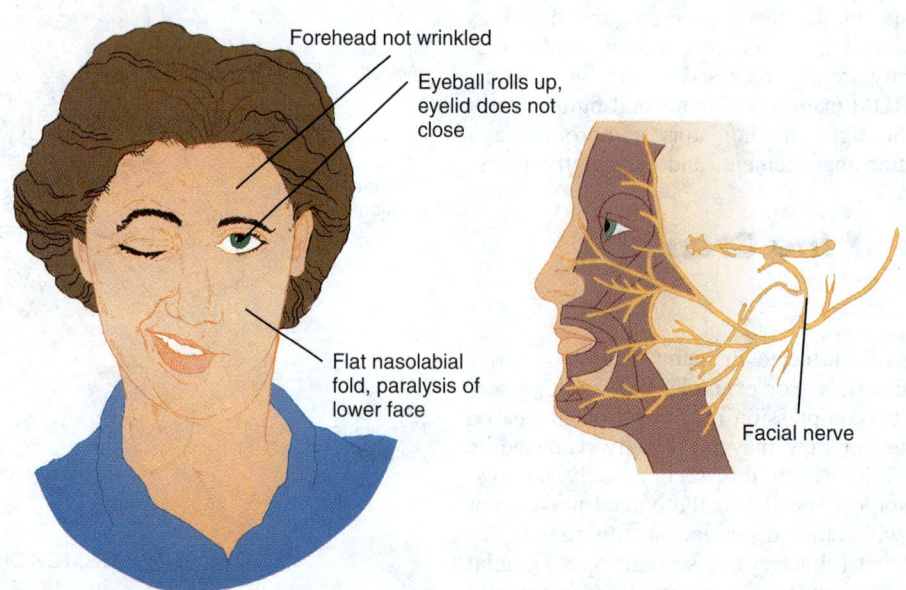

Forehead not wrinkled

Eyeball rolls up, eyelid does not close

Flat nasolabial fold, paralysis of lower face

Facial nerve

Figure 35–20. Bell's palsy.

There is no known cure for Bell's palsy. Palliative measures include the following:

- Analgesics if discomfort occurs from herpetic lesions
- Corticosteroids to decrease nerve tissue edema
- Physiotherapy, moist heat, gentle massage, stimulation of the facial nerve with faradic current
- Corneal protection with an artificial tears solution, sunglasses, an eye patch at night, and periodic gentle closure of the eye

Clients experiencing Bell's palsy often think they have had a stroke. Reassure the client that this is not the case. Most clients recover from Bell's palsy within a few weeks without residual manifestations. If permanent complete facial paralysis occurs, surgery may be necessary. Anastomosis of the peripheral end of the facial nerve with the spinal accessory or hypoglossal nerve allows closure of the eye during sleep and restores tone to the facial musculature.

Conclusions

Disorders of the spinal cord and peripheral nervous system range from life-threatening SCIs to temporary peripheral nerve compressions. The physical and psychological impairments vary with the degree of damage as well as the client's response and ability to cope with the body changes. The coping response is not always related to the degree of physiologic damage. A client can have facial paralysis or trigeminal neuralgia and be more compromised psychologically than a client with SCI who has strong coping skills. It is imperative that nurses comprehend the severity of the client's dysfunction as it relates to quality of life, as well as the impact it has on family dynamics.

Thinking Critically

1. A 23-year-old man was admitted from the emergency department (ED) following a car accident in which he sustained a concussion and thoracic injuries with thoracic cord involvement. The client's baseline data included loss of consciousness for 15 minutes, headache, nausea, and inability to move or feel any sensation from his thorax down. One hour after receiving this man in the intensive care unit (ICU), additional assessment changes included inability to move fingers and hands and flex or extend the arms. Shoulder movement was still intact. He was fully conscious and his vital signs were stable. What critical interventions initiated in the ED need to be continued in the ICU? What do these changes in data indicate? What nursing interventions are appropriate both initially and as precautions?

Factors to Consider. What are the implications when a high thoracic injury occurs? What changes indicate ascending cord dysfunction?

2. A 22-year-old man was admitted 4 hours after sustaining a C6 spinal cord compression injury. No neurologic deficits were found, but his blood alcohol level was very high on admission. Initially, he kept falling asleep after you completed your assessments. Gardner-Wells tongs with 10 lb of traction were placed. Now that the client is more awake, he has begun thrashing his arms and attempting to roll over in bed. What are the priorities for his care? What nursing interventions should be used?

Factors to Consider. What is the purpose of the Gardner-Wells tongs? How would edema and microscopic bleeding compromise his recovery?

3. The client, a 34-year-old woman, had a lumbar laminectomy done earlier today. An earlier assessment showed that movement and sensation of both lower extremities were intact. During the current postoperative assessment she stated that her right toes felt numb, and the dorsiflexion and plantar flexion of the right foot are a little weaker than earlier. She has requested an analgesic because she is starting to get a headache. What are the priorities for her care? What assessments and interventions might be used?

Factors to Consider. What assessment methods can be used to determine the extent of vascular insufficiency? What type of neurologic checks should be done?

Bibliography

1. Agency for Health Care Policy and Research (AHCPR). (1994). *Acute low back problems in adults: Assessment and treatment.* No. 95-0642. Rockville, MD: U.S. Department of Health and Human Services: Public Health Service, Agency for Health Care Policy and Research.
2. American Spinal Injury Association (ASIA). (1992). Standards for neurological and functional classification of spinal cord injury.
3. Berard, E. J. (1989). The sexuality of spinal cord injured women: Physiology and pathophysiology. A review. *Paraplegia, 27*(2), 99.
4. Berard, E. J., et al. (1989). Effects of bethanechol and adrenoblockers on thermoregulation in spinal cord injury. *Paraplegia, 27*(1), 46.
5. Beretta, G., et al. (1989). Reproductive aspects in spinal cord injured males. *Paraplegia, 27*(2), 113–118.
6. Bodner, D. R., et al. (1989). The effect of verapamil on the treatment of detrusor hyperreflexia in the spinal cord injured population. *Paraplegia, 27*(5), 364.
7. Bracken, M. B., et al. (1990). A randomized trial of methyl prednisolone or naloxone in the treatment of acute spinal cord injury. *New England Journal of Medicine, 322*(20), 1405–1411.
8. Brown, C. W., et al. (1986). The rate of pseudoarthrosis in patients who are smokers and patients who are nonsmokers: A comparison study. *Spine, 11*(9), 942–943.
9. Brown, M. D. (1991). Perioperative care in lumbar spine surgery. *Orthopedic Clinics of North America, 22,* 355–370.
10. Clark, J. C., et al. (1992). Conditions associated with carpal tunnel syndrome. *Mayo Clinic Proceedings, 67,* 541–548.
11. Clemens, S., & Foss-Campbell, B. (1993). Rehabilitation following traumatic hand injury: Hand therapist's perspective. *Plastic Surgical Nursing, 13*(3), 129–139.
12. Curry, K., & Casady, L. (1992). The relationship between extended periods of immobility and decubitus ulcer formation in the acutely spinal cord-injured individual. *Journal of Neuroscience Nursing, 24,* 185–189.

13. Davis, B., Handy, C. (1996). Cellulitis: An unreported complication of long-term SCI patients. *SCI Nursing 13*(2), 35–38.
14. Ditunno, J. F., & Formal, C. S. (1994). Chronic spinal cord injury. *New England Journal of Medicine, 330*(8), 550–556.
15. Dunnum, L. (1989). Life satisfaction and spinal cord injury: The patient perspective. *Journal of Neuroscience Nursing, 21*(6), 43.
16. Frank, R. G., & Elliott, T. R. (1989). Spinal cord injury and health locus of control beliefs. *Paraplegia, 27*(4), 250–256.
17. Gaehle, K. E., et al. (1992). Thoracolumbar burst fractures. *AORN Journal, 55*(3), 721–731.
18. Geary, S. (1996). Nursing management of cranial nerve dysfunction. *Journal of Neuroscience Nursing, 27*(2), 102–108.
19. Gianino, J. (1993). Intrathecal baclofen for spinal spasticity: Implications for nursing practice. *Journal of Neuroscience Nursing, 25*(4), 254–264.
20. Hirschfeld, A., & Young, W. (1991). Trends in spinal cord injury research. In J. D. Anderson & E. Frost (Eds.), *Spinal cord injuries* (pp. 199–225). London: Butterworths.
21. Huang, C., et al. (1990). Anemia in acute phase of spinal cord injury. *Archives of Physical Medicine and Rehabilitation, 71,* 3.
22. Kawamura, J., et al. (1989). The clinical features of spasms in patients with a cervical cord injury. *Paraplegia, 27*(3), 222.
23. Little, J. W., et al. (1989). Lower extremity manifestations of spasticity in chronic spinal cord injury. *American Journal of Physical Medicine and Rehabilitation, 68*(1), 32.
24. Maksud, D. (1993). Psychological adjustments to hand injuries: Nursing management. *Plastic Surgical Nursing, 13*(4), 72–76.
25. Maldonado, A. (1995). Comprehensive assessment of common musculoskeletal disorders. *Journal of Nurse-Midwifery, 40*(2), 202–214.
26. Marshall, S. B., et al. (1990). *Neuroscience critical care: Pathophysiology and patient management.* Philadelphia: W. B. Saunders.
27. McConaghy, D. J. (1994). Trigeminal neuralgia: A personal review and nursing implications. *Journal of Neuroscience Nursing, 26*(2), 85–89.
28. Midwest Regional Spinal Cord Injury Care System. (1992). *Annual progress report.* Chicago: Northwestern University.
29. Nayduch, D., Lee, A., & Butler, D. (1994). High-dose methylprednisolone after acute spinal cord injury. *Critical Care Nurse, 14*(4), 69–78.
30. Neatherlin, J. S., & Brillhart, B. (1996). Body image in preoperative and postoperative lumbar laminectomy patients. *Journal of Neuroscience Nursing, 27*(1), 43–46.
31. Patterson, D. R., et al. (1993). When life support is questioned early in the care of patients with cervical-level quadriplegia. *New England Journal of Medicine, 328*(7), 506–509.
32. Presksto, D. (1992). The Kaneda device: A new anterior spine stabilization system. *AORN Journal, 55*(3), 734–746.
33. Richmond, T., Metcalf, J., & Daly, M. (1995). Requirements for nursing care services and associated costs in acute spinal cord injury. *Journal of Neuroscience Nursing, 27*(1), 47–52.
34. Rivara, F., et al. (1988). The public cost of motorcycle trauma. *JAMA, 260*(2), 221–223.
35. Rose, D. D., et al. (1993). Cervical spine injury. *AORN Journal, 57*(4), 830–850.
36. Schultz, D. L. (1995). Role of the neuroscience nurse in lumbar fusion. *Journal of Neuroscience Nursing, 27*(2), 90–95.
37. Segatore, M. (1994). Understanding chronic pain after spinal cord injury. *Journal of Neuroscience Nursing, 26*(4), 230–235.
38. Shaddinger, D. E. (1996). An acute spinal cord injury: My family's perspective. *Journal of Neuroscience Nursing, 27*(4), 236–239.
39. Spica, M. M. (1989). Sexual counseling standards for the spinal cord–injured. *Journal of Neuroscience Nursing, 21*(1), 56.
40. Youmans, J. R. (1990). *Neurological surgery* (3rd ed.). Philadelphia: W. B. Saunders.

Eye and Ear Disorders

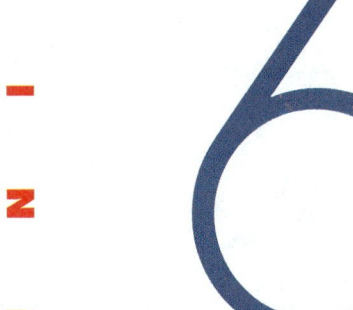

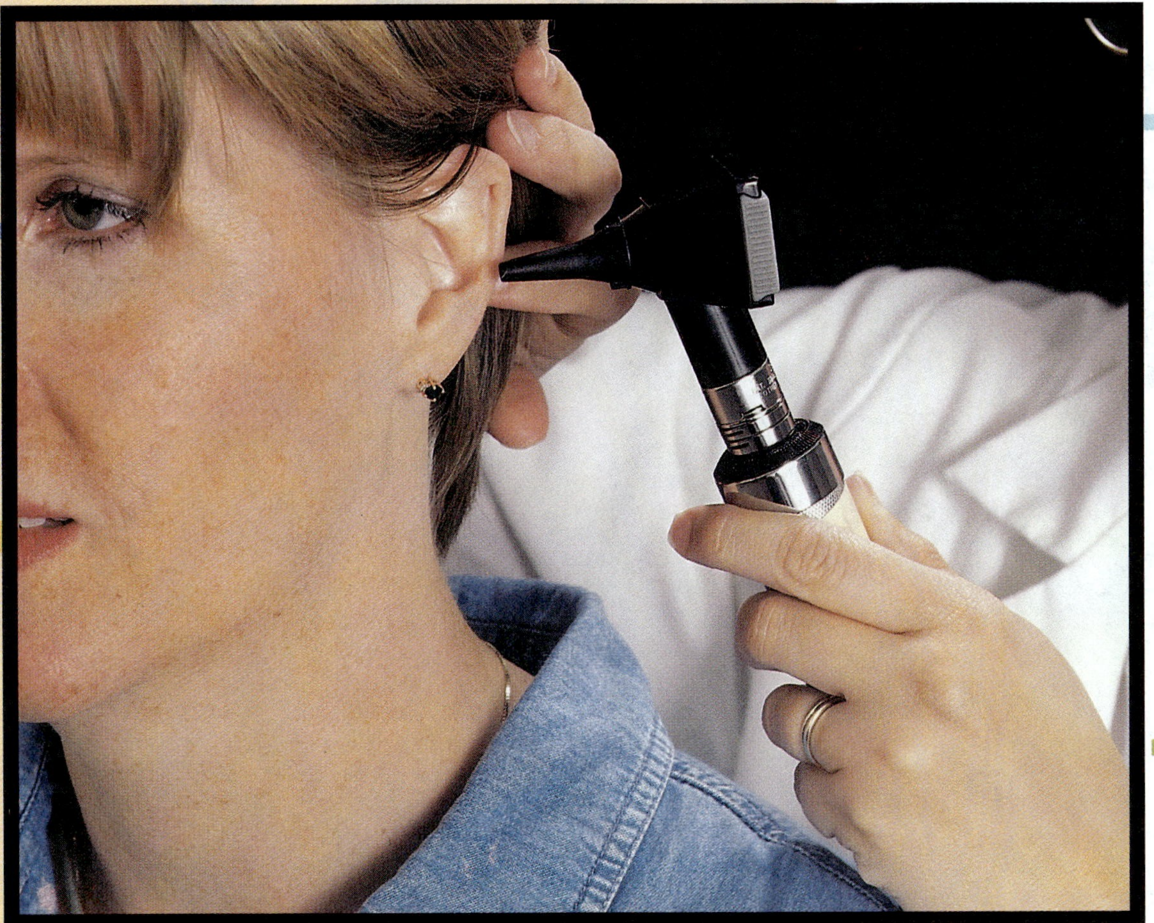

Eye Disorders

Linda A. Vader

The role that vision plays in our lives is difficult to define because it is so deeply personal and intimate. It is the connection between the mind and the body and the rest of the world. The visual pathway is a multidimensional system with many structures and processes subject to trauma or disorders. When there is a failure of any part along the visual pathway, the result is loss of vision.

Loss of vision is closely associated with the loss of independence. Even simple tasks become difficult to perform without assistance. Seeing what food is being served at the table, selecting clothes for color and design, avoiding objects while walking, and reading books, magazines, or personal mail are no longer possible. The visually impaired person must adapt to this loss in order to maintain control in the daily affairs of life.

The nursing diagnosis *Sensory/Perceptual Alterations* is commonly identified for clients with visual problems or impairment. Nursing interventions focus on providing a safe environment and education for self-care. The most important assessment you can make, however, should address your client's grieving process. Visual impairment is more than a physiologic deficit. It is a loss that has physical, emotional, and spiritual effects on the person afflicted. Even minor changes in vision can provoke feelings of anger and frustration in persons who must rely on clear and sharp vision in their work (e.g., airline pilots, artists, photographers, architects). Permanent and profound loss of vision can result in morbid grieving, where an individual is unable to cope with or adapt to life changes.

Surveys have shown that most people are more afraid of going blind than dying of cancer. Although we have made some improvements in the way our society views and provides for people who are physically challenged, blind people are frequently regarded with pity. Loss of vision is a threat to a person's independence, self-esteem, and self-control.

Structure and Function of the Eye

Structure of the Eye

The visual system is a complex group of structures that includes the eyeballs, muscles, nerves, fat, and bones. Although the eyes are intricate receptacles for light that adapt to varying conditions such as light intensity and object distance, the eyes do not actually see. The eyes are the external portion of the visual pathway to the brain. The pathway transmits and ultimately converts electrical impulses into vision. The eyes are often referred to as eyeballs or globes. They are not true spheres, however, but are actually a combination of two spheres with different curvatures.

Structure of the Ocular Adnexa

The ocular adnexa (Fig. 36–1) are the accessory structures of the eye (muscles, fat, and bone) that support and protect it. Bony orbits and pads of fat surround each eye.

Bony Orbit. The bony orbit, or eye socket, surrounds and protects most of the eye so that only a small portion is visible. The orbit is formed from portions of the frontal, lacrimal, ethmoid, maxilla, zygoma, sphenoid, and palatine bones. These bones are thin and fragile and break easily when pressure is applied to the eye (as in a fistfight). In addition to bone, the orbit contains fat, various connective tissues, blood vessels, and nerves.

Ocular Muscles. The eyeball is moved by six ocular muscles, which are attached to the surface of the globe (Fig. 36–2). The four rectus muscles (the medial, lateral,

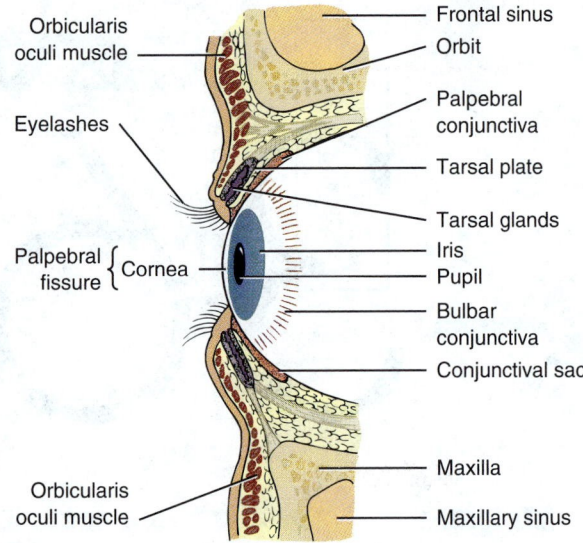

Figure 36–1. The ocular adnexa.

superior, and inferior) move the eyes horizontally and vertically. The two oblique muscles (superior and inferior) primarily rotate the eye in circular movements to allow vision at all angles. The eye moves through six cardinal gazes, which are discussed later.

Eyelids. The eyelids (upper and lower) are elastic folds of skin that close to protect the anterior eyeball. When they close, the eyelids also distribute the tear film, which prevents evaporation and drying of the surface epithelium.

The elliptic space between the two open lids is the palpebral fissure. The corners of the fissure are called the canthi. The medial, or inner, canthus is next to the nose, and the lateral, or outer, canthus is the outside corner (Fig. 36–3). Oil-secreting glands called meibomian glands are embedded in both upper and lower lids.

Lacrimal Apparatus. The lacrimal gland is in the upper lid over the outer canthus and produces tears that reach the eyeball through secretory ducts. Tiny openings called puncti in both the upper and lower lids at the inner canthus direct tears to the lacrimal sac. The nasolacrimal duct directs the flow of tears into the nose (see Fig. 36–3). The tear film is composed of lipids secreted by the meibomian glands, and dissolved salts, glucose, urea, protein, and lysozyme secreted by the lacrimal glands. Along with mucus secreted by goblet cells located in the lids, the tear film lubricates, cleans, and protects the ocular surface.

Structure of the Internal Eye

In the normal adult, the eyeball measures approximately 24 mm in diameter. It is protected by the orbital fat in the one orbit. We will examine the structure of the eye in layers (Fig. 36–4A).

Conjunctiva

The conjunctiva is a thin transparent layer of mucous membrane that lines the eyelids and covers the eyeball. The palpebral conjunctiva lines the eyelids and is contiguous with the bulbar conjunctiva, which covers the eyeball. The elasticity of the bulbar conjunctiva allows the eye to move freely; however, the continuous surface prevents the eye from coming out of its socket.

Cornea

The cornea is a transparent avascular structure with a brilliant, shiny surface. It is convex in shape and acts as a powerful lens to bend and direct (refract) rays of light to

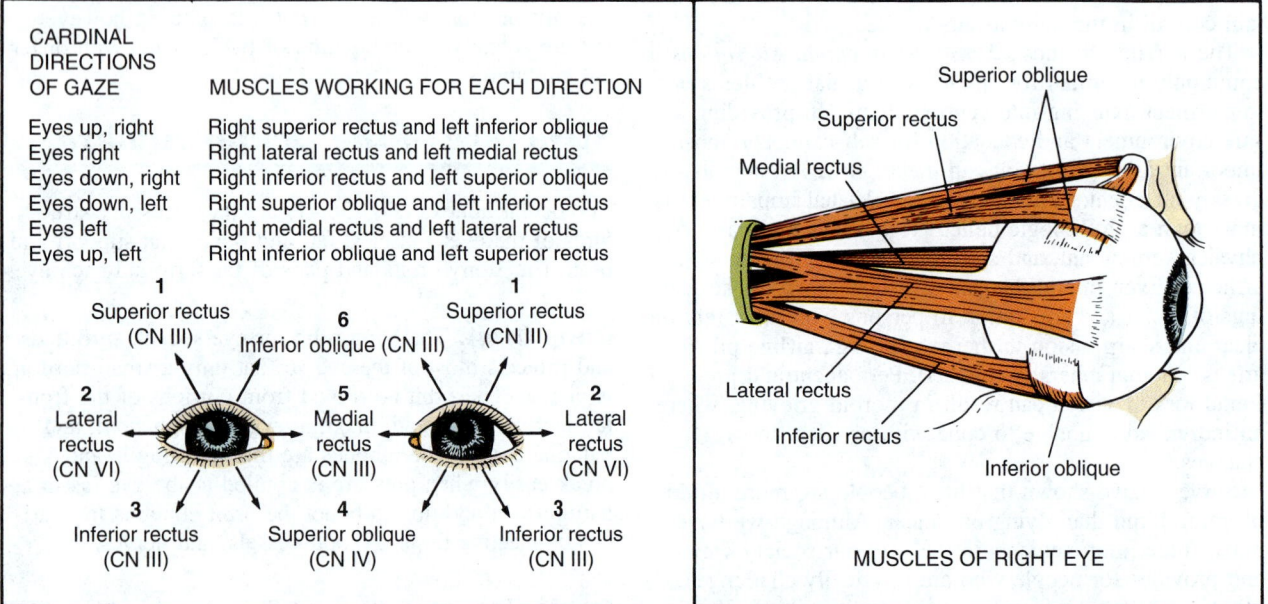

Figure 36–2. The six cardinal directions of gaze and the muscles responsible for each. The six cardinal directions are (1) right, (2) left, (3) up and right, (4) up and left, (5) down and right, and (6) down and left.

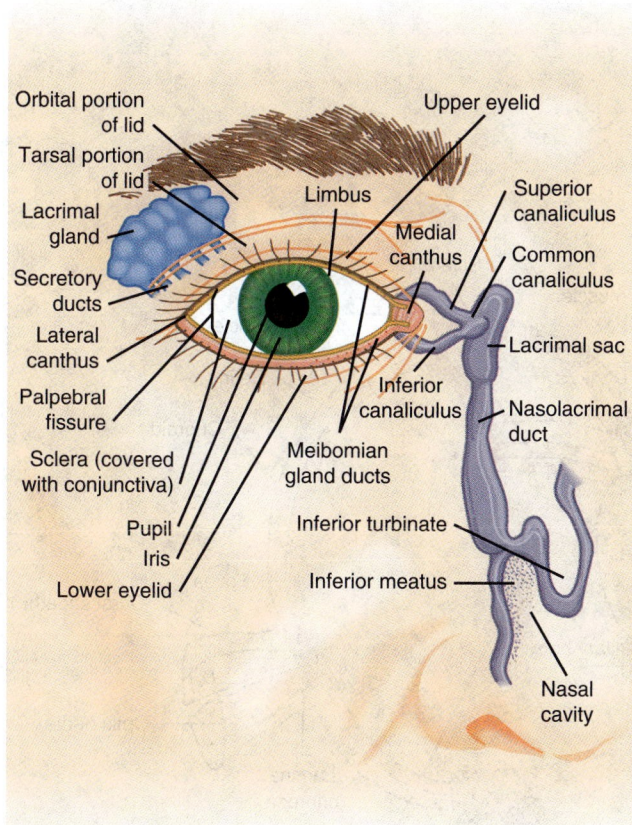

Figure 36–3. The surface anatomy of the eye, and the lacrimal drainage system.

the retina. It is about 0.5 mm thick and composed of five layers. The cornea derives oxygen from the atmosphere. A rich network of nerve fibers in the outer layer (epithelium) (Fig. 36–4B) produces a sensation of pain whenever the fibers are exposed or stimulated.

Sclera

The sclera is the fibrous protective coating of the eye. It is white, dense, and continuous with the cornea. In children, the sclera is thin and appears bluish because of the underlying pigmented structures. In old age, it may become yellowish due to degeneration.

Uveal Tract

The uveal tract consists of three structures: (1) iris, (2) ciliary body, and (3) choroid. The tract is the middle vascular layer of the eye and furnishes the blood supply to the retina.

Iris. The iris is a thin, pigmented diaphragm with a central aperture, the pupil. Iris color is determined by the degree of pigmentation in the stromal melanocytes. Pupil diameter is determined by the interaction of the two iris muscles—the sphincter and the dilator. Expansion and contraction of the iris regulate the amount of light enter-

ing the eye. As the iris contracts, it forms visible furrows on the surface. Between the iris and the cornea is a clear fluid called the aqueous humor. This fluid occupies the space called the anterior chamber of the eye.

Ciliary Body. The ciliary body is in direct continuity with the iris and is circular, surrounding the lens. It produces and secretes the aqueous humor, an alkaline fluid composed mainly of water. The ciliary body also supports the lens, because the lens' zonules insert into the ciliary body.

The aqueous humor is secreted by the ciliary body and circulates from the posterior chamber through the pupil into the anterior chamber (Fig. 36–4C). The flow continues into the anterior chamber angle and is filtered out through the trabecular meshwork into Schlemm's canal. From there the aqueous humor is channeled into a capillary network and into episcleral veins. Normal intraocular pressure is maintained as long as there is a balance between the aqueous production and the aqueous humor outflow.

Choroid. The choroid is the posterior segment of the uveal tract between the retina and the sclera. It is composed of three layers of vessels and is attached to both the ciliary body and the optic nerve.

Angle Structures

Although the angle of the anterior chamber is not really a structure, it is a critical component of the eye. The angle is formed where the cornea and the iris meet. At the apex of the angle, a filtering system called the trabecular meshwork allows the outflow of the aqueous fluid. The aqueous fluid is filtered out through the trabeculum into Schlemm's canal and then flows into the venous drainage system.

Lens

The lens is a biconvex, avascular, colorless, and almost completely transparent structure, about 4 mm thick and 9 mm in diameter. It is suspended behind the iris by ligamentous fibers called zonules, which connect to the ciliary body. The sole purpose of the lens is to focus light on the retina. The physiologic interplay of the zonular fibers and elasticity of the lens allows for focusing on nearby or distant objects. The change of focus from distant to near is called *accommodation.* There are no pain fibers or blood vessels in the lens. The lens is surrounded by a transparent envelope called the capsule. The lens of the eye consists of about 65% water and 35% protein. The protein content is the highest of any tissue in the body. Potassium, ascorbic acid, and glutathione are also present in the lens.

Vitreous Body

The vitreous body is a clear, avascular, jelly-like structure. The fluid is thick, viscous, and occupies a space

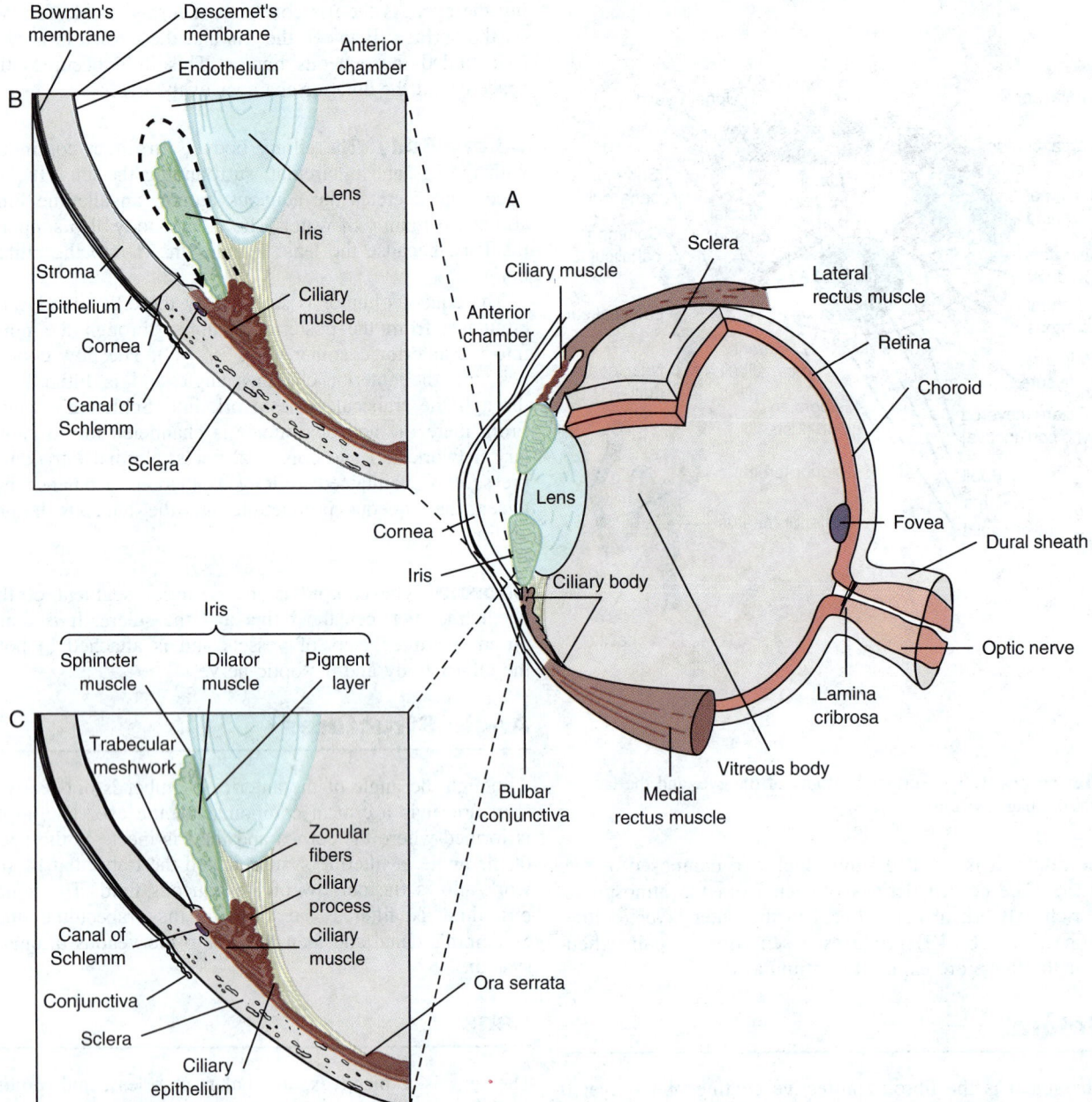

Figure 36–4. *A,* A horizontal section of the eye. *B,* The flow of aqueous humor into the anterior chamber through Schlemm's canal. *C,* Schlemm's canal.

called the vitreous chamber. It fills the largest cavity of the eye, accounting for two thirds of its volume. It helps maintain the shape and transparency of the eye.

Retina

The retina is a thin, semitransparent layer of nerve tissue that forms the innermost lining of the eye. It consists of 10 distinct layers of highly organized, delicate tissue. The retina contains all the sensory receptors for the transmission of light, and is really part of the brain. There are two types of retinal receptors—the rods and the cones. The approximately 125 million rods are distributed in the periphery of the retina and function best in dim light.

Damage to these structures results in night blindness. The cones, numbering about 6 million, provide for the resolution of small visual angles, resulting in perception of fine details. They are also responsible for color vision. The cones are concentrated in an area about 1.5 mm in diameter in the center of the retina. Damage to this area can severely reduce central vision. The center of the retina is an area about 5 mm in diameter called the macula. In an ophthalmoscopic examination, it appears as a yellowish spot with a depressed center (the fovea). The fovea, an area of 1.5 mm in diameter where only cones are present, is the point of finest vision.

The retina is composed of many fine layers or neural tissue attached to a single layer of pigmented epithelial cells. The photoreceptor cells in the retina are nourished by the capillaries of the choroid layer just beneath the pigment epithelial cell layer. Oxygen supply to these delicate structures is critical because the conversion of visual stimuli into impulses that the brain records as images requires very active metabolic processes.

Optic Nerve

The optic nerve is located at the posterior portion of the eye and transmits visual impulses from the retina to the brain. The head of the optic nerve can be seen by ophthalmoscopic examination and is called the *optic disc.* The optic nerve contains no sensory receptors (rods or cones) and represents a blind spot in the eye. The nerve emerges from the back of the eye and extends for 25 to 30 mm, traveling through the muscle cone to enter the bony optic foramen, eventually joining the other optic nerve to form the optic chiasm. One half of the visual field of each eye is projected to the other side of the brain. For example, visual impulses from the right visual field of each eye are transmitted to the left occipital lobe (Fig. 36–5).

Function of the Eye

Eyes provide us with our sense of sight. In humans, the two eyes collaborate to work as though they were one,

focusing on the same point in space and fusing their images so that a single mental impression is obtained. The ability of the eyes to fuse two images into a single image is called binocular vision.

Effects of Aging on the Eye

There are several age-related changes that occur in the structures of the eye and surrounding tissue. Eyebrows and eyelashes turn gray, and the skin around the eyelids becomes wrinkled and loosened because of loss of muscle tone and elasticity. Loss of orbital fat causes the eyes to sink deeper into the orbit and, sometimes, limits the upward gaze. Tear secretions may also diminish, resulting in the condition of dry eyes.

The most frequent and significant age-related change in the eye is the formation of a cataract. With age, the thickness and density of the lens increase and the lens becomes progressively yellowed and opaque. Throughout the lifespan, the lens continues to grow by repeated formation of new fiber cells. Although the rate of growth gradually diminishes, the accumulation of cells over the life span contributes to lens density. Loss of transparency also results from molecular deterioration from absorption of ultraviolet radiation. The yellow material is associated with the development of abnormal fluorescent substances

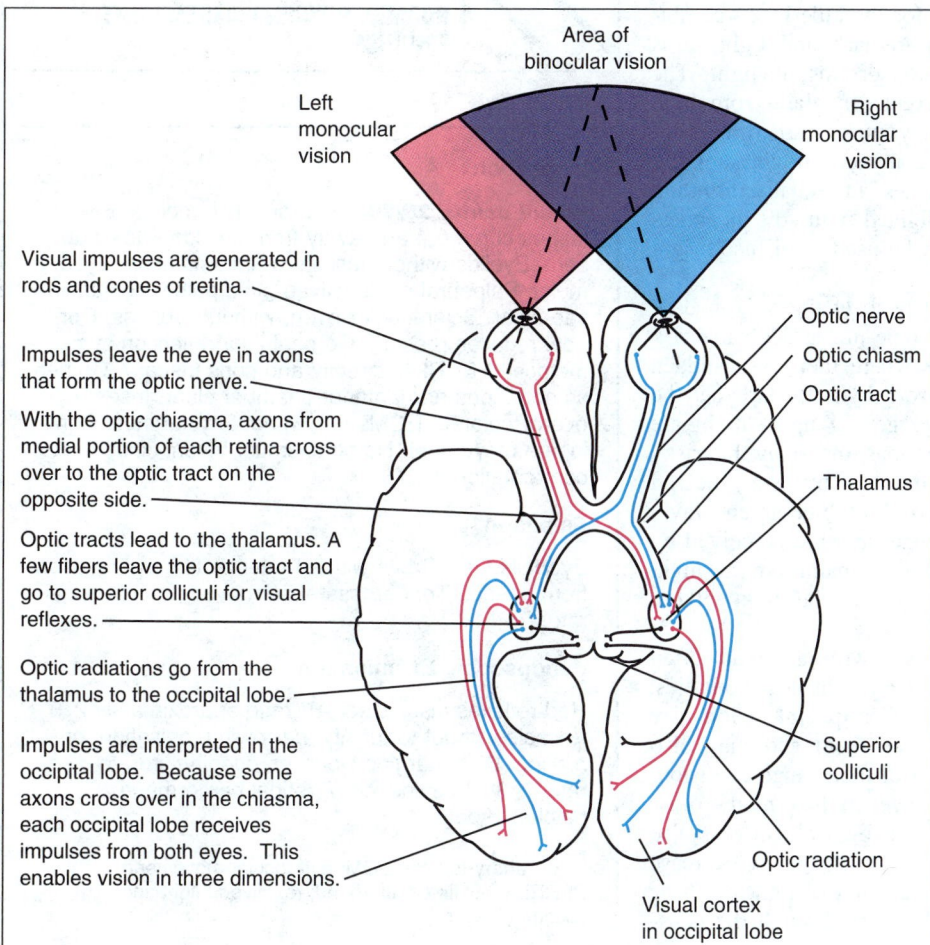

Figure 36–5. Visual pathways from the retina, where impulses are generated, to the occipital lobe, where they are interpreted. (From Applegate, E. J. [1995]. *The anatomy and physiology learning system: Textbook* [p. 195]. Philadelphia: W. B. Saunders.)

Area of binocular vision

Left monocular vision

Right monocular vision

Visual impulses are generated in rods and cones of retina.

Impulses leave the eye in axons that form the optic nerve.

With the optic chiasma, axons from medial portion of each retina cross over to the optic tract on the opposite side.

Optic tracts lead to the thalamus. A few fibers leave the optic tract and go to superior colliculi for visual reflexes.

Optic radiations go from the thalamus to the occipital lobe.

Impulses are interpreted in the occipital lobe. Because some axons cross over in the chiasma, each occipital lobe receives impulses from both eyes. This enables vision in three dimensions.

Optic nerve

Optic chiasm

Optic tract

Thalamus

Superior colliculi

Optic radiation

Visual cortex in occipital lobe

in the aging lens. Although the cloudiness of the lens that occurs with aging decreases visual acuity, it does provide a natural protection for the retina against ultraviolet light. The lens also loses its accommodative power because of ciliary muscle atrophy.

The cells of the inner layer of the cornea (endothelium) decrease in number with age. Because this layer does not reproduce lost cells, the ability of this layer to heal after injury or surgery may be compromised. The corneal reflex also may be diminished or absent. Another phenomenon characteristic of aging is the arcus senilis, which is a grayish-yellow ring found on the periphery of the cornea surrounding the iris. This ring is thought to be the result of the accumulation of lipids.

The ciliary body produces less aqueous humor during the aging process, but there is less outflow, so the intra-ocular pressure remains relatively stable or increases just slightly. The ciliary muscle tends to atrophy with age, and sometimes connective tissue replaces lost muscle tissue. The loss in muscle action, along with lens thickening, decreases the focusing ability of the lens. Decreasing ability to focus at near accommodation is called *presbyopia*.

The major visual changes with aging include a decrease in visual acuity, tolerance of glare, ability to adapt to dark and light, and peripheral vision. All of these decreases are related to changes in the eye structure, and all affect the quality and intensity of the light that is able to reach the retina.

Glare is a particular problem for the elderly. In combination with difficulty adjusting to dark and light, it is often the reason older people stop driving at night. The lights from oncoming traffic produce a glare from both the cornea and lens, which may make discernment of objects very difficult. In a similar manner, bright sunlight, either indoors or outdoors, causes an equally blinding glare. Indoor rooms should be lighted with soft incandescent light and sheer curtains can be used to diffuse bright sunlight.

Because it takes longer to adapt to changes from dark to light and vice versa, older people are at a greater risk of falls and injuries. Any place where there is a sudden change from dark to light or from light to dark can be dangerous. Entering theaters and getting up at night are two particularly hazardous situations that may be risky for older adults. Eyes adapt to the dark by using the rod receptors, which are sensitive to short blue-green wavelengths. Red wavelengths are longer and are perceived by the cones. Thus, a red light in the bathroom at night allows for enough vision to function in the dark without the need for adaptation.

Peripheral vision also decreases with age and often interferes with social interactions and physical activities. Older adults suffering from loss of peripheral vision may not notice someone sitting next to them and may also have difficulty finding objects out of their range of vision.

The iris loses pigment with age so that many older people appear to have grayish or light-blue eyes. The pupil becomes increasingly smaller with age. A decrease in pupil size results in a smaller amount of light reaching the retina, and the light must also pass through the densest and most opaque area of the lens.

In the posterior chamber, the vitreous body begins to liquify and collapse. Small pieces of debris from separation and shrinkage may become visible as floaters, and although they may not obstruct vision, they are certainly an annoyance. Vitreal shrinkage may result in retinal detachment. Additionally, the retina also may degenerate as a result of local ischemia and loss of neural function.

Assessment of Clients with Eye Disorders

One of the most important considerations in an ocular assessment is that many ophthalmic disorders are asymptomatic. The four most common preventable causes of permanent vision loss in developed nations are (1) amblyopia (reduced visual acuity that is uncorrectable with glasses in the absence of anatomic defects in the eye or visual pathways), (2) diabetic retinopathy, (3) age-related maculopathy, and (4) glaucoma. Routine eye examinations are therefore imperative.

The eye is a unique organ of the body in that the external anatomy of the eye may be easily assessed. Even

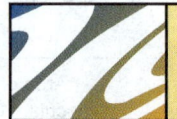

NORMAL PHYSICAL ASSESSMENT FINDINGS

The Eye

Inspection

Visual acuity 20/20. Eyebrows full, mobile. Eyelashes curve out and away from eyelids. Ptosis absent. Eyelids without lesions or inflammation. Eyes moist. Palpebral conjunctivae pink; bulbar conjunctivae clear. Scleral color even, without redness. Corneal reflexes present. Corneal light reflection symmetrical. PERRLA, directly and consensually. Cornea smooth; lens and anterior chamber clear. Irises evenly colored. EOMs full, without nystagmus. Conjugate movement. No strabismus. Visual fields full to confrontation.

Palpation

Eyeballs firm. Orbits without edema. No regurgitation from puncta. Tenderness absent over lacrimal apparatus.

Funduscopic Examination

Red reflexes visualized. AV ratio approximately 2:3. Vessels without tortuosity, narrowing, pulsation, or nicking. Disc margins clear, no cupping; cup-to-disc ratio 1:3. No evidence of retinal hemorrhage, patches, spots.

AV, artery-to-vein; EOM, extraocular movement; PERRLA, pupils equal, round, reactive to light and accommodation.

Box 36-1. Common Misconceptions About Vision and the Eyes

The following statements are often passed along as "advice." They are all false.

1. Reading in the dark is harmful to the eyes.
2. Children will outgrow crossed eyes.
3. A cataract is a film growing over the surface of the eye.
4. Cataracts must "ripen" before they are removed.
5. The surgeon takes out the eye to operate on it.
6. A person with failing eyesight should avoid reading to save the eyes.
7. Children must be cautioned not to sit too close to the television.
8. Wearing someone else's glasses may damage your eyes.
9. Misuse of the eyes in childhood results in the need for glasses later in life.
10. Cataracts can be removed by a laser.
11. Emotional stress increases intraocular pressure.

the internal eye is visible through the cornea, where blood vessels and central nervous system (CNS) tissue (the retina and optic nerve) may be visualized without the use of x-rays or invasive procedures. The effects of many systemic disorders, such as infections, neoplasms, vascular disorders, and autoimmune disorders, are detectable with an internal eye examination. Box 36-1 lists common misconceptions that clients may have about vision and the eyes. The nurse may encounter some of these misconceptions while conducting a physical assessment and should be prepared to address them.

History

An ophthalmic history includes demographic data, exploration of current symptoms, past health history, family health history, psychosocial history and life-style, and review of systems.

Biographical and Demographic Data

Demographic data relevant to ocular assessment include age and sex. The incidence of cataracts, dry eye, retinal detachment, glaucoma, entropion, and ectropion increases with age. Hereditary color vision deficits are more common in males than in females.

Current Symptoms

Ocular manifestations may be divided into three basic categories of abnormalities: (1) vision, (2) appearance, and (3) ocular sensation—pain and discomfort. These symptoms are discussed below.

Chief Complaint

The most common chief complaint is often a change or loss of vision but may also be less specific, such as headache or eyestrain. Commonly, the client is unable to verbalize a specific complaint. The chief complaint may be as vague as "something is wrong with my eyes."

Symptom Analysis

Whenever possible, clinical manifestations are characterized according to rapidity of onset, location, duration, and characteristics (such as frequency and severity). The circumstances surrounding onset are important, as well as the client's response to treatment. Record current eye and systemic medications being used and all other current and past ocular disorders.

Abnormal Vision. Visual changes or loss of vision may be caused by abnormalities in the eye or anywhere along the visual pathway. Considerations in this category include a refractive (focusing) error; interference from lid ptosis (drooping of the eyelid); clouding or interference in the cornea, lens, aqueous or vitreous space; and malfunction of the retina, optic nerve, or intracranial visual pathway.

Glare or halos may result from uncorrected refractive error, scratches on glasses, dilated pupils, corneal edema, or cataract. Flashing or flickering lights may indicate retinal traction or migraine. Floating spots may represent normal vitreous body strands or the pathologic presence of blood, pigment, or inflammatory cells in the vitreous body. Diplopia (double vision) may occur in one eye or both and may be caused by refractive correction, muscle imbalance, or neurologic disorders.

Abnormal Appearance. The most common abnormal appearance is a red eye. Causes of a red eye include minor irritation, vascular congestion, subconjunctival hemorrhage, inflammatory disorders, infection, allergy, and trauma. Box 36-2 lists eye disorders associated with a red eye. Other external changes in appearance include growths or lesions, edema, or abnormal position.

Abnormal Sensation. Eye pain is often poorly localized. Nonspecific complaints may be eyestrain, pulling, pressure, fullness, or generalized headache. The pain may be periocular, ocular, or retrobulbar (behind the globe). Foreign-body sensation produces a sharp superficial pain relieved by topical anesthesia. Deeper internal aching may indicate glaucoma, inflammation, muscle spasm, or infection. Reflex spasm of the ciliary muscle and iris sphincter that occurs with inflammation may produce browache and *photophobia* (sensitivity to light) or a constricted pupil (miosis). Itching is usually a sign of an allergic response. Dryness, burning, grittiness, and mild foreign-body sensation can occur with dry eyes or mild corneal irritation. Tearing may be due to irritation or an abnormality of the

Box 36–2. Red Eye

Nurses often encounter a client whose chief complaint is a "red eye." The condition causing the eye to be red (engorgement of the conjunctival vessels) may be a subconjunctival hemorrhage that requires no treatment or it may be a sign of a serious eye disorder requiring immediate attention. These disorders include the following:

Conjunctivitis—bacterial, viral, allergic, and irritative
Herpes simplex keratitis—inflammation of the cornea
Scleritis—inflammation of the sclera
Angle-closure glaucoma—sudden occlusion of the anterior chamber angle by iris tissue
Adnexal disease—stye, dacryocystitis, blepharitis, lid lesions (carcinoma), thyroid disease, and vascular lesions
Subconjunctival hemorrhage—accumulation of blood in the potential space between the conjunctiva and the sclera
Pterygium—abnormal growth of tissue that progresses over the cornea
Keratoconjunctivitis sicca—inflammation associated with lacrimal deficiency
Abrasions and foreign bodies—hyperemic response
Abnormal lid function—Bell's palsy, thyroid ophthalmopathy, or lesions that cause ocular exposure

To evaluate a red eye:

1. Check the client's visual acuity with Snellen's chart.
2. Inspect for a pattern of redness.
3. Observe for the presence of discharge.
4. Using a penlight or slit lamp, observe for corneal opacities.
5. Using fluorescein stain, observe corneal defects.
6. Examine the anterior chamber for depth, blood cells, or pus.
7. Examine the pupils for irregularity.
8. Check intraocular pressure.
9. Observe for the pressure of proptosis or a lid disorder.

lacrimal system. Increased ocular secretions usually indicate viral or bacterial infections and may also be present in allergic and noninfectious irritations.

Past Health History

The past health history focuses on the client's general state of health. Specifically, ask about systemic disorders commonly associated with ocular manifestations, such as diabetes mellitus, arthritis, hypertension, and thyroid disease.

Childhood and Infectious Diseases. Diseases occurring in childhood with possible ocular sequelae include diabetes mellitus, retinoblastoma, thyroid disorders, rheumatoid arthritis, exposure to sexually transmitted diseases such as syphilis and acquired immunodeficiency syndrome (AIDS), and muscular dystrophy. Inquire about immunizations, particularly for measles (rubella).

Major Illnesses and Hospitalizations. In addition to the above-mentioned systemic diseases, ask about hypertension, multiple sclerosis, myasthenia gravis, and adult onset of thyroid disorders, rheumatoid arthritis, and diabetes mellitus. Ocular diseases and structural problems include refractive errors (and corrective lenses used), strabismus, amblyopia, cataracts, glaucoma, and retinal detachment. If eyeglasses or contact lenses are worn currently, ask when the last eye examination was done and when the prescription was last changed. Inquire whether the client has been hospitalized or has had surgery related to the eyes or brain. Is there a history of head trauma or eye trauma related to motor vehicle accidents or sports injury? Has the client had surgery on the eyes, such as laser treatment?

Medications. Many medications affect the eyes. Prescription drugs include insulin, corticosteroids, oral hypoglycemics, and thyroid replacement hormones. Ask whether the client uses eye drops, and note the name, dose, and frequency taken. Specifically ask whether or not the client uses over-the-counter eye drops such as natural tears. Over-the-counter preparations that may dry the eyes include antihistamines and decongestants.

Allergies. Note allergies to medications and other substances. Has the client ever had an allergic reaction to eye drops or other medications that have affected the eyes? Allergic symptoms include eye redness, tearing, and itching. Determine past allergic reactions not only to medications but also to inhalants (dust, chemicals, or pollens) and contactants (cosmetics or pollens).

Family Health History

Because there are many ocular disorders with familial tendencies, it is important to ask questions specifically about strabismus, glaucoma, myopia (nearsightedness), and hyperopia (farsightedness). Other common familial disorders include migraine, retinoblastoma, macular degeneration, retinitis pigmentosa, sickle cell anemia, keratoconus, and diabetes mellitus. Lack of a family health history does not necessarily rule out the possibility of a genetic disorder. Some clients do not know the ocular history of family members, and some may be embarrassed or hesitant to share the information.

Psychosocial History

Psychosocial history and life-style factors data significant to the ocular health history include occupational hazards, leisure activities and hobbies, and health management behaviors. A driving history can reveal a vision problem. Ask about the nature of the client's work and hobbies. Is the client exposed to irritating fumes, smoke, or airborne particles? Are safety goggles worn in situations in which eye injury may occur from fragments of metal or sand? Is there a problem with insufficient lighting, leading to eyestrain or harsh, glaring light? Leisure and sports activities with increased incidence of eye injury include baseball, racquetball, and contact sports with a potential for head trauma such as football. Participation in active outdoor activities such as gardening, hiking, and cross-country skiing increases the risk of foreign-body injury, abrasion, or penetrating injury. Does the client wear sunglasses or other protective eye gear when outdoors?

Explore health management behaviors related to the eyes. If the client has a systemic disease that affects the eyes, are self-care measures practiced? For example, does the diabetic client aggressively manage the disease by attempting to regulate blood glucose levels with diet and medication? If the client wears contact lenses, are the lenses cleaned and stored as recommended? Is the client capable of safely taking care of the lenses?

Briefly review the client's driving history for information that can indicate a vision deficit. Ask if there is a problem driving at night because of difficulty adjusting to the glare from oncoming headlights. Does the client have trouble seeing the dashboard instrument panel at night because of dim lighting? Are traffic or street signs hard to read while driving? Is the client able to drive in conditions of reduced visibility such as rain or fog? Do other vehicles, pedestrians, bicyclists, or objects appear unexpectedly in the peripheral vision while the client is looking straight ahead? Has the client had a motor vehicle accident or "close call" within the past year?

Visual ability is one of several capabilities necessary for a person to operate a motor vehicle. Tact is needed when assessing a client who may have impaired vision. The client may not answer truthfully if he or she feels that driving privileges will be lost.

The social stigma of blindness underlies the anxiety that clients experience with actual or potential vision loss. Total loss of vision isolates an individual within a different reality. Although most clients are successfully rehabilitated, some losses are permanent. Some individuals, for a variety of reasons, remain socially isolated. The image of a blind person who is pitied and must accept the charity of others is disturbing.

Not all jobs and work environments are adaptable for a person who is visually impaired. Clients with actual or potential vision loss may be faced with barriers in their vocations that force an unwanted change. Age may be a major factor in the client's ability to meet this challenge.

Self-esteem is closely related to the roles of the client in his or her particular life-style. Loss of control in personal, family, and work situations can be devastating. The issue of dependence versus independence for an individual may also be a factor in the client's ability to cope with the stressors of vision loss.

Review of Systems

The review of systems (ROS) relevant to the eyes includes asking about systems such as headaches and problems with sinusitis. Specifically, ask whether symptoms occur in association with pain or discomfort, visual changes, swelling, redness, or drainage from the eye. Also ask about the time of day and the season of year during which symptoms occur, as well as about sensitivity to light.

Detailed questions for the ROS may be found in Box 11–2.

Physical Examination

Your role and scope of practice in ophthalmic assessment and examination varies according to state nurse practice acts, institutions, and employer guidelines. Regardless of the level of responsibility in any practice situation, you must be knowledgeable about ophthalmic clinical manifestations and diagnoses as they relate to the holistic approach to client care.

Examination of the eyes includes assessment of external structures, using inspection and palpation, extraocular movements (EOMs), visual acuity, and visual fields (peripheral vision). If you have advanced clinical assessment skills, you may perform tonometry and examine the internal eye structures with an ophthalmoscope.

Observe the client's body structure and features for obvious deformities and apparent age. For example, the hand deformities or abnormal gait of a client with arthritis may be a clue to the diagnosis of an associated eye disorder of keratoconjunctivitis sicca (dry eye syndrome) in a client who reports itching and burning eyes.

External Eye Examination

External eye structures include: the eyebrows, eyelashes, eyelids, the lacrimal apparatus, anterior portion of the eyeballs, conjunctivae, sclerae, corneas, anterior chambers, pupils, and irises. Inspect and palpate these structures while the client sits at eye level to the examiner.

Eye Position

Assess eye position for symmetry and alignment. Sunken or protruding eyes are abnormal findings, such as protrusion of one eye or both eyes, called *exophthalmos*.

Eyebrows

Inspect the eyebrows for symmetry, hair distribution, skin conditions, and movement. The eyebrows normally move up and down smoothly under control of the facial nerves. Hair loss of the lateral aspects occurs with aging. The skin may be dry and flaking (i.e., dandruff), which is abnormal.

Eyelids and Eyelashes

Examine the eyelids and eyelashes for placement and symmetry. When open, the upper lids rest at the top of the irises and the lower lids at the bottom so that the sclerae are not visible above or below the irises. Sagging of the upper lids that covers part of the pupil is abnormal and called *ptosis*. Ptosis may occur with aging but also results from edema, third cranial nerve disorders, and neuromuscular disorders. Check for effective closure by asking the client to close the eyes. Eyelids that turn inward (entropion) or outward (ectropion) can result in corneal irritation. Lid eversion and inversion are often due to aging tissues but may also be due to facial nerve paresis, scarring, or allergies. Elevate the eyebrows to inspect the upper lids for lesions. Inspect the lower lids by asking the client to open the eyes. Examine the skin of the eyelids and orbit by palpating for texture, firmness, mobility, and integrity of the underlying tissues.

Blink Response

Blinking is an involuntary reflex that occurs bilaterally up to 20 times a minute. Rapid, infrequent, or asymmetrical blinking is abnormal.

Eyeballs

The eyeballs are palpated for symmetry and firmness. Instruct the client to close the eyes and look down. Place the tip of the index fingers on the upper eyelids, over the sclerae, and palpate gently. Normally, the eyeballs feel firm and symmetrical, not asymmetrical, hard, or soft. If you have advanced clinical skills you may perform tonometry to measure ocular pressure. See under Internal Eye Examination for a discussion of tonometry.

Lacrimal Apparatus

The lacrimal apparatus is examined by retracting the upper lid and having the client look down so that part of the lacrimal gland may be visualized. Observe this area for swelling or tenderness. The eye surface should be moist, without excess tearing. Inspect the area between the lower lid and the nose, which should be free of edema. The area over the lower orbit rim near the inner canthus (over the lacrimal sac) is palpated gently. There should be no regurgitation of fluid from the sac or puncta.

Conjunctivae and Sclerae

The conjunctivae and sclerae are inspected for color changes, texture, vascularity, lesions, thickness, secretions, and foreign bodies. The bulbar conjunctivae are colorless and transparent, allowing the sclerae to be seen. Small blood vessels may be visible. In whites, the sclerae are white, whereas they may appear light yellow in people with dark skin. To inspect the palpebral conjunctivae, you may wish to wear gloves. Regardless of whether gloves are worn or not, meticulous hand washing is advised both before and after the conjunctivae are examined. The lower eyelids are retracted to expose the conjunctivae without applying pressure to the eyeballs. You (or the client) gently push the lower lids down against the bony orbit while the client looks up. Healthy conjunctivae are pink to light red; paleness or a bright-red color is abnormal. If the lower palpebral conjunctivae are normal, the upper palpebral conjunctivae usually are not inspected. If examination is necessary, the upper eyelids are everted by gently grasping the eyelashes of the upper lid and pulling down while the client looks down. Place a cotton-tipped applicator just above the lid margin and turn the upper lid inside out over the applicator. After the inspection, return the eyelid to its normal position by gently pulling the eyelashes forward while the client looks up.

Cornea

Inspect the cornea from an oblique angle while shining a penlight on the corneal surface. The irises are easily visible. In the elderly, a thin, grayish-white ring around the edge of the cornea may be seen (arcus senilis). Abnormalities include surface irregularity and cloudiness or opacity.

Corneal Reflex

The corneal reflex test is performed to assess the function of the fifth (trigeminal) cranial nerve. Instruct the client to keep the eyes open and look straight ahead. A sterile cotton wisp is brought from behind the client and lightly touched to the cornea. The client should blink and tear, indicating that the nerves are intact. A separate wisp is used for each eye. An alternative method is to use a syringe or the bulb from an otoscope to gently puff air across the cornea, eliciting the blink-and-tear response. Persons who wear contact lenses may not respond to the same degree as persons who do not wear them because they become somewhat insensitive to the stimulus.

Anterior Chamber

The anterior chamber is inspected with the cornea, using the same oblique angle and penlight. The chambers should appear clear and transparent with no cloudiness or shadows cast upon the irises. The depth of the chamber between the cornea and iris normally is about 3 mm. Shallower or deeper chambers are abnormal and the client should be referred to an ophthalmologist.

Iris and Pupil

The iris and pupil are inspected. The iris should light up with oblique lighting from the penlight and have a consistent color. Bulging or uneven coloring is abnormal. When light shines into the eyes, the iris constricts as the optic nerves are stimulated, making the pupil smaller. Dim lighting causes the pupil to dilate. Inspect the pupils for size, shape, equality, and ability to react to light and accommodation. Pupils are normally black, round, have smooth borders, and are the same size. The actual size depends on the level of lighting, effect of medications that alter iris contractility, changes in intracranial pressure, or lesions impinging on the optic nerve.

Dim the light to test pupil reactions to light and accommodation. Instruct the client to look straight ahead.

To test direct response to light, bring the penlight in from the side to shine directly over the center of the pupil. The illuminated pupil should constrict briskly and evenly. This maneuver is repeated on the other eye. Both eyes should react to the same degree. Consensual response is tested by observing one pupil while the penlight is shone on the opposite pupil. Both pupils should constrict to the same degree, although the consensual response is slightly slower.

Accommodation is tested by holding the penlight 4 to 6 inches (10–15 cm) away from the client's nose. Instruct the client to look first at the penlight, then at the distant wall straight ahead, and then back at the penlight. While the client gazes from near to far and back again, observe the pupils' response to changes in distance. They should dilate when looking at the far point and constrict when looking at the near object. Then move the penlight toward the bridge of the client's nose and observe the pupils for convergence and constriction.

Results of the pupil assessment that are normal are recorded as PERRLA (*p*upils *e*qual, *r*ound, and *r*eactive to *l*ight, and *a*ccommodation). Abnormal results include light intolerance (photophobia), irregular or unequal pupils, or pupils that do not react to light or accommodation. Abnormalities of the pupil may be caused by neurologic disease, intraocular inflammation, iris adhesions, the effect of systemic or ocular medications, or surgical alteration, or they may be benign variations of normal findings.

Ocular Motility

Evaluation of ocular motility provides information about the extraocular muscles; the orbit; the oculomotor, trochlear, and abducent nerves; their brain stem connections; and the cerebral cortex. The client is asked to track a target with both eyes as it is moved in each of the six cardinal directions of gaze (see Fig. 36–2). The examiner notes the speed, smoothness, range, and symmetry of movements and observes for unsteadiness of fixation (*nystagmus*).

The eyes normally move in parallel to each other, smoothly and in unison. To test the function of the oculomotor, trochlear, and abducent nerves, ask the client to look straight ahead while standing directly in front, holding a penlight approximately 12 inches (30 cm) from the eyes. Instruct the client to keep the head still and to follow the penlight's movements with the eyes only. Move the penlight slowly and smoothly through the six cardinal positions of gaze, being careful not to go beyond the client's field of vision. Move the penlight in an orderly manner from the center outward along each of the six directions, pause briefly to observe for nystagmus, then return to the center. Nystagmus is an involuntary rapid, oscillating movement of the eyeball and is considered an abnormal finding except for slight nystagmus in the extreme lateral gazes (e.g., endpoint nystagmus). If the eyes do not move in parallel or if the upper eyelid covers more than a tiny portion of the iris, the conditions are noted as abnormal findings.

Corneal Light Reflex Test. The corneal light reflex test (Hirschberg's test) determines eye alignment. Shine a penlight at the bridge of the client's nose from a distance of 12 to 15 inches (30–38 cm) while the client stares straight ahead. Observe where the light reflects from both corneas; the reflection should be symmetrical. Asymmetrical reflection is abnormal and may indicate strabismus. *Strabismus* is a disorder in which the eye axes cannot be directed to the same object. A constant deviation of ocular alignment is termed *tropia*. Deviation toward the nose is called *esotropia,* a deviation away from the nose is called *exotropia,* and a vertical (up or down) deviation is called *hypertropia.* Latent deviations are seen only when one eye is covered and are called *phorias (esophoria* and *exophoria*).

Cover-Uncover Test. The cover-uncover test assesses eye muscle function and alignment for tropia and phoria. The client is asked to stare straight ahead at a fixed point approximately 20 inches (51 cm) away. Cover one of the client's eyes with an opaque card while observing the uncovered eye for lateral or medial movement as it focuses on the fixed point. There should be none. Remove the eye cover and observe that eye for movement as it focuses on the fixed point. Again, there should be no movement. The maneuvers are repeated for the opposite eye. The test may need to be repeated several times to confirm abnormal findings of strabismus.

Vision

Visual Acuity. Testing visual acuity is the standard and routine method used to determine the clarity of the ocular media (cornea, lens, and vitreous) and the function of the visual pathway from the retina to the brain. Although abnormal acuity implies an uncorrected refractive error or pathologic process, normal acuity does not exclude disease of the visual system. Visual acuity is assessed in one eye at a time, then in both eyes together, with the client comfortably seated. Begin with the right eye while the left eye is covered by an occluder or an opaque card. Test visual acuity with and without corrective lenses. Visual acuity is traditionally measured with Snellen's chart (Fig. 36–6A) at a distance of 20 ft; at this distance, rays of light from an object are practically parallel and little effort of accommodation is required. In rooms that are shorter than 20 ft, mirrors or projection may be used to achieve the required distance. Charts may also be reduced proportionally to compensate for distance. Adaptations may be needed for the client who is illiterate or does not speak English; variations of Snellen's chart are available for these clients. The numbers and symbols can be used in lieu of letters. There must be adequate lighting for the client to see.

Begin by asking the client to read the smallest line of symbols or letters that is seen. The client is credited for the smallest line of print that is read with more than 50% accuracy. Record the results according to the standardized numbers printed by the lines on Snellen's chart. The sizes of the symbols are identified according to the distances at which they are normally visible. For example, the largest

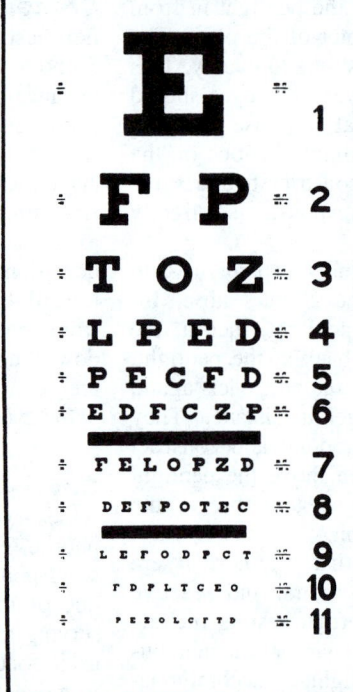

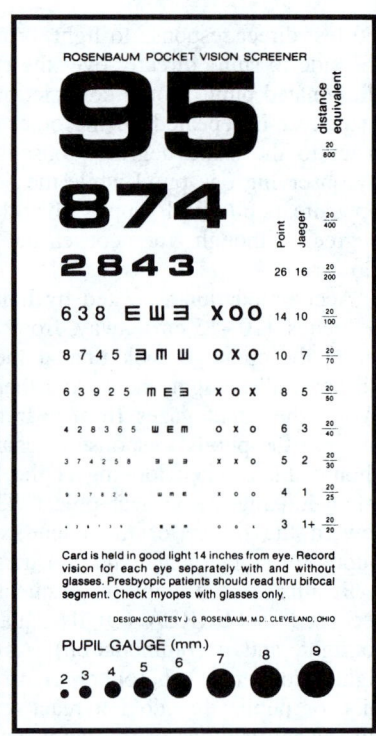

Figure 36–6. *A,* Snellen's chart, for assessment of visual acuity. *B,* A Rosenbaum pocket vision screener. (*B,* courtesy of SMP Division, Cooper Laboratories [P.R.], Inc., San German, Puerto Rico.)

symbols can be read 200 ft away by people with unimpaired vision. The results of visual acuity testing are expressed as a fraction. The numerator denotes the distance the client is from the chart letters, and the denominator denotes the distance from the chart at which a client with normal vision can see the chart letters. Vision that is 20/20 is normal, that is, the client is able to read from 20 ft what a person with normal vision can read from 20 ft. A client with a visual acuity of 20/60 can only read at a distance of 20 ft what a client with normal vision can read at 60 ft. The client with *myopia* (i.e., nearsightedness) will have results of 20/30 or greater, signifying that the client can only read at 20 ft what a person with normal vision can read at 30 ft (or greater). *Hyperopia* (i.e., farsightedness) results are 20/15 or less, meaning the client can read at 20 ft what a person with normal vision can read at 15 ft (or less). It is not uncommon for a client to have a test result of 20/15, which indicates better-than-average visual acuity. Legal blindness is defined as 20/200 or less with corrected vision (glasses or contact lenses), or less than 20 degrees of visual field in the better eye.

When a client is unable to distinguish the largest letter on the chart, vision may be assessed by asking the client to read the number of fingers held up in front of him or her at a distance of 3 ft (CF = count fingers). If the client is unable to distinguish fingers, ask whether the client perceives hand movements (HM = hand motion). Finally, determine whether the client can perceive light (LP = light perception). NLP indicates no light perception.

Near vision is tested with a card or newsprint held 12 to 14 inches (30–36 cm) from the client's eyes (Fig. 36–6B). Corrective lenses are worn if needed. The client with normal vision is able to read the material at that distance.

Complaints of blurring or attempts by the client to move the card either closer or farther away signal abnormal near vision.

If this examination is repeated many times and you know your client has become familiar with the letters, ask the person to read the letters backward. When the individual is able to read most of the letters in a particular line, but misses one or two, document the visual acuity as 20/40 − 2.

Visual Fields. Visual field testing evaluates peripheral vision. It may be accomplished by the confrontational method (Fig. 36–7) or with a computerized instrument. The confrontational method assumes that the examiner has normal peripheral vision.

The client sits facing you approximately 2 ft (60 cm) away. The eyes of the client and the nurse should be at the same level. Both you and the client cover the eyes directly opposite to one another with an opaque cover (e.g., your right eye and the client's left eye) and stare at each other's uncovered eye. Hold a small object such as a penlight in your free hand and hold it equidistant between yourself and the client, just out of view at the periphery of the visual field. Starting with the superior field, slowly bring the penlight down between the client and yourself until the client states that he or she can see it. (You should be able to see the penlight at the same time.) Repeat this maneuver at 45-degree angles, progressing through the superior, temporal, inferior, and nasal fields until all are tested. You may need to position the penlight slightly behind the client to adequately test the client's temporal fields. The test is repeated for the other eye. Normal visual fields extend approximately 50 degrees su-

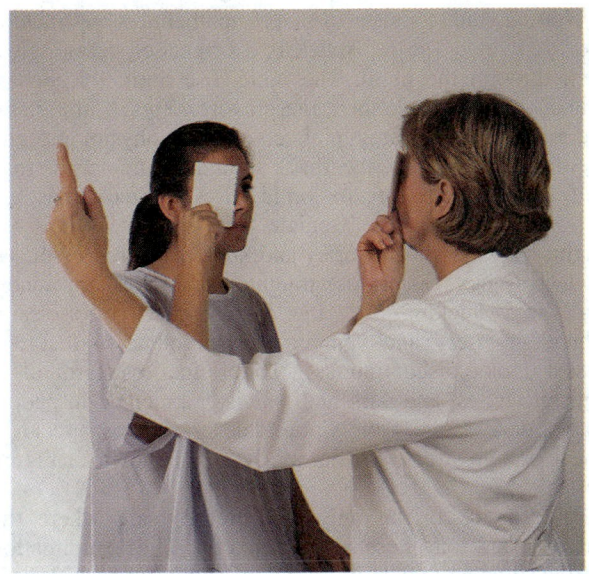

Figure 36–7. The confrontational method of assessment of visual fields. (From Jarvis, C. [1996]. *Physical examination and health assessment* [2nd ed.]. Philadelphia: W. B. Saunders.)

periorly, 90 degrees laterally, 70 degrees inferiorly, and 60 degrees medially. Gross visual field defects can be detected and, if found, the client is referred for further examination.

A variety of manual and computerized visual field testing equipment may be used to permit more accurate, reproducible detection and quantification of *scotoma* (an area of decreased visual function). Visual fields can be altered by CNS disorders, such as a brain lesion or syphilis, and ocular disorders, such as glaucoma or retinal detachment.

Special Testing of Vision

Color Vision Testing. Color vision testing is not always part of the usual eye examination. It is used most often in screening people seeking a license to operate a motor vehicle or for employment in which color discrimination is important. A common test involves the use of color plates on which numbers are outlined in primary colors and surrounded by "confusion" colors. The person with color vision problems is unable to recognize the figure. One such test consists of 84 chips of color that are matched in terms of increasing hues.

Defective Color Vision. Color vision problems are genetic and acquired in both men and women. Men are most often affected with inherited losses in color vision (7%) and women are less affected (0.5%). Nutritional problems, optic nerve disorders, and problems with the fovea centralis can also alter color perception.

Central Area Blindness Assessment

The Amsler grid is a 20-cm square that is divided into 5-mm squares with a dot in the center. The grid is used to

detect and follow the development of central area blindness (called *scotoma*). It is most often used at home by the client to follow the progress of macular degeneration. With glasses on and one eye closed, the client holds the grid at 12 inches from the face (the usual reading distance). The person fixes vision on the central dot and describes any areas of distortion of absences in the grid.

Internal Eye Examination

Internal eye structures are visible only with illumination such as that provided by an ophthalmoscope. The oph-

---

Box 36–3. Guidelines for Using an Ophthalmoscope

1. Assemble the ophthalmoscope by attaching the head to the handle.
2. Darken the room.
3. Turn on the ophthalmoscope light by depressing the rheostat button and turning the rheostat to the brightest light.
4. Turn the aperture selector to a large round circle of light.
5. Turn the lens selector dial to zero.
6. Instruct the client to stare straight ahead and to focus on a distant object.
7. Leave both of your eyes open during the examination. Learn to suppress visual stimulation from the eye that is not looking through the viewing aperture.
8. Hold the ophthalmoscope while steadying the client's head with your free hand.
9. Approach the client from the side at approximately a 45-degree angle and a distance of 15 inches. Direct the light into the client's pupil.
10. Move slowly closer to the client's eye, keeping the light directed on the pupil. If the client blinks, hold your position steady until the client's eye opens again. At approximately 15 inches, visualize the red reflex, then the anterior chamber. Moving closer, look at the lens. Finally, when very close (1–2 inches), vessels of the fundus may be seen.
11. Adjust the lens selector with your index finger to focus on a blood vessel and follow it into the optic disc.
12. Focus on the disc, adjusting the lens selector as needed to correct for visual deficits of both you and the client. Once the focus is adjusted, examine the optic disc (for color, margins, shape, and presence of physiologic cup; see Fig. 36–10).
13. Follow the major blood vessels from the disc and look for evidence of tortuosity, pulsation, diameter, ratio of arteries to veins (normally 2:3), and areas where arteries and veins cross for signs of nicking.
14. Note the retinal background color. Look for the presence of exudate or hemorrhage.
15. Last, ask the client to look into the light so that you can examine the fovea centralis. The fovea may be seen as a tiny bright light in the center of the macula. Only a very brief glimpse is possible because the light is too bright for the client to look at for long.
16. Repeat the examination for the opposite eye.

thalmoscope is used to inspect the structures posterior to the iris, including the lens and fundus (which includes the retina, retinal vessels, choroid, optic disc, macula, and fovea). The ophthalmoscope requires considerable skill and practice.

Direct Ophthalmoscopy

The handheld direct ophthalmoscope provides a magnified (×15) image of the fundus (posterior portion of the eye). It provides a detailed view of the disc and retinal vascular and is a part of a general physical examination as well as an ophthalmologic examination. Dilating the eye enhances the examiner's view, although a darkened room may cause adequate dilation. The examiner holds the ophthalmoscope 1 to 2 inches away from the client's eye and is able, through a light source and reflective mirrors, to examine the macula, optic disc, and retinal vessels (Box 36–3; Fig. 36–8). The examiner's view may be impaired by a cloudy cornea or the presence of a cataract.

Normal findings seen in direct ophthalmoscopy include the following: The red reflex is a bright red-orange glow seen through the pupil. The optic disc normally appears round, with well-defined margins (except in the nasal margin), and a creamy pink color. The physiologic cup (depressed center of the disc) should be no larger than half the diameter of the optic disc. Retinal veins are darker than arteries and radiate from the disc. Veins are slightly thicker than arteries and should be free of pulsation. Tortuous vessels or straightened arteries are abnormal, as is nicking (i.e., the disappearance of a vessel where an artery and vein cross each other so that one vessel looks discontinuous). The retinal background is pink in whites, and dark and heavily pigmented in people with a dark complexion. Choroidal vessels may appear as linear orange streaks. A normal retina is shown in Figure 36–8.

The fundus is the only site in the body where the vascular bed may be observed directly. Thus examination of the fundus yields information about many systemic diseases. Abnormal findings include an altered arteriove-

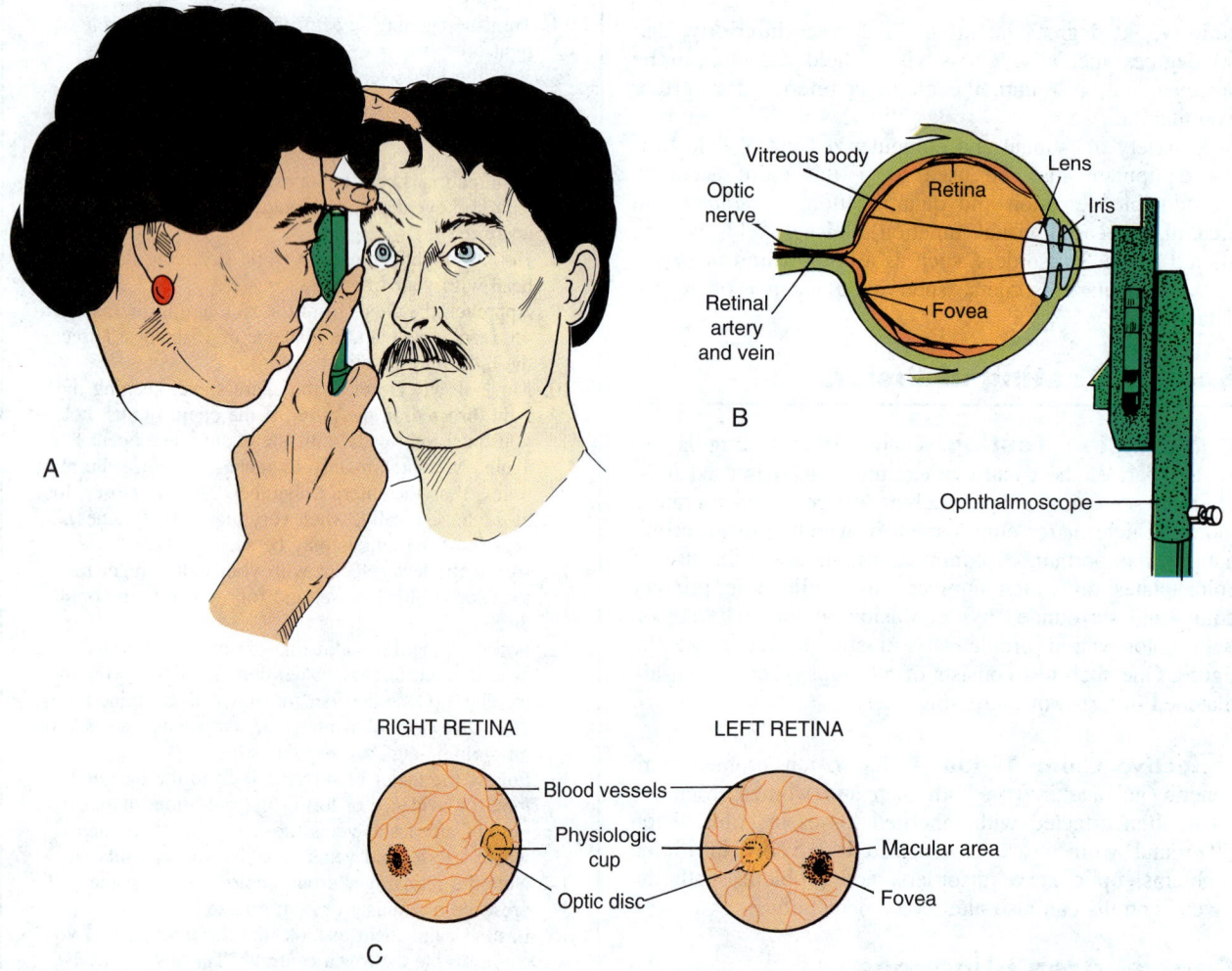

Figure 36–8. *A,* The examiner uses the right hand to hold the ophthalmoscope to the right eye to examine the client's right eye. The examiner uses the left hand and left eye when examining the client's left eye. Note the positioning of the examiner's free hand, which is placed to steady the client's head and to slightly retract the eyebrow. *B,* The examiner sees what appears in the angle of light through the viewing aperture. *C,* The actual area of retina visualized depends on the dilation of the pupil. Note the structures that may be examined.

nous (AV) ratio, narrowed arteries, widened veins, pinched-off vessels, abnormal arterial light reflex, excessive tortuosity, numerous AV nickings, exudates, white patches, and focal hemorrhage.

Indirect Ophthalmoscopy

Indirect ophthalmoscopy enables the examiner to obtain a stereoscopic picture over a large area of the retina. The light source comes from a head-mounted light. The examiner holds a convex lens in front of the client's eye, and through a viewing device attached to the headband, sees an inverted reversed image. The indirect ophthalmoscope has the advantage of binocular vision with depth perception for the examiner and permits a wider field of view.

Tonometry

Tonometry is the method of measuring intraocular fluid pressure using calibrated instruments that indent or flatten the corneal apex. The eye can be thought of as an enclosed compartment through which there is a constant circulation of aqueous humor. The aqueous humor maintains the shape of the eye with a relatively uniform pressure within the globe. As the pressure increases, the eye becomes firmer and a greater force is required to cause the same amount of indentation. Pressures between 8 and 21 mm Hg are considered within the normal range.

The two most common types of tonometers are the Schiøtz and applanation. The Schiøtz tonometer (Fig. 36–9) is a portable handheld instrument that may be used in an office, clinic, emergency room, operating room, or at the bedside. It measures the amount of corneal indentation produced by a preset weight. The softer the eye, the more a given weight will be able to indent the cornea. The examiner first anesthetizes the cornea with a topical anesthetic eye drop. With the client in a supine position and looking straight upward, the Schiøtz tonometer is placed directly on the cornea. A conversion chart is used to translate the scale reading into millimeters of mercury.

An applanation tonometer, which may either be a hand-held model or one that is attached to a slit-lamp microscope, measures the amount of force required to flatten the corneal apex by a standard amount. Anesthetic eye drops are also used prior to this examination method.

Intraocular pressure is noted in the client record with a large *T*. The top number indicates the pressure in the right eye and the bottom number indicates the pressure in the left eye.

Slit-Lamp Examination

The slit-lamp microscope is used to illuminate and examine the anterior segment of the eye under magnification. A linear slit beam of incandescent light is projected onto the globe, illuminating an optical cross-section of the anterior chamber. The angle of illumination, length, width, and intensity of the light may be adjusted. The client is seated, and the head is stabilized by an adjustable chin rest and forehead strap. Details of the lid margins, lashes, conjunctiva, tear film, cornea, iris, lens, and aqueous humor can be studied. At the highest magnification setting, the abnormal presence of red or white blood cells in the

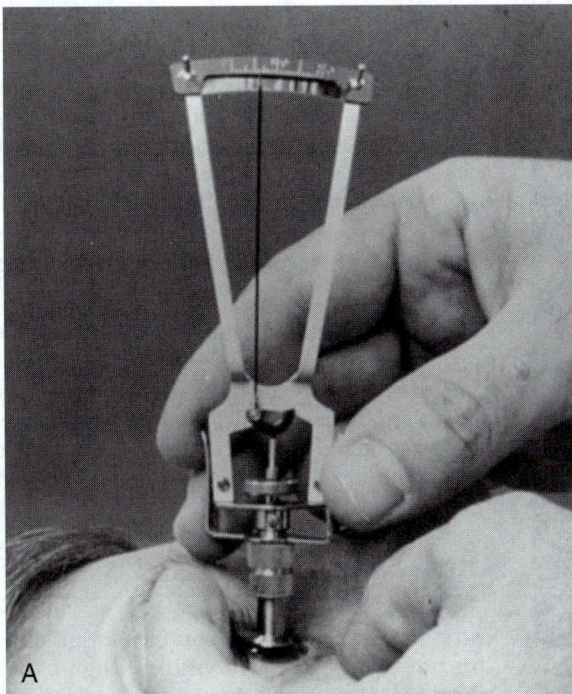
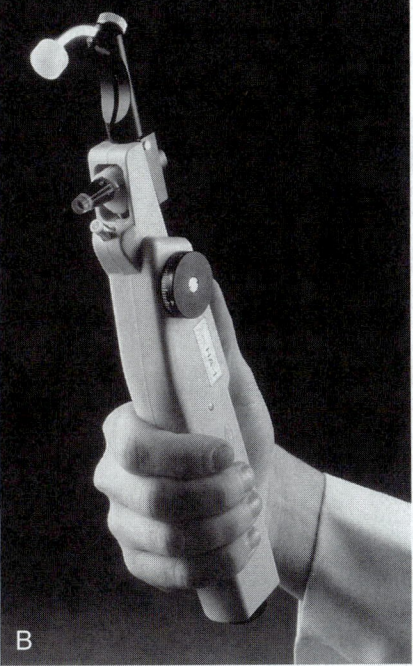

Figure 36–9. *A,* Schiøtz tonometry. *B,* A hand-held applanation tonometer. (*B,* courtesy of Kowa Optimed, Torrance, CA.)

aqueous humor may be visualized. The presence of protein (flare), called an *anterior chamber reaction,* that accompanies intraocular inflammation may also be detected. Normal aqueous humor is optically clear, without cells or flare. The presence of cells and flare is documented as 1 to 4+.

Fluorescein dye is often used in a slit-lamp examination to highlight corneal irregularities. Sterile paper strips containing fluorescein dye are wetted and touched against the inner surface of the lower lid, instilling the yellow dye into the tear film and onto the corneal surface. A blue filter is attached to the light beam, causing the dye to fluoresce. The dye highlights defects in the cornea.

In addition to the applanation tonometer, several other devices may be attached to the slit lamp to expand the scope of the examination. A gonioscope provides visualization of the anterior chamber angle. The Hruby lens permits examination of the vitreous body and fundus. A pachymeter is an instrument used to measure the thickness of the cornea and the anterior chamber.

Diagnostic Tests

Fundus Photography

Special retinal cameras are used to document fine details of the fundus for study and future comparison. One of the most common applications is the evaluation of insidious optic nerve changes in clients with glaucoma. Photographs are compared over time to identify subtle changes in disc shape and color (Fig. 36–10).

Specular Micrography

Specular micrography is a photographic technique used to count cells of the corneal endothelium. A camera is focused on the endothelial layer, and the area is magnified 200 times; the number of cells per square inch is counted. This layer of the cornea is one cell thick. Cells in this

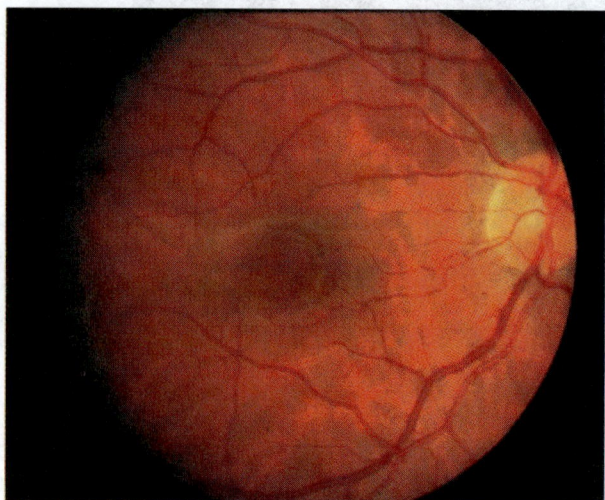

Figure 36–10. A normal fundus. (Courtesy of Ophthalmic Photography at the University of Michigan W. K. Kellogg Eye Center, Ann Arbor.)

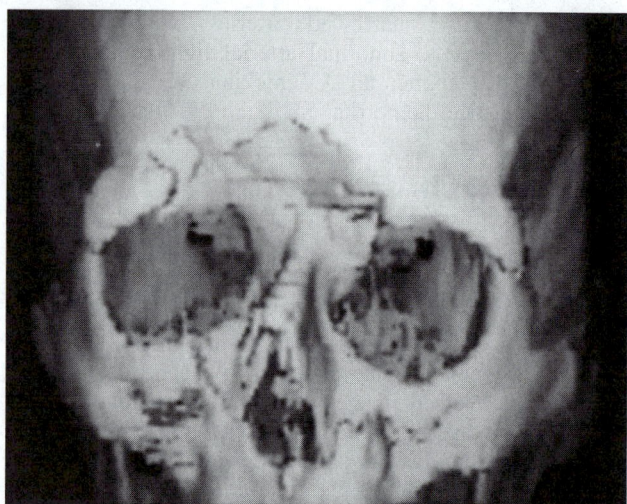

Figure 36–11. A magnetic resonance imaging (MRI) scan showing massive facial fractures. Note the three-dimensional appearance obtained with MRI.

layer do not reproduce, but rather expand to fill gaps in the endothelium. The number, or lack of number, of cells may indicate healing potential.

Exophthalmometry

The exophthalmometer is an instrument designed to measure the forward protrusion of the eye. This instrument provides a method of evaluating and recording the progression and regression of the prominence of the eye in disorders such as thyroid disease and tumors of the orbit.

Ophthalmic Radiography

X-ray study, tomography, the computed tomographic (CT) scan are useful in the evaluation of orbital and intracranial conditions. Common abnormalities evaluated by these methods include neoplasms, inflammatory masses, fractures, and extraocular muscle enlargement associated with Graves' disease. Radiography is also useful in the detection of foreign bodies.

Magnetic Resonance Imaging

Magnetic resonance imaging (MRI) has the advantage of not exposing the client to ionizing radiation. Also, multidimensional views are possible without repositioning the client (Fig. 36–11). MRI is used to image edema, areas of demyelination, and vascular lesions. However, the availability of MRI equipment is often limited and the examination takes longer.

Ultrasonography

Ultrasonography uses the principle of sonar to study structures not directly visible. High-frequency sound waves are transmitted through a probe placed directly on the eyeball. As the sound waves bounce back off the

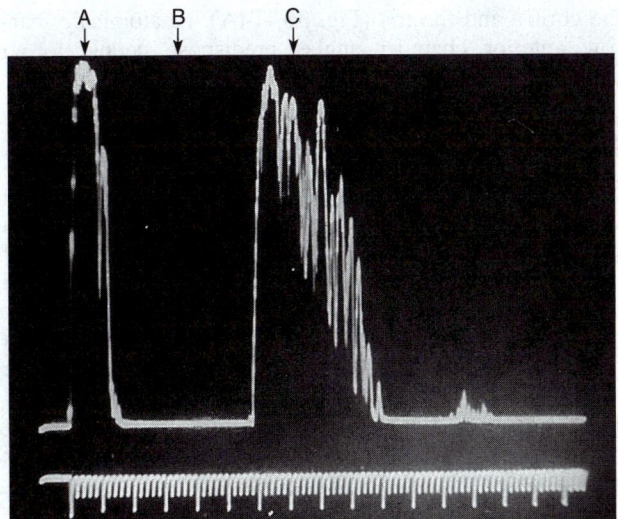

Figure 36–12. A normal A-scan ultrasound of the eye. The sound beam is aimed in a straight line, and echoes are displayed as spikes. The amplitude depends on the density of the reflecting tissue and perpendicularity of the probe. *A,* cornea and lens; *B,* clear vitreous; *C,* retina and choroid.

various tissue components, they are collected by a receiver that amplifies them on an oscilloscope screen. Sound waves derived from the most distal structures arrive last, having traveled the farthest (Fig. 36–12). A-scan ultrasonography is used to measure axial length, the distance from the cornea to the retina, to determine the refractive power of an intraocular lens in cataract surgery. B-scan ultrasonography may be used to evaluate the characteristics of a lesion, as well as its size and growth over time, or the presence of a foreign body.

Ophthalmodynamometry

Ophthalmodynamometry is a test that consists of exerting pressure on the sclera with a spring plunger while observing the central retinal vessels emerging from the disc through an ophthalmoscope. This instrument gives an approximate measurement of the relative pressures in the central retinal arteries and is an indirect method of assessing carotid arterial flow on either side. Ophthalmodynamometry is indicated in the neurologic evaluation of patients who complain of "blacking out" of vision in one eye *(amaurosis),* spells of weakness on one side of the body, or other symptoms of cerebral ischemia. A difference of more than 20% in the diastolic pressures between the two eyes suggests insufficiency of the carotid arterial system on the side with the lower pressure.

Electroretinography

An electrical potential exists between the cornea and retina of the eye. Because the retina is neurologic tissue, the normal retina exhibits certain electrical responses when stimulated by light. Electroretinography (ERG) measures the normal change in electrical potential of the eye caused by a diffuse flash of light. For this test, electrodes

incorporated into a contact lens are placed directly on the anesthetized eye. Eye movements disrupt the values of the test, so the client must be able to fixate on a target while keeping the eyes still. A normal ERG signifies functional integrity of the retina. Examples of retinal diseases that may be evaluated with ERG include retinitis pigmentosa (progressive degeneration of photoreceptor cells), massive ischemia, disseminated infection, or toxic effects from drugs or chemicals.

Visual Evoked Response

Visual evoked response (VER) is similar to ERG in that it also measures the electrical potential resulting from a visual stimulus. The entire visual pathway from the retina to the cortex may be evaluated in this examination through the placement of electrodes on the scalp. Reduced speed of neuronal conduction, as with demyelination in optic neuritis, results in an abnormal VER. Retinal or optic nerve disease may be diagnosed by stimulating each eye separately.

Fluorescein Angiography

Fundus photography is enhanced by the use of fluorescein dye whose molecules emit green light when stimulated by blue light. For this examination, the client is seated in front of a retina camera following pupillary dilation. A small amount of fluorescein dye is injected into an antecubital vein. The dye circulates throughout the body before eventually being excreted by the kidneys. As the dye passes through the retinal and choroidal circulation, it can be visualized and photographed because of its ability to fluoresce (Fig. 36–13). A rapid sequence of pictures captures the initial rapid perfusion of the retinal and choroidal vessels. Later photos may demonstrate the gradual leakage of dye from abnormal vessels. Changes in blood flow, ischemia, and hemorrhage may be detected. Because it can so precisely delineate areas of abnormality, it is an essential guide for planning laser treatment of retinal vascular disease.

You may administer the intravenous fluorescein dye injection under an ophthalmologist's direction. It is important to first assess the client's general health status and identify any allergies. Allergic reactions to other dye injections (i.e., for intravenous pyelogram [IVP] or cholangiogram) should be considered before the fluorescein injection. Diphenhydramine (Benadryl) may be prescribed prophylactically. Although anaphylactic shock is a rare occurrence, emergency equipment should be located nearby. Occasionally, clients have a vasovagal response to the dye that includes vertigo, nausea, and momentary loss of consciousness. A consent for the procedure should be obtained. Explain that during the injection, the client may experience a warm sensation. The client will also hear the mechanics of the camera taking rapid-sequence photographs and experience bright flashes of light. After the examination, encourage the client to increase intake of fluids because the dye is excreted through the kidneys. During the next 24 hours, the urine will be a yellow color and light-complexioned clients may experience a

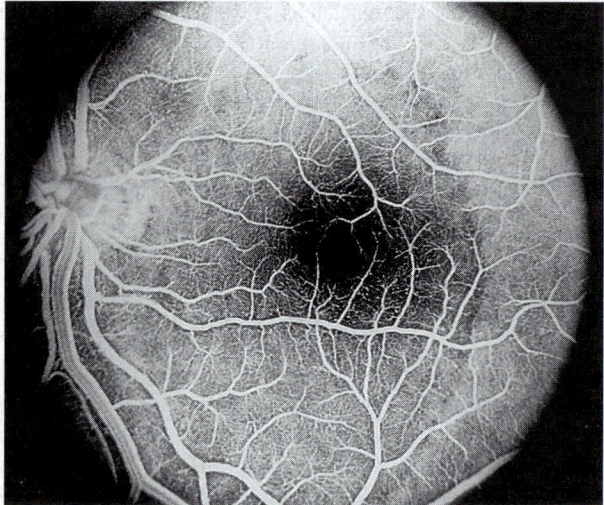

Figure 36–13. A normal fluorescein angiogram. The normal pattern of fluorescein angiography can be divided into three phases: The *filling phase* (pictured) takes 8 to 20 seconds. The *recirculation phase* starts 0.5 second after the filling phase and lasts 3 to 5 minutes. The *late phase* lasts 30 to 60 minutes. Photographs are taken prior to injection, at half-second intervals for 20 seconds, and then at intervals of 5 minutes.

temporary yellow tint to the skin that will fade within a few hours as the dye is excreted. Because the pupils are dilated before the examination, it may be necessary to wear dark glasses for several hours.

Nursing Care of Clients with Eye Disorders

Glaucoma

Glaucoma includes a group of ocular disorders characterized by increased intraocular pressure, optic nerve atrophy, and visual field loss. The individual response to intraocular pressure varies. Thus, some people sustain damage from relatively low pressures while others sustain no damage from high pressure. The degree of increased pressure that causes ocular damage is not the same in every eye, and some individuals may tolerate a pressure for long periods of time that would rapidly blind another.

It is estimated that over 50,000 persons in the United States are blind as a result of glaucoma. The incidence of glaucoma is about 1.5%, and in blacks, between the ages of 45 and 65, the prevalence is at least five times that of whites in the same age group. In most cases, blindness can be prevented if treatment is begun early.

Classification

Many terms are used to describe the various types of glaucoma. The terms *primary* and *secondary glaucoma* refer to whether the cause is the disease alone or due to another condition. *Acute* and *chronic* refer to the onset and duration of the disorder. The terms *open* (wide) and *closed* (narrow) describe the width of the angle between

the cornea and the iris (Fig. 36–14A). Anatomically narrow anterior chamber angles predispose people to an acute onset of angle-closure glaucoma.

■ Primary Open-Angle Glaucoma

Primary open-angle glaucoma is the most common form of glaucoma. It is a multifactorial disorder that is often genetically determined, bilateral, insidious in onset, and slow to progress. This type of glaucoma is often referred to as the "thief in the night" because there are no early clinical manifestations alerting the client that vision is being lost. Aqueous humor flow is slowed or stopped due to obstruction by the trabecular meshwork (Fig. 36–14B).

■ Angle-Closure Glaucoma

An acute attack of angle-closure glaucoma can develop only in an eye in which the anterior chamber angle is anatomically narrow. The attack occurs because of a sudden blockage of the anterior angle by the base of the iris (Fig. 36–14C).

■ Low-Tension Glaucoma

Low-tension glaucoma resembles primary open-angle glaucoma. The angle is normal, the optic nerves are cupped, and the visual fields show characteristic glaucomatous effects (peripheral vision deficits). These changes, however, develop in the presence of statistically normal intraocular pressures. Although the pressure readings are in the normal range, treatment is indicated to lower the pressure even further to avoid progressive optic nerve damage and visual field loss.

■ Secondary Glaucoma

Increased intraocular pressure may occur as a postoperative complication. Edematous tissue may inhibit the outflow of aqueous humor through the trabecular meshwork. Delayed healing of corneal wound edges may result in epithelial cell growth into the anterior chamber.

■ Congenital Glaucoma

Congenital glaucoma is rare. It is the result of developmental abnormalities of anterior chamber angle structures, the cornea, and the iris.

Etiology and Risk Factors

Approximately 90% of primary glaucoma occurs in people with open angles. Because there are no early warning symptoms, it is imperative that regular ophthalmic examinations include tonometry and assessment of the optic nerve head (disc). The most common cause of chronic open-angle glaucoma is degenerative change in the trabecular meshwork, resulting in decreased outflow of aqueous humor.

The cause of low-tension glaucoma is not known. Secondary glaucoma may occur as a result of trauma. Lens

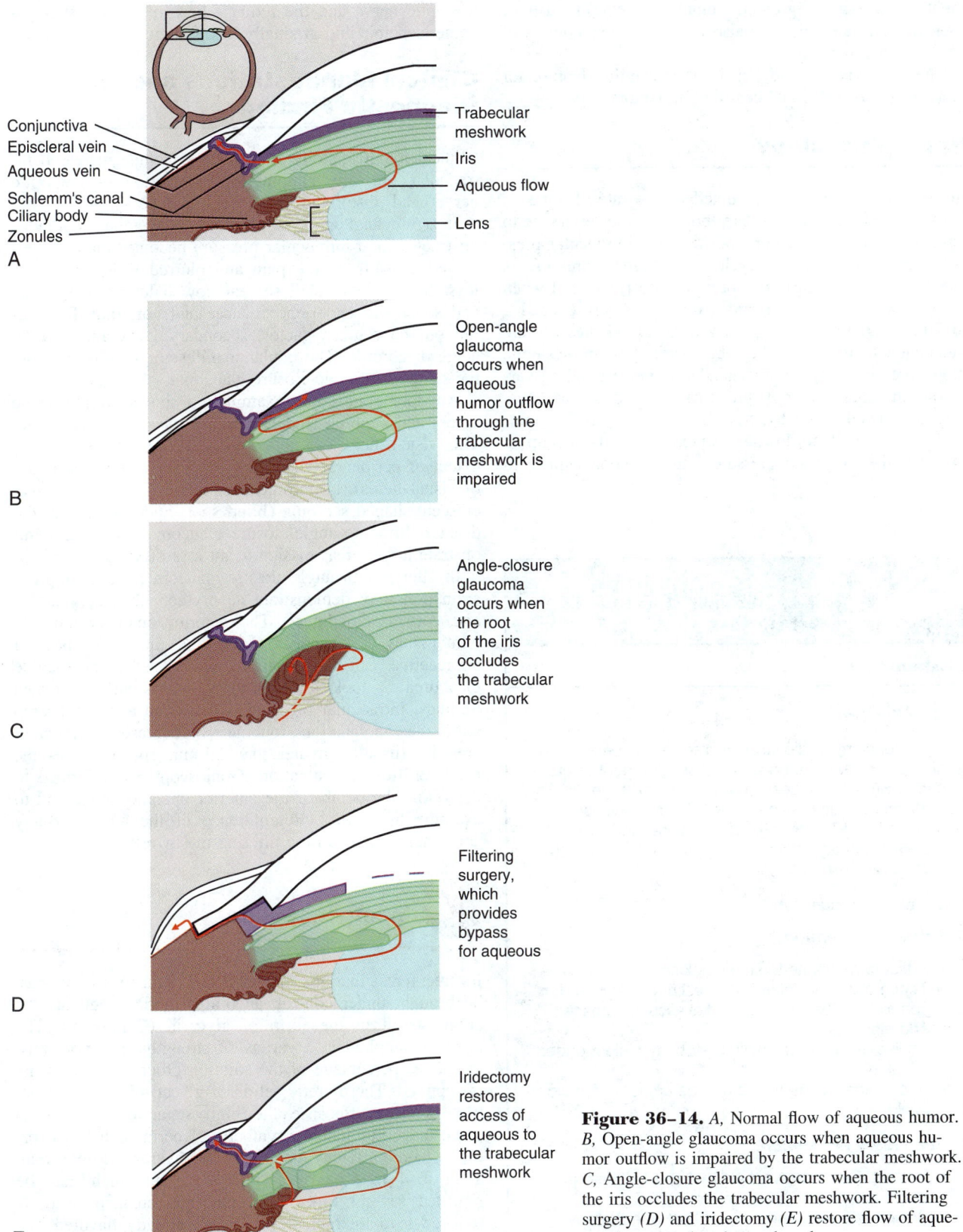

Figure 36–14. *A*, Normal flow of aqueous humor. *B*, Open-angle glaucoma occurs when aqueous humor outflow is impaired by the trabecular meshwork. *C*, Angle-closure glaucoma occurs when the root of the iris occludes the trabecular meshwork. Filtering surgery *(D)* and iridectomy *(E)* restore flow of aqueous through trabecular meshwork.

displacement, hemorrhage into the anterior chamber, lacerations, and contusions can disrupt the flow pattern of aqueous humor.

Congenital glaucoma is caused by an arrest of develop-

ment of the anterior chamber angle structures at about the seventh month of fetal life.

Other causes of increased intraocular pressure include inflammation of filtering structures in uveitis. Encroachment by a rapidly growing tumor and chronic use of topical corticosteroids may also produce the symptoms of open-angle glaucoma.

The Risk Factors and Levels of Prevention feature for glaucoma lists additional contributing factors.

Pathophysiology

Intraocular pressure is determined by the rate of aqueous humor production in the ciliary body and the resistance to outflow of aqueous humor from the eye. Intraocular pressure varies with diurnal cycles (the highest pressure is usually on awakening) and body position (increased when lying down). Normal variations do not usually exceed 2 to 3 mm Hg. Intraocular pressure and blood pressure are independent of each other, but variations in systemic blood pressure may be associated with corresponding variations in intraocular pressure. Increased intraocular pressure may result from hyperproduction of aqueous humor or obstruction of outflow. As aqueous fluid builds up in the eye, the increased pressure inhibits blood supply to the optic nerve and the retina. These delicate tissues become ischemic and gradually lose function.

Clinical Manifestations and Diagnostic Findings

Clinical manifestations of glaucoma include increased intraocular pressure, cupping or indentation of the optic nerve head (disc), and visual field defects.

In acute angle-closure glaucoma, the aqueous flow is obstructed, and intraocular pressure becomes markedly elevated, causing severe pain and blurred vision or vision loss. Some clients will see rainbow halos around lights, and some will experience nausea and vomiting. Depending on the primary factor, secondary glaucoma may be acute or chronic. The ocular manifestations, however, are the same as in angle-closure glaucoma.

An ophthalmoscopic examination shows atrophy (pale color) and cupping (indentation) of the optic nerve head. The visual field examination is used to determine the extent of peripheral vision loss (see the earlier discussion of visual fields). In chronic open-angle glaucoma, a small crescent-shaped scotoma (blind spot) appears early in the disease. In acute angle-closure glaucoma, the fields demonstrate larger areas of significant loss of vision.

In clients with angle-closure glaucoma, a slit-lamp examination may demonstrate an erythematous conjunctiva and corneal cloudiness. The anterior chamber aqueous humor may also appear turbid and the pupil may be nonreactive. Slit-lamp examination is used in open-angle glaucoma to look for secondary causes and associated findings. Intraocular pressure is measured at the slit lamp with the applanation tonometer. Increased intraocular pressure (usually greater than 23 mm Hg) indicates the need for further evaluation. Gonioscopy is performed to determine the depth of the anterior chamber angle and to examine the entire circumference of the angle for any abnormal changes in the filtering meshwork.

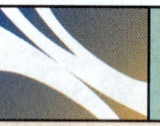

RISK FACTORS AND LEVELS OF PREVENTION

Glaucoma

Risk Factors

Hypertension, cardiovascular disease, diabetes, and obesity are associated with the development of glaucoma. Smoking, ingestion of caffeine or large amounts of fluids, alcohol, illicit drugs, corticosteroids, altered hormone levels, posture, and eye movements may cause varying transient increases in intraocular pressure.

Levels of Prevention

Primary Prevention

- Encourage clients to stop smoking.
- Teach clients to follow the prescribed regimen for control of hypertension, cardiovascular disease, and diabetes.
- Advise clients to maintain their body weight under 120% of ideal.
- Encourage clients to avoid large amounts of fluid intake.

Secondary Prevention

- Instruct clients to avoid alcohol and caffeine several hours before an eye examination.
- Review the pros and cons of hormone therapy.

Tertiary Prevention

- Teach clients to avoid activities that include prolonged bending over.
- Teach clients to avoid Valsalva's maneuver.

Emergency Care

In emergent situations in which intraocular pressure must be brought under control, an oral osmotic agent may be administered in the form of glycerin (Osmoglyn). The agent is supplied in a variety of strengths, and you must check the percentage of the solution ordered against what is supplied. The diuretic action of glycerin lowers intraocular pressure. Because the high sugar content effects some diabetic clients, a synthetic glycerin such as isosorbide (Isomotic) may be used. The average dose for an adult is 4 to 6 oz of a 50% solution, which may be repeated several times until the intraocular pressure is reduced to a tolerable level. If not already flavored, the extreme sweetness and viscosity may be made more palatable by mixing the glycerin with equal parts of a tart juice such as lemon. Serving the solution over cracked ice also makes it more palatable. After 3 hours, encourage the intake of water and other liquids to prevent mild-to-moderate dehydration and also make sure the client can get to the bathroom during the diuretic phase. Intravenous mannitol, a potent intravenous osmotic diuretic, may be used to arrest extremely high intraocular pressure. It should only be used for the management of a glaucoma crisis under close nursing and medical supervision. The client's cardiovascular and renal status should be carefully evaluated before treatment is begun. Document baseline vital signs before the treatment and frequently during the infusion. Because mannitol has a tendency to crystallize, the bottle may need to be warmed before it is administered. The vial should not be used while crystals are present. An in-line micropore filter should also be used to prevent infusion of any crystal particles.

Acute and Subacute Care

■ Medical Management

The goal of management is to facilitate the outflow of aqueous humor through remaining channels. This is achieved through the use of the following:

● Topical miotics, which constrict the pupil and increase outflow
● Topical epinephrine, which also increases outflow
● Topical beta-blockers or alpha-adrenergics, which suppress the secretion of aqueous humor
● Oral carbonic anahydrase inhibitors, which also reduce the production of aqueous humor.

Figure 36–15 shows the sites of action for various drugs. Also shown in the figure are sites of action for drugs used to treat open-angle glaucoma:

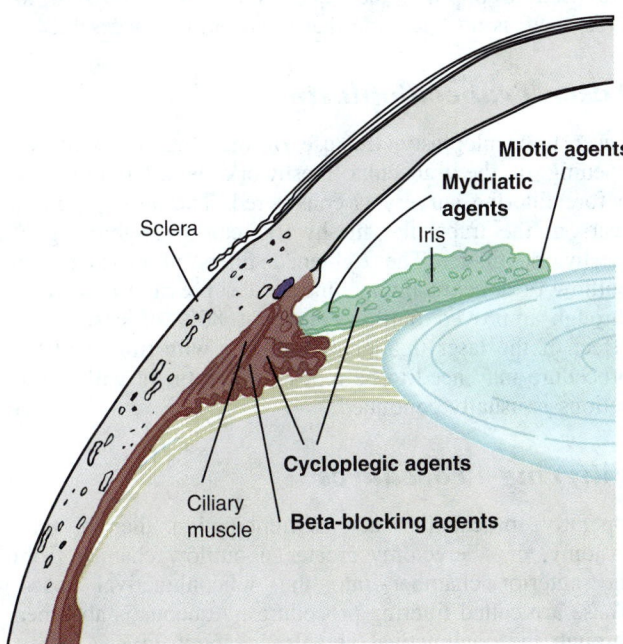

Figure 36–15. Sites of action of mydriatic, beta-blocking, cycloplegic, and miotic agents.

● Mydriatric agents dilate the pupil by inhibiting the parasympathetic nervous system and blocking acetylcholine.
● Cycloplegic agents paralyze the ciliary muscle and the dilator muscle of the iris, causing both pupillary dilation and paralysis of accommodation.

These agents, which dilate the pupil, would be contraindicated in narrow-angle glaucoma, because further dilation of the pupil restricts outflow of aqueous humor.

■ Nursing Management of the Medical Client

Assessment

The nursing assessment of the client includes establishing demographic data of age and race because open-angle glaucoma occurs most often in clients over 40 and in blacks. It is also important to determine whether there is a family history of glaucoma or other eye problems, or if the client has had ocular surgery, infections, or trauma. An accurate list of current medications is imperative because over-the-counter medications such as antihistamines may dilate the pupil, putting the client at risk for angle-closure glaucoma. A history of allergic reactions, particularly to medications or dyes, should always be noted.

Ask the client to describe any changes in vision. Although the symptoms of primary open-angle glaucoma are insidious, the client may describe blind spots in the periphery or an overall decreased visual acuity with loss of contrast sensitivity. Decreased uncorrectable visual acuity usually occurs when there has been irreversible damage to the optic nerve.

If it has been previously established that the client has visual loss from glaucoma, assess how the client is coping with the loss of vision. Although individuals adapt to the loss of vision in different ways, people usually manifest grief and loss at any stage of the disease process. Clients may be understandably anxious during examinations because it may be discovered that further vision loss has occurred. Assess the client's perception of glaucoma and the effect it has on his or her life. Assist the client in identifying effective coping skills the client may have used in the past.

Diagnosis, Planning, Implementation

Sensory/Perceptual Alterations (Visual). The increased intraocular pressure alters the function of the optic nerve, decreasing vision. The nursing diagnosis *Visual Sensory/Perceptual Alterations (visual) related to recent loss of vision* may be appropriate if the loss of vision is a new problem for the client.

Planning: Expected Outcomes. The client will maintain as much functional vision as possible. He or she will report no further loss of vision and adapt to any visual loss, demonstrate an ability to perform activities of daily living (ADLs), and recognize clinical manifestations of complications.

Implementation. Reassure the client that although some vision has been lost and cannot be restored, further loss may be prevented by adhering to the treatment plan.

Anticipatory Grieving. Vision lost to glaucoma is irreparable. Even with the most aggressive medical and surgical management, it may still be progressive. A typical nursing diagnosis would therefore be *Anticipatory Grieving related to loss of vision.* Significant loss of vision represents the need for compromise and adaptation for both the client and the family.

Planning: Expected Outcomes. The client will express grief, describe the meaning of the loss, and share the grief with significant others.

Implementation. Assess the causative and contributing factors that may delay the work of grieving and promote family cohesiveness.

The social stigma of blindness underlies the anxiety that clients experience with actual or potential loss of vision. Total loss of vision isolates an individual within a different reality. Although most clients are successfully rehabilitated, there are some losses that are permanent. There are also individuals who, for a variety of reasons, remain socially isolated. The image of a blind person who is pitied and must accept the charity of others is disturbing.

Not all jobs and work environments are adaptable for a person who is visually impaired. People with actual or potential loss of vision may be faced with barriers in their vocations that force an unwanted change. Age may be a major factor in the person's ability to meet this challenge.

Self-esteem is closely related to the roles of the person in his or her particular life-style. Loss of control in personal, family, and work situations can be devastating. The issue of dependence versus independence may also be a factor in the person's ability to cope with the stressors of vision loss.

Risk for Ineffective Management of Therapeutic Regimen (Individuals). The regimen for eye drops and oral medications to control glaucoma ranges from simple to complex. This diagnosis should be stated as *Risk for Ineffective Management of Therapeutic Regimen (Individuals) related to complex medication schedule.*

Planning: Expected Outcomes. The client will describe the disease process and the regimen for disease control. The client will also relate how the medication routine will be incorporated into the ADLs.

Implementation. The client may need to instill as many as three or four different eye drops from one to six times a day. Constricting eye drops are usually prescribed four times a day and beta-blockers are usually prescribed every 12 hours; however, there may be a need to prescribe eye drops every 4 to 6 hours. The schedule is designed to provide the best possible control of intraocular pressure around the clock. Medications are an integral part of the treatment and care of a client with glaucoma, so nursing interventions must be directed at the client's ability to understand and comply with prescribed therapy. First determine the client's current level of knowledge and then provide necessary information about glaucoma and its treatment in understandable terms. Diagrams may be helpful to the client and significant others. Because treatment for glaucoma is often complex, involving both oral and topical ophthalmic medications, review a written plan of care in large print with the client and family. In order to maximize compliance, the plan of care must fit into the client's life-style.

The administration of eye drops is a critical component of self-care for the client with glaucoma. After instructing the client and family on the technique of instillation, validate the client or family's ability to properly instill eye drops by asking for a demonstration. The discussion of side effects of medications is also very important. Table 36–1 lists additional guidelines for teaching the client about eye drops.

Evaluation

Independent self-care is the area for evaluation in the medically managed client. Evaluate the client's ability for self-care (a short-term outcome) and compliance with the medical regimen (a long-term outcome).

Modifications for Elderly Clients

Elderly clients with arthritic or shaking hands have difficulty instilling their own eye drops. Instruct the elderly client to lie down on a bed or sofa. Tilting the head back can lead to loss of balance. The eye-drop regimen for glaucoma requires accurate timing. Elderly clients may need visual reminders such as a checkoff list, and may also need to use a timer or an alarm clock to help them remember.

■ Surgical Management

When maximal medical therapy has failed to halt the progression of visual field loss and optic nerve damage, surgical intervention is recommended. Many procedures are used to improve the aqueous humor outflow; however, there is no operation that is uniformly successful.

Laser Trabeculoplasty

Laser trabeculoplasty, the use of the laser to create an opening in the trabecular meshwork, is often indicated before filtering surgery is considered. The laser produces scars in the trabecular meshwork, causing tightening of meshwork fibers. The tightened fibers allow increased outflow of aqueous humor. Intraocular pressure is reduced through improved outflow in about 80% of cases. The effect of the laser treatment decreases with time, and the procedure may need to be repeated. Treatment with medications is usually continued.

Filtering Procedures

Operative procedures such as trephination, thermal sclerostomy, or sclerectomy create an outflow channel from the anterior chamber into the subconjunctival space. These are called filtering procedures. Aqueous is absorbed through the conjunctival vessels. In about 25% of cases, the opening closes because of scar tissue formation, and reoperation is necessary.

Table 36–1. Teaching the Client About Eye Drops for Glaucoma

Medication	Usual Frequency	Teaching Aspects
Pilocarpine hydrochloride	3–4 times/day	A miotic, causes pupillary constriction to open Schlemm's canal Space out the administration, beginning on awakening and ending at bedtime May cause blurred vision after instillation Browache has been reported Consider the use of thin gel strips (a timed-release form) to improve compliance
Timolol maleate and other beta-blockers (e.g., levobunolol)	Every 12 hours	Decreases production of aqueous humor Space out administration Contraindicated in clients with asthma and chronic obstructive pulmonary disease Assess for bradycardia prior to administration
Carbonic anhydrase inhibitors (e.g., acetazolamide)		Inhibits the production of aqueous humor Available as tablets and in sustained-release capsules Side effects include anorexia and tingling in the hands and feet

A more common filtering procedure called trabeculectomy reduces some of the complications of surgery but achieves a somewhat lesser reduction in pressure. A half-thickness scleral flap is loosely sutured over the opening, through which the fluid escapes, again resulting in subconjunctival absorption of aqueous humor (Fig. 36–14C).

Glaucoma filtering procedures differ from other surgical procedures in that the goal is to prevent the newly created opening for outflow from closing. Filtering procedures are less successful in young and black clients because of their increased ability to produce thicker scar tissue. Topical corticosteroids are used postoperatively because their anti-inflammatory action inhibits the proliferation of fibroblasts at the surgical site.

5-Fluorouracil (5-FU), mitomycin, and other antimetabolites are sometimes injected subconjunctivally because they also inhibit fibroblast proliferation and thereby reduce postoperative scarring.

Ocular implantation devices such as the Molteno implant or Baerveldt seton are sometimes used to control the flow of aqueous humor in patients with complicated types of glaucoma. A device is sutured to the outer surface of the eyeball on the sclera between the ocular muscles. A tiny tube is inserted under the scleral flap directly into the anterior chamber that directs the flow of aqueous humor more posteriorly than in the more common filtering procedures.

Iridectomy

Iridectomy is the creation of a new route for the flow of aqueous humor to the trabecular meshwork. The laser is used to create the new opening (Fig. 36–14E).

Cyclodestructive Procedures

When other surgical procedures have failed, cyclocryotherapy (the application of a freezing tip) or cyclophoto-

coagulation may be used to damage the ciliary body and decrease the production of aqueous.

■ Nursing Management of the Surgical Client

Preoperative Care

Preoperative nursing care includes preparing the client for a surgical procedure that may be performed in either an outpatient or inpatient setting.

Laser therapy is most often performed in a clinic or office using a topical anesthetic. Explain not only the expected outcome of the procedure but also the popping sounds and flashing lights that the client will experience. Inform the client that there will be a waiting period (usually 1–2 hours) after the procedure to evaluate a possible rise in intraocular pressure. Because of the instability of the intraocular pressure, the client should arrange to have a friend or family member accompany him or her to provide transportation.

Postoperative Care

Postoperative nursing care may need to be accomplished in a matter of hours or days, depending on the expected length of stay. When the client returns from the operating room, the eye is covered with a patch and a metal or plastic shield for protection. Instruct the client not to lie on the operative side to avoid pressure on the operative site. When the effects of perioperative sedation have diminished, the client may walk about and eat as desired.

Complications

Frequent monitoring of intraocular pressure is necessary because the surgical site is microscopic. When healing is delayed, the anterior chamber may not re-form. Intraocular pressure readings may be 2 to 5 mm Hg, or the anterior chamber may even be flat. If the anterior chamber fails to re-form, another surgical procedure may be required. On the contrary, the wound may seal tight, causing intraocular pressure to rise above normal levels; this also requires reoperation.

Outcomes

The goal of surgical or medical intervention is to maintain intraocular pressure within a range that will prevent further damage to the optic nerve. In either case, the client should maintain a strict regimen of self-care.

Community and Self-Care

The plan for discharge must include client education and evaluation of the home environment and available care. Client and family education for postoperative eye care includes a review of the following:

- Manifestations of infection (redness, swelling, drainage, blurred vision, pain)
- Manifestations of increased intraocular pressure (unrelieved pain, nausea, decrease in vision)
- The rationale for eye protection (shield or eyeglasses at all times)
- Medications and eye-drop instillation technique
- Return visit date and time

Instruct clients to carefully clean the area around the eye with warm tap water and a clean washcloth. Special eyewash solutions of balanced saline may be used, but are not necessary. Eyewash should not be applied directly to the eye. It is important that the client understand that rubbing or applying pressure over the closed eye could damage healing tissue. Although many clients with glaucoma may undergo repeated surgical procedures, the above-mentioned information should be carefully reviewed each time.

Because the level of independence varies with individual clients, use information supplied by the client and family or friends to assess how much support may be needed. Referrals may need to be made to visiting nurses for home healthcare or social services for assistance with rehabilitation or finances. Assist the client and family to plan for housekeeping and meal preparation, safety in the home environment, transportation, and assistance with eye care. The family physician should also be informed of the medical or surgical treatment.

Cataracts

A *cataract* is an opacity of the lens. Although cataract formation is usually associated with aging, cataracts may have a variety of other causes. Some degree of cataract formation is to be expected in most persons over age 70. Over a million cataract operations are now being performed annually in the United States. A person with a normal lifespan is more likely to undergo a cataract operation than any other major surgical procedure.

Etiology and Risk Factors

The cumulative exposure to ultraviolet light over the lifespan is the single most important risk factor in the development of cataracts. People who live at high altitudes or who work in bright sunlight such as commercial fishermen appear to experience cataract formation earlier in life. Glass blowers and welders without eye protection are also at higher risk.

■ Age-Related Cataracts

The most common cataract is age-related or senile cataract. Worldwide, it is the primary cause of reduced vision and blindness. Senile cataracts usually begin around the age of 50 and consist of cortical, nuclear, or posterior subcapsular opacities. These three forms may coexist in various combinations.

In cortical cataracts, spokelike opacifications are found in the periphery of the lens. They progress slowly, infrequently involve the visual axis, and often do not result in severe loss of vision.

Nuclear sclerotic cataracts are a result of a progressive yellowing and hardening of the central lens (nucleus). Most people over the age of 70 have some degree of nuclear sclerosis.

Posterior subcapsular opacities occur centrally on the posterior lens capsule. They cause visual loss early in their development because they lie directly on the visual axis.

■ Other Forms of Cataracts

Cataracts may develop as a result of many other ocular, systemic, and congenital disorders. Systemic disorders include: diabetes, tetany, myotonic dystrophy, neurodermatitis, galactosemia, Lowe's syndrome, Werner's syndrome, and Down syndrome. Intraocular disorders that may be associated with cataract are iridocyclitis, retinitis, retinal detachment, and onchocerciasis. Blunt trauma, lacerations, foreign bodies, radiation, exposure to infrared light, and chronic use of corticosteroids may also result in cataracts. Infections (German measles, mumps, hepatitis, poliomyelitis, chickenpox, infectious mononucleosis) during the first trimester of pregnancy may cause congenital cataracts.

Pathophysiology

Cataract formation is characterized chemically by a reduction in oxygen uptake and an initial increase in water content followed by dehydration. Sodium and calcium contents are increased. Potassium, ascorbic acid, and protein are decreased. The protein in the lens undergoes numerous age-related changes, including yellowing from formation of fluorescent compounds and molecular changes. These changes, along with the photoabsorption of ultraviolet radiation throughout life, suggest that cataracts may be caused by a photochemical process.

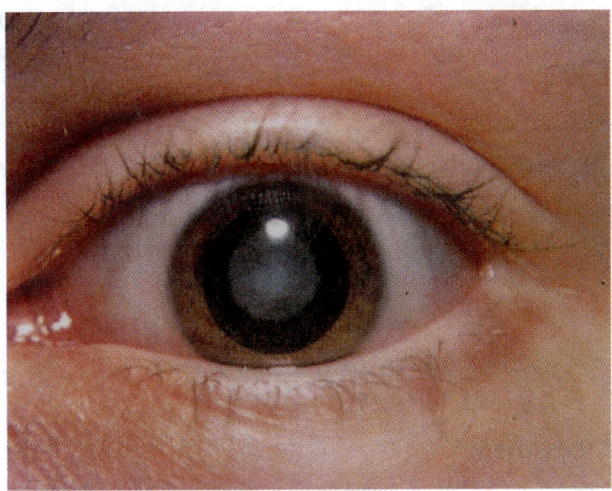

Figure 36–16. The cloudy appearance of a lens affected by cataract. (Courtesy of Ophthalmic Photography at the University of Michigan W. K. Kellogg Eye Center, Ann Arbor.)

Cataracts progress through the following clinical stages of development:

- *Immature cataracts* are not completely opaque, and some light is transmitted through them, allowing useful vision.
- *Mature cataracts* are completely opaque. The former term for this stage was *ripe.* Vision is significantly reduced.
- *Intumescent cataracts* are those in which the lens absorbs water and increases in size. The lens may be mature or immature. The increase in size may result in glaucoma.
- *Hypermature cataracts* are those in which the lens proteins break down into short-chain polypeptides that leak out through the lens capsule. The pieces of protein are engulfed by macrophages, which may obstruct the trabecular meshwork, causing phacolytic glaucoma.

Clinical Manifestations and Diagnostic Findings

Clients experience blurred vision, sometimes monocular diplopia, photophobia, and glare. Clients usually see better in low light when the pupil is dilated, which allows for vision around a central opacity. There is no complaint of pain. A cloudy lens can be observed (Fig. 36–16).

A cataract should be suspected when the red reflex seen with the direct ophthalmoscope is distorted or absent. Although cataracts can usually be diagnosed easily with the direct ophthalmoscope, an accurate determination of the type and extent of the lens change requires a slit-lamp examination.

 Acute and Subacute Care

■ Surgical Management

There is no known medical treatment to prevent or reduce cataract formation.

The objective of cataract surgery is to remove the opacified lens. Over the last two decades, cataract surgery has improved dramatically as a result of the operating microscope, new instrumentation, improved suture material, smaller incisions, and refinement of the intraocular lens implant. The lens is surgically removed by an intracapsular or extracapsular procedure (Fig. 36–17).

Intracapsular cataract extraction (ICCE) consists of removing the lens, including the lens capsule. Extracapsular cataract extraction (ECCE) consists of removing the lens and the anterior portion of the lens capsule. The posterior lens capsule is left intact. Although intracapsular surgery is highly successful and still performed, extracapsular extraction is by far the most common procedure in the United States. The primary reason for performing extracapsular surgery is to allow the insertion of a posterior chamber intraocular lens inside the remaining capsule, which results in fewer postoperative complications.

Phacoemulsification is an extracapsular technique that uses ultrasound vibrations to break up the lens material. Pieces of the anterior lens capsule and the lens are removed by suction through the phacoemulsifier tip. This technique requires a much smaller incision in the eye and is often called the small incision technique. These small incisions require only one to three sutures, and in some cases, none at all. Wound healing in small incision surgery occurs at the same rate as in larger incision techniques.

Cataract surgery is usually performed under intravenous conscious sedation. The client is given an intravenous

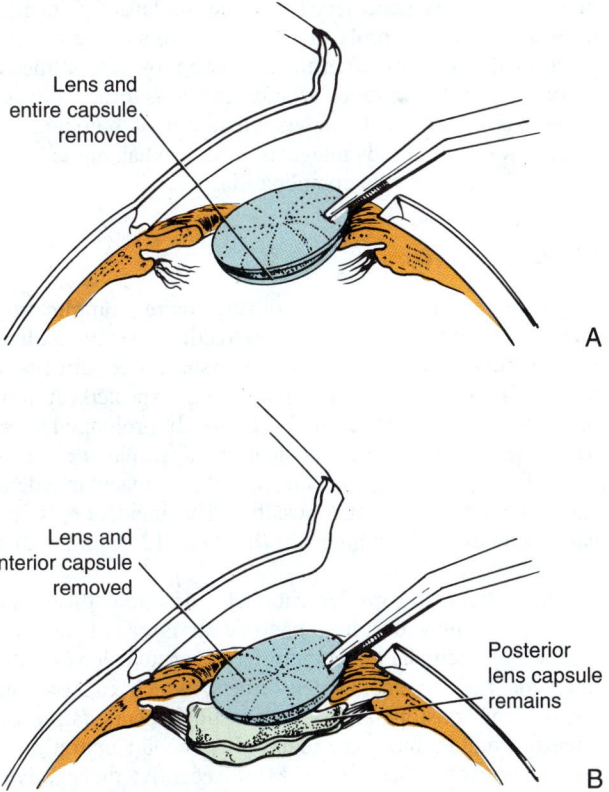

Figure 36–17. Surgical approaches to lens removal for cataracts. *A,* Intracapsular cataract extraction. *B,* Extracapsular cataract extraction.

injection of methohexital sodium (Brevital) or thiopental (Pentothol) to induce a few minutes of light anesthesia while the retrobulbar injection of local anesthetic is given. Cataract surgery is also successfully performed using topical anesthetic.

Intraocular Lens Implantation

Following extraction of the cataract, a new lens is inserted in the posterior chamber, or the client is left without a lens. Although there are many styles of intraocular lenses, they all consist of two basic parts: (1) a clear spherical optic lens usually made of polymethyl methacrylate (Plexiglas) and (2) footplates or haptic lenses to hold the lens in place. Foldable lenses made of silicone or hydrogel material have been developed to fit through the smaller incisions, but data on their long-term use are not available yet.

Management of Aphakia

Aphakia (absence of the lens) is corrected by the use of eyeglasses, contact lenses, or intraocular lenses. Without the lens, the eye has no accommodative power and has lost a great deal of its refractive power. Depth perception is greatly altered. The safest and least expensive method of correcting aphakia is with eyeglasses (with very thick lenses). The disadvantage of this correction is that the thick lenses also magnify objects. Vertical lines appear curved, and it is difficult for the person to judge distances. Contact lenses can achieve visual correction with much less distortion. The client, however, must have the manual dexterity necessary to handle the lenses. Cleaning, insertion of lenses, replacement of lenses, and the dangers of corneal abrasions often make this option less attractive to older people. Intraocular lens implants offer the best visual correction, with immediate return of binocular vision. The main disadvantage is a somewhat higher incidence of postoperative complications.

Complications

Secondary glaucoma is one of the major complications that may occur after cataract extraction. As a result of postoperative edema in the ocular tissues, a certain rise in intraocular pressure is anticipated and expected. It most often resolves within 24 to 72 hours. If prolonged intraocular pressure persists, medical therapy may be necessary. Postoperative infection, bleeding, macular edema and wound leaks are also possible. The incidence of retinal detachment is higher in the first 12 months after cataract surgery.

Following extracapsular cataract extraction, the posterior capsule may become opacified. It is called an after-cataract or secondary membrane. Subcapsular lens epithelial cells may regenerate lens fibers, which can obstruct vision. This postoperative complication occurs fairly frequently and, in the past, required a second operation to remove the opacified tissue. More recently, the neodymium:yttrium-aluminum-garnet (Nd:YAG) laser is being used to create an opening in the capsule through pulses of laser energy that cause tiny "explosions" in the target

tissue. Complications of this technique include a transient rise in intraocular pressure and possible damage to the introcular lens.

Outcomes

The Nursing Research feature discusses whether the outcome of cataract extraction is improved vision and quality of life.

■ Nursing Management of the Surgical Client

Assessment

During the history and physical examination, ask the client about any predisposing factors (trauma, systemic diseases, medications such as corticosteroids, and other ocular problems). Visual acuity (both distant and near) in each eye is documented. Ask the client to describe visual disturbances. The client's visual acuity may be relatively close to normal ranges, yet the client may experience difficulty in performing ADLs. The client's individual perception of the quality of vision is an important factor in determining the need for surgery.

NURSING RESEARCH

Does Cataract Surgery Improve the Client's Quality of Life?

Legro, M. (1991). Quality of life and cataracts: A review of patient-centered studies of cataract surgery outcomes. *Ophthalmic Surgery, 22*(8), 431–443.

The portion of the U.S. population over 50 years old is increasing. As the number of cataract operations performed approaches 1.5 million per year, it is becoming increasingly important to investigate whether this surgery improves the quality of life.

Defining "quality of life" is difficult because it depends on personal values. To one person it may mean the ability to get dressed without help. To another, it may mean the ability to drive and to work. The desired outcome of cataract surgery is improved vision; however, other factors affect the ability to see after surgery. Age, gender, socioeconomic status, attitudes and values, and the presence of other eye disease may greatly influence the outcome of the surgery.

Many recent studies have addressed the quality of life after cataract surgery, but to date, no two studies have measured quality-of-life issues in the same way. Changes in well-being or satisfaction with care have received minimal attention. The role of cataract surgery in preventing falls or other injuries caused by poor eyesight requires further investigation.

Diagnosis, Planning, Implementation

Sensory/Perceptual Alterations (Visual).
Removal of the clouded lens reduces glare and cloudy vision. Improvement in visual acuity is related to the type of correction. Intraocular lens implantation provides the best visual correction. Contact lenses provide a good correction, and eyeglasses provide functional correction. None of these corrections provide the same visual acuity as the natural lens of the eye. Although vision may be greatly improved, there may still be varying degrees of change in depth perception. Write the nursing diagnosis as *Sensory/Perceptual Alterations (Visual) related to lens extraction and replacement.*

Planning: Expected Outcomes. The client will gain improved vision and will adapt to changes in visual correction.

Implementation. Adaptation is the key issue in caring for the client having cataract surgery. Nursing interventions are based on assisting the client to gain or maintain as much independence as possible. The client's life-style, abilities, and home environment must be evaluated. A 55-year-old client who is an architect and otherwise healthy may be having an early cataract removed because it interferes with his work in areas where bright light is used. A 75-year-old diabetic client who is retired and mainly watches television will have entirely different needs.

Unless there are other ocular complications or health factors, cataract surgery is performed on an outpatient basis. At the time of admission to the hospital or surgical facility, determine the client's current level of knowledge and understanding of the perioperative events. Preoperative eye drops may include a dilating agent such as tropicamide (Mydriacyl) to dilate the pupil, facilitating the surgery. A cycloplegic, cyclopentolate (Cyclogyl), may also be administered to paralyze the ciliary muscles.

Evaluation

Assess the degree of attainment of the expected outcome. Adaptation to restored normal vision is usually rapid. Adaptation to limited vision will require more time based on individual variations.

Community and Self-Care

After cataract surgery, clients are expected to return for a follow-up visit the next morning and again at 2 weeks and at 1 month. Postoperative care includes observation of the ocular dressing, if present, and assessment of the client's ability to perform ADLs at the preoperative level. Nausea and vomiting are no longer an expected outcome of the surgical procedure and if present should be reported immediately. Prolonged vomiting could result in increased intraocular pressure and wound dehiscence. The eye patch is usually removed the next morning but may be removed after a few hours if the client has limited vision in the other eye. Instruct the client to wear a metal or plastic shield to protect the eye from accidental injury and not to rub the eye. Glasses may be worn during the day. The Client Education Guide provides instructions that the client should follow after cataract removal.

Restrictions on postoperative activity vary according to the practice of the ophthalmologist. Generally, the client should avoid heavy lifting (over 5 lbs) or straining in the early postoperative period. The client should also avoid sleeping on the side operated on.

Eye care for the client after cataract surgery is the same as that for glaucoma clients (see Glaucoma). Postoperative eye medications may include antibiotics or corticosteroids, or both. Assess the client or family's ability to instill eye drops appropriately. Also review the rationale and schedule for the medications with the client and family. Postoperative discomfort should be minimal to moderate and is usually relieved by acetaminophen. Clients commonly experience an itching sensation after cataract surgery. Instruct the client to report any pain that is unrelieved. Review the clinical manifestations of infection and increased intraocular pressure with the client and family.

Depending on the client's age, ability, and availability of assistance, make a referral for home healthcare if it is indicated. Adjustment to changes in vision also varies with the individual client.

Retinal Disorders

Retinal Detachment

Rhegmatogenous retinal detachment (secondary to a tear in the retina) is characterized by a retinal hole, liquid in the vitreous body with access to the hole, and subsequent fluid accumulation between the retina and the retinal pig-

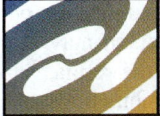

CLIENT EDUCATION GUIDE

Care after Cataract Removal

Leave the eye patch in place.
For 24 hours, limit your activity to sitting in a chair, resting in bed, and walking to the bathroom.
Do not rub your eye.
You can wear your glasses.
Do not lift more than 5 lb (the weight of a gallon of milk).
Do not strain (or bear down).
Do not sleep on the side of your body that was operated on.
Take your eye drops.
Take acetaminophen (Tylenol) as needed for pain or itching.
DO NOT take aspirin or drugs containing aspirin.
Report any pain that is unrelieved, redness around the eye, nausea, or vomiting.

ment epithelium. The liquid seeps through the hole and separates the retina from its blood supply. Without intervention, the detachment continues to spread and the detached retina will lose the ability to function. It may become increasingly detached over a period of hours to years.

Etiology and Risk Factors

Retinal detachment occurs mainly in the adult eye. The overall incidence is 1 in 15,000 people per year but the risk of detachment increases after the fourth decade and most often occurs between the ages of 50 and 70.

Predisposing factors to retinal detachment include: aging, cataract extraction, degeneration of the retina, trauma, severe myopia, previous retinal detachment in the other eye, and a family history of retinal detachment. Retinal holes and tears usually occur from spontaneous vitreous traction, but there may be abnormal adhesions between the retina and vitreous body secondary to diabetic retinopathy, injury, or other ocular disorders. Atrophy of the vitreous body may also result in a retinal tear.

Pathophysiology

If the retina is separated from its choriodal blood supply, it will die. The retinal tissues are at a high risk of avascular necrosis because they are delicate structures and have a high metabolic rate.

Clinical Manifestations and Diagnostic Findings

Characteristic clinical manifestations of retinal detachment are described by clients as a shadow or curtain falling across the field of vision (Fig. 36–18). There is no pain associated with detachment of the retina. The onset is usually sudden and may be accompanied by a burst of black spots or floaters indicating that bleeding has occurred as a result of the detachment. The person may also see flashes of light caused by separation of the retina.

Examination with a direct and indirect ophthalmoscope reveals the portion of the retina involved and the extent of the detachment (Fig. 36–19). A scleral depressor also

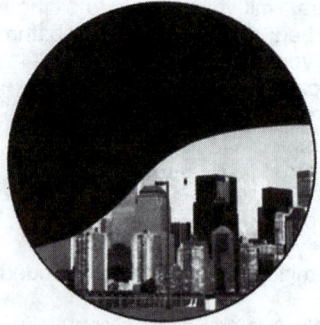

Detached Retina

Figure 36–18. Vision of a client with retinal detachment. (Courtesy of National Industries of the Blind, Wayne, NJ.)

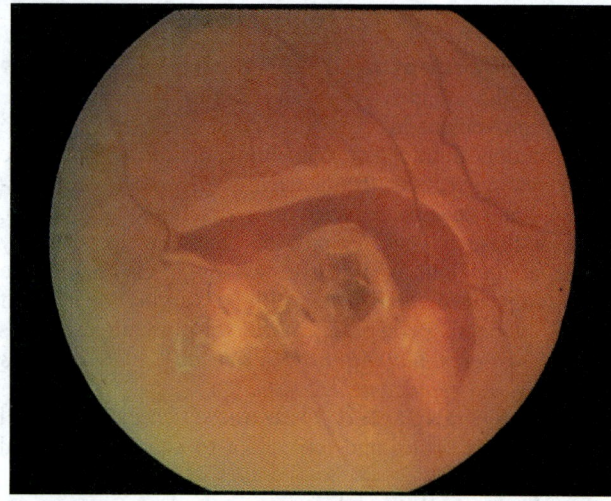

Figure 36–19. Bluish-gray appearance of areas of retinal detachment. (Courtesy of Ophthalmic Photography at the University of Michigan W. K. Kellogg Eye Center, Ann Arbor.)

may be used externally on the lid or conjunctiva to assist in rotating the eyeball and to indent the retina for increased viewing ability. Areas of detachment appear bluish-gray as opposed to the normal red-pink color. Tears are most often horseshoe-shaped but may be round.

Emergency Care

If not treated promptly, a retinal detachment may progress to involve the macula; this greatly compromises visual acuity. A retinal detachment is an ophthalmic emergency and even more so if visual acuity is still normal.

There is no known medical treatment for a detached retina.

■ Surgical Management

The goal of surgical repair of retinal detachment is to place the retina back in contact with the choroid and to seal the accompanying holes and breaks. Often cryopexy (the use of a freezing probe) or laser photocoagulation is used to seal the hole if it has not progressed to detachment. Both methods create inflammation around the area, which scars and seals the hole.

The surgical procedure to place the retina back in contact with the choroid is called scleral buckling (Fig. 36–20). The sclera is actually depressed from the outside by Silastic sponges or silicone bands that are sutured in place permanently. In addition to the buckling procedure, an intraocular injection of air or sulfahexafluoride (SF6) gas bubble, or both, may be used to apply pressure on the retina from the inside of the eye. This holds the retina in place by gravitational force during the healing phase. Postoperative positioning of the client maximizes the tamponade effect of the air or gas bubble. The bubble is slowly absorbed.

Postoperative swelling of tissues and cells in the anterior chamber caused by the inflammatory process or com-

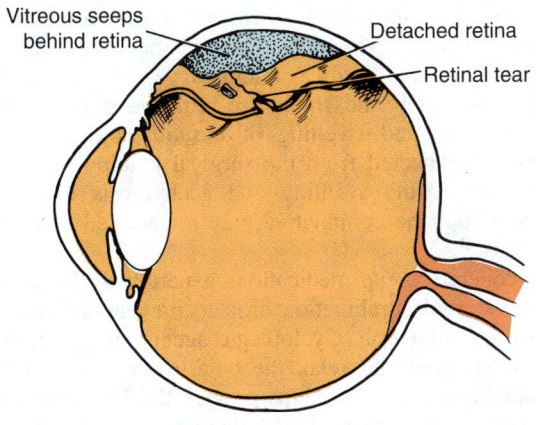

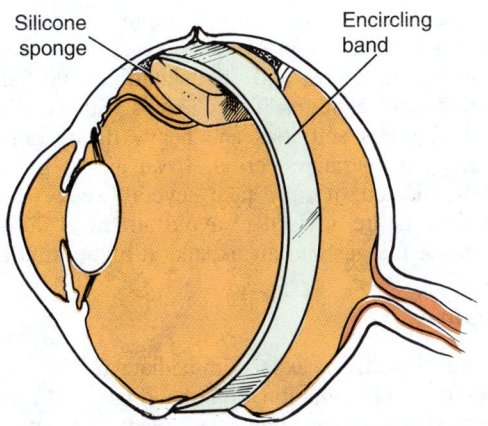

Figure 36–20. Scleral buckling to repair a detached retina. A silicone sponge implant is placed over the tear and held in place with an encircling band. When the buckle is tightened, the implant indents the sclera, holding the choroid and retina together.

promise of the venous drainage system may result in increased intraocular pressure. Because of the fragility of the tissues involved in the repair, re-detachment of the retina may occur at any time. At times, the retina has been separated from its blood supply long enough so that, even when reattached, it no longer has useful function and the client's vision does not improve significantly. Postoperative infection is also a risk.

■ Nursing Management of the Surgical Client

Assessment

When the history has been obtained and the physical examination is being performed, assess the client's visual changes in both eyes. Visual field loss is seen by the client in the opposite quadrant of the actual detachment. For example, a tear in the temporal region, which is affected more frequently, creates a visual defect in the nasal area.

The pupil must be widely dilated for a retinal examination. Explain that the client will experience an extremely bright light and be asked to change gaze frequently to facilitate the examination.

Diagnosis, Planning, Implementation

Sensory/Perceptual Alterations (Visual). The extent of loss of vision is related to the portion of the retina involved. Giant tears involving the entire retina may result in temporary blindness, whereas peripheral tears may not interfere with central vision at all. Healing involves delicate neurologic tissue and visual improvement may be gradual over several months. Write the nursing diagnosis as *Sensory/Perceptual Alterations (Visual) related to decreased retinal function.*

Planning: Expected Outcomes. The client will maintain as much functional vision as possible as evidenced by reporting no further loss of vision and adapting to any visual loss, and demonstrating an ability to perform ADLs, to instill his or her own eye medications, and to recognize clinical manifestations of complications.

Implementation. The focus of the care plan is to help the client cope with the fears and reality of loss of vision and adapt to changes in vision. The client must be aware of the clinical manifestations of further loss of vision. See the Bridge to Home Healthcare feature for suggestions on how to assist clients.

Evaluation

Determine if the client has adapted to imposed changes in vision. You may need to find help at home for independent living until sight returns or the client adapts to changes in vision.

Preoperative Care

Preoperative nursing care involves preparing the client for outpatient surgery or an overnight stay in the hospital. Assess the client's current level of knowledge and understanding of the implications of retinal detachment and the expectations for the surgical procedure. Because retinal detachment repair may take several hours, general anesthesia is used in many cases. The pupil must be widely dilated before the operation, and the client may be given a sedative.

Postoperative Care

Postoperatively, observe the eye patch for any drainage. Blood loss in retinal detachment surgery is minimal, and only serous drainage is expected on the postoperative dressing. Activity restrictions may be necessary if an air or gas bubble has been injected. The client will need to be positioned so that the bubble can apply maximal pressure on the retina by the force of gravity. The position, usually head down and to one side, is maintained for several days. Provide suggestions for comfort and support with the positioning (pillows under stomach, elbows, or ankles).

Posterior segment surgery, such as scleral buckling procedures, results in considerably more discomfort than an-

BRIDGE TO HOME HEALTHCARE

Coping with Failing Vision

Bernadette Mruz, R.N., Visiting Nurse Association of Omaha, Omaha, Nebraska

Providing a safe home environment for the client with failing vision is essential. Promoting an autonomous life-style is desirable. Assessing the client's ability to remain safely at home is an important responsibility of home healthcare nurses.

Basic emergency procedures can be implemented by the use of nationwide services such as Lifeline. This service provides a portable electronic device usually worn around the client's neck or wrist. By simply pushing the button immediate contact is made with emergency personnel. Information can be obtained by calling toll-free 1-800-852-5433.

Local telephone companies can provide special adaptive equipment for 911 access. Phones that can be programmed and have lighted or large numbers are available in most retail stores.

Home safety precautions can be simple. Burns can be prevented by color-coding water faucets. Use red for hot water and blue for cold water. Marking the "Off" dials on stoves and microwaves with colored tape or paint will reduce the chance of injury.

Adequate lighting is essential. During the day, natural light is preferable. Open drapes or shades to provide ample light. Replace light bulbs with the highest wattage recommended.

Removal of hazards, such as throw rugs, clutter, and unnecessary furniture, will provide unrestricted ambulation. Handrails can be installed in hallways, bathrooms, and on steps to prevent falls. Equipment such as canes, walkers, raised toilet seats, and bathtub rails promote safely. These items are available at medical supply stores.

Many commercial products are now marketed that can be of great assistance in the home. Pill organizers are clearly marked boxes with the day of the week and the times pills are to be taken. These can be filled by family members for a week at a time. Electronic lamp timers and voice-activated switches will allow the client to function more independently.

Access to a television and a radio are important. Large-print newspapers and reading materials will keep the client in touch with current events. The local library and the American Association for the Blind can provide assistance in obtaining needed items.

Creativity and planning can allow the client to remain at home in a safe environment for as long as possible.

pressure. The intraocular pressure is monitored closely during the first 24 hours. Encourage the client to resume a regular diet and fluids as tolerated.

The eye patch and shield are removed the next morning. Redness and swelling of the lids and conjunctiva should be expected from the surgical manipulation. After several days, the swelling and ecchymosis of the lids subsides, but the conjunctiva may remain red or pink for a few weeks.

Postoperative eye medications generally include an antibiotic-steroid combination drop to prevent infection and reduce inflammation. Cycloplegic agents are prescribed to dilate the pupil and relax the ciliary muscles, which decreases discomfort and helps prevent the formation of iris adhesions to the corneal endothelium (synechiae). Either warm or cold compresses may be applied for comfort several times a day.

Instruct the client to clean the eye with warm tap water using a clean washcloth. Warm compresses may be continued at home. Either an eye shield or glasses should be worn during the day, and the shield should be worn during naps and at night. The client is usually instructed to avoid vigorous activities and heavy lifting during the immediate postoperative period. If an air or gas bubble has been injected, it may take several weeks to totally absorb. Clients are advised to avoid air travel during this time because the gas and air expand at high altitudes.

Outcomes

The client should not expect immediate return of vision. Postoperative inflammation and the dilating drops interfere with vision. As healing takes place over weeks and months, vision may improve gradually.

Community and Self-Care

Because retinal detachment surgery is often performed on an urgent basis, the client rarely has an opportunity to plan for the surgery. It is important to evaluate the home environment and to assist the client and family in preparing for any necessary support. Assess the home for safety hazards, such as throw rugs, electrical cords, stairs, and poor lighting. Although the eye patch is usually removed early in the postoperative period, the client likely has decreased functional vision in the eye.

Diabetic Retinopathy

Diabetic retinopathy is a progressive disorder of the retina characterized by microscopic damage to the retinal vessels, resulting in occlusion of the vessels. As a result of inadequate blood supply, sections of the retina deteriorate and vision is permanently lost.

Diabetic retinopathy is one of the leading causes of blindness worldwide. All persons with diabetes are prone to develop retinopathy, although studies indicate that there is a strong correlation between the incidence and severity of retinopathy and the duration of the disease and

terior segment procedures. Ocular muscles are separated, and the globe is manipulated to reach the posterior portions of the eyeball. Narcotics may be needed during the first 24 hours after surgery. Nausea and vomiting may also require management. Intravenous acetazolamide (Diamox) may be used to reduce increased intraocular

erratic blood glucose control. Approximately 30% to 40% of the diabetic population has some degree of retinopathy. Clients who have had diabetes for 15 to 20 years have an 80% to 90% chance of developing retinopathy.

There are two types of retinopathy: (1) background, or nonproliferative diabetic retinopathy, and (2) proliferative diabetic retinopathy. In background retinopathy, early pathologic changes demonstrate the hyperpermeability and weakening of the retinal vessels. The capillaries develop tiny dotlike outpouchings called microaneurysms, and the retinal veins become dilated and tortuous. Multiple hemorrhages occur from these defective vessels. Retinal edema is caused by leaking capillaries, and after the serous fluid is absorbed, a yellowish precipitate called a "hard exudate" remains. Hemorrhages, exudates, and ischemia contribute to impaired vision, particularly if these occur on or around the macula.

Progressive retinal ischemia stimulates the growth of new but ineffective blood vessels. These new and fragile blood vessels proliferate and grow into the vitreous body. These vessels leak, hemorrhage, and undergo fibrous changes that may form bands that pull on the retina, causing detachment. This process is called *proliferative retinopathy* (Fig. 36–21). With increasing ischemia, microinfarcts of the nerve fiber layer, called cotton-wool spots, appear.

Clients experience a wide range of visual disturbances and fluctuations. Retinal vessel hemorrhage into the vitreous space obstructs vision with black spots or floaters or may result in complete loss of vision. Areas of retinal ischemia become blind spots. Macular edema causes decreased central vision.

To reduce the occurrence of hemorrhage and retinal detachment in progressive retinopathy, the argon laser is used to photocoagulate the blood vessels. Hundreds and even thousands of microscopic photocoagulation applications (burns) are systematically placed around the peripheral retina, avoiding the central area that includes the macula and the optic disc.

When a hemorrhage does not clear spontaneously over time, a vitrectomy (removal of a portion of the vitreous) may be performed. A vitrectomy may also need to be performed to release the traction of membranes on the retina.

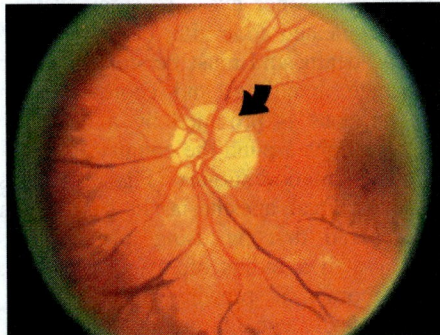

Figure 36–21. Proliferative diabetic retinopathy. Neovascularization covers one fourth to one third of the optic disc *(arrow).* (Standard photograph No. 10A of the Modified Airlee House Classification of Diabetic Retinopathy; courtesy of the Early Treatment Diabetic Retinopathy Study Research Group.)

Nursing interventions for the client with diabetic retinopathy are focused on assessment and management of diabetes. A high blood sugar level causes a temporary decrease in visual acuity. Because retinopathy is generally progressive, the client will need to cope with increasing visual deficits. Community referrals for rehabilitation and aids for low vision often provide useful assistance. Visiting nurses often prepare insulin injections for the upcoming week, as the client cannot see well enough to do this correctly.

Retinitis Pigmentosa

Retinitis pigmentosa is a genetic disorder that initially destroys the rods of the eye. Because the rods perceive black and white vision, the earliest manifestation is noticed during childhood as night blindness. Over the next several years, manifestations progress until a total loss of peripheral vision occurs. In time, central vision is also lost. No treatment is available to slow or stop this disorder. Genetic counseling is advised.

Age-Related Macular Degeneration

Previously known as senile macular degeneration, age-related macular degeneration is an atrophic degenerative process that affects the macula and surrounding tissues, resulting in central visual deficits.

Age-related macular degeneration is found to some degree in most adults over the age of 65. It is one of the most common causes of visual loss in the elderly. The exact cause is unknown, but the incidence increases with each decade over 50. It may be hereditary.

Age-related macular degeneration falls into two groups: (1) nonexudative and (2) exudative. Both are usually bilateral and progressive. Also referred to as "dry" macular degeneration, nonexudative age-related macular degeneration is characterized by atrophy and degeneration of the outer retina and underlying structures. Yellowish round spots called *drusen* may be seen on the retina and macula with an ophthalmoscope. Drusen are deposits of amorphous material from the pigment epithelial cells of the retina. Over time, these spots increase, enlarge, and may calcify.

At this "wet," exudative stage of age-related macular degeneration, Bruch's membrane, which lies just beneath the pigment epithelial cell layer of the retina, becomes compromised and this results in serous fluid leaks from the choroid, with accompanying proliferation of choroidal blood vessels. A dome-shaped retinal pigment epithelium may be seen when examining the fundus. These leaks produce a visual effect called *metamorphopsia*, which is the blurred, wavy distortion of vision. The client may also notice a blurred scotoma or decreased central visual acuity (Fig. 36–22). Fundus photography and angiography may be performed on a regular basis to document and evaluate changes.

There is no known means of medical treatment or prevention of age-related macular degeneration. Further

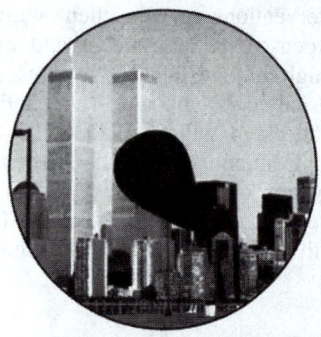

Macular Degeneration

Figure 36–22. Vision of a client with macular degeneration. (Courtesy of National Industries for the Blind, Wayne, NJ.)

damage from exudative macular degeneration sometimes may be arrested by the use of argon photocoagulation, even though laser damage to the retina in this area results in a blind spot. When the fovea is involved, central vision is lost and the only helpful measures are low-vision aids.

The client with age-related macular degeneration is threatened with the loss of central vision (see Bridge to Home Healthcare). In order to evaluate changes in vision, the client is taught to use Amsler's chart at home. You may assist the client to maximize remaining vision with low-vision aids and community referral to a low-vision specialist and low-vision support groups.

Retinal Artery Occlusion

Occlusion of the retinal artery or vein can cause loss of vision. The most common causes of occlusion are emboli from athersclerosis, valvular heart disease, and increases in blood viscosity. The retinal artery can also be occluded from embolized plaque in the carotid artery or from spasm. Retinal artery occlusion causes a sudden, unilateral, painless loss of vision. The severity of the visual loss ranges from total loss, when the central artery is occluded, to a loss of a visual field, when a branch of the artery is blocked. Retinal vein occlusion is due to systemic vascular disorders, venous stasis, hypertension, or increased blood viscosity. Manifestations of retinal vein occlusion are gradual loss of vision, occurring over several hours. Retinal artery occlusion is an emergency. Management includes intermittent massage of the eyeball by a physician to move an embolius from the central artery into a branch, and increased oxygenation (95% oxygen for 10 minutes). Surgery can include anterior chamber paracentesis to reduce intraocular pressure and to move the embolus. Anticoagulants are used in early phases of occlusion.

Corneal Disorders

Corneal Dystrophies

Corneal dystrophies are a group of hereditary and acquired disorders of unknown cause, characterized by deposits in the layers of the cornea and alteration of the corneal structure.

Specific corneal dystrophies characteristically appear at different ages. They may be stationary or slowly progressive throughout life. The most common, Fuchs' dystrophy, usually begins in the 20s or 30s, affects more women than men, and is slowly progressive.

Corneal dystrophies are associated with all five layers of the cornea. Although the disease usually originates in the inner layers (Descemet's membrane, the stroma, and Bowman's membrane), the degeneration, erosion, and deposits affect all layers.

Fuchs' dystrophy is characterized by deposits in Descemet's membrane that look like warts. Descemet's membrane becomes thickened, and defects appear in the endothelial layer. Because the integrity of the cornea is compromised, it becomes edematous and cloudy. Vision is compromised not only by the corneal deposits but by the altered structure of the cornea secondary to the edema.

The cornea is evaluated by slit-lamp examination. Fluorescein staining is used to enhance visualization of surface corneal defects. Corneal scrapings may be taken with a sterile spatula for further staining and microscopic evaluation. Specular micrography (see Diagnostic Tests) may be used to evaluate the corneal endothelium.

 Acute and Subacute Care

Because some corneal dystrophies and other disorders may progress slowly, assist the client in adapting to the loss of vision (see the discussion of nursing care for the client with cataracts).

■ Surgical Management

Corneal transplantation, or keratoplasty, may be indicated for serious corneal conditions, including corneal dystrophy. Penetrating keratoplasty denotes full-thickness corneal replacement; lamellar keratoplasty denotes a partial-thickness procedure.

Because there is a direct relationship between age and health of the endothelial layer of the cornea, young donor tissue is preferred. Donor eyes are obtained from cadavers, must be enucleated soon after death because of rapid endothelial cell death, and must be stored in a preserving solution. Storage, handling, and coordination of donor tissue with surgeons is provided by a network of state eye bank associations around the country.

Corneal transplantation surgery (Fig. 36–23) is usually performed under local anesthesia. In surgery, the donor cornea is prepared first by using a trephine to cut a corneal button with a radius of, usually, 7.0 to 8.5 mm. The recipient cornea is prepared in the same manner; however, it is usually cut 0.5 mm smaller so that there is an overlap by the donor cornea, which is then sutured into place. Figure 36–24 shows the eye after keratoplasty.

Graft rejection or failure may occur at any time after transplantation. It can result from unsuitable storage of

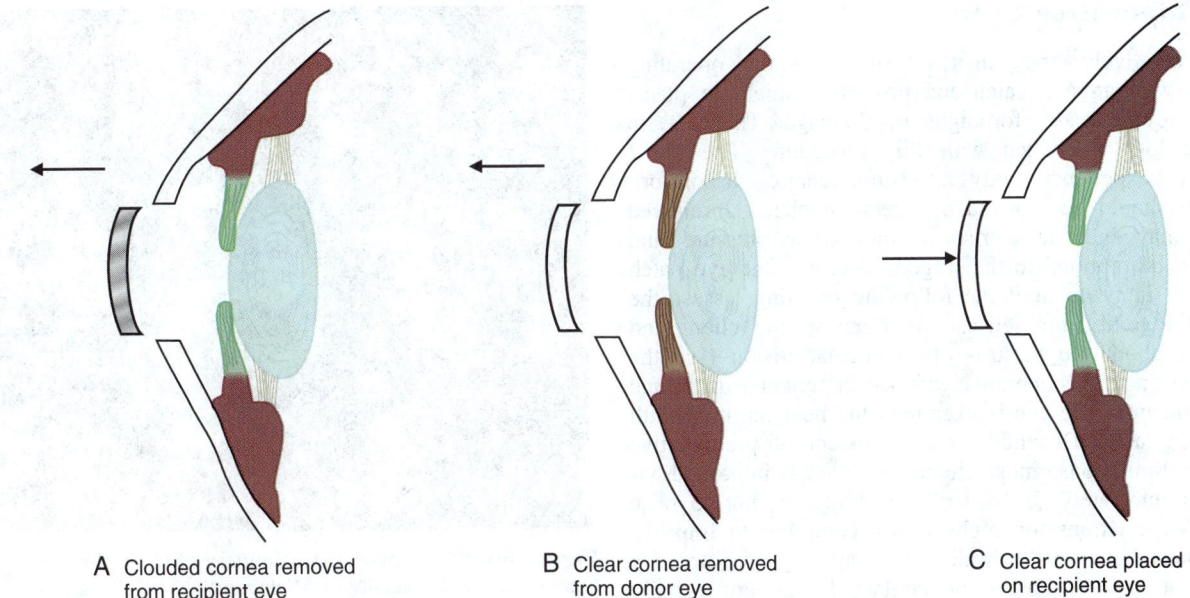

A Clouded cornea removed
   from recipient eye

B Clear cornea removed
   from donor eye

C Clear cornea placed
   on recipient eye

Figure 36–23. Steps involved in corneal transplantation (penetrating keratoplasty). *A,* The diseased cornea is removed with a trephine. *B,* A button of donor cornea is removed with the same trephine so that the cuts are identical. *C,* The donor cornea is placed on the eye and stitched in place with extremely fine suture material.

donor tissue, dystrophy of the donor's endothelium, surgical trauma, or immunologic rejection. Because the cornea is an avascular structure, blood typing, which is necessary for other types of grafts, is not necessary.

At the first sign of graft rejection, when the cornea becomes cloudy and edematous and when there is an anterior chamber reaction (presence of white blood cells or protein; Fig. 36–25), topical steroids are prescribed in frequent doses to control the inflammatory response and reverse the rejection reaction. In severe cases, a repeat transplantation may be necessary.

Wound leakage, bleeding into the anterior chamber, glaucoma, cataract, and infection are other complications that may occur.

■ Nursing Management of the Surgical Client

Preoperative Care

The client is usually notified the day before surgery that donor tissue has become available. Receiving a call with short notice for surgery usually produces a relatively high level of anxiety for the client and significant others. Assist the client in coping with the rush of preoperative activities by assuming a calm and assured manner and providing education about perioperative events. Corneal transplantation surgery is usually performed on an outpatient basis.

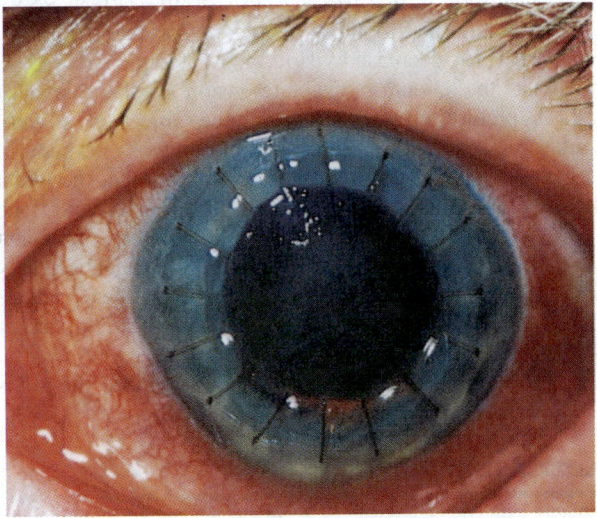

Figure 36–24. Clinical appearance of the eye after keratoplasty. (Courtesy of Ophthalmic Photography at the University of Michigan W. K. Kellogg Eye Center, Ann Arbor.)

Figure 36–25. Acute graft rejection. (Courtesy of Ophthalmic Photography at the University of Michigan W. K. Kellogg Eye Center, Ann Arbor.)

Postoperative Care

Postoperatively, the client returns from the operating room with an eye patch and protective shield in place. Observe the patch for signs of drainage. There is no blood loss associated with this procedure. The client should experience only mild-to-moderate discomfort, which should be relieved by acetaminophen. Unrelieved pain may indicate a rise in intraocular pressure and should be reported to the surgeon. Because the eye patch will be in place until the following morning, assess the client's ability for self-care and advise the client and family about the hazards of monocular vision (see the discussion of postoperative care for the client with retinal detachment). The eye is examined the next morning with the slit lamp. Depending on the extent of preoperative visual limitations, most clients experience improved vision immediately. Instruct clients, however, not to raise their expectations too high. Vision continues to improve gradually because the healing process may take up to a year or more. Glasses or contact lenses are usually needed to obtain the best result. Many months may be required for restoration of vision, so revisions in the care plan may be needed.

Community and Self-Care

Postoperative eye drops usually include an antibiotic and a corticosteroid. Topical corticosteroid therapy may be needed indefinitely. Discharge instructions include the rationale for the medications and proper instillation technique. It is important for the client to wear eye protection in the form of regular glasses, sunglasses, or a protective shield to prevent injury to the eye. The client is advised never to rub the eye. The area around the eye may be cleaned with warm tap water using a clean washcloth.

Teach the client and family to recognize the clinical manifestations of graft rejection. A mnemonic tool may be useful in teaching the client to remember the signs of graft rejection. It involves the use of the letters RSVP which are familiar to most people: *R* for redness, *S* for swelling, *V* for decreased vision, and *P* for pain.

Advise the client to evaluate vision in the eye each day. A picture on the wall or some object in a well-lighted room should be selected as a point of reference. If a change in vision from the day before is noted, the client should reevaluate his or her vision in a few hours. If no improvement is noted or if vision is worse, the client should notify the physician. Because graft rejection may occur at any time (even years) after the surgery, advise the client to make the vision check a routine part of ADLs for the rest of his or her life.

Also teach the client and family to recognize the signs of increased intraocular pressure and infection.

Keratoconus

Keratoconus is a degenerative disease of the cornea characterized by a thinning and protrusion of the cornea in

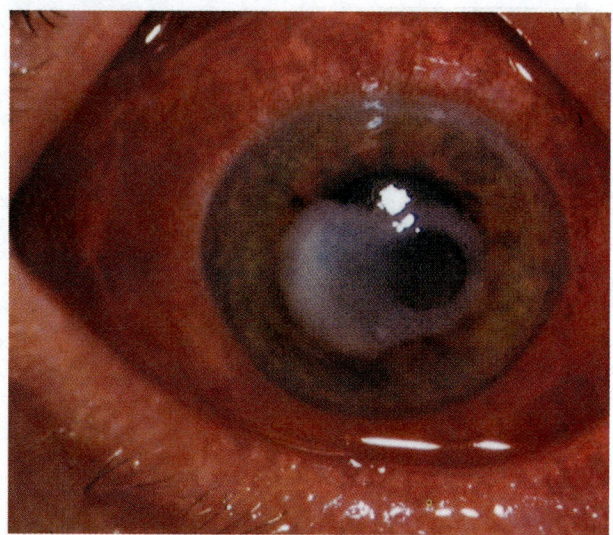

Figure 36–26. Keratoconus. (Courtesy of Ophthalmic Photography at the University of Michigan W. K. Kellogg Eye Center, Ann Arbor.)

the shape of a cone (Fig. 36–26). Blurred vision is the result of the change in the shape of the cornea, which may be corrected by contact lenses. Keratoconus is often slowly progressive with onset between the ages of 20 and 60. At some point, the conical shape of the cornea may no longer allow for contact lenses to correct vision. Corneal transplantation for keratoconus is highly successful.

Corneal Infections: Keratitis

The corneal epithelium is normally an effective barrier against microorganisms. Once it is compromised from disease or trauma, the underlying stromal layer becomes an excellent culture medium for a variety of organisms.

Dry eyes or ineffective eyelid closure predispose the eye to keratitis. Clients who have a systemic collagen disorder such as rheumatoid arthritis are particularly susceptible to corneal infections and ulceration.

Tearing and photophobia are common, and blurred vision results from inability of the cornea to provide the proper refractive surface. The client with a corneal defect from an infection will experience a great deal of discomfort, which is worsened by eyelid movement. The eye appears infected and indurated. Fluorescein staining of the cornea outlines the affected area, which can be viewed through the slit lamp or with a handheld flashlight.

Corneal infections may develop into ulcerations (Fig. 36–27) that severely compromise the integrity of the eye. Sources of infection include bacteria (e.g., *Staphylococcus aureus, Pseudomonas aeruginosa, Streptococcus pneumoniae*), fungi *(Candida, Aspergillus),* viruses (adenovirus, herpes simplex, herpes zoster), and protozoa *(Acanthamoeba).* Clinical findings under slit-lamp examination are specific to particular organisms. *Hypopyon* (a layer of white cells in the anterior chamber) may accompany corneal ulceration.

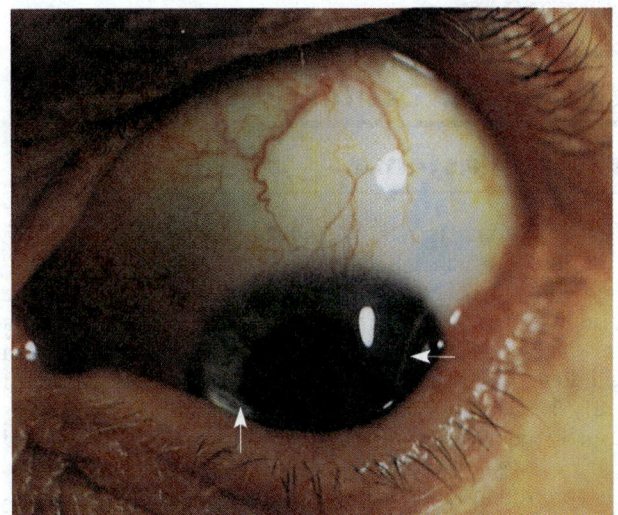

Figure 36–27. A corneal ulcer *(arrows)*. (Courtesy of Ophthalmic Photography at the University of Michigan W. K. Kellogg Eye Center, Ann Arbor.)

Topical antibiotic, antifungal, and antiviral therapy is prescribed, with the frequency of instillation based on the severity of the infection to prevent progression to perforation and to promote healing. Maximal therapy includes the alternating instillation of two broad-spectrum eye drops every 15 minutes around the clock. As the infection begins to respond to the medication, frequency of administration is gradually decreased. Systemic intravenous medication may be prescribed as well.

In order to aid the healing process, surgical intervention may be necessary. Tarsorrhaphy (suturing the eyelid shut) promotes healing by decreasing eyelid blinking and by decreasing evaporation of the corneal tear film. For corneal perforation, a conjunctival flap may be performed to cover the defect. Tissue adhesive, a kind of superglue, may also be used to seal the perforation. A soft contact lens may be used as a bandage to maintain the seal. Large perforations may require either lamellar (partial-thickness) or penetrating (full-thickness) keratoplasty.

In cases in which medical and surgical interventions fail, enucleation (removal of the entire eyeball) may be necessary (see discussion of nursing care of ocular melanoma). In some cases, evisceration (removal of only the orbital contents) may be indicated. The scleral shell is left intact along with the ocular muscles, which allows for improved ocular prosthetic fit and function.

Although the early stages of corneal infection are often managed at home, the client may need to be hospitalized for the management of a severe corneal ulcer. If the client and family have been instilling frequent eye drops at home, the client may be fatigued from lack of sleep as well as anxious about possible loss of vision. Assess the client's level of discomfort and methods of coping with the stress of pain and lack of sleep. Often at this stage, the client is not coping well at all.

When eye drops are given every 15 minutes around the clock, the schedule is a challenge not only for the client

but for you as well. Hand washing is particularly important in this situation and is carried out even if gloves are worn to instill the drops. The threat of losing eyesight compels many clients to watch the clock for fear that you will forget to administer the eye drops. You can build the client's trust and reduce anxiety by scrupulous adherence to the time schedule.

Effective sleep and rest are nearly impossible with interruptions every 15 minutes. The client rarely reaches the deeper stages of sleep and most experience restless light sleep in stages 1 and 2. In addition to the eye pain the client may already be experiencing, some eye drops, such as fortified bacitracin, may cause stinging that lasts several minutes.

You can institute several measures to comfort the client. A daily routine of care should be outlined, based as much as possible on the client's normal routine at home. Because there are so many interruptions to the client's personal time and space, it is important to identify at least two periods of time during the day when the client may rest or nap with the only interruption being the nurse who comes in to administer the eye drops. A sign should be posted on the door to the client's room for privacy during these rest times. You and the client may also agree that you will not open topics of conversation during this time but will quietly instill the eye drops. Adopt this same routine during the client's normal nighttime. Some clients are actually able to sleep during instillation of eye drops at night; however, establish this routine with the client in advance. Older clients, who are accustomed to more stage 2 sleep than younger clients, are able to rest more effectively. Because younger clients tend to become confused and irritable more often, speak to the client before touching him or her. Oral analgesics are given at regular intervals, and mild sleeping medications may be helpful at bedtime.

The client's eye may need to be cleaned frequently because the medications and excessive tearing will become dried and the lids will stick together. Warm tap water applied with soft gauze pads is used. The combination of tearing, medications, and cleaning may cause the skin of an elderly client to become excoriated. Antibiotic ophthalmic ointment may be applied to the lower lid margin and cheek to reduce irritation.

Clients usually become adapted to this regimen of interruptions after the first 48 hours. As the cornea begins to show signs of improvement, the eye drops may be reduced in frequency to every 30 minutes and then to every hour. Most clients will not notice a great deal of difference in the every-30-minute routine, but when the routine is reduced to every hour, they will begin to sleep more heavily as the body attempts to compensate for lost sleep. At the end of an hour, the client may complain to you that it has seemed like only a few minutes since the last interruption. Intense dreaming may also be experienced during this time.

At discharge, the client should be able to demonstrate how to properly instill eye drops. The client will also understand the importance of complying with the medication regimen. Instruct the client and family about the clinical manifestations of increasing infections. The eye may continue to be cleaned with warm tap water at home. Also assess the home environment if the client's vision is greatly reduced. Referrals for rehabilitation may be necessary, as well.

Uveal Tract Disorders: Uveitis

Uveitis is an inflammation of the uveal tract that can affect one or more parts (iris, ciliary body, choroid). Uveitis commonly occurs in its acute form from a hypersensitivity reaction or in its chronic form, following microbial infection. Clients with this condition complain of pain, blurred vision, and photophobia. There is marked redness of the eye, and the pupil is usually constricted. Cells (white blood cells) and flare (protein), called an anterior chamber reaction, are seen in the anterior chamber fluid with the slit lamp.

The primary cause of discomfort in clients with uveitis is ciliary body muscle spasm. A cycloplegic medication such as atropine effectively relieves the spasm, and the dilation of the pupil prevents the inflamed iris from adhering to the lens and the corneal endothelium from forming synechiae. Topical steroid drops are prescribed to reduce the inflammation.

Photophobia (sensitivity to light) and eye discomfort are the chief complaints. Advise the client to wear dark glasses and to avoid bright light. Reduced lighting at home may be hazardous because the client's pupil is dilated, causing blurred vision. Oral analgesics usually relieve the ocular discomfort.

Be sure that the client and family understand the rationale for the prescribed medications. The client should also be able to recognize signs and symptoms of increased intraocular pressure.

Acute uveitis can become severe and involve the entire eyeball (panophthalmitis). Pyogenic bacteria can penetrate the uvea during trauma or rupture of an ulcerated area or through endogenous sources, such as bacterial endocarditis, septicemia, or meningitis. Severe pain is present with visual loss and necrosis of the sclera. The globe may rupture. Infections that do not invade the sclera but remain confined to the inner globe are called *endophthalmitis*. This form of infection is less severe and responds rather quickly to antibiotics.

Sympathetic Ophthalmia

Sympathetic ophthalmia is an inflammation of the uveal tract in an uninjured eye that occurs after a penetrating injury or retained foreign body in the opposite eye. The exact cause of this problem is not known, but it may be an autoimmune response to uveal pigment. The inflammation spreads from the uvea to the optic nerve. Clinical manifestations include inflammation, photophobia, excessive tearing, decreased vision, and pain in the noninjured eye. The clinical manifestations develop 3 to 8 weeks after the injury but have been known to develop many months later. It is a rare problem.

Tumors of the Eye

Malignant Ocular Tumors

Retinoblastoma

Retinoblastoma is a highly malignant intraocular tumor. The tumor occurs in two forms: sporadic (60%) and inherited (40%). The neoplasm arises from mutations in the primitive neuroectodermal tissue of the retina. It is a relatively rare form of cancer, occurring most often in children. Clinical manifestations are difficult to detect early because they are not obvious. In children, parents usually notice a whitish appearance of the pupil (called *cat's eye reflex*) and strabismus. Decreased vision, proptosis (protruding eye), and pain are late signs. Retinoblastomas grow rapidly along the optic nerve and invade the brain. Treatment of mild or moderate forms includes radiation, photocoagulation, and/or cryotherapy to save vision. Eyes with extensive retinal destruction or glaucoma are enucleated (see following). Adults who have survived retinoblastoma are at increased risk of developing other malignancies, especially osteogenic sarcoma.

Ocular Melanoma

Although less than 1% of the population of the United States are affected by malignant ocular tumors, treatment of these tumors can be a challenge to both client and nurse. Choroidal melanomas are often detected during a routine ocular examination because there is no pain associated with the development of the tumor. By the time the tumor has grown large enough to obstruct vision, there may be involvement of the macula and metastasis.

When ocular melanoma is discovered early, radiation therapy alone may be the treatment of choice. Radiation therapy to the eye is accomplished through insertion of a tiny plate or plaque about the size of a dime that holds tiny seeds of radioactive iodine 125. The plaque is sutured to the sclera directly over the site of the tumor. It is left in place for several days, depending on the required dose, and then removed. Both insertion and removal are performed in the operating room. During treatment, a lead shield is placed over the eye. Radiation exposure to the nurse who cares for the client is minimal—a small fraction of a chest x-ray study. In spite of this extremely low exposure, the routine restrictions for hospital personnel and visitors are implemented for the sake of consistency. Hospitalization for treatment with radioactive iodine is required, depending on regulations.

During the client's hospitalization for this treatment, provide support and encouragement for the client. The plaque is only mildly to moderately uncomfortable, and discomfort should be relieved with acetaminophen. The difficult challenge for the client is confinement to his or her room with limitations on visitors at a time when support is essential. Eye medications include a cycloplegic and an antibiotic-steroid drop.

Enucleation (removal of the entire eyeball) has been the traditional method of treatment and may be combined with radiation treatments. Exenteration (removal of the eyeball and surrounding tissues and bone) may also be necessary.

Enucleation surgery is usually performed under general anesthesia. The ocular muscles are dissected from the eyeball which is removed by severing the optic nerve and vessels at the back. An acrylic sphere covered by donor scleral tissue is usually placed within the capsule of tissue that formerly held the eyeball. Scleral tissue encourages fibrovascular ingrowth, which prevents migration and extrusion of the implant. A soft plastic scleral shell is placed in the visible outer portion of the socket as a support until a permanent prosthesis can be made. More recently, a new type of implant, hydroxyapatite, which is made of the same inorganic material present in human bone, is being used. Several weeks later, a central hole is drilled into the sphere and covering tissues. A peg (which will later fit into a depression on the posterior surface of the artificial eye) is then inserted into the hole. The movement of the implant by the muscle cone is transferred directly to the prosthesis. With the artificial eye being primarily supported by the peg instead of the lids and socket tissues, there are fewer cosmetic and structural complications.

The client undergoing enucleation for a malignant tumor is stressed not only by the threat of cancer but by disfigurement of the face. Assess the client's response, home, and family for support mechanisms.

The goal for the client following enucleation is adaptation to monocular vision and return to his or her former level of independence. Nursing interventions are focused on assisting the client to grieve for the lost body part and lost vision, and to identify coping mechanisms that will facilitate rehabilitation.

Preoperatively, assist the client in preparing for the surgical procedure. Most often, the client is made aware of the tumor at a routine office visit. Surgery is usually scheduled within a few days. Recognizing that the client is most appropriately in a stage of shock and denial, carefully explain the perioperative events. Although it is possible to have an enucleation as an outpatient procedure, the client may stay overnight in the hospital.

Provide routine postoperative care. The client returns from the operating room with a pressure dressing over the eye. Periodically assess the dressing for bleeding because hemorrhage is a possibility with this surgery. Clients are understandably anxious about the removal of the dressing the next morning. Prepare the client by explaining how the eye and conformer will appear. The socket and lids will be swollen, and the white plastic conformer is visible. Also determine the client's or family's ability to care for the wound postoperatively.

Some clients are afraid that their appearance will frighten others, especially children. In this case, an eye patch may be worn during the 4 to 6 weeks before the prosthesis is fitted, but it should not be worn continuously. Eventually the eye prosthesis can be worn and looks pleasingly normal (Fig. 36–28). The Client Education Guide lists steps for insertion and removal of the prosthesis.

The area around the lids may be cleaned with warm tap water using a clean washcloth. Soap and water should

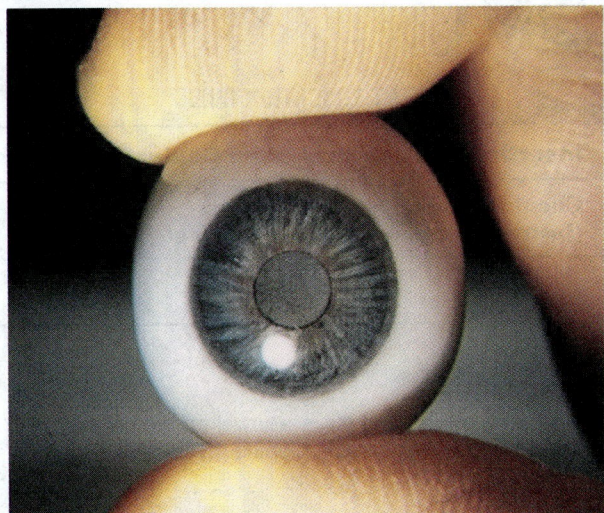

Figure 36–28. An ocular prosthesis. (Courtesy of Ophthalmic Photography at the University of Michigan W. K. Kellogg Eye Center, Ann Arbor.)

be kept away from the socket. If the plastic conformer accidentally comes out, it should be washed and replaced. Antibiotic ophthalmic ointment is usually ordered to be instilled in the socket once or twice a day.

Adjustment to monocular vision is a challenge the client begins to face immediately. Depth perception is altered, and the client will need to exercise caution in walking, crossing streets, and driving. Advise the client to practice ADLs until visual and body adjustments are made.

Emphasize the need for extra precaution with the remaining eye. Eye protection should be worn when engaging in any activity that might even remotely result in an injury. Many clients are advised to wear glasses even if no correction is needed.

Benign Lid Tumors

Benign tumors of the lids are very common and often increase in frequency with age. Melanocytic nevi (moles) and verrucae (warts) commonly appear on the lids and lid margins. Xanthelasma appears as yellow wrinkled patches, which are actually lipid deposits under the skin of the eyelids. These benign lesions may be removed for cosmetic reasons.

Malignant Lid Tumors

Basal cell and squamous cell carcinomas of the lids are the most common malignant tumors of the eyelids. These tumors appear more frequently in persons with fair complexions who have had chronic exposure to the sun. Malignant lid tumors are most often (90%–95%) of the basal cell type and frequently appear on the lower lid as nodules that gradually enlarge, becoming scaly and ulcerated.

Malignant tumors may be removed and treated by a variety of methods such as electrodessication, cryother-

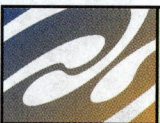

CLIENT EDUCATION GUIDE

Insertion and Removal of an Ocular Prosthesis

Client Instructions in English (*Instrucciones para el cliente en inglés*)	Client Instructions in Spanish (*Instrucciones para el cliente en español*)
Insertion	**Para ponerse la prótesis ocular**
Wash your hands.	Lávese las manos.
Work at a mirror, and place a towel on the counter to keep the prosthesis from chipping if you drop it.	Párese enfrente de un espejo y ponga una toalla sobre el mostrador para prevenir que la prótesis se dañe si se cae al suelo.
Rinse the prosthesis in lukewarm water.	Enjuage la prótesis en agua tibia.
Lift your upper eyelid with the hand that you *don't* use to write.	Levante el párpado superior con la mano que *no* usa para escribir.
With the hand that you use to write, hold the prosthesis between your thumb and index finger.	Con la mano que usa para escribir, sostenga la prótesis entre el pulgar y el índice.
Hold the notched end of the prosthesis facing the side of your nose.	Sostenga la prótesis por la parte indentada que va hacia la nariz.
Insert the top edge of the prosthesis under the upper eyelid. Continue until the colored part of the prosthesis is almost covered by your eyelid.	Meta el borde superior de la prótesis debajo del párpado superior. Continue metiéndola hasta que la parte de color esté casi cubierta por el párpado.

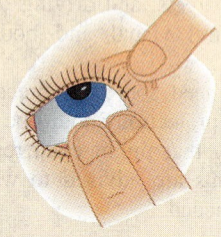

apy, or surgical removal. When the tumor is large, reconstruction may be required.

Eyelid, Lacrimal, and Conjunctival Disorders

Dacryocystitis

Dacryocystitis is an inflammation of the lacrimal sac. It can be an acute or a chronic problem and is due to blockage of tear drainage. The lacrimal system can become obstructed following bacterial infections, injuries, or nasal lesions. Management includes antibiotics, daily massage of the lacrimal drainage system, and warm compresses. Sometimes the lacrimal system needs to be opened. A probe can be used or surgery can be performed to reconstruct the lacrimal system.

Hordeolum

Hordeolum (stye) is an infection of the glands of the eyelids. It is most often caused by *Staphylococcus* infections, and clients complain of redness and pain caused by the lid swelling. A localized swelling is noted on either the external or internal margin of the lid close to the lashes. As the hordeolum forms, it may fill with purulent material, becoming reddened and painful.

Warm compresses applied several times and antibiotics are prescribed. If the hordeolum does not resolve spontaneously, incision and drainage of the purulent material is indicated.

Chalazion

A chalazion is a sterile chronic granulomatous inflammation of a meibomian gland. It is usually characterized by

Client Instructions in English *(Instrucciones para el cliente en inglés)*	Client Instructions in Spanish *(Instrucciones para el cliente en español)*
Gently release the upper eyelid.	Suelte suavemente el párpado superior.
Gently pull the lower eyelid outward until the prosthesis slips behind it. 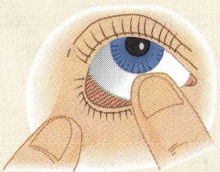	Suavemente hale el párpado inferior hasta que la prótesis se deslize detrás de él.
Removal	**Para quitarse la prótesis ocular**
Fill a container with saline (saltwater) solution to hold the prosthesis once you remove it.	Llene un recipiente con solución salina (agua con sal) para guardar la prótesis cuando se la quite.
Place a towel on the surface in front of you.	Ponga una toalla sobre la superficie delante de usted.
Wash your hands.	Lávese las manos.
Tilt your head forward slightly.	Incline un poco la cabeza hacia adelante.
Place your hand under the prosthesis.	Ponga la mano debajo de la prótesis.
Pull the lower eyelid down and to the side.	Hale el párpado inferior hacia abajo y para el lado.
Allow the prosthesis to slide out onto your hand. If necessary, pull gently on the lower edge of the eye with one finger to loosen the prosthesis.	Deje que la prótesis se le deslice en la mano. Si es necesario, hale suavemente con el dedo el borde inferior de la prótesis para aflorjarla.
Wash the prosthesis in warm water and store it in a container of saline solution.	Lave la prótesis en agua tibia y guárdela en un recipiente con solución salina (aqua con sal).

painless localized swelling along the lid margin without redness (Fig. 36–29). If the chalazion is large enough to distort vision or be a cosmetic blemish, it may be surgically excised.

Blepharitis

Blepharitis is a common chronic bilateral inflammation of the eyelid margins. Clients complain of itching and burning of the eyes and the eyes appear red, especially along the lid margins. Scales or granulations may be noted along the lashes of both the upper and lower lids. Treatment is to keep the scalp as well as the eyebrows and lid margins clean. Scales should be removed with baby shampoo, water, and cotton-tipped applicators. Infected blepharitis may be treated with antibiotic ophthalmic ointment.

Conjunctivitis

Conjunctivitis is an inflammation of the conjunctiva caused by bacterial, chlamydial (trachoma), viral, rickettsial, fungal, or parasitic infections; allergies; irritants; or secondary to systemic or other ocular diseases. Generally, the first sign of conjunctivitis is hyperemia (redness), accompanied by tearing, and exudation (flaking and sticky substances on the lid margins). Other symptoms may include pseudoptosis (drooping of the upper lid), papillary hypertrophy, follicles, pseudomembranes, and granulomas. Conjunctivitis is treated with antibiotic eye drops or systemic medications.

Episcleritis

Episcleritis is inflammation of the collagenous shell of the eye. It can be superficial (episcleritis) or deep (scleritis).

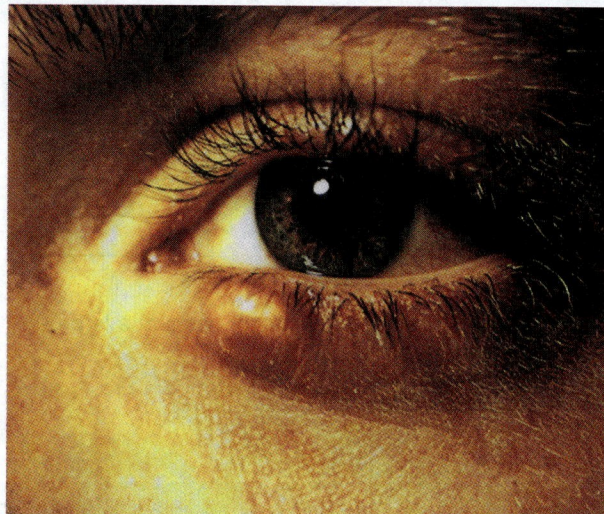

Figure 36–29. A chalazion. (Courtesy of Ophthalmic Photography at the University of Michigan W. K. Kellogg Eye Center, Ann Arbor.)

Episcleritis resembles a localized conjunctivitis. It is usually a self-limiting condition and does not damage the eye. It is often associated with autoimmune disorders.

Entropion

Entropion is the abnormal turning inward of the margin of the eyelid. The lower lid is most commonly affected. It can be caused by atrophy of the lower lid retractor muscles, spasms of the orbicularis oculi muscle, or scarring and deformity of the tarsal plate from trauma. Entropion can lead to conjunctival injury or inflammation. Medical management may consist of stabilizing the lower lid by taping it to the cheek. Surgical management corrects the underlying problem and may include resection of the orbicularis muscle, resection of a wedge of excess tissue from the eyelid, or reconstruction of the conjunctiva with mucosal grafts. Postoperative nursing care follows the standards of care for other eye surgery.

Ectropion

Ectropion is the abnormal turning outward of the margin of the lower eyelid. The most common cause is relaxation of the orbicularis oculi muscle with advancing age. Ectropion can be severe and lead to corneal drying, irritation, and conjunctivitis. Ectropion can also be caused by injury to the eye, such as burns, infections, or lacerations. This form of ectropion can involve both lids and is called *cicatricial* (meaning due to scar) *ectropion.* Ectropion is medically managed with lubricating drops during the daytime and eye ointments at night. Surgical management includes resection of the redundant tissues. Cicatricial ectropion is managed with skin grafts to replace missing tissues. Postoperative nursing care follows the standards of care for other eye surgery.

Ptosis

Ptosis (pronounced *toe'-sis*) is a drooping of the upper eyelid or eyelids. Ptosis can be congenital or acquired and constant or intermittent. Congenital ptosis involves malfunctions of the levator muscle and the client cannot move the eyelid. Acquired ptosis may be from mechanical, neurogenic, or myogenic factors. Mechanical factors include edema of the eyelid, tumors of the lid, or excess skin on the eyelids. Neurogenic factors include problems due to third cranial nerve degeneration. Nerve degeneration is seen in clients with carotid aneurysms and diabetes. Horner's syndrome is ptosis and pupil dilation seen in clients with tumors on the sympathetic nerves that control lid movement and pupillary constriction. Clients with goiter, cervical lymph node enlargement, and apical lung cancer are commonly seen with ptosis. Unilateral ptosis is one of the first signs of myasthenia gravis. It often escalates into bilateral ptosis. Ptosis can also be seen due to aging, because muscle tone is lost. Ptosis is managed primarily by surgical correction. Surgery is used to resect the levator palpebrae muscle, if it is working, or to resuspend it, if it is not working. Postoperative nursing care is the same as care needed after other eye surgery. If the client is not a candidate for surgery, ptosis can be reduced by using special glasses that lift the redundant skin.

Lagophthalmos

Lagophthalmos is inadequate closure of the eyelids. This condition may result on facial nerve weakness (cranial nerve V) or from enlargement with protrusion of the eyeball. When only a small portion of the central cornea is exposed, artificial tears should be used several times a day. Lubricating eye ointments should be used at night. Sustained-release tear inserts can also be used. Surgically, the lids can be temporarily or permanently closed to protect from corneal drying and injury.

Blinking Disorders

Blinking is both a voluntary and involuntary action. The rate of involuntary blinking varies, but the rate is rapid enough to spread tears across the surface of the eye. Reflex blinking is in response to irritants in the eye or pain in the eye. Rapid blinking also accompanies anxiety. Absence of blinking is seen in clients with Parkinson's disease and hyperthyroidism. Blinking too often is managed by removing the cause. Absence of blinking is treated with eye drops and ointments.

Dry Eye Syndrome

Dry eye syndrome is a condition in which tear production is inadequate. It most commonly occurs in women between 50 and 60 years of age. Dry eye syndrome occurs for three reasons: lacrimal gland malfunction, mucin deficiency, and mechanical abnormalities that prevent the spread of tears across the surface of the eye. The lacrimal gland can be genetically malformed or malformed due to injury or infection. Tear production is also decreased in Sjögren's syndrome, an autoimmune disorder that commonly accompanies rheumatoid arthritis. Facial nerve (cranial nerve VII) palsy disrupts tear production. Conjunctivitis and mumps can obstruct the gland. Some medications, such as antihistamines, atropine, and beta-adrenergic blocking agents, decrease tear production.

Mucin is a substance produced by the goblet cells in the eyelid; it maintains an even layer of tears across the surface of the eye. The absence of mucin allows the tear film to break up, leaving "dry spots" on the cornea. Mucin deficiency is seen with vitamin A deficiency and from medications such as antihistamines and beta-adrenergic blocking agents.

Mechanical abnormalities include problems with eyelid structure, eyeball extrusion, and misuse of contact lenses.

Clinical manifestations include burning, itching eyes and a sensation of "something" in the eye. The term *keratoconjunctivitis sicca* is used to describe the problem. Management includes determining the degree of injury to the cornea. Artificial tears can be used (drops and lubricants). In addition, some clients benefit from using airtight goggles at night to prevent tear evaporation. Postmenopausal women have found some relief from estrogen replacement. Surgery can be used to open the lacrimal duct or to repair lid problems.

Refractive Disorders

Light is bent (refracted) as it passes through the cornea and lens of the eye. Refractive errors (Fig. 36–30) exist when light rays are not focused appropriately on the retina of the eye.

There are three basic abnormalities of refraction that occur in the eye: (1) myopia, (2) hyperopia, and (3) astigmatism. Optical correction is important to distinguish between visual loss caused by disease and visual loss caused by refractive error. *Refractometry* is defined as the measurement of refractive error, and should not be confused with the term *refraction,* which is the method used to determine which lens or lenses (if any) will most benefit the client.

Myopia

Myopia, or nearsightedness, is a condition in which the light rays come into focus in front of the retina (Fig. 36–30A). In this case, the refractive power of the eye is too strong and a concave, or minus, lens is used to focus light rays on the eye. In most cases, myopia is caused by an eyeball that is longer than normal, which may be a familial trait. Transient myopia may occur with the administration of a variety of medications (sulfonamides, acetazolamide, salicylates, and steroids) and has been as-

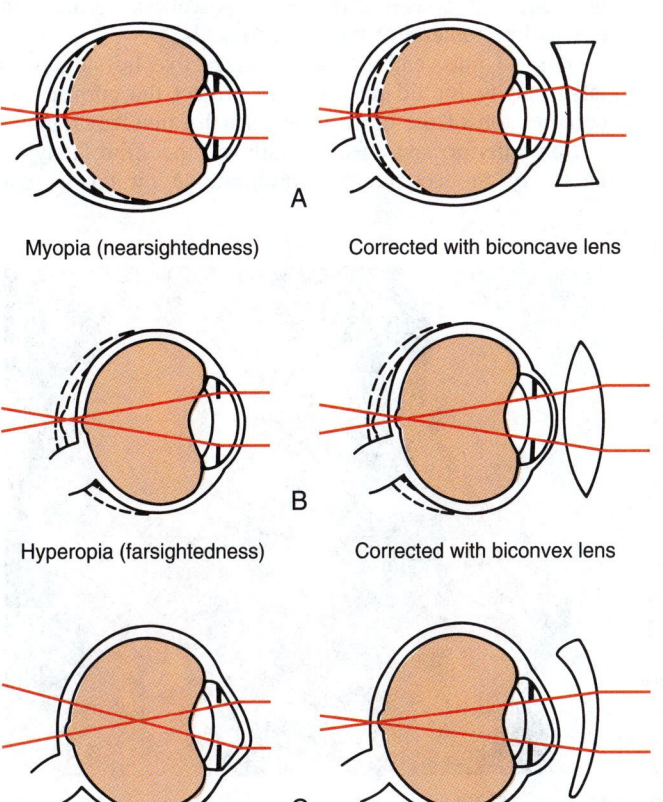

Myopia (nearsightedness)   Corrected with biconcave lens

Hyperopia (farsightedness)   Corrected with biconvex lens

Astigmatism   Corrected with astigmatic lens

Figure 36–30. *A–C,* Common refractive disorders and their correction. *Dashed lines* in *A* and *B* indicate normal eye contour.

sociated with other disorders, such as influenza, typhoid fever, severe dehydration, and large intakes of antacids (for stomach ulcers). Correction is accomplished with eyeglasses or contact lenses.

Hyperopia

The hyperopic, or farsighted, eye is one that is deficient in its ability to focus light rays. The focal point falls behind the eye (Fig. 36–30B) and consequently the image that falls on the retina is blurred. Vision may be brought into focus by placing a convex, or plus, lens in front of the eye. The lens supplies the magnifying power that the eye is lacking. Hyperopia may be caused by an eyeball that is shorter than normal or a cornea that has less curvature than normal. Because children have a greater ability to accommodate, they are less often affected than adults. Demands for close work and reading usually bring on symptoms of headache or eyestrain. Correction is based on age and individual needs and complaints.

Astigmatism

Astigmatism is a refractive condition in which rays of light are not bent equally by the cornea in all directions, so that a point of focus is not attained (Fig. 36–30C). In most instances, astigmatism is caused because the curvature of the cornea is not perfectly spherical. This is the cause of poor vision for both distant and near objects. Astigmatism is corrected with cylindrical lenses.

Surgical Management of Refractive Disorders

Refraction errors can be treated with elective surgery to reshape the cornea and change the refraction of light onto the retina. In one type of procedure, eight partial-thickness incisions are made in the cornea with a diamond blade to flatten the curvature of the cornea. Radial keratotomy is an elective procedure, and although it has been somewhat controversial over the past few years, it has been successful. Risks associated with this procedure include unsatisfactory correction, corneal glare, and postoperative infection. The excimer laser is used in this type of corneal surgery. It can evaporate tissue cleanly, with almost no damage to adjacent cells. The excimer laser is able to make extremely precise incisions in the cornea and may be useful in refractive surgery as well as keratoplasty.

Clients are assessed for degree of myopia or astigmatism prior to surgery. Advanced cases usually cannot achieve full correction. Surgery is performed on an outpatient basis under local anesthesia. After surgery, the eye is treated with steroid eye drops and most clients report watering of the eyes and minimal pain. Refraction is slow to stabilize after surgery. There is a period of adjustment during which time visual acuity waxes and wanes. Re-

duced contrast sensitivity in night vision and daytime glare is common. Visual acuity stabilizes in about 18 to 24 months. Some clients require retreatment for scarring unresponsive to topical steroids.

Ocular Manifestations of Systemic Disorders

Endocrine Disorders

Graves' disease may exist with or without any clinical evidence of thyroid dysfunction. Ocular signs include retraction of both upper and lower lids, giving a staring or frightened expression (Stellwag's sign), and lid lag (Graefe's sign), the retarded lowering of the upper lid when looking down (see Fig. 36–31). When the gaze is changed from down to up, the globe then lags behind the upper lid. Other signs are infrequent blinking, marked fine tremor with lid closure, and jerky movements on lid opening.

Infiltrative ophthalmopathy is characterized by enlargement of the extraocular muscles and edema in the extracellular tissues. Subsequent degeneration of muscle tissue leads to fibrosis, which restricts muscle movement, resulting in double vision. Proliferation of orbital fat tissue along with the enlargement of muscle tissue and edema result in proptosis (the forward protrusion of the eyeballs), which is also called exophthalmos.

As a primary measure, adequate control of thyroid abnormalities is essential. Diuretics, as well as steroid therapy and radiotherapy, may be indicated.

Surgical interventions include corrective lid surgery or tarsorrhaphy for lid retraction to protect the cornea. Decompression of the orbit, which usually involves removal of the inferior and medial walls of the orbit, may be necessary to accommodate proliferative orbital fat and

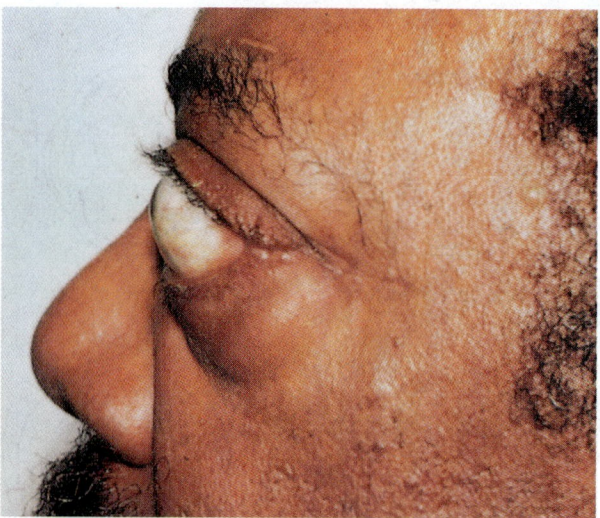

Figure 36–31. Graves' exophthalmos. (Courtesy of Ophthalmic Photography at the University of Michigan W. K. Kellogg Eye Center, Ann Arbor.)

enlarged ocular muscles. Ocular muscle surgery may also be indicated.

The extent of the surgical procedure is likely to determine whether or not the client undergoing an orbital decompression will require a hospital stay. If the surgery is extensive, the operative sites may have suction drains. Drainage is usually serosanguineous. It is important that the client sleep with the head elevated to reduce postoperative swelling. Advise the client to expect redness, swelling, and ecchymoses around the eyes and lids. In the immediate postoperative period, check the client's visual acuity with a near vision card every hour to monitor the possibility of pressure on the optic nerve (see Thinking Critically). Caution the client to modify normal activities for the first 2 weeks after surgery.

Rheumatoid and Connective Tissue Disorders

Sjögren's syndrome includes keratoconjunctivitis sicca, a common condition in which tear secretion is reduced, in association with a systemic disorder such as rheumatoid arthritis, psoriatic arthritis, connective tissue disorders, sarcoidosis, or Crohn's disease. Symptoms include ocular irritation and foreign-body sensation. Frequent instillation of lubricating eye drops or ointment is effective in most cases.

Several ocular problems may be associated with systemic lupus erythematosus, a connective tissue disorder. The eyelids may be involved with the discoid lesions characteristic of the disease. Punctate epithelial keratopathy and secondary Sjögren's syndrome may also occur. Retinopathy of systemic lupus erythematosus produces cotton-wool spots and increased retinal vessel fragility, as in diabetes. Optic neuropathy can also occur.

Neurologic Disorders

Approximately 90% of clients with myasthenia gravis have ocular involvement. In most cases, it is the presenting symptom. Ptosis (drooping of the eyelid) is bilateral, but may be asymmetrical. Diplopia (double vision) is frequently in the vertical plane. Nystagmus is also present. Ocular myopathy and cranial nerve palsy may develop later, as can opththalmoplegia (paralysis of all the extraocular muscles). Medical treatment is supportive and includes systemic steroids.

There is also a close association between optic neuritis and multiple sclerosis. Approximately three fourths of women and one third of men who develop optic neuritis are diagnosed with multiple sclerosis at 15-year follow-up. Typically, an attack of optic neuritis starts with acute onset of loss of vision in one eye, with periocular discomfort made worse by movement of the eye. Visual impairment is progressive over a 2-week period and usually recovers after 4 to 6 weeks. Recovery may take longer and may be incomplete. Medical treatment consists of oral, intravenous, and retrobulbar steroids.

Circulatory Disorders

The primary response of retinal arterioles to hypertension is narrowing. In chronic hypertension, the blood-retina barrier is disrupted in small areas, resulting in increased vascular permeability. The fundus examination reveals vasoconstriction, leakage, and arteriosclerosis. Hypertensive retinopathy is graded for severity on a scale of 1 to 4, with 4 being the most severe. Systemic hypertension is also associated with an increased risk of retinal vein occlusion. There is no known treatment for retinal vein occlusion.

Immunologic Disorders

Ocular complications affect approximately 75% of patients with AIDS. In many cases, the ocular manifestations may be the presenting symptoms that lead to diagnosis of human immunodeficiency virus (HIV) infection. Cytomegalovirus (CMV) retinitis is the most common ocular opportunistic infection. This sight-threatening condition occurs in 30% of persons with AIDS. It is often asymptomatic until it is well established, when the client begins to notice visual field loss, floaters, or other vague vision problems. A unilateral lesion with the appearance of a cotton-wool spot often develops with white irregular borders associated with hemorrhages. Small lesions may be seen beyond the edges. The retina in the center of the lesion becomes thin and tears easily. Loss of vision is involved and central vision is greatly diminished.

CMV retinitis requires intravenous therapy, usually through placement of a long-term indwelling catheter. Ganciclovir or foscarnet sodium is administered over several weeks in the hospital or through homecare. Because progression is rapid, early treatment is essential and may prevent involvement of the other eye. Careful monitoring of side effects and response to the medication is imperative.

Other infectious ocular conditions that may occur in persons with HIV disease are bacterial corneal ulcers (syphilis, staphylococcosis), fungal corneal ulcers (candidiasis, cryptococcosis, histoplasmosis, sporotrichosis), and protozoan (toxoplasmosis, pneumocystosis) and viral infections (herpes simplex).

Noninfectious ocular manifestations in persons with HIV infection include HIV retinopathy and neoplastic processes such as Kaposi's sarcoma and non-Hodgkin's lymphoma which appear around the ocular adnexa. AIDs retinopathy is seen in over 50% of clients with HIV infection. Direct ophthalmoscopy reveals the presence of cotton-wool spots, retinal hemorrhages, and other microvascular anomalies. The lesions of AIDs retinopathy are indistinguishable from the retinopathy of diabetes or hypertension. They usually occur in the superficial retina and resolve over a period of a few weeks, while CMV retinitis lesions will expand. Kaposi's sarcoma and non-Hodgkin's lymphoma present around the eyelids and orbit with diplopia, ptosis, conjunctival edema, or hemorrhage. Diagnosis is confirmed with diagnostic imaging, needle biopsy, and systemic work-up. Treatment of Kaposi's sarcoma is usually conservative and may include radiotherapy.

Evaluation of extraocular muscle function is important because lymphoma may increase intracranial pressure. This increased pressure may lead to cranial nerve palsies and alter eye position. Surgical correction of extraocular muscle position may be necessary for resolving diplopia or for cosmetic reasons.

Lyme Disease

Lyme disease, *Borrelia burgdorferi*-transmitted by the bite of a tick, has three stages. The initial stage involves a lesion and erythema around the bite, accompanied by regional lymphadenopathy, malaise, fever, headache, myalgia, arthralgia, and frequently conjunctivitis. Several weeks to months later during the second phase, there is a period associated with neurologic and cardiac problems. Along with these problems, there may also be cranial nerve palsies, uveitis, optic neuropathy, keratitis, choroiditis, and exudative retinal detachments. Tetracycline and penicillin are effective in treating the initial infection and in preventing late complications.

Conclusions

It is essential to understand the complexity of ocular structures and the physiology of vision to provide comprehensive nursing care for clients. The specialty practice of ophthalmic registered nursing is devoted to caring for clients with eye disorders. Ophthalmic registered nurses perform the roles of caregiver, advocate, educator, counselor, technician, coordinator, and researcher. Ophthalmic nursing care is directed not only at those biologic systems that are affected by an actual or potential deficit but is an integration of how actual or potential visual deficits affect the individual as an entire being.

Thinking Critically

1. Your client is a 72-year-old retired carpenter who has undergone outpatient cataract surgery. He and his wife live an hour away from the surgery center, where they received instructions to call the emergency number for any unusual pain or nausea. They have an appointment to return for a follow-up evaluation the next morning. After supper, the client's wife calls to report that her husband has a headache. She says that her husband also has an upset stomach, but thinks he feels queasy because he ate some spicy food. The client does not want his wife to drive him back at night and thinks his wife should not have bothered to call, since they have an appointment in the morning. How would you proceed? What further assessment data are needed? What are the likely complications following cataract surgery, and what are their clinical manifestations?

Factors to Consider. Could the headache and upset stomach be related to the cataract surgery, or are they likely to be unrelated?

2. Your client, a 55-year-old woman with Graves' ophthalmopathy, had surgery in the late afternoon today for a right orbital decompression. An incisional drain is in place at the right temple with a bulb attached for suction. The surgeon has ordered postoperative vision checks with a near vision card every hour throughout the night. The surgery took more than 3 hours under general anesthesia, and your client is still sedated. Her right eye is extremely swollen, so is unable to open it to read the vision card. She winces and cries when her operative eye is touched, and she is so sleepy that she cannot respond by reading the vision card. What should you do to carry out the surgeon's postoperative orders?

Factors to Consider. Are such severe eye pain and swelling normal postoperative findings? How would you assess the eye? How would you rouse the client to perform these crucial eye assessments?

Bibliography

1. Abrahamson, J., Kushnick, H., and Mayers, M. (1994). Ocular manifestations of systemic infection. *Current Opinion in Ophthalmology, 5,* 84–90.
2. Allen, M., and MacDougall, F. (1994). Origins of beliefs and attitudes toward blindness. *Journal of Ophthalmic Nursing and Technology, 13*(6), 278–280.
3. Anderson, W., et al. (1991). *Atlas of ophthalmic surgery* (Vol. 1). St. Louis: Mosby–Year Book.
4. Barraquer, R., and Barraquer, J. (1994). Corneal dystrophies and keratoconus. *Current Opinion in Ophthalmology, 5,* 53–67.
5. Berson, F., (1993). *Basic ophthalmology for medical students and primary care residents.* San Francisco: American Academy of Ophthalmology.
6. Bigar, R., and Herbort, C., (1992). Corneal transplantation. *Current Opinion in Ophthalmology, 3,* 473–481.
7. Bigerly, J., and Nozik, R. (1992). Management of uveitis. *Current Opinion in Ophthalmology, 3,* 527–533.
8. Burlew, J. (1991). Preventing eye injuries—the nurse's role. *Journal of the American Society of Ophthalmic Registered Nurses, 16*(6), 24–28.
9. Donneffel, M. (1990). Corneal transplantation. In K. Sigardson-Poor and L. Haggerty (Eds.), *Nursing care of the transplant recipient.* Philadelphia: W. B. Saunders.
10. Dinowitz, K., et al. (1994). Ocular manifestations of immunologic and rheumatologic inflammatory disorders. *Current Opinion in Ophthalmology, 5,* 91–98.
11. Duane, T., & Jaeger, E. (1990). *Clinical ophthalmology* (Vols. 1–5). Philadelphia: J. B. Lippincott.
12. Ehlers, W., and Donshik, P. (1994). Allergic diseases of the lids, conjunctiva, and cornea. *Current Opinion in Ophthalmology 5,* 31–38.
13. Fagerstrom, R. (1992). Defense mechanisms of elderly persons before and after a cataract operation, *Journal of Visual Impairment and Blindness, 86*(8), 361–363.
14. Fishbaugh, J. (1995). Look who's driving now—Visual standards for driver's licensing in the United States. *Insight, 20*(4), 11–20.
15. Garber, N. (1991). Basic ocular motility assessment. *Journal of Ophthalmic Nursing and Technology, 10*(5), 215–219.
16. Gills, J., Loyd, T., and Cherchio, M. (1995). Anesthesia, preoperative, and postoperative medications. *Current Opinion in Ophthalmology, 6,* 31–35.

17. Gold, D., (1994). Ocular manifestations of systemic disease. *Current Opinion in Ophthalmology, 5,* 63–64.
18. Gramer, E., and Tausch, M. (1995). The risk profile of the glaucomatous patient. *Current Opinion in Ophthalmology, 6,* 78–88.
19. Grehn, F. (1995). The value of trebeculotomy in glaucoma surgery. *Current Opinion in Ophthalmology, 6,* 52–60.
20. Harding, J. (1995). Epidemiology, pathophysiology, and world blindness. *Current Opinion in Ophthalmology, 6,* 27–30.
21. Hoffman, J. (1989). *Pocket glossary of ophthalmologic terminology,* Thorofare: Slack.
22. Huber-Spitzy, V., and Graner, G. (1991). Degenerative conditions, keratoconus, contact lenses, and dry eyes. *Current Opinion in Ophthalmology, 2,* 402–408.
23. Kaye, G., et al. (1990). IOL implant patients need your help. *Journal of Ophthalmic Nursing and Technology, 4*(4), 18–23.
24. Lang, G., and Lang, G. (1994). The cornea and systemic diseases. *Current Opinion in Ophthalmology, 5,* 25–30.
25. Legro, M. (1991). Quality of life and cataracts: A review of patient-centered studies of cataract surgery outcomes. *Ophthalmic Surgery, 22,* 431–443.
26. Lichter, P. (1990). Caffeine and other prescriptions for patients with glaucoma. *Ophthalmology, 97*(8), 965–966.
27. Masket, S. (1992). Complications of cataract and intraocular lens surgery. *Current Opinion in Ophthalmology, 3,* 52–59.
28. Novack, G. (1994). Ocular toxicology. *Current Opinion in Ophthalmology, 5,* 110–114.
29. Obstbaum, S. (1991). *Glaucoma surgery atlas.* Norwalk, CT: Appleton & Lange.
30. Pavan-Langston, D. (1991). *Manual of ocular diagnosis and therapy* (3rd ed.). Boston: Little, Brown.
31. Pavan-Langston, D., and Dunkel, E. (1991). *Handbook of ocular drug therapy and ocular side effects of systemic drugs.* Boston: Little, Brown.
32. Perry, A. (1990). Integrated orbital implants. *Advances in Ophthalmic Plastic and Reconstructive Surgery, 8,* 75–81.
33. Plona, R., and Schremp, P. (1992). Nursing care of patients with ocular manifestations of human immunodeficiency virus infection. *Nursing Clinics of North America, 27*(3), 793–805.
34. Rapuano, C., and Laibson, P. (1992). Corneal dystrophies. *Current Opinion in Ophthalmology, 3,* 438–444.
35. Rozakis, G. (1990). *Cataract surgery.* Thorofare, NJ: Slack.
36. Servodidio, C. (1991). Teaching aids to patients diagnosed with choroidal melanoma. *Journal of the American Society of Ophthalmic Registered Nurses, 16*(6), 21–23.
37. Singerman, L., & Jampol, L. (1991). *Retinal and choroidal manifestations of systemic disease.* Baltimore: Williams & Wilkins.
38. Slakter, J. (1992). Recent developments in ophthalmic lasers. *Current Opinion in Ophthalmology, 3,* 83–93.
39. Solomon, K., and Kostick, A. (1992). Capsular opacification after cataract surgery. *Current Opinion in Ophthalmology, 3,* 46–51.
40. Sperber, L., and Dodick, J. (1995). Laser therapy in cataract surgery. *Current Opinion in Ophthalmology, 6,* 22–26.
41. Stein, H., Slatt, B., and Stein, R. (1994). *The ophthalmic assistant* (6th ed.). St. Louis: Mosby–Year Book.
42. Stewart, W. (1995). The effect of lifestyle on the relative risk to develop open-angle glaucoma. *Current Opinion in Ophthalmology, 6,* 3–9.
43. Trobe, J. (1993). *The physician's guide to eye care.* San Francisco: American Academy of Ophthalmology.
44. Vader, L. (1992). Invisible light. *Insight 17*(2), 12–14.
45. Vaughan, D., Asbury, T., and Riordan-Eva, P. (1995). *General ophthalmology* (14th ed.). Norwalk, CT: Appleton & Lange.
46. Werner, E. (1991). *Manual of visual fields.* New York: Churchill Livingstone.
47. Wesley, R. (1994). Lacrimal disease. *Current Opinion in Ophthalmology, 5,* 78–83.
48. Williams, G. (1994). Posterior vitreous detachment. *Current Opinion in Ophthalmology, 5,* 10–13.
49. Wilson, S., & Kaufman, H. (1990). Graft failure after penetrating keratoplasty. *Survey of Ophthalmology, 34*(5), 325–356.
50. Young, R. (1991). *Age related cataract.* New York: Oxford University Press.

Joyce M. Black

Hearing and balance problems can reduce the ability to communicate, limit social activities, and hinder the constructive use of leisure time. Career options, job opportunities, and financial security can also be compromised. Ear problems can interfere with the client's ability to remain independent, which can lead to isolation. Also, the aesthetic enjoyment of life and the ability to share human experiences can be temporarily or permanently diminished. All these situations can result in feelings of anger, anxiety, frustration, uncertainty, and loneliness, which ultimately may affect the quality of life.

Structure and Function of the Ear

Structure of the Temporal Bone

The ear is housed in the temporal bone of the skull. The temporal bones are two of the eight cranial bones that form part of the base and lateral wall of the skull. The temporal bone can be divided into four parts: (1) squamous, (2) mastoid, (3) petrous, and (4) tympanic. The petrous portion of the temporal bone houses the most dense bone in the body, the otic capsule. The temporal bone articulates with the sphenoid, parietal, and occipital bones. The bony anatomy of the temporal bone is the most detailed part of the skull. If a 50¢ coin were superimposed on the external auditory canal, the following structures would all fit within the coin's circumference: the tympanic ring and tympanic membrane, the three ossicles, the jugular vein, the carotid artery, the facial nerve, and the auditory and vestibular parts of the inner ear.

Structure of the External Ear

The external ear is divided into the auricle, or pinna, and the external auditory canal, or ear canal. The ears are located on each side of the head at approximately eye level. If an imaginary line were drawn from the outer canthus of the eye to the top of the ear canal, this line should be parallel to the floor. The pinna is attached to the side of the head at approximately a 20- to 30-degree angle.

Auricle (Pinna)

The conspicuous part of the ear that projects outward is called the *auricle,* or pinna. The pinna is attached to the side of the head by skin. It is composed mostly of cartilage, except for the fat and subcutaneous tissue in the lobule. The cartilage is held to the skull by small muscles that are innervated by a branch of the facial nerve. The muscles are the posterior, anterior, and superior auricular muscles.

The parts of the pinna are illustrated in Figure 37–1. The *concha* is the deepest part and leads to the ear canal. The *helix* is the outer rim of the pinna and leads inferiorly to the lobule. The concha is bounded anteriorly by a triangular fold of cartilage called the *tragus,* which projects posteriorly over the entrance to the ear canal. Hair covers most of the ear, but it is usually rudimentary, except in the region of the tragus and antitragus. Sebaceous glands are also found on the skin surface.

In front of (anterior to) the external opening of the ear is the temporomandibular joint. The head of the mandibular condyle can be felt by the tip of a finger placed in the external meatus while the mouth is opened and closed. Very often, temporomandibular joint problems produce referred pain to the ear (otalgia) because of the same sensory nerve supply.

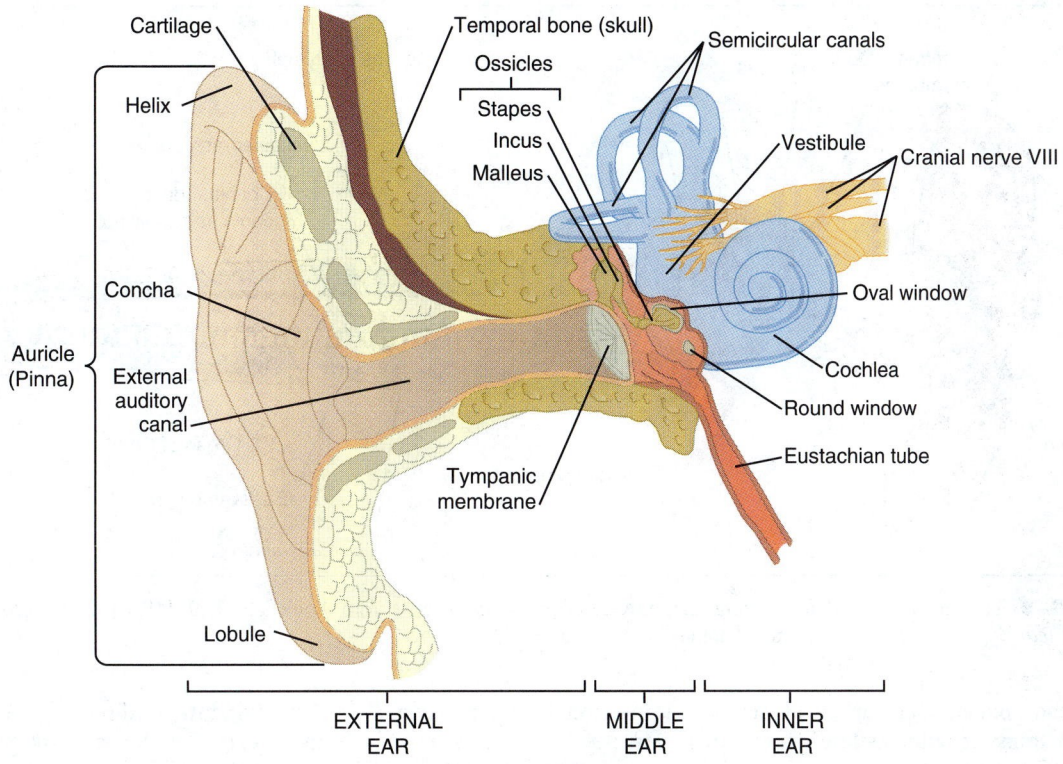

Figure 37–1. Anatomy of the ear.

External Auditory Canal or Ear Canal

The ear canal extends from the concha of the pinna to the tympanic membrane (see Fig. 37–1). This S-shaped canal is approximately 2.5 cm (1 inch) in length and follows an inward, forward, and downward path. The lumen is irregular in shape. The skeleton of cartilage in the outer third is continuous with the cartilage of the pinna. The inner two thirds is a bony canal entering the skull. The lumen of the ear canal is narrowest where the transition from cartilage to bone occurs. The skin covering the cartilage portion is thick; it contains sebaceous and ceruminous glands and hair follicles. The secretion of these cerumen glands and the fat from the sebaceous glands form a golden to black substance called *cerumen* (wax). The skin covering the bony portion is very thin.

Tympanic Membrane

The tympanic membrane, or eardrum, is an oval disc approximately 1 cm in diameter; it covers the end of the auditory canal and separates the canal from the middle ear (see Fig. 37–1). The eardrum is a thin, translucent, pearly gray membrane obliquely directed downward and inward, so that the posterior part is more accessible than is the anterior part. The eardrum consists of three tissue layers: an outer epithelial layer continuous with the skin of the ear canal, a fibrous supporting middle layer, and an inner mucosal layer continuous with the mucosal lining of the middle ear cavity.

Function of the Temporal Bone and External Ear

The ears are a pair of complex sensory organs for both hearing and balance. Their location on either side of the head produces binaural hearing, allows the detection of sound direction, and aids in maintaining equilibrium. The temporal bone provides protection for the organs of hearing and balance. It houses the external and internal auditory canals; the mastoid air cells, which provide an air reservoir for the middle ear; the blood vessels; the facial, vestibular, and auditory nerves; the labyrinth; and the cochlea.

Sound Wave Conduction

Sound is transmitted from the external ear through the middle ear (which amplifies the sound) to the inner ear (Fig. 37–2). The pinna collects and directs sound. The funnel shape of the pinna collects and directs sound to the eardrum. The tympanic membrane is a common membrane between the external ear canal and the middle ear space. The tympanic membrane protects the middle ear and conducts sound vibrations from the external ear to the ossicles. The sound pressure applied to the stapes (the smallest ossicle) in the oval window is 22 times greater than the sound pressure exerted on the eardrum. The pressure of the sound vibrations is increased as a result of transmission from a larger area to the smaller area and the lever effect of the ossicular chain.

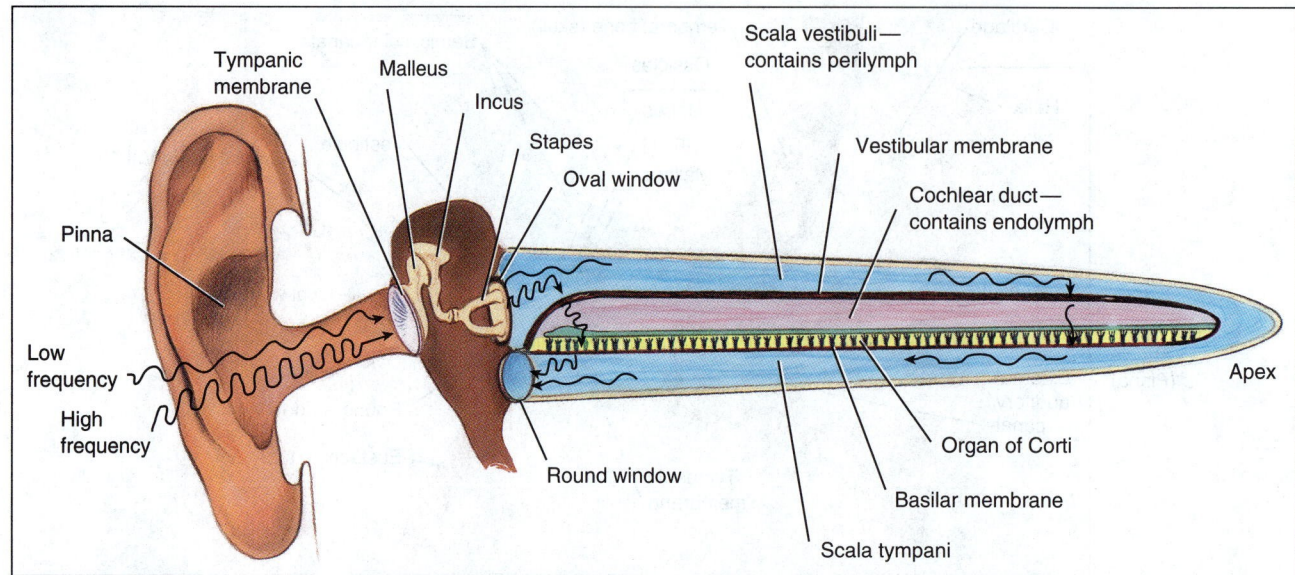

Figure 37–2. The uncoiled cochlea, showing the pathway of pressure waves. (From Applegate, E. J. [1995]. *The anatomy and physiology learning system: Textbook.* Philadelphia: W. B. Saunders.)

The head, pinna, and ear canal act as an integrated system to transmit sound vibrations on their way to the eardrum. The external ear actually amplifies certain frequencies. The sound energy, after transformation, is carried by neural elements to the brain for decoding and, thus, hearing.

Wax Production

Cerumen (wax) protects the ear. Wax is to the ear what tears are to the eyes. The sticky consistency of the wax and the fine hairs of the ear canal help cleanse the ear canal of foreign matter and protect it from water damage. The hairs become coarser during the aging process; thus, retention of wax is more of a problem in the elderly. Impacted cerumen can cause hearing losses in clients of all ages. At times, the wax must be mechanically removed.

Structure of the Middle Ear

The middle ear consists of the middle ear cleft and contents: ossicles, oval and round windows, facial nerve, and eustachian tube (see Fig. 37–1). The ear canal is external to the middle ear, and the labyrinth (inner ear) is internal to the middle ear. The middle ear cavity has a mucosal lining.

Ossicles

The middle ear contains the three smallest bones of the body. The names of these bones, or ossicles, have their origins in the bones' appearance. The outermost ossicle is the *malleus* (hammer), which is firmly attached to the tympanic membrane and is the largest of the ossicles. The innermost ossicle is the *stapes* (stirrup). The stapes foot-

plate occupies the oval window, in direct contact with the perilymph of the inner ear. The stapes is the smallest of the ossicles. The *incus* (anvil) lies between the other two and has the same shape as a tooth with two roots (see Fig. 37–1).

Windows

The middle ear contains two windows, named because of their shape. The round window is an opening into the inner ear from which sound vibrations exit. The oval window is an opening into the inner ear into which sound vibrations enter. The oval window is not a true window because the footplate of the stapes bone covers it.

Eustachian Tube

The eustachian tube is a narrow channel approximately 35 mm (1½ inch) in length and only 1 mm wide at its narrowest end. This tube connects the middle ear to the nasopharynx (see Fig. 37–1). The structure consists mostly of fibrous tissue, cartilage, and bone; it extends downward, forward, and inward from each middle ear. The lining of the eustachian tube consists of mucous membrane that is continuous with the lining of the middle ear at one end and the nasopharynx at the other end. A small section of this tube, originating in the middle ear, remains permanently open. Otherwise, the walls of the tube are lightly opposing or touching each other, closing the tube to both the throat and ear. This closure prevents the sound of normal nasal respiration and of one's own voice from passing up the eustachian tube. However, during yawning, swallowing, and sneezing, the eustachian tube is opened by the tensor veli palatini muscle, to equalize pressure. The natural opening and closing of the eustachian tube allows equalization of air pressure between the middle ear and the environment and drainage of exudate from the middle ear mucosa.

Mastoid Bone

The mastoid section of the temporal bone includes the mastoid process, which is cone-shaped; the mastoid antrum, a large cavity posteriorly continuous with the middle ear; and the mastoid air cells, which extend from the antrum and fill the temporal bone with air pockets.

The mastoid bone is located posterior to the pinna and can be felt as a bony protuberance behind the lower portion of the pinna. The mastoid cavity is close to several important cranial structures: the dura of the temporal lobe, the cerebellar dura, the sigmoid sinus, and the jugular bulb. The middle ear is also bounded by the internal carotid artery. Therefore, infection of the middle ear and mastoid cavities can also involve these structures.

Function of the Middle Ear

The ossicles transmit sound vibrations mechanically (see Fig. 37–2). The ossicles are held in place by joints, muscles, and ligaments, which also offer protective mechanisms from loud sounds. The light weight and configuration of the ossicles provide an efficient means of transmission of sound vibrations from the air molecules of the external ear to the fluid molecules of the inner ear. Fluids offer more resistance than air and need more force to transmit movement. The ossicular chain produces and magnifies this force in order to move the inner ear fluids.

The eustachian tube provides an air passage from the nasopharynx to the middle ear to equalize pressure on both sides of the eardrum. This tube allows air to enter and leave the middle ear and is responsible for ventilation and pressure regulation, both of which are necessary for normal hearing. The tube can be forcibly opened by increasing nasopharyngeal pressure. This act is called Valsalva's maneuver and is accomplished by attempting to blow air through the nose while it is held closed.

The cavity of the mastoid bone and the interconnected arrangement of the air-filled spaces aid the middle ear in adjusting to changes in pressure. The mastoid system acts as a buffer for the middle ear. The system of cavities and air cells also lightens the skull.

Structure of the Inner Ear (Labyrinth)

The inner ear, or labyrinth, is located deep within the petrous section of the temporal bone; it contains the sense organs for hearing and balance, which form the eighth cranial nerve (Fig. 37–3). The inner ear is a complicated system of intercommunicating chambers and connecting tubes composed of two structures: the bony labyrinth and the membranous labyrinth; the membranous labyrinth lies within, but does not completely fill, the bony labyrinth.

The bony labyrinth is the rigid capsule in which the membranous labyrinth lies. This otic capsule surrounds and protects the delicate membranous labyrinth. The vestibule connects the cochlea, for hearing, to the three semicircular canals, for balance. The cochlea, which looks like a snail shell with 2½ turns, is approximately 7 mm in diameter at the widest part and is structurally divided into two compartments. The upper compartment, the scala vestibuli, leads from the oval window to the apex of the cochlear spiral. The lower compartment, the scala tympani, leads from the apex of the cochlear spiral to the round window. The scala media, which contains the organ of Corti, lies between the scala vestibuli and scala tympani.

The three semicircular canals are at right angles to each other and, because of position, are named the superior, the posterior, and the lateral or horizontal canal. The horizontal canal lies closest to the middle ear.

The membranous labyrinth, within the bony labyrinth, is bathed in a fluid called perilymph, which communicates with the cerebrospinal fluid via the cochlear duct. The membranous labyrinth consists of the utricle, the saccule, the semicircular canals, the cochlear duct, and

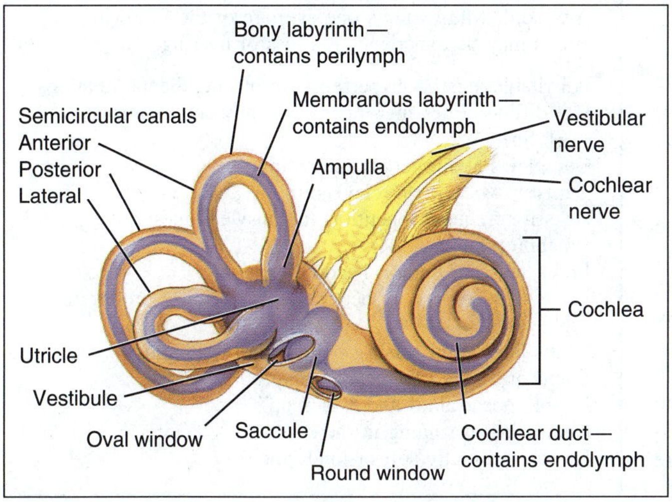

Figure 37–3. The labyrinths of the inner ear. (From Applegate, E. J. [1995]. *The anatomy and physiology learning system: Textbook.* Philadelphia: W. B. Saunders.)

Bony labyrinth— contains perilymph
Membranous labyrinth— contains endolymph
Semicircular canals
Anterior
Posterior
Lateral
Ampulla
Vestibular nerve
Cochlear nerve
Cochlea
Utricle
Vestibule
Oval window
Saccule
Cochlear duct— contains endolymph
Round window

the organ of Corti, which is the end organ for hearing. The membranous labyrinth contains a different fluid, called *endolymph*. This fluid also protects the end organ because it acts as a cushion against abrupt movements of the head.

Function of the Inner Ear

Hearing

Sound waves are transmitted by the ossicles to the delicate membrane of the oval window (see Fig. 37–2). These vibrations move the perilymph in the scala vestibuli. The perilymph of the scala vestibuli is continuous with that of the scala tympani at the extreme tip of the snail shell called the *helicotrema*. The sound energy vibrations enter through the oval window and exit through the round window.

Vibrations in the perilymph of the scala vestibuli are transmitted through the vestibular membrane, or Reissner's membrane, to the endolymph that fills the cochlear duct. The cochlear duct is located between the scala vestibuli and the scala tympani. The organ of Corti, which is bathed in the endolymph, lies on the basilar membrane in a spiral strip from the basal turn near the round window to the apex at the helicotrema. This structure transforms mechanical sound vibrations into neural activity and separates sound into different frequencies. This electrochemical impulse travels via the acoustic nerve to the brain stem and then to the temporal cortex of the brain. The acoustic nerve, or eighth cranial nerve, reaches the cochlea and vestibule via the internal auditory canal. The facial nerve, or seventh cranial nerve, courses through the same canal.

Many physiologic changes lead to changes in hearing in the elderly. *Presbycusis* is a type of hearing loss that occurs with aging, even in people living in a quiet environment. It is a gradual sensorineural loss caused by nerve degeneration in the inner ear or auditory nerve. Other anatomic and physiologic changes due to aging are shown in Table 37–1.

Balance

The utricle and saccule are vestibular receptors that position the head as it relates to the pull of gravity. The semicircular canals are arranged to sense rotational movements, such as movements or changes in position. Each of the semicircular canals connects with the utricle. Where the canals connect with the utricle, each canal contains an enlarged portion, called the *ampulla*. The ampulla contains a cluster of hair cells, called the *crista*, which are concerned with dynamic balance. For example, when the head position is changed, movement of the endolymph stimulates the hair cells, which initiates increased impulses that travel over the vestibular division of the acoustic nerve to the brain. Balance functions in the vestibular system combine with visual cues and musculoskeletal cues for balance. Hearing and balance are partially maintained with the loss of function of one ear.

Table 37–1. Changes in Auditory Acuity Caused by Aging	
Anatomic Changes	**Physiologic Changes**
Degeneration of basilar conductive membrane of cochlea	Decreased ability to hear at all frequencies but greater at higher frequencies
Degeneration of cochlear hair cells	Decreased ability to hear high-frequency sounds
Decreased vascularity of cochlea	Loss of hearing equal at all frequencies
Loss of auditory neurons in spiral ganglia of organ of Corti	Loss of ability to hear high-frequency sounds
Loss of cortical auditory neurons	Diminished hearing and speech comprehension

Loss of auditory neurons in the organ of Corti and cochlear hair cell degeneration creates an inability to hear high-frequency sounds. There may also be degeneration of the cochlear conductive membrane and decreased blood supply to the cochlea leading to inability to hear at all frequencies (but more pronounced at higher frequencies). Finally, a loss of cortical auditory neurons leads to diminished hearing and speech comprehension.

Assessment of the Ear

The otologic history can be the most important assessment tool and should be obtained before audiometric testing. Certain behavioral cues can indicate hearing loss (Box 37–1). Significant data are collected by conducting a thorough interview. Specific items that should be included in the otologic history are identified in Box 37–2.

Box 37–1. Clues Suggesting Loss of Hearing

Any adult who exhibits one or more of the following traits may be experiencing a loss of hearing:

Is irritable, hostile, hypersensitive in intercliental relations
Has difficulty hearing upper frequency consonants (Sl, Sh)
Complains about people mumbling
Turns up volume on television
Asks for frequent repetition and answers questions inappropriately
Loses sense of humor, becomes grim
Leans forward to hear better or turns head to preferred side
Shuns large- and small-group audience situations
Shuns areas with increased background noise
Might appear aloof and "stuck up"
Complains of ringing in the ears
Has an unusually soft or loud voice

Box 37–2. Otologic History Assessment Guide

Current Problem

What changes are you having in your hearing?
Do you have any of the following symptoms?

Distortion of hearing	Yes No
Differences in the pitch of sound	Yes No
Noise in your ear	Yes No
Fullness or pressure in your ear	Yes No
Pain in your ear	Yes No
Drainage from your ear	Yes No
Have you ever had a hearing examination?	Yes No

    If yes, why?
    What were the results?

Use of Hearing Aids

Are you wearing hearing aids now?	Yes No
Are your hearing aids effective?	Yes No
How old are your hearing aids?	L __ yr R __ yr

Associated Problems

Do you have any of the following symptoms?

Head noise or ringing	Yes No
Feeling dizzy or unsteady	Yes No
Blurred vision	Yes No
Double vision	Yes No
Numbness in the hands or feet	Yes No
Weakness in the arms or legs	Yes No
Tingling around the mouth or face	Yes No
Loss of consciousness or blackouts	Yes No
Fainting	Yes No
Convulsions or seizures	Yes No

Risk Factors

Have you ever worked around loud noises?	Yes No
How long? _____ yr	
Do you still work around loud noise?	Yes No
Do you wear ear protection?	Yes No

Past Medical History

Did you have hearing problems as a child?	Yes No

    Explain.

Have you had ear surgery?	Yes No

    If yes,

	Date	Operation	Surgeon
Right ear	_____	_____	_____
Left ear	_____	_____	_____

Do you have any food or medication allergies?
    Please list and describe your reaction.

Family History

Do you have family members who were hard of hearing before 50 years old?
    If yes, explain.

Have any members of your family ever had ear surgery?
    If yes, explain.

History

An otologic history includes demographic data, current clinical manifestations, past health history, family health history, psychosocial history, and review of systems. Ear problems often result from childhood illnesses or problems associated with adjacent structures. The history interview is essential for determining current problems related to the ear.

Demographic data relevant to otologic assessment include the client's age. Hearing loss occurs as a consequence of the aging process.

Current Symptoms

The most common chief complaints include the following:

Hearing loss
Pain
Tinnitus
Ear drainage
Loss of balance
Vertigo
Dizziness

The client may also complain of associated nausea or vomiting. The nurse completes a symptom analysis to determine onset, duration, frequency, and precipitating and relieving factors for the presenting symptom. Explore the client's past medical history carefully to determine the chronicity of the problem and to determine the cause.

Hearing loss may occur suddenly or gradually and vary according to whether loss is conductive, sensorineural, or related to a central nervous system disorder. The client may report inability to hear certain words or sounds or that sounds are muffled. *Pain* may be perceived by the client as a feeling of fullness in the ear. It may be intensified by movement and relieved by holding the head still or by application of heat. Ear pain may occur as a result of related problems of the nose, sinuses, oral cavity, or pharynx. *Ear drainage* can be bloody (sanguineous), clear (serous), mixed (serosanguineous), or contain pus (purulent). Drainage may also be accompanied by an odor. Tinnitus (ringing in the ears) may be reported as high- or low-pitched, roaring, humming, hissing, or loud and persistent. Tinnitus may occur more commonly at certain times of the day. Loss of balance may be accompanied by vertigo or dizziness. Vertigo is a sensation of motion while not moving. A client may feel that either he or the room is moving.

Past Health History

Childhood and Infectious Diseases

Common childhood diseases involving the ears include the following:

Acute middle ear infections (otitis media)
Eardrum perforations resulting from otitis media

Complications of ear infections such as chronic otitis media, frequent upper respiratory tract infection, and acute and chronic sinus infections.

Infectious diseases with ear problem sequelae include mumps, measles, and meningitis. Specifically inquire whether the client has been immunized for mumps, measles, and *Haemophilus influenzae* B (HIB). In utero exposure to maternal influenza or rubella may result in congenital hearing loss in the child. Premature birth is also associated with hearing problems.

Major Illnesses and Hospitalizations

Inquire about a history of upper respiratory tract infections. Has the client had a tonsillectomy or adenoidectomy? Does the history include ear surgery? Has the client had trauma to the head or ear, such as a severe blow or sustained loud noise exposure or concussion from sudden changes in air pressure (such as may occur in an explosion)? Does the history include chronic eardrum perforation?

Medications

Certain medications can damage the vestibulocochlear nerve (eighth cranial nerve), with resultant hearing loss, tinnitus, or disturbances in equilibrium. Aspirin is a common cause of tinnitus. Other drugs include aminoglycosides, analgesics, salicylates, and antiprotozoal agents. Box 37–3 lists drugs that can cause ototoxic effects. Inquire whether the client has taken or is currently taking medications and how long he or she has been taking them.

Allergies

In addition to asking about allergies to medications and other substances, inquire about allergies resulting in nasal stuffiness and congestion. Close proximity of the eustachian tubes to the nasal mucosa may also result in edema, which obstructs the flow of air between the middle ear and nose so that air pressure cannot be equalized.

Family Health History

Ask about a history of hearing loss or ear surgery among family members. Determine the age at onset for hearing loss or changes in hearing acuity.

Psychosocial History

Psychosocial and life-style factors that influence the occurrence of ear problems include occupational hazards, environmental exposure, and leisure activities and hobbies. Ask about exposure to loud noises (Table 37–1), including type, frequency, and duration. Is protective ear gear worn? Does the client swim, especially in water that

---

Box 37–3. Selected Ototoxic* Drugs

Aminoglycoside Antibiotics

Streptomycin
Neomycin
Gentamicin
Tobramycin
Amikacin
Kanamycin
Minocycline
Netilmicin

Other Antibiotics

Vancomycin
Viomycin
Polymyxin B (Aerosporin)
Polymyxin E
  (colistin; Coly-Mycin)
Erythromycin
Minocycline
Capreomycin
Ampicillin
Chloramphenicol

Other Drugs

Chemotherapeutic agents
  Bleomycin
  Cisplatin
  Nitrogen mustard
Salicylates

Quinine drugs
Quinidine
Chloroquine

Chemicals

Metals
  Lead
  Mercury
  Gold
  Arsenic
Alcohol
Aniline dyes
Caffeine
Carbon monoxide
Nicotine
Potassium
  bromate
Povidone-iodine

Diuretics

Furosemide
  (Lasix)
Ethacrynic acid
  (Edecrin)
Acetazolamide
  (Diamox)
Bumetanide
Mannitol

* Substances toxic to the ear.

---

may be contaminated? Has the client had problems with "swimmer's ear"? Does the client use earplugs to prevent water from entering the ear canal?

Ordinary speech level measures about 50 dB; heavy traffic is about 70 dB; at above 80 dB, noise becomes uncomfortable to the human ear. Exposure to levels greater than 85 to 90 dB for months or years causes cochlear damage. Participate in teaching the proper use of protective ear devices or earplugs. Courses about industrial hearing conservation requirements are available.

A client who notices tinnitus (ringing in the ear), a sensation of fullness in the ear, or a temporary hearing loss while engaged in a noise-producing activity (e.g., firing a gun) should refrain from the activity or wear suitable ear protection. Sound in front of rock band speakers can reach up to 120 dB, and hearing losses have been measured in some members of rock bands. If proximity to the high noise level cannot be avoided, earplugs should be worn during exposure. Listening to music with regular speakers or earphones seldom causes hearing loss.

Earplugs are inserted into the external auditory canal and can reduce the noise by 10 to 30 dB. Usually standardized plugs are effective, but custom-made plugs molded to the client's ear canal can also be purchased and are better tolerated. For noise levels reaching 120 dB and above, clients must wear both earmuffs and earplugs.

Explore health management behaviors the client practices regarding ear hygiene. Does the client have a habit of putting objects into the ear, such as pencils, hairpins, or cotton-tipped applicators? Instruct the client about proper ear care.

Review of Systems

The review of systems related to the ear includes asking about problems with the nose, sinuses, mouth, pharynx, and throat. Ask whether the client has experienced head trauma, loss of balance, dizziness, or vertigo. Detailed questions for the review of systems are found in Box 11–2.

Physical Examination

Physical examination of the ear includes assessment of hearing acuity, balance, and equilibrium. Because the external ear is completely visible, it is easy to identify anatomic landmarks and to assess any abnormalities. The eardrum reveals significant information regarding the middle ear. However, much of the middle ear and inner ear is inaccessible to direct examinations, and inferences must be made indirectly by testing auditory and vestibular function.

Inspection and Palpation

External Ear

Gross examination of both ears should precede individual examination of either ear. Inspection and palpation are used for assessment of the external ear. The external ear should be inspected for size, configuration, and angle of attachment to the head. The configuration of the pinna is observed for gross deformity. Whether the ears protrude (and the degree to which they protrude), the color of the skin of the ears, and whether any additional skin tags are present are noted. The skin of the ear should be smooth and without breaks or inflammation, especially in the crevice behind the ear. Note any lumps, skin lesions, or cysts, and record approximate size and location.

Palpation and manipulation of the pinna produce information regarding tenderness, nodules, or tophi. Tophi are small, hard nodules in the helix that are deposits of uric acid crystals characteristic of gout. In palpation, move the pinna, feel the mastoid area, and press on the tragus. Note whether any of the manipulations produces pain or discomfort, which could indicate inflammation or infection.

Ear Canal

Direct Observation. Inspection of the ear canal is carried out by direct observation, otoscopy, or microscopic examination. For direct observation, ask the adult to tip his or her head slightly to the opposite side while you pull the pinna up, back, and out. Then use a penlight to inspect the ear canal for any abnormalities such as extreme narrowing, excessive wax, redness, scaliness, swelling, drainage, cysts, or foreign objects. Normally, none of these signs is present. Visualization of the eardrum with this method would be unlikely.

Otoscopy. The eardrum is located at the end of the only skin-lined canal in the body. Therefore, visualization is difficult and requires illumination and magnification for accurate assessment. An otoscope is portable, and otoscopic examination is the most common method used. An otoscope is a device (Fig. 37–4) consisting of a handle, a light source, a magnifying lens, and an attachment for visualizing the ear canal and eardrum. Some otoscopes have a pneumatic device for injecting air into the ear canal to test the mobility and integrity of the eardrum.

Specula for the otoscope come in a variety of sizes. The diameter of the meatus and the length of the ear canal vary; thus, the speculum with the largest diameter that fits comfortably into the ear canal should be selected. The light source must be checked for brightness. If the light appears yellowish or dim (like a flashlight with weak batteries), the batteries must be recharged or replaced.

The otoscope is held with the dominant hand, with the hand resting against the client's head (Fig. 37–5). In this manner, if the client should move suddenly, the otoscope will also move, so that the examination will be less likely to damage the external canal. With the nondominant hand, the pinna is pulled up, back, and out (in the adult); thus, the ear canal is straightened. While this is done,

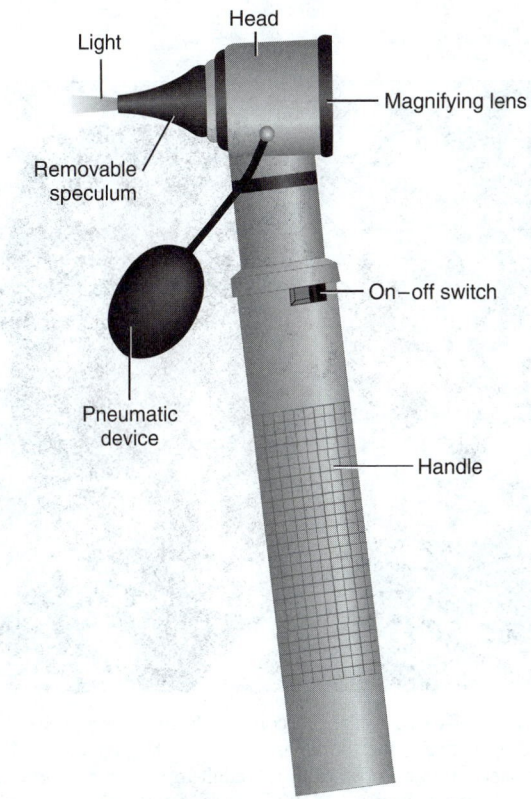

Figure 37–4. An otoscope.

gently tilt the client's head away from you, and insert the speculum slowly and carefully into the ear canal. Bring your eye close to the magnifying lens to visualize the ear canal and eardrum. When a pneumatic bulb is present, advance the otoscope far enough to make a secure seal.

The ear canal is observed while the speculum is entering and leaving. The otoscope is moved in a circular fashion to visualize the entire ear canal; abnormalities such as extreme narrowing of the ear canal, nodules, redness, scaliness, swelling, drainage, cysts, foreign objects, and excessive wax are noted. Visualization of the eardrum will be impaired by most of these abnormalities. Sometimes the ear canal must be cleaned of wax, dead skin, and other debris. Wax and debris can be removed with a cerumen spoon (wax curet), suction aspirator, or irrigation.

Cerumen should not interfere with the examination when the amount is small. Cerumen is normally present in the external ear and varies in color from light yellow to black. Cerumen that is impacted in the ear canal is a common cause of hearing loss, especially in the elderly. Therefore, assessment of the amount of cerumen is important.

Some distinguishing landmarks of the normal eardrum (Fig. 37–6) are the annulus, which is the fibrous border that attaches the eardrum to the temporal bone; the short process of the malleus, which protrudes into the eardrum superiorly; the long process of the malleus (manubrium); the umbo of the malleus, which is at the point of maximal concavity and attaches to the center of the eardrum; the pars flaccida, a small triangular area above the short process of the malleus; and the pars tensa, the remaining and largest portion of the eardrum.

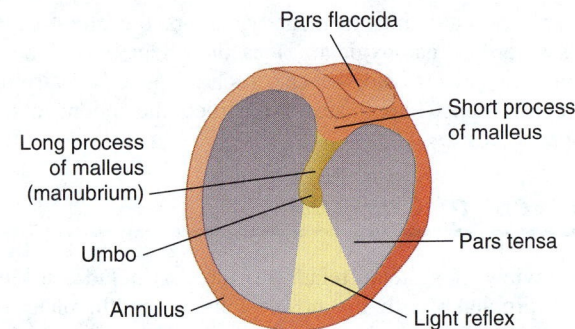

Figure 37–6. Normal right eardrum (tympanic membrane).

The normal eardrum is slightly conical, quite shiny and smooth, and pearly gray in color. The position of the drumhead is oblique with respect to the ear canal. In the presence of disease, not only does the color of the eardrum change, but also are other abnormalities manifest, such as retraction of the eardrum, bulging of the eardrum, perforation of the eardrum, or a white plaque (tympanosclerosis) in the eardrum.

Carefully inspect the entire eardrum, including the border (annulus), again rotating the otoscope as needed. The umbo and the long and short process of the malleus should be easily visible through the eardrum.

The mobility of the eardrum is tested by using the pneumatic device of the otoscope to inject a small puff of air into the ear canal. The eardrum is observed for normal movement. An adequate seal is important to perform this maneuver accurately.

Tests for Auditory Acuity

Assessment of the middle and inner ear for hearing is accomplished by sophisticated methods of indirect testing (e.g., audiometry and vestibular testing). However, a gross assessment of hearing can be made simply through conversation, by evaluating the logical sequence of replies and the appropriateness of the responses. Gross assessments can be made at the bedside or in the office.

Each ear is tested separately to estimate the hearing. Begin by occluding one of the client's ears with a finger. Then, while standing 1 foot away, whisper two-syllable numbers softly toward the unoccluded ear, and ask the client to repeat the numbers. The intensity of your voice can be increased from a soft, medium, or loud whisper to a soft, medium, or loud voice. If you suspect that the client is lip reading, the client's face should be turned away. Ask the client whether hearing is better in one ear than in the other ear. If the auditory acuity is different, the ear that hears better should be tested first. Then, noise is produced in the better-hearing ear by rapidly but gently moving the finger in the client's ear canal while the other ear is tested.

A watch tick can also be used to test hearing. However, a watch tick produces a higher-pitched sound, which is less relevant to functional hearing than is the voice test.

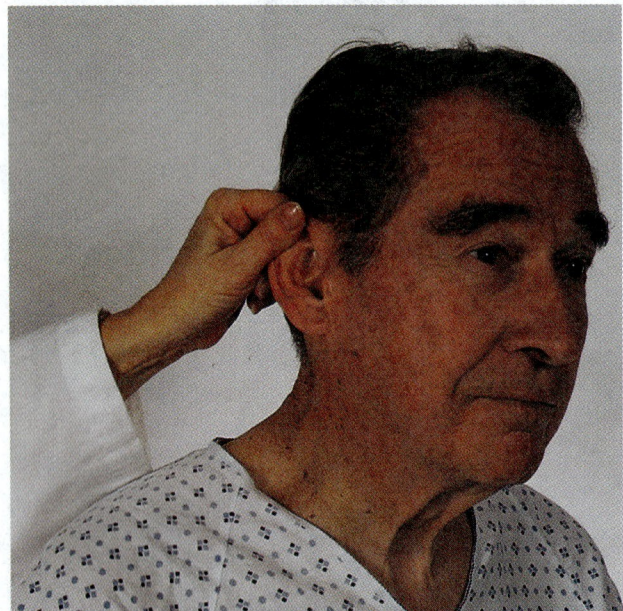

Figure 37–5. Use of the otoscope. Hold the otoscope handle pointed up between the thumb and fingers. The pinna should be pulled backward and upward in the adult to straighten the auditory canal. (From Jarvis, C. [1996]. *Physical examination and health assessment* [2nd ed.]. Philadelphia: W. B. Saunders.)

The tuning fork also provides a general estimate of hearing loss. The two major tuning fork tests date from the 19th century and are named after their originators: Weber and Rinne.

Weber Test

The tuning fork is set into vibration by striking the tines on the examiner's hand or knee. The rounded tip of the handle is placed on the center of the client's forehead or nasal bone (Fig. 37–7). Placement on the teeth (even if the client has false teeth) is a reliable option. The client is asked whether the tone is heard in the center of the head, the right ear, or the left ear. The Weber test is useful in identifying a hearing loss. Normally the sound is heard equally in both ears by bone conduction. If the client has a sensorineural hearing loss in one ear, the sound is heard in the other ear. If the client has a conductive hearing loss in one ear, the sound is heard in that ear.

Rinne Test

The vibrating tuning fork is shifted between two positions: against the mastoid bone (bone conduction) and 2 inches from the opening of the ear canal (air conduction) (see Fig. 37–7). As the position is changed, the client is asked to indicate which tone is louder (in front of the ear or behind the ear) or when one of the tones is no longer heard. The Rinne test compares air versus sensorineural conduction.

With conductive hearing loss, the pathways of normal sound conduction are blocked. However, vibrations against the mastoid bone can bypass the obstruction; therefore, bone conduction lasts longer or sounds louder than air conduction. With sensorineural hearing loss, the acoustic nerve has decreased ability to perceive vibrations from either route; therefore, normal patterns are reported by the client. Clients with normal hearing also report normal patterns.

Normally sound is heard twice as long or as loud by air conduction than it is by bone conduction. Therefore, a normal response is one in which air conduction is greater than bone conduction, or a positive Rinne test finding. With a conductive hearing loss, a client hears bone conduction sounds louder or longer than air conduction sounds, which constitutes a negative Rinne test finding. With a sensorineural hearing loss, the client hears better by air conduction, which constitutes a positive Rinne test finding.

Tests for Vestibular Acuity

Romberg Test

To assess the inner ear for balance, perform a Romberg test. Have the client stand with feet together, arms out in front, and eyes open. Note the ability to maintain an upright posture. Perform the same test with the client's eyes closed. Normally, only a minimal amount of sway-

ing exists. If the client loses balance, this may indicate a vestibular ear problem or cerebellar ataxia. A dysfunction constitutes a positive Romberg test finding.

A tandem Romberg test should also be performed. Instruct the client to walk forward and backward, heel to toe. A peripheral vestibular lesion may cause marked swaying or falling. A client without pathologic vestibular change is usually able to maintain balance, depending on age.

A past-pointing test can also indicate a labyrinthine disorder. With the client seated and facing you, hold out an index finger at the client's shoulder level. Instruct the client to touch your finger with the right index finger. Ask the client to lower the arm, close the eyes, and touch your finger again. The procedure is repeated using the left index finger. The presence or absence of, as well as the degree and direction of, past-pointing is observed and recorded. A labyrinthine disorder can lead to past-pointing when the eyes are closed. Cerebral lesions are indicated when past-pointing occurs whether the eyes are open or closed.

Test for Nystagmus

Nystagmus is involuntary, rhythmic oscillation of the eyes associated with vestibular dysfunction. Nystagmus occurs normally when a client watches a rapidly moving object or looks beyond 30 degrees laterally (endpoint nystagmus). To check a client for gaze nystagmus, place your finger directly in front of the client at eye level. Ask the client to follow the finger without moving the head. Move your finger slowly from the midline toward the right ear and then the left ear, but not more than 30 degrees laterally, superiorly, or inferiorly. Observe the client's eyes for any jerking movements. For example, if the eyes jerk quickly to the left, and drift slowly back to the right, the client has left spontaneous (horizontal) nystagmus. Nystagmus is named for the direction of the fast phase. Nystagmus can be horizontal, vertical, or rotary.

Diagnostic Tests

Tests for Structure

The temporal bone and its structures are easily examined by x-ray. The oldest, but not necessarily most useful, study is x-ray examination of the mastoid bone. More recent radiographic techniques have largely been replaced by imaging studies.

Computed Tomography

Computed tomographic (CT) scan without contrast is the most commonly ordered CT scan for the temporal bone. Contrast is not generally used, as most bony structures are well seen on CT scan. Contrast may be used to delineate vascular or soft tissue structures.

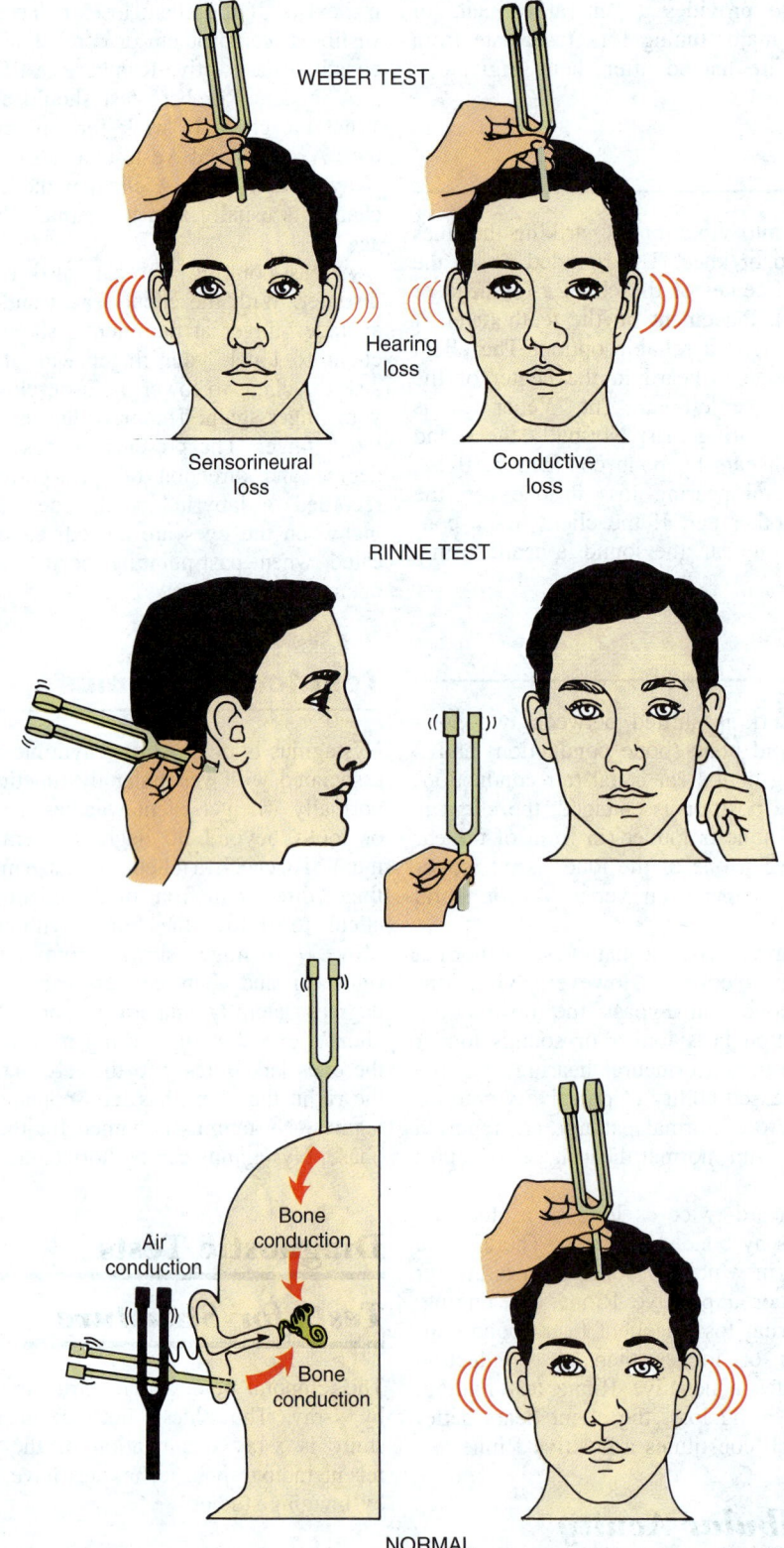

Figure 37–7. The Weber and Rinne tests for hearing loss. The Weber test is used to detect lateralization of hearing damage; the Rinne test distinguishes between conductive hearing loss and sensorineural hearing loss. The two tests should be performed consecutively. The Weber test uses a vibrating tuning fork placed on the client's head or nose to produce a centrally located stimulus. The client should hear the sound equally in both ears. The tone is louder in an ear with unilateral conductive loss and quieter in unilateral sensorineural loss. The Rinne test then characterizes the unilateral hearing loss as either conductive or sensorineural. The Rinne test is performed by holding a vibrating tuning fork about 2 inches from the external ear. When the client cannot hear the sound, the tuning fork is placed on the mastoid bone. When the tone is louder through air than through bone, the client has a positive Rinne test finding, which indicates normal hearing or a sensorineural hearing loss. A negative Rinne test finding, or louder bone conduction than air conduction, indicates a conductive loss.

Magnetic Resonance Imaging

Magnetic resonance imaging (MRI) reveals membranous organs as well as nerves and blood vessels of the temporal bone. MRI is the test of choice for tumors of the temporal bone. Again, contrast can be used for enhancement. For certain diagnostic assessments, both MRI and CT scan are obtained.

Arteriography

Arteriography is used to assess vascular abnormalities in the temporal bone.

Tests for Function

Audiometric Tests

Audiology may be broadly termed the science of hearing. Audiometric tests are performed to measure hearing and comprehension. A hearing test is performed in a sound-proof booth by an audiologist. An audiometer is an electronic instrument used to test hearing by producing sounds of varying tones and loudness. The unit of measure of hearing, the decibel (dB), is a logarithmic function of sound intensity. Earphones are used for the audiogram. The client is asked to signal the audiologist by raising a hand or pressing a button when a tone is heard; the responses are plotted on a graph called an audiogram (Fig. 37–8).

The components of hearing are tested through assessment of air conduction, bone conduction, and speech. Air conduction is assessed by presenting tones through the earphones. By varying the loudness and frequency of tones, a hearing level is established. Bone conduction is assessed by presenting tones through a bone conduction oscillator placed behind the ear on the mastoid bone. The bone conduction level is the level at which the cochlea can hear, bypassing the middle ear structures, and is referred to as the nerve hearing level. A difference between air and bone conduction signifies a conductive hearing loss. When air and bone conduction are the same, either normal hearing or a nerve (sensorineural) hearing loss exists. Speech evaluation includes speech reception threshold and speech discrimination. Speech reception threshold is the level of speech hearing and serves as a check on the reliability of the air conduction test. Speech discrimination is the ability to understand the spoken word.

Normal hearing is a range of hearing established nationally by testing the hearing levels of people of all ages. A client with normal hearing has 80% or more hearing, depending on age.

Some of these tests are performed by computer-assisted instruments. The object of these special tests is to differentiate whether a disorder is in the cochlea, acoustic nerve, or brain stem.

Tympanometry. A popular test used for differentiating problems in the middle ear is tympanometry, or im-

pedance audiometry. This test measures compliance (mobility) and impedance (opposition to movement) of the tympanic membrane and ossicles of the middle ear. It is done by applying positive, normal, and negative air pressure into the external meatus and measuring the resultant sound energy flow. The sound energy flow is traced on a graph called a *tympanogram*. Abnormalities of the tympanogram describe the function of the middle ear, eustachian tube, and ossicles. Tympanometry can also be used to measure the stapedial muscle reflex and its decay. This test also indicates the function of the acoustic nerve.

Tests for Brain Stem Response. The auditory brain stem response test is currently one of the most popular approaches to the assessment of the auditory nervous system. By presenting a sound to the ear and measuring the response (computer averaging) in the brain stem, specific diagnostic information can be obtained. Imaging tests of the head are usually ordered to confirm the abnormality. Brain stem auditory evoked responses can be recorded from scalp electrodes. The early potentials reflect activity in the cochlea, eighth cranial nerve, and brain stem. Later evoked potentials reflect cortical activity. Early evoked responses may be used to estimate the magnitude of the hearing loss and differentiate cochlea, eighth cranial nerve, and brain stem lesions.

Vestibular Tests

Electronystagmography. The vestibular system can be tested by electrophysiologic means. Although the physical assessment of balance is important, the most common objective measurement of balance is accomplished by electronystagmography (ENG). The ENG instrument was developed to measure nystagmus (involuntary, rapid eye movement) in response to stimulation of the vestibular system. This stimulation includes testing the client at rest in different positions for both the eyes and the head, and with different temperatures of air or water in the ear canals, thus stimulating the semicircular canals. The different test results give a recording (electronystagmogram) that reflects the status of each labyrinth and can point to central nervous system disorders.

Platform Posturography. Platform posturography, which is performed while the client is standing, is one of the newest computerized balance tests. This platform test helps to identify, quantify, and localize the source of balance disorders (Fig. 37–9). The client stands in a tall box-like device that provides no visual cues for balance. The floor is moved while the client stands on it, and the response to correcting balance is recorded. Most people correct posture changes with adjustments in muscles (e.g., of the feet and ankles). The client is strapped in for safety in case he or she loses balance. This test can help isolate the etiologic basis as vestibular, visual, or proprioceptive.

Rotary Chair Assessment. Rotary chair or harmonic acceleration can also be used. Rotation of the client in a chair in darkness provides information about

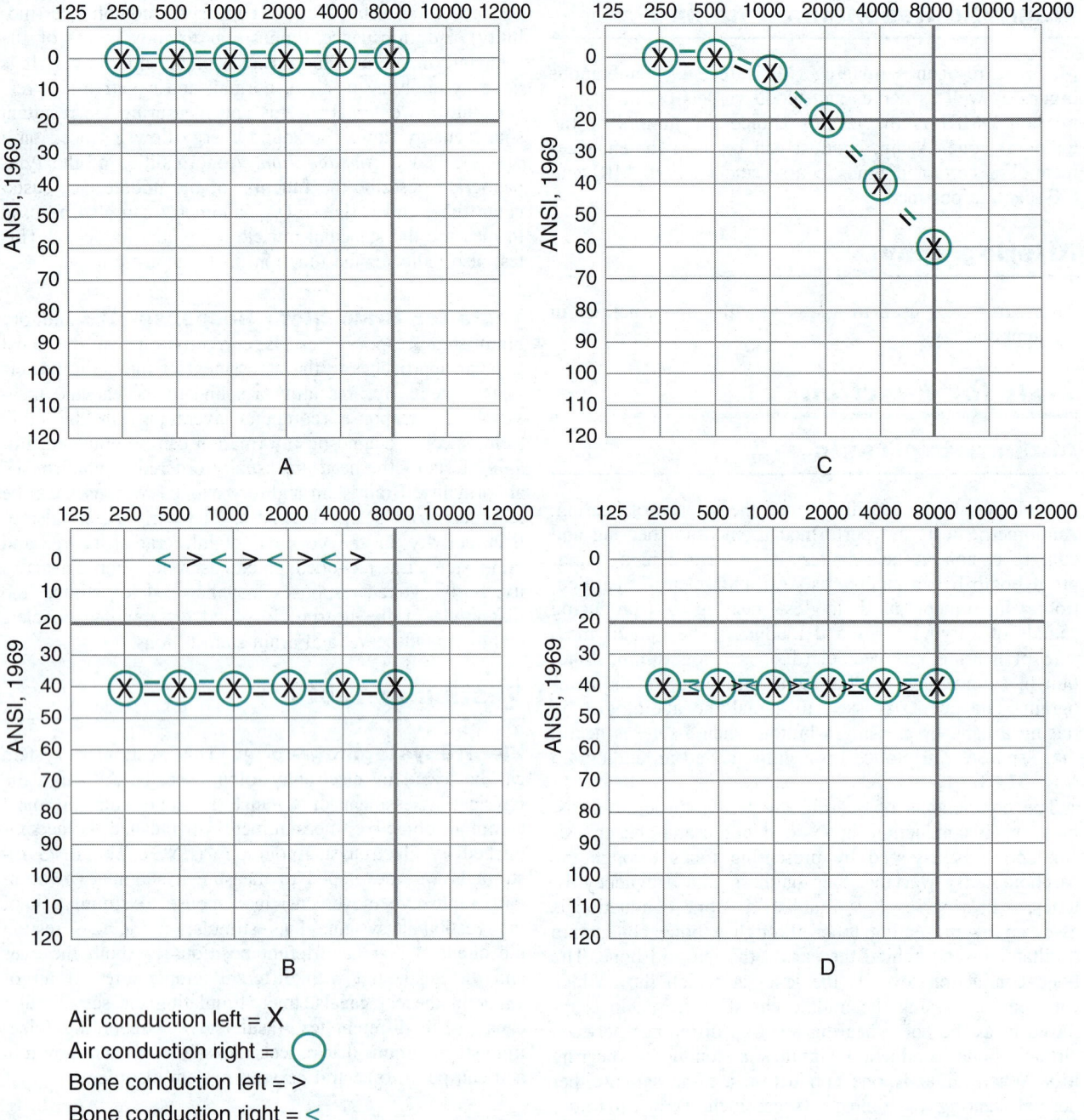

Figure 37–8. Audiograms showing types of hearing. *A,* Normal hearing. *B,* Conductive hearing loss. *C,* High-frequency hearing loss. *D,* Sensorineural hearing loss. (Courtesy of Arnold G. Schuring, M.D.)

vestibular dysfunction and the level of central compensation.

Laboratory Tests

Blood Tests

Blood tests that are diagnostic for systemic abnormalities are only secondarily significant for ear disease. For example, an elevated white blood cell count points to an infec-

tion but is not diagnostic of ear disease. However, in the presence of ear infection, and in the absence of other infection, blood tests are necessary for assessing acute ear infection. Other blood tests are useful for diagnosis of autoimmune diseases and other systemic illnesses that can affect hearing and balance.

Ear Drainage Cultures

Drainage from the ear canal or a surgical incision is usually cultured to identify an infecting organism. This is

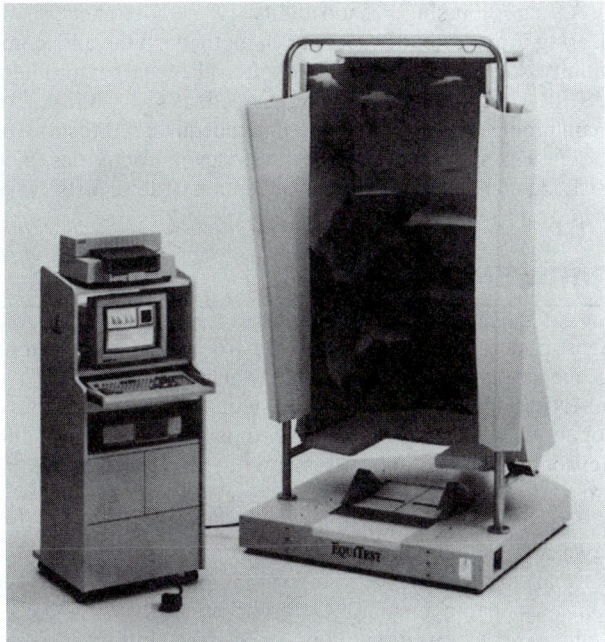

Figure 37–9. Platform posturography to assess vestibular function. The client stands on a movable platform, and vision is restricted by the panels with clouds. The platform is moved so that the client must compensate for the postural changes. Without visual cues, the vestibular system is tested for its ability to compensate. Because of the risk of falls, the client is strapped to the sides of the apparatus. (Courtesy of Neurocom International, Inc.)

especially necessary to choose the appropriate antibiotic in acute infections. When long-term drainage is present, such as in chronic otitis media, cultures are less helpful, because gram-negative bacillus growth covers up the original pathogen. In these cases, many physicians do not culture the drainage but begin administration of broad-spectrum antibiotics.

Tests for the Presence of Cerebrospinal Fluid

When clear drainage is found in the ear, a dilemma is presented. Is this fluid cerebrospinal fluid (CSF) or serous drainage? A fistula from the inner ear to the middle ear can drain CSF. This pathway can also lead to meningitis by retrograde contamination. Therefore, an analysis of clear fluid drainage from the ear or nose is often helpful in diagnosing the problem.

Tissue Specimens

Biopsies of abnormal tissue from the ear canal, or from other tissue harvested during surgery, are necessary both to rule out a malignancy and to identify unusual problems. In an infected ear, abnormal tissue is readily identified with visual assessment. If the surgeon is in doubt about the findings, a tissue sample is taken for pathologic examination.

Disorders of the Ear

Hearing Impairment

Hearing impairment ranges from difficulty in understanding words or hearing certain sounds to total deafness. Up to 80% of all hearing impairments are caused by hearing nerve disorders, for which no cure is presently available. Hearing impairments diminish the quality of life for a third of adults between ages 65 and 75 years.

Hearing impairment is the nation's number one disability; 1 of 15 Americans is affected. By the year 2050, approximately 1 of 5 clients in the United States will be age 55 years or older. Of these estimated 58 million people, 26 million are expected to have hearing impairment.

Of the 10 million people in the United States with a hearing loss who are age 65 years or older, more than 90% have a sensorineural hearing loss. Because of fear, misinformation, lack of information, and vanity, many clients do not admit that they have a hearing problem.

Etiology and Risk Factors

Many factors influence the type and amount of hearing loss. Hearing loss is not an actual disorder but is rather a clinical manifestation of many possible problems. We will examine the common and uncommon causes of hearing impairments.

Conductive hearing loss occurs in the external and middle ear and impairs sound from being conducted into the inner ear. It may be caused by anything that blocks the external ear, such as wax, infection, or a foreign body; a thickening, retraction, scarring, or perforation of the tympanic membrane; or any pathophysiologic changes in the middle ear affecting or fixing one or more of the ossicles. Otitis media is a common cause of conductive hearing loss. Otosclerosis, which leads to conductive hearing loss, is discussed in the next section.

Tympanosclerosis is a result of repeated infection and deserves special emphasis. Tympanosclerosis is a deposit of collagen and calcium within the middle ear that can harden around the ossicles, causing a conductive hearing loss. Tympanosclerotic deposits can also be found mounded in the middle ear or as plaque in the tympanic membrane.

Noise-induced hearing loss can be traumatic if it is caused by a sudden loud noise, such as a blast. More commonly, this hearing loss occurs over time from repeated injury from loud noise. The major cause is industrial noise, use of firearms, and listening to loud music.

Sensorineural hearing loss is caused by impairment of the function of the inner ear. Causes include congenital and hereditary factors, noise injury, aging, Ménière's disease, and ototoxicity. Systemic disorders, such as certain collagen disorders, diabetes, and Paget's disease, can also alter hearing.

Infection can lead to hearing loss. An infection of the inner ear called *labyrinthitis* can be either viral or bacterial in origin. Viral labyrinthitis is usually isolated to the inner ear, whereas the rarer bacterial labyrinthitis is from infection in the middle ear and mastoid.

Both benign and malignant tumors of the temporal bone can involve the inner ear and lead to hearing loss. The most common benign tumor is an acoustic neuroma of the eighth nerve arising in the internal ear canal. Spread of this tumor out of the internal ear canal toward the brain stem causes other neurologic problems and can be life-threatening. Other tumors in the cerebellar-pontine angle, likewise, involve the seventh and eighth cranial nerves as they enter the internal acoustic meatus. Malignant tumors invade the entire inner ear, spreading from the middle ear and mastoid.

Diseases that alter the central nervous system, such as cerebrovascular accidents and tumors, are the cause for central deafness, a rare form of sensorineural hearing loss. Central deafness is also known as *central auditory dysfunction*. With this phenomenon, the central nervous system cannot interpret normal auditory signals. Therefore, the hearing test findings are normal, although the client is deaf.

Different types of hearing loss are listed in Box 37–4. A client has a mixed hearing loss when both conductive and sensorineural hearing losses are present simultaneously. A functional loss is a hearing loss for which no organic lesion can be found, and special testing suggests normal hearing. A hearing loss may also be congenital or acquired. Most clients with ear problems have some degree of hearing loss.

A major nursing responsibility is the identification of hearing impairment in clients in both hospital and community settings. Detection and referral of an ear problem are the first steps in limiting the client's disability. For maintaining normal ear function, adequate protection of the ears is important and involves several activities. The Risk Factors and Levels of Prevention feature lists ways to prevent hearing loss.

Pathophysiology

Sensorineural hearing loss results from disease or trauma to the organ of Corti or auditory nerve pathways of the inner ear leading to the brain stem. Normal analysis of sound waves is disrupted. Sound is distorted and faint. Sensorineural hearing losses are usually permanent and are not correctable by medical or surgical treatment.

The inner ear is usually not involved in a conductive loss, and sound amplification can reach the inner ear. Normal movement of sound vibration through the ear canal, tympanic membrane, and/or ossicles is prevented. Sound is perceived as faint or distant, but it remains relatively clear. Most conductive hearing losses are correctable by medical or surgical treatment.

Clinical Manifestations and Diagnostic Findings

Most hearing loss is gradual and goes unnoticed by the client until several incidents of problems with communication have occurred. Significant others and co-workers are usually aware of the hearing problem long before the client is aware of or admits to the problem. Sensorineural hearing cannot be regained, so early detection of hearing loss is important to diagnose the cause of the loss and, it is hoped, treat the problem. However, a small loss of hearing goes unnoticed and does not cause manifestations. Healthcare providers should be alert for the following signs:

- Failure to respond to oral communication
- Inappropriate response to oral communication
- Excessively loud speech
- Abnormal awareness of sounds
- Strained facial expressions
- Tilted head when listening
- Constant need for clarification of conversation
- Faulty speech articulation
- Behavioral clues (see Box 37–1)

Sometimes the hard-of-hearing client may repeat the information, even incorrectly, to provoke a response and, thus, a repetition of the information. Clients with a hearing loss can also experience distorted or abnormal sounds. Sometimes a sound is heard at different pitches for each ear; this is called *diplacusis*. A sound may cause a rapid increase in loudness; this is called *recruitment*. These abnormal sounds can cause the client discomfort.

Noise-induced hearing loss is characterized by a greater loss in the higher frequencies. Sudden or fluctuating hearing loss is recognized as a separate hearing disorder because of the isolated finding and dramatic outcome. Be-

---

Box 37–4. Types of Hearing Loss

Air conduction hearing loss: Loss of hearing through the external and middle ear.

Bone conduction hearing loss: Loss of hearing through the inner ear.

Central hearing loss: Loss of hearing from damage to the brain's auditory pathways or auditory center.

Conductive hearing loss: Loss of hearing in which air conduction is worse than bone conduction and involves the external and middle ear.

Fluctuating hearing loss: A sensorineural hearing loss that varies with time.

Functional hearing loss: Loss of hearing for which no organic lesion can be found.

Mixed hearing loss: Both sensorineural and conductive hearing loss.

Neural hearing loss: A sensorineural hearing loss originating in the eighth cranial nerve or brain stem.

Sensorineural hearing loss: Loss of hearing involving the cochlea and hearing nerve; bone and air conduction equal but diminished.

Sensory hearing loss: A sensorineural hearing loss in the cochlea and involving the hair cells and nerve endings.

Sudden hearing loss: A sensorineural hearing loss with a sudden onset.

Conductive hearing loss results from interference with conduction in the external and middle ear; sensorineural hearing loss in the inner ear; and mixed hearing loss in all three areas.

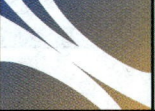

RISK FACTORS AND LEVELS OF PREVENTION

Hearing Loss

Risk Factors

Use of toxic substances (including ototoxic drugs), trauma, age, noise exposure, and infectious diseases (measles, mumps, and meningitis).

Levels of Prevention

Primary Prevention

● Teach young clients to prevent trauma to the ear by wearing protective helmets or headgear during sports.
● Teach people in occupations with high noise exposure to wear earplugs. Exposure to noise levels in excess of 80 dB over an 8-hour day is considered excessive and should be avoided (see Table 37–2).
● Teens need to be aware that excessively loud music in enclosed spaces (such as cars) can contribute to hearing loss.
● Teach clients to avoid inserting hard instruments into the ear canal and to avoid obstructing the ear canal with objects.
● Encourage clients to avoid inserting unclean articles or solutions into the ear and to avoid swimming in water identified as being polluted.

Secondary Prevention

● Encourage people to report hearing changes. A hearing loss in one ear is difficult to detect. The client can notice the loss when using a telephone or by having difficulty with the direction of sounds.
● Encourage clients to participate in screening programs for detection of hearing losses.
● Teach clients to monitor noise pollution.
● Encourage clients to have periodic ear examinations.
● Monitor side effects of ototoxic drugs. If vertigo, lessened hearing acuity, or tinnitus occurs, the next dose of the drug should be omitted and the physician should be consulted. Audiometric and vestibular testing may be necessary.
● Assess clients with prolonged ear pain, swelling, drainage, a "plugged" feeling, or decreased hearing.
● Teach clients with upper respiratory infections (colds) to blow the nose with at least one nostril open.

Tertiary Prevention

● Encourage clients to participate in hearing rehabilitation programs.
● Teach clients to avoid situations where background noise is excessive.
● Teach coping strategies, communication strategies, and care of hearing aid.

cause it is thought to be vascular in nature, attempted treatments are made to alter the vascular system in some way. Occasionally, hearing may return to normal without an understandable reason. Unfortunately, most clients do not regain normal hearing.

A characteristic of a severe hearing loss is the loss of discrimination (understanding of words). To some clients, a hearing loss feels like a blockage in the ear and/or an inability to distinguish the direction of sounds. The hearing loss may sometimes fluctuate, but a progressive hearing loss usually results.

Tinnitus accompanies most sensorineural hearing losses and is very annoying. Tinnitus actually can sound like roaring, chirping of crickets, or, occasionally, music. In some clients, the tinnitus becomes the problem, and the underlying cause may be forgotten.

Table 37–3 presents clinical manifestations of conductive and sensorineural hearing loss. Diagnostic findings include testing for hearing of pure tones on audiometry, speech reception and discrimination, and sometimes brain stem evoked responses. Tones are presented using ear-

phones (air conduction) and vibrators (bone conduction). The minimal level at which the client can hear is determined. The speech reception threshold is the intensity at which the client can correctly repeat 50% of the words presented. The speech discrimination test is a measure of the client's ability to understand speech when it is presented at a volume that is easily heard.

Community and Self-Care

Few persons are treated for hearing loss in acute care settings. Most diagnostic studies, management, and aural rehabilitation are completed in outpatient settings.

■ Medical Management

Hearing loss is assessed by history, physical examination, and audiometry. Other than giving antibiotics for infec-

Table 37–2. Decibel Ratings and Hazardous Time Exposure of Common Noises

Typical Level* (dB)	Example	Dangerous Time Exposure
0	Lowest sound audible to human ear	
30	Quiet library, soft whisper	
40	Quiet office, living room, bedroom away from traffic	
50	Light traffic at a distance, refrigerator, gentle breeze	
60	Air conditioner at 20 ft, conversation, sewing machine	
70	Busy traffic, noisy restaurant (constant exposure)	Critical level begins
80	Subway, heavy city traffic, alarm clock at 2 ft, factory noise	More than 8 hr
90	Truck traffic, noisy home appliances, shop tools, lawnmower	Less than 8 hr
100	Chain saw, boiler shop pneumatic drill	2 hr
120	Rock concert in front of speakers, sandblasting, thunderclap	Immediate danger
140	Gunshot blast, jet plane	Any length of exposure time is dangerous
180	Rocket launching pad	Hearing loss is inevitable

* Sound levels refer to intensity experienced at typical working distances. Intensity drops 6 dB with every doubling of distance from noise source. (Courtesy of American Academy of Otolaryngology–Head and Neck Surgery, Washington, DC.)

tions, the medical treatment of sensorineural hearing loss is dismal. General modalities include steroids and vasodilators, but specific treatment is still lacking. The purpose of medication is to attempt to lessen the progressive hearing loss or, it is hoped, to reverse a sudden loss. The only treatment for noise-induced hearing loss is to prevent further injury by avoiding noise or by wearing ear protection. Therefore, most clients with hearing loss require some form of rehabilitation. Conductive hearing loss, in contrast, is often amenable to surgical correction.

If hearing loss is irreversible or not amenable to surgical intervention or if the client elects not to have surgery, aural rehabilitation may improve communication. The purpose of aural rehabilitation is to maximize the hearing-impaired client's communication skills.

Hearing is one of our primary modes of communication, and rehabilitation is directed toward teaching the client more effective use of the other senses, those of vision, touch, and vibration, and maximizing the use of any remaining hearing ability. Rehabilitation is affected by all demographic variables and the severity of impairment. As with other forms of rehabilitation, success depends partly on the degree of motivation.

Hearing Aids

Because most hearing losses are permanent, the use of a hearing aid should always be considered. A client should undergo a trial period before purchasing the aid. Bilateral (binaural) aids are desirable.

Hearing aids amplify sound in a controlled manner. They are used by both hearing-impaired clients (slight or moderate hearing loss) and deaf clients (severe or profound hearing loss). Hearing aids make sound louder but may not improve the ability to hear. Therefore, clients with decreased discrimination (the ability to understand

Table 37–3. Clinical Manifestations of Conductive and Sensorineural Hearing Loss

	Conductive Hearing Loss	Sensorineural Hearing Loss
Voice quality	Soft voice	Loud voice
Effect of environmental noise on hearing	Hearing improved	Hearing made worse
Speech discrimination	Good	Poor
Ability to hear on telephone	Good	Poor
Weber test lateralization	To diseased ear	To normal ear
Rinne test	Negative, AC<BC	Positive, AC>BC

AC, air conduction; BC, bone conduction.

what is spoken) benefit less from a hearing aid. The hearing aid amplifies all background noises, such as hospital machinery, background conversation in restaurants, footsteps, and department store noises, as well as speech. These noises may mask conversation or confuse the hearing-impaired client, especially if he or she is elderly.

Several types of hearing aids are available; they vary according to size and location. Hearing aids can be worn in the following locations:

- In the ear
- In the ear canal
- Behind the ear (postauricular)
- In the middle of the chest (body-worn aid)

Regardless of the type of aid, the hearing aid consists of the following parts:

- Microphone to receive sound waves from the air and change sounds into electrical signals
- Amplifier to increase the strength of electrical signals
- Receiver (loudspeaker) to change the electrical signals into sound waves
- Battery to provide the electrical energy needed to operate the hearing aid

On all types of hearing aids but the body-worn type, all four components are housed in one small case. The louder sounds are then directed into the ear through a custom-molded earpiece (Fig. 37–10).

The evolution in hearing aid development has led to smaller and more effective aids. Small hearing aids are available that fit into the ear canal. The latest advancement in hearing aids is the ability to produce digital hearing aids, some with remote control. Other advancements include microphones that enhance the voice of a speaker in front of the client, with suppression of background noise. Hearing aids will advance even further.

Assistive Listening Devices

In addition to hearing aids, many practical devices are on the market that use hearing aid technology. These devices help the hard-of-hearing client hear the television or radio as well as use the telephone. Stationary devices called teletypewriters and portable devices called telephone devices for the deaf are used for telephone communication by the profoundly deaf. A flashing light signals the presence of a dial tone, a busy signal, or a ring. When another teletypewriter or telephone device for the deaf is reached, messages are typed and displayed on a screen or printed. Other devices, such as flashing lights that alert a deaf person to a ringing doorbell, alarm clock, or smoke alarm, are available. Hearing dogs are trained to be sensitive to certain noises, such as the telephone, doorbells, and crying children. On hearing the sound, the dog moves back and forth between the owner and the sound.

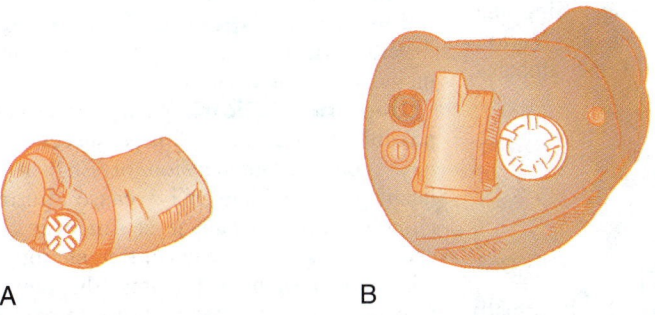

A   B

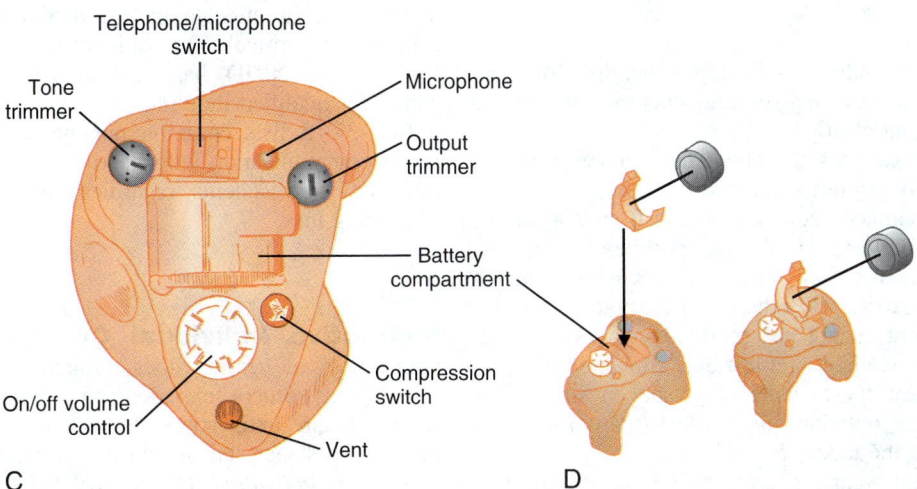

Figure 37–10. Types of hearing aids and components. *A,* In-the-canal aid. *B,* In-the-ear aid. *C,* Hearing aid components. *D,* Battery compartment. (Courtesy of Arnold G. Schuring, M.D.)

Hearing Education

Clients with a hearing loss need special education. Auditory training is an approach to enhancing listening skills. The hearing-impaired client is initially exposed to gross differences in sound, which are gradually "fine tuned" so that subtle differences in discrimination of two similar sounds can be made. The primary purpose of auditory training exercises is to help the client concentrate on the speaker. For some clients, only gross differences between sounds may be recognized.

Speech reading is the current term used for lip reading and is an important means of communication. Speech reading is the process of understanding vocal communication by the integration of lip movements with facial expressions, gestures, environmental clues, and conversation contexts. Speech reading is difficult without auditory cues. Many movements for speech are rapid, many sounds are similar (*b, m, p*), and certain sounds of any language are silent. A high percentage of words have to be guessed at by the hearing-impaired client. Knowledge of this fact alone helps you to be more understanding of the client who is using this approach.

Because of reduced auditory feedback (the inability of hearing-impaired clients to monitor their own speech), the clearness, pitch quality, or rate of the client's speech may deteriorate. These changes may alter the efficiency of communication and reduce the intelligibility of speech. The goal of speech training is to conserve, develop, or prevent deterioration of speech skills.

Last, but still important, is sign language. Sign language allows communication by hand signals. Various hand signals represent different letters of the alphabet, words, or phrases.

■ Nursing Management of the Medical Client

Assessment

The client's ability to communicate may be informally assessed during the history. Assess the client's ability to follow conversation. During the interview, the following information should be noted:

1. Does the client admit to having a hearing loss and difficulty communicating, or are other people blamed for not speaking clearly?
2. In what settings does the client have more problems with hearing or communicating?
3. Are family members, co-workers, and friends aware of the hearing problem? Are they supportive of the client, making communication easier and including him or her in conversation? Do others feel frustrated or angry when the client cannot hear correctly or does not respond? Does the client feel left out? Embarrassed?
4. Does the client try to understand spoken words? Or does he or she withdraw or refuse to participate, letting others do the talking?
5. Does the client wear a hearing aid? Does it appear to work?

Occasionally, laboratory, radiologic, and vestibular examinations will be used. In an otology office, the nurse may have the responsibility of performing the history, otologic examination, and screening audiometry. The history is often the most important part of the clinical assessment as previously described (see questionnaire in Box 37–2). The extent of assessment of the sensorineural hearing loss depends on the setting and the nurse's educational preparation and experience. Nurses should be able to inspect the outer ear and grossly assess the auditory acuity.

Identify clients with impaired hearing and encourage them to seek professional diagnosis and treatment. The Bridge to Home Healthcare feature provides suggestions for assisting hearing-impaired clients in the home environment. The impact of not hearing others may make some clients withdraw from social situations and become anxious and insecure. Important nursing assessments include the extent and duration of the hearing loss, how the client has coped with stress previously, and what support systems are available. The Nursing Research feature describes the effect of hearing impairment on the client's quality of life.

Impaired Verbal Communication. Clients who have lost their ability to hear are best managed within the nursing diagnosis *Impaired Verbal Communication related to effects of hearing loss.*

Planning: Expected Outcomes. The client will develop effective methods to communicate needs and be included in conversation.

Implementation. When normal conversation is impossible, writing may be used successfully by clients who have good comprehension of English (or their primary language). Writing may cause frustration when the client's primary language is American Sign Language because it is grammatically different from standard English. Visual aids such as pictures, diagrams, or models may also improve the nurse's ability to explain medical terminology or procedures.

An expert interpreter should be used when other attempts to communicate have failed or when speed and accuracy are critical. The National Registry of Interpreters for the Deaf (NRID) has local chapters and offers certification for qualified individuals.

Box 37–5 lists common nursing interventions to improve communication with hearing-impaired clients. They can apply to all clients, regardless of the type or severity of hearing loss.

Ineffective Individual Coping. The individual with a loss of hearing goes through the same stages of grieving as others experiencing a loss. Rehabilitation cannot begin until some degree of acceptance of the hearing loss has taken place. State this diagnosis as *Ineffective Individual Coping related to recent loss of hearing.*

BRIDGE TO HOME HEALTHCARE

Living with a Severe Hearing Loss

Gail Wilkerson, R.N., M.S.N., C.S., *Deaconess Home Health Services, St. Louis, Missouri*

Clients are often reluctant to admit that they have a hearing impairment. This reluctance results in difficulty with verbal communication, inability to follow instructions, and social isolation. To maximize communication, reduce background noise (turn off the television or radio), face the client, and speak clearly without shouting. At times, the only way to communicate is by writing. Develop written materials for repeated use. Include introduction materials (e.g., your name, your agency's name, the purpose of the visit), symptoms, and treatment regimens.

Many individuals have a hearing loss because of an accumulation of cerumen. Use an otoscope to visualize the ear canal. If cerumen is present, contact the physician to discuss a prescription for an ear irrigation solution. You are responsible for (1) instilling the solution when a normal ear irrigation medication procedure is prescribed and (2) assessing the amount and color of drainage. The cerumen often needs to be removed by a physician.

When clients experience a hearing loss, they need a medical evaluation and a hearing aid evaluation. Many older adults are reluctant to wear a hearing aid for various reasons. It is expensive, it is a visual sign of an impairment, it is expensive, and it necessitates leaving home for evaluation, fitting, and follow-up appointments. If clients are reluctant because of cosmetic reasons, show pictures of hearing aids and discuss individuals who wear hearing aids, such as former President George Bush. If cost is a problem, consider a referral to a social worker to identify local resources. Currently, Medicare will pay only for the cost of a hearing aid; Medicaid will usually pay the cost of the hearing aid. Consider other financial resources such as the American Association for Retired Persons and local hearing aid vendors. When leaving home is a problem, see if a vendor will make a home visit. If this is not possible, suggest that the client consider a head-set amplifier that can be purchased from a local electronics store.

Teaching is an important nursing intervention and includes cleaning the devices and changing the batteries. Also evaluate the client's ability to use the telephone and answer the door. Local telephone companies can equip the telephone with an adjustable volume control, hearing aid adapters, loud ringing signals, and telecommunication devices for the deaf (TDD). TDD allows the hearing-impaired individual to communicate by typing information into a specially designed device. To receive information, the receiver must have a specific TDD telephone number. Teach the client with a TDD about TDD telephone numbers for an emergency response and provide information about the home health agency and community resources.

It is important to involve caregivers, significant others, and family members in the management of a hearing impairment. Instruct these individuals about maximizing communication with a variety of techniques and adaptive equipment.

Planning: Expected Outcomes. The client will discuss and/or demonstrate problem-solving–based coping strategies as evidenced by the following:

Taking the initiative to inform others of the hearing impairment and requesting that they assist with communication by using techniques that promote comprehension

Not experiencing feelings of embarrassment, frustration, or withdrawal

Not blaming others for failure to communicate effectively

Avoiding situations and environments, such as noisy areas, that impair hearing

Implementations. Work with the client and family on methods to enhance communication and thereby enhance coping. Encourage the client to role-play how he or she might tell people that he or she has a hearing impairment and indicate what techniques should be used to help hearing.

Impaired Social Interaction. Clients with hearing losses can experience fears of inadequacy, feelings of inferiority, depression, and varying degrees of stress and isolation. The nursing diagnosis *Impaired Social Interaction related to perceived inability to interact with others secondary to hearing loss* can be used to guide interventions.

Planning: Expected Outcomes. The client will exhibit a willingness to be involved in social situations, as evidenced by attempting to become a part of social events, conversing with others, indicating lessened feelings of inadequacy, and responding appropriately to questions asked (not fabricating answers to cover hearing loss).

Implementation. The National Association of Speech and Hearing Agencies (NASHA) urges that all clients with hearing impairments *not* be grouped into one category. Each client is unique and has an individual hearing problem. The nurse is a role model in accepting the client as an individual and demonstrating effective communication techniques.

Work with the client to enhance coping, encourage continued social involvement, and advocate the use of various organizations to their fullest extent. Many agencies and associations exist for the hearing-impaired client. Services are offered by audiology clinics and sponsored

NURSING RESEARCH

How Does Hearing Impairment Affect Quality of Life in Older Clients?

Magilvy, J. K. (1985). Quality of life of hearing-impaired older women. *Nursing Research, 34*(3), 140–144.

A survey of 66 older women with impaired hearing examined the major influences on their quality of life. Deafness had occurred in early life in 27 and in older life in 39 women. The researchers recognized that regardless of age at onset, hearing impairment can have a profound impact on physiologic, psychological, and socioeconomic aspects of living. The stress-transactional framework by Lazarus and Launier was used to consider the relationships of variables.

The best predictors of quality of life were social hearing handicap (the degree of difficulty hearing social conversation), functional social support, and perceived health. Overall, the group of women who developed hearing loss later in life had a perception that the quality of their life was lowered because of their condition.

Implications for Practice

If hearing loss is perceived as a stressor, find avenues in teaching to assist clients to overcome these problems. Content on social support, aural rehabilitation, and other adaptations to hearing loss should be incorporated into nursing practice.

by universities, hospitals, community programs, state or local departments of health, the Veterans Administration, and national organizations.

Knowledge Deficit. Clients with new hearing aids need information about their care and proper use. State this diagnosis as *Knowledge Deficit related to lack of previous exposure to a hearing aid.*

Planning: Expected Outcomes. The client will have increased knowledge about the hearing aid as evidenced by being able to properly care for it.

Implementation. The hearing aid user should know how to care for the aid (Box 37–6) and what to do if the aid does not work. Nurses should also have a basic knowledge of the hearing aid to assist the client who is ill. Encourage the client to use the hearing aid and to provide safe storage when it is not in use. It should be turned off prior to removing it to prevent squealing feedback. The maintenance of a hearing aid is becoming less of a problem today. Usually, the aid is returned to the dealer for factory repair while a loaner hearing aid is worn.

Cost has been cited as a major factor in the nonuse of hearing aids. Clients needing financial assistance should

be referred to vocational rehabilitation, Lions clubs, and, in some states, Medicaid.

Evaluation

A client with a new hearing loss disorder needs frequent evaluation for determination of the degree of hearing regained as well as the coping strategies used. Because many forms of hearing loss are permanent or progressive, long-term evaluation should also be performed to be certain the client is adapting positively. Also determine whether the client has questions about the equipment used for hearing rehabilitation.

■ Surgical Management

Surgery is usually not warranted for sensorineural hearing loss. However, because mixed conductive and sensorineu-

Box 37–5. Improving Communication with Hearing-Impaired Clients

- Get the client's attention by raising your arm or hand.
- Stand with a light on your face; this will help the client to speech-read.
- Talk directly to the client while facing him or her.
- Speak clearly, but do not overaccentuate words.
- Speak in a normal tone; do not shout. Shouting overuses normal speaking movements and may cause distortion and be too loud for the client with sensorineural damage. If the client has conductive loss only, sometimes it is helpful to make the voice louder without shouting.
- If the client does not seem to understand what is said, express it differently. Some words are difficult to "see" in speech reading, such as "white" and "red."
- Move closer to the client and toward the better ear.
- Write out proper names or any statement that you are not sure was understood.
- Do not smile, chew gum, or cover the mouth when talking.
- Inattention may indicate tiredness or lack of understanding.
- Use phrases to convey meaning rather than one-word answers. State the major topic of the discussion first and then give details.
- Do not show annoyance by careless facial expressions. Clients who are hard of hearing depend more on visual clues for understanding.
- Encourage the use of a hearing aid if it is available; allow the client to adjust it before speaking.
- In a group, repeat important statements and avoid asides to others in the group.
- Avoid the use of the intercommunication system, because this may distort sound and cause poor communication.
- Do not avoid conversation with a client who has hearing loss. It has been said that to live in a silent world is much more devastating than to live in darkness, and clients with hearing loss appear to have more emotional difficulties than do those who are blind.

Box 37-6. Care of a Hearing Aid

- Turn the hearing aid off when it is not in use.
- Open the battery compartment at night to avoid accidental drainage of the battery.
- Keep an extra battery available at all times.
- Wash the earmold frequently (daily if necessary) with mild soap and warm water with the use of a pipe cleaner to cleanse the cannula.
- Dry the earmold completely before reconnecting it to the hearing aid.
- Do not wear the hearing aid during an ear infection.

What to Do if the Hearing Aid Fails to Work

- Check the on-off switch.
- Inspect the earmold for cleanliness.
- Examine the battery for correct insertion.
- Examine the cord plug for correct insertion.
- Examine the cord for breaks.
- Replace the battery, cord, or both, if necessary. The life of batteries varies according to the amount of use and power requirements of the aid. Batteries last 2 to 14 days.
- Check the position of the earmold in the ear. If the hearing aid "whistles," the earmold is probably not inserted properly into the ear canal, or you need to have a new earmold made.

ral hearing loss exists, surgery may be performed to alleviate the conductive hearing loss component. Also, some surgery is performed today to try to stop progressive hearing loss.

Surgery is also used for the treatment of acoustic neuroma, because this slow-growing tumor can cause severe problems outside the temporal bone. Preoperative hearing loss remains, but the chance for further hearing loss is reduced.

Three types of implantable hearing devices either are available for use or are in the investigation stage. They are cochlear implants, bone hearing devices, and semi-implantable hearing devices.

Cochlear implants provide auditory sensation to clients with severe to profound binaural sensorineural hearing loss who cannot benefit from a hearing aid (Fig. 37–11). This device has a small computer that changes the spoken word to electrical impulses. The impulses are transmitted across the skin to an implanted coil that carries the impulse to the hearing nerve-endings in the cochlea by an electrode introduced through the round window. The best of the cochlear implants use multichannels. In multichannel cochlear implants, 22 electrodes are inserted along the cochlear partition. The surgery for insertion of a cochlear implant is like mastoid surgery. The success of a cochlear implant varies widely and ranges from minimal improvement in auditory awareness to understanding of speech on the telephone.

In some cases of hearing loss, sound can be transmitted through the skull to the inner ear. For clients with a conductive hearing loss, a device is available in which the receiver is implanted under the skin into the skull. The external device transmits the sound through the skin. This device is worn above the ear and not in the ear canal. Because some conductive hearing losses cannot be repaired, this device may provide an alternative rehabilitative method to conventional hearing aid potential.

The implantable device with the greatest potential usage will be for those clients now using a hearing aid. Clinical research has shown that a magnet implanted in the middle ear can be stimulated by an ear canal driver that changes sound to a magnetic force. This system eliminates several bothersome problems of hearing aids, such as feedback and hearing-in noise. A semi-implantable hearing device is the first step to a totally implantable device that would eliminate any external device. However, many challenges have to be met before a workable device is available. This method of hearing aid technology is still in the research stage.

Otosclerosis

Otosclerosis, or "hardening of the ear," is a genetic disorder in which repeated resorption and redeposition of abnormal bone gradually leads to fixation of the footplate of the stapes in the oval window (Fig. 37–12A). The immobile footplate prevents transmission of sound vibration into the inner ear, leading to conductive hearing loss. It occurs twice as often in women and is ten times more prevalent in whites. The disorder is autosomally dominant, and therefore can be transmitted to offspring if only one parent has the disorder. Another form of otosclerosis that does not fix the stapes is cochlear otospongiosis, which can cause a sensorineural hearing loss.

Clinical manifestations of otosclerosis include slow, progressive hearing loss with changes noted even in adolescence. Hearing loss is usually bilateral but asymmetrical. Other manifestations include mild tinnitus, recurrent vertigo, and postural imbalance. It is common for the client to speak in a very soft voice. A reddish blush from dilated blood vessels may be noted behind the tympanic membrane when viewed through the otoscope (Schwartz's sign).

Diagnostic findings include greater bone conduction than air conduction on the Rinne test. If hearing loss is greater in one ear than the other, the Weber test shows lateralization to the more affected ear. Pure tone audiometry confirms hearing loss. Speech discrimination is usually maintained. Vestibular testing may be used for clients who report balance problems. Otosclerosis usually stabilizes when hearing levels reach 50 to 60 dB, and it rarely progresses to deafness.

The conductive hearing loss that results from otosclerosis is one of the most common correctable middle ear disorders. Because speech discrimination is usually unimpaired, simple amplification of sound is quite effective. Persons who are at high risk of otosclerosis or who are not candidates for surgery can be given some medications to reduce the severity of the bony fusion. Sodium fluoride can be given to replace the hydroxyl ion in bone and decrease resorption. In addition, calcium gluconate and vitamin D can be used to retard bone resorption. If hear-

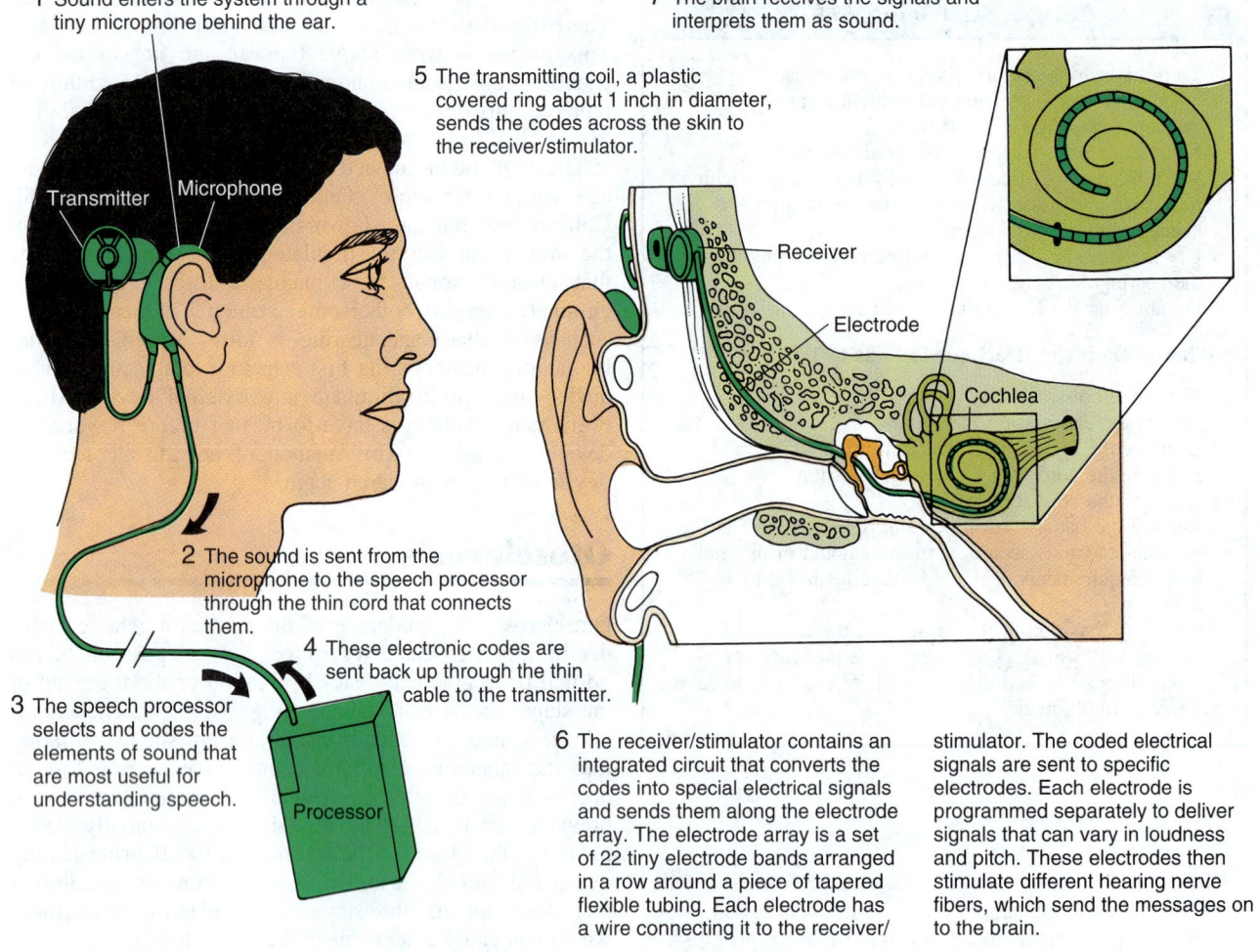

1 Sound enters the system through a tiny microphone behind the ear.

7 The brain receives the signals and interprets them as sound.

5 The transmitting coil, a plastic covered ring about 1 inch in diameter, sends the codes across the skin to the receiver/stimulator.

Transmitter   Microphone

Receiver

Electrode

Cochlea

2 The sound is sent from the microphone to the speech processor through the thin cord that connects them.

4 These electronic codes are sent back up through the thin cable to the transmitter.

3 The speech processor selects and codes the elements of sound that are most useful for understanding speech.

Processor

6 The receiver/stimulator contains an integrated circuit that converts the codes into special electrical signals and sends them along the electrode array. The electrode array is a set of 22 tiny electrode bands arranged in a row around a piece of tapered flexible tubing. Each electrode has a wire connecting it to the receiver/stimulator. The coded electrical signals are sent to specific electrodes. Each electrode is programmed separately to deliver signals that can vary in loudness and pitch. These electrodes then stimulate different hearing nerve fibers, which send the messages on to the brain.

Figure 37–11. Cochlear implant to restore hearing.

ing is stable, these minerals and vitamins are given only for 2 years.

Stapedectomy is a surgical option to remove the damaged stapes and replace it with stainless steel or plastic prosthesis (Fig. 37–12*B*). The oval window is grafted with Gelfoam or tissue grafts. Complications of the operation include granuloma formation and perilymph fistula (rupture of the oval or round window, permitting leakage of perilymph fluid). Either complication may result in profound deafness and persistent vertigo. Hearing loss may also develop after surgery from middle ear adhesions or shifting of the prosthesis. Stapedectomy was once a common middle ear procedure. However, the pool of clients with otosclerosis is dwindling, and today stapedectomy is performed less and less often.

The client must be free of otitis externa and otitis media prior to surgery. No aspirin or products with aspirin can be used for 2 weeks before surgery, to reduce the risk of bleeding.

After surgery the client lies on the nonoperative ear with the head of the bed elevated. This position helps to reduce edema and prevent dislodging of the prosthesis. Antibiotics are prescribed. The packing in the ear canal should not be disturbed. On discharge from the hospital, the client is told to report any vertigo or nystagmus. To reduce the risk of perilymph formation, the client should avoid excessive exercise, straining, and activities that may lead to head trauma. If the client needs to blow the nose, it should be done gently, one nostril at a time. Sneezing should be done with the nose open. No airplane flights are allowed for a month. Hearing aids may still be required, and the client will need to have a reevaluation of hearing.

Acoustic Neuroma

Acoustic neuroma is a tumor of the eighth cranial nerve. The tumor usually develops in the auditory canal, the bony channel through which the vestibular nerve passes as it leaves the inner ear. The tumor presses on the nerve, which sends false signals to the brain. If the vestibular portion of the nerve is compressed, the client is unable to interpret stimuli about position and movement. If the cochlear branch is compressed, the client develops tinnitus. The first clinical manifestation is partial or complete

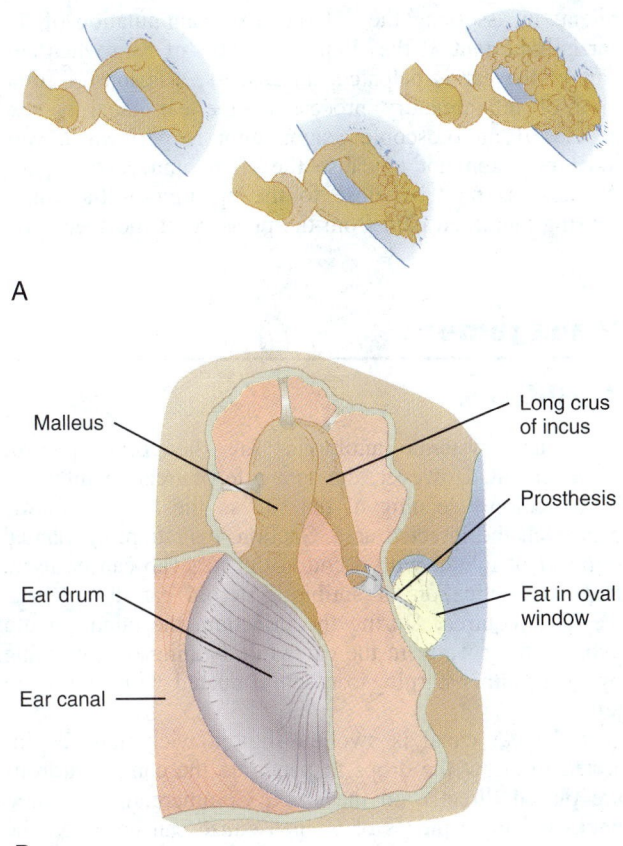

A

Malleus

Long crus
of incus

Prosthesis

Ear drum

Fat in oval
window

Ear canal

B

Figure 37–12. *A,* Stapedial otosclerosis. *B,* Stapedectomy.

sensorineural hearing loss followed by tinnitus. The client may also report dizziness. Current microsurgical techniques yield remarkably good results, usually preserving the seventh cranial nerve and, occasionally, hearing as well.

Tinnitus (Head Noises)

Tinnitus literally means "ringing." Not all ear noises are ringing sounds, but they fall under the broad classification of tinnitus. Tinnitus is not a disease but a very distressing manifestation, and it is often a warning of hearing loss or other more serious problems. Ear noise that cannot be heard by an observer is classified as subjective tinnitus, which is the most common kind. Any ear noise that can be heard by someone other than the client is called objective tinnitus. In some cases, tinnitus is so severe or disruptive that clients have attempted suicide.

The major nursing responsibility is to perform a thorough history and assessment of the onset, frequency, constancy, and level of intensity of the tinnitus. Unilateral tinnitus merits a complete neuro-otologic evaluation with the goal of ruling out the potential of a tumor, most likely an acoustic neuroma. Keep in mind that tinnitus is a manifestation of an underlying pathologic process that warrants further referral.

Many approaches have been tried to alleviate this distressing disorder, such as biofeedback, electrostimulation,

hypnosis, medication, hearing aids, and tinnitus maskers. Tinnitus maskers are quite similar to hearing aids except that they generate noise. The tinnitus masker can cause a phenomenon called residual inhibition. Residual inhibition is the absence of the tinnitus for a period of 1 minute to a few weeks after treatment. However, every approach for the relief from tinnitus is only moderately successful, at best. Educate clients to avoid unproved treatments for tinnitus. Be alert to depression if the tinnitus is chronic. The spouse's support of the client with tinnitus has been shown to be strongly correlated to role function. Be alert to spousal interaction and facilitate with problem-solving as needed.

Otalgia

Otalgia is ear pain or earache. Otalgia can be primary in origin (i.e., coming from a disorder in the ear) or referred (i.e., coming from a disorder outside the ear). Referred otalgia is pain in the ear caused by disorders in the temporomandibular joint, cranial nerves, face, scalp, pharynx, tonsils, thyroid, trachea, teeth, or cervical muscles.

When obtaining the history of the pain, ask the client about what events have triggered the pain, paying special attention to a recent history of any of the following:

1. Upper respiratory tract infection
2. Travel by airplane
3. Exposure to very loud noises
4. Trauma to the head
5. Stressors that led to teeth grinding or dental work

During physical examination, determine the presence of pain with swallowing, neck rotation, palpation of the face and head (over the sinuses), palpation of the mastoid process, and manipulation of the pinna. Assess the temporomandibular joint (TMJ) by asking the client to open and close the mouth. Place your index fingers in the external auditory canal and press anteriorly while the client opens and closes the mouth. TMJ syndrome may cause pain, clicking, or crepitation of the joint during movement.

Otalgia is managed by treating the primary problem. Comfort can be promoted by using anesthetic ear solutions or systemic analgesics. Other measures include application of heat by warm compress, eating a soft diet, providing a quiet environment, and positioning the client with affected ear down. The client with TMJ should avoid chewing and hyperextension of the jaw (e.g., for dental examination and care). He or she should also try to stop grinding the teeth. A specially fitted mouth guard to be worn while sleeping can be helpful in preventing teeth grinding at night.

Ear Infections

Otitis Externa

The most common problems found in the external ear are infections, primarily bacterial or fungal. The most frequent infection, called *external otitis,* involves the external ear canal. It is the most common cause of ear pain in adults. Infection begins when there has been damage to the protective waxy coating by dryness, wetness, or treatment. Infection can lead to edema, which can occlude the canal. External otitis occurs more frequently in the summer than in the winter. The most common form of external otitis is also called *swimmer's ear,* because it is prevalent when water remains in the ear canal. In addition, opportunistic fungal infections are common. When a debilitating systemic disease such as diabetes is present, the external otitis can spread wildly through cartilage and bone and is then named *malignant external otitis. Pseudomonas* is the usual offending pathogen.

Occasionally, infection can involve only the cartilage of the pinna (perichondritis), with resultant necrosis of the cartilage and loss of the distinctive shape of the pinna if the infection is not treated quickly. Frostbite of the pinna has findings similar to those of infection. Another form of infection is seen as an ear canal furuncle or abscess.

Clinical Manifestations and Diagnostic Findings

Pain in the external ear is the most common clinical manifestation of infection. Pain ranges from mild to severe and is generally unilateral. Pain is more intense when the ear canal is swollen. Painful sites are tender because of the close proximity of bone (a hard surface) when the ear is palpated. A clue to early external otitis is tenderness when the pinna is gently pulled on, in contrast to otitis media, in which touching the ear does not cause pain. A forerunner of pain in external otitis is itching in the ear canal. Inflammation (redness) is easily identified with an otoscope. At different stages of infection, drainage will be found from the ear canal. In early infectious disorders, the drainage may be clear and not discolored by pus.

Observe the external ear for signs of redness, swelling, lumps, scaling, crusting, or drainage, either serous or purulent. In assessing the external ear, manipulation of the ear is important. If the client complains of pain when any part of the ear is palpated, an abscess, a lesion, or some kind of inflammatory process of the ear canal is suspected. If an otoscopic examination is performed, care must be taken not to cause the client unnecessary pain. An abscess may be close to the opening of the canal, causing increased pain from the pressure of the speculum.

Management

Antibiotics

Local and systemic antibiotics are the cornerstone of management. However, the first rule of treating infection is meticulous cleaning of the site so the local antibiotic can reach the infected area. Suction, irrigation, or manual removal of matter with a cotton-tipped swab can be used. Regular application of antibiotic-steroid ear drops for a week is required. During the infection, the client should avoid getting water in the ear while bathing or showering by using either earplugs or cotton coated with petroleum jelly.

If the ear canal is swollen shut, a wick must be inserted to allow the drops to penetrate the canal. Eardrops are placed directly on the wick. Commercially prepared wicks or single pieces of ¼-inch gauze can be used. The wick serves not only as a bandage but also as an excellent vehicle to medicate the ear canal. The wick is gently inserted into the ear canal by means of forceps while the external ear is gently pulled upward and backward. The wick is usually slightly less than 1 inch in length (Fig. 37–13). The client should lie on the unaffected side for 3 to 5 minutes to allow gravity to promote movement of the medication into the ear canal.

If the infection is generalized or severe, systemic antibiotics are used. An infection that involves cartilage has to be treated aggressively and quickly with systemic antibiotics to avoid complications.

Figure 37–13. Administration of antibiotics for otitis externa. A curet with a cotton wick around it is placed into the ear canal. The wick is gently placed into the canal and an antibiotic or treatment solution is added to the wick.

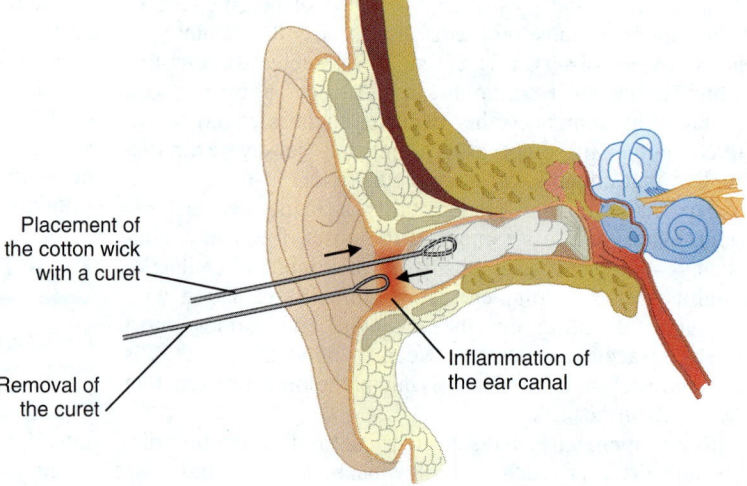

Placement of the cotton wick with a curet

Removal of the curet

Inflammation of the ear canal

Ear Irrigation

The ear is commonly irrigated to cleanse the external auditory canal or to remove impacted wax, debris, or foreign bodies. Irrigation is not used in clients with a history of, or who are suspected of having, a perforated eardrum. The irrigating solution (usually water) is warmed to body temperature and placed in the irrigating syringe. The client's clothes are protected with a plastic drape, and a kidney-shaped basin is placed below the ear to catch the irrigating solution. The client sits with the ear to be irrigated toward you, with the head tilted toward the opposite ear. The external ear is pulled upward and backward for the adult, and the tip of the syringe is directed along the upper wall of the ear canal (Fig. 37–14). The canal should not be completely obstructed by the syringe to allow the backflow of solution. When charting the ear irrigation, include the type of irrigation solution used and the nature of returned solution regarding amount, texture, color of cerumen, and type of debris. Instruct the client to report pain, vertigo, or nausea during the procedure.

Analgesics

Because external otitis is one of the most painful disorders of the ear, appropriate analgesics are required. Pain persists for 24 to 48 hours after treatment is initiated. After the physician has prescribed the analgesic, instruct the client as to the amount, frequency, and duration. Once the swelling and drainage are reduced by treatment in about 48 hours, the pain subsides. Heat may be helpful.

Surgery

The surgical treatment of infections involves incision and drainage in the acute phase for abscesses and, at times, for perichondritis. The most common surgical treatment is excision of cysts and cutaneous carcinomas. For conditions that occlude the ear canal, more extensive surgery that involves skin grafting, known as a *canalplasty,* is performed.

Tympanic Membrane Infection

Infections of the external ear canal can involve the surface of the tympanic membrane, and the tympanic membrane will be a "window" for infection of the middle ear. Infection can cause hard deposits in the tympanic membrane, known as *tympanosclerosis* (see later discussion). A specific viral infection of the tympanic membrane is bullous myringitis. This inflammatory disease forms blisters or bullae between the layers of the eardrum, which are extremely painful. Holes or perforations of the tympanic membrane can be caused by infection and can be accompanied by drainage.

Tympanic membrane disorders can lead to perforation of the membrane. A perforation may be either acute, as seen in trauma and acute infection, or chronic, as seen in repeated infection. An acute perforation has a better chance of healing spontaneously than does a chronic perforation.

Otitis Media

Otitis media is the most prevalent infectious disorder of the middle ear. It is most common in children, but it does occur in adults. When the infection is sudden in onset and short in duration, the diagnosis is acute otitis media. When the infection is repeated, usually causing drainage and perforation, the problem is called chronic otitis media. Chronic otitis media is usually due to *Pseudomonas, Staphylococcus,* or *Klebsiella. Bacteroides* has also been cultured from the ear. Infection can cause swelling of the mucosa throughout the middle ear and eustachian tube.

Figure 37–14. Ear irrigation. The tip of the syringe is directed along the upper wall of the ear canal.

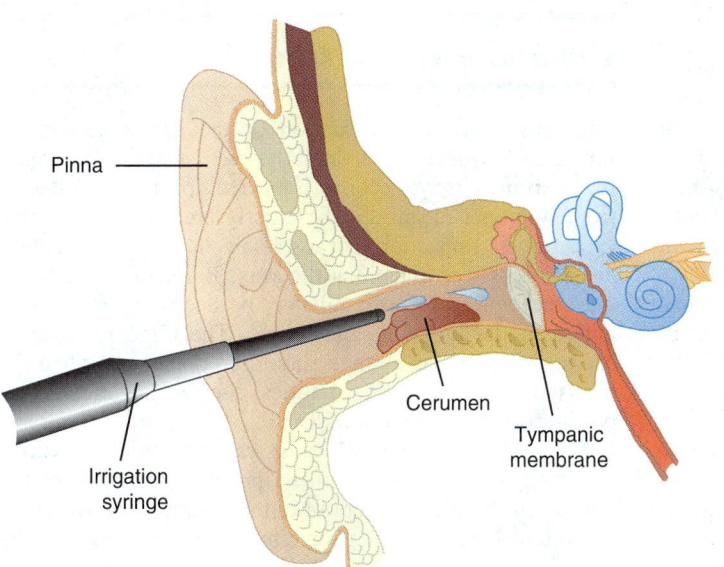

Pinna

Cerumen

Tympanic membrane

Irrigation syringe

Chronic otitis media can lead to tympanic membrane retraction, adhesive otitis media, and/or necrosis of the tympanic membrane (perforations) or of the ossicles. Both problems create a conductive hearing loss. Necrosis of the bony covering of the facial nerve may cause facial paralysis. Because of the extraordinary anatomy of the temporal bone, middle ear infection can also lead to brain abscesses that are life-threatening if not treated properly. Cholesteatoma is a complication and is discussed later.

Clinical manifestations include ear pain and an immobile tympanic membrane. Because the tympanic membrane is a semitransparent membrane, it can show what lies beneath it. It can also become discolored or displaced. Therefore, both fluid and infection can be seen in the middle ear. The tympanic membrane may be dull or red instead of the normal pearly gray. The eardrum may be normal, perforated, infected, retracted, or bulging, according to the disease process involved.

In addition, the client may report bubbling, crackling, or popping sensations in the ear, especially during swallowing. There is a sense of fullness in the ear and conductive hearing loss that fluctuates.

In between bouts of otitis media, fluid may form in the middle ear, known as *serous otitis media*. This fluid is formed when a vacuum develops in the middle ear, caused by a blocked eustachian tube. When the swelling subsides, the fluid may be too thick to drain. At times, serous otitis media is found in conjunction with upper respiratory infections or allergies. Tympanometry is a useful diagnostic assessment to distinguish a normal ear from one with middle ear effusion.

Suppurative otitis media is invasion of the middle ear by virulent organisms and formation of pus. Clinical manifestations include intense ear pain, fever, mild to moderate conductive hearing loss, thickened and bulging tympanic membrane, and occasional dizziness.

With any form of otitis media, appropriate antibiotic therapy may be necessary. If drainage is present, a culture and sensitivity study should be performed. However, most episodes of acute otitis media do not produce drainage, and the most probable bacterial cause need not be identified. Teach the client how to facilitate opening of the eustachian tube. Chewing gum, sucking hard candy and swallowing often, yawning, and flowing air out against closed nostrils help open the tube. Local heat may reduce ear discomfort also. Teach the client to complete the entire prescription of antibiotics even though symptoms have cleared. Otitis media is generally a very easily managed disease, but if it is not treated properly it can lead to sinusitis, meningitis, and brain abscess because of the proximity of the ear to other tissues.

In chronic ear discharge, the normal contaminants of the ear abound and, unfortunately, do not respond to the common antibiotics. Thus, local treatment involving ear irrigations, antibiotic drops, and antibiotic powders is used.

Suppurative otitis media is managed with systemic antibiotics and analgesics. If it becomes chronic, myringotomy may be required to ventilate the middle ear and equalize pressure between the middle and external ear.

Mastoiditis

Before the discovery of antibiotics, a mastoid infection was a life-threatening event. Now, acute mastoiditis is very rare. Still, chronic mastoiditis is present. With repeated middle ear infections, the mastoid cavity becomes a significant part of the problem, which increases the amount of drainage. A chronic infection also leads to the development of cholesteatoma.

Drainage from the mastoid cavity via the ear canal is the most likely sign to appear. The drainage courses through the middle ear and out the tympanic membrane through a perforation. Tenderness over the mastoid cavity behind the ear points to an infection but usually is caused by an acute exacerbation of chronic mastoiditis rather than an acute mastoiditis. The protrusion of the pinna as a result of swelling over the mastoid may be part of this process.

Because infection starts in the middle ear, the problems in the mastoid cavity are avoided by early use of antibiotics with otitis media. Various irrigations of the mastoid and middle ear are used in chronic infections along with antibiotic eardrops or powders.

Radical mastoidectomy removes the mastoid bone for control of infection and cholesteatoma. However, because the radical mastoidectomy sacrificed hearing, a modified radical mastoidectomy was developed that saved the remaining middle ear structures. At the onset of the period of antibiotic administration, a simple mastoidectomy was performed, which maintained a normal-appearing ear canal. Because the radical and modified mastoidectomies exteriorize the mastoid cavity to the external ear canal, they are known as *open mastoidectomies*. *Closed mastoidectomies* are simple mastoidectomies with modifications, in conjunction with tympanoplasty and ossiculoplasty to retain or regain hearing. Today, even the open mastoidectomy is performed with various tympanoplasties. Care of the client with mastoidectomy is discussed in the section on ear masses.

Ear Obstructions

Cerumen Impaction

The most frequent obstruction of the ear is caused by impacted cerumen. Although the ear canal is self-cleaning, cerumen may become impacted from a disorder or from improper cleaning. The elderly are more susceptible to cerumen impaction because hair in the ear becomes coarser with age and traps the wax. Removal of cerumen must be done carefully and may be necessary for examination of the tympanic membrane. The blind removal of earwax with an ear syringe should be done only when the ear is free of other abnormalities, such as an infection or perforation of the eardrum.

Visible wax in the ear canal can be removed with a cotton-tipped applicator. Do not put more than the cotton portion in the ear. Impacted accumulations of earwax may be softened and loosened for removal by alternate instillation of glycerin and hydrogen peroxide eardrops. The eardrops are warmed to body temperature and used daily as directed for 1 to 2 weeks. The ear is then irrigated gently with warm water for removal of the softened wax or cleaned under magnification with a cerumen spoon. Wax that is on the tympanic membrane should be removed by a physician or a clinical nurse-specialist in otology. The removal of cerumen can lead to irritation from mild caustic commercial products.

Foreign Bodies

Surprisingly, a wide array of foreign bodies fit into the ear canal. The most common foreign body found in the adult ear is either a piece of cotton or, most annoying, an insect. Equally surprising is the difficulty that can be encountered in removing a foreign body.

Ear pain from obstruction usually results from the buildup of matter in the small ear canal, which leads to pressure and pain. Clients may also report decreased hearing, a sense of fullness, a throbbing sensation, and itching. The onset, duration, frequency, and intensity of manifestations should be noted.

Removal of foreign bodies can be quite difficult. The external auditory canal is an exquisitely sensitive, elliptically shaped, cylinder-like structure. In adults, it is about 24 mm long and has two anatomic points of narrowing. Objects caught behind these narrow points create the greatest problems for removal. If perforation of the tympanic membrane is deemed unlikely and the object is not tightly wedged, you can irrigate the external canal with warm water. Direct the stream of water superiorly and anteriorly into the ear canal and around the object (see Fig. 37–14). Water pressure builds up and forces the object outward. It often takes about 200 to 300 ml of water to remove an object. Do not irrigate vegetable foreign proteins, such as beans, because they swell and become even more difficult to remove.

Insects are wily, evasive little creatures, and attempts to do battle with a live bug will most likely injure the ear canal. For removal of a live insect, the ear canal is filled with mineral oil, lidocaine, or an ether-soaked cotton ball, *not water,* to kill or stupefy the insect. Water will cause the insect to swell, and it will become more difficult to remove.

The least traumatic method of removing a foreign body is with the aid of an operating microscope. Do not spend a long time attempting to remove an object from the ear without asking for help.

After the object is removed, examine the tympanic membrane and ear canal for signs of trauma. If trauma is noted, treat the client for external otitis and see him or her again in 4 to 5 days.

Ear Trauma

External Ear Trauma

Auricular trauma is common because ears are prominent and unprotected. The pinna is subject to lacerations, blunt injury, abrasions, and burns (or frostbite). A special concern with ear trauma is that a hematoma can quickly develop between the skin and cartilage (called *perichondrial hematoma*). The hematoma exerts pressure on the cartilage, which impairs its healing. Such hematomas are common after blunt injuries, such as occur in wrestling, fighting, or boxing. Clinical manifestations include a bluish or reddish-purple tense swelling over the pinna. Perichondrial hematomas are incised and drained and then dressed in large bulky dressings. A residual finding of untreated perichondrial hematoma is hypertrophic scar formation, known as *cauliflower ear,* which is an occupational hazard for boxers. Ear trauma should be avoided by wearing headgear for contact sports, wide-brimmed hats in the summer, and earmuffs or hats in the winter; heavy pierced earrings should also be avoided because the lobule can be lacerated.

Tympanic Membrane Trauma

The tympanic membrane can be damaged by trauma. Increased pressure from a hand slap, falling in water, sports injuries, cleaning the ear with a sharp instrument, or industrial accidents involving welding sparks can rupture the thin membrane. Trauma to the tympanic membrane from a blast or blunt injury can involve the middle ear, causing a fracture or dislocation of the ossicles and tearing of the tympanic membrane. Also, the facial nerve is vulnerable to trauma. A basal skull fracture involves the temporal bone and, depending on the fracture site, causes ossicular damage as well as facial nerve paralysis and sensorineural hearing loss. Care of clients with facial fracture is discussed in Chapter 80. When the tympanic membrane is perforated, infection is a concern.

Clients often report an episode of brief but intense otalgia. However, if the tympanic membrane is ruptured from barotrauma or otitis media, the client often notes a sudden *relief of pressure and pain.* Pain is not usually elicited on palpation of the external ear; this phenomenon usually provides a differential diagnosis between problems of the external and middle ear. Disorders involving the tympanic membrane are painful, perhaps the most painful of all middle ear disorders.

Examination of the client reveals conductive hearing loss and serous drainage in the ear canal. Hearing loss found with a perforation is approximately 35 dB (one third of the hearing range). If a perforation is present, damage to the ossicles should be suspected, which will cause a greater hearing loss.

 Acute and Subacute Care

■ Medical Management

Medical management includes the use of antibiotics (see the Client Education Guide). The client may be asked to use a medicinal ear irrigation solution.

The most common solution for ear irrigation is boric acid and alcohol, which is obtained by prescription. This solution cleanses the ear of debris and infection and provides a drying agent. A 2- or 3-oz ear syringe will be needed. A family member performs the irrigation for the client. Usually, the ear irrigation is followed by the use of eardrops.

■ Surgical Management

Myringoplasty

Surgery can be performed on the tympanic membrane with use of an operating microscope for magnification. Closure of a perforation is called a *myringoplasty*. If the tympanic membrane needs to be reconstructed, temporalis muscle fascia or other connective tissue can be used.

Tympanoplasty

Tympanoplasty is the surgical correction of a perforated tympanic membrane. There are four types of corrections. When the eustachian tube is stable, hearing results worsen as one proceeds from type I to type IV. Under favorable conditions, type I tympanoplasty should result in normal or near normal restoration of conductive hearing loss, whereas type IV should result in approximately a 30-db air–bone gap. In tympanoplasty a graft is placed to restore the damaged tympanic membrane. The location of the graft depends on the original defect. Sometimes tympanoplasty (ventilation) tubes are inserted.

Type I. — Graft rests on malleus
Type II. — Graft rests on incus
Type III. — Graft attaches to head of stapes
Type IV. — Graft attaches to footplate of stapes

Ossiculoplasty

The surgical procedure of ossicular reconstruction is called *ossiculoplasty*. Reconstruction of the necrotic ossicles is not yet an exact science. Various methods of repositioning these tiny ear bones are now in use. The surgery is difficult to perform and, unfortunately, does not always prove successful over the long term. Therefore, various synthetic prostheses have been used to reconnect the ossicles to carry sound. In an attempt to prevent extrusion of the prostheses, tissue is combined with the prostheses to rebuild the ossicles. This semibiologic method is used in different forms by most otologic surgeons (Fig. 37–15).

■ Nursing Management of the Surgical Client

Preoperative Care

The scope of nursing activities for the client can be as broad as a preoperative assessment performed in an office or clinic or as limited as an assessment performed in the holding area of the surgical suite. Data are collected to assess the client's (1) knowledge of events that are going to occur, (2) mental readiness for surgery, and (3) physiologic status.

The client undergoing ear surgery should be told what to expect during surgery, because frequently only local anesthesia is given. The client is awake but sedated during surgery. Instructions should be given about the length of the procedure, the estimated length of hospital stay, and immediate postoperative instructions. Very often, fear of the unknown can be decreased by understanding of events that will occur.

Postoperative Care

Pain is not usually a major problem, but mild analgesia may be required. Vertigo or lightheadedness may occur when the client ambulates for the first time. Clients should be supervised when ambulating on the day of surgery to protect them from falling. Some clients who are quite vertiginous exhibit nystagmus from stimulation

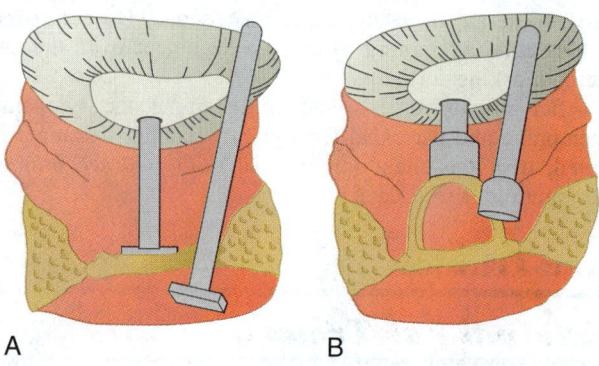

A   B

Figure 37–15. Middle ear prostheses used for reconstruction. *A,* Ossicle columella prosthesis (total ossicular replacement). *B,* Ossicle cup prosthesis (partial ossicular replacement). (Courtesy of Arnold G. Schuring, M.D.)

of the inner ear. The vertigo usually passes very quickly and seldom requires medication.

The ear rarely bleeds after surgery. A small amount of serosanguineous drainage on a cotton ball is expected. Most ear surgery requires only a cotton ball in the ear postoperatively, although a dressing over the ear may be necessary after tympanomastoidectomy. The Client Education Guide lists precautions that the client should be aware of after ear surgery.

Immediate postoperative instructions may include the following:

- Positions should be specified, such as the client lying with operated ear up for several hours after surgery.
- If necessary, blow nose gently one side at a time.
- Sneeze or cough with the mouth open.
- Participation in water sports or activities is prohibited.

Normal occurrences in the initial period may include the following:

- Decreased hearing in operated ear from surgical packing (the sound of talking in a barrel)
- Noises in the ear, such as cracking or popping
- Minor earache and discomfort in cheek and jaw
- Ear swelling

Eustachian Tube Disorders

Because the eustachian tube connects the middle ear to the nasopharynx, pharyngeal disorders also cause eustachian tube dysfunction and, thus, secondary middle ear

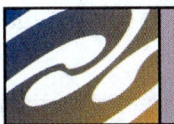

CLIENT EDUCATION GUIDE

Precautions After Ear Surgery

Continue to blow your nose gently one side at a time and to sneeze or cough with your mouth open for 1 week after surgery.
Avoid physical activity for 1 week and exercises or sports for 3 weeks after surgery.
Return to work as recommended, usually 3 to 7 days after surgery (3 weeks if work is strenuous).
Avoid heavy lifting, especially after stapedectomy.
Change the cotton ball in your ear daily as prescribed.
Keep your ear dry for 4 to 6 weeks after surgery.
Do not shampoo for 1 week after surgery.
Protect your ear when necessary with two pieces of cotton (outer piece saturated with petroleum jelly).
Avoid airplane flights for the first week after surgery.
 For sensation of ear pressure, hold your nose, close your mouth, and swallow to equalize pressure.
Wear noise defenders for loud noise environments.
Report any drainage other than a slight amount of bleeding to the physician.

problems. For example, the most common disorder is blockage of the eustachian tube by enlarged adenoid tissue in children. The most common blockage in adults is swelling of the mucosa in the eustachian tube during an upper respiratory infection that can lead to serous otitis media. In a persistent unilateral blocked eustachian tube, a malignant tumor must be ruled out as the cause.

Acute blockage from *barotrauma* (altitude changes) caused by flying or underwater diving will also cause middle ear problems. Hyperbaric oxygen treatments can also cause barotrauma. Hyperbaric oxygen treatment is common for carbon monoxide poisoning as well as other disorders. The incidence of barotrauma is increased when an upper respiratory infection is present. Aerotitis media is a form of serous otitis media in which fluid or air is trapped in the middle ear during descent in an airplane. Any long-term blockage of the eustachian tube leads to serous otitis media and a hearing loss.

Decongestants are used to decrease the swelling and to open the eustachian tube. Pain medication may be needed.

An incision into the tympanic membrane through which fluid is removed by suction is called *myringotomy*. To keep the incision open and to prevent a recurrence of fluid, various types of transtympanic tubes can be inserted into the incision. These tubes extrude by themselves in 3 to 12 months and rarely have to be removed. More permanent tubes (T tubes) with larger flanges may be used for clients who require repeated myringotomies.

Ear Masses

Cholesteatoma

Cholesteatoma is a cyst in the middle ear and/or mastoid that is lined with squamous epithelium and filled with keratin debris. Often, infection is present in the mass of the cholesteatoma. These chronic changes produce cholesterol granules, from which the term *cholesteatoma* is derived.

Cholesteatoma most often results from chronic otitis media or marginal perforation of the tympanic membrane. Clients have conductive hearing loss and foul-smelling discharge from the ears. Although it is a benign growth, the cholesteatoma causes erosion of the surrounding structures, which causes other problems. Cholesteatoma can lead to brain abscesses, vertigo, and facial paralysis. These complications are infrequent.

Other Masses

Benign masses of the external ear canal are usually cysts that arise from a sebaceous gland or, more rarely, from the cerumen glands. Cysts can also be congenital in nature. A bony protrusion seen in the lower bony portion of the ear canal is called *exostosis*. The skin covering the exostosis is normal. If the skin is red, the mass is usually an abscess. Infectious polyps found in the ear canal arise from either the tympanic membrane or, more commonly, the middle ear, through a hole in the tympanic membrane.

Malignant tumors are also found in the external ear. The cutaneous carcinomas are most often basal cell carcinoma on the pinna and squamous cell carcinoma in the ear canal. If not treated, the carcinomas can invade underlying structures; squamous cell carcinoma may spread throughout the temporal bone. Rare tumors of the cerumen glands are of the adenoma cell type. Masses of the external ear are diagnosed by physical examination and biopsy to rule out malignancy. Surgical excision may be required.

Both benign and malignant tumors can involve the tympanic membrane, but they seldom arise from it. However, an infectious glandular polyp can be isolated to the tympanic membrane. Tumors in the middle ear can be seen through or protrude through the tympanic membrane.

The most common benign growth in the middle ear is an infectious polyp. A facial nerve neuroma is found along the course of the facial nerve. Malignant tumors involving the middle ear can be primary or secondary in nature.

The same tumors that arise in the middle ear can be found in the mastoid cavity. Because the mastoid cavity is connected to other air cells throughout the temporal bone and is close to the brain, malignant tumors in the mastoid carry a poor prognosis.

Balance Disorders

Vertigo refers to the perception by a person that either he or she or the surroundings are moving. The person usually remains seated or supine to prevent falling. Vertigo is often described as "dizziness." However, dizziness, which is a feeling of disorientation in space, is different than vertigo. Vertigo results from imbalance of neural signals from the vestibular system in the ears. The imbalance of signals is interpreted by the brain as constant motion in space.

Disorders of balance and coordination result from problems of the vestibular system and righting reflexes. Balance can also be affected by problems outside of the vestibular system. Very few problems are more private than those involving one's sense of balance. Balance problems may be debilitating and also cause embarrassing gait problems, which can jeopardize safety. More than 90 million Americans age 17 years of age or older have experienced vertigo or a balance problem. Vertigo is second only to chronic pain as the most common symptom reported in America today.

Etiology and Risk Factors

Although vertigo and dizziness are not synonymous, they both relate to a sense of balance and equilibrium. Dizziness, vertigo, and syncope are all manifestations of one of the following types of problems:

● Peripheral vestibular disorders (i.e., labyrinthine/inner ear)
● Central disorders (i.e., medullary, cerebellar, and cortical)
● Systemic disorders (i.e., cardiovascular and metabolic)

Peripheral vestibular disorders involve a disorder in the labyrinth or internal ear. Central disorders result from a problem in the brain or nerves, such as a tumor of the eighth cranial nerve (acoustic neuroma) or stroke. Systemic disorders begin in a nerve or organ outside the cranium (e.g., orthostatic hypotension, hypoglycemia). Examples of common causes of vertigo and dizziness, grouped by etiology, are presented in Box 37–7.

Little can be done to reduce the risk of balance disorders. Clients should be treated early for manifestations of ear problems. Clients at high risk of falling as a result of vertigo should arise slowly to prevent injury. Finally, situations that lead to vertigo should be avoided. Motion sickness occurs normally if the provocative stimulus is present. Humans are not evolutionarily adapted to special environmental situations, such as deep-sea diving, high-speed flying, and space travel. Vertigo or dizziness may occur in these environments.

■ Peripheral Vestibular Disorders
Benign Paroxysmal Positional Vertigo

Benign paroxysmal positional vertigo (BPPV) is a common cause of vertigo. It tends to follow head injury and viral infections of the inner ear. BPPV is due to cupulolithiasis, which is the presence of calcium crystals in the semicircular canals. These crystals are normally deposited on small hair-like structures in the ear, and they slow responses to head movement. When they are dislodged, head movement creates a hypersensitive response. BPPV is provoked when the head is placed in certain positions, usually hyperextended and to one side. Clinical manifestations usually include brief attacks or rotational vertigo, a rapid head tilt to the affected ear, and a lag time of 3 to

---

Box 37–7. Disorders Associated with Vertigo and Dizziness

Peripheral Labyrinthine (Inner Ear) Disorders

Benign paroxysmal positional vertigo (BPPV)
Labyrinthitis
Ménière's disease
Cholesteatoma

Central Nervous System Disorders

Cerebellar lesions
Temporal lobe lesions
Tumors of cranial nerve VIII (e.g., acoustic neuroma)
Stroke

Systemic Disorders

Diabetes
Postural hypotension
Arthritis
Hypoglycemia
Multiple sclerosis
Parkinson's disease
Allergies

6 seconds between change of position and vertigo with nystagmus.

Labyrinthitis

Labyrinthitis is infection or inflammation of the cochlear and/or vestibular portion of the inner ear. Causes are not fully understood, but the syndrome tends to occur in spring and early summer preceded by an upper respiratory infection. Therefore, a virus has been implicated, but never isolated. Three classic manifestations are reported: vertigo, nausea, and vomiting. There are no hearing changes. Vertigo is usually in onset; it peaks in 24 to 48 hours and then gradually subsides over 1 to 2 weeks. Supportive treatment is usually given while waiting for the underlying problems to clear.

Ménière's Disease

Ménière's disease is caused by excess endolymph in the vestibular and semicircular canals. Endolymph is clear intracellular fluid in the membranous labyrinth of the inner ear. Normal vestibular activity is dependent on stability of fluid pressure. Ménière's disease is a disorder that causes hearing changes and vertigo. It is discussed under balance disorders because the vertigo is often the most troublesome manifestation in early stages. A triad of manifestations develops: paroxysmal whirling vertigo, fluctuating hearing loss, and tinnitus. Only one or two symptoms may be present initially. Vertigo is characterized by remission and relapses without apparent cause, although the manifestations become less severe in time. The initial attacks consist of approximately 30 minutes of intense vertigo, which commonly provokes nausea and vomiting. Remaining stationary reduces vertigo. Hearing loss is usually subtle and reversible in early stages. Later hearing loss becomes permanent. The client may not realize hearing has been lost because of the roaring tinnitus. Control of Ménière's episodes is usually possible, although a cure is not yet available. Clients are treated with low-sodium diets, diuretics, and balance exercises. Surgery is an option, which is discussed below.

■ Central Disorders of Balance

Dizziness may be a manifestation of a transient ischemic attack (TIA) ("a small stroke"). A temporary loss of blood flow to the brain leads to several manifestations, depending on the brain area that is not being perfused. Clients can develop momentary losses of consciousness, transient numbness, tingling, weakness, and changes in speech. TIAs should be reported and treated aggressively to prevent true ischemic changes.

■ Systemic Disorders Leading to Vertigo

Physiologic Vertigo

Physiologic vertigo includes common disorders such as motion sickness, space sickness, and height vertigo. In these conditions, vertigo is minimal or absent while autonomic manifestations are present. Motion and space sickness lead to perspiration, nausea, vomiting, increased salivation, yawning, and malaise. With height vertigo, clients report acute anxiety and panic reaction. Physiologic vertigo can usually be suppressed by supplying sensory cues that come from other stimuli. For example, motion sickness from reading in a car can be reduced by looking out the window at the moving environment.

Presbystasis

A disorder that is recognized more and more is presbystasis, or balance disorder of aging. Because of the generalized degenerative changes that occur in aging, balance and stability are also affected. In addition to the labyrinth, balance also depends on the visual system and the proprioceptive changes in the muscles. Because all three systems are involved in aging, the elderly have difficulty with stability, which results in falls and subsequent trauma.

Orthostatic Hypotension

Orthostatic hypotension is a sudden drop in blood pressure and dizziness on sitting or standing. Dizziness is due to lack of adequate cerebral blood flow. The elderly are at high risk of orthostatic hypotension because of atherosclerosis and the use of medications that lead to diuresis or hypotension (e.g., furosemide, calcium-channel blockers). Orthostasis is diagnosed by assessing positional blood pressure changes. Clients should be taught to change position slowly, and medications may require adjustment if blood pressure is too low.

Pathophysiology

The body maintains balance and equilibrium by responding to an intricate network of information. The ability to maintain balance depends on four systems being intact: (1) the vestibular system (the labyrinth or inner ear); (2) the visual system (the eyes); (3) the proprioceptive system (the somatosensors of joints and muscles); and (4) the cerebellar system (the coordinator). The sensations transmitted from the ears, the eyes, and the somatosensors are integrated in the brain stem and cerebellum and perceived in the cerebral cortex. Gradual interference of vestibular input will cause compensatory changes that allow the brain to adjust slowly. Quick changes demand more adjustments than can be made. Infections can destroy the nerve and later transmission of messages. Overproduction of lymph can slow transmission of messages and lead to the perception that the body is in constant motion. Head trauma can shake free calcium carbonate crystals on the utricular macule and alter endolymph movement.

Clinical Manifestations and Diagnostic Findings

Vertigo is the most common clinical manifestation in a client with a balance problem. The symptoms of balance disorders vary widely depending on the cause, the loca-

	Table 37–4. Vestibular and Nonvestibular Vertigo	
	Vestibular	**Nonvestibular**
Common descriptions	Spinning (environment moves), on a merry-go-round	Light-headedness, feeling of being dissociated from body, swimming, giddiness, spinning inside (environment stationary)
Clinical manifestations	Drunkenness, tilting, motion sickness, off-balance	
Course of illness	Episodic	Constant
Precipitating factors	Head movement, position change	Stress, hyperventilation, cardiac dysrhythmia
Associated manifestations	Nausea, vomiting, tinnitus, hearing loss, impaired vision, unsteadiness	Perspiration, pallor, paresthesias, palpitations, syncope, difficulty concentrating, tension headache

tion (one or both ears), the client's age at onset, the extent of the loss, and the rapidity with which damage occurs. Pathology in the external, middle, and inner ear usually leads to vertigo that is sudden, transient, and accompanied by vagal manifestations (e.g., nausea, vomiting, sweating, and pallor). The vertigo that is associated with cerebrovascular lesions does follow a pattern; however, tinnitus and hearing loss are usually not present.

An important differentiation is if the vertigo is associated with hearing loss. The close anatomic relationship between the balance and hearing systems sometimes causes the sensation of vertigo in conjunction with a hearing loss. However, in most instances, vertigo is present without a hearing loss. It is also important to distinguish between vertigo from vestibular problems and other forms of vertigo. Table 37–4 differentiates the two forms of vertigo.

Vertigo is described in such varied terms that it is almost impossible to define. Not all the terms listed below point to vertigo. The nurse should record the terms or description used to help find the actual etiology. Clinical manifestations include, but are not limited to, the following:

- Spinning vertigo
- Sensation of falling
- Imbalance
- Staggering
- Giddiness
- Lightheadedness
- Disorientation
- Visual blurring
- Veering in one direction while walking
- Unsteadiness
- Reeling
- Faintness
- Wooziness
- Shakiness
- Instability
- Wobbliness
- Bewilderment
- Confusion
- Being dazed
- Clumsiness
- Sense of floating

- Sense of falling
- Weakness
- Vague feeling of uncertainty

Even after the vertigo has abated, anxiety tends to persist. Clients are very worried about having another "attack."

For the client with vertigo, the differential diagnosis may be accomplished by a thorough medical assessment, including audiometry, vestibular tests, imaging evaluation, and, sometimes, laboratory studies. Clients who have had vertigo may become quite anxious thinking about developing vertigo again. Because vertigo is only a clinical manifestation, the diagnosis and treatment of the underlying disease are important. Unlike in vision or hearing, no single organ is responsible for balance problems. Therefore, the diagnosis, treatment, and rehabilitation of the client with a balance problem can be difficult as well as frustrating.

Community and Self-Care

■ Medical Management

Treatment of acute vertigo involves several medicines, which are called antivertigo agents. These medicines tend to suppress the balance system or the central nervous system. In chronic vertigo, vasodilators such as nicotinic acid are used. Other medicines used for specific disorders include antibiotics, steroids, diuretics, tranquilizers, and vitamins. The nonspecific nature of the medical treatment points to the fact that a curative approach does not yet exist.

Vestibular rehabilitation is now a recognized form of control for vertigo. Whereas certain forms of exercises for balance disorders have been available for decades, only now has this treatment modality been formalized. Because the balance system can compensate, head and total body exercises are performed by the client to hasten compensation. Usually, physical therapists are involved in structuring this treatment. Vestibular rehabilitation uses all three organ systems that provide balance.

The exercises include the following:

- While lying in bed, slowly then quickly turn the eyes up, down, and from side to side, and the head forward, backward, and from side to side
- Perform the same exercises while sitting; in addition, bend forward and pick up objects from the ground
- While standing, perform the previously mentioned exercises; in addition, change from sitting to standing position with the eyes open, and then closed, and turn around in between
- While moving about, walk up and down steps with eyes open and then closed, or play games involving stooping and stretching, such as basketball

It is believed that when vertigo is induced by these exercises, a tolerance for it is acquired. Clients should do these exercises from the time of the acute attack and continue until they are free of manifestations for two consecutive days. Driving a car safely will need to be addressed with clients.

■ Nursing Management of the Medical Client

Assessment

Nursing assessment of the client with a balance problem should include the following:

- A client interview to obtain a health history and specific information about the onset and characteristics of the balance problem and associated hearing problems. Attempt to distinguish the type of vertigo reported and note aggravating conditions (e.g., head movement).
- An interview with a family member to identify the effect of the client's balance problem on others
- Assess effect of vertigo on performance of activities of daily living

The importance of the history and interview cannot be overemphasized. An adequate description about vertigo should include information about the onset, exacerbating and alleviating factors, associated clinical manifestations, and predisposing factors in the medical history as previously described. All clients bring some degree of anxiety regarding this illness to the examination. Balance problems can have devastating effects on the client's behavior. The disruption of the client's routine, the severity of the "attacks," and the fear of the unknown can make the client agitated, anxious, or depressed. Be aware of these feelings and demonstrate self-confidence, patience, courtesy, and gentleness.

A structured questionnaire such as the one shown in Box 37–8 should be completed by the client. These questions can also be used to facilitate the interview. However, the interview should be guided by client cues. A gross assessment of the client's balance can be made by watching the client's gait. Evidence of instability may be noted if the client touches the wall or walks with a wide-based waddling gait.

The same inspection, palpation, and otoscopic examination should be performed for the client with a balance problem as was performed for the client with a hearing

---

Box 37–8. Assessment Guide for Clients with Balance Disorders

I. When you are dizzy, do you experience any of the following sensations? Please read the entire list first. Then circle the numbers of those sensations that describe what you experience most accurately.
   1. Lightheadedness
   2. Tendency to lose balance or to fall
   3. Objects spinning or turning around you
   4. Sensation that you are turning
   5. Headache
   6. Nausea or vomiting
   7. Pressure in the head

II. Please fill in the blank spaces.
   1. When did the dizziness first occur? _____
   2. Is your vertigo constant? _____
   3. Does it come in attacks? _____
   4. How often do attacks occur? _____
   5. How long are the attacks? _____
   6. Does vertigo occur only in certain positions? ___

      When upright? _____
      When lying flat? _____
      Turning to the right? _____
      Turning to the left? _____
   7. Have you ever stumbled or fallen because of vertigo? _____
   8. Do you know of anything that will stop the vertigo or make it better? _____

      Make your vertigo worse? _____

      Bring on an attack? _____

   9. Did you ever injure your head? _____
   10. Do you take any medications regularly (e.g., tranquilizers; oral contraceptives; barbiturates; a course of antibiotics, such as streptomycin, neomycin)? _____
   11. Do you use tobacco in any form? _____
       Alcohol? _____
   12. Have you worked for long in a noisy environment? _____
   13. Do you suffer easily from motion sickness? ___ _____

---

loss (see earlier discussion). Assess the client for the loss of hearing and tinnitus, which are symptoms that can accompany a balance problem.

Diagnosis, Planning, Implementation

Nursing care of the client with vertigo is detailed in the Care Plan.

Evaluation

Evaluate the client's ability to institute measures to prevent vertigo, remain free from injury, and have less anxiety about vertigo attacks.

CARE PLAN

The Client with Vertigo

Nursing Diagnosis. Risk for Injury related to tendency to lose balance

Planning: Expected Outcomes. The client will reduce the risk of injury by moving slowly, remaining immobile when dizzy, and using aids for ambulation if gait and balance are unstable.

Implementation: Nursing Intervention	**Rationales**
While the client is on bedrest: Encourage the client to move in bed slowly.	Slow movement allows the vestibular system time to regain balance and integrate messages.
Minimize the client's head movement during acute attacks.	Eye and head movements often aggravate vertigo.
Darken the room.	Darkness may help reduce acute vertigo.
Avoid startling the client to reduce reflexic head movement.	The risk of vertigo caused by sudden movement is reduced.
Assist the client with hygiene as needed while encouraging independence.	Assistance protects the client from slipping. Complete care may be needed.
Keep the side rails up and the bed in low position when the client is in bed. Place call light, phone, and personal articles within the client's reach.	Side rails remind the client to call for help and limit the distance to the floor in case of falls from bed. Placing articles within reach decreases the client's risk of falling when reaching for articles.
Assist with ambulation as needed.	Reduces risk of falls.

Evaluation. Expect this outcome to be met over several days. Look for small improvements and encourage the client.

Nursing Diagnosis. Risk for Impaired Adjustment related to a required change in life-style secondary to unpredictability of vertigo

Planning: Expected Outcomes. The client will adjust to or modify his or her life-style to decrease disability and exert maximal control and independence within limits imposed by vertigo and balance disorder.

Implementation: Nursing Intervention	**Rationales**
Encourage the client to identify personal strengths and roles that can still be fulfilled.	Encouragement fosters positive self-esteem.
Encourage the client to talk about feelings, personal perception of danger, and perception of his or her own coping skills and limitations.	Allows nurse to provide individualized support.
Encourage the client to make decisions and assume responsibility for self-care.	Personal responsibility helps the client to maintain a sense of control.
Provide information about vertigo and how to prepare for attacks.	Education promotes a problem-solving approach to managing the disorder.
Encourage the client to perform balance exercises.	Balance exercises reduce the severity of attacks by training the central nervous system to adjust to changes in position.
Include the clients' family and significant others in discussions.	Family involvement promotes awareness and hopefully fosters support.

Evaluation. Achievement of this outcome rests almost entirely on the client's willingness to modify a previous life-style and his or her ability to overcome limits that can be felt from vertigo.

Nursing Diagnosis. Impaired Verbal Communication related to decreased hearing and tinnitus

Planning: Expected Outcomes. The client will report satisfaction with ability to communicate.

Implementation: Nursing Intervention	**Rationales**
Assess the client's hearing acuity and audiogram results.	These results provide factual information on the degree of hearing loss.
Speak distinctly and enunciate words without shouting.	Clear speech facilitates hearing and comprehension.
Use picture boards or write to communicate.	These are alternate methods of communication.
Assess for the client for hearing aid candidacy and make needed referrals.	Hearing aids augment sound.

Evaluation. This outcome may require several days to achieve. Hearing loss is reversible in early stages but may become permanent if prolonged.

Nursing Diagnosis. Risk for Fluid Volume Deficit related to decreased oral intake and loss of fluids through emesis

Planning: Expected Outcomes. The client will maintain adequate fluid volume as evidenced by normal blood pressure, normal pulse rate, quick skin turgor, moist oral mucous membranes, and adequate urine output.

Implementation: Nursing Intervention	Rationales
Assess the client's pulse, respiration, and blood pressure every 4 hours (if stable).	Hypotension and tachycardia are indicators of dehydration.
Assess the client's skin turgor, oral mucous membranes, oral intake, and urine output every 8 hours (if stable).	Decreased skin turgor, dry mucous membranes, and oliguria are indicators of dehydration.
Compare intake with output, and consider intravenous fluids if the output is greater than intake for several hours.	Intake should equal output over 24 hours. Urine output should be 20–30 ml/hr. IV fluids are another access for fluids.
Encourage the client to drink fluids.	Lost fluids should be replaced.
Teach the client to avoid caffeinated beverages.	Caffeine is a vestibular stimulant.
Administer antiemetics as ordered and observe for side effects of medications given.	Reduces the risk of emesis and allows for increased oral intake.
Encourage the client to try resting on the unaffected ear.	Gravity facilitates drainage from affected ear.

Evaluation. If the client's nausea can be controlled, fluid balance should be achievable within 24 to 48 hours.

Nursing Diagnosis. Powerlessness related to feelings of loss of control secondary to unpredictability of vertigo

Planning: Expected Outcomes. The client will verbalize ways to maintain control and respond to vertigo.

Implementation: Nursing Intervention	Rationales
Assess the client's cognitive appraisal of his or her illness.	Cognitive appraisal of the illness provides information about the client's perception of the illness and how much control the client feels he or she has over vertigo.
Assess the client's previous coping strategies.	The client will use previous coping strategies during this new stress.
Help the client develop coping strategies based on past coping skills and situational support available to the client.	Reuse effective past coping strategies. Situation support can help bridge the client's return to society.
Stress the importance of maintaining or resuming normal activities or developing diversionary activities.	Reduces the risk that client will become disabled due to vertigo. Activity also reduces depression.
Provide needed information about vertigo:	Encourage the use of problem-solving coping.
■ Information about prescribed medications ■ Manifestations requiring medical attention (e.g., a sudden loss of hearing, a change in the current level of hearing, visual disturbances, weakness or numbness in the extremities, seizures, loss of consciousness, or progressive worsening of vertigo)	
Refer to the client to support groups in the community.	The client may benefit from interaction with others and may learn effective methods to cope with the disorder.

Evaluation. Feelings of powerlessness may require weeks to months to resolve; especially if vertigo is chronic.

■ Surgical Management

Approximately 5% of all clients with vertigo undergo surgical intervention. However, more clients will undergo surgical procedures in the future because of new surgical developments and advanced technology.

Endolymphatic Sac Surgery

The endolymphatic sac procedures include decompression and various forms of shunts to the central nervous system or mastoid cavity. The intent of these procedures is to lessen the fluid pressure within the labyrinth and control the vertigo of Ménière's disease. Outcomes of the surgery are not fully researched. One group found improvement of vertigo in 81% of clients, improvement of tinnitus in 38%, and improvement in hearing in 19%.

Labyrinthectomy

Labyrinthectomy is another form of surgery to lessen pressure within the labyrinth. It is performed through the oval or round window. This is considered a destructive procedure and removes the membranous labyrinth, either subtotally through the oval window or totally through the mastoid bone. Any remaining hearing is sacrificed.

Vestibular Nerve Resection

Vestibular nerve resection can be performed to alleviate vertigo. Vestibular nerve resection can be performed through the labyrinth (sacrificing hearing) or around the labyrinth (saving hearing). The retrolabyrinthine surgical choice is the most common form of surgical control for vertigo today. Alleviation of the client's vertigo is usually immediate. Because of the compensation by all of the other structures related to maintaining balance, a client can function with only one labyrinth.

Conclusions

Nurses caring for clients with hearing and balance problems need to focus on safety and on promoting independence. Many hearing-impaired clients live a normal life with hearing augmentation and aural rehabilitation. Clients who have decreased hearing or balance disorders are at increased risk of injury because of lack of awareness of risk or losing balance. Infections remain common, but excellent antibiotics have reduced the incidence of chronic problems caused by infections. Tumors of the ear are rare, but when they occur they are quite destructive.

Thinking Critically

1. A middle-aged client comes to the health clinic with ear pain and difficulty hearing. He had some serious drainage 1 day ago but does not recall any recent infection (throat or ear). The problem has persisted intermittently over the past 6 months and is getting progressively more painful and occurring more frequently. If surgery was deemed necessary, how would you prepare the client? What discharge teaching might need to be completed for the client after ear surgery?

Factors to Consider. What preoperative assessments are needed? How should equal pressure be maintained on the tympanic membrane? What normal occurrences might the client expect in the initial period following surgery?

2. An elderly client reveals a 10-year history of ear infection. She is experiencing sensorineural hearing loss associated with presbycusis, which affects older people. During her clinic appointment, she tells the nurse that her right ear is painful and is keeping her awake at night. She explains that she can hear most sounds, although sounds on the right side seem to be coming through a filter. She has been using her eardrops as directed but has stopped taking her antibiotic because she felt better 2 days ago. She requests information about daily medication or a surgical procedure that might alleviate the problem. How should you respond to the client's request? How do age-related changes contribute to the client's problem?

Factors to Consider. What is the assessment focus for this client? What is the prognosis for the client with presbycusis? What type of teaching does the client require?

Bibliography

1. Chipps, E., Clanin, N., & Campbell, V. (1992). *Neurologic disorders.* St. Louis: Mosby–Year Book.
2. Cohen, N. L., & Hoffman, R. A. (1992). Complications of cochlear implant surgery in adults and children. *Annals of Otorhinolaryngology, 99,* 791–795.
3. Cohen, N. L., Waltzman, S. B., Fisher, S. G., & The Department of Veterans Affairs Cochlear Implant Study Group. (1993). A prospective randomized study of cochlear implants. *New England Journal of Medicine, 328*(4), 233–237.
4. Cummings, C. W., et al. (1993). *Otolaryngology-head and neck surgery* (2nd ed.). St. Louis: Mosby–Year Book.
5. Curtin, H. D. (1991). The use of magnetic resonance imaging in otolaryngology head and neck. *Advances in Otolaryngology Head and Neck Surgery, 5*(71), 107–111.
6. Erkan, M., et al. (1994). Bacteriology of chronic suppurative otitis media. *Annals of Otorhinolaryngology, 103*(10), 771–774.
7. Fairbanks, D. N. F. (1991). *Antimicrobial therapy in otolaryngology–head and neck surgery* (6th ed.). Alexandria, VA: American Academy of Otolaryngology–Head and Neck Surgery.
8. Gershman, K., & Nielsen, C. (1995). Prevention and screening in the nursing home. *Clinics in Primary Care, 22*(4), 731–753.
9. Glasscock, M. E., & Stambaugh, G. E. (1990). *Surgery of the ear.* Philadelphia: W. B. Saunders.
10. Hughes, G. B. (1994). Surgical treatment of incapacitating peripheral vertigo: Criteria for the evaluation of surgical results. *Otolaryngological Clinics of North America, 27* (2), 301–305.
11. Jamieson, D. G., Brennan, R. L., & Cornelisse, L. E. (1995). Evaluation of speech enhancement strategy with normal-hearing and hearing-impaired listeners. *Ear and Hearing, 16*(3), 274–286.
12. Lebo, C. P., et al. (1994). Restaurant noise, hearing loss, and hearing aids. *Western Journal of Medicine, 161*(1), 45–49.
13. Meyerhoff, W. L., & Rice, D. H. (1992). *Otolaryngology–head and neck surgery.* Philadelphia: W. B. Saunders.
14. Moffat, D. A. (1994). Endolymphatic sac surgery: Analysis of 100 operations. *Clinical Otolaryngology, 19*(3), 261–266.
15. Nobel, W., Ter-Horst, K., & Byrne, D. (1995). Disabilities and handicaps associated with impaired auditory localization. *Journal of the American Academy of Audiology, 6*(2), 129–140.
16. Osterweil, D., Martin, M., & Syndulko, K. (1995). Predictors of skilled nursing placement in a multilevel long-term care facility. *Journal of the American Geriatric Society, 43*(2), 108–112.
17. Paparella, M. M., et al. (1991). *Otolaryngology* (3rd ed.). Philadelphia: W. B. Saunders.
18. Schuring, L. T. (1992). Clinical standards of practice. *ORL—Head and Neck Nursing, 10*(2), 5–10.
19. Sigler, B., & Schuring, L. T. (1993). *Ear, nose and throat disorders.* St. Louis: Mosby–Year Book.
20. Siriboonrit, U., & Jahn, A. F. (1994). Ménière's disease: Diagnosis and management. *New England Journal of Medicine, 91*(3), 171–173.
21. Smith, T. L., DiRuggiero, D. C., & Jones, K. R. (1994). Recovery of eustachian tube function and hearing outcomes in patients with

cleft palate. *Otolaryngology Head and Neck Surgery, 111*(4), 423–429.

22. Souza, P. E., & Turner, C. W. (1994). Masking of speech in young and elderly listeners with hearing loss. *Journal of Speech and Hearing Research, 37*(3), 655–661.

23. Sullivan, M., et al. (1994). Coping and marital support as correlates of tinnitus disability. *General Hospital Psychiatry, 16*(4), 259–266.

24. Yardley, L., Luxon, L. M., & Haacke, N. P. (1994). A longitudinal study of symptoms, anxiety and subjective well-being in patients with vertigo. *Clinical Otolaryngology, 19*(2), 109–116.

Respiratory Disorders

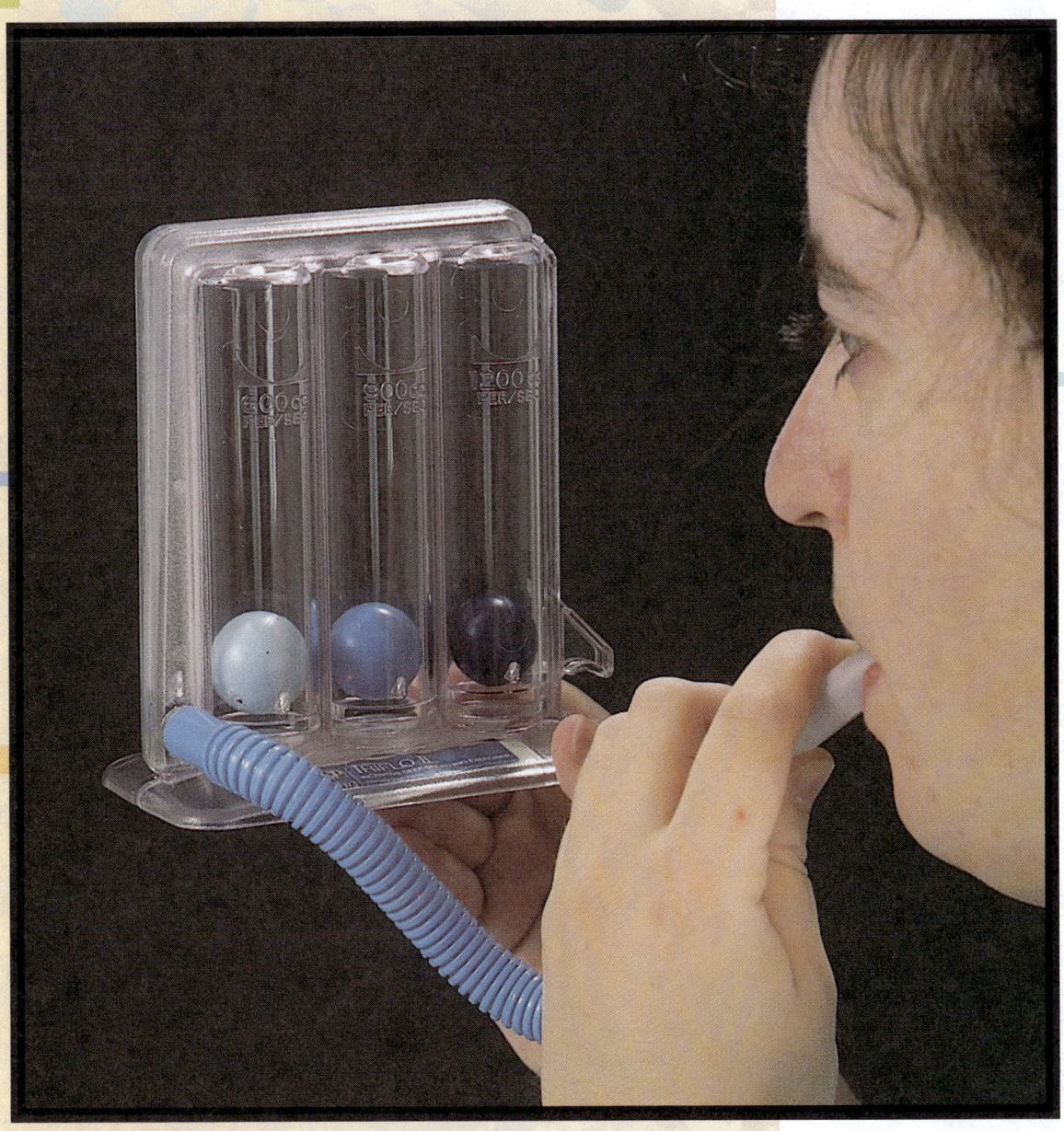

Structure and Function of the Respiratory System

Joyce M. Black

Breathing is a basic human function that we tend to be unconscious of unless we have some difficulty with it. Breathing is a physiologic function that is almost synonymous with being alive. We experience difficulty in breathing as a threat to life itself. People with respiratory disorders are often very anxious and fearful that they may die, perhaps agonizingly. Whether death is a real possibility often has nothing to do with the fear.

Respiratory problems are widespread. They may be acute (short term) or chronic (long term). Acute disorders range from minor inconveniences, such as colds or flu, to more life-threatening problems, such as asthma, some types of pneumonia, and chest trauma. Chronic respiratory problems are also widespread, and are the cause of significant disability. People who experience them often have to make radical life-style changes, often retiring from work earlier than they wish. Such disabling conditions include chronic obstructive pulmonary disease (COPD), now called *chronic airflow limitation*, and certain restrictive lung diseases.

Respiratory problems have many causes: allergies, occupational factors, genetic factors, smoking and tobacco use, infection, neuromuscular disorders, chest abnormalities, trauma, pleural conditions, and pulmonary vascular abnormalities. The most significant factor in chronic respiratory illness and lung cancer is cigarette smoking.

Nurses are involved both in providing care for clients with respiratory conditions and in preventing such problems. It is important to encourage clients to take care of their lungs and especially to stop smoking. In acute healthcare settings, significant nursing intervention is directed at relieving existing respiratory problems and preventing possible respiratory complications. Such intervention includes the following:

- Encouraging deep breathing and coughing in immobile people

This chapter incorporates material written for the fourth edition by Margaret Nield.

- Turning bedridden people at risk of developing atelectasis or pneumonia
- Preventing aspiration in people who are paralyzed or obtunded
- Determining that respiratory therapy is given in a safe, appropriate, and timely manner
- Maintaining a patent airway by measures such as suctioning, positioning, and artificial airway care
- Encouraging the alternation of active with passive activities and other forms of energy conservation in people with chronic problems
- Coordinating activities of daily living with breathing retraining techniques and goal-oriented progressive exercise
- Helping people (especially those with chronic respiratory problems) incorporate relaxation and stress-reduction activities into their daily lives
- Helping people with respiratory problems and their significant others learn ways to lessen the likelihood of further disease and disability
- Providing extensive nursing care for acutely ill people.

Gas exchange is the primary function of the respiratory system. The respiratory system takes oxygen from the atmosphere, transports it to the lungs, exchanges the oxygen for carbon dioxide in the alveoli, and returns carbon dioxide to the air. This chapter reviews the anatomy and physiology of the respiratory system so the student can see the relationship between disease and alterations in structure or function.

The Airways

The airways are commonly divided into the upper and lower airways. The upper airway consists of the nasal cavities, pharynx, and larynx.

Upper Airway

Structure

Nasal Cavity

The nose is formed from both bone and cartilage. A very small portion of the nose is bone; the nasal bone only forms the bridge of the nose. The remainder of the nose is composed of cartilage and connective tissue. The nasal cartilages form the shape of the nose (Fig. 38–1).

The openings of the nose on the face are called *nostrils* or *nares*. Each nostril leads to a cavity, called a vestibule. The vestibule is lined anteriorly with skin and hair (called *vibrissae*). The vibrissae filter foreign objects and prevent them from being inhaled. The posterior vestibule is lined

with mucous membrane. This membrane is composed of columnar epithelial cells, which secrete mucus. The portion of mucous membrane that is located at the top of the nasal cavity, just beneath the cribriform plate of the ethmoid bone, is specialized epithelium, called *olfactory epithelium,* which provides the sense of smell. The region is supplied by the olfactory nerve (cranial nerve I) which passes through holes in the cribriform plate. The olfactory epithelium does not lie along the usual path of air movement, so smell is enhanced by sniffing.

Along the sides of the vestibule are turbinates. The turbinates are mucous membrane-covered projections. They contain a very rich blood supply (from the internal and external carotid arteries), and they warm and humidify inspired air.

Paranasal sinuses are open areas within the skull. They are named for the bones in which they lie—frontal, ethmoid, sphenoid, and maxillary (Fig. 38–2). Passageways

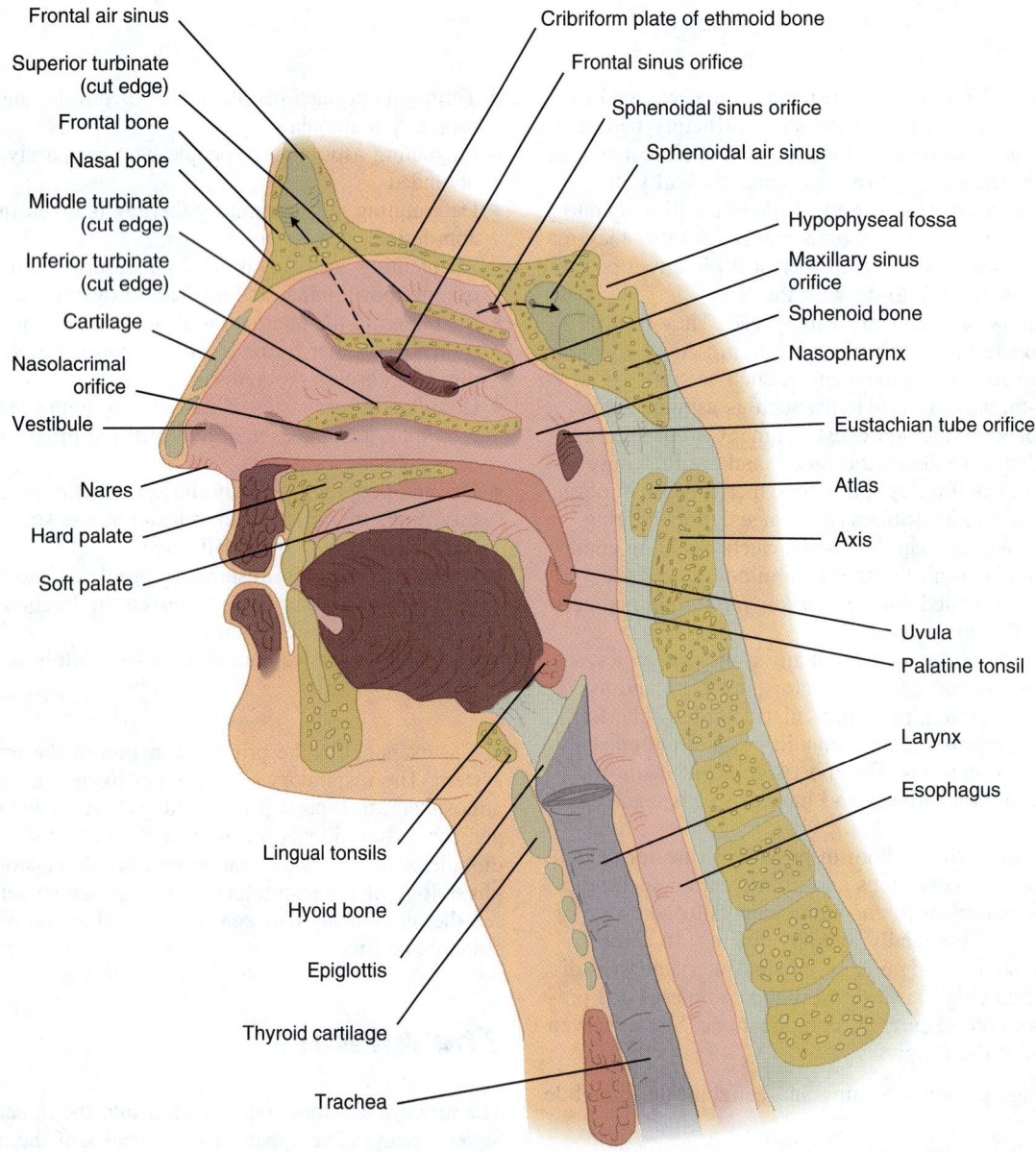

Figure 38–1. Structures of the upper airway.

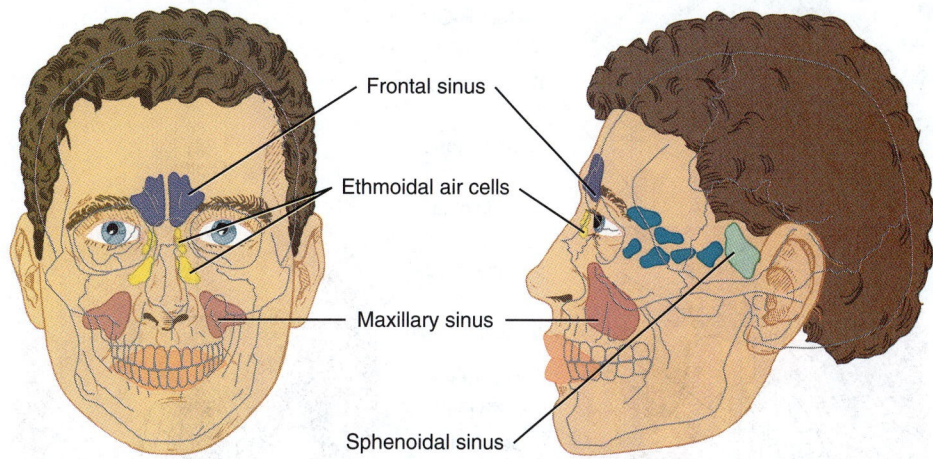

Figure 38–2. The paranasal sinuses.

from the paranasal sinuses drain into the nasal cavities. The nasolacrimal ducts, which drain tears from the surface of the eyes, also drain into the nasal cavity.

The mouth is considered part of the upper airway, but only because the mouth can be used to deliver air to the lungs. The mouth may be used for breathing when the nose is obstructed or when high volumes of air are needed, such as during exercise. The mouth does not perform the functions of the nose efficiently, especially warming, humidifying, and filtering air.

Pharynx

The pharynx is a funnel-shaped tube that extends from the nose to the larynx. It is used for digestion as well as for respiration. The pharynx is divided into three sections: (1) the nasopharynx, located above the margin of the soft palate; (2) the oropharynx, the part of the pharynx that is visible when the tongue is depressed with a tongue depressor; and (3) the laryngopharynx, located below the base of the tongue.

The nasopharynx is the upper section and receives air from the nasal cavity. The nasopharynx is lined with ciliated columnar epithelium. From the ear, the eustachian tubes open into the nasopharynx. The pharyngeal tonsils are located on the posterior wall of the nasopharynx. The tonsils are masses of lymphoid tissue; they serve as an additional defense mechanism against bacterial infection. When the pharyngeal tonsils become enlarged following repeated infections or are at their point of maximum growth during adolescence, they are called *adenoids*.

The oropharynx serves both respiration and digestion. It receives air from the nasopharynx and food from the oral cavity. Palatine (faucial) tonsils are located along the sides of the posterior mouth, and the lingual tonsils are located at the base of the tongue.

The laryngopharynx (hypopharynx) is the most inferior portion of the pharynx. It connects to the larynx and serves both respiration and digestion.

Larynx

The larynx is commonly called the *voice box*. It connects the upper (pharynx) and lower (trachea) airways. It is

located anterior to the fourth and sixth cervical vertebrae. The upper esophagus is just posterior to the larynx. The larnyx is formed by nine cartilages: three paired and three single cartilages. The three large unpaired cartilages are the epiglottis, thyroid, and cricoid; the three paired cartilages, which are smaller, are the arytenoid, corniculate, and cuneiform. The cartilages are held together and attached to the hyoid bone above the trachea and below the trachea by muscles and ligaments. The larynx consists of the endolarynx and a surrounding triangle-shaped bone and cartilage. The endolarynx is formed by two pairs of folds of tissue, which form the false vocal cords and the true vocal cords. The slit between the vocal cords forms the glottis (Fig. 38–3). The epiglottis, a leaf-shaped structure immediately posterior to the base of the tongue, lies above the larynx. When food or liquids are swallowed, the epiglottis closes over the larynx, protecting the lower airways from aspiration. The thyroid cartilage protrudes in front of the larynx, forming the Adam's apple. The cricoid cartilage lies just below the thyroid cartilage and is the anatomic site for an artificial opening into the trachea (tracheostomy). These cartilages are all connected by ligaments that prevent the larynx from collapse during inspiration and swallowing. The internal portion of the larynx is composed of muscles that assist with swallowing, speaking, and respiration, and contribute to the pitch of the voice. The blood supply to the larynx is through the branches of the thyroid arteries. The nerve supply is through the recurrent laryngeal and superior laryngeal nerves.

Function

Major functions of the upper airway are (1) air conduction to the lower airway for gas exchange; (2) protection of the lower airway from foreign matter; and (3) warming, filtration, and humidification of inspired air. It is important for the nurse to appreciate the function of the upper airway. In various disorders and in the treatment of some disorders, this function is lost or altered. For example, when a client has a cold, it is difficult to breathe through the swollen nose, and mouth breathing is common. When the client breathes through the mouth, the

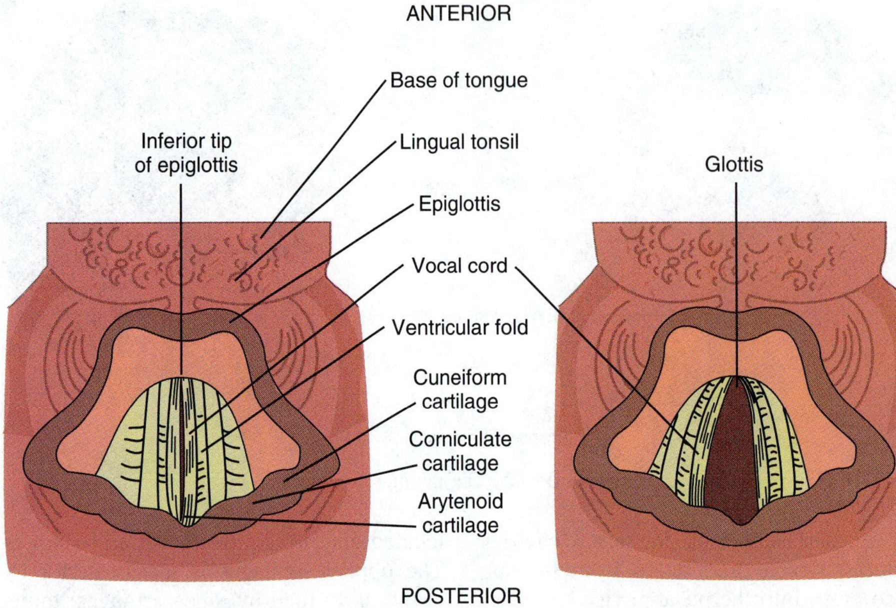

Figure 38–3. Superior view of the larynx, showing the glottis closed and open.

normal functions of the nose (smell, taste, humidification, and filtering) are lost.

The upper airway is lined with mucous membranes to assist in warming and humidifying inspired air. Regardless of the temperature of air inspired, by the time the air reaches the lung (in about 0.25 seconds) the air has been warmed to 36° to 37° C (96.8° to 98.6° F) and humidified to 70% to 80%. The mucus also helps trap foreign particles. The cilia of the membrane assist in moving the particles down into the pharynx. The posterior part of the nasal cavity opens into the internal nares and the nasopharynx. The two nasal vestibules are divided by the septum.

The nose also provides for the sense of smell and is an adjunct to taste. The part of the mucous membrane covering the cribriform plate is modified for olfaction. The nose provides a sneeze reflex, which is similar to the cough reflex. Irritation of the nasal passages causes receptors in the trigeminal nerve (cranial nerve V) to stimulate the respiratory center in the medulla. The medulla stimulates a blast of air through the nose that carries foreign matter out the nose and mouth. Sinuses lighten the weight of the skull and modify sound by acting as resonating chambers.

Lower Airway

Structure

The lower airway (tracheobronchial tree) is composed of the (1) trachea, (2) right and left mainstem bronchi, (3) segmental bronchi, (4) subsegmental bronchi, and (5) terminal bronchioles (Fig. 38–4). Smooth muscle, wound in overlapping clockwise and counterclockwise helical

bands, is found in all of these structures. This muscle is subject to spasm in many airway disorders.

Trachea

The trachea (windpipe) extends from the larynx to the level of the seventh thoracic vertebrae where it divides into two main bronchi (also called *primary bronchi*). The point at which the trachea divides is called the *carina*. The trachea rests anterior to the surface of the esophagus. The trachea is a flexible, muscular, 12-cm long air passage with C-shaped cartilaginous rings. It is lined with pseudostratified ciliated columnar epithelium that contains numerous goblet (mucus-secreting) cells. Because the cilia beat upward, they tend to carry foreign particles and excessive mucus away from the lungs to the pharynx. No cilia are present in the alveoli.

Bronchi and Bronchioles

The right mainstem bronchus is shorter and wider, and extends more vertically downward, than the left. Thus, foreign bodies are more likely to lodge in the right mainstem bronchus than in the left mainstem bronchus.

The segmental and subsegmental bronchi are subdivisions of the main bronchi and are spread in an inverted, treelike formation through each lung. Cartilage surrounds the airway in the bronchi. This structure contrasts with the bronchioles, the final pathway to the alveoli, which contain no cartilage and thus can collapse and trap air.

The terminal bronchioles are the last airways of the conducting system. This area does not have gas exchange and is called the *anatomical dead space*. Inspired air that remains in the dead space is what allows artificial respiration (mouth-to-mouth resuscitation).

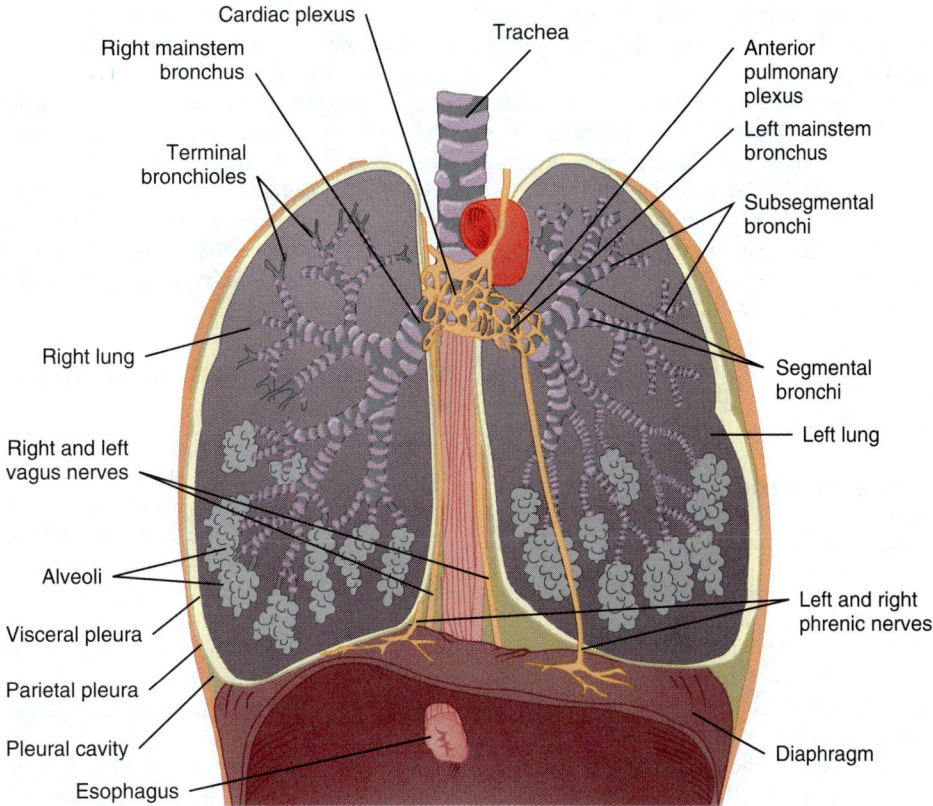

Figure 38-4. Structures of the lower airways.

Function

The lower airways continue to warm, humidify, and filter inspired air that is en route to the lungs. In addition, they provide several defense mechanisms.

The respiratory gas-exchanging membrane has a surface area that is almost the size of a tennis court. The size of the membrane of the lungs and the daily exposure of the lungs to atmospheric pollutants requires efficient protective mechanisms. The elaborate defense mechanisms of the lungs fall into three categories: (1) clearance mechanisms, (2) immunologic responses in the lung, and (3) pulmonary reaction to injury. An intact respiratory epithelium and mucociliary system are necessary for the efficient functioning of the lung defense mechanisms.

Defense by the Respiratory Epithelium

The predominant cell of the upper respiratory tract (trachea and bronchi) is a one-cell–layer thick squamous ciliated cell. The cilia are microscopic, hairlike projections that protect the airways with a rapid, coordinated, unidirectional sweeping motion toward the mouth. The movement of the cilia propels a mucus blanket toward the mouth. This blanket is produced by goblet cells located on the mucosal surface (Fig. 38–5). The mucociliary system propels debris (pollutants and infectious agents) to the mouth within 30 minutes for the large bronchi, 2.5 hours for most of the bronchial tree, and 5.6 hours for the

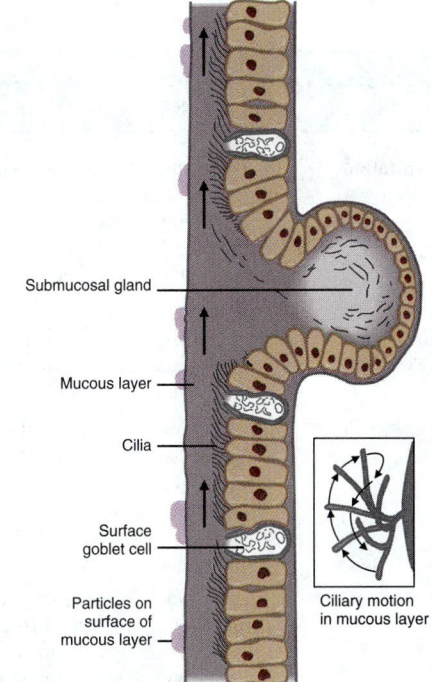

Figure 38-5. The mucociliary blanket is an important respiratory defense mechanism. Mucus is secreted by surface goblet cells. About 100 ml of mucus is normally secreted each day by the submucosal glands. Mucus covers the epithelial lining of the tracheobronchial tree in two layers—the watery solution layer close to the mucosal surface and the thicker gel layer. The cilia (hairlike projections) beat in an upward direction toward the upper airway. Particulate matter is trapped on the mucous layer and moved upward by the cilia. Debris-laden mucus is then either swallowed or expectorated as sputum.

peripheral airways. At the mouth, the debris is removed from the airways by swallowing or coughing. Sputum is mucus expelled by coughing.

The alveolar lining is made up of flat, membranous pneumocytes (type I cells). Rounded granular cells (type II) are also found there. These type II cells are resistant to injury and cover most of the alveolar surface after exposure to infectious agents. Alveolar macrophages, derived from blood monocytes that migrate into the lungs, are also found over the surface of the alveoli. Alveolar macrophages are active phagocytes that remove dead cells and protein. Macrophages are also metabolically active cells that synthesize and secrete substances that regulate the immune system. They leave the lung by either the mucociliary system or the lymphatic system.

Defense by Clearance Mechanisms

The upper airways filter particles. Inhaling air through the nose is more effective in air cleaning and conditioning than inhaling air through the mouth. The nose has a larger surface-volume ratio and a much more tortuous pathway for airflow than the mouth. Thus, particle deposition on the mucociliary system is more efficient when the client breathes by nose rather than by mouth. The larger particles (greater than 10 μm) are generally trapped, but the smaller particles (less than 1 μm) may readily enter the lower airways.

Table 38–1. Physiologic Elements of a Cough

Deep inspiration	Inhaled volume of air must be sufficient to (1) increase lung volume, (2) increase diameter of bronchi and bronchioles, and (3) move mucus up and out of airways
Inspiratory pause	A pause (inspiratory pause) allows a buildup and distribution of air and pressure distal to mucus
Closed glottis	Requires intact muscles and nerves supplying larynx. A closed glottis allows the development of high intrapleural pressures, resulting in a high air flow velocity to propel mucus out of airway
Abdominal muscles	These muscles increase intra-abdominal pressure, which forces the diaphragm upward to increase intrapleural pressure against the closed glottis
Open glottis	After intrapleural pressures increase, the glottis opens suddenly and allows a high velocity of air to leave the lungs; flow rates may be as high as 300 L/min
Mucus is expelled	Occurs because of high velocity of air leaving the airway

The lower airways have four clearance mechanisms: (1) cough (first five to eight bronchial generations), (2) mucociliary system (to terminal bronchioles), (3) macrophages (alveoli and respiratory bronchioles), and (4) lymphatics (alveoli and interstitium). The cough occurs most rapidly in the clearing process. Table 38–1 describes the physiologic elements of a cough. The cough is an automatic protective reflex used to clear the trachea. If a delayed or absent swallowing reflex is present, a cough may be stimulated to avoid aspiration of particles into the lower airways.

Defense by Immunologic Mechanisms

The systemic immune system responds to the lung during inflammatory processes by mobilizing blood neutrophils and monocytes. Recruited thymus-dependent (T) and thymus-independent (B) lymphocytes contribute to local cell-mediated immune reactions and the production of specific antibodies within the alveoli. Cell-mediated immunity is a key determinant in the resistance to organisms such as *Mycobacterium tuberculosis* and *Pneumocystis carinii*. Immune mechanisms are generally a host defense function. However, hypersensitivity immune reactions lead to tissue injury and are responsible for clinical conditions such as asthma, granuloma formation, and lung transplant rejection. (See Chapter 27 for a detailed discussion of types I, II, III, and IV hypersensitivity reactions.)

Thorax, Diaphragm, and Pleura

Structure

Thorax and Diaphragm

The bony thorax provides protection for the lungs, heart, and great vessels. The outer shell of the thorax is made up of 12 pairs of ribs. The ribs connect posteriorly to the transverse processes of the thoracic vertebrae of the spine. Anteriorly, the first seven pairs of ribs are attached to the sternum by cartilage. The 8th, 9th, and 10th ribs (false ribs) are attached to each other by costal cartilage. The 11th and 12th ribs (floating ribs) allow full chest expansion because they are not attached in any way to the sternum.

At the top of the thorax in the neck area are two accessory muscles of inspiration—the scalene and sternocleidomastoid muscles. The scalene muscles elevate the first and second ribs during inspiration to enlarge the upper thorax and stabilize the chest wall. The sternocleidomastoid muscle elevates the sternum. The parasternal, trapezius, and pectoralis muscles are also accessory inspiratory muscles and are used during increased work of breathing.

Between the ribs are the intercostal muscles (Fig. 38–6). The external intercostal muscles pull the ribs upward and forward, thus increasing the transverse and anteroposterior diameter. The internal intercostal muscles decrease the anteroposterior diameter of the chest wall.

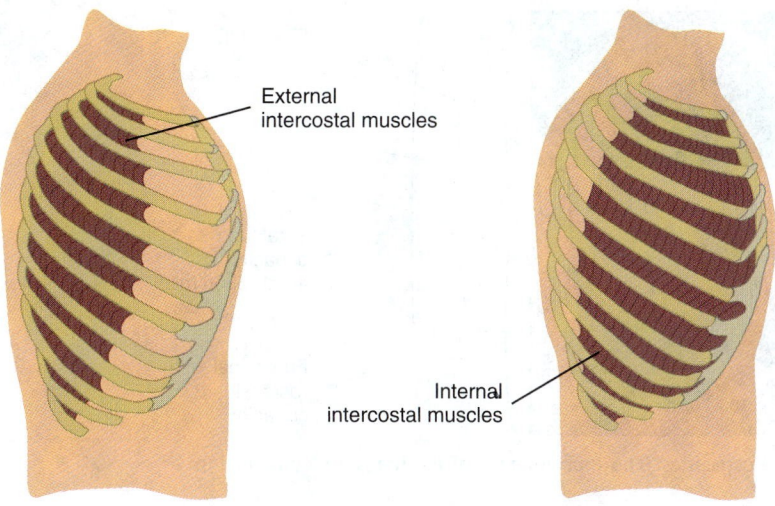

External
intercostal muscles

Internal
intercostal muscles

Figure 38–6. The intercostal muscles.

The diaphragm serves as the lower boundary of the thorax. The diaphragm is dome shaped in the relaxed position, with central muscular attachments to the xiphoid process of the sternum and the lower ribs. The diaphragm's nerve supply (phrenic nerve) comes through the spinal cord at the level of the third cervical vertebra. Thus, C3 spinal injuries impair ventilation.

Pleura

The pleura are serous membranes that enclose the lung in a double-walled sac. The visceral pleura covers the lung and the fissures between the lobes of the lung. The parietal pleura covers the inside of each hemithorax, the mediastinum, and the top of the diaphragm. The parietal pleura joins the visceral pleura at the hilus (a notch in the medial surface of the lung, where the mainstem bronchi, pulmonary blood vessels, and nerves enter the lung).

The pleural space is a potential space between the two layers of pleura. Normally, no space exists between the pleurae. A thin film (only a few milliliters) of serous fluid acts as a lubricant in the potential space. The fluid also causes the moist pleural membranes to adhere, creating a pulling force that helps to hold the lungs in an expanded position. The action of pleura is analogous to coupling two sheets of glass by a thin film of water. It is extremely difficult to separate the sheets of glass at right angles to their surfaces, even though they readily slide past each other. Because of the nature of this coupling, the movement of the lungs closely follows the movement of the thorax. If air or increased amounts of serous fluid, blood, or pus accumulates in the space, the lungs are compressed and respiratory difficulties follow. These conditions are called *pneumothorax* (air in the pleural space) or *hemothorax* (blood in the pleural space).

Function

The function of the thorax and diaphragm is to alter pressures in the thorax to move fresh air in and out. The movement of air depends on pressure differences between the atmosphere and the air in the lungs. Air flows from regions of higher pressure to regions of lower pressure.

On inspiration, the dome of the diaphragm flattens and the rib cage lifts. This action increases the transverse diameter of the thorax, which increases the volume of the thorax and the lungs. As volume increases, pressure decreases and air moves into the lungs.

Airway resistance also affects air movement. Airway resistance is affected by the viscosity of air, length of the airways, and diameter of the airways. Doubling the length of the airway doubles the resistance. You can experiment with this change by trying to breathe through a straw and noting the increased effort that is required to move air. Decreasing the diameter by half creates a 16-fold increase in resistance. Thus, a decreased diameter of the airways due to bronchial muscle contraction or to secretions in the airways increases resistance and decreases the rate of air flow. This is a common finding in obstructive airway diseases such as asthma.

During quiet breathing, expiration is usually passive, that is, expiration does not require the use of muscles. The chest wall, in contrast to the lungs, has a tendency to recoil outward. The opposing forces of lung and chest wall create a subatmospheric (negative) force of about -5 cm H_2O in the intrapleural space at the end of quiet exhalation. Exhalation is also due to the elastic recoil of the lungs, which is discussed later in the chapter.

Forced expiration and coughing bring the internal intercostal muscles and the abdominal muscles into play. The abdominal muscles force the diaphragm upward to its dome-shaped position. The intercostal muscles contract, pulling the ribs inward.

The Lungs and Alveoli

Structure

Lungs

The lungs lie within the thoracic cavity on either side of the heart (see Fig. 38–4). The lungs are cone shaped,

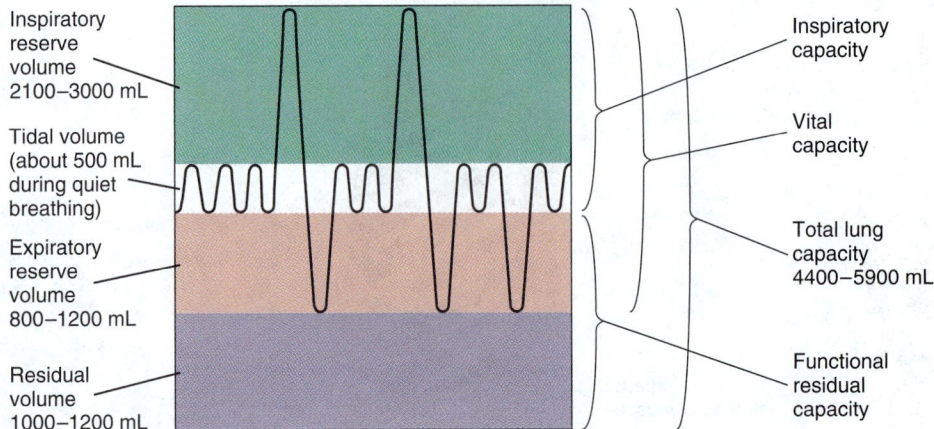

Figure 38–7. Lung volumes and capacities. The four volumes of the lungs are combined to form four capacities.

with the apex above the first rib and the base resting on the diaphragm. Each lung is divided into superior and inferior lobes by an oblique fissure. The right lung is further divided by a horizontal fissure, which bounds a middle lobe. The right lung, therefore, has three lobes, whereas the left lobe has only two. In addition to these five lobes, which are visible externally, each lung can be subdivided into about 10 smaller units called *bronchopulmonary segments.* Each bronchopulmonary segment represents the portion of the lung that is supplied by a specific tertiary bronchus. These segments are important surgically, because a diseased segment can be resected without having to remove the entire lobe or lung.

The two lungs are separated by a space called the *mediastinum.* The heart, aorta, vena cava, pulmonary vessels, esophagus, part of the trachea and bronchi, and the thymus gland are located in the mediastinum.

The lungs contain gas, blood, thin alveolar walls, and support structures of the lung. Elastic and collagen fibers contribute to the alveolar walls and form a three-dimensional basket-like structure that allows the lung to inflate in all directions. They are capable of stretching if a pulling force is exerted on them from outside of the body or if they are inflated from within. The elastic recoil helps return the lungs to their resting volume.

Nutrient blood supply to the lungs is provided by branches of the pulmonary artery; thus, the blood is oxygen poor. The alveoli are supplied by branches of the aorta; thus, the blood is oxygen rich.

In young men (19 years old), the lungs have a total capacity of about 5,900 ml. However, a person cannot exhale all the air from the lungs, and about 1,200 ml of air always remains no matter how forceful the expiration. This remaining volume is called the *residual volume,* and it prevents the collapse of the lung structures during expiration. The volume of air that moves in and out with each breath is called the *tidal volume.* During quiet breathing, tidal volume is about 500 ml. When a deep breath is taken, the lung is more fully expanded. The amount of extra air inhaled, beyond the tidal volume, is called the *inspiratory reserve volume.* Likewise, the extra air that can be exhaled after a normal breath is called the *expiratory reserve volume.* The lungs have four volumes: (1) residual, (2) tidal, (3) inspiratory reserve, and (4)

expiratory reserve. The volumes are often combined into capacities, which also number four: (1) total lung capacity (all four volumes); (2) vital capacity (all volumes except residual volume), which is the amount we can ventilate; (3) functional reserve capacity (expiratory reserve volume plus residual volume); and (4) inspiratory capacity (tidal volume plus inspiratory reserve volume). These volumes and capacities are frequently altered by disease. They can be measured by pulmonary function tests, described in Chapter 39. Lung volumes are shown in Figure 38–7.

Alveoli

The lung parenchyma is the working area of the lung tissue. The parenchyma consisting of millions of alveolar units. It is estimated that 24 million alveoli are present in humans at birth. By age 8 years, the number of alveoli has increased to the adult number of 300 million. The total working alveolar surface area is approximately 750 to 860 ft². The large number of alveoli and the large surface area are necessary to meet both resting and exercise oxygen requirements. Each alveolar unit is supplied with 9 to 11 prepulmonary and pulmonary capillaries. The blood supply for these capillaries comes from the right ventricle of the heart. The major function of the alveolar unit is the exchange of oxygen and carbon dioxide between pulmonary capillaries and alveoli. Because of the extensiveness of the capillary system, the flow of blood in the alveolar wall has been described as a "sheet" of flowing blood.

The entire alveolar unit (respiratory zone) is made up of respiratory bronchioles, alveolar ducts, and alveolar sacs. This is the region where gas exchange takes place (Fig. 38–8). The respiratory zone consists of the respiratory bronchioles, the alveolar ducts, and alveolar sacs. Alveoli, small air sacs at the end of the respiratory bronchioles, permit exchange of the oxygen and carbon dioxide. The alveolar walls are extremely thin, and within them is an almost solid network of interconnecting capillaries. Oxygen and carbon dioxide are exchanged through a respiratory membrane that is about 0.2 μm thick (Fig. 38–9). The average diameter of the pulmonary capillary is only about 5 μm, which means that a red blood cell must squeeze through it. Therefore the red blood cell

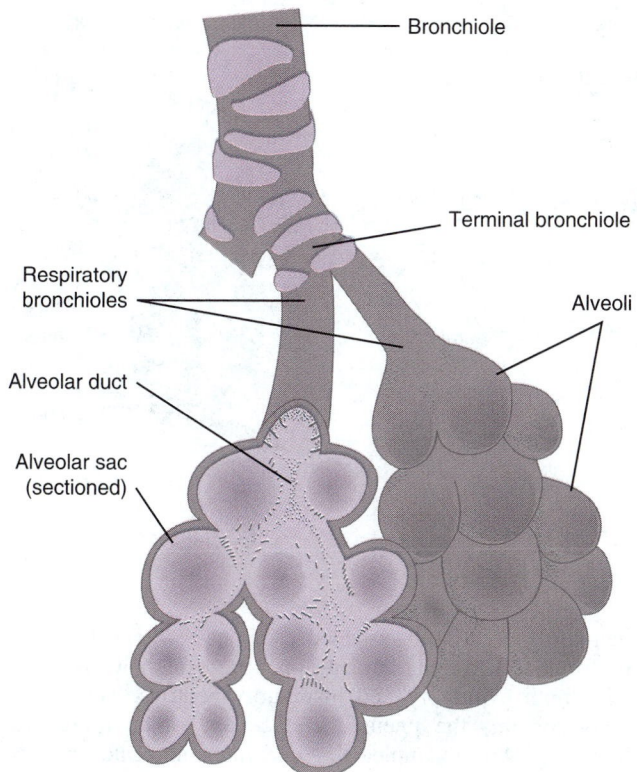

Figure 38–8. Gas exchange occurs in the respiratory zone, which consists of the respiratory bronchioles, alveolar ducts, and alveolar sacs.

actually touches the capillary wall, so that oxygen and carbon dioxide need not pass through significant amounts of plasma as they diffuse. The thickness of the respiratory membrane occasionally increases (e.g., with pulmonary edema or fibrosis). Increases in thickness of the membrane interfere with normal exchange of gases.

The alveolus is comprised of two cell types: type I and II pneumocytes. Type I pneumocytes are thin and incapable of reproduction. They line the alveolus. Type II pneumocytes are cuboidal and do not exchange oxygen and carbon dioxide well. These cells produce surfactant and differentiate into type I cells. These cells are important in lung injury and repair. When lung tissue has been damaged, type II cells are produced, which eventually differentiate into type I cells. During the transition, oxygenation is impaired due to the thickness of the cells.

Function

The function of the lungs is to deliver oxygen to the mitochondria to liberate energy stored in molecular bonds of adenosine triphosphate (ATP) and remove carbon dioxide. Cellular processes for life require ATP. Ventilation, gas exchange, the relationship of ventilation and perfusion, and oxygen transport are discussed in the following text.

Ventilation

Ventilation is the movement of air in and out of the lungs. Three forces are involved in the process of ventila-

tion: (1) the compliance properties of the lung and the thorax (chest wall), (2) surface tension, and (3) the muscular efforts of inspiratory muscles.

■ Compliance

Compliance is a term used to describe the ease with which the lung expands. The word *compliance,* when used to discuss respiration, can be confusing. Compliance is affected by elastic recoil (the tendency of the lung to contract) and surface tension.

The lungs are elastic structures that have a tendency to recoil to a volume slightly less than residual volume (volume of gas remaining in the lungs following a full exhalation). The force required to distend the lungs is the difference between the alveolar pressure and the intrapleural pressure. The relationship between volume and pressure is expressed as the compliance of the lungs, with 200 ml/cm H_2O being the average value for adults. Diseases that cause fibrosis of the lungs result in "stiff" lungs, which have low compliance; these require high inspiratory pressures to achieve a set volume of gas. In contrast, diseases that change the elastic structure of the alveolar walls result in "floppy" lungs, which have a greater compliance; thus, relatively low pressures achieve the same volume of air.

■ Surface Tension

Changes in the surface tension of the liquid film lining the alveoli also affect compliance by changing resistance. Surface tension is the result of the air-liquid interface present in each alveolus. The surface tension restricts alveolar expansion on inspiration and aids alveolar collapse on expiration. The production of surfactant by type II cells in the alveolar lining lowers the surface tension and, thus, aids ventilation. A deficiency of surfactant re-

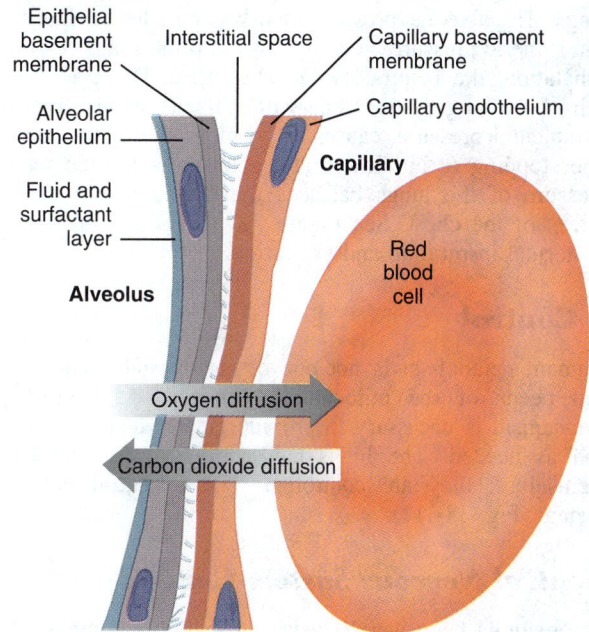

Figure 38–9. The ultrastructure of the respiratory membrane, where oxygen is exchanged.

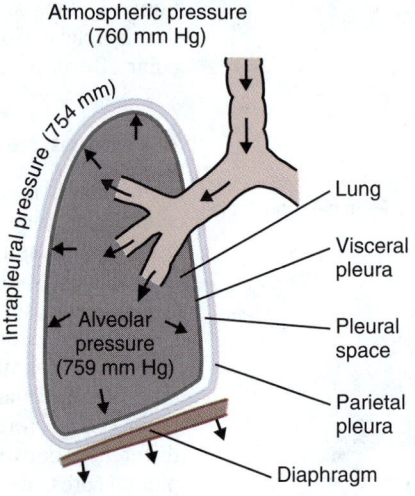
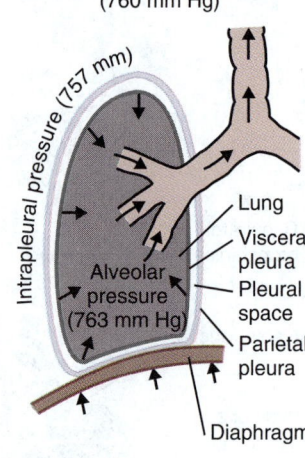

Figure 38–10. Normal inspiration and expiration.

NORMAL INSPIRATION   **NORMAL EXPIRATION**

sults in stiff lungs. A low surface tension increases compliance and, therefore, reduces the work of expanding the alveoli.

■ Muscular Effort

The elastic recoil properties of the lung and chest wall, coupled with the muscular effort required to overcome the recoil of the lungs and airflow resistance, make air movement possible. The pressure within the lungs (alveolar pressure) and between the pleura (intrapleural or intrathoracic pressure) must be less than atmospheric pressure for inspiration to occur. As the diaphragm and the external intercostal muscles work to enlarge the size of the thorax, the intrapleural and alveolar pressures decrease below atmospheric pressure. The expanding thorax creates a more negative intrapleural pressure, which expands the lungs. The alveolar pressure then becomes lower than the atmospheric pressure, and air flows into the lungs. During exhalation, the inspiratory muscles relax. The elastic recoil of the lung tissue, along with a rise (less negative) in intrapleural pressure, causes air to move out of the lungs. The stopping of air flow is the point at which the recoil pressure of the lungs balances the muscular and elastic forces of the chest. See Figure 38–10 for an illustration of normal inspiration and expiration.

■ Control

Human metabolism is not one of steady state. The oxygen needs of the mitochondria change. A controlling mechanism is necessary to provide greater intake of oxygen as needed. The lungs have no intrinsic control of themselves; they are controlled by the central nervous system (Fig. 38–11).

Central Nervous System Control

The medulla has several levels of respiratory centers. The dorsal respiratory group primarily provides for inspiration. The ventral respiratory group is normally quiet unless an

increase in ventilation is needed or if active exhalation is performed. The pons has an apneustic center, which contains both expiratory and inspiratory neurons. The upper pons contains the pneumotaxic center, which fine-tunes breathing. For example, the pneumotaxic center allows for talking and breathing.

Output from the respiratory neurons, located in the medulla, descends via the ventral and lateral columns of the spinal cord to phrenic motor neurons of the diaphragm and intercostal motor neurons of the intercostal muscles. The result is rhythmic respiratory movements.

The cortex also allows for voluntary control of breathing. We can hold our breath or alter the rate or depth of breathing.

Reflex Control

One example of a neural reflex stimulated by mechanical stimuli is the cough reflex. Inhaled irritants and mucus (mechanical stimuli) can excite rapidly adapting pulmonary stretch receptors that are concentrated in the region of the carina and the large bronchi. The stimulation of the receptors results in high-velocity expiratory gas flow (cough).

Peripheral Control

Peripheral control of respiration is due the sensing of partial pressure of oxygen (PO_2) and of partial pressure of carbon dioxide (PCO_2) in the blood. Receptors that are responsive to changes in oxygen, carbon dioxide, and pH are located in two areas in the brain and in the blood vessels. Blood vessel receptors are the carotid arteries and aorta. The carotid body receptors are located close to the carotid sinus, and the aortic bodies are located near the aortic arch. The second location of the chemical receptors is on the brain side of the blood-brain barrier. Low levels of partial pressure of oxygen in arterial blood (PaO_2) cause high receptor output from the carotid bodies to the medulla and increase the rate and depth of ventilation. The arterial pH is another major stimulus. A decrease in

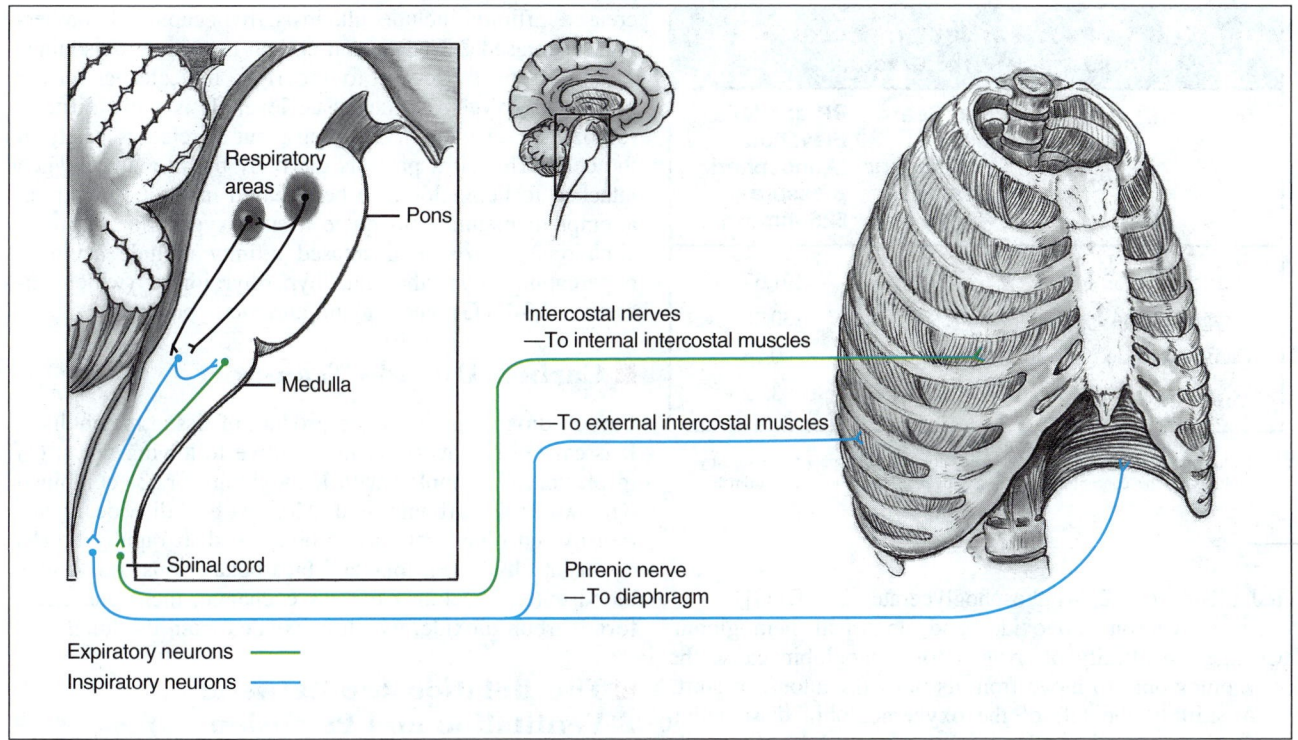

Figure 38–11. Neurologic control of respiration. (From Applegate, E. J. [1995]. *The anatomy and physiology learning system.* Philadelphia: W.B. Saunders.)

pH with acidemia increases the output from the carotid body to the central nervous system and stimulates ventilation. The partial pressure of carbon dioxide in arterial blood ($PaCO_2$) also stimulates peripheral receptors. Chemoreceptors on the brain side of the blood-brain barrier are sensitive to the hydrogen ion content of brain extracellular fluid as well as to CO_2 levels.

Gas Exchange

The exchange of gases occurs between air and blood in the respiratory membrane. Respiration is the exchange of oxygen and carbon dioxide at the alveolar-capillary level (external respiration) and at the tissue-cellular level (internal respiration). During respiration, body tissues are supplied with oxygen for metabolism and carbon dioxide is released from the tissues.

In the earth's atmosphere, air contains 20.84% oxygen, 78.62% nitrogen, 0.04% carbon dioxide, and 0.50% water vapor. Each gas exerts a pressure, called its *partial pressure*, as if it were the only gas present. The sum of the partial pressures is the barometric pressure. Table 38–2 shows the partial pressures of each of these gases in air at sea level and at a barometric pressure of 760 mm Hg (i.e., elevation of 1 mile). When a liquid is exposed to a gas, gas enters the liquid in proportion to the individual pressures. The partial pressure of oxygen (PO_2) in the alveoli is about 104 mm Hg, and the partial pressure of carbon dioxide (PCO_2) is about 40 mm Hg. Venous blood has a PO_2 of 40 mm Hg and a PCO_2 of about 45 mm Hg. These differences in concentration result in the movement of oxygen into the pulmonary capillary bloodstream and

carbon dioxide out of the pulmonary capillary bed into the alveoli, where it is exhaled. See Figure 38–12 for partial pressures of gases during normal respiration. Because gases move from an area of greater partial pressure to an area of less partial pressure, gas exchange occurs.

■ Oxygen Transport

After oxygen diffuses into the pulmonary capillaries, it is transported throughout the body by the circulatory system. The oxygen is dissolved in the plasma (3%) or bound with hemoglobin (97%) in ferrous iron. The combination of ferrous iron and oxygen forms oxyhemoglobin, which releases oxygen to tissues that have a low partial pressure of oxygen. Tissues take up oxygen at varying rates. The most metabolically active tissues receive it first. Methemoglobin, carbon monoxide, and other chemicals impair the uptake of oxygen by tissues.

The oxyhemoglobin dissociation curve represents the relationship between PaO_2 and the saturation of hemoglobin. This saturation reflects the amount of oxygen available to the tissues. In plotting the normal curve, it is assumed that the client's temperature is 37° C, pH is 7.40, and PaO_2 is 40 mm Hg. This relationship is represented in Figure 38–13 as an S-shaped curve. Changes in the PaO_2 at the flattened top portion of the curve result in small changes in oxygen saturation. The opposite is true as the slope of the curve steepens. At the steepest portion of the curve, with the PaO_2 below 60 mm Hg, small changes in the PaO_2 result in large drops in oxygen saturation.

The oxyhemoglobin curve is affected by a number of factors, including temperature, pH, PCO_2, enzymes in the

Table 38–2. Partial Pressures of Atmospheric Gases		
Gas	PP at Sea Level (Atmospheric pressure 760 mm Hg)	PP at 1 Mile Elevation (Atmospheric pressure 625 mm Hg)
Nitrogen (78.62%)	597.0	491.37
Oxygen (20.84%)	159.0	130.26
Carbon dioxide (0.04%)	0.3	0.25
Water vapor (0.50%)	3.7	3.12

Partial pressure (PP) may be calculated for any atmospheric pressure by multiplying the concentration of a gas by the atmospheric or barometric pressure.

red blood cell (2,3-diphosphoglycerate [2,3,-DPG]), presence of carbon monoxide, and abnormal hemoglobin. Changes in affinity of oxygen for hemoglobin cause the oxyhemoglobin to move from its normal contour, or shift.

A shift to the left of the oxyhemoglobin dissociation curve increases the affinity of the hemoglobin molecule for oxygen. It is easier for oxygen to bind to hemoglobin, but it is not easily released at the tissues. Thus, at any PO_2 level, oxygen saturation is greater than normal, but tissue hypoxia is present. Clinical situations that cause decreased affinity include alkalosis, hypocapnia, hypothermia, decreased 2,3-DPG, and carbon monoxide poisoning.

A shift of the curve to the right indicates an easier release of oxygen at the tissue level. It is more difficult for oxygen to bind in the lungs, but it releases easily at the cells. This shift protects the body by allowing oxygen attached to hemoglobin to be released in the tissues in an attempt to maintain adequate tissue oxygenation. Clinical situations that cause decreased affinity include acidosis, hypercapnia, hyperthermia, hyperthyroidism (which increases 2,3-DPG), anemia and chronic hypoxia.

■ Carbon Dioxide Transport

Carbon dioxide is the waste product of tissue metabolism. It is carried by the blood in the three following ways: (1) in plasma; (2) coupled with hemoglobin; or (3) combined with water as carbonic acid. Most carbon dioxide is carried by red blood cells as carbonic acid. It rapidly breaks down into hydrogen ions and bicarbonate ions. As venous blood enters the lungs for gas exchange, these chemicals form carbon dioxide, which is exhaled from the lungs.

■ The Relationship Between Ventilation and Perfusion

The relationship between ventilation (air flow) and perfusion (blood flow) determines the efficiency of gas exchange. When ventilation occurs without perfusion, a unit of dead space exists (e.g., when a pulmonary embolus

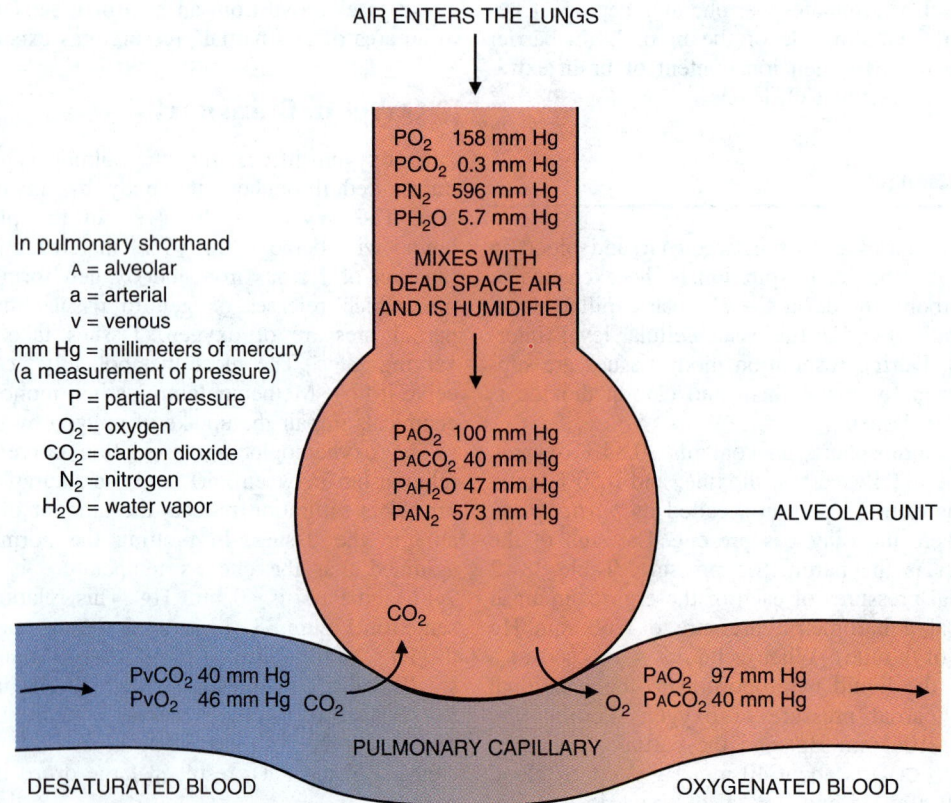

Figure 38–12. Partial pressures of gases during normal respiration.

	Factors shifting curve...	
	To the left	To the right
[H⁺], pH	↑	↓
P_{CO_2}	↓	↑
Temperature	↓	↑
2,3 DPG	↓	↑

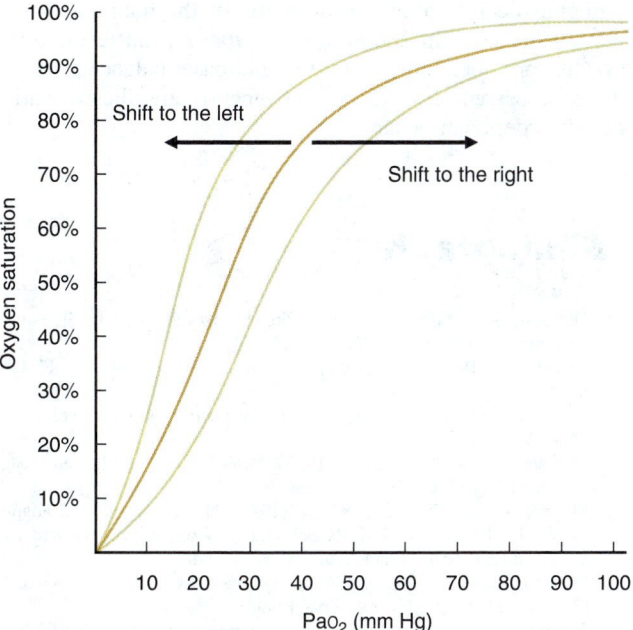

Figure 38–13. The normal oxyhemoglobin wave. Changes in the affinity of oxygen for hemoglobin shift the curve to the right or the left.

prevents blood flow through a pulmonary capillary). When no ventilation of an alveolar unit occurs, but perfusion continues, a shunt exists. This occurs with collapse of alveoli (atelectasis). Low ventilation/perfusion ratios (V/Q) and high V/Q ratios both result in lower oxygen levels in the blood. See Figure 38–14 for the relationships between ventilation and perfusion.

Gravity also affects ventilation and perfusion. Blood flows to more dependent lung segments. Air flows more easily to the upper lung segments because it is less dense than blood.

Regulation of Acid-Base Balance

The lungs, through gas exchange, have a key role in regulating the acid-base balance of the body. Pulmonary disorders that change the carbon dioxide level in the blood cause either respiratory acidemia or respiratory alkalemia. Hypercapnia (retention of excessive amounts of carbon dioxide) causes respiratory acidemia, and hypocapnia (low amounts of carbon dioxide in the blood) results in respiratory alkalemia.

The effectiveness of ventilation is best measured by the partial pressure of carbon dioxide in the arterial blood ($PaCO_2$). Because the respiratory system is normally set to maintain a $PaCO_2$ between 35 and 45 mm Hg at sea

level, a $PaCO_2$ above this range represents hypoventilation. Anesthetic agents, sedatives, and narcotics all tend to increase the resting $PaCO_2$. (For a complete discussion of acid-base balance, see Chapter 16).

Reaction to Injury

Injury to the lung barrier, inflammation, and repair are the three components of responses of the lung to injury. Any injury to the lung affects the barrier between the atmosphere and the bloodstream. This barrier, which lies within the alveolar septum, is made up of epithelial (types I and II pneumocytes) and vascular endothelial cells. Injury, as a result of airborne or bloodborne agents, may increase vascular permeability and cause pulmonary edema. Inflammatory cells (e.g., neutrophils) arrive soon

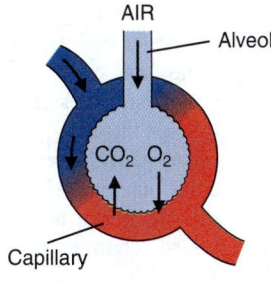

NORMAL

A normally functioning alveolus and normal pulmonary capillary flow. Ventilation and perfusion match.

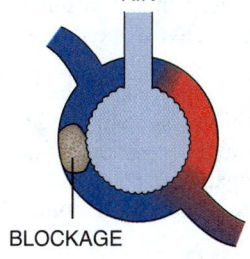

DEAD SPACE UNIT

When there is ventilation without perfusion, a dead space unit exists. Example: Pulmonary embolus preventing blood flow through the pulmonary capillary.

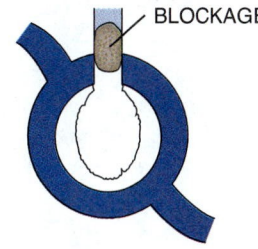

SHUNT UNIT

When there is no ventilation to an alveolar unit but perfusion continues, a shunt unit exists, and unoxygenated blood continues to circulate. Examples: atelectasis, pneumonia. The alveoli collapse.

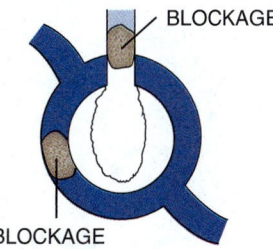

SILENT UNIT

When there is neither ventilation nor perfusion, a silent unit develops. Example: Pulmonary embolus combined with ARDS (adult respiratory distress syndrome). The alveoli collapse.

Figure 38–14. Relationships between ventilation (air flow) and perfusion (blood flow).

after acute injury. Then, the proportion of lymphocytes, monocytes, and macrophages increases.

The basic lung repair processes include lymphatic drainage of excess fluid and phagocytic removal of protein and debris. This action generally restores lung function and structure. More severe injury requires endothelial and epithelial cell regeneration and proliferation of interstitial cells (fibroblasts). Type II cells are generated and they dedifferentiate into the thin type I cells, which will permit gas exchange. The lung's ability to recreate alveolar septa determines the degree to which normal lung function and structure are restored.

Effects of Aging

Most of the changes that occur with aging are seen in the lower airway. The movement of the cilia of the upper airway slows and becomes less effective. This change predisposes the aged client to increased respiratory infections.

Changes in lung structure occur with age. One change is in the actual shape of the lung. The lungs become rounder as a result of an increase in the anteroposterior diameter, circumference, area, and height of the lung. An increase in the proportion of the lung formed by alveolar duct air and a relative decrease in alveolar air occur. Loss of alveolar wall tissue and of elastic tissue fibers in the alveolar walls is seen. The result of these changes is a deterioration of lung function.

Enlargement of air spaces occurs with old age. It is not referred to as emphysema because it is not a result of disease. These changes may be due to environmental pollutants rather than to aging alone.

An increased frequency of true emphysema and a greater prevalence of chronic cough and sputum production is seen in the elderly population. These findings also suggest that environmental or occupational pollutants, in addition to the normal aging process, may be a component in the decline of lung function.

Conclusions

The primary function of the lungs is gas exchange. The physical structure of the airways allows air to be warmed, filtered, and humidified as it enters the body. In the alveolar sacs, oxygen is exchanged for carbon dioxide. The mechanics of breathing are coordinated by the ribs, diaphragm, pleural space, elastic recoil of the lungs, and the nervous system. In addition to respiration, the respiratory system provides one form of acid-base balance. When these processes of structure and function are altered, various disorders can occur.

Bibliography

1. Dickson, S. L. (1995). Understanding the oxyhemoglobin dissociation curve. *Critical Care Nurse, 15*(5), 54–58.
2. Guyton, A. (1996). *Textbook of medical physiology* (9th ed.). Philadelphia: W. B. Saunders.
3. Kersten, L. D. (1989). *Comprehensive respiratory nursing*. Philadelphia: W. B. Saunders.
4. McCance, K., & Huether, S. (1993). *Pathophysiology* (2nd ed.). St. Louis: Mosby–Year Book.
5. Plopper, C. G., Thurlbeck, W. M. (1994). Growth, aging and adaptation. In J. Murray & J. Nadel (Eds.), *Textbook of respiratory medicine* (2nd ed.). Philadelphia: W. B. Saunders.
6. Shapiro, B., et al. (1994). *Clinical applications of respiratory care* (5th ed.). St. Louis: Mosby–Year Book.
7. Solomon, E., et al. (1990). *Human anatomy and physiology* (2nd ed.). Philadelphia: Saunders College.
8. West, J. (1990). *Respiratory physiology: The essentials* (4th ed.). Baltimore: Williams & Wilkins.
9. Wilson, S., & Thompson, J. (1990). *Respiratory disorders*. St. Louis: Mosby–Year Book.

Assessment of Clients with Respiratory Disorders

Amy Verst

General Respiratory Assessment

Nurses caring for clients experiencing respiratory disorders perform and interpret a variety of assessment procedures. This chapter discusses the physical assessment and diagnostic procedures performed for clients with respiratory disorders. The data obtained during the respiratory assessment are used to plan client care.

History

A respiratory history gathers information about a client's present condition and previous respiratory problems. Interview the client and family and focus on the clinical manifestations of the chief complaint, events leading up to the current condition, past health history, family history, and psychosocial history.

The detail and time taken for a respiratory history depend on the client's condition (e.g., acute, chronic, or emergent). State questions simply, using short, easy-to-understand sentences. Whenever necessary, reword questions to clarify statements the client seems not to understand. Ask questions in the contest of the client's daily activities (e.g., Are you able to carry the groceries in from the car? Are you able to make your bed, vacuum the house, bathe yourself, or dress yourself without stopping to rest and catch your breath?).

Biographical and Demographic Data

The history begins with obtaining biographical data. Included are the client's name, age, sex, and living situation.

Demographic data are usually recorded on a clinic or hospital assessment form. Note the client's biologic age and compare it with his or her appearance. Does the client look his or her stated age? Disorders such as lung cancer and chronic lung disorders often make the client appear older. The living situation, whether it be alone, with children, or with significant others, is important in planning for discharge.

Current Symptoms

Chief Complaint

The chief complaint is determined to establish priorities for intervention and to assess the client's level of understanding of the current condition. Common respiratory complaints include dyspnea, cough, sputum production, hemoptysis, wheezing, stridor, and chest pain. Focus on the manifestations and prioritize questions to elicit a symptom analysis (see Chapter 12).

In emergency or acute situations, simple questions are all that may be asked until the client is stable and comfortable. Whenever possible, seek further details from significant others.

Take an extensive respiratory history as the client's condition allows. Detailed questioning provides valuable clues to (1) the client's manifestations, (2) the client's degree of existing respiratory dysfunction, (3) the client and family's understanding of the condition and its management, and (4) the family's support system and ability to cope with the manifestations and management of the condition on an ongoing basis.

■ Dyspnea

Dyspnea is one of the most common manifestations experienced by clients with pulmonary and cardiac disorders. *Dyspnea* may be defined as difficulty breathing. It is a subjective symptom and a reflection of the client's assess-

This chapter incorporates material written for the fourth edition by Mary Elizabeth Egloff.

ment of the degree of work of breathing for a given task or effort. Clients may define dyspnea as shortness of breath, suffocation, tightness, being winded, or breathless.

The assessment of dyspnea involves several aspects. The subjective nature of dyspnea makes it difficult to quantify objectively. Several methods are currently used to accurately assess the level of dyspnea experienced by a client. The Visual Analogue Scale (Fig. 39–1) is used to quantify breathlessness in response to particular questions. It is easy to understand and the amount of dyspnea during various activities can be assessed. The Modified Borg Category-Ratio Scale (Table 39–1) is used to rate the intensity of dyspnea. It is simple and results from it have been reproduced in several populations.

The Pulmonary Functional Status and Dyspnea Questionnaire (PFSDQ) is used to quantify dyspnea and changes in activity with dyspnea. This instrument was developed and initially tested in a hospital-based pulmonary rehabilitation program (see Nursing Research).

In addition to subjective assessment, conduct an extensive symptom analysis to document the characteristics of the client's dyspnea. It is important to assess all the characteristics of dyspnea because it has many respiratory and nonrespiratory causes.

■ Cough

Detail the many aspects of the client's cough by conducting a symptom analysis. Note when the cough began, how it began (suddenly or gradually), and how long it has been present. Determine the frequency of the cough and the time of day in which the cough is better or worse (early morning, late afternoon, nighttime). Use the client's own words to describe the cough. A cough is often described as hacking, dry, hoarse, congested, barking, wheezy, or bubbling.

Determine what medications or treatments the client has used for the cough (e.g., antitussives, codeine, inhalers, nebulizers, rest, sitting up). Also determine what precautions are being used to prevent the spread of infection (if present). Use the opportunity to remind the person about good hand washing, proper disposal of soiled tissues, and completion of a full course of antibiotics (if prescribed).

Coughing may lead to stress incontinence and you may want to ask female clients about this embarrassing problem. The incontinence should clear once the coughing subsides; protective padding may be of some help.

■ Sputum Production

Sputum is the substance expelled by coughing or clearing the throat. The tracheobronchial tree normally produces about 3 oz of mucus a day as part of the normal cleaning mechanism. However, sputum production with coughing

is not normal. Question the client about sputum color (clear, yellow, green, rusty, bloody), odor, quality (watery, stringy, frothy, thick), and quantity (teaspoon, tablespoon, cup). Changes in color, odor, quality, or quantity are important to document in the client's medical record. Also ask if sputum is produced only after lying in a certain position. Several disorders increase the amount of sputum production. Cups of sputum can be expectorated daily with chronic bronchitis.

The sputum could actually be secretions from the oral or nasopharyngeal area or sinuses rather than from the tracheobronchial tree. For example, draining sinuses may provoke a productive cough.

■ Hemoptysis

Hemoptysis is blood expectorated from the mouth in the form of gross (visible to the naked eye) blood, frankly bloody sputum, or blood-tinged sputum. Attempt to identify the source of the blood—lungs, nosebleed, or stomach. Blood from the lungs is usually bright red because blood in the lungs usually stimulates an immediate cough reflex. However, if the blood remains in the lungs for any period of time, it may turn dark red or brown. Ask the client if the hemoptysis was produced as a result of forceful coughing. Also, an estimate of the amount of blood expectorated is obtained (teaspoon, tablespoon, cup). Pulmonary causes of hemoptysis include chronic bronchitis, bronchiectasis, pulmonary tuberculosis, cystic fibrosis, upper airway necrotizing granulomas, pulmonary embolism, pneumonia, lung cancer, and lung abscesses. Cardiovascular abnormalities, anticoagulants, and immunosuppressive drugs that cause parenchymal (lung tissue) bleeding may also cause hemoptysis.

■ Wheezing

Wheezing sounds are produced when air passes through partially obstructed or narrowed airways on inspiration or expiration. Wheezing may be audible or heard only with a stethoscope. The client may not complain of wheezing, but may complain of chest tightness or chest discomfort instead. Ask the client to identify when the wheezing occurs and if the wheezing relieves itself or if medication (such as inhaled bronchodilators) is required for relief. Not all wheezing is asthma. Wheezing can be caused by mucosal edema, airway secretions, collapsed airways due to loss of elastic tissue, and foreign objects or tumors partially obstructing air flow.

■ Stridor

Stridor is the name given to high-pitched sounds produced when air passes through partially obstructed or a narrowed upper airway on inspiration. Stridor is associ-

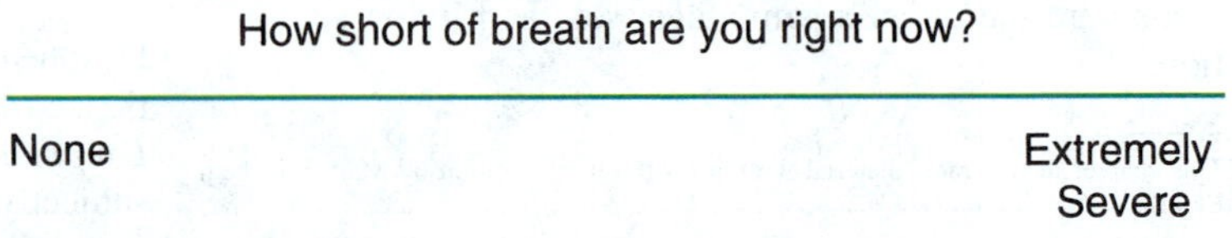

Figure 39–1. The Visual Analogue Scale of dyspnea. Although the scale can be in the form of either a vertical or a horizontal line, the most commonly used scale consists of a 100-mm horizontal line, like the one shown here.

How short of breath are you right now?

None

Extremely
Severe

Table 39–1. The Modified Borg Category-Ratio Scale for Assessment of Dyspnea	
0	Nothing at all
0.5	Very, very slight
1	Very slight
2	Slight
3	Moderate
4	Somewhat severe
5	Severe
6	
7	Very severe
8	
9	Very, very severe
10	Maximal

Modified from Burden, J., et al. (1982). The perception of breathlessness. *American Review of Respiratory Diseases, 126,* 825–828.

ated with respiratory distress and can be life-threatening because the airway is compromised. Several conditions can lead to stridor: epiglottitis, sleep apnea, congestive heart failure, and aspiration. Inquire about changes in voice character, hoarseness, difficulty swallowing, sleep-related disorders such as insomnia, degree of snoring, hypersomnolence (excessive sleepiness) in the morning, early-morning headaches, weight gain, fluid retention, apnea, and restlessness.

■ Chest Pain

Chest pain may be associated with pulmonary and cardiac problems, and differentiation between the two is important. Conduct a complete symptom analysis on any chest pain. Chest pain from angina (decreased blood flow to the heart) is a potentially life-threatening problem.

The location, duration, and intensity of the chest pain are important to obtain from the client, and provide early clues to the cause. Coughing and pleuritic infections can cause chest pain. Pleuritic chest pain is commonly a sharp, stabbing pain that occurs at one site on the chest wall and increases with chest wall movement or deep breathing. Retrosternal (behind the sternum) pain is usually burning, constant, and aching. Pain can also originate in the bony and cartilaginous parts of the thorax.

The characteristics of angina and other chest pains differ. Cardiac chest pain is usually described as an aching, heavy, squeezing sensation, with pressure or tightness in the substernal area. Angina can also radiate into the neck or arms. (See Table 44–1 for comparison of selected causes of chest pain.) Also ask what brings on the pain (activity, coughing, movement) and what relieves the pain (nitroglycerin, splinting the chest wall, heat).

Symptom Analysis

To obtain a complete history of the respiratory system, it is important to assess the characteristics of any clinical

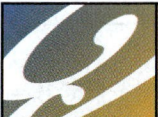

NURSING RESEARCH

Is the Pulmonary Functional Status and Dyspnea Questionnaire a Valid Measurement of Dyspnea and Activity Intolerance in Clients with Chronic Obstructive Pulmonary Disease?

Lareau, S., et al. (1994). Development and testing of the Pulmonary Functional Status and Dyspnea Questionnaire (PFSDQ). *Heart and Lung: Journal of Critical Care, 23*(3), 242–250.

Dyspnea is a common manifestation of chronic obstructive pulmonary disease (COPD). Many clients with COPD have dyspnea and activity intolerance. Acute measurements of these two manifestations are scant.

A study was conducted to test a questionnaire that measures both the intensity of dyspnea with activities and changes in the ability of clients with COPD to perform daily activities. The Pulmonary Functional Status and Dyspnea Questionnaire (PFSDQ) was developed and initially tested for validity and reliability in a hospital-based pulmonary rehabilitation program with 131 adult male clients with COPD. The PFSDQ is a 164-item paper-and-pencil self-administered questionnaire that consists of two components measuring dyspnea intensity with activities and changes in functional ability related to 79 activities of daily living. Content and initial construct validity were supported by clinical experts and findings related to expected theoretical relationships. Internal consistency reliability for both the dyspnea and functional ability components was .91.

Implications for Practice

Conclusive findings indicate that the PFSDQ can be used clinically and in research studies to assess dyspnea and changes in the functional ability of clients with pulmonary disease.

manifestation. Assessment of these characteristics will lead to a comprehensive symptom analysis. When the client describes a specific respiratory symptom, assess the setting, timing, the client's perception, the quantity and quality of the symptom, its location, aggravating and relieving factors, and associated manifestations.

Setting. In what setting does the symptom occur most often? The *setting* refers to the time and place or particular situation—physical setting and psychological environment—present when the client experiences the complaint. An example is a morning cough after the client has had a cigarette, or the employee who complains of respiratory distress at work.

Timing. *Timing* encompasses both onset (the gradual or sudden appearance of the symptom) and the period (days, weeks, months) during which the problem has occurred. Ask the client whether there is a specific time of day during which the problem occurs most frequently, for example, the morning cough or the shortness of breath associated with lying flat at night.

Client's Perception. The client's perception should be phrased in his or her own words. Note any unique properties of the complaint. Use a direct quote to document the client's complaint. For example, client reports a "catch" in the left posterior chest with deep breaths.

Quantity and Quality. The quantity and quality of the problem should be described in common language. Ask the client to report the amount, size, number, and extent of the chief complaint. Especially with sputum production, the client is asked to estimate how much sputum is produced a day—a cup, a tablespoon, or teaspoon. Avoid using terms such as "a little" or "a lot" because they have different meanings for different clients and healthcare providers. Often a scale of 1 to 10, with 1 being the least and 10 the most, is used to describe pain or distress. When assessing a cough, it may be described as being tight, loose, dry, hacking, or congested. Have the client describe in his or her own words the characteristics of the complaint.

Location. The *location* of the complaint should be noted. Ask the client to identify the exact location of the complaint. Location is especially important when the client is complaining of chest pain because it is important to differentiate whether the pain has a cardiac or respiratory origin.

Aggravating and Relieving Factors. The aggravating and relieving factors precipitate, worsen, or relieve the symptom. Environmental allergens, such as dog or cat dander, dust mites, mold, and pollen, are often described as aggravating factors. Sitting up or lying down may relieve or aggravate the symptom. Medication may also aggravate or relieve the symptom.

Associated Manifestations. Associated manifestations occur in conjunction with the chief complaint. Examples include chills, fever, night sweats, anorexia, weight loss, excessive fatigue, anxiety, and hoarseness. You may be able to recognize that chills and fever commonly accompany infectious lung disorders, whereas anorexia and weight loss can occur in clients with disorders that lead to dyspnea.

Past Health History

The past health history examines the health history of the client and family members for data related to the upper and lower respiratory systems (the upper respiratory history and physical examination are discussed later). These systems are common sources of both acute and chronic health problems. Assess clients with chronic conditions for changes in their ongoing respiratory manifestations (e.g., cough, dyspnea, sputum production, or wheezes) because these changes provide clues to the cause of the new problem. Include questions about the following areas.

Childhood and Infectious Diseases

In addition to obtaining data regarding common childhood diseases and immunizations, ask the client about the occurrence of tuberculosis, bronchitis, influenza, asthma, pneumonia, and the frequency of lower respiratory infections after upper respiratory infection. Determine the existence of congenital problems such as cystic fibrosis or premature birth history. These problems are associated with respiratory complications such as obstructive or restrictive pulmonary disease.

Immunizations

Inquire about immunization against pneumonia (Pneumovax) and influenza. Ask the client for the dates of these immunizations. Pneumovax provides lifelong immunity against pneumococcal pneumonia, whereas "flu shots" must be received annually in the fall of the year.

Major Illnesses and Hospitalizations

Ask the client about previous hospitalizations or treatment for respiratory problems. Determine dates of illnesses or hospitalization, the specific respiratory problem, medical treatment (including surgery, use of a ventilator, and inhalation treatments or oxygen therapy), and the present status of the problem. Ask whether a chest x-ray was taken and when it was taken, and if other pulmonary diagnostic tests were performed. These test results can provide baseline data for the evaluation of the current problem. Inquire about previous injuries to the mouth, nose, throat, or chest (such as blunt trauma, fractured ribs, or pneumothorax).

Medications

Obtain detailed information regarding both prescribed and over-the-counter medications because many affect the respiratory system. The client may have taken antibiotics for respiratory infections, bronchodilators, or steroids. Specify the route of administration (pill, liquid, or inhalation). Many respiratory medications are inhaled through a metered dose inhaler (MDI) or mini-nebulizer. If an MDI is used, the client may use a spacer to properly disperse the medication. Ask the client to demonstrate the use of the MDI and spacer.

Allergies

Question the client about a history of allergies and timing of manifestations in an attempt to identify a possible allergic basis for the condition. Ask about precipitating factors such as foods, medications, pollens, smoke, fumes, dust, and animal dander. Sources of molds that may cause allergic manifestations include the water reservoir of a furnace humidifier, air conditioners, and plant soil.

The client should describe the allergic symptoms experienced (e.g., chest tightness, wheezing, cough, rhinitis, watery eyes, scratchy throat) and the severity of these symptoms. Ask the client at what age allergies first occurred and whether they have become progressively more severe. Also ask if the client has been allergy-tested and when. Are medications (including allergy shots) taken prophylactically or on an as-needed basis to provide symptomatic relief?

Family Health History

Question the client about the family history of respiratory diseases. Blood relatives (genetically transmitted diseases) and family members (infectious conditions) experiencing asthma, cystic fibrosis, emphysema or chronic obstructive pulmonary disease (COPD), lung cancer, respiratory infections, tuberculosis, or allergies are identified. List the age and cause of death of each deceased family member, including mother, father, brothers, sisters, children, grandparents, aunts, and uncles. Ask whether any household members smoke. Secondary inhalation of smoke often precipitates or aggravates respiratory symptoms.

Psychosocial History

Respiratory status is affected by numerous factors that may lead to acute problems or affect the client's coping with chronic problems such as COPD. Areas to assess include the following.

Occupation

Identify any possible environmental agents that may contribute to the client's condition. Ask specifically about the work environment and hobbies; focus on exposure to dust, asbestos, beryllium, silica, and other toxins or pollutants. Farmers are exposed to airborne particles that may be inhaled, such as grain dust, fertilizers, and animal dander. Hobbies may involve chemicals, heat, dust, grinding, soldering, or welding.

Geographic Location

Ask questions related to recent travel to areas where respiratory diseases are prevalent, such as Asia, where tuberculosis is common; the Ohio River valley (histoplasmosis); or the San Joaquin valley (valley fever). Polluted city air has also been related to increasing incidence and severity of asthma.

Environment

Ask about the client's living conditions, such as the number of people in the household. Crowded living conditions increase risk of exposure to infectious respiratory diseases such as tuberculosis, cold viruses, and the like. Recent exposure to continuous air conditioning in a hotel or motel setting may relate to legionnaires' disease. Assess for environmental hazards such as stairs or poor air circulation. If the client has a chronic respiratory condition, it may be difficult for him or her to climb stairs or breathe unfiltered air.

Habits

Inquire about any history of smoking cigarettes, cigars, or pipes. Calculate the pack-years, which helps quantify the smoking history, as follows: Years of smoking × packs smoked per day = pack-years. Smoking has been associated with decreased ciliary function of the lungs, increased mucus production, and the development of lung cancer. Also ask the client about the use of smokeless tobacco (such as snuff, chewing tobacco) and smoking non-tobacco substances (such as marijuana and clove cigarettes). Ask about alcohol use. Ciliary action is slowed by alcohol, which reduces mucus clearance from the lungs. Heavy alcohol ingestion depresses the cough reflex so that risk of aspiration is increased. Clients who use and abuse recreational drugs are at risk of drug overdose and respiratory failure. If the client shares needles, the rise of human immunodeficiency virus (HIV) infection is increased, along with the development of acquired immunodeficiency syndrome (AIDS) and opportunistic infections such as *Pneumocystis carinii*.

Exercise

Clients who are active may describe the onset of coughing and wheezing when exercising. These clients need to be further evaluated for exercise-induced asthma before continuing any further workouts. Clients with chronic respiratory conditions often do not have the lung capacity to sustain even mild forms of exercise and subsequently become dyspneic. Ask whether tolerance for activity has decreased or remained stable. Ask the client to describe typical activities such as walking, light housekeeping chores, or grocery shopping that either are tolerated or, conversely, result in shortness of breath.

Nutrition

Maintaining a nutritious diet is important for clients with chronic respiratory disease. Chronic respiratory diseases result in decreased lung capacity and greater workload for the lungs and cardiovascular system. The added workload increases caloric expenditure and weight loss may occur. Clients may become anorectic secondary to the effects of medications and fatigue. The client may not have enough energy to consume the needed calories to maintain body weight. Ask the client to recall intake for the last 24 hours. Assess the amount of protein, kilocalories, and sodium intake.

Review of Systems

Ask the client to describe other manifestations associated with the respiratory system. In addition to cough, dyspnea, sputum production, hemoptysis, wheezing, stridor, and chest pain, these include breathlessness, fever, hoarseness, night sweats, anorexia, weight loss, and dependent edema. Upper respiratory manifestations include colds, nasal discharge, postnasal drip, sinus pain and swelling, epistaxis, and sinus headaches. Hypoxia may be seen as subtle neurologic changes such as restlessness, fatigue, disorientation, or personality changes. Tachycardia usually accompanies respiratory problems as the body attempts to compensate for decreased oxygen delivery. Stomach upset, nausea, and vomiting can result from accumulation of excess mucus swallowed from draining sinuses. Anorexia and weight loss are seen in many chronic respiratory conditions. Detailed questions for the review of systems may be found in Box 11–2.

Physical Examination

Physical examination follows the health history. Use the techniques of inspection, palpation, percussion, and auscultation. Successful examination requires that you be familiar with the anatomic landmarks of the posterior, lateral, and anterior thorax (Fig. 39–2). Use these landmarks to locate and visualize the underlying structures, particularly the lobes of the lungs, the heart, and major vessels. Compare the findings on one side of the thorax with the other side. Palpation, percussion, and auscultation proceed in a back-and-forth or side-to-side manner so that you continually evaluate findings by using the opposite side of the client as the standard for comparison.

The condition and color (pale, red, blue) of the client's skin is noted throughout the examination of the thorax. Note and record abnormalities. Respiratory rate, depth, and rhythm, if not assessed previously with the vital signs, are assessed during inspection of the thorax (see

Chapter 12). Assess the client's level of consciousness and orientation throughout the examination to determine adequate gas exchange. See the Normal Physical Assessment Findings feature for normal respiratory findings.

Inspection

The physical examination actually begins during the history-taking stage as you observe the client and his or her response to questions. Note manifestations of respiratory distress at this time: position of comfort, tachypnea, gasping, grunting, central cyanosis, open mouth, flared nostrils, dyspnea, color of facial skin and lips, and use of accessory muscles. Note the inspiratory-to-expiratory ratio. Because the normal length of expiration is twice that of inspiration, the normal ratio is 2:1. Observe the client's speech pattern. How many words or sentences can be said before another breath is taken? Clients who are short of breath may be able to say only three or four words before taking another breath. During the physical examination, the client should be bare to the waist while privacy and warmth are maintained. Inspection and palpation are often performed together but are discussed separately here.

Head and Neck

The key to any assessment technique is to develop a systematic approach. Logically, it is easiest to start with the head and work down the body. Inspection begins with observation of the head and neck area for any gross abnormalities that would interfere with respiration. Note the odor of the breath and whether any sputum is present. Note nasal flaring, pursed lips breathing, or cyanosis of the mucous membranes. Record the use of accessory muscles, such as flexion of the sternocleidomastoid muscle.

Chest

■ Chest Wall Configuration

Continue inspection by observing the chest wall configuration. Observe chest size and contour and note the anteroposterior (AP) diameter. Calculate the ratio of the AP diameter to the transverse diameter. The transverse diameter is generally twice the AP diameter (Fig. 39-3A).

■ Chest Deformities

Barrel Chest. Barrel chest occurs when the AP diameter is increased and equals the transverse diameter (Fig. 39–3B). It is a characteristic finding in clients with chronic disorders that interfere with ventilation (e.g., emphysema).

Pigeon Chest. Pigeon chest (pectus carinatum) is the opposite of funnel chest. The sternum juts forward and increases the AP diameter (Fig. 39–3C). Congenital atrial

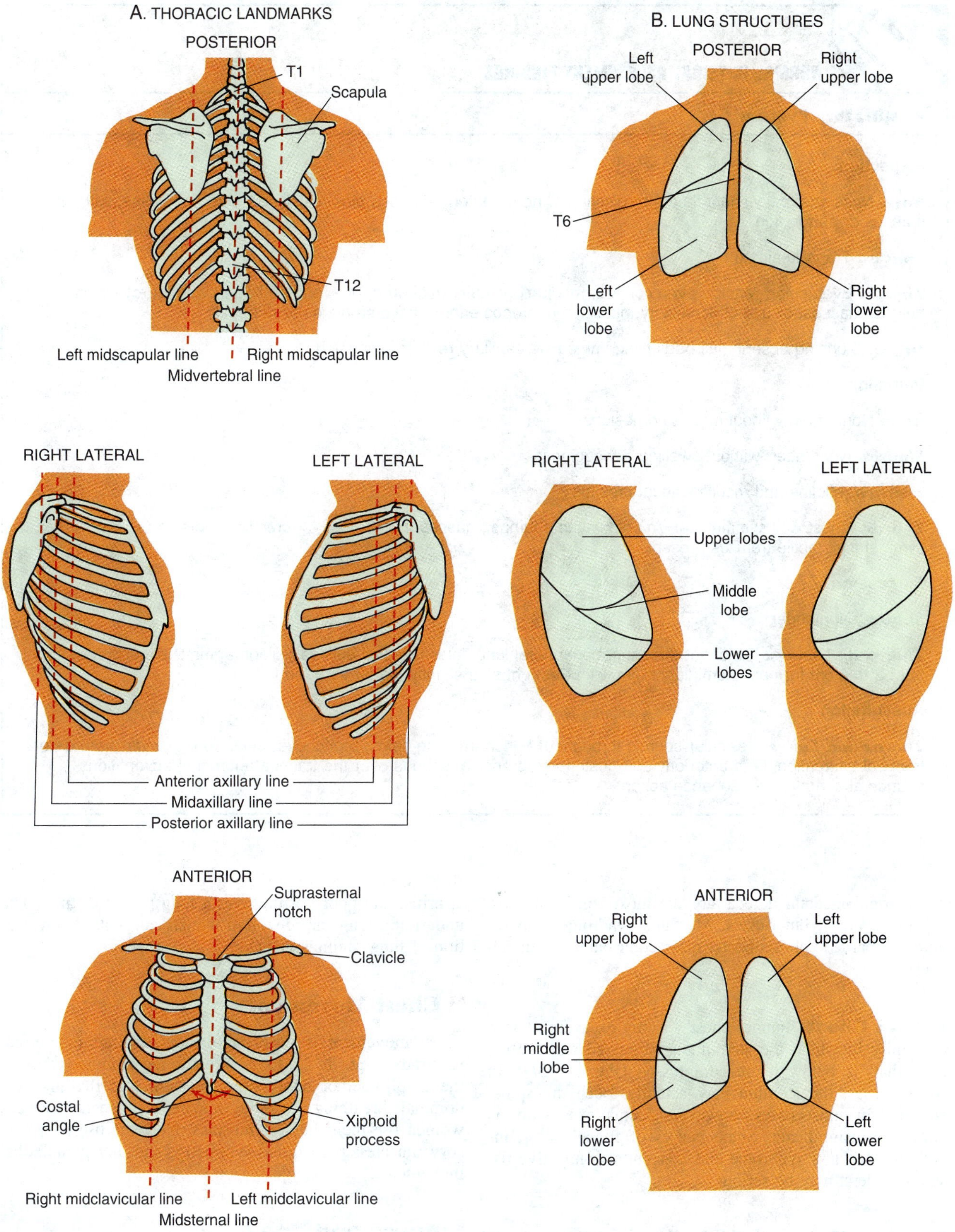

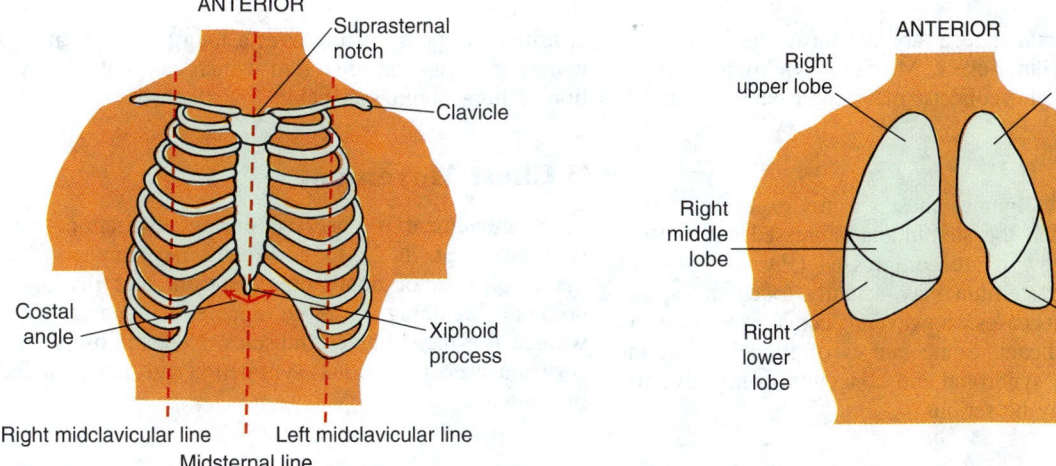

Figure 39–2. Thoracic landmarks and underlying lung structures. During chest examination, it is important to document in a universally understood manner the location of unusual or abnormal findings. Use the terminology of thoracic landmarks and lung structure to do so.

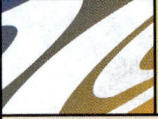

NORMAL PHYSICAL ASSESSMENT FINDINGS

Respiratory System

Inspection

Nose. Nose straight, without flaring or discharge; nares patent; mucosa pink and moist; septum midline, without masses or perforation

Sinuses. Transilluminate

Thorax. Even color; regular, even contour; respirations quit, unlabored, of even depth, and without retractions, bulges, masses, or use of accessory muscles; anteroposterior-transverse diameter ratio 1:2

Digits. Clubbing absent; nail beds pink; immediate capillary refill on blanching

Palpation

Nose. Nontender, without masses or lesions

Sinuses. Nontender, without swelling or bogginess

Trachea. Midline and mobile without crepitus

Thorax. Chest wall symmetrical, smooth, without lumps, masses, tenderness, or crepitus; thoracic excursion symmetrical; tactile fremitus present

Percussion

Sinuses. Nontender

Thorax and Lungs. Resonant throughout peripheral lung fields; cardiac dullness; diaphragmatic excursion ranges from 3 to 6 cm for each hemidiaphragm, with the right side slightly higher than the left

Auscultation

Thorax and Lungs. Vesicular sounds throughout peripheral lung fields; bronchovesicular sounds over the area of tracheal bifurcation, both anteriorly and posteriorly; bronchial sounds over the trachea anteriorly; adventitious sounds absent; vocal resonance absent

---

or ventricular septal defects are the most common cause of pigeon chest, but rickets, Marfan's syndrome, and severe primary kyphoscoliosis may contribute to pigeon chest.

Funnel Chest. Funnel chest (pectus excavatum) is a deformity in which the sternum is depressed and the organs that lie below it are compressed (Fig. 39–3D). In severe cases, the sternum may actually touch the spinal column. In most cases, however, pectus excavatum is clinically insignificant. Some causes of funnel chest, including Marfan's syndrome and congenital connective tissue disorders, may be serious.

Thoracic Kyphoscoliosis. Thoracic kyphoscoliosis is the accentuation of the normal thoracic curve (Fig. 39–3E). The client takes on a hunched-over or hunchback appearance. Causes include congenital defect, osteoporosis secondary to aging, spinal tuberculosis, rheumatoid arthritis, and poor posture over a long period of time. The underlying lungs are distorted, which can make interpretation of lung findings difficult.

■ Chest Movement

Chest movement is observed during respiration. Normal respiratory rate is 12 to 22 breaths per minute. Observe the amplitude, or depth of expansion, and rhythm. Abdominal breathing is more apparent in men, whereas women use their thoracic muscles. Note the use of accessory muscles, retractions, symmetry, and any paradoxical movements.

Fingers and Toes

Examination of the fingers and toes may reveal *clubbing,* which may be present in clients with pulmonary fibrosis, lung cancer, or bronchiectasis. Clubbing occurs as a com-

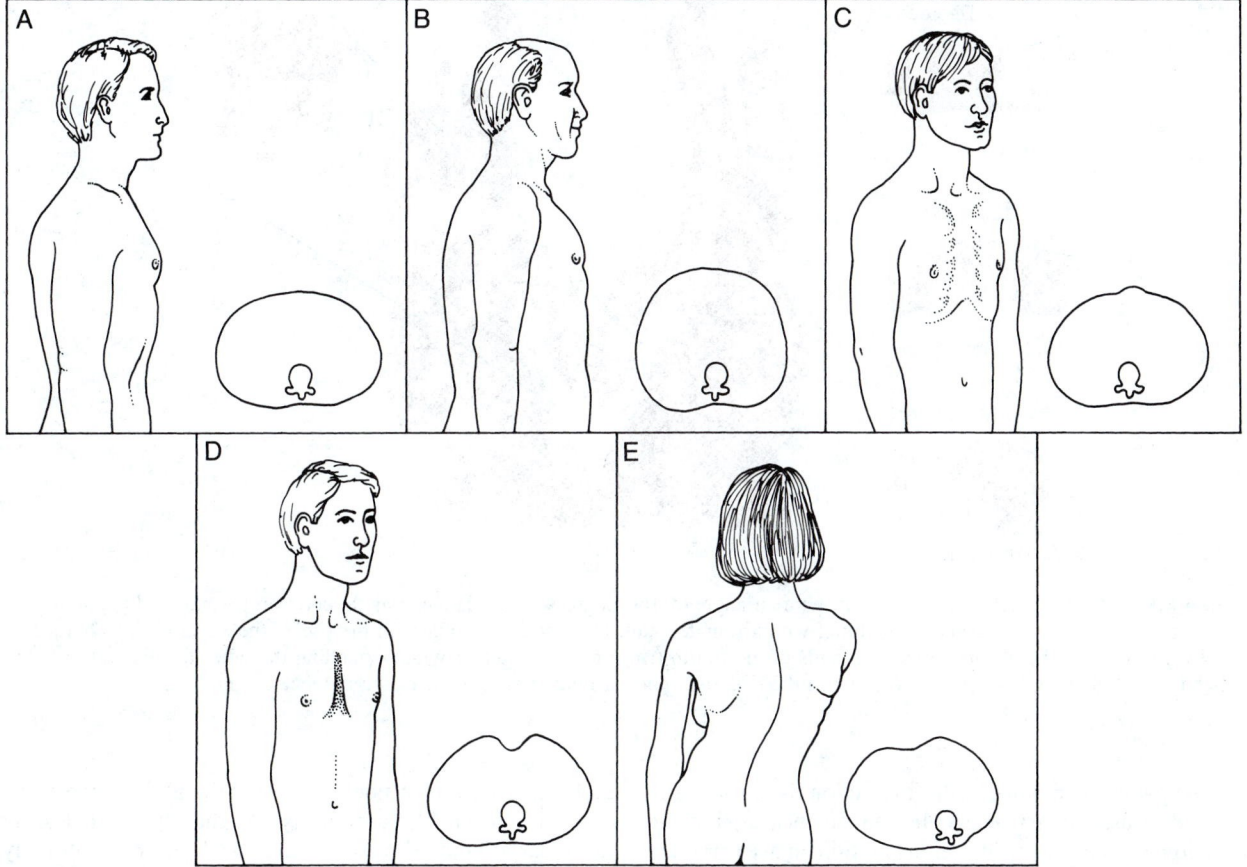

Figure 39–3. Chest deformities. *A,* Normal adult, for comparison. The ratio of anteroposterior diameter to transverse diameter can be seen here as 1 : 2 *B,* Barrel chest. The anteroposterior-transverse diameter ratio is 1 : 1. *C,* Pigeon chest (pectus carinatum). *D,* Funnel chest (pectus excavatum). *E,* Thoracic kyphoscoliosis.

pensatory measure to chronic hypoxia. The physiologic cause of clubbing has not yet been identified, although some hypotheses have been proposed. The body develops collateral circulation around areas of impaired circulation to provide more oxygen to that area. With clubbing the nail bed loses its normal angle of 160 degrees between the nail plate and the finger, and the angle increases to 180 degrees. The base of the nail bed may also feel spongy and soft. With advanced clubbing, the finger takes on a bulbous or spoonlike appearance. Early clubbing may be assessed by using the Schamroth technique (Fig. 39–4).

Note the color of the nail beds to assess the status of peripheral tissue oxygenation. Nail beds should be pink, without cyanosis or a dusky-blue color. Quickly and gently compress (between thumb and index finger) and release several of the client's nail beds on each extremity. Continuously observe for the *blanch response and capillary refill.* With compression, the nail bed becomes pale as capillary blood is squeezed from the tissue. Upon release of the pressure, oxygenated arterial blood fills the capillary bed. Normal capillary refill occurs within 3 seconds; a refill time of longer than 3 seconds is called delayed capillary refill.

Palpation

Palpation is the use of the hands to feel various structures on and below the surface of the body. The technique of palpation is described in Chapter 12.

Trachea

Gently place the thumb of the palpating hand on one side of the trachea and the remaining fingers on the other side. Move the trachea gently from side to side along its length while palpating for masses, crepitus, or deviation from the midline. The trachea is usually slightly movable and quickly returns to midline position after displacement. A chest mass, goiter, or an acute chest injury may displace the trachea.

Chest Wall

Palpate the chest wall with the heel or ulnar aspect of your hand held against the client's chest. Abnormalities found on inspection are further investigated during palpa-

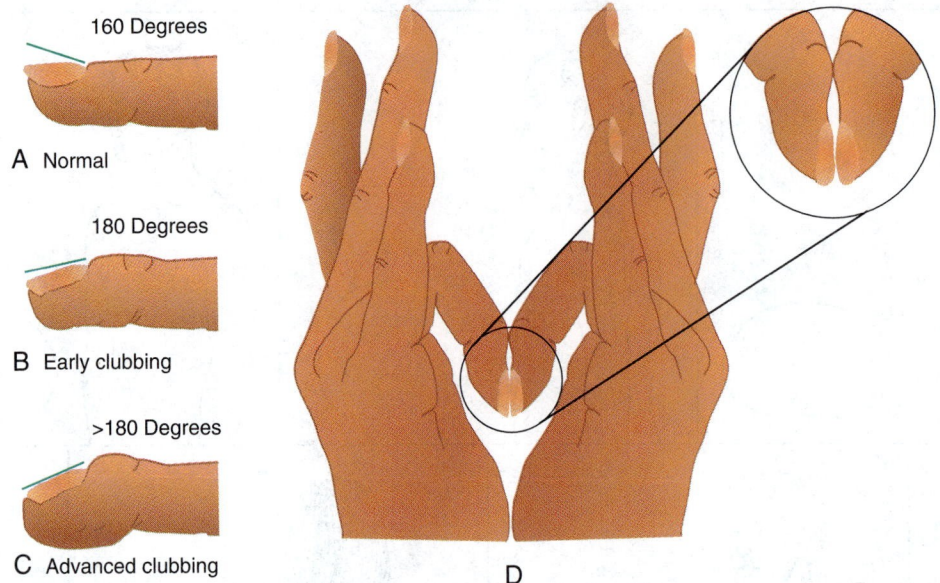

Figure 39–4. Clubbing. *A,* A normal digit, with an angle of 160 degrees. *B,* A flattened angle between the nail and the skin, exceeding 180 degrees. *C,* Advanced clubbing, with a rounded nail. *D,* Assess clubbing with the use of the Schamroth technique, whereby you instruct the client to place the nails of the fourth (ring) fingers together while extending the other fingers and to hold the hands up. A diamond-shaped space between the nails is a normal finding and indicates the absence of clubbing.

tion. Palpation combined with inspection is particularly effective in assessing whether the movements, or thoracic excursion of the chest during inspiration and expiration, are symmetrical and equal in amplitude. During palpation, assess for any crepitus (air in the subcutaneous tissues); defect or tenderness of the chest wall; muscle tone; edema; and tactile fremitus, or the vibration of air movement through the chest wall while the client is speaking.

■ Thoracic Excursion

For evaluation of thoracic excursion, the client sits upright, and the examiner's hands are placed on the client's posterior chest wall (Fig. 39–5). The thumbs oppose

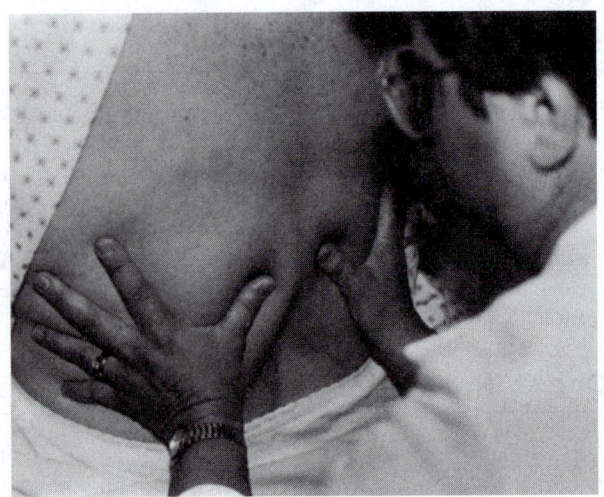

Figure 39–5. Assessment of thoracic excursion to determine the degree and symmetry of chest movement.

each other on either side of the spine, and the fingers face upward and out like a butterfly. As the client inhales, the examiner's hands should move up and out symmetrically. Any asymmetry may be indicative of a disease process in that region.

■ Tactile Fremitus

Palpate the posterior chest wall while the client says words that produce relatively intense vibrations (e.g., "ninety-nine"). The vibrations are transmitted from the larynx via the airways and can be palpated on the chest wall (Fig. 39–6). The intensity of vibrations on both sides is compared for symmetry. Stronger vibrations are felt over areas where there is consolidation of the underlying lung (e.g., pneumonia). Decreased tactile fremitus is usually associated with abnormalities that move the lung farther from the chest wall, such as pleural effusion and pneumothorax.

Percussion

Percussion is an assessment technique of producing sounds by tapping on the chest wall with the hand. Percussion technique is discussed in Chapter 12. Taping on the chest wall between the ribs produces various sounds that are described in regard to their acoustic properties—resonant, hyperresonant, dull, flat, or tympanic.

Resonant sounds are low-pitched, hollow sounds heard over normal lung tissue. *Hyperresonant* sounds indicate an increased amount of air in the lungs or pleural space. These sounds are louder and lower-pitched than resonant sounds. Emphysema and pneumothorax produce hyperresonant sounds. Hyperresonant sounds are normally heard

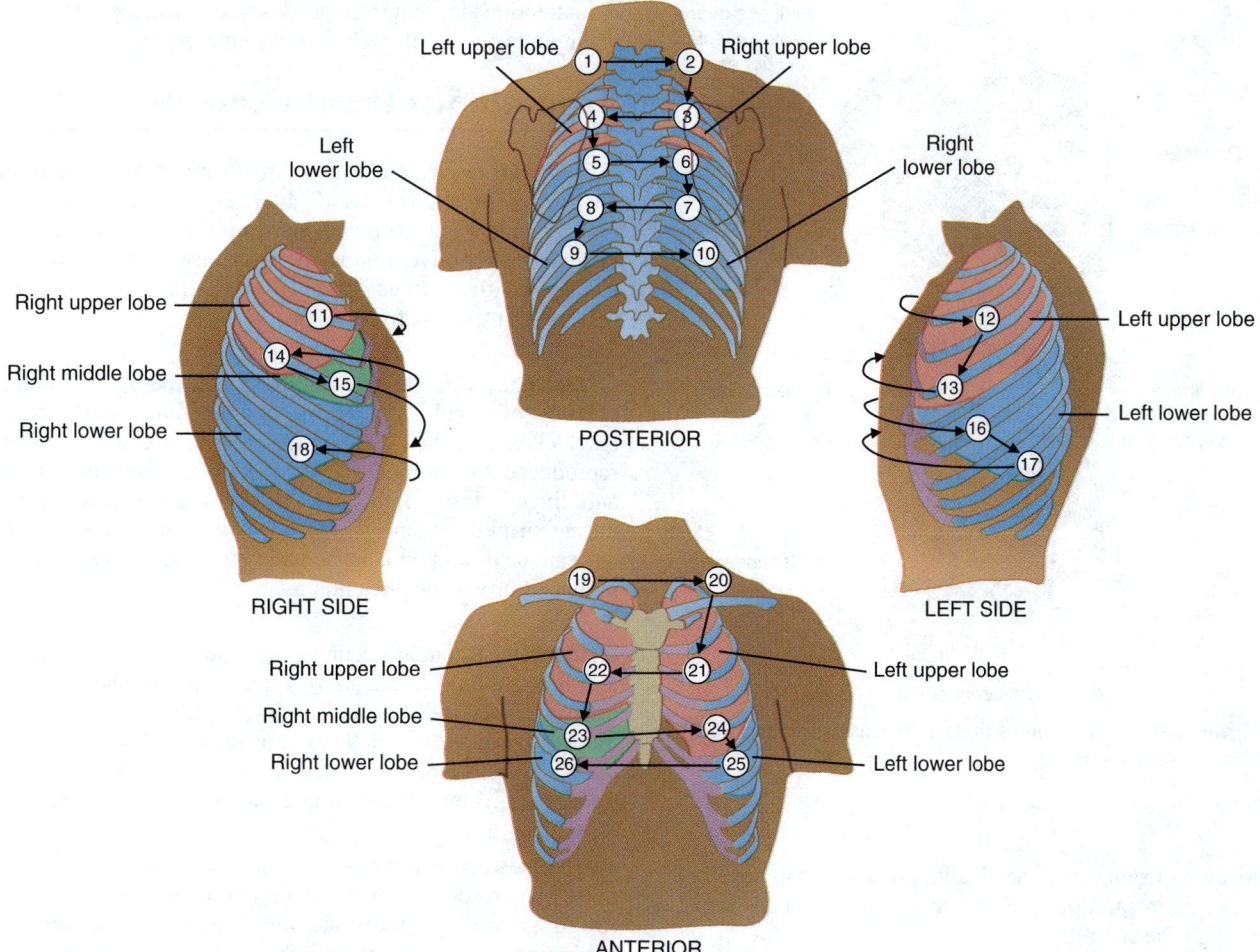

Figure 39–6. The sequence of palpation, percussion, and auscultation of the thorax (posterior, lateral, and anterior).

in children and very thin adults. *Dull* sounds occur over dense lung tissue, such as a tumor or consolidation. Dull sounds are thudlike, medium-pitched, and normally heard over the liver and heart. *Flat* notes are soft, high-pitched, and the result of percussion over airless tissue. This sound can be replicated with percussion of the examiner's thigh or bony structures. *Tympanic* notes are high, hollow, drumlike sounds heard with percussion over the stomach, a large tension pneumothorax, or a large air-filled chamber (such as the empty stomach). Figure 39–7 illustrates the location of percussion sounds of the chest.

Percussion begins at the apices and proceeds to the bases, moving from the posterior areas to the lateral areas and then to the anterior areas (see Fig. 39–7). The posterior chest is best percussed with the client in an upright position and with arms crossed to separate the scapulae.

Percussion is also used to assess diaphragmatic excursion. Ask the client to take a deep breath and hold it as you percuss down the posterior lung field and listen for the percussion note to change from resonant to dull. This area is marked with a pen. The process is repeated after the client exhales, and again the area is marked. Assess both right and left sides. The distance between the two marks should be 3 to 6 cm; smaller spans are found in

females, and larger spans in males. The marks on the right will be slightly higher because of the presence of the liver. A client with an elevated diaphragm related to a pathologic process will have a decreased diaphragmatic excursion. If the client has lung disease in the lower lobes (e.g., consolidation or pleural fluid), the same dull percussion note will be heard. When abnormalities are found, other diagnostic tests should be used to fully assess the problem.

Auscultation

Auscultation is listening to chest sounds with a stethoscope. By listening to the lungs while the client breathes through an open mouth, the examiner is able to assess three things: (1) the character of the breath sounds, (2) the presence of adventitious sounds, and (3) the character of the spoken and whispered voice. Figure 39–6 identifies a sequence for auscultation with comparison of sounds from right to left. Listen to all areas of the lungs and listen over a bare chest; do not listen to lungs over sheets, gowns, or shirts. The sounds heard may only be the movement of fabric beneath the stethoscope! At each

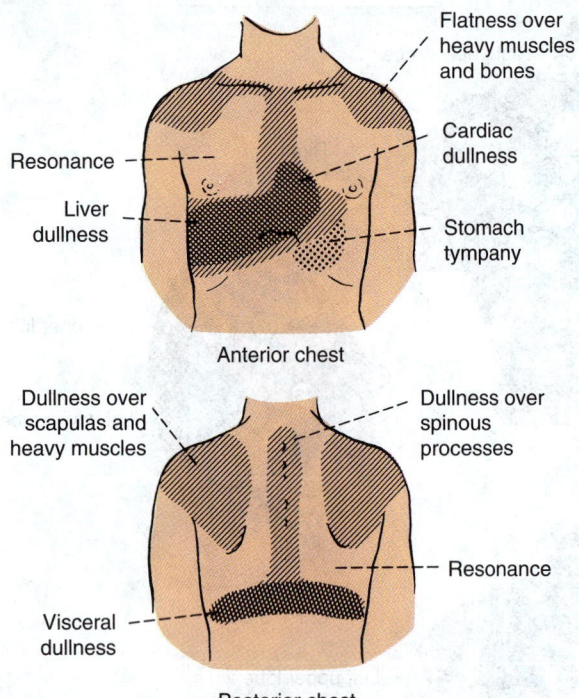

Flatness over
heavy muscles
and bones

Cardiac
dullness

Resonance

Liver
dullness

Stomach
tympany

Anterior chest

Dullness over
scapulas and
heavy muscles

Dullness over
spinous
processes

Resonance

Visceral
dullness

Posterior chest

Figure 39–7. Location of thoracic percussion sounds and their associated structures.

position, listen with the diaphragm for a full respiratory cycle of inspiration and expiration as the client breathes through the mouth.

Normal Breath Sounds

Breath sounds are noises from the transmission of vibrations produced by the movement of air in the respiratory passages. Be familiar with the sounds created by normal air exchange and their location (Table 39–2). Normal breath sounds are termed *vesicular, bronchial,* and *bronchovesicular;* they are heard in the locations identified in Figure 39–8.

Vesicular breath sounds are heard throughout the chest and heard best in the bases of the lungs. They are low-pitched, soft, "swishing" sounds best heard during inspiration, with an inspiratory-to-expiratory ratio of 5:2. *Bronchial* breath sounds are heard over the manubrium in the large tracheal airways. Bronchial sounds, heard only anteriorly, are best heard during expiration, with an expiratory-to-inspiratory ratio of 2:1. These sounds are loud and high-pitched and have a hollow or harsh quality. *Bronchovesicular* sounds are heard anteriorly and posteriorly over the central, large airways. They are heard equally during inspiration and expiration and have a tubular or breezy-sounding quality. *Absent* or *diminished* breath sounds are confirmed during deep respirations after the client has been instructed to take deep breaths and sounds cannot be heard. Shallow breaths may produce diminished sounds in the peripheral lung regions, but deep breaths should produce normal vesicular sounds. If absent breath sounds are a new finding, immediate medi-

cal attention is required because this usually indicates pneumothorax or other respiratory emergency.

Adventitious Breath Sounds

Adventitious sounds are abnormal sounds superimposed on normal breath sounds (Table 39–3 outlines adventitious sounds). The current American Thoracic Society nomenclature for adventitious sounds is used throughout this chapter. Adventitious sounds are crackles, rhonchi, wheezes, or pleural friction rub.

Crackles. Crackles are audible when there is a sudden opening of small airways that contain fluid. In the past, crackles were called rales. The sound of a crackle can be reproduced by rubbing a lock of hair between the thumb and finger close to the ear. Crackles are usually heard during inspiration and do not clear with a cough. Crackles can be found in clients with pulmonary edema, pulmonary fibrosis, or pneumonia.

Rhonchi. Rhonchi occur as the result of the passing of air through fluid-filled, narrow passages. Rhonchi sometimes are referred to as gurgles. Diseases with excess mucus production, such as pneumonia, bronchitis, or bronchiectasis, are associated with rhonchi. Rhonchi are usually heard on expiration and may clear with a cough.

Wheezes. A wheeze is a continuous musical or hissing noise that results from the passage of air through a narrowed airway. Wheezes are heard during inspiration or expiration, or both. Severe wheezes are audible without a stethoscope. Wheezing is commonly associated with asthma and its bronchoconstriction and edema, but foreign bodies can also cause airway narrowing and wheezing.

Pleural Friction Rubs. Pleural friction rubs are the result of pleural inflammation often associated with pleurisy, pneumonia, or pleural infarct. A rub is described as a creaking, grating noise similar to that made by two pieces of leather rubbing together. A rub is audible on inspiration and expiration over the area of the inflammation. Chest wall splinting can be associated with a pleural friction rub.

Voice Sounds

Assess voice sounds (vocal resonance) by auscultation if tactile fremitus is abnormal. Auscultation while the client speaks normally reveals muffled and indistinct sounds. The sound is louder medially over the larger airways and softens toward the periphery. Consolidation results in *bronchophony* or increased resonance so that when the client says "ninety-nine," it is heard clearly. If bronchophony is present, assess for egophony next. *Egophony* involves a change in the sound of the letter *e* to that of the letter *a,* indicating consolidation. The sound will also have a nasal or bleating quality. A third voice test for consolidation is *whispered pectoriloquy.* The client is

	Pitch	Amplitude	Duration	Quality	Normal Location
Table 39-2. Characteristics of Normal Breath Sounds					
Bronchial (tracheal)	High	Loud	Inspiration < expiration	Harsh, hollow, tubular	Trachea and larynx
Bronchovesicular	Moderate	Moderate	Inspiration = expiration	Mixed	Over major bronchi where fewer alveoli are located: posterior, between scapulae, especially on the right; anterior, around the upper sternum in the first and second intercostal spaces
Vesicular	Low	Soft	Inspiration > expiration	Rustling, like the sound of the wind in the trees	Over peripheral lung fields where air flows through smaller bronchioles and alveoli

From Jarvis, C. (1996). *Physical examination and health assessment* (2nd ed.) Philadelphia: W. B. Saunders.

asked to whisper "one-two-three." If the words are distinct, the abnormal finding of whispered pectoriloquy is present. Consolidation enhances the transmission of sound vibrations and results from lung tumors, pneumonia, or pulmonary fibrosis.

Assessment of the Nose, Pharynx, and Sinuses

History

Upper respiratory problems can occur alone or progress to lower respiratory complications, such as viral infections.

Current Symptoms

Chief Complaint

The client may present with a current complaint of nosebleeds (epistaxis); sinus infection; hay fever; postnasal drip; rhinitis; sneezing; or nasal, facial, or referred ear pain. Obstruction from engorged mucous membranes or nasal polyps may occlude the upper airway. A loss or decreased sense of smell may accompany manifestations of the common cold and allergies or may signal a more serious neurologic problem. Inquire whether the client has experienced these manifestations previously and, if so, when and how often. Ask the client to describe self-

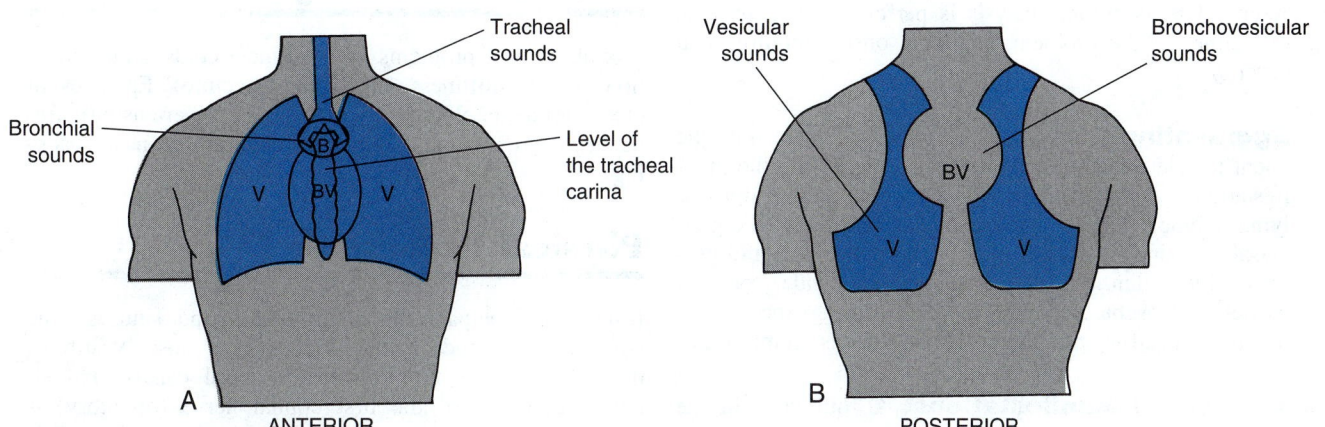

Figure 39-8. Location of normal breath sounds.

Table 39–3. Adventitious Breath Sounds			
Sound*	**Description**	**Mechanism**	**Clinical Example**
Discontinuous Sounds			
Crackles—fine (rales, crepitations) Inspiration Expiration	Discontinuous, high-pitched, short crackling, popping sounds heard during inspiration that are not cleared by coughing; this sound can be simulated by rolling a strand of hair between the fingers near the ear, or by moistening thumb and index finger and separating them near the ear	Inhaled air collides with previously deflated airways; airways suddenly pop open, creating a crackling sound as gas pressures between the two compartments equalize	*Late inspiratory crackles* occur with restrictive disease: pneumonia, congestive heart failure, and interstitial fibrosis *Early inspiratory crackles* occur with obstructive disease: chronic bronchitis, asthma, and emphysema
Crackles—coarse (coarse rales)	Loud, low-pitched, bubbling and gurgling sounds that start in early inspiration and may be present in expiration; may decrease somewhat by suctioning or coughing but will reappear shortly; sound like opening a Velcro fastener	Inhaled air collides with secretions in the trachea and large bronchi	Pulmonary edema, pneumonia, pulmonary fibrosis, and in the terminally ill who have a depressed cough reflex
Atelectatic crackles (atelectatic rales)	Sound like fine crackles, but do not last and are not pathologic; disappear after the first few breaths; heard in axillae and bases (usually dependent) of lungs	When sections of alveoli are not fully aerated, they deflate and accumulate secretions; crackles are heard when these sections reexpand with a few deep breaths	In aging adults, bedridden persons, or in persons just aroused from sleep

* Although nothing in clinical practice seems to differ more than the nomenclature of adventitious sounds, most authorities concur on two categories: (1) discontinuous, discrete crackling sounds and (2) continuous, coarse, or musical sounds.
From Jarvis, C. (1996). *Physical examination and health assessment* (2nd ed.) Philadelphia: W. B. Saunders.

treatment measures such as nasal sprays, decongestants, antihistamines, and other over-the-counter cold and allergy medications.

Symptom Analysis

A complete symptom analysis is performed to determine the nature of the problem, including onset, duration, and severity.

Aggravating and Relieving Factors. Ask the client to relate factors that alleviate or aggravate the manifestations, such as increased humidity, sitting upright, lying supine, weather and seasonal changes, or allergies. Nasal and sinus problems may be allergy-related and provoked by pollen, fumes, smoke, animal dander, or dust particles. Nosebleeds may increase during the winter months if insufficient humidity dries mucous membranes.

Associated Manifestations. A foul taste in the mouth, unpleasant breath odor (halitosis), nasal obstruction, and facial pain (particularly over the frontal and maxillary sinuses) may accompany sinusitis. Chronic sinusitis may be accompanied by headache or facial pain present on awakening and diminishing during the day (because the sinuses drain when the client sits or stands).

Past Health History

Ask about past problems with frequent colds, sinus infections, nasal stuffiness, or trauma (fracture). Episodes of epistaxis are explored for cause (e.g., hypertension), frequency, and treatment (e.g., cauterization or nasal packing).

Physical Examination

Inspect and palpate the client's nose and sinuses. The structures assessed include the external nose, vestibule, nasal mucosa, septum, turbinates, nasal canals, and sinuses. Function of the first cranial nerve (olfactory) is usually not tested unless a deficit in the sense of smell is reported or suspected.

Sound*	Description	Mechanism	Clinical Example
Pleural friction rub	A very superficial sound that is coarse and low-pitched; it has a grating quality as if two pieces of leather are being rubbed together; sounds just like crackles, but *close* to the ear; sounds louder if the stethoscope is pushed harder onto the chest wall; sound is inspiratory and expiratory	Caused when pleurae become inflamed and lose their normal lubricating fluid; their opposing roughened pleural surfaces rub together during respiration; heard best in the anterolateral wall where there is greatest lung mobility	Pleuritis, accompanied by pain with breathing (rub disappears after a few days if pleural fluid accumulates and separates pleurae)
Continuous Sounds			
Wheeze—high-pitched (sibilant rhonchi)	High-pitched, musical squeaking sounds that predominate in expiration but may occur in both expiration and inspiration	Air squeezed or compressed through passageways narrowed almost to closure by collapsing, swelling, secretions, or tumors; the passageway walls oscillate in apposition between the closed and barely open positions; the resulting sound is similar to a vibrating reed	Obstructive lung disease such as asthma or emphysema
Wheeze—low-pitched (sonorous rhonchi)	Low-pitched, musical snoring, moaning sounds; they are heard throughout the cycle, although they are more prominent on expiration; may clear somewhat by coughing	Air flow obstruction as described by the vibrating reed mechanism above; the pitch of the wheeze cannot be correlated with the size of the passageway that generates it	Bronchitis

Nose

■ External Nose

Inspect and palpate the external nose for deviations from normal alignment, symmetry, color, discharge, nasal flaring, lesions, and tenderness. Normal findings are listed. The skin color over the nose is the same as that of the facial skin. Alignment is straight and symmetrical without deviation from midline. Discharge from the nares (nostrils) should be absent, and the nares should not flare (spread) with respirations. The client is able to breathe quietly through the nose rather than mouth-breathe. Masses, lesions, and tenderness are absent. Check the nasal canals for patency by asking the client to occlude one naris with a finger and to breathe through the open naris while closing the mouth. This is repeated for the opposite naris. The client should be able to breathe without difficulty through both nares. Ask the client to tip the head back and inspect the outer nares for crusting, bleeding, or dryness, which should be absent.

■ Internal Nose

Next, inspect the vestibules with a penlight while the client's head is tipped back. Normal findings include the presence of coarse hairs, a clear passage without discharge, and a midline septum. Further examination of the internal nose requires use of a nasal speculum; this is not done unless indicated. If a detailed examination of the internal nose is done, either attach a nasal speculum tip to the otoscope head or use a metal nasal speculum (Fig. 39–9) and penlight for illumination. While the client tips the head back, gently insert the speculum into one naris, taking care not to scrape the mucosa. One naris is inspected at a time.

Hold the speculum correctly and insert the blades gently about ½ inch into the nostril. Gain additional control of the speculum by resting the index finger of the dominant hand on the side of the client's nose. Steady the client's head with the nondominant hand. Open the blades gently and vertically, avoiding pressure on the septum and turbinates. Slowly move the head to inspect all areas of the nasal chamber. Observe the condition of the mucous membrane (e.g., pallor, redness, swelling.) Normally,

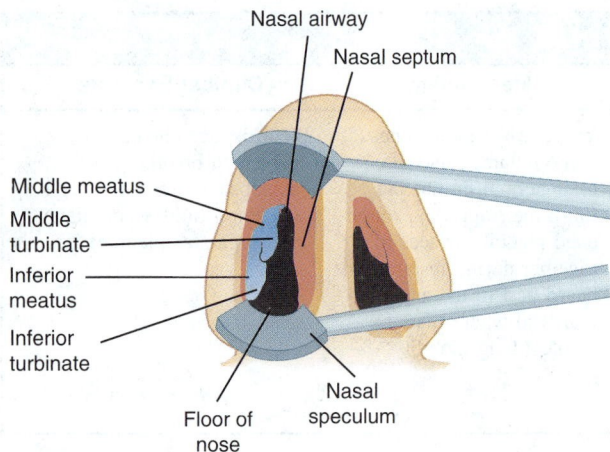

Figure 39–9. Internal inspection of the nose with a nasal speculum.

the mucosa is moist and dark pink without sign of inflammation, pallor, or a blue color. Presence of discharge is abnormal. The septum divides the nasal cavity into halves without deviation, masses, perforation, or exudate. The turbinates (only the inferior and part of the middle turbinate are visible; the superior is not) have the same color as the mucosa and should be free of exudate, swelling, or inflammation. Look for polyps and other masses. Observe mucous plugs for color, consistency, amount, and odor.

Inspection may be hampered by nasal congestion. It may be necessary to shrink the nasal mucosa with a topical vasoconstrictor (e.g., phenylephrine hydrochloride) for adequate inspection. When these agents are instilled into the nose, ask the client to say *e* and hold the sound. This technique raises the posterior tongue, occludes the upper airway, and prevents the fluid from running into the pharynx.

Nasopharynx

The nasopharynx is best examined with a mirror while the tongue is depressed with a tongue blade or pulled forward and grasped with a gauze sponge. Prevent the mirror's fogging by warming it before putting it into the mouth. Hold the mirror to one side of the uvula and focus light on it. A small part of the nasopharynx can be observed with a nasal speculum. Specialists may use a nasopharyngoscope to examine the nasopharynx.

Paranasal Sinuses

Assess the paranasal sinuses by (1) inspecting and palpating the soft overlying tissues, (2) observing any nasal secretions (it is possible to determine which sinus is infected according to where discharge appears), and (3) transilluminating the maxillary and frontal sinuses. Palpate and percuss the frontal and maxillary sinuses to assess for swelling and tenderness, which normally are absent. The frontal sinuses are palpated simultaneously by placing the thumbs above the eyes, just under the bony ridge of the orbits, and applying gentle pressure. The maxillary sinuses are palpated by use of either the index and third fingers or thumbs to gently press on each side of the nose just under the zygomatic bones. Use direct percussion over the eyebrows for the frontal sinuses and on either side of the nose below the eyes in line with the pupils for the maxillary sinuses.

Transillumination is a technique used to further access the sinuses if tenderness is present. Either a penlight or the otoscope handle fitted with a transilluminator head (see Chapter 12) is used. Darken the room. Place the light against the orbital bones immediately below the eyebrows and direct upward. Shield the light source with one hand. Normally, a reddish glow appears above the frontal sinus area. Lack of illumination may indicate sinus congestion and purulent fluid accumulation. The maxillary sinuses are assessed by placing the light beneath the center of the eyes and the zygomatic bones and directing it down and in toward the roof of the mouth. Ask the client to open the mouth. A glow should appear on the hard palate on the side being illuminated. For a more complete assessment of sinus conditions, radiologic studies may be done. Air, normally present in the sinuses, appears as a dark area on a developed film.

Smell

The senses of taste and smell are closely related. Many conditions affect taste and smell, such as viral infections, normal aging, head injuries, and local obstruction. Some medications can affect smell and taste, such as metronidazole (Flagyl), local anesthetics, clofibrate (Atromid-S), some antibiotics, some antineoplastics, allopurinol, phenylbutazone, levodopa, codeine, morphine, carbamazepine (Tegretol), lithium, and trifluoperazine (Stelazine). Smell impairment may be (1) hyposmia (decrease in smell sensitivity) or (2) anosmia (bilateral and complete absence of smell sensitivity). Smell assessment is done by having the client identify various odors. Various substances are placed in individual test tubes (covered to eliminate visual cues). Testing each nostril separately, have the client sniff the tubes (first with the eyes closed and then with the eyes open). Document whether the client can (1) perceive each odor and (2) identify each odor accurately. Smell is perceived mainly via the olfactory nerves, although some smell is perceived via the trigeminal nerves. Trigeminal irritants are perceived even by clients experiencing anosmia. (Therefore, a client who claims not to smell trigeminal irritants has a hysterical loss of smell rather than hyposmia or anosmia.) A client with a tracheostomy may not be able to smell because of limited upper airway movement. Olfactory stimulants and trigeminal stimulants commonly used to assess smell are listed in Box 39–1.

Diagnostic Tests

Diagnostic procedures augment the assessment of clients with respiratory disorders. To clarify which diagnostic test is used when and for what purpose, the tests are

Box 39–1. Substances Used in Assessing Smell	
Olfactory stimulants	**Trigeminal stimulants**
Coffee (instant powder)	Ammonia
Phenylethyl alcohol	Acetone
Almond oil	Menthol
Peppermint	Distilled water
Musk	

discussed here in the framework of what is being evaluated: functional status, anatomy, or specimens. The diagnostic test may be used for any or all of these reasons. This listing is by no means all-inclusive, but identifies the most commonly used diagnostic tests.

Tests to Evaluate Respiratory Function

The diagnostic tests that evaluate the functional status of the pulmonary system include (1) pulmonary function tests, (2) pulse oximetry, (3) capnography, (4) arterial blood gas analysis, and (5) ventilation-perfusion studies.

Pulmonary Function Tests

Pulmonary function tests (PFTs) provide information about a client's manifestation by measuring lung volumes, lung mechanics, and diffusion capabilities of the lungs (Table 39–4). PFTs performed in a pulmonary function laboratory can measure respiratory volumes and capacities. On the other hand, PFTs done outside of a laboratory are modified to include ventilation tests of forced expiratory volume, vital capacity, and maximal voluntary ventilation measures. A handheld measure of inspiratory flow is called a peak flow. Many clients with asthma use a peak flowmeter (Fig. 39–10) at home to monitor changes in their condition and responses to treatment.

Education about the purpose, procedure, and implications of the test is performed by the nurse and reinforced by the examiner. Explicit instructions for each maneuver are given during the testing. Instruct clients that it is normal to feel short of breath after the test. Clients should not smoke or use a bronchodilator 6 hours before undergoing a PFT.

■ Forced Spirometry

The flow and volume capacities of the lungs are measured with forced spirometry. This method involves the recording of the volume of air inhaled and exhaled plotted against time during a series of ventilatory maneuvers. Flow volume loops are created as visual patterns. Normal loop spirograms and spirogram patterns with obstructive and restrictive disorders are shown in Figure 39–11. Table 39–4 defines maneuvers that test lung mechanics.

■ Gas Dilution Tests and Body Plethysmography

Lung volume is measured by a gas dilution technique or body plethysmography. The two most commonly used gas dilution methods are the open circuit nitrogen method and the closed circuit helium method. These tests are most often used to measure functional residual capacity. In the open circuit method, all exhaled gas is collected while the client breathes pure oxygen. The measurement of the total amount of nitrogen washed out from the lungs permits calculation of the volume of gas present in the lungs at the beginning of the maneuver. The open circuit method also allows an assessment of the uniformity of ventilation in the lungs.

To use helium to test the lungs, the client inhales a mixture of air with a known concentration of helium. Helium will not significantly diffuse into the pulmonary bed. The helium will diffuse throughout the air in the breathing box and lungs. The client exhales and is disconnected from the box. Changes in helium concentration in the box are computed to determine total lung volume.

Body plethysmograph, or the body box (Fig. 39–12), is a device used to measure lung volumes. The lung volume changes seen with obstructive and restrictive lung disorders are shown in Table 39–5. While sitting in the airtight box, the client is instructed to perform a panting maneuver. Changes in the box pressure reflect changes in thoracic volume. Clients who cannot pant, who cannot tolerate closed spaces, or who have equipment that would interfere with the test cannot be tested by this method.

■ Tests of the Diffusing Capacity of the Lungs

Studies of the diffusing capacity of the lungs (DL or DLCO) measure gas transfer of carbon dioxide across the alveolar-capillary membrane. The DL indicates the ease with which carbon monoxide diffuses across the alveolar capillary membrane and binds with hemoglobin. (Remember that hemoglobin has 250 times greater affinity for carbon monoxide than for oxygen.) With a normal hemoglobin and normal ventilatory function, the only limiting factor to diffusion of carbon monoxide is the alveolar-capillary membrane.

Many diseases, such as sarcoidosis, systemic lupus erythematosus, and emphysema thicken the alveolar membrane and impair oxygen transfer and diffusion. They cause a decreased DL. An increased DL is found during exercise, polycythemia, and hypervolemia.

Instruct the client to hold a single breath for 10 seconds and exhale. A sample of the exhaled air is then collected for analysis.

Pulse Oximetry

Procedure. Pulse oximetry is a safe and simple method of assessing oxygenation. A distinct advantage is that the data obtained are noninvasive and continuous. Previously, the most common method of assessing oxygenation was the use of arterial blood gases. Pulse oxime-

Table 39–4. Pulmonary Function Test (PFT) Components

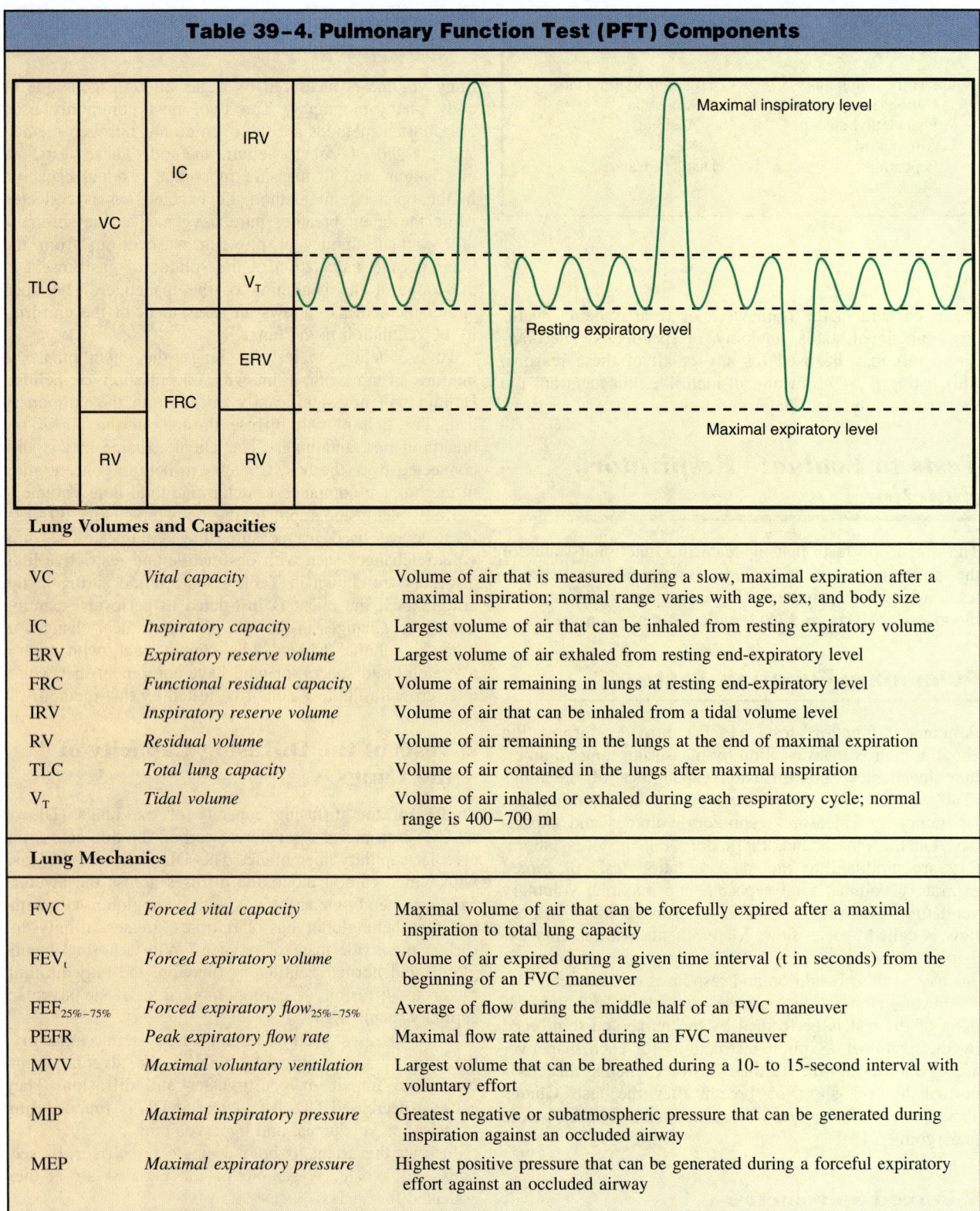

Lung Volumes and Capacities

VC	*Vital capacity*	Volume of air that is measured during a slow, maximal expiration after a maximal inspiration; normal range varies with age, sex, and body size
IC	*Inspiratory capacity*	Largest volume of air that can be inhaled from resting expiratory volume
ERV	*Expiratory reserve volume*	Largest volume of air exhaled from resting end-expiratory level
FRC	*Functional residual capacity*	Volume of air remaining in lungs at resting end-expiratory level
IRV	*Inspiratory reserve volume*	Volume of air that can be inhaled from a tidal volume level
RV	*Residual volume*	Volume of air remaining in the lungs at the end of maximal expiration
TLC	*Total lung capacity*	Volume of air contained in the lungs after maximal inspiration
V_T	*Tidal volume*	Volume of air inhaled or exhaled during each respiratory cycle; normal range is 400–700 ml

Lung Mechanics

FVC	*Forced vital capacity*	Maximal volume of air that can be forcefully expired after a maximal inspiration to total lung capacity
FEV_t	*Forced expiratory volume*	Volume of air expired during a given time interval (t in seconds) from the beginning of an FVC maneuver
$FEF_{25\%-75\%}$	*Forced expiratory flow$_{25\%-75\%}$*	Average of flow during the middle half of an FVC maneuver
PEFR	*Peak expiratory flow rate*	Maximal flow rate attained during an FVC maneuver
MVV	*Maximal voluntary ventilation*	Largest volume that can be breathed during a 10- to 15-second interval with voluntary effort
MIP	*Maximal inspiratory pressure*	Greatest negative or subatmospheric pressure that can be generated during inspiration against an occluded airway
MEP	*Maximal expiratory pressure*	Highest positive pressure that can be generated during a forceful expiratory effort against an occluded airway

try was originally used in surgery, but has been extended to most areas of acute care settings. In fact, it is so common that pulse oximetry has been called the fifth vital sign. The pulse oximeter (Fig. 39–13) passes a beam of light through the tissue, and a sensor attached to the fingertip, toe, or ear lobe measures the amount of light absorbed by the oxygen-saturated hemoglobin. The oximeter then gives a reading of the percentage of hemoglobin that is saturated with oxygen (SaO_2). SaO_2 has a close correlation with the saturations obtained from the pulse oximeter if it is above 70%. Table 39–6 provides a quick guide for comparison of SaO_2 and partial pressure of arterial oxygen (PaO_2).

Limitations of pulse oximetry are still present despite

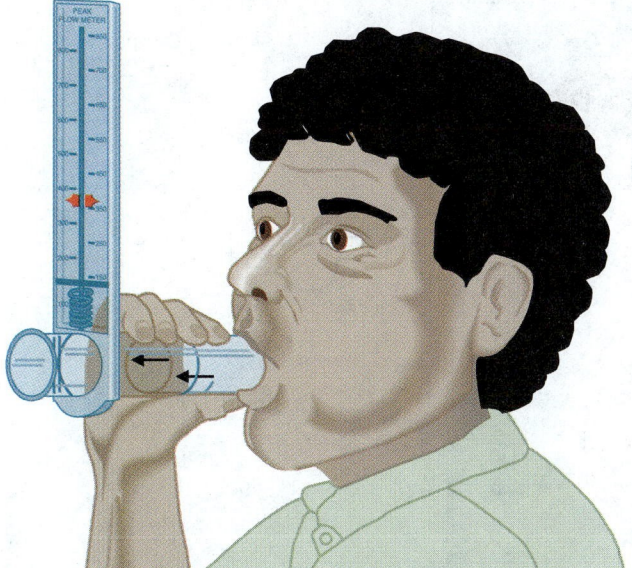

Figure 39–10. Use of a peak flowmeter to measure peak expiratory flow volume. The client stands and exhales into the mouthpiece. Normal peak flow values for adults are based on age, sex, height, and underlying lung disorder. Normal values range from 300 to 700 L/min but are best assessed when compared against a client's baseline values.

the advancement of the technology. Motion at the sensor site changes light absorption. The motion mimics the pulsatile motion of blood and because the detector cannot distinguish between movement of blood and movement of the finger, results can be inaccurate. Hypotension, hypothermia, and vasoconstriction reduce arterial blood flow to the sensor. Keeping the finger warm may help with this problem. There are also sensors for the nose which can be used to improve accuracy. The sensor should not be placed distal to blood pressure cuffs, pressure dressings, arterial lines, or any invasive catheters. The sensor should not be taped to the client's finger. Clients with severe right-sided heart failure and those on high levels of positive end-expiratory pressure (PEEP) may have inaccurate readings due to the creation of pulsatile venous blood. Dark nail polish (especially blue, green, black, and brown-red) may interfere with accuracy. Red nail polish and artificial nails do not affect accuracy. Hyperbilirubinemia can also yield false results. The nurse should continue to assess the whole patient and not just the oxygen saturation monitor. If values fall below preset norms, (usually 90%) the client should be instructed to deepbreathe (if appropriate). Sometimes the amount of inspired oxygen is increased (titrated) to keep oxygen satu-

Figure 39–11. A normal flow volume loop pattern and patterns for obstructive and restrictive lung disease. (From Kersten, L. D., et al. [1989]. *Respiratory nursing* [p. 382]. Philadelphia: W. B. Saunders.)

LOOP SPIROGRAM PATTERNS AND EXPLANATION

NORMAL PATTERN

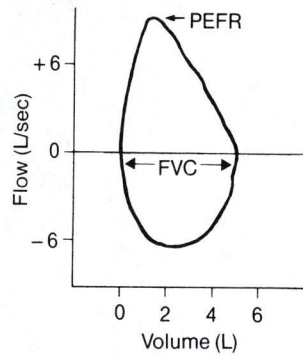

The expiratory curve shows a straight line decrease in flow after peak flow (PEFR). The inspiratory curve has a normal rounded pattern.

OBSTRUCTIVE PATTERN

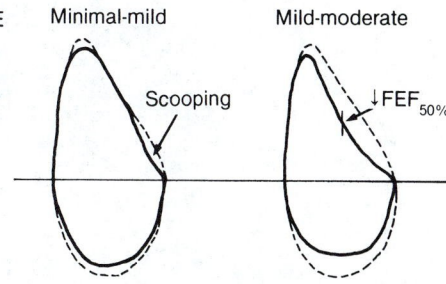

The expiratory curve shows scooping at low lung volumes (minimal to mild obstruction). As obstruction increases, the scooping becomes more marked and is accompanied by a decreased $FEF_{50\%}$ (mild to moderate obstruction).

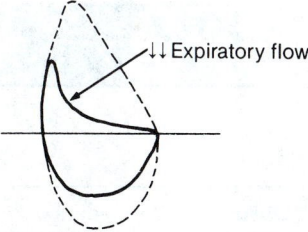

The expiratory curve shows a sudden decrease in PEFR in an "index finger" pattern, followed by a nearly horizontal line.

The inspiratory curve is normal, except for absolute decreases in flow rates.

RESTRICTIVE PATTERN

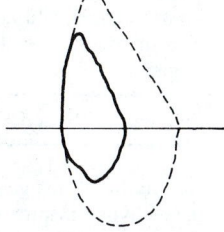

The entire loop resembles a miniature normal flow-volume loop. The FVC is markedly reduced. The expiratory curve shows a straight line decrease in flow with decreasing lung volumes. Peak flow rates may be normal, increased, or decreased, depending on the degree of respiratory impairment.

*The dotted lines represent the boundaries of the normal flow-volume loop.

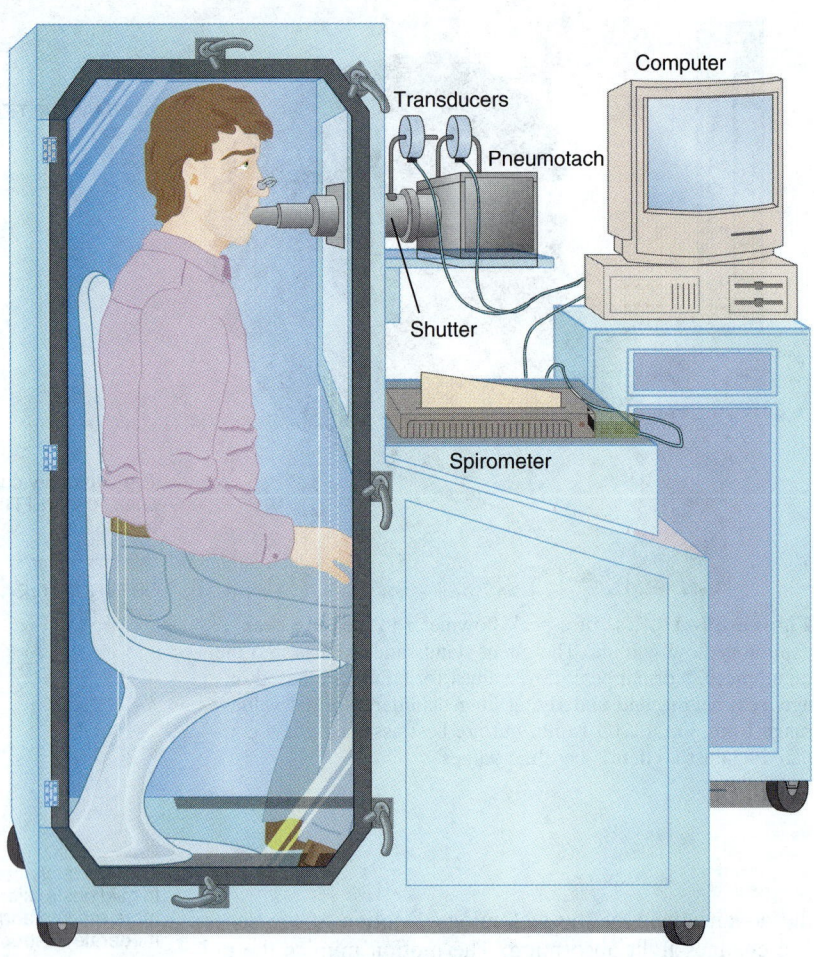

Figure 39–12. The volume plethysmograph—the "body box."

Table 39–5. Categorization of Obstructive and Restrictive Pulmonary Disorders and Pulmonary Function Test (PFT) Findings

	PFT Findings					
	VC	FEV$_1$	FEV$_+$/VC	FRC	TLC	RV
Obstructive Disorders						
Affect the patency or elasticity of the airways, leading to an increase in airway resistance; expiration is primarily affected. Obstructive disorders include emphysema, chronic bronchitis, asthma, bronchiectasis, and airway inflammation in response to irritants, infections, or allergies.	↓	↓	↓	↑	↑	↑
Restrictive Disorders						
Interfere in or change chest wall or lung parenchyma; inspiration is primarily affected. Restrictive disorders include kyphoscoliosis, pulmonary fibrosis, neuromuscular diseases and disorders, chest wall trauma, congenital chest wall changes, and tumors.	Normal or ↓	Slightly ↓	Normal or ↑	↓	↓	↓

FEV, forced expiratory volume in a unit of time; FRC, functional residual volume; RV, residual volume; TLC, total lung capacity; VC, vital capacity.

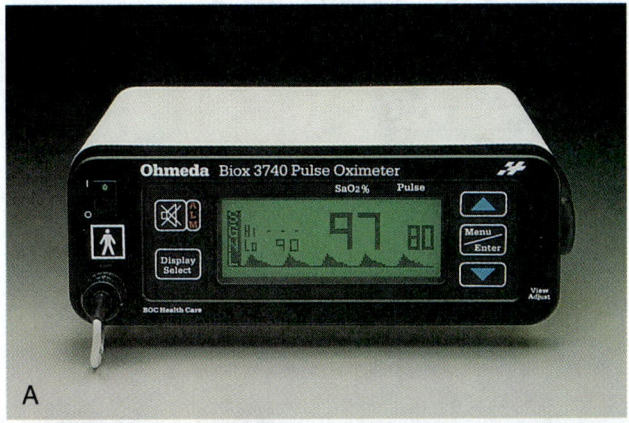

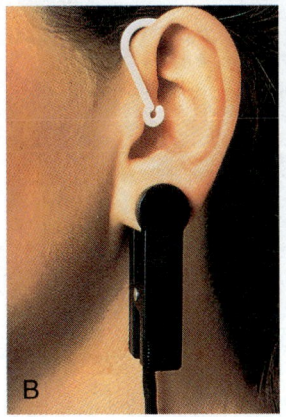

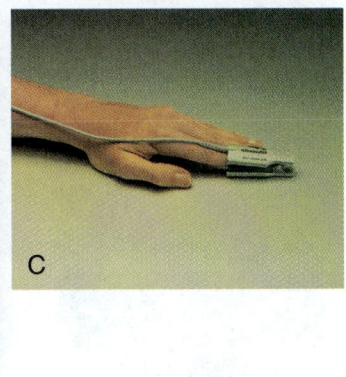

Figure 39–13. Oximetry. Noninvasive monitoring of SaO_2 (oxygen saturation) is performed with a pulse oximeter. This unit has an ear probe and a finger probe. The ear probe (B) is used during measurements of SaO_2 while the client is exercising. The finger probe (C) is most frequently used for stationary measurement. (Courtesy of Ohmeda, Boulder, CO.)

ration above 90%. If the probe comes off of the client's finger, the monitor usually indicates that the probe is off. Seldom is a loose probe the cause for readings of low levels of oxygen saturation.

Preprocedure Care. Tell the client about the need for the monitor. The test is noninvasive and painless. Instruct the client that an infrared light probe will be attached to a finger, toe, or ear lobe. The client should avoid moving the sensor because movement disrupts the sensor and gives false readings.

Table 39–6. Comparing Oxygen Saturation to Partial Pressure of Arterial Oxygen (PaO_2)		
Oxygen Saturation	**PaO_2**	**Client Status**
50%	25 mm Hg	Life-threatening hypoxemia
75%	40 mm Hg	Moderate hypoxemia
90%	55 mm Hg	Mild hypoxemia

Capnography

Procedure. Capnography, another noninvasive procedure, is the measurement of exhaled carbon dioxide concentrations for clients on mechanical ventilation. The amount of carbon dioxide found in exhaled air, end-tidal carbon dioxide ($ETCO_2$), correlates very closely with partial pressure of arterial carbon dioxide ($PaCO_2$) in clients with normal respiratory, cardiovascular, and metabolic function. The normal gradient of $PaCO_2$-$ETCO_2$ is approximately 5 mm Hg. As the $PaCO_2$ increases with hypoventilation, or decreases with hyperventilation, associated changes will be noted in $ETCO_2$. Capnography requires a continuous sampling of exhaled air.

Preprocedure Care. Explain to the client the purpose of this test. The test is noninvasive and painless. Clients who require capnography will already have an endotracheal tube or tracheostomy tube in place for mechanical ventilation or airway management. A sensor will be attached to the endotracheal tube or tracheostomy tube to measure $ETCO_2$.

Arterial Blood Gas Analysis

Arterial blood gas (ABG) analysis is the use of arterial, rather than venous, blood to directly measure PaO_2, $PaCO_2$, and pH. Other data are calculated such as bicarbonate (HCO_3^-) and SaO_2. It is an excellent diagnostic tool. PaO_2 reflects the efficiency of gas exchange, whereas $PaCO_2$ reflects the effectiveness of alveolar ventilation. The acid-base status of the body (see Chapter 16) is indicated by the pH of arterial blood. ABGs are essential for the assessment of clients who are acutely ill with pulmonary and nonpulmonary disorders, require an artificial airway, are dependent on mechanical ventilation, or are experiencing chronic respiratory diseases.

Procedure. A sample of arterial blood is obtained by arterial puncture. This procedure is done by inserting a sterile needle (connected to a heparinized syringe) into one of the superficial arteries (i.e., radial, brachial, or femoral) (Fig. 39–14). Arterial blood is differentiated from venous blood by its bright-red color. The radial artery is most commonly used because it is readily accessible, is easily palpated, and is associated with fewer complications. Low complication rates are related to ease of access and presence of collateral circulation via the ulnar artery. The sample should be sent to the laboratory immediately on ice. For serial ABG analyses or ongoing respiratory monitoring, multiple punctures may be avoided by using an arterial line (i.e., a sterile cannula inserted into one of the arteries).

A systematic approach to ABG interpretation, in conjunction with the client's overall status, can lead to the identification of potentially life-threatening abnormalities. First assess the client's oxygenation status. Acid-base interpretation follows to evaluate imbalances (see Chapter 16). The following steps are included in the ABG analysis: PaO_2, pH, $PaCO_2$, HCO_3^-, the presence and degree of compensation, and identification of the primary disorder.

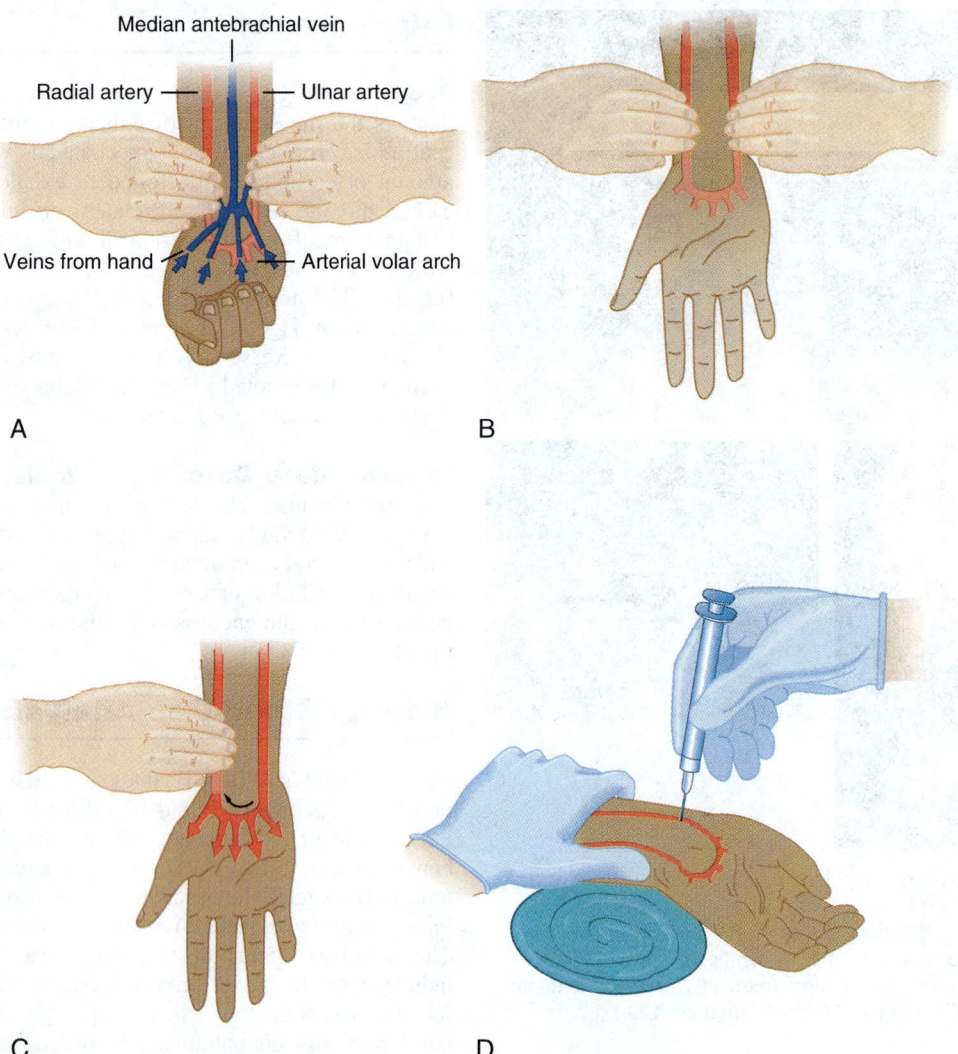

Median antebrachial vein

Radial artery — — Ulnar artery

Veins from hand → ← Arterial volar arch

A

B

C

D

Figure 39–14. Obtaining a sample of arterial blood by arterial puncture. First, perform Allen's test, a quick assessment of collateral circulation in the hand. This test is essential prior to radial artery puncture. *A,* Occlude both the radial and the ulnar arteries with your fingers. Ask the client to close the hand into a fist. *B,* When the client opens the hand with the arteries still occluded, the hand is pale. *C,* When you release either the radial or the ulnar artery, the hand should become pink because of collateral circulation. Assess the patency of each of the two arteries in this way, one at a time. *D,* If collateral circulation is adequate, you can draw arterial blood from the radial artery with a heparinized needle and syringe, as shown.

PaO₂. Evaluate PaO_2 first because of the seriousness of hypoxemia. *Hypoxemia* reflects the PaO_2 but does not reflect the status of tissue oxygenation. Normal PaO_2 is considered to be 80 to 100 mm Hg. Mild hypoxemia is a PaO_2 less than 80 mm Hg on breathing room air. Moderate hypoxemia is a PaO_2 less than 60 mm Hg; severe hypoxemia is a PaO_2 less than 40 mm Hg. Baseline normal values decrease with age at a rate of 1 mm Hg per year of age over 60. Nonetheless, the same values are used to label levels of hypoxemia. Hypoxemia is treated with oxygen. Oxygen should never be withheld from a client with severe hypoxia for fear of elevating PaO_2 levels.

pH. The pH is the alkalinity or acidity of blood. Normal values are considered to be 7.35 to 7.45. A value less than 7.35 is acidotic; a value greater than 7.45 is alkalotic. The pH must remain within the narrow limits of normal for enzymes to function and normal body metabolism to occur. If the body becomes acidotic, cardiac contractions diminish and normal vascular reactions to catecholamines decrease. In an alkalotic state, tissue oxygenation and neuromuscular functions are impaired.

PaCO₂. Normal values for $PaCO_2$ are 35 to 45 mm Hg. $PaCO_2$ indicates the efficiency of alveolar ventilation. *Alveolar ventilation* is defined as the inspired air that reaches the alveoli and participates in gas exchange. (See Chapter 38 for further details related to gas exchange.) Alveolar hypoventilation or ventilatory failure is diagnosed when a $PaCO_2$ greater than 50 mm Hg is observed. Alveolar hyperventilation, with a $PaCO_2$ less than

30 mm Hg, is the result of overbreathing. It is important to remember that CO_2 reflects acid. It normally combines with water to form carbonic acid. Therefore, when the $PaCO_2$ is high, blood is acidotic. If the $PaCO_2$ is low, the blood is alkalotic. The $PaCO_2$ is the respiratory component of ABGs. The lungs can compensate for pH abnormalities in 15 minutes to 1 hour.

HCO_3^-. Normal levels of HCO_3^- are 22 to 26 mEq/L. HCO_3^-, or bicarbonate, a base, represents the metabolic component of acid-base balance and is regulated by the kidneys. When there is too much HCO_3^- in the blood (>26 mEq/L), the blood is alkaline. The body may become acidotic if the HCO_3^- is low (<22 mEq/L).

The Presence and Degree of Compensation. To help the body remain in homeostasis and maintain a normal pH, a compensatory mechanism exists. A healthy renal or respiratory system can partially or completely offset the effects of a fluctuating pH. To determine if compensation is present, examine the $PaCO_2$ and HCO_3^- levels. Compensation is taking place if both are abnormal in opposite directions. Partial compensation exists when there is evidence of compensation but the pH remains abnormal. Complete compensation is present if the pH is normal and $PaCO_2$ and HCO_3^- are normal. Compensation is absent if one of the components ($PaCO_2$ or HCO_3^-) is normal and the other abnormal.

Identification of the Primary Disorder. To identify the primary disorder causing the acid-base imbalance, the pH level must be consistent with one of the acid-base components. For instance, if the pH is low and the $PaCO_2$ is high, respiratory acidosis is the primary disorder. Both the pH and $PaCO_2$ are acidotic and the $PaCO_2$ is the respiratory component of acid-base balance.

The lungs play a major role in acid-base balance. Changes in the retention or elimination of carbon dioxide will directly affect pH. However, the lungs may act in a compensatory manner to correct metabolic acid-base disorders with hypoventilation or hyperventilation as the compensatory mechanism. Changes in pH that correlate with changes in carbon dioxide indicate primary respiratory abnormalities. For example, an increase in $PaCO_2$ will result in a decrease in pH, as in ventilatory failure. The lungs are not able to remove carbon dioxide, and the ABG reflects hypoventilation with an increase in $PaCO_2$ and decrease in pH. The reverse is also true; as the $PaCO_2$ decreases, the pH will increase, as in a hyperventilatory state. Deep, rapid respirations "blow off" carbon dioxide, and the ABG analysis reveals a low $PaCO_2$ level with an increased pH.

The physician or other clinician skilled in arterial puncture must collect the blood sample. In most hospitals, physicians are the only personnel allowed to draw from the femoral artery, whereas nurses and respiratory therapists with special training can draw radial or brachial samples.

Preprocedure Care. Educate the client about the procedure and the need for the test. The client should be told that the needle-stick will be painful for a moment, and he or she must hold very still. The client's arm may need to be held still during the procedure to avoid inadvertent injury to the nerves, vessels, or tendons. After the test is completed, tell the client that pressure must be held at the puncture site for 5 to 10 minutes and it may be uncomfortable.

An Allen test must be completed before the procedure is initiated (Figure 39–14, A–C). Before the sample is drawn, the site must be treated with a disinfectant and allowed to dry. Position the area to facilitate the puncture. Help the client remain calm during the test by explaining what is happening. If the client is anxious about the test or other problems and hyperventilating, the results of the test may be altered. The amount of blood needed for the sample varies with each laboratory but may be as small as 0.5 ml, or as large as 10 ml.

Postprocedure Care. After the sample is drawn, continuous pressure must be applied to the site for 5 minutes for radial and brachial sites and 10 minutes for femoral sites. Pressure bandages are commonly used. If the client has a tendency to bleed, or is on an anticoagulant, pressure is needed for a longer period of time. When interpreting the results, note whether the client is receiving oxygen; the amount and source of oxygen should be recorded on the laboratory request form. The results are evaluated in light of the degree of oxygen needed. For example, if a client's PaO_2 is 85 mm Hg on 50% oxygen, the client has a more significant problem with oxygen transport than does the client whose PaO_2 is 85 mm Hg on room air (21% oxygen). Complications from arterial sampling include bleeding or hematoma formation at the site and injury to the artery and surrounding structures. Report any of these signs to the physician.

Ventilation-Perfusion Lung Scan

Ventilation-perfusion (V/Q) scanning is used to assess lung ventilation and lung perfusion. V/Q scans are valuable in diagnosing pulmonary embolism, pulmonary infarction, emphysema, fibrosis, and bronchiectasis. Quantitative perfusion scans may be helpful in preoperative assessment of clients undergoing surgical resection of thoracic malignancy.

Procedure. The test has two parts (done together or separately): (1) assessing the distribution of ventilation (ventilation scan), and (2) assessing the pulmonary vasculature (perfusion scan).

Ventilation Scan. Radioactive gas is inhaled, which produces an image of the areas where ventilation is occurring. Assessment of the pattern of deposition of radioactive gas in the alveoli is also possible.

Ventilation images are compared with the pictures taken during the perfusion scan. There should be an equal amount of radioactivity discernible on both ventilation and perfusion pictures. If there are areas in which there is ventilation but little or no perfusion, a pulmonary embolus is suspected (Fig. 39–15). Further assessment may be

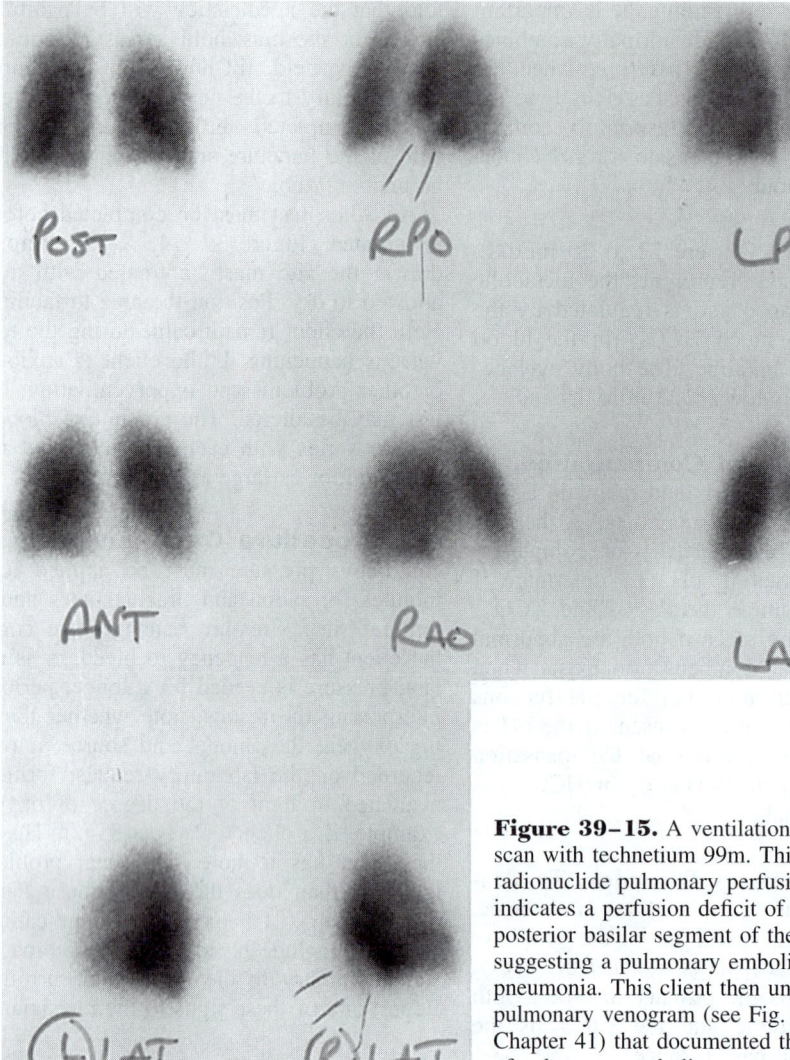

Figure 39–15. A ventilation-perfusion scan with technetium 99m. This upright radionuclide pulmonary perfusion study indicates a perfusion deficit of the right posterior basilar segment of the lung, suggesting a pulmonary embolism or pneumonia. This client then underwent a pulmonary venogram (see Fig. 41–9 in Chapter 41) that documented the presence of pulmonary embolism.

needed. If there is doubt as to the cause of impaired perfusion, pulmonary angiography may be needed.

Perfusion Scan. Radiologic material (non-iodine-based) is injected intravenously and carried into the pulmonary vasculature. Decreased blood flow to any part of the lungs is revealed as a decrease in the amount of radioactivity shown on either the x-ray film with use of a rectilinear scanner or on Polaroid film with use of a gamma or scintillation camera. Scanning is done in both the anterior and posterior views.

Preprocedure Care. Explain the procedure to the client. The test is painless with the exception of local discomfort from the injection of radiologic material for the perfusion scan. The client will hear clicking noises during the scan, but the noise is not loud. If the client has dyspnea while lying down, reassure him or her that sitting up is possible during the procedure. Radiation exposure is minimal. The client may remain dressed with all metal items removed. The procedure takes 30 to 60 minutes to complete.

Tests to Evaluate Anatomic Structures

The following diagnostic tests are done to evaluate the anatomic structures:

● Chest x-ray studies
● Ultrasonography
● Fluoroscopy
● Computed tomography (CT)
● Magnetic resonance imaging (MRI)
● Gallium scan
● Bronchoscopy
● Alveolar lavage
● Endoscopic thoracotomy
● Pulmonary angiography

Chest X-Ray Studies

Chest x-ray studies provide information about the chest that may not be available through other assessment means. Also, they often graphically illustrate the cause of respiratory dysfunction. Chest films may reveal abnormalities when there are no physical manifestations of pulmonary disease.

Chest films show the bony structures (e.g., ribs, sternum, clavicles, scapulae, and upper portion of the humerus). The vertebral column is visible vertically through the middle of the thorax. The two hemidiaphragms normally appear rounded, smooth, and sharply defined, with the right hemidiaphragm slightly higher than the left. The junction of the rib cage and the diaphragm, called the costophrenic angle, is normally clearly visible and angled. Heart tissue is dense and appears white but less intensely white than bony structures. The heart shadow is normally clearly outlined, extends primarily onto the left side of the thorax, and occupies no more than one third of the chest width. Close observation shows the trachea in the upper middle chest almost superimposed above the cervical and thoracic vertebrae. The trachea bifurcates at the level of the fourth thoracic vertebra into the right and left mainstem bronchi. The pulmonary blood vessels, bronchi, and lymph nodes are located in the hilum on both the right and left sides of the midthorax. Lung tissue appears black on x-ray film. Vascular lung structures are visible as white, thin, wispy strings fanning out from the hilum (Fig. 39–16).

Chest x-ray studies may be taken (1) as part of a routine screening procedure, (2) when pulmonary disease is suspected, (3) to monitor the status of respiratory disorders and abnormalities (e.g., pleural effusion, atelectasis, and tubercular lesions), (4) to confirm endotracheal or tracheostomy tube placement, (5) after traumatic chest injury, or (6) in any other situation in which radiographic information helps in the management of a respiratory problem.

Procedure. Routine adult chest x-ray studies are taken with the client standing or sitting facing the x-ray film, with the chest and shoulders in direct contact with the film cassette. The shoulders are rotated forward to pull the scapulae away from the lung field. The x-ray beam

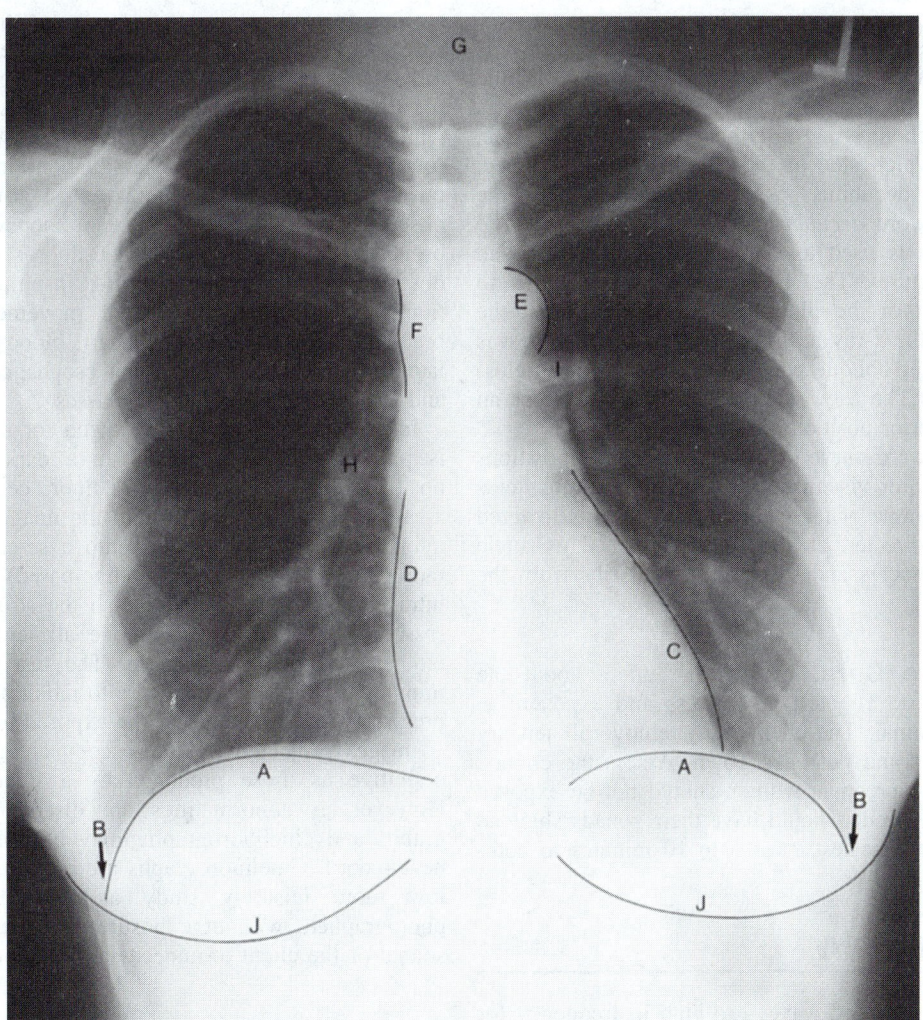

Figure 39–16. A normal chest x-ray taken from the posteroanterior view. The backward *L* in the upper right corner is placed on the film to indicate the left side of the client's chest. *A,* diaphragm; *B,* costophrenic angle; *C,* left ventricle; *D,* right atrium; *E,* aortic arch; *F,* superior vena cava; *G,* trachea; *H,* right bronchus; *I,* left bronchus; *J,* breast shadows.

penetrates from posterior. This position is called the posteroanterior (PA) position. The radiograph is usually taken at full inspiration, which causes the diaphragm to move downward. Radiographs taken on expiration are sometimes requested for demonstrating the degree of diaphragm movement or for assisting in the assessment and diagnosis of pneumothorax.

For clients unable to be transported to the radiology department, a portable chest radiograph may be taken. Portable radiographs are usually taken with the film placed behind the client, and the x-ray beam penetrates from the front of the chest—the anteroposterior (AP) position. Because the x-ray beam enters from anterior, the heart will appear larger than it really is and larger than on a PA view.

Other positions include the lateral view, which usually accompanies a standard PA view. It is taken from either the right or left side of the chest. The arms are raised above the head, and the side of the chest is placed against the film. The lateral view allows better visualization of the heart and the dome of the diaphragm. When used in conjunction with a PA film, a lateral position gives a three-dimensional view, allowing more specific identification of the location of an abnormality.

The lateral decubitus position may be used when it is necessary to determine whether opaque areas on the pleura are due to solid or liquid media. This view is taken with the client lying on either the right or left side, depending on which side of the chest is being assessed. In a left lateral decubitus position the client lies on the left side. (The word *decubitus* means "lying-down.") The oblique position is used to visualize behind and around underlying structures. The shoulders are rotated either to the right or left of the film. By turning the client, the angle at which the x-ray beam passes through the chest is shifted. In a right oblique position, the right side is closest to the film. The view may be taken from either an anterior or posterior position.

Lordotic (forward curve of the lumbar spine) positions are useful if clearer visualization of the upper lung fields is needed. The angle of the cathode x-ray tube is lowered and the beam directed at an upward angle. This angle removes the clavicles and first and second ribs from the field of vision.

Preprocedure Care. Instruct the client about the need for this test. The test is painless and exposure to radiation is minimal. The client must remove all jewelry and underclothes and put on a gown. Assess the client's pregnancy status; pregnant women should not be exposed to radiation. All clients should have their gonads shielded during the x-ray. The test takes 5 to 10 minutes to complete.

Ultrasonography

Ultrasonic waves (sound waves too high in frequency for a human ear to detect) are used diagnostically to assess various body structures. The waves are directed at the organ or structure, and as they vibrate back from the target, they are transduced into oscilloscope tracings. Sonography may be used in conjunction with other pulmonary diagnostic procedures such as thoracentesis or pleural biopsy to assess fluid or fibrotic abnormalities. Ultrasonography is especially helpful and very accurate in detecting the amount and location of 50 ml or less of pleural fluid. In comparison, a positive detection by chest radiography requires at least 500 ml of liquid. If the technique is used in combination with thoracentesis, the ultrasonographer can determine the best location for needle placement as well as the depth of the fluid. This facilitates obtaining an adequate amount of fluid for laboratory analysis without unnecessary puncturing and probing.

Instruct the client as to the need for this procedure. The test is painless. Gel is applied to the skin and it may be cool or warmed. Ultrasound is noninvasive, that is, the client is not exposed to ionizing radiation. The client may remain dressed or put on a gown. The test will take 15 to 30 minutes to complete.

Fluoroscopy

Fluoroscopy uses x-rays to observe deep structures in motion. Instead of producing a single, still image, a fluoroscopy screen registers a constant image of the chest (or other body part) being examined. This makes it possible for the chest and intrathoracic structures to be observed while they function dynamically. Fluoroscopy is not used routinely, but rather in those situations in which continuous observation of the thorax is an advantage (e.g., to observe transbronchial passage of biopsy forceps during bronchoscopy). Other uses for fluoroscopy include (1) observing the diaphragm during inspiration and expiration, (2) detecting mediastinal movement during deep breathing, (3) assessing the heart, blood vessels, and related structures, (4) identifying esophageal abnormalities, and (5) detecting mediastinal masses.

Instruct the client as to the need for this test. The test is painless. Place the client in a darkened room, and position him or her between a fluorescent screen and an x-ray source (x-ray tube), with the images of the moving internal structures projected onto a screen. Sometimes a radiopaque medium (non–iodine-based) is administered intravenously to help distinguish the structures being assessed. The client must remove all jewelry and underclothes and put on a gown. The test takes 30 to 45 minutes to complete. Exposure to radiation is minimal but pregnant women should not be exposed to fluoroscopy.

Images projected by fluoroscopy are not as clear and definitive as those produced by a standard chest film. However, if abnormalities are discovered, still photographs and cinefluorography may be done for a permanent record. Cinefluorographs are motion pictures that allow more leisurely study and restudy of the area photographed, without exposure of either radiology personnel or the client to unnecessary radiation.

Computed Tomography

Computed tomography (CT) provides more sophisticated tomography than is possible with conventional x-ray equipment. See Chapter 13 for a detailed discussion of CT and client preparation.

CT scans are particularly helpful in diagnosing peripheral (e.g., pleural) or mediastinal disorders. Special techniques can be used to view pulmonary nodules. Thin cuts of the CT are used in diagnosing interstitial lung disorders such as pulmonary fibrosis and bronchiectasis.

Magnetic Resonance Imaging

Magnetic resonance imaging (MRI) is the use of magnetic fields rather than radiation to create images of body structures. MRI is used much like the CT scan. The MRI is more definitive than CT because it creates more detailed images of anatomic structures. See Chapter 13 for a detailed discussion of MRI and client preparation.

Gallium Scans

This type of scan is usually done 24 to 48 hours after intravenous injection of radioactive gallium citrate. Many organs take up radioactive gallium, and so do some tumors and inflammations. An example of the use of a gallium scan is in differentiating embolism from pneumonitis as the cause of an infiltrate on a chest radiograph. Gallium has an affinity for areas of inflammation such as those caused by pneumonia. However, there is little inflammation involved in a nonseptic pulmonary embolism. Therefore, gallium accumulates around pneumonitis, but not around a pulmonary embolism. The usefulness of gallium scanning in clinical pulmonary assessment is limited.

Educate the client about the test and the need for it. The test is painless with the exception of local pain at the injection site. Gallium is not iodine-based and has no side effects. The client returns for serial scans at 24, 48, or 72 hours. Scanning is performed with the client supine. The client may remain dressed but must remove all metal objects. The scan takes 45 to 60 minutes to complete.

Bronchoscopy

Procedure. Bronchoscopy is the passage of a lighted bronchoscope into the bronchial tree (Fig. 39–17). Bronchoscopy may be performed with rigid steel or flexible fiberoptic instruments. Bronchoscopy may be performed for diagnostic or therapeutic purposes. The diagnostic purposes include (1) examination of tissue (2) further evaluation of a tumor for potential surgical resection, (3) collection of tissue specimens for diagnosis, and (4) evaluation of bleeding sites. Therapeutic bronchoscopy is used to (1) remove foreign bodies, (2) remove thick, viscous secretions, (3) treat postoperative atelectasis, and (4) destroy and remove lesions.

Preprocedure Care. Explain the procedure to the client and family and obtain an informed consent. Instruct

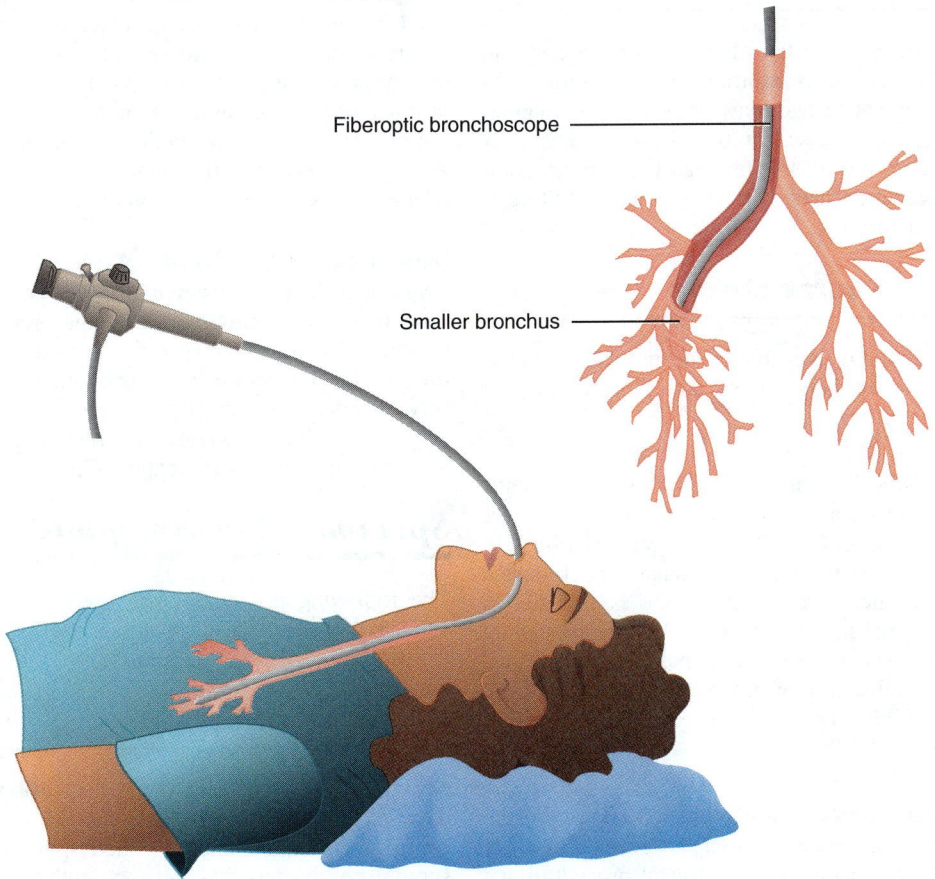

Fiberoptic bronchoscope

Smaller bronchus

Figure 39–17. Bronchoscopy.

the client not to eat or drink anything 6 hours before the test. The client is told that his or her throat may be sore after bronchoscopy, and some initial difficulty swallowing will be present. Before preprocedural sedation, dentures, contact lenses, and other prostheses are removed. The client undresses and puts on a gown. Local anesthesia and intravenous sedation are used to suppress the cough, and to relieve anxiety. A topical anesthetic is also sprayed into the back of the throat. The test takes 30 to 45 minutes to complete.

During the procedure, the client lies supine with the head hyperextended. The nurse monitors vital signs, talks to and reassures the client, and assists the physician as necessary.

Postprocedure Care. After the procedure, vital signs are monitored per agency protocol. Observe the client for signs of respiratory distress, including dyspnea, changes in respiratory rate, use of accessory muscles, and changes in or absent lung sounds. Expectorated secretions are inspected for evidence of hemoptysis. Nothing is given by mouth until the cough and swallow reflexes have returned, which is usually in 1 to 2 hours. Once the client can swallow, feeding may begin with ice chips and small sips of water. Lung sounds are monitored for 24 hours. Development of asymmetrical or adventitious sounds should be reported to the physician. Pneumothorax has been noted after bronchoscopy.

Alveolar Lavage

Sterile saline can be injected during bronchoscopy to wash tissues. The saline is aspirated and examined for atypical cells. Alveolar lavage may be used in the diagnosis of interstitial lung disease, sarcoidosis, hypersensitivity pneumonitis, and *P. carinii* pneumonia. There is no additional client preparation needed because this procedure is done during bronchoscopy.

Endoscopic Thoracotomy

Endoscopic thoracotomy is a diagnostic procedure that is an alternative to open lung biopsy and thoracotomy for pleural surface disorders.

Procedure. Typically, three small incisions are made into the middle chest wall. A scope attached to a camera and video projector is inserted through the first incision to inspect tissue, and tissues are manipulated and biopsied through the other incisions. A chest tube is inserted to promote lung reexpansion. Advantages of the procedure include reduced anesthesia time, less pain, and shortened hospital stay. In addition, biopsies may be obtained from the lower lobes, which are not routinely biopsied during open lung biopsy procedures.

Preprocedure Care. Instruct the client as to the need for this test and obtain a signed informed consent form. Endoscopic thoracotomy is a surgical procedure and the client will be receiving general anesthesia (see Chap-

ter 20 for a discussion of the needs of the surgical patient). Instruct the client that he or she will have a chest tube in place and will need to perform coughing and deep breathing exercises.

Pulmonary Angiography

Sometimes the vascular structure of the thorax needs to be assessed. Angiography and other procedures designed to examine specific vascular structures (i.e., aortography for the aorta) all use similar techniques.

Pulmonary angiography may be done to detect (1) congenital abnormalities of the pulmonary vascular tree, (2) abnormalities of the pulmonary venous circulation, (3) acquired diseases of the pulmonary arterial and venous circulation (e.g., primary pulmonary arterial hypertension), (4) the destructive effects of emphysema, (5) the potential benefit of resection for bronchogenic carcinoma, (6) peripheral pulmonary lesions, and (7) the extent of thromboembolism in the lungs.

Procedure. Contrast medium is injected into the vascular system through an indwelling catheter. During pulmonary angiography, the catheter may be inserted either peripherally or directly into the main pulmonary artery or one of its branches. The contrast medium is injected while cinefluorographs or still photographs are taken. (Pulmonary angiography is shown in Chapter 41.)

Preprocedure Care. Instruct the client as to the need for this test and obtain informed consent. The test is painless and exposure to radiation is minimal. It will be uncomfortable for the client when the indwelling catheter is placed with the insertion of a needle. The client must remove all jewelry and underclothes and put on a gown. Assess the client's pregnancy status; pregnant women should not be exposed to radiation.

Postprocedure Care. As with any procedure in which a catheter is inserted into the peripheral or central vasculature, it is important after the procedure to observe the site of catheter entry for infection, hematoma formation, or local reaction to contrast media. Continue to observe for signs of an adverse reaction to contrast media (e.g., increasing respiratory distress, hypotension, stridor, and other indications of anaphylaxis).

Specimen Recovery and Analysis

The following procedures are used for the recovery and analysis of pulmonary specimens: (1) sputum collection, (2) thoracentesis, (3) and biopsy.

Sputum Collection

Normally, the goblet cells product 100 ml of mucus a day, but an infectious process can lead to excessive mucus production, commonly called sputum. Assessment of sputum for bacteria, fungus, or cellular elements assists the practitioner in treating the underlying infection.

Procedure. The sputum is initially inspected for color, quantity, quality, presence of blood, food particles, or other unusual contents. If possible, sputum should be collected before antimicrobial treatment is begun.

Acid-fast smear and culture specimens are collected in the morning, at which time sputum is more plentiful and concentrated from pooling through the night. Sputum can be collected by the direct method, by the indirect method, or by gastric lavage.

Preprocedure Care. Instruct the client as to the need and purpose of this test. To obtain a specimen by the direct method, the client first brushes the teeth to reduce contamination, then coughs into a sputum specimen container. The client should be encouraged to cough and not spit, so as to obtain sputum. Sputum can be thinned to aid expectoration by inhaling nebulized saline or water.

Indirect techniques for obtaining sputum use a sterile suction catheter with a sputum trap attached to the catheter. Sputum can be obtained by transtracheal aspiration also. A puncture is made with a needle through the cricothyroid membrane into the trachea, and sputum is aspirated. Gastric lavage is not a common technique for obtaining sputum but can be used in uncooperative or extremely ill clients. Lavage is based on the assumption that sputum is swallowed while sleeping and sometimes after coughing. A nasogastric tube is inserted using appropriate techniques. Gastric juice is aspirated with a syringe and sent to the laboratory. The tube is then removed.

Once collected, the sputum is sent to the laboratory for Gram stain, culture, and sensitivity study. The Gram stain classifies the bacteria as gram-positive or gram-negative and provides guidelines for appropriate antimicrobial therapy, along with the sputum culture. After the Gram stain, the sputum is incubated for 24 hours or longer on the appropriate culture medium and studied by a microbiologist. The culture allows further identification of the infecting organism. Once the organism is identified, its sensitivity to antibiotic treatment is tested and an appropriate antibiotic(s) is prescribed.

Identification of organisms that cause tuberculosis and similar diseases (acid-fast bacilli) requires tests other than the Gram stain, culture, and sensitivity study.

Regardless of the technique used to obtain the specimen, the nurse notes the color, consistency, odor, and amount of sputum obtained.

Nose and Throat Cultures

Bacteria in the nose and throat can be identified by culture during assessment of the upper airway. Some bacteria are normally present (e.g., streptococci, staphylococci, pneumococci, *Haemophilus influenzae;* and *Klebsiella pneumoniae*). Other organisms are abnormal (e.g., those causing diphtheria or tuberculosis).

Swab the nose and throat using a sterile cotton swab. Place the swab in a sterile culture tube. Some laboratories require the swab to be suspended in a tube containing 2 ml of fluid (to keep air in the tube moist and prevent evaporation and drying of the specimen). The fluid is not a culture medium, so the swab should not touch the fluid. If Loeffler's medium is used in the tube (i.e., if diphtheria is suspected), the medium should touch the swab. When culture tubes without fluid are used, take the specimen to the laboratory immediately, where the swab is streaked across a culture plate.

Thoracentesis

Procedure. *Thoracentesis* is the drainage of fluid or air found in the pleural space. Therapeutic thoracentesis will remove an accumulation of pleural fluid or air that has caused lung compression and respiratory distress. When the main goal is to determine the cause of an infection or empyema, diagnostic thoracentesis is performed. The fluid collected is sent to the laboratory and assessed for specific gravity, glucose, protein, pH, culture, sensitivity study, and cytology. The color and consistency of the pleural fluid are also documented.

Preprocedure Care. Obtain informed consent and instruct the client about the procedure and the need for it. The client will need to sit upright while leaning over the tray table. Figure 39–18A shows the appropriate positioning for thoracentesis. With the client in the upright position, pleural fluid accumulates in the base of the thorax. Alternatively, place the client in a recumbent position with his or her arm resting under the head. Insertion of the needle will be painful. Instruct the client about the importance of holding still during the procedure. Sudden movement may force the needle through the pleural space and injure the visceral pleura or lung parenchyma. Tell the client that you will help hold him or her and provide reassurance. The test takes 5 to 15 minutes to complete.

During the procedure, assist the physician; monitor vital signs; and observe for dyspnea, complaints of difficulty breathing, nausea, or pain.

Postprocedure Care. After the procedure, the client is usually turned onto the unaffected side for 1 hour to facilitate lung expansion. Vital signs should be assessed according to the facility's policy. The respiratory rate and character and breath sounds should be assessed carefully. Tachypnea, dyspnea, cyanosis, retractions, or diminished breath sounds, which may indicate pneumothorax, should be reported to the physician.

The amount of fluid withdrawn should be recorded as fluid output. A chest x-ray study may be performed to evaluate the degree of lung reexpansion or pneumothorax. Subcutaneous emphysema may follow this procedure, because air in the pleural cavity leaks into subcutaneous tissues. The tissues feel like lumpy paper and crackle when palpated (crepitus). Usually subcutaneous emphysema causes no problem unless it is increasing and constricting vital organs (e.g., trachea). The client often needs reassurance about this disorder.

If the client has pleural effusion due to a malignancy, cytotoxic medications may be inserted into the pleural space after thoracentesis. Some of these agents burn, and others require the client to roll about in order to have the

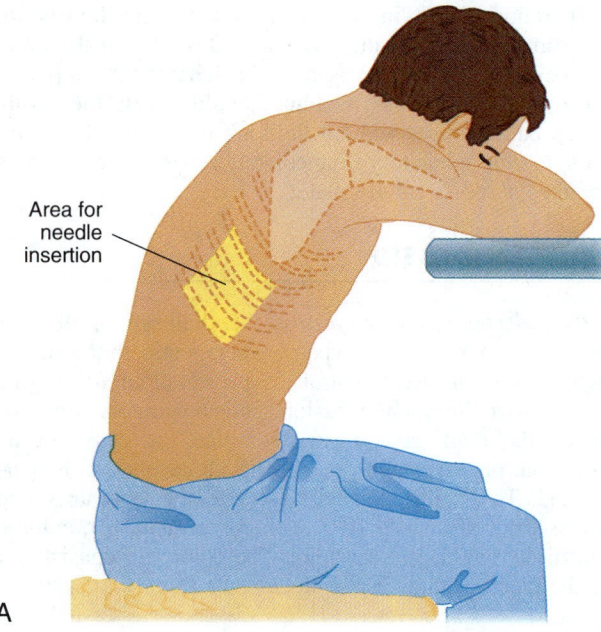

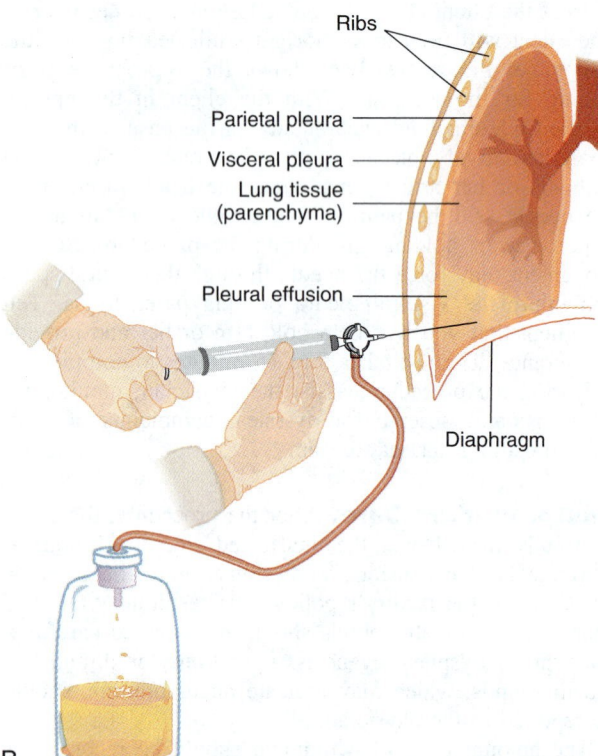

Figure 39–18. Thoracentesis. *A,* Correct position of the client for the procedure. The arms are raised and crossed. The head rests on the folded arms. This position allows the chest wall to be pulled outward in an expanded position. If an institutional overbed table is not available, you may leave the client's arms down, but position them toward the client's hips or cross them in front of the chest. *B,* Usual site for insertion of a thoracentesis needle for a right-sided effusion. The actual site varies, depending on the location and volume of the effusion. The needle is kept as far away from the diaphragm as possible, but is inserted close to the base of the effusion so that gravity can help with drainage.

medication coat the entire pleural space. Review the interventions used with the various medications.

Biopsy

Biopsy specimens may be taken from various respiratory tissues for examination. As previously mentioned, biopsy of tracheobronchial structures may be performed during bronchoscopy. Biopsies of scalene and mediastinal nodes may be done (with local anesthesia) to obtain tissue for pathologic study, culture, or cytologic assessment.

■ Pleural Biopsy

Procedure. Pleural biopsies may be performed surgically through a small thoracotomy incision or during thoracentesis, using a Cope needle. Needle biopsy is a relatively safe, simple diagnostic procedure that is useful for determining the cause of pleural effusions. The needle removes a small fragment of parietal pleura, which is used for microscopic cellular examination and culture. If bacteriologic studies are needed, the biopsy specimen should be obtained before chemotherapy is begun.

Preprocedure Care. Obtain informed consent and instruct the client as to the need and purpose of the test. The preparation and positioning of a client for pleural biopsy is similar to that for thoracentesis. The test is painful, and the client will need to hold still. Assist the client and reassure him or her. The test takes 15 to 30 minutes to complete.

Postprocedure Care. Rare complications include temporary pain from intercostal nerve injury, pneumothorax, and hemothorax. After the biopsy procedure, observe for indications of complications (e.g., dyspnea, pallor, diaphoresis, excessive pain). A pneumothorax associated with needle biopsy may develop. Chest tubes and chest drainage equipment must be available. Follow-up chest x-ray studies are usually done after the procedure. The development of hemothorax is indicated by a substantial increase in fluid in the pleural space and requires immediate thoracentesis.

■ Lung Biopsy

As with pleural biopsy, lung biopsy may be done by surgical exposure of the lung (open lung biopsy) with or without endoscopy using a needle designed to remove a core of lung tissue. Tissue is then examined for abnormal cellular structure and bacteria. Lung biopsies are most often done to identify pulmonary tumors or parenchymal changes (e.g., sarcoidosis).

■ Aspiration Biopsy of Chest Lesions

Procedure. Needle puncture (aspiration) biopsy of chest lesions is done under fluoroscopy. After a lesion is found on a chest x-ray study and localized under fluoroscopy, topical anesthesia is administered, and the needle is inserted through the chest wall into the lung tissue and lesion. A small sample of cells is aspirated for microscopic study, and the needle is withdrawn. Aspiration biopsy may enable definitive diagnosis of malignant neoplasms, granulomas, or other nonmalignant growths. Possible complications of needle aspiration lung biopsy are hemoptysis, hemothorax, and pneumothorax.

Postprocedure Care. After the procedure, examine any sputum closely for evidence of blood. Observe for respiratory distress (may indicate pneumothorax). Monitor the client's vital signs, breath sounds, skin color, and temperature.

Conclusions

Respiratory assessment begins with obtaining a thorough client history. One of the most essential aspects of history-taking is to determine the degree of dyspnea and the impact it has on activities of daily living. The client's smoking history and occupational risks should also be noted, because they are common risk factors for respiratory disorders. The chest is inspected for obvious deformity and shape. Percussion, palpation, and auscultation assist in locating areas of possible fluid accumulation or consolidation that interfere with breathing.

Chest x-ray studies, bronchoscopy, pulmonary function tests, and arterial blood gas analysis are common diagnostic assessments. Educate the client about the diagnostic assessment and monitor for potential complications after the study.

Bibliography

1. Bates, B. (1995). *A guide to physical assessment and history taking* (6th ed.). Philadelphia: J. B. Lippincott.
2. Burton, G., Hodgkin, J., & Ward, J. (1991). *Respiratory care: A guide to clinical practice.* Philadelphia: J. B. Lippincott.
3. Desai, S., & Chan, O. (1992). Interpretation of a normal chest x-ray. *Nursing Standard, 7*(7), 38–39.
4. Gift, A. G., & Nield, M. D. (1991). Dyspnea: A case for nursing diagnosis status. *Nursing Diagnosis, 2*(2), 66–71.
5. Gift, A. G., & Pugh, L. C. (1993). Dyspnea and fatigue. *Nursing Clinics of North America, 28*(2), 373–384.
6. Guyton, A. C. (1996). *Textbook of medical physiology* (9th ed.). Philadelphia: W. B. Saunders.
7. Jarvis, C. (1996). *Physical examination and health assessment* (2nd ed.). Philadelphia: W. B. Saunders.
8. Kelly-Heidenthal, P., & O'Connor, M. (1994). Nursing assessment of portable AP chest x-rays. *Dimensions of Critical Care Nursing, 13*(3), 127–132.
9. Malley, W. (1990). *Clinical blood gases: Application and noninvasive alternates.* Philadelphia: W. B. Saunders.
10. McCord, M., & Cronin-Stubbs, D. (1992). Operationalizing dyspnea: Focus on measurement. *Heart and Lung 21*(2), 167.
11. Murray, J. F., & Nadel, J. A. (1994). *The textbook of respiratory medicine* (2nd ed.). Philadelphia: W. B. Saunders.
12. Pastercamp, H. (1990). R. A. L. E. [computer disk for IBM-PC/XT/AT or compatible]. PixSoft, Inc.
13. Peters, K., et al. (1990). Increasing clinical use of pulse oximetry. *Dimensions of Critical Care Nursing, 9*(2), 107–111.
14. Pierson, D., & Kacmarek, R. (1992). *Foundations of respiratory care.* New York: Churchill Livingston.
15. Ruppel, G. (1994). *Manual of pulmonary function testing* (5th ed.). St. Louis: Mosby–Year Book.
16. Shapiro, B. A., et al. (1991). *Clinical application of respiratory care* (4th ed.). St. Louis: Mosby–Year Book.
17. Shapiro, B. A., et al. (1994). *Clinical application of blood gases* (5th ed.). St. Louis: Mosby–Year Book.
18. Speck, D., et al. (1993). *Respiratory control: Central-peripheral mechanisms.* Lexington, KY: University of Kentucky.
19. Von Rueden, K. T. (1990). Noninvasive assessment of gas exchange in the critically ill. *AACN Clinical Issues in Critical Care Nursing, 1*(2), 239–247.
20. West, J. B. (1995). *Respiratory physiology* (5th ed.). Baltimore: Williams & Wilkins.
21. Wilkins, R., & Dexter, J. (1990) Comparing RCPs to physicians for the description of lung sounds: Are we accurate and can we communicate? *Respiratory Care, 35*(10), 969–976.

Nursing Care of Clients with Upper Airway Disorders

Barbara Sigler

Clients with disorders of the upper airway will initially complain of problems with breathing. You will observe obstruction to nasal breathing in clients with nasal polyps, deviated nasal septum, or nasal fractures. Following surgical interventions, nasal breathing will continue to be compromised because of postoperative edema. Laryngeal disorders may also result in breathing problems. Tumors of the larynx create an obstruction to the flow of air entering the trachea, as well as an obstruction to the air being exhaled. Vocal cord paralysis and laryngospasm may also affect the passage of air through the larynx and vocal cords. Clients with epistaxis and sinusitis will have bleeding, drainage, and may exhibit fever and pain. Inflammation associated with these problems results in obstruction to breathing. Surgical intervention and nasal packing will further compromise these problems.

Tracheostomy

A *tracheotomy* is a surgical opening made into the trachea for airway management. A *tracheostomy* is the surgical creation of a stoma from the trachea to the overlying skin. Even though the terms indicate different procedures, they are often used interchangeably. Realizing the difference in terms, but for the benefit of simplicity, the term tracheostomy is used here.

Tracheostomy is a life-saving procedure used only when other options for airway management are not feasible. The tracheostomy also provides the best route for long-term airway maintenance. Because of its many indications it is discussed at the beginning of this chapter.

Indications for tracheostomy are the following:

- Need for long-term artificial airway
- Upper airway obstruction
- Upper airway bleeding
- Decreasing level of consciousness and inability to protect the lower airway
- Inability to clear lower airway secretions

- Need for continuous mechanical ventilation
- Prolonged endotracheal tube insertion, causing erosion or pain
- Sleep apnea
- Laryngeal or tracheal fracture
- Airway burns

Tracheostomy is by far the most satisfactory artificial airway. It totally bypasses the upper airway and glottis. Tracheostomy makes it easier to stabilize, suction, and attach respiratory equipment than other types of artificial airways. The client can eat and, with some adjustments, can talk.

A tracheostomy is performed by making an incision in the lower neck (Fig. 40–1). It can be performed as an emergency or elective procedure.

Tracheostomy Tubes

Tracheostomy tubes vary in their (1) composition, (2) number of separate parts, (3) shape, and (4) size. Tracheostomy tubes are chosen specifically for each client. Incorrectly fitted tubes can precipitate permanent or life-threatening damage.

A tracheostomy tube's diameter should be smaller than the trachea so that it will lie comfortably within the tracheal lumen. Air should be able to pass between the outer wall of the tracheostomy tube and the tracheal mucosa. Although there is no standard tracheostomy tube sizing system, all packages indicate the inner and outer diameter in millimeters.

The length and curve of a tracheostomy tube are important. Tracheostomy tubes may be long (e.g., Hollinger tube, Shiley single-cannula tube), or short. They may be angled from 50 to 90 degrees. Short to moderately short tubes with an angle of about 60 degrees are most often used. A tube must be long enough to avoid dislodgment into paratracheal tissue when the person coughs or turns the head. The lower end of a tracheostomy tube should be located above the carina. The tube's curve must allow

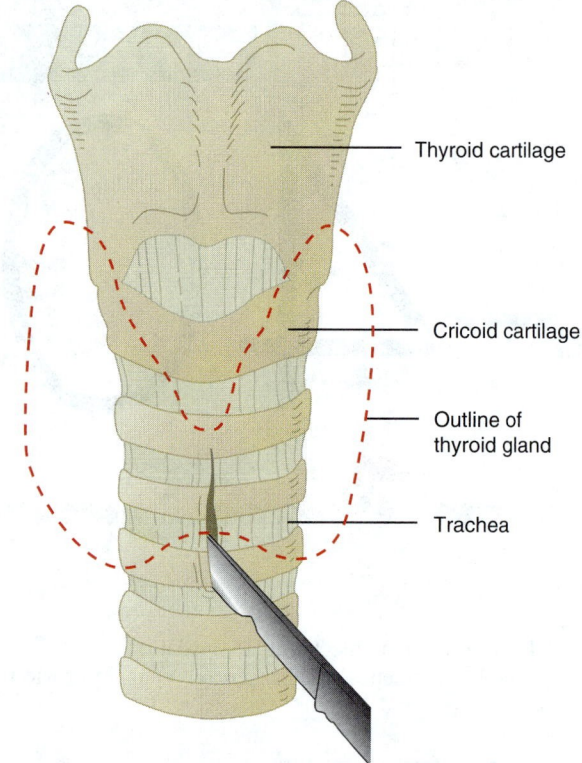

Figure 40–1. Incision for a tracheostomy is made vertically through the second, third, or fourth tracheal ring.

the tip to be in a straight line with the trachea rather than press on the anterior or posterior tracheal wall.

Tracheostomy tubes may be cuffed or uncuffed. Inflated cuffs permit mechanical ventilation and protect the lower airway by creating a seal between the upper and lower airways. Tracheostomy cuffs do not hold the tube in place. Rather, when inflated, they seal the area between the outer cannula and the tracheal wall.

Tracheostomy tubes are made of various substances (e.g., nonreactive plastic, stainless steel, sterling silver). Plastic tubes are disposable and used for only one person. Metal tubes may be reused for different people following sterilization.

Universal Tracheostomy Tube. The most common tube is a universal, or standard, tracheostomy tube (Fig. 40–2) with three parts: (1) outer cannula with cuff, flange, and pilot tube, (2) inner cannula, and (3) obturator. The parts fit together as one unit and may not be interchanged with other units. Therefore, all three parts of each individual set are kept together.

The outer cannula fits in the tracheostomy stoma to keep it open. The outer cannula has a flange or neckplate that fits flush with the neck and has holes on each side to attach the securing tapes or ties. A tracheostomy tube must be secured to prevent accidental extubation, excessive motion, or misalignment. Cloth tape or commercially available Velcro ties may be used.

The obturator fits in the outer tube before insertion. Its rounded tip smooths the end of the cannula and facilitates

nontraumatic insertion of the tube into the stoma. The obturator is removed immediately after insertion to open the tube. Place the obturator in a plastic wrapper and tape it to the head of the client's bed in a conspicuous place. If the tracheostomy tube is accidentally displaced, the obturator can be immediately placed into the outer cannula for quick reinsertion.

Once the obturator is removed, the inner cannula fits into the outer cannula. Lock it into place to prevent accidental removal (e.g., when coughing). The inner cannula maintains airway patency because it is cleaned often. It is removed easily for cleaning. At the distal end, most inner cannulas have a standard 15-mm adaptor that fits respiratory therapy and anesthesiology equipment.

Single-Cannula Tracheostomy Tube. This tube is slightly longer than a double-cannula tube. Because it does not have an inner cannula that can be cleaned to eliminate secretions, clients with a single-cannula tube must have continuous supplemental humidification to prevent obstruction by accumulated secretions. The longer single-cannula tube is used in clients with a thick neck or with an altered airway in whom routine tracheostomy tubes are too short.

Fenestrated Tracheostomy Tube. A fenestrated tracheostomy tube has an opening (*fenestration*) on the curvature of the posterior wall of the outer cannula. When the inner cannula is removed, the fenestration permits air to flow through both the upper airway and the tracheostomy opening. This permits speech and more effective coughing. This tube may be used (a) while a

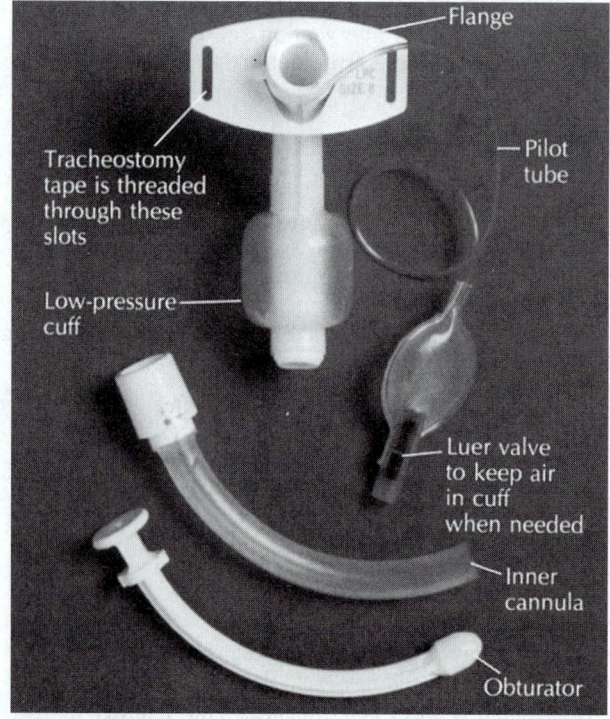

Figure 40–2. Parts of a tracheostomy tube. (Courtesy of Shiley, Inc., Irvine, CA.)

client is being weaned from a tracheostomy and (b) for a client needing long-term tracheostomy. When the inner cannula is in place, the fenestration is closed and the tube functions as a universal tracheostomy tube.

Talking Tracheostomy.

Talking Tracheostomy. This is a one-way valve in a plastic T-piece attached to the 15-mm end of the inner cannula of a universal tracheostomy tube. It permits talking without the need to plug the tracheostomy tube. The one-way valve allows air (and supplemental humidification and oxygen) to flow into the arm of the T-piece during inspiration. On exhalation, the one-way valve closes, directing air from the lungs up through the vocal cords and upper airway. Phonation and effective coughing are facilitated by this normal passage of air.

A talking tracheostomy is *never* used unless there is enough room around the tracheostomy tube to permit sufficient air flow for breathing. *Always deflate* a cuffed tracheostomy tube before using a talking tracheostomy adaptor. Cuff inflation prevents exhalation, causing suffocation.

Communitrach Tube. This tube allows speech but requires coordination. An air flow tube (which looks like a second pilot tube) runs outside the Communitrach and opens just above the cuff. There is a port at the distal end of the air flow tube. When occluded, compressed air or oxygen flow is directed through the air flow tube, generating an air flow up through the vocal cords. This air flow enables speech, although it does not sound "normal." Mucosal irritation may develop from air or oxygen flowing into the upper airway.

Tracheostomy Button. This button is sometimes used during weaning as an intermediate device between using a standard tracheostomy tube and extubation. A button is a short, straight tracheostomy tube that fits into the stoma of a tracheostomy but is not deep enough to enter the tracheal lumen. It has a removable cap with a one-way flap inside that permits inhalation but not exhalation. Exhalation occurs through the normal upper airway. When the cap is on, the person can talk.

A button cannot be used with a ventilator. It replaces a standard tracheostomy tube for people with retained secretions who do not require ventilatory assistance. A button creates less airway resistance than a plugged standard tracheostomy tube. Hence, breathing is easier. Artificial humidification of inspired air is necessary with a button (as with any tracheostomy tube), since the natural airway is bypassed.

Permanent Tracheostomy. Most clients with a permanent tracheostomy use a universal, cuffless, tracheostomy tube or an Olympic tracheostomy button. To minimize the tracheostomy's appearance, many persons prefer a low-profile inner cannula. This does not have a 15-mm adaptor incorporated. Instead, it fits into the outer cannula and lies flush with the neck. If the client has had a total laryngectomy, the cut end of the trachea is sutured to the skin creating a permanent stoma. Once healed, most laryngectomy clients will not need a tube.

Metal Tracheostomy Tube. These tubes are made of sterling silver or stainless steel. The most popular type is the Jackson tracheostomy tube. It does not have a cuff. Metal tubes are most often used following a permanent tracheostomy or laryngectomy. The inner cannula locks together with the outer cannula. Because metal tubes do not have a standard 15-mm adaptor, rapid adaptation to respiratory or anesthesia equipment is impossible unless a specific adaptor is available. The Hollinger tube is made of metal and is similar to the Jackson tube.

Potential Problems Associated with Tracheostomy Tubes and Cuffs

Most tracheostomy tube cuffs are designed to exert a low pressure against the tracheal wall through use of an easily distensible cuff that accepts a high volume of air without generating excessive force (i.e., high-volume, low-pressure cuffs). Low cuff pressure is necessary to prevent damage to the tracheal mucosa. The volume of air in the cuff determines the pressure exerted on the tracheal mucosa. Cuff pressures should not exceed 20 cm H_2O. Cuff pressure above 42 cm H_2O impairs circulation to the tracheal mucosa, resulting in ischemia of the tracheal mucosa and necrosis. This is because the normal pressure within tracheal arteries is 42 cm H_2O. In the veins and lymphatics the normal pressures are 24 cm H_2O and 7 cm H_2O, respectively.

Tracheal damage from cuff pressure is a frequent complication of intubation. Cuffed tubes can cause tracheal damage in as few as 3 to 5 days.

Tracheal Wall Necrosis. Necrosis of the tracheal wall can lead to an artificial opening between the posterior trachea and esophagus. This problem is called *tracheoesophageal fistula*. The fistula allows air to escape into the stomach, causing distention. It also promotes aspiration of gastric contents. Fistulas most often develop when a cuffed tube is used in conjunction with a standard nasogastric (NG) tube. Use of small lumen NG tubes can decrease the risk of fistula. Necrosis of the anterior trachea can lead to a rare but life-threatening complication due to erosion into the innominate artery. It is suspected when bright red blood is expelled or the tracheostomy tube pulsates. Immediate intervention is mandatory because the client can exsanguinate.

When long-term tracheostomy is required, uncuffed tracheostomy tubes are usually used unless the client is at high risk of aspiration. Some clients requiring long-term mechanical ventilation can tolerate uncuffed tracheostomy tubes. Tidal volumes and respiratory rates may be adjusted on the ventilator to produce satisfactory ventilation and arterial blood gases (ABGs) while eliminating the risks associated with tracheostomy tube cuffs.

Tracheal Dilation. Prolonged intubation can lead to dilation of the trachea from the cuff. Suspicions arise when increasing amounts of air is needed to seal the cuff, or when bulging is noted on the tracheal wall by x-ray.

Box 40–1. Inflation and Deflation of Tracheostomy Tube Cuff*

Inflation (Minimal Leak Technique)

Objective

Inflate the cuff with the minimum volume of air required to adequately seal the trachea during positive pressure ventilation and to prevent aspiration of foreign material while exerting the lowest possible cuff-to-tracheal wall pressure.

Intervention

1. Withdraw all residual air from the cuff.
2. Place 6 ml air in a syringe.
3. Place the diaphragm of a stethoscope over the client's neck in the area of the tracheostomy tube cuff.
4. On inhalation, slowly inject air through the one-way valve into the pilot line in 1-ml increments.
5. Auscultate the neck area over the cuff.
6. Apply positive pressure to the tracheostomy tube with a manual self-inflating bag. An audible air leak will be heard via the stethoscope unless the cuff is inflated.
7. Continue slowly injecting air until the air leak is no longer present during inhalation.
8. When a leak is no longer auscultated, withdraw a small amount of air from the cuff until a very small leak is heard. This is called a *minimal* leak.
9. Note the amount of air necessary to achieve the minimal leak. This is the *minimal occluding volume (MOV)*.
10. Once minimal leak is attained, measure the cuff pressure with a manometer.
11. Routinely measure and document cuff pressures.

Deflation

Objective

Allow air to flow around the tracheostomy tube to (a) permit phonation and (b) provide opportunity to blow secretions

above the cuff into the oropharynx where they may be removed by suctioning.

Intervention

Routinely deflating the cuff is not necessary provided safe cuff inflation and cuff pressure measurements are performed.

1. Remove ventilator assembly (if present), and attach a self-inflating bag to the 15-mm adaptor on the inner cannula.
2. Hyperoxygenate, hyperinflate, and suction the trachea to remove secretions below the cuff. Remove secretions above the cuff by gently applying suction deep into the oropharynx.
3. Insert an empty syringe into the one-way valve, and pull back on the plunger to remove the air in the cuff. At the same time, apply positive pressure with the manual self-inflating bag. This will blow secretions lying directly above the cuff into the mouth, which will prevent secretions accumulated above the cuff from draining into the trachea and lower airway.
4. Suction the oropharynx again.
5. If the person is ventilator-dependent, remember that with the cuff "down" or deflated, a portion of ventilation volume will not reach the lungs. Air will escape through the upper airway and may compromise the person's ventilatory status. This volume loss will create an audible leak. Phonation is possible during the exhalation phase of the ventilator.

*The same procedure is used for inflation and deflation of endotracheal tube cuffs.

Tracheal Stenosis. Tracheal stenosis is narrowing of the trachea that occurs 1 week to 2 years after intubation. It results from scar formation in the inflamed trachea. The severity of stenosis can be prevented by choosing the right size tube, maintaining adequate cuff pressure, keeping intubation time short, preventing infection, and reducing movement of the tube.

Airway Obstruction. The flow of air through a tracheostomy tube may become occluded for several reasons. The tracheostomy tube may be misaligned so its opening lies against the tracheal wall, preventing air flow. Cuff overinflation causes the cuff to herniate over the tip of the tube, obstructing air flow. Without adequate airway care, the inner cannula can become occluded with dried secretions or excessive bronchial secretions.

Infection. Tracheostomies increase the risk of bronchopulmonary infection because they (1) bypass upper airway protective mechanisms (i.e., filtering, warming, and humidifying) and (2) decrease mucociliary transport and coughing, thus increasing retained secretions. Stoma site

infection may also occur. Nosocomial infection is also a potential problem. The lower airway (below the larynx) is normally sterile. Therefore, all solutions and equipment entering the trachea must be sterile. Organisms (e.g., *Pseudomonas aeruginosa* and other gram-negative bacteria) grow readily in respiratory equipment and contaminate the lower airway. In addition, some bacteria may colonize a tracheostomy without causing infection.

Recommendations for changing tracheostomy tubes vary. Most physicians and healthcare facilities have established protocols. Although some facilities change tracheostomy tubes as often as every week, others wait longer. Ideally, the tube should be changed at least every 6 to 8 weeks, or more frequently if the person is at risk of recurrent tracheobronchial infections. Each client has a unique set of circumstances that may dictate the frequency of tracheostomy tube changes.

Accidental Decannulation (Tube Removal). A tracheostomy tube that is not properly secured may be accidentally dislodged from the stoma. Since most new tracheostomy tubes are sutured in place, decannulation is rare, but it is serious nonetheless. Decannulation may occur while changing the ties. Manipulation of a tracheostomy tube or suctioning often produces vigorous coughing which can expel the tube from the stoma unless it is held firmly. With accidental extubation, if the stoma is less than 4 days old, it may close because a tract is not yet formed.

If extubation occurs, call for help immediately. Maintain ventilation and oxygenation by bag and mask. If ventilation is impossible you must reinsert the tube. To do so, deflate the cuff, remove the tube's inner cannula, insert the obturator in the outer cannula, elevate the person's shoulders with a pillow, and gently hyperextend the neck. You may need to use tracheal dilators (spreaders) to hold the stoma open. Insert the outer cannula with obturator into the client's neck and immediately remove the obturator. Auscultate for breath sounds. If present, insert the inner cannula and reconnect to oxygen and ventilation equipment. *If the tracheostomy tube cannot be reinserted in 1 minute, call a code for respiratory arrest. Unless the client is breathing adequately, an emergency cricothyroidotomy will be necessary* (see Chapter 89).

If accidental decannulation occurs once a tract has formed following a tracheostomy, the same procedure is used however but it is generally easier to reinsert the tube. If bleeding occurs or the airway is obstructed, use emergency measures, as indicated earlier.

Subcutaneous Emphysema. Subcutaneous emphysema occurs when air escapes from the tracheostomy incision into the tissues, dissects fascial planes under the skin, and accumulates around the face, neck and upper chest. These areas appear puffy and slight finger pressure produces a crackling sound and sensation. Generally this is not a serious condition; the air will eventually be absorbed.

Weaning, Removal, and Rescue Breathing

Weaning from the Tracheostomy Tube. For clients not requiring continuous mechanical ventilation, weaning begins by deflating the cuff to determine the client's ability to manage secretions without aspirating them. A smaller, uncuffed tube may be inserted to ensure adequate ventilation around the tube. The tube can then be plugged for varying lengths of time to assess the client's ability to breathe through the upper airway. The time is gradually lengthened according to the client's respiratory status, condition, and confidence. Eventually, the tracheostomy tube can be removed. The weaning process takes a varying length of time (typically 2–5 days), depending on a person's ability to breathe through the upper airway. If the client still requires some intervention via the tracheal opening, an uncuffed tube, a fenestrated tube, or a tracheal button may be used.

Plugging a tracheostomy tube is usually done by inserting a tracheostomy plug (decannulation stopper) into the opening of the outer cannula. This closes off the tracheostomy, and air flow and respiration occur normally, through the nose and mouth. *When plugging a cuffed tracheostomy tube, the cuff must be deflated.* If the cuff remains inflated, ventilation cannot occur, and respiratory arrest could result.

Explain the process to the client and family. Naturally, most clients are anxious about weaning because they fear they may not be able to breathe. Constant, supportive observation during weaning is necessary. Encourage the client to begin to think about breathing through the nose again. This breathing is a strange sensation for people who have used a tracheostomy tube for a long time. Explain to them ways to facilitate optimal respiration and to maintain control of breathing (e.g., inhale slowly and completely through the nose; avoid holding the breath).

Arterial blood gas (ABG) analysis and measurement of spontaneous respiratory mechanics (respiratory rate, tidal volume, vital capacity, inspiratory effort, expiratory effort) are important assessments during weaning. Oximetry and other noninvasive assessment may also be used once baseline ABGs are established.

During weaning from tracheostomy, assess for indications of respiratory distress or ventilation impairment. Findings may include:

1. Abnormal respiratory rate and pattern
2. Use of accessory muscles to assist breathing
3. Abnormal pulse and blood pressure
4. Abnormal skin and mucous membrane color
5. Abnormal ABGs or oxygen saturation levels

Remove the tracheostomy plug immediately if any indication of respiratory distress or ventilation impairment appears. Also assess the client's quality of phonation and ability to deep-breathe and cough effectively. If oxygen has been administered via the tracheostomy, administer it at the prescribed liter flow with nasal prongs.

Removing the Tracheostomy Tube (Decannulation). A tracheostomy tube is removed after successful tracheostomy plugging and when the client's respiratory status and function are stable. Successful tracheostomy plugging is indicated by (1) a client's ability to breathe comfortably with the tracheostomy plugged, (2) normal ABG analysis or oxygen saturation, and (3) a client's ability to cough and raise secretions. Gradually increase the length of plugging sessions until the client is comfortable and confident with the tube plugged continuously for at least 24 hours.

After a tracheostomy tube is removed, place a dry sterile dressing over the stoma. Initially, every 8 hours, clean the skin around the stoma; remove mucus with hydrogen peroxide; rinse the area with normal saline; and apply a fresh dry dressing over the healing stoma. Document the condition of the stoma and surrounding skin. If they appear irritated or infected, notify the physician. Topical antibiotic ointment may be prescribed. A tracheostomy stoma closes gradually (over a period of several days). As long as the stoma is open, an air leak is present. To correct this the client may need to place his or her clean fingers firmly over the dressing to facilitate normal speech and coughing.

Following extubation, ongoing respiratory function assessment is necessary. Some complications of tracheostomy do not appear for months following tracheostomy tube removal, for example, tracheal stenosis.

Performing Rescue Breathing. Emergency rescue breathing, mouth to neck (mouth to tracheostomy or mouth to stoma) may be necessary if a client with a tracheostomy or laryngectomy experiences respiratory depression or respiratory arrest. If the client has a tracheostomy tube, provide ventilation by attaching a manual self-inflating bag to the standard 15-mm adaptor on the inner cannula. Some volume is lost from an uncuffed tube. Adequate ventilation can often be compensated for by altering the usual method of manual inflation (e.g., compress the bag more forcefully and quickly). If the tracheostomy tube is cuffed, inflate the cuff and maintain ventilation at the correct rate, that is, 12 to 16 breaths a minute for an adult. If inflation of the cuff impedes ventilation, immediately deflate the cuff and attempt to compensate for volume loss by compressing the bag more forcefully or quickly. If ventilation continues to be impaired or prevented and you determine the cause is a malfunction in the tube, remove the tube immediately and provide mouth-to-stoma ventilation. Keep the nose and mouth closed during mouth-to-stoma breathing to prevent air from escaping through the upper airway.

Nursing Management of the Client with a Tracheostomy

Preoperative Care

For clients having elective tracheostomy, the nurse reinforces education provided by the physician or respiratory therapist. The client's understanding of the tracheostomy tube may be enhanced by looking at and touching a tube. The changes in ability to speak and eat should also be explained. If it is expected that the tracheostomy will be permanent, information about living a productive life with modifications in clothing can be provided. A visit by a client with a permanent tracheostomy may be desired.

For clients needing emergency tracheostomy, precious seconds are all that is available for teaching. The client may be anxious or even unconscious. Education is often provided to the family in lieu of the client.

Postoperative Care

Assessment

Following tracheostomy, the frequent assessment is required, including (1) monitoring vital signs; (2) assessing amount, color, and consistency of secretions; and (3) observing for indications of shock, hemorrhage, respiratory insufficiency, or complications from the client's general condition or the surgical intervention.

Diagnosis, Planning, Implementation

Ineffective Airway Clearance. Several factors lead to ineffective airway clearance in clients with tracheostomy. For example, dehydration, fever, anesthesia, anticholinergic drugs, sedatives, and immobility. All of these factors may be experienced by a person with a tracheostomy.

Planning: Expected Outcomes. The client will have an effective airway clearance as evidenced by no retained secretions, clear (or clearing) lung sounds, and no fever.

Implementation. Promote airway clearance and pulmonary aeration by changing the client's position frequently, providing humidification and hydration, using sedatives cautiously, and performing frequent hyperinflation and suctioning to promote lung expansion and reduce the risks of atelectasis, pulmonary infection, and ineffective gas exchange. Hyperinflation creates an "artificial sigh," improving lung aeration and facilitating removal of tracheobronchial secretions by enhancing the cough effort. When the client's condition is stabilized sufficiently, coughing may be enhanced by having the client place a finger over the tracheostomy tube opening while attempting to cough. It is important that the client's hands be washed before doing this. Have the person cough into paper tissues and dispose of them carefully.

Suctioning. When a cuffed tracheostomy tube is used, secretions collect above the cuff. It is difficult to reach such secretions by oropharyngeal suctioning. However, the secretions can be "blown" into the mouth by simultaneously deflating the cuff and giving a deep manual inflation. The client may also be instructed to cough during cuff deflation to expel accumulated secretions through the tracheostomy tube. If the client is unable to produce an effective cough, the nurse should suction the tracheostomy tube during deflation to prevent aspiration of secretions into the lower airway.

Suction the airway as needed. Careful technique reduces mucosal trauma, which can lead to tracheal infection. Mucosal trauma is indicated by tracheal irritation, tracheitis, and bloody tracheal secretions. If tracheal secretions are thick and not easily removed, directly instill 3 to 5 ml of sterile normal saline into the trachea to try to reduce the viscosity of the secretions and stimulate coughing. Instill the saline directly into the tracheostomy tube during inhalation. If the client is unable to cough, suction the airway through the tracheostomy tube.

Tracheostomy Care. Tracheostomy care is detailed in a fundamentals textbook. Reinsertion of the clean inner cannula is shown in Figure 40–3.

Hydration. Provide adequate hydration. The normal hydrating mechanisms of the upper airway are bypassed by a tracheostomy. Hydration can be ensured by oral, parenteral, or inhalation routes. Inhalation may be provided by increasing the humidity of room air (room humidifier) or of dry gases (e.g., oxygen) by administering aerosols.

If humidification is insufficient, the body tries to make up the deficit by taking fluid from body water. The result is inspissated (very thick) mucus, which compromises airway patency and increases the risk of secretion pooling and subsequent infection. Dried mucus also occludes air

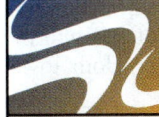

MANAGEMENT AND DELEGATION

Assisting With Respiratory Care

Assisting with respiratory care is one of the more controversial areas involving the use of assistive personnel. Opinions differ widely on the role of assistive personnel in caring for clients who need respiratory care. The performance of suctioning in particular is central to this debate. Your clinical site should provide you with clear guidelines about the role of assistive personnel in this aspect of care.

The following aspects of respiratory care are commonly delegated to unlicensed assistive personnel:

- Setting up of oxygen delivery equipment and suction equipment
- Stocking routine respiratory care supplies at the bedside
- Assisting clients with the use of an incentive spirometer (following instruction from a nurse or respiratory care clinician)
- Assisting clients with coughing and deep breathing (following instruction from a nurse or respiratory care clinician)
- Performing tracheostomy care
- Measuring peripheral oxygen saturation (SpO_2)

Controversial aspects of respiratory care less commonly delegated to unlicensed assistive personnel are as follows:

- Suctioning via an artificial airway
- Performance of chest physiotherapy to promote the loosening of secretions

Prior to the delegation of any aspect of respiratory care, consider the following:

- What is the client's respiratory status? Complete a thorough respiratory assessment.
- What is the indication for respiratory care? Is the client's condition stable? A client with acute respiratory compromise should receive your full attention and care; the care of such a client should not be delegated.
- Is your client on oxygen therapy? Oxygen is a type of medication for your client. All guidelines that pertain to medications also apply to oxygen. You may delegate the setup of oxygen delivery equipment to assistive personnel. However, you are responsible to verify that the ordered amount (dose) of oxygen is actually being delivered to the client.
- Has the client been instructed in the use of the incentive spirometer or coughing and deep breathing exercises? Does the client need reinforcement or to be instructed again? Reinforcement can be provided by assistive personnel; education and instruction should always be provided by a registered nurse or respiratory care clinician.
- Does the client have a *new* artificial airway, such as an oral airway, nasotracheal or endotracheal tube, or tracheostomy? Have you assessed the client during suctioning? How has the client tolerated suctioning previously? Well-tolerated suctioning via an existing artificial airway may be delegated to a skilled assistant, if this is consistent with training and institutional policy.
- Is this a client with a new or long-term tracheostomy? A new tracheostomy should always be managed by a registered nurse. The tracheostomy tube that has been placed through a new surgical incision should be evaluated as should any other fresh postoperative site.
- Have the client and family managed this tracheostomy at home? This is an opportunity to evaluate their sterile technique, provide reinforcement, and review instructions with the client and family. After doing so, you may choose to delegate the suctioning of this client to assistive personnel.
- Are the assistive personnel aware that suctioning and care of artificial airways are sterile procedures? The sterile technique of assistive personnel should be evaluated intermittently.

Findings that are immediately reportable to you, the registered nurse, should be described for the assistive personnel. These include any change or difficulty that they or the client experience during the provision of care, changes in the respiratory rate or pattern, and the consistency, color, and quantity of respiratory secretions.

---

passages and leads to atelectasis, pneumonia, and potentially severe gas exchange abnormalities.

Prevent tube movement. Secure a tracheostomy tube properly. If tracheostomy tube securing tapes require knotting, tie a square knot. Avoid placing the knot over the client's carotid artery or spine. Make sure the tapes are not too tight (i.e., allow room for two fingers to slide comfortably under the tape). Inspect the skin under the securing tape for skin irritation. Clients requiring a long-term tracheostomy may use more comfortable securing devices (e.g., padded straps with Velcro fasteners or intravenous tubing). Secure the tube in midline tracheal align-

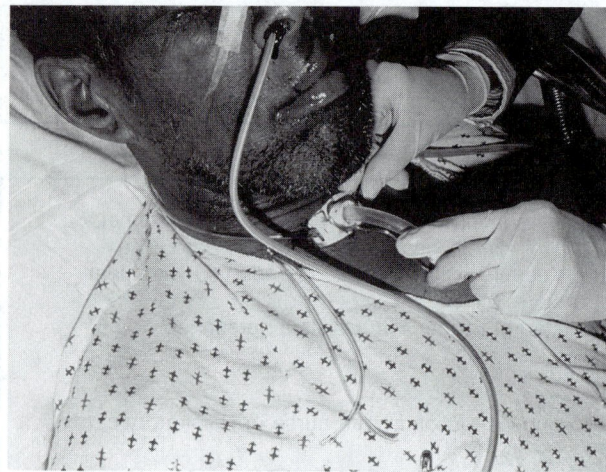

Figure 40–3. Reinserting a cleaned inner cannula.

ment. Support ventilator and aerosol tubing to prevent pulling on the tracheostomy tube. Be careful not to disconnect tubing when turning the client.

Risk for Impaired Gas Exchange.
Following tracheostomy, impaired gas exchange may occur because of various factors. Factors affecting oxygen delivery include

1. Aspiration of blood, oral secretions, or gastric contents
2. Restricted lung expansion from immobility
3. Excessive tracheobronchial secretions
4. Inability to cough and deep-breathe
5. Preexisting medical conditions (e.g., obesity, fever, inadequate hydration, pneumonia, tracheal injury such as from burns)

Factors affecting the removal of carbon dioxide include (1) sedatives or anesthesia, (2) deteriorating level of consciousness, and (3) any other condition potentially affecting ventilation efficiency and leading to hypoventilation and retention of carbon dioxide.

Planning: Expected Outcomes. The client will have adequate gas exchange as evidenced by maintaining oxygen saturation at greater than 90% (or ABGs within normal limits), and showing no manifestations of respiratory distress.

Implementation. Assessment of gas exchange by ABG analysis is important immediately following tracheostomy and whenever there is a change in the client's condition or a change in treatment. Noninvasive monitoring such as pulse oximetry is appropriate once baseline values are established by ABG analysis. Remember, if shock or hypotension exists, or if peripheral vasoconstrictive drugs are used, data provided by transcutaneous monitoring will be incorrect because an accurate reading is not possible.

Do not allow smoking in the room of a person who has a tracheostomy. Do not use aerosol spray cans (e.g., room deodorizers) near the person. Do not shake bedding or create dust clouds. Be careful when shaving or tending the person's hair that whiskers or hair do not fall into the trachea. Cover the tracheostomy with a thin cloth towel during shaving.

Risk for Infection.
The tracheostomy bypasses normal upper airway protective mechanisms. The client also has an incision. Both areas can become infected.

Planning: Expected Outcomes. The client will exhibit no indications of infection as evidenced by remaining afebrile, having a clean and dry tracheostomy site, healing incisions and clear sputum.

Implementation. Use aseptic technique when working with the tracheostomy. Careful hand washing, appropriate use of gloves, use of sterile supplies and solutions, and changing and decontaminating respiratory equipment every 24 hours are essential. Create a "loop" in the aerosol or ventilator tubing assembly; that is, let the tube loop down to catch condensate. Drain water and condensate in the tubing away from the tracheostomy into a receptacle.

Clean and inspect the skin around the stoma and the stoma itself. Observe for indications of irritation, inflammation, skin breakdown, and purulent drainage. If skin or stomal infection does occur, a topical antibacterial ointment may be prescribed.

Tracheostomy dressings (Fig. 40–4) are often used, especially in the early postoperative stage. Damp blood- and mucus-soaked dressings are a perfect medium for the growth of microorganisms. They also promote tissue irritation and breakdown. Change dressings whenever they are damp. Using hydrogen peroxide and cotton-tipped applicators, carefully clean the skin each time the dressing is changed. Rinse with normal saline and dry the area. Do not use plastic-backed or water-proofed dressings. Moisture, secretions, and blood may seep behind them, and these dressings hold warmth and moisture in. Skin then becomes irritated and macerated.

Risk for Aspiration.
The presence of a tracheostomy increases the *Risk for aspiration* because the tubes tether the larynx, preventing normal upward movement of the larynx and closure by the epiglottis when swallowing.

Planning: Expected Outcomes. The client will exhibit no evidence of aspiration by having clear lung sounds, no fever, and no choking upon swallowing.

Implementation. Intravenous fluids are usually given during the first 24 hours following tracheostomy. Then, if the client is alert and swallowing and if gag mechanisms are intact, oral fluid and food may be attempted.

If a cuffed endotracheal tube was used before the tracheostomy, assess for tracheoesophageal fistula before permitting oral feedings. To assess for fistula, give the client a "test swallow" of water (room temperature and colored blue with food coloring) before giving fluid or food. Severe coughing or blue fluid suctioned from the tracheostomy tube may indicate aspiration or a fistula. In either case, withhold oral food and fluid, and continue feeding by nasogastric tube or other methods.

A client with a long-term or permanently impaired

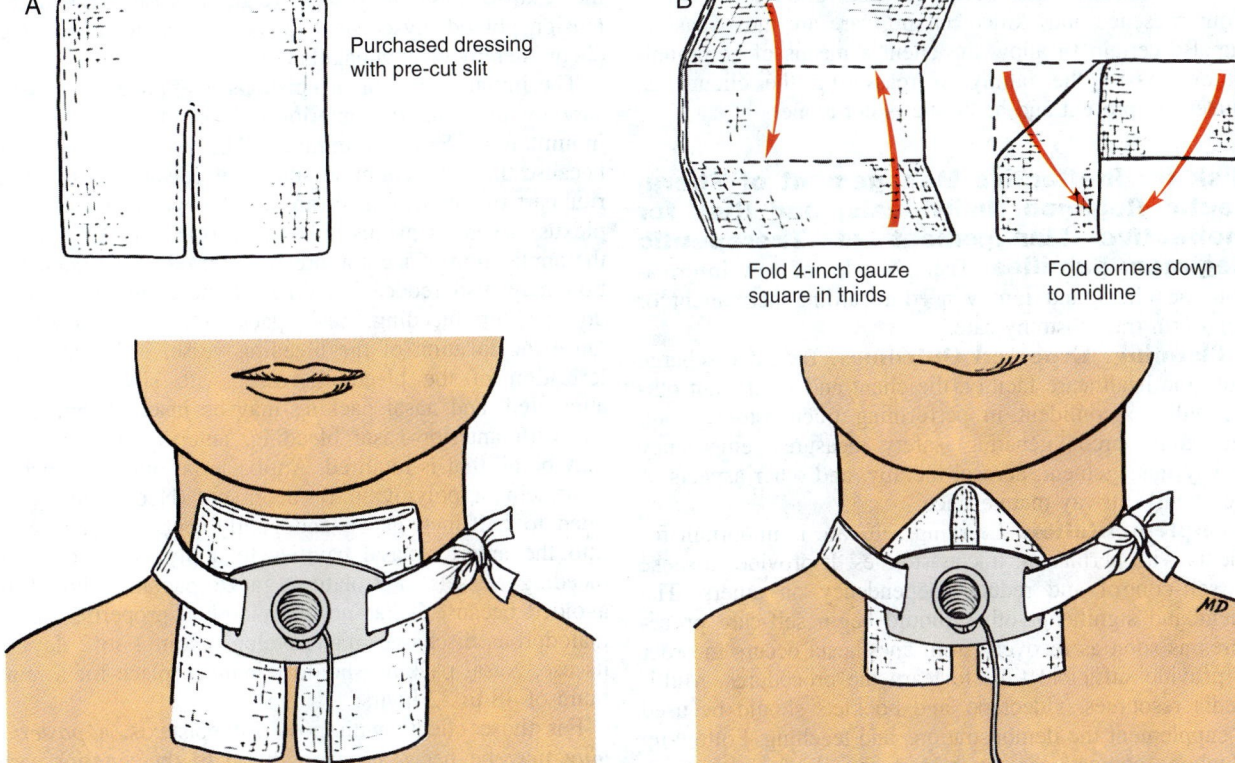

A Purchased dressing with pre-cut slit

B Fold 4-inch gauze square in thirds   Fold corners down to midline

Figure 40–4. Tracheostomy dressings. If there is significant bleeding or tracheal secretions, cleaning the skin and changing the dressing frequently may prevent infection and skin breakdown. *A,* Manufactured dressing with a precut slit has no fine threads that could unravel and enter the stoma. Place the dressing around the tracheostomy tube with the slit downward, as shown, or upward. *B,* 4 × 4 gauze pad folded and placed under the tracheostomy tube. Do not have any cut edges that could unravel.

swallowing mechanism (e.g., following a cerebrovascular accident) requires a permanent feeding tube or gastrostomy feedings (see Chapter 61). Tube feedings may cause reflux and be aspirated into the trachea. Before administering tube feedings, inflate the cuff of the tracheostomy tube. Leave it inflated for at least 1 hour after feeding. Suction above the cuff before deflating it to remove any tube-feeding material.

When feeding a client with a tracheostomy, have him or her sit upright. Often, food and fluids with semisolid consistency (e.g., pudding) are easier to swallow than water. Tipping the chin toward the chest narrows the airway and helps food enter the esophagus. Overinflation of the cuff causes swallowing difficulty. If oral fluid intake is limited, continue intravenous fluids.

Impaired Verbal Communication. Because the vocal cords are bypassed by the tracheostomy tube, the client cannot talk. This diagnosis may need to be combined with fear or anxiety, if the client feels afraid of not being able to summon help.

Planning: Expected Outcomes. The client will have a satisfactory method of communicating with the nursing staff as evidenced by being able to summon help and have needs met.

Implementation. Make sure the client can always reach an emergency call system to summon help. Do not use an intercom system because the client cannot talk. Be sure all personnel know this. Make a written list of common needs, words, and phrases so the client can point to the list to communicate needs (e.g., I want to pass urine; I need a drink; I have pain). Use a paper and pencil or picture communication board to facilitate communication.

Risk for Constipation. When the glottis and vocal cords are bypassed (as with tracheostomy), a person cannot perform Valsalva's maneuver. This impairs the person's ability to defecate.

Planning: Expected Outcomes. The client will have regular bowel movements (per usual schedule).

Implementation. Assess for most recent bowel movement. Elimination is a frequently overlooked area of client care. Use prescribed stool softeners, laxatives, and even enemas or suppositories as necessary.

Anxiety and Fear. These problems are due to various factors affecting clients with tracheostomies, for example, inability to talk, fear of suffocating, anxiety about diagnosis, fear that the tracheostomy tube will come out.

Planning: Expected Outcomes. The client will exhibit decreasing manifestations of anxiety and fear as evidenced by pulse rate within normal limits, calm facial appearance, ability to communicate, no expressed fears.

Implementation. Frequent observation is essential. Your presence and skilled nursing care are most reassuring. Be certain to allow the client a means of communication. Assist the family in reassuring the client that nurses are present and he or she is not alone.

Risk for Ineffective Management of Therapeutic Regimen (Individuals) and Risk for Ineffective Management of Therapeutic Regimen: Families.
There is a lot of new information the client and family need regarding permanent or long-term tracheostomy care.

Planning: Expected Outcomes. Before discharge from the healthcare facility, the client and significant others will be confident in performing tracheostomy care, suctioning, preoxygenating, safety measures, emergency airway management, aerosol therapy, and other aspects of the client's airway maintenance.

Implementation. Learning self-care is important for clients with permanent tracheostomies. It provides a sense of self-control and reduces dependency on others. The client and significant other should begin self-care procedures as soon as recovery from anesthesia occurs in order to provide sufficient time to learn the procedures. Multimedia resources, videotape, and booklets should be used to supplement the demonstrations and teaching. Follow-up telephone contact, contact through the physician's office, and home health nurses are necessary to identify the effectiveness of the teaching.

Evaluation. Nursing diagnoses related to airway management should be resolvable within a few days. Problems with communication, infection, constipation, and eating will remain and require long-term planning.

Significant others must also be able to provide tracheostomy care and other aspects of airway management. Teach the client's family how to provide rescue breathing using the information above.

The client and significant others are often anxious about home management. Send a duplicate tracheostomy tube for use in changing the tube or for use in the event of accidental decannulation. Close follow-up is essential. Arrange home equipment and follow-up visits by a home health agency or community health nurse with expertise in caring for people with complex airway needs. Involve a tracheostomy nurse-specialist in the teaching when available. Order home healthcare equipment from medical suppliers who employ respiratory therapists or nurses. Ideally, have the equipment initially delivered to the hospital, so the client and significant others can learn its use under the supervision of professionals.

Hemorrhagic, Infectious, and Inflammatory Disorders

Epistaxis

Epistaxis (nosebleed) may result from irritation, trauma, infection, or tumors. In addition, epistaxis may also be the result of systemic disease (e.g., atherosclerosis, hypertension, blood dyscrasias) or systemic treatment (e.g., chemotherapy or anticoagulants).

The initial treatment of epistaxis is application of pressure by pinching the anterior portion of the nose for a minimum of 5 to 10 minutes. This is often successful because the most common source of epistaxis is the anterior part of the septum in an area known as Kisselbach's plexus, a venous plexus vulnerable to trauma. In addition, the application of ice compresses to produce vasoconstriction may also reduce bleeding. If these initial measures do not stop bleeding, nasal packing may be necessary. Once the location of the bleeding vessel is located, cauterization of the bleeding vessel with silver nitrate is attempted, and nasal packing may be inserted. For a client with anterior nasal bleeding, anterior nasal packing may be all that is required. Antibacterial ointment such as bacitracin or polymyxin B–neomycin (Neosporin) is applied to half-inch gauze and gently, but firmly, inserted into the anterior nasal cavities to apply pressure to the bleeding vessels. Petrolatum gauze packing should be avoided because it has no antimicrobial properties, and a malodorous discharge may develop within 1 to 2 days of its use. Nasal packing should remain in place for a minimum of 48 to 72 hours.[19,29]

For those clients with posterior epistaxis, a *posterior plug* may be necessary in addition to the anterior nasal packing (Fig. 40–5). Insertion of a posterior plug is very uncomfortable for clients, and a mild analgesic may be required to reduce anxiety and discomfort. A small, red rubber catheter is passed through the nose into the oropharynx and mouth. A gauze pack is tied to the catheter, and the catheter is withdrawn; this moves the pack into proper placement in the nasopharynx and posterior nose to apply pressure. The nasal cavity is packed with half-inch gauze, and the strings from the posterior pack are tied around a rolled gauze or bolus to maintain its position. The ties from the oral cavity are taped to the client's face to prevent loosening or dislodgment of the plug. Clients with posterior plug and anterior nasal packing are admitted to the hospital and monitored closely for hypoxia. General comfort measures, such as humidification, the use of a drip pad to collect bloody drainage and mucus, and the use of water-soluble ointment around the nares to provide lubrication will alleviate some discomfort. The client should be monitored closely for any signs of bleeding from the anterior or posterior nares. Inspect the oral cavity for the presence of blood and proper placement of the posterior plug. If the posterior plug is visible, notify the physician for readjustment of the packing. Posterior nasal packs remain in place for 5 days.[19,29] Prophylactic antibiotics are used to prevent toxic shock syndrome and sinusitis.

If medical measures are not sufficient to eliminate epistaxis, surgical intervention may be necessary. Internal maxillary or ethmoidal *artery ligation* may be required to control nasal bleeding. An incision is made in the gum line above the incisor on the affected side, and the maxillary sinus is entered. The artery that supplies the area of bleeding is identified, and a metal clip or suture is used to ligate the artery. Clients will have nasal packing inserted for a minimum of 24 hours, during which time

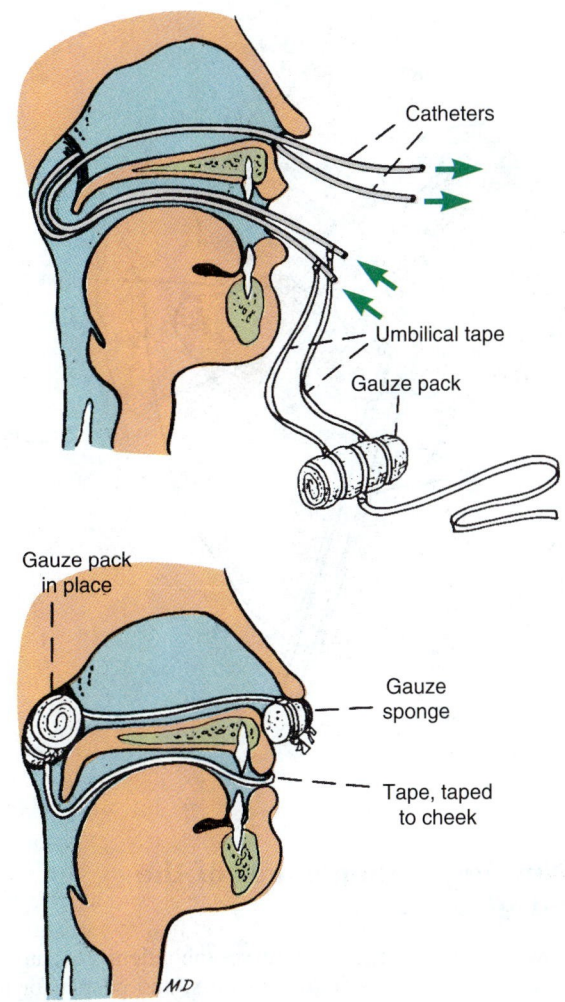

Figure 40–5. Instillation of posterior nasal pack (plug) (typically used in emergency).

they must be observed for additional bleeding, hyper- or hypotension, and infection. Upon discharge, the client is instructed to minimize activity for approximately 10 days. This is most frequently accomplished by avoiding strenuous exercise; not blowing the nose; sneezing with the mouth open; and not lifting, stooping, or straining. The use of water-soluble ointment at the entrance of the nose and around the nares may provide comfort, and mouth rinses of half-strength hydrogen peroxide mixed with water or saline should be provided for oral hygiene. The use of a humidifier or vaporizer will add supplemental moisture to prevent dryness and crusting of secretions.

Sinusitis

Sinusitis is an infection of any of the paranasal sinuses. Pansinusitis is infection of more than one sinus. It is a common medical condition that affects an estimated 35 million people a year.[28] The sinuses are protected against infection by mucociliary action. The normal mucus produced by the sinuses is removed through small openings in the nose called ostia. When the ciliary action is impaired or the ostia are obstructed, mucus can accumulate in the sinus and become infected.

Sinusitis is considered by evaluation of the client's clinical manifestations and confirmed by x-ray. Fever and chills along with pain in the sinuses that is exacerbated with bending, pain or numbness in the upper teeth, and a purulent or discolored nasal discharge may be present. Sinus radiographs or computed tomography scans may show opacification of the sinus, thickened mucous membranes, and an air-fluid level (accumulation of secretions in the sinus), all indicative of sinusitis.

Acute and Subacute Care

■ Medical Management

Medical management of sinusitis includes use of the appropriate antibiotic to manage the bacterial infection; decongestants to reduce nasal edema; corticosteroid nasal sprays to reduce mucosal inflammation; and humidification by use of normal saline solution irrigations or a vaporizer or humidifier to prevent nasal crusting and to moisten secretions.

Antral irrigation or sinus lavage may be performed in clients who are not responding to treatment or who have increased purulent exudate in the maxillary sinus. Antral irrigation is performed with the use of a local anesthetic. A trocar (a sharp metal instrument) is inserted through the ostium in the lateral wall of the nose into the sinus. Prepare the client for the procedure with thorough explanations of the anesthetic, the sensation of the trocar passing through the ostium, and feelings of pressure. Normal saline solution is then injected through the cannula to rinse the sinus of purulent exudate. The client is placed in a sitting position, leaning slightly forward with the mouth open to allow drainage of the irrigating solution through the nose and mouth. A culture of the exudate may be made to determine the causative organism for prescription of an appropriate antibiotic.[25]

■ Surgical Management
Functional Endoscopic Sinus Surgery

If nonoperative measures fail, functional endoscopic sinus surgery (FESS) may be necessary. The major objective of FESS is the reestablishment of sinus ventilation and mucociliary clearance.[8] Small sinus endoscopes are passed through the nasal cavity and into the sinuses to allow direct visualization of the sinuses in order to remove diseased tissue and enlarge sinus ostia (Fig. 40–6). The possible complications of FESS include nasal bleeding, pain, scar formation, and rarely, cerebrospinal fluid leak and blindness from intraorbital hematoma formation or direct injury to the optic nerve. After FESS, nasal packing may be inserted. Nasal packing is used to minimize

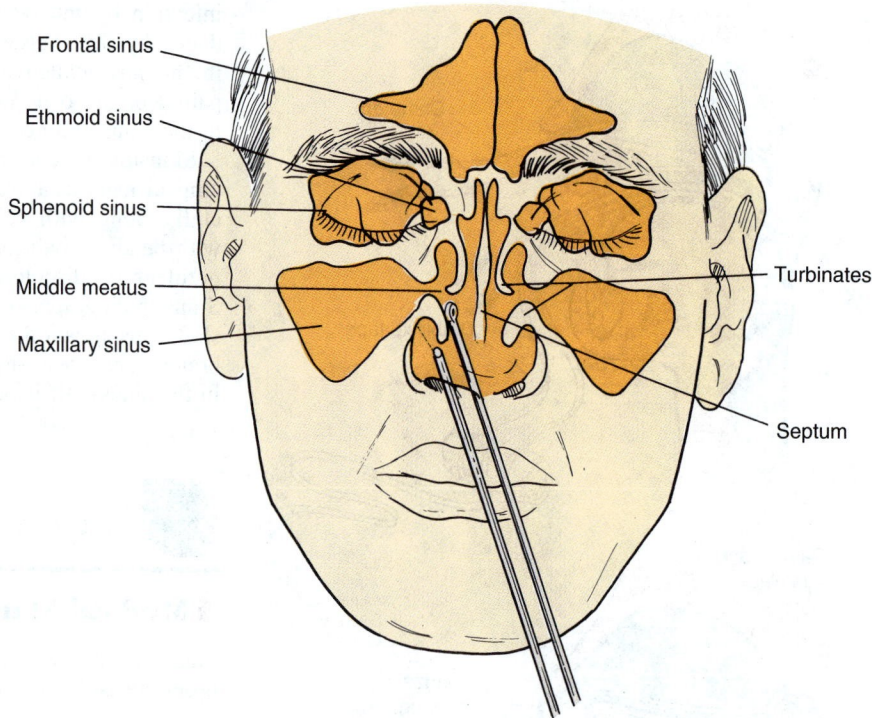

Figure 40–6. Functional endoscopic surgery. The middle meatus is the site where most of the sinuses drain and if plugged drainage is obstructed. With an endoscope the sinuses can be seen and obstructions removed.

nasal bleeding and is removed within a few hours of the surgical procedure.

Caldwell-Luc Procedure

Caldwell-Luc is another surgical procedure for maxillary sinusitis. An incision is made into the gingival buccal sulcus above the lateral incisor teeth under general or local anesthesia. Through this opening, the diseased mucous membrane is removed. In addition, an opening between the maxillary sinus and lateral nasal wall (nasal antral window) may be created to increase aeration of the sinus and permit drainage into the nasal cavity. After a Caldwell-Luc procedure, the maxillary sinus and anterior nasal cavity are packed with half-inch gauze. Because of the packing, nasal breathing is obstructed. The oral cavity is frequently evaluated for the presence of blood or packing that may have become dislodged, obstructing the pharynx. If packing is present in the pharynx, the visible portion may be held with a hemostat and cut with scissors. Be certain the hemostat is holding the trimmed gauze; otherwise it could be aspirated.[25]

External Sphenoethmoidectomy

External sphenoethmoidectomy is a surgical procedure to remove diseased mucosa from the sphenoidal or ethmoidal sinuses. A small incision is made over the ethmoidal sinus on the lateral nasal bridge, and the diseased mucosa is removed. The client will have nasal and ethmoidal packing inserted. An eye pressure patch is usually applied to decrease periorbital edema.[25]

■ Nursing Management of the Surgical Client

Following sinus surgery, observe the client for an increase in bleeding, respiratory distress, and edema for the first 24 hours after surgery. Apply ice compresses to the nose and cheek to minimize edema and control bleeding. Place the client in a semi- to high-Fowler position for 24 to 48 hours after surgery to minimize postoperative edema. The nasal packing is generally removed the morning after surgery; however, antral packing may remain in place for 36 to 72 hours. Give mild analgesics to the client to minimize discomfort after surgery and before removal of the packing.

Instruct clients to increase fluids to moisten secretions. Although there may be some pain, a mild analgesic is usually all that is required. Minimal nasal bleeding is expected for 24 to 48 hours after surgery. A "drip pad" under the nose may eliminate the need for constant wiping. (Fig. 40–7). Instruct clients to avoid blowing the nose for 7 to 10 days after surgery; tell them to sniff backward or spit, not blow. Teach the client to sneeze only with the mouth open. Nasal saline sprays may be started 3 to 5 days after surgery to moisten the nasal mucosa. Instruct clients that they are to have minimal physical exercise and avoid strenuous activity, lifting, and straining for approximately 2 weeks. After FESS, clients will be required to return to the physician's office for removal of crusts and debris and examination of the nose.

After a Caldwell-Luc procedure, the client may have temporary numbness of the upper teeth caused by interruption of sensory nerves from the mucosal incision. This sensation may remain for several weeks.[17,19,25,29,34]

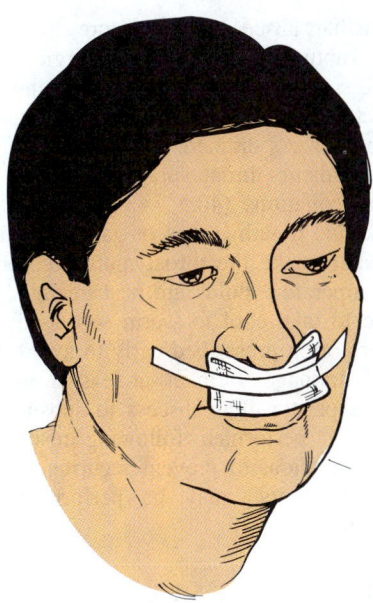

Figure 40–7. A nasal drip pad is taped beneath the nares to absorb drainage after nasal or sinus surgery. The usual technique is to fold 3 × 3 dressings into thirds and tape in place. These dressings can be changed at your discretion.

Pharyngitis

Pharyngitis is inflammation of the pharynx and may be viral or bacterial in origin. A culture of the pharyngeal mucosa is sometimes indicated before treatment is started. Clients may complain of a sore throat, difficulty swallowing, fever, malaise, and cough, and have an elevated white blood cell count. Treatment of pharyngitis depends on the causative agent. Both viral and bacterial pharyngitis are contagious by droplet spread. Good hand washing technique is essential, and the use of a mask may prevent spread. Antibiotics are used to treat the bacterial pharyngitis; comfort measures are required for viral types. Bedrest, fluids, warm saline irrigations or gargles, analgesics, and antipyretics are recommended until the clinical manifestations are alleviated.

Chronic pharyngitis (chronic pharyngeal inflammation) is most common in people who (1) habitually use tobacco and alcohol, (2) have a chronic cough, (3) are employed or live in dusty environments, or (4) use their voices excessively. Clinical manifestations vary according to the degree of irritation and inflammation.

Tonsillitis

Tonsillitis is an acute infection of the tonsils. *Streptococcus* is the most common infecting organism, although tonsillitis can be caused by *Haemophilus influenzae,* and other organisms.

The client with tonsillitis will report throat pain, difficulty in swallowing, otalgia (referred pain to the ear), and generalized malaise. Examination will disclose an acutely inflamed mucous membrane around the tonsillar

area with or without the presence of purulent exudate. In some clients, lymphadenopathy of the cervical lymph nodes may also be present.

Complications from streptococcal tonsillitis include pneumonia, nephritis, osteomyelitis, and rheumatic fever. Acute tonsillitis may become chronic. Acute otitis media, acute rhinitis, acute sinusitis, and peritonsillar abscess or other deep neck abscesses may also develop.

 ## Acute and Subacute Care

■ Medical Management

Antibiotics are used to treat acute tonsillitis. In addition, the client is instructed to minimize activity, encourage bedrest and increased fluid intake. Saline throat irrigations or gargles may relieve the discomfort. Mild analgesics such as acetaminophen, with or without codeine, may be prescribed.

■ Surgical Management

Surgical removal of the tonsils (tonsillectomy) and the adenoids (adenoidectomy) is collectively called adenotonsillectomy, or T&A. The tonsils and adenoids may be removed separately but are most often removed in the same procedure. Removal of chronically diseased tonsil or adenoid tissue is indicated in the following circumstances:

1. When there are recurrent, incapacitating episodes of acute or chronic tonsillitis
2. When tonsillar or adenoid hypertrophy causes obstruction of the airway and impairs swallowing
3. Following resolution of a peritonsillar abscess
4. When repeated ear problems related to eustachian tube obstruction occur
5. When there are sinus complications

T&A is most often done in children. Tonsillectomy may also be indicated for a carrier of diphtheria, because tonsils may "seed" the infection. Adults with recurrent sore throats, ear pain, or hearing dysfunction, or who snore because of hypertrophied adenoid or tonsillar tissue may also benefit from this procedure. Although T&A are not as routine as in the past, they are indicated in clients who have repeated episodes of infection. Tonsillectomy may be performed under general or local anesthesia, although general anesthesia is most commonly used. Surgical intervention is not used during an acute infection, that is, upper respiratory infection. Other contraindications to T&A include hematologic disorders such as hemophilia, aplastic anemia, purpura, or leukemia.

■ Nursing Management of the Surgical Client

After tonsillectomy, place the client in a lateral decubitus position until awake and alert. This will provide for drainage of blood and other secretions through the nose and mouth. Gently inspect the oropharynx and mouth for fresh blood frequently during the first several hours postoperatively. Monitor vital signs closely. Hemorrhage is the most serious complication after tonsillectomy and is most often seen during the first 12 to 24 hours. If postoperative hemorrhage occurs, resuturing or cauterization of the bleeding vessel is mandatory.

The client should begin taking oral feedings once recovery from anesthesia is complete. Encourage cool fluids, and progress the client to a soft, bland diet, as tolerated. Highly seasoned foods, as well as any food the client finds difficult to swallow, should be avoided.

Pain in the first 7 to 10 postoperative days is common after tonsillectomy. Most clients report generalized throat pain as well as otalgia. Mild analgesics such as acetaminophen with or without codeine may be required to alleviate pain. Increased swallowing of fluids will also minimize discomfort.

Encourage clients to seek immediate medical attention if bleeding occurs after hospital dismissal. Delayed bleeding may occur once the healing membrane separates from the underlying tissue (7–10 days). The surgical site is usually well healed in 14 to 21 days, and the client should have minimal difficulty after this time.[25,29]

Chronic Tonsillitis

The most frequent manifestation of chronic tonsillitis is recurrent sore throat. Between episodes of acute tonsillitis, the throat remains uncomfortable. The tonsils are often enlarged, and if they are infected, a sharp line may be seen between the color of the buccal mucosa and that of the tonsillar pillar. The most reliable indication of chronic tonsillitis is the expression of purulent material from the tonsillar crypts with a wooden tongue blade. Once chronic tonsillitis is diagnosed, surgical removal is recommended. Surgery is contraindicated during acute tonsillar infection, although tonsillectomy may be performed in a client with acute peritonsillar abscess.

Peritonsillar Abscess (Quinsy)

Peritonsillar abscess may arise from acute streptococcal or staphylococcal tonsillitis. The tissue between the tonsils and the fascia covering the superior constrictor muscles becomes infected, causing extensive swelling of the soft palate and the pharyngeal wall. The uvula may be pushed to one side, and up to half of the pharyngeal opening may be occluded. Pus formation in the fascial space pushes the tonsil forward toward the midline of the throat.

Peritonsillar abscesses typically occur several days after the onset of acute tonsillitis. As the manifestations of tonsillitis begin to resolve, increasing pain develops on one side of the throat and ear. Inflammation and edema create a partial obstruction to swallowing. Often, the client keeps the mouth partially open to allow drooling, rather than attempting painful swallowing. The voice takes on a characteristic "hot potato," or muffled sound. Thick secretions are raised with difficulty.

A peritonsillar abscess may rupture spontaneously. If spontaneous rupture does not occur, surgical intervention may be necessary. With the client in a sitting position (to allow expectoration of pus and blood), an incision is made and the abscess drained.

Topical anesthetic throat sprays, analgesic agents, hot saline throat irrigations (40.5°–43.3° C [105°–110° F]), saline or alkaline mouthwashes or gargles, and ice collars may be used to make the throat more comfortable. Cool and room temperature fluids are best tolerated. The client may be able to take cool to warm soft foods. High-dose antibiotics are often prescribed early to avoid the need for incision and drainage. It takes at least 1 month for the infection of a peritonsillar abscess to subside. Usually, a tonsillectomy is performed following resolution of the abscess and infection, to prevent recurrence. However, a "quinsy tonsillectomy" may be performed during the acute infection.[16,25,29]

Rhinitis

Rhinitis is inflammation of the nasal mucosa. Manifestations of rhinitis include increased nasal drainage. Normally this drainage is clear mucus. If the infection spreads to the sinuses, however, drainage may become yellow or green. Rhinitis may be classified as acute, allergic, vasomotor, or medicamentosa.

Acute rhinitis is also known as the common cold or coryza. Acute rhinitis may be bacterial or viral in origin; it is treated symptomatically. Acute rhinitis usually lasts 5 to 7 days, with or without treatment. Common interventions for acute rhinitis are symptomatic and include supplemental humidification, decongestants to reduce the edema of the nasal mucosa, increased fluids to prevent dehydration, and analgesics to relieve the generalized myalgia. Sometimes antibiotics are given to prevent a secondary infection by bacteria.

Allergic rhinitis is most often seen as a seasonal disorder. In addition to obstruction to nasal breathing, the client may also experience irritation of other mucous membranes (i.e., the conjunctiva, causing tearing and edema of the eyelids). Treatment is symptomatic. A complete allergy evaluation may be required to determine the offending allergen. Most clients are placed on a desensitization program, told to avoid the antigen, and treated with antihistamines, steroids or mast cell–stabilizing sprays.[3]

Vasomotor rhinitis causes the same manifestations as do acute and allergic rhinitis but has no known cause. Clients complaining of vasomotor rhinitis who have a negative culture and negative allergy evaluation are treated symptomatically. If medications have been prescribed for clients with rhinitis (especially nasal sprays), the client must be taught the use of medications, including side effects and possible interactions with other medications.

Rhinitis medicamentosa is caused by abuse or overuse of topical nasal decongestant sprays or intranasal cocaine. These substances initially cause vasoconstriction. When used frequently, however, the initial decongestion is followed by severe mucosal edema. The edema is self-treated with more medication and the rhinitis becomes cyclic. Treatment of rhinitis medicamentosa is avoidance of the causative agent and evaluation and treatment of the original problem.[25,29]

Laryngitis

Laryngitis may be caused by an inflammatory process or vocal abuse. The laryngeal membrane is continuous with the lining of the upper respiratory tract, and infections in other areas of the nose and throat may include the larynx. Edema of the vocal cords caused by the chronic irritation of an upper respiratory tract infection inhibits the normal mobility of the vocal cords, which causes an abnormal sound.

Laryngitis may also be the result of gastroesophageal reflux disorder (GERD). In this syndrome, the sphincter between the stomach and esophagus relaxes, and gastric acid is allowed to enter the esophagus. Reflux of gastric secretions, especially during sleep, may result in the aspiration of gastric secretions into the larynx, causing a chemical irritation or burning of the mucous membrane lining the larynx.[18,25,29] Clients with gastroesophageal reflux may complain of hoarseness from the chemical irritation of the gastric acid on the vocal cords, increased mucus production from the body's natural tendency to protect the irritated membrane, foreign-body sensation, or sore throat. Chronic cough and asthma may also be associated symptoms of GERD.

Hoarseness is a common manifestation of disorders of the larynx and may be caused by inflammation of the vocal cords, abnormal movements of the vocal cords, or a benign or malignant tumor of the vocal cords. All of these interfere with normal mobility of the vocal cords, which produces a change in sound. Abnormal voice may also be the result of vocal abuse. Screaming, shouting, and loud speaking over a period of time may produce edema of the vocal cords and the formation of nodules or polyps, outpouchings of inflamed mucous membranes.

The initial treatment of laryngitis is to treat the causative factors. If inflammatory laryngitis is suspected, the inflammation should be treated. Antibiotics may be used if a bacterial infection is suspected. In severe cases, systemic steroids (e.g., methylprednisolone [Medrol Dosepak]) may be prescribed to reduce inflammation and edema. Supplemental humidification may add increased moisture to liquify secretions, and mucolytic agents may be prescribed to thin and mobilize mucus. Clients with laryngitis may also be placed on voice rest to allow the edema of the vocal cords to subside without added strain. Caution the client to avoid whispering, which also causes excessive vocal cord strain.

Gastroesophageal reflux is initially treated symptomatically. The client is instructed to elevate the head of the bed to minimize reflux; to avoid eating or drinking for 2 to 3 hours before going to sleep; to avoid caffeine, alcohol, and tobacco, which are known to increase gastric secretions; and to use antacids and hydrogen inhibitors (famotidine [Pepcid], ranitidine [Zantac], omeprazole [Prilosec]) to neutralize and decrease acid production.[18,25,29]

Chronic laryngitis may stem from repeated infections, allergy, chronic irritant exposure, long-term voice abuse, and reflux esophagitis of acidic gastric contents. Chronic laryngitis is manifested by a tickling sensation in the throat, voice huskiness, and painful or difficult phonation. Management involves correction or removal of the irritation, in addition to measures to increase comfort. Long-term voice retraining may be necessary if improper use or overuse of the voice is the main cause of chronic laryngitis. This retraining includes (1) learning to use the voice without straining and (2) forming and projecting words to use the diaphragm without shouting.[18,25,29]

Diphtheria

Diphtheria is an acute, communicable disease caused by *Corynebacterium diphtheriae.* In the 1920s and 1930s, vaccination with diphtheria toxoid was introduced. In most western countries, diphtheria has been virtually eliminated. Immunity to diseases from vaccination wanes with time, and a growing number of people may be susceptible. A resurgence has occurred in the incidence of diphtheria in several countries of the former Soviet Union. Diphtheria is a highly contagious disease that is spread easily in areas with poor personal hygiene, crowding, and limited access to medical care.

Humans are the only natural reservoir for *C. diphtheriae.* *C. diphtheriae* colonizes on the mucosal surface of the nasopharynx and multiplies. The bacteria releases a toxin, which causes the tissues to necrose and form a tough pseudomembrane. Toxins can become systemic and damage distal sites such as the heart, nerves, and kidneys.

Diphtheria is spread by aerosolization of the organism (droplet infection), and when objects used by diphtheria-infected people, such as eating utensils, towels, handkerchiefs, and so forth, are used by others. Healthy people, as well as clients recovering from the disease, may harbor the organism in their throats for 2 to 4 weeks.

Diphtheria is characterized by a pseudomembrane covering the posterior pharynx. This exudate forms a dirty, gray-white, rubbery membrane that covers and adheres to the inflamed, eroded surfaces of the oropharynx, nasopharynx, and laryngopharynx. The membrane may also extend into the trachea.

Clinical manifestations can range from a single, localized lesion without systemic manifestations to a rapidly progressive fatal illness. In general, the severity of diphtheria is correlated with the site of the local lesion. Anterior nasal lesions tend to be chronic, but clients have few symptoms. People with chronic lesions are most often carriers, especially in developed countries.

There are two types: tonsillar and pharyngeal. Tonsillar diphtheria is seldom life-threatening, although it can progress rapidly to more fatal forms. A low-grade fever, fatigue, headache, and sore throat are common manifestations.

Pharyngeal diphtheria, especially when a membrane covers the larynx or bronchus, is the most serious form of diphtheria. The client is gravely ill, with a weak pulse, restlessness, and confusion. Fever may or may not be present. Because of the location of the membrane, the airway is often obstructed and the client has stridor and cyanosis. The neck may also be swollen and warm.

Diphtheria is diagnosed by culture of the material with the enzyme-linked immunosorbent assay (ELISA) or Elek test. Gram stain or fluorescent antibody stains may also be performed, and more quickly. Although cultures are used to identify the organism, treatment begins while waiting for the definitive results.

To prevent transmission of the disease, the client is placed in strict isolation. Contacts need to be identified, screened, immunized, and treated. All contacts should be cultured. Those persons immunized 5 or more years previously should receive a booster dose. Those persons who were never immunized should be treated with immunization and antibiotics. During antitoxin administration, observe the client for anaphylaxis; epinephrine is kept at the bedside.

Nursing management focuses on management of the airway obstruction. Suction equipment and a tracheotomy tray should be kept at the bedside. Oxygen is administered. Clients experience pain, especially with swallowing. In addition to analgesia, pain can be reduced by limiting the diet to liquids and soft foods. Throat irrigation and fluids may also help control pain.

Neoplastic Disorders

Benign Tumors of the Larynx

Papillomas are one type of benign tumor of the larynx. They are small wartlike growths believed to be viral in origin. Papillomas may be removed by surgical excision or laser. Surgery must be exact, because the nondiseased portion of the vocal cords needs to be retained for function. Other benign tumors of the larynx include nodules and polyps. Nodules and polyps frequently occur in people who abuse or overuse their voice.

Cancer of the Larynx

Cancer of the larynx accounts for 2% to 3% of all malignancies. Clients with these tumors present a unique challenge to the nurse because of the cosmetic and functional deformities commonly seen with the disorder and its treatment. Benign and early malignant tumors may be treated with limited surgery, and the client recovers with little functional loss. Advanced tumors require extensive treatment, including surgery, radiation treatments, and chemotherapy. At times the operation may render the client unable to speak, breathe through the nose or mouth, or eat normally. In addition, the defect left by the operation and its reconstruction may cause a significant deformity and a need for further surgery to restore appearance.

Laryngeal cancer is classified and treated by its anatomic site. Cancer of the larynx (voice box) may occur on the glottis (true vocal cords), the supraglottic structures (above the vocal cords), or the subglottic structures (below the vocal cords) (Box 40–2).

There are an estimated 12,500 cases of laryngeal cancer each year, with the majority of those afflicted being men. However, the incidence of women with cancer of the larynx is increasing.[32] If untreated, cancer of the larynx is inevitably fatal; 90% of untreated persons die within 3 years. Like other cancers, however, it is potentially curable if discovered early enough.

Etiology and Risk Factors

Considerable data indicate that the primary etiologic agent of laryngeal cancer is cigarette smoking. Three of four clients who develop laryngeal cancer have smoked or currently smoke. The use of alcohol appears to act synergistically with tobacco, increasing the risk of developing a malignant tumor in the upper airway. The inhalation of other noxious fumes, such as polluted air, chronic laryngitis, and voice abuse may also contribute to the disorder. The Risk Factors and Levels of Prevention feature for laryngeal cancer lists the warning signs for this type of cancer.

Pathophysiology

Squamous cell carcinoma is the most common malignant tumor of the larynx, arising from the membrane lining the respiratory tract. Metastasis from cancer of the glottis is unusual because of the sparse lymphatic drainage from the vocal cords. Cancer elsewhere in the larynx spreads more quickly because there are abundant lymphatic vessels. Metastatic disease often may be palpated as neck masses. Distant metastasis may occur in the lungs. Patterns of spread of head and neck cancer are shown in Figure 40–8.

Clinical Manifestations and Diagnostic Findings

The earliest clinical warning signs of laryngeal cancer (Box 40–3) are dependent on the location of the tumor. In general, hoarseness that lasts longer than 2 weeks should be evaluated. Unfortunately, most clients wait before seeking a diagnosis for chronic hoarseness.

Tumors on the glottis prevent it from closing during speech, which causes hoarseness or a voice change. Supraglottic tumors cause pain in the throat, especially with swallowing, aspiration during swallowing, a sensation of a foreign body in the throat, neck masses, and pain radiating to the ear by way of the glossopharyngeal and vagus nerves. Subglottic tumors have no early manifestations; manifestations do not appear until the tumor grows to obstruct the airway.[25]

The diagnosis of laryngeal cancer is made by visual examination of the larynx with direct or indirect laryngoscopy. The nasopharynx and posterior soft palate are inspected indirectly with a small mirror or an instrument resembling a telescope. While the mirror is inserted, slight pressure is applied to the tongue, and the client is

Box 40–2. Clinical Manifestations of Laryngeal Cancer

Area	Manifestations
Glottic Tumor 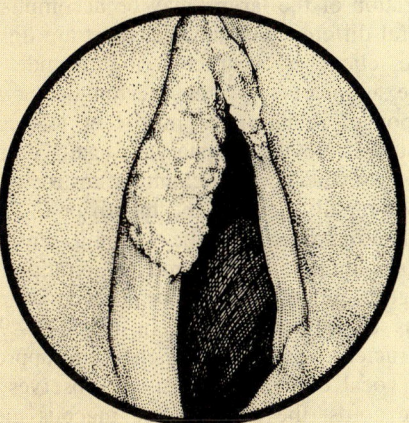 True glottic tumors interfere with normal closure and vibration of the vocal cords	*Early:* voice change, hoarseness, hemoptysis *Late:* dyspnea, respiratory obstruction, dysphagia, weight loss, pain *Metastasize:* through regional lymph nodes (rare except in superior or inferior tumors)
Supraglottic Tumor 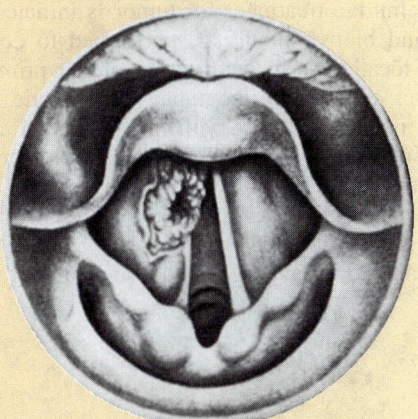 Carcinoma of the false cord partially hiding the true cord	*Early:* aspiration on swallowing (especially liquids), persistent unilateral sore throat, foreign-body sensation, dysphagia, weight loss, neck mass, hemoptysis *Late:* dyspnea, pain in the throat or referred to the ear
Subglottic Tumor 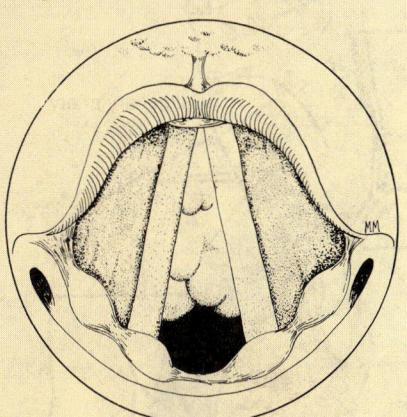 Subglottic polyp; this type of polyp can be single and smooth or lobulated as shown	*Early:* None *Late:* dyspnea, airway obstruction, dysphagia, weight loss, hemoptysis

Top and bottom figures from DeWeese, D. F., & Saunders, W. H. (1982). *Textbook of otolaryngology* (6th ed.). St. Louis: Mosby–Year Book; middle figure from Del Regato, J. A., et al. (1985). *Ackerman and Del Regato's cancer* (6th ed.). St. Louis: Mosby–Year Book.

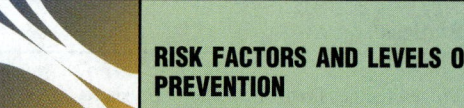

RISK FACTORS AND LEVELS OF PREVENTION

Laryngeal Cancer

Risk Factors

Smoking, alcohol abuse, inhalation of noxious fumes or polluted air, voice abuse

Levels of Prevention

Primary Prevention

- Educate the public on the hazards of smoking and alcohol abuse.
- Refer clients to smoking cessation programs.
- Refer clients to alcohol abuse programs.

Secondary Prevention

- Teach clients to recognize the early warning signs of cancer of the larynx:
  - Hoarseness or other change in voice
  - Lump in the neck
  - Persistent sore throat, cough, earache (otalgia)
  - Hemoptysis
  - Difficulty swallowing, aspiration on swallowing, weight loss
  - Difficulty breathing

Tertiary Prevention

- Intervene early to reduce the risk of progression of malignancy.

instructed to say "uh-hah," which elevates the soft palate (Fig. 40–9A). The instrument should not touch the tongue or the client will gag. The nasopharynx is then inspected for drainage, bleeding, ulceration, or masses.

Direct visualization of the larynx may be accomplished with use of several different instruments; most are lighted endoscopes. The client is instructed to protrude the tongue, and the examiner *gently* pulls the tongue forward with a gauze sponge. A laryngeal mirror or telescopic endoscope is inserted into the oropharynx; again, contact with the tongue is avoided. The client is instructed to breathe in and out rapidly through the mouth or to "pant like a puppy." Panting decreases the gagging sensation caused by the examination. During quiet respiration, the base of the tongue, epiglottis, and vocal cords are examined for signs of infection or tumor (Fig. 40–9B). The client is instructed to say a high-pitched *e* to approximate (close) the vocal cords. The examiner observes the movement of the cords, the color of the mucous membrane, and the presence of any lesions. If the client is unable to cooperate with this examination, it may be performed with a fiberoptic endoscope inserted through the nose.

Before any definitive treatment for tumor is initiated, a panendoscopy and biopsy should be performed to determine the exact location, size, and extent of the primary tumor. Sometimes computed tomography or magnetic resonance imaging is used to assist with this process. Laboratory analysis includes a complete blood count, determination of serum electrolytes and calcium levels, and kidney and liver function tests. These data help determine the physiologic state of the client for surgery. Because the airway will be altered after surgery, the client requires a

Figure 40–8. The pattern of spread of head and neck cancer. (From Black, J. [1991]. Reconstructive surgery in the elderly. *Plastic Surgical Nursing, 11;* 157.)

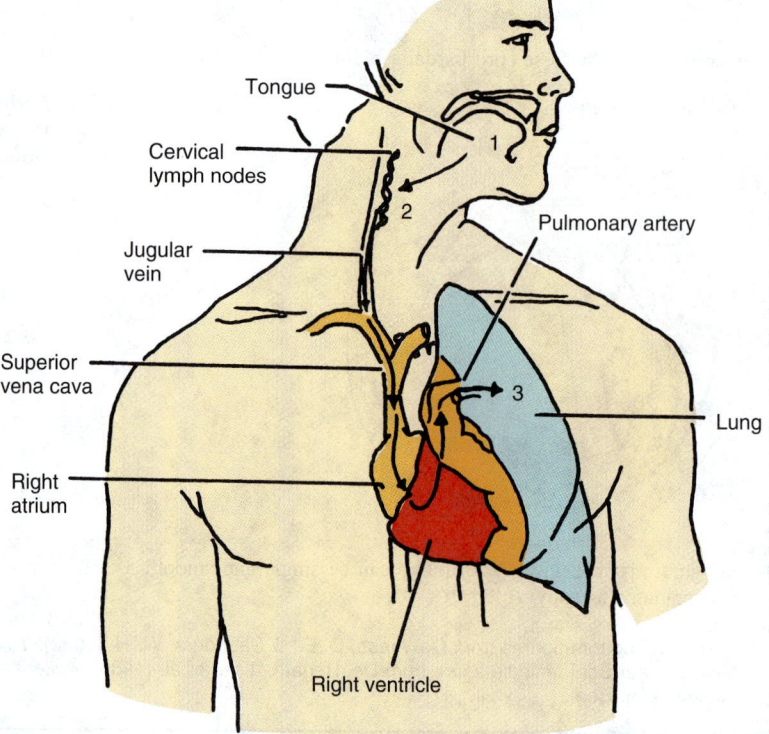

gery places clients at increased risk of aspiration, and they must be able to cough to rid the airway of aspirated secretions. Finally, for ascertaining possible tumor spread or other primary tumors, a chest radiograph and barium swallow or esophagogram are performed.

Once the tumor has been identified and a biopsy performed, the tumor can be staged. Staging has important implications for treatment choice and outcome. It is essential to determine the extent of the primary tumor in order to select the most appropriate intervention. Staging is accomplished by (1) measuring the size of the primary tumor, (2) determining the presence of enlarged lymphatic nodes, and (3) determining the presence of distant metastasis. Data obtained are called the TNM classification (T, tumor; N, nodes; and M, metastasis). The TNM classification system for laryngeal cancers is shown in Box 40–4.[23] See also Chapter 23 for more information on staging.

thorough pulmonary assessment with ABG analysis for identification of any preexisting pulmonary disorders that would interfere with breathing. Clients who will have a partial laryngectomy must have an adequate pulmonary reserve in order to produce an effective cough. The sur-

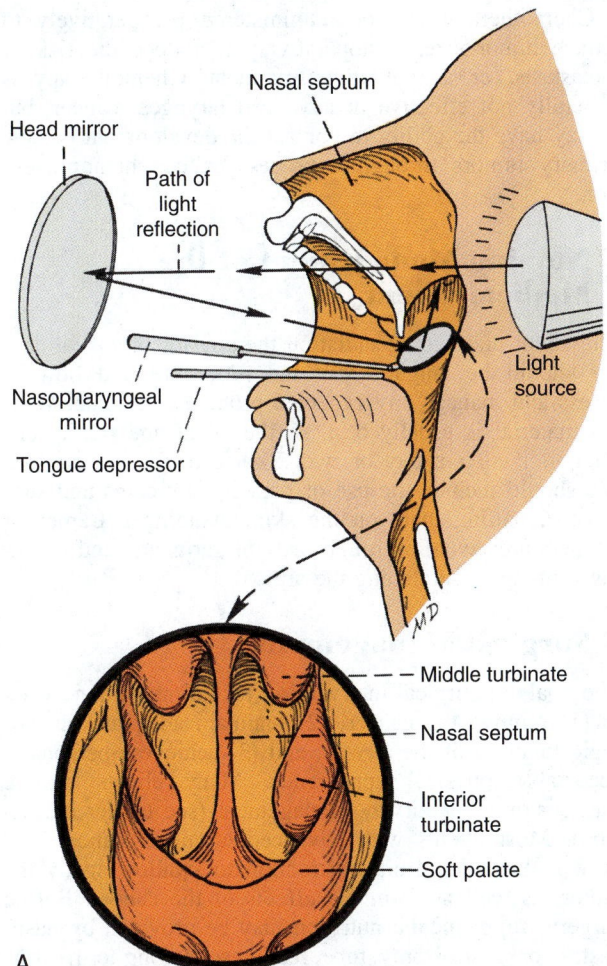

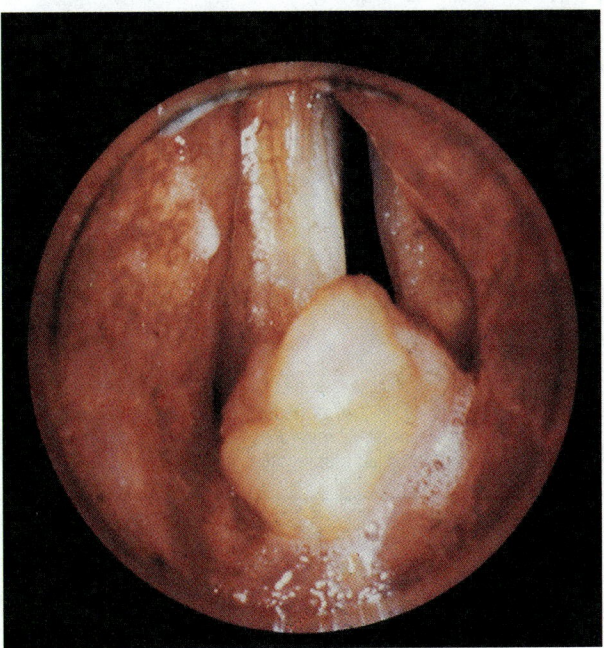

A

B

Figure 40–9. *A,* Indirect laryngoscopy enables assessment of the pharynx and buccal cavity and some visualization of the larynx. (Laryngeal structure and function are best assessed by direct visualization, such as flexible or rigid laryngoscopy or flexible fiberoptic bronchoscopy). Indirect laryngoscopy is performed using a head mirror, tongue depressor, light source, and small examining mirror. The mirror is positioned behind the soft palate after the tongue is depressed. To visualize the larynx, the tongue is gently grasped with a gauze sponge and pulled forward. A mirror is placed against the soft palate in front of the uvula and moved gently until the cords are visualized. The sound "eee" will cause the larynx to move. The larynx is assessed for symmetrical cord motion. *B,* Large granular cell tumor of the true vocal cord as seen during laryngoscopy (From Wenig, B. M. [1993]. *Atlas of head and neck pathology.* Philadelphia: W. B. Saunders.)

Acute and Subacute Care

■ Medical Management

Treatment of glottic cancer depends on the degree of tumor involvement. If the tumor is limited to the true vocal cord, without causing limitation of the cord's movement, radiation therapy is usually the best treatment, with cure rates of 85% to 95%. The dosage of radiation therapy depends on the size and location of the tumor; it is usually a minimal dose of 5500 to 6000 cGy (*gray* [Gy] is a more accurate unit than *rad*) over 5 to 7 weeks. During radiation therapy, the client needs to be assessed for signs of destruction of normal tissue, ability to eat, airway distress, and other side effects. The complications of radiation therapy to the larynx include skin irritation, xerostomia, mucositis, and laryngeal edema, and delayed healing. Radiation therapy is discussed fully in Chapter 24.

Supraglottic tumors may be treated with radiation therapy or a partial laryngectomy with or without lymph node dissection. Subglottic tumors are usually more advanced carcinomas in which the tumor has spread to surrounding tissues. Metastasis is common. Treatment requires a total laryngectomy with or without radical neck dissection on the same or both sides. (See later discussion.) The operative site may require reconstruction with pectoralis myocutaneous flaps (see Chapter 80).

Chemotherapy can be administered preoperatively to reduce tumor size, postoperatively to reduce the risk of metastasis, or as palliative treatment. Chemotherapy is generally not effective in advanced laryngeal cancer, but it may have the ability to control the development of new primary tumors through a process called chemoprevention.

■ Nursing Management of the Medical Client

The client undergoing radiation therapy for laryngeal cancer should be taught about the procedure and how to assess and manage any expected problems at home. Written material is usually best, so the client and family can refer to it after a day or two. Skin care for the radiated site should include the use of prescribed creams and sunscreens, patting them on the skin; avoiding extremes of temperature; avoiding rough or tight garments; and avoiding rubbing or scratching the area.

■ Surgical Management

The goals of surgical intervention for laryngeal cancer are to (1) remove the cancer, (2) maintain adequate physiologic function of the airway, and (3) achieve a personally acceptable physical appearance. Many clients require tracheostomy for airway management (see earlier discussion). Most clients with advanced laryngeal cancer also have malnutrition from obstruction to swallowing by the tumor, as well as from the effects of the cancer. Before surgery, supplemental nutrition may be provided by nasogastric or gastrostomy tube feedings. If long-term difficulty in swallowing is anticipated, a gastrostomy tube may be inserted at the time of surgery.

Laser Surgery

An option for small tumors is the use of laser to eradicate them. Laser surgery for vocal cord tumors can preserve much of the normal glottis and leave the client with a

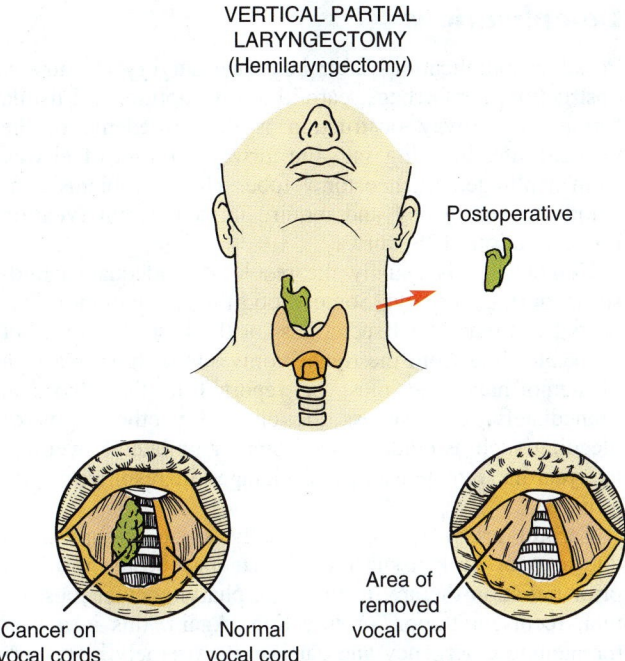

**VERTICAL PARTIAL
LARYNGECTOMY**
(Hemilaryngectomy)

Postoperative

Cancer on
vocal cords

Normal
vocal cord

Area of
removed
vocal cord

Figure 40–10. The technique of partial laryngectomy.

feasible. This operation is also called a vertical partial laryngectomy and is the removal of half or more of the larynx (Fig. 40–10). A horizontal neck incision is made, and the diseased portion of the vocal cord is removed. Sometimes up to one third of the contralateral cord is also removed. This operation is generally well tolerated, and the client has only mild difficulty swallowing and an altered, but adequate, voice.

Another form of partial laryngectomy is the supra-glottic laryngectomy. This surgery is performed for cancer of the supraglottis. The operation removes the superior portion of the larynx from the false vocal cords to the epiglottis and may extend upward to remove a portion of the base of the tongue. Lymph node dissection also may be performed. Because the true vocal cords are preserved, the voice quality is maintained. The major postoperative problem is risk of aspiration because the epiglottis, which closes over the larynx, has been removed. Airway is managed with a tracheostomy after surgery; when the edema subsides in surrounding tissues, it can usually be removed. The client will need to be taught how to swallow to avoid aspiration.

usable voice. Sometimes laser surgery is combined with radiation therapy.

Partial Laryngectomy

For cancer of one true vocal cord or one true vocal cord and a portion of the other, a partial laryngectomy is

Total Laryngectomy

For large glottic tumors with fixation of the vocal cords, a total laryngectomy is required. The larynx is the connection of the pharynx (upper airway) and the trachea (lower airway) (Fig. 40–11A). When the larynx is removed, a permanent opening is made by suturing the trachea to the neck. The esophagus remains attached to the pharynx (see Fig. 40–11B). Because no air can enter

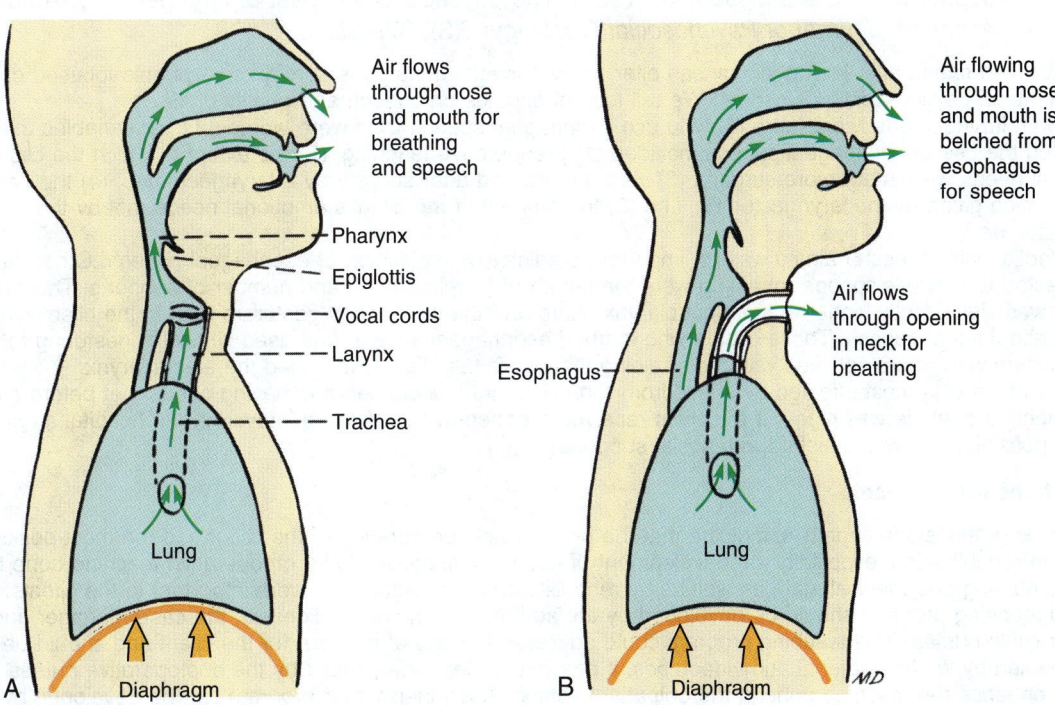

Air flows
through nose
and mouth for
breathing
and speech

Pharynx

Epiglottis

Vocal cords

Larynx

Trachea

Lung

A   Diaphragm

Air flowing
through nose
and mouth is
belched from
esophagus
for speech

Air flows
through opening
in neck for
breathing

Esophagus

Lung

B   Diaphragm

Figure 40–11. *A,* Prior to laryngectomy, air flow is through the nose and mouth. *B,* Surgical removal of the larynx requires that a new opening be made for air passage. The trachea and esophagus are separated.

the nose, the client loses the sense of smell. The biggest problem for the client after laryngectomy is loss of voice. The client should be made aware that without surgery, the voice quality will worsen as the tumor enlarges, but in any case the loss of voice is a serious psychological problem. Because the trachea and esophagus are permanently separated by surgery, there is no risk of aspiration unless a fistula forms from the trachea to the esophagus. Besides this, the potential complications of the total laryngectomy are the same as for the partial laryngectomy (see earlier discussion).

Cervical Lymph Node Dissection

Metastasis to the cervical lymph nodes is common with tumors of the upper aerodigestive tract. Surgical management of laryngeal tumors often includes neck dissection. Radical neck dissection (also called en bloc) is the removal of lymphatic drainage channels and nodes, sternocleidomastoid muscle, spinal accessory nerve, jugular vein, and submandibular area. A modified radical neck dissection spares the spinal accessory nerve and a selective neck dissection removes only the lymph nodes within the area of anticipated spread.[23,25]

Complications

Possible complications after laryngeal surgery are airway obstruction, hemorrhage, carotid artery rupture, and fistula formation. Airway obstruction is due to edema in the surgical site, bleeding into the airway, or loss of airway from a plugged tracheostomy tube. These problems constitute an emergency and require immediate intervention for restoration of the airway.

Hemorrhage is usually the result of inadequate hemostasis during surgery. Some blood-tinged sputum is expected in the tracheal secretions for the first 48 hours, but frank bleeding from the tracheotomy site or tube is a sign of hemorrhage and must be reported to the physician immediately. Also assess the client for other signs of bleeding such as evident hematoma or unilateral swelling, tachycardia, hypotension, and changes in respiratory patterns.

Carotid artery rupture is usually a late complication due to poor neck tissue integrity. It may be the result of prior radiation therapy to the area, pharyngocutaneous fistula, recurrent tumor, or infection. Again, this is a life-threatening emergency and carries an extremely high mortality rate. Mild bleeding from the oral cavity, neck, or

---

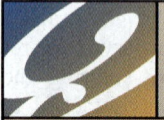

NURSING RESEARCH

What is Life Like After a Laryngectomy?

Stam, H., Koopmans, J., & Mathieson, C. (1991). The psychosocial impact of laryngectomy: A comprehensive assessment. *Journal of Psychosocial Oncology, 9*(3), 37–57.

The inability to speak after laryngectomy can alter many aspects of life. This survey of 51 people focused on components of psychosocial adjustment. We will look at findings on speech and quality of life.

Men with laryngectomy were more likely to use esophageal speech than were women. Other variables that influenced the use of esophageal speech included (1) preoperative teaching, (2) the extent to which the client's emotional needs were met before surgery, (3) visits before and after surgery by a laryngectomee, (4) the amount of information given by the laryngectomee, and (5) the amount of the client's emotional needs met by the laryngectomee.

Satisfaction with speech training was an important predictor of acquisition of esophageal speech. Other variables that affected the client's speech retraining were the length of hospitalization and number of supports. The extent of surgery was significantly higher in the electrolarynx users and the writers and gesturers than in the clients who learned esophageal speech. Those clients who learned esophageal speech and used writing or gesturing to communicate were more satisfied with their training than were the clients who used the electrolarynx.

Quality of life was most affected by a visit from a previous laryngectomee and having needs met before surgery. Adjustment as a whole was higher if the client received preoperative counseling, stayed in the hospital as brief a time as possible, and was satisfied with social supports.

Implications for Practice

The results of this study appear to indicate that the preoperative preparation of the client had the most positive impact on rehabilitation, especially the development of esophageal speech. The preoperative teaching done by both the nursing and medical staff, as well as by rehabilitated laryngectomees, were important to the clients. A planned teaching program should be developed by the staff nurses in conjunction with the case manager and office or clinic nurses. This teaching program could address all areas of concern for the client and should be accompanied by written material and videotapes, if possible. Telephone contact by the postoperative nurses can be used to enhance the teaching done in the outpatient setting. A planned visitor program can be developed by the hospital with the local Lost Cord Club or American Cancer Society.

trachea may precede an impending rupture by 24 to 48 hours. A pulsating tracheostomy tube may indicate that the tip of the tube is resting on the innominate artery and may cause injury to the artery resulting in hemorrhage.

Fistulas between the hypopharynx and the skin may also develop. Many fistulas heal on their own, but surgery may be required, depending on the location and size.

■ Nursing Management of the Surgical Client

Partial Laryngectomy

Preoperative Care

In addition to the usual preoperative assessments, assess the client's nutritional status. Compare current body weight with ideal body weight, usual caloric intake, total lymphocyte count, albumin levels, and hemoglobin value and hematocrit.[25] The client's state of dentition and oral care should also be assessed. Because many of these clients have abused tobacco and alcohol, their dentition and oral cavity are frequently in poor repair. In addition, if the client is still an active alcoholic, plans should consider support through the period of alcohol withdrawal. The ideal plan would allow some nutritional support and oral care before surgery. Unfortunately, today, few clients can be admitted before surgery and therefore this must be accomplished prior to surgery.

The client's work history and financial concerns should also be investigated during this initial assessment. A lack of medical insurance or money may account for the client's lack of personal and medical care.

The client's usual coping strategies and family support should also be evaluated. There will be some degree of cosmetic (aesthetic) change after surgery and a period of time during which the client is unable to speak.[2] Preoperative plans should consider alternative methods of communication and family support networks. The psychosocial impact of laryngectomy is discussed in the Nursing Research feature.

Because of the multiple problems common in these clients, a team approach to their care is used. Members of the team usually include physician or surgeon, nurses, social worker, dietician, speech or swallowing therapist, physical therapist, and home healthcare nurses. If extensive surgery is required, a plastic surgeon and maxillofacial prosthodontist may also care for the client during reconstruction.

Postoperative Care

Assessment

In addition to the routine assessments of any postoperative client, after a partial laryngectomy the client needs to have careful assessment of the airway, lung sounds, position of the tracheostomy tube, and potential complications of the surgery and the tracheostomy tube (see earlier discussion).

Diagnosis, Planning, Implementation

Risk for Aspiration. Because of the removal of the epiglottis (which normally acts as a trap door to close over the airway and prevent aspiration) and excessive secretions secondary to surgery, the client is a very high risk for aspiration. This is a priority probably diagnosis and remains so for about 72 hours.

Planning: Expected Outcomes. The client will not aspirate, as evidenced by clear breath sounds throughout the chest, normal (for age) respiratory rate and rhythm, chest secretions that are clear or only slightly blood-tinged, and ability to cough.

Implementation. In the immediate postoperative period, priority is given to management of the upper airway. The client should be positioned in the semi- to high-Fowler position to decrease edema of the airway, facilitate breathing, and improve comfort.

A cuffed tracheostomy tube is generally inserted during surgery and is maintained for the first several days after surgery to minimize aspiration of secretions and for assisted or controlled ventilation. Secretions collect above the cuff. For removal of secretions, the cuff should be deflated during exhalation. The client should be instructed to cough during deflation of the cuff. If the client cannot cough, suctioning should be used to prevent secretions from being aspirated. The cuff should be reinflated during inspiration.

When the edema has subsided, the tracheostomy tube may be removed. The decannulation process is slow and begins by observing the client for aspiration. The cuff of the tube is deflated, and the client is observed for ability to swallow saliva and other secretions without coughing or requiring additional suctioning. If there are increased secretions through and around the tracheostomy tube, aspiration is occurring and the cuff should be reinflated. If no aspiration is occurring, the tracheostomy tube can be replaced with a smaller uncuffed tube. If this is tolerated without aspiration, the tube is capped to determine the client's ability to breathe through the upper airway. If the client can breathe through the upper airway for 24 hours, the tracheostomy tube is removed, and the stoma is taped closed and covered with an occlusive dressing.[1,15] (Fig. 40–12).

Ineffective Airway Clearance. The physical alteration in the airway and the presence of a tracheostomy tube interfere with normal movement of mucus up and out of the bronchial tree. In addition, because of prior smoking, the cilia have become ineffective. This is also a priority diagnosis for several days.

Planning: Expected Outcomes. The client will have improved airway clearance, as evidenced by effortless, quiet respirations at baseline rate and clear breath sounds.

Implementation. The client may have copious secretions because of the presence of the tracheostomy tube, history of chronic obstructive lung disease, and aspiration. There may also be oral secretions that cannot be swallowed. In the alert and conscious client, coughing and deep breathing will mobilize and eliminate many of these

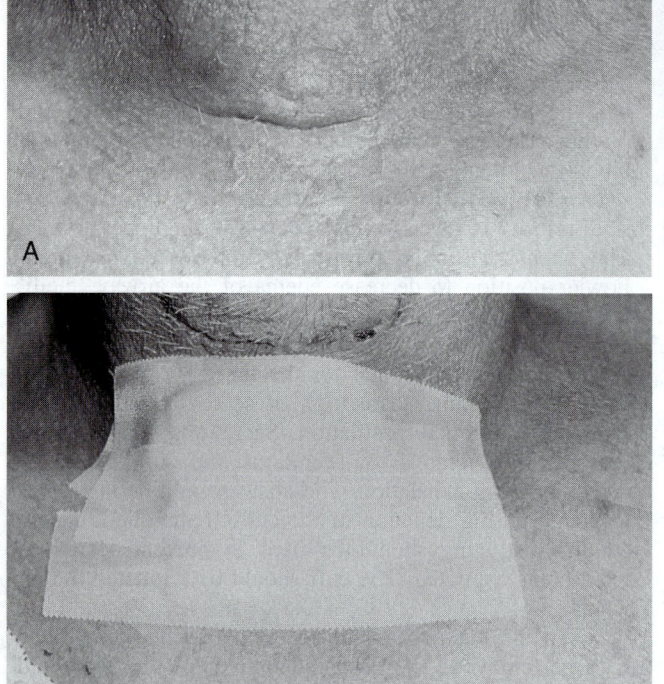

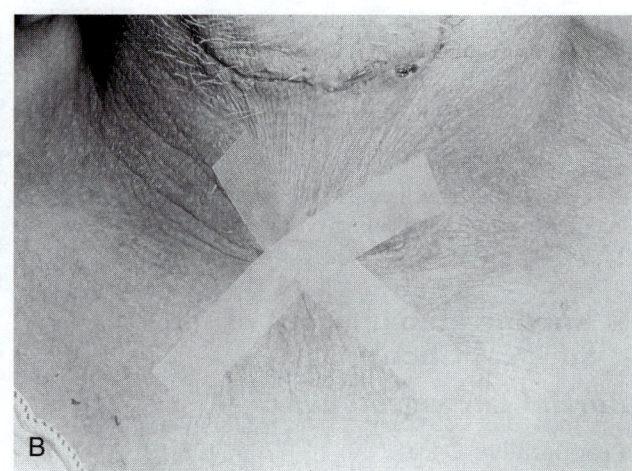

Figure 40–12. *A,* Closing stoma after decannulation. The skin is cleaned with hydrogen peroxide and protected with tincture of benzoin. *B,* The skin edges are pulled together and taped in an X. *C,* An occlusive dressing is applied.

secretions. However, in the client having head and neck surgery and just emerging from anesthesia, this may not be possible. Suctioning of the trachea will be needed for the first 24 to 48 hours after surgery. The frequency of suctioning depends on the client's needs, but suctioning every hour or more often is common for the first 24 hours. Sterile technique must be used to avoid introducing microorganisms into the tracheobronchial tree in a client with impaired immune defenses due to malignancy and surgery. (Suctioning techniques can be found in a fundamentals of nursing textbook.)

The inner cannula of the tracheostomy tube should be cleaned as often as necessary to provide a clear airway. In the immediate postoperative phase, the inner cannula is cleaned after suctioning. Once the client is ambulatory and handles secretions safely, it can be cleaned as necessary, but at least three times a day.

Chest physiotherapy, ultrasonic nebulization, or aerosol administration of medications are recommended to prevent pulmonary complications. These treatments are performed every 4 hours for the first few days after surgery and then usually decreased to four times a day once the client can ambulate.[25]

Risk for Impaired Gas Exchange. Like other postoperative clients, clients with neck surgery have high risk for atelectasis related to low tidal volume breathing secondary to pain, sedation, and increased mucus production.

Planning: Expected Outcomes. The client will have adequate oxygenation as evidenced by pulse oximetry values above 90%, ABGs within normal limits (considering any preexisting lung disorders, such as emphysema), no air hunger, and clear lung sounds.

Implementation. Oxygenation is assessed through ABGs or pulse oximetry and the fraction of inspired oxygen (FIO_2) may be adjusted. If the client has preexistent chronic air flow limitations, oxygen may have to be delivered at lower percentages or not at all. Compressed air with high humidity may be substituted for these clients.

Altered Nutrition: Less than Body Requirements. A combination of the preexisting malignancy and swallowing difficulties sets the stage for malnutrition. In addition, preexisting lung disorders and alcoholism, which are common in this population, increase the tendency for malnutrition.

Planning: Expected Outcomes. The client will have an improved nutritional status, as evidenced by maintaining baseline body weight or losing less than 5 lbs; consuming adequate fluid, protein, fat, and carbohydrate each 24 hours; swallowing without aspirating or choking; and hemoglobin, hematocrit, albumin, and total lymphocyte values remaining within normal limits.

Implementation. Immediately after surgery, it is likely the client will have a nasogastric tube inserted for removal of gastric secretions until postoperative ileus subsides. If long-term difficulty in swallowing is anticipated, a gastrostomy tube may be inserted at the time of surgery. Assess for bowel sounds, passing of flatus, and hunger as signs of returning gastrointestinal function. Some clients will be tube-fed with commercial supplements. Continually ascertain the correct presence of the tube before each feeding. (Techniques to check feeding tube placement can be found in a fundamentals of nursing textbook.) The tube feeding can be administered by pump, slow drip, or bolus feeding depending on the client's tolerance. Aspiration remains a high risk with partial laryngectomy, and precautions to guard the client from it are critical.

Because the epiglottis has been removed, when to begin oral feeding after a partial laryngectomy is controversial. One approach is to begin oral feedings with the tracheostomy tube in place when edema has subsided and the client is able to swallow secretions. The advantage of this technique is that aspirated liquid can be suctioned. A second technique is to delay oral feeding until the client has been decannulated and the stoma has healed. The advantage of this technique is that with a closed stoma, the client is able to increase intrathoracic pressure and remove any aspirated material through an effective cough.

Whenever the client eats, eating should begin with a nonpourable pureed diet; liquids are reserved until swallowing has been relearned. The Client Education Guide describes one technique for swallowing after a partial laryngectomy. Once swallowing can be accomplished without aspiration, carbonated beverages may be added. Thin liquids should be withheld until the risk of aspiration is minimal.[1,15,25]

Risk for Infection. The loss of primary defenses of the skin and delayed healing due to preexisting malignancy and malnutrition make this nursing diagnosis common.

Planning: Expected Outcomes. The client will develop no clinical manifestations of wound infection, as evidenced by incisional edges remaining approximated; amounts of wound drainage decreasing; no purulent drainage; absence of redness, swelling, tenderness, or warmth beyond the suture lines; remaining afebrile; and white blood cell count remaining within normal limits.

Implementation. During surgery, a wound drain is placed into the surrounding tissues of the neck and attached to constant suction. A common mechanism for collecting the drainage is a Hemovac container, which is

CLIENT EDUCATION GUIDE

Swallowing Technique After a Partial Laryngectomy

1. Begin with soft or semisolid foods.
2. Stay with a nurse or swallowing therapist during meals until you master the technique of swallowing without choking.
3. Be patient; learning to swallow again is frustrating.
4. Take a deep breath.
5. Bear down to close the vocal cords.
6. Place food into your mouth.
7. Swallow.
8. Cough to rid the closed cord of accumulated food particles.
9. Swallow.
10. Cough.
11. Breathe.

attached to the client's gown to prevent accidental dislodgment. Using universal precautions, assess the amount and color of the drainage every 4 hours for the first 24 hours. Assess the wound for signs of hematoma or seroma formation by noting whether the amount of drainage is increasing or if there is a change in the color or consistency of the drainage. Also assess the color of the incision lines. If the drainage is subsiding, the drain may be removed by the physician. Dressings are placed over the drain puncture sites on the skin. Small-to-moderate amounts of serosanguineous drainage should be expected for another 48 to 72 hours.

The suture lines should be cleaned at least twice daily with hydrogen peroxide followed by a water or saline rinse. A thin film of antibiotic ointment may be applied to the suture line to prevent crusting of secretions and promote healing.

Evaluation

Expect the problems with airway management to resolve within a few days. Infection, apart from atelectasis, will not arise for about 72 hours. Nutritional problems and problems with healing will require several weeks to resolve.

Total Laryngectomy

The nursing management of the client after a total laryngectomy is the same as the care given a client with a partial laryngectomy except for feeding and teaching about permanent stoma care. Clients who have a total laryngectomy will have a permanent tracheostomy and need to learn how to speak using other methods.

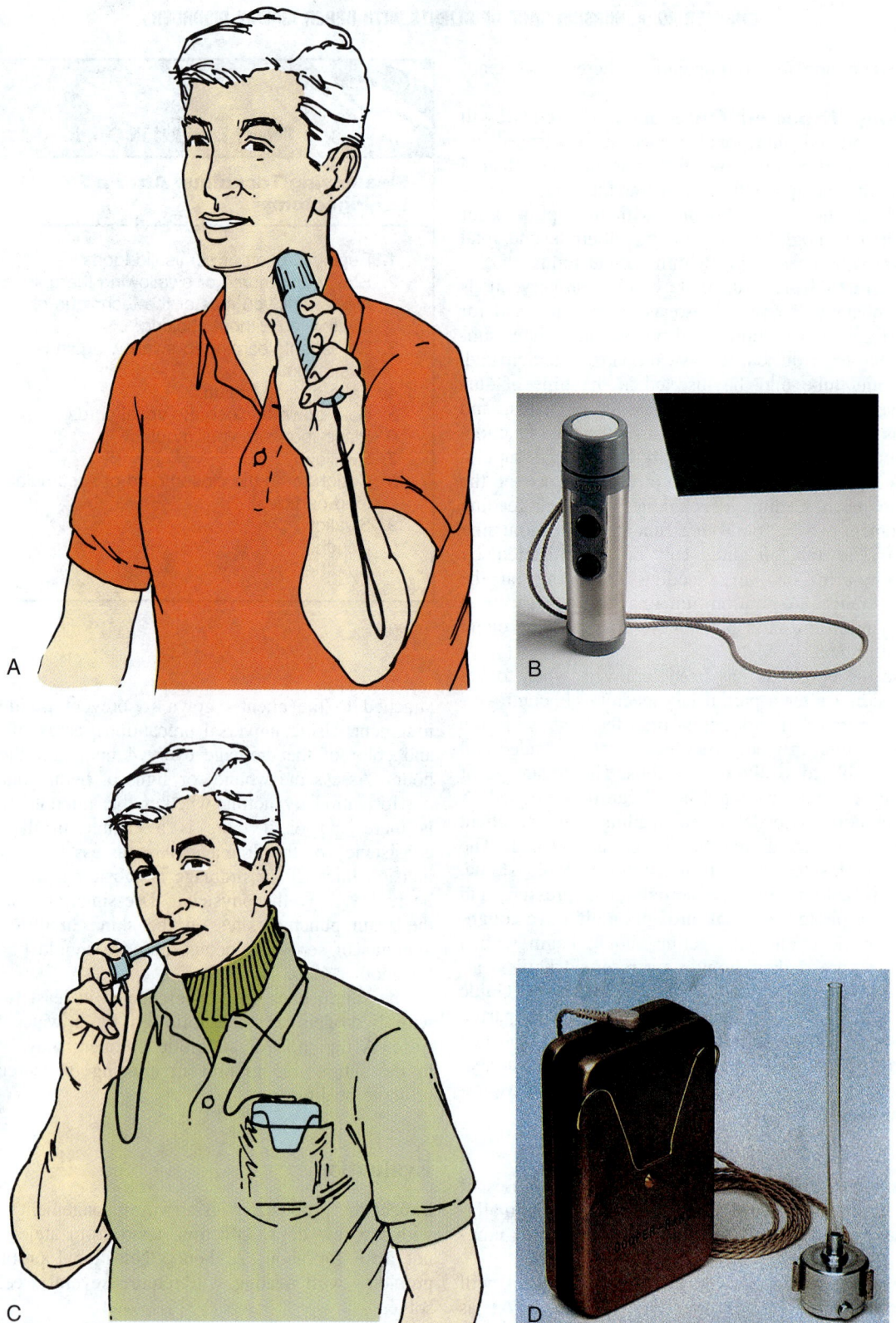

Figure 40–13. *A* and *B,* Artificial larynx (electrolarynx). This handheld, battery-powered speech aid is placed against the neck. *A,* When activated, it creates a vibration that is transmitted to the neck and into the mouth. Words silently formed by the mouth become sounds from the vibrations emitted by the device. Any type of artificial larynx requires muscle and tongue control and hand strength. It normally is not used until immediate postoperative neck tenderness has subsided. (*B,* Courtesy of Servox Electrolarynx Mfg. by Siemans Hearing Instruments, Inc., Union, NJ.) *C* and *D,* Electronic speech aid (Cooper Rand) allows the client to adjust tone, pitch, and volume. An oral connector permits speech without the necessity for placing the device against the neck. This is an advantage immediately after surgery, when the neck is too sensitive for a neck-vibrating device. (*D,* Courtesy of Luminaud, Inc., Mentor, OH.)

Nutrition. Immediately after surgery, the client's nutrition is supplemented with nasogastric feedings. When the client exhibits signs of swallowing his or her own secretions, the edema has subsided and feeding can begin. The diet usually begins with liquid or semisoft foods and progresses as healing occurs.

For the first few days after surgery, the client should communicate by writing. If the client is very fatigued, common client requests such as "I need something for pain" may be written on a pad of paper or a communication board may be used and the client can just point to the statement. Even though the client cannot speak, conversation should still include the client's input through nodding and pointing and not be directed only to others such as the family. Avoiding conversation with the client because of difficulty in communication is demeaning to the client and leads to frustration.

Artificial Larynx. An artificial larynx may be used as early as 3 to 4 days after surgery. These electronic devices are held alongside the neck, or a plastic tube is inserted in the mouth; vibration produces mechanical speech (Fig. 40–13). The air inside the mouth is vibrated, and the client articulates as usual. The speech quality is monotone and mechanical-sounding but intelligible.[14,25]

Esophageal Speech. Esophageal speech is a technique that requires the client to swallow and hold air in the upper esophagus. By controlling the flow of air, the client can pronounce as many as 6 to 10 words before stopping to reswallow air. The voice is deep but it is loud and effective once the technique is mastered.

Tracheoesophageal Puncture. Tracheoesophageal puncture (TEP) is a surgical technique that may also restore speech (Fig. 40–14). A small puncture is made into the upper tracheostoma to the cervical esophagus for creation of a fistula. Once the fistula is healed, a small one-way valve, called a voice button or trapdoor prosthesis, is inserted. By occlusion of the valve, air can be shunted into the esophagus, producing speech. These devices require maintenance; therefore, only clients who are highly motivated, are able to perform self-care, and have good manual dexterity are eligible for this procedure. Care for the tracheoesophageal puncture is presented in the Client Education Guide.

Neck Dissection

Preoperative Care

Before surgery, the client's understanding of the plans for surgery should be assessed. Determine what the surgeon has told the client and how much information has been retained or lost because of anxiety. In addition, address the fears the client has about the diagnosis of cancer and fears of deformity after surgery. The Ethical Issues in Nursing feature explores the client education that is needed for informed consent to radical procedures. Explain to the client and family what to expect after surgery

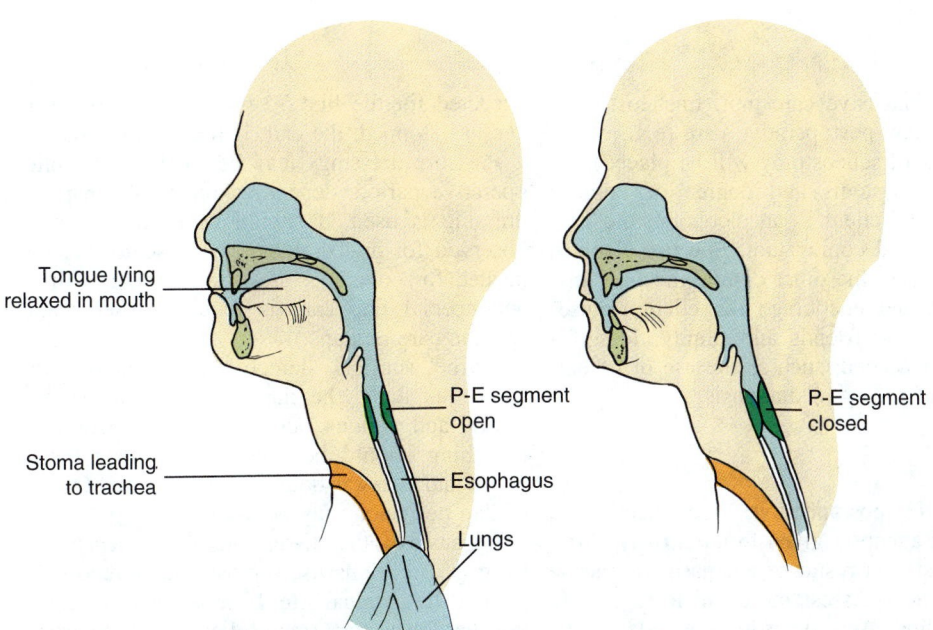

Tongue lying relaxed in mouth

P-E segment open

Stoma leading to trachea

Esophagus

P-E segment closed

Lungs

Figure 40–14. Tracheoesophageal puncture for voice rehabilitation after laryngectomy. A prosthesis is inserted into a fistula created in the neck. The prosthesis has a one-way valve that permits air to pass into the esophagus but prevents accidental aspiration. To speak, the client occludes the prosthesis with a finger or attachment. Exhaled air is then shunted through the prosthesis, where it vibrates, and exits the mouth as a spoken word.

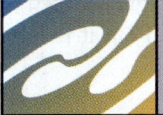

CLIENT EDUCATION GUIDE

Care of the Tracheoesophageal Puncture

1. A 10F, 12F, or 14F red rubber catheter is inserted into the puncture site to maintain the opening until a tract has formed (Fig. A).
2. Tie a knot at the end of the catheter to prevent the backflow of gastric secretions onto your chest.
3. Tape the catheter securely to your chest.
4. If the catheter comes out and cannot be reinserted, contact your physician or speech therapist immediately.
5. Once the prosthesis is able to be inserted, clean

your neck and stoma. Using the inserter, place the prosthesis into the fistula.
6. Tape the prosthesis to the skin of your neck (Fig. B).
7. To use the prosthesis, take a breath, cover your stoma with your thumb, and speak. The air from your lungs will pass through the prosthesis and vibrate the walls of the throat. The mouth is used for producing the words.
8. If food or fluid leaks around the prosthesis, it may need to be replaced.

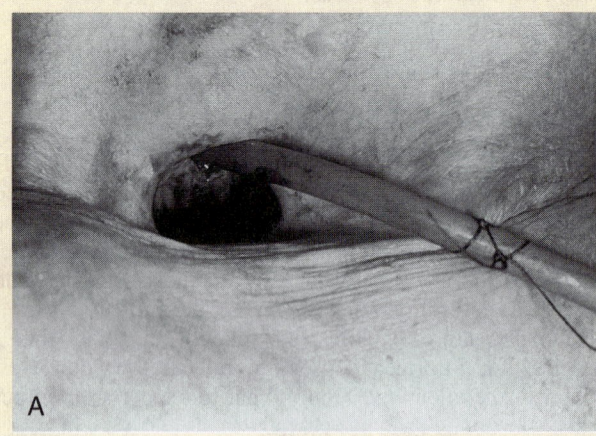

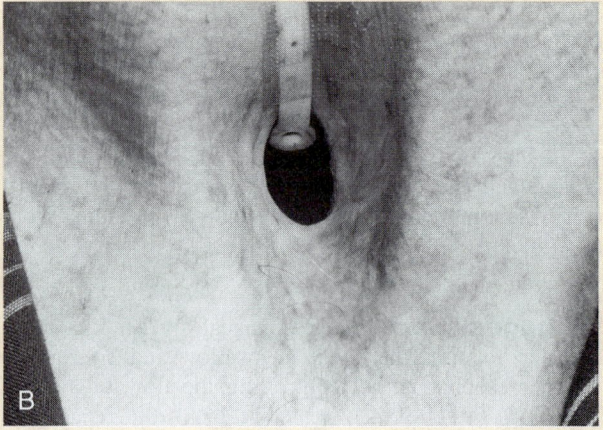

(e.g., placement in the intensive care unit, tracheostomy, drainage tubes) and review postoperative care (e.g., communication technique if a tracheostomy will be placed).

The client's support systems and degree of coping should be assessed. If the client is an alcoholic, the use of alcohol may be the usual coping tool. Because alcohol will not be available, assess the other coping mechanisms available to the client and encourage the client to use them. Sources may include friends and family. Identify new support systems, if needed, such as the use of others who have had the same surgery or diagnosis.

Postoperative Care

After surgery, the usual postoperative assessments are performed with special attention given to the airway. Airway patency can be lost as a result of edema of the neck or bleeding within the area. Assess the client for signs of airway edema or bleeding. Auscultate lung sounds every 2 hours for the first 24 hours. Report signs of airway obstruction immediately.

Place the client in a semi-Fowler position to minimize postoperative edema. Monitor neck drainage for volume and color. Sanguineous or serosanguineous drainage is

expected for the first 72 hours after surgery. Once drainage has stopped, the catheters are removed.

Pressure dressings may be used in the immediate postoperative period, depending on physician preference. If a dressing is used, it should be reinforced as needed and observed for any drainage. If musculocutaneous flaps are needed for coverage, pressure dressings will not be used, and special flap care is required. (See Chapter 80 for specific care of flaps.)

If the surgical defect was repaired with musculocutaneous flaps, the flap should be assessed for arterial inflow and venous outflow. The temperature, color, and blanching should be noted every hour for the first 24 hours and every 4 hours after that time. Other monitoring of flap perfusion may be used.

Because of the disruption of the sensory nerve fibers from the incisions used, most clients report only minimal pain at the surgical site. If an en bloc radical neck dissection has been performed, clients will experience shoulder dysfunction resulting in a forward rotation and dropping of the shoulder. Sectioning of the spinal accessory nerve during neck dissection will also interrupt innervation to the upper trapezius muscle.

Exercises to increase range of motion and muscle

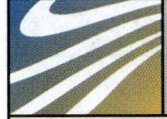

ETHICAL ISSUES IN NURSING

What Type of Client Education Is Needed for Informed Consent to Radical Procedures?

Surgical procedures for upper airway disorders may result in very extensive, aesthetically dramatic results. Clients who undergo radical tumor resection or musculocutaneous flap reconstruction procedures do so because a disease process has given them little choice—they either undergo surgery or allow the disease to cause irreversible damage and even death. Sometimes clients have time to think about their treatment options, and surgery may not be the recommended first choice. Other times, however, a client may be diagnosed with throat cancer that is compromising the airway, and surgery is indicated as soon as possible.

The question here is not what treatment is best for the client, but rather what information is given to and processed by the client so that he or she can give an informed consent to such a radical procedure. Clients who are candidates for radical procedures are most likely aware of the severity of their condition. The physician explains the diagnosis, treatment options, and treatment recommendations. Again, there are times when surgery, however radical, may be the only treatment option (unless the client opts for no treatment). Do clients really understand how their body image will change after such a procedure? Do they really understand that they may never speak in the normal way they have spoken their whole life (as with a total laryngectomy)? Do they understand that without treatment, they may not speak at all? Is there anything that can help them understand all the psychosocial implications of a radical procedure? Finally, is their consent to such procedures really informed if they do not have an understanding of these issues?

Client education is of paramount importance to these clients. Nurses who work in a surgical setting in which these kinds of clients are seen have a large responsibility in helping their clients understand the possible results of such radical procedures. Our society places great importance on the physical components of our body, in particular the face, and clients need to understand the physical changes that will take place as a result of surgery. You can help clients work through their feelings by offering supportive services such as social work, support groups, or psychiatric counseling. If possible, all of these aspects should be explored before surgery. Only through such teaching efforts in which you play a vital role can clients truly make informed decisions regarding life-altering surgery.

strength, shown in the next Client Education Guide, are encouraged to prevent a frozen shoulder and restore full movement. If a selective or modified neck dissection has been performed, minimal alterations in range of motion and muscle strength are anticipated. Encourage use of exercise to prevent permanent disability.[5,29]

Community and Self-Care

Partial Laryngectomy

The client undergoing partial laryngectomy may be discharged from the hospital prior to completion of wound healing. If upper airway edema has not subsided, the client will be discharged with a temporary tracheostomy. The client and significant other should be aware of the care of the tube, including inner cannula care, technique for insertion of the entire tube in case of accidental decannulation, suctioning, humidification techniques, and emergency resuscitation measures.

Once decannulation has occurred, the stoma must be cleaned and an occlusive dressing applied, at least once a day (see Figure 40–12). Additional wound care includes cleaning the incision area with hydrogen peroxide and water and applying an antibiotic ointment. All instructions given to the client should be in writing, with additional teaching materials used as available. Ongoing assessment for healing, recurrent tumor, or a new tumor, is required.

Total Laryngectomy

Clients should be dismissed with an extra tracheostomy tube to allow daily changes at home (Fig. 40–15). To provide supplemental humidification, normal saline may be instilled into the stoma several times each day to stimulate coughing, moisten the mucosa, and loosen dried secretions and crusts. A bedside humidifier or vaporizer will also aid in humidifying the inspired air. A stoma bib or covering should be worn to prevent foreign bodies from entering the stoma. These coverings can be purchased, or the client may improvise by using a scarf, necktie, or turtleneck shirt.[25,29]

The Bridge to Home Healthcare describes how to encourage the client to continue speech therapy as begun in the hospital. The techniques to restore speech require much time for mastery; the client is seen by a speech therapist after dismissal from the hospital. There are community support groups for clients after laryngectomy, the Lost Cord Club and International Association of Laryngectomees, which offer needed reassurance. Much patience is required by the client and family while the client is relearning to speak. The process is time-consuming and frustrating and requires time. Encourage the family to give the client enough time to formulate the words and not speak for the client.

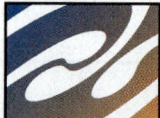

Exercises After Radical Neck Surgery

Step 1: Begin by gently moving your head from side to side, tipping your ear toward your shoulder on the same side, and moving your chin toward your chest.

Step 2: To exercise your shoulders using the hand on the nonaffected side, lean or hold onto a low table or chair. Bend your body slightly at the waist and

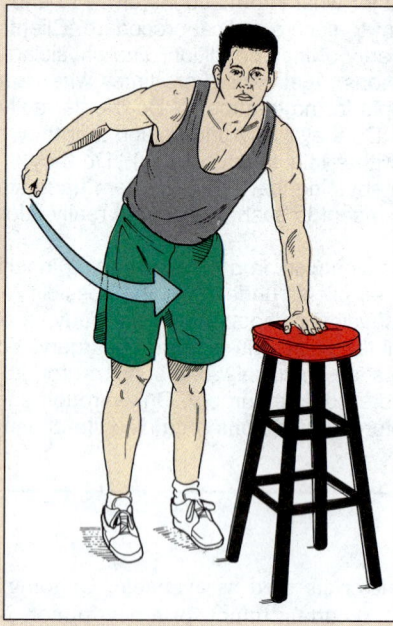

a. Swing your shoulder and arm from left to right.

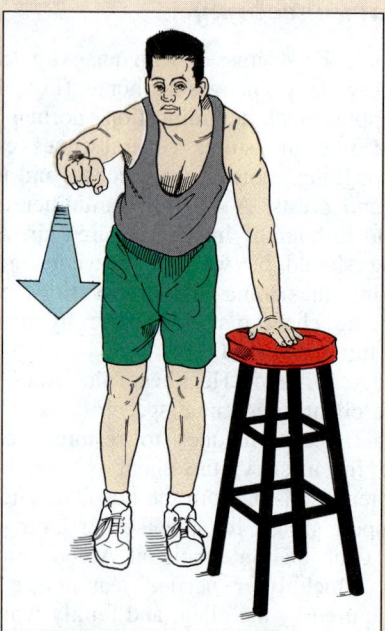

b. Swing your shoulder and arm from front to back.

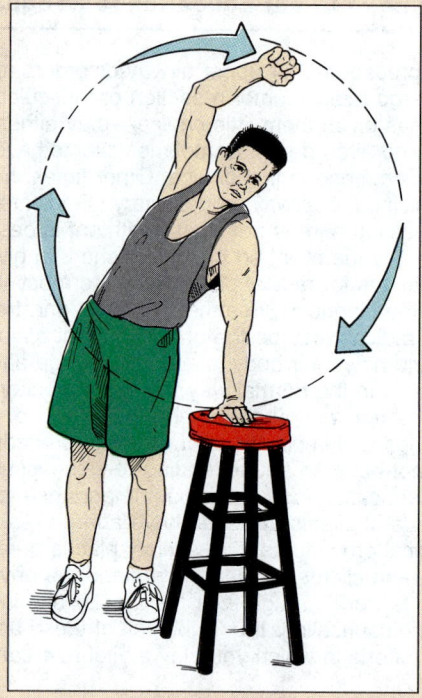

c. Swing your shoulder and arm in a wide circle, gradually bringing your arm all the way over your head.

Step 3: To strengthen your neck muscles, sit on a stool and

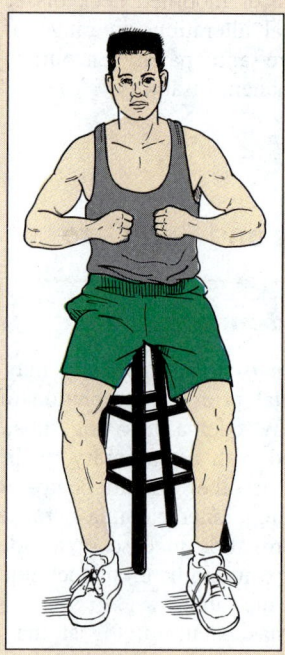

a. Place your hands in front of you with your elbows at right angles, sticking out from your body.

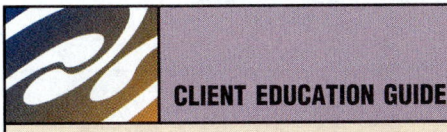
Exercises After Radical Neck Surgery *(Continued)*

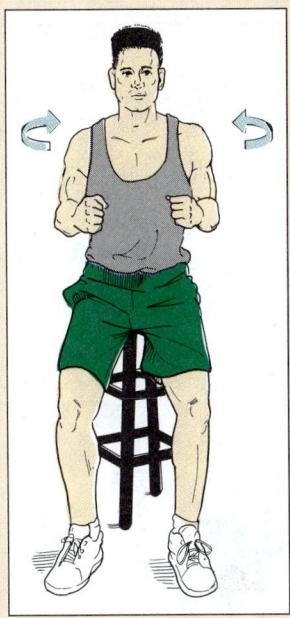

b. Rotate your shoulders back, bringing elbows to your side.

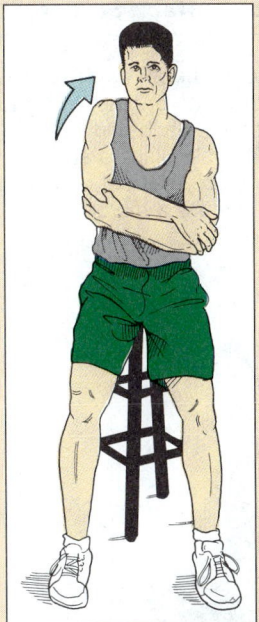

d. With your arms crossed in front of you, support the elbow on the affected side with your opposite hand, and help lift the arm and shoulder while shrugging.

Step 4: To increase motion in your shoulder, stand at a wall and

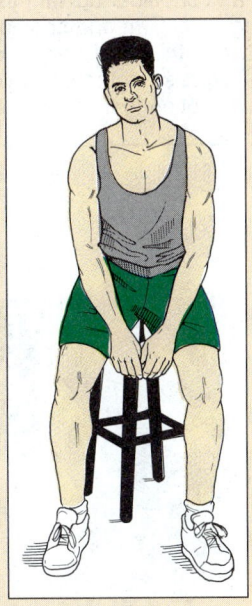

c. Relax your whole body.

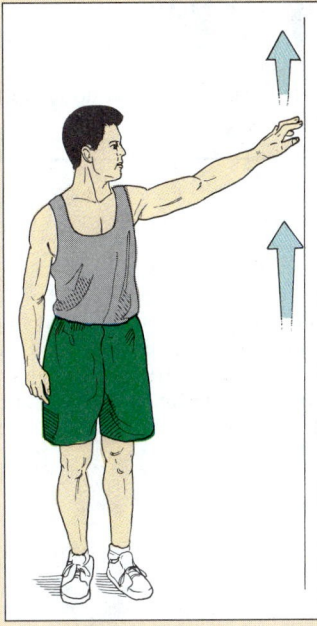

a. Walk your fingers slowly up the wall.
b. As your fingers climb up, begin to move your body closer to the wall.
c. Continue until your arm is high above your head and shoulder.

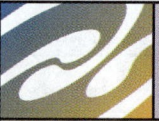

CLIENT EDUCATION GUIDE

Exercises After Radical Neck Surgery *(Continued)*

Step 5: To gain shoulder and upper arm strength, attach a hook to a wall or door. Hang a short rope knotted at each end over the hook. Under the hook, place a straight-backed chair or stool. It would be helpful to do this exercise before a mirror.

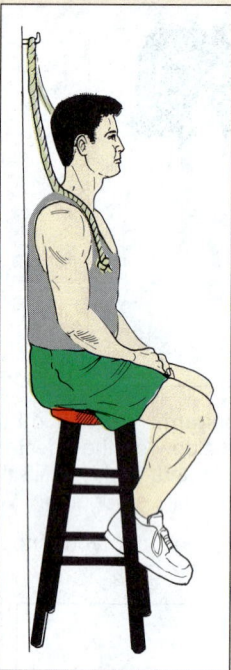

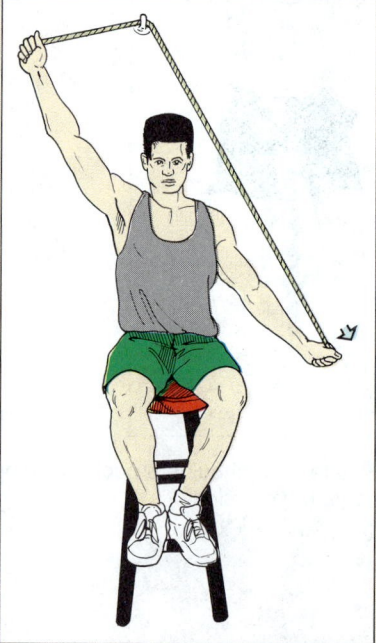

a. Sit straight, with your back against the wall.

b. Pull one arm and shoulder up with the rope by bringing the other arm and shoulder down. Repeat with the other arm. It is important in this exercise not to bend your body. Keep the motion in the shoulder.

Figure 40–15. Insertion of laryngectomy tube into a permanent tracheostoma. The obturator or guide is inserted into the outer cannula. After the tube is lubricated with water-soluble ointment, the client takes a deep breath, and the lubricated tube is inserted. The obturator is removed, and the tube is tied in place.

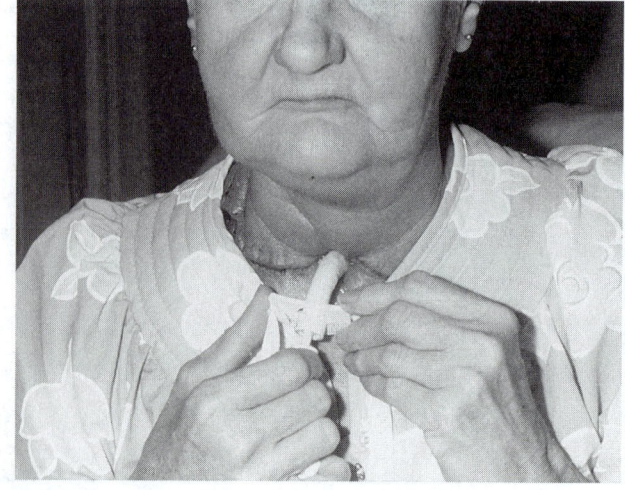

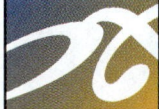

BRIDGE TO HOME HEALTHCARE

Supporting the Client at Home After a Laryngectomy
Anne Rutenbeck, R.N., B.S.N., C.E.T.N., *Visiting Nurse Service, Des Moines, Iowa*

Returning home after a laryngectomy is a frightening experience. Nurses cannot be available to the client around the clock as in the hospital. The client or caregiver is now responsible for most care. Fear and anxiety can be alleviated by letting the client know that the home care nurse is on call 24 hours a day and by writing down the nurse's telephone number.

It is critical for the nurse to help the client and caregiver get organized during initial visits. Even though teaching was done in the hospital, clients often forget important information. Continue with instructions and adjust procedures as necessary for the home situation. Reinforce learning in various ways including return demonstrations. Writing down the information, making lists, or using pictures is always a good idea. Do not rely on the client's or caregiver's memory because often the information is overwhelming.

Not all homes are suited for the "sterile" procedures done at the hospital. At home, procedures are not usually sterile but as "clean as possible." Finding adequate, clean, or pest-free space is sometimes a challenge. Using bags that can be sealed, boxes with lids, or sealable containers are good ways to keep equipment clean. Encourage meticulous hand washing with antibacterial soap.

The home care nurse may be responsible for coordinating aspects of medical care such as setting up appointments with physicians, arranging transportation, and encouraging compliance with the appointments. Speech therapy can be arranged through the hospital or an agency that provides home visits. Until the client can use a speech method, a pen and paper or wordboard may be needed.

Nutrition is very important in general recovery and healing of the surgical site. Extra protein in the form of supplements may be needed. Instant breakfast drinks are a low-cost alternative to commercially prepared supplements.

The home care nurse strives to make the client or caregiver increasingly independent and gain control of the situation. The client gains control by becoming independent with care. Having the client or caregiver assume more responsibility at each visit fosters independence. Completing those responsibilities and having even small successes encourage independence and confidence.

Some clients have inadequate insurance or money to purchase needed equipment. These clients need to be referred to appropriate resources. The U.S. Department of Health and Human Services pays for equipment, medications, and medical services for clients who qualify. The American Cancer Society (ACS) has loan equipment such as hospital beds, overbed tables, commodes, and suction equipment and, occasionally, has funding available for equipment. The ACS also has a support group called the Lost Cord Club for laryngectomy clients and caregivers.

The home care nurse's assessment of client needs and knowledge of resources are very important to the client and caregiver. Such skills and information can make the transition to home as smooth as possible.

Once the incision has completely healed, the tracheostomy tube will not be required (Fig. 40–16). This process varies but usually takes about 6 to 8 weeks. Occasionally, the tube will be required at night, if the stoma is small or the client does not get adequate air exchange during sleep. Once the tracheostomy tube has been removed, the client is able to disguise the stoma with clothing and begin to regain a sense of normalcy.

Tub baths or showers are permitted, but the client must use caution to prevent introduction of water into the stoma. Commercial stoma shower covers are available, and the water spray should be aimed at midchest. Water sports are prohibited. If the client fishes, a life preserver will need to be worn at all times on the boat.

The client should wear a medical alert bracelet or carry an emergency wallet card to identify the fact that resus-

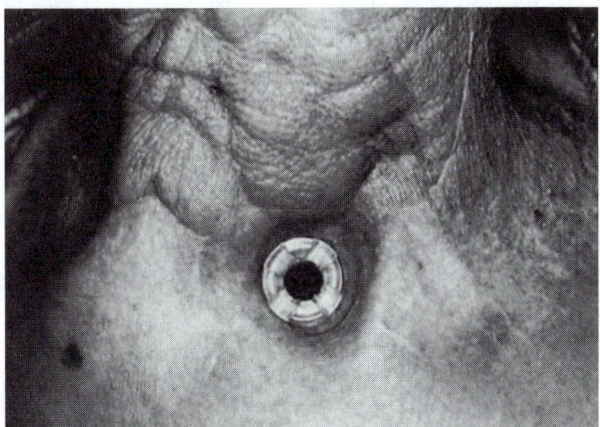

Figure 40–16. Healed tracheostomy incision.

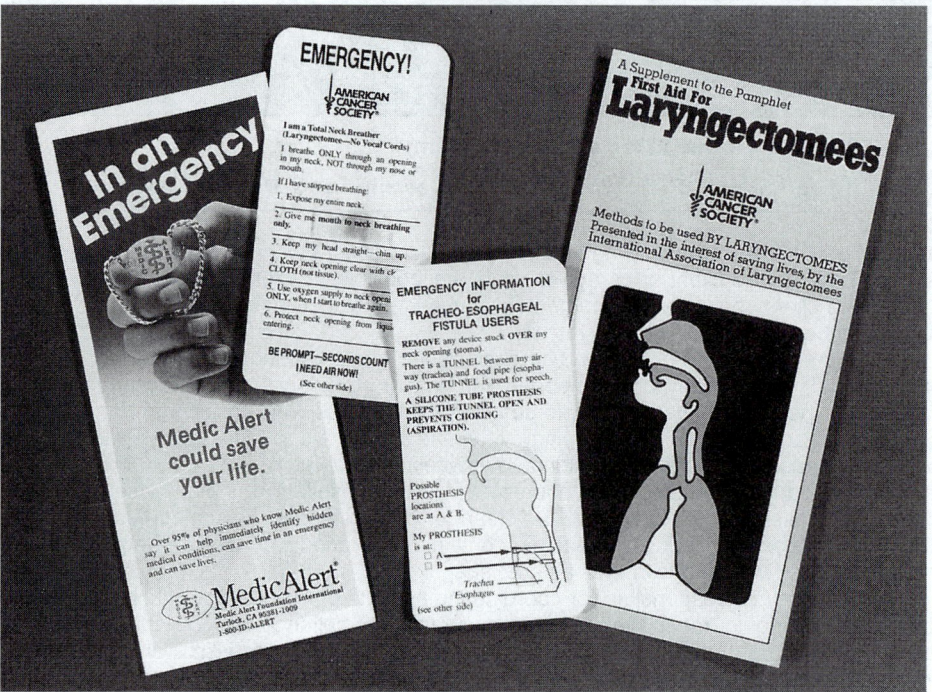

Figure 40–17. This emergency wallet card is available from the American Cancer Society. It provides vital information to a rescuer who finds a person with a laryngectomy in either respiratory or cardiac arrest. People who have had a total laryngectomy and breathe only through a stoma in the neck cannot be ventilated by mouth-to-mouth or mouth-to-nose ventilation. Mouth-to-stoma artificial ventilation is necessary.

citation cannot be performed through the mouth. The client will need mouth-to-stoma rescue breathing (Fig. 40–17).

The client may require a nutritional plan for the first few weeks at home. The dietitian should work with the client and family to determine the consistency of food easiest to swallow as well as the kinds of foods required to obtain needed protein and calories.

It is essential that the client not smoke so that lung function is preserved and the formation of other aerodigestive tract tumors is prevented. For some clients after laryngectomy, the process of smoking cessation seems pointless. Some clients continue to smoke by inhaling the cigarette smoke through the stoma. The attitude is one of Why quit now? What else could happen to me? Use extra support and encouragement with the client, remembering to be an advocate of the client's choice as well as providing assurance that the quality of life after smoking cessation improves.

Follow-up care is important to assess the healing process, evaluate coping mechanisms, and examine the client for possible metastasis or new tumors. The client should be taught to report any of these signs or symptoms to the physician:

● A lump anywhere in the neck or body
● Persistent cough, sore throat, or earache
● Hemoptysis
● Sores around the stoma or within the trachea that do not heal
● Difficulty swallowing or breathing

Neck Dissection

After neck dissection, caution clients about potential injury to neck tissue because of lack of sensation. The use of a heating pad or exposure to temperature extremes may result in tissue injury (burns, frostbite) in a client who cannot feel these temperatures. Clients with tracheostomy need specific instructions for its management. Explain ongoing evaluations and follow-up.

Obstructions of the Upper Airway

Acute Airway Obstruction

Acute Laryngeal Edema

Acute laryngeal edema may be associated with inflammation, injury, or anaphylaxis. It is manifested by an acute onset of hoarseness and dramatic shortness of breath. Dyspnea progresses rapidly, and unless a patent airway is established, respiratory arrest occurs. Endotracheal intubation may be very difficult because the larynx is edematous and is likely to bleed. Emergency tracheostomy may be required. If anaphylaxis is the precipitating cause, subcutaneous epinephrine 1:1000 is given. Intravenous corticosteroids are also used.[12]

Chronic Laryngeal Edema

Chronic laryngeal edema may occur when lymph drainage is obstructed, as with infection, tumor, or radiation therapy. If the edema is significant, an artificial airway may be required (either a tracheostomy or an endotracheal tube). The choice of route depends on the severity of the edema.

Laryngospasm

Laryngospasm, spasm of the laryngeal muscles, may occur (1) after administration of some general anesthetic agents, (2) after repeated and traumatic attempts at endotracheal intubation, (3) as a response to some inhaled agents and foreign material, such as industrial fumes, dusts, and chemicals, and (4) from hypocalcemia.

Management is directed at reestablishing the airway as quickly and efficiently as possible. Administer 100% oxygen until the airway is fully reestablished and the larynx relaxes and the spasms stop. Titrate FIO_2 according to ABG or pulse oximetry values. If the laryngospasm persists, paralysis with neuromuscular blocking agents, such as succinylcholine, may be required to allow intubation until the spasm breaks. Manual or mechanical ventilation is then necessary until the effects of the paralyzing agent have worn off. Occasionally, emergency cricothyroidotomy or tracheotomy may be necessary, and should not be delayed.

Laryngeal Paralysis

Laryngeal paralysis may be the result of neck surgery, peripheral disorders, central nervous system (CNS) disorders, tumor, viral infections, or of unknown cause. One of the most common causes of laryngeal paralysis is trauma to the recurrent laryngeal nerve during thyroidectomy. Other causes of laryngeal paralysis are aortic aneurysm; mitral stenosis; thoracic surgery; thyroid gland carcinoma; neck injuries; tuberculosis; tumors of the bronchi, lungs, and mediastinum; metallic poisons (e.g., lead); and infection (e.g., diphtheria). CNS disorders that may lead to laryngeal paralysis include cerebrovascular accident (stroke) and myasthenia gravis. Bilateral laryngeal paralysis is rare and when it occurs, the client usually exhibits difficulty breathing or stridor.

Unilateral vocal cord paralysis occurs when one vocal cord is affected. The airway is usually not impaired and the primary manifestation is hoarseness. The client may complain of a breathy quality to the voice. Aspiration of food or saliva may occur until the normal moving cord compensates by approximating the paralyzed cord. The client must be observed for manifestations of aspiration such as coughing upon swallowing, ineffective cough, decreased breath sounds, and crackles, rhonchi, or wheezes. The client with bilateral vocal cord paralysis will have a near-normal voice if the vocal cords are paralyzed in the adducted position. However, the major concern is airway compromise, especially on exertion.

Dyspnea, intercostal muscle retraction, and stridor may occur with activity or upper airway infections.[6,25,29]

If the paralyzed cords are bilaterally adducted, an emergency tracheotomy may be required. Surgery, such as *arytenoidectomy*, in which one or both arytenoid cartilages are removed and the vocal cords are held in an open position, may be used to open the glottis.

Injection of absorbable sponge (Gelfoam) (temporary) or Teflon (permanent) may be used if the client with a unilateral vocal cord paralysis exhibits signs of aspiration, or requires strength or projection of the voice. The injection is placed into the paralyzed cord to add bulk for approximation to occur by the functioning cord.

Type I thyroplasty is recommended for permanent unilateral vocal cord paralysis. A window is made in the thyroid cartilage through an external incision and a stent is inserted to move the paralyzed vocal cord into a midline position. The client may show signs of airway edema with both the injection and thyroplasty, and should be observed for distress.

Laryngeal Injury

Laryngeal injury most often results from trauma during a motor vehicle accident, when the driver's neck strikes the steering wheel. Other causes include inhalation of hot gases or aspiration of caustic liquids. If complete airway obstruction does not occur, carefully assess for post-traumatic edema, which may lead to complete obstruction. Few outward signs may be present. It is often easy to overlook potential problems in the neck structures while focusing on other, possibly more dramatic injuries. Observe for increased dyspnea, intercostal muscle retraction, stridor, inability to speak, and change in respiration patterns.

The thyroid cartilage may be fractured. This problem leads to soft tissue and laryngeal edema as well as hematoma. If airway obstruction occurs, tracheostomy may be necessary. Indications of a fractured thyroid cartilage include (1) tender, swollen ecchymotic neck; (2) stridor; (3) possible cyanosis; and (4) possible subcutaneous emphysema.

Damage to the larynx above the cricoid cartilage may lead to tracheal stenosis. The cricoid cartilage forms the only complete circle of cartilage in the upper airway, and it maintains the open lumen of the upper end of the airway.

Chronic Airway Obstruction

Nasal Polyps

Nasal polyps are outpouchings of mucous membrane lining the nose or paranasal sinuses. Polyps are most commonly seen in people with severe allergies and may be single or multiple. Most persons seek medical attention for obstruction to nasal breathing.

The medical management of clients with nasal polyps is symptomatic. Attempts are made to reduce the size of the polyps by eliminating or treating the causative factor (i.e., allergy). In many clients, surgery is needed to remove nasal polyps in order to restore nasal breathing before allergy treatment. Nasal polypectomy (removal of nasal polyps) can be done in the physician's office or in the operating room. Nasal polypectomy is usually performed with use of a local anesthetic. The anesthetic (commonly lidocaine with epinephrine) is sufficient to eliminate discomfort while also producing vasoconstriction to minimize bleeding during the procedure. A snare-like instrument is used to remove the polyps. The bleeding sites are cauterized, and intranasal packing is inserted. In some instances, intranasal splints are used to prevent formation of adhesions. The nasal packing is maintained for several hours to minimize the possibility of postoperative bleeding and is generally removed before discharge.

Because of the presence of nasal packing and edema, clients will breathe through the mouth for the first 24 to 48 hours. The use of humidification, frequent mouth care, and increasing oral fluids will help to minimize the dryness and oropharyngeal discomfort. Inspect the oral cavity frequently to evaluate the effectiveness of these measures. Clients with polyps frequently also have asthma (when combined with aspirin allergy this is called triad disease). Asthmatic symptoms may be exacerbated after surgery.[28]

The client is placed in a semi- to high-Fowler position after surgery to minimize edema. In addition, continuous ice compresses are recommended for the first 48 hours to reduce edema and control bleeding. With the proper application of nasal packing at the time of surgery and the use of ice compresses in the immediate postoperative period, nasal bleeding should be minimal. However, the client should be assessed for changes in vital signs and the oropharynx inspected for the presence of blood. Because the nasal packing absorbs anterior bleeding, it is essential to observe the client for posterior nasal bleeding. If active posterior bleeding occurs, the client will swallow frequently and blood will be present in the throat.

Most clients have only minimal discomfort after a nasal polypectomy. Mild analgesics may be used for any postoperative discomfort. The use of aspirin and aspirin-containing products should be avoided because of their anticoagulant effects. Instruct the client not to try to blow the nose or sneeze. If the client needs to sneeze, the client should sneeze through an open mouth.[25,29]

Deviated Nasal Septum and Nasal Fracture

The nasal septum, the dividing structure of the nose, is usually straight and divides the nose into two equal chambers. After trauma, the septum may become deviated, creating asymmetrical breathing passages. For some clients, the deviation may cause an obstruction to nasal breathing, dryness of the nasal mucosa causing bleeding, and occasionally a cosmetic deformity.

If a nasal fracture occurs, immediate medical management is advised. Within several hours of nasal injury, severe edema may occur, which causes difficulty in reducing the fracture. Immediately after the injury, ice should be applied. A simple nasal fracture may be reduced in an emergency facility with use of local anesthesia. If immediate reduction of the nasal fracture is not possible, it is advisable to wait several days until edema subsides but before healing begins.

Surgical management of a client for correction of a deviated nasal septum, reconstruction of a cosmetic deformity of the nose, and reduction of a nasal fracture are similar. All three procedures are usually performed under local anesthesia combined with mild sedation. Because of the vasoconstrictor properties of local anesthetics, they reduce bleeding during and immediately after surgery. Surgery to correct a deviated nasal septum is known as a nasal septoplasty and consists of making an incision on either side of the septum, elevating the mucous membrane, and straightening or removing the offending portion of the cartilage. If a cosmetic deformity is also of concern or if the deformity interferes with septal reconstruction, a rhinoplasty (reconstruction of the external nose) may be done in conjunction with the nasal septoplasty or as a separate procedure. (See also Chapter 80.)

After these three procedures, intranasal packing and internal splints may be used to maintain the position of the septum, control bleeding, and prevent hematoma formation. If the patient has had rhinoplasty or reduction of a nasal fracture, an external splint and a small dressing may also be applied. Postoperative care is directed at airway management, control of edema and hemorrhage, and pain control. Because of the presence of bilateral nasal packing, clients require the same care as discussed for the client after nasal polypectomy.

Conclusions

Disorders of the upper airway range from a simple cold to cancer of the larynx. This chapter has presented care of those clients most commonly hospitalized with upper airway disorders. Nursing management ranges from assessment of life-threatening airway obstruction to teaching techniques that reduce the spread of infection.

Thinking Critically

1. The client has had a temporary tracheostomy inserted following a supraglottic laryngectomy. The second postoperative day, the client indicates to you that he is having trouble breathing. How should you evaluate the client and eliminate the problem?

Factors to Consider. What principles are used as the basis of tracheostomy care? How does evaluation of pulse oximetry contribute to decision-making for care?

2. You walk into the room of a client who has had a total laryngectomy 12 hours ago. The client is complaining of severe nausea but has not vomited. What are the client's risks following this type of surgery? How should you respond to the present problem?

Factors to Consider. What risks are inherent when tracheal interruption occurs? How well can the client communicate with you at this time?

3. You enter the room of a client who has developed a nosebleed. Bright red blood is seeping continuously from the nares and the client states that it feels like some is going down the back of his throat. What is the priority intervention? What are the implications if the bleeding continues?

Factors to Consider. What are the causes of epistaxis? What are the psychological effects of a nosebleed?

Bibliography

1. Bryce, J. C. (1995). Aspiration: Causes, consequences and prevention. *ORL—Head and Neck Nursing, 13* (2), 14–20.
2. Dropkin, M. J. (1989). Coping with disfigurement and dysfunction after head and neck surgery: A conceptual framework. *Seminars in Oncology Nursing, 5* (3), 231–219.
3. Gibbs, L. (1992). Assessment and management of the allergic patient. *ORL—Head and Neck Nursing, 10* (3), 10–16.
4. Harris, L. L., & Kraege, J. (1986). After T-E puncture: Relearning to speak. *American Journal of Nursing, 86* (1), 55–58.
5. Hillel, A., et al. (1989). Radical neck dissection: A subjective and objective evaluation of postoperative disability. *Journal of Otolaryngology, 18* (1), 53–61.
6. Isshiri, N. (1991). Laryngeal framework surgery. In E. N. Myers et al. (Eds.), *Advances in otolaryngology—Head and neck surgery,* (vol. 3, pp. 37–57). St. Louis: Mosby–Year Book.
7. Johnson, J. T., et al. (1987). Adjuvant chemotherapy for high-risk squamous cell carcinoma of the head and neck. *Journal of Clinical Oncology, 5* (3), 456–458.
8. Kennedy, D. W., & Zinreich, S. J. (1989). Functional endoscopic surgery. In E. N. Myers et al. (Eds.), *Advances in otolaryngology—Head and neck surgery* (vol. 3, pp. 1–27). St. Louis: Mosby–Year Book.
9. Kim, M. J., McFarland, G. K., & McLane, A. M. (1993). *Pocket guide to nursing diagnosis.* St. Louis: Mosby–Year Book.
10. Krakoff, I. (1991). Cancer chemotherapeutic and biologic agents. *CA: A Cancer Journal for Clinicians, 41* (5), 264–278.
11. Lavertu, P., et al. (1989). Secondary tracheoesophageal puncture for voice rehabilitation after laryngectomy. *Archives of Otolaryngology—Head and Neck Surgery, 115* (3), 350.
12. Litwack, K. (1991). Managing postanesthetic emergencies. *Nursing 91, 21* (9), 49–51.
13. Lockhart, J., & Bryce, J. (1993). Restoring speech with tracheoesophageal puncture. *Nursing 93, 23* (1), 10–13.
14. Lockhart, J., Troff, J., & Artim, L. (1992). Total laryngectomy and radical neck dissection. *AORN Journal, 55* (2), 458–479.
15. Logemann, J. A. (1983). *Evaluation and treatment of swallowing disorders.* San Diego: College-Hill Press.
16. McCall, M. (1993). It killed George: Managing the peritonsillar abscess patient effectively. *ORL—Head and Neck Nursing, 11* (1), 10–13.
17. Miller, W. E. (1992). The role of the outpatient nurse in endoscopic sinus surgery. *ORL—Head and Neck Nursing, 10* (3), 20–24.
18. Olson, N. R. (1986). The problem of gastroesophageal reflux. *Otolaryngologic Clinics of North America, 19* (1), 119–113.
19. Petruzzelli, G. J., & Johnson, J. T. (1989). How to stop a nosebleed. *Postgraduate Medicine, 86* (4), 44–56.
20. Sievers, A. E. F., & Donald, P. J. (1989). Staging system for head and neck cancer. *Journal of SOHN, 7* (3), 5–10.
21. Sigler, B. A. (1988). Nursing care of the head and neck cancer patient. *Oncology, 8* (2), 49–59.
22. Sigler, B. A. (1989). Nursing care of patients with laryngeal carcinoma. *Seminars in Oncology Nursing, 5* (3), 160–165.
23. Sigler, B. A. (1995). Nursing care for head and neck tumor patients. In S. E. Thawley & W. R. Panje (Eds.), *Comprehensive management of head and neck tumors* (pp. 79–100). Philadelphia: W. B. Saunders.
24. Sigler, B. A., & Hooper, J. A. (1989). Nursing care of the head and neck cancer patient. In E. N. Myers & J. Y. Suen (Eds.), *Cancer of the head and neck* (pp. 1045–1071). New York: Churchill Livingstone.
25. Sigler, B. A., & Schuring, L. T. (1993). *Ear, nose and throat disorders.* St. Louis: Mosby–Year Book.
26. Singer, M. I. (1988). Surgical restoration of the voice after total laryngectomy. In E. N. Myers et al. (Eds.), *Advances in otolaryngology—Head and neck surgery* (vol. 2, pp. 141–165). St. Louis: Mosby–Year Book.
27. Singer, M. I., & Blom, E. D. (1990). Medical techniques for voice restoration after total laryngectomy. *CA: A Cancer Journal for Clinicians, 40* (3), 166–173.
28. Slavin, R. G. (1991). Recalcitrant asthma: Could sinusitis be the culprit? *Journal of Respiratory Diseases, 12* (2), 182–194.
29. Society of Otorhinolaryngology and Head and Neck Nurses: (1996). *Guidelines for otorhinolaryngology and head and neck nursing practice.* New Smyrna Beach, FL: Author.
30. Stam, H., Koopmans, J., & Mathieson, C. (1991). The psychological impact of laryngectomy: A comprehensive assessment. *Journal of Psychosocial Oncology, 9* (3), 37–57.
31. Thibodeau, G. A. & Patton, K. T. (1993). *Anatomy and Physiology* (2nd ed.). St. Louis: Mosby–Year Book.
32. Wingo, P. A., Tong, T., & Bolden, S. (1995). Cancer statistics, 1995. *CA: A Cancer Journal for Clinicians, 45* (1), 8–31.

Nursing Care of Clients with Disorders of the Lower Airways and Pulmonary Vessels

Sherill Nones Cronin

CHAPTER 41

Disorders of the Lower Airways

Asthma

Asthma is a disorder of the bronchial airways characterized by periods of reversible bronchospasm (spasms of prolonged contraction of the airway). This complex disorder involves biochemical, immunologic, endocrine, infectious, autonomic, and psychological factors. Asthma affects about 3% to 4% of the United States population, and its incidence is rising. It is the most common chronic disease in children and adults.

Etiology and Risk Factors

Asthma occurs in families, which indicates that it is an inherited disorder. Apparently, environmental factors (e.g., viral infection, allergens, pollutants) interact with inherited factors to produce disease. Other inciting factors can include excitatory states (stress, laughing, crying), exercise, changes in temperature, and strong odors. Asthma is also a component of *triad* disease: asthma, nasal polyps, and allergy to aspirin. The Risk Factors and Levels of Prevention feature describes primary, secondary, and tertiary prevention.

Pathophysiology

Asthma involves a chronic inflammatory process that produces mucosal edema, mucus secretion, and airway inflammation. When persons with asthma are exposed to extrinsic allergens and irritants (such as dust, pollen, smoke, mold, medications, foods, respiratory infections), their airways become inflamed, producing shortness of breath, chest tightness, and wheezing. Initial clinical manifestations, termed *early-phase reaction,* develop immediately and last about an hour.[28]

When a client comes in contact with an allergen, IgE is produced by B lymphocytes. IgE antibodies attach to mast cells and basophils in the bronchial walls. As shown in the Pathophysiology and Treatment algorithm, the mast cell empties, releasing chemical mediators of inflammation such as histamine, bradykinin, prostaglandins, and slow-reacting substance of anaphylaxis (SRS-A). The substances induce capillary dilation leading to edema of the airway in an attempt to dilute the allergen and wash it away. They also induce airway constriction in an attempt to close the airway to prevent inhalation of more allergen.

About half of all asthma clients also experience a delayed or *late-phase reaction.* While the symptoms of this phase are the same as in early phase, they do not begin until 4 to 8 hours after exposure and may last for hours or days.

In both phases, the release of chemical mediators produces the airway response. However, in the late-phase response, the mediators attract other inflammatory cells and create a self-sustaining cycle of obstruction and inflammation. This chronic inflammation produces hyperresponsiveness of the airways. This causes subsequent episodes in response to not only specific antigens but also to stimuli such as physical exertion or breathing cold air.[14] Thus, clinical manifestations may occur with increasing frequency and severity.

Both alpha- and beta-adrenergic receptors of the sympathetic nervous system are found in the bronchi. Stimulation of alpha-adrenergic receptors causes bronchoconstriction. Conversely, stimulation of beta-adrenergic receptors causes bronchodilation. Cyclic adenosine monophosphate (AMP) balances the two receptors. Some theories suggest that asthma may be due to lack of beta-adrenergic stimulation.

Clinical Manifestations and Diagnostic Findings

During asthma attacks, clients are dyspneic and have marked respiratory effort. The Nursing Research feature

This chapter incorporates material written for the fourth edition by Steve Alderfer.

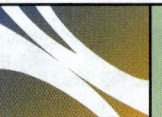

RISK FACTORS AND LEVELS OF PREVENTION

Asthma

Risk Factors

Exposure to allergens in a genetically susceptible high-risk population

Levels of Prevention

Primary Prevention

- Encourage clients to stop smoking.
- Advise clients of the dangers of secondhand smoke inhalation.
- Participate in community efforts to reduce levels of air pollution.

Secondary Prevention

- Instruct known clients with asthma in the daily monitoring of peak air flow volumes (typically, peak air flow volume decreases about 24 hours before clinical manifestations begin).
- Encourage clients to keep written records of their manifestations and the activities and circumstances surrounding them. These records will be helpful in identifying personal triggers and evaluating treatment effectiveness.
- Encourage clients to use stress reduction and relaxation techniques.

Tertiary Prevention

- Help the client plan a course of action for minimizing exposure to known triggers.
- Promote early treatment of upper respiratory infections.

describes other manifestations that may be present in clients with dyspnea. Marked respiratory effort can be seen in nasal flaring, pursed-lip breathing, and the use of accessory muscles. Cyanosis is a late development. (Table 41–1).

Auscultation of breath sounds will usually reveal wheezing, especially during expiration. The inability to auscultate wheezing in an asthmatic client with acute respiratory distress may be an ominous sign. It may indicate that the small airways are too constricted to allow any air flow. This client may require immediate, aggressive medical intervention. In addition, bronchospasm may lead to almost continuous coughing in an attempt to clear the airway.

The diagnosis of asthma is based on clinical manifestations, spirometry results, and response to treatment. Spirometry reveals decreased peak expiratory flow rate (PEFR), forced expiratory volume timed (FEV_t), and forced vital capacity (FVC). Functional residual capacity (FRC), total lung capacity (TLC), and residual volume (RV) are increased because air is trapped within the lungs. A 20% improvement in FVC, FEV, and PEFR following inhaled administration of a beta-agonist bronchodilator implies a reversible air flow obstruction, that is, asthma. Figure 41–1 shows peak flowmeters for monitoring air flow.

Baseline assessment of pulmonary status often includes pulse oximetry and arterial blood gas (ABG) analysis. Pulse oximetry usually reveals low oxygen saturation. Table 41–2 lists typical ABG changes during an asthma attack.

Status asthmaticus is a severe, life-threatening complication of asthma. It is an acute episode of bronchospasm that tends to intensify. With severe bronchospasm, the workload of breathing increases 5 to 10 times, which can lead to acute cor pulmonale. When air is trapped, a severe paradoxical pulse (i.e., drop in blood pressure of over 10 mm Hg during inspiration) develops as venous return is obstructed. Pneumothorax commonly develops. If status asthmaticus continues, hypoxemia worsens, and acidosis begins. If the condition is untreated or not reversed, respiratory or cardiac arrest will ensue.

Emergency Care

The management of asthma is based on disease severity. A severe asthma episode may constitute a medical emergency. Medical intervention for such episodes is primarily aimed at (1) maintaining a patent airway by relieving bronchospasm and clearing excess or retained secretions, (2) maintaining effective gas exchange, and (3) preventing complications such as acute respiratory failure and status asthmaticus.

Emergency management of the client begins with inhaled beta-adrenergics. Beta-adrenergic agents are the mainstay of bronchodilator therapy because they stimulate the beta-adrenergic receptors and dilate the airways. If the asthma does not abate (i.e., if FEV [forced expiratory volume in 1 second] remains less than 40% of predicted), nebulized atropine sulfate, intravenous theophylline, or intravenous steroids may be given. Atropine is an anticholinergic and therefore blocks the effect of the parasympathetic system. When the vagus nerve is stimulated, bronchial smooth muscle tone increases. Theophylline is a smooth muscle relaxant. Steroids prevent the mast cell

Understanding Asthma and Its Treatment

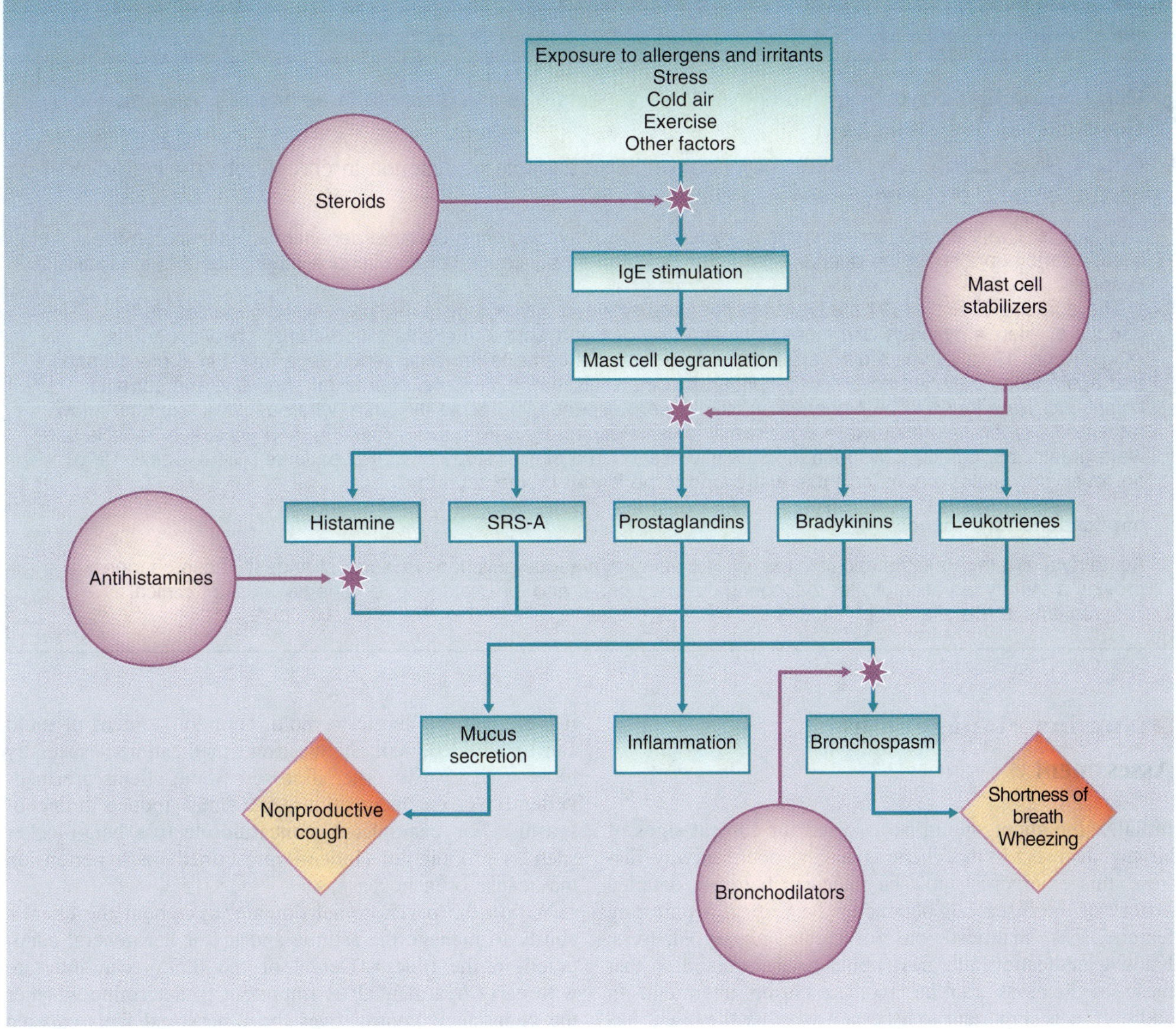

Exposure to allergens and irritants
Stress
Cold air
Exercise
Other factors

Steroids

IgE stimulation

Mast cell degranulation

Mast cell stabilizers

Histamine   SRS-A   Prostaglandins   Bradykinins   Leukotrienes

Antihistamines

Mucus secretion   Inflammation   Bronchospasm

Nonproductive cough

Bronchodilators

Shortness of breath Wheezing

---

from emptying, thereby reducing the edema and spasm. If these treatments do not reverse the symptoms, the client is usually admitted to the hospital for further treatment. If the client has an acute asthma attack and no medications are nearby, the attack can sometimes be lessened by pursed-lips breathing. Caffeine has also been used as a lay remedy to try to stop an asthma attack, but its effectiveness has not been confirmed.

Critical Care

■ Medical Management

In critical or acute care the client continues to receive bronchial dilators and steroids. Supplemental oxygen is

indicated if partial pressure of arterial oxygen (PaO_2) levels fall below 60 mm Hg. The client should be monitored closely for clinical manifestations of increasing anxiety, increased work of breathing, and indications of tiring. Endotracheal intubation and mechanical ventilation may be necessary. Sedation, and in rare cases administration of paralytic agents, may be necessary to blunt the client's respiratory effort and prevent further air trapping and pressure increases. Status asthmaticus is treated with aggressive use of intravenous corticosteroids and frequent administration of inhaled beta-adrenergics to avoid intubation and mechanical ventilation.

After the acute asthma attack is over, the client is assessed to determine the precipitating event or factors and is instructed in self-care activities. Steroids usually have to be tapered because of the induced adrenal suppression from the medication.

NURSING RESEARCH

What Clinical Indicators Can Be Assessed in Dyspneic Clients?

Gift, A. G. (1991). Psychologic and physiologic aspects of acute dyspnea in asthmatics. *Nursing Research, 40,* 196–199.

Gift, A. G., & Cahill, C. A. (1990). Psychophysiologic aspects of dyspnea in chronic obstructive pulmonary disease: A pilot study. *Heart and Lung, 19,* 252–257.

Dyspnea is a very intense sensation. Inability to breathe may also bring on other sensations. Reliance on the client's statements about the degree of shortness of breath may cause you to overlook other cues that indicate dyspnea.

The purpose of Gift's 1991 study was to compare selected psychological and physiologic variables during periods of intense dyspnea with those at times of no or low dyspnea in clients with asthma. Thirty-six adults ranging from 19 to 76 years old were tested when they first came to the emergency department in acute dyspnea and again when they had no or low dyspnea just before discharge. Anxiety, depression, hostility, and somatic complaints were found to be higher when clients were experiencing acute dyspnea, whereas peak expiratory flow rates and oxygen saturation were significantly lower. Respiratory rate, pulse, wheezing, and accessory muscle use were greater during acute dyspnea in asthmatic clients. In a similar study of COPD patients (Gift & Cahill, 1990), however, only accessory muscle use was found to be higher during acute dyspnea.

Implications for Practice

Acute dyspnea in the asthmatic client is accompanied by various psychophysiologic changes. These changes provide a variety of indicators for monitoring dyspnea onset and for evaluating the effectiveness of clinical interventions in this client population.

■ Nursing Management

Assessment

Initially, the client should be assessed for clinical signs of airway distress. If the client is having acute airway distress, this emergency must be managed before a detailed history of the disease is obtained. The Critical Monitoring feature lists manifestations of acute airway distress. Known medication allergies should be determined so that these medications can be avoided during treatment. In addition, it is important to ascertain whether the client has a history of cardiac disease, because beta-adrenergics can produce tachycardia and stress a diseased heart.

Once the acute episode is controlled, the history of the client's asthma should be explored. Assist the client to determine if there is a pattern to the manifestations. These data may help identify a trigger that precipitates the asthmatic symptoms. If an extrinsic trigger can be identified, it may be possible to reduce or eliminate it. For example,

if the client is allergic to mold. common sources of mold can be avoided. Ask about current medications, especially those used to treat other illnesses. Some clients are inadvertently given medications that may induce bronchospasms. For example, a noncardioselective beta-blocker such as propranolol (Inderal) prescribed for hypertension may cause bronchospasm.

Within the psychosocial domain, ask about the client's ability to manage the asthma and his or her general adaptation to the illness. Denial of the illness can interfere with early treatment. It is important to determine whether the client feels control over the illness and feels capable of managing it. Clients who have this feeling of control may have improved compliance with treatments. Determine whether the client is experiencing an increased number of stressors. A stressful life-style may exacerbate asthmatic symptoms.

Assess the attitude of the family. The family can be a great source of support and assist the client in recognizing early manifestations. In contrast, an unsupportive

Table 41–1. Alterations in Arterial Blood Gases Associated with Asthma				
	Mild	**Moderate**	**Severe**	**Status Asthmaticus**
PaO_2	Slightly elevated	Normal to mild hypoxemia	Hypoxemia	Severe hypoxemia
$PaCO_2$	Decreased	Decreased to normal	Elevated	Significantly elevated
pH	Alkalosis	Alkalosis	Alkalosis	Acidosis

$PaCO_2$, partial pressure of arterial carbon dioxide; PaO_2, partial pressure of arterial oxygen.

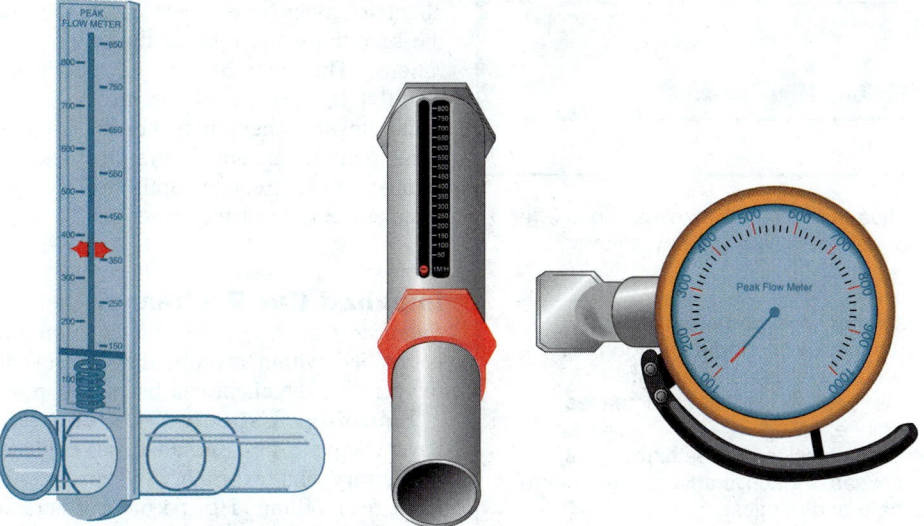

Figure 41–1. Peak flowmeters. Several types of portable meters are available for self-monitoring of air flow.

family may contribute to denial or be an additional source of stress to the client.

The client with a new diagnosis of asthma may be asked to assess the home and work environment for likely triggers of the clinical symptoms. In addition, skin testing for allergy may be performed. The presence of pets that shed hair or dander, cigarette smoke, or occupational exposure to other allergens may require some life-style changes. Teach clients and others about the dangers of secondhand smoke. Elimination of irritants is generally performed in a reasonable fashion, such as removing exposure to one allergen at a time. Improvements in a

client's symptoms that result from a major life-style change, such as job change or loss of a pet, may be quickly offset by the stress felt from such a change.

Diagnosis, Planning, Implementation

Ineffective Breathing Pattern. A typical nursing diagnosis would be *Ineffective Breathing Pattern related to impaired exhalation and anxiety.*

Because of airway spasm and edema, the client cannot move air in and out of the lungs as needed to maintain

Table 41–2. Action Plan for Adult Asthma Episodes		
Manifestations	**Peak Flow**	**Actions**
Mild episode—Mild wheeze, cough, chest tightness, shortness of breath occurring with activity but not at rest.	70%–90% of baseline (personal best or predicted, as determined by the clinician).	Take inhaled bronchodilator; if improved, continue medication on regular basis for 24–48 hours; if not improved, take action as indicated for moderate episode
Moderate episode—Wheeze, cough, chest tightness, and shortness of breath while at rest; symptoms may interfere with daily activity.	50%–70% of baseline.	Repeat inhaled bronchodilators every 20 minutes for 1 hour; if improved, continue medication every 3–4 hours for 24–48 hours; if not improved in 2–6 hours after initial treatment, begin or increase prednisone; contact your clinician.
Severe episode—Severe shortness of breath, wheeze (wheeze may disappear with very severe episode), cough, and chest tightness at rest: difficulty walking and talking; perhaps retraction of muscles in chest or neck.	<50% of baseline and little response to bronchodilator.	Repeat inhaled bronchodilator, 4–6 puffs, every 10 minutes up to three times; begin or increase prednisone; contact your clinician if available; if there is no significant improvement after 20–30 minutes, seek emergency care immediately

Adapted from Reinke, L. F., and Hoffman, L. A. (1992). How to teach asthma co-management. *American Journal of Nursing, 92,* 40–48.

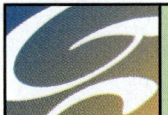

CRITICAL MONITORING

Asthma

If the client still has the following manifestations after being treated for asthma, notify the physician:

- Increased anxiety
- Increased respiratory rate and effort
- Wheezing, both inspiratory and expiratory
- Almost continuous nonproductive cough
- Nasal flaring as respiratory distress increases
- Lips pursed while exhaling
- Use of accessory muscles of breathing
- Increasing tachycardia (tachycardia is a normal response to beta-adrenergics)
- Paradoxical pulse as bronchospasm worsens
- Cyanosis and central nervous system depression as late findings

adequate tissue oxygenation. Anxiety with dyspnea is another cause of breathing pattern problems.

Planning: Expected Outcomes. The client will have improved breathing patterns, as evidenced by a decreasing respiratory rate to within normal limits; decreased signs of dyspnea, nasal flaring, and use of accessory muscles; decreased signs of anxiety; ABG levels returning to normal limits; oxygen saturation above 95%; and vital capacity measurements within normal limits or greater than 40% of predicted.

Implementation. Assess the client frequently, observing respiratory rate and depth. Assess the breathing pattern for shortness of breath, pursed-lips breathing, nasal flaring, sternal and intercostal retractions, or a prolonged expiratory phase. During an acute asthma attack, these assessments may be conducted continuously.

Monitor ABGs and oxygen saturation levels to determine the effectiveness of treatments. Compare pulmonary function test results with normal levels. The degree of dysfunction will assist you in planning client activity.

Place the client in Fowler's position and give oxygen as ordered. Bronchodilators and steroids are commonly prescribed.

Ineffective Airway Clearance. Write the nursing diagnosis as *Ineffective Airway Clearance related to increased production of secretions and bronchospasm.* The excessive production of mucus and spasm in the airway makes it difficult to keep the airway patent.

Planning: Expected Outcomes. The client will have effective airway clearance, as evidenced by decreased inspiratory and expiratory wheezing; decreased rhonchi; and decreasing dry, nonproductive cough.

Implementation. If the airway is compromised, the client may require suctioning. Some clients experience asthma episodes as a result of pulmonary infection. Monitor the color and consistency of the sputum and assist the

client to cough effectively. Encourage oral fluids to thin the secretions and replace fluids lost through rapid respirations. The humidity in the room may be increased slightly. If chest secretions are thick and difficult to expectorate, the client may benefit from postural drainage, lung percussion and vibration, and frequent position changes. Give frequent oral care, every 2 to 4 hours, to remove the taste of the secretions.

Impaired Gas Exchange. The nursing diagnosis is *Impaired Gas Exchange related to air trapping.* When air is trapped within alveoli, they are eventually drained of oxygen and the client can become hypoxic.

Planning: Expected Outcomes. The client will have adequate gas exchange, as evidenced by decreased inspiratory and expiratory wheezing; decreased rhonchi; PaO_2 over 60 mm Hg, partial pressure of arterial carbon dioxide ($PaCO_2$) equal to or less than 45 mm Hg, and pH of 7.35 to 7.45; usual skin color (no cyanosis); and decreasing dry, nonproductive cough.

Implementation. Assess lung sounds every hour during acute episodes to determine the adequacy of gas exchange. Assess skin and mucous membrane color for cyanosis. Recall that cyanosis is a late manifestation of hypoxia and an indication of serious gas exchange problems. Monitor pulse oximetry for oxygen saturations levels. Administer oxygen as ordered.

Refer to the Care Plan for the client with COPD when working with clients with diagnoses of Activity Intolerance; Anxiety; Altered Nutrition; or Sleep Pattern Disturbance.

Evaluation

Generally asthma episodes can be reversed quickly if there is no underlying problem such as infection. Expect the client to be hospitalized only briefly, so plan a coordinated approach to assessment and follow-up.

Community and Self-Care

The approach to pharmacologic therapy is often referred to as "step-care." This means that the number of medications and frequency of administration are increased as needed. Beta-adrenergic agents with varying degrees of beta-2 selectivity are given by nebulizer or metered dose inhaler (Fig. 41–2). Some beta-adrenergic agents can be administered orally also. Common agents include albuterol (Proventil), metaproterenol (Alupent), pirbuterol (Maxair), and terbutaline (Brethine).

Clients with very mild asthma (fewer than three or four attacks per year) can use the inhalers on an as-needed basis. Clients with moderate asthma (six to eight attacks annually) should use inhalers on a regular, daily basis. Clients with severe asthma combine inhalers with other agents.

In addition to beta-adrenergic agents, theophylline and aminophylline are moderately potent bronchodilators used

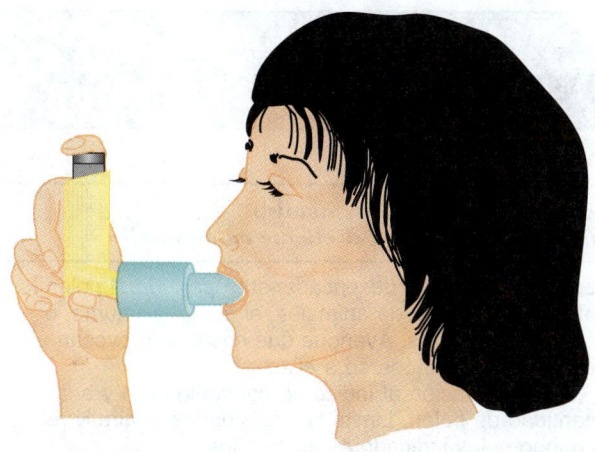

Figure 41–2. A client using a metered dose inhaler with a spacer.

to manage asthma. The use of theophylline is limited by its toxicity and by the wide variations in the rate of metabolism. Theophylline levels are monitored to evaluate the effectiveness of the drug.

Anticholinergics, inhaled and systemic corticosteroids, and mast cell stabilizers may also be used in treating asthma (Table 41–3).

Table 41–3. Pharmacologic Management of Chronic Obstructive Pulmonary Disease (COPD)	
Classification	**Rationale for Use**
Bronchodilators	Relax constricted airways and help relieve the portion of airway obstruction that is reversible
Antihistamines	Block action of histamine at H_1-receptor sites in smooth muscles of the bronchioles, thus inhibiting bronchoconstriction and increasing air flow
Steroids	Reduce inflammation and inflammatory response in bronchial walls; used for symptomatic relief and preventive care of asthma
Antibiotics	Prevent or treat respiratory infections that commonly develop with COPD as a result of alterations in the normal respiratory defense mechanisms and decreased immune resistance
Expectorants	Facilitate the removal of thick mucus from the airways by liquifying secretions
Mast cell stabilizers	Prevent the release of bronchoconstrictive and inflammatory substances when mast cells are confronted with allergens and other stimuli, thus helping to prevent asthma attacks

Nebulized medications can be difficult to learn how to use. The Client Education Guide provides directions for using an inhaler. The client must coordinate inhalation with compression of the canister. Observe the client's use of the nebulizer to ascertain whether the medication is entering the airway.

Many clients can manage their asthma effectively with a thorough action plan to guide their decisions. An action plan for asthma is presented in Table 41–2.

Chronic Obstructive Pulmonary Disease

Chronic obstructive pulmonary disease (COPD), also called chronic obstructive lung disease (COLD), refers to several disorders that affect movement of air in and out of the lungs. The most important of these disorders are obstructive bronchitis, emphysema, and asthma. Although bronchitis, emphysema, and asthma may occur in a "pure form," they most commonly coexist, and clinical manifestations overlap. Although the term COPD is commonly used, some pulmonologists think that it is not completely accurate, and you may see the term "chronic air flow limitation" (CAL) in its place.

COPD may occur as a result of increased airway resistance secondary to bronchial mucosal edema or smooth muscle contraction. It may also be a result of decreased elastic recoil, as seen in emphysema. Elastic recoil, like the recoil of a stretched rubber band, is the force used to passively deflate the lung. Decreased elastic recoil results in a decreased driving force to empty the lung.

COPD is a widespread disorder, affecting 1 in every 10 Americans. Most COPD clients are men over the age of 45. With the increase in smoking among females, however, the incidence of COPD among women is steadily rising.

Etiology and Risk Factors

The specific causes of COPD are not clearly understood. However, the effects of numerous irritants found in cigarette smoke (i.e., stimulation of excess mucus production and coughing, destruction of ciliary function, and inflammation and damage of bronchiolar and alveolar walls) make smoking the leading risk factor for the development of the disorder. Chronic respiratory infections, including sinusitis, contribute to the development of COPD, as does the aging process. In addition, heredity and genetic predisposition appear to have a role.

Pathophysiology

COPD is a combination of chronic obstructive bronchitis, emphysema, and asthma. The pathophysiology of bronchitis and emphysema is presented here. See earlier discussion on the pathophysiology of asthma.

■ Chronic Obstructive Bronchitis

Chronic obstructive bronchitis is inflammation of the bronchi. This causes increased mucus production and

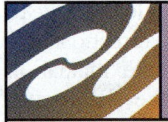

CLIENT EDUCATION GUIDE

Asthma

Client Instructions in English *(Instrucciones para el cliente en inglés)*	**Client Instructions in Spanish** *(Instrucciones para el cliente en espanol)*

Asthma may be triggered by pollen, dust, animal dander, molds, smoke, or other allergens. Learn what triggers your asthma and minimize your exposure to it.
 	
  Monitor the pollution index and pollen counts. Limit outdoor activities when these indicators are high.
 	
  Take all medications as prescribed by your physician. If you are taking both a bronchodilator and a steroid via inhaler, take the bronchodilator first to open the airways.
  Use these directions for using an inhaler:
	El asma se puede desencadenat/dispar con el polen, al polvo, la caspa de animales, el moho, eh humo, o con otros factores. Averigue qué cosas le provocan el asma y evite exponerse a ellas.
	  Ponga atención al índice de contaminación y a la cantidad de polen. Limite las actividades al aire libre cuando estos indicadores estén altos.
	  Tome todos los medicamentos como se los recetó el médico. Si esta tomando un broncodilatador y esteroides por inhalador, aplique el broncodilatador primero para abrir las vías respiratorias.
	  Siga estas instrucciones para usar un inhalador.

• Remove the cap and shake the inhaler well.
• Hold the canister upright with your index finger on the top and your thumb on the bottom.
• Breathe out through your mouth.
• Place the mouthpiece 1 to 2 inches away from your opened mouth.
• Begin with a slow, deep breath. As you breathe in, press the canister down with your finger to give yourself one puff of medication.
 	
• Hold your breath in for at least 5 to 10 seconds.
 	
• Slowly breathe out, holding your lips tight (pursed).
 	
• If your doctor has prescribed more than one puff, wait 1 minute between puffs to let the medication open up the upper airway. That way the next puff can reach lower into your lungs.
 	
  Pursed-lip breathing, progressive muscle relaxation, and tripod positioning (i.e., leaning on your arms positioned in front of you) may improve your breathing during asthma episodes.
	• Quite la tapa y agite bien el inhalador.
	• Sostenga el bote (frasco) derecho con el dedo índice sobre la tapa y el dedo pulgar en la base.
	• Exhale todo el aire por la boca.
	• Abra la boca y ponga la boquilla del inhalador a 1 ó 2 pulgadas de distancia.
	• Empiece con una respiración lenta, honda. Cuando aspire, ponga presión con el dedo hacia abajo sobre la tapa del bote (frasco) para hacer salir un soplido del medicamento.
	• Sostenga la respiración por lo menos de 5 a 10 segundos.
	• Exhale despacio, manteniendo los labios firmente cerrados (fruncidos).
	• Si el médico le recetó inhalar más de una vez, espere 1 minuto para que el medicamento le abra la porción superior de las vías respiratorias inferiores, a fin de que la segunda inhalacion pueda llegarle hasta más abajo en los pulmones.
	
	  El respirar manteniendo la boca fruncida, la relajación progresiva de los músculos, y la posición "trípode" inclinándose hacia el frente, descansando los codos sobre las rodillas) pueden mejorar la respiración durante los ataques de asma.

chronic cough. In contrast to acute bronchitis, the clinical manifestations of chronic bronchitis continue for at least 3 months of the year for 2 consecutive years. Additionally, if the client has a decreased FEV_1/FVC ratio of less than 75% and chronic bronchitis, then the client is said to have chronic *obstructive* bronchitis. This term implies that the client has obstructive lung disease combined with chronic cough. Clients with chronic bronchitis have (1) an increase in the size and number of submucous glands in the large bronchi, which increases mucus production; (2) an increased number of goblet cells, which also se-

crete mucus; and (3) impaired ciliary function, which reduces mucus clearance. Therefore, the lung's mucociliary defenses are impaired, and there is increased susceptibility to infection. When infection occurs, mucus production is even greater, and the bronchial walls become inflamed and thickened. Chronic bronchitis initially affects only the larger bronchi, but eventually all airways are involved. The thick mucus and inflamed bronchi obstruct airways, especially during expiration. The airways collapse, and air is trapped in the distal portion of the lung. This obstruction leads to reduced alveolar ventila-

Client Instructions in English *(Instrucciones para el cliente en inglés)*	**Client Instructions in Spanish** *(Instrucciones para el cliente en espanol)*
Unless your doctor has told you to limit fluids, drink 8 to 10 glasses of water every day. Water helps to thin your sputum so you can cough it up more easily.	A menos que el médico le haya dicho que limite la cantidad de líquidos que bebe, tome de 8 a 10 vasos de agua al día. El agua le ayunda a adelgazar la flema para que así pueda expectorarla más fácilmente.
Some forms of asthma may be triggered by exercise. Discuss an exercise plan with your physician before starting. Keep track of your peak flows. Often they will fall about 1 day before an asthma attack.	Algunas formas de asma se disparan con activan el ejercicio. Discuta un plan con el médico antes de empezar a hacer ejercicio. Siga con atención los medidas de su "peak flow" (aparato que indica el flujo máximo del aire). A menudo, se ven bajas un día antes de un ataque de asma.
Follow these directions on how to use a peak flow-meter: ● Attach the mouthpiece and set the pointer to zero. ● Stand up and take a deep breath. ● Put the mouthpiece in your mouth and close your lips tightly around it. ● Blow into the mouthpiece as hard and as fast as you can. ● Record the value and reset the meter. ● Repeat the procedure for a total of three readings. ● Record the highest value on your record sheet.	Siga estas instrucciones para usar el metro de su "peak flow": ● Adjunte la boquilla y fije el indicador en cero. ● Póngase de pie y respire hondo. ● Póngase la boquilla en la boca y cierre los labios firmemente alrededor de la boquilla. ● Sople en la boquilla tan duro y tan rápido como pueda. ● Apunte los resultados y regrese el indicador a cero. ● Repita el procedimiento por un total de tres medidas. ● Anote la medida más alta en su hoja del registro.
Call your physician if you experience any of the following symptoms: ● Wheezing and shortness of breath, even though you are taking your medications as prescribed ● Fever, muscle aches, chest pain, or thickening of sputum ● Sputum color changes to yellow, green, gray, or red (bloody) ● Problems that may be related to your medications (e.g., rash, itching, swelling, or trouble breathing)	Llame al médico si experimenta cualquiera de los síntomas siguientes: ● Resuallo con dificultad o silbido, faita de aliento que no se mejoren con los medicamentos acostumbrados ● Fiebre, doloras musculares, dolor en el pecho, o espesamiento de la flema. ● Flema amarilla, verde, gris, o roja (sanguinolenta) ● Salpullidos, comezón, hinchazón, o dificultad al respirar relacionada con sus medicamentos

tion. An abnormal V/Q (ventilation-perfusion) ratio develops, with a corresponding fall in PaO_2. Impaired ventilation may also result in increased levels of $PaCO_2$. As compensation for the hypoxemia, polycythemia (an overproduction of erythrocytes) occurs.

■ Emphysema

Emphysema is a disorder in which the alveolar walls are destroyed. This leads to permanent overdistention of the airspaces. Air passages are obstructed as a result of these changes, rather than from mucus production, as in chronic bronchitis. Although the precise cause of emphysema is unknown, research has shown that the enzymes protease and elastase can attack and destroy the connective tissue of the lungs. Emphysema may result from a breakdown in the lung's normal defense mechanisms (alpha₁-antitrypsin or AAT), against these enzymes. Difficult expiration in emphysema is the result of destruction of the walls (septa) between the alveoli, partial airway collapse, and loss of elastic recoil. As the alveoli and septa collapse, pockets of air form between the alveolar spaces (blebs) and within the lung parenchyma (bullae). This process leads to increased ventilatory dead space, areas that do not participate in gas or blood exchange. The work of breathing is increased because there is less functional lung tissue to exchange oxygen and carbon dioxide. Em-

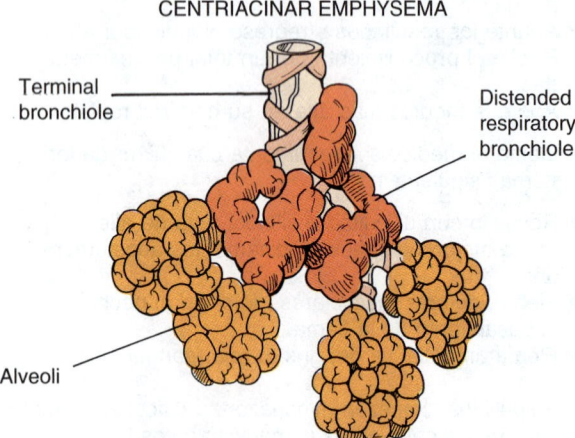

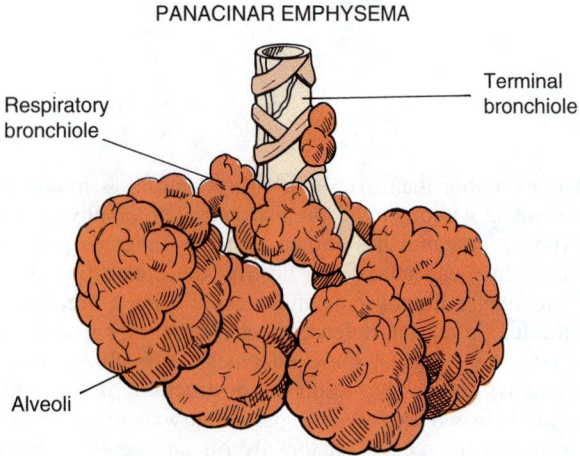

Figure 41–3. Types of emphysema.

physema also causes destruction of the pulmonary capillaries, further decreasing oxygen perfusion and ventilation.

There are three types of emphysema (Fig. 41–3). *Centrilobular emphysema,* the most common type, produces destruction in the bronchioles, usually in the upper lung regions. Inflammation develops in the bronchioles, but usually the alveolar sac remains intact. *Panlobular emphysema* affects both the bronchioles and alveoli and most commonly involves the lower lung. These forms of emphysema occur most often in smokers. *Paraseptal (or panacinar) emphysema* destroys the alveoli in the lower lobes of the lungs resulting in isolated blebs along the lung periphery. Paraseptal emphysema is believed to be the likely cause of spontaneous pneumothorax. Paraseptal emphysema occurs in the elderly and in clients with an inherited deficiency of AAT. Normally, AAT inhibits the action of enzymes that break down proteins. Clients without AAT have increased risk of COPD because the walls of the lung are at higher risk of destruction. Interestingly, cigarette smoking is thought to alter the balance of these enzymes and thus increase destruction of lung tissue.

Clinical Manifestations and Diagnostic Findings

Recall that all three disorders, asthma, chronic bronchitis, and emphysema, are present to some degree in the client with COPD. Figure 41–4 illustrates the common physical findings in the client with COPD.

■ Chronic Obstructive Bronchitis

Clients who have chronic obstructive bronchitis as their major disease have productive cough, decreased exercise tolerance, wheezing, and shortness of breath (Box 41–1). Spirometry shows airway obstruction (decreased FEV_1). The clients will have prolonged expiration and an elevated hematocrit level. Cyanosis and manifestations of cor pulmonale (right ventricular failure) are also common.

As the chronic bronchitis progresses, copious amounts of sputum are produced; pulmonary infection is common. Chronic hypoxemia and hypercapnia cause pulmonary vasoconstriction, leading to cor pulmonale. This is caused by the heart's attempts to pump against increased resistance. Cyanosis develops, along with peripheral edema caused by the heart failure (Fig. 41–5).

■ Emphysema

Clients who have primary emphysema have progressive dyspnea on exertion that eventually becomes dyspnea at rest. Cough is uncommon. The client is often thin, has tachypnea with prolonged expiration, and uses the accessory muscles for respiration (Fig. 41–6). The client often leans forward with arms braced on the knees to support the shoulders and chest for breathing. The anteroposterior diameter of the chest is enlarged (Fig. 41–7) and the

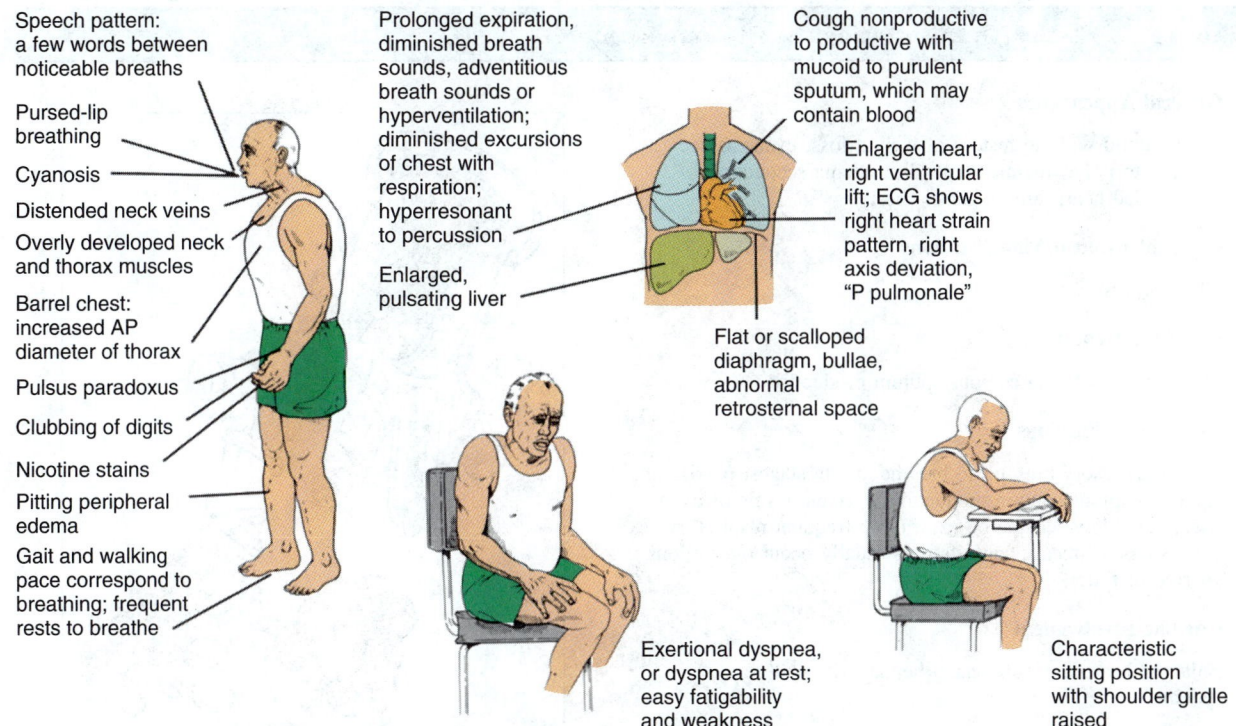

Speech pattern: a few words between noticeable breaths

Pursed-lip breathing

Cyanosis

Distended neck veins

Overly developed neck and thorax muscles

Barrel chest: increased AP diameter of thorax

Pulsus paradoxus

Clubbing of digits

Nicotine stains

Pitting peripheral edema

Gait and walking pace correspond to breathing; frequent rests to breathe

Prolonged expiration, diminished breath sounds, adventitious breath sounds or hyperventilation; diminished excursions of chest with respiration; hyperresonant to percussion

Enlarged, pulsating liver

Cough nonproductive to productive with mucoid to purulent sputum, which may contain blood

Enlarged heart, right ventricular lift; ECG shows right heart strain pattern, right axis deviation, "P pulmonale"

Flat or scalloped diaphragm, bullae, abnormal retrosternal space

Exertional dyspnea, or dyspnea at rest; easy fatigability and weakness

Characteristic sitting position with shoulder girdle raised

Figure 41–4. Clinical manifestations of chronic obstructive pulmonary disease (COPD).

chest has hyperresonant sounds to percussion. ABGs are usually normal until later stages. Box 41–2 outlines the clinical manifestations of emphysema.

Pulmonary function tests reveal decreased FVC and FEV_1. There is an increase in FRC, RV, and TLC. TLC may be twice normal, but the area for oxygen–carbon dioxide transport is greatly reduced because of the destruction of the alveolar walls. Table 41–4 contrasts common findings in chronic bronchitis and emphysema.

■ Complications

Respiratory infections commonly develop in clients with COPD. This is a result of alterations in the normal respiratory defense mechanisms and decreased immune resistance. Because respiratory status is already compromised, infection frequently leads to acute respiratory failure and is a common reason for hospitalization (see Chapter 42).

Spontaneous pneumothorax may develop from rupture of an emphysematous bleb. This results in a closed pneumothorax and requires insertion of a chest tube for reexpansion of the lung (see Chapter 42).

Like asthma, chronic obstructive bronchitis and emphysema may worsen at night. Clients often report sleep-onset dyspnea and frequent or early-morning awakenings. During sleep, there is a decrease in the muscle tone and activity of the respiratory muscles. This leads to hypoventilation, an increase in resistance of the airways, and V/Q mismatch. Eventually the client becomes hypoxemic.

Critical Care

The treatment goals for the client with COPD are as follows: (1) to improve ventilation; (2) to facilitate the removal of bronchial secretions; (3) to prevent complications and to slow the progression of clinical manifestations; and (4) to promote health maintenance and client management of the disease.

At times, the client must receive continuous mechanical ventilation (CMV) for adequate oxygenation. Ventilator-dependent clients with COPD may be managed in critical care. However, some centers have noncritical care areas for clients on ventilators.

Acute and Subacute Care

■ Medical Management

Improving Ventilation

Bronchodilators and steroids are also used in the treatment of COPD (see Table 41–3). As with asthma, they are used to stop the reversible portion of airway spasm. Narcotics, tranquilizers, and sedatives are used with caution in treatment because they depress the respiratory cen-

Box 41–1. Clinical Manifestations of Chronic Bronchitis

General Appearance

Stocky build with no history of weight loss; cyanosis secondary to polycythemia; dependent edema secondary to right-sided heart failure; barrel chest

Onset of Clinical Manifestations

40–50 years

Chief Complaint

Persistent cough and copious sputum production

Assessment Findings

Use of accessory muscles to breathe in late stages; persistent cough, copious sputum production; variable levels of dyspnea; variable wheezing on expiration; frequent respiratory infections. Clinical manifestations usually occur over a long period of time.

Cardiac Involvement

Enlarged heart; cor pulmonale; hematocrit >60%; edema

Smoking History

Invariably, a long history of smoking

Diagnostic Findings

Pulmonary Function

Small airways affected early (reduced $FEF_{25\%-75\%}$); FEV_1 reduced later as airway damage progresses; normal to variable diffusion capacity

Arterial Blood Gases

Increased $PaCO_2$ common; hypoxemia usually present and increasing in severity as disease progresses

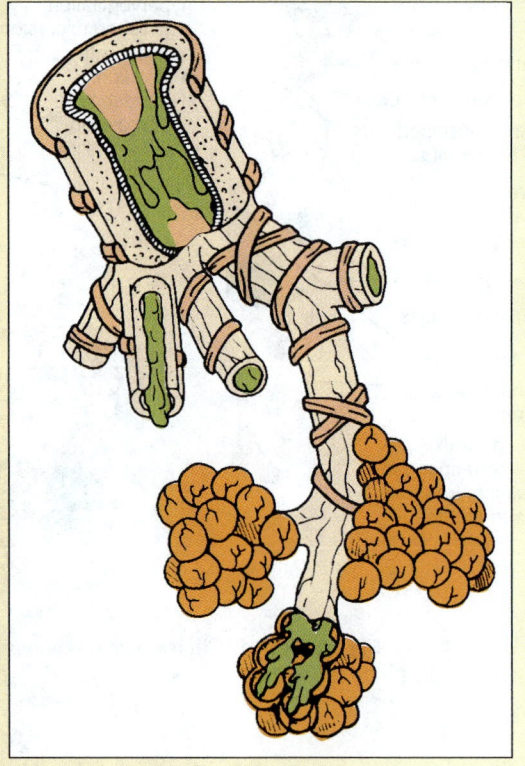

Chest Film

Chest film shows normal or "dirty" chest with increased bronchovascular markings

Clinical Course

Variable with exacerbations usually related to respiratory infections

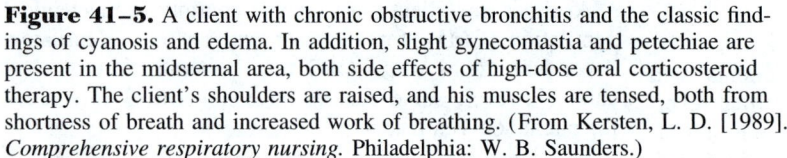

Figure 41–5. A client with chronic obstructive bronchitis and the classic findings of cyanosis and edema. In addition, slight gynecomastia and petechiae are present in the midsternal area, both side effects of high-dose oral corticosteroid therapy. The client's shoulders are raised, and his muscles are tensed, both from shortness of breath and increased work of breathing. (From Kersten, L. D. [1989]. *Comprehensive respiratory nursing.* Philadelphia: W. B. Saunders.)

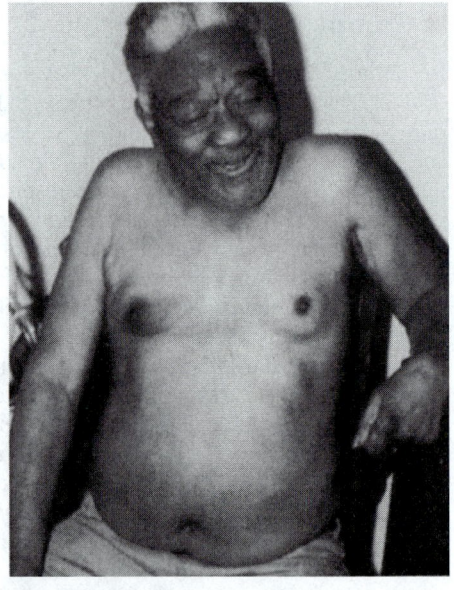

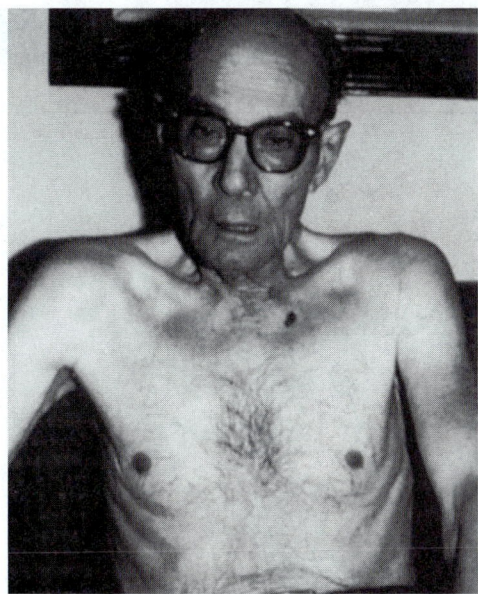

Figure 41–6. A client with emphysema and all the classic findings of the condition. Use of accessory muscles of respiration (intercostal, neck, and shoulder muscles) and the cachectic appearance reflect two factors: (1) shortness of breath (the client's most pressing complaint) and (2) the tremendously increased work of breathing necessary to increase minute ventilation and maintain normal arterial blood gases. (From Kersten, L. D. [1989]. *Comprehensive respiratory nursing.* Philadelphia: W. B. Saunders.)

ter. There are some ongoing studies examining the effect of AAT replacement therapy. The future looks promising for the treatment of early emphysema with the replacement of this protective enzyme inhibitor.

Oxygen is used when the client has severe exertional or resting hypoxemia (PaO_2 below 40 mm Hg). One to 3 L oxygen by nasal cannula may be required to raise the PaO_2 to 60 to 80 mm Hg. However, oxygen is used cautiously in clients with emphysema. Because of long-stand-

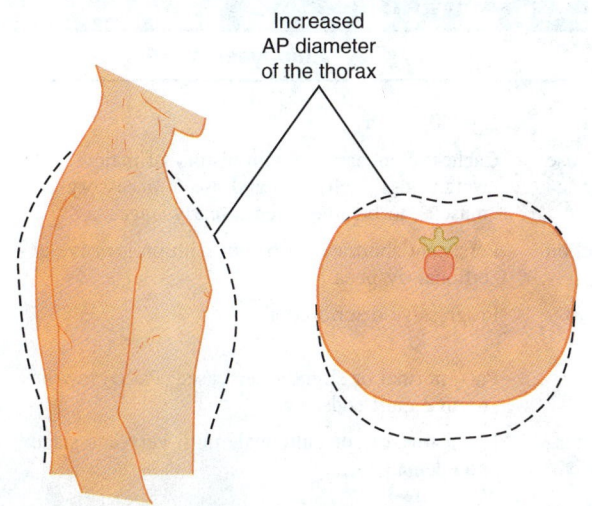

Figure 41–7. Chest wall changes associated with chronic obstructive pulmonary disease (COPD). The *dotted lines* indicate changes occurring with COPD. In COPD the chest becomes barrel-shaped.

Increased AP diameter of the thorax

ing hypercapnia, the respiratory drive in emphysematous clients is triggered by low oxygen levels rather than increased carbon dioxide levels, as is the case in a normal respiratory system. If high levels of oxygen are administered to these clients, their respiratory drive can be obliterated and carbon dioxide retention can occur.

Removing Bronchial Secretions

Pulmonary hygiene is needed to rid the lungs of secretions and reduce the risk of infection. In the hospital, the client may be treated with nebulized bronchodilators and positive-pressure air flow or positive end-expiratory pressure (PEEP) devices to increase the caliber of the airways. In addition, postural drainage and chest physiotherapy may be prescribed to move the secretions from the small to the large airways, from which they can be expelled.

Exercise

Aerobic exercise does not improve lung function. Instead, it is used to enhance cardiovascular fitness and train respiratory muscles to function more effectively. Research has shown that respiratory muscles can be strengthened even when the lungs are diseased.[18] Progressively increased walking is the most common form of exercise. Before a walking program is begun, ABGs should be assessed and compared with resting levels. Supplemental oxygen should be used during exercise if the client becomes severely hypoxemic.

Breathing exercises may also be prescribed. Encourage diaphragmatic breathing and pursed-lips breathing, and discourage rapid, shallow "panic" breathing.

Controlling Complications

Edema and cor pulmonale are treated with diuretics and digitalis. Phlebotomy may be used to reduce blood volume in clients with marked elevations in hematocrit (over 60%). Phlebotomy reduces blood volume and thereby reduces cardiac workload.

Improving General Health

The most effective way to slow disease progression is for the client to stop smoking. In addition, exposure to known allergens should be minimized. All clients with COPD should avoid high altitudes, and supplemental oxygen may be required for air travel. No specific climate has been shown to alter the course of the disorder.

Adequate nutrition is essential to maintain respiratory muscle strength. Consult a clinical dietitian to assist clients in modifying their diet to meet their caloric needs. Clients with COPD often have difficulty eating because of dyspnea. Offer the client frequent small meals, rather than large meals. Adjust oxygen delivery devices so that the mouth is not obstructed but oxygen is delivered through the nose during eating. Calculate the liter flow of the nasal cannula when converting from a mask style by using the formulas in Table 41–5. For example, if a client is using a Venturi oxygen mask at 28%, he or she

Box 41–2. Clinical Manifestations of Emphysema

General Appearance

Cachectic, with history of major weight loss; pink skin color; no signs of right-sided heart failure with dependent edema until endstage

Onset of Manifestations

50–75 years

Chief Complaint

Persistent shortness of breath with progressive exertional dyspnea

Assessment Findings

Use of accessory muscles to breathe, even in early stages; infrequent respiratory infections; on auscultation, diminished breath sounds even with deep breathing; expiratory wheezing not a prominent finding; rare sputum production and cough

Cardiac Involvement

No cardiac enlargement; cor pulmonale late; hematocrit <60%; no edema

Smoking History

Usually, but not always, a smoking history

Diagnostic Function

Pulmonary Function

Reduced $FEF_{25\%-75\%}$ and FEV_1; reduced diffusion capacity due to destruction of alveoli

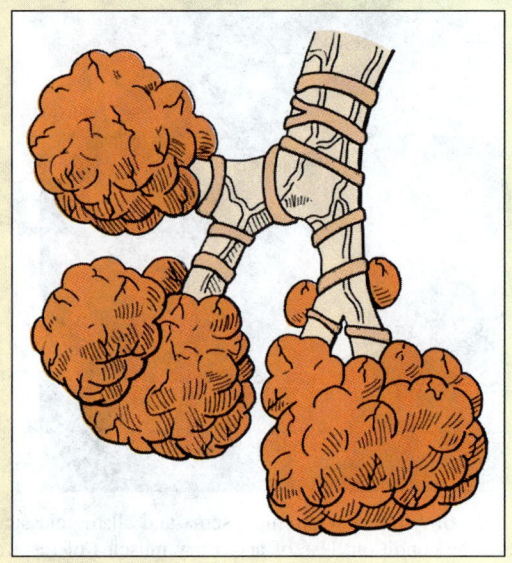

Arterial Blood Gases

$PaCO_2$ usually low or normal until endstage; PaO_2 normal or slightly decreased

Chest Film

Shows overinflation, flattened diaphragms, increased retrosternal airspace, and increased lucency of lower lung fields

Clinical Course

Progressive deterioration

Table 41–4. Common Findings in Chronic Bronchitis and Emphysema

Findings	Chronic Bronchitis	Emphysema
Onset of symptoms	Age 40–50 yr	Age 50–75 yr
Physical appearance	Stocky build with no history of weight loss; use of accessory muscles to breathe in late stages; cyanotic	Cachectic appearance with history of major weight loss; tachypnea and use of accessory muscles to breathe, even in early stages
Chief complaint	Persistent cough and copious sputum production	Persistent shortness of breath with progressive exertional dyspnea
Clinical course	Variable, with exacerbations usually related to respiratory infections	Progressive deterioration
ABGs	↓ PaO_2, ↑ $PaCO_2$	PaO_2 normal or slightly decreased; $PaCO_2$ low or normal until endstage
Associated findings	Frequent episodes of cor pulmonale with dependent edema (especially in late stage); elevated hematocrit	No history of cor pulmonale until very late stage; no edema

ABGs, arterial blood gases; $PaCO_2$, partial pressure of arterial carbon dioxide; PaO_2, partial pressure of arterial oxygen.
Adapted from Whitney, L. (1992). Chronic bronchitis and emphysema: Airing the differences. *Nursing 92, 22,* 34–41.

Table 41–5. Converting Low-Flow to High-Flow Oxygen Systems*

100% Oxygen Flow Rate (L)	FIO₂
Nasal cannula or catheter	
1	24%
2	28%
3	32%
4	36%
5	40%
6	44%
Oxygen mask	
5–6	40%
6–7	50%
7–8	60%
Mask with a reservoir bag	
6	60%
7	70%
8	80%
9	90%
10	100%

* A normal ventilatory pattern is assumed.
FIO₂, fraction of inspired oxygen.

will receive the same amount of oxygen on 2 L via nasal cannula.

Clients with COPD often continue to deteriorate despite medical care. It is difficult to cope with failing health that limits activity and employment. As much as possible, encourage the client to live an active life with daily exercise. The support of significant others is essential.

■ Nursing Management of the Medical Client

Assessment

The nursing history can ascertain whether the client's clinical manifestations are primarily those of chronic bronchitis, emphysema, or asthma. In addition, determine the client's ability to recognize manifestations that require further care. For example, if a client says, "I knew I was developing an infection and went to the doctor," the statement indicates an understanding of the disorder. In contrast, if a client does not fully understand the reasons for hospitalization, you will need to educate the client about COPD. A review of past medical history will help determine whether the client has other disorders, such as heart disease, that may affect treatment.

Complete a physical examination with an emphasis on the respiratory and cardiac system. Note the degree of dyspnea, decreased breath sounds, and clinical manifestations of congestive heart failure. Evaluate mental status, as confusion and restlessness may be early indicators of increasing hypoxia and hypercapnia.

Consider the impact of stressors that may have led to exacerbations of COPD. Possible factors include the progressive illness itself, marital or other family problems, or financial concerns. Also, review the coping strategies that the client normally uses. Determine whether these strategies are working now and if not, why not. Support systems, such as friends and family, are also important components of psychosocial stability. Determine the reliability of the client's support system.

The psychosocial impact of COPD is significant. Clients commonly have feelings of loss of control over their bodies and their social environment. These responses leave the client socially isolated and depressed. A Canadian study found that clients with poor adjustment to COPD used more healthcare dollars for disease management. Therefore, psychosocial intervention is quite important.

A thorough history may need to be delayed until the client is able to breathe comfortably, or it may be taken over short periods of time or obtained through the family. Likewise, the physical examination should not tire the client.

Diagnosis, Planning, Implementation

Common nursing diagnoses and interventions for the client with COPD are listed in the Care Plan for the client with COPD.

■ Surgical Management

Surgery is relatively uncommon in the treatment of COPD. At times, bullectomy may benefit clients who have repeated spontaneous pneumothorax. Bullectomy is the removal of large bullae that compress the lung and add to dead space.

Recent advances have been made with lung volume reduction surgery. This procedure, which involves removal of portions of diffusely emphysematous lungs, helps to restore more normal chest wall configuration and improves respiratory mechanics and functional capacity.[10] Bovine pericardium strips can be used to reinforce staple lines of resected lung tissue. This new approach has reduced the problem of air leaks that occurred in earlier lung volume reduction operations.[2]

Candidates for surgery include persons who are younger than 75 years old, weigh more than 80% of ideal body weight, and have progressive and severe dyspnea that prevents them from walking more than 100 yds or a

CARE PLAN ▰▰▰▰▰▰▰▰▰▰▰▰▰▰▰▰▰▰▰▰▰▰▰▰▰

The Client with Chronic Obstructive Pulmonary Disease (COPD)

Nursing Diagnosis. Impaired Gas Exchange related to decreased ventilation and mucous plugs

Planning: Expected Outcomes. The client will maintain adequate gas exchange as evidenced by blood gas values (i.e., PaO_2 of at least 60 mm Hg, pH within normal limits, and $PaCO_2$ at baseline).

Implementation: Nursing Intervention	Rationales
Regularly monitor the client's respiratory rate and pattern, ABG results, and signs of hypoxia or hypercapnia. Report significant changes promptly.	Prompt recognition of deteriorating respiratory function can reduce potentially lethal outcomes.
Administer low-flow oxygen therapy (1–3 L/min on 24%–31% FIO_2) as needed via nasal prongs or a high-flow Venturi mask (24%–31% FIO_2).	Oxygen corrects existing hypoxemia. Excessive increases in oxygen (55%–70% FIO_2) may diminish respiratory drive and further increase carbon dioxide retention.
Assist the client into high-Fowler position.	The upright position allows full lung excursion and enhances air exchange.
Administer bronchodilators if ordered. Monitor for side effects.	Bronchodilators relax bronchial smooth muscle, facilitating air flow. Common side effects include tremor, tachycardia, and other cardiac dysrhythmias.
Use caution when administering narcotics, sedatives, and tranquilizers.	These medications are respiratory depressants and can further impair ventilation.

Evaluation. Client's respirations are regular, unlabored, and between 12–20/minute. ABGs are within normal range.

Nursing Diagnosis. Ineffective Airway Clearance related to excessive secretions and ineffective coughing

Planning: Expected Outcomes. The client will have improved airway clearance as evidenced by effective coughing techniques and patent airways.

Implementation: Nursing Intervention	Rationales
Teach the client to maintain adequate hydration by drinking at least 8 to 10 glasses of fluid per day (if not contraindicated) and increasing the humidity of the ambient air.	Hydration helps to thin secretions.
Teach and supervise effective coughing techniques.	Proper coughing techniques conserve energy, reduce airway collapse, and lessen client frustration.
Perform chest physical therapy, if needed, and instruct the client and significant others in these techniques.	Chest physical therapy techniques utilize forces of gravity and motion to facilitate secretion removal.
Assess the client's breath sounds before and after coughing episodes.	This assessment will help in the evaluation of coughing effectiveness.

Evaluation. Client's cough is productive and breath sounds are clearer.

Nursing Diagnosis. Activity Intolerance related to inadequate oxygenation and dyspnea

Planning: Expected Outcomes. The client will have improved activity tolerance as evidenced by maintaining a realistic activity level and demonstrating energy conservation techniques.

Implementation: Nursing Intervention	Rationales
Advise the client to avoid conditions that increase oxygen demand, such as smoking, temperature extremes, excess weight, and stress.	These factors increase peripheral vascular resistance, which increases cardiac workload and oxygen requirements.
Instruct the client in energy conservation techniques such as pacing his or her activities throughout the day, interspersed with adequate rest periods, and alternating high- and low-energy tasks.	Conservation techniques allow the client to accomplish more tasks, with a limited energy supply.
Assist the client in scheduling a gradual increase in daily activities and exercise.	Gradual increases in physical activity improve respiratory and cardiac conditioning, thus improving activity tolerance.
Teach the client to use pursed-lip and diaphragmatic breathing techniques during activities.	Breathing retraining ensures maximal use of available respiratory function. Pursed-lip breathing leaves positive end-diastolic pressure in the lungs and helps keep airways open.
Schedule active exercise after respiratory therapy or medication (e.g., bronchodilator in metered dose inhaler).	Lung function is maximized during peak periods of treatment and drug effect.
Maintain supplemental oxygen therapy as needed.	Supplemental oxygen helps alleviate exercise-induced hypoxemia, thus improving activity tolerance.

CARE PLAN

The Client with Chronic Obstructive Pulmonary Disease (COPD)
(Continued)

Implementation: Nursing Intervention	Rationales
Assess the client for signs of a negative response to activity (e.g., significant change in respiratory rate, failure of pulse to return to near resting rate within 3 minutes of activity, changes in mental status).	Significant changes in respiratory, cardiac, or circulatory status signal activity intolerance.

Evaluation. Client performs ADLs and other activities with no significant deterioration in respiratory status.

Nursing Diagnosis. Anxiety related to acute breathing difficulties and fear of suffocation

Evaluation. Client performs ADLs and other activities with no significant deterioration in respiratory status.

Planning: Expected Outcomes. The client will express an increase in psychological comfort and demonstrate use of effective coping mechanisms.

Implementation: Nursing Intervention	Rationales
Remain with the client during acute episodes of breathing difficulty and provide care in a calm, reassuring manner.	Reassure the client that competent help is available, if needed. Anxiety can be contagious. Remain calm.
Provide a quiet, calm environment.	Reduction of external stimuli helps promote relaxation.
During acute episodes, open doors and curtains and limit the number of people and unnecessary equipment in the client's room.	Environmental changes may lessen the client's perceptions of suffocation.
Encourage the use of breathing retraining and relaxation techniques.	A feeling of self-control and success in facilitating breathing will help reduce anxiety.
Give sedatives and tranquilizers with extreme caution. Nonpharmaceutical methods of anxiety reduction are more useful.	Oversedation may cause respiratory depression.

Evaluation. Client's anxiety is decreased; demonstrates use of relaxation techniques and appears restful.

Nursing Diagnosis. Altered Nutrition: Less than Body Requirements related to reduced appetite, decreased energy level, and dyspnea

Planning: Expected Outcomes. The client will maintain body weight within normal limits for sex and body build and hemoglobin and albumin levels will be within the normal ranges.

Implementation: Nursing Intervention	Rationales
Assist the client with mouth care before meals and as needed.	Coughing and sputum production may impair appetite. Mouth-breathing dries mucous membranes.
Advise the client to eat small, frequent meals (e.g., six meals a day) that are high in protein and calories.	Large meals may create an excessive feeling of fullness that may make breathing uncomfortable and difficult. High protein and calorie levels are needed to maintain nutritional status in light of the increased workload of breathing.
Advise the client to avoid gas-producing foods, such as beans and cabbage.	Gas-forming foods may cause abdominal bloating and distention and thus impair ventilation.
Instruct the client in the use of high-calorie liquid supplements, if indicated.	Increased calorie intake is needed to provide energy for the increased work of breathing. Liquid supplements provide high-calorie concentrations in a relatively small volume.
Advise hypoxemic clients to use oxygen via a nasal cannula during meals.	Adequate oxygenation increases the energy available for eating.
Suggest methods to make meal preparation more convenient (e.g., a Meals on Wheels program).	Reducing the energy expenditure of preparation will maximize the energy available for eating.
Monitor the client's food intake, weight, and serum hemoglobin and albumin levels.	Changes in body weight reflect the degree of nutrition or malnutrition. Hemoglobin and albumin levels reflect protein intake.

Evaluation. Client maintains normal body weight and blood protein levels.

Care Plan continued on following page

CARE PLAN

The Client with Chronic Obstructive Pulmonary Disease (COPD)
(Continued)

Nursing Diagnosis. Sleep Pattern Disturbance related to dyspnea and external stimuli

Planning: Expected Outcomes. The client will report feeling adequately rested.

Implementation: Nursing Intervention

Promote relaxation by providing a darkened, quiet environment; ensuring adequate room ventilation; and following bedtime routines, if possible.

Schedule care activities to allow periods of uninterrupted sleep.

Instruct the client in measures to promote sleep:

- Plan physical exercise during the day and passive, non-stimulating activities in the evening.
- Avoid stimulants such as caffeine.
- Maintain a consistent bedtime and a regular bedtime routine.
- Eat a high-protein snack before bedtime.
- Use relaxation techniques (e.g., meditation, massage, warm bath, warm beverage).
- If the client awakens during the night, suggest the use of a quiet, diverting activity, such as reading, in another room.
- If dyspnea is severe, a recliner chair or hospital bed may be more comfortable than a regular bed.

Rationales

The hospital environment can interfere with relaxation and sleep. Using established bedtime rituals increases relaxation.

For most people, completing four to five complete sleep cycles (60–90 minutes) per night promotes a feeling of being rested.

- Activity increases the need for sleep and contributes to a feeling of "tiredness."
- Stimulants increase metabolism and inhibit relaxation.
- Consistency promotes relaxation and prevents disruptions of the biologic clock.
- Protein digestion produces tryptophan, an amino acid that has a sedative effect.
- Sleep is difficult unless the client is relaxed.
- Frustration over being awake will further deter sleep efforts. The bedroom should be mentally associated with sleep to enhance future sleep promotion.
- The upright position facilitates ventilation.

Evaluation. Client gets at least 4–5 hours of uninterrupted sleep per night and voices feeling of being rested.

Nursing Diagnosis. Altered Family Processes related to chronic illness of a family member

Planning: Expected Outcomes. The family will verbalize their feelings, participate in the care of the ill family member, and seek external resources as needed.

Implementation: Nursing Intervention

Plan interventions considering the client and significant others as the unit of care. Encourage participation in the planning process.

Assess family communication patterns and intervene if they are ineffective. Family counseling may be needed.

Encourage as wide a social support system as feasible.

Encourage the client and family to seek support from other sources (e.g., self-help groups and support groups such as the Better Breathers clubs sponsored by the American Lung Association).

Provide the family with anticipatory guidance as the client's COPD progresses.

Rationales

COPD affects not only the client experiencing the condition but also the client's significant others.

Effective communication helps each member to understand his or her own and others' feelings. Counseling may facilitate healthy interaction.

The use of a wide support group prevents a few family members from being overloaded with responsibility.

Clients may benefit from opportunities to share common experiences and learn from others in similar situations.

Knowing what to expect facilitates family adjustment.

Evaluation. Client's family copes effectively with stress of client's illness, communicates openly, and supports client.

Nursing Diagnosis. Sexual Dysfunction related to dyspnea, reduced energy, and changes in relationships.

Planning: Expected Outcomes. The client will report increased satisfaction with sexual function.

Implementation: Nursing Intervention

Provide an opportunity for the client to discuss concerns.

Suggest measures that may facilitate sexual activity (e.g., alternative positions, use of bronchodilator therapy before beginning sexual activity).

Rationales

Many people are embarrassed or reluctant to talk about their sexual concerns.

Such measures can reduce physical exertion and maximize available oxygen levels.

CARE PLAN

The Client with Chronic Obstructive Pulmonary Disease (COPD)
(Continued)

Implementation: Nursing Intervention	Rationales
Encourage the client and his or her partner to consider other forms of sexual expression (e.g., hugging, cuddling, stroking, kissing).	Alternative methods require less energy expenditure than does intercourse.
Refer to a professional sex therapist, if appropriate.	Talking with a skilled professional may further assist the client with constructive problem-solving.

Evaluation. Client discusses concerns and verbalizes more satisfaction with sexual relations.

---

few minutes without stopping for breath. In addition, most clients are considered candidates for surgery when their FEV is 20% to 30% of normal.[16]

After surgery, monitor closely the client's ABGs. Chest assessment and x-ray help determine if the client's lungs are expanding. Assess the chest tubes for air leaks and drainage. Most clients have chest physiotherapy every 4 hours and nebulized aerosol treatments. Clients usually ambulate soon after surgery, sometimes the same day as the operation. Manage pain aggressively to promote activity and pulmonary hygiene.

After dismissal the client is assessed for tissue oxygenation with pulse oximetry, wound healing, and ventilation. Pulmonary treatments may continue until lung sounds clear. The clients are weaned from oxygen and placed into a formal pulmonary rehabilitation program. Outcomes of the surgery have not been fully researched. See Figure 41–8 for changes in chest x-ray findings.

■ Modifications for Elderly Clients

COPD is the second most significant disorder of people in the middle to late adult years. The elderly client frequently has other problems that influence the treatment of COPD. For example, the client may have decreased exercise tolerance, impaired nutrition, or a long-standing habit of smoking that retards rehabilitation. Also consider the possibility of drug-drug interactions in elderly clients.

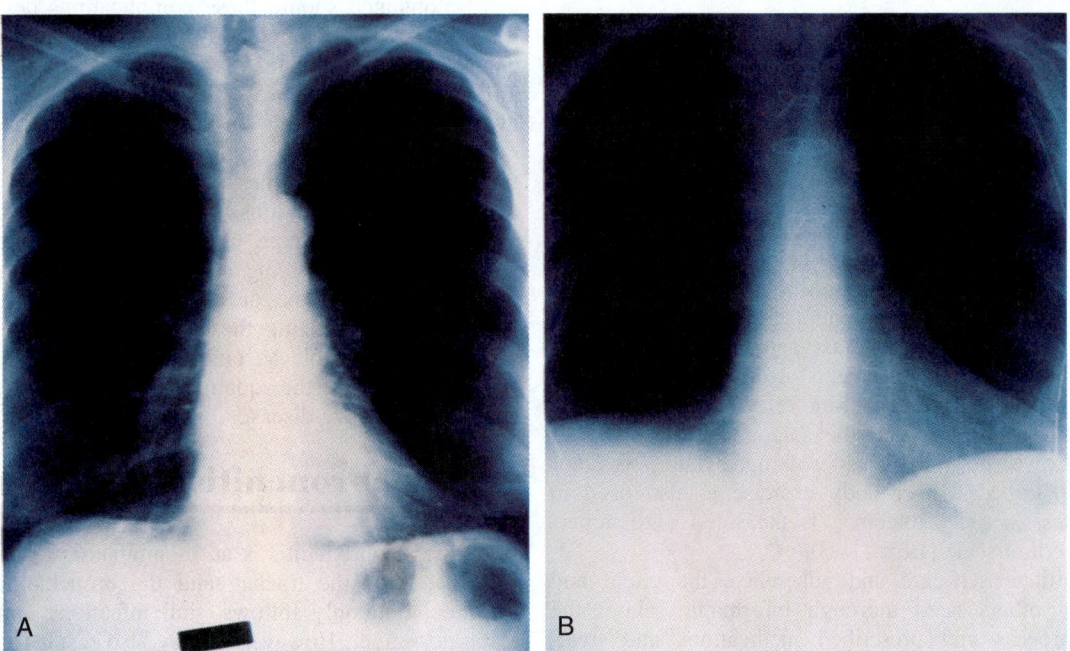

Figure 41–8. *A,* A preoperative chest x-ray of a client with emphysema. Note the flattened diaphragm and the laterally hyperexpanded chest walls. *B,* A postoperative chest x-ray of a client after lung volume reduction surgery. Note that the right side of the diaphragm is rounded and no longer flattened by emphysematous lung tissue. (From Allen, G. [1996]. Surgical treatment of emphysema using bovine pericardium strips. *AORN Journal, 63*[2], 373–388.)

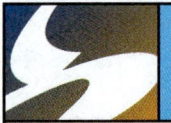

CASE MANAGEMENT

COPD/Asthma
For Clinical Pathway, see Appendix D

Clinical Pathway From Birmingham Baptist Medical Center, Birmingham, Alabama
Information provided by Kathy T. Martin, M.S.N.

Development and Revision of Pathway

- COPD is a high-volume, high-cost case type. The care of an acute asthma patient is similar, so the two case types were combined in one pathway.
- We have been using this pathway for approximately 3 years.
- The development team included pulmonary nurses, physicians, respiratory therapists, pharmacists, administration, and the case manager.
- A Continuous Quality Improvement team meets quarterly, composed of physicians, nurses, respiratory therapists, administrators, emergency physicians, clinical managers, pharmacists, microbiologist, and decision support staff. Issues related to practice patterns are discussed during this meeting. Changes may be made in the pathway at that time.
- The pathway is revised as needed. The length of stay was recently changed, necessitating a revision in the pathway.

Use and Impact of Pathway

- All patients who are admitted with either COPD or asthma are placed on this pathway.
- All nurses and assistive personnel use it daily, and the physicians use it occasionally.
- Length of stay for these patients has decreased by 2 to 3 days. There has been improved timing of antibiotic, steroid, and aminophylline administration as well as improvement in the timing of sputum collection. Nurses advance the patient's activity level sooner, and the oxygen-weaning protocol is initiated in a timely manner due to the pathway. Nurses are much more aware of the activities and expected outcomes for the entire admission and can therefore take a more proactive role in care.
- There has been a marked impact on cost per case (a decrease in cost), and the length of stay has dropped by 2 to 3 days for these patients.

Community and Self-Care

■ Medical Management

Pulmonary rehabilitation is designed to reduce the toll of pulmonary disease for the individual and the healthcare system. Pulmonary rehabilitation helps clients learn methods to control dyspnea and develop more effective breathing patterns and coughing techniques. The Bridge to Home Healthcare described oxygen conservation activities for the COPD client. Clients are also taught how to administer medications, what side effects to look for and how to manage them, and the safe and correct use of oxygen. Lower body exercise (walking, cycling) is commonly prescribed. Upper body exercise is also used in some cases. Activity tolerance is measured with a perceived exertion scale (Box 41–3).

To facilitate self-care and adherence, the client and significant others need thorough information about the disease process and prescribed medications and treatments. Review the signs of impending respiratory problems (e.g., increased confusion or drowsiness), respiratory infection, and right-sided heart failure (e.g., peripheral edema, distended neck veins) so that prompt intervention

can be obtained should these complications develop. The need for routine respiratory follow-up should also be discussed. Teaching should include a discussion of the hazards of infection and ways to decrease personal risk (i.e., avoid crowds during the flu and colds season, clean respiratory equipment well, obtain Pneumovax [pneumococcal vaccine] and flu vaccines yearly). In addition, the need for life-style modifications should also be reviewed.

Clients with endstage lung disease experience significant, intensely distressing manifestations. Whether care is provided in the home or an extended care facility, the focus is on minimizing these symptoms and making the client as comfortable as possible. The Nursing Research feature addresses the quality of life for clients with chronic respiratory disease.

Tracheobronchitis

Acute tracheobronchitis is an inflammation of the mucous membranes of the trachea and the bronchial tree. This disorder commonly follows viral infections of the upper respiratory tract. However, it may also result from inhalation of noxious or irritating gases and particulate matter (including cigarette smoke), bacterial pneumonia, overvigorous tracheobronchial suctioning, and harsh paroxysms of coughing.

BRIDGE TO HOME HEALTHCARE

Conserving Oxygen

Lois Brass-Ernst, R.N., B.S.N., *Staff Builders Health Care Services, Baltimore, Maryland*

Oxygen conservation techniques for the patient with chronic obstructive pulmonary disease (COPD) require planning and coordination. A multidisciplinary team approach offers the greatest benefit to the patient. The patient and his or her family are important members of the team and active participation in care will increase their satisfaction.

Prior to hospital discharge, the patient should have physical and occupational therapy. Upper body exercise programs can improve exhalation performance, decrease small airway atelectasis, and conserve energy expenditure. Lower body exercise programs contribute to overall endurance training and specific muscle toning. Oxygen conservation is generally included within the context of this training.

When the patient is discharged to home, work with physical, occupational, and respiratory therapists in collaboration with the physician to successfully assess, plan, intervene, and evaluate care. First determine what teaching has already occurred and the patient's level of understanding of that teaching.

Identify the patient's personal needs and priorities for oxygen conservation with a simple activity diary. Similar to a dietary diary, instruct the patient to record his or her typical daily behavior during a 24- to 48-hour period. This activity diary should account for all hours of the day; from the time the patient arises from bed through and including the hour of sleep. Evaluation of the activity diary allows you to draw conclusions about the patient's typical activities of daily living (ADLs), priorities of behavior, and areas of behavior concern.

Using the diary, work with the patient to correlate specific activities with the patient's perceptions of dyspnea throughout the day. By connecting an activity to a specific dyspnea rating, you can develop a plan for specific oxygen conservation technique training. Oxygen conservation training includes an environmental assessment for safety and appropriate modification of barriers to that safety. Consider the placement of medications and equipment such as oxygen, puffers, and nebulizers for not only ease of access but appropriateness of access. For example, early-morning ADLs are often critical respiratory effort times. By placing the puffer or nebulizer in the patient's bedroom, the patient may take a treatment before beginning early-morning ADLs.

You and the patient can develop and implement a plan to conserve energy and pace activities based on the patient's priorities and the identified oxygen demand times. Oxygen conservation techniques of pursed-lips breathing, diaphragmatic breathing, and abdominal breathing can be reviewed. By practicing pacing activities, the patient may fine-tune his or her oxygen conservation skills before they are actually needed. The use of pulse oximetry to measure oxygen saturation during the practice as well as the real-time performance of conservation techniques can be reassuring to the patient. Associating perceived dyspnea with an objective measure of oxygen saturation encourages the patient to recognize his or her own distress and act accordingly.

Oxygen conservation is a challenge for the patient as well as for you. Collaborative efforts among all team members bring about the most successful outcomes for respiratory comfort and control in the patient's ADLs.

Clinical symptoms of tracheobronchitis include a raw burning pain over the upper anterior chest wall over the midsternum. Pain is increased with exposure to cold environments, cigarette smoke, cough, and tracheobronchial suctioning. In addition, the client may have a cough that progresses from dry to productive as the irritation increases. Fever, headache, and malaise may also be present. Observe for cough-related syncope. Lightheadedness or fainting may occur with forceful coughing spells. This is caused by prolonged elevation of intrapulmonary pressure during the compressive phase of a cough. The increased pressure impairs venous return to the thorax, causing a decrease in cardiac output. Syncope may result.

Treatment is focused on the cause of the cough. Cough suppressants are rarely effective. Antibiotics, bronchodilators, corticosteroids (inhaled and systemic), and anticholinergics are the primary treatments. Sinusitis is a common accompanying finding, as well as a cause of tracheobronchitis.

Priority nursing goals include relief of pain and elimination of the tracheal irriation. Strongly advise the client to stop smoking. Whenever possible, eliminate other irritating gases or substances from the environment. Promote airway clearance by encouraging effective coughing, increased fluid intake, changing positions, and increasing inspired humidity. Inspired humidity may be increased through the use of aerosols. Tell the client to avoid cold air and to cover his or her mouth and nose before going outdoors.

Bronchiectasis

Bronchiectasis is an extreme form of bronchitis. This disorder causes permanent, abnormal dilation and distortion of bronchi and bronchioles. It develops when bronchial walls are weakened by chronic inflammatory changes in the bronchial mucosa. Bronchiectasis most often develops after recurrent inflammatory conditions. However, any condition producing a narrowing of the lumen of the bronchioles may result in bronchiectasis, including tuberculosis, adenoviral infections, and pneumonia. Some forms of bronchiectasis are congenital and are associated with cystic fibrosis, sinusitis, dextrocardia (heart located on the right side of the chest), and alterations in ciliary activity (Kartagener's syndrome). Bronchiectasis is usually localized to a lung lobe or segment rather than generalized throughout the lungs. At times, however, persistent, nonresolving infection may cause the disorder to spread to other parts of the same lung. Diagnosis may be confirmed through chest x-ray, bronchogram, or computed tomography (CT) scan.

Manifestations vary according to the etiologic agent. The main manifestations are cough and purulent sputum production in large quantities. Fever, hemoptysis, nasal stuffiness, and drainage from sinusitis are also common. The client may complain of fatigue and weakness. Clubbing of the fingers may be found on physical assessment.

Management of bronchiectasis is the same as for COPD. Most clients are managed medically to prevent progression of the disorder and control symptoms. Antibiotics, chest physical therapy, hydration, bronchodilators, and oxygen are commonly prescribed. Severe cases may be treated by surgical resection if the pathologic process is well localized in one lobe or two adjacent lobes and when no contraindications to surgery exist.

Disorders of the Pulmonary Vasculature

Pulmonary Embolism

Pulmonary embolism (PE) is an occlusion of a portion of the pulmonary blood vessels by an embolus. An embolus is a clot or other plug that is carried by the bloodstream from its point of origin to a smaller blood vessel where it obstructs circulation. Depending on its size, a PE can be a potentially lethal disorder. In fact, estimates show that 50,000 people in the United States die each year from PE and this mortality figure has remained unchanged over the past 20 years.[9]

Etiology and Risk Factors

Virtually all PEs develop from thrombi (clots), most of which originate in the deep calf, femoral, popliteal, or iliac veins. Other sources of emboli include tumors, air, fat, bone marrow, amniotic fluid, septic thrombi, and vegetations on heart valves that develop with endocarditis (see Risk Factors and Levels of Prevention).

Pathophysiology

When emboli travel to the lungs, they lodge in the pulmonary vasculature. The size and number of emboli determine the location. Blood flow is obstructed, leading to decreased perfusion of the section of lung supplied by the vessel. The client continues to ventilate the lung portion but because the tissue is not perfused, a ventilation-perfusion mismatch occurs and hypoxemia develops.

If an embolus lodges in a large pulmonary vessel, it increases proximal pulmonary vascular resistance, causes atelectasis, and eventually reduces cardiac output. If the embolus is in a smaller vessel, less dramatic clinical manifestations follow, but perfusion is still altered.

The arterioles constrict because of platelet degranulation, accompanied by a release of histamine, serotonin, catecholamines, and prostaglandins. The chemical agents result in bronchial and pulmonary artery constriction. This vasoconstriction probably plays a major role in the hemodynamic instability that follows PE.

PE can lead to right-sided heart failure. Once the clot lodges, affected blood vessels in the lung collapse. This increases the pressure in the pulmonary vasculature. The increased pressure increases the workload of the right side of the heart, leading to failure. Massive PE of the pulmonary artery can also result in cardiopulmonary collapse

NURSING RESEARCH

How Does Chronic Obstructive Pulmonary Disease Affect Quality of Life?

Berg, J. (1996). Quality of life in COPD patients using transtracheal oxygen. *MEDSURG Nursing, 5*(1), 36–40.

Clients with chronic obstructive pulmonary disease (COPD) experience numerous problems that interfere with their quality of life. The use of a nasal cannula, which is inefficient, irritating to the mucous membranes and skin, conspicuous, and embarrassing, may contribute to a decreased quality of life. Transtracheal oxygen is more efficient, reduces energy expenditure, causes less irritation, and leads to less embarrassment. This study examined clients' perceptions of the effect of transtracheal oxygen on their quality of life.

This qualitative study assessed quality of life from a client-centered view. The sample included seven subjects (four men and three women) with COPD. These subjects were part of a larger longitudinal study group. Subjects ranged in age from 54 to 76 years and had used transtracheal oxygen for as little as 22 months to as much as 40 months. The subjects were interviewed in their homes. Interviews were tape-recorded and transcribed verbatim. The transcripts were coded by two independent coders. Only themes identified and agreed on were used in analysis of the data.

Four themes emerged from the data: (1) activity, (2) failure to name the device, (3) isolation, and (4) control. All subjects described a life that grew increasingly inactive. All of the subjects were largely homebound. Typical statements about activity were "I don't do anything; I go from here into that chair and that's all." Most subjects indicated that the transtracheal oxygen made it easier to be active even if only in their home.

An interesting theme was failure to name the device and the names subjects chose to call the catheter. Most subjects called the transtracheal catheter "it" or "the thing." Some called it an elusive "you know."

Isolation from friends because of being housebound and having a chronic illness was the final pattern that emerged. Some subjects who lived with a spouse still reported that they spent a lot of time "alone." One subject stated that people who visit are afraid of the oxygen. Another stated that he did not call anyone when "down" because "they do not want to hear about his problems." Their greatest joy was when family members visited.

A positive aspect of control was related to the ability to carry out the regimen associated with the transtracheal oxygen catheter. A negative aspect was the loss of control associated with the disease. One client had recently fallen and said, "I have lost my lungs. Now I have lost my legs."

Implications for Practice

Know and appreciate the feelings of isolation and inactivity that these clients feel. Strategies to overcome isolation are especially important. The clients' inability to name the transtracheal catheter may be due to the complexity of the name of the device. Use language that is clear and specific when talking about equipment.

---

from lack of perfusion and resulting hypoxia and acidosis.

Clinical Manifestations and Diagnostic Findings

The clinical manifestations of PE are nonspecific and, in some clients, may not appear until late in the event. The most common signs of PE are tachypnea, dyspnea, and chest pain. These symptoms are similar to those seen with myocardial infarction, so a differential diagnosis is often made. However, the pain usually experienced with PE is pleuritic in nature, caused by an inflammatory reaction of the lung parenchyma, or by pulmonary infarction or ischemia, caused by obstruction of small pulmonary arterial branches. Typical pleuritic chest pain is sudden in onset and aggravated by breathing. The client is usually dyspneic, especially if the embolus has occluded major arteries or major portions of lung tissue. Apprehension, cough, diaphoresis, syncope, and hemoptysis may occur.

The presence of hemoptysis indicates that the infarction or areas of atelectasis have produced alveolar damage.

Respirations typically increase. The client may also develop crackles, an accentuated second heart sound, tachycardia, and fever. Less common findings include heart gallops, edema, heart murmur, and cyanosis.

The diagnosis of PE is suggested by the clinical picture and the results of diagnostic tests. ABG analysis indicates arterial hypoxemia (low PaO_2) and hypocapnia (low $PaCO_2$) in massive PE. There may be a severe respiratory alkalosis. Lactic dehydrogenase (LDH) isoenzymes show an increase in LDH_3 if there is lung tissue injury. A chest x-ray may help to rule out other pulmonary diagnoses.

The best noninvasive diagnostic test for PE is the ventilation-perfusion lung scan. A radioisotope lung scan is performed by intravenous injection of particles of human serum albumin that have been labeled with iodine 131 or technetium 99m. These particles are trapped in the pulmonary microvasculature and are distributed according to pulmonary flow. Both lungs are scanned with a scintillation counter, and the amount of radioactivity counted gives an indication of obstruction to flow. A lung scan can be seen in Chapter 40.

Pulmonary angiograms provide the most effective means of diagnosing PE (Fig. 41–9). This procedure is performed by injecting a radiopaque contrast agent into the right atrium and pulmonary artery via a catheter threaded through a peripheral vein. Visualization of any filling defects of the heart and right pulmonary artery is achieved by taking sequential x-rays.

Emergency Care

Successful management of PE depends on prompt recognition of the condition and immediate treatment. Medical management focuses on anticoagulation to limit further clot formation and give the body's fibrinolytic system time to dissolve the clot.

Maintenance of cardiopulmonary stability is also required. Cardiopulmonary resuscitation can help propel clots away from the central arteries. Acidosis, a potent pulmonary vasoconstrictor, must be corrected with bicarbonate. Heart rhythm must be restored and blood pressure stabilized.

About 95% of clients with PE can be treated successfully with heparin. In certain clients, however, heparin cannot be used and surgery is needed (see Surgical Management).

Acute and Subacute Care

▪ Medical Management

Anticoagulant Therapy

Anticoagulation is begun with intravenous heparin sodium to reduce the risk of further clots and prevent extension of existing clots. Heparin does *not* break up existing thrombi or emboli. Anticoagulants are administered until the partial thromboplastin time (PTT) is 2.0 to 2.5 times the control value. Administration of sodium warfarin (Coumadin) is begun about 3 to 5 days before heparin is stopped to provide a transition to anticoagulation. Because the half-life of warfarin is long, it requires about 2 to 3 days to achieve adequate anticoagulation. Clients are maintained on warfarin for 3 to 6 months.

Fibrinolytic Therapy

The use of fibrinolytic therapy in the management of massive PE is not clear but may be useful in clients who are hemodynamically unstable after PE. Thrombolytic

---

RISK FACTORS AND LEVELS OF PREVENTION

Pulmonary Embolism

Risk Factors

Hip and knee surgery without prophylactic anticoagulation; extensive pelvic or abdominal surgery for advanced malignant diseases; diagnostic or therapeutic procedures that can produce air, fat, amniotic fluid, or tumor emboli; predisposition to thrombotic diseases

Levels of Prevention

Primary Prevention

- Encourage early ambulation of all clients, especially postsurgical, post-trauma, obese, and elderly clients
- Direct bed- or chair-bound clients to perform leg exercises regularly to enhance circulation
- Discourage smoking, especially with at-risk clients, as the vasoconstriction caused by nicotine further impairs circulation
- Apply sequential compression stockings if ordered
- Administer low-dose heparin, if ordered, as prophylactic treatment
- Clients with a history of deep vein thrombosis and/or pulmonary embolus should be taught to avoid restrictive clothing on the legs and prolonged sitting or standing

Secondary Prevention

- Carefully assess clients with deep vein thrombosis for early clinical manifestations

Tertiary Prevention

- Teach clients on anticoagulant therapy about medications/side effects/follow up.
- Patients with vena caval filtering devices should be taught signs and symptoms of possible complications (e.g., wound hematoma or infection, recurrent emboli).

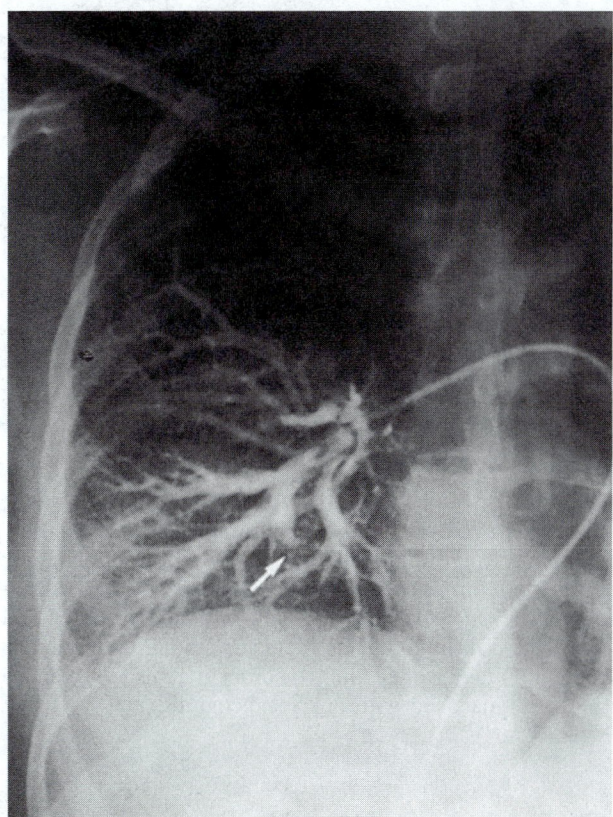

Figure 41–9. An angiogram showing a pulmonary embolus (*arrow*).

agents lyse the clots and restore right-sided heart function. However, some clinicians have found that although the clot dissolves, the mortality rate is not improved.

Cardiopulmonary Support

Cardiopulmonary support varies with the client's symptoms. Sometimes hypoxemia can be reversed with low-flow oxygen by nasal cannula. Other clients require endotracheal intubation to maintain PaO_2 over 60 mm Hg. Hypotension is treated with fluids. If fluids do not raise the preload (right ventricular end-diastolic pressure) enough to raise blood pressure, inotropic agents may be required.

Analgesia

Chest pain and apprehension are usually treated with intravenous analgesics. Morphine is the most common agent.

Positioning

The head of the bed is elevated to reduce dyspnea. Because the usual cause of PE is thrombus from the lower legs, elevate the legs with caution to avoid severe flexure of the hips. Such flexure will again slow blood flow and increase the risk of new thrombi.

■ Nursing Management of the Medical Client

Monitor the client closely for hypoxemia and respiratory compromise. Vital signs and lung sounds are assessed frequently. Monitor blood gas values. To facilitate breathing, place the client in the semi-Fowler position and apply oxygen per physician's orders.

Also monitor the client for signs of right-sided heart failure. Auscultate heart sounds frequently, assessing for murmurs or extra heart sounds. Check for peripheral edema, distended neck veins, and liver engorgement.

Assess treatment effectiveness by monitoring the PTT. The usual goal is 2.0 to 2.5 times the control value. Watch for signs of excess anticoagulation, such as blood in the urine, stool, or along the gums or teeth, subcutaneous bruising, or flank pain. When invasive studies, such as ABGs, are necessary, apply pressure for 30 minutes to the puncture site.

The client typically experiences fear with the sudden onset of severe chest pain and inability to breathe. Anxiety, restlessness, and apprehension are common. Emotional support can reduce anxiety and lessen dyspnea. Stay with the client and give calm, yet efficient, nursing care.

Analgesics are given as needed to reduce pain and anxiety. Anxiety and pain increase oxygen demand and dyspnea. Oral care with soft brushes or rinses is given while oxygen is in use, especially if the client breathes through the mouth.

The client will be discharged on oral anticoagulation. Instruct the client to monitor prothrombin times and to take precautions to prevent bleeding. Also, review methods to reduce thrombophlebitis, if that was the likely cause of the embolus (see Chapter 49).

■ Surgical Management

Surgical interventions for PE include (1) vena cava interruption, with the insertion of a filter (Fig. 41–10) and (2) pulmonary embolectomy.

The Greenfield filter, a basketlike cone of wires bent to look like an umbrella, is the filter most commonly used. The filter is inserted by threading it up the veins until it reaches the vena cava at the level of the renal arteries. The filter allows blood flow while trapping emboli.

An embolectomy involves surgical removal of emboli from the pulmonary arteries via either a thoracotomy or an embolectomy catheter. Embolectomy is used in clients with significant hemodynamic instability caused by the embolus, especially those with unstable circulation and contraindications to thrombolytic therapy.

Pulmonary Hypertension

Pulmonary hypertension is defined as a prolonged elevation of the mean pulmonary artery pressure (PAP) above 18 mm Hg (normal, 10–20 mm Hg) and systolic PAP above 30 mm Hg (normal 20–30 mm Hg) at rest or during exercise. Normally, the pulmonary circulation is a

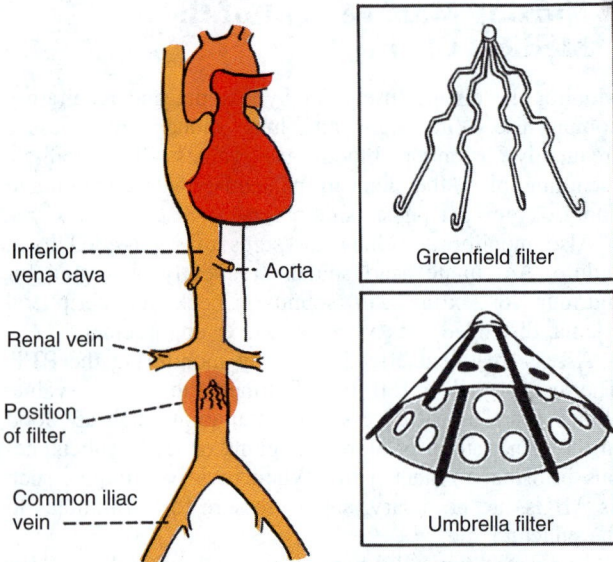

Figure 41–10. Inferior vena cava filters, such as the Greenfield and umbrella filters, prevent emboli from traveling to the lung.

low-pressure, low-resistance system. Increased cardiac output in the healthy person, as with exercise, causes minimal elevations in PAP because of the large pulmonary vascular reserve. When pulmonary vasoconstriction is present, however, pressure elevation occurs because the pulmonary vasculature cannot accommodate increased blood flow.

Mild forms of pulmonary hypertension are generally caused by pulmonary vasoconstriction due to chronic hypoxia, acidosis, or both. The administration of oxygen, correction of acid-base imbalance, and use of vasodilating medications in selected cases will generally return PAP to normal, either completely or partially.

Severe forms of pulmonary hypertension are classified as either secondary or idiopathic (primary). Secondary pulmonary hypertension is usually associated with underlying heart or lung disease (e.g., PEs, venocclusive disease, COPD). The cause of the idiopathic form is, by definition, unclear. However, it occurs most often in young adults between the ages of 30 and 40 years. Females are affected more often than males. The condition is progressive, leading to right-sided heart failure and severe dyspnea.

Clients with mild pulmonary hypertension may be relatively asymptomatic. In moderate to severe forms, the main (and occasionally only) manifestation is dyspnea. Fatigue, syncope, angina-like chest pain, palpitations, and muscular weakness may also occur. Chest x-ray reveals right ventricular hypertrophy, enlarged pulmonary arteries, prominent hilar vessels, and normal or reduced intrapulmonary vascular markings. Cardiac catheterization provides the most valuable diagnostic measurements. Typical findings include elevated PAP and increases arteriovenous oxygen differences accompanied by normal systemic blood pressure and normal-to-low cardiac output. Pulmonary wedge pressures remain normal because left ventricular function is typically unchanged.

The overall prognosis in severe pulmonary hypertension is poor. There is no known cure for the disorder, although treatment of the underlying cause of secondary forms may slow its progression. Vasodilator therapy may also be employed with some success, as may high-dose calcium channel blocker therapy.[32] Additionally, supportive intervention is used to reduce hypoxemia. A few clients with severe pulmonary hypertension have undergone heart-lung transplantation, but data regarding long-term effectiveness are not yet available. Interventions appropriate for underlying diseases and preparation for diagnostic procedures are incorporated into nursing care.

Conclusions

Lower airway disorders include asthma, chronic air flow limitations, and inflammations of the airways. Nursing care centers on reversal of any airway spasms and education of the client on how to live with the disorder and reduce the risk of future problems. Pulmonary embolus is a potentially life-threatening disorder that usually can be effectively managed with prompt recognition.

Thinking Critically

1. A 52-year-old woman is being treated at the neighborhood health clinic for chronic bronchitis. Her husband of 30 years smoked 2 to 3 packs of cigarettes a day. The client never smoked. During this exacerbation, she presents with shortness of breath; wheezing; a deep, throaty, productive cough when she tries to talk; and fatigue. Her blood pressure is 180/90 mm Hg, pulse is 90 beats/minute, respirations are 28/minute and labored, and her temperature is 99.4° F. She tells you that she tried to shovel the driveway on this cold winter day and did not wear a scarf over her mouth as she usually does. She further states that her inhalers did not seem to help her. She is on a diuretic for her hypertension with a blood pressure controlled at about 160/86. What is your priority nursing action? What teaching is appropriate at this time?

Factors to consider: What are the clinical manifestations of chronic obstructive emphysema? What nursing assessments are in order?

2. An elderly client is recovering from pelvic surgery. Because of a previous cerebrovascular accident, she is hemiplegic. She has been on bedrest since the surgery. While the nursing assistant is giving her a bath, she notices the client grimacing as if in pain. The client responds to her question by pointing to her chest and nodding when asked if the pain is severe. The nursing assistant notifies you that the client is in distress. What is the priority assessment?

Factors to consider: What complications of surgery and resulting bedrest might the client be at risk for? How would you compare and contrast the clinical manifestations for pneumonia and pulmonary embolus?

3. You enter the room of the above client and discover that she is apprehensive. She is trying to hold her breath because it hurts to breathe. She is sweating and there is frothy sputum on her lips. What nursing interventions are appropriate? What treatment might be ordered?

Factors to consider: What are the clinical manifestations of pulmonary embolus? What diagnostic studies may be ordered?

Bibliography

1. Aberman, A. (1968). Managing asthmatics. *Emergency Medicine, 18*:26.
2. Allen, G. (1996). Surgical treatment of emphysema using bovine pericardium strips. *AORN Journal, 63*(2), 373–388.
3. Andrews, L. (1994). Medical management of pulmonary emboli. *Medsurg Nursing, 3*(1), 31.
4. Bennett, J., & Plum, F. (1996). *Cecil Textbook of Medicine* (20th ed.). Philadelphia: W. B. Saunders.
5. Bone, R. C. (1993). Bronchial asthma: Diagnostic and treatment issues. *Hospital Practice, 28*, 45.
6. Brundage, D. J., et al. (1993). Self-care instruction for patients with COPD. *Rehabilitation Nursing, 18*(5), 321.
7. Carpenito, L. J. (1992). *Nursing diagnosis: Application to clinical practice* (4th ed.). Philadelphia: J. B. Lippincott.
8. Caswell, D. R. (1993). Thromboembolic phenomena. *Critical Care Nursing Clinics of North America, 5*(3), 489.
9. Cooper, J. D., et al. (1994). Bilateral pneumectomy (volume reduction) for chronic obstructive pulmonary disease. *Journal of Thoracic and Cardiovascular Surgery, 109*(1), 106.
10. Couser, J. I., et al. (1995). Pulmonary rehabilitation improves exercise capacity in older elderly patients with COPD. *Chest, 107*(3), 730–734.
11. DeVito, A., & Kleven, M. (1987). Dyspnea. *RN, 50*(6):38–46.
12. Eggland, E. T. (1987). Teaching the ABC's of COPD. *Nursing 87, 17*(1):60.
13. Ferguson, G. T., & Cherniack, R. M. (1993). Management of chronic obstructive pulmonary disease. *New England Journal of Medicine, 328*, 1017–1022.
14. Fitzgerald, S. T. (1992). National Asthma Education Program expert panel report: Guidelines for the diagnosis and management of asthma. *American Association of Occupational Health Nurses Journal, 40*(8), 376.
15. Gift, A. G. (1995). Application in research: Issues in asthma self-management. *Perspectives in Respiratory Nursing, 6*(4), 5–6.
16. Graling, P., Hetrick, V., Kiernan, P. (1996). Bilateral lung volume reduction surgery. *AORN Journal, 63*(2), 389–404.
17. Hahn, K. (1989). Sexuality and COPD. *Rehabilitation Nursing, 14*(7), 191.
18. Heslop, A., & Shannon, C. (1995). Assisting patients living with long-term oxygen therapy. *British Journal of Nursing, 4*(19), 1123–1128.
19. Janssen, W. (1996). Treatment for emphysema: An overview of lung volume reduction surgery. *Perspectives in Respiratory Nursing, 7*(1), 1–5.
20. Jess, L. W. (1992). Chronic bronchitis and emphysema: Airing the differences. *Nursing 92, 22*(3), 34.
21. Kinzel, T. (1993). Management of end-stage lung disease in the nursing home: The hospice concept. *Nursing Home Medicine, 1*(1), 23.
22. Leidy, N. K. (1995). Functional performance in people with chronic obstructive pulmonary disease. *Image, 27*(1), 23–35.
23. Lewis, D., & Bell, S. K. (1995). Pulmonary rehabilitation, psychological adjustment, and use of healthcare services. *Rehabilitation Nursing, 20*(2), 102–107.
24. McKinney, B. (1995). Under new management: Asthma and the elderly. *Journal of Gerontological Nursing, 21*(11), 39–45.
25. Pfister, S. M. (1995). Home oxygen therapy: Indications, administration, recertification, and patient education. *Nurse Practitioner, 20*(7), 44–56.
26. Preusser, B. A., Winningham, M. L., & Clanton, T. L. (1994). High- vs low-intensity inspiratory muscle interval training in patients with COPD. *Chest, 106*(1), 110–117.
27. Reid, W. D., & Samrai, B. (1995). Respiratory muscle training for patients with chronic obstructive pulmonary disease. *Physical Therapy, 75*(11), 996–1005.
28. Reinke, L. F., & Hoffman, L. A. (1992). How to teach asthma co-management. *American Journal of Nursing, 92*(10), 40.
29. Rich, S., & Rubin, L. J. (1991). New views on pulmonary hypertension. *Patient Care, 25*(9), 87.
30. Scherer, Y., Schmieder, L., & Shimmel, S. (1995). Outpatient instruction for individuals with COPD. *Perspectives in Respiratory Nursing, 6*(3), 1–8.
31. Sexton, D. L. (1990). *Nursing care of the respiratory patient.* Norwalk, CT: Appleton & Lange.
32. Shelmerdine, L. (1995). Occupational asthma: Assessing the risk. *Nursing Standard, 10*(4), 25–28.
33. Verderber, A., Gallagher, K., & Severino, R. (1995). The effect of nursing interventions on transcutaneous oxygen and carbon dioxide tensions. *Western Journal of Nursing Research, 17*(1), 76–90.
34. Weaver, T. E., & Narsavage, G. L. (1992). Physiological and psychological variables related to functional status in chronic obstructive pulmonary disease. *Nursing Research, 41*, 286–291.
35. Whitney, L. (1992). Chronic bronchitis and emphysema: Airing the differences. *Nursing 92, 22*(3), 34.

Nursing Care of Clients with Disorders of the Lung Parenchyma and Pleura

CHAPTER 42

Sherill Nones Cronin

The parenchyma of any organ, in this case the lung, is the tissue essential for the function of the organ. This chapter discusses disorders of the lung parenchyma, such as pneumonia and cancer. Disorders of the airways and vessels of the lung were discussed in Chapter 41.

Atelectasis

Atelectasis is the collapse of lung tissue at any structural level (e.g., segmental, basilar, lobar, microscopic). It develops when there is interference with the natural forces that promote lung expansion. Such interference may result from a reduction in lung distention forces, localized airway obstruction, insufficient pulmonary surfactant, or increased elastic recoil. Examples of each of these causes are given in Box 42–1. Atelectasis is particularly common in postoperative clients, especially those undergoing upper abdominal or thoracic surgeries, the elderly, and bedridden clients.

Atelectasis may be diagnosed by physical examination, although it is usually detected first by chest x-ray. Some clients are asymptomatic. However, if significant hypoxemia is present, dyspnea, tachypnea, tachycardia, and cyanosis may occur. Chest auscultation may reveal diminished breath sounds or crackles over the involved area. Fever of less than 101° F is common. However, elderly persons typically do not exhibit a fever.

If atelectasis is severe, physical assessment findings may include (1) tracheal shift toward the side of the atelectasis, (2) decreased tactile fremitus over the affected lung area, (3) dull percussion note over the atelectatic region, and (4) decreased chest movement on the involved side. However, none of these signs is specific for atelectasis, and the entire clinical picture must be considered.

One of the primary goals of nursing intervention is to prevent atelectasis in the high-risk client. Frequent position changes and early ambulation help promote drainage of all lung segments. Deep breathing and effective coughing enhance lung expansion and prevent airway obstruction. Incentive spirometry is an excellent means of encouraging clients to deep-breathe.

If atelectasis develops, treatment is directed toward the underlying cause. If the client becomes hypoxemic, oxygen should be administered as prescribed (e.g., per cannula 1–4 L/min). More aggressive measures to maintain airway patency, such as postural drainage, chest physiotherapy, or tracheal suctioning, may also be ordered. If an airway obstruction is causing atelectasis, bronchoscopy may be used to remove the material.

Infectious Disorders

Influenza

The term "flu" is often used inappropriately to describe many symptoms and disorders. Influenza actually refers to an acute viral respiratory tract infection. Influenza usually occurs seasonally in epidemic form. People most at risk include (1) very young children, (2) the elderly, (3) people living in institutional situations, (4) people with chronic diseases, and (5) healthcare personnel.

Influenza differs from a common cold primarily by its sudden onset and widespread occurrence within the population. Assessment findings with influenza include fever, myalgias (muscular pain), and cough. Influenza predisposes to complications such as viral bronchitis or pneumonia, bacterial pneumonia, and superinfections. Chest findings are usually negative unless pneumonia results. People with colds (1) are usually afebrile, (2) have malaise as a major manifestation, and (3) commonly have nasal manifestations.

Influenza is a communicable disease spread by droplet infection. Prevent the spread of this infection by encouraging clients with influenza to remain at home, practice

---

This chapter incorporates material written for the fourth edition by Steve Alderfer.

Box 42-1. Causes of Atelectasis

■ Decreased lung distention forces
　Pleural space encroachment (e.g., pneumothorax,
　　pleural effusion, pleural tumor)
　Chest wall disorders (e.g., kyphoscoliosis, flail chest)
　Impaired diaphragmatic movement (e.g., ascites,
　　obesity)
　Central nervous system dysfunction (e.g., coma,
　　neuromuscular disorders, oversedation)

■ Localized airway obstruction
　Mucous plugging
　Foreign body aspiration
　Bronchiectasis

■ Insufficient pulmonary surfactant
　Respiratory distress syndrome
　Inhalation anesthesia
　High concentrations of oxygen (oxygen toxicity)
　Lung contusion
　Aspiration of gastric contents
　Smoke inhalation

■ Increased elastic recoil
　Interstitial fibrosis (e.g., silicosis, radiation
　　pneumonitis)

---

frequent hand washing, and cover their nose and mouth when sneezing or coughing.

Encourage clients at risk of influenza to obtain annual immunization before the start of the "flu season," in the winter. Immunization controls influenza for many high risk clients. However, clients allergic to eggs or who have a history of Guillain-Barré syndrome should not receive an influenza immunization. When influenza breaks out in institutional settings, additional protection may be prescribed by the daily short-term administration of the antiviral agents amantadine hydrochloride or rimantadine. These are effective against type A influenza virus only and do not replace immunization.

Intervention in influenza is based on assessment findings as they arise (e.g., supportive measures to relieve fever, myalgia, and cough).

Pneumonia

Pneumonia (pneumonitis) is an inflammatory process in lung parenchyma usually associated with a marked increase in interstitial and alveolar fluid. Advances in antibiotic therapy have led to the widespread perception that pneumonia is no longer a major health problem in the United States. However, pneumonia is presently the sixth most common cause of death for all ages and one of the most common causes in the elderly. Among all nosocomial (hospital-acquired) infections, it has the highest fatality rate. Because of its prevalence, prevention at all

levels is very important. The Risk Factors and Levels of Prevention feature lists preventive measures.

Etiology and Risk Factors

There are many causes of pneumonia, including bacteria, viruses, mycoplasmas, fungal agents, and protozoa (Table 42-1). Pneumonia may also result from (1) aspiration of food, fluids, or vomitus, or (2) inhalation of toxic or caustic chemicals, smoke, dusts, or gases. Pneumonia may complicate immobility and chronic illnesses. It often follows influenza.

Pathophysiology

The feature common to all types of pneumonia is an inflammatory pulmonary response to the offending organism or agent. The defense mechanisms of the lungs lose effectiveness and allow organisms to penetrate the lower airways, where inflammation develops. Inflamed and fluid-filled alveolar sacs cannot exchange oxygen and carbon dioxide effectively. Bacterial pneumonia may be associated with significant ventilation-perfusion mismatch. Alveolar exudate tends to consolidate and becomes difficult to expectorate.

Clinical Manifestations and Diagnostic Findings

The onset of all pneumonias is generally marked by any or all of the following: fever, chills, sweats, pleuritic chest pain, cough, sputum production, hemoptysis, dyspnea, headache, or fatigue. The elderly client, however, may present not with fever or respiratory manifestations but with altered mental status and volume depletion.

Chest auscultation reveals bronchial breath sounds over areas of consolidation (i.e., dense areas on the chest film). Consolidated lung tissue transmits bronchial sound waves to outer lung fields. Crackling sounds (from fluid in interstitial and alveolar areas) and whispered pectoriloquy may be heard over affected areas. Tactile fremitus is usually increased over areas of pneumonia, while percussion sounds are dulled. Unequal chest wall expansion may occur during inspiration if a large area of lung tissue is involved. This is due to decreased distensibility in the affected area. Clinical manifestations seen in specific types of pneumonia are shown in Table 42-1.

Definitive diagnosis is usually determined through sputum culture and sensitivity or serologic testing. At times, fiberoptic bronchoscopy or transcutaneous needle aspiration or biopsy may be necessary for confirmation. Additional diagnostic testing may include (1) skin tests, if tuberculosis or coccidioidomycosis is suspected; (2) blood and urine cultures to assess systemic spread; and (3) arterial blood gas (ABG) or transcutaneous oxygen levels analysis to assess the need for supplemental oxygen.

Chest x-ray examination provides information about the location and extent of pneumonia. On the chest film,

RISK FACTORS AND LEVELS OF PREVENTION

Pneumonia

Risk Factors

- Smoking
- Air pollution
- Upper respiratory infection
- Altered consciousness: alcoholism, head injury, seizure disorder, drug overdose, general anesthesia
- Tracheal intubation (bypassing the upper airway)
- Prolonged immobility
- Immunosuppressive therapy: corticosteroids; cancer chemotherapy
- Nonfunctional immune system: acquired immuno-deficiency syndrome (AIDS)
- Severe periodontal disease
- Prolonged exposure to especially virulent organisms
- Malnutrition
- Dehydration
- Chronic diseases: diabetes mellitus, heart disease, chronic lung disease, renal disease, cancer
- Prolonged debilitating disease
- Inhalation of noxious substances
- Aspiration of oral or gastric material
- Aspiration of foreign material (e.g., petroleum products)
- Residing in group-living situations where there is an increased probability of respiratory disease transmission

Levels of Prevention

Primary Prevention

- Promote adequate nutrition and fluid intake and proper hygiene measures to help maintain normal defenses.
- Discourage cigarette smoking
- Advise high-risk clients to avoid exposure to infected persons.

Secondary Prevention

- Promote effective airway clearance and mobilization.
- Advocate rigorous hand washing by medical personnel in the hospital to reduce the transmission of infectious agents.
- Maintain proper infection control measures during respiratory procedures.
- Maintain a high index of suspicion for the common clinical manifestations in at-risk clients, especially the elderly.
- Assess high-risk clients for other subtle, nonspecific manifestations such as change in cognition (confusion or lethargy), anorexia, tachypnea, and exacerbation of preexisting disorders (e.g., heart failure, chronic air flow limitation).

Tertiary Prevention

- Instruct the client and family in the techniques of deep breathing and coughing.
- Teach the importance of completing antibiotics, as prescribed.
- Discuss a plan for rest and gradual resumption of activity.
- Instruct the client and family about manifestations that should be reported to the physician (i.e., fever, chills, chest pain, hemoptysis).

---

areas of pneumonia appear as white opacification, known as consolidation.

Pneumonia may involve one or more lobe segments of the lungs (segmental pneumonia), one or more entire lobes (lobar pneumonia) (Fig. 42–1A), or lobes in both lungs (bilateral pneumonia). On the basis of location and radiologic appearance, pneumonias may be classified as bronchopneumonia, interstitial pneumonia, alveolar pneumonia, or necrotizing pneumonia. Bronchopneumonia (bronchial pneumonia) (Fig. 42–1B) involves the terminal bronchioles and alveoli. Interstitial (reticular) pneumonia involves inflammatory responses within lung tissue surrounding the air spaces or vascular structures rather than the air passages themselves. In alveolar, or acinar, pneumonia, there is fluid accumulation in a lung's distal air spaces. Necrotizing pneumonia causes the death of a portion of lung tissue surrounded by viable tissue; x-ray examination may reveal cavity formation at the site of necrosis. Necrotic lung tissue, which does not heal, constitutes a permanent loss of functioning parenchyma.

Acute and Subacute Care

■ Medical Management

Clients who are ambulatory but have an ongoing health problem may require hospitalization. Similarly, clients who are already hospitalized for other reasons are at risk of developing nosocomial pneumonias because of their decreased ability to combat infection and their potential

Table 42–1. Assessment and Treatment of Pneumonias

Common Name	Clinical Manifestations	Management
Pneumococcal pneumonia (caused by *Streptococcus pneumoniae*)	Sudden onset with a single shaking chill, high fever, stabbing, pleuritic chest pain, malaise, weakness, occasional vomiting, tachypnea, dyspnea, and elevated WBC count; single or multiple lobar consolidation on the chest film; cough productive of rusty brown or blood-streaked purulent sputum that turns yellow and mucoid	Primary: penicillin G IV or penicillin V PO Alternative: erythromycin, cephalosporin Prevention: Vaccine available
Staphylococcal pneumonia (caused by *Staphylococcus aureus*)	Sudden onset with fever, multiple chills, pleuritic pain, dyspnea, rales, decreased breath sounds, elevated WBC count, and exaggerated cough productive of purulent golden-yellow or blood-streaked sputum; chest film may show patchy infiltrates, empyema, abscesses, and pneumothorax; disease may start with headache, cough, and myalgia	Primary: penicillin, cephalosporin; vancomycin for non-pencillinase–producing organism; penicillinase-resistant penicillin if organism produces penicillinase, vancomycin if methicillin-resistant organism
Influenzal pneumonia (caused by *Haemophilus influenzae*)	Similar to pneumococcal pneumonia; cough productive of apple- or lime-green purulent sputum, which may be blood-tinged	Primary: cefuroxime, chloramphenicol, ampicillin
Gram-negative bacterial pneumonia (most commonly caused by *Klebsiella pneumoniae*)	Sudden onset with high fever, multiple chills, pleuritic pain, dyspnea, cyanosis, and elevated WBC count; lobar consolidation and cavitation on the chest film; cough productive of red sputum resembling currant jelly—mucoid, sticky, and difficult to expectorate	Primary: aminoglycosides, third-generation cephalosporins, TMP-SM2, extended-spectrum penicillin, ciprofloxacin
Anaerobic bacterial pneumonia, hypostatic pneumonia (caused by normal oral flora)	Insidious onset with low-grade fever, dyspnea, crackles, cyanosis, hypertension, tachycardia, and elevated WBC count; patchy infiltrates in dependent lung segments on the chest film; cough productive of purulent greenish-yellow, foul-smelling sputum	Primary: third-generation cephalosporins (such as cefotaxime) or penicillin G Alternative: cefoxitin, clindamycin, or chloramphenicol

HIV, human immunodeficiency virus; IV, intravenous; PO, oral; TMP-SMZ, trimethoprim-sulfamethoxazole; WBC, white blood cell.

exposure to resistant strains of organisms. The Case Management Feature describes a clinical pathway for a client with pneumonia.

The primary treatment for most forms of pneumonia is antibiotic therapy. Table 42–1 lists the drugs of choice for each type, once the specific organism has been identified. However, initial therapy usually consists of broad-spectrum antibiotics.

■ Nursing Management of the Medical Client

Assessment

The following should be determined through the nursing history:

- Contact with other clients experiencing similar manifestations (suggests viral or mycoplasmal pneumonia)
- Factors suggesting the presence of noninfectious diseases that produce manifestations similar to those of pneumonia (e.g., pulmonary embolism, allergic reaction to drugs or other substances, neoplasm)
- Presence of tuberculosis or contact with others who have active tuberculosis
- Presence and character of any chest pain
- Presence and character of cough and sputum production

Physical assessment should include rate and character of respirations, auscultation of breath sounds, and assessment of skin and nail beds to determine the degree of hypoxia.

Diagnosis, Planning, Implementation

Ineffective Airway Clearance. The inflammation and increased secretions seen with pneumonia make it difficult to maintain a patent airway. Use the nursing diagnosis *Ineffective Airway Clearance related to excessive secretions* to express this client problem.

Planning: Expected Outcomes. The client will maintain effective airway clearance, as evidenced by maintaining a patent airway and effectively clearing secretions.

Implementation. Measures should be taken to promote airway patency. These may include increasing fluid

Common Name	Clinical Manifestations	Management
Legionnaires' disease (caused by *Legionella pneumophila*)	Prodrome of 24–48 hours with fever, headaches, and malaise followed by high fever with pulse-temperature dissociation, dyspnea, hypoxia, pleuritic pain, nausea, vomiting, diarrhea, confusion, and elevated WBC count; single or multilobar consolidation and small pleural effusions on the chest film; dry cough productive of scant mucoid or blood-tinged sputum	Primary: erythromycin Alternative: TMP-SM2, fluroquinolone
Mycoplasma pneumonia (caused by *Mycoplasma* microorganisms)	Insidious onset with slowly rising fever, headache, myalgia, malaise, and normal WBC count; pulmonary infiltrate—sometimes extensive—on the chest film; cough productive of scant mucoid sputum; client may show only minimal signs and symptoms	Primary: tetracycline Alternative: erythromycin, ciproflaxin
Viral pneumonia (caused by influenza A virus)	Prodrome with headache and myalgia followed by high fever, dyspnea, normal breath sounds with occasional wheezing and crackles, and normal or slightly elevated WBC count; diffuse, patchy infiltrates on the chest film; dry cough with initial mucoid sputum that later turns purulent; cough may be unproductive	Antiviral agents, symptomatic treatment
Fungal pneumonia (caused by histoplasmosis, blastomycosis, coccidioidomycosis, aspergillosis, candidiasis)	Usually asymptomatic. When manifestations occur they range from brief periods of malaise to severe, life-threatening illness; typical illness resembles influenza	Amphotericin B and other oral imidazoles (ketaconazole fluconazole)
Parasitic pneumonia (caused by protozoa, nemotodes, platyhelminths); common organism is *Pneumocystis carinii*	Clients who develop *P. carinii* pneumonia are invariably immunocompromised (HIV); cough, dyspnea, pleuritic chest pain, fever and night sweats, crackles	Diamidines, folate antagonists (TMP-SMZ), and other agents (clindamycin)

intake, teaching and encouraging effective coughing and deep-breathing techniques, and frequent turning. Clients with an altered level of consciousness should be turned at least every 2 hours and should be placed in side-lying positions, unless contraindicated, for prevention of aspiration. Administer bronchodilating medications, if prescribed. If indicated, more aggressive measures to maintain airway patency may be required (e.g., chest physiotherapy, suctioning, artificial airway).

Ineffective Breathing Pattern. Many clients develop compensatory tachypnea because of an inability to meet metabolic demands. This occurs because affected alveoli cannot effectively exchange oxygen and carbon dioxide. Increased respiratory rates can also develop from chest pain and increased body temperature. *Ineffective Breathing Pattern related to tachypnea* is the best nursing diagnosis to describe this problem.

Planning: Expected Outcomes. The client will have improved breathing patterns, as evidenced by a respiratory rate within normal limits, adequate chest expansion, clear breath sounds, and decreased dyspnea.

Implementation. Position the client for comfort and to facilitate breathing (e.g., at 45 degrees). Teach the client how to splint the chest wall with a pillow for comfort during coughing. Administer prescribed cough suppressants and analgesics. Be cautious, however, because narcotics may depress respirations more than desired. Routinely monitor respiratory rate, and transcutaneous oxygen levels, auscultate the chest, and document findings. Monitor ABGs and observe for signs of hypoxemia, hypercapnia, or acid-base imbalance.

Activity Intolerance. Depleted energy reserves due to not eating during periods of dyspnea and impaired oxygen and carbon dioxide transport leave little oxygen to meet metabolic demands. State the nursing diagnosis as *Activity Intolerance related to decreased oxygen levels for metabolic demands.*

Planning: Expected Outcomes. The client will have improved activity tolerance, as evidenced by ability to perform activities of daily living and demonstrating progressively increasing physical activity without excessive dyspnea and fatigue.

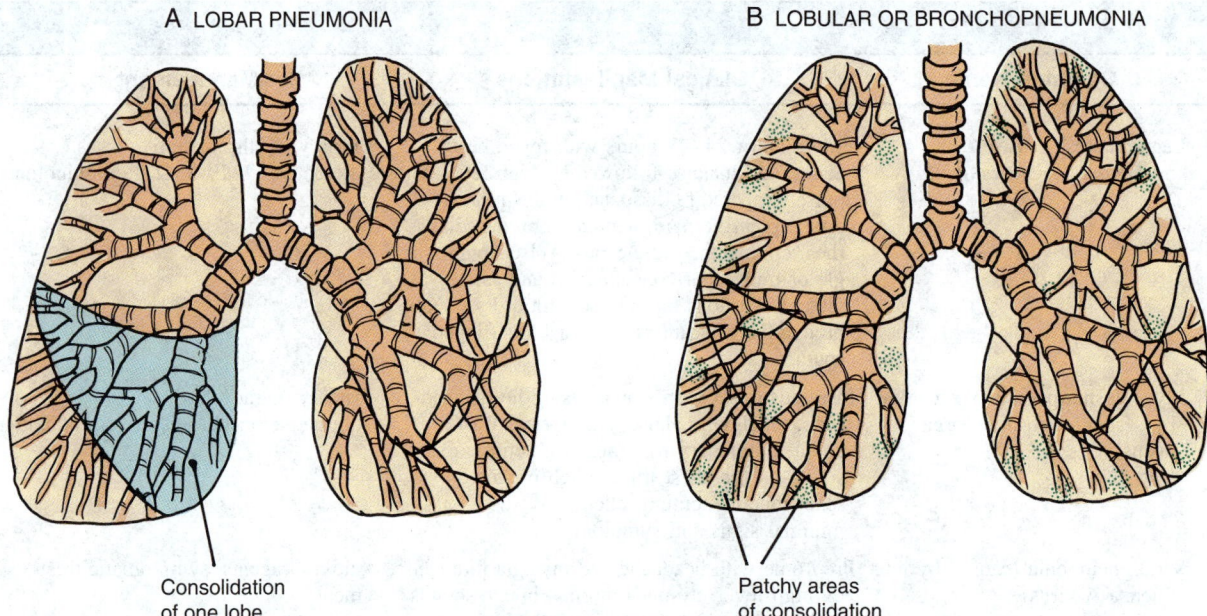

A LOBAR PNEUMONIA

B LOBULAR OR BRONCHOPNEUMONIA

Consolidation
of one lobe

Patchy areas
of consolidation

Figure 42–1. Two types of pneumonia. *A*, Lobar pneumonia with consolidation in one lobe of one lung. *B*, Lobular or bronchopneumonia with patchy consolidation throughout both lungs.

Implementation. Assess the client's baseline activity level and response to activity. Note how well the client tolerates activity by assessing for changes in respiratory and pulse rate, marked dyspnea, fatigue, pallor or cyanosis, and dysrhythmias. Schedule activity after treatments or medications. Use oxygen as needed. Gradually increase activity on the basis of tolerance. Balance activity with adequate rest periods.

Teach the client to avoid conditions that increase oxygen demand, such as smoking, temperature extremes, weight gain, and stress. Pursed-lip and diaphragmatic breathing, as well as techniques to lower energy use, should be reinforced. Activities that are tiring should be interspersed with rest.

Provide psychological support and a quiet environment to reduce anxiety and promote rest. Regulate nursing care and visitors, as warranted by the client's condition.

Other nursing diagnoses may include *Altered Nutrition: Less than Body Requirements related to dyspnea, Pain related to frequent coughing,* and *Altered Oral Mucous Membranes related to mouth breathing and frequent cough.*

Evaluation

The degree of expected outcome attainment is monitored every 2 to 3 days. Pneumonia should resolve quickly once the client is on antibiotics, provided there are no immune disorders. Elderly clients may require additional time to fully recover.

Community and Self-Care

Hospitalization is not always necessary for clients with pneumonia. If the client has intact defense mechanisms and good general health, recuperation can often take place at home with rest and supportive treatment. The term "walking pneumonia" is sometimes used to describe this situation.

Chest physical therapy may be continued for a period of time. The client is followed in a clinic setting until the chest clears as demonstrated on x-ray and clinical manifestations abate. The client is encouraged to plan for influenza immunization the next winter. People who live with the client are also monitored for the onset of pneumonia.

Lung Abscess

A lung abscess is a collection of pus within lung tissue. In its early stages, it resembles a localized pneumonia. If lung abscess is undiagnosed and untreated, tissue necrosis may occur. Lung abscesses are becoming more rare due to improved treatment of pneumonia and effective preventive care of clients at high risk of aspiration. Abscesses today are most often from anaerobic bacteria.

Single lung abscesses usually occur distal to a bronchial obstruction. They nearly always create putrid (foul) material. The bronchial obstruction may be due to:

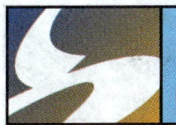

CASE MANAGEMENT

Pneumonia
For Clinical Pathway, see Appendix D.

Clinical Pathway from Birmingham Baptist Medical Center, Birmingham, Alabama
Information provided by Kathy T. Martin, M.S.N.

Development and Revision of Pathway

- Pneumonia was selected for pathway development because it is a high-volume case type with a long length of stay.
- We have been using this pathway for approximately 3 years.
- The development team included pulmonary nurses, physicians, respiratory therapists, pharmacists, administrators, and the case manager.
- A continuous quality improvement team meets quarterly. It is composed of physicians, nurses, respiratory therapists, administrators, emergency physicians, clinical managers, pharmacists, a microbiologist, and decision support staff. Issues related to practice patterns are discussed during this meeting. Changes may be made in the pathway at that time.
- The pathway is revised as needed. Last year the pathway underwent a major revision when the length of stay was reduced from 7 days to 5 days.

Use and Impact of Pathway

- All patients who are admitted with pneumonia are placed on this pathway.
- The nursing staff use the pathway daily, and the physicians use it occasionally.
- Several changes have occurred since the pathway was initiated. First, the length of stay was reduced by 2 to 3 days for acute and simple pneumonia. Second, antibiotics are started within 4 hours of triage in the emergency room or on admission to the hospital. Third, sputum is collected (or attempts made) within 2 hours of admission or triage. Fourth, nurses increase the patient's activity level much sooner than before. Fifth, there is an increased emphasis on the importance of pushing oral fluids. Finally, the pathway heightens physician and nurse awareness of, and participation in, practice changes.
- There has been a marked impact on cost per case (a decrease in cost) and the length of stay has dropped by 2 to 3 days for all pneumonia patients.

- Aspirated foreign material (e.g., vomitus, mucus, teeth, blood, food, or tissue during upper airway surgery)
- Benign or malignant tumors

Multiple lung abscesses can follow pneumonia caused by necrotizing bacteria (i.e., such as *Staphylococcus aureus*, that create necrotic lung tissue). Bacteria may also arise from septic emboli from infected foci such as septic phlebitis. Immunosuppressed clients and those who may aspirate foreign material are at high risk.

Early assessment findings in a client with a lung abscess are the same as with bronchopneumonia (i.e., chills, fever, pleuritic pain, cough of abundant sputum). The body attempts to wall off the abscess with fibrous tissue. If the attempt is unsuccessful, the abscess ruptures into a bronchus, causing a cough producing copious amounts of sputum. The sputum is purulent, foul-smelling, and foul-tasting. After bronchial rupture, hemoptysis often occurs. Chest auscultation reveals decreased breath sounds and dullness to percussion over the affected area. Crackles may be present when the abscess drains. Diagnosis is commonly made by chest x-ray or CT scan. Sputum cultures assist with identification of the organism.

Antibiotics are prescribed based upon culture results. Bronchoscopy was once believed to be essential in management of lung abscesses. Now it is reserved for clients who fail to progress and/or may have malignancy. Surgery is seldom needed due to success with antibiotic therapy.

Caring for a client with a lung abscess is similar to caring for a client experiencing pneumonia (e.g., promoting hydration, effective cough techniques, and postural drainage). Lung abscesses produce copious volumes of sputum. Nursing intervention focuses on removing sputum from the lungs through postural drainage and expectoration. Note the color, quantity, quality, and smell of the expectorated material, including the presence of blood. Use gloves when handling articles contaminated with sputum.

The sputum may have a foul taste. Provide frequent opportunities to use mouthwashes and to perform toothbrushing and flossing. Because long-term antibiotic administration is usually necessary, observe oral mucous membranes for indications of *Candida albicans* overgrowth (i.e., white, cheesy patches). Encourage long-term dental care. Oral nystatin (swish and swallow) may be ordered.

Antibiotic therapy for lung abscess may be necessary for 8 weeks or longer. Clients with lung abscesses must understand the importance of compliance with the medication schedule. The entire course of antibiotics must be taken. Teaching regarding medications includes (1) the reasons for taking them; (2) specific directions such as time of day, frequency, and when to take in relation to food; (3) potential side effects; and (4) what to do if side effects occur. Reassessment after antibiotics are completed (e.g., reculture of sputum, chest films) is essential to evaluate treatment effectiveness.

Pulmonary Tuberculosis

The mycobacteria have played an extremely important role in influencing today's society. Tuberculosis and Hansen's disease (leprosy), the two most prominent mycobacterial diseases, have been recognized as scourges of humanity since antiquity. Whereas leprosy was most apparent as a biblical metaphor for the destitute, disabled, and disfigured—tuberculosis was the "captain of these men of death," a plague that carried away young and talented members of society. Today, we are witnessing a resurgence of tuberculosis, and the disease is again prominent in the consciousness of society.[5] Each year for the past several decades, TB has caused an estimated 3 million deaths throughout the world. Nearly all these deaths are in Third World countries.

Before the development of anti-TB drugs in the late 1940s, TB was also the leading cause of death in the United States. Drug therapy, along with improvements in public health and general living standards, resulted in a marked decline in incidence over the next three decades. However, beginning in 1985, the number of reported TB cases has steadily increased. This increase has been attributed to the emergence of the human immunodeficiency virus (HIV) epidemic, recent influxes of immigrants from developing Third World nations, and the deterioration of the healthcare infrastructure.[15] Adding to the public health concern is the concurrent rise in multidrug resistant strains of tuberculosis (MDR-TB) which are more difficult to treat. It is believed that resistance develops as a result of persons who stop taking their medication once they begin to feel well or who are noncompliant due to other health problems such as substance abuse.

Etiology and Risk Factors

TB is a communicable disease caused by *Mycobacterium tuberculosis*, an aerobic, acid-fast bacillus. Tuberculosis is an airborne infection. In nearly all instances, tuberculosis infection is acquired by inhalation of a particle small enough (1–5 μm in size) to reach the alveolus. Droplets are emitted during coughing, laughing, sneezing, or singing. Infected droplet nuclei may then be inhaled by a susceptible person (host). Before pulmonary infection can occur, the inhaled organisms must resist the lung's defense mechanisms and actually penetrate lung tissue.

Brief exposure to TB does not usually cause infection. Clients most commonly infected are those having repeated close contact with an infected person who is not yet diagnosed. When a client is diagnosed as having TB, public health officials (often nurses) talk with the client and develop a contact list. Everyone with whom the client has had contact is then assessed with a tuberculin skin test and chest x-ray to determine whether he or she has been infected with TB.

In countries that do not have public health programs and those in which TB commonly occurs in cattle, humans may develop bovine TB from drinking raw milk from infected cattle. This form of TB can be prevented by pasteurizing milk and maintaining tuberculin skin-testing programs for cattle. Reducing the risk of TB is essential. The Risk Factors and Levels of Prevention feature describes persons at high risk for contracting tuberculosis. The Ethical Issues in Nursing feature considers whether the federal government should regulate testing for tuberculosis.

RISK FACTORS AND LEVELS OF PREVENTION

Tuberculosis

Risk Factors

Persons at high risk are:
- Immigrants from Asia, Africa, Latin America, and Oceania.
- Medically underserved populations (e.g., racial and ethnic minorities [African blacks, Hispanics, Native Americans, Eskimo Americans]; homeless)
- Those with HIV infection, requiring immunosuppression, with diabetes mellitus, alcoholism, or drug abuse
- Personnel and residents of long-term care facilities and congregate living settings (e.g., mental institutions, correctional facilities)
- Healthcare workers

Levels of Prevention

Primary Prevention

Give tuberculosis (TB) skin tests to persons:
- With signs, symptoms, or laboratory abnormalities suggestive of clinically active TB.
- With recent contacts with persons known to have or suspected of having clinically active TB.
- At high risk
- With abnormal chest x-rays compatible with past TB.

Secondary Prevention
- Reduce the spread of TB by teaching the client with TB to control aerosolization of the organism by wearing a mask, covering the mouth while coughing, and disposing of sputum correctly.
- Evaluate persons with positive TB skin tests who do not have active disease for isoniazid preventive therapy.

Tertiary Prevention
- Clients must finish a complete course of antituberculosis medications.
- Recognize, prevent, and manage noncompliant behavior in persons being treated for TB.

Pathophysiology

■ Primary (First) Infection

The first time a client is infected with TB, it is said to be a "primary infection." Primary TB infections are usually located in the apices of the lungs or near the pleurae of the lower lobes. Although a primary infection may be only microscopic in size (and hence not appear on x-ray), the following sequence of events typically occurs.

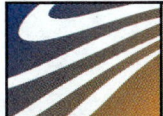

ETHICAL ISSUES IN NURSING

How Should the Federal Government Regulate Testing for Tuberculosis?

Tuberculosis (TB) is transmitted from person to person by the inhalation of infected droplets from respiratory secretions. The infecting bacterium, *Mycobacterium tuberculosis*, remains a medical problem in many developing countries. In the United States, TB is commonly associated with overcrowding and poverty conditions. Testing may not be done in these areas, often because of a lack of healthcare services provided to these areas. Immigration, either permanent or through university programs, is also a cause of TB reintroduction. Undetected, this disease can be fatal.

How should public health agencies regulate such an infectious and possibly fatal disease? A person can be infected with TB without knowing it simply by breathing in the bacterium. Should there be massive testing campaigns in which all persons must be tested? How can the United States government be responsible for testing all foreign students? What about illegal aliens who, for fear of deportation, would not seek testing even if it were legislated?

With the rise of tuberculosis in America and the ease with which it is transmitted, healthcare workers need to take special caution in their care of all clients. Healthcare providers need to think about routine testing of clients and themselves for TB. Government agencies can make rules and set guidelines, but many of the infected may slip through the cracks. Keep up with current public healthcare concerns to protect yourself and also to better serve your clients.

A small area of bronchopneumonia develops in the lung tissue. Many of the infecting tubercle bacilli are phagocytised by wandering macrophages. However, before the development of hypersensitivity and immunity, many of the bacilli may survive within these blood cells and be carried into regional bronchopulmonary (hilar) lymph nodes via the lymphatic system. The bacilli may even spread throughout the body. Thus, the infection, although small, spreads rapidly.

The primary infection site may or may not undergo a process of necrotic degeneration (caseation), which produces cavities filled with a cheeselike mass of tubercle bacilli, dead white blood cells (WBCs), and necrotic lung tissue. In time, this material liquifies and may drain into the tracheobronchial tree and be coughed up. The air-filled cavities remain and may be detected by x-ray.

Most primary tubercles heal over a period of months by forming scars and, ultimately, calcified lesions, also known as Ghon tubercles. These lesions may contain living bacilli that can be reactivated, even after many years, and cause secondary infection.

Primary TB infections cause the body to develop an allergic reaction to tubercle bacilli or their proteins. This cell-mediated immune response appears in the form of sensitized T cells and is detectable by a positive reaction to a tuberculin skin test. The development of this tuberculin sensitivity occurs in all body cells 2 to 6 weeks after the primary infection. It is maintained as long as living bacilli remain in the body. This acquired immunity usually inhibits further growth of the bacilli and the development of active infection.

The reason active TB disease develops in some clients (instead of being controlled by the acquired immune response) is poorly understood. However, factors that seem to play a role in the progression from TB infection to active disease include the following:

1. Advanced age
2. Immunosuppression
3. HIV infection
4. Malnutrition
5. Alcoholism and drug abuse
6. Presence of other disease states (e.g., diabetes mellitus, chronic renal failure, or malignancy)
7. Genetic predisposition

■ Secondary Infection

In addition to progressive primary disease, reinfection may also lead to a clinical form of active TB. Primary sites of infection containing TB bacilli may remain latent for years and then be reactivated if the client's resistance is lowered. Because reinfection is possible and because dormant lesions may be reactivated, it is extremely important for clients who have had a TB infection to be reassessed periodically for new evidence of active disease.

Clinical Manifestations and Diagnostic Findings

The detection and diagnosis of TB is achieved by objective tests and subjective assessment findings. The diagnosis can be difficult because TB mimics many other diseases. Also, TB may occur concurrently with other pulmonary diseases. Nurses and other healthcare providers should maintain a high index of suspicion for TB in high-risk groups.

History includes assessing the probability of recent or past exposure to TB, as well as the client's occupation, other usual activities, and travel or residence in countries with a high incidence of TB. A history of exposure to TB is certainly significant, but most clients are not aware of exposure. Also, during assessment for TB, it is advisable to determine whether the client has been previously tested for TB and to obtain the results of that testing.

Figure 42–2 shows the logical progression of diagnosis and management of TB. Typical findings in pulmonary TB may include nonproductive or productive cough; fatigue; anorexia; weight loss; low-grade fever; chills and sweats (often at night); dyspnea; hemoptysis; chest pain that may be pleuritic or dull; and chest tightness. Crackles may be present.

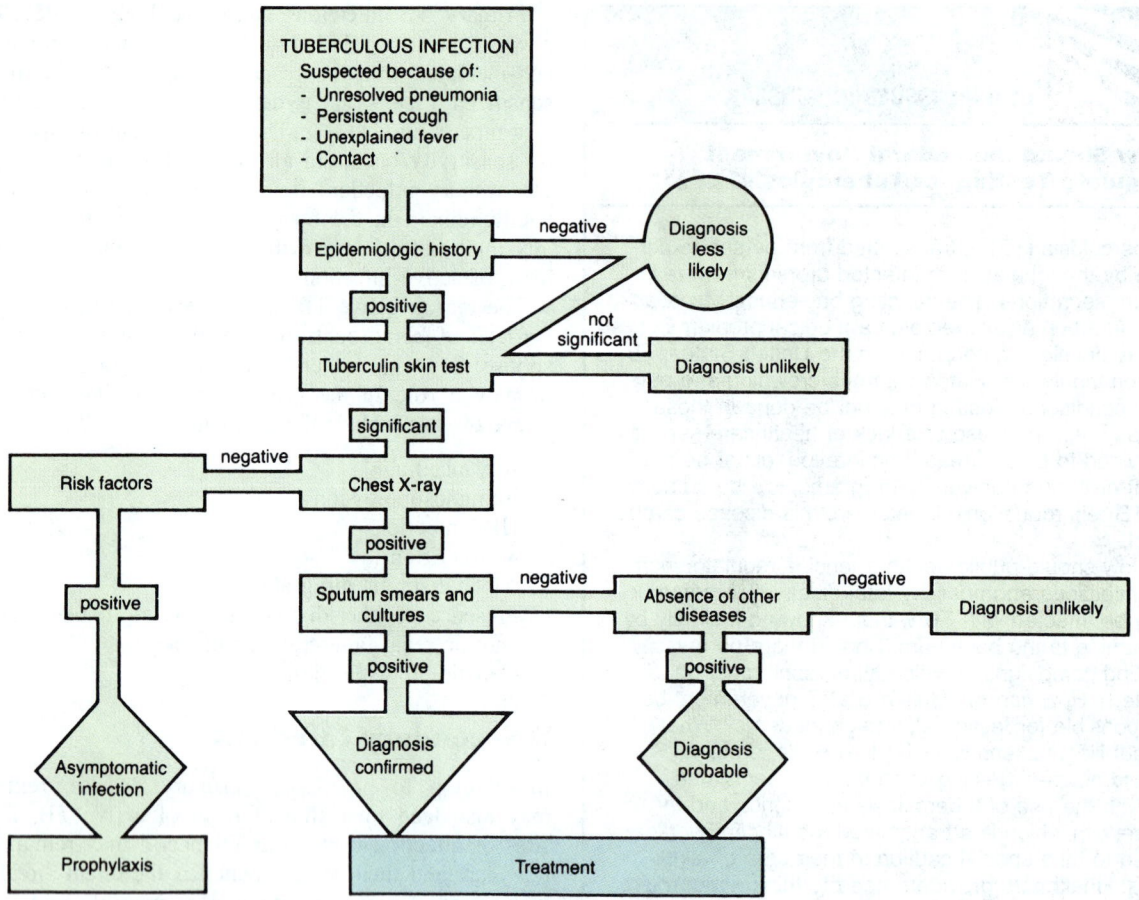

Figure 42–2. Algorithm for diagnosis and management of tuberculosis: a logical progression. (Courtesy of the American Lung Association, The Christmas Seal People).

Primary TB infections are often not recognized because usually they are relatively asymptomatic. Calcified lesions and a positive skin test are frequently the only indications that a primary TB infection has occurred. Most clients harbor tubercle bacilli for life and never develop actual disease. Usually, their body defenses are adequate to arrest primary infection, and they heal by fibrosis and calcification. However, infected persons face a 10% risk that the primary infection will progress to active disease during their lifetime. In this situation, the primary complex sites progress and worsen, possibly causing cavitation and the spread of active infection, and the client becomes clinically ill.

Routinely perform tuberculin skin testing (Mantoux test) when there is a suspicion of active TB. However, false-negative reactions are possible, especially in immunosuppressed persons. Therefore, the AFB (acid-fast bacilli) sputum smear examination and chest x-ray are also used to rapidly identify active disease. Initiate respiratory isolation until AFB sputum results are known.

The term "tuberculin converter" refers to a client who does not show radiologic or bacteriologic evidence of pulmonary TB but whose tuberculin skin test converts from a known negative reaction to a known positive reaction (i.e., from less than 5 mm of induration to 10 mm or more on the Mantoux skin test). It is important to know

that the absence of a positive (reactive) tuberculin test does not always mean that TB is absent.

Acute and Subacute Care

■ Medical Management

Most persons with newly diagnosed active TB are not hospitalized. If pulmonary TB is diagnosed in the hospitalized client, the client may be kept in the hospital until therapeutic drug levels are established. Some clients with active TB may be hospitalized for the following reasons.

1. They are acutely ill.
2. Their living situation is considered a high risk.
3. They are suspected of noncompliance.
4. There is a history of previous TB and noncompliance and the disease has been reactivated.
5. Concomitant diseases are present and acute.
6. Improvement does not occur after chemotherapy.
7. Their organisms are highly resistant to the usual treatment, requiring second- or third-line drugs. In this situation, brief hospitalization is necessary to monitor the effects and side effects of the drugs.

Antituberculosis Medications

Clients with diagnosed active TB are usually started on three or more medications to be certain the resistant organisms are eliminated. The dose of some drugs may initially be large because the bacilli are difficult to kill. Treatment continues long enough to eliminate or substantially reduce the number of dormant or semidormant bacilli. Long-term, uninterrupted chemotherapy is important.

Medications used for TB may be divided into primary agents and second-line agents. Table 42–2 lists and comments on medications in these categories. Primary agents are almost always initially prescribed until culture and sensitivity laboratory reports are available. Clients with a previous history of incomplete TB chemotherapy may have developed resistant organisms and secondary agents are used.

The duration of treatment varies. Some programs have a two-phase approach: (1) an intensive phase using two or three drugs, aimed at destroying large numbers of rapidly multiplying organisms, and (2) a maintenance phase, usually with two drugs, directed at eliminating most remaining bacilli. The recommended basic treatment regimen for previously untreated clients is 2 months of daily doses of isoniazid, rifampin, and pyrazinamide. This treatment is followed with 4 months of isoniazid and rifampin. Sputum cultures are used to evaluate the effectiveness of the therapy. If compliance with daily dosing is a problem, some TB protocols call for medication two or three times a week rather than daily. These programs are often administered in a clinic or physician's office to ensure that they are received.

If the medication regimen does not seem effective (e.g., worsening symptoms, continued AFB in sputum, increasing infiltrates, or cavity formation), the program needs reevaluation, and the client's compliance should be assessed. At least two medications (never just one) are added to a failing TB chemotherapy program.

Because medications used to treat TB have potentially serious side effects (see Table 42–2), baseline studies (depending on the specific drugs prescribed) are performed. Drug toxicity can limit the treatment of TB. Drug tolerance, drug effect, and drug toxicity depend on factors such as age, medication dosage, time since last dosage, the medication's chemical formula, renal and intestinal function, and the client's compliance.

Clients whose TB is not improving or who are unable to tolerate medication may require assessment and treatment at medical facilities specializing in the treatment of complicated pulmonary TB.

Infection Control

During hospitalization, appropriate infection control and employee health practices are essential. Private respiratory isolation rooms should be available. These rooms should be maintained at negative pressure relative to the hallway. This keeps room air from flowing out into the hallway when the door is opened and, thus, helps to avoid the spread of infectious particles. Exhaust isolation room air directly to the outside, with at least 6 air exchanges per hour. Additional equipment, such as ultraviolet lamps and high-efficiency particulate air (HEPA) filters may also be used. Healthcare workers entering the room should wear a well-fitting mask with filtration properties effective for droplet muclei.[15]

Preventive Measures

Prevention of active TB with isoniazid preventive therapy (IPT) consists of taking 300 mg of isoniazid daily for 6 to 12 months. IPT stops the growth of the bacilli, thus preventing active pulmonary or extrapulmonary TB. IPT is recommended for the following clients:

1. Newly infected (have converted tuberculin skin tests but no other indication of active disease)
2. Live or closely associate with others who have active TB
3. Have significant tuberculin skin test reactions and abnormal chest x-rays compatible with inactive TB
4. Have positive tuberculin skin tests and conditions (e.g., steroid therapy, diabetes mellitus, AIDS) placing them at increased risk for TB
5. Less than 35 years old and have significant tuberculin skin test reactions, even though they may have a normal chest x-rays and no other risk factors

■ Nursing Management of the Medical Client

Nursing management of the client with TB may include many of the interventions discussed earlier in this chapter depending on the specific nursing diagnoses identified. Possible nursing diagnoses for the client with TB include Anxiety; Ineffective Airway Clearance; Impaired Gas Exchange; Pain; Ineffective Individual Coping; Ineffective Family Coping; Altered Health Maintenance; Noncompliance; and Sleep Pattern Disturbance.

Community and Self-Care

As recently as the 1960s, clients with TB were often confined for treatment for months or years in sanatoriums. Many clients are not familiar with current treatments and still have perceptions of TB as a "shameful" disease. It is essential that clients with TB, and their significant others, receive the information in the Client Education Guide.

TB treatment is a long process. Nurses in clinics and public health facilities are often responsible for follow-up assessment and monitoring. Determining medication compliance, understanding the pharmacologic actions of medications, monitoring unwanted side effects, collecting follow-up sputum specimens, obtaining serial chest x-rays, and observing for reversal or worsening of initial assessment findings are all part of the ongoing follow-up.

Suspicion of noncompliance is dealt with in various ways. In the United States, public health departments have regulations that may be enforced regarding noncompliance with TB treatment. Directly observed therapy (i.e., observation of the client by a responsible person as the client takes the medication) may be instituted. In some

Table 42–2. Antituberculosis Agents

	Dosage	Toxic Effects	Nursing Considerations
Primary Agents			
Isoniazid	5 mg/kg/day (maximum 300 mg/day) Given PO or IM	Hepatitis Neuropathy Hepatic enzyme elevation	Monitor hepatic enzymes during the first 3 mo of treatment and in clients over the age of 50 or who are alcohol abusers Can cause fatigue, weakness, anorexia, malaise Take on empty stomach. When administered with phenytoin (Dilantin), may lead to phenytoin toxicity
Rifampin	10 mg/kg/day (maximum 600 mg/day) Given before meals	GI disturbances Orange discoloration of secretions and urine Febrile reaction	Inform client that red-orange urine, feces, saliva, sputum, sweat, and tears may occur If severe GI symptoms occur, ask if client can take medication with meals Drug is a liver enzyme inducer and may lead to more rapid excretion of methadone, oral antidiabetic agents, digitalis, oral anticoagulants, and oral contraceptives
Ethambutol	15–25 mg/kg/day for 60 days, then 15 mg/kg/day Maximum 2.5 g	Optic neuritis (decreases in visual acuity and red-green discrimination) Dermatitis	Visual testing should be done prior to and periodically during therapy. May be contraindicated in clients with ocular defects (e.g., cataracts, diabetic retinopathy, etc.) Administer cautiously in clients with renal disease
Streptomycin	15 mg/kg/day Maximum 1 g Must be given IM	Ototoxicity Nephrotoxicity	Hearing should be evaluated prior to start of treatment and periodically thereafter Observe for signs of nephrotoxicity Both ototoxicity and nephrotoxicity are more common in older patients

GI, gastrointestinal; IM, intramuscular; PO, oral.
Modified from Gray, M. A. (1993). Medication for a growing concern: Tuberculosis. *Orthopaedic Nursing, 12*(2), 75–79.

cities, a noncompliant client may be confined to a hospital or other institution for treatment, according to that city's law. Providing complete information, as outlined in the Client Education Guide, and ongoing support help. The more information clients have, and the more personal control they perceive, the more likely they are to comply with treatment.

Extrapulmonary Tuberculosis

Extrapulmonary tuberculosis (XPTB) is TB occurring anywhere outside the lungs. Although pulmonary TB is the most common form of the disease, after initial invasion tubercle bacilli can spread throughout the body via the blood and lymph. *Mycobacterium tuberculosis* thrives in oxygen-rich areas. In XPTB, it most commonly grows in highly aerobic sites, such as the renal cortex, bone

growth plates, and meninges. It may also occur in the genitourinary tract, lymph nodes, pleurae, pericardium, abdomen, and endocrine glands.

Despite the severity of the disease, XPTB is often difficult to detect. Assessment findings are frequently nondistinct. Weight loss, fatigue, malaise, fever, and sweats may or may not be present.

Widespread dissemination throughout the body is termed miliary tuberculosis. It involves the lungs and many other organs. It is more common in clients with HIV and in those 50 years or older. Older people infected with TB many years earlier may develop miliary tuberculosis from delayed or late dissemination after immune system compromise.

Assessment findings in miliary TB are usually nonspecific (e.g., anorexia, weakness, fatigue, weight loss, fever, chills, sweats, headache, and abdominal pain). The only physical finding that is specific for disseminated TB is a

	Dosage	Toxic Effects	Nursing Considerations
Primary Agents (Continued)			
Pyrazinamide	15–30 mg/kg/day Maximum dosage 2 g/day	Hepatotoxicity, dose-related Hyperuricemia	Observe for hepatotoxicity Monitor liver function tests and uric acid levels
Second-Line Agents			
Capreomycin	15–30 mg/kg/day Maximum dose 1 g/day Must be given IM	Nephrotoxicity, auditory ototoxicity Abnormal liver function tests	Observe for nephrotoxicity and oto-toxicity Observe for signs of sterile abscesses at sites of injection
Kanamycin	15–30 mg/kg/day Maximum dose 1 g/day Given IM	Ototoxicity Nephrotoxicity	Monitor hearing during use of this drug Observe for signs of renal toxicity
Ethionamide	15–20 mg/kg/day Maximum dose 1 g/day	Hepatotoxicity Excessive salivation with metallic taste in mouth Transient increase in liver enzymes	Adverse GI effects may be minimized by decreasing dosage or changing time of drug administration. Consult physician relative to dosage changes Use with caution in diabetics as it may make the diabetes more difficult to control
Para-aminosalicyclic acid	150 mg/kg/day Maximum dose 12 g/day	GI disturbances Hepatotoxicity	Moisture will cause tablets to deteriorate. Discard any tablet that becomes brownish or purple in color Use cautiously when gastric ulcers, renal disease, or hepatic disease are present
Cycloserine	15–20 mg/kg/day Maximum dose 1 g/day	Psychosis Personality changes Seizures Rash	Observe for seizures. Warn client that alcohol use may increase the potential for seizures Monitor renal and liver function tests

granuloma in the choroid of the retina. Clinical manifestations may precede changes in the chest x-ray.

The diagnosis and treatment of XPTB proceed in a similar manner to diagnosis and treatment of pulmonary TB. However, the treatment period may be longer, and more medications may be used. Treatment will depend on the extent, severity, course, and complications of the disease. Sometimes corticosteroids are used in treating severe pulmonary disease.

Nontuberculous Mycobacteria Infection

Nontuberculous mycobacteria (NTM), also known as MOTT (mycobacteria other than tuberculosis), are responsible for increasing numbers of mycobacterial infections. Although this infection is still relatively uncommon (i.e.,

approximately 1.8 cases per 100,000 in the United States), changing disease patterns have recently appeared: more cases; wider geographical distribution; and new groups of vulnerable hosts, most notably clients with HIV infection.

NTM are widely distributed in nature (i.e., in standing fresh water, salt water, animal bedding, soil, animals, and birds), and most clients acquire their infections from environmental sources rather than from other diseased clients. Infection is common in the southeastern part of the United States and more prevalent in rural areas.

The most commonly occurring NTM diseases are caused by *Mycobacterium avium* complex, *Mycobacterium kansasii*, and *Mycobacterium fortuitum*. The primary site of NTM disease is the lungs, although extrapulmonary sites (e.g., lymph nodes, skin, joints) may occur. Disseminated disease with multiple organ involvement is also possible, most commonly in immunosuppressed cli-

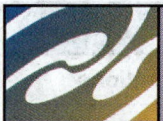

CLIENT EDUCATION GUIDE

Pulmonary Tuberculosis

Tuberculosis (TB) is infectious, but it may be cured or arrested if you take your medication as prescribed.

TB is transmitted by droplet infection and is not carried on articles such as clothing, books, or eating utensils. You do not need to dispose of any possessions.

Cover your nose and mouth when coughing, laughing, or sneezing.

Wash your hands very carefully after any contact with body substances, masks, or soiled tissues. Sputum is highly contaminated. Cough into paper tissues and dispose of them properly.

Wear a mask in appropriate situations as advised. Make sure the mask is tight-fitting, and change it frequently.

People with TB are usually not restricted in their activities for more than 2 to 4 weeks after medication is begun, and they are not isolated from others, as long as compliance is maintained. TB is no longer treated by isolation in a sanatorium.

Treatment may be necessary for a long time. Take your medication exactly as prescribed and report all side effects to your physician. Do not stop the medication for any reason without the physician's supervision. Keep an adequate supply of medication available at all times to avoid running out. Compliance with treatment is essential.

ents. Pulmonary NTM disease is very similar to TB, although the clinical manifestations may be less severe. Clients with preexisting bronchopulmonary disease (e.g., bronchiectasis, chronic obstructive pulmonary disease [COPD], or healed pulmonary TB) are at highest risk of pulmonary involvement.

Diagnosis of NTM disease is often difficult because of the widespread distribution of the organisms in the environment. Definitive diagnosis of disease is possible only if NTM are isolated from normally sterile sites (e.g., blood, cerebrospinal fluid, lymph nodes) or through biopsy. However, NTM disease is strongly suspected when a client presents with a clinical syndrome that is compatible with NTM, no other pathogens can be identified, and repeated sputum cultures reveal large numbers of NTM.

The same medications used to treat TB are prescribed for NTM disease. However, NTM are considerably more resistant to drugs than is *M. tuberculosis*. Consequently, combined drug regimens and longer treatment periods are necessary. Treatment typically includes three to six different medications and lasts for a minimum of 18 to 24 months, continuing until there are no AFB in the sputum in consecutive collections taken over a period of 1 year. As a result, medication adherence is critical.

Unsuccessful treatment may result in further lung damage and general debilitation. Regular, daily medication is essential. The more clients understand about the condition and its management, the more likely they will be to complete the full medication course.

Other aspects of the nursing management of NTM disease are the same as for pulmonary TB (see preceding discussion). However, because these diseases are not believed to be transmitted from person to person, beyond good hygiene, isolation and other measures to control infection are not necessary.

Fungal Pulmonary Infections

Most fungi that are pathogenic to humans limit their activities to the skin. However, the spores of some fungi become airborne and can be inhaled into the respiratory tract, causing pulmonary diseases that, in their chronic forms, produce granulomatous conditions similar to TB. The most common of these are coccidioidomycosis and histoplasmosis. Each has a specific geographical distribution and occurs in people living or traveling in the regions where these fungi are found. Person-to-person transmission is virtually unknown.

Coccidioidomycosis is found in the Western Hemisphere, primarily in the San Joaquin Valley of California, New Mexico, Arizona, western Texas, and northern Mexico. The disease is most likely to develop in those engaging in desert recreational activities or working in construction or other occupations that involve digging (e.g., archaeology). The disease is mild and self-limiting in 60% of those affected. Such clients are either asymptomatic or have only mild upper respiratory assessment findings. The remaining 40% develop a syndrome similar to influenza, with cough, fever, pleuritic chest pain, myalgias, and arthralgias. Erythema multiforme, which is a flat, red rash that erupts with dark red papules, occurs in some people.

The causative organism of *histoplasmosis*, the fungus *Histoplasma capsulatum*, is endemic to the central and eastern portions of North America, most notably in the Ohio, Missouri, and Mississippi River valleys. It is also found in South and Central America, India, and Cyprus. This fungus lives in moist soil of appropriate chemical composition, in mushroom cellars, on the floors of chicken houses and bat caves, and in bird droppings, especially those from starlings and blackbirds. As with coccidioidomycosis, histoplasmosis infections are usually asymptomatic or mild.

The diagnosis of fungal pulmonary diseases is usually based on history and clinical assessment findings. Skin testing is also used for coccidioidomycosis. Chest x-rays may show hilar adenopathy, small areas of infiltrates, or signs of pneumonia. Sometimes, cavities and calcified nodules may form, usually remaining in the lungs as permanent indicators of previous infection.

A few clients may develop disseminated or chronic forms of pulmonary fungal disease. When disseminated disease occurs, central nervous system, liver, spleen, gastrointestinal tract, or musculoskeletal involvement may be present. Chronic disease may result in progressive changes similar to those seen with TB. Emphysema-like pulmonary structural changes may also occur.

Mild, primary forms of fungal pulmonary disease usually do not require treatment. Progressive, disseminated, or chronic forms are usually treated with intravenous amphotericin B. This fungicidal antibiotic is quite toxic, and acute reactions (e.g., chills, fever, vomiting, headache, or decreased renal function) may occur during infusion. Antiemetics, antihistamines, antipyretics, or hydrocortisone may be prescribed as premedications. In order to reduce the common problem of thrombophlebitis at the intravenous site, a small amount of heparin may be added to the infusion. Ketoconazole, a less toxic oral medication, may also be used. If the disorder is not responsive to drug therapy, surgical removal of affected areas (e.g., lung cavities) may be necessary.

Nursing management includes providing (1) preventive education to minimize exposure of clients to infectious fungi (i.e., learning to avoid high-risk situations and to recognize early indications of infection), and (2) appropriate support and education for infected clients and their significant others, along with symptomatic management of the disease. Education involves teaching about not only the disease and intervention measures but also reportable indications of complications.

In addition to the pathogenic fungi, other common fungal spores may cause serious, potentially fatal pulmonary disease in immunocompromised persons. These fungi include *Aspergillus*, *Blastomyces dermatitidis*, *Candida*, and *Cryptococcus neoformans*. Treatment of these infections is also with amphotericin B.

Restrictive Lung Disorders

Restrictive lung disorders are a major category of pulmonary problems. The category includes any disorder that limits lung expansion and produces a pattern of abnormal function on pulmonary function tests characterized by a decrease in total lung capacity (TLC).

There are many causes of restrictive lung diseases. They may result from (1) conditions affecting lung tissues or (2) extrapulmonary causes. Extrapulmonary causes include neurologic and neuromuscular disorders and disorders affecting the thoracic cage, pleura, and movement of the diaphragm. Obesity may also lead to restrictive lung disorders. Box 42–2 lists restrictive lung disorders.

Clinical manifestations vary according to the cause of the restrictive disorder. For example, kyphosis, scoliosis, and kyphoscoliosis result in changes in the thoracic cage (Fig. 42–3). Generally, clients with restrictive lung disease exhibit a rapid, shallow respiratory pattern. Chronic hyperventilation occurs in an effort to overcome the effects of reduced lung volume and compliance. Shortness of breath is experienced, at first only with exertion, but later at rest. ABGs reveal alveolar hyperventilation (i.e., reduced partial pressure of arterial carbon dioxide [$PaCO_2$]) during the initial and intermediate phases of the disease process. As the disease progresses, respiratory muscle fatigue may occur, leading to inadequate alveolar ventilation and carbon dioxide retention. Hypoxemia is a common finding, especially in the later stages of restrictive lung disease.

Box 42–2. Restrictive Lung Diseases

Disorders affecting lung volumes and compliance of either chest wall or lung tissue

Intrapulmonary

- Pulmonary fibrosis
- Sarcoidosis and other interstitial lung diseases
- Pneumonia
- Atelectasis
- Pneumoconioses
- Surgical lung resection
- Neoplastic disease

Extrapulmonary

- Head or spinal cord injury
- Amyotrophic lateral sclerosis
- Myasthenia gravis
- Muscular dystrophy
- Congenital chest wall deformity
- Acquired chest wall changes (e.g., kyphosis or scoliosis)
- Abdominal distention restricting diaphragmatic movement
- Sleep disorders
- Poliomyelitis
- Pleural effusion
- Pleurisy
- Excessive obesity

Pulmonary function tests demonstrate impairment of the lungs' bellows action. Commonly, the ratio of forced expiratory volume in 1 second to forced vital capacity (FEV_1/FVC) will be normal or increased (i.e., 75% or more of expected values). The FEV_1/FVC ratio by itself is not an absolute indicator of restrictive lung disorders. Reduced TLC is the primary indicator of the disease. TLC is less than 80% of expected values in these clients.

Often, a specific diagnosis of restrictive lung disease is made only after extensive testing, including chest x-ray, biopsy, immunologic testing, and tests to differentiate neurologic dysfunction such as electromyography or spinal fluid analysis.

Management is based on the degree of impairment and the ability to reverse the condition. Clients with spinal deformities may be helped by corrective spinal surgery. Likewise, obese clients will breathe better after weight loss. Clients with restrictive lung disorders due to interstitial disease are discussed later in this chapter. Selected clients may benefit from the use of transtracheal oxygen administration or nighttime mechanical ventilation with a mask or cuirass respirator (a device that covers the chest and moves the chest wall out and back through changes in pressure), especially those clients with postpoliomyelitis syndrome.

The primary goals of nursing management of the client with restrictive lung disease are (1) promotion of adequate oxygenation, (2) maintenance of a patent airway, and (3) achievement of the highest possible functional level. Interventions to attain these goals are similar to those used in the treatment of chronic air flow limitation

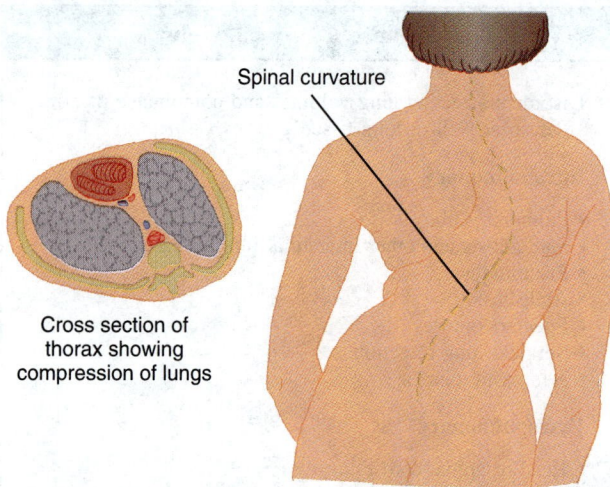

Spinal curvature

Cross section of
thorax showing
compression of lungs

Figure 42–3. Thoracic kyphoscoliosis. Note the S shape of the spine. These thoracic deformities alter the chest cage space. Lung tissue may be compressed, producing altered lung function (restrictive lung disease).

(CAL) (see Chapter 41). ABG analysis is important for monitoring oxygen needs, acid-base balance, and the effects of physical activity. $PaCO_2$ levels should be monitored because rising carbon dioxide levels are an indicator of impending respiratory failure.

Most restrictive lung disorders are not reversible. Endstage disease is characterized by the development of pulmonary hypertension, cor pulmonale (right-sided heart failure due to pulmonary problems), severe hypoxemia, and eventual ventilatory failure. Efforts should be made to maintain the client's functional status and quality of life at as high a level as possible.

Lung Transplantation

Some clients with endstage disease may be candidates for single-lung transplantation. This procedure involves replacement of one of the diseased lungs with a lung from a cadaver donor. Although the procedure is still relatively uncommon, the success of lung transplantation is increasing with advanced surgical techniques and antirejection medications, such as cyclosporine.

Following surgery, the client is observed for excessive bleeding. Monitor vital signs, hemodynamic pressures, electrocardiogram (ECG), and chest tube drainage. Pulmonary edema may develop in the denervated transplanted lung. Therefore, the client is placed on continuous mechanical ventilation with positive end-expiratory pressure (PEEP) for 24 to 48 hours. Fluids are restricted, lung sounds are auscultated, and the degree of peripheral edema is monitored. Following extubation, assist the client to cough and deep-breathe and use incentive spirometry to expand the lung.

The client is at high risk of infection and transplant rejection. Isolation is used to decrease inadvertent exposure to pathogens. Laboratory values are monitored, especially the WBC and absolute neutrophil count. Also monitor the client for clinical manifestations of infection such

as changes in vital signs, especially fever, local infections at intravenous access sites and incision lines, and changes in respiratory status (excessive secretions, tachypnea, dyspnea, fatigue). Rejection of the transplanted lung may present as dyspnea, the development of infiltrates on chest x-ray, need for ventilatory support, and fatigue.

Following the initial surgery, the client may develop alterations in self-concept related to changes in appearance from the side effects of medications such as steroids and immunosuppressants, changes in life-style, or changes in work ability and role performance. Be sensitive to these issues and encourage the client and family to discuss their feelings and explore options.

Prior to discharge, teach the client about the medication regimen and stress the need for daily medication despite a lack of manifestations. The client should report fever, dyspnea, excessive weight gain, and fatigue to the physician. In addition, the client should begin a physical rehabilitation program.

During follow-up visits the client is monitored for signs of rejection, compliance with immunosuppressive therapy, and progress in functional status.

Lung transplantation offers some hope for extended life to clients with previously fatal conditions. However, it is a very frightening and stressful surgery. Clients undergoing lung transplants are always critically ill before surgery. In addition, they must undergo a radical, major surgery and endure prolonged intensive care and isolation procedures. They may also have to tolerate a certain degree of public, and sometimes media, attention. In addition, persons with transplants must adapt to an altered self-concept. The client and significant others need constant emotional support for achievement of a successful outcome.

Cystic Fibrosis

Cystic fibrosis is a congenital restrictive lung disorder in which the secretions of the exocrine (mucus-producing) glands are abnormal. It affects the (1) sweat glands, (2) respiratory system, (3) digestive tract, particularly the pancreas, and (4) reproductive tract. Cystic fibrosis is the most common inherited genetic disease in the white population, affecting approximately 1 in 2000 white newborns in the United States. Previously, this condition was considered a "pediatric problem" because it was fatal in childhood. However, advances in treatment, including antibiotics, chest physiotherapy, and nutrition programs, have extended the median life expectancy into the late 20s, with maximum survival estimated at 30 to 40 years.

Pulmonary involvement is the most common and most severe manifestation of cystic fibrosis. Over 90% of clients with cystic fibrosis die with severe pulmonary disease. The disease process causes tracheobronchial secretions to become thick and viscous, leading to (1) interference with normal ciliary action, (2) plugging of airways, and (3) creation of a reservoir for bacterial growth and infection. Bronchiectasis may also develop, which compounds the infection risk.

The goal of pulmonary therapy is to prevent infections by removing secretions, improving aeration, and administering antimicrobial agents. Effective clearing of tracheobronchial secretions is promoted by (1) ensuring adequate hydration; (2) administering prescribed mucolytic aerosols; and (3) teaching and supervising effective coughing techniques, use of positive expiratory pressure devices, postural drainage, and chest vibration and percussion. The chest should be auscultated before and after therapy, noting quality of lung sounds and effectiveness of therapy.

Adequate aeration is maintained by (1) following the techniques for maintaining clear airways, (2) administering oxygen if hypoxemia is present, and (3) maintaining correct body position to facilitate breathing (i.e., sitting up). Recent studies have also shown that exercise can improve pulmonary function in these clients.[21] The client should be assessed for signs of hypercapnia and other indications of respiratory failure.

Antimicrobial therapy has played a significant role in extending the life expectancy of cystic fibrosis clients. Oral antibiotics may be given prophylactically on a routine basis. Intravenous antibiotics are essential during acute infections. Inhaled antibiotics are also being used on a more regular basis. The choice of antibiotic should be determined by sputum culture and sensitivity. Infections are most commonly caused by *Staphylococcus aureus* and *Pseudomonas aeruginosa*. Sputum should be assessed for color, quality, and quantity. All respiratory equipment should be thoroughly cleaned on a routine basis to prevent reinfection from contaminated equipment.

New treatments for cystic fibrosis are currently under trial. These include: (1) use of synthetically produced DNAase, an enzyme which breaks down DNA. DNA, produced by the destruction of neutrophils and bacteria, increases mucus "stickiness"; (2) anti-inflammatory drugs to decrease the inflammatory response in the respiratory tract epithelium; (3) augmentation of the immune defense with supplemental gamma globulin; and (4) drugs that alter ion movement and thin secretions. Gene therapy and lung transplantation are also being evaluated.[21,24]

Treatment of end-stage disease is primarily concerned with the management of severe complications. Obstruction of the airways leads to a state of hyperinflation. In time, restrictive lung disease is superimposed by the obstructive disease. Pneumothorax may develop, requiring lung reinflation with chest tubes.

Persistent pulmonary infection with *Pseudomonas* organisms is common in the end stages of cystic fibrosis. Treatment with continuous, large doses of intravenous antibiotics is usually indicated. Moderate-to-severe hemoptysis can occur if the infection causes erosion of pulmonary blood vessels. Blood replacement and temporary cessation of postural drainage may be required.

Over time, pulmonary obstruction leads to chronic hypoxemia, hypercapnia, and acidosis. Pulmonary hypertension and, eventually, cor pulmonale may result. Treatment may include digitalis, diuretics, and oxygen therapy.

Attention to psychosocial concerns is a nursing priority throughout the disease course. In the adult cystic fibrosis client, psychosocial concerns center around three major areas: (1) disease management (e.g., treatment compliance, sleep disturbance, hemoptysis, nutrition, and hospitalizations); (2) growth and development (e.g., daily activities, school and work, and sex and reproduction); and (3) family relations (e.g., substance abuse, depression, anxiety, and marital problems). Nursing intervention involves assisting clients to cope with these problem areas as well as providing emotional support to both the client and family.

Interstitial Lung Disease

Interstitial lung diseases (ILDs) comprise a group of diffuse, inflammatory lower respiratory tract disorders. The term *interstitial* is used to indicate that the interstitium of the alveolar walls is thickened and usually fibrotic. The alveolar walls thicken as a result of the accumulation of inflammatory cells. The thickened alveolus becomes nonfunctional.

The cause of ILD is not clearly defined. It most commonly develops from idiopathic pulmonary fibrosis, sarcoidosis, and collagen-vascular disorders. ILD can also result from the inhalation of inorganic dust, such as crystalline silica, asbestos and coal dust, and organic dust from organisms encountered in farming, air conditioner use, and animal husbandry. Other possible causes include radiation damage and infectious agents.

Clinical manifestations are insidious and nonspecific, such as fatigue, dyspnea, and nonproductive cough. Because the clinical manifestations are nonspecific, ILD may go undiagnosed for years. The client's history plays a major part in diagnosis, because it is important to determine the agents to which the client has been exposed. Clients report progressive dyspnea and often have dyspnea at rest. Chest expansion is normally reduced, reflecting a decreased TLC. Inspiratory and expiratory crackles are frequently heard. The crackles have a characteristic sound, like the sound of Velcro being pulled apart. Clubbing of the finger tips may be evident. Diagnostic assessment may include gallium ventilation-perfusion scans. These scans usually reveal impaired perfusion in the lower lobes and multiple areas of impaired ventilation. The ventilation-perfusion mismatch results in hypoxemia and carbon dioxide retention. Bronchoscopy and biopsy may also be used to confirm ILD.

Management of a client with ILD is based on the degree of impairment. Inflammation is controlled with corticosteroids. The client is taught that corticosteroids reduce further impairment, but previously damaged alveolar-capillary units are lost forever. Many clients have subjective improvement while on steroids and can eventually be tapered off the drugs. If the offending agent is known, the initial treatment is to remove the client from exposure to the agent. As the disorder progresses, clients are usually treated with inhaled corticosteroids and bronchodilators to help mobilize secretions and oxygen during periods of exercise. Nursing management is the same as for clients with restrictive lung disorders.

Sarcoidosis

Sarcoidosis is an inflammatory condition that affects many body systems. The disease is characterized by the formation of widespread granulomatous lesions. In addition to lung involvement, which occurs in over 90% of cases, clients may present with clinical manifestations involving the peripheral lymphatic system, skin, liver, eyes, spleen, bones, salivary glands, joints, and heart. The onset of sarcoidosis is generally between the ages of 20 and 40 years. The disorder is approximately 14 times more common in blacks than in whites. Although the male-female ratio is about even in the nonblack population, black females develop sarcoidosis twice as frequently as do black males.

The cause of sarcoidosis remains unknown. However, the disease itself is becoming more fully understood. Current evidence suggests that a triggering agent, which may be genetic, infectious, immunologic, or toxic, stimulates enhanced cell-mediated immune processes at the site of involvement. A series of interactions between T lymphocytes and monocytes-macrophages leads to the formation of noncaseating (i.e., no cheesy necrotic degeneration) granulomas, which are characteristic of the disease. Granuloma formation may regress with therapy or as a result of the disorder's natural course, but may also progress to fibrosis and restrictive lung disease.

About a third of the clients with sarcoidosis are asymptomatic; diagnosis is made by chest x-ray. Clients with pulmonary manifestations usually present with a dry cough and shortness of breath. Chest pain, hemoptysis, or pneumothorax may also be present. Systemic manifestations may include fatigue, weakness, malaise, weight loss, and fever. A definitive diagnosis of sarcoidosis is made by tissue biopsy. When lung involvement is suspected, bronchoscopy, bronchoalveolar lavage, mediastinoscopy, or open lung biopsy may be performed.

Medical management is primarily determined by the degree to which the client's life is disturbed by the manifestations experienced. If the client with sarcoidosis is asymptomatic, management involves ongoing assessment for further disease progression. Repeat chest films at 6-month intervals are often indicated. When manifestations are present, medical treatment usually consists of systemic corticosteroids, which often lead to dramatic improvement.

Nursing intervention in clients with sarcoidosis is the same as that for other restrictive lung diseases and hypoxemia. Assess for drug side effects, especially adverse responses to corticosteroids (such as weight gain, change in mood, development of diabetes mellitus). Also assess for signs of improvement, such as (1) increased exercise tolerance, (2) disappearance of initial assessment findings, (3) improved pulmonary function studies, and (4) improved oxygenation. If assessment findings worsen, document them and notify the physician.

Occupational Lung Diseases

Lung diseases are among the most common occupational health problems. They are caused by the inhalation of various chemicals, dusts, and other particulate matter that are present in certain settings. Not all clients exposed to occupational inhalants will develop lung disease. Harmful effects depend on the nature of the exposure, duration and intensity of the exposure, particle size and water-solubility of the inhalant (the larger the particle, the lower the probability of its reaching the lower respiratory tract; highly water-soluble inhalants tend to dissolve and react in the upper respiratory tract, whereas poorly soluble substances may travel as far as the alveoli), smoking history, and the presence of underlying pulmonary disease.

The most commonly encountered occupational lung diseases are described in Table 42–3. Acute respiratory irritation results from the inhalation of chemicals such as ammonia, chlorine, and nitrogen oxides in the form of gases, aerosols, or particulate matter. If such irritants reach the lower airways, alveolar damage and pulmonary edema can result. Although the effects of acute irritants are usually short-lived, some may cause chronic alveolar damage or airway obstruction.

Occupational asthma is defined as variable air flow obstruction caused by a specific agent in the workplace. By far the greatest number of occupational agents causing asthma are those with known or suspected allergic properties, such as plant and animal proteins (e.g., wheat flour, cotton, flax, and grain mites). In most cases, the asthma resolves after exposure is terminated. However, hyperactivity of the airways may persist for years.

Hypersensitivity pneumonitis, or allergic alveolitis, is most commonly due to the inhalation of organic antigens of fungal, bacterial, or animal origin. The nature of the exposure and the client's immunologic reactivity will determine the pulmonary response. Nonatopic persons (i.e., those with no history of allergies) develop a pulmonary response to organic dusts more often than do atopic persons, although they too may exhibit pulmonary reactions.

Pneumoconioses, or the "dust diseases," result from inhalation of minerals, notably silica, coal dust, or asbestos. These diseases are most commonly seen in miners, construction workers, sandblasters, potters, and foundry and quarry workers. Pneumoconioses usually develop gradually over a period of years, eventually leading to diffuse pulmonary fibrosis that diminishes lung capacity and produces restrictive lung disease. Early clinical manifestations may include cough and dyspnea on exertion. Chest pain, productive cough, and dyspnea at rest develop as the condition progresses.

Early detection is one way to prevent progression of occupational lung disease. The respiratory history should include a complete occupational history and questions about (1) the actual job performed rather than title or job description, (2) past as well as current occupations, and (3) exposure to organic and inorganic substances in each job. Assess dyspnea, cough, chest tightness, or other manifestations indicating potential lung disease. Some employers support ongoing assessment programs (e.g., routine pulmonary function studies or chest films) for workers at risk of occupational disorders.

Exposure precautions are essential for avoiding permanent pulmonary disability. Safety measures include adequate ventilation, wearing masks, and using care when handling garments worn in dusty environments.

Nursing intervention for clients experiencing occupational lung diseases is similar to that for clients with other restrictive lung disorders (see Restrictive Lung Disorders). Supportive measures can help these clients to adjust their life-styles to their condition.

Table 42–3. Characteristics of Occupational Lung Disease

	Onset of Symptoms	Diagnosis	Treatment	Clinical Course
Acute respiratory irritation	Usually within minutes of exposure to irritant, but pulmonary edema may be delayed several hours	Consistent history; physical findings of respiratory tract irritation and damage	Prevention of exposure; respiratory support as needed	Upper respiratory tract signs resolve in hours to days; pulmonary edema resolves in days to weeks; residual damage rare
Occupational asthma	Usually within minutes of exposure to precipitant, but possibly delayed 4–6 hr or more	PFTs show obstructive pattern during exacerbations; chest film usually normal; skin tests, IgE measurement, and history of atopy helpful only if the disorder is IgE-mediated	Prevention of exposure; asthma medications	Usually resolves within hours; airways may remain persistently hyperreactive
Hypersensitivity pneumonitis	Usually 4–8 hr after exposure to antigen; possible subacute or chronic presentation	Specific IgG antibodies; x-ray findings ranging from normal to pulmonary edema to interstitial fibrosis; PFTs present restrictive or restrictive-obstructive pattern	Prevention of exposure; respiratory support as needed; steroids helpful in some cases	Usually resolve in several days; x-ray and PFT findings normalize in a few weeks; however, there may be permanent lung damage
Pneumoconioses	Requires long-term exposure; first symptom often cough progressing to dyspnea	Restrictive pattern on PFTs; on chest film, asbestosis is associated with interstitial markings in lower lobes and silicosis with opacities in upper lobes	Prevention of exposure; cessation of smoking	Gradual worsening

PFTs = pulmonary function tests.
From Mandel, J. H., & Baker, B. A. (1989). Recognizing occupational lung disease. *Hospital Practice, 24*(1), 21.

If occupational lung disease is significant, the client may qualify for a disability allowance. Refer clients to community resources, such as federal or state departments of labor, if they have questions concerning their eligibility. Because of legal problems that may surround compensation claims, you may have to deal with hostility and resentment aimed toward the employer and the legal system. These clients may also experience anxiety and uncertainty about their future health status. Adopt a calm, positive, supportive approach.

Neoplastic Lung Disorders

Malignant Lung Tumors

Lung cancer is malignancy in the epithelium of the respiratory tract. At least a dozen different cell types of tumors are included under the classification of lung cancer. The four major types of lung cancer include small cell carcinoma (oat cell carcinoma), squamous cell carcinoma, adenocarcinoma, and large cell carcinoma. The term *lung cancer* excludes other disorders such as sarcomas, lymphomas, blastomas, and mesotheliomas.

Etiology and Risk Factors

Cigarette smoking is by far the most important risk factor in lung cancer development. Cigarette smoke contains several organ-specific carcinogens. Genetic predisposition to the development of lung cancer also plays a role in the etiology. Other carcinogens include inhaled toxins, such as asbestos, and pollutants. Finally, tuberculosis and low-level radiation are risks for lung cancer. The Risk Factors and Levels of Prevention feature lists ways to prevent lung cancer.

Pathophysiology

Lung cancers are divided into two major categories: small cell lung cancers (SCLCs) and non–small cell lung cancers (NSCLCs), which include epidermoid or squamous cell carcinoma, adenocarcinoma, and large cell carcinoma. The characteristics of each of these types are described in Table 42–4. In general, survival rates are best for NSCLC, especially with treatment in its early stages. Despite increasing knowledge and technology, however, overall survival from lung cancer remains low, especially for clients with small cell carcinomas.

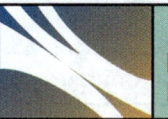

RISK FACTORS AND LEVELS OF PREVENTION

Lung Cancer

Risk Factors

Cigarette smoking, genetic predisposition, inhaled toxins such as asbestos and pollutants, TB.

Levels of Prevention

Primary Prevention

- Promote smoking cessation activities.
- Discourage smoking initiation.
- Teach clients the dangers of secondhand smoke.
- Assist with efforts to limit occupational exposure to known carcinogenic agents, such as asbestos, radioactive isotopes, polycyclic hydrocarbons, vinyl chloride, metallurgical ores, and mustard gas.
- Participate in community efforts to reduce levels of air pollution.
- Instruct clients to maintain a low fat diet rich in beta carotene, vitamin C, and vitamin E.
- Complete prescribed TB prophylaxis

Secondary Prevention

- Educate clients regarding the warning signals of lung cancer (see Box 42–4).
- Emphasize the need for an annual physical examination

Tertiary Prevention

- Provide clients and their families with information about support groups for cancer patients.
- Stress the importance of regular follow-up after treatment to detect possible recurrence.

Metastatic spread of pulmonary tumors is usually to the long bones, vertebral column (especially the thoracic vertebrae), liver, and adrenal glands. Brain metastasis is also common, occurring in as many as 50% of cases.

Clinical Manifestations and Diagnostic Findings

The warning signals of lung cancer are presented in Box 42–3. In many instances, lung cancer may mimic other pulmonary conditions. Extrapulmonary manifestations may occur before pulmonary manifestations. Specific clinical assessment findings vary according to tumor type, location, and extent, as well as preexisting pulmonary health.

Centrally located pulmonary tumors usually obstruct air flow, producing clinical manifestations such as coughing, wheezing, stridor, and dyspnea. As obstruction increases, bronchopulmonary infection often occurs distal to the obstruction. Chest, shoulder, and back pain may develop as the tumor invades the perivascular nerves. Squamous and small cell tumors often cause hemoptysis. Small cell tumors may also extend into the pericardium, causing pericardial effusion and, possibly, tamponade. Cardiac arrhythmias are also likely. Centrally located pulmonary tumors are easiest to locate and identify with fiberoptic bronchoscopy and sputum cytologic study. Positive tissue diagnosis is possible 90% of the time.

Peripheral pulmonary tumors often do not produce assessment findings initially. In time, pleural pain develops that increases on inspiration, is sharp and severe, and is usually localized. Pleural effusion also develops and, along with the pain, limits lung expansion. Only 30% of peripheral lung tumors are successfully categorized by bronchoscopic and cytologic examination.

Pancoast's tumor occurs in the apices of the lungs in both squamous cell and adenocarcinomatous cancers. The tumor is asymptomatic until it extends into surrounding structures. Clinical manifestations are caused by compression of the brachial plexus in the distribution from the eighth cervical nerve to the first two thoracic nerves. This results in arm and shoulder pain on the affected side, along with atrophy of the arm and hand muscles. With continuing tumor growth, the ribs over the tumor (usually the first and second ribs) may be invaded, resulting in bone pain. Later, involvement of the cervical sympathetic nerve ganglia may lead to Horner's syndrome. This syndrome consists of miosis (i.e., pupil contraction), partial eyelid ptosis, and anhidrosis (i.e., absence of sweating) on the affected side of the face.

The primary finding in pleural tumors (malignant mesotheliomas) is chest pain. Dyspnea, cough, weight loss, and fever may also be present. Thoracotomy is usually required for a definitive diagnosis. In addition to pulmonary manifestations, there are some rare syndromes associated with lung cancer called paraneoplastic syndromes. These usually result from the secretion of substances (e.g., hormones) by the tumor itself. These substances then act on target organs, producing a variety of clinical manifestations, such as carcinoid syndrome, clubbing of digits, Cushing syndrome, hypercalcemia, antidiuretic hormone secretion, and peripheral neuropathy.

■ Metastasis

If tumors spread, either by direct extension or metastasis, further clinical manifestations may result. Direct extension to the recurrent laryngeal nerve produces hoarseness. Compression of the esophagus may produce dysphagia. Invasion or compression of the superior vena cava produces superior vena cava syndrome, a potentially life-threatening emergency. Obstruction of venous blood flow leads to clinical manifestations that may include shortness of breath; facial, arm, and trunk swelling; distended neck veins; chest pain; and venous stasis. Immediate, palliative surgical treatment may be necessary.

Regional lymph node involvement may produce manifestations due to impaired lymph drainage. Involvement of the mediastinal lymph nodes may result in vocal cord paralysis, dysphagia, diaphragmatic paralysis on the affected side (due to phrenic nerve compression), vena cava compression, and malignant pleural effusion. When medi-

Table 42–4. Overview of Malignant Pulmonary Neoplasms

Cell Type	Approximate Incidence	Specific Characteristics	Growth Rate
Epidermoid (squamous cell)	30%–35% of lung cancer	Arises from bronchial epithelium; as growth occurs, cavitation may develop in lung distal to tumor Pancoast's tumor arises in apex and upper lung zones Secondary infections distal to obstructive tumor in bronchioles frequently occur	Slow growth, metastasis not common If tumor metastasizes, usually to lymph, adrenals, and liver, in that order
Adenocarcinoma	25%–30% of lung cancer	60%–70% arise from bronchial mucous gland Often subpleural; often difficult to distinguish from other tumors in the body; rarely cavitates; often arises in previously scarred lung tissue Incidence strongly linked to cigarette smoking Increasing incidence in women Bronchioloalveolar cell carcinoma is a subtype	Slow growth May metastasize throughout lung or to other organs of the body
Large cell	10%–20% of lung cancer	More often peripheral mass, either single or multiple masses Cavitation common May be located centrally, midlung, or peripherally Rare hilar involvement Often grows to large tumor mass before diagnosis	Slow; metastasis may occur to kidney, liver, and adrenals, in that order
Small cell (oat cell)	20%–25% of lung cancer	65%–75% present with hilar or central mass May compress bronchi Involvement of diaphragm through paralysis of phrenic nerve and hoarseness through paralysis of recurrent laryngeal nerve Pleural, pericardial effusions and tamponade Does not form cavities	Rapid growth Metastasis to mediastinum, thoracic, and extrathoracic structures occurs early

astinal lymph nodes are involved, surgical excision of the pulmonary tumor is usually no longer possible.

■ Diagnostic Assessment

Numerous diagnostic tests may be used to determine the presence and extent of the disease. Sputum cytology and chest x-ray are most commonly used. Computed tomographic (CT) scans may be used to provide detailed anatomic assessment. MRI can provide high-quality images of the lung and mediastinum to assess for tumor invasion. New imaging techniques use monoclonal antibodies that have an affinity for cancer cells. The antibodies are

tagged with technetium and injected into the client. They concentrate in the area of tumor and can be detected by single photon emission computed tomographic (SPECT) images.

Bronchoscopy may be performed with centrally located lesions; bronchial washing or brushing is done to obtain tumor cells for cytologic and pathologic study. In addition, percutaneous transthoracic needle biopsy, mediastinoscopy, or direct surgical biopsy may be required to confirm the diagnosis. Radionuclide scans may be used to detect metastasis to the bone, liver, or brain (see Chapter 23).

The TNM classification scheme is used for lung cancer staging (Box 42–4 and Fig. 42–4). Staging is performed to provide a guideline for the selection of appropriate therapies and the estimation of prognosis. Staging information is valuable for helping clients and their families to make treatment decisions and to set appropriate short- and long-term goals.

Box 42–3. Warning Signals of Lung Cancer

- Any change in respiratory patterns
- Persistent cough
- Sputum streaked with blood
- Frank hemoptysis
- Rust-colored or purulent sputum
- Chest, shoulder, or arm pain
- Recurring episodes of pleural effusion, pneumonia, or bronchitis
- Dyspnea, unexplained or out of proportion

Acute and Subacute Care

The key to increasing the survival rate of clients with lung cancer is early detection. When premalignant changes begin, dysplastic cells are identifiable with fiber-

Box 42–4. TNM Staging of Pulmonary Malignancies

Primary Tumor (T)

T_X Tumor proven by presence of malignant cells in bronchopulmonary secretions but not visualized on x-ray or during bronchoscopy, or any tumor that cannot be assessed as in a retreatment staging

T_0 No evidence of primary tumor

T_{is} Carcinoma in situ

T_1 A tumor that is 3 cm or less in greatest dimension, surrounded by lung or visceral pleura and without evidence of invasion proximal to a lobar bronchus at bronchoscopy

T_2 Tumor more than 3 cm in greatest dimension or a tumor of any size that either invades the visceral pleura or has associated atelectasis or obstructive pneumonitis extending to the hilar region; at bronchoscopy, the proximal extent of demonstrable tumor must be within a lobar bronchus or at least 2 cm distal to the carina; any associated atelectasis or obstructive pneumonitis must involve less than an entire lung

T_3 A tumor of any size with direct extension into the chest wall (including superior sulcus tumors), the diaphragm, or the mediastinal pleura or pericardium without involving the heart, great vessels, trachea, esophagus, or vertebral body; or a tumor in the main bronchus within 2 cm of the carina without involving the carina

T_4 A tumor of any size with invasion of the mediastinum or involving the heart, great vessels, trachea, esophagus, vertebral body, or carina in the presence of malignant pleural effusion

Lymph Nodes (N)

N_0 No demonstrable metastases to regional lymph nodes

N_1 Metastasis to lymph nodes in the peribronchial or the ipsilateral hilar region or both, including direct extension

N_2 Metastasis to ipsilateral mediastinal lymph nodes and subcarinal lymph nodes

N_3 Metastasis to contralateral mediastinal, contralateral hilar, ipsilateral or contralateral scalene, or supraclavicular lymph nodes

Distant Metastasis (M)

M_0 No (known) distant metastasis

M_1 Distant metastasis present; specify site(s)

Modified from the American Joint Committee on Cancer. In Harvey, J. C., & Beattie, E. J. (1993). Lung cancer. *Clinical Symposia, 45*(3), 2.

---

primary treatment modalities include surgery, radiation therapy, and chemotherapy.

■ Medical Management

Radiation Therapy

Radiotherapy may be used as a potentially curative treatment in clients with locally advanced disease who are poor surgical risks, who have technically inoperable tumors, or who refuse thoracotomy. Radiation therapy may also be used in combination with surgery or chemotherapy to improve treatment outcomes. Radiotherapy is administered over a period of 5 to 6 weeks, either consecutively or in split courses. Doses are limited by other structures in the treatment area and by normal tissue tolerance. Irreversible fibrotic changes and other pulmonary side effects may occur. To delineate the area to be irradiated precisely, CT scanning is often performed before treatment begins. This method also minimizes tissue damage to surrounding areas.

Radiotherapy may also be used for palliation of symptoms such as pain, shortness of breath, hemoptysis, and obstruction or compression of bronchi, blood vessels, or esophagus. Irradiation of metastases to the brain and bone may reduce the distressing symptoms associated with these sequelae as well.

Chemotherapy

The response of lung cancer to chemotherapy depends on the tumor's cell type. SCLC responds well to chemotherapeutic agents because of its rapid growth rate. Results of clinical trials have demonstrated that long-term survival in clients with SCLC can be improved with intensive combination chemotherapy. As a result, chemotherapy is the cornerstone of management of SCLC.

Chemotherapy's effectiveness in the treatment of NSCLC remains controversial. It is commonly used in clients treated with surgery or radiation who experience recurrent disease or distant metastasis. However, large-scale studies have failed to demonstrate a significantly improved overall survival rate for these clients. As a result, the decision to use chemotherapy is usually made on an individual basis, depending on the client's previous history, current condition, and acceptance of the risks and side effects involved.

■ Nursing Management of the Medical Client

Diagnostic Phase

The client who is undergoing diagnostic tests for lung cancer faces an uncertain future. If the diagnosis is confirmed, the client can anticipate a variety of physical difficulties, potentially extensive medical treatment, and many emotional changes. The nursing assessment plays a critical role in developing a plan of care that will provide needed support.

---

optic bronchoscopy and sputum cytologic studies. At this stage, lesions are potentially curable. However, a tumor must be at least 1 cm in diameter before it is detectable on chest film. Unfortunately, invasion and metastasis have usually already occurred. Management of the client with lung cancer depends on tumor type and stage as well as the client's underlying health status. Following diagnosis,

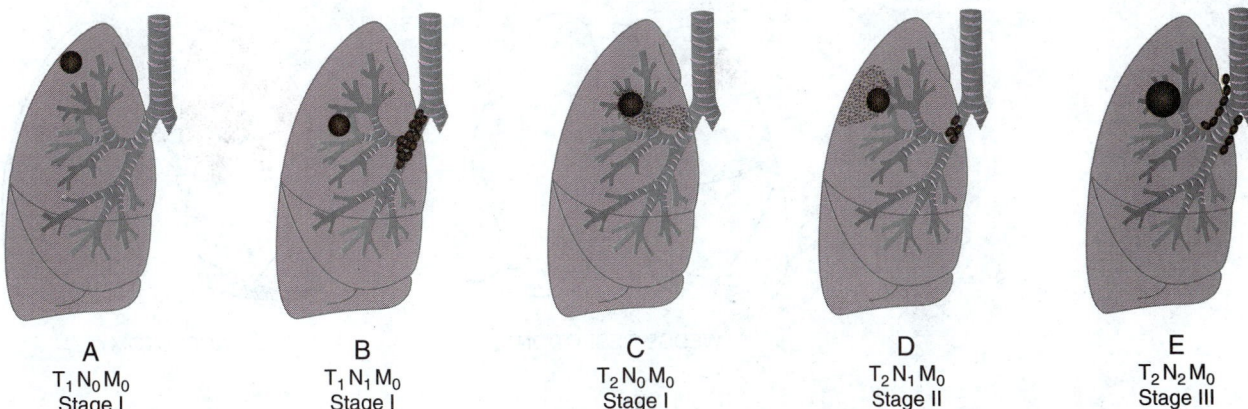

A	B	C	D	E
$T_1 N_0 M_0$	$T_1 N_1 M_0$	$T_2 N_0 M_0$	$T_2 N_1 M_0$	$T_2 N_2 M_0$
Stage I	Stage I	Stage I	Stage II	Stage III

Figure 42–4. Staging of lung cancer by the TNM classification system. *A* and *B*, Stage I disease includes tumors classified as T_1, with or without metastasis to the lymph nodes in the ipsilateral hilar region. *C*, Also included in stage I are tumors classified as T_2 but having no nodal or distant metastases. *D*, Stage II disease includes those tumors classified as T_2, with metastasis only to the ipsilateral hilar lymph nodes. *E*, Stage III includes all tumors more extensive than T_2, or any tumor with metastasis to the lymph nodes in the mediastinum or with distant metastasis.

The nursing history should include an exploration of the client's chief complaints, particularly cough (productive or nonproductive), dyspnea, pain, or recurrent infection. Ask the client about the presence of risk factors, including a smoking history, exposure to occupational respiratory carcinogens, or a family history of the disease. Also assess the client's socioeconomic situation and available social support because these factors will affect subsequent management options.

Nursing management during the diagnostic phase focuses on emotional support and client education, along with required physical care. Help clients maintain a sense of control by keeping them informed about all scheduled tests. Once a diagnosis of lung cancer is confirmed, nursing care must incorporate aspects of assisting the client to cope with anxiety and fear, family responses, financial considerations, absence from work and social activities, and possible changes in life goals.

Treatment Phase

Nursing care of the client receiving radiation and chemotherapy is fully discussed in Chapter 24.

■ Surgical Management

Surgical intervention is the treatment of choice in early-stage NSCLC. Cure is possible if the disease is still localized to the thoracic cavity and no distant metastases are present. However, only 20% to 25% of clients with NSCLC meet these criteria at the time of diagnosis. For patients who do successfully undergo surgical resection, the 5-year survival rate is approximately 25% to 35%.[27]

The role of surgical resection in the treatment of SCLC is limited. Surgery may be effective for clients in the early stages of SCLC, as a component of combined-modality therapy. For clients with more advanced disease,

surgery causes unnecessary risk and stress, with no valid benefits.

The primary aim of surgical resection is to remove the tumor completely while preserving as much of the normal surrounding lung tissue as possible. The extent of the operation will depend on the location and size of the pulmonary tumor and the degree of the underlying pathologic process. Clients with preexisting pulmonary disease may not be able to tolerate extensive lung tissue removal.

Preoperative Management

Extensive pulmonary function testing may be ordered before chest surgery to determine the client's ability to tolerate the proposed surgical intervention. Clients with impaired pulmonary function may be treated with antibiotics, bronchodilating medications, intermittent positive pressure breathing procedures, and supervised breathing exercises to improve respiratory efficiency. Clients are encouraged to refrain from smoking during the preoperative period, because smoking will increase pulmonary secretions and decrease blood oxygen saturation.

Surgical Procedures

Laser Surgery. Another surgical treatment modality is laser therapy. Currently, laser is used as a palliative measure for relief of endobronchial obstructions that are not resectable. Laser procedures do not produce systemic or cumulative toxic effects and are well tolerated. Laser therapy may be done in an outpatient setting. However, in order to use the laser, the tumor mass must be accessible by bronchoscopy. Therefore, tumors pressing on bronchial tissue from outside the bronchial lumen are not amenable to laser therapy.

Pulmonary Resection. Common pulmonary resection procedures are shown in Figure 42–5. They are also discussed here.

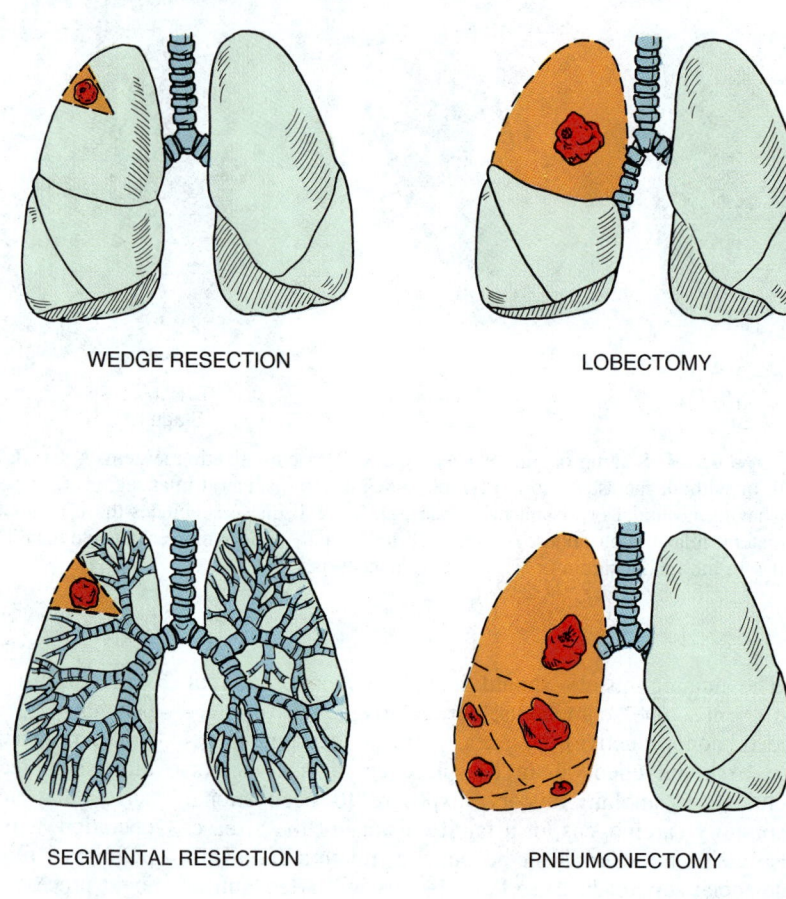

WEDGE RESECTION   LOBECTOMY

SEGMENTAL RESECTION   PNEUMONECTOMY

portion of tissue
surgically removed

Figure 42–5. Pulmonary resections.

Wedge Resection. This procedure involves removal of a small, localized area of diseased tissue near the surface of the lung. Because the resected area is small, pulmonary structure and function are relatively unchanged after healing.

Segmental Resection. This form of resection involves the removal of one or more lung segments (a bronchiole and its alveoli.) The remaining lung tissue overexpands to fill the previously occupied space.

Lobectomy. Lobectomy is the removal of an entire lobe of the lung. After lobectomy, the remaining lung overexpands to fill the open portion of the thoracic space.

Pneumonectomy. This procedure is removal of an entire lung. Once the lung is removed, the involved side of the thoracic cavity is an empty space. In order to reduce the size of the cavity, the phrenic nerve is severed on the affected side to paralyze the diaphragm in an elevated position. A thoracoplasty may also be performed, which is the removal of several ribs or portions of ribs to further reduce the thoracic space.

Closed chest drainage is usually not used after pneumonectomy. The serous fluid that accumulates in the empty thoracic cavity eventually consolidates. The consolidation prevents shifts of the mediastinum, heart, and remaining lung.

Chest Tubes. Chest tubes are usually inserted in an operating room during chest surgery. However, in some emergencies, a chest tube may be inserted in a treatment room or at the bedside.

Two catheters are usually placed in the chest following resectional surgery (except pneumonectomy). One of these (the upper, or anterior, tube) is placed anteriorly through the second intercostal space to permit the escape of air rising in the pleural space. The other catheter (the lower, or posterior, tube) is placed posteriorly through the eighth or ninth intercostal space in the midaxillary line to drain off serosanguineous fluid accumulating in the lower portion of the pleural space. The lower tube may have a larger diameter than the upper tube, to enhance fluid drainage. Chest tubes are brought out of the chest wall through stab wounds or through the incisional line. The catheters are secured to the client's skin with sutures.

The two chest tubes may be joined to each other with a plastic Y-junction (and then attached to one closed chest drainage system). However, it is preferable to leave them separate and to attach them to separate drainage systems. This makes it possible to monitor air and fluid drainage from each tube and later to remove a nondraining tube without disrupting the rest of the system. Flexible drainage tubing connects the chest tube to the drainage apparatus. Usually, chest tubes are connected to a closed chest drainage apparatus before the client leaves surgery.

■ Nursing Management of the Surgical Client

Preoperative Assessment

Preoperative preparation is the same as for any surgical client but with greater emphasis on assessment and preparation of the respiratory system (see Chapter 21 for discussion of preoperative nursing care).

Preoperative Care

Nursing interventions during the preoperative period are primarily aimed at reducing the client's anxiety level. Anxiety results from fear of cancer and its prognosis, as well as from fear of the surgical procedure and insufficient knowledge of surgical routines and postoperative self-care activities. The client and family are taught about the following:

● The anticipated surgical procedure. Assess the client's (and family's) understanding and give further information as needed.
● The early postoperative period. Talk specifically about what will be happening to the client and how he or she can participate in recovery activities. Specific explanations should be given about the presence of chest tubes (except with pneumonectomy) and drainage tubes, intubation and mechanical ventilation, oxygen therapy, and available pain relief measures.
● Postoperative exercises (Figs. 42–6 and 42–7). These include (1) respiratory exercises to maintain effective pulmonary function; (2) leg exercises to prevent thrombophlebitis; and (3) arm and shoulder exercises to maintain normal range of motion and correct posture. These exercises should be demonstrated, and opportunity should be given for practice and return demonstration.

Postoperative Assessment

During the immediate postoperative period, thorough assessment is essential. Make observations as often as the client's condition warrants. This will be determined by the following factors:

1. The amount of anesthesia received and the client's reaction to it
2. The amount of intraoperative blood loss
3. The client's preoperative condition (e.g., presence of preexisting medical conditions such as diabetes, heart disorders)
4. The client's response to pain
5. Facility protocols

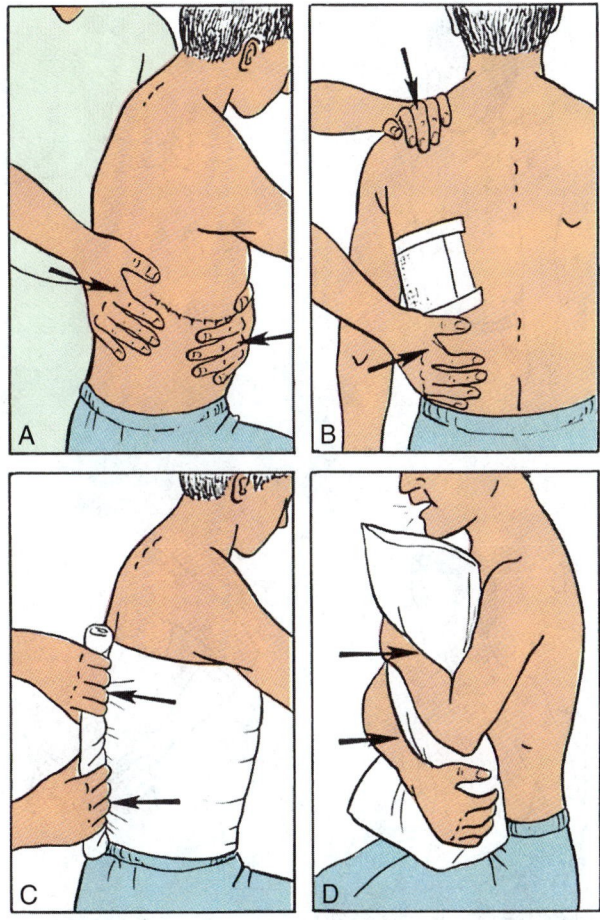

Figure 42–6. Splinting techniques to promote effective coughing and deep breathing. Apply firm, even pressure after the client has taken a deep breath and during forced expiratory cough. Do not squeeze the chest or interfere with chest inspiratory expansion. *A*, Place one hand around the client's back and the other around the incisional area. *B*, Support the area below the incision with one hand while exerting downward pressure on the shoulder on the affected side with the other. *C*, Place a towel or draw sheet snugly (but not tightly) around the chest. *D*, Have the person hug a pillow during forced expiratory cough.

In general, make assessments every 15 minutes until the client is stable, then every 30 minutes for several hours. Hourly assessment is usually indicated throughout the first postoperative night. More frequent assessments may be required if the client's condition changes.

Postoperative Care

Maintaining Closed Chest Drainage

Nursing interventions are based on careful assessment and appropriate nursing diagnoses. General postoperative nursing measures are applicable (see Chapter 21). Nursing management specific to thoracic surgery is discussed in the Care Plan.

The client will have closed chest drainage after all forms of chest surgery (except pneumonectomy) and some forms of chest trauma. Chest surgery causes a

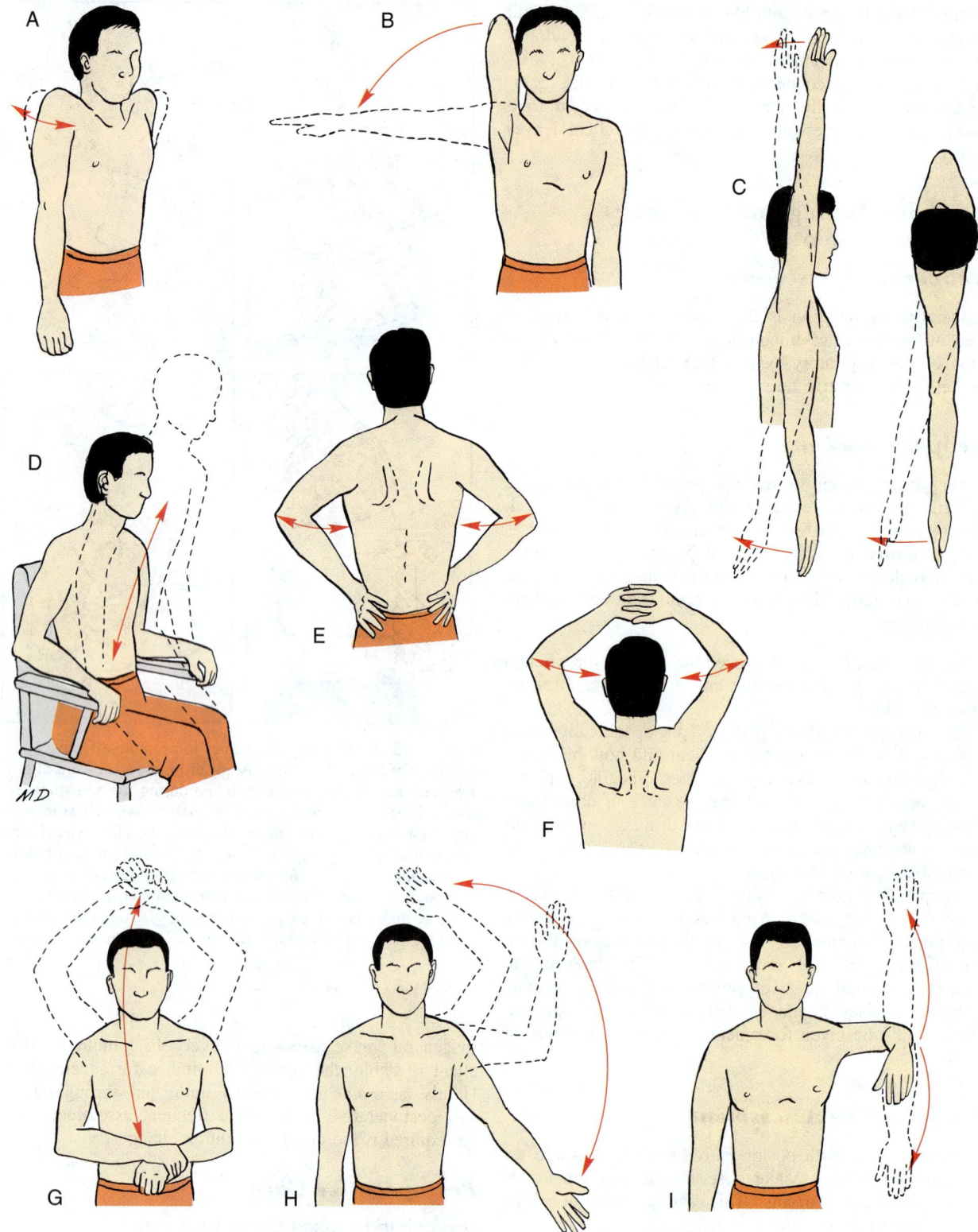

Figure 42–7. Arm and shoulder exercises often prescribed after chest surgery.

pneumothorax on the operated side. During thoracotomy, the parietal pleura is incised and the pleural space is entered. Atmospheric air rushes into the pleural space. This changes the normally negative pressure in that pleural space to a positive pressure. As a result, the lung recoils to its unexpanded size and remains collapsed. Chest trauma, such as fractured ribs, leads to pneumothorax in the same manner. This section discusses the principles and purpose of chest drainage, the specific apparatus used, guidelines for assessing the functioning of

Text continued on page 1163

CARE PLAN

The Client Undergoing Thoracic Surgery

Collaborative Problem. Potential complications of thoracic surgery: pulmonary edema; cardiac dysrhythmias; hemorrhage, hemothorax, and hypovolemic shock; and thrombophlebitis.

- Respiratory insufficiency
- Tension pneumothorax and mediastinal shift
- Subcutaneous emphysema
- Pulmonary embolus

Planning: Expected Outcomes. The nurse will monitor for respiratory, cardiac, and vascular complications.

Implementation: Nursing Intervention	Rationales
Monitor for manifestations of respiratory failure: ■ Increased respiratory rate ■ Dyspnea ■ Use of accessory muscles or retractions ■ Cyanosis ■ Decreased PaO_2 levels and increased $PaCO_2$ levels ■ Restlessness ■ Increase in adventitious breath sounds	Postoperatively, respiratory insufficiency may result from an altered level of consciousness due to anesthesia and pain medications, incomplete lung reinflation, decreased respiratory effort due to chest pain, and inadequate airway clearance.
Monitor for manifestations of tension pneumothorax: ■ Severe dyspnea ■ Tachypnea and tachycardia ■ Extreme restlessness and agitation ■ Progressive cyanosis ■ Laryngeal and tracheal deviation to unaffected side ■ PMI shift laterally or medially	Postoperative tension pneumothorax can result from air leaking through pleural incision lines if closed chest drainage fails to function properly.
Observe for subcutaneous emphysema around incision and in the chest and neck.	Subcutaneous emphysema may result from air leakage at pulmonary incision site.
■ Assess progression by periodically marking the chest with a skin-marking pencil at the outer periphery of emphysematous tissue. If neck involvement occurs, measure neck circumference at least every 2 to 4 hours. ■ Keep emergency tracheostomy tray at beside.	■ Rapid progression (i.e., an increase of more than a hand's width in 1 hour) may indicate leakage through the bronchial stump. ■ Severe subcutaneous emphysema in the neck may compress the trachea and may require tracheostomy.
Monitor for manifestations of pulmonary embolus: ■ Chest pain ■ Dyspnea and tachypnea ■ Fever ■ Hemoptysis ■ Indications of right-sided heart failure	Pulmonary embolism is a serious potential complication after chest surgery and a significant cause of postoperative hypoxemia.
Monitor for signs of acute pulmonary edema: ■ Dyspnea ■ Crackles ■ Persistent cough ■ Frothy sputum ■ Cyanosis	Circulatory overload may result from the reduced size of the pulmonary vascular bed due to surgical removal of pulmonary tissue and delayed reexpansion of the affected lung. Additionally, hypoxia increases capillary permeability, causing fluid to enter pulmonary tissue.
Monitor intravenous flow rates. Consult physician if fluid amounts (maintenance plus intermittent medications [e.g., antibiotics]) exceed 125 ml/hr.	After chest surgery, intravenous fluids should not exceed 125 ml/hr because of possible circulatory overload.
Assess cardiac monitor for the development of cardiac dysrhythmias, particularly atrial fibrillation, atrial flutter, and paroxysmal atrial tachycardia.	Cardiac dysrhythmias are fairly common after chest surgery. Rhythm disturbances result from a combination of factors, including increased vagal tone, hypoxia, mediastinal shift, and abnormal blood pH.

Care Plan continues on following page

CARE PLAN

The Client Undergoing Thoracic Surgery *(Continued)*

Implementation: Nursing Intervention	**Rationales**
Assess dressing and incisional area every 4 hours for evidence of bleeding (increase to every 1 to 2 hours if bleeding develops). Assess drainage in closed chest drainage system for signs of bleeding.	Blood loss may be great with major thoracic surgery because blood vessels in the thorax are of large diameter and the incision is often large and produces considerable capillary oozing.
Monitor for signs of hypovolemic shock: ▪ Increased pulse ▪ Decreased blood pressure ▪ Restlessness and decreased level of consciousness ▪ Decreased urine output ($<$ 30 ml/hr) ▪ Cool, pale, clammy skin ▪ Increased respirations	The body compensates for lost blood volume by increasing blood flow (through increased heart rate) to vital organs and decreasing peripheral circulation.
Monitor for thrombophlebitis: ▪ Unilateral leg edema ▪ Calf tenderness, redness, unusual warmth	Anesthesia and immobility reduce vasomotor tone, leading to decreased venous return and peripheral pooling of blood.
Encourage client to perform leg exercises. Discourage placing pillows under knees, crossing the legs, or prolonged sitting. Apply elastic hose or pneumatic compression stockings, if ordered.	These measures prevent venous stasis, thus reducing the risk of thrombophlebitis.

Evaluation. The nurse monitors for the development of these complications. Most occur early after surgery, except for pulmonary embolus.

Nursing Diagnosis. Ineffective Airway Clearance related to increased secretions and decreased coughing effectiveness due to pain

Planning: Expected Outcomes. The client will demonstrate effective airway clearance, as evidenced by clear breath sounds, effective coughing, and adequate air exchange in the lungs.

Implementation: Nursing Intervention	**Rationales**
Once the vital signs are stable, place the client in the semi-Fowler position. Assist client to cough and deep-breathe at least every 1 or 2 hours during the first 24 to 48 postoperative hours. When possible, schedule coughing and deep-breathing sessions at times when pain medication is maximally effective. Assess breath sounds before and after coughing. Provide support and reassurance:	The upright position enhances lung expansion and facilitates ventilation with minimal effort. Coughing helps to move tracheobronchial secretions out of the lung. Deep-breathing dilates the airways, stimulates surfactant production, and expands lung tissue. The less postoperative pain a client experiences, the more effective are coughing and deep-breathing. This will help in evaluation of coughing effectiveness.
▪ Explain that breathing exercises will not damage lungs or suture line. ▪ Manually splint the incision area during coughing and deep-breathing. ▪ Offer sips of warm water.	▪ Fear of "splitting open" the incision may hamper coughing efforts. ▪ Physical support of the incision is both comforting and reassuring. ▪ Warm water can aid relaxation and produce more effective coughing.
Maintain adequate level of hydration and adequate humidity of inspired air. Monitor results of chest x-rays. Evaluate need for suctioning.	Fluids and moisture help to thin secretions, making them easier to expectorate. Frequent chest films help detect atelectasis and infection. If coughing is ineffective, suctioning may be required to remove pulmonary secretions. Suctioning should be performed cautiously so that disruption of pulmonary suture lines is avoided.

Evaluation. Outcomes on effective airway clearance will require days to achieve.

CARE PLAN

The Client Undergoing Thoracic Surgery *(Continued)*

Nursing Diagnosis. Pain related to surgical procedure

Planning: Expected Outcomes. The client will have improved comfort, as evidenced by verbalizing that discomfort is reduced, using less narcotics, moving in bed with less pain.

Implementation: Nursing Intervention	Rationales
Assess pain intensity using a self-report measurement tool.	Use of a consistent, valid tool promotes communication and evaluation of pain intervention effectiveness.
Administer pain medication as ordered. Observe for side effects of medication used.	Use of narcotics is a common method of postoperative pain control. Narcotics bind to opiate receptors decreasing sensations of pain. Side effects are monitored.
Offer pain medication before pain becomes severe.	A preventive approach to pain control provides a more consistent level of relief and reduces client anxiety.
Assess medication effectiveness and avoid overmedication.	Adequate pain relief must be obtained. However, overmedication can depress respirations and the cough reflex.
Use nonpharmacologic pain relief measures concurrently.	Proper positioning, relaxation techniques, and the like can augment effects of medications.

Evaluation. Pain will be most acute for 48 to 72 hours postoperatively, requiring narcotics for pain control. Expect pain to subside after that time and offer less potent narcotics or analgesics.

Nursing Diagnosis. Impaired Physical Mobility, related to pain, muscle dissection, restricted positioning, and chest tubes

Planning: Expected Outcomes. The client will maintain physical mobility in the arm and shoulder, as evidenced by regaining preoperative arm and shoulder function.

Implementation: Nursing Intervention	Rationales
Position client as indicated by phase of recovery and surgical procedure.	
■ Nonoperative side-lying position may be used until consciousness is regained.	■ This position promotes hemodynamic stability in the immediate postoperative period and prevents aspiration.
■ Semi-Fowler position (head of bed elevated 30 to 45 degrees) is recommended once vital signs are stable.	■ The upright position enhances lung expansion and facilitates chest tube drainage.
■ Avoid positioning client on operative side if a wedge resection or segmentectomy has been performed.	■ Lying on the operative side hinders expansion of remaining lung tissue and may accentuate perfusion of poorly ventilated tissue, thus further impeding normal gas exchange.
■ Avoid complete lateral positioning after pneumonectomy.	■ Because the mediastinum is no longer held in place on both sides by lung tissue, extreme turning may cause mediastinal shift and compression of the remaining lung.
Gently turn the client every 1 to 2 hours, unless contraindicated.	Frequent turning promotes mobilization and drainage of air and fluid from the pleural space. Turning also improves circulation, promotes lung aeration, and enhances comfort.
Avoid traction on chest tubes while changing client position. Check for kinking or compression of tubing.	Traction may dislodge the chest tubes. Kinking or compression inhibits drainage and reestablishment of negative intrapleural pressure.
Encourage regular ambulation, once client's condition is stable. Maintain supplemental oxygen, if ordered.	Early ambulation improves ventilation, circulation, and morale. Oxygen therapy is used to avoid hypoxia.
Begin passive ROM exercises of the arm and shoulder on the affected side 4 hours after recovery from anesthesia. Exercises should be performed two times every 4 to 6 hours through the first 24 postoperative hours, with progression to 10 to 20 times every 2 hours.	ROM exercises help prevent adhesion formation in the operative area, which can lead to dysfunction syndrome (i.e., "frozen shoulder").
Active ROM exercises are begun once the client's condition permits (see Fig. 42–7).	Active ROM exercises prevent adhesions of the incised muscle layers.
Encourage client to use the arm on the affected side in daily activities (e.g., eating, reaching, grooming). Keep bedside stand on the operative side to encourage reaching. Teach importance of continued use after discharge.	Regular use of the affected arm and shoulder reduces the possibility of contractures.

Care Plan continues on following page

CARE PLAN

The Client Undergoing Thoracic Surgery *(Continued)*

Implementation: Nursing Intervention	Rationales
Carefully assess client's response to activity and exercise. Observe for signs of dyspnea, shortness of breath, and fatigue. Allow adequate rest periods between activities.	It may take time for the client's activity tolerance to increase, because the body must adjust to reduced respiratory capacity after resectional surgery. Adequate rest will allow the client to cooperate more fully with activities.

Evaluation. Expect the client to be able to turn independently after 24 hours. Improvement in ROM will require a few days until pain subsides and chest tube is removed.

Nursing Diagnosis. Risk for Ineffective Individual Coping related to temporary dependence and loss of full respiratory function

Planning: Expected Outcomes. The client will use adaptive coping mechanisms, as evidenced by verbalizing feelings related to emotional state and taking appropriate actions to regain self-care capabilities.

Implementation: Nursing Intervention	Rationales
Provide opportunity for client to ventilate feelings. Encourage use of positive coping strategies that have been successful in the past. Allow client to have as much control over daily activities and decision-making as is possible. Support and praise all independent activities that promote recovery.	Loss of normal body function and self-care capabilities can lead to feelings of powerlessness, anger, and grief. Open expression of these feelings can help client to begin the coping process. The use of effective coping actions can decrease feelings of hopelessness and helplessness. Active involvement in the plan of care gives the client a sense of control and promotes return to independence. Emotional support and encouragement help motivate client to continue progress toward independence.

Evaluation. The use of effective coping mechanisms is dependent on prior coping strategies. This outcome may be met quickly if the client is able to cope with a diagnosis of cancer and has hope for recovery and a support system. On the contrary, coping in the face of a dreaded diagnosis, fear of pain, little hope for recovery, and limited support systems will tax coping mechanisms.

Nursing Diagnosis. Altered Health Maintenance related to self-care after discharge

Planning: Expected Outcomes. Client will be able to maintain health, as evidenced by stating or demonstrating discharge plans.

Implementation: Nursing Intervention	Rationales
Provide thorough instruction and preparation for hospital discharge:	Thorough understanding promotes compliance and enhances self-care capabilities.
■ Proper wound care	■ Wound care will vary according to condition of incision and client.
■ Continuation of exercise program	■ Continued exercise increases activity tolerance and prevents complications.
■ Precautions regarding activity and environmental irritants	■ Heavy lifting should be avoided. Return to work will depend on client's condition and type of job. However, it is usually possible to return to work within 4 to 6 weeks. Environmental irritants can cause severe coughing episodes.
■ Clinical manifestations to be reported to healthcare professional	■ Evidence of infection, deteriorating respiratory status, or other complications should be reported promptly.
■ Importance of regular follow-up care	■ The client should be followed closely for signs of surgical complications, recurrence of malignancy, and metastasis.
■ Community agencies that can provide resources, as needed	■ Community resources can facilitate home management.

Evaluation. Client and family must demonstrate understanding of discharge teaching.

PaCO$_2$, partial pressure of arterial carbon dioxide; PaO$_2$, partial pressure of arterial oxygen; PMI, point of maximal impulse; ROM, range of motion; TED, thromboembolic disease.

closed chest drainage systems, precautions, and indications of complications.

Closed chest drainage means that the chest drainage system is closed to atmospheric pressure. Various equipment may be used. Historically, closed chest drainage was performed using a glass bottle water-seal apparatus (one, two, or three bottle setups) with or without controlled mechanical suction. Most healthcare facilities have replaced glass bottle water-seal drainage systems with disposable single units (e.g., Pleur-evac, Atrium, Thora-Seal) (Fig. 42–8). However, an understanding of the basic principles of closed chest drainage will aid understanding of any specific system.

Closed chest drainage following thoracotomy or chest trauma is used to:

- Promote evacuation of air and serosanguineous fluid from the pleural space and prevent their reflux
- Help reexpand the remaining lung tissue by reestablishing normal negative pressure in the pleural space
- Prevent mediastinal shift and pneumothorax by equalizing pressures on both sides of the thoracic cavity

Assessing Chest Drainage. It is important to measure *and* document the amount of drainage coming from the pleural space. This record helps determine the

amount of blood loss and the flow rate of drainage from the pleural space. Disposable plastic systems are manufactured with a marked write-on surface to record the amount of drainage. Drainage rates and amounts are used in planning blood replacement therapy and assessing the client's status. Usually as much as 500 to 1000 ml of drainage occurs in the first 24 hours after chest surgery. Between 100 and 300 ml of drainage may accumulate during the first 2 hours. After this, the drainage should lessen. Excessive drainage may require further surgery to determine its cause.

Chest drainage is normally grossly bloody immediately following surgery. However, it should not continue to be so for more than several hours. Assess blood loss by monitoring the rising fluid level in the collection chamber. Suspect hemorrhage if the blood pressure drops and the pulse is rapid. Check fluid in the drainage collection chamber. If the fluid level has not risen, check the tubes for patency. Notify the surgeon if the drainage remains frankly bloody for longer than the first few postoperative hours, if bleeding recurs after it has stopped, or if there are any other signs of hemorrhage.

Assessing Water Seal Function. A water seal provides a one-way valve between atmospheric pressure and subatmospheric (negative) intrapleural pressure. It allows air and fluid to leave the intrapleural space, but prevents the backflow of atmospheric air into the chest.

On expiration, air and fluid in the pleural space travel through the drainage tubing. The air bubbles up through the water seal and enters atmospheric air.

On inspiration, the water seal prevents atmospheric air from being sucked back into the pleural space (which would collapse the lung). The fluid in the water-seal compartment is not drawn into the chest cavity, because the negative pressures generated in the intrapleural space are not high enough to pull the fluid through the drainage tubing. However, fluctuation of the fluid will occur during respiration. This is known as tidaling.

A water-seal drainage system must be airtight between the pleural space and the water seal. Any air leak allows the entry of atmospheric air into the pleural space, creating a positive pressure that collapses the lung. However, a water-seal chamber *must* have an air vent to provide an escape route for air passing through the water seal from the pleural space.

Observe the water seal. Fluid in the water-seal compartment should rise with inspiration and falls with expiration (tidaling). When tidaling occurs, the drainage tubes are patent, and the apparatus is functioning properly. Tidaling stops when the lung has reexpanded or if the chest drainage tubes are kinked or obstructed. If tidaling does not occur, (1) check to be sure the tube is not kinked or compressed, (2) change the client's position, (3) have the client deep-breathe and cough, and (4) *if indicated*, milk the tube. If these measures do not restore tidaling, notify the surgeon. (*Note:* Tidaling may not occur or may be minimal in systems using suction.)

Observe for bubbling in the water-seal compartment. Bubbling in the water-seal compartment is caused by air passing out of the pleural space into the fluid in the

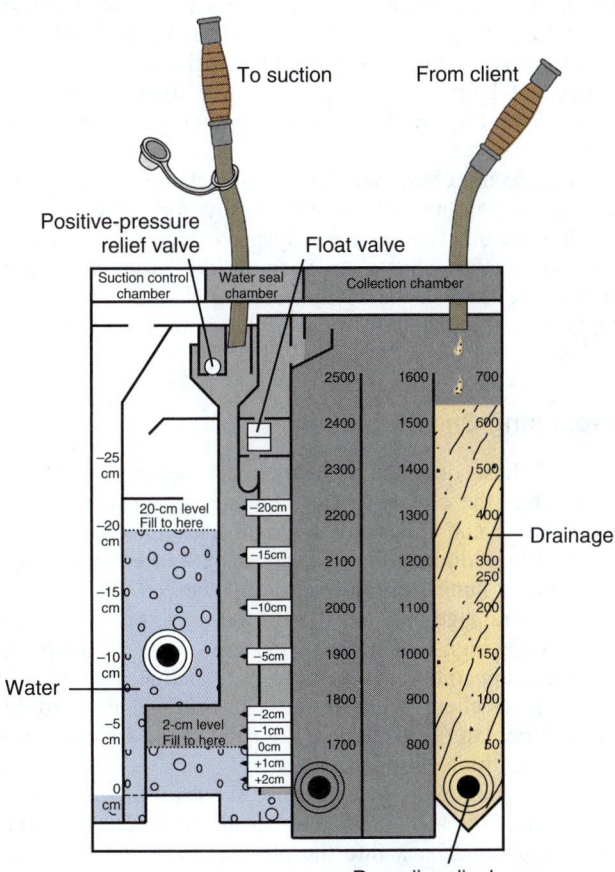

Figure 42–8. A commonly used disposable chest drainage system that combines the three bottles into a single device. (Courtesy of Deknatel, Fall River, MA.)

chamber. Intermittent bubbling is normal. It indicates that the system is accomplishing one of its purposes, that is, removing air from the pleural space.

Continuous bubbling during both inspiration and expiration indicates that air is leaking into the drainage system or pleural cavity. This situation must be corrected, because air entering the system also enters the pleural space. Locate the source of the air leak, and repair it if you can. Begin by inspecting the chest wall where the catheters are inserted. If a chest catheter is loose, gently squeeze the skin up around the catheter or apply sterile petrolatum gauze around the insertion site. Determine whether this stops the continuous bubbling in the chamber. If this does not stop it, check the tubing, inch by inch, and all the connections. A break in the tubing or a loose connection may be found that can be sealed with tape. If the leak still cannot be located, it may be necessary to replace the drainage system.

Rapid bubbling in the absence of an air leak indicates considerable loss of air, as from an incision or tear in the pulmonary pleura. When this occurs, notify the physician *immediately* so that appropriate intervention can be taken to prevent collapse of the lung or mediastinal shift. Suction may be needed, or the amount of suction may need to be increased, or thoracotomy may be necessary.

When caring for a client on water-seal drainage, find out whether this particular client's water-seal chamber should be "bubbling." Knowing this facilitates accurate assessment of the drainage pattern (e.g., if intermittent bubbling changes to constant bubbling or if the apparatus that has not been "bubbling" begins to bubble).

Suction. Suction of 10 to 20 cm H_2O may be applied to a chest drainage system if gravity drainage is not adequate or if a client's cough and respirations are too weak to force air and fluid out of the pleural space through the chest catheters. Additionally, suction may be applied to closed chest drainage (1) if air is leaking into the pleural space faster than it can be removed by a water-seal apparatus or (2) to speed up the removal of air from the pleural space. Suction is regulated by the height of the water column in the suction chamber. The more fluid in the chamber, the more suction (subatmospheric pressure) is created.

If water was not in the chamber, atmospheric air would go straight from the air vent into the suction source as fast as the suction was applied. Passing through water slows the air, and the suction force is controlled. Increasing the source of suction only causes more air to travel through the air vent. The suction applied to the client remains stable. An occluded atmospheric air vent is dangerous because it would cause the suction to be directly applied to the pleural cavity. A suction force greater than 50 cm H_2O may cause lung damage. Some newer drainage systems feature dry suction, which uses a spring or dial mechanism in place of a water column to control the suction level. The advantages include ease in setup, no noise and provision of higher, more precise levels of suction. However, because you cannot directly visualize the suction level via bubbling it is important to check the suction indicator periodically.[20]

Assessing Suction Apparatus Function. Because most suction motors can create potentially damaging amounts of suction, the amount of suction in the system must be controlled. Proper functioning of a wet suction control compartment is indicated by continuous bubbling. Vigorous bubbling does not increase the amount of suction, it just causes the water in the bottle to evaporate more rapidly.

Absence of bubbling in a suction control bottle means that the system is not functioning properly and that the correct level of suction is not being maintained. Possible reasons for malfunction of a mechanical suction apparatus include (1) large amounts of air leaking into the pleural space or into the drainage apparatus and (2) mechanical problems in the pump or suction power source. The most serious problem is air leaking into the pleural space.

If bubbling in the suction control chamber stops, check for air leaks by briefly clamping the chest drainage tube and observing the suction control chamber. If bubbling begins in the suction control chamber there is nothing wrong with either the drainage apparatus or the pump. The problem is therefore an air leak into the pleural space around the chest tubes. If the air leak cannot be sealed off (e.g., with petrolatum gauze), notify the surgeon immediately. If bubbling does not begin in the suction control chamber when the chest catheter is clamped, the problem is in the drainage connections or the pump. Check the system carefully, looking for loose connections, air leaks around compartment tops, or air leaks in the tubing (e.g., split tubing). Also, make sure that the tubing is not kinked, is correctly positioned, and has no dependent loops. If the suction power source appears to be causing the problem, obtain another pump or power source.

Because the chest catheter remains clamped during this inspection, observe the client closely for indications of tension pneumothorax (e.g., dyspnea, tachycardia, hypotension, trachea shift). As soon as the problem is corrected, the fluid in the suction control chamber will begin to bubble. Immediately remove the clamps on the chest catheter.

Promoting Chest Drainage

Closed chest drainage systems must always be placed lower than the client's chest. Drainage by gravity is thus maintained, and fluid is not forced back into the pleural space. Chest drainage systems must be placed upright on the floor or hung from the bottom of the bed.

If the drainage apparatus is on the floor, be careful not to lower a high-low bed or side rails onto it. Keep the drainage apparatus about 2 to 3 ft below the client's chest. If a client with closed chest drainage is to be moved, be careful to always keep the chest drainage system below the level of the chest.

If the apparatus is placed above the level of the client's chest, even for a moment, fluid from the drainage chamber is siphoned back into the pleural cavity. If absolutely necessary, chest tubes may be double-clamped very briefly during momentary movement of the apparatus above the level of the person's chest (e.g., when moving drainage apparatus from one side of the bed to the other if the tubing is not long enough to allow movement around an end of the bed).

Follow positioning orders carefully. If a client can be positioned on the side that has chest tubes, be sure the client is not lying on (compressing or kinking) the catheters or tubing. This could (1) impair drainage and cause retrograde pressure (forcing drainage back into the pleural cavity) and (2) increase the client's discomfort. Coil the drainage tubing on the client's mattress so it falls straight to the drainage apparatus, with no dependent loops. Dependent loops of tubing that contain fluid obstruct fluid flow and create backpressure, thus impairing air or fluid drainage.

Make sure the tubing is long enough to allow the person to turn and sit up without pulling on the chest tubes. Each time the client is turned or moved, check the chest tubes to be sure they are not being pulled or displaced, and check drainage tubing to be certain it is properly positioned.

Drainage tubing (connecting the chest tube to the drainage apparatus) should be neither too short nor too long. Excessive tubing length causes tangling and kinking.

Patency is unlikely to be a problem when chest tubes are evacuating air only or when fluid or blood is draining well by gravity. However, if fragments of a blood clot or lung tissue are visible in the tube, use of chest tube clearance techniques *may* be indicated. Traditionally, nurses have manipulated chest tubes by "milking" and "stripping" (Fig. 42–9). To strip a chest tube, gently compress it and slide your hand down the tubing, away from the client's chest and toward the drainage system. The tubing is stabilized with the other hand so that the tube will not be pulled on or displaced while stripping. To milk a chest tube compress the tube intermittently using a twisting or squeezing motion.

Theoretically, these techniques dislodge clot material from the tube lumen and propel it towards the drainage collection chamber. However, several recent studies have demonstrated no difference in tube patency with or without manipulation.[40] Additionally, stripping a chest tube may cause complications because it creates excessive negative intrapleural pressure (over -100 cm H_2O). Therefore, each patient's clinical situation should be evaluated individually before clearance techniques are used.[40]

Activity with Chest Drainage

Encourage a client on closed chest drainage to cough and deep-breathe frequently. In addition to clearing the bronchi of secretions, these activities promote lung expansion and the expulsion of air and fluid from the pleural space by increasing intrapulmonary and intrapleural pressure.

A client with a chest drainage system can sit up in bed, get in and out of bed, and ambulate without clamping the chest tubes as long as the apparatus stays upright. Do not exert traction (pulling) on the tubing. Various arrangements are used to hold a person's chest drainage system below waist level during ambulation. The device may be placed in a wheelchair in front of the client. Many disposable units have handles to allow for carrying. If the

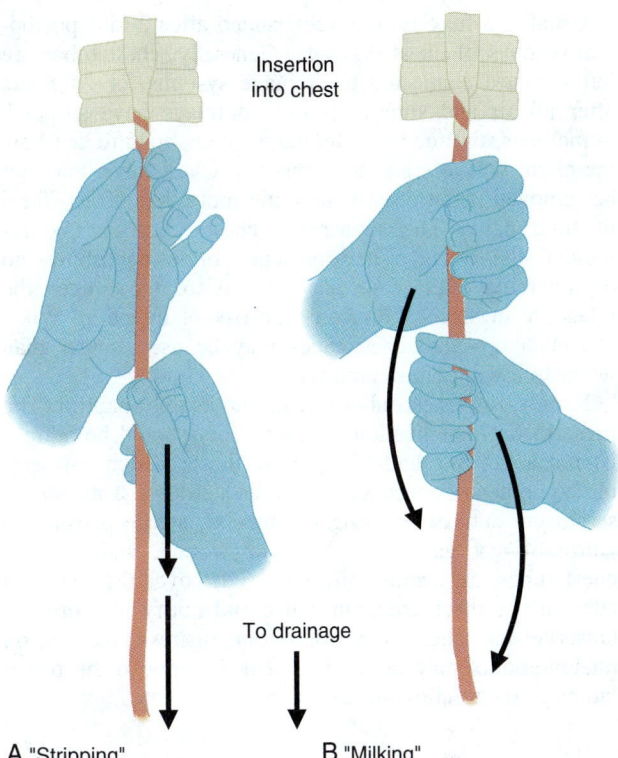

Figure 42–9. Stripping and milking of chest tubes is performed carefully to remove blood clots, but these procedures are not performed routinely.

client's condition warrants, suction may be ordered removed during ambulation.

Clamping Chest Drainage Tubing

In most situations, clamping of chest tubes is contraindicated. When the client has a residual air leak or pneumothorax, clamping the chest tube may precipitate a tension pneumothorax because the air has no escape route. If the tube becomes disconnected, it is best to immediately reattach it to the drainage system or to submerge the end in a bottle of sterile water or saline to reestablish a water seal. If fluid is not readily available, it is preferable to leave the tube open as the risk of tension pneumothorax outweighs the consequences of an open tube.[20]

However, there are occasions when clamping is appropriate. These include assessment of a persistent air leak, assessment of readiness for removal, or changing the drainage system. Except for those occasions in which clamping is clearly indicated, *never* clamp chest drainage tubes without an order to do so. If clamps must be used, the best time to apply them is following an expiration. Remove the clamps as soon as possible.

Removing Chest Tubes

The physician determines when to remove chest tubes and closed chest drainage. One indication is that the lung has reexpanded noted by the cessation of fluctuation in the water-seal chamber (if suction is not applied). Chest auscultation, chest percussion, and chest x-ray study confirm lung reexpansion.

Usually, a lung is fully reexpanded after 2 to 3 postoperative days of chest drainage. Generally, chest tubes are left in place connected to drainage systems for 24 hours after all air and significant fluid drainage have stopped. Sometimes, the tubes are temporarily clamped to see how the client will tolerate their removal. Chest tubes may not be removed if the chest is draining more than 50 to 70 ml of fluid daily. The sooner the chest tubes can be removed, the better. Their presence often contributes to postoperative pain and inactivity. Also, the longer the tubes are in place, the greater the risk of infection. When treating empyema, chest tubes may be used longer than when following chest surgery.

Removal of chest tubes can be moderately painful. The prescribed premedication for pain relief should be administered about one half-hour before the procedure. Assemble equipment as necessary, such as sterile scissors, suture set to cut sutures securing the tube(s), sterile petrolatum gauze, 4 × 4 gauze to cover the wound, and tape. If chest tubes are accidentally removed, cover the insertion site with sterile petrolatum gauze and notify the surgeon. Observe the client for respiratory distress, as tension pneumothorax may develop. If it does, remove the petrolatum gauze to allow air to escape.

Benign Lung Tumors

Benign pulmonary neoplasms account for less than 10% of all primary pulmonary tumors. The term "benign" may be misleading, because although they are not directly harmful to the body, some of these tumors may still have serious physiologic effects. Mechanical interference with lung function (e.g., obstruction of a major bronchus) may occur, depending on the tumor's location. In addition, some of these tumors may become malignant over time.

The most common benign lung tumor is the hamartoma, which usually arises in peripheral lung parenchyma. This tumor is more common in older men. Other benign tumor types include the fibroma, hemangioma, lipoma, and papilloma.

Benign lung tumors are often difficult to diagnose because clients may be asymptomatic. Unless there is preexisting lung disease or major airway obstruction, pulmonary function studies and ABGs are usually within normal limits. The tumor may be first detected by chest x-ray. Confirmatory diagnosis usually requires bronchoscopy or, more commonly, thoracotomy.

Until the diagnosis is confirmed, most clients will be quite anxious and fearful of the possibility of cancer. Emotional support is an important adjunct to the physical preparation required for diagnostic procedures.

Surgical intervention is the treatment of choice for all benign neoplasms. Tumor removal promptly alleviates any respiratory symptoms that may have resulted from pressure on lung structures. Postoperative management is the same as that used with the surgical treatment of malignant lung disease.

Disorders of the Pleura and Pleural Space

Pleural Pain

Pleural pain is a common pulmonary manifestation associated with a variety of disorders. It arises from the parietal pleura, which is richly supplied with sensory nerve endings. Pleuritic pain indicates the presence of pleural inflammation (pleurisy) due to pneumonia, pulmonary infarction, or other cause; pleural effusion; or pneumothorax. It is often accompanied by a pleural friction rub that is discovered during chest auscultation.

Pleuritic chest pain often develops abruptly and is usually severe enough that the client seeks medical attention. It frequently occurs only on one side of the chest, usually in the lower lateral portions of the chest wall, and is aggravated by deep breathing or coughing. Often the client can point directly to the exact location of the pain. However, pleural pain may also be referred to the neck, shoulder, or abdomen. Because other types of chest pain (e.g., cardiac pain, chest wall pain) may be misinterpreted as pleuritic pain, careful assessment is necessary.

Pleuritic chest pain may restrict normal respiratory efforts, leading to problems with gas exchange and airway clearance. If pain-relieving measures, including administration of prescribed analgesics, do not relieve the pain, the physician may perform an intercostal nerve block (see Chapter 17).

Pleural Effusion

A pleural effusion is an accumulation of fluid in the pleural space. Pleural fluid normally seeps continually into the pleural space from the capillaries lining the parietal pleura and is reabsorbed by the visceral pleural capillaries and lymphatics. Any condition that interferes with either secretion or drainage of this fluid will lead to pleural effusion.

Causes of pleural effusion can be grouped into four major categories. They are conditions that:

1. Increase systemic hydrostatic pressure (e.g., congestive heart failure)
2. Reduce capillary oncotic pressure (e.g., liver or renal failure)
3. Increase capillary permeability (e.g., infections or trauma)
4. Impair lymphatic function (e.g., lymphatic obstruction due to tumor)

Clinical manifestations of pleural effusion will depend on the amount of fluid present and the degree of lung compression. If the effusion is small (i.e., < 250 ml), its presence may be discovered only by chest x-ray examination. With large effusions, lung expansion may be restricted and the client may experience dyspnea, primarily on exertion, and a dry, nonproductive cough caused by bronchial irritation or mediastinal shift. Tactile fremitus may be decreased or absent, and percussion notes may be dull or flat.

Primary Pleural Effusion

Thoracentesis (see Chapter 40) is used to remove excess pleural fluid. The fluid is analyzed to determine if it is transudate or exudate. Transudates are substances that have passed through a membrane or tissue surface. They occur primarily in conditions in which there is protein loss and low protein content (e.g., hypoalbuminemia, cirrhosis, nephrosis) or increased hydrostatic pressure (e.g., congestive heart failure). Exudates are substances that have escaped from blood vessels. They contain an accumulation of cells, have a high specific gravity, and a high lactate dehydrogenase (LDH) level, and occur in response to malignancies, infections, or inflammatory processes. Exudates occur when there is an increase in capillary permeability. Differentiating between transudates and exudates helps establish a specific diagnosis. Diagnosis may also require analysis of the fluid for (1) white and red blood cells, (2) malignant cells, (3) bacteria, (4) glucose content, (5) pH, and (6) LDH.

Pleural fluid may be (1) hemorrhagic, or bloody (e.g., if tumor is present, after trauma, or after pulmonary embolus with infarction), (2) chylous, or thick and white-colored (e.g., after lymphatic obstruction or trauma to the thoracic duct), or (3) rich in cholesterol (e.g., chronic, recurrent effusions due to tuberculous or rheumatoid arthritis).

If there is a high WBC count and the pleural fluid is purulent, the effusion is called an empyema. An empyema of any amount requires drainage and treatment of the infection. If the pus is not drained, it may become thick and almost solidified or loculated (containing cavities). This is called fibrothorax. Fibrothorax may significantly restrict lung expansion and may require surgical intervention. The procedure, known as decortication, involves removal of the restrictive mass of fibrin and inflammatory cells. Decortication is usually not performed until the fibrothorax is relatively solid, so it can be easily removed. After the procedure, closed chest drainage with suction is used to reexpand the lung rapidly and fill the pleural space. If the fibrous material has restricted the lung for some time, the lung may not reexpand effectively, and further intervention (usually thoracoplasty) may be needed.

Recurrent Pleural Effusion

In some cases, pleural effusions may recur despite repeated thoracenteses (e.g., malignancy-induced effusions), with resultant compromise of lung function or persistent pleural pain. Treatment of recurrent effusions is accomplished through obliteration of the pleural space. Methods of obliterating the pleural space include the following:

● Pleurectomy (pleural stripping). This procedure consists of surgically stripping the parietal pleura away from the visceral pleura. This produces an intense inflammatory reaction that promotes adhesion formation between the two layers during healing.
● Pleurodesis. This involves the instillation of a sclerosing substance (e.g., unbuffered tetracycline, nitrogen mustard, talc) into the pleural space via a thoracotomy tube. This creates an inflammatory response that scleroses tissue together.

Because pleural space obliteration creates permanent changes, the client's existing and predicted postprocedure respiratory status must be carefully evaluated. If a large area is involved, significant alterations in ventilatory mechanics (e.g., deep-breathing, coughing) may occur, leading to compromised respiratory function.

After the procedure, closely monitor lung function, including respiratory rate and ventilation pattern. Document alleviation or persistence of pleural pain and watch for indications of a return of the pleural effusion. Pulmonary function studies (see Chapter 40) and ABGs should also be evaluated.

Bronchopleural Fistula

A bronchopleural fistula is a communication between the pleural space and a bronchus. It may occur when (1) an undrained empyema erodes into a bronchus or (2) the pleural space does not heal spontaneously after chest tube removal. A bronchopleural fistula increases the risk of pleural infection. It may also compromise ventilation and oxygenation.

The management of a client with a bronchopleural fistula is often complex. Bronchopleural fistulas may be slow to heal. The client may be discharged home with a chest tube connected to a collection system. It is important that the client and family understand how to care for the chest tube and collection system and recognize manifestations of irritation at the chest puncture site and changes in chest drainage (e.g., blood) that require the physician to be notified.

Metastatic Pleural Tumors

Primary tumors in the lungs and other organs often metastasize to the pleura. The primary tumor is usually in a lung but may occur in the breast, ovaries, liver, kidneys, uterus, testicles, or larynx, or it may result from leukemia or lymphoma. Metastatic pleural disease frequently causes pleural effusions.

Assessment findings with malignant pleural effusion are the same as for pleural effusion from other causes. Diagnosis of pleural effusion is by chest x-ray examination. The source of the effusion is determined by cytologic examination of pleural fluid obtained by thoracentesis. Intervention is the same as for any pleural effusion, along with treatment of the primary malignancy.

Disorders of the Diaphragm

Subdiaphragmatic Abscess

A subdiaphragmatic abscess may develop as a result of (1) gastrointestinal perforation; (2) surgery of the upper gastrointestinal system, liver, or biliary tract; (3) abdominal trauma; or (4) other intra-abdominal surgery. A subdiaphragmatic abscess produces abdominal and thoracic clinical manifestations that potentially compromise respiratory status.

Thoracic assessment findings may include pleuritic pain or pain referred to the shoulder on the affected side. Dyspnea and poor or no diaphragmatic movement are common. Abdominal assessment findings may include flank pain or tenderness and a palpable abdominal mass in the region of the abscess. Generalized assessment findings include fever, anorexia, weight loss, and vomiting.

A subdiaphragmatic abscess is diagnosed by chest x-ray. The diaphragm is generally elevated on the affected side. Fluoroscopic studies of diaphragmatic movement reveal limited or absent diaphragmatic movement on the affected side. Pleural effusion also commonly occurs. Thoracentesis and analysis of the pleural fluid reveal an exudate. Subdiaphragmatic abscesses may erode and perforate the diaphragm.

Intervention for subdiaphragmatic abscess includes (1) antibiotic administration, (2) draining the abscess, and (3) supportive measures to maintain ventilation and respiratory status. An untreated subdiaphragmatic abscess is nearly always fatal. With treatment, the mortality rate is still high but drops to approximately 25%.

Diaphragmatic Paralysis

Many situations may affect diaphragm function and result in paralysis, either unilateral or bilateral. Unilateral diaphragmatic paralysis is more common than bilateral. Causes of unilateral diaphragmatic paralysis include the following:

1. Severing of the phrenic nerve during surgery
2. Bronchogenic or metastatic tumors
3. Neurologic disorders such as poliomyelitis, encephalitis, herpes zoster, and diphtheria
4. Accidental or birth trauma
5. Mechanical obstruction (e.g., from aortic aneurysm)
6. Infectious processes such as tuberculosis, pneumonia, pleuritic disorders, or subdiaphragmatic abscess
7. Other disorders (e.g., pulmonary infarction, congenital abnormalities)

Causes of bilateral diaphragmatic paralysis include (1) many neuromuscular disorders, including amyotrophic lateral sclerosis, muscular dystrophy, and Guillain-Barré syndrome; (2) alcohol and lead neuropathy; (3) closed chest trauma; and (4) anatomic causes, such as congenital absence of the phrenic nerve, traumatic diaphragmatic rupture, and spinal injuries.

Although the diaphragm is the primary muscle of respiration, its role can be assumed in part by the accessory and abdominal muscles. As a result, diaphragmatic paralysis is often difficult to detect.

Unilateral diaphragmatic paralysis is diagnosed by fluoroscopy. The client is asked to "sniff" during fluoroscopy. If paralysis is present, the nonparalyzed side of the diaphragm descends during inspiration (the sniff), and the paralyzed side paradoxically rises during this maneuver. Clients with unilateral diaphragmatic paralysis usually experience dyspnea when lying on the affected side. Dyspnea on exertion is not usual unless there is underlying lung disease. Both TLC and vital capacity (VC) are reduced by about 20%. There is also less ventilation to the affected side and mild hypoxemia because of shifts of ventilation and blood flow. Preexisting lung disease combined with unilateral diaphragmatic paralysis may be disabling, depending on the extent of the lung disease.

The effects of bilateral diaphragmatic paralysis are potentially much more severe than those of unilateral paralysis. However, the problem is often subtle and overlooked, especially if the client has a neuromuscular disorder. Fatigue, disturbed sleep, and morning headache are frequently the only manifestations. A classic manifestation of bilateral paralysis of the diaphragm is increased dyspnea when lying flat on the back (supine). Paradoxical inward abdominal movement during inspiration when supine and active use of the accessory muscles of inspiration also occur. The pulmonary effects of bilateral paralysis include reduced VC and TLC when the client is upright, which are even more reduced when the client is supine. Functional residual capacity (FRC) is also decreased, as is lung compliance. In the side-lying position, ventilation is preferentially distributed to the uppermost lung tissue and away from blood flow, which leads to a significant mismatch of ventilation and perfusion. Severe hypoxemia results. Reduced tidal volume leads to retention of carbon dioxide and respiratory acidosis. Respiratory muscle function decreases during rest and sleep, further compromising respiratory status.

Little can be done to treat diaphragmatic paralysis. Management is aimed, instead, at supporting ventilatory function, as needed. If the phrenic nerve is intact, a phrenic nerve pacer may be surgically inserted. However, this is possible only if the phrenic nerve can be stimulated (this is tested by a fluoroscopic procedure). This procedure is useful primarily for clients with spinal cord injuries.

Assess the client for subjective indications of hypoxemia or hypercapnia. Monitor ventilatory mechanics (e.g., inspiratory effort, spontaneous VC) and ABGs, observing for deteriorating trends.

Nursing management focuses on maintenance of a patent airway and detection of deteriorating gas exchange. Because inspiration is impaired, the client may need assistance to cough and deep-breathe effectively. Position the client on the unaffected side in the semi-sitting or sitting position. Suction as necessary. Increase hydration to liquify secretions. Administer oxygen, as prescribed. If respiratory function declines significantly, the physician and client (or possibly significant others) must decide whether to place a permanent tracheostomy and to use mechanical ventilation or other assistance devices (e.g., rocking bed, cuirass respirator).

Acute Pulmonary Disorders

Noncardiogenic Pulmonary Edema

Pulmonary edema is the abnormal accumulation of fluid in the interstitial and alveolar spaces. It results from an imbalance between hydrostatic and colloidal osmotic pressures within the respiratory circulation. When the normal balance between these two forces is disturbed (i.e., hydrostatic pressure increases or colloidal osmotic pressure decreases), fluid leaves the pulmonary capillaries and enters interstitial spaces.

Some fluid in the interstitial spaces of the lungs is not uncommon. It normally escapes from the microcirculation and enters the interstitium, providing nutrients for the cells. The lymphatic system drains excess interstitial fluid volume. Additional fluid in the pleura drains into the hilar lymph nodes. However, if this pathway becomes overwhelmed, fluid moves from the interstitium into the alveolar walls. If the alveolar epithelium is damaged, the fluid accumulates in the alveoli. Alveolar edema is a serious late sign in the progression of fluid imbalance.

Pulmonary edema most commonly results from left-sided heart failure (see Chapter 45). When pulmonary edema does not result from heart failure, it is called noncardiogenic pulmonary edema. Several conditions may lead to noncardiogenic pulmonary edema (Box 42–5). Sometimes, the precipitating event has occurred 12 to 24 hours earlier (e.g., smoke inhalation). At other times, noncardiogenic pulmonary edema develops rapidly, as with neurogenic causes.

Box 42–5. Common Causes of Noncardiogenic Pulmonary Edema

- Aspiration of gastric contents, especially if a significant amount of hydrochloric acid is present
- Drugs (e.g., after administration of narcotics)
- Fluid overload from intravenous fluids
- Hypoalbuminemia (e.g., nephrotic syndrome, hepatic disease, malnutrition)
- Smoke inhalation (e.g., trapped in a burning building)
- Inhalation of toxic chemicals (e.g., sulfur dioxide, paraquat, phosgene, chlorine, nitrogen oxides)
- High altitudes (i.e., greater than 8000 ft)
- Neurogenic stimulus (e.g., conditions causing increased intracranial pressure, epileptic seizures, head trauma)
- Near-drowning syndrome
- Mechanical ventilation, oxygen toxicity, adult respiratory distress syndrome (ARDS)
- Malignancies blocking outflow of lymph within the lungs
- Unilaterally, after reexpansion of collapsed lung (pneumothorax)

Manifestations of pulmonary edema are the same, regardless of the cause. In the noncardiogenic form, however, no signs of cardiac involvement (i.e., cardiac enlargement, presence of S_3 heart sound, jugular vein distention, and elevated pulmonary wedge pressures) will be seen. Dyspnea will be present, usually accompanied by a cough. As fluid fills the interstitium and alveolar spaces, lung compliance decreases and oxygen diffusion is impaired. Cyanosis may be present and ABGs reveal progressive hypoxemia. Chest auscultation reveals crackles and occasional diffuse wheezing.

Medical and nursing management of noncardiogenic pulmonary edema are essentially the same as for adult respiratory distress syndrome (see later). Overall, intervention is aimed at reversing the precipitating event and providing supportive respiratory measures.

Acute Respiratory Failure

Respiratory failure is a broad, nonspecific clinical diagnosis used to indicate that the respiratory system is unable to supply the oxygen necessary to maintain metabolism or cannot eliminate sufficient carbon dioxide. Acute respiratory failure is defined as a partial pressure of arterial oxygen (PaO_2) of 50 mm Hg or less or a partial pressure of arterial carbon dioxide ($PaCO_2$) of 50 mm Hg or more. In clients with chronic hypercapnia, $PaCO_2$ elevations of 5 mm Hg or more from their previously stable levels indicate acute respiratory failure superimposed on chronic respiratory failure. Various factors may precipitate respiratory failure. If these factors are not recognized and corrected, other organ systems are affected. Box 42–6 lists some causes of acute respiratory failure.

Classically, a client in acute respiratory failure has an elevated $PaCO_2$ directly related to alveolar hypoventilation from either (1) decreased minute ventilation with normal dead space ventilation or (2) normal or increased minute ventilation with increased dead space ventilation. In the first category are clients with normal lungs whose respiratory status is impaired by drugs or diseases affecting respiration (e.g., neuromuscular disorders). In the second category are clients with intrinsic lung diseases such as COPD or severe pneumonia. Lung damage in these clients increases the amount of nonfunctional lung tissue, thus increasing dead space (or wasted) ventilation. Even with normal or increased minute ventilation, they cannot "blow off" a sufficient amount of carbon dioxide.

Diagnosis of respiratory failure is sometimes difficult. Assessment findings indicating hypoxemia and hypercapnia often occur subtly. By the time abnormalities are recognized, an emergency may exist. If respiratory failure is suspected, confirmation with ABG analysis is essential. Diagnosis is made by clinical observation, chest x-ray, and blood gas analysis.

Medical management of clients in acute respiratory failure is directed to (1) treating the underlying cause of the respiratory failure and (2) restoring gas exchange to maintain physiologic function.

Nursing intervention focuses on the following:

1. Promoting effective airway clearance and adequate gas exchange

---

Box 42–6. Causes of Acute Respiratory Failure

Factors Decreasing Ventilatory Drive

■ Depression of respiratory drive with drugs (e.g., barbiturates, sedatives, narcotics, tranquilizers)
■ Brain disorders (e.g., stroke, brain tumor, brain trauma)
■ Obstructive sleep apnea syndrome
■ Obesity

Chest Wall Dysfunction and Neuromuscular Factors

■ Anesthetic blocking agents
■ Cervical spinal cord injury
■ Neuromuscular disorders (e.g., muscular dystrophy, Guillain-Barré syndrome, amyotrophic lateral sclerosis, poliomyelitis, and post-polio syndrome)
■ Neuromuscular blocking agents (e.g., curare)
■ Kyphoscoliosis

Factors in Lung Parenchyma

■ Near drowning
■ Pneumonia
■ Interstitial lung diseases
■ Pulmonary edema
■ Chronic airflow limitation
■ Adult respiratory distress syndrome (ARDS)
■ Inhalation of toxic chemicals, gases, or smoke
■ Pulmonary contusion

Other Factors

■ Carbon monoxide inhalation
■ Upper airway obstruction (e.g., foreign body, tumor)
■ Abdominal distention due to intestinal obstruction
■ Ascites

---

2. Preventing complications of immobility
3. Monitoring and documenting indications of altered tissue perfusion
4. Monitoring and promoting effective breathing patterns
5. Reducing anxiety and fear
6. Promoting comfort

If endotracheal intubation and mechanical ventilation are required, the client must communicate nonverbally. When acute respiratory failure is superimposed on chronic respiratory disease or chronic respiratory failure, nursing intervention is directed to (1) promoting self-care and (2) performing teaching activities to prevent complications and increase treatment compliance.

Adult Respiratory Distress Syndrome

Adult respiratory distress syndrome (ARDS) is a sudden, progressive pulmonary disorder characterized by severe dyspnea, hypoxemia, and diffuse bilateral infiltrates. It follows acute and massive lung injury that results from a variety of clinical states, often occurring in previously healthy persons. The syndrome was first described in 1967 and has been alternatively referred to by a variety of terms, including shock lung, wet lung, Da Nang lung (in reference to the high number of cases observed during the Vietnam War era), post-traumatic lung, congestive atelectasis, capillary leak syndrome, and adult hyaline membrane disease. Tremendous advances in the treatment of this condition have occurred over the last two decades. However, mortality rates remain in the 40% to 60% range.[42]

Etiology and Risk Factors

ARDS develops as a result of an insult, condition, or noxious event that traumatizes the lung tissue. The insult may be directly to lung tissue or indirect, occurring in other body areas. Conditions leading to ARDS are listed in Box 42–7. Early recognition and treatment of these conditions may reduce the risk of ARDS.

Pathophysiology

The hallmark of ARDS is increased permeability of the alveolar membrane, with resultant movement of fluid into the interstitial and alveolar spaces. This leads to the development of pulmonary edema, which decreases lung compliance and impairs oxygen transport. The type II alveolar cells, which produce pulmonary surfactant, are also damaged, which leads to atelectasis and further impairment in lung distensibility and gas exchange. Inflammatory responses accompany the pulmonary parenchymal damage, leading to the release of toxic mediators, the activation of complement, the mobilization of macro-

---

Box 42–7. Clinical States That May Lead to Adult Respiratory Distress Syndrome (ARDS)

Direct Pulmonary Trauma

■ Viral, bacterial, or fungal pneumonias
■ Lung contusion
■ Fat embolus
■ Aspiration (e.g., foreign material, drowning, vomitus)
■ Massive smoke inhalation
■ Inhaled toxins
■ Prolonged exposure to high concentrations of oxygen

Indirect Pulmonary Trauma

■ Sepsis
■ Shock
■ Multisystem trauma
■ Disseminated intravascular coagulation
■ Pancreatitis
■ Uremia
■ Drug overdose
■ Anaphylaxis
■ Idiopathic
■ Prolonged heart bypass surgery
■ Massive blood transfusions
■ Pregnancy-induced hypertension
■ Increased intracranial pressure
■ Radiation therapy

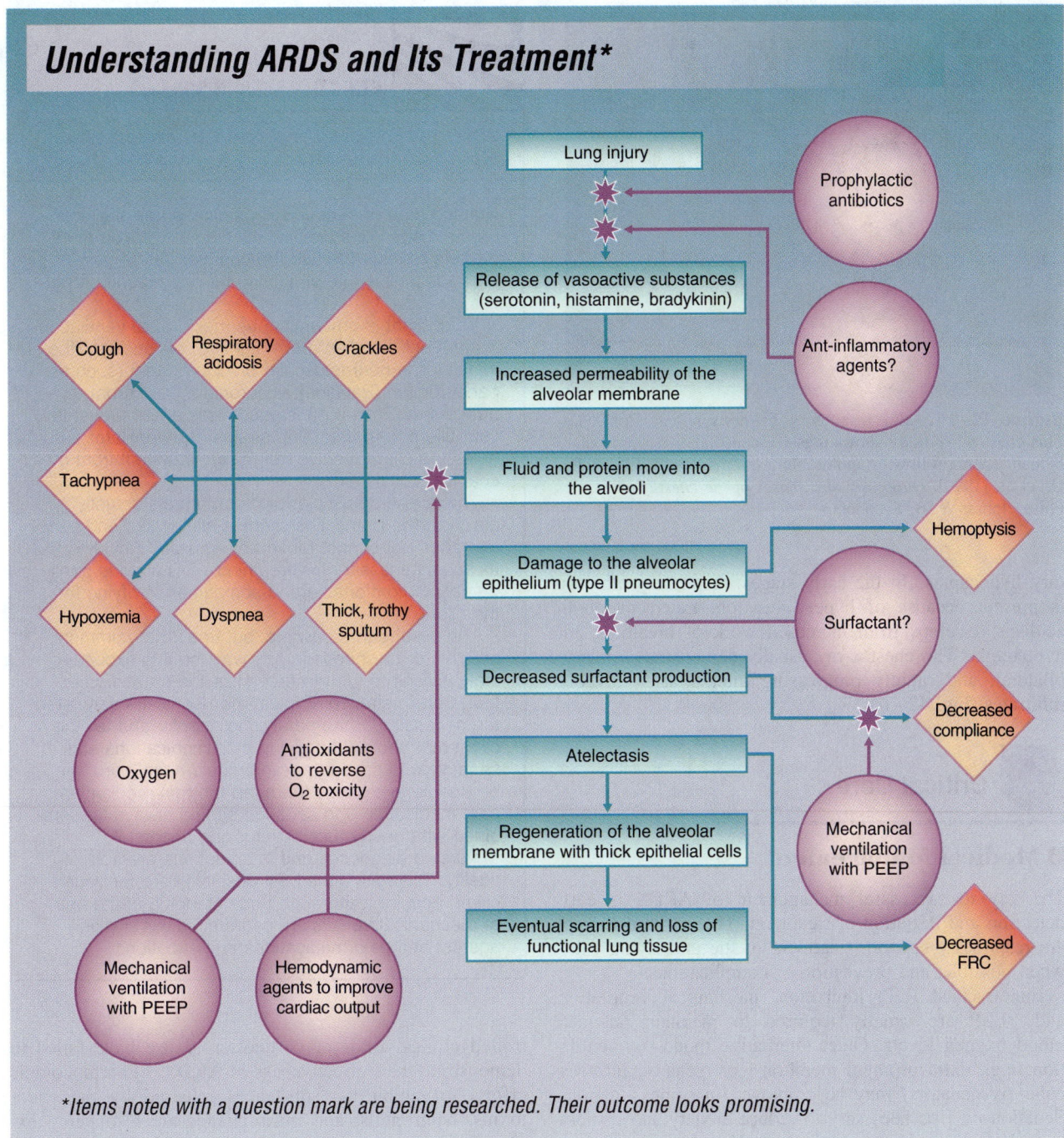

Understanding ARDS and Its Treatment*

*Items noted with a question mark are being researched. Their outcome looks promising.

phages, and the release of vasoactive substances from mast cells. These events lead to additional endothelial and epithelial injury and increased capillary permeability. The end result is a significant ventilation-perfusion imbalance and profound arterial hypoxemia (see Understanding ARDS and Its Treatment).

Clinical Manifestations and Diagnostic Findings

The initial insult is followed by a period of apparently normal lung function that may last from 1 to 96 hours.

Then hypoxemia rapidly develops and progresses, along with decreasing lung compliance and the development of diffuse lung infiltrates.

The earliest clinical sign of ARDS is usually an increased respiratory rate. Breathing becomes increasingly labored; the client may exhibit air hunger, retractions, and cyanosis. Chest auscultation may or may not reveal the presence of adventitious sounds. If present, abnormal sounds may range from fine inspiratory crackles to widespread coarse crackles.

Blood gas analysis reveals increasing hypoxemia ($PaO_2 < 60$ mm Hg) that does not respond to increased fraction of inspired oxygen levels ($FIO_2 < 40\%$) and compensa-

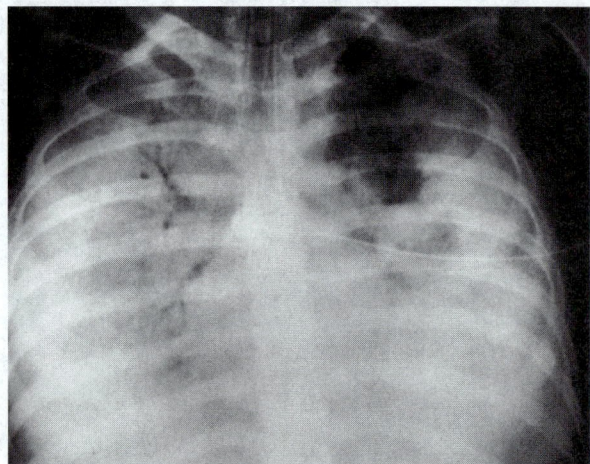

Figure 42–10. Adult respiratory distress syndome (ARDS). This chest x-ray study shows massive consolidation from pulmonary edema following multisystem trauma. (From Fraser, R. G., et al, [1990]. *Diagnosis of diseases of the chest* (3rd ed.). Philadelphia: W. B. Saunders.)

tory hypocapnia. In the early stages, respiratory alkalosis is present because of hyperventilation. Later, metabolic acidosis develops from increased work of breathing and hypoxemia. The chest x-ray usually demonstrates diffuse, bilateral, and rapidly progressing interstitial or alveolar infiltrates (Fig. 42–10).

 ## Critical Care

■ Medical Management

The key to successful management of ARDS is early detection and initiation of treatment. The goals of therapy are respiratory support, treatment of the underlying cause when possible, and prevention of complications.

Endotracheal (ET) intubation, mechanical ventilation, and PEEP are usually required to maintain adequate blood oxygen levels. Other alternative modes of ventilation (e.g., extracorporeal membrane oxygenator, intravascular oxygenators) may be employed in some situations. Sedation may be necessary to reduce anxiety and restlessness during ventilator management. If tachypnea, restlessness, or respirations out of phase with the ventilator ("bucking") cannot be managed by sedation, paralyzing agents (e.g., pancuronium bromide, curare) may be used (see Nursing Management of the Client on Mechanical Ventilation and Ethical Issues in Nursing).

The use of pharmacologic agents in the treatment of ARDS will vary according to the client's underlying disease process. Inotropic agents (e.g., dopamine, dobutamine) may be indicated to improve cardiac output and increase systemic blood pressure. Antibiotics are administered if suspected or confirmed infection is present. Although controversial, the use of large doses of corticosteroids is also common. The rationale for steroid administration is to reduce inflammatory response and promote pulmonary membrane stability. However, con-

ETHICAL ISSUES IN NURSING

What is the Nurse's Moral Obligation When Neuromuscular Blocking Agents Are Used?

Nursing care of seriously ill medical-surgical clients requires sharpened critical thinking skills. You must be able to think through the complexities of using highly technical interventions and pharmacotherapeutics.

Your client is on continuous mechanical ventilation. To prevent the client from "fighting" or "bucking" the ventilator, a neuromuscular blocking agent (such as pancuronium [Pavulon], vecuronium [Norcuron], or atracurium [Tracrium]) is used. This agent prevents your client from breathing against the ventilator and helps the client receive the maximal benefit from mechanical ventilation.

These neuromuscular blocking agents actually paralyze the client. The client is still awake and can feel pain, but cannot move any muscles including the muscles necessary for breathing. This state is extremely uncomfortable and sometimes terrifying for the client.

The client can be awake, but unable to communicate his or her needs in any way, so it is exceedingly difficult for you to recognize the client's pain, fear, and frustration. Explain the use of the ventilator, the necessity for the paralyzing agents, and tell the client that you will be giving pain medications and sedatives. Because the client could have pain, but be unable to express the need for pain medication, pain medication and sedation should always be combined with neuromuscular blocking agents.

Nursing diagnoses and interventions are acts of fidelity. To provide the best possible care for your client, acquire a thorough understanding of the use of mechanical ventilation, neuromuscular blocking agents, and pain medications and sedation.

trolled clinical trials of corticosteroid use have failed to demonstrate their effectiveness in ARDS.[13] Pharmocologic efforts to inhibit the substances released by the endotoxins, neutrophils, and macrophages are also being explored.[42]

In addition to lung fibrosis, a number of other complications may arise during supportive management of the client with ARDS. These include cardiac dysrhythmias due to hypoxemia, oxygen toxicity, renal failure, thrombocytopenia, gastrointestinal bleeding secondary to stress ulcers, sepsis from invasive lines, and disseminated intravascular coagulation (see Chapter 53).

■ Nursing Management of the Medical Client

The principles of nursing management of clients with pneumonia, pulmonary edema, and other pulmonary disorders that affect gas exchange are also appropriate in the care of the client with ARDS. Evaluation of the client's response to treatment, as well as careful monitoring for potential complications, is essential. Emotional support for the client's family and significant others is also important. The disease can progress very rapidly, leaving family members unprepared for the severity of the client's condition. Clear communications and frequent condition updates are essential to keeping the family adequately informed.

■ Nursing Management of the Client on Mechanical Ventilation

Mechanical ventilation helps to minimize the work of breathing while effectively promoting gas exchange (oxygenation and ventilation). It requires the establishment of an artificial airway (usually by ET intubation, initially) and use of a positive pressure ventilator.

Endotracheal Tube

An ET tube is a long, slender, hollow tube, usually made of polyvinyl chloride, that is inserted into the trachea via the mouth or nose. It passes through the vocal cords, and the distal tip is positioned just above the bifurcation of the mainstem of the bronchus (carina). Oral intubation is usually used for short-term airway management. Nasal intubation is generally more secure and is believed to be more comfortable because it does not move as much in the airway. However, many institutions are not using nasal intubation because of the risk of sinusitis. If prolonged intubation is required, the ET tube will be replaced with a tracheostomy.

Inserting the Tube. The client is positioned supine with all dental bridgework and plates removed. Identify loose teeth. These items can be jarred loose and aspirated during intubation. The client's head is hyperextended, the lower aspect of the neck flexed, and the mouth opened (Fig. 42–11). This position brings the mouth, pharynx, and larynx into a straight line. A laryngoscope is used to hold the airway open, expose the vocal cords, and serve as a guide for the tube into the trachea. ET tubes are inserted only by fully trained healthcare team members.

Intubation should not cause or exacerbate hypoxia. If the client's neck and mandible are mobile, the procedure usually takes about 30 seconds. Certain preexisting conditions, such as rheumatoid arthritis of the neck, can make intubation difficult. For clients with expected difficulty of intubation, an oxygen mask can be used to provide oxygen through the mouth. An oxygen saturation monitor may also be used to warn of hypoxemia. A good practice to remember during difficult intubation is to hold your breath while intubation is attempted. If you must stop to breathe before the client is intubated, the intubation is taking too long. Stop the intubation, reoxygenate the client by mask, and then reattempt intubation.

Checking Tube Placement. Immediately after an ET tube has been inserted, tube placement is verified by auscultation and chest x-ray to ensure aeration of both sides of the chest. Record in the nurses' notes and on the respiratory flow sheet the point at which the tube meets the lips or nostrils. This position can be noted by using the numbers listed on the side of the ET tube. Then, if the tube slips, its correct position can be reestablished quickly.

Securing the Tube. Secure the ET tube immediately after intubation with adhesive tape, twill tape, or specially designed ET tube holders (Fig. 42–12). Secure a nasotracheal tube in the same way, but place the second of the small strips across the bridge of the nose instead of on the upper lip. Retaping is required only if the tape becomes loose or soiled.

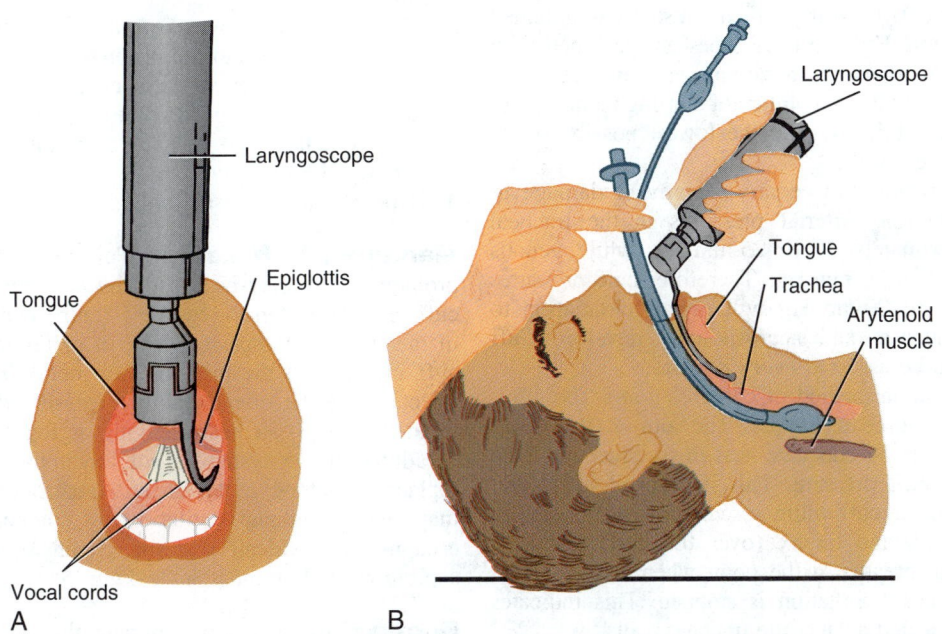

Figure 42–11. Positioning the client for endotracheal intubation.

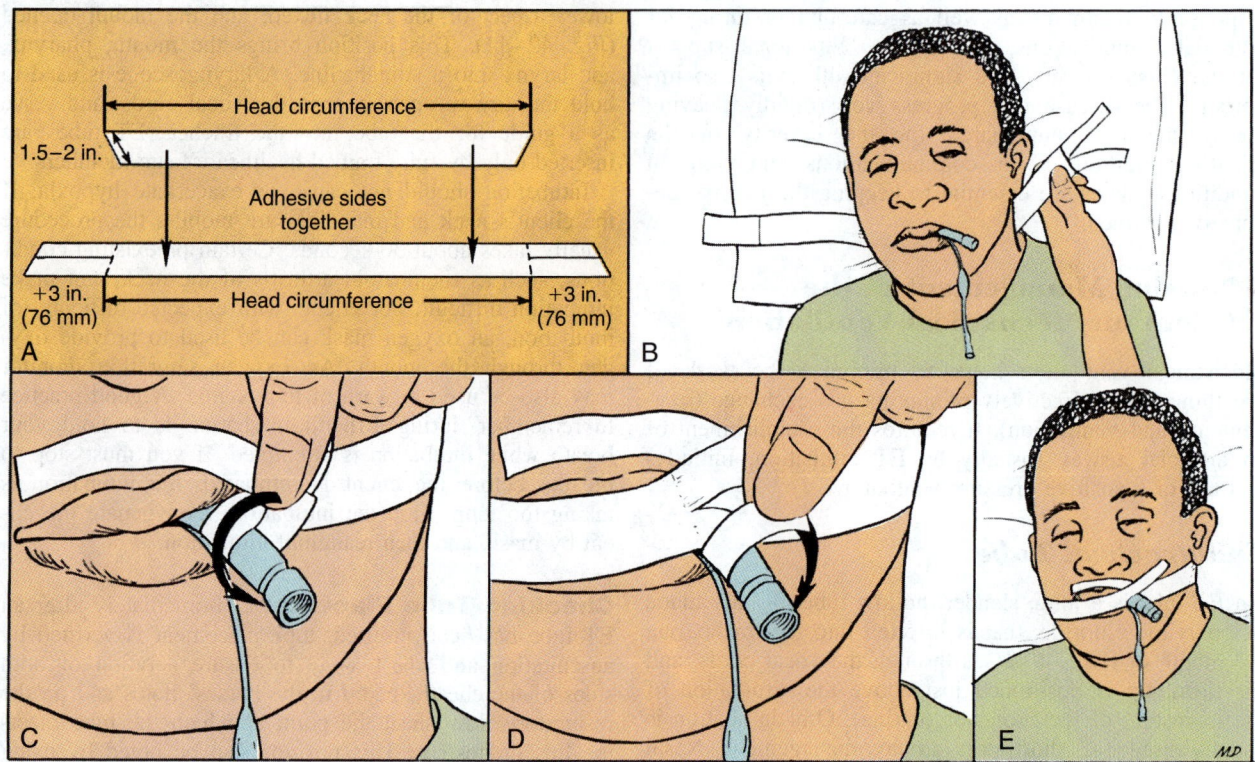

Figure 42–12. Securing a cuffed endotracheal tube with tape. *A*, Two strips of tape are torn, one measuring head circumference and the other 6 inches longer. They are placed with adhesive sides together to form a strip. *B*, Place the strip behind the head and tear one end of the strip in half. *C*, Secure the tube to the upper lip with the untorn end. *D*, Wrap the torn segments around the tube to secure it (*E*).

Caring for the Tube Cuff. The cuff of an ET tube (1) seals the tube against the tracheal wall to facilitate positive pressure ventilation and (2) protects the respiratory tract from the aspiration of foreign material.

The amount of air required to seal an ET tube cuff is reflected by the cuff pressure, which is usually maintained at less than 20 mm Hg. Most ET tubes are designed with soft plastic cuffs to use high volumes at low pressures. They are inflated with a volume of air high enough to seal the trachea while exerting the lowest possible pressure on the tracheal wall.

Low cuff pressure is necessary to prevent damage to the tracheal mucosa. Arterial pressures in the tracheal wall are approximately 20 to 25 mm Hg, while venous pressures are 18 to 20 mm Hg. Therefore, cuff pressures greater than 18 to 20 mm Hg will impair circulation to the tracheal mucosa, and necrosis may develop. Cuff pressures should be assessed every 8 hours.

The most common method of cuff inflation is the minimal occlusion volume technique. The aim of this technique is to provide an adequate seal in the trachea at the lowest possible cuff pressure. This is attained by slowly injecting air into the cuff while auscultating with a stethoscope placed over the larynx (over the cuff) during a positive pressure breath. At the point when sounds (from air movement) cease, inflation is stopped. This indicates that the cuff is sealed against the tracheal wall.

Generally, ET cuffs should remain inflated at all times.

If cuff deflation is required for any reason, use the following procedure:

1. Suction the trachea (remember to hyperventilate and hyperoxygenate client before and during this procedure).
2. Clean the area above the cuff of secretions by gently suctioning deep into the oropharynx.
3. Advance the suction catheter to the end of the ET tube. Deflate the cuff while applying suction to the suction catheter, so that any secretions lying above the cuff will be removed.
4. Repeat pharyngeal suctioning.

Managing Cuff Leaks. Cuff leaks can be a major problem. They may be caused by a rupture or tear in the cuff or pilot system or by the ET tube changing positions in the trachea. Signs of a leak in or around the ET tube cuff include (1) the pilot balloon not filling when air is injected, (2) the client's ability to talk when the cuff is inflated, and (3) air heard leaking during positive pressure breathing. If the system is not functional, the ET tube is replaced. Before replacement, increasing tidal volume may help maintain ventilation by compensating for the escaping gas. Recall that the client is at high risk of aspiration while the cuff is leaking.

Suctioning. ET tubes impair the client's ability to cough, while stimulating increased secretion formation in

Table 42–5. Complications of Tracheal Suctioning

Complication	Pathophysiologic Basis	Nursing Precautions
Hypoxemia	Suctioning removes oxygen from the airways	Preoxygenate the client with manual ventilation or ventilator sighing, to 1½ the usual tidal volume and with a high FIO_2 (0.6–1.0)
Dysrhythmias (premature ventricular contractions, tachycardia, bradycardia, asystole)	Hypoxemia can be caused by prolonged suctioning, stimulating pacemaker cells within the heart; a vasovagal response may also occur, causing bradycardia	Limit suctioning pass to 15 seconds, preoxygenate Monitor the ECG during suctioning Use extra caution in clients (1) with PaO_2 below 70 mm Hg (suctioning further reduces PaO_2, (2) with a large alveolar-arterial gradient (indicating very low cardiopulmonary reserve), and (3) in generally poor condition, e.g., with inadequate oxygenation, hypotension, arrhythmias, acid-base imbalances
Bronchospasm	Respiratory reflex caused by irritation of the tracheal membranes, improper ventilation, and coughing	Be certain to time the inflation stage of mechanical ventilation with the client's own inspiratory effort Do not forcibly inflate the bag against the client's exhalation May require bronchodilators
Airway trauma	Direct trauma to the airway or excessive pressures used to suction	Keep the suction level below 120 mm Hg Suction only as the client needs it, usually no more often than every hour
Infection	Introduction of pathogens into the sterile airway	Use sterile technique for suctioning procedures Change reservoirs of water for humidification daily Assess the color and quantity of sputum
Atelectasis, lobar collapse	Use of excessive wall suction pressure and a suction catheter that is too large for the airway causes a vacuum, collapsing the lung units distal to the tip of the catheter	Use suction catheter that does not exceed one third to one half of the diameter of the airway being suctioned (12F–14F is average size) Use smaller catheters if the ET tube size is less than a 7F Keep suction pressure less than 120 mm Hg

ECG, electrocardiogram; ET, endotracheal; FIO_2, fraction of inspired oxygen; PaO_2, partial pressure of arterial oxygen.

the lower tracheobronchial tree. As a result, ET suctioning is usually required to help maintain a patent airway.

Suctioning should be performed only when needed, as excessive suctioning can cause airway trauma, dysrhythmias, atelectasis, and other problems. (Table 42–5). Assess for clinical manifestations that indicate the need for suctioning. These include noisy, wet respirations; restlessness; increased pulse and respirations; visible mucus bubbling into the ET tube; rhonchi identified by auscultation; and an increase in peak airway pressure during continuous mechanical ventilation. A conscious client is usually aware of airway obstruction and can ask for help. Obtunded clients need careful and constant assessment with prompt suctioning when indicated.

The principles and techniques of suctioning via an ET tube are the same as for nasotracheal suctioning (Box 42–8). However, in some settings, closed system suctioning is used for mechanically ventilated clients. For this method, the catheter is enclosed in a sleeve arrangement and left attached to the artificial airway. The closed system method is designed to reduce the risks of arterial oxygen desaturation, hypotension, bradycardia, and infec-

tion by eliminating the need to disconnect the client from the ventilator for suctioning. However, more investigational evidence is needed to support the closed system method over the open system method.[6]

Communication. An ET tube passes through the vocal cords. Therefore, the client cannot cough effectively or speak. Help the client develop a means of communication. For example, keep a pencil and paper pad or a picture board readily available. Be patient and willing to spend time communicating with the client so that feelings of frustration are avoided.

Providing Oral Hygiene. Careful oral hygiene is essential every few hours for a client with an ET tube. Secretions pool in the oropharynx because of the inflated tracheal cuff. Frequent oral suctioning above the cuff is highly recommended. The client's teeth should be brushed and oral mucosa moistened with solutions without alcohol or lemon because these solutions dry mucous membranes. Apply lubricant to the lips to prevent drying,

Box 42–8. Airway Suctioning

- Assess the need for suctioning. Airway suctioning should be performed on an 'as-needed' basis, not at regularly scheduled intervals.
- Airway suctioning is a sterile procedure. Maintain sterility throughout the procedure.
- Avoid excessive vacuum pressures that may traumatize the airway. The safe range for adults is 80–120 mm Hg.
- Select an appropriately sized catheter. The suction catheter should never exceed half the diameter of an artificial airway or the natural airway it is to enter. The most commonly used sizes for adults are 12F and 14F.
- Provide oxygen before, during, and after the procedure. The vacuum removes oxygen and will intensify any preexisting hypoxemia.
- Limit the suctioning time to 15 seconds. Longer intervals increase the risk of complications.
- Watch the client closely for side effects of suctioning (hypoxemia, cardiac irregularities due to vagal stimulation, mucosal trauma, hypotension, and paroxysmal coughing). If side effects develop, especially cardiac irregularities, stop the procedure and reoxygenate the client.
- Thoroughly explain the procedure before starting. Suctioning can be an uncomfortable and frightening experience. Provide reassurance to the client throughout.

cracking, and excoriation. To reduce the risk of necrosis of the mouth and pharynx from pressure, the ET tube should be rotated from one corner of the mouth to the other at least every 24 hours.

Continuous Mechanical Ventilation

The client on continuous mechanical ventilation (CMV) is a challenge to the nurse providing care. The nurse must be familiar with the equipment, the complications of CMV, and nursing management. The goals of CMV are to (1) maintain adequate ventilation, (2) deliver precise concentrations of FIO_2, (3) deliver adequate tidal volumes to obtain an adequate minute ventilation and oxygenation, and (4) lessen the work of breathing in those clients who cannot sustain adequate ventilation on their own.

Types of Ventilators. Continuous mechanical ventilators can be either pressure-cycled or volume-cycled ventilators (Fig. 42–13). Pressure-cycled ventilators deliver a volume of gas to the airway using positive pressure during inspiration. This positive pressure is delivered until the preselected pressure has been reached. When the preset pressure is reached, the machine cycles into exhalation. Pressure-cycled ventilators are currently used in only a small portion of those clients who require CMV.

Volume-cycled (volume-controlled or volume-limited) ventilators deliver a preset tidal volume of inspired gas. The tidal volume that has been preselected is delivered to the client regardless of the pressure required to deliver this volume. A pressure limit can be set to prevent dangerously high airway pressures from occurring.

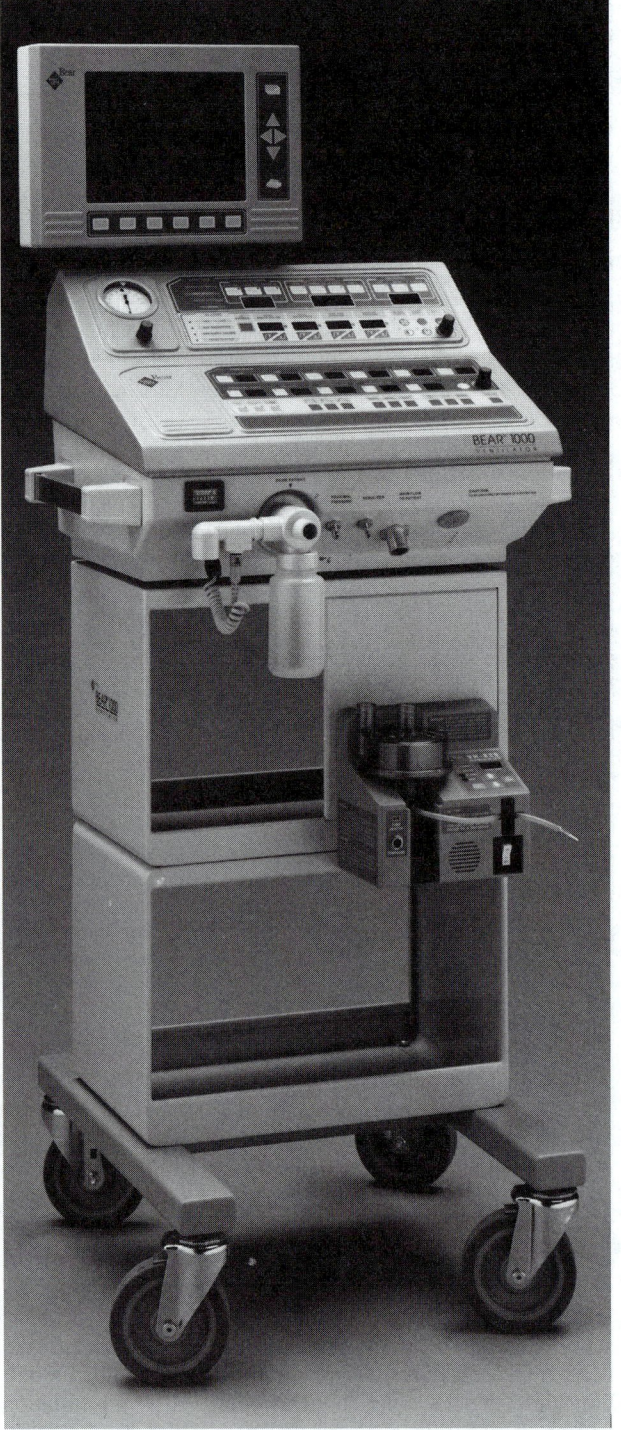

Figure 42–13. A volume-cycled mechanical ventilator. (Courtesy of Bear Medical Systems, Riverside, MA.)

Physiologic Changes with Mechanical Ventilation.

Many physiologic changes occur when a client is placed on mechanical ventilation. Decreased cardiac output is the most common of these. Normal unassisted respiration begins with subatmospheric pressure. Negative pressure increases during inhalation and decreases during exhalation. Positive pressure applied to the airway has the opposite effect. As positive pressure inflates the lungs, pressure in the thorax builds, decreasing the flow of blood to the vena cava, and reducing blood flow to the right atrium of the heart. Exhalation is passive, and pressures return to their normal, resting, subatmospheric level. Positive pressure also briefly affects the left side of the heart by increasing filling and output. This increase is due to the displacement of blood from the pulmonary system into the left ventricle. However, this effect is noted only immediately after the institution of positive pressure ventilation. If positive pressure ventilation is continued for more than a few minutes, the blood flow to and from the right ventricle is decreased. This in turn decreases the filling of the left ventricle, leading to a lowered cardiac output. The lowered cardiac output will be reflected in the hypotension that clients commonly exhibit immediately after being placed on mechanical ventilation. It is imperative that blood pressures be monitored closely.

Other body systems are also affected by positive pressure. As the diaphragm descends into the abdomen during the inspiratory phase, blood flow to the splanchnic area decreases. This decrease in splanchnic blood flow may lead to ischemia of the gastric mucosa. Ischemia of the gastric mucosa may be one of the reasons that clients who receive positive pressure ventilation for an extended period of time have a high incidence of gastrointestinal bleeding and stress ulcerations. Decreasing blood flow to the splanchnic region also results in decreased blood flow to the kidneys. This decrease in blood flow signals the posterior pituitary gland to increase secretion of vasopressin (antidiuretic hormone). Elevated vasopressin levels lead to reabsorption of free water in the renal tubular cells, thereby increasing water retention. Lymphatic flow also decreases as a result of positive pressure.

Positive pressure can also cause neurophysiologic changes. When ABG values improve in acute, uncompensated respiratory failure, improved cerebral oxygenation results. A client with compensated respiratory acidosis (chronic carbon dioxide retention) may be adversely affected by positive pressure breathing owing to blowing off of carbon dioxide. Acute alkalosis may occur, producing faintness, dizziness, lightheadedness, and anxiety. If severe alkalosis persists, convulsions, cardiac arrhythmias, and cerebral edema may occur. Cerebral edema may contribute to intensive care unit psychosis.

Modes of Ventilation. The ventilation mode refers to the way the client receives breaths from the ventilator. There are several conventional modes of CMV (See Table 42–6).

Control Mode. Controlled (machine-cycled) ventilation governs a client's rate of ventilation by automatically cycling the ventilator at a predetermined number of cycles per minute; the ventilator does all of the work of breathing, and the client does none. This mode is independent of the client's efforts or pattern of breathing. This mode of ventilation is used only if the client is chemically paralyzed with neuromuscular blocking agents, such as vecuronium bromide (Norcuron) or pancuronium bromide (Pavulon). Clients who are on controlled mechanical ventilation and have spontaneous respirations

may "fight" or "buck" the ventilator because they cannot synchronize their respirations with the machine's cycle.

Assist/Control Mode. In this mode, the client's own inspiratory effort "triggers" the ventilator, thus initiating the mechanical inspiratory phase. If, after a period of delay, the client does not spontaneously trigger the machine, the ventilator will automatically give a breath at a set rate. This ensures continued ventilation if the inspiratory efforts cease or the client becomes too weak to trigger the machine regularly. Assist/control ventilation allows the client to take as many breaths as he or she desires. Every breath received will be delivered by the machine at the same preset tidal volume and FIO_2. Assisted ventilation is indicated for clients who can control their own respiratory rate and pattern.

Intermittent Mandatory Ventilation (IMV). In the IMV mode, the ventilator delivers a preset number of mechanical breaths. However, it also allows the client to breathe spontaneously in between with no assistance from the ventilator (i.e., no "triggered" breaths) and at varying tidal volumes. For example, if a ventilator is set on the IMV mode, rate of 8, and tidal volume of 800 ml, then it will deliver eight breaths each minute at a volume of 800 ml. However, if the client breathes two additional breaths in that minute, these breaths will be at whatever tidal volume the client can obtain. As the client is increasingly able to breathe on his or her own, the IMV rate is slowly reduced until all breaths are spontaneous and ABGs are within the normal range for that client.

Synchronized Intermittent Mandatory Ventilation (SIMV). This mode is essentially the same as IMV, except the mandatory (preset) breaths are activated by the client's inspiratory efforts and are synchronized with his or her underlying breathing pattern.

IMV and SIMV are currently the preferred modes of CMV. They are frequently used as weaning modes. Some clients have special ventilatory needs that cannot be met adequately by conventional modes of CMV. New trends in ventilatory support have helped to address these needs.

Pressure Support Ventilation. Pressure support ventilation (PSV) is a form of ventilation that augments spontaneous inspiratory effort with a preset level of positive airway pressure. When the client on PSV initiates a breath, the machine is triggered and delivers a flow of gas at the preset pressure. This pressure is maintained as long as minimal inspiratory flow is occurring. Theoretically, this permits a more even distribution of inspired gas. PSV has been shown to reduce the work of breathing in postoperative and critically ill clients.[6] Clients on IMV report greater comfort with PSV, as well. Pressure support is also useful for clients who are having difficulty weaning from CMV.

High-Frequency Ventilation. High-frequency ventilation (HFV) is another mode of mechanical ventilation used for clients who cannot be adequately ventilated with conventional techniques. HFV is often useful for clients

Table 42–6. Modes of Mechanical Ventilation

Mode	Description	
Spontaneous ventilation	Normal breathing	
Controlled mechanical ventilation (CMV)	Ventilator delivers preset tidal volume and respirator rate. No allowance for spontaneous breaths	
Assist/control ventilation (A/C)	Spontaneous inspiratory effort of client triggers ventilator to deliver preset tidal volume. If client does not trigger an assisted breath, ventilator delivers breaths at preset respiratory rate	
Intermittent mandatory ventilation (IMV)	Ventilator delivers preset tidal volume and respiratory rate. Client can take unassisted spontaneous breaths between preset breaths	
Synchronized intermittent mandatory ventilation (SIMV)	Similar to IMV except that present ventilator breaths are synchronized with client's spontaneous breaths to avoid "stacking" of breaths (i.e., ventilator breath delivered before client has time to exhale fully)	
Positive end-expiratory pressure (PEEP)	Preset amount of pressure stays in the lungs at the end of exhalation, keeping the alveoli open. Used in conjunction with CMV, A/C, IMV, or SIMV	
Continuous positive airway pressure (CPAP)	Similar to PEEP, but for the client who is breathing entirely on own (i.e., no ventilator-generated breaths)	
Pressure support ventilation (PSV)	Client breathes spontaneously but ventilator provides a preset level of pressure assistance with each spontaneous breath (inspiration only)	

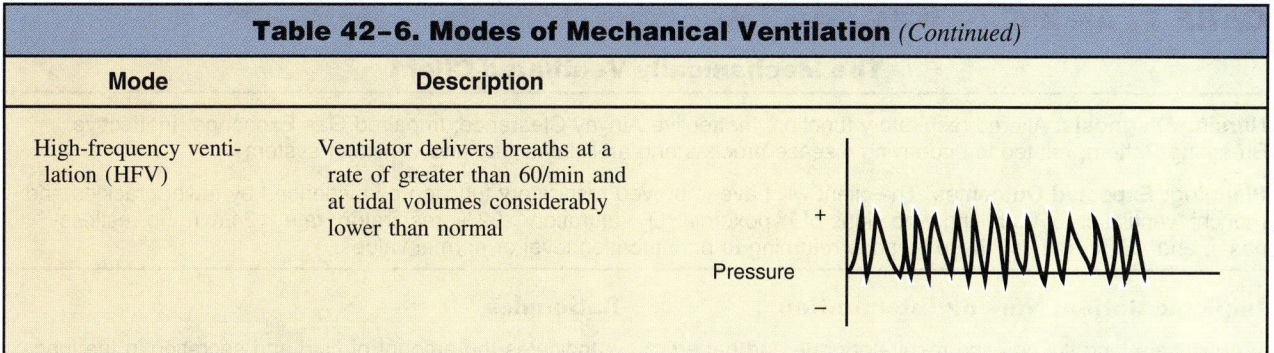

Table 42–6. Modes of Mechanical Ventilation (*Continued*)		
Mode	**Description**	
High-frequency venti-lation (HFV)	Ventilator delivers breaths at a rate of greater than 60/min and at tidal volumes considerably lower than normal	+ Pressure −

Adapted from Boggs, R. L., & Wooldridge-King, M. (1993). *AACN procedure manual for critical care.* Philadelphia: W. B. Saunders.

with severely noncompliant lungs. HFV uses respiratory rates of 60 to 100 breaths per minute with considerably lower tidal volumes than those used in CMV. Although the results are not completely understood, apparently with HFV the fast jets of air cause increased turbulence and enhance diffusion in the lungs. The theoretical advantage of HFV over conventional forms of ventilation is that with HFV there is a reduction in peak and mean airway pressure, resulting in better ventilation of noncompliant lungs, for example, as in ARDS.

Positive End-Expiratory Pressure and Continuous Positive Airway Pressure. PEEP and continuous positive airway pressure (CPAP) are techniques applied during expiration whereby intrathoracic pressures are not allowed to return to ambient atmospheric pressure. This increased pressure helps to keep the alveoli open, increase FRC, and enhance oxygenation as a result of the enlarged surface area that is available for diffusion. With the implementation of PEEP or CPAP, oxygenation is improved, thus allowing the use of lower levels of FIO_2. In this way, the body's metabolic oxygen requirements are met without the toxic effects of higher concentrations of oxygen.

CPAP is applied to a client with spontaneous respiration. PEEP, on the other hand, is applied during mechanical ventilation.

FRC is the volume of air remaining in the lung after normal expiration. When end-expiratory alveolar volumes remain above their critical closing point, the alveoli remain open and functioning, allowing oxygen to diffuse into the bloodstream. However, if they fall below the closing point, the alveoli have a tendency to collapse. When alveoli collapse, oxygenation of blood flow to the alveoli does not occur (Fig. 42–14). The residual volume is decreased, as is the FRC. This results in a true intrapulmonary shunt (perfusion without oxygenation). Lung compliance is also affected. Once alveolar collapse occurs, reinflation requires very high opening pressures, the generation of which significantly increases the work of breathing. The hypoxemia resulting from alveolar collapse and the increased oxygen consumption caused by the increased work of breathing may severely compromise the client.

The aim of PEEP and CPAP is to apply positive airway pressure that keeps the alveoli open and reduces the amount of shunting. Positive pressures of +5 to +20 cm H_2O are typically used in adults. Pressures may be adjusted until the level is found that produces the best PaO_2 without producing adverse effects. This level is called best PEEP.

The physiologic effects of positive airway pressure on inspiration and expiration are basically the same as those effects discussed for CMV. There are a few added risks, such as the following:

1. Rupture of the lung from increased intrathoracic and intra-airway pressures (barotrauma)
2. Pneumothorax
3. Subcutaneous emphysema

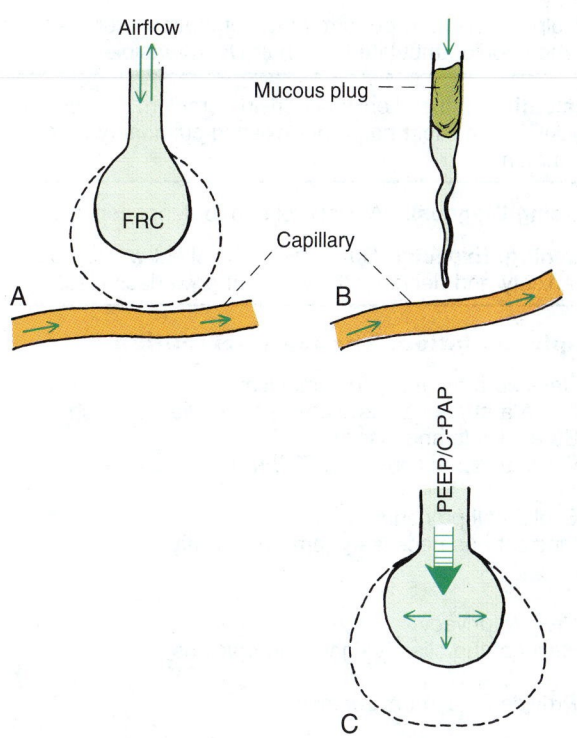

Figure 42–14. Effects of positive airway pressure on alveolus. *A,* Normal alveolus. *Dotted line* represents expansion during inspiration. *B,* Collapsed alveolus. Perfusion continued. *C,* Alveolus opened by positive pressure. *Dotted line* indicates alveolus during inspiration and *solid line* indicates end-expiratory alveolar volume.

CARE PLAN

The Mechanically Ventilated Client

Nursing Diagnosis. Altered respiratory function: Ineffective Airway Clearance; Impaired Gas Exchange; Ineffective Breathing Pattern; related to underlying disease process and artificial airway and ventilator system

Planning: Expected Outcomes. The client will have improved respiratory function as evidenced by fewer crackles and rhonchi, ventilation of both lungs, no signs of hypoxemia (O_2 saturation >92%, respiratory rate <24/min, no restlessness), and ABGs and acid-base balance returning to preintubation level or normal values.

Implementation: Nursing Intervention	**Rationales**
Auscultate lung sounds and respiratory rate and pattern every 1 to 2 hours as needed.	Indicates the amount of fluid and secretion in the lungs; validates that the endotracheal (ET) tube is placed correctly so that both lungs can be ventilated; determines ventilatory effectiveness.
Check ventilator settings, alarms, and connections at least hourly and after any removal of ventilator from client (e.g., after suctioning).	Ensures that ventilator values are set as ordered and that the monitoring and warning functions of the ventilator are operational (see Troubleshooting Mechanical Ventilator Alarms in Bridge to Critical Care).
Suction as needed; provide pre- and post-hyperinflation and hyperoxygenation.	Suctioning removes airway secretions, facilitating ventilation; oxygen and inflation reduce hypoxia during suctioning.
Provide adequate humidity via the ventilator or nebulizer.	Replaces the function of the upper airway to warm and humidify the inspired air; thins secretions to facilitate their removal.
Turn and reposition the client every 2 hours.	Allows both lungs to be fully ventilated, mobilizes secretions.
Secure the ET tube properly.	Prevents accidental dislodgement.
Use a bite-block or oral airway.	Prevents ET tube compression. If the client is biting it, the bite-block is more comfortable for the conscious client.
Monitor arterial blood gas (ABG) values and arterial oximetry.	Indicates the degree of oxygenation; lack of improvement in ABGs may require a change in interventions.
Help the client to perform range-of-motion exercises; he or she should ambulate to a chair when feasible.	Immobility leads to decreased respiratory muscle strength.

Evaluation. If the client's underlying problem was corrected by mechanical ventilation, these outcomes will be met quickly. If the client has a pre-existing pulmonary disease or is acutely ill, the outcomes may require several days for attainment.

Nursing Diagnosis. Anxiety related to dependence while on CMV

Planning: Expected Outcomes. The client will exhibit decreased anxiety as evidenced by reduction in the level of stress or anxiety and decreased feelings of powerlessness.

Implementation: Nursing Intervention	**Rationales**
Develop a means of communication.	Allows the client to have needs met.
Place a nurse call device within the client's reach.	Allows the client to contact you.
Be available and visible.	Reduces anxiety in the client.
Provide distractions (e.g., TV, radio).	Reduces anxiety because the client does not focus on the ventilator and noises.
Explain all procedures.	Allows the client to feel respected and alleviates fears.
Medicate as necessary (prn) for anxiety.	Antianxiety medications and narcotics may be needed but use them with caution in clients being weaned because these drugs suppress respiratory drive.
Provide privacy.	Demonstrates respect for the client.
Respect the client's rights and opinions.	Demonstrates respect for the client and maintains dignity.
Provide a calm environment.	A frenzied environment engenders anxiety, and if the client becomes anxious, ventilation will be more difficult and oxygen needs will increase.
Explain to the client and family that the client's vocal cords have been bypassed, which prevents talking; encourage them to use other modes of communication.	Clients can hear and respond even though they cannot talk.

Evaluation. Expect client to remain moderately anxious while on CMV.

CARE PLAN

The Mechanically Ventilated Client

Collaborative Problem. High Risk for Complications of Continuous Mechanical Ventilation and Positive-Pressure Ventilation

Planning: Expected Outcomes. The nurse will monitor the client for pulmonary barotrauma, cardiovascular depression, inadvertent extubation, and malposition of the ET tube.

Implementation: Nursing Intervention	**Rationales**
Assess for acute, increasing, or severe dyspnea; agitation; panic; decreased or absent breath sounds; localized hyperresonance; increased breathing effort; tracheal deviation away from the side with abnormal findings; subcutaneous emphysema; and decreasing PaO$_2$ levels.	Barotrauma can lead to pneumothorax or tension pneumothorax.
Assess for an acute or gradual fall in blood pressure, tachycardia (early sign), bradycardia (late sign), dysrhythmias, weak peripheral pulses, acute or gradual increase in pulmonary capillary wedge pressure, and respiratory "swing" (depression) in arterial or pulmonary artery wave forms during inspiration.	Cardiovascular depression can occur after an increase in tidal volume, PEEP, CPAP, or with hyperinflation; positive pressure decreases venous return and cardiac output because of an increase in intrathoracic pressure.
Monitor for signs of inadvertent extubation: vocalization, low-pressure alarm, bilateral decrease in upper lobe airway sounds, gastric distention, clinical manifestations of inadequate ventilation; change in length of portion of ET tube that extends beyond the lip. If inadvertent extubation occurs, notify the physician, because reintubation is necessary; manage ventilation and oxygenation with a self-inflating resuscitation bag.	Inadvertent extubation can be obvious, as when the tube is found in the client's hand; it can also be obscure, as when the tube slips into the hypopharynx or esophagus.
Keep an intubation tray readily available.	Intubation supplies may be needed quickly.

Evaluation. Most complications of positive-pressure ventilation occur within 48 hours after intubation. Inadvertent extubation can occur at any time.

Nursing Diagnosis. Risk for Infection related to impaired primary defenses in respiratory tract

Planning: Expected Outcomes. The client will remain free of infection as evidenced by clear sputum, no fever, clear lung sounds, no increased difficulty with ventilation (e.g., increased peak inspiratory pressure), white blood cell count within normal limits, and respiratory rate less than 24 breaths per minute.

Implementation: Nursing Intervention	**Rationales**
Wash your hands thoroughly.	Hand washing reduces the spread of infection.
Use sterile technique for suctioning.	The respiratory tract is considered sterile.
Monitor the client for increased breathing effort, localized changes in auscultation, and changes in PaO$_2$.	Infected lung segments transmit sound differently (more solid) and do not permit gas exchange.
Provide oral care every 2 hours.	The client's mouth becomes dry, and stomatitis may develop from lack of oral secretions.
Drain water from ventilator tubing; do not drain water back into the humidifier.	Water may become a source of contamination, especially with *Pseudomonas*.
Monitor laboratory values, white blood cell count, and differential.	White blood cell increases may indicate pulmonary infection.
Monitor sputum for changes in color, consistency, amount, and odor.	Infection may cause sputum to increase, darken, thicken, and become malodorous.

Evaluation. Infection usually develops after 72 hours of intubation unless the client is immunosuppressed.

Nursing Diagnosis. Altered Nutrition: Less than Body Requirements related to lack of ability to eat while on a ventilator and increased metabolic needs

Planning: Expected Outcomes. The client will exhibit adequate nutritional intake as evidenced by:

▪ Stable weight, or weight appropriate to height
▪ Intake of adequate calorie levels
▪ No signs of catabolism
▪ Wound healing

▪ No infection
▪ Laboratory values within normal limits (prealbumin, total protein, transferrin)

Adequate muscle strength to breathe spontaneously.

Care Plan continues on following page

CARE PLAN

The Mechanically Ventilated Client (Continued)

Implementation: Nursing Intervention	Rationales
Provide adequate nutrition (high calorie intake, protein, vitamins, and minerals); provide a nutrition consult, as needed.	Intake of 1200 kcal (approximate) is adequate to maintain weight; inadequate nutrition decreases diaphragmatic muscle mass, decreases pulmonary function, and increases mechanical ventilation requirements.
Begin tube feeding as soon as it is evident that the client will remain on CMV for a length of time (usually 2–3 days).	The client should not be allowed to develop a catabolic state.
Avoid excessive carbohydrate loads.	Carbohydrate loads may increase carbon dioxide production to the point of producing hypercapnia.
Weigh the client daily.	Changes in body weight are a reliable indicator of nutritional balance.
Monitor intake and output.	Fluids are still required, and output should match intake.
Assess for complications of tube feeding: aspiration, diarrhea, constipation.	Feed the client while he or she is sitting upright, with the cuff inflated. Check for residual tube feeding every 4 hours (continuous feeding) or before beginning another feeding (intermittent feeding). Diarrhea is often caused by osmotic changes from an excessive concentration of tube feeding or the use of sorbitol-based elixirs; consider reducing the concentration or changing to crushed pills. Constipation is caused by a lack of free water within the feeding; add 100 ml of water every 4 to 6 hours if allowable.
If the client is unable to tolerate enteral feeding, total parenteral feeding (TPN) should be considered.	Clients with decreased gastrointestinal function may require parenteral nutrition to meet metabolic needs.
Monitor bowel sounds.	Bowel obstruction and ileus present as changes in bowel sounds.
Before tube feeding or between bolus feedings, obtain pH and guaiac test every 8 hours.	A change in pH may indicate an increased risk of gastric stress ulcer. A positive guaiac test indicates bleeding.

Evaluation. Malnutrition is preventable. Expect the client's weight to stabilize (unless there is fluid imbalance).

ABG, arterial blood gas; CMV, controlled mechanical ventilation; CPAP, continuous positive airway pressure; PaO_2, partial pressure of arterial oxygen; PEEP, positive end-expiratory pressure.

---

4. Pneumomediastinum
5. Cardiovascular embarrassment

Cardiovascular embarrassment results from the increased intrathoracic pressure caused by the PEEP, which leads to a decrease in cardiac output. If cardiac output cannot be improved with vasopressors or increased blood volume, hepatic and renal function become compromised. CPAP and PEEP also increase intracranial pressure. In neurologically injured clients, this is an added risk.

Nursing Management. Management of the client on CMV is primarily a nursing responsibility. The nurse coordinates efforts of the healthcare team, teaches and supports the client and family, monitors and intervenes in the client-ventilator system, and ensures that the client's complex needs are met during CMV. The Nursing Care Plan for the Mechanically Ventilated Client discusses appropriate nursing care. The Bridge to Home Healthcare describes ways to assist the ventilator-dependent client at home.

Weaning. The physician decides when to begin gradually removing, or "weaning," the client from CMV. The decision is usually based on assessments made by nurses and respiratory therapists. The length of time required for successful weaning generally relates to the underlying disease process and to the client's state of health before the ventilator was used. For example, a young client who is recovering from an overdose of drugs usually weans rapidly. However, a client with COPD who develops acute respiratory failure and has little or no pulmonary reserve often takes longer and requires much professional patience and skill.

Criteria for a weaning trial are as follows:

● Improvement, correction, or stabilization of the active disease process
● Nutrional and fluid status sufficient to maintain the increased metabolic needs and demands of spontaneous respiration
● Adequate physical strength and mental alertness
● Afebrile status, that is, any infections controlled
● Stable cardiovascular, renal, and cerebral status
● Optimal levels of ABGs, electrolytes, hemoglobin, and other laboratory tests
● Achievement of the physiologic parameters listed in the Bridge to Critical Care

BRIDGE TO HOME HEALTHCARE

Living with a Ventilator

Terri Brown, R.N., B.S.N., *Bergan Home Health Care, Omaha, Nebraska*

Good communication between the ventilator-dependent client, family members and caregivers, and the home health nurse, the physician, and community resources is essential. As soon as you obtain physician's orders and establish a plan of care, call the durable medical equipment (DME) supplier to review all of the equipment that will be required by the client in the home setting. You may want to plan a shared home visit with the DME supplier to evaluate and coordinate all of the client's medical needs. Next, check with the local electric company to ensure that they will put your client on a list of persons to receive priority to get service turned back on immediately in case of an electrical failure. It is very important to have a portable battery-operated ventilator in the home in case of a power failure.

Plan to spend several hours with the family and caregivers on your initial home visit. They need to be instructed about the equipment, ventilator alarms, suctioning devices, dressing changes, and other care requirements. Be certain that caregivers give satisfactory return demonstrations to you. Often, the equipment is very intimidating to the family. Write down as much information as possible, such as the telephone numbers of the home health agency, yourself, the equipment supplier, the physician, and other pertinent emergency phone numbers. Also write down instructions about the the use of the equipment in terms that the caregivers and family understand. Writing this information on a large piece of paper in large print makes the information easily accessible and will prevent the caregiver or family from shuffling through various papers or pamphlets to obtain pertinent information. It is not unusual to have families or caregivers forget most of the information you have given or demonstrated after you leave. Remember, the client is probably happy to be back in the home environment, but the family may be very anxious and frightened. Also address the availability of respite care or other community resources to provide the family with periods of rest and relaxation.

Equipment noise may be a nuisance for clients and caregivers. Suggest a radio, television, or cassette player with earphones. If clients can communicate through writing, make sure they have a small chalkboard or dry erase board on which to communicate messages or needs to others. The family and client may want to hire a tutor to teach sign language, but most persons learn to read lips. Keep the room light and open; a bed by a window serves as extra sensory stimuli. Be sure to caution the family to avoid irritants or pollutants such as smoke, animal fur or dander, bird feathers, and heavy dust in the environment. Use creativity and imagination to provide a safe and secure home setting for your client and his or her family when a ventilator is needed.

Scales have been developed to provide weaning scores that can assist in predicting the success of a weaning effort. However, little research is available to validate their accuracy with various client populations.

Careful assesment of ventilatory status before and during weaning is necessary, including spontaneous tidal volume; VC; maximal voluntary ventilation, inspiratory effort, breath sounds, cardiovascular, renal, and cerebral status; and ABGs.

Weaning from mechanical ventilation can be accomplished in two ways. The first is called "rapid" or T-piece weaning. This technique is often used when mechanical ventilation has been instituted for only a brief period of time. Start in the morning after the client has had a good night's rest. Place the client in the semi-Fowler position. The mechanical ventilator's respiratory rate may be reduced to half the original rate. (In some cases, this step may be eliminated.) Obtain ABGs in 30 minutes. If the ABGs are at or near the client's baseline, place the client on a T-piece at the same FIO_2. Obtain ABGs in 30 minutes. If the ABGs are again at or near the baseline and the respiratory rate is below 25 to 30 breaths per minute, extubate. Place on a face tent for high humidity. The practice of beginning a weaning program in the morning is being questioned by nurse researchers. You may see

changes in practice in the next few years based upon the correlation of circadian rhythms with ideal timeframes for weaning.

The second method of weaning is called "gradual" or "slow" weaning. This technique is utilized when prolonged mechanical ventilation has been used or a neuromuscular disorder is present. The first step in this technique is to ascertain whether or not spontaneous breathing is present. Once spontaneous breathing has been established, slowly reduce the amount of ventilatory support. Continue to reduce ventilatory support until the client is able to accept full responsibility for his or her own ventilatory requirements. This may be accomplished through increasingly longer periods of time on a T-piece (followed by periods of CMV support) or by decreasing the rate of IMV or SIMV breaths. This technique may take weeks or even months. Patience is critical.

A first weaning attempt may not be successful. Failure in weaning may be due to the following:

1. Decreased muscular strength caused by protein-carbohydrate malnutrition or certain disease processes, or incoordination of respiratory muscles due to disuse from prolonged CMV
2. Increased work of breathing due to increased airway

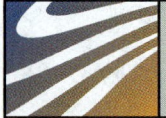

ETHICAL ISSUES IN NURSING

How Should the Decision to End Continuous Mechanical Ventilation Be Made?

Continuous mechanical ventilation (CMV) is used for many different reasons. Ventilator support may be needed for short-term care, as in certain cases of severe pneumonia, or for more long-term care, as in some stroke patients. In some emergency cases, ventilator support is required to stabilize a client's condition. No matter why CMV is initiated, it offers degrees of benefit to the patient. A positive benefit is that CMV allows the lungs to rest so that healing may take place (as in severe pneumonia). However, CMV may artificially prolong death and cause suffering, as with severe stroke patients or patients in terminal states.

The decision to place a person on CMV is made by the client, or his or her surrogate, and the medical team. This decision may be a very difficult one, for example, when a client is in a persistent vegetative state, and the wishes of the client regarding CMV are not known. However, it is even more difficult for persons to decide for another whether to discontinue CMV. To many persons, this decision is viewed as somehow causing the person's death and this is very uncomfortable for them.

The best alternative to this dilemma is for all persons to decide, while in a state of good health, what they would want done should a situation arise requiring resuscitative measures, including CMV. Advance directives such as a living will or a durable power of attorney for healthcare can help people guide their own treatment should critical healthcare situations arise. As of December 1991, all healthcare facilities that take Medicare or Medicaid reimbursement must include, on admission, an advance directive assessment of all their clients.

You have a great deal of influence over the healthcare teaching of your clients. Information about advance directives may be shared with clients, community members, family members, and friends. The more the public is made aware of such directives, the easier it is for healthcare professionals to guide their care. In many cases, people have strong feelings about the initiation of certain treatments, such as CMV. Advance directives allow all persons to decide, in advance of crisis situations, what they wish to have done in such situations. By allowing all persons to exercise advance directives, healthcare providers may avoid many legal and ethical dilemmas that occur in the initiation, continuation, or discontinuation of certain treatments.

resistance, abdominal distention, a small-diameter artificial airway, upper airway obstruction, or unresolved acute lung diseases
3. Increased ventilation requirements
4. Problems with secretion management
5. Psychological factors, such as fear

If the first attempt at weaning is not successful, it is important to determine the reasons and try to eliminate them in subsequent attempts. Clients who require prolonged ventilatory support and extended periods of weaning often do best in a setting that promotes rehabilitation concepts. These clients will usually be transferred to subacute or extended care facilities.

Extubation. Once the client has been weaned successfully and has demonstrated adequate ventilatory effort and an acceptable level of consciousness to sustain spontaneous respiration, the ET tube may be removed. ET tubes are removed on physician's orders and only by healthcare team members qualified to reintubate if necessary. The occurrence of laryngospasm and tracheal edema after extubation may occlude the airway and require reintubation.

The ET tube is suctioned, the cuff deflated, and the tube removed. Immediately after extubation, the client is usually placed on oxygen. The client is also assessed for signs of respiratory distress and hypoxemia as evidenced by restlessness, irritability, tachycardia, tachypnea, and decreased PaO_2 or increased $PaCO_2$. If these signs are noted, the physician should be notified, and the nurse should prepare for reintubation.

Some clients are restless and extubate themselves. Because the cuff is not deflated, there can be damage to the tracheal wall and bleeding. In most cases, the client requires reintubation, and this is done swiftly to prevent hypoxemia and to avoid having to insert the ET tube through swollen tissues. Sometimes, however, the client will be monitored and not reintubated, especially if the client was nearing the time for extubation.

Conclusions

Clients with lung disorders are a challenge to the nurse providing care. In addition to common nursing diagnoses centering on *Impaired Gas Exchange and Ineffective Airway Clearance,* the client is often anxious due to feelings of dyspnea and air hunger. Management of lung disorders includes methods to open the airway (bronchodilators), clear infection (antibiotics), and improved oxygenation (position, oxygen).

Thinking Critically

1. **Your postoperative thoracotomy client has a pleural chest tube in place, connected to water-seal**

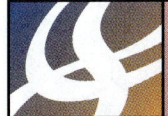

BRIDGE TO CRITICAL CARE

The Ventilator-Dependent Client

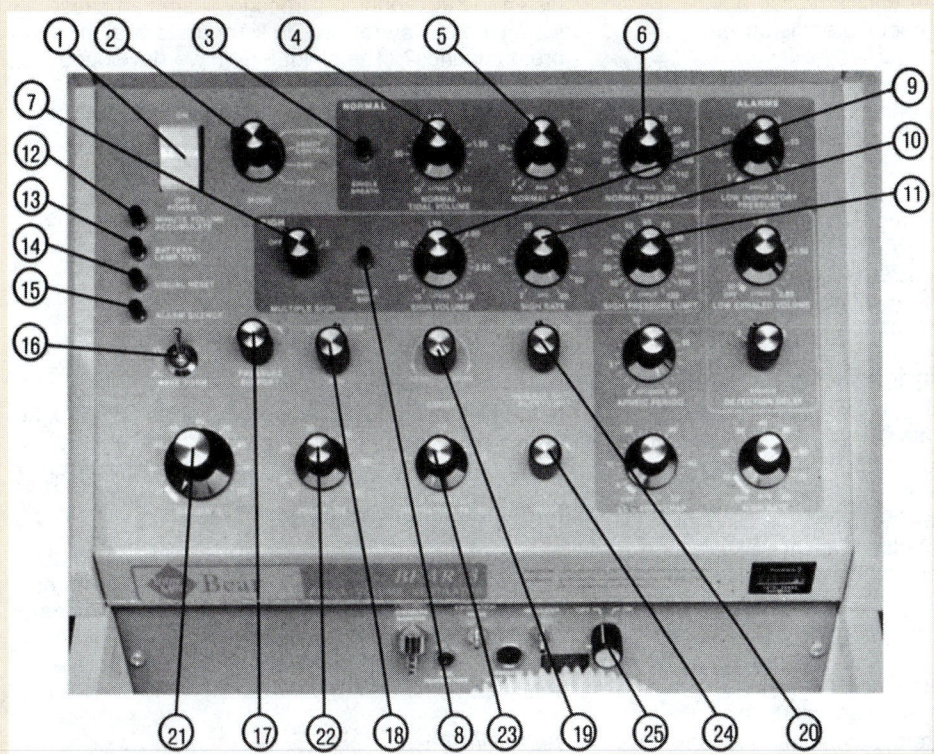

① **POWER ON/OFF**—Controls electrical power to the ventilator.

② **MODE CONTROL**—Selection of mode of operation.

③ **NORMAL SINGLE BREATH**—Delivers a single manual breath when pressed. Operates in all modes.

④ **TIDAL VOLUME**—Sets amount of air to be delivered with each breath. When tidal volume is delivered, inspiration ends. (Exhaled tidal volume and minute volume are displayed.)

⑤ **NORMAL RATE**—Sets the number of ventilator-generated breaths.

⑥ **NORMAL PRESSURE LIMIT**—Sets a limit on amount of pressure used to ventilate client. When the selected pressure is reached, inspiration ends and terminates volume delivery. (Audio-visual alert, PRESSURE LIMIT on display panel shows that pressure limit was reached.)

⑦ **MULTIPLE SIGH**—Number of sighs to be delivered in succession at preset intervals. (CONTROL and ASSIST/CONTROL modes only.)

⑧ **SINGLE SIGH**—Delivers a single manual sign when pressed.

⑨ **SIGH VOLUME**—Sets amount of air to be delivered with each sigh. When sigh volume is delivered sigh breath ends.

⑩ **SIGH RATE**—Sets number of sighs delivered

each hour. (CONTROL and ASSIST-CONTROL modes only)

⑪ **SIGH PRESSURE LIMIT**—Sets limit on amount of pressure used to sigh client. When the selected sigh pressure is reached, inspiration ends and terminates volume delivery. (Audio-visual alert, PRESSURE LIMIT on display panel shows that pressure limit was reached.)

⑫ **MINUTE VOLUME ACCUMULATE**—Tidal volume accumulates for 1 minute, displays for second minute, and then automatically returns to tidal volume. (MINUTE VOLUME ACCUMULATE indicator blinks during accumulation and remains lit during the display of minute volume.)

⑬ **BATTERY/LAMP TEST**—Activates all digital and LED displays, as well as testing the battery-powered, power-loss sensing circuit.

⑭ **VISUAL RESET**—All activated visual alarm/alert indicators remain on, until the VISUAL RESET button is pushed.

⑮ **ALARM SILENCE**—Allows silencing of all audible alarms except the VENT INOPERATIVE alarm. The alarm system will reset automatically in 60 seconds or can be reset manually by depressing the ALARM SILENCE pushbutton (display panel light shows ALARM SILENCE on).

⑯ **WAVE FORM**—Control flow pattern delivered during positive pressure breaths.

Feature continued on following page

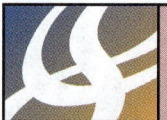

BRIDGE TO CRITICAL CARE

The Ventilator-Dependent Client *(Continued)*

⑰ **PRESSURE SUPPORT**—Adjusts pressure support levels during spontaneous breaths only in SIMV and CPAP.

⑱ Activates pressure support in SIMV and CPAP modes only. *Note: if on during assist/control or control ventilation, PSV indicator on display panel will flash.*

⑲ **ASSIST/SENSITIVITY**—Determines the level of effort required by client to trigger ventilator breath. Senses client effort in ASSIST/CONTROL and SIMV modes to deliver synchronized positive pressure breaths. (Display light shows inspiratory source.)

⑳ **INVERSE RATIO ALERT/LIMIT**—OFF: Allows INVERSE I/E RATIO (visual alert only; display panel light indicates INVERSE RATIO is OFF). ON: Prevents inverse ratio, 1:1 ratio terminates inspiration (audio-visual alert).

㉑ **OXYGEN %**—Controls concentration of oxygen delivered through ventilator.

㉒ **PEAK FLOW**—Regulates the speed at which air flows into the lungs. Controls initial flow rate during positive pressure breaths; no effect on spontaneous flow.

㉓ **INSPIRATORY PAUSE**—Delays the beginning of exhalation.

㉔ **PEEP**—Regulates the amount of pressure applied during expiration to keep alveoli open.

㉕ **NEBULIZER**—Allows intermittent administration of medication during positive pressure breaths. Does not alter oxygen concentration or tidal volume (display panel light shows NEBULIZER ON).

Troubleshooting Mechanical Ventilator Alarms

High-Pressure Alarms

1. Check to see whether the client is biting on the endotracheal tube.
2. Check to see whether the ventilator tubing is kinked.

3. Listen to lung sounds. (Bronchospasm can cause increased airway resistence.) Are there bilateral breath sounds? (The client may have developed pneumothorax.)
4. Question the possibility of mucus plugging. Suction vigorously.
5. Is the client coughing?
6. Check for water in the tubing.
7. Is the client out of rhythm with the ventilator? The client may be breathing against an incoming mechanical breath.

Low-Pressure/Low Exhaled Tidal Volume Alarms

1. Check for disconnected tubing.
2. Listen for a cuff leak.
3. Is the client on an IMV mode of ventilation? If so, he or she may need a higher flow rate if more air is being drawn in than the ventilator is set to deliver.

Minute Ventilation Alarms

1. Assess the client's respiratory rate. If it is rapid, this may produce a larger minute ventilation than normal, especially if the client is on an assist/control mode of ventilation.
2. The alarms may not have been reset after a rate or volume change on the ventilator.

Oxygen Alarms

1. Check the oxygen to ensure that it is set on the proper amount.
2. Check to make sure that the alarms were changed after a change in FIO_2 on the ventilator.

Note: If at any time an alarm is sounding and you cannot quickly ascertain the problem, disconnect the client from the ventilator and use a manual resuscitation bag to support him or her until the problem can be corrected.

CPAP, continuous positive airway pressure; IE, inspiration-expiration; IMV, intermittent mandatory ventilation; LED, light-emitting diode; PEEP, positive end-expiratory pressure; PSV, pressure supported ventilation; SIMV, synchronized intermittent mandatory ventilation.

---

drainage. While your client is being positioned for a bedside chest x-ray, the drainage tubing is inadvertently disconnected from the chest drainage apparatus. What actions should you take?

Factors to Consider. What happens to the normally negative pressure in the pleural space when it is exposed to room air? Is this a dangerous problem?

2. You are caring for a client who is on a mechanical ventilator. You have just suctioned the client and

begin to leave the room when the high-pressure alarm on the ventilator goes off. What should you do?

Factors to Consider. What changes in the client can set off the high-pressure alarm? What changes in the ventilator can cause high pressure?

3. A client with exertional dyspnea is admitted to the unit with a diagnosis of pleural effusion. He has difficulty breathing during the transfer from the cart to bed. You are asked to prepare the client for a

thoracentesis. How would you prioritize care? What preparations are necessary for a thoracentesis?

Factors to Consider. What is the purpose of a thoracentesis? How are complications avoided? What clients are at risk for pleural effusion?

Bibliography

1. American Thoracic Society. (1992). Control of tuberculosis in the United States. *American Review of Respiratory Disease, 146*(6), 1623.
2. American Thoracic Society. (1993). Guidelines for the initial management of adults with community-acquired pneumonia: Diagnosis, assessment of severity, and initial antimicrobial therapy. *American Review of Respiratory Disease, 148*, 1418.
3. Bates, D. V., et al. (1992). Prevention of occupational lung disease. *Chest, 102*(3), 257S.
4. Berk, S. L., et al. (1994). Respiratory pathogens: Something old, something new. *Patient Care, 28*(9), 65.
5. Bloom, B. R., & Murray, C. J. (1992). Commentary on a reemergent killer. *Science 257*, 1055.
6. Boggs, R. L., & Wooldridge-King, M. (1993). *AACN procedure manual for critical care.* Philadelphia: W. B. Saunders.
7. Burns, S. M., Clochesy, J. M., & Hanneman, S. K. G., et al. (1995). Weaning from long-term mechanical ventilation. *American Journal of Critical Care, 4*, 4.
8. Butler, K. (1995). Psychological care of the ventilated patient. *Journal of Clinical Nursing, 4*, 398.
9. Carpenito, L. J. (1993). *Nursing diagnosis: Application to clinical practice* (5th ed.). Philadelphia: J. B. Lippincott.
10. Carroll, P. (1991). What's new in chest tube management. *RN, 54*(5), 34.
11. Carroll, P. (1992). Nursing the thoracotomy patient. *RN, 55*(6), 34.
12. Carroll, P. (1995). A med/surg nurse's guide to mechanical ventilation. *RN, 58*(2), 26.
13. Case, S. C., & Sabo, C. E. (1992). Adult respiratory distress syndrome: A deadly complication of trauma. *Focus on Critical Care, 19*(2), 116.
14. Curry, J. L. (1994). Identifying the patient with tuberculosis and protecting the emergency department staff. *Journal of Emergency Nursing, 20*(4), 293.
15. Daugherty, J. S., et al. (1993). Prevention and control of tuberculosis in the 1990's. *Nursing Clinics of North America, 28*(3), 599.
16. Davidson, P. T. (1989). The diagnosis and management of disease caused by *M. avium* complex, *M. kansasii*, and other mycobacteria. *Clinics in Chest Medicine, 10*(9), 431.
17. Freichels, T. (1993). Orchestrating the care of mechanically ventilated patients. *American Journal of Nursing, 93*(10), 26.
18. Gray, J. E., et al. (1990). The effects of bolus normal saline instillation in conjunction with endotracheal suctioning. *Respiratory Care, 35*(8), 785.
19. Gray, M. A. (1993). Medications for a growing concern: Tuberculosis. *Orthopaedic Nursing, 12*(2), 75.
20. Gross, S. B. (1993). Current challenges, concepts, and controversies in chest tube management. *AACN Clinical Issues, 4*(2), 260.
21. Hardy, K. A. (1993). Advances in our understanding and care of patients with cystic fibrosis. *Respiratory Care, 38*(3), 282.
22. Harvey, J. C., & Beattie, E. J. (1993). Lung cancer. *Clinical Symposia, 45*(3), 2.
23. Hee, M. K., et al. (1992). Intubation of critically ill patients. *Mayo Clinic Proceedings, 67*(6), 569.
24. Hopkins, S. (1995). Advances in the treatment of cystic fibrosis. *Nursing Times, 91*(39), 40.
25. Jenkinson, S. G. (1993). Lung transplantation: An update. *Respiratory Care, 383*, 278.
26. Johns, C. J., Scott, P. P., & Schonfeld, S. A. (1989). Sarcoidosis. *Annual Review of Medicine, 40*, 353.
27. Langston, W. G. (1992). Surgical resection of lung cancer. *Nursing Clinics of North America, 27*(3), 665.
28. Leffert, C. C., & Luecke, L. (1993). Assessing and treating pulmonary edema. *Nursing 93, 23*(7), 54.
29. Lekander, B. J. (1988). Preventing complications for the heart and lung transplant recipient. *Dimensions of Critical Care Nursing, 7*(1), 18.
30. Long, C. O., Ismeurt, R., & Wilson, L. W. (1995). The elderly & pneumonia: Prevention and management. *Home Healthcare Nurse, 13*(5), 43.
31. Mandel, J. H., & Baker, B. A. (1989). Recognizing occupational lung disease. *Hospital Practice, 24*(1), 21.
32. Mathewson, H. S. (1994). Drugs for pulmonary mycoses. *Respiratory Care, 39*(6), 652.
33. O'Brien, R. J. (1989). The epidemiology of nontuberculous mycobacterial disease. *Clinics in Chest Medicine, 10*(9), 407.
34. Pierce, J. D., et al. (1991). Effects of two chest tube clearance protocols on drainage in patients after myocardial revascularization surgery. *Heart and Lung, 20*(2), 125.
35. Ramsey, B. W. (1996). Management of pulmonary disease in patients with cystic fibrosis. *New England Journal of Medicine, 335*(13), 179.
36. Rice, R. (1995). Home mechanical ventilator management. *Home Healthcare Nurse, 13*, 73.
37. Ruppert, S. D., Kernicki, J. G., & Dolan, J. T. (1996). *Critical Care Nursing* (2nd ed.). Philadelphia, F. A. Davis.
38. Seale, D. D., & Beaver, B. M. (1992). Pathophysiology of lung cancer. *Nursing Clinics of North America, 27*(3), 603.
39. Stone, K. S., & Turner, B. (1989). Endotracheal suctioning. *Annual Review of Nursing Research, 7*(1), 27.
40. Teplitz, L. (1991). Update: Are milking and stripping chest tubes necessary? *Focus on Critical Care, 18*(6), 506.
41. Tobin, M. J. (1994). Mechanical ventilation. *New England Journal of Medicine, 330*(15), 1056.
42. Vollman, K. M. (1994). Adult respiratory distress syndrome: Mediators on the run. *Critical Care Nursing Clinics of North America, 6*(2), 341.
43. Von Nessen, S. (1995). Exercise for patients with cystic fibrosis. *Perspectives in Respiratory Nursing, 6*(2), 5.
44. Wade, J. F., & King, T. E. (1993). Infiltrative and interstitial lung disease in the elderly patient. *Clinics in Chest Medicine, 14*(3), 501.
45. Webb, A. K., & David, T. J. (1994). Clinical management of children and adults with cystic fibrosis. *British Medical Journal, 308*, 459.
46. Weilitz, P. B. (1993). Weaning a patient from mechanical ventilation. *Critical Care Nurse, 13*(4), 33.

Cardiac Disorders

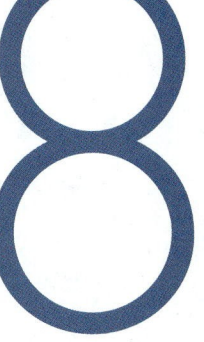

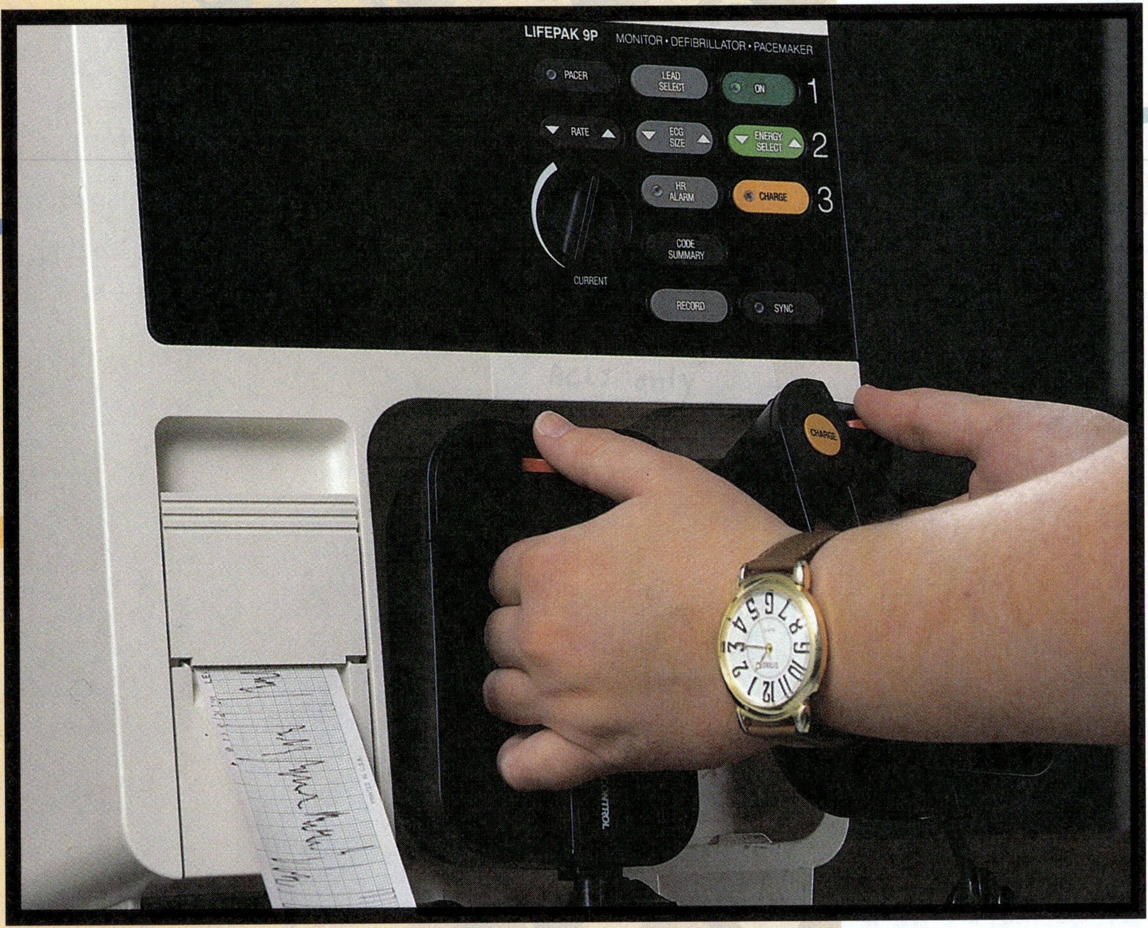

Structure and Function of the Heart

Barbara B. Ott

The human heart beats approximately 72 times per minute, 100,000 times a day, and 22.5 billion times in a lifetime. This small pump, weighing approximately 11 oz, pumps approximately 5 qt of blood each minute and 75 gal/hour. With computer-like efficiency, it pumps oxygen-rich blood into the arterial system. This pump contracts every second of every day throughout a lifetime, resting only 0.4 seconds between beats.

The heart beats continuously, and unlike other muscles of the body, it cannot stop to rest when tired and worn from work. Instead, it must keep pumping continuously with sufficient force to circulate blood properly to all parts of the body. And, amazingly, it must increase its work output by four or five times its resting level if it is to sustain the body during periods of stress (e.g., hard exercise, emotions, and illness).

When the heart does not work efficiently, the client's life may be threatened. This normally efficient and remarkably durable structure can develop structural defects and functional disturbances. What happens to the body when this mechanism begins to weaken and fail? What happens to the tissues and cells when the heart cannot pump oxygenated blood to them in adequate amounts? To understand cardiac disease, one must first examine normal cardiac function.

This chapter reviews normal cardiac structure, function, and control as a basis for understanding pathologic conditions presented in the following chapters.

The function of the heart is to pump oxygenated blood into the arterial system, which carries it to the cells, and to collect deoxygenated blood from the venous system and deliver it to the lungs for reoxygenation (Fig. 43–1).

The heart is located within the mediastinum, which is the space between the lungs in the thoracic cavity. The heart is cone-shaped and lies on the diaphragm. It is tilted forward and to the left. The apex of the heart (tip of the cone) is at its bottom and lies left of the midline. The base is at the top of the heart, where the great vessels enter the heart, and it lies posterior to the sternum.

The Layers of the Heart

The heart consists of three distinct layers of tissue: epicardium, myocardium, and endocardium (Fig. 43–2). The *epicardium* covers the outer surface of the heart. It has the same thin, transparent structure as the visceral pericardium. The *myocardium,* the middle layer, consists of striated muscle fibers forming interlaced bundles. It is the actual contracting muscle of the heart. The *endocardium,* the innermost layer, consists of thin endothelial tissue. It lines the inner chambers and the heart valves.

The Chambers of the Heart

Each side of the heart consists of two chambers, an upper collecting chamber (atrium) and a lower pumping chamber (ventricle). A muscular wall, the septum, separates the chambers of the right side of the heart from those of the left side of the heart. The *right atrium* receives deoxygenated blood from the body via the superior and inferior vena cava. The blood then flows into the right ventricle. The *right ventricle,* a flat muscular pump, receives blood from the right atrium and pumps it to the lungs against low resistance, via the pulmonary artery. The *left atrium* receives oxygenated blood from the lungs via the four pulmonary veins. The blood then flows into the left ventricle. The *left ventricle,* the heart's largest, most muscular chamber, receives oxygenated blood from the lungs via the left atrium and pumps it out into the systemic circulation via the aorta. The left ventricle pumps against high systemic pressure.

The heart is actually two pumps working in unison. The right side receives deoxygenated blood from the body and pumps it to the lungs via the pulmonary arteries. At the same time, the left side receives oxygenated blood from the lungs and pumps it out through the aorta to all parts of the body (Fig. 43–3).

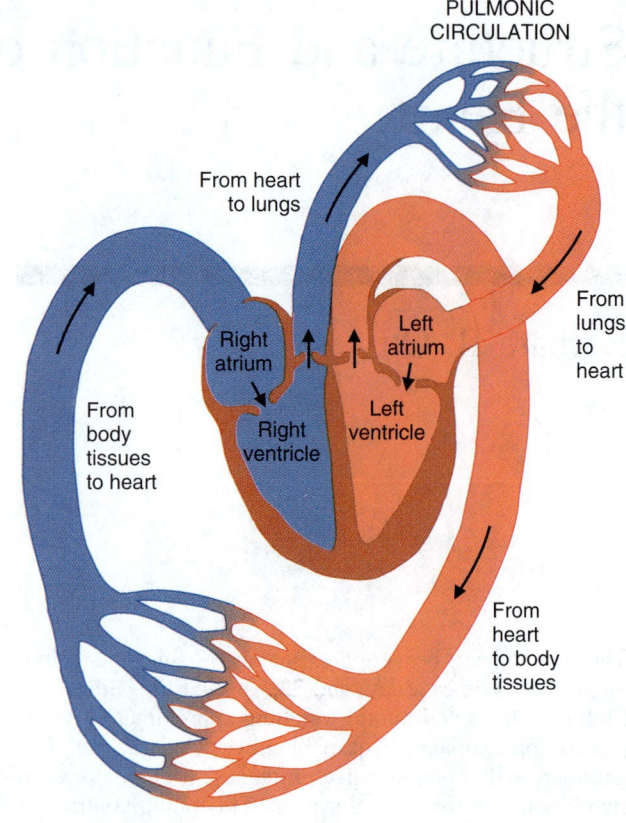

PULMONIC
CIRCULATION

From heart
to lungs

From
lungs
to
heart

Right
atrium

Left
atrium

From
body
tissues
to heart

Right
ventricle

Left
ventricle

From
heart
to body
tissues

SYSTEMIC CIRCULATION

Figure 43–1. Functions of the heart. In the peripheral capillaries, blood oxygen is exchanged for carbon dioxide. The deoxygenated blood returns to the right atrium and right ventricle to be pumped into the lungs, where carbon dioxide is exchanged for oxygen. Oxygenated blood from the lungs enters the left atrium and left ventricle of the heart to be pumped once again into the systemic circulation.

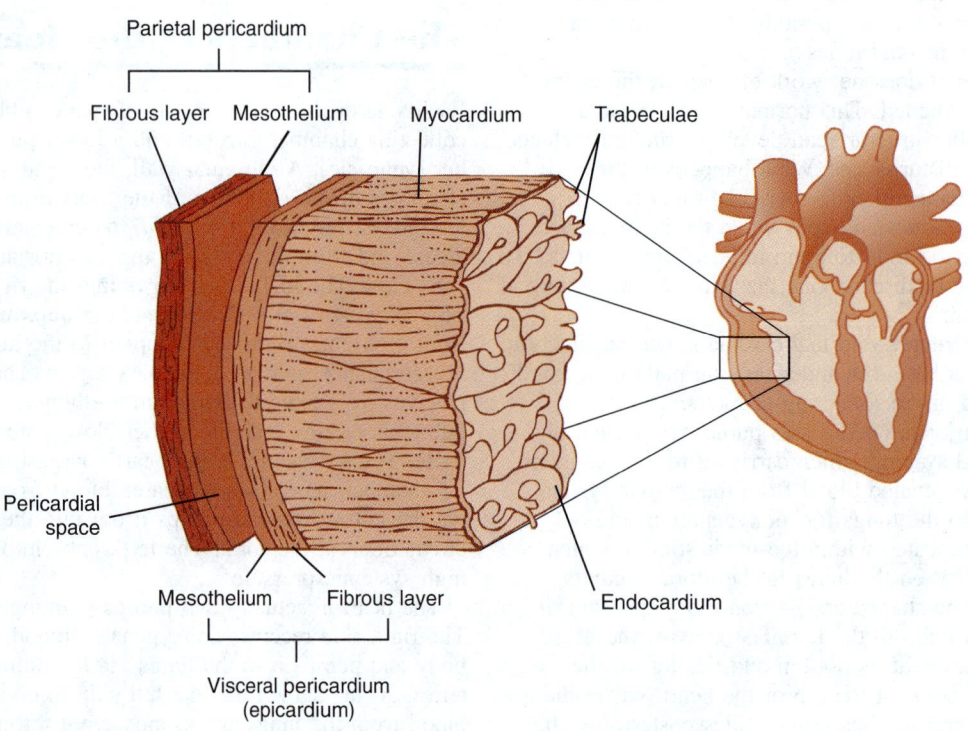

Parietal pericardium

Fibrous layer   Mesothelium   Myocardium   Trabeculae

Pericardial
space

Mesothelium   Fibrous layer   Endocardium

Visceral pericardium
(epicardium)

Figure 43–2. The three layers of the heart.

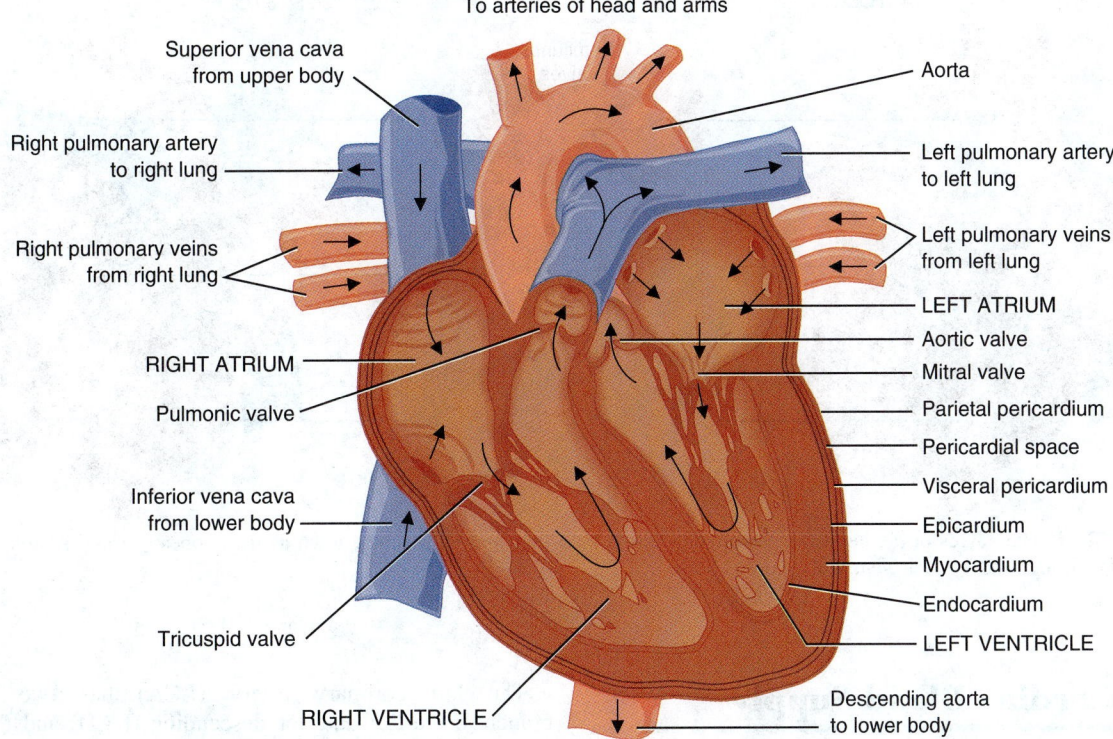

To arteries of head and arms

Superior vena cava
from upper body

Aorta

Right pulmonary artery
to right lung

Left pulmonary artery
to left lung

Right pulmonary veins
from right lung

Left pulmonary veins
from left lung

LEFT ATRIUM

RIGHT ATRIUM

Aortic valve

Pulmonic valve

Mitral valve

Parietal pericardium

Pericardial space

Visceral pericardium

Inferior vena cava
from lower body

Epicardium

Myocardium

Endocardium

LEFT VENTRICLE

Tricuspid valve

Descending aorta
to lower body

RIGHT VENTRICLE

Figure 43–3. The structure of the heart and the circulation of blood through the heart. Blood entering the left atrium from the right and left pulmonary veins flows into the left ventricle. The left ventricle pumps blood into the systemic circulation through the aorta. From the systemic circulation, blood returns to the heart through the superior and inferior venae cavae. From there, the right ventricle pumps blood into the lungs through the right and left pulmonary arteries.

The Pericardium

Encasing the heart is the pericardium, a loose-fitting covering that protects the heart from trauma and infection. It consists of two layers, one sac inside another: the parietal pericardium and the visceral pericardium. The *parietal pericardium* is the tough, fibrous outer membrane that is attached anteriorly to the lower half of the sternum, posteriorly to the thoracic vertebrae, and inferiorly to the diaphragm. It provides an effective barrier to infection from surrounding structures. The *visceral pericardium* is the thin, inner layer, which closely adheres to the heart and to the first several centimeters of the pulmonary artery and aorta.

The pericardial space is between the visceral and parietal layers and holds 5 to 20 ml of pericardial fluid. The fluid lubricates the pericardial surfaces as they slide over each other when the heart beats, and it cushions the heart against external trauma.

The Cardiac Valves

The cardiac valves are delicate, flexible structures that consist of endothelium covered by fibrous tissue. They permit only unidirectional blood flow through the heart, from right to left. The valves open and close passively, and these movements depend on pressure gradients in the cardiac chambers (Fig. 43–4).

Cardiac valves are of two types: atrioventricular (AV) and semilunar.

The Atrioventricular Valves

Atrioventricular valves lie between the atria and ventricles. The tricuspid valve, on the right side, is composed of three leaflets. The mitral (bicuspid) valve is on the left and is composed of two leaflets. Attached to the edges of the AV valves are strong, fibrous filaments called *chordae tendineae*, which arise from papillary muscles on the ventricular walls. The papillary muscles and chordae tendineae work together to prevent the AV valves from opening during ventricular contraction (systole). These valves prevent backflow of blood during periods of high-pressure blood flow.

The Semilunar Valves

The semilunar valves consist of three cuplike cusps that prevent blood from flowing back into the ventricles during relaxation (diastole). Unlike AV valves, semilunar valves are open during ventricular contraction. The pulmonic semilunar valve lies between the right ventricle and the pulmonary artery. The aortic semilunar valve lies between the left ventricle and the aorta. These valves do not have papillary muscles because they regulate blood flow during diastole, which is a low-pressure flow.

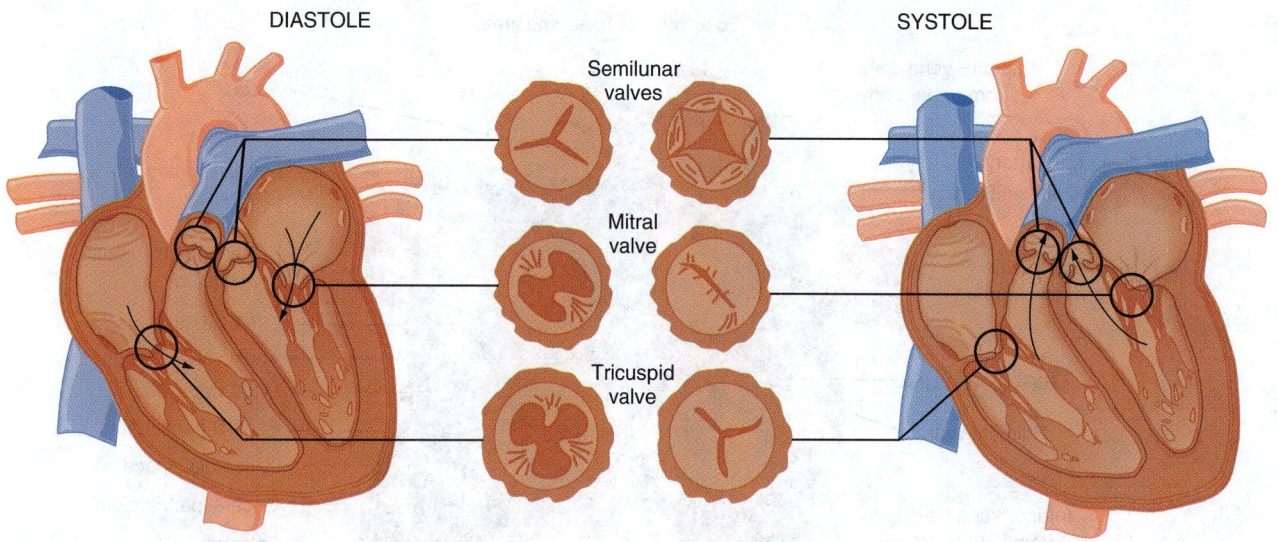

Figure 43–4. The valves of the heart. The semilunar, mitral, and tricuspid valves are shown as they appear during diastole (ventricular filling) and systole (ventricular contraction).

The Cardiac Blood Supply

The heart muscle requires a rich oxygen supply to meet its own metabolic needs. The coronary arteries (right and left) branch off the aorta just above the aortic valve, encircle the heart, and penetrate the myocardium (Fig. 43–5). They supply the capillaries of the myocardium with blood.

The right coronary artery (RCA) and its branches perfuse the right atrium, the right ventricle, the inferior portion of the left ventricle, and the posterior septal wall, as well as the sinoatrial (SA) node and the atrioventricular (AV) node.

The left coronary artery (LCA) has two major branches, the left anterior descending (LAD) and the circumflex arteries. The LAD supplies blood to the anterior wall of the left ventricle, the anterior ventricular septum, and the apex of the left ventricle. The circumflex artery provides blood to the left atrium, the lateral and posterior surfaces of the left ventricle, and, occasionally, the posterior interventricular septum. In some clients, the circumflex artery supplies the SA and AV nodes.

Unlike other arteries, in the coronary artery 75% of blood flow occurs during diastole, when the heart is relaxed.[1] For adequate blood flow through the coronary arteries, the diastolic blood pressure must be at least 60 mm Hg. Coronary blood flow increases with increased

Figure 43–5. The coronary arteries. The right and left coronary arteries branch off the aorta just above the aortic valve; they normally supply the myocardium with oxygenated blood.

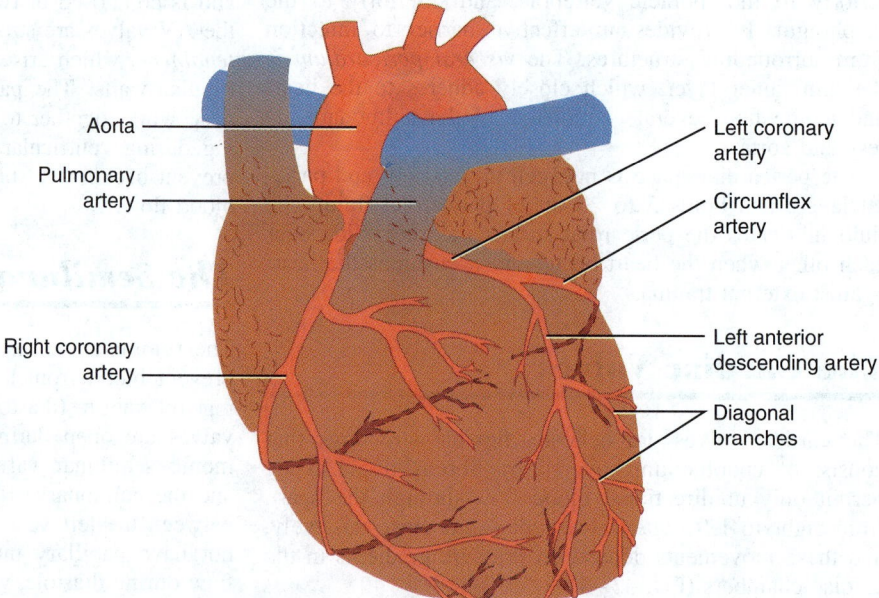

activity (i.e., exercise) and with increased stimulation of the sympathetic nervous system.

The coronary veins return blood from the myocardium to the right atrium. These veins usually run parallel to the arteries.

Electrophysiologic Properties of the Heart

The electrophysiologic properties of cardiac muscle regulate the heart rate and rhythm. These properties include excitability, automaticity, conductivity, and refractoriness.

Excitability

The ability of cardiac muscle cells to depolarize in response to a stimulus is called *excitability*. Once stimulated, the whole heart muscle contracts. In contrast, skeletal muscle contracts partially to produce a graded force. If the heart contracted only partially, it would not effectively pump blood. Excitability is influenced by hormones, electrolytes, nutrition, oxygen supply, medications, infection, and nerve characteristics.

In myocardial cells, as in neurons, differences in intracellular and extracellular ion concentrations create electrical and concentration gradients for ionic movement across the semipermeable cell membrane. At rest, the inside of a myocardial cell is more negative than the outside. This "resting membrane potential" primarily results from the differences in concentrations of sodium (Na+) and potassium (K+). Although both ions are present on either side of the cell membrane, potassium has a greater intracellular concentration and sodium has a greater extracellular concentration. A lowered intracellular concentration of cations (positive ions) results when the cell membrane allows movement of potassium out of the cell, yet remains relatively impermeable to sodium.

When the cardiac cell is stimulated to a certain threshold, the transmembrane potential undergoes a dramatic change, known as an *action potential* (Fig. 43–6). The action potential consists of depolarization and repolarization phases. The ECG reflects these waves of depolarization and repolarization sweeping over the heart.

Stimulation of the cardiac cell initiates depolarization and the subsequent change in transmembrane potential. The intracellular electrical potential shifts from negative to positive. This change results from an increase in cell membrane permeability to sodium, with resultant rapid influx of sodium ions. The wave of depolarization spreads to adjacent cells and through the whole heart.

The cell returns to its resting (relaxed) state during repolarization. Sodium permeability drops sharply, and potassium and chloride move out of the cell, returning the membrane to resting potential. In the process of depolarization and repolarization, small amounts of sodium leak into the cell and potassium leaks outward. The cell membrane monitors this balance, actively pumping sodium back out and potassium inward.

Other ions, such as calcium, chloride, and magnesium, also play a role in the action potential and the contraction

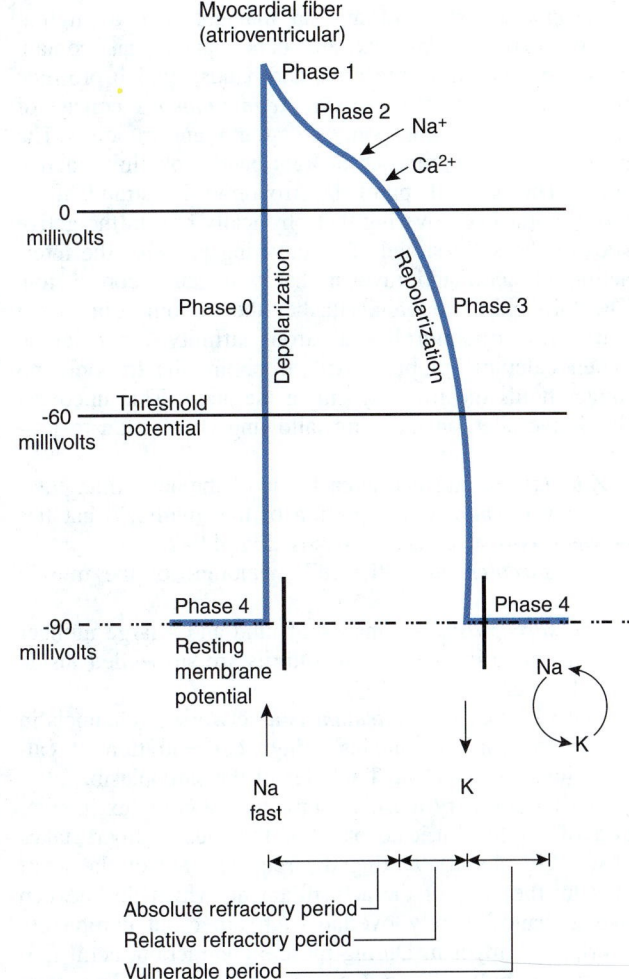

Figure 43–6. The action potential of cardiac cells has five phases: *Phase 0:* Sodium rapidly enters the cell through fast sodium channels, and cell depolarization (contraction) begins. *Phase 1:* The fast sodium channels close. *Phase 2:* Sodium continues to enter along with calcium, but it does so more slowly. *Phase 3:* Potassium enters the cell. *Phase 4:* The cell returns to its resting potential, sodium is pumped out of the cell, and potassium is pumped into the cell through the cell's sodium-potassium pump. In all cardiac cells, a period occurs during which the cells cannot be stimulated to fire another action potential. During the end of the action potential, the membrane is relatively refractory and can be reexcited only by a larger than usual stimulus. Immediately after the action potential, the membrane has transitory hyperexcitability and is said to be in a vulnerable state.

it causes. The most important ion is calcium. During depolarization, myocardial cell membrane permeability to calcium increases and calcium moves into the cell. As the intracellular concentration of calcium increases, calcium reacts with contractile elements and myocardial muscle fibers contract.

The heart muscle is composed of long, narrow cells or *fibers*. Coronary muscle fibers contain myofibrils, Z bands, sarcomeres, sarcolemmas, sarcoplasm, and sarcoplasmic reticulum.

Myofibrils consist of myosin filaments and actin filaments. *Myosin filaments* are dark bands that contain cross-bridges (similar to arms and hands), which protrude from the side of the myosin. *Actin filaments* consist of three parts: actin, a tropomyosin strand, and troponin. The actin portion is composed of light bands containing active sites. The second part, the tropomyosin strand, is a loosely attached covering that physically covers the active sites of the actin strand. This covering prevents the interaction of actin and myosin that will cause contraction. The third part, troponin, attaches the tropomyosin to the actin. But troponin has a strong affinity for calcium. When calcium combines with troponin, the troponin no longer holds the tropomyosin in the actin. This uncovers the active sites on the actin, allowing contraction to proceed.

Z bands are attached at each end of the actin filament.

The *sarcomere* is the portion of the myofibril that lies between two successive Z bands (Fig. 43–7).

The *sarcolemma* is the cell membrane of the muscle fiber.

The *sarcoplasm* is a matrix of fluid and a large number of mitochondria in which myofibrils are suspended inside muscle fiber.

The *sarcoplasmic reticulum* is a network of channels in the sarcoplasm. It contains a high concentration of calcium ions stored in the T tubules of the sarcoplasm.

During coronary muscle contraction, a complex interaction of all the intricate parts of the muscle fibers takes place (Fig. 43–8). During the relaxed state of the heart muscle, the ends of the actin filament, which lie between two Z bands, barely overlap each other but completely overlap the myosin. During muscle contraction, actin filaments are pulled inward among the myosin. The actin filaments now overlap each other. The Z bands are smaller, too, as they are pulled up by the action of the actin and the myosin. Muscle contraction occurs as a result of this sliding filament mechanism.

The action potential initiates the muscle contraction by releasing calcium through the T channels of the sarcoplasm. The calcium diffuses to the myofibrils, where it binds with troponin. As soon as the actin filaments become activated by calcium, the heads of the cross-bridges from the myosin filaments immediately become attracted to the active sites of the actin. Contraction then occurs.

After contraction, free calcium ions are actively pumped out of the cell back into the sarcoplasmic reticulum, and muscle relaxation begins.

Automaticity

The ability of cardiac cells to initiate an impulse spontaneously and repetitively, without external neurohormonal control, is known as automaticity, or rhythmicity. Given the proper laboratory conditions, the heart can continue to beat outside of the body by means of its intrinsic control system. In contrast, skeletal muscle must be stimulated by a nerve to depolarize and contract. Heart muscle can depolarize spontaneously and stimulate its own contraction. Pacemaker cells have the highest rate of automaticity of all cardiac cells. The conduction tissue area with the highest automaticity, or rate of spontaneous depolarization, assumes the role of pacemaker. In normal circumstances, this is the SA node. Electrophysiology of the heart is discussed in more detail in Chapter 46.

Conductivity

Conductivity is the ability of heart muscle fibers to propagate electrical impulses along and across cell membranes. The heart muscle must conduct the action potential from its origin throughout the heart both rapidly and in a coordinated manner, so that the heart contracts as a unit. Intercalated disks join adjacent myocardial cells, allowing the action potential to travel over the entire muscle mass.

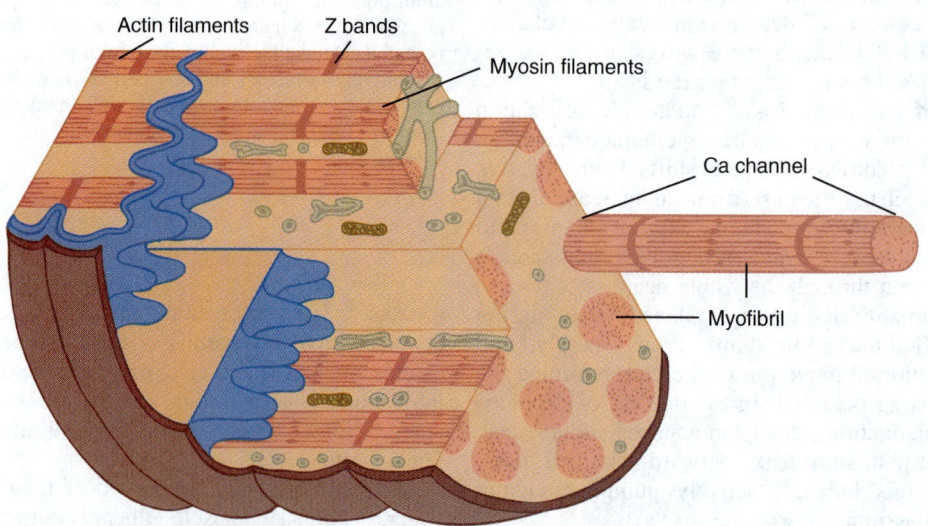

Figure 43–7. The sarcomere, the functional unit of the cardiac muscle. Ca^{2+} enters through calcium ion channels on the surface of the sarcomere.

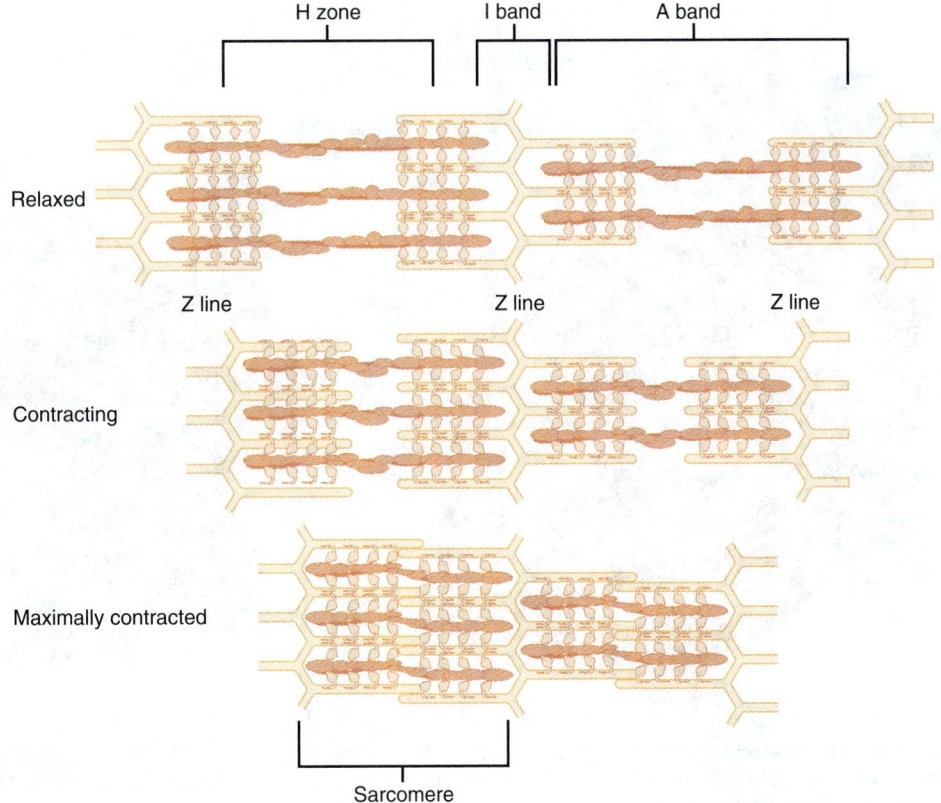

Figure 43–8. The actin filaments are pulled along the myosin, causing the heart muscle to contract.

Refractoriness

Refractoriness is the heart's inability to respond to a new stimulus while still in a state of contraction from an earlier stimulus. Thus, the heart muscle does not respond to restimulation during the action potential, preventing the possibility of tetanic contractions seen in skeletal muscle. Such sustained contractions of the heart would be fatal, because sufficient time would not be allowed for ventricular filling. Refractoriness develops because the sodium channels of the cardiac cell membrane become inactivated during an action potential (depolarization).

Refractoriness occurs in two periods. The absolute refractory period occurs during depolarization and the first part of repolarization. During this period, cardiac cells do not respond to any stimuli, however strong. Then, in the final stages of repolarization, refractoriness diminishes and depolarization can occur once again. During this period, known as the *relative refractory period*, only a stronger-than-normal stimulus can excite the heart muscle to contract. At the end of the refractory period, the sodium channels are restored and the cardiac cells can again conduct action potentials.

Normally, the ventricles have an absolute refractory period of 0.25 to 0.3 seconds, which approximates the duration of the action potential. The relative refractory period for the ventricles lasts about 0.05 seconds. The atria have a refractory period of about 0.15 seconds, which is much shorter than for the ventricles. This means that the atria can rhythmically contract much faster than the ventricles.

Refractoriness of the myocardium normally prevents uncontrolled rapid cardiac contractions. Thus, refractoriness helps to preserve the heart rhythm.

The Cardiac Conduction System

The cardiac conduction system (Fig. 43–9) consists of modified cardiac muscle cells. These cells are characterized by their ability to conduct electrical impulses very rapidly. The conduction system acts to spread the action potential, initiated in one area of the myocardium, rapidly through the whole heart. Spread of the action potential stimulates synchronized contraction of the atria and ventricles. The conduction system consists of the following major parts.

The Sinoatrial Node

The sinoatrial node (SA node) or pacemaker, is located at the junction of the superior vena cava and right atrium. Under normal circumstances, the SA node initiates each heartbeat. It generates electrical impulses approximately 60 to 100 times per minute but can adjust its rate. Internodal and interatrial tracts carry the wave of depolarization through the right atrium and left atrium, respectively.[10] The sympathetic and parasympa-

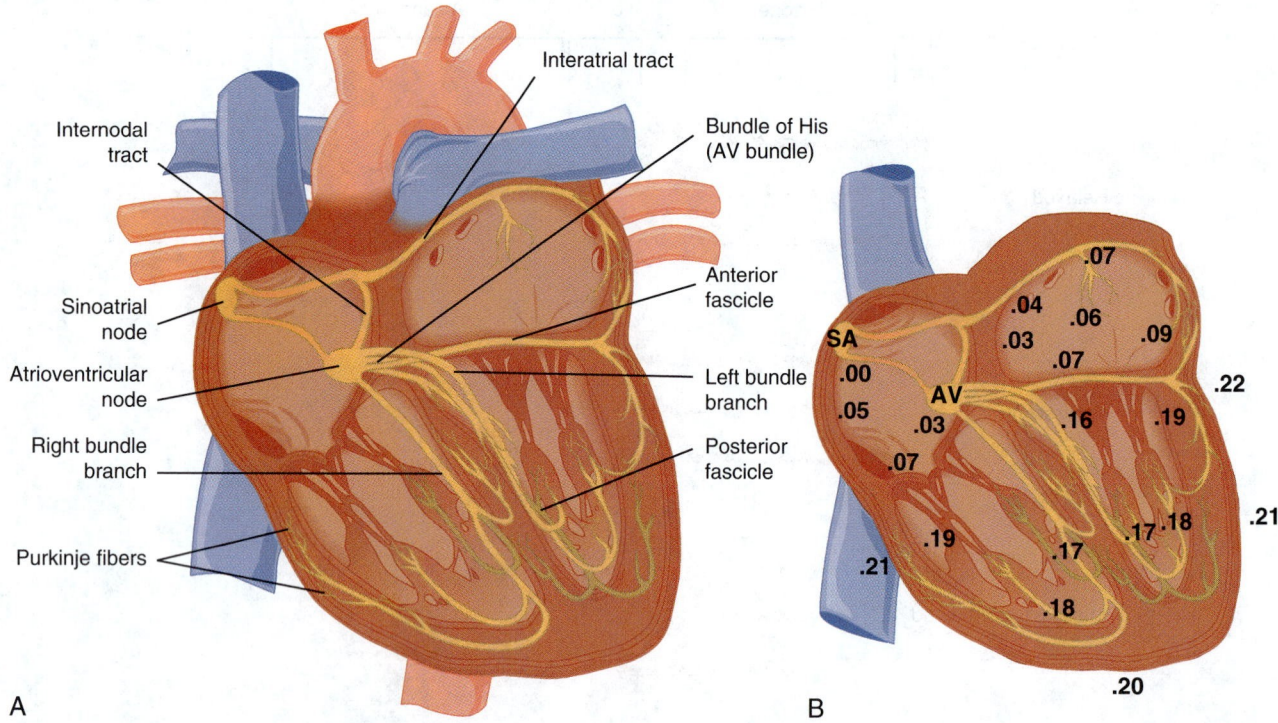

Figure 43–9. *A,* The cardiac conduction system. *B,* Transmission of the cardiac impulse through the heart, showing the time of appearance (in fractions of a second) of the impulse in different parts of the heart. (*B* after Guyton, A. C. [1996]. *Textbook of medical physiology* [9th ed.]. Philadelphia: W. B. Saunders.)

thetic nervous systems control the SA node. Any myocardial tissue in the atria, AV bundle, or ventricles has the capability of taking over the role of pacemaker if that tissue generates impulses at a higher rate than the SA node.

The Atrioventricular Node

The AV node, or AV junction, is located in the lower aspect of the atrial septum. The AV node receives electrical impulses from the SA node. Within the AV node, the impulse is delayed 0.07 seconds while the atria contract. This delay enables atrial contraction to be completed before the ventricles are stimulated and contract.

The Bundle of His

The bundle of His (AV bundle) fuses with the AV node to form another pacemaker site. If the SA node fails, the bundle of His can initiate and sustain a heart rate of 40 to 60 beats/minute. The bundle of His is relatively short, branching into right and left segments. The right bundle branch (RBB) courses down the right side of the interventricular septum. The left bundle branch (LBB) bifurcates into anterior and posterior fascicles, both of which extend into the left ventricle. The right and left bundle branches terminate in Purkinje's fibers.

Purkinje's Fibers

Purkinje's fibers are a diffuse network of conducting strands beneath the ventricular endocardium; they rapidly spread the wave of depolarization through the ventricles. Activation of the ventricles begins in the septum and then moves from the apex of the heart upward. Within the ventricular walls, depolarization proceeds from endocardium to epicardium. Repolarization is a passive event that occurs in each cell and does not involve the conduction system. Repolarization occurs in reverse order, so that the last cells to depolarize are the first to repolarize.

The Cardiac Cycle

One cardiac cycle (Fig. 43–10) is equivalent to one complete heartbeat. The sequence of events in the cardiac cycle is divided into two parts: systole (contraction) and diastole (relaxation).

Ventricular Systole

In the isovolumetric contraction phase, the ventricles begin to contract, closing the AV valves and building up pressure within the ventricles. As the aortic and pulmonic valves also remain closed at this point, no blood leaves the ventricle. As the AV valves close, the first heart sound (S$_1$) is heard. The ejection phase begins when pressure in the ventricles exceeds the aortic and pulmonic

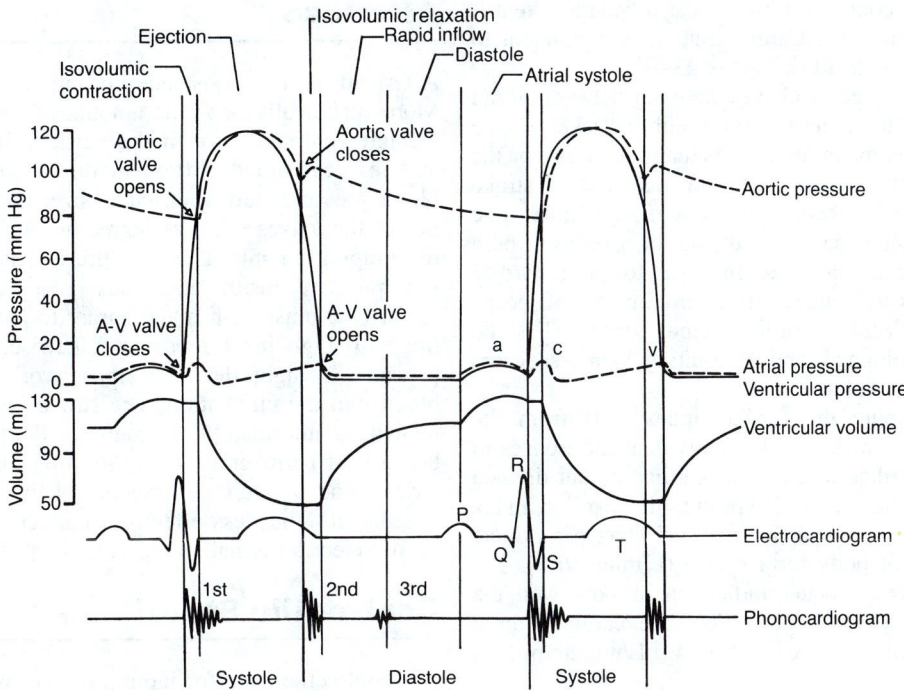

Figure 43–10. Changes that occur during the cardiac cycle in left atrial pressure, left ventricular pressure, aortic pressure, ventricular volume, the electrocardiogram, and the phonocardiogram. (From Guyton, A. C. [1996]. *Textbook of medical physiology* [9th ed.]. Philadelphia: W. B. Saunders.)

pressures. The semilunar valves open, and the ventricles pump blood into the systemic and pulmonary circulations.

Ventricular Diastole

In early diastole, as the ventricles begin to relax, aortic and pulmonic pressures exceed ventricular pressures, and the semilunar (aortic and pulmonic) valves close. The valve closure causes the second heart sound (S₂). The AV valves remain closed; all four valves are closed again, and no blood moves in or out of the ventricles. This is called *isovolumetric relaxation.* As the ventricles continue to relax, the AV valves open and blood rushes into the ventricles, initiating the rapid ventricular filling phase.

Extra Heart Sounds

Because blood rapidly fills the ventricles, the ventricular wall must expand suddenly to accommodate it. If ventricular wall compliance is decreased (as in congestive heart failure or valvular regurgitation), structures within the ventricular wall vibrate and a third heart sound (S₃) may be heard. An S₃ heart sound may be a normal finding in people younger than 30 years. During the last phase of ventricular diastole, atrial contraction (atrial systole or atrial kick) occurs, contributing 20% to 30% more blood volume to the ventricles. A fourth heart sound (S₄) may be heard on atrial systole if resistance to active ventricular filling is present. This is not a normal finding, and its

causes include hypertrophy, disease, or injury of the ventricular wall.

Mechanical Properties of the Heart

The heart propels blood throughout the body. It can perform this task because it is able to contract. Myocardial contraction, as stated earlier, occurs in response to depolarization and the diffusion of calcium into myocardial cells, where it combines with troponin to activate contractile elements. Proper contractility depends on intact electrophysiologic stimuli and conduction and on a functional myocardium. If the heart muscle is damaged (e.g., following a myocardial infarction), contractile units fail to function properly. Hence, the strength of contraction decreases. One way to measure myocardial contractility is by the cardiac output.

Cardiac Output and Cardiac Index

Cardiac output is the volume of blood ejected by each ventricle into the pulmonic and systemic circulations per minute by rhythmic ventricular contraction. At the end of ventricular diastole (filling phase), each ventricle contains approximately 120 ml of blood (end-diastolic volume). Normally, during systole, the heart ejects approximately two thirds of its end-diastolic volume (EDV). The volume ejected with each contraction (heartbeat) of the left ventricle is the *stroke volume*. Cardiac output is equivalent to stroke volume times heart rate (Box 43–1).

Cardiac output ranges widely, averaging between 4 and 8 L/minute in adults. Adjustments in either stroke volume or heart rate can compensate for fluctuations in one or the other, or both can rise or fall. For instance, if stroke volume decreases, as occurs in hemorrhage, heart rate increases to sustain cardiac output. In exercise, both stroke volume and heart rate increase to raise cardiac output. Decreases in heart rate to approximately 50 beats/minute may not decrease cardiac output because diastolic filling time is prolonged, and a resulting increase occurs in EDV and stroke volume.

Clinicians compute the cardiac index (CI) from the cardiac output to compensate for individual differences in body size. The cardiac index is the cardiac output divided by the body surface area. Therefore, the cardiac index describes the cardiac output in terms of liters per minute per square meter of body surface area (L/minute/m²). The cardiac index gives a better indication of how well the tissues are being perfused than does the cardiac output alone. Normal cardiac index is 2.5 to 4.0 L/minute/m².

Stroke Volume

Stroke volume has a major influence on cardiac output. Several determinants influence stroke volume; these include preload, afterload, and the contractile state of the heart.

Preload

Preload is the myocardial fiber length of the left ventricle at end diastole. It is determined by the end-diastolic volume. The Frank-Starling law of the heart states that the greater the myocardial fiber length, or stretch, the greater will be its force of contraction. This phenomenon is similar to the increased recoil of a rubber band when subjected to greater stretching. Preload therefore increases when increased end-diastolic blood volume (e.g., from increased venous return) subjects myocardial fibers to greater stretch. The ventricles respond with a greater force of contraction, producing a larger stroke volume and increased cardiac output. This phenomenon, however, has limits. After a point, further stretching of the myocardium does not improve stroke volume; indeed, it may actually decrease stroke volume (Fig. 43–11).[3] This concept can be demonstrated by an overstretched rubber band.

Box 43–1. Calculating Cardiac Output

Cardiac output (CO) = stroke volume (SV) × heart rate (HR)*

---

* For a normal 150-lb [70-kg] adult at rest, CO is 5 to 6 L/min

---

Afterload

Afterload is the resistance to left ventricular ejection. More specifically, it is the amount of tension required by the left ventricle to open the aortic valve during systole and to eject blood. Afterload directly relates to arterial blood pressure, left ventricular size, and the characteristics of the valves.[6] A low degree of afterload is analogous to pumping air into a bicycle tire that is flat; the tire has low pressure inside and, thus, requires little pumping force. One must push much harder to pump air into a full tire with high inner pressure. Likewise, if arterial blood pressure is high, the heart must work harder to pump blood into the circulation. The stroke volume is inversely related to afterload. For example, if afterload increases because of peripheral vasoconstriction (thus increasing arterial blood pressure), shortening of the myocardial fibers is reduced. With less effective contractions, the ventricles cannot eject a normal stroke volume.

Contractile State

The contractile state (or inotropic state) refers to the vigor of contraction generated by the myocardium regardless of its blood volume (preload). The ability to alter contractile force and velocity is an inherent property of the myocardium. Sympathetic stimulation increases myocardial contractility and ventricular pressure, thereby ejecting blood more rapidly, and increasing stroke volume. Metabolic abnormalities (e.g., hypoxemia) and metabolic acidosis decrease myocardial contractility, therefore reducing stroke volume.

Cardiac Pressures

With the use of a pulmonary artery pressure catheter (Swan-Ganz), pressures inside the cardiac chambers can be measured. These pressures are useful in determining factors such as preload, afterload, volume, filling pressures, and resistance. Normal cardiac pressures are shown in Figure 43–12. The technique and nursing implications are discussed in the Bridge to Critical Care in Chapter 45.

Heart Rate

The normal heart rate is 60 to 100 beats/minute. *Sinus tachycardia* is defined as a rate of more than 100 beats/minute; it can follow exercise or emotional upset. *Sinus bradycardia* is defined as a rate of fewer than 60 beats/minute. Variations in heartbeat are normally caused by exercise, size of the individual, age, sex, hormones, temperature, blood pressure, anxiety, stress, and pain.

Exercise causes increased need for oxygen and elimination of CO_2, which in turn causes increased heart rate. The conditioned athlete, however, usually has a lower heart rate at rest. The size of the individual also affects heart rate. A larger person has a slower heart rate. *Age* affects heart rate, which is fastest in the fetus (120 to 160 beats/minute) and lowest in adults (65 to 80 beats/min-

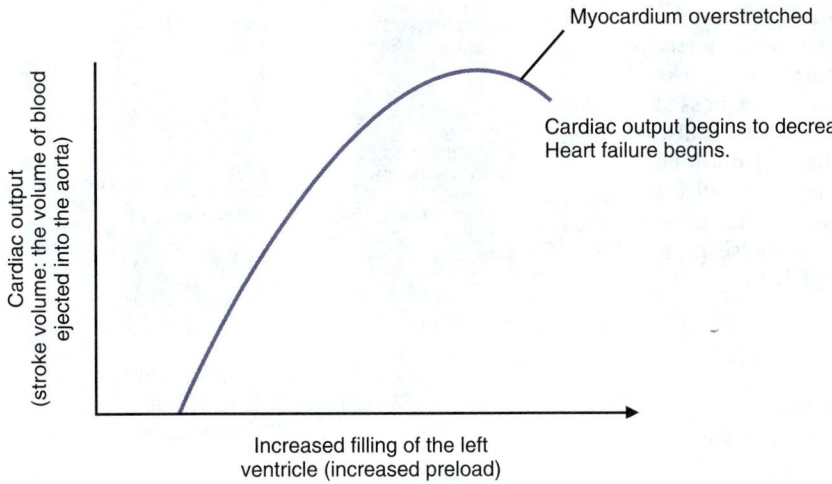

Myocardium overstretched

Cardiac output begins to decrease.
Heart failure begins.

Cardiac output
(stroke volume: the volume of blood
ejected into the aorta)

Increased filling of the left
ventricle (increased preload)

Figure 43–11. According to the Frank-Starling law, the more the left ventricle fills with blood (preload), the greater is the quantity of blood ejected into the aorta. If the left ventricle fills to such an extent that it overdistends the myocardium *(arrow)*, cardiac output begins to decrease, and the heart begins to fail.

ute). *Sex* affects heart rate. Women have a faster rate than men. The hormones epinephrine and thyroxine cause increased heart rate. Temperature also affects heart rate. Fever causes an increased heart rate; hypothermia causes a decreased heart rate. Blood pressure, too, affects the heart rate. Hypotension causes increased heart rate. Finally, *anxiety* and *stress* as well as *pain* can cause increased heart rate.

Arterial Pressure

Arterial pressure is the pressure of blood against arterial walls. Types of arterial pressure include systolic pressure, diastolic pressure, pulse pressure, and mean arterial pressure. Systolic pressure is the maximum pressure of the blood exerted against the artery walls when the heart

Figure 43–12. Normal cardiac pressures.

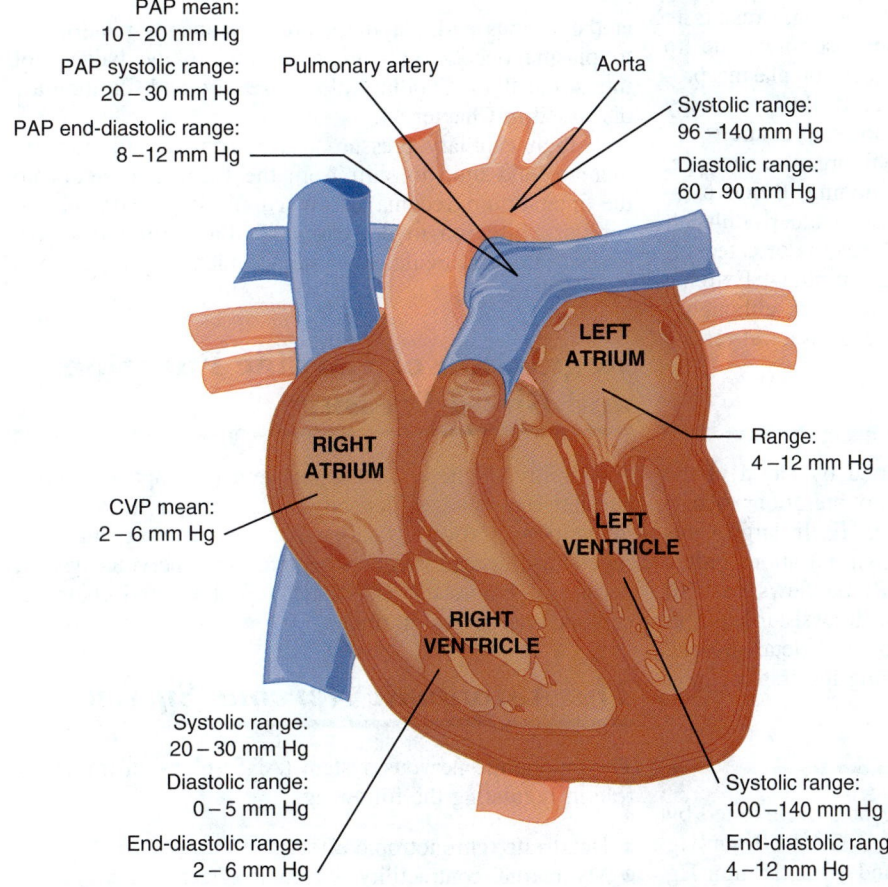

PAP mean:
10 – 20 mm Hg

PAP systolic range:
20 – 30 mm Hg

PAP end-diastolic range:
8 – 12 mm Hg

Pulmonary artery

Aorta

Systolic range:
96 – 140 mm Hg

Diastolic range:
60 – 90 mm Hg

LEFT
ATRIUM

RIGHT
ATRIUM

Range:
4 – 12 mm Hg

CVP mean:
2 – 6 mm Hg

LEFT
VENTRICLE

RIGHT
VENTRICLE

Systolic range:
20 – 30 mm Hg

Diastolic range:
0 – 5 mm Hg

End-diastolic range:
2 – 6 mm Hg

Systolic range:
100 – 140 mm Hg

End-diastolic range:
4 – 12 mm Hg

contracts. It is normally 100 to 140 mm Hg. Diastolic pressure is the force of blood exerted against the artery walls during the heart's relaxation (or filling) phase. It is normally 60 to 90 mm Hg. Blood pressure is expressed as systolic pressure/diastolic pressure (e.g., 120/80). Pulse pressure is the difference between systolic and diastolic pressures. It is normally 40 to 60 mm Hg and reflects stroke volume and arterial elasticity. Mean arterial pressure (MAP) is equivalent to one third of the pulse pressure (PP) plus the diastolic blood pressure (DBP):

$$MAP = 1/3\ PP + DBP$$

MAP may be used in hemodynamic monitoring.

The two determinants of blood pressure are cardiac output (CO) and peripheral vascular resistance (PVR), and can be shown through the following formula:

$$BP = CO \times PVR$$

Circulatory factors that influence arterial pressure include cardiac output, peripheral vascular resistance, arterial elasticity, blood volume, and blood viscosity (Fig. 43–13). Increased cardiac output increases arterial pressure. Decreased cardiac output decreases arterial pressure. Increased peripheral vascular resistance, such as from narrowed arterioles, increases blood pressure. Dilated arterioles decrease blood pressure. Arterial elasticity affects blood pressure. Elastic vessels accommodate changes in blood flow. Rigid, sclerotic vessels cause increases in systolic pressure and pulse pressure. Decreased blood volume (e.g., as a result of hemorrhage) results in decreased pressure. Increased blood viscosity, due to overabundance of red blood cells (RBCs) or plasma proteins, results in high pressure. Decreased blood viscosity from anemia or lack of RBCs causes lower pressure.

Other factors that influence arterial pressure are age, weight, emotions, and physical conditioning. Blood pressure is lowest in neonates and highest in older adults. It increases with excess weight and with release of catecholamines in response to strong emotions or stress. Extreme physical activity may increase blood pressure, although a conditioned person often has low blood pressure at rest.

Venous Pressure

Venous pressure is the pressure exerted by blood in the veins. In small veins and venules, no pulsations occur; venous pressure is about 12 to 15 mm Hg. In large veins leading to the heart (e.g., jugular veins), pulsations reflect back from right atrial contractions. Blood flows back to the heart via the venous system with assistance from vessel wall tone, the pumping action of skeletal muscle, and the negative thoracic pressure during inspiration.

Capillary Pressure

Capillary (hydrostatic) pressure is the pressure exerted by the blood against the capillary wall. It is 25 to 30 mm Hg at the arterial end of the capillaries and 10 to 15 mm Hg

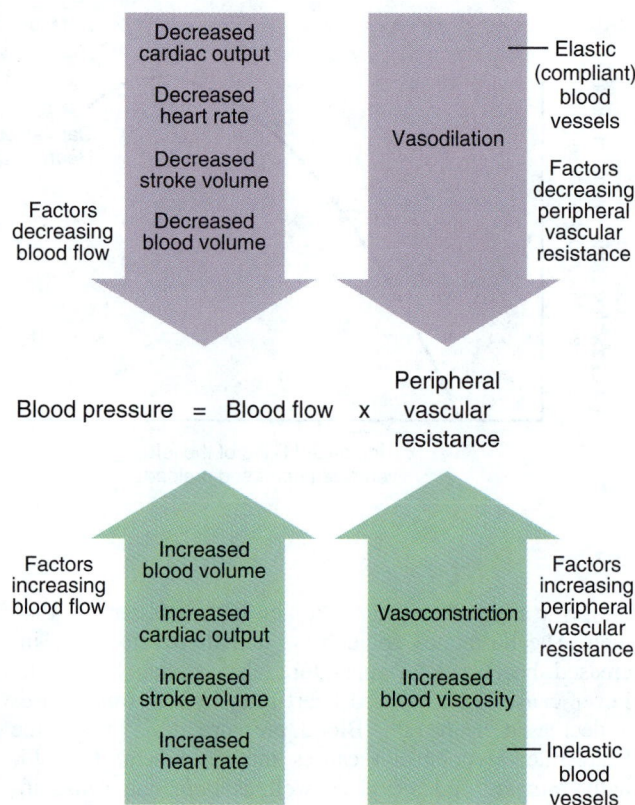

Figure 43–13. Factors affecting blood pressure.

at the venous end. Capillary pressure and its relationship to plasma oncotic pressure contribute to the balance of interstitial fluid. Capillary blood pressure and filtration are discussed in Chapter 44.

A high capillary pressure causes capillary filtration to increase and fluid to shift from the vascular system into the interstitium (edema). Low capillary pressure causes capillary filtration to decrease and draws fluid from the tissues into the circulatory system, which may raise blood pressure.

Regulation of Cardiac Function and Blood Pressure

The ability of the circulatory system to adapt to internal and external changes depends on the proper function and integration of several factors. Among the most important regulatory mechanisms are the autonomic nervous system; peripheral baroreceptors, stretch receptors, and chemoreceptors; and several hormones.

The Autonomic Nervous System

The autonomic nervous system (ANS) plays an important role in regulating the following:

● Heart rate (chronotropic effect),
● Myocardial contractility (inotropic effect),

- Conduction velocity
- Peripheral vascular resistance (arterial and venous constriction and dilation)

The two subdivisions of the autonomic nervous system are the sympathetic and parasympathetic nervous systems. These systems, with opposing influences, balance their activities to promote cardiovascular adaptation to internal and external demands. Autonomic nervous system responses are involuntary. These responses are not preceded by thought.

Parasympathetic nerves arise from the dorsal motor nucleus of the vagus nerve, located in the medulla oblongata. They innervate the atria, ventricles, and conduction system. When stimulated, parasympathetic nerve endings release the neurotransmitter acetylcholine, which produces inhibitory effects opposite to those of norepinephrine. Parasympathetic stimulation decreases the rate of SA node firing, thus lowering heart rate. Atrial and ventricular contractility and conductivity lessen as well.

Sympathetic nerve fibers originate between the first thoracic and second lumbar vertebrae and terminate in all areas of the heart. With stimulation, the nerve endings release the neurotransmitter norepinephrine, producing the following acceleratory effects on the heart: increased heart rate, increased conduction speed through the AV node, increased atrial and ventricular contractility, and peripheral vasoconstriction.

The sympathetic nervous system influences adrenal activity. The adrenal medulla responds to stimulation by secreting catecholamines (norepinephrine and epinephrine) into the circulation. Norepinephrine and epinephrine exert their influences by interacting with adrenergic receptors found within cell membranes of the heart and blood vessels. The response to stimulation depends on the type and location of adrenergic receptors involved. The four types of receptors are $alpha_1$, $alpha_2$, $beta_1$, and $beta_2$.

Alpha$_1$-adrenergic receptors are located in peripheral arteries and veins. When stimulated, alpha receptors produce a dramatic vasoconstrictive response.

Alpha$_2$-adrenergic receptors are located in several tissues. Their actions include contraction of some vascular smooth muscle, inhibition of lipolysis, inhibition of neurotransmitters, and promotion of platelet aggregation.

Beta$_1$-adrenergic receptors are predominantly located in the heart. When stimulated, beta-1 receptors cause an increase in heart rate, AV node conduction, and myocardial contractility. This may result in increased cardiac output and blood pressure.

Beta$_2$-adrenergic receptors are found in the arterial and bronchial walls. Stimulation of beta-2 receptors causes smooth muscles to dilate, producing vasodilation of arterial vessels and bronchodilation.

In general, epinephrine influences alpha$_2$ and beta$_2$ receptors, whereas norepinephrine predominantly affects alpha$_1$ and beta$_1$ receptors.

Dopamine receptors are found in the smooth muscle of renal blood vessels and in nerve endings. When stimulated, they cause dilation of renal arteries and modulate transmitter release.

Baroreceptors, Stretch Receptors, and Chemoreceptors

Changes in sympathetic and parasympathetic activity occur in response to messages sent from sensory receptors involved in various parts of the body. Important receptors involved in cardiovascular reflexes include the baroreceptors, the stretch receptors, and the chemoreceptors.

Baroreceptors (also called *pressoreceptors*) are specialized nerve endings affected by changes in arterial blood pressure. They are located in the walls of the aortic arch and carotid sinuses. Increases in arterial pressure stimulate baroreceptors, which send impulses to the medulla oblongata. As a result, heart rate and arterial pressure decrease (also called the vagal response). When arterial pressure decreases, baroreceptors receive less stimulation and thus send fewer impulses to the medulla oblongata. Then sympathetic-mediated vasoconstriction occurs, and heart rate increases.

Stretch receptors are located in terminal sections of the vena cava and the right atrium. These receptors respond to pressure changes, which reflect circulatory volume status. When blood pressure decreases in the vena cava and the right atrium (e.g., hypovolemia), stretch receptors send fewer impulses than usual to the central nervous system (CNS). This process results in a sympathetic response, which causes increased heart rate and blood vessel constriction. Hypervolemia produces the opposite effects.

Chemoreceptors, found in the aortic arch and carotid bodies, are primarily sensitive to hypoxemia and secondarily to increased CO_2 and decreased arterial pH (acidemia). These changes stimulate chemoreceptors that transmit impulses to the CNS.

Hormonal Influences

In addition to epinephrine and norepinephrine from the adrenal medulla, several other hormones regulate cardiovascular activity. The most important hormones include antidiuretic hormone (ADH) and the renin-angiotensin-aldosterone mechanism.

Several studies have shown that increases in central venous volume (such as those that occur with hypervolemia) result in decreased ADH release from the posterior pituitary gland.[1, 3] Inhibition of ADH secretion, in turn, increases diuresis, which decreases blood volume. Hence, ADH influences blood pressure indirectly by regulating vascular volume.

Renin is an enzyme that is synthesized, stored, and released from the kidney. It is secreted in response to a decrease in renal blood flow and to sympathetic stimulation. The major function of renin is the conversion of angiotensinogen to angiotensin I. Angiotensin I is then converted to angiotensin II in the lungs. This last substance, a potent vasoconstrictor, causes blood pressure to increase. Angiotensin II also stimulates the release of aldosterone, which promotes water and sodium retention by the kidneys. Blood volume and blood pressure increase as a result.

Other hormonal regulators of blood pressure include the following:

- *Histamine*, which is a potent vasodilator of small blood vessels, although it may also constrict the large arteries
- *Bradykinin,* which is one of a group of vasoactive peptides and is a powerful vasodilator, especially of cutaneous vessels
- *Muscle metabolites* (lactic acid), which have a strong vasodilator action
- *Serotonin,* which is liberated from platelets that stick to the vessel wall in the injured area; although this is a powerful constrictor of cutaneous arterioles, it dilates capillaries.

Other factors also influence cardiac activity and blood pressure. For example, cerebral cortical input from anger, fear, pain, or excitement can augment the effects of the sympathetic nervous system. Increased activity and exercise cause an increased need for oxygen and the elimination of metabolic wastes, which in turn cause an increased heart rate and force of contraction. The conditioned athlete, however, usually has a lower heart rate. Body temperature can also affect heart activity. Fever increases the metabolic needs of the body, thereby necessitating an increase in heart rate to increase blood flow to the tissues. The opposite is true in hypothermia, when metabolic needs of tissues decline. Other factors influencing cardiac activity and blood pressure include serum electrolyte levels and medications.

Effects of Aging

The heart muscle also undergoes changes with aging that lead to dilation of the cardiac chambers and lessening of contractility. This has little effect on stroke volume, but it reduces cardiac reserve. The conduction system is replaced with fibrous tissue. This nonconducting tissue reduces the effectiveness of the pacemaker cells, decreases conduction, and leads to dysrhythmias. Coronary arteries become thickened and rigid. These changes decrease the ability of the heart to respond to additional demands and increase the likelihood of coronary artery disease. Heart valves thicken and become incompetent, resulting in a systolic ejection murmur.

Conclusions

Although the heart can be viewed as simply a pump, this remarkable, durable organ is much more than just a pump. The heart is a continuously beating organ that never rests. It moves blood throughout the body to oxygenate cells for energy. Blood is propelled through the four chambers of the heart in one direction, from right to left. It is then delivered to the body through a system of arteries. In the capillaries, nutrients are exchanged for waste, and the deoxygenated blood returns through the veins to the right side of the heart. Heart disease remains the major cause of death and is a result of disorders of structure or function of the heart. These disorders are studied in the following chapters in this unit.

Bibliography

1. Ahrens, T., & Taylor, L. (1992). *Hemodynamic waveform analysis.* Philadelphia: W. B. Saunders.
2. Berne, R. M., & Levy, M. N. (1993). *Physiology* (3rd ed.). St. Louis: Mosby–Year Book.
3. Braunwald, E., et al. (1992). Normal and abnormal circulatory function. In E. Braunwald (Ed.), *Heart disease: A textbook of cardiovascular medicine* (4th ed.). Philadelphia: W. B. Saunders.
4. Guyton, A. C. (1996). *Textbook of medical physiology* (9th ed.). Philadelphia: W. B. Saunders.
5. Hollenberg, N. K., & Hollenberg, I. B. (1989). *The heart facts.* Glenview, IL: Scott, Foresman.
6. Hurst, J. W. (1990). *The heart.* New York: McGraw-Hill.
7. Hurst, J. W., et al. (1988). *Atlas of the heart.* New York: McGraw-Hill.
8. Jarvis, C. (1996). *Physical examination and health assessment* (2nd ed.). Philadelphia: W. B. Saunders.
9. McCance, K. L., & Richardson, S. J. (1990). Structure and function of the cardiovascular and lymphatic systems. In K. L. McCance & S. E. Huether (Eds.), *Pathophysiology.* St. Louis: Mosby–Year Book.
10. Solomon, E. P., Schmidt, R. R., & Adragna, P. J. (1990). *Human anatomy and physiology* (2nd ed.). Philadelphia: Saunders College.

Assessment of Clients with Cardiac Disorders

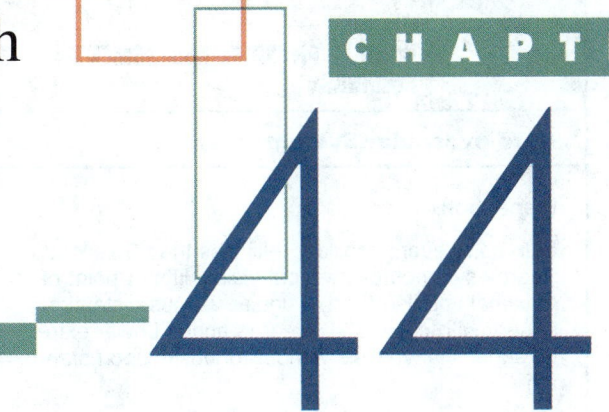

CHAPTER 44

Pamela Shumate

Cardiovascular disease remains the most common cause of death in the United States, taking nearly 1 million lives each year.[19] Cardiovascular disease is not just a disease of the elderly. Forty-five percent of all heart attacks occur in people under age 65.[3] Nor is cardiovascular disease a male disease. More than half of all deaths from cardiovascular disease occur in females.[3] Because of the high incidence of heart disease and the seriousness of its complications, nurses must know how to assess the cardiovascular system. Assessment of the cardiovascular system incorporates data obtained from history-taking, physical examination, and diagnostic studies. Normal findings are described in the Normal Physical Assessment Findings feature.

History

Assessment is a dynamic process. It begins during the initial visit with the client and continues throughout the course of intervention. A health history includes information about the following three areas: (1) the client's chief complaint, (2) current health status, and (3) past health history.

Chief Complaint

Inquire about the client's chief complaint(s) to establish priorities for intervention and to evaluate how well the client understands the presenting condition.

Common clinical manifestations of cardiovascular disorders include shortness of breath, chest pain or discomfort, dyspnea, palpitations, fainting, fatigue, and peripheral skin changes, such as edema. A client may have more than one major symptom. When this occurs, assess them in their order of importance.

A symptom analysis is performed on the chief complaint, using the following questions:

● How long has the symptom been experienced?

This chapter incorporates material written for the fourth edition by Laura Haynes Jacobson.

● How much does the symptom bother the client?
● Does any particular type of incident or episode trigger the symptom?
● What activities or interventions alleviate the symptom?
● What is the perceived cause of the symptom (heart attack, heartburn, indigestion)?
● What impact does the symptom have on the client's life-style?

Chest Pain

Pain in the chest is a common symptom, occurring in such cardiac disorders as angina, myocardial ischemia, myocardial infarction, and pericarditis. Chest pain may also be present in pulmonary diseases such as pleurisy, pneumonia, and pulmonary embolism. Cardiac pain most often results from myocardial ischemia, that is, lack of blood supply to the myocardial tissues. Because chest pain is caused by a number of different conditions, it is highly variable. Evaluate chest pain and its cause by obtaining descriptive data in the following areas.

Characteristics. Chest pain may be described as a "strange feeling," as indigestion, a dull heavy pressure, burning, crushing, constricting, aching, stabbing, or a tightness.

Location. Chest pain occurs in the substernal or precordial areas. It may be diffuse or localized. The pain may also radiate to the jaw, teeth, neck, one or both shoulders, arms, elbows, or the back. If the pain radiates down the arm, it may cause a sensation of numbness or tingling. Sometimes the client feels only the radiated pain and no precordial (lower part of chest) pain.

Duration. Note the time the pain begins and ends to determine the duration of discomfort. Several intermittent small episodes of chest pain are not considered as one long period of pain. Generally, the pain of myocardial

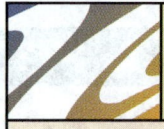

NORMAL PHYSICAL ASSESSMENT FINDINGS

Cardiovascular System

Inspection

Skin color even; capillary refill less than 3 seconds. Thorax symmetrical, without visible lifts or point of maximal impulse (PMI). Jugular venous distention absent with client at 45-degree angle. Lower extremity superficial vessels without tortuosity upon standing.

Palpation

Skin warm. PMI palpable in fifth intercostal space at left midclavicular line, approximately 1 cm in diameter. Forceful thrusts, heaves, and pulsations absent. No palpable thrills. Abdominal aorta pulsations slightly palpable over epigastrium, without lateral radiation. Carotid and peripheral pulses equal bilaterally at 2+ (on scale of 0 to 3+). Evidence of unimpeded arterial flow and venous return in upper and lower extremities. No edema evident.

Percussion

Right heart border not discerned.

Auscultation

S_1 and S_2 heard without splitting. Apical rate, 72 BPM, regular. Murmurs and extra heart sounds absent.

---

infarction lasts longer than 30 minutes, or until intervention is instituted. Conversely, anginal pain typically lasts less than 20 to 30 minutes.

Severity. To assist the client to better quantify the chest pain, ask him to use a scale of 1 (least severe) to 10 (most severe). This recorded scale can then be used to compare future episodes of chest pain. For example, the client may report 10/10 pain on admission and then report 3/10 pain the following day.

Precipitating or Aggravating Factors. The pain may sometimes be associated with certain factors or conditions. Emotional excitement, temperature extremes, exertion, deep sleep, position changes, deep breathing, straining during bowel movements, or eating may trigger the onset of chest pain.

Associated Symptoms. Ask the client whether other symptoms accompany the onset of chest pain, for example, anxiousness, shortness of breath, nausea, diaphoresis, vertigo, or palpitations.

Alleviating Factors. Anginal pain may be relieved by resting, sublingual nitroglycerin, oxygen, and a change in position. Pain that is not relieved with these interven-

tions and lasts 20 minutes or longer highly suggests myocardial infarction.

Table 44–1 compares selected cardiac, pulmonary, gastrointestinal, musculoskeletal, neurologic, and anxiety-related conditions in relation to the assessment of chest pain (see p. 1208).

Shortness of Breath

Labored breathing, or shortness of breath, is termed *dyspnea*. Like chest pain, this common symptom affects clients with cardiac and pulmonary disorders. Dyspnea also may occur in clients experiencing anxiety, depression, and various psychosomatic conditions.

Although dyspnea can develop in any form of heart disease, it usually occurs in conjunction with cardiac enlargement and other pathologic, cardiovascular, structural, and physiologic changes. Dyspnea develops when the left ventricle fails and the lungs become congested with fluid.

There are several forms of dyspnea: exertional dyspnea, orthopnea, and paroxysmal nocturnal dyspnea.

Exertional Dyspnea. This is the most common form of cardiac-related dyspnea. Exertional dyspnea occurs during mild-to-moderate exercise or activity and disappears with rest. If severe, exertional dyspnea can greatly limit activity tolerance. Ask the client to describe the degree of activity that typically precipitates the onset of dyspnea, for example, walking up one flight of stairs, or walking to the mailbox. Noncardiac conditions such as obesity, poor physical conditioning, anemia, asthma, and obstructions of the nasal passages may also lead to dyspnea on mild exercise. This form of dyspnea is abbreviated DOE (dyspnea on exertion).

Orthopnea. Orthopnea is difficult breathing that occurs when the person is lying flat and is relieved when the person assumes an upright or semivertical position. Ask clients what actions they take to facilitate breathing. Do they sit up in a chair or dangle their feet at the bedside? What position do they sleep in? How many pillows do they sleep on? Record the degree of head elevation the client requires to breathe. Orthopnea usually indicates a more serious compromise of the cardiovascular system than does exertional dyspnea.

Paroxysmal Nocturnal Dyspnea. This is a form of difficult breathing that occurs in terrifying "attacks" during the night, awakening the sleeper. Paroxysmal nocturnal dyspnea is associated with severe left ventricular failure.

Fatigue

Easy fatigability on mild exertion is a frequent problem for clients experiencing cardiac disease. Progressive deterioration in activity tolerance results from the heart's inability to pump an effective volume of blood to meet the varying metabolic demands of the body.

Palpitations

The word "palpitation" is derived from the Latin *palpitare*, "to throb." Palpitation is a common symptom in heart disease. It is a sensation of rapid heartbeats, skipping, irregularity, thumping, or pounding, and may be accompanied by anxiousness. Tachycardia (rapid heart rate), increased force of myocardial contraction (as can occur with ingestion of caffeine or with emotional or physical stress), or premature ventricular beats may cause palpitations. The onset and termination of palpitations are often abrupt.

Syncope

Syncope, or fainting, is a momentary loss of consciousness resulting from a reduction in cerebral blood flow. Certain cardiac disorders, especially cardiac dysrhythmias (irregular heart rhythm), can precipitate a sudden decrease in cardiac output. Valvular disorders may also cause an adverse change in circulatory hemodynamics and cause syncope or vertigo. Clients who are prone to syncopal episodes (e.g., those with Stokes-Adams syndrome) should wear medical alert bracelets to inform emergency healthcare providers.

Weight Gain

Because of fluid accumulation, an expanded blood volume may result when the heart fails. An increase in body weight of 3 lbs or more within 24 hours results from fluid rather than body mass changes. Ask the client about weight change. Body weight is a sensitive indicator of water and sodium retention and will increase even before edema occurs. Methods to ensure accurate measurement of weight are discussed in basic nursing texts.

Past Health History

The past health history explores the health history of the client and his or her family. Information acquired here reveals the lifelong health record of the client, past experiences in the healthcare system, attitudes regarding health, and nonmodifiable and modifiable risk factors that may have contributed to the development of cardiovascular symptoms. The client is asked questions about the following areas.

Childhood and Infectious Diseases

In addition to the usual data regarding common childhood diseases and immunizations, ask about the client's experiences with rheumatic fever and severe streptococcal infections. These two conditions are associated with structural heart disease. The presence of known congenital anomalies is also ascertained.

Major Illnesses and Hospitalizations

The history or presence of any major illness is determined. Pay attention to those conditions that have the greatest influence on the client's current cardiovascular performance, that is, diabetes mellitus, chronic obstructive lung disease, kidney disease, anemia, hypertension, stroke, gout, thrombophlebitis, collagen diseases, and bleeding disorders. Explore previous hospitalizations, pregnancies, and outpatient interventions. Inquire about previously performed cardiovascular diagnostic studies, such as an electrocardiogram (ECG) or an exercise stress test. The results of such studies provide baseline data for comparative analysis when later studies are performed.

Medications

Prescription as well as over-the-counter and recreational drug use is evaluated. Whenever possible, use brand names or simple descriptors instead of generic names. For example, ask if the client is currently taking "water pills," "heart pills," or "blood pressure" medications. Numerous medications can affect the overall performance of the cardiovascular system. Ask specifically about the use of the following agents: antihypertensives, diuretics, vasodilators (nitroglycerin), cardiotonic drugs, (digoxin), anticoagulants, bronchodilators, contraceptives, and steroids. Noncardiac medications can also have profound secondary effects on cardiovascular performance. For example, tricyclic antidepressants and other psychotropic medications can potentiate dysrhythmias. Oral contraceptives increase the incidence of thrombophlebitis. Steroid use may cause hypertension and increases fluid retention. Various antineoplastic agents may be cardiotoxic, causing dysrhythmias and cardiomyopathy.

Discuss the use of recreational drugs with the client. Cocaine toxicity is a major threat to the cardiovascular system. Its systemic sympathomimetic effects result in a "fight or flight" reaction that increases heart rate, contractility, blood glucose levels, and peripheral vasoconstriction. Cocaine also potentiates the effects of circulating catecholamines (epinephrine and norepinephrine).

Finally, discuss the use of over-the-counter drugs such as aspirin and cold remedies. While investigating the use of these drugs, note the dose and times of administration.

In addition to discovering the types and names of the medications the client takes, ask the client to describe how many pills he or she takes and how often, and if he or she is currently taking these medications. Clients with cardiac disease will occasionally cease taking prescribed medications because of unwanted side effects, or in the belief that the problem has resolved, or for economic reasons. The client to whom diuretics are prescribed may fail to take the medication because it "makes him go to the bathroom all the time." Clients on antihypertensive medications may stop taking their medication once their blood pressure reaches a normal range because they perceive that the problem has resolved. Identify areas for client teaching with these sorts of questions.

Table 44-1. Assessment of Chest Pain

Condition	Location	Quality	Severity	Course	Aggravating or Relieving Factors	Symptoms or Signs
Angina	Retrosternal region; radiates to neck, jaw, epigastrium, shoulders, arms (left common)	Pressure, burning, squeezing, heaviness, indigestion	Moderate to severe	<10 min	Aggravated by exercise, cold weather, emotional stress, or after meals; relieved by rest or nitroglycerin; atypical (Prinzmetal's) angina may be unrelated to activity and caused by coronary artery spasm	S_4, paradoxical split S_2 during pain
Intermediate syndrome or coronary insufficiency	Same as angina	Same as angina	Increasingly severe	>10 min	Same as angina, with gradually decreasing tolerance for exertion	Same as angina
Myocardial infarction	Substernal; may radiate like angina	Heaviness, pressure, burning, constriction	Severe, sometimes mild (in 25% of patients)	Sudden onset; lasting longer than 15 min	Unrelieved	Shortness of breath, sweating, weakness, nausea, vomiting, severe anxiety
Pericarditis	Usually begins over sternum and may radiate to neck and down left upper extremity	Sharp, stabbing, knifelike	Moderate to severe	Lasts many hours to days	Aggravated by deep breathing, rotating chest or supine position; relieved by sitting up and leaning forward	Pericardial friction rub, syncope, cardiac tamponade, pulsus paradoxus (Kussmaul's sign)
Dissecting aortic aneurysm	Anterior chest; radiates to thoracic area of back; may be abdominal; pain shifts in chest	Tearing	Excruciating, tearing, knifelike	Sudden onset, lasts for hours	Unrelated to anything	Lower blood pressure in one arm, absent pulses, paralysis, murmur of aortic insufficiency, pulsus paradoxus, stridor; myocardial infarction can occur
Mitral valve prolapse syndrome	Substernal; sometimes radiates to the left arm, back, jaw	Stabbing, sharp	Variable; generally mild but can become severe	Episodes are paroxysmal, may be prolonged	Not related to exertion, not relieved by nitroglycerin or rest	Variable palpitations, dizziness, syncope, dyspnea, late systolic or pansystolic murmur

Condition	Location	Quality	Severity	Duration	Aggravating factors	Associated findings
Pulmonary embolism (many pulmonary emboli do not produce chest pain)	Substernal	Deep, crushing; if pulmonary infection, may be pleuritic	Can be absent, mild, or severe	Sudden onset; lasts minutes to <1 hr	May be aggravated by breathing	Fever, tachypnea, tachycardia, hypotension, elevated jugular venous pressure, right ventricular lift, accentuated pulmonary valve (P_2) sound during S_2, occasional murmur of tricuspid insufficiency and right ventricular S_4; with infarction usually in the presence of congestive heart failure; crackles, pleural rub, hemoptysis, clinical phlebitis present in minority of cases
Pulmonary hypertension	Substernal	Pressure; oppressive	Variable		Aggravated by effort	Pain usually associated with dyspnea; right ventricular lift, accentuated P_2
Spontaneous pneumothorax	Unilateral	Sharp, well localized		Sudden onset; lasts many hours	Painful breathing	Dyspnea, hyperresonance, and decreased breath and voice sounds over involved lung
Pneumonia with pleurisy	Localized over area of consolidation	Pleuritic, well localized	Moderate		Painful breathing	Dyspnea, cough, fever, dull-to-flat percussion, bronchial breathing, crackles, occasional pleural rub
Gastrointestinal disorders	Lower substernal area, epigastric, right or left upper quadrant	Burning, colic-like aching			Precipitated by recumbency or meals	Nausea, regurgitation, food intolerance, melena, hematemesis, jaundice
Musculoskeletal disorders	Variable	Aching		Short or long duration	Aggravated by movement, history of muscle exertion	Tender to pressure or movement
Neurologic disorders (herpes zoster)	Dermatomal in distribution			Prolonged period of time	Unassociated with external events	Rash appears in area of discomfort with herpes
Anxiety states	Usually localized to a point	Sharp burning; commonly location of pain moves from place to place	Mild to moderate	Varies; usually very brief	Situational anger	Sighing respirations, often chest wall tenderness

P_2, pulmonic second sound.
From Andreoli, K., et al. (1987). *Comprehensive cardiac care* (6th ed., pp. 54–55). St. Louis: Mosby–Year Book.

Psychosocial History

Information in this area provides abundant data about risk factors for the development of cardiovascular disease. From this background information, formulate a plan to assist the client in making necessary life-style adaptations to promote health and lessen disease.

The client's age, sex, race, and family history are non-modifiable risk factors. These factors are discussed in Chapter 45 as risk factors for coronary artery disease. Nevertheless, the relationship of these risk factors to cardiovascular disease is sensitively discussed when the client asks, Why did my heart condition happen? Information about marital status, household members, children, the living environment, employment, spiritual orientation, and hobbies helps in the identification of support systems and coping mechanisms.

Include information about the following modifiable risk factors in history-taking.

Stress. Research indicates a strong correlation between stress response and the manifestations of various cardiac disorders. Chronic stress stimulates an overactive fight or flight reaction. This response may have an adverse effect on circulating catecholamines and on blood clotting.[22] Common stressors include a change in job, residence, health, or marital status. Chapter 2 discusses stress response in detail.

Personality Type. Much has been written about the relationship between the so-called type A personality and the development of coronary artery disease. Early studies intimated a positive correlation between the two; more recent studies have failed to confirm an association.[15,22]

Exercise. Ask the client about the type and amount of exercise routinely engaged in during an average week before and after the onset of current symptoms. Several studies suggest that effective, routine aerobic exercise may lower the likelihood of a coronary event. Research confirms that a sedentary life-style potentiates the lethality of a myocardial infarction, and it is considered a significant risk factor in the development of coronary artery disease. To be effective, aerobic exercise should raise the heart rate from 50% to 100% of baseline (depending on age and prior physical conditioning) for at least 20 to 30 minutes. Such exercise must be performed at least three times a week to be beneficial. The prevailing wisdom is that aerobic exercise, along with general body conditioning, makes the heart more efficient in its use of oxygen. Examples of aerobic exercise are swimming, jogging, brisk walking, bicycling, and rowing. But advise clients over the age of 40 and any client with a history of cardiovascular disease to consult their physician before beginning an exercise program.

Nutrition. A dietary history assesses excess or deficit caloric intake and the approximate intake of foods high in sodium, cholesterol, saturated fat, and caffeine. Although these are common components of the average American diet, they have been linked to the development of atherosclerosis and hypertensive disease. Elevated serum cholesterol levels have a clear association with coronary artery disease (CAD). This correlation diminishes with age, but still remains.[23] Elevated serum triglyceride levels are positively related to the development of CAD, especially in women. Examine not only the client's daily food habits but also his or her attitudes toward food and resistance to therapeutic alterations in diet. Cultural beliefs and economic status greatly affect the choice of foods. Therefore, clinicians must consider these factors before prescribing changes in diet. In addition, identify and include the primary food purchaser and preparer in dietary instruction.

Habits. If the client smokes, inquire about the duration of the smoking habit and the number of cigarettes smoked daily. Cigarette smoking increases the risk of CAD and worsens hypertension. Nicotine, a major ingredient in cigarettes, probably causes peripheral vasoconstriction, increasing resistance to left ventricular emptying and thus increasing the myocardial workload. Smoking increases the mortality rate of middle-aged clients with diagnosed CAD and greatly potentiates the development of peripheral vascular disease. Cigarette smokers have a 70% higher death rate from coronary heart disease than do nonsmokers. Clients who stop smoking will, after several years, experience a death rate from heart attack almost as low as that of people who never smoked.[19]

There is no conclusive evidence to show that caffeine and alcohol increase the risk of developing atherosclerosis. Nevertheless, caffeine is a stimulant that, in excessive amounts, can increase heart rate and blood pressure (BP), both of which can raise the myocardial workload and precipitate angina pectoris, heart failure, and some dysrhythmias. Therefore, assess caffeine intake and caution those with known heart disease to limit the use of caffeine to the equivalent of two 8-oz cups of coffee per day.

Researchers state that only excessive alcohol intake has deleterious effects on the cardiovascular system and its performance. An intake of 100 g of pure (100%) alcohol may slightly increase BP and heart rate. This amount is approximately equal to three beers or one mixed drink. Alcoholism, in contrast, has been associated with the development of hypertension and damage to the heart muscle, leading to congestive cardiomyopathy. Ask the client to approximate daily and weekly alcohol consumption, bearing in mind that the alcoholic client may lie about his or her consumption.

Review of Systems

Ask the client about past problems involving the cardiovascular system, including paroxysmal nocturnal dyspnea, chest pain, palpitations, shortness of breath, fatigue, edema, orthopnea, wheezing, fainting (syncope), weight gain, heart murmurs, hypertension, and history of rheumatic fever.

Cardiovascular problems also affect the pulmonary, renal, and neurologic systems. Ask about productive cough, decreased urination, dark or concentrated urine, edema of the legs, dizzy spells, and memory loss.

Detailed questions for the review of systems are found in Table 11–4.

Physical Examination

Nurses, especially those who care for the critically ill or who are family nurse-practitioners, should be able to perform a basic cardiovascular examination. Assessment of the client's cardiovascular status must be ongoing, because the underlying condition can change dramatically within minutes. A physical examination involves obtaining objective data via observation, palpation, and auscultation. Percussion is rarely performed to assess cardiovascular status.

The order of the examination proceeds in logical fashion from head to foot. It is often performed routinely along with vital signs.

General Appearance

Much may be learned through simple observation. Before beginning the examination, look at the client and consider the following:

● Does the client lie quietly in bed or is he or she restless and moving about continuously?
● What is the client's posture? Can he or she lie flat in bed or tolerate only an upright and erect position?
● What is the facial expression? Are there grimaces of pain or obvious signs of respiratory distress?
● Are there signs of significant cyanosis or pallor?
● Can the client answer questions without dyspnea during the interview?

Level of Consciousness

Note the client's general level of consciousness. This assessment reflects the adequacy of cerebral perfusion and oxygenation. Also assess whether the client is manifesting appropriate behavior based on the surroundings:

● What is the client's affect?
● Are there obvious signs of anxiety, fear, depression, or anger?
● How does the client react to those in the immediate vicinity, including significant others?
● Assessment of the client's general appearance and level of consciousness provides an initial composite picture of the client and indicates the level of comfort and distress.

Blood Pressure

Measure the BP of both arms during the initial examination to rule out dissecting aortic aneurysm, coarctation of the aorta, vascular obstruction, vascular outlet syndromes, and errors in measurement. If the client's arms are inaccessible, pressures are obtained using the thighs and popliteal artery or the calves and posterior tibial artery. If

pressures are difficult to auscultate, systolic pressures can be determined through palpation or by Doppler ultrasonography.

When recording BP measurements, note both systolic and diastolic pressures, for example, 120/70 mm Hg. However, the muffling of Korotkoff's sounds may also be included and recorded as 120/80/70. The American Heart Association recommends recording the point at which the sound disappears (fifth Korotkoff's sound) as the diastolic pressure in adults. Record in which arm the BP measurement was taken and the position of the client at the time of the reading.

Postural Blood Pressure

A postural BP reading is taken when an extracellular volume depletion or decreased vascular tone is suspected. BP is recorded in relation to the client's position (Fig. 44–1).

Paradoxical Blood Pressure (Pulsus Paradoxus)

Paradoxical BP is frequently found in clients with pericardial tamponade, constrictive pericarditis, and pulmonary hypertension. It is an abnormal fall in systolic BP of greater than 10 mm Hg during inspiration. To check for a paradoxical pulse, place a sphygmomanometer on the client's arm and a stethoscope over the brachial artery and instruct the client to breathe normally. The cuff is inflated 20 mm Hg above the systolic BP. Slowly deflate the cuff (1–2 mm Hg/sec) and listen for Korotkoff's sounds to appear only during expiration. (Sounds are first heard during expiration and then during inspiration.) Then deflate the cuff until Korotkoff's sounds are heard equally well during inspiration and expiration. The degree of paradoxical BP is the difference between the BP level when the sounds are first heard during expiration and the BP level when the sounds are heard on both expiration and

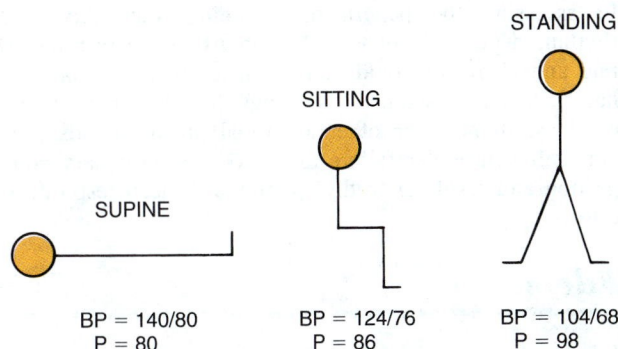

Figure 44–1. Recording postural blood pressure (BP). After measuring the client's BP and pulse in the supine position, leave the BP cuff in place and assist the client to sit. Then measure the BP within 15 to 30 seconds. Assist the client to stand, and measure again. A BP drop of more than 10 to 15 mm Hg systolic and more than 10 mm Hg diastolic indicates postural hypotension. Postural hypotension is typically accompanied by a 10% to 20% increase in heart rate (pulse). Sample measurements given earlier indicate postural hypotension.

inspiration. Normally, this difference is less than 10 mm Hg. If the client has normal breathing and a systolic difference of greater than 10 mm Hg, possible cardiac compression, such as cardiac tamponade, may exist.

Pulse

Pulses can have varying characteristics. If the pulse is irregular, assess for a pulse deficit by taking apical and radial pulses simultaneously, noting differences in rate. Peripheral pulse assessment is discussed in Chapter 49.

Water-hammer pulse is a large, bounding pulse with a rapid rise and fall. It is associated with an increased stroke volume and widened pulse pressure, as occurs with emotional excitement. It may be seen in aortic regurgitation and patent ductus arteriosus.

Pulsus tardus is a weak and feeble pulse, with a slow upstroke and prolonged peak. It is associated with a decrease in stroke volume and diminished pulse pressure, as seen in hypovolemic shock.

Pulsus alternans has a regular rhythm along with alterations in pulse amplitude. Strong beats alternate with weak ones. This type of pulse may be seen in myocardial infarction or congestive heart failure when left ventricular function is depressed.

Bigeminal pulse primarily results from an underlying rhythm disturbance, which is most commonly associated with premature ectopic beats. A strong beat alternates with a premature (early), weak beat. The irregularity of the pulse differentiates this type of pulse from pulsus alternans.

Pulsus bisferiens is characterized by a rapid upstroke and has two systolic peaks. This pulse may be present in aortic regurgitation (with or without stenosis), with large left-to-right shunts, and in idiopathic hypertrophic subaortic stenosis (hypertrophic obstructive cardiomyopathy). This pulse is best felt in the carotid artery.

Respirations

In assessing the pattern of breathing, note the rate, rhythm, depth, and quality. Variations in the respiratory rate and character could indicate heart failure or pulmonary edema. Auscultate the lungs for the presence of crackles, rhonchi, or other abnormal breath sounds. Severe left ventricular failure may produce pulmonary congestion and resulting frothy sputum with deep respiratory efforts.

Edema

Edema occurs in right-sided heart failure when the excess intravascular volume begins to increase capillary hydrostatic pressure and force fluid out into the interstitium.

Inspect dependent areas for edema. In the mobile client, edema is best seen in the feet, ankles, and lower legs. In the chair- or bedridden client, edema may be best discerned over the sacrum, abdomen, or scapula. Assess the severity of edema by pressing a thumb or finger carefully into the area. A depression that does not rapidly resume its original contour is noted as orthostatic, or pitting, edema. Because such a wide discrepancy exists in edema grading scales, you may best describe the edema by describing the actual depth of the indentation.

Head and Neck

In examining the head, pay particular attention to the lips, ear lobes, and buccal mucosa. The presence of a bluish tinge or duskiness is indicative of central cyanosis. Central cyanosis implies serious heart or lung disease in which hemoglobin is not fully saturated with oxygen. Peripheral cyanosis usually accompanies this condition.

Examination of Neck Veins

Examine the neck veins to estimate central venous pressure (CVP). The distensibility of the neck veins reflects pressure and volume changes within the right atrium. The internal jugular veins, although harder to detect than the external jugular veins, are more reliable indicators of CVP. The external jugular vein can be easily engorged with only slight provocation, for example, by holding the breath, twisting the neck, and constrictive clothing. Exceptions are weightlifters, football players, and professional speakers and singers, who have overdeveloped neck muscle tendons. The vessels are prominent and visible, but soft and compressible.

To measure jugular vein distention, the following protocol is suggested.

1. Have the client assume a relaxed supine position with the head of the bed inclined between 15 and 30 degrees to maximize jugular vein prominence. In clients with greatly increased right atrial pressure, head elevations from 45 to 90 degrees may be required.
2. Use a small pillow to support the client's head, avoiding sharp neck flexion. The head should be turned slightly away from the examiner. Remove any clothing that compresses the neck or upper thorax.
3. Use tangential (oblique) lighting so that small shadows make the veins more apparent. Observe both sides of the neck. The internal jugular vein lies deep to the sternocleidomastoid muscle and runs parallel along its length to the jaw and ear lobe (Fig. 44–2). Identify the pulsations of the internal jugular. The external jugular vein may be used if the internal jugular is not visible.
4. Note the highest point at which the internal jugular pulses can be seen (the meniscus). Use the sternal angle (manubrial joint) as a reference point to measure the height of venous pulsation. This point is approximately 4 to 5 cm above the center of the right atrium. Using a centimeter ruler, measure the vertical distance between the sternal angle and the point of highest venous pulsations. Figure 44–3 demonstrates the method of jugular vein measurement.
5. Normally, the value is less than 3 or 4 cm above the sternal angle with the head of the bed elevated at 30 to 40 degrees. Higher values indicate increased right atrial or right ventricular pressure, as seen in right

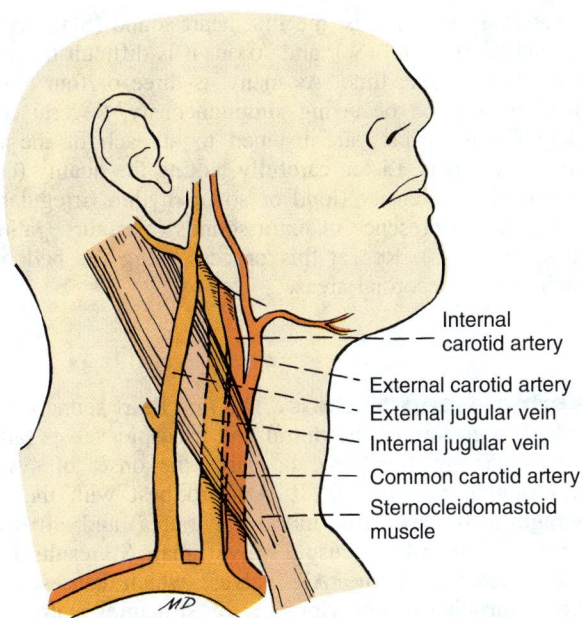

Figure 44–2. Location of internal jugular vein.

ventricular failure, tricuspid regurgitation, and pericardial tamponade. Flat jugular veins noted with the client supine suggest extracellular volume depletion. Unilateral distention may indicate vessel obstruction on that side.

The timing and amplitude of the jugular vein pulsations may also be assessed to evaluate right-sided heart function, tricuspid valve performance, and the presence of certain dysrhythmias.

Examination of Carotid Arteries

Examining the carotid arteries provides evidence regarding the adequacy of stroke volume and the patency of the

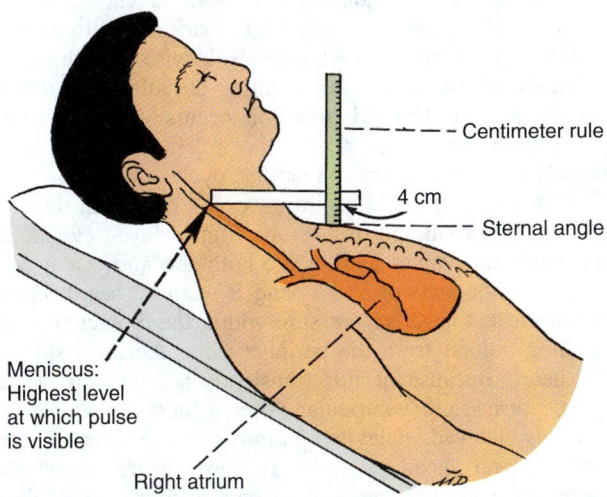

Figure 44–3. Estimation of jugular vein measurement to assess central venous pressure.

arteries. With the finger tips, gently palpate the carotid arteries one side at a time, checking and comparing the rate, rhythm, and amplitude of the pulse. A bruit (a blowing sound) may be heard by listening to the carotid arteries with the diaphragm of a stethoscope while the client holds his or her breath. Tracheal breath sounds are heard if respiration is ongoing. A bruit generally indicates that the carotid artery has narrowed. Bruits typically result from atherosclerosis or radiation of sounds from an aortic valve murmur.

Chest

Inspection and Palpation of the Precordium

Inspection and palpation of the precordium are performed together to determine the presence of normal and abnormal pulsations. For more efficient assessment of the precordium, the client should be supine with the chest exposed. The left lateral position is also used as it allows the heart to move closer to the chest wall. This position accentuates precordial movements and certain heart sounds. The examination area should have good lighting and be warm and quiet. Stand at the client's right side and observe the anterior chest for size, shape, symmetry of movement, and any evident pulsations. Record the location of pulsation in relation to the intercostal space and the midclavicular line. Confirm the observed phenomenon by palpation. When palpating, use the fingers and palm of the hand.

Normally, the point of maximum intensity (PMI) or apical impulse is seen at the apex. The PMI is associated with left ventricular contraction and should appear at the fifth intercostal space medial to the left midclavicular line. It is most prominent in thin people and may be obscured in those who are obese or who have large breasts. It is palpated as a single, faint, instantaneous tap beneath the fingers and is no more than 2 cm in diameter. Turning the client onto his or her left side may assist in locating the PMI, but this maneuver will displace its location. With left ventricular enlargement and aneurysm, the PMI is more diffuse, sustained, and displaced downward and to the left of the midclavicular line.

Right ventricular enlargement can produce an abnormal pulsation that is viewed as a sustained thrust along the left sternal border. Termed "heaves" or "lifts," these pulsations may be found in association with various disorders, such as valvular disease and pulmonary hypertension. Thrills represent turbulent blood flow through the heart, especially across abnormal heart valves. The best way to feel thrills is to use the heel or ulnar surface of the hand to palpate the precordium over each of the five cardiac landmarks (Fig. 44–4). Thrills are perceived as a rushing vibration, much like feeling the throat of a purring cat. Thrills are associated with significant heart murmurs. They may also be palpated over partially obstructed blood vessels.

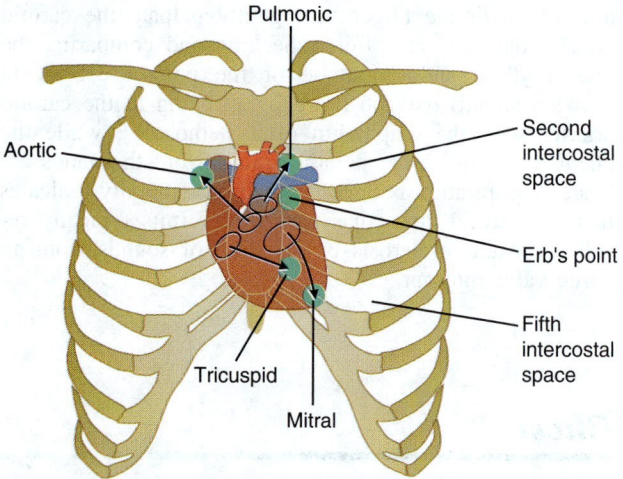

Figure 44–4. Precordial locations for cardiac palpation and auscultation of heart sounds. Closure of mitral and tricuspid valves produces the S_1 heart sound; closure of pulmonic and aortic (semilunar) valves produces the S_2 heart sound.

Auscultation of Heart Sounds

Auscultation of the precordium yields valuable information about the presence of normal or abnormal heart rate and rhythm, ventricular filling, and blood flow across heart valves. Assessment of heart sounds is a sophisticated skill, requiring study of heart sound characteristics and extensive clinical practice. It is important you become thoroughly familiar with the techniques of auscultation of normal cardiac sounds. With practice and experience, you will be able to detect abnormal heart sounds.

Discerning abnormal heart sounds is difficult even for skilled practitioners under ideal circumstances. The sensitivity of the human ear falls sharply when the frequency of sound vibrations is below 1000 Hz. Most cardiac murmurs and sounds are below that frequency. Therefore a reliable stethoscope is a must, and take care when selecting one (see discussion of auscultation and choice of a stethoscope in Chapter 12).

The environment is key to successful auscultation. The surroundings should be warm and quiet. An exposed chest is ideal, but prevent shivering, which can greatly distort heart sound transmission. Instruct the client to breathe through the nose while supine. Again, use of the left lateral position may facilitate auscultation. Having the client assume an upright position, lean forward, and hold the breath after exhalation helps when assessing for early diastolic murmurs and pericardial friction rubs.

A systematic approach should always be used in evaluating heart sounds. Methods vary, and examiners should develop their own routine to ensure a thorough assessment each time cardiac auscultation is performed.

Examination of heart sounds may progress from the base (right second intercostal space) of the heart to the apex, or from the apex to the base. Whichever approach is used, pay special attention to each of the precordial locations diagrammed in Figure 44–4. Each area corresponds to a specific valvular outflow tract. In auscultating each area, concentrate on one component of the cardiac

cycle at a time, that is, the first heart sound (S_1) then the second heart sound (S_2), and so on. It is difficult to assess everything at one time. As many as three or four abnormalities may be occurring simultaneously. Several complete cardiac cycles are listened to at each of the five precordial areas. Listen carefully, noting the quality (crisp or muffled), intensity (loud or soft); rhythm (irregular or regular), and presence of extra sounds (murmurs, gallops, rubs, or clicks). Repeat this process using the bell over each of the precordial areas.

Normal Heart Sounds. The first heart sound (S_1) is linked to closure of the mitral and tricuspid valves (atrioventricular [AV] valves). It marks the onset of systole (ventricular contraction). It is heard best with the diaphragm at the apex (the mitral valve area) and left lower sternal border (the tricuspid valve area). S_1 results from abrupt closure of the AV valves, which causes some blood turbulence and vibration of structures within the ventricles. This vibration is transmitted across the chest wall as a heart sound. Phonetically, if both heart sounds are appreciated as "lub-dup," S_1 is "lub." Although closure of both mitral and tricuspid valves is heard as a single sound, mitral valve closure occurs a fraction of a second earlier. The intensity of S_1 may vary in certain pathologic conditions. Diseased and stiffened AV valves (as seen in rheumatic heart disease) may augment S_1, while rhythms of asynchrony between the atria and ventricles (as in atrial fibrillation and AV block) will cause varying intensity to the first heart sound.

The second heart sound (S_2) relates to closure of the pulmonic and aortic (semilunar) valves and is heard best with the diaphragm at the base of the heart. Phonetically, it is the "dup" of the heart sound. It signifies the end of systole and the onset of diastole (ventricular filling). At the base of the heart, normal S_2 is always louder than S_1, whereas both sounds usually are of nearly equal intensity at the left sternal border over Erb's point. Usually S_1 is the louder of the two sounds at the apex and occurs just after or along with the carotid pulse.

Knowing the usual quality of sounds at various points on the precordium can help in the differentiation of S_1 and S_2 during rapid heart rates. Likewise, simultaneous palpation of the carotid pulse during auscultation helps to discern sounds. Carotid pulsation occurs with systole or S_1. Figure 44–5 illustrates the relationship of heart sounds to events during the cardiac cycle.

Physiologic (normal) splitting of S_2 occurs during inspiration. Normal splitting results from delayed closure of the pulmonic valve. During S_2, both the aortic and pulmonic components of S_2 (A_2 and P_2) can be heard. Inspiration creates negative pressure within the thoracic cavity, "pulling" blood from the periphery into the right side of the heart. Because of this transient augmentation in venous return, right ventricular volume increases and emptying is delayed, delaying pulmonic valve closure. The "split-second heart sound" is best heard over the pulmonic area. The two components of S_2 occur so close together that the pause between them produces a phonetic gap similar to the "pl" sound in the word "split."

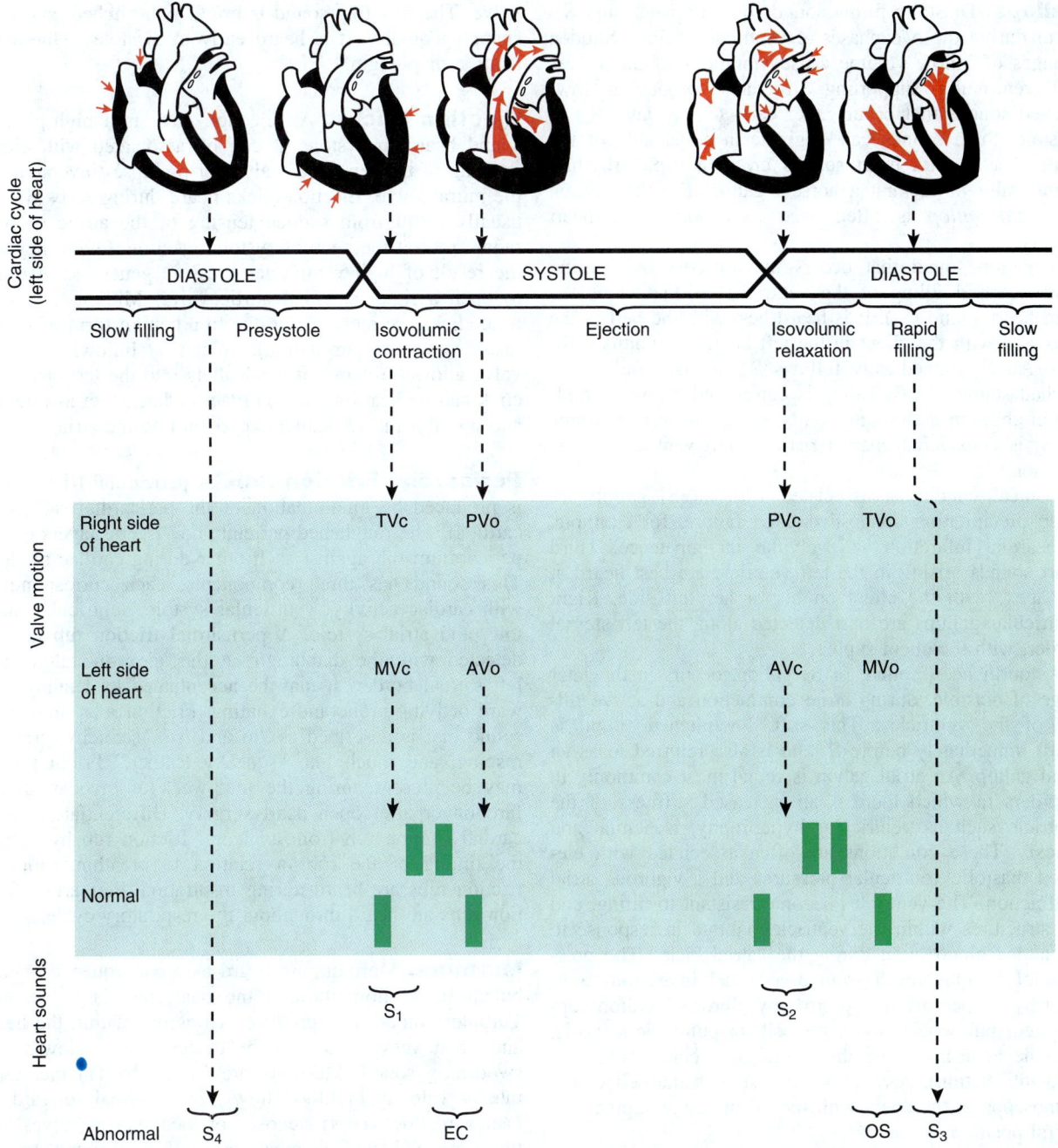

Figure 44–5. Relationship of heart sounds to events during the cardiac cycle. Understanding heart sounds is facilitated when they are correlated with cardiac cycle events and valvular movements. MVc, mitral valve closing; TVc, tricuspid valve closing; PVo, pulmonic valve opening; AVo, aortic valve opening; AVc, aortic valve closing; PVc, pulmonic valve closing; TVo, tricuspid valve opening; MVo, mitral valve opening; EC, ejection click; OS, opening snap.

Abnormal Heart Sounds. There are many abnormal heart sounds that may indicate a serious heart disorder or change in cardiac function. You may not be able to label each abnormality, but with a thorough understanding of the normal sounds, you should be able to recognize the various abnormal sounds and refer the problem to the physician.

Pathologic Splitting of S_2. A wide splitting of S_2 may be heard during both inspiration and expiration, with an increase during inspiration. This form of splitting occurs in right bundle branch block, due to delay in depolarization of the right ventricle and late closure of the pulmonic valve. Fixed splitting is the hallmark of atrial septal defect. This form of S_2 split is continuous and does not vary with respirations. Fixed splitting occurs because the emptying of the right ventricle is prolonged. Paradoxical splitting occurs from a delay in closure of the aortic valve due to aortic stenosis, left bundle branch block, or patent ductus arteriosus. In paradoxical splitting, the S_2 split is heard during expiration rather than inspiration.

Gallops. Diastolic filling sounds or gallops (S_3 and S_4) occur during the two phases of ventricular filling. Sudden changes of inflow volume cause vibrations of the valves and ventricular supporting structures, producing low-pitched sounds that occur either early (S_3) or late (S_4) in diastole. Such sounds can originate in either side of the heart. These extra heart sounds create a triplet rhythm, acoustically mimicking a horse's gallop. For that reason the term *gallop* is often used to denote these heart sounds.

A gallop sound that occurs in early diastole, during passive, rapid filling of the ventricles, is known as the third heart sound (S_3). It is heard best with the bell at the apex and with the client in the left lateral decubitus position. An S_3 immediately follows S_2 and is a dull, low-pitched sound. An S_3 gallop is considered a normal finding in children and young adults. In adults over 30 years, an S_3 is considered characteristic of left ventricular dysfunction.

Clinical conditions associated with an S_3 gallop are those precipitating congestive heart failure, for example, myocardial infarction and valvular incompetence. Third heart sounds arising in the left ventricle are best heard at the apex, with the client on his or her left side. Right ventricular gallops are best detected along the left sternal border, with the client supine.

A fourth heart sound, or S_4 gallop, occurs in the later stage of diastole, during atrial contraction and active filling of the ventricles. This soft, low-pitched sound is heard immediately before S_1 and is also referred to as an atrial gallop. An atrial gallop is found most commonly in disorders in which there is an increased stiffness of the ventricle such as ventricular hypertrophy, ischemia, and fibrosis. These conditions are often associated with elevated diastolic ventricular pressures and a vigorous atrial contraction. The ventricles become resistant to filling, and the structures within the ventricles vibrate in response to the added blood input during the "atrial kick." The presence of S_4 may result from myocardial infarction (transient S_4), hypertension, hypertrophy, fibrosis, cardiomyopathy, cor pulmonale, aortic stenosis, or pulmonic stenosis. S_4 is never heard in the absence of atrial contraction (i.e., atrial fibrillation). A S_4 is heard best with the bell of the stethoscope at the apex, with the client in the supine, left lateral position.

Quadruple Rhythm. At times a quadruple rhythm is noted when both S_3 and S_4 become audible. Clients manifesting this unusual heart sound often have tachycardia, which causes the diastolic filling sounds to fuse, forming a summation gallop that may be louder than S_1 or S_2. It can be heard best at the apex and resembles the sound of a galloping horse.

Opening Snaps. These high-pitched sounds heard in diastole are produced by the opening of certain stenosed valves. Valves normally open silently, but when they become calcified or rigid from disease, greater pressure is required to force them open. When they do "pop" open, they produce a characteristic sound. Opening snaps occur with the opening of a stenotic mitral and (rarely) tricuspid valve. The resulting sound is brief, high-pitched, and of a snapping quality. It is heard early in diastole at the apex using a diaphragm.

Ejection Clicks. An ejection click is a high-pitched sound heard in systole. It can be associated with either opening of the semilunar valves or prolapse (inversion) of the mitral valve. Ejection clicks heard during early systole usually result from sudden tensing of the aortic or pulmonic root at the peak of systolic ejection. Often they are the result of high ventricular pressure generated in order to open a rigid, calcified aortic valve. Mid- to late systolic clicks are more likely due to a benign form of mitral insufficiency (regurgitation). When a billowing mitral valve allows prolapse of the leaflets into the left atrium, a click can be heard as the chordae tendineae act as a tether and prohibit further leaflet excursion into the atria.

Pericardial Friction Rub. A pericardial friction rub is produced by inflammation of the pericardial sac (pericarditis). The roughened parietal and visceral layers of the pericardium rub against each other during cardiac motion. This sound has three components, each corresponding with cardiac activity: ventricular systole, ventricular diastole, and atrial systole. A pericardial friction rub is best detected with the diaphragm at the apex and along the left sternal border. It may be accentuated by leaning forward or lying prone and exhaling. Friction rubs produce a sound that is described as "to and fro," scratchy, grating, rasping, and much like "squeaky leather." Friction rubs may be present during the first week of myocardial infarction or after open heart surgery. Differentiate a pericardial friction rub from a pleural friction rub by noting the timing of the rub in relation to breathing. Pleural friction rubs are heard during inspiration. Pericardial friction rubs are heard throughout the respiratory cycle.

Murmurs. Murmurs are heard as a consequence of turbulent blood flow through the heart and large vessels. Turbulent blood flow produces vibrations within the heart and great vessels that can be detected as a blowing or swooshing sound. Murmurs are caused by (1) increased rate or velocity of blood flow, (2) abnormal forward or backward flow across stenosed or incompetent valves, (3) flow into a dilated chamber, or (4) flow through an abnormal passage between heart chambers. Bruits are due to turbulence in vessels.

The following characteristics help identify the various types of murmurs and their origins.

Timing. When does the murmur occur during the cardiac cycle? Is it in the systolic phase or the diastolic phase? It is imperative to identify S_1 and S_2 to determine the phase. The murmur is then described as occurring in early, mid-, or late systole or diastole. A murmur that is heard throughout the systolic phase is described as pansystolic or holosystolic.

Quality. What is the quality or sound of the murmur? Is it blowing, harsh, rumbling, or musical? For example, the murmur of mitral stenosis is described as rumbling, whereas the murmur of mitral regurgitation creates a blowing sound.

Pitch. What is the frequency (pitch) of the murmur? Is it high and heard best with the diaphragm or low and heard best with the bell?

Location. Where is the murmur loudest? Murmurs, like all sounds, are loudest at their point of origin. Is the murmur of highest intensity over the aortic, pulmonic, tricuspid, or mitral valve outflow tract? The location is usually described in terms of its position in relation to intercostal spaces.

Radiation. The sound of the murmur is transmitted in the direction of blood flow. It may be transmitted upstream, as with regurgitant murmurs, or downstream, as noted in stenotic murmurs. Therefore, the sound may be transmitted to the axilla, neck, back, and other locations on the chest.

Configuration. Note the shape of the sound. Does the sound begin soft and become louder (crescendo)? Does it do just the opposite (decrescendo)? Does it seem to have a "diamond shape" (crescendo-decrescendo)? The sound may be fairly constant (plateau). Table 44–2 compares selected heart murmurs.

Intensity. The degree of intensity (loudness) is typically measured using a rating system that does not necessarily reflect the seriousness of disease. Six grades (I–VI) of intensity are noted (Box 44–1). A grade II murmur is recorded as II/VI.

Examination of the Lungs

Because of the intimate relationship between the cardiovascular and respiratory systems, assessment of the cardiovascular system must include evaluation of the respiratory system. A more thorough discussion of respiratory assessment may be found in Chapter 39. Some common respiratory findings related to cardiovascular disease are as follows.

Tachypnea. Tachypnea, or rapid respirations, is often associated with the pain and anxiety that may accompany myocardial ischemic pain. Tachypnea also commonly occurs as a compensatory mechanism in congestive heart failure and pulmonary edema.

Crackles. Rales or crackles are a frequent sign of left ventricular failure and usually occur just after the onset of an S_3 gallop. As pulmonary capillary pressure rises from the backward pressure of left ventricular failure, fluid shifts into the intra-alveolar spaces and crackles can be auscultated. Crackles may also result from atelectasis due to limited chest wall excursion from prolonged bedrest, chest splinting from pain, and the effects of sedatives and narcotics. Crackles are high-pitched, noncontinuous sounds. Crackles are best heard at the lung bases (gravitational effects on the fluid) during late inspiration.

Blood-Tinged Sputum. A pink frothy sputum may indicate acute pulmonary edema. This symptom accompanies diffuse pulmonary crackles and denotes very serious left ventricular failure. Frank hemoptysis may be associated with pulmonary embolus. A cough frequently occurs in association with hemoptysis.

Cheyne-Stokes Respirations. These abnormal respirations are characterized by abnormal periods of deep breathing alternating with periods of apnea. This is a common finding in heart failure, anemia, and brain damage (from anoxic encephalopathy).

Abdomen

Examination of the abdomen provides data regarding cardiac competence. It is, however, of less value than other areas discussed in this section. Abdominal assessment is discussed in Chapter 59.

Inspection and Palpation

Upon inspection, you may note abdominal distention. Palpation may confirm the presence of ascites (fluid accumulation within the peritoneal cavity) and an enlarged liver. Both of these findings indicate liver failure, which can be a sequela of chronic right ventricular failure. In addition, you may elicit a hepatojugular reflex in the client with right ventricular distention. After assessing the client for jugular vein distention, apply mild pressure with one hand over the liver for 1 minute. An increase in jugular vein distention during and immediately after liver compression indicates chronically elevated right ventricular pressure.

Auscultation

Auscultation can yield the following clues about cardiovascular function:

- Decreased bowel tones can accompany potassium (K^+) depletion. K^+ depletion can complicate chronic diuretic use without sufficient K^+ replacement.
- Increased bowel tones, indicative of hypermotility, may result from laxative use or may be a side effect of certain antiarrhythmics (such as quinidine).
- Loud bruits, heard with the bell just over or above the umbilicus, may herald the presence of an aortic obstruction or aortic aneurysm (the latter can be detected by a palpable abdominal pulsation). Bruits heard over the upper midline or toward the back typically arise from renal arterial stenosis.

Diagnostic Tests

The four most common types of diagnostic procedures used to diagnose cardiovascular disease are laboratory

Table 44–2. Heart Murmurs

Type of Heart Sound	Origin	Preferred Method of Auscultation
Systolic murmurs Ejection type S₁ ∙∙᳁ᴵᴵᴵᴵᴵ᳁∙ S₂	Systolic ejection murmurs are associated with forward blood flow during ventricular contraction across stenotic aortic or pulmonic valves	Use the stethoscope diaphragm. Ejection murmurs are typically of medium pitch and harsh quality and may be associated with early ejection click. Aortic ejection murmurs are best heard over aortic valve and radiate into the neck, down left sternal border, and occasionally to apex. May be accompanied by decreased S₂. Pulmonic ejection murmurs are heard best over pulmonic valve, and radiate toward left shoulder and left neck vessels. May be accompanied by a wide split S₂
Pansystolic regurgitant murmurs S₁ ᴵᴵᴵᴵᴵᴵᴵᴵᴵᴵᴵ S₂	Pansystolic murmurs occur when blood regurgitates through incompetent mitral and tricuspid valves (AV valves) or ventricular septal defect as pressures rise during systole and blood seeks chambers of lower pressure. Damage to valve leaflets, papillary muscles, and chordae tendineae results in mitral valve insufficiency (blood regurgitates from left ventricle to left atrium) and tricuspid valve insufficiency (blood regurgitates from right ventricle to right atrium). Ventricular septal defect results in blood regurgitation from left ventricle to right ventricle	All regurgitant murmurs are high-pitched, and those of AV valve incompetence have blowing quality. Mitral regurgitant murmurs are heard at apex and radiate into left axilla and may be accompanied by ejection click and signs of left ventricular failure. Tricuspid regurgitant murmurs are heard loudest over the tricuspid area, and radiate into the sternum. Ventricular septal defects are usually loud, harsh, and heard best over left sternal border in fourth, fifth, and sixth intercostal spaces and radiate over the precordium but not the axilla
Early systolic murmurs S₁ ᴵᴵᴵᴵᴵ᳁.. S₂	Early systolic (innocent) murmurs are associated with high cardiac outputs, as blood flow velocity is increased across normal semilunar valves. Causes include anemia, tachycardia, thyrotoxicosis, and fever. Murmur disappears with correction of underlying condition. Normal variant in children	These are best heard with bell over base of heart or along lower left sternal border. Are usually no greater than grade II, are of medium pitch, and have blowing quality. Intensity may increase during inspiration with patient in left recumbent position or with increased heart rates
Late systolic murmurs S₁ EC ᴵᴵᴵᴵᴵ S₂	These imply mild mitral regurgitation as mitral valve balloons into left atrium late in ventricular systole	Best heard with diaphragm of stethoscope over apex and are often preceded by mid- or late systolic ejection click
Diastolic murmurs Early diastolic murmur S₁ S₂ ᴵᴵᴵᴵᴵ.. S₁	These (decrescendo murmurs) are usually caused by semilunar valve insufficiency, with regurgitation due to valvular deformity or dilation of valvular ring. Are heard immediately following S₂ and then diminish in intensity as pressure in aorta or pulmonary artery falls and ventricles fill	Heard best with diaphragm at base of heart while the patient leans forward in deep expiration. Are high-pitched and blowing and radiate down left sternal border, perhaps to apex or down right sternal border. Accompanying signs of heart failure may be present
Diastolic filling rumbles S₁ S₂ ᴵᴵᴵᴵᴵᴵᴵᴵᴵ S₁	Caused as blood flows across stenotic AV valves (more often mitral). May also occur during augmented blood flow across normal AV valves. Murmur has two phases, becoming louder as the blood flow from the atrium to ventricle increases with passive ventricular filling just after AV valve opening and again during atrial contraction (presystole)	With the bell, this murmur is heard over only a small area at and just medial to the apex. Exercise and a left lateral position of the patient increase the intensity of the sound. It is a low-pitched, rumbling sound often accompanied by an augmented S₁ and an opening snap

AV, atrioventricular; EC, ejection click.
From Huang, S. L., et al. (1989). *Coronary care nursing* (2nd ed., p. 19). Philadelphia: W. B. Saunders.

Box 44–1. Grading of Heart Murmurs

Grade I   Faint; heard after listener has "tuned in"
Grade II   Faint murmur heard immediately
Grade III   Moderately loud, with accompanying thrill
Grade IV   Loud
Grade V   Very loud; heard only with the stethoscope
Grade VI   Very loud; heard without the stethoscope

tests, graphic procedures, x-ray studies, and hemodynamic studies.

Nursing responsibilities in diagnostic testing include the following:

- Explaining the purpose and the procedure and answering any questions
- Scheduling the test
- Performing any necessary preliminary care (e.g., adjustments in medications and special diets)
- Promoting maximal emotional and physical comfort.

Laboratory Tests

Data obtained from laboratory tests are used to diagnose a variety of cardiovascular ailments (e.g., myocardial infarction), to screen persons considered at risk of cardiovascular disease, to determine baseline values, to identify the presence of concurrent conditions (e.g., diabetes mellitus, electrolyte imbalance) that may affect the course of intervention, and to evaluate the effectiveness of intervention. We consider here only those tests that are more commonly used to determine cardiovascular function and disease.

To prepare the client for the laboratory test, explain the procedure. Determine whether the client should fast or refrain from the intake of any particular substances before blood is drawn. If so, provide clear instructions to the client.

Handle the blood sample carefully. Laboratory tubes should be gently inverted to prevent clotting of the specimen for a complete blood cell count (CBC). Vigorous handling of the specimen may lead to hemolysis, which will falsely elevate the levels of intracellular ions such as potassium and magnesium.

Apply pressure to the puncture site until bleeding stops. Assess the site for any hematoma formation.

Complete Blood Cell Count

The erythrocyte red blood cell count usually decreases in rheumatic fever and infective endocarditis. It usually increases in heart diseases characterized by inadequate oxygenation of tissues, for example, right-to-left congenital shunts and heart conditions accompanied by obstructive lung disease.

Measuring the packed cell volume, or hematocrit, is the easiest way to ascertain the concentration of red blood cells in the blood. An elevated hematocrit can result from obstructive lung disease and conditions of vascular vol-

ume depletion with hemoconcentration (e.g., hypovolemic shock and excessive diuresis). Decreases in hematocrit and hemoglobin indicate anemia, which is commonly caused by hemorrhage, hemolysis (from prosthetic valves), and chronic disease states. Patients with anemia have a significant reduction in red blood cell mass and a decrease in oxygen-carrying capacity. Anemia can manifest as angina or aggravate congestive heart failure and produce heart murmurs.

The white blood cell (WBC) count is elevated in infectious and inflammatory diseases of the heart (e.g., infective endocarditis and pericarditis). It is also elevated following myocardial infarction because large numbers of WBCs are necessary to dispose of the necrotic tissue resulting from the infarction.

Cardiac Enzymes

Enzymes are special proteins that catalyze chemical reactions in living cells. Cardiac enzymes are specific enzymes that are present in high concentrations in myocardial tissue. Tissue damage causes release of enzymes from their intracellular storage areas. For example, myocardial infarction causes cellular anoxia, which alters membrane permeability and causes spillage of enzymes into the surrounding tissue. This leakage of enzymes can be detected by rising plasma levels.

The enzymes most commonly used to detect myocardial infarction are creatine kinase (CK) and lactic acid dehydrogenase (LDH). Serum elevations of these two enzymes following myocardial insult occur in sequence. Because these enzymes are also found in other organs and tissues (e.g., skeletal muscle and liver), cardiac specificity must be determined by measuring isoenzyme activity. Isoenzymes are the various forms of CK and LDH, identified by a process known as electrophoresis. There are three isoenzymes of CK: CK-MM (skeletal muscle), CK-MB (myocardial muscle), and CK-BB (brain). An elevated CK-MB, then, indicates myocardial damage. Elevation of CK-MB may occur within 4 to 6 hours and peaks 18 to 24 hours after the acute ischemic event. Of particular importance is the fact that up to a threefold elevation of CK may follow an intramuscular injection. Therefore the level of CK-MB is much more helpful in documenting myocardial infarction than the total CK value.

There are five isoenzymes for LDH (numbered 1–5), of which only LDH_1 and LDH_2 are cardiac-specific. If the serum concentration of LDH_1 is higher than the concentration of LDH_2, the pattern is said to have "flipped," signifying myocardial necrosis. Eighty percent of clients demonstrate elevations in LDH within 48 hours after myocardial infarction.

As well as indicating the presence of myocardial damage, these elevations in serum cardiac enzymes can reveal the timing of the acute cardiac event. This is discussed in further detail in Chapter 45.

Blood Coagulation Tests

Blood coagulation tests are used to examine the ability of the blood to clot. It is important to evaluate coagulation tests such as prothrombin time and partial thromboplastin time in persons with a greater tendency to form thrombi, for example, clients with atrial fibrillation, infective endocarditis, or prosthetic valves. Research has shown an increase in coagulation factors during and after a myocardial infarction. Therefore, the client is at greater risk of thrombophlebitis and extension of clots in the coronary artery. Chapter 52 discusses coagulation tests in detail.

Serum Lipids

Serum lipids play a major role in the development of atherosclerosis. Serum lipids are composed of fatty substances that are insoluble in water. They are derived from dietary intake of fats or synthesized in the liver. The lipid profile measures serum cholesterol, triglycerides, and lipoprotein levels and is used to assess the risk of developing coronary artery disease. Serum lipids are discussed in Chapter 49.

Serum Electrolytes

Cardiovascular disorders may affect fluid and electrolyte regulation. In addition, certain medications alter electrolyte balance.

Potassium. The serum potassium level lowers as a result of diuretic therapy, vomiting, diarrhea, and alkalosis. Cardiac effects of hypokalemia include increased electrical instability, ventricular dysrhythmias, and increased risk of digitalis toxicity. Characteristic changes on the ECG include flattening and inversion of the T wave, the appearance of a U wave, and sagging of the ST segment.

A high serum potassium level is usually associated with kidney and endocrine disorders. The cardiac effects of hyperkalemia include asystole and ventricular dysrhythmias.

Sodium. The serum sodium level reflects water balance and may decrease (indicating water excess) in congestive heart failure, stress, excessive intravenous (IV) infusion of hypotonic fluids, and vomiting. Extensive use of diuretics and severely restricted sodium intake also lower serum sodium.

Calcium. The serum calcium level decreases as a result of multiple transfusions of citrated blood, renal failure, alkalosis, and laxative and antacid abuse (phosphate excess). Cardiac manifestations of hypocalcemia include serious ventricular dysrhythmias, prolonged Q–T interval, and cardiac arrest. Hypercalcemia occurs in thiazide diuretic use, acidosis, adrenal insufficiency, immobility, and vitamin D excess. A high serum calcium level shortens the Q–T interval and causes AV block, tachycardia, bradycardia, digitalis hypersensitivity, and cardiac arrest.

Magnesium. Magnesium helps regulate intracellular metabolism, activates essential enzymes, and aids in the transport of sodium and potassium across the cell membrane. It plays a vital role in neuromuscular excitability.

Low magnesium levels may result from prolonged use of diuretics, malnutrition, chronic alcoholism, severe diarrhea, and dehydration. Symptoms include mental apathy, facial tics, leg cramps, respiratory depression, and severe cardiac dysrhythmias, including ventricular tachycardia and fibrillation.

High magnesium levels may develop in the client with chronic renal failure. Symptoms include profound muscle weakness, hyporeflexia, hypotension, and bradycardia with a prolonged P-R interval and wide QRS complex.

Phosphorus. Most extracellular phosphorus is found in the bone with calcium (85% of the body's total phosphorus). A small amount of phosphorus is found in intracellular fluid. There it helps regulate energy formation (adenosine triphosphate, ATP), maintain acid-base balance, and maintain neuromuscular excitability. Phosphate levels should be interpreted with serum calcium levels, as the kidneys retain or excrete one electrolyte in an inverse relationship to the other.

Hypophosphatemia may result from hyperparathyroidism, diabetic ketoacidosis, prolonged use of IV dextrose infusions, or renal tubular acidosis. Symptoms of hypophosphatemia include bleeding, decreased WBC levels, muscular weakness (including respiratory muscles), and nausea and vomiting.

Hyperphosphatemia usually occurs in clients with chronic renal failure; clients with skeletal disease, including healing fractures; and clients undergoing chemotherapy. Symptoms are similar to those of hypocalcemia, with muscle tetany being the most common finding.

Blood Urea Nitrogen

Blood urea nitrogen (BUN) is a test of renal function, specifically, the ability of the kidney to excrete urea and protein. The BUN level is elevated in kidney diseases, during water and saline depletion, and heart disorders that adversely affect renal circulation, for example, congestive heart failure and cardiogenic shock.

Blood Glucose

Diabetes mellitus is a major risk factor in the development of atherosclerosis. In addition, the stress of an acute cardiac event can greatly elevate blood glucose, causing unstable hyperglycemia in clients with latent diabetes mellitus. For these reasons, blood glucose is routinely assessed in all clients with acute cardiovascular disorders.

Electrocardiogram

Each heartbeat is the result of an electrical impulse. This impulse, which begins in the sinoatrial node of the right atrium, is conducted through a network of fibers (the conduction system) within the heart and causes the heart to contract. This same electrical impulse spreads outward from the heart to the skin, where it can be detected by electrodes attached to the skin. The ECG is a display of the electrical action of the heart. There are several types of ECG: continuous monitoring, 12-lead, and signal-averaged ECG. Through analysis of the ECG wave forms, disorders of cardiac rate, rhythm, or conduction can be identified.

ECG is a common test. It is performed on clients over the age of 40 prior to surgery to assess for unknown heart disease and is a frequent noninvasive diagnostic test in clients with known or suspected heart disease.

To prepare the client for a 12-lead ECG, explain the procedure. Tell the client that this test helps evaluate the heart's function by recording its electrical activity. Note any recent cardiac medications.

During the procedure, advise the client to lie still and breathe normally. Ask the client to refrain from talking during the procedure.

After the procedure, disconnect the equipment. If using conductive gel, wipe the gel from the client's skin. If using conductive stickers, remove them unless serial ECG readings are to be done. If serial ECGs are ordered, leave the stickers in place to assure consistent lead placement.

Continuous Electrocardiogram Monitoring

Four steps are required for ECG monitoring: (1) attaching the electrodes to the client's skin, (2) connecting the electrodes to the monitor by way of a cable, (3) adjusting the monitor to obtain a readable ECG, and (4) setting the alarms for desired high and low rates. Assure the client that the ECG does not cause electrical shock and does not hurt.

Attaching the Electrodes. Electrodes pick up electrical impulses from the heart on the skin. It is appar-

ent that unless the signal is detected accurately, the remaining phases of ECG monitoring have little value. The most common form of electrodes are disc-type or floating electrodes, which are deliberately separated from direct contact with the skin by a spacer filled with conductive gel. The gel is used to improve the signal by reducing local electrical interference on the skin. The gel is surrounded by a ring of adhesive. By peeling a paper backing off the pad, the electrode can be immediately applied to the skin. Three electrodes are required for continuous ECG monitoring. Two of these serve to detect the heart's activity; the third is an electrical ground.

Attach the electrodes to the lead wires before they are applied to the chest wall. This process avoids applying pressure to the electrode, which could hurt the client and squeeze the gel outward, reducing contact.

Good skin preparation improves impulse conduction. Thoroughly clean the skin areas where electrodes will be applied. Wipe the skin with alcohol and allow this to air-dry before applying the electrodes. If the client has a lot of chest hair, clip it to improve contact.

In positioning the electrodes on the chest wall, select locations that will provide the clearest ECG wave forms. Two of the most common positions are the conventional position and the modified chest lead position (Fig. 44–6). The lead II wave form (shown) is the most common rhythm strip lead. MCL$_1$ (shown), V$_1$, or V$_6$ are more helpful, however, for dysrhythmia detection. When close monitoring of ST segments is essential, such as after thrombolytic therapy or coronary angioplasty, the lead most closely associated with the area of heart muscle involved should be monitored. Change electrodes if the tracing is not clear or if they become dry or lose skin contact. In addition, electrodes should be routinely changed every 48 hours to avoid skin irritation and to ensure that electrode gel is sufficient for good conduction.

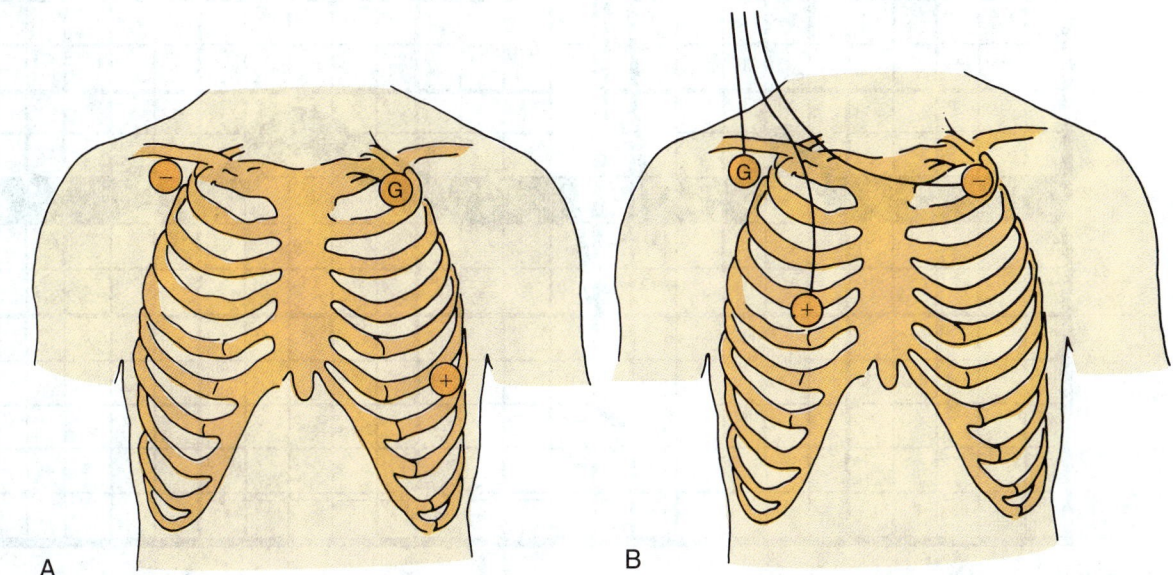

Figure 44–6. Common positions for continuous monitoring lead placement. Use lead II (*A*) or lead V$_1$ (*B*). (From Phillips, R. E., & Feeney M. K. [1990]. *The cardiac rhythms: A systematic approach to interpretation* [3rd ed.]. Philadelphia, W. B. Saunders.)

Connecting the Monitor. The electrodes are connected to the monitor by lead wires. These wires are 12 to 18 inches in length. One end snaps onto the electrodes, and the other end is attached to a cable that is connected to the monitor. At the cable is a cable receptacle for the attachment of each wire. The receptacle and lead wires are color-coded to facilitate connection.

Adjusting the Monitor. The ECG pattern should be clear and distinct. If the pattern is not clear, recheck the first steps. Monitor adjustments will vary with the brand of monitor in use. Refer to the operating instructions for assistance.

Setting the Alarms. Alarm limits should be set at levels appropriate to alert the nurse to any acute changes. Many monitors have default alarm settings. These should be verified as appropriate for the client. If no default settings or institutional standards are present, alarm limits should be set approximately 20 beats above and below the client's typical heart rate.

At times, false alarms may occur due to poor electrode contact or client movement. You may be tempted to set the alarm limits widely apart (e.g., 40–180 beats per minute [BPM]) or, worse, to turn the alarm off completely. This practice defeats the purpose of the alarm system and should never be adopted.

Electrocardiogram Tracings

Once the client is attached to continuous ECG monitoring, the heart rhythm is assessed hourly. Rhythm strips are logged into the medical record routinely as well as when dysrhythmias are noted. Dysrhythmias are discussed in Chapter 45.

The impulse waves, recorded by the ECG machine onto graph paper, are arbitrarily designated by the letters P, Q, R, S, and T. The QRS letters are generally referred to as the QRS complex. Figure 44–7 depicts the typical ECG pattern formed by these waves.

The components of the ECG are defined as follows:

The P wave represents depolarization of the atria.
The P–R interval represents the time it takes for the impulse to spread from the atria to the ventricles.
The QRS complex represents depolarization of the ventricles.

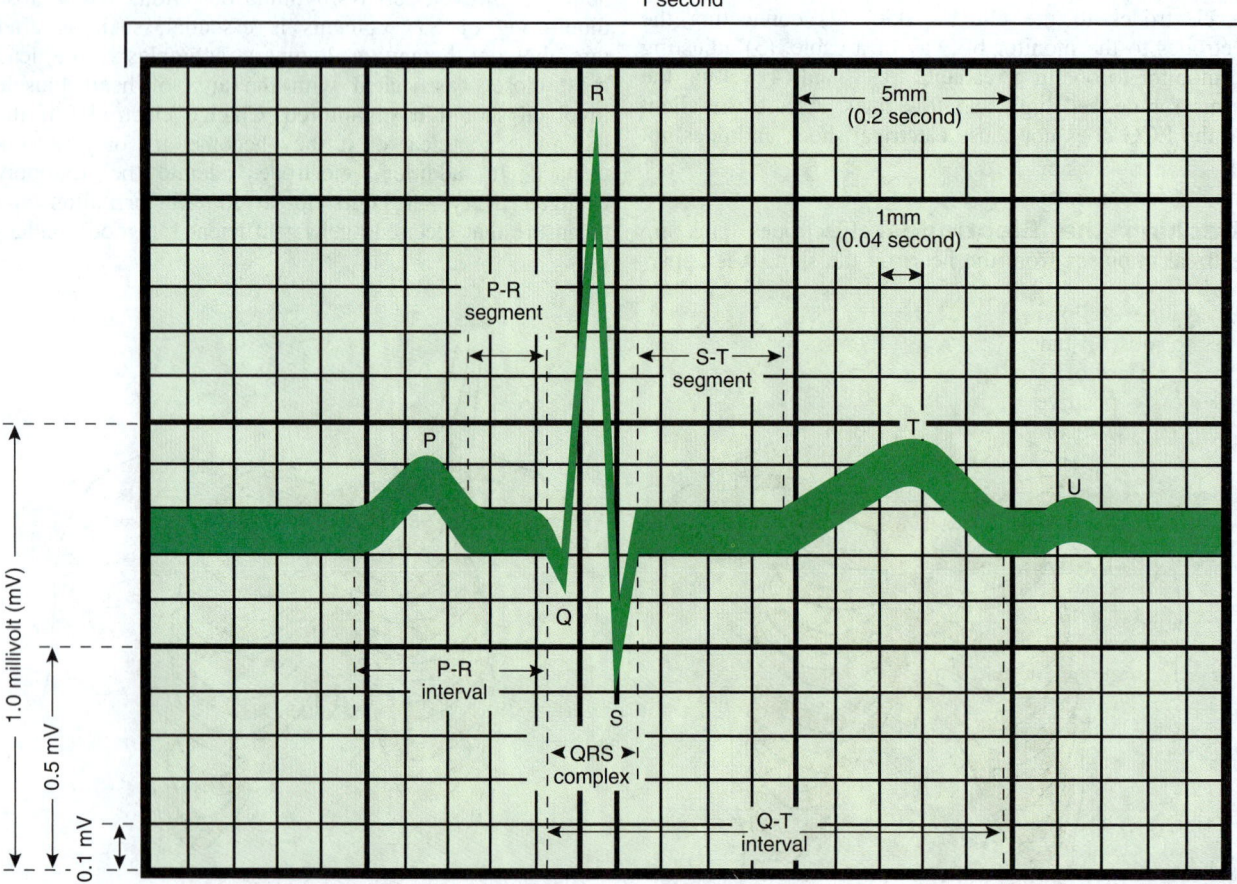

Figure 44–7. Normal electrocardiographic (ECG) pattern. The P wave represents depolarization of the atria to the ventricles. The QRS complex represents depolarization of the ventricles, and the T wave represents repolarization of the ventricles. The small U wave is sometimes seen following the T wave. Time and voltage lines of ECG paper: *vertically*, 1 mm = 0.1 mV; 5 mm = 0.5 mV; 10 mm = 1.0 mV; *horizontally*, 1 small box = 0.04 second; 5 small boxes = 0.20 second; 25 small boxes = 1 second.

The T wave represents repolarization of the ventricles.

The ST segment indicates completion of ventricular depolarization and that repolarization is about to begin.

The Q–T interval represents electrical systole, and varies with age, sex, and heart rate.

The U wave is a small wave that sometimes follows the T wave. It may indicate hypokalemia.

An ECG tracing also shows the voltage of the waves and the duration of both the waves and the intervals. Note that ECG graph paper is divided into horizontal lines and vertical lines, large squares and small squares. Voltage is represented on the vertical axis of the ECG paper. Each small square is 1 mm in height. Five small squares are equivalent to 5 mm, which, in turn, is equivalent to 0.5 mV. Voltage yields information regarding the presence and degree of atrial or ventricular hypertrophy. Time duration is measured on the horizontal axis. Each small square signifies the passage of 0.04 second. Each large square indicates the passage of 0.20 second. By studying the duration of the waves and intervals, the examiner can diagnose abnormal impulse formation and conduction. Normal time durations for waves and intervals are as follows:

P wave: less than 0.11 second

P–R interval: 0.12 to 0.20 second (average, 0.16 second)

QRS complex: 0.4 to 0.11 second

Q–T interval: in women, up to 0.43 second; in men, up to 0.42 second (normal duration is inversely related to heart rate)

Because of its normal variation in configuration, more must be said about the QRS complex. The Q wave is always the first downward (negative) deflection of the complex. The R wave is always the first upward (positive) deflection. If there is a negative deflection (below the baseline) following an R wave, it is labeled an S wave. In most instances, a Q wave is not obvious on the ECG of the normal heart. The QRS complex may appear as a mostly positive or mostly negative deflection, depending on the recording electrode used.

Electrocardiogram Variations

■ The 12-Lead Electrocardiogram

Indications for a 12-lead ECG are listed in Box 44–2.

The standard ECG has a 12-lead system, offering 12 points of reference for recording the electrical activity of the heart. This can be conceptualized as 12 different views of the heart, looking in both horizontal and vertical planes. The standard 12-lead ECG has six limb leads (used to view the heart in a frontal or vertical plane) and six precordial leads (used to view the heart in a horizontal plane). The limb leads are composed of three bipolar leads (leads I, II, and III) and three unipolar leads (leads aVR, aVL, and aVF). The bipolar leads consist of two electrodes and measure the difference in electrical potential flowing through the heart between two extremities. The unipolar leads compare the electrical potential of a

---

Box 44–2. Indications for a 12-Lead Electrocardiogram

Dysrhythmias
Chest pain
Myocardial infarction
Heart rate determination
Chamber dilation or hypertrophy
Preoperative assessment
Pericarditis
Effect of medications (especially cardiac)
Effect of systemic disease on the heart (i.e., renal or pulmonary disease)
Effect of electrolyte disturbances (especially potassium)

---

positive electrode, placed on one limb, and a negative pole within a central terminal that averages the potential of the other two limb leads.

Standard bipolar limb leads are called I, II, and III. Lead I measures the difference in electrical potential between the left arm and right arm; lead II measures the difference in potential between the left leg and right arm; and lead III measures the difference in potential between the left leg and left arm (Fig. 44–8).

Augmented unipolar limb leads measure as follows: aVR measures electrical potential between the center of the heart and the right arm; aVL measures electrical potential between the center of the heart and the left arm; and aVF measures electrical potential between the center of the heart and the left leg (see Fig. 44–8).

The precordial leads (V_1, V_2, V_3, V_4, V_5, and V_6) provide six views of the heart from the anterior and left lateral vantage points. These unipolar leads compare the electrical potential between a positive electrode (in the six different chest locations) and a central, negative terminal that represents an average potential of the three standard limb leads (Fig. 44–9).

Together the 12 leads permit multidirectional examination of the electrical events in the heart. The location of pathologic change within the heart, which alters electrical activity, can be pinpointed. Table 44–3 correlates the area of infarct with expected ECG changes and coronary artery lesion location. Views from the different leads are oriented to various surfaces of the myocardium:

● Leads I, aVL, V_5, and V_6 record electrical events occurring on the lateral surface of the left ventricle.
● Leads II, III, and aVF record electrical events occurring on the inferior surface of the left ventricle.
● Leads V_1 and V_2 record electrical events occurring on the surface of the right ventricle and anterior surface of the left ventricle.
● Leads V_3 and V_4 record electrical events occurring within the septal region of the left ventricle.

The placement of 12-lead electrodes is shown in Figures 44–8 and 44–9.

It is important that good contact be made between the skin and the electrodes. To facilitate this, the electrodes are placed firmly on the flat surface just above the wrists and ankles. There are many varieties of electrodes: adhesive back, foam, cloth, plastic, and suction cups. In clients with an amputation, the electrodes are applied to the stump of the affected extremity. Note that the leg and arm electrodes must remain attached in order to obtain the precordial leads. Some ECG machines are able to record only one lead at a time, while others can record 3, 6, or all 12 leads simultaneously.

Note any unusual chest deformities, respiratory distress, or tremors that may account for alterations in the recording and whether the client experiences angina pectoris or chest discomfort at the time of the ECG.

■ Signal-Averaged Electrocardiogram

A signal-averaged ECG is used to identify the presence of electrical impulses called late potentials. These im-

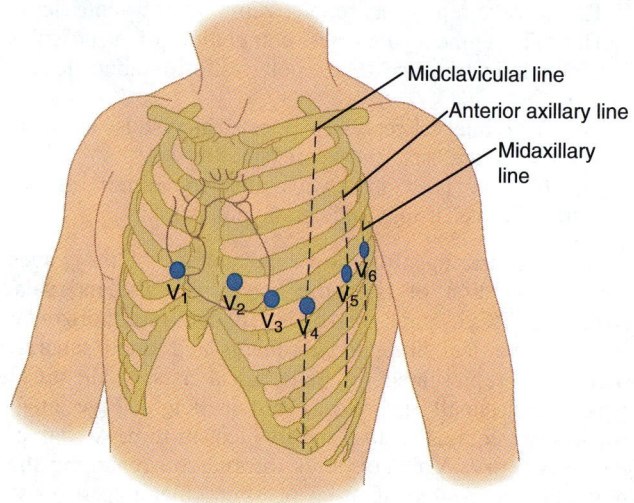

A

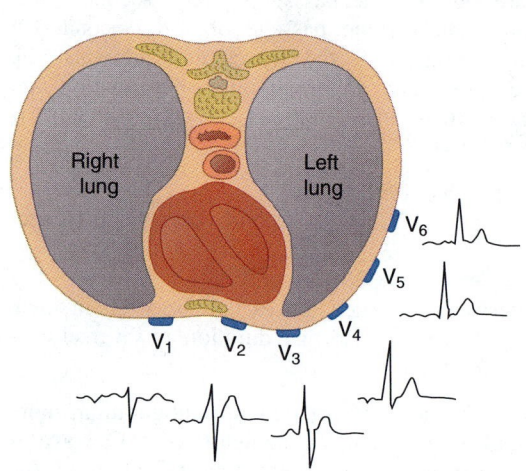

B

Figure 44–9. Placement of chest (*V*) leads. *A,* Precordial (chest) lead placement. *B,* Normal electrocardiographic findings with corresponding chest leads to cross-section at fourth rib level.

pulses occur during diastole late into the QRS complex and ST segment. This noninvasive test may be done at the bedside and is used to predict which clients may be prone to ventricular tachycardia resulting in sudden death. In a signal-averaged ECG, a computer is used to record and process low-level signals that are not detected by a traditional ECG. This technique allows detection of signals that may otherwise be masked by noise that conceals the small electrical events of the heart. Late potentials are multiphasic, low-amplitude, high-frequency spikes that appear after the terminal portion of the QRS complex and extend into the ST segment. They are thought to be generated by delayed activation in an abnormal area of the heart. The presence of late potentials in clients with normal sinus rhythm identifies the risk of ventricular tachycardia and sudden cardiac death.[20]

■ Holter Monitoring

When the client wears a portable Holter monitor, an ECG tracing may be recorded continuously over a period of a

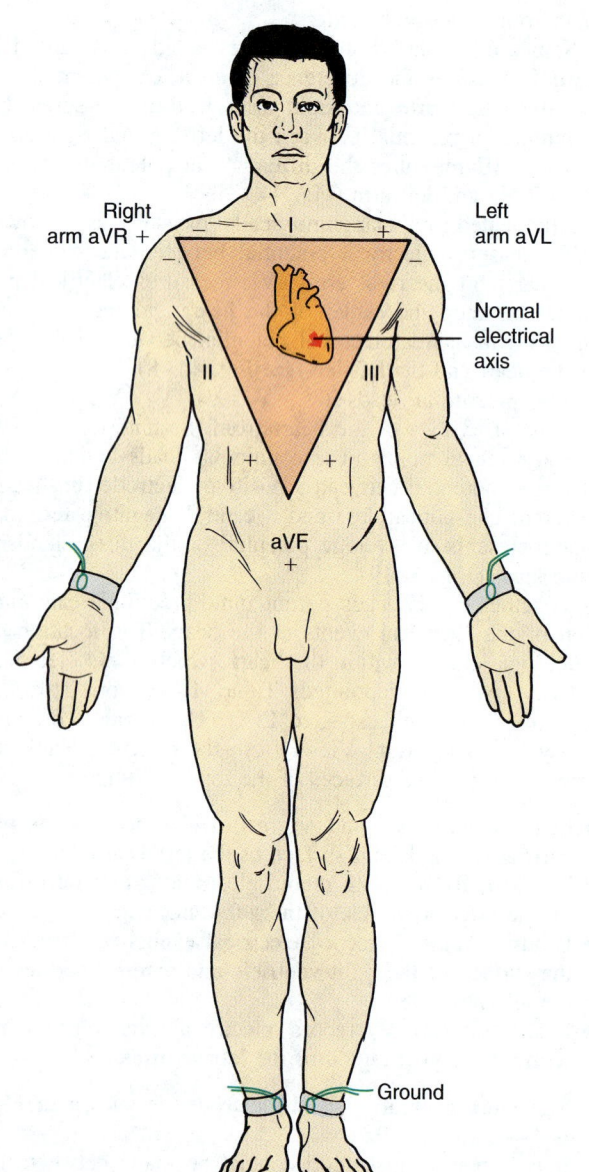

Figure 44–8. Standard positions for electrocardiogram leads. Bipolar limb leads are I, II, and III (Einthoven's triangle). Augmented unipolar limb leads: aVR (right arm), aVL (left arm), and aVF (left leg).

Table 44–3. Coronary Artery Lesion Location, Area of Infarct, and Electrocardiographic (ECG) Changes

Coronary Artery	Area of Infarct	ECG Leads	Dysrhythmias
LAD	Anterior	V_{2-4}	RBBB, LAH, Mobitz type II, CHB
	Septal	V_{1-2}	
	Anteroseptal	V_{1-4}	
Circumflex	Lateral	I, aVL	Ventricular and possibly SA and AV node conduction disturbances
	Anterolateral	I, aVL, V_{5-6}	
	Inferolateral	aVF, II, III, V_{5-6}	
	Posterior	Reciprocal, V_{1-3}	
RCA	Inferior	II, III, aVF	SA node, AV node, and His bundle conduction disturbances
	Right ventricle	II, III, aVF, V_{4-6R}	

AV, atrioventricular, CHB, complete heart block; LAD, left anterior descending, LAH, left anterior hemiblock; RBBB, right bundle branch block; RCA, right coronary artery; SA, sinoatrial.
From Alspach, J. G. (Ed.) (1992). *Instructor's resource manual for the AACN core curriculum for critical care nursing.* Philadelphia: W. B. Saunders.

day or longer on an outpatient basis. Whereas a standard ECG is obtained over a relatively short time period, Holter monitoring continues for an extended period. Thus, Holter monitoring is done to determine which dysrhythmias may be causing clinical manifestations that may not occur during a routine ECG but do occur when the client is ambulating at home or work. Holter monitoring is also useful in evaluating the effectiveness of antiarrhythmic or pacemaker therapy. The monitoring system records at preset time intervals and when it senses an unusual event.

To prepare the client, place two to three electrodes on the chest and attach them to the telemetry unit. This unit is not much larger than a beeper and is worn in a sling fashioned about the chest or waist. Encourage the client to go about his or her daily activities normally and keep a written account of these activities along with any symptoms that may develop. These data are used to document transient dysrhythmias and correlate the client's perceived symptoms with the underlying rhythm. Holter monitoring also helps clinicians evaluate the effectiveness of pacemaker and pharmacologic antiarrhythmic therapy.

■ Exercise Electrocardiogram (Stress Testing)

Exercise ECGs, referred to as stress testing, are valuable tools for detecting and evaluating coronary artery disease. Stress testing involves (1) using controlled and carefully supervised exercise to increase myocardial oxygen demands and (2) evaluating the coronary arteries' ability to meet the increased demands successfully. Its greatest advantage is that it provides information about the cardiovascular system in a dynamic state. A study of the heart during activity cannot be duplicated by the resting, recumbent position typically used in routine physical examination. Stress testing may be used in conjunction with myocardial radionuclide testing.

Exercise testing may have single or multiple stages. A single-stage test is one in which the exercise workload is constant throughout. Multiple-stage testing involves increasing the exercise workload in increments until a de-

sired point is reached. These incremental increases in workload may occur every 1 to 5 minutes. The duration of testing varies with the type of test being used and the client's tolerance for testing.

The two major modes of exercise used for stress testing in the United States are bicycle ergometry and the treadmill. Bicycle ergometry uses a device equipped with a wheel operated by pedals that can be adjusted to increase the resistance to pedaling (multistage testing). It can be used for arm cranking, foot pedaling, or both. Bicycle ergometry has the advantage of being a relatively inexpensive test and portable. It does, however, require frequent recalibration and can induce localized muscle group fatigue.

Treadmill testing is the most commonly used mode of stress testing, especially when used in conjunction with thallium 201 imaging. The treadmill is a motorized device that has an adjustable conveyor belt able to reach speeds of 1 to 10 miles per hour. The conveyor belt can be adjusted from a horizontal position to a 20% gradient, allowing the client to walk or run on slopes at all different angles.

Prior to stress testing, inform the client of the purposes and risks of exercise testing and obtain a signed consent. The client must have a detailed physical examination before testing. In addition, the examiner must take a baseline resting ECG immediately before testing begins. Prepare the skin for electrode placement as previously described. Secure electrodes to the chest with tape or a belt. Drape lead wires, cable, and BP cuff to allow maximal freedom of movement. Refer to the Client Education Guide for further client instructions. During the exercise test, the client's BP (using an automatically inflating cuff) and ECG are closely monitored by a physician or appropriately trained person.

During the procedure, perform the following:

● Obtain baseline BP, heart rate, and rhythm strip.
● Observe the ECG monitor constantly for changes.
● Record the client's BP, heart rate, rhythm strip, and activity level and time at specified intervals.

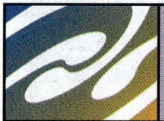

CLIENT EDUCATION GUIDE

Stress Testing

Get sufficient rest the night before the test.

Avoid eating a heavy meal just prior to the test, although it is advisable to eat a light meal 1 to 2 hours before the test.

Avoid smoking, alcohol, and beverages containing caffeine during the day of testing.

Wear nonconstrictive, comfortable clothing and rubber-soled, supportive shoes during testing. Only a loose-fitting, front-buttoning shirt (or blouse) should be worn. (Women should wear a brassiere.)

Continue all usual medications unless specified otherwise by the physician. (An inquiry about this should be made to the physician.)

Following the test, rest and keep the physician informed of any lingering symptoms of cardiovascular distress, that is, chest pain, shortness of breath, or dizziness.

Avoid taking a hot shower for 1 to 2 hours following the test because this may potentiate hypotension, resulting in a fainting episode. If bathing is desired, use only tepid water.

- Monitor the client for chest pain, arrhythmias, ST segment changes, unexpected changes in BP, or other cardiac symptoms (extreme dyspnea, claudication, vertigo).

A multilead monitoring system is most often used to provide maximal views of the heart wall. The examiner makes frequent observations throughout testing for any untoward manifestation related to impaired cardiovascular performance. These symptoms include chest pain, ventricular arrhythmia, extreme dyspnea, claudication (leg pain due to peripheral vascular disease), vertigo, and a sudden drop in BP. Reasons for terminating the test are as follows:

- Chest pain or fatigue
- Greatly increased heart rate (age-related):
    - 20–29 years: 170 BPM
    - 30–39 years: 160 BPM
    - 40–49 years: 150 BPM
    - 50–59 years: 140 BPM
    - 60–69 years: 130 BPM
- Untoward signs and symptoms of myocardial ischemia or heart failure
- Failure of systolic BP to rise or a drop in BP (below resting levels)
- Sudden development of bradycardia
- Serious cardiac dysrhythmia
- Severe hypertension
- Severe dyspnea
- ST segment depression (greater than 2–4 mm)
- A sudden loss of coordination (cerebral ischemia)

Because these symptoms occur with some frequency, an emergency cart containing cardiac drugs and resuscitation equipment is kept close at hand at all times. Clients rarely die from this procedure.

A positive exercise test is one that must be terminated before the predicted maximal (or submaximal) limits have been achieved because of manifestations of cardiovascular intolerance. Generally, the earlier these symptoms appear, the more serious is the extent of the disease. Alterations in the ST segment and T wave on the ECG during exercise and recovery are often considered diagnostic of coronary artery disease. This is because these alterations reflect an imbalance between myocardial oxygen demand and supply. There is, however, controversy about what extent of ST segment change constitutes an abnormal response to exercise. Currently, the most widely held position is that the stress test is positive when the configuration and magnitude of the ST segment fulfill any of the following criteria:

- A 1-mm flat (horizontal) ST segment depression lasting for 0.08 second
- A 1-mm downsloping ST segment depression lasting for 0.08 second (this has the highest predictive value)
- A 1.5- to 2.0-mm upsloping ST segment depression lasting for 0.08 second (this characteristic alone does not constitute a positive response)

Although the exercise test is very helpful as an adjunct diagnostic study for coronary artery disease, it can produce false-positive findings in some cases, especially in women. In some persons, alterations in ST segment may occur during exercise, even though no coronary artery disease exists. Hyperventilation, certain drugs, and electrolyte imbalances can produce false-positive readings. For this reason, diagnosis cannot be made on the basis of exercise findings alone.

False-negative findings can also occur, although with less frequency. Medications such as beta-blocking agents and nitrates are capable of producing false-negative results. Another limitation of the study is that it is absolutely contraindicated in various cardiovascular and noncardiac conditions. See Box 44–3 for contraindications to exercise testing.

Become familiar with the stress testing procedure to provide clear teaching guidelines for clients scheduled to undergo exercise testing. Many clients harbor misconceptions and unnecessary fears about the procedure. Although the procedure is not painful, it can produce a great deal of fatigue. Warn the client that this test may trigger chest pain and dyspnea. Along with this warning, point out that the procedure is performed in a controlled environment with prompt nursing and medical attention close at hand. It is very important that the client arrive for the exercise testing appointment relaxed and well rested. Teaching guidelines to stress testing are given in the Client Education Guide.

After the procedure, assist the client to a chair or bed for recovery. Periodically monitor the client's BP, heart rate, and rhythm strip for a least 15 minutes after test completion or until the ECG returns to baseline.

phology and rate of the induced tachycardia are compared with the morphology and rate of the client's own spontaneous ventricular tachycardia. The ventricular tachycardia is often terminated by rapid ventricular decremental pacing. If the tachycardia cannot be stimulated, IV isoproterenol may be infused to simulate stress or exercise, which may produce the tachycardia.

Antiarrhythmic drugs may be administered during the study to evaluate their effect. After the initial antiarrhythmic has been given, induction of ventricular tachycardia is attempted. If ventricular tachycardia is induced, the dosage may be increased or other drugs administered and the electrophysiologic studies repeated in several days to determine the effectiveness of antiarrhythmic drug therapy.

Frequently when the irritable focus has been identified (e.g., accessory pathway or bundle of His), an ablation may be performed. Ablation of the irritable focus may be accomplished by the use of radiofrequency, direct current, ethyl alcohol, or cryosurgery. Radiofrequency ablation is the most popular method because its effect may be localized, with less damage to surrounding tissue.

Nursing care of the client undergoing electrophysiologic studies is similar to that of the client undergoing cardiac catheterization and is discussed in that section. Since the study attempts, under controlled circumstances, to induce potentially lethal arrhythmias, it is imperative that emergency drugs, equipment, and a defibrillator be immediately accessible.

Electrophysiologic Studies

The electrophysiologic study is an invasive method of recording intracardiac electrical activity. It is used to shed light on the mechanisms of dysrhythmias, to differentiate between supraventricular and ventricular dysrhythmias, to evaluate sinoatrial (SA) or AV node dysfunction, to determine the need for a pacemaker, and to evaluate the effect of antiarrhythmic agents used to prevent the occurrence of tachycardias.

An electrophysiologic catheter has four electrodes at the distal tip that record or stimulate (pace). Under fluoroscopy, the catheter is threaded into the heart via the femoral, basilica, or subclavian vein. The catheter sites selected depend on the purpose of the examination. One catheter is left at the bundle of His just beneath the AV node as a point of reference. An additional catheter is introduced high in the right atrium. If Wolff-Parkinson-White syndrome is suspected, a catheter may be placed in the coronary sinus. A catheter may also be placed in the right ventricle. During mapping of ventricular tachycardia, a catheter may be introduced into the left ventricle via an artery.

The procedure is designed to reproduce any dysrhythmia so that its origin may be isolated. Ventricular tachycardia is induced by using programmed stimulation to fire an impulse at different times during the cardiac electrical cycle. If the dysrhythmia is induced, the client's BP and hemodynamic responses are observed. It is possible for arterial pressure, surface ECGs, and ECGs from intracavitary catheters to be recorded simultaneously. The mor-

Chest X-Ray Studies

The physician routinely orders posteroanterior, lateral, and oblique chest x-ray films to determine the size, silhouette, and position of the heart. In the acutely ill client, an anteroposterior x-ray film is taken at the bedside. Specific pathologic changes of the heart are difficult to determine on x-ray examination, but anatomic changes in the heart and pulmonary sequelae of various cardiac conditions can be seen. Valvular and pericardial calcifications; pulmonary congestion (from heart failure); pericardial effusion; and placement of central lines, endotracheal tubes, hemodynamic monitoring devices, and intra-aortic balloon catheters are all assessed on x-ray film.

Magnetic Resonance Imaging

Although magnetic resonance imaging (MRI) is one of the most expensive noninvasive diagnostic options, a variety of information may be obtained in a single image. MRI provides the best information on chamber size, wall motion, valvular function, and great vessel blood flow. The MRI is commonly used for examination of the aorta, detection of tumors or masses, cardiomyopathies, and pericardial disease. In MRI, a strong magnetic field and radio waves are used to detect and define the differences between healthy and diseased tissue. MRI is able to image over three spatial dimensions and over time. It can actually show the heart beating and the blood flowing in any direction. All standard quantitative functional indices can be obtained from an MRI study with the exception of transstenotic gradients.

Information obtained from MRI includes the following:

- Normal morphology and structural changes
- Wall thickness, chamber volumes, valve areas, vessel cross-sections, and extent, location, and size of lesions
- Global and regional biventricular function, including ejection fraction, stroke volume, and cardiac output
- Blood flow quantifications within vessels over the cardiac cycle
- Tissue characterization of para- and intracardiac masses, pericardial effusions, and myocardial infarction

The average length of the procedure ranges from 45 minutes to 1 hour. The client must remove all metal items such as a watch, zipper, and eyeglasses before the procedure. Clients with pacemakers, prosthetic valves, or recently implanted clips or wires cannot undergo MRI scans. Prepare the client for the fact that lying on the table inside the MRI is very confining and that the scanner makes a loud knocking noise. Any client who is claustrophobic may need sedation. The client may choose to wear mirrored glasses that allow visualization outside the magnet. A family member may remain in the room during the procedure if the client is particularly apprehensive.

Positron Emission Tomography

The positron emission tomographic (PET) scanner is a diagnostic imaging tool that allows visualization of regional physiologic function and images biochemical changes that often separate normal from diseased myocardium. Cellular metabolic information is obtained by mapping regional myocardial glucose metabolism. Combining information from the perfusion and the metabolism images provides a thorough assessment of regional cardiac viability. For a more complete discussion of positron emission tomography, see Chapter 13.

The scanning procedure takes about 2 to 3 hours. An IV radiopharmaceutical, (N)-ammonia, is administered and a 20-minute blood flow image is begun. Next an IV injection of glucose follows. It takes this about 40 minutes to localize in the myocardium. Final uptake of this tracer is proportional to the glucose metabolic activity of myocardial cells and provides an excellent indication of regional tissue viability.

The following are clinical indications for PET scanner use:

- Detection of coronary artery disease
- Assessment of myocardial viability
- Assessment of progression of coronary artery stenosis
- Documentation of collateral coronary circulation
- Differentiation of ischemia and dilated cardiomyopathy

The terms "match" and "mismatch" describe the relationship between the perfusion and the metabolism studies. Similarities between a perfusion study with poor blood flow and a metabolic study showing decreased glucose uptake of necrotic tissue is described as a "match." A perfusion study that shows poor blood flow and a metabolic study that shows only stunned viable myocardium that has survived the initial insult is described as a "mismatch."

Echocardiography

The echocardiogram, a noninvasive diagnostic procedure based on the principles of ultrasound, is used to evaluate structural and functional changes in a wide variety of heart ailments. It is one of the mainstays of diagnostic cardiology because it is noninvasive, can be used at the bedside, and provides accurate information at no risk to the client.

An echocardiogram is performed by placing a transducer on several areas of the chest wall. This transducer emits short pulses of high-frequency sound through the chest wall and heart. Wave pulses bounce off tissues of varying densities and are reflected back to the transducer as a series of echoes, thus creating an image via an oscilloscope graph. The bursts of ultrasound are directed at the part of the heart under investigation. The echocardiogram records the structure and motion of that area in relation to its distance from the anterior chest wall (Fig. 44–10). An ECG is recorded simultaneously on the graph. Two-dimensional echocardiography generates a continuous picture of the beating heart. These images are recorded on videotape for analysis.

Echocardiograms are used to help assess and diagnose pericardial effusion, cardiomyopathy, valvular disorders (including prosthetic valves), cardiac shunts, myocardial ischemia, chamber size, left ventricular function, ventricular aneurysms, and cardiac tumors (atrial myxoma). In addition, they are very useful during heart biopsies because the physician can view the heart on a monitor while taking tissue samples.

Nursing intervention for clients undergoing echocardiography involves explaining the procedure and reassuring the client that the study is noninvasive, painless, and without complication. An echocardiogram can be performed at the bedside, although it is preferable to send the client to the echocardiography laboratory.

Transesophageal Echocardiography

Transesophageal echocardiography (TEE) gives a higher-quality picture of the heart than does a regular echocardiogram. It is especially useful in clients who have thickened lung tissue or thick chest walls or are obese. The procedure may also be used intraoperatively where conventional echocardiography is ineffective. The client needs to be in bed or on a table with ECG leads attached. ECG and BP are monitored. The throat is anesthetized and sedation is given. An esophageal scope is inserted through the mouth and passed into the esophagus by the physician. Because the probe is placed behind the heart, it allows the left atrium to be viewed. TEE allows clearer visibility of the heart and its structures and is most useful in diagnosis of cardiac masses, prosthetic valve function, aneurysm, and posterior effusions.

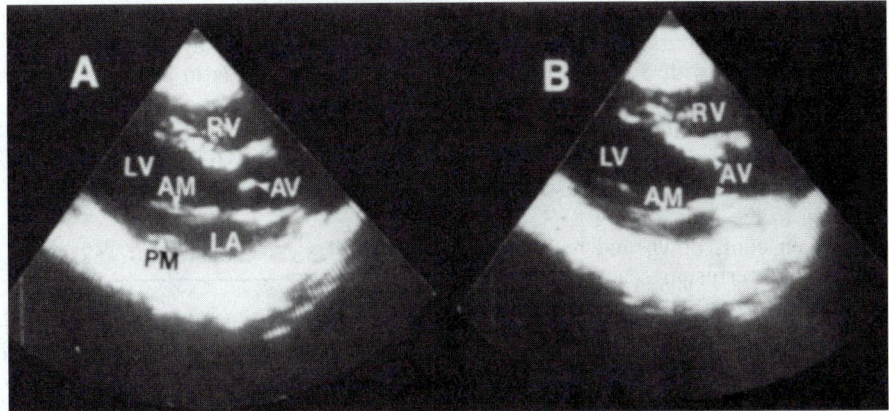

Figure 44–10. Long-axis cross-sectional echocardiographic images of the left ventricle (*LV*), right ventricle (*RV*), mitral valve, aortic valve, and left atrium (*LA*) during diastole (*A*) and systole (*B*). During diastole, the anterior (*AM*) and posterior (*PM*) mitral leaflets are apart and the aortic valve leaflets (*AV*) come together as a single echo in the midportion of the aorta (*A*). With systole (*B*) the mitral leaflets come together and the aortic valve leaflets separate. (From Braunwald, E. [1992]. *Heart disease*, [4th ed., p. 67]. Philadelphia, W. B. Saunders.)

The procedure lasts approximately 15 minutes to 1 hour. No food or liquids should be taken for 8 to 10 hours before the procedure. The client is not to eat or drink anything following the procedure for at least 2 hours or until the effects of the anesthetic wear off.

Explain the procedure to the client. Assure the client that he or she will feel only mild discomfort from the passage of the scope into the throat. See that the client signs a consent form. Instruct the client to refrain from eating or drinking the day of the procedure.

During the procedure, do the following:

- Administer sedation and topical anesthetic as ordered.
- If the client has a nasogastric tube in place, remove this before the esophageal scope is inserted.
- Monitor the client's vital signs and respiratory status throughout the procedure.

After the procedure, keep the client NPO (fasting) until the gag reflex is fully restored. Instruct the client that there may be mild throat discomfort for a day or two, but to report significant discomfort or any hemoptysis to his or her physician immediately.

Phonocardiography

Phonograms are recordings of audible vibrations coming from the heart and great vessels. Phonograms are used to assist in diagnosing the timing of cardiac sounds and murmurs. Microphones are placed under elastic straps, usually at the base and apex of the heart. No preparation is required for this assessment.

Myocardial Scintigraphy

Myocardial function, motion, and perfusion may be studied by a method called scintigraphy, which involves the IV injection of a radioactive isotope. As the isotope is absorbed by the blood cells of the heart muscle, photons are emitted. These photons are detected by an external gamma camera, which produces a radionuclide image. Because these nuclear imaging techniques are relatively noninvasive, they are frequently used diagnostic tools.

Thallium 201 Scintigraphy

Thallium 201 is the most widely used isotope for myocardial perfusion because of its short (73 hours) half-life and low total body radiation dose. Thallium 201 is a radioactive analog of potassium, which is easily extracted by smooth skeletal and cardiac muscle fibers that possess the potassium active transport system. Eighty-eight percent of bloodborne ^{201}Tl is taken up on its first pass through the heart. The amount of ^{201}Tl found in the myocardium after an IV injection depends on the regional myocardial perfusion and the efficiency of cellular extraction. Regional perfusion is dependent on coronary artery patency. Areas of the myocardium that receive less blood flow also receive less thallium.

A high concentration of ^{201}Tl is present in well-perfused cells, and a lower concentration remains in the blood, setting up a concentration gradient for the diffusion of ^{201}Tl. Infarcted or scarred myocardium does not extract any ^{201}Tl, showing up as "cold spots." If the defective area is ischemic, the cold spots fill in or become "warm" on the delayed images. Infarcts continue to appear cold with little or no perfusion of ^{201}Tl either during a stress test or with delayed images.

The perfusion scanning is performed with a special camera that is capable of showing the source of emitted low-energy photons on a screen. Each photon detected by the camera is recorded on film and a computer screen over a half-hour period. The computer refines and enhances the images and then provides quantitative information about the myocardial walls.

Thallium 201 imaging can be performed before or after an exercise ECG study or as a resting study only. Ischemic myocardium may show up on a resting ^{201}Tl study. Two sets of images are taken 3 hours apart and compared. The ^{201}Tl stress test begins with a graded exercise protocol on a treadmill. The client has a slow infusion of IV normal saline. The ECG is monitored continuously. About 1 minute before the peak of the stress test, ^{201}Tl is injected IV. The client should exercise for the last minute to ensure ^{201}Tl distribution to the heart during 85% maximum stress. The client then cools down and reclines on an examination table for the perfusion scan. Continuous imaging in a 180-degree arc over the chest is obtained. The client then waits for 3 hours and returns for repeat films. Before the delayed images are obtained, the client receives additional ^{201}Tl by IV injection. The two sets of images are then carefully compared.

Dipyridamole Thallium 201 Test

This test may be used as an alternative to standard treadmill exercise when the client is not able to achieve a vigorous level of exercise. Dipyridamole (Persantine) serves as a pharmacologic stress agent. It is given IV to dilate the coronary arteries, which would normally dilate during the stress of exercise. Arteries that are narrowed as a result of coronary artery disease do not expand as much as normal arteries. Infusion of dipyradimole for 5 minutes is followed by injection of ^{201}Tl. Thallium 201 travels easily through normal arteries that have dilated and travels less freely through narrowed arteries. At 7 minutes, images are taken.

Any form of caffeine as well as medications for asthma, such as theophylline or aminophylline, should be omitted prior to this test. Aminophylline is the antagonist to dipyradimole and may be given slowly IV to reverse any adverse side effects.

Technetium 99m Ventriculography (Multiple Gated Acquisition Scanning)

This test studies the motion of the left ventricular wall and measures the ventricle's ability to eject blood (ejection fraction). If a coronary artery is narrowed, causing ischemia, the segment of the myocardium it serves exhibits diminished wall motion or contractility. In addition, hemodynamic changes may be measured by observing the actual filling and emptying of the cardiac chambers. Changes in cardiac output as well as ejection fraction may be obtained. Multiple gated acquisition (MUGA) scans represent the blood pool within the ventricular and atrial chambers.

Stannous pyrophosphate (PYP) is given IV to allow the red blood cells to tag onto the ^{99m}Tc. Approximately 20 minutes after the PYP is injected, the ^{99m}Tc is injected. The client is then placed on a heart monitor and images are begun.

MUGA scans use counts from any one of a number of consecutive beats. Multiple serial images are obtained using a gamma camera. The cardiac cycle is broken into intervals, with counts taken during these intervals for a number of beats. These counts are stored and then displayed in a weighted average picture.

If a stress study is to be performed, the client is put on a bicycle ergometer with a gamma camera positioned to project the right and left blood pools. The ECG is monitored continuously. Images are obtained at rest and during each stage of exercise.

First-Pass Cardiac Study

During a first-pass study, a single IV injection of ^{99m}Tc is administered and traced as it passes through the heart. Only the initial pass of the ^{99m}Tc is recorded as it passes through the cardiac chambers. Ejection fraction and information about ventricular wall motion are obtained. A first-pass study may be performed during exercise or rest.

Before the procedure, ask female clients if they are pregnant or suspect pregnancy, because these studies involve radiation exposure (although minimal).

Explain the purpose of the procedure to the client and tell him or her what to expect during the procedure. Explain that electrodes will be placed on the chest and an IV line will be inserted for the administration of the radioisotope. Generally, total exposure to radiation during these scans is less than or equal to that of one chest x-ray study.

Instruct the client to wear walking shoes if exercise on the treadmill or bicycle is anticipated.

Follow the diet protocol of the institution. Some tests may require fasting. A light meal is preferred over a heavy meal if the scan will be taken during exercise. This prevents nausea and stomach cramping during exercise and allows for better uptake of the radioisotope. Instruct the client to avoid alcohol and smoking on the day of the procedure.

Check the physician's orders for omission of any medications. Usually beta-blockers, calcium channel blockers, and xanthines are prohibited prior to the procedure.

Ensure that the client signs a consent form.

During the procedure, ask the client to notify the nurse or technologist of any chest pain (ischemia).

After the procedure, again ask the client to report any chest pain to the nurse or technologist. If the client must return for follow-up scanning, instruct the client to rest between studies.

Cardiac Catheterization

This complex procedure involves the insertion of a catheter into the heart and surrounding vessels to obtain detailed information about the structure and performance of the heart, the valves, and the circulatory system. Specifically, cardiac catheterization is performed to:

● Confirm a diagnosis of heart disease and determine the extent to which the disease has affected the structure and function of the heart.
● Determine congenital abnormalities.
● Obtain a clear picture of cardiac anatomy prior to heart surgery.
● Obtain pressures within the heart chambers and the great vessels (aorta and pulmonary artery [PA]).

- Measure blood oxygen concentration, tension, and saturation within the heart chambers.
- Determine cardiac output.
- Perform angiography for better coronary artery visualization.
- Obtain endocardial biopsies.
- Allow infusion of fibrinolytic agents directly into an occluded coronary artery in an attempt to restore coronary blood flow.

Cardiac catheterization is usually performed in the controlled environment of a cardiac catheterization laboratory. Typically, only one side of the heart is catheterized, although it is sometimes necessary to insert the catheter into both sides of the heart.

Right-Sided Catheterization

For right-sided cardiac catheterization, the physician inserts a sterile, radiopaque catheter through the antecubital or femoral vein. Under fluoroscopic guidance, the catheter is advanced slowly to the right atrium and right ventricle and is finally wedged in a small branch of the PA. Clinicians continuously monitor the ECG during the procedure. Premature ventricular contractions may occur as the catheter is being passed through the ventricles. If they occur frequently, cardiac output falls and the physician may need to withdraw the catheter temporarily or order administration of lidocaine (an antiarrhythmic).

Left-Sided Catheterization

This procedure is far more difficult to perform than right-sided catheterization. There are two major methods of catheter introduction: (1) The catheter can be passed retrograde (backward) from the brachial or femoral artery into the aorta and then to the left ventricle, or (2) rarely during right-sided catheterization, the middle or lower third of the atrial septum is punctured and the catheter is passed transseptally into the left atrium.

As the catheter is passed through the venous or arterial system and into various heart chambers, the desired studies are performed. The catheter has several end or side holes that allow blood withdrawal for oxygen analysis from the various cardiac chambers. Pressures can be obtained by attaching the catheter to a transducer with its connecting amplifier and recording device. Radiopaque contrast materials and indicator solutions can be injected via the catheter into the left ventricle to examine the mitral valve, the left ventricular outflow tract, wall motion and thickness, left ventricular end-diastolic volume, and ejection fraction.[7]

Complications

Although cardiac catheterization has become a safer and more useful diagnostic tool in recent years, it is far from innocuous and has inherent complications. Most complications are related to the puncture site. Clot formation during catheterization may be prevented by administering moderate amounts of anticoagulant (usually 4000–5000

units of heparin), which increases the risk of bleeding at the insertion site or into the retroperitoneal area. In addition, trauma from arterial cannulation may potentiate vasospasm or clot formation, causing temporary or permanent arterial occlusion of the affected extremity. Dysrhythmias frequently develop during catheterization because of direct catheter stimulation of the atrium and ventricle. In addition, the client may experience anginal pain. Pain occurs when contrast dye replaces the blood flowing through the coronary arteries under study. Lack of blood flow causes a painful regional cardiac hypoxia. Occasionally, clients have an allergic reaction to the iodine-based contrast medium. Allergic symptoms include flushing, nausea and vomiting, tingling and numbness, weakness, and urticaria. Fortunately, anaphylactic shock is rare. Osmotic diuresis following injection of hypertonic radiographic contrast agents can produce significant dehydration. Finally, myocardial and aortic perforations are rare but potentially deadly complications of cardiac catheterization.

Prior to cardiac catheterization, prepare the client both physically and emotionally. Cardiac catheterization is an important and frightening procedure. Major steps in preparing the client are as follows:

1. Explain the procedure, its purpose, and its hazards.
2. Explain that the procedure will be carried out in a special cardiac catheterization room and that the client will be lying on an x-ray examination table with ECG leads attached to the extremities. The physician and cardiac nurses will be wearing scrub gowns and masks and the room will be darkened at some point to take x-ray films.
3. Tell the client that there is little or no pain associated with the procedure, because a local anesthetic is used to numb the catheter insertion site. However, the client may feel fatigue and various aches, because it will be necessary to lie quietly for up to 2 hours on a hard table. The client may also, at times, experience certain sensations: a fluttery feeling as the catheter passes through the heart; a flushed, warm feeling when the dye is injected; a strong desire to cough (with right heart angiography); and palpitations caused by transient heart irritability. The client should also be forewarned about the sound made by the x-ray apparatus during the procedure.
4. Have the client sign an informed consent for the procedure after his or her questions have been answered satisfactorily.
5. Ask if there is any history of allergies, particularly to iodine-containing substances or shellfish. The physician may order a skin test with an iodine-containing solution the day before the procedure.
6. Withhold solid food for 6 to 8 hours and liquids for at least 4 hours prior to the procedure to prevent vomiting and aspiration.
7. Be sure that the client's height and weight are recorded in the chart. This is needed for calculating the amount of dye that will be administered.
8. Mark the peripheral pulses distal to the probable cannulation sites with a felt-tipped pen and record the quality of the pulses in the chart. This will aid in

locating the pulses after the procedure. Pulses are checked at this time for postprocedure comparisons and to detect possible occlusion of the vessel that will be undergoing cannulation.

9. Administer the prescribed medications (often a sedative and sometimes an antibiotic). The insertion site may be prepared by shaving and cleaning it with an antiseptic solution.

10. Insert an IV line.

During the procedure, perform the following:

- Monitor vital signs.
- Monitor for ventricular dysrhythmias, which are especially prevalent when the catheter is passed through the ventricle.
- Watch for signs of an allergic reaction to the contrast dye.
- Instruct the client to inform the physician, nurse, or technologist of any chest pain.
- Have emergency equipment readily available during the procedure.

Following cardiac catheterization, assessment, prevention, and early detection of complications are the primary goals. Postcatheterization care varies, depending on the institution, but the following are basic:

1. Assess vital signs every 30 minutes for 2 hours initially and then less frequently, as specified by institution policy.

2. Keep the extremity in which the catheter was inserted straight for 4 to 6 hours after the procedure. If the antecubital vessel was used, immobilize the arm on an arm board. If the femoral artery was used, enforce strict bedrest for 6 to 12 hours following the procedure. The client may turn from side to side. To keep the leg straight at the groin and prevent arterial occlusion, do not elevate the head of the bed more than 15 degrees.

3. Check the pressure dressing over the puncture site for intactness and for evidence of bleeding. Occasionally a sandbag is applied to the insertion site for 4 to 6 hours. Monitor the site for hematoma formation and ask the client about the presence of increasing pain or tenderness.

4. Check the pulses, color, warmth, and sensation of the extremity distal to the insertion site every 30 minutes during the first hour and then as specified by healthcare facility policy. Notify the physician at once if the client experiences numbness or tingling. Also note if the extremity becomes cool, pale, or cyanotic or if sudden loss of peripheral pulses occurs. These manifestations represent serious impairment of circulation.

5. Monitor cardiac rhythm for the occurrence of dysrhythmias. Also assess the client for chest pain. If either is found, notify the physician and intervene per ordered protocols.

6. Encourage fluid intake (if the underlying condition allows) for adequate fluid replacement and renal elimination of the contrast.

7. Observe for nausea, vomiting, rash, and other signs of hypersensitivity to the contrast.

8. Because the procedure is lengthy as well as a psychological drain on the client, institute supportive measures to promote comfort. Whatever the findings of the procedure, the client needs clear explanations of the significance and consequences of these findings.

9. Sometimes cardiac catheterization is an emergency procedure and not elective. In such instances, the client gets caught in a whirlwind of activity that ends not on completion of the catheterization but on completion of either balloon angioplasty or cardiac surgery. Provide emotional support to the client and significant others.

Angiography

Angiography is an invaluable tool in cardiac diagnosis and offers great assistance in understanding heart and vascular disease. The physician injects contrast agents IV at the location under study. These contrast materials, which are usually iodinated water-soluble compounds, are given in doses determined by the client's weight.

Angiocardiography is the IV injection of contrast into the heart during cardiac catheterization. Immediately after the contrast is injected, a series of x-ray films are taken that reveal the course of the contrast as it circulates through the heart, lungs, and great vessels.

Cineangiography involves taking moving pictures during cardiac catheterization. This is particularly valuable because the examiner can view the film at both rapid and slow speeds, permitting detailed and unlimited review of the study.

Coronary angiography refers to the injection of contrast directly into the coronary arteries (via the coronary ostia) during cardiac catheterization. Table 44–4 outlines the various forms of angiocardiography.

Table 44–4. Major Types of Angiocardiography	
Angiocardiography Procedure	**Method Employed**
Right-sided angiocardiography	Contrast medium is injected into the right heart chambers and pulmonary artery by means of a catheter threaded up a vein and into the heart during cardiac catheterization
Left-sided angiocardiography	Contrast medium is injected into the left side of the heart through a transvenous catheter passed through the atrial septum during cardiac catheterization or via a catheter passed retrograde through an artery into the left heart
Selective coronary artery angiocardiography	Contrast medium is injected directly into the ostium of each coronary artery via a catheter that is placed retrograde through an artery into the aorta

Hemodynamic Studies

Four important parameters are used to assess hemodynamic status: CVP, PA pressure, cardiac output, and intra-arterial pressure. Each of these parameters requires an invasive procedure. Critical care nurses perform all of these routinely at the bedside. Hemodynamic studies provide a wealth of information reflecting the earliest changes in the circulatory system that are not yet clinically detectable.

The monitoring of hemodynamic pressures provides information about blood volume, fluid balance, and how well the heart is pumping. Current technology allows us to measure right atrial pressure (CVP), PA pressures during systole and diastole (reflecting right and left ventricular pressures), and pulmonary capillary wedge pressure (PCWP) (an indirect indicator of left ventricular pressure).

The Pulmonary Artery Catheter. Development of the balloon-tipped, flow-directed catheter has enabled continuous direct monitoring of PA pressure (see the Bridge to Critical Care).

This catheter has four lumina. The proximal lumen terminates in the right atrium, allowing CVP measurement, fluid infusion, and venous access for blood samples. The distal lumen terminates in the PA and measures PA systolic pressure, PA diastolic pressure, PA mean pressure, and PCWP. There is a small lumen that is used for inflation and deflation of the balloon. The fourth lumen is the thermistor port and permits measurement of cardiac output. In addition, some catheters have an additional port for infusion of fluids and capabilities for cardiac pacing and measuring of oxygen saturation of the blood. Five-lumen catheters also exist.

Inserting the Catheter. Insertion of a PA catheter is not risk free for the client. The potential complications of the catheter are PA infarction, pulmonary embolism, injury to the heart valves, and injury to the myocardium. In addition, while the catheter is in place, the heart valves have less ability to close completely.

PA monitoring must be carried out in a critical care unit under careful scrutiny of an experienced nursing staff. Prior to insertion of the catheter, explain to the client that (1) the procedure may be uncomfortable but not painful, and (2) a local anesthetic will be given at the catheter insertion site. Your support of the critically ill client at this time helps promote cooperation and lessens anxiety.

Using sterile technique, the physician inserts the PA flow-directed catheter at the bedside via percutaneous puncture of the brachial, subclavian, jugular, or femoral vein. The catheter is connected to a transducer and a fluid-filled pressure monitoring system. Pressure levels and fluctuations are monitored both graphically and by numerical display.

The inflated balloon follows the direction of blood flow through the right ventricle into the PA, where it finally wedges in the right or left branch of the PA. Clinicians can follow the path of the balloon by observing wave forms and pressure readings on the monitor (see Bridge to Critical Care).

When wedged, the catheter is "pointing" indirectly at the left end-diastolic pressure. PCWP therefore is the most accurate, though indirect, indicator of left ventricular end-diastolic pressure or left ventricular preload available at the bedside. The normal PCWP is 8 to 13 mm Hg. Elevations in PCWP (greater than 18–20 mm Hg) therefore indicate increased left ventricular pressure, as seen in left ventricular failure, and they may coincide with the onset of pulmonary congestion. Pressures climbing to more than 30 mm Hg generally herald the onset of pulmonary edema. Conversely, low PCWP suggests insufficient volume and pressure in the left ventricle, as seen in hypovolemic shock. Pressure changes commonly related to various cardiac conditions are discussed in the Bridge to Critical Care.

Central Venous Pressure

Central venous pressure is the pressure within the superior vena cava, reflecting the pressure under which the blood is returned to the superior vena cava and right atrium. CVP is determined by vascular tone, blood volume, and the ability of the right heart to receive and pump blood. When the tricuspid valve is open at the end of diastole, the atrium and ventricle are, in effect, one chamber. At this time, the CVP is equal to the pressure in the right ventricle and is a good indicator of right ventricular function (Table 44–5).

CVP can also be seen as a measurement of preload on the right side of the heart. Preload is the amount of blood presented to the heart, or when the ventricle is full prior to the next ejection. Preload is the right ventricular end-diastolic pressure. (Preload is also discussed in Chapter 45.)

CVP can be measured with a central venous line placed in the superior vena cava or a balloon flotation catheter in the PA. Normal CVP pressure is 2 to 12 mm Hg. A drop in CVP pressure indicates a decrease in circulating volume, which may result from fluid imbalance, hemorrhage, or severe vasolidation and pooling of blood in the extremities with limited venous return. A rise in CVP indicates an increase in blood volume due to a sudden shift in fluid balance, excessive IV fluid infusion, renal failure, or sodium and water retention.

For an accurate CVP measurement, a baseline must be established for the transducer position. The zero point on the transducer needs to be at the level of the right atrium. The right atrium is located at the midaxillary line at the fourth intercostal space. The client should be supine with the head of the bed up to 45 degrees for the most accurate reading.

In measuring CVP, make certain that the client is relaxed at the time of the measurement. Straining, coughing, or any other activity that increases intrathoracic pressure causes falsely high measurements. If the CVP is measured while the client is on a ventilator, the readings should always be taken at the point of end expiration for greatest accuracy.

BRIDGE TO CRITICAL CARE

Swan-Ganz Monitoring

Positioning the Swan-Ganz Catheter

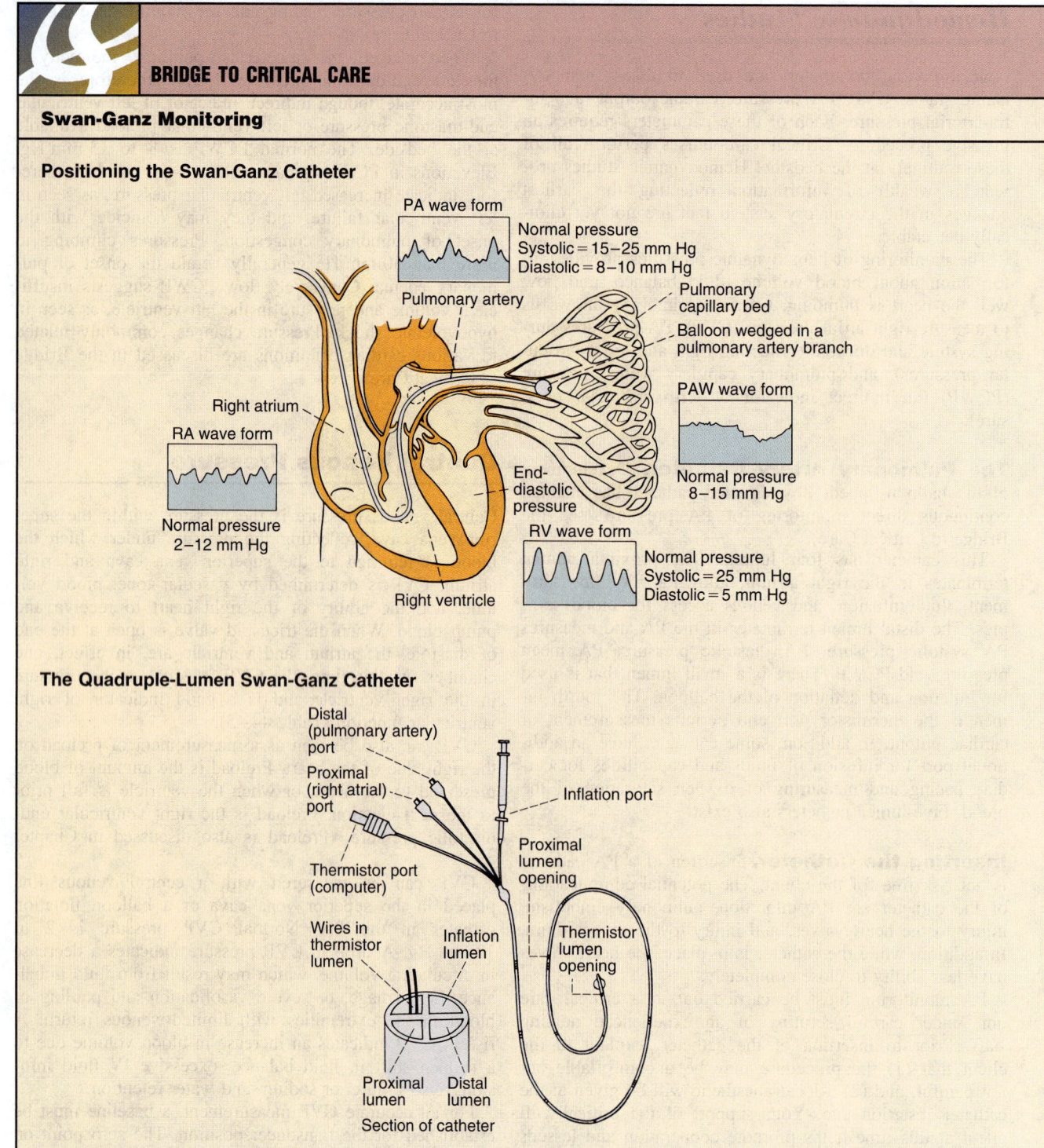

PA wave form

Normal pressure
Systolic = 15–25 mm Hg
Diastolic = 8–10 mm Hg

Pulmonary artery

Pulmonary capillary bed

Balloon wedged in a pulmonary artery branch

Right atrium

RA wave form

Normal pressure
2–12 mm Hg

PAW wave form

Normal pressure
8–15 mm Hg

End-diastolic pressure

RV wave form

Normal pressure
Systolic = 25 mm Hg
Diastolic = 5 mm Hg

Right ventricle

The Quadruple-Lumen Swan-Ganz Catheter

Distal (pulmonary artery) port

Proximal (right atrial) port

Inflation port

Thermistor port (computer)

Proximal lumen opening

Wires in thermistor lumen

Inflation lumen

Thermistor lumen opening

Proximal lumen

Distal lumen

Section of catheter

The connections between the catheter and the attachments must be checked frequently to make certain that they are secure (in order to prevent air embolism). The dressing at the insertion site is changed according to healthcare facility policy to prevent infection. Complications of the procedure include pneumothorax, phlebitis, air emboli, pulmonary emboli, fluid overload, dysrhythmia, sepsis, and microelectric shock.

In order to maintain patency of the system, a small amount of fluid is delivered under pressure at a constant rate of flow. This fluid may or may not be heparinized.

Pulmonary Artery Pressure

The CVP is not a satisfactory means of determining the status of left-sided heart function, especially in critically ill persons, for example, those who are immediately re-

Measuring Cardiac Output by Thermodilution

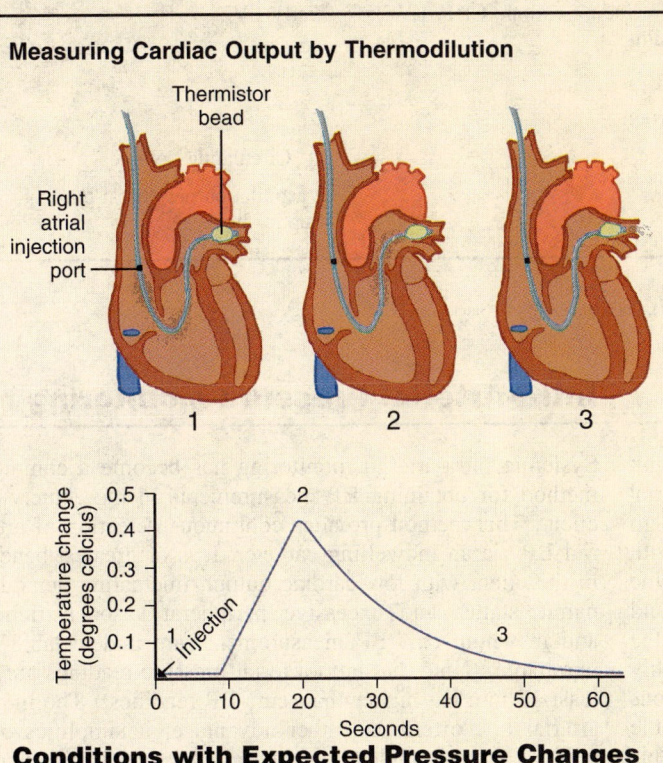

Conditions with Expected Pressure Changes

Condition	Pressure Changes			
	RAP	*RVP*	*PAP*	*PAWP*
Heart failure (volume overload)	↑	↑	↑	↑
Hypovolemia	↓	↓	↓	↓
Cardiogenic shock*	—or ↑	—or ↑	—or ↑	—or ↑ (diastolic)
Pulmonary hypertension	↑	↑	↑	—or ↑
Cardiac tamponade	↑	↑	↑	↑ (diastolic)
Pulmonary emboli	↑	↑	↑	↑ (systolic)
Mitral valve stenosis/insufficiency†	↑	↑	↑	↑

PAP, pulmonary artery pressure; PAWP, pulmonary artery wedge pressure; RAP, right atrial pressure; RVP, right ventricular pressure.
* Pressure readings depend on the heart's ability to handle circulating volume. Chronic lung disease elevates all readings.
† Mitral valve disease produces unreliable pressure readings.

covering from cardiac surgery, have experienced myocardial infarction, have cardiomyopathy, or are in cardiogenic shock. Significant changes can occur in the left side of the heart without being reflected for some time in the right side of the heart. This can lead to a delay in intervention or even inappropriate intervention.

During diastole, blood flows freely from the PA through the pulmonary capillaries, left atrium, and open mitral valve to the left ventricle. Therefore, the pressure in the left ventricle at the end of diastole approximates the diastolic pressure in the PA, pulmonary capillaries, and left atrium.

Starling's principle tells us that the heart muscle contracts most effectively when under slight stretch. PA pressure measurements can assist in determining whether the ventricle is understretched and the client needs fluids, overstretched and the client needs diuretics, or appropriately stretched and at maximal function.

Table 44–5. Indications for Central Venous Pressure (CVP) and How They May Affect the Readings		
To Assess	**↑ CVP (>11 cm H$_2$O)**	**↓ CVP (<3 cm H$_2$O)**
Right-sided heart hemodynamics	Right heart failure (including chronic CHF, LVF) Constrictive pericarditis Cardiac tamponade Valvular stenosis Pulmonary hypertension	Early LVF
Blood volume	↑ Circulating volume	↓ Circulating volume
Vascular tone	Vasoconstriction Hypertension	Vasodilation/peripheral pooling Septic shock

CHF, congestive heart failure; LVF, left ventricular failure.
From Huange, S. H., et al. (1989). *Coronary care nursing* (2nd ed., p. 101). Philadelphia: W. B. Saunders.

Cardiac Output Measurement

As detailed in Chapter 43, cardiac output is the amount of blood pumped out of the left ventricle into the arterial system every minute: that is, cardiac output is equal to the stroke volume (volume of blood pumped out with each beat) multiplied by the heart rate. Therefore, if the stroke volume of the left ventricle is between 50 and 90 ml (average, 70 ml), and the heart rate is 80 BPM, the normal cardiac output of the left ventricle is roughly between 4 and 8 L/min. Table 44–6 lists the conditions that change cardiac output. The cardiac output of the right ventricle is considered equal to that of the left. This is because the right ventricle, although not as muscular as the left ventricle, pumps against less resistance.

Table 44–6. Conditions that Cause a Change in Cardiac Output

Conditions That Decrease Cardiac Output	Conditions That Increase Cardiac Output
Acute congestive heart failure	Hypoxia
Pericarditis with effusion	Hyperthyroidism
Old age	Excitement
Arterial hemorrhage	Exercise
Standing motionless, which decreases venous return to the heart	Food intake
Myxedema	Oral and intravenous fluid intake
Shock	Early stage of septic shock
Valvular heart disease	Pregnancy
Myocardial ischemia	
Dysrhythmias	
Paroxysmal atrial tachycardia (PAT)	
Atrial fibrillation	
Heart block	
Ventricular tachycardia	
Heat stroke	

Intra-Arterial Pressure Monitoring

Systemic intra-arterial monitoring has become a common method for obtaining BP measurements in the acutely ill client. This method provides continuous detection of arterial BP via an indwelling catheter. It is of greatest benefit in the client with low cardiac output, fluctuating hemodynamic status, and excessive peripheral vasoconstriction and in whom cuff BP measurements are undetectable or unreliable. (Note that intra-arterial pressure readings are at least 10 mm Hg higher than cuff BP readings.) The intra-arterial line offers one other advantage: it simplifies obtaining blood samples for arterial blood gas and blood studies, minimizing the need for arterial or venous punctures.

The physician introduces a short, nonreactive Teflon catheter into an artery (radial, brachial, axillary, femoral, or even the dorsalis pedis) using sterile technique.

Prior to catheter insertion, the examiner must assess the adequacy of circulation in the chosen extremity. If the radial artery is chosen as the site for insertion, the physician evaluates blood flow to the hand by performing Allen's test. The examiner first instructs the client to hold out the hand, then checks for obstruction of the ulnar artery by placing one thumb lightly over the radial artery and one thumb over the ulnar artery. The client is then instructed to make a tight fist for 1 minute. After 1 minute, the client is directed to open the hand and extend the fingers. The examiner releases the pressure over the ulnar artery. If the fingers become pink rapidly (within 6 seconds), adequate ulnar circulation exists. If pallor of the hand persists, the examiner should suspect ulnar artery obstruction, and thus not perform cannulation of the radial artery. Radial artery patency may be checked by the same method, but by releasing pressure over the radial, rather than the ulnar, artery.

The major complications of intra-arterial monitoring include hemorrhage caused by loose connections of the monitoring system, hematoma at the insertion site, infection (local or systemic), and embolization of the artery that supplies the distal portion of the cannulated extremity.

Besides accurate monitoring and recording of arterial

pressure, nursing responsibilities focus on preventing complications of arterial cannulation. Do the following:

● Check all connections frequently to ensure that they remain tight and secure. Accidental blood loss from a disconnected catheter can be as much as 200 ml in 4 to 5 minutes.
● Evaluate the cannulated extremity for neurovascular function every 2 hours. Assess color, temperature, capillary filling, and sensation distal to the site of cannulation.
● Check the insertion site for redness or signs of infection daily and change dressing per institutional policy.

Conclusions

Cardiovascular assessment can range from taking BP to the insertion of hemodynamic monitors. Even though the use of invasive diagnostic tests is increasing, the nurse needs to be able to accurately assess heart sounds, BP, and client history. These data are just as important as the invasive studies, and frequently it is the nurse who identifies early signs of heart disease in the client through routine screening.

Bibliography

1. Adler, L., Brundage, B., & Shapiro, B. (1991). Tomorrow's cardiac imaging—today. *Patient Care, 25*(11), 143–161.
2. Ahrens, T. & Taylor, L. (1992). *Hemodynamic waveform analysis.* Philadelphia: W. B. Saunders.
3. American Heart Association (1991). *Heart and stroke facts.* Dallas: Author.
4. American Heart Association (1994). *Textbook of basic life support for health care providers.* Author.
5. Bates, B. (1995). *A guide to physical examination and history taking* (6th ed.). Philadelphia: J. B. Lippincott.
6. Bentley, L. (1987). Radionuclide imaging techniques in the diagnosis and treatment of coronary heart disease. *Focus on Critical Care, 14*(6), 27–31.
7. Braunwald, E., et al. (Ed.) (1990). *Harrison's principles of internal medicine* (12th ed.). New York. McGraw-Hill.
8. Canobbio, M. (1990). *Cardiovascular disorders.* St. Louis: Mosby–Year Book.
9. Castelli, W. P. (1992). Using cardiac leads the right way. *Nursing 92, 22,* 50–54.
10. Dennison, R. (1990). Understanding the four determinants of cardiac output. *Nursing 90, 20*(7), 35–42.
11. Drew, B., & Tisdale, L. (1993). ST segment monitoring for coronary artery reocclusion following thrombolytic therapy and coronary angioplasty: Identification of optimal bedside monitoring leads. *American Journal of Critical Care, 2*(4), 280–283.
12. Ehman, R. L., & Julsrud, P. R. (1989). Magnetic resonance imaging of the heart: Current status. *Mayo Clinic Proceedings, 64*(9), 1134–1146.
13. Fahey, V. (1995). *Vascular nursing* (2nd ed.). Philadelphia: W. B. Saunders.
14. Friedman, M., & Rosannea, R. H. (1959). Association of a specific overt behavior pattern with blood and cardiovascular findings: Blood, cholesterol levels, blood clotting times, incidence of arcus senilis and clinical coronary heart disease. *JAMA, 169,* 1286–1296.
15. Goodman, M., et al. (1996). Hostility predicts restenosis after percutaneous transluminal angioplasty. *Mayo Clinic Proceedings, 71*(8), 729–734.
16. Huang, S., (1989). *Coronary care nursing* (2nd ed.). Philadelphia: W. B. Saunders.
17. Izor-Povenmire, K., & House, M. A. (1989). Acute crack cocaine intoxication: A case study. *Focus on Critical Care, 16*(2), 112–119.
18. Loveys, B., & Woods, S. (1986). Current recommendations for thermodilution cardiac output measurements. *Progress in Cardiovascular Nursing, 1*(4), 242–247.
19. National Heart, Lung, and Blood Institute (1990). *Morbidity and mortality chartbook on cardiovascular, lung, and blood diseases 1990.* Bethesda, MD. Author.
20. Nelson, S. (1989). Clinical utility of signal averaged electrocardiography. *Practical Cardiology, 15*(3), 59–72.
21. Purcell, J. (1990). Advances in treatment of dilated cardiomyopathy. *AACN Clinical Issues in Critical Care Nursing, 1*(1), 31–45.
22. Ragland, D. R., & Brand, R. J. (1988). Type A behavior and mortality from coronary heart disease. *New England Journal of Medicine, 318,* 65–69.
23. Rubes, S. M., et al. (1990). High blood cholesterol in elderly men and the excess risk for coronary heart disease. *Annals of Internal Medicine, 113,* 916–920.
24. Schelbert, H. (1989). Myocardial ischemia and clinical applications of positron emission tomography. *American Journal of Cardiology, 64,* 46–52.
25. Thelan, L. A., et al. (1990). *Critical care nursing.* St. Louis: Mosby–Year Book.
26. Toto, K. H., & Yucha, C. B. (1994). Magnesium: Homeostasis, imbalances, and therapeutic uses. *Critical Care Nursing Clinics of North America, 6*(4), 767–783.
27. Wolf, G. (1989). Magnetic resonance imaging and the future of cardiac imaging. *American Journal of Cardiology, 64,* 60–63.
28. Yucha, C. B., & Toto, K. H. (1994). Calcium and phosphorous derangements. *Critical Care Nursing Clinics of North America, 6*(4), 747–766.

45

Nursing Care of Clients with Disorders of Cardiac Function

Peggy Gerard

Kathleen A. Ringel

The heart muscle must have an adequate blood supply to contract properly. The coronary arteries carry oxygen and blood to the myocardium. When a coronary artery is narrowed or blocked, the area of the heart muscle supplied by that artery becomes ischemic and injured, and infarction may result. The major disorders due to insufficient blood supply to the myocardium are angina pectoris, myocardial infarction (MI), and congestive heart failure (CHF). Recent work by the Agency for Health Care Policy and Research (AHCPR) refers to congestive heart failure as heart failure because not all forms are congestive. We also use the term *congestive failure*.[27] These disorders are collectively known as coronary artery disease (CAD), also called coronary heart disease or ischemic heart disease.

Coronary Artery Disease

CAD is the leading cause of death in the United States. Nearly 1 million Americans died in 1993 from cardiovascular diseases.[4, 7] As high as these figures may seem, mortality from cardiovascular disease, including coronary heart disease and stroke, has declined by more than 50% over the past 30 years.[59] Contributing to this decline in mortality are factors such as improved technologies and therapies for treatment of cardiovascular disease, use of thrombolytic drugs in acute MI, interventional therapies and improved surgical techniques, and modification of risk factors in populations at risk.

Etiology and Risk Factors

Although CAD claims more lives each year than does any other disease, its causes are poorly understood. CAD results from the development of obliterative atherosclerotic lesions within the coronary arteries that narrow

This chapter incorporates material written for the fourth edition by Juanita Reigle.

or obstruct these vessels. Atherosclerosis, a disorder of lipid metabolism, is characterized by (1) deposits of fat-containing substances within the intima of blood vessels and (2) smooth muscle cell proliferation. It underlies most causes of cardiovascular disease and death.

Although all the causes of CAD are not known, clinical evidence suggests that many factors contribute to the onset of atherosclerosis. The Risk Factors and Levels of Prevention feature lists these factors. Risk factors that precipitate CAD can be presented in three categories: (1) nonmodifiable risk factors, (2) modifiable risk factors, and (3) contributing factors (Box 45–1).

■ Nonmodifiable Risk Factors

Heredity. Genetic factors contribute to four traits that increase the incidence of atherosclerosis: hypertension, dyslipidemia, diabetes, and obesity. In the Framingham study, a longitudinal study of CAD, a family history of heart disease was found to be an independent predictor of CAD in men but not in women.[6, 7]

Age. Symptomatic CAD appears predominantly in people over 40 years old. However, persons in their 30s, and even in their 20s, sometimes suffer anginal attacks or MI.

Sex. Women of childbearing age display one-fourth the risk of developing CAD compared with men of the same age. This obvious difference in susceptibility diminishes after menopause; however, even after age 65 years, women continue to be less likely than men to develop CAD. Women who take oral contraceptives are more likely to develop CAD. This risk is particularly significant in women who smoke. Once oral contraceptives are discontinued, the increased risk of CAD does not continue. Women with an early menopause have three times the risk of CAD as women with a normal or late menopause.[17, 43, 55, 65, 100, 122, 143]

Two life-style changes during the past decade may

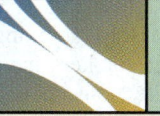

RISK FACTORS AND LEVELS OF PREVENTION

Coronary Artery Disease

Risk Factors

Women. *Modifiable:* Natural or surgical menopause without estrogen replacement; oral contraceptive use combined with cigarette smoking

Men. *Nonmodifiable:* Sex (more men develop coronary heart disease and develop it at an earlier age than women)

Both. *Modifiable:* Hypertension (systolic pressure > 140 mm Hg; diastolic pressure > 90 mm Hg), smoking, disorders of lipid metabolism (total cholesterol > 200 mg/dl, HDL < 35 mg/dl, LDL > 130 mg/dl, total cholesterol-to-HDL ratio > 7.5); physical inactivity)

Nonmodifiable: Increasing age, family history of coronary heart disease, race (black Americans have a greater risk most likely due to higher incidence of hypertension).

Contributing: Diabetes, obesity, individual response to stress

Levels of Prevention

Primary Prevention

- Provide health education on cardiovascular risk factor reduction. Address the need to avoid smoking, to eat a balanced diet low in saturated fats, and maintain a moderate level of physical activity.
- Teach stress reduction techniques such as progressive muscle relaxation and guided imagery.
- Participate in cardiovascular risk factor screening for children and adults.
- Instruct postmenopausal women to discuss the need for estrogen replacement therapy with their physician.
- Monitor BP control in clients with diagnosed hypertension.
- Monitor blood glucose levels of clients with diabetes mellitus.

Secondary Prevention

- Assess cardiovascular risk factors and provide individualized education on risk reduction.
- Teach clients the signs and symptoms of angina and myocardial infarction.
- Emphasize the need to seek prompt treatment if signs and symptoms of coronary artery disease occur.
- Provide information related to diagnostic tests and medical and surgical treatment of coronary artery disease (CAD).

Tertiary Prevention

- Emphasize the importance of adopting risk reduction behaviors to prevent the recurrence or progression of CAD through participation in cardiac rehabilitation.
- Teach clients about the importance of taking prescribed medications such as aspirin, beta-blockers, nitrates, and calcium channel blockers.
- Monitor therapeutic drug levels.
- Teach client about the side effects of, and adverse reactions to, cardiac medications.
- Emphasize the importance of follow-up appointments with healthcare practitioners.
- Instruct clients to seek prompt medical attention if symptoms of CAD return.

BP, blood pressure; HDL, high-density lipoprotein; LDL, low-density lipoprotein.

---

increase the incidence of CAD among women. More women (many with full responsibility for the household and children) have entered the work force. Also, more women have begun to smoke at an earlier age. The Diversity in Healthcare feature describes the "silent epidemic" of CAD in women.

Race. Although CAD is more prevalent in non-Hispanic whites, the death rate from CAD is highest in blacks. In 1992, the death rate for black males was 2.4% higher than that for white males, while the death rate for black females was 33% higher than that for white females.[5]

■ Modifiable Risk Factors

Environment, smoking, hypertension, elevated serum cholesterol levels, and physical inactivity constitute other major risk factors.[7, 55] The role that some of the modifiable risk factors have in precipitating heart disease is controversial. Cigarette smoking, hypertension, and hyperlipidemia have been objectively identified as predictive of CAD.[65, 71, 80, 92]

Environment. CAD is seven times more prevalent in North America, Australia, Europe, and New Zealand than

Box 45–1. Risk Factors for Coronary Artery Disease

Nonmodifiable Risk Factors

Heredity
Age
Male
Race

Modifiable Risk Factors

Environment
Cigarette smoking
Hypertension
Elevated serum cholesterol
Physical inactivity

Contributing Factors

Obesity
Diabetes
Stress response

Cigarette Smoking. One of the three major risk factors for CAD is cigarette smoking. How smoking causes CAD remains unknown. Male adult smokers have a 70% higher mortality rate than do male nonsmokers, and all smokers have more than twice the risk of heart attack of nonsmokers. Clients who smoke have two to four times the risk of sudden cardiac death.

The three substances thought to increase the prevalence of CAD are tar, nicotine, and carbon monoxide. Tar contains hydrocarbons and other carcinogenic substances. Nicotine increases the release of epinephrine and norepinephrine, which results in peripheral vasoconstriction, elevated blood pressure and heart rate, greater oxygen consumption, and increased likelihood of dysrhythmias. In addition, nicotine activates platelets and stimulates smooth muscle cell proliferation in the arterial walls. Carbon monoxide reduces the amount of blood available to the intima of the vessel wall and increases the permeability of the endothelium.[152] Clients who quit smoking lose their increased risk in 2 to 3 years.[7]

Hypertension. High blood pressure afflicts nearly 50 million American adults and children. Men over 45 years of age with blood pressure exceeding 140/90 mm Hg, and all adult women with pressures above 160/95 mm Hg, have a 50% greater mortality rate.[22] As blood pressure increases, the risk of a serious cardiovascular event also escalates. Although hypertension cannot always be pre-

in Japan, Switzerland, and Italy. Also, urban populations have a higher incidence of CAD than do rural populations. In developing countries, CAD is most prevalent in the affluent; in Great Britain and the United States, the reverse is true.[6]

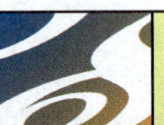

DIVERSITY IN HEALTHCARE

Coronary Artery Disease in Women

Although coronary artery disease (CAD) is the leading cause of death and disability in women over 40 years of age, the epidemic of CAD in women has been a silent one until recent years. Despite the fact that about 200,000 of the 500,000 heart attack deaths per year occur in women, until recently neither women nor their healthcare providers recognized the incidence and severity of CAD in women. Consequently, most of the research on heart disease and treatment was focused primarily on men and studies included few, if any, women. Our current knowledge of CAD in women comes from data pooled from previous studies, each having small numbers of women, and from studies that have reexamined spe-

cific issues related to women. Their data indicate that there are important sex-related differences in coronary anatomy, the relative importance of CAD risk factors, diagnostic tests, and treatment. In addition, recovery from coronary bypass graft (CABG) surgery differs for men and women.

In 1995, Artinian and Duggan[1] studied recovery patterns after CABG surgery in a sample of 132 men and 47 women. They collected data on physical, psychological, and social recovery at discharge, and at 1, 3, and 6 weeks following discharge. Although both men and women recovered well after surgery, there were some important sex-related differences in recovery in all three areas.

Women reported slower physical recovery, more physical clinical manifestations, and more difficulty walking than did men. Women also rated their health lower than did men. Although both men and women reported their mental health was very good overall, scores on a depression inventory indicated that more women had signs of mild depression. In the area of social recovery, women reported more difficulty with managing household chores than did men. However, social recovery improved for both men and women over time. These results indicate that women have special healthcare needs after CABG surgery that should be addressed in discharge teaching and follow-up care.

[1] Artinian, N. T., & Duggan, C. H. (1995). Sex differences in patient recovery patterns after coronary artery bypass surgery. *Heart and Lung, 24*(6), 483–494.

vented, it should be treated to lower the risk of CAD and premature death.[7, 22, 46]

Elevated Serum Cholesterol.

An elevated serum cholesterol level definitely increases the risk of developing CAD. A person with a serum cholesterol level greater than 259 mg/dl is three times more likely to develop CAD than a person with a serum level of 200 mg/dl.

Cholesterol, a sterol found in animal tissue, circulates in the blood in combination with triglycerides and protein-bound phospholipids. This complex is called a lipoprotein. There are four basic groups of lipoproteins, all produced in the intestinal wall. Elevation of lipoproteins is called hyperlipoproteinemia. Elevation of lipids, a component of lipoproteins, is called hyperlipidemia.

Lipoproteins and their functions are as follows:

- Chylomicrons primarily transport dietary triglycerides and cholesterol.
- Very-low-density lipoprotein (VLDL) mainly transports the triglycerides synthesized by the liver.
- Low-density lipoprotein (LDL) has the highest concentration of cholesterol and transports endogenous cholesterol to body cells.
- High-density lipoprotein (HDL) has the lowest concentration of cholesterol and transports endogenous cholesterol to body cells.

Recent investigations have documented how the presence of lipoproteins may predispose the body to the development of CAD. People with high levels of HDL in proportion to LDL are less likely to develop CAD than people with low HDL. High concentrations of HDL seem to protect against the development of CAD. Experts believe that the cholesterol in HDL does not become incorporated into the fatty plaques that develop in the lining of the artery wall, as does LDL. The ratio of total cholesterol to HDL or of LDL to HDL is the best test for predicting the risk of CAD. Exercise and low fat, low cholesterol diets increase the amount of HDL in the blood. Current recommendations for cholesterol and lipoproteins are total blood cholesterol less than 200 mg/dl; LDL less than 130 mg/dl; and HDL more than 35 mg/dl.[18, 152]

In the average American diet, approximately 45% of the total calories come from fat. This level is in excess of the so-called prudent diet recommended by the American Heart Association. Dietary fat comes in many forms and disguises. A high intake of cholesterol and saturated fats is associated with the development of coronary heart disease, whereas a proportional intake of polyunsaturated and monounsaturated fats is linked with lower risk. The so-called prudent diet should include no more than 30% of calories from fat, 55% from carbohydrate (at least half of these should be complex carbohydrates), and 15% from protein. When fat intake does not exceed 30% of total calories, the expected rise in triglycerides from a high carbohydrate diet is minimal. Saturated fats should account for no more than 10% of caloric intake.[71, 80, 92, 109, 118]

Physical Inactivity.

Regular aerobic exercise is important in preventing heart and blood vessel disease. The Framingham study has demonstrated an inverse relationship between exercise and the risk of CAD. Exercise may lower the risk of CAD by lowering weight and blood pressure, and elevating the protective lipoprotein HDL.[48, 65, 80, 107]

■ Contributing Factors

Obesity, diabetes, and response to stress also increase the risk of CAD.

Obesity.

Obesity places an extra burden on the heart, requiring the muscle to work harder to pump enough blood to support added tissue mass. In addition, obesity is often associated with a sedentary life-style, elevated serum cholesterol, and high blood pressure.

Diabetes.

Diabetes frequently appears in middle-aged, overweight people. A fasting blood sugar of more than 120 mg/dl, or a routine blood glucose of 180 mg/dl and glucosuria signals the presence of diabetes and represents an increased risk of CAD. Diabetes leads to early atherosclerosis. For women in particular, diabetes is a contributing factor to the development of CAD.[7]

Response to Stress.

Stress appears to be associated with elevated blood pressures. Although stress is unavoidable in modern life, an excessive response to stress can be a health hazard. Significant stressors include major changes in residence, occupation, or status.

Type A behavior is characterized by aggressiveness, ambition, competitiveness, and a preoccupation with deadlines. Although type A behavior has not been correlated with an increased incidence of CAD in men, it may be a significant factor in working women. The anger component in the stress response is also important. Recent studies have questioned type A behavior as a risk factor. Scientists now believe that the amount of stress and the psychological impact of the stress are more important than specific behavior patterns (such as type A).[44, 53, 55]

The electrocardiographic (ECG) abnormality seen with left ventricular hypertrophy is independently associated with CAD. The mechanism that accounts for this is unknown.[73, 80]

Pathophysiology

There are three layers in the arterial wall: (1) the intima, (2) the media, and (3) the adventitia (Fig. 45–1A). The intima, a single layer of cells on the inner surface of the artery, normally provides an impermeable barrier to proteins in the blood. The media (middle layer) is made up almost entirely of smooth muscle cells. The adventitia consists mainly of smooth muscle cells, fibroblasts, and loose connective tissue.

Atherosclerosis primarily affects the intima of the arterial wall. It normally takes years to develop. When clinical manifestations develop, the disorder is usually well advanced. CAD progresses through developmental stages:

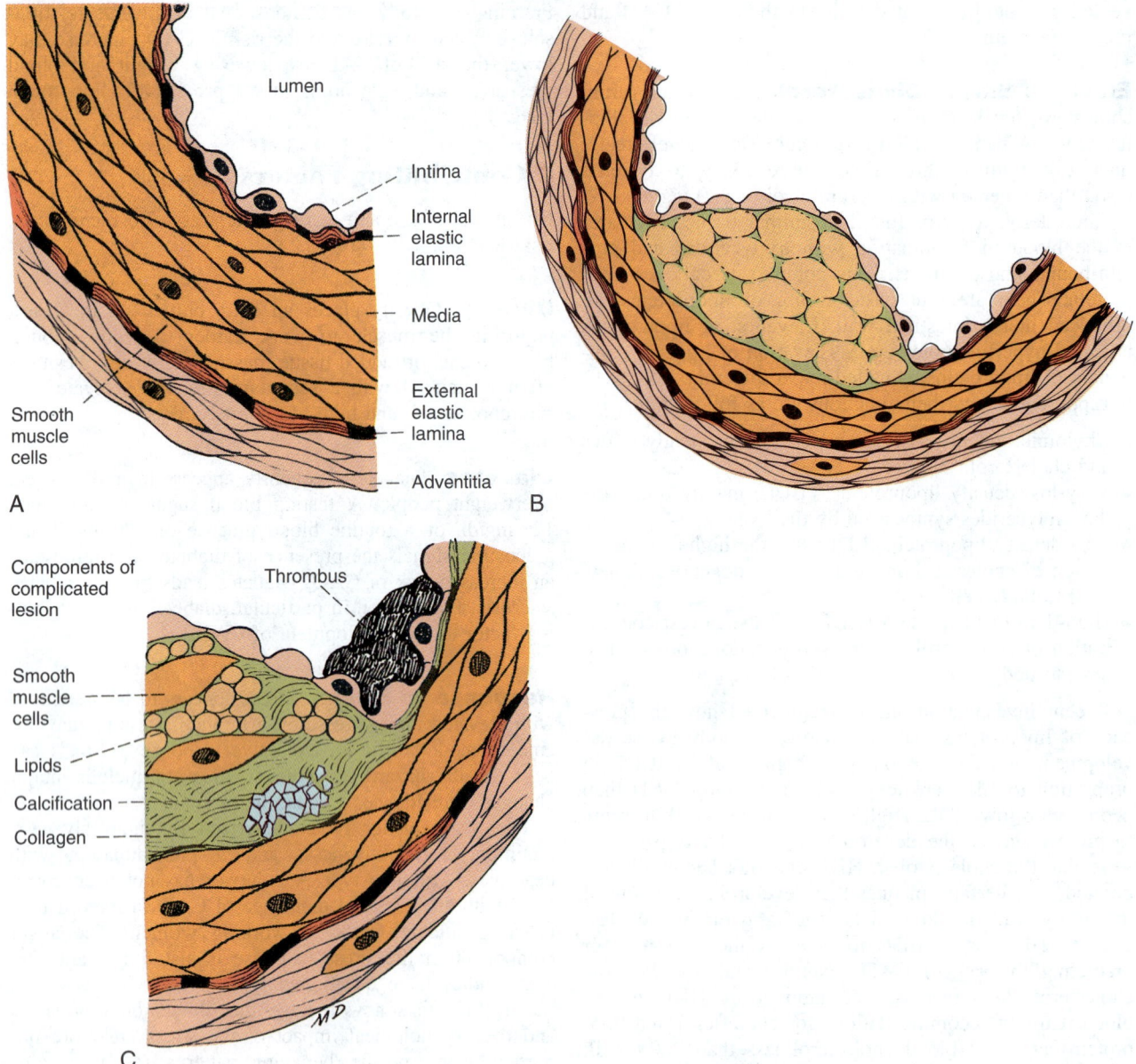

Figure 45–1. Cross-section of an artery. *A,* Normal. *B,* With a fatty lesion. *C,* With a complicated lesion. As CAD progresses, the lumen becomes smaller.

(1) the fatty streak, (2) the fibrous plaque, and (3) the complicated lesion.

The fatty streak (Fig. 45–1B) appears as a smooth, yellowish, slightly raised streak on the inner surface of the artery. It is characterized by the presence of lipoprotein deposits (mostly cholesterol). Fatty streaks have been seen in infants as young as 1 month old. Researchers have not yet determined whether they are reversible or are a precursor to plaque formation.

The raised fibrous plaque appears as a yellowish-gray bump on the surface of the artery. It is the beginning of progressive changes in the arterial wall. They appear by the age of 30. Nonspecific injury to the wall produces more plaque formation. (See Theories of Pathogenesis on the next page.) The plaque is made up of three types of material: (1) smooth muscle cells from the medial layer, (2) collagen, and (3) accumulated lipid within the intimal layer.

A complicated lesion, as shown in Figure 45–1C, contains the fibrous plaque, calcium deposits, and a thrombus formed by hemorrhage into the plaque.[147, 152] It is the final stage of development and the most dangerous. The lesion becomes rigid and may partially or totally block the artery. Once the artery is blocked and stiff, it cannot provide an increased blood supply to muscles demanding blood flow. When metabolic needs of active muscle cannot be supplied, the muscle reverts to anaerobic metabolism. Lactic acid is produced, which leads to pain and decreases muscle efficiency. This process is called *angina* in the myocardium and it is discussed later in the chapter.

■ Collateral Circulation

Collateral circulation is the presence of more than one artery supplying a muscle. There is normally some collateral circulation in the coronary arteries, especially in older persons. Collateral vessels develop when a muscle is chronically ischemic. Extra blood vessels are developed to meet metabolic demands. The development of collateral circulation takes time. Therefore, an occlusion of a coronary artery in a younger person is more likely to be lethal because there are no collateral arteries present to supply the myocardium with blood.

■ Theories of Pathogenesis

Over the last 10 years, our understanding of the atherosclerotic process has changed. A number of currently popular theories attempt to explain the development of atherosclerosis. These theories, although still controversial, endeavor to trace the formation of the fatty streak and raised fibrous plaque. Many of these theories have been integrated into the response-to-injury hypothesis. This theory suggests that certain changes occur in response to a nonspecific injury to the inner surface of the arterial wall. These changes then produce a raised fibrous plaque (Fig. 45–2). Nonspecific injury (mechanical, chemical, hormonal, or immunologic) may arise from hypertension, hydrocarbons from smoking, cholesterol, catecholamines, angiotensin, or hormones. In turn, nonspecific injury results in the shedding or desquamation of the superficial layer of the artery. Continued exposure to the source of intimal injury results in continued lipid deposition and proliferation of smooth muscle cells.

Other theories to explain the development of CAD include the monoclonal hypothesis, the senescence hypothesis, the thrombogenic hypothesis, the lipid-irritation hypothesis, and the hemodynamic hypothesis.

According to the monoclonal hypothesis, the primary process of proliferation of smooth muscle cells arises from the unchecked multiplication of a single cell.

The senescence hypothesis suggests that the development of atherosclerosis occurs with age. Smooth muscle cell proliferation results from an age-dependent decline in control over replication of intimal smooth muscle cells. This results in the characteristic increase in smooth muscle cell proliferation.

According to the thrombogenic hypothesis, the aggregation of platelets at the site of injury stimulate proliferation of smooth muscle cells and migration into the intima. Fibrin is stimulated, and small thrombi begin to form at the site of endothelial injury.

The lipid-irritation hypothesis holds that the deposit of lipids from the blood in the arterial wall acts as an irritant that induces proliferation of smooth muscle cells.

The hemodynamic hypothesis attempts to explain why plaques commonly appear in arterial branchings. According to the hemodynamic hypothesis, plaque formation results from turbulence, pressures, and stresses that all act as irritants on the endothelial wall.

In general, most theories include the following major events in the development of atherosclerotic plaque[16, 152]:

- Endothelial injury
- Platelet-fibrin interaction
- Smooth muscle cell proliferation
- Lipid entry and accumulation
- Fibrosis
- Thrombus formation
- Ulceration and calcification

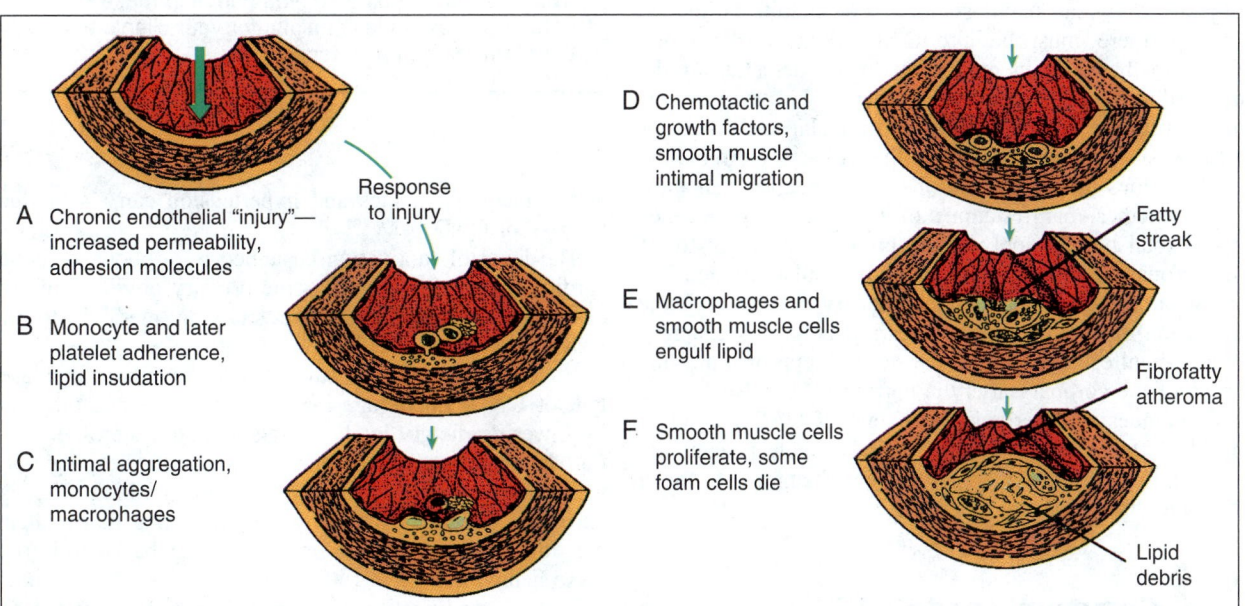

Figure 45–2. The response-to-injury theory of atherogenesis. *A,* The process begins with focal areas of endothelial injury—usually very subtle—that result in increased endothelial permeability. *B,* Lipids and platelets aggregate in the area. The lipoproteins commonly include low-density lipoproteins (LDLs) and very-low-density lipoproteins (VLDLs). *C,* Oxidized LDL attracts monocytes and macrophages to the site. *D,* Plaques begin to form foam cells that embed in the endothelium. *E,* Lipids are engulfed by the cells, and smooth muscle cells develop, leading to a fatty atheroma (*F*). (From Kumar, V., et al. [1992]. *Basic pathology* [p. 281]. Philadelphia: W. B. Saunders.)

■ Sudden Cardiac Death

CAD is a progressive disorder; if not prevented or treated in the early stages, it will progress to a more severe form of cardiac disorder. Common sequelae of CAD include sudden cardiac death, angina pectoris, and MI. In addition, clients may develop heart failure, chronic arrhythmias, conduction disturbances, and unstable angina. Sudden cardiac death is presented here; the other sequelae are the focus of the rest of this chapter.

Sudden cardiac death is a descriptive term for death from cardiac causes within 24 hours of the onset of symptoms. CAD makes up 75% of all causes of sudden cardiac death. Other risk factors of sudden cardiac death include the following[11, 14, 41, 140]:

● Hypertrophic and dilated cardiomyopathies
● Wolff-Parkinson-White syndrome
● Long QT syndrome
● Valvular abnormalities
● Electrolyte abnormalities (hypomagnesemia and hypokalemia)

Primary ventricular fibrillation is the major cause of sudden cardiac death. Dyspnea and fatigue are the most commonly reported symptoms experienced immediately preceding sudden cardiac death. Angina is a primary symptom in less than 35% of cases.[37, 114, 124]

The Ethical Issues in Nursing feature addresses your role in "do not resuscitate" decisions.

Clinical Manifestations and Diagnostic Findings

Atherosclerosis, by itself, does not necessarily produce subjective clinical manifestations. For manifestations to develop, there must be a critical deficit in the blood supply to the heart in proportion to the demands of the myocardium for oxygen and nutrients. In other words, there must be a supply-and-demand imbalance. When atherosclerosis progresses slowly, the collateral circulation that develops generally can meet the heart's demands. Thus, whether manifestations of CAD develop depends on the total blood supply to the myocardium (by way of the coronary arteries and collateral circulation) and not solely on the condition of the coronary arteries (see the discussion of angina, which appears later in this chapter). Often, manifestations of CAD do not appear until the lumen of the coronary artery is narrowed by 75%.

Techniques to determine the extent of CAD and identify the affected vessels include ECG, nuclear scanning, and angiography.[2, 29, 138, 153, 154] (See Chapter 44 for a complete discussion.)

Community and Self-Care

Prevention, rather than treatment, is the goal with regard to CAD. Fatty streaks are capable of regressing and disappearing entirely if cholesterol and fat intake are reduced. Cessation of cigarette smoking, controlling diet,

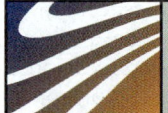

ETHICAL ISSUES IN NURSING

What Is Your Role in a "Do Not Resuscitate" Decision?

Cardiopulmonary resuscitation (CPR) upon cardiac arrest may prolong life, if it is successful; but with no corrective treatment options left for such a client, should CPR be performed at all? When medical-surgical science and technology can no longer ward off death, a "do not resuscitate" (DNR) order by the physician appears to be the logical course. Should the client need to consent to such a DNR order? Should the client or family members have a right to refuse a DNR order even if the physicians believe that all resuscitative measures would be futile? What is your role in a DNR decision?

All clients have a right to autonomy, that is, they have a right to direct their care as they wish. If certain treatment choices are considered futile, should clients be allowed to choose them? Healthcare providers have an obligation to act beneficently toward their clients. Could the withholding of CPR or other resuscitative measures ever be of benefit to the client?

Nurses see their clients in all stages of health and illness. The dying process is perhaps the most difficult stage to deal with. Dealing with clients who are not to be resuscitated can be very stressful for the nurses caring for them. The natural defense mechanism is to keep distance between yourself and the client. This may make you feel better but may also make the client feel alienated. Come to terms with your own feelings about DNR clients and death and dying issues. In doing so, you can help make such natural processes less painful for your clients and their families and also for yourself.

and managing diabetes and hypertension can also reduce the risk of CAD.[71, 80, 101]

The level of motivation sustained by a client to reduce cardiovascular risk factors is the primary predictor of success. Nursing researchers are studying methods to improve motivation.[49, 99, 106]

Have a high index of suspicion for clients at increased risk of CAD. Encourage these clients to reduce their risk by lowering dietary intake of fats and cholesterol, exercising, controlling diabetes and hypertension, keeping body weight at near-ideal levels, and ceasing smoking. The risk and incidence of CAD are so pervasive that many clients are doing these activities on an ongoing basis. Reinforce these behaviors.[55, 65, 92, 100]

Dietary modification is an initial step. Instruct the client to alter his or her diet so that saturated fats compose less than 10% and nonsaturated fats less than 30% of daily food intake. Cholesterol intake should be reduced to 250 to 300 mg/day.[109, 118]

Medications can be given to reduce cholesterol levels and reduce the risk of clotting. Cholestyramine (Questran) and colestipol (Colestid) inhibit the reabsorption of bile acids in the intestine, which increases fecal excretion of bile acids. With the increase in fecal excretion of bile acids, the liver increases production of bile acids from cholesterol, thereby lowering serum levels. Gemfibrozil (Lopid) and Simvastatin (Zocor) block lipolysis of stored triglycerides in adipose tissue and inhibit hepatic uptake of fatty acids.

Acute and Subacute Care

■ Interventional Cardiology

Since the first percutaneous transluminal coronary angioplasty (PTCA) was performed in 1977, many new techniques of coronary revascularization have been developed. Although PTCA remains the most common intervention, directional coronary atherectomy, intracoronary stents, and laser ablation are being performed with increased frequency. These nonsurgical interventions are examples of interventional cardiology.[3, 21, 45, 57]

Percutaneous Transluminal Coronary Angioplasty

Percutaneous transluminal coronary angioplasty is a technique in which a balloon-tipped catheter is inserted into a leg artery and threaded under x-ray guidance into a blocked coronary artery. The balloon is inflated to reshape the lumen by stretching it and flattening the atherosclerotic plaque against the arterial wall, thus opening the artery (Fig. 45–3). In 1993, over 369,000 PTCA procedures were performed. The success rate (defined as a greater than 20% reduction in stenosis) is reported as 82%. PTCA is less invasive, less expensive, and therefore an attractive alternative to open heart surgery.[92, 139]

The guidelines for selection of clients for PTCA are rapidly changing. Clients with no or mild manifestations to clients with unstable angina may be suitable candi-

dates. PTCA may also be successful in single-vessel or multiple-vessel disease.[93, 98] However, balloon angioplasty is most successful in clients who are male, are less than 70 years of age, have normal pumping ability, who have no more than two blocked arteries and have no history of diabetes, heart attack, or coronary artery bypass surgery.[21, 47, 131] A recent study indicated that clients with type A behavior, specifically hostility, had increased risk of restenosis after PTCA.[59] In addition to PTCA, new therapeutic devices for coronary application continue to evolve as alternatives to bypass surgery.[117]

Directional Coronary Atherectomy

Atherectomy was designed to overcome two of the most significant complications of PTCA: restenosis and abrupt closure of the coronary artery.[30, 133] Restenosis occurs in 25% to 50% of cases within 2 to 6 months after PTCA while abrupt closure resulting from plaque fracture, coronary artery dissection, localized thrombus, or coronary artery spasm occurs in 2% to 6% of clients after PTCA. Directional coronary atherectomy (DCA) reduces coronary stenosis by excising and removing atheromatous plaque. The DCA cutter consists of a catheter that contains a rigid cylindrical housing with a central rotating blade (Fig. 45–4). The blade shaves off the atherosclerotic material and deposits it in the nose cone of the housing for later histopathologic study. Since the spinning of the cutter can cause vibrations that can irritate the vessel wall and cause coronary vasospasm, calcium channel blockers are usually given before the procedure.[23, 74]

DCA is most appropriate for lesions in medium-to-large coronary arteries located in the proximal or middle portions of the vessel. It is not recommended for use with tortuous vessels, distal lesions, or heavily calcified lesions. The large size of the catheter limits the usefulness of DCA in treating women.[17, 43] The use of DCA has decreased recently because of the increasing use of stents and recent reports that the results are not comparable to PTCA.[21] Complications of DCA include embolus formation, acute vessel occlusion, vessel perforation, and arte-

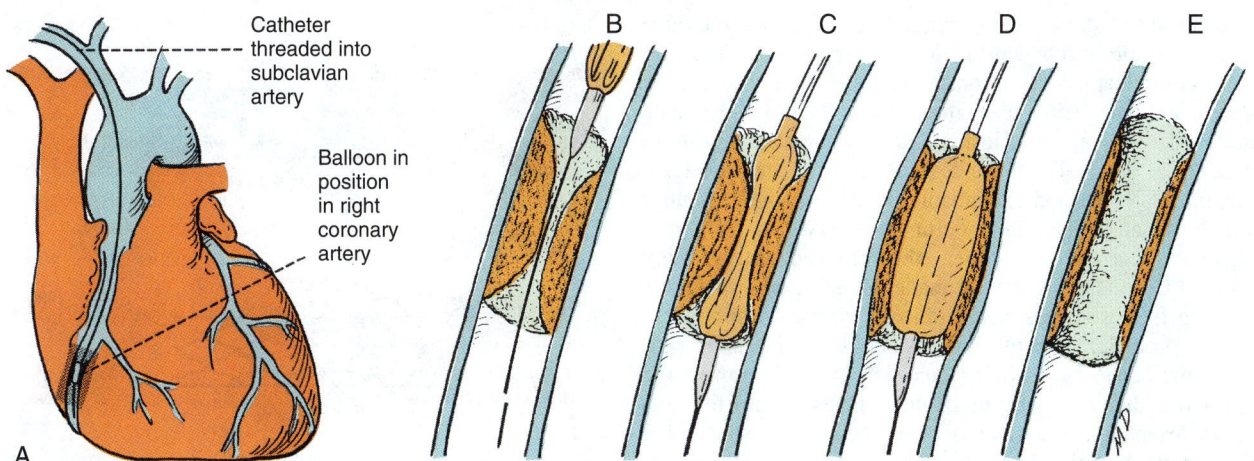

Figure 45–3. Percutaneous transluminal coronary angioplasty (PTCA). *A,* A balloon-tipped catheter positioned in a blocked artery. *B,* The balloon is centered. *C,* The balloon expands to (*D*) compress the blockage. *E,* The artery is restored to its original diameter.

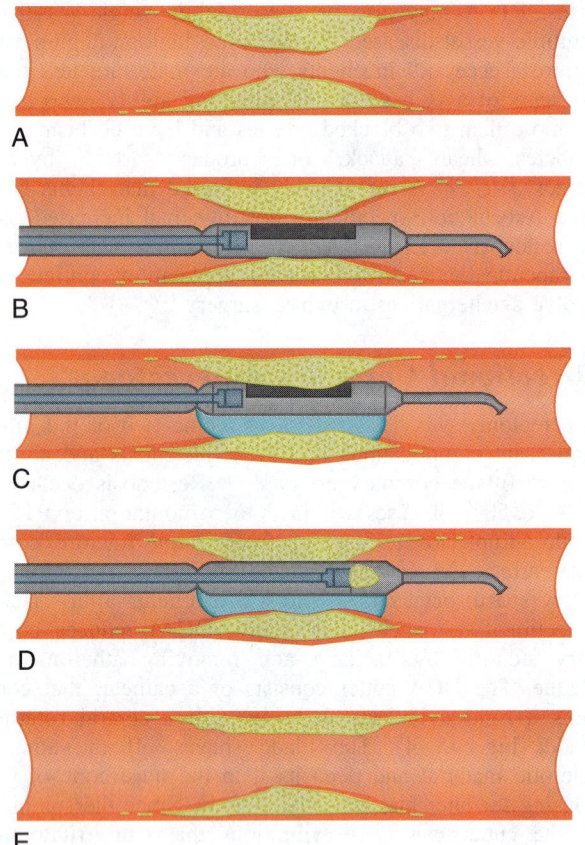

Figure 45–4. Atherectomy. *A*, Lesion. *B*, The atherectomy catheter is advanced through the artery so that the cutting device is positioned over the lesion. *C*, The balloon on the device is inflated to stabilize the catheter. *D*, The cutting portion of the catheter is advanced, cutting away the lesion and trapping it in the cylindrical housing. Then the balloon is deflated, and the catheter is removed. *E*, Result of the procedure.

rial spasm. Following DCA, clients are given enteric-coated aspirin to prevent thrombosis.[74]

Intracoronary Stents

Intracoronary stents were originally designed to reduce restenosis and abrupt closure of coronary vessels resulting from complications of coronary angioplasty. Intracoronary stents are now being used instead of PTCA to eliminate the risk of acute closure and improve long-term patency.[47, 137, 148] There are several different stent designs, but most are balloon-expandable or self-expandable tubes which, when placed in a coronary artery, act as a mechanical scaffold to reopen the blocked artery (Fig. 45–5). Coronary stents are made of numerous materials ranging from stainless steel to bioabsorbable compounds.

The procedure for placing a stent is similar to PTCA. Once the coronary lesion is identified by angiography, the balloon catheter bearing the stent is inserted into the coronary artery and the stent is positioned at the site of the occlusion. A major concern with stent placement is prevention of acute thrombosis, especially during the first several weeks after the procedure. To prevent thrombosis, combined antiplatelet and anticoagulant therapy is used

before, during, and after the procedure. Aspirin, dipyridamole, heparin, and dextran are used before and during stent placement.

Following stent placement, clients take aspirin, dipyridamole, and warfarin for at least several months. Complications include stent occlusion, bleeding secondary to anticoagulation, and coronary artery dissection.[3, 19, 21]

Laser Ablation

Lasers are used with balloon angioplasty to vaporize atherosclerotic plaque. After the initial balloon angioplasty, a brief burst of laser radiation is administered, and additional remaining plaque is removed.[39] Results of clinical trials indicate that laser ablation combined with balloon angioplasty is more effective in treating lesions that typically respond poorly to angioplasty alone.[39] Complications include coronary dissection, acute occlusion, perforation, and embolism.

■ Nursing Management of the Client Undergoing Interventional Cardiology

Prior to interventional procedures, the client is usually given an antiplatelet medication such as aspirin. The client is also given anticoagulants (heparin) to prevent occlusion and calcium channel blockers or nitrates to reduce coronary spasm during the procedure. Following the procedure, the client may continue with this drug regimen to prevent reocclusion or arterial spasms.[86, 112] Interventional procedures are very common. Many hospitals have developed clinical pathways to facilitate hospital stays (see Appendix D).

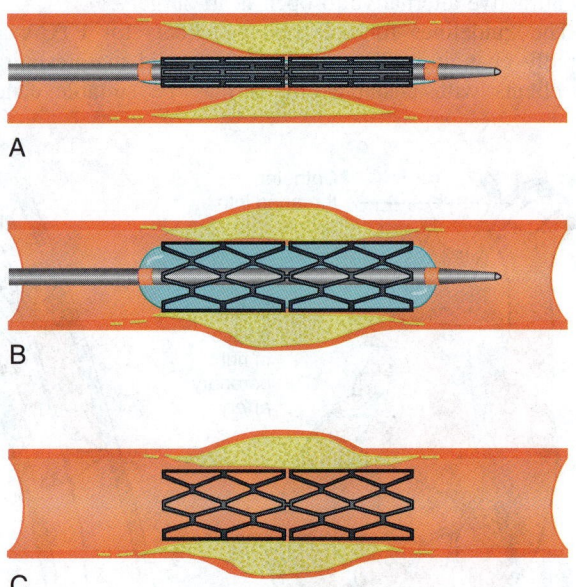

Figure 45–5. Placement of a coronary artery stent. *A*, The stent is positioned at the site of the lesion. *B*, The balloon is inflated, expanding the stent. The balloon is then deflated and removed. *C*, The implanted stent is left in place.

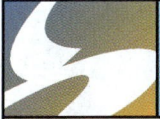

CASE MANAGEMENT

**Percutaneous Transluminal Coronary Angioplasty and Arteriography
For Clinical Pathway, see Appendix D.**

Clinical Pathway from Montclair Baptist Medical Center, Birmingham, Alabama.
Information provided by Karen Tauxe, M.S.N.

Development and Revision of Pathway

- Percutaneous transluminal coronary angioplasty (PTCA) is a high-volume case type. Since so many patients undergo this procedure, a pathway was developed.
- The pathway was initiated in August 1992.
- The development team included the nurse-manager, registered nurses, the clinical pharmacist, catheter laboratory staff, dietician, and physicians.
- A multidisciplinary task force meets two to four times per year to discuss the care of these patients. Pathway revision could take place at these meetings.
- During the meetings mentioned above there is opportunity to revise the pathway. At a minimum, the pathway is revised annually.

Use and Impact of Pathway

- All patients who undergo a PTCA or arteriogram are placed on the pathway for the preoperative and postoperative period related to this procedure. (Sometimes patients are admitted for other procedures or conditions. If they require PTCA during their stay, this pathway will be used for the procedure episode only.)
- The nursing staff use the pathway daily.
- By documenting the expected plan of care for the entire episode on a pathway and using that plan to deliver care to PTCA patients, nurses and physicians have been encouraged to collaborate closely.
- Increased awareness of the appropriate plan of care for these patients has reduced the variable cost of care. Physicians have been made very aware of the costs of the care they order since the pathway was developed and as the outcomes are reviewed quarterly within the multidisciplinary team.

The client is also typed and crossmatched for blood in the event that emergency coronary artery bypass grafting (CABG) is needed. A consent is signed for the interventional procedure and surgery if required for spasm, perforation of the artery, or acute occlusion. The Nursing Research feature addresses the needs of families of clients who are undergoing this procedure.

Following interventional procedures, monitor the client for changes in vital signs, especially the quality and rhythm of pulse, and ECG. Report any indication of coronary ischemia to the physician. ST segment monitoring is frequently used to detect ischemia. If the client complains of chest pain, obtain a 12-lead ECG immediately. Force fluids, orally or intravenously, to assist the body to excrete contrast and because the contrast causes diuresis and may cause acute tubular necrosis (ATN). Monitor the puncture site for hematoma, and palpate pulses to assess peripheral perfusion. Complications include bleeding and hematoma formation at the puncture site, acute MI resulting from perforation of an artery, refractory spasm, or occlusion. Bedrest may be ordered for longer periods for clients undergoing stent placement and DCA because of the larger sheaths used to dilate the vessels in these procedures.

Nursing considerations specific to the care of the client with a coronary stent include close monitoring of anticoagulation status and ongoing assessment for bleeding. Un-til the sheath is removed, instruct the client to limit movement of the sheathed leg, and keep the head of the bed below 30 degrees to prevent bleeding and hematoma formation at the site. Clients with coronary stents usually have longer hospital stays than with other interventional procedures because their antithrombin therapy must be monitored closely.[144, 148, 151]

■ Surgical Management

Coronary Artery Bypass Graft

Coronary artery bypass graft (CABG) surgery involves the bypass of a blockage in one or more of the coronary arteries using the saphenous veins or mammary artery as replacement vessels. Prior to surgery, coronary angiography precisely locates lesions and points of narrowing within the coronary arteries.

During CABG surgery, the surgeon harvests a length of saphenous vein from the thigh. The heart is accessed through a median sternotomy. With the client on cardiopulmonary bypass, the distal end of the vein is sutured to the aorta and the proximal end is sewn to the coronary vessel distal to the blockage (Fig. 45–6). The veins are reversed so that their valves do not interfere with blood flow. The cardiopulmonary bypass machine is discussed in Chapter 46. In some cases, the internal mammary ar-

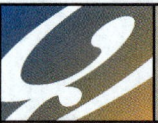

NURSING RESEARCH

What Are the Needs of Families of Clients Having Cardiac Catheterization?

Miracle, V. A., & Hovekamp, G. (1994). Needs of families of patients undergoing invasive procedures. *American Journal of Critical Care,* 3(2), 155–157.

Although nurses are responsible for providing care to families of clients undergoing invasive cardiac procedures, little research-based information is available to guide their interventions. The purpose of this descriptive study was to identify the needs of families of clients undergoing percutaneous transluminal coronary angioplasty (PTCA) or cardiac catheterization. Following completion of the procedure, 95 family members completed a 25-item questionnaire adapted from Molter's Critical Care Family Needs Inventory. The study sample had a mean age of 50 years. Sixty-one percent of the subjects were waiting for clients undergoing cardiac catheterization; 62% were clients' spouses, and 62% had no prior experience with the procedure. Subjects were asked to rate each need on a scale of 1 to 4, from not important (1) to very important (4). Family members rated all but four items as "important" and rated informational needs and concern needs the highest. Family members were less concerned with personal comfort.

Implications for Practice

These results suggest that you can best meet family members' needs by allowing them to see the client immediately before and after the cardiac procedure, explaining the procedure to them, answering questions, and providing frequent condition reports during the procedure.

---

tery (IMA) can be grafted to a coronary artery. The disadvantage of the IMA is that more time is required to remove it and it is shorter. It is used only to revascularize the portion of the myocardium supplied by the left anterior descending (LAD) artery. An advantage is that IMA grafts have a greater chance of remaining patent. Surgical methods only ease the manifestations. Surgery cannot halt the process of atherosclerosis, although it may prolong life in some cases. The surgical management of CAD in women is being studied. At this time, women appear to have less short-term benefit from surgery (i.e., suffer more immediate complications) but have similar, if not better, long-term results than men.[10, 17, 43, 45]

Possible complication of CABG include the following[87, 98]:

- Postoperative bleeding
- Wound infection and dehiscence
- Intraoperative stroke
- Myocardial infarction
- Blood clots
- Multiple system organ failure
- Death

The development of calcium channel blockers and nonsurgical interventional techniques such as PTCA, atherectomy, and stents have reduced the number of CABG surgeries performed. Also, survival rates in CABG have not been found to be significantly better than survival rates of medically treated people. CABG nevertheless remains a common surgery, and because it can reduce angina in 80% to 90% of clients refractory to medical management, it will continue as an important intervention in the management of coronary heart disease. Benefits from CABG surgery also include prolongation of life, increased exercise tolerance, reduced need for medication, and ability to resume former activities. The Nursing Research feature on p. 1251 describes sex differences in physical activity after bypass surgery.

Transmyocardial Revascularization

A new procedure that is still experimental shows promise for clients with widespread atherosclerosis involving vessels that are too small and numerous for replacement or balloon catheterization. Transmyocardial revascularization (TMR) uses a high-powered laser to open up channels in the heart through a relatively small chest incision by punching holes in a fraction of a second in the beating heart. The laser beam is applied between heart beats when the ventricle is filled with blood. The laser creates from 15 to 30 holes in the heart. Blood enters these small channels, providing the affected region of the heart with oxygenated blood. The opening on the heart's surface heals over; however, the main channels remain and perfuse the myocardium. To date, approximately 200 TMPs have been performed in the United States in clinical trials since 1990. TMR promises to help in severe angina unhelped by PTCA or CABG surgery. The procedure is estimated to cost $15,000, slightly more than angioplasty but much less than CABG. Sustained improvement has been seen up to 27 months after the operation.[1, 93, 126] Atrial fibrillation is a common complication after CABG. Clients with atrial fibrillation require longer hospitalization in most cases.[104]

Modifications for Elderly Clients

Over half of all CABGs are performed on people over 65, and 73% of them on men.[8] Elderly clients have a postoperative recovery similar to younger clients, but the pace is slower. Elderly clients typically remain hospitalized for 2 to 4 more days on average. They also have a higher mortality rate.[11]

Postoperative complications that are more prevalent in the elderly include dysrhythmias related to aged sinoatrial node cells, drug toxicity related to impaired hepatic and renal perfusion, multiple drug-drug interactions, and decreased physical stamina. These complications contribute to a 15-day mean length of hospital stay for clients over the age of 80 years.

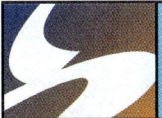

CASE MANAGEMENT

Coronary Artery Bypass Graft
For Clinical Pathway, see Appendix D.

Clinical Pathway from Birmingham Baptist Medical Center, Birmingham, Alabama
Information provided by Paula Midyette, M.S.N., and Nancy Meisler, M.S.N.

Development and Revision of Pathway

- In addition to being a high-volume, high-cost case type, a great deal of physician practice variability existed for this diagnosis. We believed there was high potential for cost savings if such variation in practice could be decreased. The cardiovascular surgeons had already initiated some cost containment measures within their practice, which set the stage for the development of a CareMap.
- This pathway was initiated in 1990. There have been several revisions as practice changes occur.
- The case manager worked with registered nurses, licensed practical nurses, nursing assistants, unit secretaries, cardiac rehabilitation, respiratory therapists, the chaplain, cardiovascular surgeons, and the clinical nurse specialist to develop the first map.
- Process and outcome data are collected and analyzed by the case manager and representatives from various departments. Recommendations for practice changes are presented at the quarterly continuous process improvement meeting. The case manager is responsible for updating the map and implementing educational activities relating to practice changes.
- Maps are reviewed quarterly through the continuous improvement methods outlined above.

Use and Impact of Pathway

- All patients admitted for this procedure are placed on the pathway. In addition, all patients receive a copy of the patient pathway which explains various aspects of care to the patient and their family members in terms they can understand.
- Registered nurses, licensed practical nurses, nursing assistants, surgeons, case managers, cardiac rehabilitation staff, and the cardiovascular educator use the map daily. The dietitian uses the map periodically during the patient's stay.
- Nurses are more aware of the whole episode of care, including postdischarge issues. They are also more autonomous in directing patient care. CareMaps have enhanced collaborative practice and therefore improved job satisfaction.
- Cost savings of greater than $3000 per case have been realized. The average postoperative length of stay is 5 days (it used to be 7 days), and 45% of patients are being discharged on postoperative day 4.

During the first and second weeks after discharge, depression, fatigue, incisional chest discomfort, dyspnea, and anorexia are common. By the fourth to fifth weeks, elderly clients report improved mood, comfort, and appetite. At 1 year, almost all (93%) were pleased with the outcome and improved quality of life.[64]

■ Nursing Management of the Surgical Client

Many hospitals have initiated rapid recovery programs for cardiac surgery clients; these programs reduce the hospital stay to 4 days. With rapid recovery programs, most of the client's recovery takes place in the home with the client and family assuming primary responsibility for many aspects of care. Discharge planning begins on admission to the hospital, activity progression in the postoperative period is accelerated, and client and family education continues on a daily basis throughout hospitalization. Many hospitals have developed clinical pathways for CABG. Use the clinical pathway in Appendix D to assist you in planning your clients' care. In addition, a three-phase program of activity is implemented (see below).

Phase I (In-Hospital) Rehabilitation Programs. Most CABG clients participate in cardiac rehabilitation following surgery. Phase I begins immediately after the client returns to surgery. The goals of phase I inpatient rehabilitation are the following:

- To prevent the negative effects of prolonged bedrest
- To assess the client's physiologic response to exercise
- To manage the psychosocial issues related to recovery from CABG surgery
- To educate the client and family concerning recovery and adoption of risk reduction behaviors.

While in the intensive care unit, clients are turned every 2 hours during the first several hours after surgery. Once extubated, clients get up in a chair and ambulate in the room. After transfer to the intermediate care unit, clients continue to walk three to four times per day, increasing the distance walked each time.

Assess the client's blood pressure, heart rate, ECG, and oxygen saturation before, during, and after activity.[12] Systolic blood pressure should not increase more than 20 mm Hg or decrease more than 10 to 15 mm Hg after exercise. Heart rate should not increase more than 20

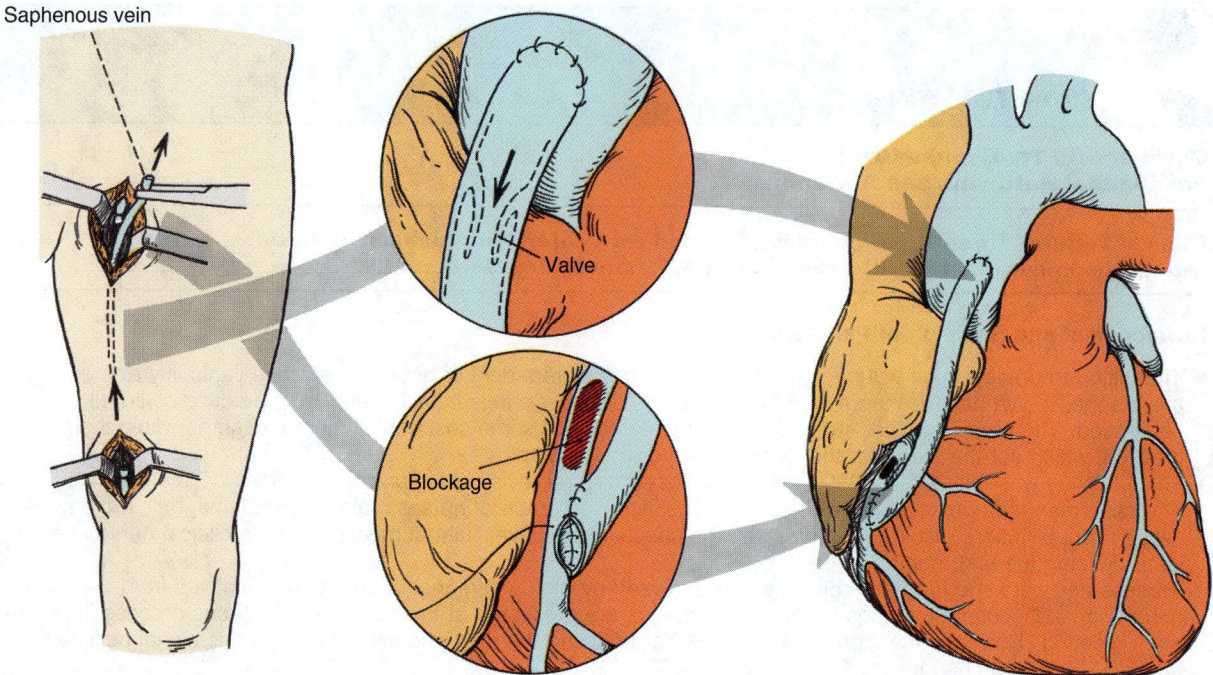

Figure 45–6. Coronary artery bypass grafting (CABG). A section of saphenous vein is harvested from the leg and anastomosed (upside down, because of its directional valves) to a coronary artery to bypass an area of occlusion.

beats per minute above resting and no significant arrhythmias should occur. Activity levels will be reduced if clients respond negatively to exercise. Clients are seated for all meals. Research has demonstrated that early mobilization improves cardiac function and benefits the client psychologically.

Education for a healthier life-style is an important part of each phase of cardiac rehabilitation. The emphasis in phase I is on the identification and modification of reversible risk factors to prevent further deleterious cardiac events.

Community and Self-Care

Before discharge, instruct the client and family (or significant other) in medication actions and side effects, dietary restrictions, physical activity restrictions and progression, and wound care. Since it is not always possible to anticipate all the problems clients may encounter the first few days at home, instruct the client who to call when there is an emergency or when there are questions or concerns. If possible, introduce the client to the home health nurse who will be supervising home care. Following discharge, the home healthcare nurse provides additional education and counseling, and assesses the client for complications.[111, 113, 146] In addition, instruct the client on how to assess response to exercise and activity.[127, 128, 129, 135]

Prior to discharge, a low-level symptom-limited exercise test may be performed. The purpose of this test is to evaluate the client's ability to perform activities of daily living and exercise. The results of this test are used to

prescribe a safe and effective exercise program for the first few weeks at home and serve as a basis for the initial exercise prescription in phase II.[21]

Phase II (Outpatient Exercise Training) Rehabilitation Programs.
Outpatient (phase II) exercise training usually takes place in a facility that provides continuous ECG monitoring, emergency equipment, and medically supervised exercise. Outpatient treatment usually begins 10 to 14 days after discharge and requires physician referral.

The goals of phase II are as follows:

- To restore clients to a desirable exercise capacity appropriate to their health status, life-style, and occupation
- To provide additional education and support to the client and family for adoption of risk-reduction behaviors
- To meet the psychosocial needs of clients and families, restore confidence, and minimize anxiety and depression
- To promote early identification of medical problems through close observation and monitoring of clients during exercise
- To assist clients to return to occupational and leisure activities

Exercise therapy is conducted three times per week for a period of 2 to 3 months. The duration of the aerobic exercise session ranges from 20 to 40 minutes at an intensity of 70% to 85% of the baseline exercise heart rate. During each exercise session, the client's blood pressure, heart rate, respiratory rate, and ECG are monitored before, during, and after exercise. Activity levels are in-

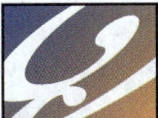

NURSING RESEARCH

Are Factors That Predict Physical Activity After Bypass Surgery Different for Women and Men?

Gerard, P. S. (1994). *Gender differences in predictors of physical activity following coronary artery bypass surgery.* Purdue University, Hammond, IN.

Adoption of a physically active life-style is recommended for secondary prevention of coronary artery disease. Knowledge of factors that influence physical activity, however, is based on studies conducted on men. The purpose of this study was to examine sex differences in long-term activity following cardiac surgery.

Gerard used several tools to collect data from 104 subjects (60% female) on their activity, locus of control, social support, and exercise benefits and barriers. Activity was grouped into general activity, activity associated with sports and exercise, and home activities.

There were sex differences in predictors of total activity and sports and exercise activity. Perceived benefits and barriers were the best predictors of both men's and women's activity patterns for general activity and sports activities. However, age at time of surgery was a significant predictor of women's general activity, whereas a man's weight influenced his exercise habits.

Implications for Practice

These results suggest that you should consider sex differences when designing activities for men and women after coronary bypass surgery.

creased gradually, based on the client's response. A nutritionist may counsel clients about proper diet, and a psychologist or social worker may work with clients on stress management and adoption of other risk prevention behaviors. At the end of the program, clients are given a symptom-limited exercise test and are reevaluated. Decisions regarding progression to a phase III or home program are based on the results of the stress test, the client's ability to self-monitor his or her response to exercise, the stability of the client, and the client's psychological or emotional status. Periodic evaluations are scheduled so that activity progression and cardiopulmonary function can be assessed.[26, 39, 64]

Phase III (Community) Rehabilitation Programs. Phase III programs are conducted in community settings such as the YMCA or a health club.

The goals of phase III are as follows:

● To maintain and, if possible, increase exercise capacity
● To institute long-term follow-up of risk-reduction behavior change

● To encourage clients to take responsibility for continuing life-style changes

Exercise consists of walking, jogging, weight training, and recreational games. Clients are usually not monitored while exercising, although some facilities obtain exercise ECGs on a monthly basis. Clients are responsible for monitoring their own heart rate response to exercise, although blood pressure can be taken by program personnel if indicated.[26, 155, 156]

Home Exercise Rehabilitation Programs. For CABG clients, a home exercise program is usually prescribed in conjunction with or in place of the outpatient program. Clients are given detailed exercise instructions and are told to keep a log of heart rates, perceived exertion rates, exercise parameters, and any problems that may occur during the home program. Cardiac rehabilitation staff members or the client's physician should analyze the data and adjust the home exercise program if necessary. Once clients reach their optimal level of functional capacity, they should be instructed to continue to exercise at least three times per week so that cardiopulmonary exercise capacity can be maintained.[26, 60, 130, 155, 156]

Angina Pectoris

As vessels become lined with atherosclerotic plaques, clinical manifestations of inadequate blood supply develop in the tissues supplied by these vessels. Problems such as cerebrovascular accident (CVA or stroke), claudication, and angina develop. This section discusses angina. Discussion of CVA may be found in Chapter 32, and of claudication in Chapter 50.

Angina pectoris is chest pain resulting from myocardial ischemia (inadequate blood supply to the myocardium).[132] Angina pectoris is common, although its incidence is not recorded. The cause of angina pectoris is CAD (discussed in the preceding section). Angina can occur in clients with normal coronary arteries also, but is less common. Clients with aortic stenosis, hypertension, and hypertrophic cardiomyopathy can have angina pectoris.

Etiology and Risk Factors

Exertion, emotion, and exposure to cold precipitate angina. Primary prevention is through the lifelong commitment to reducing the risk factors of CAD (see earlier). Secondary prevention is through recognition and early treatment of anginal attacks. Tertiary prevention is resolution of angina before myocardial damage occurs.

Pathophysiology

The coronary arteries normally supply the myocardium with blood to meet its metabolic needs during varying workloads (Box 45–2). The coronary vessels are normally efficient and perfuse the myocardium during diastole. When the heart needs more blood, the vessels dilate. As the vessels become lined and eventually occluded with

BRIDGE TO HOME HEALTHCARE

Rehabilitation After Coronary Artery Surgery

Peggy Gerard, D.N.S., R.N., *Hammond, Indiana,* **and Kathleen A. Ringel, D.N.S., C.F.N.P.,** *Omaha, Nebraska*

Successful cardiac rehabilitation can be done in the home setting. Bridging hospital care to home care involves continuing the exercise program and nursing assessments implemented in the hospital; the home health nurse serves as a facilitator and communicator. Increasingly, home healthcare of coronary artery bypass surgery clients is coordinated through the use of clinical pathways which identify critical assessments, teaching needs, and rehabilitative interventions.

Cardiac assessment of the client includes, but is not limited to, vital signs, lung sounds, peripheral pulses, and auscultation of heart sounds. Other important assessments include wound healing, diet history, and current weight and height measures. The home health nurse should possess knowledge of basic arrhythmias, murmurs, and extra heart sounds. The detection of an S_3 or S_4 heart sound is critical to detecting impending complications. Orthostatic blood pressure readings are assessed because of side effects precipitated by antihypertensive drugs, diuretics, vasodilators, and antianginal agents. Occasionally, portable electrocardiograms and chest films are done by home radiology companies.

Teaching medication actions, side effects, and methods of administration is more successful in the home, where stress levels are usually lower. Written medication sheets can be individualized for each client, with dosage and time of administration written in by you. You can also assess the client's understanding of wound care instructions and can correct any misconceptions.

Ambulation in the home should be equivalent to levels achieved at the hospital. If exercise equipment is absent in the home, creative ideas are necessary for bridging the gap between hospital and home care. The client and family are taught to measure blood pressure and pulse before and after an exercise session. The home health nurse teaches when to stop exercise, what signs and symptoms are critical, and when to schedule rest periods and pace daily activities. Recording vital signs, activities, and tolerance is essential. Perhaps most important of all is to establish goals with the client according to life-style and needs.

The home health nurse often refers clients to community resources such as the American Heart Association and the Red Cross. Encouraging participation in lifeline services can increase the sense of security of those clients who live alone. When possible, a family member should be encouraged to take courses in cardiopulmonary resuscitation.

Finally, the home health nurse is in a unique position to reinforce teaching about healthy heart strategies. These include reducing weight, continuing a lifelong exercise program, decreasing dietary intake of sodium and fats, reducing stress levels, and ceasing smoking. Family members should be included in the teaching, when appropriate. A written contract can be used as a tool for help in establishing goals with the client and identifying steps toward these goals. These goals are still the cornerstone of any successful cardiac rehabilitation program.

---

atherosclerotic plaques, the vessels cannot dilate. As the vessels become occluded, they cannot supply the myocardium with blood for normal workloads. A growing mass of plaque in the vessel collects platelets, fibrin, and cellular debris. Platelet aggregations release prostaglandins capable of causing vessel spasm. This in turn promotes platelet aggregation, and a vicious circle begins.

Myocardial ischemia develops if the blood supply through the coronary vessels or oxygen content of the blood is not adequate to meet metabolic demands. Disorders of the coronary vessels, the circulation, or the blood may lead to deficits in supply.

Disorders of the coronary vessels include atherosclerosis, arterial spasm, and coronary arteritis. Atherosclerosis increases resistance to flow. Arterial spasm also increases resistance. Coronary arteritis is inflammation of the coronary arteries due to infection or autoimmune disease.

Disorders of circulation include hypotension and aortic stenosis or insufficiency. Hypotension may be due to spinal anesthesia, potent antihypertensive drugs, blood loss, or other factors that result in decreased blood return to the heart. Aortic valve stenosis or insufficiency results in decreased filling pressure of the coronary arteries.

Blood disorders include anemia, hypoxemia, and polycythemia. Anemia and hypoxemia result in decreased oxygen flow to the myocardium. Polycythemia causes increased blood viscosity, which slows blood flow through the coronary arteries.

The opposite of supply is demand, and increased demands can be placed on the heart. Conditions that increase demands on the myocardium include conditions that increase cardiac output and that increase myocardial need for oxygen. Conditions that increase cardiac output or myocardial need for oxygen are listed in Box 45–2.

Myocardial ischemia occurs when either supply or demand is altered. In some persons, the coronary arteries can supply adequate blood when the person is at rest; but when the person attempts activity or is taxed in some other manner, angina develops. Myocardial cells become ischemic within 10 seconds of coronary artery occlusion. After several minutes of ischemia, the pumping function of the heart is reduced. The reduction in pumping de-

---

Box 45–2. Factors Influencing Myocardial Supply and Demand

Factors That Decrease Supply

Coronary Vessel Disorders

Atherosclerosis
Arterial spasm
Coronary arteritis

Circulation Disorders

Hypotension
Aortic stenosis
Aortic insufficiency

Blood Disorders

Anemia
Hypoxemia
Polycythemia

Factors That Increase Demand

Increased Cardiac Output

Exercise
Emotion
Digestion of a large meal
Anemia
Hyperthyroidism

Increased Myocardial Need for Oxygen

Damaged myocardium
Myocardial hypertrophy
Aortic stenosis
Aortic insufficiency
Diastolic hypertension
Thyrotoxicosis
Strong emotions
Heavy exertion

---

prives the ischemic cells of much-needed oxygen and glucose. The cells convert to anaerobic metabolism, which leaves lactic acid as a waste product. As lactic acid accumulates, pain develops. Angina pectoris is transient, lasting for only 3 to 5 minutes. If blood flow is restored, no permanent myocardial damage occurs.[9, 27]

Clinical Manifestations and Diagnostic Findings

■ Characteristics of Angina

Angina pectoris produces transient paroxysmal attacks of substernal or precordial pain with the following characteristics:

Onset. Anginal attacks can develop quickly or slowly. Some clients ignore the chest pain thinking it will go away or that it is indigestion. Ask what the client was doing when pain began.

Location. Eighty percent to 90% of clients experience the pain as retrosternal or slightly to the left of the sternum.

Radiation. The pain usually radiates to the left shoulder and upper arm. It may then travel down the inner aspect of the left arm to the elbow, wrist, and fourth and fifth fingers. The pain may also radiate to the right shoulder, neck, jaw, or epigastric region. On occasion, the pain may be felt only in the area of radiation and not in the chest. Rarely is the pain localized to any one single small area over the precordium.[9]

Duration. Anginal attacks usually last a short time, typically less than 5 minutes. However, attacks precipitated by a heavy meal or extreme anger may last 15 to 20 minutes.

Sensation. The sensation of anginal pain is described as "squeezing," "burning," "pressing," "choking," "aching," or "bursting" pressure. The client often says the pain feels like "gas" or "heartburn" or "indigestion." Clients do not describe anginal pain as sharp or knifelike.

Severity. The pain of angina is usually mild or moderate in severity. Rarely is the pain described as severe.

Associated Characteristics. Other manifestations accompanying the pain include: dyspnea, pallor, sweating, faintness, palpitations, dizziness, and digestive disturbances.

Relieving/Aggravating Factors. Angina is aggravated by continued activity, and most anginal attacks quickly subside with the administration of nitroglycerin and rest. The typical "exertion—pain, rest—relief" pattern is the major clue to the diagnosis of angina pectoris.

Treatment. Has the client treated the pain with nitroglycerin? Did it work? Angina should subside after nitroglycerin use.

■ Patterns of Angina

Classic angina pectoris may be subdivided into the following basic patterns.

Stable Angina. Stable angina is paroxysmal chest pain or discomfort triggered by a predictable degree of exertion or emotion. Stable angina characteristically has a stable pattern of onset, duration, severity, and relieving factors.

Unstable Angina. Unstable angina (preinfarction angina, crescendo angina, or intermittent coronary syndrome) is paroxysmal chest pain triggered by an unpredictable degree of exertion or emotion, which may occur at night. Unstable angina attacks characteristically increase in number, duration, and severity over time.

Variant Angina. Variant angina (Prinzmetal's angina) is chest discomfort that is similar to classic angina but is of longer duration and may occur while at rest. These attacks tend to happen in the early hours of the day. Variant angina may result from coronary artery spasm and may be associated with elevation of the ST segment on the ECG.

Nocturnal Angina. Nocturnal angina is possibly associated with rapid eye movement (REM) sleep during dreaming.

Angina Decubitus. Angina decubitus is paroxysmal chest pain that occurs when the client reclines and lessens when the client sits or stands up.

Intractable Angina. Intractable angina is chronic incapacitating angina unresponsive to intervention.

Postinfarction Angina. Postinfarction angina occurs after MI, when residual ischemia may cause episodes of angina.

■ Diagnostic Tests

Electrocardiography. The ECG tracings remain normal in 25% to 30% of clients with angina pectoris. An ECG taken in the presence of pain may document transient ischemic attacks with ST segment elevation or depression. An ECG taken during an episode of pain may also suggest coronary artery involvement and the extent of cardiac muscle affected by the ischemic event.[9]

Exercise Electrocardiography (Stress Testing). The client exercises on a treadmill or stationary bicycle, until reaching 85% of maximal heart rate. ECG or vital sign changes may indicate ischemia.[52]

Radioisotope Imaging. Various nuclear imaging techniques are used to evaluate the myocardial muscle. Regions of poor perfusion or ischemia appear as areas of diminished or absent activity (cold spots).

Coronary Angiography. Angiography provides the most accurate information about the patency of the coronary arteries. This diagnostic assessment allows visualization of the artery and any partial or complete blockages.[27]

These diagnostic tests are described fully in Chapter 44.

Emergency Care

■ Medical Management

Medical management of clients with angina pectoris focuses on two goals: (1) relief of the acute attack and (2) prevention of further attacks to reduce the risk of MI.

Angina pectoris is diagnosed by history and various diagnostic tests. A complete history of the pain and its pattern is taken. Clients are encouraged to describe the pain in their own words. A complete symptom analysis is recorded. This description provides a baseline that can be used in ongoing care.

Most physical findings are transient. The client exhibits pallor or has cold and clammy skin. Tachycardia and hypertension may be recorded. Pulsus alternans (force of each beat varies) may be present at the onset of ischemia attacks. On auscultation, an S_3 or S_4 gallop or a paradoxical split of S_2 may be noted. If the client has mitral regurgitation from ischemia of the papillary muscle, a murmur will be heard.

The primary goal of pharmacologic treatment of angina is to balance the supply and demand of the myocardium by altering the various components of the process increasing oxygen supply to the myocardium or reducing myocardial oxygen demand. The components of myocardial oxygen consumption that can be pharmacologically treated are blood pressure, heart rate, contractility, and left ventricular volume. The agents used in the treatment of angina are listed in Table 45–1.[9, 27, 89]

The major types of medications used in angina pectoris are (1) opiate analgesics, (2) vasodilators, (3) beta-adrenergic blocking agents (e.g., propranolol), (4) calcium-channel blockers, and (5) antiplatelet medications.[27, 82, 123, 125]

Vasodilators

Nitroglycerin, a short-acting nitrate, has been the medication of choice against anginal attacks since 1867. Today, nitroglycerin remains the major weapon against acute attacks. Administered sublingually, per tablet, or via translingual spray, nitroglycerin acts to relieve the pain of angina within 1 to 2 minutes.

Nitroglycerin reduces the oxygen requirements of the myocardium by causing coronary and systemic vasodilation, a decrease in blood pressure, and a decrease in left ventricular wall tension (preload), which consequently decreases the cardiac workload.[27]

Long-acting nitrates act to maintain coronary artery vasodilation, thereby promoting a greater flow of blood and oxygen to the heart muscle. Currently, the most frequently prescribed nitrates are isosorbide dinitrate (Isordil) and long-acting nitroglycerin preparations (e.g., nitroglycerin ointment or transdermal patch).

Nitroglycerin is also available as a sustained-release concentrated patch that can be worn for 10 to 12 hours. Long-acting nitrates produce the same general side effects as nitroglycerin (i.e., severe headache, flushing of the skin, nausea and vomiting, hypotension, vertigo, and syncope). Approximately two thirds of clients taking long-acting nitrates develop a tolerance to the medication. Therefore, maintain a 12-hour drug-free interval to preserve responsiveness. For most clients, this drug-free time is at night.[82, 89, 103]

Beta-Adrenergic Blockers

Administration of a beta-adrenergic blocking agent will reduce the workload of the heart and may decrease the number of anginal attacks. Propranolol reduces the oxygen requirements of the myocardium by blocking beta-receptors, inhibiting catecholamine action at these sites, and reducing cardiac contractility, sinus node rate, and atrioventricular (AV) conduction velocity. These actions, in turn, raise the exercise tolerance of clients with reduced coronary blood flow. (See Table 45–1).

Because of the adverse effects of propranolol on the bronchial tree, pharmaceutical companies have developed other beta-blockers that act more specifically on the heart. Examples of beta-blocking agents that are cardioselective are metoprolol (Lopressor) and atenolol (Tenormin). In small doses, these medications can induce full cardiac beta-blockage without causing wheezing in clients with pulmonary disease. At larger doses, cardioselective beta-blockers may become nonselective and block both the heart and bronchial beta-receptors.[82, 89]

Calcium-Channel Blockers

Calcium plays a major role in the electrical excitation of cardiac cells and in the contraction of vascular and cardiac muscle cells. The Food and Drug Administration has accepted several calcium-channel blockers for use in the United States; some examples are amlodipine, nifedipine (Procardia, Norvasc, Cardene), verapamil (Calan, Isoptin), and diltiazem (Cardizem). The clinical use of these drugs varies with the way each agent affects the heart. Nifedipine and amlodipine have the largest peripheral arterial vasodialting effect, verapamil has a moderate effect, and diltiazem has the least effect. Physicians usually order nifedipine to treat angina. Nifedipine appears to complement the antianginal action of the vasodilators and beta-blockers.[51, 82, 89, 125] (See Table 45–1.)

Antiplatelet Medications

Antiplatelet drugs such as aspirin (acetylsalicylic acid) inhibit platelet aggregation by inhibiting the formation of thromboxane A_2. When used to treat clients with unstable angina, aspirin lowers the chance of developing an acute MI and reduces mortality by 50%. Recommended dosage is from 80 to 325 mg/day for prevention of MI in clients with unstable angina. Aspirin is currently the only antiplatelet drug recommended for the prevention of acute MI in clients with unstable angina. Because it can cause gastrointestinal bleeding, gastric ulcers, and erosive gastritis, instruct clients to take the enteric-coated form. Researchers have not found other antiplatelet medications to be as effective as aspirin in preventing MI. In the treatment of unstable angina, antiplatelet drugs should be used only in addition to risk reduction interventions such as control of hypertension, diabetes, and hyperlipidemia.[125, 141]

Antiplatelet drugs are also used to prevent restenosis and thrombosis in clients who have undergone an interventional procedure such as DCA or stent placement. In addition to aspirin, other antiplatelet drugs such as dipyridamole (Persantine) and sulfinpyrazone (Anturane) are used occasionally in these clients.[16, 22, 39]

Outcomes

The goal of therapy in the treatment of angina is to prevent the progression of the disease and the development of MI. At present, the most effective treatment is to eliminate or reduce known cardiovascular risk factors. Stopping smoking reduces the risk of coronary heart disease by 37%; a 10% reduction in cholesterol lowers the risk of coronary heart disease by 20%; and a 6-mm reduction in diastolic blood pressure lowers the risk of coronary heart disease by 10%.[129] The American Heart Association recommends that persons with angina control their modifiable risk factors and seek prompt treatment for episodes of chest pain.

■ Nursing Management of the Medical Client

In addition to documenting the clinical manifestations of angina, ascertain how long the client has had angina, whether he or she has risk factors for CAD, and his or her emotional reaction to chest pain. Start cardiac monitoring, obtain a 12-lead ECG, and control ongoing angina. Until the angina is controlled and coronary blood flow reestablished, the client is at risk of myocardial damage from myocardial ischemia. If the client reports angina, assess the pain and ask the client whether it is the same pain experienced in the past. Note new characteristics or increased pain. Give sublingual nitroglycerin tablets or spray as prescribed. Because nitroglycerin causes vasodilation and hypotension, monitor blood pressure. If the pain is not relieved after three nitroglycerin tablets 5 minutes apart or morphine, notify the physician. In addition, an environment that provides rest and security as well as allays fear and anxiety will help reduce pain.[9, 27, 75]

Community and Self-Care

The client must be knowledgeable in the care of episodes of angina and how to reduce the risk factors that exacerbate the process. The following information should be used as needed to help clients control risk factors for angina pectoris.

First, educate the client to avoid activities or habits that precipitate angina, such as eating large meals, drinking coffee, smoking, exercising too strenuously, going out in cold weather, and excessive stress. If an attack begins, the client should stop the activity and sit down. An antianginal medication, for example, nitroglycerin, should be taken. Three pills can be taken sublingually 5 minutes apart. If the pain does not subside, or worsens, or radiates, the client should be taken to an emergency department (not drive himself or herself).

Second, explain the importance of daily management of hypertension. It is important that the client take daily medication even if no clinical manifestations are evident (see also Chapter 50).

Third, encourage and help plan a regular program of daily exercise to promote improved coronary circulation and weight management.

Fourth, instruct clients who smoke to quit smoking at once. Smoking cigarettes raises carboxyhemoglobin levels

Table 45–1. Antianginal Agents

Class	Example	Action	Common Side Effects	Nursing Implications	Contraindications
Opiate analgesic	Morphine sulfate	Relieves severe pain and anxiety associated with acute MI Reduces venous return: thereby, myocardial workload is decreased	Sedation, confusion, hypotension, nausea and vomiting, constipation, dry eyes, and respiratory depression	When administering IV, administer slowly over 3–5 min; monitor closely for hypotension and respiratory depression	Hypersensitivity; use cautiously in clients with head injury, pulmonary disease, undiagnosed abdominal pain, liver disease, or history of addiction
Vasodilators	Nitrates/nitrites; nitroglycerin SL, translingual spray, and nitroglycerin IV Long-acting; isosorbide dinitrate Nitroglycerin, topical	Relax smooth muscle of coronary and peripheral blood vessels, causing an increase in their diameter; blood flow is improved and resistance is decreased As peripheral resistance decreases, workload on heart is reduced, and oxygen supply–demand ratio improves	Flushing, headache, dizziness, hypotension Tolerance to topical long-acting nitrates	Assess baseline cardiac function, heart rate, and blood pressure Postural hypotension may occur, caution clients to change position slowly, especially when taking NTG tablets SL Can take up to 3 NTG tablets SL at 5-min intervals if necessary; if pain is not relieved after 15 min, physician should be contacted immediately or client should report to hospital Tablets are inactivated by light, heat, air, and moisture; store at room temperature, in tight-fitting amber glass container A potent NTG tablet should produce a burning sensation under tongue when taken SL: check expiration date When administering IV, titrate in 5 μg/min every 3–5 minutes until pain free or hypotensive Maintain a 12-hr drug free interval when using topical long-acting nitrates (usually at night)	Hypersensitivity, severe anemia, pericardial tamponade, and constrictive pericarditis; use cautiously with head trauma, cerebral hemorrhage, glaucoma, hypertrophic cardiomyopathy, and severe liver impairment
Calcium channel blockers	Diltiazem Nifedipine Verapamil Bepridil Nicardipine	Reduce vascular smooth muscle tone by interfering with the ability of free calcium ions to initiate muscular contraction Causes vasodilation, increased myocardial oxygen supply, and decreased peripheral resistance	Dizziness, hypotension, bradycardia with diltiazem, diarrhea, abdominal cramps, nausea, vomiting, rash, dermatitis	Assess baseline cardiac function, ECG, heart rate, and blood pressure Monitor hepatic and renal function Food delays absorption and reduces plasma levels Decrease dosage gradually Administer slowly IV	Hypersensitivity, bradycardia, second- or third-degree heart block, uncompensated heart failure; use cautiously in liver disease and uncontrolled arrhythmias

	Drugs	Action	Side Effects	Nursing Implications	Contraindications/Cautions
Beta blockers	Selective beta-adrenergic blockers: acebutolol, atenolol, metoprolol Nonselective beta-blockers: labetolol, nadolol, pindolol, propranolol, timolol	Competes with adrenergic neurotransmitters at beta$_1$ and beta$_2$ nerve or cellular receptor sites Blunts sympathetic effect and prevents increases in heart rate, force of contraction, and myocardial oxygen requirements	Bradycardia and heart block, bronchospasm, altered glucose metabolism, diarrhea, hypotension, heart failure, CNS-fatigue, malaise, sexual dysfunction in males, withdrawal, insomnia, and hypertriglyceridemia	Monitor BP and pulse frequently during dosage adjustment and periodically thereafter Monitor I&O, daily weights, signs of heart failure, and bronchospasm Assess frequency and severity of chest episodes during therapy Instruct client to continue taking even if feeling well and not to abruptly discontinue medication Teach client how to take BP and pulse and instruct to monitor on regular basis Caution client to make position changes slowly to avoid dizziness	Asthma, aortic valvular disease, bradyarrhythmias, heart block, brittle diabetes, MAO inhibitor use; use in heart failure controversial.
Antiplatelet agents	Acetylsalicylic acid (aspirin, ASA); if ASA-intolerant, use ticlopidine	Decreases platelet aggregation and reduces thrombus formation Used to prevent coronary heart disease, and as adjunctive treatment in angina and acute MI	Most common are gastric irritation and GI bleeding; other reported side effects include tinnitis, hearing loss, anemia, hemolysis	Teach client and family about dosing, drug interactions, and potential side effects Suggest that elderly clients and those with dyspepsia or heartburn use enteric-coated aspirin	Clients with aspirin intolerance, hypersensitivity, peptic ulcer disease, recent GI bleeding, history of coagulation disorders or bleeding problems, uncontrolled hypertension
	Dipyridamole	Decreases platelet aggregation by inhibiting phosphodiesterase Also causes coronary vasodilation by inhibiting adenosine uptake	Headache, dizziness, flushing, hypotension and nausea; when administered IV can cause MI and arrhythmias Risk of bleeding may be increased when used with anticoagulants/thrombolytics	Monitor BP and pulse during period of dosage adjustment Administer full glass of water 1 hr before or 2 hr after meals for faster absorption May be administered with meals if GI irritation develops Tablets may be crushed and mixed with food if needed Instruct client to take medication at evenly spaced intervals as prescribed Caution client to make position changes slowly to avoid dizziness Advise client to check with pharmacist before taking over-the-counter medications Teach client to notify physician if unusual bleeding or bruising occurs	Hypersensitivity Use with caution in clients with hypotension or platelet defects

BP, blood pressure; CNS, central nervous system; ECG, electrocardiogram; GI, gastrointestinal; I&O, intake and output; IV, intravenous; MI, myocardial infarction; SL, sublingual; MAO, monoamine oxidase; NTG, nitroglycerin.

in the blood, which reduces the amount of oxygen available to the myocardium, and can precipitate an anginal attack. Clients with angina pectoris exposed for 2 hours to cigarette smoke suffer elevations in carboxyhemoglobin concentration; decreased exercise time, and increased heart rate and blood pressure. Also, advise clients to avoid "passive smoking" (i.e., being with a smoker or in a smoke-filled room).

Fifth, urge overweight clients to lose excess weight. Encourage them to eat small meals, avoid high calorie and high cholesterol diets, abstain from gas-forming foods, and rest for short periods after meals. In addition, recommend a high fiber diet, which may not only prevent constipation and other intestinal tract ailments but also decrease the number and severity of anginal attacks. Diets high in fiber may also lower serum cholesterol and triglyceride levels. CAD is less common among clients with high intake of dietary fiber than in those with low intake. High fiber diets can also decrease hypertension.

Finally, help the client who leads an active, hectic life to adjust activities to a level below that which precipitates anginal attacks. Encourage brief rest periods throughout the working day, an early bedtime, and longer or more frequent vacations. Advise clients who are anxious and nervous to consider counseling. Relaxation techniques may also be used.[9, 29, 40]

Acute Myocardial Infarction

Acute myocardial infarction (MI), also known as a heart attack, coronary occlusion, or simply a "coronary," is a life-threatening condition characterized by the formation of localized necrotic areas within the myocardium.[29] MI usually follows the sudden occlusion of a coronary artery and the abrupt cessation of blood and oxygen flow to the heart muscle. Because the heart muscle must function continuously, blockage of blood to the muscle and the development of necrotic areas can be lethal.

Every year approximately 1.5 million Americans have heart attacks. MI is the leading cause of death in America. Heart attacks cause an estimated 500,000 deaths each year. About 240,000 women die of MI.[8, 41, 129] Approximately 250,000 people die before they reach the hospital. Studies indicate that, half of all heart attack victims wait more than 2 hours before getting help. On the basis of data from the Framingham study, approximately 45% of all heart attacks are in people under the age of 65 years, and 5% are in people under age 40 years. Four out of five people who die of myocardial infarction are 65 years or older.[7, 8, 115]

Etiology and Risk Factors

The most common cause of MI is complete or nearly complete occlusion of a coronary artery, usually the result of atherosclerosis. The vessel lumen slowly occludes and is often blocked by a thrombus. When blood flow ceases abruptly, the myocardial tissue supplied by that artery dies. Other causes of acute occlusion include coronary artery spasm and hemorrhage into a plaque. The risk factors that predispose a client to a heart attack are the same as for all forms of CAD (see earlier).[19]

Pathophysiology

MI can be considered the endpoint of CAD. Unlike the temporary ischemia that occurs with angina, prolonged unrelieved ischemia causes irreversible damage to the myocardium. Cardiac cells can withstand ischemia for about 20 minutes before cellular death occurs. Because the myocardium is metabolically active, signs of ischemia can be seen within 8 to 10 seconds of decreased blood flow. When the heart is not sustained by blood and oxygen, it converts to anaerobic metabolism. This form of metabolism creates less adenosine triphosphate (ATP) and more lactic acid as a by-product. Myocardial cells are very sensitive to changes in pH and become less functional. Acidosis makes the myocardium more vulnerable to the effects of the lysosomal enzymes within the cell. Acidosis leads to conduction system disorders, and dysrhythmias develop. Contractility is also reduced, decreasing the heart's ability to pump. As the myocardial cells necrose, intracellular enzymes are introduced into the bloodstream, where they can be detected by laboratory tests.

Figure 45–7 illustrates the depth of various types of infarctions in the wall of the ventricle. Cellular necrosis occurs in one layer of myocardial tissue in subendocardial, intramural, and subepicardial infarctions. In a transmural infarction, cellular necrosis is present in all three layers of myocardial tissue. The infarct site is called the zone of infarction and necrosis. Around it is a zone of hypoxic injury. This zone is able to return to normal but may also necrose if blood flow is not restored. The outermost zone is called the zone of ischemia; damage to this area is reversible.

The most common site of MI is the anterior wall of the left ventricle near the apex. Infarction of the anterior left ventricle results from thrombosis of the descending branch of the left coronary artery (Fig. 45–8). Other common sites are (1) the posterior wall of the left ventricle near the base and behind the posterior cusp of the mitral valve and (2) the inferior (diaphragmatic) surface of the heart. Infarction of the posterior left ventricle results from occlusion of the right coronary artery or circumflex branch of the left coronary artery. An inferior infarction occurs when the right coronary artery is occluded. In nearly one fourth of inferior wall MIs, the right ventricle is the site of infarction. Atrial infarctions develop less than 5% of the time.[147, 153]

Clinical Manifestations and Diagnostic Findings

The major clinical manifestation of MI is chest pain (Fig. 45–9), similar to angina pectoris but more severe and unrelieved by nitroglycerin. The pain may radiate to the neck, jaw, shoulder, back, or left arm. Also, the pain may present near the epigastrium, simulating indigestion.

Understanding Myocardial Infarction and Its Treatment

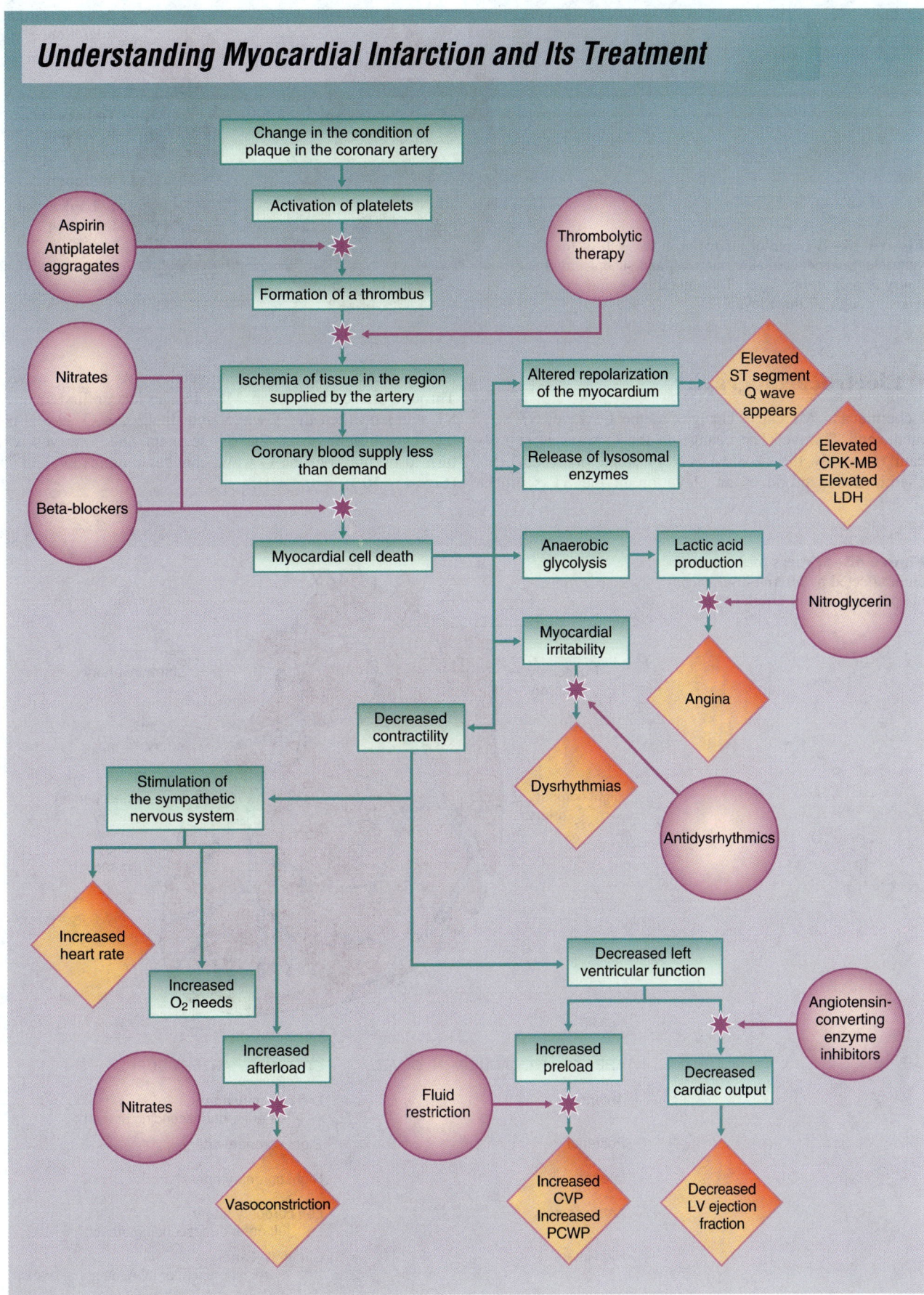

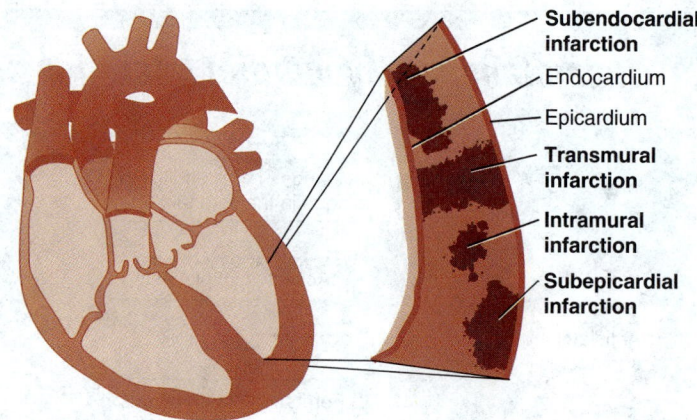

Figure 45–7. Depth of infarction in the wall of the ventricle. Subendocardial, intramural, and subepicardial injury is only in one layer. Transmural infarction extends through all three layers.

■ Electrocardiography

Ischemia and MI cause changes in the Q wave, ST segment, and T wave. The change in the Q wave is significant (normally the Q wave is very small or absent). Ischemic tissue produces an elevation in the ST segment and a peaked T wave or inversion of the T wave. Through the course of an MI, changes occur first in the ST segment, then the T wave, and finally the Q wave. As the myocardium heals, the ST segment and T waves return to normal, but the Q wave changes remains evident.[26] (Fig. 45–10.)

Figure 45–8. Areas of the myocardium affected by arterial insufficiency of specific coronary arteries.

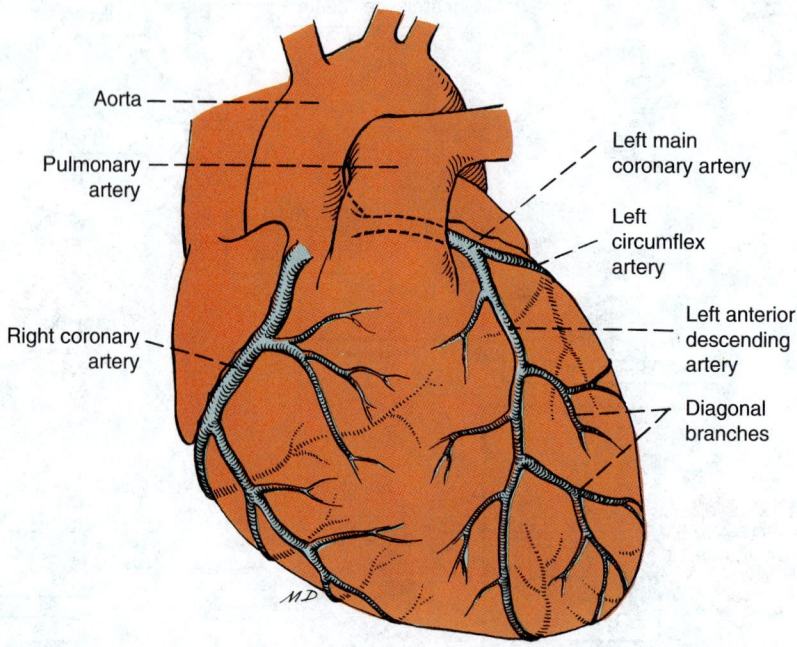

AREA OF MYOCARDIUM INVOLVED	CORONARY ARTERY SUPPLY
Anterior	Left coronary artery, left anterior descending branch
Posterior	Right coronary artery
Inferior	Right coronary artery
Anteroseptal	Left coronary artery, left anterior descending branch
High lateral	Circumflex artery, marginal branch, or LCA, diagonal branch
Apical	Usually LCA, left anterior branch, may be RCA, posterior descending branch

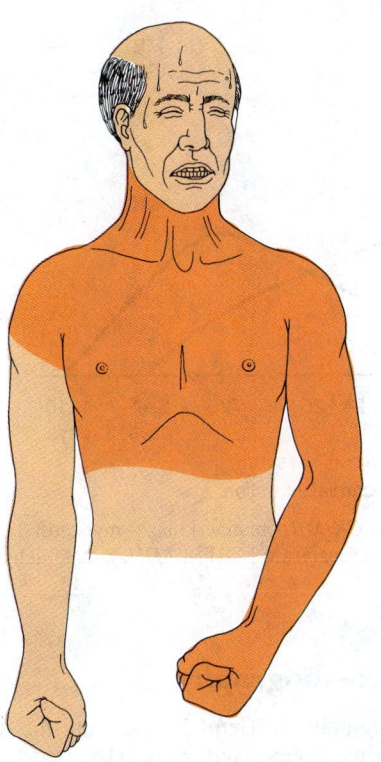

Figure 45–9. Possible extent of pain from a myocardial infarction.

■ Laboratory Tests

Laboratory findings include an elevated serum creatine kinase (CK) MB isoenzyme, elevated lactate dehydrogenase (LDH) M_1 isoenzyme, elevated serum aspartate aminotransferase (AST), and leukocytosis, and elevated erythrocyte sedimentation rate.

Serum levels of CK-MB (an isoenzyme of CK found primarily in cardiac muscle) increase 3 to 6 hours after the onset of chest pain, reach a peak in 12 to 18 hours, and return to normal levels in 3 to 4 days.[26]

The LDH_1 subunit is plentiful in heart muscle and is released into the serum when myocardial damage occurs. Serum levels of LDH elevate 14 to 24 hours after onset of myocardial damage, peak within 48 to 72 hours, and slowly return to normal over the next 7 to 14 days. See Figure 45–11.

Serum levels of AST rise within several hours after the onset of chest pain, peak within 12 to 18 hours, and return to normal within 3 to 4 days.

Leukocytosis of 10,000 to 20,000 mm^3 appears on the second day after MI and disappears in 1 week.

■ Radionuclide Imaging

Radionuclide imaging is a new method of diagnosing MI. A scintigraphic camera records gamma rays emitted by a radioisotope. Technetium 99m–tagged pyrophosphate

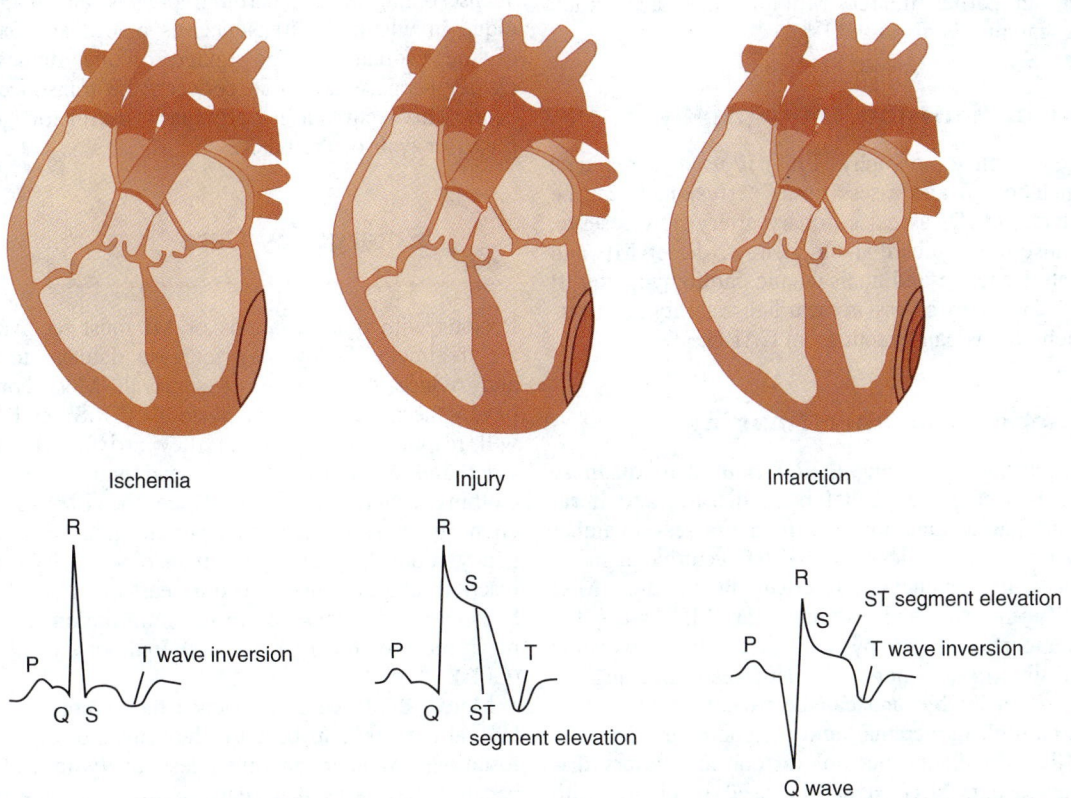

Ischemia Injury Infarction

Figure 45–10. Zones of hypoxic injury, zone of infarction, and zone of necrosis and the electrocardiographic patterns that accompany these changes during myocardial infarction.

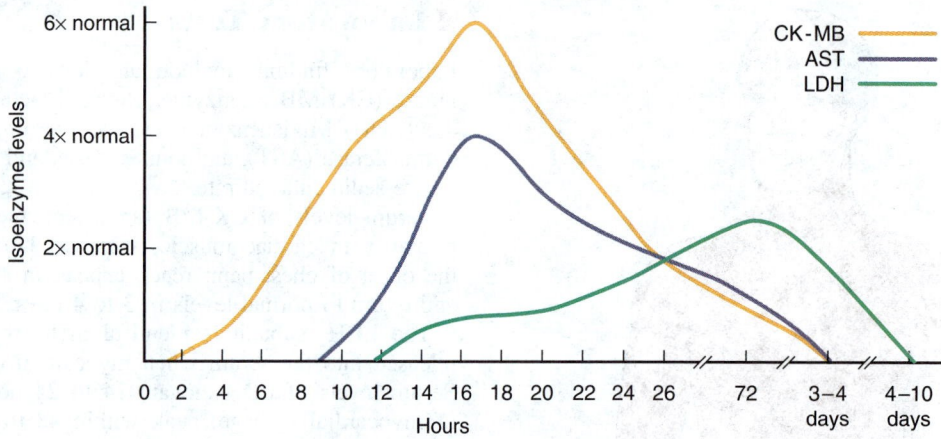

Figure 45–11. Isoenzyme alterations in acute myocardial infarction. *CK-MB*, creatine kinase–myocardial band; *SGOT*, serum glutamic oxaloacetic transaminase (aspartate aminotransferase [AST]); *LDH*, lactate dehydrogenase.

binds with calcium in areas of myocardial necrosis. Areas of uptake (hot spots) seen on nuclear imaging indicate areas of infarction. However, because this test does not give positive results for 24 hours, it cannot be used to diagnose an acute MI during the early stage. Radiolabeled antimyosin is another agent used for hot spot imaging.[33] As mentioned earlier, thallium 201, another radioisotope, produces a cold spot on an area of infarction or ischemia. It has limited diagnostic value, however, because it cannot be used to differentiate between a new infarct and a scar from an earlier infarct. Multiple-gated acquisition (MUGA) scanning is also used.[154]

■ Positron Emission Tomography

Positron emission tomography (PET) is used to evaluate cardiac metabolism and assess tissue perfusion. It can be used to detect CAD, assess coronary artery flow reserve, measure absolute myocardial blood flow, detect MI, and differentiate ischemic and nonischemic cardiomyopathy. It can also be used to assess myocardial viability to determine which clients can benefit from CABG.[2, 154]

■ Magnetic Resonance Imaging

Magnetic resonance imaging (MRI) is used to diagnose great vessel disease, congenital heart disease, and intracardiac and paracardiac masses. It can assess chamber size, wall motion and thickness, and left ventricular mass, and evaluate the patency of CABGs. In addition, MRI can identify the site and extent of an MI, assess the effects of reperfusion therapy, and differentiate reversible and irreversible tissue injury. Magnetic resonance angiography is now available and can be used to evaluate the coronary, carotid, intracranial, and peripheral arteries. The use of MRI as a diagnostic tool for coronary artery disease is increasing. MRI cannot be used in clients with implanted metallic devices such as pacemakers or defibrillators.[2]

■ Echocardiography

Echocardiography is useful in assessing the ability of the heart walls to contract and relax. The transducer is placed on the chest, and images are relayed to a monitor screen.[154]

■ Transesophageal Echocardiography

Transesophageal echocardiography is an imaging technique in which the transducer is placed against the wall of the esophagus. The image of the myocardium is clearer because no air is between the transducer and the heart. This technique is particularly useful for viewing the posterior wall of the heart.[2, 153]

Emergency Care

Persons with manifestations of MI must receive immediate treatment. Delay may increase damage to the heart and reduce the chance of survival. Most communities have emergency medical systems (EMS; call 911) that will respond quickly. Until they arrive, keep the client quiet and calm. Elevate the head and loosen any tight clothing around the neck. Once the EMS arrives, the client is assessed and transported quickly to an emergency room. The client is given oxygen, has an IV line inserted, and is connected to a heart monitor. Clients who become unconscious before reaching the emergency room may receive emergency cardiopulmonary resuscitation (CPR).[1, 7, 142]

Many people who experience the symptoms of MI delay calling for help because they misinterpret their manifestations. Women are even less likely to call for help because they think that heart disease is a male problem.[41] Community education to "call first, call fast" is important.[108]

Critical Care

Major goals of care for clients with acute MI are (1) Successful treatment of the acute attack and prompt alleviation of manifestations, (2) prevention of complications and further attacks, and (3) rehabilitation and education of the client and significant others.

The client who suffers an acute MI needs immediate admission to a hospital with a coronary care unit, if possible. The first 24 hours after an MI is the time of highest risk of sudden death. Invasive monitoring (arterial and pulmonary artery pressure lines) is commonly used.[115, 117] (See The Bridge to Critical Care on arterial lines and Chapter 46 for the Bridge to Critical Care on pulmonary artery pressure lines.)

The first 6 hours after the onset of pain is the crucial time frame for salvage of the myocardium. Pain control is

---

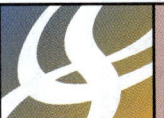

BRIDGE TO CRITICAL CARE

Arterial Lines

Insertion of a catheter into an artery for direct measurement of systolic, diastolic, and mean blood pressure readings.

Insertion Sites

- Radial
- Brachial
- Axillary
- Femoral
- Dorsalis pedis

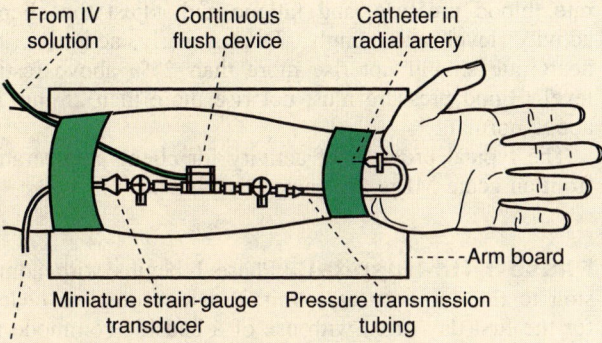

Indications for Use

- Monitoring any major medical or surgical condition that compromises cardiac output or fluid volume status
- Continuous assessment of arterial perfusion to the major organ systems
- Continuous measurement of systole, diastole, and mean arterial blood pressure (MAP)
  MAP = (2 × diastolic + systolic)/ ÷ 3
- Direct arterial access—blood gas measurements
- Assessment of arterial compliance and stroke volume
  Pulse pressure = (systolic − diastolic)

Nursing Precautions

- Access collateral circulation prior to arterial cannulation
- Allen's test to assess radial and ulner arteries
- Continued assessment of tissue perfusion at arterial site
- Maintenance of arterial line patency (pressure tubing, heparinized solution, pressure bag)

Complications

- Blood back-up from improper setup
- Thrombus formation
- Embolization
- Arterial spasm
- Ischemic damage
- Amputation
- Hemorrhage
- Infection

Typical Arterial Waveform

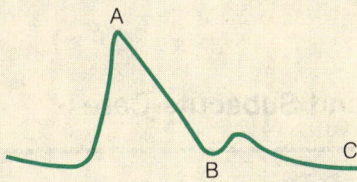

The three components of a typical waveform:
A, systolic peak; B, dicrotic notch; and C, end-diastole.

Effect of Premature Ventricular Contractions on Arterial Pressure

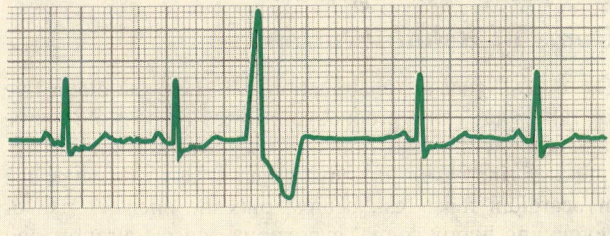

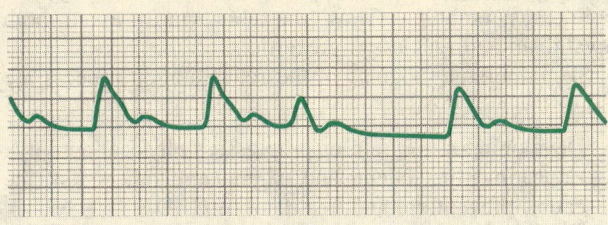

a priority. Continued pain is a manifestation of myocardial ischemia. Pain also stimulates the autonomic nervous system and increases preload, increasing myocardial demands. Oxygen is used to treat tissue hypoxia. Because dysrhythmias are common, ECG monitoring is essential. Antiarrhythmics are begun. Anticoagulants are given to reduce the risk of embolism.[1, 5, 32, 68, 76] Stool softeners are used to relieve constipation and to lower the risk of bradycardia from straining.[1, 32]

Recently clinicians have treated acute MI with medications that lyse or dissolve the clot that forms part of the blockage of the coronary artery. Thrombolytic therapy includes streptokinase, urokinase, tissue-plasminogen activator (t-PA), and anisoylated plasminogen streptokinase activator complex (anistreplase, APSAC). To be most effective, thrombolytic agents must be given within 3 to 6 hours after the onset of chest pain.[1] After the thrombolytic agent is administered, IV heparin is usually continued for 5 to 7 days. All of these thrombolytic agents can be given IV, and some clinicians initiate the infusions at the scene of the infarction.[95, 96, 119] The Pathophysiology/ Treatment Algorithm depicts the management of MI.

Not all clients with MI are suitable candidates for thrombolytic therapy. Complications of thrombolytics include bleeding, allergic reactions, and stroke.[35] Successful reperfusion of the coronary arteries is evidenced by return of the ECG changes to normal; relief of chest pain; presence of reperfusion dysrhythmias (usually sudden onset of frequent premature ventricular contractions [PVCs] or short runs of PVCs); and a rapid, early peak of the CK MB isoenzyme ("washout").[115] An aspirin (80- to 325-mg tablets) a day should be continued once the client returns home.[20, 115]

Acute and Subacute Care

A successful rehabilitation program begins the moment the client enters the coronary care unit for emergency care and continues for months and even years after discharge home from the healthcare facility.[26]

■ Medical Management
Goals of Rehabilitation

The overall goal of rehabilitation is to help the client live as full, vital, and productive a life as possible while remaining within the limits of the heart's ability to respond to increases in activity and stress. Although the myocardium must rest, bedrest puts the client at risk of developing hypovolemia, hypoxemia, muscle atrophy, and pulmonary embolus. Thus, the client must avoid both invalidism and reckless overexertion.

Six important subgoals of the rehabilitation process are as follows:

1. Developing a program of progressive physical activity
2. Educating the client and significant others on the cause, prevention, and treatment of CAD
3. Helping the client accept the limitations imposed by illness

4. Aiding the client in adjusting to changes in occupational goals
5. Lessening exposure to risk factors
6. Changing the psychosocial factors adversely affecting recovery from CAD.[155, 159]

Program of Physical Activity

Clients who have suffered a heart attack usually remain on bedrest for less than 24 hours unless complications such as congestive heart failure (CHF) or dysrhythmias develop. Remember that protracted bedrest produces severe problems. The client loses 10% to 15% of skeletal muscle and contractile strength within the first week of bedrest, and 20% to 25% after 3 weeks of bedrest.

The client must increase activities gradually to avoid overtaxing the heart as it pumps oxygenated blood to the muscles. The METs (metabolic equivalents) system provides one way of measuring the amount of oxygen needed to perform an activity: 1 MET equals 3.5 ml of oxygen per kilogram of body weight per minute. One MET is approximately equivalent to the oxygen uptake a client requires when resting. Early mobilization activities after an acute MI should not exceed 1 to 2 METs (e.g., shaving, washing, and self-feeding). Later activities can increase up to 10 or 11 METs (e.g., cycling, running).

With each activity level increase, monitor the heart rate, blood pressure, and fatigue and adjust the client's activity level accordingly. During early activities, the heart rate should not rise more than 25% above resting level. Blood pressure must not rise more than 25 mm Hg above normal.[155]

The typical program of activity for clients recuperating from an acute MI is designated by phases.

Phase I (In-Hospital). Phase I begins with admission to the coronary care unit. Provide complete bedrest for the first day or so with use of a bedside commode for bowel movements. Most clients receive a 2-g sodium diet. If nausea is present, provide a clear liquid diet until it subsides. A coronary care nurse or physiotherapist should start passive exercises. As strength is regained, have the client sit for brief periods on the side of the bed and dangle the feet. Allow the client to ambulate to a bedside chair for 15 to 20 minutes if permissible after the first day.

When the client is transferred from the coronary care unit to an intermediate or regular unit, bathroom privileges and self-care activities are encouraged. Wireless heart monitoring (telemetry) may continue. Allow brief walks in the hall with supervision. The length and duration of these walks are increased progressively according to the client's endurance.

Help the client avoid fatigue. Dyspnea, chest pain, tachycardia, and a sense of exhaustion warn that the client is attempting to do too much. Instruct the client regarding these warning signs of overexertion.

Client education during phase I should include anatomy and physiology of the heart and CAD, risk factors and management of CAD, behavioral counseling, and home activities.

Phase II (Intermediate). If no complications arise, the physician will discharge the client home by the end of the second week. Nearly 50% of people who suffer an acute MI have an uncomplicated hospital course without evidence of angina, heart failure, or major arrhythmias. There is a growing trend toward early discharge of clients with uncomplicated MI. A team at one healthcare facility discharges post-MI clients at the end of the fourth day. However, they allow clients to go home early only if their households have adequate help and are conducive to rest. Also, such clients are followed carefully by trained nurse-clinicians who come to their homes and supervise their physiologic status, exercise, and diet on an alternate-day basis. Researchers hope that earlier discharge after MI will reduce depression as well as the expense of hospitalization.[50] The Bridge to Home Healthcare provides suggestions for helping the client to adjust to convalescence at home.

Resuming sexual activity may be one of the most difficult aspects of returning to normal life after an MI. One study reports that over 50% of a group of women reported fear of resuming sexual activity after an MI (44% of their partners reported similar concerns). Sexual intercourse may resume 4 to 8 weeks after an MI if the physician agrees. A good rule of thumb to use is that the client should be able to climb two flights of stairs before resuming sexual activity. Caution clients not to eat or drink alcoholic beverages immediately before intercourse. Taking nitroglycerin before intercourse may help prevent exertional angina.[105, 107, 146]

Advise the client to stop smoking. Encourage frequent walks, but the client must avoid strenuous activities such as shoveling snow. The walking program aims toward a goal of 2 miles in less than 60 minutes. A monitored group program may help the client achieve the best possible physical conditioning. These programs offer a variety of training devices, such as treadmills, stationary bicycles, and rowing machines, to facilitate fitness. In addition, clients are trained in warm-up and stretching exercises.[106]

After an acute MI, many clients are instructed to take one aspirin daily. Aspirin inhibits platelet aggregation and may be useful in preventing MIs. Side effects include epigastric distress, gastrointestinal bleeding, and nausea.

Some clients may be able to return to work at the end of 8 or 9 weeks if they remain asymptomatic. Clients with less physically strenuous jobs can sometimes work full-time, but manual laborers may have to work part-time or find less taxing work.[66]

Between the 8th and 10th weeks, the client requires a complete physical examination, including ECG, exercise

---

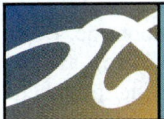

BRIDGE TO HOME HEALTHCARE

Myocardial Infarction: Convalescence and Home Care

Pamela Singh, M.S., R.N., P.H.N., *San Diego, California*

Helping the postmyocardial client to adjust his or her life-style by teaching healthy heart living is the role of the home care nurse. During the acute episode of myocardial infarction (MI), stress is high and the client may recall very little of what was taught. Teaching is focused on those areas that will assist the client to perform self-care.

Instruct the client and significant other to monitor for clinical manifestations that may indicate extensions and reoccurrences of MI. Clients need to report indigestion, shortness of breath, increased edema, and palpitations. Learning when to call the physician or nurse for these physical problems is very important.

Assessment of what the client knows about his or her medications is paramount. Knowing what the medication is called, its function, the schedule for taking it, and its side effects is required for patient safety. Generally, multiple medications are prescribed and you give the client written instructions and information about each medication. Many pharmacists provide a computer printout of medications and interactions for the client to keep. Daily medication planners that have compartments for various times of day allow the patient to prefill medications for a week at a time and may prevent errors.

The convalescence period for the client and significant other creates anxiety about daily activities. Instruct the client that to prevent vasodilation baths or showers should not be prolonged. Use of tepid water and a stool or bath chair in the shower is recommended. Encourage the use of energy conservation techniques such as keeping the arms at waist level and getting enough rest to prevent fatigue. Routine household activities and mild recreational activities such as playing golf are usually permitted. Climbing more than two flights of stairs and lifting more than 20 lb are restricted.

An appropriate unsupervised exercise is a prescribed indoor walking program. Exercising after a heavy meal or during mild illness is contraindicated. Instruct the client to begin each exercise session with a warm-up period (which may be as long as 15 minutes) and to end with a cool-down period. Walking should be constant and last long enough to increase blood flow to the muscles.

The client or caregiver should have an emergency plan that includes having someone available to drive if necessary and someone in the home who knows basic cardiopulmonary resuscitation (CPR). A personal emergency response system may be appropriate for clients who live alone. Some emergency response systems are worn around the neck, and the push of a button will summon medical assistance. Caregiver stress, communication problems, and fear of the unknown are valid concerns. Community resources and additional information can be obtained by calling the American Heart Association toll-free at 1-800-242-8721.

stress tests, lipid analysis, and chest x-ray. Clinicians need to correct pre-existing health problems that might have contributed to the development of CAD (e.g., hypertension, anemia, hyperthyroidism).[85, 156]

Psychosocial Rehabilitation. Recovery after an MI may be lengthy and difficult. The client may have undergone surgery or have been managed medically. In either case, a serious threat to integrity occurred. Four stages of recovery have been documented:[79] (1) "Defending oneself" occurs for up to 7 days after MI. During this period, clients attempt to prove that they are not seriously ill. Coping strategies include denial and minimization. Some clients conceal the recurrence of chest pain. (2) "Coming to terms" with MI is a process of comprehending that a heart attack really occurred, understanding why it happened, and considering its impact on the future. Clients face their own mortality during this phase, which takes place over 3 to 8 days. (3) "Learning to live" is the process of life adjustment to find a life-style that can be tolerated and maintained while preserving a sense of self-worth. A variety of strategies are used to regain self-control, such as gauging progress, seeking reassurance, learning about health, and being cautious. (4) "Living again" is the last stage when clients come to terms with the fact that they will not be living life to its fullest. Clients learn to accept limitations and to refocus on other aspects of life. Some clients are unable to adjust. They are caught between stages 2 and 3. Sometimes the client finds he or she has had too many setbacks and is powerless to make changes or gain control.[63, 155]

Phase III (Long-Term). Clinicians trained in cardiac rehabilitation may provide detailed, written instructions for a long-term exercise program. Various methods are used to determine the appropriate exercise routines. Periodic evaluation is necessary to assess the client's endurance and tolerance to the prescribed exercise program. See description of phase III under Surgical Treatment.

Complications

The possibility of death from complications always accompanies an acute MI. Thus, prime collaborative goals include prevention of life-threatening complications or at least recognition of them.[153]

Dysrhythmias. Dysrhythmias are the major cause of death after an MI; 40% to 50% of deaths occur because of dysrhythmias. Ectopic rhythms arise in or near the borders of intensely ischemic and damaged myocardial tissues. Damaged myocardium may also interfere with the conduction system, causing dissociation of the atria and ventricles (heart block). Supraventricular tachycardia sometimes occurs as a result of heart failure. Spontaneous or pharmacologic reperfusion of a previously ischemic area may also precipitate ventricular arrhythmias.

Provide continuous cardiac monitoring and frequent counts of PVCs (many monitoring systems count continuously). Notify the physician if more than six PVCs occur per minute and the client is symptomatic (e.g., hypotension, chest pain). Provide prompt intervention for dysrhythmias per protocol or orders. Clients with new-onset, symptomatic ventricular ectopy (runs, couplets, salvos) may benefit from lidocaine. For ventricular tachycardia, administer lidocaine, procainamide, bretyllium, or provide elective cardioversion.[15, 160] For ventricular fibrillation, provide immediate defibrillation. For supraventricular tachycardia, administer a vagal maneuver, adenosine, verapamil, or lidocaine, and provide elective cardioversion. For heart block, administer atropine or isoproterenol (with caution) and use a temporary pacemaker.[146] Dysrhythmias are discussed in Chapter 46.

Cardiogenic Shock. Cardiogenic shock accounts for only 9% of the deaths from MI. Despite its low incidence, an estimated 80% of clients who develop shock die from it. Causes include decreased myocardial contraction and diminished cardiac output, undetected dysrhythmias, and sepsis.[147]

Clinical manifestations include systolic blood pressure significantly below the client's normal blood pressure, diaphoresis, rapid pulse, restlessness, cold clammy skin, and gray skin color.

Shock can be prevented with rapid relief of pain and sufficient IV fluids to prevent circulatory collapse. It is also vital to identify dysrhythmias rapidly.

Administer vasopressors such as, norepinephrine, dopamine, dobutamine, and metaraminol (Aramine) as prescribed to raise blood pressure by increasing peripheral resistance. In other cases, vasodilators such as nitroprusside promote better blood flow in the microcirculation. Positive inotropic agents such as dobutamine, epinephrine, and isoproterenol increase cardiac contractility and cardiac output and improve tissue perfusion. Administer oxygen therapy and antiarrhythmic agents as prescribed, and continuously monitor arterial and pulmonary artery pressures. Chapter 22 discusses shock in detail.

Heart Failure and Pulmonary Edema. The common cause of in-hospital death in clients with cardiac disorders is heart failure. Heart failure will disable 20% of clients who experience an MI and is responsible for one third of deaths after an MI.[66]

Heart failure may develop at the onset of the infarction, or it may occur weeks later. Clinical manifestations include dyspnea, orthopnea, weight gain, edema, enlarged tender liver, distended neck veins, and crackles. It is managed by correcting the underlying cause, relieving clinical manifestations, and enhancing cardiac pump performance.[55, 115] Heart failure is discussed later in this chapter. The Case Study presents a scenario involving cardiogenic shock, tachycardia, and heart failure.

Pulmonary Embolism. Pulmonary embolism (PE) may develop secondary to phlebitis of the leg or pelvic veins (venous thrombosis), or from atrial flutter or fibrillation. PE occurs in 10% to 20% of clients at some point, either during the acute attack or in the convalescent period. PE is discussed in Chapter 41.

Recurrent Myocardial Infarction. Within 6 years after an initial MI, 23% of men and 31% of women will have recurrent MI.[7] Possible causes include overexertion, embolization, or further thrombotic occlusion of a coronary artery by an atheroma. The clinical manifestation is the return of angina. Management is the same as for acute MI.[115]

Complications Due to Myocardial Necrosis. Complications due to necrosis of the myocardium include ventricular aneurysm, rupture of the heart (also called *myocardial rupture*), ventricular septal defect (VSD), and ruptured papillary muscle. These problems are infrequent but serious complications that usually occur 7 to 10 days after an MI. Weak, friable necrotic myocardial tissue increases vulnerability to these complications (Fig. 45–12).

Manifestations of CHF develop with ventricular aneurysm, rupture of the ventricular septum, and rupture of the papillary muscle. Symptoms of severe mitral insufficiency often develop when the papillary muscle of the left ventricle ruptures. Ventricular dysrhythmias (e.g., frequent PVCs and ventricular tachycardia) occur often in the presence of a ventricular aneurysm (the necrotic tissue is very irritable). Signs of cardiac tamponade develop with rupture of the heart.

The goal of treatment is to decrease the workload of the heart and increase the oxygen supply to keep the area of infarction and necrotic tissue as small as possible.

Surgery is performed to (1) excise the ventricular aneurysm, (2) replace the mitral valve if the papillary muscle is ruptured, or (3) repair the VSD. Pericardiocentesis and immediate surgery help relieve cardiac tamponade occurring after rupture of the heart.[115]

Pericarditis. Up to 28% of clients suffering an acute transmural MI will develop early pericarditis (within 2–4 days). The inflamed area of the infarction rubs against the pericardial surface and causes it to lose its lubricating fluid. A pericardial friction rub can be auscultated across the precordium. The client complains of chest pain that is aggravated with movement, deep inspiration, and cough. The pain of pericarditis is relieved by sitting up and leaning forward.

Frequent assessment may lead to early identification and intervention. Relieve pain with analgesics such as acetaminophen, nonsteroidal anti-inflammatory agents, or other anti-inflammatory agents. Reduce the client's anxiety by differentiating the pain of pericarditis from the pain of MI.[115]

Dressler's Syndrome (Late Pericarditis). The form of pericarditis known as Dressler's syndrome can occur as late as 6 weeks to months after an MI. Although the etiologic agent is unknown, current research suggests an autoimmune cause. The client usually presents with a fever lasting 1 week or longer, pericardial chest pain, pericardial friction rub, and occasionally pleuritis with pleural effusions. This is a self-limiting phenomenon, and no prevention is known. Treatment includes aspirin, prednisone, and narcotic analgesics for pain. Anticoagulation therapy may precipitate cardiac tamponade and should be avoided in these clients.[115]

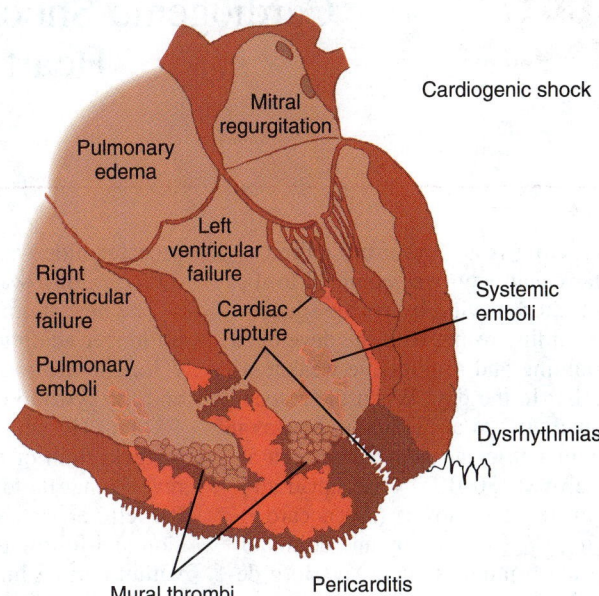

Figure 45–12. Major complications of acute myocardial infarction. (From O'Rourke, R. A. [1982] The bedside diagnosis of the complications of myocardial infarction. In R. S. Eliot [Ed.], *Cardiac emergencies*. Mt. Kisco, NY: Futura.)

Outcomes

Since the advent of coronary care units and devices that aid in promptly recognizing and treating life-threatening arrhythmias, 70% to 80% of those suffering from an acute MI survive the initial attack. Chances for survival greatly diminish with the presence of the following:

● Old age (clients 80 years or older have a 60% mortality rate)
● Evidence of other cardiovascular disease, respiratory disease, or uncontrolled diabetes mellitus (concomitant angina or previous MI carries a mortality rate of greater than 30%).
● Anterior location of MI (anterior MI is associated with a 30% mortality rate)
● Hypotension (a systolic blood pressure of less than 55 mm Hg on admission betokens a 60% mortality rate)

Deaths generally result from severe dysrhythmias, cardiogenic shock, congestive-heart failure (CHE), rupture of the heart, and recurrent MI.

Clients fortunate enough to avoid complications after MI still require a period of 6 to 12 weeks for complete recovery. Unfortunately, however, 50% of those who completely recover from their first coronary will die within 5 years; 75% will die within 10 years from massive infarctions.[145]

■ Nursing Management of the Medical Client

The goals of nursing management for the MI client is as follows:

1. Recognition and treatment of potentially life-threatening dysrhythmias

Text continues on p. 1276

Cardiogenic Shock, Tachycardia, and Heart Failure

Mr. Borg is a 70-year-old retired black man who was admitted to the ER after arriving by rescue squad. According to his wife, he developed vomiting and progressive weakness earlier in the day. When the rescue squad arrived at his home, he was in supraventricular tachycardia with a rate over 180 BPM. The squad administered adenosine (Adenocard) 6 mg IV, followed by an additional 12 mg 3 minutes later. Mr. Borg denied the presence of chest pain or shortness of breath upon admission to the ER. He was cyanotic with no palpable blood pressure and a regular heart rate of 160 BPM. A bolus of diltiazem (Cardizem) 10 mg was administered IV push and he converted briefly to normal sinus rhythm. When he went back into supraventricular tachycardia, a diltiazem drip was initiated. Blood gases drawn in the ER showed a pH of 7.3 and a $PaCO_2$ of 55 mm Hg. Mr. Borg was transferred to the ICU with the diltiazem drip and oxygen at 4 L per nasal cannula.

In ICU, Mr. Borg's hypotension and tachycardia persisted and a low-dose dopamine drip was initiated at 2 μg/kg/min. Mr. Borg became more hypotensive, tachycardic, and hypoxic. He was then intubated and placed on a ventilator with 100% oxygen. A Swan-Ganz catheter was placed, and his initial PA wedge pressure was 30 mm Hg. Furosemide (Lasix) 80 mg and procainamide (Pronestyl) 500 mg IV bolus were administered. A 2 mg/min IV drip of procainamide was continued, and the diltiazem drip was discontinued.

The next morning, Mr. Borg was no longer acidotic, with a pH of 7.36. His heart rate was 140 BPM, and the systolic BP was around 100 mm Hg while he was on 9 μg/kg/min of dopamine. The ECG reveals that the distal two thirds of the left ventricle is akinetic. Admission and follow-up CPK levels were within normal limits, which indicates that Mr. Borg had an extensive anterior MI at an earlier date. Mr. Borg is scheduled to have a right and left heart catheterization at 1:00 PM today. Given his condition, he is not considered a candidate for PTCA at this time.

Selected Laboratory Values	
RBC	4.08 million/mm³
Hgb	14.2 g/dl
Hct	41.7%
WBC	20,500/mm³
Sodium	135 mEq/L
Potassium	3.3 mEq/L
Chloride	94 mEq/L
Cholesterol	264 mg/dl
Triglycerides	334 mg/dl

Nursing Admission Assessment

Mr. Borg is a former mail carrier who retired 10 years ago. He and his wife recently celebrated their 50th wedding anniversary. Their two sons live in cities 1500 miles away, and they will be flying in to visit their father as soon as possible. His wife reports that he stopped smoking 20 years ago and continues to drink two to four alcoholic beverages per day. He has gained 40 lbs during the past 10 years. His wife is concerned that he eats and drinks too much and that he spends most of the day sitting in front of the television. Mr. Borg's wife also reports that he has been taking benazepril (Lotensin) 10 mg/day.

Nursing Physical Examination

Height: 5'11" Weight: 210 lbs (95.45 kg)
Vital signs: BP = 90/40; TPR = 101, 135, 20
LOC: Sedated and intubated
EENT: Within normal limits
Cardiac: S_1, S_2 audible without murmur, questionable S_3 regular rate, unable to assess neck vein distention
Pulmonary: Rhonchi present throughout lungs with fine basilar rales bilaterally
Abdominal: Within normal limits
Genitourinary: Foley catheter in place draining clear yellow urine.
Peripheral pulses: 1/1 with 1+ pitting edema which extends to midcalf

Current Treatment Plan

Meds: Dopamine 1600 mg in 500 ml D5W; titrate to keep systolic BP >90 mm Hg

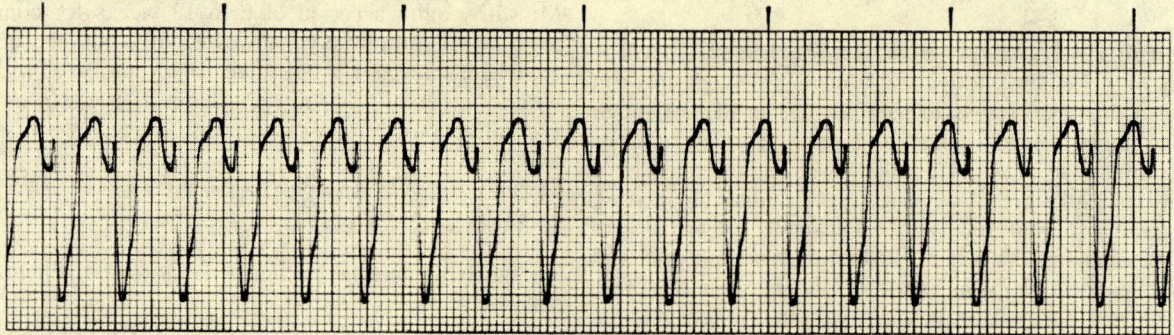

■ When the rescue squad arrived at Mr. Borg's home, he was in supraventricular tachycardia, with a rate of more than 180 BPM.

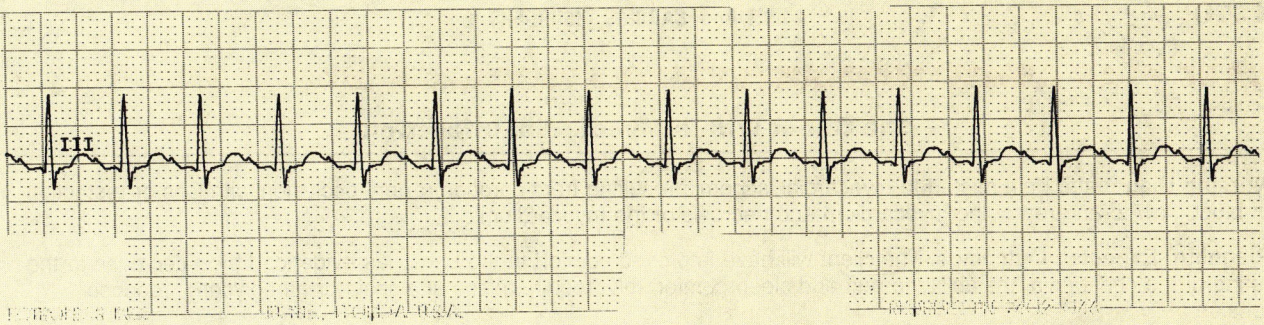

■ After initial treatment, Mr. Borg was still in supraventricular tachycardia, but his heart rate had dropped to 140 BPM.

Furosemide 40 mg IV tid
Potassium 40 mEq in 100 ml
  D5W over 4 hours bid
Thiamine 100 mg IM qd
MVI 1 ampule IV qd
Methylprednisolone (Solu-
  Medrol) 100 mg IV q 8 h
Ceftriaxone (Rocephin)
  1 g q 12 h IV
Saline lock as needed for
  medications, flush bid, prn
Diet: NPO
Activity: Bedrest
Respiratory treatments: 70% FIO_2,
  IMV = 10, tidal volume = 750 ml
  with 5 cm PEEP
Diagnostic tests: Repeat chest x-ray,
  ECG, CBC, metabolic profile, car-
  diac enzymes this AM

The results of the cardiac catheteri-zation reveal 100% occlusion of the left coronary artery and severe diffuse disease of the left anterior descending coronary artery. The physicians have determined that he is a poor surgical risk and plan to treat him medically. Mr. Borg has interpreted this as an indication that his problem is temporary and states, "You can't keep a good man down."

Over the next several days, Mr. Borg's blood pressure stabilizes and he is weaned off the dopamine. The furosemide is changed to an oral dose and the potassium is reduced to 10 mEq PO tid. The IV procainamide is discontinued after oral procainamide (Procan SR) is initiated at 250 mg bid. Mr. Borg is also digitalized and will be maintained on digoxin 0.25 mg qd. His resting heart rate has been approximately 70 BPM. A nitroglycerin (Nitro-Dur) patch is ordered daily to be applied in AM and removed at HS. Mr. Borg is also extubated and placed on a no added salt, low fat diet. He is to begin a cardiac rehabilitation program. The physician is planning to discharge him tomorrow following a recovery treadmill test.

Discharge Criteria

Average LOS: 7 days
Cardiac rehabilitation initiated and
  follow-up appointments scheduled
  (includes diet, exercise, stress management, and medication teaching)

Questions to Be Considered

1. Compare and contrast left versus right ventricular, backward versus forward, and high- versus low-output heart failure. Given the information provided, how would you categorize Mr. Borg's heart failure?
2. Compare and contrast the effects of Mr. Borg's cardiac medications: dopamine, diltiazem, adenosine, procainamide, digoxin, nitroglyc-erin. Why are the furosemide and potassium ordered?
3. According to the four stages of psychosocial recovery outlined under community and self-care for the MI client, what stage is Mr. Borg in? Discuss examples of behavior that indicate that he is progressing through the other stages of recovery.
4. What ramifications do Mr. Borg's life-style have on the success of his cardiac rehabilitation program? How might a home health nurse facilitate Mrs. Borg's participation in his rehabilitation program?
5. Eight weeks after discharge, Mr. Borg asks the cardiac rehabilitation nurse if new lights have been installed because "they all have a yellow ring round them and the edges are fuzzy." Upon further investigation the nurse determines that Mr. Borg has also had a decreased appetite, intermittent nausea and vomiting, and decreased ability to complete his entire exercise protocol. What should the nurse suspect? What recommendations should she make?
6. Six months after discharge, the physician resumes Mr. Borg's medication orders for benazepril 10 mg PO qd. Describe the pharmacodynamics of this drug and how it compares with furosemide.

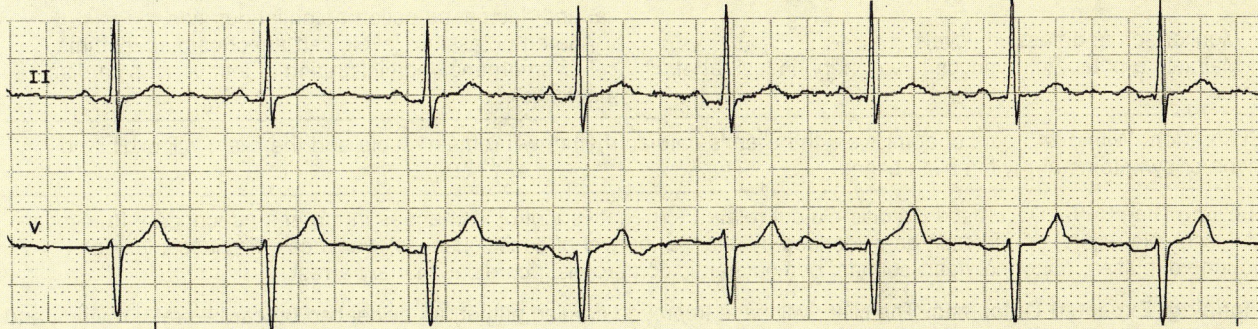

■ After several days of treatment, Mr. Borg is in normal sinus rhythm, with a resting heart rate of approximately 70 BPM.

CARE PLAN

The Client with a Myocardial Infarction

Nursing Diagnosis. Pain related to myocardial ischemia resulting from coronary artery occlusion with loss or restriction of blood flow to an area of the myocardium and necrosis of the myocardium.

Planning: Expected Outcomes. The client will have improved comfort in the chest, as evidenced by a decrease in the rating of the chest pain, the ability to rest and sleep comfortably, requiring less analgesia or nitroglycerin, reduced tension.

Implementation: Nursing Intervention	Rationales
Assess characteristics of chest pain, including location, duration, quality, intensity, presence of radiation, precipitating and alleviating factors, and associated symptoms; have client rate pain on a scale of 0 to 10 and document findings in nurses' notes.	Pain is an indication of myocardial ischemia. Assisting the client in quantifying pain may differentiate pre-existing and current pain patterns as well as identify complications. Usually a scale of 0 to 10 is used, 10 being the worst pain, 0 being none.
Assess respirations, blood pressure, and heart rate with each episode of chest pain.	Respirations may be increased as a result of pain and associated anxiety; release of stress-induced catecholamines will increase heart rate and blood pressure.
Obtain a 12-lead electrocardiogram (ECG) on admission, then each time chest pain recurs for evidence of further infarction.	Serial ECG and stat ECGs record changes that can give evidence of further cardiac damage and location of myocardial ischemia.
Monitor response to drug therapy. Notify physician if pain does not abate within 15 to 20 minutes.	Pain control is a priority because it indicates ischemia.
Provide care in a calm, efficient manner that will reassure the client and minimize anxiety; stay with the client until discomfort is relieved.	External stimuli may aggravate anxiety and cardiac strain and limit coping abilities.
Limit visitors.	Limiting visitors prevents overstimulation and promotes rest.

Evaluation. Client will be pain free within 15 to 20 minutes after administration of drug therapy. Client will verbalize relief of pain and will not exhibit associated signs and symptoms of pain.

Collaborative Problem. Dysrhythmias related to electrical instability or irritability secondary to ischemia or infarcted tissue as evidenced by increase or decrease in heart rate, change in rhythm, dysrhythmias.

Planning: Expected Outcomes. The client will have no dysrhythmias, as evidenced by normal sinus rhythm or return to client's own baseline rhythm, normotension.

Implementation: Nursing Intervention	Rationales
Teach the client and family about the need for continuous monitoring; keep alarms on and limits set at all times.	Continued monitoring keeps staff aware of myocardial changes. Family anxiety is decreased.
Assess the apical heart rate; auscultate for change in heart sounds (murmurs, rub, S_3 and S_4).	The apical heart rate is indicative of early cardiac decompensation and potential loss of cardiac output.
Document the rhythm strip every shift and prn (as needed) if dysrhythmias occur; measure the pulse rate and QRS segments with each strip; note and report any deviations from the client's baseline.	Dysrhythmias are the most common complication after a myocardial infarction (MI).
Report six or more multifocal premature ventricular contractions (PVCs) per minute to the physician.	Multifocal PVCs indicate ventricular irritability, which decreases cardiac output and may lead to life-threatening dysrhythmias.
Give antidysrhythmics as ordered.	Antidysrhythmics reduce myocardial irritability.
Monitor the effects of antidysrhythmic agents.	The desired result is increased diastolic threshold potential and decreased action potential duration.
Monitor serum potassium levels.	Altered potassium levels can affect cardiac rhythms.
Maintain a patent intravenous line or heparin lock at all times.	For emergency administration of intravenous cardiac medications.

Evaluation. Within 24 hours of admission, the client's cardiac rhythm will remain stable and the client will exhibit no signs or symptoms of rhythm disturbance.

Nursing Diagnosis. Decreased Cardiac Output related to negative inotropic changes in the heart secondary to myocardial ischemia, injury, or infarction as evidenced by change in level of consciousness; weakness, dizziness; loss of peripheral pulses; abnormal heart sounds; hemodynamic compromise; cardiopulmonary arrest.

Planning: Expected Outcomes. The client will have improved cardiac output, as evidenced by cardiac rate, rhythm, and hemodynamic parameters within normal limits; dysrhythmias controlled or absent; absence of angina.

CARE PLAN

The Client with a Myocardial Infarction (Continued)

Implementation: Nursing Intervention	Rationales

Assess for and document the following as evidence of myocardial dysfunction with decreasing cardiac output.
  Mental status—be alert to restlessness and decreased responsiveness.
  Lung sounds—monitor for crackles and rhonchi.
  Heart sounds—note the presence of gallop, murmur, and increased heart rate.
  Urinary output—be alert to output less than 30 ml/hr.
  Peripheral perfusion—monitor for pallor, mottling, cyanosis, coolness, diaphoresis, and peripheral pulses.
  Vital signs—note any abnormalities in the client's vital signs.
  Presence of jugular neck vein distention.
  Dependent edema (sacral).
  Weakness, fatigue.
  Decreased activity level.
  Shortness of breath with activity.
  Monitor arterial blood gases.
	Cerebral perfusion is directly related to cardiac output and aortic perfusion pressure and is influenced by hypoxia and electrolyte and acid-base variations; crackles may develop, reflecting pulmonary congestion related to alterations in myocardial function; hypotension related to hypoperfusion, vagal stimulation, or ventricular dysfunction may occur; hypertension may be related to pain, anxiety, catecholamine release, or pre-existing vascular problems; urinary output less than 30 ml/hr may reflect reduced renal perfusion and glomerular filtration as a result of reduced cardiac output.

If the client has a pulmonary artery catheter, record hemodynamic parameters every 2 to 4 hours and prn; be alert to pulmonary capillary wedge pressure greater than 18 mm Hg, cardiac output less than 4 L/min, and cardiac index less than 2.5 L/min.	Hemodynamic pressures reflect intravascular responses and ventricular function; use to assess drug therapy and for prevention or early detection of complications of MI (i.e., extension, heart failure, cardiogenic shock).
Maintain hemodynamic stability by monitoring the effects of beta-blockers and inotropic agents.	Assess the effect of drug therapy on myocardial contractility and function.

Evaluation. Within 2 to 3 days of admission, client will have normal hemodynamic pressures, normal vital signs, clear breath sounds, no shortness of breath, and normal blood gas values. Client's rhythm will be normal sinus and rate will be controlled between 60 to 100 BPM.

Nursing Diagnosis. Impaired Gas Exchange related to decreased cardiac output as evidenced by increased or decreased heart rate, decreased blood pressure, decreased temperature, dusky color, impaired capillary refill, reduced arterial oxygen tension (PaO_2), dyspnea.

Planning: Expected Outcomes. Client will have improved gas exchange, as evidenced by vital signs within normal limits for client, absence of cyanosis, absence of dyspnea, arterial blood gases within normal limits.

Implementation: Nursing Intervention	Rationales
Administer oxygen as ordered; maintain continuous oximetry.	Increases the amount of oxygen available for myocardial uptake; oximetry measures peripheral oxygen saturation.
Monitor arterial blood gases as ordered. Continue to assess the client's skin, capillary refill, level of consciousness, and vital signs every 2 to 4 hours and prn.	The presence of hypoxia indicates a need for supplemental oxygen. Monitoring provides data on the adequacy of tissue perfusion and oxygenation.
Prepare for intubation and mechanical ventilation if hypoxia increases.	With increasing hypoxia, mechanical ventilation may be necessary to oxygenate the client adequately.

Evaluation. Within 2 to 3 days of admission, client's vital signs will be within normal limits (for client), breath sounds will be clear, and blood gas values will be within normal limits (for client).

Nursing Diagnosis. Powerlessness related to hospital environment and anticipated life-style changes as evidenced by verbalized "feelings of doom," crying, anger.

Planning: Expected Outcomes. The client will have an improved feeling of control, as evidenced by verbalizing feelings of powerlessness, verbalizing a sense of control over the present situation and future outcomes.

Implementation: Nursing Intervention	Rationales
Provide opportunities for the client to express feelings about self and illness.	These opportunities create a supportive climate and send the message that caregivers are willing to help.
Explore reality perceptions and clarify if necessary.	Listening to the feelings as well as to the words of the client can help the client acquire a more hopeful outlook.

Chart continued on following page

CARE PLAN

The Client with a Myocardial Infarction (Continued)

Implementation: Nursing Intervention

Eliminate the unpredictability of events by allowing adequate preparation for tests and procedures.

Reinforce the client's right to ask questions.

Allow choices when possible.
Provide positive reinforcement for increased involvement in self-care.

Help the client identify strengths and areas of control.

Rationales

Information can help the client or family feel more hopeful about the situation and more willing to participate in care.
Maintain a supportive climate to let the client feel free to ask questions or have information repeated.
Self-care allows the client to feel independent.
When clients participate in planning for care, they are more apt to feel a sense of control and to follow through with actions.
Self-confidence and security come with a sense of control; foster full client participation.

Evaluation. Within 24 hours of admission, client will verbalize a feeling of control over current situation and will actively participate in decisions regarding care.

Nursing Diagnosis. Anxiety and Fear related to hospital admission and fear of death as evidenced by client and family appear restless, hostile, or withdrawn; client and family verbalize fatalism or act extremely emotional as if in the grieving process.

Planning: Expected Outcomes. The client will have reduced feelings of anxiety and fear, as evidenced by demonstrating appropriate range of feelings and initial signs of effective coping, such as participation in treatment regimen, ability to rest, and the client and family ask fewer questions.

Implementation: Nursing Intervention

Limit nursing personnel; provide continuity of care.

Allow and encourage the client and family to ask questions; do not avoid questions. Bring up common concerns.

Allow the client and family to verbalize fears.

Stress that frequent assessments are routine and do not necessarily imply a deteriorating condition.

Repeat information as necessary because of the reduced attention span of the client and family.
Provide a comfortable, quiet environment for the client and family.

Rationales

Continuity of care promotes security and development of rapport with and trust of healthcare providers.
Accurate information about the situation reduces fear, strengthens the client-nurse relationship, and assists the client and family to deal realistically with the situation.
Sharing information elicits support and comfort and can relieve tension and unexpressed worries.
The client may feel reassured to know that frequent assessments may prevent development of more serious complications.
The client's attention span is short, and time perception may be altered. Anxiety decreases learning and attention.
A comfortable environment enhances coping mechanisms and reduces myocardial workload and oxygen consumption.

Evaluation. Within 2 days of admission, client will exhibit signs of effective coping and progression through stages of recovery.

Nursing Diagnosis. Risk for constipation related to bedrest, pain medications, and NPO (nothing by mouth) or soft diet as evidenced by subjective feeling of fullness, abdominal cramping, painful defecation, palpable impaction.

Planning: Expected Outcomes. The client will have improved bowel elimination, as evidenced by eliminating a stool without straining or having a vasovagal response (bradycardia).

Implementation: Nursing Intervention

Ensure that the client has adequate bulk in diet and adequate fluid intake (without violating fluid restrictions).
Monitor the effectiveness of softeners or laxatives; instruct the client on prevention of straining and avoiding Valsalva's (vasovagal) maneuver.
Encourage the client to use a bedside commode rather than a bedpan.

Rationales

Bulk and fluid within the colon prevent straining.

Stool softeners decrease the myocardial workload of straining; Valsalva's maneuver causes bradycardia, decreasing cardiac output.
Bedpan use requires more straining and increases the vasovagal response.

Evaluation. Within 2 to 3 days of admission, client will have normal bowel function.

Nursing Diagnosis. Altered Health Maintenance related to MI and implications for life-style changes

CARE PLAN

The Client with a Myocardial Infarction *(Continued)*

Planning: Expected Outcomes. The client and family will have improved knowledge of medical regimen and life-style changes, as evidenced by verbalizing an understanding of a heart attack and the necessary life-style changes regarding diet, medications, stress reduction, quitting smoking, and cholesterol, weight, and blood pressure reduction

Implementation: Nursing Intervention	Rationales
Discuss the following with clients and family, providing both oral instructions and written materials: Anatomy and functions of the heart muscle, coronary arteries and the atherosclerotic process, definition of a "heart attack," the healing process of the heart and the role of collateral circulation.	Use of multiple learning methods enhances retention of material; information helps the client understand the underlying problems or overall heart functions.
Assist the client with identifying his or her own risk factors.	Risk factor identification is the first step before changes can be implemented.
Assist the client in devising a plan for risk factor modification (e.g., diet; smoking cessation; cholesterol, stress, and blood pressure reduction).	This information is helpful in providing opportunity for the client to identify risk factors, assume control, and participate in a treatment regimen.
Provide guidelines for a diet low in cholesterol and saturated fat; arrange for dietary consultation before the client is discharged from hospital.	Consultation with other health professionals enhances client learning from others; guidelines developed with the client and family before discharge will help once they are home.
Teach the client and family about medications that will be taken after hospital discharge, including name, purpose, dosage, schedule, precautions, and potential side effects.	The more the client understands the medical regimen and potential side effects, the more adept he or she will be in monitoring for them.
Discuss post-MI activity progression; arrange for a cardiac rehabilitation consultation.	Continued follow-up will let the client know how he or she is doing; outpatient cardiac rehabilitation will support and assist the client in the life-style changes necessary for a healthy recovery and life.

Evaluation. Within 2 days of admission, the client and family will be able to verbalize understanding of heart attack and identify personal risk factors and necessary life-style changes.

Nursing Diagnosis. Risk for Activity Intolerance related to an imbalance between oxygen supply and demand as evidenced by weakness, fatigue; change in vital signs; dysrhythmias; dyspnea; pallor; diaphoresis.

Planning: Expected Outcomes. The client will have improved activity tolerance, as evidenced by participating in desired activities, meeting his or her own activities of daily living, reduced fatigue and weakness, vital signs within normal limits during activity, absence of cyanosis, diaphoresis, and pain.

Implementation: Nursing Intervention	Rationales
Monitor vital signs before and immediately after activity, and 3 minutes later.	Data on client's response to increase in activity. Vital signs should return to baseline in 3 minutes. Pulse rate over established limits and development of chest pain or dyspnea may indicate a need for alterations in exercise regimen or medication changes.
Monitor for tachycardia, dysrhythmias, dyspnea, diaphoresis, or pallor after activity.	These are indicators of myocardial oxygen deprivation that may require decrease in activity, changes in medications, or use of supplemental oxygen.
Encourage verbalization of feelings or concerns regarding fatigue or limitations.	Knowing limitations prevents exertion and increasing myocardial workload.
Provide assistance with self-care activities and provide frequent rest periods, especially after meals.	Large meals may increase myocardial workload and cause vagal stimulation, with resultant bradycardia or ectopic beats; caffeine, a cardiac stimulant, increases heart rate.
Increase activity per cardiac rehabilitation nurse and physician orders.	Gradual increase in activity increases strength and prevents overexertion, enhances collateral circulation, and restores a normal life-style as far as possible.

Evaluation. Within 3 to 4 days of admission, client will be progressing normally through steps of phase I cardiac rehabilitation without signs or symptoms of exercise intolerance.

Chart continued on following page

CARE PLAN

The Client with a Myocardial Infarction *(Continued)*

Collaborative Problem. Risk for Heart Failure related to disease process as evidenced by tachycardia, hypotension or hypertension, S_3 or S_4 heart sounds, dysrhythmias, ECG changes, decreased urine output, decreased peripheral pulses, cool ashen skin, diaphoresis, orthopnea, rales, crackles, jugular vein distention, edema, and chest pain.

Planning: Expected Outcomes. The nurse will monitor for clinical manifestations of heart failure by assessing cardiac rate, rhythm, hemodynamic parameters, skin perfusion, renal perfusion, and CNS perfusion.

Implementation: Nursing Intervention	Rationales
Auscultate the apical pulse.	Atrial (S_4) or ventricular (S_4) gallop rhythms are common and reflect noncompliance or distention of chambers.
Assess heart rate and rhythm.	Sinus tachycardia, paroxysmal atrial contractions tachycardia, (PACs), paroxysmal atrial tachycardia, multifocal atrial tachycardia, and PVCs are frequently seen with congestive heart failure.
Document dysrhythmias if present prn.	Dysrhythmias reduce ventricular filling time, decrease myocardial contractility, and increase myocardial oxygen demands, which further compromises cardiac output.
Note heart sounds every 2 to 4 hours and prn (especially S_3 and S_4).	Crackles may develop; they reflect pulmonary congestion related to alterations in myocardial function.
Palpate peripheral pulses every 2 to 4 hours and prn.	Pulses may be weak, thready, or difficult to obtain when cardiac output is decreased.
Monitor blood pressure every 2 to 4 hours and prn.	Hypotension related to hypoperfusion, vagal stimulation, or ventricular dysfunction may occur; hypertension may be related to pain, anxiety, catecholamine release, or pre-existing vascular problems.
Inspect the client's skin for pallor, cyanosis, and diaphoresis every 2 to 4 hours and prn.	Pallor is associated with vasoconstriction, reduced cardiac output, and anemia; cyanosis may develop during severe episodes of pulmonary edema; dependent areas are often blue or mottled as venous congestion increases.
Monitor urine output, noting changes or decreasing output and dark or concentrated urine every 2 to 4 hours and prn.	Urinary output less than 30 ml/hr may reflect reduced renal perfusion and glomerular filtration as a result of reduced cardiac output.
Assess changes in sensorium.	Cerebral perfusion is directly related to cardiac output, and mentation may be a sensitive indicator of deterioration.
Assess the client's lung sounds every 2 to 4 hours and prn.	Rhonchi, wheezes, and moist crepitant crackles reflect pulmonary congestion that may develop rapidly.
Provide frequent rest periods.	Physical rest decreases the production of catecholamines, which raises heart rate, myocardial oxygen demand, and blood pressure.
Provide for rest by maintaining a calm, quiet environment; explain medical and nursing management; help the client avoid stressful situations; allow the client to ventilate fears or concerns.	A calm environment prevents overstimulation and allows rest; when clients participate in planning of care, they are more apt to feel a sense of control and to follow through with actions.
Instruct the client on avoidance of activities that increase cardiac workload.	Avoidance of activities provides the opportunity for myocardial recovery and decreases workload and myocardial oxygen consumption.
Provide a bedside commode; avoid Valsalva's response.	Valsalva's maneuver causes bradycardia and temporarily decreases cardiac output.
Elevate the client's legs and avoid pressure under his or her knees; permit increase in activity as tolerated.	This position enhances venous return and reduces dependent swelling, decreases venous stasis, and may reduce the incidence of thrombus and embolus formation.
Assess for calf tenderness; diminished pedal pulses; swelling, redness, or pallor of extremities.	These are indicators of thrombophlebitis.
Monitor for digitalis toxicity (i.e., decreased heart sounds, hypokalemia, first-degree heart block).	These factors may be present in various stages of congestive heart failure and may cause a cumulative effect in the digitalis level.

CARE PLAN

The Client with a Myocardial Infarction *(Continued)*

Evaluation. Expect dysrhythmias to be present during acute phase of MI recovery. Cardiac output should stabilize over 72 hours once infarction abates.

Nursing Diagnosis. Fluid Volume Excess related to reduced glomerular filtration rate, decreased cardiac output, increased antidiuretic hormone production, and sodium and water retention as evidenced by orthopnea; S_3 heart sound; oliguria; edema, jugular neck vein distention; increased weight; increased blood pressure; respiratory distress; abnormal breath sounds.

Planning: Expected Outcomes. The client will have an adequate fluid volume balance, as evidenced by balanced intake and output, clear or clearing breath sounds, vital signs within normal limits, stable weight, absence of edema.

Implementation: Nursing Intervention	Rationales
Monitor the client's intake and output (especially note color, specific gravity, and amount) every 2 to 4 hours and prn and 24-hour totals.	Diuretic therapy resulting in sudden or excessive fluid reduction may cause hypovolemia.
Maintain chair or bedrest in the semi-Fowler position.	This position promotes diuresis by recumbency-induced increase of glomerular filtration and reduction of antidiuretic hormone production.
Involve the client and family in fluid schedule, especially if restricted, and provide frequent oral care.	Involvement of the client in the therapy regimen may enhance his or her sense of control and cooperation with restrictions.
Weigh the client daily.	Documents the increase or decrease in congestion and edema in response to therapy; a gain of 5 lb represents approximately 2 L of fluid.
Assess for jugular neck vein distention, edema, peripheral pulses, and the presence of anasarca.	Excessive fluid retention may be demonstrated by venous engorgement and edema formation; peripheral edema often begins in the feet and ascends upward as failure worsens.
Auscultate breath sounds; note adventitious sounds and monitor for dyspnea or tachypnea.	These are symptoms of pulmonary congestion reflecting increased vascular volume and pulmonary hypertension, or worsening of heart failure.
Monitor for sudden extreme shortness of breath and feelings of panic.	These are signs of extreme pulmonary capillary hypertension (pulmonary edema).
Palpate for hepatomegaly; note complaints of right upper quadrant pain or tenderness.	Advancing heart failure leads to venous congestion, which results in liver engorgement and altered organ function (i.e., impaired drug metabolism, prolonged drug half-life).

Chart continued on following page

The Client with a Myocardial Infarction (*Continued*)

Implementation: Nursing Intervention	**Rationales**
Note increased lethargy, hypotension, and muscle cramping.	These are signs of hypokalemia and hyponatremia that may occur because of fluid shifts and diuretic therapy.
Evaluate the effectiveness of diuretics and potassium supplements.	Fluid shifts and use of diuretics can alter electrolytes, especially potassium and chloride, which affects cardiac rhythm and contractility.
Assess the need for dietary consultation as needed.	Restrictions of foods high in sodium may be necessary. The client may need to eat foods enriched with potassium when taking loop diuretics.

Evaluation. Within 3 days of admission, client will have a normal fluid volume. Client's intake and output will be balanced, breath sounds will be clear, vital signs will be normal, and weight will be stable, with no signs of peripheral or central edema.

Nursing Diagnosis. Risk for Impaired Skin Integrity related to bedrest, edema, and decreased tissue perfusion as evidenced by reddened areas and the presence of areas of breakdown.

Planning: Expected Outcomes. The client will have intact skin integrity, as evidenced by no reddened areas and no areas of breakdown.

Implementation: Nursing Intervention	**Rationales**
Inspect the client's skin (noting bone prominences, edema, altered circulation, pigmentation, obesity, or emaciation).	Altered skin color in isolated areas may indicate damage caused by pressure or decreased circulation.
Assist with active or passive range-of-motion exercises.	These exercises enhance venous return; isometric exercises may adversely affect cardiac output by increasing myocardial work and oxygen consumption.
Reposition the client every 2 hours in a bed or chair.	Repositioning increases circulation and reduces the time that weight deprives any one area of blood flow.
Provide pressure-reducing devices, sheepskin, or elbow and heel protectors if needed.	These devices reduce pressure to bone prominences and improve skin integrity.
Assess and provide special air or flotation beds for clients with special needs.	These beds reduce pressure to skin and may improve circulation.

Evaluation. Within 2 to 3 days of admission, client will have intact skin integrity and will not have any reddened areas or skin breakdown.

2. Monitoring for complications of reduced cardiac output
3. Maintenance of a therapeutic critical care environment
4. Identification of the psychosocial impact of MI on the client and family
5. Education of the client in life-style changes and rehabilitation

Nursing diagnoses or collaborative problems that may apply to the client after acute MI are discussed in the Care Plan.

Heart Failure

Heart failure is a physiologic state in which the heart is unable to pump enough blood to meet the metabolic needs of the body (determined as oxygen consumption) at rest or during exercise even though filling pressures are adequate. The heart fails when, owing to intrinsic disease or structural defects, it cannot handle a normal blood volume or, in the absence of disease, it cannot tolerate a sudden expansion in blood volume (e.g., during exercise). Heart failure is not a disease itself; instead, the term denotes a group of manifestations related to inadequate pump performance from either the cardiac valves or myocardium. Whatever the cause, pump failure results in hypoperfused tissue followed by pulmonary and systemic venous congestion. Because heart failure causes vascular congestion, it is often called *congestive heart failure,* although this term is no longer advised by most cardiac specialists. Other terms used to denote heart failure include *cardiac decompensation, cardiac insufficiency,* and *ventricular failure.*[90]

Estimates from the American Heart Association[7] indicate 4.7 million Americans have heart failure and are

Table 45–2. Terms Used to Describe Cardiac Function	
Term	**Function**
Afterload	Force that the ventricle must develop during systole in order to eject the stroke volume
Cardiac output	Stroke volume × heart rate
Inotropic state	A measure of contractility
Preload	Stretch of myocardial fibers at end-diastole
Stroke volume	The amount of blood ejected from the ventricle with each contraction

alive. The incidence of new cases is around 400,000 annually. Annually, about 39,387 clients die from heart failure. The incidence of heart failure approaches 10 in 1000 people after age 65.[70, 77, 78]

Etiology and Risk Factors

The performance of the heart depends on two essential components: fiber length (Frank-Starling mechanism) and the inherent contractility (inotropic state) of the muscle. The normal heart automatically responds to maintain cardiac output. Several factors automatically adjust the extent of shortening of myocardial fibers and, consequently, the stroke volume and cardiac output. Five interrelated factors are involved: preload, afterload, contractility, the coordinated pattern of contraction, and the heart rate. Table 45–2 lists and defines the terms commonly used to describe cardiac function. Adverse changes in these determinants of myocardial performance ultimately cause the heart to fail. The causes of heart failure can be divided into three subgroups: (1) abnormal loading conditions, (2) abnormal muscle function, and (3) conditions or diseases that precipitate or exacerbate heart failure. Conditions that damage the heart include atherosclerosis, a congenital heart defect, high blood pressure, pulmonary hypertension, MI, or valvular disorders.[90]

Table 45–3. Abnormal Loading Conditions of the Heart	
Increased Preload	**Increased Afterload**
Regurgitation of any of the four valves	Aortic valvular stenosis
Hypervolemia	Mitral valvular stenosis
Congenital defects (left-to-right shunts)	Pulmonic valvular stenosis
Ventricular septal defect	Systemic hypertension
Atrial septal defect	Pulmonary hypertension
Patent ductus arteriosus	High peripheral vascular resistance
Heart failure	

■ Abnormal Loading Conditions

Recall the analogy that the heart muscle is like a stretched rubber band. When the rubber band is stretched it contracts with more force. The heart muscle does the same. Venous return stretches the heart and improves contractility. Extending the analogy, when the rubber band is overstretched it becomes limp and cannot contract. Likewise, when the heart is overloaded with blood, excessive stretch and decreased contraction occurs. Overload develops because blood does not leave the ventricles during contraction. Therefore, cardiac workload increases to try to move blood.

Preload refers to the stretch of the ventricular myocardial fibers just before ventricular contraction. The load or stretch placed on the ventricular fibers corresponds to the end-diastolic ventricular volume and pressure. Preload is determined by the condition of the heart valves (especially the mitral valve), blood volume, ventricular wall compliance, and venous tone. Increased preload usually increases contractility (more stretch on the rubber band) and stretch due to filling pressures from venous return and previous volume. Stretch and filling pressures may rise beyond the capabilities of the normally compliant heart. This increased preload lessens the force and efficiency of ventricular contraction. Cardiac output decreases. Under the strain of this load, the heart will fail. Table 45–3 lists conditions that may result in increased preload.

Afterload corresponds to the amount of tension that the heart must generate to overcome systemic pressure and allow adequate ventricular emptying. In other words, afterload indicates how "hard" the heart must pump to force blood into the circulation. The tone of systemic arterioles, the elasticity of the aorta and large arteries, the size and thickness of the ventricle, the presence of aortic stenosis, and the viscosity of the blood all determine afterload. High peripheral vascular resistance and high blood pressure force the ventricle to work harder to eject blood. Subjected to prolonged high pressures, the ventricle will eventually fail.[90] Table 45–3 lists conditions that increase afterload.

■ Abnormal Muscle Function

There are certain conditions that directly interfere with myocardial contractility. Intrinsic conditions are inherent in the cardiac muscle and include MI; myocarditis, an inflammation of the myocardium associated with viral, bacterial, fungal, or parasitic diseases or toxic chemical injury; cardiomyopathy; and ventricular aneurysm. Such disorders impair the contractile function of the myocardial fibrils, which reduces ventricular emptying and stroke volume.

After MI, some of the heart muscle is replaced by noncontracting scar tissue, and the ventricles pump less efficiently. Some degree of heart failure, either chronic or transient, appears in over half of clients after MI.

Sometimes certain conditions externally compress the heart, thereby hampering ventricular filling and myocardial contractility. Disorders that greatly restrict cardiac chamber filling and myocardial fiber stretch include constrictive pericarditis, which is an inflammatory and fibrotic process of the pericardial sac; and cardiac tamponade, which involves the accumulation of fluid or blood within the pericardial sac. Because the pericardium encloses all four heart chambers, compression of the heart (1) decreases diastolic relaxation and thereby elevates diastolic pressure and (2) hampers forward blood flow through the heart.

Some clients have pre-existing mild-to-moderate heart disease with no evidence of heart failure. In these clients, adequate cardiac output depends on functional compensatory mechanisms. When the heart undergoes undue stress, these compensatory mechanisms may prove inadequate, and the heart fails. Careful assessment helps identify precipitating causes of the great increase in cardiac workload. Recognition of these factors allows prompt treatment and long-term prevention.[90] Precipitating factors are described in the following section.

■ Conditions That Precipitate or Exacerbate Heart Failure

Physical or Emotional Stress. Strenuous physical exercise and strong emotions (fear, excitement, anxiety) increase sympathetic nervous tone and catecholamine release. This increases myocardial work by increasing heart rate, myocardial contractility, and blood pressure.

Dysrhythmias. Cardiac dysrhythmias, most notably tachycardia (rapid heart rate), are the most common factors precipitating heart failure. A rapid heartbeat shortens the time for ventricular filling (diastole), which in turn reduces cardiac output and decreases myocardial perfusion. In addition, the workload and oxygen requirements of the myocardium increase.

Infections. Any systemic infection increases the oxygen demands of the body tissues. The heart must keep pace with these demands. Fever and hypoxemia, which occur in some pulmonary infections, further tax the ailing heart and may precipitate failure.

Anemia. Reduction in the oxygen-carrying capacity of the blood, as in anemia, necessitates increased cardiac output to meet the body's need for oxygen. Whereas a normal heart may adjust to the increased workload, a compromised heart cannot, and failure ensues.

Thyroid Disorders. Thyrotoxicosis, associated with hyperthyroidism, augments the metabolic needs of the body, accelerating heart rate and the workload of the heart. If thyrotoxicosis is untreated, heart failure may occur. In hypothyroidism, the thyroid produces an inadequate amount of thyroxine (thyroid hormone). This can indirectly lead to heart failure by predisposing the client to coronary atherosclerosis.

Pregnancy. Heart failure ranks high among causes of death during pregnancy. Like anemia and hyperthyroidism, pregnancy increases the metabolic needs of the body, thereby increasing the workload of the heart. Pregnant

women with rheumatic valvular disease are particularly prone to heart failure.

Paget's Disease. In some cases, Paget's disease also increases myocardial workload. This disease causes vascular proliferation in the bones. When the disease involves over one third of the skeleton, a high cardiac output state exists and may tax the compromised heart (see Chapter 74).

Nutritional Deficiency. Thiamine (vitamin B_1) deficiency causes beriberi. It occurs in cultures in which polished rice constitutes the primary food source. Alcoholism (especially with Wernicke's syndrome) is also associated with thiamine deficiency. Thiamine deficiency interferes with cardiac function by reducing myocardial contractility and causing tachycardia and ventricular dilation.

Pulmonary Disease. Increased pressure in the pulmonary system due to chronic obstructive lung disease, severe pulmonary embolization, or primary pulmonary artery hypertension can produce sizable resistance to right ventricular emptying. Such resistance may lead to right ventricular hypertrophy and failure.

Hypervolemia. An excess in circulating blood volume can result from poor renal function, cardiac disease, medications (such as steroids), or excessive intake of sodium (promoting water retention). Iatrogenic causes include overadministration of IV fluids. Expanded circulatory volume augments venous return, increasing preload. A diseased heart may not be able to pump the increased load, and cardiac decompensation occurs.

Pathophysiology

The healthy heart can meet the demands of life through the use of cardiac reserve. Cardiac reserve is the heart's ability to increase output in response to stress. The normal heart can increase its output up to five times the resting level. However, the failing heart, even at rest, is pumping near its capacity and thus has lost much of its reserve. The compromised heart has a limited ability to respond to the body's needs for increased output in situations of stress.

The heart in failure has recourse to three main compensatory mechanisms to meet the body's demands: (1) ventricular dilation, (2) ventricular hypertrophy, and (3) increased sympathetic nervous system stimulation (tachycardia).[90, 158]

■ Ventricular Dilation

Ventricular dilation refers to lengthening of the muscle fibers, which increases the volume of the heart chambers. Dilation causes an increase in preload and thus cardiac output, because a stretched muscle contracts more forcefully (Starling's law). However, dilation has limits as a compensatory mechanism. Muscle fibers, if stretched beyond a certain point, become ineffective. Second, a dilated heart requires more oxygen. Thus, the dilated heart with a normal coronary blood flow can suffer from a lack of oxygen. Hypoxia of the heart further decreases the muscle's ability to contract.[158]

■ Ventricular Hypertrophy

Ventricular hypertrophy is an increase in the diameter of the muscle fibers in order to increase the contractile power of the muscle fibers. Like dilation, hypertrophy has limits as a compensatory mechanism. A hypertrophied heart does far greater work than a normal-sized heart and, as a consequence, has a greater demand for oxygen. Unfortunately, as the heart's muscle mass increases, the number of capillaries supplying the muscle fibers remains the same. Thus, the hypertrophied heart may simply outgrow its coronary blood supply and become hypoxic. As the myocardium becomes hypoxic, the contractile force of the heart decreases. Ventricular hypertrophy may also impede ventricular emptying if the enlarged muscle blocks the valve areas.[158]

■ Increased Sympathetic Nervous System Stimulation

Increased sympathetic nervous system stimulation is the least effective compensatory mechanism and often proves to be more of a burden than a blessing. Sympathetic activity produces venous and arteriolar constriction, thus increasing peripheral vascular resistance (afterload) and

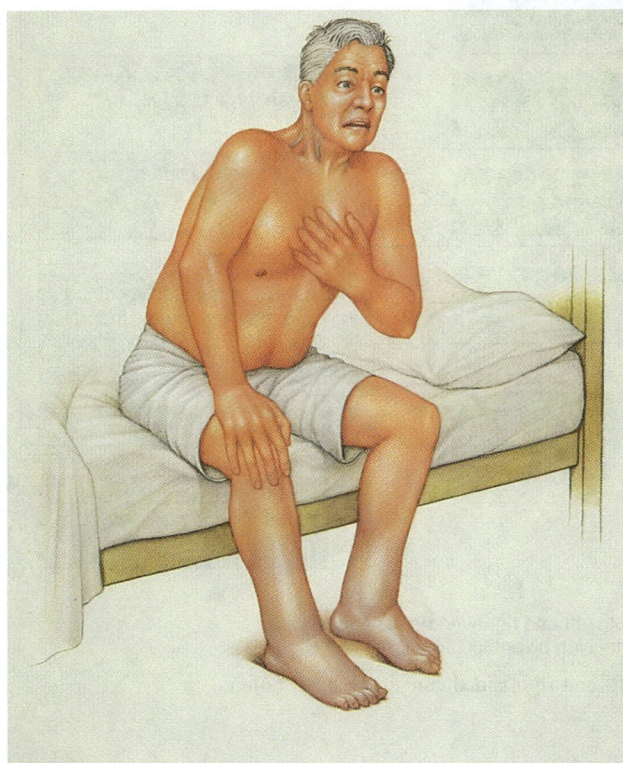

Figure 45–13. Appearance of a client with both right- and left-sided heart failure. (Courtesy of *Mayo Clinic Health Letter* with permission of Mayo Foundation for Medical Education and Research, Rochester, MN 55905.)

myocardial workload. In addition, sympathetic stimulation reduces renal blood flow, and the kidneys respond by retaining water and sodium. The expanded blood volume increases the load on an already compromised heart. Finally, tachycardia occurs as a cardiac response to distention of the great veins at their atrial attachment as well as to an increase in circulating catecholamines.

The myocardium of the left ventricle may either (1) be diseased and unable to meet normal circulatory demands or (2) be intrinsically normal but unable to meet increased circulatory needs. When failure first begins, the left ventricle fails to eject a sufficient amount of blood. At this point, the compensatory mechanisms of sympathetic nervous system activation (tachycardia, dilation, and hypertrophy) maintain perfusion. When these mechanisms fail, the amount of blood remaining in the left ventricle at the end of diastole increases. This increase in residual blood in turn decreases the ventricle's capacity to receive blood from the left atrium. The left atrium, having to work harder to eject blood, dilates and hypertrophies. It is unable to receive the full amount of incoming blood from the pulmonary veins, and left atrial pressure increases. This leads to pulmonary edema (Fig. 45–13).

The right ventricle, because of the increased pressure in the pulmonary vascular system, must now dilate and hypertrophy in order to meet its increased workload. It too eventually fails. Engorgement of the venous system then extends backward to produce congestion in the gastrointestinal tract, liver, viscera, kidneys, legs, and sacrum, with edema as the main manifestation. Right ventricular failure results.

Right ventricular failure usually follows left ventricular failure. Occasionally, right ventricular failure develops independently of left ventricular failure.

Cardiac compensation exists when these three mechanisms—ventricular dilation, ventricular hypertrophy, and sympathetic nervous system stimulation—succeed in maintaining an adequate cardiac output and blood flow to the tissues in the presence of pathologic changes. Cardiac decompensation occurs when the heart, despite these mechanisms, fails to cope with the demands put on it and must expend most of its reserve. At this point, symptoms of heart failure develop because the heart cannot maintain adequate circulation.[158]

Clinical Manifestations and Diagnostic Findings

The manifestations of heart failure depend on the specific ventricle involved, the precipitating causes of failure, the degree of impairment, the rate of progression, the duration of the failure, and the client's underlying condition. Manifestations of pulmonary congestion and edema dominate the clinical picture of left ventricular failure. Right ventricular failure is associated with signs of abdominal organ distention and peripheral edema.[90]

■ Types of Heart Failure

Heart failure may be categorized as left ventricular versus right ventricular, backward versus forward, and high-output versus low-output.[158]

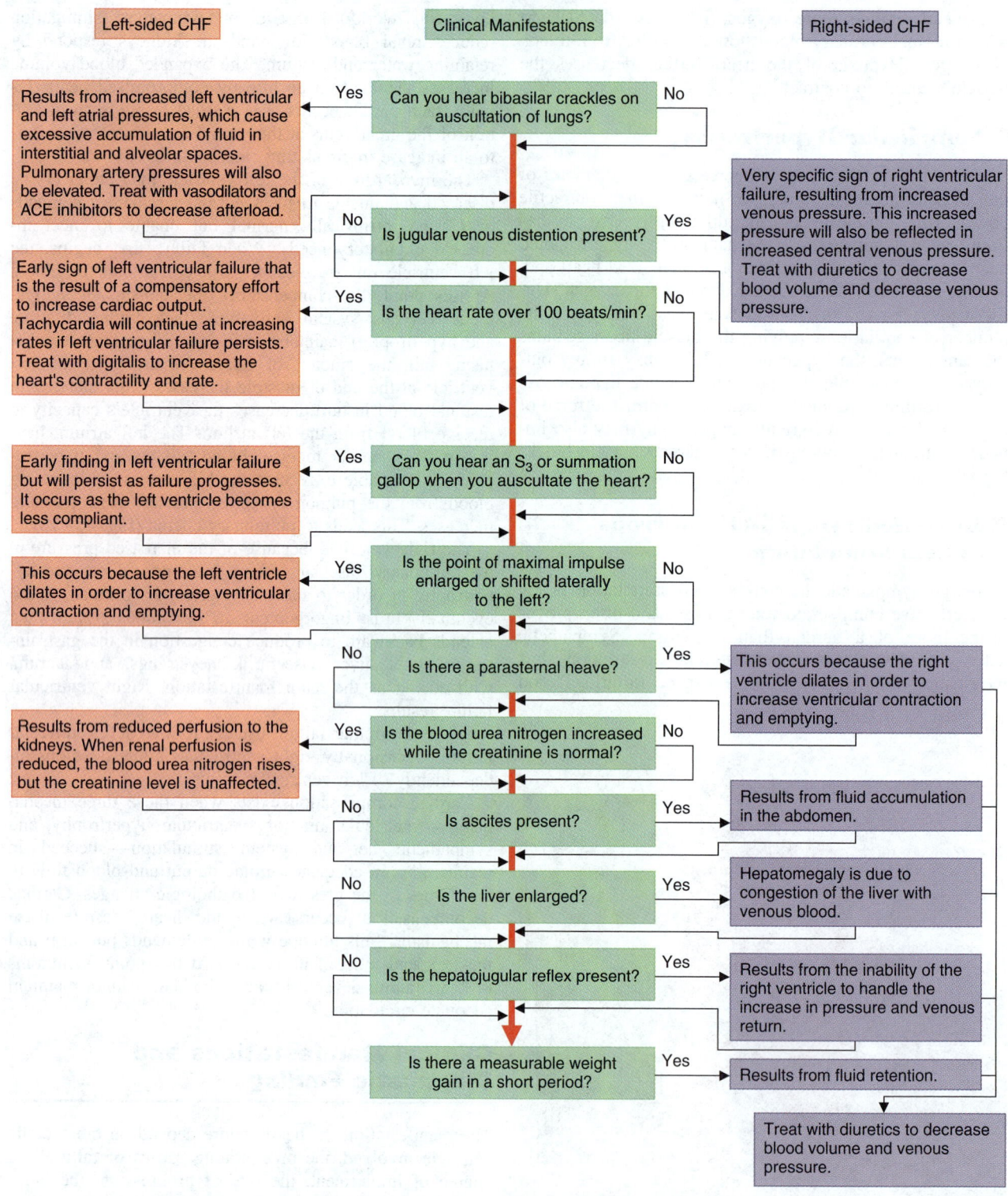

Figure 45–14. Clinical manifestations of left- and right-sided congestive heart failure.

Left Ventricular Versus Right Ventricular Failure

The theory of left-sided (LVF) versus right-sided (RVF) failure is based on the fact that fluid accumulates behind the chamber that first fails. However, because the circulatory system is a closed circuit, impairments of one ventricle will frequently progress to failure of the other. This is referred to as ventricular interdependence. See Figure 45–

14 for clinical manifestations that differentiate LVF from RVF.

Left Ventricular Failure

LVF causes either pulmonary congestion or a disturbance in the respiratory control mechanisms. These problems in turn precipitate respiratory distress. The degree of distress varies with the client's position, activity, and level of stress.

Dyspnea is a subjective problem, and it does not always correlate with the extent of heart failure. Because breathing is usually effortless at rest, the feeling of breathlessness can mean anything from an awareness of breathing to extreme distress. An apprehensive client with only moderate ventricular failure may be more aware of dyspnea than a client with advanced disease. To some degree, exertional dyspnea occurs in all clients. Therefore, elicit from the client a description of the degree of exertion that results in the sensation of breathlessness. The mechanism of dyspnea may be related to the decrease in the lung's air volume (vital capacity) as the air is displaced by blood or interstitial fluid. Pulmonary congestion can eventually reduce the vital capacity of the lungs to 1500 ml or less.

Cheyne-Stokes respirations sometimes occur in clients with severe forms of heart failure. Cheyne-Stokes respirations probably result from the prolonged circulation time between the pulmonary circulation and the central nervous system.

Cough is a common symptom of LVF. The cough, often hacking, may produce large amounts of frothy, blood-tinged sputum. The client coughs because a large amount of fluid is trapped in the pulmonary tree, irritating the lung mucosa. On auscultation, bilateral crackles may be heard.

Orthopnea is a more advanced stage of dyspnea. The client often assumes a "three-point position," sitting up with both hands on the knees and leaning forward. Orthopnea develops because the supine position increases the amount of blood returning from the lower extremities to the heart and lungs (preload). The client learns to avoid respiratory distress at night by supporting the head and thorax on pillows. In severe heart failure, the client may resort to sleeping upright in a chair.

Paroxysmal nocturnal dyspnea (PND) resembles the frightening sensation of suffocation. The client suddenly awakens with the feeling of severe suffocation and seeks relief by sitting upright or opening a window for a "breath of fresh air." Respirations may be labored and wheezing (cardiac asthma). PND represents an acute aggravation of pulmonary congestion. It stems from (1) a combination of increased venous return to the lungs due to recumbency and (2) suppression of the respiratory center to sensory input from the lungs during sleep. Once the client is in the upright position, relief from the attack of PND may not occur for 30 minutes or longer.

Acute pulmonary edema, a medical emergency, usually results from left ventricular failure. In clients with severe cardiac decompensation, the capillary pressure within the lungs becomes so elevated that fluid is pushed from the circulating blood into the interstitium, then into the alve-

oli, bronchioles, and bronchi. The resulting pulmonary edema, if untreated, may cause death from suffocation. Clients with pulmonary edema literally drown in their own fluids.

The dramatic symptoms of acute pulmonary edema terrify the client and significant others. Typical manifestations include the following:

Severe dyspnea
Orthopnea
Pallor
Tachycardia
Expectoration of large amounts of frothy, blood-tinged sputum
Fear
Wheezing
Sweating
Bubbling respirations
Cyanosis
Nasal flaring
Use of accessory breathing muscles
Tachypnea
Vasoconstriction
Hypoxia in arterial blood gas findings

Cardiovascular signs also denote LVF. Inspecting and palpating the precordium may reveal an enlarged or left laterally displaced apical impulse. This occurs because the left ventricle dilates in an effort to augment ventricular contraction and emptying. Also, heart gallop (S_3 or S_4) sounds may be an early finding in heart failure as the left ventricle becomes less compliant and its walls vibrate in response to filling during diastole. The appearance of pulsus alternans (alternating strong and weak heartbeats) may also herald the onset of LVF.

Cerebral hypoxia may occur as a result of a decrease in cardiac output causing inadequate brain perfusion. Depressed cerebral function can cause anxiety, irritability, restlessness, confusion, impaired memory, bad dreams, and insomnia. Impaired ventilation with resultant hypercapnia may also be a precipitant.

Fatigue and muscular weakness are often associated with LVF. Inadequate cardiac output leads to hypoxic tissue and slowed removal of metabolic wastes, which in turn causes the client to tire easily. Disturbances in sleep and rest patterns may aggravate fatigue.

Renal changes can occur in both RVF and LVF, but are more striking in the latter. Nocturia occurs early in heart failure. During the day, the client is upright, blood flow is away from the kidneys, and the formation of urine is reduced. At night, urine formation increases as blood flow to the kidneys improves. Nocturia may interfere with effective sleep patterns, which may contribute to fatigue. As cardiac output falls, decreased renal blood flow may result in oliguria, a late sign of heart failure.

In addition, if renal artery pressure falls, lowered glomerular filtration increases retention of sodium and water. In response to a continued reduction in renal blood flow, the renin-angiotensin-aldosterone mechanism is activated. Aldosterone, released from the adrenal cortex, promotes further retention of sodium and water by the renal tubule. This results in an expansion in blood volume of up to 30% and edema. As the sodium concentration in the extracellular fluid increases, so also does the osmotic pressure of the plasma. The hypothalamus responds to the higher osmotic pressure by releasing antidiuretic hormone (ADH) from the posterior pituitary. This, in turn, promotes renal tubular reabsorption of water. However, aldosterone is more important than is ADH in the production of edema.[90, 158]

Right Ventricular Failure

When the right ventricle fails, peripheral edema and venous congestion of the organs develop. Liver enlargement (hepatomegaly) and abdominal pain occur as the liver becomes congested with venous blood. If this occurs rapidly, stretching of the capsule surrounding the liver causes severe discomfort. The client may notice either a constant aching or a sharp pain in the right upper quadrant. In chronic heart failure, abdominal tenderness generally disappears.

In severe RVF, the lobules of the liver may become so congested with venous blood that they become anoxic. Anoxia leads to necrosis of the lobules. In long-standing heart failure, these necrotic areas may become fibrotic and then sclerotic. As a result, a condition called *cardiac cirrhosis* develops, manifested by ascites and jaundice.

In chronic heart failure, the increased workload of the heart and the extreme work of breathing increase the metabolic demands of the body. Anorexia, nausea, and bloating develop secondary to venous congestion of the gastrointestinal tract. The combination of increased metabolic needs and decreased caloric intake results in a marked wasting of tissue mass and cardiac cachexia.[158] Anorexia and nausea may also result from digitalis toxicity. This is a common problem because digitalis is usually prescribed for heart failure.[102]

Dependent edema is one of the early signs of RVF. Venous congestion in the peripheral vascular beds causes increased capillary hydrostatic pressure. Capillary hydrostatic pressure overwhelms the opposing pressure of plasma proteins, and fluid shifts out of the capillary beds into the interstitial spaces, with resultant pitting edema. Edema is usually symmetrical and occurs in the dependent parts of the body where venous pressure is highest. In ambulatory clients, edema begins in the feet and ankles and ascends up the lower legs. It is most noticeable at the end of the day and often subsides after a night's rest. In the recumbent client, pitting edema may develop in the presacral area and, as it worsens, progress to the genital region and medial thighs. Concurrent jugular vein distention differentiates the edema of heart failure from that of lymphatic obstruction, cirrhosis, and hypoproteinemia. Anasarca, a late sign in heart failure, is substantial and generalized edema. It can involve the upper extremities, genital area, and thoracic and abdominal walls. Cyanosis of the nail beds appears as venous congestion reduces peripheral blood flow.

Clients with heart failure often feel anxious, frightened, and depressed. Almost all clients realize that the heart is a vital organ and that when the heart begins to fail, health also fails. As the course of the disease progresses and manifestations worsen, the client may develop an over- whelming fear of permanent disability and death. Clients express their fears in varying ways: nightmares, insomnia, acute anxiety, depression, or withdrawal from reality.

Backward Versus Forward Failure

The clinical presentation of heart failure arises from inadequate cardiac output or the pooling of blood behind the failing chamber, or both. Backward failure is venous congestion arising from the damming of blood behind the failing chamber. Forward failure is a problem of inadequate perfusion. It results when reduced contractility produces a decrease in stroke volume and cardiac output. As cardiac output falls, blood flow to vital organs and peripheral tissues diminishes. This causes mental confusion, muscular weakness, and renal retention of sodium and water. Extracellular fluid retention increases circulating blood volume, further taxing the ailing heart.

High-Output Versus Low-Output Failure

High-output failure occurs when the heart, despite normal- to high-output levels, is simply not able to meet the accelerated needs of the body. Causes of high-output failure include sepsis, Paget's disease, beriberi, anemia, thyrotoxicosis, arteriovenous fistula, and pregnancy.

Low-output failure occurs in most forms of heart disease. Low-output failure results in hypoperfused tissue cells. The underlying disorder is related not to increased metabolic needs of the tissues but to poor ventricular pumping action and a low cardiac output.[158]

■ Diagnostic Tests

The diagnosis of heart failure rests primarily on presenting manifestations and pertinent data from the client's health history. Diagnostic studies assist in determining the underlying cause and the degree of heart failure. Such studies include a chest x-ray, ECG, and echocardiogram.[90]

In LVF, chest x-ray often depicts an enlarged cardiac silhouette, pulmonary and venous congestion, and interstitial edema. Interstitial edema on x-ray produces images called Kerley B lines. Pleural effusions may develop and generally reflect biventricular failure.

Arterial blood gases are drawn. Early heart failure with pulmonary edema may lead to respiratory alkalosis due to hyperventilation. However, as the disorder progresses and oxygenation becomes more impaired, acidosis will develop. Pulse oximetry values will show decreased oxygen levels.

Liver enzymes document the degree of liver failure. Elevated blood urea nitrogen and creatinine levels reflect decreased renal perfusion.

An ECG may give clues to the cause of LVF. Abnormalities in the ECG arise from the underlying cardiac disorder and from therapeutic agents. For instance, cardiac dysrhythmias may occur due to myocardial ischemia or electrolyte imbalance induced by diuretics or digitalis excess. Therefore, the ECG plays an important role in the management of heart failure.

Echocardiography provides information about cardiac chamber size and ventricular function and aids in assessing myocardial, valvular, congenital, and pericardial heart disease.

Critical Care

■ Medical Management

Clients with acute heart failure are usually admitted to an intensive care unit where they receive continuous assessment and intervention. The goals in the management of heart failure are to improve ventricular pump performance and reduce myocardial workload.

Positioning the Client

The client is placed in a high Fowler position or chair to reduce pulmonary venous congestion and relieve the dyspnea. The legs are maintained in a dependent position as much as possible.[83] Recognize that even though the legs are edematous, they should not be elevated. Elevating the legs would rapidly increase venous return.

Administering Oxygen

Administer oxygen in high concentrations by mask or cannula to (1) relieve hypoxia and dyspnea and (2) improve oxygen-carbon dioxide exchange. For hypoxemia, the physician may order a partial rebreathing mask with a flow rate of 8 to 10 L/min to deliver oxygen concentrations of 40% to 70%. A nonrebreathing mask can achieve higher oxygen concentrations. If these methods fail to raise the arterial oxygen tension (PaO_2) above 60 mm Hg, the client may need intubation and ventilatory management. Intubation provides a route for removing secretions from the bronchi. Should severe bronchospasm or bronchoconstriction present, bronchodilators are given. Monitor the client's heart rhythm because some bronchodilators also stimulate the myocardium and may lead to dysrhythmias.[83]

Improving Ventricular Pump Performance

Digitalis. Digitalis exerts a direct and beneficial effect on myocardial contraction in the failing heart. Digitalis does the following:

- Increases ventricular contractility (inotropic effect)
- Increases ventricular emptying and the capacity of the heart for work
- Slows conduction of impulses through the AV node and Purkinje fibers
- Increases the AV nodal refractory period
- Augments stroke volume
- Increases cardiac output

Improved cardiac output enhances kidney perfusion, which may create a mild diuresis of sodium and water.

A number of digitalis and cardiac glycoside preparations are available, and all have approximately the same effect on the heart. However, these medications differ significantly in their potency, speed of action, elimination from the body, and gastrointestinal irritation. Table 45–4 compares two cardiac glycosides.

The effectiveness of digitalis in heart failure depends on the severity and underlying cause of the condition. It is most effective in heart failure associated with low cardiac output caused by ischemic, rheumatic, hypertensive, or congenital heart disease. Digitalis may also be initiated to control the ventricular response in atrial fibrillation, which is the most common dysrhythmia in heart failure.[12] Digitalis is not given for heart failure associated with high cardiac output states, such as anemia and thyrotoxicosis. Digitalis is contraindicated in constrictive pericarditis or cardiac tamponade. Digitalis should be used with caution in acute MI because it increases myocardial oxygen demand.

When administering digitalis, assess for signs of digitalis toxicity. Digitalis has a relatively long half-life: 1.6 to 2.0 days in uncomplicated clients and over 4.4 days in clients with renal failure. Digitalis levels can become elevated as a result of medication interactions. The most common medications that increase digoxin levels are quinidine, verapamil, and amiodarone. Antibiotics may

			Onset of Action	Peak Effect	Half-Life	Therapeutic Plasma Level	Toxic Plasma Levels
Agent	**Absorption**	**Excretion**					
Digoxin	55%–75% gastrointestinal	Principally renal; some hepatic	5–30 min	1–5 hr	30–40 hr	0.5–2.0 ng/ml	2.4 ng/ml
Digitoxin	90%–100% gastrointestinal	Principally hepatic; some renal excretion	30 min–2 hr	4–12 hr	5–7 days	14–26 ng/ml	35 ng/ml

Table 45–4. Pharmacologic Properties of Selected Cardiac Glycosides

IV, intravenous.
Data from Kuhn, M. (1991). *Pharmacotherapeutics.* Philadelphia: F. A. Davis.

Table 45–5. Digitalis Toxicity

System	Clinical Manifestations
Gastrointestinal tract	Anorexia, nausea, vomiting, diarrhea, abdominal cramps (these symptoms are common in 50% of clients with digitalis toxicity and are often the first indication of toxicity)
Central nervous system	Headache, fatigue, lethargy, depression, restlessness, irritability, drowsiness; profound manifestations may include convulsions, neuralgia, delusions, hallucinations, aphasia, memory loss
Cardiovascular system	Bradycardia, ventricular bigeminy or trigeminy, ventricular tachycardia, atrioventricular block, atrial tachycardia with block, sinus arrest
Eyes	Flickering flashes of light; "colored vision," usually yellow or blue; halo vision; photophobia; blurring; diplopia; scotomata (blind spots in visual field)

Treatment
Hospitalization and administration of intravenous digoxin immune Fab (Digibind) in a dosage equimolar to the amount of digitalis in the body; 40 mg of Digibind = 0.5 mg of digoxin or digitoxin

raise digitalis levels by decreasing gastrointestinal flora and preventing bacterial inactivation of digitalis. Anticholinergic agents, which decrease gastric motility, may also result in increased digitalis levels. Digitalis dosage may need to be reduced if the client is taking any of these medications.[88] Clients most prone to the toxic effects of digitalis are the elderly and those with advanced heart disease, severe arrhythmias, or acute MI. Also, clients with cor pulmonale, hypothyroidism, hepatic disease, renal disease, metabolic alkalosis, or hypokalemia (lowered serum potassium) more readily develop toxic effects.

Digitalis toxicity occurs in approximately one in five clients. It may present with systemic or cardiac manifestations. The major clinical manifestations and treatment of digitalis toxicity are outlined in Table 45–5. Digitalis toxicity is more prevalent when serum concentration is equal to or greater than 2 μg/L, serum potassium is less than 3.0 mEq/L, or serum magnesium is low. If any of these manifestations are present, notify the physician, withhold digitalis, and initiate interventions to abate the undesirable symptoms.

Digitalis toxicity may be a life-threatening condition. Carefully follow the guidelines in Box 45–3 for prevention of toxicity.[84, 90, 102]

Dopamine and Dobutamine. Other inotropic agents (e.g., dopamine, dobutamine, and amrinone) may be ordered for clients with severe low-output heart failure. These medications facilitate myocardial contractility and enhance stroke volume.

Dopamine is a naturally occurring catecholamine with alpha-adrenergic, beta-adrenergic, and dopaminergic activity. When given in small doses (<4 μg/kg/min), dopamine stimulates the dopaminergic receptors in the renal, mesenteric, cerebral, and coronary vascular beds, which causes vasodilation. The primary result is an increase in renal blood flow, glomerular filtration rate, and sodium excretion. The alpha- and beta-adrenergic receptors in the vasculature and myocardium are affected by moderate doses of dopamine (4–8 μg/kg/min). The results are increases in heart rate, stroke volume, and cardiac output.

Alpha-adrenergic effects, such as intense vasoconstriction, dominate when dopamine is given in doses larger than 8 μg/kg/min.[151] Although dopamine may effectively improve cardiac output, it may do so at the expense of the myocardium and renal blood flow. An increase in heart rate may increase myocardial oxygen demands and decrease myocardial oxygen supply, which may prove costly to the already ischemic myocardium.

Another inotropic agent is dobutamine, a synthetic derivative of dopamine that has strong beta-stimulatory effects within the myocardium; it increases heart rate, AV conduction, and myocardial contractility. Dobutamine is capable of increasing cardiac output without increasing myocardial oxygen demands or reducing coronary blood flow.[90]

Amrinone is also used to increase cardiac output in severe heart failure. In addition to the positive inotropic effects, amrinone increases renal blood flow and glomerular filtration rate.[13, 90]

Box 45–3. Guidelines for Digitalis Preparations

1. Read the labels of all digitalis preparations with care. Digitalis preparations have similar names but different strengths and dosages.
2. Always take the client's pulse for 1 full minute *apically* before giving a dose of digitalis.
3. Carefully note the rate and rhythm of the pulse and chart them.
4. If the heartbeat is very rapid, below 60, or irregular (if it is normally regular), withhold the drug and notify the physician.
5. Observe the client carefully for signs of digitalis toxicity. When severe symptoms present, call the physician before administering the drug.
6. Advise the client and significant others to monitor the pulse rate daily. Also reinforce the importance of taking prescribed potassium supplements.

Diuretic	Effects on Serum Electrolytes	Action		Duration (hr)
		Onset (hr)	*Peak (hr)*	
Thiazides—Carbonic anhydrase inhibitors inhibit NaCl reabsorption from the luminal side of distal tubule				
Chlorothiazide (Diuril)	↓ Cl⁻ ↓ K⁻ ↑ HCO₃⁻	2 (PO) ¼ (IV)	4 ½	6–12 2
Hydrochlorothiazide (Hydro-DIURIL)		2 (PO)	4	6–12
Chlorthalidone (Hygroton)		2 (PO)	6	48–72
Loop Diuretics—Short-acting agents inhibit NaCl reabsorption in the thick ascending loop of Henle				
Furosemide (Lasix)	↓ Cl⁻ ↓ K⁺ ↑ HCO₃⁻ ↓ Na⁺	1 (PO) 5 min (IV)	1–2 ½	6–8 2
Bumetanide (Bumex)				
Ethacrynic acid (Edecrin)		½ (PO) 5 min (IV)	2 ½	6–8 2
Potassium-Sparing Diuretics—Antagonize the effects of aldosterone at the cortical tubule				
Spironolactone (Aldactone)	↑ K⁺	Gradual (PO)	3 days after starting therapy	2–3 days after ending therapy
Triamterene (Dyrenium)		2–4 (PO)	6–8	7–24
Osmotic Diuretics—Increase water excretion over sodium excretion				
Mannitol Urea	↓ Na⁺ ↓ K⁺	30–60 min (IV)	1	6–8
Sucrose		30–45 min (IV)	1	5–6
		10–30 min (IV, PO)	30 min	4–5

Table 45–6. Characteristics of Some Commonly Used Diuretics

IV, intravenously; PO, orally.
Adapted from Kuhn, M. M. (1991). *Pharmacotherapeutics.* Philadelphia: F. A. Davis; Katzung, B. G. (1992). *Basic and clinical pharmacology.* Norwalk, CT: Appleton & Lange; Koda-Kindle et al. (1994). *Handbook of applied therapeutics.* Vancouver, WA: Applied Therapeutics.

Reducing Myocardial Workload

Reducing Preload. Diuretic therapy plays an integral part in the successful management of heart failure. Diuretics enhance renal excretion of sodium and water, which reduces circulating blood volume, diminishes preload, and lessens systemic and pulmonary congestion. Table 45–6 describes the characteristics of commonly used diuretics.

Although they are effective, diuretics should be administered cautiously because they have side effects. First, diuretics can produce mild to severe electrolyte imbalance. Hypokalemia, a particularly dangerous problem, potentiates digitalis toxicity and can cause myocardial weakness and cardiac arrhythmias. Second, vigorous diuresis may produce hypovolemia and hypotension, jeopardizing cardiac output.[13, 90]

Reducing Afterload. Vasodilating agents have become an increasingly important intervention in heart failure. Vasodilators vary in their mechanisms of action, which include (1) direct dilation of veins, (2) dilation of arterioles, (3) combined action on veins and arterioles, and (4) inhibition of angiotensin-converting enzyme (ACE). Closely assess the client receiving vasodilators because they can cause rapid drops in blood pressure.

Venous dilators relax venous smooth muscle and increase the capacity of the systemic venous bed; blood is "trapped" in the veins, and venous return to the heart is decreased. This increased venous capacity reduces preload. Examples of venous dilators are nitroglycerin and isosorbide dinitrate.

Arteriolar dilators reduce systemic arteriolar tone, which decreases peripheral vascular resistance and afterload. Reduction in afterload reduces the left ventricular workload and increases cardiac output. Improved renal perfusion may initiate diuresis. Hydralazine is the most commonly used arterial dilator. Be aware that hydralazine may precipitate reflex tachycardia.

Combined venous and arteriolar dilators decrease both preload and afterload. Sodium nitroprusside helps manage severe heart failure. A potent vasodilator, sodium nitroprusside relaxes the smooth muscles of both veins and arterioles. It does not directly affect the heart muscle or heart rate.

ACE inhibitors suppress the renin-angiotensin-aldosterone system, blocking production of the potent vasoconstrictor angiotensin II. This results in an increase in renal blood flow and a decrease in renal vascular resistance, which enhances diuresis. ACE inhibitors, such as captopril, improve hemodynamic status and have been shown to prolong the survival of clients with CHF.[13, 90]

Researchers are studying the use of beta-adrenergic receptor antagonists in heart failure. Traditionally, these agents were contraindicated in heart failure, but recent studies have shown that administration of beta-blockers may result in improved symptomatic and functional status.[90]

Managing the Client's Diet

The two major objectives in the treatment of heart failure are to improve cardiac efficiency and control sodium and water retention. Sodium restrictions are placed on the diet to prevent, control, or eliminate edema. Two- to 4-g sodium diets are usually prescribed (Table 45–7).

From the use of some loop diuretics, potassium is lost via the kidneys, which can lead to dysrhythmias and electrolyte imbalances. Hypokalemia sensitizes the myocardium to digitalis and therefore predisposes the client to digitalis toxicity. Potassium supplements and adequate dietary potassium are important.

It is usually not necessary to restrict fluid intake in clients with mild or moderate heart failure. However, with more advanced failure, it is beneficial to limit water to 1000 ml/day. The reason for this restriction is that excessive water intake tends to dilute the amount of sodium in body fluids and may produce a low salt syndrome (hyponatremia). Hyponatremia is characterized by lethargy and weakness. It results more often from the combination of a restricted sodium diet, increased sodium loss during diuresis, and excessive water intake.[90, 110]

Reducing the Client's Stress and Risk of Injury

In addition to improving ventricular pump performance and reducing myocardial workload, the client also needs to reduce physical and emotional stress. Sometimes clinicians overlook rest to diminish the workload of the heart as an intervention. The client must rest both physically and mentally. The proper use of rest as the initial step in management offers many benefits. Rest can promote diuresis, slow the heart rate, and relieve dyspnea, all of

Table 45–7. Sodium Content of Selected Foods

Foods Low in Sodium	
Dairy products	Skim milk, eggs, cottage cheese, cream cheese, ice cream
Meats*	Turkey, chicken, veal, lamb, liver, fresh fish, tuna packed in water (meats should be unprocessed)
Fruits and vegetables*	Any fresh or frozen food in this group
Beverages	Any juice (except tomato or V-8), coffee, tea, Poland Spring water
Breads	Some breads and cereals
Seasonings	Garlic, onion, bay leaf, pepper, dill, nutmeg, rosemary, allspice, thyme, sage, caraway, cinnamon, almond and vanilla extract, fresh dried herbs
Fats	Margarine, oils, shortening, unsalted salad dressings
Desserts	Sherbet, fruit ice, gelatin, fruit drinks
Miscellaneous	Unbuttered, unsalted popcorn; unsalted nuts; vinegar

Foods High in Sodium	
Milk and dairy products	Aged, hard cheese; pasteurized processed cheese; buttermilk
Meats	Sausage, frankfurters, ham, bacon, corned beef; all smoked, pickled, or cured meats; canned meats, "TV dinners," salami, most luncheon meats, beef jerky
Fruits and vegetables	Pickled or canned fruits and vegetables, olives, sauerkraut, pickles
Breads and cereals	Salted crackers, macaroni and cheese, pretzels, rye rolls, pizza, commercial pancake mixes
Beverages	Tomato juice, V-8 juice, beef broth, bouillon
Fats	Commercial salad dressings, dips and party spreads, peanut butter
Seasonings	Garlic, celery, or onion salt; Accent, monosodium glutamate (MSG), meat tenderizer, soy sauce, catsup, steak sauce, mustard, canned soup
Desserts	Fruit pies, doughnuts, cake, commercial puddings
Miscellaneous	Baking soda, baking powder, salted popcorn, salted nuts, potato chips

* Food sources high in potassium.

which allow more conservative use of pharmacologic agents (e.g., digitalis, diuretics, and vasodilators).[54, 110]

Whether the physician prescribes complete bedrest or a program of modified bedrest depends on the seriousness of the client's condition. Clinicians may use the New York Heart Association functional classification of cardiovascular disability as a guide to activity prescription (Box 45–4).

The physician may prescribe a mild sedative or small doses of barbiturates and tranquilizers to promote rest and overcome problems of restlessness, insomnia, and anxiety.

The client may also be at risk of injury because of immobility. The client should be confined to bed only long enough to regain cardiac reserve, but not so long as to promote the complications of immobility. The client confined to bedrest should be given specific teaching and learning guidelines to prevent the harmful effects of immobility. Passive leg exercises should be performed several times daily to prevent venous stasis, which may lead to the formation of venous thrombi and pulmonary emboli. The physician may also initiate anticoagulant therapy to prevent these potentially deadly complications.[42, 67, 81, 88, 97]

■ Nursing Management of the Medical Client

Assessment

Assess the client for the clinical manifestations of CHF, especially the high-risk client. Use Figure 45–14 to help differentiate right and left-sided failure. Also consider the psychosocial affect of heart failure on the client and family.

Diagnosis, Planning, Implementation

Decreased Cardiac Output. When the heart can no longer effectively pump blood, cardiac output falls. Write the diagnosis as *Decreased Cardiac Output related to heart failure or dysrhythmias, or both*.

Planning: Expected Outcomes. The client will have increased cardiac output, as evidenced by regular cardiac rhythm, heart rate within normal limits, and hemodynamic parameters within normal limits.

Implementation. Assess vital signs and heart rhythm every 15 minutes to 1 hour, depending on the stability of the client's vital signs. Tachycardia is a common compensatory mechanism, but it further taxes the myocardial oxygen supply. Monitor dysrhythmias hourly. Most intensive care units have a central area of monitors for all clients in the unit. Common dysrhythmias include premature atrial contractions, PVCs, and paroxysmal atrial tachycardia. Dysrhythmias reduce ventricular filling time, decrease myocardial contractility, and increase myocardial oxygen demands. All of these conditions further compromise cardiac output. Respirations are usually rapid and labored, and the client is orthopneic. Hypotension, if present, is due to decreased perfusion, vagal stimulation, and dysrhythmias. Hypertension is usually due to pain, anxiety, or previous history of hypertension.

Monitor lung and heart sounds every 2 to 4 hours.

Box 45–4. New York Heart Association Classification of Cardiovascular Disability

Class I

No limitation on physical activity. Ordinary physical activity does not cause undue fatigue, palpitation, dyspnea, or anginal pain.

Class II

Slight limitation of physical activity. Comfortable at rest, but ordinary physical activity results in fatigue, palpitation, dyspnea, or anginal pain.

Class III

Marked limitation of physical activity. Comfortable at rest, but less than ordinary physical activity causes fatigue, palpitation, dyspnea, or anginal pain.

Class IV

Unable to carry on any physical activity without discomfort. Symptoms of cardiac insufficiency or of the anginal syndrome may be present even at rest. If any physical activity is undertaken, discomfort is increased.

From Konstam, M., Drakup, K., Baker, D. et al. (1994). Heart failure: Evaluation and care of patients with left-ventricular systolic dysfunction. Clinical Practice Guideline No. 11. AHCPR publication 94–0612. Rockville, MD: Agency for Health Care Policy and Research, Public Health Service.

Crackles are common, and respirations may be wet and frothy as pulmonary congestion develops. Heart sounds may be distant and include an S_3 or S_4 as filling and ejection times are delayed. Administer oxygen as prescribed to improve tissue hypoxia.

Monitor urine output hourly, noting changes in color and volume of output. Oliguria may reflect decreased renal perfusion. Diuresis is expected once the client is digitalized and given diuretics. For many clients fluid balance and left ventricular function are managed with a pulmonary artery catheter. The catheter and nursing responsibilities are discussed in Chapter 47.

Assess for changes in mental status every 4 hours. Adequate cerebral perfusion requires adequate cardiac output. The client may exhibit changes in problem solving as an early indicator of cerebral hypoxia.

Feed the client small meals and provide a rest period after meals. Large meals increase myocardial workload and cause vagal stimulation, which results in bradycardia. If caffeine causes tachycardia or ectopic beats, it should be avoided.

Fluid Volume Excess. When cardiac output falls, the kidneys attempt to increase cardiac output by retaining sodium and water; this can lead to a condition of fluid overload. Write the diagnosis as *Fluid Volume Excess related to reduced glomerular filtration, decreased cardiac output, increased ADH production, and sodium and water retention*.

Planning: Expected Outcomes. The client will have an adequate fluid balance, as evidenced by output exceeding intake if on diuretics, clearing breath sounds, stable vital signs, decreasing weight, and resolving edema.

Implementation. Monitor intake and output every 2 hours during acute phases of heart failure. Maintain Fowler's position to facilitate breathing. Provide frequent oral care, at least every 4 hours. Clients need oral care more often if they are breathing through the mouth. Weigh the client daily to monitor response to diuretic therapy. Body weight is a more sensitive indicator of fluid balance than is intake and output.

Monitor for signs of increasing peripheral edema. Assess jugular neck vein distention, peripheral edema in the legs or sacrum, and hepatic engorgement or pain in the right upper quadrant.

Provide the client with a low sodium diet. Physicians commonly order a 2- to 4-g diet. Fluid restrictions may also be used until diuresis is achieved.

Impaired Gas Exchange.
When the left ventricle fails, intravascular pressure in the heart and lungs increases. This increase in pressure can cause fluid to leave the vascular space and enter the interstitial spaces in the lungs. Write the diagnosis as *Impaired Gas Exchange related to fluid in alveoli.*

Planning: Expected Outcomes. The client will have improved gas exchange, as evidenced by vital signs within normal limits for the client's age and condition, skin and mucous membranes without cyanosis or pallor, decreased dyspnea, and arterial blood gases within normal limits.

Implementation. Auscultate breath sounds every 2 to 4 hours, noting adventitious sounds indicating congestion. Encourage the client to turn, cough, and deep-breathe to clear the airway and facilitate oxygen delivery. Maintain the client in Fowler's position to facilitate diaphragmatic expansion and ventilation. Administer oxygen as ordered to improve tissue oxygenation. Monitor arterial blood gas and pulse oximetry results; changes may reveal severe hypoxia or acidosis. If respiratory failure develops, the client may require intubation and continuous mechanical ventilation.

Altered Peripheral Tissue Perfusion.
When the left ventricle fails, cardiac output falls and perfusion to organs and tissues is decreased. Write the diagnosis as *Altered Peripheral Tissue Perfusion related to decreased cardiac output and vasoconstriction.*

Planning: Expected Outcomes. The client will have adequate peripheral tissue perfusion, as evidenced by warm, dry skin, the presence of peripheral pulses, and rapid blanching.

Implementation. Monitor the client's peripheral pulses every 4 hours. Note the color and temperature of the skin. Keep the extremities warm to promote vasodilation to decrease preload. Be alert for the development of thrombophlebitis, because the legs are commonly kept flat or dependent to decrease venous return. Encourage active range-of-motion exercise or provide passive range-of-motion exercise to decrease venous pooling. Clinical manifestations of thrombophlebitis include unilateral swelling, calf pain, and pallor. Homans' sign, which is pain in the calf with dorsiflexion of the foot, is not a reliable indicator of thrombophlebitis.

Risk for Activity Intolerance.
With LVF, the heart is unable to increase cardiac output and oxygen delivery in response to increases in activity. Write the diagnosis as *Risk for Activity Intolerance related to decreased cardiac output.*

Planning: Expected Outcomes. The client will have improved tolerance and levels of activity without dyspnea.

Implementation. Intersperse nursing care activity with rest periods. During the acute stages of heart failure, provide all self-care activity for the client and allow the client to participate as dyspnea allows. Monitor the client's response to each activity, noting the development of dyspnea, tachycardia, angina, hypotension, diaphoresis, and dysrhythmias. Assess vital signs prior to any major activity (i.e., getting into a chair, walking), immediately after activity and 3 minutes later. The time required for vital signs to return to baseline indicates the degree of cardiac deconditioning. Increase the client's activity levels according to the cardiac rehabilitation nurse or physician orders.

Instruct the client to avoid activities that increase cardiac workload during acute stages of care. Activities that precipitate fatigue may demand more cardiac output than the ailing heart can supply.

Risk for Impaired Skin Integrity.
When cardiac output falls, perfusion to peripheral tissues is decreased. Write the diagnosis as *Risk for Impaired Skin Integrity related to decreased peripheral tissue perfusion and immobility.*

Planning: Expected Outcomes. The client will maintain intact skin and will not exhibit any stage I or greater pressure ulcers.

Implementation. If possible, turn the client from side to side every 2 hours. If the client is too dyspneic to turn, provide a pressure reduction mattress. Use heel protectors or elevate the client's calf. Wash the client's lower legs carefully, and apply lotion to maintain skin integrity.

Risk for Digitalis Toxicity.
A collaborative problem is *Risk for Digitalis Toxicity related to impaired drug excretion from hepatic and renal involvement.*

Planning: Expected Outcomes. The nurse will monitor the client for signs of digitalis toxicity.

Implementation. Assess the client for decreased heart sounds, hypokalemia, and first-degree heart block. Monitor serum digitalis levels and potassium.

Anxiety.
When cardiac output falls, the sympathetic nervous system is stimulated and this results in the flight

or fight reaction. Write the diagnosis as *High Risk for Anxiety related to decreased cardiac output, hypoxia, and fear of death or serious consequences.*

Planning: Expected Outcomes. The client will have few signs of anxiety, as evidenced by being able to rest calmly in bed, being able to ventilate fears, and vital signs becoming stable.

Implementation. Provide for psychological rest by maintaining a calm environment; anxiety is contagious. Explain in advance the routine regimens and management strategies. Solicit the client to ask questions. If the client seems reluctant, impart the common fears and questions expressed by other clients. This strategy often encourages the client to ask questions that were thought of but not spoken.

Anxiety often develops as a result of the diagnosis of heart failure, the presenting manifestations, and the fear of death. Provide emotional support for both the client and significant others. Intervention in heart failure involves a long, often difficult period of adjustment. The initial fear of death, brought on by the dramatic symptoms of acute heart failure, can evolve into a long-term strain on coping resources. Remember that anxiety and fear further tax the client's failing heart. Take time to talk with the client about his or her concerns and anxieties. Many clients with heart failure fail to cope. They need your skill and emotional support as well as the additional support of a cardiovascular clinical specialist, counselor, social worker, religious leader, or other appropriate person.

Evaluation

Heart failure is not resolved quickly. The client will often make initial strides once diuresis begins and be able to breathe more easily. But the disorder is usually chronic, and much more time is required for complete resolution. Many times, the goal of less than full resolution must be accepted.

The outcome for the client with heart failure depends on (1) the degree of cardiac hypertrophy, (2) the amount of cardiac reserve, and (3) the presence of other heart or associated disorders. The prognosis can generally be predicted by the client's response to therapeutic measures. A very slow or inadequate response to prescribed medications, special diets, activity limitations, and so forth signals a poor prognosis. Nevertheless, thorough ongoing assessments, early intervention, therapeutic compliance, and prevention of complications can control this disorder.[90]

Acute and Subacute Care

Heart failure is termed *refractory* or *intractable* when recommended diet, medications, and interventions fail to alleviate symptoms and restore partial cardiac reserve. To treat refractory heart disease, the physician usually (1) reviews the client's entire course, (2) reassesses the medical intervention, and (3) prescribes the following interventions:

- A prolonged course of therapy and rest in a healthcare facility or under the close supervision of a home healthcare nurse
- Severe sodium restriction (e.g., 250-mg sodium diet)
- Fluids restricted to less than 500 ml/day
- Diuretic therapy using several different types of diuretics
- IV dobutamine therapy[14]

Some clients with heart failure need additional monitoring and nursing care following hospital discharge. Increasingly, these clients are being transferred to subacute units before returning home. While in the subacute care unit, the client may receive additional rehabilitation, monitoring, and discharge teaching.[148]

■ Medical Management

The use of a variety of drugs is typically the mode of therapy in treatment of heart failure. However, attempts are under way to provide respite for the heart in acute failure. The common feature of the different approaches is to unload the heart for hours to days while it is recuperating. The most popular devices are (1) venoarterial bypass, which assists the heart by diverting blood to a pump that returns it to the arterial tree; and (2) counterpulsation, which operates in synchrony with the heartbeat to adjust the aortic blood pressure by rhythmically changing either the volume of blood in the aorta (with use of an external pump) or the capacity of the aorta (with use of an internal balloon). Counterpulsation is discussed in Chapter 47. All methods aim to reduce the external work of the heart and the tension during systole and to decrease myocardial oxygen consumption while improving coronary arterial perfusion.[14]

Ventricular Assist Devices

For the last few decades, when conventional therapy, such as medications and the intra-aortic balloon pump (IABP) became ineffective, there was little hope for the client with myocardial failure. Advances continue to be made in perfecting methods of mechanical ventricular support until a client stabilizes or receives a heart transplant. If the client is likely to recover in 5 to 7 days or will be ready for transplant, a ventricular assist device (VAD) can be used.

VADs are devices with the capability to support circulation, either partially or totally, until the heart recovers or is replaced. Various devices are available and can be inserted in the cardiac catheterization laboratory, the emergency department, or the intensive care unit (ICU).

Extracorporeal membrane oxygenation (ECMO) systems are widely used for short-term hemodynamic stabilization. These devices remove blood from the inferior vena cava to a centrifugal pump that pumps the blood to an oxygenator. The oxygenated blood is returned to the client via the femoral artery. Long-term use, over 48 hours, has not been shown to promote recovery. In addition, bleeding is a concern because anticoagulation is needed.

External centrifugal and roller pumps are positioned outside the body. Cannulas are inserted into any heart chamber (except the right ventricle) and can provide cardiac output for both the right and left side of the heart. Cardiac outputs of 2 to 6 L/min have been reported. The client is immobile and anticoagulated while the pump is in use.

Implantable left VADs are designed for clients with isolated left ventricular end-stage heart disease. This device is inserted into the heart while the client is on cardiopulmonary bypass. The pump is powered by electrical or pneumatic pumps inserted in the abdominal or peritoneal wall. The pump is powered externally by using an external power cable, which allows for greater client mobility (e.g., sitting in a chair or walking). A battery-powered system has recently been developed so that the client need not remain hospitalized.

As the number of donor organs shrinks and the options for mechanical assist devices grow, the nurse needs to become more aware of these devices for clients with end-stage heart diseases. Traditionally clients were cared for in the ICU, but today a critical care environment is not needed once the client is stabilized (except for clients on ECMO).

■ Surgical Management

Heart Transplantation

When the heart is irreversibly damaged and can no longer adequately function, and the client is at risk of dying, cardiac transplantation and the use of an artificial heart to assist or replace the failing heart are last measures. With the development of cyclosporine and with improvements in the procurement and preservation of donor hearts, cardiac transplantation has become an accepted therapeutic procedure. One-year survival rates after transplantation are greater than 85%. Although transplantation may not be appropriate for all clients, it may be the only option available to some. Heart transplantation is discussed in Chapter 47.

Cardiomyoplasty

For clients with low cardiac output who are not candidates for cardiac transplantation, a new procedure called cardiomyoplasty may support the failing heart. Initially developed in 1985, this procedure involves wrapping of the latissimus dorsi muscle around the heart and electro-stimulating it in synchrony with ventricular systole. In 1994 the Food and Drug Administration approved expansion of cardiomyoplasty clinical trials; to date over 200 clients have undergone this procedure.

Preoperative preparation involves an extension evaluation of the client to reveal associated medical conditions that would exclude them from the procedure. Preoperative assessments include the following:

- A New York Heart Association functional class assignment
- Twenty-four-hour Holter monitoring study
- Left ventricular ejection fraction
- Exercise stress test
- Left and right heart catheterization
- Chest radiographs
- Computed tomography of the chest
- Pulmonary function tests

Throughout this evaluation, clients and their families need education as well as psychological support.

The cardiomyoplasty procedure is performed by a team of surgeons and completed in two stages that can last more than 5 hours. Initially a plastic surgeon dissects the latissimus dorsi muscle from the lower five or six thoracic vertebrae, lower ribs median ridge of the sacrum, and outer lip of the iliac crest. Next, two intramuscular pacing electrodes are implanted in the proximal portion of the latissimus dorsi, allowing the distal and middle portions, which will be wrapped around the heart, to be free of electrodes.

In the second stage, a cardiothoracic surgeon performs a median sternotomy. The surgeon lifts the heart and sutures the posterior ventricular area to the larger border of the latissimus dorsi muscle flap. The lateral and anterior walls of the left and right ventricles are then sutured to the borders of the latissimus dorsi to complete the wrapping. Once the wrapping is completed, an intramyocardial sensing electrode is placed to ensure long-term synchronization between the heart and the latissimus dorsi. The muscle-stimulating device (Cardiomyostimulator, Medtronic, Minneapolis) is then placed in a small pocket in the rectus abdominis muscle, and the sensing electrodes are connected to it.

Immediate postoperative care is similar to that of any cardiac surgery client. Continuous cardiac and hemodynamic monitoring is initiated. Inotropic and vasopressor agents are administered to maintain cardiac output until the pulse generator is activated (within 2–3 weeks). Since the muscle flap obliterates the left upper lobe and can reduce vital capacity by as much as 20%, aggressive pulmonary hygiene and judicious pain management are essential to prevent atelectasis or pneumonia. In addition, an upper extremity exercise regimen is prescribed.

Stimulation of the latissimus dorsi muscle begins 2 weeks after surgery. At this time the client may be dismissed from the hospital and is seen in the cardiologist's office. The electrical stimulation phase is a long and gradual 7-week process of retraining. Impulses are initiated with every other cardiac cycle and are slowly increased to several with each cardiac cycle. Amplitude and the number of impulses are increased until a train of impulses is generated to contract with substantial force. Electrical stimulation bursts are timed to occur with mitral valve closure. The ECG shows spikes similar to pacemaker spikes with each impulse from the muscle stimulator. The client will require the muscle stimulating device for the rest of his or her life.

Follow-up care involves ECGs, chest films, and at 6 weeks a 24-hour Holter monitoring study. Every 6 months these tests are repeated to assess cardiac function. The client should begin to feel the effects of the wrap and improved left ventricular function 6 months after surgery. A 5-year survival rate of 47% was reported in 1991, similar to early heart transplant statistics.[24, 32]

Community and Self-Care

When the client leaves the healthcare facility and returns home, schedule adjustments to help avoid overexhaustion. The client may require a nap in the afternoon, shorter working hours, more sleep at night, and frequent vacations. With growing strength and improvement, the client may gradually undertake mild exercise (e.g., walking short distances on level ground, playing a few holes of golf, and simple calisthenics). Such exercises, when performed sensibly, can strengthen the heart muscle and improve its performance.

The client will need instruction before discharge on measures to prevent the recurrence of heart failure. Such measures include the following:

- Take digitalis and all other medications exactly as prescribed.
- Stay on the sodium-restricted diet.
- Adhere to the program of diuretic therapy.
- Treat all infections promptly.

Have medical follow-up as ordered, usually every 2 weeks until stable.[29, 83, 97]

Serum potassium is closely monitored. The combination of hypokalemia and digitalis therapy can lead to lethal dysrhythmias.

Sodium is controlled in the diet, whereas the intake of cholesterol in the elderly usually is not reduced. Trace elements lost in diuresis are usually replaced with a multivitamin.[70, 77, 78]

■ Modifications for Elderly Clients

Heart failure is becoming increasingly a disorder of the very old. Cardiac decompensation can be triggered by seemingly minor illnesses and dietary indiscretions.[12, 72, 77, 130]

Medications commonly used by the elderly may have an impact on heart performance even though they pose little risk of interaction with cardiovascular medications. Nonsteroidal anti-inflammatory agents tend to worsen heart disease because they promote sodium retention; tricyclic antidepressants and neuroleptic agents lead to orthostatic hypotension. Conversely, cardiac performance can have an impact on the medication's action also. The development of RVF can markedly increase the prothrombin time and thereby increase the action of anticoagulants.

Conclusions

Disorders of cardiac function are the leading causes of death in the industrialized world. It is imperative that you fully understand the care of clients with heart disease to improve outcomes and quality of life and reduce morbidity and mortality. Coronary artery disease is the precursor to several problems. The development of occlusive plaque damages the myocardium. MI, permanent damage to the myocardium, may be the first indicator of how serious the heart disease is. Your role in the care of these clients is to improve cardiac output and educate the client about risk reduction. Heart failure is a frequent endpoint of cardiac disease. Again, it is important to maximize cardiac output and reduce system demands on the heart.

Thinking Critically

1. Your client is a 67-year-old man with newly diagnosed insulin-dependent diabetes in end-stage heart failure. The client was recently released from the hospital. You are to begin intravenous dobutamine therapy during this initial home visit. What assessment should be made prior to initiating dobutamine therapy? What other assessment interventions might be done?

Factors to Consider. How does heart failure respond to the administration of dobutamine? What teaching or learning needs might be assessed in the client?

2. A client with long-standing coronary artery disease experiences severe chest pain unrelieved by nitroglycerin. He is admitted with an acute myocardial infarction to the coronary care unit. What are the priorities on admission? What medical treatment may be instituted in the first hours following the infarction?

Factors to Consider. What time frame is considered most crucial to the salvage of myocardial muscle. What care is given to the newly admitted client?

3. A 70-year-old man is scheduled for a coronary artery bypass graft (CABG). What postoperative complications are most prevalent in the elderly?

Factors to Consider. How is CABG surgery accomplished? Why is the CABG surgery popular option?

Bibliography

1. Abou-Awdi, N. L., & Samuels, W. L. (1995). Transmyocardial laser revascularization. *Seminars in Perioperative Nursing, 4,* 173.
2. Adler, L. P., Brundage, B. H., & Shapiro, E. H. (1991). Tomorrow's cardiac imaging—today. *Patient Care, 25,* 143–146, 149–154, 156.
3. Albert, N. M. (1994). Laser angioplasty and intracoronary stents: Going beyond the balloon. *AACN Clinical Issues in Critical Care Nursing, 5,* 15.
4. American Heart Association. (1994). *Advanced cardiac life support.* Dallas: Author.
5. American Heart Association. (1994). Randomized trial of intravenous heparin versus recombinant hirudin for acute coronary syndromes. In *The global use of strategies to open occluded coronary arteries (GUSTO) IIa investigators.* Dallas: Author.
6. American Heart Association. (1996). *Research facts—update 1996.* Dallas: Author.
7. American Heart Association. (1996). *Heart and stroke facts.* Dallas: Author.

8. American Heart Association. (1996). *Heart and stroke facts: 1996 statistical supplement.* Dallas: Author.

9. Angina Guideline Panel. (1994). Quick reference guide for clinicians: Diagnosing and managing unstable angina. *Journal of the American Academy of Nurse Practitioners, 6,* 585.

10. Artinian, N. T., & Duggan, C. H. (1995). Sex differences in patient recovery patterns after coronary artery bypass surgery. *Heart and Lung, 24,* 483.

11. Assey, M. E. (1993). Heart disease in the elderly. *Heart Disease and Stroke, 2,* 330.

12. Atkins, P. J., Hapshe, E., & Riegel, B. (1994). Effects of a bedbath on mixed venous oxygen saturation and heart rate in coronary artery bypass graft patients. *American Journal of Critical Care, 3,* 107.

13. Baker, D. W., et al. (1994). Management of heart failure: I. Pharmacologic treatment. *JAMA, 272,* 1361.

14. Baker, D. W., et al. (1994). Management of heart failure: III. The role of revascularization in the treatment of patients with moderate or severe left ventricular systolic dysfunction. *JAMA, 272,* 1528.

15. Barbiere, C. C., & Liberatore, K. (1992). Automated external defibrillators: An update of additions to the ACLS algorithms. *Critical Care Nurse, 12,* 17.

16. Baxendale, M. (1992). Pathophysiology of coronary artery disease. *Nursing Clinics of North America, 27,* 143.

17. Beery, T. A. (1995). Gender bias in the diagnosis and treatment of coronary artery disease. *Heart and Lung, 24,* 427.

18. Bergstrom, D. L., & Keller, C. (1992). Drug induced myocardial ischemia and acute myocardial infarction. *Critical Care Nursing Clinics of North America, 3,* 273.

19. Bevans, M, & McLinmore, B. (1992). Intracoronary stents: A new approach to coronary artery dilatation. *Journal of Cardiovascular Nursing, 7,* 34.

20. Beyers, J. F. (1993). The use of aspirin in cardiovascular disease. *Journal of Cardiovascular Nursing, 8,* 1.

21. Bittl, J. A., & Thomas, P. (1996). Beyond the balloon. *Harvard Health Letter, 21,* 4.

22. Blumenfeld, J. D. (1995). Renal and cardiac complications of hypertension. *Clinical Symposia, 46,* 3.

23. Borriello, S. L., Siegel, S. C., & Fishman, R. F. (1994). Directional coronary atherectomy: A new treatment for coronary artery disease. *Heart and Lung, 23,* 199.

24. Bove, L. A., et al. (1995). Nursing care of patients undergoing dynamic cardiomyoplasty. *Critical Care Nurse, 15,* 96.

25. Bousquet, G. L. (1990). Congestive heart failure: A review of nonpharmacologic therapies. *Journal of Cardiovascular Nursing, 4,* 35.

26. Brannon, F. J., et al. (1993). *Cardiopulmonary rehabilitation: Basic theory and application* (2nd ed.). Philadelphia: F. A. Davis.

27. Braunwald, E., Mark, D. B., Jones, R. H., et. al. (1994). *Diagnosing and managing unstable angina. Clinical practice guideline—Quick reference guide for clinicians.* No. 10. Rockville, MD: U. S. Department of Health and Human Services. Agency for Health Care Policy and Research.

28. Carson, P. (1996). Pharmocologic treatment of congestive heart failure. *Clinical Cardiology, 19* (4), 271.

29. Cason, C. L., et al. (1992). Preparatory sensory information for cardiac catheterization. *Cardiovascular Nursing, 28,* 41.

30. The CAVEAT investigators. (1992). The coronary angioplasty versus excisional atherectomy trial-preliminary results (abstract). *Circulation, 86,* 374.

31. Chase, S. L. (1996). Critical care drug update; part II. *RN, 59* (6), 49.

32. Chyun, D. (1993). The cutting edge in cardiovascular medicine. *Critical Care Nurse, 13,* (Suppl.) 16.

33. Cimini, D. M. (1992). Indium-111 antimyosin antibody imaging. *Critical Care Nurse, 12,* 44.

34. Cohn, J. N. (1996). The management of chronic heart failure. *The New England Journal of Medicine, 335* (7) 490–498.

35. Collins, E. G., Pfeifer, P. B., & Mozdzierz, G. (1995). Decisions not to transplant: Futility or rationing. *Journal of Cariovascular Nursing, 9,* 23.

36. Corley, M. C., et al. (1995). Patient and nurse criteria for heart transplant candidacy. *Medsurg Nursing, 4,* 211.

37. Craney, J. M. (1993). Radiofrequency catheter ablation of supra-

ventricular tachycardias: Clinical consideration and nursing care. *Journal of Cardiovascular Nursing, 7,* 26.

38. The Criteria Committee of the New York Heart Association (1979). *Nomenclature and criteria for diagnosis of the diseases of the heart and great vessels.* Boston: Little, Brown.

39. Daumer, R., & Miller, P. (1992). Effects of cardiac rehabilitation on psychosocial functioning and life satisfaction of coronary artery disease clients. *Rehabilitation Nursing, 17,* 69.

40. Deelstra, M. H. (1993). Coronary rotational ablation: An overview with related nursing interventions. *American Journal of Critical Care, 2,* 16.

41. Dempsey, S. J., Dracup, K., & Moser, D. K. (1995). Women's decision to seek care for symptoms of acute myocardial infarction. *Heart and Lung, 24,* 444.

42. Dracup, K., et al. (1994). Management of heart failure: II. Counseling, education, and lifestyle modifications. *JAMA, 272,* 1442.

43. Eaker, E., et al. (1994). Special report: Cardiovascular disease in women. *Heart Disease and Stroke, 3,* 114.

44. Engler, M. B., & Engler, M. M. (1995). Assessment of the cardiovascular effects of stress. *Journal of Cardiovascular Nursing, 10,* 51.

45. Eysmann, S. B., & Douglas, P. S. (1992). Reperfusion and revascularization strategies for coronary artery disease in women. *JAMA, 268,* 1903.

46. *Fifth Report, Joint National Committee on Detection, Evaluation, and Treatment of High Blood Pressure.* (1993). Bethesda, MD: National Heart, Lung, and Blood Institute.

47. Fischman, D. L., et al. (1994). A randomized comparison of coronary-stent placement and balloon angioplasty in patients with coronary artery disease. *New England Journal of Medicine, 331,* 496.

48. Fletcher, G. F. (1993). The value of exercise in preventing coronary atherosclerotic heart disease. *Heart Disease and Stroke, 2,* 183.

49. Fleury, J. (1992). The application of motivational theory to cardiovascular risk reduction. *Image, 24,* 229.

50. Foley, J. J. (1994). Pharmacologic management of hypertensive crisis in the emergency department. *Journal of Emergency Nursing, 20* (2), 134.

51. Fowles, R. E. (1995). Myocardial infarction in the 1990s: Complications, prognosis, and changing patterns of management. *Postgraduate Medicine, 97,* 155.

52. Franklin, B. A. (1995). Diagnostic and functional exercise testing: Test selection and interpretation. *Journal of Cardiovascular Nursing, 10,* 8.

53. Friedman, M. M. (1993). Stressors and perceived stress in older women with heart disease. *Cardiovascular Nursing, 29,* 25.

54. Friedman, M. M. (1995). Correlates of fatigue in older women with heart failure. *Heart and Lung, 24,* 512.

55. Froelicher, E. S., et al. (1995). Risk profile screening. *Journal of Cardiovascular Nursing, 10,* 30.

56. Futterman, L. G. (1995). Presumed consent: The solution to the critical organ donor shortage? *American Journal of Critical Care, 4,* 383.

57. Gist, H., Mesrobian, H. D., & Ziskind, A. A. (1993). New interventional techniques for coronary revascularization. *Heart Disease and Stroke, 2,* 198.

58. Go, R. T. (1994). Current status of the clinical applications of cardiac positron emission tomography. *Radiologic Clinics of North America, 32* (3) 501.

59. Goodman, M., et al. (1996). Hostility predicts restenosis after percutaneous transluminal coronary angioplasty. *Mayo Clinic Proceedings 71* (8), 729–734.

60. Goodman, S. G., et al. (1994). Safety and anticoagulation effect of a low-dose combination of warfarin and aspirin in clinically stable coronary artery disease. *American Journal of Cardiology, 74,* 657.

61. Granger, C. B., et al. (1994). A pooled analysis of coronary arterial patency and left ventricular function after intravenous thrombolysis for acute myocardial infarction. *American Journal of Cardiology, 74,* 1220.

62. Gunnar, R. M., et al. (1990). ACC/AHA guidelines for the early management of patients with acute myocardial infarction. *Journal of the American College of Cardiology, 16,* 249.

63. Hamilton, G. A., & Seidman, R. N. (1993). A comparison of the

recovery period for women and men after an acute myocardial infarction. *Heart and Lung, 22,* 308.

64. Hanisch P. (1993). Informational needs and preferred time to receive information for phase II cardiac rehabilitation patients: What CE instructors need to know. *Journal of Continuing Education in Nursing, 24,* 82.

65. Hanson, M. J. S. (1994). Modifiable risk factors for coronary heart disease in women. *American Journal of Critical Care, 3,* 177.

66. Hartley, L. H., et al. (1995). Physical work capacity after acute myocardial infarction in patients with low ejection fraction and effect of captopril. *American Journal of Cardiology, 76,* 857.

67. Hawthorne, M. H., & Hixon, M. E. (1994). Functional status, mood disturbance and quality of life in patients with heart failure. *Progress in Cardiovascular Nursing, 9,* 22.

68. Hirsh, J., & Fuster, V. (1994). Guide to anticoagulant therapy. Part 1: Heparin. *Circulation, 89,* 1449.

69. Hirsch, J., & Fuster, V. (1994). Guide to anticoagulant therapy. Part 2: Oral anticoagulants. *Circulation, 89,* 1469.

70. Hixon, M. E. (1994). Aging and heart failure. *Progress in Cardiovascular Nursing 9,* 4.

71. Hodis, H. N., Cashin-Hemphill, L., & Mack, W. J. (1994). Prevention of coronary atherosclerosis. *Heart Disease and Stroke, 3,* 182.

72. Horvath, K. A., et al. (1996). Transmyocardial laser revascularization: Operative techniques and clinical results at two years. *Journal of Thoracic and Cardiovascular Surgery, 111* (15), 1047.

73. Hudgins, C., & Sorenson, G. (1994). Directional coronary atherectomy: A new treatment for coronary artery disease. *Critical Care Nurse, 14,* 61.

74. Hylton-Rushton, C. (1996). Creating an ethical practice environment: A focus on advocacy. *Critical Care Nursing Clinics of North America, 1* (2), 387–398.

75. Jacavone, J., & Dostal, M. (1992). A descriptive study of nursing judgment in the assessment and management of cardiac pain. *Advances in Nursing Science, 15,* 54.

76. Jafri, S. M., & Borzak, S. (1995). Medical therapy of acute myocardial infarction: Part II. The role of adjunctive medical therapy. *Journal of Intensive Care Medicine, 10,* 109.

77. Jessup, M., et al. (1992). CHF in the elderly: Is it different? *Patient Care, 26,* 40.

78. Jessup, M., et al. (1992). Managing CHF in the older patient. *Patient Care, 26,* 65.

79. Johnson, J. L., & Morse, J. M. (1990). Regaining control: The process of adjustment after myocardial infarction. *Heart and Lung, 19,* 126.

80. Jones, P. H., & Gotto, A. M. (1994). Prevention of coronary heart disease in 1994: Evidence for intervention. *Heart Disease and Stroke, 3,* 290.

81. Karmilovich, S. E. (1994). Burden and stress associated with spousal caregiving for individuals with heart failure. *Progress in Cardiovascular Nursing 9,* 33.

82. Katzung, B. G. (1992). *Basic and clinical pharmacology,* (5th ed.). Norwalk, CT: Appleton & Lange.

83. Kayser, S. R. (1994). Management of chronic congestive heart failure: Part I—General introduction to treatment. *Progress in Cardiovascular Nursing 9,* 39.

84. Kelly, R. A., & Smith, T. W. (1992). Use and misuse of digitalis blood levels. *Heart Disease and Stroke, 1,* 117.

85. Keresztes, P., et al. (1993). Measurement of functional ability in patients with coronary artery disease. *Journal of Nursing Measurement, 1,* 19.

86. King, K. B. (1994). Preparing patients and families for health care procedures. *Heart Disease and Stroke, 3,* 95.

87. King, K. B., et al. (1992). Patient perceptions of quality of life after coronary artery surgery: Was it worth it? *Research in Nursing and Health, 15,* 327.

88. Kinney, M. R. (1995). Assessment of quality of life in recovery settings. *Journal of Cardiovascular Nursing, 10,* 88.

89. Koda-Kimble, M. A., et al. (1992). *Handbook of applied therapeutics* (2nd ed.). Vancouver, WA: Applied Therapeutics.

90. Konstam, M., et al. (1994). *Heart failure: Evaluation and care of patients with left-ventricular systolic dysfunction. Clinical practice guideline* No. 11, AHCPR Publication No. 94-0612, Rockville, MD: Agency for Health Care Policy and Research, Public Health Service, U.S. Department of Health and Human Services.

91. Kop, W. J., et al. (1994). Vital exhaustion predicts new cardiac events after successful coronary angioplasty. *Psychosomatic Medicine, 56,* 281–287.

92. Krepostman, A., & Borzak, S. (1993). Coronary heart disease: Seven steps to primary prevention. *Consultant, 33,* 33, 39, 49.

93. Landau, C., Lange, R. A., & Hillis, L. D. (1994). Percutaneous transluminal coronary angioplasty. *New England Journal of Medicine, 330,* 981.

94. Larson, G. C., et al. (1994). Recurrent cardiac events in survivors of ventricular fibrillation or tachycardia. *JAMA, 271,* 1335.

95. Lee, K. L., et al. (1994). Holding GUSTO up to the light. *Annals of Internal Medicine, 120,* 876.

96. Lemmon, P. N., Kalman, J., & Zamary, K. (1994). Tissue plasminogen activator: The nurse's role. *Critical Care Nurse, 14,* 22.

97. Letterer, R. A., et al. (1992). Learning to live with congestive heart failure. *Nursing 92, 22,* 34.

98. Little, T., & Lindsay, J. (1994). Percutaneous transluminal coronary angioplasty and coronary artery bypass graft surgery in octogenarians: Indications and outcomes. *Heart and Stroke, 3,* 261.

99. Luepker, R. V. (1993). Patient adherence: A "risk factor" for cardiovascular disease. *Heart Disease and Stroke, 2,* 418.

100. Manson, J. E., et al. (1990). A prospective study of obesity and risk of coronary heart disease in women. *New England Journal of Medicine, 322,* 882.

101. Manson, J. E., et al. (1992). The primary prevention of myocardial infarction. *New England Journal of Medicine, 326,* 1406.

102. Marcus, F. I. (1992). Use and toxicity of digitalis. *Heart Disease and Stroke, 1,* 27.

103. Mark, D. B., et al. (1994). Continuing evolution of therapy for coronary artery disease. *Circulation, 89,* 2015.

104. Matthew, J. P., et al. (1996). Atrial fibrillation following coronary artery bypass graft surgery. *JAMA, 276* (4), 300–306.

105. McCauley, K. M. (1995). Assessing social support in patients with cardiac disease. *Journal of Cardiovascular Nursing, 10,* 73.

106. McSweeney, J. C. (1993). Making behavior changes after a myocardial infarction. *Western Journal of Nursing Research, 15,* 441.

107. Mellion, M. B. (1994). Exercise: How much is enough, and how much is too much? *Heart Disease and Stroke, 3,* 2.

108. Melschke, H., Eisengerg, M. S., & Larson, M. D. (1993). Prehospital delay interval for patients who use emergency medical services: The effect of heart-related medical conditions and demographic variables. *Annals of Internal Medicine, 22,* 1597.

109. Milander, M. M., & Kuhn, M. (1992). Lipid-lowering drugs. *AACN—Clinical Issues in Critical Care, 3,* 494.

110. Miller, M. M. (1994). Current trends in the primary care management of chronic congestive heart failure. *Nurse Practitioner, 19,* 64.

111. Miller, P., et al. (1990). Marital functioning after cardiac surgery. *Heart and Lung, 19,* 55.

112. Miracle, V. A., Hovekamp, G. (1994). Needs of families of patients undergoing cardiac procedures. *American Journal of Critical Care Nursing, 3,* 155.

113. Moore, S. M. (1995). A comparison of women's and men's symptoms during home recovery after coronary artery bypass surgery. *Heart and Lung, 24,* 495.

114. Moser, S. A., Crawford, D., & Thomas, A. (1993). Updated care guidelines for patients with automatic implantable cardioverter defibrillators. *Critical Care Nurse, 13,* 62.

115. Moss, A. J., & Benhorin, J. (1990). Prognosis and management after a first myocardial infarction. *New England Journal of Medicine, 322,* 743.

116. Murphy, M. C., et al. (1994). Differences in symptoms during post PTCA versus rotational ablation. *Progress in Cardiovascular Nursing 9,* 4.

117. Nara, A. R., et al. (1989). *Biophysical measurement series: Blood pressure.* Redmond, WA: SpaceLabs.

118. National Cholesterol Education Program Adult Treatment Panel II: Summary of the second report of the National Cholesterol Education Program (NCEP) Expert Panel on Detection, Evaluation, and Treatment of High Blood Cholesterol in Adults. (Adult Treatment Panel II). (1993). *JAMA, 269,* 3015.

119. Navarra Lemmon, P, Kalman, J., & Zamary Sefcik, K. (1994). Tissue plaminogen activator: The nurse's role. *Critical Care Nurse, 14,* 22.

120. Owens, M. W., & Daniel, J. L. (1993). IV magnesium sulfate in the treatment of ventricular tachycardia and acute myocardial infarction. *Critical Care Nurse, 13*, 83.

121. Peppers, M. (1995). Drug watch: Treating hypertensive crisis. *Emergency, 27* (9), 18.

122. Peberdy, M. A., & Ornato, J. P. (1992). Coronary artery disease in women. *Heart Disease and Stroke, 1*, 315.

123. Porter, L. A. (1995). Drug profiles: Maximizing therapeutic effectiveness. *Journal of Cardiovascular Nursing, 10*, 64.

124. Porterfield, L. M., Porterfield, J. G., & Collins, S. W. (1993). The cutting edge in arrhythmias. *Critical Care Nurse*, Suppl. June 8–9.

125. Rakel, R. E. (1992). Use of antiplatelet medication for prevention of myocardial infarction and stroke. *Heart and Stroke, 1*, 2.

126. Rebenson-Piano, M. (1989). The physiologic changes that occur with aging. *Critical Care Nursing Quarterly, 12*, 1.

127. Redeker, N. S., et al. (1995). Women's patterns of activity over 6 months after coronary artery bypass surgery. *Heart and Lung, 24*, 502.

128. Riddle, M. M., Dunston, J. L., & Castanes, J. L. (1996). A rapid recovery program for cardiac surgery patients. *American Journal of Critical Care, 5*, 152.

129. Riegel, B., & Gocka, I. (1995). Gender differences in adjustment to acute myocardial infarction. *Heart and Lung, 24*, 457.

130. Ringel, K. (1991). *Effects of time on lifestyle adjustments following a cardiac event as influenced by an outpatient cardiac rehabilitation program.* Unpublished dissertation, Rush University, Chicago.

131. Rodeheffer, R. J. (1996). Congestive heart failure: Current clinical issues. *Circulation, 93* (1), 196.

132. Ryan, T., & Skolnick, A. E. (1994). Indications for coronary angioplasty. *Heart Disease and Stroke, 3*, 29.

133. Saatvedt, K., Dragsund, M., & Nordstrand, K. (1996). Transmyocardial laser revascularization and coronary artery bypass grafting. *Annals of Thoracic Surgery, 62* (1), 323.

134. Safian, R. D., et al. (1996). Do excimer laser angioplasty and rotational atherectomy facilitate balloon angioplasty? *Journal of the American College of Cardiology, 27* (3), 552.

135. Sauve, J., & Fortin, F. (1996). Factors related to the recovery of women following coronary artery bypass surgery. *Cardiovascular Nursing, 32*, 1

136. Schron, E. B., et al. (1996). Relation of sociodemographic, clinical, and quality of life variables to adherence in the cardiac arrhythmia suppression trial. *Cardiovascular Nursing, 32*, 1.

137. Serruys, P. W., et al. (1994). A comparison of balloon-expandable-stent placement and balloon angioplasty in treatment of coronary artery disease. *New England Journal of Medicine, 331*, 489.

138. Sheldon, W. C. (1993). Indications for coronary arteriography. *Heart Disease and Stroke, 2*, 192.

139. Simari, R. D., et al. (1994). Coronary angioplasty in acute myocardial infarction: Primary immediate adjunctive, rescue, or deferred adjunctive approach? *Mayo Clinic Proceedings, 69*, 346.

140. Simons, L. H., Cunningham, S., & Catanzaro, M. (1992). Emotional responses and experiences of wives of men who survive a sudden cardiac death event. *Cardiovascular Nursing, 28*, 17.

141. Sommers, M. S. (1992). The near-death experience after cardiopulmonary arrest. *Med-Surg Nursing Quarterly, 1*, 55.

142. Sommers, M. S. (1992). Preventing complications of CPR. *Med-Surg Nursing Quarterly, 1*, 44.

143. Speroff, L., & Lobo, R. A. (1994). Postmenopausal hormone therapy and the cardiovascular system. *Heart Disease and Stroke, 3*, 173.

144. Speroni, R., et al. (1992). Coronary atherectomy: Overview and implications for nursing. *Journal of Cardiovascular Nursing, 7*, 17.

145. Stahl, D. (1994). Subacute care: The future of healthcare. *Nursing Management, 25*, 35.

146. Steinke, E. E., & Patterson, P. (1995). Sexual counseling of MI patients by cardiac nurses. *Journal of Cardiovascular Nursing, 10*, 81.

147. Stewart, S. L. (1992). Acute MI: A review of pathophysiology, treatment, and complications. *Journal of Cardiovascular Nursing, 6*, 1.

148. Strimike, C. L. (1995). Caring for a patient with an intracoronary stent. *American Journal of Nursing, 95*, 40.

149. Sugarman, D. I., & Brozovich, F. V. (1995). Cardiac imaging and assessment of left ventricular function. *Physical Medicine and Rehabilitation Clinics of North America, 6*, 97.

150. Sullivan, M. J. (1994). New trends in cardiac rehabilitation in patients with chronic heart failure. *Progress in Cardiovascular Nursing, 9*, 13.

151. Sulzbach, L. M., Hazard Munro, B., & Hirshfield, J. (1995). A randomized clinical trial of the effect of bed position after PTCA. *American Journal of Critical Care, 4*, 221.

152. Teplitz, L., & Siwik, D. (1994). Cellular signals in atherosclerosis. *Journal of Cardiovascular Nursing, 8*, 28.

153. Thompson, E. J. (1993). Transesophageal echocardiography: A new window on the heart and great vessels. *Critical Care Nurse, 13*, 55.

154. Velas, J. C. (1991). A review of cardiac imaging modalities. *Nurse Practitioner Forum, 2*, 231.

155. Wenger, N. K., et al. (1995). *Cardiac rehabilitation as secondary prevention (Clinical practice guideline: Quick reference guide for clinicians)*, No. 17. Rockville, MD: U. S. Department of Health and Human Services, Public Health Service, Agency for Health Care Policy and Research and National Heart, Lung, and Blood Institute.

156. Wilbur, J., Holm, K., & Dan, A. (1993). A quantitative survey to measure energy expenditure in midlife women. *Journal of Nursing Measurement, 1*, 29.

157. Wingate, S. (1995). Quality of life for women after a myocardial infarction. *Heart and Lung, 24*, 467.

158. Wright, S. M. (1990). Pathophysiology of congestive heart failure. *Journal of Cardiovascular Nursing, 4*, 1.

159. Wu, C. Y. (1995). Assessment of postdischarge concerns of coronary artery bypass graft patients. *Journal of Cardiovascular Nursing, 10*, 1.

160. Zipes, D. P. (1992). Management of cardiac arrhythmias: pharmacological, electrical and surgical techniques. In E. Braunwald (Ed.), *Heart disease* (4th ed.) Philadelphia: W. B. Saunders.

Nursing Care of Clients with Disorders of Cardiac Rhythm

Kathleen A. Ringel

Peggy Gerard

The heart is endowed with a specialized system for (1) generating rhythmical impulses to cause rhythmical contraction of the heart muscle and (2) conducting these impulses rapidly throughout the heart. When this system functions normally, the atria contract about one-sixth of a second ahead of the ventricles. This orderly electrical activity must precede contraction to provide adequate cardiac output for perfusion of all body organs and tissues.

The rhythmical and conduction systems of the heart are susceptible to damage by heart disease, especially by ischemia of the heart tissues resulting from decreased coronary artery blood flow. The consequence is often a bizarre heart rhythm or abnormal sequence of contraction through the heart chambers. The abnormal rhythms, called dysrhythmias or arrhythmias, can decrease the pumping effectiveness of the heart severely, even to the extent of causing death.

Before reading about dysrhythmias, you may want to review the electrical conduction system of the heart in Chapter 43 and/or the electrocardiogram in Chapter 44.

A *normal sinus rhythm* is a heart rhythm that begins in the sinoatrial (SA) node and is between 60 and 100 beats per minute (BPM), with normal intervals and no aberrant or ectopic beats (Fig. 46-1). Characteristics of normal sinus rhythm are shown in Table 46-1.

Dysrhythmias

Dysrhythmias are abnormal heart rhythms. Dysrhythmias are common in persons with cardiac disorders, but also occur in persons with normal hearts. The most serious complication of a dysrhythmia is sudden death.[1,9] Since seconds can literally make the difference between life and death for the person who is experiencing a serious dysrhythmia, evaluating responsiveness, quickly activating

the emergency medical service (EMS), and initiating cardiopulmonary resuscitation (CPR) can determine the outcome.

Etiology and Risk Factors

Dysrhythmias result from disturbances in three major mechanisms: automaticity, conduction, and problems with reentry of impulses.[6,8,35]

■ Disturbances in Automaticity

Automaticity is a term used to describe alterations in the normal heart rates produced by various pacemaker cells in the myocardium. Recall that the SA node is the pacemaker of the heart because it possesses the highest level of automaticity. It normally produces a rhythm of 60 to 100 BPM. The SA node is regulated by the nervous system through the vagus nerve. Sympathetic stimulation increases the rate of firing; lack of sympathetic stimulation or vagal stimulation (which is parasympathetic) decreases the rate.

If the SA node does not initiate an impulse, every other muscle cell in the myocardium can start the impulse. This fail-safe mechanism is crucial during heart disease. Latent pacemaker cells in the atrioventricular (AV) junction will usually assume the role of pacemaker of the heart but at a slower rate (40–60 BPM). Such a pacemaker is called an escape pacemaker. If the AV junction is unable to take over as the pacemaker because of disease, an escape pacemaker in the electrical conduction system below the AV junction (i.e., in the bundle branches or Purkinje fibers) may take over at a still lower rate (< 40 BPM). In general, the farther the escape pacemaker is from the SA node, the slower it generates electrical impulses.

These impulses can also occur prematurely, that is, before the SA node would normally fire again. Premature impulses occur when the heart is ischemic; as with coro-

---

This chapter incorporates material written for the fourth edition by Juanita Reigle.

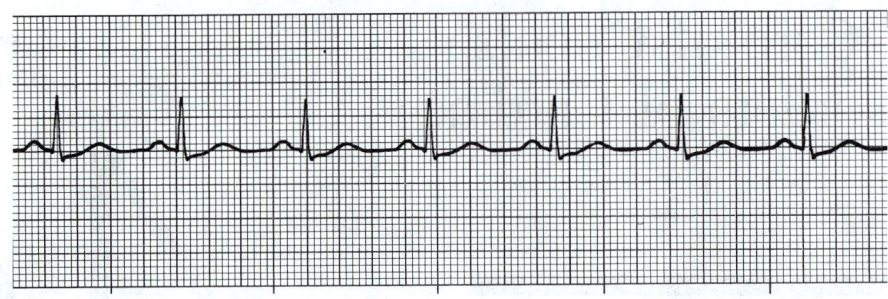

Figure 46–1. Normal sinus rhythm as seen on an ECG strip. Note the regular R–R interval, a rate of 80 beats per minute, and a P–R interval of 0.16 second.

nary artery disease. Myocardial infarction or heart failure has areas of calcification along different points in the heart, as a normal variant, or has irritation of the AV node, Purkinje system, or myocardium from drugs, nicotine, or caffeine.

Under a variety of circumstances, cardiac cells in any part of the heart, whether they be latent pacemaker cells or nonpacemaker myocardial cells, may take on the role of a pacemaker and start generating extraneous electrical impulses. When impulses begin from other sites, the sites are called ectopic pacemakers. For instance, if the SA node fails to fire, other sites in the atria can fire. If the atria do not initiate a beat, it can begin in the AV node, and if the AV node does not initiate a beat, one can start in the ventricles. When an ectopic pacemaker initiates a beat, the electrocardiographic (ECG) tracing appears different from the way it looks with a normal sinus rhythm beat.

Each of these areas of myocardium (atria, AV node, ventricles) have their own intrinsic rates:

Sinus node 60–100 BPM
Atria 60–100 BPM
AV node 40–60 BPM
Ventricles 20–40 BPM

When rates exceed these beats per minute, the rhythm is called accelerated and classified as a problem due to altered automaticity. When the rhythm is slower than the intrinsic rate, it is called bradycardia. A rhythm faster than the intrinsic rate is called tachycardia. Therefore sinus bradycardia is identified as a heart rate below 60 BPM. Sinus tachycardia is defined as a heart rate above 100 BPM.

Latent pacemaker cells can also fire at increased rates beyond their inherent rate. For example, an accelerated

Table 46–1. Characteristics of Normal Sinus Rhythms

Rhythm	Regular, P–P intervals and R–R intervals may vary as much as 3 mm and still be considered regular
Rate	60–100 beats per minute
P waves	One P wave preceding each QRS complex
P–R interval	0.12–0.20 second, consistent with each complex
QRS complex	0.04–0.10 second, consistent with each complex
Q–T interval	<0.40 second

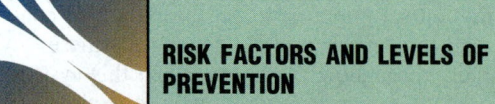

RISK FACTORS AND LEVELS OF PREVENTION

Dysrhythmias

Risk Factors

Myocardial ischemia (e.g., during angina, myocardial infarction, or heart failure); hypoxia; autonomic nervous system imbalances; lactic acidosis; electrolyte imbalances (especially potassium); drug toxicity; hemodynamic abnormalities; alterations in conduction, automaticity, or reentry.

Levels of Prevention

Primary Prevention

• Reduce the risk of myocardial disorders by curtailing intake of fats, cholesterol, limiting consumption of alcohol, exercising regularly, controlling stress responses.
• Prevent potassium imbalances in persons taking potassium-wasting diuretics.
• Monitor clients taking digitalis closely.

Secondary Prevention

• Monitor heart rhythm continuously in clients with chest pain of unknown origin, myocardial disease, advanced respiratory disease, multiple injuries.
• Stabilize hemodynamic abnormalities (fluid losses).
• Use antidysrhythmic medications to control dysrhythmias.

Tertiary Prevention

• Treat lethal dysrhythmias without delay. Defibrillate ventricular fibrillation quickly.
• Consider pacemakers or implantable defibrillators for clients with chronic dysrhythmias.

junctional tachycardia can develop with a rate higher than 60 (the inherent AV node rate). Abnormal automaticity is commonly caused by ischemia, hyperkalemia, hypocalcemia, hypoxia, increase in catecholamines, digitalis toxicity, and administration of atropine.

■ Disturbances in Conduction

Conduction is the speed the impulse travels through the sinus node, AV node, and Purkinje fibers. Conduction may be either too rapid or too slow. Blocks that slow or stop an impulse can occur anywhere along the pathway. Blocks develop as a result of ischemia of the tissues, scarring of conduction pathways, compression of the AV bundle by scar tissue, inflammation of the AV node, extreme vagal stimulation of the heart, electrolyte imbalances, increased atrial preload, digitalis toxicity, beta-blocking agents, impaired cellular metabolism, myocardial infarction (MI) (especially inferior), and valvular surgery.

Blocks result in changes in the appearance of the ECG. The blocked impulse needs more time to travel to its destination; therefore the wave is wider than normal. Disturbances in conduction can also lead to decreased cardiac output and life-threatening dysrhythmias.

Reentry is activation of muscle for a second time by the same impulse. The waves of electrical impulse are not extinguished. They keep going due to a combination of slow conduction and blocks. Therefore the conduction system is delayed or blocked (or both) in one or more segments while being conducted normally through the rest of the conduction system.

The problem occurs when some cells have been repolarized sufficiently so that they can prematurely depolarize again, producing ectopic beats and rhythms. Hyperkalemia and myocardial ischemia are the two most common causes of delay or block in the conduction system responsible for the reentry mechanism. The reentry mechanism can result in atrial fibrillation and ventricular fibrillation.

Clinical Manifestations and Diagnostic Findings

The significance of all dysrhythmias is the effect they have on cardiac output and vascular perfusion. During normal sinus rhythm, the atria fill and stretch the ventricles with about 30% more blood. This process is called the *atrial kick*. The extra stretch improves contractility of the ventricles and thereby increases cardiac output. When the impulse starts in the AV node or in the ventricles, atrial and ventricular contraction are no longer coordinated. Atrial kick is lost and cardiac output falls. For example, during contractions initiated in the ventricle the impulse begins in the ventricle and travels backward up the heart. Therefore the atria fill the ventricles while they are contracting or even afterward. Obviously, the efficiency of the heart as a pump is restricted during dysrhythmias and the clinical manifestations noted are due to changes in cardiac output.

The clinical manifestations of dysrhythmias include palpitations, dizziness or syncope, pallor, diaphoresis, altered mentation (restlessness and agitation to lethargy and coma), hypotension, sluggish capillary refill, swelling of the extremities, and diminished urinary output. Palpitations, dizziness, and syncope are the clinical symptoms that are most effectively evaluated by ambulatory ECG monitoring. The client wears a portable ECG monitor and records worrisome manifestations. The correlation of manifestations to the heart rhythm can be assessed. Shortness of breath, chest pain, and fatigue may also be caused by dysrhythmias. However, these manifestations are more likely to be caused by other factors, such as myocardial ischemia or heart failure.

Physical assessment findings may reveal a heart rate below 50 or above 140 BPM; an extremely irregular heart rhythm or pulse; a first heart sound that varies in intensity; sudden appearance of heart failure, shock, and angina pectoris; and a slow, regular heart rate that does not change with activity or medications such as atropine or epinephrine.

Diagnostic findings include abnormalities on the ECG. The key to dysrhythmia interpretation is the analysis of the form and interrelations of the P wave, the P–R interval, and the QRS complex. The ECG should be analyzed with respect to its rate, its rhythm, and the site of the dominant pacemaker, and the configuration of the P and QRS waves. Always remember that any ECG findings should be correlated with clinical observations of the client. A good admonition to remember is "treat the client, not the monitor."

It is necessary that the student develop a method of analysis of ECG strips that allows him or her to consistently identify the rhythm demonstrated. The analysis of rhythms is one of two types: sight reading and paper analysis. Sight readers identify the ECGs by looking at the whole rhythm. This technique requires much experience and continued regular viewing of rhythm strips. It is of little use to the beginner. Those with less experience need to develop a method of ECG analysis (Box 46–1).

Management

The management of dysrhythmias depends upon the type of dysrhythmia present and the client's response to the dysrhythmia. Ventricular dysrhythmias can be life-threatening, demanding immediate treatment. All dysrhythmias can reduce cardiac output and the client may be asymptomatic or very symptomatic from the decreased cardiac output. We will discuss the dysrhythmias and their management progressing from problems arising in the atria, then the AV junction and finally the ventricles.

Atrial Dysrhythmias

Disturbances in Automaticity

Sinus Tachycardia

Sinus tachycardia is characterized by a rapid, regular rhythm at a rate of 100 to 180 BPM with a normal P wave and QRS complex (Fig. 46–2A). It often occurs in

Box 46–1. Electrocardiographic Interpretation of Dysrhythmias

There are seven basic steps that assist you in the identification of dysrhythmias. The electrocardiogram (ECG) should be studied in an *orderly* fashion in the following manner.

Step 1

Calculate the heart rate. The simplest method for obtaining the rate is to count the number of R waves in a 6-inch strip of the ECG tracing (which equals 6 seconds). Multiply this sum by 10 to get the rate per minute (BPM). Because the ECG paper is marked into 3-inch intervals (at the top margin), the approximate heart rate can be rapidly calculated. Another method is to count the number of large squares between R waves. Find an R wave crossing a large square. Count the number of large squares until the next R wave. The approximate heart rate is

1 large square	= 300 BPM
2 large squares	= 150 BPM
3 large squares	= 100 BPM
4 large squares	= 75 BPM
5 large squares	= 60 BPM
6 large squares	= 50 BPM
7 large squares	= 43 BPM
8 large squares	= 37 BPM
9 large squares	= 33 BPM
10 large squares	= 30 BPM

Step 2

Measure the regularity (rhythm) of the R waves (ventricular rhythm). This can be done by gross observation or actual measurement of the intervals (R–R). If the R waves occur at regular intervals (with a variance of less than 0.12 second between beats), the ventricular rhythm is normal. When there are differences in R–R intervals (greater than 0.12 second), the ventricular rhythm is said to be irregular. The division of ventricular rhythm into regular and irregular categories assists in identifying the mechanism of many dysrhythmias.

Note atrial regularity and measure the atrial rate. Measure the regularity (rhythm) of the P waves (P–P). Use the above method, but calculate the distance between the same point on two consecutive P waves.

Step 3

Examine the P waves. If P waves are present and precede each QRS complex, the heartbeat originates in the sinus node, and a sinus rhythm exists. The absence of P waves or an abnormality in their position with respect to the QRS complex indicates that the impulse started outside the sinoatrial node and that an ectopic pacemaker is in command.

Step 4

Measure the P–R interval. Normally, this interval should be between 0.12 and 0.20 second. Prolongation or reduction of this interval beyond these limits indicates a defect in the conduction system between the atria and the ventricles.

Step 5

Measure the duration of the QRS complex. If the width between the onset of the Q wave and the completion of the S wave is greater than 0.12 second (three fine lines on the paper), an intraventricular conduction defect exists.

Step 6

Examine the ST segment. Normally this segment is isoelectric, meaning it is neither elevated nor depressed because the positive and negative forces are equally balanced during this period. Elevation or depression of the ST segment indicates an abnormality in the onset of recovery of the ventricular muscle, usually because of injury (e.g., acute myocardial infarction).

Step 7

Examine the T wave. Normally the T wave is upright and one-third the height of the QRS complex. Any condition that interferes with normal repolarization (e.g., myocardial ischemia) may cause the T waves to invert. An abnormally high serum potassium level will cause the T wave to become very tall—sometimes the height of the QRS complex.

---

response to an increase in sympathetic stimulation or decreased vagal (parasympathetic) stimulation. Causes of sinus tachycardia include fever; emotional and physical stress; heart failure; fluid volume loss; hyperthyroidism; hypercalcemia; medications, including, atropine, nitrates, epinephrine, and isoproterenol; caffeine; nicotine; and exercise. Most clients do not experience clinical manifestations except for occasional palpitations. However, the clinical manifestations are also dependent upon the heart rate and the effect it has on cardiac output. There is little time for ventricular filling and atrial contraction between these quick beats. Clients with underlying heart disease may not tolerate the increased myocardial workload and reduced and coronary artery filling time that accompanies the increased heart rate. These clients may experience hypotension and angina pectoris.

Management focuses on alleviating the underlying cause and reducing further demands on the heart. Medications such as digitalis, beta-adrenergic blocking agents (e.g., propranolol), and calcium channel blockers may be prescribed.[1,25,35] The client is placed on bedrest to reduce metabolic demand. Oxygen may be prescribed to supply the myocardium adequately.

Sinus Bradycardia

Sinus bradycardia occurs when the SA node fires at a rate of less than 60 times per minute. There is a normal P wave and QRS complex (Fig. 46–2*B*). Sinus bradycardia may result from increased vagal (parasympathetic) tone,

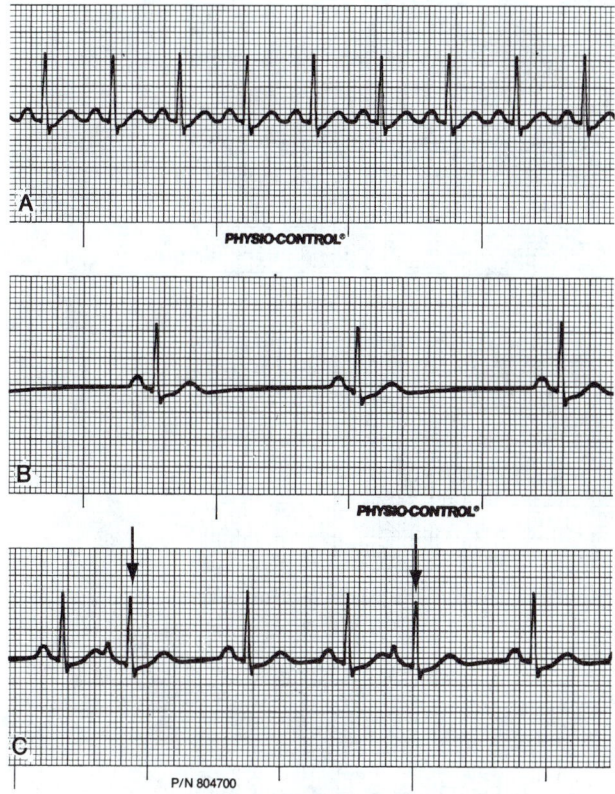

Figure 46-2. Atrial dysrhythmias. *A,* Sinus tachycardia— regular R–R interval, rate 125 beats per minute (BPM); P–R interval, 0.16 second. *B,* Sinus bradycardia—regular R–R interval, rate 40 BPM; P–R interval, 0.16. *C,* Premature atrial contractions. The second and fifth beat are premature atrial contractions (PACs). Note the difference in appearance of the P wave and the shortened R–R interval.

as occurs with Valsalva's maneuver (e.g., straining while moving bowels). Other causes of sinus bradycardia include drugs (especially digitalis, propranolol, or verapamil), MI (most often inferior MI), hyperkalemia, and various diseases such as hypothyroidism, myxedema, and obstructive jaundice.

Sinus bradycardia can be normal in some people. Athletes often have sinus bradycardia because their heart is an effective pump with a greater than normal stroke volume. Because cardiac output is the product of stroke volume and heart rate, the heart rate decreases and yet cardiac output is adequate.

Sinus bradycardia may be asymptomatic. When manifestations develop, it is because cardiac output decreased. Fatigue, hypotension, lightheadedness, syncope, shortness of breath, decreased level of consciousness, pulmonary congestion, or congestive heart failure may develop. The slowed rate of SA discharge may allow junctional or ventricular pacemakers to take over, thereby producing ectopic beats.

Management aims to correct the underlying cause of sinus bradycardia. The goal of intervention is to increase the heart rate just enough to relieve manifestations but not enough to cause tachycardia. The intervention sequence for treating symptomatic bradycardia is atropine,

transcutaneous pacing if available, dopamine, epinephrine, and isoproterenol, or insertion of a temporary transvenous pacemaker.[1,25,35]

Sinus Dysrhythmia

Sinus dysrhythmia is characterized by phasic changes in the automaticity of the SA node, which cause it to fire at varying speeds. The heart rate generally ranges between 60 and 100 BPM. The ECG has a normal P wave, P–R interval, and QRS complex; the only abnormality is an irregular P–P interval. Sinus dysrhythmia may develop from alterations in vagal tone and in response to delayed atrial filling with inhalation. During inspiration, venous return to the right atrium is delayed because of increased intrathoracic pressure. In quiet respiration, the heart rate can decrease about 5%. It can decrease up to 30% with deep respiration Sinus dysrhythmia does not usually require intervention other than alleviation of the underlying cause. It has no effect on cardiac output.

Disturbances in Conduction: Sinoatrial Node Conduction Defects

Under certain circumstances, the impulse from the SA node is either (1) not generated in the SA node (SA arrest) or (2) not conducted from the SA node (sinus exit block). Causes of SA node conduction abnormalities include conditions that increase vagal tone, coronary artery disease (CAD), MI, digitalis and calcium channel blocker toxicity, and hypertensive disease. These dysrhythmias may also occur from tissue hypoxia, scarring of intra-atrial pathways, or electrolyte imbalances.

During SA arrest, neither the atria nor the ventricles are stimulated, which produces a pause in the rhythm. An entire PQRST will be missing for one or more cycles. After the pause of sinus arrest, a new pacemaker focus assumes the pacing responsibility. The new pacer paces the heart at its inherent rate (see earlier discussion), which is usually slower than the original SA node rate. The most likely new pacer site is another atrial focus, but the junction or ventricle can also assume pacing responsibility.

In sinus exit block, there is a conduction delay between the sinus node and the atrial muscle. Unlike SA arrest, the rhythm of SA node discharge in sinus exit block remains constant and uninterrupted. The ECG characteristically displays a normal sinus rhythm that is interrupted intermittently by pauses. This creates a pattern of pauses that, when measured, are multiples of the underlying P–P interval. Sinus arrest differs from SA exit block in that the SA node intermittently fails to fire at all. The result is the occurrence of pauses that are longer and not a multiple of the underlying P–P interval. These pauses are also frequently terminated by escape ectopic beats. Sinus arrest often has a more serious prognosis.

The client usually remains asymptomatic, depending on the duration and frequency of the pauses. However, lengthy pauses can cause lightheadedness or syncope. In-

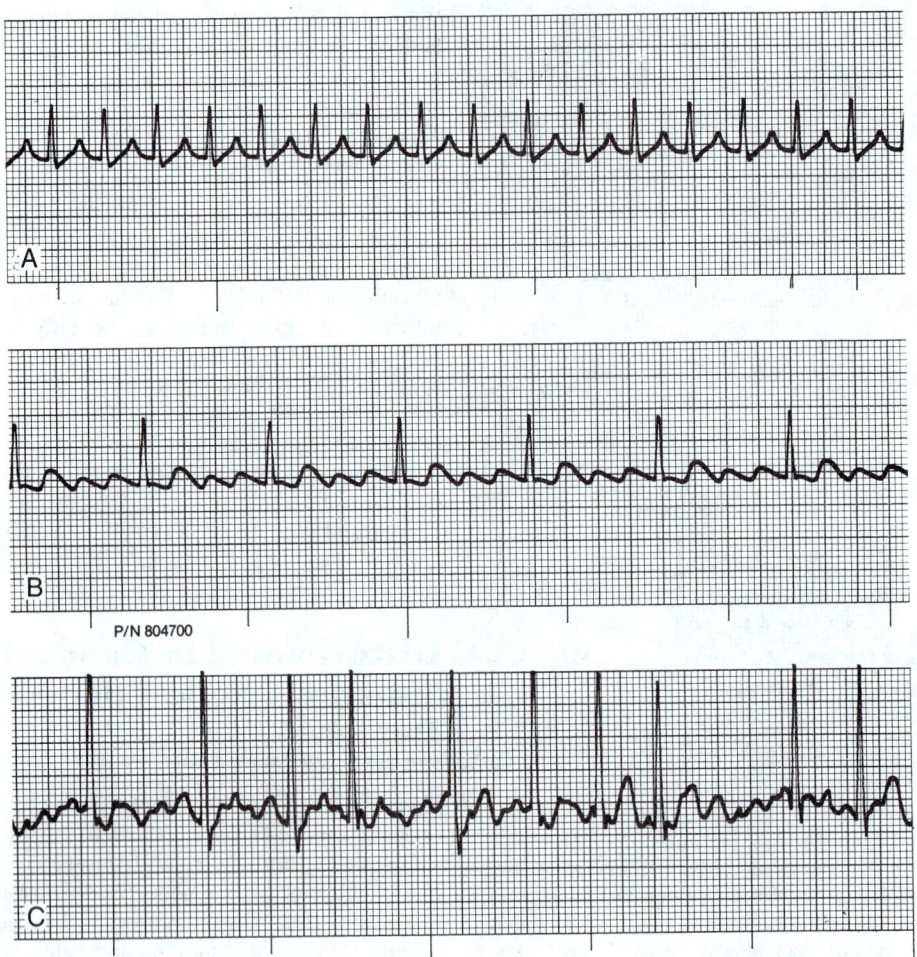

P/N 804700

Figure 46–3. *A*, Paroxysmal atrial tachycardia (PAT). The rate is rapid, about 175 BPM. The P wave is not distinguishable, but the QRS complex is narrow, indicating that the impulse began above the atrioventricular node. *B*, Atrial flutter. Note the saw-toothed appearance of the P waves. There are three P waves for every QRS complex, indicating a 3:1 block. Atrial rate is 75 BPM. *C*, Atrial fibrillation is identifiable by a chaotic P wave, not one clear P wave, and an irregular R–R interval.

tervention is unnecessary unless the client becomes symptomatic and exhibits signs of decreased cardiac output. An irregular pulse can be palpated or auscultated. Clinicians can only infer impulse formation within the SA node from the appearance of P waves, which reflect atrial depolarization. Intervention may include administration of vagolytics (atropine) or sympathomimetics (isoproterenol) to increase the rate of SA node firing. If pharmacologic measures fail, a pacemaker may be required. Finally, the physician needs to determine and treat the underlying cause of the dysrhythmia.[1,25,35]

Disturbances in Impulse Generation

Recall that the usual pacemaker of the heart is the SA node. Impulses can also be generated from other cells in the atria at an intrinsic rate of 60 to 100 BPM. An atrial ectopic focus may become so irritable that it produces impulses in rapid succession, thereby totally taking over the role of pacemaker. Such rapid rates of impulse formation occur in paroxysmal atrial tachycardia (PAT), atrial flutter, and atrial fibrillation (AFib). Atrial and junctional dysrhythmias are sometimes called supraventricular dysrhythmias because the abnormal foci for ectopic beats originate at a site above the ventricles. We will look at several forms of impulse generation problems in the atria.

Premature Atrial Contractions

Premature atrial contractions (PACs) are early beats arising from ectopic atrial foci interrupting the normal rhythm. They most often result from enhanced automaticity of the atrial muscle. They occur in normal and diseased hearts. PACs are associated with valvular disease and atrial chamber enlargement and also can be seen with stress, fatigue, alcohol, smoking, CAD, cardiac ischemia, heart failure, cardioactive medications (digitalis, quinidine, procainamide), pulmonary congestion, and pulmonary hypertension. Frequent PACs may mark the onset of AFib, heart failure, or reflect electrolyte imbalances.

PACs have premature P waves that differ from the normal sinus P wave in appearance, size, or shape (Fig. 46–2C). Premature beats from any ectopic focus can be palpated as skipped or irregular beats. The client who experiences numerous PACs may note palpitations, or "missed beats." PACs are usually benign. However, if the client has increasing numbers of "skipped beats" or feels palpitations often, the problem should be evaluated. Intervention usually focuses on correcting the underlying cause and may include quinidine or procainamide.

Paroxysmal Atrial Tachycardia

Paroxysmal atrial tachycardia is the sudden onset and sudden termination of a rapid firing from an ectopic atrial pacemaker (Fig. 46–3A). PAT is due to the reentry phenomenon. This allows (1) the atrial impulses to travel down less refractory conduction pathways to the bundle of His and (2) retrograde conduction through previously refractory parallel fibers. A circular circuit for rapid repetitive depolarizations results from these events.

PAT occasionally appears in clients with normal hearts, it most often develops in clients with cardiac disease. Cardiac problems precipitating PAT include MI, cardiomyopathy, extreme emotions, caffeine ingestion, fatigue, smoking, and excessive alcohol intake. Rheumatic heart disease, valvular disease, pulmonary emboli, cor pulmonale, thyrotoxicosis, digitalis toxicity (PAT with block), and cardiac surgery are less common causes.

Clinicians identify PAT by three or more consecutive atrial ectopic beats occurring at a rate greater than 150 BPM alternating with normal sinus rhythm. The P waves are usually upright, narrow, and peaked in lead II. At faster atrial rates, the P waves may become lost in the preceding T wave. The P–R intervals may be normal. However, rapid atrial rates may overcome the conduction limits of the AV node, causing varying degrees of AV block. Atrial tachycardia with 2:1 block (i.e., two P waves for every QRS complex) most often results from digitalis toxicity. The QRS complexes are usually normal, although aberrant ventricular conduction may occur at very rapid atrial rates, or when a conduction defect exists within the ventricle.

PAT decreases ventricular filling time and mean arterial pressure. It also increases myocardial oxygen demand. Clients may report palpitations and lightheadedness. Management of PAT varies with the severity of manifestations. Clients with extremely rapid heart rates or significant underlying cardiovascular disease may develop syncope and heart failure. The heart rate must be immediately reduced. Any maneuver that stimulates the vagus nerve can successfully terminate PAT or increase AV block. The vagus nerve can be stimulated by carotid sinus massage and Valsalva's maneuver (bearing down). Useful pharmacologic agents include adenosine, verapamil, and beta-blockers. Sedatives may also be used to reduce sympathetic stimulation. The physician may also employ cardioversion (see later discussion) as an effective means of terminating PAT if medications and vagal stimulation are not effective. Ablation procedures that destroy a part of the reentrant path are increasing in use. Such procedures can result in a long-term cure in appropriate clients.[1,6,23,25,35]

Atrial Flutter

Atrial flutter is dysrhythmia arising in an ectopic pacemaker or the site of a rapid reentry circuit in the atria, characterized by rapid "saw-toothed" atrial wave formations and, usually a slower, regular ventricular response. Atrial flutter differs from PAT in that it produces a much more rapid atrial rate. The P waves are actually inverted or bidirectional, producing a "picket fence" or saw-toothed pattern of "flutter waves" (Fig. 46–3B). The atrial rate generally ranges from 220 to 350 BPM. The AV node cannot conduct all of the atrial impulses that bombard it; that is, the AV node blocks a 1:1 conduction. Therefore, the ventricular rate will always be slower than the atrial rate. Thus, the pulse, which reflects the ventricular rate, may be normal even though the atrial rate is quite rapid. The ratio of atrial to ventricular beats may be constant (2:1, 3:1, 4:1, and 7:1, and so forth), or it may vary. A variable degree of block produces an irregular ventricular rhythm.

Atrial flutter most commonly occurs in association with organic diseases such as CAD, mitral valve disease, pulmonary embolus, and hyperthyroidism. In addition, it may follow cardiac surgery. The client may sense occasional palpitations and chest pain, especially when rapid ventricular rates exist.

Intervention aims at controlling rapid ventricular rates. Cardioversion is used (see later discussion). Medications used to treat atrial flutter include digitalis, quinidine, verapamil, propranolol, and procainamide, especially if cardioversion is not successful. Carotid sinus massage helps temporarily slow the ventricular response so that flutter waves can be identified.[1,25,35]

Atrial Fibrillation

Atrial fibrillation is characterized by rapid, chaotic atrial depolarization from a reentry disorder. Ectopic atrial foci produce impulses between 400 and 700 BPM. However, at extremely rapid rates, the entire atrium may not be able to recover from one depolarization wave before the next begins. This results in mechanical and electrical disorganization of the atria. As with atrial flutter, the AV node is bombarded with more impulses than it can conduct. Most of these impulses are blocked, which results in a very irregular ventricular rhythm. The ventricular rate ranges from 160 to 180 BPM. Examination of the ECG reveals erratic or no identifiable P waves and a baseline that appears to be irregular and undulating (Fig. 46–3C). Because of atrial disorganization, there is no "atrial kick." This can decrease cardiac output by as much as 20% to 30%. With increasing ventricular rates, cardiac output falls even further and may result in angina pectoris, heart failure, and shock.

AFib may be associated with sick sinus syndrome, hypoxia, increased atrial pressure, pericarditis, and many other conditions. Clients may be asymptomatic, or they may note an irregular pulse and palpitations. The client may have a pulse deficit between apical and radial pulses.

Mural thrombi formation can severely complicate AFib. Blood pools in the "quivering" atria because of lack of adequate contraction of atrial muscle. This blood can clot, which increases the potential for cerebral and pulmonary vascular emboli. Most clients with sudden onset of AFib are given heparin as an anticoagulant until the AFib is controlled.

Rate control is the initial treatment goal, using drugs such as diltiazem, verapamil, beta-blockers, or digoxin. Chemical cardioversion, usually after a period of anticoagulation, can then be attempted with procainamide or quinidine. Electrical cardioversion is the third therapeutic option.[1,25,35] It is discussed later in this chapter.

Atrioventricular Junctional Dysrhythmias

If the SA node fails to fire and an impulse is not initiated in other ectopic sites in the atria, the AV junction is the next pacemaker for the heart. An impulse begins in the junction and simultaneously spreads up to the atria and down into the ventricles. During junctional rhythms there is decreased cardiac output due to a lack of atrial kick to the ventricles. Junctional rhythms are also not dependable for a long-term cardiac pacemaker, because the rate is slow and more irritable ectopic foci may fire, such as from the ventricles. Consider junctional rhythms to be a warning or forerunner of more serious dysrhythmias.

Two major types of dysrhythmias arise in the AV junction: (1) disturbances in automaticity, that is, the AV junctional tissue assumes the role of the pacemaker; and (2) disturbances in conduction, that is, the AV junction blocks impulses journeying from the atria to the ventricles. Both of these types of dysrhythmias may result from ischemia or trauma in the area of the AV junction, that is, after MI or cardiac surgery. Digitalis toxicity, quinidine toxicity, and hyperkalemia may also cause junctional dysrhythmias.

Junctional rhythms produce abnormal upward direction of impulse (e.g., in lead II the P waves are inverted). This is because the impulse is traveling through the atria in a direction opposite to that found in normal sinus rhythm. Also, the P–R interval shortens to less than 0.12 second. The impulse may spread through the atria at the same time that the ventricles are being activated by the AV junction. In this instance, the P wave will be buried in the QRS complex and not observed. Also, the atria may contract after the ventricles. In this case, the P wave follows the QRS complex. The QRS complex will be normal if ventricular conduction is normal.

Disturbances in Automaticity

The major junctional dysrhythmias due to changes in automaticity are premature junctional contractions (PJCs), junctional escape rhythm, and junctional tachycardias. As occurs with PACs, an ectopic focus in the AV junctional tissue may develop increased automaticity and discharge prematurely, initiating depolarization of the heart.

Premature Junctional Contractions

A premature junctional contraction (PJC) is the single, early firing of a junctional ectopic focus (Fig. 46–4). PJCs are slower due to lower intrinsic rates. Usually, clients can tolerate junctional rhythms. However, clients with severe forms of cardiac disease may not tolerate junctional rhythms because cardiac output decreases.

Paroxysmal Junctional Tachycardia

A junctional rhythm with a rate that exceeds 60 BPM is termed a junctional tachycardia. It usually stops and starts abruptly, thereby getting the name paroxysmal junctional tachycardia, or PJT. The usual rate is 140 to 220 BPM. Causes of PJT include metabolic imbalances and increased sympathetic stimulation. Rapid ventricular rates can lead to left ventricular failure due to increased myocardial oxygen demand and decreased blood supply. If PJT cannot be distinguished on the ECG from PAT, it is called supraventricular tachycardia (SVT).

Management of rapid junctional rhythms begins with vagal stimulation such as carotid sinus massage. If clini-

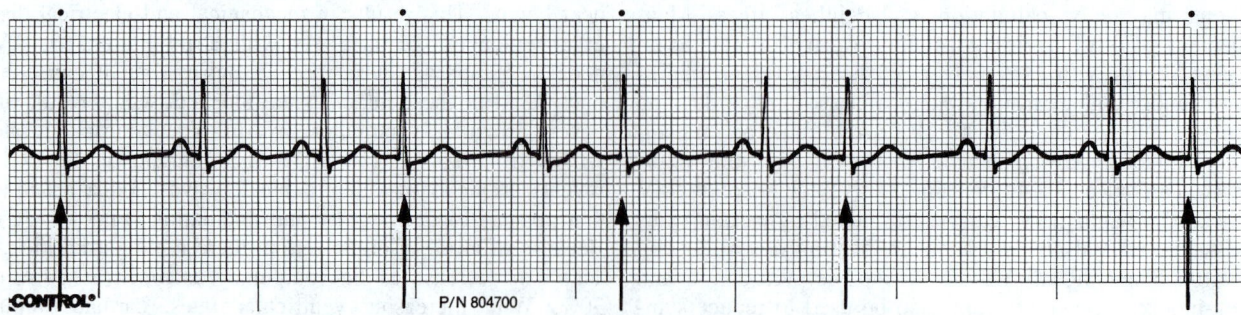

Figure 46–4. A premature junctional contraction. The beats marked with *arrows* are premature junctional contractions. Note the absence of a P wave, but otherwise normal deflection indicating the impulse was initiated above the ventricles.

cal manifestations develop, treatment is pharmacologic agents and cardioversion. Common medications used in the treatment of PJT include propranolol, quinidine, and digitalis. Evaluation of digitalis intoxication and potassium levels may also be indicated.[1,35]

Disturbances in Conduction

Atrioventricular block comprises the second group of disturbances arising in the area of the AV junction. Impulses passing through the AV junction are blocked to varying degrees. Therefore, the conduction of impulses from the atria to the ventricles slows or stops entirely, depending on the degree of the AV block. Normally the impulse coming from the SA node is delayed at the AV junction for less than 0.20 second before traveling on to the bundle of His. However, when the AV junction has been damaged by ischemia, rheumatic fever, or drug toxicity, impulses are delayed or completely blocked at the AV junction for abnormally long periods of time.

First-Degree Atrioventricular Block

First-degree AV block is a delay in passage of the impulse from atria to ventricles. This delay usually occurs at the level of the AV node. The rhythm is regular, each P wave is followed by a QRS complex, and the P–R interval is prolonged beyond the normal 0.20 second. It usually remains constant (Fig. 46–5A). This is an important differentiation between first-degree AV block and the other AV blocks. This block is often associated with CAD, increased vagal tone, and congenital anomalies. It may also result from digitalis administration.

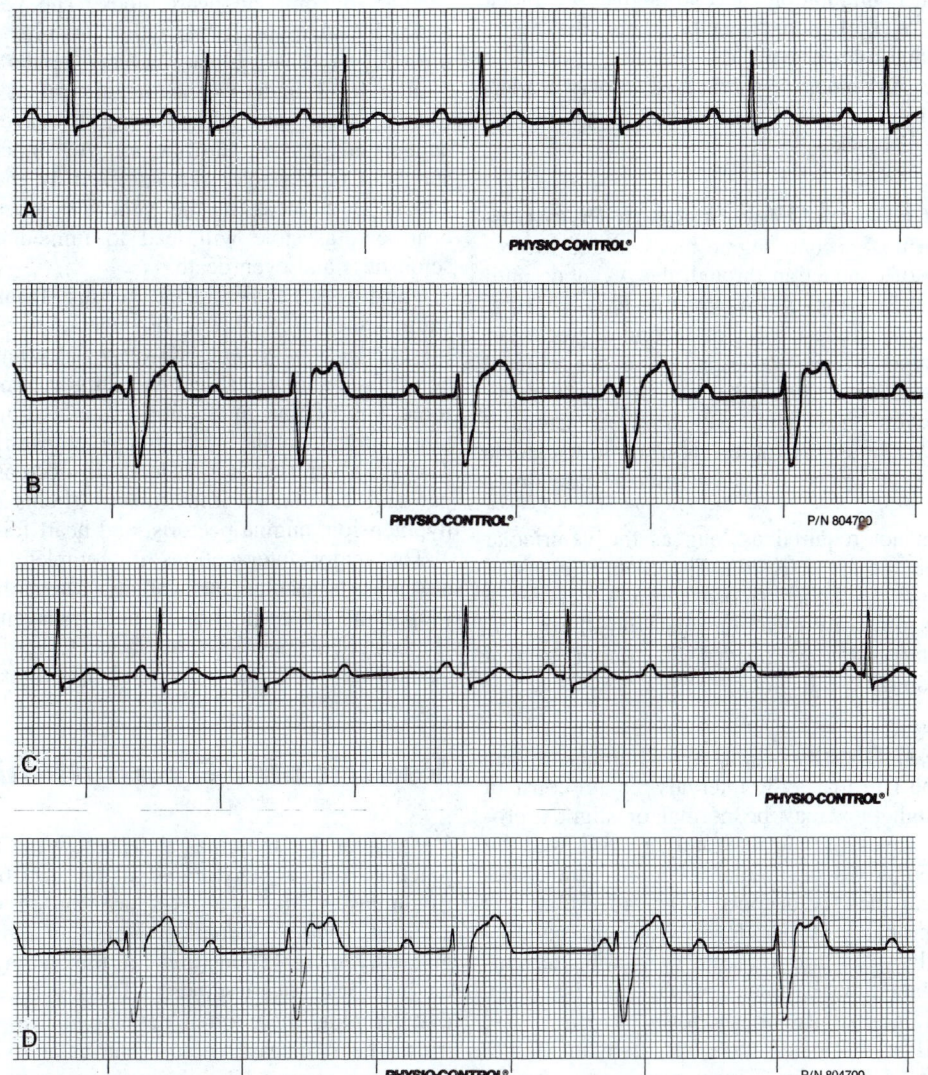

Figure 46–5. Junctional dysrhythmias. *A*, First-degree atrioventricular (AV) block. *B*, Second-degree AV block (Mobitz type I, Wenckebach phenomenon; note the regularly occurring P waves and the increasing P–R intervals). *C*, Second-degree AV block (Mobitz type II). *D*, Third-degree AV block (note the variable P–R interval and the lack of association of the P wave with the QRS complex).

First-degree AV block, existing alone as the only abnormal feature of a client's ECG, produces no clinical manifestations and requires no intervention. If the block is due to digitalis, the medication may be discontinued. Because it can progress to a higher-degree AV block, the client requires observation and ECG monitoring.[1,35]

Second-Degree Atrioventricular Block

Second-degree AV block is a more serious form of conduction delays in the heart. In this dysrhythmia some impulses are conducted and others are blocked. Second-degree block results in intermittently dropped QRS complexes. Atrial depolarization continues without disturbance, and normal-appearing P waves occur at regular intervals. Second-degree AV block does not usually affect conduction through the ventricles, and QRS complexes appear normal in configuration. Second-degree AV block develops from CAD, digitalis toxicity, rheumatic fever, viral infections, and inferior wall MI.

Second-degree AV block is subdivided into two additional types—Mobitz type I (Wenckebach phenomenon) and Mobitz type II block.

Mobitz Type I Block (Wenckebach Phenomenon).
This form of second-degree block is due to progressive slowing of conduction through the AV node until eventually no QRS complex follows the P wave (Fig. 46–5B). This is the mildest form of second-degree heart block. Mobitz type I does not usually produce clinical manifestations because the client has an adequate ventricular rate. However, the client may have an irregular pulse. Vertigo, weakness, or other signs of low cardiac output may be experienced if the ventricular rate drops precipitously.

Intervention is not required as long as the ventricular rate remains adequate for perfusion. The client is assessed for progression to a higher (more serious) degree of block. Clinicians primarily focus on managing the underlying cause. Intervention, if needed, is similar to that described for Mobitz type II block.[1,25,35]

Mobitz Type II Block.
Mobitz type II block differs from Mobitz type I in that P–R intervals remain constant in length, although they may be normal or slightly prolonged. The P waves are normal and are followed by normal QRS complexes at regular intervals, until suddenly a QRS complex is dropped (Fig. 46–5C). This dysrhythmia is probably farther down within the conduction system, perhaps residing close to or within the bundle of His. Mobitz type II blocks result from ischemia, digitalis or quinidine toxicity, or anterior wall MI.

Mobitz type II is considered more serious than Mobitz type I AV block. Mobitz type II more often progresses to third-degree AV block, especially in clients with an anterior wall MI. Clients with second-degree AV block require close ECG monitoring for possible progression to complete heart block. Intervention includes (1) administration of atropine and isoproterenol (which speed the rate

of impulse conduction), (2) insertion of a temporary or permanent pacemaker, and (3) withholding cardiac depressant drugs (e.g., digitalis). Second-degree block, which occurs after MI, particularly an inferior MI, may be reversible as the injury of ischemia heals.[1,25,35]

Third-Degree Atrioventricular Block

Third-degree AV block is the complete absence of conduction of the electrical impulses due to a block in the AV node, bundle of His, or bundle branches. Third-degree heart block is sometimes called AV dissociation, because the two halves of the heart are working independently of each other. The atria are paced by the SA node, but since the message is blocked, the ventricles are being paced by a ventricular ectopic pacemaker (Fig. 46–5D). The atrial rate is always equal to or faster than the ventricular in complete heart block. The ventricular rate is typically 40 to 60 BPM. Other features of the ECG in third-degree heart block include regular P–P intervals, regular R–R intervals, no meaningful or consistent P–R intervals, and normal-appearing P waves. The greatest danger inherent in third-degree AV block is ventricular standstill or asystole, characterized by the Stokes-Adams attack. If a focus in the ventricles does not initiate a heartbeat, asystole will lead to immediate loss of consciousness and even death.

Third-degree AV block results from a variety of causes, including fibrotic or degenerative changes within the conduction system, MI (especially anterior wall MI), congenital anomalies, cardiac surgery, myocarditis, viral infections of the conduction system, drug toxicity (digitalis, procainamide, quinidine, verapamil), and trauma. The slow ventricular rate leads to decreased cardiac output and circulatory impairment. Clients may experience hypotension, angina pectoris, and heart failure.

The major interventions in complete heart block are atropine, transcutaneous pacing, catecholamine infusions (dopamine or epinephrine), and transvenous pacemaker. If the client develops asystole, CPR is used until a pacemaker can be inserted. Isoproterenol is rarely indicated.[1,25,35]

Ventricular Dysrhythmias

Ventricular dysrhythmias arise below the level of the AV junction. Like dysrhythmias in the atria or junction, dysrhythmias in the ventricles are caused of problems of automaticity or conduction. Ventricular dysrhythmias are generally more serious and life-threatening than are atrial or junctional dysrhythmias. This is because ventricular dysrhythmias more often develop in association with intrinsic heart disease. Also, ventricular dysrhythmias usually cause greater hemodynamic compromise (e.g., hypotension, heart failure, and shock). The independent contraction of the ventricles results in a reduced stroke volume and therefore a reduced cardiac output. Rapid ventricular rates prevent optimal filling of the ventricular chambers and reduce stroke volume even further. At rates of less than 40 per minute, cardiac output is simply not sufficient to support the body's vital functions.

The ECG tracing of ventricular dysrhythmias reveals wide and bizarre QRS complexes. Normally, impulses traverse the ventricles via the shortest, most efficient route. This normal pathway results in a narrow QRS complex. When an impulse originates in the ventricles, however, the impulse follows an abnormal pathway through the ventricular muscle tissue. This abnormality appears as a wide (greater than 0.12 second) complex on the ECG.

Disturbances in Automaticity

Dysrhythmias due to problems in automaticity are characterized by ectopic impulses, which result from either myocardial irritability or the phenomenon of reentry. The four ventricular dysrhythmias due to automaticity are (1) premature ventricular contractions (PVCs), (2) ventricular tachycardia (VT), (3) ventricular fibrillation (VFib), and (4) torsades de pointes.

Premature Ventricular Contractions

Premature ventricular contractions, also called ventricular premature beats, are the most common of all dysrhythmias other than those of the sinus node. They are usually caused by the firing of an irritable pacemaker in the ventricle. PVCs result from enhanced ventricular automaticity or reentry. Factors promoting PVCs include myocardial hypoxia, hypokalemia, hypocalcemia, acidosis, alcohol, caffeine, nicotine, CAD, heart failure, toxic agents (e.g., digitalis, tricyclic antidepressants), exercise, hypermetabolic states, and intracardiac catheters.

PVCs produce easily recognized ECG changes. They occur earlier than the expected beat of the underlying rhythm and are usually followed by a compensatory pause. On the ECG, an unusually wide and bizarre QRS appears, interrupting the underlying rhythm (Fig. 46–6A).

Isolated PVCs are usually not treated. If the client becomes symptomatic of decreased cardiac output, the PVCs can be treated with lidocaine or any of the other class I antidysrhythmics. In clients with acute MI, the development of PVCs indicates that the myocardium is ischemic. When the myocardium becomes ischemic, ectopic foci become irritated and fire more often.

PVCs are dangerous when they are as follows:

- Frequent (more than six per minute)
- Coupled with normal beats (bigeminy)
- Multiform (Fig. 46–6B)
- Occur in pairs after every third beat (trigeminy) (Fig. 46–6C)
- Occur as a result of acute MI
- Fall on the T wave (Fig. 46–6D).

Clinicians refer to "falling on the T wave" as the R on T phenomenon. The downward slope of the T wave is the most vulnerable period of the cardiac cycle. If the heart is stimulated at this time, it often cannot respond to the stimulus in an organized fashion because the muscle fibers are in various stages of repolarization. Therefore, PVCs occurring during this vulnerable period can precipitate the more life-threatening dysrhythmias of VT (Fig. 46–6E) and VFib.

Management of dangerous PVCs involves administration of antidysrhythmic agents that have myocardial depressant actions. In acute situations, the clinician may administer class I and class II antidysrhythmic agents intravenously (IV), followed by a continuous IV drip. Table 46–2 describes a variety of antidysrhythmic agents.[1,15,17,21,24,25,35]

Ventricular Tachycardia

Ventricular tachycardia (VT) is a life-threatening dysrhythmia that occurs when an irritable ectopic focus in the ventricles takes over as the pacemaker. VT occurs in the presence of significant cardiac disease: in clients with CAD, cardiomyopathy, mitral valve prolapse, heart failure, acute MI experiencing hypoxia and acidosis, and digitalis toxicity.

VT is characterized by rapidly occurring series of PVCs (three or more) with no normal beats in between (see Fig. 46–6E). P waves are absent, and the P–R interval is absent. The QRS complex is wide (greater than 0.12 second) and bizarre. The ventricular rate ranges between 100 and 220 BPM, usually 130 to 170 BPM. The ventricular rhythm is slightly irregular. VT produces a very low cardiac output that can quickly lead to cerebral and myocardial ischemia. At any time, VT can develop into VFib. Clients with VT often express they are experiencing feelings of impending death.

VT when sustained but hemodynamically stable is initially treated with antidysrhythmics (i.e., lidocaine, procainamide, or bretylium). It may require cardioversion to convert to sinus rhythm. VT that causes loss of consciousness must be terminated immediately with defibrillation. The physician may also order IV administration of antidysrhythmic agents, usually lidocaine. Another drug gaining favor is magnesium sulfate, particularly if the client has low magnesium levels.[1,20,25,35]

Ventricular Fibrillation

Ventricular fibrillation is a life-threatening dysrhythmia characterized by extremely rapid, erratic impulse formation and conduction. This lethal dysrhythmia causes abrupt cessation of effective cardiac output. It usually results from severe myocardial damage, hypothermia, R on T phenomenon, hypoxia, contact with high-voltage electricity, electrolyte imbalance, and toxicity from quinidine, procainamide, or digitalis. The ECG tracing displays bizarre, fibrillatory wave patterns, and it is impossible to identify P waves, QRS complexes, or T waves (Fig. 46–7A). VFib may be either coarse or fine. Death results within minutes without immediate intervention (i.e., defibrillation, CPR, and medications).

When VFib appears, the clinician must immediately initiate CPR until the defibrillator is attached. Defibrillate

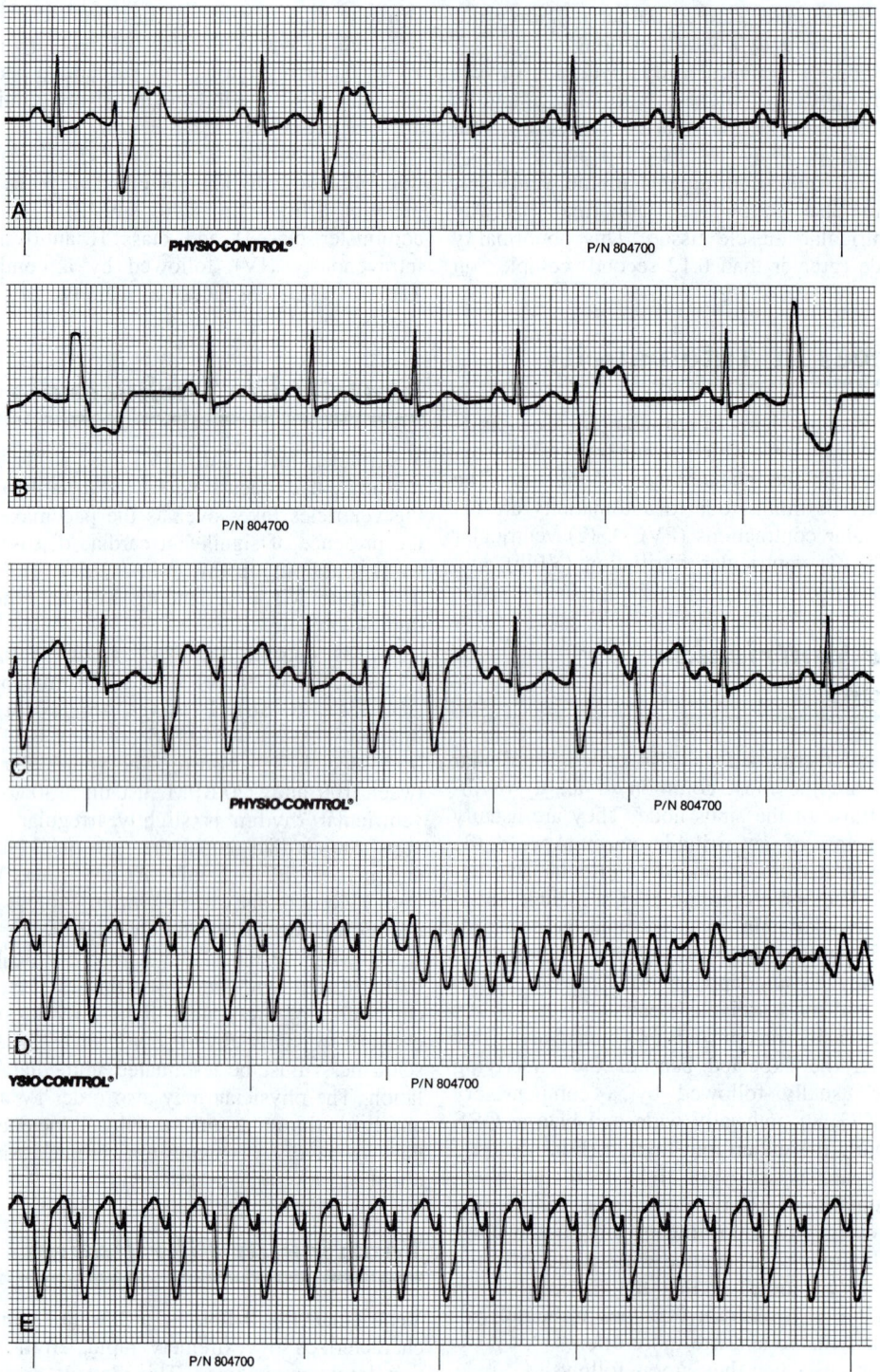

Figure 46–6. Ventricular dysrhythmias. *A*, Beats 2 and 4 are unifocal premature ventricular contractions (PVCs). *B*, Multifocal PVCs. *C*, Paired PVCs. *D*, R on T phenomenon leading to ventricular fibrillation. *E*, Ventricular tachycardia.

up to three times if needed. Defibrillation can be performed by nurses who have advanced training. A standard pattern of energy and current is used: It begins with 200 Joules (J); if not successful it is advanced to 300 J, and then to 360 J. With persistent VFib, epinephrine is given and the clinician defibrillates at 360 J. Other medications are alternated with defibrillation (lidocaine, bretylium, magnesium sulfate, sodium bicarbonate) depending on the client's cardiac rhythm, and electrolyte and acid-base balance.[1,25,35]

Table 46–2. Dysrhythmia Medications

Class	Example	Action	Common Side Effects	Nursing Implications
Class I Antidysrhythmics				
Drugs with local anesthetic effects and membrane-stabilizing properties. Affect upstroke velocity of phase 0. They are subdivided based on the magnitude of effects on phase 0, action potential duration, and effective refractory period				
Type IA				
Moderate slowing of phase 0 upstroke; moderate effects on action potential duration and effective refractory period ↑ QRS complex and Q–T interval	Quinidine Procainamide (Pronestyl) Disopyramide (Norpace)	Prolongs refractoriness and slows conduction velocity Decreases membrane responsiveness by increasing effective refractory period in Purkinje fibers to decrease automaticity and reentry disturbances Used in treatment of AFib, PVCs, and VT	Prolongs QRS complex or Q–T interval, which increases vulnerable period in ventricle Can cause tinnitus, vertigo, visual disturbances, loss of hearing, confusion, delirium, and gastrointestinal symptoms May also cause sinus arrest, SA block, and AV block	Monitor vital signs and ECG, especially Q–T interval Give with meals Monitor plasma levels Avoid excessive citrus fruits, which increase urine pH and decrease excretion
Type IB				
Minimal effect on phase 0 upstroke, little effect on effective refractory period, decrease action potential duration, and no change in QRS complex and Q–T interval	Lidocaine (Xylocaine) Tocainide (Tonocard) Mexiletine (Mexitil)	Depresses the phase 4 stage of the action potential and increases the VFib threshold In Purkinje fibers, action potential, effective refractory period, and automaticity are decreased Used in treatment of reentry disturbances, including PVCs and VT	Because lidocaine is an anesthetic, it can cause paresthesia, numbness, agitation, and disorientation May lead to hallucinations, decreased hearing, twitching, seizures, confusion, and respiratory arrest	Monitor vital signs and ECG continuously Therapy usually initiated with a bolus and then maintained with an IV infusion Common infusion rate is 1–4 mg/min Monitor kidney and liver function tests
Type IC				
Marked slowing of phase 0 upstroke, minimal effects on action potential duration, and effective refractory period ↑ QRS complex width, and no change in Q–T interval	Flecainide (Tambocor) Encainide (Enkaid) Indecainide (Decabid)	Depresses sinus node automaticity and prolong conduction in the atria, AV node, ventricle, and Purkinje fibers	Can aggravate existing dysrhythmias and precipitate new ones May lead to dizziness, visual disturbances, headache, fatigue, palpitations, chest pain, and gastrointestinal distress	Monitor vital signs and ECG continuously Use cautiously in clients taking digitalis and propranolol Usual blood level is 0.2–1.0 mg/ml
Class II Antidysrhythmics				
Beta-adrenergic blocking agents. General myocardial depressants for both supraventricular and ventricular rhythm disturbances				

Table continued on following page

Table 46–2. Dysrhythmia Medications (Continued)

Class	Example	Action	Common Side Effects	Nursing Implications
	Propranolol (Inderal) Atenolol (Tenormin) Labetalol (Normodyne) Metoprolol (Lopressor) Esmolol	Blocks sympathetic stimulation at the sinus node Reduces automaticity in Purkinje fibers Used to treat AFib, atrial flutter, SVT	Can cause bronchospasm Contraindicated in bronchial asthma, bronchospasm, and chronic obstructive pulmonary disease	Monitor vital signs and ECG Administer with food

Class III Antidysrhythmics

No membrane-stabilizing properties. Selectively increases action potential duration

Class	Example	Action	Common Side Effects	Nursing Implications
	Bretylium (Bretylol) Amiodarone (Cordarone)	Increases action potential duration and refractory period in Purkinje fibers Increases threshold for developing VFib	Hypotension, nausea, and vomiting Neurologic symptoms	Monitor vital signs and ECG closely Potentiate effects of digoxin and warfarin Hypotension more common in clients receiving quinidine or procainamide Monitor liver enzymes Clients on amiodarone need pulmonary function tests with diffusion capacity

Class IV Antidysrhythmics

Calcium-channel blockers

Class	Example	Action	Common Side Effects	Nursing Implications
	Verapamil (Calan)	Blocks slow calcium channel and has slight nonspecific sympathetic depressant effect Increases relative refractory period through AV node Interferes with reentry of impulses at AV node Used in treating PSVT, AFib, and atrial flutter	Hypotension, syncope, peripheral edema, constipation, bradycardia, AV blocks May precipitate or worsen CHF Reduces clearance of digitalis	Monitor vital signs and heart rhythm Monitor lung sounds and liver function tests Administer with food Monitor blood pressure and P–R interval

Unclassified Antidysrhythmics

Class	Example	Action	Common Side Effects	Nursing Implications
	Digoxin	Decreases AV node conduction to control ventricular response to AFib	Increases irritability and automaticity of ectopic sites in atria and ventricles	Given as rapid IV bolus to convert PSVT to NSR
	Adenosine (Adenocard)	An endogenous nucleoside, decreases AV node conduction and interrupts AV reentry pathways		

AFib, atrial fibrillation; AV, atrioventricular; CHF, congestive heart failure; ECG, electrocardiogram; IV, intravenous; NSR, normal sinus rhythm; PSVT, paroxysmal supraventricular tachycardia; PVCs, premature ventricular contractions; SA, sinoatrial; SVT, supraventricular tachycardia; VT, ventricular tachycardia. Data from Katzung, B. G. (1992). *Basic and clinical pharmacology* (5th ed.). Norwalk, CT: Appleton & Lange; Koda-Kimble, M. A., et al. (1992). *Handbook of applied therapeutics* (2nd ed.). Vancouver, WA: Applied Therapeutics.

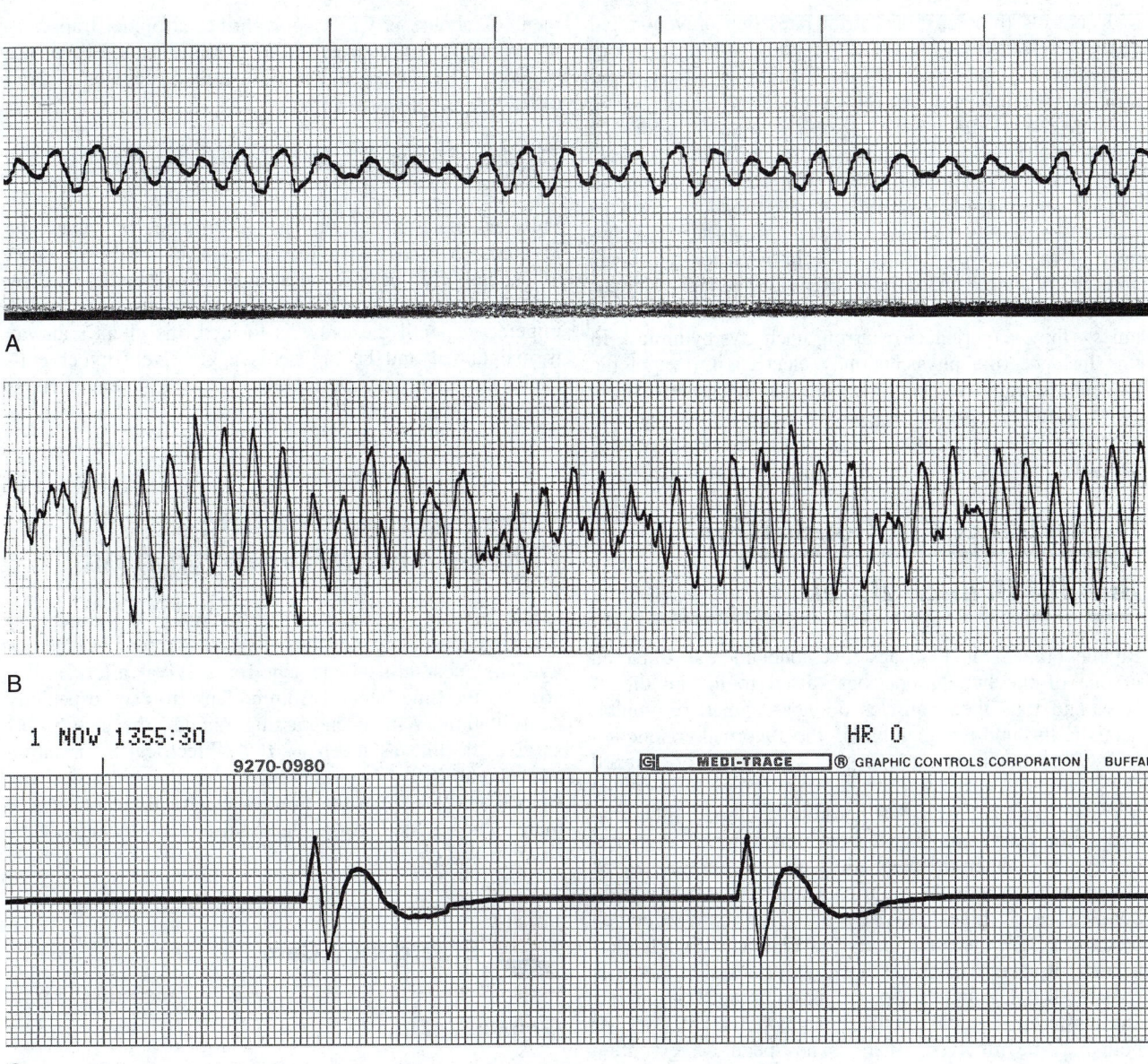

Figure 46–7. *A,* Coarse ventricular fibrillation. *B,* Torsades de pointes. *C,* Ventricular asystole in a dying heart. (*B* from Phillips, R. E., & Feeney, M. K. [1990]. *The cardiac rhythms: A systematic approach to interpretation.* [3rd ed.; p. 393]. Philadelphia: W. B. Saunders.)

Torsades de Pointes

Torsades de pointes is a form of VT in which the QRS complexes appear to be constantly changing. It has delayed repolarization of the ventricle revealed as a prolonged Q–T interval and a broad flat T wave in preceding sinus rhythm. The rhythm is regular or irregular with a ventricular rate of 150 to 300 BPM (Fig. 46–7*B*). The QRS complex is wide and bizarre. Torsades de pointes is usually due to drug toxicity (procainamide, quinidine, disopyramide) or electrolyte imbalances (hypokalemia or hypomagnesemia). Clinical manifestations begin with palpitations and syncope. This rhythm often precedes VFib and sudden death. Torsades de pointes is treated only if the Q–T interval is prolonged with temporary overdrive ventricular or atrial pacing. Discontinuation of offending agents is also crucial. Magnesium sulfate IV is considered the treatment of choice.[1,20,35]

Preexcitation Syndromes

Preexcitation syndromes occur when part or all of the ventricle is reentered by a depolarization wave traveling down a congenital or acquired accessory conducting pathway between the atrium and ventricle.

An accessory pathway is abnormal conductile tissue connecting the atria and ventricle. Normally the AV node is the only connection between the atria and ventricles and controls (blocks) rapid atrial rates that prevent rapid ventricular rates (e.g., atrial fibrillation). When accessory pathways are present, there is nothing to block rapid atrial rates, and ventricular rates soar.

There are several types of disorders in this category, of which Wolff-Parkinson-White syndrome (WPW) appears most frequently. Clients with WPW frequently develop sudden attacks of very rapid supraventricular dysrhythmias. Most adults with WPW have normal hearts. However, if the tachydysrhythmias occur persistently, clients with WPW may develop myocardial fatigue and ventricular failure. Clients with WPW do not require intervention unless they experience recurring tachydysrhythmias. In this instance, the physician may elect to use vagotonic maneuvers, cardioversion, adenosine, amiodarone (Cordarone), esmolol administration, or chemical, mechanical, or radiofrequency ablation. Ablation cuts the accessory pathway.

Disturbances in Conduction

Bundle Branch Block

Bundle branch block means that conduction is impaired in one of the bundle branches (distal to the bundle of His), and thus the ventricles do not depolarize simultaneously. In bundle branch block, the abnormal conduction pathway through the ventricles causes a wide or notched QRS complex. The defect may result from myocardial fibrosis, chronic CAD, MI, cardiomyopathies, inflammation, pulmonary embolism, severe left ventricular hypertrophy, or congenital anomalies. These disturbances of conduction through the ventricles result in either a right bundle branch block (RBBB) or a left bundle branch block (LBBB). Because of its association with left ventricular disease, LBBB has a worse prognosis than does RBBB. The left bundle branch is composed of anterior and posterior fascicles (little bundles) of which one or both may be involved. There is no specific intervention for this conduction defect. However, if RBBB exists along with block in one of the fascicles of the left bundle, the one remaining fascicle represents the only conduction pathway to the ventricles. Therefore, in this situation a pacemaker is required.[1,34,35]

Ventricular Asystole

Ventricular asystole (cardiac standstill) represents the total absence of ventricular electrical activity (Fig. 46–7C). The client has no palpable pulse (no cardiac output) and a rhythm is absent if the client is monitored. The occurrence of sudden ventricular asystole in a conscious person results in faintness, followed within seconds by loss of consciousness, seizures, and apnea, and if the dysrhythmia remains untreated, death. Ventricular asystole must be treated immediately.

Cardiac standstill can occur as a primary event or it may follow VFib, or pulseless electrical activity. Asystole can occur also in clients with complete heart block (CHB) in whom there is no escape pacemaker. The treatment of choice is CPR, epinephrine, atropine, transcutaneous pacing, and correction of possible causes (hypoxia, hyperkalemia, hypokalemia, pre-existing acidosis, drug overdose, hypothermia).[1,25,35]

Pulseless Electrical Activity

Pulseless electrical activity is the presence of some type of electrical activity in the heart seen on the monitor, other than VFib or VT, but a pulse cannot be detected by palpation of any artery. Rapid searching for the cause is imperative. Until the cause is located, the client's airway is maintained and he or she is aggressively hyperventilated. Common causes include hypoventilation, hypoxemia, and hypovolemia.

Management of Life-Threatening Dysrhythmias

Life-threatening dysrhythmias can often be effectively managed with exogenously delivered currents of electricity. The most crucial element for survival after cardiac arrest is the time interval from collapse to care, especially defibrillation. With each passing minute, the chances of survival decline as much as 10%. Electrical intervention can (1) abruptly stop the heart's erratic electrical discharge or (2) resume the flow of electrical current where there is none. Methods of electrical therapy include defibrillation and cardioversion.

 ### Emergency Care

Defibrillation

Defibrillation delivers an electrical current (shock) of preset voltage to the heart through paddles placed on the chest wall (closed chest procedure). This causes the entire myocardium to completely depolarize at the very moment of shock. That will produce transient asystole and allow the heart's intrinsic pacemakers to regain control. The amount of energy required to produce this effect is largely determined by the client's transthoracic impedance, or resistance to current flow. Because of this factor, the amount of energy that reaches the heart is less than the amount that the defibrillator is charged to deliver.[1,15,18] Defibrillation has potential hazards, particularly myocardial damage. Research has shown that the higher the amount of energy or frequency of the shocks, the greater the risk of injury. Advances in defibrillators allow measurement of transthoracic impedance. Once impedance is determined, the defibrillator automatically selects the amount of current needed that can restore rhythm and cardiac output. It is hoped this mode of defibrillation will reduce the risk of complications.[1,35]

The degree of transthoracic resistance depends on several variables:

Energy level. The higher the energy level selected, the more current will follow.

Number and frequency of shocks. The more shocks administered and the shorter the time interval between them, the lower the transthoracic resistance.

Ventilation phase. Resistance is lower when shocks are delivered during exhalation, when there is less air (and therefore less diameter) in the lungs.

Paddle size. The larger the paddle, the lower the resistance.

Chest size. The smaller the distance between the defibrillator electrodes once they are in place, the lower the resistance.

Paddle-skin interface material. Conductive material between the skin and paddles reduces transthoracic impedance.

Paddle pressure. Applying firm pressure increases contact between the skin and the paddles, helping to overcome transthoracic resistance. Exert about 25 lb of pressure on each paddle.

Paddle placement. Place one paddle on the upper chest, to the right of the sternum; place the other on the lower left chest, to the left of the nipple, with the center of the paddle in the midaxillary line.

If the client has a permanent pacemaker or an internal cardiac defibrillator, place the paddles at least 5 inches away from the generator to avoid damaging it. If a temporary pacing system is in use, disconnect the pacing lead from the pulse generator immediately before defibrillation and reconnect it after the shock.[1,5,7,10,11,19]

Most defibrillators can be used to perform either synchronized cardioversion or unsynchronized cardioversion—commonly called defibrillation. Defibrillation is always indicated in VFib. It is also used in VT when the client is unconscious and pulseless. Specially trained nurses, emergency medical technicians, and physicians perform this procedure in emergency settings.

Care Before Defibrillation. Immediately before defibrillation, do the following:

1. Assess the client's responsiveness.
2. If not responsive, activate the EMS system.
3. Call for the defibrillator.
4. Assess the client's airway, breathing, and circulation (ABCs). Open the airway. Look, listen, and feel.
5. If the client is not breathing, give two slow breaths.
6. Assess the client's circulation; if no pulse, start CPR.
7. Perform CPR until the defibrillator is attached.
8. Check the ECG to verify the presence of VFib or pulseless VT.
9. Check leads for any loose connections.
10. Remove any nitroglycerin patch.

On confirmation of the emergency, the code alarm is given over the healthcare facility intercom system or to their pagers to summon the emergency team (e.g., "Code 99, Dr. Blue"). In the meantime, CPR measures are started by the first person on the scene. The clinician turns on the defibrillator and sets it at 200 J. In the presence of VFib, the synchronous mode must not be used. Start an IV line as needed for administration of resuscitation medications. Intubation is completed with oxygen supplementation.

Care During Defibrillation. When VFib develops, clinicians must attempt defibrillation at the earliest opportunity. The paddles are lubricated with electrode paste or conducting pads to enhance conduction and prevent burning of the skin. The paste should not extend beyond the paddles, and the paddles must lie flat against the body in order to avoid burns. The clinician places the paddles firmly against the chest. Clinicians often use a transverse (anterolateral) position for paddle placement. One paddle is placed at the second intercostal space, at the right of the sternum, and the other paddle is positioned at the fifth intercostal space on the anterior axillary line (Fig. 46–8). To ensure safe defibrillation, people who perform defibrillation must always announce when they are about to shock. The phrase "One. I'm clear. Two. You're clear. Three. All clear." is recommended. Because electricity is carried along metal devices and the client, all personnel, including the clinician administering the shock, must stand back from the bed. Open chest defibrillation occurs in an operating room setting where electrical current may be applied directly to the heart.

Care After Defibrillation. The clinician immediately assesses the ECG and pulse after defibrillation. If the first countershock is unsuccessful, then the client must be immediately defibrillated again at a higher energy level (300 and 360 J). Defibrillate up to three times (200, 300, 360 J) if needed for persistent VFib or pulseless VT. Defibrillators are frequently equipped with paddles that are capable of monitoring the ECG, even immediately after defibrillation. Therefore, if the paddles are left in place after the shock has been delivered, the cardiac response can be quickly evaluated.

CPR should be continued if the three defibrillations were not successful. A member of the healthcare team administers appropriate medications again before the next defibrillation attempt. A successful response is indicated by cessation of fibrillation, restoration of sinus rhythm, and palpation of a regular pulse. After successful defibrillation, the client requires continuous ECG monitoring. The client must also be continuously assessed—vital signs along with neurologic status.

For clients with a pacemaker or an automatic implantable cardioverter-defibrillator (AICD), a programmer-analyzer should be readily available to examine the system for damage and erroneous reprogramming after defibrillation. Continue to monitor for pacemaker malfunction for at least the next 24 hours.

In documenting the outcome of defibrillation, record the following points:

- Preprocedure rhythm
- Times and voltage of shocks delivered
- Postdefibrillation rhythm pattern
- Names, times of administration, and doses of administered medications
- Other hemodynamic data available before, during, and after defibrillation

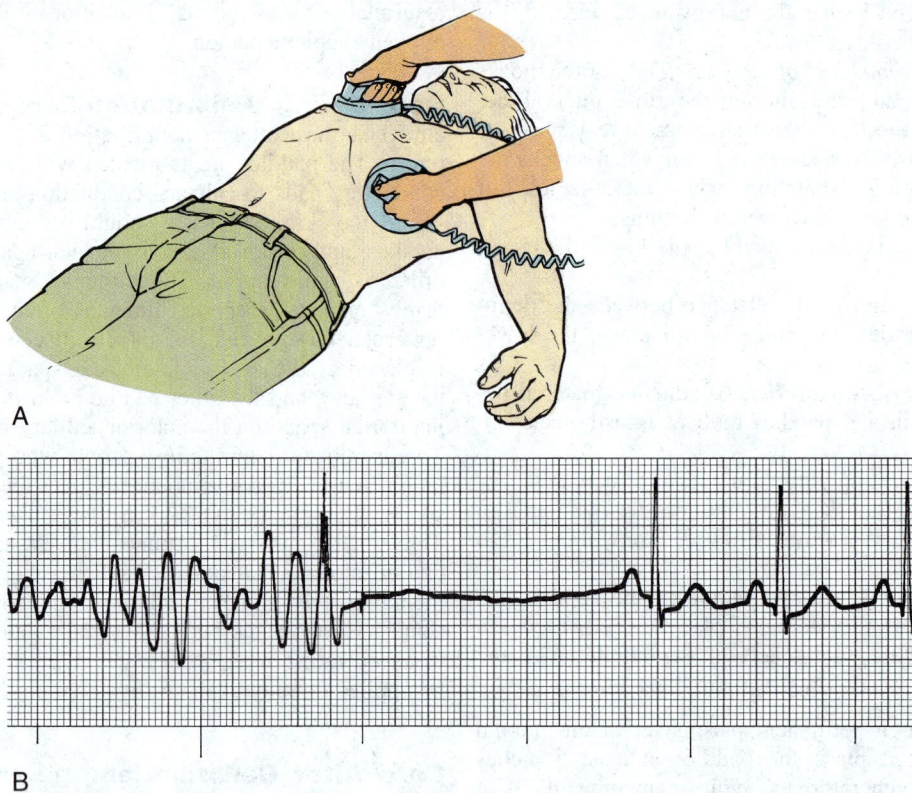

Figure 46–8. *A*, Anterolateral paddle placement for external countershock. External paddles are placed at the second right intercostal space and at the anterior axillary line in the fifth left intercostal space. *B*, Ventricular fibrillation converted to normal sinus rhythm.

Termination of Resuscitation. In general, if an organized rhythm and pulse have not returned, the advanced cardiac life support team leader can cease efforts to resuscitate clients from confirmed and persistent asystole when the client has received successful endotracheal intubation, successful IV access, suitable basic CPR, and all rhythm-appropriate medications. Always consider any pre-existing problems that may make the client less responsive to defibrillation—acidosis, hypokalemia, hyperkalemia, hypoxia, or hypovolemia—and treat them appropriately. Many times the client has other, noncardiac, disorders that make resuscitation attempts futile.

The 1994 American Heart Association guidelines to advanced cardiac life support do not state a specific time limit beyond which rescuers can never have a successful resuscitation.[1] Cardiac arrests in special situations such as hypothermia, electrocution, and drug overdose present exceptions to any rules. Special situations call for common sense and clinical judgment.[1,25,35] Television portrayal of defibrillation and CPR contribute to many misconceptions about these treatments (see Nursing Research).

Other Forms of Defibrillation

Automated External Defibrillators. Automated external defibrillators (AEDs) deliver electrical shocks to clients after the AED identifies VT or VFib. Automated external defibrillators are attached to the client through adhesive sternal-apex pads on flexible cables. This allows "hands-free" defibrillation, a feature available with conventional defibrillation as well. The AEDs also have an internal microprocessor-based detection system that analyzes the rhythm for the characteristics of VFib or VT. When VFib or VT is present, the AED "advises" the operator to deliver a shock. AEDs are "automated" in the sense that the device, and not the operator, analyzes the rhythm and determines the presence of VFib or VT.[1,5] The most common cause of unconsciousness in an adult is VFib. Defibrillation is the only effective treatment. Therefore, these devices are common in emergency response units.

Automatic Implantable Cardioverter-Defibrillators. The AICD consists of a pulse generator and a sensor that continuously monitors heart rhythm. When it detects a dysrhythmia, it automatically delivers a countershock. For VFib, the AICD will give an electrical countershock within 15 to 20 seconds. It can also detect and treat VT with cardioversion. This implanted system does not require as much energy as external defibrillation does because less energy is lost when the impulse is applied directly to the heart. In addition, a back-up pacemaker will help control the rhythm.

The AICD is implanted surgically into a pouch into the abdominal wall through a thoracotomy incision or trans-

NURSING RESEARCH

What Is the Influence of CPR as Seen on Television on the Public's Perception of the Use of and Outcomes from CPR?

Diem, S., Lantos, J., & Tuklsy, J. (1996). Cardiopulmonary resuscitation on television: Miracles and misinformation. *New England Journal of Medicine, 334*(24), 1578–1582.

Television is an important source of information for clients and their families. Is the portrayal of CPR on television providing accurate information? Three television shows that often depict CPR were viewed (*ER, Chicago Hope,* and *Rescue 911*). The cause of cardiac arrest, the demographics of the client, the underlying illness, and the outcomes were recorded. A total of 97 episodes of the three shows were reviewed.

Of the 60 clients who had CPR, 46 (77%) survived the immediate cardiac arrest. Survival rates for CPR on these television programs is significantly higher than the highest rates reported in the literature. (Note: *Rescue 911* has a 100% survival rate because, by intention, the program presents successful rescues). Most people resuscitated were children, teenagers, and young adults. In the hospital, cardiac arrest is most common in the aged. On television, most cardiac arrests were caused by trauma. In real life, most cardiac arrests are due to heart disease. During the same episodes, 37 clients died. In only eight of the situations in which persons died was there any discussion about the use of CPR or reference to do-not-resuscitate orders.

Implications for Practice

Clients participate in discussions about their health-care today more than ever before. Many people have few resources from which to learn about acute care, because for many people death is no longer part of everyday life. Therefore, images in the media strongly shape the public's belief about medical care, illness, and death. The portrayal of CPR and death on three popular programs is misleading. Misrepresentation of CPR on television may lead people to generalize the outcomes seen there to real life. Nurses need to be able to clarify misconceptions and to provide actual data on CPR as seen on television and as it occurs in real life.

venously. The latter is a new procedure that has been approved by the Food and Drug Administration for two types of conditions: (1) survival of one or more episodes of sudden cardiac death resulting from VT or VFib; and (2) recurrent, refractory, life-threatening ventricular dysrhythmias that can develop into VT or VFib, or both, despite antidysrhythmic therapy.[1,5,35]

Clients who require AICDs have a great deal of anxiety. Anxiety can develop from past episodes of near death as well as from feelings of not ever being able to die. Other patients fear that the AICD will not be able to reverse their dysrhythmia. The nurse is sensitive to these thoughts and facilitates their discussion.[1,5,7,10,13,19]

Cardioversion

Cardioversion, most often an elective procedure, is the use of a synchronized direct current (DC) electrical countershock that depolarizes all the cells simultaneously, allowing the SA node to resume the pacemaker role. The electrical discharge is synchronized with or triggered by the client's QRS complex for avoidance of accidental discharge during the repolarization phase when the ventricle is vulnerable to the development of VFib. A QRS complex must be present for successful conversion of the dysrhythmia. Low voltages are tried initially using 50 to 100 J. If unsuccessful, cardioversion can be repeated using larger voltages. Only specially trained physicians can perform this procedure.[1,25,35]

Cardioversion is used to treat SVT, AFib, and atrial flutter that is resistant to medication, and VT in an unstable patient. The unstable client may be hypotensive, dyspneic, experiencing chest pain, or have evidence of heart failure, MI, or ischemia. Analgesia or sedation may be provided before the electrical shock.

Care Before Cardioversion. The physician evaluates the ECG to diagnose the type of dysrhythmia present. The client must sign an informed consent, and then the intervention is scheduled. The client and family must receive a full explanation of cardioversion.

Cardioversion is typically performed at the client's bedside in the critical care unit. However, in case the client develops a life-threatening dysrhythmia after cardioversion, emergency equipment and trained clinicians must be in the room.

If the client has been taking a digitalis preparation, a therapeutic drug level must be present. Digitalis toxicity may predispose the client to the development of ventricular dysrhythmias during cardioversion. In addition, a low serum potassium level also increases the risk of lethal dysrhythmias. Premedicate the client with prescribed antidysrhythmics to ensure maintenance of postconversion rhythms. Administer oxygen before cardioversion and discontinue if oxygenation saturations are within normal limits. Keep the client NPO (fasting) for several hours before cardioversion. Start an IV line for medication delivery. To reduce fear and promote amnesia, administer an antianxiety medication IV as prescribed.

Care During Cardioversion. The physician does the following:

1. Sets the machine within a range of 50 to 200 J (more or less depending on the underlying impedances)
2. Turns the synchronizer switch to "on" to deliver the shock during the QRS complex and not on the downslope of the T wave
3. Lubricates the paddles and places them exactly as described for defibrillation

4. Calls for all healthcare personnel to stand back from the bed
5. While standing back from the bed, depresses and holds the buttons on the paddles until the shock is delivered

Newer equipment for cardioversion includes the use of adhesive skin paddles that are attached to the client's chest and back.

Care After Cardioversion. Clinicians immediately assess the ECG and pulse after cardioversion. In some cases, VFib or VT occurs, demanding emergency action. Monitor the client's ECG rhythm and vital signs continuously for at least 2 hours and carefully assess for rhythm changes and complications. A successful response to cardioversion resolves the dysrhythmia and restores normal sinus rhythm. With a good response and no complications, the client may be discharged later that day when fully awake and able to eat.

Acute and Subacute Care

■ Medical Management

Oxygen Administration

Oxygen is an essential component of dysrhythmia management, especially for dysrhythmias that occur due to irritable foci in ischemic myocardium. These include PVCs and other ventricular dysrhythmias. Oxygen should be given to all persons at risk of ventricular dysrhythmias, such as persons with chest pain, hypoxemia, or during cardiac arrest.

Antidysrhythmic Therapy

Table 46–2 reviews the classes of medications used to treat dysrhythmias. The student should not attempt to memorize the table, but rather commit a few drugs to memory, including atropine, lidocaine, epinephrine, verapamil, and procainamide. These medications may be administered orally or by continuous IV infusion. Nurses must be diligent in monitoring for the intended effect and side effects of the medication.

Ablation Therapies

A variety of procedures can be used to treat dysrhythmias when medications fail to convert the abnormal rhythm. Interventions include chemical and mechanical ablation, or radiofrequency of the abnormal pathway. These procedures involve risk to normal conduction tissue and a pacemaker may be needed either temporarily or permanently.[5,23,35]

Chemical Ablation. Alcohol or phenol is inserted into involved areas of the myocardium through an angioplasty catheter. Test injections with saline or lidocaine are given to determine whether the dysrhythmia ceases prior to the final injection. Postoperative care is the same as that for angioplasty.

Mechanical Ablation. The abnormal pathway is surgically dissected or treated with a cryoprobe to interrupt its effect on heart rhythms. SVT, AFib, atrial flutter, and WPW syndrome are dysrhythmias that may be treated with this method when they fail to respond to medication. Prior to the procedure, the myocardium is mapped to determine whether other forms of surgery (e.g., coronary bypass grafting or valve replacement) may correct the dysrhythmia. The mapping also isolates the area to be treated. The procedure may be performed through open heart or closed heart methods. Postprocedure care and recovery are similar to those following cardiac catheterization.

Radiofrequency Ablation. Radiofrequency catheter ablation (RFA) is a nonsurgical treatment used primarily for SVT associated with WPW or AV nodal reentry, although it has also been used successfully to treat refractory VT. In RFA a steerable pacing catheter directs low-power, high-frequency current to a localized accessory pathway and necroses a small portion of the heart. When this current is applied, the temperature of the contact tissue rises, water is driven out, and coagulation necrosis results. The amount of tissue injury depends on the amount of energy delivered (5–50 W), the length of time it is delivered (10–90 seconds), and the resistance at the end of the catheter. RFA produces lesions that are smaller and more controllable than DC catheter ablation lesions. The major advantage of RFA is the high rate of success (99% at some centers) and low morbidity. RFA is more successful than conventional medical therapies or DC ablation, but equal in success to surgical treatment.

Although RFA is a relatively safe procedure, the following complications can occur: cardiac tamponade (<1%), deep vein thrombosis (<1%), trauma to vessel (<1%), transient ischemic attack or stroke (<0.5%), perforation of AV leaflet (extremely rare), hematoma at introducer site (common), and unintentional AV block requiring pacemaker implantation (up to 10%). Postprocedure nursing care and recovery are similar to those following cardiac catheterization. Specific nursing responsibilities include preprocedure education of client and family, interventions to reduce anxiety before and during the RFA procedure, monitoring of vital signs and lower extremity perfusion during and after the procedure, and discharge instructions. Clients are usually discharged within 24 hours after RFA and are instructed to gradually resume normal activities but to avoid strenuous activities for 7 to 10 days. ECGs are obtained routinely at 1, 3, 6, and 9 months after RFA. Aspirin 325 mg is prescribed for 14 days after RFA to prevent clot formation and platelet aggregation at the ablation site.[5,35]

■ Surgical Management

Pacemakers

Surgical management includes the use of pacemakers to take over the role of the SA node or the Purkinje system. Pacemakers can be permanent or temporary.

An artificial pacemaker is indicated if the conduction system fails to transmit impulses from the sinus node to

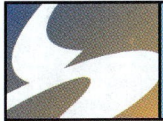

CASE MANAGEMENT

Pacemaker
For Clinical Pathway, see Appendix D.

Clinical Pathway from Birmingham Baptist Medical Center, Birmingham, Alabama Information provided by Karen Tauxe, M.S.N.

Development and Revision of Pathway

- Pacemaker insertion is a low-volume procedure at our hospital, but it is a high-cost case. Therefore, a pathway was initiated to try to reduce the cost of this procedure.
- The pathway was initiated in May 1995.
- The development team included the nurse-manager, registered nurses, the clinical pharmacist, catheter laboratory staff, dietitian, and physicians.
- A multidisciplinary task force meets two to four times per year to discuss the care of these patients. Pathway revision could take place at these meetings.
- During the meetings mentioned above there is opportunity to revise the pathway. At a minimum, the pathway is revised annually.

Use and Impact of Pathway

- All patients who have a pacemaker implanted are placed on the pathway for the preoperative and postoperative period related to this procedure. (Sometimes patients are admitted for other procedures or conditions. If they need a pacemaker implanted during their stay, this pathway will be used for the procedure episode only.)
- The nursing staff use the pathway daily.
- By documenting the expected care plan for the entire episode on a pathway and using that plan to deliver care to pacemaker patients, nurses and physicians have been encouraged to collaborate closely.
- Increased awareness of the appropriate plan of care for these patients has reduced the variable cost of care. Physicians have been made very aware of the costs of the care they order since the pathway was developed. The outcomes are reviewed quarterly by the multidisciplinary team.

Box 46–2. Conditions That May Necessitate a Pacemaker

- Acute myocardial infarction
- Myocardial ischemia
- Electrolyte imbalance
- Autonomic nervous system failure
- Drug toxicity (antiarrhythmics)
- Cardiac surgery
- Ablation

An artificial pacemaker is intended to provide a physiologic back-up for the heart during failure of the conduction system to depolarize the myocardium and maintain adequate cardiac output. When cardiac output is diminished because of lack of depolarization of the ventricles, artificial pacing will provide the necessary stimulus directly to the atria or ventricles, or both, for contraction to occur. If cardiac output is compromised because an ectopic pacemaker is causing the ventricles to depolarize and contract at a rate that does not promote adequate ventricular filling, artificial pacing will compete with the ectopic pacemaker to assume the primary pacing function of the heart.

Pacemaker Design

An artificial pacemaker provides an external source of energy for impulse formation and delivery, and stimulation of myocardial tissue. Whereas there are numerous pacemaker models, each with unique capabilities, every pacemaker consists of a pulse generator with circuitry, the lead, and the electrode system.

The pulse generator is essentially the pacemaker's power source. It houses the electronic circuitry responsible for sending out appropriately timed signals and for sensing cardiac activity. The output circuit controls the current pulse delivery rate, pulse duration, and refractory period. The sensing circuit is responsible for identifying and analyzing any spontaneous intrinsic electrical activity and responding appropriately. The pulse generator can be external or internal. The external unit is designed for temporary pacing, primarily for support of transient dysrhythmias that impair cardiac output. The unit is the size of a small transistor radio and operates by dry-cell batteries (Fig. 46–9). The unit has dials for adjustment of power, rate of discharge, and mode. The pulse generator can also be permanently implanted. The surgeon places the permanent pulse generator into a small tunnel burrowed within the subcutaneous tissue below the right (Fig. 46–10) or left clavicle or in the abdominal cavity. The pulse generator is a small—about the size of a stethoscope head—hermetically sealed (to prevent exposure to body fluids) lithium battery. Most of the new generators can be reprogrammed after insertion, as needed.

The lead delivers the electrical impulse from the pulse generator to the myocardium. The leads consist of flexible conductive wires enclosed by insulating material. The electrode is the end of the lead that delivers the impulse

the ventricles, to generate an impulse spontaneously, or to maintain primary control of the pacing function of the heart. There are many conditions a client can encounter clinically that affect the ability of the heart's conduction system to function normally, creating circumstances for which pacing is indicated (Box 46–2). Pacemakers can be used temporarily or prophylactically until the condition responsible for the rate or conduction disturbance resolves. Pacemakers also can be used on permanent basis if the client's condition persists despite adequate therapy.

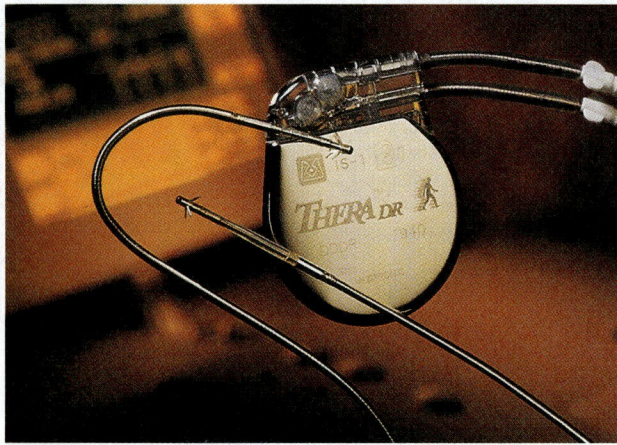

Figure 46–9. A permanent pacemaker (pulse generator). (Courtesy of Medtronic, Inc., Minneapolis, MN.)

directly to the myocardial wall. It is usually made of platinum-iridium, a highly conductive material that also deters the adherence of platelets. Not only does this system deliver electrical impulses but it relays information about spontaneous intracardiac signals back to the sensing circuit within the pulse generator.

Electrodes can be unipolar or bipolar. Unipolar designs incorporate the cardiac electrode as the negative terminal of the electrical circuit with the metallic shell or second wire of the impulse generator as the positive electrode. Bipolar systems use two wires, each ending in an electrode a short distance apart. Pacemakers can be either single-chamber pacemakers that pace either the ventricles

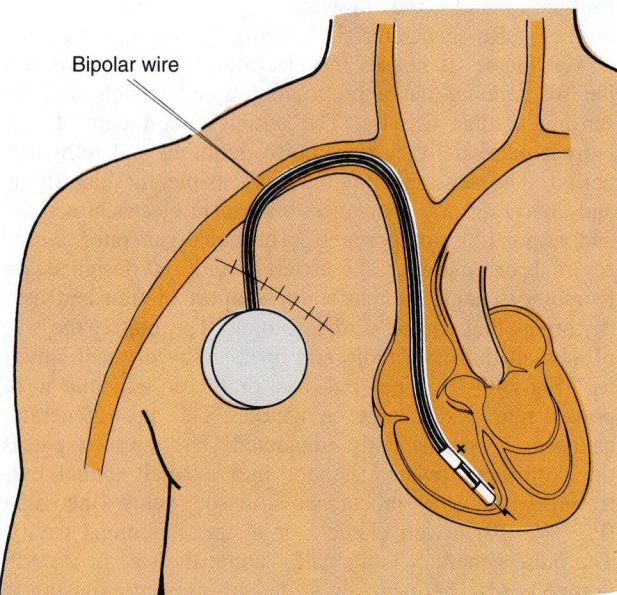

Figure 46–10. Transvenous catheter placement for dual-chamber pacing. Separate electrodes in the atrium and ventricle allow synchronized contraction, and thus stroke volume is improved. (From Phillips, R. E., & Feeney, M. K. [1990]. *The cardiac rhythms: A systematic approach to interpretation* [3rd ed.]. Philadelphia: W. B. Saunders.)

or atria or dual-chamber pacemakers that pace both the atria and ventricles.

Pacemaker Methods

There are three major modes of delivering energy to the myocardial tissue for the purpose of artificial pacing: (1) external (transcutaneous), (2) epicardial (transthoracic), and (3) endocardial (transvenous).

External. In external (transcutaneous) pacing the heart is stimulated through large gelled electrode pads placed anteriorly and posteriorly and connected to an external transcutaneous pacemaker. Transcutaneous pacing is the treatment of choice in emergency cardiac care (ECC) because it can be instituted quickly while a temporary transvenous pacemaker is being inserted or as prophylaxis against warning dysrhythmias. It is also the least invasive pacing technique. Because no vascular puncture is needed for electrode placement, transcutaneous pacing is preferred in clients who are anticoagulated or who may require thrombolytic therapy. Since the anterior electrode is placed to the left of the sternum and centered close to the point of maximal impulse (PMI), excessive chest hair must be clipped or shaved to ensure good contact, or alternative pacing electrode positions must be used. The pacing device is usually activated at a rate of 80 BPM. Electrical capture is characterized by widening of the QRS complex and broadening of the T wave. Many clients feel extreme discomfort with each paced beat; this is a significant limitation to transcutaneous pacing. Narcotic analgesia and sedation may be given to clients who are conscious, or who regain consciousness, to reduce discomfort and anxiety. Additional complications of external transcutaneous pacing can be skin burns, muscular twitching, psychological reactions, failure to capture (inability of the impulse to initiate a contraction), and failure to sense (inability of the pacemaker to sense intrinsic electrical activity) (Table 46–3).

Epicardial. Epicardial (transthoracic) pacing is another method of artificial pacing in which the electrical energy travels from an external pulse generator through the thoracic musculature directly to the epicardial surface of the heart via lead wires. This method of pacing is most common during and immediately following open heart surgery, since there is direct access to the epicardium at this time. Some complications sometimes seen with an epicardial pacemaker are lead dislodgement, microshock, cardiac tamponade, infection, psychological reactions, failure to capture, and failure to sense.

Endocardial. Endocardial (transvenous) pacing provides the most common means of pacing the heart in emergency situations. The surgeon (1) inserts the pacing electrode via the transvenous route (via the antecubital, femoral, jugular, or subclavian vein) and (2) threads the electrode into the right atrium or right ventricle so that it comes into direct contact with the endocardium. This procedure can be done at the bedside under fluoroscopic control or in a cardiovascular laboratory. Major draw-

Table 46–3. Pacemaker Malfunctions and Nursing Interventions

Problem	Possible Cause	Nursing Interventions*
Failure to Pace Properly		
Intermittent or complete absence of pacing artifact Rapid, inappropriate firing of pacemaker (pacemaker-mediated tachycardia)	Battery failure A break or loose connection anywhere along the system Pulse generator failure Circuitry failure "Oversensing" or "undersensing" by the pacemaker	Replace pulse generator Replace battery unit Check and tighten all connections between pulse generator and leads Reduce or increase sensitivity threshold of pacemaker unit Assess client's tolerance of pacemaker failure; have emergency drugs on hand; perform CPR as indicated
Failure to Capture		
Pacing artifact present but is not followed by a QRS complex or P wave	Decreased conductivity by the myocardial tissue due to electrolyte imbalance, infarction, drug toxicity, perforation, or excessive fibrosis of tissue at electrode site Lead displacement due to migration, or idle manipulation of pulse generator ("twiddler's syndrome")	Increase voltage by 1–2 mA (temporary pacemaker) Increase amplitude of pacemaker output/pulse width Reposition client to either side in attempt to improve contact of electrode with endocardium; in temporary pacemaker, try moving arm if lead wire is inserted in antecubital area Obtain chest film to determine pacemaker position Have emergency drugs on hand; initiate CPR if necessary
Failure to Sense		
Pacing artifact present despite the presence of QRS complexes and P waves A competitive rhythm may develop	Sensitivity threshold set too low Intrinsic beats are of too-low voltage and go undetected by pacemaker's sensing mechanism Dislodged or fractured lead Circuitry failure Electromagnetic interference	Increase sensitivity threshold on pulse generator Reposition client If client's intrinsic rhythm or rate is adequate, turn off pacemaker Increase pacing rate to overdrive client's intrinsic heart rate Give antidysrhythmics to decrease ectopy Notify physician Obtain chest film to determine electrode placement
Oversensing		
Pacemaker senses electrical activity within the myocardium (which should be ignored) or myopotentials	Sensitivity threshold set too high T wave sensing myopotentials Electromagnetic interference Two leads touching	Decrease sensitivity threshold Correct conditions that produce large T waves

CPR, cardiopulmonary resuscitation.
* For all problems, document malfunction by an electrocardiogram. If pacemaker is programmable, have reprogramming machine available. Monitor client's tolerance to pacemaker malfunction (vital signs, chest pain).
From Huang, S. H., et al. (1989). *Coronary care nursing* (2nd ed.). Philadelphia: W. B. Saunders.

backs include thrombophlebitis, infection at the insertion site, sepsis from unsterile technique, increased chance of lead displacement as the client changes position, and the discomfort of having the extremity nearest the insertion site immobilized (Fig. 46–11). Other additional complications occasionally seen are pacer-induced dysrhythmias, hiccups, abdominal twitching, myocardial irritability, and perforation of chamber or septum, in addition to failure to capture, and failure to sense.

Temporary Pacing

Temporary pacing may be used in emergent or elective situations that require limited, short-term pacing (under 2 weeks). In this form of pacing, the pulse generator is external. Temporary pacemakers can be applied transcutaneously, and inserted transthoracically or, more commonly, transvenously.

Although the principles of cardiac pacing are the same whether a temporary or permanent pacemaker is used, each type has distinct issues for nurses to assess in the client and teach to the client and family. The client having a temporary pacemaker needs:

- An explanation about the procedure and the purpose of the pacemaker
- Monitoring for the response to the pacemaker
- Maintenance of electrical safety

- Monitoring for pacing parameters (sensing, capturing, threshold)
- Protection against injury and infection

Before the procedure, explain the purpose of the temporary pacemaker to the client and family. Ensure that a permit for the procedure has been signed and that all questions have been answered. Necessary equipment is gathered, and the functioning of the external generator is checked (battery and sense and pace modes). Assess the client's vital signs, and obtain a rhythm strip.

During the procedure, monitor the client's ECG and vital signs continuously. Large P waves are seen as the catheter passes through the atrium, and larger QRS complexes are seen in the ventricles. Set and maintain the stimulus and sensitivity settings according to the physician's orders. Tape or suture the electrode at the insertion site.

After the procedure, assess vital signs routinely along with heart rhythm and emotional reactions to the procedure and pacing. Secure and check all connections. Monitor battery and control settings. Clean and dress the incision site according to protocols. Keep the generator dry and protect the controls from mishandling. The client must be protected from electromicroshocks and electromagnetic interference. Wear rubber gloves when exposed wires are handled. Check electrical equipment for adequate grounding. Limit motion of the extremity at the insertion site. Stabilize arm, catheter, and pacemaker to an arm board and avoid movement of the arm above shoulder level. Do not lift the client from under the arm. If the leg is the insertion site, likewise limit its motion, especially hip flexion and outward rotation.

In addition to protecting the client from injury, monitor pacemaker function. Document the location and type of pacing lead. Note the pacing mode, stimulus threshold, sensitivity setting, pacing rate and intervals, and intrinsic rhythm. Pacing intervals are shown in Figure 46–12.

Permanent Pacing

Permanent pacing is indicated for chronic or recurrent dysrhythmias that are severe, unresponsive to antiarrhythmic medication, and caused by AV block or sinus node malfunction. The need for permanent pacemakers is confirmed through ECGs, electrophysiology studies, and Holter monitoring.

In 1984 the American College of Cardiology/American Heart Association (ACC/AHA) Task Force on Assessment of Diagnostic and Therapeutic Cardiovascular Procedures issued guidelines for permanent cardiac pacemaker implantation to ensure cost-effective optimal medical care. These recommendations were instrumental in the development of guidelines for Medicare and Medicaid and have contributed substantially to their reimbursement schedules. The guidelines were revised in 1991 and are grouped into three classes. Class I criteria are identified in Box 46–3.[34,35]

Central to the ACC/AHA committee recommendations is the presence of clinical manifestations associated with bradycardia or conduction disorder. Significant manifestations are defined by the committee as "clinical manifesta-

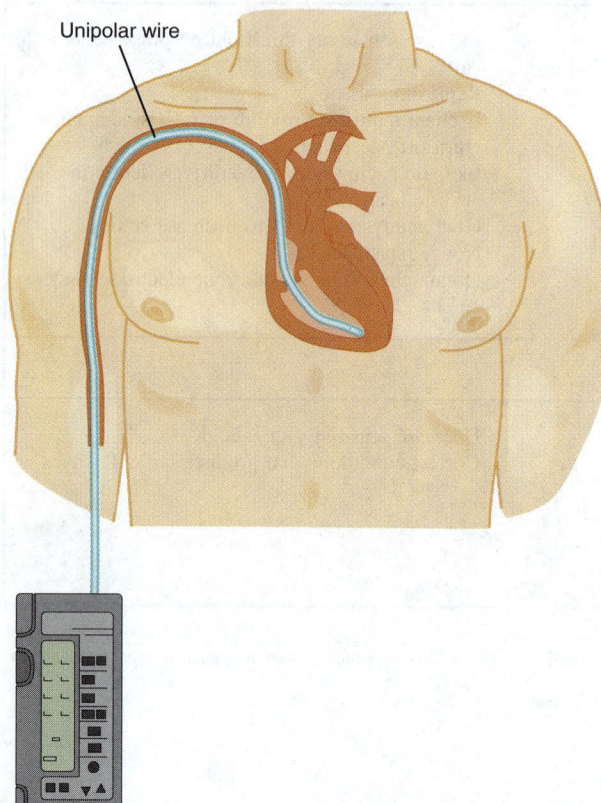

Unipolar wire

Figure 46–11. A temporary endocardial pacemaker.

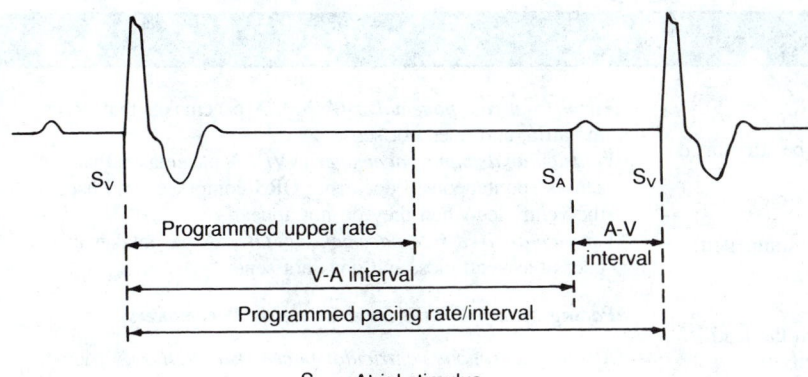

S_A = Atrial stimulus
S_V = Ventricular stimulus

Figure 46–12. Pacing intervals. The atrioventricular (A–V, delay) interval can be thought of as an artificial P–R interval. The programmed pacing rate or interval is also called the ventriculoventricular (V–V) interval. Ventricular pacing will occur if intrinsic ventricular activity does not occur within the V–V interval. (From *Symbiotics series: Selecting the DDD patient* [1984]. Minneapolis: Medtronic.)

tions that are directly attributable to the slow heart rate: transient dizziness, lightheadedness, near syncope or frank syncope as manifestations of transient cerebral ischemia, and more generalized manifestations such as marked exercise intolerance or frank heart failure.[12,34,35]

Pacemaker Modes

There are two basic kinds of pacemakers: fixed-rate (asynchronous or nondemand) and demand.

Fixed-rate pacemakers are designed to fire constantly as a preset rate without regard to the client's own electrical activity of the heart. This mode of pacing is appropriate in the absence of any electrical activity (asystole), but is dangerous in the presence of an intrinsic rhythm because of the potential of the pacemaker to fire during the vul-

nerable period of repolarization and initiate lethal ventricular dysrhythmias.

Demand pacemakers have a sensing device that senses the heart's electrical activity and fires at a present rate only when the heart's electrical activity drops below a predetermined rate level (Fig. 46–13). In addition to a variety of capabilities, permanent pacemakers now have special programmable and antitachyarrhythmic functions that are quite complex. In order to communicate all the functions of the individual pacemakers, in 1974 international codes were developed by the Inter-Society Commission for Heart Disease (ICHD). The coding system has gone through two revisions since 1974. Pacemakers now can be identified with a five-digit letter code. Although the last two letters contain pertinent information, commonly a pacemaker will be referred to only by its first three letters (Box 46–4).

Pacemaker Function

Because there are so many types of pacemakers with greater than 250 programs, the general function of pacemakers is discussed first. A simple demand pacing system functions in the following manner. The cardiac cycle normally begins with the client's own beat. The pacemaker has a sensor that senses if the intrinsic beat has occurred; if not, the pacer sends out an impulse to begin myocardial depolarization through a pulse generator. The impulse generator is said to capture the myocardium and thereby maintain heart rhythm.

Box 46–3. Clinical Conditions Warranting Permanent Pacemakers (Class I Criteria)

A. Complete heart block (permanent or intermittent), associated with the following complications:
   1. Symptomatic bradycardia
   2. Left ventricular heart failure
   3. Ectopic rhythms that suppress the automaticity of escape pacemakers and result in symptomatic bradycardia
   4. Documented periods of asystole greater than 3 seconds or any escape rate less than 40 beats per minute in a symptom-free client
   5. Confusional states that clear with temporary pacing
   6. Post-AV (atrioventricular) junctional ablation
B. Second-degree AV block, permanent or intermittent, with symptomatic bradycardia
C. Atrial fibrillation, atrial flutter, supraventricular tachycardia with complete heart block or advanced AV block, bradycardia (the bradycardia must be unrelated to digitalis or drugs known to impair AV conduction)

From Zaim, B, Zaim, S., & Kutalek, S. (1994). Indications for use of permanent cardiac pacemakers. Heart Disease and Stroke, 3, 71–76.

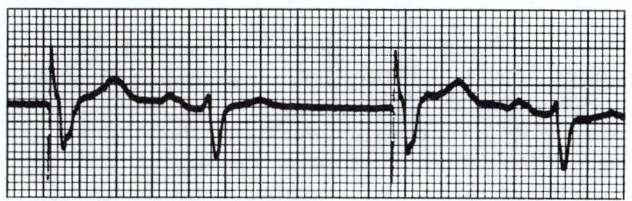

Figure 46–13. Demand pacing. The pacemaker initiates an electrical impulse when the sinus node fails to pace the heart. (From Phillips, R. E., & Feeney, M. K. [1990]. *The cardiac rhythms: A systematic approach to interpretation* [3rd ed.]. Philadelphia: W. B. Saunders.)

Box 46–4. Classification System for Pacemakers

First Letter: Chamber-Paced

Indicates which chamber(s) of the heart will be stimulated.

V = Ventricle
A = Atrium
D = Dual-chamber (both atria and ventricles stimulated)

Second Letter: Chamber-Sensed

Indicates the chamber(s) of the heart in which the lead is capable of recognizing intrinsic electrical activity.

V = Ventricle
A = Atrium
D = Dual-chamber (sensing capabilities in atria and ventricles)
O = No sensing capability

Third Letter: Mode of Response

Indicates how the pacemaker will act based on the information it senses.

T = Triggered (may have energy output triggered)
I = Inhibited (pacing output inhibited by intrinsic activity)
D = Dual-chamber (may be either inhibiting or triggering of both chambers)

Fourth Letter: Programmable Functions

Indicates ability to change function once the pacemaker has been implanted.

P = Programmable for one or two functions
M = Multiprogrammable ability to change functions other than the rate or output

Fifth Letter: Tachyarrhythmic Functions

Indicates specific methods of interrupting tachyarrhythmias.

B = Bursts of pacing
N = Normal rate competition
S = Scanning

Examples

Pacing Modes Within Single-Chamber Pacemakers

Atrial demand pacemaker (AAI). A pacemaker that senses spontaneously occurring P waves and paces the atria when they do not appear.

Atrial fixed-rate pacemaker (AOO). A pacemaker that paces the atria, and does not sense.
Ventricular demand pacemaker (VVI). A pacemaker that senses spontaneously occurring QRS complexes and paces the ventricles when they do not appear.
Ventricular fixed-rate pacemaker (VOO). A pacemaker that paces the ventricles, and does not sense.

Pacing Modes Within Dual-Chamber Pacemakers

Atrial synchronous ventricular pacemaker (VDD). A pacemaker that senses spontaneously occurring P waves and QRS complexes and paces the ventricles when QRS complexes fail to appear after spontaneously occurring P waves, as in complete atrioventricular (AV) block. In this type of pacemaker, the pacing of ventricles is synchronized with the P waves, so that the ventricular contractions follow the atrial contractions in a normal sequence. A major benefit is that it permits the heart rate to vary, and AV synchrony occurs, depending on the physiologic demands of the body. A built-in safety mechanism causes ventricular depolarizations to occur at a fixed rate should atrial rates become too fast.
AV synchronous pacemaker (VAT). A pacemaker that has ventricular pacing, atrial sensing, and triggered response to sensing. The ventricular pacing stimulus will fire at a set time after sensing of a spontaneous atrial depolarization.
AV sequential pacemaker (DVI). A pacemaker that senses spontaneously occurring QRS complexes and paces both the atria and ventricles (the atria first, followed by the ventricles after a short delay) when QRS complexes do not appear.
AV sequential fixed-rate pacemaker (DOO). A pacemaker that paces both the atria and ventricles, but does not sense.
Optimal sequential pacemaker (DDD). A pacemaker that senses spontaneously occurring P waves and QRS complexes and (1) paces the atria when P waves fail to appear, as in sick sinus syndrome, and (2) paces the ventricles when QRS complexes fail to appear after spontaneously occurring or paced P waves. In this type of pacemaker, like the VDD pacemaker, the pacing of ventricles is synchronized with the P waves, so that the ventricular contractions follow the atrial contractions in a normal sequence.

For a predetermined amount of time after the pacemaker impulse, the pacemaker is incapable of sensing incoming signals. This process prevents the pacer from sensing its own generated electrical current and acting again. The refractory period is followed by the noise-sampling period. If any electromagnetic interference is sensed during this phase, the pacemaker goes into a fixed-rate mode of operation and remains in this mode until the source of interference is removed. At the end of the noise-sampling period, the alert period begins, and the cycle starts over again. If a PVC or PAC occurs during the alert period, the pacemaker will sense it and start its cycle over again without emitting any impulse.

Electrocardiography of Paced Beats

The ECG of a paced rhythm appears different from that of a normal sinus rhythm. A pacing artifact is seen. With atrial pacing, a P wave follows the artifact but may be hidden in some leads. Leads II and V1 are best for deciding whether a P wave follows a pacer spike. The

QRS complex appears normal with atrial pacing; the impulse travels through usual conduction systems.

The ECG with ventricular pacing shows an abnormal QRS complex because the impulse begins in the ventricle. With right ventricular endocardial pacing, a pseudo-LBBB ECG wave is created. If the left ventricle is paced, a pseudo-RBBB is created.

Assess the ECG strip for pacer spikes followed by the expected appearance of a P wave or QRS complex. Spikes not followed by depolarization waves or paced beats that appear too early or too late may signal pacemaker failure.

Teach the client and family how to care for the pacemaker and the precautions to follow, as shown in the Client Education Guide.[11,32]

Transtelephonic Pacemaker Monitoring

Special telephone monitoring of the client's ECG may be done from time to time on an outpatient basis. Telephone ECG systems are designed for follow-up monitoring of a pacemaker client. Via finger tip, wrist, or ankle electrodes, the transmitter detects, amplifies, and converts a client's electrical activity and pacemaker artifacts to frequency-modulated audio tones for transmission, via the telephone, to an ECG receiver. From the transmitted signals, the ECG receiver provides an ECG strip recording and printout of the rate and pulse width of a client's implanted pacemaker.

Pacemaker Failure

Pacemakers can develop malfunctions in the sensor or pulse generator. Complications associated with the components of the pacemaker system itself include failure to sense, pace, or capture (see Table 46–3).

Failure to sense is the inability of the sensor to detect the client's intrinsic beats, and thus the pacemaker sends out impulses too early (Fig. 46–14*A*). This may be due to improper position of the catheter, tip or lead dislodgement, battery failure, the sensitivity being set too low, or a fractured wire in the catheter.

Failure to pace is a malfunction of the pulse generator. The ECG shows a lack of any impulse (Fig. 46–14*B*). Component failure to discharge (pace) can be due to battery failure, lead dislodgement, fracture of the lead wire inside the catheter, disconnections between catheter and generator, and a sensing malfunction.

Failure to capture is a disorder in the pacemaker electrodes; the impulse does not generate depolarization (Fig. 46–14*C*). Failure to capture can occur with low voltage, battery failure, faulty connections between the pulse generator and catheter, improper position of the catheter, catheter wire fracture, fibrosis at the catheter tip, or a fracture of the catheter.

Clinical manifestations of pacemaker malfunctioning include syncope, bradycardia or tachycardia, and palpita-

tions. When this occurs the malfunctioning leads or pacemaker needs to be replaced.

■ Nursing Management

Assessment

Assess the client for subjective clinical manifestations of dysrhythmias and alterations in cardiac output. These include palpitations, syncope, fatigue, shortness of breath, chest pain, or skipped beats felt in the chest. The client may also feel anxiety about the heart disorder and manifest nervousness, fear, sleeplessness, uncertainty, or hopelessness. Objective clinical manifestations may include diaphoresis, pallor or cyanosis, variations in radial and apical pulses such as bradycardia or tachycardia, rhythm changes, hypotension, crackles, or decreased mental acuity. The client may be anxious and exhibit a fear of being left alone. The client is placed on a monitor, and heart rhythm is monitored continuously by the nurse, a computer, and a monitor technician. Rhythm strips are examined at least every shift.

Explain to the client and family the purpose of the pacemaker and the experience of having a pacemaker inserted. Most permanent pacemakers are inserted transvenously. Try to keep the ECG leads off the possible insertion site. The insertion site is prepared according to hospital policy. A preoperative ECG is obtained, and a patent IV line is maintained. Prophylactic antibiotics may be given.

After insertion, monitor vital signs and pacemaker function. Pain can usually be managed with oral analgesics if the transvenous approach was used. Initially, instruct the client to avoid excessive extension or abduction of the arm on the operative side. Perform passive range-of-motion exercises on the arm.

Paced and nonpaced ECGs are obtained. A magnet may be placed over the pulse generator, converting it to a fixed-rate pacing mode, so that the client's intrinsic rhythm can be determined. The location of the pacemaker electrodes is determined by x-ray. The model and serial numbers of the pulse generator and leads are recorded along with the date of implantation and programmed functions of the initial implant.

Diagnosis, Planning, Implementation

Decreased Cardiac Output. Dysrhythmias often lead to decreased ventricular filling due to rapid rate or from not being coordinated to allow for atrial kick. Express this common nursing diagnosis as *Decreased Cardiac Output related to decreased ventricular filling time secondary to (name the rhythm).*

Planning: Expected Outcomes. The client will have an adequate cardiac output, as evidenced by heart rate, rhythm, palpable pulse, and blood pressure returning to baseline; level of consciousness returning to baseline; warm and dry skin; clear lung sounds; no S_3 or S_4; no dysrhythmias; and adequate urine output.

Implementation. Monitor heart rate and rhythm and vital signs continuously, many times with the aid of the

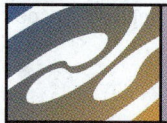

CLIENT EDUCATION GUIDE

The Client with a Permanent Pacemaker

Wound Care

Assess your wound daily. Report any signs of inflammation (fever, redness, tenderness, discharge, or warmth) to the physician. Avoid constrictive clothing (e.g., tight brassiere straps), which puts excessive pressure on the wound and the pulse generator. Avoid extensive "toying" with the pulse generator, because this could cause pacemaker malfunction and local skin inflammation.

Pacemaker Management

Take your pulse daily in your wrist or on your neck. You will be taught how to do this before leaving the hospital. Notify the physician if the pulse is slower than the set rate; also report sensations of feeling your heart race, beating irregularly, or dizziness.

Avoid being near areas with high voltage, magnetic force fields, or radiation; this can cause pacemaker problems. Things to avoid include large running motors (gas or electric), standing near high-tension wires, power plants, radio transmitters, large industrial magnets, and arc welding machines. Riding in a car is safe, but avoid bringing the pacemaker to within 6 to 12 inches of the distributor coil of a running engine.

You can continue to safely operate most appliances and tools that are properly grounded and in good repair, including the following: microwave ovens, televisions, VCRs, AM and FM radios, electric blankets, lawn mowers, leaf blowers, and cars. You can safely operate the following office and light industrial equipment that is properly grounded and in good repair: electric typewriters, copying machines, and personal computers.

The airport's metal detector may be triggered by the pacemaker's metal casing and the programming magnet. This should be mentioned to the security guards. The metal detector itself will not harm the pacemaker.

Carry a pacemaker identity card (along with programming information—the pacemaker manufacture and emergency phone numbers) at all times; and wearing a medical alert bracelet is also recommended.

Avoid activity that could damage the pulse generator; such as playing football or firing a rifle with the butt end against the affected shoulder.

Some stores have antitheft devices that may affect pacemaker function. If symptoms suddenly arise, move away from the area and notify the store clerk about the pacemaker.

If radiation therapy has been prescribed to the area in which the pulse generator was implanted, a relocation of the pulse generator will be necessary.

Do not lift more than 5 to 10 lb (this equals a full grocery sack or a gallon of milk) for the first 6 weeks after surgery. Do not move your arms and shoulders vigorously for the first 6 weeks. Normal activities can be resumed in 6 weeks, including sexual activity.

The purpose, dose, schedule, and possible side effects of prescribed medications should be thoroughly discussed. Written information sheets can reinforce learning.

Plan to see your physician to test your pacemaker. Your cardiologist will periodically reevaluate pacemaker function and reprogram it if needed. You may also be able to check your pacemaker by telephone. If this is possible, you will receive instructions.

---

computer. Assess skin temperature, lung sounds, heart sounds, and peripheral pulses every 2 to 4 hours. Monitor laboratory studies, especially if the client is suspected of having an MI. Give antidysrhythmic medications according to orders. Use blood levels as a guide to dosage. Many medications, especially antidysrhythmics, can rise to toxic levels, especially if the client has a pre-existing liver, renal, or electrolyte disorder.

Maintain a quiet atmosphere and administer analgesics to control pain. Stimulation can lead to increased levels of catecholamine release and trigger tachycardias and increased oxygen demand.

Apply oxygen with nasal prongs to supplement serum levels. Hypoxia can lead to further myocardial ischemia and dysrhythmias.

If life-threatening dysrhythmias develop, many nurses are trained to defibrillate the client. Other emergency in-terventions include CPR, various medications, and preparation of the client for a transcutaneous or permanent pacemaker.

Anxiety. The risk of death from sudden onset of life-threatening dysrhythmias weighs heavily on most clients. Express this nursing diagnosis as *Anxiety related to fear about unknown outcome.*

Planning: Expected Outcomes. The client will have a reduced level of anxiety, as evidenced by stating he or she feels less anxious and not voicing feelings of helplessness or hopelessness; increased ability to sleep and rest; return of heart rate to baseline; and reduction of dyspnea.

Implementation. Identify the client's anxiety and assist the client in discussing sources of fear. Clarify

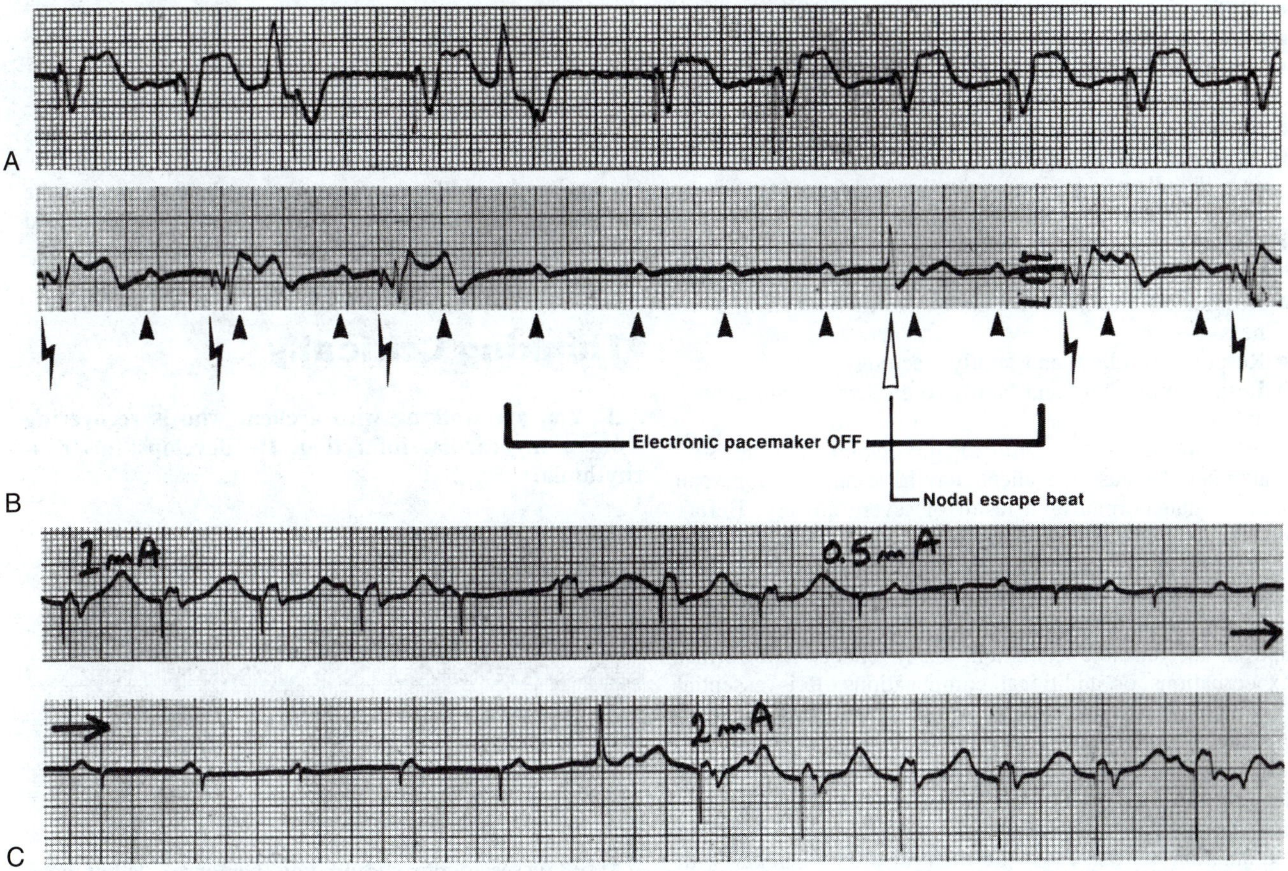

Figure 46–14. Pacemaker failures. *A*, Failure to sense. *B*, Failure to pace. *C*, Failure to capture. (From Phillips, R. E., & Feeney, M. K. [1990]. *The cardiac rhythms: A systematic approach to interpretation* [3rd ed.]. Philadelphia: W. B. Saunders.)

misconceptions. Commonly, the client or a member of the family has had a heart condition and the client's ability to cope may be directly influenced by that experience. Explain the equipment present in the room. Most rooms are stocked with various equipment, and its presence does not always indicate the severity of the client's condition. Remain with the client and tell the client and family what is happening now and what will be happening (e.g., blood will be drawn soon). Finally, explore the usual coping methods with the client. Positive coping methods are usually supported; discuss maladaptive coping mechanisms, and suggest substitutions. For example, smoking may be a common coping mechanism, but it is not permitted with cardiac disorders, nor is it permitted in most hospitals. Therefore, if smoking is the client's coping mechanism when stressed, a substitute will need to be found such as nicotine patches or chewing gum. Be aware that these patches actually can increase the levels of nicotine because they provide constant levels of the drug. Light smokers will require less nicotine. Adjust the dose of the patch, beginning with the lowest levels.

Evaluation

The degree of expected outcome attainment is assessed hourly (or more often) if the client has life-threatening dysrhythmias. Dysrhythmias are treated promptly and usually stop quickly once treatment is begun. Recalcitrant dysrhythmias may require several medications. Anxiety can sometimes abate quickly, but commonly it requires several days. Some clients remain anxious for their entire hospital stay.

Community and Self-Care

With limited resources, lack of adequate insurance coverage, early discharge, and shorter allotted hospital days for various diagnoses, nursing units may develop and utilize client and family discharge teaching checklists. These list the issues needed to be reviewed before discharge. They also provide documented evidence that the client and family discussed the issue before discharge or transfer to an extended-care facility. Upon discharge from the hospital, documentation should show evidence of the following:

● Vital signs stable
● Stable cardiac rhythm with dysrhythmias controlled
● Absence of fever, pulmonary, or cardiovascular complications
● Laboratory values within expected levels

- Ability to tolerate adequate nutritional intake
- Absence of urinary or bowel dysfunction
- Ability to perform activities of daily living (ADLs) and ambulate as before hospitalization
- Mental status within normal limits for client
- Adequate home support system, or referral to home care if indicated by inadequate home support system or client's inability to perform ADLs
- Referral to community support group for cardiac conditions
- Response of family or significant other to client's illness
- Response of client and family teaching
- Response of client and family to discharge planning

Teaching about the nature of the disorder is done several times, because the client may have an attention span shorter than normal as a result of severe anxiety. Before discharge, make certain clients appreciate the importance of taking antidysrhythmic agents as prescribed. Include details concerning medication administration, dosage, and side effects in the discharge plan. If dismissed too early and in an unstable condition, many clients risk further exacerbations or additional complications. It is essential that nursing discharge criteria are met and documented.

Clients who have experienced cardiac dysrhythmias while at a healthcare facility may be apprehensive about leaving the facility. Those who have experienced innocuous dysrhythmias may need only calm reassurance and an explanation of the cause of their disorder. Clients with recurring life-threatening dysrhythmias such as VT will require comprehensive and specialized attention. These clients may have experienced many frightening events in the course of their hospitalization.

When a client is at risk of developing a life-threatening dysrhythmia, check if the client's housemates and significant others know how to perform CPR. Refer these persons to community agencies that provide CPR training (e.g., the American Heart Association, the American Red Cross, local fire departments, and some local hospitals).

Sometimes clients with serious, chronic, or potential dysrhythmias use portable telemetry units for self-monitoring at home after discharge. This allows resumption of daily activities while providing continuous 24-hour surveillance of cardiac rhythm. Nurses are often responsible for instructing clients in the use of these units. Ask these clients to keep a diary of their daily activities so that clinicians can correlate factors in the client's life that may be contributing to the development of dysrhythmias.

Finally, instruct clients concerning the importance of regular medical follow-up. Advise them to keep regular appointments with their physician after discharge. Also, the client and significant others should know how to obtain emergency medical attention if necessary.

Living under the constant threat of sudden death provokes anxiety, depression, and, occasionally, dependent behavior. In some cases, psychological counseling may bolster coping resources. Significant others also benefit from counseling. The nurse can recommend community and private counseling services for the client and significant others.

Conclusions

Common dysrhythmias usually do not interfere with everyday activities. In fact, most people with dysrhythmias are able to lead a productive and relatively normal life. Clients need to follow a prescribed medical regimen, take medications as directed, and report any symptoms and side effects along with continued follow-up medical care.

Thinking Critically

1. You are walking with a client who is recovering from a myocardial infarction. He develops this dysrhythmia:

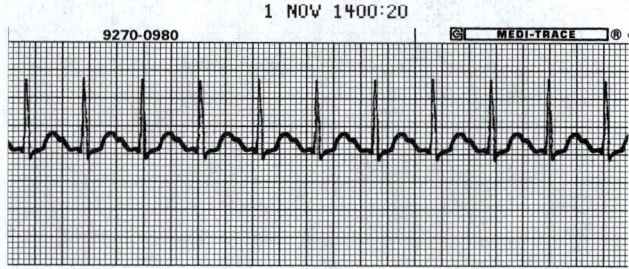

What assessments should you perform? What care does the client need?

Factors to Consider. What is the usual heart rhythm response to activity? How can you assess if he is tolerating this rhythm? How should the client be returned to his room?

2. An 82-year-old woman is brought to the emergency department by her son after losing consciousness and hitting her head on falling. She is now awake and states that she has been having periods of dizziness and blackouts for the past few weeks. During your physical examination, you notice what appears to be a pacemaker device implanted under her left clavicle. What additional assessments should you make? What information should you obtain about the pacemaker?

Factors to Consider. What might have happened to the pacemaker during the fall? Could a faulty pacemaker be responsible for the loss of consciousness?

Bibliography

1. American Heart Association. (1994). *Advanced cardiac life support.* Dallas: Author.
2. American Heart Association. (1994). *Research facts—Update 1994.* Dallas: Author.

3. American Heart Association. (1995). *Heart and stroke facts*, Dallas: Author.

4. American Heart Association. (1995). *Heart and stroke facts: 1994 statistical supplement*, Dallas: Author.

5. Barbiere, C. C., & Liberatore, K. (1992). Automated external defibrillators: An update of additions to the ACLS Algorithms. *Critical Care Nurse, 12*(5), 17–20.

6. Bubien, R., et al. (1993). What you need to know about radiofrequency ablation. *American Journal of Nursing, 93*(7), 30–36.

7. Collins, M. A. (1994). When your patient has an implantable cardioverter defibrillator. *American Journal of Nursing, 94*(3), 34–39.

8. Drew, B. J. (1992). Using cardiac leads: The right way. *Nursing 92, 22*(5), 50–54.

9. Dunn, F. G. (1990). Prevention of sudden cardiac death. *Cardiovascular Clinics, 20*(3), 95–109.

10. Harper, P. (1993). Implantable cardioverter defibrillator: A patient education model for the illiterate patient. *Critical Care Nurse, 13*(2), 62–71.

11. Hasemeier, C. S. (1996). Permanent pacemaker. *American Journal of Nursing, 96*(2), 30–31.

12. Hayes, D. L. (1992). The next 5 years in cardiac pacemakers: A preview. *Mayo Clinic Proceedings, 67*(4), 379–384.

13. Higgins, C. A. (1990). The AICD: a teaching plan for patients and families. *Critical Care Nurse, 10*(6), 69–74.

14. Kater, K. M., et al. (1992). Corralling atrial fibrillation with "maze" surgery. *American Journal of Nursing, 92*(7), 34–38.

15. Katzung, B. G. (1992). *Basic and clinical pharmacology* (5th ed.). Norwalk, CT: Appleton & Lange.

16. King, K. B. (1994). Preparing patients and families for health care procedures. *Heart Disease and Stroke, 3*(2), 95–97.

17. Koda-Kimble, M. A., et al. (1992). *Handbook of applied therapeutics* (2nd ed.), Vancouver, WA: Applied Therapeutics.

18. Meek, J. (1991). The dreaded defibrillator. *American Journal of Nursing, 91*(5), 32–33.

19. Moser, S. A., Crawford, D., & Thomas, A. (1993). Updated care guidelines for patients with automatic implantable cardioverter defibrillators. *Critical Care Nurse, 13*(4), 62–71.

20. Owens, M. W., & Daniel, J. L. (1993). IV magnesium sulfate in the treatment of ventricular tachycardia and acute myocardial infarction. *Critical Care Nurse, 13*(12), 83–85.

21. *Physicians' desk reference*. (50th ed.). (1996). Montvale, NJ: Medical Economics Data.

22. Porter, L. A. (1995). Drug profiles: Maximizing therapeutic effectiveness. The *Journal of Cardiovascular Nursing. 10*(1), 64–72.

23. Porterfield, L. M., Porterfield, J. G., & Collins, S. W. (1993). The cutting edge in arrhythmias. *Critical Care Nurse, 13*(Suppl. 6), 8–9.

24. Rakel, R. E. (1992). *Conn's current therapy*. Philadelphia: W. B. Saunders.

25. Saver, C. L. (1994). Decoding the ACLS algorithms. *American Journal of Nursing, 94*(1), 26–36.

26. Schron, E. B., et al. (1996). Relation of sociodemographic, clinical, and quality of life variables to adherence in the cardiac arrhythmia suppression trial. *Cardiovascular Nursing, 32*(2), 1–5.

27. Simons, L. H., Cunningham, S., & Catanzaro, M. (1992). Emotional responses and experiences of wives of men who survive a sudden cardiac death event. *Cardiovascular Nursing, 28*(2), 17–21.

28. Sirles, A. T., & Selleck, C. S. (1989). Cardiac disease and the family: Impact, assessment, and implications. *Journal of Cardiovascular Nursing, 3*(2), 23–32.

29. Sommers, M. S. (1992). Preventing complications of CPR. *Medical-Surgical Nursing Quarterly, 1*(1), 44–54.

30. Sommers, M. S. (1992). The near-death experience after cardiopulmonary arrest. *Medical-Surgical Nursing Quarterly, 1*(1), 55–62.

31. Stahl, D. (1994). Subacute care: The future of health care. *Nursing Management, 25*(10), 35–37.

32. Stuart, J. V., & Sheehan, A. M. (1991). Permanent pacemakers: The nurse's role in patient education and follow-up care. *Journal of Cardiovascular Nursing, 5*(3), 32–43.

33. Thompson, E. J. (1993). Transesophageal echocardiography: A new window on the heart and great vessels. *Critical Care Nurse, 13*(5), 55–66.

34. Zaim, B., Zaim, S., & Kutalek, S. P. (1994). Indications for use of permanent cardiac pacemakers. *Heart Disease and Stroke, 3*(2), 71–76.

35. Zipes, D. P. (1992). Management of cardiac arrhythmias: Pharmacological, electrical and surgical techniques. In Braunwald, E. (Ed.), *Heart disease* (4th ed.) Philadelphia: W. B. Saunders.

Nursing Care of Clients with Disorders of Cardiac Structure

Barbara B. Ott

Adequate tissue perfusion is essential to life and good health. There are many disorders of the heart that can cause varying degrees of inadequate tissue perfusion. Specifically, disorders that affect the structure of the heart may decrease the heart's pumping ability and thus lead to inadequate tissue perfusion.

Infectious Disorders

Bacteria and other microbes are found in abundance in our environment. The heart can become infected by these microbes, with the initiation of an inflammatory response. Involvement of the heart can be lethal during the acute stage or lead to structural damage.

Rheumatic Fever

Rheumatic fever is a diffuse inflammatory disease. It is a delayed response to an infection by group A beta-hemolytic streptococcus. Although these infections remain common, the incidence of rheumatic fever has declined dramatically in the United States. This decline is due to an emphasis on prevention. In many parts of the world, rheumatic heart disease is still the leading cause of death from heart disease in the 5- to 24-year-old group.

Etiology and Risk Factors

Rheumatic fever develops in only a relatively small percentage of people (3%), even after a virulent bout of streptococcal infection; there is, therefore, some evidence of host predisposition. Genetic links have been studied with no clear correlation to the incidence of disease.[18] Once rheumatic fever is acquired by a person, he or she becomes more susceptible than the general population to recurrent infection. Poor hygiene, crowding, and poverty are risk factors for acute rheumatic fever. If appropriate antibiotic therapy for group A beta-hemolytic streptococ-

cal infections is given within the first 9 days of the infection, rheumatic fever is usually prevented.[59]

Prevention of rheumatic fever is the best treatment. The most effective measures against rheumatic fever are probably socioeconomic. In the affluent neighborhoods of Western cities, where there is spacious housing and no crowding, the incidence of rheumatic fever is low.

Pathophysiology

Rheumatic fever produces a diffuse, proliferative, and exudative inflammatory process. In rheumatic fever, there is involvement of the heart, joints, subcutaneous tissue, central nervous system, and skin. Although the cellular disease processes are not clear, it is probably through an abnormal humoral and cell-mediated response to streptococcal cell membrane antigens. These antigens bind to receptors on the heart, other tissues, and joints, which begins the autoimmune response. The inflammatory process often produces permanent and severe heart damage.

Rheumatic fever produces carditis, or inflammation of the heart. Carditis affects the pericardium, epicardium, myocardium, and endocardium. There may be Aschoff's bodies, minuscule nodules with localized fibrin deposits surrounded by areas of necrosis in the myocardium, which are due to the inflammation of rheumatic fever. Endocardial inflammation causes swelling of the valve leaflets, which leads to valve dysfunction and murmurs. Small bacterial vegetations form on the valve tissues. Rough eroded areas of the valves attract platelets, which adhere and form platelet-fibrin clumps that eventually cause scarring and shortening of the valve. The valves lose their elasticity, and cardiac function is impaired. First, the damaged valve may become stenosed. This increases the cardiac workload, because higher pressure must be generated to propel blood through the narrow valve. Second, the valve leaflets may become so short that they cannot close securely. As a result, blood regurgitates (leaks backward) through the damaged valve into

Table 47–1. Effects of Rheumatic Fever on the Myocardium, Endocardium, and Pericardium			
Condition	**Characteristic Lesion**	**Cause of Lesion**	**Significance of Pathophysiologic Involvement**
Rheumatic myocarditis	Aschoff's bodies (minute nodules in connective tissue around small arteries in myocardium)	Formed by leukocytes that mass in inflamed tissues	Nodules may eventually become fibrotic; damage from fibrosis may eventually damage arteries in myocardium; myocarditis may cause temporary loss in contractile power of heart; permanent damage rarely results
Rheumatic endocarditis	Tiny vegetations resembling little beads form along line of closure of valve leaflets (primarily mitral and aortic valves)	Probably result from inflammation, ulceration, and erosion of valve leaflets	Progressive fibrosis, scarring, and calcification of valve leaflets result in valvular incompetence and stenosis
Pericarditis	Nonspecific lesions	Result from diffuse, nonspecific fibrinous or serofibrinous inflammatory reaction	May cause pericardial friction rub; usually no serious sequelae

the chamber from which it was ejected. Both valvular stenosis and regurgitation eventually cause heart failure from the high workload (Table 47–1).

Complications of rheumatic fever include valvular disorders, cardiomegaly, and congestive heart failure (see Risk Factors and Levels of Prevention: Rheumatic Valvular Disease). These complications may be fatal.

Clinical Manifestations and Diagnostic Findings

Rheumatic fever almost always follows a streptococcal infection of the nasopharynx. Clinical manifestations usually include arthritis, carditis, fever, subcutaneous nodules, erythema marginatum, chorea, abdominal pain, weakness, malaise, weight loss, and anorexia.

Arthritis. Arthritis, a prominent finding, is painful and migratory. It most often affects the larger joints, such as the ankles, knees, elbows, shoulders, and wrists. The arthritis may or may not be symmetrical. If the client takes aspirin early in the course of the disease, arthritis manifestations may not be as apparent. Joint manifestations may last hours or days.

Carditis. Carditis, one of the most common manifestations of rheumatic fever, is the most destructive consequence of this disease. Characteristics include a significant murmur, cardiomegaly, pericarditis that produces a significant friction rub, and heart failure. Chest pain due to pericardial inflammation may be present. Sometimes there is myocardial involvement that produces atrioventricular (AV) conduction defects or atrial fibrillation.

Fever. Fever, with a temperature of 38° C (100.4° F) or higher, alternates with normal temperature.

Subcutaneous Nodules. Subcutaneous nodules are small, painless, firm nodules that adhere loosely to the tendon sheaths (especially in knees, knuckles, and elbows). They are usually evident only during the first week or so of the disorder and usually only in children.

Erythema Marginatum. Erythema marginatum is an unusual rash seen primarily on the trunk. The lesions are crescent-shaped and have clear centers. The rash is transitory and may change in appearance in minutes or hours.

Chorea. Chorea is a disorder of the central nervous system. It is manifested by sudden, irregular, aimless, involuntary movements. The chorea disappears without treatment and has no permanent sequelae.

Abdominal Pain. Abdominal pain, a common clinical manifestation, varies in site and severity. The pain may be related to engorgement of the liver.

Weakness, Malaise, Weight Loss, and Anorexia. Weakness, malaise, weight loss, and anorexia probably develop as a result of fever, pain, and the general debilitation associated with serious illness.

No single diagnostic feature identifies rheumatic fever. Many of the common clinical manifestations are associated with other disorders as well as rheumatic fever. The Jones criteria were developed to assist in diagnosis (Box 47–1). The clinical manifestations of rheumatic fever may last 3 months.

A positive throat culture for group A beta-hemolytic streptococci can help with the diagnosis. An elevated white blood cell (WBC) count, erythrocyte sedimentation rate, and C-reactive protein indicate inflammation and these may also be increased.

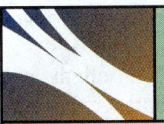

RISK FACTORS AND LEVELS OF PREVENTION

Rheumatic Valvular Disease

Risk Factors

β-Hemolytic streptococcal infection, mitral valve prolapse, and an altered immune response are risk factors.

Levels of Prevention

Primary Prevention

● Decrease risk of rheumatic fever by adequate housing and sanitation for all socioeconomic levels and adequate education on hygiene and infection control.

Secondary Prevention

● Identification of individuals with beta-hemolytic streptococcal infections by nurses in community settings.
● Careful treatment of rheumatic fever and infective endocarditis will help decrease valvular disease.
● Refer individuals with beta-hemolytic streptococcal infections for appropriate diagnosis and medical treatment.
● Evaluate and treat individuals with mitral valve prolapse early to prevent valvular disease.
● Teach that adherence to dietary restriction of sodium is appropriate in some clients with valvular disorders.

Tertiary Prevention

● Monitor carefully for side effects of multiple cardiac drugs that may be prescribed for clients with valvular disease.
● Prophylactic antibiotics should be administered before surgery, other invasive procedures, and dental work.

Acute and Subacute Care

■ Medical Management

The medical therapy for acute rheumatic fever depends on the manifestations and severity of the attack. The first priority is to eradicate the streptococcal infection. Usually this can be accomplished with oral administration of penicillin or erythromycin. Clients with arthritic symptoms are clinically relieved with salicylates; however, because these drugs can confuse the diagnosis, a firm diagnosis should be in place before the administration of salicylates.

Corticosteroids are used to treat carditis, especially if there is evidence of heart failure. If heart failure develops, treatment, including cardiac glycosides and diuretics, is effective.

Bedrest is usually prescribed to reduce cardiac work until evidence of inflammation has subsided. For clients with rheumatic valvular heart disease, bacterial endocarditis prophylaxis is necessary (see Infective Endocarditis).

■ Nursing Management of the Medical Client

Assessment

Nursing assessment involves gathering subjective and objective data concerning the following:

● Cardiac function
● Tolerance to activity and feelings regarding restrictions on activity
● Support systems
● Coping strategies
● Nutritional status
● Level of discomfort
● Knowledge (the client's and significant others') concerning the nature of, and intervention for, rheumatic fever

Diagnosis, Planning, Implementation

Pain. The inflammatory response in the joints can lead to pain. The nursing diagnosis statement would be *Pain related to the inflammatory response in the joints.*

Box 47–1. Guidelines for the Diagnosis of Initial Attack of Rheumatic Fever (Jones Criteria)*

Major Manifestations

Carditis
Polyarthritis
Chorea
Erythema marginatum
Subcutaneous nodules

Minor Manifestations

Clinical findings
　Arthralgia
　Fever
Laboratory findings
　Elevated acute phase reactants
　　Erythrocyte sedimentation rate
　　C-reactive protein
　Prolonged P–R interval

Supporting Evidence of Antecedent Group A Streptococcal Infection

Positive throat culture or rapid streptococcal antigen test
Elevated or rising streptococcal antibody titer

---

*If supported by evidence of preceding group A streptococcal infection, the presence of two major manifestations, or of one major and two minor manifestations, indicates a high probability of acute rheumatic fever.
Modified from Diagnosis of Rheumatic Fever—Special Writing Group (1992). *JAMA, 268*(15), 2069–2073.

Planning: Expected Outcomes. The client will experience increased comfort, as evidenced by reports of restful sleep and reduced discomfort; reports of joint pain relief; reduced use of pain medications; and a relaxed body posture and calm facial expression.

Implementation. Obtain a clear description of the pain or discomfort. Identify the source of greatest discomfort as a focus for intervention. Administer analgesics as needed. Balance rest and activity based on degree of pain and activity tolerance. Other pain interventions are discussed in Chapter 17.

Activity Intolerance. A reduced cardiac reserve and enforced bedrest can quickly lead to activity intolerance. The nursing diagnosis statement would be *Activity Intolerance related to reduced cardiac reserve and enforced bedrest.*

Planning: Expected Outcomes. The client will demonstrate progression toward an optimal level of physical activity tolerance, based on underlying cardiovascular status and psychosocial readiness, as evidenced by ability to pace activity; to verbalize improvement in fatigue; to express acceptance of any imposed activity restrictions; and to steadily increase his or her activity level to include climbing one flight of stairs without chest pain or electrocardiographic (ECG) changes, while the heart rate remains under 90 beats per minute.

Implementation. Bedrest is important in the acute phase because it reduces myocardial oxygen demand. Bedrest usually continues until the following criteria are met:

- Temperature remains normal without the use of salicylates
- Resting pulse remains under 100 beats per minute
- ECG tracings show no signs of myocardial damage
- Sedimentation rate returns to normal
- No pericardial friction rub is present

Once ambulatory, the client must still be careful not to overdo it. The nurse should assess the client's stamina and response to exercise to gauge the degree of gradual activity progression. Assess vital signs before and after exercise. After 3 to 5 minutes of rest, repeat vital signs. The client should reduce or discontinue activity if chest pain, vertigo, dyspnea, confusion, a drop in blood pressure, or an irregular pulse develops. The length of activity restriction depends on whether carditis develops and the extent of permanent heart damage. Restrictions may extend for months. In severe cases of rheumatic carditis, clients may be forced to undergo restrictions on a permanent basis. Encourage a gradual increase in activity within the limits of the client's condition.

The client experiencing chorea requires sedatives, bedrest, and protection from self-injury. A carefully planned and supervised activity schedule should be maintained and evaluated.

Altered Nutrition: Less than Body Requirements. Hypermetabolism seen with fever and inflammation and other factors in rheumatic fever can lead to impaired nutrition. This diagnosis is stated as *Altered Nutrition: Less than Body Requirements, related to fever, inflammation, anorexia, and fatigue.*

Planning: Expected Outcomes. The client will maintain or restore adequate nutritional balance, as evidenced by resumption of ideal weight (based on premorbid status), no further weight loss, normal serum albumin, and a positive nitrogen balance.

Implementation. A high protein, high carbohydrate diet helps maintain adequate nutrition in the presence of fever and infection. Hypermetabolic states (fever and infection) can induce a catabolic state, thus delaying healing. Vitamin and mineral supplements may also benefit the client. Oral hygiene every 4 hours, small attractive meal servings, and foods that are not overly rich, sweet, or greasy stimulate the appetite. Adequate fluid intake prevents dehydration due to fever. If the client shows signs of severe carditis or heart failure, sodium and fluids must be restricted. Daily weights can serve as an indication of nutritional and fluid status and the effectiveness of nursing interventions.

Risk for Ineffective Management of Therapeutic Regimen (Individuals). Following rheumatic fever the client must follow a lifelong regimen to reduce risk of rheumatic heart disease. This diagnosis is stated as *Risk for Ineffective Management of Therapeutic Regimen (Individuals), related to a need for lifelong therapy.*

Planning: Expected Outcomes. The client and family will demonstrate adequate knowledge of rheumatic fever and its cause, course, and therapy, as evidenced by the ability to accurately describe the causes and process of rheumatic fever, its clinical manifestations, its prevention, and the rationale for prescribed interventions.

Implementation. Today, streptococcal infections do not have to develop into rheumatic fever if the client seeks immediate assessment and begins antibiotics. Also, clients who have recovered from an attack of rheumatic fever may prevent subsequent attacks by taking prophylactic doses of antibiotics and observing good health practices. Because repeated attacks may lead to serious heart disease and permanent cardiac disability, the importance of avoiding subsequent attacks of rheumatic fever must be emphasized.

Penicillin is the prophylactic medication of choice. For penicillin-allergic clients, the physician will usually prescribe erythromycin.

The client typically takes prophylactic agents for rheumatic fever for 5 years after the initial attack. After 5 years, recurrences rarely occur. Clients who have had rheumatic fever remain vulnerable to bacterial endocarditis. Therefore, in addition to the antibiotics they take to prevent rheumatic fever recurrence, they must take prophylactic medications before and after any surgical procedure or dental work. Advise clients that they must adhere to this practice permanently.

The client should be taught how to reduce exposure to streptococcal infection:

- Take good care of teeth and gums and obtain prompt dental care for cavities and gingivitis. Prophylactic medication may be needed before teeth are cleaned by a dentist.

- Avoid people who have an upper respiratory infection or who have had a recent streptococcal infection.
- Notify the physician if any of the manifestations of streptococcal sore throat (pharyngitis) develop. It is extremely important to begin antibiotic therapy promptly for any infection. The clinical manifestations include an elevated temperature (102°–104° F), chills, sore throat, and enlarged, painful lymph nodes. Instruct clients who have had rheumatic fever that they must guard against infections for the rest of their lives to avoid possible development of heart disease.

Evaluation

Rheumatic fever is treated over 10 days or so. The nurse should expect activity tolerance to improve once fever and pain are controlled. Altered nutrition may require more than 2 weeks to be improved, depending on the severity of anorexia and the fever.

Infective Endocarditis

Endocarditis is an inflammatory process of the endocardium, especially the valves. This disorder was once lethal, but morbidity and mortality have been greatly reduced with the use of antibiotics and advanced diagnostic procedures.

In the past, many different terms and classifications were used to describe infective endocarditis. The nurse may still see these terms used or find them in old medical records. Some are defined here.

Subacute bacterial endocarditis (SBE) develops gradually over several weeks or months and is usually caused by organisms of low virulence, such as *Streptococcus viridans,* which has a limited ability to infect other tissues.

Acute bacterial endocarditis develops over days or weeks with an erratic course and earlier development of complications. It is frequently caused by *Staphylococcus aureus,* which is capable of infecting other body tissues.

Native valve endocarditis is an infection of a previously normal or damaged valve.

Prosthetic valve endocarditis is an infection of a prosthetic valve.

Nonbacterial thrombotic endocarditis is caused by sterile thrombotic lesions (frequently aggregates of platelets), which may develop in people with malignancies or other chronic diseases.

Changes in the population at risk are currently altering the classic picture of endocarditis. The proportion of acute cases is rising. Five of every 1000 patients admitted to a hospital have endocarditis. Overall mortality is 20% to 30% and as high as 70% in the aged.[19] Fewer patients are developing the classic physical signs of advanced endocarditis, such as Osler's nodes, finger clubbing, or Roth's spots (see Fig. 47–3). The proportion of cases due to streptococci has fallen slightly. The proportion of cases caused by gram-negative bacilli, fungi, and other unusual microbes is increasing.

The changes are traced to several notable alterations in the population. The increase in the incidence of endocarditis caused by yeasts and fungi is attributable to the increased number of persons with valve prostheses, to the increased number of persons using intravenous (IV) drugs, and rising use of long-term antimicrobial therapy or immunosuppression.

The decrease in the incidence of rheumatic fever lowers the incidence of endocarditis, whereas the number of children surviving congenital heart disease raises the incidence of endocarditis. The growing elderly population also increases the number of endocarditis episodes.

Etiology and Risk Factors

Circulating microorganisms in the bloodstream attach to the endocardial surface and multiply. Usually the multiplication of these organisms requires a rough or abnormal endocardium. IV drug abusers may be injecting particulate matter into the bloodstream, with damage to the previously normal endocardium that allows the organism to adhere, thereby initiating acute bacterial endocarditis.

Defective heart valves causing changes in blood flow and pressures encourage the proliferation of vegetations. Open heart surgery to replace damaged valves increases the risk of endocarditis. Fortunately, coronary artery bypass grafting, one of the most frequently performed surgeries in the United States, carries a low risk of infective endocarditis. This is because the endocardium is not invaded during the operation.

Most people who develop endocarditis have a pre-existing heart condition, but some cases develop even though there is no known heart disease. Acquired valvular disease (especially mitral valve prolapse) and heart valve prostheses can lead to infective endocarditis. In some cases, endocarditis follows an invasive procedure, such as minor surgery, dental procedures, or insertion of renal shunts, urinary catheters, or long-term indwelling catheters (for dialysis, hemodynamic monitoring, or hyperalimentation).

Not unlike most disorders, identification of high-risk clients is the key to prevention. (See Risk Factors and Levels of Prevention for infective endocarditis).

Pathophysiology

Microorganisms are able to enter the bloodstream in many ways. Once the colonization process begins on the endothelium, replication occurs, and bacterial colonies form within layers of platelets and fibrin. As the colonies become entangled within the tight layers of fibrin and platelets, the colony becomes less and less vulnerable to the body's defense mechanisms. The bacteria stimulate the humoral immune system to produce nonspecific antibodies, but the bacteria are protected by the fibrin-platelet aggregation. It is not uncommon for these vegetations to form clots that travel to other organs, forming abscesses. The vegetations can severely damage heart valves by perforating and deforming the valve leaflets (Fig. 47–1).

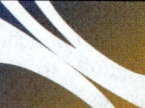

Infective Endocarditis

Risk Factors

Rheumatic heart disease, valve replacement, bacteremia, IV drug abuse, previous episode of endocarditis, prolonged indwelling intravenous catheters, cardiomyopathy, congenital heart disease, mitral valve prolapse, cardiomyopathy, immunocompromise, previous cardiac surgery.

Levels of Prevention

Primary Prevention

- Encourage adequate sanitation
- Decrease crowded housing

Secondary Prevention

- Educate concerning opportunities for infection in clients with preexisting heart conditions.
- Teach preventive strategies to clients with preexisting heart conditions.
- Use prophylactic antibiotics in high-risk clients (especially those with congenital heart defects, mitral valve prolapse, prosthetic heart valves, or a previous case of endocarditis).
- Prophylactic antibiotic therapy is used in conjunction with dental procedures; surgical procedures; and invasive procedures, such as insertion of renal shunts, urinary catheters, and intravenous catheters.
- Ensure that specific prophylactic regimen is easily accessible and well understood by clients at risk.

Tertiary Prevention

- Obtain blood cultures from all clients with fever and heart murmur.
- Adhere to antibiotic regimen.
- Antibiotic therapy is usually intravenous. This can be accomplished at home with in-depth teaching, careful supervision, and professional back-up.

Extensions of the bacteria may invade the aorta or pericardium. The amount of damage depends on the type and virulence of the organisms causing the infection.

There are many possible complications. Heart failure may develop due to structural valvular damage. Arterial emboli can occur from the vegetation. Systemic embolization occurs in 30% of clients with left-sided infective endocarditis. Locations and manifestations of these emboli are shown in Figure 47–2. Common infarction sites are the kidney, spleen, and brain. Pulmonary embolus is associated with right-sided infective endocarditis. Emboli can also travel to the brain and produce a myriad of symptoms. Occasionally, a client will develop immune complex glomerulonephritis. Renal function will usually return to normal after the infection has been controlled.

Clinical Manifestations and Diagnostic Findings

Clinical manifestations of infective endocarditis vary according to its acute or subacute nature, but many manifestations are common to all types. Clinical manifestations can be divided into three groups:

1. Evidence of systemic infection includes fever, chills, sweats, malaise, weakness, anorexia, weight loss, backache, and splenomegaly.
2. Evidence of an intravascular lesion includes dyspnea, chest pain, murmurs, cold and painful extremities, petechiae, Roth's spots, Osler's nodes, splinter hemorrhages, and stroke.
3. Evidence of an immunologic reaction to infection includes arthralgia, proteinuria, hematuria, casts, and acidosis.[60]

General malaise, fatigue, weakness, and anorexia are common. Headaches and musculoskeletal complaints are frequent. Clients with infective endocarditis often feel as if they have the flu.

In the acute type of infective endocarditis, the clinical manifestations occur more quickly and are more severe. Clients appear very ill. Fever, chills, and prostration are so severe that admission to a hospital usually occurs within a few days.

Cardiac failure may develop suddenly in either acute or subacute endocarditis. Mechanical complications include perforation of a valve leaflet, rupture of one of the chordae tendineae, or development of a functional stenosis from obstruction of blood flow by large vegetations. Myocardial infarction may develop as a result of coronary artery embolism.

Unusual findings may be present on physical examination, including splinter hemorrhages, Osler's nodes, finger

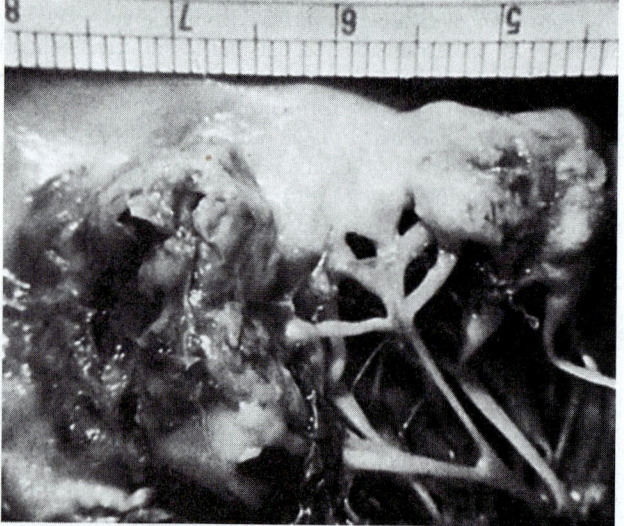

Figure 47–1. Vegetations of the heart valves resulting from infective endocarditis. This client had large vegetations on the leaflets of the mitral valve. (From Braunwald, E. [1992]. *Heart disease: A textbook of cardiovascular medicine* [4th ed.]. Philadelphia: W. B. Saunders.)

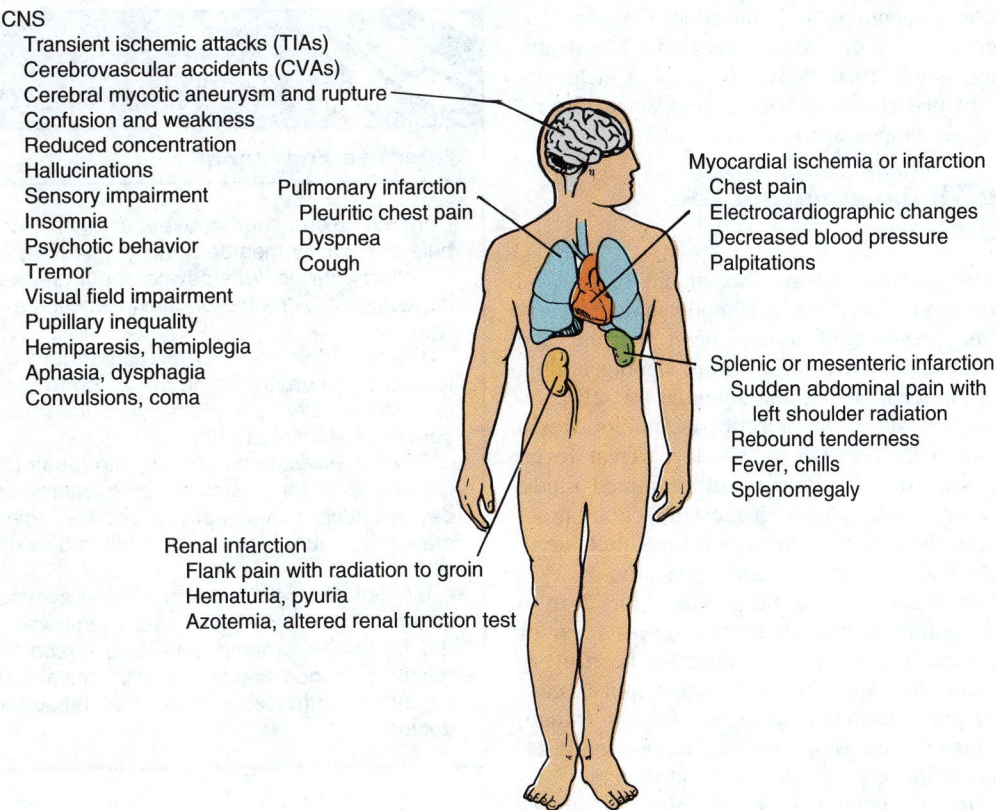

CNS
Transient ischemic attacks (TIAs)
Cerebrovascular accidents (CVAs)
Cerebral mycotic aneurysm and rupture
Confusion and weakness
Reduced concentration
Hallucinations
Sensory impairment
Insomnia
Psychotic behavior
Tremor
Visual field impairment
Pupillary inequality
Hemiparesis, hemiplegia
Aphasia, dysphagia
Convulsions, coma

Pulmonary infarction
Pleuritic chest pain
Dyspnea
Cough

Myocardial ischemia or infarction
Chest pain
Electrocardiographic changes
Decreased blood pressure
Palpitations

Splenic or mesenteric infarction
Sudden abdominal pain with
left shoulder radiation
Rebound tenderness
Fever, chills
Splenomegaly

Renal infarction
Flank pain with radiation to groin
Hematuria, pyuria
Azotemia, altered renal function test

Figure 47–2. Locations and clinical manifestations of the emboli associated with infective endocarditis. (Data from Guzzetta, C., & Dossey, B. [1984]. *Cardiovascular nursing: Bodymind tapestry.* St. Louis: Mosby–Year Book.)

clubbing, Janeway's lesions, ocular signs, and splenomegaly.

Splinter hemorrhages are caused by microembolization and are characterized by linear subungual hemorrhages that look like tiny splinters under the nail.

Osler's nodes are painful, erythematous, pea-sized nodules in the skin of the extremities, usually on the finger tips. They are due to inflammation around a small, infected embolus.

Finger clubbing is found less frequently now but is common in long-standing infective endocarditis. The pathogenesis remains unclear.

Janeway's lesions are flat, small, nontender red spots on the palms of the hands and the soles of the feet.

Ocular signs are sometimes present, including the following:

● Conjunctival petechiae—small, bright-red hemorrhages that are easily seen if the eyelids are everted
● Roth's spots, visualized by funduscopic examination as a white or yellow center surrounded by a bright-red, irregular halo
● Loss of vision, which can occur during the course of endocarditis from embolization to the brain or to the retinal artery

Splenomegaly is an enlarged spleen that is soft and may or may not be tender.

Blood cultures for bacteria, fungus, and yeast are the most important diagnostic tests. ECG, complete blood count, and other routine diagnostic procedures are helpful.

Because the clinical manifestations of endocarditis are numerous and often nonspecific, several modalities are employed for differential medical diagnosis. Blood cultures should be obtained for all clients with both fever and heart murmur. ECGs should be done on admission to the hospital and repeated during the hospital stay. Although a negative ECG does not rule out endocarditis, transesophageal echocardiography can be useful in diagnosis. Chest x-ray is useful for determining early heart failure.

 Acute and Subacute Care

■ Medical Management

The chief aims of management are to eradicate the infecting organism and to treat complications. Antimicrobial therapy has changed this disorder from one that was almost always fatal to one that is rarely fatal. The choice of antibiotic depends on the organism involved. Penicillin and streptomycin are commonly used. Therapy is usually continued IV for 4 to 6 weeks. This is usually begun in the hospital but is occasionally continued at home with extensive discharge planning and education. Occasionally, after the infection is under control (negative blood cultures, no fever, and normal WBC count) it is necessary for the client to undergo heart valve replacement for reversal of newly developed heart failure.

■ Nursing Management of the Medical Client

In infective endocarditis, nursing assessment focuses on gathering data about the client's hemodynamic stability (particularly the presence of a new heart murmur and embolic complications), level of comfort, coping ability, support from significant others, and potential for self-care.

Administer antibiotics IV as prescribed. Antibiotics will relieve most discomfort within a few days. Treat fever, when present, with rest, cooling measures, forced fluids, and sometimes salicylates. As with most infectious processes, encourage the client to eat a nutritious diet, drink sufficient fluids, and rest mentally and physically.

The client may need to be hospitalized for 2 to 6 weeks. Do not enforce complete bedrest unless fever or signs of heart damage develop. Auscultate the heart every 8 hours for heart murmurs. Assess for rapid pulse, easy fatigability, dyspnea, restlessness, signs of heart failure, and embolic manifestations. Document these manifestations if they occur and report them to the physician.

When the client's condition improves, plan and implement a progressive activity schedule. As activity increases, monitor the client's physical response to exercise. For example, assess blood pressure, heart rate, diaphoresis, vertigo, and weakness.

Prior to discharge, educate the client and family about:

- The cause of infectious endocarditis
- The purpose of long-term antibiotic administration and the need to comply with the entire course of therapy
- The need for prophylactic antibiotics when undergoing dental procedures and surgical interventions or instrumentation
- The importance of ongoing assessments to determine the efficacy of treatment and to identify the early signs of complications (see the Client Education Guide for infective endocarditis)

Community and Self-Care

The trend toward early hospital discharge has changed the course of treatment for those clients with infective endocarditis. IV therapy may now be routinely done in the home. Clients who are alert, cooperative, and reasonably stable and who want to return home may be allowed to do so. Typically, the nurse, pharmacist, and physician teach the techniques of self-administered IV antibiotics. Before discharge, the client must demonstrate the knowledge and technique required for antibiotic administration. The physician's office or home healthcare nurses often monitor the client's progress.

Home IV antibiotic therapy offers many benefits. It is less costly, motivates clients to become active participants

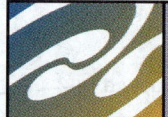

CLIENT EDUCATION GUIDE

Infective Endocarditis

Continue taking your intravenous antibiotics with the help of a family member after you leave the hospital.

Follow your doctor's advice about gradually resuming activities. A month of convalescence at home is typical.

Tell your doctor and dentist about having had infective endocarditis. If you are going to have surgery or extensive dental work, be sure you take a full course of antibiotics first.

Floss every day, and brush with a soft toothbrush. Consult your dentist before using water-jet cleaning devices such as a Water Pik, because these devices may cause gum bleeding and put you at risk of infection.

Monitor yourself for the signs and symptoms of infective endocarditis. Take your temperature every day for the next month; and keep a record of your readings. Report any fever, chills, malaise, loss of appetite, weight loss, or increased fatigue to your doctor.

in their own care, reestablishes a more normal life-style, and promotes a sense of control that aids in psychosocial and physiologic recovery. To be effective, this program requires exceptional communication and cooperation between healthcare team members and the client.[44]

Myocarditis

Myocarditis is an inflammation of the myocardial wall. It can be caused by almost any bacterial, viral, or parasitic organism, as well as by radiation, toxic agents such as lead, and drugs such as lithium and cocaine. Myocarditis affects people of all ages and may be acute or chronic. An immunodeficient person is at greater risk of myocarditis. Frequently, the inflammation is not limited to the myocardium but extends to the pericardium, with production of an associated pericarditis. The incidence of myocarditis is not possible to ascertain. The incidence varies with the age of clients and various etiologic agents.

In the United States, most cases of myocarditis are due to viral infections. Viruses associated with this disorder include coxsackieviruses A and B, mumps, influenza virus serotypes A and B, rubella virus, measles virus, adenoviruses, echoviruses, cytomegalovirus, and Epstein-Barr virus. Other causes of myocarditis include the following:

- Bacterial infections: diphtheria, typhoid fever, staphylococcal, pneumococcal, tetanus, and tuberculosis
- Hypersensitive immune reactions: acute rheumatic fever and postcardiotomy syndrome
- Toxins and chemicals: alcohol

- Radiation: large doses of radiation therapy to the chest for the treatment of malignancy
- Parasitic infections: Chagas' disease and toxoplasmosis

Myocardial damage from acute myocarditis is usually the result of the direct invasion or the toxic effects of the microorganism in cardiac myocytes. This can cause an alteration in cellular energy systems and cellular damage. The virus is only rarely isolated from human hearts in acute myocarditis; even in the laboratory during experimental infections, it is never isolated after 3 weeks. This does not prevent the infection from becoming subacute or chronic or from causing dilated cardiomyopathy.[105] Usually myocarditis involves both ventricles. If there is impairment of myocardial contractility, there may be an elevation of ventricular diastolic pressures and volumes in order to maintain stroke volume. Disruptions leading to cardiac dysrhythmias can decrease cardiac output.

Complications that may develop from myocarditis include heart failure, dilated cardiomyopathy, and sudden death from lethal arrhythmias or rupture of a myocardial aneurysm.

Myocarditis displays a wide variation in clinical manifestations. There may be no clinical manifestations at all. The health history may reveal a recent upper respiratory infection, a viral pharyngitis, or tonsillitis. The most frequent symptoms, however, are fatigue, dyspnea, palpitations, and chest pain. The client often experiences chest pain as a mild continuous pressure or soreness in the chest. Thus, the chest pain of myocarditis can be distinguished from the effort-induced pain of angina pectoris. Tachycardia, if present, may be disproportionate to the degree of fever, exertion, or illness. Dysrhythmias can also occur, sometimes producing a fatal circulatory collapse. There may be a pericardial friction rub if the client has pericarditis.

In most cases, myocarditis is self-limiting and uncomplicated. If myocardial involvement becomes extensive or prolonged, myofibril degeneration can produce heart failure, with pulmonary congestion, dyspnea, neck vein distention, peripheral edema, and cardiomegaly. Recurrent myocarditis can produce cardiomyopathy.

The chest x-ray may show an enlarged cardiac silhouette due to ventricular enlargement or pericardial effusion. Blood tests may show a moderate leukocytosis and elevated cardiac enzymes. Echocardiography is helpful in determining heart chamber size and ventricular functioning. Gallium scan shows regional wall abnormalities, dilated ventricles, and hypokinesis of the left ventricle.

ECG abnormalities and elevated serum levels of cardiac enzymes are helpful to the physician diagnosing this illness. The ECG may show a bundle branch block or complete AV heart block, ST segment elevation, or T wave flattening.

An endomyocardial biopsy may be done during the acute phase of the illness to help with the diagnosis.

Clients with acute myocarditis are usually admitted to the hospital for observation. Clients with pericardial effusion, dysrhythmias, heart failure, or hypotension are usually admitted to the intensive care unit (ICU). Medical management begins with specific therapy for the underlying infection. Bedrest is suggested to decrease cardiac work. Supplemental oxygen may be prescribed for clients with low cardiac output or dysrhythmias. Immunosuppressive therapy is currently being investigated; initial reports are favorable in the treatment of myocarditis.[100] Antipyretic agents are helpful for the fever and the hemodynamic effects of fever that increase myocardial work. Clients who remain at home may use Holter monitoring of the heart. This provides continuous surveillance of the client's heart rhythm.

The outlook for clients with myocarditis is generally good. Most patients recover rapidly. Some have recurrent or chronic myocarditis, and some become very ill and die.

Nursing management for the client experiencing myocarditis is essentially the same as that provided to clients with infective endocarditis and rheumatic fever. Review those sections within this chapter.

Teaching begins when acute manifestations have subsided and the client has demonstrated physical and emotional readiness. Teach clients with myocarditis how to monitor their pulse rate and rhythm. Instruct them to immediately report any sudden changes in heart rate, rhythm, or palpitations. Encourage family members to take CPR training. They can obtain this training from groups such as the local fire department, the American Red Cross, or the American Heart Association. Educating family members about CPR can enhance their sense of preparedness for an emergency.

Because the myocardial infectious process resolves slowly and late complications can occur, advise clients to continue self-monitoring and to schedule clinical follow-up appointments, even after apparent recovery.

The potential of lethal arrhythmias may frighten the client and significant others. The client who is experiencing extreme anxiety, fear, and ineffective coping may manifest insomnia, tearfulness, somatic complaints, inability to problem-solve, and agitation. Determine with the client (and family) the specific focus of anxiety. Clarify any misconceptions that arise. Speak slowly and calmly and focus on the present situation, giving feedback about current reality. Encourage the use of relaxation techniques to help allay stress. Schedule activities around periods of undisturbed sleep.

Pericarditis

Pericarditis may be either acute or chronic (recurrent). It is not known why pericarditis may be an acute illness in some clients and recurrent in others. Chronic pericarditis is usually called constrictive pericarditis. Constrictive pericarditis is present when a fibrotic, thickened, and adherent pericardium restricts diastolic filling of the heart.[15] This eventually results in cardiac failure.

Acute Pericarditis

Acute pericarditis is a syndrome that is caused by inflammation of the parietal and visceral pericardium. This inflammatory process may develop either as a primary condition or secondary to a number of diseases and circumstances (Box 47–2).

Box 47–2. Causes of Pericarditis

Infections
    Viral: coxsackie, influenza
    Bacterial: tuberculosis, staphylococcus, streptococcus,
        meningococcus, pneumococcus
    Parasitic
    Fungal
Myocardial injury
    Myocardial infarction (Dressler's syndrome)
    Cardiac trauma: blunt or penetrating
    Post cardiac surgery
    Hypersensitivity
Collagen diseases: rheumatic fever, scleroderma, systemic
    lupus erythematosus, rheumatoid arthritis
Drug reaction: procainamide, methysergide, hydralazine
Radiation therapy
Cobalt therapy
Metabolic disorders
    Uremia
    Myxedema
Chronic anemia
Neoplasm: lymphoma
Aortic dissection

Acute pericarditis may be either dry (fibrinous) or exudative. The exudate that is present with acute pericarditis may be serous, purulent, or hemorrhagic. This exudate can accumulate in the pericardial sac, causing cardiac tamponade that restricts cardiac filling and emptying. Without prompt treatment, shock and death can result from decreased cardiac output.

Dry pericarditis can follow a common viral infection, myocardial infarction, tuberculosis, bacteremia, or renal failure. Delicate adhesions form within the pericardial space along with serous fibrin deposition, hemorrhage, and calcification. Adhesions may eventually obliterate the pericardial sac. Inflammation of the pericardium frequently penetrates the myocardium to some degree, which produces myopericarditis.

The characteristic subjective clinical manifestation of pericarditis is chest pain. The nature of this pain varies with the client. Sometimes the pain is similar to the pain of myocardial infarction; at other times, it mimics the pain of pleurisy. The pain is exacerbated with respiration and rotating the trunk but usually does not radiate to the arms. Sitting up frequently relieves the pain.

Pericardial friction rub is a classic objective manifestation of acute pericarditis. The rub is produced by inflamed, roughened pericardial layers that create friction as their surfaces rub together during heart movement. Auscultation over the precordium reveals a scratchy, leathery, or creaky sound that is heard anywhere over the precordium but most frequently at the third intercostal space left of the sternal border. The rub is best heard with the diaphragm of the stethoscope and with the client holding his or her breath. In some clients, it is best heard with the client sitting up. Pericardial friction rubs vary with intensity from hour to hour and from day to day.

Fever is another common finding in pericarditis. The client's temperature may rise to 39.4° C (103° F). Chills, malaise, joint pain, anorexia, nausea, and weight loss accompany the fever. Dyspnea and chest pain can potentiate anxiety. An increase in heart rate usually corresponds to the degree of fever and anxiety.

Chest x-ray studies help little in detecting acute pericarditis. ECG changes provide more distinctive evidence of the underlying inflammatory process. The rhythm may be bradycardic or show atrial fibrillation. The ECG frequently shows a decrease in the amplitude of the QRS complex and changes in the ST segment elevation and the T wave.[68]

Laboratory studies show an elevated erythrocyte sedimentation rate and may show an elevated WBC count. Cardiac enzymes are usually normal but may be elevated.

When the cause of acute pericarditis is known, treatment of the cause is indicated. If no causal agent is known, symptomatic intervention for acute dry pericarditis is provided. Pain and fever, usually self-limited, may be eased by aspirin given in maximally tolerated doses. The physician may prescribe a nonsteroidal anti-inflammatory agent. Stronger analgesia, such as morphine sulfate, may be necessary if chest pain becomes severe.

If acute pericarditis is present after the client has suffered a myocardial infarction, it is important to reassure the client that the pain experienced with pericarditis is not to be associated with another infarction. If the client becomes anxious, thinking that this pain is the pain of another infarction, oxygen demand increases and myocardial ischemia may develop.

The focus of nursing care related to pericarditis is the same as that described for the other inflammatory cardiac diseases discussed in this chapter. Nursing assessment of the client with pericarditis also includes scrutiny for the presence of pericardial tamponade (pulsus paradoxus, distended neck veins). Vigilance is necessary. Provide reassurance concerning the temporary nature of the disease.

Acute Pericarditis with Effusion

Acute pericarditis with effusion results when fluid accumulates within the pericardial sac. Rapid or excessive fluid accumulations may compress the heart and reduce ventricular filling and cardiac output. When fluid accumulates slowly, the fibrous pericardium is better able to stretch and accommodate its presence. One to 2 L of fluid can be tolerated without increase in intrapericardial pressure if accumulation is slow. However, the normal unstretched pericardial sac can accommodate the rapid addition of only 80 to 200 ml of fluid without decrease in cardiac output.

Pericardial effusion may be asymptomatic. If dry pericarditis precedes the condition, the friction rub will often disappear. Fever may develop. Heart sounds may be muffled because the pericardial fluid further separates the stethoscope and the heart chambers.

Pulsus paradoxus can be present. If the client has normal breathing and a systolic difference of greater than 10 mm Hg, evaluation for cardiac compression and possibly cardiac tamponade should be done.[74]

Echocardiography is the most accurate technique for evaluating pericardial effusion. The test is sensitive enough to detect as little as 20 ml of pericardial fluid.[4,68] Pericardiocentesis is not indicated unless there is evidence of cardiac compression caused by cardiac tamponade.[4,68] (See the next section.)

Care of the client with pericardial effusion is similar to the plan of intervention for dry pericarditis. Bedrest, analgesia, and proper positioning can help alleviate symptoms. Psychological support is very important.

Chronic Constrictive Pericarditis

Chronic constrictive pericarditis is a chronic inflammatory condition in which the pericardium changes into a thick, fibrous band of tissue. This tissue encircles, encases, and compresses the heart, preventing proper ventricular filling and emptying. Cardiac failure eventually results from this slow compression.

Chronic constrictive pericarditis usually begins with an episode of acute pericarditis characterized by fibrin deposition, often with pericardial effusion. In the majority of cases, the visceral and parietal layers become completely fused. Constrictive pericarditis is usually symmetrical scarring that causes uniform constriction of all heart chambers. The heavily fibrosed pericardium restricts diastolic filling in all chambers and decreases systolic ejection.

Clinical manifestations include right ventricular failure first, and decreased cardiac output that is manifested by fatigue on exertion, dyspnea, leg edema, ascites, low pulse pressure, distended neck veins, and delayed capillary refill time.

Constrictive pericarditis is a progressive disease without spontaneous reversal of symptoms. A minority of clients survive for many years with minor symptoms. The majority of clients become progressively more disabled over time. Treatment is both surgical and medical. Medical treatment includes digitalis, diuretics, and sodium restriction to relieve manifestations of right ventricular failure. Surgical intervention involves the excision of the damaged pericardium (pericardiectomy) and should be performed early in the course of the disease.[4,68]

Cardiac Tamponade

Cardiac tamponade is a life-threatening complication due to accumulation of fluid in the pericardium. This fluid can be blood, pus, or air in the pericardial sac that accumulates fast enough and in sufficient quantity to compress the heart and restrict blood flow in and out of the ventricles. *This is a cardiac emergency!* Large or rapidly accumulating effusions raise the intrapericardial pressure to a point at which venous blood cannot flow into the heart, which decreases ventricular filling. As a result, venous pressure rises, and cardiac output and arterial blood pressure fall. A narrowing pulse pressure signals cardiac tamponade. The heart attempts to compensate by beating rapidly (tachycardia). Tachycardia cannot sustain cardiac output for very long. Prompt intervention is necessary to prevent shock and death.

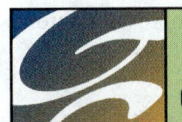

CRITICAL MONITORING

Cardiac Tamponade

Report the following manifestations of cardiac tamponade immediately!

Elevated venous pressure (increased central venous pressure)
Distended neck veins
Kussmaul's sign (distended neck veins on inspiration)
Hypotension
Narrowed pulse pressure
Tachycardia
Dyspnea
Restlessness, anxiety
Cyanosis of lips and nails
Diaphoresis
Muffled heart sounds
Pulsus paradoxus
Decreased friction rub
Decreased QRS voltage and electrical alternans

In cardiac tamponade, assessment reveals hypotension, tachycardia, jugular venous distention, cyanosis of lips and nails, dyspnea, muffled heart sounds, diaphoresis, and paradoxical pulse. The client may be comfortable and quiet one minute and then very restless with a feeling of impending doom the next minute. Clients may panic when fluid accumulates rapidly. Slowly developing tamponade has manifestations resembling those of heart failure: nonspecific ECG changes, decreased voltage, and visualization of fluid in the pericardial sac on echocardiogram (see the Critical Monitoring feature).

Cardiac tamponade requires immediate intervention. The emergency intervention of choice is pericardiocentesis, which involves aspirating the fluid or air from the pericardial sac (Fig. 47–3). This emergency procedure

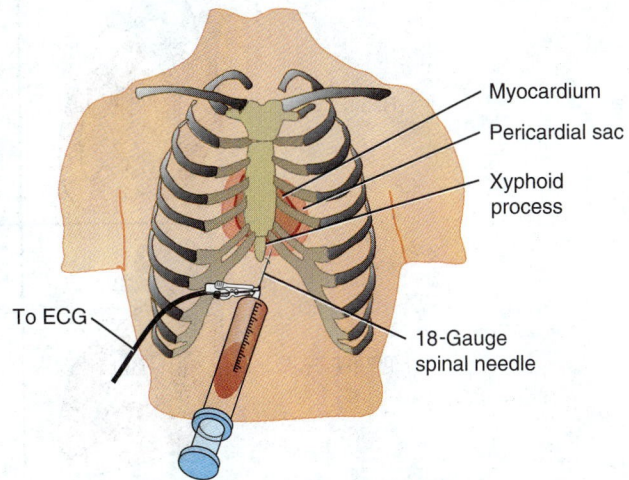

Figure 47–3. Pericardiocentesis.

relieves pressure on the heart, thereby improving cardiac function and perhaps saving the client's life.

Cardiomyopathy and Valvular Disease

Cardiomyopathies are acquired disorders in which disease of the cardiac muscle fibers reduces myocardial contractility or distensibility. Valvular disorders may be either congenital or acquired.

Cardiomyopathy

Cardiomyopathy is a heart muscle disorder of unknown cause (idiopathic). The dominant feature of cardiomyopathy is the involvement of the heart muscle itself. The definition excludes structural and functional abnormalities due to valvular disorders, coronary artery disease, and systemic and pulmonary vascular disorders.[104] Idiopathic cardiomyopathies can be classified according to the ventricular changes they cause (Fig. 47–4).

Four conditions seem to lower the threshold for the development of cardiomyopathy: (1) chronic ingestion of excessive alcohol, (2) pregnancy, (3) systemic hypertension, and (4) a variety of infections. Health promotion for cardiomyopathy is shown in Risk Factors and Levels of Prevention: Cardiomyopathy.

The three major classes of cardiomyopathy are:

1. Dilated (congestive) cardiomyopathy
2. Hypertrophic cardiomyopathy (also called hypertrophic subaortic stenosis)
3. Restrictive cardiomyopathy

Table 47–2 compares diagnostic data for the three types of idiopathic cardiomyopathy. We will examine the forms of cardiomyopathy separately.

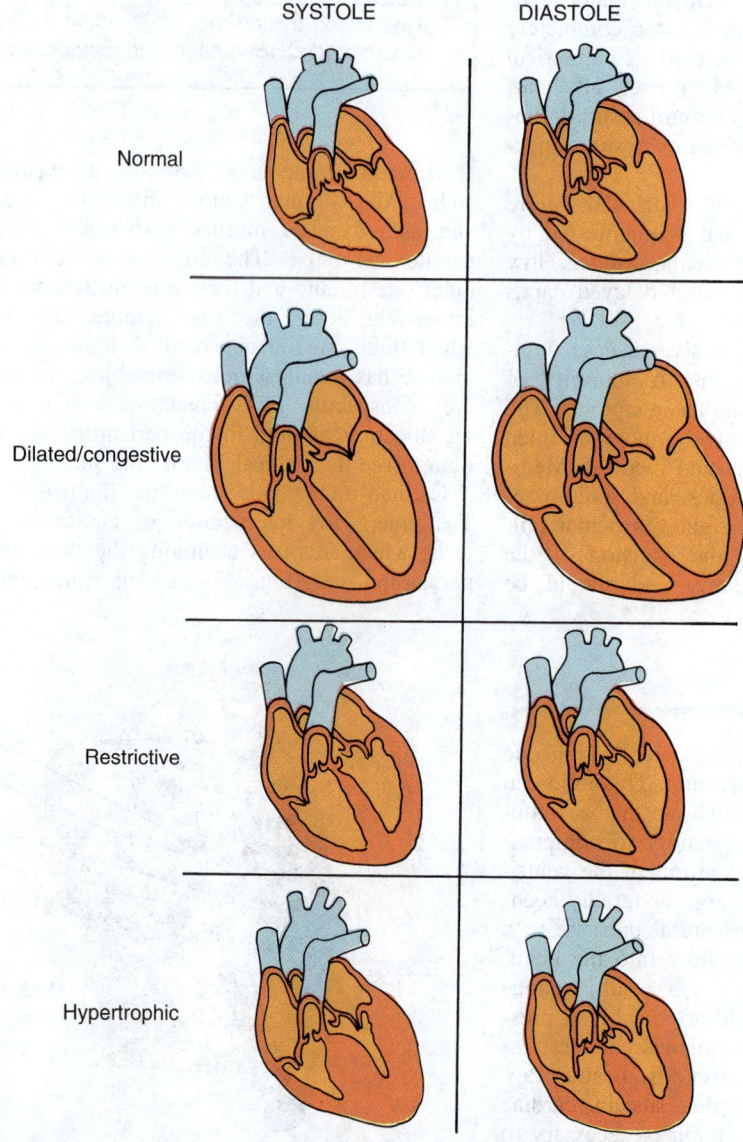

SYSTOLE   DIASTOLE

Normal

Dilated/congestive

Restrictive

Hypertrophic

Figure 47–4. The four types of cardiomyopathy.

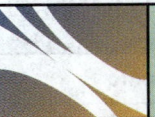

RISK FACTORS AND LEVELS OF PREVENTION

Cardiomyopathy

Risk Factors

The cause of cardiomyopathy is unknown, but it has been associated with the following conditions: cardiac ischemia, viral infections, alcohol intake, drug abuse, pregnancy, genetic predisposition, amyloidosis, and sarcoidosis.

Levels of Prevention

Primary Prevention

- Advise clients to reduce alcohol consumption. Chronic ingestion of excessive alcohol increases the risk of cardiomyopathy.
- Prevent infectious processes. Infections can lower the threshold for the development of cardiomyopathy.
- Monitor for systemic hypertension. Hypertension can increase the risk of cardiomyopathy.
- Monitor women during pregnancy. Pregnancy increases the risk for cardiomyopathy.

Secondary Prevention

- Monitor for early signs of congestive heart failure.
- Evaluate clients with dysrhythmias for cardiomyopathy.

Tertiary Prevention

- Carefully adhere to specific drug protocols. Because treatment may be less than satisfactory, multiple cardiac drugs may be used. This increases the risk of side effects.
- Consider heart transplant. Some clients with cardiomyopathy are candidates for transplantation.
- Evaluate for anticoagulation therapy to decrease risk of systemic embolism.

Dilated Cardiomyopathy

Dilated cardiomyopathy is a syndrome characterized by cardiac enlargement. The first abnormality noted is ventricular enlargement followed by ventricular contractile dysfunction. This eventually leads to heart failure. Many clients with idiopathic dilated cardiomyopathy die within 5 years after the onset of manifestations.[105]

Etiology and Risk Factors

The cause of idiopathic dilated cardiomyopathy is not known. Dilated cardiomyopathy associated with pregnancy can disappear. There may be spontaneous rapid improvement in some women and early fatality in others.

Pathophysiology

Whatever the cause of dilated cardiomyopathy, it results in a diffuse degeneration of myocardial fibers, with a decrease in contractile function. There is enlargement and dilation of all four chambers. Left ventricular filling pressures are generally elevated because of poor contractile function.

Clinical Manifestations and Diagnostic Findings

Clinical manifestations usually develop gradually in clients with congestive cardiomyopathy. Fatigue and weakness are common. Chest pain may be present and may be associated with ischemic heart disease. Right-sided heart failure is a late and ominous sign.

Systemic blood pressure is usually normal or low. Heart failure develops steadily and is seen as dyspnea, orthopnea, tachycardia, palpitations, peripheral edema, enlarged jugular veins and liver engorgement. An S_4 gallop often precedes the development of congestive heart failure, and an S_3 gallop generally occurs with heart failure. If the heart rate is rapid, both S_4 and S_3 may fuse to form a summation gallop sound. There may be a systolic murmur of mitral or tricuspid insufficiency, because ventricular dilation prevents sufficient closure of those valves. Gallop sounds and regurgitant murmurs may be intensified by an isometric handgrip exercise because of the increase it causes on systemic vascular resistance. Pulmonary crackles become audible as failure progresses.

Diagnostic tests, including ECG, cardiac biopsy, echocardiography, chest radiography, and blood chemistries, are useful for diagnosis. ECG findings include sinus tachycardia, ventricular dysrhythmias, ST segment changes, and left bundle branch block.

Management

Because the cause of idiopathic dilated cardiomyopathy is not known, there is no specific therapy. Treatment is similar to that for heart failure. Intervention focuses on enhancing myocardial contractility and unloading the heart. Digitalis preparations, angiotensin converting enzyme (ACE) inhibitors, vasodilators, diuretics, and sodium-restricted diets provide the major means for achieving these objectives. Antiarrhythmic agents may help suppress ventricular irritability. In appropriate candidates, the implantation of the automatic internal cardiac defibrillator may be used to prevent sudden cardiac death.[105] (See Chapter 46.)

The combined problem of ventricular dilation and ineffective myocardial contractility also increases the risk of pooled blood within the heart and subsequent clot formation. Anticoagulants may help prevent clots and emboli.

Rest improves cardiac function and reduces heart size. Most clients experience severe activity intolerance during the later stages of the disease, which automatically limits their activities. However, during the earlier stages of the disease, most clients find it difficult to accept rigidly imposed restrictions on activity. Clients should avoid

Table 47–2. Diagnostic Data for the Three Types of Cardiomyopathy

	Dilated	Restrictive	Hypertrophic
Symptoms	Heart failure, particularly left-sided Fatigue and weakness Systemic or pulmonary emboli	Dyspnea, fatigue Right-sided heart failure Signs and symptoms of systemic disease: amyloidosis, iron storage disease, etc.	Dyspnea, angina pectoris Fatigue, syncope, palpitations
Physical examination	Moderate to severe cardiomegaly: S_3 and S_4 Atrioventricular valve regurgitation, especially mitral	Mild to moderate cardiomegaly: S_3 or S_4 Atrioventricular valve regurgitation; inspiratory increase in venous pressure (Kussmaul's sign)	Mild cardiomegaly Apical systolic thrill and heave; brisk carotid upstroke S_4 common Systolic murmur that increases with Valsalva's maneuver
Chest radiograph	Moderate-to-marked cardiac enlargement, especially left ventricular Pulmonary venous hypertension	Mild cardiac enlargement Pulmonary venous hypertension	Mild-to-moderate cardiac enlargement Left atrial enlargement
Electrocardiogram	Sinus tachycardia Atrial and ventricular arrhythmias ST segment and T wave abnormalities Intraventricular conduction defects	Low voltage Intraventricular conduction defects Atrioventricular conduction defects	Left ventricular hypertrophy ST segment and T wave abnormalities Abnormal Q waves Atrial and ventricular arrhythmias
Echocardiogram	Left ventricular dilation and dysfunction Abnormal diastolic mitral valve motion secondary to abnormal compliance and filling pressures	Increased left ventricular wall thickness and mass Small or normal-sized left ventricular cavity Normal systolic function Pericardial effusion	Asymmetrical septal hypertrophy Narrow left ventricular outlfow tract Systolic anterior motion of the mitral valve Small or normal-sized left ventricle
Radionuclide studies	Left ventricular dilation and dysfunction (RVG)	Infiltration of myocardium (thallium 201 scan) Small or normal-sized left ventricle (RVG) Normal systolic function (RVG)	Small or normal-sized left ventricle (RVG) Vigorous systolic function (RVG) Asymmetrical septal hypertrophy (RVG ^{201}Tl scan)
Cardiac catheterization	Left ventricular enlargement and dysfunction Mitral/tricuspid regurgitation Elevated left- and often right-sided filling pressures Diminished cardiac output	Diminished left ventricular compliance Square root sign in ventricular pressure recordings Preserved systolic function Elevated left- and right-sided filling pressures	Diminished left ventricular compliance Mitral regurgitation Vigorous systolic function Dynamic left ventricular outflow gradient

RVG, Radionuclide ventriculogram.
From Braunwald, E. (1992). *Heart disease: A textbook of cardiovascular medicine* (4th ed.). Philadelphia: W. B. Saunders.

poorly tolerated activities. Advise clients that physical and emotional stress exacerbate the disease. Because alcohol depresses myocardial contractility, the client should abstain from drinking alcoholic beverages.

Only transplantation and specific vasodilator therapy (hydralazine plus nitrates) have prolonged life.[105] Heart transplantation shows a 1-year survival rate of over 80% and a 3-year survival of 70% in appropriate clients. The 1-year survival in nontransplanted clients is 5%.[98, 99]

Hypertrophic Cardiomyopathy

Hypertrophic cardiomyopathy is disproportionate thickening of the interventricular septum, compared with the free wall of the ventricle. The overgrowth of the wall leads to rigidity in the wall and thereby increases resistance to blood flow from the left atrium. There is also obstruction of left ventricular outflow.

Although this disease is also known as idiopathic hypertrophic subaortic stenosis, many clients do not have the obstructive or stenotic component of the disease. Therefore, it is more accurate to use the term *hypertrophic cardiomyopathy* to describe this disease.

Etiology and Risk Factors

Hypertrophic cardiomyopathy appears to be a genetically transmitted disease of the heart muscle, but its cause remains a mystery. It appears most often in young adults, both men and women.

The predominant feature of hypertrophic cardiomyopathy involves unexplained myocardial hypertrophy, which typically appears with disproportionate thickening of the interventricular septum. The term *asymmetrical septal hypertrophy* is sometimes used to describe the disorder.

Pathophysiology

In its severest form, the left ventricular wall reaches tremendous dimensions and encroaches on the left ventricular chamber, which becomes small and elongated. Septal hypertrophy may obstruct the left ventricular outflow tract during systole. Frequently, there is diastolic dysfunction in the form of stiffness of the left ventricle during diastolic filling. This stiffness raises left ventricular end-diastolic pressure, which eventually results in elevation of left atrial, pulmonary venous, and pulmonary capillary pressures.

Clinical Manifestations and Diagnostic Findings

Clients with hypertrophic cardiomyopathy most commonly present with clinical manifestations in late adolescence or early adulthood, but symptoms may appear at any age. Many clients with hypertrophic cardiomyopathy are asymptomatic and can lead long lives. Interestingly, they often have relatives with incapacitating manifestations of the disease. Sadly, sudden death is frequently the first clinical manifestation of the disease in asymptomatic clients. Sudden death appears more often in younger clients and, if the presence of the disease is known, may be avoided by eliminating strenuous exercise.

The most common manifestation of the disease is dyspnea. Dyspnea is due to the high pulmonary pressures produced by the elevated left ventricular end-diastolic pressure. Angina pectoris, fatigue, and syncope are also common clinical manifestations. Cardiac dysrhythmias are frequently present. Palpitations, paroxysmal nocturnal dyspnea, and frank heart failure are less common. Many clients complain of dizzy spells. Exertion tends to worsen most symptoms.

Physical examination may be normal in asymptomatic clients. The appearance of a fourth heart sound may be the only sign of the disease. An increase in the intensity of the heart murmur usually suggests progression of the condition. ECG, chest film, echocardiogram, and radionuclide scanning are very useful in diagnosing hypertrophic cardiomyopathy.

Management

The goals of intervention are to reduce ventricular contractility and to relieve left ventricular outflow obstruction. Beta-adrenergic blocking agents, such as propranolol, provide the mainstay of medical intervention for hypertrophic cardiomyopathy. These medications reduce myocardial contractility. With decreased vigor of ventricular contraction, outflow obstruction diminishes. Beta-ad-

renergic blockade also reduces heart rate (which further reduces myocardial workload) and prevents arrhythmias. Calcium channel blocking agents such as verapamil are also used to relieve clinical manifestations and improve exercise tolerance.

Restrictive Cardiomyopathy

Restrictive cardiomyopathy is the least common form of cardiomyopathy. This form is characterized by excessively rigid ventricular walls. The rigid walls impair filling during diastole; however, contractility with systole is usually normal.

Etiology and Risk Factors

Any infiltrative process of the heart that results in fibrosis and thickening can cause restrictive cardiomyopathy. The most frequently associated disease is amyloidosis (deposition of eosinophilic fibrous protein in the heart). Other disorders include glycogen storage disease, hemochromatosis, and sarcoidosis.

Pathophysiology

In restrictive cardiomyopathy, the ventricular walls are excessively rigid and impede ventricular filling. Myocardial contractility is usually unaffected. Fibrotic infiltrations into the myocardium, endocardium, and subendocardium cause the ventricles to lose their ability to stretch. The tight heart muscle hampers ventricular diastolic filling. Filling pressures increase, and cardiac output falls. Eventually, cardiac failure and mild ventricular hypertrophy occur.

Clinical Manifestations and Diagnostic Findings

Restrictive cardiomyopathy causes clinical manifestations of decreased cardiac output. As cardiac output falls and intraventricular pressures rise, manifestations of congestive heart failure appear. The earliest manifestations may include exercise intolerance, fatigue, and shortness of breath, followed by neck vein distention, peripheral edema, and ascites. In severe or endstage disease, the clinical manifestations of restrictive cardiomyopathy are indistinguishable from those of chronic constrictive pericarditis. (See preceding text for a more complete discussion of pericarditis.) Cardiac murmurs are usually minimal or absent. Heart failure without cardiac enlargement indicates restrictive cardiomyopathy.

 ## Acute and Subacute Care

■ Medical Management

Currently there are no specific interventions for restrictive cardiomyopathy. Intervention aims at diminishing congestive heart failure. Diuretics, vasodilators, and salt restriction help accomplish this goal. Digitalis may help in some forms of restrictive cardiomyopathy.

Death due to dysrhythmia from restrictive cardiomyopathy may occur suddenly; or a more progressive course may be followed by eventual, intractable heart failure. The prognosis largely depends on the underlying cause. Unfortunately, intervention rarely brings about long-term improvement.

■ Surgical Management

Surgical intervention for hypertrophic cardiomyopathy may become necessary if medical management is ineffective. Several surgical procedures have been developed to reduce the outflow gradient. The most popular surgical treatment involves an incision into the ventricular septum with or without resection of part of the septum.

The excision of fibrotic endocardium is successful in a limited number of clients with restrictive cardiomyopathy. Recent advances in surgical treatment have had some success. Surgery has been effective in treating some arrhythmias. Cardiac transplantation is becoming an increasingly common surgery for dilated cardiomyopathy. Valve replacement may also be required, but it is not commonly performed.

■ Nursing Management

Nursing assessment of clients with cardiomyopathy focuses on the following:

● The duration and extent of manifestations
● Limitations on activity and life-style
● Coping strategies
● The client's and family's understanding of, perception of, and reaction to the illness
● Genetic counseling

The management of the client with cardiomyopathy is outlined in the Care Plan. In addition, clients who are acutely or chronically ill with cardiomyopathy require strong psychosocial support. The uncertain and serious consequences of the disease create fear and anxiety. The chronic nature of the disorder can deplete coping resources, leaving those afflicted with feelings of helplessness and hopelessness. As physical capabilities diminish, feelings of inadequacy, frustration, and poor self-esteem grow. Clients may become irritable, angry, withdrawn, or dependent.

Even though their prognosis is often poor, help those who suffer from this debilitating disorder to maintain hope and dignity. Encouragement, a caring touch, a listening ear, and attainable goals can promote a high quality of life. Create an environment in which clients can openly express concerns and acknowledge fears. Acceptance, empathy, and kindness can help clients with cardiomyopathies adopt more successful coping strategies.

The poor prognosis for these disorders need not lead to frustration and despair. With an optimistic outlook and conscientious effort, you can assist the client with cardiomyopathy to maintain a reasonable level of health and achieve a satisfying quality of life.

Community and Self-Care

With hypertrophic cardiomyopathy, syncope or sudden death may follow physical exertion. Therefore, warn the client with hypertrophic cardiomyopathy to avoid strenuous physical exercise such as running or active competitive sports. In addition, encourage household members to learn CPR. Although chest pain often accompanies this disease, nitroglycerin can worsen obstruction. Instead, clinicians treat chest pain with reduced activity and beta-blocking agents.

Hypertrophic cardiomyopathy predisposes the client to the risk of infective endocarditis. Advise clients with this cardiomyopathy always to take prophylactic antibiotics before and after dental and surgical procedures. (See earlier discussion of prevention of and intervention for infective endocarditis.) Also, relay this vital information to the client's family.

All clients with cardiomyopathy need clear, honest education concerning the disease and its cause and intervention. Both the nurse and the client must be watchful for untoward effects of therapy. Clients with restrictive cardiomyopathy are especially prone to the toxic effects of digitalis (see Chapter 45).

Valvular Heart Disease

The four heart valves maintain a one-way flow of blood. When the valves are healthy, the blood flows through the heart and lungs in one direction. Dysfunction occurs when the heart valves are unable to fully open or fully close. A stenosed valve may impede the flow of blood from one chamber to the next; an insufficient (incompetent) valve may allow blood to regurgitate (flow backward) (Fig. 47–5). Valvular heart disease remains fairly common in the United States even though the incidence is steadily decreasing as the incidence of rheumatic fever decreases. Mitral valve prolapse syndrome is one of the most common cardiac abnormalities; as much as 5% to 10% of the population is affected.[13]

Mitral Valve Disease

Disorders of the mitral valve obstruct the flow of blood from the atrium to the ventricle (stenosis) or allow blood to leak back from ventricle to atrium (regurgitation). Mitral regurgitation overworks the left atrium and left ventricle; mitral stenosis overworks the left atrium.

Mitral Stenosis. Mitral stenosis is a block in blood flow resulting from an abnormality of the mitral valve leaflets that prevents proper opening of the valve during diastole.

Mitral Regurgitation. Mitral regurgitation occurs when blood from the left ventricle is ejected back into the left atrium during systole because of abnormalities in the mitral valve. Regurgitation of the mitral valve sometimes occurs with mitral stenosis.

Text continues on page 1344

CARE PLAN

The Client with Cardiomyopathy

Collaborative Problem. Risk for Heart Failure related to mechanical dysfunction of the heart

Planning: Expected Outcomes. The nurse will monitor for the following clinical manifestations of heart failure:

- Peripheral edema
- Pulmonary edema
- Decreased renal perfusion
- Decreased CO
- Diaphoresis
- Dyspnea, orthopnea
- Anxiety
- Frothy, pink sputum

Implementation: Nursing Intervention

Assess the client every 4–8 hours for

- Neck vein distention
- Peripheral edema
- Altered lung sounds
- Dyspnea or orthopnea
- Tachycardia
- Hypotension
- Confusion
- Urine output > 30 ml/hr

Monitor BUN, bilirubin, liver enzymes, and creatinine
　Monitor fluid balance every 8–24 hours
　Daily weights

Rationales

These assessments will detect early signs of heart failure; as the heart muscle fails to pump effectively, falling cardiac output stimulates the adrenergic system and the renin-angiotensin-aldosterone system. These changes lead to tachycardia and oliguria. Increased preload and afterload lead to neck and vein distention, peripheral edema, altered lung sounds, dyspnea, and orthopnea. Hypoxia may lead to confusion.

These laboratory studies indicate liver congestion.
Clients are treated with potent diuretics to reduce pulmonary and peripheral edema. Accurate assessment of fluid balance and weight assist in determining the effectiveness of the treatment.

Evaluation. Heart failure will remain an active problem. Some clients will have improvement of heart failure after diuresis. Others have such severe cardiomyopathy that a goal is to have no further deterioration.

Nursing Diagnosis. Decreased Cardiac Output related to alterations in cardiac structure and function

Planning: Expected Outcomes. The client will demonstrate improved cardiac output, as evidenced by

- Clear lung sounds
- Vital signs WNL
- Warm, dry skin
- Normal sinus rhythm
- Absence of S_3 or S_4
- Urine output > 30 ml/hr
- Decreased peripheral edema, neck vein distention, and ascites

Implementation: Nursing Intervention

Monitor for clinical manifestations of decreasing CO.

Encourage bedrest during acute phase; limit self-care.

Avoid Valsalva's maneuver (with hypertrophic cardiomyopathy).
Observe and record dysrhythmias every 4–8 hours.
Monitor intake and output every 1–8 hours.
Restrict intravenous and oral fluids as ordered.

Administer unloading and inotropic agents.

Administer calcium antagonists as ordered.

In hypertrophic cardiomyopathy, avoid nitrates, beta-adrenergics, and cardiac glycosides.

Rationales

Early detection of decreasing CO improves treatment options.
Rest decreases oxygen consumption and demand on myocardium.
Valsalva's maneuver impedes venous return and impairs outflow.
Dysrhythmias may further impair CO.
Fluid retention may occur with decreased CO and CHF.
This restriction decreases the amount of circulating fluids.
These agents are used to improve ejection, reduce preload, and improve contractility.
These are used to decrease LV outflow obstruction and increase LV compliance to improve ventricular filling.
These agents increase contractility and increase obstruction.

Care Plan continued on following page

CARE PLAN

The Client with Cardiomyopathy *(Continued)*

Implementation: Nursing Intervention	Rationales
Hemodynamic monitoring: monitor arterial pressure, RAP, PAP, PCWP, CO/I every 2–4 hours as indicated.	These monitor the degree of CHF and the response to therapy.

Evaluation. Like heart failure, decreased cardiac output will remain an active problem. Degree of outcome attainment varies greatly.

Nursing Diagnosis. Intolerance related to mechanical dysfunction of the heart and decreased cardiac reserve.

Planning: Expected Outcomes. The client will have an improved activity tolerance, as evidenced by

■ Demonstrating a progression of activity appropriate to the disorder
■ Showing a willingness to combine rest and activity
■ Demonstrating minimal change in pulse or BP during activities
■ Having pulse, respirations, and BP return to normal range within 3 minutes of the activity
■ Accepting any imposed restrictions

Implementation: Nursing Intervention	Rationales
Assess the tolerance to activities in bed before ambulating.	This provides a baseline to plan activity.
During activity, monitor pulse, respiration, color, and ECG.	Early detection of orthostatic changes as well as data on the ability of the diseased myocardium to meet oxygen demand.
Discontinue activity if chest pain, dyspnea, cyanosis, dizziness, hypotension, sustained tachycardia, or dysrhythmias develop.	These manifestations are evidence of myocardial hypoxia.
Monitor pulse, respirations, and BP 3 minutes after activity.	These will evaluate tolerance of activity.
Explore which sedentary activities client may enjoy.	Sedentary activities may provide diversion, if activity is not permitted; sedentary activities do not place a demand on the diseased myocardium.

Evaluation. If the cardiomyopathy is severe, plan to achieve only small increments in activity tolerance. This problem will remain active since the condition is not curable.

BP, blood pressure; BUN, blood urea nitrogen; CO, cardiac output; CO/I, cardiac output/cardiac index; ECG, electrocardiogram; LV, left ventricular; PAP, pulmonary artery pressure; PCWP, pulmonary capillary wedge pressure; RAP, right atrial pressure; WNL, within normal limits.

Mitral Valve Prolapse. In mitral valve prolapse, one or both of the valve leaflets bulge into the left atrium during ventricular systole. Various names have been given to the disorder: late apical systolic murmur, Barlow's syndrome, and floppy mitral valve syndrome. Usually a benign disorder, it may progress to a stage of pronounced regurgitation and ventricular dilation. Although it is often an isolated abnormality, this syndrome is associated with a number of other conditions, such as endocarditis, myocarditis, atherosclerosis, systemic lupus erythematosus, muscular dystrophy, acromegaly, and cardiac sarcoidosis. In addition, there may be a genetic component. It tends to be more common in young women.[17]

Etiology and Risk Factors

Factors leading to the development of acquired valvular disease include acute rheumatic fever, infectious endocarditis, and connective tissue abnormalities. Rheumatic heart disease, the most common cause of valvular heart disease, is preventable. Community health nurses working in healthcare centers or schools can often detect people with beta-hemolytic streptococcal infections (the precursor to rheumatic heart disease). The nurse needs to refer these clients for appropriate diagnosis and intervention.

Pathophysiology

Acquired valvular dysfunction is usually caused by inflammation of the endocardium due to acute rheumatic fever or infectious endocarditis. The inflammation causes the valve leaflets and chordae tendineae to become fibrous. The chordae tendineae shorten, which narrows the outflow tract.

The aortic and mitral valves become dysfunctional more often than the pulmonary and tricuspid valves do.

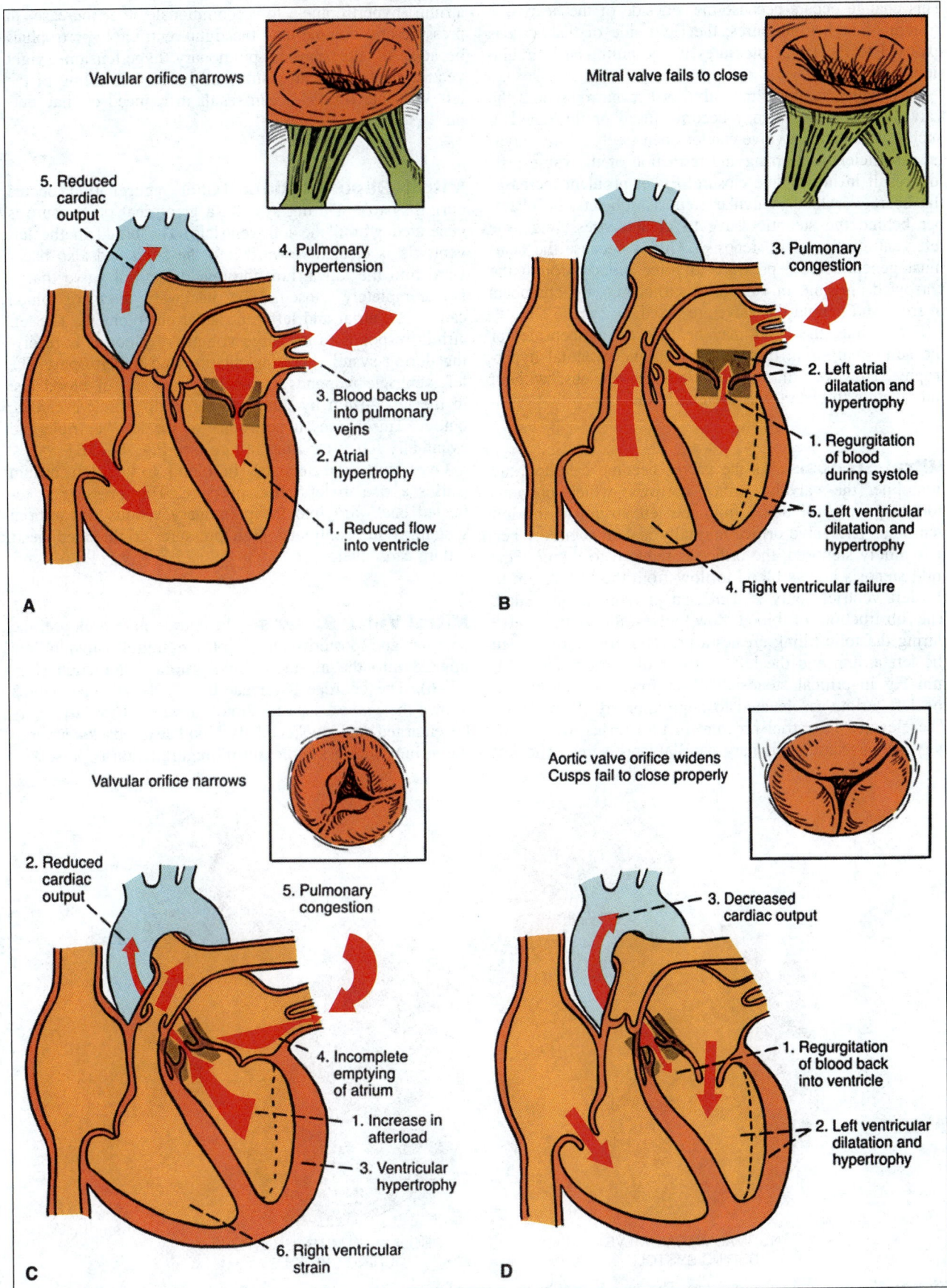

Figure 47–5. Dysfunctions of the cardiac valves. *A,* Mitral stenosis. *B,* Mitral regurgitation. *C,* Aortic stenosis. *D,* Aortic regurgitation.

This change occurs because the left side of the heart is a system of higher pressures; the right side of the heart is exposed to the lower pressures in the pulmonary circulation.

In valvular stenosis, the valve orifice narrows, and the valve leaflets (cusps) may become fused or thickened in such a way that the valve cannot open freely. With valvular insufficiency, scarring and retraction of the valve leaflets result in incomplete closure. Either problem increases the heart workload. Valvular stenosis subjects the chamber behind the stenotic valve to greater stress (e.g., the left ventricle in aortic stenosis). This is because the heart must generate more pressure to force blood through the narrowed opening. In valvular insufficiency, the chambers in front and behind the valve are taxed.

For a time, the heart may be able to compensate for the additional strain through dilation and eventual hypertrophy. However, if valvular damage worsens, without intervention the heart will eventually fail.

Mitral Stenosis.
As the valves become calcified and immobile, the valvular orifice narrows, which prevents normal passage of blood from the left atrium to the left ventricle. The valve orifice normally is 4 to 6 cm². When it is mildly stenosed, the orifice is reduced to 2 cm². This mild stenosis allows blood to flow from the left atrium to the left ventricle only if increased pressure is generated. The obstruction of blood flow across the mitral valve during diastolic filling creates a pressure gradient between the left atrium and the left ventricle of approximately 20 mm Hg in critical stenosis.[21] Therefore, the pressure in the left atrium is elevated to approximately 25 mm Hg. The elevated left atrial pressure in turn raises the pulmonary venous and pulmonary capillary pressures. The left atrium hypertrophies to accommodate the increase in pressure and volume, and the right ventricle hypertrophies because of the chronic pulmonary hypertension. Right ventricular failure can result, and inadequate filling of the left ventricle (preload) can result in reduced cardiac output[43] (see Fig. 47–5A).

Mitral Regurgitation.
Mitral regurgitation occurs during systole. During systole, a great deal of pressure is generated within the left ventricle. The blood in the left ventricle is ejected forward into the aorta and also backward into the left atrium through the mitral valve that is not completely closed. The backward flow of blood causes left atrial and left ventricular enlargement. The left atrium responds to the large volume of blood it is receiving during systole, causing dilation and hypertrophy. The left ventricle responds to the large amount of blood lost to the left atrium by pumping harder to preserve cardiac output. This causes hypertrophy of the left ventricle and eventually left ventricular failure (see Fig. 47–5B).

Over time, the increase in blood to the left atrium causes a rise in left atrial pressure. This pressure is reflected backward into the pulmonary venous and arterial system. With continued high pressures, right-sided heart failure can develop.

Mitral Valve Prolapse.
In mitral valve prolapse, the anterior and posterior cusps of the mitral valve billow upward into the atrium during systolic contraction (Fig. 47–6). The chordae tendineae can be lengthened, which allows the valve cusps to stretch upward. The cusps may be enlarged and thickened. If blood leaks backward into the atrium during systole, mitral regurgitation is present.

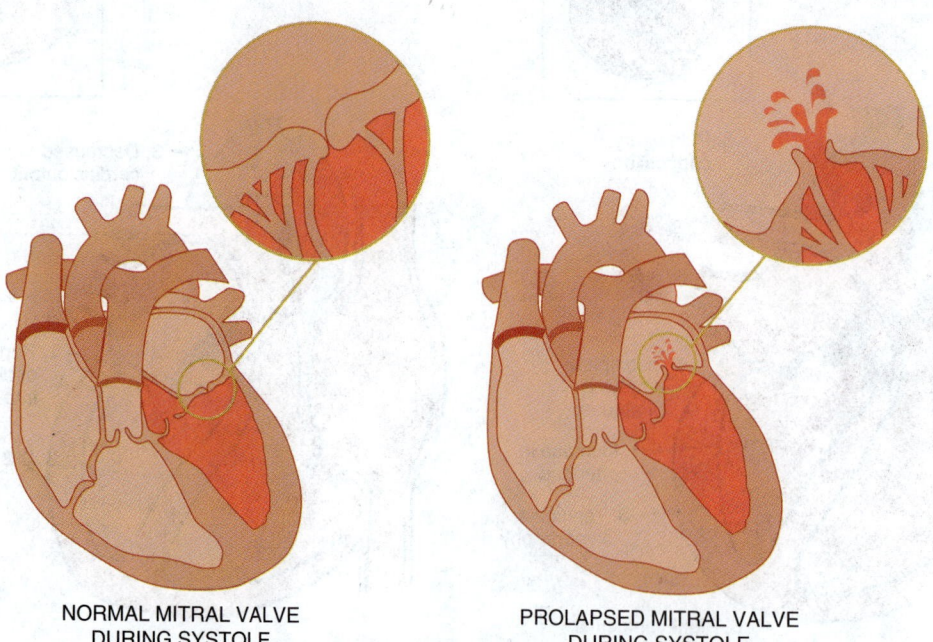

NORMAL MITRAL VALVE
DURING SYSTOLE

PROLAPSED MITRAL VALVE
DURING SYSTOLE

Figure 47–6. Mitral valve prolapse. The main figure shows a normal mitral valve, and the *inset* shows a prolapsed mitral valve. Prolapse permits the valve leaflets to billow back into the atrium during left ventricular systole. The billowing causes the leaflets to part slightly, permitting regurgitation of blood into the atrium.

Clinical Manifestations and Diagnostic Findings

The clinical manifestations of valvular heart disease may appear gradually or suddenly.

Mitral Stenosis. On auscultation, a loud first heart sound and then an opening snap that ushers in a low-pitched, rumbling diastolic murmur will be heard. The opening snap is best heard at the apex with the diaphragm of the stethoscope. The diastolic murmur is best heard at the apex using the bell of the stethoscope while the client is in a left lateral recumbent position.[45]

Atrial fibrillation is a common finding in persons with mitral stenosis. During episodes of atrial fibrillation, the pulse becomes irregular and faint, and the blood pressure often drops.

Up to 20% of clients with mitral stenosis will develop systemic embolization.[60] Ineffective atrial contractions allow some stagnation of blood in the left atrium and encourage the formation of mural thrombi. These thrombi easily break away and travel as emboli throughout the arterial system, causing tissue infarction.

Mitral Regurgitation. Clients with mitral regurgitation may be asymptomatic, but if cardiac output falls, symptoms will develop. When cardiac output falls, fatigue and dyspnea are the first symptoms. Clinical manifestations gradually increase to include orthopnea, paroxysmal nocturnal dyspnea, and peripheral edema. Pulmonary symptoms are less severe than in mitral stenosis because changes in the mean pulmonary capillary pressure are less exaggerated. However, when the right side of the heart is affected the symptoms are the same as in mitral stenosis.

Auscultation reveals a blowing, high-pitched systolic murmur with radiation to the left axilla, heard best at the apex. The first heart sound may be diminished, and often a splitting of the second sound will be heard. Severe regurgitation is associated with a third heart sound (S_3).

Vital signs are usually normal unless the client has severe mitral regurgitation. Atrial fibrillation is common in clients with this condition. However, emboli and hemoptysis occur far less often than in mitral stenosis.

Mitral Valve Prolapse. It is not uncommon for many clients with mitral valve prolapse to be completely asymptomatic. In a healthy client, a physical examination may reveal a regurgitant murmur or a midsystolic click on auscultation. If symptoms are present, they may include tachycardia, lightheadedness, syncope, fatigue, weakness, dyspnea, chest discomfort, anxiety, and palpitations related to dysrhythmias.[60] Symptoms may be vague. Mitral valve prolapse has recently been associated with an autonomic dysfunction in which large quantities of catecholamines are produced, with or without adrenergic stimulation. This may help explain the vague and various symptoms.[13] There is minimal morbidity and mortality associated with mitral valve prolapse. Clinically, clients have no physical limitations.[17]

Various diagnostic assessments are used to detect valvular lesions or structural heart changes. These studies include echocardiography, chest radiography, and cardiac catheterization.

Management

■ Medical Management

Mitral Stenosis. Untreated mitral stenosis can progress from mild disability to severe disability in about 5 years.[13] Improvement of symptoms can be achieved with oral diuretics and a diet restricted in sodium. Digitalis is useful in clients with atrial fibrillation for slowing the ventricular heart rate. Beta-blockers may decrease the heart rate and therefore increase exercise tolerance. Anticoagulants are helpful in clients who are not anticipating surgical intervention.

Mitral Regurgitation. Symptomatic reduction is the aim of nonsurgical treatment of mitral regurgitation. The client should restrict physical activities that produce fatigue and dyspnea. Reducing sodium intake and promoting sodium excretion with diuretics will lessen the work of the heart. Nitrates and ACE inhibitors have demonstrated hemodynamic improvement and symptomatic relief in clients with chronic mitral regurgitation.[13]

Mitral Valve Prolapse. Treatment of mitral valve prolapse depends on the symptoms. Beta-blockers are helpful in relieving syncope, palpitations, and chest pain. For preventing infective endocarditis, the client is given antibiotics prophylactically before any invasive procedures.

■ Surgical Management

When conservative medical intervention fails to improve hemodynamics in valvular disorders, surgical intervention is indicated. The surgeon usually performs valve repair or replacement for severe valvular defects that are accompanied by left ventricular dysfunction and heart failure. Valvular surgery must be performed at an appropriate time during the course of the disease. The projected natural history of the condition, its impact on the client's lifestyle, and the projected performance of the artificial valve are factors that the surgeon and the client consider before valvular surgery is performed. Valvular repairs are discussed later in the chapter.

Aortic Valve Disease

Aortic valve disease is far less common than mitral valve disease. However, it often occurs in conjunction with mitral valve disease. Aortic stenosis obstructs the forward flow of blood during systole from the left ventricle into the aorta and systemic circulation. This obstruction to flow creates a resistance to ejection and increased pressure in the left ventricle. Aortic regurgitation allows blood to leak back from the aorta into the left ventricle.

During systole, blood that is ejected into the aorta re-enters the left ventricle. In order to maintain normal pressures, the left ventricle hypertrophies. Both aortic stenosis and regurgitation overwork the left ventricle.

Etiology and Risk Factors

Aortic stenosis can be caused by several congenital defects of the aortic valve. It can also be caused by two degenerative processes: (1) calcification of the valve in the elderly, and (2) retraction and stiffening of the valve from rheumatic fever. As the population in the United States ages, there is a rising incidence of aortic stenosis from calcification.[55]

Aortic regurgitation is most often due to infectious disorders such as rheumatic fever, syphilis, and infective endocarditis. Connective tissue disorders can also lead to aortic regurgitation.

Pathophysiology

Aortic Stenosis. In aortic stenosis, the orifice of the aortic valve becomes narrowed, which causes a decrease in the blood flow from the left ventricle into the aorta. The pressure within the left ventricle rises as the blood is ejected through the narrowed opening. A pressure gradient develops between the left ventricle and the aorta. The elevation of pressure in the left ventricle during systole causes the ventricle to hypertrophy. Dilation of the left ventricle occurs over time when there is a deterioration of the contractility of the hypertrophied muscle. Eventually, dilation and hypertrophy of the left ventricle are unable to maintain adequate cardiac output. There is a rise in left ventricular end-diastolic pressure, a decrease in cardiac output, and an increase in pulmonary hypertension (Fig. 47–5C).

Aortic Regurgitation. Aortic regurgitation (aortic insufficiency) is a diastolic event in which blood that is propelled forward into the aorta regurgitates back into the left ventricle through an incompetent valve. This causes abnormal filling and a volume overload of the left ventricle. The magnitude of the overload depends on the severity of the incompetence. However, a small incompetent area can result in significant aortic regurgitation over time.

Because the left ventricle receives blood from both the atrium and the systemic circulation, aortic regurgitation will gradually increase left ventricular end-diastolic volume. Left ventricular stroke volume is increased to produce an effective forward-moving volume into the systemic circulation. There is a compensatory dilation of the left ventricle but minimal increase in left ventricular end-diastolic pressure.[13] As much as 60% of the stroke volume can be regurgitated, markedly increasing left ventricular workload. The compensatory mechanisms of dilation and hypertrophy help maintain an adequate cardiac output. However, as the condition progresses and the contractile state of the myocardium declines, cardiac output falls (Fig. 47–5D).

Clinical Manifestations and Diagnostic Findings

Aortic Stenosis. Clinical manifestations of aortic stenosis tend to occur gradually and late in the course of the disease. There is usually a long latent period in which the client is asymptomatic. Symptoms begin to appear as the obstruction and ventricular pressure increase to critical levels. Angina pectoris is a frequent symptom in approximately 60% of clients. The character of the angina is similar to that in clients with coronary artery disease. The angina commonly is brought on by exertion and relieved by rest. Myocardial oxygen consumption is higher in clients with aortic stenosis because of the hypertrophy of the left ventricle, and this probably accounts for the angina.[13]

Syncope is another frequent clinical manifestation. It also occurs during exertion because of a fixed cardiac output and an increased demand.[5] Syncope at rest may be due to arrhythmias. Exertional dyspnea, paroxysmal nocturnal dyspnea, and pulmonary edema occur with increasing pulmonary venous hypertension due to left ventricular failure.

In severe aortic stenosis, additional symptoms may include palpitations, fatigue, and visual disturbances. Sudden death occurs in 15% to 20% of symptomatic clients as a result of dysrhythmias and myocardial ischemia.[13]

On auscultation, the systolic murmur may be associated with a diminished second heart sound and an early ejection click. There is a systolic thrill over the aortic areas.

Aortic Regurgitation. Clients with chronic severe aortic regurgitation may have a long period of time with no symptoms. During this time, the left ventricle gradually enlarges. Clients may complain of an uncomfortable awareness of the heartbeat and palpitations. These symptoms are due to the large left ventricular stroke volume with rapid diastolic runoff. This is also apparent with prominent pulsations in the neck and even head-bobbing with each heartbeat. Sinus tachycardia or premature ventricular contractions may make palpitations more pronounced.

On physical examination, the client may have an increased systolic blood pressure due to the large stroke volume and a decreased diastolic blood pressure due to the regurgitation and distal runoff. Carotid artery pulsations may be exaggerated. The arterial pulse pressure widens, and palpable pulse amplitude increases. This may be noted as a sudden sharp pulse, followed by a swift collapse of the diastolic pulse (Corrigan's or water-hammer pulse). Auscultation reveals a soft, high-pitched, blowing decrescendo diastolic murmur heard best at the second right intercostal space and radiating to the left sternal border.

Management

■ Medical Management

Aortic Stenosis. Noninvasive assessment of clients with Doppler echocardiography should be done. Those clients with known or suspected critical obstruction of the aortic valve should be told to avoid vigorous physical activity. Clients with mild obstruction may continue exercise if it is tolerated.

Prophylactic antibiotics should be given for invasive medical or dental procedures for prevention of infective endocarditis. Digitalis and diuretics that are usually used for ventricular failure will not help in aortic stenosis because the mechanical obstruction to outflow will not be reduced.[17] Beta-blockers are not usually used because they can depress myocardial function and induce left ventricular failure. Cardiac dysrhythmias should be treated pharmacologically.

Aortic Regurgitation. Medical intervention for aortic regurgitation is the same as for aortic stenosis: relieve the manifestations of congestive heart failure and prevent infection of the already deformed aortic cusps.

■ Surgical Management

Aortic Stenosis. Surgical intervention should be considered for aortic stenosis when the pressure gradient is greater than 50 mm Hg or the valve orifice is less than 0.8 cm^2. Clients with symptomatic aortic stenosis have a poor prognosis without surgical intervention. There is an increased incidence of sudden death once myocardial failure develops.[43]

Aortic Regurgitation. Surgical replacement of the incompetent valve provides the only effective long-term intervention for aortic regurgitation. The surgeon's critical concern involves the proper timing of the surgery. In clients with acute, severe aortic regurgitation and left ventricular failure, early valve replacement can be life-saving. A high percentage of clients with aortic regurgitation and aortic stenosis show striking clinical improvement with valve replacement.[55]

Tricuspid and Pulmonic Valve Disease

Tricuspid stenosis or regurgitation usually develops in combination with other structural disorders of the heart. Lesions of the tricuspid valve are relatively rare occurrences that stress the right side of the heart and produce right ventricular failure.

Abnormalities of the pulmonic valve are usually congenital defects. Few lesions develop after birth. Pulmonary hypertension, caused by mitral stenosis, pulmonary emboli, or chronic lung disease, can precipitate functional pulmonary regurgitation.

Tricuspid disorders usually develop in combination with other structural disorders of the heart. Pulmonic valve disorders are commonly due to congenital defects.

Because the tricuspid valve is on the right side of the heart, the major hemodynamic alteration with tricuspid stenosis is a decrease in cardiac output and increased right atrial pressure. The inability of the right atrium to propel blood across the stenosed valve explains these changes. Likewise, with tricuspid regurgitation, pressure in the right atrium is elevated. In this situation, however, it is due to regurgitation of the blood volume in the right ventricle back into the right atrium during systole.

Pulmonic stenosis and regurgitation lead to a decrease in cardiac output because blood does not reach the left side of the heart in adequate supply for metabolic demands. Right-sided heart failure can also develop.

Clinical manifestations of tricuspid stenosis are dyspnea and fatigue, pulsations in the neck, and peripheral edema. Physical assessment reveals prominent waves in the neck veins as the atrium vigorously contracts against the stenotic valve. A diastolic murmur is heard best along the left lower sternal border. The murmur increases with inspiration. The ECG reveals tall, tented P waves in leads II, III, and aV.

Tricuspid insufficiency causes hepatic congestion and peripheral edema. The client often has atrial fibrillation and evident jugular waves. The murmur is holosystolic along the left sternal border.

Pulmonic regurgitation may lead to dyspnea and fatigue. The murmur is a high-pitched diastolic blow along the left sternal border. There are no significant changes in the ECG. Pulmonic stenosis causes similar clinical manifestations except that the murmur is often a crescendo-decrescendo type.

Tricuspid stenosis usually responds well to diuretics and digitalis therapy. If the leaflets are severely stenotic, surgery may be required. Intervention in pulmonic valve disease focus on ameliorating the underlying cause and the presenting signs of right-sided heart failure.

Nursing Management of the Client with Valvular Heart Disease

Nursing assessment involves gathering subjective and objective data concerning the following:

1. The type, severity, and progress of the valvular disorder
2. The degree of heart failure
3. The client's tolerance for activity
4. The client's support systems
5. The degree of knowledge that the client and family have concerning the nature of and intervention in the disorder

The main focus of nursing intervention in valvular heart disease is to help the client maintain a normal cardiac output, thereby preventing manifestations of heart failure, venous congestion, and inadequate tissue perfusion. To evaluate the effectiveness of therapeutic interventions, perform ongoing hemodynamic assessment. Monitor vital signs closely every 1 to 4 hours. A decrease in cardiac output is manifested in a compensatory rise in heart rate, a drop in blood pressure, or a decrease in urinary output. Carefully auscultate the chest every 4 hours to identify the presence of adventitious breath sounds (crackles, rhonchi) or heart gallops (S$_3$, S$_4$).

Clients may find it difficult to cope physically and psychosocially after discharge. The chronicity of valvular heart disease and its potential complications can create an atmosphere of uncertainty, fear, and frustration. Take time to help the client identify support persons, personal strengths, and coping strategies. Assess how the client handles frustration or anger and what activities are particularly relaxing. Address the client's fears and misconceptions. In some instances, counseling referrals may help. Stress the importance of follow-up physical examinations and intervention.

Valvular heart disease requires lifelong management. With a sincere desire to understand and accept each client's response to chronic illness, you can help the client with valvular heart disease adapt to difficult life-style changes and achieve a positive sense of well-being.

Before discharge, prepare detailed teaching material for the client and family concerning the therapeutic regimen, the disease process, factors contributing to symptoms, and the rationale for intervention.

Give information concerning prescribed medications. Medications frequently prescribed include digoxin, quinidine, diuretics, beta-blockers, potassium supplements, anticoagulants, and prophylactic antibiotics. Explain their rationale, dosages, side effects, and special considerations in their use.

Review exercise prescriptions with the client. Clients with aortic stenosis often require activity restrictions. The client should demonstrate ability to pace activity, verbalize improvement in fatigue, and accept activity restrictions.

Address dietary restrictions and plan interdisciplinary follow-up. Make sure the client knows whom to call when questions arise.

Congenital Disorders

There have been significant advances in the medical and surgical treatment of people with congenital heart disease. Congenital heart disorders result from faulty development of the heart's structures in utero. Congenital disorders include septal defects, vessel stenosis, abnormally positioned vessels, and patency of the ductus arteriosus. These advances have assisted an ever-growing number of clients to survive into adulthood. As their number grows, medical and nursing support has grown also.

With current available treatments, it is estimated that 85% of children with congenital heart disease will survive into adulthood.[95] Currently, there are approximately 500,000 adults with congenital heart disease in the United States. Each congenital defect brings its own morbidity and mortality statistics, but normally, the people with the less complex defects will have a longer survival than those with the more complex defects. The latter will have an uncertain course.

Surgical procedures may be palliative or corrective. Most adult patients today went through their surgical procedures many years ago during the developmental phase of the surgical interventions. Their course may be quite different from the course of those having surgery today. Many refinements in surgical techniques have been developed and continue to be developed so that clinical outcomes vary significantly.

Many people have remained asymptomatic. Others have had varying levels of functional ability. Clients may have both residua and sequelae. Residua are problems that are not corrected or improved at the time of the surgical repair and sequelae are problems that are the result of the surgical procedure.[43, 80]

The risk of infective endocarditis is increased in clients with artificial valves or with suture repair of an atrial septal defect.

It is not uncommon for a client with a repaired coarctation of the aorta to find that the aorta has gradually become narrowed again. Frequently, these clients may develop essential hypertension.

Clients who have had cyanotic defects repaired as children are likely to have sequelae and complications in adulthood.[79] There may be some degree of exercise intolerance that can be better managed after proper stress testing.

Arrhythmias frequently present a lifelong complication. Clients who have had intraventricular repairs may present with ventricular arrhythmias or complete heart block. A 24-hour Holter monitor and stress testing may help evaluate the client's tolerance for activity.

Many people will have had surgical procedures as infants and children and then had repeated surgeries as they "outgrew" their repairs or prosthetic devices. Many women are of childbearing age. The pregnancy outcome of women with known heart disease seems to be related to their functional ability. The health of the mother and the infant is good if the mother's functional ability is good.[51] There is also a growing geriatric population that may have unknown late consequences of congenital heart disease or surgical repair. It is important to encourage these people to participate in long-term follow-up.

The role of the nurse who is caring for the adult with congenital heart disease varies with the setting. However, nurses play an integral role in helping these patients achieve optimal health and functioning. Nursing assessment, intervention, education, and follow-up are directed toward improving functional levels, managing medications, psychosocial adjustment, and preventing complications.

Cardiac Surgery

Cardiac surgery is performed when the probability of survival with a useful life is greater with surgical treatment than with nonsurgical treatment. The first heart surgery was performed in 1923 by Cutler and Levine.[43] That procedure was repair of a stenosed mitral valve. Since that time, heart surgery has been revolutionized by the development of open heart techniques that allow surgeons to visualize the heart directly while they explore, cut, repair, and sew. These improved operating conditions have enabled today's surgeons to replace diseased valves with prosthetic valves, repair severe congenital lesions, and perform heart transplants. Today, under ideal conditions, cardiac surgery should have a hospital mortality approaching zero. However, a description of the results of cardiac surgery by hospital mortality alone is not sufficient. The preoperative condition of the client's heart and other body systems greatly influences the results of cardiac surgery. The identification of incremental risk factors will continue to improve results.

Types of Heart Surgery

There are three types of cardiac surgery: (1) reparative, (2) reconstructive, and (3) substitutional. Reparative surgeries are likely to produce cure or excellent and prolonged improvement. These operations include closure of a patent ductus arteriosus, atrial septal defect, and ventricular septal defect; repair of mitral stenosis; and simple repair of tetralogy of Fallot. Reconstructive procedures are more complex. They are not always curative procedures, and reoperation may be needed. Reconstructive procedures include coronary artery bypass grafting and reconstruction of an incompetent mitral, tricuspid, or aortic valve. Substitutional surgeries are not usually curative because of the preoperative condition of the client. Examples of substitutional surgeries include valve replacement, cardiac replacement by transplantation, ventricular replacement or assistance, and cardiac replacement by mechanical devices.

Valvular Surgery

The repair or replacement of cardiac valves with acquired stenosis or incompetence is not considered curative, but the results are generally good and long-lasting. Cure is usually unable to be obtained because of the preoperative condition of the heart or other body systems. Indications for surgery include the following:

- Progressive impairment of cardiac function due to scarring and thickening of the valve with either (1) impaired narrowing of the valvular opening (stenosis) or (2) incomplete closure (insufficiency, regurgitation)
- Gradual enlargement of the heart with symptoms of

decreased activity, shortness of breath, and heart failure.

Surgical therapy for mitral valve stenosis can include valve commissurotomy or valve replacement. Commissurotomy or valve reconstruction can be accomplished if the preoperative assessment indicates that the valve is pliable. If the valve is not pliable, valve replacement is necessary. In clients with mitral regurgitation, valve reconstruction or annuloplasty may be done. This may include the use of a flexible ring that is sewn into the valve for stabilization. Aortic stenosis may be surgically treated with valve replacement or balloon aortic valvuloplasty. The valvuloplasty procedure uses a catheter with a balloon to dilate the valve orifice (Fig. 47–7). Surgical treatment for the client with aortic regurgitation is not always the treatment of choice, but may be considered.

Artificial cardiac valves are continuing to show improvements in design, safety, function, and durability. Mechanical and tissue prosthetic valves are currently available. The type of valve prosthesis used is based on a number of considerations. The surgeon primarily considers the client's tolerance of anticoagulation and the durability of the valve. Clients with mechanical valves require continuous anticoagulation therapy for the remainder of their lives. Therefore, if the client has a preoperative history of bleeding or noncompliance with pharmacologic regimens, the surgeon may decide to use a tissue valve. The overall advantages and disadvantages of tissue and mechanical valves are almost equal. The mechanical valves are very durable but require anticoagulant therapy; the tissue valves may not require anticoagulation therapy but are less durable. Some physicians recommend mechanical valves in clients under 65 or 70 years of age and tissue valves in clients 70 years or older.[75] Artificial valves are shown in Figure 47–8.

Potential complications of heart valves include a risk of thrombus formation, especially in mechanical valves. Newer types of heart valves have reduced rates of throm-

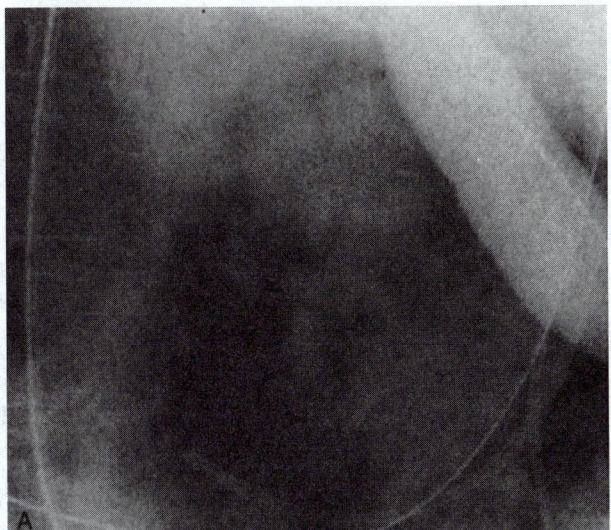
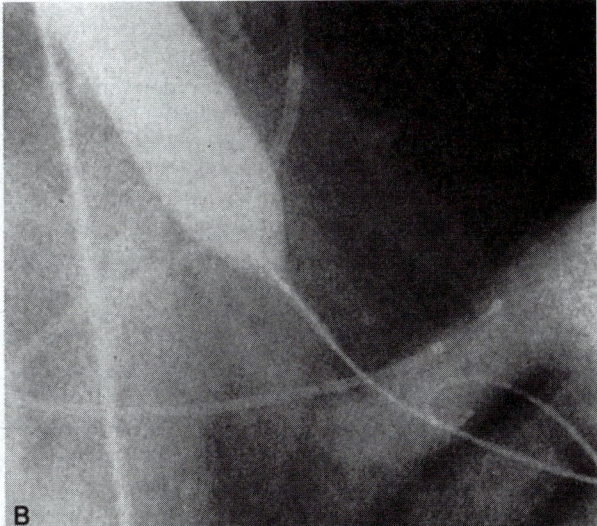

Figure 47–7. Valvuloplasty. *A,* The valvuloplasty balloon is inflated across the aortic valve. Note the indentation ("waist") in the balloon. *B,* The valvuloplasty balloon inflated across the aortic valve after dilation. Note the disappearance of the indentation seen in *A.* (From Barden, C., et al. [1990]. Balloon aortic valvuloplasty: Nursing care implications. *Critical Care Nurse, 10*(6), 26.)

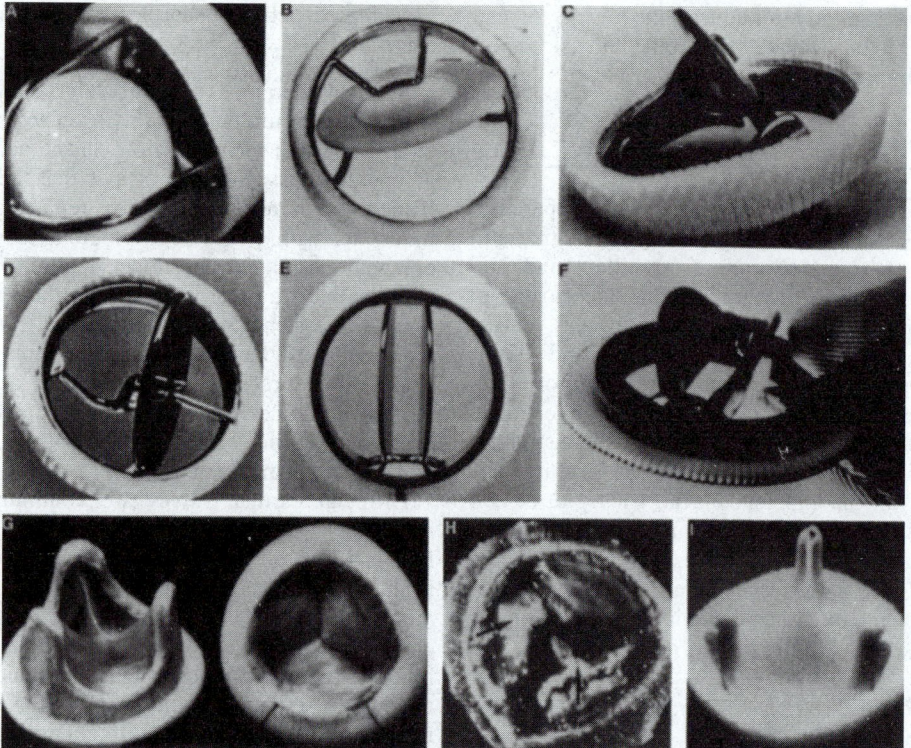

Figure 47–8. Prosthetic heart valves. *A,* The Starr-Edwards caged-ball valve with a cloth sewing ring and bare struts. *B,* The Björk-Shiley tilting disc valve. *C,* The Omniscience tilting disc valve. *D,* The Medtronic-Hall tilting disc valve. *E,* The St. Jude medical bileaflet valve as viewed end-on. Note the large size of the effective orifice area compared with the potential orifice area and the minimal obstruction to flow by the leaflets. *F,* The Duromedics bileaflet valve. *G,* The Carpentier-Edwards prosthetic valve. *H,* A porcine valve removed several years after implantation because of primary valve failure; *arrows* point to areas of calcification and destruction of leaflets. *I,* The Ionescu-Shiley pericardial valve. (*A* from Starek, P. J. K., and *F* from Clark, R. E. [1987]. *Heart valve replacement and reconstruction.* St. Louis: Mosby–Year Book; *B* from Björk, V.; *C* from Austin, E. H., III; *E* and *I* from Crawford, F. A., Jr.; *G* and *H* from Magilligan, D. J., Jr., [1987]. In F. A. Crawford [Ed.], *Cardiac surgery: Current heart valve prostheses* [vol. 1]. Philadelphia: Hanley & Belfus; *D* from Cobanoglu, A., & Brockman, S. K. [1986]. In W. S. Frankl & A. N. Brest [Eds.], *Valvular heart disease: Comprehensive evaluation and management.* Philadelphia: F. A. Davis.)

bosis. Most clients require long-term anticoagulation. The major risk with tissue valves is durability. The leaflets of these valves may degenerate, calcify, or develop structural abnormalities. Mitral valves tend to fail most often because of the higher stress on the valve. The rate of tissue valve failure is 2% to 5% for the first 6 years, and then the rate accelerates. Almost every client with a tissue valve will require replacement eventually.[75]

Management of the client after heart surgery is discussed later in this section.

Heart Transplantation

Cardiac transplantation is now a standard and effective treatment for clients with endstage cardiac disease. The first human heart transplant was performed in 1967 in South Africa by Dr. Christiaan Barnard. Much publicity and discussion throughout the world has surrounded heart transplantation since that time. Between 1967 and 1970,

about 150 heart transplants were performed with a dismal 85% mortality rate.[98] Almost all institutions stopped performing the operation for several years while advances in the laboratory continued.

In the 1980s, heart transplants were being performed on a routine basis. In 1990 the Registry of the International Society for Heart Transplantation listed more than 13,000 cardiac transplant procedures performed in more than 230 transplant centers.[65] Widespread application of heart transplantation had depended upon the development of better immunosuppressive therapy. The use of cyclosporine has resulted in superior results. Later favorable results resulted from the rapidly accumulating experience.

Currently, 80% of heart transplant patients survive 1 year, 75% survive 3 years,[8] and approximately 70% survive 10 years.[54] Heart transplant recipients who die following the procedure usually do so within the first 30 days postoperatively. Those at greatest risk are those who deteriorate rapidly before the transplant procedure. Infection, cardiac failure, or rejection is usually the cause of death.

Box 47–3. Selection Criteria for Heart Transplantation

- End-stage heart disease
- Current medical management is unsuccessful
- New York Heart Association class III or IV
- Prognosis of less than 1 year to live
- Under 65 years of age
- Nonsmoker
- No drug or alcohol abuse
- Client is well motivated and will follow postoperative instructions and medications
- No underlying condition that would limit survival:

   Systemic infection
   Irreversible hepatic insufficiency
   Irreversible renal insufficiency
   Malignancy
   Active peptic ulcer
   Recent pulmonary embolus
   Irreversible pulmonary insufficiency

Those wanting a heart transplant must be evaluated and screened. Their cardiac status is evaluated to determine the need for transplant. They are also evaluated for underlying conditions that predispose to an unfavorable outcome. Selection criteria for heart transplantation are shown in Box 47–3.

The current orthotopic technique for heart transplant retains a large portion of the right and left atrium in the recipient and implants the donor heart to the atria (Fig. 47–9). Cardiopulmonary bypass is used during the operation (see later discussion). Temporary pacemaker wires and chest drainage catheters are inserted.

Another type of heart transplant is the heterotopic transplant, although this procedure is done rarely. In this technique the donor heart is placed parallel to the recipient's heart (Fig. 47–10). The right side of the client's heart can continue to function while the dysfunctional left side of the heart is bypassed.

Recognition and treatment of rejection are the most difficult tasks of heart transplantation. The most reliable technique used to assess rejection is the endomyocardial biopsy. The biopsy technique enables identification of the diffuse interstitial infiltrate associated with rejection.

Drug therapy is adjusted to give the maximum amount of immunosuppression with the minimum amount of side effects. This is a very individualistic regimen. There is a higher risk of acute rejection soon after transplantation that decreases dramatically after 3 months. Immunosuppression treatment relies on four main drugs: cyclosporine, prednisone, azathioprine, and OKT3 (Box 47–4). Even with this intense drug therapy, 84% of heart transplant clients have at least one episode of rejection during the first 3 months.

For these rejection episodes, pulse therapy with methylprednisolone is used. High doses are given for 3 consecutive days, then gradually reduced over the next 2 weeks. Because of the side effects of increased steroid therapy, the client must be monitored carefully for infections. If the steroid therapy has not been successful in reversing the rejection, other, more aggressive therapy is begun. Equine antithymocyte globulin or OKT3 monoclonal antibody therapy may be used. Some clients have persistent recurrent rejection episodes, which have been treated with total lymphoid irradiation.

In the long term, survival and rehabilitation can be expected in most recipients.

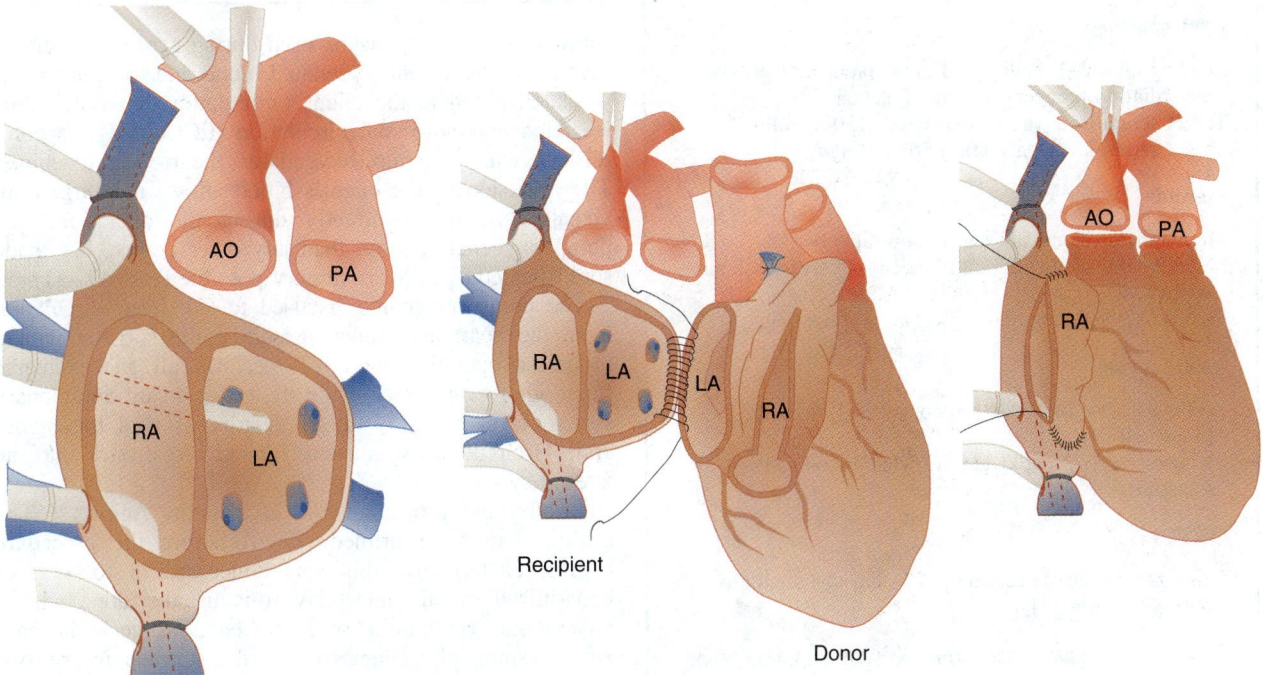

Figure 47–9. The orthotopic technique of heart transplantation.

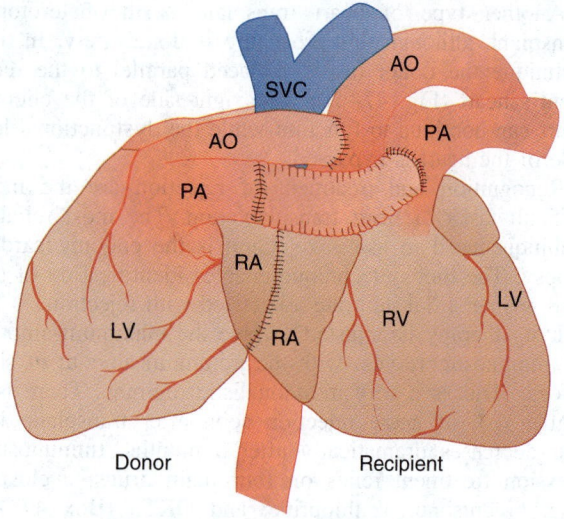

Figure 47–10. The heterotopic technique of heart transplantation.

Assisted Circulation and Mechanical Hearts

Cardiac failure leads to multisystem organ failure if it is not reversed. Sometimes, despite maximal therapy, the failing heart will not adequately respond to therapy. If, for various reasons, cardiac transplantation is not an immediate option, other therapies are sought. It is in these cases that assisted circulation devices or mechanical

---

Box 47–4. Stanford University Immunosuppressive Protocol for Heart Transplantation—1988

Cyclosporine

Loading dose 2–8 mg/kg 2–3 hours preoperatively (dose according to preoperative renal function)
Target serum level (first month) 100–150 ng/ml
Target serum level (thereafter) 50–150 ng/ml

Steroids

Methylprednisolone 500 mg intraoperatively
Methylprednisolone 125 mg intravenously every 8 hours × 3
Prednisone beginning 0.6 mg/kg/day + tapering

Azathioprine

Loading dose 4 mg/kg intravenously 2–3 hours preoperatively
Maintenance 1–2 mg/kg/day (to white blood cell tolerance)

OKT3

5 mg intravenously every day × 14 days beginning on postoperative day 1

From Hurst, J. W. (1990). *The heart* (7th ed.). New York: McGraw-Hill.

---

hearts seem like the only option. Intra-aortic balloon counterpulsation is discussed elsewhere in this chapter. Other devices that are currently being used in practice or tested include external centrifugal and roller pumps, external pulsatile ventricular assist devices, implantable left ventricular assist systems, and orthotopic biventricular replacement prostheses (artificial hearts). Many of these devices offer a bridge to transplantation when the client's heart is failing and a donor heart is not readily available. These devices will maintain a client until transplant surgery is able to be performed.

The artificial heart is a commercially made device implanted in place of the failing heart. These hearts are made of rubber, silicone, and Teflon and are air-powered through a life-support console. The artificial heart is attached surgically in an operation similar to that described in the heart transplant procedure. Major complications (hemorrhage, infection, acute tubular necrosis, and neurologic disturbances) have been encountered frequently, and the permanent use of the artificial heart is currently not recommended. There is some use of the artificial heart as a bridge to transplantation, helping patients survive until a donor heart is available.

The greatest single problem in performing heart transplants is not the surgical procedure itself but the rejection process by which the client's body rejects the donor heart. Allograft rejection, discussed in Chapter 27, remains poorly understood. The recipient forms antibodies against the foreign heart tissue, which leads to an antigen-antibody reaction. As a result, the heart lining hemorrhages, walls thicken, and the myocardium assumes a mottled appearance. Because of rejection, the new heart fails to function altogether, and circulatory collapse ensues.

Technique of Open Heart Surgery

Cardiopulmonary bypass is used during cardiac surgery to divert the client's unoxygenated blood and to return reoxygenated blood to the client's circulation. This technique is called extracorporeal circulation (ECC) and is accomplished with a pump oxygenator (heart-lung machine). The diversion of the client's blood allows the surgeon to visualize the heart directly during the operation. The pump oxygenator, more than any other device, has made sophisticated open heart surgery possible (Fig. 47–11).

The pump oxygenator is used to (1) divert circulation from the heart and lungs, providing the surgeon with a bloodless operative field; (2) perform all gas exchange functions for the body while the client's cardiopulmonary system is at rest; (3) filter, rewarm, or cool the blood; and (4) circulate oxygenated, filtered blood back into the arterial system.

Briefly, the procedure for ECC is as follows.[12] The machine must be primed (filled) before the procedure begins. Historically, this was done with 3 to 4 L of heparinized blood, but today it is usually done with a physiologic crystalloid solution (e.g., Ringer's lactate). After opening the client's chest, the surgeon inserts two large-bore cannulas through the right atrium into the superior and inferior venae cavae and suction catheters into

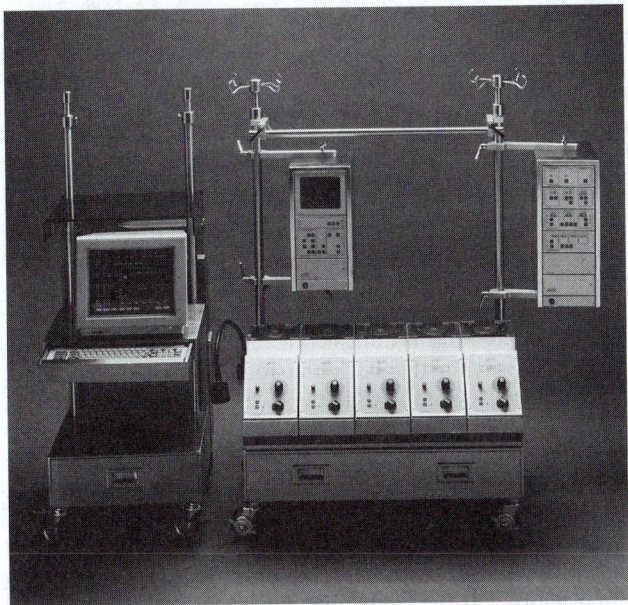

Figure 47–11. The Stöckert heart-lung bypass machine with a computer-aided perfusion system—a type of pump-oxygenator, or heart-lung bypass machine. Machines like this are used during open heart surgery to circulate oxygenated blood while the heart is unable to pump. (Courtesy of Sorin Biomedical, Irvine, CA.)

the thoracic cavity and ventricles. Blood is next pumped from the venae cavae, the thoracic cavity, and the ventricles into the pump oxygenator. In the machine, a heat exchanger rewarms (or cools, if the surgeon wants hypothermia) the blood. An oxygenator then removes carbon dioxide from the blood and adds oxygen. Finally, the blood passes through a filter that removes air bubbles and other emboli before returning to the body via either the aorta or the femoral artery.

Although the pump oxygenator is considered safe, it does have risks. The pump can crush and destroy blood cells; sludging of cells can lead to thrombus formation; or air emboli can form. Other complications related to ECC are shock, hemorrhage, fluid overload, hemolysis, and kidney or lung damage.

The extracorporeal membrane oxygenator (ECMO) is a more expensive but improved method of ECC. The advantages include less trauma to blood cells and prolonged pump time (up to several days). However, the clinical benefits are still being evaluated.[12]

 Acute and Subacute Care

■ Medical Management Before Cardiac Surgery

Clients may enter the healthcare facility a few days before surgery for a thorough medical evaluation. Preoperative laboratory tests include urine tests and blood electrolyte, enzyme, and coagulation studies. Important diagnostic studies that give valuable information about cardiac status include the ECG, phonocardiogram, echo-

cardiogram, vectorcardiogram, chest x-ray films, and cardiac catheterization.

Any physiologic imbalance or problem in cardiac or respiratory status is corrected when possible by means of rest, diet, medication, or other appropriate therapy. Physiologic baselines should be established for postoperative comparison of vital signs, weight, and laboratory values.

■ Nursing Management Before Cardiac Surgery

Preparation for surgery is discussed in Chapter 21. However, the client undergoing the stress of heart surgery needs some special preparation and instruction.

Assessment

The client undergoing heart surgery has probably experienced cardiopulmonary clinical manifestations for months or years. Data to collect during the initial assessment include the following.

- The primary cardiovascular problem that requires surgical correction and its duration
- The purpose of the surgery and the risk involved
- Past cardiopulmonary illnesses that may predispose the client to postoperative complications (e.g., bacterial endocarditis, pulmonary embolus, allergy, abnormal bleeding)
- The degree of cardiac impairment (e.g., does the client have symptoms when at rest or only during exertion?)
- The types of medications and interventions that the client has received or is currently receiving (e.g., digitalis, quinidine, oxygen)

The nurse should note the client's psychological readiness for surgery and his or her reaction to the need for heart surgery. Typically, the client will pass through three psychological stages when preparing for heart surgery:

1. Confrontation. The client may initially experience shock and grief over the impending surgery. Chief concerns may be helplessness and fear of disability or death.
2. Self-reflection. The client may try to explain or justify the cause of the problem.
3. Resolution. Finally, if the client successfully negotiates the first two stages, the meaning of the surgery will be internalized and incorporated into the "self."

Psychological Preparation

The psychological preparation of the cardiac surgery client is very important. Many hospitals around the country have quite extensive preoperative education programs that greatly reduce client and family anxiety. A program to reduce preoperative anxiety should include a thorough explanation of the preoperative, intraoperative, and postoperative procedures. Also helpful is the introduction of the client to involved healthcare team members and the healthcare facility environment. Box 47–5 provides a list of topics for education. Your institution probably has written material for you to use.

Box 47–5. Guidelines to Preparing the Client Undergoing Cardiac Surgery

Plan teaching well in advance of the surgical date, if possible. By the time of surgery, the client should be prepared by the following:

1. Describe the surgical procedure:

   - The surgical procedure, including heart-lung machine
   - Review of the anatomy and physiology of the heart and valves
   - Brief definition of unfamiliar technical terms
   - Length of time in surgery and approximate time of first visit by family
   - Giving the client pictures of the heart and involved valve for future reference

2. Describe the intensive care unit (ICU) environment and monitoring equipment:

   - Cardiac monitor and alarm
   - Endotracheal (ET) tube and projected length of time with ET tube in place
   - Mechanical ventilator and alarm
   - Suctioning procedure
   - Arterial line and automatic blood pressure cuff
   - Any limitation on visits from family
   - Chest tubes or mediastinal tubes
   - Nasogastric tube and length of NPO (nothing by mouth) status
   - Urinary catheter
   - High noise level in ICU
   - Multiple intravenous lines and fluids

3. Describe preoperative preparation:

   - Shower with antimicrobial soap
   - Shaving of chest, abdomen, neck, and groin
   - Special cardiac studies: echocardiogram, electrocardiogram, cardiac catheterization

4. Describe comfort measures:

   - Pain relief
   - Turning, range-of-motion exercises
   - Out of bed next morning
   - Medication for sleep, if needed

Allow clients to tell you in their own words about their heart problem and the surgery. Correct any misconceptions, using pictures and a model of the heart. Clients tend to ask the greatest number of questions about what will happen to them in the recovery room and intensive care unit (ICU). Prepare them to awaken from anesthesia with a chest tube in place. Also discuss the ventilator that will assist the client's breathing for the first 8 to 24 hours. Remind clients that during this time they will be unable to talk. Explain that an IV line for fluid or blood will be inserted in an arm, and various equipment that continuously monitors vital signs will be attached to their skin. Questions concerning the necessity of using blood products should be answered. Use these facts to respond to concerns about transfusion. Blood transfusions postoperatively are used only as needed; blood is screened carefully, so there is very little risk of contracting acquired

immunodeficiency syndrome (AIDS). Family members can be screened for possible donation. Emphasize that although the client will experience pain, the pain will be swiftly relieved by medication and comfort measures.

Finally, explain that the client will be awakened frequently in the ICU for vital nursing assessments and interventions. Give examples of scheduled activities: vital signs every 15 minutes; temperature every 2 hours; frequent turning, coughing, and deep breathing; blood draws for tests every morning.

Clients also need information concerning discharge from the ICU and healthcare facility. Explain the average length of stay in the ICU, the room to which the client will return from the ICU, the average length of stay in the healthcare facility, and the diet and activities permitted once the client is back home. Be general in the discussion. Remember that many unforeseen events can arise and greatly alter the postoperative course.

Give verbal and written information concerning (1) healthcare facility services, rules, and regulations; (2) visiting hours; (3) the chaplain's name and visiting hours (if appropriate); and (4) names of clinical nurse-specialists and other healthcare professionals who can be contacted for information.

Most clients benefit from a tour of the recovery room and ICU. (If they are not physically able to participate in a tour, audiovisual material is helpful.) Familiarize the client with the equipment that will be used in the ICU (e.g., chest drainage tubes, oxygen apparatus, ventilators, cardiac monitors, and IV setups). Reassure the client that lights and alarm noises are part of the critical care environment and are not indicators that something is wrong.

Preoperative Care

Preparation the evening before and the day of surgery is essentially the same as the preparation of clients for any thoracic surgery (see Chapter 42). The client may often take several showers with an antimicrobial soap; skin preparation (shaving) for a thoracotomy is performed in the operating room. If the surgeon plans a coronary artery bypass graft, the legs may also be prepared in the operating room (see Chapter 21).

■ Nursing Management After Cardiac Surgery

Assessment

The most reliable measures of cardiovascular function and tissue perfusion are the vital signs, including arterial blood pressure, pulses, venous and left heart filling pressures, and temperature. Heart sounds are monitored and continuous ECG monitoring is also performed. Stabilization of vital signs after heart surgery usually indicates adequate cardiovascular function. Conversely, severe deviations indicate complications such as hemorrhage, shock, cardiac tamponade, or infection. The normal ranges for each vital sign after cardiac surgery and the meaning of deviations follow.

Arterial Blood Pressure. To obtain an accurate blood pressure reading postoperatively, an 18- or 20-gauge Teflon catheter is (1) inserted into an artery, usually the radial artery, and (2) attached to a strain-gauge transducer via stiff connecting tubing called pressure transmission tubing. This is connected to an electronic pressure monitor and oscilloscope. The monitor provides numerical pressure readings and produces a continuous tracing of the arterial pressure wave form as shown in the Bridge to Critical Care in Chapter 45. The arterial line is usually irrigated (continuously or at intervals) with heparinized water or saline. The arterial line is sometimes used as a route for obtaining blood for laboratory studies.

Most pressure monitors are able to monitor the pulmonary artery, arterial pressures, and ECG tracing simultaneously. This assists in determining the effect that the surgery may have had on hemodynamic status and cardiac output. It can also demonstrate the effect a dysrhythmia or body temperature change may have on cardiac output.

In general, the physician will request that the blood pressure be maintained between 20 mm Hg above and 20 mm Hg below the baseline blood pressure. Frequently, this will be a mean arterial pressure of 70 mm Hg or above. After mitral and aortic valve surgery, clients may tolerate a low systolic blood pressure of 90 mm Hg without difficulty. After coronary artery surgery, clients may not tolerate systolic blood pressure drops of more than 10 mm Hg below preoperative baseline because the myocardium may not be adequately perfused. Maintaining a sufficient diastolic blood pressure is also very important because the myocardium receives 70% of its blood supply during this phase of the cardiac cycle. Careful assessment and monitoring of the client's hemodynamic status is essential.

Hypertension is also dangerous in a client who has undergone a coronary artery bypass graft because the high blood pressure may cause the new graft to break loose or leak. Vasoactive medications can be used to improve cardiac functioning (e.g., vasodilators such as sodium nitroprusside).

Pulses. Check radial pulse for rate, rhythm, and volume. A rapid radial pulse may indicate dysrhythmia, shock, fear, fever, hypoxia, congestive heart failure, or hemorrhage. A slow radial pulse may indicate heart block or severe anoxia.

Check the apical radial pulse for a pulse deficit. Pulse deficit may indicate atrial fibrillation, a frequent complication of mitral stenosis.

Assess peripheral pulses. Absence of pedal pulses may indicate the presence of peripheral emboli blocking a blood vessel in the extremity. Report this finding immediately to the surgeon. If pulses are absent, assess all pulses in the extremity and check the lower extremities for coldness, pallor, or cyanosis.

Venous and Left Heart Filling Pressures. The central venous and pulmonary artery pressures are usually monitored postoperatively. A pressure higher than normal may be acceptable after open heart surgery. This is be-

cause a heart that has been diseased and then is subjected to surgical trauma is weak and needs a higher filling pressure to (1) strengthen the force of myocardial contraction and (2) maintain an adequate cardiac output. Therefore, the surgeon will usually specify values for venous and pulmonary artery pressures that address this problem.

If the client has a pulmonary artery catheter in place, a pulmonary artery wedge pressure (PAWP) can be obtained and cardiac output measured by the thermodilution method. The PAWP is a reflection of the left atrial filling pressure (see Bridge to Critical Care in Chapter 45 for a discussion of the Swan-Ganz catheter and these measurements).

Causes of abnormally elevated central venous pressure and left heart filling pressure include hypervolemia and ineffective myocardial contractions. Abnormally decreased central venous pressure and left heart filling pressure result from hypovolemia.

Body Temperature. Initially, the client has a low temperature of 35° to 36° C (95° to 96.8° F) because of hypothermia induced during surgery. With careful warming in a heating blanket, the client may reach a normal temperature within 4 hours. Be aware that the blood pressure may drop as body temperature rises due to vasodilation.

The temperature may rise 1° to 1.5° C (2° or 3° F) above normal during the first or second day postoperatively and may remain elevated for 3 to 4 days. Treat this with acetaminophen suppositories as prescribed and minimal bed covering. For persistent elevations, apply ice bags or use a hypothermia blanket, if prescribed.

Report abnormal findings, such as an elevated temperature to 38.5° C (101° F) or higher or an elevation that persists for more than 4 or 5 days. Abnormal temperature elevation may result from infection, dehydration, hemolysis due to transfusion reaction, or atelectasis. The untoward effects of the elevated temperature include increased metabolic demands (which increase the work of the heart), dehydration, and hypovolemia.

Abnormally low temperatures ranging from 34.4° C (94° F) to 36° C (96.8° F) result from shock or cardiac decompensation. The physician may order a warming blanket to increase temperature. The Nursing Research feature compares five methods of measuring temperature in the ICU.

Respirations. To assess respiratory function, prevent respiratory complications, and provide appropriate intervention, closely monitor the rate and depth of respirations, the presence of dyspnea, and the presence of wheezing.

Make certain the ventilator is set at a rate that adequately ventilates the client and delivers an appropriate tidal volume and oxygen percentage. A conscious client may initiate respirations in addition to those delivered by the ventilator (usually the assist light will come on). Adjust the rate, tidal volume, and oxygen level so that adequate ventilation of the lungs and oxygenation of the blood are ensured. Adjustments are usually determined by

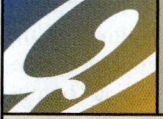

NURSING RESEARCH

How Do Different Methods of Measuring Temperature Compare?

Schmitz, T., et al. (1995). A comparison of five methods of temperature measurement in febrile intensive care patients. *American Journal of Critical Care, 4*(4), 286–292.

Thirteen intensive care patients with temperatures of 37.8° C were studied. Temperature readings in rapid succession were taken using an electronic thermometer for oral and axillary temperatures, a rectal probe, an infrared ear thermometer on core setting, and a pulmonary artery catheter. Temperature readings were obtained every hour during the day and every 4 hours at night.

The results showed that rectal temperatures correlated most closely with pulmonary artery temperatures, followed by oral, ear-based, and axillary temperatures.

Implications for Practice

If the rectal site is contraindicated, oral or ear-based temperatures are acceptable. Axillary temperatures do not correlate well with pulmonary artery temperatures. This should remind nurses of the importance of consistency in method when establishing temperature trends.

arterial blood gas analysis and the assessments by the physician and the nurse.

Assessment of depth of respiration may reveal shallow respirations, which may be due to pain. Give a narcotic if vital signs are stable.

Assessment of dyspnea may reveal that the client is "fighting" the ventilator, in other words, breathing against instead of with the machine. This can lead to inadequate ventilation. The client may feel short of breath. Airway obstruction (possibly due to excessive secretions), pain, fear, anoxia, acidosis, hemorrhage, and improper placement of the tube may cause the client to have difficulty in breathing and must be investigated immediately. The physician usually orders arterial blood gas studies and a chest film. The ventilator settings may need adjustment, and the client may require sedation. (See Bridge to Critical Care for ventilators in Chapter 42.) While the client is on the ventilator, make sure the ventilator alarms are functioning. Never turn off the alarms, not even during suctioning.

Wheezing results from pulmonary edema, bronchospasm, or airway obstruction. It may be treated with bronchodilators.

Assess the amount of pulmonary secretion: copious or scant.

Assess color. Sputum is normally white and translucent. A yellow color suggests infection and represents the presence of WBCs. Green represents old retained secretions with the breakdown of WBCs. Green and foul-smelling secretions usually suggest *Pseudomonas* infection. Red denotes fresh blood. Streaking with red suggests upper airway or tracheal bleeding. Brown represents old blood residue.

Assess for accompanying signs of retained secretions: apprehension, perspiration, rapid pulse, dyspnea, cyanosis, and gurgling respirations.

Assessment of respiration in the preextubation period involves drawing blood for arterial blood gas analysis and obtaining respiratory values, including inspiratory effort and tidal volume. The client is ready for extubation if these values are within normal limits.

Respiratory assessment in the postextubation period begins with careful assessment of clinical manifestations of respiratory distress. Check the rate, depth, and character of respirations frequently. Note the client's skin color and vital signs; changes may indicate inadequate ventilation and the need for reintubation. Arterial blood gases should be analyzed to determine whether the client is breathing adequately after extubation.

Heart Sounds. For the first 2 days postoperatively, assess heart sounds at least every 4 hours. Pericardial rubs are commonly caused by the irritation and inflammation from surgery. A new murmur may indicate valve problems. Notify the physician if one develops. A gallop probably indicates hypervolemia. See discussion of cardiovascular assessment in Chapter 44.

Electrocardiogram Tracings. Monitor the electrical activity of the client's heart continuously for at least 3 or 4 days after surgery. Observe carefully for abnormal ECG tracings; heart block, ventricular tachycardia, and atrial fibrillation commonly complicate open heart surgery. The physician requests 12-lead ECGs preoperatively, immediately postoperatively, and before discharge to observe for signs of perioperative infarction.

Most dysrhythmias can be treated effectively with antiarrhythmic medications. These medications are listed in Chapter 46. Some life-threatening dysrhythmias require defibrillation or cardioversion (see Chapter 46).

Often the surgeon implants atrial or ventricular pacing wires during surgery. These are small wires that lead from the myocardium through the chest wall. They can be connected to an external pacemaker and used to treat bradycardia or heart block. These wires should always be insulated. When connecting them to a pacemaker, wear rubber gloves. Microshocks to these wires could result in atrial or ventricular fibrillation. Atrial pacing wires can also be connected to the chest leads of an ECG machine for differential diagnosis of atrial arrhythmias.

Chest Drainage. Check chest drainage from chest tubes. The surgeon inserts chest tubes to drain air and fluid from the pleural cavity, thereby allowing the lungs to respond after surgery. Chest tubes can also drain the pericardial sac. These tubes are called mediastinal tubes.

Measure and observe chest drainage by collecting drainage in a calibrated cylinder. (Most hospitals use disposable chest drainage setups that are clearly calibrated.)

Measure findings and record hourly. Up to 100 ml of drainage may be lost during the first hour postoperatively as a result of reexpansion of the lungs, which forces drainage through the chest tube. There will be approximately 500 ml of drainage over the first 24 hours. Large gushes of drainage are sometimes expelled when the client coughs or turns. Drainage, usually dark red during the early postoperative phase, gradually becomes more serous as time passes. Chest tubes are fully discussed in Chapter 42.

Bloody mediastinal drainage that is collected from the chest tubes can be transfused back into the client (autotransfusion). This transfused blood has the advantage of being the client's own blood and not blood from the blood bank. There is less risk to the client and less cost. The bloody drainage is infused into the client with the use of filtered IV tubing. Different manufacturers make disposable chest drainage systems that have this autotransfusion capability.

Fluid Balance. Carefully measure and record intake and output. Obtain daily weights to determine whether the client is retaining fluids within tissues or losing excessive fluid rapidly. Significant fluctuations in weight act as a guide to fluid replacement.

Renal Function. Measure volume hourly for the first 8 to 12 hours after surgery. The client almost always has an indwelling urinary catheter. Normal output is greater than 30 ml/hr. Urine may be bloody as a result of hemolysis of erythrocytes during ECC.

The urine 24-hour specific gravity should be assessed. Normal value is 1.015 to 1.020. Specific gravity may rise because of oliguria or the presence of red blood cells. Lowered specific gravity results from overhydration or inability of kidney tubules to filter waste products.

Electrolyte Balance. Daily electrolyte studies are performed to determine blood levels of sodium, potassium, and chloride. The physician replaces electrolytes parenterally if they are deficient. If diuretics are given to reduce volume overload, monitor potassium closely and replace as prescribed. The heart may be particularly sensitive to hypokalemia soon after surgery. Obtain hematocrit, hemoglobin, and prothrombin time daily to determine extent of blood loss or hemorrhage, and daily blood gases to determine the pH, and partial pressures of arterial carbon dioxide ($PaCO_2$) and oxygen (PaO_2) (see Chapter 16).

Neurologic Response. After heart surgery, carefully observe the client's level of consciousness, pupil size and reaction, orientation, and ability to move extremities.

The client should awaken within 1 to 2 hours after surgery. Failure to awaken may result from embolization of air, calcium, fat, or thrombotic particles to the brain. Slow return to consciousness (over 2–4 days) may result from a diffuse neurologic deficit due to poor cerebral capillary perfusion during ECC.

Check pupils hourly during the early postoperative period for size, equality in size, and reaction to light. Pupils dilate when blood contains excess carbon dioxide.

Disorientation and restlessness may indicate anoxia or embolization to the brain. Also, fatigue or fear can produce mental confusion.

Hemiplegia, inability to move an extremity, or extreme weakness of an extremity may indicate embolization to the motor area of the brain.

After cardiac surgery, clients may become disoriented, delusional, and psychotic. Severe depression is not uncommon. Causes of confusion, hallucinations, and psychotic behavior include (1) isolation within the ICU, (2) sensory deprivation, (3) lack of rest and sleep over an extended period, (4) fear and anxiety, (5) an impersonal environment if care providers are preoccupied with monitors and machines, and (6) desynchronization of circadian rhythm (ICUs are active and well-lighted 24 hours a day). Causes of postoperative depression include (1) fatigue and debility after surgery and (2) resumption of responsibilities.[53]

Diagnosis, Planning, Implementation

Risk for Decreased Cardiac Output. Heart failure, metabolic acidosis, weakening of the left ventricle, dysrhythmias, and cardiac tamponade can decrease cardiac output. State this diagnosis as *Risk for Decreased Cardiac Output related to* (choose the appropriate cause).

Planning: Expected Outcomes. The client will have improved cardiovascular function, as evidenced by adequate tissue perfusion, stabilization of vital signs, clear lung sounds on auscultation, stable body weight, adequate urine output (30 ml/hr or greater), no reported or observed dyspnea or orthopnea, regular heart sounds without S_3 or S_4, and decreased or absent peripheral edema (blood pressure within 20 mm Hg of baseline values).

Implementation. Intervention for a failing heart muscle often involves administration of inotropic agents (e.g., dopamine, isoproterenol, or epinephrine), which increase cardiac contractility. Administer inotropic agents cautiously because they also increase the work of the heart and its need for oxygen.

Complications resulting from persistent hypotension are cerebral ischemia, renal shutdown, myocardial infarction, and shock. To correct these complications, the surgeon may use a mechanical device to support the failing heart if medications are unsuccessful.

The intra-aortic balloon pump (IABP) is a counterpulsation device that supports the failing heart by increasing coronary artery perfusion during diastole and reducing afterload. It consists of a sausage-shaped balloon catheter that is passed through the femoral artery and positioned in the descending thoracic aorta just distal to the subclavian artery. The catheter is attached to a power console that inflates and deflates the balloon in time with the heart. The balloon is inflated during diastole: blood is pushed back into the aorta, and coronary artery perfusion is improved. The balloon is deflated during systole: resistance is decreased, and thereby the workload of the heart is reduced (see Bridge to Critical Care). The timing of the balloon inflations and deflations is critical. A nurse educated in the use of the balloon pump is assigned to

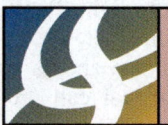

BRIDGE TO CRITICAL CARE

Intra-Aortic Balloon Pumping (IABP)—Counterpulsation

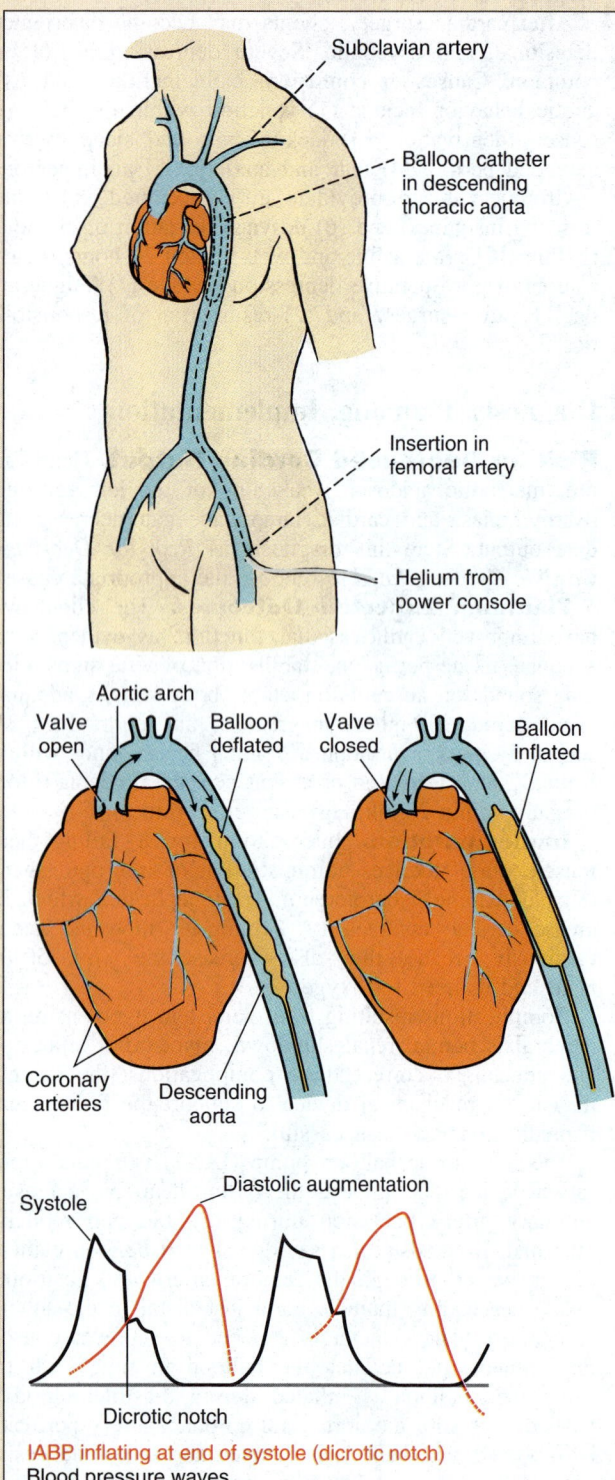

Subclavian artery

Balloon catheter
in descending
thoracic aorta

Insertion in
femoral artery

Helium from
power console

Aortic arch

Valve open | Balloon deflated | Valve closed | Balloon inflated

Coronary arteries | Descending aorta

Systole | Diastolic augmentation

Dicrotic notch

IABP inflating at end of systole (dicrotic notch)
Blood pressure waves

When the left ventricle fails to support adequate circulation and perfusion, intra-aortic balloon pumping can be used in both medical and surgical settings to support the injured or ischemic myocardium. The device consists of a polyethylene balloon that is inserted via the femoral artery into the descending thoracic aorta distal to the left subclavian artery, and is connected to an external pneumatic pumping system. The pump inflates the balloon with helium or carbon dioxide during diastole, and deflates it during systole. The inflation-deflation cycle is triggered by the client's ECG, specifically by the R wave, which signals the beginning of systole. Balloon deflation during diastole augments coronary artery filling. Systolic balloon deflation decreases afterload.

Guidelines for Management of IABP

Indications for Use

- Complications of acute myocardial infarction
  Cardiogenic shock
  Papillary muscle rupture or dysfunction with severe mitral valve regurgitation
  Ventricular septal defect
  Refractory ventricular arrhythmias related to ischemia
- Left ventricular failure
- Unstable angina refractory to medications
- Preoperative open heart surgery or cardiac transplantation
- Prophylaxis, noncardiac surgeries, high-risk PTCA
- Septic shock
- Low cardiac output syndromes

Complications

- On insertion, dissection of the arterial system (femoral, iliac, aorta)
- Plaque dislodgment causing embolization
- Balloon rupture
- Arterial occlusion
- Mechanical destruction of RBCs
- Inability to wean from IABP
- Hematoma at insertion site

Nursing Precautions

- Select an ECG lead that optimizes the R wave
- Time the IABP using arterial waveform
- Monitor perfusion in extremity with IAB
- Maintain immobility in cannulated extremity
- Monitor for balloon rupture and misplacement
- Monitor for pain, bleeding disorders, and aortic dissection
- Clarify and/or reinforce client and family understanding of IABP

ECG, electrocardiogram; PTCA, percutaneous transluminal coronary angioplasty; RBCs, red blood cells.

care for the client. Monitoring the effects of the pumping on the client's vital signs requires special skills.

Risk for Ineffective Airway Clearance.
Retained secretions are common after open heart surgery. State the diagnosis as *Risk for Ineffective Airway Clearance related to retained secretions.* Also consider using the diagnosis of *Impaired Gas Exchange* if the client has marginal levels of oxygen saturation.

Planning: Expected Outcomes. The client will exhibit improved airway clearance, as evidenced by clear lung sounds, afebrile state, strong nonproductive cough, and arterial blood gas values within normal limits.

Implementation. Turn and suction the intubated client frequently. Today, most clients are extubated within hours of surgery. Skilled nursing care to promote pulmonary hygiene is critical. Help the nonintubated client to turn, take deep breaths, and cough every 1 to 2 hours; suction the trachea if the temperature rises to about 38.5° C (101° F) and the client is coughing ineffectively. In addition, the client can wear a high-humidity oxygen mask after removal of the endotracheal tube for help in loosening secretions. Chest physiotherapy may be used to loosen secretions. In rare cases, bronchoscopy may be indicated for removal of secretions. Complications of retained secretions include atelectasis, pneumonia, and subsequent inadequate oxygenation of the tissues. Monitor oxygen saturation continuously.

Hemorrhage.
State the collaborative problem as *Hemorrhage related to surgical trauma or slipped ligature* (suture).

Planning: Expected Outcomes. Collaborative problems are only monitored by the nurse. Therefore, the expected outcome addresses the nurse's actions, not the client's goals. The nurse will monitor the client for amounts of drainage in excess of 2 ml/kg body weight per hour or a sustained period of bleeding through the chest tube.

Implementation. If bleeding is noted, the physician should be notified because the client may need to be returned to the operating room for repair of the bleeding sites. Replace blood by transfusion as prescribed. The chest drainage may be autotransfused back into the client from the chest drainage system through an IV line. The use of blood transfusions has decreased dramatically since the onset of HIV. However, sometimes it is necessary to replace blood lost during surgery. If the client's hematocrit is adequate, albumin or high-molecular-weight plasma expanders, such as hetastarch, may be prescribed in place of blood.

Risk for Cardiac Tamponade.
Occlusion in the pericardial drainage system can lead to cardiac tamponade. State this collaborative problem as *Risk for Cardiac Tamponade related to occlusion of the pericardial drainage system.*

Planning: Expected Outcomes. The nurse will monitor the client for sudden cessation of chest drainage with an increase in venous pressure, pulsus paradoxus,

dyspnea, oliguria, distant or inaudible heart sounds, or lowered left atrial pressure.

Implementation. Pericardial chest tube stripping is no longer performed. Gentle milking of the chest tube to express clots that could block drainage may be performed. If clots cannot be removed by gentle milking of the tube, the physician may need to declot the tube using a long catheter with an inflatable balloon on the end. The client may need to be returned to the operating room or have a pericardial tap for removal of fluid.

Risk for Renal Failure.
State this collaborative problem as *Risk for Renal Failure related to* (add specific risk). Hypovolemia, decreased cardiac output, or hemolysis of erythrocytes during cardiopulmonary bypass can lead to acute renal failure.

Planning: Expected Outcomes. The nurse will monitor urinary output, expecting output greater than 30 ml/hr. Laboratory values for blood urea nitrogen (BUN), creatinine, and potassium should also be monitored.

Implementation. A client with decreased urine output may be treated with extra fluids (sometimes called a fluid challenge) if dehydration is the probable etiologic factor. Other interventions may include correcting shock or low output failure and administering a diuretic (e.g., furosemide) IV. The client who develops renal failure requires peritoneal dialysis or hemodialysis.

During the course of surgery, the client typically receives 3 to 4 L of extra fluid. Often this fluid accumulates as edema and does not increase the vascular volume very much. However, the fluid does place the client at high risk of circulatory overload. Because of this, IV fluids are administered judiciously for the first 3 days postoperatively to avoid overwork of the heart. Typically, 500 to 700 ml/m² body surface/24 hr including oral intake (normal surface area is 1.5–2.0 m²) will be given. Administer sodium-containing fluids cautiously to prevent circulatory overload and heart failure.

Risk for Paralytic Ileus.
Sympathetic responses leading to shunting of blood from the gastrointestinal tract during surgery, side effects of anesthesia and narcotics, and immobility lead to paralytic ileus. State this collaborative problem as *Risk for Paralytic Ileus* (choose the appropriate cause; all may apply in this case).

Planning: Expected Outcomes. The nurse will monitor the client for clinical manifestations of ileus, as evidenced by hypoactive or absent bowel sounds, abdominal distention, nausea, vomiting, lack of appetite, and no passing of flatus.

Implementation. Give sips of water 4 hours after extubation if the client is fully responsive and not nauseated. The client may have clear liquids next, followed by solid foods. Watch for signs of abdominal distention and paralytic ileus (see Chapter 21). If either of these conditions develops, stop oral fluids and notify the physician.

Risk for Pain.
Sternal and leg incisions cause intense pain after surgery. Express this common diagnosis as *Risk for Pain related to sternal and leg incision.*

Planning: Expected Outcomes. The client will have increased comfort, as evidenced by normal heart rate, no restlessness, normal respiratory rate, reports of comfort, decreasing use of narcotics, and periods of rest.

Implementation. Give narcotic analgesics for pain postoperatively as ordered. Avoid overmedicating a client who is recovering from hypothermia because narcotic metabolism is slowed and the medication may not be excreted. Attempt to relieve the pain and restlessness with comfort measures before administering a narcotic. Most clients have more pain in the legs than sternum.

Risk for Altered Cerebral Tissue Perfusion.

The surgical procedure, hemodynamic stability, electrolyte imbalances, hypoxia, medications, and several other potential problems can lead to impaired cerebral circulation. Use this nursing diagnosis early after surgery. Later, if confusion develops, use *Risk for Injury or Acute Confusion* as the best diagnosis.

Planning: Expected Outcomes. The client will demonstrate adequate cerebral tissue perfusion, as evidenced by continuous progress toward an alert level of consciousness.

Implementation. To prevent mental confusion, undue fear, anxiety, and tension, consider the following:

- Always address the client by name and introduce yourself by name.
- Place a calendar and clock at the bedside to orient the client to the date and time of day.
- Take an interest in the client. Do not ignore the client while working with monitors and equipment.
- Position the cardiac monitor so that it is out of the client's view. Many clients become nervous watching their own heart action.
- Schedule the day so that periods of nursing intervention alternate with periods of rest and relaxation.
- Encourage the client to freely discuss fears and anxieties.
- Prepare significant others for changes in the client's sensorium after surgery. Before visiting times, warn visitors if the client is hallucinating or is severely depressed so that they know what to expect.
- Explain all interventions to the client and allow time for questions.

Risk for Impaired Physical Mobility.

Prolonged bedrest after surgery and a weakened condition before surgery lead to impaired physical mobility. State this diagnosis as *Impaired Physical Mobility related to prolonged bedrest or weakened condition before surgery* (or both).

Planning: Expected Outcomes. The client will demonstrate postoperative mobility, as evidenced by having mobility that is equal to or greater than preoperative mobility.

Implementation. Prolonged periods of bedrest after heart surgery (or any surgery) may cause weakness, pooling of respiratory secretions, atelectasis, thrombophlebitis, osteoporosis, urinary retention, renal calculi, and a negative nitrogen balance. Planned activity is the most important single factor in preventing the complications of bedrest. The type and amount of activity allowed for each client depend on the type of surgery and the client's general postoperative condition.

Turning and Exercising. If the client is stable, turn him or her from side to side at intervals for back care. Perform passive exercises and leg flexion every 2 hours to prevent thrombosis of lower extremities.

Typical Ambulation Schedule. The day after surgery, the client usually dangles the legs over the side of the bed for a short period. That evening or on postoperative day 2, the client usually sits in a chair for a brief time. On day 3 to 5, the client begins to ambulate in the room and up and down the hallway. By the day 8 to 10, the client is usually fully ambulatory. Cardiac monitors are used to evaluate the client's response to increasing activity.

It usually takes 8 to 10 weeks for clients to fully regain strength after surgery. On discharge home, the client gradually increases activity until moderate walks and climbing stairs do not cause undue fatigue. The client usually returns to work 2 months after surgery.

Risk for Transplant Rejection.

Recall that the body's normal response to foreign protein is to recognize and destroy it. Rejection of the transplanted heart is a common concern with transplantation. State this collaborative problem as *Risk for Transplant Rejection related to immune response after surgery.*

Planning: Expected Outcomes. The nurse will monitor for clinical manifestations of rejection, as evidenced by decreases in oxygenation, fever, malaise, anxiety, and infiltrates on chest film.

Implementation. Rejection and infection are the most common complications of cardiac transplantation. The prevention of rejection with immunosuppression is continually being examined (see immunosuppressive protocol, Box 47–4). Cyclosporine has been helpful in preventing rejection but is toxic. Renal failure, hypertension, liver toxic effects, and neurologic disturbances are not uncommon.

Risk for Infection.

The loss of primary defenses and use of immunosuppressive agents in clients with transplants makes them excellent candidates for infections. State this common nursing diagnosis as *Risk for Infection related to loss of primary defenses (skin incision) and use of immunosuppression.*

Planning: Expected Outcomes. The client will exhibit no clinical manifestations of infection, as evidenced by remaining afebrile and having WBC levels within normal limits, no malaise, and no abnormal heart sounds.

Implementation. Infection remains the major cause of death in the early postoperative period as well as a major cause of death after 1 year in heart transplant clients. Clients are treated prophylactically with antibiotics. Nonhealing sternal wounds are treated promptly. Myocutaneous flaps may be required (see Chapter 80).

Evaluation

Clients who have open heart surgery for coronary bypass may have a leg incision from a saphenous vein graft. These long incisions can be slow to heal, in part due to decreased peripheral circulation. Delayed leg wound healing is a very common problem. Wounds are usually cleaned twice daily with povidone-iodine and redressed.

The degree of expected outcome attainment should be examined frequently. Some of the problems discussed in the care of the client after heart surgery require prompt treatment (e.g., dysrhythmias); others can be evaluated over longer periods of time.

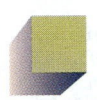

Community and Self-Care

As the client returns home, his or her activity level will continue to increase. It takes approximately 6 weeks postoperatively for the sternum to heal. During that time, advise the client to lift nothing heavier than 5 lb. Also, the client must not drive, because driving can strain the incision. As the client gets into and out of bed or a chair, the arms should not bear weight; the arms are used only for balance. Teach the client and significant others to inspect the incision daily. Care of the incision may include swabbing with povidone-iodine and applying dry dressings over oozing areas.

Some cities have developed exercise rehabilitation programs for clients who have had heart attacks or heart surgery. These programs involve supervised, closely monitored exercise sessions and teaching.

Low sodium and low cholesterol diets are often prescribed for clients after cardiac surgery. In order for the client to be able to comply with dietary instruction, the diet must be carefully planned. Diets for clients with heart disease are discussed in Chapter 45.

Teach the client or significant other to check the pulse daily for rate and regularity and to call the physician if the resting heart rate rises by more than 20 beats per minute or a new irregularity is present. The client can also use heart rate to monitor responses to exercise. Authorities usually recommend a rise of not more than 20 beats per minute for the immediate postoperative period.

Make sure the client knows how and when to schedule follow-up appointments. Instruct the client to report the following to the primary healthcare provider:

- Signs or symptoms of infection, including fever, and increased redness, tenderness, or swelling of incisions
- Palpitations, tachycardia, or irregular pulse (if normally regular)
- Dizziness or increased fatigue
- Sudden weight gain or peripheral edema
- Shortness of breath

Modifications for Elderly Clients

Elderly clients often have many other disorders that interfere with or delay their ability to respond to the hemodynamic changes of surgery and recovery. The elderly client is also more prone to problems of skin breakdown and renal impairment. Fluids must be closely titrated because there are often preexistent heart disorders.

Conclusions

The client with a cardiac disorder frequently has activity intolerance, decreased cardiac output, and ineffective coping due to the seriousness of the disorder. Nurses must be skilled in the physical and psychosocial aspects of disease when providing care.

Thinking Critically

1. A 45-year-old man arrives in the emergency department from an automobile accident. Initially, the client does not complain about himself, but is more concerned about his daughter who was injured in the accident. Neither the child nor the client were wearing seat belts when their car was struck from behind. While sitting at his daughter's bedside in the emergency department, the client becomes more and more anxious; his respiratory rate increases, and he becomes restless. The vital signs reveal a blood pressure of 88/72, pulse of 118, and respirations of 28. What other assessments are needed to rule out cardiac tamponade? What intervention will relieve pressure on the heart and improve cardiac function?

Factors to Consider. What are the clinical manifestations of cardiac tamponade? How is cardiac output affected by cardiac tamponade?

2. The client is a 60-year-old man with dilated cardiomyopathy. His prognosis is very poor. He is able only to tolerate minimal amounts of activity: using the bedside commode, feeding himself, and shaving himself in bed. Today, he continues to be short of breath but seems particularly withdrawn. Repeated physical assessment to identify cardiovascular status shows no change in assessment findings. He continues to take his medications at the proper dosages. His physician thinks these medications are at their maximal levels. Repeated psychosocial assessment would show that the client is withdrawn because he is anxious that he will become physically worse, hospitalized, and placed on a ventilator again. He does not wish to be placed on a ventilator. He was terrified the last time and sees no purpose in just prolonging his dying. What nursing actions might help your client?

Factors to Consider. What are the clinical manifestations of cardiomyopathy? What are the psychologic considerations for the client's care?

3. A 52-year-old man with a lengthy history of mitral valve prolapse is recovering from kidney transplantation surgery. This is his fourth postoperative day and he and his spouse are asking questions about

care at home. What priorities for client education should be established?

Factors to Consider. What complication is associated with mitral valve prolapse? How does the medication regimen following transplantation surgery further place the client at risk?

Bibliography

1. Antman, E. M. (1992). Medical management of the patient undergoing cardiac surgery. In E. Braunwald (Ed.). *Heart disease* (pp 1670–1693). Philadelphia: W. B. Saunders.
2. American Heart Association, (1993). *Heart and stroke facts.* Dallas: Author.
3. Assey, M. (1993). Heart disease in the elderly. *Heart Disease and Stroke, 2,* 330.
4. Barbiere, C. C. (1990). Cardiac tamponade: Diagnosis and emergency intervention. *Critical Care Nurse, 10*(4), 20–22.
5. Barden, C., et al. (1990). Balloon aortic valvuloplasty: Nursing care implications. *Critical Care Nurse, 10*(6), 22–30, 86.
6. Bates, B. (1995). *A guide to physical examination and history taking.* Philadelphia: J. B. Lippincott.
7. Baumgartner, W. A. (1990). Comparative results and future implications of heart transplantation. In W. A. Baumgartner, B. A. Reitz, & S. C. Achuff (Eds.). *Heart and heart-lung transplantation.* Philadelphia: W. B. Saunders.
8. Baumgartner, W. A. (1990). Evaluation and management of the heart donor. In W. A. Baumgartner, B. A. Reitz, & S. C. Achuff (Eds.). *Heart and heart-lung transplantation.* Philadelphia: W. B. Saunders.
9. Berne, R. M., & Levy, M. N. (1992). *Cardiovascular physiology.* St. Louis: Mosby–Year Book.
10. Billingham, M. E. (1990). The pathology of transplanted hearts. *Seminars in Thoracic and Cardiovascular Surgery, 2,* 233–237.
11. Bisno, A. L., et al. (1990). Antimicrobial treatment of infective endocarditis due to *viridans* streptococci, enterococci, and staphylococci. *JAMA 261,* 1471.
12. Blanche, C., et al. (1990). Technical aspects of cardiopulmonary bypass. In R. J. Gray & J. M. Matloff (Eds.). *Medical management of the cardiac surgery patient.* Baltimore: Williams & Wilkins.
13. Braunwald, E. (1992). Valvular heart disease. In E. Braunwald (Ed.). *Heart disease* (pp. 1007–1077). Philadelphia: W. B. Saunders.
14. Burge, D. J., & DeHoratius, R. J. (1993). Acute rheumatic fever. *Cardiovascular Clinics, 23,* 3.
15. Cardin, S. (1992). The person with pericarditis, pericardial effusion, and cardiac tamponade. In C. E. Guzzetta & B. M. Dossey (Eds.). *Cardiovascular nursing.* St. Louis: Mosby–Year Book.
16. Carpenito, L. J. (1995). *Nursing diagnosis.* Philadelphia: J. B. Lippincott.
17. Cavallo, G. O. (1992). The person with valvular heart disease. In C. E. Guzzetta, & B. M. Dossey (Eds.). *Cardiovascular nursing.* St. Louis: Mosby–Year Book.
18. Chan, J. C., & Bisno, A. L. (1991). Rheumatic fever and rheumatic heart disease. *Practical Cardiology, 17*(4), 25–42.
19. Child, J. S. (1991). Infective endocarditis: Risks and prophylaxis. *Journal of the American College of Cardiology, 18*(2), 337–338.
20. Craver, J. M. (1990). Surgical reconstruction for regurgitant lesions of the mitral valve. In J. W. Hurst (Ed.). *The heart.* New York: McGraw-Hill.
21. Dalen, J. E. (1990). Valvular heart disease, infected valves and prosthetic heart valves. *American Journal of Cardiology, 65*(6), 29c–31c.
22. Daljani, A. S. (1990). Prevention of bacterial endocarditis: Recommendations by the American Heart Association. *JAMA, 264*(22), 2919–2922.
23. Deanfield, J. E., Gersh, B. J., & Mair, D. D. (1994). Adult congenital disease (pp. 1829–1856). In J. W. Hurst (Ed.). *The heart.* New York: McGraw-Hill.
24. Decker, C. F., & Trazon, C. V. (1994). *Staphylococcus aureus* pericarditis in HIV-infected patients. *Chest, 105*(2), 615–616.
25. Dressler, D. K. (1992). The person undergoing cardiac transplant surgery. In C. E. Guzzetta & B. M. Dossey (Eds.). *Cardiovascular nursing.* St. Louis: Mosby–Year Book.
26. Dressler, D. K. (1993). Transplantation in end-stage heart failure. *Critical Care Nursing Clinics of North America, 5*(4), 635–648.
27. Durack, D. T. (1990). Infective and noninfective endocarditis. In J. W. Hurst (Ed.). *The heart.* New York: McGraw-Hill.
28. Eagan, J. S., Stewart, S. L., & Vitello-Cicciu, J. M. (1991). *Quick reference to cardiac critical care nursing.* Gaithersburg, Md: Aspen.
29. Eisenberg, M. J., Gordon, A. S., & Schiller, N. B. (1992). HIV-associated pericardial effusion. *Chest, 102*(3), 956–958.
30. Enfanto, P. A., Pickett, S., Pieczek, A. M., et al. (1994). Percutaneous laser myoplasty: Nursing care implications. *Critical Care Nurse, 14*(3), 94–101.
31. Feldman, T. (1993). Rheumatic mitral stenosis: On the rise again. Part 3. *Postgraduate Medicine, 93*(6), 93–94, 99–104, 195–197.
32. Fifth report of the Joint National Committee on Detection, Evaluation and Treatment of High Blood Pressure. (1993). *Archives of Internal Medicine, 153,* 154.
33. Fragomeni, L. S., et al. (1990). Donor identification and organ procurement for cardiac transplantation. In M. E. Thompson (Ed.). *Cardiac transplantation.* Philadelphia: F. A. Davis.
34. Furst, E. (1992). Cardiovascular technology. *Journal of Cardiovascular Nursing, 4*(3), 59–70.
35. Futterman, L. G., & Lemberg, L. (1995). New indications for dual chamber pacing: Hypertrophic and dilated cardiomyopathy. *American Journal of Critical Care, 4*(1), 82–87.
36. Gallo, J. A., & Todd, B. A. (1990). Mediastinitis after cardiac surgery. *Critical Care Nurse, 10*(6), 64–68.
37. Ganz, N. M. (1991). Geriatric endocarditis: Avoiding the trend toward mismanagement. *Geriatrics, 46*(4), 66–68.
38. Gillis, C. L., Gortner, S. R., Hauck, W. W. et al. (1993). A randomized clinical trial of nursing care for recovery from cardiac surgery. *Heart and Lung, 22*(2), 125–133.
39. Giuliani, E. R., et al. (1991). *Cardiology: Fundamentals and practice.* St. Louis: Mosby–Year Book.
40. Gortner, S. R., Jaeger, A. A., Harr, J., et al. (1994). Elder's expected and realized benefits for cardiac surgery. *Cardiovascular Nursing, 30*(2), 9–14.
41. Griffith, D., Hampton, D., Switzer, M., et al. (1996). Facilitating the recovery of open heart surgery patients through quality improvement efforts and careMAP implementation. *American Journal of Critical Care, 5*(5), 346–352.
42. Guyton, A. C. (1991). *Textbook of medical physiology.* Philadelphia: W. B. Saunders.
43. Guyton, R. A., & Hatcher, C. R. (1990). Techniques of valvular surgery. In J. W. Hurst (Ed.). *The heart.* New York: McGraw-Hill.
44. Guzzetta, C. E. (1992). The person with infective endocarditis. In C. E. Guzzetta & B. M. Dossey (Eds.). *Cardiovascular nursing.* St. Louis: Mosby–Year Book.
45. Guzzetta, C. E., & Casey, P. (1992). Cardiovascular assessment. In B. M. Dossey, C. E. Guzzetta, & C. V. Kenner (Eds.). *Critical care nursing: Body-mind-spirit.* Philadelphia: J. B. Lippincott.
46. Guzzetta, C. E., & Dossey, B. M. (1990). Cardiovascular assessment. In B. M. Dossey et al. (Eds.). *Essentials of critical care nursing.* Philadelphia: J. B. Lippincott.
47. Guzzetta, C. E. & Seifert, P. C. (1991). Cardiovascular assessment. In M. R. Kinney, et al. (Eds.). *Comprehensive cardiac care.* St. Louis, Mosby–Year Book.
48. Guzzetta, C. E., & Whitman, G. (1992). Cardiac surgery. In B. M. Dossey, C. E. Guzzetta, & C. V. Kenner (Eds.). *Critical care nursing: Body-mind-spirit.* Philadelphia: J. B. Lippincott.
49. Halm, M. A. (1996). Acute gastrointestinal complications after cardiac surgery. *American Journal of Critical Care, 5*(2), 109–117.
50. Hastillo, A., & Hess, M. L. (1990). Selection of patients for cardiac transplantation. In M. E. Thompson (Ed.). *Cardiac transplantation.* Philadelphia: F. A. Davis.
51. Hess, D. B., & Hess, L. W. (1992). Management of cardiovascular disease in pregnancy. *Obstetrics and Gynecological Clinics of North America, 19,* 679–684.
52. Heyd, J. W. (1994). Comparison of blood glucose levels in the

cardiac surgical patient. *American Journal of Critical Care, 3*(5), 387–388.

53. Hudak, C. M., et al. (1990). *Critical care nursing.* Philadelphia: J. B. Lippincott.

54. Hurst, J. W. (1994). *The heart* (8th ed.). New York: McGraw-Hill.

55. Hurst, J. W. (1991). *Current therapy in cardiovascular disease.* Philadelphia: B. C. Decker.

56. Johnston, J. (1991). A new beginning: Current trends in pediatric heart transplantation. *Focus on Critical Care, 18*(1), 23–28.

57. Julian, D. G. (1990). *Current status of clinical cardiology.* Boston: Kluwer Academic Publishers.

58. Kaplan, E. L. (1994). Acute rheumatic fever. In R. E. Schlant & R. W. Alexander (Eds.). *Hurst's the heart.* New York: McGraw-Hill.

59. Keiser, H. D. (1993). Acute rheumatic fever. *Hospital Medicine, 29*(4), 60, 65–68, 73–75.

60. King, K. M. (1994). Valve disorder: Theoretical and practical nursing perspectives. *Canadian Journal of Cardiovascular Nursing, 5*(1), 13–17.

61. Kinney, M. R., et al. (1991). *Comprehensive cardiac care.* St. Louis: Mosby–Year Book.

62. Kinney, M. R., & Craft, M. S. (1992). The person undergoing cardiac surgery. In C. E. Guzzetta & B. M. Dossey (Eds.). *Cardiovascular nursing.* St. Louis: Mosby–Year Book.

63. Kochar, M. S. (1992). Hypertension in elderly patients: The special concerns in this growing population. *Postgraduate Medicine, 91,* 393.

64. Korzeniowski, O. M., & Kaye, D. (1992). Infective endocarditis. In E. Braunwald (Ed.). *Heart disease* (pp. 1078–1105). Philadelphia: W. B. Saunders.

65. Kriett, J. M., & Kaye, M. P. (1990). The registry of the International Society for Heart Transplantation: Seventh Official Report— 1990. *Journal of Heart Transplantation, 9,* 323–328.

66. Lange, S. S., et al. (1992). Infection control practices in cardiac transplant recipients. *Heart and Lung, 21*(2), 101–105.

67. Lee, R. E., & Ramos, R. (1990). Nursing care of the cardiac surgical patient. In R. J. Gray & J. M. Matloff (Eds.). *Medical management of the cardiac surgery patient.* Baltimore: Williams & Wilkins.

68. Lorell, B. H., & Braunwald, E. (1992). Pericardial disease. In E. Braunwald (Ed.). *Heart disease* (pp. 1465–1516). Philadelphia: W. B. Saunders.

69. Mahon, P. M. (1991). OKT3 and cardiac transplantation: An overview. *Critical Care Nurse, 11*(8), 42–50.

70. Mann, S. F. (1992). Systolic hypertension in the elderly: Pathophysiology and management. *Archives of Internal Medicine, 152,* 1977.

71. Mason, J. W. (1994). Classification of cardiomyopathy. In J. W. Hurst (Ed.). *The heart.* (pp. 1585–1590). New York: McGraw-Hill.

72. Miner, P. D. (1994). Infective endocarditis: Implications for care of the adult with congenital heart disease. *Nursing Clinics of North America, 29*(2), 269–283.

73. Nair, C. K., et al. (1992). Ten years' experience with mitral valve replacement in the elderly. *American Heart Journal, 124,* 154–159.

74. National Heart, Lung, and Blood Institute. (1992). Morbidity and mortality: Chart book on cardiovascular, lung and blood diseases. Bethesda, MD: Author.

75. Olsson, M., et al. (1992). Aortic valve replacement in octogenarians with aortic stenosis: A case-control study. *Journal of the American College of Cardiology, 20*(7), 1512–1516.

76. Ostrow, C. L., Hupp, E., & Topjian, D. (1994). The effect of Trendelenburg and modified Trendelenburg positions on cardiac output, blood pressure and oxygenation: A preliminary study. *American Journal of Critical Care, 3*(5), 382–386.

77. Pennington, G., & Swartz, M. T. (1992). Assisted circulation and the mechanical heart. In E. Braunwald (Ed.). *Heart disease* (pp. 535–550). Philadelphia: W. B. Saunders.

78. Parker-Cohen, P. D., et al. (1990). Alterations of cardiovascular function. In K. L. McCance & S. E. Huerther (Eds.). *Pathophysiology.* St. Louis: Mosby–Year Book.

79. Perloff, J. K. (1991). Congenital heart disease in adults: A new cardiovascular subspecialty. *Circulation, 84*(5), 1881.

80. Perloff, J. K. (1992). Congenital heart disease in adults. In E. Braunwald (Ed.). *Heart disease* (pp. 966–991). Philadelphia: W. B. Saunders.

81. Piano, M. R., & Schwertz, D. W. (1994). Alcoholic heart disease: A review. *Heart and Lung, 23*(1), 3–20.

82. Pratt, N. G. (1993). Neurohormonal response to ventricular failure: Pharmacologic management. *Journal of Cardiovascular Nursing, 8,* 49.

83. Quaal, S. (1993). *Cardiac mechanical assistance beyond balloon pumping.* St. Louis: Mosby–Year Book.

84. Rackley, C. E., et al. (1990). Mitral valve disease. In J. W. Hurst (Ed.). *The heart* (7th ed.). New York: McGraw-Hill.

85. Rackley, C. E., et al. (1990). Aortic valve disease. In J. W. Hurst (Ed.). *The heart* (7th ed.). New York: McGraw-Hill.

86. Reitz, B. (1992). Heart and heart-lung transplantation. In E. Braunwald (Ed.). *Heart disease* (pp. 520–534). Philadelphia: W. B. Saunders.

87. Relf, M. V. (1993). Surgical intervention for tricuspid valve endocarditis: Vegetectomy, valve excision, or valve replacement? *Journal of Cardiovascular Nursing, 7*(2), 71–79.

88. Riddle, M. M., Dunstan, J. L., & Castanis, J. L. (1996). A rapid recovery program for cardiac surgery patients. *American Journal of Critical Care, 5*(2), 152–159.

89. Sanford, S. J., & Disch, J. A. (1989). *American Association of Critical-Care Nurses: Standards for nursing care of the critically ill.* East Norwalk, Conn: Appleton-Lange.

90. Shively, M., Verderber, A., & Fitzsimmons, L. (1994). Caring for patients with ventricular assist devices. *Journal of Cardiovascular Nursing, 8,* 91.

91. Simpson, T., & Lee, E. R. (1996). Individual factors that influence sleep after cardiac surgery. *American Journal of Critical Care, 5*(3), 182–189.

92. Simpson, T., Lee, E. R., & Cameron, C. (1996). Patients' perceptions of environmental factors that disturb sleep after cardiac surgery. *American Journal of Critical Care, 5*(3), 173–181.

93. Snelson, C., Cline, B. A., & Luby, C. (1993). Infective endocarditis: A challenging diagnosis. *Dimensions of Critical Care Nursing, 12*(1), 4–20.

94. Spaniol, S. E. (1994). Shivering following cardiac surgery: Predictive factors, consequences, and characteristics. *American Journal of Critical Care, 3*(5), 356–367.

95. Sparacino, P. A. (1994). Adult congenital heart disease. *Nursing Clinics of North America, 29*(2), 213.

96. Stovsky, B., Dehner, S. (1994). Patient education after valve surgery. *Critical Care Nurse, 14*(2), 117–123.

97. Templin, K., Shively, M., & Riley, J. (1993). Accuracy of drawing coagulation samples from heparinized arterial lines. *American Journal of Critical Care, 2*(1), 88.

98. Thompson, M. E. (1990). *Cardiac transplantation.* Philadelphia: F. A. Davis.

99. Uszenski, H. J., Booker, S. M., Goliash, I. B., et al. (1993). Hypertrophic cardiomyopathy: Medical, surgical and nursing management. *Journal of Cardiovascular Nursing, 7*(2), 13–22.

100. Valle, B. K., Valle, G. A., & Lemberg, L. (1995). Volume control: A reliable option in the management of 'refractory' congestive heart failure. *American Journal of Critical Care, 4*(2), 169–173.

101. Verderver, A., & Gallagher, K. J. (1994). Effects of bathing, passive range of motion exercises, and turning on oxygen consumption in healthy men and women. *American Journal of Critical Care, 3*(5), 374–381.

102. Wahl, M. J. (1994). Myths of dental-induced endocarditis. *Archives of Internal Medicine, 154,* 137.

103. Wakowski, C. A., & Bierman, P. Q. (1995). Dual chamber pacing in patients with hypertrophic obstructive cardiomyopathy: A case study. *American Journal of Critical Care, 4*(2), 165–168.

104. Wingate, S. (1992). The person with cardiomyopathy or myocarditis. In C. E. Guzzetta & B. M. Dossey (Eds.). *Cardiovascular nursing.* St. Louis: Mosby–Year Book.

105. Wynne, J., & Braunwald, E. (1992). The cardiomyopathies and myocarditides. In E. Braunwald (Ed.). *Heart disease* (pp. 1394–1450). Philadelphia: W. B. Saunders.

Peripheral Vascular Disorders

UNIT 9

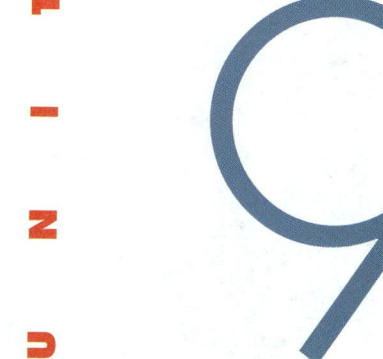

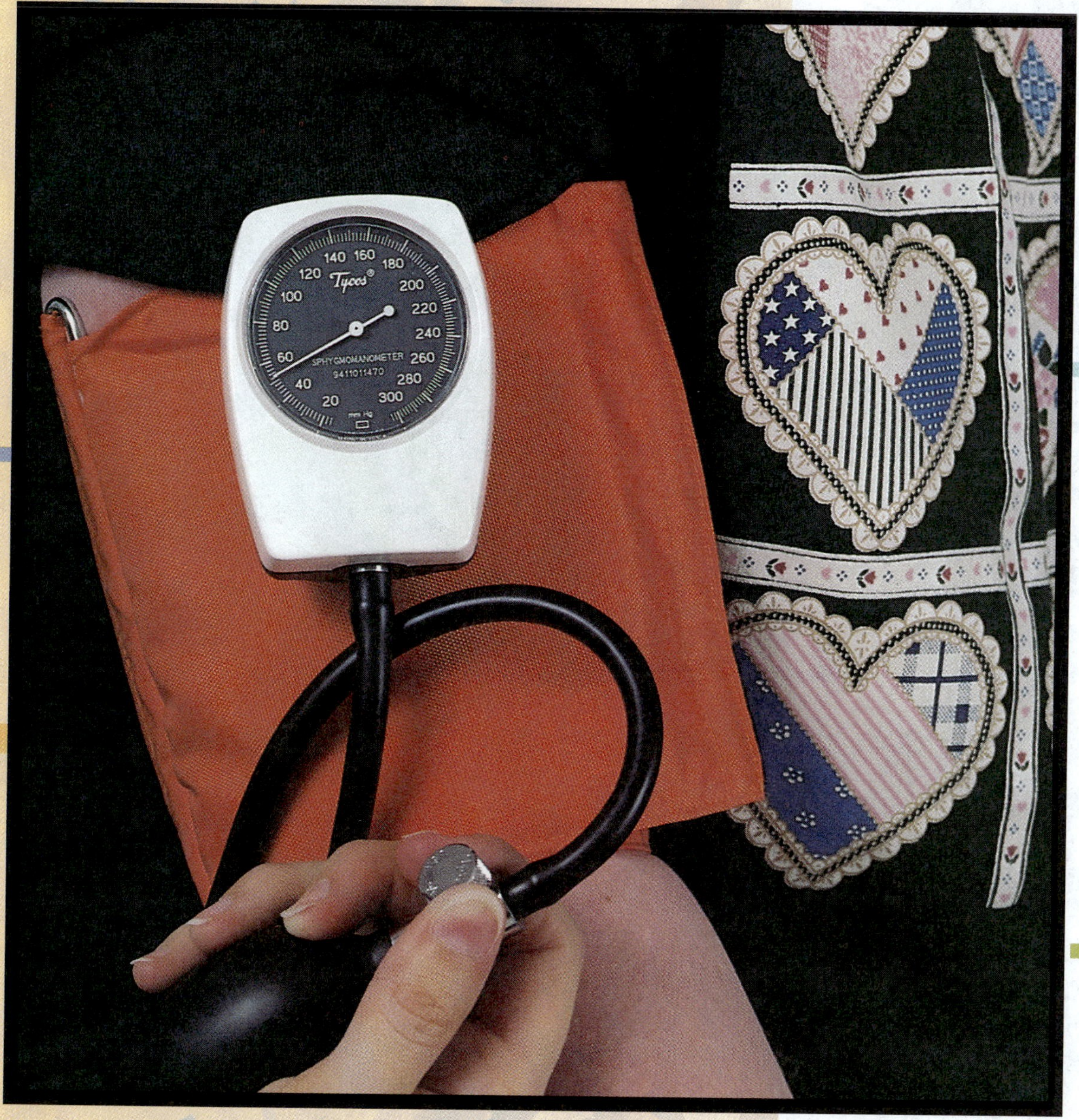

Structure and Function of the Peripheral Vascular System

Joyce M. Black

The flow of blood is essential for sustaining human life. When blood leaves the heart it enters the vascular system, which is composed of numerous vessels. The vascular system provides conduits for blood to travel from the heart to nourish cells, to carry away metabolic wastes to the excretory organs, to deliver hormones to target organs, to exchange substances between the interstitial fluid and blood, to allow lymph fluid to return into circulation, and to return blood to the heart for recirculation (Fig. 48–1).

Blood flow depends on the efficiency of the heart as a pump and the patency of the blood vessels. Circulation is influenced by blood viscosity (thickness), hydration, mechanisms affecting coagulation and fibrinolysis of blood, and local changes in the size of the vessels.

Components of the Vascular System

The vascular system is composed of arteries, arterioles, capillaries, venules, veins and lymphatic channels. The structure and function of these components are examined in this chapter.

Structure of the Blood Vessels

Arteries carry blood *away* from the heart after it has been oxygenated in the pulmonary circulation. Major arteries divide into smaller arteries, which divide into arterioles, which finally divide into capillaries.

Blood vessel walls vary in thickness. The variation is due to the presence or absence of one or more thicknesses of tissues.

This chapter incorporated material written for the fourth edition by Pamela D. Dennison.

Arteries are composed of the following three distinct layers (Fig. 48–2):

1. Tunica intima, the innermost layer, provides a smooth passageway through which blood flows. It is present in all blood vessels. It is continuous with the endocardium of the heart.
2. Tunica media, the middle layer, is composed of elastic connective tissue and circular smooth muscle. It is a thick layer of smooth muscle and elastic fibers. The tunica media is responsible for regulating the diameter of the vessel by dilation and constriction.
3. Tunica adventitia is a relatively thin layer of connective tissue that runs parallel to the long axis of the vessel. This outermost layer gives support to the vessel and maintains its shape.

Arteries can be classified into two categories:

1. First are the elastic arteries, such as the aorta and its major branches. The vessels consist of the three layers just described. The vessels stretch and recoil to accommodate the flow of blood. They expand with each surge of blood ejected from the heart during systole and then resume their original diameter. This recoil propels blood forward to all parts of the body, and it is the basis of the pulse that is felt on palpation. During diastole, the elastic nature of these arteries helps maintain pressure within the vessels. Elastic arteries follow relatively straight courses and have comparatively few branches. These arteries are most severely affected by atherosclerosis, particularly at branch points.
2. Muscular arteries are the second type of artery. The walls of these arteries are smaller and muscular and contain few elastic fibers. They distribute blood throughout the body. Each branch divides into further branches of smaller-caliber arteries until the blood passes from the smallest arteries into the arterioles and then into the capillaries, where it nourishes the tissues.

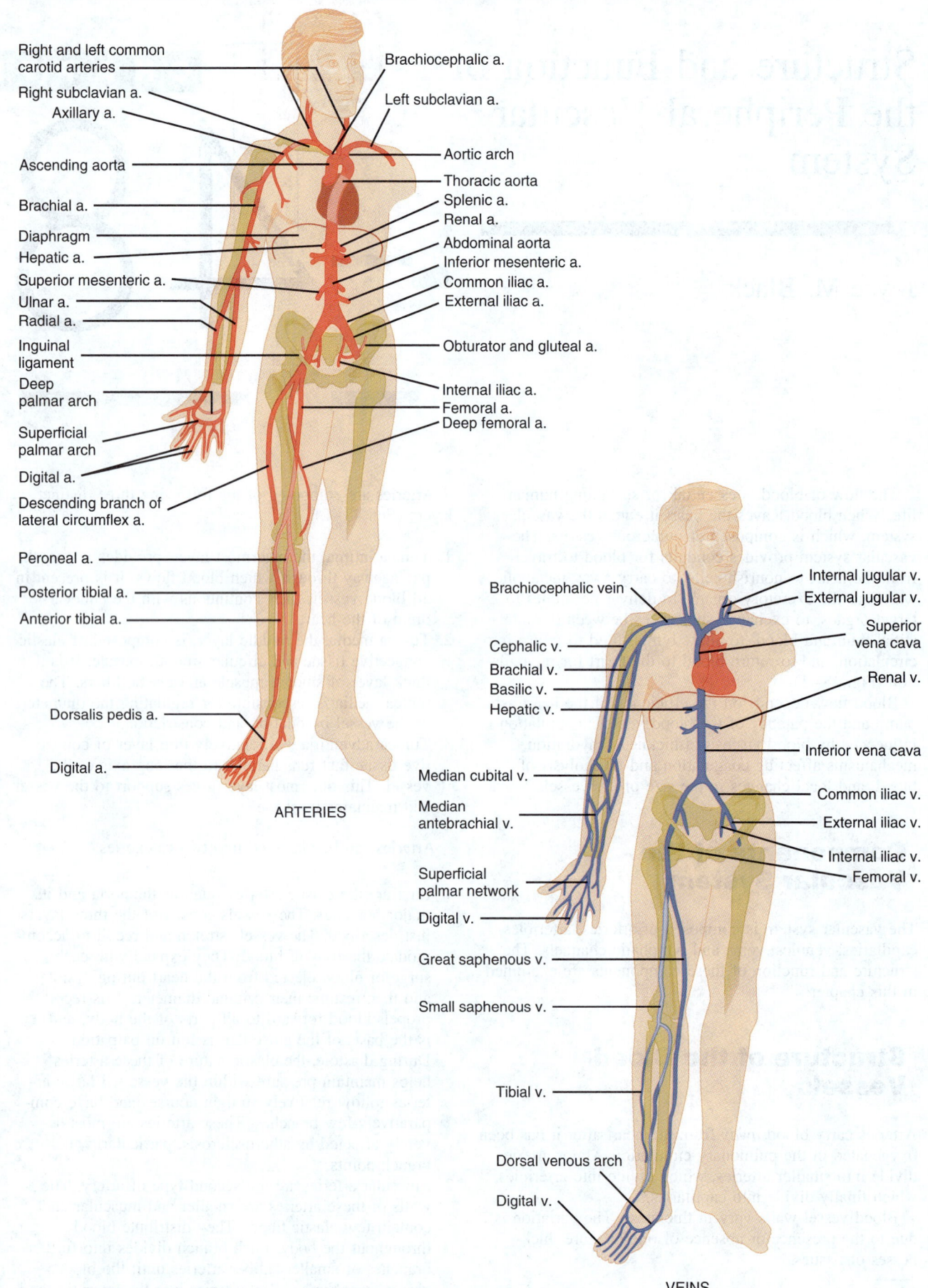

Figure 48–1. Major arteries and veins.

Right and left common carotid arteries

Right subclavian a.

Axillary a.

Ascending aorta

Brachial a.

Diaphragm

Hepatic a.

Superior mesenteric a.

Ulnar a.

Radial a.

Inguinal ligament

Deep palmar arch

Superficial palmar arch

Digital a.

Descending branch of lateral circumflex a.

Peroneal a.

Posterior tibial a.

Anterior tibial a.

Dorsalis pedis a.

Digital a.

Brachiocephalic a.

Left subclavian a.

Aortic arch

Thoracic aorta

Splenic a.

Renal a.

Abdominal aorta

Inferior mesenteric a.

Common iliac a.

External iliac a.

Obturator and gluteal a.

Internal iliac a.

Femoral a.

Deep femoral a.

ARTERIES

Brachiocephalic vein

Cephalic v.

Brachial v.

Basilic v.

Hepatic v.

Median cubital v.

Median antebrachial v.

Superficial palmar network

Digital v.

Great saphenous v.

Small saphenous v.

Tibial v.

Dorsal venous arch

Digital v.

Internal jugular v.

External jugular v.

Superior vena cava

Renal v.

Inferior vena cava

Common iliac v.

External iliac v.

Internal iliac v.

Femoral v.

VEINS

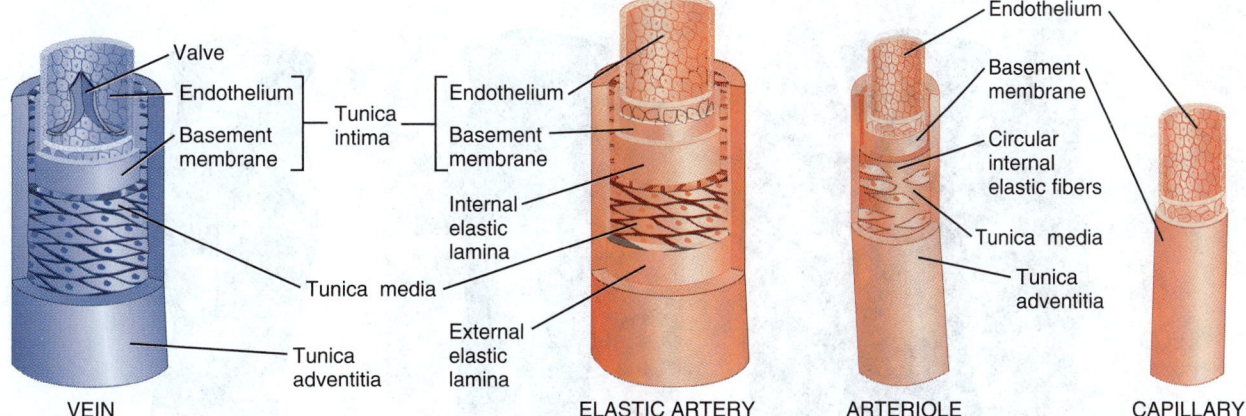

Figure 48–2. Cross sections of an artery and a vein, an arteriole, and a capillary. Note the thickness of the elastic arterial and vein walls compared with those of the capillary walls. The arteriole is the major controller of peripheral vascular resistance.

Structure of the Arterioles

When arteries are less than 0.5 mm thick, they are called *arterioles*. Arterioles are small, thick-walled vessels. Arterioles are important regulators of the peripheral circulation because they are innervated with sympathetic nerves in the muscle of the tunica media. Therefore, the arteriole constricts and dilates to regulate peripheral vascular resistance, a component of blood pressure. If the arteriole constricts, that is, the lumen (opening) becomes smaller, blood flow is restricted beyond the point of constriction. When the lumen dilates, blood flow can enter the capillaries freely.

Structure of the Capillaries

Before blood enters the capillary network, it passes through structures called *precapillary sphincters*. These sphincters work in conjunction with the autonomic nervous system to relax and constrict capillary openings. The precapillary sphincters can also be influenced by local changes in temperature, pH, and oxygen.

The capillaries are the functional units of the vascular system because they are the vessels that allow substances to diffuse to and from the blood into the interstitial space (Fig. 48–3). The capillary network is composed of a single layer of endothelial cells.

Structure of the Venules and the Veins

From the capillaries, blood flows into venules. Venules are tiny veins that have extremely thin walls that allow the passage of substances and serve to remove waste products from capillaries. The venules merge to form veins, which eventually combine to form larger veins that carry deoxygenated blood back to the heart. Approximately 75% of the total blood volume at any given time can be found in the venous system. Veins are also known as *capacitance vessels* because of their ability to stretch.

Veins lie closer to the skin's surface than arteries do, and although they are composed of three layers, their walls are thinner and contain less smooth muscle and less elastic tissue than arteries do. Most veins also contain valves that prevent the backflow of venous blood (Fig. 48–4). Valves break the hydrostatic column of blood into small units, thereby reducing the hydrodynamic load in the propulsion of blood toward the heart. A valve consists of two frail cusps composed of endothelial folds. Valve competence depends on the integrity of the vein wall.

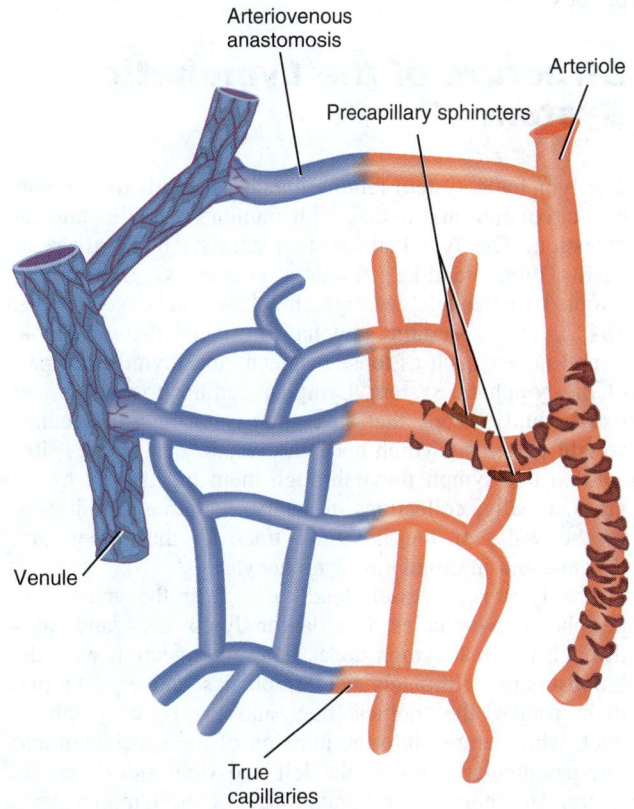

Figure 48–3. Capillary bed. Many substances move across the capillary walls into the tissues and cells. Precapillary sphincters help regulate flow.

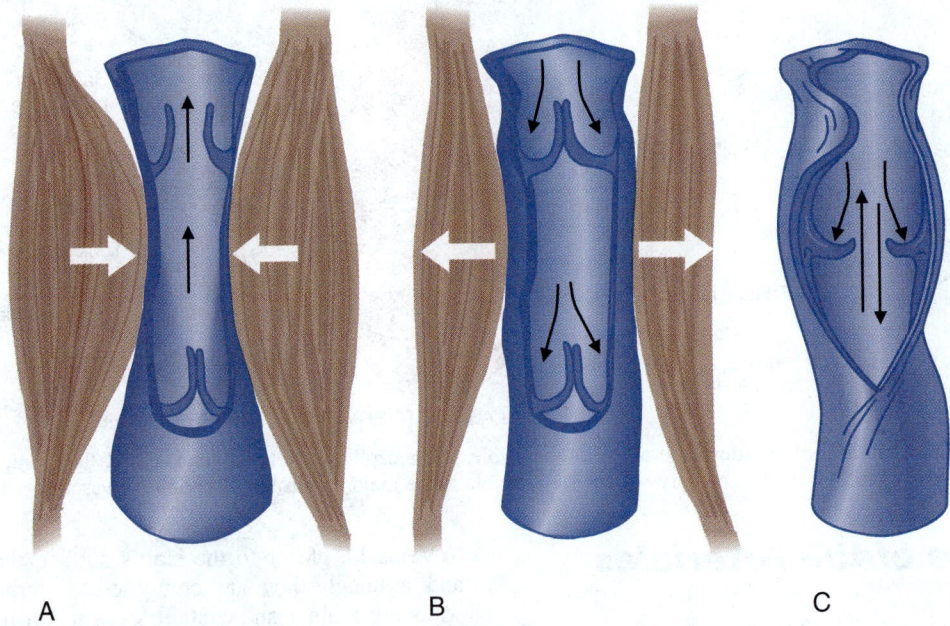

A   B   C

Figure 48–4. One-way venous valves (*A*). Valves allow blood to be pumped back to heart, but prevent it from draining back into periphery (*B*). *C,* Incompetent valves permit the column of blood to fall to the lower legs.

The valve becomes incompetent when the cusps no longer meet at the midline. Valvular incompetence develops when veins have been overstretched by excess venous pressure for a prolonged period of time, as occurs during pregnancy or when a person stands still for long periods.

Structure of the Lymphatic System

The lymphatic system returns interstitial fluids to the general circulation and assists with immune reactions and fat digestion. The lymphatic system consists of plexuses of small, thin, veinlike vessels (lymphatics) that empty lymph into the left and right brachiocephalic veins (Fig. 48–5). Also, certain lymphatic organs that resemble lymph nodes, such as tonsils, spleen, and thymus, are part of the lymphatic system. Lymph is similar to plasma and tissue fluid except that it contains no high-molecular-weight proteins. Lymph nodes are small, oval bodies situated so that lymph flows through them on its way to the veins. Finally, collections of lymphoid tissue are situated in the walls of the intestinal tract, in the spleen and thymus, and in circulating lymphocytes.

The lymphatic vessels tend to lie near the veins. The peripheral lymphatics join larger lymphatics and pass through regional lymph nodes before connecting with the bloodstream. Ultimately, all lymphatics converge at two main trunks, the thoracic duct and the right lymphatic duct, which empty into the junction of the subclavian and internal jugular veins of the left and right sides, respectively. The thoracic duct drains most of the lymph vessels of the body: lower extremities, pelvis, abdominal cavity, left arm, and the left side of the neck, thorax, and head. The right lymphatic duct is the common trunk for lymph flow from the right arm and the right side of the head, neck, and thorax.

Active and passive mechanisms transport the lymph along the lymphatic vessels. Valves in the lymphatics promote proximal flow. Lymph flow results from a combination of interstitial pressure, negative and positive pressure in the thoracic and abdominal cavities, compression of adjacent muscles, and arterial pulsation (Fig. 48–6).

Function of the Blood Vessels

Effective circulation requires an adequate blood volume, blood vessels that are intact and in good condition, and a heart that functions forcefully as a pump to propel the blood. Blood volume remains adequate as a result of continuous production by the bone marrow and distribution of plasma to and from the interstitial spaces. Healthy blood vessels without layers of plaque provide the best conduits for blood flow. The ability of the heart to pump can be affected by many variables. Some of the variables are discussed here; others are discussed in Chapter 43. Blood vessels play a major role in homeostasis. Several major aspects of circulation and the impact of peripheral vascular resistance on blood flow are examined in this chapter.

Blood Flow Through the Large Arteries

Arterial blood pressure is the pressure within the large systemic arteries. It is essentially equal to the pressure

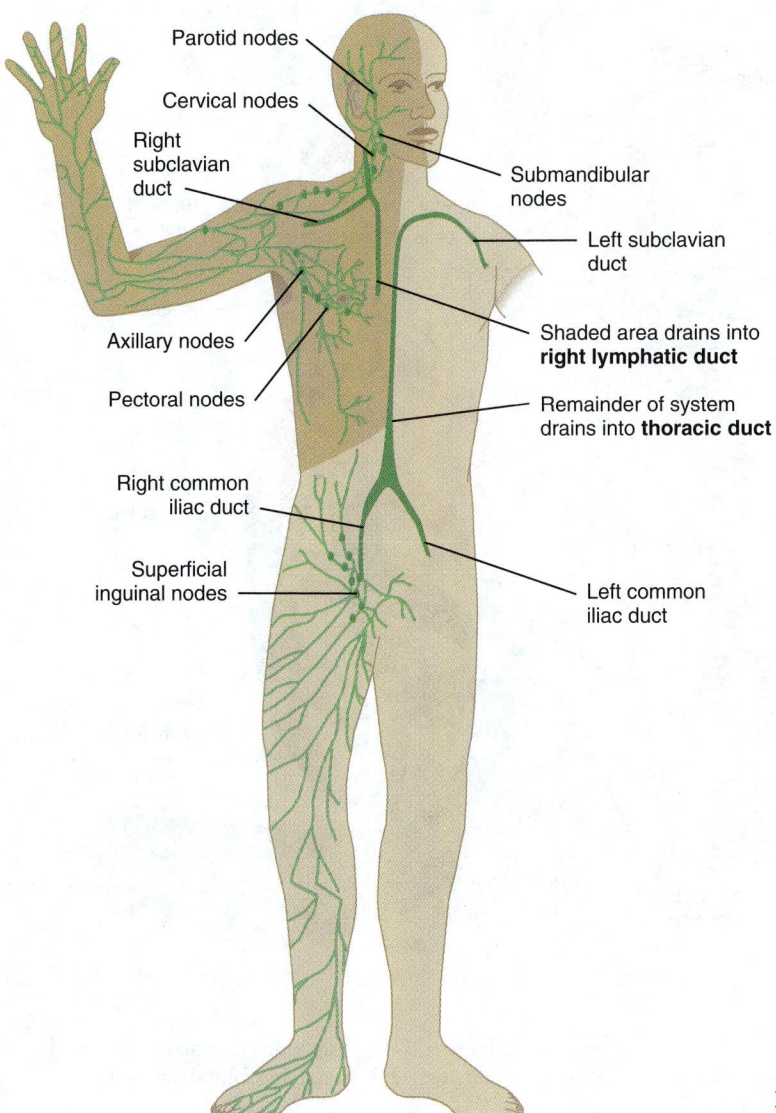

Figure 48–5. Superficial lymphatic collecting channels and nodes.

generated by the left side of the heart and serves as the driving force to propel blood. Therefore, it must be maintained to ensure adequate blood delivery. Several factors can influence arterial blood pressure.

Vasomotor Nerve Fibers

Vasomotor nerve fibers are efferent fibers (moving away from the brain) that regulate the diameter of blood vessels. The arterioles are the major arteries that are influenced by vasomotor nerve fibers. Sympathetic nervous system nerves contain both vasodilator and vasoconstrictor vasomotor fibers. The vasoconstrictor fibers are most common. They rest on the blood vessel walls and release norepinephrine, which causes vasoconstriction. Vasodilator fibers are found in the skeletal muscle. At the points at which they form junctions with blood vessels in the muscles, they release acetylcholine, which leads to vessel dilation.

Vasomotor Center

The vasomotor center is located in the lower third of the pons and medulla oblongata of the brain. It senses carbon dioxide partial pressure in the blood. When carbon dioxide pressures rise, vasoconstriction occurs.

Baroreceptors

Baroreceptors sense the pressure in the aortic arch, in the carotid sinus in the internal carotid artery, and in the right atrium. Baroreceptors send blood pressure impulses to the medulla. The medulla can increase or decrease sympathetic nervous system stimulation to cause vasoconstriction or vasodilation, respectively. When arterial pressure rises, the rate of nerve transmission from the baroreceptors increases. As a consequence, blood vessels dilate and the heart rate and contractile force of the heart decreases. Blood pressure is lowered.

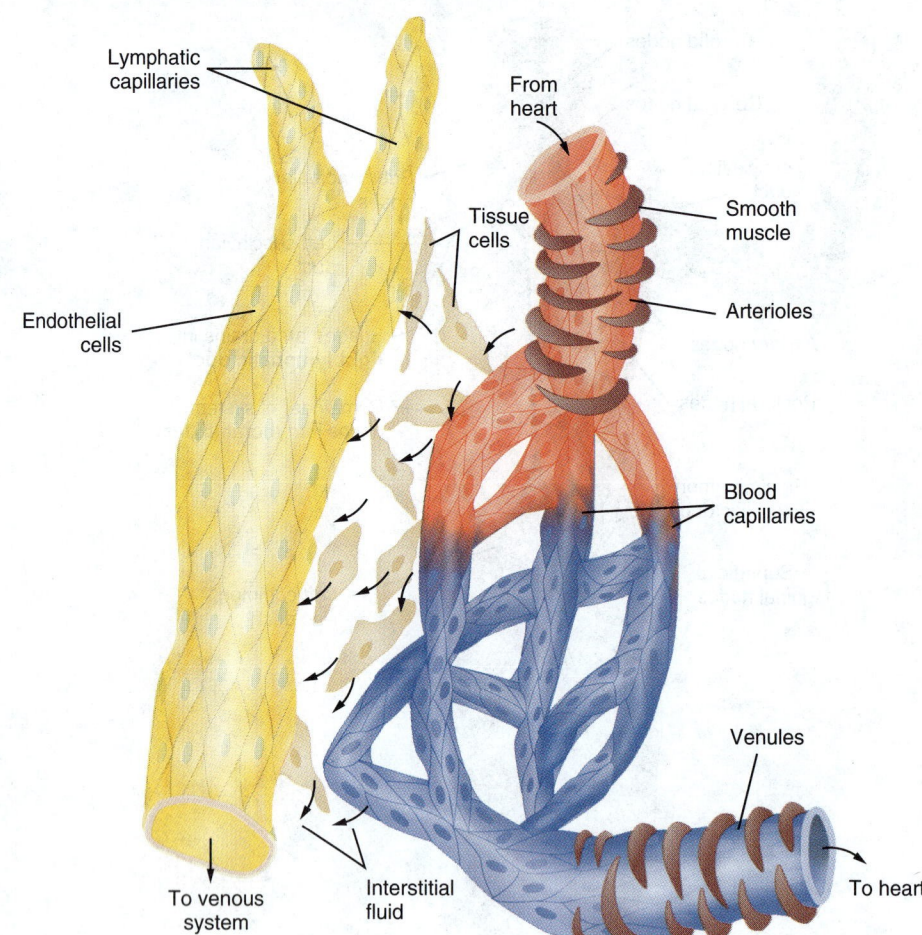

Figure 48–6. The lymphatic capillaries lie next to arteries and veins, where they collect interstitial fluids. The *arrows* indicate movement of interstitial fluid. Note that lymphatic channels begin as dead-end vessels.

Aortic and Carotid Bodies

The aortic and carotid bodies, which are located in the aortic arch and branchings of the common carotid arteries, sense pressures of arterial oxygen, carbon dioxide, and hydrogen ions. Falls in arterial oxygen pressure cause an increase in arterial pressure.

Influence of Chemicals and Hormones

Three powerful substances within the blood help to regulate the diameter of blood vessels: epinephrine, norepinephrine, and angiotensin II. Epinephrine constricts superficial blood vessels, but in small doses it dilates vessels that supply the muscles, brain, and heart. Norepinephrine constricts all blood vessels. It particularly affects the peripheral vessels. Renin is a substance formed by the activation of the renin-angiotensin system of the kidney, and it is a powerful arterial vasoconstrictor.

Vasopressin, often called antidiuretic hormone (ADH), is secreted into the bloodstream by the hypothalamus. When blood pressure falls below normal, stretch receptors in the wall of the heart relax. The hypothalamus is trig-

gered to release ADH. Vasopressin causes the body to conserve water, thereby increasing blood pressure.

Blood Flow Through the Tissues

Velocity of Blood Flow

In general, the velocity of blood flow is inversely related to the cross-sectional area of the vessels of the segment through which it flows. The larger the cross-sectional area, the lower the velocity. Consider a small tributary: it runs much faster than a large river when trying to move the same amount of river water. The largest vascular cross-section is in the aorta. It may seem that as blood flow channels into arterioles and capillaries it should flow faster and faster because of the change in diameter of the vessels. Just the opposite is true. There is only one aorta, but it channels its blood into hundreds of smaller vessels. If you were to add up the cross-sectional area of the arterioles, it would be much larger than that of the aorta. The same process occurs as blood flow is divided further at the capillaries. Therefore, blood velocity slows as it moves from the great vessels into the capillaries.

Resistance to Blood Flow

As the blood flows through the vessels, it encounters some resistance. Resistance can be thought of as friction. In general, the greater the resistance offered by the vessels to blood flow, the harder the heart must pump to overcome the resistance and still have enough energy left to propel blood forward.

Factors Affecting Resistance

Blood Viscosity. *Blood viscosity*, or the thickness of the blood, causes adjustments in flow. Proteins and cells within the blood make it thick. Thicker blood moves more slowly.

Vessel Length. The longer the blood vessel, the greater the amount of resistance that is met as the blood courses through it.

Vessel Diameter. The smaller the diameter of the vessel, the greater its resistance to flow. The resistance of a vessel is inversely related to the fourth power of the diameter. For example, if the diameter of a vessel is decreased by half, its resistance is increased 16 times!

Alterations in Resistance

The length of a blood vessel does not change greatly. Neither does the viscosity of blood show much variance. Therefore, the major influence on resistance is the diameter of a vessel. The resistance to the flow of blood offered by the entire systemic circulation is called *total peripheral resistance*. The resistance offered by the entire pulmonary system is called *total pulmonary resistance*.

There are many influences on resistance. The role of norepinephrine, acethycholine, renin, and carbon dioxide on vessel diameter have already been discussed. Local factors in the cells themselves can alter blood flow to the tissues.

The body's main method of regulating heat is vasoconstriction and vasodilation. The regulators of this response are called *vasomotor reflexes*.

When tissues are metabolically active, they have a greater need for blood. The tissue can alter blood flow by increasing supply or by slowing transit through the capillary bed.

Substances produced by the body that increase blood supply to an injured area include the following:

- Histamine, which is a potent vasodilator of small blood vessels, although it may also constrict the large arteries
- Bradykinin, which is one of a group of vasoactive peptides and is a powerful vasodilator, especially of cutaneous vessels

- Serotonin, which is liberated from platelets that stick to the vessel wall in the injured area. Although a powerful constrictor of cutaneous arterioles, it dilates capillaries
- Tissue oxygen levels, carbon dioxide tension, and potassium and lactic acid levels also affect arterial flow

Capillary Exchange

In the capillary bed, oxygen and carbon dioxide are exchanged, nutrients are delivered, and waste products are collected. The movement of substances across the capillary wall is the result of a *gradient*. The concentration of one substance is higher on one side of the capillary wall (gradient), and the substance therefore moves to the area of lesser concentration. Small holes (called *fenestrations*) in the capillary wall allow movement. Protein is the only substance that does not normally move in peripheral tissue. To transport all of these substances across the wall, blood moves slowly through the capillary. The volume of fluid that moves out of the capillaries into the interstitial spaces is about 3 L/day. The fluid is picked up by the lymphatic system and returned to circulation.

Venous Return

Blood that leaves the capillaries flows into venules and then into veins on its way back to the heart. The volume of blood that flows from the systemic circulation to the right atrium at any time is called the *venous return*. Many factors, which are examined here, can influence venous return.

When a person is in an upright position, blood return from the lower limbs to the heart depends almost entirely on the contraction of the calf muscles and the competence of the valves. When a leg muscle contracts, it presses against the veins in the leg, thus compressing them and pumping blood toward the heart. Whan a person is standing still, this "muscle pump" does not work, and the venous pressures in the lower part of the leg rise to about 90 mm Hg. When a person is sitting or lying down, the calf muscle pump is not activated, especially if the calf muscles are not flexed. In the recumbent position, the pressure gradient between the peripheral venous circulation and right atrium provides the major driving force for propulsion of the blood. The valves allow blood flow in one direction only.

Breathing also affects venous return. When a person inhales, pressure in the thoracic cavity decreases. This opens the diameter of the vena cava and blood flows in. Expiration decreases the inflow. If intrathoracic pressure is increased by contraction of the thoracic muscles (as in forced expiration, lifting a heavy weight, or Valsalva's maneuver), the intrathoracic pressure rises enough to compress the vena cava.

Disorders of the vein valves can decrease venous blood flow. The blood may actually pool, or collect, in the feet and lower legs.

Function of the Lymphatic System

The lymphatic system is related both by structure and function to the vascular system. As previously mentioned, the volume of fluid that moves into the interstitial spaces is about 3 L/day. Ordinarily, the volume of lymph represents the difference between capillary filtration and reabsorption. If this fluid were allowed to accumulate, tissues would swell, producing edema. The lymphatic system returns this fluid to the bloodstream.

Interstitial fluid enters the lymphatic channels through very thin walls with open spaces in them. Once the fluid enters the system it is called *lymph*. The lymphatic system is a one-way system, carrying lymph only to the heart at the thoracic duct.

Lymphatic capillaries permit free entry of fluid, small and large molecules, and cellular elements from the interstitial space. Any increase in the interstitial pressure increases lymph flow, as does any agent or procedure that increases the rate of filtration from the capillaries. Interstitial pressures and lymphatic flow can be increased by raising venous pressure, reducing plasma oncotic pressure, or altering capillary permeability. A general increase in systemic arterial pressure does not significantly increase lymph flow, but hypotension decreases or stops lymph flow.

Effects of Aging on the Vascular System

The changes in intima and media that are a result of aging most often affect the larger and medium-sized vessels. The most prominent changes are intimal thickening, loss of elasticity, and an increase in both diameter and calcium content. These changes are referred to as *arteriosclerosis*, or hardening of the smaller arteries/arterioles. Atherosclerosis involves the deposit of plaque composed of cholesterol and lipids within the intima of large and medium-sized arteries. Thickened intima inhibits the diffusion of nutrients from the vessel.

Effects of Aging on the Lymphatic System

Lymphatic tissue diminishes in older people, which results in a decrease in the number of lymph nodes and in the size of the remaining nodes. The lymph nodes in the elderly may also tend to be fatty and fibrotic compared with those in the young; thus, the ability to fight infection is reduced.

Introduction to Disorders of the Vascular System

Disorders of the cardiovascular system are major killers of U.S. citizens. Arteriosclerosis can plug arteries and arterioles and increase total peripheral resistance (TPR). This is manifested as hypertension, or increased arterial blood pressure. Increased TPR places a greater demand on the heart and causes stress as the heart tries to pump blood into the tight vessels.

In conditions such as shock, when there has been a loss of blood, the cardiovascular system plays a major role in preserving life. Peripheral vascular resistance rises to move blood from the abdominal organs, skin, and muscles to the brain and heart. This movement of blood is completed by the action of norepinephrine and renin, which cause vasoconstriction.

The most common venous disorder is varicose veins. The valves in such veins are incompetent, and the blood cannot move upward toward the heart.

Lymphatic systems can be destroyed with infection, especially from parasites. The role of the lymphatic system is evident in the client with cancer. Unfortunately, neoplastic cells are transported into the lymphatics. From there, cancer cells can invade lymph nodes and distant organs, a process called *metastasis*.

Conclusions

The vascular system is a series of conduits that move blood from the heart to the cells. Delivery of the blood is controlled by the pressure in the left ventricle and by the muscular action of the arterioles. Veins and lymphatic vessels return blood and plasma to the heart for reoxygenation and recirculation.

Bibliography

1. Berne, R., & Levy, M. (1993). *Physiology*. St. Louis: Mosby–Year Book.
2. Fahey, V. (1994). *Vascular nursing*. Philadelphia: W. B. Saunders.
3. Guyton, A., & Hall, J. (1996). *Textbook of medical physiology* (9th ed.). Philadelphia: W. B. Saunders.
4. McCance, K., & Huether, S. (1994). *Pathophysiology*. St. Louis: Mosby–Year Book.
5. Solomon, E., Schmidt, R., & Adranga, P. (1990). *Human anatomy and physiology*. Philadelphia: W. B. Saunders.
6. Spence, A., & Mason, E. (1983). *Human anatomy and physiology* (2nd ed.). Menlo Park, CA: Benjamin-Cummings Publishing Co.

Assessment of Clients with Peripheral Vascular Disorders

CHAPTER 49

Barbara Harrison

Peripheral vascular disease is common among elderly and diabetic clients. It is characterized by disturbances of blood flow through the peripheral vessels. These disturbances eventually result in damage to tissues of the extremities as a result of (1) ischemia and (2) excessive accumulation of waste and fluid due to venous or lymphatic stasis. Damage can be due to any disorder that narrows, obstructs, or damages blood vessels, thus impeding blood flow. Without intervention, tissue damage may advance to the point of ulceration or gangrene. The limb may have to be amputated. Assessment of the peripheral vascular system includes collection of data through history and physical examination of the arterial and venous circulation.

History

While assessing the client, the nurse should be alert to risk factors for atherosclerosis (see Chapter 44), diabetes (see Chapter 69), and venous disorders (see Chapter 50). In addition, note any medications that the client is taking; they may increase the risk of vascular disease (e.g., birth control pills, cortisone) or of circulatory disorders (e.g., vasodilators, anticoagulants). Some clients are reluctant to mention what they believe to be minor symptoms. Consequently, perform a careful assessment, ask specific questions skillfully, and be alert for important information concerning early manifestations of these insidious conditions.

Clients with normal peripheral vasculature display characteristics like those listed in Normal Physical Assessment Findings.

Biographical and Demographic Data

When assessing biographical data of the client with peripheral vascular disease, note the client's age. Athero-

sclerosis is more prominent in the elderly. Ask about occupation and clarify whether the occupation adds risk for cardiovascular disease. If the client is retired, ask about previous employment.

Current Symptoms

When assessing for vascular disease, ask for specific data to determine the frequency and duration of clinical manifestations and to indicate whether the client has arterial or venous disease. This section describes the typical chief complaints of clients with arterial and venous disorders.

Symptoms of Arterial Disorders

With arterial disorders, the chief complaint is usually cramping leg pain on walking, which disappears with 1 to 2 minutes of rest. (Rarely, a client is noted to limp.) The pain is called *intermittent claudication*. The pain can be localized or can radiate from the calf to the thigh.

Intermittent claudication results from inadequate oxygenation of the tissues (or ischemia) due to progressive occlusion of the vessels from atherosclerosis. It is a pathologic process similar to angina. Initially, the pain is predictable, and it develops after a fixed amount of activity (e.g., walking around the block).

As the ischemia becomes more severe, the pain also becomes more severe, and it reaches a point at which the client has distal forefoot burning, numbness, and tingling pain at rest or during the night (known as *rest pain*). This pain is due to decreased cardiac output during sleep and to the relative elevation of the legs while the client is in a supine position. The pain is relieved when the client stands up. Even during non-sleep hours, elevation of the legs decreases blood flow and increases pain. Clients of-

This chapter incorporates material written for the fourth edition by Pamela D. Dennison and Joyce M. Black.

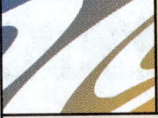

NORMAL PHYSICAL ASSESSMENT FINDINGS

Peripheral Vascular System

Inspection

Extremities of normal contour, without edema. Even hair distribution; symmetrical venous pattern. Varicosities, skin lesions, and ulcers absent. Capillary refills immediate on blanching.

Palpation

Extremities warm and dry without areas of localized heat or tenderness. Peripheral pulses (temporal, carotid, brachial, radial, ulnar, femoral, popliteal, posterior tibial, dorsalis pedis) are even and regular, and are rated +2 (normal) on a scale of 0 to +3. Homans' sign absent bilaterally.

Auscultation

Blood pressure equal in both upper extremities. Orthostatic hypotension absent. Bruit over peripheral pulses absent.

---

ten report that they sleep upright with legs dangling to control pain.

Obtain information from the client regarding the sequence, duration, and persistence of the discomfort, manner of onset, and associated symptoms. Document the amount of activity required to cause pain. The extent of the disease can be gauged by the distance the client is able to walk without pain, or *claudication distance*. For example, one client may develop claudication after walking one block, whereas another may walk six blocks before experiencing pain.

Disorders of the aorta and iliac vessels, such as atherosclerosis, can lead to impotence. If you suspect the client has aortoiliac disease, ask about sexual changes. Sexuality is a sensitive issue, and although these questions raise the risk of embarrassment to the client, ask them nonetheless.

Symptoms of Venous Disorders

In contrast to clients with arterial disorders, those with chronic venous disease report that pain has a slow onset and is not associated with exercise or rest. These clients have typically worked at a job involving many hours of standing in one place, have had multiple pregnancies, or display abdominal obesity. The client may also have varicose veins and a history of phlebitis. In these clients, the leg veins have been subjected to increased pressure gradients, and return of venous blood has been obstructed. The vein wall eventually loses competence. An incompetent vein lets the column of blood fall downward, which increases the hydrostatic pressure in the venous end of the

capillary. This increase in pressure leads to leg edema. As the process continues, blood flow is slowed and the tissues become hypoxemic. Ulcerations develop in the lower third of the leg, where the pressure is highest. The client often reports a feeling of heaviness in the legs and nighttime cramping. Exercise and elevation generally relieve the pain and swelling as venous return is improved.

In more severe forms of chronic venous disorders, lower extremity edema is the usual initial complaint. The edema gets worse as the day wears on and diminishes after a night's sleep. Pitting edema may be seen at first, but as the edema becomes more chronic, scarring develops and the pitting disappears.

Skin changes noted with chronic venous disorders include erythema in early stages, followed by development of brawny, thick skin with pigmentation of the skin. The skin becomes very dry and flaky, which leads to itching and scratching. Continued irritation results in stasis dermatitis, and the skin eventually ulcerates. The medial malleolus is the most common site of occurrence.

Lymphatic disorders lead to edema. If the lymphatic accumulation is prolonged, edematous tissue becomes stiff and almost impossible to compress. Lymphedema tends to be unilateral and may follow damage to lymphatic channels.

Symptom Analysis

Vascular disease in the extremities may affect the arterial system or the venous system. Table 49–1 compares and contrasts the clinical manifestations of arterial and venous disorders.

Clients with venous disease present with dilated, tortuous, cordlike superficial veins. Assessment also reveals aching pain when the legs are in a dependent position. Edema, dependent cyanosis, brown discolorations of the skin, possible ulcers of the ankle, pruritus, and paresthesia are noted with chronic venous insufficiency. Skin temperature remains normal, and pulses are present (although they may be hard to palpate through the edema).

Hallmarks of arterial insufficiency include the following:

1. Decreased or absent arterial pulses
2. Possible systolic bruit over involved arteries
3. Muscular atrophy
4. Thin, shiny, hairless skin
5. Thick, ridged toenails
6. Cool skin temperature
7. Ulcers on pressure points of the feet
8. Pain with leg elevation

The skin is pale gray when the legs are elevated above heart level and dusky red after they are placed in a dependent position. Edema, if present, is mild.

Past Health History

Note any medical history of vascular impairment. Ask specifically whether the client has had a history of hypertension, diabetes, phlebitis, extremity blood clots, pulmo-

Table 49-1. Clinical Manifestations in Arterial and Venous Disorders

Manifestation	Arterial Disorders	Venous Disorders
Pain	Intermittent claudication Cramping Worsening with elevation	Aching pain Exercise improves pain Better with elevation Nocturnal cramping Pruritus, paresthesias Heaviness in the legs at end of day
Skin	Absence of hair Small, painful ulcers on pressure points, especially lateral malleolus and toes (surrounding skin is normal) Thin, shiny skin Thick toenails	Brown discoloration Broad, shallow, slightly painful ulcers of the ankle and lower leg (surrounding skin is damaged) Normal toenails
Color	Pale, dependent cyanosis	Brown discoloration Dependent cyanosis
Temperature	Cool	No change
Sensation	Decreased; sometimes itching, tingling Numbness	Pruritus
Pulses	Decreased to absent Possible systolic bruit over involved arteries	Usually unaffected, but may be difficult to palpate if legs edematous
Edema	May be present	Present, worse at end of day, improved with elevation
Muscle mass	Reduced	Unaffected

nary emboli, cerebrovascular accidents, edema, varicose veins, leg ulcers, pain in legs during activity, leg cramps, or extremities that are cold, pale, or blue. Ask about any past medical tests, surgery, or treatments involving the cardiovascular system, and about prior treatment for diabetes mellitus, collagen disorders, or hypertension. It is also important to know if the client smokes. Nicotine is a potent vasoconstrictor.

Family Health History

Family history helps to determine risk factors and provides clues about reported and observed signs and symptoms. A family history of diabetes, hypertension, coronary artery disease, collagen diseases, and peripheral vascular disease is assessed.

Psychosocial History

An occupational history should be recorded. If the client's occupation is unfamiliar to you, ask questions about the number of hours spent in various positions (e.g., standing, walking). In addition, some occupations involve contact with chemicals or are associated with cold environments. These should also be noted.

Assess for proper nutrient and fluid intake. Determine the usual intake of protein and calories. Clients should also be asked about sodium, cholesterol, and fat intake.

The client's activity, rest, and sleep habits should be assessed. The nurse also assesses the degree to which clinical manifestations interfere with activities of daily living. Obtaining information about the frequency and duration of clinical manifestations, precipitating activities, and the influence of manifestations on daily life enables the nurse to understand the severity of the disease. Assessment of the client's stress level, emotional state, and coping mechanisms (including the use of tobacco products, alcohol, or recreational drugs) is also important.

Remain sensitive to the emotional effect of peripheral vascular disorders. Clients with visible lesions may fear embarrassment. Those with severe claudication may resent the imposed restriction on activities. Clients also have concern about the inability to perform self-care and about changes in role performance and sexual performance. Losing the involved extremity is a significant fear.

Physical Examination

Physical examination of the peripheral vascular system involves inspection, palpation, and auscultation. Before starting the physical examination, it is important to have a well-lighted and warm room. Natural lighting is the best, as it allows the examiner to assess for subtleties in skin color. Warm the room to minimize cutaneous and small artery vasoconstriction. A quiet room is also needed; decreased sound is helpful when auscultating the low-pitched sounds commonly found in the blood vessels.

Inspection

Observe the lower extremities, noting skin color, ulcerations, hair distribution, venous pattern, turgor, capillary refill, and presence of muscle atrophy or edema. These are reviewed in detail in the following text.

Skin Color

The range of normal skin color, from pink to deep brown, is noted. The presence of localized areas of cyanosis, rubor (redness), or pallor is easily noticed in a person with fair skin. It is harder to see in persons with darker skin tones. For these clients, the changes in skin color are best assessed in the conjunctiva, tongue, buccal mucosa, and palms. Clients with vascular disorders may have cold and pale extremities (arterial disorders) or edematous, cyanotic, or red extremities (venous disorders).

Ulcerations

The presence of skin lesions, ulcerations, or scar tissue (indicating healed ulcers) is also noted; ischemic fissures of the feet and ulcers of ankles and heels are reliable signs of arterial insufficiency. Tissue necrosis and gangrene may be present with severe arterial disease. Areas of tissue necrosis may degenerate into wet or dry gangrene. It is very important to examine between the toes for signs of tissue loss. Scars indicating healed ulcers over the medial malleolus can indicate chronic venous insufficiency.

Hair Distribution

Lack of hair growth may indicate inadequate circulation to an area. It is common to note a clear line of demarcation on the leg where hair has been lost. The loss of hair on the legs is a fairly good indicator of the level of impaired arterial supply.

Venous Pattern

Varicosities indicate venous insufficiency. Angiomas (benign tumors of blood and lymph vessels) and petechiae (small, purplish spots on the skin from several causes, including hemorrhage) are also noted.

Turgor

Turgor reflects the elasticity and the water content of the skin and subcutaneous tissues. It is assessed by lifting a fold of skin and observing how quickly it returns to a flat position after being let go. Skin turgor is slowed in dehydrated clients, but is also normally slower in older clients.

Capillary Refill

Capillary refill time is an evaluation of peripheral perfusion and cardiac output. This assessment is usually completed while pulses are assessed. The nail bed of the toe or finger is depressed until it blanches (becomes pale). Pressure on the blanched nail bed is released, and the

nurse observes the length of time required for usual skin color to return. Normal capillaries refill in a fraction of a second, but "normal" findings include up to 3 seconds. With diminished blood flow, the return to normal color is delayed, and a refill time of more than 3 seconds is sometimes called "sluggish." Note whether the environment is cold, because external temperatures can delay capillary refill.

Muscle Atrophy

If atrophy is suspected, it may represent long-standing arterial insufficiency. The nurse measures the muscle and compares it with the measurement of the muscle on the opposite side.

Edema

To assess edema of the leg, the examiner pushes with the thumb on the skin over the the client's foot or tibia for 5 seconds. Edematous skin may leave an indentation or pit (thus the term *pitting edema*). The degree of edema is often graded; however, the scale used to grade pitting edema is variable. It may be based on the time for the pitting to resolve and for the skin surface to return to baseline or on the depth of the indentation created by the thumb's pressure. A commonly used scale is shown in Figure 49–1.

Edema resulting from cardiac disease is generally bilateral and occurs in dependent areas (in the legs of a client who is ambulatory and the sacrum of a client who is bedridden). Edema tends to be unilateral when the client has occlusion of a deep vein. With lymphatic obstruction, edema may be unilateral or bilateral. This long-standing edema destroys the structure of the skin. The skin becomes hard. It is called *brawny edema*.

Additional Inspections

If the examiner suspects, but cannot confirm, venous or arterial disease, some additional assessments can be performed.

Elevation Pallor. If an arterial defect is suspected, the leg can be elevated 30 cm (12 inches). Pallor occurring within 60 seconds indicates arterial insufficiency. Next, have the client dangle his or her legs from the side of the bed or examination table. Normally, the color returns within 10 seconds. Severe arterial insufficiency causes dependent rubor (red-purple color).

Because the leg elevation can cause pain, it should be performed only as needed. Note the degree of pallor at rest and use the test only to assist with determining the severity of ischemia.

Trendelenburg's Test. Intended to help detect abnormal venous filling time, Trendelenburg's test reveals whether valves have become incompetent in varicose veins. Superficial varicose veins are usually easy to rec-

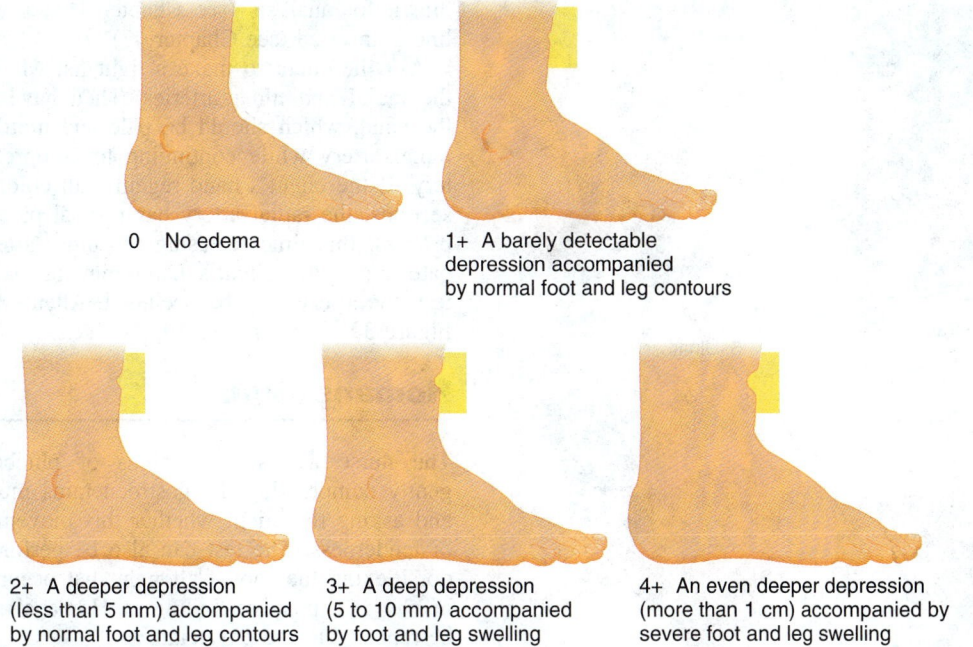

0   No edema

1+ A barely detectable depression accompanied by normal foot and leg contours

2+ A deeper depression (less than 5 mm) accompanied by normal foot and leg contours

3+ A deep depression (5 to 10 mm) accompanied by foot and leg swelling

4+ An even deeper depression (more than 1 cm) accompanied by severe foot and leg swelling

Figure 49–1. To assess peripheral edema, press a finger into the skin over the client's tibia and note the depth and persistence of the resulting depression. Use the numerical scale to record your findings.

ognize. They appear as dilated, tortuous (twisting) veins. The client lies down with the leg elevated until the veins are empty. A tourniquet is applied at midthigh, snugly enough to occlude the superficial veins. With the tourniquet in place, the client stands. The examiner then notes the time required for the veins to fill from below. Normally, veins fill in about 30 seconds. After 60 seconds, the tourniquet should be released. Normally, when the tourniquet is released, no further blood fills the veins from above. Additional blood flowing into the vein from above indicates that a valve is incompetent and has allowed backflow of blood. A vein normally fills from below; a varicose vein fills from above because incompetent valves allow blood to flow backward.

Palpation

Temperature

Palpate the legs with the dorsal surface of your hand and notice the temperature. Temperature and vascular tone should be the same in both legs. Vasoconstriction produces cold, pale, moist skin with collapsed superficial veins. Bilateral vasoconstriction may be caused by smoking, temperature of the room, apprehension, or generalized arterial disease. Unilateral or localized vasoconstriction indicates peripheral vascular disease. Venous disorders seldom alter the temperature of skin.

Pulses

Palpate the pulse by placing the first three fingers of your dominant hand along the length of the selected artery.

Apply gentle pressure against the bone or firm surface, followed by a gradual release. Palpate temporal, carotid, brachial, radial, and ulnar pulses (upper extremities) and femoral, popliteal, posterior tibial, and dorsalis pedis pulses (lower extremities) as shown in Figure 49–2. Pulses should be palpated bilaterally and simultaneously except for the carotid pulse. Carotid pulses should be palpated sequentially to avoid stimulation of the carotid sinus, which may produce bradycardia or sinus arrest. Ulnar pulse assessment is performed during Allen's test, as described in the following section.

Always note rhythm, amplitude, and symmetry of pulses. Do not count the rate of peripheral pulses. Peripheral pulses should be compared for rate, rhythm, and quality, then graded as follows:

  0 Absent
+1 Weak and thready
+2 Normal
+3 Full and bounding

Be sure to record the scale used to assess pulse quality. Several scales are used in clinical practice. A common method of documentation is to use a stick figure labeled with graded pulses.

Note whether a pulse is absent or feels unequal bilaterally. The dorsalis pedis pulse is congenitally absent in approximately 10% to 17% of the normal adult population. The posterior tibial pulse is absent congenitally in 9% of the black adult U.S. population. In the elderly client, dorsalis pedis and posterior tibial pulses may be more difficult to palpate. If they occur, the site at which they were found should be marked with a pen to facilitate later examinations.

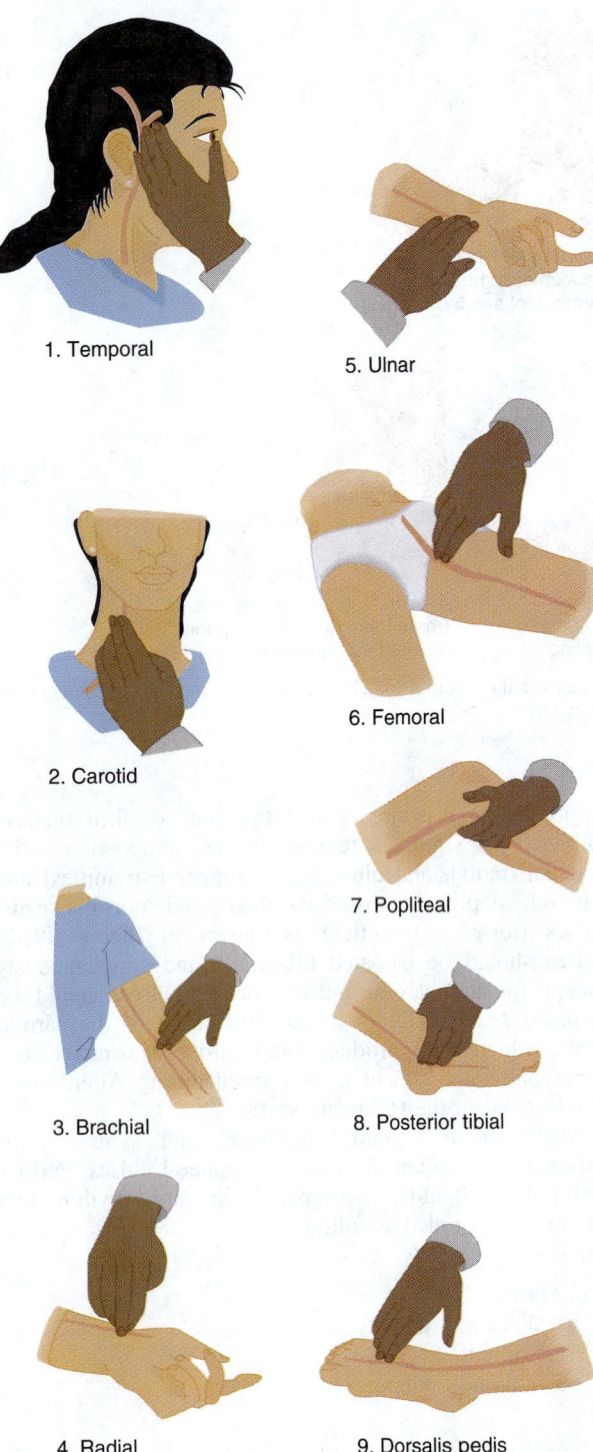

1. Temporal

5. Ulnar

2. Carotid

6. Femoral

7. Popliteal

3. Brachial

8. Posterior tibial

4. Radial

9. Dorsalis pedis

Figure 49–2. Assess peripheral pulses bilaterally (except carotid) from head to toe, comparing one side to the other for amplitude, rhythm, and symmetry.

Allen's Test

Blood flow to the hand normally is supplied by both the ulnar and the radial arteries, which join at the volar arch in the palm. Allen's test is used to assess the patency of the radial and ulnar arteries distal to the wrist. It is commonly performed before arterial blood samples are

drawn for analysis (see Chapter 16) or when an arterial line is inserted (see Chapter 47).

Ask the client to make a tight fist while you compress the radial and ulnar arteries. Then have the client open the hand, which should be pale and mottled. Release the radial artery while continuing to compress the ulnar artery. If the client's hand regains full color within about 6 seconds, the radial artery has normal patency. Repeat the process, this time releasing the ulnar artery to assess its patency. If the client's hand remains pale during either test, the artery may be occluded. Allen's test is shown in Figure 39–5 in Chapter 39.

Homans' Sign

The nurse assesses for signs of phlebothrombosis by gently compressing the gastrocnemius muscle of the calf and asking the client whether this movement causes pain or tenderness. The test can also be performed quickly by dorsiflexing the foot. Calf pain that occurs with this maneuver is a positive finding of Homans' sign and should be reported to the physician.

Keep in mind that the value of Homans' sign is limited. Studies indicate that only about 35% of people with deep venous thrombosis (DVT) have a positive response to Homans' test. Superficial phlebitis, Achilles tendinitis, and plantar muscle injury can also elicit a positive Homans' sign. Therefore, 50% of the people who have a positive response to Homans' test do not have DVT. Doppler studies are more accurate.

Auscultation

Auscultation of the peripheral vascular system typically is done with a stethoscope, but the best results are obtained with a Doppler ultrasonographic flowmeter. Measurement of arterial blood pressure is done by sphygmomanometry with a properly fitting cuff. For an accurate reading, the cuff must be placed on the client's arm at the level of the heart; it should be wide enough to transmit pressure to the center of the arm and long enough to encircle the arm firmly. Measurement should be recorded in both arms. A few points' difference in readings is normal. If there is a 15 to 20 mm Hg difference in extremity readings, it may indicate aortic dissection, subclavian artery atherosclerosis, or arterial thromboembolic events. Asymmetry of blood pressure readings should be documented so that all subsequent measurements are made on the arm with the higher reading. The blood pressure is measured with the client in supine, sitting, and standing positions, when possible, and documentation should include the position of the client and the site used. Orthostatic (positional) changes in blood pressure should be noted.

Auscultation over each pulse point should be done to assess for the presence of bruits. A bruit, (pronounced brew-ée) is described as a "whooshing" sound, soft or loud in pitch; it results from turbulent blood flow caused by irregularities in the vessel wall. The presence of a bruit is considered abnormal, but its importance in indicating severity of vascular disease is not well demonstrated. Bruits usually occur in the carotid, aortic, femoral, and popliteal arteries and indicate some degree of arterial narrowing. These arterial sounds are best heard with the bell of the stethoscope. Severity of disease is determined by Doppler flow studies and angiography.

Diagnostic Tests

Noninvasive Techniques

Noninvasive diagnostic techniques have assumed an increasingly important role in the management of vascular disease. The purpose of noninvasive diagnostic tests is to provide reliable, relevant data that can be used to evaluate the extent of the disease process. Variables include the amount of blood flow through the affected limb, abnormality of blood flow, and some measure of the degree of functional limitations.

Limb Blood Pressure

The measurement of blood pressure is the most commonly applied noninvasive test of cardiovascular function. It may be the best single indicator of how well perfusion is being maintained. Acute and chronic arterial occlusion produce regional hypotension.

Doppler Ultrasonography

Hand-held Doppler instruments permit assessment of peripheral arterial disease by audible evaluation of arterial signals or measurement of limb blood pressures (Fig. 49–3). This test is simple and inexpensive, but the technique may not detect minor disease, and it is less accurate than duplex scanning.

Brightness mode (B-mode) ultrasound refers to the creation of a two-dimensional image from ultrasound waves. It can be used to assess vein size, compressibility, flow patterns, presence of thrombus, and valve function.

Ankle-Brachial Index

The ankle-brachial index (ABI) is a commonly used parameter for overall evaluation of extremity status. A regular arm blood pressure cuff is applied above the malleoli. Doppler probes are used to identify the systolic endpoint at both the dorsalis pedis and the posterior tibial site (see Fig. 49–3). The higher of the two pressures is used as the indication of leg blood pressure status. This number is then divided by the higher of the two brachial artery pressures:

$$\text{Ankle-brachial index} = \frac{\text{Higher systolic ankle pressure}}{\text{Higher systolic brachial pressure}}$$

For example, a systolic ankle pressure of 60 mm Hg with a systolic brachial pressure of 120 mm Hg gives an ankle-brachial index of 0.5. With normal circulation, ankle pressure is the same as or higher than the brachial pressure. Thus, an ABI of 1 or more is considered a normal finding; the client with an ABI of 0.3 to 0.8 typically experiences claudication, and the client with an ABI of 0.3 or less typically experiences rest pain.

Ultrasonic Duplex Scanning

Ultrasonic duplex scanners are used to localize the site of vascular obstruction and to evaluate the degree of narrowing and the amount of vascular reflux. The technique is the most sensitive and specific noninvasive modality for detecting deep vein thrombosis. This device provides both an ultrasonographic image of the vessel and a Doppler signal that characterizes the flow pattern at a given site. The anatomic data allow more specific localization of the level of stenosis than is possible with simple pressure or waveform techniques. The major limitations to these devices are their cost, complexity, and lack of portability.

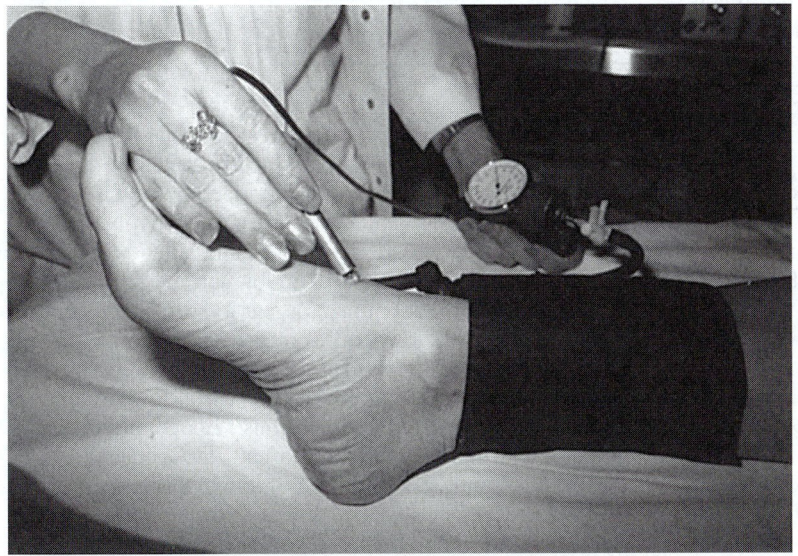

Figure 49–3. Measurement of ankle pressures with a Doppler probe placed over the dorsalis pedis artery. (From Fahey, V. [1994]. *Vascular Nursing.* Philadelphia: W. B. Saunders.)

Computed Tomography

Computed tomography (CT) allows visualization of the arterial wall and its structures. CT scans can be used in the diagnosis of abdominal aortic aneurysms and postoperative complications, such as graft infection, graft occlusion, hemorrhage, and abscess. If contrast dye is to be used, steroids or antihistamines may be given before the scan to clients with a history of allergic reaction to the dye, iodine, or seafood. Clients must lie still while a long tube passes over them. If the client cannot lie still or is claustrophobic, sedation may be necessary.

Magnetic Resonance Imaging

Magnetic resonance imaging (MRI) uses magnetic fields, rather than radiation, to obtain cross-sectional images of the body. MRI is used to detect aneurysms and deep vein thrombosis from the pelvic iliac veins and leg veins. Clients with implanted metal devices, such as aneurysm clips, pacemakers, implantable cardioverter defibrillators, or iron or steel foreign objects in their bodies (e.g., shrapnel) cannot undergo MRI. The client is placed in a long magnetic tube. Clients who cannot lie still or who have claustrophobia should use relaxation techniques, or they may require sedation. For evaluation of blood flow in the extremities, the limb to be examined is placed in a cradle-like support in a flow cylinder. Examination of an extremity requires approximately 15 minutes.

It is likely in the future that MRI techniques will supply much of the information currently available only with angiography. MRI has the double advantage of not requiring ionizing radiation and not using any form of injection into the arterial system. The expense and time required for the procedure will make it a less than optimal technique for routine screening and follow-up.

Air Plethysmography

Air plethysmography (APG) uses a pneumatic plethysmograph to measure volume changes in the legs. Venous reflux, venous obstruction, calf muscle pump function, and venous volume can be measured. A large cuff is applied to the client's calf and a known volume of air is instilled to calibrate the cuff. Venous volume, ejection fraction, and residual volume fractions are then measured.

Impedance Plethysmography

Impedance plethysmography (IPG) and photoplethysmography are also used to measure venous blood volume changes in the extremities. These tests are not as complete as air plethysmography. During the procedure, electrodes from a plethysmograph are applied to a limb along with a pressure cuff. As pressure is increased, electrical resistance is increased; thus, the quality of venous blood flow is revealed.

The client is informed about the purpose of the procedure and is told that a technique similar to blood pressure measurement will be used, which lasts 30 to 60 minutes.

Clients must be able to assume a supine position with the involved extremity elevated above the level of the heart.

Exercise Testing

Exercise testing provides an objective measurement of the severity of intermittent claudication and it suggests the extent to which it interferes with the client's life-style. The most commonly used method for stress testing is the treadmill exercise test. The treadmill test is similar to that used for clients who have had a myocardial infarction, except that walking speed is usually 1.5 to 2 miles/hour, with a grade elevation of 10% to 20% and a time limit of 5 minutes. If a client can walk 5 minutes, he or she is considered mildly symptomatic; a walking time of 1 minute represents severe disease. Test performance is also gauged by measurement of ankle systolic pressure. In normal clients, the time required for return to preexercise ankle pressure is usually less than 3 minutes with a drop from baseline of 20% or less. In clients with intermittent claudication, the recovery time is longer; ankle pressure is usually less than 50 mm Hg and may be unrecordable during recovery.

Clients undergoing stress testing should wear loose-fitting clothes and comfortable walking shoes. The procedure should be explained so the client knows what to expect. The client should also know that exercise will be stopped at the maximal level of exertion or when clinical manifestations become disabling.

Intravascular Ultrasonography

Intravascular ultrasonography provides information about the atherosclerotic intima beneath the luminal surface. It can thus determine the thickness of the arterial wall and can distinguish thrombus and calcium from vascular tissue, allowing more exact removal of lesions. One current limiting factor is the need for specialized interpretation of the scans.

Invasive Techniques

Contrast Angiography

Contrast angiography is the most invasive of the diagnostic procedures for arterial disorders and has the greatest risk for the client. It is frequently performed before vascular surgery and can be used intraoperatively to evaluate the results of an operation. The procedure involves injecting contrast into the arterial system and performing radiographic studies (Fig. 49–4). Angiography is performed in a catheterization laboratory or in a special procedures room in the radiology department. The client is given nothing by mouth (NPO) for 2 to 6 hours before the procedure. A mild sedative may be used. Angiography is performed under sterile conditions. Local anesthesia is given at the injection site, and a catheter is placed percutaneously. Contrast is injected through the catheter, and then fluoroscopy may be done. Serial pictures of the movement of the dye are taken by cameras positioned

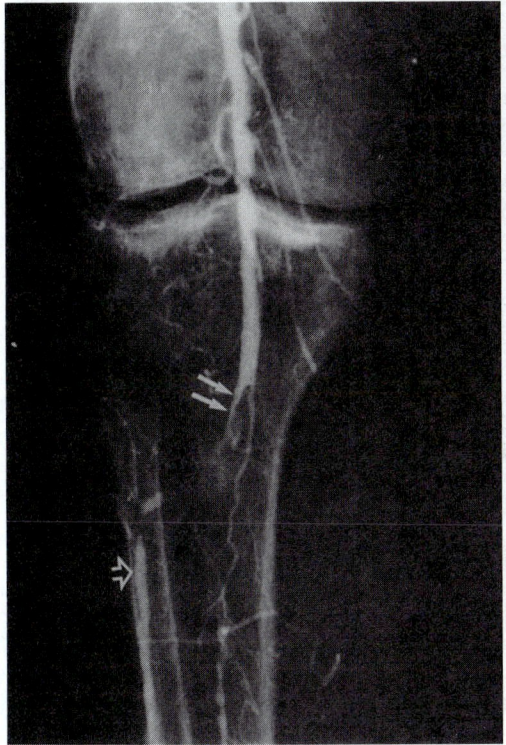 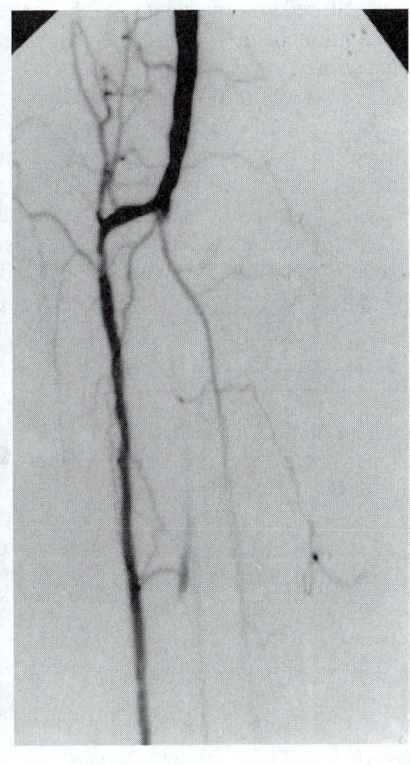

Figure 49–4. Angiograms from an 82-year-old woman with acute onset of right lower-leg rest pain. The first angiogram (*A*) shows an occluded distal popliteal artery. The second angiogram (*B*) shows complete resolution of the occlusion after overnight treatment with urokinase; this is an excellent clinical result. (From Fahey, V. [1994]. *Vascular nursing*. Philadelphia: W. B. Saunders.)

over the study field. Most angiograms take 30 to 90 minutes.

Nursing care after angiography usually involves routine postprocedural orders, including the following:

- Frequent assessment of vital signs, neurologic function, and pulses in both extremities, with particular attention to the extremity that has been punctured (every 15 minutes for 1 hour and then every hour for 2 hours)
- Assessment of the puncture site for hematoma and the appearance of the extremity distal to the puncture site
- Bedrest for 6 to 8 hours, with the punctured extremity kept straight (with translumbar aortography, supine bedrest is indicated for the same period of time)
- Continuous intravenous hydration for 6 to 8 hours to assist with contrast excretion
- Assessment of blood urea nitrogen (BUN) and creatinine levels the next day (a complete blood count should be obtained for translumbar approach)
- Resumption of preprocedural diet and medications. If the client is receiving heparin, its administration is not resumed for a minimum of 4 hours.

The nurse also assesses motor and sensory function, especially following angiography of the upper extremity. Bleeding can compress the brachial plexus, resulting in permanent neurologic deficits.

Pain at the injection site is fairly common and can usually be managed with mild analgesics. More severe pain or pain distal to the puncture site requires further assessment of peripheral pulses, neurovascular assessment, and palpation for masses. Notify the physician of abnormal assessment data.

Complications of angiography, in addition to allergic reaction to the contrast medium, include thrombi, perfora-

tion of the vessel, emboli, and renal failure. Creatinine levels should be monitored. Pseudoaneurysm is a significant complication and may extend the hospital stay. Pseudoaneurysm is a contained outpouching of the arterial wall with persistent communication between the artery and the fluid component of an adjacent mass. Pseudoaneurysms (also called false aneurysms) generally result from arterial trauma (after arterial puncture) or occur at the surgical site. They provide a site of infection and a source of emboli and are associated with intravascular thrombosis. They can enlarge, compress an adjacent structure, and even rupture, although rupture is rare.

Contrast Venography

Venography is performed in a manner similar to angiography, but it is used to examine the venous system. Venograms can be used to detect deep vein thrombosis or other abnormalities, such as incompetent valves. For an ascending venogram, dye is injected into a vein in the foot to record venous patency. A descending venogram involves injecting contrast into the femoral vein at the groin to evaluate vein reflux and valve incompetence.

It is important to document the presence and quality of peripheral pulses before the procedure. The client should be informed that the procedure may involve multiple attempts to find and puncture a vein. The client is usually given clear liquids for 3 to 4 hours before the procedure to help maintain adequate hydration. Procedures for the use of contrast were discussed under Contrast Angiography.

After the procedure, a pressure dressing is placed on the injection site. The client should remain at bedrest for 2 hours after the procedure if the femoral vein was punctured. Pulses distal to the site are monitored for the next 4 to 6 hours. Intravenous fluids are continued for 8 to 24 hours after the procedure to help with dye excretion. Fluid status is assessed; observe for signs of fluid overload. On the client's return to the nursing unit, the nurse monitors vital signs, palpates pulses, and observes the insertion site frequently for bleeding or hematoma formation. Postangiography protocols vary, but generally vital signs, pulses, and the insertion site are monitored every 15 minutes for the first hour and every hour for 2 to 6 hours. The client is on bedrest for 2 hours.

Vascular Endoscopy (Angioscopy)

Vascular endoscopy permits imaging of intra-arterial disease in color and in three dimensions through the use of fiberoptic technology. Equipment consists of a flexible fiberoptic angioscope, a light source, an irrigation system, a camera, a video recorder, and a monitor. The major asset of angioscopy is visualization of the surface of the vessel, which enables identification of thrombus, plaque, hemorrhage, ulceration, or embolus. Angioscopes can be used to remove debris from a vessel and to check the integrity of an anastomosis from within a vessel. They may also be used to remove the valves from veins to prepare them for use as bypass grafts. Complications are rare, but they may include intimal damage, vessel spasm, thrombosis or embolism, perforation, fluid overload, and infection. Postprocedural care is similar to that for clients who have had angiography.

Conclusions

Assessment of the peripheral vascular system centers on evaluating signs and symptoms and on distinguishing venous disorders from arterial disorders. Diagnostic assessments can range from simple noninvasive tests to invasive angiography. The most common assessment techniques include inspection of the skin and palpation of edema and blood flow. Applying these and other assessments properly is instrumental in providing clients with the appropriate diagnosis and care.

Bibliography

1. Baker, J. D. (1991). Assessment of peripheral arterial occlusive disease. *Critical Care Nursing Clinics of North America, 3*(3), 493–498.
2. Barnes, R. W. (1991). Noninvasive diagnostic assessment of peripheral vascular disease. *Circulation, 83*(Suppl. I), I-20–I-27.
3. Bright, L. D., & Georgi, S. (1992). Peripheral vascular disease: Is it arterial or venous? *AJN 92*(9), 34–43.
4. Fahey, V. (1994). *Vascular nursing.* Philadelphia: W. B. Saunders.
5. Hall, L. T. (1990). Endovascular surgery: An overview. *Progress in Cardiovascular Nursing, 5*(2), 43–49.
6. Massey, J. A. (1986). Diagnostic testing for peripheral vascular disease. *Nursing Clinics of North America, 21*(2), 207–218.

Nursing Care of Clients with Peripheral Vascular Disorders

Barbara Harrison

CHAPTER

50

Hypertension

Arterial hypertension, or high blood pressure, is generally defined as a persistent elevation of systolic blood pressure of 140 mm Hg or above and of diastolic pressure of 90 mm Hg or above. The fifth report of the Joint National Committee on Detection, Evaluation, and Treatment of High Blood Pressure notes the remarkable changes in the control of hypertension since the mid-1970s. Members of the public are more knowledgeable about high blood pressure, more likely to visit a healthcare provider for hypertension, and more likely to follow medical advice. These practices have contributed to a 50% decline in coronary artery disease mortality.[39]

Hypertension remains, however, a major contributor to morbidity and mortality in the United States. Arterial hypertension affects nearly 50 million persons in the United States. Prevalence of hypertension increases with advancing age, and blacks are affected more often than whites. It is especially significant in lower socioeconomic groups of all races.[39] Hypertension is the single most important predictor of cardiovascular risk. Increased blood pressure level is related to increased severity of atherosclerosis, stroke, nephropathy, peripheral vascular disease, aortic aneurysms, and congestive heart failure.

The advent of effective antihypertensive agents has dramatically reduced the mortality rate associated with hypertension. Still, if hypertension is untreated, nearly half of hypertensive clients die of heart disease, a third die of stroke, and the remaining 10% to 15% die of renal failure. Hypertension may also be a silent factor in many deaths attributed to stroke or heart attacks. When hypertension arises as a secondary process, death usually results from the primary disease.

Classification of Hypertension

Hypertension may be classified according to type, cause, and degree of severity.

This chapter incorporates material written for the fourth edition by Pamela D. Dennison and Joyce M. Black.

Systolic and Diastolic Hypertension. Systolic hypertension is systolic pressure of 140 mm Hg or higher. Diastolic hypertension is diastolic pressure of 90 mm Hg or higher.

Primary and Secondary Hypertension. Primary hypertension, also known as essential or idiopathic hypertension, constitutes more than 90% of all cases of hypertension. The etiology of primary hypertension is multifactorial; several interacting homeostatic forces are involved. Secondary hypertension results from an identifiable cause. A variety of specific disease states or problems are responsible. Fewer than 10% of the population of adult hypertensive clients has secondary hypertension. The importance of identifying clients with secondary hypertension centers on the fact that sometimes the disorder that creates the hypertension can be corrected.

"White Coat" Hypertension. "White coat" hypertension is defined as hypertension in persons who are actually normotensive except when their blood pressure is measured by a healthcare professional. The prevalence of white coat hypertension is unknown, but may be as high as one-third of diagnosed hypertensive individuals.[65] It has not yet been determined if this represents a variant form of hypertension or if this can be considered a normal finding. Twenty-four hour ambulatory blood pressure monitoring is recommended if white coat hypertension is suspected.

Isolated Systolic Hypertension. Isolated systolic hypertension (ISH) occurs when the systolic blood pressure is 140 mm Hg or higher, but the diastolic blood pressure remains below 90 mm Hg. It occurs primarily in people older than 50 years, with almost 24% of people affected by age 80 years. It is thought to occur because of atherosclerosis-induced changes in blood vessel compliance. The decreased vessel elasticity causes the systolic pressure to rise but does not affect the diastolic pressure.

Treatment for ISH is the same as for hypertension of both systolic and diastolic blood pressure.

Malignant Hypertension. Malignant hypertension is an emergency condition characterized by diastolic blood pressures above 120 mm Hg, retinal hemorrhage and exudates with papilledema, acute renal failure, and rapid vascular deterioration. Malignant hypertension has a peak incidence at age 40 to 50 years; its occurrence in clients younger than 30 or older than 60, should raise the suspicion of a secondary cause of hypertension. Without treatment, malignant hypertension results in a 90% mortality rate within 1 year secondary to renal or congestive heart failure, cerebrovascular accident, myocardial infarction, or aortic dissection. Blood pressure control reduces the chances of these complications.

Etiology and Risk Factors

Primary hypertension has no single or specific cause; it is multifactorial. It develops in response to increased cardiac output or to a rise in peripheral resistance. Factors that affect these two forces include the following:

- Genetic propensity to a heightened neurologic response to stress or for a defect in renal excretion or cellular transport of sodium
- Obesity associated with high levels of insulin (hyperinsulinemia) that lead to raised blood pressure
- Environmental stress
- Loss of elastic tissue and arteriosclerosis of aorta and other large arteries
- Secondary hypertension can result from a variety of identifiable primary causes (Box 50–1).

The most common cause of malignant hypertension is untreated hypertension. Other causes include eclampsia, dissecting aortic aneurysms, pyelonephritis, sudden catecholamine release (pheochromocytoma), drug or toxic substance ingestion/exposure, or food and drug interactions (e.g., monoamine oxidase inhibitors and aged cheeses). The relative risk for hypertension depends on the number and severity of nonmodifiable and modifiable risk factors.

■ Nonmodifiable Risk Factors

Family History. The genetic predisposition that makes certain families more susceptible to hypertension seems to be associated with elevated intracellular sodium levels and lowered potassium-to-sodium ratios. This is found more often in blacks. Clients with parents who have hypertension have a greater risk of developing hypertension at a younger age. This has not been demonstrated to be solely genetic; environmental factors may also be involved.

Age. The incidence of hypertension increases with age; 50% to 60% of clients older than 60 years have a blood pressure over 140/90 mm Hg. However, epidemiologic studies have shown a poorer prognosis in clients whose hypertension began at a young age.

Sex. Men experience hypertension at higher rates and at an earlier age than do women. Men also have greater risk of cardiovascular morbidity and mortality. After age 50 years, hypertension is more prevalent in women. The reasons are not clear.

Box 50–1. Causes of Secondary Hypertension

Renal Disorders

Renal parenchymal disease
    Acute glomerulonephritis
    Chronic nephritis
    Polycystic disease
    Connective tissue diseases
    Diabetic nephropathy
    Hydronephrosis
Renal artery stenosis
Renin-producing tumors

Endocrine Disorders

Acromegaly
Hypothyroidism
Hyperthyroidism
Adrenal
    Cortical
        Cushing's syndrome
        Primary aldosteronism
    Medullary
        Pheochromocytoma

Neurologic Disorders

Increased intracranial pressure
    Brain tumor
    Encephalitis
Sleep apnea
Autonomic dysreflexia

Medications

Oral contraceptives
Glucocorticoids
Mineralcorticoids
Cyclosporine
Erythropoietin
Monoamine oxidase inhibitors
Tricyclic antidepressants

Tyramine-Containing Foods

Aged cheeses (esp. cheddar)
Chicken liver
Yeast extract
Beer, wine

Acute Stress

Psychogenic hyperventilation
Hypoglycemia
Burns
Pancreatitis
Alcohol withdrawal
Sickle cell crisis

Vascular Disorders

Arteriosclerosis
Coarctation of the aorta

Pregnancy

Increased Intravascular Volume

Cocaine

Ethnic Group. Hypertension is more prevalent in blacks than in whites in the United States. Target organ damage is more severe in blacks than in other Americans from European or Hispanic backgrounds or native Americans. The reason for the increased prevalence of hypertension among blacks is unclear, but it has been attributed to lower renin levels, greater sensitivity to vasopressin, higher salt intake, and greater environmental stress.

■ Modifiable Risk Factors

Stress. Stress increases peripheral vascular resistance and cardiac output and stimulates sympathetic nervous system activity. Stress may be associated with occupational factors, socioeconomic levels, and personality characteristics.

Obesity. Obesity, especially in the upper body with increased amounts of intra-abdominal fat, is associated with hypertension. The combination of obesity and hypertension may be related to hyperinsulinemia secondary to insulin resistance.

Nutrients. Sodium is an important cause of essential hypertension. A high-salt diet may induce excessive release of natriuretic hormone, which may indirectly increase blood pressure. Sodium loading also has been shown experimentally to stimulate vasopressor mechanisms within the central nervous system. Potassium deficiency has been implicated as a cause of hypertension. Also, calcium intake may be lower among hypertensive than among normotensive clients. The impact of caffeine is controversial. It raises blood pressure acutely but does not have sustained effects.

Pathophysiology

■ Primary (Essential) Hypertension

The actual pathogenesis of hypertension remains unknown. Arterial blood pressure is a product of cardiac output and total peripheral resistance. Cardiac output is determined by stroke volume and heart rate. Control of peripheral vascular resistance is maintained by the autonomic nervous system and circulating hormones. Therefore, any factor producing an alteration in peripheral vascular resistance, heart rate, or stroke volume affects systemic arterial blood pressure.

Four control systems play a major role in maintaining blood pressure. These include the arterial baroreceptor system, regulation of body fluid volume, the renin-angiotensin system, and vascular autoregulation. Probably no single defect causes essential hypertension in all clients.

Arterial baroreceptors are found in the carotid sinus, aorta, and wall of the left ventricle. These baroreceptors monitor the level of arterial pressure and counteract rises through vagally mediated cardiac slowing and vasodilation with decreased sympathetic tone. The role of the arterial baroreceptors in hypertension is not well under-

stood. The sensitivity of the baroreceptors may be "reset" so that pressure rises are sensed inadequately; or the mechanism may be excessive central nervous system (CNS)-mediated stimulation of adrenergic nerves.

Changes in fluid volume affect systemic arterial pressure. Thus, an abnormality in the transport of sodium in the renal tubules may cause essential hypertension. When sodium and water are in excess, total blood volume increases, thereby increasing blood pressure. In functional kidneys, a rise in pressure leads to diuresis. Pathologic changes that alter the pressure threshold at which kidneys excrete salt and water alter systemic blood pressure. In addition, the overproduction of sodium-retaining hormones has been implicated in hypertension.

Renin and angiotensin play a role in blood pressure regulation. Renin is an enzyme produced by the kidney that catalyzes a plasma protein substrate to split off angiotensin I, which is removed by a converting enzyme to the lung to form angiotensin II, then angiotensin III (Fig. 50-1). Angiotensin II and III act as vasoconstrictors and control aldosterone release. With increased sympathetic nervous system activity, angiotensin II and III also seem to inhibit sodium excretion, which results in elevated blood pressure. Increased renin secretion has been investigated as a cause of increased peripheral vascular resistance in primary hypertension.

Clients also may develop hypertension from deficiencies in vasodilators, such as prostaglandins, or congenital abnormalities in resistance vessels.

■ Secondary Hypertension

The primary mechanisms involved in producing secondary hypertension include the following:

1. Increased secretion of catecholamines (e.g., pheochromocytoma)
2. Increased release of renin (e.g., renal artery stenosis)
3. Expansion of sodium and blood volume (e.g., Cushing's syndrome)

Chronic renal disease, mainly chronic glomerulonephritis and renal artery stenosis, is the most common cause of secondary hypertension. Any serious insult to the kidney that interferes with sodium excretion, renal perfusion, or the renin-angiotensin-aldosterone mechanism may elevate blood pressure.

The adrenal glands cause secondary hypertension as a result of primary excesses of aldosterone, cortisol, and catecholamines. Primary aldosteronism usually arises from solitary benign adenomas of the adrenal cortex that release excess aldosterone. Excess aldosterone causes renal retention of sodium and water, expands blood volume, and elevates blood pressure. Other adrenal cortical problems can result in excess production of cortisol (Cushing's syndrome). Clients with Cushing's syndrome have an 80% risk of developing hypertension. Cortisol increases blood pressure by increasing renal sodium retention, angiotensin II levels, and vascular reactivity to norepinephrine. Pheochromocytoma, a small tumor of the adrenal medulla, can cause dramatic hypertension because of the release of excessive amounts of epinephrine and norepinephrine.

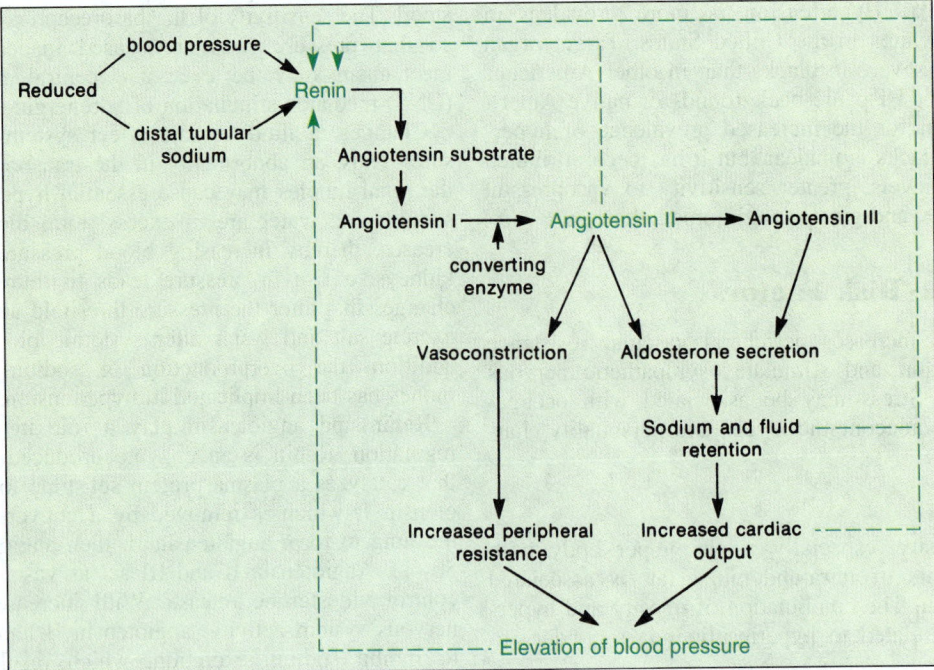

Figure 50–1. The role of the renin-angiotensin-aldosterone system in the regulation of blood pressure. *Solid lines* represent positive interactions; *broken lines* show negative interactions or feedback inhibition. (From Kumar, V., Cotran, R. S., & Robbins, S. L. [1992]. *Basic pathology* [5th ed.]. Philadelphia: W.B. Saunders.)

■ Vessel Changes

Early in the course of primary or secondary hypertension, there may be no obvious pathologic changes in the blood vessels and organs. The client may experience few or no symptoms other than intermittent elevations of blood pressure (labile hypertension). Slowly, widespread pathologic changes take place in both the large and small blood vessels and in the heart, kidneys, and brain.

The large vessels, such as the aorta, coronary arteries, basilar artery to the brain, and peripheral vessels in the limbs, become sclerotic, tortuous, and weak. Their lumina narrow, with resultant decreased blood flow to the heart, brain, and lower extremities. As the damage continues, large vessels may occlude or hemorrhage.

Small vessel damage, equally dangerous, causes structural changes in the heart, kidneys, and brain. Elevated diastolic blood pressure damages the intima of the small vessels. Because of intimal damage, fibrin accumulates in the vessels, local edema develops, and intravascular clotting may occur. The net result of these changes involves (1) a decreased blood supply to the tissues of the heart, brain, kidneys, and retina and (2) progressive functional impairment of these organs.

In the development of hypertensive cardiovascular disease, a vicious circle of pathologic changes occurs in which each new manifestation of the disease complicates other manifestations of the disease. When arterioles are constricted, the heart must increase its contractility to maintain normal cardiac output and overcome elevations in "afterload." This chronic overwork leads to hypertrophy of the heart, primarily the left ventricle. Hypertrophy

may lead to coronary insufficiency and myocardial infarction if the enlarged heart muscle outgrows its blood supply. If the hypertrophied heart cannot maintain sufficient cardiac output, left ventricular failure ensues. Left ventricular hypertrophy is a major risk factor for cardiac arrhythmias and sudden death.

As diastolic pressure rises in the failing left ventricle and atrium, the congestion extends back to involve the entire pulmonary tree; this, in turn, may lead to right ventricular failure. Blood may back up into the systemic circulation, causing systemic venous pressure to rise. Venous congestion and reduced arterial blood flow decrease renal perfusion. The kidneys may then fail, which further aggravates the hypertension. The increased arterial pressure in the arteries, coupled with arteriosclerotic weakening of the blood vessels, can cause aneurysms to develop and blood vessels to rupture.

Clinical Manifestations and Diagnostic Findings

The early stages of hypertension have no clinical manifestations, other than elevations in blood pressure. This unfortunate fact means that there are no clinical manifestations to lead a person to seek healthcare. As hypertension advances, without treatment, clients may report morning occipital headache, fatigue, dizziness, palpitations, flushing, blurred vision, and epistaxis. The presenting manifestations of malignant hypertension include hypertensive retinopathy. The retinopathy is characterized by arteriolar constriction, flame-shaped hemorrhages resulting from damaged capillary endothelium, and soft exudates secondary to transudation of protein from ischemic infarction of nerve fibers. Papilledema results from obstruction of venous outflow from the optic discs because of intracranial hemorrhage.

Additional clinical manifestations include hypertensive encephalopathy manifested by restlessness, changes in level of consciousness (e.g., confusion, somnolence, lethargy, memory defects, coma, seizures), blurred vision, dizziness, headache, nausea, and vomiting. Assessment may also reveal renal insufficiency, proteinuria, hematuria, urinary sediment casts, hemolytic anemia, left ventricular failure, and pulmonary edema. Severe headache may be occipital or anterior in location, is steady and throbbing in quality, and is often worse in the morning. Visual blurring, reduced visual acuity, and even blindness can occur.

The diagnosis of hypertension in the adult is determined when the average of two or more diastolic blood pressure readings, on at least two separate visits at least 1 week apart, is 90 mm Hg or higher, or when the average of multiple systolic blood pressure readings over several visits is 140 mm Hg or higher.

The 1992 Joint National Committee on Detection, Evaluation, and Treatment of High Blood Pressure has revised the classification of diastolic and systolic blood pressure readings (Table 50–1). Because the traditional terms of "mild" and "moderate" hypertension may not have conveyed the seriousness of hypertension at those levels, the terms were eliminated. High-normal was added as a category because people to whom this applies are at an increased risk of developing hypertension. Clinicians can use this classification to categorize blood pressure readings and to diagnose hypertension in clients age 18 years or older. Risk related to hypertension continues to increase as systolic and diastolic pressures rise. Classifying hypertension according to blood pressure readings reflects the degree of risk and helps determine intervention. Stage 1 is the most common form of hypertension and leads to much of the morbidity and mortality of hypertension. The Joint National Committee used these same clas-

sifications to develop follow-up criteria for first-occasion measurement (Table 50–2).

Table 50–1. Classification of Blood Pressure in Adults Aged 18 Years and Older*		
Category	**Systolic (mm Hg)**	**Diastolic (mm Hg)**
Normal	<130	<85
High normal	130–139	85–89
Hypertension		
Stage 1 (mild)	140–159	90–99
Stage 2 (moderate)	160–179	100–109
Stage 3 (severe)	180–209	110–119
Stage 4 (very severe)	≥210	≥120

* Not taking antihypertensive medications and not acutely ill. When systolic and diastolic pressures fall into different categories, the higher category should be selected to classify the individual's blood pressure status. For example, 170/96 would be classified as stage 2, and 184/122 would be classified as stage 4.

From the 1992 Joint National Committee. (1993). The fifth report of the Joint National Committee on the Detection, Evaluation, and Treatment of Hypertension. *Archives of Internal Medicine, 153,* 161.

 ## Community and Self-Care

Primary Prevention

Hypertension presents a national problem that individual interventions alone cannot counter. Prevention of hypertension and early discovery of new cases depend on a national public health effort. To be successful, this national effort needs to enlist government support and involve such nationwide structures as business and industry, labor organizations, healthcare institutions, voluntary associations, and local communities.

Table 50–2. Follow-up Criteria for First-Occasion Measurement		
Initial Screening Blood Pressure (mm Hg)*		
Systolic	**Diastolic**	**Follow-up Recommended†**
<130	<85	Recheck in 2 yr
130–139	85–89	Recheck in 1 yr
140–159	90–99	Confirm within 2 mo
160–179	100–109	Evaluate or refer to care within 1 mo
180–209	110–119	Evaluate or refer to care within 1 wk
≥210	≥120	Evaluate or refer to care immediately

* If the systolic and diastolic categories are different, follow recommendation for the shorter follow-up time.
† The scheduling of follow-up should be modified by reliable information about past blood pressure, other cardiovascular risk factors, or target-organ disease.

From the 1992 Joint National Committee. (1993). The fifth report of the Joint National Committee on the Detection, Evaluation, and Treatment of Hypertension. *Archives of Internal Medicine, 153,* 162.

Because the exact cause of primary hypertension remains unknown, it has been difficult for public health services to develop a comprehensive primary prevention program. However, several risk factors associated with the development of hypertension are known. Once high-risk clients are identified, clinicians can teach them how to modify certain risk factors such as diet, sodium intake, and exercise.

Hypertensive clients usually find out about their condition through incidental screening in healthcare facilities or organized community screening in public settings (e.g., shopping malls, schools, the workplace). Nurses are actively involved in both approaches. About 80% of Americans come into contact with some aspect of the healthcare system at least once a year (e.g., in a physician's office, clinic, or hospital). Each encounter with the healthcare system presents an opportunity for incidental blood pressure screening. Blood pressure measurement should be a routine procedure at every initial encounter with a healthcare practitioner and annually thereafter.

Organized community screening programs help assess the remaining 20% of Americans not in contact with any part of the healthcare system. Such programs identify not only untreated hypertensive clients but also those who have discontinued intervention or whose hypertension is not adequately controlled by current intervention. In addition, screening programs provide an opportunity to educate the public. It is particularly important to screen high-risk "target groups," such as black and elderly populations. Community services need to keep target groups in mind when choosing the setting for blood pressure screenings. Those who take blood pressure readings need to inform clients in writing of their blood pressure, its significance, and, if necessary, the importance of follow-up evaluation.

Secondary Prevention

Because the beginnings of adult hypertension often lie in childhood and adolescence, children over the age of 3 years need yearly blood pressure determinations. Asymptomatic youngsters who have an elevated blood pressure reading on three separate occasions require a careful work-up and follow-up program.

Of national concern is the rise in childhood obesity. In the past 20 years, obesity among 6- to 11-year-old American children increased 54%; among the 12- to 17-year-old population, the increase was 39%. Obese teenagers have an 80% chance of becoming obese adults. Obesity in children is a major cause of hypertension, so these statistics dramatically demonstrate the need for attention to this issue.

Tertiary Prevention

Once diagnosed, hypertension requires ongoing management despite the absence of manifestations. The many sequelae of unmanaged hypertension (e.g., stroke, myocardial infarction) can be prevented or their severity reduced if hypertension is well managed. Because of the cost of antihypertensives, side effects, and lack of symptoms, many clients do not manage the disorder well.

■ Medical Management

The goal of treating clients with hypertension is to prevent morbidity and mortality associated with high blood pressure. The objective is to achieve and maintain arterial blood pressure below 140/90 mm Hg, if possible.

Normalizing high blood pressure may involve psychosocial and economic stressors for the client. These stressors are considered when intervention is initiated. As mentioned earlier, most hypertensive clients do not have clinical manifestations and are not aware that they have hypertension. The long-term nature of intervention along with the high costs and untoward side effects of pharmacologic interventions promote poor adherence to therapeutic regimens. Poor adherence has great impact on the effectiveness of intervention.

Intervention for secondary hypertension involves treating the underlying disorder, whereas intervention for primary hypertension aims directly at reducing blood pressure. Careful differential diagnosis of primary versus secondary causes of high blood pressure must precede any intervention.

Life-Style Modifications

Life-style modifications are widely advocated as initial therapy for most clients, at least for the first 3 to 6 months after initial diagnosis. These interventions do not include medication and are used as treatment only if the diastolic blood pressure is below 100 mm Hg. This therapy may be effective for many of the 40% of clients with stage 1 hypertension (diastolic levels between 90 and 94 mm Hg). For the remainder of clients with hypertension, life-style modifications may aid in reducing blood pressure such that less drug therapy is needed.

Weight Reduction. The relationship between obesity and blood pressure has been clearly established from numerous studies. For many people with hypertension who are more than 10% over ideal body weight, weight reduction will lower blood pressure. Weight reduction also enhances the effectiveness of antihypertensives. Therefore the client's blood pressure should be reassessed during weight loss and appropriate changes made as needed.

Sodium Restriction. An estimated 40% of persons with hypertension are sodium sensitive. Studies demonstrating the antihypertensive efficacy of moderate sodium restriction to a level of 2.3 g of sodium or 6 g of salt have been reported since the early 1970s. This degree of sodium restriction may control blood pressure in some people with stage 1 hypertension. In others, the amount of medication needed may be decreased if sodium intake is lowered. In addition, this moderate sodium restriction may reduce the degree of potassium depletion that often accompanies diuretic therapy. Most dietary sodium intake comes from prepared foods rather than from added table salt, so teach clients to read and understand food labels.

Dietary Fat Modification. Modification of dietary intake of fat by decreasing the fraction of saturated fat and increasing that of polyunsaturated fat may decrease blood pressure and will decrease the cholesterol level, which is an important risk factor for coronary artery disease. The use of fish oil supplements to lower cardiovascular risk has been shown to lower blood pressure in preliminary studies, but fish oil supplementation may cause deficient blood clotting and excessive bleeding in some clients. Therefore, this therapy alone for hypertension is not recommended until long-term results are known.

Exercise. A regular program of aerobic (isotonic) exercise facilitates cardiovascular conditioning, can aid the obese hypertensive client in weight reduction, and may provide some benefit in reducing blood pressure. Heavy isometric exercises, such as weight lifting, may be harmful; blood pressure often rises to very high levels because of vasovagal reflexes that occur during an isometric contraction. Advise hypertensive clients to initiate exercise programs gradually and to receive ongoing professional surveillance of their condition.

Alcohol Restriction. The consumption of more than 1 oz of alcohol per day is associated with a higher prevalence of hypertension, poor adherence to the antihypertensive therapy, and, occasionally, refractory hypertension. Carefully assess alcohol intake. Advise those who do drink to do so in moderation (i.e., less than 1 oz of ethanol per day). There is 1 oz (28 g) of ethanol in 2 oz of 100-proof whiskey, 8 oz of wine, or 24 oz of beer.

Caffeine Restriction. Although acute ingestion of caffeine may raise blood pressure, chronic moderate caffeine ingestion appears to have no significant effect on blood pressure. Therefore, caffeine restriction is not necessary unless cardiac or other excessive sensitivity to caffeine is present.

Relaxation Techniques. A variety of relaxation therapies, including transcendental meditation, yoga, biofeedback, and psychotherapy, reduce blood pressure in hypertensive clients at least transiently. Although each has its advocates, none has been conclusively shown to be either practical for the majority of hypertensive clients or effective in maintaining a significant long-term effect.

Smoking Cessation. Smoking has not been statistically linked to the development of hypertension. However, nicotine definitely increases heart rate and produces peripheral vasoconstriction, which does raise arterial blood pressure for a short time. Smoking cessation is strongly recommended, however, to reduce the client's risk for cancer, pulmonary disease, and cardiovascular disease. Smokers appear to have a higher frequency of malignant hypertension and subarachnoid hemorrhage. In addition, risk reduction brought about by antihypertensive therapy may not be as great in smokers as in nonsmokers.

Potassium Supplementation. The high ratio of sodium to potassium in the modern diet has been held responsible for the development of hypertension. However, even though potassium supplements may lower blood pressure, they are too costly and potentially too hazardous for routine use. A reduction of high-sodium, low-potassium processed foods with an increase in low-sodium, high-potassium natural foods may be all that is needed to achieve the potential benefits.

Calcium Supplementation. The most recent studies examining the antihypertensive effects of calcium supplements demonstrate that this therapy may be helpful for a small portion of the population with hypertension. Clients should ensure a reasonable dietary calcium intake rather than using calcium supplements for preventing or treating hypertension.

Magnesium Supplementation. The antihypertensive effect of supplemental magnesium has been less well studied than that of potassium or calcium. Lower magnesium levels have been noted in hypertensive clients, and diuretic therapy may induce hypomagnesemia. In the presence of documented hypomagnesemia, supplementation may be considered.

Pharmacologic Intervention

Considerable debate continues regarding the appropriate time and circumstances for the initiation of pharmacologic management of hypertension. Clinicians sometimes question whether the benefits of medications outweigh their risks and inconveniences, particularly in mildly hypertensive clients. However, antihypertensive agents do decrease cardiovascular mortality and morbidity associated with hypertension.

Once a decision has been made to use pharmacologic intervention, one of several drugs can be used. If therapy is chosen carefully, more than half of mild hypertension cases can be controlled with a single drug, and more than 90% should be controlled with no more than two drugs. Long-term compliance has emerged as an essential element in reducing morbidity and mortality associated with hypertension. Several factors related to specific drug use, including side effects, interference with life-style, cost, and inconvenience of use, play an important role in noncompliance. Thus, drug selection is a critical part of the management of the client with hypertension. The ultimate factors in determining whether a correct choice has been made are that the medication controls the blood pressure, is tolerated, is safe, and is a drug that the client is willing to take over the long term.

Antihypertensive medications can be classified by mode of action into the following categories: diuretics, adrenergic inhibitors, vasodilators, angiotensin-converting enzyme (ACE) inhibitors, and calcium antagonists. Table 50–3 outlines major antihypertensive agents.

Diuretics are used to initiate and maintain antihypertensive therapy. Thiazide diuretics have been used for more than 30 years in the treatment of hypertension. Their efficacy and safety are well demonstrated. They are most effective in older and in black clients who tend to have a low-renin type of hypertension. Diuretics lower blood pressure by reducing extracellular fluid volume.

Text continued on p. 1397

Table 50–3. Antihypertensive Medication Therapy

Medication	Actions	Comments	Contraindications	Side Effects	Nursing Considerations
Diuretics					
Thiazide and Related Agents					
Bendroflumethiazide (Naturetin) Benzthiazide (Exna, Aquatag) Chlorothiazide (Diuril) Chlorthalidone (Hygroton) Hydrochlorothiazide (Esidrix, HydroDIURIL) Hydroflumethiazide (Diucardin, Saluron) Indapamide (Lozol) Methyclothiazide (Enduron) Metolazone (Zaroxolyn) Polythiazide (Renese) Quinethazone (Hydromox) Trichlormethiazide (Metahydrin, Naqua)	Promote renal excretion of sodium, water, and potassium Blood volume and cardiac output are decreased at first; with continued therapy, levels rise to normal Peripheral vascular resistance is increased at first, then drops below normal	All thiazides have a comparable effect on blood pressure, differing mainly in potency and duration Alone, thiazides can control hypertension in 40% of clients; in combination, they permit smaller doses of other antihypertensive agents Inexpensive	Known sensitivity to sulfonamide-derived drugs; renal insufficiency or failure; hepatic disease; lactation; blood urea nitrogen 40% or higher	Hypokalemia, hyperglycemia, hyperuricemia, hypercalcemia, lethargy, dry mouth, thirst, restlessness, muscle cramps, hypotension, polyuria, fatigue, tachycardia, gastrointestinal disturbances, vertigo, gout, leukopenia, and agranulocytosis Sexual dysfunction may occur May increase cholesterol, low-density lipoprotein, and triglyceride levels	Warn client that orthostatic hypotension may be potentiated by alcohol, barbiturates, and narcotics Monitor serum electrolytes, blood urea nitrogen, uric acid Teach client which foods are high in potassium and low in sodium Daily weight monitoring Resulting hypokalemia can potentiate digitalis toxicity Monitor diabetic clients closely
Loop Diuretics					
Bumetanide (Bumex) Ethacrynic acid (Edecrin) Furosemide (Lasix)	Comparable to thiazides Act on loop of Henle to minimize sodium and water reabsorption	Drug of choice in clients with renal failure	Comparable to thiazides; not recommended for pregnant women	Same as thiazides, hyponatremia, plus dehydration, vascular thrombosis, and embolism in elderly Can cause side effects, oral and gastric burning, and a sweet taste	Comparable to thiazides May avoid taking drug before bedtime to prevent frequent urination and loss of sleep May need to increase dose of hypoglycemic agents
Potassium-Sparing Diuretics					
Amiloride (Midamor) Spironolactone (Aldactone) Triamterene (Dyrenium)	Block action of aldosterone in distal loop, promoting excretion of sodium and water and retention of potassium Action of triamterene is unknown	These are weak diuretics that potentiate other antihypertensive drugs	Acute renal insufficiency, rapidly progressing impaired renal function, and hyperkalemia Avoid concomitant use with calcium-channel blocking agents	Hyperkalemia, hyponatremia, elevated blood urea nitrogen, gynecomastia, menstrual irregularity, hirsutism, headache, urticaria, impotency, and ataxia (with spironolactone) Blood dyscrasias with triamterene	Administer after meals to reduce nausea Potassium supplementation not required Closely monitor potassium, especially in those with renal insufficiency

Table 50–3. Antihypertensive Medication Therapy *(Continued)*

Medication	Actions	Comments	Contraindications	Side Effects	Nursing Considerations
Adrenergic Inhibiting Agents					
Beta-Blockers					
Atenolol (Tenormin) Betaxolol (Kerlone) Bisoprolol (Zebeta) Metoprolol (Lopressor, Toprol XL) Nadolol (Corgard) Propranolol (Inderal, Inderal LA) Timolol (Blocadren)	Block beta-receptors in the heart and peripheral vessels to reduce peripheral vascular resistance	These agents vary in their effects on beta-receptors: some (e.g., propranolol) affect $beta_1$- and $beta_2$-receptors; others (e.g., atenolol and metoprolol) are cardioselective, affecting only $beta_1$-receptors	Bronchial asthma, allergic rhinitis, chronic obstructive pulmonary disease, bradycardia, heart block, pulmonary hypertension, congestive heart failure Do not give with (or <2 wk after) therapy with monoamine oxidase inhibitors	Bradycardia, congestive heart failure, bronchospasm, hypoglycemia, fatigue, vivid and colorful dreams, insomnia, Raynaud's phenomenon, depression, nausea, vomiting, diarrhea, fluid retention, and (rarely) impotence	Avoid use in clients with bronchial asthma Assess for signs of heart failure Instruct client to take own pulse daily for evidence of bradycardia or irregularity Warn diabetics that these medications may mask signs of hypoglycemia Do not stop abruptly; this may exacerbate myocardial ischemia Toxic effects are reversed with isoproterenol or dopamine
Beta-Blockers with Intrinsic Sympathomimetic Activity (ISA)					
Acebutolol (Sectral) Carteolol (Cartrol) Penbutolol (Levatol) Pindolol (Visken)		No clear advantage for agents with ISA except for those with bradycardia who must take a beta-blocker; they produce fewer or no metabolic side effects			
Alpha-Beta Blocker					
Labetalol (Trandate, Normodyne)	Same as beta-blockers plus alpha blocking	May be more effective in blacks than other beta-blockers		Postural effects; titrate based on standing blood pressure	
Alpha₁-Receptor Blockers					
Doxazosin (Cardura) Prazosin (Minipress) Terazosin (Hytrin)	Block alpha-1 receptors and cause vasodilation			Titrate based on standing blood pressure	

Table continued on following page

Table 50–3. Antihypertensive Medication Therapy (Continued)

Medication	Actions	Comments	Contraindications	Side Effects	Nursing Considerations
Angiotensin-Converting Enzyme (ACE) Inhibitors					
Benazepril (Lotensin) Captopril (Capoten) Enalapril (Vasotec) Fosinopril (Monopril) Lisinopril (Prinivil, Zestril) Quinapril (Accupril) Ramipril (Altace)	Inhibit conversion of angiotensin I to angiotensin II May also inactivate the vasodepressor bradykinin Reduce peripheral vascular resistance without changing cardiac output	Extremely effective in clients with high-renin, severe hypertension Reduce or discontinue diuretic dose before starting ACE inhibitors	Use with caution in clients with pre-existing renal insufficiency and renal artery stenosis Not recommended for pregnant women	Fever, rash, stomatitis, taste loss, tongue ulceration, hyperkalemia, granulocytopenia, hemolytic anemia, renal damage with proteinuria, hyperkalemia in clients with renal impairment	Monthly urine protein analysis recommended along with a leukocyte count to detect renal damage Taste loss is a frequent side effect and may decrease desire for eating Hypotension may accompany first dose
Calcium Antagonists					
Diltiazem (Cardizem, Cardizem SR, Cardizem ER) Verapamil (Calan, Calan LA, Isoptin) Dihydropyridines Amlodipine (Norvasc) Felodipine (Plendil) Isradipine (DynaCirc) Nicardipine (Cardene) Nifedipine (Procardia)	More potent vasodilators than diltiazem or verapamil Block entry of calcium into smooth muscle cells and may interfere with the intracellular release of calcium Cause arteriolar vasodilation and decreased peripheral vascular resistance	Nifedipine has the most potent vasodilating effect Nifedipine and diltiazem are preferred agents in this group	Severe congestive heart failure, sick sinus syndrome, or progressive heart block Avoid use with beta-blocking agents	May cause more headaches, dizziness, peripheral edema, and tachycardia than diltiazem and verapamil Headache, dizziness, palpitations, weakness, nausea, flushing, hypotension, arrhythmia, constipation, diarrhea, rash, fluid retention, and edema Verapamil can cause bradycardia	Watch for sudden hypotension, especially with the administration of nifedipine; this can occur 5 minutes after sublingual administration and 20 minutes after oral administration Monitor pulse for bradycardia with use of verapamil May exacerbate asthma, peripheral vascular disease, and diabetes
Supplemental Antihypertensive Agents					
Centrally Acting Alpha₂ Agonists					
Clonidine (Catapres) Guanabenz (Wytensin) Guanfacine (Tenex) Methyldopa (Aldomet)	Suppress central nervous system sympathetic outflow Cardiac output decreases at first, then returns to normal Peripheral vascular resistance and heart rate decrease	An extremely effective medication, especially in clients with severe hypertension or renin-dependent disease Replace clonidine patch once a week	Tricyclic antidepressants may block drug's effect	Dry mouth, sedation, dizziness, constipation, headache, fatigue, bradycardia, and some sodium and water retention (transient), hyperglycemia	Action potentiated by alcohol, sedatives, digitalis, propranolol, and guanethidine Diabetics may require more insulin Drug should be discontinued over 2 to 4 days to prevent rebound hypertension

Table 50–3. Antihypertensive Medication Therapy *(Continued)*

Medication	Actions	Comments	Contraindications	Side Effects	Nursing Considerations
Centrally Acting Alpha₂ Agonists Continued					Recommend periodic eye examinations Chewing gum or hard candy may relieve dry mouth
Peripheral-Acting Adrenergic Antagonists					
Guanadrel (Hylorel) Guanethidine (Ismelin) Rauwolfia (Raudixin) Reserpine (Serpasil)	Deplete brain and peripheral nerve tissues of norepinephrine Decrease peripheral vascular resistance, heart rate, and standing blood pressure	Has same actions as other rauwolfia alkaloids Seldom used alone but in combination with a diuretic and beta-blocker	Mental depression, especially with suicidal tendencies; peptic ulcer disease, ulcerative colitis	Depression, weight gain, nasal stuffiness, peptic ulceration, postural hypotension, drowsiness, constipation, bizarre dreams, bradycardia, and impotence	Observe for signs of depression; instruct client to notify physician or you if "low mood" sets in Deplete catecholamines, so stop reserpine 2 weeks before elective surgery Concurrent use with digitalis and quinidine may potentiate arrhythmias
Vasodilators					
Hydralazine (Apresoline) Minoxidil (Loniten)	Direct action on smooth muscle walls of arterioles causing arteriolar vasodilation Cardiac output increases initially, then returns to normal Peripheral vascular resistance is decreased Some vasodilation	Most commonly used in combination with a beta-blocking agent and a diuretic with good results. Antihypertensive effects can be counteracted by the increase in cardiac output	Coronary artery disease, mitral valvular rheumatic heart disease, and hypersensitivity to drug	Minimal side effects Headache, palpitation, flushing, dyspnea, angina pectoris, and lupus-like syndrome (after prolonged use)	Monitor for reflex tachycardia Treat headache with acetaminophen, cold packs, or relaxation techniques

Stepped-Care Therapy. The goal of antihypertensive therapy is to control blood pressure with a minimum of side effects. The Joint National Committee on Detection, Evaluation, and Treatment of High Blood Pressure has recommended the stepped-care approach to the treatment of hypertension (Box 50–2). The 1992 report expands the pharmacologic choices available for initial and subsequent therapy and encourages substituting drugs as well as adding or reducing drugs to improve blood pressure control or to reduce side effects. Clinicians are encouraged to adopt an individualized approach to drug therapy, considering demographic concerns, the presence of concomitant diseases or therapies, and quality of life in selecting drugs for individual clients.

Step-Down Therapy. Once a client with stage I hypertension has been controlled for 1 year and at least four visits, medication dosages can be decreased slowly. Regular follow-up is essential.

Combination Therapy. In more than 50% of clients with mild hypertension, the condition can be controlled with one drug; the remaining clients will require combination therapy. If more than one drug is necessary, several combination therapies have proved effective. The combination of a diuretic with a beta-adrenergic blocker or other adrenergic inhibitor has been effective in both blacks and whites, unlike the responses to the individual drugs. The combination of diuretic and ACE inhibitor is

Box 50–2. Stepped-Care Approach to Management of Hypertension

Step 1: Life-style modifications

Weight reduction
Moderation of alcohol intake
Regular physical activity
Reduction of sodium intake
Smoking cessation

If there is inadequate blood pressure control, move to Step 2

Step 2: Continue life-style modifications, make initial pharmacologic selection: diuretics or beta-blockers recommended because of studies that demonstrate reduced
morbidity and mortality

If there is inadequate blood pressure control, move to Step 3

Step 3: Increase drug dose
OR
Substitute another drug
OR
Add a 2nd drug from a different class

ACE inhibitors
Calcium antagonists
Alpha-receptor blockers
Alpha-beta blockers

If there is inadequate blood pressure control, move to Step 4

Step 4: Add 2nd or 3rd drug and/or diuretic if not already prescribed

From the 1992 Joint National Committee. (1993). The 5th report of the Joint National
Committee on the Detection, Evaluation, and Treatment of Hypertension. *Archives of
Internal Medicine, 153,* 164.

---

synergistic because diuretics create high-renin hypertension, a milieu in which ACE inhibitors are effective. The
combination of a diuretic and calcium-channel blocker
has additive effects on blood pressure. Orthostatic hypotension can be a problem, especially in older clients or in
clients with acute volume depletion.

■ Nursing Management of the Medical Client

Assessment

Assessment of the client with hypertension involves the
following three main objectives:

1. To determine the extent of target organ involvement
2. To ascertain the presence of other cardiovascular risk
   factors
3. To identify the type of hypertension (primary or secondary) involved

Clinicians can obtain information relevant to these areas from the history, physical examination, and laboratory
studies.

History. Note the following points when interviewing
the hypertensive client:

- Family history of hypertension, diabetes mellitus, cardiovascular disease, hyperlipidemia, or renal disease.
- Previous documentation of high blood pressure, including age at onset, level of elevation, and currently prescribed medical regimen.
- History of any disease or trauma to target organs.
- Results and side effects of previous antihypertensive
  therapy.
- Clinical manifestations of cardiovascular disorders, such
  as angina, dyspnea, or claudication.
- History or presence of weight gain, exercise activities,
  sodium intake, fat intake, alcohol use, and smoking.
- Psychosocial and environmental factors (e.g., emotional
  stress, cultural food practices, and economic status) that
  may influence blood pressure control.
- Presence of other cardiovascular risk factors, including
  smoking, obesity, hyperlipidemia, and exercise levels.
- History of all prescribed and over-the-counter medications. Medications that may either raise blood pressure
  or interfere with the effectiveness of antihypertensive

medications include oral contraceptives, steroids, non-steroidal anti-inflammatory agents, nasal decongestants, appetite suppressants, cyclosporine, tricyclic antidepressants, monoamine oxidase inhibitors, and erythropoietin.

Physical Examination. Physical assessment should include accurate determination of blood pressure as well as evaluation of target organs.

Because blood pressure is variable and can be affected by multiple factors, it should be measured so that readings are representative of the client's usual level. The following techniques are strongly recommended:

1. The client should be seated with the arm bared, supported, and positioned at heart level. The client should not have smoked tobacco or ingested caffeine within the past 30 minutes.
2. Measurement should begin after 5 minutes of quiet rest. The client's back should be supported, and both feet should be flat on the floor with the legs uncrossed. The client should not speak while blood pressure is being monitored.
3. Use the appropriate cuff size to ensure an accurate measurement. The rubber bladder should encircle at least 80% of the limb being measured. The bladder's width should be one third to one half the circumference of the limb. Several sizes of cuffs (e.g., child, adult, and large adult) should be available. If the cuff is too wide, the blood pressure reading will be falsely low. If the cuff is too narrow, the reading will be falsely high. Inaccurate cuff size is the most common error in taking blood pressure measurement.
4. Measurements should be taken with a mercury sphygmomanometer, a recently calibrated aneroid manometer, or a validated electronic device. Aneroid gauges should be calibrated every 6 months against a mercury manometer.
5. Both the systolic and diastolic blood pressure should be recorded. The disappearance of sound (phase V) should be used for the diastolic reading.
6. Two or more readings should be averaged. If the first two readings differ by more than 5 mm Hg, additional readings should be obtained.

Clients should be informed of their blood pressure reading and advised of the need for periodic remeasurement. When working with lay clients, the examiner should refer to hypertension as *high blood pressure* to help allay confusion associated with the term *hypertension*. Many clients unfamiliar with medical terms may believe that hypertension denotes a state of being hypertense, that is, being worried or agitated. For these clients, the term *high blood pressure* more accurately conveys the nature of the health problem.

Evaluation of target organs typically includes the following data:

1. Funduscopic examination for retinal arteriolar narrowing, hemorrhages, exudates, and papilledema
2. Examination of the neck for distended veins, carotid bruits, and enlarged thyroid
3. Examination of the heart for increased heart rate, arrhythmias, enlargement, precordial impulses, murmurs, and S_3 and S_4 heart sounds
4. Examination of the abdomen for bruits, aortic dilation, and enlarged kidneys
5. Examination of extremities for diminished or absent peripheral pulses, edema, and bilateral inequality of pulses
6. Neurologic evaluation for signs of cerebral thrombosis or hemorrhage

Be especially alert to assessment findings that suggest secondary hypertension. These include headache, palpitations, and excessive perspiration (pheochromocytoma); leg claudication and diminished or absent lower extremity pulses (aortic coarctation); truncal obesity with pigmented striae (Cushing's syndrome); and polyuria, fatigue, and muscle cramps (hyperaldosteronism).

Laboratory Studies. A few general laboratory tests are usually done before intervention begins. These tests provide useful information in determining the severity of vascular disease, the extent of target organ damage, and the possible causes of hypertension. Studies used in the routine evaluation of hypertension include a complete blood count, urinalysis, determinations of levels of serum potassium and sodium, fasting blood glucose, serum cholesterol, blood urea nitrogen, and serum creatinine, electrocardiogram, and chest x-ray. Clients with potential for secondary hypertension may need more extensive studies.

Diagnosis, Planning, Implementation

Ineffective Management of Therapeutic Regimen (Individuals). Use the nursing diagnosis *Ineffective Management of Therapeutic Regimen (Individuals)* to identify the learning needs of the newly diagnosed hypertensive client. The diagnosis can be written *Risk for Ineffective Management of Therapeutic Regimen (Individuals) related to a new diagnosis, no previous learning about the disease process, potential consequences, the rationale for intervention and proper administration of prescribed medications.*

Planning: Expected Outcomes. The client and significant others will demonstrate knowledge required for self-care. This knowledge will be demonstrated by the ability to do the following:

Describe the disease process and factors contributing to its symptoms and risks and reasons that management of this disease is important

Describe the proper administration of prescribed medication therapy, including drug name, rationale for use, dosage, frequency, potential side effects, and measures to minimize side effects

Demonstrate proper blood pressure measurement technique for home blood pressure monitoring

Discuss the importance of lifelong medical follow-up for hypertension control

Implementation. Because of the chronicity of hypertension and its dangerous complications, clients with hypertension need clear, practical, and realistic learning guidelines. Guidelines should include information concerning the disease and its management. Use written materials with clear illustrations to introduce the subject of hypertension to the newly diagnosed client. Teach the client to monitor and record his or her own blood pressure at home at least once a week and to record the findings in a diary.

Altered Nutrition: More than Body Requirements.

Because dietary adjustments can reduce the severity of hypertension and may reduce the need for medications, this is an important aspect of nursing care. Write the diagnosis as *Altered Nutrition: More than Body Requirements related to high sodium, calorie, and fat intake.*

Planning: Expected Outcomes. The client will demonstrate knowledge of and adherence to the nutritional regimen by

Describing specific dietary modifications including sodium, fat, and calorie restrictions and their rationale
Listing common foods to be avoided
Reducing levels of urine sodium and blood cholesterol
Losing weight

Implementation. The two most important aspects of dietary intervention for hypertension are weight reduction (for overweight clients) and mild to moderate sodium restriction. Therefore, advise the client with hypertension to eat a diet low in salt, calories, cholesterol, and saturated fat. Discuss the prescribed diet with those in the household who prepare food. If possible, enlist the aid of a dietitian to provide detailed dietary instructions. Before dietary intervention begins, assess the client's patterns of food intake, life-style, food preferences, and ethnic, social, cultural, and financial influences. A highly individualized approach to dietary counseling is critical.

Restrict Sodium. Sodium is a hidden ingredient in many processed foods, beverages (including water), and

---

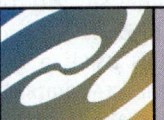

CLIENT EDUCATION GUIDE

Low-Sodium Diet

Client Instructions in English *(Instrucciones para el cliente en inglés)*	**Client Instructions in Spanish** *(Instrucciones para el cliente en español)*
Avoid Foods High in Sodium Read labels of foods carefully for "sodium," "Na+," "salt," "NaCl," "bicarbonate of soda," and "MSG" because these are all sources of sodium. If these words appear in the first four to five ingredients listed on the package, avoid the food item. Avoid common commercial preparations that are high in sodium, including baking powder, baking soda, monosodium glutamate, meat tenderizer, and soy sauce. Avoid canned, boxed, and some frozen foods to which sodium has been added. (Frozen fruits and vegetables are okay.) Avoid canned, smoked, pickled, or cured meat and fish products. (Canned tuna in water is okay.) Pickled or preserved vegetables always contain salt. Be aware that not all dietetic foods are sodium-free; read the labels before purchasing and using. In restaurants, choose foods that are baked, broiled, boiled, or roasted and without salted gravies or juices. Avoid soups and salted or cheesy dressings. Carry your own salt substitute if desired. Be aware that "fast foods" also tend to be high in sodium.	**Evite Alimentos con Mucho Sodio** Lea cuidadosamente las etiquetas para ver el contenido de "sodio," "Na+," "sal," "NaCl," "bicarbonato," y "MSG" porque estos son todos fuentes de sodio. Si estas palabras aparecen en el paquete entre los primeros cuatro o cinco ingredientes de la lista, evite esos alimentos. Evite las preparaciones comerciales comúnes que tengan mucho sodio, incluso la levadura en polvo, el bicarbonato, el glutamato de monosodico, el elblandador de carne, y la salsa de soya (soy sauce). Evite alimentos enlatados, envasados, y algunos alimentos congelados a los cuales se les ha agregado sal. (Puede comer frutas y verduras congeladas). Evite alimentos enlatados, ahumados, encurtidos, o carne y pescado curados. (Puede comer el atún enlatados en agua.) Las verduras encurtidas o en conserva siempre contienen sal. Debe saber que no todos los alimentos para régimen de dieta están libres de sodio; léa las etiquetas antes de comprarlos y usarlos. En el restaurante, escoja alimentos que estén cocinados al horno, hervidos, asados a la parrilla, sin jugos o salsas con sal. Evite las sopas y los salsas saladas o preparadas con queso. Si desea, lleve su propio salero con sustitución de sal. Reconozca que las "comidas rapidas" (fast-foods) tienden a contener gran cantidad de sodio.

over-the-counter drugs (particularly antacids, cough remedies, and laxatives). It cannot be seen and is often not tasted. Whereas the average adult daily intake of salt is 5 to 15 g, the therapeutic effects of sodium reduction on blood pressure do not occur until salt intake is reduced below 5 g/day. Low-salt diets can be very difficult to adhere to, at least initially. Reassure the client that it becomes easier as taste adjusts to decreased salt over a period of several weeks to months. When someone becomes fully accustomed to the low-salt diet, unsalted foods usually cease to taste bland. Research has suggested a relationship between lower blood pressure and increased intake of the minerals calcium, potassium, and magnesium, but the data are not yet conclusive.[41] The Client Education Guide presents guidelines for teaching clients about sodium reduction.

Reduce Fat and Cholesterol. Hypertension and high serum cholesterol (>250 mg/dl) seem to be linked risk factors in the development of coronary artery disease. The level of serum cholesterol is partly determined by the consumption of cholesterol, saturated and polyunsaturated fats, and total calories. Cholesterol is contained in animal fats and dairy products. Saturated fats occur predominantly in animal fats and tropical oils (e.g., coconut and palm oils). Unsaturated fats predominate in most plant-derived fats. Polyunsaturated fats occur predominantly in vegetable and seed oils. A diet low in saturated fats and high in polyunsaturated fats is beneficial in reducing blood pressure. The Client Education Guide entitled Low-Fat, Low-Cholesterol Diet provides guidelines for teaching clients about fat and cholesterol reduction.

Reduce Calories and Weight. Weight reduction in the overweight hypertensive client can significantly reduce blood pressure and decrease workload of the heart. Ideally, weight loss should be no more than 0.5 kg (~1 lb) a week. Advise the average adult with hypertension to reduce caloric intake by at least 250 calories/day. The overall goal should be achievement and maintenance of a weight that is within 15% of desirable weight. Caution clients to avoid over-the-counter appetite suppressants,

Client Instructions in English *(Instrucciones para el cliente en inglés)*	**Client Instructions in Spanish** *(Instrucciones para el cliente en español)*
Know that "lite" salt has half the sodium of table salt per unit. Nonsodium salt substitutes have a high potassium content and may be used to help prevent potassium deficiency if you are taking a thiazide diuretic.	Sepa que la sal ligera ("lite") contiene la mitad del sodio de la sal de mesa. Los sustitutos de sal monosódicos tienen un contenido alto en potasio y pueden usarse para prevenir deficiencias de potasio si se esta tomando un diurético thiazide (Diuril).
Prepare Low-Sodium Meals	**Prepare Comidas Bajas en Sal**
Do not add salt at the table.	No agregue sal cuando coma.
Use no salt during food preparation (2-g sodium diet) or use only half the salt called for in the recipe (4-g sodium diet).	No use sal durante la preparación de la comida (dieta baja en sal, 2 gramos de sodio) o use solo la mitad de la sal que indique la receta (dieta de 4 gramos de sodio).
Prepare canned vegetables (if they are to be eaten at all) by draining off the canned liquid and heating the food in tap water.	Prepare verduras enlatadas (si es que tiene que comerlas) escurriendo todo el líquido y calentandolas con el agua de la llave.
Liberally use natural spices, herbs, and condiments like pepper, parsley, chili, horseradish, lemon, and cloves, which contain negligible amounts of salt. Onion or garlic powder (dehydrated or pulverized) is also useful in low-salt cooking. Steak sauce, catsup, marinade, hot pepper sauce, and soy sauce are all high in sodium.	Use especias naturales, hierbas, y condimentos tales como pimienta, perejil, chile, rábano picante, limón o clavo de olor que casi no contienen sal. La cebolla o el ajo (en polvo o seco) también son buenos para cocinar con poco sodio. Las salsas para bistec o el adobo, salsa de tomate, salsa de pimienta picante, y la salsa de soya contienen gran cantidad de sodio.
Do not use herb salts (celery, onion, garlic), which are high in sodium.	No use sales de hierbas (apio, cebolla, ajo), que contienen mucho sodio.
Obtain low-sodium cookbooks from bookstores and from heart associations.	Obtenga recetarios de cocina en las librerias o en las asociaciónes del corazón.

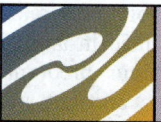

CLIENT EDUCATION GUIDE

Low-Fat, Low-Cholesterol Diet

Client Instructions in English *(Instrucciones para el cliente en inglés)*	Client Instructions in Spanish *(Instrucciones para el cliente en español)*
Avoid Foods High in Saturated Fats and Cholesterol	**Evite Alimentos Altos en Colesterol y Grasas Saturados**
Use margarine and vegetable oils instead of butter.	Use margarina y aceites vegetales en lugar de mantequilla
Avoid gravies, creams, and cheese sauces.	Evite comer salsas, cremas y aderezos de queso.
Avoid fried foods; instead, eat broiled, baked, or boiled foods	Evite las comidas fritas; en su lugar cocine al horno, ase a la parrilla o hierva los alimentos.
Use skim or low-fat milk and milk products.	Use leche o productos desnatados o descremados.
Choose lean cuts of meat. Trim off all visible fat. Remove all poultry skin.	Use trozos de carne delgados. Quiteles toda la grasa que les vea. Quitele el cuero al pollo.
Use a wire rack when roasting, broiling, or baking meats so that the fat can drip off.	Use una rejilla de alambre cuando ase a la parilla o cuando cocine carnes en el horno para que se escurra la grasa.
Keep in mind that poultry, fish, and veal have a relatively low fat content. Chicken and turkey breasts are the leanest poultry available. Avoid duck and goose. Haddock, cod, and water-packed tuna are the leanest fish available.	Recuerde que las aves, el pescado, y la ternera tienen contenido de grasa relativemente bajo. Las pechugas de pollo y de pavo son las carnes de ave que tienen menos grasa. No coma carne de pato o ganso. El bacalao, el abadejo y el atun enlatado en agua son los pescados más magros (sin grasa) que hay.
Use Teflon-coated pans when cooking to reduce the need for oil or shortening.	Cuando cocine, use cacerolas de teflón para reducir la necesidad de usar aceite o manteca.
Prepare meat stews, soups, and gravies in advance and chill them until the fat hardens. Then skim off the fat.	Prepare de antemano, el estofado, caldos, sopas, y salsas, y enfriels (en el refrigerador) hasta que la grasa se endurezca. Después, saque la grasa que cubre la comida.
Eat no more than three egg yolks per week. Egg whites are low in cholesterol, as are many egg substitutes.	No coma más de tres yemas de huevo a la semana. Las claras de huevo y otros sustitutos de huevo tienen poco colesterol.
Limit your intake of organ meats and shellfish.	Limite los alimentos de carnes de órganos (e.j.: higado, riñónes) y mariscos (e.j.: camarónes, cangrejo).

which often contain sympathomimetic agents that elevate blood pressure. The Client Education Guide entitled Calorie-Restriction Diet provides advice on regulating caloric intake.

Altered Health Maintenance. Exercise is like dietary management: a regular exercise program can lower blood pressure. This diagnosis can be written as *Altered Health Maintenance related to a lack of regular exercise regimen.*

Planning: Expected Outcomes. The client will begin and maintain an appropriate exercise program, as evidenced by self-report, demonstration of ability to monitor heart rate during exercise, sensation of reduced physical and emotional stress, and reduced blood pressure.

Implementation. Exercise programs may heighten the client's sense of well-being, provide an outlet for emotional tensions, and raise the levels of high-density lipoproteins relative to total blood cholesterol. Elevated high-density lipoprotein levels are associated with a decreased risk of cardiovascular morbidity and mortality. Instruct the client, however, to avoid heavy weight-lifting, isometric exercises, and other activities inappropriate to the client's physical limitations. A modest but consistent

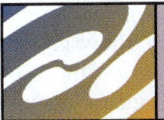

CLIENT EDUCATION GUIDE

Calorie-Restriction Diet

Client Instructions in English *(Instrucciones para el cliente en inglés)*	**Client Instructions in Spanish** *(Instrucciones para el cliente en español)*
To Regulate Your Caloric Intake Never eat when you are doing something else, such as watching television or reading. Chew properly and slowly and always sit down to eat. Begin each meal with raw vegetables or salad. Do not eat more than one slice of bread at a time. Except for a piece of toast with breakfast or a sandwich at lunch, do not eat bread with meals. Do not put butter or margarine on bread. Stop eating when you feel not quite full. (A feeling of satiety will usually occur about 20 minutes after eating.) Never wait until you are very hungry before you eat. Eat low-calorie, between-meal snacks if necessary. Eat something before going to parties. Avoid high-calorie party snacks, such as potato and corn chips and peanuts, almonds, and other nuts. Drink only low-calorie beverages, such as coffee or tea (decaffeinated). Avoid adding sugar to them, although nonfat milk may be added. Do not quench your thirst with milk; use water. Drink one to two glasses of water before drinking an alcoholic beverage. Alcoholic beverages are high in calories (7 kcal/ml). Avoid sugar; use artificial sweeteners instead. To appease an irresistible urge to eat something sweet, take ⅕ teaspoon of sugar or a tiny bite from a toffee. Leave the sugar on your tongue for as long as possible. Doing this even up to six times a day will provide fewer calories than a piece of cake or several cookies.	**Para Regularizar la Ingestión de Calorías** Nunca coma cuando esté haciendo otras cosas tales como ver la televisión o leer. Mastique despacio y bien y sientese siempre a comer. Empiece cada comida con verduras crudas o ensalada. No coma más de una rebanada de pan en cada comida. A parte de una rebanada de pan tostado en el desayuno y un sandwich para el amuerzo, no coma pan con las comidas. No le ponga mantequilla o margarina al pan. Deje de comer cuando se sienta casi lleno (casi siempre ocurre más o menos 20 minutos después de comer). Nunca se espere para comer hasta que tenga mucha hambre. Coma bocadillos que contengan poca grasa entre las comidas, si es necesario. Coma algo antes de asistir a fiestas. Evite comer bocadillos que tengan muchas calorías tales como papitas, fritos, cacahuates, almendras, u otras nueces. Tome bebidas de pocas calorías tales como el café o el té (descafeinádo). Evite agregarles azúcar, pero puede agregarles leche descremada. No se quite la sed tomando leche; tome agua. Beba uno o dos vasos de agua antes de tomar bebidas alcohólicas. Las bebidas alcohólicas tienen gran contenido de calorías (7 C/ml). Evite el azúcar; en su lugar use los sustitutos de azúcar. Para calmar un impulso irresistible de comer algo dulce, comase ⅕ de cucharita de azúcar o un pedacito de caramelo. Deje que se derrita el azúcar lentamente en la lengua. El hacer ésto un máximo de seis veces diarias le dá menos calorías que un pedazo de pastel o varias galletas.

exercise program provides greater benefits than do spurts of strenuous activity mixed with periods of inactivity. A gradually increasing program of aerobic activity such as walking, jogging, or swimming can thus be recommended. Current recommendations include aerobic exercise, maintaining 70% to 80% of maximal heart rate for 20 to 30 minutes, three times a week. Maximal heart rate is calculated by subtracting age from 220.

Risk for Noncompliance. Many aspects of hypertension management set the stage for noncompliance. After you fully understand the reasons for your client's noncompliance, the diagnosis can be stated as *Risk for Noncompliance related to a lack of understanding about the seriousness of high blood pressure, cost of therapy, side effects of medications, complexity of management, multiple changes in life-style.*

Planning: Expected Outcomes. The client will demonstrate understanding of the seriousness of high blood pressure and accept the treatment plan, as evidenced by active participation in creating a treatment plan, description of underlying causes of hypertension and self-care strategies, adherence to scheduled follow-up appointments, description of actions and side effects of current medications, and expression of commitment to and self-responsibility for controlling hypertension.

Implementation. The greatest problem in the management of chronic hypertension involves the client's lack of adherence to nonpharmacologic and pharmacologic intervention. An estimated 40% to 60% of clients with hypertension fail to comply with prescribed therapy. There are several reasons that hypertensive clients fail to follow prescribed regimens. The asymptomatic nature of the disease tends to minimize the perceived seriousness of the problem and importance of intervention. Also, therapeutic regimens often demand difficult life-style changes, such as low-sodium diets, weight loss, and smoking cessation. Many hypertensive agents have annoying side effects, and clients who require antihypertensive medication may consider the intervention worse than the disease. The high cost of prescribed medications and the inconvenience of obtaining healthcare also contribute to noncompliance. Nursing interventions for promoting compliance with the antihypertensive treatment regimen include individualizing care, ensuring adequate follow-up, communicating often with the client, and teaching the client and family. Compliance usually improves dramatically when the client understands the causative factors underlying hypertension as well as the consequences of inadequate intervention and health maintenance.

Antihypertensive medications may cause emotional lability, sleep disturbances, and sexual changes, including impotence. Discuss these potential problems with the hypertensive client and significant others. Counseling may help the client to cope.

Evaluation

The client's blood pressure should be reduced to less than 140/90 mm Hg. Medications can bring blood pressure down quickly. The remainder of interventions, such as exercise and smoking cessation, are more difficult to implement and maintain. Expect the client to struggle with compliance with all of the necessary changes. Ask specific questions in a nonjudgmental manner. Offer various self-help group involvement as needed, such as smoking cessation groups.

■ Modifications for Elderly Clients

Hypertension is one of the most prevalent cardiovascular diseases among the elderly. Research has provided conflicting findings on the effectiveness of treating hypertension in older adults. Because of this disagreement, a wide range of therapy is given to elderly hypertensive people, who consequently require extensive support, detailed advice, and careful follow-up. Older adults are also more likely to experience adverse reactions to antihypertensive

drugs and therefore need to be monitored more closely. Blood pressure readings in older adults may show greater variability from one reading to the next than do those of younger clients. The examiner must thus guard against making a diagnosis based on too few readings.

Emergency Care

■ Medical Management

Malignant hypertension constitutes a true medical emergency, and any delay in initiating intervention can be catastrophic. The seriousness of the crisis correlates not so much with the level of blood pressure elevation as with the extent of target organ damage. Intervention relies almost entirely on parenteral administration of medications. Most often, the physician orders concurrent administration of two or three agents (Table 50–4).

Clients with malignant hypertension require monitoring in an intensive care unit. Parameters that require close scrutiny include urinary output, blood pressure (via an intra-arterial catheter), central venous pressure, and pulmonary capillary wedge pressure. Continuous electrocardiographic (ECG) monitoring helps to assess for ischemic myocardial changes and arrhythmias.

The treatment goal is to lower blood pressure, but as blood pressure decreases, evidence of target organ impairment (especially of kidneys) may appear. Consequently, restoration of normal blood pressure must be done slowly and with care. Once the client is out of immediate danger, oral medications are administered while vital signs are monitored continuously. The physician typically prescribes a combination of diuretic, beta-blockers, and hydralazine. With better surveillance and control of hypertensive clients, hypertensive crisis is becoming less common.

■ Nursing Management of the Medical Client

Monitor blood pressure frequently (every 15 minutes) and titrate the medications to manage the blood pressure. Raise the client's head to decrease the risk of cerebral bleeding. Anxiety is reduced, and urinary output is also closely monitored.

Syncope

Syncope (fainting) is defined as generalized muscle weakness and inability to stand erect accompanied by loss of consciousness. It is a good measure of cardiovascular status, because it may indicate decreased cardiac output, fluid volume deficits, or defects in cerebral tissue perfusion. Syncope is a common occurrence when a person tries to stand after being bedridden for a time. This form of syncope, called *postural hypotension,* can be seen in clients attempting to ambulate for the first few times after surgery, clients who have been on prolonged bedrest, and

Table 50–4. Parenteral Drugs for Treatment of Hypertensive Emergency (in Order of Rapidity of Action)

Drug	Dosage	Onset of Action	Adverse Effects
Vasodilators			
Nitroprusside (Nipride, Nitropress)	.25–10 μg/kg/min as IV infusion	Instantaneous	Nausea, vomiting, muscle twitching, sweating, thiocyanate intoxication
Diazoxide (Hyperstat)	50–100 mg/IV bolus repeated, or 15–30 mg/min by IV infusion	1–2 min	Nausea, hypotension, flushing, tachycardia, chest pain, aggravation of angina
Nitroglycerin	5–10 μg/min as IV infusion	2–5 min	Tachycardia, flushing, headache, vomiting, methamoglobinemia
Hydralazine (Apresoline)	10–20 mg IV / 10–40 mg IM	10 min / 20–30 min	Tachycardia, flushing, headache, vomiting, aggravation of angina
Enalaprilat (Vasotec IV)	0.625–1.25 mg every 6 hr IV	15–60 min	Precipitous fall in blood pressure in high renin states; response variable
Adrenergic Inhibitors			
Trimethaphan (Arfonad)	0.5–1.0 mg/min as IV infusion (500 mg in 500 ml d₅w)	Immediate	Paresis of bowel and bladder, orthostatic hypotension, blurred vision, dry mouth
Labetalol (Normodyne, Trandate)	20 mg slow IV over 2 min / 40–50 mg IV every 10 min up to 300 mg *or* 2 mg/min by continuous IV infusion	5–10 min	Vomiting, scalp tingling, burning in throat, postural hypotension, dizziness

From the 1992 Joint National Committee. (1993). The 5th report of the Joint National Committee on the Detection, Evaluation, and Treatment of Hypertension. *Archives of Internal Medicine, 153,* 172.

clients who have dysrhythmia or take potent diuretics. When a person quickly moves to a standing position, blood normally pools in the lower legs. The arterial pressure receptors in the aortic arch detect the fall in cardiac output due to lack of venous return and increase sympathetic tone to compress arterioles to improve venous return. If the sympathetic response is not adequate, the person becomes dizzy due to decreased cerebral perfusion.

Syncope can usually be managed by anticipating it. Expect clients who have been on bedrest for a day or more to become dizzy when first sitting up. Have the client make slow movements and stop to rest in a sitting position before standing. Moving slowly allows time for the sympathetic tone to be reestablished. If the client becomes dizzy, instruct him or her to breathe deeply and to keep both eyes open. Syncope should resolve within moments. If it is prolonged, place the client back in bed. Assess for orthostatic hypotension by checking blood pressure in supine, sitting, and standing positions. Assess fluid volume status and pulse for irregularities. Use leg exercises to improve venous return. Have the client attempt to get up in a few hours; do not have the client rest in bed as a treatment for simple syncope. Bedrest increases poor sympathetic tone.

Arterial Disorders

Chronic Arterial Occlusion

Peripheral arterial occlusive disorders involve narrowing of the arterial lumen or damage to the endothelial lining. They are sometimes classified according to duration of the problem: acute or chronic.

Etiology and Risk Factors

Peripheral arterial occlusive diseases can be caused by atherosclerosis, embolism, thrombosis, trauma, vasospasm, inflammation, or autoimmunity. The cause of some disorders remains unknown. Most of the pathologic changes that occur in peripheral arterial occlusive disease are caused by atherosclerosis. Atherosclerosis is considered in detail in Chapter 45.

Pathophysiology

The peripheral arterial system delivers oxygen-rich blood to the peripheral vascular beds. Any alteration in blood flow disrupts the balance between oxygen supply and demand. Prolonged reduction in blood flow or the involvement of large areas of decreased perfusion initiates the compensatory mechanisms of vasodilation, collateralization, and utilization of anaerobic pathways for metabolic demands to be met. These compensatory mechanisms are useful in protecting blood supply to the peripheral vascular bed but are limited by certain factors. Vasodilation has a limited effect because arteries that become oxygen-deprived quickly dilate fully. The diffuse network of collateral vessels needed to protect blood supply develops slowly over time. Cellular anaerobic metabolism tries to meet the basic requirements, but the waste products of lactic acid and pyruvic acid build up quickly, are extremely toxic, and are excreted slowly. Significant increases in these two acids change the body's acid-base balance. As the compensatory mechanisms prove inadequate to meet peripheral vascular needs, and without medical or surgical intervention, the eventual result is pain. The pain is analogous to anginal pain, and is called *intermittent claudication*. Intermittent claudication occurs when a muscle is forced to contract without an adequate blood supply to meet the metabolic needs of exercise. It is the only specific manifestation of peripheral arterial disease and it results from muscular hypoxia and metabolite accumulation. If untreated it can lead to peripheral gangrene.

The physiologic effect of any given stenosis is unpredictable because it is determined not only by the extent to which the blood vessel is narrowed, but also by the effectiveness of collateral vessels that have developed in response to the gradually increasing pressure gradient. The lower limbs are far more susceptible to arterial occlusive disorders and atherosclerosis than are the upper limbs.

The most common locations for stenosis in a lower extremity are the aortoiliac bifurcation and the femoral bifurcation (Fig. 50–2). These lesions cause narrowing of the arterial lumen and slowly, but critically, reduce blood flow.

Clinical Manifestations and Diagnostic Findings

The most important manifestations of chronic arterial occlusive disease are *intermittent claudication and rest pain*. The client typically complains of pain described as tightening pressure in the calves or buttocks or a sharp, cramplike sensation that occurs during walking and disappears quickly with rest. As the disorder progresses, the client develops the same pain while at rest.

Another hallmark of chronic arterial insufficiency is a dusky, purplish discoloration of the foot and leg when the foot is placed in a dependent position. This *dependent rubor* changes to white pallor when the leg is elevated.

Intermittent claudication is influenced by the speed, incline, or surface of the walk. The client's exercise tolerance decreases over time; episodes of claudication occur more frequently with less exertion. In most clients, the clinical manifestations are constant and reproducible. Reproducible means that the same situation produces the same response almost every time. The client who cannot walk the length of a house because of leg pain one day but can walk indefinitely the next day does not have intermittent claudication. In most clients with arterial insufficiency, the onset of manifestations is gradual.

Clinical manifestations of chronic arterial occlusion may not appear for 20 to 40 years. Claudication, usually

Figure 50–2. Major sites of peripheral atherosclerotic occlusive disease.

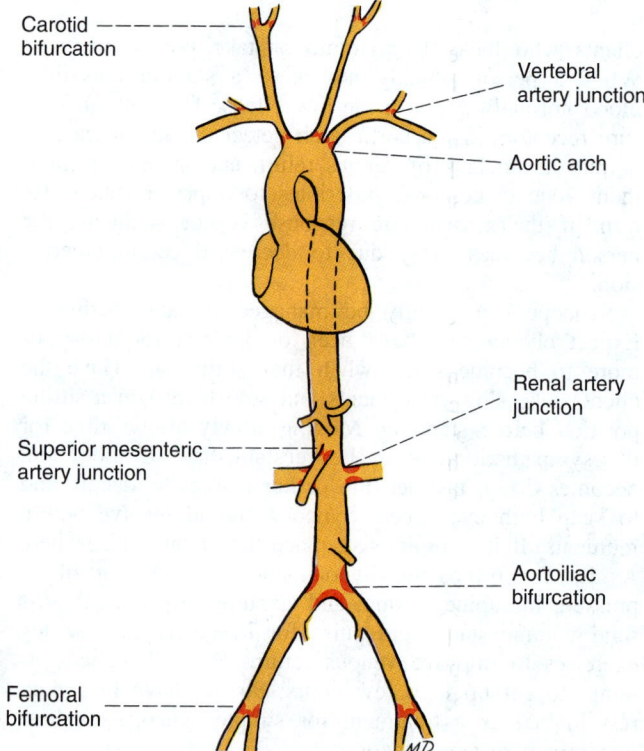

Carotid bifurcation

Vertebral artery junction

Aortic arch

Renal artery junction

Superior mesenteric artery junction

Aortoiliac bifurcation

Femoral bifurcation

MD

insidious in onset, generally occurs in men, although there is an increased incidence in women after menopause. Usually, claudication strikes males in their sixth or seventh decade. Nearly half of clients who experience claudication have associated severe coronary artery disease.

The development of pain at rest, usually occurring at night when the client lies supine, indicates progressive disease. Usually described as a dull aching in the toes or forefoot, this sensation may awaken the client from sleep and cause him or her to hang the foot over the side of the bed or get up and walk around for relief. As manifestations progress, the client may start to sleep in a chair with legs dependent. This often results in a moderate degree of lower extremity edema. The affected foot usually demonstrates dependent rubor.

Manifestations of cutaneous arterial insufficiency are nonspecific. Their presence, however, in combination with claudication indicates advanced disease. Skin and subcutaneous tissues require little blood flow for maintenance of normal nutrition. Coldness of feet is an unreliable sign, but a sudden onset of coldness is indicative of acute arterial insufficiency or occlusion. Clinical signs associated with arterial insufficiency include weak or absent peripheral pulses, color changes associated with position changes, hypertrophied toenails, tissue atrophy, ulceration, and gangrene. Paresthesias with exertion indicate ischemia of the peripheral nerves because of the phenomenon of *arterial steal*. This phenomenon occurs as arterioles of the muscles are maximally dilated because of hypoxia. To meet muscular metabolic needs, these arterioles steal from cutaneous and peripheral nerve vessels, which results in coldness and a pins-and-needles sensation.

Lower extremity pain may also appear in several other disorders unrelated to arterial disease. Other conditions that cause a similar type of pain include arthritis, lumbar disc protrusion, neuritis, and muscle cramps. Other forms of chronic arterial disease include aortoiliac and aortofemoral disorders.

Aortoiliac disorders are a form of chronic arterial occlusive disease characterized by aortoiliac stenosis and occlusion. Assessment reveals hip, thigh, and buttock claudication with absent or diminished femoral and distal pulses. Dependent rubor is common when aortoiliac and femoropopliteal disorders are combined.

A femoropopliteal disorder refers to an occlusion in the chief arteries of the proximal leg or thigh. The most common symptom of superficial femoral artery and popliteal disease is calf claudication, which will either improve or develop into rest pain. Popliteal artery disease and stenosis in the anterior or posterior tibial artery results in claudication in the distal leg and foot.

Since 1985, the use of noninvasive methods of circulatory assessment has increased dramatically. Techniques range from simple measurement of ankle/arm blood pressure index to the use of magnetic resonance imaging to measure arterial blood flow. Whereas the recording of ankle/arm index provides information at the bedside, segmental Doppler systolic blood pressure and pulse waveform analysis, via plethysmography, provide more objective information about the level and severity of oc-

clusive disease. Arteriography is the definitive examination when surgery is being considered. Arteriography reveals the lumen of the blood vessels. It is not a measurement of actual blood flow like the noninvasive assessment.

Community and Self-Care

■ Medical Management

Medical management of clients with chronic arterial occlusive disease is recommended for those with intermittent claudication and, in general, mild to moderate disease.

Nonpharmacologic Intervention

Weight Reduction. Obesity is a risk factor for arterial disorders. However, no evidence has indicated that a special diet alters the course of atherosclerosis once it has appeared. Nevertheless, encourage overweight clients to reduce and improve dietary habits in conjunction with activity as tolerated. Encourage clients to follow a low-fat, low-cholesterol diet containing more fruits and vegetables. Weight management and dietary reduction of fat and cholesterol are included in the previous discussion of hypertension.

Exercise. A prescribed moderate program of exercise and rest helps increase circulation. Several studies have shown that clients involved in an exercise program generally feel better and can slowly improve their walking distance. Instruct the client to walk every day, provided no ulcerations are present. The exercise program should begin judiciously and progress gradually until the client has substantially lengthened walking distances. For obese and chronically ill clients, it is important that an exercise program (1) be individually tailored to the client's abilities, goals, interests, and resources and that it (2) be written with specific instructions.[20]

Remind clients that at first it may be painful to walk any distance, and that they may need to stop frequently to rest. Also encourage them to walk in enclosed shopping malls in the winter for safety from falls on icy pavement and to avoid vasoconstriction from the cold outdoors.

Some clients are not aware of chest pain, shortness of breath, or fatigue because their attention is focused on leg discomfort. Question them carefully about these discomforts. Medical or surgical intervention may reduce pain and thus improve walking ability. Daily walking exercise has been shown to be beneficial to clients with intermittent claudication, although the mechanism by which it improves clinical manifestations is controversial. It probably combines "training effect" and an increase in collateral blood supply to the extremity. Many clients can significantly increase their walking distance, and most can avoid surgery if they exercise regularly and stop smoking.

Smoking Cessation. Cigarette smoking influences vascular disability. It is a potent vasoconstrictor. Clients who are able to stop smoking successfully improve their treadmill walking distance. Smoking cessation is extremely difficult, because nicotine is a highly addictive chemical. Social support, especially of friends and family members, seems to be an important factor in assisting smokers to quit their habit. Educate clients about the dangers of cigarette smoke, encourage them to stop, act as role models for nonsmoking, and support policies to prohibit smoking in the workplace.

Blood Lipid Level Reduction. Interventions for lowering blood lipid levels are recommended for those clients with hyperlipidemia. The initial steps for lowering cholesterol involve dietary intervention.

1. For obese clients, the first goal is to reduce calories to achieve ideal body weight. If weight loss is seen as improbable, the client should try to maintain current weight.
2. The next major step is to reduce the total fat intake in the diet to 30% or less of total calories. Saturated fat intake should be reduced. The most common sources of saturated fat in the American diet are red meat, fried foods, and dairy products, especially whole milk and cheese. Increasing the quantity of fish and poultry and changing to skim milk and nonfat cheese may be sufficient to meet saturated fat recommendations.
3. The third major goal is to reduce the amount of sources of cholesterol, including egg yolks, organ meats, shellfish, and animal meats. Increasing dietary fiber, especially soluble fiber, such as that found in oats, lentils, and beans, has a beneficial effect on lipid levels. Fast foods, snack foods, and restaurant dining account for a large amount of the increased fat intake in the United States. Dietary counseling by a registered dietitian is a helpful intervention for clients and families who are attempting to change eating habits.

Pharmacologic Intervention

Pharmacologic intervention may be needed for clients with high levels of hyperlipidemia and for those for whom dietary changes have been less than successful. The major drug groups include nicotinic acid, fibrin acid derivatives, bile acid resins, meglutol (hydroxymethylglutaryl), coenzyme A (CoA)-reductase inhibitors, and probucol. These medications have varying degrees of effectiveness, and each has important side effects.

Vasodilators have been popular in the past, although no convincing studies have supported their use. Pentoxifylline (Trental) has been introduced and shown to be effective in some clients in combination with conditioning exercise. Pentoxifylline is reported to act by reducing blood viscosity and enhancing oxygen delivery to the muscle of the affected limb. The major side effect is gastrointestinal upset, which may be avoided by taking the medication with meals.

■ Nursing Management of the Medical Client

Assessment

Assess the client with arterial disorders for a past history of arterial problems, surgery, medications, and ulcerations. Because of the chronic nature of the problem, perform a psychosocial assessment. Feelings of powerlessness may exist.

Diagnosis, Planning, Implementation

Altered Peripheral Tissue Perfusion. The ideal nursing diagnosis for clients with arterial disorders is *Altered Peripheral Tissue Perfusion.* Write the diagnosis as *Altered Peripheral Tissue Perfusion related to interruption of blood flow secondary to arterial occlusion.*

Planning: Expected Outcomes. The client will maintain adequate peripheral tissue perfusion to affected extremities. He or she will have warm, dry skin with normal peripheral pulse, color, temperature, motor and sensory function, and capillary filling.

Implementation
Position the Client. For safe positioning of a client with peripheral vascular disease, first learn whether the disorder is arterial or venous in nature. Because blood flows to dependent parts of the body (i.e., parts lower than the heart), position clients with arterial disease so that blood flows toward the legs and feet. In severe cases of arterial insufficiency, the physician may order the head of the client's bed to be elevated on 6-inch blocks so that blood from the heart flows more easily to the extremities whenever the client sleeps or rests. When placing the client in a reverse Trendelenburg position, watch for dependent edema. In milder cases, clients can benefit from simply sitting for periods of time with their feet flat on the floor. Remind clients with arterial insufficiency to avoid raising their feet above heart level unless the physician has specifically prescribed this as an exercise. Authorities vary in their opinion as to the best position for enhancing arterial flow to the feet.

Provide Warmth. Warmth can be both a blessing and a curse for clients with vascular disease. Warmth is beneficial for clients only when it acts as insulation against cold and chilling. For example, encourage the client with vascular disease to set the thermostat at home at around 70° to 72° F (21° to 22° C). If possible, keep the client's room comfortably warm. Teach the client to enter warmed cars in the winter.

Applying any source of heat directly to the extremities is especially dangerous. Heat increases tissue metabolism. If the arteries are unable to dilate normally, blood flow to the extremities becomes inadequate, and the tissues in turn become ischemic. The use of hot water bottles, heating pads, and hot foot soaks is strictly contraindicated unless specifically ordered by the physician, especially for diabetics with peripheral neuropathies and for paraplegics.

Prevent Vasoconstriction. Factors that cause vasoconstriction include nicotine and caffeine ingestion (cause vasospasm), high emotion (stimulates the sympathetic nervous system), and chilling. Perform the following actions to help clients to avoid the damaging effects of prolonged vasoconstriction:

● Explain the dangers of smoking to the client who uses tobacco. Encourage the client to stop smoking completely. The client who realizes that smoking literally threatens life and limbs may develop sufficient motivation to abstain permanently. Help the client locate therapy groups or biofeedback training. Do not advise the use of nicotine patches. Patches provide continuous administration of nicotine and thereby can cause continuous vasospasm.

● Protect the client whenever possible from upsetting, emotionally charged situations. Encourage the client to try to relax, both mentally and physically. Counseling services may be indicated for nervous, high-strung clients. Offer information regarding stress reduction classes. Remember to involve significant others.

● Prevent the client from becoming chilled, using the methods previously described.

Risk for Impaired Skin Integrity.
Because of altered peripheral tissue perfusion, the client is at risk of arterial ulceration and skin infection. Write the diagnosis as *Risk for Impaired Skin Integrity related to decreased peripheral circulation.* If the client has an arterial ulcer, this diagnosis can still be used for the remaining intact skin.

Planning: Expected Outcomes. The client will maintain intact skin surfaces, with healed skin surfaces, freedom from signs of infection, and signs of wound healing.

Implementation. Prevent injury to the extremities, particularly the feet. Excellent foot care should be an integral part of the daily routine of clients with peripheral vascular disorders, because prevention is easier to initiate and maintain than is correction.

Important points concerning foot care include the following:

1. No foot problems are minor for clients with peripheral vascular disease, especially clients with diabetes mellitus.
2. Ascertain whether the client is wearing adequate footwear and hosiery and whether nails and skin on the feet are cared for properly. The client should wear supportive shoes that have adequate room and closed toes. Clothing that constricts blood flow, especially tight socks and garters, must be avoided.
3. Be careful when referring clients to a podiatrist. Not all podiatrists are vascular specialists.
4. Refer the client with corns, calluses, and ingrown toenails to a physician who specializes in peripheral vascular disease.
5. Inspect the feet daily. Use a mirror. Teach the client to inspect the feet and to wash and dry them well.

The Client Education Guide entitled Foot Care presents guidelines for clients with vascular disorders.

Pain. The pain from arterial disease is called intermittent claudication and is caused by ischemia. The diagnosis can be written *Pain related to inadequate arterial blood supply to the legs.*

Planning: Expected Outcomes. The client will experience increased comfort, as evidenced by self-report and demonstrated knowledge of pain relief measures, both pharmacologic and nonpharmacologic. In most cases, total relief of pain is unrealistic.

Implementation. The pain of ischemia is usually chronic, continuous, and difficult to relieve. Leg ulcers are also typically very painful. Because of pain, clients with arterial disorders are often depressed and irritable. Pain limits their activities, disturbs their sleep, saps their energy, and has a demoralizing emotional effect. Thus, pain must be relieved if the client is to rest and improve.

Help clients assess and plan ways of correcting the position of their beds at home. The head of the bed can be elevated to promote blood flow to the legs. Remind the client with arterial insufficiency of the following points:

1. Avoid standing in one position for more than a few minutes
2. Avoid crossing the legs at the knees
3. In general, seek the most comfortable position
4. Watch for and report edema

Any measure that increases circulation to the extremities will help alleviate ischemic pain. Although pain also can be subdued by analgesics, interventions that augment circulation are best. For more information on pain control, see Chapter 17.

When strong analgesics, such as morphine, are necessary around the clock, the client may come to accept amputation. Amputation can improve the quality of life by diminishing pain and improving mobility with a prosthesis.

Risk for Activity Intolerance.
The pain (intermittent claudication) the client experiences may greatly deter activity. This common diagnosis is written as *Risk for Activity Intolerance related to leg pain after walking.*

Planning: Expected Outcomes. The client will tolerate appropriate levels of activity free from pain and excess fatigue, as evidenced by normal vital signs, absence of pain, and verbalized understanding of benefits of gradual increase in activity and exercise.

Implementation. Although exercise helps most clients with vascular disorders, some clients *must not exercise.* These clients have leg ulcers, pain at rest, cellulitis, deep vein thrombosis, or gangrene. Exercise and activity increase the metabolic needs of tissues and, consequently, tissue requirements for oxygenated blood. Thus, clients with tissue breakdown or necrosis must remain for a period on complete bedrest. Even minimal activity raises the oxygen requirements of the tissues above that which damaged arteries can provide.

When assisting the client with a walking program, assert that *pain* should be the guide to the amount of

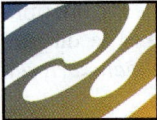

CLIENT EDUCATION GUIDE

Foot Care

Client Instructions in English *(Instrucciones para el cliente en inglés)*	**Client Instructions in Spanish** *(Instrucciones para el cliente en español)*
Daily Hygiene	**Higiene Diaria**
Do not soak your feet; use mild soap and a washcloth to clean them.	No remoje los pies; use un jabón suave y una toallita para limpiarlos.
Dry well between your toes.	Sequese bien entre los dedos de los piés.
Check water temperature with a bath thermometer or your elbow, not your toes, to prevent burns; 32.2° to 35° C (90° to 95° F) is safe.	Compruebe la temperatura del agua con un termómetro de baño o con el codo, no con los dedos de los piés, para prevenir asi las quemaduras. No hay peligro con temperaturas de 32.2° a 35° C (90° a 95° F).
Gently rub corns or calluses. Avoid cutting, digging, or using harsh commercial products.	Frote suavemente los callos. Evite cortar, escarbar, o usar productos comerciales ásperos.
Daily Inspection and Lubrication	**Inspección y Lubricación Diaria**
Use good lighting.	Use buena iluminación.
Put on your glasses or contacts, if you wear them.	Pongase las gafas o los lentes de contacto, si los usa generalmente.
Promptly report ulcerations, redness, calluses, blisters, or cracking of the skin on the feet, or thickening of the nails, to the physician.	Informele inmediatamente al médico si tiene ulceraciones, enrojecimiento, callos, ampollas, agrietamientos el la piel de los pies, o engrosamiento de las uñas.
Rub soothing lotions or lanolin on your hands, feet, legs, and arms to prevent dryness.	Frote lanolina o cremas suaves en las manos, los brazos, los pies y las piernas para prevenir la sequedad.
Do not use lotion on sores or in between your toes.	No se ponga lociones en las heridas o entre los dedos del pie.
Do not use perfumed lotions.	No use lociones que contienen perfume.
Dust your feet lightly with cornstarch if they sweat.	Si le sudan los pies, apliquese polvos de maicena ligeramente.
Care of Toenails	**Cuidado de las Uñas de los Pies**
Use clippers, not scissors or razor blades.	Use un cortauñas, no use tijeras o navajas de afeitar.
Cut straight across the nail.	Corte la uña en linea recta.
Do not perform "bathroom surgery."	No se haga "cirugia en el baño."
If your eyesight is poor or if you are unable to reach your toes, find qualified assistance.	Si no puede ver bien o si no se alcanza a tocar los dedos de los pies, busque a alguien que esté capacitad para ayudale.
Place lamb's wool between overlapping toes.	Pongase lana de cordero entre los dedos de los pies que se sobrepongan.
Proper Footwear	**Calzado Apropiado**
Never go barefoot, not even at the beach or at home.	Nunca ande descalzo(a), niqun en la playa o en la casa.
Avoid high heels and shoes with pointed toes.	Evite usar zapatos puntiagudos y de tacón alto.

Client Instructions in English *(Instrucciones para el cliente en inglés)*	Client Instructions in Spanish *(Instrucciones para el cliente en español)*
Make sure nothing is in your shoes before putting them on your feet.	Asegurese que no haya nada dentro de los zapatos antes de ponerselos.
Avoid tight socks and shoes.	Evite usar zapatos y calcetines apretados.
Wear cotton socks for absorbency. Change your socks daily.	Use calcetines de algodón que tienen más absorbencia. Cambiese diariamente de calcetines.
Alternate several pairs of comfortable, firm, well-made shoes during the week.	Durante la semana, varié el uso de zapatos bien hechos, comodos, y firmes.
Avoid shoes that cause your feet to perspire (for example, canvas shoes and rubber boots).	No use zapatos que le aumenten la transpiración (por ejemplo, zapatos de lona o botas de caucho/plástico).
Make sure that your shoes and slippers fit well and are sturdy enough to prevent foot injury.	Asegurese de que los zapatos y las pantunflas le queden bien y de que sean lo suficientemente firmes para prevenir lesiones del pie.
Safety	**Seguridad**
Avoid sunburn.	Evite las quemaduras del sol.
Avoid scratching insect bites on your legs, to avoid creating open lesions.	No se rasque las picaduras de insectos en las piernas para evitar crear abrir lesiones en la piel.
Do not use heating pads.	No use almohadillas eléctricas.
Wear adequate foot protection on cold days.	Protéjase los pies cuando hace frio.
Turn on the lights before entering a dark hallway or room.	Encienda las luces antes de entrar a un pasillo o a un cuarto oscuro.
Avoid sitting with your legs crossed.	Evite cruzar las piernas al sentarse.
Use a cane or walker, if indicated.	Use bastón o andador, si se lo indican.
When in doubt, ask for help. Have phone numbers of people who can assist you handy.	Busque ayuda cuando tenga dudas. Tenga a la mano los números de teléfono de personas que le puedan ayudar.
Activity	**Actividad**
Walking is good, but get your physician's permission before beginning a regular program.	El caminar es buen ejercicio, pero obtenga permiso de médico antes de empezar un programa.
Do not walk if you have open ulcerations.	No camine si tiene ulceraciones abiertas.
Walk until pain begins, stop and rest, then begin again.	Camine hasta que le empiese el dolor, pare y descanse, luego vuelva a caminar.
Elevate your feet if they swell.	Suba los pies si se le hinchan.
Find a nurse and a physician who will get to know you and your foot problems and will take the time to talk with you when you need help.	Busque a un(a) enfermero(a) y a un médico que lleguen a concerlo a usted y a concerle los pies y quienes se den tiempo para hablar con usted cuando necesite ayuda.

activity to be undertaken. Intermittent claudication signals that the muscles and tissues of the legs are not receiving enough oxygen. Before the client begins a walking program, take a careful history and perform a physical assessment. Establish a cardiopulmonary profile and carefully examine the client's feet and legs to locate open ulcerations or anatomic deformities. The client should have sturdy shoes to prevent foot trauma. Again, a client with open ischemic ulcerations should not walk.

A popular form of exercise for clients with vascular disorders is the Buerger-Allen routine. These exercises are divided into three parts, as shown in Figure 50–3.

Health Seeking Behaviors. Health-conscious clients may request information about self-improvement and interventions to reduce the severity of manifestations. Write the diagnosis as *Health Seeking Behaviors related*

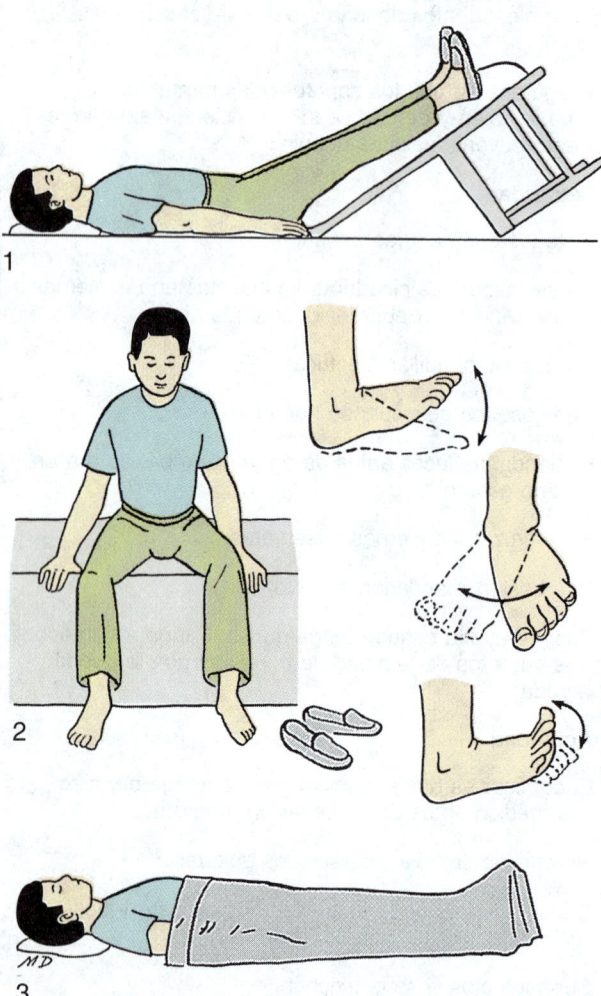

Figure 50–3. Buerger-Allen exercises. *1*, Have the client elevate his or her feet on a padded chair or board for ½ minute to 3 minutes. *2*, Have the client sit in a relaxed position while he or she flexes and extends, then pronates and supinates each foot for 3 minutes. The client's feet should become entirely pink. If the feet are blue or painful, have the client elevate them and relax as necessary. *3*, Have the client lie quietly for 5 minutes, keeping his or her legs warm with a blanket.

to lack of knowledge about the role of exercise, weight reduction, and smoking cessation in management of arterial disease.

Planning: Expected Outcomes. The client will begin and maintain the chosen health promotion program, as evidenced by demonstrated knowledge of the specific activities of the program, regular evaluation of goals against performance, and verbalized feelings of increased well-being.

Implementation. Instruct the client in areas of concern or interest. Refer to the nonpharmacologic intervention methods described earlier. Refer the client to groups in the community if available.

The client with intermittent claudication caused by arterial disease should have a check-up at least every 3 months. At this time, document the following:

1. Extent of claudication
2. Impact on life-style
3. Manifestations of ischemia
4. Pulses
5. Ankle/arm indices
6. Condition of the feet
7. Venous filling time to determine improvement, stability, or progression of the disease

Evaluation

Arterial disorders are chronic, so do not expect to see reversal of the problems. Write outcomes that allow for time and client adjustments.

■ Modifications for Elderly Clients

Age-related changes and impairments of physiologic function concomitant with arterial disease will affect the nursing diagnoses of *Activity Intolerance* (possibly increased), *Altered Peripheral Tissue Perfusion* (possibly reduced), and *Pain*. Recognition of pain may be complicated by physical or cognitive impairments, ongoing drug therapy, and psychosocial factors (e.g., depression or social isolation).

Acute and Subacute Care

■ Surgical Management
Endovascular Interventions

Endovascular interventional therapies use angioscopy, intraluminal ultrasonography, balloon angioplasty, laser, mechanical atherectomy, thrombolytic therapy, and stents to treat vascular disorders. The goal is to operate from within the artery to remove partial or total blockages. Most of the procedures can be done in the radiology department or in cardiac catheterization laboratories. Additional benefits of endovascular interventions include the following:

1. A puncture wound replaces a long incision
2. Significant reduction in postoperative care

3. Reduction in cardiac and pulmonary complications from general anesthesia, because most of these procedures are done with local or regional anesthesia
4. Reduction in hospital costs and hospital stay

Percutaneous Transluminal Angioplasty.

Percutaneous transluminal angioplasty (PTA, balloon angioplasty) is a procedure that uses a catheter with a distal inflatable balloon to mechanically dilate stenotic vessels. Angioplasty causes a controlled injury to the vessel wall by stretching the artery, thereby enlarging the lumen. Observation of a segment of an arterial wall that has undergone PTA reveals rupture of the plaque at the thinnest place, stretching of the artery wall away from the plaque, and rupture of the media with the lumen of the artery being maintained by the adventitia. The enlarged vessel's new dimensions are maintained by the hydrostatic pressure of the increased luminal blood flow. PTA has been used successfully, in varying degrees, for treatment of hemodynamically significant stenoses in the coronary, aortic, iliac, femoral, popliteal, tibial, mesenteric, and renal circulations as well as for stenoses in arteriovenous dialysis shunts.

Complications of balloon angioplasty include bleeding, hematoma and thrombus formation at the insertion site, perforation, and dissection of the artery. Reocclusion that occurs over a longer period of time is caused by accelerated cell growth of the intima (intimal hyperplasia), which occurs in response to injury.

Nursing care is similar to that for routine diagnostic arteriography (Chapter 13). Major nursing concerns are acute reocclusion and bleeding. Clients are given heparin as an anticoagulant during the procedure; thus, the arterial puncture site requires frequent assessment for swelling, bleeding, ecchymosis, or hematoma formation. Peripheral pulses are usually assessed every 15 to 30 minutes during the first post-procedure hour, then hourly for the next 4 to 8 hours. Report clinical manifestations of circulatory compromise immediately (e.g., sudden change in limb color or temperature, increasing muscle discomfort, pain at rest, and motor or sensory paresthesias). Long-term aspirin or dipyridamole administration is prescribed to PTA clients.

Laser-Assisted Balloon Angioplasty.

Laser-assisted balloon angioplasty (LABA) uses laser energy and balloon catheters to reverse ischemia by re-forming the diseased artery. LABA is used for high-grade and total occlusions that are difficult or impossible to cross. In these situations, laser recanalization is used to cross lesions to allow subsequent balloon angioplasty. After access is gained to the artery in the same fashion as for PTA, the laser probe or fiber is advanced to the obstructing lesion under fluoroscopy. The catheter tip is placed as close to the center of the occlusion as possible. Very gentle pressure is then applied to the catheter until it has passed through the occluding lesion. Standard balloon angioplasty is then used to enlarge the channel to its full diameter. After the procedure is completed, antiplatelet or anticoagulant therapy is given.

LABA carries a higher incidence than PTA of arterial wall perforation or dissection. Nursing responsibilities are much the same as for the care of the client after PTA.

Peripheral Atherectomy.

Atherectomy selectively removes atheroma from atherosclerotic diseased arteries. The advantages of this technique over PTA are (1) decreased risk of arterial rupture because the vessel is not stretched as much and (2) decreased risk of thrombus formation because the arterial surface is smoother after the procedure.

Many atherectomy devices have been created, and each offers its own unique features with advantages and disadvantages. The devices use various high-speed rotating drills, circular cutters or blades, or a football-shaped metal burr studded with diamond chips that serve as microblades. The plaque is pulverized into small particles. Most of the devices provide for particle retrieval, which allows examination to determine whether the occlusion consisted of plaque or thrombus. Atherectomy devices require fluoroscopy and contrast for visualization of the lesion. The restenosis rate is about the same as for angioplasty. The major complications are perforation and arterioembolization.

Nursing care for the atherectomy client is the same as for the angioplasty client.

Intravascular Stents.

The recognized problem of restenosis after PTA has led to the development of intravascular stents. Stents are designed to provide a scaffold to maintain the intraluminal structure and patency of the artery. So far, stents have been used mostly to treat residual stenoses or dissections after balloon angioplasty. Several types of stents have been developed, including flexible, rigid, balloon-expandable, and self-expanding varieties. After a stent has been in place for about 8 months, it becomes covered by a thin neointimal layer. After the procedure, clients are treated with aspirin and dipyridamole.

Nursing care includes client education regarding medications as well as information about the procedure and the stent.

Thrombolytic Therapy.

Thrombolytic therapy is an important aspect of management of extensive venous or arterial thrombosis. Streptokinase and urokinase are used to treat acute arterial emboli and arterial graft occlusion. Contraindications to therapy include surgery within the past 10 days (including arteriogram, lumbar puncture, or paracentesis), recent trauma (including cardiopulmonary resuscitation [CPR]), renal or liver biopsy, and pregnancy. Renal function must be adequate because of the amount of contrast given during thrombolytic therapy.

Thrombolytic agents are given through a peripheral vein or through an intra-arterial catheter. A test dose is given; then, if it is determined to be safe, it is followed by a loading dose and then by continuous infusion. The agents have a half-life of 16 to 18 minutes. Thrombin times, fibrinogen levels, or both may be monitored to be certain that the thrombolytic system has been activated.

Major adverse reactions include hemorrhage, allergic reactions, and fever.

Nursing management is related to the stage of fibrinolytic therapy: preinfusion, intrainfusion, and postinfusion. Prior to infusion, the client is monitored closely (commonly in intensive care). Baseline values are obtained for partial thromboplastin time, prothrombin time, thrombin time, platelet count, hematocrit, and white blood cell count. Because of the risk of hemorrhage, if data reveal a bleeding disorder, the physician is notified. A history of recent streptococcal infection may diminish the drug's effects. Baseline pulses and assessments are performed in each extremity, using Doppler ultrasonography if needed.

During infusion, vital signs, pulses, skin color, movement, and sensation are assessed frequently. Assess for clinical manifestations of bleeding and hematoma formation. If bleeding does occur, direct pressure is applied, the infusion is stopped, and the physician is notified. Bleeding typically is from the gastrointestinal or genitourinary tract or is intramuscular, intracerebral, or retroperitoneal.

No intramuscular injections are given for 24 hours after infusion, and any medications that have bleeding as a side effect are used with caution. There is also a chance that a partially lysed thrombus will embolize. After infusion, pressure is continued on the puncture site. The involved extremity is positioned in straight alignment to facilitate perfusion. The client's leg remains immobile. Heparin therapy in low doses is also begun. Streptokinase is administered from glass bottles because it is inactivated by plastic containers. Administration is regulated by a volume-control pump.

Arterial Bypass

Arterial obstruction can be reconstructed with bypass operations. Selecting the client for surgery follows careful history, physical and diagnostic assessments, including arteriography. Arteriography provides a necessary road map to indicate the level of obstruction, because it is essential to reconstruct the arterial inflow to the legs before correcting the outflow. This process prevents newly placed bypass grafts from thrombosing because of inadequate blood supply to the graft. During the operation the surgeon assesses inflow, and after it is ascertained that inflow to the femoral system is adequate, a distal site is chosen for outflow.

Various locations along the arterial system can be reconstructed as follows:

1. Femoral artery bypass grafting or axillofemoral reconstruction (Fig. 50–4) is used if the aortoiliac segment is obstructed. Operative mortality is 1%. The patency rates of aortofemoral grafts are 80% to 90% at 5 years.
2. Axillofemoral grafting is reserved for people who have increased operative risk, usually because of their cardiopulmonary status. The graft starts at the axillary artery and travels subcutaneously along the lateral chest wall to the femoral artery. It may then be combined with a femorofemoral graft to revascularize both extremities. Axillofemoral grafts have a higher incidence of occlusion than aortofemoral grafts and carry

a mortality rate of 4% to 5%, but the necessary anesthesia time is greatly reduced. The patency rates are 60% to 70% at 5 years, in part because thrombi are easily removed from axillofemoral grafts.

3. The femoral artery can be bypassed with grafts anastomosed (surgically connected) to any one of three lower leg arteries (posterior tibial, anterior tibial, or peroneal artery). The success of bypass grafts of the legs depends largely on what material is used for grafting. The client's own saphenous vein remains the most successful grafting material used today. Seventy-five percent of saphenous vein grafts are patent after 5 years; in contrast, only 12% of synthetic material (polytetrafluoroethylene [PTFE]) is patent after the same length of time. (Gore-Tex is a common brand name for PTFE.) Unfortunately, the client's own saphenous vein is not always large enough or long enough for the surgery, or it may have been removed during another operation. In these cases, PTFE is used. In situ grafts can also be used for reconstruction. In situ grafting uses the client's own vein for a bypass of the artery. A section of vein is anastomosed proximally and distally and then stripped of its valves. The vein then becomes an artery.

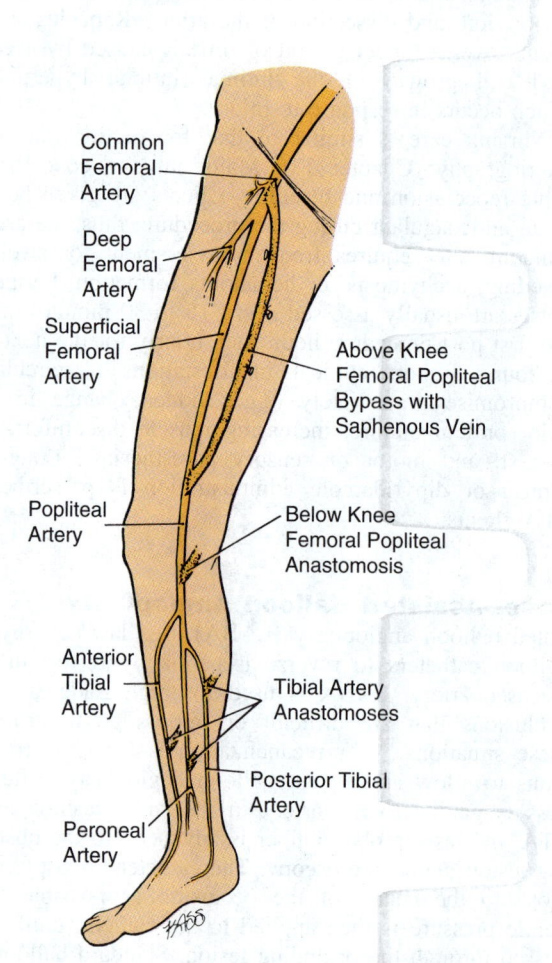

Figure 50–4. Femoral artery bypass grafts. The anastomosis can be to any one of three tibial arteries. (From Fahey, V. A. [1994]. *Vascular nursing.* Philadelphia: W.B. Saunders.)

■ Nursing Management of the Surgical Client

Arterial Bypass

Preoperative Care

Preoperatively, obtain baseline vital signs and document the character of peripheral pulses, comparing one side to the other. Know exactly which pulses are palpable and which pulses can be assessed only with the Doppler. Mark with ink the sites where peripheral pulses can be palpated, to assist with postoperative assessment.

Before the client goes to surgery, it is common to begin administration of intravenous fluids, insert a urinary catheter, and weigh the client. Just before surgery, arterial and central venous pressure lines may be inserted.

In addition, broad-spectrum antibiotics normally are prescribed for 48 hours preoperatively. All infections (e.g., tooth abscesses, urinary tract infections, respiratory infections) must be resolved, especially if the surgeon plans to use a synthetic graft. Adequate circulating blood volume must be maintained to permit good perfusion throughout the period of arterial repair.

As with any preoperative assessment, perform careful cardiac and pulmonary evaluation. Even though the incision for a femoral artery bypass is peripheral, and major complications are infrequent, the client probably has other manifestations of atherosclerosis (such as heart and kidney disease) that may complicate the surgery. If the operation is not an emergency, malnutrition can be reversed and open wounds cleaned.

The client and family are taught the various procedures involved and are offered psychological support. First assess the client's readiness and desire to learn about the surgery.

Postoperative Care

The client is placed on bedrest for the evening after surgery, with the leg flat in bed. The leg is wrapped with light dressings or a vascular boot. Boots are commonly used in clients who had a loss of sensation prior to surgery or who are at risk of pressure ulcers. Elastic wraps are not used if vein grafts have been used for reconstruction. Leg swelling is common after revascularization related to the reperfusion of ischemic muscles and surgical dissection around lymphatic drainage systems in the leg. If edema worsens when the client's leg is dependent, elastic wraps and a mild diuretic can be used. Edema usually resolves within 4 to 8 weeks.

Anticoagulant medications (e.g., heparin) are used in clients who have had previously thrombosed femoral bypass grafts. It is also possible to treat some clients with fibrinolytics. Three drugs, streptokinase, urokinase, and tissue plasminogen activator, are in current clinical use. All three drugs convert the client's plasminogen to the active molecule plasmin, which instigates fibrinolysis. The client is eventually given warfarin sodium (Coumadin) based on coagulation studies, especially prothrombin, partial thromboplastin times, and international normalized ratio (INR). Dextran is sometimes used to improve blood flow in the microcirculation. Medications that decrease platelet aggregation, aspirin and dipyridamole (Persantine), are also used to increase the length of graft patency. Oxygen saturation monitors may also be used to measure tissue perfusion. Daily aspirin is usually required after surgery.

Broad-spectrum antibiotics are used before and after surgery. Carefully monitor clients for clinical manifestations of infection (e.g., elevated white blood cell count, fever, changes in wound appearance). The Care Plan describes care of the client after bypass surgery.

Most clients are discharged to home. Because activity was limited by claudication prior to surgery, the client needs to begin regular permissible exercise, including climbing stairs and going out of doors. The client is taught that swelling of the operative leg is normal. Elastic wraps can be used when the client is ambulating, but they should not be worn continuously. Elastic wraps are usually not permitted on clients with in situ grafts.

Complications

Bleeding may develop along the suture line and can indicate a disruption in the suture line, pseudoaneurysm formation, or a slipped ligature (suture). These problems require additional surgery. Reclotting of the graft is also possible. Peripheral tissue perfusion is monitored and noninvasive follow-up studies are performed to assess patency.

Infection is not a common complication after bypass surgery, but it can occur, especially when synthetic grafting material is used. Because infection in a synthetic graft necessitates its removal, infection often results in the loss of a limb. Poorly nourished clients appear to be at highest risk of infection and delayed healing.

Compartment syndrome may also develop from swelling around the fascial compartments of the leg. In addition to loss of sensation and function, muscle cells can die and release myoglobin, which can cause acute tubular necrosis in the kidney.

Amputation

Extremity amputation is the surgical removal of all or part of an extremity. Clients with peripheral vascular disease are the most frequent candidates for amputation of the lower extremities. Diabetes mellitus is a major etiology of arterial occlusion and has been associated with more than 50% of major amputations in clients with lower extremity occlusive disease.

Improvements in vascular surgery have provided outstanding examples of long-term limb salvage in clients who in the past would have required amputation. Current data indicate that revascularization should be the first option considered in clients with critical limb ischemia. This recommendation is based on the following observations:

1. Previous revascularization does not raise the level of amputation
2. Mortality rates for amputation are at least as high as for arterial bypass

CARE PLAN

Postoperative Care of the Client Who Has Had Arterial Bypass Surgery of the Lower Extremity

Nursing Diagnosis. Risk for Fluid Volume Deficit related to hemorrhage, hematoma, third spacing of fluid, or diuresis from contrast given during angiography

Planning: Expected Outcomes. The client will maintain adequate vascular fluid volume as evidenced by the following:

- Hemodynamic stability
- Urine output ≥30 ml/hr
- Warm, dry skin
- Being alert, awake

- No excess drainage on dressings
- Intake that equals output
- Stable hemoglobin and hematocrit

Implementation: Nursing Intervention	Rationales
Observe the client for an increase in pulse, decrease in blood pressure, anxiety, restlessness, pallor, cyanosis, thirst, oliguria, clammy skin, venous collapse, and decreasing level of consciousness.	Hemorrhagic shock can develop from surgical or postoperative blood loss.
Check the client's dressings for excessive drainage.	Incision drainage first appears on dressings.
Assess the client's pulmonary artery pressures and cardiac output if parameters are available.	Pulmonary artery pressures and cardiac output parameters are reliable indicators of hemodynamic stability.
Check the client's daily weights; monitor intake and output closely.	Intake should equal output. Weight is a reliable indicator of fluid balance.
Check hematocrit and hemoglobin values and notify the physician if they are abnormal.	Hematocrit and hemoglobin normally fall slightly because of surgical blood loss. Transfusion may be required.
Check the client's creatinine level after angiography.	Contrast is excreted by the kidneys.

Evaluation. This outcome should be attainable within 24 hours.

Nursing Diagnosis. Altered Tissue Perfusion related to graft thrombosis, compartment syndrome, progressive arterial disease, or inadequate anticoagulation

Planning: Expected Outcomes. The client will maintain adequate tissue perfusion to the lower extremities, as evidenced by full pedal pulses, intact sensory and motor function, and minimal swelling.

Implementation: Nursing Intervention	Rationales
Check the client's pedal pulses every hour for 24 hours, then every shift, unless otherwise ordered. Obtain Doppler pressures per doctor's orders.	Pedal pulses indicate graft patency.
Check the sensory and motor function of the client's extremities.	Compartment syndrome may develop because of bleeding.
Check the client's leg for hematoma or severe swelling.	Severe swelling may impede the flow through the graft.
Monitor creatine phosphokinase levels when appropriate.	Enzymes are released from ischemic muscle.
Observe for a change in color and the presence of red blood cells in the client's urine.	These manifestations may be caused by a release of myoglobin secondary to muscle ischemia.
Avoid raising the knee section of the Gatch bed and placing pillows under the client's knees.	Pressure may increase the risk of thrombosis.

Evaluation. Outcomes related to tissue perfusion should be met within 48 hours.

Nursing Diagnosis. Risk for Impaired Skin Integrity related to altered circulation, altered nutritional state, infection, and multiple surgical procedures

Planning: Expected Outcomes. The client will maintain adequate skin integrity.

Implementation: Nursing Intervention	Rationales
Inspect the client's lower extremities on daily basis.	Early detection of ulceration will improve the chances of healing
Provide proper skin care using lanolin-based creams.	Soft skin does not crack open.
Protect the client's lower extremities from trauma.	Tissue perfusion is decreased and injured sites heal poorly.
Use sheepskin, a bed cradle, or heel protectors when appropriate.	These devices are used to protect the skin from breakdown.
Check the sensory and motor function of the client's extremities.	Compartment syndrome may develop because of bleeding or edema.
Avoid using tape on the skin below the client's knee.	Tape burns from tape removal may be slow to heal.

CARE PLAN

Postoperative Care of the Client Who Has Had Arterial Bypass Surgery of the Lower Extremity (Continued)

Implementation: Nursing Intervention

Monitor the client's nutritional status and albumin level. Obtain a dietitian's consultation, if necessary.

Observe strict aseptic technique during dressing changes.

Monitor the client for low-grade fever, elevated white blood cell count, any drainage from the wound, and graft exposure at each shift.

If ordered, apply 4-inch Ace bandages below the knee to the affected extremity when the client is out of bed.

Instruct client to inspect feet and incisions daily. (See Foot Care Guide.)

Assess for presence of footdrop.

Rationales

Malnutrition is the most common cause of delayed healing.

Aseptic technique reduces risk of infection.

These are clinical manifestations of wound infection.

Edema, although normal after surgery, can inhibit wound healing.

Circulation to the legs and feet is impaired from arteriosclerosis. Daily assessment and proper care can lead to early intervention.

Nerve injury due to ischemia can lead to footdrop.

Evaluation. Expect the wound to heal slowly over 10 days if arteriosclerosis is extensive.

Nursing Diagnosis. Impaired Physical Mobility related to a surgical procedure, pain, or nerve injury secondary to ischemia

Planning: Expected Outcomes. The client will maintain intact motor function, will avoid potential complications of immobility, and will demonstrate use of adaptive devices to increase mobility.

Implementation: Nursing Intervention

Assess the causative factors for immobility and the patient's range of motion and ability to ambulate.

Encourage progressive ambulation and range of motion while the client is in bed.

Request a physical therapy consult when appropriate.

Encourage independence in the client's activities of daily living.

Rationales

Mobility can be facilitated once the cause is known.

These activities promote venous return and muscle strength.

Assistive devices may be necessary for ambulation.

Independence improves both physical and psychological recovery

Evaluation. Outcomes related to mobility may require several days, depending on initial physical status.

Nursing Diagnosis. Pain related to surgical incision

Planning: Expected Outcomes. The client verbalizes and demonstrates an increased level of comfort.

Implementation: Nursing Intervention

Assess the client's level of pain: type, duration, and location.

Provide comfort measures and means of distraction.

Medicate with prescribed analgesics as needed.

Evaluate the effectiveness of pain medication after each administration.

Rationales

This assessment provides baseline data to evaluate the effectiveness of treatment.

Distraction is a nonpharmacologic method of pain management.

Adequate pain management promotes healing.

This evaluation determines the adequacy of analgesics.

Evaluation. Acute pain should subside over 48 to 72 hours.

Adapted from Fahey, V. A. (1994). *Vascular nursing.* Philadelphia, W. B. Saunders.

3. There is no difference in cost between amputation and successful bypass

Amputations are classified as primary or secondary. Primary amputations are undertaken as definitive surgical treatment for lower extremity ischemia. Secondary amputations are those that follow a previous vascular reconstructive procedure. Amputations may also be required for acute limb-threatening conditions, mainly trauma, and for malignant tumors and congenital deformities.

Amputation of a limb is an emotional issue for clients and families. To many clients the word *amputation,* like the word *cancer,* is thought more often than spoken. Some clients are willing to endure multiple attempts at revascularization or extended periods of intense pain in an effort to avoid amputation. You can play an integral role in assessing client and family fears and concerns, in promoting the use of positive coping mechanisms, and in coordinating efforts of the rehabilitation team toward a positive outcome. The rehabilitation team must design a total care plan tailored to the client's personality and needs. Intervention focuses on the whole client rather than on a diseased or missing limb.

Before amputation, the surgeon and rehabilitative team consider the following:

The client's physical condition. The following physical conditions may determine the need for amputation: ischemic gangrene, rest pain, infection, and massive injury.

The type of amputation to be performed. There are two types of amputation procedures: the open, or guillotine, amputation; and the closed, or "flap," amputation (Fig. 50–5). The major indication for guillotine amputation is infection. In open amputation, the surgeon does not close the stump with a skin flap immediately but leaves it open, allowing the wound to drain freely. Antibiotics are used. Once the infection is completely eradicated, the client undergoes another operation for stump closure.

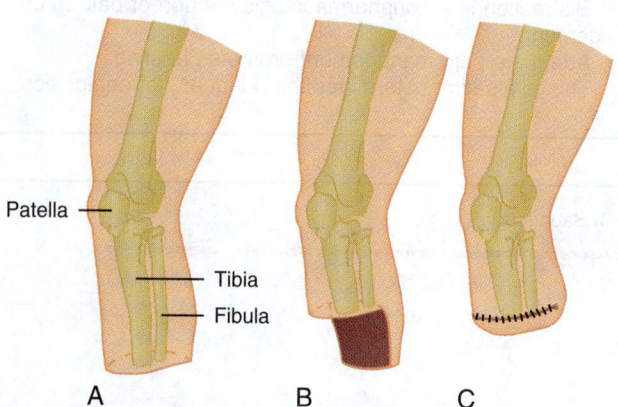

Figure 50–5. Open and closed amputations. *A,* Step 1 of open amputation; this technique is used when infection complicates amputation. *B,* Closed amputation (or step 2 of open amputation, performed when infection has resolved). *C,* Stump closure.

Labels in figure: Patella, Tibia, Fibula, A, B, C

During a "flap" amputation, the surgeon closes or covers the stump with a flap of skin sutured over the end of the stump. This type of amputation is performed when there is no evidence of infection and, consequently, no need for open drainage. However, the surgeon may insert small drains to promote wound healing.

The level of amputation required. The level of amputation for any extremity should be as distal as possible (Fig. 50–6). Clients with below-knee amputations (even bilateral) more successfully achieve independent function with a prosthesis than do those with above-knee amputations (Fig. 50–7).

Peripheral vascular function test results. Angiography is used to determine vascular patency. It commonly reveals a range of problems, from marked reduction of to absence of blood flow.

The client's general attitude toward amputation. Attitude toward amputation depends to a large degree on the client's age and maturity. Young clients may resist amputation even though it would greatly improve their function. For some, the thought of amputation dramatically conflicts with their ideal self-image. Conversely, some clients who suffer from the agonizing pain of chronic ischemia may welcome amputation. These clients are more concerned with removing the source of their pain than they are with altering their body image or function.

The client's rehabilitation potential. Ideally, clients should attain independent function with the use of a prosthesis. However, prosthetic rehabilitation requires cooperation, commitment, good coordination, and a tremendous amount of energy. Most clients may be expected to regain ambulatory status after ischemic amputation. Not all amputees, however, are candidates for prostheses. General contraindications may involve concurrent medical conditions (e.g., chronic and progressive mental deterioration; advancing neurologic problems; chronic obstructive pulmonary disease; or cardiac disease with congestive heart failure or angina). The use of a prosthesis increases energy requirements and workload.

The type of postoperative prosthetic-fitting and rehabilitation program. Clients are fitted immediately with a temporary prosthesis and then fitted a week or two later when the stump wound has healed and the sutures have been removed. The surgeon decides on the type of prosthetic fitting before surgery. Ideally, the client facing amputation goes to surgery expecting some functional restoration of the limb. Carefully describing the prosthesis to the client helps pave the way to successful rehabilitation.

Types of Prostheses

Temporary Prostheses. After the operation is completed, the surgeon applies an occlusive dressing (such as silk or Telfa) and places a small amount of fluffed gauze over the end of the stump. The surgeon or prosthetist then applies the rigid dressing (usually a cast), carefully distributing pressure evenly over the end of the stump. The cast protects the stump from injury and re-

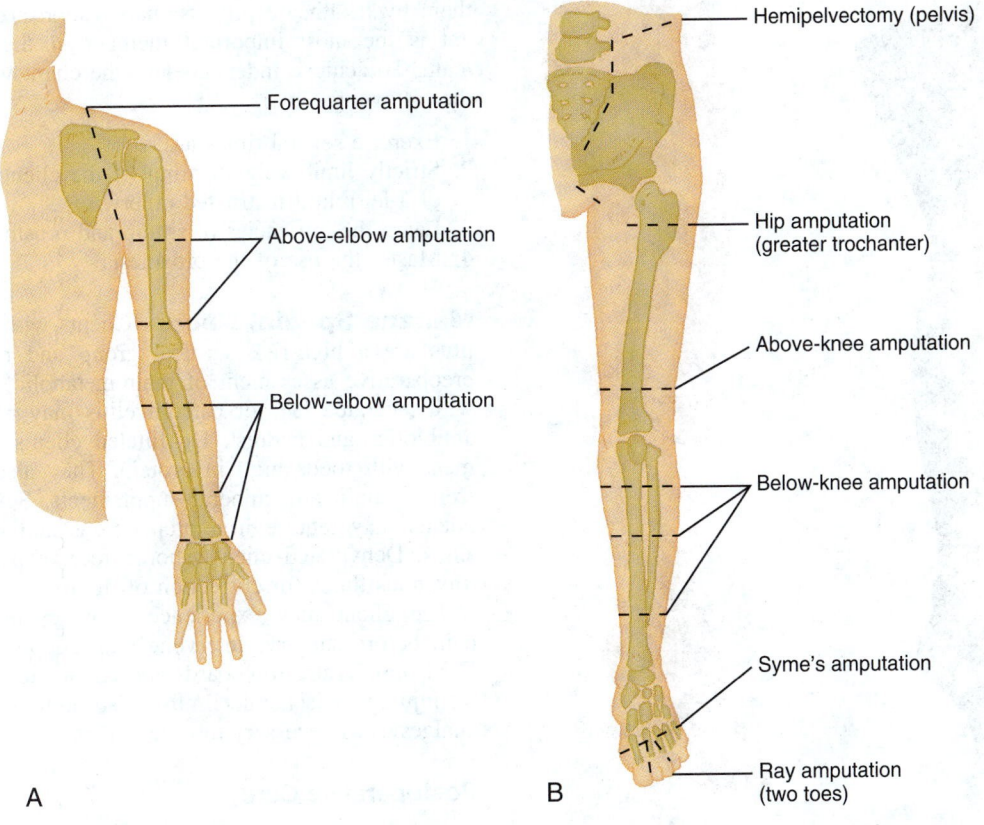

Figure 50–6. Common sites of amputation: *A*, upper extremity; *B*, lower extremity.

duces swelling by gently compressing the tissues. Controlling edema enhances wound healing, comfort, and freedom of movement. In below-knee amputations, the surgeon immobilizes the knee to eliminate joint flexion.

The socket of the distal end of the cast connects to a pylon. A pylon is an adjustable rigid support, the proximal end of which attaches to the below-knee socket or to the knee unit of an above-knee prosthesis. The distal end connects to a foot-ankle assembly.

The rigid dressing is usually changed three to four times before application of a permanent prosthesis. Cast changes are necessary because the stump tends to shrink as it heals and, consequently, is no longer adequately compressed by the original cast.

Permanent Prostheses. Immediate prosthetic fitting is not always possible. However, anyone with a new amputation who is capable of ambulating should receive a temporary prosthesis as soon as possible after surgery. When a conventional delayed prosthesis fitting is anticipated, the client returns from surgery with the stump dressed and covered with elastic bandages or stump socks (Fig. 50–8).

Soft dressings may be used whenever the wound requires frequent inspection. The dressings may be accompanied by external anteroposterior splints for prevention of joint contractures. However, soft dressings poorly control wound pressure and pain. Also, some healthcare pro-

fessionals believe that soft dressings risk greater wound contamination because of repeated wound inspections.

When the sutures are removed 2 to 3 weeks after surgery, the surgeon or prosthetist fits the client with a provisional temporary prosthesis made of plaster of Paris or plastic. A permanent prosthesis is fitted once the stump is healed and molded (Fig. 50–9).

Preoperative Care

Address Fears and Worries. Clients fear amputation because it destroys a familiar body image, imposes physical and social limitations, and temporarily upsets personal life-style. Such fears and anxiety must be resolved during the preoperative period to ensure successful postoperative recovery.

Fear of the impending amputation may lead the client to experience anticipatory grief. Establish open, honest communication. Allow the client to freely express fears and negative feelings about the loss of a limb. Ask significant others how they feel about the amputation and how they perceive the client to be responding. The social worker or psychologist may need to be involved if the client is responding poorly.

The client may also be anxious about unknown consequences and sensations after the amputation. Provide and reinforce information. Most clients feel less anxious when

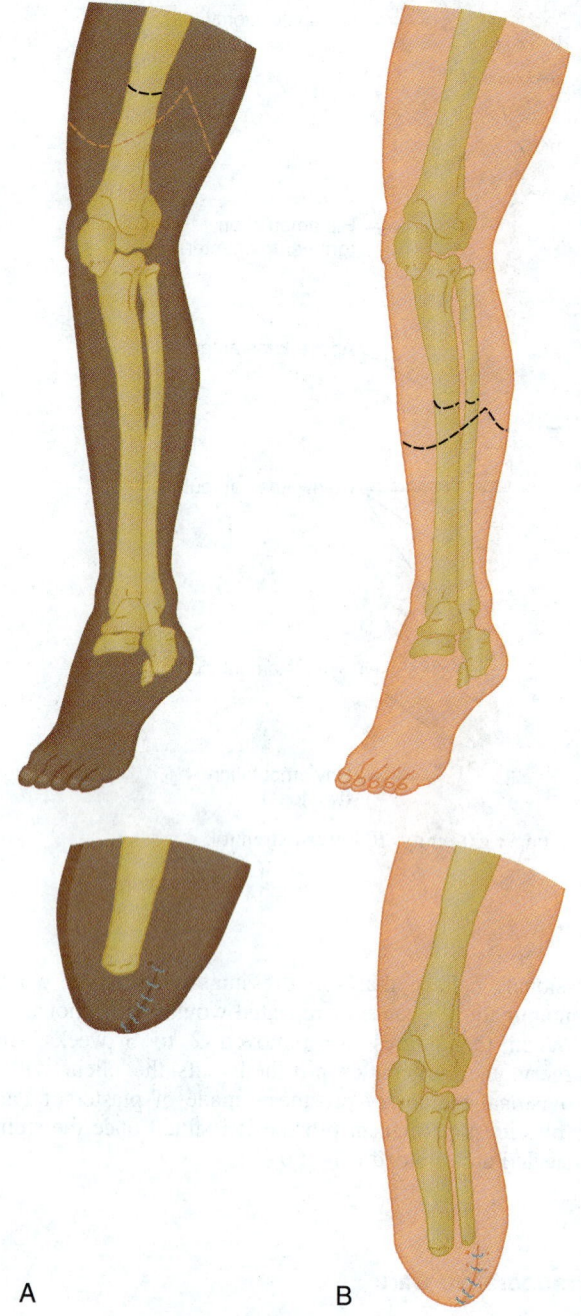

A   B

Figure 50–7. *A,* Above-knee amputation. *B,* Below-knee amputation.

they know what to expect on awakening from surgery. Prepare the client for *phantom limb sensation.* Most clients with new amputations experience the peculiar sensation that their missing limb is still present. This phantom limb sensation may or may not be painful. Also, it may either disappear within hours after surgery or persist for years. Its cause is unknown. To avoid misunderstandings, inform clients that phantom limb sensations occur and are normal.

Establish Expectations. Clients want to know what to expect after surgery and what will be expected of

them by healthcare professionals. Emphasize that the client is the most important member of the rehabilitation team. To achieve independence, the client will need to do the following:

1. Exercise several times a day
2. Strictly limit weightbearing (if the client is losing part of a leg) until instructed otherwise
3. Learn the intricacies of stump and prosthesis care
4. Master the use of the prosthesis

Manage Special Needs. Clients with diabetes mellitus are a high-risk surgical group and require careful preoperative assessment of their metabolic status. Clients with ulcerated legs or osteomyelitis may be treated with antibiotics and bedrest. Debilitated clients need nourishment with foods high in protein. They also may benefit from vitamin and mineral supplements. Severely anemic clients may require iron preparations and blood transfusions. Dehydrated clients should receive preoperative intravenous fluids for correction of fluid imbalances.

The client may experience very severe to moderate pain before surgery. Intervene with supportive measures. For example, use footboards and cradles to avoid pressure on injured or ischemic limbs. Also administer prescribed analgesics as necessary to relieve pain.

Postoperative Care

Following an amputation, the usual postoperative care is given. Special attention is given to the following:

- Bleeding: Look for signs of obvious bleeding or oozing. Outline the drainage including the time on the temporary prosthesis or soft dressing. If drains were placed in the wound, carefully monitor the amount and type of drainage.
- Edema: Edema is controlled by elevating the stump for the first 24 hours after surgery. Then, the stump is placed flat on the bed to reduce hip contracture. Edema is also controlled by stump wrapping techniques.
- Healing: Assess the incision for indications of healing or lack of healing. The incision should be dry, slightly red along the suture line, and intact.

Provide Psychological Support. Following surgery several psychological responses can be noted. The client with unrelenting pain before surgery may feel relief that the pain is finally gone. For clients with some chronic disorders, such as diabetes, the amputation may signal further losses in their battle. These clients may express anger openly or covertly.

Individuals whose limbs were amputated because of trauma have had no time prior to surgery to grieve the loss or adjust to their perceived alterations in body image. They may express sadness or anger, or may show a strong determination not to let the amputation alter their ability to function.

Many clients express depression after amputation. The client may cry easily, eat little, sleep poorly, sleep more, or avoid interactions with others. Many times depression is a reaction to the fear that the client will never walk again, and therefore, early ambulation is therapeutic.

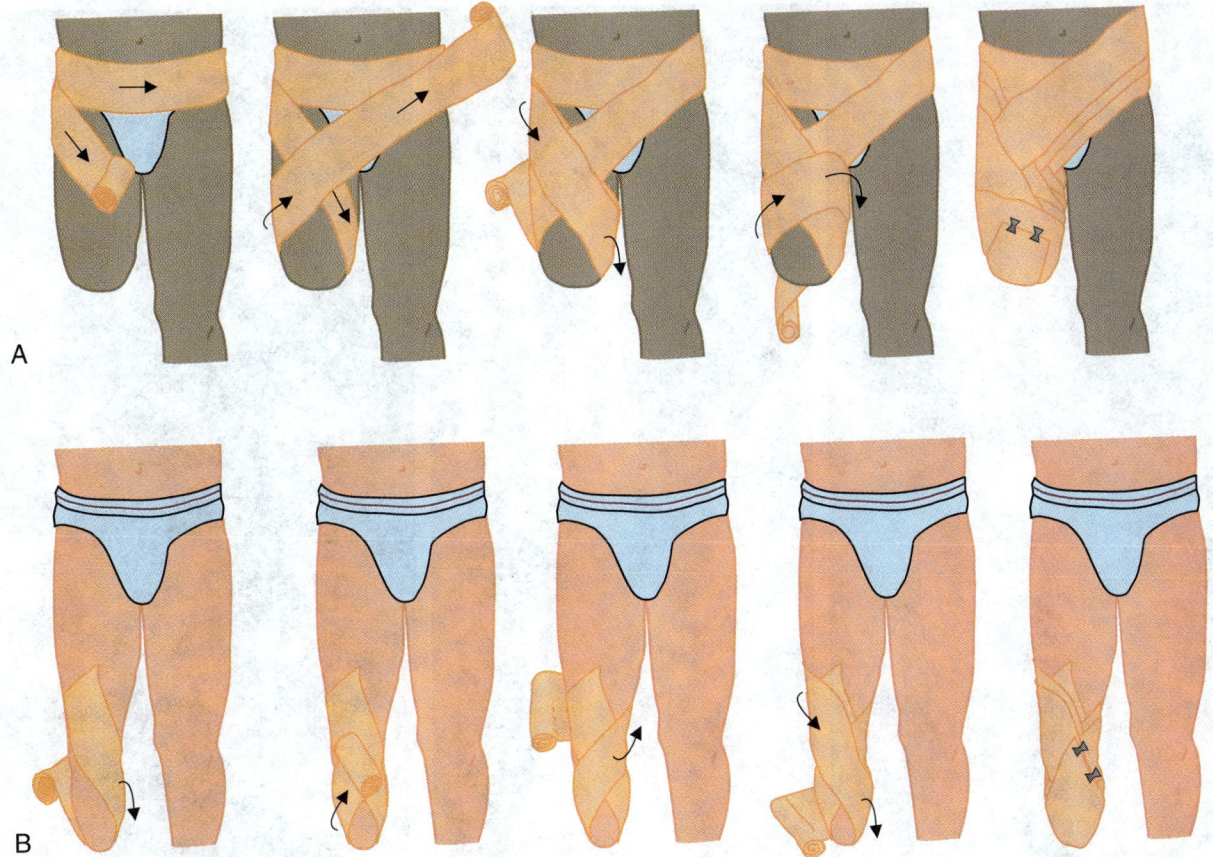

Figure 50–8. Common methods of stump wrapping. *A*, For an above-knee stump, two bandages are required. *B*, For a below-knee stump, one bandage is usually sufficient.

Assist the Client in Adjusting to Phantom Sensations. Phantom sensations are feelings that are perceived in the area of the amputated limb. Although these sensations are often referred to as *phantom pain*, not all of the sensations are painful. The client may describe sensations of warmth, cold, itching, or pain, especially in amputated fingers or toes. Phantom sensations are caused by intact peripheral nerves proximal to the amputation site that carried messages between the brain and the now amputated part. These sensations are normal, and the client should be prepared for them. Phantom sensations often are felt immediately after surgery, and gradually decrease over the next 2 years.

Phantom pain is an awareness of actual pain. The pain is usually burning, cramping, squeezing, or shooting in nature. Phantom pain is less well understood and may occur in a large percentage of clients. It is thought to be caused by a combination of physiologic and psychological components. However, no research has identified a link between phantom pain and any clinical psychological disorder. Phantom pain occurs most often in clients who have had pain in the limb prior to the amputation. Interventions that may reduce phantom pain include range of motion exercises, visual imaging, and other interventions for chronic pain.

Assist the Client in Adjusting to the Prosthesis. The focus of subacute care is the rehabilitation of the client. Physical therapists usually work with the client twice daily for strengthening and gait training.

When making discharge plans for the client with a new amputation (and probably a prosthesis), consider the client's ambulatory level and the tasks with which the client may need help. Frequently, by the time clients with amputations are aware of their changed circumstances, they are at home, alone, and without the informed and professional advice that can prepare them for their altered lives. Schedule home visits from community healthcare nurses until such clients have adjusted to their new situation and feel reasonably comfortable and confident in their ability to provide self-care.

The most common prosthesis for clients with a below-the-knee amputation is a patellar tendon-bearing limb prosthesis. The interior of the prosthesis contacts all surfaces of the stump and weightbearing is on several areas. Clients with above-the-knee amputation are fitted with either a quadrilateral socket or an ischial containment prosthesis. Weight is borne on the ischial tuberosity and the soft tissues of the proximal stump, respectively.

Prostheses for the upper extremity consist of a hook or hand device, a harness to supply force to the hand, and a

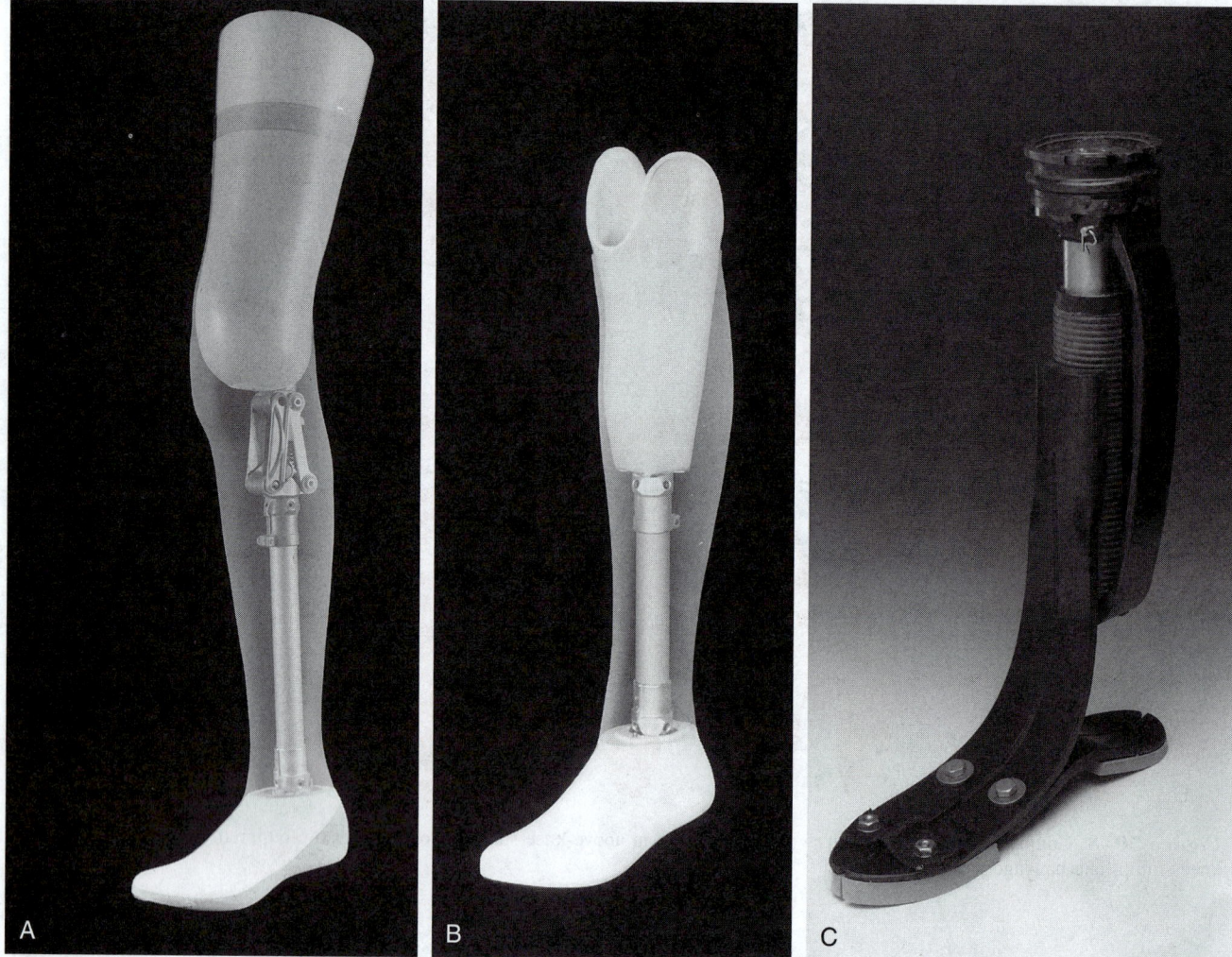

A

B

C

Figure 50–9. Permanent lower-extremity prostheses. *A*, Above-knee prosthesis. *B*, Below-knee prosthesis. *C*, Flex-foot prosthesis, which connects to the distal end of the pylon of an above-knee or below-knee prosthesis and provides increased flexibility for people who want to be more active than they are able to be with a traditional foot-ankle assembly. (*A* and *B*, Courtesy of Otto Bock Orthopedic Industry, Inc., Minneapolis, MN; *C*, courtesy of Flex Foot, Inc., Mission Viejo, CA.)

socket for attachment. The client coping with an upper extremity amputation must be highly motivated to master the prosthesis and achieve independence. For successful rehabilitation, the client must integrate the prosthetic arm and hand into the total body image.

Cosmetic prostheses are primarily used to enhance self-esteem and make reentry into society minus a limb more tolerable for clients who are not candidates for a functioning prosthesis. Because the construction of cosmetic prostheses does not allow weightbearing, caution the client never to attempt transfers or ambulation with a cosmetic prosthesis.

The client coping with a new amputation must adjust to the prosthesis physically as well as psychologically. Physically, the client increases strength and endurance with regularly scheduled exercise; controls weightbearing until the wound completely heals; and practices ambulating with the new prosthesis until a skillful, automatic gait is developed.

Psychologically, clients must integrate the new prosthesis into their self-image if they are to become truly independent again. Psychological adjustment to a prosthesis is often more difficult and may take longer than physical adjustment. Some clients may benefit from talking with others who have mastered the use of their prostheses and have attained independent function. Support groups may be helpful in this endeavor.

Assist the Client with Stump and Prosthesis Care. The Client Education Guide suggests ways for clients who have had lower limb amputation to care for their stump and prosthesis in the healthcare facility or at home.

Physical mobility will be compromised for the client who has just experienced an amputation. Amputating a limb displaces the center of gravity, normally located just below the umbilicus. A client coping with an amputation

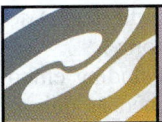

CLIENT EDUCATION GUIDE

Stump and Prosthesis Care

Client Instructions in English *(Instrucciones para el cliente en inglés)*	**Client Instructions in Spanish** *(Instrucciones para el cliente en español)*
Stump Care	**Cuidado del Muñón**
Inspect the stump daily for redness, blistering, or abrasions.	Inspeccione diariamente el muñón para ver si hay enrojecimiento, ampollas, o abrasiones.
Use a mirror to examine all sides and aspects of the stump. Skin breakdown on the stump is extremely serious because it interferes with prosthesis training and may prolong hospitalization and recovery. If you have diabetes mellitus, you are particularly susceptible to skin complications, because changes in sensation may obliterate your awareness of stump pain.	Use un espejo para examinar todos los lados del muñón. Las lesiones o la piel partida en el muñón son muy serias porque interfieren con el entrenamiento para la prótesis y pueden prolongar la hospitalización y la recuperación. Si tiene diabetes, está muy susceptible a desarrollar complicaciones de la piel, porque los cambios de sensibilidad pueden destruir el sentido del dolor en el muñón.
Perform meticulous daily hygiene. Wash the stump with a mild soap, then carefully rinse and dry it. Apply nothing to the stump after it is bathed. Alcohol dries and cracks the skin, whereas oils and creams soften the skin too much for safe prosthesis use.	Mantenga diarriamente una higiene meticulosa. Lave el muñón con un jabón suave, enjuagelo cuidadosamente y séquelo. No aplique nada al moñón después de lavarlo. El alcohol seca y parte la piel, mientras que los aceites y las cremas suavizan demasiado la piel para lograr el uso seguro de la prótesis.
Wear woolen stump socks over the stump for cleanliness and comfort. Wash woolen socks in cool water and mild soap to prevent shrinkage. To prevent stretching, wash socks gently. Dry stump socks flat on a towel. Replace torn socks; mending creates wrinkles that irritate the skin.	Use calcetines de muñón de lana sobre el muñón para limpieza y comodidad. Lave los calcetines de lana en agua fria con jabón suave para prevenir que se encojan. Para prevenir se agranden, lave los calcetines suavemente. Seque los calcetines del muñón sobre una toalla. Reemplace los calcetines rotos; al remendarlos se hacen plieges que irritan la piel.
Put on the prosthesis immediately when arising and keep it on all day (once the wound has healed completely) to reduce stump swelling.	Pongase la prótesis inmediatamente después de que se levante y usela todo el día (una vez que la herida haya sanado completamente) para reducir la hinchazón en el muñón.
Continue prescribed exercises to prevent weakness.	Continue los ejercicios que le recetaron para evitar que se la debilite.
Prosthesis Care	**Cuidado de la Prótesis**
Remove sweat and dirt from the prosthesis socket daily by wiping the inside of the socket with a damp soapy cloth. To remove the soap, use a clean damp cloth. Dry the prosthesis socket thoroughly.	Quitele el sudor y el polvo a la cavidad de la prótesis, que acopla el muñón con una toallita húmeda enjabonada. Para sacarle el jabón, use una toallita limpia húmeda. Seque completamente la cavidad de la prótesis.
Never attempt to adjust or mechanically alter the prosthesis. If problems develop, consult the prosthetist.	Nunca intente adaptar o alterar mecanicamente la prótesis. Si se le presentan problemas, consulte al técnico de prótesis.
Schedule a yearly appointment with the prosthetist.	Haga una cita cada año con el técnico de prótesis.

must relearn balance because the prosthesis, however similar, will not be an exact replica in weight and movement of the lost limb. Adapting to a change in the center of gravity occurs slowly but progressively until the conscious effort of maintaining balance comes under unconscious control.

When the prosthesis is not worn (e.g., during the night), turning also requires a readaptation in body balance. Consequently, the client may need assistance while turning until the new center of gravity is comfortable.

Acute Arterial Occlusion

Acute occlusion of a limb's main artery may be caused by trauma, embolism, or thrombosis and may occur in a healthy or diseased artery; about 90% occur in the lower limbs. In arterial embolism, the wall of the artery is often healthy; the obstruction in the artery arises most frequently from a thrombus within the heart. Causative factors include atrial fibrillation, myocardial infarction, prosthetic heart valves, and rheumatic heart disease. Sometimes, portions of a blood clot, such as platelet emboli, form at points of turbulence, lodge at a bifurcation, and initiate a thrombus. Atheromatous emboli sometimes block small arteries. In the lower extremity, over half the emboli lodge in either the superficial femoral or the popliteal artery. Other noncardiac causes of emboli are abdominal aortic aneurysm, peripheral aneurysm, and diabetes mellitus. Most of these emboli lodge in the lower extremities. About 15% travel to the arms. Arterial thrombosis is usually superimposed on atherosclerosis and consequently develops in a damaged vessel.

The circulatory changes that follow arterial occlusion and that predict the outcome are complex and depend on a variety of factors. Acute occlusion produces a fall in mean and pulse pressures in the distal arteries and a decrease in tissue perfusion and oxygenation. In a normal artery, blood flow is restored by collateral channels, but with acute emboli, collateral vessels have not had time to develop.

It is important to differentiate between arterial thrombosis and arterial embolism. Acute arterial thrombosis is usually caused by arterial obstruction by a blood clot that forms in an artery that has been damaged by atherosclerosis. Arterial thrombosis may also develop in an arterial aneurysm, especially aneurysms that form in the popliteal artery.

The classic manifestations of acute ischemia caused by peripheral thrombus or embolism, which are known as the *six Ps*, are as follows:

1. *Pain* or loss of sensory nerves secondary to ischemia
2. *Paresthesias* and loss of position sense; the client is unable to detect pressure or to sense a pinprick; the client cannot tell if toes are flexed or extended
3. *Poikilothermia* (coldness)
4. *Paralysis*
5. *Pallor* caused by empty superficial veins and no capillary filling; pallor can progress to a mottled, cyanotic, cadaverous, cold leg
6. *Pulselessness*

Muscle necrosis may start as early as 2 to 3 hours after occlusion. Complete paralysis with stiffness of muscles and joints (rigor mortis) indicates irreversible damage. The leg must be amputated to prevent systemic reaction to the products of massive muscle destruction and systemic sepsis.

Surgery is required to correct arterial embolism. Surgery for thrombosis usually involves an arterial reconstructive procedure for revascularization of the leg. Arterial emboli can be removed by an embolectomy.

If the decision is made to remove the occluding embolus or thrombus, surgery should be performed as quickly as possible, generally under local anesthesia. If hours have elapsed since the occlusion occurred, the viability of the limb will determine whether embolectomy should be attempted.

While decisions about surgery are being made, put the client to bed in a comfortable, warm room. Protect the limb from pressure and other trauma and keep it at room temperature, neither warm nor chilled. The best position for the limb is level or slightly dependent.

If medical intervention is selected or the surgeon is delayed, anticoagulants are generally started. Heparin is usually continued for a minimum of 2 to 7 days, after which a change to an oral anticoagulant may be made. The prevailing practice is to treat all clients who have a definite source of embolism and who have satisfactorily recovered from the acute episode of occlusion with long-term anticoagulant therapy.

Aside from surgery, fibrinolytic agents may be used to dissolve a thrombus or embolus.

Arterial Ulcers

Areas of an ischemic foot subjected to local pressure may have skin breakdown. The usual sites of arterial ulcers are the medial and lateral metatarsal heads and the tip of the heel. The ulcers are very painful, which distinguish them from venous stasis ulcers. Arterial ulcers also have a "punched out" look, again in contrast to venous stasis ulcers, which are broad and flat.

Sadly, once an ulcer develops, it tends to heal poorly or not at all (especially in diabetics). Without normal vessels and adequate blood flow, the damaged tissues fail to receive needed oxygen, nutrients, antibodies, and protective leukocytes, and the process of tissue damage continues. Eventually, the client may be forced to undergo limb amputation.

Although skin grafting may ultimately be required to cover the site of arterial ischemic leg ulcers (once the ulcerated area is free from infection and granulation tissue is evident), intervention for the skin lesion does not cure the underlying disease. Most ulcers require revascularization to heal. Arterial bypass surgery improves circulation when the client has an aortoiliac or femoropopliteal occlusion. For this surgery to be successful, however, the arteries in the leg must be healthy enough to carry sufficient blood to the foot once the block has been removed or bypassed.

General intervention involves keeping the area of ulceration clean and free from pressure and irritation. Bedrest reduces the oxygen needs of the impaired tissues. Debridement followed by application of wet-to-damp saline dressings is also a standard intervention for leg ulcers. Whirlpool treatments also provide good debridement. If the ulcer is clean and granulating, healing is enhanced with damp normal saline dressings or a moist occlusive dressing, such as DuoDerm.

Aneurysms

An aneurysm is a permanent localized dilation of an artery. A 50% increase in the size of a vessel is the usual criterion. Once initiated, an aneurysm tends to enlarge gradually; this, along with the thrombus that develops within the aneurysm, leads to the usual complications of aneurysms: rupture, pressure on surrounding structures, thrombosis, and distal embolization. Atherosclerotic aneurysms occur about 10 times more often in men than in women and, for the most part, occur after age 50 years.

The most common cause of arterial aneurysm is atherosclerosis. Less common causes include congenital defects of the arterial wall (e.g., Marfan's disease), trauma (both blunt and penetrating types), infection (including syphilis), polyarteritis, and hereditary abnormalities of connective tissue. Hypertension seems to enhance aneurysm formation.

A combination of factors, such as "wear and tear" and impaired nutrition, results in weakening of the arterial wall over time, which leads to tortuosity, dilation, and aneurysm formation in atherosclerotic arteries. Atherosclerotic aneurysms tend to develop where the artery is not supported by skeletal muscle or where it is subject to frequent bending with physical activity. The most common locations for arteriosclerotic aneurysms are the thoracic and abdominal aorta, the iliac arteries, and the femoral and popliteal arteries.

Classification of Aneurysms

Aneurysms may be classified according to the following characteristics:

Location. Aneurysms are designated as being either *venous* or *arterial*. They are also described according to the specific vessel in which they develop (e.g., aortic, iliac artery) and, more precisely, according to the exact area of the vessel that they affect (e.g., thoracic aortic aneurysm, abdominal aortic aneurysm).

Etiology. Aneurysms can be classified according to the cause, such as atherosclerotic aneurysm, mycotic aneurysm (caused by bacterial infection), hypertensive aneurysm, or syphilitic (luetic) aneurysm.

Gross Appearance. Classification of aneurysms is sometimes based on their shape, anatomic features, and size. Fusiform aneurysms are localized, rather uniform dilations of an artery; the term *saccular* is used to describe an outpouching of an artery at a point at which the medial coat is thinned (Fig. 50–10). A dissecting aneurysm occurs as the hematoma in the arterial wall forms a localized enlargement of the involved artery, separating the layers of the arterial wall. A dissecting aneurysm may be either acute or chronic. A *pseudoaneurysm*, or false aneurysm, results from the development of a sac around a hematoma that maintains a communication with the lumen of an artery whose wall has been ruptured or penetrated.

Abdominal Aortic Aneurysms

Abdominal aortic aneurysms (Fig. 50–11A) occur about four times more often than thoracic aneurysms. The natural course of an untreated abdominal aortic aneurysm is to expand and rupture.

The aorta is under greater stress than the rest of the arterial system because of its large diameter and its exposure to high pressure during each systolic ejection of blood. Abdominal aneurysms may extend into the iliac arteries. When the aneurysm reaches about 5 cm in diam-

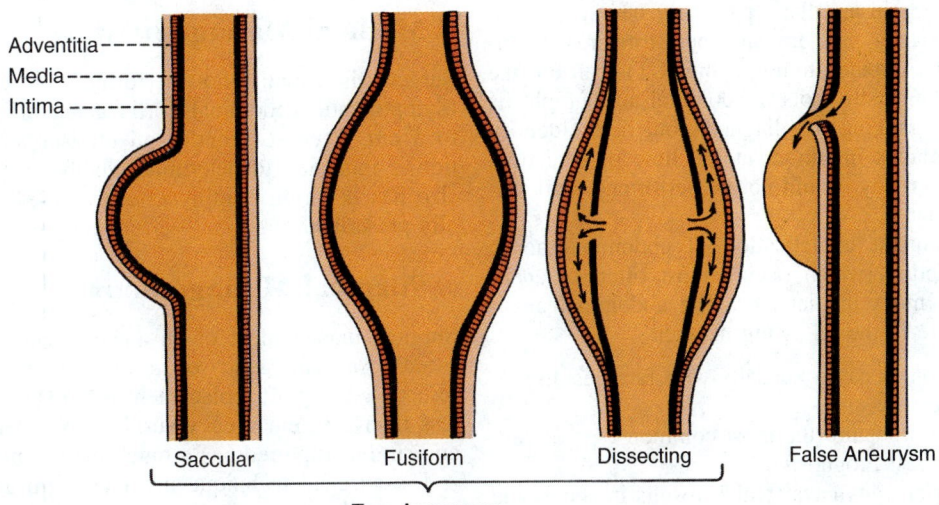

Figure 50–10. Classification of aneurysms. In a true aneurysm, layers of the vessel wall dilate in one of the following ways: *saccular,* a unilateral outpouching; *fusiform,* a bilateral outpouching; or *dissecting,* a bilateral outpouching in which layers of the vessel wall separate, with creation of a cavity. In a false aneurysm, the wall ruptures, and a blood clot is retained in an outpouching of tissue.

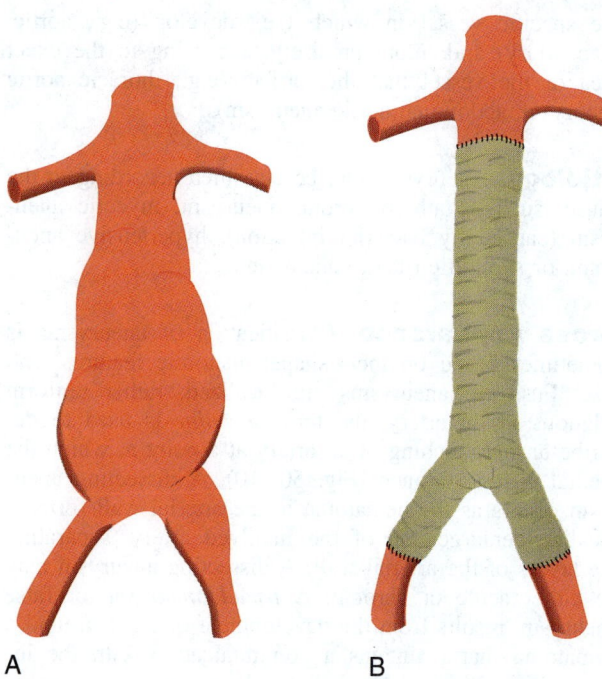

A   B

Figure 50–11. *A*, An abdominal aortic aneurysm. *B*, A bifurcated synthetic graft in place.

eter, it can usually be palpated. An abdominal aneurysm measuring 6 cm or more in diameter has a 20% chance of rupturing in 1 year.

Most abdominal aneurysms are asymptomatic; discovery is usually made on physical or x-ray examination of the abdomen or lower spine for other reasons. Smaller aneurysms and aneurysms in obese clients may be more difficult to confirm. The most common clinical manifestation is awareness of a pulsating mass in the abdomen, with or without pain, followed by abdominal pain and back pain. Groin pain and flank pain may be experienced because of increasing pressure on other structures. Ultrasonography and computed tomographic (CT) scan are the most accurate diagnostic tools. Abdominal aortography is not essential for making the diagnosis but helps identify circulatory anomalies important at the time of resection. Therefore, angiography should not be performed until surgery is contemplated.

The most frequent complication of abdominal aortic aneurysm is rupture, which occurs most often in aneurysms 5 cm or more in diameter. The abdominal aneurysm may rupture in the following manner:

1. Into the peritoneal cavity (usually with fatal results)
2. Into the mesentery
3. Behind the peritoneum (the most common type of rupture with the best prognosis)
4. Into the inferior vena cava (which results in shock and heart failure due to massive arteriovenous fistula)
5. Into the duodenum or rectum, causing severe gastrointestinal hemorrhage

Ruptured abdominal aortic aneurysm presents with a triad of manifestations, including the following:

1. Abdominal pain combined with intense back and flank pain and possible scrotal pain
2. A pulsating abdominal mass
3. Shock, with systolic blood pressure below 100 mm Hg and apical pulse rate greater than 100 per minute

Other manifestations include ecchymosis in the flank and perianal area; severe sudden pain in the abdomen, paravertebral area, or flank; lightheadedness; and nausea with sudden hypotension. In addition, the red blood cell count falls and the white blood cell count rises. These are also the signs of a ruptured postoperative abdominal bypass graft.

After the initial rupture, the blood is walled off in the retroperitoneal space, or tamponaded, for a period. If the ruptured abdominal aortic aneurysm can be identified during this phase, the client has a much greater chance of survival. Once the aorta ruptures anteriorly into the peritoneal cavity, death is almost certain.

Surgery is the only intervention for clients with ruptured abdominal aortic aneurysm. New surgical and grafting techniques and faster methods for transport (e.g., helicopters) now permit rapid resection of ruptured abdominal aortic aneurysm and sometimes save the client's life. The operative mortality rate for repair of ruptured abdominal aneurysm may be as high as 35%.

About 4% of all ruptured abdominal aortic aneurysms rupture into the inferior vena cava, producing aortocaval fistula. Manifestations include intractable congestive heart failure because of the right-to-left shift, massive lower extremity edema, acute abdominal pain, ascites, pleural effusions, and hepatomegaly. The abdominal aortic aneurysm may rupture into the duodenum, producing aortoenteric fistula. Gastrointestinal bleeding, which may progress to shock, is the presenting sign.

Acute and Subacute Care

■ Medical Management

Surgery is usually not performed on clients with an asymptomatic abdominal aortic aneurysm smaller than 4 to 5 cm. Every 6 months, an ultrasonographic examination is indicated to determine whether any change in the size has occurred. Antihypertensive medications are usually prescribed.

■ Surgical Management

Surgical management of an aneurysm may be performed as either an emergency or an elective procedure. Elective resection and graft replacement has a surgical mortality of less than 5%; emergency surgical treatment after the aneurysm has ruptured has a much higher mortality.

The surgical technique involves exposure of the aneurysm, application of clamps just above and below the aneurysm, excision of the aneurysm, and replacement of the excised segment with a Dacron graft (see Fig. 50–11*B*). Excision of an abdominal aneurysm is done through a midline incision that extends from the xiphoid process to the symphysis pubis.

Abdominal aortic aneurysm repair is considered a major operation, and many specific postoperative complications can develop. Complications after abdominal aortic aneurysm repair are generally caused by underlying coronary artery disease and chronic obstructive pulmonary disease. These conditions decrease metabolism of anesthetic, increase the risk of postoperative atelectasis, and decrease the client's tolerance of hemodynamic changes from blood loss and fluid shifts.

One of the most serious complications is acute myocardial infarction. To reduce the risk of this complication, many clients undergo coronary artery bypass prior to aneurysm repair.

Renal failure can develop for several reasons. The kidney can sustain ischemia from decreased aortic blood flow, decreased cardiac output, emboli, inadequate hydration, or the need for clamps on the aorta above the renal arteries during surgery.

Emboli can also develop and lodge in the arteries of the lower extremities or mesentery. Clinical manifestations include those of acute occlusion in the leg. Bowel necrosis is exhibited as fever, leukocytosis, ileus, diarrhea, and abdominal pain.

The spinal cord can also become ischemic, resulting in paraplegia, rectal and urinary incontinence, or loss of pain and temperature sensation. Spinal cord ischemia tends to occur more commonly when an abdominal aortic aneurysm has ruptured.

Changes in sexual function may also develop following repair of an abdominal aortic aneurysm. Retrograde ejaculation occurs in about two-thirds of male clients, and loss of potency occurs in one-third of males who have undergone repair of abdominal aortic aneurysm.

■ Nursing Management of the Surgical Client

Preoperative Care

Abdominal aortic surgery is major surgery; it lasts approximately 4 hours. During the hours under anesthesia, the client faces a great risk of pulmonary and cardiac complications developing. Preoperative assessment must include detection of concurrent coronary artery disease and cerebrovascular disease. Also assess all peripheral pulses for baseline comparison postoperatively. If dissection or rupture has occurred, the client may receive intravenous fluids (often in large volumes) for maintenance of tissue perfusion.

Postoperative Care

Assessment

Postoperative assessment of the client after abdominal aortic aneurysm repair is essential. Potential complications are many, because of the seriousness of the problem and the complexity of the repair. Even though extracorporeal perfusion (cardiopulmonary bypass) is not needed for the surgery, arterial flow to tissues distal to the aneurysm is reduced during the time required to perform the surgery.

Diagnosis, Planning, Implementation

Risk for Hemorrhage. Because of the risk of bleeding at the graft site, the client is at risk for hemorrhage. Use the collaborative problem *Risk for Hemorrhage*. You can also use the nursing diagnosis *Risk for Fluid Volume Deficit*, but recognize that the "fluid" that can be lost is blood.

Planning: Expected Outcome. The nurse will monitor for manifestations of hemorrhage and notify the physician if any signs occur.

Implementation. Monitor the client for increase in pulse rate, decrease in blood pressure, clammy skin, anxiety, restlessness, decreasing levels of consciousness, pallor, cyanosis, thirst, oliguria less than 30 to 50 ml/hr, increase in abdominal girth, increased chest tube output greater than 100 ml/hr for 3 hours, and back pain (from retroperitoneal bleeding). Monitor central venous pressure, left atrial pressure, pulmonary artery pressure, and pulmonary capillary wedge pressure continuously. Assess for changes indicating hypovolemia. Report any of these manifestations immediately.

Risk for Impaired Gas Exchange. The large abdominal incision impairs deep inspiration and usually reduced effective coughing. Write the diagnosis as *Risk for Impaired Gas Exchange related to ineffective cough secondary to pain from large incision.*

Planning: Expected Outcome. The client will have improved gas exchange as evidenced by oxygen saturation or PaO$_2$ greater than 95%, increasing effectiveness in coughing, and clearing of lung sounds.

Implementation. Monitor settings on ventilator to ensure that client is adequately oxygenated. Assess lung sounds every 1 to 2 hours. Report any adventitious sounds. Monitor oxygen saturation continuously. Report any desaturation. After extubation, assist with coughing by using incentive spirometry, provide splinting pillows before coughing, encourage ambulation, and provide adequate analgesia.

Risk for Altered Peripheral Tissue Perfusion. During the operation, the aorta is clamped to stop bleeding while the graft is placed. During that time, peripheral tissues are not perfused. The graft site can also become occluded with thrombus. In addition, the client often has pre-existing arterial disease. Write the diagnosis as *Risk for Altered Peripheral Tissue Perfusion related to temporary decrease in blood supply.*

Planning: Expected Outcomes. The client will maintain adequate tissue perfusion as evidenced by pedal pulses, warm feet, capillary refill of less than 5 seconds, absence of numbness or tingling, and abililty to dorsiflex and plantar flex both feet equally.

Implementation. Assess dorsalis pedis and posterior tibial pulses every hour for 24 hours. Report changes in pulse quality or absent pulses (assess with Doppler if needed). Assess dorsiflexion and plantar flexion and sensation (needles-and-pins sensation) every hour for 24 hours. Inspect lower extremities for mottling, cyanosis, coolness or numbness every 4 hours.

Pain. Abdominal aortic aneurysm repair necessitates a long incision. Write this common postoperative diagnosis as *Pain related to surgical incision.*

Planning: Expected Outcomes. The client will have increased comfort as evidenced by self-report of decreasing levels of pain, use of decreasing amounts of narcotic analgesics for pain control, and ambulating and/or coughing without extreme pain.

Risk for Ischemia of the Bowel. If the client undergoes extensive aortic procedures that involve clamping the mesenteric vessels, ischemic colitis can develop. In addition, the inferior mesenteric artery can embolize. The lack of blood supply can lead to ischemia and ileus.

Planning: Expected Outcomes. The nurse will monitor the client for abdominal distention, diarrhea, severe abdominal pain, sudden elevations in white blood cell count, and bowel sounds.

Implementation. Maintain accurate intake and output. Tally and analyze hourly for 24 hours. Notify physician if output falls below 30 to 50 ml/hr. Assess urine specific gravity and daily weight. Monitor blood urea nitrogen (BUN) and creatinine levels. Assess bowel sounds every 4 hours. Keep NPO (nothing by mouth), provide oral care every 2 to 4 hours. Provide routine nasogastric (NG) tube care, assess nares for tissue impairment. Perform guaiac tests of NG drainage every 4 hours or if bleeding is suspected (i.e., drainage has dark, coffee-ground appearance or is bright red).

Risk for Spinal Cord Ischemia. A rare but devastating effect of aortic abdominal aneurysm repair is spinal cord ischemia leading to paralysis, with or without bowel and bladder involvement. It appears to be most common in clients who have suprarenal aortic reconstruction.

Planning: Expected Outcomes. The nurse will monitor for manifestations of spinal cord damage and report any abnormal data.

Implementation. Monitor ability to move lower extremities (dorsiflexion and plantar flexion) and sensation in both legs every 1 to 2 hours.

Community and Self-Care

Most clients who require abdominal aortic aneurysm repair have significant degrees of arterial disease. Many of the postoperative instructions should address care of clients with arterial disorders, such as avoiding foot injury by having a podiatrist perform foot care, avoiding hot water bottles or heating pads, and doing daily foot inspection. Have the client avoid clothing that constricts the abdomen and legs, which would decrease blood supply. Review all medications to be used by the client to be

certain that he or she understands their purpose, schedule, and side effects. Instruct the client about incision care and manifestations of infection.

Prepare the client and family for specific discharge needs by educating them about the following:

■ Activity

The client should ambulate as tolerated, including climbing stairs and walking outdoors. If leg swelling develops, the leg should be wrapped in elastic bandages or support stockings should be used. Activities that involve lifting heavy objects, usually more than 15 to 20 lb, are not permitted for 6 to 12 weeks postoperatively. Activities that involve pushing, pulling, or straining may also be restricted. Driving may also be restricted because of postoperative weakness.

■ Sexual Activity

The client can resume sexual activity as soon as he or she is able to walk without shortness of breath (e.g., two flights of stairs). This will take about 4 to 6 weeks. The risk of impotence in male patients should be discussed before discharge. Causes vary from pre-existing aortoiliac disease or diabetes to side effects from aortic cross-clamping. Referral may be appropriate if the client is amenable.

Aortic Dissection

Aortic dissection is the longitudinal splitting of the medial (muscular) layer of the aorta by blood flowing through it. It is the most common catastrophe involving the aorta. Dissection occurs following a tear in the intima, or inner lining, of the aorta, which allows blood to dissect between it and the medial layer. As the dissection progresses, blood flow through the arterial branches of the aorta becomes blocked, and blood flow to the organs that are served by these branches is reduced. Aortic dissections occur more often in men between ages 50 and 70 years, the majority of whom are hypertensive. Aortic dissections differ from aneurysms in that a false lumen is formed by separation of the intima from the medial layers of the aorta. An aneurysm is a dilation of the entire aortic wall.

Etiology and Classification

The exact cause of dissection is not known. The medial layer of the aorta can become necrotic and thereby lose strength. Clients with Marfan's syndrome (a hereditary condition of connective tissue that predisposes it to aneurysm formation) have a high incidence of dissection. Blunt trauma to the chest wall, such as impact on the steering wheel during a car accident, can also lead to tearing of the aorta.

Dissections are classified by the anatomic location and by time of occurrence. Type I starts above the aortic valve and extends to the iliac bifurcation, traversing the entire aorta. This type of dissection is most common and most lethal. Type II is confined to the ascending aorta and proximal transverse arch and is most often seen in conjunction with Marfan's syndrome. Type III dissections have the best prognosis. They begin just distal to the left subclavian artery and extend to the iliac bifurcation and are usually treated medically. Dissections are also classified as acute (those that have occurred during the 2 preceding weeks) and chronic (those that have persisted for more than 2 weeks). If untreated, 50% of clients will die within the first 48 hours, 60% to 70% within the first week, and 90% within 3 months after dissection.

Clinical Manifestations

Abrupt, excruciating pain is the most common presenting manifestation in clients with aortic dissection. Clients describe the pain as ripping or knife-like tearing sensations that radiate to the back, abdomen, extremities, or anterior part of the chest. Hypertension is a common finding, although the client looks "shocky," is sweating profusely, is severely apprehensive, and has diminished peripheral pulses. Other manifestations from decreased perfusion include unequal pulses, different blood pressures in the arms, paraplegia or hemiplegia, decreased urine output or hematuria, mental status changes, and chest pain. A murmur of aortic regurgitation can be heard if the dissection proceeds proximally.

Chest x-ray reveals a widened mediastinum and may show fractured ribs. Echocardiogram can be used to determine the size, shape, and location of the tear. Laboratory tests during emergency settings are usually not helpful, except for hemoglobin and hematocrit assays to calculate blood loss and transfusion needs. If the client's condition is stable, aortography can be used to determine the extent of the dissection.

Complications

Cardiac tamponade can develop when the client has dissection of the ascending aortic arch. This life-threatening complication occurs when blood escapes from the area of dissection into the pericardial sac. Clients will have pulsus paradoxus, muffled heart sounds, narrowed pulse pressure, and distended neck veins. Pulsus paradoxus occurs when beats are weaker in amplitude during inspiration and are stronger with expiration. Blood pressure readings decrease more than 10 mm Hg during inspiration and increase with expiration.

Because the dissection decreases blood supply to many vital organs, ischemic changes in many organs can develop. The spinal cord, kidneys, and abdominal organs are most commonly affected. Ischemia of the spinal cord can lead to manifestations ranging from weakness to paralysis. Renal ischemia can lead to oliguria. Ileus is the most common sign of decreased bowel perfusion.

Management

Emergency management is directed at lowering the blood pressure to decrease the force of the blood tearing the aorta. Potent vasodilators, such as trimethaphan and nitroprusside, are used to quickly reduce blood pressure. Beta-blockers can also be used to decrease myocardial contractility.

If the client's condition is stable, management is directed at pain reduction, blood transfusion (as needed), and management of heart failure (as needed). Pain levels are used as a guide for needed treatment. Pain subsides when the dissection stabilizes.

Surgery is used for clients whose condition is unstable, who develop severe heart failure, who have leaking blood, or who have occlusion of arteries to major organs. During surgery, the torn area is resected and repaired with synthetic graft materials.

Nursing care is directed at reducing blood pressure. The client is kept at bedrest in a semi-Fowler's position. Unnecessary environmental stresses (e.g., noise) should be minimized. Use narcotics to reduce pain; tranquilizers may also be needed. If the client is receiving potent antihypertensive agents, blood pressure should be monitored continuously with an arterial line. Usually the desired parameters for blood pressure are maintained by titrating the vasodilators. Observe the client often for signs of further tearing or rupture. Monitor peripheral pulses, level of anxiety, level of pain, and pulse pressure and check for pulsus paradoxus.

If the client is being managed medically, teach the client about the need for antihypertensive agents and beta-blocker drugs. The client and family should understand that if pain returns, they should immediately return to the emergency room.

Thoracic Aortic Aneurysms

Aneurysms of the thoracic aorta appear most often in hypertensive men between the ages of 40 and 70 years. The aneurysms can develop in any portion of the aorta (ascending, transverse, or descending) and are the most common aneurysms to dissect. The thoracic aorta is relatively out of the reach of physical examinations unless the aorta becomes large enough to be palpable above the clavicle. Therefore, the aneurysm is usually asymptomatic early. If the mass presses on other structures in the chest, various manifestations develop. Respiratory manifestations are a result of compression of the trachea or bronchus and can include cough, dyspnea, and hemoptysis. Respiratory arrest can develop. Pressure on the recurrent laryngeal nerve can lead to hoarseness. Dysphagia can develop from pressure on the esophagus. Upper extremity and head swelling can ensue from superior vena cava obstruction. Aortic valve insufficiency can occur if the aneurysm is located in the ascending aorta. The aneurysm can be seen on chest x-ray and by angiography.

If the aneurysm ruptures, the client reports intense chest pain, hemoglobin is decreased, and hemodynamic instability develops. The pain is described as a ripping sensation up or down the aorta, and it is more intense when the client lies supine. The pain is usually substernal, but it may be noted in the back, lower back, shoulders, or abdomen. An increase in the intensity of pain usually indicates rapid enlargement or imminent rupture and is a sign of extreme peril. Unless fortuitous tamponade develops in local tissue, death ensues rapidly.

Surgery for repair requires use of extracorporeal circulation. The aorta is clamped and the aneurysm is resected and replaced with a Teflon or Dacron prosthesis. Postoperative nursing care is the same as for clients having open heart surgery (see Chapter 45). Operative mortality is the highest in clients who have an acute onset of symptoms because of rupture and in clients with aortic valve insufficiency.

Peripheral Aneurysms

Aneurysms are found more commonly in the lower extremities than in the upper extremities. The most common site is the popliteal space. Popliteal aneurysms cause ischemic manifestations in the lower limbs and have an easily palpable pulse. Although the client may be aware of an enlarged area behind the knee, discomfort is seldom present. Peripheral aneurysm is differentiated from other swellings by the presence of expansile pulsation. Thrombosis may occur and possibly result in severe ischemia with gangrene and loss of the limb.

Bypass operations are the only satisfactory intervention for aneurysms of the popliteal artery and must be performed before emboli develop. Results are excellent in uncomplicated cases.

Subclavian Steal Syndrome

Subclavian steal syndrome produces arm ischemia arising from subclavian artery blockage. The arm is perfused from the carotid artery as blood is taken from the brain to supply the arm. The most prevalent physical finding is a significant difference in blood pressure of the right and left arms. Other manifestations include dizziness, syncope, and arm paresthesias. Intervention is surgical, by carotid-subclavian bypass, transluminal dilation of the subclavian artery, or endarterectomy of the subclavian artery.

Thoracic Outlet Syndromes

Thoracic outlet syndromes are a group of disorders that produce symptoms affecting the neck, shoulder, and upper extremities by compression or mechanical irritation of the brachial plexus, subclavian artery, or subclavian vein as these structures pass through the thoracic outlet. There are three types of syndrome: (1) neurologic, which affects 95% of all clients with thoracic outlet syndrome; (2) arterial, which affects 1% to 2% of clients, but is the most serious form; and (3) venous, which affects 3% to 4% of clients.

Aching or throbbing pain and paresthesias of the neck and upper limb are the most prominent symptoms of the neurologic type syndrome. In more than half of the clients, the symptoms appear to follow a hyperextension injury to the neck or upper back. Intervention is usually nonsurgical and involves physical therapy. The syndrome

in some clients has been treated by surgical removal of the first rib, but this intervention is controversial.

Arterial thoracic outlet syndromes result from chronic compression of the subclavian artery. This leads to the formation of intimal and mural thrombus and, eventually, to peripheral embolization. This type of syndrome is more serious because it frequently results in severe ischemia of the upper extremity. Diagnosis is made by arteriography; treatment is the surgical excision of the anatomic abnormality and removal of the emboli.

Venous thoracic outlet syndrome is caused by external compression of the axillosubclavian vein that results in thrombosis. The primary symptoms are sudden swelling, pain, and cyanosis of the upper extremity. Treatment choices are conservative and include arm elevation and anticoagulation, thrombectomy, or thrombolytic therapy.

Vasculitis

Vasculitis is a grouping of disorders characterized by inflammation and necrosis of blood vessel walls. Most forms of vasculitis are thought to be immunologic in origin. Therefore, most of the discussion of vasculitis is found in Chapter 28.

Thromboangiitis Obliterans (Buerger's Disease)

Etiology and Risk Factors

Thromboangiitis obliterans is a vasculitis of small and medium-sized veins and arteries in the extremities of young adults. The disease process starts distally and progresses cephalad, involving both upper and lower extremities. It is a disease of the second through fourth decades, seen predominantly in men, although the incidence in women is increasing.

The cause of Buerger's disease remains unknown. Almost all clients are moderate to heavy smokers. Many clients have a hypersensitivity reaction to intradermal injection of tobacco products. Therefore, the probable etiology is an exaggerated autoimmune reaction.

Clinical Manifestations and Diagnostic Findings

Pain is the outstanding clinical manifestation. Intermittent claudication is a common problem that occurs in almost all clients at some stage of the disease. It is often the first manifestation noted by the client, usually in the arch of the foot. It is somewhat less common in the calf of the leg but may be noted in both sites. Rest pain with persistent ischemia of one or more digits and coldness or cold sensitivity may be early manifestations. Various types of paresthesias may occur. Pulsations in the posterior tibial and dorsalis pedis arteries are weak or absent. In advanced cases, the extremities may be abnormally red or cyanotic, particularly when dependent. Advanced forms of the disorder occur when color or temperature changes involve only one extremity, only certain digits, or only portions of digits.

Ulceration and gangrene are frequent complications and may occur early in the course of the disease. These lesions can appear spontaneously but often follow trauma. Gangrene usually occurs in one extremity at a time. Edema of the legs is fairly common in advanced cases. Changes in the nails and skin appear, and segmental thrombophlebitis affects the smaller veins in about 40% of clients. The primary diagnostic study is leg arteriography. Biopsy may also be used; inflammatory lesions are usually noted.

Thromboangiitis is usually not life threatening. It does, however, result in disability from pain and amputation.

Management

Intervention is generally the same as for atherosclerotic peripheral arterial disease, and is aimed at the following results:

1. Arresting progress of the disease
2. Producing vasodilation
3. Relieving pain
4. Providing emotional support

The need for smoking cessation must be clearly and unequivocally conveyed to the client and family. Information about programs to promote abstinence from tobacco should be provided.

For clients with rest pain and ischemic lesions, adequate pain control is essential. Vasodilation by calcium-channel blockers or prazosin may be helpful for a few clients. Regional sympathetic ganglionectomy also produces vasodilation and may be recommended. Because of vasoconstriction, the client should be taught to avoid exposure to cold. Work-related exposure to cold should be considered. Ulcerations will need wound care to facilitate healing.

Amputation should be deferred until conservative interventions have failed. However, it is unwise to delay amputation of the leg when the following signs are present:

1. Gangrene extends well into the foot
2. Pain is severe and cannot be controlled
3. Severe infection or toxic effects occur

Amputation above the knee is seldom necessary.

Raynaud's Syndrome

Etiology and Risk Factors

Raynaud's syndrome is a condition in which the small arteries and arterioles constrict in response to various stimuli. It is classified as either vasospastic or obstructive. Manifestations of vasospastic Raynaud's syndrome can be induced by cold, nicotine, caffeine, and stress. Obstructive Raynaud's syndrome is often found in association with autoimmune disorders such as systemic lupus erythematosus, scleroderma, or rheumatoid arthritis.

Raynaud's syndrome may be a benign primary disorder (previously called *Raynaud's disease*) or secondary to another disease or underlying cause (previously called *Raynaud's phenomenon*). It can be difficult to distinguish between the two forms, because symptoms of Raynaud's can occur as much as 10 years before the onset of the underlying condition. People, therefore, with symptoms of Raynaud's syndrome should be carefully evaluated for inflammatory disorders.

Because there is no standard definition or test for Raynaud's syndrome, it is difficult to determine the incidence. It is known to be more common in women than in men, and it is more likely to occur in areas with a cool, damp climate.

Clinical Manifestations

Raynaud's syndrome causes classic color changes in the hands. Exposure to causative stimuli leads to spasm of the digital arteries, which results in pallor. The resulting tissue hypoxia causes the arteries to dilate slightly. Because they carry mainly deoxygenated hemoglobin, the fingers look cyanotic. Finally, rubor develops when arterial spasms stop completely. Criteria for diagnosing primary Raynaud's disease include the following:

● Intermittent attacks of pallor or cyanosis of the digits by exposure to cold or from emotional stimuli
● Bilateral or symmetrical involvement
● No evidence of occlusive disease in the digital arteries or of any systemic disease that might be the cause of the changes
● Gangrene, which (when it occurs) is limited to the skin of the tips of the digits
● A history of manifestations for at least 2 years

Management

Conservative measures are helpful for most clients with primary or secondary Raynaud's syndrome. These measures include keeping hands and feet warm and dry, protecting all parts of the body from cold exposure to prevent reflex sympathetic vasoconstriction of the digits, and cessation of tobacco use. Biofeedback has been of help to some clients.

Pharmacologic management is begun when the vasospastic attacks interfere with the client's ability to work or to perform activities of daily living. Individuals with vasospastic Raynaud's syndrome are more likely to benefit from medication than those with the obstructive form. The aim of drug therapy is to induce smooth muscle relaxation, to relieve spasm, and to increase arterial flow. Calcium antagonists, such as nifedipine, are currently the drugs of first choice because they have been shown to decrease the frequency, duration, and intensity of vasospastic attacks. Other categories of drugs used in treatment include alpha-adrenergic receptor blockers, vasodilators, and agents that interfere with sympathetic nerve activity (sympatholytic drugs). Medications may be necessary only during the winter months. Individuals who rarely go out in the cold weather may take medications prophylactically 1 to 2 hours before exposure to the cold.

Sympathectomy is sometimes performed. It seems to be most effective in primary Raynaud's syndrome and in the treatment of lower extremity disease. The long-term results of sympathectomy are disappointing. The duration of benefit is limited as peripheral nerves regenerate.

The manifestations of Raynaud's syndrome may be alarming, so reassure the client that the condition is not likely to lead to a serious disability. Advise the client to stay warm by wearing wool gloves and turtleneck sweaters, turning up the thermostat at home if necessary, and staying out of drafts. Teach the client to warm up a cold car before driving. Body core heating is important to prevent chilling and the shunting of blood from the extremities to the trunk. Encourage clients to limit their intake of caffeine or chocolate. They must stop smoking to control the disease. Stress can also bring on vasospasm, so stress management workshops and biofeedback programs may prove beneficial. Also, teach the client about any prescribed medications.

Venous Disorders

Venous disorders can be separated into acute and chronic conditions. Chronic venous disorders can be further separated into varicose vein formation and chronic venous insufficiency. Acute venous disorders include thromboembolism. Acute venous disorders are discussed first.

Acute Venous Disorders

Acute venous disorders are caused by thrombus (clot) formation. Thrombus formation obstructs venous flow. Blockage may occur in both the superficial and deep veins.

Superficial thrombophlebitis is usually an easily diagnosed condition; it is often iatrogenic, resulting from careless insertion of intravenous catheters or inattentive care of intravenous sites. Clinical manifestations include a raised, red, slightly indurated, warm, tender cord along the course of the involved vein. Relieve discomfort by applying heat.

Deep vein thrombosis is thrombophlebitis of the deep veins. Veins and valves permanently damaged by deep vein thrombosis increase the risk for another deep vein thrombosis, pulmonary embolism, and venous stasis ulcers. Deep vein thrombosis is a common disorder, more so in women than in men, and more so in adults than in children. It is particularly common among hospitalized clients. Around one third of clients older than 40 years who have had either major surgery or an acute myocardial infarction develop deep vein thrombosis.[58]

Etiology and Risk Factors

Thrombus formation is usually attributed to Virchow's triad:

1. Venous stasis

2. Hypercoagulability
3. Injury to the venous wall

At least two of the three preceding conditions must be present for thrombi to form.

Venous stasis is usually caused by immobilization or absence of the calf muscle pump. Other conditions that may cause stasis are surgery, immobility, obesity, pregnancy, paralysis, and congestive heart failure.

Hypercoagulability often accompanies malignant neoplasms (especially visceral and ovarian tumors). Dehydration and blood dyscrasias may raise the platelet count, decrease fibrinolysis, increase the clotting factors, or increase the viscosity of the blood. Oral contraceptives and hematologic disorders may also increase the coagulability of the blood.

Conditions that may cause vein wall trauma are intravenous injections, thromboangiitis obliterans (Buerger's disease), fractures and dislocations, chemical injury from sclerosing agents, contrast x-rays, and certain antibiotics (such as chlortetracycline). The resulting damage to the vein wall attracts platelets, and blood debris accumulates. This, in combination with low blood flow and a hypercoagulable state, results in thrombus formation.

Box 50–3 presents common clinical risk factors for venous thrombosis and pulmonary thromboembolism. In addition to those listed, varicose veins appear to be associated with the development of thrombosis.[18]

Immobile clients with deep vein thrombosis have a lower risk of developing pulmonary embolism than do clients who are ambulatory. Thus, the risk of pulmonary embolism is often underestimated after hospital discharge in clients who have "low-risk" surgery. Presumably, hospitalized clients are treated prophylactically with antiembolism stockings and anticoagulants. Clients discharged to their homes seldom receive this prophylaxis.

Prevention is geared toward promoting venous return, avoiding injury to the endothelial wall, and maintaining normal coagulability. Prevention methods generally used for the high-risk hospitalized client have included mechanical methods such as devices that elevate the foot of the bed, compression stockings, motorized foot movers, and intermittent calf muscle compressors. Pharmacologic

---

Box 50–3. Common Conditions Associated with Venous Thrombosis and Thromboembolism

Age >40 years
Surgery requiring more than 30 minutes of general, spinal, or epidural anesthesia
Venous stasis (bedrest, prolonged travel, stroke)
Previous deep vein thrombosis
Cardiac disease (heart failure, myocardial infarction, cardiomyopathy)
Pregnancy
Trauma, especially of the lower extremities
Estrogen therapy or oral contraceptives
Malignancy
Obesity

prevention has included warfarin, platelet antiaggregation agents (aspirin being the most common), heparin, and dextran.

Additional nursing measures for prevention of venous stasis include the following:

● Facilitating active and passive range-of-motion exercises for postoperative, postpartum, and immobilized clients
● Using intermittent sequential pneumatic compression (IPC) devices (Fig. 50–12). Use of these devices is initiated at the time of many operations and continued until the client is ambulatory. The leggings or boots are attached by polyethylene tubing to an electric pump attached to the foot of the bed. Air is pumped sequentially into three chambers (ankle, calf, and thigh) at a pressure of 45 to 60 mm Hg for 15 to 20 seconds. The compression is followed by deflation and a 45-second resting period. Research has shown that IPC is clinically effective in reducing the incidence of deep vein thrombosis. It is also a good alternative for clients who cannot tolerate any anticoagulation. These devices augment the leg muscle pumps to move blood from venous stores
● Encouraging early ambulation, especially for postoperative and postpartum clients
● Encouraging postoperative deep-breathing exercises to promote thoracic pumping action
● Avoiding use of pillows under the client's knees postoperatively to facilitate venous return
● Teaching the client to avoid sitting or standing in one position for prolonged periods

Nursing interventions for prevention of hypercoagulability include the following:

● Administering prophylactic, preoperative, low-dose heparin therapy for elderly clients with hip fractures, obese clients undergoing surgery, all clients undergoing major surgery, and clients on bedrest
● Teaching clients about risk of oral contraceptives
● Maintaining adequate hydration

Nursing interventions for preventing injury to the vein wall include the following:

● Avoiding infiltration during intravenous therapy

Pathophysiology

Thrombus development is a local process. It begins by platelet adherence to the endothelium. Several factors promote platelet aggregation, including thrombin, fibrin, activated factor X and catecholamines. In addition, where the platelets adhere to collagen, adenosine diphosphate (ADP) is released. ADP is also released from the damaged tissues and disrupted platelets. ADP produces platelet aggregation that results in a platelet plug.

Deep vein thrombi vary from 1 mm in diameter to long tubular masses filling main veins. Small thrombi are found commonly in the pocket of deep vein valves. As thrombi become larger in diameter and length, they obstruct the veins. The resulting inflammatory process can destroy the valves of the veins; thus, venous insufficiency and postphlebitic syndrome are initiated.

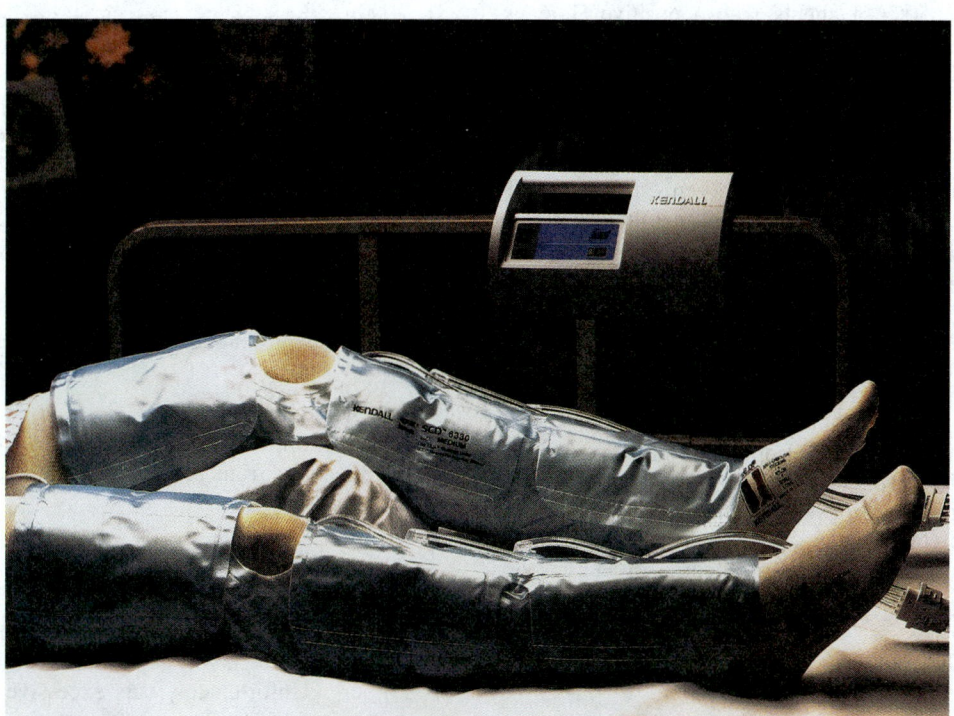

Figure 50–12. Pneumatic compression devices, such as the Kendall sequential compression device, are commonly used to prevent deep vein thrombosis in high-risk clients. (Courtesy of Kendall Company, Mansfield, MA.)

Newly formed thrombi may become pulmonary emboli. Probably 24 to 48 hours after formation, thrombi undergo lysis or become organized and adhere to the vessel wall. This diminishes the risk of embolization.

If a thrombus occludes a major vein (e.g., femoral, vena caval, axillary), the venous pressure and volume rise distally. Conversely, if a thrombus occludes a deep small vein (e.g., tibial, popliteal), collateral venous channels usually relieve the increased venous pressure and volume.

Pulmonary emboli, most of which start as thrombi in the large deep veins of the legs, are an acute and potentially lethal complication of deep vein thrombosis. Pulmonary embolism is discussed in Chapter 41.

Clinical Manifestations and Diagnostic Findings

The presence of superficial thrombophlebitis is easily ascertained by finding the inflamed vein. In contrast, the clinical manifestations of deep vein thrombosis are less distinctive; about half of clients are asymptomatic. The most common clinical manifestations are pain in the region of the thrombus and unilateral swelling distal to the site. Other clinical manifestations include redness or warmth of the leg, dilated veins, or low-grade fever. Unfortunately, the first clinical manifestation may be pulmonary embolism. Frequently, clients have thrombi in both legs even though the symptoms are unilateral.

Homans' sign—discomfort in the upper calf during forced dorsiflexion of the foot—is commonly assessed during physical examination. Unfortunately, it is insensitive and nonspecific. It is present in less than a third of clients with documented deep vein thrombosis. In addition, more than 50% of clients with a positive Homans' sign do not have venous thrombosis.

The Doppler ultrasonographic flowmeter determines blood flow in the larger blood vessels and the patency of vessels. Reliability of the test is directly related to the skill of the examiner; its accuracy is affected by inability to detect partially or totally occluded veins, inaccessibility of deep pelvic and thigh veins, and inability to distinguish collateral circulation from that in native veins.

Venous duplex scanning has become the primary diagnostic test of deep vein thrombosis because it allows visualization of the vein, which provides an extremely reliable diagnosis of venous thrombus.

Plethysmographic examination of the venous system entails the recording of volume changes in a limb during venous filling and emptying. Impedance plethysmography measures maximal venous filling capacity by applying a pneumatic cuff at thigh level and then recording the rate of venous emptying after cuff release. The rate of venous emptying correlates well with the degree of venous obstruction and is also a very good indicator of deep vein thrombosis.

Plethysmography may produce false-negative results if the following conditions are present:

1. The client cannot sustain deep inspiration long enough to cause pooling of blood in the deep veins
2. The client is unable to lie flat and laterally rotate the hip and bend the knee

3. The client has congestive heart failure
4. The client has peripheral arterial occlusion

The client must lie perfectly still during plethysmography because any movement can cause distortion and false readings. Venography can be performed to locate the thrombus, but its use is rare.

Acute and Subacute Care

■ Medical Management

Superficial thrombophlebitis can be managed with local measures, such as warm packs and elevation of the extremity. Sometimes anti-inflammatory medications are required.

Deep vein thrombosis is treated with bedrest, elevation of the leg, and anticoagulation. The client is closely assessed for pulmonary embolism. Five to seven days of bedrest allows the thrombus to adhere to the vein wall and decreases embolization. After 5 to 7 days, the client is usually allowed to ambulate wearing elastic stockings.

Anticoagulant therapy is based on the premise that the initiation or extension of thrombi can be prevented by inhibiting the synthesis of clotting factors or by accelerating their inactivation. The anticoagulants heparin and warfarin do not induce thrombolysis, but they effectively prevent clot extension.

Anticoagulation. Heparin is the drug of choice for the treatment of thromboembolic disease. Heparin prevents the activation of clotting factor IX and inhibits the action of thrombin in forming fibrin threads. An intravenous bolus of 5000 to 10,000 units followed by 750 to 1000 units/hour can be given via continuous intravenous infusion. Heparin's effect is measured by activated partial thromboplastin time. During treatment, activated partial thromboplastin may be monitored every 4 hours and the heparin infusion rate adjusted accordingly. Therapeutic activated partial thromboplastin values are usually 1.5 to 2.5 times normal control levels. Platelet counts should be done before beginning heparin and every 5 days after that time while the client is receiving medication.

Heparin is contraindicated in the following conditions:

Severe hypertension
Cerebrovascular hemorrhage
Active gastrointestinal ulceration
Overt bleeding from the gastrointestinal, genitourinary, or respiratory tract
Recent neurosurgery
Recent childbirth
Heparin allergy

The specific antidote to heparin is protamine sulfate. It neutralizes the effects of heparin immediately and lasts for 2 hours. Unfortunately, an excessive dose of protamine may actually prolong clotting.

Warfarin. Warfarin (Coumadin) inhibits hepatic synthesis of the vitamin K–dependent clotting factors. The effect of the warfarin is determined by measurement of the prothrombin time (PT). PT must be measured every day before warfarin is administered. Generally, a PT of 1.5 times the normal reading is desired. If INR is used to monitor, the therapeutic level is an INR of 2.0 to 3.0. The antidote for the warfarin derivatives is vitamin K (Mephyton). If bleeding occurs, the physician will discontinue the medication for a period.

The warfarin derivatives require 24 to 48 hours to take effect. Therefore, heparin, which is fast-acting, is used initially with warfarin and discontinued when the warfarin begins to take effect. Anticoagulation is usually continued about 3 months after an acute venous thrombosis and after pulmonary embolism.

Low Molecular Weight Heparin. Low molecular weight heparins are a new class of anticoagulants. They produce less bleeding than equivalent doses of the standard heparin. They are given once or twice daily and require no laboratory monitoring. These agents may easily replace standard heparin as the standard therapy.

Fibrinolytic Agents. Fibrinolytic medications (e.g., streptokinase and urokinase) dissolve thrombi by stimulating the conversion of plasminogen to plasmin, an enzyme that decomposes fibrin. (Fibrinolytic therapy is discussed earlier in the chapter.)

■ Nursing Management of the Medical Client

Goals of nursing management are to prevent existing thrombi from becoming emboli and to prevent new thrombi from forming. The following measures should be undertaken when caring for the client with deep vein thrombosis:

1. Protect the client from thromboemboli and bleeding caused by anticoagulant therapy
2. Teach the client about deep vein thrombosis and anticoagulation therapy
3. Provide analgesia
4. Assess for pulmonary embolism
5. Reduce anxiety

Promote Bedrest. Bedrest is indicated to prevent emboli. Bedrest also prevents pressure fluctuations in the venous system that occur with walking. Because clients with thrombi will be on bedrest for about 5 to 7 days, provide them with an orthopedic overbed frame and a trapeze, a pressure-reduction mattress, and heel protectors. Have a nightstand, over-the-bed table, call light, and telephone within easy reach. Stool softeners, coughing, and deep-breathing exercises are also recommended.

Elevate the Client's Legs. Elevation of the legs above the level of the heart facilitates blood flow by the force of gravity. The increase of blood flow prevents venous stasis and the formation of new thrombi. Eleva-

tion of the legs also decreases venous pressure, which in turn relieves edema and pain. Elevate the foot of the bed 6 inches (Trendelenburg's position), with a slight knee bend to prevent popliteal pressure. The veins of the legs should be level with the right atrium. The head of the bed may be raised to facilitate eating and bathing. Various forms of elastic support are used to promote venous return. Elastic bandages are advantageous for clients with large or misshapen legs. Apply elastic wraps snugly from toe to groin. Rewrap them every 4 to 8 hours. If compression stockings are prescribed, they must be fitted correctly and removed for a short time every day.

Relieve Discomfort. Bedrest, elevation of the extremity, and application of warm packs usually relieve discomfort. Some clients need a mild sedative or analgesic.

Monitor Anticoagulant Therapy. Intravenous heparin followed by oral anticoagulation medication is used to decrease the risk of new thrombi. Assess for effectiveness by monitoring the activated partial thromboplastin time and PT. Also, monitor for the following:

Manifestations of excess anticoagulation
Bleeding, evidenced by blood in the urine, stool, and along the gums or teeth
Subcutaneous bruising
Flank pain

When invasive studies are necessary (e.g., arterial blood gas analyses), apply pressure for 30 minutes to the puncture site.

Monitor the Client for Development of Pulmonary Embolism. Pulmonary embolism is an acute and potentially lethal complication of deep vein thrombosis. Chest pain is the most common clinical manifestation of pulmonary embolism, but it is not diagnostic of the condition. The pain most often associated with pulmonary embolism is pleuritic. Pleuritic pain is caused by an inflammatory reaction of the lung parenchyma or by pulmonary infarction or ischemia caused by obstruction of small pulmonary arterial branches. Pleuritic chest pain is typically sudden in onset and is aggravated by breathing.

Hemoptysis occurs in about 30% of clients. The presence of hemoptysis indicates that pulmonary infarction or atelectasis has produced alveolar hemorrhage. Other clinical manifestations may include cough, diaphoresis, dyspnea, and apprehension. Because of the seriousness of pulmonary embolism, promptly notify the physician of these clinical manifestations. Pulmonary embolism is fully discussed in Chapter 41.

■ Surgical Management

Surgical measures for deep vein thrombosis fall into two categories: (1) intervention for the thrombus itself and (2) surgical prophylaxis against pulmonary embolism involving ligation or interruption of the inferior vena cava with a filter or an "umbrella."

Venous Thrombectomy

The direct removal of venous thrombi was previously recommended. Now it is rarely performed because of the high incidence of recurrent postoperative thrombosis.

Umbrella Procedure

During this procedure, a filter on an umbrella is inserted in the vena cava to trap large emboli. Some types of umbrellas can be inserted under local anesthesia by threading the device through the femoral or jugular vein. A rare complication of this technique is the migration of the filter into the iliac vein, renal vein, right atrium, right ventricle, or pulmonary artery. Such migrations may be fatal.

Community and Self-Care

When teaching clients about deep vein thrombosis, first assess their learning abilities. Many clients with thrombophlebitis are older and may suffer from sensory loss or limited mobility. Begin teaching on the first day of heparinization, discussing reasons for anticoagulants and bedrest. Also inform the client about the complications of therapy and emphasize manifestations to report. Prevention is the key to deep vein thrombosis. Therefore, teach risk factors of deep vein thrombosis and how to avoid them. Continue teaching with explanations of medications being taken, actions, doses, timing, adverse effects, and importance of monitoring coagulation status. Clients need to know who to contact and how to reach a healthcare practitioner in the event that problems develop.

Chronic Venous Insufficiency

Chronic venous insufficiency is marked by the following characteristics:

1. Chronically swollen limbs
2. Thick, coarse, brownish skin around the ankles (referred to as the "gaiter" area)
3. Venous stasis ulceration

Chronic venous insufficiency, also known as *postphlebitic syndrome*, follows most severe cases of deep vein thrombosis but may take as long as 5 to 10 years to manifest. However, about 20% of clients with chronic venous insufficiency have no history of deep vein thrombosis. Within 5 years of a known deep vein thrombosis, almost 50% of clients develop chronic induration and stasis dermatitis, and 20% suffer from venous stasis ulcer. Therefore, clients with a history of deep vein thrombosis must be monitored periodically for life. Alert them to observe for the slightest skin changes. Once the skin is broken and a venous ulcer develops, the client faces a frustrating chronic problem. Venous stasis ulcers do not heal well.

Chronic venous insufficiency results from dysfunctional valves that reduce venous return, which thus increases venous pressure and causes venous stasis. Skin ulcerations also occur. Because existing valves are destroyed, venous blood flow is bidirectional, resulting in inefficient venous outflow. The net effect of this change is that the weight of the venous blood column from the right atrium is transmitted along the full length of the veins. Very high venous pressure is exerted at the ankle and the venules become the final pathway for the highest venous pressure.

Important management goals are to increase venous blood return and to decrease venous pressure. Antigravity measures increase blood return to the heart. They include elevating the clients legs above the heart level and avoiding prolonged standing or sitting. Advise the client to avoid the following:

1. Crossing the legs
2. Sitting in chairs that are too high to allow the feet to touch the floor or that are too deep (and press on the popliteal area)
3. Wearing garters
4. Sources of pressure above the legs (e.g., tight girdles)

Encourage the client to sleep with the foot of the bed elevated 6 inches. At least one third of every 24 hours should be spent with the feet and legs elevated above the heart.

The Bridge to Home Healthcare feature describes how increased venous pressure on the tissues of the leg can be counteracted by the compression of elastic support hose. Ideally, this support should just balance the increased venous pressure. Thus, hose should be fitted individually to the client's legs. Measurements of the ankle and calf circumference and from 1 inch below the knee or 1 inch below the groin to the bottom of the foot are usually taken. Measure after the client has been recumbent and leg edema is minimal. Stockings that extend above the knee often bind the popliteal space and act as a tourniquet, especially when the knee is bent. Knee-length elastic stockings are preferable. Elastic wraps are often preferable for clients who have periods of leg swelling. Wrap the stocking using a graded technique, placing more tension on the lower leg.

After thrombosis of a deep calf vein, clients should wear elastic support for at least 6 to 8 weeks and probably for life. Elastic support compresses the superficial veins when the client walks, and blood flow in the larger veins is increased while venous pressure is kept to a minimum. Standing and sitting are not allowed during the acute phase because they increase the hydrostatic pressure in the capillaries, which promotes edema. Once the threat of embolization is over, encourage walking and exercises in bed to decrease venous pressure and to promote blood flow. Also recommend that the client who is on bedrest dorsiflex the feet against a footboard for exercise. Sometimes intermittent pneumatic compression devices are ordered to aid blood flow. Use of these leggings is usually discontinued when the client starts walking.

Venous Stasis Ulceration

Venous stasis ulceration is the end stage of chronic venous insufficiency. Over a period of years, the ex-

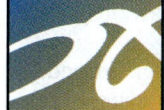

BRIDGE TO HOME HEALTHCARE

Managing Peripheral Vascular Disease

Jodi Cotton, R.N., B.S.N., *Maximus, Omaha Office, Omaha, Nebraska*

Preventing further complications is a priority when you are working with a home care client who has peripheral vascular disease. Specifically, the client needs to learn how to prevent edema and to avoid trauma. Properly fitted antiembolic hose, Jobst stockings, or elastic wraps (Ace wraps) can reduce edema in the lower extremities. The measurements required for antiembolic hose are the ankle, calf, thigh, and length from heel to thigh. Use a regular tape measure and report the measurement to the supply company or pharmacy to obtain the correct size. Jobst stockings are specially fitted; the client needs to be measured by the company that supplies the stockings. When choosing the type of treatment intended to reduce edema, consider the cost, the client's ability to apply or use the treatment independently, and the client's likelihood of using the treatment as prescribed. Sometimes elastic wraps do not stay up and may be removed too easily by the client, but they conform well to the leg and provide gradient support when applied correctly. Elastic wraps are also inexpensive.

Assess the client's lower extremities during each home visit to evaluate the condition and to observe for signs of stasis ulcers. Assess for the following:

Pain in the extremities
Color changes of the skin or nails
Impaired growth of the nails
Shiny, taut skin
Discrepancy in the size of one extremity
Enlarged veins
Temperature variations
Ulcerations

Measure the lower extremities on each home visit. You must report pertinent and unusual assessment information to the physician quickly.

When you detect a stasis ulcer—no matter how small it is—begin treatment. Treatment may include an Unna boot, damp-to-dry dressings, occlusive dressings, foam, Duoderm, and Duoderm compression wraps. Clean an open and draining wound with saline and dry it well; then apply an appropriate dressing. Some physicians have a preferred dressing procedure. If the physician does not have a preference, consult your agency's wound specialist, enterostomal therapist, or a local supply company's nurse. If a managed care company is responsible for the client's bills, the case manager will request the most cost-effective treatment with the fewest visits.

The frequency of home visits for changing the dressing depends on the amount of drainage and the treatment selected. Duoderm compression dressings are expensive but heal a wound quickly by keeping edema to a minimum. A damp-to-dry dressing with saline can be used for a smaller wound if edema is not a problem. Usually, stasis ulcers are not debrided because of poor circulation and tissue loss. However, new ointments, such as Santyl, can produce debridement in 3 to 7 days.

Teaching is an essential nursing intervention. Teach the client to call you about specific clinical manifestations. Involve the client and family members in client care and teach them how to change dressings when possible; this will be a goal of managed care companies. Remember, prevention is the key for a client with peripheral vascular disease. Instruct the client about preventive measures such as:

Limiting or stopping smoking
Elevating the legs
Avoiding constrictive clothing
Avoiding standing in one place for long periods of time
Avoiding excessive heat to the extremities (by a hot water bottle or heating pad)
and maintaining daily hygiene and proper foot care

Health education is important for preventing further complications of peripheral vascular disease, which does not have a cure.

---

cess venous pressure causes small skin veins and venules to rupture, which creates stasis ulcers. Subcutaneous fibrosis, cutaneous atrophy, and lymphatic obstruction contribute to the development of stasis ulcers, characteristically located in the malleolar area. Once the skin is broken, infection occurs, usually caused by either *Staphylococcus* or *Streptococcus* bacterial species.

Management of venous stasis ulceration includes leg elevation, wound care, moist dressings, and support stockings. Gravity is the major enemy of venous stasis disease.

The client should rest with his or her legs elevated 6 inches. Supply stool softeners and encourage the client to do deep-breathing exercises.

When ulcers are present, cultures should be taken. Antibiotics may be required to treat infection or cellulitis. Local wound care begins. Some ulcers require debridement of eschar, whereas others require protection.

Debridement techniques include the following:

- Application of wet-to-dry dressings with saline (use coarse mesh gauze with no cotton filler)
- Whirlpool therapy once a day with saline
- Use of enzymatic debriding agents such as collagenase or Elase
- Surgery

Hydrocolloid dressings are used to protect epithelialization. Protect granulation tissue with wet-to-wet saline dressings, Vaseline gauze, or moist occlusive dressings. Almost all ointments, creams, powders, and local antibiotics are harmful to ulcers. They contribute to skin sensitivity problems, which complicate healing. To clean the ulcer, use sterile normal saline. The surrounding skin is probably dry and scaly. Gently clean the area and apply Alpha Keri Oil or a lanolin-containing lotion, such as Eucerin, every day. Avoid lotions containing alcohol and perfumes because they dry and irritate the skin. Solutions such as povidone-iodine (Betadine) can be used to control infection, but any solution other than normal saline retards healing. (Wound care is discussed in Chapter 20.)

An Unna boot is a popular form of bandage impregnated with calamine, zinc oxide, and glycerin. When wrapped snugly around the leg, it provides excellent compression during ambulation and applies minimal pressure during limb elevation. An Unna boot is a permeable dressing that can be applied directly over skin ulcers, thereby allowing drainage of exudate. It creates a moist and warm interface between the ulcerated skin and the bandage. It can be changed on a weekly or biweekly basis, which forces the client to wear it without interruption and thereby improves compliance. Disadvantages of the Unna boot include allergy, skin irritation, discomfort, difficulty in bathing, and pain while changing the boot. The Unna boot has been shown to achieve healing rates of 70%.

If arterial supply to the client's leg is adequate, wrap the lower leg, starting just behind the toes, to just below the popliteal space. Wrap tightly at the ankle with a gradual lessening of pressure toward the knee. Teach the client to rewrap the legs twice daily.

Skin grafting may be necessary to achieve healing. Surgery to remove incompetent, varicose veins or to improve perfusion may also be necessary.

Varicose Veins

Varicose veins are a common complaint of clients with venous insufficiency. The loss of valvular competence and the constant elevation of venous pressure cause distention and tortuosity of the superficial veins. The greater and lesser saphenous veins and perforator veins in the ankle are common sites of varicosities.

Varicose veins may be either primary or secondary. Primary varicose veins often result from a congenital or familial predisposition that leads to loss of elasticity of the vein wall. Secondary varicosities occur when trauma, obstruction, deep vein thrombosis, or inflammation causes damage to valves.

Varicose veins are a prevalent problem that continues to rise in incidence and affects a large percentage of the adult population. An estimated 24 million Americans have varicose veins. The prevalence increases with age and peaks between the fifth and sixth decades of life. Varicose veins are more common in women; however, the sex ratio decreases with advancing age and almost disappears in clients older than 70 years. Prolonged standing has been implicated as a cause of varicose veins, but epidemiologic studies have not demonstrated an association between standing at work and an increased incidence of varicose veins.

Clients with varicose veins often complain of aching, a feeling of heaviness, itching, moderate swelling, and, frequently, the unsightly appearance of their legs. Severity of discomfort is difficult to assess and does not seem related to the size of varicosities. A superficial inflammation may develop along the path of the varicose vein and may be associated with complaints of fever and malaise.

To assess for varicose veins, carefully examine both of the client's legs in good lighting. Varicosities appear as dilated, tortuous skin veins (Fig. 50–13). Check for patency with a Doppler flowmeter.

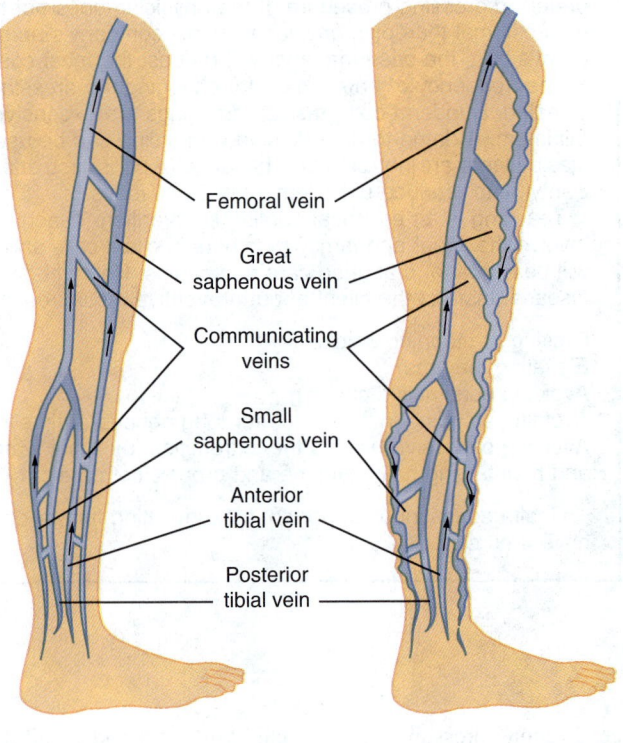

A   B

Figure 50–13. Venous return from the legs. *A,* Normal flow. *B,* Varicosities and retrograde venous flow.

Incompetency of the deep and superficial veins can be diagnosed by the following measures and tests:

1. Noting venous pressure changes during walking
2. Trendelenburg's test
3. Phlebography,
4. Doppler flowmetry
5. Plethysmography

These are discussed in Chapter 49.

■ Medical Management

In early stages of varicose veins, the goal is to reduce venous pooling, prevent complications, and improve appearance. The simplest form of treatment is the application of below-the-knee compression stockings. These stockings are designed to apply the greatest amount of pressure over the ankle. The client should be taught to avoid standing still in one position for extended periods of time. For example, a clerk in a grocery store should shift weight, flex the knees, and walk for short distances often. Clients should also avoid wearing constricting garments, elevate the legs, and walk for exercise.

■ Surgical Management

Sclerotherapy is the injection of a sclerosing agent into varicose veins. The agent damages the vein and endothelium, causing an aseptic thrombosis that closes the vein. Sclerotherapy is palliative, not curative, and is usually performed for cosmetic reasons. It is most effective in closing small, residual varicosities after surgical intervention for varicose veins. (Sclerotherapy is contraindicated before such surgery, because it makes vein stripping more difficult.) Within minutes after injection of the sclerosing agent, elastic compression and active walking should commence. Elastic bandages are worn for about 6 weeks.

Surgical management of varicose veins consists of ligation (tying off) of the greater saphenous vein with its tributaries at the saphenofemoral junction, combined with saphenous vein stripping and ligation of incompetent perforator veins. Removal of the vein is performed through multiple, short incisions. An incision is made at the ankle over the saphenous vein and a nylon wire is threaded up the vein to the groin. The wire is brought out through the groin, capped, and then the wire and vein are pulled out through the ankle incision.

Elastic compression bandages are applied from foot to groin. The client is usually hospitalized overnight. Complications are rare. They include the usual surgical complications, bleeding, infection, and nerve damage. Hemorrhage most commonly occurs at the surgical wound site in the groin. Bleeding comes primarily from the stripped canal. The risk of serious bleeding can be decreased by carefully wrapping the leg from foot to groin and by applying compression, especially to the upper thigh and groin. Some discoloration and bruising along the stripped tract are normal. One week after stripping, the client's leg looks ecchymotic.

Saphenous nerve damage may occur with surgery. In the distal third of the leg, the saphenous nerve runs close to the saphenous vein. Thus, risk of nerve injury increases when the distal part of the vein is involved.

Deep vein thrombosis, embolism, and infection are rare following varicose vein surgery, especially if postoperative precautions (e.g., bandaging, movement, exercise) are taken.

■ Nursing Management of the Surgical Client

Three important postoperative nursing objectives are as follows:

1. To maintain firm elastic pressure over the whole limb
2. To promote regular movement and exercise of the legs
3. To elevate the foot of the bed 6 to 9 inches so that the legs are above the heart level when the client is in bed

The client ambulates for short periods, starting 24 to 48 hours after surgery. Instruct clients to walk rather than to stand or sit. After ambulation, elevate the client's legs again.

Also assess for complications after varicose vein surgery. The major problems are hemorrhage, infection, nerve damage, and deep vein thrombosis.

Lymphatic Disorders

Lymphedema

Lymphedema is swelling caused by impaired transcapillary fluid transport and transportation of lymph. Failure of lymph transport allows the plasma proteins in the interstitial fluid to accumulate. The increase in fluids increases interstitial colloid osmotic pressure. The osmotic pressure is reduced by drawing water into interstitial areas. In addition, as the lymph channels dilate, valves become incompetent. The fluid seeks new pathways through the tissues, which causes inflammation, lymphatic thrombosis, and, eventually, fibrosis. Lymphedemas are best classified into primary and secondary forms.

Etiology and Risk Factors

■ Primary Lymphedema

Primary lymphedema may be classified according to age at onset: congenital (present at birth), praecox (before age 35), or tarda (after age 35). Congenital and familial lymphedema is also called Milroy's disease. It is inherited as an autosomal dominant trait.

Of the primary forms, lymphedema praecox encompasses the largest group of clients; it peaks in the teenage years and is more common in females than in males. The edema usually appears spontaneously and without known cause (Fig. 50–14).

■ Secondary Lymphedema

Secondary lymphedema occurs because of some damage or obstruction to the lymph system by another disease

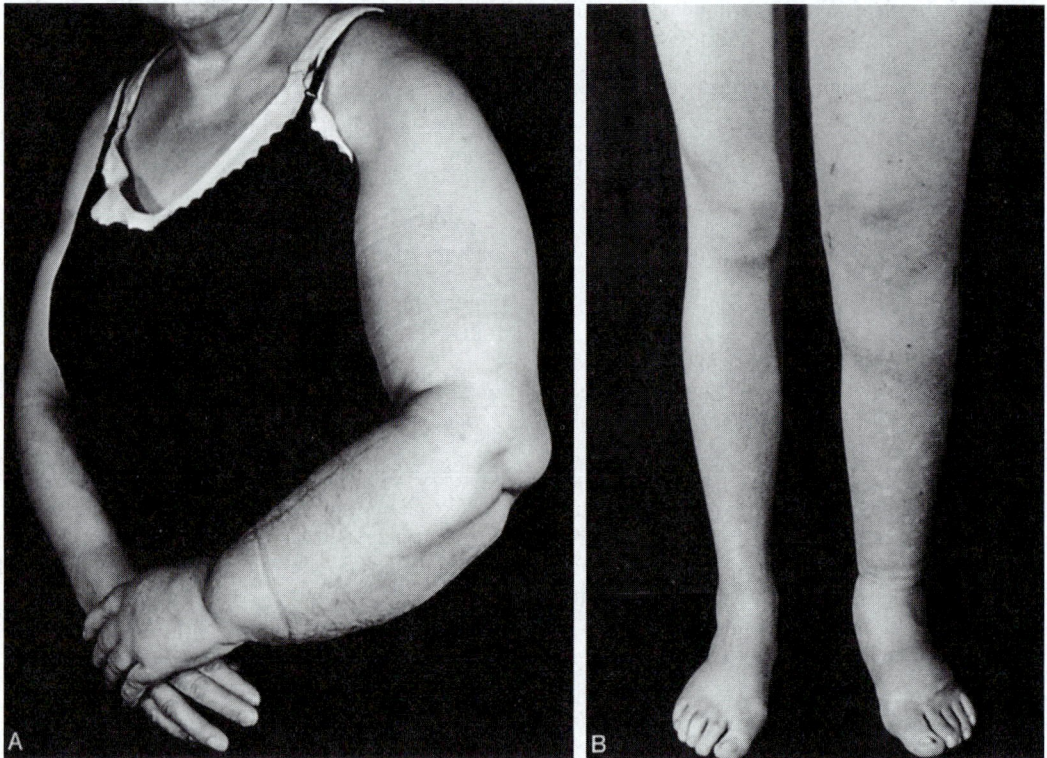

Figure 50–14. Types of lymphedema. *A*, Secondary lymphedema of the arm following mastectomy. *B*, Primary lymphedema.

process or by a procedure: trauma, neoplasms (primary or metastatic), filariasis, inflammation, surgical excision, or high doses of radiation.

Postsurgical lymphedema is usually seen after surgical excision of axillary, inguinal, or iliac nodes, usually performed as a prophylactic or therapeutic measure for metastatic tumor. For example, lymphedema of the arm is encountered after mastectomy (see Fig. 50–14).

Filariasis, caused by the filarial nematode *Wuchereria bancrofti* (and others), is one of the most common diseases in undeveloped nations; it is transmitted by mosquitoes from human to human. The living embryos (microfilariae) of the adult worms are found in the bloodstream. The larvae migrate to the lymphatics, where they mature into adult worms. Adult worms in the lymph nodes and lymphatics lead to obstruction, lymphedema, and elephantiasis. Most clients have intermittent attacks of high fever, chills, malaise, fatigue, tender regional lymphadenopathy, severe muscle pain, and areas of erythema with increased edema. For clients with advanced disease, little can be offered in terms of cure.

Lymphedema secondary to neoplasms in the lymph nodes is common. The malignant disease may be primary (lymphoma or Hodgkin's disease) or metastatic from another site.

Chronic lymphedema secondary to inflammation is relatively uncommon, probably as a result of early control with antibiotics. Chronic lymphedema because of recurrent lymphangitis and cellulitis is caused by bacterial organisms.

Radiation in moderate amounts does not appear to damage the lymph vessels. However, heavy radiation for a particularly resistant tumor usually leads to lymphatic obstruction.

Clinical Manifestations and Diagnostic Findings

Presentation of primary lymphedema is as follows:

1. Bilateral mild edema of ankles and legs in women at puberty or shortly after
2. Unilateral edema of the entire leg in men and women (see Fig. 50–14)
3. Bilateral edema present at birth or early age

The skin of clients with congenital lymphedema contains vesicles (blisters) filled with lymph.

A dull, heavy sensation is present, but actual pain is absent. Elevation of the limb and rest in bed cause a reduction but not disappearance of the sensation. Smooth skin becomes roughened; the edema is nonpitting. Acute lymphangitis and cellulitis are infrequent. Ulceration of the skin does not occur. However, the limb becomes greatly enlarged, uncomfortable, and unsightly.

Lymphedema can be diagnosed with isotopic lymphography, lymphangiography, and phlebography.

Management

There is no known cure for lymphedema once the swelling appears. The goal of treatment is to remove as much fluid as possible from the affected extremity and to maintain as normal-appearing an extremity as possible.

Physical therapy for arm or leg lymphedema involves mechanical or manual squeezing of the tissue in order to press the stagnant lymphatic fluid to the proximal part of the limb. This is followed by specific active and passive exercises to transport the lymph farther into the lymphatic system and finally into the bloodstream. Many pneumatic pumping devices for intermittent compression are available. Diuretics may also be prescribed. Elastic stockings are used to maintain the effects of the pneumatic pump.

To reduce the swelling, the extremity is elevated above the right atrium. Pneumatic pumps may be used to reduce the extremity size. If pumps are used, teach the client how to apply the device, the frequency of application, and the reasons for its use. When stockings are used, ascertain that the stockings fit and do not gather behind the knee. Activity such as walking, rather than sitting or standing, should be promoted. For bedridden clients, teach bed exercises to promote venous and lymphatic return and to maintain muscle strength.

The client with lymphedema is at high risk for infection. Therefore, monitor the affected extremity for clinical manifestations of infection such as redness, warmth, pain, and fever. Meticulous skin care is given to the extremity using mild soaps and lotions. Nails are kept trimmed.

Clients with lymphedema may suffer from disturbances in self-concept because of the visibility of their deformity. Encourage the client to discuss these feelings and help the client understand that such feelings are normal. Variations in clothing style may be suggested to disguise the deformity.

Finally, when caring for clients with lymph disorders, remember that these clients must cope with difficult, chronic diseases. Take time to give emotional support to the client and the family. Emphasize the possible need for lifelong follow-up.

When lymphedematous limbs are massively swollen to the point that compression devices or stockings are no longer beneficial, surgery may be required. The most common surgical procedure for lymphedema is excisional, in which all skin, subcutaneous tissue, and deep fascia in the leg are removed. The leg is covered with skin grafts. Scarring is evident, and the cosmetic appearance may not be acceptable to all clients. Another form of surgery is the removal of the bulk of edematous tissues. This form of surgery is not curative, but the final appearance may be more acceptable.

Lymphadenitis

Lymph nodes act as defense barriers and are secondarily involved in virtually all systemic infections and in many neoplastic disorders arising elsewhere in the body. Generalized lymphadenopathy (enlargement of two or three regionally separated lymph node groups) is usually the result of inflammation, neoplasm, or immunologic reactions.

The infections that lead to lymphadenitis are so numerous and varied that a detailed description would involve a list of all systemic microbiologic diseases. The specific node or nodes affected in an infectious disease depend on the location of the infection, the nature of the invading organism, and the severity of the disease. Lymphadenitis can be classified nonspecifically as either acute or chronic.

Acute Lymphadenitis

Acute lymphadenitis usually follows one of two pathologic patterns: (1) suppuration in lymph nodes that drain infections, caused by pyogenic organisms, or (2) reticuloendothelial hyperplasia, edema, and leukocyte infiltration of the nodes caused by nonpyogenic organisms, such as spirochetes, rickettsiae, and viruses.

Acutely inflamed lymph nodes are most common locally in the cervical region in association with infections of the teeth or tonsils or in the axillary or inguinal regions secondary to infections of the extremities. Generalized lymphadenopathy is characteristic of the secondary stage of syphilis, viral infections, and bacteremia. Clinically, in acute lymphadenitis, the lymph nodes are enlarged, tender, warm, and reddened.

Chronic Lymphadenitis

In the course of long-standing infection, the lymph nodes frequently become scarred with fibrous replacement connective tissue. Clinically, these nodes are enlarged, firm to palpation, and not tender or warm. The management of lymphadenitis is treatment of the underlying disorder.

Conclusions

Clients with vascular diseases can challenge a broad range of the nurse's capability and skill, from monitoring a client with malignant hypertension in an intensive care unit, to performing and teaching meticulous foot care, to educating and counseling a client to make significant lifestyle changes. Vascular diseases involve a broad spectrum of arterial, venous, and lymphatic problems. Nursing care for clients with arterial disorders centers on promoting circulation and adequate tissue perfusion, protecting against skin breakdown and injury, managing pain, and encouraging positive life-style changes. Nursing care for clients with venous disorders focuses on monitoring therapeutic regimens such as thrombolytic therapy, controlling and preventing thrombus formation, and promoting circulation by increasing venous blood return and decreasing venous pressure. Nursing care for clients with infectious lymphatic processes targets the primary infection; nursing care for lymphedema is palliative. Limb amputation requires particularly sensitive assessment, teaching, and counseling skills. The unique nursing care needs of clients with vascular disorders along with the exploding knowledge base that nurses need to command has led to the growth of vascular nursing as a recognized area of specialty practice. The Society for Peripheral Vascular Nursing was founded in 1982.

Thinking Critically

1. **A 50-year-old man in the hypertension clinics was diagnosed with hypertension 1 month ago; a regimen of antihypertensive medication was started. He returns to the clinic today for a follow-up visit. His blood pressure is higher than it was initially. What could explain his continued elevated blood pressure?**

Factors to Consider. What conditions affect compliance? What diseases worsen hypertension?

2. **The client is admitted to the hospital for the care of leg ulcers. He is homeless and usually wanders the streets, sleeping on external heating grates in the sidewalk. He has large, irregularly shaped ulcers covered with thick, yellow, devitalized tissue. The ulcers are weeping and his stockings have adhered to the ulcers. What type of ulcers are present? What type of wound care will he need? How can he continue to do wound care after discharge?**

Factors to Consider. How are arterial and venous ulcers distinguished? Is it important to remove the devitalized tissue? If so, how? How does his life-style influence his recovery?

Bibliography

1. Anderson, K. (1992). Thrombolytic therapy for treatment of acute peripheral arterial occlusion. *Journal of Vascular Nursing, 10*(3), 20–24.
2. Baker, J. D. (1991). Assessment of peripheral arterial occlusive disease. *Critical Care Nursing Clinics of North America, 3*(3), 493–498.
3. Barnes, R. W. (1991). Noninvasive diagnostic assessment of peripheral vascular disease. *Circulation, 83*(suppl. I). I-20–I-27.
4. Bloomfield, R., et al. (1993). Hypertension: Practical recommendations for evaluation and nonpharmacologic intervention. *Consultant, 33*(3), 47–60.
5. Braunwald, E. (1992). *Heart disease: A textbook of cardiovascular medicine* (4th ed.). Philadelphia: W. B. Saunders.
6. Bright, L. D., & Georgi, S. (1992). Peripheral vascular disease: Is it arterial or venous? *AJN, 92*(9), 34–43.
7. Bright, L. D., & Georgi, S. (1994). How to protect your patient from DVT. *AJN, 94*(12), 28–32.
8. Bunt, T. J. (1995). Revascularization versus amputation for elderly patients. *AORN Journal, 62*, 433–435.
9. Butler, L, & Fahey, V. (1993). Acute arterial occlusion of the lower extremity. *Journal of Vascular Nursing, 11*(1), 19–22.
10. Cahall, E., & Spence, R. (1994). Nursing management of venour ulceration. *Journal of Vascular Nursing, 12*(2), 48–56.
11. Cameron, J. (1994). Venous leg ulcers. *Nursing Standard, 8*(22), 31–36.
12. Cameron, J. (1994). Arterial leg ulcers. *Nursing Standard, 8*(24), 31–36.
13. Carroll, P. (1993). Deep venous thrombosis: Implications for orthopaedic nursing. *Orthopaedic Nursing, 12*(3), 33–42.
14. Coen, S. D, & Silverman, E. (1994). Peripheral intra-arterial thrombolytic therapy for acute arterial occlusion. *Critical Care Nurse, 14*(5), 23–29.
15. Collins, J. W. (1991). The treatment of mild to moderate hypertension in patients with diabetes mellitus. *Nurse Practitioner, 16*(6), 28–40.

16. Cookingham, A. (1995). Peripheral vascular disease: Educational concerns for patients with a chronic disease in a changing health-care environment. *AACN Clinical Issues, 6*, 670–676.
17. Cottrell-Ikerd, V. (1994). The Syme's amputation: A correlation of surgical technique and prosthetic management with an historical perspective. *The Journal of Foot and Ankle Surgery, 33*(4), 355–364.
18. Copstead, L. C. (1995). *Perspectives on pathophysiology.* Philadelphia: W. B. Saunders.
19. Crosby, F., et al. (1993). Well-being and concerns of patients with peripheral arterial occlusive disease. *Journal of Vascular Nursing, 11*(1), 5–11.
20. Davis, E., (1993). The diagnostic puzzle and management challenge of Raynaud's syndrome. *Nurse Practitioner, 18*(3), 18–25.
21. Devine, C. E., & Reifschneider, E. (1995). A meta-analysis of the effects of psychoeducational care in adults with hypertension. *Nursing Research. 44*, 237–245.
22. Dowdell, H. R. (1995). Diabetes and vascular disease: A common association. *AACN Clinical Issues, 6*, 526–535.
23. Elizaga, A. M., et al. (1994). Continuous regional analgesia by intraneural block: Effect on postoperative opioid requirements and phantom limb pain following amputation. *Journal of Rehabilitation Research and Development, 31*(3), 179–187.
24. Epstein, M. (1995). Calcium antagonists should continue to be used for first-line treatment of hypertension. *Archives of Internal Medicine, 155*, 2150–2156.
25. Eton, D., & Ahn, S. S. (1991). Trends in endovascular surgery. *Critical Care Clinics of North America, 3*(3), 535–547.
26. Fagan, T. C. (1995). Calcium antagonists and mortality: Another case of the need for clinical judgment. *Archives of Internal Medicine, 155*, 2145.
27. Fahey, V. A., (1994). *Vascular nursing* (2nd ed). Philadelphia: W. B. Saunders.
28. Fatourechi, V., et al. (1996). A practical guideline for management of hypertension in patients with diabetes. *Mayo Clinic Proceedings, 71*, 53–58.
29. Fleg, J. L., et al. (1992). Hypertension therapy: The first steps. *Patient Care, 26*(9), 161–180.
30. Fowler, S. F., & Murray, K. M. (1995). Torsemide: A new loop diuretic. *American Journal of Health-System Pharmacists, 52*, 1771–1780.
31. Furberg, C. D. (1995). Should dihydropyridines be used as first-line drugs in the treatment of hypertension: The con side. *Archives of Internal Medicine, 155*, 2157–2161.
32. Fuster, V., & Verstraete, M. (1992). *Thrombosis in cardiovascular disorders.* Philadelphia: W. B. Saunders.
33. Graor, R. A. (1991). Deep vein thrombosis. In J. R. Young, et al. (Eds.), *Peripheral vascular disease* (pp. 403–422). St. Louis: Mosby–Year Book.
34. Gullickson, C. (1993). Client-centered drug choice: An alternative approach in managing hypertension. *Nurse Practitioner, 18*(2), 30–41.
35. Hatswell, E. M. (1994). Abdominal aortic aneurysm surgery, Part I: An overview and discussion of immediate perioperative complications. *Heart and Lung, 23*(3), 228–240.
36. Hatswell, E. M. (1994). Abdominal aortic aneurysm surgery, Part II: Major complications and nursing implications. *Heart and Lung, 23*(4), 337–343.
37. Heafy, M. L., et al. (1994). Using nursing diagnoses and interventions in an inpatient amputee program. *Rehabilitation Nursing, 19*(3), 163–168.
38. Hildreth, C. (1992). Hypertension in blacks: Disease characteristics and unique needs. *Consultant, 32*(2), 109–115.
39. Huber, C., et al. (1992). Postoperative pulmonary embolism after hospital discharge. *Archives of Surgery, 127*(3), 310–313.
40. Jarvis, C. (1996). *Physical examination and health assessment* (2nd ed.). Philadelphia: W. B. Saunders.
41. Johannsen, J. M. (1993). Update: Guidelines for treating hypertension. *AJN, 93*(3), 42–53.
42. Joint National Committee. (1993). The fifth report of the Joint National Committee on Detection, Evaluation, and Treatment of High Blood Pressure. *Archives of Internal Medicine, 153*, 154–183.
43. Kaplan, N. (1991). Long term effectiveness of non-pharmacological treatment of hypertension. *Hypertension, 18*(3), I-153–I-160.
44. Karch, A. M. (1995). Pain, pills, and possibilities: Drug therapy in peripheral vascular disease. *AACN Clinical Issues, 6*, 614–630.

45. Keller, C., Fleury, J., & Bergstrom, D. L. (1995). Risk factors for coronary heart disease in African-American women. *Cardiovascular Nursing, 31*(2), 9–14.

46. Laino, C. (1993). The TOMHS trial. *Medical World News, 34*(9), 32–35.

47. Lamont, L. J. (1994). Venous ulcers: A nursing challenge. *Journal of the American Academy of Nurse Practitioners, 3*(4), 158–165.

48. Lehne, R. A., et al. (1994). *Pharmacology for nursing care* (2nd ed.). Philadelphia: W. B. Saunders.

49. Lever, A. F., & Ramsay, L. E. (1995). Treatment of hypertension in the elderly. *Current Science, 13,* 571–579.

50. Levinson, P. D. (1994). Insulin resistance and hypertension. *Consultant, 34*(2), 254–263.

51. Lovell, M. B., et al. (1994). Peripheral aneurysms. *Journal of Vascular Nursing, 12*(2), 44–47.

52. Lovel, M. B., et al. (1993). The management of chronic venous disease. *Journal of Vascular Nursing, 11*(2), 43–47.

53. Mahan, L. K., & Arlin, M. (1996). *Krause's food, nutrition and diet therapy* (9th ed.). Philadelphia: W. B. Saunders.

54. Markel, A., et al. (1992). Pattern and distribution of thrombi in acute venous thrombosis. *Archives of Surgery, 127*(3), 305–309.

55. Massie, B. M. (1994). First line therapy for hypertension: Different patients, different needs. *Geriatrics, 49*(4), 22–30.

56. McCuistion, L. E. (1994). Treatment algorithm for hypertension. *Medsurg Nursing, 3,* 487–490.

57. McCulloch, J. M., et al. (1994). Intermittent pneumatic compression improves venous ulcer healing. *Advances in Wound Care, 7*(4), 22–26.

58. Monreal, M., et al. (1992). Deep venous thrombosis and the risk of pulmonary embolism. *Chest, 102*(3), 677–681.

59. Murphy, C. (1995). Hypertensive emergencies. *Emergency Medicine Clinics of North America, 13,* 973–1007.

60. Nash, C. A. & Jensen, P. L. (1994). When your surgical patient has hypertension. *AJN, 94*(11), 39–45.

61. National High Blood Pressure Education Program Working Group. (1993). National High Blood Pressure Education Program Working Group report on primary prevention of hypertension. *Archives of Internal Medicine, 153,* 186–208.

62. Neaton, J. D., et al. (1993). Treatment of mild hypertension study. *JAMA, 270*(6), 713–724.

63. Notowitz, L. B. (1993). Normal venous anatomy and physiology of the lower extremity. *Journal of Vascular Nursing, 11*(2), 39–42.

64. Patterson, J. W. (1994). Banishing phantom pain. *Nursing 94, 24*(9), 64.

65. Pinkowish, M. D. (1995). What is white-coat hypertension? *Patient Care, 23*(2), 15.

66. Pinzur, M. S. (1994). Functional outcome following traumatic upper limb amputation and prosthetic limb fitting. *The Journal of Hand Surgery, 19*(5), 836–839.

67. Porsche, R. (1995). Hypertension: Diagnosis, acute antihypertension therapy, and long-term management. *AACN Clinical Issues, 6,* 515–525.

68. Poskus, D. B. (1995). Revascularization in peripheral vascular disease: Stents, atherectomies, lasers, and thrombolytics. *AACN Clinical Issues, 6,* 536–546.

69. Rounsevall, C., (1992). Phantom limb pain: The ghost that haunts the amputee. *Orthopaedic Nursing, 11*(2), 67–73.

70. Schneider, R. H., et al. (1995). A randomized controlled trial of stress reduction for hypertension in older African Americans. *Hypertension, 26,* 820–827.

71. Setara, J. F., & Black, H. R., (1992). Refractory hypertension. *New England Journal of Medicine, 327*(8), 543–547.

72. Solomon, J. (1994). Hypertension: New drug therapies. *RN, 57*(1), 26–33.

73. Stovsky, B. (1992). Nursing interventions for risk factor reduction. *Nursing Clinics of North America, 27*(1), 257–270.

74. Tanji, J. L., & Batt, M. E. (1995). Management of hypertension: Adapting new guidelines for active patients. *The Physician and Sportsmedicine, 23*(2), 47–55.

75. Thacker, H. L., & Jahnigen, D. W. (1991). Managing hypertensive emergencies and urgencies in the geriatric patient. *Geriatrics, 46*(10), 26–36.

76. Trottier, D. J., & Kochar, M. S. (1993). Managing isolated systolic hypertension. *AJN, 93*(10), 51–53.

77. Weber, M. A., & Laragh, J. H. (1993). Hypertension: Steps forward and steps backward. *Archives of Internal Medicine, 153,* 149–152.

78. Whitaker, L., & Kelleher, A. (1994). Raynaud's syndrome: Diagnosis and treatment. *Journal of Vascular Nursing, 12*(1), 10–13.

79. Wyngaarden, J. B., et al. (1992). *Cecil textbook of medicine* (19th ed.). Philadelphia: W. B. Saunders.

Hematologic Disorders

UNIT 10

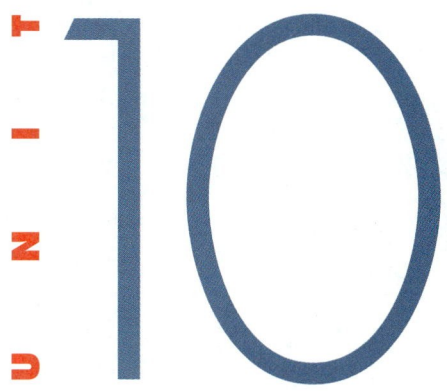

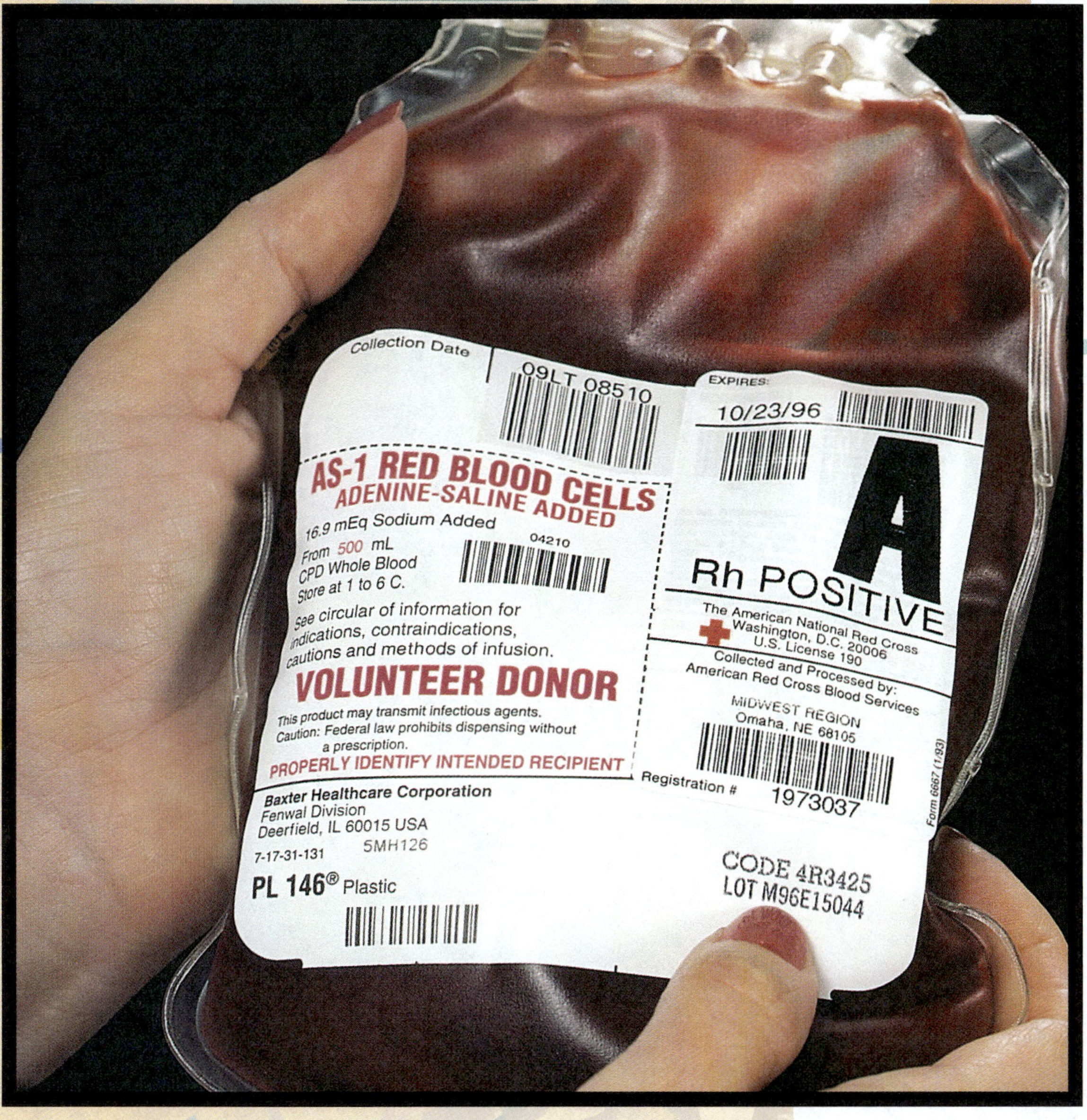

Structure and Function of the Hematologic System

R. B. Boley
Arlene L. Polaski

Blood is a mixture of cells (red blood cells, white blood cells, and platelets) and plasma. It circulates continuously through the heart and vascular system. Propelled through the body by the heart's pumping action, the blood performs many vital functions (Table 51–1), such as the following:

- Supplying oxygen from the lungs and absorbed nutrients from the gastrointestinal tract to cells
- Removing waste products from tissues to the kidney, skin, and lungs for excretion
- Transporting hormones from their origin in the endocrine glands to other parts of the body
- Protecting the body from dangerous microorganisms
- Promoting hemostasis (the arrest of bleeding)
- Regulating body temperature by heat transfer

Characteristics of Blood

The major characteristics of blood are color, viscosity, pH, volume, and composition.

Color. Arterial blood is bright red due to the oxygen bound to hemoglobin and oxygen within red blood cells. Venous blood is dark red because it has a lower oxygen content than arterial blood.

Viscosity. Blood is three to four time more viscous than water. Blood has a specific gravity of 1.048 to 1.066.

pH. Blood is slightly alkaline, with a pH of 7.35 to 7.45 (neutral pH is 7.0).

This chapter incorporates material written for the fourth edition by Janet Pavel, Ann Plunkett, and Bonnie Sink.

Volume. An adult has about 70 to 75 ml of blood/kg of body weight. Thus, the average adult body contains about 4 to 5 L of blood.

Composition. Plasma makes up about 55% of the blood, and solid suspended particles (blood cells and platelets) compose the other 45%.

Plasma is the liquid portion of the blood. Its major function is to maintain the blood volume within the vascular compartment. A straw-colored, watery substance, plasma is composed of 92% water, 7% proteins, and less than 1% nutrients, metabolic wastes, respiratory gases, enzymes, hormones, clotting factors, and inorganic salts. The proteins include serum albumin (α_1-globulin, and α_2-globulin, β-globulin, and γ-globulin) as well as fibrinogen, prothrombin, and protein essential for blood coagulation. Serum albumin and gamma globulin are necessary for maintaining colloidal osmotic pressure (see Chapter 15). γ-Globulin also contains the antibodies (immunoglobulins) IgM, IgG, IgA, IgD, and IgE, which are essential in the body's defense against microorganisms (see Chapters 25 and 26).

Hematopoiesis: Formation of Blood Cells

Hematopoiesis is the process of formation and development of blood cells. This important process begins very early in the development of the human embryo and it must persist unabated throughout the lifetime of the individual. The demands made on this function are enormous, cells in the peripheral blood have a finite life span and must be continuously renewed at a rate estimated to be greater than 10 billion cells per day. For a 100-year-old individual this would amount to more than 10^{14} cells being made during his or her lifetime.

In the adult human all blood cells are produced in microenvironments in marrow tissue that is contained in the medullary cavities of bone. Bone marrow is one of

	Table 51–1. Functions of Blood		
Component	**Function**	**Diagnostic Tests**	**Survival**
Red blood cells	Mediate the exchange of oxygen and carbon dioxide between lungs and tissue	Red blood cell count Hemoglobin Hematocrit Reticulocyte count Blood indices: mean corpuscular hemoglobin, concentration, mean corpuscular volume, mean corpuscular hemoglobin Red cell fragility Morphologic description in stained smear	120 days
Platelets	Form platelet plug to arrest bleeding Promote thrombin production	Platelet aggregation Platelet count Bleeding time	7–10 days
White blood cells	Protection from bacteria and other foreign substances	White blood cell count with differential	
Granulocytes	White cells containing granules broken down into three subcategories		6–8 hr circulating in the blood and 2–3 days in the tissues
Neutrophils	Phagocytosis		
Eosinophils	Allergic and inflammatory reactions		
Basophils	Prevention of clotting in microcirculation Allergic reactions		
Lymphocytes	Formation of immunoglobins	Immunoglobins Cell markers (T cell, B cell, etc.)	
	Cellular immunity	Mixed lymphocyte culture	
Monocytes	Phagocytosis	White blood cell count with differential	
Plasma			
Water	Liquid in which cells circulate		
Proteins		Total protein	
Albumin	Maintains colloidal osmotic pressure	Albumin level	
γ-Globulins	Contains antibodies for body's defense	Quantitative immunoglobulins	
Fibrinogen	Blood coagulation	Fibrinogen level	

the largest organs in the body with an aggregate weight in the adult of about 3000 (comparable in mass to the liver).

Ontogeny of Hematopoiesis

Blood cell production begins during embryogenesis. In humans, by the end of the second week of development, primitive red blood cells can be detected in the yolk sac. After about 6 weeks of development the formed fetal liver has begun to produce most of the erythroid cells, possibly as a result of being seeded with precursor cells from the yolk sac. In the middle of the first trimester granulocytes and megakaryocytes begin to appear. Lym-

phocyte production starts in the third trimester, and shortly afterward, monocytes are being produced. By the fifth month of fetal development, the marrow in the developing bones has become the exclusive site of production of granulocytes, megakaryocytes, and lymphocytes (some erythrocytes are still being produced in the fetal liver). The bone marrow becomes the exclusive site of hematopoietic function only at the end of fetal development.

During childhood all blood cells are essentially produced in marrow sites of the flat bones of the skull, clavicle, sternum, ribs, vertebrae, and pelvis. After puberty, hematopoietic function becomes localized within the flat bones of the sternum, ilium, ribs, and vertebrae with some production in the proximal ends of long bones (humerus and femur).

Structural and Organizational Features of Bone Marrow

■ Anatomic Compartments in Bone Marrow

Based on visual appearance the marrow mass was originally described as being either red or yellow. The yellow marrow has a large number of adipose cells which accounts for its characteristic light color. This portion, or compartment, of the marrow is generally not active in hematopoiesis in a normal healthy person. However, following severe blood loss or the development of a sustained state of hypoxia, the yellow marrow can be converted into a red marrow state and production of blood cells initiated.

The red marrow consists of a mass of supporting cells surrounding aggregates of hematopoietic cells and interspaced with sinusoidal capillaries.

The red marrow ground structure includes fibers produced by reticulum cells which together provide interstices that are occupied by hematopoietic cells and adipocytes. These cell masses, called cords, are surrounded by the thin-walled venous sinuses. In addition to the reticular fibers, the extracellular matrix includes molecules of collagen, proteoglycans, fibronectin and laminin. These components have roles in cell-cell interactions, cytokine presentation, and cell differentiation.

■ Functional Compartments in Bone Marrow

Available data give only a partial picture of the hematopoietic process, especially in the early stages. The means by which constituents from the local or distant environments induce activation and differentiation of stem cells are slowly being unraveled, but many details remain obscure. The functional compartments that are generally recognized within mammalian bone marrow provide for the following:

1. Maintenance of a self-renewing pluripotent stem cell population from which all blood cells are derived.
2. An environment for the differentiation and maturation of blood cells.
3. A storage site for large numbers of neutrophils.
4. Transformation of undifferentiated lymphocytes into mature B cells.
5. A defensive action based on the phagocytic activity of the macrophages attached to the luminal side of the marrow sinuses. These phagocytes, part of the reticuloendothelial system (RES) or mononuclear phagocytic system, monitor the blood for the presence of foreign particulate matter, remove it, and destroy it.
6. Service in a limited role as a peripheral lymphoid tissue site for humoral antibody production in some secondary immune responses.

Events in Hematopoiesis

■ Stem Cells

The stem cell population is a group of poorly characterized undifferentiated cells that exists within the red marrow. This totipotent, or pluripotent, stem cell is self-replicating and maintains a small population throughout the lifetime of the individual. Following stimulation by one or more signal molecules called poietins, the stem cell is capable of undergoing differentiation into erythrocytes, megakaryocytes, and leukocytes.

The derivational relationships between the stem cell and the various subsequent cell types during hematopoiesis are shown in Figure 51–1.

When the stem cell population is damaged by genetic changes, tumor development, chemical or radiation treatment, its ability to undergo differentiation and proliferation is compromised and may be destroyed. When this occurs, the affected individual is not able to replace blood cells eliminated by normal attrition or that are destroyed while responding to injury or infection. Such persons are at great risk and most will die unless the lost function(s) can be compensated for or restored in a timely manner.

■ Erythrocytes

The production of erythrocytes is termed *erythropoiesis*. Erythrocytes are produced in the bone marrow. The general requirements for this process are precursor cells; a proper microenvironment; and adequate supplies of iron, vitamin B_{12}, folic acid, protein, pyridoxine, and traces of copper. If any of these factors is missing, the resultant erythrocytes will be fragile, misshapen, abnormally large or small, deficient in hemoglobin, or too few in number.

Erythrocytes arise from a undifferentiated progenitor cell in the bone marrow called a pluripotent stem cell. Development of an erythrocyte from its stem cell–derived precursor involves several changes that include loss of cell volume, decrease in size of the nucleus, compression of chromatin and extrusion of the nuclear remnant, disappearance of mitochondria, and an increase in intracytoplasmic hemoglobin. This process takes about 7 days and involves about six stages in the differentiation process (see Fig. 51–1).

Immature erythrocytes leave the bone marrow via veins in the marrow and enter the general circulation as reticulocytes. After being released from the marrow sites, the reticulocytes travel to the spleen where they undergo conditioning and evolve into mature erythrocytes before being released to the general circulation.

As erythrocytes age, they become increasingly fragile and eventually rupture. The released hemoglobin and the empty membranes (called ghost cells) are taken up by macrophages within the liver, spleen, lymph nodes, and bone marrow. The hemoglobin is broken down into heme (iron and porphyrin) and globin (polypeptide chain) fractions. The iron of the heme fraction is returned to the liver, spleen, and bone marrow to be reused in making hemoglobin. The liver converts the porphyrin of the heme fraction into bilirubin, an orange pigment, and secretes it into the bile to be excreted from the body in the feces

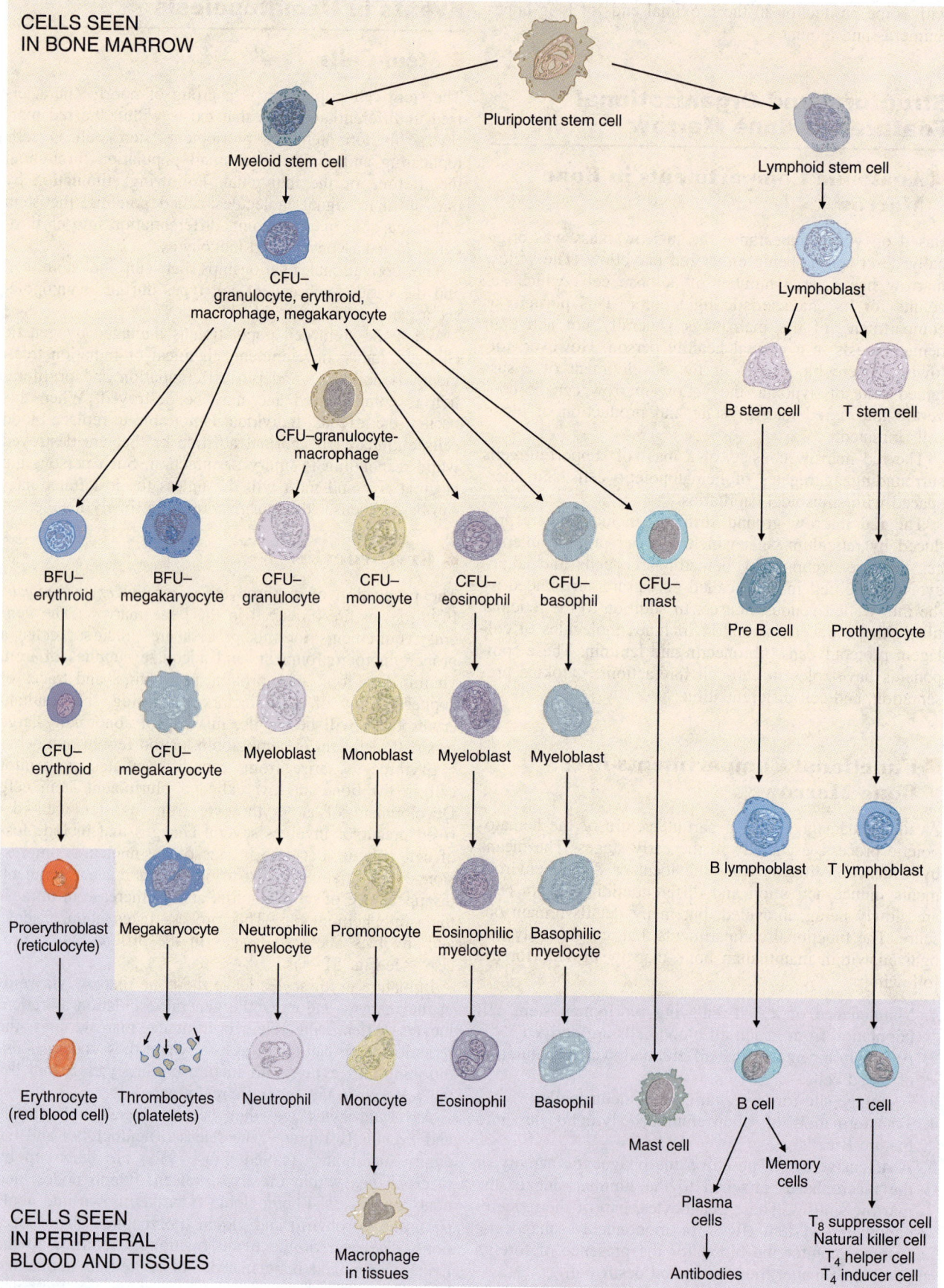

Figure 51–1. Origin, development, and structure of thrombocytes, leukocytes, and erythrocytes from pluripotent stem cells. BFU, burst-forming unit; CFU, colony-forming unit.

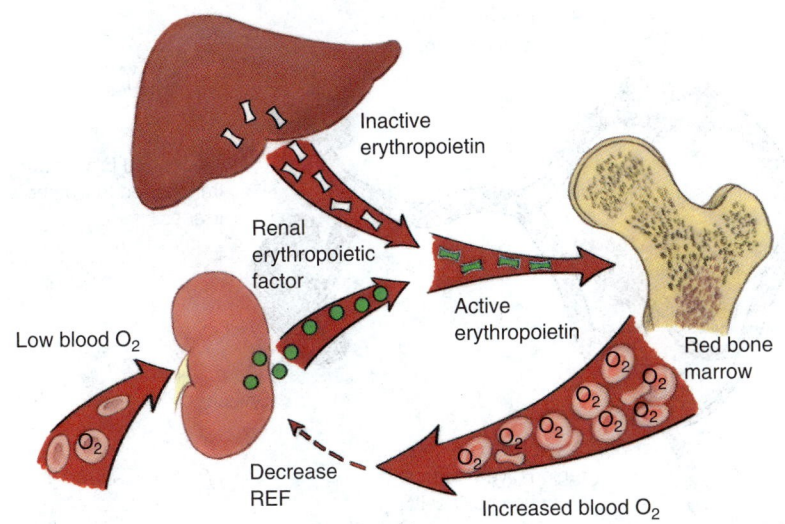

Figure 51–2. Regulation of erythrocyte production. (From Applegate, E. J. [1995]. *The anatomy and physiology learning system: Textbook.* Philadelphia: W. B. Saunders.)

and urine (Fig. 51–2). During periods of increased red blood cell destruction (e.g., in hemolytic anemia), excessive amounts of bilirubin are formed which may accumulate in the body's tissues.

Normally, about 180 million effete erythrocytes are destroyed and replaced each minute in humans. When the loss of erythrocytes exceeds production of replacements inadequate amounts of oxygen are delivered to the tissues. The resultant hypoxia (low blood oxygen) stimulates cells in the kidneys to release erythropoietin, which is transported via the blood to the bone marrow where it acts on hematopoietic stem cells to increase the production of red blood cells. Healthy bone marrow has the capacity to increase its production of erythrocytes six to eight times over the normal rate and is thus readily able to keep pace with increased destruction or loss of red blood cells. This response mechanism is able to maintain a remarkably constant number of erythrocytes within each individual.

A significant structural feature of the red blood cell is a high degree of plasticity, which enables the cell to carry out its most important function: transporting oxygen. A normal erythrocyte has the shape of a biconcave disc and the ability of the red blood cell to alter its shape is essential to movements through capillaries and splenic channels since the diameter of the human red blood cell (8 μm) far exceeds that of the capillaries (2 to 3 μm).

■ Granulocytes

A myeloblast is produced from a stem cell and undergoes further differentiation into three types of myelocytes: (1) neutrophilic, (2) eosinophilic, and (3) basophilic (see Fig. 51–1). As these cells mature their nucleus changes in morphology and the cytoplasm becomes filled with membrane-bounded vesicles containing enzymes and other types of molecules. The mature forms of these cells, collectively called granulocytes, are found in different body sites. About 90% of mature neutrophils remain in the bone marrow, a storage arrangement that enables the body to quickly release large numbers of these cells when

inflammation occurs in perimeter tissues. The neutrophils in the peripheral blood are subdivided, about half and half, into a circulating cell group and a marginated cell group (adherent to endothelial linings in small blood vessels). Thus a complete blood count for a healthy person accounts for only about 5% of the total number of mature neutrophils actually present in the body at that time. The neutrophil is the primary responding cell during an acute inflammatory response. The increases seen in peripheral white blood cell counts during episodes of inflammation are the result of large numbers of neutrophils being released from the bone marrow reserve. If the inflamed state is prolonged, the supply of mature cells with lobed nuclei will be exhausted, and immature neutrophils with a banded nucleus will appear in the circulating blood (shift to the left).

Under normal circumstances, mature eosinophils do not remain long in the marrow, and are present in only small numbers in the peripheral blood (less than 3% of the total white blood cell count in a healthy person). These cells exit the peripheral blood compartment and accumulate in extravascular sites near epithelial surfaces whence they can be recruited to protect against worm infections and to modulate IgE-mediated allergic responses.

The basophil is an enigmatic cell type. Details of its normal role in body homeostasis are lacking. The intracytoplasmic granules (storage vesicles) include heparin, histamine, and a chemotactic factor for eosinophils. There is general disagreement as to whether this cell is a precursor to a similar cell found in solid tissues: the mast cell. Vesicular contents in the mast cell are similar to those found in the basophil, and the human mast cell is known to bind IgE and be a primary participant in the induction of IgE-mediated allergic cascades.

■ Monocytes

The monocyte is derived from a precursor cell that is indistinguishable from a myeloblast. Subsequent differentiation, however, leads to a cell structure that is markedly different from the granulocyte. The monocyte released

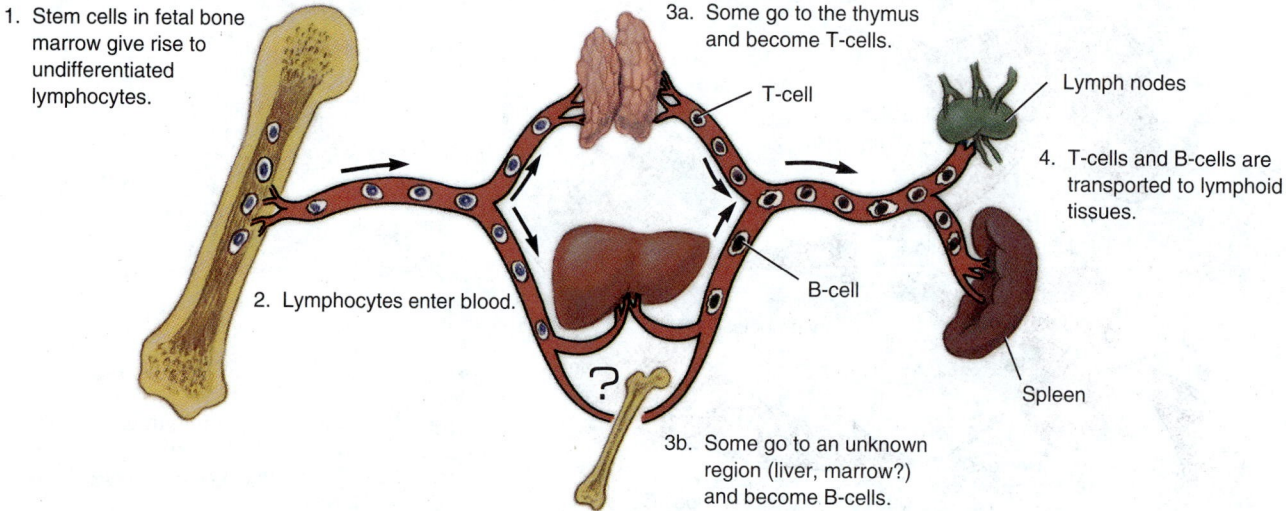

1. Stem cells in fetal bone marrow give rise to undifferentiated lymphocytes.

2. Lymphocytes enter blood.

3a. Some go to the thymus and become T-cells.

T-cell

Lymph nodes

4. T-cells and B-cells are transported to lymphoid tissues.

B-cell

Spleen

3b. Some go to an unknown region (liver, marrow?) and become B-cells.

Figure 51–3. Development of lymphocytes. (From Applegate, E. J. [1995]. *The anatomy and physiology learning system: Textbook.* Philadelphia: W. B. Saunders.)

from the bone marrow into the circulation is a hypoactive phagocytic cell. After becoming attached to sinusoidal endothelium in the spleen, bone marrow, and liver, or after emigrating from the blood into lung, connective, lymphoid tissue, this cell becomes transformed into a macrophage with full phagocytic function. Some macrophages were given special names when discovered in earlier times: alveolar macrophages (dust cells) in the lungs, histiocytes in connective tissues, and Kupffer cells in the liver. In the 1920s, it was recognized that all of these cells formed a large dispersed cell population whose major functional feature was phagocytosis. These cells constitute the RES and are charged with the responsibility for removing all foreign particulate material entering the body. The macrophage is attracted secondarily to acute inflamed sites and are the characteristic cell in chronic and in many secretory T cell–orchestrated inflammatory lesions. Some of the macrophages also participate in immune function by serving as antigen processing and antigen-presenting cells.

■ Lymphocytes

Lymphocytes in their mature form are assigned to one of three groups depending on the presence of characteristic surface markers and on the cell function (Fig. 51–3). One group of lymphocytes is programmed in the thymus to become T cells; another is programmed in the bone marrow to become B cells, and the third population, which are not identifiable as either T or B cells, are called *null cells.* The B cells function in antibody-mediated immune responses helping to defend the body against invasive types of bacteria, bacterial toxins, and some viruses. T cells are the basis of cell-mediated immune functions that defend against facultative and obligate intracellular pathogens, fungi, and viruses. The null lymphocytes, some called natural killer cells, defend against some viral infections and are able to kill some tumor cells. Cell-mediated immunity is pictured in Figure 51–4.

■ Megakaryocytes and Platelets

Platelets (thrombocytes) have essential roles in hemostasis. One action is the physical occlusion of small openings in blood vessels (a hemostatic function), and the other is to provide chemical components in the molecular cascade leading to coagulation (a thromboplastic function).

Individual platelets are produced by a fragmentation process from giant multinucleated cells in the red bone marrow called megakaryocytes (see Fig. 51–1). The earliest precursor in this transformation sequence is called a megakaryoblast. This differentiating cell is large (about 30 μm in diameter), has a basophilic cytoplasm, and, when mature, will contain multiple nuclear equivalents. The time required for the formation of human platelets has been estimated at about 5 days. Cytoplasmic extensions from megakaryoblasts are extruded into sinusoids, and platelets are formed by fragmentation at the terminal ends of the filaments. Normal human marrow may have up to 6 million megakaryocytes per kilogram of body weight, with each megakaryocyte being able to give rise to a thousand or more individual platelets. Platelet production in a normal person appears to be under tight control and is remarkably consistent since the numbers in a healthy person often remain constant for years.

Roles of the Liver and Spleen in Hematopoiesis

The spleen and liver both have important roles in the hematopoietic system. The spleen is a fist-sized organ located in the upper part of the abdominal cavity on the left side. The action of the spleen in sequestering some of the peripheral blood erythrocytes provides for a ready reserve supply of these cells that can rapidly enter the circulation whenever the red blood cell count drops significantly below normal levels (e.g., during pregnancy and emergencies such as hemorrhage or carbon monoxide poisoning). Other functions of the spleen include (1) assisting in recycling iron by capturing hemoglobin released

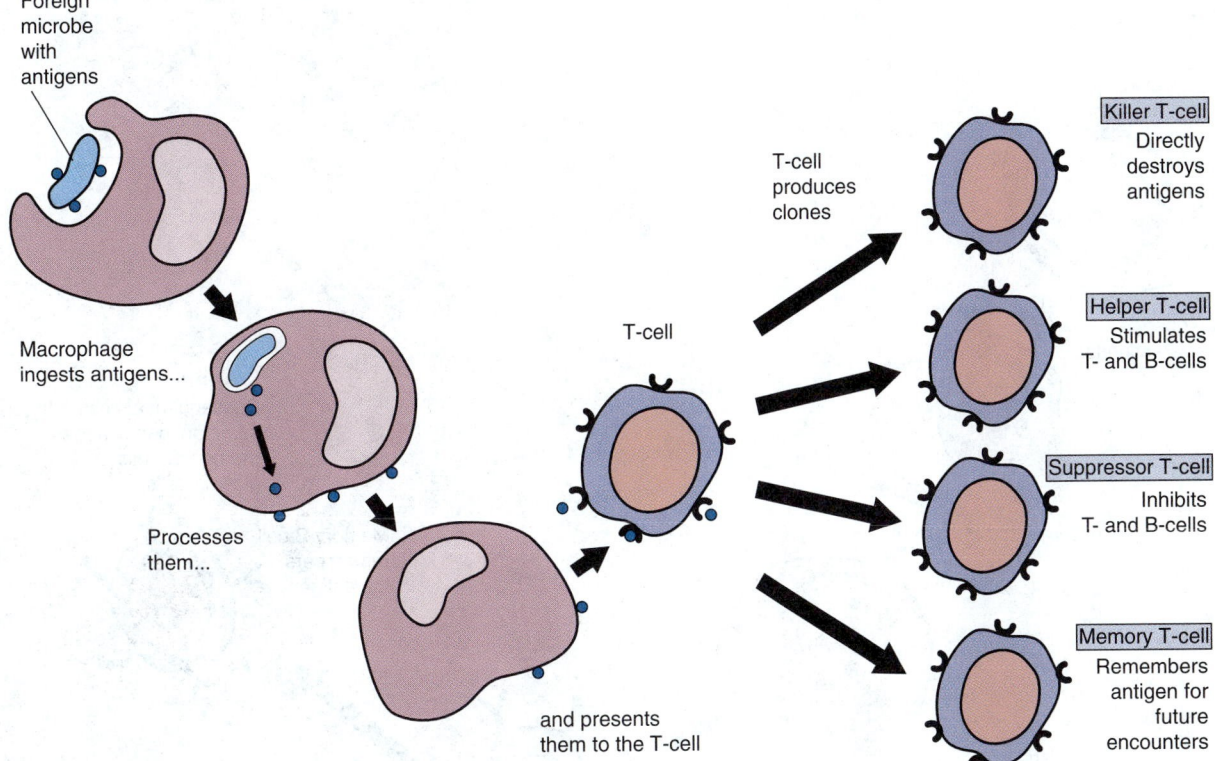

Figure 51–4. Cell-mediated immunity. (From Applegate, E. J. [1995]. *The anatomy and physiology learning system: Textbook.* Philadelphia: W. B. Saunders.)

from destroyed red cells, and (2) performing pitting (removal of particles from a red blood cell without destroying the cell itself). The spleen also functions in defense. Foreign particulate material (including bacteria) is removed from the circulating blood by macrophages attached to the luminal surfaces of sinusoid walls (part of the blood-clearing process). Antigens present in the blood are removed by cells in the white pulp areas of the spleen, processed, and presented to T and B cells to stimulate antibody production (Fig. 51–5). In these contexts, splenectomy often increases the risk of the individual for infection with extracellular bacteria.

The liver is also important in the blood-clearing process. Fixed macrophages (called *Kupffer cells*) remove inanimate particulates and bacterial cells that appear in the peripheral blood. The roles of the liver in hematopoiesis are mostly indirect and consist of the following: production of small quantities of erythropoietin, synthesis of plasma proteins and clotting factors, decomposition of hemoglobin into bilirubin, and storage of iron in the form of ferritin.

Control of Hematopoiesis

■ Nutritional Factors and Metabolites

Vitamin B_{12} is essential for normal red blood cell maturation and normal nervous system function. Because it is not synthesized in the body, vitamin B_{12} must be a component of the daily diet. Animal products such as meat and dairy products are the only sources of this vitamin. In this context, vitamin B_{12} is called *extrinsic factor* (meaning outside the body). When released from food during gastric digestion, vitamin B_{12} binds with an autogenous glycoprotein called *intrinsic factor* (inside the body) present in the duodenum and the complex is transported to the distal ileum, where specific receptors in the mucosa bind vitamin B_{12} for absorption into the blood.

Folic acid, a B-group vitamin, is necessary for red cell formation and maturation but, unlike vitamin B_{12}, does not play a role in nervous system function. The molecule is synthesized by many plants and bacteria. The major dietary sources of folic acid are vegetables and fruits. Cooking destroys some forms of folic acid.

Iron is essential to hemoglobin production. The adult human body contains about 50 mg of iron per 100 ml of blood. Total body iron ranges between 2 and 6 g, depending on the size of the person and the amount of hemoglobin sequestered within his or her cellular compartment. Hemoglobin accounts for about two thirds of the total iron (called *essential iron*). The other third resides in the bone marrow, spleen, liver, and muscle. When a person develops an iron deficiency, the latter iron stores are depleted first, followed by a gradual loss of the iron contained in hemoglobin.

■ Physiologic Control: Cytokine Regulation

Much of the mechanism of hematopoietic regulation that stimulates the initial differentiation of stem cells and con-

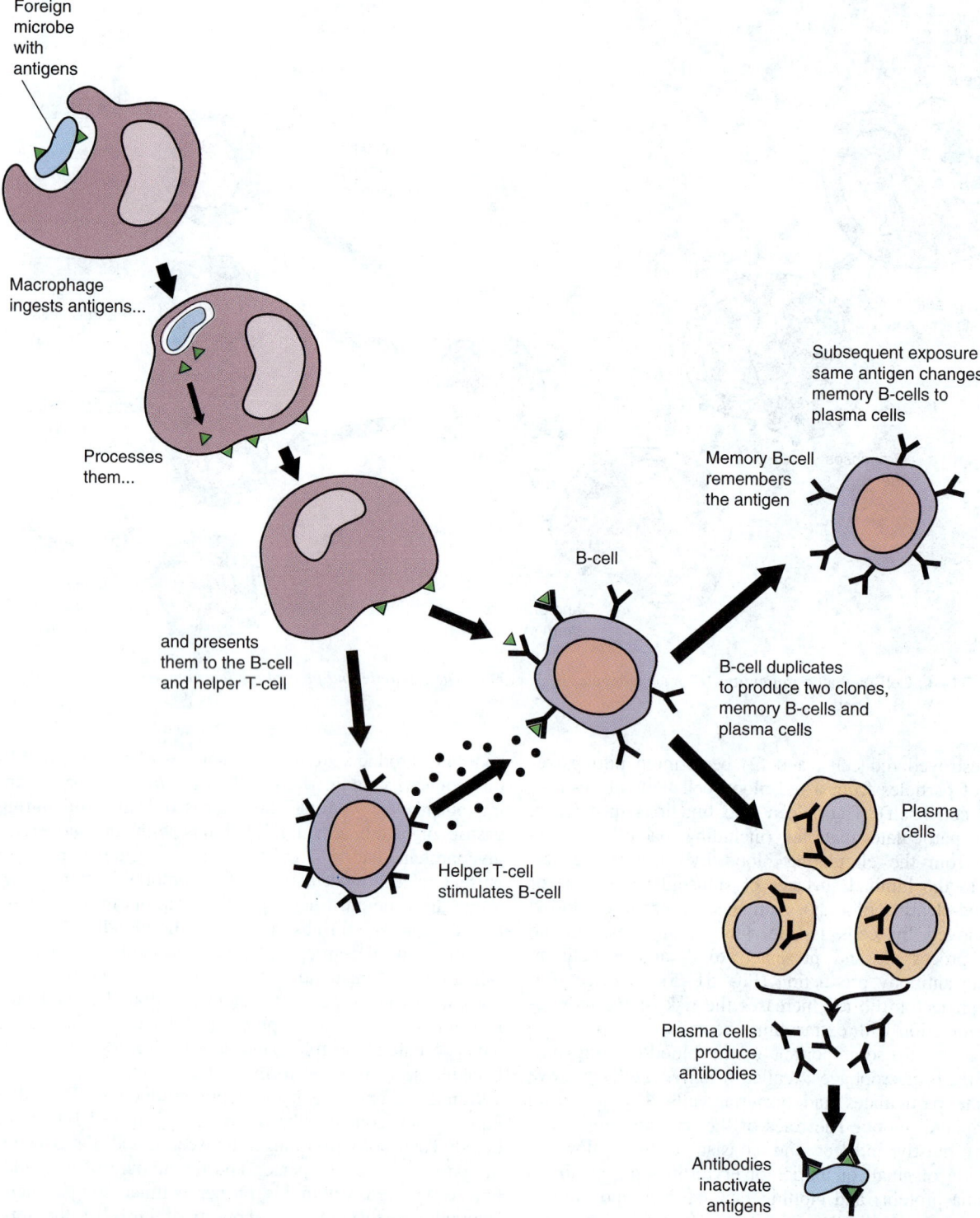

Foreign
microbe
with
antigens

Macrophage
ingests antigens...

Processes
them...

and presents
them to the B-cell
and helper T-cell

Helper T-cell
stimulates B-cell

B-cell

Subsequent exposure to
same antigen changes
memory B-cells to
plasma cells

Memory B-cell
remembers
the antigen

B-cell duplicates
to produce two clones,
memory B-cells and
plasma cells

Plasma
cells

Plasma cells
produce
antibodies

Antibodies
inactivate
antigens

Figure 51–5. Antibody-mediated immunity. (From Applegate, E. J. [1995]. *The anatomy and physiology learning system: Textbook.* Philadelphia: W. B. Saunders.)

trols the early differentiation of the expanding cell lines is either not known or poorly characterized. The so-called hematopoietic inductive environment is provided mainly by cellular elements: fibroblasts, fat cells, endothelial cells, and T cells, which, along with macrophages, are the main sources of growth factors necessary for cell replica-tion and differentiation. The noncellular component composed of fibronectin, laminin, and complex mucopolysaccharides has an important role in concentrating and presenting the growth factors to progenitor and other cells undergoing differentiation.

Cell growth, proliferation, and differentiation are all

under the control of regulatory molecules called growth factors, or cytokines. These molecules are produced by certain cell lines and act on a variety of target cells. They have a number of features, which follow, in common:

● Glycoprotein composition
● Multiple biologic activities
● Active in all stages of hematopoiesis
● When two or more are involved, the interaction may be synergistic or antagonistic
● Any abnormality in production or function of receptors on target cells will have a marked impact on hematopoiesis.

Growth factors are usually identified by using acronyms that are a legacy from original studies on colony-forming cells. The suffix "-CSF" (colony stimulating factor) is used to describe the growth factor that stimulates or regulates the growth and development of the corresponding cell type identified with the prefix "CFU-." For example, G-CSF is the growth factor for CFU-G (colony forming unit-granulocytic series), and M-CSF is the growth factor regulating the development of monocytes (CFU-M). Other growth factors are designated as interleukins (IL) and are given numbers to distinguish between different molecules: IL-1 derived from macrophages and IL-3 from activated T cells, and so forth.

The method of production of the growth factors is multifactorial and involves a complex series of interactions between producing and responding cells. A common pathway leading to the synthesis and secretion of these substances involves the macrophage and the T cell. The macrophage is activated by engaging in phagocytosis or by stimulation with endotoxin from gram negative bacteria and begins to secrete IL-1 and tumor necrosis factor (TNF) which, in turn, bind to receptors on the surfaces of T cells, fibroblasts, and endothelial cells causing them to synthesize and secrete other growth factors.

Blood Groups and Blood Typing

Human RBCs display antigens that are either glycoproteins or glycolipids on the surface of the membrane. Together the various blood group systems contribute more than 400 characterized antigens. Antigens are inherited from the parents. Less than a dozen of these blood group antigens attract frequent clinical notice, and of these only the ABO and rhesus (Rh) systems are major determinants of compatibility testing.

Antibodies are proteins (immunoglobulins) that float freely in the plasma. Antibodies are usually produced following exposure to an antigen that the person does not have. The body recognizes the antigen as foreign, and the immune system responds by producing an antibody. Combining an antigen on the surface of a cell with an antibody initiates a series of immune responses that can result in the destruction of the cell.

The ABO Blood Group System

The ABO blood type is inherited as an autosomal trait. The four major blood types of clinical importance in this genetic system are A, B, AB, and O. Blood is typed according to the antigens found on the RBC and the antibodies found in the serum.

Usually, for the antibodies to be formed, there must be exposure to foreign or homologous red cell antigens through pregnancy or transfusion. The major exceptions are the A and B antigens, for which there are structurally similar proteins in the environment, resulting in antibody formation against the missing A or B or AB antigen by the age of 3 months.

The two major antigens within the blood group system are antigens A and B. A client may have one (type A or type B), both (type AB), or neither (type O) antigen on his or her RBCs. There also are two major antibodies found in the serum, anti-A and anti-B. A client with type A blood has anti-B antibodies; a client with type B blood has anti-A antibodies, a client with type O blood has anti-A and anti-B antibodies, and group AB has neither antibody (Table 51–2).

The Rh System

The Rh blood groups are nearly equal in clinical importance to the ABO groups. The Rh factor was named for the rhesus monkey used in the initial experiments by Landsteiner and Weiner in 1940. Although Rh serology involves more than 20 different antigens, the D antigen has the most clinical significance because of the high risk of formation of an anti-D in an Rh-negative recipient. The term *Rh-positive* means the client has the D antigen, whereas the Rh-negative client has no D antigen.

The incidence of Rh antigens varies widely among different populations. About 85% of whites are Rh-positive, and about 95% of blacks are Rh-positive.

The most striking difference between the ABO and Rh systems is that in the ABO system, there is spontaneous development of antibodies directed against A and B antigens not present on the RBC. In the Rh system, antibody formation is never spontaneous. Instead, a client must first be exposed to the Rh antigen, for example, through a blood transfusion or pregnancy. This means that clients with Rh-negative blood, transfused for the first time with Rh-positive blood, do not experience a reaction because their blood does not yet contain anti-Rh antibodies (anti-

Table 51–2. The ABO Blood Group System			
Blood Type	Agglutinogens on RBS	Agglutinins in Plasma	Frequency in United States
A	A	Anti-B	41%
B	B	Anti-A	10%
AB	A and B	None	4%
O	None	Anti-A and anti-B	45%

D). About 50% of people, however, develop sensitivity and form antibodies against the D as a result of exposure to the D antigen from transfusion or pregnancy. Should a sensitized client receive a second transfusion or have a second pregnancy with exposure to the D antigen, some degree of RBC destruction will occur. However, it is usually possible to prevent sensitization from occurring the first time by administering a single dose of anti-Rh antibodies in the form of $Rh_o(D)$ immune globulin (RhoGAM) immediately following exposure to the D antigen.

The HLA System

Human leukocyte antigens (HLAs) are also called *histocompatibility antigens* because the antigens (glycoproteins) are found on the surface of most cells in the body except RBCs (including circulating and tissue cells). The HLA system is a series of closely linked genes located on the short arm of chromosome 6. The major function of

the HLA antigen is regulation of the immune response, distinguishing self from nonself. This plays a major role in the rejection of transplanted tissues when donor and recipient HLA antigens do not match. There also is an association between HLA antigens and some diseases. For example, in ankylosing spondylitis, the association with HLA factor is so strong that HLA typing can be used diagnostically.

Hemostasis

Normal hemostasis is a process that repairs vascular breaks to reduce blood loss from blood vessels while maintaining the flow of blood through the vascular system. The three components of the hemostatic mechanism are the blood vessels, platelets (or thrombocytes), and coagulation factors. These components accomplish hemostasis in three phases (Fig. 51–6): (1) the vascular phase, in which vasoconstriction of the vessels occurs; (2) the

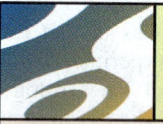

DIVERSITY IN HEALTHCARE

Blood Groups and Rh Factor in Diverse Cultures

Differences in blood groups and Rh factor have been noted in people from various racial and ethnic backgrounds. Among Native-Americans type O blood is the most prevalent, with some type A blood and virtually no type B blood. Almost equal prevalence of types A, B, and O blood are found in Japanese and Chinese, but only 10% have type AB blood. Blacks and whites have equal prevalence of A, B, and O blood types. Types A and O predominate, while types AB and B occur less frequently. Statistically, women with type O blood are less likely to get thromboembolic disease, particularly when taking birth control pills.[1-4]

ABO incompatibility can lead to *spontaneous abortion* when the fetus is A or B blood type and the mother is O blood type. Fetal wastage caused by ABO incompatibility occurs in approximately 18% of maternal-fetal ABO-incompatible pregnancies. At term, about 1% of the surviving infants are affected with ABO hemolytic disease. Here is where the racial differences become apparent. Black infants are more than twice as likely to manifest the disease as those in the general population.[1-4]

Because neonatal jaundice is harder to detect in blacks and because black infants have a greater risk of developing ABO hemolytic disease, all mothers and infants should be ABO blood-typed at the time of delivery. Infants from incompatible pregnancies should be tested for bilirubin levels prior to hospital discharge. Phototherapy is usually needed to reduce the bilirubin level.

The Rh-negative factor in blood is most common in whites, much rarer in other groups, and absent in Eskimos. Although there are at least 27 different antigens in the Rh system, the D antigen has clinical significance in immunogenic disease. When antigen D is present, the term *Rh-positive* is used. Approximately 85% of all people in the world have Rh-positive blood. The D antigen is usually involved in hemolytic disease of the newborn when an Rh-positive infant is born to an Rh-negative mother.

When an Rh-negative client is exposed to Rh-positive blood, the Rh antibody will bind to corresponding antigens on the surface of red blood cells that contain the Rh antigen. Ordinarily, Rh antibodies do not fix complement. As a result, there is no

immediate hemolysis, as occurs with ABO incompatibility. Rather, Rh-antigen red blood cells are broken down by macrophages in the spleen, resulting in conversion of hemoglobin to bilirubin. The clinical manifestation of the conversion is jaundice. When Rh-negative women with Rh-positive mates deliver Rh-positive infants, the infant is susceptible to jaundice. This condition can be prevented in subsequent pregnancies if the Rh-negative woman is given Rh_o (D) immune globulin (RhoGAM) immediately after delivering an Rh-positive infant.

1 Andrews, M. M. (1995). Transcultural perspectives in the nursing care of children and adolescents. In M. M. Andrews, & J. S. Boyle (Eds.), *Transcultural concepts in nursing care* (pp. 123–180). Philadelphia: J. B. Lippincott.

2 Giger, J. N., & Davidhizar, R. E. (1995). *Transcultural nursing: Assessment and intervention.* St. Louis: Mosby–Year Book.

3 Huether, S. A., & McCance, K. L. (1996). *Understanding pathophysiology.* St. Louis: Mosby–Year Book.

4 Overfield, T. (1985). *Biologic variation in health and illness: Race, age, and sex differences.* Menlo Park, CA: Addison-Wesley.

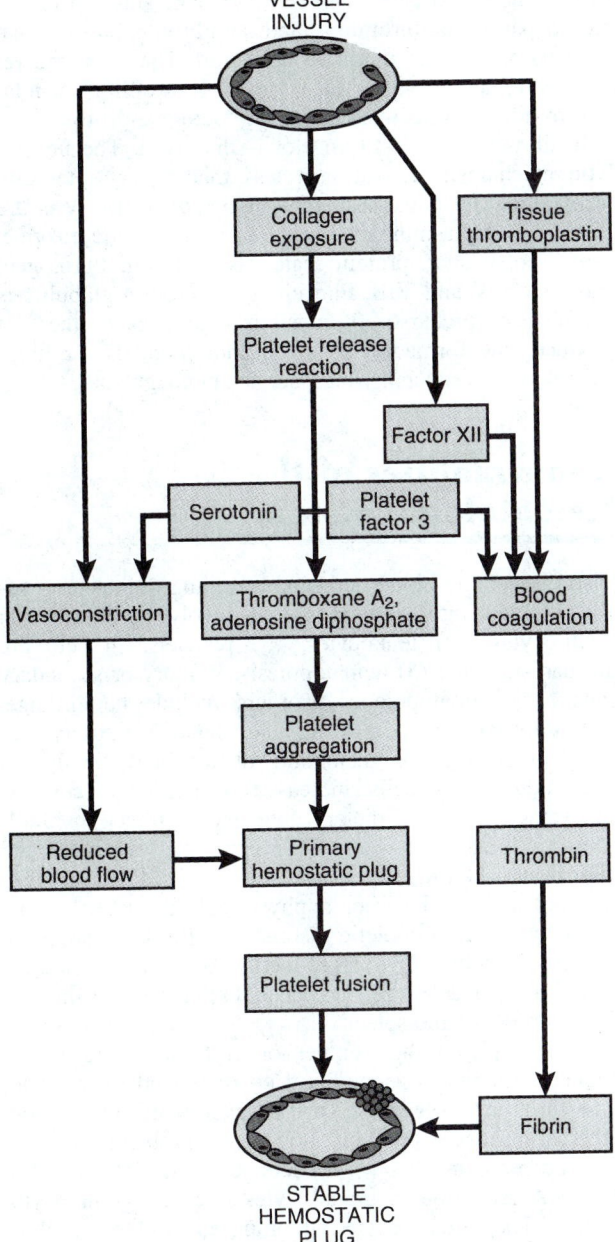

Figure 51–6. Mechanism of normal hemostasis.

formation of a platelet plug; and (3) the coagulation or formation of a fibrin clot. Once the fibrin clot has served its purpose, it is balanced by fibrinolysis (clot dissolution), thus preventing thrombosis.

The Role of Blood Vessels

Whenever bleeding results from injury or disease, the blood vessels that supply the damaged site constrict. This is helpful because vasoconstriction slows the flow of blood to the injured area, decreasing blood loss. Vasoconstriction results from muscular tissue and reflex nervous system reactions. Serotonin is a potent local vasoconstrictor that is secreted by cells in the small intestine and promotes blood vessel constriction on injury.

The Role of Platelets

Adequate numbers of cells (150,000 to 400,000/mm³) are required in the peripheral blood to play the role of hemostasis. When platelets come into contact with an alteration of the endothelial cell lining of a blood vessel, they become sticky and adhere to one another, thus sealing the surface of the vessel lining. Along with these adhesive reactions, the platelets have a secretory response resulting in the release of intracellular storage granules from within the platelet. Granule constituents include substances that can stimulate circulating platelets and cause them to acquire new adhesive properties. These platelet constituents can activate additional platelets that aggregate to form a thrombus.

Platelets control hemostasis unless large blood vessels have been damaged. If bleeding is severe, coagulation factors must join with platelets to form a permanent clot.

The Role of the Coagulation System

The coagulation system consists of a series of interactions that result in the formation of a fibrin clot. The system consists of clotting proteins (except factor IV), that is, factors that circulate in the plasma (except factor III, which is released from damaged cells) in an inactive state (see Fig. 51–6).

The formation of a fibrin clot can result from activation of one of two pathways: the intrinsic or the extrinsic pathway. Various factors are needed by these two pathways for completion of a final common pathway that results in a fibrin clot (Fig. 51–7).

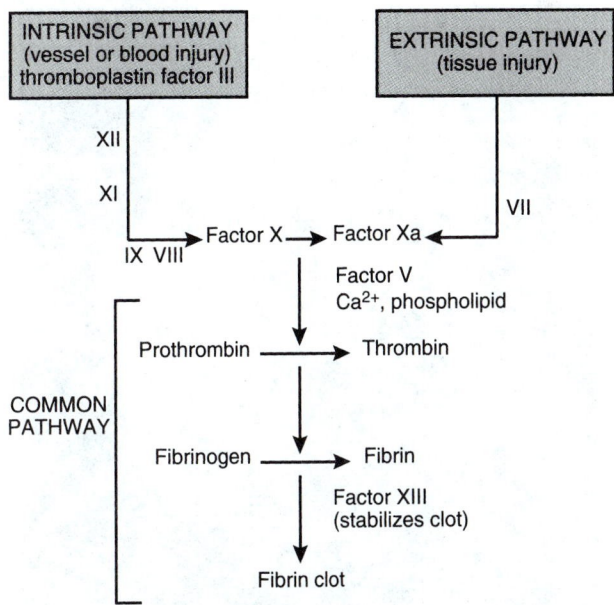

Figure 51–7. The coagulation process. The intrinsic and extrinsic pathways lead to activation of factor X. Activated factor X along with factor V leads to the common pathway and formation of a stable clot.

The extrinsic pathway is initiated when tissue injury occurs outside the vessels, such as a burn. Damaged tissues release factor III (tissue thromboplastin), which initiates the clotting cascade to form activated factor X, which leads to the final common pathway of clot formation.

The intrinsic pathway involves the blood itself (i.e., antigen-antibody reactions and endotoxins) or damage to the blood vessels. All factors for the intrinsic system are present in the plasma. This pathway is initiated when factor XII is exposed to a foreign surface, which initiates a cascade of enzymatic reactions to activate factor X, leading to the common pathway.

Activated factor X is responsible for the conversion of prothrombin to thrombin and soluble fibrinogen to an insoluble fibrin clot. The protein fibrin forms dense interlacing threads that entrap erythrocytes and platelets (Fig. 51–8). The platelets then release a contractile protein, which causes shrinkage and retraction of the clot into a firm, insoluble fibrin mass. The process of retraction squeezes out the clear yellow serum. Serum differs from plasma in that it does not contain clotting factors.

In some cases, the formation of a fibrin clot is unnecessary because hemostasis occurs at an early stage. Temporary clots are sometimes insufficient. For example, bleeding from a small pin prick can normally be ended by a platelet plug, while more serious cuts require the interaction of the various coagulation factors.

The Role of Fibrinolysis and Anticoagulants

The coagulation system is controlled by several mechanisms to maintain a flow of blood through the vascular space. The blood carries natural anticoagulants, for example, heparin, antithrombin, and antithromboplastin, that act continuously to inhibit coagulation. The liver and reticuloendothelial system also aid in controlling coagulation by removing activated clotting factors and fibrin.

In fibrinolysis, the fibrin clot is dissolved. The fibrinolytic mechanism activates in less than a day after clot formation. The two substances involved in clot lysis are plasmin and plasminogen. Plasmin, a proteolytic enzyme, can dissolve such protein materials as fibrin, fibrinogen, and factors V and VIII. Plasminogen, a serum globulin, is the inactive precursor of plasmin. The lysis of the clot produces the formation of fibrin split products (or fibrin degradation products), which act as anticoagulants.

Abnormalities of the Hematologic System

Disorders of the blood and blood-forming organs are usually divided into categories that involve primarily (1) erythrocytes, (2) leukocytes, (3) platelets, (4) clotting mechanisms, and (5) hematopoiesis. Primary or secondary causes of hematopoietic disorders include hemorrhage, malabsorptive disorders, drug and chemical toxicity, genetic predisposition, metabolic disturbances, malignant overproduction of cells, increased destruction of cells by an overactive spleen, dietary deficiencies, infections, radiation, immunologic defects, autoimmune response, and idiopathic (unknown) factors.

There are four basic pathophysiologic disturbances that characterize hematopoietic disorders: (1) a decrease in the number of cells, (2) overproduction of normal or defective cells, (3) defects in the coagulation mechanism, and (4) disorders of the spleen.

A decrease in the number of erythrocytes results in anemia. Anemia is a condition characterized by a reduction in the oxygen-carrying capacity of the blood: Hypoxia produces fatigue, among other problems.

A decrease in all types of leukocytes is termed leukopenia. A reduction in granulocytes is called granulocytopenia. The granulocytes (composed of neutrophils, eosinophils, and basophils) work with monocytes and lymphocytes to guard the body against invasion by foreign materials. Therefore, granulocytopenia and neutropenia (decrease in the number of neutrophils) predispose a person to severe infections.

A decrease in the thrombocyte, or platelet, count is called *thrombocytopenia*. Because thrombocytes are an important component in the clotting mechanism, hallmarks of thrombocytopenia are easy to spot: bruising; petechiae (fine red hemorrhagic rash); and a tendency to bleed readily from the perianal area, gastrointestinal tract, and mucous membranes.

An abnormal increase in erythrocyte production is called *polycythemia*. Increased manufacture of abnormal, immature leukocytes is termed *leukemia*. The abnormal malignant proliferation of plasma cells results in plasma cell myeloma or multiple myeloma. These conditions (polycythemia, leukemia, and plasma cell myeloma) are usually classified as myeloproliferative diseases because

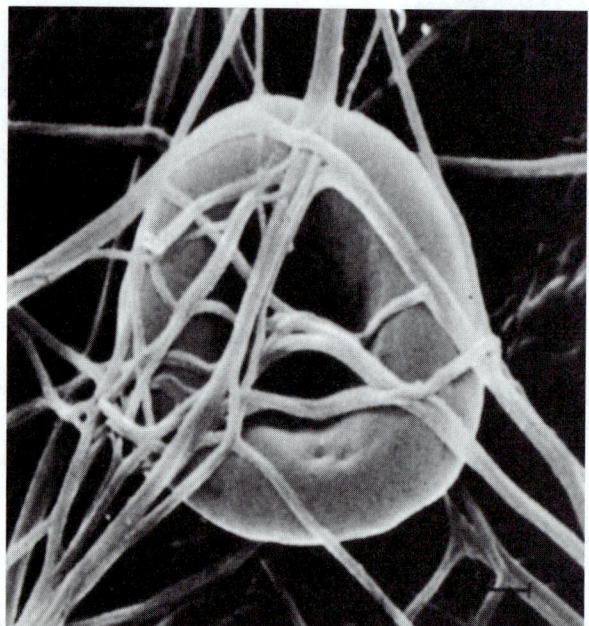

Figure 51–8. Fibrin enmeshing a red blood cell. (From Page, J., et al. [1981]. *Blood: The river of life* [p. 79]. Washington, DC: U.S. News Books.)

the malignant overproduction of cells takes place within the bone marrow.

Overproduction of cells within the lymphatic tissues results in lymphoproliferative disorders. Examples include (1) Hodgkin's disease and non-Hodgkin's lymphomas, characterized by malignant proliferation of lymphocytes and other cells within the lymph nodes, and (2) lymphocytic leukemia, characterized by an overproduction of lymphoblasts within the lymph nodes and bone marrow that are released into the blood.

Effects of Aging

The effects of aging on function of the hematopoietic system are not well documented. Bone marrow cellularity decreases as a person becomes older, but this may reflect only the increase in adipose tissue associated with decreased bone mass in the elderly. There is a gradual but progressive loss of defensive functions that is related to decreased functions in the T cell series and in macrophages. Whether this phenomenon is associated with altered function(s) in the bone marrow or is consequential to as yet unidentified factors arising in peripheral solid tissues is open to question. Total red blood cell hemoglobin values appear to remain unchanged or be minimally affected by age, and platelet counts remain unchanged.

Conclusions

Blood cell formation is a vital homeostatic function that must start early in embryogensis and continue unabated until life ceases. Any significant deficiency or alteration in this procedure during an individual's lifetime will have grave consequences. Several of the more serious diseases afflicting humans are derived from or are related to pathologic changes in the blood-forming system.

Bibliography

1. Adams, S. (1992). The HLA system: Seminar, 1992.
2. Alkire, K., & Collingwood, J. (1990). Physiology of blood and bone marrow. *Seminars in Oncology Nursing, 6,* 99–107.
3. Amino, N. (1990). Receptors in disease: An overview. *Clinical Biochemistry, 23,* 31–36.
4. Baldwin, J. G. (1988). Hematopoietic function in the elderly. *Archives of Internal Medicine, 148,* 2544–2546.
5. Bottema, C. D. & Sommer, S. S. (1993). PCR amplification of specific alleles: Rapid detection of known mutations and polymorphisms. *Mutation Research, 288,* 93–102.
6. Carlson, K., & Golub, A. (1987). *Autologous and directed blood programs.* Arlington, VA: American Association of Blood Banks.
7. Corbett, J. V. (1992). *Laboratory tests and diagnostic procedures with nursing diagnoses.* East Norwalk, CT: Appleton & Lange.
8. DiJulio, J. (1991). Hematopoiesis: An overview. *Oncology Nursing Forum, 18,* 3–6.
9. Duguid, J. K. M. (1990). Developing techniques in blood transfusion. *Bailliere's Clinical Haematology, 3* (1), 999–1017.
10. Ganong, W. F. (1995). *Review of medical physiology.* (17th ed.). Norwalk, CT: Appleton & Lange.
11. Golde, D. W. (1991). The stem cell. *Scientific American, 265* (6), 86–93.
12. Henney, C. S. (1989). Interleukin-7. Effects on early events in lymphopoiesis. *Immunology Today, 10,* 170.
13. Hoffbrand, A. V. (1995). *Recent advances in hematology.* (25th ed.). Edinburgh: Churchill Livingstone.
14. Hoffbrand, A. V., & Pettit, J. E. (1994). *Color atlas of clinical hematology.* (2nd ed.). London: Gower Medical Publishing.
15. Hoffman, R., et al. (1991). *Hematology: Basic principles and practice.* Edinburgh: Churchill Livingstone.
16. Ikuta, K., et al. (1992). Lymphocyte development from stem cells. *Annual Revue of Immunology, 10,* 759–784.
17. Jandl, J. H. (1991). *Blood: Pathophysiology.* Cambridge, England: Blackwell Scientific Publications.
18. Kruger, B. (1989). Toward an understanding of structure and function of ion channels. *FASEB Journal, FASEB 3,* 1906–1914.
19. Lehrer, R. I., et al. (1988). Neutrophils and host defense. *Annals of Internal Medicine, 109,* 127.
20. Metcalf, D. (1992). The hematopoietic regulators—an embarassment of riches. *Bioessays, 14,* 799–805.
21. Ogawa, M. (1993). Review: Differentiation and proliferation of hematopoietic stem cells. *Blood, 81,* 2844–2854.
22. Perez, W. E., & Viets, J. L. (1990). Transfusion and coagulation: An overview and recent advances in practice modalities. *Nurse Anesthetist, I,* 149–161.
23. Quinton, P. (1990). Cystic fibrosis: A disease of electrolyte transport. *FASEB Journal, 4,* 2709–2717.
24. Read, E. L., & Klein, H. G. (1986). Hematological effects of aging: Considerations for clinical trials. In N. R. Cutler & P. K. Narang (Eds.), *Drug studies in the elderly* (pp. 123–144). New York: Plenum.
25. Salmon, C., et al. (1984). *The human blood groups.* New York: Masson.
26. Sherman, J. L. (1988). *Guide to patient evaluation: History taking, physical examination, and the nursing process.* New York: Medical Examination.
27. Stiehm, E. R. (1993). New and old immunodeficiencies. *Pediatric Research, 33,* (Suppl.), S2.
28. Spivak, J. L., et al. (1996). Cell cycle-specific behavior of erythropoietin. *Experimental Hematology, 24*(2), 141–150.
29. Till, J. E., & McCulloch, E. A. (1980). Hematopoietic stem cell differentiation. *Biochemical and Biophysical Acta, 605,* 431–459.
30. Valent, P., & Bettelheim, P. (1990). The human basophil. *Critical Reviews in Oncology/Hematology, 10,* 327.
31. Williams, W. J., et al. (1995). *Hematology* (5th ed.). New York: McGraw-Hill.
32. Yang, K. D., & Hill, H. R. (1991). Neutrophil functional disorders: Pathophysiology, prevention and therapy. *Journal of Pediatrics, 119,* 343.

Assessment of Clients with Hematologic Disorders

Esther Matassarin-Jacobs

CHAPTER 52

History

Biographical and Demographic Data

In taking the history of the client with a hematologic disorder, note the client's age and sex, because the activity of the bone marrow decreases with aging and women normally have a blood count lower than men. During the years when women experience menses, the blood counts may be even lower. Other important data to collect from the client includes occupation, housing, hobbies, and areas of possible exposure to chemicals.

Chief Complaint

Clients present with many vague and nonspecific manifestations, including chills, fever, chronic fatigue, weight loss, and physical discomfort. Conduct a symptom analysis (see Chapter 11) to determine whether the onset was sudden or gradual and whether it was associated with trauma or a known disease. Disorders of the hematologic system often affect all organs and tissues of the body, resulting in widespread pathophysiologic manifestations. The review of systems (ROS) outlines the systems and their common hematologic findings as well as their possible pathophysiologic bases.

Past Health History

Major Illnesses and Hospitalizations

Ask the client about previous hematologic problems that may provide clues to the current problem. Inquire about

anemia, recurrent infections, delayed wound healing, thrombophlebitis, deep vein thrombosis, liver disease, or excessive bleeding. Has the client been diagnosed previously with a hematologic disorder?

Surgical procedures that may affect the hematologic system include splenectomy, tumor removal, cardiac valve replacement, and resections of the gastrointestinal tract. For example, loss of duodenal tissue results in decreased iron absorption, partial or total gastrectomy reduces intrinsic factor production and vitamin B_{12} absorption, and loss of the terminal portion of the ileum leads to inability to absorb vitamin B_{12}.

Ask the client whether he or she has received a blood or blood product transfusion. If so, what was the reason for the transfusion? Were there any problems or reactions to the blood or blood products? Does the client know his or her blood type, including Rh factor? This information is particularly important for the client who may be pregnant and is Rh-negative (see Chapter 51).

Health problems involving the liver, such as cirrhosis or hepatitis, can disrupt production of several clotting factors. These problems increase the client's risk of bleeding disorders. Other causes of bleeding disorders include genetic factors and chemical toxicity. Ask the following questions when assessing the client with a bleeding disorder:

- How long has the client had a bleeding problem? Was it present in childhood, or has it appeared only recently? Do any members of the family have a history of bleeding disorders?
- Is the bleeding linked to any specific event or procedure? For example, does severe bleeding occur with menses or following minor trauma, a tooth extraction, minor surgery, shaving, or participation in contact sports? Does the client have frequent nosebleeds (epistaxis)? Is there a history of bleeding into the joints or cavities? Does the client bruise easily? Does the client report petechiae?
- How severe are any bleeding episodes, and what is their duration? More precisely, is there prolonged oozing of blood from a site or sudden massive bleeding?

This chapter incorporates material written for the fourth edition by Janet Pavel, Ann Plunkett, and Bonnie Sink.

(Sudden bleeding is far less common than prolonged slow hemorrhage.)

● Does the client have a history of hepatic, splenic, or renal disease? These three conditions are often characterized by hemorrhagic manifestations. Has the client recently taken anticoagulants or medications that may suppress bone marrow activity (e.g., chloramphenicol, antineoplastic agents) or medications that interfere with platelet function?

Medications

Ask the client what medications are being taken for either a hematologic condition or some other disorder. This includes over-the-counter medications; for example, aspirin or aspirin-containing compounds and nonsteroidal anti-inflammatory agents can interfere with platelet aggregation and cause prolonged bleeding.

A variety of medications can lead to bone marrow suppression. Ask the client about a history of having received chemotherapeutic agents. Many of these agents are powerful bone marrow suppressants with the effects continuing for a significant time after the medications have been stopped.

Ask the client about the use of medications such as chlorpropamide (Diabinese), glyburide (Micronase), or tolbutamide (Orinase), antidiabetic agents that may cause hemolysis. Also ask about cardiovascular medications such as mefenamic acid (Ponstel), methyldopa (Aldomet), and procainamide (Pronestyl), and a variety of antibiotics, including sulfonamides and penicillins.

Allergies

Specifically inquire about known allergies and allergic reactions, particularly anaphylaxis. If not previously determined, ask the client for a history of blood or blood product transfusions, as well as any complications from the transfusions, such as fever, chills, back or flank pain, shock, wheezing, headache, vomiting, or urticaria (hives).

Family Health History

A family history of bleeding disorders can be important. Ask about a family history of jaundice, anemia, bleeding disorders (hemophilia or thrombocytopenia), malignancies, or congenital blood dyscrasias, such as sickle cell disease.

Psychosocial History

Hematologic disorders can result in many physiologic changes that affect the client's psychosocial status and ability to perform activities of daily living (ADLs).

Occupation and Environment

Ask the client about previous exposure to toxic chemicals or radiation, either occupation- or treatment-related. Radi-ation and chemicals such as benzene, lead, and phenylbutazone can increase the incidence of hematologic problems, particularly anemia. Does the client have sufficient energy to perform ADLs and occupational tasks? Are there problems with fatigue, dyspnea, or other manifestations that interfere with a productive life-style? Has the client missed time from work or school, resulting in financial loss or other economic concerns, such as health or life insurance eligibility?

Geographical location and environment may affect potential hematologic disorders. Some of these disorders predispose the client to blood dyscrasias. Ask the client about exposure to possible health hazards in the environment such as pollutants, high levels of hydrocarbons, or excessive radiation.

Nutrition

Nutritional habits have a significant effect on the hematologic system. The hematologic system is very dependent on nutritional status. Malnutrition can lead to anemia and immunosuppression.

A dietary history is important when assessing whether there may be any vitamin deficiencies causing anemia. Weight loss may indicate hematologic alterations or deficits in nutrients. Ask the client whether he or she is eating foods that contain iron, folic acid, and vitamin B_{12}, all necessary for the development of red blood cells.

Habits

Carefully explain to the client the importance of asking about the use or abuse of alcohol and other recreational drugs. Chronic substance abuse is often accompanied by malnutrition and vitamin deficiency. Many substances, most notably alcohol, damage the structure and function of liver cells, resulting in decreased clotting factor production and bleeding tendencies.

Review of Systems

Manifestations related to disorders of the hematologic system can be general as well as specific. Conduct a symptom analysis and a focus assessment (see Chapter 11) for all reported manifestations.

General manifestations include fatigue, apathy, lethargy, malaise, weakness, heat intolerance (anemia), chills, fever, night sweats (infection, particularly recurrent infections, and Hodgkin's disease), and delayed wound healing (leukopenia).

Integumentary manifestations may be pruritus (lymphoma), jaundice (hemolytic anemia and pernicious anemia resulting in bile pigment accumulation), pallor, flushing (iron deficiency anemia), petechiae, ecchymoses, and prolonged bleeding (thrombocytopenia and clotting disorders).

Delayed wound healing, lymph node swelling, and infections (leukopenia) may be immunologic manifestations. The client may exhibit neck lymphadenopathy, which is particularly significant if painful (lymphoma and leukemia).

Sensory effects on the eyes include visual disturbances (anemia and polycythemia), blindness (thrombocytopenia and retinal hemorrhage related to anemia), and yellowed sclerae (jaundice). If the hematologic disorder affects the ear, the client might experience vertigo or tinnitus (severe anemia). Manifestations affecting the nose include epistaxis (thrombocytopenia and clotting disorders). Oral manifestations include smooth tongue (pernicious anemia, iron deficiency anemia, nutritional deficiencies), gingival bleeding (thrombocytopenia, clotting disorders), sores, and ulcerations (leukemia and neutropenia).

Respiratory manifestations include fatigue, dyspnea, and orthopnea (anemia).

Cardiovascular manifestations include tachycardia, palpitations (compensatory mechanism to increase cardiac output secondary to anemia); murmurs, particularly systolic (increased volume and velocity of blood through valves related to anemia); and angina (decreased oxygen supply to the heart related to rapid-onset anemia).

The client's gastrointestinal system may be affected by dysphagia (mucous membrane atrophy related to iron deficiency anemia), abdominal pain (intestinal obstruction related to lymphoma, retroperitoneal bleeding, acute hemolysis, allergic purpura, and sickle cell disease), hepatomegaly, splenomegaly (hemolytic anemia resulting in increased need for removal of erythrocytes), hematemesis, and melena (thrombocytopenia and clotting disorders).

Urinary manifestations include hematuria (hemolysis and clotting disorders).

Reproductive manifestations are amenorrhea and menorrhagia (iron deficiency and clotting disorders).

Musculoskeletal manifestations are back pain (hemolysis), sternal tenderness (leukemia and sickle cell disease), bone pain (blast crisis in leukemia and multiple myeloma resulting in pathologic fractures), and joint pain (hemarthroses or bleeding into joints, often related to hemophilia).

Systemic neurologic manifestations are confusion (severe anemia and malignant process or infections in the brain), headache (anemia, polycythemia, invasion or compression of the brain related to leukemia, lymphoma, infection, or brain hemorrhage caused by thrombocytopenia or a clotting disorder), syncope (severe anemia and polycythemia), and paresthesias (peripheral neuropathy secondary to pernicious anemia or hematologic malignancy and a side effect of vincristine therapy). In addition, the client may experience mental depression (hematologic disorders that cause fatigue, discomfort, and acute and chronic problems related to a disease process, or coping difficulties related to a diagnosis of cancer).

Physical Examination

The physical examination of the hematologic system can entail both a complete head-to-toe examination and examinations of specific systems, depending on the nature of the client's problem. For example, the client who presents with abdominal pain and absent bowel sounds related to intraluminal hemorrhage needs a complete gastrointestinal examination, as well as a hematologic assessment. Similarly, the client with hemarthrosis needs a complete ex-

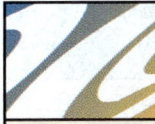

NORMAL PHYSICAL ASSESSMENT FINDINGS

Hematologic System

Inspection

Client alert and oriented; afebrile; skin color even, without pallor, flushing, jaundice, bruises, or petechiae; lumps or masses absent; sclerae white; lingual papillae visible; oral lesions absent; eupneic; joints have full range of motion

Palpation

Lumps, masses absent; lymph nodes, liver, and spleen nonpalpable and nontender; joints nontender

Auscultation

Heart sounds regular, without murmurs or palpitations

amination of the affected joint, as well as a hematologic assessment.

The portions of the physical examination specifically related to the hematologic system include the lymphatic system, liver, and spleen. Lymph node assessment is discussed in Chapter 26, and assessment of the liver and spleen is described in Chapter 64. The Normal Physical Assessment Findings feature outlines normal findings on inspection, palpation, and auscultation. Findings from the history and physical examination are supplemented by laboratory tests and specific diagnostic studies.

Diagnostic Tests

Diagnosis of a blood disorder depends primarily on laboratory analysis. Although dozens of specific tests are used to diagnose individual disorders, all cases generally call for (1) a complete blood count (CBC) to determine the number of leukocytes and erythrocytes; (2) a total differential count to indicate the relative percentages of the different leukocytes; (3) coagulation studies such as prothrombin time (PT) or partial thromboplastin time (PTT) and bleeding time; (4) a bone marrow aspiration and biopsy to determine both the cellularity of the bone marrow and the morphology of the cells present; and (5) a peripheral blood smear (a blood cell morphology to differentiate various anemias and blood dyscrasias). The results of laboratory tests also guide treatment for the client receiving chemotherapy or radiation therapy.

There is no particular preprocedure or postprocedure care associated with the simple blood tests that are involved in most hematologic assessments.

Complete Blood Count

The CBC includes the red blood cell (RBC) count, hemoglobin, hematocrit, red cell indices, white blood cell

Table 52–1. Normal Values for Adult Complete Blood Counts

Measure	Value*
Erythrocytes	
Hemoglobin (oxygen-carrying pigment of the red blood cells)	Women: 12.0–15.5 g/dl of blood Men: 13.0–16.5 g/dl of blood
Red blood cell count	Women: 4.0–5.0 million/mm³ Men: 4.8–5.5 million/mm³
Hematocrit (% volume of red cells in whole blood)	Women: 37%–45% Men: 40%–45%
Leukocytes	
White blood cell (WBC) count (number of cells/mm³ of blood)	4000–9000/mm³
Differential count	
Granulocytes	
Neutrophils	60%–70%
Eosinophils	0%–5%
Basophils	0%–3%
Agranulocytes	
Lymphocytes	30%–40%
Monocytes	0%–5%
Thrombocytes (platelets)(number of cells/mm³ of blood)	150,000–450,000/mm³

* Normal values may differ significantly between laboratories.

(WBC) count with or without differential, and platelet count. Table 52–1 presents reference values for the CBC. Table 52–2 reviews the effects of blood dyscrasias on the CBC.

Red Blood Cell Count

The RBC count measures the number of RBCs per cubic millimeter (mm³) of blood. These values are useful in verifying findings from other hematologic tests for diagnosing anemia and polycythemia. Normal values vary with age and sex.

Hemoglobin Level

The hemoglobin determination evaluates the hemoglobin content of erythrocytes by measuring the number of grams of hemoglobin per 100 ml of blood. This measurement helps to indicate anemias and polycythemia. Normal hemoglobin levels vary with age and sex.

Hematocrit Level

Often used in place of the RBC count, hematocrit measures the volume of RBCs in whole blood, expressed as a percentage. This test is useful in the diagnosis of anemia,

polycythemia, and abnormal hydration states. The hematocrit value is roughly three times the hemoglobin concentration. Normal values also vary with age and sex.

Red Blood Cell Indices

RBC indices measure erythrocyte size and hemoglobin content. These values derive from the RBC count and hemoglobin level. Table 52–3 describes the three RBC indices: mean corpuscular volume, mean corpuscular hemoglobin, and mean corpuscular hemoglobin concentration. The indices are helpful in assessing the various anemias.

White Blood Cell Count

The WBC count measures the number of WBCs in a cubic millimeter (mm³) of blood. It helps detect infection or inflammation and is useful in monitoring a client's response to chemotherapy or radiation therapy.

White Blood Cell Differential

The WBC differential determines the proportion of each of the five types of WBCs in a sample of 100 WBCs. To figure the actual (absolute) count of a specific cell, multiply the total WBC count by the cell percentage reported in the differential. The differential helps in evaluating the body's capacity to resist and overcome infection and in detecting and classifying leukemias.

Platelet Count

The platelet count evaluates thrombocyte (platelet) production, which has a role in blood clotting. The count is valuable in assessing the severity of thrombocytopenia (abnormally low platelet count), which could result in spontaneous bleeding.

Peripheral Blood Smear

A peripheral blood smear is an examination of the peripheral blood to determine variations and abnormalities in erythrocytes, leukocytes, and platelets. Cells of normal size and shape are termed *normocytes*. Cells of normal color are called *normochromic*. Abnormalities of erythrocyte size, shape, and color usually indicate some form of anemia (Table 52–4).

Direct and Indirect Antiglobulin Tests

The direct antiglobulin test (Coombs' test) is used to (1) detect certain antigen-antibody reactions between serum antibodies and RBC antigens, (2) differentiate between various forms of hemolytic anemia, (3) determine unusual

Table 52-2. How Blood Dyscrasias Affect the Complete Blood Count

Increased by	Decreased by
Red blood cell count Polycythemia vera, cardiac and pulmonary disorders characterized by cyanosis, dehydration, acute poisoning	Anemia, fluid overload, recent hemorrhage, leukemia
Hemoglobin Hemoconcentration from polycythemia or dehydration	Hemodilution (fluid overload), anemia, recent hemorrhage
Hematocrit Hemoconcentration from loss of fluid, dehydration, polycythemia	Hemodilution, anemia, acute massive blood loss
Mean corpuscular volume Pernicious anemia, macrocytic anemia, folic acid or vitamin B_{12} deficiency anemias	Microcytic anemia, iron deficiency anemia, hypochromic anemias, thalassemia, lead poisoning
Mean corpuscular hemoglobin Macrocytic anemia	Microcytic anemia
Mean corpuscular hemoglobin concentration Spherocytosis	Microcytic, hypochromic anemia; thalassemia; iron deficiency anemia
White blood cell count Infection, leukemia, tissue necrosis	Bone marrow depression
Neutrophils Inflammatory disease or response, tissue necrosis (burns, myocardial infarction), granulocytic leukemia and other malignancies, acute stress response, bacterial infection	Bone marrow depression, viral diseases, drugs (chemotherapy, some antibiotics, psychotropics)
Eosinophils Allergic reactions, parasitic infestations, skin diseases, neoplasms, pernicious anemia	Stress response, Cushing's syndrome
Basophils Leukemia, some hemolytic anemias, polycythemia vera	Corticosteroids, allergic reactions, acute infections (note: decline is unlikely to be detected because normal count is 0%–2%)
Lymphocytes Viral infections (infectious mononucleosis, pertussis, tuberculosis), lymphocytic leukemia, chronic bacterial infections	Acquired immunodeficiency syndrome (AIDS), adrenal corticosteroids, immunosuppressive drugs
Monocytes Infections (tuberculosis, malaria, Rocky Mountain spotted fever), collagen-vascular diseases, monocytic leukemia	Drug therapy, prednisone
Platelet count Malignancies, polycythemia vera, splenectomy	Idiopathic thrombocytopenic purpura, viral infection, AIDS, anemias, hemolytic disorders, chemotherapeutic drugs or radiation, hypersplenism or splenomegaly, infiltrative bone marrow disease, disseminated intravascular coagulation

blood types, and (4) test for hemolytic disease in newborns. The direct antiglobulin test examines erythrocytes for the presence of antibodies (agglutinins) that damage erythrocytes without causing clumping or hemolysis. It is used to crossmatch blood for blood transfusions, test umbilical cord blood for erythroblastosis fetalis, and diagnose acquired hemolytic anemia.

The indirect antiglobulin test identifies antibodies to erythrocyte antigens in the serum of clients who have a greater than normal chance of developing transfusion reactions. Both tests are agglutination procedures that use a suspension of RBCs.

Reticulocyte Count

A reflection of RBC production, the reticulocyte count measures the responsiveness of the bone marrow to a diminished number of circulating erythrocytes. Specifically, this test measures the number of reticulocytes released from the bone marrow into the blood. An increase in the reticulocyte count indicates an increase in erythrocyte production, probably because of excessive RBC destruction (e.g., hemolytic anemia) or loss (e.g., hemorrhage). A decrease in the reticulocyte count may indicate

Table 52–3. Red Blood Cell Indices

Mean Corpuscular Volume (MCV)	Mean Corpuscular Hemoglobin (MCH)	Mean Corpuscular Hemoglobin Concentration (MCHC)
Measures average size or volume of individual erythrocytes	Measures hemoglobin content within erythrocyte of average size	Measures average hemoglobin concentration within 100 ml of packed red cells
Formula: $\dfrac{\text{Hct}}{\text{RBC}}$	Formula: $\dfrac{\text{Hb}}{\text{RBC}}$	Formula: $\dfrac{\text{Hb}}{\text{Hct}}$
Normal value: $87 \pm 5\ \mu g^3$	Normal value: 29 ± 2 pg	Normal value: 30–36 g/dl of packed RBCs
MCV <80 means abnormally small (i.e., *microcytic*) cells	MCH <27 indicates hemoglobin deficiency (*hypochromic* cells)	MCHC <32 indicates hemoglobin deficiency
MCV >94 means abnormally large (i.e., *macrocytic*) cells	MCH >32 indicates *macrocytic* cells with abnormally large volume of hemoglobin	MCHC remains normal when MCH >32 because cells are oversized (i.e., fewer cells can be packed together within 1 dl)

Hb, hemoglobin; Hct, hematocrit; RBC, red blood cells.

bone marrow failure or pernicious anemia. In addition, it is used to evaluate the effectiveness of treatment of pernicious anemia and bone marrow failure.

Bone Marrow Aspiration

Procedure. Bone marrow aspiration is used to assess and diagnose most blood dyscrasias (e.g., aplastic anemia, leukemias, pernicious anemia, thrombocytopenia). Examination of the bone marrow reveals the number, size, and shape of the RBC, WBC, and platelet precursors. Hematologists study marrow cells for various maturational ab-

normalities. Bone marrow samples are most commonly taken from the posterior iliac crests. Other sampling sites include the sternum and the anterior iliac crests.

The procedure for a bone marrow aspiration is as follows:

1. The physician or nurse cleans the client's skin with an antiseptic solution such as povidone-iodine (Betadine).
2. The physician anesthetizes the client's skin and subcutaneous tissue down to the periosteum with a local anesthetic.

Table 52–4. Abnormalities of the Erythrocyte

Abnormality	Characteristics of Abnormal Cell	Conditions Characterized by Abnormality
Anisocytes	Vary from normal in size	Any of the anemias
Poikilocytes	Abnormally shaped (e.g., tear- or club-shaped)	Any of the anemias; most bizarre shapes seen in the severe anemias
Microcytes	Abnormally small (<6 μm)	Microcytic anemias (e.g., iron deficiency anemia, thalassemia major)
Macrocytes	Abnormally large (>9 μm)	Macrocytic anemias (e.g., pernicious anemia, folic acid deficiency anemia)
Hypochromic cells	Appear pale because of abnormally low hemoglobin content	Any of the anemias
Spherocytes	Relatively small and round rather than biconcave	Hereditary spherocytosis, warm antibody-induced immunohemolytic disease
Schistocytes	Fragmented, with bizarre shapes (e.g., triangles, spirals)	Hemolytic anemia (e.g., thrombotic thrombocytopenic purpura)
Sickle cells	Crescent- or sickle-shaped owing to presence of abnormal hemoglobin (Hb S)	Sickle cell anemia
Target cells	Thin with small amount of hemoglobin in center	Hemoglobin C diseases, thalassemia major, sickle cell anemia
Metarubricytes	Nucleated	Severe anemia

Table 52–5. Laboratory Tests Used in the Diagnosis of Hemorrhagic Disorders

Name of Test	Purpose	Normal Values	Interpretation of Findings
Bleeding time	Measures the ability to stop bleeding after a small puncture wound	3–8 min in adults (varies with test method)	Prolonged bleeding time occurs in vascular maladies and after aspirin ingestion
Platelet count	Measures number of circulating platelets in venous or arterial blood	150,000–450,000/mm^3	Low count results in prolonged bleeding time and impaired clot retraction; diagnostic of thrombocytopenia
Partial thromboplastin time (PTT)	Complex method for testing normalcy of intrinsic coagulation process; employed to identify deficiencies of coagulation factors, prothrombin, and fibrinogen; used to monitor heparin therapy	25–38 sec	Prolongation of time indicates coagulation disorder due to deficiency of a coagulation factor; not diagnostic for platelet disorders
Prothrombin time (PT)	Determines activity and interaction of factors V, VII, X, prothrombin, and fibrinogen; used to determine dosages of oral anticoagulant drugs	11–15 sec (one-stage)	Prolongation of time indicates person receiving anticoagulants; abnormally low fibrinogen concentration; deficiencies of factors II, V, VII, and X; presence of circulating anticoagulants as seen in lupus erythematosus; impaired prothrombin activity
Activated clotting time	Crude measure of coagulation process in venous blood; used to control heparin therapy; commonly used during cardiovascular surgery and in ICU	7–120 sec (depends on type of activator used)	Prolonged time occurs in severe coagulation problems; therapeutic administration of heparin
Thrombin time	Measures functional fibrinogen available, as shown by time needed to form fibrin clot after thrombin is added	10–15 sec	Prolonged time indicates DIC or hypofibrinogenemia; presence in blood of excess heparin or other anticoagulants
Thromboplastin generation test (TGT)	Measures generation of thromboplastin; if result abnormal, second stage is done to identify missing coagulation factor	≤12 sec (100%)	Abnormal values found in hemophilia
Fibrinogen level	Measures level of fibrinogen	200–400 mg/dl	Abnormally low values may indicate liver disease, congenital afibrinogenemia, acquired afibrinogenemia, or DIC
Clot retraction	Indicates function and number of platelets; measures time needed for contraction of an undisturbed clot	50%–100% in 24 hr	Clot retraction retarded in thrombocytopenia; clot is small and soft in thrombasthenia (functional disturbance of platelets)
Capillary fragility test (tourniquet test, Rumpel-Leede test)	Crude test of vascular resistance and platelet number and function; done by placing blood pressure cuff on arm for 5 min and then counting petechiae	No petechiae	Petechiae appear in thrombocytopenia and vascular purpura
Fibrin split products (FSPs) test	Measures the products that result from the breakdown of fibrin clots	Screening assay <10 μg/ml of FSPs Quantitative assay <3 μg/ml	Abnormally high levels helpful in diagnosis of DIC; monitoring of fibrinolytic therapy

DIC, disseminated intravascular coagulation; ICU, intensive care unit.

3. Apply ice on the contralateral site to help with pain control.
4. The physician inserts a short, sharp, beveled needle containing a stylus through the bone cortex into the marrow space. Once the needle is in the marrow space, the stylus is removed. A syringe is then attached to the needle and about 1 ml of marrow is withdrawn. Because the marrow space itself cannot be anesthetized, removal of the marrow usually produces moderate to severe pain of short duration. It stops as soon as suction on the marrow space is stopped.
5. The marrow is ejected onto slides.
6. Slides are labeled and sent to the laboratory immediately.

Preprocedure Care. To prepare the client for a bone marrow aspiration, (1) explain the purpose and procedure of the examination, (2) make sure the client has signed an informed consent form before aspiration, (3) obtain an order for sedation if the client is extremely apprehensive, and (4) position the client according to the healthcare policy of your facility.

Postprocedure Care. Following the procedure, apply pressure until the bleeding stops. Most clients require only a small bandage over the site because there is usually minimal bleeding. However, many clients who require bone marrow aspiration are thrombocytopenic and may need a longer period of pressure to stop bleeding. A pressure dressing and sandbag also may need to be applied in these cases. Tell the family to observe the site frequently on the day of the procedure and for several days following for clients with an increased risk of bleeding. There may be some discomfort or pain that requires a mild analgesic.

A bone marrow biopsy may be taken at the time of marrow aspiration. This bone specimen is ejected into a jar containing a preservative and is sent to the laboratory with the marrow.

Coagulation Screening Tests

Laboratory studies provide the most crucial evidence for pinpointing the type and cause of a bleeding disorder (Table 52–5). Initially, four basic laboratory tests are performed to discern whether the bleeding problem is due to a vascular, coagulation, or platelet defect. These tests are (1) bleeding time, (2) PT, (3) platelet count, and (4) PTT. Ninety-nine percent of all bleeding disorders are diagnosed by the PT and PTT.

Conclusions

Understanding the structure, function, and assessment of the hematologic system will help you care for clients with any of the wide variety of disorders that affect this highly complex system. You are faced with complex assessments and treatments in the care of these clients.

Bibliography

1. Barkauskas, V., Stoltenberg-Allen, K., & Darling-Baumann, C. (1994). *Health and physical assessment.* St. Louis: Mosby–Year Book.
2. Bates, B. (1995). *A guide to physical examination and history taking.* Philadelphia: J. B. Lippincott.
3. Bower, A., & Thompson, J. (1992). *Clinical manual of health assessment* (3rd ed.). St. Louis: Mosby–Year Book.
4. Chernecky, C. C., Krech, R. L., & Berger, B. J. (1993). *Laboratory tests and diagnostic procedures.* Philadelphia: W. B. Saunders.
5. Colman, R., et al. (1994). *Hemostasis and thrombosis: Basic principles and clinical practice* (3rd ed.). Philadelphia: J. B. Lippincott.
6. Copstead, L. (1995). *Perspectives on pathophysiology.* Philadelphia: W. B. Saunders.
7. Fischbach, F. (1992). *A manual of laboratory diagnostic tests* (4th ed.). Philadelphia: J. B. Lippincott.
8. Fuller, J., & Schaller-Ayers, J. (1994). *Health assessment: A nursing approach* (2nd ed.). Philadelphia: J. B. Lippincott.
9. Grimes, J., & Burns, E. (1992). *Health assessment in nursing practice* (3rd ed.). Boston: Jones & Bartlett.
10. Jarvis, C. (1996). *Physical examination and health assessment* (2nd ed.). Philadelphia: W. B. Saunders.
11. Kee, J. L. (1995). *Laboratory and diagnostic tests with nursing implications* (4th ed.). Norwalk, CT: Appleton & Lange.
12. Kenny, R. A. (1992). *Physiology of aging: A synopsis.* St. Louis: Mosby–Year Book.
13. Pagana, K., & Pagana, T. (1993). *Diagnostic testing and nursing implications: A case study approach* (4th ed.). St. Louis: Mosby–Year Book.
14. Treseler, K. M. (1995). *Clinical laboratory and diagnostic tests* (3rd ed.). Norwalk, CT: Appleton & Lange.
15. Watson, J., & Jaffee, M. S. (1995). *Nurse's manual of laboratory and diagnostic tests* (2nd ed.). Philadelphia: F. A. Davis.

Nursing Care of Clients with Hematologic Disorders

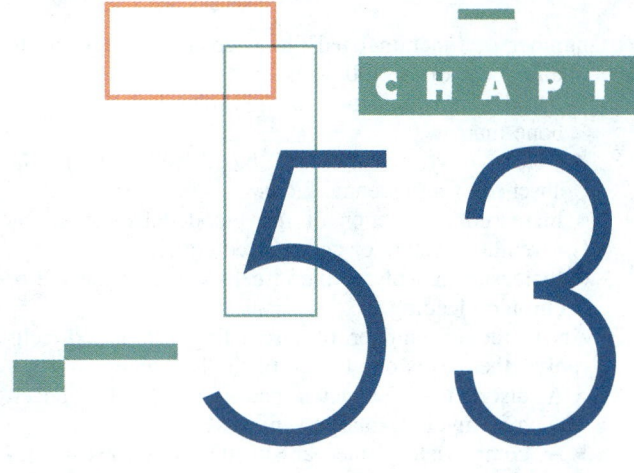

Esther Matassarin-Jacobs

This chapter discusses disorders affecting red blood cells (erythrocytes), white blood cells (leukocytes), the lymph system and spleen primarily, and platelets and clotting factors. There are a variety of concepts appropriate to these disorders, but many are related to the nursing diagnoses Impaired Gas Exchange, Fluid Volume Deficit, or Risk for Infection. The most common collaborative problems associated with the hematologic system are Hemorrhage, Sepsis, and Thrombus Formation.

Red blood cell disorders include anemias and polycythemias. Major disorders that affect white blood cells are (1) the leukemias (acute and chronic), (2) agranulocytosis, and (3) multiple myeloma (plasma cell myeloma). Disorders primarily affecting the lymph nodes and spleen are the lymphomas, classified as either (1) Hodgkin's disease or (2) non-Hodgkin's lymphoma. Disorders affecting platelets and clotting factors include (1) hemorrhagic disorders, (2) purpura, (3) coagulation disorders, and (4) leukemias.

Disorders Affecting Red Blood Cells

The Anemias

Anemia is a reduction in red blood cells (erythrocytes), which in turn decreases the oxygen-carrying capacity of the blood. Not a disease in itself, anemia reflects an abnormality in red blood cell number, structure, or function.

Anemia is the principal manifestation of many abnormal conditions, such as (1) deficiency states caused by a dietary lack of iron, vitamin B_{12}, and folic acid; (2) hereditary disorders of red blood cells; (3) disorders involving the hematopoietic tissues (bone marrow damage or a hyperactive spleen); and (4) bleeding from the gastrointestinal tract or any organ secondary to cancer or trauma.

This chapter incorporates material written for the fourth edition by Janet Pavel, Ann Plunkett, and Bonnie Sink.

Increased destruction of red blood cells can also result from extrinsic sources, physical causes such as prosthetic heart valves, or thrombotic thrombocytopenic purpura. It can also result from antibodies, as in immune thrombotic thrombocytopenia; from infectious agents and toxins; or from other causes, such as hypersplenism, vasculitis syndromes, or osmotic and physical injury.

Studies suggest that the prevalence of anemia increases with age; an estimated average of 20% of the elderly are anemic. However, anemia cannot be assumed to be caused simply by aging without the exclusion of reversible causes. The elderly client should be fully assessed for an underlying cause of anemia.

The incidence of anemia is high, especially in underdeveloped countries where nutrition is poor and in tropical regions where the hookworm (a parasite that extracts blood from the intestinal wall of its host) is endemic. Some epidemiologists calculate that at least one half of the world's population suffers from anemia sometime in their lives.

Etiology and Risk Factors

Major causes of anemia are (1) excessive blood loss, (2) deficiencies and abnormalities of red blood cell production, and (3) excessive destruction of red blood cells.

Poor nutrition, blood loss, and conditions that cause excessive red blood cell destruction are risk factors for the development of anemia. Proper nutrition will obviously help prevent anemia. With the other risk factors, early detection can help reduce the severity of the anemia.

Pathophysiology

Two basic pathophysiologic alterations underlie all red blood cell disorders:

1. A decrease in the hemoglobin concentration or the

number of functional red blood cells (anemia) due to one or more of the following:

- Insufficient production of red blood cells by the bone marrow
- Defective synthesis of red blood cells due to the absence of an essential factor
- Increased destruction of red blood cells caused by hereditary factors or an acquired condition
- Increased loss of red blood cells caused by acute or chronic bleeding

2. An increased number of circulating red blood cells (polycythemia) is due to one of the following:

- A disorder of unknown cause, similar to cancer, such as myelodysplastic syndrome
- A compensatory mechanism that develops in response to tissue hypoxia (secondary polycythemia)

Anemias are classified according to either the morphologic features of the red blood cell (e.g., normocytic, microcytic) or the cause of the condition (e.g., hemolytic, hemorrhagic). It is important to be familiar with the more accurate and commonly used morphologic classification system. However, it is more practical to relate nursing assessment, diagnosis, and treatment of an anemia to the classification shown in Box 53–1 than to its cellular characteristics. Box 53–1 divides the anemias into acquired anemias (common to uncommon), anemias due to excessive blood loss, and congenital anemias.

Clinical Manifestations and Diagnostic Findings

Manifestations accompanying anemia differ, depending on the severity and chronicity of the anemia, the age of the person, and the presence of other disorders. Tissue hypoxia is the underlying cause of all manifestations accompanying anemia. Respiratory and cardiovascular compensatory mechanisms produce many of the manifestations. Persons with mild anemia (hemoglobin of 10–12 g/dl) are usually asymptomatic. If manifestations do occur, they typically follow strenuous exertion. Some persons may have a severe anemia but be asymptomatic if their anemia develops gradually.

Persons with moderate anemia also suffer from dyspnea, palpitations, diaphoresis with exertion, and chronic fatigue.

Severely anemic persons (those with a hemoglobin well below 8 g/dl) appear pale and always feel exhausted. They may have severe palpitations, sensitivity to cold, loss of appetite, profound weakness, dizziness, and headaches. Severely anemic persons, particularly the elderly, can eventually develop serious cardiac complications. Congestive heart failure may arise as a result of increased demands on the heart to beat faster and harder (to transport more oxygen to the tissues). Angina pectoris may also develop, either alone or with congestive heart failure. In severe anemia, angina pectoris results from insufficient oxygenation of the myocardium. Persons with preexisting heart conditions, in addition to anemia, are particularly vulnerable to circulatory and pulmonary complications.

Box 53–1. Classification of Anemias

Acquired Anemias

Anemias resulting from reduced red blood cell production
  Anemias due to deficiencies of factors necessary for red blood cell production
    Iron deficiency anemia
    Anemias due to deficiencies of vitamin B$_{12}$ and folic acid (megaloblastic anemias)
    Pernicious anemia
    Other anemias due to vitamin B$_{12}$ deficiency
    Anemia caused by folic acid deficiency
    Anemias due to bone marrow failure
      Aplastic anemia

Hemolytic anemias
  Anemias resulting from excessive red blood cell destruction
    Hemolysis caused by trauma
    Hemolysis caused by chemical agents and medications (toxic hemolytic anemia)
    Hemolysis caused by infectious agents
    Hemolysis caused by systemic diseases (secondary hemolytic anemia)
    Hemolysis caused by isoimmune hemolytic reactions
    Hemolysis caused by autoimmune disorders
    Paroxysmal hemoglobinurias

Secondary anemias

Hemorrhagic Anemias

Acute hemorrhagic anemia

Chronic hemorrhagic anemia

Congenital Anemias

Hemoglobinopathies
  Sickle cell anemia and sickle cell trait
  Thalassemia

Hemolytic anemias caused by intrinsic red blood cell defects
  Glucose-6-phosphate dehydrogenase (G6PD) deficiency
  Hereditary spherocytosis

Other manifestations of anemia associated with specific systems include the following:

- *Integumentary:* pallor (particularly of palm lines, nail beds, conjunctivae, and circumoral area), delayed wound healing, sore mouth and tongue, jaundice, spider angiomas, sensitivity to cold
- *Respiratory:* shortness of breath, dyspnea on exertion, orthopnea
- *Cardiovascular:* palpitations, angina, tachycardia, cardiomegaly, claudication, dependent edema, bruits, tachypnea, fatigue, weakness
- *Gastrointestinal:* beefy red tongue, anorexia, nausea, dietary change (clay-eating, pica), tarry stool, constipation, diarrhea, hemorrhoids, hematemesis, weight loss
- *Genitourinary and reproductive:* hematuria, menstrual irregularity, loss of libido, impotence

- *Neurologic:* headache, dizziness, sternal tenderness, numbness, tingling of extremities, irritability, paralysis
- *General:* chronic fatigue, malaise

The diagnosis of anemia relies on blood tests, physical assessment, and examination, psychosocial assessment, and the health history. The red blood cell count, hemoglobin level, and hematocrit confirm the presence of anemia. To determine the specific type of anemia present, the hematologist examines a bone marrow specimen and a peripheral blood smear and calculates red cell indices and, in some cases, the rate of red blood cell destruction.

A thorough history, physical examination, observation, and review of records are essential in evaluating the client suspected of having a red blood cell abnormality. Elicit a database from the client that provides information about the possible cause of the disease process, the manifestations, and the pathophysiologic mechanism. Specifically ask about the history of the present illness, significant past medical history, and current medications.

Community and Self-Care

■ Medical Management

The goals of care for clients with anemia include (1) alleviating or controlling the causes, (2) relieving the manifestations, and (3) preventing complications.

Management of the anemias ranges from specific treatments to symptomatic care. Treatment also varies in intensity and duration because some anemias resolve within a few weeks or months, whereas others require lifelong intervention.

The anemias caused by deficiency states respond best to specific intervention. For example, iron preparations and diet can cure iron deficiency anemia; injections of vitamin B_{12} control pernicious anemia.

Other anemias (e.g., aplastic anemia due to bone marrow failure and some of the acquired hemolytic anemias) may be successfully treated by stopping a cytotoxic medication or avoiding a dangerous chemical agent.

Oxygen Therapy. Oxygen therapy may be prescribed for clients with severe anemia, because their blood has a reduced capacity for oxygen. Oxygen helps prevent tissue hypoxia and lessens the workload of the heart as it struggles to compensate for the lower hemoglobin levels.

Blood Transfusions. Blood transfusions are valuable in treating anemia due to acute blood loss. They may also benefit clients with severe chronic anemia (hemoglobin less than 6 g/100 ml) who have responded poorly to other forms of therapy. Transfusion therapy, in which the specific blood components required are transfused, supports clients until they spontaneously recover or respond to treatment.

Long-term red blood cell support, however, carries with it the potentially fatal complication of iron overload. The normal iron level of 2 to 3 g usually remains constant because iron is metabolized at a fixed rate. Each unit of red blood cells contains an additional 200 mg of iron. Clients who receive more than 100 units of red blood cells frequently develop excess iron stores in major organs. Complications of iron overload include cardiac myopathies (pericarditis, arrhythmias, congestive heart failure), thyroid insufficiency, endocrine and pancreas malfunction (glucose intolerance), liver fibrosis, profound anemia, and skin discoloration. Cardiomyopathies related to iron overload are a frequent cause of death in the chronically transfused client.

Iron Chelating Agents. Deferoxamine (Desferal) is an iron chelating agent that can prevent iron overload when it is properly administered. However, the short half-life of this agent requires intravenous (IV) infusion over a prolonged period. A common treatment regimen is a continuous pump infusion 12 hours a day, 5 days a week. With new, lightweight infusion pumps, transfusions can be given without severely impairing mobility or they can be given overnight so the client is more independent.

Erythropoietin. Subcutaneous injections of erythropoietin can be given to treat anemia of chronic disease. For this to be effective, however, the client must have a bone marrow capable of producing red blood cells and sufficient nutrients to produce red blood cells.

Iron and Vitamin B_{12}. Iron and vitamin B_{12} can be given when the client has anemia due to deficiency of these elements.

Iron-Rich Diet. When the anemia is related to poor nutrition, or when the cause is blood loss, proper nutrition can improve red blood cell production. A diet high in iron, vitamin B_{12}, and folic acid will help increase red blood cell production if a deficiency of these nutrients is present.

■ Nursing Management of the Medical Client

The general nursing care of clients with anemia includes adequate assessment by the nurse to help identify the cause of the anemia and client education. The nurse can help in diagnosis by taking a complete health history focusing on the elements outlined in Chapter 52. Client teaching is extremely important in treating the anemias because most of the care will take place in the clinic or the client's home. The nurse must help the client become knowledgeable about self-care in both preventing and treating anemia.

Acquired Anemias

As stated in Chapter 52, effective erythropoiesis depends on adequate intake and proper assimilation of iron, vitamin B_{12}, folic acid, protein, pyridoxine, and traces of copper. The most common deficiency state is iron deficiency. In addition, deficiencies of vitamin B_{12} and folic acid are prevalent. Protein deficiency is also frequently seen. Pyridoxine (vitamin B_6) and copper deficiencies occur infrequently in humans.

Iron Deficiency Anemia

Iron deficiency anemia is defined as anemia associated with either inadequate absorption or excessive loss of iron; it is a chronic, microcytic, hypochromic anemia.

The worldwide incidence of iron deficiency anemia is high. It is common in countries where nutrition is poor; it is also prevalent in tropical zones and in the southern United States, Mexico, and Puerto Rico, where blood-sucking parasites such as the hookworm are endemic. The poor of all nations suffer far more frequently from iron deficiency than do the middle and upper classes.

Menstruating and pregnant women and young children also are vulnerable to iron deficiency, whereas adult men and postmenopausal women rarely develop this problem. Iron deficiency anemia also occurs with chronic blood loss.

Etiology and Risk Factors

Iron deficiency anemia is caused by an inadequate supply of iron needed to synthesize hemoglobin. This results in a decreased supply to the developing red blood cells of a crucial component of hemoglobin—iron—essential to the oxygen-carrying function of heme. When these disorders of heme synthesis become severe, the marrow produces red blood cells that are deficient in hemoglobin concentration and that are hypochromic and microcytic.

The major risk factors for iron deficiency anemia are blood loss and poor nutrition. An adequate intake of iron with normal absorption should prevent the disorder.

Pathophysiology

An average diet supplies the body with about 12 to 15 mg/day of iron, of which only 5% to 10% (0.6–1.5 mg) is absorbed. The amount of iron normally absorbed daily is sufficient for meeting the needs of women past childbearing age and healthy men. However, it does not meet the greater needs of menstruating and pregnant women, adolescents, children, and infants. These five groups must have a higher daily intake of iron for prevention of deficiency. Economic constraints, poor dentition, and lack of interest in food preparation commonly lead to iron deficiency in elderly people. Fortunately, the gastrointestinal tract can increase its absorption of iron from 10% daily to about 20% to 30% daily. In this way, the body often compensates for diminishing iron stores due to inadequate iron intake or excessive iron loss.

Iron is stored in the form of ferritin, an iron-phosphorus-protein complex that contains about 23% iron. It is formed in the intestinal mucosa when ferric iron joins with the protein apoferritin. Ferritin is stored in the tissues, primarily in the reticuloendothelial cells of the liver, spleen, and bone marrow.

Normal iron excretion is less than 1 mg/day. Iron is excreted in urine, sweat, bile, and feces and from the skin in desquamated cells. The average woman loses another 0.5 mg of iron daily or 15 mg monthly during menses. Menstruation is the most common cause of iron deficiency in women.

Gastrointestinal tract bleeding is a common etiologic factor in men; it may result from peptic ulcers, hiatal hernia, gastritis, cancer, hemorrhoids, diverticula, ulcerative colitis, or salicylate poisoning. It may also be associated with the use of aspirin, steroids, or nonsteroidal anti-inflammatory agents. Bleeding from the gastrointestinal tract is usually chronic and occult (too small to be seen). A chronic blood loss of as little as 2 to 4 ml/day can result in iron deficiency anemia, because every 2 ml of blood contains 1 mg of iron. The body can compensate for such losses to some degree by excreting less than 0.5 mg of iron daily rather than the normal 1 mg.

Alteration in the mucosa of the duodenum and proximal jejunum (as in chronic diarrhea, malabsorption syndromes such as celiac disease, and gastrectomy) affects iron absorption, predisposing to iron deficiency states. Tannates (in tea and coffee), carbonates, the chelating agent ethylenediaminetetraacetic acid (EDTA), and the medicinal antacid magnesium trisilicate all hinder non-heme iron absorption. Clay-eating (pica), a practice of women and children in socioeconomically disadvantaged areas, causes iron to precipitate as an insoluble substance within the intestinal tract.

Clinical Manifestations and Diagnostic Findings

In mild cases of iron deficiency anemia, the client is asymptomatic. However, in more severe cases, assessment reveals the general manifestations of anemia (e.g., palpitations, dizziness, and sensitivity to cold).

Later during the disease, hair and nails usually become brittle. In severe cases, dysphagia (difficulty in swallowing), stomatitis (inflammation of the mucosa of the mouth), and atrophic glossitis (the tongue is inflamed and smooth due to atrophy of papillae) may appear. This triad of manifestations is known as the Plummer-Vinson syndrome, a condition that primarily affects middle-aged women who have recently had their teeth extracted. Despite the weakness and discomfort associated with iron deficiency anemia, death rarely occurs unless severe cardiac complications develop.

Examinations of the blood and bone marrow form the basis for diagnosing iron deficiency anemia. Because they are deficient in hemoglobin, the red blood cells are small (microcytic) and pale (hypochromic), morphologic characteristics of iron deficiency. Other indications of anemia are a hemoglobin level decreased to as low as 6 to 9 g/dl; total red blood cell count moderately reduced, rarely dropping below 3 million cells/mm³, mean corpuscular volume (MCV), mean corpuscular hemoglobin (MCH), and mean corpuscular hemoglobin concentration (MCHC) reduced; serum iron level (normally 50–150 μg/dl) may be decreased to 10 μg/dl; total iron-binding capacity elevated to 350 to 500 μg/dl (normal is 250–350 μg/dl); hemosiderin (an insoluble form of storage iron) completely absent from the bone marrow; and immunoradiometric serum ferritin assay below normal.

Once the diagnosis of iron deficiency anemia is confirmed, studies are conducted to find the cause of the anemia. If gastrointestinal tract bleeding is suspected, approximate the amount of blood lost daily and the site of bleeding. X-ray studies (gastrointestinal tract series), stool examination for occult blood, esophagoscopy, gastroscopy, and sigmoidoscopy are commonly done to identify the site of blood loss.

Community and Self-Care

■ Medical Management

Therapeutic goals for clients with iron deficiency anemia are to (1) diagnose and correct the underlying cause of the anemia and (2) treat the iron deficit through diet and supplemental iron preparations.

Supplemental iron is usually administered to increase iron available in the blood. The medications of choice are ferrous sulfate (Feosol), 0.325 g orally three times a day with meals; ferrous gluconate (Fergon), 0.3 g orally twice a day; and iron dextran (Imferon), 100 to 250 mg intramuscularly. Figure 53–1 illustrates the Z-track technique for administration of iron dextran. Clients usually receive iron supplements for at least 6 months for repletion of the body stores.

Parenteral iron therapy is administered to clients who (1) have an intolerance to oral iron preparations, (2) habitually forget to take their medications, or (3) continue to suffer blood losses. Iron dextran is the parenteral drug of choice. The client typically feels more energetic and has an increased appetite within 48 hours. Peak reticulocytosis occurs about day 10. Red blood cell indices and hemoglobin content gradually return to normal. Because of the high risk of allergic reaction, if iron is to be given intravenously, the physician usually administers the first dose.

■ Nursing Management of the Medical Client

Assessment

Nursing assessment of iron deficiency anemia focuses on data collection of causative and risk factors, dietary history, family history, psychosocial problems, and medications. Common physical manifestations are integumentary—stomatitis; smooth red beefy tongue, cold sensitivity, brittle hair, and spoon-shaped brittle nails (*koilonchychia*); respiratory—dyspnea on exertion; cardiovascular—tachycardia; and neurologic—dizziness, dysphagia, numbness, tingling, decreased concentration, headache, and fatigue.

Diagnosis, Planning, Implementation

Altered Nutrition: Less than Body Requirements. Write the nursing diagnosis as *Altered Nutrition: Less than Body Requirements:* related to disease, treatment, or lack of knowledge of adequate nutrition.

Planning: Expected Outcomes. The client will have nutritional deficiencies corrected and optimal nutrition will be achieved, as evidenced by blood tests reaching normal range, improved tolerance for activity, and anemia resolved.

Implementation. Teach the basics of good nutrition; encourage a diet high in protein, iron, and vitamins with frequent small meals. Encourage foods cooked in iron pots and ingestion of foods such as liver (the richest source), oysters, lean meats, kidney beans, whole wheat bread, kale, spinach, egg yolk, turnip tops, beet greens, carrots, apricots, and raisins. Document the client's weight. Encourage good oral hygiene.

Risk for Ineffective Management of Therapeutic Regimen (Individuals). The nursing diagnosis *Risk for Ineffective Management of Therapeutic Regimen (Individuals)* is related to the client's ability to care for himself or herself and take iron preparations.

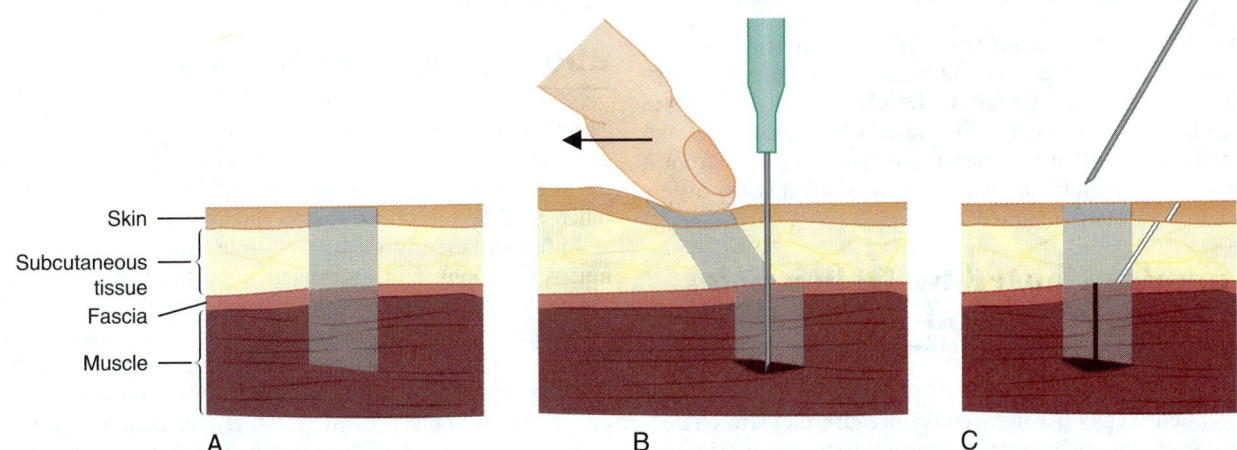

Figure 53–1. Z-track technique used for administration of iron dextran. *A,* Normal tissue relationships before injection. *B,* Altered tissue relationships during injection. Retract tissue, insert needle, administer medication, remove needle, and release tissue. *C,* Normal tissue relationships after injection. Note angled Z-track left by needle.

Planning: Expected Outcomes. The client will verbalize correct dosage of, route of, and indications for iron preparations, as evidenced by correct administration of iron medications and no complications developing.

Implementation. Inform the client that iron salts are gastric irritants and should always be taken after meals. Liquid iron preparations should be well diluted and taken through a straw (undiluted liquid iron stains teeth). Constipation, commonly seen during iron therapy, will be avoided by a high fiber diet and use of stool softeners or laxatives as required.

To administer parenteral iron medications as ordered, see Figure 53–1. Iron dextran causes darkening and discoloration of the skin around the injection site unless it is administered properly. Therefore, when administering this medication:

- Use one needle to withdraw iron dextran and another needle to administer it; thus, staining from iron that adheres to the needle is avoided.
- Give the injection with a 2- or 3-inch, 19- or 20-gauge needle, deep into the upper outer quadrant of the buttock. Never use the arm or any other exposed area.
- Use the Z-track and air-lock injection techniques to prevent medication leakage.
- Never massage the site of injection.
- Throughout therapy, observe for pain at the injection site, abscesses, lymphadenitis, fever, headache, urticaria, hypotension, and anaphylactic shock.

The client will have to be followed with frequent blood counts to determine whether the anemia is resolving. Once the anemia has resolved, the client will still need to be followed to ensure that the anemia does not recur.

Evaluation

Resolution of anemia requires time and the eventual evaluation will be that the client's anemia is resolved and did not recur. It takes weeks for anemia to resolve, so the client will need assessments at intervals to monitor the progress of therapy.

■ Modifications for Elderly Clients

The older client is more prone to iron deficiency anemia because of poor nutritional intake and a decreased absorption of iron in the intestine. Older clients will also require complete assessment for diagnosis of the cause of the anemia. They often experience chronic blood loss from a variety of diseases that also may cause anemia, so differential diagnosis is required.

Anemias Caused by Deficiencies of Vitamin B_{12} and Folic Acid

Anemias due to deficiencies of vitamin B_{12} and folic acid are called megaloblastic anemias because they are characterized by the appearance of megaloblasts (large primitive red blood cells) in the blood and bone marrow.

Other common features of the megaloblastic anemias are leukopenia (decrease in white blood cells) and throm-bocytopenia (decrease in platelets); oral, gastrointestinal, and neurologic manifestations; and favorable response to injections of either vitamin B_{12} or folic acid.

The underlying defect in the megaloblastic anemias is disturbed DNA synthesis. Deficiencies of either vitamin B_{12} or folic acid impede the formation of DNA precursors, which causes abnormal maturation of red blood cells, leukocytes, and platelets. The same basic etiologic factors—dietary inadequacies, impaired absorption, and metabolic disturbances—underlie both vitamin B_{12} and folic acid deficiency. In the former, the diet is deficient in meat and dairy products; in the latter, vegetables are lacking.

The principal cause of impaired vitamin B_{12} absorption is intrinsic factor deficiency. The small intestine cannot absorb vitamin B_{12} (extrinsic factor) unless intrinsic factor (i.e., a substance of internal origin) combines with it. When intrinsic factor is missing, pernicious anemia develops. Conditions such as tapeworm, overgrowth of intestinal bacteria, or intestinal diverticula may also impair vitamin B_{12} absorption. Folic acid antagonists, anticonvulsants, or liver disease may inhibit folic acid uptake. Intestinal malabsorption of both vitamins may result from any of a group of disorders such as sprue, celiac disease, steatorrhea, or surgical resection of the small intestine. Metabolic changes, such as those that occur in hyperthyroidism, pregnancy, or cancer, can lead to additional requirements for both vitamin B_{12} and folic acid.

Pernicious Anemia

Pernicious anemia is a type of anemia due to failure of absorption of vitamin B_{12}. It is the most prevalent form of vitamin B_{12} deficiency in the United States and Canada. The most common megaloblastic anemia, pernicious anemia occurs in only 0.1% of the population. It mainly strikes men and women age of 50 to 70 years and primarily people of northern European origin. Occasionally, it develops in southern Europeans, Asians, and blacks. Although rare, juvenile pernicious anemia has been found in children under 10 years of age. Juvenile pernicious anemia is a congenital disorder in which the stomach secretes abnormal intrinsic factor.

Etiology and Risk Factors

This chronic, progressive, megaloblastic anemia of adults is caused by a deficiency of intrinsic factor. Lack of intrinsic factor due to atrophy of the stomach's glandular mucosa is the basic defect in pernicious anemia.

Although heredity may play a role, the exact reason for mucosal atrophy and associated hypochlorhydria remains unknown. Pernicious anemia may be inherited as a single dominant autosomal factor. Prolonged iron deficiency, which may cause gastric atrophy, is a second possible predisposing factor. However, pernicious anemia may also be an autoimmune disorder. Ninety percent of persons with pernicious anemia have autoantibodies that react specifically against parietal gastric cells, and 60% have anti-intrinsic factor antibody.

One major risk factor for the development of pernicious anemias is gastric resection. The parietal cells in the stomach secrete the intrinsic factor required for vitamin B_{12} absorption. The disease can also be congenital as a result of absence of intrinsic factor.

Pathophysiology

The four major characteristics of pernicious anemia are the following:

1. Abnormally large red blood cells (macrocytic anemia)
2. Hypochlorhydria (deficiency of gastric hydrochloric acid)
3. Neurologic and gastrointestinal manifestations
4. A fatal outcome unless the client receives lifelong injections of vitamin B_{12}

Unless it is controlled with vitamin B_{12}, pernicious anemia inevitably develops after total gastrectomy. Also, 15% of clients develop pernicious anemia after partial gastrectomy or gastrojejunostomy for a peptic ulcer.

Pathologic consequences of vitamin B_{12} deficiency are macrocytic anemia and gastrointestinal disorders. Both problems respond to injections of vitamin B_{12}. Clients with pernicious anemia have a high incidence of benign gastric polyps and gastric carcinoma; they require routine assessment for gastric bleeding and tumor growth.

Lack of vitamin B_{12} also alters the structure and disrupts the function of the peripheral nerves, spinal cord, and brain. Thus, the third major consequence of this disorder is disturbed nervous system function and, in extreme cases, permanent neurologic damage unresponsive to vitamin B_{12} therapy. Central nervous system manifestations, such as paresthesias of the hands and feet and problems with balance and gait, develop in three fourths of clients with pernicious anemia. Clients with this anemia tend to be fair-haired or prematurely gray.

Untreated pernicious anemia causes death; delayed intervention results in permanent disabilities. In addition to the nervous system damage already mentioned, severe macrocytic anemia of long duration can trigger congestive heart failure and angina pectoris in the elderly.

Clinical Manifestations and Diagnostic Findings

The major manifestations of pernicious anemia are low hemoglobin, hematocrit, and red blood cell levels. Diagnosis of pernicious anemia is based on the presence of anemia, gastrointestinal manifestations, and neurologic disorders; laboratory blood and bone marrow tests; the absence of gastric hydrochloric acid; and a favorable response to a vitamin B_{12} "therapeutic trial."

Low hemoglobin levels and consequent hypoxemia may trigger congestive heart failure because of increased demands on the heart to transport oxygen to the tissues. Angina pectoris also may develop from insufficient oxygenation of the myocardium.

Laboratory findings that confirm a diagnosis of pernicious anemia include the following:

● Red blood cells are usually decreased to less than 3

million/mm³, MCV and MCHC are likely to be elevated, with white blood cells and MCH decreased.
● On peripheral blood smear, red blood cells are oval, macrocytic, and hyperchromic.
● The bone marrow contains high numbers of megaloblasts (a precursor of red blood cells in an abnormal blood erythropoietic process).
● Unconjugated bilirubin (a product of hemoglobin breakdown) is usually elevated due to hemolysis of defective red blood cells.
● Serum lactate dehydrogenase is extremely high. (Lactate dehydrogenase is an enzyme present in many tissues that is released into the circulation when tissues are damaged.)
● The Schilling test measures the absorption of orally administered radioactive vitamin B_{12} (tagged with cobalt 60) before and after parenteral administration of intrinsic factor. This procedure detects lack of intrinsic factor and is the definitive test for pernicious anemia.
● Gastric secretion analysis to check for the presence of free hydrochloric acid is another important test; most clients with pernicious anemia have low-volume gastric secretions with a high pH and free hydrochloric acid. Furthermore, these findings do not change, even after the administration of histamine, which normally stimulates gastric secretion.

Community and Self-Care

■ Medical Management

Vitamin B_{12}. Clients with pernicious anemia need both immediate treatment and lifelong therapy with maintenance vitamin B_{12}. During the acute phase of illness, the client may be given vitamin B_{12} injections. The response to vitamin B_{12} injections is usually quick and dramatic, often occurring within 24 to 48 hours. Within 72 hours, reticulocytes begin to increase; by the end of the first week, the total red blood cell count rises significantly. Cardiovascular involvement usually lessens with improved erythropoiesis. Although peripheral nerve function may improve with treatment, spinal cord and brain damage usually persist.

Iron Supplements. Additionally, the client may need oral iron supplementation if the hemoglobin level fails to rise in proportion to an increased red blood cell count. As stated earlier, iron deficiency may be an etiologic factor in pernicious anemia and must be corrected if it is present. Iron deficiency anemia can also develop during treatment of pernicious anemia. Injections of vitamin B_{12} may cause a rapid regeneration of red blood cells that depletes iron. As a result, the hemoglobin level remains low, although the total red blood cell count rises.

Folic Acid. Folic acid is sometimes given with vitamin B_{12} to clients with a history of poor nutrition. Folic acid can be dangerous, however, because it may intensify neurologic problems and large doses of folate may obscure a vitamin B_{12} deficiency. Therefore, a therapeutic trial of folate should never be given without pernicious anemia first being ruled out.

Digestants. Digestants (to enhance metabolism of vitamins), such as hydrochloric acid diluted in water and given with meals, are often used during the first few weeks of vitamin B_{12} therapy.

Blood Transfusions. Blood transfusions are usually unnecessary, because clients with pernicious anemia respond to vitamin B_{12} injections. Occasionally, however, blood transfusions may be life-saving.

Nutritional Support. The client should be encouraged to eat a diet high in folic acid and iron to supplement the medication used to treat the anemia. If the cause involves altered absorption of vitamin B_{12}, then nutritional supplements are useless. If the disease is related to decreased intake of the vitamin, then a diet high in vitamin B_{12} is encouraged.

■ Nursing Management of the Medical Client

Once the acute stage of the illness is past, the client with pernicious anemia must undertake a lifelong program of maintenance therapy. Monthly injections of vitamin B_{12} are needed to avoid relapse. The nurse plays a vital role in educating clients with this disorder on the importance of continuous care.

In addition to medications, clients with permanent neurologic disabilities need an intensive program of physical therapy and rehabilitation. Because clients with pernicious anemia are at risk of developing gastric carcinoma, encourage them to see their physician at least twice a year for a complete physical examination.

If therapy remains adequate and uninterrupted, the client with pernicious anemia can expect a life free of anemic manifestations, without further manifestations of neuropathy.

Other Anemias Due to Vitamin B_{12} Deficiency

Whereas pernicious anemia arises from lack of intrinsic factor, another group of anemias results from lack of extrinsic factor (vitamin B_{12}). This problem may be caused by faulty diet, defective absorption from intestinal disease, or by a metabolic disturbance. The megaloblastic anemia that characterizes these conditions is the same as that seen in pernicious anemia. However, hypochlorhydria and degenerative neurologic changes do not occur.

Treatment of vitamin B_{12} deficiency depends on the cause. Oral administration of 25 μg of vitamin B_{12} daily, with a more balanced diet, corrects inadequate dietary intake.

Extremely deficient diets are rarely seen in developed countries except among the very poor who cannot afford meat and among some vegetarians. However, inadequate diets are common in India and other countries with large populations of poor people.

Poor absorption of vitamin B_{12} results from (1) an overgrowth of intestinal bacteria due to intestinal stasis, (2) infestation with the fish tapeworm, or (3) one of the malabsorption syndromes such as sprue and celiac disease. Bacteria that proliferate within intestinal blind loops and diverticula (small blind pouches that form in the walls of the colon) compete with the host for available vitamin B_{12}. This problem can be corrected by (1) surgical removal of the pouches or blind loops and (2) administration of broad-spectrum antibiotics to control infection. The tapeworm eaten in raw fish also competes with its host for vitamin B_{12}. Treatment involves removal of the tapeworm and the temporary administration of vitamin B_{12} until the anemia resolves.

Treatment of anemia caused by malabsorption syndromes (e.g., sprue and celiac disease) consists of administering 100 μg of vitamin B_{12} intramuscularly daily for 10 days followed by 100 μg of vitamin B_{12} monthly until the absorption dysfunction clears.

Clients who have an increased need for the vitamin because of metabolic changes (e.g., in pregnancy or hyperthyroidism) may take oral vitamin B_{12} as a supplement.

Anemia Due to Folic Acid Deficiency

Anemia associated with folic acid deficiency is very common. This condition has many causes, most of which are the same as the causes of vitamin B_{12} deficiency. Usually, folic acid deficiency results from a diet lacking in such foods as green leafy vegetables, liver, citrus fruits, and yeast. Clients with chronic alcoholism, because of their typically inadequate diets, are particularly susceptible to this problem. High levels of alcohol in the blood also partially block the response of the bone marrow to folic acid, which thereby interferes with erythropoiesis.

Folic acid deficiency, like vitamin B_{12} deficiency, can develop with malabsorption syndromes (e.g., sprue, celiac disease, steatorrhea). Certain medications can also impede folic acid absorption and utilization. For example, a serious anemia may develop with (1) the long-term use of anticonvulsant medications (e.g., primidone, diphenylhydantoin, and phenobarbital), (2) the administration of antimetabolites (e.g., folic acid antagonists, purine and pyrimidine analogs) to clients with cancer and leukemia, or (3) the administration of certain oral contraceptives.

Finally, folic acid deficiency may occur with increased demands for folate, such as during the growth spurts of infancy and adolescence. During the third trimester of pregnancy, expectant mothers need six times the normal amount of folic acid because of the increased demands of the developing fetus.

Folic acid, like vitamin B_{12}, is necessary for DNA synthesis. Both vitamin B_{12} and folic acid deficiencies cause manifestations of megaloblastic anemia (fatigue, cardiac manifestations, slight jaundice) and gastrointestinal tract disturbances (e.g., dyspepsia; smooth, beefy tongue). However, unlike pernicious anemia, folic acid deficiency does not cause neurologic manifestations.

Anemia due to folic acid deficiency has a slow and insidious onset. The client, often thin and emaciated, usually appears quite ill. The client's malnourished and debilitated state frequently leads to other deficiencies, for example, of iron, protein, minerals, and other vitamins. Some clients may also have an electrolyte imbalance and may develop neurologic manifestations as a result of thiamine, calcium, or magnesium deficiencies (problems frequently linked with alcoholism). Cirrhosis of the liver and bleeding varices further complicate anemia for the alcoholic client. Women planning a pregnancy should increase intake of folic acid before the pregnancy to prevent neural tube defects.

The megaloblastic anemia caused by folic acid deficiency is the same as that seen in pernicious anemia. It is diagnosed by blood smear and bone marrow examinations. On confirmation of macrocytic anemia, the physician must decide whether it results from folic acid or vitamin B_{12} deficiency. In folic acid deficiency, the serum folate level is less than 4 ng/ml (normal is 7–20 ng/ml): the Schilling test is normal; hydrochloric acid is probably present in the gastric juice; neurologic manifestations are absent; and the client responds favorably to a therapeutic trial of 50 to 100 μg folic acid administered intramuscularly daily for 10 days.

For correction of anemia due to folate deficiency, the client receives oral doses of folic acid 0.1–5.0 mg/day until the blood picture improves or until the cause of intestinal malabsorption is corrected. Clients with malabsorption syndromes may need parenteral folic acid initially, followed by maintenance therapy with oral doses.

Folic acid is administered intramuscularly in the form of folinic acid (leucovorin calcium injection). Additionally, vitamin C is sometimes prescribed because it increases the role of folic acid in promoting erythropoiesis.

Anemias Due to Bone Marrow Failure

The anemias due to bone marrow failure have several names, each of which is descriptive of some aspect of the disease (aplastic, hypoplastic, regenerative, or primary refractory anemia). *Aplastic anemia,* the most commonly used term, describes bone marrow that is severely hypoplastic (underdeveloped), that is, devoid of erythroid, myeloid, and megakaryocytic cell lines. Hypoplastic bone marrow results in anemia, leukopenia, and thrombocytopenia. When all three cellular elements are suppressed, the condition is known as pancytopenia.

Aplastic anemia affects people of all ages, and both sexes are equally susceptible. The incidence of aplastic anemia is about four cases per million population. Congenital aplastic anemia (Fanconi's anemia) usually occurs in childhood.

Etiology and Risk Factors

In about half of cases, the cause of aplastic anemia is unknown. Acquired aplastic anemia may result from either an autoimmune mechanism or a direct injury by myelotoxins. Three groups of myelotoxins are (1) agents that always cause marrow damage when received in sufficiently large doses, such as radiant energy (x-rays, radium, and radioactive isotopes of gold or phosphorus), benzene and its derivatives, alkylating agents, and antimetabolites used to treat malignant tumors; (2) agents that occasionally cause marrow failure, such as chloramphenicol (Chloromycetin, the drug most commonly linked with aplastic anemia), sulfonamides, quinacrine, phenylbutazone, the anticonvulsants diphenylhydantoin and mephenytoin, and gold compounds; and (3) agents that have been linked with aplastic anemia in only a few cases, such as streptomycin, tripelennamine, DDT, meprobamate, hair and aniline dyes, and carbon tetrachloride. Some of the newer psychotropic medications can cause neutropenia. Occupational exposure to many of these agents should also be considered. If clients are receiving or expected to receive any of these agents, they must have their blood count monitored at frequent intervals.

Pathophysiology

The etiologic agents cause the bone marrow to stop producing blood cells when radiant energy inhibits mitosis, or cell division, and antimetabolites used in cancer therapy block the synthesis of purines or nucleic acids. Usually, however, the mechanism of marrow failure from these agents is unknown. Why certain drugs and chemicals cause pancytopenia in some clients and not in others also is mysterious. Current thought is that some clients are hypersensitive to certain agents, and the development of bone marrow failure in these cases is an idiosyncratic reaction.

The onset of aplastic anemia may be insidious or rapid. In idiopathic or hereditary cases, the onset is usually gradual. When bone marrow failure results from a myelotoxin, however, the onset may be explosive, with quickly developing manifestations. If the condition does not reverse itself when the offending agent is removed, it can be fatal.

Clinical Manifestations and Diagnostic Findings

Manifestations of pancytopenia are particularly severe. Not only does the red blood cell count fall, but so do the leukocyte and platelet counts. The client consequently develops the following three conditions: (1) normocytic anemia, (2) neutropenia, and (3) thrombocytopenia.

■ Normocytic Anemia

The red blood cell count is usually below 1 million/mm³, with a low reticulocyte count. The client reports progressive fatigue, lassitude, and dyspnea.

■ Neutropenia

The leukocyte count may be less than 1000/mm³ (normal is 5000–10,000/mm³). The client, therefore, suffers from an increased susceptibility to infection, because without leukocytes, the body cannot adequately battle bacteria and other invading organisms. If the absolute neutrophil count (ANC) drops below 500/mm³, the client may develop a fulminating bacterial infection, often from the client's own normal flora. The ANC is calculated by multiplying the total white blood cell count by the percentage of neutrophils. Many health professionals use the terms *neutropenia* and *granulocytopenia* interchangeably although neutropenia is a more precise term.

■ Thrombocytopenia

The platelet count may fall below 30,000 to 15,000/mm³ (normal is 150,000–450,000/mm³), which usually causes bleeding into the skin and mucous membranes. The client is also at risk of retinal hemorrhage and intracranial hemorrhage. If platelets are severely reduced, the client may hemorrhage spontaneously.

The diagnosis of aplastic anemia and pancytopenia is based on the differential blood count, the client's manifestations, history of exposure to a myelotoxin, and bone marrow examination. In pancytopenia, the bone marrow is fatty and contains very few developing blood cells.

Acute and Subacute Care

■ Medical Management

The client with pancytopenia is often critically ill. Prompt medical attention and skillful nursing care are necessary. The first step in halting the process of aplastic anemia is immediate withdrawal of the offending agent or drug.

Any client undergoing radiotherapy or receiving a medication that is a suspected myelotoxin must be monitored for marrow failure by frequent complete blood counts (CBCs). A significant drop in the red blood cell, leukocyte, or platelet count signals the need to stop the drug. Usually, stopping a suspicious agent is followed by a rise in the blood count. Unfortunately, chloramphenicol marrow failure may progress despite discontinuation of the drug.

If aplastic anemia develops from a suspected myelotoxic agent, blood transfusions are the mainstay of therapy until bone marrow activity signals recovery. If the marrow fails to recover and long-term red blood cell support is required, iron overload often results. This complication was a leading cause of death before iron chelating therapy became available.

Bone marrow transplantation is now the treatment of choice in aplastic anemia when (1) an autoimmune phenomenon is suspected or (2) the bone marrow fails to regenerate after discontinuation of myelotoxic agents. Currently, transplantation can take place only if the client has an HLA (human leukocyte antigen)-matched donor.

Because the marrow of the aplastic client is so severely depressed, cellular blood components should be irradiated prior to transfusion to inactivate lymphocytes and prevent transfusion-associated graft-versus-host disease (GVHD) (see Chapter 27).

Comparing the results of clients treated by bone marrow transplantation with conventional therapy of steroids and androgens reveals a 2-year survival rate of 60% to 80% with bone marrow transplantation versus 25% for those treated conventionally.

Corticosteroids and androgens are sometimes prescribed to stimulate bone marrow activity; unfortunately, these drugs often fail to work as desired or produce only transient increases.

■ Nursing Management of the Medical Client

Preventing and treating complications resulting from pancytopenia is of major importance in caring for the client with aplastic anemia. The two main complications of this anemia are infection and bleeding.

Hemolytic Anemias

Major hallmarks of hemolytic anemia are the following:

- A shortening of the red blood cell life span
- An abnormal increase in the number of red blood cells destroyed by macrophages
- Failure of the bone marrow to replace destroyed red blood cells

Premature hemolysis of red blood cells results from either (1) an intracorpuscular defect within the erythrocyte itself, a defect that is sometimes triggered by an extracellular agent (e.g., drugs, plasma components, or splenic hyperactivity); or (2) an extracorpuscular factor (e.g., infections and chemical or physical agents).

Hemolytic anemia may be acute or chronic. Severe, acute episodes of hemolysis, known as hemolytic crises, punctuate some chronic forms of hemolytic anemia. The client with hemolytic anemia suffers from all the general manifestations of anemia discussed earlier (lassitude, fatigue, etc.). The clinical manifestations that characterize hemolytic anemia are listed and the pathophysiology is explained in Table 53–1. Renal failure may be a complication of severe hemolysis. It is caused by excretion of an increased load of red blood cell degradation products.

Laboratory findings indicative of hemolytic anemia usually include normocytic anemia, reticulocytosis due to increased efforts of the bone marrow to compensate for excessive erythrocyte destruction, increased red blood cell fragility, shortened erythrocyte life span, hyperbilirubinemia, increased fecal and urinary urobilinogen, and (in cases of massive intravascular hemolysis) hemoglobinemia.

Treatment of hemolytic anemia includes the following steps.

1. Pinpoint and eliminate, whenever possible, causative factors that precipitate episodes of hemolysis (e.g., infections, exposure to certain chemicals).
2. Maintain fluid and electrolyte balance.

Table 53–1. Hemolytic Anemia: Clinical Manifestations and Pathophysiologic Bases

Clinical Manifestation	Pathophysiologic Bases
Jaundice	Accumulation of bilirubin within the blood due to excessive destruction of erythrocytes
Splenomegaly, hepatomegaly	Macrophages within the spleen and liver become hyperactive because of increased demands to phagocytose defective erythrocytes
Cholelithiasis (pigment gallstones)	Excessive accumulation of bilirubin within the gallbladder due to erythrocyte destruction

3. Administer oxygen, because a decreased number of red blood cells may cause hypoxia.
4. Maintain renal function. In cases of severe hemolysis, infusions of either sodium bicarbonate or sodium lactate are administered to alkalize the urine, which decreases the likelihood of precipitation in the renal tubules.
5. Combat anemia and shock with the cautious administration of blood transfusions. Caution is necessary because the transfused cells are rapidly destroyed in the presence of autoimmune hemolytic disease.
6. If corticosteroids fail to halt hemolytic reactions in autoimmune disorders, splenectomy is usually the treatment of choice.

The major extracorpuscular factors that cause hemolytic anemia include trauma, chemical agents and medications, infectious agents, systemic disease, isoimmune reactions, and autoimmune disorders.

Hemolysis Caused by Trauma

When red blood cells are exposed to excessive turbulence in the circulation, they may fragment. Fragmented erythrocytes (schistocytes) are quickly destroyed by phagocytes, which results in anemia.

Hemolytic anemia may develop after external trauma or severe burns. In addition, hemolysis sometimes occurs after prosthetic cardiac valve replacement or cardiac septal defect repair.

Clinical findings include hemoglobinemia, hemoglobinuria, and a drop in the erythrocyte count. Treatment is directed toward correcting the underlying problem.

Hemolysis Caused by Chemical Agents and Medications

Hemolytic reactions are usually due to one of the following factors: the oxidant effects of the medication or chemical, or an immune reaction caused by the medication. Chemical oxidants vary in their potency and in their ability to destroy red blood cells. Some mild chemical oxidants cause hemolytic reactions in a small segment of the world population (e.g., people with glucose-6-phosphate dehydrogenase [G6PD] deficiency). Other, very potent oxidants cause hemolytic reactions in anybody exposed to a sufficient amount (e.g., benzene, phenylhydrazine, nitrites, potassium chlorate, arsenic, colloidal silver, lead). These powerful compounds can damage the red blood cell membrane, resulting in a fragile cell that is quickly destroyed.

A common example of hemolysis due to contact with a chemical agent is lead poisoning (plumbism). Lead poisoning causes characteristic changes in the brain, nervous system, spinal cord, and digestive tract. Industrial workers who are exposed daily to lead vapors, mist, or dust may become victims of plumbism. Also, small children develop lead poisoning if they chew on furniture or windowsills covered with lead-based paint. Flakes of lead-based paint found in older, deteriorating buildings also are a hazard.

Between 1976 and 1980 in the United States, the mean blood lead level declined by about 35%, apparently because of the reduced use of leaded gasoline, stricter controls in industry, and the growth of widespread screening programs. Nevertheless, researchers estimate that 1.5 million Americans are exposed to potentially dangerous levels of lead while on the job. Clinicians have also discovered that blood lead levels once thought safe and even normal are dangerous and result in many metabolic and neurologic disorders. A lead level higher than 40 μg/dl in adults and 25 μg/dl in children now is considered unsafe. Treatment in this condition usually involves administration of chelating agents such as edetate calcium disodium.

An immune response, the second major cause of toxic hemolysis, is the result of an antigen-antibody reaction (see Chapter 26). Medications that can precipitate antigen-antibody reactions in susceptible persons are quinine, quinidine, methyldopa, sulfonamides, phenacetin, and penicillin.

The most common example of an immune response to a drug is the "penicillin reaction." Penicillin is a potentially dangerous drug because it is a hapten. A hapten is a substance that is normally nonantigenic but can combine with a body protein. When penicillin combines with a body protein, the protein is modified so it can act as a foreign antigen. The body builds antibodies that react with the altered body protein in an antigen-antibody reaction. Because of the danger of triggering an immune response, always take a careful medication history before administering any medication (e.g., penicillin) that is a hapten.

Finally, certain snake and spider venoms, as well as some vegetable poisons and fungi (e.g., some mushrooms), cause hemolytic reactions that frequently are fatal.

Hemolysis Caused by Infectious Agents

Bacterial endocarditis, malaria, miliary tuberculosis, infectious hepatitis, infectious mononucleosis, gram-negative sepsis, and meningococcemia may be complicated by hemolytic anemia. Infectious organisms can cause hemolytic anemia in three ways: (1) by releasing toxins that cause hemolysis; (2) by entering the red blood cell and destroying it; and (3) by promoting antigen-antibody reactions. For example, an organism may attach itself to the surface of a red blood cell, so altering it that it acts as a foreign antigen. In response, antibodies form against the altered red blood cells, and an immune reaction takes place.

Hemolysis Caused by Systemic Disease

Hemolytic anemia sometimes complicates the following systemic conditions: Hodgkin's disease, leukemias, renal cortical necrosis, lymphomas, and systemic lupus erythematosus.

Hemolysis Caused by Isoimmune Hemolytic Reactions

An isoimmune hemolytic reaction is an antigen-antibody reaction that destroys red blood cells. Antibodies develop in response to antigens from another individual of the same species. An example is a transfusion reaction due to ABO incompatibility. The most severe transfusion reactions involve hemolysis of the donor's red blood cells by the recipient's antibodies. Erythroblastosis fetalis, a disorder of the newborn, is an example of a hemolytic isoimmune reaction resulting from incompatibility between the blood of an Rh-positive fetus and an Rh-negative mother.

Hemolysis Caused by Autoimmune Disorders

Autoantibodies, like isoantibodies, can destroy red blood cells. Unlike isoantibodies, they arise in response to autoantigens that have developed within the client's own body.

Autoimmune hemolytic anemia is a disorder of the immune mechanism in which the immune system produces antibodies that agglutinate the client's own red blood cells in an antigen-antibody reaction. As a result, the agglutinated cells are phagocytosed within the spleen.

This condition arises in two ways. First, it may develop secondary to other autoimmune disorders or follow the administration of certain drugs. Autoimmune conditions such as systemic lupus erythematosus and the lymphoproliferative diseases (leukemia, lymphoma) are sometimes complicated by hemolytic anemia.

Second, this disease can develop spontaneously without a history of prior autoimmune disease. This form, known as idiopathic autoimmune anemia, is characterized by a mild-to-moderate hemolysis; the red blood cells become coated with IgG antibodies that arise spontaneously or after ingestion of one of the above-mentioned medications.

The manifestations of autoimmune hemolytic anemia differ little from those of other hemolytic anemias. Pro-

found, sporadic, and sometimes fatal hemolytic crises are common. Other complications include gallstones and thrombocytopenic purpura. Autoimmune hemolytic anemia is diagnosed by a positive direct antiglobulin test. The direct antiglobulin test detects whether the client's red blood cells are coated with antibodies.

Treatment of secondary autoimmune hemolytic anemia includes treating the underlying autoimmune condition and stopping the use of any suspicious medications. The idiopathic form of the disease is treated with steroids, transfusions, and splenectomy when indicated. The steroid of choice is prednisolone. Recently, clients refractory to steroids have been treated with immunosuppressive agents (e.g., cyclophosphamide and azathioprine) with some success.

Transfusion may give temporary relief from manifestations. However, special crossmatching is required because clients often have developed sensitivities to many blood antigens, and donor cells may be rapidly destroyed by the client's antibodies. Administer red blood cells slowly, and be aware of the chance of an immediate transfusion reaction (see discussion under Blood Transfusions).

Splenectomy is indicated if medications fail to produce a remission or if steroid therapy produces severe side effects. Once the spleen is removed, recurrences of hemolytic anemia may develop, but they are less severe and can be controlled with steroid therapy.

Paroxysmal Hemoglobinemias

Paroxysmal hemoglobinuria is a rare but serious condition involving acute episodes of intravascular hemolysis that result in passing of hemoglobin into the urine.

Episodes of paroxysmal hemoglobinuria mass occur chiefly at night (paroxysmal nocturnal hemoglobinuria), follow exposure to cold temperatures (paroxysmal cold hemoglobinuria), or after extreme exertion, as in running a marathon or marching (march hemoglobinuria).

Paroxysmal nocturnal hemoglobinuria (PNH), the most common of these three conditions, produces severe manifestations (e.g., jaundice, chronic fatigue, scleral icterus, and splenomegaly). In addition, the client's urine often has a dark-brown or port-wine color after sleep. If hemoglobinuria continues for days or weeks, substantial iron losses eventually result in iron deficiency anemia.

Laboratory results in PNH include the following: red blood cell count indicating normocytic anemia, increased reticulocyte count, increased red blood cell fragility, and shortened red blood cell life span; increased bilirubin; increased fecal and urinary urobilinogen; and bone marrow hyperplasia.

Treatment of PNH is symptomatic. Most clients with PNH eventually require blood transfusions. Donor red blood cells initially survive normally and suppress the production of the client's abnormal red blood cells, with resultant marked clinical improvement. After repetitive transfusions, however, alloimmunization is likely to occur, which makes further transfusion therapy difficult. If evidence of increased hemolysis follows transfusion of packed donor red blood cells, administration of washed, frozen red blood cells, or leukocyte-poor blood may stop this problem. Clients with iron deficiency anemia also receive iron.

The course of PNH is exceedingly variable. Clients experience waxing and waning hemolysis, which may be exacerbated by infection, transfusion, and immunization. Although a client with PNH may have a normal life span, debilitating attacks of hemolytic anemia can occur at any time. Many clients lead an active, normal life between attacks.

Secondary Anemias

The secondary anemias, as the name implies, arise in association with other conditions. These include the following:

1. Chronic systemic disease (e.g., rheumatoid arthritis, leukemia)
2. The lymphomas and multiple myeloma
3. Chronic infections (lung abscess, empyema, pelvic inflammatory disease)
4. Acute and chronic renal disease complicated by uremia
5. Cirrhosis of the liver
6. Endocrine disorders (myxedema)
7. Cancer

Although the cause of the secondary anemia varies according to the primary condition, all have two factors in common: (1) the red blood cells have a shortened life span, and (2) the bone marrow fails to produce enough red blood cells to compensate for losses.

The anemia that develops in these conditions may be moderate to severe, depending on the associated condition, and treatment involves correcting the condition. Packed red blood cell transfusions are sometimes given when hemoglobin levels fall below 8 to 9 g/dl.

Hemorrhagic Anemias

Acute Hemorrhagic Anemia

Acute hemorrhagic anemia is a normocytic, normochromic anemia that develops after rapid loss of red blood cells from hemorrhage.

Common causes of acute bleeding are severed blood vessels due to trauma, spontaneous rupture of an aneurysm, hemorrhagic disorders, and erosion of an artery by a cancerous growth or ulcerative lesion.

The adverse effects of acute hemorrhage result from a rapid decrease in blood volume and red blood cells: the oxygen-carrying capacity of the blood is reduced. The severity of the manifestations of and the prognosis for acute hemorrhage depend on (1) the rate of bleeding, (2) the site of the hemorrhage, and (3) the volume of blood lost. A gradual loss of even a large amount of blood is usually less threatening than the rapid loss of a smaller volume.

Manifestations of acute blood loss are restlessness, dizziness, syncope, thirst, pallor, diaphoresis, rapid thready pulse, a dramatic drop in blood pressure, rapid deep respirations that later become shallow, and disorientation or coma indicative of cerebral hypoxia or anoxia.

In addition to these manifestations, internal hemorrhage into body organs and tissues causes fever, pain in the area of bleeding due to distention of tissues, and manifestations of organ displacement (e.g., hemothorax can result in a mediastinal shift). If internal or external hemorrhage remains uncontrolled, the blood pressure continues to drop, and hypovolemic shock develops (see Chapter 22).

After hemorrhage, the red blood cell count, hematocrit, and hemoglobin values appear to be high (although they are actually low) because of vasoconstriction and loss of plasma volume. These tests return to a lower level after infusion of IV fluid and restoration of intravascular volume from extracellular fluids.

Chronic Hemorrhagic Anemia

Chronic hemorrhagic anemia is a microcytic, hypochromic anemia, following chronic loss of blood.

The major causes of chronic blood loss are bleeding peptic ulcers, prolonged or excessive menses, bleeding hemorrhoids, and cancerous lesions within the gastrointestinal tract.

The results of chronic bleeding are (1) continuous loss of small numbers of erythrocytes, usually replaced by the bone marrow; and (2) continuous loss of iron, which results in a total depletion of iron stores.

Because of this iron loss, the anemia of chronic bleeding closely resembles iron deficiency anemia. Correction of the anemia involves locating and controlling the site of bleeding and replacing iron with a proper diet and iron supplements.

Manifestations of anemia due to chronic blood loss are the same as those associated with iron deficiency anemia. In mild cases of anemia, the client is asymptomatic. However, in more severe cases, assessment reveals the general manifestations of anemia (palpitations, dizziness, sensitivity to cold, etc.).

IV infusions of fluids, electrolytes, and packed red blood cells should be administered if manifestations of anemia cannot be managed with oxygen therapy, sedation, and rest. Oral fluids should be encouraged for maintenance of tissue hydration and renal perfusion.

Iron intake may be supplemented by the administration of ferrous sulfate, 325 mg orally three times daily with meals. It is also important to institute a bowel program at the same time to prevent constipation. A diet high in iron, protein, and fiber is needed. Surgery may be needed to stop the chronic loss of blood.

Congenital Anemias

Hemoglobinopathies

In abnormal hemoglobin synthesis, the globin portion of the hemoglobin molecule is defective. Any deviation in the polypeptide chain results in a disorder of hemoglobin synthesis.

Hemoglobinopathies are a group of conditions characterized by formation of abnormal hemoglobin. Specifically, they result from abnormalities of the α- and β-chains in globin, the protein of hemoglobin. Usually, β-globin is defective. The abnormalities resulting in defective hemoglobin usually consist of minute variations in the amino acid residue sequence.

The three major forms of normal hemoglobin are hemoglobin A (Hb A), hemoglobin A_2 (Hb A_2), and fetal hemoglobin (Hb F). Ninety-seven percent of normal hemoglobin is composed of Hb A, and 2% to 3% is Hb A_2 and F. Variants of Hb A number over 100, including Hb C, D, E, G, H, I, J, K, L, M, N, O, P, Q, and S. Fortunately, most of these abnormal hemoglobins are not detrimental and cause neither anemia nor any manifestations.

In the United States, the only abnormal hemoglobins of consequence are Hb S (sickle cell hemoglobin), Hb C, and Hb D. These forms of abnormal hemoglobin produce a mild disorder in people who are heterozygous carriers of the trait (those who inherit the gene from only one parent), but cause a profound, sometimes fatal anemia in homozygous carriers (those who inherit the gene from both parents). For a discussion of sickle cell anemia, see Congenital Disorders.

Hemoglobin C disease, the homozygous state of Hb, (1) occurs in 1 in 6000 blacks. Two percent to 3% of blacks carry the Hb C trait only. Although their erythrocytes do not assume a sickle shape, persons with Hb C disease suffer from a severe anemia accompanied by manifestations similar to those of sickle cell anemia. Persons who carry the trait (i.e., they have Hb A, B, and C) usually remain asymptomatic.

Treatment consists of relief of manifestations. Occasionally, blood transfusions are required.

Individuals heterozygous for both Hb C and Hb S (Hb SC disease) are seen more often than those with Hb C disease because so many blacks are heterozygous carriers of the sickle cell trait. Manifestations of this condition include sicklemia, anemia, and splenomegaly. Hematuria, retinal hemorrhages, and aseptic necrosis of the femoral head may also be present.

Hb SD disease is rare. Apparently, it affects all races alike. Manifestations are similar to those of sickle cell anemia but less severe.

The Thalassemias

The thalassemias are a group of inherited, chronic, hemolytic anemias. These anemias were first discovered among people living around the Mediterranean, hence the Greek *thalassa,* meaning "sea." Other names are Mediterranean anemia and Cooley's anemia.

Etiology and Risk Factors

The most common genetic variety of thalassemia is prevalent in areas around the Mediterranean, especially Italy, Greece, and the Mediterranean islands. High prevalence is also noted in India, Southeast Asia, Turkey, the Sudan,

Israel, and West Africa. From 3% to 8% of Americans of Italian or Greek ancestry and 0.5% of blacks carry a gene for thalassemia minor. The incidence in most non-Mediterranean people is very low, but cases have been reported in many ethnic groups. Like the sickle cell gene, that of thalassemia appears to be associated with increased resistance to malaria, which may account for its geographical distribution.

Pathophysiology

The severity of the anemia produced by the thalassemias depends on whether the afflicted person is homozygous or heterozygous for the thalassemia trait. Thalassemia major and intermedia, both characterized by a profound anemia, appear in homozygotes. Thalassemia minor, characterized by a mild anemia, develops in heterozygotes.

Unlike the α- and β-globin chains in sickle cell anemia, the chains in the thalassemias are completely normal in structure but insufficient in number because of a genetic alteration.

Either α- or β-chains can be affected by diminished synthesis. In α-thalassemia, α-chain synthesis slows. In β-thalassemia, β-chain synthesis diminishes. Because β-thalassemia is more common, it is called classic thalassemia, or simply thalassemia.

The outlook for clients with thalassemia major is usually poor. Children are retarded in their growth and development. Many fail to live through puberty. Thalassemia minor, on the other hand, does not affect life expectancy.

Clinical Manifestations and Diagnostic Findings

The manifestations of thalassemia major resemble those of other hemolytic anemias (e.g., jaundice, cholelithiasis, leg ulcers, and enlarged spleen). In addition, thalassemia is characterized by a pronounced bone hyperactivity that causes a thickening of the cranium and mongoloid facies.

Thalassemia minor is usually asymptomatic, except for a mild anemia. Blood smears of persons with this condition contain small, defective red blood cells.

Diagnostic findings in β-thalassemia include the following: target cells (cells that resemble a shooting target) and other bizarrely shaped red blood cells appear in the circulation; serum bilirubin and fecal and urinary urobilinogen are elevated because of the severe hemolysis of abnormal cells; an elevated fetal hemoglobin is present, in some cases as high as 90%; and an elevated Hb A_2 (a normal variant of Hb A), as high as 6% instead of the normal 1.5% to 3.0%, is found.

The high percentages of Hb F and Hb A_2 result from the decrease in β-chains characteristic of this anemia. The bone marrow compensates by producing abnormally large numbers of α-chains, γ-chains (normally made only during fetal life), and δ-chains. Hb F results from the combination of α- and γ-chains. Hb A_2 results from the combination of α- and δ-chains.

Management

Transfusion therapy is the only treatment available. Clients with thalassemia major receive packed red blood cells, which may be given (1) on a monthly or bimonthly basis (regular transfusion regimen), (2) whenever the hemoglobin falls below 3 to 4 g/dl (nonsystemic transfusion), or (3) every 15 days to maintain the hemoglobin at 12 to 15 g/dl (hypertransfusion regimen). When it becomes clear that transfused cells are being rapidly destroyed by the spleen (causing a severe hemolytic anemia), splenectomy is necessary.

Because clients with thalassemia must receive many transfusions, they can develop an iron overload, which may eventually cause myocardial hemosiderosis and cardiac arrhythmias. Excessive iron can to some extent be removed from the blood by chelating agents such as deferoxamine.

Thalassemia minor is usually so mild that treatment is not required. However, clients who carry the thalassemia trait need genetic counseling.

Hemolytic Anemias Caused by Intrinsic Red Blood Cell Defects

Glucose-6-Phosphate Dehydrogenase Deficiency

Glucose-6-phosphate dehydrogenase (G6PD) is an important red blood cell enzyme. G6PD deficiency can be classified as an enzymopathy, a genetic defect that involves the partial or complete deficiency of certain essential enzymes.

Etiology and Risk Factors

A deficiency of G6PD makes red blood cells more susceptible to hemolysis after ingestion of medications and foods classified as chemical oxidants. An X-linked disorder, G6PD deficiency affects at least 100 million people in the world. Among Americans, G6PD deficiency affects about 20% of blacks and about 1% to 2% of whites. It is common among Sephardic Jews, Greeks, Italians, and Arabs.

Pathophysiology

G6PD catalyzes about 10% of the glucose metabolized by red blood cells. When exposed to oxidative medications and foods, red blood cells require even more glucose for energy. If a G6PD deficiency exists, the red blood cells cannot adequately metabolize more glucose and so cannot cope with the oxidative effects of certain substances. As a result, hemolysis occurs. Because young, newly released red blood cells contain a large amount of G6PD, only aging red blood cells are destroyed upon exposure to oxidative agents.

Clinical Manifestations and Diagnostic Findings

Persons with this enzymopathy may remain completely asymptomatic throughout their lives. Typically, manifestations develop only after viral or bacterial infection or certain medications or toxins. Occasionally, however, spontaneous attacks of hemolytic anemia develop that are not precipitated by a known external factor.

More than 40 oxidative medications and foods produce hemolytic anemia in people with G6PD deficiency (e.g., primaquine, quinine, aspirin, sulfonamides, phenacetin, vitamin K derivatives, chloramphenicol, thiazide diuretics, and the fava bean). After exposure to any of these agents, the person with G6PD deficiency develops acute intravascular hemolysis lasting about 7 to 12 days. During this acute phase, the client suffers from anemia and jaundice.

Diagnostic findings include moderate hemoglobinemia and hemoglobinuria, elevated serum bilirubin, reticulocytosis, and Heinz bodies (small particles of denatured hemoglobin) within the red blood cell. After the acute hemolytic stage, the blood picture begins to improve whether the offending drug is stopped or not. The hemolytic reaction is self-limiting, because only older red blood cells in contact with a chemical oxidant are destroyed. However, if drug exposure continues for a long period, the client will develop chronic hyperhemolysis until contact with the offending agent ceases.

Management

Correcting the anemia primarily involves identifying and removing the medication or food precipitating the hemolytic reaction. Care of the client during the week of acute hemolysis is purely symptomatic (rest, fluids, and nutritious diet).

Because medications that precipitate hemolytic reactions in G6PD deficiency are common (e.g., aspirin), and because G6PD has a high worldwide incidence, screening tests for this enzymopathy should be a part of every public health program. Careful screening is particularly important for the black population. Tests performed during hemolytic episodes may be falsely negative because of the increased proportion of young red blood cells.

Hereditary Spherocytosis

Etiology and Risk Factors

Hereditary spherocytosis (congenital hemolytic jaundice or congenital spherocytic anemia) is a common form of chronic hemolytic anemia found in all races and ages. A simple mendelian dominant trait, spherocytosis can be inherited even if only one parent carries the abnormal gene. In about 20% of cases, hematologic abnormalities are absent in other family members, which suggests that a spontaneous mutation in the client caused the illness.

Pathophysiology

The two most distinctive characteristics of hereditary spherocytosis are (1) the appearance of large numbers of spherical red blood cells (spherocytes) and (2) an enlarged spleen. Spherocytosis develops because the red blood cells have a defective cellular membrane that is extremely permeable to the influx of sodium ions. To curtail the flow of sodium ions through its defective membrane, the red blood cell must increase its metabolic work and, so, its use of glucose.

When glucose and cellular energy become depleted, sodium ions flow through the cellular membrane without resistance. Thus, the red blood cell interior becomes hypertonic; water is drawn into the cell, which causes the red blood cell to swell and become spherical. Spherocytes, thick and rigid, are easily trapped within the splenic venous sinusoids, where they are phagocytosed. As a result, the spleen becomes enlarged, and the client suffers from anemia and jaundice because of the massive red blood cell hemolysis within the spleen.

Clinical Manifestations and Diagnostic Findings

Manifestations of hereditary spherocytosis are the same as the manifestations of hemolytic anemia discussed earlier (e.g., malaise, mild anemia, jaundice, gallstones, and splenomegaly). Splenomegaly is particularly pronounced, and clients may experience left upper quadrant fullness and abdominal pain. In the presence of systemic infection, the hemolytic rate may increase, inducing further splenic enlargement. Occasionally, acute abdominal pain results from splenic infarction. Such severe hemolytic crises are sometimes fatal.

Diagnostic findings are distinctive and include spherocytes in the blood smear; reticulocytosis; lowered red blood cell count and hemoglobin values; positive direct antiglobulin test; and increased osmotic fragility.

Osmotic fragility is increased (greater than 0.5%) because the spherocyte, already swollen and hypertonic, cannot tolerate a further influx of water, and it ruptures quickly when placed in hypotonic saline solutions.

Acute and Subacute Care

■ Surgical Management

Although blood transfusions may benefit a client in hemolytic crisis, the only treatment indicated in all cases of hereditary spherocytosis is splenectomy. Ninety percent of clients who undergo splenectomy experience complete reversal of manifestations. Although spherocytes continue to circulate, these misshapen cells usually have a longer life span once the spleen is removed.

■ Nursing Management of the Surgical Client

Assessment

See each discussion under The Anemias for the appropriate assessments. The surgical client with acute anemia is at greater risk of problems associated with oxygenation and oxygen transport and with wound healing. This client may also be at risk of difficulties associated with transfusion of large amounts of red blood cells. These problems put the client at higher risk of multiple complications after surgery.

Diagnosis, Planning, Implementation

Iron Overload. The collaborative problem may be written as *Iron Overload related to chronic infusion of iron through red blood cell transfusions.*

Planning: Expected Outcomes. The nurse will recognize the potential for iron overload, as evidenced by implementation of preventive therapy and monitoring of treatment compliance.

Implementation. Monitor for manifestations of iron overload by performing routine assessment of cardiac status and observing for manifestations of liver dysfunction, diabetes related to pancreatic malfunction, and thyroid insufficiency. Because there is no effective means for removal of the iron stores causing these complications, the primary goal is early detection, treatment of manifestations, and prevention.

Educate the client about the importance of iron chelation therapy, which will prevent this complication. An opportune time for routinely assessing treatment compliance is during periodic clinic visits for red blood cell transfusions. Referrals to home healthcare agencies and other groups who may help with financial aid and emotional support may also be appropriate.

Hypoxemia. Another collaborative problem is *Hypoxemia related to the decreased oxygen-carrying capacity of blood.*

Planning: Expected Outcomes. The client will have maintained adequate organ oxygenation, as evidenced by limiting activities or by receiving supplemental agents to enhance red blood cell function, production, or replacement.

Implementation. The nurse will administer blood according to policy and teach the client about possible side effects (see Blood Transfusions). Educate the client about the cause of anemia, preventive and treatment measures, diet therapy, and proper administration of iron supplements and their effect on stools. Provide oxygen therapy if ordered. Pace activities and schedule rest periods to prevent fatigue.

Altered Tissue Perfusion. One nursing diagnosis is *Altered Tissue Perfusion related to deficit or malfunctioning red blood cells.*

Planning: Expected Outcomes. The client will experience optimal peripheral tissue perfusion, as evidenced by warm, pink extremities; adequate pulses noted in extremities; and no complaints of tingling or numbness.

Implementation. Monitor for manifestations of oxygen deprivation: increased pulse and respirations, decreased blood pressure, and shortness of breath. Report manifestations immediately to the physician and start appropriate medical support. Keep the extremities warm to prevent vasoconstriction. Bathe the client in warm, *not* hot, water.

Altered Nutrition: Less than Body Requirements.
The nursing diagnosis is *Altered Nutrition: Less than Body Requirements related to anorexia, stomatitis, knowledge deficit, and inability to get proper foods* (physical and financial problems).

Planning: Expected Outcomes. The client will maintain proper nutrition, as evidenced by maintenance of or increase in body weight and intake of proper nutrients.

Implementation. Assess the client's usual diet and eating pattern. Make referrals when necessary (e.g., social worker, dietitian, home healthcare aide). Provide symptom management for the anorexia. Administer vitamin B_{12} and other medication as ordered. Encourage a diet high in iron, protein, and vitamins.

Ineffective Individual Coping.
The nursing diagnosis is *Ineffective Individual Coping related to the chronic status of the disease.*

Planning: Expected Outcomes. The client will cope effectively with the chronic nature of the illness, as evidenced by statements and demonstration of effective coping behaviors such as maintaining usual activities and ability to establish positive relationships.

Implementation. Provide the client with opportunities to express concerns, fears, feelings, and expectations. Encourage the client to develop realistic goals and activity levels. Instruct the client in the need for rest periods and adequate diets. Collaborate with the client to establish follow-up appointments that will enable him or her to lead a more normal life. Use other resource persons such as support systems, clinical specialists, social workers, and psychiatric liaison personnel.

Evaluation

The evaluation of care is based on the client's recovery from surgery, adequate nutritional intake, and return of the CBC to normal levels. Since surgery usually corrects the problem within 2 to 3 months afterwards, the client should return to having a normal blood profile.

■ Modifications for Elderly Clients

The nursing care plan for the aged client should include consideration of problems related to poor dentition, economic constraints, lack of interest in food preparation, or simple inability to shop and prepare nutritious meals.

Polycythemias

Polycythemia is defined as an increase in both the number of circulating erythrocytes and the concentration of hemoglobin within the blood.

Polycythemia Vera

Polycythemia vera is classified as a myeloproliferative disorder (meaning overgrowth of bone marrow). It usually develops in middle age, particularly among Jewish men.

Etiology and Risk Factors

Although the cause remains unknown, it is possibly a form of malignancy similar to leukemia and is often considered a premalignant condition, sometimes referred to as myeloproliferative dysplasia.

Pathophysiology

The three hallmarks of the condition are (1) relentless, unrestrained production of erythrocytes; (2) production of excessive myelocytes (leukocytes occurring normally in the bone marrow); and (3) overproduction of platelets.

Clinical Manifestations and Diagnostic Findings

The inordinate mass production of these three cell lines results in the following pathologic consequences: (1) an increase in blood viscosity; (2) an increase in the total blood volume, which may be twice or even three times greater than normal; and (3) severe blood congestion of all tissues and organs. Because of these problems, the client suffers many manifestations, including an increased risk of clot formation.

Diagnostic findings include a red blood cell count as high as 8 to 12 million/mm³; hemoglobin level of 18 to 25 g/dl; hematocrit greater than 54% in men and 49% in women; platelet count usually increased; normal arterial blood gases; hyperplastic bone marrow; and serum uric acid level three to four times normal.

 Acute and Subacute Care

■ Medical Management

The goals of care in polycythemia vera are twofold: (1) reduction of blood volume and viscosity and (2) reduction of bone marrow activity. These are accomplished through phlebotomy, the administration of myelosuppressive agents, and radiation therapy.

Phlebotomy. Emergency treatment involves removing 500 to 2000 ml of blood until the hematocrit reaches

45%. Once the hematocrit has been reduced, subsequent phlebotomies should be carried out as frequently as necessary to maintain the hematocrit at about 45%. As iron deficiency supervenes, red blood cell production will be retarded, so that clients managed by phlebotomy alone may require as few as two or three phlebotomies a year.

Myelosuppressive Agents. These include radioactive phosphorus, which sometimes produces remissions that last from 6 months to 2 years (see Chapter 24). Other drugs useful for combating polycythemia are chlorambucil, busulfan, and hydroxyurea.

Radiation Therapy. Radiation therapy may be used to reduce the production of red blood cells in the marrow.

Complications. Thrombotic complications claim the lives of about 30% of those affected with polycythemia vera; another 10% to 15% die from hemorrhage. Finally, for obscure reasons, about 15% die from either myelogenous leukemia or myelofibrosis accompanied by pancytopenia. Prognosis depends on age at diagnosis, treatment used, and complications.

■ Nursing Management of the Medical Client

Assessment

In its early stages, polycythemia usually remains asymptomatic (an increased hematocrit level may be an incidental finding). However, as altered circulation secondary to increased red blood cell mass leads to hypervolemia and hyperviscosity, the client may complain of a feeling of fullness in the head, dizziness, headache, tinnitus, visual disturbances, and other manifestations, depending on the body system affected. Manifestations include the following: integumentary—ruddy complexion (plethora) and dusky, red mucosa; cardiovascular—hypertension (with dizziness, headache, and a sense of fullness in the head) and congestive heart failure (shortness of breath, orthopnea); increased clotting leading to cerebrovascular accident, myocardial infarction, or peripheral gangrene; and bleeding (hemorrhage in capillaries, venules, and arterioles), which causes rupture of vessels; gastrointestinal—peptic ulcers, enlargement of liver and spleen; and skeletal—gout (painful swollen joints, usually the big toe) characterized by an increased uric acid level.

Diagnosis, Planning, Implementation

Altered Tissue Perfusion. Write the nursing diagnosis as *Altered Tissue Perfusion related to hypervolemia and hyperviscosity.*

   Planning: Expected Outcomes. The client will experience optimal peripheral tissue perfusion, as evidenced by warm, pink extremities; adequate pulses noted in extremities; and no complaints of tingling or numbness.

   Implementation. Administer medications as prescribed. Monitor vital signs and breath sounds. Notify the physician immediately if any manifestations of a thrombotic event are present. For reducing the blood viscosity, encourage intake of oral fluids. Monitor intake and output. Administer anticoagulants as ordered and monitor for manifestations of bleeding. Monitor blood studies. For preventing the development of thrombi from circulatory stasis, encourage the client to ambulate if possible, elevate the feet when seated, and wear support hose. Turn bedridden clients frequently, and provide passive exercise to their extremities. Caution clients undergoing phlebotomy to avoid foods high in iron (clams, oysters, liver, legumes), because a high iron intake counteracts to some degree the therapeutic effects of phlebotomy.

Evaluation

Since polycythemia vera is a chronic disease, control and prevention of long-term complications is the desired outcome.

Secondary Polycythemia

When the body's demand for oxygen increases for any reason, the bone marrow must produce more red blood cells to prevent tissue hypoxia. This compensatory response to tissue hypoxia is called secondary polycythemia.

Hypoxia that is sufficiently prolonged to cause polycythemia results from chronic lung disease (particularly emphysema), congenital heart disease, and prolonged exposure to altitudes of 10,000 ft or more. People who live in mountainous areas are not hypoxic because their blood has "thickened." These mountain dwellers produce high numbers of red blood cells increasing the oxygen-carrying capacity of their blood, enabling them to live at an altitude that would incapacitate a newcomer.

The manifestations and laboratory findings in persons with secondary polycythemia are the same as those in persons with polycythemia vera, except the white blood cell and platelet counts are normal and the spleen is not enlarged.

Medical management of secondary polycythemia involves treating the underlying disease or condition causing hypoxia.

Relative Polycythemia

Whenever the body loses plasma without losing red blood cells, the concentration of red blood cells increases relative to the amount of plasma remaining in the vascular system. Some causes of relative polycythemia are fluid loss and dehydration as a result of inadequate fluid intake, diarrhea, vomiting, burns, and excessive administration of diuretics. Treatment simply involves the reestablishment of fluid and electrolyte balance.

Disorders Affecting White Blood Cells

White blood cells (leukocytes) are divided into two groups: (1) granulocytes (polymorphonuclear leukocytes) and (2) agranulocytes (mononuclear cells). Granulocytes, in turn, are divided into three groups: neutrophils, basophils, and eosinophils. The names denote affinity for the dyes used in staining.

Agranulocytes include lymphocytes (B and T) and monocytes. Plasma cells, or plasmacytes, are derived from B lymphocytes. Plasma cells, formed within the bone marrow and lymph nodes, are active in producing immunoglobulins (antibodies). Pathologic conditions involving plasma cells are called plasma cell dyscrasias.

Major defects that affect leukocytes and plasma cells are (1) the leukemias, acute and chronic; (2) agranulocytosis; and (3) multiple myeloma (plasma cell myeloma).

The Leukemias

Leukemia is a malignant disease of the blood-forming organs. Leukemia accounts for 8% of all human cancers and is the most common malignancy in children and young adults. One half of all leukemias are classified as acute, with rapid onset and progression of disease resulting in 100% mortality within days to months without appropriate therapy. The remaining leukemias, classified as chronic, have a more indolent course. In childhood, 80% of the leukemias are lymphocytic with only 20% nonlymphocytic. In the adult, the percentages are reversed, with 80% being nonlymphocytic.

Etiology and Risk Factors

Acute leukemia is characterized by the proliferation of large numbers of abnormal, immature leukocytes in the bone marrow, lymph nodes, liver, spleen, and eventually all body systems. In addition, the production of other blood cells (i.e., red blood cells, platelets, neutrophils) is inhibited by a mechanism not clearly understood, resulting in inadequate oxygen transport, thrombocytopenia, and immune system malfunction (Fig. 53–2).

The French-American-British (FAB) Cooperative Group developed a system for classifying acute leukemias based on morphologic characteristics and the percentage of immature cells in the bone marrow (Table 53–2).

For the leukemic process to be termed acute, at least 50% of the marrow cells must be immature. Acute lym-

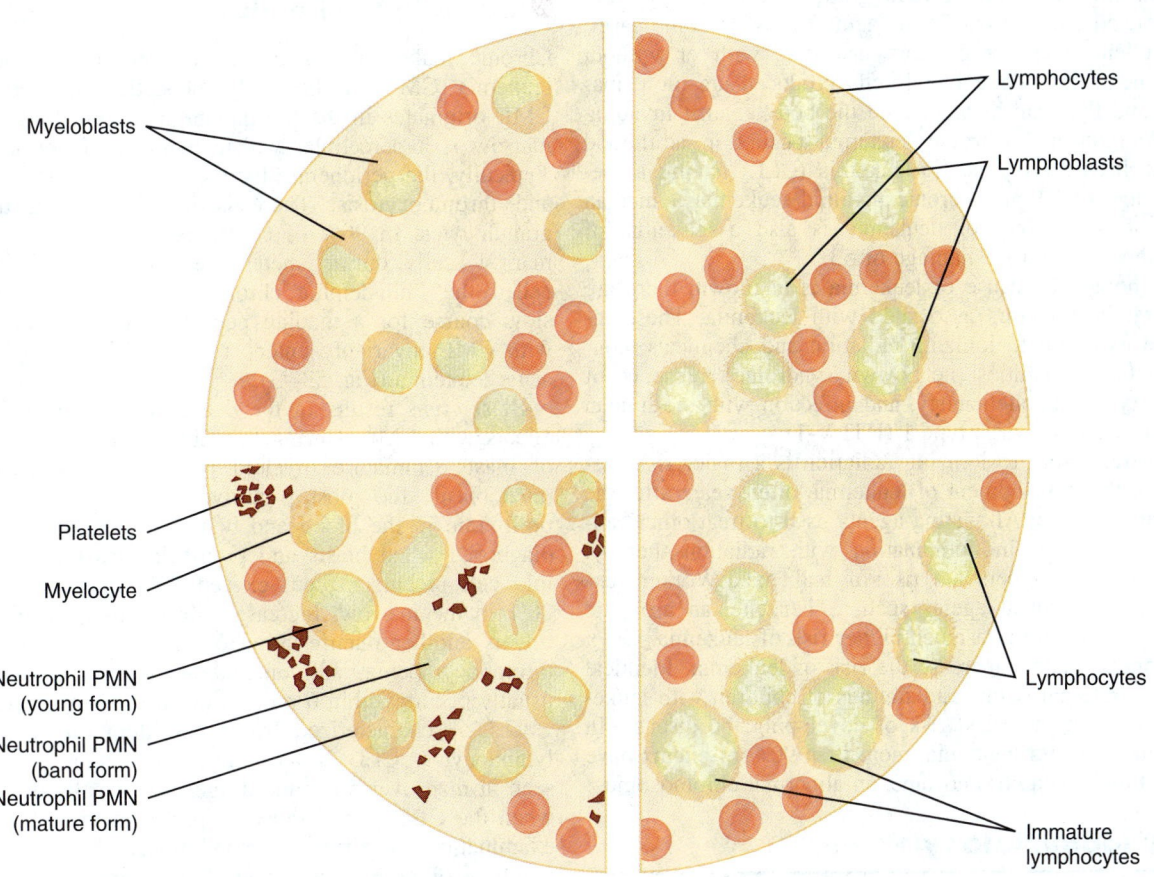

A Acute nonlymphocytic leukemia (ANLL)

B Acute lymphocytic leukemia (ALL)

Myeloblasts

Lymphocytes

Lymphoblasts

Platelets

Myelocyte

Neutrophil PMN (young form)

Neutrophil PMN (band form)

Neutrophil PMN (mature form)

Lymphocytes

Immature lymphocytes

C Chronic myelogenous leukemia (CML)

D Chronic lymphocytic leukemia (CLL)

Figure 53–2. Types of leukemia: a comparison.

Table 53–2. French-American-British (FAB) Classification of Acute Leukemia

Acute lymphocytic leukemia
- L1 Common childhood leukemia
- L2 Adult acute lymphocytic leukemia
- L3 Rare subtype, blasts resembling those in Burkitt's lymphoma

Acute myeloblastic leukemia

Granulocytic
- M1 Myeloblastic leukemia without maturation
- M2 Myeloblastic leukemia with maturation
- M3 Hypergranular promyelocytic leukemia

Monocytic
- M4 Myelomonocytic leukemia
- M5 Monocytic

Erythroid
- M6 Erythroleukemia

phoblastic leukemia is most common in children, with a median age of 11 years. Acute nonlymphocytic leukemia is more common in adulthood, with a median age of 67 years.

Chronic leukemias have a gradual onset and a more protracted course than do the acute forms. In some cases, the client lives for 5 years or more, with or without treatment. The white blood cells produced are more mature and thus can better defend the body against invading microorganisms. Chronic leukemia occurs in adulthood with chronic lymphocytic leukemia (CLL) having a median age of 71 and chronic myeloid leukemia a median age of 67. Hairy cell leukemia is also a leukemia of adulthood with a median age of 53.

Although the cause of leukemia is unknown, there are several host factors associated with leukemia. These include exposure to ionizing radiation and chemicals, congenital abnormalities (i.e., Down syndrome), presence of primary immunodeficiency, and infection with the human T-cell leukemia virus type 1 (HTLV-1).

Overexposure to ionizing radiation is a major risk factor for the development of leukemia, often years after the initial exposure. Alkylating agents used to treat other cancers, especially in combination with radiation therapy, also increase a person's risk of leukemia. Workers exposed to chemical agents such as benzene, an aromatic hydrocarbon, are at a much higher risk of leukemia.

Genetic factors increase the risk of leukemia. Identical twins, fraternal twins, and siblings of children with leukemia have an increased risk of developing the disease. In chronic myeloid leukemia, more than 90% of clients have the Philadelphia chromosome, an abnormal chromosome.

Pathophysiology

■ Acute Leukemia

There are two major forms of acute leukemia: *lymphocytic leukemia*, which involves the lymphocytes and lymphoid organs; and *nonlymphocytic leukemia*, which involves hematopoietic stem cells that differentiate into myeloid cells: monocytes, granulocytes, erythrocytes, and platelets.

From these two broad categories, leukemias are further classified according to the specific malignant cell line. Ninety percent of acute leukemia is acute-lymphoblastic, caused by the malignant proliferation of precursor lymphocytes called lymphoblasts. Acute lymphoblastic leukemia presents most often in children 2 to 10 years of age. Advances in therapy during the last several decades have significantly improved the chances for remission and even a cure. Acute lymphoblastic leukemia was one of the first human cancers to be cured by combination chemotherapy.

Acute nonlymphocytic leukemia (ANLL, formerly known as acute myelogenous leukemia, or AML) is characterized by aberrations in the growth of megakaryocytes, monocytes, granulocytes, and erythrocytes. Typically, however, aberrations in one cell type predominate. The most common type of ANLL involves maturational arrest and proliferation of cells in the myeloblastic and monoblastic stages of development. The prognostic factors are less clearly defined in ANLL, and the long-term prognosis is usually poor. Bone marrow transplantation is currently the best treatment option.

■ Chronic Leukemia

Chronic leukemia is classified as chronic myelogenous leukemia (CML) or chronic lymphocytic leukemia (CLL). CML originates in the pluripotent stem cell. Initially, the marrow is hypercellular with a majority of normal cells. Typically, the peripheral blood smear reveals leukocytosis and thrombocytosis. There is increased production of granulocytes. In 90% of cases, examination of the bone marrow cells during metaphase shows a translocation called the Philadelphia chromosome. After a relatively slow course for a median period of 4 years, the client with CML invariably enters a blast crisis that resembles acute leukemia (Fig. 53–3).

Blast crisis results in the death of more than 70% of clients with CML. During this phase, increasing numbers of blasts (immature myeloid precursor cells, especially myeloblasts, the most primitive granulocyte precursors) proliferate in the blood and bone marrow. Blast crisis is diagnosed when blasts and promyelocytes (another myeloid cell precursor type) exceed 20% in the blood and 30% in the marrow. Increased fibrotic tissue in the marrow is another manifestation of blast crisis. Leukopenia, thrombocytopenia, and anemia are also evident. Death usually occurs within 6 months of onset if not treated.

CLL is characterized by the proliferation of early B lymphocytes. CLL is an indolent leukemia most often seen in men over 50 years of age. It is usually discovered when the CBC is performed as part of a routine physical examination. A peripheral blood smear reveals increased numbers of both mature and slightly immature lymphocytes.

As the disease progresses, lymphocytes infiltrate the lymph nodes, liver, spleen, and ultimately the bone marrow. A staging system has been developed that correlates

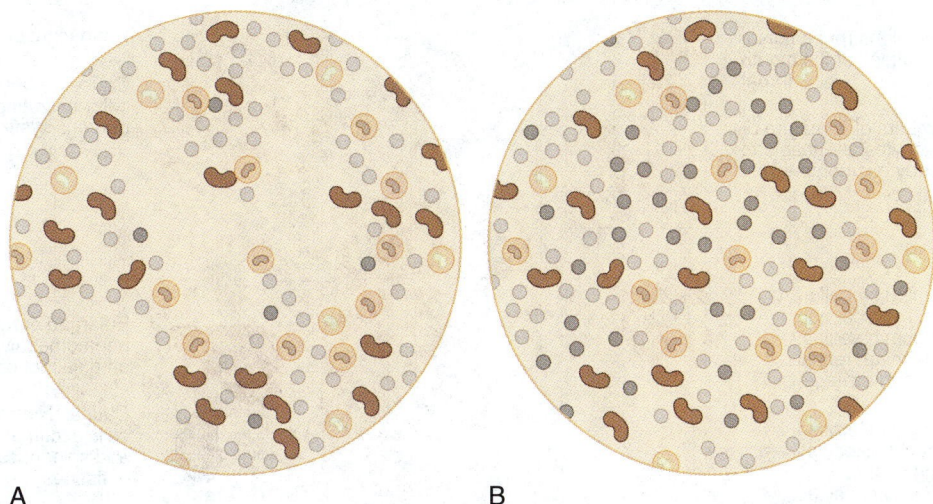

Figure 53–3. *A,* This microscopic view of a normal bone marrow specimen shows a normal distribution of blood cell types and fatty spaces. Blast cells appear as round, dark gray circles. *B,* During blast crisis, the number of blast cells increases, and fatty spaces shrink.

stage with the extent of lymphocyte infiltration. Progression of the disease may take as long as 15 years.

Clinical Manifestations and Diagnostic Findings

The manifestations of all types of leukemia are similar. The clinical history will usually reveal manifestations characteristic of anemia, thrombocytopenia, and leukopenia. Clients often complain of fatigue, weakness, easy bruising, bleeding gums, epistaxis, fever, headache, and generalized pain. In some types of leukemia (most frequently CML), the client may have a feeling of abdominal fullness and early satiety as a result of splenomegaly. On physical examination, pallor, scattered petechiae and ecchymoses, generalized lymphadenopathy, hepatosplenomegaly, bone and joint pain, and fever may be found. Assessment data for leukemia and the pathophysiologic bases may be found in Figure 53–4.

A comprehensive evaluation of all body systems is necessary to establish the treatment plan. Tests most often included in the initial evaluation are the CBC, bone marrow aspiration, lumbar puncture, radiographic tests, and lymphangiograms.

Complete Blood Count. CBC values vary greatly. The total white blood cell count may be normal, abnormally low (less than 1000/mm³), or extremely high (greater than 200,000/mm³). The differential may reveal that one type of leukocyte is overwhelmingly predominant. There may be abnormal leukocytes, including immature blast forms, noted on the peripheral smear. The platelet count and hemoglobin level are usually low.

Bone Marrow Aspiration. Bone marrow aspiration or biopsy is a key diagnostic tool for confirming the diagnosis and identifying the malignant cell type. If an adequate sample of marrow cannot be obtained by aspira-

tion, a fragment of bone can be removed for a bone marrow biopsy. Typical findings on the bone marrow aspirate and biopsy are an overall increase in the number of marrow cells with an increase in the proportion of earlier forms.

Lumbar Puncture. Lumbar puncture determines the presence of blast cells in the central nervous system; 5% of cases present with this abnormality.

Radiographic Tests. Radiographic tests may include radiographs of the chest and skeleton; magnetic resonance imaging and computed tomographic scans of the head and body detect lesions and sites of infection.

Lymphangiography. Lymphangiography or lymph node biopsy may be performed to locate malignant lesions and accurately classify disease.

The treatment of all classifications of leukemia is targeted at destroying neoplastic cells and maintaining a sustained remission. During each phase of therapy, the medical treatment may vary, but the basic nursing principles are the same.

Acute and Subacute Care

■ Medical Management

Acute Leukemia

The treatment plan for leukemia is determined by disease classification, presence or absence of prognostic factors, and disease progression. The goal of treatment is complete remission with restoration of normal bone marrow function. This means that the level of blast cells in the marrow is less than 5%. Approximately 60% to 80% of adults with acute lymphocytic leukemia will achieve com-

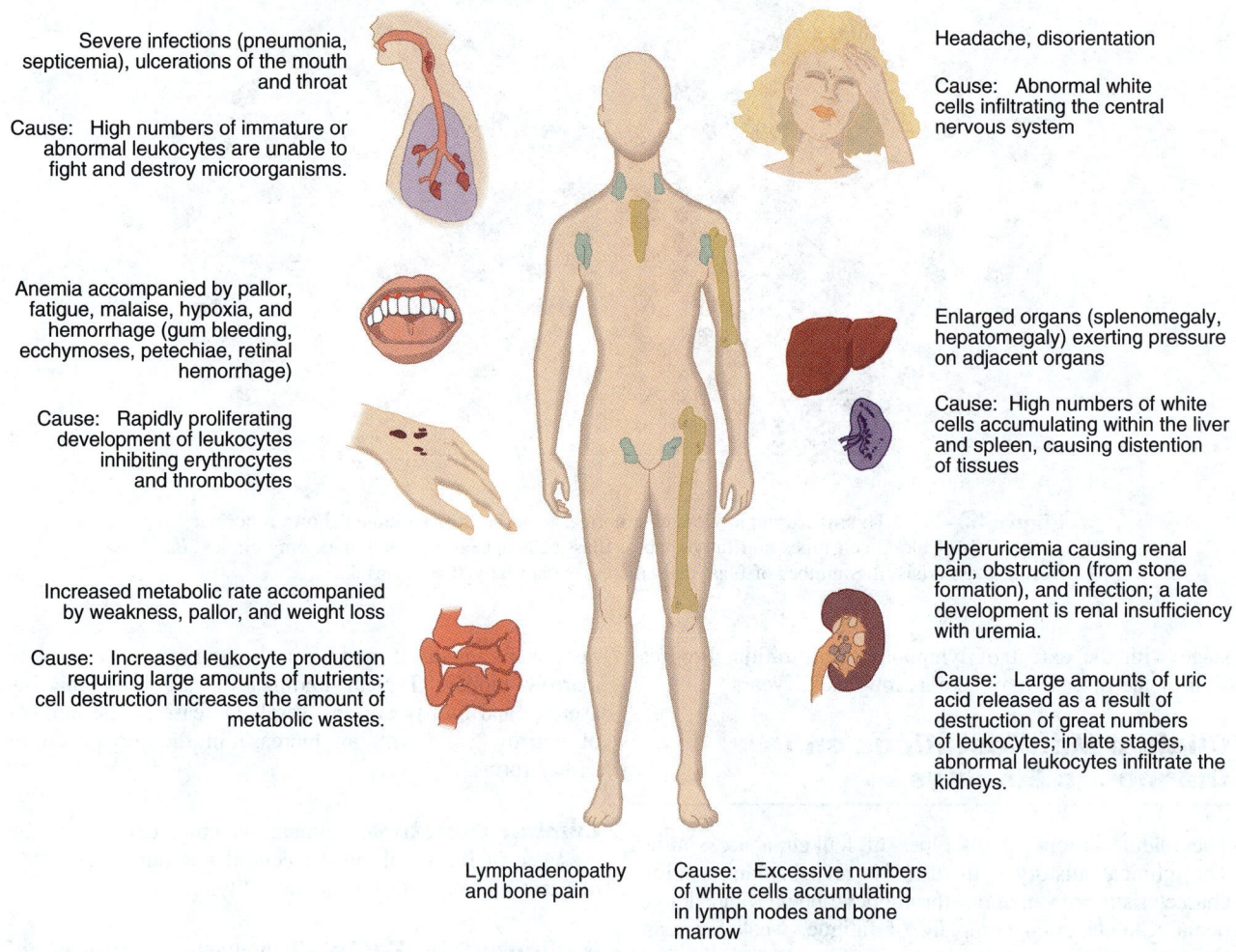

Severe infections (pneumonia, septicemia), ulcerations of the mouth and throat

Cause: High numbers of immature or abnormal leukocytes are unable to fight and destroy microorganisms.

Anemia accompanied by pallor, fatigue, malaise, hypoxia, and hemorrhage (gum bleeding, ecchymoses, petechiae, retinal hemorrhage)

Cause: Rapidly proliferating development of leukocytes inhibiting erythrocytes and thrombocytes

Increased metabolic rate accompanied by weakness, pallor, and weight loss

Cause: Increased leukocyte production requiring large amounts of nutrients; cell destruction increases the amount of metabolic wastes.

Headache, disorientation

Cause: Abnormal white cells infiltrating the central nervous system

Enlarged organs (splenomegaly, hepatomegaly) exerting pressure on adjacent organs

Cause: High numbers of white cells accumulating within the liver and spleen, causing distention of tissues

Hyperuricemia causing renal pain, obstruction (from stone formation), and infection; a late development is renal insufficiency with uremia.

Cause: Large amounts of uric acid released as a result of destruction of great numbers of leukocytes; in late stages, abnormal leukocytes infiltrate the kidneys.

Lymphadenopathy and bone pain

Cause: Excessive numbers of white cells accumulating in lymph nodes and bone marrow

Figure 53–4. Leukemia: assessment data and pathophysiologic bases.

plete remission, with 35% to 45% surviving 2 years. The cure rate, however, remains low without bone marrow transplantation. Sixty percent to 70% of adults with ANLL achieve complete remission, with about 25% surviving 5 years or more.

Chemotherapy. Chemotherapy is given to destroy the malignant cells of the bone marrow. The treatment protocol for acute leukemia involves three phases: (1) induction, (2) consolidation, and (3) maintenance.

Induction Phase. During the induction phase, the client receives an intensive course of chemotherapy designed to induce a complete remission of the disease. The usual criteria for complete remission are blast cells less than 5% of the bone marrow cells and normal peripheral blood counts. Both conditions must be sustained for at least 1 month. Once remission is achieved, the consolidation phase begins.

Consolidation Phase. During the consolidation phase, modified courses of intensive chemotherapy are given to eradicate any remaining disease. This usually involves giving a higher dose of one or more chemotherapeutic agents.

Maintenance Phase. During the maintenance phase, small doses of different combinations of chemotherapeutic agents are given every 3 to 4 weeks. This phase may continue for a year or more and is, therefore, structured to allow the client to live as normal a life as possible. This is used more commonly with ALL.

Complications. Tumor lysis syndrome is a group of metabolic complications associated with the rapid destruction of a large number of white blood cells. If the white blood cell count is high when chemotherapy is initiated, rapid cell lysis can lead to increased serum uric acid, phosphate, and potassium levels and decreased serum calcium. Manifestations include confusion, weakness, numbness, bradycardia, electrocardiographic (ECG) changes, and dysrhythmias (hyperkalemia); numbness, tingling, muscle cramps, seizures, tetany, and ECG changes (hypocalcemia); and uric acid crystalluria, renal obstruction, and acute renal failure (hyperuricemia). Acute tumor lysis syndrome can be prevented by increasing IV hydration, alkalizing the urine, and administering allopurinol (Zyloprim).

Current treatment modalities for acute leukemia destroy both normal and aberrant cells. Therapy is aimed at preventing and resolving complications of acquired and induced pancytopenia, which are anemia, bleeding, and infection. Transfusions of red blood cells and platelets are required until the marrow can produce mature cells.

Reduced exposure to microorganisms helps prevent infection, but laminar flow rooms and reverse isolation have minimal benefits. The client must be watched closely for manifestations of infection, which may be inhibited because of the severely compromised state of the immune system. Therefore, broad-spectrum antibiotics and antifungals must be started at the first manifestations of infection.

It is important to note that if the client requires IV infusions of red blood cells and amphotericin B, an antifungal agent, they should be separated by at least 1 hour so that adverse reactions, such as allergic reactions, can be detected.

Currently, clients with bone marrow suppression after chemotherapy can receive granulocyte colony-stimulating factor (G-CSF) and granulocyte-macrophage colony-stimulating factor (GM-CSF). These are given either right after the client receives chemotherapy or when the client's white blood cell count drops. These agents may induce flulike symptoms and fatigue. The colony-stimulating factors increase the white blood cell count and decrease the risk of infection.

Radiation Therapy. Radiation therapy may be administered as an adjunct to chemotherapy when leukemic cells infiltrate the central nervous system, skin, rectum, and testes, or when a large mediastinal mass is noted at diagnosis (as may occur in acute lymphocytic leukemia).

Chronic Myelogenous Leukemia

The goal of therapy in the chronic phase of CML is to control leukocytosis and thrombocytosis. Leukapheresis (Fig. 53–5) may be performed to lower an extremely high peripheral leukocyte count quickly and prevent acute tumor lysis syndrome, but the results are temporary. Likewise, thrombocytosis as high as 2 million/mm³ may require thrombocytopheresis. Apheresis is usually performed with use of automated blood cell separators designed to selectively remove the desired blood element and return remaining cells and plasma to the client. If painful splenomegaly develops, irradiating or removing the spleen relieves this manifestation.

The most widely used medications are busulfan (Myleran) and hydroxyurea, which are given orally. A blast crisis (see Fig. 53–3B) requires intensive chemotherapy with agents used in acute leukemia. These drugs can destroy leukemic blast cells, transform them into normal granulocytes, or prevent leukemic cells from inhibiting formation of normal granulocytes. Unfortunately, they have been ineffective in achieving long-term remission.

Chronic Lymphocytic Leukemia

The goal of therapy in CLL is palliation. Total body irradiation or local radiation to the spleen may also be given as a palliative treatment to reduce complications. Two complications seen during the later stages are hemolytic anemia due to autoimmune disorder and hypogammaglobulinemia, which further increases susceptibility to infection. Antibiotics, transfusions of red blood cells, and

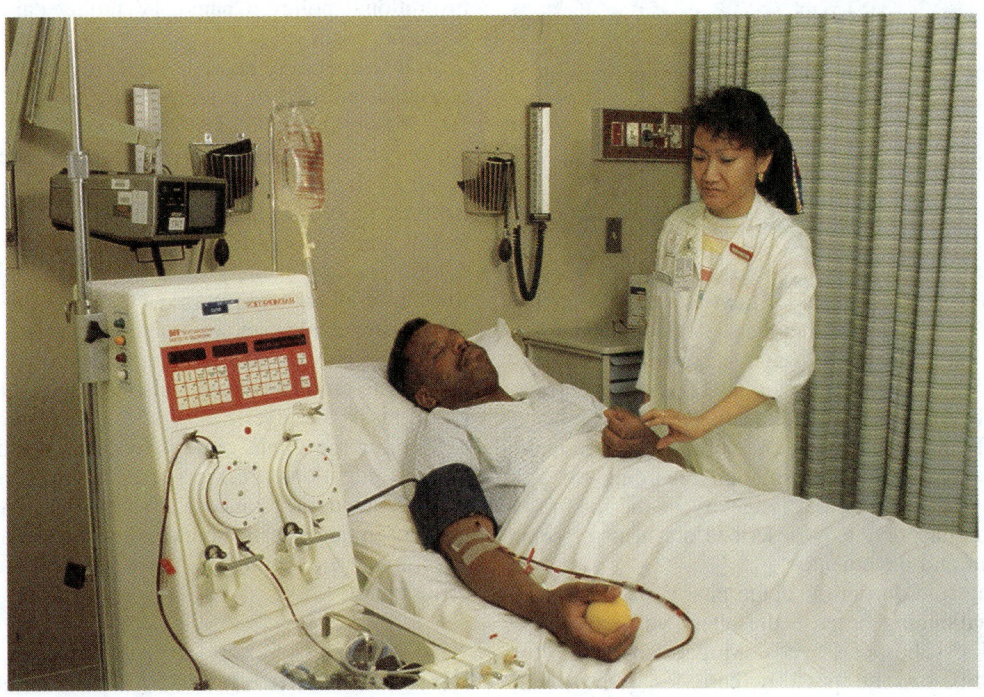

Figure 53–5. The white blood cell level can be temporarily lowered by leukapheresis. Several automated blood cell separators effectively remove large numbers of white cells and return red cells and plasma to the client. The Haemonetics V50 is a cell separator commonly used to perform this procedure.

injections of γ-globulin concentrates may be required for these clients.

Chemotherapy.
Chlorambucil (Leukeran) or cyclophosphamide (Cytoxan) may be given orally to reduce manifestations. Chemotherapy is generally given for 2 weeks of every month. When anemia (stage III) and thrombocytopenia (stage IV) develop, daily oral prednisone is given as an adjunct to the alkylating agents. Prednisone has a marked lymphocytolytic effect and may stimulate the production of red blood cells and platelets. Fludarabine is a new chemotherapeutic agent that appears effective in treating CLL.

Bone Marrow Transplantation.
In order to achieve cure with the acute leukemias, bone marrow transplantation is the current recommended treatment. Allogeneic bone marrow transplantation presents a treatment option for clients under about 50 years of age who have a suitable HLA-matched donor. Studies indicate that transplant performed during the first remission has a higher success rate than does transplant performed during repeat remissions or the blast phase of chronic leukemia.

■ Nursing Management of the Medical Client

Assessment

Nursing care for leukemia focuses on the following:

- Obtaining a thorough health history to aid in diagnosis and treatment
- Recognizing, preventing, and treating complications of ablative chemotherapy and radiation therapy
- Teaching to increase understanding of the disease, obtains compliance with treatment, and ability for self-care
- Supporting psychosocial needs of clients with a life-threatening illness

It is imperative to obtain a thorough health history from the client and family members. A family history of exposure to chemical toxins (e.g., benzene and arsenic), viral infection (Epstein-Barr virus, HTLV-1), chromosomal abnormalities, use of medications such as phenylbutazone and chloramphenicol, chemotherapy, or radiation therapy may provide key information regarding the type of leukemia. The severity and longevity of the manifestations of leukemia previously described are also important facts to obtain and document.

The nursing role during the acute phases of leukemia is extremely challenging because the client will have many physical and psychosocial needs. Modern therapy offers hope for remission and possibly cure for some clients with leukemia, but it is still a diagnosis equated with pain, expensive long-term therapy, and potential death.

Diagnosis, Planning, Implementation

Risk for Sepsis.
One collaborative problem is *Risk for Sepsis related to neutropenia or leukocytosis secondary to leukemia or treatment.*

Planning: Expected Outcomes. The healthcare team will prevent infection or will diagnose infection early and treat it effectively, as evidenced by a neutrophil count greater than 1000/mm³, no evidence of fever or respiratory difficulty, and decrease of manifestations and increase of neutrophil count with treatment.

Implementation. The nurse should institute good hand-washing technique for everyone coming in contact with the client. The client should be in a private room with protective isolation or laminar flow if the absolute neutrophil count is less than 500/mm³. Visitors with possible communicable diseases should be screened for the presence of infection and any visitors or staff with colds or respiratory infections should not be allowed near the client. Avoid all live plants, flowers, and stuffed animals in the client's room.

The client should be on a low-bacteria diet that excludes raw fruits and vegetables. Assist the client with a daily bath using antimicrobial soap. Assist, if the client is unable, with meticulous oral hygiene several times a day.

Female clients should not douche and should avoid the use of tampons. Daily stool softeners are ordered to reduce the risk of anal fissures. Insertion of rectal suppositories, rectal thermometers, and other invasive procedures should be avoided.

Provide meticulous skin decontamination before venipunctures. Maintain sterile occlusion of central venous catheters and perform routine dressing care according to institutional policy. Change IV tubing daily or according to agency policy.

Oral temperature should be taken every 4 hours and the physician notified of a temperature over 38° C (100.5° to 101° F) or under 36° C (97° to 97.5° F). Fever may be the only manifestation in a neutropenic client. Assess the cause of fever before initiation of therapy by obtaining cultures of blood, urine, central line sites, and other potential sources of infection. Administer antibiotics as ordered. Therapy usually consists of multiple broad-spectrum antibiotics administered IV on alternating schedules. Administer analgesics as ordered for relief of discomfort, avoiding aspirin if the client is thrombocytopenic. Aspirin or aspirin products should also be avoided because they might mask the fever.

Monitor the client closely for manifestations of fungal or viral infections (i.e., increased respirations, rales, dyspnea, changed oral mucosa). Monitor the respiratory rate and auscultate breath sounds regularly. Viral and fungal pneumonia are common causes of death in the neutropenic client.

Risk for Hemorrhage.
Another collaborative problem is *Risk for Hemorrhage related to thrombocytopenia secondary to either leukemia or treatment.*

Planning: Expected Outcomes. Bleeding as a result of injuries such as falls, punctures, cuts, or other environmental hazards will be prevented or will be diagnosed and treated successfully, as evidenced by absence of bleeding and platelet count greater than 20,000/mm³.

Implementation. Institute bleeding precautions:

- Provide cotton swabs or sponges for oral hygiene, avoiding flossing, hard toothbrushes, and commercial mouthwashes.
- Instruct the client to avoid blowing or picking the nose, straining at bowel movements, douching or using tampons, or using razors.
- Do not give any injections, intramuscularly or subcutaneously, or insert rectal suppositories.
- Do not give aspirin or medications containing aspirin. Instruct the client not to take these products.
- Avoid catheters whenever possible. If a catheter must be inserted, use the smallest size possible, lubricate it well, and insert it gently. Avoid mucosal trauma during suctioning.
- Both men and women should avoid shaving during the neutropenic phase.
- Pad the bed rails and remove all hazards and sharp objects from the environment.
- Use an air mattress and turn the client frequently to avoid pressure sores. Use bed cradles to protect extremities.
- Avoid overinflation of the blood pressure cuff and rotate the cuff to different sites.
- Avoid prolonged use of tourniquets.
- Use only paper tape, avoiding all strong adhesives.

Teach the client and significant others to institute bleeding precautions during periods of thrombocytopenia.

Monitor the client every 4 hours for manifestations of bleeding, such as ecchymoses, petechiae, epistaxis, gingival bleeding, hematuria, occult blood in stools, enlarged abdominal girth, disorientation, confusion, and changes in level of consciousness. All urine, stools, and emesis should be tested for blood. Take and record vital signs routinely, noting manifestations of altered tissue perfusion related to anemia (increased respirations and pulse; decreased blood pressure).

Check the platelet count, hemoglobin level, and hematocrit daily. Report a hemoglobin level of less than 10 g/dl and a platelet count of less than 20,000/mm³. Administer packed red blood cells and platelet concentrates as ordered. Keep a current blood sample in the laboratory for crossmatching if needed in an emergency.

Altered Nutrition: Less than Body Requirements.
The nursing diagnosis is *Altered Nutrition: Less than Body Requirements related to gastrointestinal tract effects of radiation therapy and chemotherapy.*

Planning: Expected Outcomes. The client will maintain body weight and adequate nutritional status, as evidenced by stable weight, adequate caloric intake, and maintenance of fluid and electrolyte balance.

Implementation. Administer antiemetics as ordered around the clock to prevent nausea and vomiting. Premedicate the client before meals to encourage food and fluid intake. Administer local and IV analgesics as ordered to relieve pain caused by mucositis. Allow the client to make food selections. Small, frequent feedings may be tolerated better than three large meals a day. Monitor weight daily. If the client cannot tolerate food for an extended period, begin total parenteral nutrition as ordered and monitor intake. Use antidiarrheals as needed to treat any diarrhea. The Bridge to Home Healthcare describes other ways to help immunosuppressed clients maintain good nutritional status.

Body Image Disturbance.
The nursing diagnosis is *Body Image Disturbance related to alopecia, weight loss, and fatigue.*

Planning: Expected Outcomes. The client will cope effectively with disturbed body image, as evidenced by the client's understanding of the disease condition and the temporary nature of changes in body image and energy.

Implementation. Inform the client before treatment of the potential for hair loss. Encourage the use of scarves, hats, or wigs as desired. Explain the temporary nature of alopecia, although the hair may have a different color or texture when it returns.

Encourage the client to balance rest with exercise and activities so that muscle tone can be maintained without the client's developing severe fatigue. Discuss daily dietary requirements with the client and provide high carbohydrate meals and oral supplements.

Risk for Sexual Dysfunction.
The nursing diagnosis is *Risk for Sexual Dysfunction related to the effects of chemotherapy or radiation therapy on reproductive organs.*

Planning: Expected Outcomes. The client will understand the potential for sterility that may result from therapy, as evidenced by his or her ability to state outcomes from therapy and their effect on sexuality.

Implementation. Describe to the client the normal cellular destruction that might lead to temporary or permanent destruction of reproductive function. Inform the client that sexual libido may be altered after the acute phase of the illness. Provide the client with emotional support and references to support groups. In appropriate cases, inform the client of reproductive alternatives, such as sperm banking and artificial insemination.

Risk for Ineffective Individual Coping.
The nursing diagnosis is *Risk for Ineffective Individual Coping related to chronic disease and possible denial of a terminal prognosis.*

Planning: Expected Outcomes. The client will cope effectively with the chronic condition and potentially fatal prognosis, as evidenced by appropriate verbalization of fears and concerns and maintenance of effective communication with significant others.

Implementation. Offer the client the opportunity to discuss fears and concerns about the disease process and

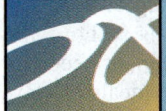

BRIDGE TO HOME HEALTHCARE

Managing Immunosuppression and Nutrition

Judy Aufenthie, R.N., *Shamrock In-Home Nursing Care, Inc., Rochester, Minnesota*

The immunosuppressed client may have great difficulty attaining and maintaining good nutritional status because of fatigue, weakness, and anorexia. To restore energy, the client should eat easily prepared and digested nutrient-dense meals. Encourage the client to add nonfat milk powder, pureed meats, whole milk, ice cream, yogurt, or nut butters to foods to increase their nutrient and caloric value. He or she should fix simple nutritious snacks rather than meals to decrease energy expenditure and deal with tiredness. Other easily prepared, nutrient-dense snacks are peanut butter and whole wheat crackers or bread with a glass of milk and fruit, or yogurt with nuts, dried fruit, and granola. Adding wheat germ or brewer's yeast to these snacks increases nutrients without undesirable flavor or texture. Teach clients to ingest foods in small amounts every 1 to 2 hours whether they are hungry or not. They should avoid or limit quantities of fat-free, low calorie foods to ensure adequate intake.

Suggest that clients use paper cups and dishes, or when possible, cook in the packages that the food comes in. On high-energy days, they can prepare extra servings and freeze them in small serving–sized containers to use on low-energy days. Individual food items or whole meals can be pureed in the blender. Such foods make foods easy to swallow when mouth or throat ulcers are present. When clients' appetites are poor or throats are particularly sore, cool nutritious blender drinks can provide alternative nutritional intake.

Two tablespoons of dry milk can be added to each serving for extra protein. Teach clients to make a tasty drink by blending 8 oz of vanilla yogurt with 3 oz of frozen orange juice concentrate and a banana. A two-cup portion of the drink can be frozen for later. Tell clients to place frozen drinks at the bedside to allow for thawing while taking a nap. Upon awakening, a small serving is ready to drink.

Safe food handling techniques are essential. Hand washing with antibacterial soap is important for all food handlers. Fresh fruits and vegetables can harbor bacteria and should be avoided or eaten infrequently. Teach clients to thoroughly wash fruits with thick skins (e.g., bananas, oranges) before peeling. Other fruits and all vegetables should be cooked, frozen, or canned. Cook all meats until well done. Food should be stored in the refrigerator as soon as possible after preparation. Encourage clients to observe expiration dates on labels and dispose of opened containers of food within 48 hours. They should not eat food that has an off odor or flavor or food that is discolored or moldy. Clients should clean counters and sinks with a solution of 1 part bleach to 10 parts water before and after food preparation and wash dishes in hot, soapy water. Dishwashers disinfect dishes with high water temperature, chlorinated detergent, and high drying temperature.

Teaching clients these principles can help them to become more independent at home. They also will develop feelings of participation rather than isolation.

---

potentially fatal prognosis. Use other members of the healthcare team (clergy, social workers) to provide emotional support throughout the disease process. Include significant others in client education and care. Inform the client of support groups, financial aid resources, and other sources of assistance.

Risk for Ineffective Management of Therapeutic Regimen (Individuals) and Risk for Ineffective Management of Therapeutic Regimen: Families.
Additional nursing diagnoses are *Risk for Ineffective Management of Therapeutic Regimen (Individuals)* and *Risk for Ineffective Management of Therapeutic Regimen: Families related to the chronic nature of the disease process and the risk for complications.*

Planning: Expected Outcomes. The client and family will manage the therapeutic regimen as evidenced by effective medication administration, no infections, no hemorrhage, and the client's ability to remain independently at home.

Implementation. After the induction phase of therapy has been successfully completed, the client frequently

returns home to recover and await subsequent courses of therapy that may be given on an outpatient basis if no serious complications arise. It is not uncommon, then, for clients to return home with anemia and thrombocytopenia. They may also suffer from the residual effects of chemotherapy or radiation therapy such as loss of appetite, nausea, and mucositis. Some clients find it difficult to leave the security of the hospital setting because of significantly altered body image, fatigue, and fear.

The client and significant others should be taught how to recognize manifestations of complications as well as appropriate actions to take. It is imperative that they be well informed of measures to ensure safety and reduce risks of bleeding and infection.

Evaluation

The desired outcome for the client with leukemia is that it will become a chronic condition that the client and family cope with in a positive manner. If acute leukemia does not respond to therapy, the client's life expectancy is very short. A successful outcome of a bone marrow transplantation is engraftment with no recurrence of disease. Engraftment can occur as early as 21 days post transplant or may take weeks longer.

■ Modifications for Elderly Clients

Elderly clients, as stated earlier, are more prone to chronic leukemia. The use of chemotherapy is less vigorous than with acute leukemia. Bone marrow transplantation is an investigational option in the elderly. Some elderly persons have done quite well with a bone marrow transplant, however, it is still under investigation as a primary treatment.

Bone Marrow Transplantation

In the last 25 years, bone marrow transplantation has progressed from a treatment of last resort to a viable therapeutic modality for a variety of hematologic, malignant, and nonmalignant disorders. Whereas the basic procedures involved in transplantation are well established, many of the techniques used to purify bone marrow to reduce complications and improve prognosis are still investigational. Peripheral stem cell transplantation and autologous transplants have further revolutionized the field.

Indications

Bone marrow transplant may be considered as a treatment for clients with the following:

- Aplastic anemia
- Malignant disorders, specifically myelodysplastic syndromes, leukemia (certain types of acute, chronic, and preleukemic states), lymphoma, multiple myeloma, neuroblastoma, and selected solid tumors (breast cancer, ovarian cancer, poor-risk germ cell tumors)
- Nonmalignant hematologic disorders, such as Fanconi's anemia, thalassemia, and sickle cell anemia
- Immunodeficiency disorders, such as severe combined immunodeficiency disease (SCID) and Wiskott-Aldrich syndrome

Bone Marrow Harvesting

Sources of Bone Marrow

There are three classifications of bone marrow donors: (1) allogeneic, (2) syngeneic, and (3) autologous.

Allogeneic Bone Marrow. Allogeneic bone marrow is obtained from a relative or unrelated donor having a close HLA type. This was the most common type of marrow transplant, but it has the highest rate of morbidity and mortality because of complications of incompatibility such as GVHD (see Chapter 26). The rate of allogeneic transplants has dropped over the last 10 years with the drop in the birth rate and the increased use of autologous and peripheral stem cell transplants.

Syngeneic Bone Marrow. Syngeneic marrow is donated by an identical twin. Although syngeneic marrow is a perfect HLA match, which eliminates the risks of marrow rejection, the incidence of leukemic relapse is higher than when an allogeneic donor is used since GVHD is considered to have an antileukemic effect.

Autologous Bone Marrow. Autologous marrow is removed from the intended recipient during the remission phase to allow another course of ablative therapy to be given if a relapse occurs. Whereas autologous marrow eliminates the risk of adverse immunologic responses such as GVHD and graft rejection, relapse after autologous bone marrow transplant is a frequent occurrence. This may be due to contamination of the harvested bone marrow by malignant cells or to failure of pretransplant chemotherapy to completely eradicate the tumor cells from the body. Techniques to purge residual tumor cells from marrow (chemotherapy, monoclonal antibodies) are currently under investigation.

Histocompatibility Testing for Allogeneic and Syngeneic Transplants

Immunologic recognition of the differences in HLA antigens is the first step in host transplant rejection. As described in Chapters 25 and 26, the HLA system antigens are a complex set of protein structures found on the surface membrane of all human nucleated cells, solid tissues, and circulating blood cells except red blood cells. This genetically inherited mixture of antigens is considered representative of the tissue type of each person.

Siblings have a 1 in 4 chance of having identical sets of HLA antigens. This would provide the optimally matched allogeneic bone marrow donor. Because of the complexity of the HLA system, nonrelated clients have less than a 1 in 5000 chance of having identical HLA types. The establishment of the National Bone Marrow Donor Registry in 1987 has given hope to many clients who do not have a compatible relative donor. More than 500,000 donors have now been typed as potential bone marrow donors for unrelated clients who require transplants. This has increased the use of unrelated donors for allogeneic transplants.

Allogeneic Donor Preparation

An extensive work-up is performed for ensuring compatibility and the mental and physical well-being of the prospective donor. This evaluation includes histocompatibility testing, medical history and physical examination, chest film, ECG, laboratory evaluation (CBC, chemistry profile, viral testing, rapid plasma reagin test [syphilis], ABO and Rh blood typing, coagulation studies), and psychological evaluation (may include psychiatric consultation).

Before marrow harvest, an informed consent, including potential donor complications (pain, fever, hematoma), must be obtained. In rare instances, the donor may experience serious adverse effects from general anesthesia. Because of the significant loss of red blood cells during the harvesting process, syngeneic and allogeneic donors are required to donate autologous blood before the procedure.

Newborns are currently being used as potential donors through the use of their cord blood, which is very rich in stem cells. Some parents are now being encouraged to freeze their newborn's cord blood for future use, especially if there is a history of cancer in the family.

Marrow Collection

When collecting marrow, the client or donor is given general or spinal anesthesia in the operating room. The marrow is obtained in 2- to 5-ml aliquots from the marrow spaces of the posterior and, occasionally, anterior iliac crest and sternum. Numerous skin punctures are required; the aspiration needle is redirected to various marrow spaces without being withdrawn (Fig. 53–6). A total of 400 to 800 ml of marrow is obtained. The blood is

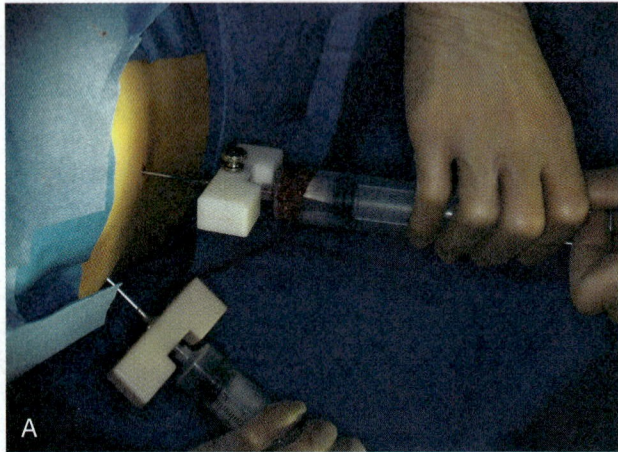

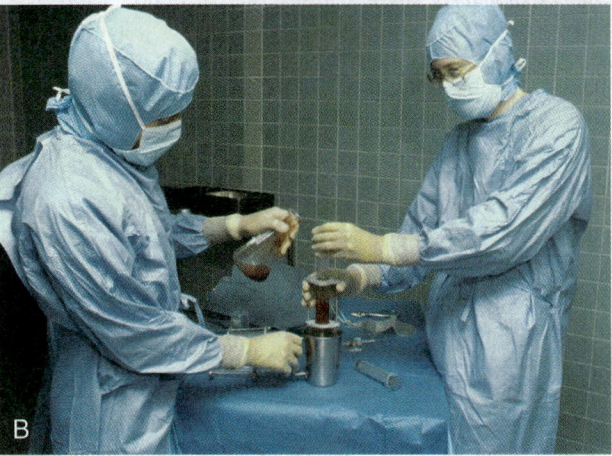

Figure 53–6. Bone marrow aspiration for bone marrow transplant. *A,* Aspiration. *B,* Collection and preservation of marrow.

placed in heparinized tissue culture media and filtered for removal of fat and bone particles. Marrow can be infused immediately or frozen in a solution containing dimethyl sulfoxide (DMSO), which preserves stem cells in the frozen state.

Peripheral Stem Cell Collection

Peripheral stem (progenitor) cells are harvested by apheresis or leukapheresis. This process involves removing blood through a large-bore catheter and running it through a machine that removes the stem cells before returning the blood to the client. Since stem cell concentration is much lower in peripheral blood compared with bone marrow, a process to increase the concentration in the peripheral blood must be done first. In order to increase the number of circulating stem cells, a stimulus such as colony-stimulating factor, interleukins, or some chemotherapeutic agents may be given to the donor before the stem cell harvest. As mentioned earlier, the umbilical cord of newborns is also rich in stem cells.

Once the stem cells have been harvested, they are preserved in the same manner as bone marrow. The engraftment of stem cells occurs at approximately the same rate as or slightly faster than with marrow transplantation. It is not known whether stem cells are less likely to contain malignant cells than marrow or whether the likelihood of relapse is the same for both types of transplant.

The Allogeneic Transplant

Recipient Preparation

The physical and psychological evaluation of the recipient is similar to that of the donor. Additional testing may be required to stage existing disease accurately. The recipient must receive immunoablative therapy before transplant. This serves three purposes: (1) malignant cells are destroyed; (2) the immune system is inactivated, which reduces the risk of GVHD; and (3) the marrow cavities are emptied to provide space for implantation of the transfused stem cells.

Common protocols combine total body irradiation and very high doses of a single chemotherapeutic agent or fractionated doses of multiple agents. A multilumen central venous catheter is inserted to provide suitable access for marrow infusion as well as for antibiotics, blood products, hyperalimentation, and frequent blood sampling.

Bone Marrow Infusion

The infusion of the marrow is often anticlimactic after the client has undergone the rigorous preparatory chemotherapy and radiation therapy. The marrow is usually administered immediately after the conditioning regimen is complete. Marrow is administered from a large blood infusion bag equipped with a standard blood filter via a multilumen catheter. Small volumes may also be prefiltered and given by IV push by a physician.

Potential immediate adverse reactions are allergic (urticaria, chills, fever), volume overload, and pulmonary complications secondary to fat emboli. Renal damage may occur from too many erythrocytes. The period immediately after transplant is critical. Multisystem failure related to ablative therapy is common, as are immune reactions caused by the transplanted cells.

The most common and potentially disastrous complication of bone marrow transplant is GVHD, which may occur acutely 7 to 30 days after infusion of viable lymphocytes. The donor T lymphocytes form an immunologic reaction against the host cells. Acute GVHD is staged according to the organ system affected. It usually affects the gut, skin, or liver. Maculopapular rash involving less than 25% of the body surface, moderate manifestations of liver dysfunction, and mild gastrointestinal manifestations are classified as stage I. This occurs in the majority of allogeneic transplant clients. Stages II to IV are classified by increasing degrees of erythema with bullous formation and desquamation, hepatic coma, and more than 200 ml of stool per day. Localized skin involvement may resolve without treatment. Systemic complications may be treated with immunosuppressive drug therapy. The prognosis and treatment depend on the severity of the syndrome. Acute GVHD that does not respond to treatment greatly increases the morbidity and mortality of bone marrow transplantation.

Chronic GVHD, a long-term form of the disease with less acute manifestations, may occur even if the client has not experienced acute GVHD. Chronic GVHD resembles autoimmune collagen-vascular disorders, such as systemic lupus erythematosus. It is characterized by scleroderma-like skin fibrosis and Sjögren's syndrome, in which the mucosa and lacrimal ducts are abnormally dry.

Diagnosis of chronic GVHD is confirmed by skin and oral mucosal biopsy. Chronic GVHD appears approximately 100 days after transplantation; it may affect the liver, gastrointestinal system, oral mucosa, and lungs, as well as the skin.

Whereas severe GVHD is usually fatal, researchers believe that a complete absence of this immune reaction increases the risk of leukemic relapse. This may be due to a beneficial graft-versus-leukemic reaction that mild GVHD stimulates. Studies are in progress to determine the number of T cells that must be purged from the marrow to reduce the risk of severe GVHD but not destroy the antileukemic effects of mild disease.

The client will remain pancytopenic until the transplanted stem cells make their way to the medullary cavities, where subsequent growth and reconstitution of the marrow are confirmed. Indications of successful engraftment are an increase in platelets and red blood cells in the peripheral blood count. This may occur as early as 14 days after marrow infusion. Each day that recovery is delayed places the client at added risk. Graft rejection is evident if the bone marrow fails to produce peripheral blood cells after several weeks.

Nursing management of bone marrow transplant clients follows the plan of care for any completely immunosuppressed client. In addition, those receiving allogeneic transplant must be closely observed for manifestations of GVHD. Therapy to treat GVHD includes high doses of methylprednisolone, antithymocyte globulin (ATG), antilymphocyte globulin (ALG), cyclosporine, and anti-T cell immunotoxins. These also leave the client immunosuppressed and vulnerable to infection.

Agranulocytosis

Agranulocytosis (granulocytopenia, malignant neutropenia) is an acute, potentially fatal blood dyscrasia characterized by profound neutropenia. Neutropenia is a reduction in the number of circulating neutrophils. Because neutrophils make up roughly 93% of all granulocytes, the terms neutropenia and agranulocytosis are often used interchangeably.

Agranulocytosis is a fairly rare condition. For unknown reasons, females are much more susceptible to this condition than are males. However, even among females, agranulocytosis is relatively rare.

Etiology and Risk Factors

The most common cause of agranulocytosis is drug toxicity or hypersensitivity. Two groups of agents are capable of suppressing granulocyte production:

1. Agents that always produce neutropenia when given in sufficiently large doses over time, such as many cancer chemotherapeutic agents, ionizing radiation, and benzene
2. Agents that produce neutropenia only in clients particularly sensitive to the drug, such as tranquilizers (chlorpromazine), antithyroid agents (propylthiouracil), anticonvulsants (phenytoin), antibiotics (chloramphenicol), and phenylbutazone

Agranulocytosis can occur in clients who have anemias related to diminished erythropoiesis (such as aplastic anemia, megaloblastic anemia). It may also accompany certain diseases, such as tuberculosis, typhoid fever, malaria, and uremia.

Exposure to any of the etiologic factors increases the client's risk of developing agranulocytosis. Avoidance of these agents, whenever possible, helps prevent the development of the condition.

Pathophysiology

Agranulocytosis results either from the failure of neutrophil production to keep pace with destruction of the cells or from increased destruction of neutrophils, which removes them from circulation. Chemotherapy, radiation, and aplastic anemia all reduce or stop neutrophil production through interference with granulopoiesis.

Accelerated destruction of the neutrophils can result from infection, autoimmune disease, and idiosyncratic reactions to many drugs. The destruction may be so rapid that production cannot keep up with it. If agranulocytosis is not reversed when the cause is removed, the client will require an allogeneic bone marrow transplant for survival.

Clinical Manifestations and Diagnostic Findings

The manifestations of agranulocytosis result from the neutropenia. Neutrophils constitute a swift and powerful defense against invading microorganisms. Consequently, decreases in their number result in a greater susceptibility to bacterial invasion, especially when the client's absolute neutrophil count (ANC) drops below 500/mm³. The mucous membranes of the throat and mouth are particularly vulnerable.

Typically, the onset of this acute disease is rapid. For the first 2 or 3 days, there is severe fatigue and weakness. Next, the client develops a sore throat, ulcerations of the pharyngeal and buccal mucosa, dysphagia, high fever, weak and rapid pulse, and severe chills. Without prompt antibiotic treatment, the disorder usually causes death within a week.

Diagnosis of agranulocytosis rests on the following:

- Leukopenia evidenced by white blood cell counts of 500 to 3000/mm³ with extreme reduction in polymorphonuclear cells (0%–2%)
- Bone marrow examination revealing an absence of granulocytes, a maturational arrest of young developing cells, or an increased number of myeloid precursors (signifying peripheral granulocyte destruction)
- Cultures of urine, blood, and ulcerative lesions in the throat and mouth that are positive for bacteria (usually gram-positive cocci)
- A history of exposure to an offending agent, plus all the above findings; because many clients medicate themselves with potentially dangerous drugs, investigate all drugs taken within the past 6 to 12 months

Acute and Subacute Care

■ Medical Management

Treatment of clients with agranulocytosis involves eliminating potentially toxic agents that may be responsible for marrow suppression. Agranulocytosis caused by toxic substances is usually reversed within 2 to 3 weeks after their elimination.

Surveillance cultures of blood, throat, sputum, urine, and stool should be taken at frequent intervals to monitor the status of infections.

Antibiotics. Pharmacologic treatment includes antimicrobial therapy in the event of positive cultures, fever, or manifestations of impending shock. Combinations of broad-spectrum antibiotics are usually administered until the offending organism is identified. Untreated infectious processes in this situation carry a mortality rate of 80%.

Colony-Stimulating Factors. A newer treatment for agranulocytosis are the variety of colony-stimulating factors such as G-CSF, GM-CSF, and erythropoietin

(EPO). These are given after the offending agent has been eliminated.

■ Nursing Management of the Medical Client

Assessment

Physical assessment should include vital signs with attention paid to a high fever or a weak, rapid pulse. Any complaints of a sore throat, dysphagia, or mouth sores should be examined. The client's history should include names of all drugs the client is presently taking (prescription or nonprescription) or has taken in the past 6 months.

Diagnosis, Planning, Implementation

Knowledge Deficit. The nursing diagnosis is *Knowledge Deficit related to toxic agents that cause agranulocytosis.*

Planning: Expected Outcomes. The client will have knowledge of agranulocytosis, as evidenced by the client's verbalization of understanding of the cause of the disorder, the need to avoid self-medication, and the importance of follow-up examinations.

Implementation. An important aspect of nursing management is to prevent agranulocytosis by providing clients with education regarding potentially dangerous medications and chemicals. To enhance awareness, encourage the client to avoid self-medication without a physician's order, to schedule frequent follow-up by a physician when medications known to cause granulocytopenia are prescribed, and to realize that repeated exposure to toxic chemicals such as benzene may cause agranulocytosis.

Evaluation

The client and significant others should understand the condition, its causes, and treatments prior to discharge. If questions still exist, try other teaching methods. If the client still requires follow-up, refer the client to a visiting nurse agency for further care and teaching.

Multiple Myeloma

Multiple myeloma is a B-cell neoplastic condition characterized by abnormal malignant proliferation of plasma cells secreting a monoclonal paraprotein, accumulation of mature plasma cells in the bone marrow, and complications throughout the body as a result of dissemination of the disease (such as lytic bone lesions and osteoporosis, hematopoietic suppression, hypercalcemia, proteinuria, and renal failure).

The condition commonly occurs in people over 40 years of age; the average age is 60 years. It is more common in males and blacks. Multiple myeloma is considered a lymphoid malignancy. Its incidence is about 1% of that of all malignant diseases.

Etiology and Risk Factors

Risk factors include an increased incidence in some families, ionizing radiation, and occupational chemical exposures.

Pathophysiology

Multiple myeloma is characterized by an abnormal proliferation of plasma cells. With this overproduction of plasma cells, bone destruction also occurs. In addition to bone destruction, multiple myeloma is characterized by disruption of red blood cell, leukocyte, and platelet production, which results from plasma cells crowding the bone marrow. Impaired production of these cell forms causes anemia, increased vulnerability to infection, and bleeding tendencies, respectively.

Complications of multiple myeloma include hypercalcemia, renal problems, and neurologic disorders. Hypercalcemia resulting from the release of calcium during bone destruction is present in 30% of newly diagnosed clients with multiple myeloma. It causes confusion, anorexia, nausea, vomiting, constipation, abdominal pain, ileus, and impairment of renal concentrating mechanisms that can eventually lead to irreversible renal failure. In addition, renal disease results from particles of coagulated protein that block the convoluted tubules. The major neurologic complications entail compression of the spinal cord, sometimes followed by paraplegia. Pain secondary to lytic bone lesions also is common.

Clinical Manifestations and Diagnostic Findings

The onset of multiple myeloma is usually gradual and insidious. Most people pass through a long presymptomatic period that lasts 5 to 20 years. Only 10% of clients are diagnosed at this stage, usually only by chance as a result of an elevated serum protein level found during a screening examination.[3]

Once manifestations appear, they typically involve the skeletal system, particularly the pelvis, spine, and ribs. Some clients have backache or bone pain that worsens with movement. Others suffer sudden pathologic fractures accompanied by severe pain. In time, skeletal destruction increases and the client may develop sternum and rib cage deformities. Diffuse osteoporosis usually appears, accompanied by a negative calcium balance. The skull shows multiple osteolytic lesions. Loss of calcium and phosphorus from damaged bones eventually leads to the development of renal stones, particularly in immobilized clients.

Diagnosis of multiple myeloma rests on x-ray studies, bone marrow biopsy, and blood and urine examination. X-ray studies reveal diffuse lesions in the bone, widespread demineralization, and osteoporosis. The bone marrow contains large numbers of immature plasma cells. Normally, plasma cells constitute 5% of the bone marrow

cell population. Because of the abnormal number of plasma cells producing immunoglobulins, peripheral blood samples sent for plasma electrophoresis reveal a large amount of abnormal immunoglobulins. Another diagnostic manifestation of multiple myeloma is the appearance of Bence Jones protein in the urine, consisting of monoclonal immunoglobulin light chains.

Acute and Subacute Care

■ Medical Management

Not all clients diagnosed with multiple myeloma should be treated. Manifestations, physical findings, and laboratory data must be considered. In some cases, treatment might be withheld and the client reevaluated in 2 to 3 months. If overt manifestations are present, chemotherapy is the preferred initial treatment. Palliative radiation should be limited to clients with disabling pain from a well-defined location that has not been responsive to chemotherapy. Autologous or allogeneic bone marrow transplantation is also an option.

Management is aimed at early recognition and treatment of complications of the disease. Clients with hypercalcemia often become anorectic, nauseated, drowsy, confused, and disoriented and may require hospitalization.

Chemotherapy. There is some controversy over the most effective chemotherapy regimen. Melphalan and prednisone or a combination of alkylating agents has shown objective responses. Prednisone and melphalan given orally for a period of 7 days and repeated at 6-week intervals produces positive results in 50% to 60% of clients. Leukocyte and platelet counts are be monitored regularly and doses adjusted until modest cytopenia occurs. Combination chemotherapy, commonly melphalan, cyclophosphamide, carmustine (BCNU), vincristine (Oncovin), and prednisone, has shown a 70% to 75% response rate. This therapy may continue for 1 to 2 years, but relapse almost always occurs when chemotherapy is discontinued. Interferon appears to be beneficial in prolonging the duration of remission.

Anticalcium Agents. Corticosteroids such as high-dose dexamethasone, mithramycin, furosemide, and IV hydration were commonly prescribed for hypercalcemia; however, newer agents now exist. Etidronate disodium (Didronel) or gallium nitrate (Ganite) and IV hydration are now used to effectively treat the hypercalcemia. The newest and most effective agent is pamidronate sodium (Aredia).

In addition, be alert to the possibility of spinal cord compression, another complication of multiple myeloma. Treatment usually consists of radiation therapy and large doses of steroids, although a laminectomy may be indicated.

■ Nursing Management of the Medical Client

Assessment

Clients with multiple myeloma must be closely assessed for the development of hypercalcemia so that it can be treated adequately. Also monitor the client's pain so that pain medications can be administered as needed.

Diagnosis, Planning, Implementation

Risk for Injury. Because of the hypercalcemia secondary to bone destruction, write the nursing diagnosis as *Risk for Injury related to bone destruction.*

Planning: Expected Outcomes. The client will not suffer injury from hypercalcemia, as evidenced by initiation of treatment before serum calcium levels are excessively elevated; absence of renal stones; no permanent renal damage; absence of nausea, vomiting, constipation, abdominal pain, or ileus; and no evidence of confusion or disorientation.

Implementation. Administer fluids in adequate amounts to maintain an output of 1.5 to 2.0 L/day. Clients with multiple myeloma usually require about 3 L of fluid per day. The client needs sufficient fluid not only to dilute the calcium overload but also to prevent protein from precipitating in the renal tubules, even after being effectively treated with chemotherapy. Administer medications to increase calcium excretion and decrease calcium loss from bone such as furosemide (Lasix), steroids, and plicamycin, etidronate, gallium, or pamidronate.

If the client is able, encourage activity that places stress on the long bones to increase calcium resorption. Antiemetics may be required for relief of nausea and vomiting. Small, frequent feedings may be better tolerated, and stool softeners may be routinely required. Closely monitor intake, output, and blood studies to determine effectiveness of treatment. Weigh the client daily so that any significant loss can be noted and corrected.

If disorientation or confusion occurs, remove sharp objects and other potentially hazardous items from the environment. The side rails should be raised, and light restraints may be required. Monitor the client's mental status closely.

Teach significant others the manifestations of hypercalcemia and to report them immediately to the physician. Also instruct the significant others on how to institute safety measures to prevent falls and injuries. The client may need some assistive devices at home, such as a toilet riser and handhold bars in the bathroom.

Measure the client's calcium level at regular intervals for assessment of the development of hypercalcemia.

Pain. Another nursing diagnosis is *Pain related to bone degeneration and possible pathologic fractures.*
Planning: Expected Outcomes. The client will have pain controlled and fractures prevented, as evidenced by his or her report of pain relief and absence of pathologic fractures.
Implementation. Clients with multiple myeloma suffer from bone pain and pathologic fractures. Administer adequate amounts of prescribed analgesics to control the client's pain. The client may be referred to the physical therapist for establishing an exercise and activity plan that will reduce the incidence of fractures. Braces may be prescribed to help control pain, especially a brace for the spine.

Evaluation

Even if the disease is only controlled by the treatments, a successful outcome would be that the client did not develop pathologic fractures and that the pain was well controlled.

Disorders of the Lymphoid System

Lymphoma is a diverse group of lymphoid neoplasms that results in uncontrolled proliferation of lymphocytes. It arises in the lymphoid tissues, that is, lymph nodes, thymus, spleen, and lymphoid tissue of the gastrointestinal tract. Lymphomas include a number of diseases that have different manifestations, treatments, and prognoses, depending on the lymphocyte type and stage of differentiation. Lymphomas are classified as either (1) Hodgkin's disease or (2) non-Hodgkin's lymphoma. Lymphomas that contain Reed-Sternberg cells (multinucleated giant cells) are termed Hodgkin's disease; those without Reed-Sternberg cells are called non-Hodgkin's lymphoma.

Hodgkin's Disease

Hodgkin's disease is a chronic, progressive, neoplastic disorder of lymphoid tissue characterized by the painless enlargement of lymph nodes with progression to extralymphatic sites such as the spleen and liver. The pathologic involvement of tissues and organs throughout the body follows.

A disorder of young adults, Hodgkin's disease principally occurs between the ages of 20 and 40 years. Among those affected, men outnumber women, and boys are stricken five times more often than are girls. Hodgkin's disease involves the proliferation of abnormal histiocytes called Reed-Sternberg cells, which are part of the tissue macrophage system. As these atypical glial cells multiply, they replace other cellular elements normally found within the lymph nodes.

Etiology and Risk Factors

The cause of lymphoma is unknown. However, persons who develop long-term immunosuppression due to illness, therapeutic treatment, or drug abuse suffer an increased incidence of the disease. There appears to be a higher risk of Hodgkin's disease in persons with high titers of Epstein-Barr virus or a history of mononucleosis.

Immunosuppression due to therapy or as a result of disease is a major risk factor for the development of Hodgkin's disease. This risk is usually not preventable, so clients should be carefully monitored for the development of this disease. Drug abuse is the most preventable cause of the disease.

Pathophysiology

The mechanism of growth and spread of Hodgkin's disease remains unknown. Some have suggested that the disease progresses by extension to adjacent structures. It may also disseminate via the lymphatics, because lymphoreticular cells inhabit all tissues of the body except the central nervous system. Hematologic spread may also occur, possibly by means of direct infiltration of blood vessels.

Hodgkin's disease is divided into categories or stages according to the microscopic appearance of the involved lymph nodes, the extent and severity of the disorder, and the prognosis. Table 53–3 shows one method of staging.

The complete remission rate for clients with Hodgkin's disease is 75% to 90%. The recurrence rate varies with the stage of disease from 10% to 20%. If untreated, clients with Hodgkin's disease have a life expectancy of 5 years.

Clinical Manifestations and Diagnostic Findings

Hodgkin's disease usually presents as a painless enlarged lymph node, often in the cervical region. The client may experience unexplained fevers, night sweats, and weight loss (B manifestations). Many clients also experience pruritus. Hepatosplenomegaly may be present, although it usually does not cause manifestations. Likewise, although disease may be present in the bone marrow, it often does not cause pancytopenia.

In addition, some clients with Hodgkin's disease experience pain over the involved nodes after ingesting alcohol. Others may have a nonproductive cough, and the chest film may reveal a mediastinal mass. Other manifestations arise when enlarged lymph nodes obstruct or compress an adjacent structure (e.g., edema of the face, neck, and right arm secondary to superior vena cava compression; or renal failure secondary to urethral obstruction). Figure 53–7 outlines the major assessment data and physiologic bases for Hodgkin's disease.

If the tumor infiltrates the spine and presses on the spinal cord, the client can develop manifestations of spinal cord compression. Manifestations range from early back pain with motor weakness and sensory loss to loss of motor function, urinary retention, constipation, and other manifestations of compression of the cord late in the disease. Treatment includes radiation therapy to the area, surgical decompression with a laminectomy, chemotherapy, and IV steroids. If all function is lost, the client will be paralyzed below the area of infiltration.

Lymph node biopsy provides a definitive test for diagnosing Hodgkin's disease. With peripheral lymph node enlargement, one entire node is removed and examined for the presence of Reed-Sternberg cells. Some clients do not have enlarged peripheral lymph nodes but may simply notice pruritus, intermittent fever, and weakness. In these cases, chest films or computed tomographic scans may reveal evidence of mediastinal or hilar adenopathy. However, Hodgkin's disease can be definitely diagnosed only by pathologic examination of tissues. Also, because of immune system disturbances, clients with Hodgkin's disease usually react abnormally to tuberculin skin testing.

Table 53–3. Cotswolds Staging Classification for Hodgkin's Disease

Stage I:	Involvement of a single lymph node region or a lymphoid structure (e.g., spleen, thymus, Waldeyer's ring).
Stage II:	Involvement of two or more lymph node regions on the same side of the diaphragm (i.e., the mediastinum is a single site, hilar lymph nodes are lateralized). The number of anatomic sites should be indicated by a subscript (e.g., II_2).
Stage III:	Involvement of lymph node regions or structures on both sides of the diaphragm: III_1: With or without involvement of splenic, hilar, celiac, or portal nodes. III_2: With involvement of para-aortic, iliac, or mesenteric nodes.
Stage IV:	Involvement of extranodal site(s) beyond that designated E.

Designation Applicable to Any Disease Stage

A:	No manifestations
B:	Fever, drenching sweats, weight loss
X:	Bulky disease: > $\frac{1}{3}$ the width of the mediastinum < 10 cm maximal dimension of nodal mass
E:	Involvement of a single extranodal site, contiguous or proximal to a known nodal site.
CS:	Clinical stage
PS:	Pathologic stage

Data from Bennett, J. C., et al. (1996). *Cecil textbook of medicine* (20th ed.). Philadelphia: W. B. Saunders.

Acute and Subacute Care

■ Surgical Management

As stated above, a lymph node biopsy is the definitive method of diagnosing Hodgkin's disease. This may be followed by a staging laparotomy with liver and lymph node biopsies. A splenectomy may also be done. This procedure can be used to stage the disease to determine the appropriate therapy.

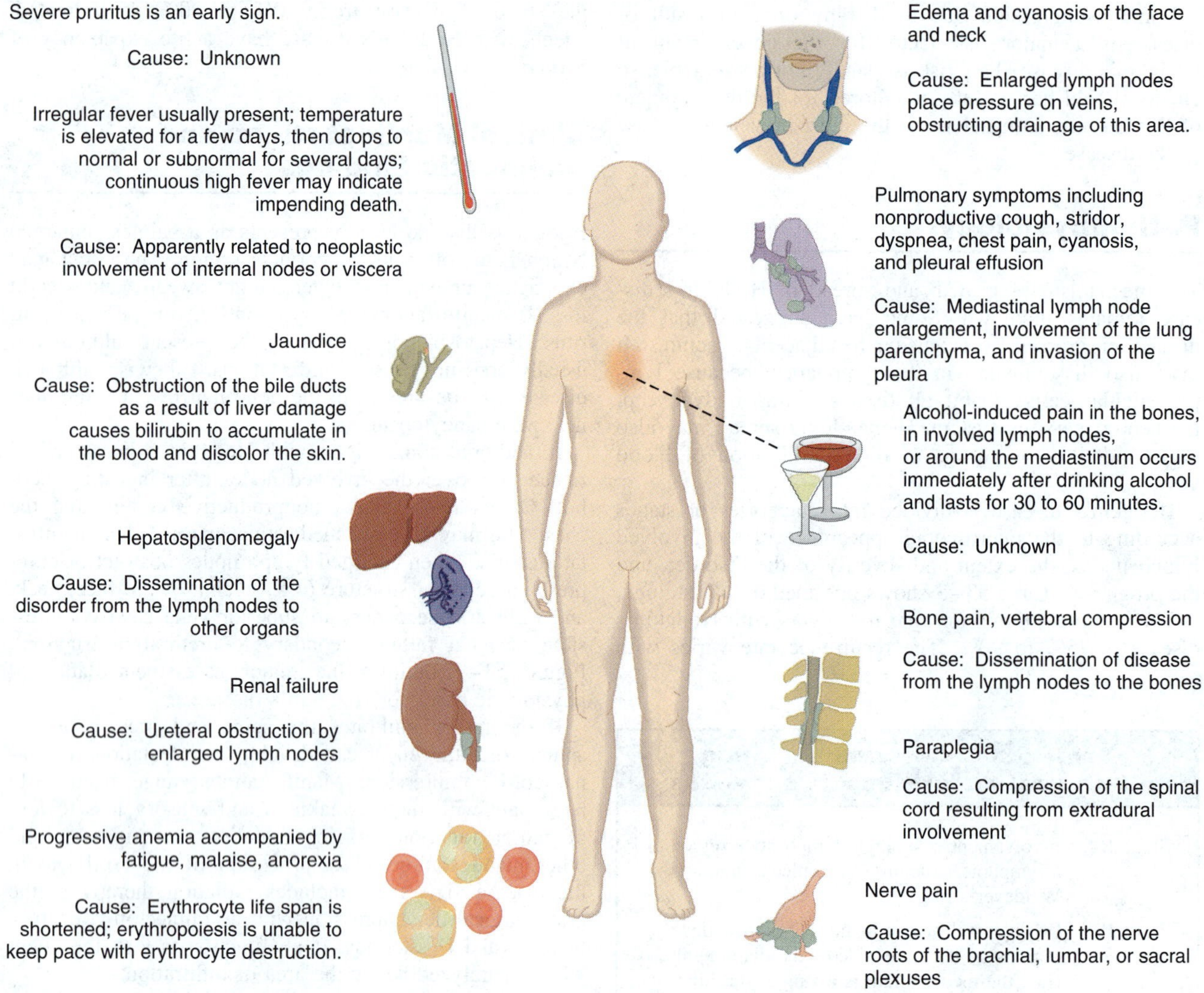

Severe pruritus is an early sign.

Cause: Unknown

Irregular fever usually present; temperature is elevated for a few days, then drops to normal or subnormal for several days; continuous high fever may indicate impending death.

Cause: Apparently related to neoplastic involvement of internal nodes or viscera

Jaundice

Cause: Obstruction of the bile ducts as a result of liver damage causes bilirubin to accumulate in the blood and discolor the skin.

Hepatosplenomegaly

Cause: Dissemination of the disorder from the lymph nodes to other organs

Renal failure

Cause: Ureteral obstruction by enlarged lymph nodes

Progressive anemia accompanied by fatigue, malaise, anorexia

Cause: Erythrocyte life span is shortened; erythropoiesis is unable to keep pace with erythrocyte destruction.

Edema and cyanosis of the face and neck

Cause: Enlarged lymph nodes place pressure on veins, obstructing drainage of this area.

Pulmonary symptoms including nonproductive cough, stridor, dyspnea, chest pain, cyanosis, and pleural effusion

Cause: Mediastinal lymph node enlargement, involvement of the lung parenchyma, and invasion of the pleura

Alcohol-induced pain in the bones, in involved lymph nodes, or around the mediastinum occurs immediately after drinking alcohol and lasts for 30 to 60 minutes.

Cause: Unknown

Bone pain, vertebral compression

Cause: Dissemination of disease from the lymph nodes to the bones

Paraplegia

Cause: Compression of the spinal cord resulting from extradural involvement

Nerve pain

Cause: Compression of the nerve roots of the brachial, lumbar, or sacral plexuses

Figure 53–7. Hodgkin's disease: assessment data and pathophysiologic bases.

■ Nursing Management of the Surgical Client

Nursing care of the client following a staging laparotomy and biopsy is the same as for any client following major abdominal surgery. The nursing care of a client with a splenectomy is discussed later in this chapter. In addition, you should be sensitive to the anxiety the client may be experiencing since the final diagnosis may take several days.

■ Medical Management

Treatment of Hodgkin's disease varies according to its stage at diagnosis. Stages I and II are treated with radiation therapy and chemotherapy. Clients with stages III and IV disease may receive radiation coupled with an aggressive multiagent chemotherapy regimen. Bone marrow transplantation may also be used to treat Hodgkin's disease.

Chemotherapy. In stage IIB, III, and IV disease, a multiagent drug regimen is the treatment of choice. MOPP (*m*echlorethamine, *O*ncovin [vincristine], *p*rocarbazine, and *p*rednisone) is the most widely used regimen (Table 53–4). Other chemotherapeutic regimens have also been used with success such as ABVD (*A*driamycin [doxorubicin], *b*leomycin, *v*inblastine, and *d*acarbazine).

The most distressing and immediate side effect of the chemotherapeutic agents used to treat Hodgkin's disease is severe nausea and vomiting. Manifestations may be controlled with agents such as ondansetron or ganisetron, new antiemetic agents that work well against nausea. Pancytopenia, a toxic effect of these agents, usually occurs 10 to 14 days after IV therapy. Any significant degree of anemia, leukopenia, or thrombocytopenia indicates that treatment must be delayed or the medication dosage adjusted. However, since this treatment is often for cure, these complications will not cause therapy to be stopped.

Radiation Therapy. Radiation therapy was the primary therapy for Hodgkin's disease. It was found, however, that the dosage of radiation used to "cure" Hodgkin's was found to predispose the client to the development of leukemia approximately 20 years after the radiation treatments. It was found that combining it with chemotherapy lowered the amount of radiation needed to achieve the same results.

■ Nursing Management of the Medical Client

Caring for the client with Hodgkin's disease revolves around control of complications associated with the pancytopenia. Supportive measures to prevent or control bleeding and infection are important. If these complications can be avoided during the treatment regimen for Hodgkin's disease, the client has a good chance for survival. A good antiemetic regimen is also instituted to prevent or treat nausea.

Non-Hodgkin's Lymphoma

Non-Hodgkin's lymphomas are a group of lymphoid disorders. Involvement starts in the lymph nodes, although a significant number, more than in Hodgkin's disease, arise outside the lymphoid system. Non-Hodgkin's lymphoma is more common in adults in their middle and older years; it is more common in males than in females in a ratio of 5:3. Many classification systems are used to differentiate non-Hodgkin's lymphoma according to histologic type and cytologic characteristics. Treatment protocols and prognosis for clients with non-Hodgkin's lymphoma vary greatly. Without effective treatment, non-Hodgkin's lymphomas are very quickly fatal.

Treatment consists of radiation therapy, chemotherapy, or a combination of both, and possibly bone marrow transplantation. Overall, the prognosis of non-Hodgkin's lymphoma is poorer than that of Hodgkin's disease. Stage I is rarely observed, because it is not usually diagnosed at this stage. If the disease is detected during this early stage, remissions have been achieved by use of involved field radiotherapy alone. In stage II disease, if the involved areas are contiguous and together, radiotherapy proves effective. Clients with stage III and stage IV disease will probably benefit more from combination chemotherapy with or without radiation therapy.

The cure rate for aggressive tumors with treatment is significantly better than for the slower-growing, low-grade type, presumably because rapidly growing cells are more susceptible to chemotherapy and radiation therapy. In some clients with large masses, surgical removal or debulking of the mass may be required before chemotherapy or radiation therapy.

Infectious Mononucleosis

Infectious mononucleosis (also known as glandular disease and the "kissing disease") is a self-limiting condition characterized by painful enlargement of the lymph nodes, lymphocytosis, sore throat, and fever.

Primarily a disease of the young, infectious mononucleosis usually strikes children between the ages of 3 and 5 years and young adults between the ages of 15 and 25 years. The greatest incidence occurs among college students, medical students, and nurses. Although this disease usually occurs sporadically, epidemic forms may sweep through colleges and children's homes.

Etiology and Risk Factors

The cause of infectious mononucleosis is a herpesvirus, the Epstein-Barr virus. Although the mode of transmission remains unknown, the disease may be transmitted through the oropharyngeal route during close contact, as with kissing.

Pathophysiology

Infectious mononucleosis is a relatively mild disorder but has widespread effects on the body. For example, the

Day of Cycle	M Mechlorethamine	O Oncovin (Vincristine)	P Procarbazine	P Prednisone †
1, 8	IV	IV	PO	PO
2, 9			PO	PO
3, 10			PO	PO
4, 11			PO	PO
5, 12			PO	PO
6, 13			PO	PO
7, 14			PO	PO

Table 53–4. MOPP Combination Chemotherapy Regimen for Hodgkin's Disease*

* Therapy consists of at least six 14-day cycles with 14 days' rest between cycles. Intravenous (IV) or oral (PO) medication doses are adjusted according to laboratory test results of white blood cells and platelets.
† In first and fourth cycle only.

lymph nodes enlarge, lymphocytosis occurs, the spleen may swell to two to three times its normal size, liver function is sometimes impaired, and both peripheral and central nervous system involvement can develop.

Clinical Manifestations and Diagnostic Findings

The onset of infectious mononucleosis follows an incubation period of 2 to 6 weeks. Before frank clinical manifestations present, the person may experience fatigue, headaches, malaise, and myalgias. Subsequently, assessment reveals temperatures up to 39° C (102.2° F), pharyngitis, and lymphadenopathy that is more pronounced in the cervical regions. Ten percent to 15% of those affected develop a maculopapular rash that closely resembles the rash of rubella. Splenic enlargement causes left upper quadrant pain. Nervous system involvement may lead to severe headache. In rare cases, liver involvement may develop into a hepatitis-like syndrome. When infectious mononucleosis is severe, the client may develop the following two complications:

1. Splenic rupture resulting from the infiltration of the spleen by massive numbers of lymphocytes
2. Streptococcal pharyngitis or Vincent's angina secondary to bacterial invasion of the throat

The diagnosis of infectious mononucleosis is based on three criteria: (1) physical assessment, (2) laboratory tests, and (3) the Paul-Bunnel test.

History and Physical Examination. Physical assessment typically reveals fever, lymphadenopathy, sore throat, and splenomegaly.

Laboratory Tests. The white blood cell count usually ranges from 12,000 to 20,000/mm³, of which 50% are lymphocytes and monocytes and 10% to 20% are large, atypical lymphocytes.

Paul-Bunnell Test. In 1932, Paul and Bunnell discovered that the blood of persons with infectious mononucleosis contained heterophil antibodies that would agglutinate the red blood cells of sheep. Humans normally do not produce agglutinins against sheep erythrocytes. Consequently, the Paul-Bunnel test helps confirm a diagnosis of infectious mononucleosis; clients usually test positive within 5 to 7 days of acute onset. However, positive tests sometimes occur in other conditions.

Community and Self-Care

■ Medical Management

No specific intervention either mitigates or shortens the disease process. Because infectious mononucleosis must simply run its course, treatments are directed at control of manifestations. Bedrest is recommended until fever is re-

solved. Salicylates, cool sponge baths, and a large fluid intake help control fever. Warm saline throat irrigations may relieve the sore throat. Steroids do not in any way alter or accelerate the course of the disease. Physicians may prescribe them, however, to promote a sense of well-being.

■ Nursing Management of the Medical Client

In addition to providing symptomatic relief, work toward preventing complications and administering treatment. When caring for clients with infectious mononucleosis, do the following:

● Caution the client against engaging in excessive activity for a period of at least 1 month, especially contact sports, which could result in splenic rupture or lowered resistance to infection.
● Watch closely for and report the two manifestations of splenic rupture: abdominal pain and shock.
● If throat pain worsens, report it immediately so that appropriate antibiotic therapy can be started.

Although complications sometimes develop, the prognosis for clients with infectious mononucleosis is generally excellent. The febrile phase of this disorder typically lasts 2 to 4 weeks. During the long convalescence, the client slowly regains strength and energy.

Splenic Rupture and Hypersplenism

Despite the important functions of the spleen, it can be removed (splenectomy) without harm in adults. Its role can be taken over completely by other organs (e.g., liver, lymph nodes, and bone marrow). The most frequent indication for splenectomy is rupture of the spleen complicated by severe hemorrhage. Splenic irradiation may achieve a reversal of cytopenia without the risk of surgery.

Etiology and Risk Factors

Causes of splenic rupture include (1) trauma (e.g., automobile accidents, bullet or knife wounds, severe blows to the spleen), (2) accidental tearing of the splenic capsule during surgery on neighboring organs, and (3) disease of the spleen that causes softening or damage (e.g., infectious mononucleosis and malaria).

In hypersplenism, a second important indication for splenectomy, the spleen destroys, in excessive numbers, one of the blood cell types (i.e., erythrocytes, leukocytes, or platelets). Primary hypersplenism occurs in idiopathic thrombocytopenic purpura and congenital spherocytosis. Some etiologic factors associated with secondary hypersplenism include lymphomas (including Hodgkin's disease), leukemia, polycythemia vera, acute infections (including infectious mononucleosis), chronic infections, malaria, syphilis, the hemoglobinopathy, and cirrhosis of the liver.

Clinical Manifestations and Diagnostic Factors

Manifestations of hypersplenism include moderate to massive splenomegaly, anemia, leukopenia, or thrombocytopenia, and a compensatory increase in the production of the affected cell line by the bone marrow. Overactivity of the spleen develops either as a primary condition of unknown origin or as a condition secondary to another disease.

Laboratory indications for splenectomy include granulocytopenia of less than 500/mm^3 and thrombocytopenia of less than 20,000/mm^3. The surgery itself is relatively simple unless the spleen is greatly enlarged or surrounded by adhesions.

Acute and Subacute Care

■ Surgical Management

Primary hypersplenism can be alleviated by splenectomy. Splenectomy is only palliative for clients with secondary hypersplenism, because the surgery has little or no effect on the course of the primary illness. When hypersplenism is diagnosed, it is important to teach the client to prevent complications associated with the specific cytopenia.

The spleen has an important role in the phagocytosis of circulating opsonized organisms. After splenectomy, young children are at high risk of fulminant infections due to *Streptococcus pneumoniae, Haemophilus influenzae, Neisseria meningitidis,* and other encapsulated organisms. Continuous prophylactic antibiotics may be advisable during the early years or indefinitely. Adults are also at increased risk of infection, especially during the first 3 years after surgery. The splenectomized client should be advised to seek medical treatment at the earliest manifestations of infection.

■ Nursing Management of the Surgical Client

Assessment

The unique functions performed by the spleen are eventually taken over by other organs. However, the loss of the spleen due to cessation of function or splenectomy does require the client to be monitored for potentially serious complications. The nursing care of the client undergoing splenectomy is generally the same as that discussed in Chapter 21 for any client undergoing surgery.

Diagnosis, Planning, Implementation

Risk for Hemorrhage. A collaborative problem is *Risk for Hemorrhage related to surgical procedure.*

Planning: Expected Outcomes. The client will not suffer from hemorrhage or will have hemorrhage detected early, as evidenced by normal blood pressure and pulse, no evidence of bleeding, and absence of manifestations of shock.

Implementation. The client should be carefully monitored for the development of hemorrhage by frequently taking and recording vital signs and measuring the abdominal girth. Clients undergoing splenectomy for thrombocytopenia are still at increased risk for hemorrhage in the postoperative period. Platelet transfusions may be given before or after surgery if the platelet count is less than 100,000/mm^3.

Risk for Infection. A nursing diagnosis is *Risk for Infection related to loss of macrophage activity after splenectomy.*

Planning: Expected Outcomes. The client will not develop an infection or will have infection detected and treated early, as evidenced by absence of fever, no rales or manifestations of pneumonia, and wound healing without difficulty.

Implementation. Teach the client to recognize early manifestations of infection (fever, chills, productive cough, shortness of breath, myalgia, neck stiffness) and to seek medical treatment immediately. Be sure the client and significant others understand the importance of prophylactic antibiotics; monitor compliance. If prophylactic antibiotics are not being taken routinely, advise the client to obtain a limited supply when traveling to locations where medical care is not immediately available. Routine immunizations against influenza and pneumococci are also recommended.

Risk for Thrombus Formation. The increased platelet count after surgery leads to the collaborative problem *Risk for Thrombus Formation related to increased platelet counts after surgery.*

Planning: Expected Outcomes. Thrombi will not occur or will be detected early as evidenced by the absence of Homans' sign, and no redness, tenderness, or swelling in the lower extremity.

Implementation. Following surgery, the platelet count often rebounds and sometimes reaches a level above the norm. Institute activities to help prevent the formation of thrombi, including pressure stockings, leg exercises, early ambulation, and prevention of pressure on the extremities. If aspirin is ordered as a mild anticoagulant, this should be administered and the client taught the importance of continuing this at home as prescribed.

Evaluation

An appropriate outcome for the client after splenectomy would be that the client's platelet count return to normal limits after a brief increase and that the client not suffer from any infections.

Disorders of Platelets and Clotting Factors

Disorders of hemostasis affecting platelets and clotting factors include (1) hemorrhagic disorders, (2) purpura, and (3) coagulation disorders. The three components of the hemostatic mechanism are the blood vessels, platelets (thrombocytes), and coagulation factors.

Hemorrhagic Disorders

Normal clot formation and lysis depend on intact blood vessels, an adequate number of functioning platelets, sufficient amounts of the 12 clotting factors, and a well-controlled fibrinolytic system. Consequently, the four basic problems underlying hemorrhagic (bleeding) disorders are as follows:

1. Weak, damaged vessels that rupture easily or spontaneously
2. Platelet deficiency (thrombocytopenia) due to hypoproliferation, excessive pooling of platelets in the spleen, or excessive platelet destruction
3. Deficiency or total lack of one of the clotting factors
4. Excessive or insufficient fibrinolysis

Disorders of hemostasis fall into two major categories: purpura and coagulation disorders. Box 53–2 outlines the types of bleeding disorders in these two categories.

The diagnosis of a hemorrhagic disorder depends on a complete health and family history, physical examination, and laboratory tests for platelet and clotting defects. The history usually offers numerous clues to the type of bleeding problem and its cause.

If the history indicates a bleeding disorder, examine the client for overt manifestations of bleeding. Petechiae (tiny hemorrhagic spots caused by intradermal or submucosal bleeding) are usually present in vascular and thrombocytopenic purpuras. The presence of ecchymoses (large, blotchy, subcutaneous hemorrhagic areas), hematomas (subdermal hemorrhage), and hemarthrosis (blood within the joints) points to hemophilia. However, ecchymoses may develop in any hemorrhagic disorder. Clients who hemorrhage severely from several areas during childbirth or a major surgical procedure may have a fibrinogen deficiency. In addition to any evidence of bleeding, search for manifestations of hepatic cirrhosis (hepatomegaly, jaundice, and so forth) and splenomegaly.

Laboratory studies provide the most crucial evidence for pinpointing the type and cause of a bleeding disorder.

Clients with hemorrhagic disorders need to understand (1) why they are at risk of bleeding, (2) the manifestations of bleeding, and (3) preventive measures to avoid bleeding. Those who can be managed by home healthcare should be referred to appropriate healthcare agencies. Clients with bleeding disorders should carry an identification card at all times that indicates their diagnosis, name of physician or healthcare agency, and blood type. It is important to assess each client before even minor invasive procedures, such as dental extractions, to rule out a history of bleeding disorders.

Purpura

Idiopathic Thrombocytopenic Purpura

Purpura is defined as the extravasation of small amounts of blood into the tissues and mucous membranes. Bleeding results from vessel damage (vascular purpura) or a platelet deficiency (thrombocytopenic purpura). A third type is thrombocytic thrombocytopenic purpura. In this condition, platelets clump together inappropriately in the microcirculation reducing the number of circulating platelets.

The term *thrombocytopenia* means a reduction in platelets below 100,000/mm³. The two major problems that characterize thrombocytopenia are (1) spontaneous bleeding into any part of the body (such as the central nervous system, muscle, joints) when the platelet count is less than 20,000/mm³ (in some cases, the count may drop to 5000/mm³ before manifestations occur) and (2) prolonged oozing from sites despite local measures to curtail bleeding. The two principal types of thrombocytopenia are idiopathic thrombocytopenic purpura (ITP) and secondary thrombocytopenia. ITP refers to thrombocytopenia caused by an unknown, possibly autoimmune cause.

Ninety percent of adults with ITP are under 40 years of age; the ratio of women to men is 3 : 1 to 4 : 1. In afflicted children, 85% of whom are under 8 years of age, the disease is self-limiting.

Etiology and Risk Factors

Childhood ITP is usually acute and follows recovery from a viral infection. In adults, the onset of ITP is usually gradual, without a preceding illness, and with a chronic

---

Box 53–2. Classification of Disorders of Hemostasis

Purpura

Vascular defect purpura
  Familial hemorrhagic telangiectasia
  Anaphylactoid purpura (allergic purpura)
  Toxic purpura

Platelet disorder purpura
  Idiopathic thrombocytopenic purpura
  Secondary thrombocytopenias

Coagulation Disorders

Hemophilia

Hypoprothrombinemia

Disseminated intravascular coagulation (DIC)

course. In a small percentage of adult cases, the disease has an acute onset.

Pathophysiology

ITP is characterized by the development of antibodies to one's own platelets, which are then destroyed by phagocytosis in the spleen and, to a lesser extent, in the liver. Normally, platelets survive 8 to 10 days within the circulation. However, platelet survival in ITP is as brief as 1 to 3 days or less. In adults, indications for treatment depend on severity of bleeding and the degree of thrombocytosis.

Clinical Manifestations and Diagnostic Findings

In most cases, ITP takes a course of remissions and exacerbations that, in untreated cases, may continue for years. Assessment reveals petechiae, ecchymosis, epistaxis, bleeding from the gums, and easy bruising. Women may have extremely heavy menses or bleeding between periods.

Complications of ITP include cerebral hemorrhage, which proves fatal in 1% to 5% of clients with ITP; severe hemorrhages from the nose, gastrointestinal tract, and urinary system; bleeding into the diaphragm, which can result in pulmonary complications; and nerve pain, extremity anesthesia, or paralysis resulting from the pressure of hematomas on nerves or brain tissues.

Diagnostic findings that confirm the presence of ITP include the following:

1. A platelet count below 100,000/mm³
2. Prolonged bleeding time with normal coagulation time (all coagulation factors are present and normal)
3. Increased capillary fragility as demonstrated by the tourniquet test
4. Positive platelet antibody screening
5. Bone marrow aspirate containing normal or increased numbers of megakaryocytes

Clients with ITP have a good prognosis: 80% of children and 10% to 20% of adults recover spontaneously without treatment.

Acute and Subacute Care

▪ Surgical Management

The treatment of choice for clients with ITP is splenectomy (see earlier). In 60% to 80% of cases, removal of the spleen results in complete and permanent remission. The effectiveness of splenectomy is believed to be related to the removal of the site of premature destruction of the antibody-sensitized platelets. Because young children often recover spontaneously from ITP, pediatricians do not usually recommend splenectomy unless the child is over 6 years of age.

▪ Nursing Management of the Surgical Client

The nursing care of a client after splenectomy is found earlier in this chapter (Splenic Rupture and Hypersplenism).

Community and Self-Care

▪ Medical Management

The medical interventions for ITP are immunosuppressant therapy and platelet transfusions. Clients suffering from severe bleeding of short duration receive steroids (such as prednisone). The purpose of steroid therapy in ITP is to suppress the phagocytic response of splenic macrophages. However, steroids rarely produce a permanent cure. Clients also receive steroids before splenectomy. Plasmapheresis is sometimes used as short-term therapy until the steroid therapy takes effect. IV infusion of γ-globulin in combination with plasmapheresis is used for clients whose condition is refractory to other treatments. Plasmapheresis plus prosorba leads to immunoadsorption and is used sometimes in refractory cases. Danazol (Danocrine) has recently been used with success in some clients. Immunosuppressive therapy used in refractory cases includes vincristine, vinblastine (Velban), azathioprine (Imuran), and cyclophosphamide.

▪ Nursing Management of the Medical Client

Assessment

Clients with ITP usually present with easy bruising, petechiae, and purpura. Platelet counts are well below normal limits. Assess clients for any manifestation of hidden bleeding.

Diagnosis, Planning, Implementation

Risk for Injury. The risk of bleeding secondary to low platelet count leads to a nursing diagnosis for *Risk for Injury related to the low platelet count.*

Planning: Expected Outcomes. The client will not suffer injury, as evidenced by absence of bleeding or bleeding that was diagnosed early and treated effectively.

Implementation. During the acute phase, teach the client oral hygiene measures to prevent gum bleeding. The client should not use a hard toothbrush and should refrain from flossing during this phase. The client should not receive any injections, aspirin, or nonsteroidal anti-inflammatory drugs. Monitor the client's platelet count, vital signs, and manifestations of bleeding or increased intracranial pressure. Teach the client to avoid Valsalva's maneuver and to use stool softeners. Safety precautions to prevent injury from falls are also indicated.

Impaired Tissue Integrity. A common nursing diagnosis is *Impaired Tissue Integrity related to intradermal bleeding, petechiae, and purpura.*

Planning: Expected Outcomes. The client will not develop impaired tissue integrity, as evidenced by early detection and treatment of any bleeding and no apparent alteration in tissue integrity.

Implementation. Carefully inspect and monitor the client's skin condition, noting petechiae, purpura, and bruising. Apply an ice bag or manual pressure over any bleeding site to promote hemostasis. Teach the client and significant others to implement bleeding precautions when the platelet count is low and how to institute immediate medical care for hemorrhage.

Pain. Another common nursing diagnosis is *Pain related to bleeding into the tissues.*

Planning: Expected Outcomes. The client will have pain controlled or eliminated, as evidenced by the client's statements of relief.

Implementation. The nurse should position the client comfortably, using pillows, a bed cradle, lightweight blankets, and other measures to reduce pressures on the tissues. Ask the client what pain is being felt and use that information to determine the need for analgesics as prescribed.

Evaluation

The outcomes are varied in clients with this condition. Some clients will recover following splenectomy, with minimal problems. Clients who do not respond to splenectomy may be placed on long-term steroid therapy. Clients with refractory disease may respond well to plasmapheresis and medications.

▪ Modifications for Elderly Clients

Elderly clients are less likely to develop ITP. If they do, bleeding can be more severe because of their already fragile capillaries. Steroids are used, and surgery is avoided unless necessary.

Vascular Defect Purpura

The major characteristic of vascular defect purpura is easy rupture of small blood vessels upon any undue pressure, with resultant bleeding into the tissues. The causes are many (e.g., heredity, allergy, exposure to poisons, drug hypersensitivity, poor nutrition, infection, and hypertension). Major forms are (1) familial hemorrhagic telangiectasia, (2) anaphylactoid purpura (allergic purpura), and (3) toxic purpura.

Familial Hemorrhagic Telangiectasia

This hereditary condition is characterized by multiple, thin, dilated capillaries and arterioles. These fragile vessels are usually found on the oral and nasal mucosa and in the gastrointestinal and renal tracts. Fragility of the vessels leads to spontaneous bleeding or bleeding with minimal trauma. Small red-to-violet lesions are often seen on the lips, oral and nasal mucosa, tongue, toes, and finger tips. These lesions blanch when pressed and bleed spontaneously.

Diagnosis is made solely by identification of characteristic lesions. Treatment is symptomatic. Treatments include topical hemostatics and administration of estrogens. Severe gastrointestinal tract hemorrhage warrants treatment with iron therapy and transfusions. Because this condition is hereditary, genetic counseling is advisable.

Anaphylactoid Purpura

This form of vascular purpura, also called allergic purpura, arises from an allergic reaction that damages the vascular epithelium. It causes acute or chronic inflammation of blood vessels supplying the skin, joints, gastrointestinal tract, and kidneys. Typically, attacks of the disease subside spontaneously within 1 to 6 weeks. However, episodes of bleeding tend to recur over the years.

Assessment reveals joint pain, abdominal pain, hematuria, gastrointestinal tract hemorrhage, fever, and malaise. Skin lesions occur in the form of erythema, urticaria, and pruritus.

Treatment primarily involves elimination of possible allergens and alleviation of manifestations. Immunosuppressive therapy (e.g., steroids, cyclophosphamide) and exchange plasmapheresis have been tried with some success.

Toxic Purpura

This condition is characterized by damage to blood vessels after exposure to certain medications and poisons (such as snake venom). Treatment involves identification of the offending agent when possible.

Symptomatic or Secondary Purpuras

These disorders arise secondary to other disorders and are not caused by intrinsic or inherited disorders of the vasculature. Such conditions include the following:

- Serious tissue trauma arising from a blow or a burn
- Arterial hypertension resulting in increased capillary pressure
- Bloodstream infections that damage the vascular epithelium, such as subacute bacterial endocarditis
- Scurvy (the result of vitamin C deficiency), which causes increased capillary fragility
- Uremia and cachexia, which, for unknown reasons, result in vessel weakness

Unlike ITP, the secondary thrombocytopenias have

identifiable causes. For example, these types of purpura may arise secondary to viral infections, bone marrow failure, the defibrination syndrome, disseminated lupus erythematosus, lymphoproliferative disorders, infectious mononucleosis, and drug hypersensitivity. Common offending drugs include quinidine, quinine, the sulfonamides, phenylbutazone, and chlorothiazide derivatives. Assessment data and diagnostic findings are the same as those found in ITP.

Treatment focuses on mitigating the underlying causes as well as controlling bleeding. All potentially toxic drugs must be identified and discontinued. The platelet count usually begins to rise within a few days, reaching normal values within a week after removal of toxic agents. To control bleeding, the physician may order the administration of corticosteroids.

Platelet transfusions are given when the platelet count falls below 20,000 to 30,000/mm³, when an invasive procedure is to be done, or as needed for treatment of hemorrhage. In some clients, a platelet count of 5000/mm³ is the critical value for deciding to use platelet transfusions. Clients can be supported with platelet transfusions for weeks to years. Although transfused platelets have a shortened life span, they may function effectively for 5 to 6 days.

Long-term platelet therapy leads to the development of platelet antibodies. The use of single-donor platelet transfusions from the onset, however, helps prevent the development of alloimmunization that occurs with the use of random-donor, pooled platelets. The use of white blood cell filters may also help decrease the development of antibodies by decreasing the infusion of white blood cells. If alloimmunization has occurred, platelet counts obtained 10 to 60 minutes after transfusion show no rise in the peripheral platelet count, or even a decrease, indicating the presence of platelet antibodies. Platelet therapy can sometimes be continued by finding specially matched donors who are able to provide HLA-matched platelets. Premedication with diphenhydramine hydrochloride (Benadryl), acetaminophen, or hydrocortisone may decrease the possibility of reactions to platelet transfusions.

Clients who have been repeatedly exposed to foreign HLA antigens may develop antibodies. Should this occur, the client usually becomes nonresponsive or refractory to platelet concentrates possessing those antigens. If testing confirms the presence of HLA antigens, single-donor platelets obtained by apheresis from a donor with identical HLA antigens may improve platelet responsiveness. Because the HLA system consists of a large number of potential antigens, the chance of locating an identical match from an unrelated donor pool is remote (1 in 5000–20,000). A family member, such as a sibling, is the most likely suitable match; however, transfusion should be avoided if there is any chance that this donor may be needed as a bone marrow donor for this client.

Clients undergoing immunosuppressive treatment who may require platelet therapy should have samples collected for HLA typing (30 ml of heparinized blood) before the onset of leukopenia. Identifying a donor and performing apheresis can be a labor-intensive process requiring advanced planning.

Coagulation Disorders

The coagulation disorders stem from a defect in the clotting mechanisms. One or more of the clotting factors is depleted or absent. The three important coagulation disorders discussed here are hypoprothrombinemia, disseminated intravascular coagulation (DIC), and the hemophilias (see also Congenital Disorders).

Hypoprothrombinemia

The term *hypoprothrombinemia* refers to a deficiency in the amount of circulating prothrombin. Prothrombin is a protein produced in the liver and normally found in the blood. For prothrombin synthesis to take place, vitamin K (a fat-soluble vitamin) must be present in the liver to act as a catalyst. Hypoprothrombinemia develops from a vitamin K deficiency or liver disorder or from an overdose of aspirin, coumarin, or coumarin-derivative anticoagulant (such as warfarin), which antagonizes the action of vitamin K.

The fat-soluble vitamin K is largely synthesized by bacteria in the small intestine—a classic example of symbiosis. The bacteria do more than their share since we excrete large amounts. There is no standard dietary daily allowance. Because it is fat-soluble, vitamin K depends on the presence of bile for absorption. Once absorbed, vitamin K catalyzes prothrombin synthesis within the liver cells. Vitamin K deficiency is seen in newborns who arrive with a limited supply and a largely sterile digestive tract, and in clients with gastrointestinal tract disorders interfering with the absorption of vitamin K, such as malabsorption syndrome and jaundice due to bile duct obstruction; liver damage so extensive that liver cells cannot produce bile or synthesize prothrombin; and prolonged sulfonamide or antibiotic administration that sterilizes the bowel, thereby halting vitamin K manufactured by gastrointestinal tract bacteria.

Dicumarol is an effective anticoagulant used to reduce clot formation in heart disease and peripheral vascular disorders. It acts by interfering with vitamin K in prothrombin synthesis. In excessive doses, prothrombin time is prolonged. If the prothrombin time is too long, the danger of bleeding or spontaneous hemorrhage increases.

The major manifestations of hypoprothrombinemia are ecchymosis after minimal trauma, epistaxis, postoperative hemorrhage from the incision, hematuria, gastrointestinal tract bleeding, and prolonged bleeding from a venipuncture. The outstanding laboratory finding is a prolonged prothrombin time.

Treatment for hypoprothrombinemia aims at the underlying cause. For example, vitamin K deficiency resulting from malabsorption is corrected through intramuscular or IV administration of vitamin K, such as menadione sodium bisulfite (Hykinone) or menadiol sodium diphosphate (Synkayvite).

If overdosage with a coumarin anticoagulant is the underlying problem, anticoagulant therapy is stopped. In order to normalize the prothrombin time, phytonadione (fat-soluble vitamin K) is administered orally for minor bleeding problems or IV for hemorrhage.

Finally, if prothrombin deficiency results from liver disease, concentrates of prothrombin or of prothrombin and factors VII, IX, and X may be transfused.

Disseminated Intravascular Coagulation

Disseminated intravascular coagulation (DIC) occurs following activation of clotting factors and fibrinolytic enzymes throughout arterioles and capillaries.

Etiology and Risk Factors

DIC is a complex and important coagulation disorder characterized by two apparently conflicting manifestations: (1) diffuse fibrin deposition within arterioles and capillaries, with resultant widespread clotting, and (2) hemorrhage from the kidneys, brain, adrenals, heart, and other organs.

The causes of DIC are many, and there is considerable overlap among the syndromes that precede its occurrence. Four categories of causative factors are (1) introduction of tissue coagulation factors into the circulation, (2) damage to vascular endothelium, (3) stagnant blood flow, and (4) infection.

Box 53–3 lists conditions that may precipitate DIC. Be alert for manifestations of DIC in caring for clients with any of these conditions.

Pathophysiology

The pathologic chain of events characterizing DIC is as follows:

1. Certain disease states cause the release of thromboplastic substances that result in activation of thrombin, which in turn activates fibrinogen and results in deposition of fibrin throughout the microcirculation.
2. Platelet aggregation or adhesiveness is increased; this enables fibrin clots and microthrombi to form in the brain, kidneys, heart, and other organs, causing microinfarcts and tissue necrosis.
3. Red blood cells become trapped in the fibrin strands and are destroyed (hemolysis). The resultant sluggish circulation of blood reduces the flow of nutrients and oxygen to the cells.
4. Platelets, prothrombin, and other clotting factors are consumed in the process, which compromises coagulation and predisposes to bleeding.
5. Excessive clotting activates the fibrinolytic mechanism, which causes the production of fibrin degradation products.
6. Fibrin degradation products act to inhibit platelet clotting functions, which causes further bleeding.
7. Ultimately, with lysis of clots and depletion of clotting factors, the blood loses its ability to clot.

The prognosis for clients with DIC varies. The condi-

Box 53–3. Conditions That May Precipitate Disseminated Intravascular Coagulation

Shock

Cirrhosis

Purpura fulminans

Glomerulonephritis

Acute fulminant hepatitis

Acute bacterial and viral infections

Conditions that may cause the release of platelet factor III
  Fat emboli
  Snakebites

Hemolytic processes caused by

■ Infection
■ Transfusion reactions
■ Immunologic disorders

Tissue damage caused by

■ Trauma
■ Heat stroke
■ Extensive burns
■ Transplant rejections
■ Surgery—particularly if extracorporeal circulation was used

Conditions that may cause the release of thromboplastin from tissues

Neoplastic growths

■ Acute leukemias
■ Prostatic cancer
■ Bronchogenic cancer
■ Giant cavernous hemangioma

Obstetric conditions

■ Abruptio placentae
■ Retained dead fetus
■ Amniotic fluid embolism

---

tion may be self-limiting. On the other hand, hemorrhage, organ damage, or even death may occur within a few days or even a few hours if associated with gram-negative sepsis.

Clinical Manifestations and Diagnostic Findings

The onset of DIC is usually acute and develops within days to hours after an initial assault to the body system, such as shock syndrome. Subacute DIC may not be apparent initially but may become fulminant as the clinical course progresses. Chronic cases of DIC characteristically develop in clients with cancer or in women carrying a dead fetus. Manifestations may be mild or extremely severe.

Assessment of clients with DIC reveals purpura, pete-

Understanding DIC and Its Treatment

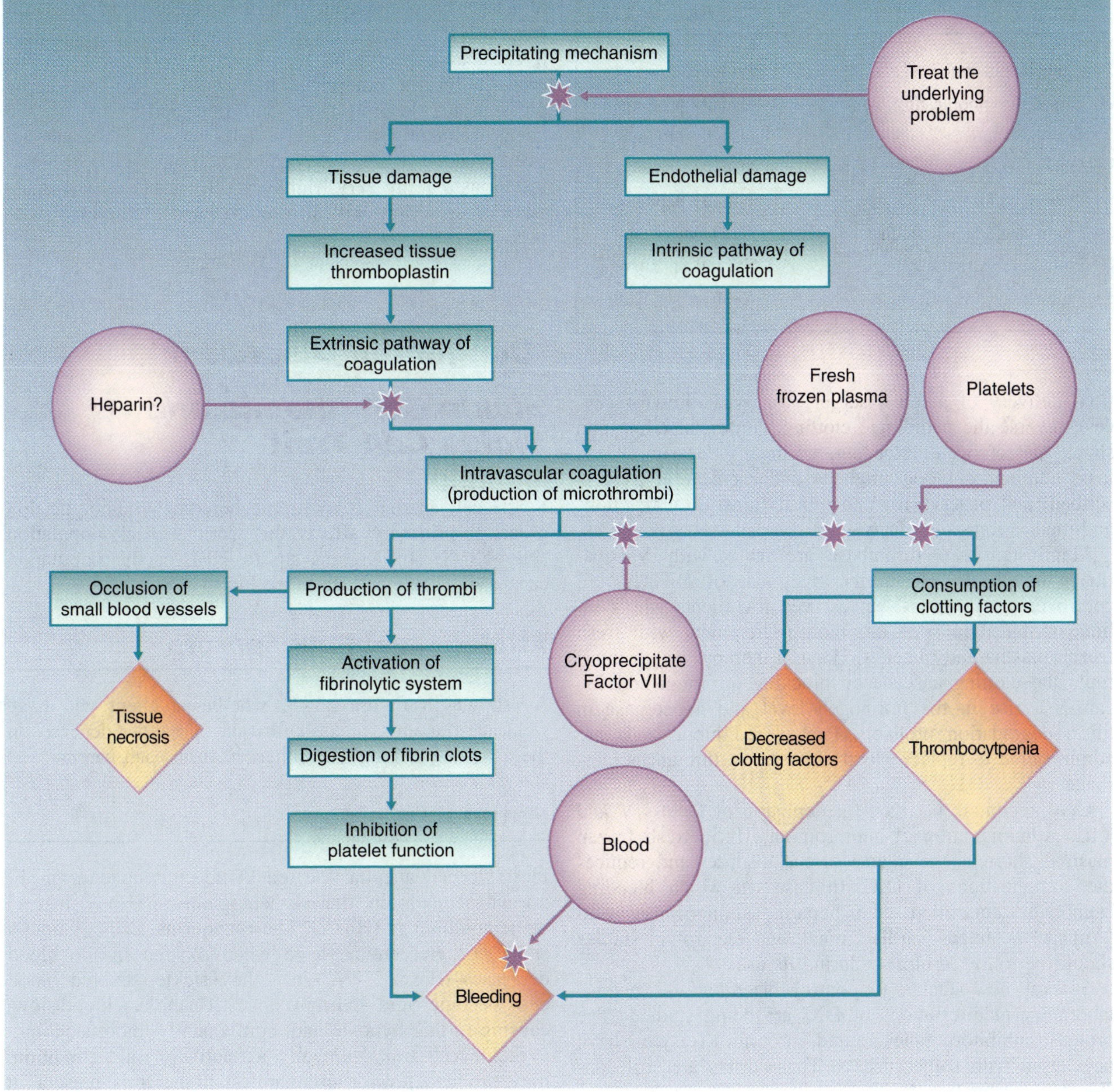

Precipitating mechanism

Treat the underlying problem

Tissue damage

Endothelial damage

Increased tissue thromboplastin

Intrinsic pathway of coagulation

Extrinsic pathway of coagulation

Heparin?

Fresh frozen plasma

Platelets

Intravascular coagulation (production of microthrombi)

Occlusion of small blood vessels

Production of thrombi

Consumption of clotting factors

Tissue necrosis

Activation of fibrinolytic system

Cryoprecipitate Factor VIII

Decreased clotting factors

Thrombocytpenia

Digestion of fibrin clots

Inhibition of platelet function

Blood

Bleeding

chiae, and ecchymoses on the skin, mucous membranes, heart lining, and lungs; prolonged bleeding from venipuncture; severe, uncontrolled hemorrhage during surgery or childbirth; oliguria and acute renal failure; and convulsions and coma, which may terminate in death.

Diagnostic findings in severe cases of DIC indicate that the hemostatic mechanism has failed totally. A prolonged prothrombin time, very low platelet count, and incoagulable blood are typical findings. Table 53–5 lists the laboratory tests used in the diagnosis of DIC.

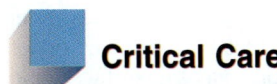

Critical Care

■ Medical Management

The treatment of DIC is currently under investigation as researchers attempt to validate the most suitable means of managing this syndrome. To treat DIC successfully, clinicians must correct the basic problem (such as infec-

Table 53–5. Laboratory Tests Used in Diagnosis of Disseminated Intravascular Coagulation

Test	Results
Prothrombin time	Prolonged
Partial thromboplastin time	Usually prolonged
Thrombin time	Usually prolonged
Fibrinogen level	Usually depressed
Platelet count	Usually depressed
Fibrin degradation products	Elevated
Protamine sulfate test	Strongly positive
Factor assays II, V, VII	Reduced

tion, delivery of a fetus, surgery, or irradiation for cancer), reverse the pathologic clotting, control bleeding and shock, detect occult bleeding, accurately measure blood loss, administer blood products and medication as prescribed, and observe for and report transfusion reactions and medication side effects.

Manifestations of thrombosis are treated with IV heparin, although its use in the treatment of DIC is still controversial. It should be reserved for clients who continue to bleed in spite of vigorous treatment with fresh frozen plasma and platelets. Heparin therapy, which interrupts the clotting cascade by blocking thrombin activity, causes a rise in the fibrinogen level and a decrease in fibrin degradation products. Packed red blood cells are administered to replace blood volume lost through hemorrhage.

Cryoprecipitate is given for depletion of factors V and VIII. Administration of antithrombin III (in fresh frozen plasma) shortens the course of the disorder and reduces the complications of DIC. In cases in which bleeding cannot be controlled with heparin, aminocaproic acid (Amicar) is given. Cardiac, renal, and electrolyte studies should be followed closely during its use.

Several new agents to control bleeding and reverse laboratory manifestations of DIC are being studied. The protease inhibitors gabexate and aprotinin (Trasylol) have been used with some success. These drugs are still considered investigational.

■ Nursing Management of the Medical Client

It is important to assess all body systems for the effect DIC has had: integumentary—bleeding or oozing of blood from venipuncture sites or mucosal surfaces and wounds, pallor, petechiae, ecchymoses, and hematomas; respiratory—tachypnea, hemoptysis, orthopnea, and basilar rales; cardiovascular—tachycardia and hypotension; gastrointestinal—abdominal distention, guaiac-positive stools or gastric contents; genitourinary—hematuria and oliguria; and neurologic—vision changes, dizziness, headache, changes in mental status, and irritability.

Nursing care of clients with DIC will vary, depending on the severity of the process. Generally, the goal is to monitor and quantify blood loss and provide supportive therapy with blood components to resolve manifestations of hemorrhage and control further bleeding. Monitor appropriate laboratory values to determine treatment effectiveness and observe for manifestations of thrombosis. To prevent further complications, avoid injections, apply pressure to bleeding sites, and turn and reposition the client frequently and gently. DIC sometimes results in overt bleeding from body orifices and other clinical manifestations that are very frightening to the client and significant others. They will all require intense emotional support.

Congenital Disorders

Sickle Cell Anemia and Sickle Cell Trait

Sickle cell anemia is a chronic hereditary hemolytic disorder. It primarily affects the world's black population (Fig. 53–8). In Nigeria, up to 30% of the population carries the sickle cell trait (see Fig. 53–8).

Etiology and Risk Factors

As shown in Figure 53–8, whether a client will have sickle cell anemia, sickle cell trait, or neither depends on the genes for hemoglobin inherited from each parent.

Pathophysiology

In sickle cell anemia, the red blood cells contain an abnormal hemoglobin, that is, hemoglobin S (Hb S) instead of hemoglobin A (Hb A). These abnormal cells assume a sickle, or crescentic, shape when oxygen in the blood decreases (Fig. 53–9). Once they sickle, the red blood cells become rigid and may obstruct capillary blood flow, causing further hypoxia and, consequently, more sickling.

Sickle cell trait, generally a relatively mild condition, may produce few or no manifestations. It is present in clients who are heterozygous for Hb S.

Hb S results when valine replaces glutamic acid on each β-chain of the hemoglobin molecule. Valine is an amino acid that tends to form strong hydrophobic bonds. This valine substitution causes an abnormal bonding between Hb S molecules when oxygen in the blood decreases.

The mechanisms that precipitate the various forms of sickling crises remain unclear. However, two major factors are definitely linked with the sickling of cells: (1) hypoxia, due to low oxygen tension, and (2) an increased blood viscosity, due to an increased concentration of sickled cells.

Exposure to low oxygen tensions (e.g., at high altitudes, flying in nonpressurized planes, exercising strenu-

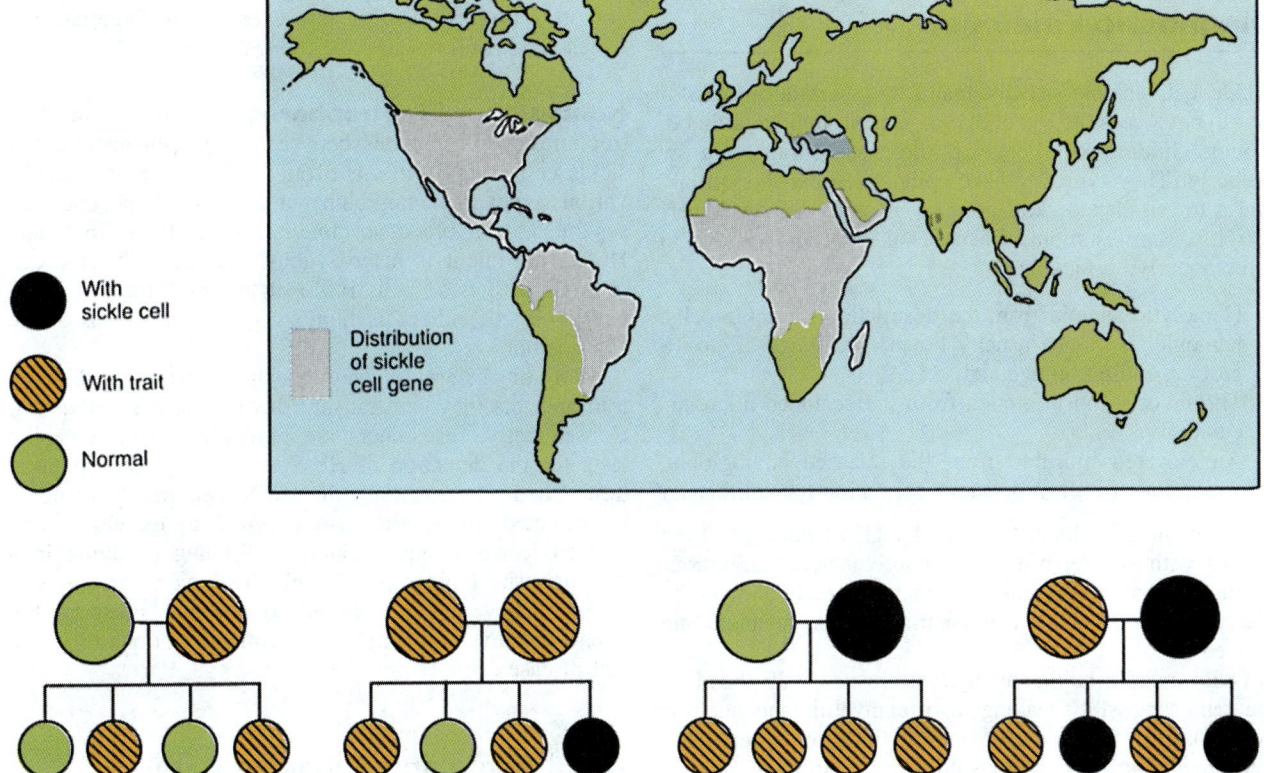

Figure 53–8. Geographical distribution and inheritance pattern of sickle cell gene. (Redrawn from Page, J., et al. [1981]. *Blood: The river of life.* Washington, D. C.: Torstar Books.)

ously, or undergoing anesthesia without receiving adequate oxygenation) results in hypoxia. Although both Hb S and Hb A have the same solubility when oxygenated, deoxygenation of the blood drastically affects Hb S.

When normal hemoglobin gives up its oxygen, it becomes only half as soluble as when it is oxygenated, whereas Hb S becomes 50 times less soluble. The decreased solubility of Hb S causes it to crystallize, thereby deforming the cell's shape. The heavy concentration of misshapen cells during a sickling crisis makes the blood abnormally viscous, which results in an extremely sluggish circulation. The pathologic situation is compounded if dehydration is present.

Owing to the increased viscosity and the irregular shape of the cells, the sickle cells tend to pack together within the smaller blood vessels. Occlusion of the microcirculation increases hypoxia, which causes more erythrocytes to sickle. Thus, a vicious circle ensues. The organs most vulnerable to infarction and necrosis are the brain and kidneys, because of their constant demand for oxygen, and the bone marrow and spleen, because of their normally sluggish circulation.

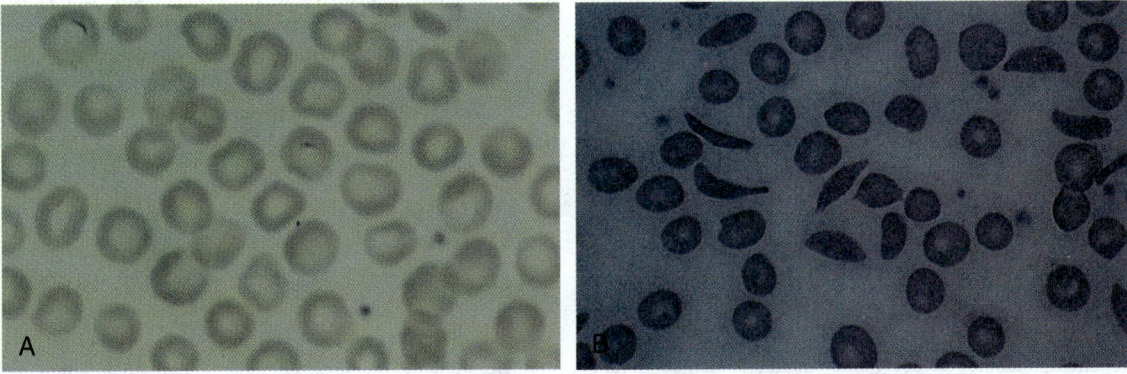

Figure 53–9. Erythrocytes. Comparison of normal red blood cells *(A)* and sickle cells *(B)* (magnification × 875.) (From Rodak, B. F. [1995]. *Diagnostic hematology.* [pp. 83, 257]. Philadelphia: W. B. Saunders.)

Clinical Manifestations and Diagnostic Findings

Sickle cell anemia usually manifests itself during childhood, but occasionally does not appear until adulthood. Young children who develop the disease fail to grow properly. They typically have spindly legs, a short trunk, and a tower-shaped skull because of bone marrow hyperactivity. Manifestations, whenever they occur, are due to three underlying factors:

1. Hemolytic anemia from the destruction of sickle cells; hemoglobin values usually lie in a range of 12 to 18 g/dl depending on age and sex
2. Thrombosis and infarction from the occluded microcirculation
3. An elevated bilirubin from the released hemoglobin, which may result in gallstone formation (cholelithiasis)

These three problems profoundly affect all organs and tissues with severe, often fatal consequences. Infarctions in the spleen are so common that, after childhood, the spleen of most sickle cell anemia clients is small and scarred.

Other manifestations include necrosis of the head of the femur, possibly leading to osteomyelitis and necrotic bone marrow with development of infection, joint pain, renal medullary ischemia resulting in diminished capacity to concentrate urine, priapism, pulmonary infarctions, myocardial infarctions, and cerebrovascular accidents. Leg ulcers are found in about 75% of older children and adults with the disease.

Thrombotic episodes often cause moderate to severe pain of the extremities, joints, and abdomen. Proliferation of the bone marrow, in an attempt to compensate for the chronic anemia, leads to osteoporosis and, later, osteosclerosis. These are only a few of the complications of sickle cell anemia.

Cerebral hemorrhage, or shock, claims the lives of many children with this disorder. However, some people survive until age 50 or older. Death usually results from uremia due to progressive renal damage.

Four laboratory procedures demonstrate the presence of Hb S in either homozygous or heterozygous carriers: (1) stained blood smear; (2) sickle cell slide preparation; (3) sickle-turbidity tube test; and (4) hemoglobin electrophoresis.

Stained Blood Smear. A stained blood smear is examined for the presence of sickle cells.

Sickle Cell Slide Preparation. A blood specimen is observed for the sickling phenomenon after deoxygenation of the blood. This test is accurate but time-consuming.

Sickle-Turbidity Tube Test. This is an excellent mass screening test to detect Hb S. After a finger prick, blood is mixed with Sickledex solution in a test tube. Five minutes later, the specimen is observed for cloudiness, which indicates the presence of Hb S. Solutions mixed with normal hemoglobin remain clear. Although demonstrating Hb S, this test does not differentiate between sickle cell disease and the trait.

Hemoglobin Electrophoresis. Hemoglobin electrophoresis differentiates between sickle cell anemia and sickle cell trait. By means of an applied electric field, the various types of hemoglobin within a blood specimen are separated. If a blood specimen contains both Hb S and Hb A, the client is heterozygous, that is, has sickle cell trait. If Hb S is 75% to 100% of the total, the rest Hb F or Hb A₂, the client is homozygous, that is, has sickle cell anemia.

Many blacks are unaware that they carry the sickle cell trait and that they can transmit this trait to their offspring. Consequently, researchers are perfecting mass screening tests for the detection of Hb S among the black population. Clients having only the sickle cell trait may never be detected unless they are exposed to extremely low oxygen tensions (e.g., mountain climbing or flying in a nonpressurized plane), extremely hard work or exercise, or pregnancy. When exposed to extreme stressors, the client with the trait may develop manifestations of sickle cell disease.

Acute and Subacute Care

■ Medical Management

Treatment of sickle cell anemia consists chiefly of supportive care (e.g., rest, oxygen, IV administration of fluids and electrolytes to ensure adequate hydration, sedation, and analgesics).

In some cases, the slow administration of packed red blood cells or partial exchange transfusion helps relieve severe anemic manifestations. During episodes of increased risk (e.g., surgery, pregnancy), some clients benefit from hypertransfusion (transfusions until more than 50% of the circulating red blood cells are of donor origin).

Anticoagulants, steroids, and cobalt treatments have all been used to reverse the sickling process without success. Clients with sickle cell disease have an increased need for folic acid and therefore usually receive a daily oral supplement to prevent increased anemia from folate deficiency. Prophylactic penicillin may also be ordered.

Hydroxyurea and erythropoietin are being used in clinical trials in an attempt to increase fetal hemoglobin in persons diagnosed with sickle cell disease.

■ Nursing Management of the Medical Client

Assessment

Assessment findings are integumentary—jaundice or pallor and ulceration; skeletal—joint swelling, disproportionately long arms and legs, fragility, and bone pain; developmental—delayed sexual maturity and retarded growth; gastrointestinal—enlargement of liver and spleen; and psychosocial—self-esteem disturbance, ineffective family coping, altered family processes, anticipatory grieving, noncompliance with health regimen, powerlessness, hopelessness, self-care deficit in activities of daily living, and altered thought processes.

Assessment findings during *sickle cell crisis* are cardiac—systolic murmurs, arrhythmias, and heart enlargement; respiratory—shortness of breath, chest pain, and cyanosis; sensorimotor—manifestations of increased intracranial pressure due to cerebral hemorrhaging; and renal—manifestations of uremia, such as decreased urinary output and edema.

Diagnosis, Planning, Implementation

Pain. Because of the joint swelling secondary to sickling crisis, one nursing diagnosis is *Pain related to joint swelling.*

Planning: Expected Outcomes. The client will have pain relieved, as evidenced by verbalization of pain relief.

Implementation. Assess for pain every 2 to 4 hours and administer analgesics as needed according to orders; monitor for effectiveness of analgesia. Apply heat to joints as ordered. Provide rest periods. Administer fluids to prevent dehydration and recurrence of pain crisis. Increase oral fluid intake. Monitor intake and output. Provide the client with information on how to prevent crises, such as (1) to avoid high altitudes and flying in nonpressurized planes, because oxygen tension is lowered under these conditions; and (2) to take caution against becoming dehydrated and to call a physician if vomiting, diarrhea, high fever, or any other cause of water loss develops.

Knowledge Deficit. Another nursing diagnosis is *Knowledge Deficit related to disease, treatment, and prevention of crises.*

Planning: Expected Outcomes. The client will understand the disease, treatment, and prevention of crises, as evidenced by the client's statements and the absence of crises.

Implementation. When educating clients about sickle cell anemia or sickle cell trait, include the following points in the discussion:

● Explain the nature of the disease, and give the client a chance to express feelings and ask questions.
● Encourage black parents to have themselves and their children tested for the presence of Hb S.
● Encourage the client to have routine medical examinations that include a red blood cell count.
● Encourage young adults who carry Hb S to ask their physician for genetic counseling before marrying or having children.
● Warn young women with sickle cell anemia that pregnancy carries a very high risk for them. They may develop pulmonary or renal complications, or both.

Evaluation

An appropriate outcome for the client with sickle cell disease is that the disease will remain in remission as long as possible. It is impossible to prevent every crisis, but, with education and an effort by the client, the number of attacks can be reduced.

The Hemophilias

There are three major types of hemophilia: hemophilia A (classic hemophilia), hemophilia B (Christmas disease), and von Willebrand's disease. Their major characteristics are compared in Table 53–6. Because classic hemophilia makes up 80% of all hemophilias, the discussion of manifestations and treatment refers only to this type.

The hemophilias are relatively common disorders. Within the United States alone, an estimated 25,000 clients are afflicted with a form of hemophilia. The hemophilias are characterized by prolonged bleeding, particularly after accidental, surgical, or dental trauma.

Table 53–6. Comparison of the Three Forms of Hemophilia

Form of Hemophilia	Etiology	Transmission	Major Laboratory Findings
Hemophilia A (classic hemophilia)	Inherited factor VIII (antihemophilic globulin) deficiency	Transmitted as sex-linked *recessive* trait; transmitted by females; occurs in males and, rarely, homozygous females	Coagulation time prolonged but bleeding time normal; factor VIII missing from plasma
Hemophilia B (Christmas disease)	Inherited factor IX (plasma thromboplastin component) deficiency	Transmitted as sex-linked *recessive* trait; transmitted by females; occurs in males and, rarely, homozygous females	Laboratory findings and symptoms same as in hemophilia A; factor IX missing
von Willebrand's disease	Inherited factor VIII deficiency and defective platelet dysfunction	Transmitted as autosomal *dominant* trait to both sexes; occurs in both males and females	Both coagulation time and bleeding time prolonged; low factor VIII levels; platelet adhesiveness decreased

Etiology and Risk Factors

Hemophilia is genetically transmitted in a sex-linked (X chromosome) recessive pattern. Females usually transmit the defective gene, but males develop the bleeding disorder. Females rarely have hemophilia. Female hemophilia carriers transmit the gene to half of their daughters. They transmit the disorder to half of their sons. Males with hemophilia transmit the gene to all of their daughters but to none of their sons.

Because this is a hereditary disease, the only way to control the risk is through genetic testing and counseling for decreasing the transmission.

Pathophysiology

Hemophilia A, the most common of the congenital coagulation disorders, is due to a deficiency in the procoagulant protein factor VIII (Table 53–7).

Clinical Manifestations and Diagnostic Findings

Hemophilia may be mild or severe, depending on the level of factor VIII or IX coagulant activity. Usually diagnosed in childhood, this disorder is manifested in the

Table 53–7. Coagulation Factors

Factor	Name	Source	Function	Comments
I	Fibrinogen	Liver	Produces fibrin	Protein found in plasma at average level of 300 mg/dl
II	Prothrombin	Liver (requires vitamin K)	Produces thrombin	Glucoprotein found in plasma
III	Thromboplastin			
	Incomplete form	Tissues and platelets		Requires factors V, VII, X
	Complete form	Plasma	Acts on prothrombin to produce thrombin	A product of interaction between factors VIII, IX, XI
IV	Calcium	Diet	Activates enzymes	Inorganic ion required in all stages of coagulation
V	Labile factor	Plasma	Accelerates conversion of prothrombin to thrombin	Deteriorates rapidly at room temperature; used up in clotting process
VI	Unassigned			In early studies was thought to be the active form of factor V
VII	Stable factor	Liver	Accelerates conversion of prothrombin to thrombin	Stable to heat and storage; not consumed in clotting
VIII	Antihemophilic globulin	Plasma globulin	Essential to thromboplastin formation and conversion of prothrombin to thrombin	Unstable at room temperature; completely consumed in clotting
IX	Plasma thromboplastin component (Christmas factor)	Liver	Influences amount of thromboplastin made	Not consumed during clotting
X	Stuart-Prower factor	Liver? (requires vitamin K)	Essential to thromboplastin formation and conversion of prothrombin to thrombin	Stable at room temperature; similar to factor VII
XI	Plasma thromboplastin antecedent	Unknown	Essential to thromboplastin formation	Stable at room temperature
XII	Hageman factor	Unknown	Uncertain	Relatively stable; activated on contact with glass
XIII	Fibrin stabilizing factor	Unknown	Maintains clot after formation	High levels in plasma; deficiency associated with mild bleeding tendency, poor wound healing

following ways: slow persistent bleeding from cuts, scratches, and other minor traumas; delayed hemorrhage that follows minor injuries—bleeding may not start from a site until hours or even days after the traumatic event; severe hemorrhaging from the gums after dental extraction or even brushing the teeth with a hard toothbrush; severe, sometimes fatal, epistaxis after injury to the nose; overwhelming gastric hemorrhage, which may be linked to gastric disorders such as ulcers; recurrent hematoma formation in the deep subcutaneous tissue, in the intramuscular tissues, and around the peripheral nerves. If nerves are compressed by hematomas, the client suffers severe pain, anesthesia of the innervated part, nerve damage, and paralysis. In addition, muscular atrophy sometimes results. Finally, there is recurrent hemarthrosis (bleeding into the joints), which is common in untreated cases and may result in serious joint deformity and permanent crippling. Hemarthrosis affects the knees, ankles, elbows, wrists, fingers, hips, and shoulders, in that order. All of this bleeding can be controlled with the administration of the missing factor (VIII or IX).

Platelet function, platelet count, bleeding time, and prothrombin time are normal. The activated partial thromboplastin time is prolonged. Quantitative assays for factor VIII determine the severity of the disease.

Acute and Subacute Care

■ Medical Management

The goals of care for clients with hemophilia are to stop topical bleeding as quickly as possible; to raise the level of antihemophilic factor (AHF) in the plasma, thereby temporarily supplying the missing factor causing hemorrhage; and to prevent complications leading to and caused by bleeding.

Immediate transfusion of factor VIII or IX concentrate is the primary treatment. Although plasma and cryoprecipitate contain factor VIII, concentrates have a known AHF content and carry less risk of blood volume overload. Hepatitis and human immunodeficiency virus (HIV) infection represent the major infectious risks, but improved purification techniques now used routinely in the preparation of concentrated factors have virtually eliminated this risk. Because the procoagulant activity of AHF disappears rapidly, clients need transfusions every 12 hours until bleeding stops.

Transfusion of packed red blood cells or white blood cells are used only to replace blood volume when there has been severe loss. Prophylactic transfusion of factor VIII to a level of 50% above normal is recommended in cases of minor injury, surgery, and dental extractions.

One major complication is linked to repeated transfusions and AHF therapy. About 5% of persons with hemophilia become sensitized to AHF and develop autoimmune anti-AHF antibodies. In clients with low titers of factor VIII antibodies, major and life-threatening hemorrhages are treated with massive doses of factor VIII from animal sources (bovine and porcine), inactivated pro-

thrombin complex concentrates (Konyne 80, Proplex T), or activated prothrombin complex concentrates (Feiba VH Immuno, Autoplex T). Clinicians are using various experimental treatments such as immunosuppressive therapy to combat this problem. Topical bleeding can usually be temporarily controlled by applying pressure to the injured site, packing the area with a fibrin foam, and applying topical hemostatics such as thrombin.

Hemarthrosis may be controlled if the client receives AHF in the early stages of bleeding. Joint immobilization and local chilling (such as packing ice around the joint) may bring relief. If pain is severe, it may be necessary to aspirate blood from the joint. Once bleeding stops and swelling subsides, the client should perform active range-of-motion exercises without weightbearing to prevent further complications, such as deformity and muscle atrophy.

The prognosis for persons with hemophilia has greatly improved since the discovery of AHF. Before this, 50% of persons with hemophilia died before they reached their fifth birthday. Today, death rarely occurs after minor trauma. Home infusion of AHF ensures that treatment is instituted at the first manifestation of bleeding, and complications are thus prevented. Clinicians have developed training programs with strict guidelines: When these guidelines are carefully followed, persons with hemophilia lose less time from work or school and need fewer emergency room visits. Fatalities mainly follow the development of autoimmune antibodies (anti-AHF) and retroperitoneal bleeding after internal hemorrhage.

Analgesics and corticosteroids often reduce joint pain and swelling. In mild hemophilia, the use of IV desmopressin may eliminate the need for AHF. Desmopressin acts by causing an increase in plasma factor VIII activity.

■ Nursing Management of the Medical Client

Assessment

Although most clients with hemophilia are successfully maintained with home healthcare, they may be seen in the hospital during acute bleeding episodes or for nonrelated treatments. If even a minor invasive procedure is planned, it is crucial to assess the factor VIII level and administer a sufficient quantity of factor concentrate before the procedure.

During routine medical examinations, these clients should be assessed for frequency of bleeding episodes and effectiveness of home therapy. Examine joints for manifestations of bleeding and related atrophy.

Diagnosis, Planning, Implementation

Knowledge Deficit. The nursing diagnosis is *Knowledge Deficit related to increased risk for bleeding.*

Planning: Expected Outcomes. The client will understand how to prevent or immediately treat bleeding, as evidenced by the client's ability to describe precautions, absence of injury, or rapid treatment of unavoidable injury.

Implementation. Provide teaching about bleeding precautions for prevention of injury or trauma that may precipitate a bleeding episode. Effective and prompt administration of factors to reduce the incidence of bleeding episodes and resultant complications, such as joint atrophy, is a priority. The client should avoid activities that may induce bleeding. Genetic counseling (if the client has the hereditary form of hemophilia) and teaching of the client and significant others should be done.

During client teaching, review routine situations that increase the client's risk of bleeding, such as contact sports, minor invasive procedures, falls, and cuts. Teach the client to recognize early manifestations and why it is critical to intervene with treatment immediately. Discuss situations that require medical consultation.

The client requires a great deal of instruction in managing the disease independently at home. The client will need to learn IV infusion administration techniques to control the bleeding.

Evaluation

Although it will not be possible to prevent all episodes of bleeding, an appropriate outcome would be that preventable bleeding does not occur. With teaching and effort by the client, bleeding can be prevented or at least minimized.

Blood Transfusions

Hematologic disorders or the aggressive ablative therapy used to treat some hematologic diseases can require acute or chronic support with a variety of blood components. Technological advances to improve the quality and safety of transfusions have caused a revolution in blood banking. This field has evolved into a broader specialty of transfusion medicine wherein the administration of blood components is considerably more complex and tightly regulated. The Joint Commission on Accreditation of Healthcare Organizations requires that all blood transfusions be evaluated to confirm that clear medical indications for the transfusion exist and that the client responds as expected. The transfusionist plays a critical role in this process. It is the nurse's responsibility to administer appropriate blood components in a manner that will ensure safety and efficacy.

Preparing for Transfusion

Assessment

The physician's order for transfusion should specify blood component, volume, and rate of infusion. However, as with all potentially hazardous biologics, the nurse must confirm that the drug being given is safe and appropriate in the present clinical situation. Table 53–8 describes blood components (see pp. 1520–1523).

Informed Consent and Client Teaching

In recent years, failure to disclose information and obtain consent for transfusion has resulted in litigation when transfusion complications occurred. Informed consent involves explaining medical indications for transfusion, and its benefits, risks, and alternatives.

Two alternatives to homologous (random) blood transfusion should be considered: autologous and directed (or designated) donation. Clients who do not have leukemia or bacteremia should be offered the option of donating their own blood before a scheduled surgical procedure if there is a reasonable expectation that blood will be required. Although the risk-benefit ratio should be evaluated, experience to date indicates that even clients with heart disease and other high-risk conditions tolerate the procedure well. The elimination of disease transmission, alloimmunization, and other potential transfusion complications makes this a reasonable option for many surgical clients.

Autologous donations can be made every 3 days if the donor's hemoglobin remains at or above 11 g/dl. For the blood to be maintained in a liquid state, donations should begin within 5 weeks of the transfusion date. Red blood cells can be stored frozen for 10 years, but the expense involved and time required for final preparation limit this practice to those who have extremely rare blood types. Donations should cease at least 3 days before the date of transfusion.

Another frequently used method of autologous blood collection is intraoperative, postoperative, or post-traumatic blood salvage. This procedure involves suctioning blood from body cavities, joint spaces, and other closed operative or trauma sites. Tissue debris and other sterile contaminants may necessitate special processing such as washing. Salvaged blood must be reinfused within 6 hours of collection.

A second option is for transfusion recipients to designate their own donors. Directed donations have not been shown to decrease the risk of contracting HIV infection. In fact, some evidence indicates that directed donors have a higher incidence of hepatitis. This is probably due to the fact that a large percentage of directed donors are giving blood for the first time, and it is well documented that first-time donors more frequently test positive for hepatitis surrogate markers. In spite of this evidence, clients frequently feel more comfortable identifying their donors. It is essential to discuss all of these options with the client in sufficient time to permit donation and blood testing.

Documentation of informed consent may consist of a form in the medical record stating that this information was presented in a manner understandable to the client (e.g., "Risks of and alternatives to blood transfusion were explained, and the client consented"). If the client is clinically unable to consent to transfusion, a reasonable effort should be made to secure consent from a family member. If no family member is available or time does not allow, a note to this effect should be placed in the chart. As described in the Ethical Issues in Nursing feature, institu-

ETHICAL ISSUES IN NURSING

Should Parents Who Are Jehovah's Witnesses Have the Right to Refuse a Life-Saving Transfusion for Their Child?

Blood transfusions are a common and effective treatment for many disorders that may be life-threatening. In the past, there was never much controversy over the transfusion of blood products. Currently, however, because of acquired immunodeficiency syndrome (AIDS), transfusions are a little more risky even though testing is done on all donor blood for the AIDS virus and for hepatitis. Even so, transfusions are common, and although concern over safety remains, the receiving of blood products is not considered highly controversial.

Controversy does exist regarding blood component therapy for those who are members of Jehovah's Witnesses. The belief among these members is that they should receive no blood components donated from another person. There is hardly a dilemma when a competent adult Jehovah's Witness refuses blood component therapy (although there might be some issues that could cause controversy). However, should a Jehovah's Witness parent have the right to refuse perhaps a life-saving transfusion for a minor child? Minors are not legally competent to make most healthcare decisions and thus rely on their parents as surrogate decision-makers. These paternal decisions in most cases are thought to be out of beneficence in the best interest of the child. Is the refusal of a life-saving treatment for a child, such as a blood transfusion, on the basis of religious beliefs of the parents ethical? Should these parents have such a surrogacy right regarding their own beliefs when the children may or may not wish to exercise the same beliefs of their Jehovah's Witness parents?

Be aware of clients who hold such religious restrictions on certain treatments. In dealing with competent adults, such decisions may not be truly understood by the healthcare providers, but they should be respected as a right of freedom of religion. The ethical and legal issues arise in dealing with minor children of parents who refuse physically beneficent treatments for their children on the basis of their religious beliefs. Be aware of your institution and state policies regarding such situations. In life-or-death situations, you can truly make a difference by being informed of such policies and by acting responsibly no matter what personal feelings may be at hand.

tional policy will vary regarding who is permitted to obtain consent. Some facilities restrict this responsibility to the physician; others allow both nurses and physicians to perform this procedure. Regardless of the degree of nursing involvement in the formal process, the nurse is the client's most readily available source of information.

The client's understanding of the transfusion should be assessed and accurate responses should be made to questions and concerns. If questions are outside the nurse's area of expertise, transfusion medicine staff can serve as a valuable resource.

It is also the transfusionist's responsibility to describe the details of the transfusion procedure. Venous access, length of transfusion, and expected outcomes should be explained. The client should be informed of normal physiologic responses to transfusion and manifestations to be reported immediately. Clients released from care after transfusion should be given written information, including the name and telephone number of a person to contact.

Pretransfusion Testing

In today's climate, the client's major concern is likely to be the safety of the transfusion, specifically the risk of contracting acquired immunodeficiency syndrome (AIDS). The transfusionist should dispel misconceptions and provide factual information. Efforts to ensure a safe and effective transfusion begin before the blood or component is collected. For many decades, prospective donors have been asked two categories of questions: (1) those intended to protect the donor from possible risks of donation, and (2) those intended to protect the recipient from risks of transfusion.

In order to reduce the risk of HIV transmission to blood recipients, there has been a marked increase in the second group of questions. In addition, donors are required to read information about behaviors known to increase the risk of HIV infection and, in most collection centers, they are questioned directly about their involvement in such activities.

Finally, a method must be made available for donors to indicate anonymously that their unit is or is not safe for transfusion. In addition to obtaining a thorough donor history, many serologic and infectious disease tests are routinely performed on the donor's blood. Table 53–9 provides an overview of these tests.

When a need for blood is identified, several tests are done to confirm that the client's blood is compatible with that of the donor. First, the recipient's ABO and Rh type are identified. To determine the presence of antibody other than anti-A or anti-B, an antibody screen is performed. This test (also referred to as the indirect antiglobulin test) is done by adding the recipient's serum to donor red blood cells known to have a certain set of minor blood group antigens. Coombs' serum (antihuman globulin) is added to facilitate visibility of cellular agglutination, an indicator of antigen-antibody complex formation. The results are viewed macro- and microscopically. More than 400 minor red cell antigens have been identified on red blood cells, each of which can stimulate the production of an antibody. However, only the few (approximately 30) that are of sufficiently potent antigenicity to be clinically significant are included in the routine antibody screen.

It is not uncommon for chronically transfused clients to develop multiple antibodies. Identifying the antibodies and obtaining blood from donors who do not possess the

Text continued on page 1524

Table 53–8. Blood Components

	Whole Blood	Red Blood Cells	Platelet Concentrates	Fresh Frozen Plasma	Cryoprecipitate	Granulocyte Concentrates	Plasma Derivatives	Coagulation Factor Concentrates
Composition	RBC, plasma, plasma proteins (globulins, antibodies), 63 ml of anticoagulant-preservative	RBC with CPDA-1 solution (anticoagulant-preservative only), final hematocrit no higher than 80% (80% RBC, 20% plasma) RBC with 100 ml additive solution, final hematocrit about 55%–60%	Single-unit platelets contain a minimum of 5.5 × 10^{10} (1 unit) platelets in 50–70 ml of plasma obtained by separating platelet-rich plasma from 1 unit of fresh whole blood; 6–10 units may be pooled for 1 transfusion Single-donor platelets contain a minimum of 3.0 × 10^{11} platelets (6 units) obtained from single donor by use of automated cell separator during apheresis; recipient exposed to fewer donors, which decreases complications	91% water, 7% protein (globulin, antibodies, clotting factors), and 2% carbohydrates Freezing within 8 hr of collection preserves all clotting factors	Each unit contains about 80–120 units of factor VIII (antihemophilic factor) that represents 50% of antihemophilic factor originally present in unit, vWF, 250 mg of fibrinogen, and 20%–30% of factor XIII present in a unit of whole blood, suspended in 10–20 ml of plasma	Unit obtained by granulocytapheresis contains a minimum of 1.0 × 10^{10} granulocytes, variable amounts of lymphocytes (usually <10%), 30–50 ml of RBC and 100–400 ml of plasma, and 6–10 units of platelets; the platelets can be separated from the unit if the granulocyte recipient is not thrombocytopenic	*Albumin:* 96% albumin, 4% globulin and other proteins extracted from plasma; available as a 5% solution, oncotically equivalent to plasma, and also a concentrated 25% solution *Plasma protein fraction:* 83% albumin and 17% globulins extracted from plasma; less pure than albumin and has higher degree of contamination with other plasma proteins; in 5% solution only	*Factor VIII:* Lyophilized concentrate containing large quantities of factor VIII; prepared from large pools of donor plasma, but heat treatment during fractionation process significantly reduces risk of transmitting viral disease *Factor IX:* Lyophilized concentrate containing large quantities of factor IX; also contains factors II, VII, and X; product prepared from large pools of donor plasma, but heat treatment during fractionation process significantly reduces risk of transmitting viral disease
Volume	500 ml/unit	250–350 ml/unit 350–400 ml/unit	50–70 ml/unit 200–400 ml/unit	200–250 ml	5–10 ml/unit	200–400 ml with platelets 100–200 ml without platelets	Albumin: 250 and 500 ml (5%); 50 and 100 ml (25%)	Multiple-dose vial

Equipment							
19- to 20-gauge needle, standard straight or Y-type blood administration set with minimum 170-μm filter, 0.9% saline	19- to 20-gauge needle, standard straight or Y-type blood administration set with minimum 170-μm filter, 0.9% saline	19- to 21-gauge needle, component administration set with standard 170-μm filter, 0.9% saline	19- to 23-gauge needle, component administration set with standard 170-μm filter, 0.9% saline	19- to 21-gauge needle, component administration set with standard 170-μm filter, 0.9% saline	19- to 21-gauge needle, component administration set with standard 170-μm filter, 0.9% saline *Never* use a leukocyte-depleting filter to infuse granulocytes	19- to 21-gauge needle and standard IV infusion set. A filter may be required by some manufacturers; check product insert for specific instructions. Administration set with filter may be supplied with the albumin	IV push through filtered needle or IV drip using component recipient set

ABO/Rh Compatibility

ABO/Rh Compatibility							
The ABO type of the donor should be identical with the recipient's. Rh− blood can be given to an Rh− or Rh+ recipient	A can match with A or O; B can match with B or O; O can match only with O; AB can match with A, B, or O. Rh− blood can be given to either Rh+ or Rh− recipient	Whereas platelets have no ABO or Rh antigens, they are suspended in 200–400 ml of plasma containing donor antibodies and a small number of RBC. There is evidence that platelet survival decreases if donor plasma is incompatible, and large volumes of incompatible plasma may cause a positive direct Coombs' test. It is also possible for even a small number of Rh+ RBC to stimulate anti-D in an Rh− recipient; therefore, plasma ABO and Rh compatibility is recommended	A can match with A or AB; B can match with B or AB; AB can match only with AB; O can match with A, B, AB, or O. Rh− and Rh+ blood can be given to either Rh+ or Rh− recipient	Cryoprecipitate contains no RBC and a small volume of plasma. ABO crossmatching not needed, and plasma compatibility preferred but not required	Granulocytes contain a significant number of RBC and plasma; therefore, ABO of donor should be identical with recipient's. Rh− components may be transfused to an Rh+ recipient	Antibodies destroyed during processing; therefore, compatibility not a factor	Antibodies destroyed during processing, so compatibility not a factor

Table continued on following page

Table 53–8. Blood Components (Continued)

	Whole Blood	Red Blood Cells	Platelet Concentrates	Fresh Frozen Plasma	Cryoprecipitate	Granulocyte Concentrates	Plasma Derivatives	Coagulation Factor Concentrates
Special Considerations	Whole blood transfusion is rarely indicated Treatment with specific blood components is usually recommended	RBC may be viscous, so 0.9% saline may be added to achieve optimal flow rates For some clients, a leukocyte depletion filter may be used to prevent complications	Because platelet concentrates contain few RBC, crossmatch testing is not required Plasma ABO and Rh compatibility is recommended, especially when the total volume of the transfusion exceeds 150–200 ml Only filters specially designed for platelet transfusion should be used	Plasma carries same risk of disease transmission as does whole blood If only volume expansion is required, products of choice are crystalloid or colloid solutions, such as saline or albumin Plasma contains no RBC, and Rh compatibility and crossmatching are not required ABO compatibility must be confirmed before administration	Single units of cryoprecipitate may be pooled into 1 container by the blood collection center If individual bags are issued, 0.9% saline may need to be added to rinse residual cryoprecipitate from bags and tubing	Granulocytes have short survival (<24 hr); infuse as soon as possible Granulocyte concentrates contain a significant number of RBC; pretransfusion testing ordinarily the same as for RBC transfusion Increased incidence of febrile, non-hemolytic reactions with granulocyte transfusions; infuse slowly, observe client closely; premedication with an antihistamine, acetaminophen, steroids, or meperidine may be indicated to prevent repeat reactions Do *not* administer amphotericin B within 4 hr of granulocyte transfusion (pulmonary insufficiency seen with concurrent administration)	PPF and albumin cannot transmit hepatitis or HIV infection; the pasteurization process used to prepare the products destroys such viruses Hypotension has been associated with rapid infusion of PPF; 25% albumin can cause a significantly increased blood pressure because of its ability to draw fluid into the intravascular space	Factor VIII and factor IX assays should be performed at appropriate intervals to assess response Factor VIII concentration lacks vWF and should not be used in treatment of von Willebrand's disease

Expected Outcomes

Prevention or resolution of hypovolemic shock and anemia

In a nonbleeding adult, 1 unit of whole blood should increase hematocrit by 3% and hemoglobin by 1 g/dl

Resolution of symptoms of anemia

In a nonbleeding adult, 1 unit of RBC should increase hematocrit by 3% and hemoglobin by 1 g/dl

Prevention or resolution of bleeding due to thrombocytopenia or platelet dysfunction

1 unit should raise peripheral platelet count 5000–10,000/mm³ if underlying cause is resolved or controlled

Efficacy of platelet transfusion can be determined by obtaining platelet counts at 1 hr and 18–24 hr after infusion

Treatment effectiveness is assessed by monitoring coagulation function, specifically, PT and PTT, or by specific factor assays

Correction of factor VIII, vWF, factor XIII, and fibrinogen deficiency; cessation of bleeding in uremic clients

Laboratory values required to assess effectiveness of treatment

Improvement in or resolution of infection

No increase in peripheral WBC count usually seen after granulocyte transfusion in adults, although increase may be seen in children

An improvement in clinical condition because of resolving infection is the only measure of treatment effectiveness

The client will acquire and maintain adequate blood pressure and volume support

The client will develop hemostasis because of increased levels of factor VIII and factor IX activity

CPDA-1, citrate-phosphate-dextrose-adenine; FFP, fresh-frozen plasma; HIV, human immunodeficiency virus; IV, intravenous; PPF, plasma protein fraction; PT, prothrombin time; PTT, partial thromboplastin time; RBC, red blood cells; vWF, von Willebrand's factor; WBC, white blood cells.

Table 53–9. Routine Donor Infectious Disease Testing

Test	Purpose	Confirmatory Test	Follow-up/Deferral
RPR (rapid plasma reagin)	Determines presence of *Treponema pallidum* infection (syphilis)	FTA (fluorescent treponemal antibody)	Blood discarded; donor deferred for 1 year; treponemes die in blood after 5 days of refrigeration
ALT (alanine aminotransferase)	Surrogate test for hepatitis C	None	Blood discarded if ALT out of range; donor deferred for repeat mild elevations or single gross abnormality
Anti-HBc	Surrogate test for antibody to hepatitis B core antigen (HBc); high incidence in HIV-positive donors	None	Blood discarded; donor may be permanently deferred
Anti-HCV	Determines presence of antibody to hepatitis C virus (HCV)	None	Blood discarded; donor permanently deferred
HBsAg	Determines presence of hepatitis B surface antigen (HBsAg)	Repeat test procedure after neutralization of HBsAg in sample with anti-HBsAg; results unaffected if false-positive, at least 50% reduction if true-positive	On confirmation, blood discarded; donor permanently deferred
Anti-HIV	Determines presence of antibody to human immunodeficiency virus (HIV)	Western blot, 0.5% false-positive rate	Blood discarded if enzyme-linked immunosorbent assay (ELISA) positive twice; donor permanently deferred if repeat ELISA positive, Western blot positive or indeterminant
Anti-HTLV-1	Determines presence of antibody to human T-cell lymphotropic virus, type 1 (HTLV-1)	Western blot and RIPA (radioimmunoprecipitation assay)	Infection may cause T-cell leukemia in 10–15 yr; confirmed positive donors permanently deferred

antigens can significantly complicate the testing procedure and lengthen the time required for blood preparation.

Blood products containing red blood cells may be further tested for compatibility to crossmatch testing. For this procedure, donor red blood cells are combined with the recipient's serum and Coombs' serum. After an inoculation period, the results are viewed microscopically. If no red blood cell agglutination has occurred, the crossmatch is compatible. Studies indicate that crossmatching adds very little to the safety of transfusion (0.01%–0.1%) if a negative antibody screen is initially obtained.[18] In these situations, the Coombs' phase can be eliminated to shorten the procedure and reduce cost.

Routine serologic testing requires a 10-ml clotted sample and a 7-ml citrated sample. Approximately 1 hour is required for testing in routine situations. In the event of a medical emergency, O-negative red blood cells and AB plasma can be safely administered to most clients without serologic testing.

Failure to correctly label the samples used for blood bank testing could lead to fatal errors. Several precautionary measures should be taken to reduce this risk. Samples must be labeled at the bedside after asking the client to state his or her name and comparing it with that on the identification bracelet. If the client is unable to state his or her name, identity should be confirmed by a family member or other person familiar with the client whenever possible. The date and initials of the phlebotomist must be written on the sample label. Many institutions have adopted a secondary identification system. Several commercial systems are available; each is designed to ensure that the sample used for crossmatch has been drawn from the client who receives the transfusion.

Obtaining Venous Access

Suitable venous access for transfusion varies with the product being infused. When packed red blood cells weighing less than 300 g are infused, a 20-gauge or larger needle will be needed to achieve maximal flow rate. If a smaller-gauge needle must be used, the red blood cells can be diluted with 0.9% saline. No solution other than normal saline should be added to blood components.

Components containing a significant volume of plasma or other diluent can be safely infused at a rapid rate through smaller-gauge needles or catheters. A central venous catheter is an acceptable access option for blood transfusion. It should be noted, however, that a large volume of refrigerated blood infused rapidly into the ventricle of the heart has been known to cause cardiac arrhythmias. Warming the blood can reduce the risk of this complication. Another issue of concern is the use of multilumen catheters which may allow blood to mix with incompatible solutions and medications as they exit the catheter tips. Experience indicates that the circulation achieved through a blood vessel suitable for central line placement results in rapid mixing of fluids. As a result, no harmful effects have been reported.

Requesting Blood Release

Blood bank regulations state that refrigerated components may not be returned to inventory if they have been warmed to more than 10° C (50° F). To meet this requirement, most transfusion medicine services consider 30 minutes to be the maximal allowable time out of monitored storage. For avoiding delays that may result in the waste of a scarce commodity, certain procedures should be performed before blood is requested.

An IV catheter appropriate for transfusing the requested component should be functional, flushed with normal saline, and maintained at a keep-vein-open (KVO) rate. Vital signs should then be taken and recorded. Fever may be a reason for delaying the transfusion. In addition to masking a possible manifestation of an acute transfusion reaction, fever can also compromise the efficacy of platelet transfusions.

Premedication may also be required if the client has a history of adverse reactions. In many cases, febrile reactions can be prevented by administering acetaminophen or diphenhydramine hydrochloride. Steroids have been used to avoid severe fever, rigors, and chills that accompany granulocyte transfusions (although these are rarely used). A history of allergic reactions may require prophylactic administration of antihistamines. For effectiveness to be ensured, oral medication should be administered 30 minutes before the transfusion is started. IV medication may be given immediately before the transfusion is initiated.

Blood should be released from the blood bank only to adequately trained personnel. The name and identification number of the recipient must be provided and a permanent record of this information maintained in the blood bank. So that delivery to the wrong client is avoided, blood should be transported to only one client at a time.

Beginning the Transfusion

Confirming Blood Acceptability

The most critical phase of transfusion is confirming product compatibility and verifying client identity. Before going to the client's bedside, the nurse should verify ABO and Rh compatibility. This can usually be done by comparing the bag label with the medical record and forms issued from the blood bank. The bag label should also be checked to ensure that the correct component has been

issued and for date of expiration. Components expire at midnight of the day marked on the bag unless otherwise specified.

Inspect the unit for leaks, abnormal color, clots, excessive air, and bubbles. Check carefully for important labels (such as autologous, directed) or instructions (such as "use leukocyte-depleting filter"). Cellular components (whole blood, red blood cells, and platelets) for an immunosuppressed client should be clearly marked *irradiated*. Clients with Hodgkin's or non-Hodgkin's lymphoma, acute leukemia, or congenital immunodeficiency disorders and bone marrow transplant recipients may develop posttransfusion GVHD if lymphocytes contaminating cellular components engraft and divide. Transfusions from firstdegree family members have also been known to cause fatal GVHD. A small dose of radiation delivered to the component before release from the blood bank renders the lymphocytes incapable of mitotic action without presenting a radiation risk to the recipient or transfusionist.

At the bedside, ask clients to state their name and compare it with the name on the identification bracelet. As with sample collection, clients unable to state their name should be identified by a person who knows them well. Compare the name and number on the identification bracelet with the tag on the blood bag. If applicable, check the secondary identification system. The American Association of Blood Banks recommends that two qualified people perform this critical step.

Blood Infusion Equipment and Devices

Most blood products should be infused through administration sets designed specifically for this use. The set usually contains a 170-μm filter designed to trap fibrin clots and other debris that accumulate during blood storage. Most standard filters have a four-unit capacity. Tubing is available in two basic configurations: straight or Y-type. The use of Y-type tubing simplifies the process of adding normal saline to red blood cells and provides ready access to a saline flush if the transfusion must be interrupted. Straight tubing usually has a medication injection site a few inches from the needle. If an adverse reaction develops, a KVO saline drip initiated at this site will maintain patency of the IV line but avoid exposure to the 30 to 50 ml of blood remaining in the tubing and filter. The administration set should be changed every 4 to 6 hours, or according to institution policy, to reduce the risk of septicemia.

Many devices are available for increasing the safety of transfusion. Special filters, electromechanical devices, and blood warmers are frequently used at the bedside. The transfusionist should be familiar with how and why special equipment is used.

Nonstandard Filters

The physician or nurse may determine that the standard 170-μm filter is not adequate in certain clinical situations. The transfusion medicine service may also recommend the use of a nonstandard filter to decrease the risk of transfusion complications. Several types of specialty filters are described in Table 53–10. Although each is technically easy to use, inappropriate use can significantly compromise desired results. It is, therefore, critically important to follow the manufacturer's instructions exactly. An insert may be found inside the package, or the instructions may be printed on the outside of the packaging container.

Electromechanical Infusion Devices

Several types of infusion devices are available to regulate and monitor the flow of IV solutions. There are basically two types: (1) infusion controllers, which monitor flow by gravity, and (2) infusion pumps, which deliver solutions under pressure. Infusion controllers may be used with all blood products if they are designed to function with opaque solutions. However, the negative pressure exerted by the peristaltic or syringelike cassette action of infusion pumps could cause red blood cell hemolysis. If the transfusion product contains a significant number of red blood cells, the manufacturer should be consulted before a pump designed for crystalloid and colloid solutions is used.

Many studies have been done to determine the effect of mechanical devices on red blood cells. They clearly indicate that in addition to pump action, there are other factors that affect the degree of red blood cell hemolysis. These include length of tubing, diameter of tubing, type of filter, infusion rate, needle gauge, blood age, temperature, and viscosity. Therefore, it is imperative that machines tested and approved for the infusion of red blood cells be used exactly as recommended by the manufacturer.

If manual pressure cuffs are used to increase red blood cell flow rate, the pressure should not exceed 300 mm Hg. Standard sphygmomanometers should not be used for this purpose because they do not exert uniform pressure against all parts of the bag.

Blood Warmers

Blood warmers may be used to prevent hypothermia, which can be induced by rapid infusion of large volumes of refrigerated blood. Neonatal exchange transfusion, plasma exchange, surgery, and trauma are all clinical situations that may require the use of a blood warmer. Other clients of concern are those with cold agglutinin disease. These clients have antibodies that react at temperatures under 37° C (98.6° F). Systemic circulatory cooling can cause intravascular agglutination. This condition may be detected during serologic testing. Once this client has been identified, the transfusion service may recommend the use of a blood warmer for all transfusions.

There are two types of devices approved by blood bank regulatory agencies for warming blood. For dry heating, a bag is placed between two aluminum heating

Table 53–10. Nonstandard Filters			
Filter	**Design Features**	**Recommended Use**	**Special Considerations**
High-flow filter	Standard pore size, large surface area; filters up to 10 units at high flow rate	For massive transfusions primarily in critical care units, operating and emergency rooms	Appropriate for adults only
Pediatric filter	Standard pore size; small surface area reduces priming volume; may contain intermediate storage container for precise volume control	For small-volume transfusions; primarily neonates, children, geriatric clients	
Microaggregate filter	Plastic chamber containing mesh or fiber that effectively removes particles 20–40 μm in size	For preventing fibrin, leukocytes, or platelets from migrating to lungs during massive transfusion; marginally effective for preparation of leukocyte-reduced red blood cells	Instruction for use varies with manufacturer; follow priming and flushing instructions exactly to optimize effectiveness
Leukocyte-reducing filter	Chamber containing synthetic fibers treated to capture leukocytes; priming volume 20–40 ml; expensive ($20–$60/filter)	For removal of 95%–99%+ of leukocytes from red blood cells or platelets to reduce incidence of febrile reactions, HLA alloimmunization, cytomegalovirus infection	Platelet and red blood cell filters are *not* interchangeable; follow manufacturer's instructions for priming, flushing, and rinsing, because failure to do so can severely compromise efficacy

plates, or a disposable cuff-style bag is wrapped around a cylindrical aluminum heating element. A second type uses warm water to increase the temperature of the blood. Water baths containing water warmed to 37° C (98.6° F) may be used only if they have been specifically designed for warming blood. The blood bag should never be fully immersed in water. Studies indicate that water baths create an optimal medium for the growth of harmful organisms, which can contaminate the blood bag port and cause septicemia. Two transfusion-related deaths were traced to a water bath contaminated with *Pseudomonas*.

Conventional blood warmers have some limitations. The rate of infusion can be impeded by the additional tubing and blood warming bags required for conventional warming devices. Standard blood warmers also require substantial priming volume, which makes them inappropriate for small-volume transfusions. Devices have been designed specifically for these situations, but care must be taken to use only equipment tested and approved for use with blood components. Acceptable devices must have a visible thermometer and an audible or visible alarm to alert the user if the temperature exceeds 38° C (100.4° F).

Monitoring During the Transfusion

The first 10 to 15 minutes of any transfusion are the most critical. If a major ABO incompatibility exists or a severe allergic reaction such as anaphylaxis occurs, it is usually evident within the first 50 ml of the transfusion. Therefore, it is recommended that the transfusion begin slowly, under close observation of medical personnel. If no evidence of a reaction is noted within the first 15 minutes, flow can be increased to the prescribed rate. Before leaving the client unattended, instruct the client to report anything unusual immediately. It is advisable to take and record vital signs before the transfusion begins, after the first 15 minutes, and every hour until 1 hour after the transfusion has been discontinued. The vital signs should be checked immediately if the client displays any untoward manifestations.

The recommended rate of infusion varies with the blood component being transfused. Components containing few red blood cells, such as platelets, plasma, and cryoprecipitate, may be infused rapidly, but care should be taken to avoid circulatory overload. This is of particular concern in neonatal, pediatric, and geriatric clients and in clients with cardiac disease. For avoiding the risk of septicemia, infusions should not exceed 4 hours. If the client's size or medical condition does not allow infusion within 4 hours, the unit may be split into smaller aliquots in the blood bank.

Regulatory agencies require complete documentation of the transfusion, including identification of personnel starting and ending the transfusion, unique product number, and outcome (e.g., "no reaction noted"). If an adverse reaction does occur, the manifestations, actions taken, and future recommendations should also be recorded in the client's medical record.

Exposure to foreign blood elements may mediate immunologic and nonimmunologic reactions affecting all major body systems, as described in Box 53–4. Any unusual manifestation occurring during or immediately after a transfusion should be considered a potential reaction. Unconscious clients should be monitored closely because manifestations of a reaction may be inhibited in the unconscious state (Box 53–5). The acute reactions most frequently seen are described in Table 53–11.

Whereas treatment may vary depending on the manifestations, certain standard procedures should be followed when a reaction is suspected. In all cases, stop the transfusion and keep the IV line open with normal saline. Treat life-threatening manifestations, such as respiratory or circulatory failure, immediately. Contact the client's physician and the blood bank. According to institutional policy, obtain appropriate laboratory samples. Samples used to evaluate a reaction include blood and urine. Free hemoglobin found in either indicates that red blood cells have hemolyzed, the most serious serologic finding. To avoid clouding the diagnostic picture by venous trauma, obtain blood samples from a large peripheral vein using at least a 19-gauge needle. The blood sample is also used to repeat ABO and Rh typing, antibody screening, and direct antiglobulin testing. A discrepancy between initial and repeat testing may indicate that incompatible blood was transfused. After laboratory testing, a physician specializing in transfusion medicine will evaluate the clinical and laboratory evidence to determine whether the client's manifestations were caused by the transfusion. The physician may then make recommendations for reducing the risk of complication in the future.

Transfusion services are required to maintain records of reaction evaluations and future transfusion restrictions. These records are consulted when future transfusions are required. Special processing, such as washing, may then be performed in the blood bank to reduce the risks of another adverse reaction. In some cases, instructions may be placed on the unit informing the transfusionist that a special filter or infusion device should be used at the bedside.

Delayed Transfusion Complications

Complications can occur days to years after a transfusion. Fever, mild jaundice, and decreased hematocrit may indicate a delayed hemolytic reaction. Hemolysis of red blood cells may occur 3 days to several months after the transfusion if an antibody was undetected during crossmatch testing and red blood cells containing that antigen were transfused. Usually no medical treatment is required. Iron overload may occur in clients receiving more than 100 units of blood over a period of time, such as clients with aplastic anemia.

Clinical manifestations are congestive heart failure, arrhythmias, impaired thyroid and gonadal function, diabetes, and cirrhosis. Deferoxamine, which chelates and removes accumulated iron via the kidneys, may be administered IV or subcutaneously to prevent this poten-

Box 53–4. Possible Manifestations of a Transfusion Reaction

General

Fever (rise of 1° C or 2° F)
Chills
Muscle aches, pain
Back pain
Chest pain
Headache
Heat at site of infusion or along vein

Nervous System

Apprehension, impending sense of doom
Tingling, numbness

Respiratory System

Changes in respiratory rate
   Tachypnea
   Apnea
   Dyspnea
   Cough
   Wheezing
   Rales

Gastrointestinal System

Nausea
Vomiting
Pain, abdominal cramping
Diarrhea (may be bloody)

Cardiovascular System

Heart rate
   Bradycardia
   Tachycardia

Blood pressure
   Hypotension, shock
   Hypertension

Peripheral Circulation

Color
   Cyanosis
   Facial flushing
Temperature
   Cool, clammy
   Hot, flushed, dry
Edema

Bleeding

Generalized (disseminated intravascular coagulation)
Oozing at surgical site

Renal System

Changes in urine volume
   Oliguria, anuria
   Renal failure
Changes in urine color
   Dark, concentrated
   Shades of red, brown, amber
   May indicate the presence in urine of red blood cells
     (hematuria) or of free hemoglobin (hemoglobinuria)

Integumentary System

Rashes, hives (urticaria), swelling
Itching
Diaphoresis

---

tially fatal complication. Post-transfusion GVHD can occur if donor lymphocytes engraft and divide in the marrow spaces of an immunocompromised recipient. Manifestations are fever, rash, diarrhea, and hepatitis. This frequently fatal complication can be prevented by irradiation of all cellular components prior to administration to high-risk clients.

Box 53–5. Manifestations of Transfusion Reaction in an Unconscious Client

Weak pulse
Fever
Hypotension
Visible hemoglobinuria
Increased operative bleeding (oozing at surgical site)
Vasomotor instability (tachycardia, bradycardia, or hypotension)
Oliguria, anuria

Many diseases can be transmitted through blood transfusion. The most common is hepatitis C. Although manifestations are milder than those seen with hepatitis B, chronic liver disease and cirrhosis may develop. Hepatitis B should be considered if the recipient develops anorexia, malaise, nausea, vomiting, dark urine, and jaundice within 4 to 6 weeks of transfusion. An elevated alanine aminotransferase and aspartate aminotransferase are frequently seen, indicating liver damage that may be permanent. Hepatitis B and C are treated symptomatically. With advances in donor testing and screening in the United States, the risk of hepatitis has decreased to about 3%.

On rare occasions, HIV-1 is transmitted from an infected donor to a blood recipient. The client may be asymptomatic for several years or develop flulike manifestations in 2 to 4 weeks. Whereas more than 25,000 cases of transfusion-associated AIDS were reported before routine donor testing in 1985, the incidence has decreased to 1 in 100,000 to 150,000 as a result of careful donor screening and testing.[127] Other infectious viruses and diseases that may be transmitted through blood transfusion are HIV-2, HTLV-1, Chagas' disease, Lyme disease, babesiosis, syphilis, Epstein-Barr virus, cytomegalovirus in-

Table 53–11. Acute Transfusion Reactions

Reaction	Cause	Clinical Manifestations	Management	Prevention
Immunogenic				
Allergic Incidence: 1%	Sensitivity to foreign proteins in plasma	Urticaria, flushing, itching (no fever)	Administer antihistamines as directed. If symptoms mild and transient, transfusion may resume	Treat prophylactically with antihistamines
Febrile, nonhemolytic Incidence: 0.5%–1.0%	Sensitization to donor white blood cells, platelets, or plasma proteins	Sudden chills and fever (rise in temperature $>1°$ C [$1.8°$ F]), headache, flushing, anxiety, muscle pain	Give antipyretics as prescribed; avoid aspirin in thrombocytopenic clients	Consider leukocyte-poor blood products (filtered, washed, or frozen) if fever occurs more than once
Acute hemolytic Incidence: 1:25,000 Fatal: $2:1 \times 10^6$	Infusion of ABO-incompatible red blood cells	Chills, fever, low back pain, flushing, tachycardia, tachypnea, hemoglobinuria, hemoglobinemia, hypotension, vascular collapse, bleeding, acute renal failure, shock, cardiac arrest, death	Treat shock. Maintain blood pressure with IV solutions. Give diuretics as prescribed to maintain urine flow. Insert indwelling catheter or measure hourly output. Dialysis may be needed	Meticulously verify recipient from sample collection to transfusion
Anaphylactic Incidence: 1:150,000	Infusion of IgA proteins to IgA-deficient recipient who has developed anti-IgA antibodies	Anxiety, urticaria, wheezing progressing to cyanosis, shock, and possible cardiac arrest	Initiate CPR if indicated. Have epinephrine ready for injection (0.4 ml of a 1:1000 solution subcutaneously)	Give blood components from IgA-deficient donors or remove *all* plasma by washing
Nonimmunogenic				
Circulatory overload Estimated Incidence: 1:10,000 (not usually reported to blood bank)	Infusion of blood at a rate too rapid for size, cardiac status, or clinical condition of recipient	Cough, dyspnea, pulmonary congestion (rales), headache, hypertension, tachycardia, distended neck veins	Place client in upright position with feet in dependent position. Administer diuretics, oxygen, and morphine as prescribed. Phlebotomy may be required	Adjust transfusion volume and flow rate on basis of client size and clinical status. If slow transfusion will exceed 4 hr, request that unit be aliquoted into smaller volumes
Septicemia Incidence: very rare	Transfusion of component contaminated with microorganism	Rapid onset of chills, high fever, vomiting, diarrhea, marked hypotension, and shock	Treat symptoms and administer antibiotics, IV fluids, vasopressors, and steroids as directed. Obtain culture of client and blood containers	Collect, process, store, and transfuse blood according to industry standards. Infuse within 4 hr of starting time

CPR, cardiopulmonary resuscitation; IV, intravenous.

fection, and malaria. Blood donors are questioned or tested for potential exposure to these diseases.

Conclusions

Hematologic diseases are complex disorders that require the nurse to understand the hematopoietic system. The nurse is often involved in the administration of blood and blood products for treatment of a wide variety of these disorders. Many of the blood disorders are life-threatening (such as acute blood loss and leukemia), whereas others are easily controlled with proper nutrition or regular medication (such as pernicious anemia or iron deficiency anemia).

Because blood and blood product transfusions are used so commonly in the treatment of hematologic disorders, it is vital that the nurse understand this procedure. The nurse must understand the implications of these procedures and the proper techniques of administration so the client will receive safe and effective care.

Thinking Critically

1. The client had a gastric resection for peptic ulcer disease 3 months ago at a hospital in another state. She comes to the nursing clinic complaining of shortness of breath and fatigue with minimal physical exertion. She currently takes ranitidine (Zantac). What assessments should you make now?

Factors to Consider. What is the significance of the history of gastric resection? How might this contribute to the client's lethargy? What could be causing the shortness of breath and fatigue? What laboratory results would be appropriate to evaluate? What teaching should you consider with this client?

2. A 34-year-old man comes to the outpatient oncology facility for his second round of chemotherapy for acute myelogenous leukemia. Three days after this, the client calls the clinic nurse complaining of bleeding gums. What is the priority problem you should address? What instructions should the clinic nurse give the client at this time?

Factors to Consider. What pathologic process underlies the client's manifestations? Are there laboratory results you would want to check? What other precautions should you institute based on the client's other manifestations and the laboratory data? What other data are significant to collect at this time?

3. The client was recently diagnosed with multiple myeloma and admitted to the oncology inpatient unit for initial evaluation and treatment. On her fourth day after admission, she becomes confused and difficult to arouse. Her bowel sounds are diminished, and she begins to vomit. What priority assessment should you make now?

Factors to Consider. What might predispose the client

to this change in her level of consciousness? What additional assessments would you need to make? What interventions should you anticipate at this time?

Bibliography

1. Acevedo, M. (1992). Blood dyscrasias: Polycythemia, idiopathic thrombocytopenic purpura, and thrombotic thrombocytopenic purpura. *Journal of Intravenous Nursing, 15*(1), 52–57.
2. Afessa, B., et al. (1992). Outcome of recipients of bone marrow transplants who require intensive-care unit support. *Mayo Clinic Proceedings, 67*, 117–122.
3. Alexanian, R., et al. (1994). Early myeloablative therapy for multiple myeloma. *Blood, 84*(12), 4278–4282.
4. Anderson, J. E., et al. (1993). Allogeneic bone marrow transplantation for 93 patients with myelodysplastic syndrome. *Blood, 82*(2), 677–681.
5. Andrews, M. M. (1995). Transcultural perspectives in the nursing care of children and adolescents. In M. M. Andrews & J. S. Boyle (1995), *Transcultural concepts in nursing care* (pp. 123–180). Philadelphia: J. B. Lippincott.
6. Ballas, S. K., & Smith, E. D. (1992). Red blood cell changes during the evolution of the sickle cell painful crisis. *Blood, 79*(8), 2154–2163.
7. Bennett, J. C., et al. (1996). *Cecil Textbook of Medicine* (20th ed.). Philadelphia: W. B. Saunders.
8. Beutler, E. (1993). Platelet transfusions: The 20,000/μL trigger. *Blood, 81*(6), 1411–1413.
9. Bortin, M. M., et al. (1992). Changing trends in allogeneic bone marrow transplantation for leukemia in the 1980s. *JAMA, 268*(5), 607–612.
10. Bortin, M. M., et al. (1992). Increasing utilization of allogeneic bone marrow transplantation: Results of the 1988–1990 survey. *Annals of Internal Medicine, 116*(6), 505–512.
11. Bradfield, V. (1991). Thrombotic thrombocytopenic purpura. *Journal of Intravenous Nursing, 14*(4), 271–273.
12. Buchsel, P. C., & Whedon, M. B. (1995). *Bone marrow transplantation: Administrative and clinical strategies.* Boston: Jones & Bartlett.
13. Butturini, A., et al. (1994). Hematologic abnormalities in Fanconi anemia: An International Fanconi Anemia Registry study. *Blood, 84*(5), 1650–1655.
14. Cain, J., et al. (1991). Myelodysplastic syndromes: A review for nurses. *Oncology Nursing Forum, 18*, 113–117.
15. Charache, S., et al. (1995). Effect of hydroxyurea on the frequency of painful crises in sickle cell anemia. Investigators of the Multicenter Study of Hydroxyurea in Sickle Cell Anemia. *New England Journal of Medicine, 332*(20), 1317–1322.
16. Chipps, E., & Skinner, C. (1994). Intravenous immunoglobulin: Implications for use in the neurological patient. *Journal of Neuroscience Nursing, 26*(1), 8–17.
17. DeLuca, V. A., Jr. (1992). *Helicobacter pylori* gastric atrophy and pernicious anemia. *Gastroenterology, 102*(2), 744–745.
18. DeVita, V. T., Hellman, S., & Rosenberg, S. A. (Eds.). (1993). *Cancer: Principles and practice of oncology.* Philadelphia: J. B. Lippincott.
19. DiJulio, J. (1991). Hematopoiesis: An overview. *Oncology Nursing Forum, 18*, 3–6.
20. Ellenberger, B., Haas, L., & Cundiff, I. (1993). Thrombotic thrombocytopenia purpura: Nursing during the acute phase. *Dimensions of Critical Care Nursing, 12*(2), 58–65.
21. Epstein, C., & Bakanauskas, A. (1991). Clinical management of DIC: Early nursing interventions. *Critical Care Nursing, 11*, 42–54.
22. Ersek, M. (1992). The process of maintaining hope in adults undergoing bone marrow transplantation for leukemia. *Oncology Nursing Forum, 19*(6), 883–889.
23. Farhi, D. C., Odell, C. A., & Shurin, S. B. (1993). Myelodysplastic syndrome and acute myeloid leukemia after treatment for solid tumors of childhood. *American Journal of Clinical Pathology, 100*(3), 270–275.

24. Ferrara, J. L. M., & Deeg, H. J. (1991). Mechanisms of disease: Graft-versus-host disease. *New England Journal of Medicine, 324*(10), 667–674.

25. Ferrell, B., et al. (1992). The meaning of quality of life for bone marrow transplant survivors: The impact of bone marrow transplant on quality of life, part 1. *Cancer Nursing, 15*(3), 153–160.

26. Ferrell, B., et al. (1992). The meaning of quality of life for bone marrow transplant survivors: Improving quality of life for bone marrow transplant survivors, part 2. *Cancer Nursing, 15*(4), 247–253.

27. Folkes, M. E. (1990). Transfusion therapy in critical care nursing. *Critical Care Nursing, 13*, 15–28.

28. Freedman, S., et al. (1990). Nursing considerations in the administration of blood component therapy. *Seminars in Oncology Nursing, 6*, 155–162.

29. Furlong, T. G., & Gallucci, B. B. (1994). Pattern of occurrence and clinical presentation of neurological complications in bone marrow transplant patients. *Cancer Nursing, 17*(1), 27–36.

30. Garry, P. J., et al. (1991). A prospective study of blood donations in healthy elderly persons. *Transfusion, 31*, 686–697.

31. Gautier, M., & Cohen, H. J. (1994). Multiple myeloma in the elderly. *Journal of the American Geriatrics Society, 42*(6), 653–664.

32. Gertz, M. A., et al. (1995). Refractory and relapsing multiple myeloma treated by blood stem cell transplantation. *American Journal of the Medical Sciences, 309*(3), 152–161.

33. Giger, J. N., & Davidhizar, R. E. (1995). *Transcultural nursing: Assessment and intervention.* St. Louis: Mosby–Year Book.

34. Gilyon, K., & Kuzel, T. (1991). Cutaneous T-cell lymphoma. *Oncology Nursing Forum, 18*, 901–908.

35. Gloe, D. (1991). Common reactions to transfusions. *Heart and Lung, 20*, 506–512.

36. Gobel, B. H. (1990). Plasma and plasma derivative therapy for coagulation disorders. *Seminars in Oncology Nursing, 6*, 129–135.

37. Graham, D. L., et al. (1992). Cytogenetic and molecular detection of residual leukemic cells after allogeneic bone marrow transplantation in chronic granulocytic leukemia. *Mayo Clinic Proceedings, 67*, 123–127.

38. Greifzu, S. (1991). Helping cancer patients fight infection. *RN, 54*, 24–29.

39. Griffin, K. B. (1990). Postoperative bleeding, current nursing management. *Critical Care Nursing Clinics of North America, 2*, 549–557.

40. Guyatt, G. H., et al. (1990). Diagnosis of iron-deficiency anemia in the elderly. *American Journal of Medicine, 88*, 205–209.

41. Haberman, M. (1995). The meaning of cancer therapy: Bone marrow transplantation as an exemplar of therapy. *Seminars in Oncology Nursing, 11*(1), 23–31.

42. Harmening, D. (1992). *Clinical hematology and fundamentals of hemostasis.* Philadelphia: F. A. Davis.

43. Hassell, K. L., Eckman, J. R., & Lane, P. A. (1994). Acute multiorgan failure syndrome: A potentially catastrophic complication of severe sickle cell pain episodes. *American Journal of Medicine, 96*(2), 155–162.

44. Hernandez, J. A., Land, K. J., & McKenna, R. W. (1995). Leukemias, myeloma, and other lymphoreticular neoplasms. *Cancer, 75* (Suppl. 1), 381–394.

45. Hoffman, R., et al. (1995). *Hematology: Basic principles and practice* (2nd ed.). New York: Churchill Livingstone.

46. Hsing, A. W., et al. (1993). Pernicious anemia and subsequent cancer: A population-based cohort study. *Cancer, 71*(3), 745–750.

47. Huether, S. A., & McCance, K. L. (1996). *Understanding pathophysiology.* St. Louis: Mosby–Year Book.

48. Huff, N. L. (1990). Sickle cell anemia: an I. V. nursing challenge. *Journal of Intravenous Nursing, 12*, 245–250.

49. Hughes, D. B., et al. (1995). Treatment planning for Hodgkin's disease: A pattern of care study. *International Journal of Radiation Oncology, Biology, and Physics, 33*(2), 519–524.

50. Isaacs, P. (1994). Combined therapy management for patients with thrombolytic thrombocytopenic purpura. *ANNA Journal, 21*(4), 196–197, 199.

51. Iserson, K. V., & Huestis, D. W. (1991). Blood warming: Current applications and techniques. *Transfusion, 31*, 558–568.

52. Jassak, P., & Riley, M. B. (1994). Autologous stem cell transplant: An overview. *Cancer Practice, 2*(2), 141–145.

53. Karnad, A. B., & Krozser-Hamati, A. (1992). Pernicious anemia. Early identification to prevent permanent sequelae. *Postgraduate Medicine, 91*(2), 231–234, 237.

54. Kernan, N. A., et al. (1993). Analysis of 462 transplantations from unrelated donors facilitated by the National Marrow Donor Program. *New England Journal of Medicine, 328*(9), 593–602.

55. Kessinger, A., & Armitage, J. The use of peripheral stem cell support of high-dose chemotherapy. In V. T. DeVita, et al. (1993), *Important advances in oncology 1993.* Philadelphia: J. B. Lippincott.

56. King, C. R., et al. (1995). Nurses' perceptions of the meaning of quality of life for bone marrow transplant survivors. *Cancer Nursing, 18*(2), 118–129.

57. Kirchner, J. T. (1992). Acute and chronic immune thrombocytopenic purpura: Disorders that differ in more than duration. *Postgraduate Medicine, 92*(6), 112–118, 125–126.

58. Kolb, H. J., et al. (1995). Graft-versus-leukemia effect of donor lymphocyte transfusions in marrow grafted patients. European Group for Blood and Marrow Transplantation Working Party Chronic Leukemia. *Blood, 86*(5), 2041–2050.

59. Kotwas, L., et al. (1990). Blood collection techniques. *Seminars in Oncology Nursing, 6*, 109–116.

60. Kupiec-Weglinski, J. W. (1994). *New immunosuppressive modalities and anti-rejection approaches in organ transplantation.* Austin, TX: R. G. Landes.

61. Kurtz, A. (1993) Disseminated intravascular coagulation with leukemia patients. *Cancer Nursing, 16*(6), 456–463.

62. Larson, P. J. (1995). Perceptions of the needs of hospitalized patients undergoing bone marrow transplant. *Cancer Practice, 3*(3), 173–179.

63. Larson, P. J., et al. (1993). Comparison of perceived symptoms of patients undergoing bone marrow transplant and the nurses caring for them. *Oncology Nursing Forum, 20*(1), 81–88.

64. Lawrence, J. (1994). Critical care issues in the patient with hematologic malignancy. *Seminars in Oncology Nursing, 10*(3), 198–207.

65. Letendre, L., et al. (1992). Mayo Clinic experience with allogeneic and syngeneic bone marrow transplantation, 1982 through 1990. *Mayo Clinic Proceedings, 67*, 109–116.

66. Linden, J., et al. (1988). In vitro and in vivo evaluation of an electromechanical infusion pump. *Laboratory Medicine, 19*, 574–576.

67. Litwack, K. (1991). Bleeding and coagulation in the PACU. *Critical Care Nursing Clinics of North America, 3*, 121–127.

68. Litwack, K. (1992). Practical points for transfusion therapy. *Journal of Post Anesthesia, 2*, 257–261.

69. Maloney, P. A., & Ryan, L. (1990). Hyperviscosity-polycythemia syndrome: A case study. *Journal of Perinatology Neonatal Nurse, 4*, 64–70.

70. Mansouri, A. (1990). Acquired hemostatic abnormalities in the elderly. *Journal of the American Gerontologic Society, 38*, 809–816.

71. Mansouri, A., & Lipschitz, D. (1992). Myelodysplastic syndromes in the elderly. *Journal of the American Gerontologic Society, 40*(4), 386–391.

72. Marelli, T. (1994). Use of a hemoglobin substitute in the anemic Jehovah's Witness patient. *Critical Care Nurse, 14*(1), 31–38.

73. Martinelli, A. M. (1991). Sickle cell disease. *AORN Journal, 53*, 716–724.

74. McFadden, M. E. (1993). Commentary on thrombotic thrombocytopenia purpura: nursing during the acute phase. *ONS Nursing Scan in Oncology, 2*(6), 4.

75. McVay, P. A., et al. (1991). Probable reasons that autologous blood was not donated by patients having surgery for which cross-matched blood was ordered. *Transfusion, 31*, 810–813.

76. Meehan, K. R., et al. (1995). Autologous bone marrow transplantation versus chemotherapy in relapsed/refractory non-Hodgkin's lymphoma: Estimates of long-term survival from the recent literature. *American Journal of Hematology, 50*(2), 116–123

77. Meropol, N. J., et al. (1992). High-dose chemotherapy with autologous stem cell support for breast cancer. *Oncology, 6*(12), 53–63.

78. Molassiotis, A., et al. (1995). Comparison of the overall quality of life in 50 long-term survivors of autologous and allogeneic bone marrow transplantation. *Journal of Advanced Nursing, 22*(3), 509–516.

79. Morse, L. K. (1992). Commentary on the meaning of quality of

life for bone marrow transplant survivors: The impact of bone marrow transplant on quality of life . . . part 1; Improving quality of life for bone marrow transplant survivors . . . part 2. *ONS Nursing Scan in Oncology, 1*(4), 10–11.

80. Mundt, A. J., et al. (1995). Patterns of failure following high-dose chemotherapy and autologous bone marrow transplantation with involved field radiotherapy for relapsed/refractory Hodgkin's disease. *International Journal of Radiation Oncology, Biology, and Physics, 33*(2), 261–270.

81. Neumann, M., & Urizar, R. (1994). Hemolytic uremic syndrome: Current pathophysiology and management. *ANNA Journal, 21*(2), 137–145.

82. Nistico, A., & Young, N. S. (1994). γ-Interferon gene expression in the bone marrow of patients with aplastic anemia. *Annals of Internal Medicine, 120*(6), 463–469.

83. Nolan, M. T., & Augustine, S. M. (1995). *Transplantation nursing: Acute and long-term management.* Norwalk, CT: Appleton & Lange.

84. Ong, S. T., & Larson, R. A. (1995). Current management of acute lymphoblastic leukemia in adults. *Oncology, 9*(5), 433–442.

85. Overfield, T. (1985). *Biologic variation in health and illness: Race, age, and sex differences.* Menlo Park, CA: Addison-Wesley.

86. Paquette, R. L., et al. (1995). Long-term outcome of aplastic anemia in adults treated with antithymocyte globulin: Comparison with bone marrow transplantation. *Blood, 85*(1), 283–290.

87. Parsons, L., & Klopovich, P. (1990). Immune globulin therapy. *Seminars in Oncology Nursing, 6,* 136–139.

88. Paschall, F. E. (1993). Thrombotic thrombocytopenic purpura: The challenges of a complex disease process. *AACN Clinical Issues in Critical Care Nursing, 4*(4), 655–663.

89. Pavel, J. (1990). Red blood cell transfusions for anemia. *Seminars in Oncology Nursing, 6,* 117–122.

90. Pavel, J. N., et al. (1990). *Transfusion therapy guidelines for nurses.* Bethesda, MD: National Blood Resource Education Program, No. 90-2668. National Heart, Lung, and Blood Institute, National Institutes of Health.

91. Perez, W. E., & Viets, J. L. (1990). Transfusion and coagulation: An overview and recent advances in practice modalities. *Nurse Anesthetist, 1,* 149–161.

92. Peterson, K. (1992). Nursing management of autologous blood transfusion. *Journal of Intravenous Nursing, 13*(3), 128–134.

93. Phillips, J. M. (1993). Commentary on hair dye use and multiple myeloma in white men. *ONS Nursing Scan in Oncology, 2*(4), 10.

94. Picard, V. T., et al. (1990). Transfusion therapy: Associated risks and alternative approaches. *American Nephrology Nurses' Association, 17,* 457–464.

95. Platt, O. S., et al. (1994). Mortality in sickle cell disease. Life expectancy and risk factors for early death. *New England Journal of Medicine, 330*(23), 1639–1644.

96. Poe, S. S., et al. (1994). A national survey of infection prevention practices on bone marrow transplant units. *Oncology Nursing Forum, 21*(10), 1687–1694.

97. Pruthi, R. K., & Tefferi, A. (1994). Pernicious anemia revisited. *Mayo Clinic Proceedings, 69*(2), 144–150.

98. Querin, J. J., & Stahl, L. D. (1990). 12 simple, sensible steps for successful blood transfusions. *Nursing 90, 20,* 68–81.

99. Rayfield, S., & Theriot, B. L. (1990). Maximizing safe blood transfusions. *Advances in Critical Care, 5,* 17–19.

100. Rivers, R., & Williams, N. (1990). Sickle cell anemia: Complex disease nursing challenge. *RN, 53,* 24–29.

101. Rosenfeld, C. S., et al. (1995). Cyclophosphamide-mobilized peripheral blood stem cells in patients with lymphoid malignancies. *Bone Marrow Transplantation, 15*(3), 433–438.

102. Rostad, M. (1990). Management of myelosuppression in the patient with cancer. *Oncology Nursing Forum, 17,* 4–8.

103. Rosvoll, R. V., et al. (1990). *Accreditations requirements manual* (pp. 4–59). Arlington, VA: American Association of Blood Banks.

104. Rutman, R., et al. (1990). The transfusion service and nursing. *Seminars in Oncology Nursing, 6,* 152–154.

105. Rutman, R., et al. (1990). Home transfusion for the cancer patient. *Seminars in Oncology Nursing, 6,* 163–167.

106. Sandler, D. P., et al. (1993). Cigarette smoking and risk of acute leukemia: Associations with morphology and cytogenetic abnormalities in bone marrow. *Journal of the National Cancer Institute, 85*(24), 1994–2003.

107. Schilling, R. F., & Williams, W. J. (1995). Vitamin B$_{12}$ deficiency: Underdiagnosed, overtreated? *Hospital Practice (Office Edition), 30*(7), 47–52; discussion 52, 54.

108. Schmidt, U., Metz, K. A., & Leder, L. D. (1995). T-cell-rich B-cell lymphoma and lymphocyte-predominant Hodgkin's disease: Two closely related entities? *British Journal of Hematology, 90*(2), 398–403.

109. Schwartzberg, L., et al. (1993). Rapid and sustained hematopoietic reconstitution by peripheral blood stem cell infusion alone following high-dose chemotherapy. *Bone Marrow Transplantation, 11*(5), 369–374.

110. Semenciw, R. M., et al. (1993). Multiple myeloma mortality and agricultural practices in the prairie provinces of Canada. *Journal of Occupational Medicine, 35*(6), 557–561.

111. Seo, I. S., Li, C. Y., & Yam, L. T. (1993). Myelodysplastic syndrome: Diagnostic implications of cytochemical and immunocytochemical studies. *Mayo Clinic Proceedings, 68*(1), 47–53.

112. Socie, G., et al. (1993). Malignant tumors occurring after treatment of aplastic anemia. European Bone Marrow Transplantation–Severe Aplastic Anaemia Working Party. *New England Journal of Medicine, 329*(16), 1152–1157.

113. Storb, R., et al. (1994). Cyclophosphamide combined with antithymocyte globulin in preparation for allogeneic marrow transplants in patients with aplastic anemia. *Blood, 84*(3), 941–949.

114. Sveningson, L. (1993). Commentary on cigarette smoking and adult leukemia: A meta-analysis. *ONS Nursing Scan in Oncology, 2*(4), 11.

115. Tate, D. J., & Hoppe, R. T. (1995). Pelvic relapse following subtotal lymphoid irradiation in early stage Hodgkin's disease: An analysis of risk, management, and outcome. *International Journal of Radiation Oncology, Biology, and Physics, 32*(4), 1239–1244.

116. Thorne, A. C., et al. (1993). Harvesting bone marrow in an outpatient setting using newer anesthetic agents. *Journal of Clinical Oncology, 11*(2), 320–323.

117. Timmerman, P. R. (1993). Intravenous immunoglobulin in oncology nursing practice. *Oncology Nursing Forum, 20*(1), 69–75.

118. Treleaven, J., & Barrett, J. (1992). *Bone marrow transplantation in practice.* Edinburgh: Churchill Livingstone.

119. U. S. Department of Health and Human Services (1994). *Bone marrow transplantation and peripheral blood stem cell transplantation.* NIH Publication No. 95-1178: Washington, DC: Author.

120. Vichinsky, E. P., et al. (1995). A comparison of conservative and aggressive transfusion regimens in the perioperative management of sickle cell disease. The Preoperative Transfusion in Sickle Cell Disease Study Group. *New England Journal of Medicine, 333*(4), 206–213.

121. Viel, J. F., & Richardson, S. T. (1993). Lymphoma, multiple myeloma and leukaemia among French farmers in relation to pesticide exposure. *Social Science and Medicine, 37*(6), 771–777.

122. Whedon, M. B. (1991). *Bone marrow transplantation principles, practice and nursing insights.* Boston: Jones & Bartlett.

123. Widmann, F. K., et al. (1992). *Standards for blood banks and transfusion services* (pp. 1–58). Arlington, VA: American Association of Blood Banks.

124. Winters, G., et al. (1994). Provisional practice: The nature of psychosocial bone marrow transplant nursing. *Oncology Nursing Forum, 21*(7), 1147–1154.

125. Workman, M., Ellerhorst-Ryan, J., & Koertge, V. (1993). *Nursing care of the immunocompromised patient.* Philadelphia: W. B. Saunders.

126. Wroblewski, S. (1994). Commentary on high-dose chemotherapy and autologous transplant with peripheral-blood stem cells. *ONS Nursing Scan in Oncology, 3*(1), 17.

127. Wujcik, D., & Downs, S. (1992). Bone marrow transplantation. *Critical Care Nursing Clinics of North America, 4*(1), 149–166.

128. Yap, P. L. (1990). Transfusion transmitted viral infections—recent developments in blood donor screening. *Postgraduate Medical Journal, 66,* 906–909.

129. Yee, W. (1993). The utilization of plasma in the treatment of thrombotic thrombocytopenic purpura. *Canadian Journal of Medical Technology, 55*(2), 97–101.

130. Zahm, S. H., et al. (1992) Use of hair coloring products and the risk of lymphoma, multiple myeloma, and chronic lymphocytic leukemia. *American Journal of Public Health, 82*(7), 990–997.

Urinary Disorders

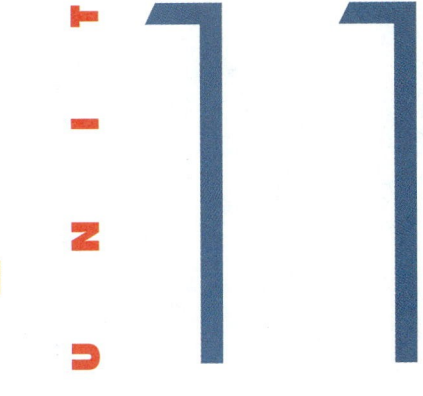

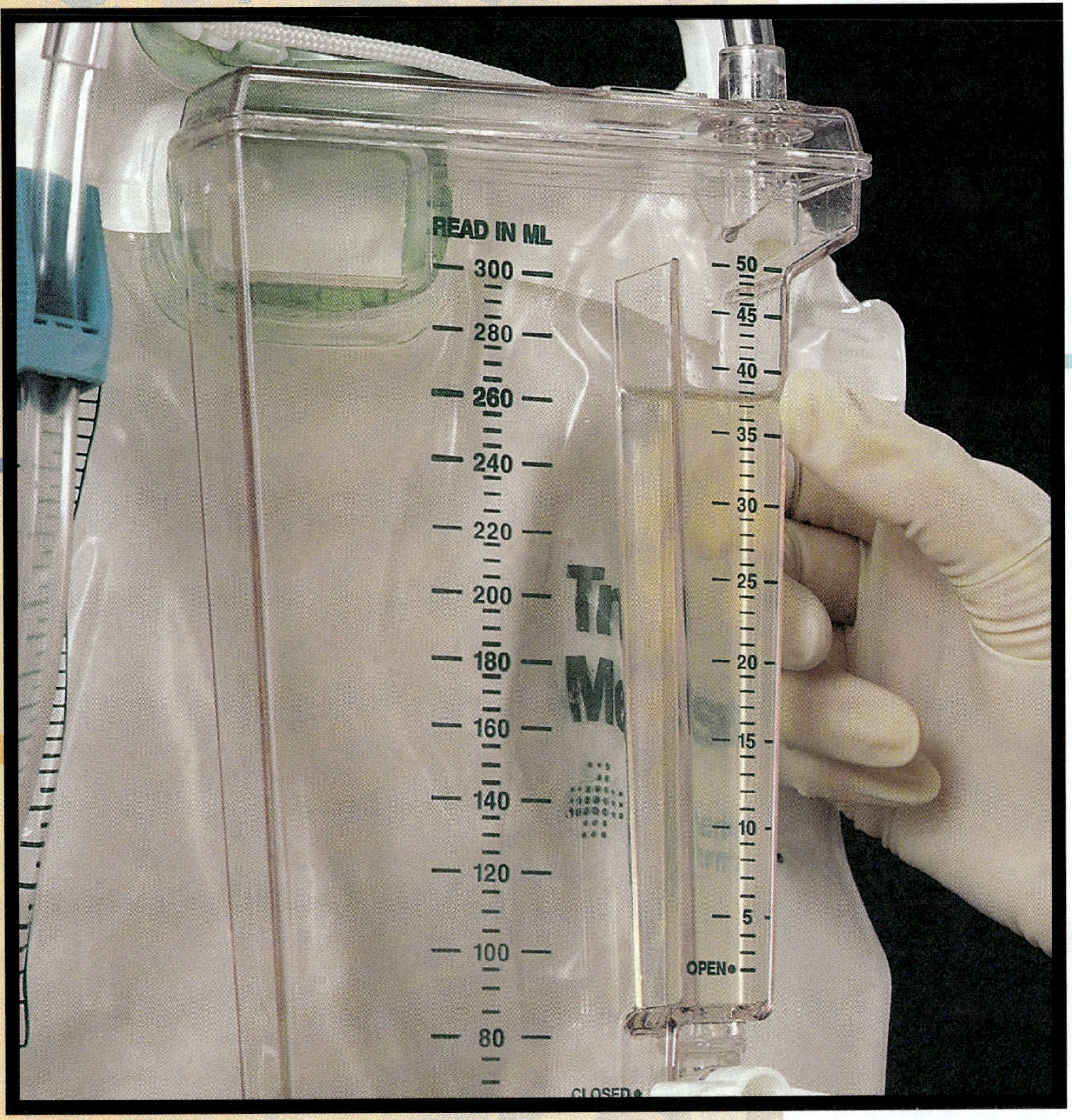

Structure and Function of the Urinary System

CHAPTER 54

Esther Matassarin-Jacobs

Structure

The urinary tract is composed of four organs: (1) kidneys, (2) ureters, (3) bladder, and (4) urethra. Figure 54–1 illustrates the anatomic location of these four organs.

Kidneys

The kidneys are located retroperitoneally, in the posterior aspect of the abdomen, on either side of the vertebral column. They lie between the twelfth thoracic and the third lumbar vertebrae. The left kidney is usually positioned slightly higher than the right. Adult kidneys average approximately 11 cm in length and 5 to 7.5 cm in width and are 2.5 cm thick. Affixing the kidneys in position behind the parietal peritoneum is a mass of perirenal fat (adipose capsule) and connective tissue called *Gerota's* (subserosa) *fascia*. A fibrous capsule (renal capsule) forms the external covering of the kidney itself, except the hilum. The kidney is further protected by layers of muscle of the back, flank, and abdomen, as well as layers of fat, subcutaneous tissue, and skin.

Each organ has a characteristic curved shape, with the distal edge being convex and the medial boundary being concave. In the innermost part of the concave section is the hilus, through which pass the renal artery, renal vein, lymphatics, nerves, and the renal pelvis, which is the natural upper extension of the ureter. A firm, tough, fibrous capsule surrounds and adheres to the renal parenchyma. Inside this capsule, each kidney is divided into three major areas: (1) cortex, (2) medulla, and (3) pelvis. Figure 54–2 demonstrates the anatomy of the kidney.

The cortex of the kidney lies just under the fibrous capsule, and portions of it extend down into the medullary layer to form the renal columns (columns of Bertin) or cortical tissue that separates the pyramids. The medulla is divided into 8 to 18 cone-shaped masses of collecting ducts called *renal pyramids*. The bases of the pyramids

are positioned on the corticomedullary boundary. Their apices extend toward the renal pelvis, forming *papillae*. The papillae each have 10 to 25 openings on the surface, through which the urine empties into the renal pelvis. The inset in Figure 54–2 shows the anatomy of a renal pyramid. Eight or more groups of papillae are present in each pyramid; each empties into a minor calix, and several minor calices join to form a major calix. The two to three major calices are outpouchings of the renal pelvis. They serve to channel the urine from the pyramids to the renal pelvis. The inner area of the kidney, or renal pelvis, is a cavity lined with transitional epithelium. The combined volume of the pelvis and calices is approximately 8 ml. Volumes in excess of this amount damage the renal parenchymal tissue. The renal pelvis narrows as it reaches the hilus and becomes the proximal end of the ureter.

The functioning unit of the kidney is the nephron. Each kidney contains more than a million of these units. A nephron is a microscopic structure consisting of a glomerular (Bowman's) capsule and tubular system that empty into the renal pelvis and the ureter. Figure 54–3 illustrates a functioning nephron.

Located in the cortex of the kidney is a double-walled cup, which is the glomerular or Bowman's capsule (see Fig. 54–3). It is lined with simple squamous epithelium that allows easy filtration of blood. Inside the capsule is the glomerulus, which is a tuft of non-anastomosing capillaries fed by an afferent arteriole and drained by an efferent arteriole. The proximal tubule is a convoluted portion with millions of microvilli lining its lumen, forming a brush border, thereby vastly increasing its membrane surface area. As it nears the medullary layer, the tubule abruptly narrows and forms the descending loop of Henle. This then turns back on itself as the ascending limb of the loop of Henle, the latter being larger in diameter than the descending limb. The loop of Henle, as it moves back into the cortex of the kidney, becomes the distal convoluted tubule, which joins a collecting duct. Each collecting duct receives the terminal end of several nephrons as it courses through the cortex and medulla of

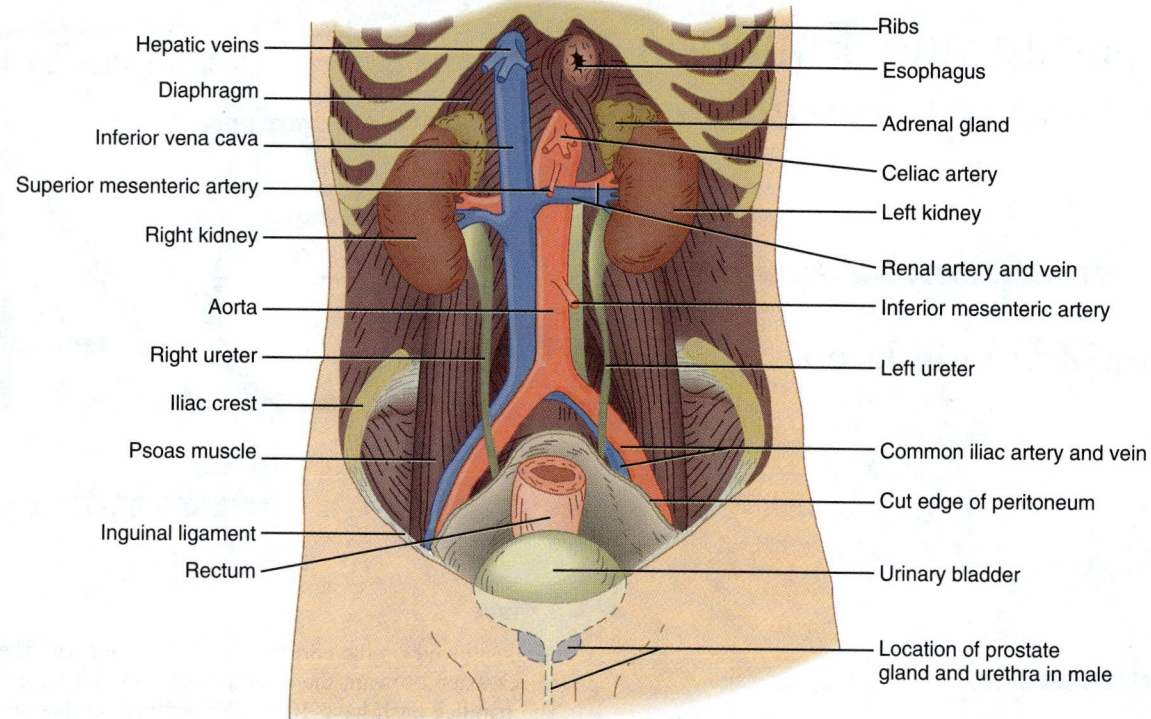

Figure 54–1. Anatomic relationships of kidneys and related structures.

the kidney. As the collecting ducts within a renal pyramid get closer to the apex of the pyramid, several coalesce to form a larger duct of Bellini, which opens onto the surface of a papilla (see Fig. 54–2).

The macula densa lies between the afferent arteriole and the distal convoluted tubule, where it passes close to the arteriole. These closely packed cells, which are located in the distal tubular epithelium of each nephron,

may function as chemoreceptors. The juxtaglomerular cells are found between the macula densa and the afferent arteriole just before it enters the glomerular capsule. Together these two cellular structures form the juxtaglomerular apparatus, which is thought to play a major role in the renin-angiotensin system. The enzyme renin helps to regulate water and sodium retention and, consequently, blood pressure.

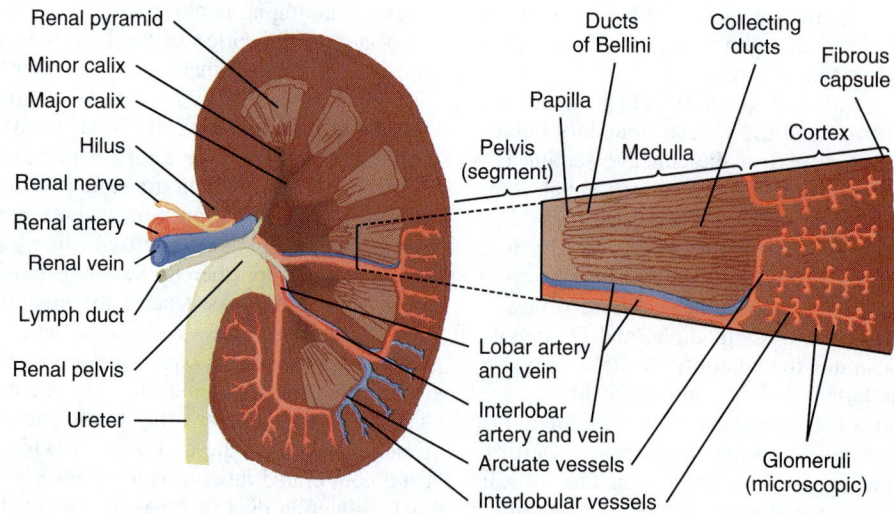

Figure 54–2. Anatomy of the kidney. *Inset*, Enlargement of a segment of the kidney.

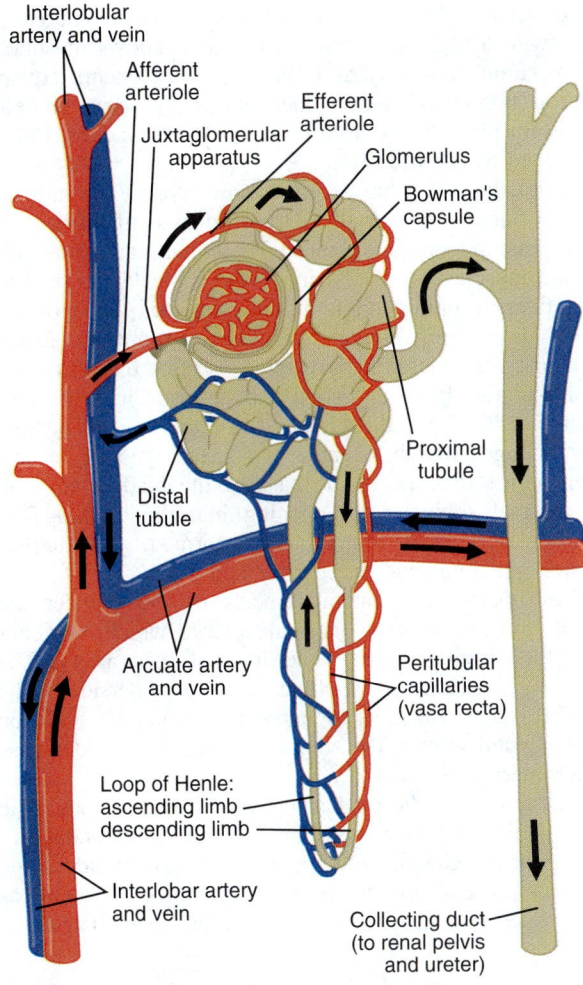

Figure 54–3. Nephron.

Circulation

The kidneys receive 20% to 25% of the cardiac output under resting conditions, averaging more than 1 L of arterial blood per minute. The renal arteries (see Fig. 54–2) branch from the abdominal aorta at the level of the second lumbar vertebra. Passing laterally to the hilus of the kidney, each artery usually divides into the anterior and posterior branches, which supply the anterior and posterior portions of the kidney, respectively. Further subdivisions of the primary branches of the renal artery are called *lobar arteries*. These vessels supply the papillae. The lobar arteries further divide into interlobar arteries, which run between the renal pyramids until they reach the corticomedullary zone. Here, they form incomplete arches called *arcuate arteries* around the bases of the pyramids. Branching from the arcuate arteries are the interlobular arteries, which supply the cortical substance and the renal capsule. The interlobular arteries also give rise to the afferent arterioles (see Fig. 54–3), which become the glomerulus.

The efferent arterioles carry blood from the glomerulus. They then divide into a network of peritubular capillaries.

These capillaries supply the tubules and receive the material reabsorbed by the tubular structures. This segment of renal circulation, in which blood in the capillaries empties into other arterioles and then proceeds to a second set of capillaries, is a unique arrangement that allows a high filtration pressure in the glomerulus. Some of the efferent arterioles from juxtamedullary glomeruli do not form a peritubular capillary network, but instead drain into a network of vessels forming hairpin loops called the *vasa recta*. These loops dip into the medulla for variable distances and play a role in the renal concentrating mechanism. The blood then leaves the kidney in a venous system closely corresponding to the arterial system: interlobular veins to arcuate veins to interlobar veins to the renal vein. The renal circulation then empties into the inferior vena cava.

Innervation

The kidney receives both *sympathetic* and *parasympathetic* innervation. The renal nerves course along the renal blood vessels as they enter the hilus of the kidney. The sympathetic nerve supply comes from the twelfth thoracic to the second lumbar nerves via the splanchnic nerves and the celiac plexus. Contributions are also made by the superficial hypogastric plexus and intermesenteric, upper splanchnic, and thoracic nerves. The nerves terminate primarily on the walls of the blood vessels, rather than in the tubules; thus, they are believed to have a vasomotor function. Adrenergic fibers also end in close proximity to the juxtaglomerular cells and renal tubes. A completely denervated kidney continues to form urine.

Ureters

The ureters form the medial tapering of the renal pelvis at the hilus of the kidney. They are 25 to 35 cm long in the adult. Ureters lie in the extraperitoneal connective tissue and descend vertically along the psoas muscle toward the pelvic cavity (see Fig. 54–1). After dipping into the pelvic cavity, the ureters course anteriorly to join the bladder in its posterolateral aspect. At each ureterovesical junction, the ureter runs obliquely through the bladder wall for about 1.5 to 2 cm before opening into the lumen of the bladder. Three points of potential obstruction exist: (1) at the ureteropelvic junction, (2) at the pelvic brim (where ureters cross iliac arteries), and (3) at the ureterovesical junction. The ureter is much narrower at these points. Because it is difficult for them to traverse these narrow passageways, calculi typically lodge here. This anatomic arrangement usually functions as a valve that prevents the backward flow, or reflux, of urine into the kidney.

Each ureter has definite elastic characteristics and is made of three tissue layers: (1) an inner mucosa (transitional epithelial membrane) lining the lumen, (2) a muscular layer, and (3) a fibrous outer layer. When cancer of the bladder or ureter is diagnosed, the potential for recurrence exists in either structure. Half of clients with ureteral cancer experience spread of the cancer to the bladder. Only about 3% of clients with bladder cancer experience spread of cancer to the ureter.[48] The musculature is generally designated as *inner longitudinal* and *outer circular*. However, along most of the ureter, the muscle fibers actually run obliquely and blend with one another to form a meshlike tissue. The muscle arrangement allows urine to be propelled down the ureter by peristaltic action. This peristalsis is probably regulated by a myogenic pacemaker located near the renal calices.

Blood is supplied to the ureters by one or more vessels that run longitudinally along the tube. The number and assortment of arteries anastomosing with the ureteric vessels vary with each individual. Because the ureters travel through several anatomic areas, the ureteral vessels are fed by several of the following arteries: (1) renal (frequently), (2) testicular or ovarian, (3) aorta and common iliac, (4) internal iliac (frequently), (5) vesical, (6) umbilical, and (7) uterine.

The ureter's innervation comes from the eleventh thoracic to the first lumbar nerves. The network of nerves becomes progressively more dense toward the terminal end of the ureters.

Bladder

The urinary bladder is a hollow organ located in the anterior half of the pelvis behind the symphysis pubis. Figures 54–4 and 54–5 illustrate the position in the female and male, respectively, of the bladder and urethra in relation to the other anatomic structures of the pelvis. The

space between the bladder and the symphysis pubis is filled with a loose connective tissue that allows the bladder to stretch cranially as it fills. The peritoneum covers the top border of the bladder, while the base is held loosely in place by the true ligaments. The bladder is also enveloped by a loose fascia.

The bladder wall has several tissue layers. The internal lining of the vesical wall is transitional epithelium with some mucus-secreting glands. Then there are three ill-defined muscle layers. The inner and outer layers tend to have fibers running longitudinally, whereas those of the middle layer are circular. The fibers from these layers exchange with each other frequently so that the result is a meshlike muscle layer called the detrusor muscle. This arrangement allows the bladder wall to be elastic while maintaining strength. Bundles of these smooth muscle layers come together at the base of the bladder to form the internal sphincter, or opening into the urethra. The *trigone* describes the triangular area formed by the ureterovesical junctions and the internal sphincter.

The superior and lateral aspects of the bladder are served by the superior vesical artery, which branches from the umbilical artery and internal iliac artery. The inferior vesical artery, which supplies the underside of the bladder, may arise independently or in common with the middle rectal artery. The veins draining the bladder pass to the internal iliac trunk.

Innervation for the bladder comes from the hypogastric sympathetic, pelvic parasympathetic, and pudendal somatic nerves. Ganglia are most commonly found in the bladder base and around the urethral orifice. These areas tend to act in continuity with each other, and their func-

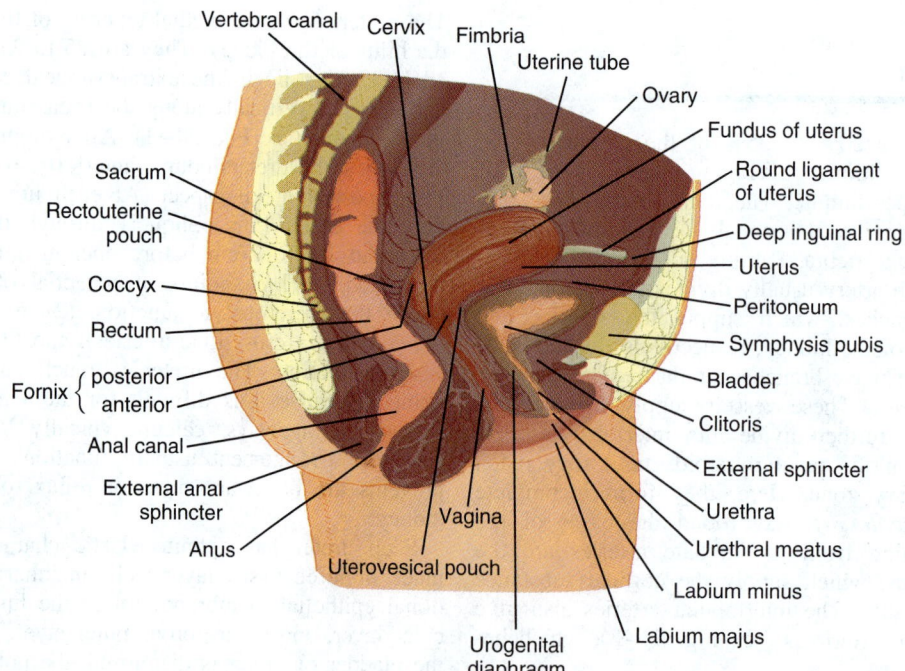

Figure 54–4. Sagittal section of the female pelvis. (From Jacob, S. W., et al. [1982]. *Structure and function in man* [5th ed.]. Philadelphia: W. B. Saunders.)

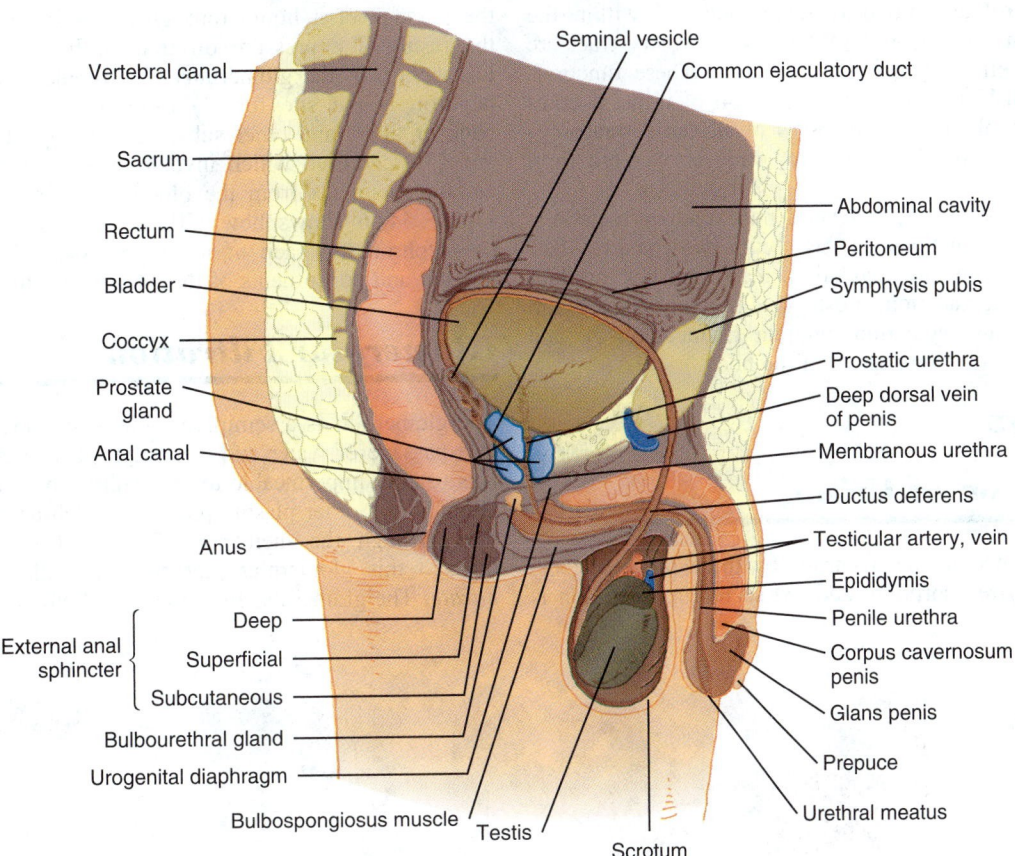

Figure 54–5. Sagittal section of the male pelvis and external genitalia. (From Jacob, S. W., et al. [1982]. *Structure and function in man* [5th ed.]. Philadelphia: W. B. Saunders.)

Urethra and Meatus

The urethra is a tube that extends from the base of the bladder to the surface of the body. The female and male urethras are greatly different. The female urethra is approximately 4 cm in length and curves slightly forward as it reaches the external opening or *meatus*. The meatus is located between the clitoris and the vaginal orifice. It is lined with epithelium, which contains some mucus-secreting glands. The longitudinal muscle layer is a continuation of longitudinal layer of bladder muscle. The circular muscle fibers encompass the urethra and meet with the circular bladder muscle. This muscle thins out near the meatus. As the urethra passes through the urogenital diaphragm, the circular muscle fibers form the external sphincter.

In males, the reproductive system is anatomically connected to the urinary tract. Both systems share the same outlet from the body, the urethra. The prostate gland, although not a direct part of the urinary system, is a major cause of urinary dysfunction in men. This gland is located below the bladder neck and completely surrounds the urethra. Normally, this relationship causes no prob-

lem, but if the gland enlarges, it constricts the urethra and obstructs the outflow of urine. Further discussion of the male reproductive system is found in Chapter 83. The male urethra is about 20 cm long and is divided into three main sections. The prostatic urethra extends about 3 cm below the bladder neck, through the prostate gland, to the pelvic floor. The ejaculatory ducts of the reproductive system empty into its posterior wall. The membranous urethra is about 1 to 2 cm in length and ends where the muscle layer forms the external sphincter. The distal portion is the cavernous, or penile, urethra. It is approximately 15 cm long and travels through the penis to the urethral orifice at the tip of the penis. It is also lined with epithelial cells.

The urethral blood supply is provided primarily by the internal pudendal artery and the urethral artery. This supply of blood is supplemented by vessels feeding the surrounding anatomic structures. Innervation arises from sources similar to those that supply the bladder.

Function

The urinary tract plays a major role in the maintenance of homeostasis. The main functions of the kidneys are (1) to remove waste products from the body and (2) to regulate fluids, electrolytes, blood pressure, and pH within the body. The main functions of the lower urinary tract are storage and elimination of formed urine. These functions are accomplished through the formation of urine, a complex task involving the processes of filtration, reabsorption, and secretion. Once formed, urine is excreted from the body.

The kidneys also have several nonexcretory metabolic and endocrine functions. In this section we consider their role in blood pressure regulation, red blood cell production, insulin degradation, prostaglandin synthesis, calcium and phosphorus regulation, vitamin D metabolism, and regulation of other substances in the body.

Kidneys

Formation of Urine

Urine is formed in the nephrons by three processes: (1) filtration, (2) reabsorption, and (3) secretion. Filtration is the passage of a liquid through a filtering membrane as the result of a pressure differential. In the kidney, this takes place in the glomerulus. The tubular portion of the nephron is the site for (1) *reabsorption*, or the taking back of fluids and other substances through body tissues, and (2) *secretion*, which involves the active transport of certain chemicals from the bloodstream into the tubules. Figure 54–6 shows how different anatomic portions of the nephron use each of these processes to regulate the amount and constituents of the urine being formed.

Glomerular Filtration

The glomerulus is a semipermeable membrane that allows free passage of water and electrolytes across it. However, it is usually impermeable to molecular substances, such as albumin and other plasma proteins, which are too large to pass through the membrane. The fluid that is filtered through this glomerular membrane is called *glomerular filtrate*. The glomerular filtration rate (GFR) is the amount

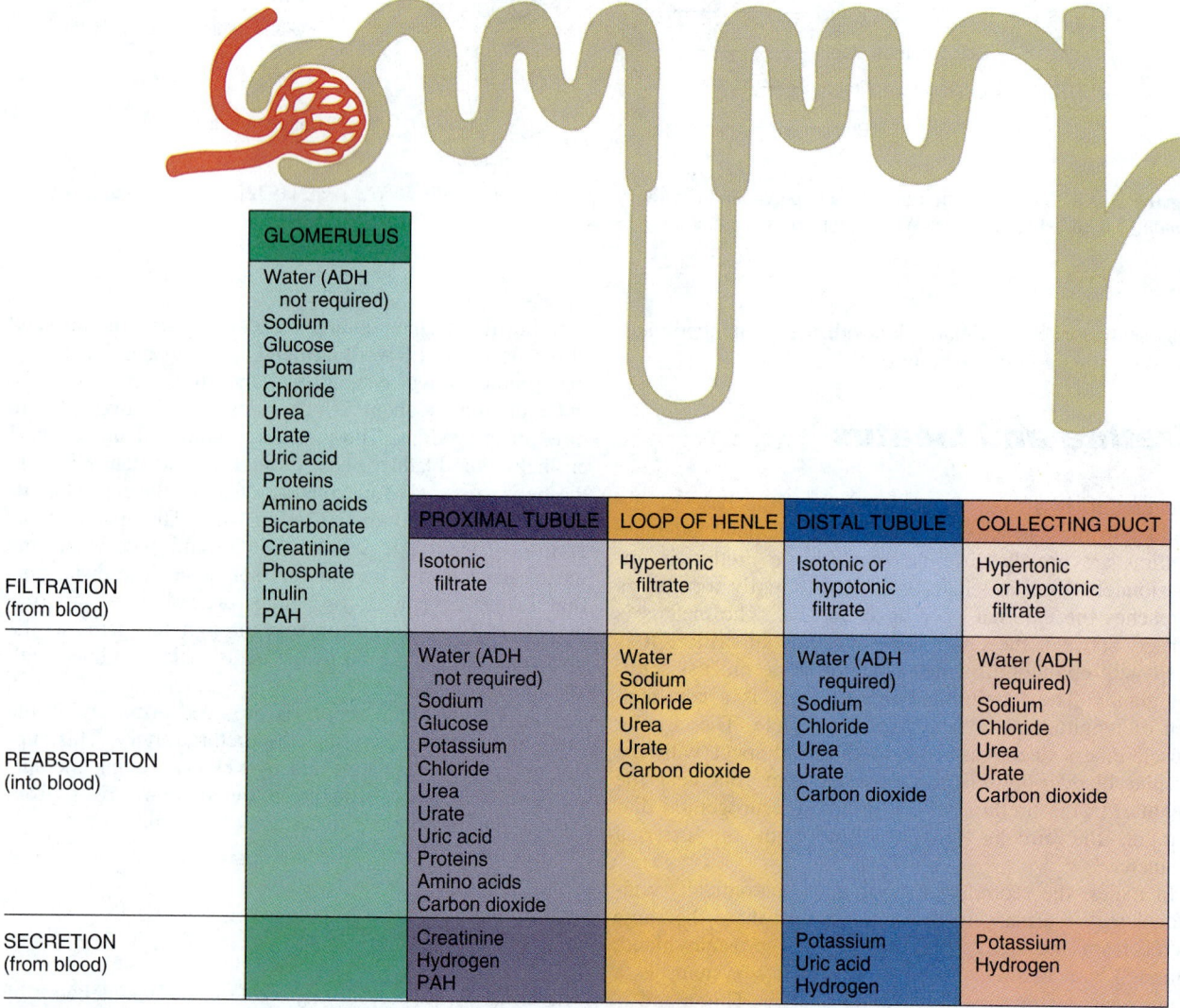

Figure 54–6. Normal physiologic function of the nephron in urine formation. Although inulin and para-aminohippuric acid (PAH) are not normally present, they are important test substances.

of glomerular filtration that occurs within a given period of time. The GFR for a normal adult male of average size is approximately 125 ml/minute.

Several factors can influence the GFR. These include (1) hydrostatic and oncotic pressure gradients between the glomerular capillaries and Bowman's capsule, (2) rate of renal blood flow, (3) permeability of the glomerular membrane, and (4) changes in the total area of the glomerular capillary bed. Most important is the amount and pressure of the blood supply reaching the glomerulus, because without blood flow no glomerular filtration can occur.

Pressure within the glomerular capillaries is usually higher than that in other capillary beds in the body. Whereas hydrostatic pressure in other capillaries is normally 15 to 20 mm Hg, glomerular capillary pressure is 70 mm Hg. The higher pressure is caused by the unique anatomic structure of the afferent arterioles and the high resistance in the efferent arterioles. The "pushing out" of fluid from the glomerular capillaries through the semipermeable membrane into Bowman's capsule results from the high pressure. Because filtration occurs under exceedingly high pressure and is a result of the hydrostatic pressure differential, this process is called *ultrafiltration*.

Changes in the GFR occur when this pressure gradient is altered (1) in the glomerular capillaries (e.g., changes in the systemic blood pressure), (2) in Bowman's capsule (e.g., renal edema), or (3) when ureteral obstruction occurs. The kidney does have some resistance to changes in systemic blood pressure through autoregulation. This capability allows the kidney, through intrinsic regulation of renal circulation, to maintain a relatively constant renal blood flow. Autoregulation also enables the GFR to remain relatively stable over a range of arterial blood pressure readings varying from 70 to 200 mm Hg. Outside of this range, the pressure of the blood flow and GFR vary with the systemic blood pressure. It is important to note that certain medications can modify the kidney's autoregulatory ability.

The oncotic pressure is the pulling pressure exerted by the plasma proteins within the capillaries (see Chapter 15). This force works in opposition to the capillary hydrostatic pressure, so the GFR is the result of the hydrostatic pressure minus the oncotic pressure. Changes in the concentration of the plasma proteins, such as occurs with fluid depletion and hypoproteinemia, alter the influence of this force.

Closely allied with the pressures affecting GFR is the amount of renal blood flow reaching the glomerulus. Anything enhancing or interfering with renal circulation alters the GFR. The list of influential factors is long. Such things as direct trauma to, or obstruction of, blood vessels interrupts this flow. Medications may alter blood flow. For instance, glucagon (a protein substance produced by the islands of Langerhans in the pancreas) and low levels of dopamine (a catecholamine precursor of norepinephrine) produce direct renal vasodilation without apparent effect on the systemic blood pressure. Other vasopressors, such as norepinephrine bitartrate, cause renal vasoconstriction; at high rates, they may drastically reduce GFR and cause acute renal failure. Some diuretics cause vasoconstriction whereas others increase renal

blood flow. Activation of the adrenergic nervous system (e.g., by a stressful event) may decrease blood flow through release of either norepinephrine from the renal sympathetic nerves or epinephrine from the adrenal medulla. Bacterial pyrogens, as occur in sepsis, prompt vasodilation. Also, a high-protein diet increases renal blood flow.

As mentioned earlier, normal capillary permeability interferes with the passage of plasma proteins into the filtrate. Any pathologic process that changes this relationship interferes with the normal oncotic pressure gradient. For example, if plasma proteins escape across the membrane, such as occurs in nephrotic syndrome, the oncotic "pull" is reduced, resulting in increased water filtration.

Changes in the total area of the capillary glomerular bed modify the structures filtering the blood. These changes usually involve a reduction in the functioning area and they result from glomeruli-destroying diseases or partial nephrectomy.

The results of the filtration process represent the first stage in the formation of urine. The composition of this ultrafiltrate is approximately 94% water and 6% solutes. The list of normal solutes is shown in Figure 54–6.

Tubular Reabsorption

Although the kidneys initially filter 180 L/day, this does not represent the daily urine output of the normal adult. The main reason for this is the reabsorptive function of the renal tubular system, which returns about 99% of the glomerular filtrate to the body. Reabsorption takes place through active transport, passive diffusion, and osmosis. Active transport is a process in which substances are moved across the tubular membranes into the interstitial space by the expenditure of metabolic energy. Once in the interstitial tissues, these substances are picked up by the capillaries.

Substances reabsorbed in this manner are shown in Figure 54–6. Blood and tissue levels of these elements regulate the rate of their active transport.

Water passively moves across the semipermeable tubular membranes by diffusion and osmosis, according to the concentration gradient. As solutes are transported into the interstitial spaces, the concentration of solutes outside the tubules rises, causing water to shift out of the tubular system. This obligatory water reabsorption is thus not dependent on the body's state of hydration, but rather on the osmotic forces. The process of reabsorption occurs without the aid of antidiuretic hormone (ADH) in the proximal tubules. However, as illustrated in Figure 54–6, ADH is required in the distal tubule and collecting duct. ADH increases the permeability of these membranes, allowing the water to move more freely along its concentration gradient.

Some substances are poorly reabsorbed through the tubular membranes. These include urea, phosphate, sulfate, uric acid, nitrate, and phenols, all waste products that need to be excreted from the body. As water is reabsorbed by osmosis, the concentration of these substances inside the tubule rises, causing some of the molecules to pass through to the interstitial spaces. However, because this process is very inefficient, the body is able to excrete these metabolic wastes.

Tubular Secretion

In addition to reabsorption, tubular cells are also capable of secretion. Secretion is a chemical activity that allows transport of substances from the blood into the tubules. The two physiologic elements most involved in this process are potassium and hydrogen, although ammonia and uric acid are also included. Some drug metabolites are excreted through this mechanism, such as acetaminophen, probenecid, and penicillin.

Regulation of Fluids and Electrolytes

The regulation of fluids and electrolytes in the body occurs primarily because of the feedback systems between the nephrons and the body fluids and tissues. These systems alter the processes described earlier—filtration, reabsorption, and secretion—thereby determining the amount and composition of the urine excreted from the body.

Assuming that the renal blood flow is adequate, the fluid volumes are maintained principally through the diluting and concentrating mechanisms of the nephrons. Dilution occurs as a result of reabsorbing solute without water, and concentration is produced by reabsorbing water without solute. The process, which allows the production of hyperosmolar urine, is called the *countercurrent* mechanism. This mechanism arises from the anatomic arrangement of the loop of Henle and the peritubular capillaries. A countercurrent system occurs when a tube or vessel makes a hairpin turn and one section travels parallel to, opposite to, and in close proximity to the other section over some distance. There continues to be debate about how this mechanism works, but the end result is concentration of the urine. Physiologists hypothesize that as the filtrate travels through the ascending loop of Henle, where the membrane is impermeable to water, sodium and chloride are moved out into the interstitial space by active transport. This reduces the salt concentration in the distal tubule and increases the concentration in the interstitium. Because of the concentration gradient, some of the interstitial salt diffuses back into the descending loop of Henle, where it moves around the hairpin turn and is again actively transported into the interstitial tissues. Because the medullary salt concentration was already slightly higher, the additional transport of salt raises the osmolarity even more. This continuing process is known as *countercurrent multiplication*.

The resulting hypertonicity of the interstitial fluid is maintained because the vasa recta, tiny capillaries that ascend and descend with the loop of Henle, operate as countercurrent exchangers. Solutes move out of the blood vessels going toward the cortex and into vessels descending into the pyramids. At the same time, water diffuses out of the descending vessels and into the ascending vessels. This recirculation preserves the solute concentration in the interstitium.

If this process were to continue unmediated, the urine produced would be very dilute. This is because the membranes of the distal tubule and collecting ducts are relatively impermeable to water without the activity of ADH. The excretion of dilute urine is desirable when body fluid volume is too high. In the presence of ADH, however, these membranes become permeable to water and allow water reabsorption to take place freely. Thus, the hypoosmolar fluid delivered to the distal tubule becomes isoosmolar with the interstitial spaces by the time it reaches the papillae. The fluid reabsorbed in this manner diffuses into the vasa recta and is returned to the general circulation through the renal circulation. Therefore, the presentation of dilute urine to the distal tubule allows regulation of water balance in the body. If the body needs to conserve fluids, such as in dehydration, ADH is released and water is reabsorbed.

Because of this influence of ADH on the concentrating and diluting abilities of the nephrons, anything that affects the release of ADH also affects the amount of urine produced. ADH release is regulated by variation in serum osmolality (state of hydration) and blood volume. As osmolality increases, ADH release increases. As osmolality decreases, ADH release decreases. The effect of changes in circulating ADH occurs within a matter of minutes.

Of lesser influence is the loss of blood volume. Usually, ADH is not released until a serious loss of circulating blood volume occurs, which then stimulates a stress response. The stress response usually causes a release of ADH, leading to water conservation. One example is the release of ADH that occurs postoperatively, which is caused by surgical stress and some anesthetic agents. Alcohol intake and a cold environment also may cause ADH release.

Urea augments the concentration of urine. As water is reabsorbed from the tubule, the concentration of urea increases. The inner medullary portion of the collecting duct is permeable to urea and thus reabsorbs it freely along the concentration gradient into the interstitium. This helps maintain the high osmolarity of the interstitial space so that more water is reabsorbed in the presence of ADH.

Electrolyte excretion by the kidney is influenced by a variety of factors, including hydrostatic and osmotic pressures and the circulating effect of aldosterone and other adrenocortical hormones. The movement of sodium also affects the regulation of several other electrolytes. For instance, the active reabsorption of sodium causes passive reabsorption of chloride and bicarbonate. The reabsorption of potassium usually decreases the reabsorption of sodium. If body levels of potassium are too high, excess potassium is secreted into the tubules. Chapter 15 further discusses the role of the kidney in water and electrolyte regulation.

Regulation of Hydrogen Ion Balance

Regulation of pH within the body is performed primarily by the kidney. Metabolic acids such as phosphoric, keto, uric, and sulfuric acids are normally excreted as they are formed. Then, in the presence of acid-base imbalances, the kidneys excrete either hydrogen or bicarbonate ions to restore balance. In response to acidotic states, the kidneys may also form new bicarbonates that are released in the blood.

Normally, the cells of the renal tubules secrete equivalent amounts of hydrogen and bicarbonate. Hydrogen ions are secreted into the proximal and distal tubules and the collecting ducts through the hydration of carbon dioxide in the presence of carbonic anhydrase. The carbonic acid then splits into carbon dioxide and water. The carbon dioxide is reabsorbed from the tubules, carried through the body, and excreted by the lungs. The water is excreted in the urine.

In acidosis, excess hydrogen ions are secreted into the proximal and distal tubules and collecting ducts and excreted in the urine. The hydrogen gradient has a limit, and without buffers to tie up the free hydrogen in the urine, this limit is reached rapidly. As mentioned earlier, hydrogen reacts with bicarbonate to form carbon dioxide and water. It also reacts with diphasic phosphate to form monobasic phosphate and with ammonia to form ammonium ion. The formation of these compounds allows the secretion of more hydrogen. The excess acid is excreted in the urine.

When needed, the kidneys can also regenerate new bicarbonate. Carbon dioxide is converted into carbonic acid, which dissociates into hydrogen and bicarbonate. The hydrogen ion is excreted in the urine and the bicarbonate is reabsorbed into the interstitial fluid.

With alkalosis, the excretion of hydrogen ions ceases. At higher levels of bicarbonate concentrations in the body, bicarbonate may actually be excreted in the urine, resulting in increased systemic pH levels. Further discussion of the kidney's contribution in hydrogen ion regulation is included in Chapter 15.

Regulation of Blood Pressure

Recall from Chapter 15 that in the event of blood volume depletion, the renin-angiotensin-aldosterone system works to maintain the blood pressure. As arterial blood pressure drops, reflex vasoconstriction in the splanchnic circulation effectively reduces renal blood flow and, thus, GFR. This stimulates the release of renin from the juxtaglomerular cells.

The mechanisms regulating the release of renin may be classified as (1) intrarenal, which includes baroreceptors in the afferent arterioles and natrioreceptors in the macula densa that are sensitive to changes in sodium concentration; (2) sympathetic, which includes renal nerves as well as the action of catecholamines; and (3) humoral, which includes the effects of sodium, potassium, vasopressin, and angiotensin II. The renin is released into the bloodstream, where it acts on *angiotensin I*. This substance is produced in the liver, and it has a weak vasoconstrictive effect on peripheral vessels. As angiotensin I passes through the lungs, it is converted by an enzyme into angiotensin II, a powerful vasoconstrictor that exerts its effects on the smooth muscle of arteriolar walls. *Vasocon-*

striction increases the peripheral resistance and, thus, the blood pressure, which in turn causes a drop in renin secretion in the kidney.

In addition, aldosterone production may be stimulated by angiotensin I. It may raise the blood pressure by facilitating the reabsorption of sodium and water from the distal tubule, resulting in increased blood volume.

Kallikrein, an enzyme found in the urine, catalyzes the formation of vasodilator hormones. Urinary kallikrein may be produced in the kidney and is therefore different from plasma kallikrein. No one knows exactly what role kallikrein plays in blood pressure regulation.

Other Metabolic and Endocrine Functions

In addition to the production of renin, the kidney has several other metabolic and endocrine functions. These include the synthesis of 1,25-dihydroxycholecalciferol, biogenesis of erythropoietin, degradation of insulin, synthesis of prostaglandins, and provision of the energy required to perform its own functions.

1,25-Dihydroxycholecalciferol is a hormone derived from vitamin D. It helps stimulate absorption of calcium from the intestine and works with parathyroid hormone to encourage osteoclastic bone activity. Thus, 1,25-dihydroxycholecalciferol helps maintain calcium homeostasis in the body. Cholecalciferol, obtained through diet or from ultraviolet light, is first hydroxylated in the liver and then again in the kidney to form 1,25-dihydroxycholecalciferol.

Erythropoietin is a glycoprotein that induces the production of red blood cells in the bone marrow. Since the 1950s, debate has taken place as to the source of this hormone. The current theory reestablishes the kidney as the point of origin. The synthesis of erythropoietin seems to be stimulated by an *oxygen deficit* in the kidney. Scientists hypothesize that anemia, hypoxia, renal ischemia, and circulatory alterations caused by vasoconstrictors prompt the synthesis of the enzyme erythrogenin. This enzyme, in turn, acts as a catalyst in the formation of erythropoietin from a circulating substrate. Although extrarenal oxygen sensors may be present in the pituitary gland, hypothalamus, and carotid bodies, the principal sensors are probably located in the cortex or medulla of the kidney.

Insulin is deactivated by the renal tubular cells. Approximately 20% of the insulin secreted by the pancreas is removed from the circulation by the kidneys and then degraded in the tubules.

Prostaglandins are a series of closely related fatty acids that have a great variety of proven and hypothesized physiologic actions. They are formed in most, if not all, organs of the body. In the kidney, prostaglandins are synthesized in the collecting tubules and medullary interstitial cells and are removed from the kidney through the renal vein and in the urine. Their synthesis is stimulated by a number of factors, including angiotensin, vasopressin, bradykinin, alpha-adrenergic catecholamines, calcium, loop diuretics, renal ischemia, unilateral ureteral obstruction, cirrhosis with ascites, glomerulonephritis, hypertension, and acute renal failure. They are inhibited by anti-inflammatory agents, especially nonsteroidal agents.

Medullary prostaglandins regulate urine concentration by increasing sodium excretion, inhibiting sodium and urea reabsorption, and antagonizing the action of ADH. Cortical prostaglandins regulate GFR, vascular resistance, and the secretion of renin. It appears that prostaglandins are not essential for renal function in healthy people, but that their actions become important when renal function is compromised. For instance, renal prostaglandins contribute to the excretion of excess sodium in hypertensive, but not in normotensive, people.

The active transport system of the kidney requires significant energy production. The provision of this energy is probably the major metabolic activity of the kidney. Because the active transport of sodium is the primary cause for energy use in the kidney, a close correlation exists among (1) the sodium reabsorption rate, (2) the renal blood flow rate, (3) the GFR, and (4) the renal oxygen consumption rate. The kidneys extract relatively little oxygen from the renal blood flow, and this rate remains stable even in states of low blood flow.

Movement of Urine Through the Kidneys

As the previously mentioned functions are carried out, the forming urine moves through each nephron. It travels through the collecting ducts toward the apex of the pyramids, where it flows through the openings in the papillae into the renal pelvis. As the urine enters and distends the pelvis, the muscle wall contracts, propelling the urine across the ureteropelvic junction into the ureter. This movement of urine into the ureter is a relatively constant process, because the maximum safe capacity of the adult renal pelvis is 3 to 5 ml. Amounts greater than this cause renal tissue damage as a result of pressure.

Ureters

The chief function of the ureter is to transport urine from the renal pelvis to the bladder. Peristaltic waves, which occur from one to five times per minute, move the urine down the ureter into the bladder through the ureterovesical junction. Although controversy exists about the mechanism that initiates these contractions, it appears that pacemaker sites are located in the calices, and that waves are propagated along the ureters from muscle cell to muscle cell by means of intracellular junctions. Generally, these contractions move from the kidney toward the bladder, but retrograde peristalsis can also occur.

Recall that the main function of the ureterovesical junction is to prevent the backflow of urine to the kidney during voiding or when the bladder becomes overdistended. Thus, this structure prevents damage to renal tissue from pressure and from the instillation of microorganisms that would ordinarily be washed out of the bladder.

In addition to its anatomic placement, the valve works because of the lack of smooth muscle in its wall just proximal to its entry into the bladder. Thus, the usual intravesical pressure tends to keep the valve collapsed except when urine is spurting through it. During micturition, the ureters are closed off by the muscular contractions of the bladder.

Bladder

The bladder stores urine received from the ureters until it is passed from the body. A slight increase occurs in the intravesical pressure for approximately the accumulation of the first 25 ml of urine. Then the pressure stays relatively stable until about 400 to 500 ml has been collected. This accommodation occurs because of the slow stretching of the detrusor muscle. The pressure curve rises markedly as the bladder fills with more than 500 ml of urine, and it soars as micturition is initiated.

Electromyographic (EMG) tracings do not measure or demonstrate activity of the bladder muscle related to filling; rather, they show the increased electrical response of the urethral sphincter to increased bladder pressure and volume. The bladder is composed of smooth muscle, whereas the urethral sphincter is composed of striated muscle and is the only area commonly monitored by EMG.

Micturition, also called *urination* and *voiding*, is the act of emptying the bladder. As the bladder fills and the muscle fibers expand, stretch receptors in the bladder wall are stimulated. The first urge to void is felt at about 150 ml, and a marked feeling of fullness usually occurs around 400 ml, although this level can be increased or decreased through habit patterns. Impulses are sent to the sacral portion of the spinal cord, where the micturition reflex is initiated; this causes the bladder to contract and the urethral sphincters to open. As the bladder musculature contracts, the pressure forces the urine out through the urethra. The bladder muscle fibers extend longitudinally down the urethra, and as they contract, they shorten the urethra and pull the bladder down toward a point of fixation at the distal portion of the pubis. Unless the reflex is mediated at this point, urination occurs immediately.

The impulses initiating the micturition reflex are also sent to the cerebral cortex. After a period of successful toilet training in early childhood, the external sphincter is usually under voluntary control. If the client feels that environmental conditions are not right for urination, the external sphincter contracts, stopping the flow of urine. The micturition reflex also can be initiated by the cerebral cortex.

Voluntary contraction of the abdominal muscles (in addition to contraction of the detrusor muscle and relaxation of the sphincters) facilitates micturition by increasing pressure on the bladder wall. During urination, the perineal muscles must be relaxed. Voluntary contraction (or exercising) of the perineal muscles assists the external sphincter to resist the outflow of urine.

In essence, this voluntary contraction is the Valsalva maneuver.

Urethra and Meatus

The urethra is the pathway through which the urine normally leaves the body. The detrusor contraction during micturition is preceded for about 5 seconds by a significant fall of pressure within the urethra. This facilitates movement of urine from the bladder, with its higher pressure, into the urethra. Following the act of micturition, the female urethra empties by gravity, whereas the male urethra empties by several contractions of the bulbocavernous muscle.

The female urethra is about 3.5 to 4.0 cm long, and it exits the urinary bladder through the pelvic floor. The urethral meatus is located anterior to the vagina and slightly below the clitoris.

The male urethra is about 15 to 20 cm long, with the urethral meatus located at the tip of the penis. The male urethra is divided into three sections. The prostatic urethra is about 3.75 cm long and passes through the prostate gland after leaving the bladder. The next portion is the membranous urethra, about 1.25 cm in length, which passes along the wall of the pelvic floor. The remainder of the urethra is called the *bulbar cavernous urethra*, and it extends the length of the penis, ending in the urethral meatus.

The urethra ends in the meatus, which is under voluntary control in the adult. When voiding is not appropriate, the external sphincter contracts, holding back the flow of urine until the reflex stimulation ceases.

Effects of Aging

As a part of the natural aging process, the kidney becomes smaller. The cause of this loss of tissue, which occurs especially in the renal cortex, is unknown. It may be focal, as the result of scarring, or diffuse, as a result of renal blood vessel changes.

Because of the loss of functioning nephrons and generalized circulatory changes, renal function decreases with advancing age. The glomerular filtation rate, tubular reabsorption, and ability to concentrate the urine are affected. All normal regulatory and metabolic functions of the kidney become less efficient, and little or no reserve remains with which to respond to periods of increased stress.

The aging process also affects the act of micturition. The bladder becomes funnel shaped as a result of alterations in the connective tissue and weakening of the pelvic floor muscles. Irritability of the bladder wall often increases, adding more urgency to the normal desire to void. Finally, impairment of the detrusor muscle's ability to elongate results in decreased bladder capacity. Because of these changes, the elderly person may have problems with incontinence, frequency, retention, and dysuria.

Conclusions

An understanding of the structure and function of the renal and urinary system is needed before the nurse can adequately care for clients experiencing disorders in this system. Once the nurse has a thorough understanding, appropriate interventions can be taken to provide comprehensive client care.

Bibliography

1. Beck, L. H. (1990). Kidney function and disease in the elderly. *Hospital Practice, 26,* 75–90.
2. Berne, R. M., & Levy, M. N. (1993). *Principles of physiology* (3rd ed.). St. Louis: Mosby–Year Book.
3. Bennett, J. C., & Plum, F. (Eds.). (1996). *Cecil textbook of medicine* (20th ed.). Philadelphia: W. B. Saunders.
4. Bower, A., & Thompson, J. (1992). *Clinical manual of health assessment* (3rd ed.). St. Louis: Mosby–Year Book.
5. Brenner, B. M. (Ed.). (1996). *Brenner & Rector's the kidney* (5th ed.). Philadelphia: W. B. Saunders.
6. Brundage, D. (1992). *Renal disorders.* St. Louis: Mosby–Year Book.
7. Burrows-Hudson, S. (Ed.). (1993). *Standards of clinical practice for nephrology.* Pittman, NJ: American Nephrology Nurses Association.
8. Chmielewski, C. (1992). Renal anatomy and overview of nephron function. *American Nephrology Nurses Association Journal, 19*(1), 34–40.
9. Christiansen, J. L., & Grzbouski, J. M. (1993). *Biology of aging.* St. Louis: Mosby–Year Book.
10. Copstead, L. C. (Ed.). *Perspectives on pathophysiology.* Philadelphia: W. B. Saunders.
11. Cotran, R. S., Kumar, V., & Robbins, S. L. (1994). *Robbins pathologic basis of disease* (5th ed.). Philadelphia: W. B. Saunders.
12. Glassock, R. J. (1992). *Current therapy in nephrology and hypertension* (3rd ed.). St. Louis: Mosby–Year Book.
13. Gray, M. (1992). *Genitourinary disorders.* St. Louis: Mosby–Year Book.
14. Guyton, A. C. (1992). *Human physiology and mechanisms of disease* (5th ed.). Philadelphia: W. B. Saunders.
15. Guyton, A. C., & Hall, J. E. (1996). *Textbook of medical physiology* (9th ed.). Philadelphia: W. B. Saunders.
16. Holechek, M. J. (1992). Glomerular filtration and renal hemodynamics. *American Nephrology Nurses Association Journal, 19*(3), 237–245.
17. Holechek, M. J. (1992). Renal physiology series: Glomerular filtration and renal hemodynamics: Part 2. *American Nephrology Nurses Association Journal, 19*(3), 237–248.
18. Jacobson, H. R., Striker, G. E., & Klahn, S. (1991). *The principles and practice of nephrology.* St. Louis: Mosby–Year Book.
19. Jeter, K., Faller, N., & Norton, C. (1990). *Nursing for continence.* Philadelphia: W. B. Saunders.
20. Karlowicz, K. A. (Ed.). (1995). *Urologic nursing: Principles and practice.* Philadelphia: W. B. Saunders.
21. Kee, C. C. (1992). Age-related changes in the renal system: Causes, consequences, and nursing implications. *Geriatric Nursing, 13*(2), 80–83.
22. Kenny, R. A. (1992). *Physiology of aging: A synopsis.* St. Louis: Mosby–Year Book.
23. Koeppen, B. M., & Stanton, B. A. (1992). *Renal physiology.* St. Louis: Mosby–Year Book.
24. Lancaster, L. E. (Ed.). (1994). *Core curriculum for nephrology nursing* (2nd ed.). Pitman, NJ: American Nephrology Nurses' Association.
25. Lindeman, R. D. (1993). Renal physiology and pathophysiology of aging. *Contributions to Nephrology, 105,* 1–12.
26. Llach, F. (1993). *Popper's clinical nephrology* (3rd ed.). Boston: Little, Brown.

27. Lote, C. J. (1994). *Principles of renal physiology* (3rd ed.). London: Chapman & Hall.

28. Ludlow, M. (1993). Renal handling of potassium. *American Nephrology Nurses Association Journal, 20*(1), 52–56.

29. Massry, S. G., & Glassock, R. J. (Eds.). (1995). *Massry and Glassock's textbook of nephrology* (3rd ed.). Baltimore: Williams & Wilkins.

30. McCance, K. L., & Huether, S. E. (1994). *Pathophysiology: The biologic basis for disease in adults and children* (2nd ed.). St. Louis: Mosby–Year Book.

31. Moffett, D., Moffett, S., & Schauf, C. (1993). *Human physiology: Foundations and frontiers* (2nd ed.). St. Louis: Mosby–Year Book.

32. Porcush, J. G., & Faubert, P. F. (1991). *Renal disease in the aged.* Boston: Little, Brown.

33. Preisig, P. (1994). Renal physiology series: Renal acidification, part 7. *American Nephrology Nurses Association Journal, 21*(5), 251–259.

34. Preisig, P. (1992). Renal physiology series: Urinary concentration and dilution, part 3. *American Nephrology Nurses Association Journal, 19*(4), 351–355.

35. Radke, K. J. (1994). Renal physiology series: The aging kidney: Structure, function, and nursing practice implications, part 6. *American Nephrology Nurses Association Journal, 21*(4), 181–190; quiz 191–193.

36. Schrier, R. W. (Ed.). (1995). *Manual of nephrology.* Boston: Little, Brown.

37. Schrier, R. W., & Gottschalk, C. W. (Eds.). (1993). *Diseases of the kidney* (5th ed.). Boston: Little, Brown.

38. Seeley, R., Stephens, T., & Tate, P. (1995). *Anatomy and physiology* (3rd ed.). St. Louis: Mosby–Year Book

39. Seidman, E. J. (Eds.). (1994). *Current urologic therapy.* Philadelphia: W. B. Saunders.

40. Selkin, D. W., & Giebisch, G. (Eds.). (1992). *The kidney: Physiology and pathophysiology.* New York: Raven Press.

41. Smith, D. R. (1992). *General urology* (13th ed.). Los Altos, CA: Lange.

42. Solomon, E. P. (1992). *Introduction to human anatomy and physiology.* Philadelphia: W. B. Saunders.

43. Tanagho, E. A., & McAninich, J. W. (1992). *Smith's general urology* (13th ed.). Norwalk, CT: Appleton & Lange.

44. Thibodeau, G. A., & Patton, K. T. (1992). *Anatomy and physiology* (2nd ed.). St. Louis: Mosby–Year Book.

45. Thibodeau, G. A., & Patton, K. T. (1992). *The human body in health and disease.* St. Louis: Mosby–Year Book.

46. Valtin, H., & Schafer, J. A. (1995). *Renal function: Mechanisms preserving fluid and solute balance in health* (3rd ed.). Boston: Little, Brown.

47. Vander, A. (1995). *Renal physiology* (5th ed.). New York: McGraw-Hill.

48. Walsh, P. C., et al. (1992). *Campbell's urology* (6th ed.). Philadelphia: W. B. Saunders.

49. Yucha, C. B. (1993). Renal physiology series: Renal control of calcium, part 5a. *American Nephrology Nurses Association Journal, 20*(4), 440–446.

50. Yucha, C. B. (1993). Renal physiology series: Renal control of phosphorus and magnesium, part 5b. *American Nephrology Nurses Association Journal, 20*(4), 447–452.

Assessment of Clients with Urinary Disorders

Esther Matassarin-Jacobs

Accurate diagnosis of urinary problems depends on complete and thorough assessment. For most people, however, urinary elimination is a private matter. Discussing urinary elimination with others can be embarrassing, making nurses less likely to ask important questions and causing clients to delay seeking medical attention until the urinary disorder is advanced. In men, the urinary and reproductive systems are combined, often creating even greater fears. When clients do come for help, their humiliation may continue to interfere with their ability to express the information necessary for an accurate history and description of their problem.

The physical examination and specific diagnostic studies used to assess urinary function can also be distressing. For example, providing a urine specimen may be embarrassing, especially if the client has to carry the full container down the hall or bring it from home. Some studies require the client to urinate in front of others, as with a voiding cystourethrogram. When assessing the client, keep in mind the client's likely embarrassment or discomfort and be understanding. Provide as much privacy as possible.

Use of good communication skills is the key to obtaining complete and accurate information. Allow the client to express anxiety and, in turn, try to make the client comfortable and at ease. Be aware of what the client communicates nonverbally, because subtle clues may be crucial to diagnosing the problem.

History

As with other systems, history taking is probably the most important part of the assessment process. Many problems are discovered at this point. A urologic history consists of the chief complaint and current health history, past medical history, family history, psychosocial history and life-style, and review of systems (ROS). If the client reports urologic manifestations, a detailed symptom analysis is performed (see Chapter 11).

Biographical and Demographic Data

A review of biographical and demographic data such as age, sex, ethnicity, and occupation are important assessments because many urinary problems are specific to a particular group. Problems such as incontinence may be age-associated or postmenopausal, while certain occupations may increase the risk of bladder cancer.

Current Manifestations

Chief Complaint

Common major manifestations in urologic disorders include a change in the usual pattern of voiding such as frequency, urgency, or dysuria, urinary incontinence, pain, hematuria, and associated manifestations. There is often more than one manifestation present, and each must be explored with the client.

Symptom Analysis

Timing
Onset. When was the problem first noted? Was the onset gradual or sudden? What was the client doing when the problem was first noticed? Is it related to fluid intake?

Duration. How long does the problem last? Does it occur occasionally, or is it persistent? Is there a pattern to the problem? If the problem is pain, note whether the pain is continuous or intermittent.

Quality and Quantity. Ask the client to describe the problem. Common major manifestations in urologic disorders include a change in the usual patterns of voiding, urinary incontinence, pain, and associated gastrointestinal manifestations. There may be more than one manifestation present, and each is explored with the client.

Change in Urinary Patterns. The client is asked to describe his or her patterns of voiding, including *frequency,* amounts, and the usual times of day and night. Ask if the client has to rely on methods to stimulate urination, such as listening to running water, applying pressure over the lower abdomen, or performing Valsalva's maneuver. Does the client have trouble starting or maintaining the urine stream *(hesitancy)*? Has there been a change in the force or shape of the stream? Does the client have feelings of *urgency* or difficulty controlling voiding? If so, is the urgency associated with a known factor such as consuming caffeine or, for women, following pregnancy and vaginal delivery? Older men may report gradually diminishing force and hesitancy of the urinary stream if they have enlargement of the prostate gland.

The client also should be assessed for changes in urinary volume. Normal output for adults with average fluid intake is between 1200 and 1800 ml/day, or about two thirds of the total fluid intake for the day. The usual amount for each voiding is about 400 ml. Adults urinate more often during the day than at night. Question the client for the presence of *nocturia* (voiding more than twice at night), which may occur in clients with benign prostatic hyperplasia (BPH) or cystitis. Ask if the client is experiencing any changes in urinary volume unrelated to intake. *Polyuria,* or increased urine output, may be related to conditions such as hyperglycemia or *nocturia,* which is common in older people and those with edema, insulin-dependent diabetes, and those who take diuretics. Decreased urine output may be a manifestation of poor fluid intake or renal failure. You should also ask the client about the presence of diarrhea or severe vomiting, which may also predispose to a decreased urinary output. *Oliguria* is a total urinary output of less than 400 ml/day, whereas *anuria* is a total urinary output of less than 100 ml/day.

Changes in the characteristics of urine are explored in detail. Ask the client what the urine usually looked like before manifestations were present. What was the usual color? What is the color now? Is the urine clear, cloudy, or bloody *(hematuria)*? Blood-tinged or bloody urine is never normal, although blood may contaminate the voided urine of women during menses. The color of urine may be altered by foods, drink, and medications. Are there particles present, such as clots, mucus, or shreds of tissue? Infection of the urinary tract results in inflammation so that the urine becomes cloudy with debris. Urine should be odor-free, although after standing for a time, an odor of ammonia is normal. If the urine does have a foul odor, this frequently is a manifestation of infection, although it may also be due to medications such as antibiotics or a high glucose content in the urine.

Urinary Incontinence. Urinary incontinence is the loss of control over the release of urine from the bladder. There are several types of urinary incontinence: stress incontinence, urge incontinence, reflex incontinence, func-

tional incontinence, and total incontinence. The nurse asks the client to describe the onset and manifestations that occur with incontinence. How often does it occur? Is there dribbling of urine between voidings? If so, how much? A teaspoonful or a great deal? Does incontinence occur in predictable situations, as with coughing, sneezing, and laughing? Does the client have an awareness of the need to void prior to incontinent episodes? How long has the client had difficulty with incontinence? Is the problem getting worse? Has there been any change in medications? (Many medications, such as diuretics, may increase incontinence.) What methods does the client use to cope with incontinence? The client may have concerns about strikethrough wetness on clothing or odor being noticeable to others and may resort to using pads or shields for protection. Many of these clients also limit their social activities and some even become homebound for fear of embarrassing situations.

Pain. If pain is present, ask the client to describe any pain associated with the urinary tract, including its location, type, severity, and duration (see Chapter 17 for further information on pain assessment). Is the pain getting worse or better? Is the client able to relate factors that may have precipitated the pain? What makes the pain better? What makes it worse? Is the pain accompanied by uncomfortable or painful urination *(dysuria)*? If dysuria is present, when during voiding does it occur, at the beginning, middle, or end of voiding?

Location. A careful description of the pain may help pinpoint the source of the problem. Kidney pain, which is usually caused by sudden distention of the renal capsule from calculi blocking the outflow of urine, produces a dull, constant ache in the costovertebral angle (CVA) lateral to the sacrospinalis muscle just below the 12th rib. This pain often spreads along the subcostal area to the umbilicus.

Radiculitis often mimics renal pain, so it is important to differentiate between the two. Radicular pain is a hyperesthesia of the skin supplied by an irritated peripheral nerve. This nerve can be stimulated by pinching both the skin and fat of the abdominal and flank regions. Exerting pressure over the CVA with the thumb may elicit local tenderness of the involved peripheral nerve at its point of emergence, whereas gentle fist percussion over the angle may be necessary to elicit renal pain, indicating a deeper, more visceral sensation. Figure 55–1 illustrates percussion over the CVA.

Ureteral pain, as would be experienced when calculi obstruct the ureter, is exhibited as back pain from distention and as colicky pain caused by spasm of the renal pelvis and ureteral muscle. It radiates from the CVA down across the abdomen to the genital area. In males, pain originating in the upper ureter is referred to the scrotum. Females describe ureteral pain in the ipsilateral labium. Ureteral pain is often sharp and excruciating and may result in a generalized systemic shock syndrome (see Chapter 22 for more information on shock).

The most common bladder discomfort arises from overdistention and is felt in the suprapubic area. The

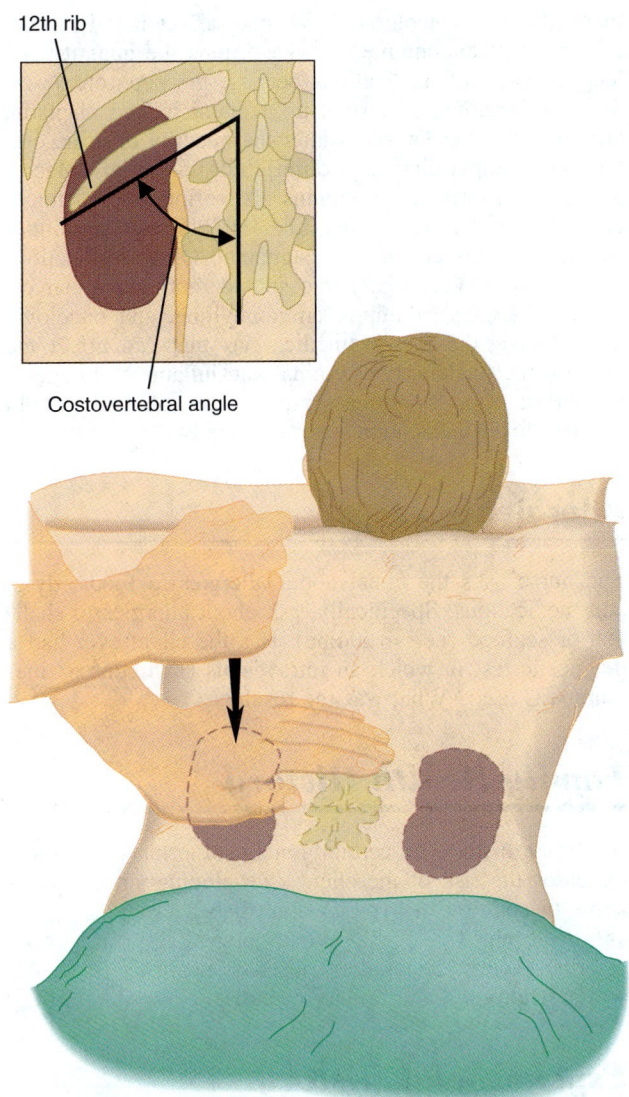

12th rib

Costovertebral angle

Figure 55–1. Percussion over the costovertebral angle (CVA).

client should be asked if dysuria occurs at the beginning, during, or at the end of urination. This often indicates the presence of a bladder infection. *Strangury* (frequent, painful urination in small amounts, with bladder spasms) is often associated with *tenesmus* (ineffectual attempts to void with painful straining). These manifestations are often associated with acute bladder or prostate infections. A bladder infection causes feelings of urgency or a burning pain, or both, during micturition in the distal urethra in females and in the prostatic urethra in males. Urethral pain is usually felt along the course of the urethra or at the meatus. Determining precisely when during the act of micturition burning occurs helps differentiate between bladder and urethral origins. Burning at the beginning of urination (as the bladder contracts the inflamed tissue as it drains into the urethra) indicates urethritis. Suspect bladder infection when the burning occurs during and after the voiding process, accompanied by suprapubic pain.

Precipitating Factors. Urinary problems are more likely to occur in the presence of low fluid intake or dehydration. Infections and calculi are much more likely to occur in the presence of low intake, dehydration, or both. Renal function also decreases when volume is low. Renal failure has many precipitating factors, such as hypovolemia, renal obstruction, and ingestion of nephrotoxic substances.

Carefully assess the client's fluid intake and fluid balance. Ask about the recent ingestion of any substnaces that are nephrotoxic (see Table 57–1). Ask the client with urinary calculi about dietary intake such as of foods high in calcium.

Aggravating and Relieving Factors. Decreased fluid intake is an agravating factor for many urinary disorders, whereas increased intake can be a relieving factor. If the client has experienced this particular urinary problem previously, ask what factors have made the problem better or worse.

Associated Manifestations. Urinary tract disorders, such as calculi and pyelonephritis with ureteritis, may be accompanied by gastrointestinal manifestations, such as anorexia, nausea, vomiting, diarrhea, or a metallic taste in the mouth. The unpleasantness of these manifestations may lead the client to alter the amount and type of fluids consumed. Ask the client to describe how much fluid is consumed in a day and types of liquids drunk. How does the fluid intake compare with the urinary output? Does the client have unusual fluid loss from diarrhea, vomiting, or excess perspiration? Have there been weight changes (loss or gain) of 2 lbs or more within a 24-hour period? Such weight fluctuations are usually related to a change in fluid balance.

Renointestinal reflexes may cause gastrointestinal and renal manifestations to occur simultaneously. Afferent stimuli originating in the renal capsule or pelvic musculature may cause pylorospasm or other changes in the smooth muscle of the enteric tract and adnexa. Additionally, the anatomic proximity of the kidneys and gastrointestinal structures may mean that intestinal disturbances will mimic renal disorders. The right kidney lies close to the hepatic flexure of the colon, duodenum, head of the pancreas, common bile duct, liver, and gallbladder, whereas the left kidney is bordered by the splenic flexure of the colon, stomach, pancreas, and spleen. This partially explains why clients may experience nausea and vomiting, anorexia, diarrhea, and abdominal discomfort concomitantly with urinary tract manifestations. Renal inflammation may also produce manifestations of peritoneal irritation. Inflammation of the peritoneum (covering the anterior surface of both kidneys) causes involuntary muscle rigidity and rebound tenderness.

Past Health History

The past medical history should include the client's experiences with disorders of the urinary tract and other disorders. These data may be linked to current health problems or may be associated with increased risk for the client of developing urinary tract disorders. Other past medical problems that may be significant include cancer of the reproductive organs, especially if radiation was used; recent surgery or trauma; systemic diseases such as hypertension and diabetes; allergies; a history of sexually transmitted disease; and medication usage (both prescription and over-the-counter).

Childhood and Infectious Diseases

Ask the client to relate incidences of urinary tract infection (UTI), particularly in females, during childhood. UTIs in male children are rare, so a history of these in men is very significant. Frequent UTIs can result in structural changes from chronic inflammation and strictures. Chronic or inadequately treated kidney infections can lead to more serious sequelae such as hydronephrosis. Skin or upper respiratory infections of streptococcal origin can result in acute glomerulonephritis, as can infectious mononucleosis, mumps, measles, cytomegalovirus infection, and other primary infections. Ask about the presence of congenital anomalies that may have affected the urinary tract, such as spina bifida causing a neurogenic bladder.

Major Illnesses and Hospitalizations

The client is asked about previous hospitalizations or treatment of urinary problems. Determine the dates of illnesses or hospitalizations, the specific urinary problems, medical treatments (including surgery or manipulation of the urinary tract such as catheterization), and the present status of the problem. Ask if the client has had diagnostic studies of the urinary tract such as a renal ultrasound, intravenous pyelogram (IVP), or cystogram. Results of these studies can provide baseline data for assessment of the current problem.

Ask the client whether there has been trauma to the urinary tract such as a direct blow to the flank or falls with resulting contusion over the lower posterior thorax. How was the problem treated and what was the result? Specific surgical procedures to ask about include any type of urinary diversion. Why was the surgery necessary? Is the diversion temporary or permanent? How does the client manage the diversion or are there problems with its management?

Major illnesses and diseases linked to urinary tract problems include hypertension, diabetes mellitus, gout, neurologic disorders such as multiple sclerosis, and connective tissue disorders (e.g., scleroderma, systemic lupus erythematosus). Ask the client about problems with urinary tract calculi, previously mentioned UTIs, and systemic infections.

Medications

A complete medication history (both prescription and over-the-counter) is obtained, including past use, because many drugs are nephrotoxic or may affect bladder function, such as anticholinergics. Determine the quantity and length of use of medications because the nephrotoxic effects of certain drugs, such as gentamicin and cisplatin, are dose-specific. Diuretics alter the quantity of urine output. Phenazopyridine (Pyridium), nitrofurantoin (Macrodantin), and even multivitamins alter urine color. Anticoagulants can cause hematuria, and many antibiotics enhance the effects of anticoagulants. Other medications that can affect the urinary tract include antibiotics, narcotics, cholinergics, rifampin, aminophylline, and oncologic agents. Over-the-counter medications that can affect the urinary tract include nonsteroidal anti-inflammatory agents (NSAIDs; e.g., ibuprofen), phenacetin, salicylates, cold and hay fever medications, and sleep aids.

Allergies

The nurse asks the client about allergies to foods, dyes, and medications. Specifically, ask about allergies to shellfish or seafood (i.e., to iodine). Has the client ever had a diagnostic test in which an intravenous (IV) contrast medium was used? What was the result?

Family Health History

A family history of certain renal and urinary disorders increases the risk of the client's developing similar problems. In addition to hypertension, diabetes mellitus, gout, and recurrent UTIs, ask about congenital urinary tract disorders, polycystic kidney disease, nephritis (e.g., Alport's syndrome), and urinary calculi.

Psychosocial History

Occupation

What kind of work does the client do? Are there barriers in the work place to allowing the client to take time for urinary elimination? Are there hazards in the work place setting that increase the client's risk of developing urinary problems such as exposure to nephrotoxic chemicals (e.g., carbon tetrachloride, phenol, and ethyl glycol)?

Urinary elimination problems may cause a change in life-style. To assess the kind and extent of changes that may occur, baseline data are collected in the following areas.

Environment

Does the client live alone or with others? How many people live in the household? How many bathrooms are there, and where are they located? For example, does the client have to negotiate stairs to gain access to the toilet? Does this present a physical limitation to the client with impaired mobility? Does the client need a bedside commode or a bedpan to facilitate urinary elimination?

Support Systems

Are others available to help the client who is dependent on help with urinary elimination? Can the client rely on family members, or is a referral needed to a community agency?

Financial Status

If the client needs special equipment (e.g., ostomy supplies), are there resources to help pay for it? Is a source of supplies accessible?

Nutrition

Ask about dietary intake. A diet high in calcium or purines in a client with gout and with low fluid intake can contribute to calculi formation. Dehydration also increases the client's risk of UTI and renal failure.

Habits

Ask about activity and exercise, smoking, and use of recreational drugs. Does the client participate in hobbies or recreational activities, or has a urinary problem resulted in a reluctance to participate? Has the client had to give up favorite activities because of incontinence? The client's activity level may indicate a risk of developing urinary stasis if the client is sedentary. Urinary stasis, in turn, predisposes the client to UTI and calculi formation. The client with impaired physical mobility is at even greater risk if bone demineralization is an accompanying factor. Cigarette smoking has been linked to the occurrence of bladder tumors, particularly in women. Drug use may expose the client to nephrotoxic agents and subsequent renal damage.

Urinary tract disorders affect and are affected by many aspects of the client's life, including psychological, social, occupational, and physical factors.

Psychological Factors

Assess the client's emotional reaction to the history-taking process and to the physical examination. Just as people are emotionally affected by the performance of the urinary system, the urinary system is affected by emotions in many ways, as by (1) past experiences, (2) the power of suggestion, (3) anxiety and fear, (4) depression, (5) changes in body image, and (6) the fear of death.

■ Past Experiences

A client's past experiences produce various effects on the process of voiding. As mentioned earlier, cultural teachings lead most people to consider the act of urination a private matter. Western society and childrearing practices support this viewpoint by providing locks on bathroom doors, separate public restrooms for men and women, and so forth. This attitude may inhibit the micturition reflex if the client is in an environment where privacy is missing, such as a commode behind the curtain in a multibed hospital room.

Experiences linked with childhood toilet training can have long-lasting effects. A client's negative or positive attitudes toward bladder elimination can sometimes be traced back to this developmental period. Reinforcement of positive behavior tends to result in continued, problem-free elimination patterns. Punishment as the primary motivator during toilet training, however, may carry over into adulthood, producing guilt or anxiety expressed in micturition problems. The guilt or shame from prolonged *enuresis* (involuntary discharge of urine, usually during sleep at night, i.e., bed-wetting) may cause voiding dysfunction long after the enuresis has been cured. In addition, to punish their parents, children may not use the toilet and this behavior may appear again in adult life when severe stress occurs.

■ Power of Suggestion

The micturition control center is connected to the various sensory portions of the brain, allowing micturition to be initiated by any number of auditory, visual, or somesthetic stimuli, such as running water in a sink. In fact, the mere act of thinking about voiding may be enough to stimulate the reflex.

■ Anxiety and Fear

Anxiety may stimulate or hinder micturition. The most noticeable effect of anxiety is to increase the frequency of voiding and produce urgency. Very commonly, people have a strong urge to void when facing stressful situations, even though they may have urinated just moments before. Conversely, anxiety characterized by general muscle tension can interfere with urination, because relaxing the perineal muscles is essential to completing micturition. Anxiety also may intensify the manifestations of urinary tract disorders. Fear of the unknown or concern about the disorder's prognosis, for instance, makes pain seem worse. Also, moderate-to-severe burning pain on urination will cause the client to inhibit micturition to avoid discomfort and to decrease the amount of fluid to produce less urine (this actually makes the dysuria worse).

There is also a great deal of anxiety and fear associated with the possible diagnosis of cancer. This may be associated with both the fear of death and the possible results of treatment, such as a urinary diversion.

■ Depression

Incontinence is not the result of depression; rather depression is the result of long-standing, untreated, unmanaged urinary incontinence. Urinary incontinence is a manifestation of an underlying physiologic problem. The isolation and changes in the client's social patterns caused by incontinence can easily lead to a sense of worthlessness, depression, and withdrawal from social activities. It is not the depression, however, that needs to be treated; the incontinence needs to be corrected so that the depression will disappear.

■ Changes in Body Image

Many urinary disorders, such as renal failure or urinary diversion, result in a change in body image and life-style, which, in turn, may lead to anxiety, depression, or anger. Changes that affect body image include an inability to control body functions such as urination, a dependence on others, and a dependency on machines, as with dialysis. Anatomic alterations that change the way urine leaves the body are sometimes surgically created. If the client is unable to produce urine at all, a machine may perform this vital blood-cleaning function. These dramatic and often permanent alterations can have a major effect on a client's usual body image.

Adapting to a serious disruption of body image often leads the client and significant others along a path of denial, anger, and depression before they finally accept the new self-concept. During this time, the client who has the dysfunction can suffer a loss of self-esteem. Additional conflicts involve dependence and independence. Changes in life role and responsibilities, life-style, and interpersonal relationships may develop. The client and significant others may need support, including long-term counseling.

■ Fear of Death

The possibility of impending death is a real concern for clients with some urinary tract problems, because most realize that a functioning urinary system is necessary to life. Urinary tract cancers, such as bladder or renal cancer, and renal failure are problems that are most likely to cause fear of death. Whether the problem is large or small, it is always possible that a urinary disorder may become terminal. Some clients can discuss this fear openly, whereas others are not able to admit such a possibility. Often, this fear is suggested by behavior such as acting out, denial, and social withdrawal.

Learn as much as possible about the client's psychological disposition. *Carefully listen to your conversation with the client* and observe behavior patterns. Sometimes a client may voice fear directly by openly saying, "I'm afraid of dying." However, some people are unable to express their fears directly. In this case, look for indirect cues in the way the client answers questions or initiates conversation. Subtle cues may be camouflaged in seemingly unconscious statements.

Whatever communication techniques are used, the nurse should consciously assess the client's emotional state, because no one else on the healthcare team may be assisting the client and significant others in this crucial area.

Review of Systems

Urinary function affects and is affected by other body systems. The nurse asks questions about the general status and specific body systems because the resulting data may reveal related renal problems. For example, assessing the neuromuscular system provides information about the client's ability to control urination. Gastrointestinal manifestations (bleeding or a metallic taste in the mouth) may indicate renal disease. Assessing the client's immune system for the presence of allergies can help determine which diagnostic tests and medications will cause allergic reactions and are thus contraindicated.

Specifically, ask the client about fatigue, headaches, blurred vision, changes in mentation, elevated blood pressure, changes in body weight, itching, numbness or tingling of the extremities, excessive thirst, chills, bleeding tendencies, anorexia, nausea and vomiting, and edema of the face or extremities. Additional questions for the ROS may be found in Table 11–2.

Physical Examination

The physical examination is based on information obtained from the history. Although most of the data needed come directly from examining the urinary system, consider other systems, too.

Urinary Tract Organs

Kidneys

Inspect for masses in the upper abdomen and flank areas. Typically, because of the location of the kidneys, only the lower pole of the right kidney can be felt on deep palpation. Normally, this is usually felt only in thin people. It is difficult to palpate the kidneys of obese or very muscular clients. With the client lying supine on a hard surface, deep palpation is accomplished in the following manner: For the right kidney, stand on the right side of the client, place the right hand on the abdomen between the rib cage and the iliac crest, and position the left hand posteriorly in the costovertebral angle (Fig. 55–2). Support the area from below with the left hand and have the client take a deep breath. As the client inhales, use the right hand to compress the tissue in deep palpation. Instruct the client to exhale and then hold the breath. Slowly release pressure with the right hand; the pole, if felt, is a smooth, firm rounded mass that descends on inspiration and slips upward and away on exhalation. Instruct the client to breathe normally and remove both hands. Palpate the left

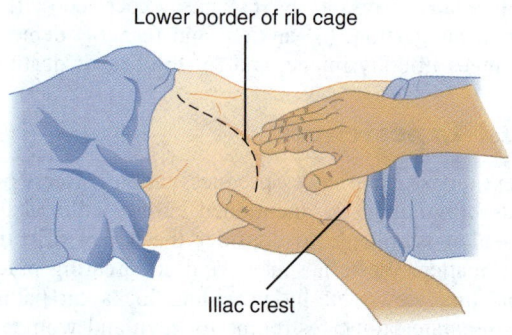

Lower border of rib cage

Iliac crest

Figure 55–2. Palpating the kidneys.

kidney while standing on the client's right side. Reach across with the left hand and place it under the client and use the right hand to palpate. The left kidney should not be felt because it lies higher up in the rib cage. In older adults, the muscles lose tone and elasticity, so the kidneys drop and may be palpated more readily.

Depending on the size of the client and the skill of the examiner, it may be possible to outline both kidneys anteriorly and posteriorly by percussion (see Fig. 55–1). This technique is particularly helpful when pain and muscle spasm prevent proper palpation. Assess costovertebral angle tenderness by placing the left hand over the area and striking it with the ulnar side of the right fist. Ordinarily, this percussion produces a dull sound and no discomfort. With inflammation, there is exquisite tenderness.

Auscultation is performed in the CVA and upper abdominal quadrants. There is normally no sound unless aortic pulsations are heard. A systolic bruit heard over the renal artery is often associated with stenosis or an aneurysm of the renal artery.

Bladder

As the bladder distends, it rises out of the pelvic cavity above the pubic symphysis. In a very thin client or one with a distended bladder, it may be visible on inspection and be palpable. When a distended bladder is palpated, it is felt as a smooth, round, and rather tense mass. The adult bladder can be percussed if it contains at least 150 ml of urine. Percussion is accomplished in the normal manner, with the sound of the bowel often being tympanic and the sound of the distended bladder being duller. The bladder can be outlined and may extend as high as the umbilicus. After the initial assessment, have the client void, and then palpate and percuss again to distinguish the bladder from a possible mass. Residual urine can also be measured at this point. This test is discussed later in this chapter.

Urethra

Urethral examination primarily involves inspecting the external meatus and the perineal area for manifestations of discharge, abnormal tissue growth, cleanliness, and anatomic integrity. Note any aberrant location of the meatus. Palpate the penis for masses along the distal portion of the male urethra, and palpate the perineal area for tenderness. In uncircumcised men, observe the urethra by having the client pull his foreskin back, if possible, and look for discharge or irritation. In the female, the posterior urethra is examined vaginally for masses, tenderness, or expressed discharge from the urethra.

The size and patency of the meatus and the urethra may be evaluated by the urologist's passing instruments of varying diameter through the urethra. This evaluation is performed with different sizes of rubber or plastic catheters or, if preferred, special urologic instruments. A *sound* is a smooth, cylindrical rod with a rounded tip. Its size ranges from 8F to 32F. Figure 55–3 illustrates examples of sounds. The urethra and meatus may be dilated using sounds. Xylocaine jelly or other local anesthetic is

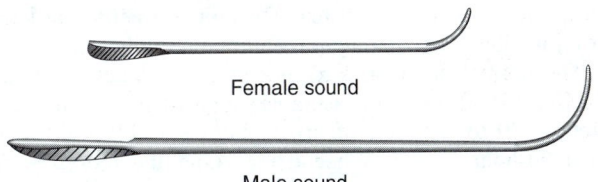

Figure 55–3. Sounds used to calibrate the diameter of the urethra, to determine patency, and (if necessary) to dilate strictures.

applied before the sound is passed under aseptic conditions, beginning with a small-sized sound and increasing in diameter until the largest caliber is found that can be easily inserted. Strictures, which are discussed in Chapter 56, may make insertion more difficult.

Alternative Urinary Outlet

The client who has had a urinary diversion created surgically, such as an ileal conduit or continent urinary reservoir, will have an opening in the abdominal wall. Assess this stoma, and note its location, size, shape, color, patency, and the odor of the urine. Observe the quality and quantity of the drainage. In addition, evaluate the condition of the periostomal skin for color, cleanliness, intactness, and the absence of lesions such as maceration and irritation. For the client with an ileal conduit, observe the cleanliness and appropriateness of the ostomy pouching system to assess the client's educational needs. Finally, assess the client's responses during this part of the examination, for these may indicate the client's acceptance of the urinary diversion.

The client may have a catheter that partially or completely drains the urine from the body. The catheter may be inserted into the bladder, a ureter, or a kidney and may come out of the body through the urethra, the abdomen, or flank. Inspect these catheters during the examination, checking them for patency, location, and cleanliness. Palpate the tubing for sedimentation by rolling it between the thumb and fingers and feeling for a sensation of grit. Observe the tissues around the catheter where it enters the body for cleanliness and the absence of lesions such as inflammation and ulceration. Evaluate the drainage bag for cleanliness and to ensure that a closed system is being maintained.

Related Body Systems

Selected information from other body systems is crucial for correctly assessing urinary tract problems and planning interventions.

Fluid Balance

Accurate *intake* and *output* measurements helps determine the client's fluid status. Intake or output of disproportionate amounts of fluid may indicate volume excess or depletion. Keeping track of intake and output helps identify the presence of important manifestations of abnormal kidney function, such as oliguria, anuria, and polyuria.

The normal adult on a regular diet who takes in about 1200 to 1800 ml of measurable fluids daily should excrete 1200 to 1800 ml of urine plus insensible fluid loss in a 24-hour period. When determining the presence of oliguria, anuria, or polyuria, remember that the output is in relation to intake. *Oliguria* is a urine volume significantly below this amount, usually 400 ml/24 hours (134 ml/8 hours). *Anuria* means the absence of urine production (or less than 100 ml/24 hours). These two conditions may indicate shock, poisoning, or any other process that would interfere with urine formation in the kidney. Anuria could be a normal finding in most clients undergoing renal dialysis. *Polyuria* is significantly larger than normal amounts of urine output when compared with fluid intake. It can be caused by disorders such as acute or chronic renal failure, diabetes mellitus, or diabetes insipidus; following correction of acute renal failure; after an obstruction is removed; or by interventions such as diuretic administration.

When polyuria is present, it is important to distinguish between water diuresis and solute diuresis. *Water diuresis* is characterized by a low urine specific gravity, a low urine osmolality, and a normal-to-elevated serum sodium level. It indicates either a lack of antidiuretic hormone (ADH), as after trauma to the posterior pituitary gland, or unresponsiveness of the renal tubules, as with hypokalemia or hydronephrosis. *Solute diuresis* results from impaired tubular absorption of a particular solute, as may accompany diabetes mellitus or relief of an acute bladder obstruction, as occurs when a client with acute retention has it relieved with a catheter. It is characterized by a high urine specific gravity, an elevated urine osmalality, and a normal or low serum sodium level.

Body weight is a good indicator of fluid gains and losses, provided it is carefully measured daily at the same time and preferably on the same scale and compared with previous findings. A gain or loss of more than 2 lb in 24 hours is considered related to fluid retention or loss. Dry mucous membranes may signal volume depletion, whereas the presence of edema may be a manifestation of volume excess. When assessing edema, it is important to determine its progression or recession. Measuring the girth of an edematous extremity daily provides accurate, objective documentation. See Chapter 15 for more information on fluid balance.

Fluid status assessment also needs to include blood pressure, heart rate, orthostatic vital signs, neck vein distention, and auscultation of lung sounds. Postural pulses taken in the supine position, followed by pulses taken while the client stands, is an objective measurement of dehydration if the standing pulse is greater than 10 beats above the supine pulse.

Nervous System

Renal dysfunction may interfere with normal activity within the nervous system, as when a buildup of calcium causes tetany, decreased calcium produces weakness, or the accumulation of toxins in acute and chronic renal failure causes lethargy. Conversely, the urinary tract depends on an intact nervous system to carry out its main function: removing waste from the body. Any abnormality in nervous stimulation of the urinary organs or their surrounding tissue interferes with the propulsion and expulsion of urine. In addition to assessing gross nervous function (e.g., the ability to walk and maintain balance), the examiner may test the intactness of innervation specific to urinary tract function. Because the anal and urinary sphincters are supplied by branches of the same nerve, the intactness of one may indicate that the other sphincter functions as well. Stroke the perianal skin to test for the presence of the anal sphincter reflex; the sphincter should respond by contracting.

To evaluate anal sphincter tone, insert a gloved, lubricated finger into the anus and note the amount of resistance felt. With the finger still in the rectum, test the bulbocavernosus reflex. Squeeze the glans penis or clitoris or gently jerk on an indwelling catheter. If the S2–4 nerves are intact, this maneuver will contract the external anal sphincter and bulbocavernosus muscle. This is a test for an intact reflex arc, that is, motor function. Other tests evaluating relevant neurologic activity are described later in this chapter.

Integumentary System

Note the color of the skin when assessing renal dysfunction. For instance, erythropoietin deficiency anemia may cause pallor. Deposits of a carotene-like substance, caused by renal excretion failure, may give the skin a yellowish-gray cast. *Dry skin* may indicate chronic renal failure and may also suggest volume depletion, especially in the elderly. Bruises or petechiae may represent bleeding tendencies. Uremic frost, crystal deposits on the skin (found primarily in areas of concentrated perspiration), is a rare, secondary manifestation of severe, prolonged renal failure.

Musculoskeletal System

Assess the client's movements during the examination to (1) determine general body tone and (2) judge the client's physical ability to handle urinary elimination needs and the ability to get to the toilet and manipulate clothing. The muscle groups involved in micturition are the perineal and abdominal muscles. To assess their strength, have the client consciously contract or tighten the perineal and abdominal muscles. Changes in tautness can then be seen and palpated. The ability to purposely interrupt the flow of urine midstream by perineal muscle contraction also indicates adequate perineal musculature.

Cardiovascular System

Monitoring the cardiovascular system can identify fluid and electrolyte imbalances. Most specific to the urinary tract is blood pressure measurement. Hypertension is a finding in many renal diseases and may result from fluid volume overload or disturbance of the renin-angiotensin system. Increasing hypertension can possibly lead to irreversible renal shutdown, and it therefore requires immediate medical action. Assess for the presence of a pericardial friction rub, a common occurrence in the client with pericarditis secondary to uremia.

Respiratory System

To some extent, the quality of respirations reflects the client's fluid and acid-base balance. Respiratory assessment is discussed further in Chapter 39. Assess the lungs for the presence of fluid, which may be associated with fluid excess secondary to renal failure. In addition, during renal failure, the breath may have an odor of urine or fruit-flavored gum, *uremic fetor,* which is the result of toxins built up in the bloodstream.

Other Examinations

Vaginal and rectal examinations are routinely performed to assess urinary problems. If appropriate, inspect and palpate the vagina and rectum to help identify fistulas, masses, prolapses, and diverticula. In the male, because of its proximity to the rectum, the posterior lobe of the prostate can be examined for enlargement, tenderness, or masses. In the female, a vaginal examination can detect prolapse of the bladder. (See Chapter 82 for assessment of male and female genitalia.)

Diagnostic Tests

A number of diagnostic tests are available to evaluate the status of the urinary system. They include laboratory tests; x-ray, ultrasound, and radioisotope studies; pressure profiles; endoscopy; and surgical exploration. The history, physical examination, and results of previous studies determine which procedures to use.

During diagnostic testing, the nurse has many roles. The nurse may be directly involved in collecting and testing specimens and in helping the examiner during certain procedures. The nurse prepares the client for testing and assesses the client after the procedures. Specific studies require particular post-test care, such as monitoring for hemorrhage after a kidney biopsy. The nurse also encourages the client to express concerns and answers questions about the test. Finally, the nurse must be able to incorporate test results appropriately in the client's care plan.

Laboratory Tests

Urine Collection

The accurate outcome of any laboratory test depends on collecting the right kind of specimen in the proper manner, in the right container, and at the right time. Once the specimen has been collected, it must be stored properly until the correct testing procedure is performed and the findings are accurately interpreted. The nurse and appropriate others—the client, people in the household, laboratory personnel—all share this responsibility.

The types of urine specimens include random, voided, clean-catch (midstream), catheter, and timed specimens such as 12-hour or 24-hour collections.

■ Random Specimens

A random specimen is one that can be collected at any time. However, an *early-morning* specimen gives more definitive results for some values such as the kidney's ability to concentrate urine or to identify substances that may not be present in dilute specimens. Generally, the client needs no special preparation, although the female may be asked to wash the perineal area to clean away any collected debris. The specimen is then collected in a clean container. This type of specimen cannot be used for culture and sensitivity tests, because the lack of specific perineal cleaning and the use of an unsterile container contaminate the specimen. Specimens for urine culture and sensitivity tests are often collected as clean-catch specimens.

■ Clean-Catch Specimens

The goal of a clean-catch, or midstream specimen is to reduce as much as possible the contamination of the specimen by external organisms. This type of specimen is usually collected if the urine is to be cultured. Female clients are asked to clean the perineal area. Uncircumcised men are asked to retract (pull back) the foreskin and clean the glans penis before voiding to decrease the risk of contamination. Circumcised men, however, may not need to follow this procedure because there is little difference in urine collected in this way versus a simple voided urine. A midstream specimen is obtained by having the client start the stream of urine in the toilet, then pass the container into the stream to collect about 50 ml of urine, and finish voiding in the toilet. Female clients and uncircumcised men are asked to clean the area around the meatus before starting this procedure.

■ Catheter Specimens

A catheter specimen may be used for culture. Avoid this procedure when possible because of the increased risk of introducing organisms into the urethra or bladder during catheterization. In clients with renal failure especially, there may not be enough urine produced to flush bacteria out, thus increasing the risk of UTI. When catheterization is used, a straight catheter of the smallest size, usually 12F to 14F, is inserted into the bladder under aseptic conditions, either through the urethra or as a suprapubic tap, allowing urine to flow directly from the end of the catheter into a sterile specimen container.

A specimen also may be collected from an indwelling catheter. Urine standing in the collection bag undergoes several chemical changes, may be contaminated with bacteria, and does not reflect the client's current urinary status. For these reasons, it should never be used for urine specimens. Instead, obtain the specimen directly from the catheter or drainage tubing. Opening the drainage system to the air can introduce microorganisms. Most urinary drainage systems have a specimen collection port built into the top of the drainage tubing. The tubing may need to be clamped for 15 to 20 minutes below the port to allow enough urine to accumulate. This self-sealing rubber-covered area is cleaned by rubbing it vigorously with an iodophor or alcohol wipe, and the urine is aspirated with a sterile needle and syringe. If there is no collection port and the catheter is latex, use a small-gauge (25) needle and syringe to aspirate urine from the catheter itself. After cleaning the site with alcohol or iodophor, insert the needle into the catheter distal to the sleeve leading to the balloon, slanting the needle tip toward the drainage tubing to avoid entering the balloon lumen. Puncture the catheter at an angle to allow resealing after the needle is withdrawn. This cannot be performed with a Silastic catheter because it will not reseal after being punctured.

A special procedure is used to obtain a specimen for culture from a person with an ileal conduit, a type of urinary diversion created from segments of the ileum. It is virtually impossible to insert a catheter directly into the conduit without contaminating it with organisms from the stoma or from the first few centimeters of the ileum. Therefore, clean the stomal area with soap and water and rinse it with sterile water. Next, using sterile technique, lubricate the tip of an 8F to 14F straight catheter with water-soluble lubricant and insert it into the stoma about 2 to 5 cm (1–2 inches), gently rotating it if any resistance is felt. Put the connector end of the catheter into a test tube or specimen container and allow the urine to flow by gravity. If there is no urine flow within several minutes, have the client move around or apply gentle suction on the catheter with a 5-ml syringe. Once the specimen is collected, remove the catheter and replace the urine collection bag. Some physicians recommend a two-catheter technique for obtaining a specimen. This requires insertion of a larger outer catheter into the stoma to be used as a protective sheath against contamination. A second, smaller catheter is passed through the larger catheter to collect the urine specimen.

■ Twelve- or 24-Hour Specimens

A 12- or 24-hour specimen is usually collected in one large container. Some of the specimens may need a chemical preservative in the container and refrigeration during the collection process. If refrigeration is not available, the specimen container may be packed in ice or insulated ice packs. In this case, make sure the cooling agent is replaced frequently enough to maintain the specimen at the necessary temperature. When the specimen collection begins, the person voids and this specimen is discarded. All urine voided in the next 12 or 24 hours, as appropriate, is placed in the container. Twelve or 24 hours from the time of the first voiding, instruct the client to void again and add this urine to the specimen. One of the major needs during this collection process is careful communication among all persons involved. If any single urine specimen is inadvertently discarded, the entire procedure must begin again.

Urine Examination

Urine can be examined by direct visualization, microscopy, dipstick, or laboratory tests. The results of these examinations may indicate pathologic changes in the urinary tract as well as in other parts of the body.

■ Routine Urinalysis

A routine urinalysis is usually performed on a single, random specimen, although a midstream or catheter specimen may be used. The Normal Physical Assessment Findings feature summarizes the usual observations made during this test and the normal findings.

Color

The color of urine normally ranges from pale yellow to deep amber, depending on its concentration. Some color changes occur because of medications or food ingested, whereas other colors may indicate pathologic processes. Foods that often cause red urine include blackberries, rhubarb, beets, and foods containing red dyes. Ingesting large amounts of carotene causes a bright-yellow urine. Table 55–1 shows some common medications producing urinary color changes.

The most common significant color change indicating a pathologic disorder results from bleeding in the urinary tract. Bleeding in the upper tract produces dark-red or smoky-gray urine, whereas bleeding in the lower tract

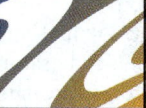

NORMAL PHYSICAL ASSESSMENT FINDINGS

Urinary System

Inspection

Urinary tract organs are not visible except for a distended bladder. The external urethral orifice should be pink without discharge.

Auscultation

No renal bruit is apparent abdominally or over the right or left costovertebral angle (CVA) on the back.

Percussion

Bladder with more than 150 ml urine can be percussed above the pubic symphysis. Kidneys can be percussed using fist percussion on the back at the right and left CVA. Kidneys should not exhibit tenderness.

Palpation

Each kidney may be identified by bimanual palpation. The lower pole of each kidney can be palpated between the left and right CVA on the back and left and right lower rib margins anteriorly. No tenderness should be elicited.

Table 55-1. Common Medications that Produce Urine Color Change	
Medication	**Color Change in Urine**
Amitriptyline	Blue or green
Anthraquinone laxatives	Reddish-brown in acid urine; red in alkaline urine
Chloroquine	Rusty-yellow
Chlorzoxazone	Orange or purple-red
Diuretics	Colorless or pale yellow
Levodopa, methyldopa	Red or brown in hypochlorite toilet bleach
Methylene blue	Green
Multiple vitamins (with riboflavin)	Bright yellow
Nitrofurantoin	Dark amber to orange; may be dark brown to black
Phenazopyridine	Orange-brown, orange-red, or red
Phenolphthalein	Pink-red in alkaline urine
Phenothiazines	Red, red-brown, or pink
Phenytoin	Red, red-brown, or pink
Rifampin	Bright orange-red
Sulfasalazine	Orange-yellow
Triamterene	Blue or green

appears as red urine. Other color changes from pathologic conditions include red-brown or tea-colored urine, due to the release of myoglobin from severely damaged muscle tissue; dark-yellow or green urine indicating the presence of urobilinogen or bilirubin; and blue-green urine produced by *Pseudomonas* organisms.

Opacity

Freshly voided urine is normally transparent. It becomes cloudy on standing, but this can be reversed by adding a few drops of acid. Increases in opacity, denoting a pathologic condition, usually result from the presence of bacteria, crystals, or other foreign material in the urine.

Specific Gravity

Specific gravity indicates the concentration of the urine. This test can be used to estimate the client's general fluid balance status and the kidneys' ability to concentrate urine. Because one of the major functions of the kidney is to maintain fluid balance, typically the more concentrated the urine, the greater the fluid depletion. Conversely, well-hydrated persons have more dilute urine, with specific gravities as low as 1.002. Typically, clients with a history of infections or other problems are encouraged to be very well hydrated to maintain dilute urine and a high output. For renal function, specific gravity primarily indicates the ability of the kidneys to concentrate and dilute urine. When the kidneys lose these abilities, the urine no longer reflects physiologic stimuli and the specific gravity becomes fixed at a level equal to that of the plasma, usually 1.010 (isosthenuria). This occurs with tubular disease or endocrine disease involving ADH insufficiency. Contrast media used during x-ray procedures can produce specific gravity readings above 1.040. Other substances in the urine, such as molecules of glucose or protein, also can cause high values.

Osmolality

Urine osmolality is more precise than specific gravity for measuring the concentrating ability of the kidneys. This is because the former is a constant weight-to-weight relationship and is not unduly affected by the presence of glucose or protein. Urine osmolality increases in hypernatremia, acidosis, and shock. It decreases in diabetes insipidus, hypercalcemia, excessive fluid intake, renal tubular acidosis, severe pyelonephritis, and sometimes hyperglycemia.

pH

Urinary pH usually reflects the plasma pH, with alkalinization or additional acidification occurring to maintain the body's acid-base balance. Metabolic alkalosis, low protein diets high in vegetables and citrus fruits, large amounts of carbonated beverages, alkalinizing medications such as sodium bicarbonate and acetazolamide, and ammonia-splitting bacteria all produce alkaline urine. Urinary pH also indicates renal tubular acidosis in which tubular reabsorption is impaired. Strongly acid urine results from metabolic acidosis, metabolic alkalosis in potassium deficiency, a high protein diet, uncontrolled diabetes, and some medications, such as ammonium chloride and mandelic acid.

Glucose

Glycosuria (glucose in urine) depends on the plasma glucose level and the renal threshold. The level of sugar in the urine indicates the point at which the blood sugar level exceeds the reabsorptive capacity of the kidneys and glucose is excreted. Glycosuria normally results from eating a heavy meal or from emotional stress. IV solutions containing glucose may also raise the serum glucose level above the renal threshold. Hyperalimentation solutions always breach this threshold, so clients who receive this form of nutrition frequently need supplemental insulin. Abnormal findings of glucose in the urine appear with uncontrolled diabetes, other pancreatic disorders, and impaired proximal tubular reabsorption.

Ketones

Ketones are found in the urine when the body's fat stores are metabolized for energy, thus producing an excess of metabolic end products. This occurs with uncontrolled diabetes and other states of altered carbohydrate metabolism, fasting, pregnancy and lactation, excessive lipid metabolism, and severe infections accompanied by vomiting and diarrhea. False-positive findings may be caused by levodopa and phenolphthalein as well.

Protein

The protein usually measured during a routine urinalysis is albumin. Although frequently a benign finding, *proteinuria* often denotes abnormal glomerular permeability, decreased tubular reabsorption, or an overflow of protein in the plasma. Factors influencing glomerular basement membrane permeability include exercise, vasoactive substances such as norepinephrine, and diseases that hinder normal renal microarchitecture. Examples of systemic diseases that may cause proteinuria are diabetes mellitus, systemic lupus erythematosus, lymphoma, solid tumors, hypertension, preeclampsia, hepatitis, sickle cell disease, secondary syphilis, febrile diseases, and physical stress, such as trauma or surgery. Medications that may cause a false-positive result include penicillamine, gold, captopril, probenecid, and fenoprofen.

One of the proteinurias not attributed to albumin is Bence Jones protein, which is found in multiple myeloma. Bence Jones protein is not included in a routine urinalysis but is detected either by heating the specimen or by electrophoresis. Other protein components may be found in the macroglobulinemia and various tubular defects.

There are three main categories of *benign proteinuria*: (1) functional (associated with high fever, exposure to cold, emotional stress, and strenuous exercise), (2) idiopathic transient, and (3) orthostatic (protein appears in the urine only when the person is standing). Proteinuria usually disappears when the predisposing factor is removed.

Pathologic proteinuria usually indicates serious renal disease. In the absence of other abnormal findings, the follow-up of an isolated instance of proteinuria may consist of serial urinalyses to make sure the proteinuria does indeed disappear. However, if proteinuria persists, there may be further evaluation of the urinary system.

Bilirubin

Bilirubinuria, the presence of bilirubin in the urine, usually indicates extrahepatic biliary tract obstruction. Other causes include hepatitis, portal inflammation, and hepatocellular damage. Use a fresh urine specimen for this test. When a urine specimen containing bilirubin is shaken, a yellow foam is produced. A false-positive finding may occur in a person taking chlorpromazine.

Red Blood Cells

Hematuria, or the presence of red blood cells, in the urine, can be either microscopic (seen only under the microscope) or gross (obviously bloody to the naked eye). Hematuria is sometimes accompanied by other manifestations. Asymptomatic hematuria often presents a challenging diagnostic problem and requires meticulous evaluation. The cause may be benign or may indicate a pathologic condition. Although the cause of the hematuria may never be found, rigorous investigation is required. Hematuria is always considered a manifestation of urinary tract carcinoma until proved otherwise. Hematuria also may appear in renal tuberculosis, sickle cell anemia (or sickle cell trait), IgA and IgG nephropathy, systemic lupus erythematosus, and polyarteritis nodosa.

A study involving 200 clients with asymptomatic hematuria found that 20% had significant lesions, usually low-stage, low-grade vesical neoplasms; renal parenchymal disease; or ureteral calculus; 32% had moderately significant findings such as renal calculi, bacterial cystitis, vesicoureteral reflux, and vesical diverticulum; and 55% had insignificant lesions, with their hematuria resulting from prostatic hyperplasia, urethrotrigonitis, renal cyst, and cystocele.[8]

Hemolytic anemia and hemolytic transfusion reactions produce detectable hemoglobin in the urine. Anticoagulants and the long-term use of analgesics leading to papillary necrosis also can produce hematuria. Hematuria following trauma, especially in the abdominal or pelvic area or a direct blow to the kidneys, may indicate injury to the urinary tract. Long-distance runners frequently exhibit hematuria (often with clots), which disappears as they recover from the run.

When collecting urine from a woman, note whether she is menstruating, because menstrual blood contaminating the specimen will give a false-positive result. Povidone-iodine washed into the urine specimen will give a false-negative result for occult blood. Finally, it is helpful to determine when during voiding blood appears: (1) bleeding only at the onset of micturition usually indicates lesions below the bladder; (2) constant bleeding throughout voiding denotes a bladder or upper urinary tract lesion; and (3) terminal bleeding, occurring only during the last few drops of voiding, localizes the bladder neck or prostate as the site. As with proteinuria, asymptomatic hematuria may be monitored initially with repeat urinalyses to determine whether the finding is indeed transient. If bleeding persists, further evaluation is necessary.

White Blood Cells

White blood cells in the urine usually indicates an infectious process somewhere in the urinary tract. When accompanied by casts, renal epithelial cells, a few red blood cells, or bacteria, the leukocytosis is usually the result of a kidney infection. Bladder infections give rise to leukocytosis with red blood cells and bladder epithelial cells, but no casts. Noninfectious inflammatory diseases of the urinary tract may also produce white blood cells in the urine.

Pyuria means pus, or a large collection of white blood cells, in the urine. A quantitative determination of more than five clumps of white blood cells per high-powered field indicates urinary pathogens. A large collection of pus may make the urine turbid and foul-smelling. Although most pyuria is caused by UTI, it also may result from renal calculi, obstruction, irritation of the urothelium by a foreign body, tumors, or renal tuberculosis.

Bacteria

Because urine is normally sterile, *bacteriuria* represents infection within the urinary tract or contamination of the specimen. The presence of multiple organisms usually denotes contamination. Bacteria in the urine, whether accompanied by physical manifestations of UTI or not, needs further evaluation with urine cultures (see p. 1560).

Casts

Casts are formed elements organized in the nephrons (especially the tubules) by agglutination of protein. They most likely are formed in the distal tubules and the collecting ducts. Casts usually indicate tubular or glomerular disease. There are several varieties of casts and the identification of the specific type helps pinpoint the contributing problem.

A few hyaline casts can be found normally, especially after strenuous exercise. Some experts hypothesize that their presence in persons at rest may indicate future renal or cardiovascular disease. Casts also are found in acute glomerulonephritis, acute pyelonephritis, malignant hypertension, chronic renal disease, congestive heart failure, and diabetic nephropathy. Contrary to expectations, casts may not be present in advanced renal disease.

Red blood cell casts denote bleeding within the nephron as the result of glomerulonephritis, acute renal allograft rejection, or acute tubular necrosis. Red blood cell casts may be the only manifestation of renal involvement in pathologic conditions such as systemic lupus erythematosus, subacute bacterial endocarditis, arteritis, and diabetic nephropathy.

White blood cell, or leukocyte, casts indicate bacterial infection and noninfective inflammatory disease. They often are hard to distinguish from epithelial casts, which denote, among other conditions, sloughing of renal tubular epithelium due to eclampsia, poisoning with heavy metals, amyloidosis, and acute renal allograft rejection. White blood cell casts and epithelial casts are frequently intermixed.

Granular casts indicate conditions such as renal parenchymal disease, acute renal transplant rejection, pyelonephritis, chronic lead poisoning, and viral disease. Granular casts also may be found in the urine after strenuous exercise. The final stages of tubular inflammation and degeneration produce waxy casts. Chronic renal failure and chronic and acute renal allograft rejection cause the formation of waxy casts. Fatty casts represent the degeneration of cellular casts incorporated with fat droplets or cholesterol esters. They indicate a nephrotic syndrome or diabetic nephropathy.

Crystals

Crystalluria (crystals in the urine) may or may not indicate disease. Common findings are calcium oxalate, uric acid, and urate crystals in acid urine, and phosphate, carbonate, and amorphous crystals in alkaline urine. The presence of crystals in the urine is an important predisposing factor in *calculus formation.*

In addition to the routine urinalysis, several other tests may be performed to examine the urine. Twelve- and 24-hour urine specimens determine the secretion rate of a number of elements. Tests measuring urinary levels of sodium, potassium, calcium, chloride, phosphorus, and uric acid and quantitative determination of proteins help diagnosis and treat renal problems.

Serial Urine Tests

Serial urines are collected to determine whether hematuria is increasing or decreasing. The procedure is simple. When the client voids, save a sample of the urine in a cup labeled 1. Do the same for the next two voidings, labeling the cups 2 and 3, respectively. When the client voids a fourth time, discard sample 1, and the new sample becomes sample 3. In this way, the nurse or physician can examine the samples and note any change in the hematuria over time and voidings. The voidings are usually collected on a daily basis.

An alternative way to obtain serial urines is by collecting three specimens from the same voiding. The initial voiding goes in cup 1, the midstream urine in cup 2, and the remainder of urine in cup 3. Urine collection in this manner permits an assessment of the source of the bleeding (i.e., kidney, bladder, or urethra).

Urine Cultures

Because the kidneys, ureters, and bladder normally are sterile, the urine formed and transported in them also is sterile. Organisms typically colonize the distal portion of the urethra, but these bacteria ordinarily do not reach further up the urinary tract. Therefore, the presence of organisms in the urine is an abnormal finding. Any clinical manifestations reported by the client or the presence of significant bacteriuria or urinary leukocytosis indicates the need to examine the urine further.

Urine cultures are done to identify the specific organisms and to estimate the number of bacteria that are present. Urine cultures should always be collected before antibiotics are started. Most cultures are done using the midstream clean-catch method. If the client is unable to cooperate or if vaginal contamination occurs, a catheterized specimen may be obtained. If there are a large number of different organisms in a voided specimen, contamination of the specimen probably has occurred.

The significance of the number of bacteria present depends on how the urine was collected. A low colony count in a catheterized specimen is more significant than a similar count in a voided specimen. In general, any colony count of 10^5 or more bacteria per millimeter is considered diagnostic of an infection. Even if the culture shows a lower number of bacteria, infection should be considered if the client is symptomatic.

Once the causative organisms are identified, sensitivity tests are performed to determine the proper antibiotics to combat their growth. Once the urine has been obtained for the culture and sensitivity, the client may be started on a broad-spectrum antibiotic until the final sensitivity report is available. The determination of sensitivity tests is becoming even more important as the number of resistant organisms increases. Treatment with an ineffective antibiotic is costly in terms of lost time and money and of continued discomfort and possible injury to the client. Be aware of culture and sensitivity reports. If these reports are overlooked, treatment with nonspecific broad-spectrum antibiotics may continue longer than is necessary. The culture and sensitivity report is usually obtained within 72 hours.

Clearance Studies

Although direct examination of the urine gives a gross estimate of renal function, more definitive measures, such as clearance studies, sometimes are necessary. Clearance is the amount of plasma totally cleared of a given substance in 1 minute.

The kidneys clear the blood of certain substances by means of filtration and excretion. Clearance studies determine the glomerular filtration rate and tubular excretory ability by measuring clearance rates of creatinine, urea, insulin, para-aminohippuric acid, phenolsulfonphthalein, and radioactive isotopes (Fig. 55–4). Quantitative renal excretory function is the difference between the filtration rate of any given substance across the glomerular wall and the rate at which the substance is then excreted in the urine.

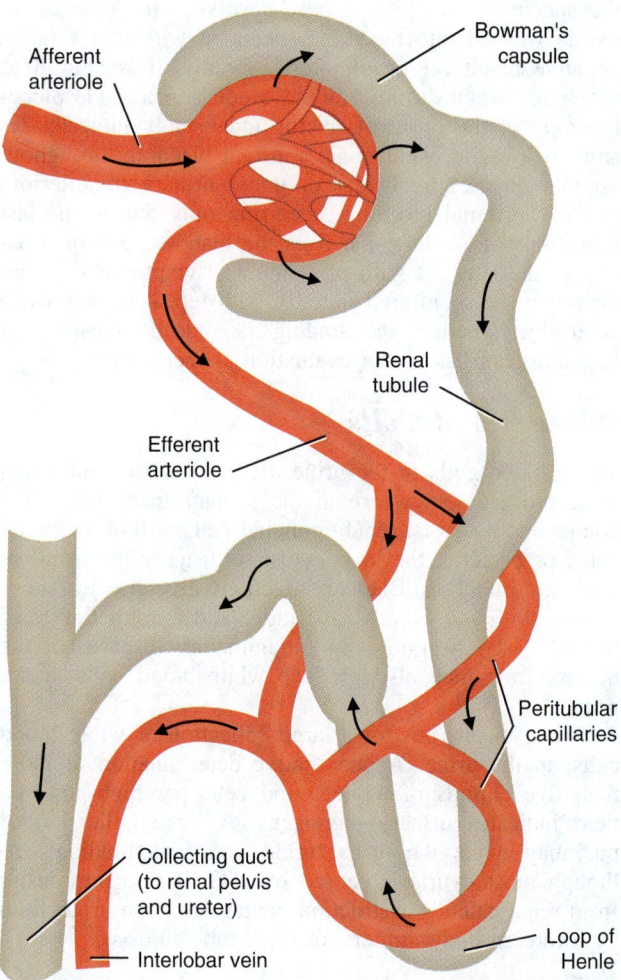

Figure 55–4. Renal clearance measures the kidney's ability to remove a substance from the plasma in 1 minute. It is measured by assessing the quantity of the substance in urine collected over a specific period of time.

In order to measure the glomerular filtration rate of a substance, the substance must be one that is filtered freely in the glomerulus but not reabsorbed or secreted in the tubule. The creatinine clearance test is generally used to reflect the glomerular filtration rate.

Creatinine clearance is currently the most accurate measure of the glomerular filtration rate. Virtually all formed creatinine, a product of muscle metabolism, is filtered by the glomerulus, and as the glomerular filtration rate falls, the serum creatinine rises. Urine for this test is collected over a 12- or 24-hour period, although a 24-hour specimen is preferred.

The test may begin any time, although it is best to begin and end the test in the early morning. A fasting blood sample is drawn sometime during the collection period. An adult female normally excretes 0.8 to 1.7 g/24 hours and a male excretes 1.0 to 1.9 g/24 hours. Use caution when applying these values to people older than 40 years of age. Longitudinal studies demonstrate declining creatinine clearance rates after age 34, with the rate of decline speeding up after age 65. This decline probably is due to reduced muscle mass and renal blood flow.

Urea clearance is used sometimes. Because the rate of tubular secretion varies with the rate of urine flow, it is not as useful as creatinine clearance. To perform this procedure, ensure a urine flow of at least 2 ml/minute. Have the client fast for several hours before the test. The client empties the bladder and then drinks two or more glasses of water. Exactly 1 hour later, the client voids and a blood sample for blood urea nitrogen (BUN) is taken. At this point, the client drinks another two or more glasses of water, and in exactly 1 hour voids again. At each voiding, the entire specimen is kept, carefully labeled with the time, and sent to the laboratory. If necessary, the bladder is catheterized to obtain an accurate specimen. The normal clearance is 65 to 99 ml/minute or 40 to 69 ml/minute if the urine flow rate is below 2 ml/minute.

Radioisotopes may be used to determine clearance rates. This procedure, called a *renogram,* involves the IV injection of a minute amount of a radioactive compound. The client is positioned supine, prone, or sitting with a scintillation camera placed posterior to the kidneys. A third radiation counter may be placed over the chest to monitor the disappearance of the isotope from the blood. The radioactive emission rate is recorded on videotape over a period of 15 to 30 minutes. A recording also may be made over the bladder just prior to and just after voiding at the end of the test. The test does not require special preparation of the client. Also, because the dose of radioactivity is so low, there are no special precautions to observe in caring for the client or the urine specimen.

This test measures renal blood flow and active tubular transport, glomerular filtration, tubular secretion, and excretion. Each kidney can be compared with the other in terms of these measurements. There is no particular follow-up care. The client can void into a commode or toilet. Although a small amount of radiation may be present, it is not dangerous.

Other techniques using radioisotopes to measure renal function use blood determination to calculate clearance rates; for example, a radioisotope is injected and plasma samples are drawn to determine the amount of remaining isotope.

■ Concentration and Dilution Tests

The loss of the kidney's ability to concentrate and dilute urine indicates significant renal tubular damage. Normally, as the body becomes fluid-depleted, larger volumes of water are reabsorbed, resulting in more concentrated urine with a specific gravity greater than 1.020. Conversely, with increased fluid intake, more water is excreted, causing more dilute urine with a specific gravity often as low as 1.002. One of the first kidney functions to be lost is this ability to concentrate and dilute urine. In severe renal damage, the specific gravity may become fixed at a level of 1.008 to 1.012, regardless of the amount of fluid intake.

Several tests can be performed to evaluate this aspect of renal function. The Fishberg and Addis tests frequently are used to measure concentration ability. The Fishberg concentration test (a 12-hour test) involves withholding all food or fluid after the evening meal. An early-morning urine specimen is collected, and the specific gravity is determined. A reading of less than 1.024 suggests renal function impairment. The Addis concentration test calls for severe fluid restriction for 24 hours. The amount of fluid allowed the client differs with each laboratory. A 12-hour specimen is collected during the last half of the fluid-restricted period. A possibility of vascular collapse exists during the period of water deprivation, so observe the client closely. Because of the risk to already compromised kidneys, clients with renal failure are not subjected to these tests. Factors that can interfere with the kidney's normal concentrating ability include decreased sodium intake, a low protein diet, and glycosuria.

For dilution tests, the client first empties the bladder and then receives a measured amount of fluid either (1) by drinking 1200 ml of water or fruit juice within 30 minutes or (2) through a rapid IV infusion. Physical activity is kept to a minimum during the test to prevent fluid losses through other routes. Urine specimens are collected at specified intervals—usually every 30 minutes—for 3 hours. The volume is measured and the specific gravity determined for each specimen. With normal renal function, the entire 1200 ml should be voided, and the specific gravity will be about 1.002. This test is risky for people with compromised cardiac and renal systems because of the large volume of fluid taken.

■ Cytologic Examination

Examining cells exfoliated from the urinary tract can be useful in diagnosing cellular problems. The specimen needs good cellular content, so an early-morning specimen is preferred. If the specimen is obtained through catheterization, be sure to note this information on the specimen container, because epithelial cells from the urethra or bladder may have been added to the urine by the catheter. If the specimen will not be examined immediately, it may be refrigerated for up to 48 hours or mixed with an appropriate fixative agent. Usually, three random specimens are collected for cytologic evaluation and compared before concluding the presence or absence of disease in the urinary tract. The three specimens may be obtained from three different times within 1 day, 3 days in a row at the same time, or three times in the course of a month.

Cytologic examination may help in identifying and monitoring the progress of inflammatory processes resulting from chemical toxins, autoimmune disease, or bodily substances (e.g., hemoglobin and myoglobin); infectious processes (including bacterial, fungal, and viral); and neoplastic disease. Although it is not effective in the early detection of renal neoplasms, cytologic examination is very accurate in identifying urinary tract malignancies below the renal parenchyma, frequently demonstrating the presence of tumors before they are visible endoscopically.

Blood Studies

■ Blood Chemistry

Measuring selected components in the blood aids in evaluating renal function. Probably the most frequently used determinant is the BUN. Urea is the end product of protein metabolism and is normally excreted from the body through the kidneys. Therefore, any renal function impairment causes an increase in the plasma urea level. The BUN starts to rise when the glomerular filtration rate falls below 40% to 60%. Unfortunately, the BUN also can be elevated by such nonrenal factors as hypovolemia, excessive protein intake, starvation, bleeding into the gut, surgery or trauma, fever, exertion, or corticosteroids. Therefore, this value must be evaluated very cautiously.

The serum creatinine level usually is measured along with the BUN. Because creatinine also is excreted through the kidneys, increased serum levels indicate decreased renal function. Creatinine excretion is not affected significantly by dietary or fluid intake, and it is thought to be a more accurate indicator of renal function than the BUN. A rising serum creatinine level indicates nephron loss. A normal creatinine level can be found with up to a 25% nephron loss. Twice the normal creatinine level signifies a 50% nephron loss and the beginning of diminished renal reserve. A creatinine level eight times the normal value indicates a 75% nephron loss with definite renal insufficiency. A creatinine level 10 or more times normal signals at least a 90% nephron loss and indicates end-stage renal disease.

Sometimes a BUN-creatinine ratio is used as a renal function indicator, with the normal ratio being $10:1$. BUN elevations in relation to serum creatinine denote renal impairment due to prerenal causes such as blood loss, severe diarrhea, heart failure, and liver disease. With prerenal causes the ratio increases to $20:1$ or higher.

There are specific tests associated with other portions of the urinary tract. Prostate-specific antigen, other prostate diagnostic tests, and testicular markers are discussed in Chapters 82 and 83.

■ Hematology

Inspecting a random blood sample provides some data about renal function as well as the progress of disease processes within the urinary tract. A reduced red blood cell count, hemoglobin, and hematocrit may indicate bleeding from the urinary tract or may signal reduced erythropoietic function by the kidney. An increased white blood cell count with increased neutrophils may denote an infectious process, whereas a return to normal values represents recovery from infection.

Radiologic Studies

In most diagnostic protocols, examining the urinary tract by radiographic study is the next step in identifying actual or potential malfunction. These studies may be performed with or without the use of contrast material and may involve static or dynamic films, or both. Because these examinations are performed in the x-ray department, the nurse's primary responsibility is to prepare the client physically and mentally for the procedure. This helps ensure accurate results.

X-Ray Study of the Kidneys, Ureters, and Bladder

An x-ray study of the kidneys, ureters, and bladder (KUB) is a plain film of the lower abdomen. It involves no contrast medium, poses no risk to the client, and can be performed without considering the remaining kidney function. The outline of these organs demonstrates their size, shape, and location. This helps identify soft tissue masses, malformation, and radiopaque calculi.

Intravenous Pyelography

Intravenous pyelography (IVP) involves the IV injection of a radiopaque contrast medium that is filtered by the kidneys and excreted through the urinary tract. This examination helps identify the absence or presence, location, size, and configuration of the kidneys, ureters, and bladder. The IVP also helps determine filling of the renal calices and pelvis. A postvoiding film is obtained to assess the efficiency of bladder emptying. If bladder emptying is incomplete, a voiding cystourethrogram (VCUG) helps determine the cause of retention. The VCUG is obtained to evaluate the size and shape of the bladder showing trabeculations; diverticuli; urethral abnormalities, especially in men; and urethral reflux. Clients with an elevated serum creatinine cannot have an IVP performed.

During the examination, the client is placed supine on the x-ray table. Initially, a KUB film is taken as a scout film. This helps to ensure the bowel is clear enough to continue with the procedure. It also screens for calculi in the renal collecting system. Because the contrast medium in the collecting ducts is the same density as any calcification in this area, some types of stones can be missed easily during the IVP. The radiopaque contrast medium is injected IV as a bolus or through an infusion drip. The contrast medium normally produces a flushed face, a warm feeling in the body, nausea, and a salty taste in the mouth. These are transitory effects and do not mean the study should be stopped.

The iodine in the substance, however, may cause severe allergic reactions in hypersensitive clients. Before the examination begins, carefully question the client about any history of allergies. A known sensitivity to iodinated contrast media is an absolute contraindication to continuing the procedure unless the client has been premedicated with a steroid infusion. If the client is unsure about an iodine allergy, ask the client about an allergy to shellfish. The presence of allergy to shellfish requires skin testing before IV injection.

A negative skin test or history, however, does not guarantee there will be no reaction. If any manifestations of allergic responses such as itching, hives, wheezing, or other manifestations or respiratory distress appear, call for immediate discontinuation of the injection. Antihistamine, epinephrine, vasopressors, oxygen, and cardiopulmonary resuscitation equipment must be available to halt the anaphylactic response.

In addition to possible anaphylactic reactions from the contrast medium, cases of acute renal failure following injection of the contrast medium have been documented. Although the incidence is low, assess carefully for this adverse effect. Predisposing factors include vascular disease, multiple myeloma, diabetes mellitus, and preexisting renal insufficiency. These factors, besides the fluid depletion, markedly increase the risk of renal failure. Following the test, the nurse should force fluids while carefully monitoring renal function and output.

After the contrast medium is injected, films are taken at regular intervals, usually at 2 minutes, 5 minutes, 15 minutes, 20 minutes, 30 minutes, and 60 minutes. The client is usually kept supine throughout this time, although upright, oblique, and lateral films may be obtained as well. Ureteral compression is frequently performed to enhance distention of the collecting system and upper ureters. A compression band with inflatable balloons or sandbags is applied across the client's lower abdomen after the 5-minute film and is left in place until the 10-minute films are obtained. Sometimes, with delayed renal functioning, additional x-ray studies may be needed 1 to 2 hours later.

In advanced renal failure or with a unilateral, nonvisualized kidney, a large bolus of undiluted contrast medium may be used to better visualize the urinary system. This technique is called high-bolus urography. In preparing the client for this examination, it is usually unnecessary to restrict fluids. Risk increases slightly with this technique. Potentially serious electrocardiographic abnormalities have occurred in older people with evidence of previous heart disease. Identified risk factors include a previously abnormal electrocardiogram, coronary artery disease, and congestive heart failure.

Preprocedure Care. Physical preparation of the client for an IVP generally involves restricting fluids and cleaning out the bowel. The client should not eat or drink after midnight before the examination. This relative fluid depletion allows the radiopaque contrast medium to be more concentrated when it enters the kidney, thus providing clearer films. If the person is receiving IV fluids, the infusion rate may be slowed for several hours before the study. Fluid depletion is contraindicated in clients with multiple myeloma, severe diabetes mellitus, or uric acid nephropathy. These conditions can seriously compromise the renal function of clients with reduced renal perfusion due to decreased renal blood flow, predisposing them to the development of acute renal failure. If these clients must have an IVP, they should be well hydrated.

Because the kidneys are located retroperitoneally, the bowel must be cleared of gas and fecal material that may partially or totally obscure the kidneys. Cathartics are usually taken the evening before the examination. This part of the preparation, however, may be omitted in clients with suspected or known inflammatory bowel disease, or when vigorous colonic activity is otherwise contraindicated. If cathartics were not effective or not given for any reason, the client will need an enema or a rectal suppository early in the morning before the x-ray study.

Postprocedure Care. When the client has completed the examination, continue to observe for reactions to the contrast medium. Counteract the fasting and fluid depletion with food and increased fluids.

Retrograde Pyelography

Retrograde pyelography involves passing a small-caliber catheter through a cytoscope into the ureters and into the renal pelvis. (Cystoscopy is described later in this chapter.)

A small amount of contrast medium is injected into the kidney through the catheters, and x-rays are taken to delineate the collecting system. The client may feel some discomfort in the kidney region when the contrast medium is injected, but there is no actual pain unless the renal pelvis has been overdistended. As the catheters are withdrawn, more contrast medium is injected, and films are taken to record the outline of the ureters.

Retrograde pyelography is indicated when the renal collection system or ureters have not been satisfactorily visualized during IVP. It is also helpful in assessing the degree of ureteral obstruction. It can be used in clients who are hypersensitive to IV contrast media because the contrast medium is not absorbed through the mucous membranes.

There are no particular contraindications to this procedure, although it does have some risk. Entering the urinary tract occasionally causes primary UTI or aggravates preexisting infections. Manipulating the ureters also may cause edema, resulting in temporary obstruction to urine flow.

Preparing and caring for the client during and after this procedure is the same as that for the client undergoing an IVP and a cystoscopy.

Computed Tomography

This procedure, also called a CT or CAT scan, involves an x-ray beam sweeping around the body and taking multiple, thin, cross-sectional pictures of the internal structure. This procedure allows measurement of various tissue densities. The computer then uses these density readings to reconstruct visual images of the body structures. IV administration of contrast medium, using either bolus technique or IV infusion, may be used to enhance the image. This contrast medium is the same as that used in the IVP, so a potential for an anaphylactic reaction or for acute renal failure exists.

There are several indications for CT scanning. These include examining the renal and urinary tract when excretory urography and ultrasound have been unsatisfactory; characterizing renal retroperitoneal and pelvic masses; staging and monitoring renal tumors; evaluating a nonfunctioning kidney, urinary tract trauma, a transplanted kidney, suspected renal calculi, or gas-forming infections; and CT-guided procedures.

Other than preparing for potential complications, there is no special preparation or postprocedure care for the client. If a contrast medium is to be used, question the client concerning possible allergies to the media.

Magnetic Resonance Imaging

Magnetic resonance imaging (MRI) provides coronal, sagittal, or transverse views of the kidney, bladder, or prostate. It provides exceptionally clear images of the tissue, allowing visualization of small abnormalities. MRI is used to identify soft tissue masses either inside the urinary tract or impinging upon it. It also is used to assess the bladder and prostate for malignancies.

Preparation of the client for an MRI requires that anything metal be removed prior to the examination. Although it is not a painful examination, some clients complain of a claustrophobic feeling associated with the test. Often music is piped into the scanner and there is usually an intercom in the machine so the client can communicate with the technician. There are no complications associated with an MRI, although clients with pacemakers, surgical clips, or any metallic foreign body cannot undergo the procedure. Grossly obese clients may be difficult to scan and may even have trouble fitting into the scanner itself.

Cystography

Procedure. X-ray examination of the bladder or urethra can be performed separately or together. During cystography, contrast medium is injected into the bladder through a urethral catheter. When the bladder is full, films are taken to profile the size and shape of the bladder and detect the presence of any vesicoureteral reflux. It also can be used to detect the presence of extravasation from a puncture or fistula of the bladder, large tumors, or bladder diverticula. This examination may be used in clients with pelvic trauma to assess for injury to the bladder. The client is frequently asked to void, which may reveal a voiding problem, and a follow-up x-ray is performed to measure the amount of residual urine.

Preprocedure Care. There is no particular preparation for this test. It should be thoroughly explained to the client prior to the test.

Postprocedure Care. There are no specific post-test nursing interventions aside from assuring the client has voided.

Urethrography

A retrograde urethrogram outlines the inner size and shape of the urethra and checks for extravasation and strictures. In males, x-ray studies are performed after a thick, jelly-like radiopaque substance is injected via a wide-mouthed syringe placed in the urethral meatus. This material usually reaches only as far as the urogenital diaphragm. In females, the procedure requires a less viscous contrast medium and a special urethral catheter.

Voiding Cystourethrography

The VCUG provides visualization of urethral lesions or diverticula, vesicoureteral reflux, and bladder and urethral obstructions. The radiopaque material is instilled into the bladder through a uretheral catheter. Then the catheter is removed and the client is asked to void. Films are taken during the voiding process to observe the contrast medium flow. The micturition process may be recorded on film to better visualize the movement of the contrast medium. Voiding in the presence of other people can be very embarrassing for the client and may even interfere with the ability to void. Giving emotional support and screens placed judiciously may help put the client at ease.

Renal Angiography

Procedure. Renal angiography makes it possible to visualize the renal vasculature. It is used to (1) diagnose renal artery stenosis or renal vein thrombosis, (2) study renovascular hypertension, (3) demonstrate vascular damage after trauma, (4) investigate causes of acute renal failure, and (5) differentiate highly vascular tumors from avascular cysts.

Renal angiography involves injecting a radiopaque contrast medium into the renal vascular tree and taking serial x-rays to outline blood vessels. Access to the circulation is usually through the femoral artery. A guidewire is threaded into the artery through an arterial needle. The needle is then removed, leaving the guidewire in place, and a radiopaque flexible catheter is passed over the guidewire. Using fluoroscopy, the catheter and wire are advanced through the femoral and iliac arteries into the aorta. When the catheter is in position at the renal arteries, the guidewire may be removed and contrast medium injected; or the wire and catheter may be guided into the renal artery itself before the contrast medium is injected. The latter procedure is called selective renal arteriography. Once the contrast medium has been injected, films are taken at the rate of two to three per second for several seconds to show filling and emptying of the renal artery tree. Delayed films are usually performed to visualize the function of the renal veins.

There are alternative sites for vascular access. A translumbar aortogram involves direct puncture of the aorta at the renal arteries with a long needle. Puncturing the axillary artery or antecubital vein also may be done.

In addition to anaphylactic reactions and possible renal damage due to the radiopaque contrast medium, several other serious potential complications may result from this procedure. Hemorrhaging along the route of the vessel puncture may be external or, especially with a translumbar aortogram, internal. Vascular injury may occur at the puncture site or anywhere along the path of the guidewire and catheter. Thrombosis or embolism can occur as a result of plaque dislodging from the vessel walls during the procedure.

Preprocedure Care. Circulation and sensation should be carefully assessed prior to the procedure in the leg that will be used for the test. Unless careful pretest assessments are made, postprocedure changes might be overlooked. Pre-examination preparation is the same as for the IVP, including testing the client for hypersensitivity to the contrast medium. This procedure is usually performed under local anesthesia, although preprocedure sedation frequently is given. A consent is required.

Postprocedure Care. One of the chief potential side effects of this examination is post-vessel puncture hemorrhage. Pressure dressings are applied over the puncture site immediately after the catheter is removed. Observe the area frequently for several hours for manifestations of fresh bleeding. The client usually is placed on bedrest for several hours to allow complete sealing of the puncture site. If a femoral puncture has been performed, check the dorsalis pedis and posterior tibial pulses frequently to detect paresthesias, warmth or coolness, numbness, or pain, which may indicate altered circulation to the feet from vascular injury. Monitor vital signs closely to check for the presence of internal hemorrhage, particularly after a translumbar aortogram.

Radioisotope Studies

In addition to renal function tests performed with radioisotopes described earlier, radioactive compounds can be used to evaluate renal structures, ureters, and the bladder. For renal studies, as with clearance studies, a radioisotope is injected IV and a scintillation camera or probe or computer, or both, are used to record the size and shape of the kidneys. The isotope compounds used are retained in the kidneys for several hours or days. Lesions in the kidney, such as tumors or infarcts, do not absorb the radioactivity and thus appear as "cold" or "blank" spots on the scanner. In this case, the diagnostician needs to investigate further to determine the actual cause of the cold spot. Indications for this procedure include renal hypertension, renal masses, trauma, obstruction, and evaluating transplanted kidneys.

To evaluate the effectiveness of the vesicoureteral valves and the bladder, the radioactive agent is instilled into the bladder through a urethral catheter. Recording the radioactivity is conducted as described earlier. This procedure is performed primarily to evaluate vesicoureteral reflux, but it may also be used to detect large bladder defects.

Ultrasonography

Ultrasonography, or ultrasound, projects high-frequency waves into the abdomen. These waves are reflected back from the surfaces of retroperitoneal structures and converted into electrical energy that is shown on an oscilloscope. Instant-developing pictures are taken of the oscilloscope image to record the outline of the structures. The client lies on a table, and a lubricant, such as mineral oil, is applied to the skin over the area to be examined. This oil promotes contact between the skin and the transducer used to administer and receive the ultrasonic waves.

Ultrasonography of the kidneys has many uses. Its prime value may be in determining the size of the kidneys and differentiating between fluid-filled cysts and solid masses. Other applications include localizing and mapping out the kidneys before biopsy by percutaneous aspiration, evaluating transplanted kidneys, determining hydronephrosis, demonstrating papillary necrosis, identifying calculi, describing diverticula, measuring residual urine in the bladder, and demonstrating parenchymal changes resulting from urinary tract infections.

An ultrasound study of the bladder is frequently done to determine postvoid residuals. Ultrasonography is entirely safe. It is noninvasive, involves no contrast medium, and has produced no ill effects in anyone, including the offspring of women pregnant at the time of the examination. The technique is also considered highly accurate, although several factors can cause scanning artifacts. For instance, sound waves penetrate bone and gas very poorly, so the ribs, bowel, and lung limit the amount of kidney that can be scanned effectively.

There is minimal preparation for ultrasonography. Clients may require enemas or laxatives to clear the bowel prior to the test so the kidneys can be visualized. This is not necessary for ultrasound of the bladder.

Urodynamic Studies

Urodynamic studies evaluate the motor and sensory functioning of the bladder and the efficiency of micturition. These tests are used primarily to diagnose voiding problems or loss of bladder control, as with incontinence, and to evaluate the effectiveness of therapies implemented to treat voiding disorders or reconstructive bladder surgery. A series of measurements provides diagnostic information about bladder function.

Urine Flow Rate (Uroflowmetry)

Uroflowmetry, measurement of urine flow rates, is a simple, noninvasive procedure in which the client voids into a special commode equipped with a load cell mechanism that measures weight over time and records the findings on graph paper. This information can be used to calculate the urine flow rate (in milliliters per minute). The client should have a full bladder for the test or, if this is not

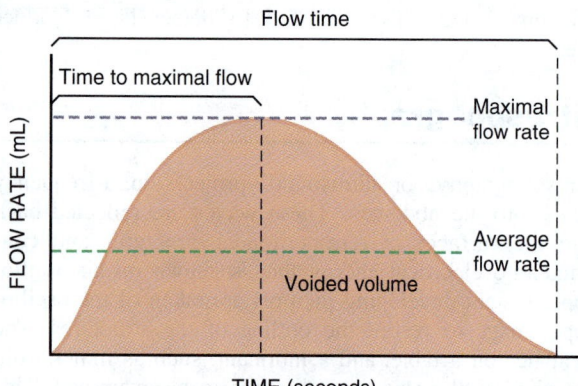

Figure 55–5. Diagram of terminology used in urodynamic studies. *Shaded area* shows voided volume. *Dotted lines* show how voided volume is divided into time and flow rate.

possible, a urethral catheter can be inserted to fill the bladder with sterile water. The client is then asked to void and the measurements are retaken. Figure 55–5 depicts the normal urinary flow rate and the parameters used to describe and assess the flow of urine during voiding.

Once the client has emptied the bladder by voiding, a urethral catheter may be inserted to determine if the client has a postvoid residual urine. More recently, bladder ultrasonography is being performed to determine residual urine after measurement of the urinary flow rate so this urodynamic procedure may remain totally noninvasive. Minimal client preparation is required. The client should be completely informed about the procedure and the need to be able to void when requested. Inform the client if catheterization is to be done. If the client experiences any discomfort after the catheterization, a warm sitz bath often relieves the pain.

Cystometrography

Procedure. A cystometrogram measures bladder pressures during filling and voiding. It is a measure sensitive to filling compliance, capacity, and detrusor contraction. No preprocedure preparation is needed other than client education.

In some institutions, at the beginning of the examination, the client voids while the examiner notes (1) the time and effort needed to initiate voiding; (2) caliber, force, and continuity of the stream; and (3) whether dribbling occurs after voiding ceases. A urethral catheter is then passed into the bladder and any residual urine is drained and measured. The distal end of the catheter is attached to an apparatus that will deliver saline or carbon dioxide to the bladder while intravesical pressures are recorded. The distending agent is infused into the bladder at a constant rate. The intravesical pressure is continuously recorded, and the client is asked when the urge to void is first felt, then when the bladder feels full, and when the need to void urgently is felt. The pressures at which these sensations are noted are recorded on the intravesical pressure tracing.

The client may be asked to cough or perform other maneuvers at specified points during the examination to evaluate the resulting pressure changes. Bladder filling also may be repeated in several different positions in order to reproduce the client's manifestations, including sitting or standing. For a study to be valid, the client's manifestations must be replicated. When filling has been completed, the catheter is removed and the client is allowed to empty the bladder while the examiner makes the same observations made during the initial voiding. The amount of residual urine is again determined. To measure bladder pressure during voiding, a tiny urethral catheter may be inserted and left in place during voiding. Intra-abdominal pressure can be measured using a small rectal catheter.

Preprocedure Care. The preparation is similar to that for the urine flow rate study. The procedure is explained to the client. The client is asked to void prior to the test.

Postprocedure Care. After the procedure, the client is monitored for the development of a UTI and may be given prophylactic antibiotics to prevent infection. The nurse also should monitor the client's voiding to make sure that the client does not develop urinary retention.

Electromyography

An *electromyogram (EMG)* measures striated perineal muscle activity, including the sphincters, during bladder filling and micturition. Several methods can be used to measure this activity, including an anal plug, urethral and anal catheter electrodes, paste-on electrodes, or needle electrodes. Because the purpose of the study is to compare perineal muscle activity with detrusor contractions, EMG is not performed alone but usually together with a cystometrogram or other pressure profile studies.

Urethral Pressure Profile Studies

Urethral pressure profile studies primarily determine the resistance to urine flow in the urethra and are especially useful in evaluating stress incontinence and the coordination, during voiding, of bladder contractions and relaxation of the external urethra. The three main methods used for determining urethral pressures are (1) resistance to fluid or gas infusion; (2) small, inflated intraluminal balloons, which provide pressure on the urethral walls; and (3) catheter tip transducers, which directly measure pressure resistance. In the infusion method, a small catheter with multiple holes along its length is inserted into the urethra with the distal end connected to a pressure transducer. As the catheter is very slowly withdrawn, fluid or gas is instilled into the urethra. Urethral pressures are determined at several levels of bladder fullness, including maximum capacity. The main factors measured are the intraluminal closing forces, urethral pressures lower than bladder pressures during voiding, and effective urethral length.

Direct Visualization

Cystoscopy

Procedure. The oldest method of direct visualization of the urinary tract is cystoscopy, which involves inserting a cystoscope into the bladder via the urethra. This procedure may be useful for diagnostic as well as therapeutic purposes. Its five major diagnostic uses include (1) directly inspecting the bladder, making it possible to see the ureteral orifices to determine tumors, calculi, ulcers, or other abnormalities or problems such as the source of the hematuria; (2) collecting urine directly from each ureter or kidney; (3) radiographic visualization by retrograde pyelography, as described earlier; (4) measuring bladder capacity and looking for evidence of vesicoureteral reflux; and (5) biopsy of the renal pelvis, ureters, bladder, and urethra. It also provides endoscopic access to the upper urinary tract. The cystoscope is used in intervention for (1) resecting tumors, (2) removing stones and foreign bodies, (3) fulgurating bleeding areas, (4) dilating the ureters, (5) emptying the renal pelvis, (6) implanting radium seeds, (7) performing bladder suspension surgery, and (8) bladder dilations for interstitial cystitis.

The rigid cystoscope consists primarily of a sheath and an optical lens system. The sheath is a solid metal tube that, when the obturator (a core that prevents trauma) is in place, can be passed through the urethra into the bladder. Once the cystoscope is in position, the obturator is removed from inside the sheath and the lighted lens system is introduced. Figure 55–6 shows a cystoscope in place. The rigidity of the standard cystoscope often prevents the examiner from visualizing some parts of the bladder. The evolution of flexible endoscopic instruments has helped solve this problem. The client being examined is in a supine position.

Several functions may be accomplished through the sheath of the scope. Forceps may be passed through the sheath to get tissue samples for biopsy or to remove foreign bodies. A guide can be used to help direct small catheters into and up the ureters to the renal pelves so specimens can be obtained from each kidney separately. Scissors, needles, and electrodes also may be introduced into the bladder or urethra as needed.

During the procedure, which is performed under surgically aseptic conditions, the nurse assists the physician and supports the client being examined, especially if the client has not had general anesthesia. In placing the client in the lithotomy position, the nurse ensures the client's protection from musculoskeletal and nerve damage. The client must be comfortable enough to maintain the desired position throughout the examination. Verbal progress reports and reassuring words during the procedure help reduce anxiety. The nurse also must alert the physician to any manifestation of developing complications. Sudden pelvic or lower abdominal pain may indicate perforation of the urethra, bladder, or ureters.

Preprocedure Care. Cystoscopy may be performed in the physician's office or outpatient surgery setting. It may be performed under local, light general anesthesia, or without medications, especially in the female. The client must remain still during the examination to avoid trauma. Therefore, the type of anesthesia used may depend on whether the client can maintain the necessary position.

Physiologic and psychosocial preparation is needed before cystoscopy. Cathartics or enemas, or both, may be taken before the procedure to clear the bowel, especially if a retrograde pyelogram is also being performed. Some clients, especially those receiving general anesthesia, may be required to fast for several hours beforehand. Clients having local anesthesia may be instructed to maintain an adequate fluid intake to ensure an effective urine flow for specimen and for retrograde pyelography, if it is to be performed. Clients who cannot have anything by mouth

Figure 55–6. Cystoscope in the male bladder.

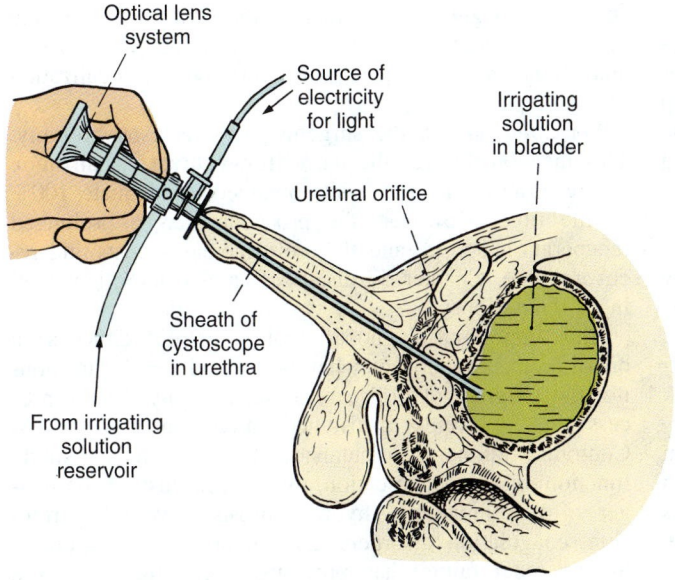

Optical lens system

Source of electricity for light

Irrigating solution in bladder

Urethral orifice

Sheath of cystoscope in urethra

From irrigating solution reservoir

will receive IV fluids. A sedative or narcotic, and sometimes an anticholinergic, typically is administered before the procedure.

As with any procedure, effective teaching helps to alleviate anxiety and ensure optimum cooperation. This is particularly important if cystoscopy is performed under local anesthesia. Because the procedure is usually performed with the client in the lithotomy position, it can be very tiring and uncomfortable, but it is essential to remain still throughout the examination. The nurse can help the client with deep breathing and general relaxation exercises to decrease discomfort as the cystoscope is introduced. The desire to void will be pronounced as the cystoscope passes the neck of the bladder and when the bladder is filled with fluid for optimal visualization. The nurse also should warn the client that this procedure is performed with the room lights off so the physician can better visualize the internal bladder.

Postprocedure Care. Care after a cystoscopy may include bedrest for a short time. If general anesthesia is used, the client needs the usual postanesthetic monitoring (see Chapter 21). Even if the procedure was performed on an ambulatory basis under local anesthesia, the client should not stand immediately after removing the legs from the stirrups, because a sudden position change may cause dizziness and syncope. This is especially true for the elderly.

Pink-tinged urine is common after cystoscopy, but any bright-red bleeding or clots in the urine should be reported to the physician. Advise the client that the urine may have an unusual color if a contrast medium such as methylene blue is used. Back pain, bladder spasms, feeling of fullness and burning in the bladder, and burning on urination also may be experienced. Warm tub baths and mild analgesics usually bring sufficient relief. Belladonna and opium (B&O) suppositories or antispasmodics such as propantheline bromide (Pro-Banthine) may relieve bladder spasms.

Urinary retention sometimes occurs from edema following instrumentation. Men with BPH are at particularly high risk. Hot sitz baths and relaxants often relieve the problem, although catheterization may be necessary. Encourage the client to drink large amounts of fluids after the procedure. Diluting the urine in this way will help prevent further tissue irritation and will decrease the burning sensation when the client voids. Some chilling and a rise in temperature often occur following cystoscopy. If these manifestations do not subside readily after providing extra warmth and offering frequent fluids, investigate the client's condition further. Cystoscopy may inoculate the bladder with bacteria, so the risk of bacteremia is present. Although the practice is controversial, some authorities recommend using prophylactic antibiotics after urinary tract instrumentation because of the risk of infection.

Clients are discharged almost immediately or within several hours after cystoscopy. Give the client written instructions as well as oral instructions, because clients may not remember the instructions later, after they have gone home.

Ureteroscopy and Nephroscopy

Ureteroscopes have been developed to examine the ureter and kidneys. Ureteroscopy evaluates tumors, obstruction, calculi, and the presence of foreign bodies. General or regional (spinal or epidural) anesthesia is used for these procedures because the dilation of the ureteral orifice causes considerable discomfort.

Performed under strict aseptic technique, nephroscopy allows the physician to observe the renal pelvis, calices, fundus, and collecting system. It can be performed to (1) locate and remove calculi; (2) identify the source of hematuria; and (3) biopsy, fulgurate, and resect tumors. Nephroscopy is not associated with any significant complications except possible infection. Nursing care for the client before and after the procedure is similar to that needed by clients having a renal biopsy (discussed later).

Renal Biopsy

Procedure. A renal tissue specimen for biopsy may be obtained using an open or closed technique. Although this procedure is not common, it may be used if other examinations are not adequate to identify renal problems.

One method of *closed biopsy* is the retrograde renal and ureteral brush procedure. This technique collects tissue specimens from the renal pelvis and ureters, particularly from areas of radiolucent filling defects found during excretory urography. The initial part of the procedure is conducted as a cystoscopy under general anesthesia. A whistle-tip ureteral catheter is introduced, and its proper positioning is guided by fluoroscopy or serial x-rays. A biopsy brush is then passed through the catheter, and the lesion is brushed several times. The brush is removed and any tissue adhering to its bristles is sent to the laboratory. If no tissue is found on the brush, 24- to 48-hour urine specimens may be collected to catch any cells that may have been dislodged by the bristles.

The *percutaneous renal biopsy* is perhaps the most frequently used procedure. During this examination, a specially designed needle pierces the skin and enters the kidney to obtain a small sample of tissue. Fluoroscopy and ultrasound techniques allow more precise localization of the biopsy needle.

For *open biopsy,* the surgeon performs a nephrotomy. This incision through the flank allows direct visualization of the kidney, and the tissue obtained is adequate 100% of the time. However, the procedure has a prolonged recuperation period, and therefore increases costs and recovery time. Chapter 57 discusses care of the client having a renal biopsy.

This important diagnostic tool is helpful either as a one-time examination or when performed serially to monitor the progress of a disease, especially any disease process that is evenly distributed throughout the kidney. Contraindications to percutaneous biopsy include a single functioning kidney, infection, tumors (because of the danger of dissemination), hydronephrosis, severe hypertension, coagulation disorders, and an uncooperative client. Severe renal failure has previously been regarded as a contraindication. However, better procedures for localizing the kidney have reduced the dangers associated with this technique. Pregnancy usually is considered a contraindication because of the high doses of radiation that may be necessary during localization of the needle. Using ultrasound instead eliminates this risk.

The procedure usually is performed under local anesthesia with little or no premedication. The client is placed in a prone position with a firm pillow or sandbag under the abdomen to straighten the spine's natural lordosis. The kidney to be biopsied is located with ultrasound or fluoroscopy and contrast medium is injected IV. After careful skin preparation, the skin is infiltrated with the anesthetic. The client is instructed to take in as deep a breath as possible and hold it. The probe needle then is (1) inserted through the skin, midway between the 12th rib and the iliac crest (Fig. 55–7), and (2) positioned inside the renal (fibrous) capsule slightly lateral to the midline of the kidney. After the correct position of the distal end of the needle has been confirmed, the probe needle is removed and the biopsy trocar is inserted. The client may now be allowed to breathe normally, but he or she must inspire deeply each time a tissue specimen is taken. When enough tissue is obtained, the trocar is removed and firm pressure is applied immediately to the site. After several minutes, a pressure dressing is applied.

Hemorrhage is a major potential complication. It may be suggested by gross or microscopic hematuria, flank or abdominal pain, hypotension, and a decreasing hematocrit. However, low hematocrit and hypotension alone are not sufficient indicators of hemorrhage, because some people develop these conditions without significant bleeding.

Continued bleeding or the resulting hematoma may require surgical exploration, and these problems may necessitate removal of the involved kidney. Intrarenal arteriovenous fistulas may occur, causing an audible bruit over the kidneys, and may lead to hypertension. Because of the chances of pneumothorax, especially when the upper pole of the kidney is biopsied, some authorities recommend a routine expiratory chest x-ray after the procedure. This precaution is especially important for elderly persons with an already compromised cardiopulmonary reserve. Other complications include infection, traumatic urinoma, and laceration or perforation of the kidney or adjacent structures.

Preprocedure Care. Prior to the procedure, the client needs to have clotting ability carefully assessed since hemorrhage post procedure is a real concern. The type of biopsy to be done (open or percutaneous) should be explained to the client. The client is NPO for 6 to 8 hours prior to the procedure.

Before the biopsy begins, a battery of radiologic and laboratory studies is done. These include excretory urography; urine culture; hematocrit; blood chemistry, including BUN and creatinine; and bleeding time and coagulation studies. If an aneurysm is suspected, renal arteriography is mandatory to avoid puncture of this vascular defect. Blood for transfusion may be ordered as standby.

Postprocedure Care. Postoperatively, the client may be given IV fluids at a rapid rate to reduce the possibility of clots forming at the biopsy site and to foster specimen collection. Unless contraindicated, at least 3000 ml of fluid should be taken in the first 24 hours after the procedure. Some oozing of blood may be expected for 24 to 48 hours at the biopsy site and in the urine. Moreover, some people experience severe renal colic, which is usually relieved by narcotics and fluids.

After the percutaneous biopsy, the client may remain prone for approximately 30 minutes or immediately be turned onto the back after completing the procedure. Monitor vital signs and the puncture site every 5 to 10 minutes. The client then may be transferred to bed and should remain on bedrest and avoid straining for at least 24 hours. Check vital signs and the puncture site regularly during this time. Obtain serial urines, keeping a sample of each voiding in consecutive order for comparison and to evaluate bleeding. Use dipsticks to determine the presence of hematuria, and send specimens to the laboratory to determine more precisely the amount of bleeding. Encourage the client to drink large amounts of fluid, 2500 to 3000 ml, to avoid clot formation and retention, which could obstruct urine flow. The period of bedrest will likely be extended in the presence of continued bleeding. A serum hematocrit and hemoglobin usually is drawn within 8 to 10 hours to test for bleeding. The client may also need emotional support while waiting for the diagnosis and its implications.

Advise the client to avoid strenuous activity for approximately 2 weeks. Also, instruct the client about the manifestations of hemorrhage and what to do if hemorrhage occurs. Bleeding may develop several days after the biopsy.

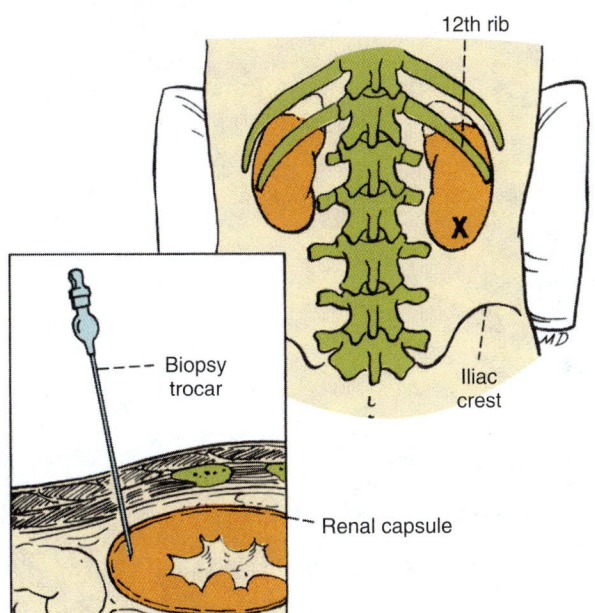

Figure 55–7. Percutaneous renal biopsy showing trocar location.

Conclusions

Care of a client with disorders of the urinary and renal system mandates that the nurse be aware of the assessments needed to determine proper functioning of the system. Clients may find some assessment embarrassing, so sensitive care is required to reassure them. The nurse must carefully explain the diagnostic tests to clients and prepare them adequately for the examinations. The nurse also provides the client with emotional support to complete the diagnostic process so that appropriate treatment may be initiated.

Bibliography

1. Beck, L. H. (1990). Kidney function and disease in the elderly. *Hospital Practice, 26,* 75–90.
2. Bower, A., & Thompson, J. (1992). *Clinical manual of health assessment* (3rd ed.). St. Louis: Mosby–Year Book.
3. Brenner, B. M. (Ed.). (1996). *Brenner & Rector's the kidney* (5th ed). Philadelphia: W. B. Saunders.
4. Chadwick, A. T. (1989). BV 2000: A noninvasive technique to assess bladder function. *Journal of Neuroscience Nursing, 21,* 256–257.
5. Chernecky, C. C., Krech, R. L., & Berger, B. J. (1993). *Laboratory tests and diagnostic procedures.* Philadelphia: W. B. Saunders.
6. Fuller, J., & Schaller-Ayers, J. (1994). *Health assessment: A nursing approach* (2nd ed.). Philadelphia: J. B. Lippincott.
7. George, N., & Samntook, P. (1991). *Diagnostic picture tests in urology.* St. Louis: Mosby–Year Book.
8. Greene, L. (1980). Management of gross and microscopic hematuria. *Consultant, 20,* 95.
9. Karlowicz, K. A. (1995). *Urologic nursing: Prevention and practice.* Philadelphia: W. B. Saunders.
10. Kee, J. L. (1995). *Laboratory and diagnostic tests with nursing implications* (4th ed.). Norwalk, CT: Appleton & Lange.
11. Kenny, R. A. (1992). *Physiology of aging: A synopsis.* St. Louis: Mosby–Year Book.
12. Kunin, C. M. (1987). *Detection, prevention, and management of urinary tract infections* (4th ed.). Philadelphia: Lea & Febiger.
13. Mackety, C. J. (1990). Lasers in urology. *Nursing Clinics of North America, 25,* 697–709.
14. Rebensen-Piano, M. (1989). The physiologic changes that occur with aging. *Critical Care Nursing Quarterly, 12*(1), 1–14.
15. Resnick, N. M. (1989). Diagnosis and treatment of the institutionalized elderly. *Seminars in Urology, 7,* 117–123.
16. Sabiston, D. C. (1991). *Textbook of surgery: The biological basis of modern surgical practice* (14th ed.). Philadelphia: W. B. Saunders.
17. Schrier, R., & Gottschalk, C. (1988). *Diseases of the kidney* (4th ed.). Boston: Little, Brown.
18. Smith, D. R. (1992) *General urology* (13th ed.). Los Altos, CA: Lange Medical.
19. Strasinger, S. K. (1994). *Urinalysis and body fluids.* Philadelphia: F. A. Davis.
20. Urinary Incontinence Guideline Panel. (March, 1992). *Urinary incontinence in adults: A patient's guide.* AHCPR Publications No. 92-0040. Rockville, MD: Agency for Health Care Policy and Research, Public Health Service, U.S. Department of Health and Human Services.
21. Urinary Incontinence Guideline Panel. (March, 1992). *Urinary incontinence in adults: Clinical practice guideline.* AHCPR Publications No. 92-0038. Rockville, MD: Agency for Health Care Policy and Research, Public Health Service, U.S. Department of Health and Human Services.
22. Urinary Incontinence Guideline Panel. (March, 1992). *Urinary incontinence in adults: Quick reference guide for clinicians.* AHCPR Publications No. 92-0041. Rockville, MD: Agency for Health Care Policy and Research, Public Health Service, U.S. Department of Health and Human Services.
23. Watson, J., & Jaffee, M. S. (1995). *Nurse's manual of laboratory and diagnostic tests,* (2nd ed.). Philadelphia: F. A. Davis.
24. Wyngaarden, J. B., & Smith, L. H. (1996). *Cecil textbook of medicine* (20th ed.). Philadelphia: W. B. Saunders.

Nursing Care of Clients with Disorders of the Ureters, Bladder, and Urethra

Esther Matassarin-Jacobs

The diagnosis of *Altered Urinary Elimination* is a common theme throughout this chapter. Dysfunction anywhere within the urethra, bladder, or ureters has the potential to alter urinary elimination. You should always keep this fact in mind when working with clients with these disorders. It is important to remember that alterations in urinary elimination can lead to a multitude of other problems such as fluid volume and electrolyte changes and all the associated problems.

Because of the private nature of the urinary system, its proximity to the reproductive system in females, and the shared urinary and reproductive system of males, urinary disorders can also lead to *Sexual Dysfunction* and *Body Image Disturbance*. In women, the development of cystitis (one of the most common urinary disorders) may be directly related to sexual intercourse. It is therefore vital that the nurse be sensitive to the psychosocial needs of the client with disorders of the urinary system.

Infectious and Inflammatory Disorders

Urinary Tract Infection (Cystitis)

Urinary tract infection (UTI) refers to an infection (presence of 10^5 organisms) within the urinary tract, usually affecting the bladder, although the urethra, ureters, and kidneys may be involved. *Cystitis* is an inflammation of the bladder wall, usually caused by ascending bacteria. The term "cystitis" is often used to refer to a UTI that is symptomatic. Abacterial or interstitial cystitis is an inflammation of the bladder mucosa that occurs without the presence of bacteria. This disorder is discussed later.

UTIs are a common health problem. The bladder is the most frequent site of infection within the urinary tract. At least 25% of women develop UTI or cystitis sometime in their lives.[63] Men rarely develop UTIs before the age of 50 because of the length of their urethra and possibly the antibacterial properties of prostatic fluid.

Acute UTIs account for 6 to 7 million office visits a year for young women, second only to treatment of upper respiratory infections.[67] Recurrence is common after treatment for an initial UTI for a variety of reasons; about 20% of women with UTIs have frequent recurrences.

Etiology and Risk Factors

The most common UTI-causing organisms are the gram-negative organisms *Escherichia coli, Enterobacter, Pseudomonas,* and *Serratia*. These organisms, normally found in the gastrointestinal tract, contaminate the urine because of the proximity of the urethral orifice and the anus. *Escherichia coli* itself is responsible for about 90% of UTIs in women. *Staphylococcus saprophyticus,* an organism recognized in Europe for some time, is now drawing more attention in the United States. It especially affects young women, occurs most often in the summer and early autumn, and has a high propensity for ascending into the upper urinary tract.

Candida is another cause of UTIs. It is associated with sepsis and death, especially in debilitated clients who are already experiencing one or more of these conditions: blood dyscrasia, diabetes mellitus, cancer, drug addiction, immunosuppression, and persistent UTI that has been treated with a variety of antibiotics. Any *Candida* found in the urine is significant, although the laboratory must determine that the organism is actually colonized and not simply a contaminant from the vagina at the time of specimen collection.

Women are more susceptible to cystitis because of the short female urethra and its proximity to the anus; sexually active and pregnant women are the most vulnerable.

The short female urethra reduces the distance between the bladder and the external environment. The location of the external meatus makes it very vulnerable to vaginal and fecal contamination. Colonization of the vaginal introitus (opening) and urethral meatus with *E. coli* is a significant variable characteristic of women who suffer recurrent UTIs. Hormonal changes in postmenopausal women alter the vaginal pH and thus the vaginal flora. Changes in the flora allow abnormal levels of normal bacteria to grow. Decreased urethral and vaginal lubrication from decreased estrogen also increases the risk of urethral irritation during intercourse.

Sexual intercourse increases the occurrence of UTIs in women; the thrusting motion during coitus "milks" the organisms up the urethra and into the bladder, which can lead to cystitis if the woman does not void after intercourse. "Honeymoon cystitis" is a term frequently used to describe this phenomenon. Poorly fitting diaphragms used for contraception are also linked to UTI because of pressure against the urethra, which prevents complete bladder emptying. Spermicides are also associated with an increase in UTIs. These agents appear to increase the vaginal pH, alter the normal vaginal flora, and are associated with increased colonization of *E. coli.*

In women, clothing such as synthetic underwear and pantyhose, tight jeans, and wet bathing suits can contribute to the development of cystitis. Allergens or irritants, such as feminine hygiene sprays, bubble baths, perfumed toilet paper and sanitary napkins, and soaps, contribute to the development of cystitis in some women.

The presence of an indwelling urethral catheter dramatically increases the occurrence of UTIs. UTIs are the most frequent nosocomial infections. The rates for UTIs in most hospitals are well above 50% in catheterized clients, with some reports as high as 100%. Indwelling catheters often introduce bacteria into the urinary tract because of poor technique of insertion, inflammation of the urethra, and ascension of bacteria along the length of the catheter. If a closed system is not maintained, infection is even more likely.

Anything that breaks down the integrity of the bladder lining opens the way to possible infection. Loss of integrity of the mucosal lining may be caused by an indwelling catheter, calculus, tumor, or parasites. Also, standing urine is an incubator for organism growth. Therefore, anything that contributes to urinary stasis significantly increases the risk for development of UTI. Distention of the bladder leads to UTIs. As the bladder wall expands, blood flow decreases. Ischemic tissue becomes more vulnerable to organism invasion. Common causes of bladder distention include urethral obstruction caused by a full rectum or benign prostatic hypertrophy (BPH) and subsequent suppression of voiding or incomplete emptying of the bladder. Infection also can occur from the client's own colon via the hematogenous or lymphatogenous routes.

In older men, obstructive uropathy, loss of the bactericidal properties of prostatic secretions, poor bladder emptying, and other medical disorders contribute to the development of UTIs. It is estimated that the incidence of UTI in older men is approximately 15%. (See Risk Factors and Levels of Prevention: Cystitis.)

Pathophysiology

Several pathophysiologic mechanisms are involved in the development of UTIs. The principal factor is the host's loss of resistance to invading organisms. The bladder and urine are normally resistant to infection. The lining of the bladder is composed of mucin-producing cells, which help maintain the integrity of the bladder lining and prevent cellular inflammation and damage. Although many pathogens reach the bladder, the sterility of the urine is quickly reestablished. The bladder's resistance to infections is due to the antibacterial properties of the bladder mucosa and urine as well as to phagocytosis. The normal acidity of the urine is a poor medium for growth of gram-negative organisms. Also, voiding washes organisms out of the lower urinary tract, helping to prevent ascending bacterial infections.

The most common organism responsible for urinary tract infections is *E. coli.* Research is being done on the presence of receptors in the uroepithelium which have a higher affinity for *E. coli.* These receptors are found in higher numbers in persons with frequent infections. These receptors may predict the susceptibility of an individual to UTIs.

Clinical Manifestations and Diagnostic Findings

The cardinal clinical manifestations of cystitis are burning pain on urination (dysuria), frequency, urgency, voiding in small amounts, inability to void, and incomplete emptying of the bladder. Low back pain is also a common problem, as is suprapubic pain. Assessment may reveal hematuria, cloudy urine, abdominal and flank pain (which may indicate pyelonephritis), malaise, chills, fever, and nausea and vomiting. About 10% of clients with bacteriuria will be asymptomatic. Lack of assessment findings, therefore, should not preclude the diagnosis of UTI. In elderly people, the only manifestation of infection may be a change in the person's mental status.

Most of the manifestations are due to the irritation of the bladder and urethral mucosa. The bacteriuria causes inflammation, fever, and chills. If the ureters become inflamed also, abdominal manifestations such as distention, nausea, and diarrhea may occur.

Definitive diagnosis should be based on a urine culture. However, the dipstick test for leukocyte esterase and nitrate activity is increasingly used to determine bacteriuria early so that interventions can begin promptly. This method is 100% sensitive and 76% specific. A urine culture is essential to identifying the causative organism. Sensitivity tests are also done routinely on the urine specimens for identifying the antibiotics that can be used to treat the infection successfully. Follow-up cultures are also used to determine the effectiveness of medications used to treat the infection. Because the potential is high for contamination and false-positives during specimen collection, some individuals require a catheterized urine specimen before organisms can definitively be identified. Asymptomatic clients with high bacterial counts in the

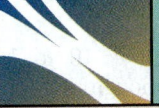

RISK FACTORS AND LEVELS OF PREVENTION

Cystitis

Risk Factors

Women: Short urethra in close proximity to vagina and anus; coitus; use of diaphragm and spermicide; pregnancy; menopause

Men: Age (incidence is 15% in older men); loss of bactericidal properties of sperm; obstructive uropathies such as benign prostatic hyperplasia (BPH)

Both: Previous UTI; catheterization; presence of indwelling Foley catheter

Levels of Prevention

Primary Prevention
- Increase fluid intake to at least 3 L/day, especially of acid-ash foods to acidify urine (cranberry juice, vitamin C) and water
- Teach women the proper way to wipe after urination (front to back)
- Teach women to shower instead of bathing in a tub, to void and drink a glass of water after intercourse, and to avoid bubble baths
- Teach women to wear cotton pants, not to wear pantyhose with slacks, and to avoid tight jeans or sitting around in a wet bathing suit
- Advise women to avoid feminine hygiene sprays and other irritants such as perfumed toilet paper or sanitary pads
- Teach pregnant women to void at least every 2 hours
- Encourage menopausal woman to use estrogen vaginal creams to restore vaginal pH
- Teach women to use water-soluble lubricants for coitus, especially after menopause
- Maintain closed urinary drainage for hospitalized clients with an indwelling catheter
- Provide daily, meticulous perineal care with mild soap and water for clients with an indwelling catheter
- Use strict aseptic technique when inserting a catheter

Secondary Prevention
- Monitor pregnant women for the presence of infection
- Teach high-risk clients the clinical manifestations of infection
- Monitor older male clients, especially those with BPH, for the presence of infection
- Closely monitor clients with an indwelling catheter for the presence of an infection

Tertiary Prevention
- Emphasize the prevalence of recurrence of infection and ways to prevent recurrence
- Ensure that clients understand the importance of taking all antibiotics and of having repeat cultures and sensitivities done

urine should have three consecutive positive cultures before a final diagnosis of UTI is established. Asymptomatic clients with indwelling urethral catheters with high bacterial counts may not be treated until the catheter is removed or manifestations develop. Cultures must be done before antibiotics are started.

The traditional bacterial count benchmark of greater than 100,000/ml for voided specimens may not be appropriate. Bacterial counts as low as 1000 to 10,000/ml (for voided specimens) may indicate an active infectious process in the lower urinary tract, especially if the client has manifestations of cystitis. This area is still unclear, and further research is needed. A colony count of 10,000/ml indicates an active infectious process in a catheterized specimen. Even a low colony count in a catheterized specimen, however, is significant and should be investigated.

In some cases of severe or recurrent cystitis, an intra-venous pyelogram (IVP), voiding cystourethrogram, retrograde pyelogram, or cystoscopy might be done to detect any abnormalities. Congenital anomalies, foreign bodies, calculi (stones), and tumors can be detected as well as abnormalities such as strictures secondary to scarring, which repeated infections may have caused. These tests will also detect obstruction such as those from an enlarged prostate—a common cause of UTI in men older than 55.

Acute and Subacute Care

■ Medical Management

Management of UTI is multifaceted, and an initial, acute infection may be treated differently from recurrent infections. The principal intervention for an initial infection is the administration of antibiotics specific for the causative organisms. Acute bacterial cystitis can often be treated with single-dose antibiotic therapy. The client must always return for a follow-up culture to ascertain the elimination of bacteria from the urine.

A urine culture must be obtained approximately 1 week after completed pharmacologic therapy to determine whether the medication has eradicated the bacteriuria. If the urine is not yet sterile, the physician may continue antibiotic therapy with the same or another antibiotic. The course of antibiotics may need to be extended a few additional weeks. Persistent infections may require therapy for months. When the infection flares up each time therapy is discontinued, suppression therapy may be prescribed to keep the urine sterile. This consists of a small dose of antibiotics that the client takes once daily or several times a week, usually at bedtime, often for years.

Frequent recurrent infections are a frustrating problem. Three or more UTIs a year are considered frequent, whether they involve the same or different organisms. Each infection must be treated with antibiotics. Caution the client against self-diagnosis and self-treatment of recurrent UTIs. Each infection requires culture and sensitivity and specific treatment. The physician may prescribe either continuous suppression therapy or continue episodic administration of antibiotics when a UTI recurs.

There is a growing trend to give the client control over the medication regimen when identical recurrent infections have occurred. For example, women whose occurrences relate to sexual activity may be provided with a supply of antibiotics, with instructions to take a prescribed dose after coitus. Others with frequent recurrences are (1) given a prescription for medication, (2) taught to recognize early manifestations of UTI, (3) instructed to begin antibiotic therapy at the first hint of infection, (4) reminded to complete the full course of antibiotics even if the manifestations have disappeared, and (5) advised to come in 1 week after completing the regimen for a follow-up urine culture.

Treating the client with asymptomatic bacteriuria is yet another problem. In general, physicians currently suggest that an asymptomatic infection be treated only if it is certain that intervention will prevent further morbidity or if the client has other medical conditions that may lead to problems.

Antibiotic Therapy

Broad-spectrum antibiotics are started even before the culture and sensitivity results are known, because medication should begin as soon as possible. Later, based on sensitivity reports, the exact medication for this infection can be prescribed. Commonly used pharmacologic agents include trimethoprim-sulfamethoxazole (Bactrim, Septra), nitrofurantoin (Macrodantin), sulfisoxazole (Gantrisin), ciprofloxacin (Cipro), ampicillin, methenamine mandelate (Mandelamine), and cephalexin (Table 56–1). Medications containing azo dyes, such as phenazopyridine (Pyridium) or phenazopyridine-sulfisoxazole (Azo Gantrisin), are believed to have an anesthetic effect on the urinary tract mucosa and are used to treat the burning sensation often felt with cystitis.

The typical course of antibiotic therapy is 10 to 14 days. However, a single *large* dose, although not accepted by all authorities, is effective in many clients, especially women with an initial uncomplicated infection of the lower urinary tract. Large single-dose therapy does not suppress the client's normal flora, including altered vaginal flora leading to yeast infections, to the same degree as long-term therapy, and reduces the development of resistant organisms.[63]

Urinary Acidification

Acidifying the urine decreases the rate of bacterial multiplication. Traditionally, cranberry juice and ascorbic acid (vitamin C) have been used to acidify the urine. However, current studies show that neither adequately reduces the urinary pH and therefore they are not as reliable as was previously thought. Although cranberry juice can acidify the urine, commercial products do not contain a sufficiently high concentration of pure juice to reduce the pH unless the client can drink a large amount.

An acid-ash diet is more effective in acidifying the urine (Table 56–2). Encourage a diet of meats, eggs, cheese, prunes, cranberries, plums, and whole grains. Cranberries and cranberry concentrate pills may increase the acidity of the urine. Foods not included on the diet include carbonated beverages, anything containing baking soda or powder, fruits other than those listed, all vegetables except corn and legumes, olives, pickles, and nuts other than peanuts.

Remember that acidifying the urine may or may not be advantageous, depending on the specific antiseptic or antibiotic being used. For instance, methenamine mandelate and methenamine hippurate (Hiprex) require acid urine to be effective. On the other hand, the action of aminoglycosides, nitrofurantoin (Macrodantin), and sulfonamides are diminished by acidic urine.

Promoting Fluid Intake

Fluid intake should also be increased to at least 3 L/day, unless contraindicated, to maintain a good urine output and to flush the urinary tract. The increased fluid intake is extremely important when the client is taking sulfa drugs because these can form crystals in concentrated urine.

Complications

Antibiotic therapy can cause problems related to the destruction of normal flora in the body with resultant overgrowth of opportunistic organisms. Clients often develop diarrhea and associated bowel problems and female clients may develop vaginitis. Some antibiotics, such as trimethoprim-sulfasoxazole, reduce the effectiveness of oral contraceptives, while sulfa drugs increase the sensitivity to the effects of the sun.

Complications can occur if the infection is not completely eradicated. An ascending infection can migrate from the bladder to the kidneys, resulting in the development of pyelonephritis. Recurrent pyelonephritis can pre-

Table 56–1. Medications Used to Treat Cystitis and Other Urinary Disorders

Agent	Action	Dosage	Side Effects	Nursing Implications
Urinary Antiseptics				
Cinoxacin (Cinobac)	Effective against *Escherichia coli, Klebsiella, Enterobacter, Proteus, Serratia, Citrobacter*	1 g/day in 2 to 4 divided doses for 7–14 days	Dizziness, headache, photosensitivity, nausea and vomiting, abdominal pain, diarrhea, rash	Contraindicated in clients who are hypersensitive to nalidixic acid; warn client about photophobic effect; give with meals to decrease GI side effects
Nalidixic acid (NegGram)	For acute and chronic UTIs, especially gram-negative bacterial infections	1 g qid for 7–14 days for acute or 2 g/day for long-term use	Drowsiness, weakness, headache, photophobia, diplopia, abdominal pain, nausea and vomiting, rash, angioedema	Use with caution in clients with liver or renal disorders; contraindicated in clients with a history of convulsions; instruct client to report visual disturbances; encourage client to drink fluids and closely monitor output; warn client to avoid sunlight
Norfloxacin (Noroxin)	For complicated and uncomplicated UTIs caused by gram-negative organisms, including *Pseudomonas;* especially useful for clients allergic to penicillin, cephalosporin, and sulfa drugs	400 mg PO bid for 7–10 days for mild infections and for 10–21 days for severe infections	Fatigue, somnolence, headache, nausea, constipation, elevated liver function tests, rash	Encourage high fluid intake to ensure high urine output; advise client to take medication 1 hr before or 2 hr after meals because food may hamper absorption
Nitrofurantoin (Macrodantin, Macrobid)	For acute and chronic UTIs in clients with adequate creatinine clearance	*Macrodantin:* 50–100 mg PO qid for 10–14 days, after meals, for acute UTI: chronic therapy, 50–100 mg PO as needed; 180 mg IV bid for adults > 120 lb; *Macrobid:* 100 mg bid	Nausea and vomiting, GI upset, diarrhea, rash, asthma, peripheral neuropathies, drug-induced fever, anaphylaxis, dizziness, hypotension	Maintain adequate intake/output; use caution in clients with anemia, diabetes, vitamin B deficiency, electrolyte imbalances, or debilitating diseases; watch for hypersensitivity; keep urinary pH in acid range with vitamin C and cranberry juice; give with food; warn client drugs may discolor urine
Methenamine mandelate (Mandelamine)	Effective in acid urine against gram-positive and gram-negative organisms for chronic UTIs	1 g PO qid pc	Nausea and vomiting, diarrhea, elevated liver enzymes, rash, dysuria, frequency in high doses	Contraindicated in clients with renal or hepatic disease or severe dehydration; maintain high urine output; warn client to limit intake of alkaline foods and increase intake of cranberry juice and foods that acidify urine; administer with food or after meals, but warn client to avoid antacids
Sulfonamides				
Co-trimoxazole, Sulfamethoxazole-trimethoprim (Bactrim, Septra)	For acute UTIs	160 mg trimethoprim/800 mg sulfa or double with double strength tablet for 10–14 days	GI distress, agranulocytosis, allergic reactions, headache, glossitis, stomatitis, hepatitis, pruritus, photosensitivity, arthralgia, peripheral neuritis, hearing loss, crystalluria, hypoglycemia	Administer with large amounts of fluid; monitor serum glucose levels; monitor for allergies (occur more commonly in AIDS); client should maintain alkaline pH because these drugs are more soluble in alkaline urine; do not use in last trimester of pregnancy; warn client to avoid sun

Table continued on following page

Table 56–1. Medications Used to Treat Cystitis and Other Urinary Disorders (Continued)

Agent	Action	Dosage	Side Effects	Nursing Implications
Sulfisoxazole (Gantrisin)	For acute UTIs	Initially 2–4 g PO, then 1–2 g qid for 10–14 days	Agranulocytosis, aplastic anemia, headache, depression, nausea and vomiting, diarrhea, toxic nephrosis, crystalluria, erythema multiforme, epidermal necrolysis, exfoliative dermatitis, hypersensitivity, anaphylaxis, serum sickness	Monitor closely for allergy; give each dose with full glass of water; maintain high fluid intake; monitor intake/output; (drug is more soluble in alkaline urine); monitor CBC; instruct client to take full dose; if Azo Gantrisin given, urine will be dark brown to red
Urinary Analgesics				
Phenazopyridine (Pyridium)	For pain of urinary tract irritation or infection	100–200 mg PO tid until pain disappears, usually about 2–3 days	Nausea, headache, vertigo	Warn client urine will be red to orange; contraindicated in renal or hepatic disease; always give with antibiotic; does not treat infection, only pain
Cholinergics				
Bethanechol chloride (Urecholine)	For acute postoperative or other nonobstructive urinary retention and neurogenic atony of bladder with retention	2.5–10 mg SQ, never IM or IV; 10–30 mg PO tid or qid; all doses should be determined individually	Cardiac arrest and vascular collapse if given IM or IV; headache, hypotension, abdominal cramps, diarrhea, nausea and vomiting, urinary urgency, flushing, bronchoconstriction	Never used in clients with any possibility of bladder obstruction; never give IM or IV, can lead to circulatory collapse; watch closely for cholinergic overdose; atropine antidote; have bedpan readily available, works within 15 min after injection or 60 min after oral dose; give on empty stomach to decrease nausea and vomiting
Antispasmotics				
Oxybutynin chloride (Ditropan)	Relaxes smooth muscles of urinary tract	5 mg bid or tid, not more than 5 mg qid	Leukopenia, eosinophilia, anxiety, dizziness, convulsions, palpitations, sinus bradycardia, nausea, vomiting, anorexia	Do not use in clients with known hypersensitivity, GI or GU obstruction, glaucoma, severe colitis, or myasthenia gravis; warn client to avoid hazardous activities
Propantheline bromide (Pro-Banthine)	Decreases bladder muscle spasms	Up to 60 mg PO qid	Palpitations, blurred vision, confusion in elderly clients, dry mouth, constipation, urinary hesitancy and retention, decreased sweating	Do not use in clients with narrow-angle glaucoma, obstructive uropathy, GI disease, or ulcerative colitis; monitor urine output closely; provide gum or hard candy for dry mouth
Antibiotics				
Ciprofloxacin (Cipro)	For severe or complicated UTIs	500 mg PO q 12 h	Headache, restlessness, tremor, light-headedness, seizures, nausea, diarrhea, vomiting, oral candidiasis, crystalluria	Contraindicated in clients allergic to quinolone antibiotics, pregnant women, children; give 2 hr after meals; may cause CNS stimulation, seizures; drink plenty of water with medication; prolonged use may result in overgrowth of resistant organisms

Table 56–1. Medications Used to Treat Cystitis and Other Urinary Disorders *(Continued)*				
Agent	**Action**	**Dosage**	**Side Effects**	**Nursing Implications**
Cephalexin monohydrate (Keflex)	For GU infections	250 mg to 1 g PO q 6 h	Transient neutropenia, anemia, pseudomembranous colitis, nausea, anorexia, diarrhea, dyspepsia, urticaria, hypersensitivity	Use carefully in clients with a history of renal insufficiency or previous hypersensitivity to penicillin or cephalosporins; prolonged use may lead to overgrowth of resistant organisms; taken with food to decrease GI distress; be sure client takes full dose of medication; obtain cultures before starting medication

dispose the client to renal scarring and the development of chronic renal failure if the damage to the kidneys is frequent and severe enough.

■ Nursing Management of the Medical Client

Assessment

The nurse should start by assessing the client's risk factors for the development of cystitis. This involves obtaining a detailed history and physical examination. The nurse should have the client describe his or her symptoms in detail.

The nurse must also collect the necessary urine culture and sensitivity specimen. Instruct the client on the proper procedure for collection so that contamination from other surface organisms is minimized.

Diagnosis, Planning, Implementation

Altered Urinary Elimination. The primary diagnosis when a client is experiencing problems related to the

cystitis is *Altered Urinary Elimination related to irritation of the bladder mucosa.*

Planning: Expected Outcomes. The client will have urinary elimination return to normal within 3 days of the start of treatment, as evidenced by absence of fever, pain, burning, frequency, and urgency; have a normal white blood cell count; and have negative urine cultures 1 week after the course of antibiotics is completed.

Implementation. The nurse should assess the client's voiding, noting problems such as frequency, urgency, retention, and dysuria. The manifestations need to be treated immediately so the client can return to normal urinary function. Encourage the client to increase fluid intake to at least 3 L/day to help wash out the bacteria. Remind the client that diluting the urine will also decrease pain on voiding.

The nurse can help the client to reestablish a normal urinary pattern. One of the best ways to do this is through administration of the prescribed anti-infective agents (see Table 56–1) and education of the client to complete the entire course of treatment. The problems of dysuria, urgency, frequency, and possibly incontinence

Table 56–2. Acid-Ash Diet		
Foods Allowed	**Foods Prohibited (Basic Foods)**	**Neutral Foods**
Meat, fish, poultry, shellfish, cheese, eggs Grains: bread, cereals, crackers, rice, whole grains, pasta, corn Vegetables: corn, lentils Fruits: cranberries, prunes, plums, and their juices Foods with large amounts of chlorine, phosphorus, and sulfur	All milk and milk products All vegetables except corn and lentils All fruits except cranberries, plums, and prunes Foods containing large amounts of potassium, sodium, calcium, and magnesium	Coffee and tea Butter, margarine, oils White sugar, honey Cornstarch, tapioca Pure fats Pure carbohydrates

will decrease within 24 hours after beginning medication. The nurse should also check the culture and sensitivity report to be sure that the proper anti-infective agents are being administered.

Pain. Another common nursing diagnosis for clients with cystitis is *Pain related to irritation of bladder and urethral mucosa.*

Planning: Expected Outcomes. The client will be able to urinate without discomfort within 24 hours of treatment, as evidenced by absence of pain and burning on urination.

Implementation. The nurse should administer any medications prescribed specifically to treat pain, such as phenazopyridine or phenazopyridine-sulfasoxazole. Again, forcing fluids will also help relieve the pain by diluting the urine, making it less irritating to the mucosa. A warm sitz bath may help the pain by decreasing smooth muscle spasms, especially if the urethra is irritated. Baking soda can be added to the sitz bath water to produce a greater soothing effect. Some clients find that a heating pad applied to the suprapubic area helps reduce bladder spasms and suprapubic pain.

Evaluation

The nurse should assess the client for complete elimination of the infection. The client should have a negative urine culture on completion of the antibiotic therapy. Pain relief is another important evaluation. The best method for controlling pain is elimination of the infection.

Modifications for Elderly Clients

In older people, cystitis may occur more often, but for different reasons. Causes may include immobility, constipation, fecal and urinary incontinence, urinary retention, altered mental status, or systemic disease. In older women, atrophy of the vagina, decreased urethral and vaginal secretions, and muscle weakness in the vagina and bladder predispose this population to infection. In older men, benign prostatic hyperplasia (BPH) is one of the main risk factors for UTI, and the incidence of BPH increases with age. The causes of UTIs in this group will alter both prevention and treatment. In men, the best treatment for recurrent UTI is to treat the BPH. Once this problem is eliminated, the infections should be eliminated.

■ Surgical Management

Surgery is very uncommon and done only to treat any anomalies that may be causing repeated infections. Bladder neck or urethral strictures are the most common problems. BPH, the common cause of cystitis in older men, can also be treated surgically. When these disorders are corrected, the infections should stop.

■ Nursing Management of the Surgical Client

The nursing care for clients after surgery is discussed under the specific disorder. Chapter 83 discusses nursing care of men following surgery for BPH.

Community and Self-Care

■ Medical Management

Chronic or recurrent cystitis may require the prolonged use of antibiotics to eradicate the organisms. This therapy can last from 6 to 24 months. Women who experience recurrence related to sexual intercourse may be given antibiotics such as nitrofurantoin, trimethoprim-sulfamethoxazole, or cephalexin to be taken following coitus.

■ Nursing Management of the Medical Client

Assessment

The nurse needs to assess the client's ability to perform self-care in relation to chronic cystitis and to the risk of future infections.

Diagnosis, Planning Implementation

Risk for Ineffective Management of Therapeutic Regimen (Individuals). Clients with chronic cystitis or the potential to develop chronic cystitis may have a diagnosis of *Risk for Ineffective Management of Therapeutic Regimen (Individuals) related to prevention, medications, hygiene, and fluid intake.*

Planning: Expected Outcomes. The client will be able to describe ways to prevent UTI, the correct method for taking medication, multiple hygienic suggestions, and the required fluid intake.

Implementation. The nurse can do much to help the client learn to prevent cystitis. After analyzing the client's risk factors, the nurse can devise specific ways to help the client prevent cystitis from occurring or to treat it if it has occurred. Increased fluid intake to wash bacteria out of the bladder is one of the simplest ways to help prevent the infections. The nurse should instruct the client to drink at least eight 8-oz glasses of water a day and to avoid caffeine and alcohol, which can irritate the bladder. Remember, coffee, tea, chocolate, and some over-the-counter medications contain caffeine.

Many nursing interventions are directed at preventing the initial infection or recurrences. The nurse should teach all clients at risk to maintain a fluid intake of at least 3000 ml/day unless contraindicated. Remind the client to void at the first urge (unless the bladder program is planned otherwise) and at least every 2 to 3 hours during the day and once or twice at night to prevent bladder distention. Encourage women to void immediately after coitus and to drink at least two glasses of water as soon as possible. Recommend that women use a position for sexual intercourse, such as the missionary position, that minimizes pressure on the anterior vaginal wall. The nurse should emphasize the need for women to maintain good perineal hygiene and teach them to wipe the meatus from front to back. Advise the use of tampons rather than sanitary pads.

There are several ways women can compensate for the proximity of the urethra and the anus. Women who experience frequent UTIs are encouraged to shower rather than take a tub bath, because a bath is more likely to cause irritation and contamination of the urethra. Avoiding bubble baths is another way to decrease irritation. Wearing cotton underpants, which are more absorbent and breathable, and avoiding pantyhose with slacks, which traps more moisture in the perineal region, are two ways to lower a woman's risk of UTI.

To help decrease the risk associated with coitus, a woman should wash well before and void immediately after intercourse, and drink at least one to two glasses of water. She also should drink at least 3000 ml of fluid per day, preferably fluids that acidify the urine. Proper fitting of a diaphragm and correct use of spermicide also help decrease the risk. Encourage the client to take suppressive antibiotics after intercourse if ordered by the physician.

For decreasing UTI risk during pregnancy, a woman should increase her fluid intake to at least 3 L/day and void at least every 2 to 3 hours. She should have her urine monitored frequently for the development of an infection and have that infection treated immediately.

Strict asepsis is vital in decreasing the incidence of UTI in catheterized clients. Nurses must maintain a closed urinary system in all clients unless it is absolutely necessary to disrupt the system. Most specimens can be obtained from a closed system via the aspiration port on the drainage tube. Daily, meticulous perineal care and care after a bowel movement is important, although the agent to be used is controversial. The Centers for Disease Control (CDC) recommends soap and water as the best agent to use for cleaning the perineum and meatus.

The nurse should teach all high-risk clients the clinical manifestations of cystitis, instructing the client to seek healthcare assistance as soon as possible if these occur. When administering medication, make sure that the client understands the drug and its side effects, emphasizing the importance of taking the full course of the drug, even after the manifestations of infection disappear.

Finally, because of the high risk for more serious or recurrent infection and the possible need to begin further intervention early, emphasize the importance of complying with the recommended schedule of follow-up urine cultures.

Evaluation

The client's ability to manage the therapeutic regimen must be carefully evaluated. The client is often followed in the clinic to assess the effectiveness of treatment and the client's ability to provide self-care. If the infection persists or recurs, ask the client to describe self-care and monitor its effectiveness.

Modifications for Elderly Clients

When administering medications to older adults, the nurse must consider the renal and hepatic status of the client. Many of the drugs used to treat UTIs require the client to have adequate renal and hepatic function, particularly with long-term administration. There are often changes in the cardiovascular system such as congestive heart failure which prevent treatments such as forcing fluids. Recent studies have shown that for elderly women, 10 oz of cranberry juice is effective in lowering the urinary pH.

Interstitial Cystitis

Cystitis may also be noninfectious or abacterial. One type is interstitial cystitis (IC), also called Hunner's ulcer, a possible autoimmune disorder. This disorder is also called painful bladder disease (PBD). Another form of abacterial cystitis is hemorrhagic cystitis, usually secondary to radiation therapy and to certain chemotherapeutic drugs such as cyclophosphamide (Cytoxan).

Etiology and Risk Factors

IC occurs mainly in women (90%–95%). Although at one time it was considered a disease of menopause, it actually occurs more frequently in younger women.

Pathophysiology

IC is a poorly understood disorder with an unclear pathophysiology. It has been thought to be a type of local autoimmune phenomenon. One factor that is clear, however, is that, in spite of the manifestations, the urine is usually sterile. The current theory is that there seems to be some change in the permeability of the glycosaminoglycan layer of the bladder mucosa, which is usually impermeable by urea and bacteria. This theory has been questioned in some recent studies which suggest that permeability of the bladder in clients with IC is no greater than that in normal persons.[97]

There are characteristic pathologic changes found in IC, including nonspecific chronic inflammatory infiltrate, edema, vasodilation, and eventually fibrosis of the submucosa and detrusor layers of the bladder wall. Mast cell infiltrates have been identified in the bladders of clients with interstitial cystitis, particularly in the detrusor layer. Since mast cells are associated with allergic reactions, it is worth noting that approximately half the clients with interstitial cystitis are reported to have allergies and 30% have inflammatory bowel disease.[101]

Questions have been raised about the possibility that IC is an infectious disease, one where the agent has simply not been identified. The corollary used is the discovery of *Helicobacter pylori* with chronic gastritis. It is possible that the bacteria are found only in the wall of the bladder, not in the urine itself.[120]

Clinical Manifestations and Diagnostic Findings

The clinical manifestations of IC are severe lower abdominal or pelvic pain, urgency, frequency (up to 60 times a day in some clients), nocturia, and, in some women, dyspareunia (painful intercourse). Some clients may exhibit only frequency and pain; others will have all manifestations. Some women find the disorder extremely debilitating with manifestations so severe that they find life miserable. In the past, especially when this condition occurred in menopausal women, physicians often felt that it was a psychosomatic disorder. This assumption is much less prevalent today, but the nurse should be aware that it can exist. Manifestations are often present for 3 to 5 years before an accurate diagnosis is made.

In order to diagnose interstitial cystitis, the National Institute of Arthritis, Diabetes, Digestive, and Kidney Diseases (NIDDK) recommends a specific set of criteria. This includes a detailed client history, urodynamic evaluation, cystoscopy under anesthesia with hydrodistention of the bladder, and bladder biopsy.[48]

During cystoscopy and hydrodilation of the bladder, glomerulations (outpouches) in the bladder wall, Hunner's ulcers, and a severely decreased bladder capacity are noted. The presence of these findings is considered diagnostic by many physicians, whereas others believe the condition is present even without these findings. This second group bases the diagnosis on the absence of any other disease of the bladder that could cause the manifestations.

Acute and Subacute Care

■ Surgical Management

Surgery is not usually the preferred treatment for IC because IC is a chronic, but in no way life-threatening, disease. A transurethral resection (TUR) or laser surgical resection of lesions may be done. The traditional therapy is hydraulic distention of the bladder, with or without instillation of dimethyl sulfoxide (DMSO) to increase the bladder's functional capacity. Clients with severely reduced bladder capacity and incapacitating manifestations may be candidates for either partial or complete cystectomy and urinary diversion.[58]

■ Nursing Management of the Surgical Client

Care for the client who has a TUR or cystectomy and urinary diversion is covered in detail under Bladder Neoplasms.

Community and Self-Care

■ Medical Management

Since this problem is not caused by infection, the treatment is different from that for bacterial cystitis. Antibiotics may actually cause further bladder irritation. The treatment for IC is controversial, with no one accepted treatment. Drugs such as anti-inflammatories, antispasmodics, tricyclic antidepressants, and antihistamines are used, as well as tranquilizers and occasionally narcotics.

Recently, a study looking at the effectiveness of cimetidine (Tagamet), the H_2-receptor antagonist, found that it provided symptomatic relief for clients with refractory cystitis.[106] It has only been used in small groups, but since the side effects of the medication are minimal, it may offer a safe, effective treatment alternative.

Another oral agent that has shown promise in the treatment of IC is the calcium channel blocker nifedipine. Treatment with this agent for a minimum of 3 months has been effective in many clients. Hydroxyzine, a tricyclic, H_1-receptor antagonist, has also shown effectiveness against IC. The low cost and minimal side effects, mainly dry mouth and mild sedation, makes it an effective alternative to more costly and riskier treatments.

Other treatments include instillation of a variety of agents into the bladder to promote healing and pain relief. These include agents such as sodium oxychlorosene (Clorpactin), silver nitrate, and DMSO. Oral sodium pentosan polysulfate (Elmiron), a heparin analog, is given to create a mucin layer in the bladder. Heparin itself has been instilled in the bladder three times a week for 3 months with good results. Some clients continue the treatments for up to a year. A significant number of those using the heparin instillations remained in remission after 1 year.[87] All of these treatments are designed to decrease the permeability of the bladder mucosa so that urea and bacteria have more difficulty penetrating the lining.

Although the mechanism of action is unclear, bacille Calmette-Guérin (BCG) has been effective as an intravesicle agent administered weekly. BCG instillations for 6 weeks have led to a decreased need for pain medications, a doubling of cystometric capacity, and a decrease in client discomfort.[132]

■ Nursing Management of the Medical Client

The major nursing responsibility associated with this syndrome is supporting the client through diagnosis and treatment. Because the cause of this disorder is unclear, there is little the nurse can teach the client about preventive measures. It is a chronic disorder requiring long-term client support. Clients require a great deal of reassurance because the diagnosis and treatment are so uncertain. The nurse should become familiar with the national and local resources for clients with IC or PBD (Interstitial Cystitis Association) and refer clients as appropriate.

Urosepsis

Urosepsis is defined as a gram-negative bacteremia originating in the genitourinary tract. The most common predisposing factor is the presence of an indwelling catheter or preexisting and untreated UTI in a client already medically compromised. It is a common diagnosis in nursing home clients admitted to the hospital. The most common organism responsible for gram-negative bacteremia is *E. coli*. A major problem associated with urinary infection is the ability of this bacterium to develop resistant strains.

The actual pathophysiologic mechanisms of urosepsis are complex and not fully understood. Urosepsis can lead to septic shock if not treated aggressively. The cell wall of the gram-negative bacillus is composed of a lipid-carbohydrate complex. Bacteria release endotoxins which damage cells. The cells release lysosomes which further damage tissues and set off the kinins and complement cascade. Cellular metabolism becomes anaerobic, and lactic acidosis develops. Fever is the most common early manifestation observed.

Treatment of gram-negative urosepsis must be prompt and aggressive following specimen collection for culture and sensitivity to prevent sepsis and shock. It is initially treated with intravenous aminoglycosides, β-lactam antibiotics, such as aztreonam, or the third-generation cephalosporins until culture results are available. As soon as culture and sensitivity results are obtained, the antibiotic is changed if indicated. Intravenous treatment is continued until the client has been afebrile for 3 to 5 days; then oral antibiotics are used. See Chapter 22 for information on septic shock.

It is important for the nurse to be aware of the potential for hospitalized clients with indwelling catheters to develop urosepsis so that diagnosis and treatment can be made early. This is vital because of the possibility that it can progress to septic shock. The nurse needs to obtain a urine culture and sensitivity as soon as possible so that the appropriate medication can be started.

Urethritis

Urethritis is inflammation of the urethra. It is a common problem associated with sexually transmitted diseases (STDs) (see Chapter 86 for incidence) and may be seen with cystitis. The most common causes of urethritis in men are gonorrhea and chlamydial infection. In women, it is often caused by feminine hygiene sprays, perfumed toilet paper and sanitary napkins, spermicidal jellies, UTIs, and changes in the vaginal mucosal lining.

Any irritant in contact with the urethra has the potential of causing urethritis. In men, prevention of gonorrhea and other STDs is the primary way to prevent urethritis. In women, avoidance of perfumed toilet paper and sanitary napkins and of feminine hygiene sprays helps prevent the development of urethritis. If the woman uses spermicidal jelly, she should be aware of the risk of developing urethritis. Coitus itself has not been shown to cause urethritis.

With exposure to the irritant, the mucosal lining of the urethra becomes highly inflamed. The mucosa becomes swollen and painful, and pus may be produced. The presence of pus cells in the urine is called *pyuria*. The urethral lining is red and irritated, and the meatus may be swollen.

As with cystitis, assessment reveals dysuria, frequency, urgency, and nocturia. In women, a history reveals exposure to the causative agents. The client may also complain of very low abdominal or perineal pain or discomfort. Male clients frequently exhibit a urethral discharge, but not females.

Culture and sensitivity testing of the urine may be negative. If the cause is an STD, then tests for this are positive. The diagnosis is often made on the basis of the client's history and the clinical manifestations.

Management of urethritis includes removing its cause and, if it is caused by microorganisms, administering systemic and topical antibiotics. Sitz baths, especially with baking soda in the water, and high fluid intake are also helpful. The client should be told to avoid coitus until the manifestations subside or treatment of the STD is completed, although the use of lubricants with intercourse seems to decrease irritation in women who have had frequent attacks. See Table 56–1 for common medications. The physician may also prescribe topical estrogens.

Urethritis is usually not treated surgically. If strictures occur, then the urethra is dilated with sounds. If the strictures are severe, surgical correction is warranted. If there is scarring at the meatus, a meatotomy may be done.

Ureteritis

Ureteritis is an inflammation of the ureter commonly associated with pyelonephritis (see Chapter 56). Once the kidney infection is cured, ureteral inflammation usually subsides. Unfortunately, chronic pyelonephritis causes the ureter to become fibrotic and narrowed by strictures.

Genitourinary Tuberculosis

Mycobacterium tuberculosis is increasing in occurrence, especially in the poor, the malnourished, those living in close quarters, and the immunosuppressed. Genitourinary tuberculosis is usually a late manifestation of tuberculosis (TB) caused by spread from the lungs through the bloodstream. Genitourinary TB occurs in about 20% of clients with TB. The bacillus may infect the kidney, ureter, bladder, testes, epididymis, and occasionally the prostate, penis, and urethra.

The medical management of genitourinary TB is the same as that for systemic disease (see Chapter 42). Antitubercular agents include medications such as isonicotinic acid hydrazide (INH), ethambutol, and rifampicin.

The nurse should use precautions when handling urine specimens from the client since the bacillus in the urine is infectious. The nurse must also teach the client precautions to avoid the spread of the disease to significant others. Male clients should be taught to use condoms during intercourse to prevent spread of the organism.

Obstructive Disorders

Bladder Neoplasms

Most bladder cancers are papillomatous growths in the bladder urothelium, although these growths may infiltrate the bladder wall. Bladder cancer is the most frequent neoplasm of the urinary tract, accounting for approximately 3% of all deaths due to cancer. It occurs most frequently in those age 40 to 60 years. Also, it appears in men two to three times more often than in women, although the incidence in women is rising. This cancer is now the 5th most common cancer in men and the 10th most common cancer in women. It affects whites twice as often as blacks. It is more common in people living in the urban, industrialized northern states as opposed to those living in the southern states.[29]

Etiology and Risk Factors

The disease process has several possible causes. There seems to be a strong correlation between cigarette smoking and the incidence of bladder cancer. Industrial exposure to certain substances or conditions also may cause bladder cancer. These include aniline dyes, aromatic amines like benzidine and naphthylamine, leather finishings, metal machinery, and processing petroleum products. The latency period for this industrial exposure can be as long as 20 to 45 years. Attempts to connect coffee consumption and bladder cancer produced contradictory findings. Another controversy relates artificial sweeteners to the incidence of bladder cancer, although recent studies find no significant increase in bladder cancer from these. Some authorities believe that clients with recurrent bladder tumors should avoid artificial sweeteners since these may act as cancer promoting agents.[61] See Risk Factors and Levels of Prevention.

Pathophysiology

Cigarette smoking or passive receipt of secondhand smoke may result in carcinogenic metabolites produced by abnormal tryptophan metabolism, with the metabolite excreted in the urine. Cigarette smoke also contains nitrosamines as well as 2-naphthylamine, both carcinogens, which are also excreted in the urine.

Most bladder cancers start as papillomas that undergo malignant changes. Nodular tumors occur less frequently but may also invade the bladder wall. Cellular proliferation is chiefly in the transitional epithelium (90%), although squamous cell (6%) or adenocarcinoma (2%) may occur.

Staging of the tumor indicates the depth of penetration into the bladder wall and its degree of metastasis. Staging must be done before selection of the treatment mode. For clinical staging, the physician needs to review at least the results from an excretory urogram, cystoscopy, biopsy, and bimanual examination under anesthesia. To check for specific areas of metastasis as well as for staging, chest

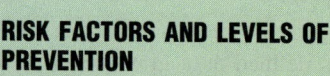

RISK FACTORS AND LEVELS OF PREVENTION

Bladder Cancer

Risk Factors

Long-term industrial exposure to aniline dyes and aromatic amines; dry cleaning chemicals; leather finishing; metal machinery; processing petroleum products; pelvic radiation; cyclophosphamide; Other Factors: smoking; chronic cystitis; chronic bladder calculi; cyclamates; large doses of phenacetin; schistosomiasis; male gender; age (over 60); low intake of retinoids

Levels of Prevention

Primary Prevention
- Stop smoking
- Limit industrial exposure as much as possible
- Avoid ingestion of large amounts of phenacetin
- Increase intake of retinoids

Secondary Prevention
- Monitor high-risk clients for development of hematuria
- Encourage high-risk clients to see a physician regularly, especially after age 60

Tertiary Prevention
- Teach clients to care for urinary diversion
- Encourage clients to return for regular cystoscopy follow-up after transurethral resections of superficial bladder tumors

radiography, lymphangiography, isotope bone scans, computed tomography (CT), and liver function analysis are needed. Figure 56–1 illustrates the usual staging schema.[63]

- Stage 0 $(T_{IS}N_0M_0)$ tumor is limited to the mucosa, includes carcinoma in situ
- Stage A $(T_1N_0M_0)$ tumor indicates invasion no farther than the submucosa
- Stage B_1 $(T_2N_0M_0)$ tumor extends not more than halfway through the muscle layer
- Stage B_2 $(T_{3a}N_0M_0)$ tumor penetrates more deeply into the muscle layer but not into the fat
- Stage C $(T_{3b}N_0M_0)$ tumor has infiltrated beyond the muscle layer but is not metastatic, nor is it invading adjacent structures
- Stage D_1 $(T_{4a}N_{1-3}M_0)$ tumor metastasizes to the pelvic lymph nodes
- Stage D_2 $(T_{4a}N_4M_1)$ tumor metastasizes beyond the pelvis

Common sites for metastasis include liver, bones, and lungs. As the tumor progresses, it can extend into the rectum, vagina, other pelvic soft tissues, and retroperitoneal structures. The prognostic "dividing line" lies between stages B_1 and B_2; tumors staged C or D on the scale have a much poorer prognosis. Less than 25% of

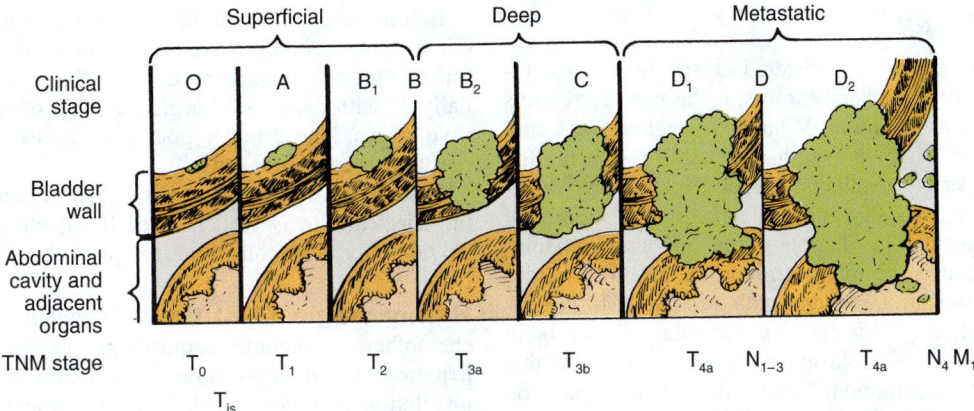

Figure 56–1. The Jewett-Marshall clinical staging of bladder cancer. Diagram shows degree of tumor infiltration at each stage and compares it with the TNM system. (Adapted from Karlowicz, K. A. (Ed.). (1995). *Urologic nursing: Principles and practice.* Philadelphia: W. B. Saunders.)

clients with deeply invasive tumors have a 5-year survival rate; aggressive adenocarcinoma results in an average survival rate of 21 months.

Superficial tumors have a good chance of being eradicated or stabilized, although recurrence is frequent. Because recurrence is high, it is crucial to do follow-up examinations with cystoscopy every 3 months. In a study of 114 clients, the interval between the original intervention and the recurrence of tumor ranged from 3 months to 27 years. Nineteen percent involved a new tumor of a higher grade, and 22% of the tumors were of a more advanced stage. Most recurrences of superficial tumors represent lesions that can be controlled by TUR.[63]

Clinical Manifestations and Diagnostic Findings

Gross painless hematuria is most frequently the first manifestation of bladder cancer, occurring in 75% of all cases. Unfortunately, the bleeding is usually intermittent initially, which often causes a delay in seeking healthcare. As the disease progresses, the client may experience frequent bladder irritability with dysuria and frequency. Finally, gross hematuria or a clot-induced obstruction forces the client to seek help. The amount of hematuria, however, does not correlate directly with the stage of disease.

The most basic test for bladder cancer is urinalysis. The presence of blood in the urine, especially if no other cause is apparent, warrants extensive work-up. Cystoscopy should be done to visualize the tumor directly and to biopsy the lesion for cytologic study. Flow cytometry can be done to examine the DNA content of the cells in the urine. Cytology on a total voided urine specimen, obtained in the late morning and sent immediately to the laboratory, is done to check for the presence of malignant cells. Cytology can also be done on specimens obtained during cystoscopy. The specimen is obtained when the bladder is irrigated with a solution of Ringer's lactate.

Another examination is the intravenous pyelogram (IVP), which evaluates not only the bladder but also the ureters and kidneys looking for filling defects. CT, mag-

netic resonance imaging (MRI), and ultrasonography also may be done to assess the bladder and surrounding structures, such as the rectum or uterus, possible sites of spread. A tumor marker, the serum carcinoembryonic antigen (CEA) level, present with adenocarcinomas of the bladder, can also be evaluated.

Acute and Subacute Care

■ Medical Management

Several forms of intervention are used in the acute medical management of bladder cancer, including chemotherapy and radiation therapy. Radiation therapy is more acceptable for advanced disease that cannot be eradicated by radical surgery. Most bladder cancers are poorly radiosensitive and therefore require higher doses of radiation.

Radiation Therapy

Intracavitary radiation applies radiation to the bladder malignancy while the adjacent tissues are protected. Radium seeds are inserted through a cystoscope or through a suprapubic opening in the bladder and placed directly in the tumor. Other methods of administering radiation therapy are through an indwelling catheter, its balloon filled with isotopes, or through planting of seeds in the uterus or vagina.

External supervoltage radiation, rather unsuccessful by itself, is effective when used in combination with surgery or chemotherapy. It may be used preoperatively to inactivate tumor cells that might disseminate during surgery and to control micrometastasis. Hyperbaric radiation therapy increases the oxygen tension of the tumor cells and therefore their radiosensitivity. Palliative radiation may be used to relieve pain, bowel obstruction, control potential hemorrhage, and leg edema secondary to venous or lymphatic obstruction.

Chemotherapy

Chemotherapy can be administered at any time, even replace surgery for superficial tumors, or be used for clients when cure is not an option. Vitamin A analogs are being investigated for "chemoprevention" capabilities during the preneoplasia period. Antineoplastic chemotherapy is administered both topically and systemically for superficial tumors. Intravesical instillation of an alkylating chemotherapeutic agent is the most common method; it provides concentrated topical treatment with relatively little systemic absorption. Thiotepa, mitomycin, doxorubicin (Adriamycin), and cyclophosphamide are all used for this purpose. After instillation, rotate the client's position every 15 to 30 minutes, starting in the supine position to avoid lying on a full bladder.

More recently, BCG has been used as an intravesical agent. It is now considered more effective than the older agents and is being used more commonly than even thiotepa, especially in carcinoma in situ and superficial tumors. Usually the medication is injected into the bladder through a urethral catheter, the catheter is clamped or removed, and the client is asked to retain the fluid for 2 hours and to change position every 15 to 30 minutes from side to side and from supine to prone or simply to resume all activity immediately. The client then voids in a sitting position (or the catheter is unclamped) and is then instructed to drink two glasses of water to help flush the bladder.

Systemic agents, including cisplatin (Platinol), doxorubicin, methotrexate, cyclophosphamide, and pyridoxine, are also used to treat inoperable or late tumors.

Complications

Abacterial Cystitis and Proctitis. The client receiving radiation therapy is at increased risk of developing complications. The most frequent complications include severe manifestations of cystitis and proctitis causing dysuria, frequency, urgency, nocturia, and diarrhea. Delayed adverse effects, such as ileitis, colitis, persistent cystitis, and bladder ulceration and hemorrhage, may occur as late as 6 to 12 months after radiation, with hemorrhagic cystitis possibly occurring 10 years after pelvic radiation.

Fistula Formation. Radiation therapy also increases the risk of fistula formation. A fistula is an abnormal passage between two organs or between an organ and the skin. This allows intercommunication of secretions and other substances. After radiation to the bladder, a vesicovaginal fistula (in women) or a colovesical fistula (in men) may develop.

A fistula is suspected when urine leaves the body from an unnatural site such as the vagina, when fecal material or air appears in the urine, or when the client suffers from recurrent UTIs. Diagnosis is confirmed by IVP, cystography, cystoscopy, or sigmoidoscopy. To further delineate the path of a fistula, a dye such as Congo red or indigo carmine is instilled into the bladder, and all outlets are identified.

Before surgical repair of the fistula is undertaken, the client must maintain a continuous flow of urine from the kidney through temporary urinary diversion, either externally or with catheters. Surgical repairs often require multiple stages. The primary goal is to excise the fistula and reestablish tissue integrity.

Postoperatively, urinary diversion is maintained until the surgical site is well healed. If catheters are in place, irrigate only after consulting the physician.

Hemorrhagic Cystitis. The major side effects of chemotherapy include hemorrhagic cystitis and bladder irritation. Local application of formalin through bladder instillation may control bladder hemorrhaging that results from the cancer or the treatments.

Outcomes

Intravesical BCG therapy appears to be quite successful in treating carcinoma in situ and in slowing the recurrence of early bladder cancers, more so than intravesical treatment with thiotepa. Systemic chemotherapeutic agents have been shown to be effective in prolonging life in clients with metastatic disease. Radiation therapy alone is not as effective a treatment for invasive bladder cancer as surgery and chemotherapy, with a 5-year survival of 20% to 39%.[49]

■ Nursing Management of the Medical Client

Assessment

The nurse should begin the assessment of the client being evaluated for bladder cancer with a careful history, looking especially for exposure to known risk factors. The nurse should also question the client about changes in urine or in urination, noting changes in color, frequency, and amount. Any abnormal passage of urine, especially vaginally, suggests the development of a fistula (a late development). Hematuria should always be investigated further.

Diagnosis, Planning, Implementation

Risk for Injury. The client who undergoes either chemotherapy or radiation therapy is at a *Risk for Injury related to side effects of radiation therapy and chemotherapy.*

Planning: Expected Outcomes. The client will not develop sequelae to radiation therapy or chemotherapy, as evidenced by absence of hemorrhagic cystitis or proctitis.

Implementation. Interventions for the side effects of radiation therapy include administering antispasmodics, increasing the client's fluid intake, and administering urinary tract antiseptics or analgesics for the cystitis. The client with proctitis requires a low residue diet and agents to decrease intestinal motility. Complete information on nursing care for clients receiving radiation therapy is covered in Chapter 23. Save the urine from clients undergoing this intervention and send it to the radioisotopes laboratory for monitoring. Learn your healthcare facility's policies about isolation of the client and the precautions to be taken. In general, clients with implants are put in a private room with limited visiting.

Nursing care for the client receiving chemotherapy is also covered in Chapter 23. If the client has intravesical chemotherapy, the nurse should remember to treat the agent and the urine as a biohazard, the same as for any other chemotherapy that needs to be disposed of properly. For 6 hours after intravesical chemotherapy, disinfect the urine and toilet with household bleach. Increase fluids to help flush all the medication out of the bladder following the period of retention. These treatments are typically repeated weekly for 4 to 8 weeks and then monthly for varying periods. Follow-up cystoscopies are always done to monitor tumor growth.

Evaluation

These problems are difficult to control since they are actually complications of treatment. Hemorrhagic cystitis or proctitis should resolve as the treatment is completed. Late effects of treatment should be explained to the client, including actions to take if these complications develop. Although prevention is not always possible, a successful outcome would be resolution of the complication.

■ Surgical Management

Surgical therapy is commonly used to treat bladder cancer. Surgical intervention ranges from local resection and fulguration (destruction of tissue by electrical current through electrodes placed in direct contact with the growth) of the tumor to total cystectomy, which requires diversion of normal urinary flow.

Transurethral Resection

The simplest procedure is TUR of the tumor and fulguration, done for very early superficial tumors for cure or sometimes for inoperable tumors for palliation.

Partial Cystectomy

A segmental or partial cystectomy may be done for clients who cannot tolerate a radical cystectomy and for early tumors. Up to half of the bladder can be removed. During the initial postoperative period, bladder capacity is markedly reduced. The postoperative bladder may be able to hold no more than 60 ml. However, over several months, bladder tissue expands, increasing its capacity from 200 to 400 ml.

Radical Cystectomy and Urinary Diversion

When the client is determined to have potentially curable stage B disease that is too advanced for TUR and intravesical chemotherapy, the treatment of choice is a radical cystectomy and urinary diversion. Radical cystectomy entails removal of the bladder and urethra in women and the bladder, urethra, and usually the prostate and seminal vesicles in men. Radical cystectomy also involves the removal of perivesical fat and dissection of the pelvic lymph nodes and, in women, includes the removal of the anterior vaginal wall, uterus, fallopian tubes, and ovaries. This procedure is necessary when the tumor has invaded the bladder wall, involves the trigone, or whenever the malignancy cannot be treated adequately by less radical methods.

When the bladder and urethra are removed, permanent urinary diversion is required. Several alternatives are possible. The entire surgery may be done in one step with urinary diversion and cystectomy performed at the same time. The surgery may be done in two stages when there is extensive tumor, with urinary diversion performed during the first operation and cystectomy done several weeks later. Radiation therapy may be given between surgeries.

Creation of an Ileal Conduit

An ileal conduit, also called ureteroileostomy, ileal bladder, or Bricker's procedure, was the most common urinary diversion alternative. Using a segment of the intestine as a conduit, this procedure constructs a system in which urine is emptied through an artificial opening in the skin (stoma) (Fig. 56–2). Usually, a portion of the terminal ileum, which has the least reabsorptive power, is isolated for the conduit, although transverse colon has been used. After the continuity of the remaining intestine is reestablished with end-to-end anastomosis, the proximal end of the segment is closed. The distal end is brought out through a hole created in the abdominal wall, folded back, and sutured to the skin to form a stoma. The ureters are then implanted into the ileal segment. The urine flows into the conduit and is continually propelled out through the stoma by peristalsis. Because the ileal segment is not a reservoir there is minimal absorption of electrolytes. An ileal conduit requires the client to wear an appliance over the stoma to collect the urine.

Creation of a Kock Pouch

Another procedure is the Kock pouch or continent internal ileal reservoir which is created from a segment of ileum and ascending colon made into a reservoir. Once the reservoir has been created, the ureters are implanted into the side of the reservoir. A special nipple valve is then constructed and used to attach the reservoir to the skin. Several weeks after surgery, the client is taught to use a catheter to drain the reservoir at 4- to 6-hour intervals. Electrolyte reabsorption is minimal with this diversion as long as the urine is drained regularly.

Creation of an Indiana Pouch

An even newer procedure, similar to the Kock pouch, is the Indiana pouch. During this procedure, a reservoir is created from the ascending colon and terminal ileum, making a larger pouch than the Kock pouch (Fig. 56–3). Clients learn how to self-catheterize and empty the pouch at 4- to 6-hour intervals. There are other continent reservoir surgeries, varying slightly in surgical technique and the portion of the colon and ileum used.

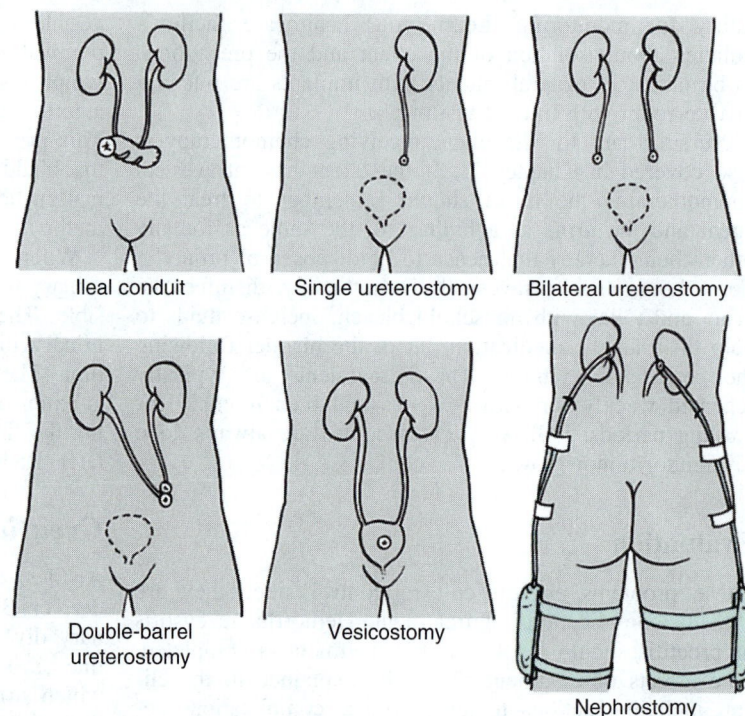

Figure 56–2. Some older surgical alternatives for urinary diversion.

Ileal conduit   Single ureterostomy   Bilateral ureterostomy

Double-barrel ureterostomy   Vesicostomy   Nephrostomy

Creation of a Neobladder

At times the urethra can be spared allowing the creation of a *neobladder*. This surgery is similar to the creation of an internal reservoir, the difference being that instead of emptying through an abdominal stoma, it empties via a pelvic outlet to the urethra. Continence can be a problem unless the lower portion of the bladder can be spared; otherwise continence depends on the urethra and external sphincter. Male clients tend to achieve better continence,

although many clients report continuing problems with nocturnal enuresis.

Many surgeons believe the urethra should be removed since there is a risk of tumor recurrence. If the urethra is resected, a reconstructed neourethra together with an artificial sphincter is created. This procedure is more successful in males than in females.

Several weeks after surgery, the catheter is removed and the client empties the neobladder with a combination of relaxing the external sphincter and creating abdominal

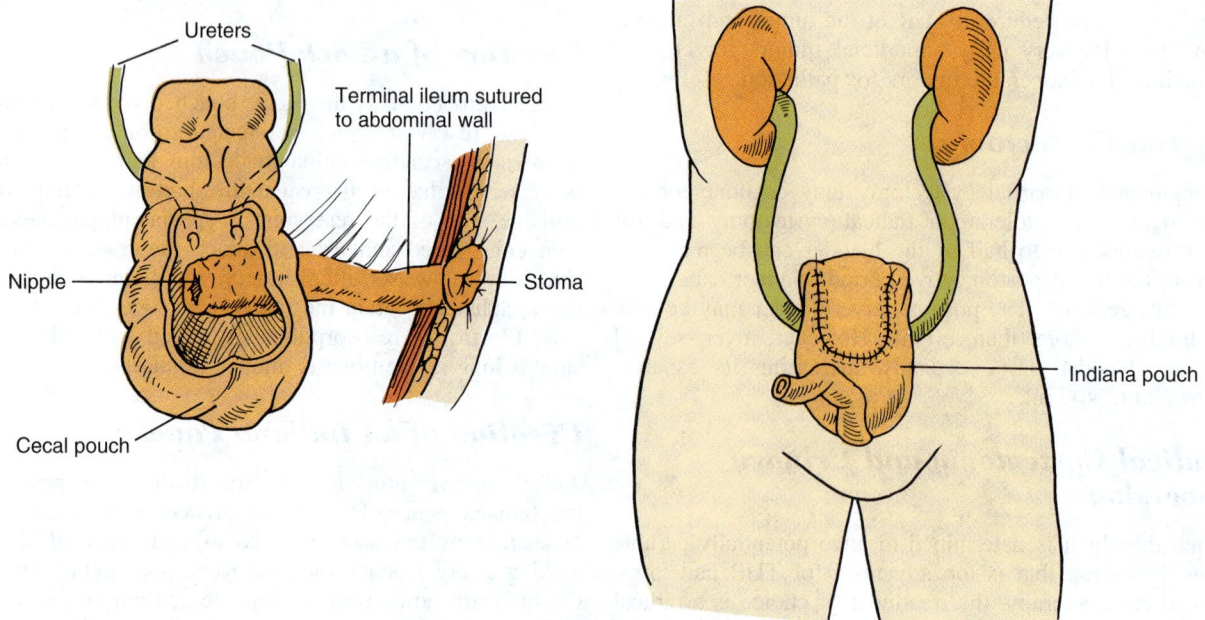

Ureters

Terminal ileum sutured to abdominal wall

Nipple

Stoma

Cecal pouch

Indiana pouch

Figure 56–3. Indiana pouch procedure.

pressure. If this technique of emptying the bladder is unsuccessful, the client will have to learn intermittent self-catheterization. Even with possible difficulties the client may encounter, acceptance of this procedure is very high since it maintains a more normal anatomy for the client.

Palliative Procedures

Percutaneous Nephrostomy or Pyelostomy

With inoperable bladder cancer, a percutaneous nephrostomy (see Fig. 56–2) or pyelostomy may be inserted to prevent obstruction. This procedure is an insertion of a catheter into the renal pelvis by surgical incision or more likely, a percutaneous puncture procedure. In the surgical approach, a balloon- or mushroom-tipped catheter is connected to an external drainage system. In percutaneous nephrostomy, a trocar is inserted under fluoroscopy by direct puncture into the renal pelvis or calix. Then a flexible small-gauge needle is used to instill contrast material to verify proper location. By use of angiographic wire as a guide, the nephrostomy tube is placed and connected to a closed drainage system. The entire procedure is done under local anesthesia. It is important to stabilize the tube to prevent dislodgement.

Ureterostomy

A ureterostomy may be performed as a palliative procedure if the ureters are obstructed by tumor. A cutaneous ureterostomy attaches the ureter to the surface of the abdomen where urine flows directly into a drainage appliance without an intermediary conduit. For clients with ureterostomies, infection, obstruction to urine flow secondary to strictures at the opening, and skin irritation are potential problems. There are several variations of this procedure (see Fig. 56–2).

- A single or bilateral ureterostomy (brings the distal end of the ureter out through the abdominal wall, creating one or two stomas as appropriate)
- A transureteroureterostomy produces only one stoma, because one ureter is connected to the other ureter
- A double-barreled ureterostomy forms two stomas in very close proximity as both ureters are brought to the surface together
- A loop ureterostomy is usually a temporary diversion that brings the midsection of the ureters to the skin surface for drainage; the rest of the urinary tract is left intact, allowing normal urinary functioning to be reestablished later

Vesicostomy

A vesicostomy (Fig. 56–4) produces a hold in the abdomen directly over the bladder. After suturing the bladder to the abdominal wall, the surgeon forms a stoma in the bladder wall. Through this stoma, the bladder can be emptied.

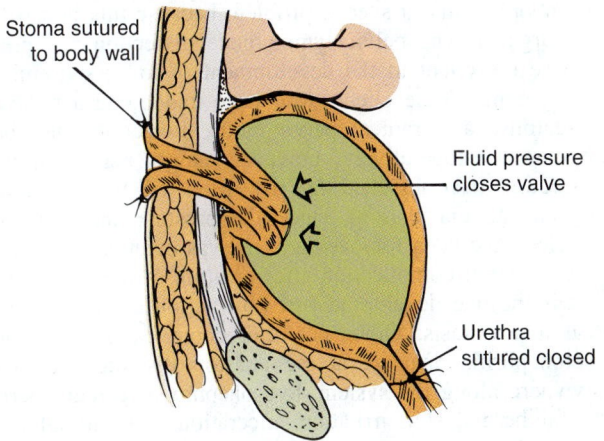

Figure 56–4. A continent vesicostomy.

Postoperative Management

Postoperative care includes the usual care for a client after major abdominal surgery. If there is a stoma, assessment of that stoma is vital postoperatively. The stoma should be red and moist. Any sign of darkness or duskiness may mean loss of vascular supply and must be corrected immediately or necrosis can occur. Peristalsis will be absent for several days on account of the manipulation and resection so the client will be NPO (nothing by mouth) with intravenous lines.

Urine flow never stops after surgery. Ureteral stents originating in the renal pelves extend through the ureters and through the reservoir, conduit, or neobladder. The stents usually exit through the stoma and are usually contained in the pouch. With the continent reservoirs, a catheter is placed through the stoma to drain the internal reservoir for 2 to 3 weeks until healing occurs. In the case of the neobladder, a catheter may be placed through the abdominal wall into the reservoir to keep it drained, while another catheter is placed through the urethra to be used as a stent to protect the anastomosis of the urethra and neobladder. The stents and catheter are removed once adequate healing has occurred.

With the reservoirs, clients must learn, prior to discharge from the hospital, to irrigate the reservoir at regular intervals. With the neobladder, the client will have to learn new ways of voiding, relaxing the external sphincter and performing abdominal straining.

Complications

Hematuria, a common problem after TUR, is controlled with a three-way indwelling catheter and, if necessary, bladder irrigation.

The greatest potential problem after a segmental resection is bladder distention, which can put too much pressure on the suture line, causing leakage and possible rupture of the bladder.

A radical cystectomy can cause several complications. It is a very invasive surgery, lasting 5 to 7 hours, which leaves the client at risk for most of the usual postoperative complications, including shock, hemorrhage, and thrombophlebitis (a special problem because this is a pelvic surgery). The pelvic lymph node dissection can predispose the client to the development of lower extremity lymphedema. Male clients who have undergone a radical cystectomy and radical pelvic node dissection may be impotent postoperatively; however, newer nerve-sparing procedures have lessened this risk. Men will have a "dry" orgasm (no ejaculation), since the prostate and seminal vesicles have been removed and the vas deferens ligated.

A potential complication after creation of the ileal conduit is the late development of obstruction at the uretero-ileal anastomosis. Other potential complications include pyelonephritis, leakage at the anastomosis site, stenosis anywhere along the system, hydronephrosis, calculi, peristomal hernia, skin irritation, ulceration, and stomal defects.

Stenosis of the stoma may occur from scarring during stomal maturation. If the opening on the faceplate is too large, epithelial hyperplasia or thickening of the peristomal skin may contract the stoma. Clients with urinary diversion are also prone to uric acid and calcium stone disease. The onset of urinary stone development usually occurs at least 2 years postoperatively and sometimes as long as 5 to 10 years later. UTI is a perpetual threat because of the exposure of the urinary tract. Obstruction anywhere in the urinary tract will interfere with normal urine flow.

The potential complications of continent reservoirs include incontinence, difficult catheterization, urinary reflux and possible pyelonephritis, obstruction, bacteriuria, electrolyte imbalances, urinary lithiasis, or absorptive problems. A major problem that can develop is rupture of the reservoir if the client is not compliant with the self-catheterization protocol.

Outcomes

Carcinoma in situ is considered curable with a simple TUR. BCG may be combined to decrease risk of recurrence. Even with a radical cystectomy, the 5-year survival rate for clients with muscle invasive tumor (stage C or later) is only 40% to 50%.

■ Nursing Management of the Surgical Client

Assessment

It is important for the nurse to assess the client's level of knowledge concerning the disease, diagnostic evaluation, and particularly his or her understanding of the surgical procedure to be done and the outcome of that procedure.

Postoperative assessment of urinary output, wound healing, the stoma, return of bowel function, and the outcome of the surgical procedure is vital. Assessing the client for the occurrence of postoperative complications also is of great importance. If the client has some form of urinary diversion, the nurse must assess the client's ability to provide self-care (see Ethical Issues in Nursing). The client also should be assessed for alterations in sexuality and body image that may occur following surgical intervention.

Diagnosis, Planning, Implementation

Knowledge Deficit. *Knowledge Deficit related to lack of information about diagnostic tests, surgery, and type of urinary diversion* is the highest-priority nursing diagnosis in the preoperative client since fear of the unknown is one of the most common fears.

Planning: Expected Outcomes. The client will understand the diagnostic tests, surgery, and care of the urinary diversion, as evidenced by his or her statements and demonstrations of self-care.

Implementation. Preoperative preparation of clients undergoing diversionary surgery includes (1) helping the client understand the surgical treatment options, (2) giving teaching guidelines concerning the urinary diversion decided upon, and (3) encouraging acceptance of the fact that diversion (other than the neobladder) results in the elimination of urine through a stoma and not through the urethral meatus as was once "normal." The enterostomal therapy nurse is an excellent resource for the nursing staff.

Since a segment of bowel will be used to create the conduit or reservoir, the client will have to undergo bowel preparation (see Chapter 62 for a complete discussion of colon surgery). This procedure includes a clear liquid diet, cleaning the bowel through laxatives and enemas, and antibiotics to lower the bacterial count within the bowel.

If the surgeon plans to construct a stoma, the site is selected during the preoperative period. An enterostomal therapy nurse should be involved in the care at this point and throughout the care of this client. The main criterion for stomal placement is that the site allow the faceplate of the drainage appliance to bind securely to the abdominal surface as well as be clearly visible to the client. This means that the surgeon must avoid the umbilicus, rib margins, pubis, iliac crests, and any pre-existing scars, wrinkles, or crevices. Placing the stoma directly on the client's waistline can cause excessive pressure by clothing. The client is observed in the supine, standing, and sitting positions during the selection process. Stoma placement is usually on the right lower quadrant of the abdomen, in the abdominal rectus muscle, about 2 inches below the waist and 2 inches from the midline. The client also will need to be taught the proper way to care for the urinary diversion.

Risk for Body Image Disturbance. The client who is to undergo a urinary diversion is likely to be at *Risk for Body Image Disturbance related to urinary diversion and altered urinary route and pattern.*

Planning: Expected Outcomes. The client will develop a positive self-concept, body image, and self-esteem after the urinary diversion, as evidenced by the client's acceptance of diversion (often measured by client's ability to perform total self-care) and ability to return to usual activities of daily living (ADL).

Implementation. Whatever diversion alternative is selected, assume that the client and significant others will need a great deal of emotional support. Changing the normal route of urine flow and the client's usual micturi-

ETHICAL ISSUES IN NURSING

What Can You Do to Prevent a Premature Hospital Discharge?

You are caring for Mr. Howard, a 75-year-old man who has recently been diagnosed with bladder cancer. He is a retired Air Force pilot who lives alone. He has had good preoperative teaching, and preoperatively he appeared to be physically and psychologically prepared to undergo bilateral ureterostomy surgery. Postoperatively, however, Mr. Howard is not recovering well. He has a great deal of pain and is very slow to ambulate. Although the nurses have been spending a lot of time with Mr. Howard on postoperative teaching, he seems uninterested in caring for his stoma and is unable to demonstrate the procedures necessary for his home care. He is scheduled for discharge today, and you feel strongly that he needs to stay in the hospital for continued teaching and possible psychological evaluation.

Nurses are the people best able to determine the amount of nursing care that a client needs, and when this need has diminished enough for discharge from the hospital. However, physicians and third-party payors are frequently the ones to decide whether a client is ready for discharge. Unfortunately, some clients are discharged too early, and this seems to be true in the case of Mr. Howard.

Being certain of Mr. Howard's understanding of his home care needs, and of the level of his ability for self-care, is a necessary part of discharge planning. Because clients are being discharged "quicker and sicker" in today's healthcare environment, they may not be able to learn at their regular pace. In fact, their need for complete and accurate home care instruction may be greatly increased at the same time as their ability to learn may be greatly decreased. In acute care facilities, nurses should take special care before discharge to ensure that clients understand the instructions of their physicians, how to take their medications, and how to execute specific home care procedures. Take special care to ensure that all written material is at a reading level that the client can easily understand. Discharge teaching takes on an especially important role in this era of tightening budgets and earlier discharge.

Too often, you may feel powerless in the decision to discharge a client. However, information that you alone may have about the client's condition and ability for self-care may be essential to the decisions about the timing of the client's discharge. As a profession, nursing must begin to establish nursing discharge criteria and to communicate the criteria to other disciplines to ensure safe patient care. Then, collaborative, client-centered discharge planning will meet client needs.

Mr. Howard could clearly benefit from additional evaluation and teaching. Calling Mr. Howard's psychological state and his lack of ability for self-care to the attention of the attending physician may change the timing of Mr. Howard's discharge. And changing that timing may be the difference between a full recovery and a readmission for complications.

---

tion pattern will change the client's self-image, including alterations in emotional, psychosocial, and perceptual reactions. Preoperative counseling should include explanations about the expected anatomic and physiologic alterations, including their possible effects on the client. Counseling should also include ways to maintain the client's current life-style. Community associations, such as the United Ostomy Association and the American Cancer Society, are a tremendous help to the client undergoing diversion. Remember that some clients experience denial as a defense mechanism both pre- and postoperatively. Thus, the nurse must share hope and faith when guiding the client and significant others through their initial unwillingness to accept the changes. The nurse may need to restrict teaching content to essentials and frequently repeat instructions before learning actually takes place. Most hospitals have educational materials available for the client and family. Postoperatively, the client and significant others may need help with looking at and touching the stoma and accepting it as part of the client's total self.

Hemorrhage. A potential collaborative problem in the postoperative client is *Hemorrhage related to surgical procedure.*

Planning: Expected Outcomes. The health team will diagnose and treat bleeding early so hemorrhage does not occur, as evidenced by the absence of hemorrhage.

Implementation. Nursing care after TUR is covered in detail in Chapter 83. The client will have some hematuria and, until the bleeding ceases, an indwelling urethral catheter. The catheter will be attached to a continuous or intermittent closed bladder irrigation system to prevent blood clots. Nursing intervention is similar to that after TUR of the prostate. This includes high intake of fluids, and analgesics and antispasmodics as needed.

As with all major abdominal surgeries, clients who have undergone a radical cystectomy and urinary diversion are at risk for hemorrhage, even more so because of the extensive nature of the surgery. The nurse should monitor vital signs, incision, and drainage closely for early manifestations of excessive bleeding. Manifestations of hemorrhage and shock are detailed in Chapter 22.

Occlusion of Urinary Drainage Device. After most types of bladder surgery the client will have a catheter, therefore *Occlusion of Urinary Drainage Device related to hematuria and clot formation* is a common problem that must be addressed through collaborative management.

Planning: Expected Outcomes. Catheters will not become obstructed or causative factors for potential obstruction will be identified before problems can occur, as evidenced by free flow of urine.

Implementation. Nursing care for the client who has had segmental bladder resection centers on maintaining constant urinary drainage so the remaining bladder does not become distended, putting strain on the suture line. The client usually has both urethral and suprapubic catheters. The suprapubic catheter is usually left in for 2 weeks, until complete healing has occurred, so the client will be discharged with the catheter in place.

Following a continent diversion it is very important to ensure that the catheter is draining urine freely. If any obstruction were to occur, the newly created reservoir could be damaged and internal leakage along the suture line could occur. The nurse should monitor output closely from the catheter and irrigate it at regular intervals as ordered. Irrigation is performed gently in the immediate postoperative period with approximately 60 ml of normal saline to avoid stress on the new suture line. Irrigation must be done to help prevent obstruction from clots or the large amount of mucus.

A neobladder also will have one or two catheters in place to prevent overdistention of the newly created bladder. These catheters are treated as any other, with a closed system. The neobladder also needs to be carefully monitored for possible obstruction. Regular irrigation must be done to rid the neobladder of mucus.

Paralytic Ileus, Stomal Ischemia, and Blockage of Ureteral Catheters. Following surgery the client must be closely monitored for the collaborative problems of *Paralytic Ileus, Stomal Ischemia, and Blockage of Ureteral Catheters related to surgery and postoperative status.*

Planning: Expected Outcomes. The client will not develop postoperative injury or have the complications diagnosed early, as evidenced by vital signs within preoperative norms, presence of active bowel sounds within 3 to 4 days postoperatively, a red moist stoma, and at least 30 to 60 ml urine output per hour via ureteral catheters.

Implementation. Postoperative nursing management of the client includes routine monitoring of the vital signs, intake and output, inspection of the incision and the stoma, and other postoperative interventions as described in Chapter 21. The client often has a nasogastric tube in place, because of the anticipated postoperative ileus. The client is kept NPO until bowel sounds return.

If the client has a stoma, there will be a temporary, clear urostomy pouch over the stoma which is connected to a gravity drainage system. Sometimes ureteral catheters are used to splint the ureters while they heal. These catheters, usually removed before the client is discharged,

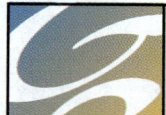

CRITICAL MONITORING

Postoperative Monitoring After Urinary Diversion Procedures

- Measure urine output every hour for the first 24 hours, and at least every 8 hours thereafter; report any amount less than 30 mL/hr or no output for more than 15 minutes
- Check the ostomy pouch for leaks and the skin under it for irritation every 4 hours initially, then every 8 hours
- Inspect the stoma every hour for the first 24 hours after surgery (this will give you a baseline from which you can quickly detect deviations. The stoma should be red and moist). If there are no problems, extend intervals to every 4 hours, and then to every 8 hours
- Note the stoma's size, shape, and color. Expect the stoma to be edematous in the immediate postoperative period. However, other changes may indicate complications, warranting action from the physician. A dusky or cyanotic color of the stoma may denote an insufficient blood supply and the onset of necrosis. This is an emergency! The reduced blood supply may result from (1) surgical technique, (2) an appliance faceplate that is too small or improperly centered, or (3) peristomal protective materials that have been poorly applied. Other complications with the stoma include prolapse (protrusion from the skin) or retraction into the abdomen beneath the skin
- Watch for manifestations of peritonitis, such as fever and abdominal pain and rigidity; leakage at the site of the anastomosis or ureteral separation from the conduit may allow urine to seep into the peritoneal cavity, leading to peritonitis
- Observe for bleeding: although bleeding from the stoma may indicate a surgical defect, it is also common for the intestinal mucosa, which is very fragile, to bleed during a change of appliance or because of a poorly fitted collection pouch

may extend through the stoma. (See Critical Monitoring feature.)

Risk for Ineffective Management of Therapeutic Regimen (Individuals). The placement of any type of urinary diversion, even the neobladder which has no external pouches, will require the client to learn new self-care strategies. The nursing diagnosis of *Risk for Ineffective Management of Therapeutic Regimen related to complexity of therapeutic regimen* is appropriate for this client.

Planning: Expected Outcomes. Client will effectively manage therapeutic regimen as evidenced by client's ability to describe regimen and successfully perform required care of diversion.

Implementation. *Ileal Conduit.* Clients with an ileal conduit will need to learn care of the stoma and skin

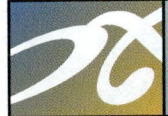

BRIDGE TO HOME HEALTHCARE

Caring for an Ileal Conduit at Home

Ethel Sharasheff, R.N., B.S.N., C.E.T.N., *Enterostomal Nurse Therapist, Bloomfield, Connecticut*

When initiating the care of a client who has just been sent home with an ileal conduit, gather information about what in-hospital teaching took place, the size of the client's stoma, what supplies were sent home with the client, and the names and numbers of the suppliers. If you cannot determine ahead of time how well the client is adjusting or what success the client has had with the appliance, call the staff of the referring facility before your first home visit. Before that visit, be certain that you are comfortable with the procedures to be performed and with the equipment that you will use; if you are hesitant, you will reinforce fears that may already be building in the client.

Plan your first visit based on all the information that you obtained prior to the visit. However, be prepared that anxiety and physical weakness, which are barriers to learning, may force you to revise your plans. Assess the client and significant others for readiness to learn. Do not be surprised if the client and others cannot perform as expected. If the client has a number of tubes still in place, consider waiting to initiate teaching until the tubes are removed. Also, instruction is easier for the client when mucus that collects around the tubes at the stoma has gently been removed.

During home visits, make certain that the client is able to satisfactorily manage the nighttime drainage system. The client must be able to detach it, clean it, and replace it. Where to hand or hold the collector at home is often an issue; consider using a wastepaper basket.

Also be sure to discuss whether the client plans to shower or bathe in a tub. Most clients will want to use one or the other shortly after returning home. Advise the client to leave the pouch in place initially while showering or bathing, so that the client becomes confident that it will not fall off during showering and bathing. Then, on the scheduled change day, the client should remove the pouch just prior to leaving the shower or tub. If the client plans to shower, advise him or her to face away from the direct flow of water. If the client plans to bathe in a tub, advise him or her to keep the water level below the stoma. The client should use only nonoily soaps and should rinse thoroughly.

If peristomal skin problems develop, the client should use only "vanishing"-based creams or powders and use them sparingly. Oil-based products will interfere with adhesion of barriers and tapes. The client should use "skin prep" only under tape. If the skin prep contains alcohol, the client should not use it over red or weepy tissue.

Additional supplies should be ordered only when you are certain that the fit is correct. Be aware that you will need to reduce the flange size as the stoma shrinks.

Evaluate the success of stoma care by establishing a schedule for changing the system every 5 to 7 days and then observing for leakage or signs of impending leakage. If you detect a problem, try changing the system 1 day earlier, or try a different system.

To evaluate the success of a particular system, consider having the client sit on the toilet, then stand, while you observe the movement of the stoma and the peristomal skin. If you notice retraction or dimpling, the client may need a convex appliance and a belt. For complex problems like these, you and the client may benefit from consulting with an enterostomal nurse. Many enterostomal nurses recommend appliance support belts, which come in a variety of widths and can be custom-designed for special needs.

Urine cultures are an important part of home care of the client with an ileal conduit. Usually, they are obtained by catheterization of the conduit; however, some physicians prefer clean-catch specimens. To obtain a urine specimen, clean the stoma and peristomal skin with the solutions normally used in catheterization. Then, adhere a new, clean appliance and collect the specimen within 15 to 30 minutes. Never collect urine from a pouch that is already in use. Transport the specimen to the laboratory as soon as possible.

Assume that clients with new stomas—and even clients with established stomas—*will have problems*. All clients will therefore benefit from contact with the United Ostomy Association. Call 1-800-826-0826 to request information about the association's volunteer visitors, local chapters, and literature. Manufacturers of barriers and pouches are additional excellent sources of information, especially for you. Also consider obtaining specialty journals such as the *Journal of ET Nursing and Ostomy and Wound Management*.

and proper application of a urinary pouch (see Bridge to Home Healthcare: Caring for an Ileal Conduit at Home). The stoma opening of the skin barrier is cut just large enough to fit over the stoma and is applied next to the skin before attaching the pouch or faceplate. A skin cement or adhesive disc may help the faceplate stick more securely to the skin. A non-water-soluble adhesive spray will allow the client to go swimming. Many pouches

today come as two pieces, a faceplate or wafer and a removable pouch. Not having to remove the faceplate or wafer as frequently makes care much easier for many clients.

Skin irritation or breakdown is a constant threat to the client who has undergone urinary diversion. Advise the client to prevent urine from contacting the skin. This can be achieved in part by using a well-fitted and properly

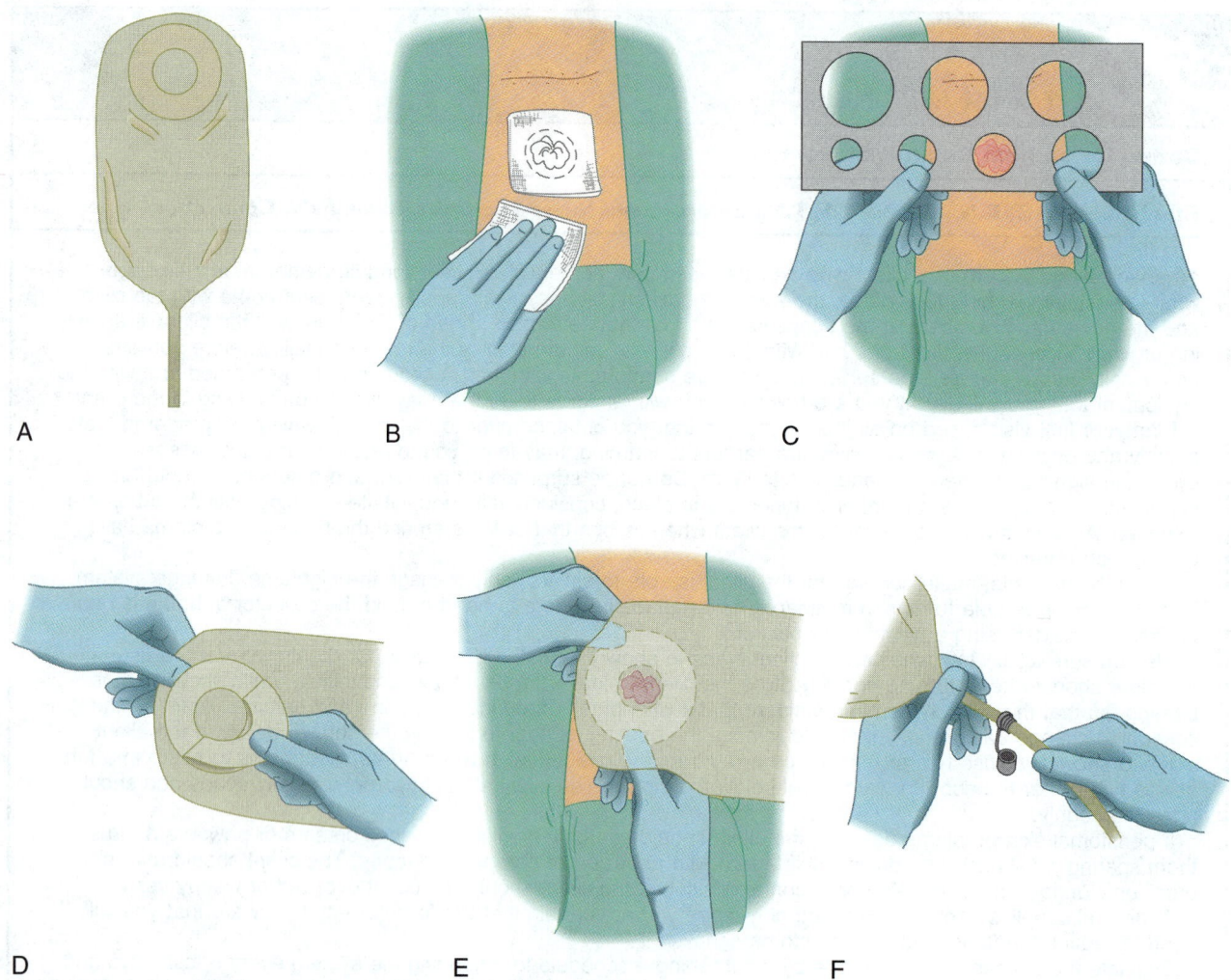

A B C

D E F

Figure 56–5. Applying a disposable ostomy pouch. *A,* Gather supplies: ostomy pouch, ostomy belt, skin barrier, stoma template, gauze pads, pouch clip or rubber band, safety pin, and clean gloves. Clamp or wrap rubber band around the end of the pouch to prevent leakage during the procedure. Make sure that lighting is adequate and that the client is comfortable and understands the procedure. Wash hands and don clean examining gloves. *B,* Gently remove the old pouch, using warm water or an adhesive solvent around the seal if necessary. Place gauze pad over stoma to prevent leakage as you gently clean peristomal area with moist gauze. *C,* Measure stoma with the stoma template. Trace the shape onto the skin barrier and adhesive, using the template. Cut openings no more than 3 mm larger than the stoma. *D,* Remove backing from the adhesive surface of the disposable ostomy pouch. *E,* Center pouch opening over stoma with pouch drain pointing to floor. (If client ambulates frequently, the pouch drain should point to the client's feet.) Make sure seal is complete. *F,* Connect drainage tubing to ostomy pouch if appropriate. Secure tubing (with rubber band around tubing, pin rubber band to sheets if client is immobile).

attached appliance (Fig. 56–5). The opening in the adhesive backing of the faceplate or wafer should be cut so it is not more than 3 mm larger than the stoma. This opening will need to be remeasured after the edema in the stoma recedes. Each time the faceplate or wafer is changed, the skin around the stoma should be cleaned with a mild, nonresidue soap and water, and thoroughly dried. A gauze pad or tampon should be held over the stoma during cleaning to prevent urine from flowing out over the skin. Remove this pad or tampon just as the appliance is reapplied. The appliance should be changed early in the morning, because urine production is slowest at this time.

Urinary pouches have a valve in the bottom for intermittent draining of urine. Alternatively, the pouch may be drained by gravity into a bedside bag, especially at night,

or a leg bag. The self-contained pouch drainage system allows the client to resume most, if not all, former activities with very little or no change in style of dress. However, caution the client to empty the pouch when it is one-third to one-half full; the weight of accumulating urine may pull the faceplate away from the skin and cause leakage. Advise the client also to check the seal often if he or she is perspiring heavily.

Urine odor is a common problem with urinary stomas. Noxious odors result mostly from poor hygiene, alkaline urine, normal breakdown of urine (ammonia), concentration of urine with insufficient intake, and the ingestion of certain foods, such as asparagus. Because diluted urine is less odoriferous, adequate fluid intake is most helpful in preventing odor. Although permanent appliances are rarely used today, to control odors in them wash reusable appliances thoroughly with soap and lukewarm water. The pouch can also be soaked in dilute white vinegar or in a commercial deodorant product for 20 to 30 minutes. Rinse the pouch and allow it to dry. For all appliances, deodorant tablets are available that can be placed in the pouch while it is being worn. Ingestion of methionine can alleviate the smell of ammonia, and acidifying the urine reduces odor.

Long-term nursing intervention aims to maintain a functional urinary system and prevent complications. It takes time for the client and significant others to adjust to the urinary diversion. Even though counseling may have been excellent during the preoperative period, the reality of the diversion often produces further anxiety, depression, and anger. The client may need help at first to look at or even talk about the stoma. As soon as possible after surgery, the client must begin to help care for the stoma, peristomal skin, and drainage system, gradually assuming more responsibility until achieving independence. (See the Client Education Guide: Learning to Care for a Urinary Diversion.)

The client with bladder cancer must be followed at regular intervals to assess for recurrence of the cancer. The client should also continue to be seen by an enterostomal therapy nurse, especially at the postoperative office visit, to be sure that no problems have arisen concerning the ostomy.

Continent Diversion. Postoperative care for the client with a Kock or Indiana pouch is similar to that for any client with a urinary diversion, except there is no

---

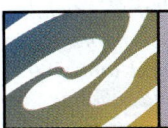

CLIENT EDUCATION GUIDE

Learning to Care for a Urinary Diversion

Client Instructions in English (*Instrucciones para el cliente en inglés*)	Client Instructions in Spanish (*Instrucciones para el cliente en español*)
Take an active role in your care as soon as possible.	Tome un rol activo en su auto-cuidado lo más pronto posible.
Learn how to remove and reapply the appliance, empty the pouch, and attach it to the night drainage system.	Aprenda como quitar y como fijar el accesorio, vaciar la bolsa, y sujetarla al sistema de derivación urinaria nocturno.
Learn about adaptations that you may need to make while traveling.	Aprenda las adaptaciones que pueda hacer cuando salga de viaje.
If necessary, select new clothing that will not constrict your drainage pouch.	Si es necesario, escoga ropa nueva que no apriete la bolsa de desagüe.
Be sure to maintain a daily fluid intake of at least 3 L (~3 qt).	Beba al menos 3 litros de líquidos diarios.
At home, select the foods and fluids recommended for people with urinary diversions.	En casa, seleccione comidas y bebidas que se recomiendan para personas que usan accesorios de derivación urinaria.
Know when to contact your enterostomal nurse therapist or physician (e.g., when you notice changes in the color or quantity of your urine, cloudy or foul-smelling urine, or changes in the color of your stoma).	Aprenda cuando llamar a su enfermera terapeuta en enterestomía o al médico (por ejemplo, cuando empiece a notar cambios en el color o la cantidad de orina, orina turbia o maloliente, o cambios en el color de la estoma).
If you have a suprapubic catheter or Medena tube, be sure you know how to care for it before you leave the hospital. You may go home with a urinary pouch on and will continue to wear it until the surgically created pouch completely heals.	Si tiene un catéter suprapúbico o un tubo "Medena", aprenda como limpiarlo antes de ser dado de alta. Es posible que salga del hospital con una bolsa urinaria fija. Usela hasta que la bolsa que se le hizo durante la cirugía cicatrize por completo.
Know where to obtain the supplies needed to care for your urinary diversion.	Aprenda donde obtener las provisiones necesarias para dar cuidado a su derivación urinaria.
Know how to contact your local ostomy association for follow-up support.	Aprenda como ponerse en contacto con la asociación local de enterestomía para que le presten apoyo.

external pouch. The client will have a 24F to 26F catheter in place to drain the urine continuously until the pouch has healed. The reservoir will be irrigated with normal saline to wash out any clots or mucus that might plug it. Following a radiographic study to ensure the system has no leaks, the catheter is removed, and the client is taught the self-catheterization procedure, a clean, not sterile, procedure.

The client is taught to insert the catheter every 2 to 3 hours to drain the reservoir. Each week thereafter, the interval is increased by 1 hour, until finally the catheterization is only done every 4 to 6 hours during the day. Regular fluid intake and adherence to the catheterization is important because a full reservoir puts pressure on the nipple valve making catheterization much more difficult. The principles of catheterization of a urinary reservoir are the same as for clean, intermittent urinary self-catheterization. Never force the well-lubricated (water-soluble lubricant only) catheter into the reservoir. If there is resistance, pause, and then apply only gentle pressure, slightly rotating the catheter. If this does not work, the client should call the physician. Once the urine has stopped flowing, the client should take several deep breaths and move the catheter in and out 2 to 3 inches to be sure that the pouch is fully emptied. Withdraw the catheter slowly so any additional urine can drain and pinch the end of the catheter before removing it so that it does not drip. Clients should be taught to carry catheterization supplies with them so that they are able to empty the reservoir whenever it is needed. Most clients gain a sensation of abdominal pressure when they need to self-catheterize.

It also is important for the client to learn proper techniques for irrigation of the stoma. Again, principles are the same as for irrigating any catheter, only it is a clean, not sterile, procedure. Using a catheter and syringe, the client should instill about 60 ml of normal saline or water into the reservoir. The fluid can either be gently aspirated or allowed to drain from the catheter. The irrigations are done until the drainage returns free of mucus. Do not overirrigate the reservoir since only enough fluid to remove the mucus is needed. The irrigations are done to break up and flush out mucus that might lead to obstruction of the reservoir. If the mucus is very thick, increasing fluid intake can decrease the viscosity. Clients should be given opportunities to practice both these skills, with supervision, before discharge, if possible, or they should be closely followed by a visiting nurse to ensure that proper techniques are being used.

Risk for Impaired Skin Integrity.
If the client has an ileal conduit, the nursing diagnosis of *Risk for Impaired Skin Integrity related to irritation of peristomal skin* is a potential problem.

Planning: Expected Outcomes. The client will not develop altered skin integrity or irritation of peristomal skin, as evidence by intact, clear skin.

Implementation. Interventions for any skin irritation must begin promptly. Check the pH of the urine (do not place dipstick in stoma); strongly alkaline urine irritates the skin and facilitates crystal formation. If urine cultures identify UTI, it may be treated. The appliance should be checked carefully to find any leakage and to determine whether the skin is sensitive to anything used in the process of application. Skin irritation may result from changing the pouch too frequently. A general recommendation is that the pouch be left in place as long as it is not leaking. During changes of the appliance, leave the skin open to the air as much as possible. When the appliance is reattached, dust the skin with a non-karaya powder and apply a pouch with a non-karaya skin barrier. Karaya cannot be used with urinary pouches because urine erodes karaya.

Skin irritation around the stoma can be caused by a yeast infection. Nystatin creams or powders are used to treat this. Nystatin powder is applied directly over the irritated skin area and then sealed to the skin with a liquid skin barrier.

Risk for Altered Sexuality Patterns.
Many of the surgeries performed to treat bladder cancer alter the reproductive anatomy so that *Risk for Altered Sexuality Patterns related to potential postoperative impotence in men after radical cystectomy, possible painful intercourse in women after a radical cystectomy, and changes in body image affecting sexuality* is a common nursing diagnosis that must be addressed.

Planning: Expected Outcomes. The client will accept and adopt alternative methods of sexual expression as evidenced by the client's statements.

Implementation. Male clients have a risk of impotence after a radical cystectomy that is related to the extent of the resection. It is important for them to receive counseling both before and after the surgery so they can begin to adjust to any alterations. Chapter 83 discusses in detail alterations in male sexuality.

Female clients often have a total abdominal hysterectomy, bilateral salpingo-oophorectomy, and anterior vaginal resection. This can result in shortening and tightening of the vagina leading to painful intercourse. Alternative positions, adequate use of lubricants, and possible vaginal dilation may decrease the discomfort of sexual intercourse. Booklets discussing both female and male sexual dysfunction are available from the American Cancer Society.

For partners of any client, encourage holding, touching, kissing, and other activities to promote intimacy. Partners are often afraid to touch the client for fear of inflicting hurt. Embarrassment may also be an issue and open discussions should be encouraged.

Evaluation

If the care of the client has been successful, the client will be able to make the transition to community and self-care with minimal difficulty. The nurse must evaluate the client's ability to engage in self-care so the possible need for further follow-up with home health nurses can be initiated.

Modifications for Elderly Clients

The major modification for older clients with urinary diversion centers around possible difficulties they may have with self-care of the appliance. Changing the appliance requires some degree of dexterity, and older clients are more likely to have arthritis and other disabilities that limit their ability to manipulate the pouches. They may require assistance or modification of teaching so they can be independent. Decreased visual acuity is often a reason why some elderly people cannot handle the devices. These problems must be closely assessed so that appropriate assistance can be offered.

Ureteral Tumors

Tumors that arise primarily in the ureter are rare. In men, ureteral cancer occurs predominantly in their 50s and 60s. This form of cancer rarely affects women. Ureteral neoplasms usually extend from renal or bladder neoplasms or from tumors originating in the bowel, uterus, or ovary. Those primary neoplasms that do occur usually first appear as a papillary transitional cell or squamous cell carcinoma. These tumors are most frequently found in the lower third of the ureter. In later stages of ureteral cancer, there is extension outside the ureter to adjacent structures and regional lymph nodes or distant metastasis. Common sites for metastasis include the lungs and liver.

Usually, the first sign of ureteral malignancy is gross hematuria. The tumor normally develops painlessly until obstruction occurs. At this point, the client may experience flank pain. Diagnosis is made through urine cytology, IVP, cystoscopy, ultrasonography, and CT scan.

Treatment of ureteral cancer almost exclusively involves surgical excision and resection, although radiation may also be used in advanced cases with local extension. When the lesion is located in the middle or proximal third of the ureter, the surgical procedure usually involves nephroureterectomy, which removes the kidney, ureter, and attached segment of the bladder on the affected side. However, if the tumor is in the distal third of the ureter and noninvasive, a more conservative procedure may be used. In this case, just the distal portion of the ureter is resected with ureteral reimplantation. Silicone rubber, Teflon, polytetrafluorourethane, and bovine carotid heterograft are used to replace the resected ureter, thereby facilitating reimplantation in the bladder. A ureter-ureter anastomosis also may be preformed. Preoperative and postoperative intervention is similar to that for clients undergoing nephrectomy, ureteral reimplantation, or segmental resection of the bladder.

If the decision is made not to perform any of these procedures, some palliative measure may be needed to prevent or alleviate ureteral obstruction. Urinary diversion may be performed, as described previously, or a ureteral stent catheter may be placed into the ureter during cystoscopy to maintain its patency. The older catheter, a flanged, winged stent (Gibbon's stent), or the newer double J stent is made to prevent migration up the ureter or dislodgement by ureteral peristaltic waves or gravity.

Urinary Calculi

Urinary calculi (urolithiasis) are calcifications within the urinary system. Calculi, commonly called stones, form primarily in the kidney, but can migrate to the ureters and bladder. This section discusses only ureteral and bladder stones; nephrolithiasis is discussed in Chapter 57. Primary bladder calculi are rare and usually develop because of urinary stasis or infection. Kidney stones may pass through the ureters and into the bladder and remain there, growing larger.

Etiology and Risk Factors

Infection, presence of a foreign body, failure to empty the bladder completely, and obstruction within the urinary tract all contribute to the formation of calculi. The two primary causative factors are urinary stasis and supersaturation of urine with poorly soluble crystalloids, such as calcium crystals, which precipitate easily in the urine. Hypercalcemia predisposes to calculi formation by the increased calcium excreted in the urine. The presence of a continent urinary diversion also increases the risk of calculi resulting from both the increased excretion of calcium and the potential stasis of urine within the pouch. Some regions of the country have a higher frequency of stone formation, such as the southern states and the Great Lakes region. It is more common in men than in women and occurs more frequently in young adults and in early middle age. Once a client has had calculi, they tend to recur at a rate of 50% in 5 to 10 years. (See Risk Factors and Levels of Prevention: Urinary Calculi.)

Pathophysiology

The exact mechanism of stone formation has not been clearly defined, although it is a process of crystallization. A primary factor in stone formation is the supersaturation of the urine with elements such as calcium, phosphate, and oxalate. Certain factors contribute to the ease of stone formation. These factors include the pH of the urine, the amount of solute in the urine, and the amount of solution or urine. Problems with purine metabolism predispose to the formation of uric acid stones, as in gout.

Prolonged immobility leads to urinary stasis and because of calcium resorption from the bones, an increase in serum and urine calcium. If the fluid intake is also inadequate, then the calcium saturating the urine is more likely to precipitate and form stones.

The pH of the urine also contributes to stone formation or stone dissolution. Uric acid and cystine stones are more likely to precipitate in acid urine; calcium phosphate and struvite stones are more common in alkaline urine. Oxalate stones are not affected by urine pH.

Clinical Manifestations and Diagnostic Findings

Calculi range in size from almost undetectable to several centimeters in diameter. Ureteral stones cause severe pain in the flank and abdomen. This pain may radiate down to the ipsilateral hemiscrotum or labia. When stones move through the ureters, gastrointestinal manifestations (colic)

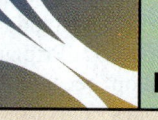

RISK FACTORS AND LEVELS OF PREVENTION

Urinary Calculi

Risk Factors

Family history of stone formation; male sex; more common in young adults and early middle adulthood; chronic dehydration leading to a high urine concentration and decreased pH; urinary stasis due to obstruction or immobility; metabolic disturbances such as gout and hyperparathyroidism that increase stone-forming solutes; Crohn's disease; living in southern states or Great Lakes region; high mineral content in drinking water; diet high in purines, oxalates, calcium, animal proteins; sedentary occupation or life-style; previous history of stones; neurogenic bladder; urinary tract infections; prolonged indwelling catheterization

Levels of Prevention

Primary Prevention
- Prevent immobilization
- Encourage active and passive range of motion in immobilized clients
- Promote high fluid intake in at-risk clients
- Reduce level of stone-forming solutes in the diet such as calcium, oxalates, purines, animal proteins

Secondary Prevention
- Monitor high-risk clients, such as those with indwelling catheters or obstructions, for development of stones
- Teach high-risk clients the clinical manifestations of calculi

Tertiary Prevention
- Encourage clients to maintain high fluid intake (at least 3 L/day) and adopt dietary modification
- Teach clients how to monitor urinary pH
- Teach clients the importance of continuing medications such as allopurinol for gout to decrease risk of stones

may occur. Colic occurs when the muscular lining of the ureters undergoes spasm in response to the movement of the stone. Normal peristalsis within the ureter propels the stone, resulting in trauma leading to hematuria. Stones that are too large to pass the length of the ureter may lodge, leading to obstruction. If the right ureter is affected, the manifestations may mimic appendicitis. The client will complain of distention, constipation, and right lower quadrant pain. If the left ureter is affected, manifestations range from nausea and vomiting to diarrhea. The pain from a left ureteral calculus is usually in the left lower quadrant.

A stone formed in the kidney may continue to grow in the bladder. As long as these stones remain in the bladder, the client will probably be asymptomatic, because pain is associated with stones that obstruct or migrate. However, some people do experience manifestations of cystitis. A very large stone lodged against the bladder neck during micturition may cause a heavy feeling in the suprapubic region, a decreased bladder capacity, and an intermittent urinary stream. The stone may partially or totally obstruct urine flow or cause mucosal trauma if it enters the urethra.

The major diagnostic examination for radiopaque stones is a simple radiograph, a flat plate of the abdomen, a kidney, ureter, and bladder (KUB) x-ray (see Chapter 57). Uric acid stones are not radiopaque (cannot be seen on x-ray); however, an elevated serum uric acid, with manifestations of stones, may be diagnostic. An IVP can also be done, which will show a filling defect at the site of the stone.

When the stones are passed in voided urine or retrieved, they are analyzed for their components. It is important to identify the exact stone composition so exact preventive measures can be implemented.

Acute and Subacute Care

■ Medical Management
Fluids and Ambulation

Medical management is often directed at facilitating the passage of small stones through simply forcing fluids and encouraging the client to ambulate. Treatment of obstructions is also important in the prevention of complications. Later medical management is directed toward preventing recurrent stone formation. Pharmacologic treatments and dietary modifications may effectively prevent many stones from re-forming.

The client should drink 3000 to 4000 ml of fluid per day (unless contraindicated) to flush the urinary tract and hinder stone formation by diluting the urine. The type of fluid is dependent on the type of stone; if it is calcium, acid-ash fluids should be taken to help the calcium remain in solution.

Sometimes just waiting for a time will allow the stones to pass naturally from the ureter and bladder. The client should ambulate, which may help gravity move the stone. However, if this does not occur, or if a cystogram shows that the calculus is too large (>4 ml) to pass safely through the urethra, more invasive treatment is necessary.

There are no particular medications used to treat calcium stones, although watching over ingestion of vitamin supplements or antacids containing calcium may increase the risk of calculi. If the client has uric acid stones, medications to lower uric acid, such as allopurinol (Zyloprim), should be given. Clients with severe colic require narcotics and antispasmodics.

Stone Prevention Diet

Once the components of the stone have been identified, dietary modification may be used to help prevent recurrence. A low calcium, low oxalate diet is used for calcium or oxalate stones, and a low purine diet for uric acid stones.

■ Nursing Management of the Medical Client

If urinary stones are suspected, the client should strain all urine through a urine strainer or at least four layers of gauze pads. After straining, inspect the filter or pads carefully for stones, which are less than 4 mm; if any are found, send them to the laboratory for stone analysis. Clients should be instructed to force fluid to wash out the stones, if possible. It is also important to teach the client stone prevention, including diet, fluid intake, and avoidance of urinary stasis (see the Client Education Guide: Preventing Recurrence of Urinary Stones).

■ Surgical Management

It has been estimated that 20% of stones will require surgical or endourologic management. Open surgery is used currently only for those clients who are unable to tolerate endourologic procedures.

Endourologic Procedures

Endourologic procedures are used whenever possible since these are less invasive procedures. The physician removes small bladder stones transurethrally with a cystoscope. Large stones may be broken up with an instrument called a lithotrite (stone crusher). This procedure is called a *cystolitholapaxy*, followed by irrigation of the bladder to wash out stone fragments. In cystoscopic lithotripsy, an ultrasonic lithotrite placed against a stone pulverizes it. Possible complications associated with this procedure include hemorrhage, urinary retention, infection, and possibly retained stone fragments.

Stones in the lower ureter, and sometimes in the middle and upper ureter, can often be removed using a flexible ureterscope passed through a cystoscope. Ureteroscopy may be used to retrieve stones (<4 mm) or, combined with ultrasonic lithotripsy, to remove fragments after treatment. This procedure is usually performed with conscious sedation or general anesthesia. Postoperative complications are usually minimal.

The newest treatment for calculi is laser lithotripsy.

Lasers are used together with a ureteroscope to remove or loosen impacted stones. The procedure requires constant water irrigation of the ureter to dissipate the heat. Complications from this procedure are the same as those from any endourologic procedure.

Lithotripsy

A newer method, begun in the early 1980s, is the use of sound waves applied externally to break up stones in the kidney or ureter. *Extracorporeal shock wave lithotripsy* (ESWL) has drastically decreased the need for surgery to remove calculi. This procedure uses high-energy shock waves transmitted through water to the stone, accurately pinpointed through fluoroscopy. These shock waves cause the stones to rupture into small fragments that can be passed or retrieved endoscopically. The procedure is usually done under conscious sedation. Complications following ESWL include retained fragments, urosepsis, and perinephric hematoma. Stone fragments may bunch up in the distal ureter obstructing the kidney. To avoid this, a double J stent is often placed via cystoscopy prior to ESWL for stones greater than 6 mm to prevent this collection and obstruction. The stent is removed during a follow-up visit.

Open Surgical Procedures

A *ureterolithotomy* is the surgical removal of a stone from the ureter through a flank incision for higher stones and an abdominal incision for lower ones. A Penrose drain and ureteral catheter are usually in place postoperatively for healing and drainage of urine. A *cystolithotomy* is the removal of bladder calculi through a suprapubic incision. This procedure is used only when stones cannot be crushed and removed transurethrally. A stricture is the most common postoperative complication.

■ Nursing Management of the Surgical Client

When a client is admitted with a diagnosis of urolithiasis, the major nursing responsibilities center on maintaining adequate urine output. The nurse should force fluids up to 4000 ml/day, unless otherwise contraindicated, so that good output is ensured. If the stone does not pass, the nurse should prepare the client for a more invasive procedure.

Postoperatively, after litholapaxy, the nurse must monitor for manifestations of hemorrhage, urinary retention, infection, and stone recurrence. Maintain the client on a high fluid intake and, if prescribed, administer intermittent bladder irrigations to wash out possible stone fragments. The nurse should continue to strain all urine.

Nursing care after cystolithotomy is similar to the care of a client after suprapubic prostatectomy (see Chapter 83). Nursing care after a ureterolithotomy may involve care of a ureteral catheter. The nurse must closely monitor the output of the ureteral catheter. Because the renal pelvis holds only 5 ml, ureteral catheters must be kept patent. Ureteral catheters are never clamped. Any unexpected reduction in urine flow requires prompt intervention.

Several conditions can interfere with the flow of urine through these catheters. The catheters are easily plugged with mucus shreds, blood clots, and chemical sediment. Also, ureteral peristalsis occasionally pushes the catheters out of the ureter into the bladder.

Monitor the output from these catheters closely. Each ureteral and urethral catheter should drain into its own collection bag so the source of the reduced flow will be noticed immediately. Measure and record the output of each catheter every hour for the first 24 hours and then every 4 to 8 hours until they are removed. Most of the urine will drain from the ureteral catheters for the first 48

to 72 hours postoperatively. As the inflammation decreases, urine flows around ureteral catheters and is drained by the urethral or suprapubic catheters. Urine output of less than 30 ml/hr or lack of output from the ureteral catheters for more than 15 minutes should be reported to the physician immediately.

If catheter irrigation is ordered by the physician, use strict aseptic technique. A maximum of 5 ml of irrigating solution, usually normal saline, should be allowed to flow in by gravity, or irrigated with *very* gentle force. Never irrigate this catheter with force. If patency cannot be established, notify the physician immediately. Take special care not to dislodge the catheter accidentally. If the catheter is not sutured in place, secure it carefully to the skin with tape.

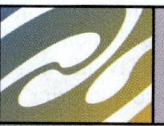

CLIENT EDUCATION GUIDE

Preventing Recurrence of Urinary Stones

Client Instructions in English *(Instrucciones para el cliente en inglés)*	**Client Instructions in Spanish** *(Instrucciones para el cliente en español)*
Increase your fluid intake to at least 3 L (~3 qt) every day.	Aumente las bebidas de líquidos al menos 3 litros por día.
Be sure to urinate at least every 2 hours.	Trate de orinar al menos cada dos horas.
Remember the early symptoms of urinary stones. If the symptoms occur again, see your physician promptly.	Recuerde los síntomas de cálculos urinarios. Sí los síntomas ocurren otra vez, vea pronto a su médico.
Monitor the pH of your urine with pH paper. If you had calcium stones, keep your urine acidic. If you had uric acid stones, keep your urine basic. Keep urine acidic with high-protein diet. Keep urine basic with low-protein diet, plenty of vegetables, and citrus fruits.	Monitoreé el pH de la orina con papel de pH. Si ha tenido cálculos de calcio, mantenga la orina más ácida. Sí ha tenido cálculos úricos, mentenga la orina básica.
Be sure to follow your physician's instructions for follow-up urinalysis and blood tests to detect factors that can cause urinary stones.	Siga las instrucciónes del médico y vaya a que le saquen muestras de orina y de sangre para detectar factores que puedan causar cálculos urinarios.
If you develop manifestations of urinary tract infection, see your physician promptly for diagnosis and treatment. Manifestations include pain and burning when you urinate, a sense of urgency to urinate, having to urinate frequently, and a fever.	Si desarroya síntomas de infección en la vía urinaria, acuda a su médico lo más pronto possible para hacerle un diagnóstico y darle tratamiento. Los síntomas incluyen dolor y ardor al orinar, urgencia al orinar, orinar con mucha frequencia, y fiebre.
For Clients with Stones Other than Uric Acid Stones: Follow your physician's instructions for keeping your urine acidic.	***Para Pacientes con Otros Cálculos que No Sean de Acido Urico:*** Siga la recomendación del médico para mantener la orina ácida.
For Clients with Calcium Stones: Follow a diet low in calcium and phosphate.	***Para Pacientes con Cálculos de Calcio:*** Siga una dieta baja en calcio y fosfatos.
For Clients with Uric Acid Stones: Follow a low-purine diet.	***Para Pacientes con Cálculos de Acido Urico:*** Siga una dieta baja en purinas.
For Clients with Uric Acid Stones: Take the medications, such as Zyloprim, prescribed to improve your excretion of uric acid.	***Para Pacientes con Cálculos de Acido Urico:*** Tome medicamento como el Zyloprim, recetado para mejorar la excreción del ácido úrico.

Urinary Reflux

Urinary reflux, or the backward flow of urine within the urinary tract, usually begins at the vesicoureteral junction, so urine flows back into the ureter and frequently upward into the renal pelvis. The severity of vesicoureteral reflux is stated as grade I (least severe) through grade V (most severe). If BPH is the cause, then the rate increases in men over 50 years of age. If congenital vesicoureteral junction abnormalities are the cause, the problem occurs in younger children or young adults.

Etiology and Risk Factors

Reflux can be caused by congenital abnormalities such as ectopic ureter, and chronic bladder infections secondary to dysfunctional bladder or outlet obstruction can contribute to the increase of intravesical pressure until it finally overwhelms the resistance of the intramural ureteral sphincters allowing reflux to occur. There is no primary prevention of reflux; however, clients with obstructions must have the cause for obstruction treated to prevent and relieve the intravesical pressure.

Pathophysiology

If there is bladder outlet obstruction, the main result is an ever-present residual urine that often leads to the development of UTIs. Continual overdistention of the bladder can also decrease detrusor tone, thereby increasing the bladder's capacity and raising the threshold required to initiate the micturition reflex.

Renal damage and pyelonephritis are the two primary problems resulting from vesicoureteral reflux. Because the capacity of the renal pelvis is only 5 ml, any larger amounts of urine can cause renal parenchymal changes, hydronephrosis or hydronephroureterosis, whether they result from ureteral obstruction or reflux. The increased hydrostatic pressure leads to renal cortical atrophy from ischemia and hypoxia and to *calicectasis* (dilation of the renal calices). The destruction of kidney tissue, often asymptomatic and undetected, can progress to end-stage renal disease. The kidneys are usually protected from ascending infections by the intramural portion of the distal ureter. However, with reflux, any pathogens in the bladder are carried through the ureters to the kidney. This problem leads to recurrent pyelonephritis (kidney infection), which, if untreated, eventually causes renal failure, with or without increased hydrostatic pressure.

Clinical Manifestations and Diagnostic Findings

The major manifestation of reflux is pyelonephritis. The bladder will be distended if the obstruction is in the bladder neck but not if the obstruction is in the vesicoureteral junction or higher. If the obstruction is higher and bilateral, then the client may exhibit clinical manifestations of renal failure.

The major diagnostic studies are cystoscopy to look for manifestations of obstruction, ureteroscopy to look at the vesicoureteral junction, ultrasound to assess for hydronephrosis, and IVP to look at the entire collecting system. Blood studies such as blood urea nitrogen (BUN) and creatinine determinations are done to assess renal function.

Acute and Subacute Care

■ Surgical Management

Since there are no medical regimens to prevent or treat reflux caused by ectopic ureter, the primary therapy is surgical. The presence of renal damage from the reflux usually calls for surgical intervention. Surgery is also indicated for obstruction at the ureteropelvic junction, for intractable infection, and if the problem is not resolved by maturation. Because the most common causes of reflux are ureteral defects, surgical procedures that focus on correcting reflux involve the ureter (e.g., reimplantation of the ureter).

Postoperatively, a urethral or suprapubic catheter keeps the bladder empty to reduce tension on the suture line. A ureteral catheter will also be inserted into the ureter involved in the surgical procedure. This tiny, semirigid catheter is inserted into the ureter with its tip frequently placed in the renal pelvis. The distal end extends through the bladder and out through the urethra or through an abdominal incision. A ureteral catheter (1) splints the ureter to facilitate healing, (2) prevents obstruction from edema after surgery or other trauma in the area, and (3) drains urine.

The major complications to monitor are problems associated with the ureteral catheter postoperatively, which was discussed earlier in the section on urolithiasis.

■ Nursing Management of the Surgical Client

The nurse should carefully assess clients who are at high risk of obstruction for any manifestation of urinary reflux. The client who is being evaluated for urinary reflux will require support during this diagnostic process.

Preoperative preparation for ureteral surgery is similar to that required by any client requiring surgery (see Chapter 21). See the earlier discussion under Urinary Calculi for the postoperative nursing care of a client with a ureteral catheter.

Postoperatively, assess the color of the urine frequently. Expect that the color will progress from bright red to clear yellow over a matter of days. Discharge teaching is dependent on a variety of factors: (1) the cause of the reflux, (2) the treatment done, and (3) the amount of renal damage that occurred.

If reflux is caused by BPH, the probable treatment would be prostatectomy and the discharge instructions would be based on the exact type of surgery done (see Chapter 83). If the cause is a problem with the vesicoureteral junction, then the teaching will possibly include information about catheter care at home, because these clients have a catheter in place longer.

If there is permanent renal damage, then the teaching will be similar to that given to a client with chronic renal failure (see Chapter 57). The client with renal involvement should have renal function closely monitored at regular intervals for about 1 year, so that any changes can be detected early.

Voiding Disorders

Urinary Retention

Urinary retention means that the urine is retained in the bladder. urine production continues, but accumulated urine is not released. The incidence of retention varies with the cause. More than 50% of men over 50 years of age experience BPH, a common cause of retention. Neurologic injury may also cause retention, and most spinal cord injuries occur in young adults. In postoperative clients, 10% to 15% of those receiving general anesthesia require catheterization because of an inability to void, and 20% to 25% of those who receive spinal anesthesia require a catheter.

Etiology and Risk Factors

Obstruction at or below the bladder outlet is the most common cause of urinary retention. This retention can be caused by a variety of disorders, including BPH, urethral strictures, urethral valves (now considered to be congenital diaphragms in the urethra), phimosis, meatal stenosis, fibrosis, calculi, blood clots, tumors, and bladder neck contractures.

Retention may also be caused by decreased sensory input to and from the bladder, muscle tension, and anxiety. Surgery has traditionally been a factor; spinal anesthesia causes retention more than does general anesthesia.

Other causes include medication that may interfere with the micturition reflex and neurologic injuries due to diabetes, strokes, and spinal cord injuries that also interfere with this reflex. Anorectal problems predispose to retention by applying pressure on the urethra. Decreased intake can also lead to retention through slowed production of urine and failure of normal detrusor reflexes.

One of the major risk factors for retention is BPH. This is not a preventable problem, although the client with an enlarged prostate should be monitored closely for the development of an obstruction secondary to the enlargement. Clients with a history of chronic UTIs that may have caused scarring of the bladder neck or urethra are also at greater risk.

Pathophysiology

Retention is a hazardous condition because the resulting urinary stasis contributes to the evolution of UTI and stone formation. There is also the potential for long-term structural damage to the bladder, ureters, or kidneys. Continued bladder distention may lead to loss of bladder tone.

The pathologic effects of any obstruction produce a snowballing effect; retained urine increases hydrostatic pressure against the bladder wall. This results in hypertrophy of the detrusor muscle, formation of trabeculae (development of connective tissue in the bladder wall), or development of diverticula. At the same time, peristalsis in the ureteral musculature increases against the pressure of the accumulating urine. The ureter gradually becomes elongated, tortuous, and fibrotic. The increasing pressure is also transmitted through the renal pelves and calices into the renal parenchyma. The resulting hydronephrosis also exerts pressure on the blood vessels, causing ischemia and adding to the renal damage. If the process is not interrupted, it can proceed to renal failure and death. Figure 56–6 demonstrates the sequence. Even after the retention is relieved, in later stages of pressure-related damage, there may be permanent damage.

Medications, such as opiates, sedatives, antispasmodics, antiparkinsonians, beta-adrenergic blockers, and psychotropic agents, can interfere with normal neurologic

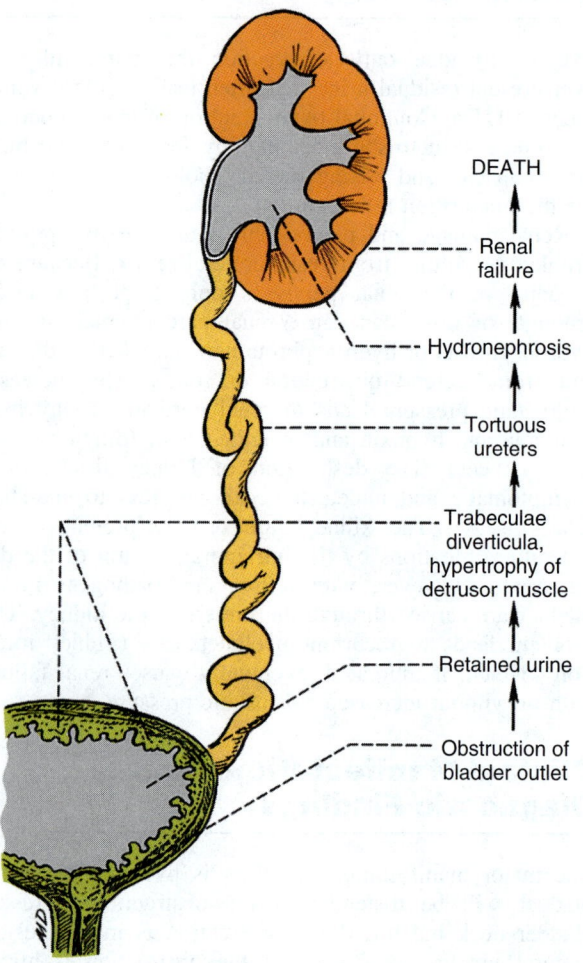

Figure 56–6. Potential effects of urinary tract obstruction.

function and the micturition reflex. Diseases with neurologic impact, such as diabetes mellitus, tabes dorsalis, and spinal cord lesions, also interfere with the micturition reflex.

Anorectal problems, such as hemorrhoids, abscess, or fecal impaction, contribute to urinary retention, either from obstruction or from secondary spasms of the perineal musculature, hampering the ability to relax.

Decreased fluid intake, either oral or intravenous, reduces the glomerular filtration rate, and very slow urine production causes the bladder to fill slowly. This may allow the detrusor muscle to accommodate the increased volume until the muscle's fibers are stretched beyond their ability to contract. When this happens, micturition cannot occur.

Retention with overflow results from the following events. As the bladder continues filling, the intravesical pressure rises. Eventually, this pressure overcomes the restraint of the sphincter. Urine flows out of the bladder until it reduces the intravesical pressure, but only to the level at which the external sphincter can again control the flow of urine. The client reports that the bladder does not feel really empty. The bladder overfills again, and the cycle is repeated.

Prolonged obstruction leads to high pressures in the urinary tract and may predispose to the development of bladder diverticula. A diverticulum is a pouch or sac resulting from the herniation of the mucous membrane lining due to a weakness in the muscular wall of an organ. Many diverticula are asymptomatic and found only accidentally during investigation of other conditions. Bladder diverticula can cause two major problems: (1) UTIs due to stasis of the urine and (2) malignancies probably related to chronic irritation from a persistent infection. Intervention involves removing the obstruction and relieving the retention, followed by surgical excision of the pouch and reestablishing normal patency of the urinary tract. Postoperatively, the client requires catheter drainage of urine to allow complete tissue healing. Because these clients have had a long-term infection, they will probably require antibiotics for months after surgery.

Clinical Manifestations and Diagnostic Findings

The primary manifestation of urinary retention is a distended bladder and the client's inability to void. A high fluid intake but low urinary output record documents that fluid either is not being converted to urine (oliguria or anuria) or is being retained in the bladder. If the client voids more than once per hour, and releases only 25 to 50 ml at any one time, the problem may be retention with overflow.

The major diagnostic test for retention is catheterization. If there is more than 250 to 500 ml of urine in the bladder and the client has not been able to void, retention is present. If the cause is thought to be an obstruction, cystoscopy may be done to determine the cause of that obstruction.

Acute and Subacute Care

■ Medical Management
Dilators

If obstruction causes the urinary retention, the urethra will need to be dilated or the occlusion removed for long-term relief. For dilation of the urethra, progressively larger indwelling catheters may be inserted each day. The urethra can be dilated more quickly with size-graded sounds, filiforms or following bougies, or other dilating instruments, usually under local or sometimes general anesthesia. The insertion of sounds should be performed only by trained professionals because perforation of the urethra can occur. Urinary catheterization with either a straight catheter or a retention catheter is commonly used to treat retention.

Cholinergics

Cholinergic medications help stimulate bladder contraction, but these drugs must never be used if a mechanical obstruction is present. In this instance, intravesical pressure increases against an obstructed outlet, which may cause ureterovesical reflux or a ruptured bladder. Although their effect is somewhat controversial, bethanechol (Urecholine) and neostigmine (Prostigmin) are often administered. Bethanechol improves detrusor tone but also increases bladder outlet and urethral resistance. In order to counteract this, it is sometimes combined with phenoxybenzamine (Dibenzyline), prazosin (Minipress), and terazosin (Hytrin), potent alpha-adrenergic blockers.

■ Nursing Management of the Medical Client

It is important for the nurse to distinguish retention from oliguria and anuria. In urinary retention, the kidneys are producing a normal amount of urine, but it is not voided. Thus, the bladder fills with urine and is raised above the level of the pubic symphysis, sometimes being displaced to either side of midline. Any percussion over the bladder produces a dull sound. The client may experience increasing discomfort and the need to urinate. Assessment may reveal restlessness and diaphoresis.

Nursing interventions may be used initially to treat retention. Provide privacy, warm the bedpan, and place the client in a normal sitting or standing position, using gravity and increased intra-abdominal pressure to help relieve the problem. Make use of the power of suggestion by running water or flushing the toilet within earshot of the client. Tape-recorded aquatic sounds may be effective. A warm bath or pouring warm water over the perineum often promotes muscle relaxation. Immersing the hands in water sometimes works, as does blowing bubbles with a straw in a glass of water. Applying ice to or gently stroking the inner thigh will stimulate trigger points that may activate the micturition reflex. Anal dilation with a

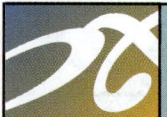

BRIDGE TO HOME HEALTHCARE

Inserting Urinary Catheters

Sue Anderson, R.N., *Shamrock In-Home Nursing Care, Inc., Rochester, Minnesota*

Inserting urinary catheters in the home may be a real challenge and may require you to improvise and adapt. You are responsible for identifying what supplies and equipment are needed and for obtaining them. When changing the catheter, have a flashlight, bed lamp, or small table lamp in the work area to provide proper lighting. Explain the procedure in a simple way to help the client relax during insertion.

For women, use multiple pillows for proper positioning. If the client is obese or arthritic, try a posterior approach and have her turn on her side away from you. If the client is agile, try a supine position with her knees flexed and separated and her feet flat on the bed. An alternative is to have her flex the knee opposite the working side of the nurse and keep the other leg extended. Using sterile technique and supplies, cleanse the meatal area, one side only; use a single downward stroke. Repeat on the opposite side. The last swab may be slightly inserted into the vagina to identify the vaginal opening. Insert a 16F or 18F well-lubricated catheter into the meatal opening as the client breathes deeply. If you accidentally insert the catheter into the vagina, leave it there as a marker to avoid vaginal reinsertion. Never reuse a catheter. Insert a new lubricated catheter. When urine returns, advance the catheter another inch, inflate the balloon with an attached saline syringe, and gently pull the catheter back. If no urine returns, gently insert a gloved, lubricated little finger into the vagina to assess for catheter slippage into the vagina.

For men, use a supine position with the legs extended. Verify with the physician the use of anesthetic gel (Xylocaine) to relieve insertion pain and to aid relaxation. Insert the prefilled gel syringe directly into the meatus, inject the gel, and remove the syringe. Wait 3 minutes. Using sterile technique, hold the penis with your nondominant hand, retract the foreskin, and lift and stretch the penis to a 60- to 90-degree angle. Cleanse the tip with a circular motion. Holding the well-lubricated catheter tip, insert it into the meatus in a small rotating motion and advance it until urine flows. Never force a catheter. Maneuver it gently as the client breathes deeply, bears down, or coughs. If resistance is met, stop and notify the physician. Never inflate the catheter balloon without establishing urine flow. Once placement is verified, inflate the balloon with a saline syringe. Tape the catheter securely with a Velcro strap attached to the thigh, to minimize pulling or stretching the catheter. Always hang the drainage bag below the level of the bladder, free of kinks. Kinks allow urine backflow into the bladder.

Whether the client is a woman or a man, your goal is to increase client independence. Teach about the use and care of equipment, skin care, and the need to increase oral fluids, such as water and cranberry juice. Also, give information about clinical manifestations in relation to pain, fever, urine color, sediment, blood, odor, and changes in output. Provide instructions about reporting changes to the nurse or physician. Leave written information with the client and family members for future reference.

---

gloved finger is sometimes helpful. If the client is tense and anxious, any measure that induces relaxation may aid in relieving the situation (e.g., a backrub or soothing music).

With appropriate training and a physician's prescription, a straight or retention catheter is inserted through the external meatus, into the urethra beyond the internal sphincter, and into the bladder. Use the straight catheter when it is to be removed as soon as the bladder is drained. Use the retention, or indwelling, catheter for undetermined time periods, keeping it in place by inflating the balloon near the catheter's tip. Regardless of the type of catheter, use strict aseptic techniques for insertion. One exception is the use of a clean technique for those clients on an intermittent self-catheterization program. (See further discussion under Neurogenic Bladder Dysfunction.)

The retention catheter is attached to either a bedside drainage bag or a leg bag. A leg bag is frequently used with long-term catheterization, especially for the client going home with an indwelling catheter. This device allows the client more mobility and eliminates the embarrassment of carrying a drainage bag in public view. Figure 56–7 shows a leg bag in position. Because of the bag's small capacity, it must be emptied frequently. At

night, a conventional drainage system is used so that the client can sleep through the night without needing to empty the leg bag. Instruct the client to avoid attaching the leg bag too tightly because the rubber straps can lead to skin irritation, thrombophlebitis, and ulcer formation. Even loose straps tend to tighten as the bag fills. Newer models have Velcro leg straps for clients with circulatory problems, for those allergic to latex, and for those at high risk of skin breakdown. Meticulous skin care and periodic removal of the bag help prevent these problems. Cleanliness and odor control are managed by washing the apparatus with soap and water and soaking it in a 1% acetic acid (white vinegar) solution overnight.

Using indwelling catheters involves several physical hazards, including UTI and tissue trauma. Over 80% of people who develop nosocomial UTIs have undergone urologic instrumentation of some kind. It is well documented that bacteriuria increases in direct relationship to duration of catheter placement. Estimates of infection rates range between 4% (within 24 hours) and 95% (within 4 weeks). The most common causative organisms are *E. coli, Proteus, Klebsiella, Aerobacter, Pseudomonas aeruginosa, Streptococcus, Staphylococcus, Providencia,* and *Serratia marcescens.* These organisms may enter the

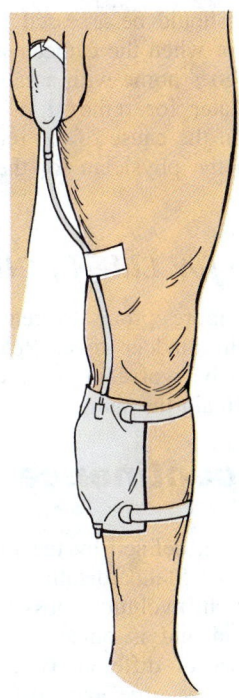

Figure 56–7. Condom drainage and leg bag. The bag may be attached to the calf of the leg, as shown, or to the thigh.

urinary drainage system when it is opened for any reason, or they may intrude via the thin layer of fluid and exudate that forms around the exterior of the catheter. The development of and intervention for UTI are discussed earlier in this chapter.

Probably the most important weapon in preventing infection is not inserting a catheter at all or, if it must be inserted, using conscientious hand washing before and after any handling of the catheter or drainage system.

To aid in preventing infection if a catheter must be used:

- Maintain a closed drainage system
- Avoid backflow of urine
- Avoid unnecessary manipulation of the catheter during perineal cleaning
- Prevent microbial invasion and colonization in the urine collection bag
- Maintain patency of the catheter
- Encourage a high fluid intake
- Provide urine acidification

Because of the potential development of resistant organisms and possible adverse reactions, antibiotics should not be used prophylactically to prevent bacteriuria.

Tissue trauma may occur during the catheterization procedure. Tissue irritation or necrosis may result from (1) using an oversized catheter, (2) continuous pressure, for example, not leaving enough slack in the catheter between the meatus and the site of taping on the leg or abdomen, or (3) using indwelling catheters that continually move in and out of the distal urethra causing tissue breakdown and enhancing encrustation on the outside of the catheter. Local irritation or systemic allergic reactions may occur when using a rubber catheter in clients with a

history of latex allergy. Clients with urinary tract disorders are at high risk of developing latex allergy due to the repeated use of latex catheters. Silicone catheters are available for these clients.

There is still some misunderstanding about what is referred to as bladder decompression drainage. This is really an older concept based on a faulty assumption that emptying a distended bladder rapidly through a catheter could result in bladder hemorrhage and hypotension. This procedure involved clamping the catheter after 1000 ml had been drained and then reopening it after an hour to drain another 1000 ml, until the bladder was decompressed. Cystometric studies have shown that this problem does not occur with retention. The current thinking is that any amount can be drained. Drainage does not occur rapidly because the usual size of a catheter does not allow rapid drainage. If the client's catheter does drain large amounts of urine, over 3000 ml, assess the client's fluid volume status; if volume depletion is indicated, fluid replacement is important. If the client has a large urine output after initial catheterization, it may be postobstruction diuresis. In this situation, one half of the urine output volume must be replaced.

■ Surgical Management

Bladder Neck Repair

Surgical intervention is sometimes necessary for obstructions below the bladder. If the bladder neck becomes rigid owing to inflammation, cystoplasty may be done to insert an elastic wedge into the area. A transurethral incision of the bladder neck might also be done. Excising urethral strictures, sometimes with a *urethroplasty* (plastic repair of the urethra), helps return it to proper functioning. A meatotomy may be done to better open the urethral meatus.

Suprapubic Cystotomy

Suprapubic catheterization is sometimes used to relieve urinary retention, especially in instances in which urethral catheterization is difficult or dangerous, as with severely enlarged prostates, urethral strictures, or in quadriplegic clients. The suprapubic catheter is inserted by the physician, often under local anesthesia and frequently in the client's room. General anesthesia may be used if another surgical procedure is also performed. To facilitate proper placement of the catheter, the bladder must be distended with fluid before the catheter is inserted. If the bladder is insufficiently distended with urine, additional fluid is instilled through a catheter or cystoscope.

The suprapubic skin is prepared. With use of sterile technique, the catheter may be inserted through a small surgical incision or by passing a trocar through the skin into the bladder. Once the trocar is in place, the pointed core of the cannula is removed. The catheter then is threaded through the cannula and attached to a closed drainage system. It may be sutured in place or secured with a commercially made retention seal.

When the suprapubic catheter is removed, the muscle

layers of the bladder immediately contract over the puncture site and shrink the surface wound, precluding any need for sutures. Advantages of the suprapubic over the urethral catheter include a lower rate of UTIs, ease in evaluation of the client's ability to void normally, and increased comfort.

Potential complications of the suprapubic catheter include dislodgement of the catheter, hematuria (especially after the use of a large-bore catheter), bowel perforation during trocar insertion, and failure of the wound to close with the development of a urinary fistula.

■ Nursing Management of the Surgical Client

The client with a suprapubic catheter requires care similar to that needed with a urethral catheter. The most frequent problem is catheter obstruction due to (1) twisting or kinking or (2) sediment or clots. Disconnecting the catheter from the drainage tubing can disrupt the siphon drainage.

When the suprapubic catheter is removed, frequent dressing changes may be needed to protect the skin from urinary leakage from the site. As the site of the suprapubic catheter heals, less drainage will occur.

The client who goes home with an indwelling suprapubic or urethral catheter needs to know how to care for the catheter at home. The family and significant others should learn the proper ways to empty the drainage bag and ways of preventing infection, such as forcing fluids and an acid-ash diet. They should also be taught the clinical manifestations of UTI and instructed to call the physician if one occurs.

The client may need an extra leg bag or drainage bag.

The client's home should be assessed for the availability of toilet facilities for when the catheter is removed.

The client who goes home with a catheter in place will need to be seen later for removal of the catheter; this varies depending on the cause of the retention. The nurse should check with the physician for the timing of a follow-up visit.

Modifications for Elderly Clients

Older clients are more prone to retention because of chronic decrease in bladder tone. Retention leading to infection may also be worse in older clients. The treatments, however, remain the same.

Urinary Incontinence

Incontinence has been defined by the International Continence Society for the Standardization of Terminology as "a condition in which involuntary loss of urine is a social or hygienic problem and is objectively demonstrable."[60] There are a number of different types of incontinence, such as enuresis, stress, urge, paradoxical (overflow), reflex, environmental (functional), and psychological (Table 56–3). The society divides it into five categories on the basis of anatomic or physiologic dysfunction. These are stress, urge, overflow (paradoxical), reflex, and functional (environmental) incontinence.

The Agency for Health Care Policy and Research (AHCPR) published a collection of booklets on urinary incontinence in 1992. The problem of urinary incontinence is a major health problem. It is estimated that 15% to 30% of noninstitutionalized adults over age 60 and at

| Table 56–3. Types of Incontinence ||
Type	Description
Stress	Increased intra-abdominal pressure caused by activities such as coughing, laughing, sneezing, walking, or running leads to involuntary loss of urine; intravesicular pressure increases to overcome resistance of internal sphincter in urethra
Enuresis	Nighttime incontinence (bed-wetting) usually associated with childhood, although problem can extend into adulthood
Urge	Inability to hold back flow of urine when feeling urge to void; spasmodic bladder contractions accentuate problem
Overflow (paradoxical)	Retention with overflow of small amounts of urine; occurs when intravesical pressure exceeds maximal urethral pressure without detrusor activity
Reflex	Caused by spinal cord injury or congenital conditions such as spina bifida leading to loss of voluntary control of bladder
Psychological	Client aware of need to urinate, but unable to respond appropriately to urge because of dementia or confusion
Environmental (functional)	Client aware of need to urinate, but physically unable to reach the toilet unaided

least half of the nursing home residents have problems with continence.[118]

Etiology and Risk Factors

Incontinence is often caused by interference with sphincter control. This includes anatomic, physical, physiologic, psychosocial, and pharmacologic factors. Anatomic and physiologic incontinence results from sphincter weakness or damage, urethral deformity, alteration of the urethrovesical junction, detrusor instability, and weak abdominal and perineal muscle tone.

Sphincter weakness or bladder neck strictures are often caused by obstetric trauma, postoperative weakness, and congenital weakness. After a suprapubic prostatectomy, men often experience some leakage for several days after the postoperative catheter is removed. A transurethral prostatectomy may cause bladder neck damage, with a longer period of incontinence or possibly permanent incontinence. A radical perineal or retropubic prostatectomy may cause permanent incontinence if the bladder neck is partially damaged during the operation.

Alteration of the *urethrovesical junction* occurs mainly in women. This angle, between the bladder and the posterior urethra, is important to continence in women. Common causes of the loss of this angle include multiple pregnancies, aging, and surgical procedures resulting in abdominal perineal weakness. This leads to stress incontinence of varying degrees. Figure 56–8 shows how the alteration of the urethrovesical angle from 90 to 100 degrees to less than 90 degrees reduces the competence of the internal sphincter.

Detrusor instability is commonly caused by

- Bladder lesions (e.g., infection, neoplasms, and senile trigonitis)
- Lower motor neuron spinal lesions (e.g., tumor, prolapsed disc, complications of pelvic surgery, and osteoarthritis of the spinal cord)
- Upper motor neuron spinal lesions (e.g., tumor, cerebrovascular accident, multiple sclerosis, and transection of the spinal cord)
- Large bowel diseases, spastic colon, and diverticulosis

Weak abdominal and *perineal muscle tone* are caused by obesity, lack of exercise, and loss of tone after childbirth or prostatectomy.

Physical causes of incontinence are those independent of the urinary tract. These are related to physical immobility, especially with the elderly. These clients are often physically unable to get to the toilet or bedpan independently because of strokes, fractures, or weakness. Failing vision can also contribute to this if the client is unable to see the commode or bedpan.

Psychosocial causes of incontinence range from true psychological problems such as dementia to simple confusion. Clients may be unaware of the need to void or simply unable to know what to do when they feel the urge. Other possible causes include regression, dependence, rebellion, insecurity, manipulative attention seeking, sensory deprivation, and the disturbance of conditioned reflexes.

Various medications also contribute to incontinence, especially overflow incontinence. These include (1) narcotics, tranquilizers, sedatives, and hypnotics, all of which affect bladder fullness cues and the ability to attend to them; (2) alcohol; (3) rapid-acting diuretics; (4) anti-histamines; (5) atropine and atropine-like substances; (6) hypotensives; (7) alpha-adrenergic blockers; (8) beta-adrenergics; and (9) ganglionic blockers.

Other factors contributing to the development and maintenance of incontinence include fecal impaction, bladder scarring, urethral adhesions, diabetes mellitus, and obesity. Incontinence may also be a sign of "giving up." Frequent voiding by clients who fear "accidents" leads to decreased bladder capacity, increased detrusor tone, and thickening of the bladder wall, which results in a vicious cycle of dysfunction. (See Risk Factors and Levels of Prevention: Urinary Incontinence.)

Pathophysiology

The pathophysiologic changes associated with incontinence are related to the specific causes. *Stress* incontinence occurs when the intravesical pressure exceeds the maximum urethral pressure in the absence of detrusor

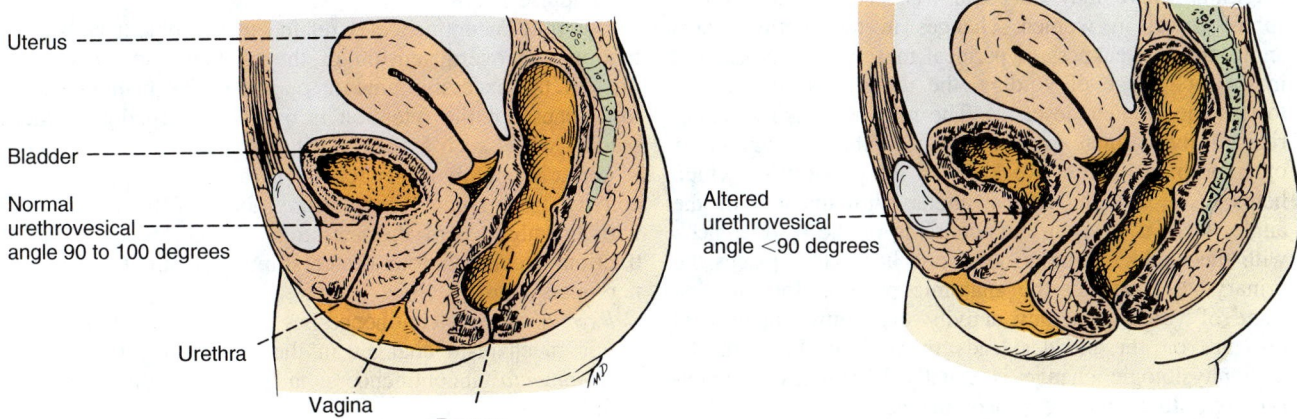

Uterus

Bladder

Normal urethrovesical angle 90 to 100 degrees

Urethra

Vagina

Rectum

Altered urethrovesical angle <90 degrees

Figure 56–8. Alteration in the normal urethrovesical angle contributes to incontinence in women. *A,* Normal angle. *B,* Altered angle.

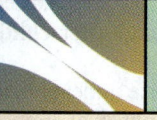

RISK FACTORS AND LEVELS OF PREVENTION

Urinary Incontinence

Risk Factors

Stress: Loss of correct posterior urethrovesical angle in women, decreased muscle tone surrounding the bladder, urethral irritation from infection, radiation damage to the bladder, prostatectomy in men

Enuresis: Causes in adulthood not clearly identified

Urge: Multiple sclerosis, urinary tract infections, strokes, arthritis, or medications that interfere with mobility

Overflow: Retention with bladder distention from atonic bladder caused by nervous system lesions, obstruction of bladder outlet (e.g., by benign prostatic hypertrophy), fecal impaction

Reflex: Spinal cord injury or congenital lesions of the cord such as spina bifida leading to complete loss of voluntary control of the bladder

Psychological: Altered mental status wherein the client loses the ability to act on the urge to void

Environmental: Inability to use the toilet independently because of poor lighting, poor access to the toilet, inaccessible clothing, inaccessible or unanswered call light, high side rails, or restraint

Levels of Prevention

Primary Prevention
- Prevent impaired mobility
- Avoid muscle weakness through exercise
- Prevent development of urinary tract infections
- Assist clients to the bathroom by the clock to avoid environmental incontinence

Secondary Prevention
- Thoroughly assess clients who report incontinence
- Monitor high-risk clients for development of incontinence

Tertiary Prevention
- Teach clients to do pelvic muscle exercises (Kegel exercises) to improve muscle tone
- Institute bladder training
- Teach clients to decrease incontinence by regulating fluid intake (e.g., not drinking large amounts of fluid at bedtime)

---

activity. This increased vesical pressure is often associated with activities such as sneezing, coughing, and laughing. There may be some weakness in the urethral sphincter or, in women, changes in the urethrovesical angle due to weakness of perineal musculature. Normally, in the first stage of voiding, the urethrovesical angle is lost as the bladder descends. The muscle weakness experienced by women as a result of childbirth, aging, or other problems causes weakness of the pelvic floor which helps to destroy the critical angle. With the loss of the angle, there is descent and funneling of the bladder neck with the bladder rotating down and back. This places the urinary structures in the anatomic position for the first stage of voiding, so any activity that causes downward pressure on the bladder leads to voiding. In men, the pathophysiologic change is usually BPH causing retention, overflow, and stress incontinence.

Urge incontinence is associated with several pathophysiologic changes. One problem is uninhibited detrusor contraction associated with motor disorders. Another cause is decreased mobility from an upper motor neuron spinal lesion combined with an inability to stop voiding once the impulse is felt.

Overflow incontinence is related to a problem with retention and overdistension of the bladder with an overflow of the excessive amount of urine. The pathophysiologic cause of the retention is usually obstruction at the bladder outlet such as with BPH.

Reflex incontinence is related to abnormal spinal cord activity from spinal cord lesions above T10, associated with the absence of the sensation to void. Bladder contraction occurs without direct stimulus from the central nervous system.

Psychological incontinence has as its basic pathophysiologic mechanism changes in the client's mental status; *environmental* incontinence is a problem with impaired mobility.

If incontinence is not controlled, it can lead to both psychological and physical problems. The psychological consequences of incontinence are serious. It can cause clients to isolate themselves and avoid going anywhere. The embarrassment associated with incontinence makes many clients sink into a world of isolation and depression. They often become dependent and almost helpless. This is also a leading cause of nursing home placements. The physical complications of incontinence include infection, skin breakdown, and permanent bladder changes.

Clinical Manifestations and Diagnostic Findings

The major manifestation of incontinence is stated in the definition: involuntary loss of control of voiding. If it is urge incontinence, it may be associated with bladder spasms. The amount of urine expelled can help differentiate whether it is overflow or stress incontinence, because these usually produce small amounts of urine.

Urodynamic evaluation is the major diagnostic test for incontinence. In order to determine the precise cause of the client's incontinence, the incontinence should be reproduced during the examination. These tests can also assess detrusor function and the likelihood that treatment will be successful. The degree of pelvic floor prolapse can be assessed by physical examination and radiologic tests.

The variety of urodynamic examinations, including cystometrogram and electromyogram, are described in Chapter 55. Cystometry can help to determine the cause of incontinence. Urine flow rate studies help identify prob-lems with the external sphincter and detrusor muscle hypotonia. The urethral pressure profile helps to determine possible incompetence of the external urinary sphincter, a common cause of stress incontinence in women. Ultrasonography of the bladder or kidneys can detect residual urine. A cystoscopy with cystography also may be useful in diagnosing this problem.

Acute and Subacute Care

■ Surgical Management

Although surgical management is not the primary therapy used to treat most incontinence, these clients require acute and subacute management.

Electrical Stimulation

Electrical inhibition of the micturition reflex has been successful for many clients. These devices, which deliver barely perceptible electrical stimulation, effect improved urethral closure by direct and reflexogenic contraction of the striated paraurethral musculature. They also may increase bladder volume through bladder inhibition and may stabilize detrusor activity. Figure 56–9 shows the three main types of electrical devices. Electrodes may be implanted surgically within the pelvic muscles for direct stimulation; indirect stimulation may be achieved by using either intravaginal or anal devices. The intravaginal

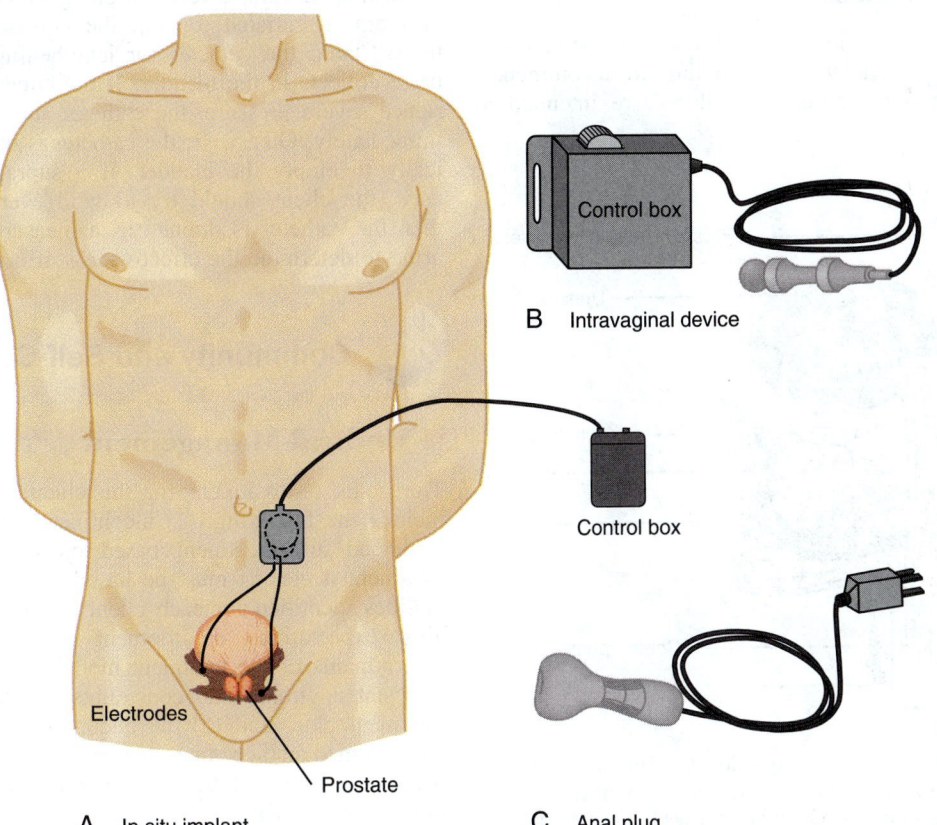

Figure 56–9. Electrical devices used to control incontinence.

device or anal plugs can be removed and reinserted as necessary. The anal plug must be removed for defecation and frequent cleaning. Once chosen, the apparatus is attached to a control box. The client can then activate the system as desired to relieve incontinence.

Implantation of an Artificial Urinary Sphincter

The implantation of an artificial urinary sphincter may help some clients achieve continence. This surgical procedure is usually reserved until after all else has failed. Figure 56–10 shows a sphincter device consisting of an inflatable cuff, a reservoir, and a control pump. The surgeon implants the cuff around the bladder neck or urethra, the deflation (or control) pump in the scrotum or labia, and the fluid reservoir in the abdomen. The cuff keeps the urethra closed until the client manually squeezes the pump, thereby moving the fluid from the cuff to the reservoir. The bladder will then drain. The cuff automatically refills after 7 to 10 seconds, again occluding the urethra. This method has been successful with many clients. However, candidates must have an obstructed lower urinary tract, no detrusor hyperreflexia, no progressive neurologic disease affecting bladder function, and the manual dexterity and motivation to manage the system. Failure of the device poses a long-term risk of reoperation. Clients must be absolutely compliant or the upper tracts will be damaged because the full bladder obstructs the kidneys.

Other Procedures

Other surgical procedures are used to correct or compensate for anatomic defects contributing to incontinence. The most common surgical procedures are intended to restore the normal urethrovesical angle or to lengthen and support the urethra. Reestablishing the urethrovesical angle allows the internal sphincter to function normally. A variety of sling procedures can be done that place material beneath the urethra to increase urethral compression.

In the Marshall-Marchetti-Krantz procedure, one of several common older techniques, the bladder neck and urethra are sutured to the perichondrium of the symphysis pubis or the periosteum of the superior pubic ramus. Newer procedures, such as the Raz procedure, are now being done transvaginally. This repair process involves elevation and suspension of the bladder with the use of tissue or inorganic materials for support. Postoperatively, clients undergoing this surgery need a suprapubic or urethral catheter for 5 to 8 days. During this time, they require a high fluid intake to prevent infection. Also, the drainage system must always be patent, because the pressure of a filling bladder inhibits the healing process.

Other surgical procedures aim to provide an intact, patent route for the transport of urine. Scar tissue that interferes with normal bladder neck function must be removed. If urethral or sphincter narrowing contributes to the problem of incontinence, it must be dilated.

■ Nursing Management of the Surgical Client

Nursing care of clients undergoing surgery centers around maintaining adequate urinary drainage. With bladder suspension, preventing distention is a priority to help avoid excessive pressure on the healing surgical procedure. After healing occurs, a reconditioning or clamp and release program is initiated to help the detrusor muscle regain tone. Clamp the catheter for lengthening intervals while urine collects in the bladder. If the client begins to experience severe pressure, the catheter should be unclamped immediately. Otherwise, the catheter is unclamped periodically to empty the bladder. If a suprapubic catheter is used, the client should try to void every 3 to 4 hours; then the catheter is drained as a measure of the residual urine to determine the effectiveness of bladder emptying.

Community and Self-Care

■ Medical Management

The goals of treatment for the client with incontinence include the following: (1) incontinence must be carefully evaluated and treatment based on this evaluation; (2) treatment decisions must be based on the specific abnormalities identified for each client; (3) the client's personality, expectations, environment, and clinical status are determinants of the treatment modalities; (4) plans to circumvent environmental constraints should be part of the treatment plan; and (5) the client must be able to make an informed choice among treatment options. The three major categories of treatment are behavioral, pharmacologic, and surgical.

There are many noninvasive, behavioral-type therapies that may be effective in controlling some types of incon-

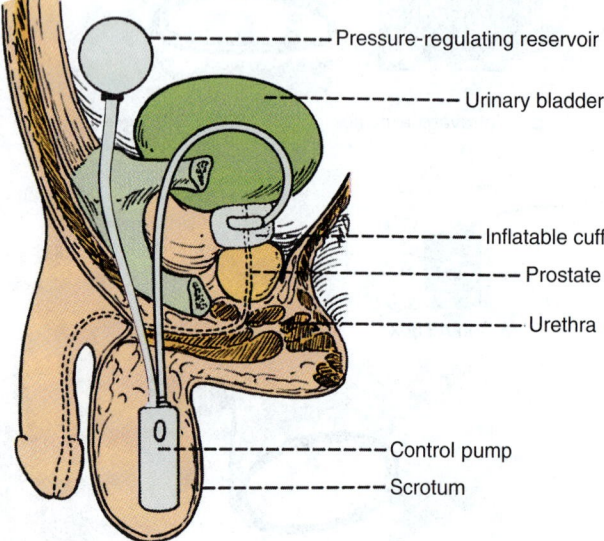

Figure 56–10. Artificial urinary sphincter. This surgically implanted urethral sphincter restores continence. To urinate, the client deflates the cuff around the bladder neck by squeezing the control pump within the scrotum. The cuff reinflates automatically.

Pressure-regulating reservoir

Urinary bladder

Inflatable cuff

Prostate

Urethra

Control pump

Scrotum

tinence. These are usually low-risk treatments that are effective in most clients when they receive care from knowledgeable healthcare professionals. The AHCPR guideline provides numerous algorithms that detail the diagnosis and treatment of a variety of forms of incontinence.[120]

Bladder Neck Support

For women, a Bladder Neck Support Prosthesis, a Silastic vaginal device, has been developed that elevates and supports the urethrovesical junction during physical exercise. This ring-shaped device is fitted into the vagina and the prongs elevate the urethrovesical junction in a manner similar to a urethropexy. It is fitted for each woman so that the device is the proper diameter and the prongs are the required length. This device appears to offer an easy and inexpensive alternative to surgery for selected women.

Pelvic Muscle Exercises

Pelvic muscle exercises, the Kegel exercises designed for postpartum women, have long been the technique used to improve control (see Nursing Research feature). Reports of success utilizing Kegel exercises range from 30% to 90%. Recently, a new device, the Femina cones, has improved the success of these exercises. These cones are weighted and inserted into the vagina. Correct muscle contraction is required to keep them in place. Early re-

---

NURSING RESEARCH

Is There a Simple, Accurate Way to Determine Whether Kegel Exercises Are Making a Difference in Pelvic Muscle Strength?

Brink, C. A., et al. (1989). A digital test for pelvic muscle strength in older women with urinary incontinence. *Nursing Research, 38*(4), 196–199.
Brink, C. A., et al. (1994). A digital test for pelvic muscle strength in women with urinary incontinence. *Nursing Research, 43*(6), 352–356.

In 1989, Brink and colleagues published the results of a study conducted on older women who were experiencing incontinence. The goal of the research was to determine whether primary care nurses could objectively measure pelvic muscle strength with a simple manual assessment technique. Such simple, objective measures are important. Pelvic muscle exercises such as Kegel exercises are believed to increase pelvic muscle strength and thereby reduce stress incontinence. With a simple, accurate measure of pelvic muscle strength, clients could fine-tune their pelvic muscle exercises and more quickly achieve improved continence.

The 1989 study compared the accuracy of digital assessment of pelvic muscle strength by primary care nurses against vaginal myography (perinometry). The study found that digital assessment of pelvic muscle strength by the primary care nurses accurately measured pelvic muscle strength. The results of this study supported the use of a digital measure of pelvic muscle strength in incontinent older women.

The researchers went on to develop and validate a scale describing these measures. The goal was to create a scale that could then be used to assess improvement in muscle strength after pelvic muscle exercises. However, the researchers found that the lower end of the scale was less useful than the rest of the scale in assessing muscle strength, so they developed and tested a new scale. This new scale measured not only the pressure exerted by the pelvic muscles but also the amount of vertical displacement and the duration of pressure during contraction of the pelvic muscles.

In 1994, Brink and colleagues published the results of a study in which they applied this new scale to 208 women, aged 25 to 87, who were suffering from incontinence, to determine their pelvic muscle strength. Unfortunately, the study found that this second version of the scale had lower reliability than the first, probably because of the added dimensions of vertical displacement and duration of pressure. The researchers believed, however, that the added dimensions increased the conceptual clarity of assessment of pelvic muscle function. They also pointed out that the added measures allow for more individualization of pelvic muscle exercises, so that the specific component needed by any given client could be emphasized.

Brink and colleagues then developed a third version of the scale, based on the limitations found in the second version. This third version will increase the increments in the subscales to allow for better differentiation. This should lead to better individualization of exercise regimens.

Implications for Practice

It has long been believed that increasing pelvic muscle strength can help decrease the occurrence of incontinence. Nurses teach clients pelvic muscle strengthening exercises to improve pelvic muscle strength. There is no easy way, however, to measure pelvic muscle strength. It is difficult, therefore, for nurses to assess the effectiveness of their teaching. If a simple test can be identified that measured this, it could improve teaching and assessment of success.

ports are that they dramatically improve the effectiveness of pelvic muscle exercises.

Behavioral Techniques

Behavioral techniques to increase the client's awareness of the need to void can also be initiated. Biofeedback has been used with clients experiencing stress or urge incontinence. Clients are trained to control sphincter, detrusor, and abdominal muscles. It is not a technique that all clients are comfortable with and does require extensive training. The use of biofeedback has been shown to be successful in eliminating incontinence in about 20% to 25% of clients and provided significant improvement in another 30%.

Bladder Training

With this technique, the client first voids at short intervals throughout the day, usually hourly or less if necessary. The client then tries to lengthen the time between voiding to intervals up to 3 hours. This seems to eliminate the problem in about 10% to 15% of clients with urge and stress incontinence, and most clients find at least some improvement.

Institutionalized clients can also use a form of bladder training. With these clients, healthcare workers check the clients at hourly intervals, urging use of the bedpan and praising success. The time between voiding can often be increased to every 2 hours with success.

UTIs must be eliminated to reduce irritation of the detrusor muscle. In the case of stress incontinence, it is important to suppress a chronic cough.

Pharmacologic Treatment

Pharmacologic intervention for incontinence is primarily guided by the following. During the urine collection phase, the detrusor relaxes because of beta-adrenergic activity. At the same time, the bladder outlet contracts in response to alpha-adrenergic stimulation. When these actions are insufficient to maintain urine storage in the bladder, medications can be prescribed as supplements or replacements for these physiologic activities.

A variety of medications have been tried to control incontinence. Table 56–4 summarizes these medications. Medications are used mainly with urge and reflex incontinence and sometimes with stress incontinence to relax the bladder and possibly to increase bladder capacity. These medications are contraindicated in clients with bladder outlet obstructions or weak detrusor muscles.

Propantheline, dicyclomine, imipramine, flavoxate, or oxybutynin chloride may decrease detrusor hyperactivity. Alpha-adrenergic agents that increase urethral resistance include phenylephrine, ephedrine, phenylpropanolamine, and imipramine. Calcium channel blockers, which antagonize transmembrane movement of calcium, are being used with some success. If external sphincter spasticity (dyssynergia) is the problem, the physician may order baclofen, dantrolene, or diazepam. Topical and systemic estrogens help relieve estrogen-deficiency urethral problems in postmenopausal women.

Controlling Fluid Intake

The major nutritional alteration involves controlling fluid intake, especially after dinner, so the client will have less incontinence during the night. For obese clients, weight reduction programs may help decrease stress incontinence. The client should avoid bladder irritants such as alcohol, chocolate, and caffeinated drinks.

■ Nursing Management of the Medical Client

Independent nursing interventions for incontinence include weight reduction, establishment of an exercise program, and institution of a bladder training program. Weight reduction, if necessary, and pelvic exercises not only help regain bladder control but may prevent recurrence of the problem.

A successful bladder training program requires a great deal of patience on everyone's part. The client has to accept this program and be a willing and active participant. The first step in instituting the program is to discuss all procedures and the expected outcome with the client. The sensitive nurse tries to inspire a sense of hope and the attitude that something indeed can be done about incontinence.

A bladder training program involves (1) adequate fluid intake, (2) accessibility to a toilet, (3) muscle-strengthening exercises, and (4) carefully scheduled voiding times. To implement this program, you will need to have well-organized teaching guidelines. If the program involves behavioral modification or intermittent catheterization, these are discussed in the paragraphs that follow. Although the bed and clothing may be padded to protect them from becoming wet during the program, avoid diapering the client, as this is demeaning and may give "permission" to be incontinent.

Many clients suffering from incontinence reduce their *fluid intake,* thinking this will decrease urine production and result in better control. Actually, adequate urine production is necessary to stimulate the micturition reflex. Therefore, unless it is contraindicated by the client's physical status, encourage a daily fluid intake of 2000 to 2500 ml. Carefully space these fluids throughout the day and limit them in the evening to allow longer sleep periods at night. Have the client avoid beverages containing caffeine, because they contribute to bladder irritability.

Kegel exercises strengthen the pubococcygeal muscle and resolve stress incontinence with diligent hard work. To teach Kegel exercises, ask the client to stop urine flow several times during voiding. Once there is full awareness of the muscles needed to do this, have the client contract these muscles three to four times a day for 5- to 10-minute sessions each. If back pain occurs during the exercises, the client is probably contracting the wrong muscles and thus needs to go back to step 1 of the exercise program. The program is involved and may take months to get the muscles strong.

Meanwhile, develop a *voiding schedule* with the client. Determine how often the client urinates during the day by maintaining a voiding record. Check frequently for wetness and document results. Depending on the voiding

Table 56-4. Medications Used to Treat Urge, Reflex, and Stress Incontinence

Agent	Action	Dosage	Side Effects	Nursing Implications
Propantheline bromide (Pro-Banthine)	Anticholinergic that inhibits detrusor contraction and may increase bladder capacity, delay and decrease in amplitude of involuntary contractions	15 mg PO tid; higher doses produce too much drying of mouth	Dry mouth, dry eyes, constipation, confusion or excitement in elderly; precipitation of glaucoma, blurred vision, mydriasis, palpitations, urinary retention or hesitancy	Do not use in clients with narrow-angle glaucoma, obstructive uropathy or GI disease, arteriosclerotic heart disease, hypertension, hiatal hernia, or hepatic or renal disease; monitor vital signs and urinary output; sugarless gum or hard candy will alleviate dry mouth
Oxybutynin chloride (Ditropan)	Direct smooth muscle relaxant that works directly on bladder muscle; helps with detrusor instability	Up to 5 mg PO qid	Drowsiness, dry mouth, palpitations, tachycardia, blurred vision, mydriasis, constipation, urinary hesitancy or retention	Contraindicated in clients with myasthenia gravis, GI obstruction, and obstructive uropathy; use cautiously in elderly; stop therapy at intervals to see if problem resolved; rapid onset of action, peaks at 3–4 hr and lasts 6–10 hr; monitor with periodic cystometry; store in tightly closed container
Verapamil hydrochloride (Calan)	Depressant effect on bladder muscles; use for incontinence not well documented	80 mg PO tid	Dizziness, hypotension, heart failure, constipation, nausea, urinary retention, peripheral edema	Use with incontinence not well studied; use cautiously in elderly clients and clients with existing heart disease; monitor urinary output; check pulse and blood pressure regularly
Imipramine hydrochloride (Tofranil)	Anticholinergic and direct relaxant effect on detrusor and contracting effect on bladder outlet (alpha-adrenergic effect)	25–75 mg/day PO	Drowsiness, dizziness, orthostatic hypotension, tachycardia, urinary retention, sweating, blurred vision, constipation, mydriasis	Do not use in clients recovering from myocardial infarction, with BPH, or history of glaucoma or seizure disorders; reduce dosage in elderly or debilitated clients; monitor for urinary retention or constipation; warn client to avoid alcohol and Sudafed and other OTC cold or hay fever medications
Phenylpropanolamine hydrochloride (Acu9trim)	Alpha- and beta-adrenergic antagonist used to treat stress incontinence; produces smooth muscle contraction at bladder outlet	25 mg q 4 h	Hypertension, tachycardia, palpitation, insomnia, nervousness, restlessness	Monitor effectiveness; check blood pressure frequently; warn client against use of OTC drug that may interact, especially Sudafed; store in light-resistant, tight container
Estrogens	Works by improving vaginal muscle tone; for postmenopausal women with urge incontinence, but ineffective against stress incontinence	Varies with agent used	Headache, increased risk of thromboembolism, nausea and vomiting, breakthrough bleeding, hyperglycemia, hypercalcemia, urticaria	Do not use in clients with history of thromboembolic disease of any kind; monitor effectiveness in reducing incontinence; warn client about possible increased risks of cancer

pattern, help the client to the toilet or commode every 30 minutes to 2 hours. As the program progresses, encourage the client to hold the urine longer and thus increase voiding intervals.

Biofeedback and *behavior modification* may be included in this bladder training program. Use biofeedback techniques to help the client regain control over the external urethral sphincter and pelvic floor musculature. This will increase relaxation of the bladder neck and pelvic muscles during voiding, reducing dyssynergia. Biofeedback involves attaching electrodes to the perianal skin and lateral thigh, then to a sequential light display mechanism. As the client contracts the pelvic floor, the lights indicate the strength or duration of the muscle contraction. Thus the lights give immediate feedback concerning progress. The device can be used at home.

Behavior modification is a variation of the voiding schedule. This program conditions the bladder to empty when the client sits on the toilet or commode. First, either by frequent assessment or by using an alarm device that sounds when the client voids, determine when incontinence consistently occurs during the day. Then place the client on the commode or toilet just before the usual time of incontinence. The theory is that gradual conditioning through use of the commode or toilet stimulates micturition. Once a stimulus-response pattern has been established, it can help achieve continence throughout the day. Programs are more successful when bladder capacity is at least 150 to 200 ml. With a capacity below this level, the client voids too frequently to achieve an optimal outcome.

Mechanical pressure is sometimes used to interfere with the outflow of urine. For example, a pessary is inserted into the vagina, where it exerts pressure on the bladder neck area. Some of these devices have inflatable balloons that are periodically released to permit voiding. However, the use of pessaries is associated with complications, including discomfort, leukorrhea, ulceration, fistulas, and malignancy. A penile clamp, as illustrated in Figure 56–11, is used to compress the urethra in the male. The use of this appliance is controversial. It should be used only temporarily as the man does pelvic muscle exercises to overcome stress incontinence. It must be removed and repositioned frequently to prevent pressure sores and ischemic necrosis of the penis.

Psychotherapy and *hypnosis* also help manage incontinence. Psychotherapy may aid the client whose incontinence has a psychogenic origin as well as assist clients in dealing with embarrassment, increased dependence, and self-image problems that may accompany incontinence.

Sometimes none of these measures are effective. Nursing interventions must then be aimed at protecting the client's skin, clothing, bed linen, and so on. Adult-sized disposable pads or briefs help protect and increase the social mobility of clients experiencing chronic incontinence. These commercially available undergarments, with elasticized legs, have a cellulose padding that draws fluid away from the skin by capillary action. Some brands include an odor-reducing agent. If the skin does become wet, it must be meticulously cleaned with a pH-balanced cleaner, dried to prevent serious rashes and skin breakdown resulting from maceration and ammonia production, and carefully moisturized. Use indwelling catheters to drain urine only as a last resort to help avoid UTIs.

External condom catheter drainage (see Fig. 56–7) involves putting a thin rubber or plastic sheath over the penis and connecting it to either a leg bag or a bedside drainage bag. When the bladder releases urine, the urine runs down the tube into the collecting device. Problems with this system include leakage (with or without detachment of the condom), twisting of the condom, and stasis of urine, which can macerate the penis. If the bladder does not empty with urination, postvoiding residual (PVR) leads to UTIs and associated complications.

Select the correct size of sheath and attach it so that it stays in place without compromising circulation to the distal penis. Make sure that the sheath is not too tight, particularly at the ring. You may need to remove the pubic hair before preparing the skin. Wash the penis with soap and water and allow it to dry thoroughly to remove skin oils from the penis. If appropriate, apply an adhesive paste or commercial skin barrier. Many commercially prepared condom systems contain a double-sided adhesive liner that is applied to the penis before the condom. Many newer devices are self-adhesive. When rolling the condom sheath over the penis, take care to allow at least 1.5 cm between the distal end of the penis and the internal end of the sheath. This will reduce skin irritation. Make sure the foreskin is over the glans. Use only elastic tape (to allow for expansion or erections). Apply this tape in a spiral only. To avoid impaired circulation, never encircle the penis completely with tape. Frequently monitor the patency of the system and remove the condom at least daily to clean and dry the skin.

The client needs to be followed at regular intervals to be sure that the interventions are working and the incontinence remains under control. Referral to continence clinics may be appropriate for some clients to ensure close follow-up of continuing problems. Help for Incontinent Persons (HIP) and the Simon Foundation for Continence both publish newsletters containing important information for the incontinent client and family.

Modifications for Elderly Clients

Incontinence is a common problem among the elderly. The elderly can be treated with any of the previously mentioned treatments. The elderly are more sensitive to many medications, so care should be used when administering them. The nurse should also remember that muscle weakness, with external factors such as decreased mobility and dependency, is a major cause of incontinence. See Figure 56–12 for an algorithm concerning incontinence in the elderly developed by the panel on urinary incontinence in the AHCPR guideline.[118] This algorithm provides a protocol for diagnosis and treatment of incontinence in this age group.

Neurogenic Bladder Dysfunction

The term "neurogenic bladder" refers to several bladder dysfunctions, all of which are caused by lesions of the central or peripheral nervous systems. Their manifestations depend on the site of the lesion.

There are five major types of neurogenic bladder dysfunction (Fig. 56–13): (1) uninhibited, (2) sensory para-

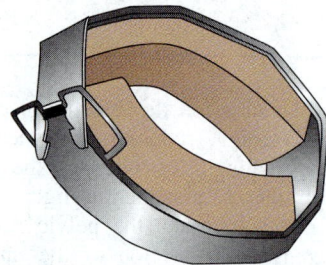

Figure 56–11. A penile clamp compresses the urethra to prevent incontinence.

lytic (detrusor muscle hyperreflexia), (3) motor paralytic (detrusor muscle areflexia), (4) autonomous, and (5) reflex.

Neurogenic bladder dysfunctions may also be classified according to the level of the lesion within the CNS. Dysfunctions related to lesions in the upper motor neuron occur above the sacral segments of the spinal cord; lesions in or below the sacral vertebrae produce lower motor neuron bladders. Upper motor neuron bladders are spastic or characterized by exaggerated reflexes (hyperreflexia); lower motor neuron bladders are lacking reflexes (areflexic) or atonic.

The incidence of neurogenic bladder dysfunction is dependent on the incidence of the various neurologic injuries or disorders that cause these problems. With certain disorders, 100% of clients will develop a neurogenic bladder (as with transection of the cord); with other neurologic disorders, fewer clients will be affected (as with multiple sclerosis).

Etiology and Risk Factors

The uninhibited neurogenic bladder produces "infantlike" or uninhibited voiding. The urge to void causes urine

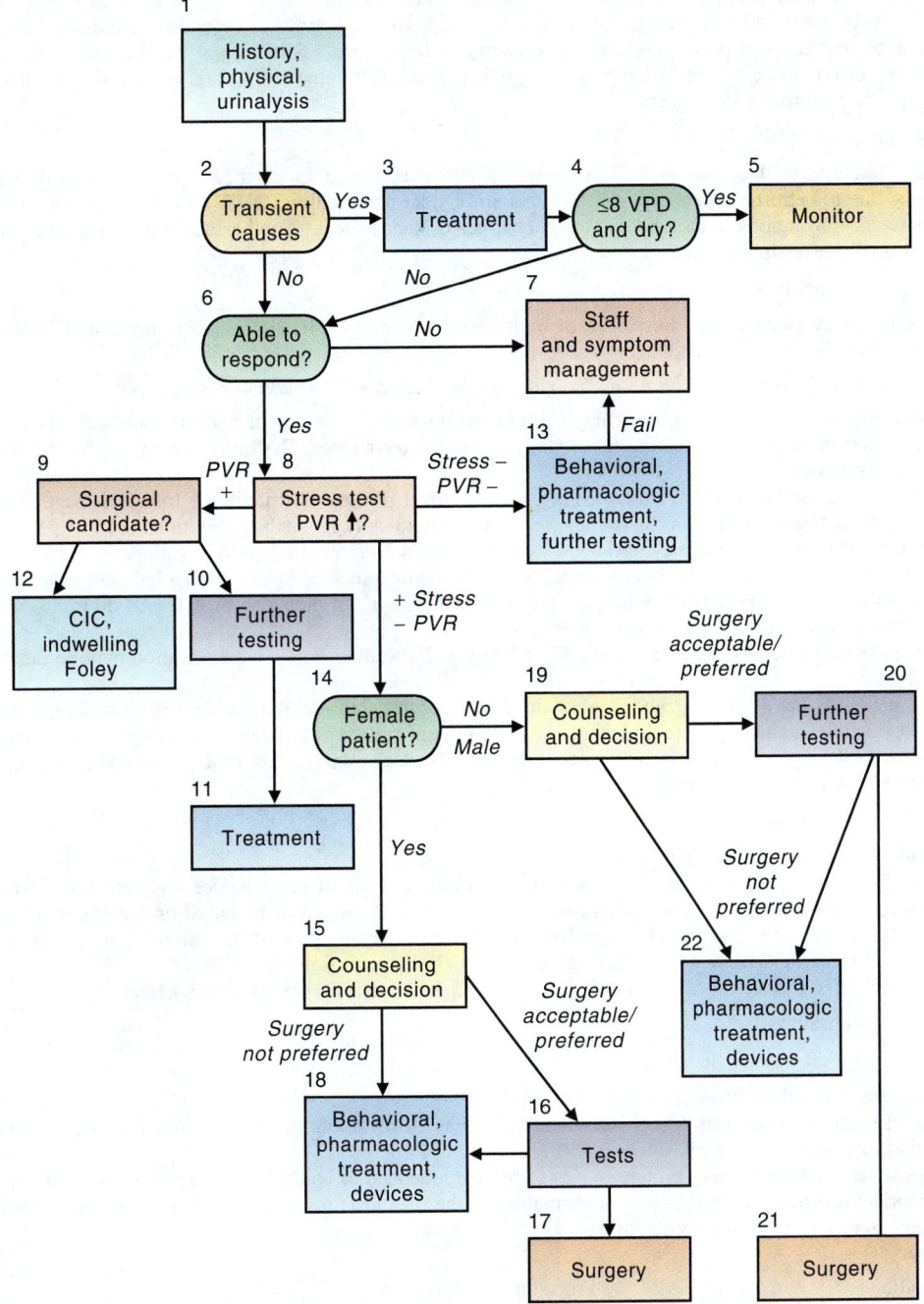

Figure 56–12. Algorithm for urinary incontinence (UI) in the elderly. (From Urinary Incontinence Guideline Panel. (1992). *Urinary incontinence in adults: Clinical practice guideline.* AHCPR Publications No. 92–0038. Rockville, MD: Agency for Health Care Policy and Research, Public Health Service, U.S. Department of Health band Human Services.)

Illustration continued on following page

Frail Elderly Male or Female (All Types of UI)

  1. History, physical, and urinalysis.
2. and 3. Identify and treat transient causes of UI.
  4. Bladder record to document voiding frequency and continence status. If record demonstrates ≤8 voids per day and dry, continue to monitor patient. If not, proceed to node 6.
  5. Staff and supervisors monitor with regular checks of wetness/dryness.
  6. Check patients with established UI for their ability to respond to toileting needs. This can be assessed by holding up two objects and asking the patient to point to or look first at one object and then the other. Patients are not eligible for incontinence rehabilitation if they fail to respond correctly to the instructions on three separate trials, preferably administered on at least two separate days. This screening must be modified for blind subjects. Similarly, blind subjects who fail to follow appropriate and simple one-step instructions are not candidates for the incontinence rehabilitation program.
  7. Patients with established UI who are unable to respond to questions regarding toileting needs will be referred for staff and symptoms management. However, many demented patients will be able to respond appropriately.
  8. Patients who are able to respond to simple questions regarding toileting are potential candidates for specific treatment, regardless of presence or degree of cognitive impairment. Therefore, it will be important to rule out overflow incontinence by determining the postvoiding residual volume (PVR) and to identify patients with stress leakage by performing stress tests.

Female patients with abnormal PVR

  9. This is likely to be due to an underactive detrusor, either neurogenic or nonneurogenic. Overflow UI in women may also be due to detrusor hyperactivity with impaired bladder contractility (DHIC) or, in those with previous anti-incontinence operations, it may be due to an obstructed bladder neck. Another possibility is the presence of an anatomically reversible condition.

Male patients with abnormal PVR

  9. In men with overflow UI, the likelihood of both obstruction and DHIC are high. Further testing should be undertaken if the patient is a surgical candidate.

     Evaluate surgical candidates based on their overall medical condition and anesthesia risk.

  10. Before surgery is selected, test to distinguish underactive detrusor from outlet obstruction and DHIC. These include voiding cystometrography (pressure flow) study or videourodynamics. Cystourethroscopy is helpful to confirm the site of obstruction.
  11. In men, based on the result of further testing in node *10,* if prostate obstruction is found, manage in accordance with existing BPH treatment criteria. In women, repair of anatomically reversible conditions such as pelvic prolapse or obstructed bladder neck may be considered if obstruction is confirmed by further testing.
     Regardless of gender, if DHIC is diagnosed, treatment options include behavioral techniques with or without bladder relaxants and clean intermittent catheterization (CIC). If CIC is not indicated or not used during the initial treatment, monitor the patient closely for urinary retention.
     If an underactive detrusor is found, use CIC if feasible. Indwelling Foley catheterization may be the option if CIC is not feasible.
  12. If the patient is not a surgical candidate, or there is no obstruction and the problem is an underactive detrusor, options include augmented voiding techniques, intermittent catheterization, or indwelling Foley catheter.
     If DHIC is the cause, treat as for urge incontinence; if bladder relaxants are required in addition to behavioral interventions, monitor closely for urinary retention.

Stress test negative and PVR normal

  13. Negative stress test and normal PVR.
     Although stress UI and urethral obstruction may still be the cause of incontinence, they are less likely. Options include behavioral techniques and pharmacologic trials. The decision will be based on the symptoms of UI and the general condition of the patient. Prompted voiding is the preferred option if the patient is not capable of independent toileting. Further testing may be considered if the initial treatment fails.
  7. If the trial fails in node *13,* the patient can be referred for staff and symptom management.

Frail Elderly Female with Stress UI

Stress test positive and PVR normal (female)

  14. Female patient with positive stress test and low PVR.
  15. Counsel regarding treatment options for presumed stress UI including behavioral, pharmacologic (alpha-adrenergic agonist), or surgical treatment.
  16. Surgical candidate or surgery preferred. Tests are recommended to confirm the diagnosis and to determine the appropriate approach and prognosis. Confirmation of the diagnosis is needed because other diagnoses may mimic simple stress UI in nursing home patients.
  17. Surgery.

Condition	Procedure
Hypermobility	Bladder suspension procedure
Internal Sphincter Device	Sling, bulking, artificial sphincter
Anatomically reversible conditions	Pelvic surgeries

Figure 56–12 *Continued*

18. Nonsurgical treatment preferred such as behavioral, pharmacologic, devices.

Frail Elderly Male with Stress UI

Stress test positive and PVR normal (male)

14. Male patient with stress UI. Possibilities include postprostatectomy incontinence and low spinal lesions (rarely). If there is no history of urethral surgery, referral should be sought unless it is not justified by the patient's condition.
19. If there is no history of prostate or urethral surgery, further investigation is warranted to confirm stress UI and determine the cause. Treatment options for men with stress UI include behavioral techniques, pharmacologic agents, surgery, or devices. Decision should be made according to patient preference.
20. If patient is a surgical candidate and prefers surgery, tests should be done to confirm the diagnosis since other diagnoses may mimic test UI in nursing home patients.
21. Surgical options for intrinsic sphincter deficiency in men include bulking and artificial sphincter.
22. Nonsurgical options include behavioral and pharmacologic treatments and devices.

Figure 56–12 *Continued*

excretion. This type is caused primarily by lesions in the corticoregulatory tracts (e.g., cerebrovascular accidents, multiple sclerosis).

The sensory paralytic bladder results from an interruption in the lateral spinal tracts (e.g., tabes dorsalis, diabetic neuropathy, and pernicious anemia). Because of the sensory loss, the client cannot perceive bladder filling. This lack of perception leads to atonic bladder and retention with overflow incontinence.

A motor paralytic bladder is the most uncommon type and is caused by lesions in the motor outflow from S2 to S4. Disease processes that cause this dysfunction include poliomyelitis, tumor, trauma, spina bifida, and infection. This dysfunction may be temporary if it is caused by a bacterial or viral infection. Although there is full sensation of bladder filling, even to the point of pain, the client is unable to initiate micturition.

The person with an autonomous neurogenic bladder can neither perceive bladder fullness nor initiate or maintain urination without some type of "assistance" (such as applying external pressure on the abdomen). Retention and incontinence are common problems. This type occurs after destruction of all nerve connections between the bladder and the CNS at S2, S3, or S4 (e.g., trauma, inflammatory processes, spinal anesthesia, or malignancy).

Finally, transection of the spinal cord above the sacral segments causes a reflex neurogenic bladder. There is no sensation, and the bladder contracts reflexively but does not empty completely. A client's neurogenic bladder may involve a combination of one or more nervous system dysfunctions.

Risk factors for neurogenic bladder disorders include tumors, neurologic disorders, and trauma to the nervous system. Accidents are the most preventable cause of this problem; tumors and many neurologic diseases are not preventable.

Pathophysiology

Lesions at the lower motor neuron level of the spinal cord often directly interfere with the reflex arc and lead to inappropriate interpretation of efferent and afferent impulses. When the bladder fills, the message is transmitted through afferent fibers to the brain cortex. The injury, however, keeps these impulses from being correctly interpreted, leading to no impulse for micturition. A flaccid bladder with urinary retention is the result.

With upper motor neuron lesions, impulses are not transmitted to or from the lower spinal areas to the cortex. When the client's bladder distends, no sensation is transmitted. Because the lower cord is intact, however, activity of the reflex arc can occur, and the client will have reflex incontinence of urine.

When the damage is to the cortical area itself, as with a stroke or trauma, the client cannot correctly interpret the impulses that are being transmitted.

Unless the client is evaluated and treated appropriately, the client with a dysfunctional bladder is more likely to develop serious UTIs, skin breakdown associated with incontinence, and even renal failure due to chronic overdistention of the bladder.

Clinical Manifestations and Diagnostic Findings

The major clinical manifestation of neurogenic bladder dysfunction is retention or incontinence. The client may or may not feel a need to void or may not even feel a sense of bladder distention. The diagnosis is often made from the type of neurologic dysfunction that has occurred.

Urodynamic studies including an electromyogram should be done to help determine the extent of neurologic involvement to help with the diagnosis of specific dysfunction so appropriate treatment can be initiated.

Acute and Subacute Care

■ Surgical Management

Surgery is not the primary therapy for the client with incontinence. It is, however, a more acute form of therapy. If conservative measures are ineffective in treating the neurogenic bladder, surgical intervention may be necessary. External sphincterotomy or incision of the bladder

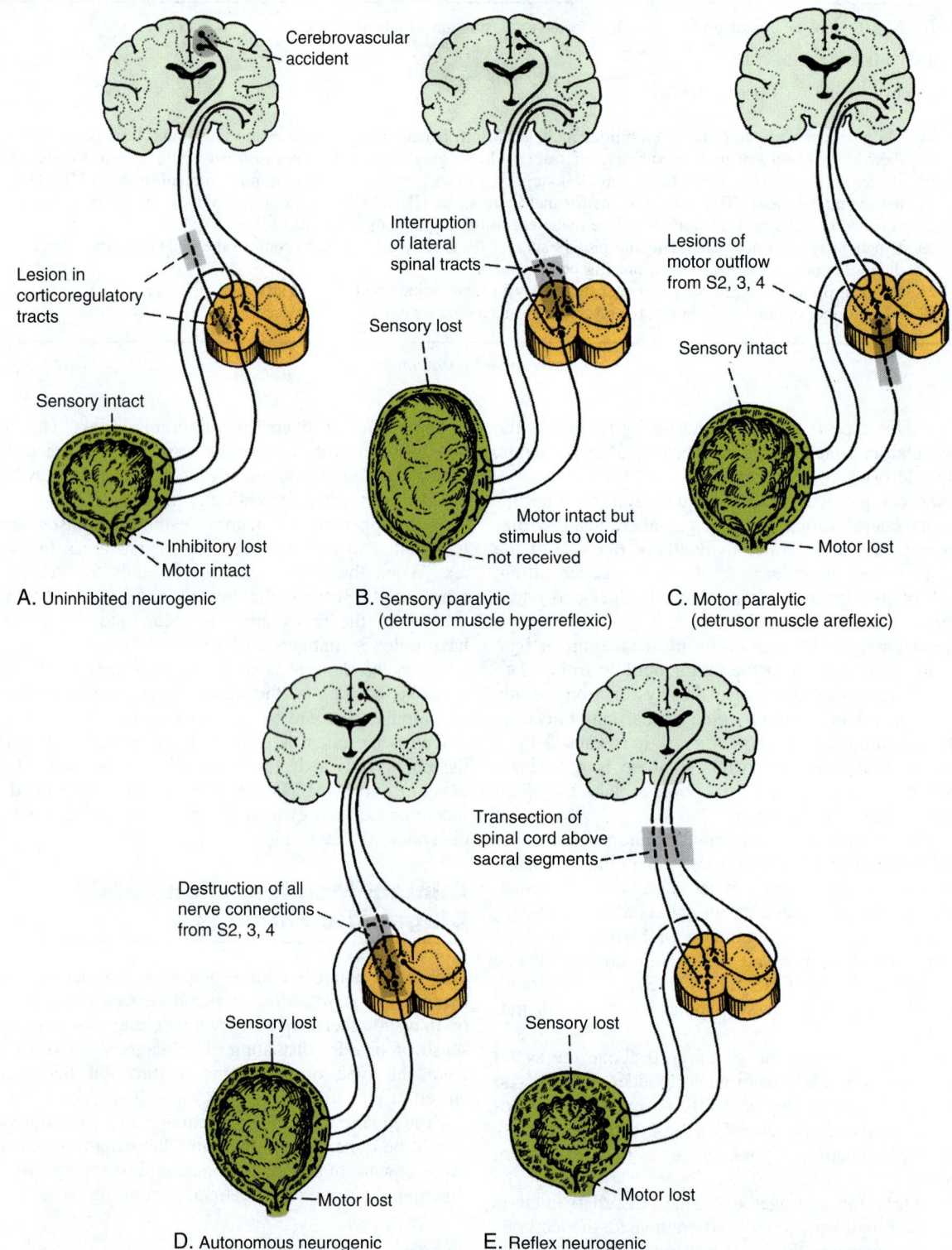

Figure 56–13. Types of neurogenic bladder dysfunction.

neck may restore normal bladder emptying. Interrupting innervation to the bladder reflex can aid an uninhibited bladder. Injection of alcohol into the subarachnoid space or rhizotomy (cutting) of the sacral nerves increases bladder capacity by inhibiting reflex bladder contractions, without interfering with normal sphincter function. Some-times the physician will do a temporary sacral nerve block before surgery to evaluate the potential candidate. Also, electrodes may be implanted in the thoracic or cervical levels of the spinal epidural space and then at-tached to a percutaneous stimulator. As soon as the client learns to regulate the electrical stimulation properly, the device can be used to interfere with the reflex bladder contractions.

Continuous intrathecal baclofen administered through an implanted infusion pump is another method of treating a neurogenic bladder. Baclofen helps decrease the spasms and detrusor sphincter dyssynergia. Clients report improvement in bladder compliance and capacity.

Finally, and only if all else fails, urinary diversion may be performed to provide the client with a more manageable urinary system.

Surgery is not always successful in alleviating the problems associated with neurogenic bladder dysfunction. Some clients cannot be helped surgically; therefore, learning other methods of bladder control is important.

■ Nursing Management of the Surgical Client

Nursing care of the client undergoing surgery for a neurogenic bladder with either an external sphincterotomy or a revision of the bladder outlet is the same as for any client undergoing bladder surgery. Urinary output maintenance is the priority of these clients. A suprapubic or urinary catheter may be needed until healing occurs.

As with the other surgical procedures, care is focused on teaching the client self-care. The client needs to learn to regulate electrical stimulation appropriately to interfere with the reflex bladder contractions. Proper care of the implantable infusion pump is another important area of client education. Care of clients undergoing urinary diversion is discussed under Bladder Neoplasms.

Community and Self-Care

■ Medical Management
Bladder Training

If possible, some form of bladder training is attempted for the client with neurogenic bladder dysfunction. This includes a bladder training program with or without intermittent catheterization, pharmacologic therapy, and sometimes surgical intervention.

Medications

A number of medications are used to treat neurogenic bladder dysfunction (see Tables 56–1 and 56–4). Antispasmodics and anticholinergics (e.g., dicyclomine, propantheline, and flavoxate) are given to relieve uninhibited or reflex bladder contractions. Phenoxybenzamine and other alpha-adrenergic blocking agents may be used. Bethanechol chloride may help stimulate an atonic bladder. Other pharmacologic agents, described in the discussion of incontinence, may be useful.

Complications

Autonomic dysreflexia is a serious, potentially life-threatening complication that can affect spinal cord–injured clients during a bladder training program if their urinary system or bowel becomes obstructed from UTIs or pressure sores. This condition results from excessive autonomic response to normal stimuli and affects primarily clients with upper motor neuron lesions. The most frequent cause is bladder distention or feces in the rectum, although autonomic dysreflexia can be triggered by visceral distention or stimulation of pain receptors in the skin.

The most common manifestations are hypertension, bradycardia, throbbing headache, flushing, diaphoresis above the level of the lesion, blurred vision, nasal congestion, nausea, and pilomotor spasm ("goose bumps") above the lesion. If left untreated, this problem can lead to retinal hemorrhage, seizures, or stroke. Teach the client to recognize its earliest manifestations and summon help immediately because this is a medical emergency. Prevention of distention of the bladder can prevent the occurrence of this emergency. If stool is accumulating in the rectum, it needs to be carefully evacuated to avoid either overdistention or overstimulation.

Medications such as diazoxide (Hyperstat), phenoxybenzamine hydrochloride (Dibenzyline), guanethidine monosulfate (Ismelin), propantheline bromide (Pro-Banthine), phentolamine mesylate (Regitine), and mecamylamine hydrochloride (Inversine) relieve both acute manifestations and the chronic recurrence of episodes.

■ Nursing Management of the Medical Client

The nurse should always be prepared for the development of autonomic dysreflexia. If the client suddenly develops manifestations of severe hypertension (sometimes >300/180 mm Hg), flushing, and a pounding headache, the nurse must act immediately. Nursing interventions involve removing the triggering stimuli, for example, reestablishing urine flow, or removing fecal impaction if necessary. Removal of a fecal impaction should be done only after a topical anesthetic has been inserted into the rectum to avoid further stimulation. In addition, a catheter may be necessary, or if one is already in place, patency of the system must be restored by irrigating or removing kinks and obstructions. Monitor vital signs every 5 minutes and raise the head of the bed to the semi-Fowler position. Administer medications as ordered.

Neurogenic bladders are difficult to control, so you will need to teach many clients with this problem how to stimulate the micturition reflex and maintain urination. Assist the client by providing external pressure on the abdomen, which helps contract the detrusor muscle. Have the client lean forward or try pushing on the abdomen with the hand or arm. Have the client breathe deeply to force the diaphragm downward. In addition, wearing a corset or girdle provides an extra source of external pressure. The Valsalva maneuver is another method of increasing intra-abdominal pressure and therefore pressure on the urinary bladder.

Another method to help the client learn to empty the bladder is the Credé maneuver. The Credé maneuver involves placing the fingers over the bladder and pressing downward slowly toward the symphysis pubis as though "milking" the urine out of the urinary system. The nurse or client should use caution when performing this technique. If the client suffers from sphincter dyssynergia (failure of muscular coordination) or if the sphincter does not readily relax, the Credé manuever can lead to sphincter damage. This maneuver also could result in ureteral reflux if there is any obstruction of outflow. It is often combined with intermittent self-catheterization.

The client can use several other methods to initiate and maintain micturition. Locate trigger points on the body (e.g., lower abdomen, inner thighs, and pubic area) and explain how to stimulate them by stroking, pinching, or applying ice. Stretching the anal sphincter also relaxes the reflexes of the external urethral sphincter because they are both innervated by the pudendal nerve. The client leans forward while sitting on the toilet and inserts two gloved fingers into the anus. The fingers are then either widened apart or pulled posteriorly. The male must be careful to avoid touching the glans penis, which stimulates the bulbocavernosus reflex, contracting the external sphincter.

For the treatment of long- or short-term bladder atony, an intermittent catheterization program is an alternative to long-term indwelling catheterization. This program consists of inserting a straight urethral catheter into the bladder at specified intervals, draining the urine, and removing the catheter. The catheter may be inserted by the client (self-catheterization), by a significant other, or by anyone properly trained. Encourage clients with bladder atony to learn self-catheterization as soon as possible because it increases independence and mobility.

Sterile catheterization technique is necessary in healthcare facilities because of the high risk of nosocomial infections. However, authorities recommend that clean, rather than sterile, technique be used for catheterization outside healthcare facilities. Studies show no increase in the rate of UTIs in comparing clean with sterile technique. Clean technique may also be easier and less expensive for the client. For reducing the risk of bacteriuria, urinary antiseptics and acidification or bladder irrigations with antibiotics and antiseptics are used with each catheterization.

The main procedural differences between clean and sterile technique are the following:

- Gloves are not worn for clean technique; thus, the client must wash the hands thoroughly before starting
- A clean rather than sterile catheter is used
- The catheter is washed and reused indefinitely
- Females may choose not to use a lubricant because the urethra is short and they are less susceptible to traumatic urethritis; they may, however, use one

The catheter should be washed thoroughly after use with soap and water and stored in a plastic sandwich bag or other clean container.

During self-catheterization, the client may sit or stand. When the female stands, she should keep one foot on the floor while placing the other on a chair or toilet seat to help her identify the meatus. The female may use a mirror while learning her anatomy, but ideally she should not become dependent on it.

Timing is the key factor for success in intermittent catheterization programs. Catheterization must be carried out at specified intervals throughout the day until bedtime. A client who is incapable of adhering to this schedule is not an appropriate candidate for the program. The interval between catheterization is set according to the degree of continence. The average interval for adults is every 3 to 4 hours, but the client usually has to start at intervals of 2 to 3 hours. Clients should catheterize so that they get about 350 to 400 ml each time.

There are various opinions concerning the amount of fluid intake allowed. Some programs allow fluid as desired, whereas others restrict fluid intake to varying degrees. This aspect of the program requires systematic investigation. Clinicians generally recommend that the client drink small amounts of fluid at regular intervals (e.g., 250 ml or less within 2 hours for an adult). Ingestion of large amounts of fluid within a short period can cause bladder distention and reflux. Most clients are urged to drink 2 L/day of fluid at regular intervals.

Two main findings indicate the success of an intermittent catheterization program: a catheter-free bladder and absence of symptomatic bacteriuria. As long as the bacteriuria remains asymptomatic, it is not treated with antibiotics. A successful program may be due to several factors, including intermittent bladder distention, which stimulates the normal micturition reflex, and reactivation of the bladder's normal antibacterial properties. Other advantages include continence, independence, good hygiene, prevention of complications arising from urinary stasis or a retention catheter, decreased cost, and ease of sexual relations.

Intermittent catheterization is not a panacea, however. The program requires that the client assume a great deal of personal responsibility. Some clients are not sufficiently motivated to fulfill the responsibilities involved in self-catheterization. Also, some problems can occur when the client is away from home, for instance, at a movie, in a restaurant, or without access to facilities in which the catheterization can be easily performed, as on an airplane.

Clients with high resting pressures in the bladder and who are wet between catheterizations are likely to have difficulty with intermittent self-catheterization. All clients should be evaluated before the initiation of intermittent self-catheterization. If urodynamic evaluation reveals high pressure, anticholinergic medications are administered to lower the resting pressures.

The focus of discharge teaching is self-care. The nurse must teach the client and significant others a bladder training program and, if appropriate, self-catheterization. The nurse needs to assess the client's ability to perform self-care procedures and ensure that the client understands the how, what, why, when, and where of the program. Written materials, teaching videos, and diagrams can be used for teaching and given to the client to reinforce the teaching.

The client needs to be assessed in the home setting to ensure that he or she is able to function there as well as in the hospital. A visiting nurse may be needed to complete the client's education of self-catheterization or bladder training.

The client should have urinary function monitored at regular intervals, including renal function tests and yearly renal ultrasound studies. The client should also be taught to call the healthcare provider if a symptomatic UTI develops.

Modifications for Elderly Clients

Older clients are more likely to have other medical problems such as arthritis and visual difficulties that may interfere with their ability to use the self-catheterization program to control bladder dysfunction. They may still be able to use this method if they have a significant other who can help with the catheterization process. Be careful, however, not to force the older client into a dependent state if this is inappropriate.

Traumatic Disorders

Bladder Trauma

Bladder trauma is defined as a blunt or penetrating injury to the bladder that may or may not cause bladder rupture. Bladder trauma is often related to automobile accidents, when the seat belt compresses the bladder, especially a distended one.

Etiology and Risk Factors

A bladder distended by urine can rupture with a direct blow to the lower abdomen. This injury commonly occurs from wearing a seat belt in an automobile accident. The bladder may also be punctured by bullets, knives, bony splinters from a fractured pelvis, or internal instruments such as a catheter, sound, or cystoscope. Accidents are the greatest risk factor for bladder trauma and, when possible, should be prevented.

Pathophysiology

When the bladder ruptures, whatever the cause, urine spills into the periotoneal cavity and continues to leak while the bladder is not intact. Urine leaking into the periotoneal cavity causes peritonitis or pelvic cellulitis to develop.

Clinical Manifestations and Diagnostic Findings

Bladder injuries usually produce a pain low in the abdomen or pain referred to a shoulder, and hematuria. If the client has a history of an injury or blow to the abdomen, this should arouse suspicion of bladder injury. The client may also demonstrate difficulty voiding (e.g., small amounts of bloody urine or inability to void at all).

Diagnostic tests to assess bladder trauma include an IVP with lateral views or a CT scan with the bladder full and empty, or both; a cystogram; and a voiding cystourethrogram. If blood is coming from the meatus, urethral disruption may be present. In this case, the client should not be catheterized until it is determined whether the urethra is disrupted. This allows assessment of both the intactness of the bladder and the bladder's ability to empty.

Acute and Subacute Care

■ Medical Management

The first treatment for suspected bladder injury is insertion of a Foley or suprapubic catheter to monitor for hematuria or a complete lack of urine and to keep the bladder empty until it has healed. Any injury other than a simple contusion or very small perforation will require surgical repair.

■ Nursing Management of the Medical Client

Assessment of the client with suspected bladder injury is very important. The nurse should closely monitor the client's urine output for both amount and presence of hematuria. The nurse should report any decreased urine output in relation to fluid intake to the physician immediately. Catheter insertion must be done very carefully in the client with suspected bladder trauma, usually by the physician.

■ Surgical Management

Bladder injuries usually require surgical intervention. After a urethral or suprapubic catheter has been inserted, surgical repair of the damaged bladder wall is performed. The extravasated urine in the perivesical is drained. If the pelvis is fractured, this is repaired before the bladder to prevent further injury.

If urinary drainage is not maintained, healing is delayed, and fistulas or leakage may develop.

■ Nursing Management of the Surgical Client

Postoperatively, the nurse must maintain urinary drainage to prevent tension on the sutures in the bladder. A Penrose drain is left in place to allow drainage of any urine remaining in the pelvis, which will necessitate dressing changes.

Because the client may be discharged with an indwelling or suprapubic catheter, it is important that the client and significant others be taught how to care for the catheter. The client's self-care abilities should be assessed for the possible need for assistance at home. If the client or significant others are unable to care for the catheter, a visiting nurse must be arranged.

The client will need to be seen by the physician after discharge for assessment of healing with a cystogram and to have the catheter removed. A suprapubic catheter allows the client to begin to void normally before the catheter is removed. If the client has a urethral catheter, this will have to be removed before the client can begin to void normally. If clients do not void within 8 hours of removal of the catheter, the catheter will not need to be reinserted.

Urethral Trauma

The urethra, as well as the bladder, may be injured in pelvic fractures. Falling astride an object, such as the bar on a boy's bike, with sudden force to the groin may cause urethral contusion and laceration. Injury may occur during medical or surgical interventions or be self-inflicted. Penetrating wounds also cause urethral damage.

Urethral damage is indicated if the client is unable to void, has an altered urine stream, or if blood is visible at the meatus. Even if the client can pass some urine through the urethra, voiding will cause urinary extravasation resulting in swelling of the scrotum or inguinal areas, which can result in sepsis and necrosis. Blood may appear at the external meatus, and blood may also extravasate into the surrounding tissues, giving the area an ecchymotic appearance. The two most common complications of urethral trauma are (1) the development of urethral strictures and (2) the risk of impotence. Impotence occurs because the corpora cavernosa of the penis, blood vessels, or nerves supplying this area are damaged.

Proper management of urethral injuries is controversial. Clinicians generally agree that urinary drainage must first be established with either a urethral or suprapubic catheter; some physicians suggest an immediate primary surgical repair of the urethra, whereas others prefer to wait 2 to 3 weeks to see if the urethra will heal around the urethral catheter without surgery. During any waiting period, the client must be monitored for manifestations of developing infection and continuing extravasation of urine.

Ureteral Trauma

The ureters are located deep within the abdomen and are protected by the spine and surrounding musculature, so ureteral injury from trauma is not common. Most accidental injury to the ureters occurs during surgery. Perforation or tearing may occur during manipulation of intraureteral catheters or other instruments. The ureters may be occluded by ligating sutures or a misplaced clamp or may be transected during pelvic surgery; many surgeons insert ureteral stents before pelvic procedures to easily identify the ureters and thus prevent trauma. Gunshot and stab wounds may also traumatize the ureters; although uncommon, blunt trauma or rapid deceleration, as in a car accident, can tear these structures.

Trauma is frequently not discovered until clinical manifestations develop. Hematuria may be present, but the most common indications are flank pain or manifestations of extravasation of urine. As the urine seeps out into the tissues, pain may develop in the lower abdomen and flank. As extravasation continues, there may be sepsis, paralytic ileus, a palpable intraperitoneal mass, and the appearance of urine in an external wound. An IVP and ultrasound are the most definitive means of diagnosis.

Surgical intervention primarily involves repair of the defect, preferably with end-to-end anastomosis. However, more radical procedures such as cutaneous ureterostomy, transureteroureterostomy, and reimplantation may be necessary. The surgeon may use prostetic ureteral implants. A nephrectomy is performed if obstruction or sepsis has caused severe renal damage. It is essential to treat sepsis aggressively. Significant extravasation of urine may require the surgeon to open the abdomen and drain the urine. However, some physicians believe that such urine will be reabsorbed within sequelae as long as it is sterile.

Congenital Anomalies

Congenital Anomalies of the Bladder

Exstrophy of the bladder is an anomaly that develops when the symphysis pubis fails to close in utero, and it is often associated with epispadias in males. With this condition, the lower anterior abdominal wall and anterior bladder wall are absent. The open bladder protrudes through the abdominal surface. In some children, especially females, the bladder can be reconstructed to a normal anatomic position, although further revision as the child grows may be needed. In males especially, urinary diversion after surgical removal of the bladder is done at an early age. The diversion may require revision as the child grows, and children who had the diversion in the past can have it revised to a continent diversion today. Urinary diversions are discussed earlier in this chapter.

Congenital Anomalies of the Urethra

Urethral anomalies are not common. Those that do occur include absence or atresia of the urethra, urethral stricture, fistulas, and misplacement of the meatus. Misplacement of the meatus (hypospadias and epispadias) is discussed in Chapter 83.

Congenital Anomalies of the Ureters

Ectopic Ureter

Ectopic ureter occurs when a ureter follows an abnormal course or has an abnormal distal opening. It is the most common congenital ureteral anomaly. For example, a retrocaval ureter hooks around the vena cava before it returns to the proper side of the pelvis and enters the bladder appropriately. In women, the ureters may open directly into the urethra or vagina, rather than opening into the bladder. Also, ureteral openings into the bladder may connect to abnormal portions of its wall outside the trigone region. During micturition, this anomaly often results in a backflow of urine. Treating these problems usually requires reimplanting the distal ends of the ureter(s).

Other anomalies include duplicate ureters, abnormal dilation of the ureters, and congenital narrowing of the ureter(s) and the junction of the pelvis of the kidney, which causes obstruction to the flow of urine.

Duplicate Ureters

Duplicate ureters, arising from the same renal pelvis, occur in several variations:

● The ureters on one side may unite at some point along the way
● Both may open in the normal portion of the trigone
● Both may open into the urethra or vagina

This anomaly is not usually recognized unless a radiographic study is done for another reason, the client develops pyelonephritis and the evaluation reveals the anomaly, or urine leakage develops in female infants. Surgical intervention is usually not necessary unless complications develop such as obstruction, infection, and inadequate renal function. Persistent enuresis is a manifestation of ectopic ureter which opens into the urethra or vagina.

Abnormal Dilation of the Ureter (Megaureter)

Abnormal dilation of the ureter (megaureter) is characterized by dilation and pouching of the ureteral wall just adjacent to the vesicoureteral junction. It causes problems because of its refluxing or obstructive effects. Although it may be asymptomatic, the defect can result in flank pain due to backflow pressure on the kidney. The condition predisposes the client to recurrent UTIs.

Congenital Ureteropelvic Obstruction

Congenital ureteropelvic obstruction occurs at the junction of the renal pelvis and the ureter. This anomaly is usually bilateral. A mild obstruction may never cause manifestations of a urinary tract disorder. As long as the kidney produces urine at a rate below 6 ml/minute the ureter can generally handle the flow. However, urine production above this rate causes urinary stasis in the kidney, which results in hydronephrosis. Assessment reveals nausea, vomiting, and abdominal or flank pain in response to fluid back-up, diuretic therapy, or uncontrolled diabetes mellitus. If the condition is symptomatic, treatment is surgical repair of the narrowed section at the ureteropelvic junction.

Conclusions

Urinary system disorders can be extremely problematic for clients, and the nurse can play a major role in the prevention and treatment of these disorders. Many of the disorders of the urinary system are chronic or lead to chronic problems. Some of the problems can drastically alter the client's self-concept and life-style. These problems range from incontinence to urinary diversions. Clients experiencing these problems require a great deal of support from the nurse so that they can adapt to the changes in their lives. Problems also can be life-threatening, and the nurse must help ensure that the client receives prompt treatment.

Thinking Critically

1. A 28-year-old newlywed woman has been experiencing pain and burning with urination for the past 24 hours. This is the third episode of urinary manifestations she has had in the past 3 months. What is the probable cause of the urinary manifestations? What further information do you need to assess her problem? What can you do to help her treat this problem and prevent further difficulties?

Factors to Consider: For what urinary tract problems does the client's status as a newlywed place her at risk? What tests would help differentiate an infectious problem from a noninfectious one?

2. The client had a radical cystectomy with formation of an Indiana pouch 12 hours ago. He has a catheter in place, which has drained 10 ml in the last hour. The stoma is a very pale pink. His vital signs are elevated from their preoperative levels. His pulse rate is 100 BPM, and he has a slightly increased temperature. What actions would be appropriate at this point in the client's care?

Factors to Consider: Is the client's urinary output within expected limits? What color should a fresh stoma normally be?

Bibliography

1. Abel, N. A., & Smith, R. A. (1994). Intrathecal baclofen for treatment of intractable spinal spasticity. *Archives of Physical Medicine and Rehabilitation, 75*(1), 54–58.
2. Adams, M. C., et al. (1992). Conversion of an ileal conduit to a continent catheterizable stoma. *Journal of Urology, 147*(1), 126–128.
3. Ahlering, T. E., et al. (1991). A comparative study of the ileal conduit, Kock pouch and modified Indiana pouch. *Acta Urology Belgica, 59*(2), 303–313.
4. Akaza, H., et al. (1995). Bacillus Calmette-Guérin treatment of existing papillary bladder cancer and carcinoma in situ of the bladder: Four-year results. *Cancer, 75*(2), 552–559.
5. Akerlund, S., et al. (1994). Bacteriuria in patients with a continent ileal reservoir for urinary diversion does not regularly require antibiotic treatment. *British Journal of Urology, 74*(2), 177–181.
6. Alemayehu, H. M., Hornak, M., & Bardos, A. (1994). Chronic ischaemia of the ileal neobladder: Clinical manifestations and management. *International Urology and Nephrology, 26*(4), 443–446.
7. Amling, C. L., et al. (1994). Radical cystectomy for stages T_a, T_{is}

and T$_1$ transitional cell carcinoma of the bladder and discussion. *Journal of Urology, 151*(1), 31–36.

8. Babaian, R. J., & Smith, D. B. (1991). Effect of ileal conduit on patients' activities following radical cystectomy. *Urology, 37*(1), 33–35.

9. Bejany, D. E., & Politano, V. A. (1993). Modified ileocolonic bladder: Five years experience. *Journal of Urology, 149*(6), 1441–1444.

10. Bejany, D. E., & Politano, V. A. (1995). Ileocolic neobladder in the woman with interstitial cystitis and a small contracted bladder. *Journal of Urology, 153*(1), 42–43.

11. Benson, M. C., & Olsson, C. A. (1992). Advanced bladder cancer: Urinary diversion. *Urologic Clinics of North America, 19*(4), 779–795.

12. Bernier, F., & Harris, L. (1995). Treating stress incontinence with the bladder neck support prosthesis. *Urologic Nursing, 15*(1), 5–9.

13. Bernstein, I. T., et al. (1991). Bricker's ileal conduit urinary diversion with a simple non-refluxing uretero ileal anastomosis. *Scandinavian Journal of Urology and Nephrology, 25*(1), 29–33.

14. Bissada, N. K., Marshall, I. Y., & Kaczmarek, A. (1993). Continent urinary diversion and bladder substitution. *Journal of South Carolina Medical Association, 89*(9), 435–438.

15. Bjerre, B. D., Johansen, C., & Steven, K. (1994). Health-related quality of life after urinary diversion: Continent diversion with the Kock pouch compared with ileal conduit. A questionnaire study. *Scandinavian Journal of Urology and Nephrology, 157*(Suppl.), 113–118.

16. Blaivas, J. G. (1990). Diagnostic evaluation of urinary incontinence. *Urology, 36*(Suppl. 4), 11–20.

17. Brink, C. A., et al. (1994). Digital test for pelvic muscle strength in women with urinary incontinence. *Nursing Research, 43*(6), 352–356.

18. Burgers, J. K., et al. (1990). Improved technique for creation of ileal conduit stoma. *Journal of Urology, 44*(5), 1188–1191.

19. Burns, P. B., & Swanson, G. M. (1991). Risk of urinary bladder cancer among blacks and whites: The role of cigarette use and occupation. *Cancer Causes and Control, 2*(6), 371–379.

20. Bushman, W., et al. (1994). Abnormal flow cytometry profiles in patients with interstitial cystitis. *Journal of Urology, 152*(6, Pt. 2), 2262–2266.

21. Bushman, W., Steers, W. D., & Meythaler, J. M. (1993). Voiding dysfunction in patients with spastic paraplegia: Urodynamic evaluation and response to continuous intrathecal baclofen. *Neurourology and Urodynamics, 12*(2), 163–170.

22. Cammu, H., & Van Nylen, M. (1995). Pelvic floor exercises: Five years later. *Urology, 45*(1), 113–118.

23. Childs, S. J. (1994). Dimethyl sulfone (DMSO) in the treatment of interstitial cystitis. *Urologic Clinics of North America, 21*(1), 85–88.

24. Choi, B. C., Connolly, H. G., & Zhou, R. H. (1995). Application of urinary mutagen testing to detect workplace hazardous exposure and bladder cancer. *Mutation Research, 341*(3), 207–216.

25. Choi, B. C., & Nethercott, J. R. (1991). A proportionate mortality study on risk of bladder cancer among rubber workers. *Cancer Detection and Prevention, 15*(5), 403–406.

26. Chyou, P. H., Nomura, A. M. Y., & Stemmermann, G. N. (1992). A prospective study of the attributable risk of cancer due to cigarette smoking. *American Journal of Public Health, 82*(1), 37–40.

27. Costello, A. J., & Bowsher, W. G. (1992). Radiotherapy as a treatment for bladder cancer. *Australia and New Zealand Journal of Surgery, 62*(1), 81–83.

28. Decter, R. M., Snyder, P., & Laudermilch, C. (1994). Transurethral electrical bladder stimulation: A follow-up report. *Journal of Urology, 152*(2, Pt. 2), 812–814.

29. Devesa, S. S., Grauman, D. J., & Blot, W. J. (1994). Recent cancer patterns among men and women in the United States: Clues for occupational research. *Journal of Occupational Medicine, 36*(4), 832–841.

30. Diamond, D. A., & Ransley, P. G. (1994). Improved glanuloplasty in epispadias repair: Technical aspects. *Journal of Urology, 152*(4), 1243–1245.

31. Dressnandt, J., Auer, C., & Conrad, B. (1995). Influence of baclofen upon the alpha-motoneuron in spasticity by means of F-wave analysis. *Muscle and Nerve, 18*(1), 103–107.

32. Duns, J., et al. (1994). Organ-sparing treatment of advanced bladder cancer: A 10-year experience. *International Journal of Radiation Oncology and Biology and Physics, 30*(2), 261–166.

33. Erickson, D. R., Simon, L. J., & Belchis, D. A. (1994). Relationships between bladder inflammation and other clinical features in interstitial cystitis. *Urology, 44*(5), 655–659.

34. Eure, G. R., et al. (1992). Bacillus Calmette-Guérin therapy for high risk stage T1 superficial bladder cancer. *Journal of Urology, 147*(2), 376–379.

35. Fall, M., & Lindrsröm, S. (1994). Transcutaneous electrical nerve stimulation in classic and nonulcer interstitial cystitis. *Urologic Clinics of North America, 21*(1), 131–140.

36. Faro, S. (1992). New considerations in treatment of urinary tract infections in adults. *Urology, 39*(1), 1–11.

37. Felsen, D., et al. (1991). Inflammatory mediators and interstitial cystitis. *Seminars in Urology, 9*(2), 102–107.

38. Fisch, M., et al. (1994). Ileocecal valve reconstruction during continent urinary diversion. *Journal of Urology, 151*(4), 861–865.

39. Fleischmann, J. (1994). Calcium channel antagonists in the treatment of interstitial cystitis. *Urologic Clinics of North America, 21*(1), 107–111.

40. Freeman, J. A., et al. (1994). Management of the patient with bladder cancer: Urethral recurrence. *Urologic Clinics of North America, 21*(4), 645–651.

41. Frye, K. (1993). Understanding interstitial cystitis. *Journal of Urological Nursing, 12*(1), 367–371.

42. Ghoneim, M. A., et al. (1992). Further experience with the urethral Kock pouch. *Journal of Urology, 147*(2), 361–365.

43. Gianino, J. (1993). Intrathecal baclofen for spinal spasticity: Implications for nursing practice. *Journal of Neuroscience Nursing, 25*(4), 254–264.

44. Gowing-Farhat, C. (1994). The Florida pouch. *Urologic Nursing, 14*(1), 1–5.

45. Grace-Louthen, C. L. (1993). Commentary on treating bladder cancer. *ONS Nursing Scan in Oncology, 2*(5), 19.

46. Hampton, B. G., & Bryant, R. A. (1992). *Ostomies and continent diversions: Nursing management.* St. Louis: Mosby–Year Book.

47. Hanno, P. M. (1994). Amitriptyline in the treatment of interstitial cystitis. *Urologic Clinics of North America, 21*(1), 89–91.

48. Hanno, P. M. (1994). Diagnosis of interstitial cystitis. *Urologic Clinics of North America, 21*(1), 63–66.

49. Hanno, P. M., & Wein, A. J. (1991). Conservative therapy of interstitial cystitis. *Seminars in Urology, 9*(2), 143–147.

50. Hasan, S. T., Marshall, C., & Neal, D. E. (1994). Continent urinary diversion using the Mitrofanoff principle. *British Journal of Urology, 74*(4), 454–459.

51. Hautmann, R. E., et al. (1993). The ileal neobladder: 6 years of experience with more than 200 patients. *Journal of Urology, 150*(1), 40–45.

52. Herbert, J. R., & Miller, D. R. (1994). A cross-national investigation of diet and bladder cancer. *European Journal of Cancer, 30A*(6), 778–784.

53. Hermann, G. G., et al. (1992). Recombinant interleukin-2 and lymphokine-activated killer cell treatment of advanced bladder cancer: Clinical results and immunological effects. *Cancer Research, 52*(3), 726–733.

54. Herzog, A. R., & Fultz, N. H. (1990). Epidemiology of urinary incontinence: Prevalence, incidence, and correlates in community populations. *Urology, 36*(Suppl. 4), 2–10.

55. Hooton, T. M., et al. (1991). Single-dose and three-day regimens of ofloxacin versus trimethoprim-sulfamethoxazole for acute cystitis in women. *Antimicrobial Agents and Chemotherapy, 35*(7), 1479–1483.

56. Hossan, E., & Striegel, A. (1993). Carcinoma of the bladder. *Seminars in Oncology Nursing, 9*(4), 252–266.

57. Howard, J., et al. (1992). A collaborative study of differences in the survival rates of black patients and white patients with cancer. *Cancer, 69,* 2349–2360.

58. Irwin, P. P., & Galloway, N. T. (1994). Surgical management of interstitial cystitis. *Urologic Clinics of North America, 21*(1), 145–151.

59. Iwakiri, J., et al. (1993). Functional and urodynamic characteristics of an ileal neobladder. *Journal of Urology, 149*(5), 1072–1076.

60. Jeter, K., Faller, N., & Norton, C. (1990). *Nursing for continence.* Philadelphia: W. B. Saunders.

61. Johnson, D. E., Swanson, D. A., & von Eschenbach, A. C. (1992). Tumors of the genitourinary tract. In E. A. Tanagho & J. W. McAninich (Eds.), *Smith's general urology* (13th ed.). Norwalk, CT: Appleton & Lange.

62. Jolleys, J. V. (1991). Factors associated with regular episodes of dysuria among women in one rural general practice. *British Journal of General Practice, 41*(347), 241–243.

63. Karlowicz, K. A. (Ed.). (1995). *Urologic nursing: Principles and practice.* Philadelphia: W. B. Saunders.

64. Keller, M. L., McCarthy, D. O., & Neider, R. S. (1994). Measurement of symptoms of interstitial cystitis: A pilot study. *Urologic Clinics of North America, 21*(1), 67–71.

65. Klein, E. A. (1992). Options in the surgical treatment of bladder cancer. *Journal of ET Nursing, 19*(4), 122–125.

66. Koziol, J. A. (1994). Epidemiology of interstitial cystitis. *Urologic Clinics of North America, 21*(1), 7–20.

67. Krieger, J. N. (1990). Urinary tract infections in women: Causes, classification, and differential diagnosis. *Urology, 35*(Suppl. 1), 4–7.

68. Kuroda, M., et al. (1994). Adjuvant and neoadjuvant chemotherapy for invasive bladder cancer. *Cancer Chemotherapeutic Pharmacology, 35*(Suppl.), S9–13.

69. Lampel, A., et al. (1995). In situ tunneled Bower flap tubes: 2 new techniques of a continent outlet for main pouch cutaneous diversion. *Journal of Urology, 153*(2), 308–315.

70. Landau, E. H., et al. (1994). The sensitivity of pressure specific bladder volume versus total bladder capacity as a measure of bladder storage dysfunction. *Journal of Urology, 152*(5, Pt. 1), 1578–1581.

71. Leaver, R. B. (1994). The Mitrofanoff pouch: A continent urinary diversion. *Journal of Professional Nursing, 9*(11), 748–753.

72. Lynch, C. F., & Cohen, M. B. (1995). Urinary system. *Cancer, 75*(1 Suppl. 1), 316–329.

73. Malloy, T. R., & Shanberg, A. M. (1994). Laser therapy for interstitial cystitis. *Urologic Clinics of North America, 21*(1), 141–144.

74. Mark, S. D., & Webster, G. D. (1995). Simplified urinary drainage following orthotopic or continent bladder replacement. *Journal of Urology, 153*(2), 334–335.

75. Matsui, U., et al. (1993). Metabolic long-term follow-up of the ileal neobladder. *European Journal of Urology, 24*(2), 197–200.

76. Matsuura, T., et al. (1991). Assessment of the long-term results of ileocecal conduit urinary diversion. *Urology International, 46*(2), 154–158.

77. McDougall, E. M., et al. (1995). Laporascopic retropubic auto-augmentation of the bladder. *Journal of Urology, 153*(1), 123–126.

78. Meek, D. (1994). BCG in bladder cancer. *Nursing Times, 90*(43), 34–35.

79. Mizutani, Y., et al. (1992). Effects of bacille Calmette-Guérin on cytotoxic activities of peripheral blood lymphocytes against human T24 lined and freshly isolated autologous urinary bladder transitional carcinoma cells in patients with urinary bladder cancer. *Cancer, 69*(2), 537–545.

80. Montie, J. E. (1994). Follow-up after cystectomy for carcinoma of the bladder. *Urologic Clinics of North America, 21*(4), 639–643.

81. Moore, S., et al. (1993). Treating bladder cancer: New methods, new management. *American Journal of Nursing, 93*(5), 32–41.

82. Navon, J. D., Weinberg, A. C., & Ahlering, T. E. (1994). Continent urinary diversion using a Modified Indiana Pouch in elderly patients. *American Surgeon, 60*(10), 786–788.

83. Nordstrom, G. M., & Nyman, C. R. (1991). Living with a urostomy: A follow up with special regard to the peristomal-skin complications, psychosocial and sexual life. *Scandinavian Journal of Urology and Nephrology 138* (Suppl.) 247–251.

84. Nurse, D. E., et al. (1991). Problems in the surgical treatment of interstitial cystitis. *British Journal of Urology, 68*(2), 153–154.

85. O'Grady, H. M., et al. (1994). An early detection assay for occupational bladder cancer. *Proceedings of the Annual Meeting of the American Association of Cancer Research, 35*, A3136.

86. Oliver, J. R., et al. (1991). Correction of incontinent ileocolic urostomy with Kock's nipple valve. *Gynecologic Oncology, 43*(2), 178–181.

87. Parsons, C. L., et al. (1994). Treatment of interstitial cystitis with intravesical heparin. *British Journal of Urology, 73*(5), 504–507.

88. Perry, J. J., & Muss, H. B. (1994). Management of disseminated disease in the patient with bladder cancer. *Urologic Clinics of North America, 21*(4), 661–672.

89. Pow-Sang, J. M., et al. (1992). Conversion from external appliance wearing or internal urinary diversion to a continent urinary reservoir (Florida pouch I and II): Surgical technique, indications and complications. *Journal of Urology, 147*(2), 356–360.

90. Ratliff, T. L., Klutke, C. G., & McDougall, E. M. (1994). The etiology of interstitial cystitis. *Urologic Clinics of North America, 21*(1), 21–30.

91. Ratner, V., Slade, D., & Greene, G. (1994). Interstitial cystitis: A patient's perspective. *Urologic Clinics of North America, 21*(1), 1–5.

92. Razor, B. R. (1993). Continent urinary reservoirs. *Seminars in Oncology Nursing, 9*(4), 272–285.

93. Richmond, J. (1994). The tyranny of interstitial cystitis. *Nursing Times, 90*(43), 72.

94. Rink, R. C., Adams, M. C., & Keating, M. A. (1994). The flip-flap technique to lengthen the urethra (Salle procedure) for treatment of neurogenic urinary incontinence. *Journal of Urology, 152*(2, P. 2), 799–802.

95. Rowland, R. G., & Kroop, B. P. (1994). Evolution of the Indiana continent urinary reservoir. *Journal of Urology, 152* (6, Pt. 2), 2247–2251.

96. Ruder, A. M., Ward, E. M., & Brown, D. P. (1994). Cancer mortality in female and male dry-cleaning workers. *Journal of Occupational Medicine, 36*(8), 867–874.

97. Ruggieri, M. R., et al. (1994). Current findings and future research avenues in the study of interstitial cystitis. *Urologic Clinics of North America, 21*(1), 163–176.

98. Salle, J. L., et al. (1994). Urethral lengthening with anterior bladder wall flap for urinary incontinence: A new approach. *Journal of Urology, 152*(2, Pt. 2), 803–806.

99. Samodai, L., et al. (1991). The efficacy of intravesical BCG in the treatment of patients with high risk superficial bladder cancer. *International Urology and Nephrology, 23*(6), 559–567.

100. Sant, G. R., & LaRock, D. R. (1994). Standard intravesical therapies for interstitial cystitis. *Urologic Clinics of North America, 21*(1), 73–83.

101. Sant, G. R., & Theoharides, T. C. (1994). The role of the mast cell in interstitial cystitis. *Urologic Clinics of North America, 21*(1), 41–53.

102. Scher, H. I. (1995). Neoadjuvant chemotherapy for invasive bladder cancer: Prognostic factors for survival of patients treated with M-VAC with 5 year follow-up. *Journal of Urology, 153*(2), 545–546.

103. Schurch, B., Yasuda, Y., & Rossier, A. B. (1994). Detrusor bladderneck dyssynergia revisited. *Journal of Urology, 152*(6, Pt. 1), 2066–2070.

104. Seidman, A. D., & Scher, H. I. (1991). The evolving role of chemotherapy for muscle infiltrating bladder cancer. *Seminars in Oncology, 18*(6), 585–595.

105. Seidmon, E. J., & Hannon, P. M. (1994). *Current urologic therapy* (Vol. 3). Philadelphia: W. B. Saunders.

106. Seshadri, P., Emerson, L., & Morales, A. (1994). Cimetidine in the treatment of interstitial cystitis. *Urology, 44*(4), 614–615.

107. Silverman, D. T., et al. (1992). Epidemiology of bladder cancer. *Hematologic/Oncology Clinics of North America, 6*(1), 1–30.

108. Spinelli, J. J., et al. (1991). Mortality and cancer incidence in aluminum reduction plant workers. *Journal of Occupational Medicine, 33*(11), 1150–1155.

109. Stein, R., et al. (1994). The fate of the adult exstrophy patient. *Journal of Urology, 152*(5, Pt. 1), 1413–1416.

110. Stone, A. R., et al. (1991). Role of the immune system in interstitial cystitis. *Seminars in Urology, 9*(2), 108–114.

111. Stone, N. N. (1994). Nalmefene in the treatment of interstitial cystitis. *Urologic Clinics of North America, 21*(1), 101–106.

112. Takeda, M., et al. (1994). Correlation of upper and lower urinary tract function in patients with neurogenic bladder: Evaluation using simultaneous measurement of cystometry and diuresis renography with full and empty bladder. *Neurology and Urodynamics, 13*(3), 243–253.

113. Terai, A., et al. (1995). Effect of urinary intestinal diversion on urinary risk factors for urolithiasis. *Journal of Urology, 153*(1), 37–41.

114. Theoharides, T. C. (1994). Hydroxyzine in the treatment of inter- stitial cystitis. *Urologic Clinics of North America, 21*(1), 113–119.

115. Trifillis, A. L., et al. (1995). Culture of bladder epithelium from cystoscopic biopsies of patients with interstitial cystitis. *Journal of Urology, 153*(1), 243–248.

116. Trump, D. L. (1994). Retinoids in bladder, testis, and prostate cancer. *Leukemia, 8*(Suppl. 3), S50–54.

117. Urinary Incontinence Guideline Panel. (1992). *Urinary inconti- nence in adults: A patient's guide.* AHCPR Publications No. 92- 0040. Rockville, MD: Agency for Health Care Policy and Re- search, Public Health Service, U.S. Department of Health and Human Services.

118. Urinary Incontinence Guideline Panel. (1992). *Urinary inconti- nence in adults: Clinical practice guideline.* AHCPR Publications No. 92-0038. Rockville, MD: Agency for Health Care Policy and Research, Public Health Service, U.S. Department of Health and Human Services.

119. Urinary Incontinence Guideline Panel. (1992) *Urinary incontinence in adults: Quick reference guide for clinicians.* AHCPR Publications No. 92-0041. Rockville, MD: Agency for Health Care Policy and Research, Public Health Service, U.S. Department of Health and Human Services.

120. Warren, J. W. (1994). Interstitial cystitis as an infectious disease. *Urologic Clinics of North America, 21*(1), 31–40.

121. Warren, J. W. (1994). Is interstitial cystitis an infectious disease? *Medical Hypotheses, 43*(3), 183–186.

122. Waxman, J., & Wasan, H. (1994). Platinum-based chemotherapy for bladder cancer. *Seminars in Oncology, 21*(5 Suppl. 12), 54–60.

123. Webster, D. C. (1990). Comparing patients' and nurses' views of interstitial cystitis: A pilot study. *Urologic Nursing,* 10–13.

124. Webster, D. C. (1993). Reframing women's health. Tension and paradox in framing interstitial cystitis. *Journal of Women's Health, 2*(1), 81–84.

125. Webster, D. C., & Brennan, T. (1994). Use and effectiveness of physical self-care strategies for interstitial cystitis. *Nurse Practi- tioner, 19*(10), 55–61.

126. Wein, A. J., & Broderick, G. A. (1994). Interstitial cystitis. Cur- rent and future approaches to diagnosis and treatment. *Urologic Clinics of North America, 21*(1), 153–161.

127. Whitmore, K. E. (1994). Self-care regimens for patients with inter- stitial cystitis. *Urologic Clinics of North America, 21*(1), 121–130.

128. Wilson, T. G., et al. (1994). Late complications of the modified Indiana pouch. *Journal of Urology, 151*(2), 331–334.

129. Wishnow, K. I., et al. (1992). Stage B (P2/3A/N0) transitional cell carcinoma of bladder highly curable by radical cystectomy. *Urol- ogy, 39*(1), 12–16.

130. Woodhouse, C. R. (1994). The sexual and reproductive conse- quences of congenital genitourinary anomalies. *Journal of Urol- ogy, 152*(2, Pt. 2), 645–651.

131. Woodhouse, C. R., & MacNeily, A. E. (1994). The Mitrofanoff principle: Expanding on a versatile technique. *British Journal of Urology, 74*(4), 447–453.

132. Zeidman, E. J., et al. (1994). Bacillus Calmette-Guérin immuno- therapy for refractory interstitial cystitis. *Urology, 43*(1), 121–124.

Nursing Care of Clients with Renal Disorders

Esther Matassarin-Jacobs

By producing urine, the kidneys regulate the body's fluid, electrolyte, and acid-base balances while removing toxic substances from the blood. The kidneys play a significant role in erythropoietin and prostaglandin synthesis, in insulin degradation, and in the renin-angiotensin-aldosterone system.

This chapter identifies the common disease processes and injuries that interfere with normal renal function. Although the effects of extrarenal influences on the kidneys are briefly described, the primary purpose of this chapter is to discuss specific renal pathologic processes. Because of the potential seriousness of any renal problem, the client and significant others will have physical as well as psychological needs. Nurses should know about both aspects and be constantly aware of the need for appropriate intervention.

Renal Disorders Associated with Extrarenal Conditions and Nephrotoxins

Many conditions primarily located in other parts of the body affect the kidneys. Examples of these include sepsis, hypertension, and diabetes mellitus. Description of the renal implications of these conditions is brief here. For further discussion, see Chapters 15, 22, 45, and 69.

Extrarenal Conditions

Diabetes Mellitus

One of the most common extrarenal diseases affecting the kidney is diabetes mellitus. Diabetic nephropathy, a pro-

gressive process, frequently leads to renal failure. Approximately 30% of clients with end-stage renal disease have diabetes mellitus. Researchers estimate that 25% to 50% of clients with insulin-dependent diabetes mellitus (IDDM or type I) will develop end-stage renal disease within 10 to 20 years of beginning insulin therapy. Renal disease can also develop in the non–insulin-dependent diabetic client. The incidence of proteinuria is about 25% after 20 years of diabetes.[8]

Several pathologic changes lead to renal failure in clients with diabetes mellitus. The most frequent is a characteristic intercapillary glomerulosclerosis, or scarring of the capillary loops. Progressive microangiopathy, nephrosclerosis, affects the afferent and efferent arterioles and eventually causes scarring of the glomerulus, tubules, and interstitium. Pyelonephritis, kidney infection, may cause scarring and subsequent ischemia in the renal parenchyma. It may also lead to renal papillary necrosis and sloughing of the papillae. Neurogenic bladder dysfunction may contribute to renal failure. The high incidence of urinary tract infection or the increased pressure in the kidney caused by the back-up of urine may be the cause.

Initially, the sclerotic, or hardening, process of glomerulosclerosis increases renal vascular resistance, contributing to systemic hypertension. This does not cause renal insufficiency. Indeed, the glomerular filtration rate (GFR) may increase as much as 20% to 50% above the GFR of normal persons during this early, or "silent," phase. It is now recognized that microalbuminemia (measurable by assay) occurs quite some time before clinical proteinuria. If diagnosed, this may be a much earlier harbinger of eventual renal failure. As more nephrons are destroyed, available functioning renal tissue decreases, and the client begins to demonstrate clinical proteinuria (a key sign), hypertension, edema, and manifestations of renal failure.

The kidney metabolizes 30% to 40% of insulin, so as renal function diminishes, the degradation of insulin also decreases, which results in a lower insulin requirement for the client. Renal failure may be initially identified when the client is undergoing evaluation for recurrent

This chapter incorporates material written for the fourth edition by Evelyn Butera.

insulin reactions. Researchers hope the sclerotic process can be slowed by (1) carefully controlling hypertension, (2) appropriately adjusting insulin therapy, and (3) restricting dietary protein. However, the client inevitably develops renal failure within 5 to 10 years after the appearance of significant proteinuria, regardless of diabetic control.

Hypertension

Because the kidneys receive such a large share of the cardiac output, renal function can affect or be affected by alterations within the cardiovascular system. The renal blood flow determines the GFR, which directly affects renal function. Hypertension is one condition that can either cause or be affected by renal disease. For example, renovascular hypertension results from renal artery stenosis or renal infarction, a condition that activates the renin-angiotensin-aldosterone system and increases systemic blood pressure. Renal hypertension arising from parenchymal renal disease (e.g., glomerulonephritis, polycystic disease, pyelonephritis) usually results from the kidney's decreasing ability to excrete salt and water. Other causes include increased renin release due to increased glomerular perfusion and inadequacy of renal vasodilating substances, as occurs with analgesic nephropathy. Whereas renovascular hypertension accounts for up to 15% of all systemic hypertension, in renal failure clients 80% to 85% of hypertension is a result of excess salt and water retention.[8]

On the other hand, sustained systemic high blood pressure adversely affects the kidneys. Researchers estimate that microscopically evident nephrosclerosis is present in clients with uncontrolled hypertension for more than 5 years, although all other renal diagnostic tests may be normal. This kidney damage is the direct result of degenerative changes in the arterioles and interlobular arteries caused by increased blood pressure. There is a direct correlation between the duration and degree of elevated blood pressure and the severity of renal vascular disease. However, progression of the disease frequently can be halted or slowed by bringing the hypertension under control. This means that client teaching is vital to controlling the hypertension and preventing renal failure.

Hypotension

Cardiovascular shock, or hypotension, also affects renal function. Renal vasoconstriction reduces renal blood flow. However, because of the autoregulation capabilities of the kidneys (see Chapter 54), GFR remains at a functional level until the advanced stages of systemic shock, at which time acute renal failure develops. Restoring the systemic blood pressure usually reverses the renal vasoconstriction, and kidney function returns, generally within 2 to 8 weeks as long as ischemia has not occurred. A period of polyuria may follow the correction of hypovolemia, although the mechanisms for this are unclear. Before renal function returns to normal, another oliguric period may occur, followed by a "mobilization phase" that shifts sequestered fluid into the intravascular space. This may cause some hypertension until the kidneys can remove the extra fluid. Careful assessment of the client's fluid status and meticulous fluid management are crucial during these recovery phases.

Cardiovascular Disease

Cardiac disease influences kidney function primarily through its effect on cardiac output and circulating blood volume. The hemodynamic and hormonal changes of cardiac disease may decrease the kidneys' ability to excrete sodium and water. This, in turn, increases intravascular congestion and edema and establishes a pathologic cycle.

Hemodynamic changes also occur with normal aging. Blood flow to the kidneys decreases by up to 50% by 70 years of age, and GFR decreases by up to 40% to 50%. Renal function deteriorates as glomeruli become sclerotic and atrophy.

Peripheral Vascular Disease

Thromboembolic disease can affect the renal circulation and cause infarction of the tissue supplied by the affected blood vessel. The interstitial hypertonicity and low oxygen pressure found in the renal medulla seem to favor sickling of red blood cells in the kidney's juxtamedullary region in persons with sickle cell disease. These cell masses cause gross hematuria as venules rupture; papillary necrosis; renal infarction; concentrating disturbances due to interference with the "countercurrent mechanism"; nephrotic syndrome; pyelonephritis; and, finally, renal failure. The kidney is the organ most affected in disseminated intravascular coagulation, in which diffuse clotting consumes clotting factors and causes hemorrhage in affected areas throughout the body.

Sepsis

Extrarenal sepsis may affect kidney function either through its effect on the systemic circulation or through its stimulation of the immune system. Renal reactions to septic shock are similar to those described under Hypotension. Immunologic injury leading to glomerulonephritis is described later. Occasionally, pathogens may break away from extrarenal foci of infection and travel to the kidney to establish additional sites.

Pregnancy

Pregnancy has a definite influence on kidney function. Collecting system dilation and kidney enlargement begin during the first trimester of pregnancy and may persist 9 to 12 weeks after delivery. Renal blood flow and GFR increase by 30% to 50% during pregnancy, contributing to increased creatinine clearance and decreased uric acid excretion. These normal changes must be taken into account when laboratory findings are interpreted in pregnant women. Pregnancy also increases the likelihood of proteinuria (usually transient), polyuria, and nocturia. These disorders are possibly caused by external bladder compression and alterations in antidiuretic hormone metabolism.[8]

Other Causes

Many other extrarenal disease processes influence kidney function. These include neoplastic disease, connective tissue disorders, and metabolic disturbances.

Nephrotoxins

Nephrotoxins are substances that have specific, destructive effects on renal cells. They can cause the following five types of renal injury:

1. Acute tubular necrosis
2. Defects in the tubular transport system
3. Interstitial nephritis
4. Vasculitis
5. Nephrotic syndrome

Nephrotoxic substances found in the environment include heavy metals, such as mercurial compounds, lead, cadmium, bismuth, arsenic, copper, and phosphorus; carbon tetrachloride; ethylene glycol; trichloroethylene; carbon monoxide; and chlorinated hydrocarbons. Exposure to many of these substances occurs in industrial locations. Other environmental nephrotoxins include snake venom and certain mushrooms. Their most frequent renal result is acute tubular necrosis. Some also cause tubular transport defects and nephrotic syndrome. Box 57–1 shows some of the common nephrotoxic agents.

All five types of kidney damage may result from nephrotoxic reactions to medications (see Box 57–1). The two most common medications causing renal damage are antibiotics and certain analgesics. Because the kidneys are the major route of excretion for many antibiotics, renal tissue is directly exposed to these compounds. The longer the exposure, the higher the risk of renal toxic effects. Pre-existing renal disease, decreased renal blood flow, electrolyte imbalances, and concurrent use of other nephrotoxic medications enhance a medication's nephrotoxic effect. High-risk antibiotics include cephalosporins, sulfonamides, polymyxins, aminoglycosides, and amphotericin B. Careful monitoring of renal function tests identifies early nephrotoxic reactions so causative medications can be discontinued or the dose decreased. Besides using these medications as briefly as possible, maintaining a high fluid intake and carefully maintaining only a therapeutic blood level may prevent nephrotoxic effects. A high urine output keeps the medication dilute within the kidney and helps prevent any crystallization of the compound.

The risk of renal damage from excessive use of certain analgesics has received more attention in recent years. Salicylates, acetaminophen, phenacetin, and nonsteroidal anti-inflammatory drugs are the most common causative agents. Short-term overdose or long-term consistent use of these medications may cause acute tubular necrosis or chronic renal failure. Researchers estimate that between 5% and 10% of all clients with end-stage renal disease have analgesic nephropathy.

Anesthesia reduces the kidney's vasoconstrictive ability, which helps protect it against systemic blood pressure drops; thus, the kidney is made more vulnerable to the effects of shock. In addition, certain anesthetics, particularly methoxyflurane, have a direct nephrotoxic effect. Administering this general anesthetic can cause acute tubular necrosis and has been associated with fatal acute renal failure. Halothane may also adversely affect renal function. Higher serum concentrations of sodium thiopental have been found in clients with renal disease than in clients with normal kidney function who receive an equal dose.

Other common medications that may have nephrotoxic effects include aggressive use of diuretics that cause hypovolemia, probenecid, phenytoin, low-molecular-weight dextran, rifampin, phenindione, lithium, and gold therapy. Nurses must know the possible adverse effects of any medication a client takes so proper assessments and intervention may be initiated.

Radioiodinated contrast agents used in radiographic and computed tomographic (CT) studies have been associated with acute tubular necrosis. Risk factors include being over 60 years old; pre-existing renal insufficiency, especially diabetic nephropathy; dehydration; low cardiac output with pre-existing renal disease; proteinuria; hypoalbuminemia; multiple myeloma; and multiple contrast studies within a 24-hour period. Using nondye studies whenever possible and keeping the client well hydrated throughout the test reduce the incidence of acute renal failure. Baseline renal function tests before the contrast study should be available to compare with post-test findings. Monitor urine output carefully for several hours after the study is completed.

Box 57–1. Nephrotoxins

Antibiotics	Anesthetics
Aminoglycosides	**Contrast Dyes**
Tetracyclines	
Amphotericin B	**Organic Solvents**
Cephalosporins	
Sulfonamides	Glycols
(co-trimoxazole)	Gasoline
Bacitracin	Kerosene
Polymyxin	Turpentine
Colistin	Tetrachloroethylene
Heavy Metals	**Other Drugs**
Lead	Acetaminophen
Mercury	Nonsteroidal anti-
Arsenic	inflammatory medications
Copper	Salicylates
Gold	Heroin
Lithium	Dextran
	Mannitol
Poisons	Interleukin-2
	Cisplatin
Mushrooms	Amphetamines
Insecticides	
Herbicides	
Snake bites	

Acquired Disorders

Pyelonephritis

Pyelonephritis is an inflammation of the renal pelvis and the parenchyma caused by a bacterial infection. This may be from an active infection in the kidney or the remnants of a previous infection. There are two main types of pyelonephritis: acute and chronic. They differ, primarily, in their clinical picture and long-term effects.

Etiology and Risk Factors

Sometimes an infection may be a primary disease, as happens with calculus, malignancy, hydronephrosis, or trauma that has reduced host resistance. However, most kidney infections appear to be extensions of infectious processes located elsewhere; the bladder is the most common site. Chapter 56 discusses the etiology and pathogenesis of infections in the lower urinary tract. The bacteria spread to the kidney primarily by traveling up (ascending) the ureter to the kidney. Blood and lymphatic circulation also provide channels for the organisms. Ureteral reflux, which allows infected urine back into the ureter, and obstruction, which causes urine to back into the ureter and allows organisms to multiply, are the most common causes of ascending urinary tract infections. *Escherichia coli* is the most common bacterial organism causing pyelonephritis.

Acute Pyelonephritis. Acute pyelonephritis often occurs after bacterial contamination of the urethra or after instrumentation such as catheterization or cystoscopy.

Chronic Pyelonephritis. Chronic pyelonephritis is more likely to occur after chronic obstruction with reflux or chronic disorders. It is a slowly progressive disease that is usually associated with recurrent acute attacks, although there may be no history of acute pyelonephritis.

Pathophysiology

Pyelonephritis occurs when bacteria enter the renal pelvis, causing an inflammatory response and an increase in white blood cells. The inflammation leads to edema and swelling of the involved tissue, beginning at the papillae and sometimes spreading to the cortex. The infection can be either ascending, that is, following cystitis or prostatitis, or descending, from the bloodstream, as with streptococcal infections.

As the infection is treated and the inflammation recedes, fibrosis and scar tissue may develop. The calices become blunted with scarring in the interstitial tissues. If the infections recur, more and more scar tissue develops; fibrosis and altered tubular reabsorption and secretion lead to decreased renal function.

Acute Pyelonephritis. Acute pyelonephritis is associated with the development of renal abscesses, perineph-

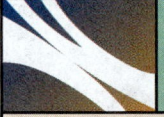

RISK FACTORS AND LEVELS OF PREVENTION

Pyelonephritis

Risk Factors

Diabetes mellitus, hypertension, chronic renal calculi, chronic cystitis, structural abnormalities of the urinary tract, presence of urinary stones, indwelling or frequent catheterization (mechanical drainage)

Levels of Prevention

Primary Prevention

● Teach clients how to prevent the primary condition, such as calculi or infection.
● Control hypertension and diabetes.
● Avoid catheterization and mechanical drainage whenever possible.
● Prevent stone formation.

Secondary Prevention

● Screen for renal problems in high-risk clients.
● Ensure that clients take a complete course of antibiotics to treat cystitis.
● Teach high-risk clients the manifestations of the development of pyelonephritis.

Tertiary Prevention

● Encourage high fluid intake.
● Encourage clients to maintain their prescribed diets.
● Encourage clients to keep their diabetes and hypertension under good control.

ric abscesses, emphysematous pyelonephritis, and chronic pyelonephritis that can lead to renal failure.

The course of acute pyelonephritis is usually short. However, it often recurs, either as a relapse of a previous infection not eradicated or as a new infection; 20% of these recurrences take place within 2 weeks of completion of therapy.[38] A client must be treated adequately to prevent the development of chronic pyelonephritis. The infection may also progress to bacteremia.

Chronic Pyelonephritis. This disease is characterized by a combination of caliceal abnormalities and overlying cortical scarring. The kidney becomes contracted, and the number of functioning nephrons decreases as they are replaced by scar tissue. Renal failure may ensue, although the development of uremia is less frequent than is commonly thought.

Clinical Manifestations and Diagnostic Findings

Acute Pyelonephritis. Acute pyelonephritis is characterized by enlarged kidneys, focal parenchymal abscess formation, and accumulation of polymorphonuclear lymphocytes around and within the renal tubules. It may cause minimal manifestations or may be asymptomatic. Typically, however, the client seems in acute distress and appears intoxicated.

Assessment reveals high fever, chills, nausea, flank pain on the affected side (costovertebral angle [CVA] tenderness), headache, muscular pain, and general prostration. The pain often radiates down the ureter or toward the epigastrium and may be colicky if the infection is complicated by calculi or sloughed renal papillae. Percussion or deep palpation over the costovertebral angle elicits marked tenderness. Frequently the client has experienced dysuria, frequency, urgency, and other manifestations of cystitis for several days. The urine may be cloudy or bloody, is foul-smelling, and demonstrates a marked increase in white blood cell casts and white blood cells.

Urine culture and sensitivity studies are the primary diagnostic tests with a physical examination. Studies may be done for calculi, especially with recurrent infections, because calculi may seed and cause reinfection, particularly with *Proteus*. X-ray studies, such as of the kidney, ureter, and bladder (KUB), and intravenous pyelography (IVP) are also done. A cystourethrogram is often done, especially after an initial episode of pyelonephritis, to look for underlying defects, particularly any cause of reflux. Magnetic resonance imaging (MRI) or CT scan may also be used to evaluate the kidney size or the presence of other problems.

Chronic Pyelonephritis. This disease has no specific manifestations of its own. Thus, it is frequently diagnosed incidentally when the client is being evaluated for hypertension or its complications. Hypertension itself is the most frequent manifestation of the disease.

Abnormal laboratory studies may show azotemia, pyuria, anemia, acidosis, and proteinuria. They may also demonstrate a poor urine-concentrating ability.

Community and Self-Care

■ Medical Management

Acute Pyelonephritis. Intervention aims at (1) eliminating the pathogenic organisms with appropriate antibiotics as identified by urine culture and sensitivity study and (2) removing any component contributing to decreased host resistance. If calculi are found during the work-up for the cause of recurrent infection, appropriate treatment is instituted.

Chronic Pyelonephritis. Medical management focuses on preventing further renal damage. If bacteria are found, appropriate antibiotics are given, as in acute pyelonephritis. Above all, hypertension must be controlled. Additional intervention depends on the degree of renal failure that has already occurred.

Antibiotics, specific to the bacteria present, are given to treat pyelonephritis (see Table 56–1). Although they may be administered orally or by use of the single large-dose method described in Chapter 56, the usual method involves parenteral antibiotics for 3 to 5 days until the client has been afebrile for 24 to 48 hours; oral administration follows for 2 to 4 weeks. The client must understand that prolonged antibiotic therapy suppresses recurrent infections, so completing therapy is of vital importance. Additional pharmacologic therapy may be needed to correct any predisposing factors.

■ Nursing Management of the Medical Client

Assessment

Assessment of the client with pyelonephritis begins with a thorough history and physical examination, with close attention paid to the presence of risk factors, recurrent UTIs, hypertension, and CVA tenderness. Look for the presence of the manifestations of pyelonephritis.

Diagnosis, Planning, Implementation

Risk for Fluid Volume Deficit. A common diagnosis is *Risk for Fluid Volume Deficit related to fever, nausea, vomiting, and possible diarrhea.*

Planning: Expected Outcomes. The client will not develop fluid volume deficit, as evidenced by balanced intake and output, maintenance of adequate hydration, and no manifestations of dehydration.

Implementation. Prepare the client for the diagnostic tests and probable antibiotic therapy. Clients with severe nausea and vomiting may require intravenous fluids. Overhydration may dilute antimicrobials, diminishing the effectiveness of these drugs. See Chapter 56 for specific information on the nursing care of the client with cystitis.

Pain. Another common diagnosis is *Pain related to an inflammatory process in the kidney and possible colic.*

Planning: Expected Outcomes. The client will have no pain or have pain controlled, as evidenced by saying so.

Implementation. Medications can be given to control the pain caused by calculi that may have precipitated the problem. The CVA tenderness should decrease as the antibiotics control the infection. Medication for nausea can be given as needed with antipyretics for high fevers. Adequate treatment of the infection quickly reverses the dysuria, pyuria, and frequency. Urinary analgesics described in Chapter 56 can also help the client with these problems.

Knowledge Deficit. Client teaching is important here. Write the diagnosis *Knowledge Deficit related to prevention of recurrent infections.*

Planning: Expected Outcomes. The client will understand how to prevent recurrent infections, as evidenced by the client's statements and no recurrence of infection.

Implementation. The preventive measures for acute and chronic pyelonephritis are similar to those for cystitis (see Chapter 56). It is important to prevent permanent renal damage. Make sure that the client understands the manifestations of a urinary tract infection. Teach the client to seek prompt medical attention when manifestations of a urinary tract infection occur.

When the acute infection subsides, instruct the client to continue to follow-up care. This includes completing the full course of antibiotic therapy and repeating urine cultures. Also, teach ways of preventing further infections in the urinary tract (see Chapter 56).

It is vital that the client return for follow-up urine cultures and possibly for other diagnostic tests if the cause of the pyelonephritis is not clear. The client needs to understand the importance of follow-up cultures because bacteriuria may be present but asymptomatic. The client must also be told to report any manifestations of recurrence immediately so re-treatment can be initiated.

Evaluation

The infections should subside with adequate antibiotic treatment for 14 days or more. The client must also be made aware of the cause of this infection and ways to prevent further infections (see Chapter 56).

■ Modification for Elderly Clients

The major difference for older clients is that their kidneys may be less able to recover from a severe infection. Antibiotic therapy should be monitored closely, because the older adult's sensitivity and response to the medication may vary. Older adults may also have altered blood levels of antibiotics because perfusion changes with age.

Acute Glomerulonephritis

Glomerulonephritis is a term that encompasses a variety of diseases, most of which are caused by an immunologic reaction that, in turn, results in proliferative and inflammatory changes within the glomerular structure.

Two forms of glomerulonephritis are included in the category of acute glomerulonephritis: postinfectious glomerulonephritis and infectious glomerulonephritis. Of the two, postinfectious glomerulonephritis, also called acute poststreptococcal glomerulonephritis, is the more common.

Etiology and Risk Factors

Box 57–2 presents a classification system based on etiology. Classically, the causative factor is a beta-hemolytic streptococcal infection elsewhere in the body, although other organisms may be responsible. Typically, it occurs about 21 days after a respiratory or skin infection.

Postinfectious glomerulonephritis is primarily a disease of children, 95% of whom recover fully. It does, how-

---

Box 57–2. Classification of Glomerulonephritis Based on Etiology

Primary Glomerulonephritis—Immune Response to Pathogens

■ Acute glomerulonephritis
■ Postinfectious glomerulonephritis
■ Group A beta-hemolytic streptococcus
■ Other infectious conditions such as cytomegalovirus infection, measles, mumps, staphylococcus or pneumococcal bacteremia
■ Infectious glomerulonephritis
■ Membranoproliferative glomerulonephritis
■ Rapidly progressive glomerulonephritis
■ Idiopathic membranous glomerulonephritis
■ IgA nephropathy
■ Chronic glomerulonephritis
■ Lipoid nephrosis
■ Focal glomerular sclerosis

Secondary Glomerulonephritis—Related to Systemic Disease

■ Goodpasture's syndrome
■ Hemolytic-uremic syndrome
■ Henoch-Schönlein purpura
■ Polyarteritis
■ Progressive systemic sclerosis
■ Systemic lupus erythematosus
■ Wegener's granulomatosis
■ Thrombocytopenic purpura
■ Postpartum renal failure

---

ever, sometimes occur in adults. Approximately 30% of adults with this disease progress to chronic renal failure.

Infectious glomerulonephritis is also associated with bacterial, viral, or parasitic infections elsewhere in the body. It differs from postinfectious glomerulonephritis in that it occurs during or within a few days of the original infectious process.

There are no specific risk factors for this disorder because it is actually an immunologic disorder that occurs in response to either endogenous (those already in the body) or exogenous (those associated with infections) antigens.

Pathophysiology

Glomerulonephritis is an immunologic disorder that results in inflammatory and proliferative changes within the glomerulus. Because the primary function of the glomerulus is to filter blood, most cases of glomerulonephritis result from trapping of circulating antigen-antibody complexes, produced from an infection elsewhere in the body, within the glomerulus. This causes inflammatory damage and impedes glomerular function, reducing the glomerular membrane's capacity for selective permeability. The source of the antigens may be either exogenous (e.g., poststreptococcal infection) or endogenous (e.g., systemic lupus erythematosus). Evidence also indicates that some antigen-antibody complexes may form in situ within the kidney.

In addition to this immune complex nephritis, glomerulonephritis may also be produced by the fixing of antibodies to the glomerular basement membrane. An example of this is Goodpasture's syndrome, which involves pulmonary hemorrhage and glomerulonephritis.

The primary pathologic process of glomerulonephritis, lipoid nephrosis, and focal glomerular sclerosis is proliferation and inflammation. However, lipoid nephrosis and focal glomerular sclerosis are characterized by degeneration.

Acute glomerulonephritis can become a fulminant process, proceeding quickly to uremia or to chronic glomerulonephritis. However, most clients start to recover within 14 days. Most clinical manifestations return to normal within several weeks, although the hematuria and proteinuria may be present for longer periods. If complete recovery does not occur within 2 years, it probably will not occur at all. Some use the term "subacute glomerulonephritis" to designate disease that lasts more than 6 to 8 weeks. Although most of the manifestations of the acute disease have disappeared, the client is still very susceptible to exacerbation of glomerulonephritis. The term "latent glomerulonephritis" refers to an asymptomatic condition characterized by the presence of significant albumin and cast levels in the urine for more than 1 year after the acute onset. These findings indicate continued but slow parenchymal changes.

Clinical Manifestations and Diagnostic Findings

The development of acute glomerulonephritis may be insidious or sudden. Classic manifestations of sudden onset include hematuria with red blood cell casts and proteinuria. Fever, chills, weakness, pallor, anorexia, nausea, and vomiting may be present. Generalized edema, particularly facial and periorbital swelling, is a typical finding. The client may have ascites, pleural effusion, and congestive heart failure.

The client frequently has headache and moderate to severe hypertension. Visual acuity may be reduced because of retinal edema. Abdominal or flank pain, probably caused by kidney edema and distention of the renal capsule, may be present. Oliguria, and even anuria, may be present for several days; the longer this persists, the more irreversible the kidney damage.

In contrast, the disease may be so mild that the client reports vague weakness, anorexia, and lethargy.

Diagnosis is usually based on the presence of an underlying infection and an elevated antistreptolysin O titer. The disease, however, may even be discovered on the basis of a routine urinalysis.

Examining the urine usually provides the information necessary for a definitive diagnosis of acute glomerulonephritis. Gross hematuria and proteinuria are the cardinal findings. The urine, which may be scanty in amount, is typically dark, smoky or cola-colored, or red-brown in hue. The proteinuria produces a persistent and excessive foam. There is a low pH and a specific gravity in the

mid- to high-normal range due to the kidneys' decreased ability to concentrate.

There are other studies that assist in the diagnosis. Serum urea nitrogen and creatinine levels will be elevated, and creatinine clearance rates will be down. C-reactive proteins and antistreptolysin O titer are usually elevated, and the serum complement level is low. Hematocrit and hemoglobin studies indicate anemia.

Acute and Subacute Care

■ Medical Management

Medical intervention aims to eliminate antigens, to alter the client's immune balance, and to inhibit or alleviate the inflammation for prevention of further renal damage and improvement of kidney function. Although some clients may require initial hospitalization, most treatment will occur on an outpatient basis.

Plasmapheresis may be used in some research protocols for certain types of glomerulonephritis, including rapidly progressive glomerulonephritis. This intervention is used in conjunction with immunosuppressive therapy. This technique is designed to remove the specific circulating antibody or mediators of the inflammatory response. Large volumes of the client's plasma are cyclically removed and replaced with fresh frozen plasma by use of a continuous-flow blood cell separator.

Antibiotic therapy (e.g., penicillin for streptococcal organisms) is used to treat the predisposing infections as well as prophylactically post streptococcal infections. Volume overload and hypertension are treated with diuretics, antihypertensives, and restriction of dietary sodium and water. Corticosteroids and immunosuppressive agents (e.g., azathioprine and cyclophosphamide) may be used.

Common complications are congestive heart failure with pulmonary edema, and increased intracranial pressure. Renal failure may develop. Appropriate monitoring, including vital signs, intake and output, and weight, is essential. Recognizing complications early facilitates prompt medical intervention.

■ Nursing Management of the Medical Client

Assessment

A comprehensive history should be taken from the client with suspected glomerulonephritis about recent upper respiratory tract (such as strep throat), skin infections, or a history of glomerulonephritis. The client should also be questioned about systemic disorders that might be present, such as lupus. Any recent invasive procedures should also be noted.

Physical examination may reveal ascites, pleural effusion, and manifestations of congestive heart failure with pulmonary edema. The urine should be closely examined for color, amount, and presence of any abnormal substances. The vital signs should be closely checked, especially blood pressure.

Diagnosis, Planning, Implementation

Altered Nutrition: Less than Body Requirements. If the client has diminished appetite or aversion to food, write the diagnosis *Altered Nutrition: Less than Body Requirements related to anorexia and increased metabolic demands.*

Planning: Expected Outcomes. The client will maintain adequate nutritional intake, as evidenced by no weight loss, absence of a negative nitrogen balance, and normal electrolytes.

Implementation. It is important to protect the kidneys while they are recovering their function. The diet prescribed by the physician is generally high calorie and low protein. This diet avoids protein catabolism and allows the kidney to rest because it handles fewer protein molecules and metabolites. The degree to which protein is restricted depends on the amount excreted in the urine and the client's individual requirements. Sodium is also restricted, depending on the amount of edema present. Anorexia, nausea, and vomiting may interfere with adequate intake, requiring creative intervention on the part of the nurse. A dietitian can help plan the client's diet around these restrictions.

Fluid Volume Excess. A common diagnosis in glomerulonephritis is *Fluid Volume Excess related to reduced urine output.*

Planning: Expected Outcomes. The client will maintain balanced intake and output, as evidenced by no manifestations of edema or fluid overload.

Implementation. Appropriate fluid balance is important. Careful monitoring of daily weight and intake and output helps determine the progress of the edema and thus provides an estimate of renal function. Daily measuring of edematous parts (e.g., legs and abdomen) also provides useful, objective data. The client's allowable fluid intake is based on the intake and output measurements. Fluid intake is usually restricted. Thirst may be relieved by sucking on hard candies, lemon slices, or by using ice chips rather than a glass of water. Assist the client to "plan" fluid distribution during the day (e.g., with meals).

Fatigue. Another common diagnosis is *Fatigue related to increased metabolic demands from disease.*

Planning: Expected Outcomes. The client will obtain an adequate balance of rest and activity, as evidenced by absence of complaints of fatigue.

Implementation. Rest is essential—both physical and emotional. As mentioned, there is a direct correlation between activity and the amount of hematuria and proteinuria. Exercise also increases catabolic activity. The allowable amount of activity depends on the results of serial urinalyses. Bedrest, followed by a period of very limited activity, may continue for several weeks to months. Therefore, the client may need assistance in arranging personal matters, such as family, home, job, finances, and community responsibilities. Encourage the client to talk about any fears or concerns and, if necessary, help the client deal with the emotional reactions expected during a long-term illness with a questionable prognosis. Only after handling these problems will the client be able to rest emotionally. Appropriate diversionary activities may help the client cope with prolonged physical immobility.

Risk for Impaired Skin Integrity. A typical diagnosis is *Risk for Impaired Skin Integrity related to edema.*

Planning: Expected Outcomes. The client will not develop skin breakdown, as evidenced by continued intact skin.

Implementation. Edema interferes with cellular nutrition, which makes the client more susceptible to skin breakdown. Take precautions to prevent this complication. Interventions include good hygiene, massage, and position changes, as well as the use of other prophylactic measures, such as mattress devices. Use research-based tools to assess the client's risk of breakdown.

Risk for Infection. Another diagnosis following immunosuppressive therapy is *Risk for Infection related to altered immune response secondary to treatment.*

Planning: Expected Outcomes. The client will not develop an infection, as evidenced by normal temperature.

Implementation. Glomerulonephritis markedly diminishes a client's natural defenses to infection, especially to streptococcal organisms. Moreover, immunosuppressives and corticosteroids further reduce host resistance. Although isolation is not necessary, take care to protect the client from people with obvious infectious processes. General supportive measures help boost the client's defense mechanisms. Client teaching should involve appropriate ways to avoid infections, especially respiratory and urinary tract infections.

Evaluation

The client must be able to understand his or her condition, and the reasons for limited activity, and dietary and fluid restrictions. It is important that the client comply with all postinfection treatments so that recurrence does not develop. The client's learning needs will depend on the amount of renal damage done by the disease. If it is minimal, the client will need to be told to avoid infections and avoid kidney stressors.

■ Modifications for Elderly Clients

The older client is at greater risk of renal damage because of the pre-existing effects of age on the kidneys. The older client is also more likely to have concurrent chronic diseases such as hypertension and diabetes that may have affected the kidneys. Treatment is the same, however.

Chronic Glomerulonephritis

Chronic glomerulonephritis is a heterogeneous category of diseases with varying causes. All the previously described forms of glomerulonephritis can progress to a chronic state. Sometimes, glomerulonephritis is first seen as a chronic process.

As the glomeruli and tubules are destroyed by the pathologic process, the kidneys shrink and become severely contracted. Fibrous and scar tissue replaces functioning renal tissue. Sclerosis of renal blood vessels also occurs. The destruction rates vary.

The disease has an insidious onset. In fact, many years may pass before findings of renal insufficiency or renal failure appear. Common manifestations include malaise; weight loss; edema; increasing irritability and mental cloudiness; metallic taste in the mouth; polyuria and nocturia due to the kidney's inability to concentrate urine; headache; dizziness; and digestive disturbances. As the disease progresses, these manifestations intensify, and the client may experience respiratory difficulty and angina.

The cardinal manifestation of this disease is hypertension. It is not uncommon for the client to experience complications such as nosebleed, manifestations of arteriosclerosis, cardiomegaly, and hemorrhage into the kidneys, lungs, retina, or cerebrum. Edema increases as heart failure becomes more severe and the serum albumin decreases. Examination of the eyegrounds shows vascular changes and edema of the discs. Urinalysis shows a fixed specific gravity, small amounts of proteinuria except during exacerbation, casts, white blood cells, renal tubular cells, and consistent hematuria. Anemia tends to be severe.

Chronic glomerulonephritis progresses over an extended period, often as long as 30 years. When it progresses to end-stage renal failure, dialytic therapy must be instituted or the client will die.

Medical treatment involves dialysis, transplant, and control of the accompanying manifestations. Chemotherapy with anti-inflammatory agents and anticoagulants may be used. Controlling edema and hypertension with diet and reduced fluid intake is imperative.

Nursing interventions focus on the need for consistent monitoring, symptomatic relief, education of the client about the disease and its management, and helping the client and significant others cope with a long-term illness.

Tubulointerstitial Disease

Traditionally, the term "interstitial nephritis" has been used to designate a category of renal disease characterized by the presence of inflammatory cells in the spaces between the renal tubules. However, not all disease processes included in this classification are inflammatory. Therefore, the term *tubulointerstitial disease* is being advocated as the label for this category of renal disorders.

Tubulointerstitial diseases are commonly classified as either acute or chronic. The acute form usually represents an allergic reaction and has a rapid onset. Assessment findings typically are the result of tubular injury. Manifestations often include fever, skin rash, eosinophilia, oliguric renal failure, and occasionally gross hematuria. The disease may progress along any of three courses: (1) complete recovery, (2) rapid progression to renal failure

and death, or (3) movement to the chronic form. Although corticosteroids are frequently used, their value is unclear. Treatment is similar to that for acute renal failure.

In chronic tubulointerstitial disease, there is progressive interstitial fibrosis and usually chronic inflammatory cell infiltration with tubular atrophy. In the terminal stages, the altered renal vasculature and renal structure make the disease indistinguishable from chronic pyelonephritis.

The morphologic findings in tubulointerstitial disease include interstitial edema, cellular infiltration of the interstitium, tubular cellular atrophy and flattening, and interstitial fibrosis. As the disease progresses, renal involvement extends beyond the tubules to progressive fibrosis of Bowman's capsule with secondary involvement of the glomeruli.

Potential causes of this pathologic process are many: acute pyelonephritis; septicemia; analgesic abuse, especially with phenacetin, aspirin, and acetaminophen; immunologic mechanisms, for example, renal allograft, systemic lupus erythematosus, and Sjögren's syndrome; heavy metal toxicity; drug toxicity; hypercalcemia; and hypocalcemia.

Additionally, several medication hypersensitivities may contribute, for example, rifampin, penicillin and its analogs, sulfonamides, cephalosporins, allopurinol, captopril, cimetidine, azathioprine, phenytoin, thiazide, lithium, nonsteroidal anti-inflammatory agents, and possibly furosemide.

An early sign of tubulointerstitial disease is a sudden, unexplained decrease in renal function that may be mild to severe. Specifically, there is an inability to concentrate urine, salt wasting, and poor acidification of the urine leading to metabolic acidosis. Finding a variety of urine sediment abnormalities is common, too. Because they are not effectively reabsorbed in the tubules, glucose, uric acid, phosphates, amino acids, and bicarbonate will appear in the urine. Severe bicarbonaturia is an indicator of renal tubular acidosis. Proteinuria is less severe than with other renal disease. Systemic hypertension is a common finding.

Membranoproliferative Glomerulonephritis

As with acute glomerulonephritis, membranoproliferative glomerulonephritis is most common in children and young adults. Although it may be preceded by a streptococcal infection, more frequently the antigen is not identified. Its indications generally are nephrotic syndrome, microscopic or gross hematuria, and proteinuria. Although remissions may occur, they tend to be short-lived; the general course of the disease is a gradual progressive chronic renal failure.

Medical treatment so far has been disappointing. Renal transplants have been performed, but the disease almost always recurs. Chronic renal dialysis therapy is necessary. Nursing interventions are a combination of those for acute and chronic glomerulonephritis.

Rapidly Progressive Glomerulonephritis

Rapidly progressive glomerulonephritis is a fulminant variation of the disease. Its stimulus may be a streptococcus, staphylococcus, pneumococcus, virus, or collagen disease—or something thus far unidentified. More frequent among men, it strikes at any age but has a peak incidence between the ages of 40 and 60 years. It often begins insidiously and, without effective intervention, relentlessly progresses to renal failure and death within a period of weeks to months.

Initial manifestations include hematuria, edema, hypertension, nausea, vomiting, abdominal pain, diarrhea, proteinuria, oliguria or anuria, and acidosis. On morphologic examination, this condition is a diffuse proliferative inflammation that encircles the glomerulus, encroaches on Bowman's capsule, and apparently compresses the glomerular tufts.

Intravenous methylprednisone has been successful in treating some clients. Immunosuppression and anticoagulant therapy have also been used with inconsistent results. Nursing interventions are similar to those for other forms of glomerulonephritis.

Idiopathic Membranous Glomerulonephritis

Idiopathic membranous glomerulonephritis is primarily a disorder of adults; peak onset is between the ages of 40 and 70 years. Immunologic challenge is less frequent than with other types, and the antigen source may not be known. Most clients present with asymptomatic proteinuria or nephrotic syndrome, and at least half of them have impaired renal function when the disease is first identified through renal biopsy. The prognosis for these clients is mixed: approximately 25% experience spontaneous remission, 25% have a persistent nephrotic syndrome, 25% have persistent proteinuria, and 25% progress to renal failure despite all treatment. Later stages of this disease become indistinguishable from chronic glomerulonephritis.

IgA Nephropathy

IgA nephropathy, also called Berger's disease, was first described in 1968. It is a focal proliferative process occurring most frequently in children and young adults. There is still much to learn about this disease. Originally, it was believed to be relatively benign because of its seemingly nonprogressive nature. However, evidence suggests it may be chronic; approximately 25% of clients demonstrate deteriorating renal function. The effectiveness of various treatments is still being studied.

Lipoid Nephrosis

Lipoid nephrosis, also called minimal change glomerulonephritis, is similar to the forms of glomerulonephritis described previously except that instead of proliferative and inflammatory changes, the pathologic change is degenerative. Although it can occur at any age, it is primarily a childhood disease and is the most common cause of nephrotic syndrome in children.

Its main morphologic finding is marked lipid accumulation in the proximal tubules and large numbers of fat bodies excreted in the urine. Overall, this disease has a good prognosis, especially when corticosteroids are given. There is, however, a tendency for spontaneous remission and repeated relapses. More information can be found in a pediatric nursing text.

Focal Glomerular Sclerosis

Some authorities believe that focal glomerular sclerosis is a form of lipoid nephrosis, whereas others consider it a separate entity. Although it is primarily a disease of young children, its incidence in adults peaks between the ages of 30 and 50 years.

Histopathologic features include segmental or glial sclerosis. The initial clinical presentation shows nephrotic syndrome or persistent proteinuria. Adults commonly demonstrate hypertension and renal insufficiency.

The prognosis of this disease is poor, although the rate of deterioration varies widely. Complete remissions are rare. Steroids and immunosuppressive agents have been used, but with disappointing results. Renal transplants have been successful temporarily, but the original disease almost invariably recurs. Therefore, the client may require chronic renal dialysis therapy.

Nephrotic Syndrome

The nephrotic syndrome is a set of clinical manifestations arising from protein wasting secondary to diffuse glomerular damage. Because of the multiple causes of this syndrome, it is a frequent sequela of both renal disorders and systemic diseases such as diabetes and lupus.

Etiology and Risk Factors

The causes of nephrotic syndrome are numerous; the most common is glomerulonephritis or some systemic disorder such as diabetes mellitus, lupus erythematosus, amyloidosis, hepatitis B, syphilis, carcinoma, leukemia, infectious disease, or preeclampsia. Other predisposing factors include allergic reactions; medication and drug reactions, for example, penicillamine, anticonvulsants, probenecid, captopril, gold salts, heroin, and nonsteroidal anti-inflammatory medications; renal vein thrombosis; sickle cell disease; and congestive heart failure. Primary prevention, other than avoidance of medications that predispose to the condition, is limited.

Pathophysiology

The pathophysiologic mechanism of this disorder is the abnormal permeability of the glomerular basement membrane to protein molecules, particularly albumin. These proteins are excessively filtered into the tubules and excreted into the urine. The resultant hypoalbuminemia alters the oncotic pressure within the vascular tree, and fluid moves into the interstitial spaces, initiating the development of edema. This stimulates plasma renin activity and augments aldosterone production so the kidney retains sodium and water, thus adding to the accumulation of extracellular fluid.

Potential complications include the effects of extracellular fluid accumulation and the progressive development of renal failure. The client may also experience severe hypovolemia, thromboembolism, secondary aldosteronism, abnormal thyroid function, and increased susceptibility to infections. Osteomalacia may also occur.

Clinical Manifestations and Diagnostic Findings

On the basis of this pathophysiologic mechanism, the clinical picture of nephrotic syndrome presents a classic constellation: proteinuria, hypoalbuminemia, and edema. Hyperlipidemia is usually found and is thought to result from increased hepatic lipoprotein synthesis in response to decreased serum albumin. Depending on the degree of renal failure, some level of normocytic anemia is common. Edema is usually the client's chief problem. Although its onset may be insidious, it becomes massive, and complications of the swelling may be seen. The skin frequently has a characteristic waxy pallor due to the edema rather than to the anemia. Other manifestations include anorexia, malaise, irritability, and amenorrhea or abnormal menses. The amount of proteinuria may account for losses of 4 to 30 g/day. Serum albumin concentrations may drop as low as 1.0 to 2.5 g/dl. The urine typically contains granular and epithelial cell casts and fat bodies. Some hematuria may be present. High amounts of protein are found in the urine.

Community and Self-Care

■ Medical Management

The primary aim of medical treatment is to heal the leaking glomerular basement membrane and to stop loss of protein in the urine. The cycle of edema would then be broken. Much of the intervention concentrates on decreasing the client's edema.

Unless the client is hyponatremic, fluids are not usually restricted. The client's fluid balance should, however, be carefully monitored via daily weights, girth measurements, and intake and output determinations. These data are important because weight loss may represent true tissue loss from protein rather than from lost fluid.

Pharmacologic Management

Steroids are successful with some clients, depending on the cause of their disease. Cytotoxic agents such as cyclo-

phosphamide and chlorambucil, indomethacin, anticoagulants, and antiplatelet agents may be used.

Loop diuretics, such as furosemide, are typically included in the medication regimen. Plasma volume expanders, such as albumin, plasma, and dextran, may be administered to raise the oncotic pressure within the vascular tree. This pulls fluid from the extracellular spaces, making it available for kidney filtration. Diuresis in elderly clients must be handled with particular caution because of their reduced capability to tolerate sudden shifts in intravascular volume.

There is a significant incidence of renal vein thrombosis among clients with nephrotic syndrome. Because of this, some clients are placed on long-term anticoagulation. The client needs to know how to monitor for possible hemorrhage and should be encouraged to carry identification describing medications being taken.

Dietary Management

Although some physicians recommend a diet containing a normal level of protein with good biologic value, others prescribe a diet of high-biologic-value protein with adequate carbohydrate and calorie intake. A daily protein intake of 1.0 to 1.5 g/kg/day with over 35 kcal/kg/day for prevention of further protein breakdown is generally recommended.[16] It is important to continually assess the amount of protein being lost in the urine to maintain a better balance.

Because the kidneys have a reduced capacity to excrete sodium, mild sodium restriction is usually instituted. The level and duration of salt restriction are controversial issues. Because the client must take in the necessary protein and calories, the diet needs to be as palatable as possible. Potassium may also be restricted as serum potassium rises.

■ Nursing Management of the Medical Client

Nursing interventions are designed to help the client maintain health, manage the edema, cope with long-term illness, and learn about the disease and its treatment.

In addition to helping the client comply with the medication regimen, nursing interventions assist the client to achieve and maintain maximal health. Much of this is accomplished through presenting learning materials to the client and significant others. For example, teach the client that the amount of exercise allowed is based, at least in part, on the severity of the edema. Bedrest is imposed only during severe edema, and as the fluid level moves toward normal, the client is allowed more activity. Other important areas of teaching include nutrition, prevention of infection, and methods of careful self-assessment.

Because edema interferes with cellular nutrition, skin care is vital. During acute stages, the client and significant others may need help dealing with the accompanying malaise, anorexia, and depression. Also assess for manifestations of electrolyte imbalance associated with aggressive diuresis required for the client with central edema, especially sodium and potassium loss.

Hydronephrosis

Hydronephrosis is the distention of the renal pelvis and calices by an obstruction of normal urine flow. Urine production continues, and the urine is trapped proximal to the obstruction. The cause of the occlusion includes calculus, tumor, scar tissue, or a kink in the ureter.

Whatever the cause, the accumulating urine exerts pressure on the renal pelvis wall. At low to moderate pressures, the kidney may dilate with no obvious loss of function. Over time, sustained or intermittent high pressure causes irreversible nephron destruction. In addition to the pressure-related problems, pyelonephritis is always a risk because of urinary stasis.

Medical treatment aims to relieve the obstruction permanently and prevent infection. After the obstruction is relieved, postobstructive diuresis occurs, possibly leading to fluid and electrolyte imbalances, including dehydration. Removal of the obstruction results in a sudden release of the pressure on the renal parenchyma caused by the trapped urine, which leads to diuresis. The kidney will gradually begin to concentrate urine appropriately. Diuresis can, however, lead to fluid depletion if it continues.

Potential fluid volume deficit related to increased urine output is the most important nursing problem. Because of the dangers involved in postobstruction diuresis, it is crucial to monitor the client closely after an obstruction is released. Make frequent assessments, including hourly outputs; daily weights; vital signs every 30 minutes for the first 4 hours and then every 2 hours; urine for specific gravity, albumin, and glucose; and edema. Make periodic serum electrolyte and glucose determinations as well. Consider the expected presence of severe fatigue caused by urinary losses and the need for frequent observation. Fluid management during this period is crucial; hourly fluid replacement is based on the previous hour's output.

Uremic Syndrome

Uremia literally means "urine in the blood." This term and the term *uremic syndrome* describe a set of manifestations that result from loss of renal function. This loss may be sudden or may develop over a long period. It may be self-limiting or irreversible. Sudden loss of kidney function, as occurs in damage from trauma, shock, toxins, or acute glomerulonephritis, brings on uremia rapidly and usually causes a severe deterioration of the client's condition. Gradual loss of kidney function over an extended period may occur with glomerulonephritis, hypertension, chronic pyelonephritis, and other diseases.

Because the kidneys perform a wide variety of functions, the effects of uremia occur not only within the kidneys themselves but also within other organ systems. Because of the time factor, chronic renal failure produces more degenerative changes in the body than does acute uremia. However, both types have many of the same consequences, and unless the process can be halted, coma, convulsions, and death result.

Acute Renal Failure

Acute renal failure (ARF) refers to the abrupt loss of kidney function. Over a period of hours to a few days, the GFR falls, accompanied by concomitant rise in serum creatinine and urea nitrogen. A healthy adult eating a normal diet needs a minimum daily urine output of approximately 400 ml to excrete the body's waste products through the kidneys. An amount lower than this indicates a decreased GFR. Oliguria refers to daily outputs of urine between 100 and 400 ml; anuria refers to outputs less than 100 ml.

Etiology and Risk Factors

The incidence of ARF will depend on the underlying cause. The most common causes of ARF are hypotension and prerenal hypovolemia. The numerous causes of ARF can be categorized into three major areas: (1) prerenal, (2) renal, and (3) postrenal (Fig. 57–1).

■ Prerenal Causes

Prerenal causes interfere with renal perfusion. The kidneys depend on an adequate delivery of blood to be filtered by the glomeruli. Therefore, a reduced renal blood flow obviously lowers the GFR. Conditions that contribute to decreased renal blood flow include the following:

- Circulatory volume depletion, as may occur with diarrhea, vomiting, hemorrhage, excessive use of diuretics, burns, renal salt-wasting conditions, and glycosuria
- Volume shifts (for example, third-space sequestration of fluid, vasodilation, and gram-negative sepsis)
- Decreased cardiac output, as during cardiac pump failure, pericardial tamponade, and acute pulmonary embolism
- Decreased peripheral vascular resistance (for example, spinal anesthesia, septic shock, and anaphylaxis)
- Vascular obstruction (for example, bilateral renal artery occlusion or dissecting aneurysm)

■ Renal Causes

Renal causes refer to parenchymal changes from disease or nephrotoxic substances. Acute tubular necrosis is the most frequent renal cause of ARF, accounting for approximately 75% of cases.[3] This destruction of the tubular epithelial cells is the result of impaired renal perfusion or direct damage from nephrotoxins. In addition to the nephrotoxins described previously, acute tubular necrosis may also be caused by the presence of heme pigments, such as myoglobin and hemoglobin, which are liberated from damaged muscle tissue. This release may result from trauma (rhabdomyolysis) such as surgery, crush injury, and electric shock, or from nontraumatic conditions such as severe muscle exertion, genetic conditions (e.g., diabetes mellitus and malignant hyperthermia), infectious

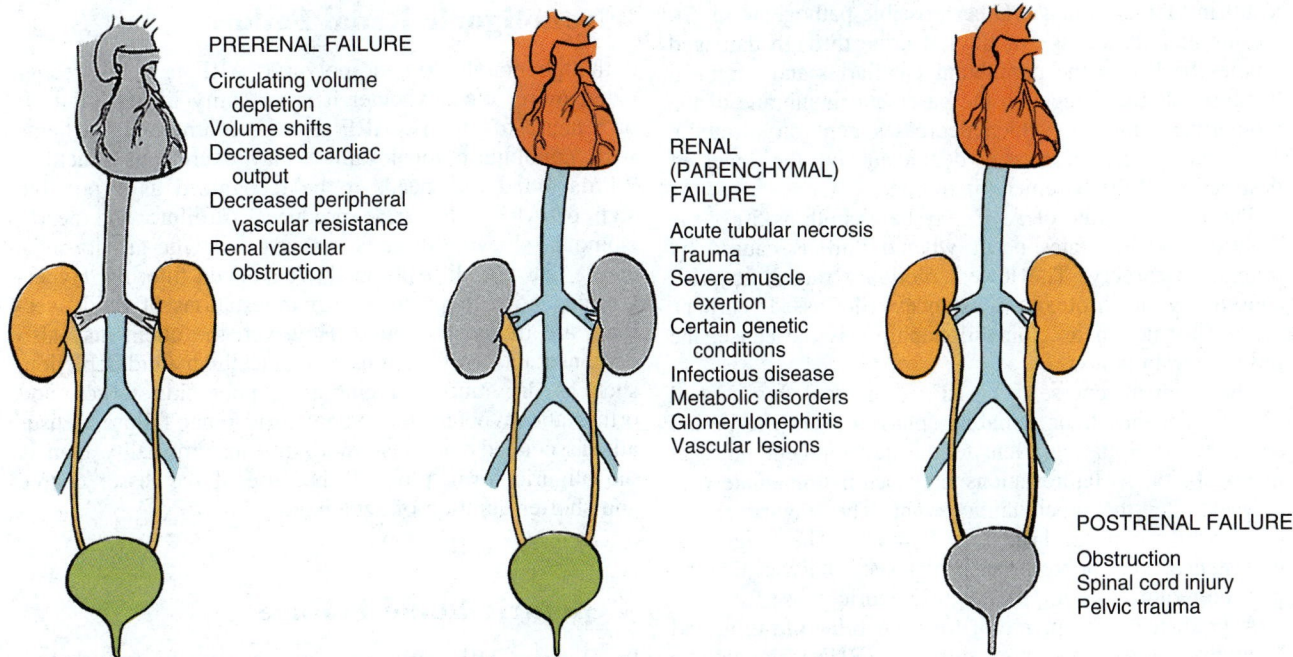

Figure 57–1. Causes of acute renal failure: prerenal, renal, and postrenal.

disease, metabolic conditions (e.g., hypokalemia, phosphatemia, and heat stroke), and from rejection of a transplanted kidney.

Additional renal causes of ARF include glomerulonephritis; microvascular and large vascular lesions, as in hemolytic-uremic syndrome; thrombosis; vasculitis; scleroderma; trauma; atherosclerosis; tumor invasion; and cortical necrosis, which is caused by prolonged vasospasm of the cortical blood vessels.

■ Postrenal Causes

Postrenal causes leading to ARF arise from obstruction in the urinary tract, anywhere from the tubules to the urethral meatus. Common sources of obstruction include prostatic hypertrophy, calculi, invading tumors, surgical accidents, ureteral or urethral strictures or stenosis, and retroperitoneal fibrosis. Obstruction caused by retroperitoneal fibrosis is difficult to identify unless it is bilateral. This is because the unobstructed kidney continues to function normally, and if the affected kidney is only partially obstructed, it may even become polyuric as it loses its ability to concentrate. Spinal cord injury may lead to decreased bladder emptying and a functional obstruction.

In managing the client with ARF, it is important to determine whether the disorder originates in the prerenal, renal, or postrenal area before intervention begins. Appropriate interventions require determining the origin of the disorder.

This condition may be preventable with close monitoring by the nurse of the client at risk. Because hypotension and hypovolemia are the two causes with the highest mortality rate, early diagnosis and reversal of these prob-

lems can save the client's life. Carefully monitor the vital signs and urine output of clients at risk of development of ARF.

Nephrotoxic agents are another risk factor for this condition. Always be aware of the action and potential side effects and toxicity of any medication administered to the client.

Pathophysiology

The pathogenesis of ARF is not clear. One hypothesis is that the damaged tubules cannot conserve sodium normally, which leads to renin-angiotensin-aldosterone system activation. This redistributes the renal vascular supply by increasing the tone of both the afferent and efferent arterioles. The resulting ischemia may cause an increase in vasopressin, cellular swelling, inhibition of prostaglandin synthesis, and further stimulation of the renin-angiotensin system. The reduced blood flow decreases glomerular pressure, GFR, and tubular flow; thus, oliguria occurs.

There is also a theory that cellular and protein debris within the tubule obstructs the lumen, which raises the intratubular pressure. This increasing oncotic pressure opposes filtration pressure until glomerular filtration stops. A biochemical theory claims that decreased renal blood flow leads to decreased oxygen delivery to the proximal tubules; this causes reduction in cellular adenosine triphosphate (ATP), which increases cytosolic and mitochondrial calcium concentrations. The result of this process is cell death and tubular necrosis. Vasomotor nephropathy, causing spasms of peritubular capillaries, may result in tubular damage. Other possible pathogenic mechanisms include leakage of filtered urine through damaged tubules back into the peritubular capillaries and chemical or morphologic changes in the basement membrane of the glomerular capillary, which decreases nephron filtration. The reversibility of this is dependent on the level of destruction of the basement membrane.

The mortality rate of ARF may be as high as 50%; the highest mortality rates occur when failure is caused by trauma or surgery. The lowest mortality rate is in ARF caused by nephrotoxic substances (discussed earlier). When obstruction or glomerulonephritis is the cause, the mortality rate is low.

The clinical course of ARF is marked by several phases. The onset, or initiating, phase covers the period from the precipitating event to the development of renal manifestations. Manifestations may begin immediately or a week after the precipitating event. The oliguric-anuric or nonoliguric phase lasts 1 to 8 weeks. The longer the persistence, the poorer the prognosis. Dialytic therapy may be required during the oliguric-anuric phase.

A gradual or abrupt return to glomerular filtration and leveling of the blood urea nitrogen (BUN) signals the diuretic phase. Urine output may be 1000 to 2000 ml/day, which may lead to dehydration; 25% of the deaths from ARF occur during this phase. The recovery phase lasts 3 to 12 months. During this time, the client often returns to a prerenal failure activity level. In actuality, mild tubular abnormalities, including glycosuria and decreased concentrating ability, may continue for years, and the client will continually be at risk of fluid and electrolyte imbalance, especially during times of stress.

The effects of ARF are widespread. The major consequences include the following:

● Fluid and electrolyte imbalances (fluid overload or depletion, hyperkalemia, hyponatremia, hypocalcemia, and hypermagnesemia)
● Acidosis
● Increased susceptibility to secondary infections
● Anemia
● Platelet dysfunction
● Gastrointestinal complications (anorexia, nausea, vomiting, diarrhea or constipation, and stomatitis)
● Increased incidence of pericarditis
● Uremic encephalopathy characterized by apathy, defective recent memory, episodic obtundation, dysarthria, tremors, convulsions, and coma

Wound healing is impaired. Other manifestations are usually a result of these sequelae.

Clinical Manifestations and Diagnostic Findings

The most common overall sign of ARF is alteration in the expected urine output. Usually this is oliguria or anuria, but polyuric ARF accounts for 30% of the cases.[31]

There are two varieties of ARF: nonoliguric and oliguric.

■ Nonoliguric Renal Failure

Although nonoliguric, or polyuric, ARF is being recognized more often, whether it is an entity in and of itself or a phase of oliguric ARF remains controversial. Clients with nonoliguric renal failure may excrete as much as 2 L/day, and this needs to be recognized as a possible sign of ARF. The urine produced is dilute and nearly isomolar, showing up as a low urine specific gravity indicating that not all nephrons have stopped filtering. Hypertension and tachypnea, with manifestations of fluid overload, are frequently found. However, the client may also demonstrate manifestations of extracellular fluid depletion, such as dry mucous membranes, poor skin turgor, and orthostatic hypotension. Nonoliguric renal failure is usually associated with less morbidity and mortality than is the oliguric form, probably because of the lesser degree and shorter duration of azotemia.

■ Oliguric Renal Failure

In oliguric ARF, urine production usually falls below 400 ml/day. However, remember that the aging kidney normally loses its concentrating ability, and the renal function becomes more susceptible to insult. Therefore, the older client may have developed oliguria at urine volumes of 600 to 700 ml/day.

The clinical manifestations of oliguric ARF depend on the cause. In prerenal failure, assessment findings are quite diverse, depending on the underlying condition. The client will frequently have a history of a precipitating event, such as hemorrhage or cardiac insult. The urine has a high specific gravity and osmolarity, and there is little or no proteinuria. Urine sediment is usually normal, although it may contain a few hyaline and granular casts. There is very little urinary sodium excretion. The BUN-creatinine ratio is significantly elevated, reaching levels of 10:1 to 40:1.

Systemic manifestations of intrinsic renal failure may include edema, weight gain, hemoptysis from elevated left ventricular end-diastolic pressure, weakness from anemia, and hypertension. The urine has a fixed specific gravity, a high sodium concentration, and definite proteinuria. In the case of glomerulonephritis, there will be hematuria and red blood cell and hemoglobin casts. Acute tubular necrosis will cause muddy-brown granular casts. If there has been significant tissue damage, elevated levels of serum creatinine, phosphokinase, and potassium can be expected.

Urine produced in postrenal failure may have fixed specific gravity and elevated sodium concentration with little or no proteinuria. Urine sediment is generally normal. The most definitive manifestations are those indicating obstruction, as described with calculi and neoplasms. Wide fluctuations between anuria and polyuria may indicate intermittent urinary tract obstruction.

Urinalysis, urine specific gravity and sodium levels, and serum creatinine and urea nitrogen are common diagnostic tests for ARF. The amount of urine in relation to intake is also important in formulating the diagnosis. To measure the exact amount of urine output or to obtain a specimen for culture and sensitivity, the client may need to be straight-catheterized.

Acute and Subacute Care

■ Medical Management

The medical management of ARF is largely based on preventing and treating its effects. As with any disease process, prevention is the primary intervention. Attaining and maintaining adequate hydration and diuresis in high-risk clients is crucial, as is the prevention of contributing factors. Once ARF has developed, prompt recognition and action facilitate restoration of optimal renal function. Correction of the underlying condition such as hydration in a client with hypovolemic shock may be all that is necessary in ARF due to prerenal disorders. Postrenal causes must be rectified. In the meantime, the sequelae of ARF require specific intervention.

Treatment of ARF may take place in an intensive care unit or other critical care unit, depending on the cause. Much of the care revolves around physiologic monitoring and interventions that center primarily on maintenance of fluid and electrolyte balance and nutrition.

Dialysis is frequently required for treatment of ARF. Indications for dialysis include significant volume overload, uncontrolled hyperkalemia or acidosis, progressive uremia as evidenced by rising BUN and creatinine concentrations, altered central nervous system function, and pericarditis. Dialysis is discussed later in this chapter.

Secondary infections are a significant cause of death in clients with ARF. The client must be monitored carefully for infectious processes; if these occur, they should be treated aggressively. Indwelling urethral catheters are avoided because of their great potential for introducing infection.

Pericarditis occurs in as many as 18% of clients with renal failure. Assessment findings include pleuritic pain that may be relieved by an upright position, pericardial friction rub, tachycardia, and fever. Treatment is usually begun with steroids or nonsteroidal anti-inflammatory agents. Pericardiocentesis and pericardiectomy may be necessary if cardiac function is compromised.

Other problems call for symptomatic relief. There is a rise in the number of seizures resulting from a decrease in the seizure threshold secondary to the rising BUN. These seizures may be relieved by intravenous phenytoin or phenobarbital. Anemia is treated by transfusions or the use of recombinant erythropoietin. Erythropoietin is the hormone produced by the kidney to stimulate red blood cell production. Erythropoietin is used in chronic renal failure, although its use in ARF has not been studied extensively. Bleeding tendencies may be minimized by correcting vitamin K deficiencies, as well as by lowering the serum BUN level, because BUN interferes with platelet aggregation.

Fluid Replacement

Fluid replacement must be done very carefully to avoid fluid overload. Fluid replacement volumes are usually calculated on the basis of some fraction of the previous day's urine output plus an amount (e.g., 400 ml) to account for the usual insensible loss that occurs during a 24-hour period. Losses from other sources, such as vomiting and diarrhea, are added to the daily allotment. Unless the client is on total parenteral nutrition, some physicians use a daily weight loss of 0.2 to 0.5 kg/day as a measure of the success of the fluid replacement program. This represents the usual daily weight loss from catabolism and loss of lean body mass.

Administration of Diuretics

Diuretic therapy may be used, although it remains controversial. Furosemide and mannitol are the pharmacologic agents most frequently used, and they must be administered cautiously. It is important to replace fluids as needed to maintain adequate blood flow and perfusion to the kidneys. These diuretics may affect the outcome of nonoliguric ARF, which generally has a better prognosis than does anuric or oliguric renal failure.

Electrolyte Replacement

Electrolyte replacement is based primarily on urine and serum electrolyte concentrations. Hyperkalemia is probably the most dangerous imbalance because of its contribution to cardiac arrhythmias and arrest. In addition to the kidney's inability to excrete potassium, this electrolyte is released in greater quantities from the body cells when acidosis is present and is further increased by rapid tissue catabolism. Electrocardiographic monitors are frequently used. Cation exchange resins may be administered orally or rectally to facilitate excretion of potassium through the gastrointestinal tract. Sorbitol, an osmotic cathartic, is given with cation exchange resins to induce a diarrhea to eliminate the potassium ions that were exchanged for sodium ions in the resins. Sorbitol can be given orally, as an enema, or via a nasogastric tube. Potassium-containing foods and medications should be avoided. The administration of 50% glucose and regular insulin, with sodium bicarbonate if necessary or calcium gluconate intravenously, can temporarily prevent cardiac arrest in an emergency by moving potassium into the cells and temporarily reducing serum potassium levels.

Hyponatremia is usually an effect of dilution rather than a true lack of sodium. Therefore, intervention is actually a matter of proper fluid replacement (i.e., fluid restriction and self-correction). Hyperphosphatemia is treated with reduced dietary intake and phosphate binders such as aluminum-based antacids (Alucaps). Antacids containing magnesium should be avoided since they will increase magnesium and phosphate levels. Physostigmine may be used for hypermagnesemia, and intravenous magnesium sulfate for hypomagnesemia.

Metabolic acidosis usually results from the accumulation of acid waste products. Sodium bicarbonate, sodium lactate, or sodium acetate may be used on a short-term basis to correct this condition. Dialysis is usually used for severe acidosis.

Maintenance of a High Calorie, Low Protein Diet

Proper nutrition is crucial. A high calorie, low protein diet is usually prescribed. It may also be low in sodium and potassium. The protein must be of high biologic value (complete), containing the essential amino acids to reduce the nitrogenous waste products. Adequate carbohydrate intake reverses the process of gluconeogenesis. During the acute phases, intake should be 135 to 150 nonprotein kcal for each 6.25 g of protein ingested; this ratio is considered adequate for prevention of protein catabolism. Low potassium liquid supplements may also be used. If oral intake is not sufficient to meet requirements, tube feedings or total parenteral nutrition, including intralipids, may be instituted.

■ Nursing Management of the Medical Client

Assessment

Assess the client for the presence of risk factors for the development of ARF. Carefully monitor the client for the development of ARF. Because hypovolemia is a common cause, assess the client closely for this problem. The most important assessment is, therefore, fluid balance.

Once the client has been diagnosed with ARF, carefully assess the client for the development of complications such as pleural effusion, pericarditis, acidosis, and uremia.

Diagnosis, Planning, Implementation

Fluid Volume Deficit. A common diagnosis in ARF is *Fluid Volume Deficit related to fluid loss from a variety of reasons*, followed by *Fluid Volume Excess related to inability of kidneys to produce urine secondary to ARF.*

Planning: Expected Outcomes. The client will not develop fluid volume deficit and ARF; if ARF does occur, the client will not develop fluid volume excess or will have it managed with dialysis, as evidenced by return to balanced intake and output.

Implementation. Careful monitoring of fluid balance indicators is crucial to the management of ARF. Accurate intake and output measurements guide the fluid replacement regimen. It is important to compare these values, looking for 24- to 48-hour trends. Vital signs, including postural blood pressures, apical pulses, skin turgor, and mucous membranes, are checked approximately every 4 hours depending on the severity of the illness. Daily weights are carefully obtained. Internal blood pressure measurements may be done. Urine specific gravity, usually an indication of fluid balance, may be negated by intrinsic renal disease. Heart sounds, lung sounds, and mental status may indicate the presence of fluid imbalances.

Once the physician has determined the client's fluid allotment, make sure that the regimen is followed. This means carefully monitoring fluid intake to make certain that the prescribed amount is taken. Many times, this amount represents a fluid restriction for the client, which causes a problem with thirst. Help the client stay within the prescribed restriction with careful oral hygiene, judicious use of ice chips, lip ointments, and appropriate diversionary activities. Placing the allotted water in a spray bottle may help to spread out the amount taken. Fluid from nutrition must be taken into account. To conserve fluids for the client, administer medications with meals, if possible.

Altered Nutrition: Less than Body Requirements. Another common diagnosis in clients with this disorder is *Altered Nutrition: Less than Body Requirements, related to anorexia and altered metabolic state secondary to renal failure.*

Planning: Expected Outcomes. The client will maintain adequate nutrition, as evidenced by sufficient intake to prevent protein catabolism.

Implementation. The client frequently experiences anorexia, nausea, and stomatitis accompanying renal failure. That combined with the general unpalatability of the diet makes adequate nutrition a challenge for nurse and client. Working with the client to plan a diet that is most acceptable is important. The therapeutic dietitian is a good resource. Provide a pleasant environment at mealtime. Food prepared in an attractive manner and presented in small amounts may help. Medications to alleviate the discomfort of nausea and stomatitis are useful. Parenteral nutrition may be instituted if the client's nutritional status cannot be maintained with oral intake.

Risk for Impaired Skin Integrity. Often, clients are at *Risk for Impaired Skin Integrity related to poor cellular nutrition and edema.*

Planning: Expected Outcomes. The client will not develop impaired skin integrity, as evidenced by intact skin.

Implementation. The poor systemic nutrition and edema accompanying renal failure may cause skin breakdown. Meticulous skin care, frequent turning, and special mattresses are very important. Range-of-motion exercises facilitate movement and increase circulation.

Risk for Infection. A disorder such as this always entrains *Risk for Infection related to lowered resistance.*

Planning: Expected Outcomes. The client will not develop infection, as evidenced by normal vital signs and white blood cell count.

Implementation. The client with ARF is compromised and very susceptible to secondary infection, which represents a stress that the kidneys cannot handle. Urethral catheters are avoided if possible. If they must be used, provide meticulous catheter care. Nursing intervention must be designed to prevent infection in the usual high-risk sites (e.g., respiratory tract, wounds, central catheters, and mouth). Also be alert to early manifestations of infection so that aggressive medical treatment may be instituted.

Anxiety. Inevitably, the client will evince *Anxiety related to unknown outcome of disease process.*

Planning: Expected Outcomes. The client will not exhibit manifestations of anxiety, as evidenced by calmness and ability to focus on the disease and its outcome (within the limits of altered mental status related to elevated BUN).

Implementation. Because the client's physical needs are so obvious, it is easy to forget that the client, as well as significant others, will be anxious and frightened. Give frequent, careful explanations and remain cognizant of the need for emotional and psychological support. Be aware that the client may be mechanically ventilated and not able to articulate feelings and fears.

Evaluation

The goal is to reverse the cause of the renal failure. Once this is accomplished and the client supported with fluids and electrolytes, the client should recover from ARF. It is important for the client to understand the implications of ARF and the vital importance of compliance with the therapeutic regimen.

The client and significant others will require a great deal of education about renal failure, and the need for possibly ongoing treatment. The client and significant others will have to understand what manifestations might indicate further renal damage or that the client has developed chronic renal failure. The client will need to be closely followed by a nephrologist at frequent intervals

for at least a year after ARF is reversed so that deterioration of renal function can be monitored.

■ Modifications for Elderly Clients

The major difference with older clients is their increased risk of developing ARF because of their cardiovascular instability. The older adult has more difficulty maintaining a homeostatic fluid balance. There is also a greater likelihood that older clients have some pre-existing renal damage, especially men in relation to benign prostatic hypertrophy and the obstruction it causes.

Chronic Renal Failure

Chronic, or irreversible, renal failure (CRF) is a progressive reduction of functioning renal tissue such that the remaining kidney mass can no longer maintain the body's internal environment. It can develop insidiously over many years or can occur as a result of a bout of ARF from which the client fails to recover.

Etiology and Risk Factors

The causes of CRF are numerous. Throughout this section, various injuries and disease processes that may potentially end in renal failure have been discussed. Chronic glomerulonephritis, acute renal failure, polycystic kidney disease, obstruction, repeated bouts of pyelonephritis, and nephrotoxins are examples of causes. Systemic diseases such as diabetes mellitus, hypertension, lupus erythematosus, polyarteritis, sickle cell disease, and amyloidosis may produce renal failure.

Hypertension and diabetes are the most common causes of CRF, accounting for over 60% of the clients seen on dialysis. Men and women are equally affected by the problem; the incidence is highest among middle-aged people.

In order to reduce the risk that these diseases will lead to CRF, the client should be closely followed and receive adequate treatment to control or slow the progress of these problems before they progress to end-stage renal failure. Some conditions, such as lupus and diabetes, however, can progress to failure despite close treatment.

Pathophysiology

The pathogenesis of CRF portrays deterioration and destruction of nephrons with progressive loss of renal function. As the total GFR falls and clearance is reduced, the serum urea nitrogen and creatinine clearance levels rise. Remaining functioning nephrons hypertrophy, as they are required to filter a larger load of solutes. One of the consequences of this is that the kidneys lose their ability to concentrate urine adequately. In an attempt to continue excreting the solutes, a large volume of dilute urine is passed, which makes the client susceptible to fluid depletion. The tubules gradually lose their ability to reabsorb electrolytes. Occasionally, this can result in salt wasting, in which the urine contains very large amounts of sodium, which leads to more polyuria.

CLIENT EDUCATION GUIDE

Acute Renal Failure

Learn the basic facts about renal function. Simple drawings and printed material are available to help you.

Watch for and report manifestations that indicate further renal damage.

Watch for the possibility of chronic renal failure developing.

Weigh yourself at regular intervals (same time of day, same scale, same clothing) and record intake and output.

Follow specific dietary restrictions. Learn the reasons for the restrictions and the need to comply with them.

See your nephrologist for follow-up within 1 year after acute renal failure reversal so that renal function can be more closely monitored.

Understanding Chronic Renal Failure and Its Treatment

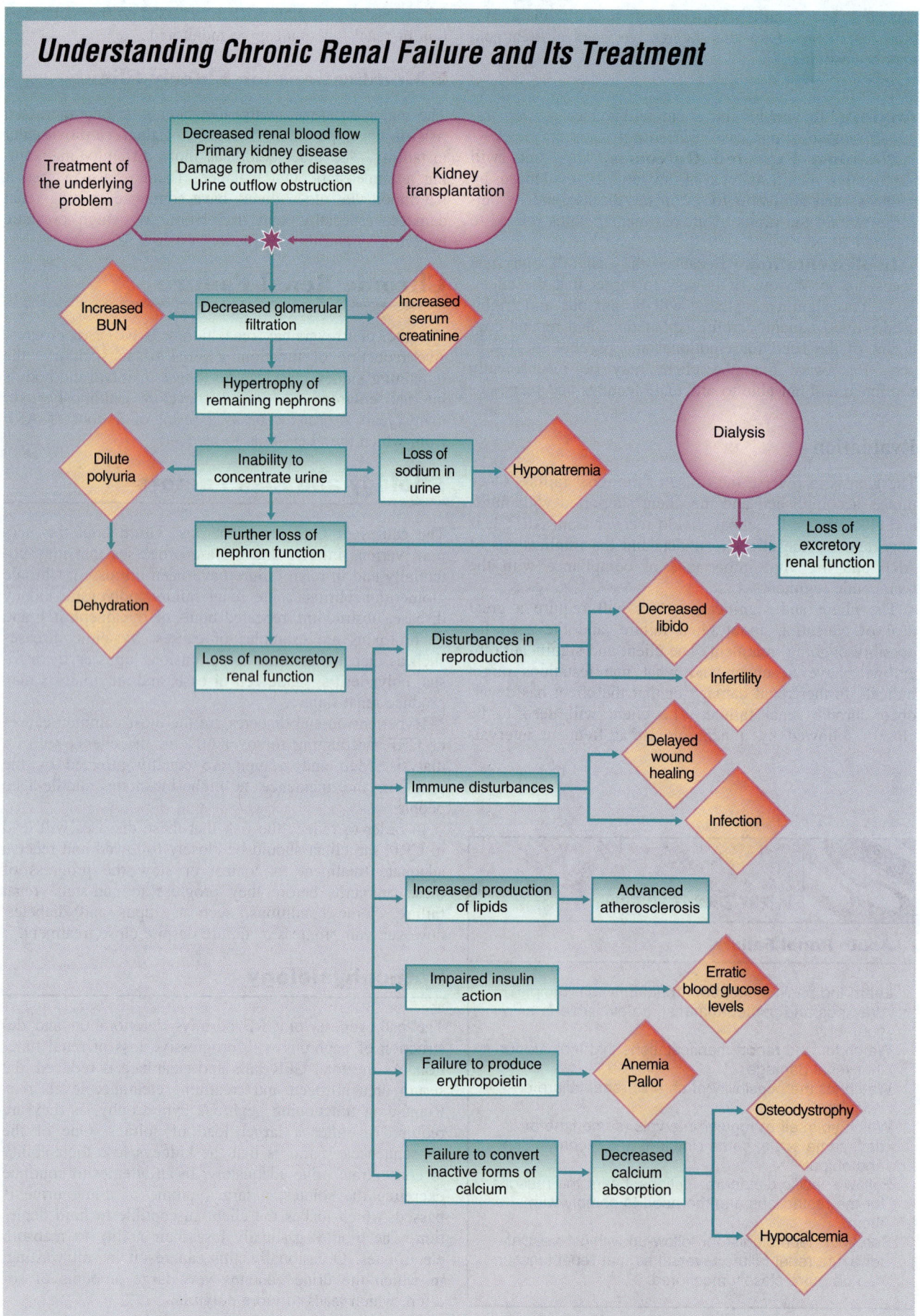

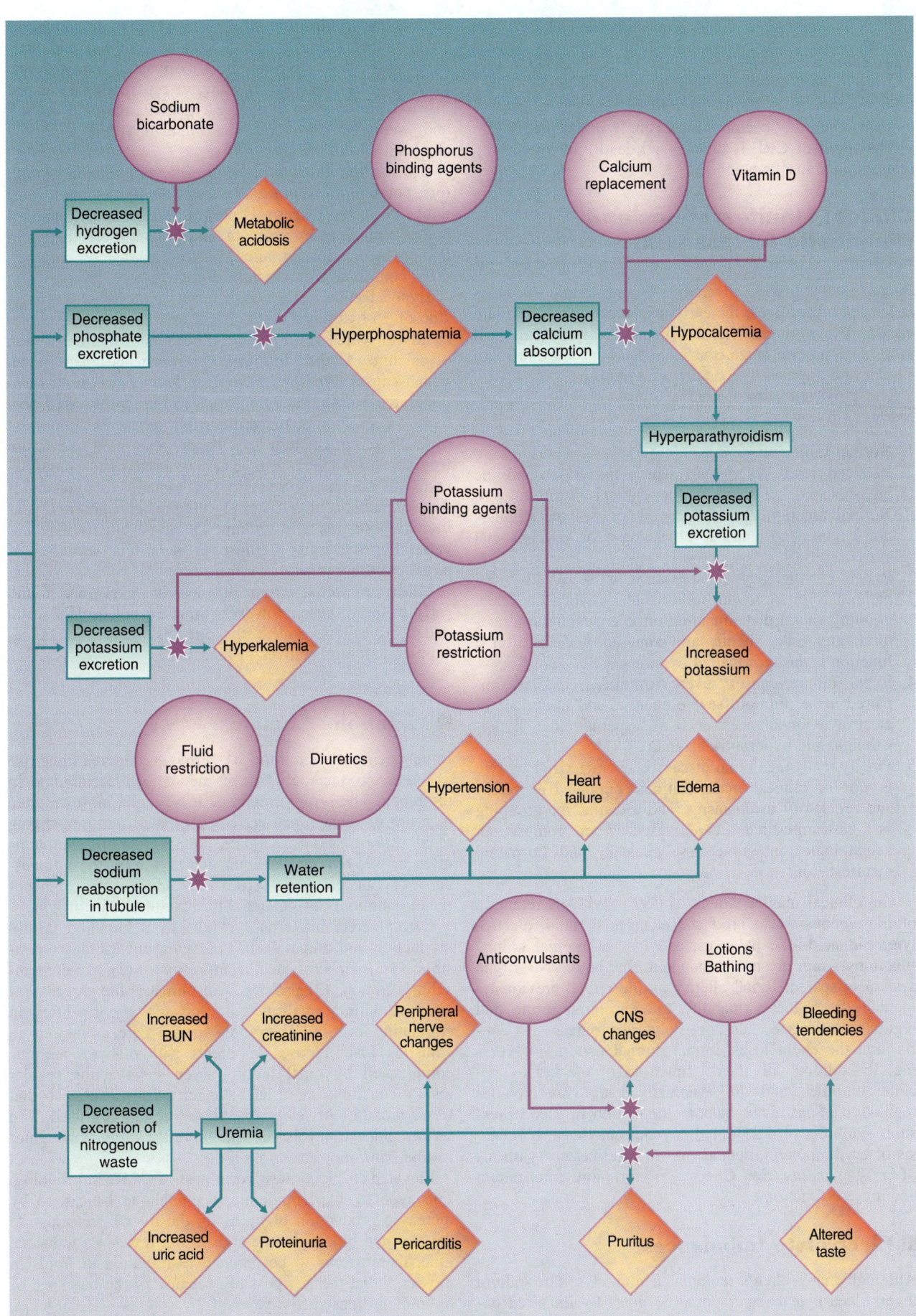

As renal damage advances and the number of functioning nephrons declines, the total GFR decreases further. Thus, the body becomes unable to rid itself of water, salt, and other waste products through the kidneys. When the GFR is less than 10 to 20 ml/min, clinical uremia is evident. The body becomes increasingly intoxicated.

The result of CRF is uremia and death, treatment with dialysis, or transplantation.

Clinical Manifestations and Diagnostic Assessment

Because of the wide diversity of contributing elements and disease processes, the early stages of renal failure are varied. However, as the destruction of nephrons progresses to its end stage, the manifestations become very similar and are classified as uremic syndrome.

The projected clinical course of irreversible renal disease is as follows:

1. Normal functioning.
2. Reduced renal reserve, in which the BUN may be high-normal, but there are no clinical manifestations. Normal functioning is evident as long as the client is not exposed to unusual physiologic or psychosocial stress.
3. Renal insufficiency demonstrates a more advanced pathologic process with mild azotemia when the client is on a general diet. Impaired urine concentration, nocturia, and mild anemia are common findings. Renal function is easily impaired by stress.
4. Renal failure causes severe azotemia, acidosis, impaired urine dilution, severe anemia, and a number of electrolyte imbalances, such as hypernatremia, hyperkalemia, and hyperphosphatemia.
5. Finally, end-stage renal disease is characterized by two groups of clinical manifestations: deranged excretory and regulatory mechanisms; and a distinctive grouping of gastrointestinal, cardiovascular, neuromuscular, hematologic, integumentary, skeletal, and hormonal manifestations.

The clinical manifestations of CRF—with its retention of nitrogenous waste products; changes in fluid, electrolyte, and acid-base balances; and loss of normal kidney functions—are present throughout the body. No organ system is spared. Renal alterations (described previously) include the kidney's inability to concentrate urine and regulate electrolyte excretion. Polyuria progresses to anuria, and the client loses normal diurnal patterns of voiding. In addition, all normal functions of the kidney become curtailed and are eventually lost. This includes regulation of acid-base balance, regulation of blood pressure, synthesis of 1,25-dihydroxycholecalciferol, biogenesis of erythropoietin, degradation of insulin, and synthesis of prostaglandins. See Chapter 54 for more information about these functions.

■ Electrolyte Imbalances

Although many clients maintain a normal serum sodium level, electrolyte balances may be upset by impaired excretion and utilization. The salt-wasting properties of some failing kidneys, in addition to vomiting and diarrhea, may cause hyponatremia. Apparent hyponatremia may be a dilutional effect of water retention. Late in the disease, the problem becomes hypernatremia, and the salt and water retention often contribute to hypertension and congestive heart failure.

Because the kidneys are very efficient potassium excretors, potassium levels usually remain within normal limits until late in the disease. However, hyperkalemia then becomes a challenging problem. Catabolism, potassium-containing medications, trauma, blood transfusions, and acidosis contribute to potassium excess.

Hypocalcemia occurs as a result of decreased conversion of 25-hydroxycholecalciferol to 1,25-dihydroxycholecalciferol which results in a reduced intestinal absorption of calcium. At the same time, phosphate is not excreted, which causes hyperphosphatemia. This combination stimulates the parathyroid glands to secrete parathyroid hormone in an attempt to facilitate phosphate excretion and raise the serum calcium level by the resorption of calcium from bone. Osteomalacia, osteitis fibrosa, and osteosclerosis are commonly seen in CRF clients as a result of these metabolic alterations in calcium, phosphorus, parathyroid hormone, and vitamin D. Some clients may develop hypercalcemia because of persistent secretion of parathyroid hormone.

Mildly elevated serum magnesium levels are found early in the disease. However, these do not usually reach a dangerous level unless the client is receiving magnesium-containing laxatives or antacids.

■ Metabolic Changes

In advancing renal failure, BUN and serum creatinine rise as waste products of protein metabolism accumulate in the blood. The serum creatinine level is the most accurate measure of renal function. The proteinuria accompanying renal disease and inadequate dietary intake of proteins often causes hypoproteinemia, which lowers the intravascular oncotic pressure. Serum uric acid is often high but is not commonly associated with manifestations of gout.

Carbohydrate intolerance results from impaired insulin production and metabolism. Four mechanisms are responsible: (1) peripheral insulin antagonism, (2) impaired insulin secretion, (3) prolonged insulin half-life directly related to kidney malfunction, and (4) abnormalities in circulating insulin. Therefore, special care is needed in adjusting insulin doses in clients with diabetes mellitus complicated by renal failure. Even short acting regular insulin functions more as a longer acting insulin so that lesser amounts or fewer injections per day are used. The serum glucose levels are monitored closely for tighter insulin control.

Elevated triglycerides is almost a universal finding. This type IV hyperlipidemia is thought to be caused by increased production of lipids by the liver in response to the elevated blood glucose and insulin levels. At the same time, there seems to be reduced assimilation of lipids in the peripheral tissues, possibly because of the blockage of lipoprotein lipase activity.

Metabolic acidosis occurs because of the kidney's inability to excrete hydrogen ions as a result of decreased reabsorption of sodium bicarbonate and decreased formation of dihydrogen phosphate and ammonia. This condition accentuates hyperkalemia and the reabsorption of calcium from the bones.

Pericarditis is usually related to accumulation of uremic toxins and is rarely due to infection. Manifestations include pericardial pain (often relieved by an upright position), tachycardia, pleural friction rub, and fever. The condition may progress to pericardial effusion and cardiac tamponade, a life-threatening complication.

■ Hematologic Changes

The primary hematologic effect of renal failure is anemia, usually normochromic and normocytic. Left untreated, hematocrit levels can drop below 20%. Frequently, it is the fatigue, weakness, and cold intolerance accompanying the anemia that initiate the evaluation leading to a diagnosis of renal failure. The mild anemia found in the early stages is usually due to reduced erythropoiesis. Later, hemolysis, gastrointestinal losses, and clotting abnormalities may add to the severity of the condition. Occasionally, the client will be iron- or folate-depleted from nutritional deficiencies. Bleeding tendencies become apparent as the disease progresses. Platelet abnormalities are the primary defect responsible for bleeding in the uremic client. The accumulation of uremic toxins interferes with platelet adhesiveness.

■ Gastrointestinal Changes

The entire gastrointestinal system is affected. Transient anorexia, nausea, and vomiting are almost universal. Clients often experience a constant, bitter, metallic, or salty taste, and their breath commonly smells fetid, fishy, or ammoniacal. Stomatitis, parotitis, and gingivitis are common problems due to poor oral hygiene and the formation of ammonia from salivary urea. Accumulations of gastrin (due to increased secretion abnormalities of gastric acid physiology) may be a major cause of ulcer disease. Esophagitis, gastritis, colitis, gastrointestinal bleeding, and diarrhea may be present. Serum amylase levels may be increased, although they may not indicate actual pancreatitis.

Constipation is a common problem. It is often the result of phosphate-binding agents; restriction of fluids and high fiber foods, many of which are potassium- and phosphorus-rich; and decreased activity. Constipation provides a particular challenge, because the usual interventions for prevention and treatment are contraindicated in the client with renal failure.

■ Immunologic Changes

Impairment of the immunologic system makes the client very susceptible to infection. Several factors are involved, including depression of humoral antibody formation, suppression of delayed hypersensitivity, and decreased chemotactic function of the leukocytes. Immunosuppression is an important part of the medical management of CRF.

Immunosuppression after transplantation is discussed later in this chapter.

■ Changes in Medication Metabolism

Finally, renal failure has a serious effect on medication metabolism. The uremic client is at very high risk of medication toxicity because of the effect of renal changes on the pharmacokinetics (absorption, distribution, metabolism, and excretion) of otherwise therapeutic medications. There are three main causes of this toxicity: (1) a high plasma level of the medication due to low serum albumin, decreased binding sites, impaired renal excretion, or impaired hepatic metabolism of the medication; (2) increased sensitivity to the medication due to uremia-induced changes in the target organ; and (3) a metabolic load because of the administration of the medication; for example, hypoalbuminemia means less protein available for binding. There are various tables and formulas that help guide dosage decisions. Remember that medication dosages must be altered and that the usual dosage ranges in the medication literature are not safe for the client with CRF. Assess the client carefully for toxic reactions.

■ Cardiovascular Changes

At least 50% to 65% of deaths occurring during CRF result from cardiovascular complications.[44] The most frequent clinical manifestation is hypertension (which may also be the cause of renal failure) produced through (1) the mechanisms of volume overload; (2) stimulation of the renin-angiotensin system; (3) sympathetically mediated vasoconstriction; for example, increased levels of dopamine β-hydroxylase; and (4) the absence of prostaglandins. Any of the many systemic complications of prolonged high blood pressure may be found.

The effects of volume overload on the heart are seen, including left ventricular hypertrophy and congestive heart failure. Heart failure may also result from anemia, arteriovenous shunt, complications of coronary artery disease, electrolyte imbalance, acidosis, myocardial calcification, and thiamine depletion. Arrhythmias may be caused by hyperkalemia, acidosis, hypermagnesemia, and decreased coronary perfusion.

Atherosclerosis is accelerated because of (1) abnormal carbohydrate and lipid metabolism; (2) impaired fibrinolysis, which leads to the development of microemboli; and (3) hyperparathyroidism. Arterial calcifications have been identified, the ankles being the most common early location. Other sites include the abdominal aorta, feet, pelvis, hands, and wrists. These vascular calcifications also occur within the heart itself, particularly at the mitral valve.

■ Respiratory Changes

Some of the respiratory effects, such as pulmonary edema, can be attributed to fluid overload. Pleuritis is a frequent finding, especially when pericarditis develops. A characteristic condition called uremic lung is a type of pneumonitis that responds well to fluid removal. Metabolic acidosis causes a compensatory increase in respiratory rate as the lungs try to eliminate excess hydrogen ions.

■ Musculoskeletal Changes

The musculoskeletal system is affected fairly early in the disease process, and bone reabsorption found on x-ray examination may be the first sign of renal failure in some clients. The most prevalent problem, affecting up to 90% of clients with CRF, is renal osteodystrophy. This condition develops insidiously and takes several forms: osteomalacia, osteitis fibrosis, osteoporosis, or osteosclerosis. The development of this manifestation results from interrelationships between the kidney-bone-parathyroid and calcium-phosphate-vitamin D connections. As the GFR decreases, phosphate excretion decreases, and calcium elimination increases. The abnormal levels of calcium and phosphate stimulate the release of parathyroid hormone, which mobilizes calcium from the bones and facilitates phosphate excretion.

As renal failure progresses, the kidney no longer converts vitamin D to its active form, 1,25-dihydroxycholecalciferol. The lack of this substance interferes with calcium absorption from the intestine and paradoxically facilitates phosphate retention. Thus, mineralization of the bone with calcium and phosphate is impaired. Demineralization of the bone frees more calcium and phosphorus into the blood. As the disease progresses even further, the parathyroid gland may become unresponsive to the normal feedback system and continue to produce parathyroid hormone, causing acceleration of renal osteodystrophy. A partial parathyroidectomy is the treatment of choice when hypercalcemia and high plasma levels of parathyroid hormone cannot be controlled with medication.

In addition to bone demineralization, this process also leads to calcification deposits in the subcutaneous, vascular, and visceral tissues throughout the body. In the advanced stages of this process, joint pain is severe. The client may also report diffuse and generalized bone and muscle pain. Bone deformities and frequent fractures are common. In children, bones fail to calcify, causing growth retardation. Tissue calcifications may be lethal if they develop in vital tissues, such as cerebral, coronary, or pulmonary vessels.

Some clients complain of muscle cramps. These may be due to osmolarity changes of the body fluids.

■ Integumentary Changes

Integumentary problems are particularly uncomfortable for some clients with CRF. Severe and intractable pruritus may be due to secondary hyperparathyroidism and calcium deposits in the skin. The skin is also often very dry because of atrophy of the sweat glands. Pruritus can lead to excoriated skin because of continued scratching.

Several color changes are found in renal failure. The bleeding tendency often results in increased bruising, petechiae, and purpura. These do not usually cause problems themselves, but their presence may be alarming to the client. The pallor of anemia is evident. The cause of retained urochrome pigments, making the skin orange-green or gray in color, is not clear.

Hair is brittle and tends to fall out, and nails are thin and brittle. Characteristic red bands that develop on the nails are called Muercke's lines. Another nail pattern that has been observed is a "half-and-half" nail with the proximal half normally white and the distal portion brown.

■ Neurologic Changes

Although dialysis has reduced the incidence of neurologic changes, some clients experience these problems early in the disease process. Peripheral neuropathy causes many manifestations such as burning feet, inability to find a comfortable position for the legs and feet (restless legs syndrome), gait changes, footdrop, and paraplegia. These manifestations move up the extremities and may extend to include the upper extremities. Initially, it is primarily a problem of the sensory system, but if left untreated, it may progress to the motor system. Nerve conduction becomes slower, and deep tendon reflexes and vibratory sense are diminished.

Central nervous system involvement is demonstrated through forgetfulness, inability to concentrate, short attention span, impaired reasoning ability and judgment, increased nervous irritability, nystagmus, twitching, dysarthria, seizures, central nervous system depression, and coma. Involvement of the cranial nerves may alter any of the senses. Hearing threshold levels show a definite high-frequency deficit early in the disease, and hearing progressively deteriorates. Uremic amaurosis is a very sudden onset of bilateral blindness, which seems to reverse itself in hours to days. Eyes often contain calcium salts, which give them an irritated appearance.

■ Reproductive Changes

Reproductive system changes can be very alarming. Women often experience menstrual irregularities, particularly amenorrhea, and infertility. However, there have been women with CRF who have conceived and successfully carried their pregnancies to term. Men frequently report impotence resulting from both physiologic and psychological causes. They may also experience testicular atrophy, oligospermia, and reduced sperm motility. Both sexes report decreased libido, which may be due to both physiologic and psychological factors.

■ Endocrine Changes

CRF also affects the endocrine system. The effect on insulin utilization has been discussed earlier, as has parathyroid function. Pituitary hormones, such as growth hormone and prolactin, may be increased in some people. The levels of luteinizing hormone and follicle-stimulating hormone vary greatly from client to client. Thyroid-stimulating hormone is usually at a normal level, but it may demonstrate a blunted response to thyrotropin-releasing hormone; this results in the common finding of hypothyroidism.

■ Psychosocial Changes

Psychosocial changes occur, probably as a result of both the physiologic alterations and the extreme stress placed on the client by the presence of a chronic, life-threatening disease. Behavior changes are greatly influenced by the client's personality. Expected alterations include marked personality changes, labile emotions, increased demand on others, withdrawal, depression, agitation, delusions, and psychosis.

Psychosocial changes in the client are among the biggest and hardest problems the nurse must deal with. Clients often suffer from role reversal, loss or curtailing of employment, and multiple life-style changes. Scheduling dialysis can create many difficulties. Both the client's self-concept and body image may be altered leading to further problems with work and relationships. Depression can be very severe and in some clients may precipitate in suicide.

Diagnostic Findings

Many laboratory tests are performed, including serum sodium, potassium, urea nitrogen, creatinine, phosphorus, creatinine clearance, calcium, and pH levels; urinalysis and urine creatinine clearance; and complete blood count. The normal ratio of BUN to creatinine is 20:1. This ratio remains the same as both the creatinine and BUN rise.

A KUB radiograph is usually done first to determine whether there is a problem with the structure of the renal system. An IVP and CT scan can be done to assess renal structure and function. Renal angiography may also be done to assess the blood supply to and through the kidneys.

Community and Self-Care

■ Medical Management

Conservative intervention does not cure the disease but may retard its progress. Eventually, most clients will require renal replacement therapy. However, even successful dialysis and transplant do not preclude the potential for death from complications of renal failure or its treatment.

After the correction of contributing factors, control of blood pressure and fluid and dietary adjustments are the mainstays of conservative intervention for the client with CRF. The five goals of medical management are the following:

1. Preservation of renal function
2. Delay of the need for dialysis or transplant as long as feasible
3. Improvement of body chemistry, values
4. Alleviation of extrarenal manifestations, as far as possible
5. Providing an optimal quality of life for the client and significant others

Pruritus can be very aggravating. Many interventions have been tried, including topical emollients and lotions, antihistamines, intravenous lidocaine, and ultraviolet B light, but relief has been inconsistent and often tempo-

rary. Subtotal parathyroidectomy has helped some, but there have been reports of recurrence. Effective dialysis seems to relieve the manifestations for many clients.

Neurologic manifestations require safety measures to protect the client from injury. Anticonvulsants and sedatives may be used. Phenothiazines are potentiated by uremia and should be avoided. Reduction in mental function, related to the rising BUN, requires more patience in explaining and reexplaining things to the client.

The hematologic changes can also be treated medically. Current therapy with epoetin alpha (EPO) three times a week helps to stimulate the production of red blood cells. Supplemental iron, B_{12}, and folic acid are usually administered as well.

Dialysis

There are two types of dialysis: peritoneal dialysis and hemodialysis. Each may be used to relieve manifestations of renal failure temporarily until the client regains kidney function or to sustain life in the client with irreversible kidney disease. In the latter case, the dialysis must continue for the rest of the client's life unless a successful kidney transplantation is done. Dialysis is also used to control uremia and to physically prepare the client to receive a transplanted kidney. Dialysis is frequently necessary to keep the client alive until a suitable donor kidney is found. If the transplanted kidney does not immediately function adequately, dialysis may help prevent uremia until the kidney functions sufficiently.

Dialysis is usually accomplished through both ultrafiltration and diffusion. Ultrafiltration refers to the removal of fluid from the blood by the use of either osmotic or hydrostatic pressure to produce the necessary gradient. Diffusion is the passage of particles (ions) from an area of high concentration to an area of low concentration. Both processes occur across a semipermeable membrane, one with pores large enough to allow certain particles to pass through but too small to allow the passage of larger particles. When the two solutions are separated by a semipermeable membrane, solute particles will move toward the solution with lesser concentration. Simultaneously, water will move toward the solution in which the solute concentration is greater.

When dialysis is used as a substitute for kidney function, the semipermeable membrane in the dialyzer or "artificial kidney" used is either the peritoneal membrane (for peritoneal dialysis) or an artificial membrane (for hemodialysis). This membrane must have pores large enough to allow the passage of electrolytes, urea, and creatinine, but too small to allow passage of blood cells and other protein molecules. The blood and a specially prepared electrolyte solution called dialysate are placed in compartments on opposite sides of the membrane.

Goals of Dialysis

The four basic goals of dialysis therapy are the following:

1. Removal of the end products of protein metabolism, such as urea and creatinine, from the blood
2. Maintenance of a safe concentration of serum electrolytes

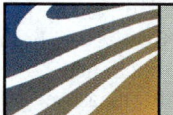

3. Correction of acidosis and replenishment of the blood's bicarbonate buffer system
4. Removal of excess fluid from the blood

Remember that solute particles and water can move freely across the membrane in either direction between the blood and the dialysate. With this in mind, note that if the client's blood has a higher concentration of urea, creatinine, and certain electrolytes than does the prepared dialysate solution, these particles will move into the dialysate solution, thus lowering the level in the blood. Likewise, if the blood is deficient in a substance such as bicarbonate, a higher concentration of this substance in the dialysate will cause it to move into the blood, raising the blood level. Excess fluid can be removed from the blood by increasing the particle concentration of the dialysate with a component such as dextrose. This increased particle concentration will cause water to move into the dialysate while at the same time the dextrose moves into

the blood. The tendency is always toward an equalization of concentration of the two solutions.

Peritoneal Dialysis

Peritoneal dialysis involves repeated cycles of instilling dialysate into the peritoneal cavity, allowing time for substance exchange, and then removing the dialysate. The procedure is useful for both ARF and CRF and for fluid and electrolyte imbalances. It has been used for overdoses of drugs and toxins, but because its clearance is much slower than that with hemodialysis, it may not be satisfactory for this purpose. One of the primary advantages of peritoneal dialysis is its relative ease, which allows it to be used in community healthcare facilities without all the sophisticated equipment needed for hemodialysis. It can be easily managed at home and often provides the client more independence and mobility than hemodialysis does.

Peritoneal dialysis may be used for clients with severe cardiovascular disease, especially those whose problems would be worsened by the rapid changes in urea, glucose, electrolytes, and fluid volume that occur during hemodialysis. Some physicians prescribe peritoneal dialysis for their diabetic patients to reduce the risk of retinal hemorrhage from the heparin used during dialysis treatment and because you can control their blood sugar by adding insulin to the dialysate. Peritoneal dialysis is the dialytic treatment of choice for children since it does not interfere with growth.

Contraindications to peritoneal dialysis include hypercatabolism, in which peritoneal dialysis is unable to adequately clear uremic toxins, and poor condition of the peritoneal membrane due to adhesions and scarring. Certain other conditions may be relative contraindications to peritoneal dialysis; these include obesity, history of ruptured diverticuli, abdominal disease, respiratory disease, recurrent episodes of peritonitis, abdominal malignancies, severe vascular disease, back problems since the increased weight from fluid may increase back strain, and extensive abdominal surgery with drains or tubes that may increase risk of infection.

Types of Peritoneal Dialysis

There are two types of peritoneal dialysis used today: continuous ambulatory and automated peritoneal dialysis.

Continuous Ambulatory Peritoneal Dialysis.
In continuous ambulatory peritoneal dialysis (CAPD), 1.5 to 3.0 L of dialysate is instilled into the abdomen approximately four times daily and left in place for 4 to 10 hours. The empty dialysate bag is folded up and carried in a pouch or pocket until it is time to drain the dialysate. The bag is later unfolded and placed lower than the insertion site so the fluid drains by gravity flow. When full, the bag is changed, and new dialysate is instilled into the abdomen as the process continues. In CAPD, there are usually four dialysis cycles every 24 hours, including an 8-hour dwell overnight. There are two major advantages to this procedure: (1) because there is no need for machinery, electricity, or a water source, the client

can go about almost any desired activity during dialysis; and (2) because the continuous exchange process closely resembles normal renal function, the body more easily maintains homeostasis, and there are fewer dietary and fluid restrictions. For diabetic management, insulin can be added to the dialysate.

Automated Peritoneal Dialysis. Automated peritoneal dialysis (APD) is similar to CAPD in that it is a continuous dialysis process but different in that it requires a peritoneal cycling machine. It can be done as continuous cyclic (CCPD), intermittent (IPD) or nightly (NPD).

Continuous Cyclic Peritoneal Dialysis. In CCPD, there are usually three cycles done at night and one cycle with an 8-hour dwell done in the morning. The advantage of this procedure is that the peritoneal catheter is opened only for the on-and-off procedures, which reduces the risk of infection. Another advantage is that the client isn't bothered by exchanges at work or school.

Intermittent Peritoneal Dialysis. IPD is not a continuous dialysis procedure like CAPD and CCPD. Dialysis is performed for 10 to 14 hours, three to four times a week, with use of the same peritoneal cycling machine as in CCPD. Hospitalized patients may be dialyzed up to 24 to 48 hours at a time if they are catabolic and require additional dialysis time.

Nightly Peritoneal Dialysis. In NPD, treatment is performed for 8 to 12 hours each night with no daytime dwells.

Procedure for Peritoneal Dialysis

The dialysate is usually allowed to run into the peritoneal cavity by gravity flow. The dialysate is warmed slightly to prevent chilling of the client and to dilate the peritoneal blood vessels, thus facilitating substance exchange. Two liters are usually instilled in adults, although smaller amounts may be needed at first until the client adjusts. Care must be taken to prevent air from entering the peritoneal cavity throughout the entire procedure.

"Dwell time" is the period during which the dialysate is left in the cavity. In IPD, equilibrium between the dialysate and the body fluids usually occurs within 15 to 30 minutes, with the maximum exchange happening within the first 5 minutes. Therefore, the solution is typically left in place 30 to 45 minutes for manual dialysis or 10 to 20 minutes when an automatic cycler is used. The fluid is then allowed to run out through the catheter by gravity. In CAPD and APD procedures, the dwell time is prolonged to 4 to 8 hours with a solution that allows continuous exchange and better clearance of certain elements.

The number of dialysis cycles depends on the normalization of body fluids and blood chemistries, as indicated by laboratory studies. Peritoneal clearance is influenced by several factors, including the size of the membrane area, blood flow to the peritoneum, and alterations in the permeability of the peritoneal membrane.

Preparation. Before catheter insertion, the client must be fully prepared. The client needs to know exactly what will happen and what to do during the dialysis process, and what kinds of results can be expected from the treatment. Obtain informed consent. Baseline weight, vital signs, and blood chemistries provide important data for later comparison. Mild sedation may be provided. The bladder and bowel should be emptied. The abdomen is shaved and prepared. If dialysis is to begin immediately, the equipment needs to be entirely ready with the dialysate warmed to 37°C (98.6°F) in order to optimize clearance of uremic metabolites; all tubing is flushed to prevent air from entering the cavity.

Catheter Insertion. Catheter insertion may be performed in the operating room or at the bedside under local anesthesia. The preferred insertion site is 3 to 5 cm below the umbilicus, an area that is relatively avascular and has less fascial resistance. For the placement of an acute rigid stylet catheter, an incision is made, and a stylet or large bore needle is inserted through the incision. Fluid is infused to expand the peritoneal cavity, and the catheter is inserted with the tip in the pelvic gutter.

There are several types of soft catheter that are inserted for acute or chronic peritoneal dialysis. These are generally inserted in the operating room under local anesthesia. The client is medicated before the procedure to relax him or her and reduce discomfort. The catheters are tunneled under the skin before they enter the peritoneal cavity to stabilize the catheter and reduce the risk of infection.

Figure 57–2 illustrates three types of peritoneal catheters. The Tenckhoff catheter has two Dacron felt cuffs bonded to the catheter. Over a period of 1 to 2 weeks, there is an ingrowth of fibroblasts and blood vessels into the cuffs, which fix the catheter in place and provide an effective barrier against dialysate leakage and bacterial invasion. Note in Figure 57–2 that a subcutaneous tunnel is created for the catheter to further reduce direct bacterial invasion into the peritoneum. The other catheters illustrated also have cuffs that provide stable placement.

Complications of Peritoneal Dialysis

Although peritoneal dialysis is considered a safe procedure, there are a number of complications that can be attributed to it.

Peritonitis. Peritonitis is the major concern; therefore, meticulous aseptic technique must be adhered to in handling the catheter, tubing and dialysate solution. Manifestations include fever, rebound tenderness, nausea, malaise, and a cloudy dialysate output. If peritonitis develops, appropriate antibiotics are added to the dialysate; in addition, systemic antibiotics may be used. Bacteria may enter the peritoneal cavity through contaminated dialysis fluid, a contaminated catheter lumen, or the catheter insertion site.

Laboratory tests routinely used to diagnose peritonitis include white blood cell counts with differential, culture, and sensitivity, and Gram stain of the peritoneal fluid. Peritonitis is diagnosed when the dialysate white blood

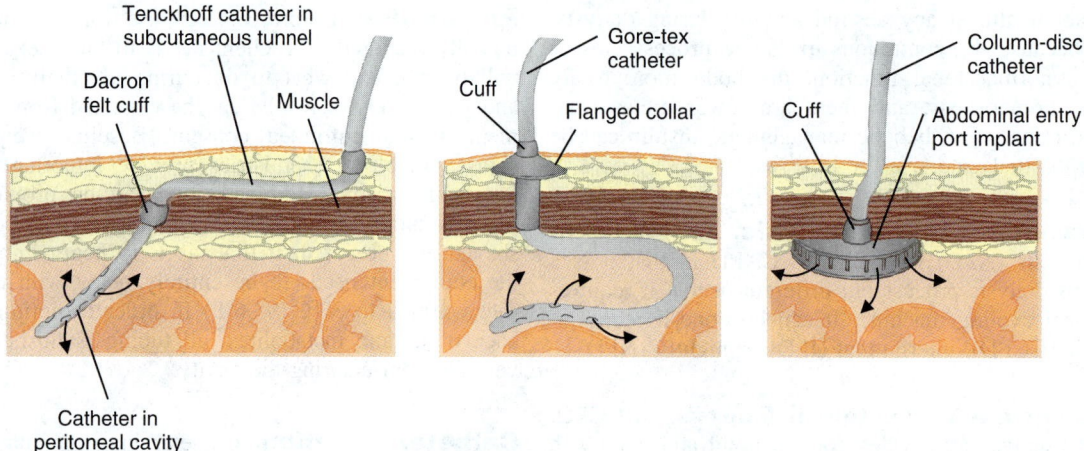

Figure 57–2. Three types of peritoneal dialysis catheter. The Tenckhoff catheter has two Dacron felt cuffs that hold the catheter in place and prevent dialysate leakage and bacterial invasion; a subcutaneous tunnel also helps to prevent infection. The Gore-Tex catheter has a Dacron cuff above a flanged collar. The column-disc catheter has a cuff and a large abdominal entry port implant.

cell count is greater than $100/mm^3$ and neutrophils are greater than 50%. Routine cultures may not grow the causative organism, but a Gram stain will be positive in 9% to 40% of the samples.

Catheter-Related Complications.

Catheter problems include displacement and plugging. Obstruction may be due to malposition, adherence of the catheter tip to the omentum, or infection. Constipation can reduce catheter flow, possibly because peristalsis facilitates outflow. A bisacodyl suppository may be used prophylactically even if the client is not constipated. Fluid leakage may indicate improper catheter function, incomplete healing of the insertion site, or excessive instillation. Especially in the early stages, it is sometimes necessary to use small-volume instillations. Bloody effluent is usually insignificant and will disappear spontaneously. However, it may indicate bowel perforation, which is most likely to occur in cachectic clients or where there are abdominal adhesions. Fecal material returned in the dialysate or massive diarrhea after instillation may also signal perforation. Bladder perforation can also occur if the bladder has not been emptied before catheter insertion.

Dialysis-Related Complications.

Pain during dialysis may result from rapid instillation, incorrect dialysate pH or temperature, dialysate accumulation under the diaphragm, or excessive suction during outflow. Some pain is expected in the early stages but should disappear after 1 to 2 weeks. Low back pain may develop with continuous dialysis procedures because of the abdominal weight affecting posture; appropriate exercises help relieve this problem. Hernia may occur. Systemic cardiovascular and neurologic effects are usually the result of fluid and electrolyte imbalances. Especially during small-volume exchanges, a significant amount of the dialysate fluid may be absorbed by the body.

Hypotension may result from too rapid removal of fluid. Overhydration, from insufficient fluid removal, may

be manifested as congestive heart failure and pulmonary edema. Hypoalbuminemia leading to hypovolemia often occurs because the peritoneal membrane allows the passage of albumin, as much as 100 g/day if the client is infected. This is especially a problem if dietary intake of protein is poor, the client is infected, or dialysis treatment is used for several consecutive days. Hyperglycemia may occur in diabetic clients as a result of absorption of glucose from the dialysate and electrolyte changes. These clients require extra insulin. Respiratory difficulties may occur during dwell time because of pressure on the diaphragm. Weight gain may occur in any client due to the high concentration of glucose in the dialysate.

Hemodialysis

Hemodialysis is used for clients with acute or irreversible renal failure and fluid and electrolyte imbalances. It is usually the treatment of choice when toxic agents, such as barbiturate overdose, need to be removed from the body quickly.

Historical Overview

The first "artificial kidney" was developed in 1943 in the Netherlands. In 1960, the first successful treatment of clients with CRF was reported. In the early years, although the technology was available, the exorbitant cost and the lack of equipment required that a stringent selection process be followed in choosing clients for hemodialysis. Clients were screened as to their motivation, intelligence, emotional stability, and rehabilitative potential. In essence, it had to be decided who among the many potential candidates would best be able to cope with the program and who would make the biggest contribution to society.

In 1972, an amendment to the Social Security Act required that anyone with CRF would be able to have any life-saving treatment needed. In 1973, Medicare took over the financial responsibility for many clients on hemodialysis. Thus, the availability of this treatment mode for clients with end-stage renal failure has become more prevalent. Generally self-selection is the only criterion used now. As a result, the population receiving hemodialysis now represents a wide cross-section in terms of age, rehabilitative potential, and socioeconomic status. There continue to be problems with selection of appropriate candidates, when to start, and when and how to stop. With the decrease in health care dollars, the problems associated with selection criteria will only increase.

Procedure for Hemodialysis

The procedure for hemodialysis involves diverting toxin-laden blood from the client into a dialyzer and then returning the clean blood to the client. Figure 57–3 schematically illustrates a typical hemodialysis system. While the blood is within the dialyzer, the dialysis fluid is delivered by a mechanical proportioning pump to flow on the other side of the membrane. Toxins diffuse across the membrane from the blood to the dialysate. Strict asepsis must be maintained throughout the procedure.

One of the vital aspects of hemodialysis is the establishment and maintenance of adequate blood access. Without it, hemodialysis cannot be done. The major routes of access are external arteriovenous shunts and subclavian catheters for acute dialysis and internal arteriovenous fistulas and grafts for chronic dialysis.

The external arteriovenous shunt requires the surgical placement of two Silastic cannulas into the forearm or leg. The two cannulas are connected to form a U shape. Blood flows from the client's artery through the shunt into the vein.

When the client is to be connected to the hemodialyzer, a tube leading to the membrane compartment is connected to the arterial cannula. Blood then fills the membrane compartment and flows back to the client by way of a tube connected to the venous cannula. When the dialysis is completed, the arterial cannula is clamped. Once the blood in the membrane compartment has been returned to the body, the venous cannula is clamped, and the ends of the two cannulas are reattached to form their U. This access can be created quickly and so is particularly suited to situations in which dialysis must be started immediately. Infection at the site of insertion and clotting are frequent complications that often necessitate moving the cannula sites. Other problems that occur with shunts are accidental dislodgement, hemorrhage, and skin erosion.

The internal arteriovenous fistula is the access of choice for chronic dialysis clients. The fistula is created through a surgical procedure in which an artery in the arm is anastomosed to a vein in an end-to-side, side-to-side, side-to-end, or end-to-end fashion (Fig. 57–5A). This creates an opening or fistula between a large artery and a large vein. The flow of arterial blood into the venous system causes the veins to become engorged (Fig. 57–5B). These fistulas require 1 to 2 weeks to mature before they can be used, which makes this approach inap-

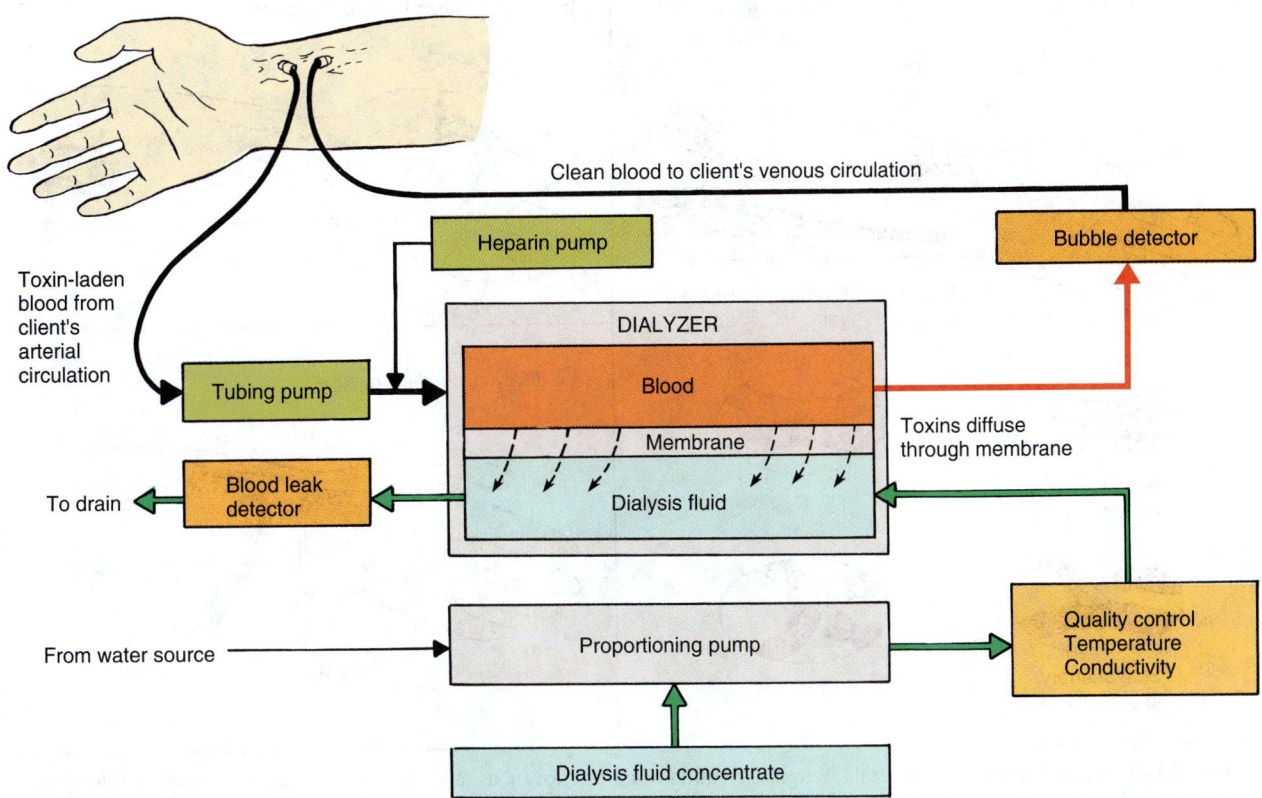

Figure 57–3. Typical hemodialysis system. Toxin-laden blood from the client diffuses across the membrane within the dialyzer into the dialysis fluid. Clean blood is returned to the client.

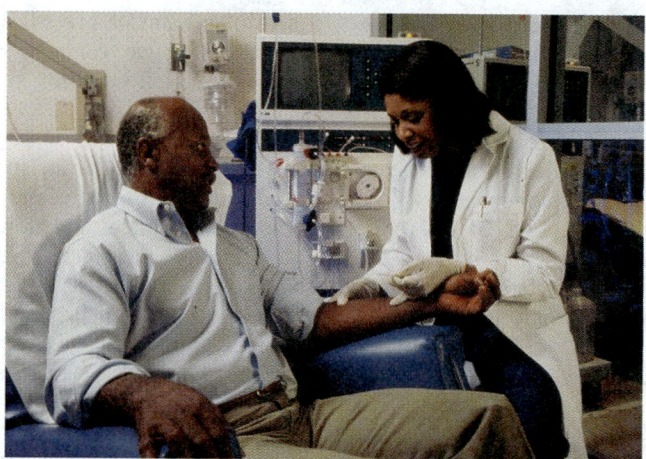

Figure 57–4. A client undergoing outpatient hemodialysis.

propriate for immediate hemodialysis. Peritoneal dialysis or external arteriovenous shunts may be used while the fistula is maturing.

The internal arteriovenous graft is used primarily for chronic dialysis. This access uses an artificial graft made of Gore-Tex or a bovine carotid artery to create an artifi-

cial vein for blood flow. The graft is used in clients who do not have adequate blood vessels for surgical creation of a fistula. One end of the artificial graft is anastomosed to an artery, tunneled under the skin, and anastomosed to a vein. The graft can be used 2 weeks after insertion. Complications include clotting, aneurysms, and infection.

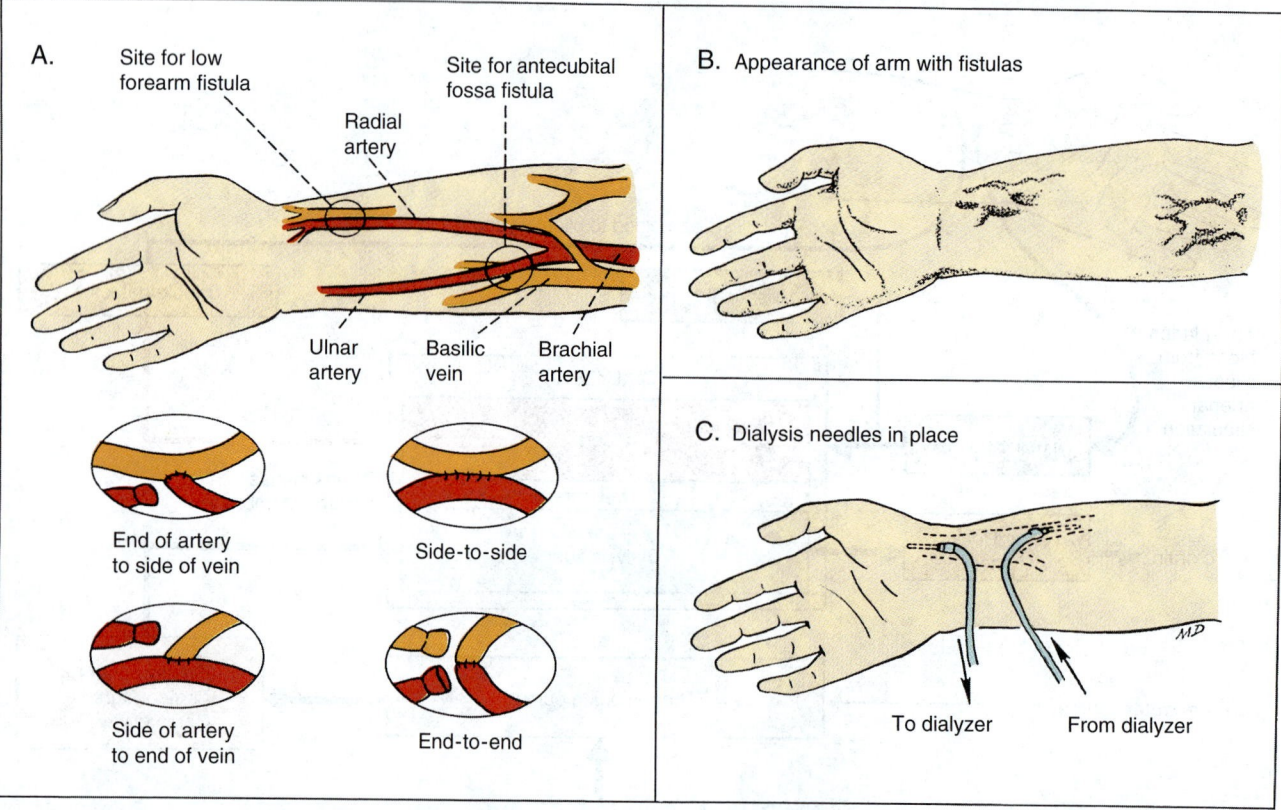

Figure 57–5. Internal arteriovenous fistula. Surgical creation of an arteriovenous anastomosis provides easy access to blood for hemodialysis. This method reduces the risk of infection and makes external shunts unnecessary except during hemodialysis. The internal fistula must be created 2 to 6 weeks before it can be used. Note that in this illustration, arteries, not veins, are toned. *A*, Types of fistulas. *B*, Appearance of arm with fistula. *C*, Dialysis needles in place.

Once the access is placed and ready for use, two 15- or 16-gauge needles are placed in the vein at each dialysis treatment (Fig. 57–5C). A pump pulls arterial blood out of the vein by way of the fistula and into the hemodialyzer. Blood returns to the client by a tube connected to the other needle. Another method of accessing the fistula is with single-needle dialysis. This device means that only one puncture is required each time, but there may be significant recirculation of dialyzed blood, meaning that clearance rates are decreased. Internal arteriovenous accesses may cause hand swelling or ischemia (steal syndrome), carpal tunnel syndrome, hemorrhage, thrombosis, and aneurysms.

Besides the arm, the ankle is the most common site used for venous access (Fig. 57–6). Figure 57–6 also shows two alternative sites—the subclavian area and the thigh.

Subclavian and femoral catheters can be inserted at the bedside for use as a vascular access. Subclavian catheters may be used as a temporary or permanent access for hemodialysis. Permanent catheters are surgically placed in the operating room and have Dacron cuffs that are implanted under the skin to anchor the catheter in place. Femoral catheters are always a temporary source of blood flow and must be replaced frequently to prevent infection.

Dialyzers

There are several types of dialyzers available. These include flat plate and hollow fiber mold. Choice of a particular system is mostly a matter of preference. Many chronic dialysis centers now reprocess and disinfect the unit and reuse it on the same client as a way to reduce costs. The dialysate solution is altered to fit the client's need.

Hemodialysis Schedules

Hemodialysis as a treatment of irreversible renal failure must be continued intermittently for the client's lifetime, unless a successful kidney transplant is done. A typical schedule is 3 to 4 hours of treatment 3 days per week. This schedule will vary with the size of the client, the type of dialyzer used, the rate of blood flow, the personal preference of the client, and other factors.

Therapeutic Effects of Hemodialysis

The overall therapeutic effect of hemodialysis is to clear waste products from the body; restore fluid, electrolyte, and acid-base balances; and reverse some of the untoward manifestations of irreversible renal failure. Success is varied. Excess fluid, potassium, urea nitrogen, and acid ions are removed but only temporarily; between dialyses, these elements will build up again. Nutritionally, carbohydrate intolerance is usually reduced. Amino acids, protein, glucose, and water-soluble vitamins are lost. The anemia is generally enhanced. The predialysis causative factors are still present, and additional losses occur during dialysis because of blood sampling, residual blood left in the dialyzer, and bleeding secondary to anticoagulation during dialysis. Serum iron stores are also further depleted. Hyperlipidemia seems to increase and is associated with accelerated atherosclerosis. Renal osteodystrophy usually improves, and this can be further enhanced by adding calcium to the dialysate. Pruritus may occur for reasons not yet understood. Men on maintenance dialysis often develop gynecomastia, which is usually transient. This occurs because of low testosterone levels. Many other sexual manifestations of uremia are reversed after a period of adaptation.

The usual effect of hemodialysis on serum concentration of medications is increased clearance. This is therapeutic in the case of overdose. Dosage schedules are altered to prevent, as much as possible, loss of medications through dialysis. Supplemental doses may be necessary to maintain therapeutic levels of certain medications.

Complications of Long-Term Hemodialysis

In addition to the therapeutic effects, there are a number of complications involved with chronic hemodialysis. These include technical problems, such as blood leaks, overheating of the dialysate solution, insufficient loss of fluid, improper concentration of salts in the dialysate, and clotting; hypotension or hypertension; cardiac arrhythmias from potassium imbalance; air embolus; hemorrhage from heparinization with particular concern for subdural, retroperitoneal, pericardial, and intraocular bleeding; restless legs syndrome; and pyrogenic reactions. Gastrointestinal ulcer disease is often complicated by hemorrhage. Muscle cramps may occur as a result of hyponatremia or hypo-

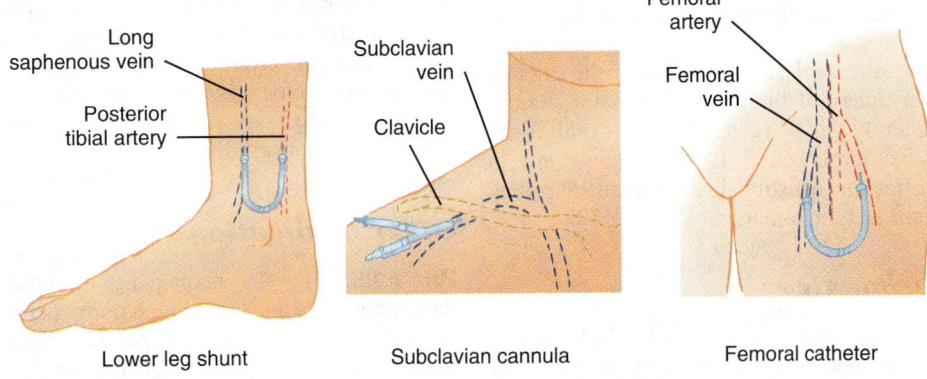

Figure 57–6. Alternative access areas for hemodialysis: ankle, clavicle, and thigh.

osmolality and too rapid removal of fluid. Infection is a significant complication, with hepatitis B being most common. Frequent infectious processes include local access infection, bacteremia, and infectious endocarditis.

Dialysis equilibrium syndrome is a complication that can occur, particularly during the client's first few dialysis episodes. It is characterized by mental confusion, deterioration of the level of consciousness, headache, and seizures and may last for several days. Rapid solute removal from the blood probably causes a relative excess of solutes interstitially or intracellularly (an osmotic gradient). This causes organ swelling, which interferes with normal physiologic function. Many dialysis centers avoid this complication by first-time dialyzing for shorter time periods at a reduced blood flow rate.

Aluminum intoxication occurs because of aluminum accumulation from phosphate binders. It leads to mental cloudiness, dementia, and infiltration of the bone with aluminum leading to significant pain. Aluminum chelating agents may be administered so that aluminum is freed up and dialyzed from the body.

Diuretics

Diuretics may be used early to stimulate excretion of water by the kidneys. The appearance of edema indicates fluid overload, but some physicians prefer to have a little end-of-the-day edema so that it is more evident that fluid depletion is not a danger. Thirst is not a reliable indicator; if thirst were used as a guide, fluid overload would be inevitable. As renal failure progresses, it usually becomes necessary to restrict fluid intake. Although authorities differ in their exact amounts, daily fluid allowances may be 400 to 1000 ml plus measured output. Diuretics are not given prior to dialysis because of potential problems with hypotension. Anti-hypertensive medications are also held until after dialysis.

Vitamins and Minerals

Vitamin supplements of water-soluble vitamins (e.g., folic acid, pyridoxine, ascorbic acid) are usually given because low protein diets are typically deficient in these. Water-soluble vitamins may need to be replaced in clients on dialysis therapy. Vitamin A supplements should be avoided unless total parenteral nutrition is to be used exclusively for several weeks. Vitamin D supplements may be necessary. Work is being done to determine the efficacy of replacing trace elements, such as iron and zinc.

Iron sulfate and folic acid are used only if the anemia is caused by a deficiency of the respective factor. Parenteral iron is frequently given rather than the oral form. Androgens may be administered if the kidneys are in place, but their effect is questionable. Transfusions may be used if the client is symptomatic.

Sodium Bicarbonate

Acidosis contributes to many of the undesirable effects of CRF. Sodium bicarbonate may be used to correct this imbalance. Shohl's solution, a mixture of sodium citrate

and citric acid, may be administered, although it may also promote stomatitis.

Erythropoietin

The primary treatment of anemia in CRF clients is erythropoietin, a hormone produced in the kidney to stimulate red blood cell production. Erythropoietin has been produced by recombinant DNA and is available for intravenous and subcutaneous administration. Epoetin alpha (EPO) is usually given subcutaneously three times a week. With adequate iron stores, vitamin B_{12}, and folic acid, anemia can be corrected in most clients within 3 to 4 months.

Calcium Preparations and Phosphorus Binders

Much of the treatment of renal osteodystrophy involves dietary and medication regulation of calcium, phosphorus, and acidosis, as directed. The hyperparathyroidism must also be brought under control. Vitamin D in its active form may be used, although it must be administered with care because of its severe side effects from metastatic calcifications. Calciferol helps promote bone mineralization by increasing the intestinal absorption of calcium and decreasing circulating parathyroid hormone and alkaline phosphatase. Some advocate subtotal parathyroidectomy if all other methods fail.

Phosphorus intake is limited to less than 1000 mg/day. To improve excretion of phosphorus, the client is given an aluminum hydroxide antacid such as Alu-Cap, Amphojel, or Basaljel with meals to bind the phosphorus so it can be excreted in the feces. Recently, calcium-based phosphate binders such as calcium carbonate in the form of Tums or calcium acetate are being administered. This reduces the risk of developing dementia related to excessive absorption of aluminum, which can occur when aluminum-based products are used.

Antihypertensives

Fluid and sodium regulation are the major interventions in congestive heart failure. Other cardiovascular manifestations are managed much the same as for clients without CRF, but diuretics are not used except in the very early stages of conservative management. Hypertension must be aggressively controlled with stronger medications such as angiotensin-converting enzyme (ACE) inhibitors and calcium channel blockers. Antihypertensive drugs are administered as necessary in relation to renal function and nephrotic response.

Other Medications

Pericarditis may be managed with nonsteroidal anti-inflammatory agents but may require pericardial aspiration or pericardial window. Tamponade (fluid in the pericardium) necessitates pericardial drainage. Some work is being done with local steroid instillation through an indwelling pericardial catheter. If conservative methods are unsuccessful, cardiac surgery to achieve revascularization or to replace a diseased valve may be performed.

Dietary Management

Dietary adjustment is dictated by many components of CRF, including accumulation of nitrogenous waste products, impaired excretion of electrolytes, vitamin deficiencies, and continued catabolism. The wasting syndrome is a major problem. The client with renal failure constantly loses body weight, muscle mass, and adipose tissue.

Specific adjustments of dietary elements often depend on the results of blood chemistry studies. Although there is some debate concerning whether and how to restrict proteins, studies are now indicating that maintaining a daily intake of high-biologic-value protein below 50 g may slow the progression of renal failure. Generally, recommendations range from no restriction other than avoiding high protein fad diets to restrictions of 1 g/kg/day. This protein must be of high biologic value so that the essential amino acids can be used more efficiently with less nitrogenous waste. This restriction of proteins also limits accumulation of acid, potassium, and phosphate.

It is also important to provide adequate nonprotein calories to prevent or reduce catabolism. One recommendation is 40 to 50 kcal/kg/day of carbohydrates and fats. As the renal disease progresses, the client's ability and willingness to take in adequate nutrition diminishes, and the challenge becomes not only to maintain appropriate intake of nonprotein calories but to satisfy protein needs as well. In these instances, elemental diets, enteral feedings, or total parenteral nutrition may be used instead of or in addition to regular food intake.

Dietary electrolytes may be encouraged or restricted. The regulation of sodium is a delicate matter. At times the kidneys are salt wasters, and sodium must be encouraged to replace that which is lost. More frequently, however, the kidneys retain sodium and dietary intake. Some believe there should be a moderate restriction with careful monitoring of urinary sodium excretion as a guideline. Serial monitoring of data indicating fluid status also gives important information about sodium needs. Many regimens are used.

Potassium is frequently restricted. Clients must be reminded not to use salt substitutes because they contain potassium chloride. When *hyperkalemia* becomes evident, restriction of potassium in food and fluids is instituted. In an emergency situation, when the serum potassium is above 7.0, intravenous glucose ($D_{50}W$), insulin, and calcium gluconate or oral or rectal sodium polystyrene sulfonate (Kayexalate), a cation exchange resin, may be given. Dissolving the resin in ginger ale helps to (1) prevent it from sticking to the teeth and (2) mask its gritty texture. Sorbitol is usually given with the resin to avoid constipation and counteract the sodium retention that can occur. Dialysis is also effective in removing potassium from the blood.

If serum calcium levels are low, adequate calcium intake is important. Dietary sources may be supplemented with calcium carbonate, calcium lactate, or calcium gluconate. Supplements are definitely needed for clients receiving dialysis therapy. However, if serum calcium levels are high, dietary restriction may be recommended. Phosphorus is restricted. In addition, phosphate-binding gels such as aluminum hydroxide, aluminum carbonate, and calcium carbonate may be used to further reduce phosphorus levels. These agents must be administered cautiously in clients who have had a parathyroidectomy for secondary hyperparathyroidism, because aluminum deposition on bony surfaces is enhanced. Aluminum intoxication also leads to encephalopathy and osteomalacia. Finally, a mild magnesium restriction may be imposed.

■ Nursing Management of the Medical Client

Assessment

When the client is suspected of having CRF, take a complete history and look closely for the presence of risk factors. It is important to question clients about past and present medications, diet and weight changes, energy levels and unexplained fatigue, and the pattern of urinary elimination.

Assess the client for the presence of the multiple effects of CRF on all body systems, such as the presence of cardiovascular or respiratory abnormalities, neurologic changes, gastrointestinal problems, or skin changes.

Also assess the client's understanding of CRF, the diagnostic tests that will be done, and the possible treatment regimens. Assess the client's level of anxiety and his or her ability to cope. Also involve the family in the assessment to determine *their* ability to cope with the disease and treatments.

When the client has been diagnosed with CRF and is being treated by peritoneal dialysis, assess the client's and significant others' understanding of the treatment regimen. The client and significant others, the nephrologist, and the nephrology nurse discuss the use of peritoneal dialysis and decide which type most meets the client's needs. The client's understanding of the treatment is also important to assess, as is the client's ability to cope with the treatment regimen. The family's ability to cope and their ability to support the client is also vital.

Once the client has begun peritoneal dialysis, the priority assessment for the nurse is the presence of an infection. Inspect the insertion site carefully for redness or other manifestations of infection. Carefully assess the effluent after it is drained for the presence of cloudiness, fibrin streaks, or blood. Monitor vital signs and weight closely.

If the client is undergoing hemodialysis, the priority assessment becomes the patency of the venous access site. It is vital that this site be assessed for possible occlusion or, if it is an external site, for the presence of infection. The client's understanding of the access site and care of it should be ascertained.

Diagnosis, Planning, Implementation

Fluid Volume Deficit or Fluid Volume Excess. As with all renal disorders, a common diagnosis is *Fluid Volume Deficit* or *Fluid Volume Excess related to impaired renal function.*

Planning: Expected Outcomes. The client will develop neither a fluid volume deficit nor excess, as evidenced by no manifestations of edema or dehydration.

Implementation. A fluid volume deficit or overload is a cardinal problem. The current fluid status must be known and fluid intake carefully regulated, depending on the status. Monitor fluid status by observing daily weight, orthostatic blood pressure, skin turgor, and mucous membrane moistness and by meticulous intake and output comparisons. Give learning guidelines to clients being followed on an ambulatory basis concerning (1) how to weigh themselves and (2) how to interpret the relationship of daily weight loss or gain to their need for sodium and water. Help clients understand that vomiting, diarrhea, and working or playing in a hot environment may cause excessive fluid loss and must be prevented or controlled. Teach clients how to take their blood pressure.

Once the fluid allowance for the day has been determined, help the client follow the recommendation. The assistance needed usually concerns restricting fluid intake. Offer suggestions about reducing thirst and moistening dry mucous membranes with lip balms, frequent oral hygiene, ice chips, or spray bottles. Spread out fluid intake over a longer period of time. If intravenous fluids are used, carefully attend to them to ensure proper administration rates. Water is often restricted so that clients will drink more nutritious liquids such as apple or cranberry juice or milk.

Altered Nutrition: Less than Body Requirements.
Yet another common diagnosis in CRF is *Altered Nutrition: Less than Body Requirements, related to anorexia, nausea.*

Planning: Expected Outcomes. The client will maintain adequate nutrition, as evidenced by maintenance of weight without loss of muscle mass.

Implementation. Dietary management is vital to the conservative management of CRF. Anorexia results from many of the manifestations of irreversible renal failure, emotional depression, and a frequently unpalatable diet. Thus, a major nursing challenge is helping the client take in adequate nutrition while minimizing uremic toxicity. This problem grows as the disease progresses and clients may develop an aversion to meat and other sources of protein. To help stimulate the client's appetite, take measures to relieve nausea and vomiting, stomatitis, and other gastrointestinal manifestations. Diet counseling is essential for compliance. Arrange for dietary consultation if appropriate. The client needs to know how to translate the dietary regimen into a palatable, understandable food program. Help the client select and prepare foods and learn where to obtain special foods if necessary. Exercise may also improve appetite.

Constipation.
The treatment of CRF leads to the predictable diagnosis of *Constipation related to medications, fluid and dietary restrictions, and decreased activity level.*

Planning: Expected Outcomes. The client will not develop constipation, as evidenced by a bowel movement at least every other day.

Implementation. Constipation is almost a universal problem for clients with CRF. Fluid restrictions, inability to eat most high fiber foods, and activity intolerance reduce the ability to use customary measures for preventing constipation. In addition, phosphate-binding agents contribute to this problem. Bran, which is not rich in potassium or phosphorus, can be used. Stool softeners are often administered on a regular basis, although care must be taken with those agents containing significant calcium and sodium. If necessary, bulk laxatives (e.g., psyllium hydrophilic mucilloid) may be given. It is important that the recommended amount of fluid be taken with the powder, and this amount subtracted from the day's fluid allotment. Stimulant and lubricant laxatives should be used only if necessary, especially compounds containing magnesium or phosphorus, such as Fleet enema. If none of these measures is effective, small-volume, gentle stimulant enemas may be used sparingly, but large-volume enemas must be avoided because of possible fluid and saline absorption. Renal failure clients are at risk for the development of diverticular disease.

Fatigue.
The physiologic alterations and the stress can be summed up as *Fatigue related to anemia and altered metabolic state.*

Planning: Expected Outcomes. The client will have a balance of rest and activity, as evidenced by the client's statement of decreased fatigue.

Implementation. Rest is important to any client whose body is under a great deal of stress. Encourage frequent naps. Insomnia is frequently a problem, and you may need to make suggestions about how to solve this problem (e.g., presleep quiet time and establishing a presleep routine). Hypnotics and sedatives must be used very cautiously because they may alter mentation. The client also needs to establish and maintain an appropriate exercise program. Discourage strenuous exercise, however, because it increases catabolism. Treat anemia to increase energy levels.

Risk for Impaired Skin Integrity.
The edema and integumentary changes presage a *Risk for Impaired Skin Integrity related to edema, dryness of skin, and pruritus.*

Planning: Expected Outcomes. The client will not develop impaired skin integrity, as evidenced by intact skin.

Implementation. Dry skin is a common problem. Moisturizing oils in the bath water or applied directly to the skin help correct this problem. Whereas the use of soaps may need to be curtailed, keep the skin clean, because the client is susceptible to secondary infection. Avoid any products containing alcohol or perfumes; these increase dryness and pruritus. If edema is present, avoid sustained pressure on the area. The potential for skin breakdown is particularly acute in the diabetic patient. Observe for poor circulation and areas of breakdown or infection.

Risk for Ineffective Family Coping.
Inevitably, the diagnosis *Risk for Ineffective Family Coping related to chronic illness, uncertain future of the client, and role reversal* must be dealt with.

Planning: Expected Outcomes. The family will cope with the client's chronic illness and future deterioration, as evidenced by acceptance of the client's problems and ability to support the client.

Implementation. Clients with CRF face a future that promises continued deterioration, but with an unknown course and timetable. In addition, the disease itself produces behavioral manifestations that contribute to the client's susceptibility to stress. Clients are often required to make important decisions about the choice of treatment modes at a time when they do not feel well. The client and significant others have many questions about such things as family, job or school, dependency, and sex life. The client may suffer from reduced self-esteem. Encourage the client and significant others to discuss their feelings and concerns, using therapeutic communication techniques. To develop an individualized nursing care plan, the nurse also needs to assess how the client handled change and stress before onset of the illness.

Knowledge Deficit. A commonplace is the diagnosis *Knowledge Deficit related to the disease process and its treatment.*

Planning: Expected Outcomes. The client will understand the disease process and treatment regimen, as evidenced by his or her ability to describe the disease and its treatment and to participate in the treatment regimen.

Implementation. Teaching is a crucial part of the nursing management plan. Most of the time, the client will be followed on an ambulatory basis and will be responsible for following the recommended treatment regimen. The client and significant others must know about normal renal function and how the disease has altered it, the details of the management protocol and how to follow it, a number of self-assessment skills as described earlier, and when to seek professional consultation for possible complications.

Although clients with renal disease need to learn about their disorder, they may not always be ready to learn.

Anxiety itself interferes with learning. In addition, the disease retards normal mental functioning; memory deficits and a short attention span may require simple presentations and frequent repeating of information. Retained learning must be continually evaluated.

Significant others may be especially frustrated during teaching sessions by the client's inability to grasp the concepts being presented. The client may seem out of touch with reality. Significant others need reassurance that this is an effect of the disease itself and that the client will become more capable of learning, especially after institution of dialysis.

With the exception of insertion and removal of the peritoneal catheter, peritoneal dialysis is primarily a nursing intervention. The nurse monitors the client, plans care, and, in many instances, teaches the client how to do the procedure independently.

Risk for Ineffective Management of Therapeutic Regimen (Individuals) and Risk for Ineffective Management of Therapeutic Regimen: Families. There is always a *Risk for Ineffective Management of Therapeutic Regimen (Individuals) and Risk for Ineffective Management of Therapeutic Regimen: Families related to nutritional needs during dialysis.*

Planning: Expected Outcomes. The client will understand nutritional needs during dialysis and the possible home dialysis program, as evidenced by discussions with the client.

Implementation. Providing adequate nutrition is often easier during dialysis and for a time afterward. Dialysis usually relieves many of the gastrointestinal problems that frequently interfere with adequate intake. Food and fluid restrictions are usually liberalized just before dialysis but must be reimposed afterward. As a result, sodium and water are metabolized and ready to be dialyzed during actual dialysis.

Dietary noncompliance remains a major problem during maintenance dialysis, and it may require all the nurse's knowledge and creativity to help the client follow the recommended regimen.

CLIENT EDUCATION GUIDE

Chronic Renal Failure

Learn about your medications: purpose, dosage, administration, side effects, and toxic effects.

Learn the manifestations of infection, venous access blockage, and graft rejection.

Learn how to avoid infections and how to manage them when they occur.

Follow your dietary regimen, learn the rationale for it, and learn how to prepare meals.

Learn about the possibility of transplantation and the implications associated with this treatment.

Enlist in an exercise program to help maintain body functions.

Fluid Volume Excess or Fluid Volume Deficit. A problem in dialysis is *Fluid Volume Excess or Fluid Volume Deficit related to fluid shifts between blood and dialysate* and blood loss associated with hemodialysis.

Planning: Expected Outcomes. The client will not develop fluid volume excess or deficit, as evidenced by absence of disequilibrium syndrome.

Implementation. Throughout the process, carefully monitor the client's vital signs, including postural blood pressure, pulse, weight, and intake and output. Fingersticks for blood glucose are done. Watch for the development of hypovolemia and the retention of dialysate. The amount of desired fluid loss will be determined by the dialysis physician. If fluid cannot be drained during dialysis, check the system for kinks or other obstructions. Report fluid accumulations exceeding the limits set in the dialysis orders to the physician. For clients undergoing hemodialysis, monitor the effects of anticoagulants and blood clotting during dialysis. When the dialysis is completed, make sure that all fluids are returned to the client.

Risk for Infection. Indwelling catheters carry a high *Risk for Infection related to the presence of an indwelling peritoneal catheter and instillation of dialysate* and related to venipuncture or connection of tubing during hemodialysis.

Planning: Expected Outcomes. The client will not develop an infection, as evidenced by a normal white blood cell count, absence of fever, and clear dialysate.

Implementation. Because peritonitis is the main complication of peritoneal dialysis, strict aseptic technique must be used throughout the procedure. Masks are worn by the nurse and client when the peritoneal dialysis circuit is opened. Gloves are worn by anyone touching the catheter during all connections and disconnection procedures. The catheter is soaked before and after these procedures in a povidone-iodine solution. Dressing changes around the catheter site are ordered per specific unit protocol. Be sure dressings are kept dry at all times. With hemodialysis, use strict aseptic technique during venipuncture or when attaching the tubing and solution.

Risk for Ineffective Breathing Pattern. Dialysis also entails *Risk for Ineffective Breathing Pattern related to pressure of dialysate* during peritoneal dialysis.

Planning: Expected Outcomes. The client will have an effective breathing pattern, as evidenced by absence of shortness of breath.

Implementation. Because of pressure on the diaphragm by the dialysate, its full excursion may be reduced. The immobilized client may be at risk for the development of respiratory problems. Encourage the client to cough and deep-breathe regularly. Keep the client in a semi-Fowler position to ease breathing. The client also needs to be alert for early manifestations of compromised respiratory function.

Knowledge Deficit. A common diagnosis is *Knowledge Deficit related to peritoneal dialysis and its impact.*

Planning: Expected Outcomes. The client will understand peritoneal dialysis and its impact, as evidenced by client discussion.

Implementation. The client and significant others may have meaningful levels of anxiety and many concerns about peritoneal dialysis and its impact on their lives. Therapeutic communication by the nurse helps them cope with these concerns. If the client will be having long-term dialysis, the client and significant others may have a prolonged relationship with the nurse, and the nurse should be constantly working to establish and maintain a supportive, therapeutic rapport with them. If the client is immobilized during the day for treatment, the nurse may need to help the client develop appropriate diversionary activities.

The client and significant others need to know about peritoneal dialysis and how to work with its ramifications.

Because so many clients continue this treatment mode in their homes, this knowledge needs to be complete and detailed. They require a complete training program so they can handle the entire dialysis process independently.

Continuous monitoring during dialysis provides vital information about the progress of the treatment and allows early diagnosis of potential complications. There should be a well-organized plan for observing and recording vital signs, dialysate composition and temperature, and functioning of the entire dialysis system and blood flow. The client should also be alert to early manifestations of potential complications, as listed earlier. The nurse often serves as case manager and coordinates the services provided by the nephrology team, which includes the physician, nurses, social worker, and dietitian.

Risk for Ineffective Family Coping. Peritoneal dialysis requires the diagnosis *Risk for Ineffective Family Coping related to chronic treatment and possible home dialysis program.*

Planning: Expected Outcomes. The client will cope with chronic treatment, as evidenced by the family's ability to work with the client and offer support.

Implementation. The number of clients availing themselves of home dialysis is about 15% of all clients receiving dialysis. The cost of this type of program is less than in-center dialysis, and usually the client's quality of life is improved. Home dialysis offers the client more access to significant others and greater feelings of independence and control. However, this type of treatment also produces stress on personal relationships, especially on the person who becomes the "dialyzer helper" during home hemodialysis. Some spouses have voiced concern about the lack of free time and increased responsibility; others see it as an opportunity to give something back to their spouse or loved one. Some states have funding available to pay for a non–family member to serve as dialysis helper. In some instances, this may reduce tension and improve the quality of life for the family.

Clients for home dialysis programs must be selected carefully. Criteria might include stability of relationships, psychological stability, financial support, and lack of severe physical complications. A successful program requires care providers who are advocates of home dialysis, a good training program, and the provision of good support services (e.g., nursing, medical, and social services; provision of supplies; equipment maintenance; dietary counseling; home visits; and retraining as necessary).

Risk for Injury. Trauma may occur. Write the diagnosis *Risk for Injury related to trauma to hemodialysis venous access site.*

Planning: Expected Outcomes. The client will not suffer injury to the venous access site, as evidenced by continued patency of site.

Implementation. Careful attention to the access site is important to its life expectancy. Care of the access site is designed to prevent infection and clotting. A dressing is used to protect cannulas and subclavian catheters from infection. The access must also be protected from trauma

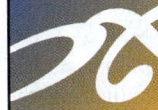

BRIDGE TO HOME HEALTHCARE

Living with Peritoneal Dialysis

Susan Belport-Williams, R.N., B.S.N., C.N.N., C.E.S., *St. Mary Corwin Regional Medical Center, Pueblo, Colorado*

Most clients who begin peritoneal dialysis at home have a real need to take control of their lives. They usually feel better because the process is slower and more natural than the intense hemodialysis treatments, and the fluid and diet restrictions are not as strict. Peritoneal dialysis gives clients the ability to conduct their own treatments in the privacy of their home and travel without the inconvenience of finding a hemodialysis unit in the new area.

The home health nurse or nurse case manager must balance the need for control with the client's other needs, especially in relation to the coordination of healthcare services. Clients and their families who have early warnings of the need for dialysis treatment tend to have a smoother transition physically, emotionally, and financially. They have the opportunity to attend renal dialysis education classes and receive dietary and social work consultation. These clients may have a peritoneal catheter in place and attend clinic sessions 5 days a week for 2 to 3 weeks at the peritoneal dialysis unit. For those clients who have little or no warning about the need for dialysis, the physical and psychosocial impact can be so traumatic that they feel helpless and even depressed. If they lack confidence to perform the procedures at home, their desire to regain control of their lives is threatened. After hospitalization, the client will need to continue hemodialysis until a peritoneal catheter can be placed, and may receive both treatments to allow for healing and the gradual increase of fluid instillation into the peritoneum.

Clients with end-stage renal disease who are on dialysis are eligible for Medicare benefits. The social worker in the dialysis unit can provide information and assistance regarding eligibility and other concerns, such as the cost of medications. The peritoneal dialysis unit is designated as the provider of total services, including nursing services. The clinic nurses can and do make home visits on a limited basis. A peritoneal dialysis nurse is on 24-hour call. If the nurse cannot coach the client or caregiver in resolution of a problem, the client will be asked to go to the emergency room. Therefore, clients who receive Medicare-reimbursed home healthcare must be homebound and require services in addition to their dialysis treatments. For example, a home health nurse may need to assess barriers in the home environment, especially if the client lives in a rural area, some distance from the peritoneal dialysis unit. Also, a home health referral is appropriate if the client and caregiver did not acquire expertise with the treatments at the clinic training sessions. The home health nurse needs to ask questions and listen. Ask the client, "What is a typical day for you?" "What was life like for you before dialysis?" "What do you think life will be like 6 months from now?" and "What would you like to be doing 6 months from now?" The client and family may benefit from joining support groups or obtaining other services locally; consider resources such as the National Kidney Foundation (1–800–638–8299) or the American Kidney Fund (1–800–622–9010). The home health nurse also needs to assess and teach about the clinical manifestations of hypotension, hypertension, fever, and cardiac changes. Such information needs to be communicated to the clinic nurses quickly. Because the last thing that these clients need are staff who "take care" of them, nurses need to consider clients and their families as "self-care" true partners. The sooner the client or family performs the dialysis exchanges and experiences the need to use precautionary processes and procedures, the more confident and successful they will be in regaining control of their lives.

that could cause clotting, bleeding, or physical disruption of the access site. Blood pressure measurement should not be taken on, or blood drawn from, the limb containing the access site. Between dialysis periods, the skin over the fistula or graft requires only routine care with soap and water. The site of a fistula should be carefully assessed. To assess patency, palpate over the fistula for a "thrill," and auscultate for a bruit at regular intervals. The client must also learn to assess for patency.

Risk for Ineffective Individual Coping. Hemodialysis is a lifetime program. Write the diagnosis *Risk for Ineffective Individual Coping related to effects of long-term hemodialysis.*

Planning: Expected Outcomes. The client will cope effectively with the effects of long-term hemodialy-

sis, as evidenced by client's ability to look at alternatives and discuss plans.

Implementation. Much of the care required by clients on chronic peritoneal dialysis and hemodialysis and their significant others revolves around the psychological aspects of dialysis. Clients on maintenance dialysis often have ambivalent feelings. On the one hand, they realize that hemodialysis is their tie to life. Yet, the many restrictions and life-style changes imposed on them make continuation of the program extremely difficult. Clients often report that they feel in limbo between the worlds of life and death.

The process of adaptation to a loss is part of adjustment. It is not uncommon for clients to feel quite grateful and optimistic at the start of their dialysis treatments. Usually they have felt ill for some time, and they view the intervention as a route to survival and a hope for feeling well again. It takes a few days or weeks for them to fully realize the permanent place of dialysis in their lives. Depression during this period is expected. The suicide rate among clients on dialysis has been estimated at 100 times that of the general population.

Three of the most common psychological problems are change in body image, the dependence-independence conflict, and facing, daily, potential death. The client's own feelings of weakness and illness plus the presence of the arteriovenous fistula and dialysis equipment are constant reminders that the client is no longer a "whole person." These clients often play one of three roles: (1) professional patient, in which all of life revolves around the dialysis; (2) rebel, in which the client acts noncompliant or mischievous; or (3) adult, in which the client uses appropriate coping skills and is able to focus outward. Relationships with relatives and friends, job, and community roles and responsibilities will probably be altered. Changes in sexuality emphasize the problem even further. The client's normal need for independence is continually threatened by dependence on the dialysis equipment and care providers. This is especially true of adolescents and young adults. Other emotional problems that have been identified include the need for identity, safety, control of the environment, love, esteem, and communication. The stress on marital relationships and significant others is extreme.

Assistance for the client and significant others must begin before dialysis is started. They need to fully understand the intervention and its implications. Encourage them to discuss their feelings. It is often difficult for clients to voice concerns about continuing dialysis because of its significance. These feelings are often, albeit subconsciously, supported by the nurses; it is sometimes difficult for care providers to accept a client's decision to stop treatment and choose death instead. The nurses, who often become a kind of family to the client, must provide a continued, unified, supportive approach and be ready to accept the whole gamut of reactions to dialysis by the client and significant others. It is helpful to know the client's usual patterns of response to stress. If clients have sound psychosocial coping mechanisms and help from those around them, they usually accommodate themselves to the situation and plan their lives realistically. Clients who handle stress poorly or who have little support from others may never make an adequate adjustment. Active participation by clients in their care is a valuable tool in helping to meet several of the needs identified here.

Evaluation

The expected outcome is that the client is successfully maintained on peritoneal dialysis or hemodialysis. With excellent nursing care aimed at helping the client understand and comply with the therapeutic regimen, the client can learn to manage and cope with the condition.

■ Modifications for Elderly Clients

The types of dialysis for the elderly client will be evaluated on the basis of the presence of other chronic disorders the client may have that would limit the ability to comply with any treatment.

Older clients may have had multiple abdominal surgeries with the development of adhesions that will limit the usefulness of peritoneal dialysis. They are more likely to have pre-existing cardiovascular problems that may limit the usefulness of many venous access sites.

Renal Transplantation

Renal transplantation is the surgical implantation of a human kidney from a compatible donor in a recipient. This procedure is performed as an intervention in irreversible kidney failure.

The first successful kidney transplant was performed in the early 1950s, and transplantation has long since been accepted as a viable alternative for the treatment of end-stage renal disease. A successful transplant prolongs life and markedly improves the quality of life. The client is freed from the restrictions of dialysis and from the reversible manifestations of uremia. However, the procedure is certainly not without risk. In addition to the surgical risks, the immunosuppressive medications that must be taken for the life of the kidney have some potentially serious complications that are discussed later in this chapter.

Over the years, both recipient and graft survival rates have greatly improved. One-year graft survival rates are 85% to 90% in living related donor transplants and 75% to 80% with cadaver kidneys.

The primary limiting factor to the number of transplants done is the availability of kidneys. The Uniform Anatomical Gift Act allows clients to give permission before their own death for the use of their organs for transplantation after their death (requires family consent at the time of potential donation). In 1992, required request legislation was passed, which mandates that hospitals ask family members of dying clients who may be suitable organ donors if they would consider donation. There are also regional and national networks known as Organ Procurement and Transplant Networks (OPTNs) and the United Network of Organ Sharing (UNOS) that have been organized to coordinate the recovery and distribution of organs and tissue for transplantation. Despite these efforts to increase donation, the loss of potentially suitable organs is still very high primarily because of lack of awareness and acceptance by healthcare professionals, families, and the community as a whole. Solution of this problem will require extensive professional and public education about donation and perhaps more legislation enabling organ donation.

Acute and Subacute Care

■ Surgical Management

Selection of a transplant recipient is based on careful evaluation of the client's medical, immunologic, and psychosocial status. The decision is usually made by the client, significant others, and physician working together. Recipient selection is usually from the group less than 70 years of age who have an estimated life expectancy of 2 years or more and in whom the transplant will improve the quality of life.[63] Important psychosocial concerns include the client's (1) feelings about the transplant, (2) understanding and acceptance of the risks and chances of graft survival, and (3) family and social obligations.

Although there are few absolute contraindications to transplantation, some physical conditions markedly increase the risk for the client, primarily because long-term immunosuppressive medications are necessary to avoid graft rejection. Infection and active malignancy are the only absolute contraindications to transplantation. Clients with liver disease, psychological disorders, advanced atherosclerosis, hypertension, respiratory disease, and gastrointestinal bleeding need particular consideration.

Living Related Donors

Because of the higher graft survival rates, the most desirable source of kidneys for transplant is a living related donor who matches the client closely. Willing family members are screened for ABO blood group, tissue-specific antigen, and human leukocyte antigen (HLA) histocompatibility (mixed lymphocyte culture stimulation test). The donors are carefully screened and must be in excellent health. Living related donors are also carefully assessed for emotional well-being and complete understanding of the donation process and outcome. However, the logistic problem of obtaining suitable living related donors for clients needing transplants is extremely difficult. Therefore, most kidneys for transplantation are cadaver organs.

Cadaver Donors

Potential cadaver renal donors must meet the criteria for brain death and the following criteria: under 60 years of age, normal renal function, no malignant disease outside the central nervous system, no generalized infection, no significant hypertension, no abdominal or renal trauma, negative hepatitis B antigen and human immunodeficiency virus (HIV) antibody, and continuous ventilation and heartbeat until the kidneys are surgically removed from the body. Warm ischemic time is the time elapsed between cessation of perfusion and cooling of the kidney plus the time required for anastomosis of the renal artery to the recipient's iliac artery. Maximum allowable warm ischemic time for a usable kidney is 30 to 60 minutes. The kidney can be cooled and the maximum time for transplantation increased to 24 to 48 hours. Once a potential donor has demonstrated cerebral death, it is crucial to restore intravascular volume, wean from vasopressors, and establish diuresis.

Transportation of the Kidney

Once permission has been obtained to remove a suitable cadaver kidney, the major problem becomes one of preserving the kidney during transportation to the recipient so that maximal renal function is maintained. Preservation times also allow adequate time for (1) tissue typing and (2) preparation of the recipient for surgery. Commonly used methods of preservation include simple cold storage, in which the kidney is flushed with a chilled electrolyte solution, and hypothermic pulsatile perfusion. If properly preserved, kidneys can now be kept for 72 hours before implantation, although most kidneys are transplanted within 48 hours.

If the potential donor is a living relative, careful physical and psychosocial assessment is necessary. After histocompatibility has been established, probably the main criterion is that the donor have two properly functioning kidneys, because continued life after the unilateral nephrectomy depends on adequate function of the remaining kidney. Full evaluation of the entire urinary tract is done. The donor also receives a complete examination to rule out any systemic disease that may render the donor unsuitable. Potential family donors must be psychologically evaluated as to their real desire to donate a kidney and their ability to make a lifelong adjustment to having one kidney. Frequently, to avoid conflict of interest, evaluation of the donor is done by a team different from that caring for the recipient. Discussions with the donor should be held in strict confidence; if the donor decides not to donate, the medical team frequently cites a physical contraindication to help ensure continued acceptance of the potential donor by the other family members.

Personal and family relationships are very important factors in the decision to accept a potential donor. A variety of motivations have been reported, including strong altruistic drives, hopes to restore previously destroyed family ties, and religious beliefs. Tremendous pressure may be brought to bear on the potential donor by the recipient and the rest of the family.

If the potential donor is a minor, special legal precautions must be taken during the evaluation period. To neutralize conflict of interest, the court may assign guardians *ad litem* for the child. The final decision is made by these people and the court. The use of young children is controversial; strong opinions are found on both sides of the issue.

The kidney is surgically placed extraperitoneally in the iliac fossa. The renal artery is anastomosed to the recipient's hypogastric artery and the renal vein to the recipient's iliac vein. Figure 57–7 illustrates this.

Usually the kidney begins to function immediately. Sometimes adequate functioning is delayed a few days. Hemodialysis may be performed until good function is established.

Complications

Graft Rejection

Except for the identical twin donor and recipient, the major postoperative complication is graft rejection. This is an immunologic attack against the foreign donor organ that the body has recognized as foreign tissue. The reaction is stimulated by foreign histocompatibility antigens (see Chapter 25). There are three main types of clinical rejection: hyperacute, acute, and chronic. Hyperacute rejection (rare now) occurs at any time, from the moment

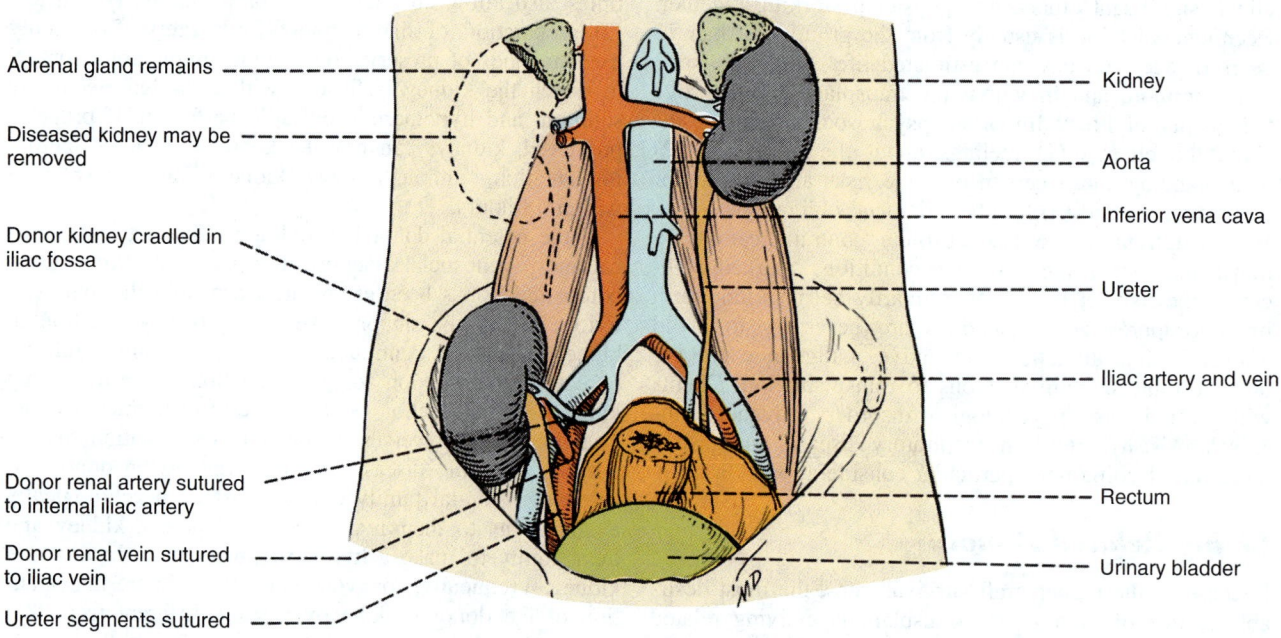

Adrenal gland remains

Diseased kidney may be removed

Donor kidney cradled in iliac fossa

Donor renal artery sutured to internal iliac artery

Donor renal vein sutured to iliac vein

Ureter segments sutured

Kidney

Aorta

Inferior vena cava

Ureter

Iliac artery and vein

Rectum

Urinary bladder

Figure 57–7. Transplanted kidney placement.

of revascularization of the kidney to 48 hours postoperatively. It appears to be caused by circulating cytotoxic antibodies in a presensitized client or transmitted by staphylococcus α-hemolysin toxin or streptococcal infection. The result is destruction of the kidney, and the intervention is immediate donor nephrectomy to avoid development of disseminated intravascular coagulopathy and microangiopathic hemolytic anemia.

Acute rejection usually occurs within 6 weeks after transplant; 3 months is the most common time, but rejection can occur as late as 2 years after transplantation. A cell-mediated process, it produces interstitial edema and vasculitis within the kidney (acute tubular necrosis). Clinical manifestations of this reaction include fever, malaise, elevated white blood cell count, acute hypertension, graft tenderness, and manifestations of deteriorating renal function. Treatment is usually initiated with high-dose steroids. If steroids are ineffective, treatment is instituted with a monoclonal antibody called OKT3 or polyclonal antibodies antithymocyte globulin (ATG), antilymphocyte globulin (ALG), or antilymphocyte serum (ALS) (see Chapter 27).

Chronic rejection occurs slowly over a period of months to years. It mimics CRF, although it is mediated differently in relation to the immunologic process and is resistant to therapy.

The manifestations of transplant rejection include fever, graft tenderness at the site of the transplanted kidney, anemia, and malaise. Urography, renal scan, ultrasonography, and CT scan are among the diagnostic tools used, mainly to rule out other causes of the manifestations.

Antirejection therapy revolves around the use of immunosuppressive drugs, which block the body's normal immune responses. A combination of azathioprine, cyclosporine, and prednisone is used most frequently for

maintenance. See Chapter 27 for a discussion of transplant and antirejection medications.

Cyclophosphamide is sometimes used in place of azathioprine. The use of monoclonal antibodies for acute rejection, with prednisone and either cyclophosphamide or azathioprine, is generally effective. ALG is a horse serum that has antibodies useful in the rejection process. It can be used prophylactically or during rejection episodes. In the case of documented, and sometimes suspected, graft rejection, daily doses of the immunosuppressive drugs may remain the same with the addition of intravenous methylprednisone or OKT3 or ATG or a combination of these. The administration of immunosuppressants continues for the lifetime of the kidney transplant. Sudden discontinuance, as may happen when the client independently decides to stop taking the medication, triggers a vigorous rejection episode.

Immunosuppressive therapy has three potential serious consequences: (1) increased susceptibility to infection, (2) increased risk of malignancy, and (3) degenerative bone disease often necessitating total hip or knee replacement. These sequelae account for many of the short- and long-term complications of renal transplant. Balancing immunosuppressive therapy to reduce the risk of infection while preventing rejection is the primary goal of post-transplant follow-up and monitoring.

Infection

Mortality rates for infectious disease in renal transplant clients have decreased dramatically over the past 6 to 8 years. However, infection remains a potential problem and represents the most serious life-threatening complication in the early transplant period. Urinary tract infections, pneumonia, and sepsis are most commonly seen.

Causative agents include bacteria (especially in the early postoperative period), viruses, and fungi. Viral and fungal complications include herpes and, more commonly, cytomegalovirus infection, which can occur in more than 50% of clients who receive transplants. Immunosuppressive drugs can mask early manifestations of infection, so by the time infections are recognized, they may be well advanced. Sometimes immunosuppressive therapy is reduced for a short time while the infection is brought under control.

Urinary Tract Complications

There are several complications that may occur within the urinary tract. Although rare, spontaneous rupture of the kidney may occur, usually within 14 days of the transplant. It is probably caused by rejection or ischemic damage or by some intrinsic renal disease. Leaking of urine from the ureteral-bladder anastomosis causes the development of a urinoma, which eventually puts pressure on the kidney and ureter, reducing renal function. Fistula formation includes the caliceal-cutaneous, ureteral, and vesical. Long-term uremia and steroid therapy may be predisposing factors. Surgical repair may be undertaken as well as tapered alternate-day steroid therapy. Other urinary tract complications include ureteral, bladder, or pelvic leaks; obstruction; reflux; and lymphoceles. A ureteral catheter is used early in the postoperative period to decompress the bladder and monitor urine output.

Cardiovascular Complications

Cardiovascular complications may be local or systemic. Hypertension occurs in 50% to 60% of adult recipients and may be caused by renal artery stenosis, acute tubular necrosis, acute and chronic graft rejection, hydronephrosis, hyperaldosteronism, large-dose steroids, and cyclosporine. Cardiac dysrhythmias and congestive heart failure may occur as a result of fluid and electrolyte imbalances. Plasma erythropoietin titers return to normal when the graft is functioning properly.

Respiratory Complications

Pneumonia caused by bacteria and fungi is the most frequent respiratory complication. Cytomegalovirus and *Pneumocystis* pneumonias are particularly serious. Respiratory infections often represent a crisis situation and should be treated immediately with appropriate antimicrobial, antiviral, and antifungal agents. Other respiratory problems include pulmonary edema, pulmonary emboli, and reactivated tuberculosis.

Gastrointestinal Complications

Infections, especially oral and esophageal, are common gastrointestinal sequelae. Hepatitis B and cirrhosis occur and may be associated with the use of hepatotoxic medications such as azathioprine. Peptic ulcer disease is a particularly problematic consequence in the presence of prednisone. Impaired gastric metabolism and increased secretion due to stress-induced epinephrine release enhance the development of ulcers. Elevated histamine levels, hyperparathyroidism, and hypercalcemia may also contribute. Histamine receptor antagonist and antacid therapy are always instituted after transplant. Pancreatitis may also occur, although its pathogenesis is not entirely clear.

Integumentary Complications

Skin carcinomas are particularly common. Other dermatologic sequelae include infection, purpura, acne, and alopecia. Wound healing may be slowed because of poor nutritional status, low serum albumin, and steroid therapy.

Other Complications

Other systems are also affected by post-transplant complications. Steroid-induced diabetes mellitus may develop. Musculoskeletal sequelae include osteoporosis and myopathy. Aseptic bone necrosis is primarily due to corticosteroid therapy. The reproductive problems described in CRF frequently disappear after transplantation. The incidence of gynecologic malignancies is higher than in the general population, with cervical cancer dominating. Successful pregnancies have been completed after transplant, although this is a risk for both the fetus and for the transplanted kidney. Steroid-induced cataracts, glaucoma, and retinitis secondary to cytomegalovirus infection may occur.

Death

The overall mortality rate 2 years post transplant is about 10%.[38] This represents a dramatic decrease in the past two decades, when 2-year survival was 40% to 50%. In particular, the decreased death rate due to infection in the first 2 years after transplant has been dramatic. Advances in immunosuppressive therapy and the treatment of infectious diseases have contributed to the overall improvement. Cardiovascular deaths remain the leading cause of death in the late transplant period. Myocardial infarction, stroke, and congestive heart failure are the primary causes of death.

■ Nursing Management of the Surgical Client

Assessment

If the client is to receive a renal transplant, the client's understanding of the procedure and follow-up regimen must be assessed. The client's ability to cope with a complex medication regimen after the transplant must also be assessed.

Diagnosis, Planning, Implementation

Knowledge Deficit. Renal transplant is a complex subject and the diagnosis *Knowledge Deficit related to renal transplant and therapeutic regimen* is germane.

Planning: Expected Outcomes. The client will understand the transplant and therapeutic regimen, as evidenced by discussion with the client and his or her compliance with the therapeutic regimen.

Implementation. The donor and recipient must be prepared for postsurgical psychological reactions. Strong emotional ties often develop between donor and recipient during the evaluation period, and the donor frequently feels responsible for the success or failure of the graft postoperatively. Graft rejection is usually devastating to these clients. Also, the need to protect the remaining kidney may give rise to later feelings of anger. Postoperative traumatic reactions by the donor are less likely in clients who have good inner resources, flexible defense mechanisms, and good mental health. Another source of postoperative stress for the donor is the fact that families tend to pay more attention to the recipient because of the continued possibility of graft rejection. The donor often feels abandoned. However, strong, long-lasting, positive effects include identification of a source of inner strength, a more positive self-image, and a general "sense of feeling good" about saving someone's life.

The donor may be assured that the remaining kidney will assume adequate total renal functioning. The renal blood flow and GFR of the remaining kidney have been reported to increase to 70% to 80% of the preoperative levels of both kidneys together. Within 2 to 6 years, the 24-hour creatinine clearance levels often recover 85% to 87%. This increased function is probably facilitated by tubular hypertrophy and hyperplasia.

Preoperative preparation of both the living donor and the recipient includes all aspects of general preoperative care as outlined in Chapter 21. In addition, there are several concerns unique to the recipient. Adequate conservative management and dialysis should have placed the client in as close to a nontoxic state as possible. All infections must be eradicated, gastrointestinal ulcers treated, and any lower urinary tract malfunctions corrected. Sometimes, when the bladder is unable to receive urine from the transplanted kidney, a urinary diversion procedure, such as an ileal conduit, may be done before the transplant itself. Immunosuppressive therapy may be started at least 24 hours before surgery.

Bilateral nephrectomy may be performed before the transplantation procedure if any of the following conditions are present: persistent or active bacterial pyelonephritis, infected stone disease, uncontrolled renin-mediated hypertension, polycystic kidneys, selected rapidly progressive glomerulonephritis, or renal malignancy. The decision to do a nephrectomy can be safely delayed until the post-transplant period when surgeons may determine it is necessary because of recurrent urinary tract infection.

Postoperative nursing care is discussed in depth in Chapter 21. The function of the transplanted kidney is a primary concern after surgery. Remember that a cadaver donor may not function immediately and the client may be maintained on hemodialysis until adequate function occurs.

Risk for Infection. The use of immunosuppressants mandates the diagnosis *Risk for Infection related to immunosuppressive therapy.*

Planning: Expected Outcomes. The client will not develop an infection, as evidenced by absence of fever and no manifestations of infection (which may be masked by steroids).

Implementation. Much of nursing management is aimed at prevention, early recognition, and treatment of complications plus measures to facilitate maximal renal function and help the client attain an optimal quality of life. Immediate postoperative care of both the donor and recipient encompasses the care required by anyone having surgery, as described in Chapter 21. Care of the donor resembles that of anyone having a nephrectomy. The additional care required by the recipient is partially suggested by the potential complications. Be constantly aware of the manifestations of these sequelae. Hand washing and universal precautions are measures taken to protect the client from potential sources of infection within the hospital environment.

Because of the high incidence and seriousness of pneumonia to the client with a renal transplant, preventive respiratory treatment is essential. Coughing and deep-breathing exercises are started immediately. These exercises are painful. Use analgesics judiciously and put external pressure over the incision to help the client cough and breathe more effectively.

Wound care must be done with use of the strictest aseptic technique because the client does not have much resistance to bacterial invasion. Delayed wound healing makes the client susceptible to dehiscence longer than usual. If the client has a fistula or graft for hemodialysis, it is left in place in case dialysis is needed postoperatively.

Oral hygiene is important because of the high incidence of stomatitis and bacterial and fungal infections. Antifungal mouthwashes may be used. Oral fluids are usually instituted after 12 to 24 hours.

Economic concerns also need to be addressed. Immunosuppressive medications, particularly cyclosporine, are expensive. Currently, Medicare covers payment of these drugs for 365 days after the client is discharged from transplant admission. After that time, other sources of funding need to be explored to ensure compliance with medications.

Peritonitis. A common collaborative problem is *Peritonitis related to surgical procedure.*

Planning: Expected Outcomes. Postoperative infection will be prevented as evidenced by vital signs within preoperative range, return of normal bowel function, and return of urinary function.

Implementation. Maintain circulatory function. Frequently monitor blood pressure, pulse, respiration, central venous pressure (CVP), weight, and hourly or half-hourly intake and output. For monitoring renal function and maintaining electrolyte balance, obtain serial laboratory determinations of hemoglobin, hematocrit, BUN, creatinine, electrolytes, white blood cell count, and platelets. Postoperatively, manage intravenous fluids carefully; the amount of fluid infused is frequently based on the previous hour's output. A high urine output is usually desired.

Carefully assess bowel function before oral intake is allowed. As bowel peristalsis returns, the diet will be advanced. Unless the client is demonstrating rejection or hypertension, there may be no dietary restrictions. As soon as the client begins taking oral food and fluids, antacid therapy is begun.

Body Image Disturbance. Although the transplanted kidney is not visible, the client may have *Body Image Disturbances related to side effects of medications and the presence of a transplanted kidney.*

Planning: Expected Outcomes. The client will acknowledge body changes and incorporate them into his or her body image, as evidenced by the client's statements about self and his or her willingness to be with others.

Implementation. Psychologically, the client must be helped to incorporate the new kidney as a part of the whole being. Provide education and counseling to enhance changes in life-style that will promote health-seeking behavior and compliance with transplant medications. If the graft fails, expected reactions include anger, hostility, guilt, and a helplessness-hopelessness syndrome. Relatives and friends may mirror these feelings. Role changes, so well established during the chronic illness period, may be difficult, such as the family member who no longer feels needed as the "caregiver." Likewise, the client may have difficulty giving up the sick role.

Evaluation

There are actually potential positive outcomes for this client: First, that the client is successfully maintained on hemo- or peritoneal dialysis with minimal side effects and complications; second, that the client receives a renal transplant and renal function returns.

■ Modifications for Elderly Clients

One of the major modifications for the older client will be the possible limits of options available for treatment. Renal transplant is not routinely done on elderly clients. Clients over age 60 years are evaluated on an individual basis; clients as old as 75 years have been successfully transplanted. One problem for elderly clients is the reduced immune system in conjunction with immunosuppressants can lead to further complications.

Renal Calculi

Although calculi (stones) can form anywhere in the urinary tract, the most frequent site is the kidney. These stones may travel down the urinary tract with or without resultant damage, may lodge anywhere along the tract, or may stay within the kidney.

Researchers estimate that approximately 12% of the male population will develop a renal stone by the age of 70 years. The incidence rate in males in the United States is 123.6 per 100,000.[8] Also, more than 200,000 Americans each year are admitted to hospitals because of nephrolithiasis (kidney stones). Many more people pass urinary stones without even knowing it, and others are treated on an ambulatory basis in emergency rooms and clinics.

Etiology and Risk Factors

A number of etiologic factors influence renal stone formation. The presence of precipitators in the urine includes protein matrix and bacteria or inflammatory elements. Increased solute concentration occurs because of fluid depletion or an increased solute load. This increased concentration predisposes to the precipitation of crystals, such as calcium, uric acid, and phosphate. Urinary pH influences the solubility of certain crystals, with some crystal types precipitating readily in acid urine and some in alkaline urine. Abnormal pH levels occur (1) in renal tubular acidosis, with the administration of carbonic anhydrase inhibitors, (2) in the presence of urea-splitting organisms, and (3) in severe, chronic diarrhea.

Not only does the deficiency of inhibitors predispose the client to develop renal stones but there may be "anti-inhibitors" in the urine, such as aluminum, iron, and silicone. Drinking water and magnesium trisilicate are common sources of silicone. Certain medications may induce stone formation. Those include acetazolamide, absorbable alkali (e.g., calcium carbonate and sodium bicarbonate), and aluminum hydroxide. Massive doses of vitamin C increase urinary oxalate concentration. Anything that results in urinary stasis predisposes to stone formation, because the crystals in unmoving urine precipitate more readily. Common conditions include urinary tract obstruction and immobilization.

Development of urinary lithiasis is probably the result not of any single factor but of multiple phenomena. One of the questions still unanswered is why some clients form stones whereas others do not. This problem is particularly important with recurrent "stone-formers."

Risk factors for stone formation include anything that causes either stasis or supersaturation of the urine. This includes stressors such as immobility, which increases stasis; dehydration, which leads to supersaturation; and an increase in calcium or other ion in the urine. Another major risk factor is having had urinary calculi previously.

These risk factors have primary preventions that can be implemented. Frequent turning of immobilized clients, a high fluid intake, and decreased calcium in the diet in susceptible individuals help prevent stones. These will also help prevent the recurrence of stones.

The prime risk factor for uric acid stones is an alteration in purine metabolism, as seen with gout. Controlling the production and excretion of uric acid can help prevent these. See Chapter 56 for more information on risk factors for and prevention of urinary calculi.

Pathophysiology

Regardless of the specific type of calculus, the process of stone formation is one of crystallization. Current theory identifies three factors that may be involved in this process: (1) urine saturation, (2) inhibitor deficiency, and (3) the production of matrix. Generally, crystal growth involves nucleation, in which crystallites are formed from supersaturated urine. Growth proceeds by aggregation to form larger particles. One of these particles may travel down the urinary tract until it is trapped at some narrow point where it becomes the nidus for stone formation. Substances such as citrate, pyrophosphate, magnesium, and glycosaminoglycans have been identified that chelate stone constituents so that they are not available for stone formation. These are called inhibitors; when present in adequate amounts, they interfere with crystal aggregation. Also, a fibrous matrix of urinary organic matter (mostly mucoproteins) may form in the kidney or bladder, producing a substance into which crystallites are deposited and trapped. This, then, becomes the nidus for a stone.[1] The excessive production of this mucoprotein may, in part, account for a family history of renal stones among clients with calculi.

Renal calculi may be of one crystalline type only or a combination of types. Approximately 80% of all urinary tract stones contain calcium, usually as calcium phosphate or calcium oxalate. Calcium stones may range from very small particles, often called sand or gravel, to giant staghorn calculi, which may fill the entire renal pelvis and extend up into the calices (Fig. 57–8). They have a peak onset in people in their 20s and primarily afflict males.

Hypercalciuria, or an increased solute load of calcium in the urine, is caused by four main components: (1) a high rate of bone reabsorption, which liberates calcium (hyperparathyroidism; Paget's disease; immobility; osteolysis caused by malignant tumors of the breast, lung, and prostate; Cushing's disease); (2) gut absorption of abnormally large amounts of calcium (milk-alkali syndrome, sarcoidosis, excessive intake of vitamin D); (3) impaired renal tubular absorption of filtered calcium (renal tubular acidosis), and (4) structural abnormalities such as sponge kidney. About 35% of all clients who form calcium stones do not have high serum levels of calcium and have no apparent cause for their hypercalciuria. This condition is called idiopathic hypercalciuria.

There are two variants of hypercalciuria. In one, the primary abnormality is increased intestinal absorption of calcium or increased bone reabsorption. The resulting higher serum calcium level triggers increased renal filtration of calcium and parathyroid hormone suppression. This in turn decreases tubular reabsorption, thereby increasing the concentration of calcium in the urine. The other abnormality involves "renal leak" of calcium caused by a tubular defect. The resulting mild hypocalcemia stimulates parathyroid hormone production, which increases intestinal absorption of calcium. This cycle then

fits into the previous one, causing an increased solute load of calcium. Clients with this problem are often called "calcium wasters."

The second most frequent stone is oxalate, which is relatively insoluble in urine. Its solubility is only slightly affected by changes in urinary pH. The mechanism for oxalate availability is unclear but may be closely related to diet. The disease is most common in areas where cereals are a major dietary component and least common in dairy-farming regions. Some conditions in which the incidence of oxalate stone increases may be related to hyperabsorption of oxalate (e.g., inflammatory bowel disease); postileal resection or small bowel bypass surgery; overdose of ascorbic acid, which metabolizes to oxalate; familial oxaluria; and administration of a methoxyflurane anesthetic. There is also some thought that a concurrent fat malabsorption causes calcium binding, which frees oxalate for absorption.

Struvite stones, also called triple phosphate, are composed of magnesium and ammonium phosphate. Their cause is certain bacteria, usually *Proteus*, which contain the enzyme urease. This enzyme splits urea into two ammonia molecules, which raises the urine pH. Phosphate precipitates in alkaline urine. This action is responsible for the label "urea-splitter" given to these organisms. The stones formed in this manner are staghorn calculi (see Fig. 57–8). Abscess formation is common, sometimes the result of erosion into the perinephric space. These stones are particularly difficult to eliminate because the hard stone forms around a nucleus of bacteria, protecting them from antibiotic therapy. Any small fragment left after surgical removal of the stone begins the cycle again.

Uric acid stones are caused by increased urate excretion, fluid depletion, and a low urinary pH. Hyperuricuria is the result of either increased uric acid production or the administration of uricosuric agents. Approximately 25% of persons with primary gout and about 50% of persons with secondary gout develop uric acid stones. A high dietary intake of purine-rich foods may predispose to uric acid stone formation. Also, treating neoplastic disease with agents that cause rapid cell destruction may increase the urine's uric acid concentration. Moreover, a link between hyperuricuria and calcium stone formation may exist. It seems uric acid crystals absorb some of the crystal inhibitors normally found in urine.

Cystinuria is the result of a congenital metabolic error inherited as an autosomal recessive disorder. Cystine stones typically appear during childhood and adolescence; development in adults is very rare.

Xanthine stones also occur as the result of a rare hereditary condition in which there is a xanthine oxidase deficiency. This crystal precipitates readily in acid urine.

Despite the type of stone that forms, the potential damage is essentially the same: pain, obstruction, and tissue trauma with secondary hemorrhage and infection.

Clinical Manifestations and Diagnostic Findings

The most characteristic manifestation of renal or ureteral calculi is a sharp, severe pain of sudden onset. Depending

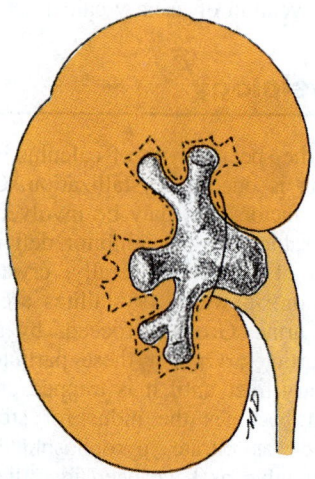

Figure 57–8. Staghorn calculus.

on the site of the stone, this pain may be called either renal colic or ureteral colic. Renal colic originates deep in the lumbar region and radiates around the side and down toward the testicle in the male and the bladder in the female. Ureteral colic radiates toward the genitalia and thigh. When the pain is severe, the client will usually exhibit nausea, vomiting, pallor, and diaphoresis and be quite anxious. Urinary frequency may occur. The pain lasts for minutes to days and can be somewhat resistant to narcotic intervention. Pain may be intermittent, which usually means that the stone has moved. Physicians hypothesize that the ureter dilates just proximal to the calculus, which allows urine to pass, relieving the ureteral distention. Then, as the stone moves into a new obstruction site, the pain returns. The pain subsides when the stone reaches the bladder.

Pain caused by renal stones is not always severe and colicky. In fact, it may be a dull, aching, or heavy feeling. This is particularly true during the early stages of hydronephrosis. Sometimes, there may be no sensation, and the first clue the client has is when a "clink" sounds against the toilet when the stone passes.

The major diagnostic test is a KUB radiograph or plain film of the abdomen to visualize the stone. An IVP is also done to determine if any obstruction is present and, if it is, how severe it is.

Acute and Subacute Care

■ Medical Management

Conservative management is described in Chapter 56. Conservative management is appropriate if (1) there is no obstruction, (2) the pain is managed, (3) the client can be hydrated with oral fluids, and (4) the stone is under 5 mm.

Two objectives are essential to the total preventive regimen. First, any underlying contributing problem must be corrected (e.g., metabolic and anatomic). Parathyroidectomy may be performed in the case of intractable hypercalcemia. Second, infection must be avoided or aggressively treated for all stone types because it places additional stress on the kidneys.

Pharmacologic Management

There are no particular medications used to treat calcium stones. If the client has uric acid stones, medications to lower uric acid such as allopurinol (Zyloprim) should be given. The client is treated with narcotics and antispasmodics.

Dietary Management

Once the components of the stone have been identified, diet modification is used to help prevent recurrence. A low calcium, low oxalate diet is used to prevent calcium or oxalate stone recurrence, and a low purine diet is used to prevent uric acid stone recurrence. See Chapter 56 for more information on dietary management.

■ Nursing Management of the Medical Client

Assessment

As with any disease, the history the client gives is very important in identifying the problem. Full information about the onset of manifestations and the pattern of pain is vital. A family history of calculi is suggestive. Evaluate recent dietary habits. For instance, a large intake of purines may be significant, and drinking large amounts of fruit juices or tea facilitates oxalate precipitation. Ask the client about recent medications and the presence of any contributing factors, such as urinary tract infection, immobility, or gout.

Physical findings primarily center on two things: the urine and x-ray studies. Be certain to strain all urine being voided through several layers of gauze or through a commercial urine strainer. Carefully examine all debris in the bedpan or urinal. Save any stone material so the stone's composition can be analyzed as a basis for treatment and to show how much has passed through the urinary tract. Also, monitor urine for hematuria. A routine urinalysis gives important information about the pH, specific gravity, and presence of red blood cells, white blood cells, crystals, and casts. Collect 24-hour urine specimens, if necessary, to determine the daily output of possible causative crystals. A urine culture will help identify urinary tract infection. Blood levels of constituent elements, such as calcium, phosphorus, and uric acid, may be determined. Stones containing calcium and cystine are radiopaque and will show up on a KUB x-ray film. IVP and retrograde pyelography are an important part of the evaluation process.

Diagnosis, Planning, Implementation

Pain. Pain is the cardinal subjective manifestation of renal calculus. Write the diagnosis *Pain related to irritation from stone movement.*

Planning: Expected Outcomes. The client will have pain relieved or controlled, as evidenced by the client's statement.

Implementation. Controlling the client's pain is a primary objective of nursing intervention. Large doses of narcotics and possibly antispasmodics are given to control the client's pain because the client cannot force fluids and ambulate if the pain is too severe.

Risk for Injury. Stones may cause tissue trauma. Hence, the diagnosis *Risk for Injury related to possible obstruction.*

Planning: Expected Outcomes. The client will not suffer an injury from an obstruction, as evidenced by normal output.

Implementation. All urine must be strained. Whenever the client voids, the urine is strained through a strainer or a gauze pad so any stones or sediment can be saved and analyzed. The stone analysis will help determine what measures are needed to prevent recurrence. Push fluids, up to 3 L or more per day.

Evaluation

Another aspect of intervention is preventing stone recurrence. Although many people with a urinary stone will never have another, researchers estimate that 25% to 30% of them will develop recurrent lithiasis. (The recurrence rate is reported by some to be as high as 60%.) The ability to predict who will and who will not have a recurrence is unreliable. Stone recurrence usually happens within 2 to 3 years, but may occur as long as 20 years later. As the number of recurrences increases, the intervals between stone formation tend to become shorter. Thus, prevention is a lifelong program.

■ Surgical Management

Mechanical Intervention

If it is decided that the stone will not pass before complications occur, mechanical intervention may be used. Depending on the position of the calculus, cystoscopy may be done. Additionally, one or two ureteral catheters may be inserted past the stone. From this point, several different interventions are appropriate. The catheters may be left in place for 24 hours. Their presence drains the urine trapped proximal to the stones and dilates the ureter, which may prompt spontaneous movement of the calculus. Otherwise, the catheters may mechanically guide the stones downward as they are removed. A continuous chemical irrigation may be established to dissolve the stone. Finally, an attempt may be made to manipulate or dislodge the stone. A variety of special catheters with loops and expanding baskets may be inserted through the cystoscope and used to snare the stone. The postprocedure care of these clients is the same as that following cystoscopy (see Chapter 55). Chapter 56 describes the care of a client with an indwelling catheter.

Endourologic Procedures

Extracorporeal Shock Wave Lithotripsy

A noninvasive mechanical procedure for breaking up stones so they can pass spontaneously or be removed by other methods is extracorporeal shock wave lithotripsy (ESWL). Figure 57–9 shows how this procedure works. The client is placed in a specially designed tub with the trunk submerged in water. Then, an underwater electrode generates shock waves via a reflector that fragments kidney stones. The client is strapped to a frame and may be sedated during the procedure, because it usually lasts for 30 to 40 minutes and immobility is essential. After the procedure, the client may experience some renal colic that needs spasmolytics. Early ambulation and adequate diuresis by increasing fluid intake are important to fully "wash out" the stone fragments.

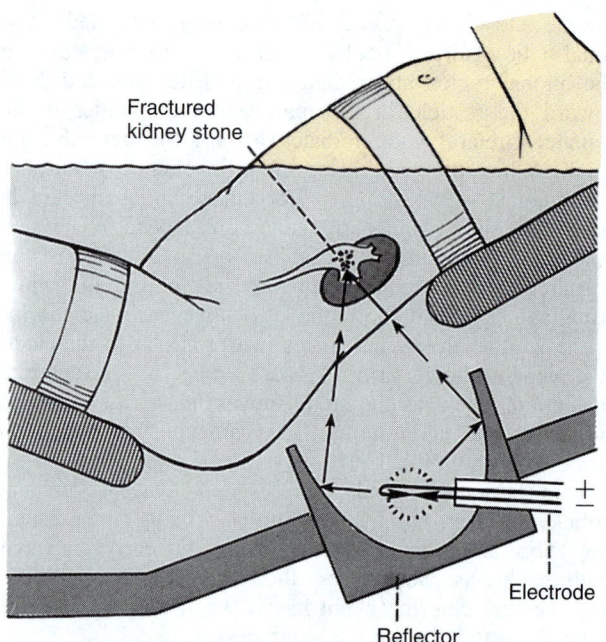

Figure 57–9. Extracorporeal lithotripsy. Electrically generated shock waves fracture kidney stones.

Percutaneous Lithotripsy

Percutaneous lithotripsy is an invasive procedure in which a guide is inserted via the percutaneous route under fluoroscopy near the area of the stone. An ultrasonic wave is then aimed at the stone to break it into fragments.

Surgical intervention may be performed through a percutaneous approach or by open procedures. The development of advanced fiberoptic equipment has made the percutaneous route the more common. Because the incision is so small, surgical risk is minimal, and the client recuperates quickly. If the client has a significant infection, antibiotics probably will be given for at least 1 day before the procedure. Small, free-lying stones may simply be retrieved by use of a nephroscope. In this instance, a needle is inserted through the skin into the kidney. The tract into the kidney is dilated, and the nephroscope is inserted through the tract. Figure 57–10A shows a nephroscope in place. The stone may be removed by alligator forceps or a stone basket. Irrigation to flush the stone out of its resting place may be done.

If the stone is too large, one of several methods may be used to break it up into smaller fragments (litholapaxy). A punch lithoclast helps to fragment the stone. An ultrasound nephroscope may be inserted into the kidney and subharmonic sound waves used to shatter the stone. Electrohydraulic lithotripsy involves inserting an electric probe through the nephroscope to produce shock waves to break up the stone. Chemolysis may also help break up the stone, especially with uric acid, struvite, and cystine stones. A nephrostomy tube is inserted and connected to a three-way connector with a central venous pressure CVP, manometer attached to measure pressure in the kidney. Fluid is instilled into the tube and is passed by urinating. If intrarenal pressure goes above 15 mm H_2O

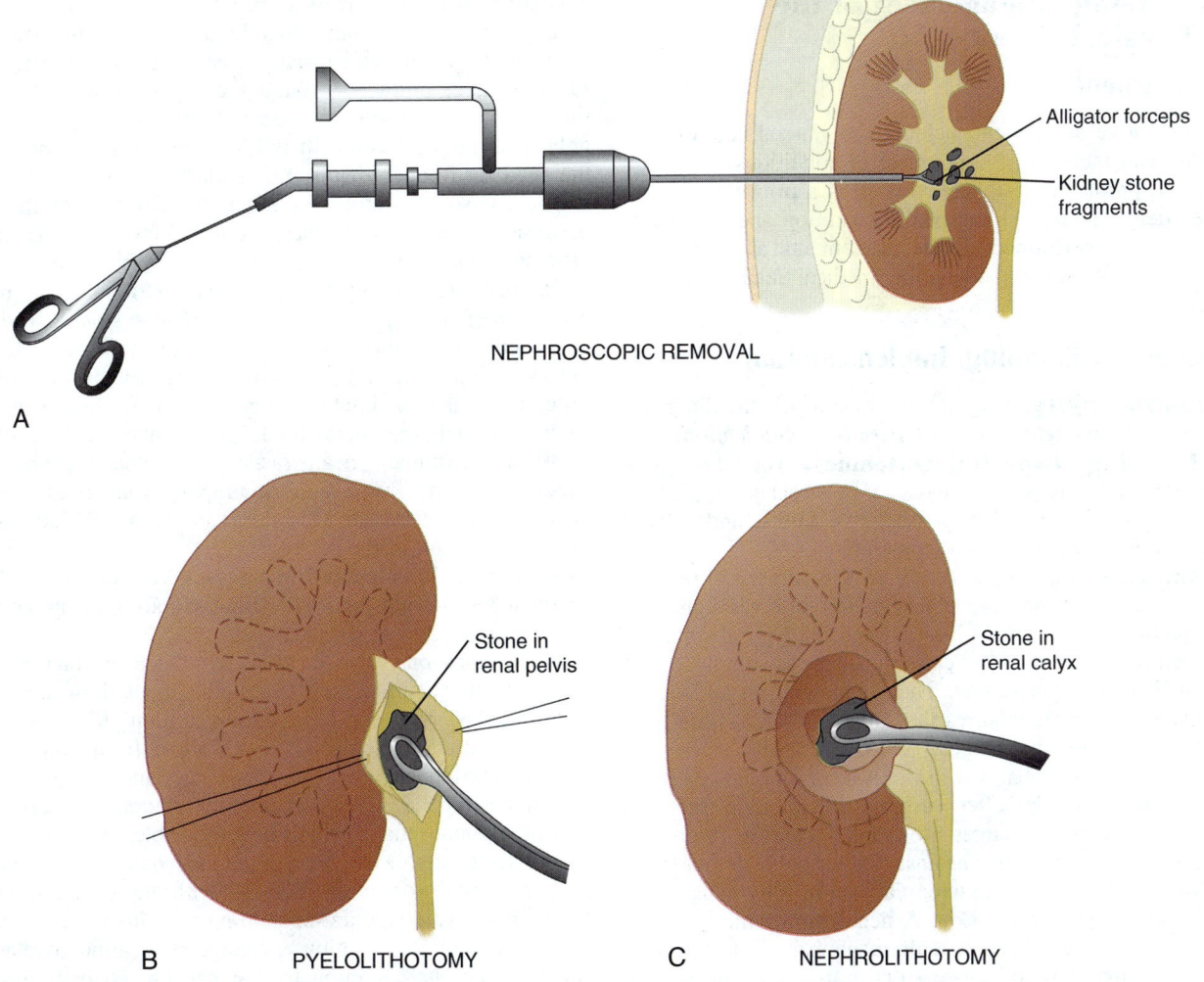

Figure 57–10. *A–C,* Surgical techniques for removal of kidney stones.

or pain or fever occurs, the tubing is opened and drained and the irrigation stopped. The irrigation is done via a volumetric pump to maintain a steady flow. Sodium bicarbonate, organic acids, and chelating solutions are the most common irrigating solutions.

After the procedure, a nephrostomy tube remains in place for 1 to 5 days. The client may be sent home with the nephrostomy tube. A nephrotomogram is then done to determine whether all stone fragments were removed. If the kidney is clear, the tube will be removed and a bulky dressing placed over the site. Be certain that a high fluid intake is maintained during the postprocedure period to flush out any fragments. Recommended daily amounts are 3000 to 4000 ml. Monitor for, or teach the client to monitor for, complications such as infection, hemorrhage, and extravasation of fluid into the retroperitoneal cavity.

If these procedures do not successfully remove the stone, an open surgical procedure may be required. A stone lodged in the ureter will require a ureterolithotomy, which involves incision into the affected ureter. The approach may be through a lower abdominal or flank incision. The stone is removed, any strictures are repaired, and the incision is closed. The stone is removed from the renal pelvis by a pyelolithotomy, and from the renal calix

by a nephrolithotomy. Figure *57–10B* and *C* illustrates these two procedures.

If constricted or tortuous ureters cause recurrent calculi, one of two procedures may be used to correct the problem. An ileal ureter, using a segment of the ileum between the renal collecting system and the bladder, may be constructed. This creates a wide-bore passage that replaces the original ureter. A renal autotransplant may also be performed. Here the kidney is transplanted to the ipsilateral or contralateral pelvis. A flap of bladder tissue is raised, formed into a large-caliber tube, and anastomosed to the renal pelvis. The bladder wall is then sutured to reestablish its continuity. These procedures are used very selectively.[59]

The physician may decide that a partial or total nephrectomy is necessary because of extensive kidney damage, overwhelming renal infection, or severe ureteropelvic junction obstruction or, in the case of an abnormal renal parenchyma, to prevent stone recurrence. This procedure is used much less now than in the past and is usually considered a "last resort" intervention.

Possible complications after litholapaxy include hemorrhage, urinary retention, infection, and possible stone recurrence.

■ Nursing Management of the Surgical Client

Assessment

Preoperative assessment includes the general condition of the client, including the presence of conditions that could present problems postoperatively. It is a priority to assess the client's understanding of the condition and the procedure to be performed. Other assessments are similar to those for the client undergoing medical management of calculi.

Diagnosis, Planning, Implementation

Risk for Injury. Surgery always compels the diagnosis *Risk for Injury related to postoperative complications.*

Planning: Expected Outcomes. The client will not develop injury, as evidenced by absence of hemorrhage, vital signs within preoperative limits, and normal white blood cell count and temperature.

Implementation. If the client had surgery to remove the stone, then postoperative nursing interventions will depend on the incision's location and the type of drainage tubes present. With a flank incision, care is similar to that needed after nephrectomy. The client with an abdominal incision, however, requires the same care as anyone having major abdominal surgery (see Chapter 21).

The incision probably will drain large amounts of urine for days to weeks after surgery. Intervention includes frequent dressing changes around the Penrose drain and protection of the skin against the urinary drainage. If urinary drainage is excessive, place an ostomy pouch over the drain to protect the skin. A nephrostomy tube may be left in place attached to a drainage bag. Take care to ensure a free flow of urine. Always use sterile technique to prevent infection.

Knowledge Deficit. Teaching will be required, so write the diagnosis *Knowledge Deficit related to fluid requirements, dietary restrictions, and medications.*

Planning: Expected Outcomes. The client will understand fluid requirements, dietary restrictions, and medications, as evidenced by discussion with client.

Implementation. The nurse has a major role in helping the client develop and maintain an effective, individual regimen to prevent recurrence. The nurse should help the client establish health habits that prevent renal stone recurrence, provide education about the disease and its implications, and provide support during the follow-up period. The three main components of a preventive regimen are (1) fluids, (2) diet, and (3) medications.

The client's fluid intake should be high enough to ensure 2500 to 3000 ml or more of urine output per day. This requires at least 3000 to 4000 ml of fluid daily; more will be needed under certain situations (e.g., hot weather, fever, diarrhea). The increased urine volume resulting from this high fluid intake decreases the concentration of solutes and alleviates urinary stasis. The kind of fluid the client drinks depends on dietary restrictions. At least half of the fluid should be water, which usually has a low calcium content. The fluid intake needs to be as consistent as possible throughout the 24-hour period. Cli-

ents are usually advised to drink one glass of water every hour during the day and two large glasses just before going to bed. This will usually mean that they will need to void about midway through the night, at which time they drink another glass of water. These clients will probably need help adjusting their life-styles to accommodate the need for frequent bathroom breaks.

There is some controversy regarding dietary restrictions because of the uncertain therapeutic effectiveness of, and problems with, long-term compliance with this regimen.

For planning recommended dietary restrictions, the results of a stone analysis are essential. Some stone constituents require specific diet adjustments to avoid stone formation. Hypercalciuria may be controlled by limiting excessive calcium intake. Clients with oxalate stones should avoid high-oxalate foods: tea, instant coffee, cola drinks, beer, rhubarb, beans, asparagus, spinach, cabbage, chocolate, citrus fruits, apples, grapes, cranberries, peanuts, and peanut butter. Megadoses of vitamin C increase oxalate excretion in the urine.

If the stone is composed of uric acid, the client should be on a low purine diet. This limits foods such as aged cheeses, wine, and organ meats.

Medications may also be used to reduce the incidence of recurrent calculi. Teach the client about these agents and the need for long-term administration. Medications frequently used to control calcium stone formation may include phosphates, thiazide diuretics, and allopurinol. Phosphates reduce urinary calcium and increase the excretion of pyrophosphate, which is responsible for inhibiting crystal formation. Methylene blue may decrease calcium oxalate crystal formation. Clients with these conditions should also avoid calcium-containing antacids.

Cholestyramine, an anion exchange resin, binds oxalate and promotes its excretion by the intestine. It does have the potential side effect of severe vitamin K deficiency. Because pyridoxine (vitamin B_6) deficiency increases crystal excretion, vitamin B_6 may be given to clients who have oxalate stones. Magnesium oxide also lowers oxalate excretion, and isocarboxazid apparently blocks the metabolism of oxalate. Allopurinol, a xanthine oxidase inhibitor, may be used to prevent oxalate and uric acid stone formation. Uricosuric agents should be avoided; they increase uric acid excretion in the urine, thus increasing the solute concentration.

One of the most frequent components of the medication regimen for triple phosphate or struvite stones is long-term antibiotic administration to control infection. Acidification of the urine, administration of phosphate-binding gels, and dietary restrictions of phosphate are also used. Cystine stone-formers are treated with D-penicillamine or mercaptopropionylglycine, which transforms L-cystine into a water-soluble disulfide derivative. Clients treated with these medications usually need supplemental vitamin B_6.

Adjusting the urinary pH as a means to control precipitation of crystals is a possible treatment. An acidic urine, with a pH below 6, is used to prevent possible calcium and triple phosphate or struvite stones. Chapter 56 describes methods of acidifying the urine. Additionally, methionine or ammonium salts may be used. Uric acid and xanthine stones are inhibited in alkaline urine; alkalinization of the urine is usually accomplished with sodium bicarbonate, citrate, or acetazolamide.

Evaluation

The outcome is usually that each individual episode of stone formation is resolved without long-term complications. The goal, however, is that the nurse and client working collaboratively will be able to prevent further stone formation.

Renal Cancer

Benign kidney tumors are rare. Classifications include lymphangioma, lipoma, medullary fibroma, adenoma, leiomyoma, and oncocytoma. When large benign tumors occur, it is relatively impossible to distinguish them from a malignant tumor by x-ray examination. If other diagnostic tests are also inconclusive, nephrectomy may be done.

At least 85% of all renal tumors are malignant. There are approximately 5000 to 7000 deaths yearly as a result of adult kidney cancer. The figure represents 1% to 3% of all malignancies. The tumors are most frequently found between the ages of 50 and 70 years. They affect men more frequently than women.

Etiology and Risk Factors

The exact cause of renal tumors is unknown. There have been some links established between kidney cancer and tobacco, lead, cadmium, and phosphates. A genetic link has also been postulated.

Pathophysiology

Renal cell carcinoma, or adenocarcinoma, is the most frequent type of tumor; it accounts for 90% of all kidney neoplasms. Tumor growth begins in the renal cortex and usually continues for some time before it produces manifestations. It can grow very large and tends to compress the adjacent renal parenchyma rather than infiltrate it. The tumor, usually avascular, tends to surround blood vessels and stenose them. The lungs and mediastinum are the most frequent metastatic sites for this tumor. Liver, bone, skin, spleen, renal vein, and brain are other common sites.

Other types of renal cancer include nephroblastoma, sarcoma, and epithelial tumors within the renal pelvis. Nephroblastoma, or Wilms' tumor, is primarily a childhood disease, although it occasionally occurs in adults. The prognosis for adults is worse than for children, with some sources reporting only a 25% survival rate. For further discussion of this type of tumor, see a pediatric nursing text. Sarcoma is infrequent, typically arising in the renal capsule. Most tumors of the renal pelvis are primarily urolithelial in origin and include three different tissue types: (1) transitional cell, (2) squamous cell, and (3) adenocarcinoma.

Staging of the tumor helps delineate the appropriate treatment to be used. Figure 57–11 illustrates the typical staging system for renal carcinoma.

Spontaneous regression of renal adenocarcinoma reportedly occurs in less than 1% of all cases. Most of these regressions develop after nephrectomy and involve metastatic areas. However, authorities consider these episodes as more evidence the disease has a definite immunologic or hormonal link.

The prognosis partially depends on the stage at time of treatment. Five-year survival rates for stage I are about 65%; for stage II, about 40%; 10-year rates drop to 40% and 35%, respectively. Five-year survivals are rare in stages III and IV.

Clinical Manifestations and Diagnostic Findings

Manifestations of renal malignancies vary, and tumor growth may advance significantly before the disease is discovered. It is not uncommon for the client to demonstrate manifestations apparently unrelated to renal disease. Frequently, a palpable abdominal mass found during a routine physical examination arouses the first suspicion. The average time between the onset of hematuria and the onset of pain is 9 months, and 14 months between initial pain and diagnosis. Many times, extrarenal manifestations are found before a diagnosis of renal cancer is confirmed. As many as 35% of all clients have metastasis when the final diagnosis of a renal neoplasm is made.

The common triad of manifestations includes hematuria, flank pain, and a palpable abdominal or flank mass. The hematuria is usually gross and intermittent, which helps explain the client's delay in seeking medical advice. The clinical picture also contains a combination of the following usual findings: fever, weight loss and cachexia, fatigue, hypertension, amyloidosis, thrombophlebitis, anemia, erythrocytosis, hypercalcemia, abnormal serum liver profile, and an elevated sedimentation rate. Less frequent findings include peripheral neuropathy, inferior vena cava obstruction, priapism, and varicocele. Hydronephrosis may occur if the tumor obstructs the ureteropelvic junction. The incidence of pulmonary embolus as a presenting manifestation may be more frequent than has been previously thought because of the high rate of vena cava and renal vein involvement. Plasma erythropoietin, renin, and chorionic gonadotropin levels are elevated, and prostaglandin production increases in renal cell carcinoma.

Several diagnostic tests help confirm a diagnosis of renal cancer. IVP is probably the most helpful in identifying a space-occupying lesion. Ultrasonography helps differentiate between a cyst and a solid mass. Other noninvasive procedures include CT scan, nephrotomography, and radioisotope studies. Arteriography evaluates the renal vascular system. Renal biopsy, usually done percutaneously, provides definitive data about the lesion.

■ Acute and Subacute Care

■ Surgical Management

The conventional and principal intervention for renal cancer is nephrectomy (either complete or heminephrec-

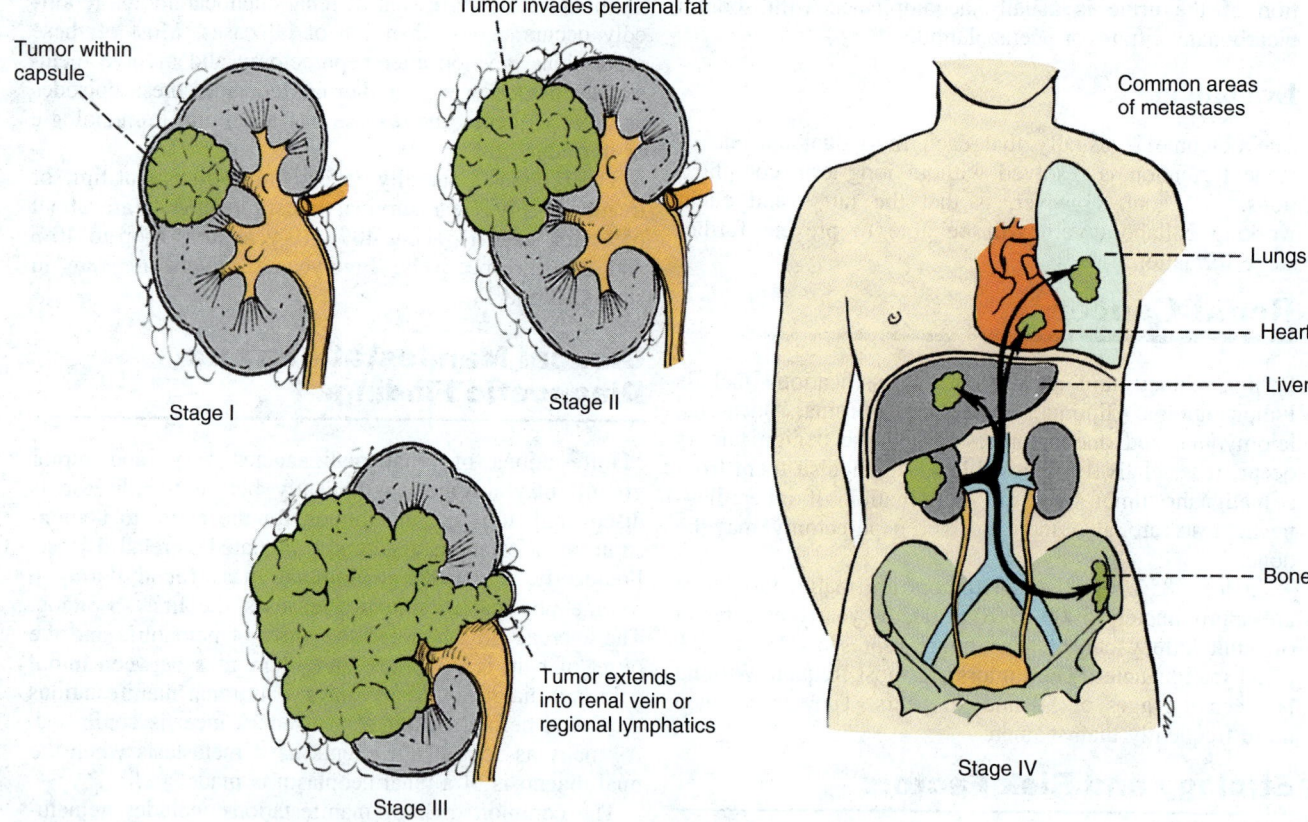

Figure 57–11. Staging system for renal carcinoma. Stage I tumor is confined within the renal capsule; stage II tumor extends beyond the renal capsule, with invasion of local perinephric fat, but no metastasis; stage III tumor extends into the renal vein or involves local lymphatics; and stage IV tumor has metastasized to other parts of the body.

tomy). Radiation and chemotherapy may be part of the medical regimen but are usually adjuncts to surgical kidney removal. For renal cell carcinoma, the surgical procedure of choice is generally radical nephrectomy, including removal of the kidney, the adrenal gland, and perinephric fat with the retroperitoneal lymphatics. Lymphadenectomy remains controversial. When the tumor is located in the renal pelvis, a nephroureterectomy is usually performed because of a tendency for transitional cell cancer to "seed" down the ureter into the bladder. With nephroureterectomy, a cuff of the adjacent bladder is removed. Even in advanced cases, when the prognosis is poor, nephrectomy may be done to relieve pain and for hematuria. If the neoplastic disease is bilateral, or if there is a solitary functioning kidney, a partial nephrectomy may be done on at least one kidney, leaving enough renal tissue to support life without long-term dialysis. If partial nephrectomy is not possible in either instance, the entire kidney is removed and the client is placed on dialysis. These clients may be candidates for renal transplant, but they are usually maintained on dialysis for about a year to observe for recurrence of the disease.

Preoperative intervention may help shrink the tumor, making it easier to resect during surgery. Irradiation helps reduce the size of the tumor, although slowly. Renal artery embolization of the affected kidney may be done to obstruct the tumor's blood supply and reduce its vascularity, thereby reducing the risk of hemorrhage. This is usu-

ally done by occluding the renal artery using an absorbable gelatin sponge (Gelfoam), metal coil, barium, subcutaneous fat, isobutyl-2-cyanoacrylate, absolute ethanol, or a balloon. This procedure may also be performed to control hemorrhage in an inoperable kidney. In addition, some researchers believe embolization may stimulate an immune response against the dying cancer cells.

Preoperative preparation of the client having renal surgery includes the general guidelines described in Chapter 21. Increase fluid intake if indicated to ensure adequate excretion of waste products before surgery. Give emotional support because the client may be anxious, not only about the surgery but about the prospects for adequate postoperative urinary function. If the remaining kidney functions adequately, assure the client that this kidney will fully meet the body's needs. (See Renal Transplantation for more information about this.)

■ Nursing Management of the Surgical Client

Surgery is often nephrectomy or nephroureterectomy. Postoperative care is similar to that for laparotomy. One of the biggest challenges is reestablishing effective breathing patterns. Deep breathing and coughing are very difficult because the incision is so close to the diaphragm. The jackknife position of the client on the surgical table increases the pain and soreness in the thoracic region, limiting respiratory excursion. Liberal use of narcotics (including the use of patient-controlled analgesia) to relieve pain and external mechanical support to the chest and abdomen with pillows or hands helps the client to do deep-breathing and coughing exercises more effectively. Incentive spirometers provide immediate feedback regarding the effectiveness of the deep breathing. Surgically induced or spontaneous pneumothorax does occur occasionally after nephrectomy, so be prepared for this possibility by assessing for sudden shortness of breath and loss of breath sounds on the affected side.

Careful monitoring of urine output is essential. Measure output hourly to identify renal failure as early as possible. Meticulous catheter care is necessary to prevent postoperative urinary tract infection.

The incision used for nephrectomy is extensive and causes significant discomfort. Muscular pain may develop as a result of the prolonged position maintained during surgery. This pain may be relieved by analgesics (including the use of patient-controlled analgesia), proper positioning, massage, and heat. Epidural fentanyl or morphine sulfate can provide effective analgesia.

Paralytic ileus is a common problem. Interventions include carefully assessing the client's gastrointestinal status postoperatively, beginning oral intake only after adequate bowel function has been established, and early exercise (i.e., ambulation).

The skin impairment depends on the size and location of the surgical incision and the number and type of drains present. Wound care is routine; dressing changes are performed as needed for the amount of drainage.

To help reduce feelings of anxiety, continue to keep the client and significant others informed about the progress made. Encourage them to express their concerns and to talk with one another. This need for support will continue throughout the follow-up period.

■ Medical Management

Radiation Therapy. Radiation may be used as adjunct therapy with chemotherapy and surgery. Irradiation is most useful in preoperative preparation of the tumor. It is sometimes also used postoperatively to (1) destroy residual or recurrent tumor cells, (2) treat lymphatic involvement, and (3) treat metastatic sites, such as the bones, palliatively.

Chemotherapy. Clinical investigation continues to search for an effective chemotherapeutic regimen. Medroxyprogesterone and testosterone have been used as hormonal therapy, but their effectiveness has been short-lived. Vinblastine seems to be the most effective single agent, with response rates of 25%. Combination regimens seem to raise toxic effects without improving response rates. Many agents are being studied, but renal cancer cells seem insensitive to chemotherapeutic or hormonal agents, possibly because of their slow growth rate.

Immunotherapy. Immunotherapy seems to have some promise in treating renal cancer. Stimulants of the immune system have shown some positive results as long as the tumor is not too large and the immunodepression is not too severe. Natural and recombinant interferon-α both show some response in treatment as well. Interleukin-2 has been approved by the Food and Drug Administration for expanded clinical trials in renal cancer.

■ Nursing Management of the Medical Client

Nursing management of the client with renal cancer must include general aspects of care for any neoplastic disease (see Chapters 23 and 24).

Renal Candidiasis

Bacteria cause most instances of pyelonephritis. However, the incidence of renal candidiasis is increasing. Primary renal candidiasis is most common in women with diabetes mellitus. Manifestations of this disease include obstruction secondary to a bezoar (tangled hyphae or clumps of yeast cells) in the ureter; progressive oliguria, sometimes alternating with episodic diuresis; ureteral colic; passing tissue- or stonelike material; pyuria; and progressive renal failure. Diagnosis is based on the presence of fungi in several properly collected urine cultures; the presence of serum *Candida precipitins*; and selected radiologic findings, such as hydronephrosis, caliceal erosion, and the presence of filling defects called fungus balls. Amphotericin B and flucytosine are the keys to medical management, although these medications present problems of dosage and nephrotoxicity. Surgery to remove obstruction or nephrectomy may be needed for severe disease.

Renal Abscess

A renal abscess (or renal carbuncle), a localized infection within the cortex of the kidney, usually forms when smaller infectious foci or microabscesses combine in the renal parenchyma. It is usually secondary to urinary tract infection with a species of Enterobacteriaceae, often complicated by renal calculi and obstruction. Other organisms, coming from extrarenal sites, may also cause this infectious process. For example, the client will frequently give a history of recent cutaneous furuncles.

Clients with renal abscess typically have high fever and moderate-to-severe pain. This pain is usually constant and is felt in either the upper quadrant of the abdomen or in the costovertebral area; it sometimes resembles renal colic. Unlike pyelonephritis, the urine is usually sterile, because the abscess does not reach into the urinary collecting system. Other manifestations of this infectious process include weakness, anorexia, weight loss, night sweats, and leukocytosis.

Medical and nursing interventions for renal abscess resemble those for acute pyelonephritis. Aggressive antibiotic therapy is usually successful. Needle aspiration of the abscess may be done for culture and sensitivity study on the contents. These help pinpoint the appropriate antimicrobial to be used. Surgical incision and drainage of the abscess sometimes is necessary. If so, nursing intervention expands to include postoperative care of the incision. A drain is left in place for some time.

Perinephric Abscess

A perinephric abscess involves the fatty tissue surrounding the kidney. It may be an extension of a renal infectious process (most common) or may have spread hematogenously from an extrarenal infection. The abscess may spread in several directions, extending to the peritoneal cavity, chest, or skin.

Assessment findings are the same as with a renal abscess—fever, tenderness, flank or loin pain, and other manifestations of sepsis—with the possible addition of swelling over the site.

Medical and nursing interventions are almost identical to those for renal abscess. Appropriate antibiotics are administered, and symptomatic interventions are undertaken. Because of the nature of a perinephric abscess, incising and draining are needed more frequently than with renal abscess. After this surgical procedure, there may be profuse drainage from the wound; frequent dressing changes and nursing interventions are required to prevent or treat skin excoriation.

Renal Trauma

Serious kidney injury is relatively rare because of the protection afforded by the rib cage, the back's heavy muscles, and the tough capsule surrounding the kidney. Traffic accidents and falls wherein the client lands on the abdomen, flank, or back are the most common cause of injury, usually resulting in blunt trauma. Kidney lacerations are also associated with fractures of the spine and ribs as well as penetrating injuries from bullets and knives.

Clinical Manifestations and Diagnostic Findings

The type of injury the client has suffered gives the first real key to identifying renal trauma. There frequently are multiple serious injuries, and renal trauma may not be immediately apparent. Hematuria (gross or microscopic) is a cardinal manifestation and is found in approximately 80% of cases. Remember, however, that serious renal injury can occur without hemorrhage, so clear urine should not negate a possible diagnosis. Other findings include shock, flank pain, and the development of a palpable mass in the affected flank area or over the 11th or 12th rib. Paralytic ileus may also occur. Grey Turner's sign refers to bruises over the flank and lower back secondary to retroperitoneal hemorrhage. A KUB film, IVP, retrograde pyelography, renal scan, ultrasonography, CT scan, and renal arteriography all help confirm the kind and amount of kidney injury.

Classification

Figure 57–12 illustrates the five categories of traumatic injury that can occur to the kidney: (1) contusion with intrarenal hemorrhage, (2) minor laceration (rupture with subcapsular hemorrhage), (3) major laceration (rupture into the renal pelvis), (4) "fractured" kidney (shattered rupture), and (5) vascular (pedicle) injury. A contusion involves development of a hematoma that remains confined within the renal parenchyma. Rupture of the kidney may cause hemorrhage between the capsular walls; bleeding may or may not reach into the renal pelvis. A shattered or "fractured" kidney results in hemorrhage throughout the renal tissue. The pedicle holds the renal artery and other vital circulatory and nervous system connections to the kidney. Injury to the pedicle may well jeopardize the life of the kidney. A pedicle injury may occur with or without intrarenal hemorrhage.

Complications

In addition to the immediate problems of hemorrhage and loss of functioning renal tissue, kidney trauma makes the client highly susceptible to a number of other problems. Even in closed injuries, there is a high risk of sepsis leading to the development of kidney and perinephric abscesses. Secondary hemorrhage is not uncommon. Other complications include hypertension due to fibrosis and ischemic kidney; renal artery thrombosis; arteriovenous aneurysms; fistula formation due to extravasation of urine; and the development of urinomas and pseudocysts.

Acute and Subacute Care

Intervention in renal trauma is controversial and centers on whether to pursue a conservative or a surgical path. Most physicians agree that kidney contusion calls for conservative treatment. Other minor injuries, such as small subcapsular hematomas and minor lacerations without extravasation, may also be better followed conservatively. Major injuries, such as renal fracture, parenchymal injury with major arterial occlusion, avulsion injuries or tears in the renal artery or vein, and parenchymal lacerations with extending perirenal hematomas or urinary extravasation, may require surgical exploration. Possible indicators to exploration include continued moderate-to-severe hemorrhage and continued urinary extravasation. Urinary extravasation itself is not definite grounds for surgery, because sterile urine usually resolves or encapsulates spontaneously. However, it sometimes produces a severe tissue reaction and causes fistula formation. The pocket of extrarenal urine may also become obstructive.

■ Medical Management

Medical management, which primarily involves waiting and watching, is possible because the retroperitoneal space allows tamponade. In the absence of other injuries,

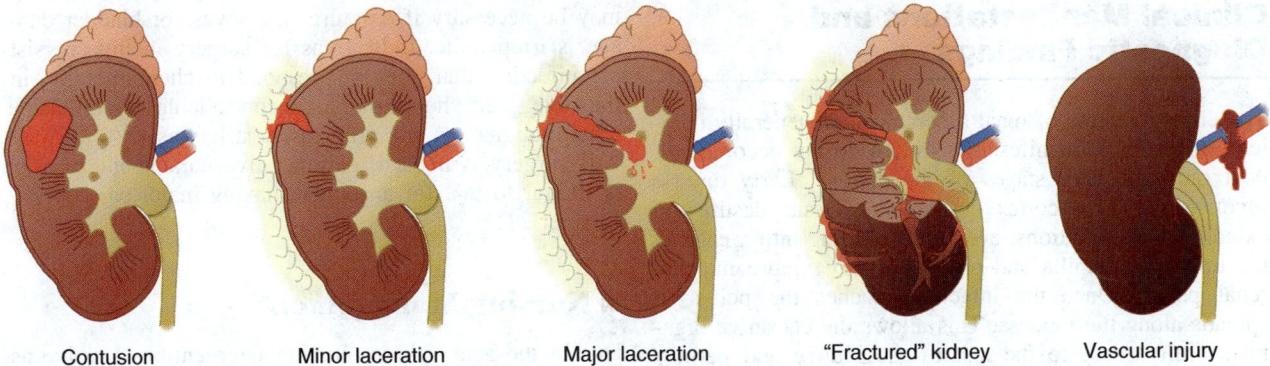

| Contusion | Minor laceration | Major laceration | "Fractured" kidney | Vascular injury |

Figure 57–12. Categories of renal trauma: contusion (intrarenal hemorrhage); minor laceration (subcapsular hemorrhage); major laceration (hemorrhage into renal pelvis); fractured kidney (shattered rupture); and vascular (pedicle) injury (damaging renal blood supply).

a client with microscopic hematuria and normal IVP may be followed on an ambulatory basis with careful instructions about activity restrictions and the need for adequate hydration. If there is gross hematuria, the client is placed on bedrest until the urine clears. Serial observations of the urine, hematocrit, and vital signs are made to watch the progress of the hemorrhage. Sequential urine specimens may be collected to compare current and previous urine color and turbidity. Even if replacement fluids are not needed, a prophylactic intravenous line may be established, and a type and crossmatch for blood may be done. If a hematoma is present or the IVP demonstrates extravasation of the urine, the client may receive antibiotics to prevent sepsis. The physician prescribes blood transfusions if the hematocrit is low. After the urine is cleared, the client will be allowed to be more active. After discharge from the healthcare facility, the client needs follow-up blood pressure checks and IVPs to rule out the development of secondary hypertension and anatomic derangement of the renal system.

■ Surgical Management

The greatest diversity of opinion concerns proper handling of the renal damage discovered during exploration. When the other kidney is functioning effectively, some physicians recommend free use of nephrectomy to avoid later sequelae, whereas others believe the goal should be salvaging maximal renal function. The latter group advocates giving the conservative approach a fair trial and, if surgery is necessary, attempts to repair the kidney before deciding to remove it. With renal vascular injury, less than 50% of kidneys can be salvaged if the injury is 18 hours old; there is virtually no chance of renal recovery after 24 hours.

Renal hemorrhage may be controlled by injecting an autologous clot into the secondary arteries supplying the bleeding site. Blood is drawn from the client and allowed to clot. The clot is then injected angiographically. Normal endothelium has a strong clot-lysing effect, so the clot disappears after a period of several hours from the normal adjacent vasculature and affects only the damaged portion.

If kidney repair is attempted rather than nephrectomy, the surgical procedure aims to debride devitalized tissue, achieve hemostasis, establish a watertight seal of the collecting system, approximate the renal parenchymal edges, and drain the renal fossa. Two surgical techniques increase the successful outcome of repair. Extracorporeal or bench surgery allows the kidney to be removed from the body so as to better visualize and manipulate the organ during the repair process; the kidney is returned by autotransplantation. During its time outside the body, the kidney is maintained either by hypothermia or by a perfusate mechanically pulsed through it. The slush technique, involving immersing the kidney in iced saline slush, slows down the metabolism and oxygen requirement of the renal tissue, allowing longer intraoperative ischemic times. This does cause some systemic hypothermia, but it is not significant. Pedicle vascular injury may also be repaired. If these techniques fail, nephrectomy is necessary. Postoperative nursing diagnoses and interventions are as described previously.

■ Nursing Management

Nursing interventions during conservative treatment center on monitoring urinary elimination patterns and helping the client to cope and comply with the medical regimen. Anxiety is common and requires supportive intervention. Imposed activity restrictions may result in problems with bowel elimination and adequate fluid intake, circulation, and respiratory function. The client being followed on an ambulatory basis needs an appropriate teaching plan covering health maintenance activities and the need for a follow-up program.

Renal Tuberculosis

Tuberculosis of the kidney, which affects men more frequently than women, occurs when the causative organism, *Mycobacterium tuberculosis*, reaches the kidney via the bloodstream from another source in the body, usually the lungs. Once the organism arrives at the kidney, it may become dormant for many years. By the time it again becomes active, the original infection is often well healed. Frequently, the primary tubercular site was asymptomatic, which makes it difficult to identify renal tuberculosis on the basis of history.

Clinical Manifestations and Diagnostic Findings

The clinical course of renal tuberculosis is generally indolent, and clinical manifestations often do not become evident until the later stages of the disease. Early disease involves the renal cortex or medulla. Tissue destruction extends in all directions, eventually eroding into a calix at the tip of the papilla and progressing to rupture into the renal pelvis. Once the infection reaches the pelvis, it spreads along the mucosa. This allows the causative organisms full access to the rest of the kidney and permits them to move down the urinary tract where they can infect any of the urinary organs. If untreated, this destructive process will continue to form large, caseating masses, which coalesce to destroy kidney tissue. X-ray examination at this time shows the kidneys to have a motheaten appearance.

Organisms reaching the lower urinary tract usually result in fibrosis and stricture formation and destruction of the ureterovesical valve. If these processes stenose the ureter, thus reducing the exit for pus and urine from the infected kidney, renal destruction will accelerate. Descending tubercle bacilli may also lodge in the male reproductive organs, causing reduced function.

When renal tuberculosis becomes evident, assessment findings are often nonspecific. Renal manifestations may be preceded by general malaise, weight loss, low-grade fever, and night sweats, but these are not as frequent as with pulmonary tuberculosis. Manifestations of cystitis, as described in Chapter 56, are often the presenting indications. Flank pain may be present, and hematuria and pyuria are common. Males frequently have manifestations of epididymitis. A culture of *M. tuberculosis* grown from the urine confirms a definitive diagnosis. The specimens for culture are collected on at least three successive mornings. Because tubercle bacilli shed intermittently, 3 to 12 negative cultures are needed to exclude the diagnosis of active renal tuberculosis absolutely.

Management

■ Medical Management

Chemotherapy with antitubercular agents has reduced the need for surgical intervention. Multiple therapy that typically combines several medications (rifampin, ethambutol, isoniazid, and pyridoxine; streptomycin, cycloserine, and sodium para-aminosalicylate) is the most common intervention. Because tubercle bacilli divide slowly, the medications are usually given in a single daily dose. However, if side effects develop, the day's dose may be divided. See Chapter 42 for further information on antitubercular medications.

■ Surgical Management

Surgical intervention includes total or partial nephrectomy or cutaneous ureterostomy. Permanent urinary diversion may be necessary if strictures are severe or bladder damage is irreparable. Indications for surgery include persistent infection that does not respond to chemotherapy, intractable pain, hemorrhage, uncontrollable hypertension, renal malignancy, and progressive strictures.

If surgery is needed, perioperative nursing intervention is similar to that for any client having major surgery (see Chapter 21).

■ Nursing Management

During the acute phase, nursing interventions involve assisting with diagnostic procedures, protecting against the spread of causative organisms, providing relief of manifestations, and assisting the client with the medication regimen. Because tuberculosis arouses a great deal of fear and a feeling of social isolation, expect your nursing diagnoses to include fear and anxiety for the client as well as for the significant others. Help these clients to discuss and work through their feelings. Listen to their concerns and help them seek additional counseling if necessary.

Renal tuberculosis is a prolonged illness that requires long-term care and support. Because the client is usually followed on an ambulatory basis, instruction in self-care frequently is the primary nursing intervention. One of the biggest problems with clients recovering from renal tuberculosis is continued compliance with the prescribed medical and nursing regimens, especially when the client begins to feel better. Help the client understand the need for continual medication therapy and continuing follow-up examinations. The client must also understand the importance of maintaining general good health, such as proper nutrition, adequate rest, and good hygiene. During recovery, give the client positive feedback for adhering to the regimens, if appropriate. If not, use problem-solving techniques to help the client reestablish compliance with the regimens.

Renal Vascular Abnormalities

The kidneys depend on adequate blood circulation to nourish tissues and provide blood for filtration so they can perform their intended functions. Anything that interferes with the normal circulatory flow significantly reduces renal capabilities.

Renal Artery Disease

Ninety percent of all renal artery disease is caused by one or two progressive disease processes: atherosclerosis or fibromuscular dysplasia. Atherosclerosis affects males more often than females and usually involves the proximal third of the artery. Fibromuscular dysplasia is an alternating stenosis and dilation; arteriographic studies demonstrate a "string-of-beads" appearance in the artery. This condition affects females four to five times as often as males; the cause is unknown.

There are several other, less common, causes of renal artery disease. Neoplasms may obstruct the vessels. Embolism or thrombosis can cause acute obstruction. Trauma, as described earlier, can interrupt blood flow. The renal artery may be purposely occluded to produce a "medical nephrectomy," or total renal infarction; this may be done preoperatively in the case of renal adenocarcinoma or to control proteinuria or hypertension. Shredded Gelfoam may be used, or a liquid substance that polymerizes instantly when it contacts blood may be injected into the renal artery. A dissecting aneurysm in the renal artery may also interrupt renal circulation.

The end result of any of these conditions, if severe enough, is reduced renal blood flow. This, in turn, causes renal parenchymal ischemia and, finally, renal atrophy. The role of renal artery disease in renovascular hypertension is also well documented, and hypertension alone may indicate treatment of the condition.

Because of the kidney's compensatory mechanisms, the gradual development of renal artery stenosis from atherosclerosis and neoplasms may give rise to very few manifestations, at least until the resulting hypertension and decreasing renal function become evident. However, acute obstruction makes itself known relatively quickly. Manifestations of this sudden episode include flank pain over the affected kidney or abdominal pain and fever. Atrial arrhythmias are a frequent finding; however, because they often alternate with periods of normal sinus rhythm, this manifestation can be missed. Urinalysis may be normal, and blood chemistries may show an elevated aspartate aminotransferase and lactic dehydrogenase. An IVP will demonstrate a nonfunctioning kidney, and a renal scan will show no arterial blood flow.

In response to reduced renal circulation, collateral circulation helps preserve the kidney if sufficient development takes place before total obstruction. Collateral circulation, in addition to a marked reduction in filtration, renal work, and oxygen requirements, allows the kidney to tolerate ischemic periods for up to several weeks. In acute total occlusion, a normal kidney can remain viable for approximately 2 hours before infarction and tissue necrosis begin.

Treatment of the ischemic kidney usually involves surgical revascularization. Arterial endarterectomy may be done with follow-up anticoagulant or antiplatelet therapy. Percutaneous transluminal renal angioplasty is a procedure in which the vessel is cleared using a balloon catheter. If the vessel cannot be recanalized, a renal artery resection with end-to-end anastomosis or an aortorenal bypass graft procedure may be performed.

In the postoperative period after an aorto-renal bypass graft procedure, the client may experience an initial exacerbation of hypertension. The cause of this development is unclear, but researchers believe it is related to systemic vasoconstriction secondary to general anesthesia and intraoperative hypothermia, severe pain, or transient renin secretion caused by the clamping of the aorta and manipulation of the kidney. This episode usually lasts no more than 48 hours, but it can be significant and may require medical intervention. You must monitor the blood pressure frequently.

Renal Vein Disease

The primary pathologic process involving the renal vein is thrombosis. Obstruction in venous drainage increases interstitial pressure, which reduces renal function. Findings include severe lumbar pain, renal enlargement, proteinuria, and hematuria. If the obstruction is bilateral, oliguria and azotemia occur. Contributing factors include diabetic nephropathy, chronic glomerulonephritis, and renal amyloidosis.

Kidney survival depends, in large part, on the development of collateral circulation before the vessel is totally occluded. Embolectomy or ligation of the renal veins may be done, and anticoagulants may be prescribed. Intravenous streptokinase is used to lyse the occluding clot. If enough renal damage has occurred, nephrectomy is an option.

Congenital Disorders

Renal congenital anomalies usually refer to the number, position, form or size, and structure of the kidneys. There may be an abnormal blood supply, although malformations that significantly affect renal function are rare. Anomalies of the ureteropelvic junction usually obstruct at that point and result in hydronephrosis. Typically, this situation is diagnosed and treated during childhood.

Anomalies Involving Kidney Number and Position

Renal agenesis indicates the absence of one or both kidneys. Having only one kidney presents no difficulty if it functions adequately. A client can live normally with one properly functioning kidney, as kidney donors aptly demonstrate. Bilateral agenesis, on the other hand, is fatal. In unilateral agenesis, the functioning kidney is at high risk of additional anomalies.

Supernumerary kidneys, or the presence of more than two kidneys, is usually asymptomatic and is found during IVP. The extra ureter enters either the ipsilateral ureter or the bladder.

Ectopic, or malpositioned, kidneys are usually found in the pelvis, although thoracic kidneys have been documented. Problems associated with this anomaly include respiratory difficulties, pain from pressure on nerves or surrounding structures, and difficulty in childbirth. Occasionally one kidney may be across the midline so that both kidneys are on the same side. This condition usually remains undiscovered until infection or obstruction requires x-ray examination.

Anomalies Involving Kidney Form and Size

Anomalies of kidney form and size include aplasia, hypoplasia, dysplasia, and horseshoe kidney. Aplastic kidneys are small and contracted and contain no functioning renal tissue. Renal hypoplasia produces miniature kidneys with some functioning tissue. Although clinically this condition may be completely asymptomatic, it may be the origin of hypertension and recurrent urinary tract infection.

Horseshoe kidney results when two kidneys are joined into a single organ whose shape somewhat resembles a horseshoe (Fig. 57–13). The kidneys are connected, usually at the lower poles, by an isthmus of tissue. Because the developmental error interferes with normal ascent and medial rotation, the kidney is usually located in the lower lumbar region with its pelvis facing anteriorly. Although horseshoe kidney may be asymptomatic, it carries with it a predisposition to hydronephrosis and infection secondary to ureteropelvic junction obstruction and calculus formation.

Anomalies Involving Cystic Disease

A congenitally abnormal kidney structure usually denotes the presence and progression of cysts within the renal tissue. This disorder ranges from a simple, solitary cyst to almost complete replacement of the functioning renal structures by cystic tissue. A simple renal cyst commonly originates superficially within the renal parenchyma. It is slow-growing and usually produces no manifestations until adulthood, when it may cause heaviness and pain in the abdomen and become a palpable mass. Diagnosis may be complicated because renal cysts closely resemble malignant tumors; differentiation between the two is vital. As long as a simple renal cyst remains asymptomatic, intervention usually is unnecessary. If needed, the cyst may be aspirated with a needle, or a partial nephrectomy to remove the cyst may be performed.

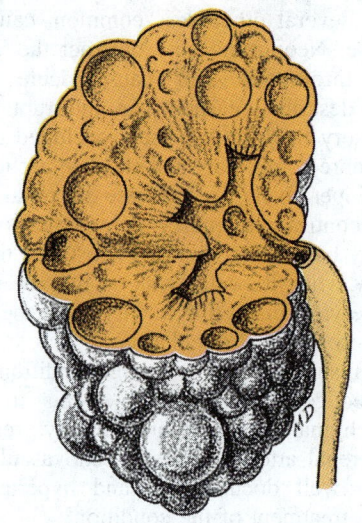

Figure 57–14. Polycystic kidney disease.

Polycystic Kidneys

Polycystic disease of the kidney is a hereditary disorder in which grapelike cysts containing serous fluid, blood, or urine replace normal kidney tissue (Fig. 57–14). The condition may strike at any age. In infancy, the disease usually results in death within days, although in milder forms the disease will not appear until childhood. Infantile polycystic kidney disease is inherited as an autosomal recessive trait, requiring both parents to carry the gene. It is a very rare disorder that affects both kidneys and often the liver.[16] Adult polycystic disease has an incidence rate of 1/250 to 5000 and accounts for about 10% of the clients receiving dialysis or transplantation. It is inherited as an autosomal dominant trait. It usually appears after 40 years of age, although it may begin as early as age 20 or as late as age 80 years.

Adult polycystic disease displays diverse manifestations. The most common manifestations are dull, aching lumbar or flank pain, which may be colicky, and hematuria. Other common urinary tract findings are proteinuria, palpable kidney masses, pyuria, calculi, and uremia. Early in the disease, the ability to concentrate urine decreases. Hypertension with resultant cardiac enlargement and heart failure are classic findings. Polycystic liver disease occurs in approximately one third of the cases, and cystic lesions are sometimes found in the thyroid, lung, pancreas, spleen, ovary, testis, epididymis, uterus, and bladder. Cerebral aneurysms occur in about 2% of clients with polycystic kidney disease.

The kidney can become so enlarged that it causes severe pressure on other organs, with production of additional extrarenal manifestations. The ultimate result of this disease is renal failure. As the disease slowly progresses, renal nephrons are destroyed, renal function deteriorates, and uremia ultimately results. The mean duration of polycystic kidney disease from onset of manifestations to development of uremia varies a great deal and may be 15 to 30 years or more. It is impossible to predict who of

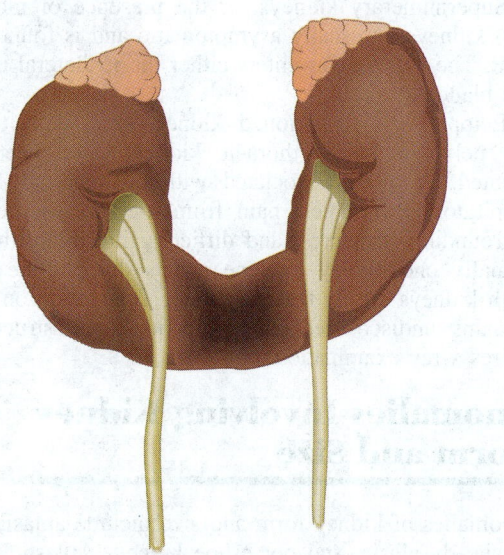

Figure 57–13. Horseshoe kidney.

those carrying the gene will go on to develop end-stage renal disease.[8]

There is no known way to arrest the progress of the destructive cysts, so conservative medical treatment deals with preserving kidney function. Urinary tract infection is the most common complication because of the distorted renal architecture, and chronic infection may occur because of the development of resistant bacteria. Aggressive control of hypertension is essential.

Unlike clients with increasing creatinine clearance rates caused by other kidney diseases, those with polycystic kidney disease seem to waste rather than retain sodium. Thus, they need an increased sodium and water intake. Percutaneous cyst puncture may bring palliative relief of obstruction or aid in draining an abscess. Once end-stage renal disease develops, hemodialysis or renal transplantation may be used. Nursing interventions for clients with renal failure are discussed earlier.

Genetic counseling is advisable because of the hereditary nature of the disease. This is particularly recommended if the disease is diagnosed during the childbearing years. However, because the disease typically appears after the childbearing period, the likelihood of transmitting the disease to another generation is greatly increased. Therefore, counseling the extended family is essential once the disease has been identified.

Adult-Onset Medullary Cystic Disease

Adult-onset medullary cystic disease, sometimes called uremic sponge kidney or medullary polycystic disease, is also an autosomal dominant disorder. It is similar to polycystic disease in all aspects except that it progresses to uremia very rapidly after its onset in the teenage years or in the 20s. Prognosis is poor, although hemodialysis and renal transplantation may be successful.

Medullary Sponge Kidney

Medullary sponge kidney is a cystic disorder that produces spaces at the apex of the renal pyramids. Onset peaks during adolescence or between the ages of 30 and 40 years. Infection, calculi, pain, and hematuria are potential complications. However, renal function usually remains adequate unless the client develops uncontrolled infection or calculi.

Other Hereditary Renal Disorders

Other hereditary renal disorders include chronic nephritis, congenital nephrotic syndrome, distal renal tubular acidosis, idiopathic hypercalciuria, and nephrotic diabetes insipidus. Many of these conditions are fatal during childhood, but some persist into adulthood and are discussed in the appropriate parts of this text.

Conclusions

Renal disorders are highly complex diseases. The nurse must have a clear understanding of the structure and function of the renal system in order to care for clients with these conditions. Treatment of renal disease may require the client to undergo many life-style changes, and the teaching provided by the nurse can influence the success of the client's adaptation. Clients requiring renal transplantation may be critically ill and need complex nursing interventions. Clients undergoing dialysis require long-term management. It is important for the nurse to be able to work with clients whatever treatments they are receiving. It is vital that the physician, nurse, and other health care professionals work together with the client toward a positive outcome.

Thinking Critically

1. **A 35-year-old newlywed woman enters the emergency room with acute abdominal pain and a fever of 101.8° F. Her abdomen is distended and she has not had a bowel movement today even though she is usually regular. The abdominal pain is diffuse and on the right side, although she is negative for rebound tenderness and has no pain at McBurney's point. Her white blood cell count is 15,000/mm³. What problems other than appendicitis might she be experiencing? What other assessments should be made—laboratory data such as a urinalysis, further assessments of her pain?**

Factors to Consider. What type of renal problem might she be experiencing? What teaching would she need once the diagnosis is made? What medication might be prescribed and why? What follow-up is needed?

2. **A 69-year-old man with diabetes is admitted with severe left flank pain, nausea, vomiting, and diarrhea. His abdomen is soft and only slightly tender. His urinalysis reveals increased red blood cells and his plain film shows a large staghorn calculus in the left kidney with hydronephrosis of the left kidney. What would be a priority assessment for this client?**

Factors to Consider. What other renal function tests should be done? What are the treatment options for large renal calculi?

3. **You are caring for a 74-year-old man who is 1 day post coronary artery bypass surgery. His urine output is about 15 ml/hr. He has a long history of hypertension (controlled) and his usual pressure still ranges from 180 to 190 over 90 to 100 mm Hg. His blood pressure since surgery ranges from 120 to 130 over 70 to 76 mm Hg. His serum sodium is 145 mEq/L and potassium is 4.9 mEq/L. His skin turgor is poor and his mucous membranes dry. What is your priority assessment and action?**

Factors to Consider. What is his intake since surgery? What are the possible causes of his low blood pressure, increased electrolytes, and decreased urine output? If he is in renal failure, what is the probable cause? What other assessments should you make?

Bibliography

1. Arnold, R. M. (Ed.). (1995). *Procuring organs for transplant: The debate over non-heart-beating cadaver protocols.* Baltimore: Johns Hopkins University Press.
2. Bach, F. H., & Auchincloss, H. Jr. (1995). *Transplantation immunology.* New York: Wiley-Liss.
3. Baer, C. L., & Lancaster, L. E. (1992). Acute renal failure. *Critical Care Nursing Quarterly, 14*(4), 1–21.
4. Bancroft, B. (1994). Immunology simplified. *Seminars in Perioperative Nursing, 3*(2), 70–78.
5. Bauer, C. L. (1993). Commentary on differences in immunosuppressant agents. *AACN Nursing Scan in Critical Care, 3*(4), 14.
6. Bennett, J. C., & Plum, F. (Eds.). (1996). *Cecil textbook of medicine* (20th ed.). Philadelphia: W. B. Saunders.
7. Bratton, L. B., & Griffin, L. W. (1994). A kidney donor's dilemma: The sibling who can donate—but doesn't. *Social Work in Health Care, 20*(2), 75–96.
8. Brenner, B. M. (Ed.). (1996). *Brenner and Rector's the kidney* (5th ed.). Philadelphia: W. B. Saunders.
9. Brundage, D. (1992). *Renal disorders.* St. Louis: Mosby–Year Book.
10. Brunier, G. M. (1994). Calcium/phosphate imbalances, aluminum toxicity, and renal osteodystrophy. *ANNA Journal, 21*(4), 171–179.
11. Burrowes, J. D., Alto, A., & Kaufman, A. M. (1993). Intradialytic parenteral nutrition: A practical approach—the malnourished patient undergoing maintenance hemodialysis. *ANNA Journal, 20*(6), 671–677.
12. Burrows-Hudson S. (Ed.). (1993). *Standards of clinical practice for nephrology.* Pitman, NJ: American Nephrology Nurses Association.
13. Busson, M., et al. (1995). Analysis of cadaver donor criteria on the kidney transplant survival rate in 5,129 transplantations. *Journal of Urology, 154*(2, Pt. 1), 356–360.
14. Chambers, J. K. (1993). Renal insufficiency: Implications for care of the medical-surgical patient. *MEDSURG Nursing, 2*(1), 33–40.
15. Chmielewski, C. (1992). Renal anatomy and overview of nephron function. *American Nephrology Nurses' Association Journal, 19*(1), 34–40.
16. Christiansen, J. L., & Grzbouski, J. M. (1993). *Biology of aging.* St. Louis: Mosby–Year Book.
17. Courts, N. F. (1994). Psychosocial interventions for patients receiving hemodialysis. *Urologic Nursing, 14*(3), 79–81.
18. Cunningham, N., & Smith, S. L. (1990). Postoperative care of the renal transplant patient. *Critical Care Nursing, 10*(9), 74–80.
19. Dolleris, P. M. (1992). Diuretic and vasopressor usage in acute renal failure: A synopsis. *Critical Care Nursing Quarterly, 14*(4), 28–31.
20. Duffy, M., & Uber, L. (1994). Immunosuppressive medications. *Dialysis and Transplant, 23*(6), 303–305.
21. Dunn, S. A. (1993). How to care for the dialysis patient. *American Journal of Nursing, 23*(6), 26–33.
22. Erikson, P. (1993). Idiopathic glomerulonephritis: Is it IgA nephropathy? *ANNA Journal, 20*(2), 127–134, 153.
23. First, M. R. (1993). Long-term complications after transplantation. *American Journal of Kidney Disease, 22,* 477.
24. Flye, M. W. (Ed.). (1995). *Atlas of organ transplantation.* Philadelphia: W. B. Saunders.
25. Glassock, R. J. (1992). *Current therapy in nephrology and hypertension* (3rd ed.). St. Louis: Mosby–Year Book.
26. Gray, M. (1992). *Genitourinary disorders.* St. Louis: Mosby–Year Book.
27. Guyton, A. C. (1992). *Human physiology and mechanisms of disease* (5th ed.). Philadelphia: W. B. Saunders.
28. Guyton, A. C., & Hall, J. E. (1996). *Textbook of medical physiology* (9th ed.). Philadelphia: W. B. Saunders.
29. Haddad, A. (1995). Ethics in action: What would you do? *RN, 58*(1), 21–23.
30. Helderman, J. H., & Frist, W. H. (Eds.). (1995). *Grand rounds in transplantation.* New York: Chapman & Hall.
31. Higashihara, E., et al. (1993). Clinical aspects of polycystic kidney disease. *Journal of Urology, 147*(2), 329–332.
32. Holechek, M. J. (1992). Glomerular filtration and renal hemodynamics. *ANNA Journal, 19*(3), 237–245.
33. Holechek, M. J. (1992). Renal physiology series: Glomerular filtration and renal hemodynamics, part 2. *ANNA Journal, 19*(3), 237–248.
34. Hricik, D. E., et al. (1995). Detiminants of long-term allograft function following steroid withdrawal in renal transplant recipients. *Clinical Transplantation, 9*(5), 419–423.
35. Hussar, D. A. (1994). Immunosuppressant: Tacrolimus. *Nursing, 24*(12), 54.
36. Jacobson, H. R., Striker, G. E., & Klahn, S. (1991). *The principles and practice of nephrology.* St. Louis: Mosby–Year Book.
37. Johnson, C. C. S. (1994). Knowledge of immunology is essential to plan effective nursing for immunocompromised patients. *Intensive and Critical Care Nursing, 10*(2), 121–126.
38. Karlowicz, K. A. (Ed.). (1995). *Urologic nursing: Principles and practice.* Philadelphia: W. B. Saunders.
39. Kee, C. C. (1992). Age-related changes in the renal system: Causes, consequences, and nursing implications. *Geriatric Nursing, 13*(2), 80–83.
40. Kenny, R. A. (1992). *Physiology of aging: A synopsis.* St. Louis: Mosby–Year Book.
41. King, C. R., Hoffart, N., & Murray, M. E. (1992). Acute renal failure in bone marrow transplantation. *Oncology Nursing Forum, 19*(9), 1327–1335.
42. Kleinpell, R. M. (1993). Commentary on transplantation immunology. *AACN Nursing Scan in Critical Care, 3*(4), 15.
43. Koeppen, B. M., & Stanton, B. A. (1992). *Renal physiology.* St. Louis: Mosby–Year Book.
44. Kroniewicz, D. M., & O'Brien, M. E. (1994). Evaluation of a hemodialysis patient education and support program. *ANNA Journal, 21*(1), 33–39.
45. Lancaster, L. E. (Ed.). *Core curriculum for nephrology nursing* (2nd ed.). Pitman, NJ: American Nephrology Nurses Association.
46. Levine, D. Z. (Ed.). (1991). *Care of the renal patient.* Philadelphia: W. B. Saunders.
47. Lewandowski, J. (1993). Issues in renal nutrition. *Nephrology Nursing Today, 3*(4), 1–8.
48. Lindeman, R. D. (1993). Renal physiology and pathophysiology of aging. *Contributions to Nephrology, 105,* 1–12.
49. Llach, F. (1993). *Popper's clinical nephrology* (3rd ed). Boston: Little, Brown.
50. Lote, C. J. (1994). *Principles of renal physiology* (3rd ed.). London: Chapman & Hall.
51. Ludlow, M. (1993). Renal handling of potassium. *ANNA Journal, 20*(1), 52–56.
52. Martinelli, A. M. (1993). Organ donation: Barriers, religious aspects. *AORN Journal, 58*(2), 236–252.
53. Massry, S. G., & Glassock, R. J. (Eds.). (1995). *Massry and Glassock's textbook of nephrology* (3rd ed.). Baltimore: Williams & Wilkins.
54. Neuman, M., & Urizar, R. (1994). Hemolytic uremic syndrome: Current pathophysiology and management. *ANNA Journal, 21*(2), 137–145.
55. Nichols, L. (1992). Future trends in transplantation. *Seminars in Perioperative Nursing, 1*(1), 55–57.
56. Nolan, M. T., & Augustine, S. M. (Eds.). (1995). *Transplantation nursing: Acute and long-term management.* Norwalk, CT: Appleton & Lange.
57. Oberley, E. T., & Comptom, A. (1994). Nursing interventions for rehabilitating renal patients. *ANNA Journal, 21*(7), 419–426.
58. Olbrisch, M. E., & Levenson, J. L. (1995). Psychosocial assessment of organ transplant candidates: Current status of methodological and philosophical issues. *Psychosomatics, 36*(3), 236–243.
59. Peterson, R. (1993). An emerging cancer risk: Organ transplantation. *Cancer Nursing, 16*(6), 468–472.
60. Porcush, J. G., & Faubert, P. F. (1991). *Renal disease in the aged.* Boston: Little, Brown.

61. Premminger, G. M. (1992). Renal calculi: Pathogenesis, diagnosis, and medical therapy. *Seminars in Nephrology, 12*(2), 200–216.

62. Preisig, P. (1992). Renal physiology series: Urinary concentration and dilution, part 3. *ANNA Journal, 19*(4), 351–355.

63. Preisig, P. (1994). Renal physiology series: Renal acidification, part 7. *ANNA Journal, 21*(5), 251–259.

64. Pudelski, B., & Bednarz, D. (1992). Nursing intervention to improve dialysis adequacy of intensive care patients in acute renal failure. *ANNA Journal, 19*(20), 163.

65. Radke, K. J. (1994). Renal physiology series: The aging kidney: Structure, function, and nursing practice implications, part 6. *ANNA Journal, 21*(4), 181–190, 191–193.

66. Schrier, R. W. (1992). *Renal and electrolyte disorders* (4th ed.). Boston, Little, Brown.

67. Schrier, R. W. (Ed.). (1995). *Manual of nephrology.* Boston: Little, Brown.

68. Schrier, R. W., & Gottschalk, C. W. (Eds.). (1993). *Diseases of the kidney* (5th ed.). Boston: Little, Brown.

69. Seidman, E. J. (Ed.). (1994). *Current urologic therapy.* Philadelphia: W. B. Saunders.

70. Selkin, D. W., & Giebisch, G. (Eds.). (1992). *The kidney: Physiology and pathophysiology.* New York: Raven Press.

71. Shapiro, R. S., Deshetter, N., & Stockand, H. E. (1994). Fluid overload again! A technique to enhance fluid compliance. *Dialysis and Transplantation, 23*(10), 571–574.

72. Shoop, K. L. (1994). Pruritus in end stage renal disease. *ANNA Journal, 21*(2), 147–153.

73. Sketris, I., et al. (1995). Optimizing the use of cyclosporine in renal transplantation. *Clinical Biochemistry, 28*(3), 195–211.

74. Smith, D. R. (1992). *General urology* (13th ed.). Los Altos, CA: Lange Medical.

75. Stark, J. (1994). Acute renal failure in trauma: Current perspectives. *Critical Care Nursing Quarterly, 16*(4), 49–60.

76. Starzomski, R. (1994). Ethical issues in palliative care: The case of dialysis and organ transplantation. *Journal of Palliative Care 10*(3), 27–34.

77. Steen, G. (1993). Maintaining near-normal life style for ESRD patients. *ANNA Journal, 20*(5), 593–594.

78. Stein, P. (1994). Perioperative considerations of vascular access for dialysis. *AORN Journal, 60*(6), 947–949, 951–952, 955–956.

79. Strohschein, B. L., Caruso, D. M., & Greene, K. A. (1994). Continuous venovenous hemodialysis. *American Journal of Critical Care, 3*(2), 92–101.

80. Suthanthran, M., & Strom, T. B. (1995). Immunobiology and immunopharmacology of organ allograft rejection. *Journal of Clinical Immunology, 15*(4), 161–171.

81. Tanagho, E. A., & McAninich, J. W. (1992). *Smith's general urology* (13th ed.). Norwalk, CT: Appleton & Lange.

82. Tarantino, A., Montagnino, G., & Ponticelli, C. (1995). Corticosteroids in kidney transplant recipients: Safety issues and timing of discontinuing. *Drug Safety, 13*(3), 145–156.

83. Valtin, H., & Schafer, J. A. (1995). *Renal function: Mechanisms preserving fluid and solute balance in health* (3rd ed.). Boston: Little, Brown.

84. Vander, A. (1995). *Renal physiology* (5th ed.). New York: McGraw-Hill.

85. Walsh, P. C., et al. (1992). *Campbell's urology* (6th ed.). Philadelphia: W. B. Saunders.

86. Wahrenberger, A. (1992). Differences in immunosuppressive agents. *ANNA Journal, 19*(6), 566–567.

87. Wood, J. M., & Bosley, C. L. (1995). Acute postrenal failure: Reversing the problem. *Nursing, 25*(3), 48–50.

88. Workman, M. L. (1995). Essential concepts of inflammation and immunity. *Critical Care Nursing Clinics of North America, 7*(4), 601–615.

89. Yucha, C. B. (1993). Renal physiology series: Renal control of calcium, part 5a. *ANNA Journal, 20*(4), 440–446.

90. Yucha, C. B. (1993). Renal physiology series: Renal control of phosphorus and magnesium, part 5b. *ANNA Journal, 20*(4), 447–452.

Gastrointestinal Disorders

Unit Editor: **BETTY BLAKE**

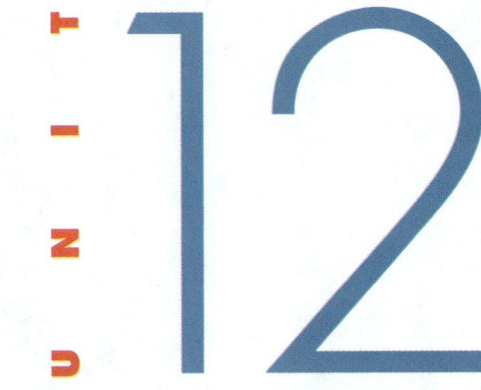

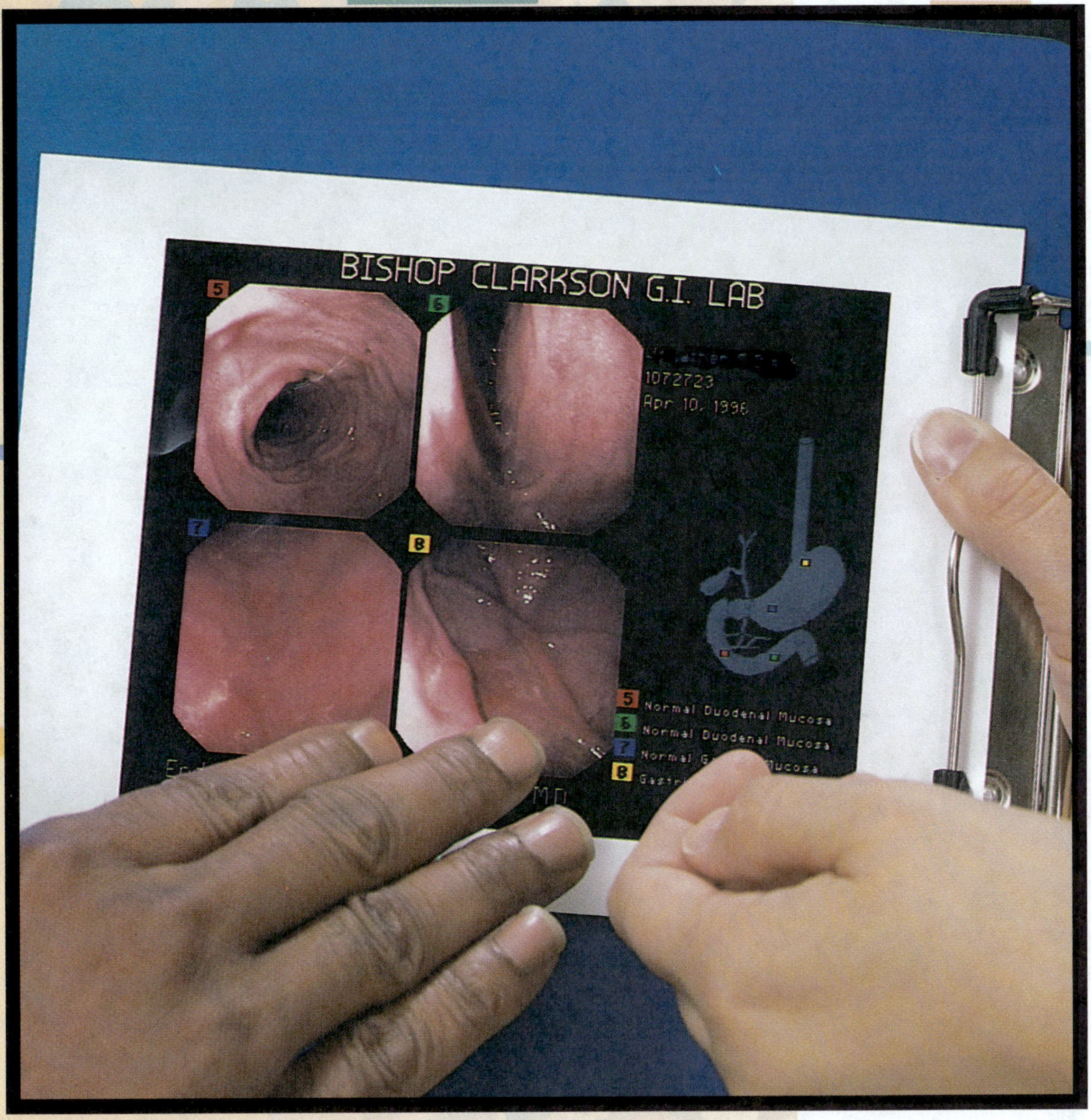

Structure and Function of the Gastrointestinal System

Esther Matassarin-Jacobs

The gastrointestinal tract, also called the digestive tract or alimentary canal, is a hollow muscular tube that extends from the mouth to the anus (Fig. 58–1). Its principal function is to provide the body with fluid, nutrients, and electrolytes.

Normally, the gastrointestinal tract is the source of intake for the body. Raw materials taken in through the mouth are metabolized for energy, tissue building, and so forth. The gastrointestinal tract also disposes of the wastes from this digestive process.

The Gastrointestinal Tract

Activities of the Tract

The four major activities of the gastrointestinal tract are (1) secretion of electrolytes, hormones, and enzymes to be used in breakdown of the ingested materials; (2) movement of ingested products; (3) digestion of food and fluids; and (4) absorption of end products into the bloodstream.

Secretion

There are two general types of secretions in the gastrointestinal tract: (1) mucous secretions, which are produced throughout the entire length of the tract; and (2) digestive secretions, which are produced in the mouth, stomach, duodenum, and jejunum. Mucous secretions protect and lubricate the walls of the tract. Digestive secretions (enzymes and electrolytes) break down ingested food so that it can be absorbed.

Movement

There are two types of movements in the gastrointestinal tract: mixing and propulsive. Both are produced by rhyth-

mic contractions of the smooth muscle fibers that lie in the walls of the stomach and gut. These fibers vary somewhat from one segment of the tract to another. However, they usually consist of an outer longitudinal layer, an inner circular layer, and a thin layer in the deeper portion of the mucosa. See Figure 58–2 for a typical cross-section of the gut.

Mixing movements, sometimes called segmentation contractions, are rhythmic contractions between individual segments of bowel that alternate with contractions occurring at the midpoint of each segment. Peristalsis is a wave of muscle contraction in the bowel wall that pushes the bolus of food ahead of it (Fig. 58–3). This type of movement occurs in all smooth muscle tubes of the body and can go in either direction from the point of stimulation. In the bowel, the waves usually move toward the anus.

Digestion and Absorption

During digestion, food is broken down into chemical compounds small and simple enough to be absorbed into the bloodstream by diffusion or active transport. The digestive process begins in the mouth.

The Mouth

Structure

The mouth (also called the oral or buccal cavity) is formed by the cheeks, the hard palate (anterior portion of the roof of the mouth), the soft palate (posterior portion of the roof of the mouth), and the tongue. The lips are folds of flesh that surround the opening of the mouth.

Chewing and Its Functions

Chewing begins digestion by preparing food for swallowing. It is controlled by reflex activity via the fifth cranial

This chapter incorporates material written for the fourth edition by Shirley M. Ruder.

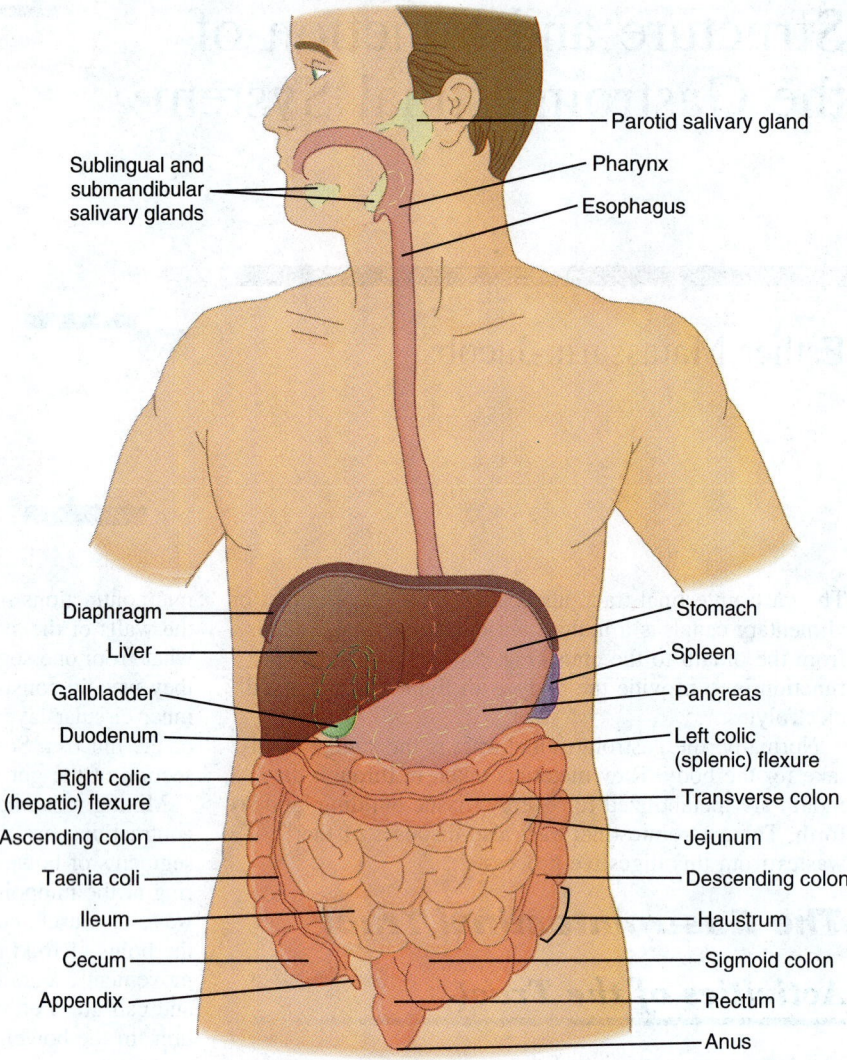

Figure 58–1. The digestive system.

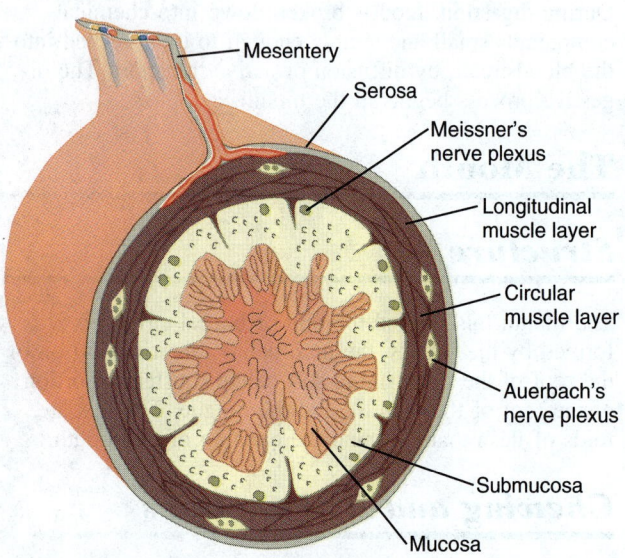

Figure 58–2. Typical cross-section of the gastrointestinal tract.

nerve. Chewing is stimulated by the presence of food in the mouth. The functions of chewing are as follows:

- To break food products into smaller portions
- To break down any fibrous coverings to allow digestive enzymes access to the food particles
- To prevent trauma to the mucous lining of the esophagus by making the food smoother

To preserve chewing capabilities, a person must maintain dental health. An individual exerts pressures ranging from 25 to 275 lb during the chewing process, depending on the nature of the food and the teeth involved. Dentures are not as effective for chewing as natural teeth, and poorly chewed foods are not readily digested.

Saliva and Its Functions

Saliva is secreted by the sublingual and submandibular glands under the tongue and by the parotid glands near the ears, opposite the second molars.

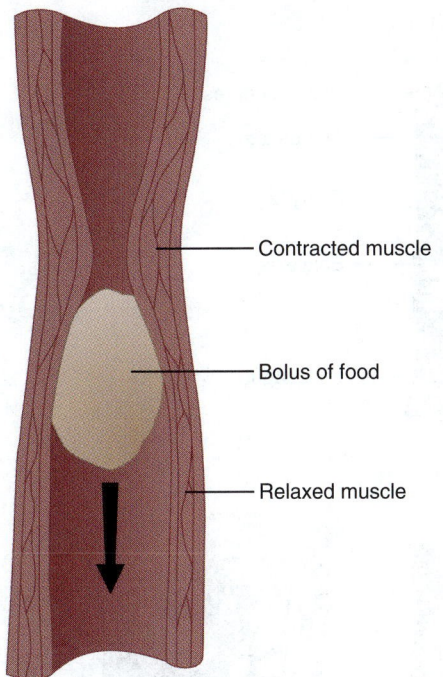

Figure 58–3. Peristalsis moves food through the gastrointestinal tract by pushing the bolus ahead of a wave of muscle contraction.

Saliva lubricates and softens the food mass and dissolves the most soluble components of food, thus stimulating the taste buds. Saliva contains the enzyme ptyalin (amylase), which breaks down starches to maltose. The action of ptyalin continues in the fundus of the stomach, where food is mixed with gastric secretions.

Swallowing (Deglutition)

Food in the mouth, called a bolus, is swallowed in three phases: (1) the oral phase, (2) the involuntary pharyngeal phase, and (3) the esophageal phase.

The time it takes for the bolus to reach the stomach depends on the consistency of the bolus and the individual's body position. Fluids tend to arrive ahead of the peristaltic wave, and the more solid masses may arrive after it. The bolus travels faster when the individual is in a vertical position. Esophageal transport requires the coordination of peristalsis with relaxation of the lower esophageal sphincter (Fig. 58–4).

The Esophagus

Structure

The esophagus, a hollow muscular tube, lies posterior to the trachea and larynx at the level of C6. It extends vertically through the mediastinum and diaphragm to the level of T11. The esophagus connects the hypopharynx with the stomach and serves as a passage for food from mouth to stomach.

The esophageal wall consists of four layers: (1) mucosa, (2) submucosa, (3) muscularis, and (4) serosa. These four basic layers compose the entire gastrointestinal tract, although slight modifications occur in different regions.

In the upper esophagus, the muscle is striated but acts like smooth muscle, contracting and relaxing as the bolus travels through the tube. The body of the esophagus is composed of smooth muscle that serves to propel food toward the stomach. The areolar layer connects the muscular and mucous layers and contains the blood and lymph vessels. The mucous layer in the proximal half of the esophagus contains glands that secrete mucus to lubricate the bolus. Mucus also protects the esophageal mucous membrane from trauma resulting from passage of partially chewed food products.

The body of the esophagus is composed of cervical and thoracic segments. At the proximal end is the upper esophageal sphincter (UES). The distal segment is composed of the ampulla and vestibule and includes the lower esophageal sphincter (LES). The LES is not a distinctive sphincter but a zone of increased pressure that provides a physiologic barrier to protect the esophageal mucosa from the effects of gastric reflux (the return or backflow of gastric secretions).

The pressure and competence of the LES is normally increased by gastrin and parasympathetic drugs. Substances such as secretin, cholecystokinin (CCK), anticholinergics, cigarettes, fatty foods, and alcohol decrease LES pressure.

Decreased sphincter pressure can cause gastric reflux, resulting in epigastric pain and indigestion. On the other hand, increased pressure can be manifested as dysphagia (difficulty swallowing).

Function

The esophagus (1) receives a bolus from the oropharynx, (2) transports the bolus along its length, (3) propels the bolus into the stomach when the LES opens, (4) provides an antireflux barrier, and (5) acts as a vent for increased intragastric pressure.

Blood Supply and Lymphatic Drainage

The esophageal arteries, the inferior thyroid artery, and the left gastric artery provide the esophagus with its arterial blood supply. The left gastric and inferior phrenic arteries supply the gastroesophageal area. Venous blood is returned via the azygos, thyroid, and left gastric veins.

Lymphatic drainage from the cervical esophagus and from the tracheal and postmediastinal nodes flows to the internal jugular vein, while intercostal nodes drain the thoracic esophagus. The lymphatic drainage of the lower esophagus occurs through the diaphragmatic, intracardiac, and left gastric lymph nodes.

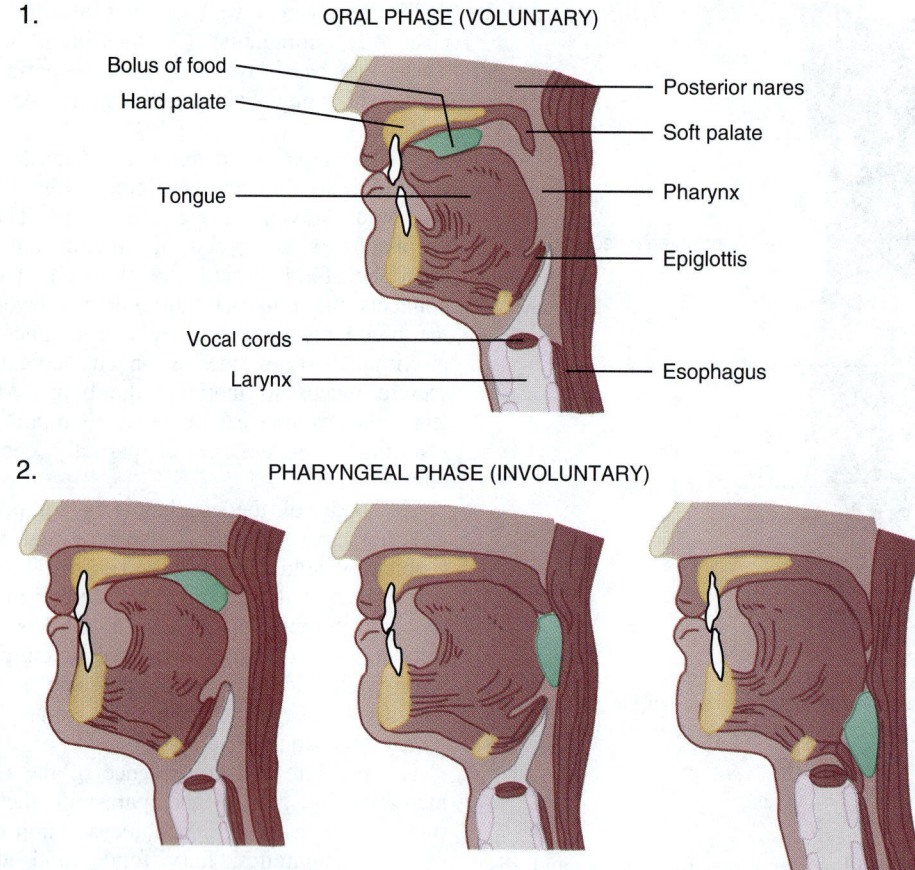

1. ORAL PHASE (VOLUNTARY)

Bolus of food
Hard palate
Posterior nares
Soft palate
Tongue
Pharynx
Epiglottis
Vocal cords
Larynx
Esophagus

2. PHARYNGEAL PHASE (INVOLUNTARY)

Early   Middle   Late

3. ESOPHAGEAL PHASE (INVOLUNTARY)

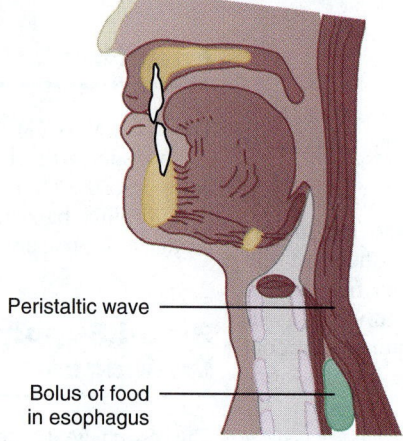

Peristaltic wave

Bolus of food
in esophagus

Figure 58–4. Swallowing occurs in three phases: (1) Voluntary or oral phase. The tongue presses food against the hard palate, forcing it toward the pharynx. (2) Involuntary, pharyngeal phase. Early: wave of peristalsis forces bolus between tonsillar pillars. Middle: soft palate draws upward to close posterior nares, and respirations cease momentarily. Late: vocal cords approximate and larynx pulls upward, covering the airway and stretching the esophagus open. (3) Involuntary, esophageal phase. Relaxation of the upper esophageal (hypopharyngeal) sphincter allows a peristaltic wave to move the bolus down the esophagus.

Innervation

Both the sympathetic and parasympathetic fibers of the autonomic nervous system provide innervation to the esophagus. The sympathetic fibers emanate from cervical and thoracic ganglia and from preganglionic fibers of the greater and lesser splanchnic nerves. Parasympathetic innervation from the vagus nerve extends along the anterior and posterior esophageal walls. Both sympathetic and parasympathetic stimuli are received by the LES.

Motor Activity

Peristaltic waves are an involuntary reflex of the glossopharyngeal nerves stimulated by the act of swallowing. Secondary stimulation of peristalsis occurs with dilation of the lower half of the esophagus and is probably reflex in origin.

The Stomach

Structure

The stomach is located in the upper portion of the abdomen, to the left of the midline. The lower esophageal, or cardiac, sphincter divides the esophagus and stomach, which, on contraction, closes the stomach off from the esophagus. The stomach has a capacity of approximately 1500 ml and has three anatomic divisions (Fig. 58–5):

1. The fundus, which lies above and to the left of the cardiac sphincter
2. The body or central area
3. The lower area, called the antrum or pyloric region

The outlet from the distal end of the stomach and the duodenum is called the pyloric sphincter. It permits the flow of chyme from the stomach.

The stomach wall has four layers: (1) serosa, (2) muscularis, (3) submucosa, and (4) mucosa. The serosal outer layer is the visceral peritoneum. The muscular layers (tunica muscularis) produce peristaltic activity of the stomach as it churns food during digestion. The submucosa (or tela submucosa) connects the muscular and mucous layers of the stomach wall and contains the blood, lymph channels, and nerve plexus.

The epithelial lining of the stomach contains many microscopic glands:

● Cardiac glands secrete mucus.
● Peptic (chief) cells secrete mucus and pepsinogen. Pepsinogen is converted to pepsin, a proteolytic enzyme.
● Parietal (oxyntic) cells secrete hydrochloric acid and water. The parietal cells are stimulated by gastrin to produce hydrochloric acid, which helps digestion of protein. These cells also produce the intrinsic factor, which allows vitamin B_{12} to be absorbed.
● Neck cells secrete mucus.
● Pyloric glands secrete gastrin and mucus.

Function

The functions of the stomach include storage, mixing, liquification of the bolus of food into chyme, and control of passage of food into the duodenum. The first stage of protein breakdown occurs in the stomach. The major portion of the mechanical breakdown of food occurs in the antrum (see Fig. 58–5). At the distal end of the stomach, the pyloric sphincter permits the flow of chyme from the stomach into the duodenum. Digestion of starches, which

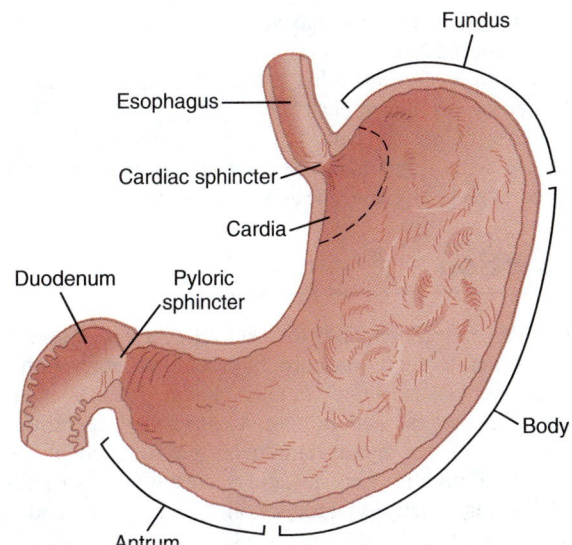

Figure 58–5. Anatomy of the stomach.

begins in the mouth by the action of ptyalin, continues in the stomach. Digestion can last for as long as 30 minutes, or until the mixing function of the stomach allows its acid contents to inactivate the ptyalin. Digestion of fats in the stomach is minimal. Small quantities of water, alcohol, glucose, and some drugs may be absorbed through the gastric mucosa. Most organisms are destroyed by the acidic gastric juice.

Blood Supply

The stomach's arterial blood supply is from the celiac artery, which branches off the lesser and greater curvatures. Gastric arteries, from the splenic artery, supply the fundus. The portal vein provides the venous drainage of the stomach. The right and left gastroepiploic veins drain the greater curvature, while the right gastric and coronary veins drain the lesser curvature. Lymph nodes of the stomach arise in the submucosa and drain into the thoracic duct.

Innervation

The stomach is innervated by both the sympathetic and parasympathetic systems. The vagus nerve supplies parasympathetic innervation. When stimulated, the vagus nerve causes (1) increased gastric secretion of acid, gastrin, and pepsin; and (2) increased gastric motor activity.

The greater splanchnic nerves and the celiac ganglia supply the sympathetic innervation. The sympathetic nerves inhibit gastric secretion and motility. They are stimulated by muscle contraction, distention, and inflammation.

Auerbach's plexus (motor function) and Meissner's plexus (sensory function) lie within the gastric wall. These nerve plexuses provide intrinsic innervation for the stomach. Both begin in the esophageal wall and extend the length of the gut. Auerbach's plexus lies between the longitudinal and circular muscle layers; Meissner's plexus is in the submucosa.

Stimulation of Auerbach's plexus generates gastric motility, increasing the intensity and rate of contractions and the release of gastrin from the antrum. Meissner's plexus functions with Auerbach's plexus to coordinate the motor and secretory activity of the gastric mucosa.

Secretion

The stomach secretes 1500 to 3000 ml of gastric juice per day. Its major secretions are hydrochloric acid, pepsin, and mucus. Gastric juice contains mucin, intrinsic factor, lipase, pepsinogen, and protein. Gastric acid secretion is directly stimulated by distention of the stomach and the presence of protein. Gastric acid secretion is also stimulated by vagal activity, acetylcholine, histamine, and the hormone gastrin (Table 58–1). Gastrin is released when the stomach becomes distended with food.

Hydrochloric acid and pepsin provide the corrosive power of gastric secretions. Pepsin is the most active factor in the digestive process of the stomach, acting to break down proteins to polypeptides, proteases, and peptones (Table 58–2). Peptic activity is greatest at pH levels less than 3.5. Pepsin is stimulated by food, whereas mucus has a neutralizing effect, which protects the stomach mucosa.

The three phases of gastric secretion are cephalic, gastric, and intestinal.

1. The cephalic (nervous) phase of digestion is dependent on stimulation of gastric secretions by receptors in the brain that are mediated by the vagus nerve. This phase is stimulated by hunger and by the sight, smell, thought, and discussion of food. The cephalic phase results in secretion of acid, pepsin, and mucus.
2. The gastric (hormonal) phase of secretion occurs when the bolus of food reaches the antrum. This phase consists of three mechanisms. When the food enters the stomach, the long vagovagal reflex, local enteric reflexes, and gastrin mechanisms are excited. These mechanisms lead to secretion of gastric juice. This phase continues for several hours, until the acidity of the gastric contents reaches 1.5 or less.
3. The intestinal phase includes both nervous and hormonal mechanisms. This phase is stimulated by food entering the duodenum, resulting in the secretion of a small amount of gastrin by the intestine. This process, in turn, stimulates gastric secretion of pepsin and mucus. The duodenal pH then decreases, resulting in the release of secretin, which inhibits gastric secretion and slows gastric emptying.

Gastric secretions are decreased by (1) vagal stimulation, (2) increased osmolality of food, (3) fat, (4) enterogastrone, (5) alterations in blood flow, and (6) inflammation, such as gastritis. Decreased gastric secretion also results from a duodenal acid pH of 1.5 or less and an antrum pH of 3.0, both of which block the release of gastrin.

In addition, hormonal mechanisms in the small bowel may inhibit gastric secretion. The presence of acid, fat, and protein breakdown products, or any irritating factor, in the duodenum causes the release of secretin and CCK. These substances are especially important for control of pancreatic secretion, and CCK promotes emptying of the gallbladder. The release of these substances inhibits gastric secretion of the parietal cells and the stomach's motor activity. Also, they decrease gastric emptying, inhibit peptic digestion, and facilitate pancreatic enzyme activity. Stimulation of the duodenum—by distention, or the presence of acid, hypotonic or hypertonic substances, carbohydrates, fats, or protein products—causes the enterogastric vagus reflex arc to slow gastric motility and secretions. Digestive hormones and enzymes are listed in Tables 58–1 and 58–2.

Motor Activity

The stomach empties slowly, accommodating itself to the ability of the duodenum to receive and act on the contents. Tonic contraction of the stomach musculature causes the pressure within it to remain almost constant, whether it be empty or full. Mixing of chyme and emptying of the stomach occur by means of slow, mild, rhythmic peristaltic waves that begin about every 30 seconds at the fundus and continue over the antrum to the pylorus. The rugae of the stomach walls also contribute to the mixing of chyme.

As chyme is ready to be discharged through the pyloric sphincter into the duodenum, pressure builds up within the pylorus. The pyloric sphincter opens, allowing chyme to pass through. The sphincter then closes to prevent backflow. This process is repeated until all the food in the stomach is emptied into the duodenum. The pressure and rate of emptying are affected by viscosity, volume, physical state, osmotic activity, acidity of the food, and receptivity of the small bowel, as well as by exercise, drugs, emotions, pain, position, and other chemical and mechanical factors. The enterogastric reflex and enterogastrone (the hormone secreted by the small bowel) both act to inhibit emptying of the stomach.

The greater the acidity and caloric density, and the more the osmolarity varies from that of body fluids, the more slowly the stomach empties. Fats move more slowly than any other dietary constituents.

The Small Intestine

Structure

The small intestine is about 22 ft long and about 1 inch in diameter. It is divided into three segments:

1. The *duodenum* begins at the pyloric valve of the stomach and extends about 25 cm (10 inches) until it joins the jejunum.
2. The *jejunum*, 2.5 m (8 ft) long, is the middle section of the small intestine and extends to the ileum.
3. The *ileum*, 3.6 m (12 ft) long, is the terminal section. The ileum joins the colon at the ileocecal valve. This valve controls flow into the large intestine and prevents reflux into the small intestine.

Table 58–1. Digestive Hormones

Hormone	Source	Stimulating Factors	Action
Gastrin	C cells of gastric antrum; duodenal mucosa	Distention of stomach by food, presence of products of protein digestion, vagal stimulation, elevated blood levels of calcium and epinephrine	Stimulates secretion of HCl, pepsin, pancreatic enzyme, and growth of gastric mucosa; relaxes ileocecal sphincter; promotes digestion; increases flow of bile and gastric and intestinal motility; increases tone of lower esophageal sphincter; inhibits gastric emptying
Enterogastrone	Duodenal mucosa	Fats, sugars, and acids in small intestine	Inhibits gastric acid secretion and motility
Secretin	Duodenal mucosa	Fats and sugars in small intestine	Stimulates secretion of watery alkaline pancreatic fluid; augments CCK; decreases gastric acid secretion; stimulates secretion of pancreatic digestive enzymes and bile from liver; stimulates pepsinogen release
Cholecystokinin (CCK)	Duodenal and jejunal mucosa	Products of fat digestion in duodenum	Augments secretin in stimulating secretion of alkaline pancreatic juice and digestive enzymes; stimulates gallbladder contraction; inhibits gastric emptying; stimulates pepsin secretion; stimulates motility of small bowel
Gastric inhibitory peptide (GIP)	Duodenal and jejunal mucosa	Presence of glucose, fat, and amino acid in duodenum	Inhibits gastric acid and pepsin secretion and gut motility; stimulates secretion of intestinal juice and insulin
Vasoactive intestinal peptide (VIP) (structurally related to secretin)	Intestinal mucosa, central nervous system, genitourinary system	None known	Stimulates insulin release, pancreatic enzyme secretion, and intestinal secretion of electrolytes and water; inhibits gastric acid secretion; dilates peripheral blood vessels and lowers blood pressure
Motilin	Small intestine, especially duodenum and upper jejunum	None known	Diminishes speed of gastric emptying and stimulates gastric acid secretion and pepsin; stimulates bicarbonate secretion of pancreas
Somatostatin	Hypothalamus and pineal gland, stomach, intestine (duodenum), Auerbach's plexus, pancreas	Secretin, CCK, glucagon; acid in duodenum	Inhibits secretion of gastrin, VIP, GIP, secretin, and motilin; inhibits gastric duodenal, gallbladder motility, and intestinal motility, and intestinal Na^+ and Cl^- absorption Inhibits gastric acid, pancreatic enzyme, and bicarbonate secretion, and intestinal motility

Table 58–2. Digestive Enzymes

Enzyme	Source	Action and Products
Carbohydrates		
Ptyalin (salivary amylase)	Parotid and submaxillary glands	Break starch into maltose and limit dextrins (polysaccharides into disaccharides)*
Pancreatic amylase (more potent than ptyalin)	Pancrease	
Maltase†	Intestinal mucosa	Breaks maltose into glucose
Dextrinase	Intestinal mucosa	Breaks alpha limit dextrins into glucose*
Lactase†	Intestinal mucosa	Breaks lactose into galactose and glucose
Sucrase†	Intestinal mucosa	Breaks sucrose into glucose and fructose
Proteins		
Pepsin I, II, III	Chief cells of gastric mucosa	Breaks dietary proteins into polypeptides of various sizes
Enterokinase	Duodenal mucosa	Activates trypsin
Trypsin	Pancreas	Splits polypeptide chains
Peptidases† (several)	Intestinal glands	Splits polypeptides into amino acids
Fats		
Gastric lipase (tributyrase)	Gastric mucosa	Digests butterfat
Pancreatic lipase	Pancreas	Splits emulsified fats into monoglycerides
Intestinal lipase†	Intestines	Splits neutral fats into glycerol and fatty acids

* Small polymers present when starch is broken down.
† Secreted mainly in brush border of epithelial cells; digests food substances on outside surfaces of microvilli before or during absorption through epithelium.

Four coats cover the small intestine: (1) an outer serous layer (tunica serosa), (2) a muscular layer (tunica muscularis), (3) a submucous layer (tela submucosa), and (4) an inner mucous layer (tunica mucosa) (Fig. 58–6).

The tunica serosa of the small intestine constitutes the peritoneum. This serous membrane lines the walls of the abdominal and pelvic cavities. The tunica muscularis is subdivided into the outer longitudinal and inner circular muscle layers. The tela submucosa contains blood vessels, lymphatics, Meissner's nerve plexus, and Brunner's glands (in the duodenum), which secrete mucus. Glands in the tunica mucosa also secrete mucus. The mucosal and submucosal layers are arranged in folds that provide a surface for secretion, digestion, and absorption.

The circular folds of the mucosa and submucosa are large and permanent. The villi, small, fingerlike projections, are in continuous motion, stirring the intestinal contents. The villi are composed of columnar cells under which lie blood capillaries and a lymph channel called a lacteal. Digested food is absorbed from the villi. Fats are absorbed from the lacteals. The microvilli are microscopic processes on the surface of the epithelial cells. Together, these structures increase the surface area of the small intestine 600-fold, enlarging its total surface area to equal approximately 250 m^2, the size of a tennis court! This area is also known as the brush border.

Solitary and aggregated lymph nodes (Peyer's patches) are present in the small intestinal mucosa. Solitary nodes are small and connect directly with lymph vessels in deeper tissues. The aggregated lymph nodes occur mainly in the ileum.

Function

The small intestine (1) completes digestion of foods, (2) absorbs the products of digestion, and (3) secretes hormones that help control the secretion of bile, pancreatic juice, and intestinal secretions. The residues are then moved on into the large intestine.

Blood Supply

Except in the duodenum, arterial blood supply to the small intestine is derived from the superior mesenteric artery. Arterial blood from the hepatic artery supplies the duodenum. Venous drainage is via the superior mesen-

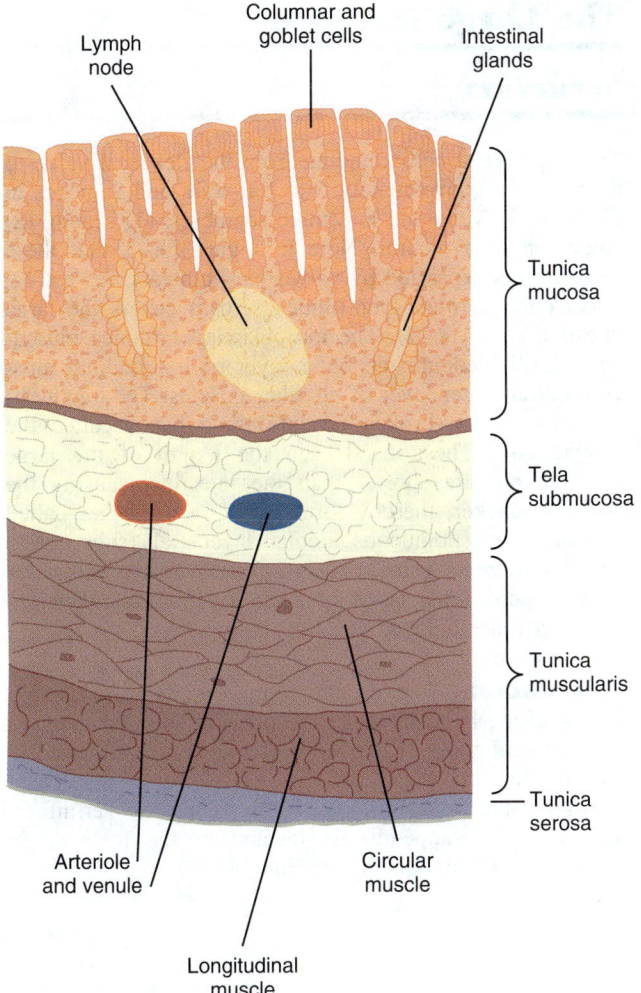

Figure 58–6. Cross-section of wall of small intestine.

teric vein, which unites with the inferior mesenteric, splenic, and gastric veins and then empties into the portal system.

Innervation

Stimulation of the sympathetic system inhibits the motility of the small intestine. Stimulation of the parasympathetic system increases intestinal tone and motility. The nerve supply to the small intestine passes through Auerbach's plexus within the intestinal wall. As within the other sections of the gastrointestinal tract, the sensory fibers of the sympathetic system carry pain, whereas those of the parasympathetic system regulate intestinal activity.

Secretion

Hormonal secretion in the small intestine helps control bile, pancreatic juice, and intestinal secretions. The duodenal (Brunner's) glands are stimulated by glucagon and duodenal mucosa. These glands produce and release mucus not only in response to intestinal hormones but also in the presence of chyme and vagal stimulation. Sympathetic stimulation inhibits the secretion of mucus by Brunner's glands, which may explain the high incidence of peptic ulcers in this area of the gastrointestinal tract. The goblet cells of the intestinal mucosa also secrete mucus.

The crypts of Lieberkühn are small pits that line the entire surface of the small intestine. These cells secrete about 2 L/day of clear, yellowish, almost pure extracellular fluid with a slightly alkaline pH of 7.5 to 8.0. This fluid is absorbed rapidly by the villi. The epithelial cells of the mucosa covering the villi contain digestive enzymes. The enzymes found in the small intestine include (1) enterokinase, which activates trypsin; (2) maltase, lactase, and sucrase, which change disaccharides into simple sugars; and (3) nuclease, which facilitates hydrolysis of nuclein and nucleic acids. Other enzymes that hydrolyze peptides also are present.

In addition to the secretions from the small intestine, the pancreas secretes enzymes, bicarbonate, and water into the duodenum which act on chyme to digest substrates. Pancreatic secretion depends on the action of two duodenal hormones, secretin and CCK.

Secretin stimulates secretion of watery alkaline pancreatic fluid and also augments CCK. CCK stimulates bile secretion from the gallbladder. The gallbladder serves as a reservoir for bile after its manufacture in and secretion from the liver. Bile secretion from the liver is stimulated by vagal stimulation, secretin, increased liver blood flow, and high levels of bile salts in the blood. Bile aids fat digestion (see Chapter 63).

Flora

The small intestine flora are predominantly gram-positive lactobacilli, streptococci, and staphylococci. *Aerobacter aerogenes, Bacteroides, Candida albicans, Escherichia coli, Proteus, Pseudomonas,* and *Streptococcus faecalis* are also found. Bile acids and gastric acid may inhibit bacterial proliferation in the intestine.

Absorption

During the process of digestion and the preparation of end products for absorption, the following transformations occur in the small intestine:

● Carbohydrates are changed to monosaccharides and a few disaccharides. Carbohydrate digestion takes place primarily in the jejunum.
● Proteins are changed to amino acids and a minute quantity of dipeptides.
● Fats are changed to fatty acids, monoglycerides, diglycerides, and a few triglycerides.

The end products of digestion are absorbed along with water and electrolytes by diffusion and by active transport. Carbohydrates and proteins are absorbed by active transport along with sodium in a mutually dependent relationship in which neither material is transported without the other. Fatty acids are absorbed by diffusion, whereas most of the electrolytes are absorbed actively. Water diffuses by osmosis as a result of these other transport systems. Diffusion, active transport, and osmosis are discussed in Chapter 15.

Absorption of up to 8 L of fluid daily occurs in the small intestine. Glucose, water-soluble vitamins, protein, and fat are absorbed primarily in the jejunum. The ileum acts mainly as a reserve to absorb these substances, and it is also the site of bile salt absorption. The duodenum and ileum share the functions of active sodium transport. Vitamin B_{12} absorption takes place in the ileum, provided the stomach has secreted intrinsic factor and calcium ions are present. Iron absorption occurs in the duodenum and jejunum.

Digestion and absorption in the small bowel are very efficient. The chyme obtained from the terminal ileum contains no digestible carbohydrates, very few lipids, and only 15% to 17% nitrogen-containing substances, most of which are bacteria or desquamated epithelial cells and the remains of digestive secretions. Generally, only 500 to 1000 ml of fluid passes into the large intestine.

Motor Activity

The motility of the small intestine is a result of the autorhythmicity of the smooth muscle, the intrinsic nerve impulses, and the hormonal effects of intestinal secretions. The chyme normally moves forward at an average rate of about 1 to 2 cm/min, and remains in the small intestine for 3 to 10 hours.

As in other parts of the gastrointestinal tract, the principal movements of the small intestine are (1) peristalsis and (2) mixing (or segmental) contractions. Although movements are divided into two categories, each type of contraction results in both mixing and propulsive activity.

Peristalsis or propulsive activity waves propel the chyme through the tract. Rhythmic segmental peristaltic waves are circular contractions that occur in the jejunum, resulting in mixing and absorption.

Peristalsis occurs by reflex as a result of mucosal stretching of the longitudinal and circular muscle layers when the chyme enters a segment of the intestine. Serotonin, produced by the intestinal glands, and acetylcholine cause contraction of the longitudinal muscle. Contraction of the circular muscle occurs through Meissner's plexus, and motor stimulation through Auerbach's plexus. This activity results in emptying of the intestinal segment.

A peristaltic rush is a powerful peristaltic wave that begins in the duodenum and passes to the ileocecal valve in a few minutes. Its purpose is to relieve the intestine of an irritating substance. A peristaltic rush can be caused by an intense chemical or mechanical irritation or by extreme distention.

Mixing movements consist of the alternate contraction of circular muscle fibers. They bring the chyme into close contact with (1) the glands and secretions involved with digestion and (2) the villi for absorption.

The Large Intestine

Structure

The large intestine, extending from the ileocecal valve to the anus, is approximately 5 to 6 ft long and 2 inches in diameter. It is divided into three segments: (1) cecum, (2) colon, and (3) rectum. Note in Figure 58–1 that these parts are not separated by valves or sphincters.

An outer serous layer (tunica serosa) covers the large intestine (Fig. 58–7). The muscular layer (tunica muscularis) is divided into an outer layer of longitudinal muscles and an inner layer of circular muscles. The longitudinal muscles are broken up into three bands called the taeniae coli. These bands run the length of the large intestine but are shorter than the intestine, causing the colon to pucker, thereby forming sacs or pouches called *haustra*. The submucous areolar layer (tela submucosa) contains arteries, veins, and lymphatic vessels, and it secretes mucus. This layer connects the muscular layer to the inner mucous layer.

The Cecum. The cecum comprises the first 2 to 3 inches of the large intestine. It connects with the ileum at the ileocecal valve. Relaxation of the cecum allows ileal contents to enter the cecum. The distal end of the cecum forms a blind pouch to which is attached the vermiform appendix. The appendix is located in the lower right quadrant of the abdomen (see Fig. 58–1).

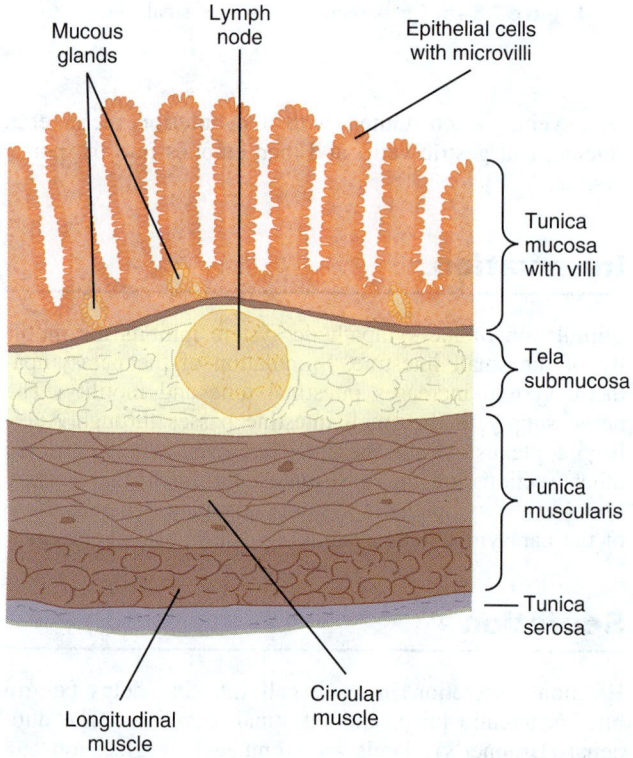

Figure 58–7. Cross-section of wall of large intestine.

The Colon. The colon is divided into four sections: (1) ascending, (2) transverse, (3) descending, and (4) sigmoid colon. The ascending colon lies just above the ileocecal valve. It continues up the right side of the abdomen to the lower border of the liver, where the section known as the hepatic flexure bends to the left. Extending horizontally from the liver across the abdomen is the transverse portion of the colon. At the spleen, the splenic flexure bends downward. Extending from the spleen down the left side of the abdomen is the descending colon. The S-shaped turn, the sigmoid colon, lies within the pelvis.

Anatomically, the colon is larger in diameter than the small bowel and does not contain villi. The only significant secretion is mucus.

The major functions of the colon are to (1) absorb the remaining water, urea, and electrolytes (sodium and chloride); (2) secrete mucus in the proximal half; and (3) store the feces in the distal half until defecation.

The Rectum and Anus. The final segments of the large intestine, the rectum and the anus, extend from the sigmoid colon to the anus. Two sphincter muscles (internal and external) control the opening of the anus.

The distal portion of the rectal walls form longitudinal folds, called rectal or anal columns. These folds terminate about ½ inch from the anus and are connected to one another by transverse folds of tissue called valves. Pockets formed by the valves are called sinuses or crypts. Because the external portion of the anal opening is lined with skin that changes at this point to mucosa, this area is sometimes called the mucocutaneous border.

The venous drainage and nerve supply also change at this point. Above this line, venous drainage is into the portal system. Below this line, drainage is into the vena cava. The autonomic nervous system supplies innervation above the line, and the somatic nervous system supplies innervation below it.

The anal canal is about 1 inch long. At the level of the crypts lies the dentate or pectinate line. This important landmark divides the (1) squamous epithelium (below) and columnar epithelium (above), and (2) the somatic nerve supply (below) and autonomic supply (above). The line also marks the division between internal and external hemorrhoids. Lymphatic drainage below the pectinate line goes largely to the inguinal nodes, while lymphatic drainage above this line goes to the pararectal and lateral pelvic (obturator) plexuses.

Function

The major functions of the large intestine are the following:

- Complete absorption of water, chloride, and sodium
- Reduction in the volume of chyme
- Manufacture of vitamins, including some B vitamins and vitamin K
- Formation of feces
- Expulsion of feces from the body

Blood Supply

The cecum and colon receive their arterial blood supply from branches of the superior and inferior mesenteric arteries. The rectum and anal canal receive arterial blood from the superior, middle, and inferior rectal arteries. The superior and inferior mesenteric veins carry venous blood from the large intestine to the hepatic portal vein and then to the liver.

Innervation

The intramural nerve plexuses that lie within the layers of the bowel wall are responsible for nervous stimulation of the large intestine. Recall that these are known as Auerbach's and Meissner's plexuses. These nerves maintain the continuous tone of the bowel and also stimulate movements.

The plexuses are stimulated by the parasympathetic nervous system and, in general, cause an increase in tone of the gut, a decrease in tone of the sphincters, and an increase in frequency, volume, and velocity of contractions. The cranial division of the parasympathetic nervous system mediates impulses via the vagus nerve from the esophagus to the proximal colon. The distance from the midcolon to the anus is controlled by the sacral division of the parasympathetic nervous system.

Sympathetic innervation comes via nerve fibers that leave the spinal cord between T8 and L3. The nerve impulses then pass through ganglia, such as the celiac and mesenteric, and spread to all parts of the gut. In general, they reduce peristaltic activity and increase the tone of the sphincters. Sympathetic effects on the bowel are minimal; this is known because denervation has only short-term effects.

Motor Activity

As food passes through the ileocecal valve, it accumulates in the proximal haustrum of the ascending colon. When the haustrum is completely distended, the walls contract and squeeze the contents into the next haustrum. This process continues, thereby moving the food through the colon. This movement is called haustral churning.

Mass peristalsis involves slow, forceful waves that occur when the bowel is evacuated. Mass peristalsis occurs two or three times a day and is stimulated by the gastrocolic reflex. Distention of a segment of the bowel or any irritation of the bowel mucosa may initiate a peristaltic wave.

Secretion

The mucosa of the large bowel contains the crypts of Lieberkühn. Secretion consists of water, mucus, potassium, and bicarbonate, resulting in alkaline secretions. Mucus is the major secretory product. It lubricates, allows passage of the fecal residue, protects the mucosa from injury, and binds fecal particles into a formed mass.

Mucus production is stimulated by the parasympathetic nervous system and is increased by bacterial, mechanical, or chemical colonic irritation. Its alkalinity helps to counteract the effects of acid formation from bacterial action.

Flora

The alkaline reaction of the large intestine permits the growth of organisms whose main functions are to putrefy and break down remaining proteins and indigestible residue. These organisms include *E. coli, A. aerogenes, Clostridium perfringens,* and *Lactobacillus.*

Intestinal bacteria convert urea to ammonium salts and ammonia. Bacterial action in the large bowel causes the formation of gases, which provide bulk and help propel the feces. This action also synthesizes nutritional factors such as vitamin K, thiamine, riboflavin, vitamin B_{12}, folic acid, biotin, and nicotinic acid.

Absorption

Absorption of sodium, chloride, and water occurs in the large bowel and reduces the volume of chyme from 500 ml in the cecum to 100 ml of fluid in the feces. The colon is capable of absorbing 90% of the sodium and water it receives.

Feces

Feces are three-fourths water and one-fourth solid matter. The solid matter includes food residues, digestive enzymes, dead cells, bile pigments, salts, and mucus. Thirty percent of the fecal mass consists of bacteria, and another 30% is fat. The outer surface of feces is usually basic, and the inner part is acidic. The nature of the diet does not change the stool's content except for the amount of cellulose.

Substances that absorb water or prevent the movement of water form a soft bulky mass of fecal material and stimulate colonic movement. The feces are expelled through the act of defecation.

Defecation

The defecation reflex is stimulated by distention of the rectum, which occurs when feces and gas are propelled into the rectum from the descending colon. As the pressure within the rectum rises and the internal and external sphincters relax, distention sets the defecation reflex in motion.

Voluntary suppression of defecation is achieved by contracting the striated muscles of the pelvic floor and external sphincter. On the other hand, if a person elects to defecate on stimulation of the reflex, performance of Valsalva's maneuver will augment the pressure within the colon by increasing intra-abdominal pressure. Specifically, the person increases the pressure by contracting the abdominal muscles and exhaling against a closed glottis. This strain causes cardiovascular alterations. There is a slight bradycardia at the beginning of the maneuver, which changes to tachycardia during Valsalva's maneuver, and then reverts to bradycardia. Intrathoracic pressure increases, thus inhibiting venous return. Blood pools in the extremities, thereby reducing cardiac filling and output. This cardiovascular effect sometimes makes a person feel lightheaded. In extreme cases, some people feel faint. When the urge to defecate is voluntarily suppressed, the rectum relaxes and the desire to defecate disappears.

Effects of Aging

Physiologic changes in the gastrointestinal tract are known to occur with aging. In the mouth, teeth may loosen from loss of supporting gums and bone. Circulation in the gums is reduced, and aging teeth darken and may become uneven and fracture. Decreased output of the salivary glands leads to dryness of mucous membranes and increased susceptibility to breakdown. This decrease can cause difficulty swallowing and decreased stimulation of taste buds.

Changes also occur in the ability to digest and absorb food because of a decrease in the secretion of digestive enzymes and bile. In the stomach, atrophy of gastric mucosa leads to a decreased secretion of hydrochloric acid. A decrease in hydrochloric acid causes a decrease in the absorption of iron and vitamin B_{12}, and leads to a proliferation of bacteria. This decrease in iron and vitamin B_{12} leads to the development of anemia. An increase in bacteria in the gut can lead to diarrhea and infection. With a decrease in bile secretion, absorption of fats and fat-soluble vitamins (A, D, E, and K) becomes impaired. This decreased absorption of fat can lead to weight loss, and the decrease in fat-soluble vitamins can lead to a variety of problems such as altered calcium metabolism and bleeding from the decrease of vitamin K (needed to synthesize prothrombin).

In the large intestine, peristalsis decreases and nerve impulses are dulled. In addition, the muscular tone of the intestinal wall and abdominal muscle strength are reduced. These changes can result in a decreased sensation to defecate and an increased incidence of constipation.

Conclusions

A thorough knowledge of the structure and function of the gastrointestinal system helps the nurse provide knowledgeable care to clients with disorders in these areas. In order to provide effective interventions, the nurse must understand the normal physiology of this system and the digestive organs.

Bibliography

1. Beck, M., & Evans, N. G. (Eds.). (1992). *Gastroenterology nursing: A core curriculum.* St. Louis: Mosby–Year Book.
2. Bennett, J. C., & Plum, F. (Eds.). (1996). *Cecil textbook of medicine* (20th ed.). Philadelphia: W. B. Saunders.

3. Christiansen, J. L., & Grzbouski, J. M. (1993). *Biology of aging.* St. Louis: Mosby–Year Book.

4. Cotran, R.S., Kumar, V., & Robbins, S. L. (1994). *Robbins pathologic basis of disease* (5th ed.). Philadelphia: W. B. Saunders.

5. Drossman, D. (Ed.). (1992). *Manual of gastroenterologic procedures* (3rd ed.). New York: Raven Press.

6. Doughty, D. B., & Jackson, D. B. (1993). *Mosby's clinical nursing series: Gastrointestinal disorders.* St. Louis: Mosby–Year Book.

7. Gitnick, G. (1994). *Current gastroenterology* (Vol. 14). St. Louis: Mosby–Year Book.

8. Grendell, J. H., McQuaid, K. R., & Friedman, S. L. (1995). *Current diagnosis and treatment in gastroenterology.* Norwalk, CT: Appleton & Lange.

9. Guyton, A. C. (1992). *Human physiology and mechanisms of disease* (5th ed.). Philadelphia: W. B. Saunders.

10. Guyton, A. C., & Hall, J. E. (1996). *Textbook of medical physiology* (9th ed.). Philadelphia: W. B. Saunders.

11. Hambrich, W. S., et al. (1994). *Bockus gastroenterology.* Philadelphia: W. B. Saunders.

12. Heatley, R. V. (Ed.). (1994). *Gastrointestinal and hepatic immunology.* New York: Cambridge University Press.

13. Johnson, L. R. (Ed.). (1994). *Physiology of the gastrointestinal tract.* New York: Raven Press.

14. Kumar, D., & Wingate, D. L. (1994). *An illustrated guide to gastrointestinal motility* (2nd ed.). New York: Churchill Livingstone.

15. McCance, K. L., & Huether, S. E. (1994). *Pathophysiology: The biologic basis for disease in adults and children* (2nd ed.). St. Louis: Mosby–Year Book.

16. Ming, S. C., & Goldman, H. (Eds.). (1992). *Pathology of the gastrointestinal tract.* Philadelphia: W. B. Saunders.

17. Porth, C. M. (1994). *Pathophysiologic concepts of altered health states* (4th ed.). Philadelphia: J. B. Lippincott.

18. Schaffer, E., & Thomson, A. B. (Eds.). (1992). *Modern concepts in gastroenterology.* New York: Plenum Press.

19. Seeley, R., Stephens, T., & Tate, P. (1995). *Anatomy and physiology* (3rd ed.). St. Louis: Mosby–Year Book.

20. Shils, M. E., Olson, H. A., Shike, M. (Eds.). (1993). *Modern nutrition in health and disease* (8th ed.). Philadelphia: Lea & Febiger.

21. Sleisenger, M. H., & Fordtran, J. S. (Eds.). (1993). *Gastrointestinal disease: Pathophysiology, diagnosis, management* (5th ed.). Philadelphia: W. B. Saunders.

22. Solomon, E. P. (1992). *Introduction to human anatomy and physiology.* Philadelphia: W. B. Saunders.

23. Thibodeau, G. A., & Patton, K. T. (1992). *Anatomy and physiology* (2nd ed.). St. Louis: Mosby–Year Book.

24. Thibodeau, G. A., & Patton, K. T. (1992). *The human body in health and disease.* St. Louis: Mosby–Year Book.

25. Townsend, C. D. (1994). *Nutrition and diet therapy.* Albany, NY: Delmar Publishers.

59

Assessment of Clients with Gastrointestinal Disorders

Jane Hokanson Hawks

Assessment of the gastrointestinal (GI) tract involves a detailed health history as well as a comprehensive physical examination of the client's oral cavity, abdomen, rectum, and anus. The goal is to collect sufficient history, physical assessment, and diagnostic test data to identify and treat the client's medical and nursing diagnoses.

History

Biographical and Demographic Data

A review of the client's demographic data, such as age, sex, culture, religion, and occupation, is helpful when assessing the GI tract. Many GI disorders are associated with age and sex. For example, some GI cancers occur more frequently in the elderly and in males, whereas others are more common in women. Sexual abuse may play a role in some women's GI problems.[13] Reproductive cycling in women may contribute to other GI manifestations.[9] Diverticulosis and hiatal hernias appear more frequently in older adults. Duodenal ulcers develop in young adults, whereas gastric ulcers are more common in middle-aged and older adults.

Ulcerative colitis occurs more frequently in young and middle-aged adults and in people of Jewish descent.[11] Japanese and Chinese people have a greater risk for development of upper GI cancers because of their intake of raw fish and of foods with a high nitrosamine content.[11] Other diets, such as those high in fat, increase the risk of development of colorectal cancer in all people as they age (see Diversity in Healthcare feature).

Chief Complaint

A thorough assessment of the client's current health problem is necessary and is often a key component of the

health history. Many GI manifestations are vague and have baffling causes, so the nurse must explore each manifestation in detail. Begin by asking the client why he or she is seeking healthcare. When conducting a symptom analysis, ask the client the following questions about the chief complaint and present illness:

Onset. When was the problem first noted? Was the onset gradual or sudden? What was the client doing when the problem was first noticed? Was it related to food intake?

Duration. Does the problem occur occasionally or is it persistent? Is there a pattern to the problem's occurrence? If the problem is pain, note whether the pain is continuous or intermittent.

Quality and Characteristics. Ask the client to describe the problem. If the problem is diarrhea, ask the client to describe the stool's appearance, odor, color, and consistency.

Severity. Ask the client to describe, on a scale of 1 to 10, how bad the problem is. Does it interfere with his or her ability to perform usual daily activities?

Location. Where does the client feel the problem occurs? Does the pain spread to other areas of the body? What happens to the client when the manifestations occur?

Precipitating Factors. Is there anything that seems to bring the problem on? Does anything make it worse or better? When does it occur? Is it related to eating, drinking, or activity? Does eating precipitate or increase the pain?

Relieving Factors. Is there anything the client can do to relieve the problem? Has he or she tried medica-

This chapter incorporates material written for the fourth edition by Shirley M. Ruder.

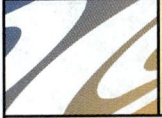

NORMAL PHYSICAL ASSESSMENT FINDINGS

Gastrointestinal System

Inspection

Mouth. Lips symmetrical, pink, moist, without lesions. Buccal mucosa and gingivae pink, moist, intact, without lesions. Hard and soft palates pink, intact. Tonsils behind pillars, without inflammation. Posterior pharynx pink, without exudate. Uvula rises midline with phonation. Tongue midline, mobile, without deviation or fasciculations.

Abdomen. Flat, symmetrical, with umbilicus inverted, centered, and midline. No scars, lesions, dilated veins, visible peristalsis or pulsations, or separation of rectus muscles at rest or with straining.

Anus and Rectum. Perianal area free of lesions, inflammation, fissures, bulges, or external hemorrhoids.

Auscultation

Abdomen. Bowel sounds present in all four quadrants with liver and splenic dullness.

Percussion*

General tympani throughout, with liver and splenic dullness. Liver span 10 cm at right midclavicular line.

Palpation*

Abdomen. Liver and spleen nonpalpable. Abdomen soft, nontender, no masses or rebound tenderness; muscle tone firm, relaxed.

Anus and Rectum: Anus and rectum without tenderness, masses, hemorrhoids, or prolapse. Rectal mucosa smooth. Stool negative for occult blood.

_____
* In assessment of the abdomen, palpation is performed *after* auscultation, so that the bowel is not stimulated.

---

tions, position changes, or anything else for relief? Does eating relieve the pain?

Associated Manifestations. Are there any other manifestations that bother the client when the problem is present? Does the client lose appetite, become nauseated, vomit, or have diarrhea?

Common GI manifestations include nausea, vomiting, stomach pain (gastritis), abdominal pain, diarrhea, constipation, abdominal distention, flatulence, dysphagia, anorexia, early satiety, heartburn, and indigestion (dyspepsia). The client may also report manifestations such as dry mouth, halitosis, sore mouth, difficulty chewing or swallowing, food intolerance, vomiting of blood (hematemesis), belching, bloody stool (melena), abdominal cramping, anal pruritus or burning, or rectal bleeding. Manifestations associated with the hepatic, biliary, and pancreatic systems may also be reported as GI disturbances (see Chapter 60).

While conducting the health history interview, the nurse notes the client's general health status. A *diet history* and *nutritional assessment* as well as assessment of the client's *elimination patterns* are important data, both for baseline information and for future comparisons. Ask

the client what foods are usually consumed on a daily basis. Note whether there are differences in the diet on weekends and holidays. Determine whether the client is knowledgeable about basic human nutrition and whether the client's diet is nutritionally sound. Specifically inquire about snacks, intake of fluids, sugar, salt, and fiber. Many GI problems are a result of dietary habits; for example, inadequate fiber intake is a factor in constipation, diverticular disease, and colorectal cancer, and inadequate fluid intake may precipitate or aggravate constipation. See Chapter 11 for a discussion of diet history and nutritional assessment. Note whether the client reports a *change* in elimination patterns (see Chapter 11). For example, has the client noticed changes in bowel habits? If so, what are they? It may be helpful to have the client describe bowel movement patterns (e.g., after every meal, daily, every other day) and shape, consistency, color, and odor of stools.

Past Health History

The nurse collects data about previous hospitalizations, major illnesses, surgery, use of medications, and allergies as part of the past medical history.

Text continued on page 1704

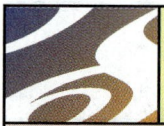

DIVERSITY IN HEALTHCARE

Nutrition and Culture

Among the most important factors in promoting, maintaining, and restoring the client's health is the nurse's ability to encourage the intake of the right types and quantities of foods. The degree to which the nurse is successful may make the difference between a rapid return to health, a slow and prolonged recovery, or none at all. For centuries, diet has been used by many cultures to promote health and prevent disease. The best way to learn about the eating patterns of the client is to conduct a comprehensive nutrition assessment.

Nutrition Assessment

When assessing the client's nutritional state and food intake, the nurse must consider the role of culture. Among those factors that must be examined are the frequency and number of meals eaten away from home, form and content of ceremonial meals, and the regularity of food consumption. Because inaccuracies may occur, the 24-hour dietary recalls or 3-day food records used traditionally for assessment may be inadequate when assessing clients from diverse cultural backgrounds. Another potential source of error is overreliance on dietary handbooks, because information and exchange tables are frequently based on Western diets and meal patterns. For example, among some low-income urban black families, weekend meals are frequently elaborate, whereas weekday dietary intake is generally quite moderate.[1]

Although it may seem self-evident, the nurse needs to arrive at a common understanding of what is meant by food. For example, certain Latin American groups do not consider greens, an important source of vitamins, to be food. For Vietnamese Americans, the dietary intake of calcium may appear inadequate, particularly with the low consumption of dairy products common to members of this group. Pork bones and shells are commonly consumed however, thus providing adequate quantities of calcium to meet daily requirements. Although milk is the only food used by everybody worldwide, many cultures consider it appropriate only for infants and children.[1,2]

Nutritional assessment is sometimes affected by biocultural variations, even when dietary intake itself does not vary. For example, the urinary nitrogen excretion in healthy Taiwanese and American college students fed similar protein-free diets is markedly different.[3] Wide variation in absorption and metabolism of alcohol has been studied extensively, especially among Native Americans. According to the Indian Health Service, the incidence of alcoholism is four times as high in Native Americans as in the general population, and evidence is considerable that members of some tribes have a genetic predisposition to this condition.[4]

Health-Related Dietary Beliefs and Practices

Diet is used by many cultures in the prevention and treatment of illness. Many people of the world believe that the key to health lies in balancing foods with opposite properties. Among some cultures, common practice to prevent and cure disease involves the balancing of body fluids between hot and cold. These beliefs and practices originated in ancient Greece during the time of Hippocrates, who considered illness to be the result of humoral imbalance, causing the body to become too hot or too cold.

Health is conceived in this system as a state of balance among the body humors (blood, phlegm, black bile, and yellow bile), which manifests itself in a somewhat wet, warm body. Illness is believed to result from a humoral imbalance that causes the body to become excessively dry, cold, hot or wet, or a combination of these states. Food, herbs, and other medications, which are also classified as wet or dry, hot or cold, are used therapeutically to restore the body to its natural balance. According to this system, a cold disease, such as arthritis, is cured by administering hot foods or medications.

Clients from Hispanic and Middle Eastern cultures are particularly likely to believe in the hot-cold theory of health and diet. Although the terminology of the hot-cold system suggests that it is based on the thermal state of the substance ingested, temperature and spiciness are not the qualities that determine the classification of specific substances. The hot-cold theory describes intrinsic properties of a food, beverage, or medicine and its effect on the body.

Hot-Cold Theory. The classification of foods, beverages, and medicines as hot or cold varies within each cultural group. In general, warm or hot foods are believed to be easier to digest than cold or cool foods. To achieve balance, illnesses are treated with substances that possess the opposite property of the illness. Conditions thought to be caused by exposure to cold or chilling are cured by taking hot medicines as well as by ingesting hot foods and beverages. The reverse is true of illnesses believed to be caused by exposure to heat. For example, an upset stomach may be attributed to eating too many foods that are classified as cold, thus chilling the stomach.

New foods or medicines are incorporated into the hot-cold system according to the effect they have on the body. The fact that new items are still being incorporated into the hot-cold system attests to its vitality among members of certain cultural groups.

Yin-Yang Theory. For more than 3,000 years, the Chinese have used health foods and herb tonics to prevent and cure illness. These treatments originated in ancient tradition and have been woven into philosophy, religion, and folklore. Diet therapy is an important part of Chinese traditional medicine, and is integrated with other forms of healing, including meditation, acupuncture, and martial arts. According to the ancient philosophy of *Tao,* the balance of the two elements *yin* and *yang* maintains harmony in the universe. Yin represents female, cold, and darkness, whereas Yang represents male, hot, and light. When foods are digested, they turn into air, which is either yin or yang.

The terms yin and yang are often, though somewhat inadequately, translated into English as cold and hot. The balance of yin and yang components in the diet is considered essential to good health because excesses of either are believed to result in body imbalances recognized as diseases. Yin conditions require yang foods or treatment and vice versa. Some neutral foods (those that are neither yin nor yang) may be used to treat either type of condition. Nutritionally, the yin-yang system has been beneficial, creating variety in the diet and balancing the amounts of animal protein, grains, and vegetables.

Religion, Culture, and Diet

Through the symbolic attachment of meanings to food and drink, some religions provide members with required or recommended practices that govern the preparation and consumption of food and drink. Religious dietary practices of selected groups are summarized in the following table.

Dietary Practices of Selected Religious Groups: Prohibited Foods and Beverages

Mormonism (Church of Jesus Christ of Latter-Day Saints)

- Alcohol
- Tobacco
- Stimulants and beverages containing caffeine (coffee, tea, colas, and selected carbonated soft drinks) are avoided by some members

Seventh Day Adventism

- Pork or pork products
- Certain seafoods including shellfish
- Fermented beverages

Note: A vegetarian diet is encouraged and snacking between meals is discouraged.

Islam

- Pork and pork products, including animal shortenings
- Regular gelatin made with pork, marshmallow, and other confections made with pork are prohibited
- Alcoholic products and beverages (including extracts such as vanilla or lemon)

Note: Only meat from four-footed animals that have been blessed by a Muslim is eaten.

Judaism

- Pork
- Predatory fowl

- Shellfish and scavengers (shrimp, crab, lobster, escargot, catfish); fish with scales and fins are permissible
- Mixing milk and meat dishes at same meal
- Blood by ingestion (e.g., blood sausage, raw meat); blood by transfusion is acceptable

Notes

Only meat from cloven-hoofed animals that chew cud (cattle, sheep, goat, or deer) is allowed

All animals must be slaughtered ritually by a *sochet* (quickly, with the least pain possible) to be *kosher*. Two methods are used to prepare kosher meats: (1) To remove the maximum amount of blood after slaughtering, meat is soaked in cold water, salted, and drained. The preparation increases the natural sodium content of the food. (2) Meat is quickly seared and cooked over an open flame, which permits liver to be eaten.

Commercially prepared foods contain labels identifying them as kosher. Products made without meat or milk are designated *parve* and labeled accordingly.

Meat and dairy products cannot be served at the same meal, nor can they be cooked or served on the same dishes. Milk or milk products may be consumed just before a meal but not until 6 hours after eating a meal with meat. Fish or eggs can be eaten with dairy products or meat.

Hinduism

- All meats

The nurse needs to be aware of religious practices that influence the client's nutritional state, such as fasting and the consumption of special foods. The following religious observations require that the client limit food or liquid intake during specified times. Observant Catholics fast and abstain from meat on Ash Wednesday and the Fridays of Lent. Muslims refrain from eating during the daytime hours for the entire

Continued on following page

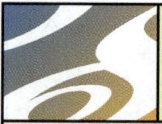

DIVERSITY IN HEALTHCARE *(Continued)*

month of Ramadan, but they are permitted to eat after sunset during this time. For Mormons, all solid foods and liquids are avoided on the first Sunday of each month. During Yom Kippur, observant Jews fast for 24 hours.

Beyond the scope of this text is a discussion of special foods eaten by members of many religions during special religious holidays. For exam-ple, Christmas, Easter, and other celebrations may be observed with foods and drinks that reflect both re-ligious and ethnic traditions of mem-bers. In general, during special cele-brations people tend to consume more calories and foods with higher levels of cholesterol and/or fat. Dur-ing some religious observances, however, very specific dietary prac-tices are expected. For example, during the 8 days of Passover, foods with leavening (bread, cakes made with baking soda or powder) or foods made with grain products are prohibited. This prohibition in-cludes many medications, such as those containing starch or grain al-cohol. Jewish clients may refuse drugs containing prohibited sub-stances unless they are urgently needed.[2,5,6]

Dietary Practices of Specific Cultural Groups

Asian. Asian food traditions are an-cient and complex. Diet is intimately associated with health, and in a complex manner with the condition of the cosmos. The diets of Chi-nese, Hindus, and many other Asians are intimately linked philo-sophically to all other aspects of so-ciety and influence the individual's state of health. Although food pat-terns have been modified signifi-cantly in the United States, clients of Asian descent generally have maintained strong ties to their native foods.[2]

Asian cookery is characterized by mixed dishes with the ingredients cut into small pieces. Although prep-aration is lengthy, the actual cook-ing time is usually brief; thus, es-sential vitamins are generally retained. Characteristic foods in-clude rice and wheat, pork, chicken, a variety of vegetables, eggs, vari-ous soy preparations, and tea. A fa-vorite sauce combines sweet and sour flavors. Sodium intake is high, whereas fat consumption is typically very low. With adult lactase defi-ciency being virtually universal, milk use is rare. The prevalence of dia-betes mellitus in Asians increases following relocation into Western so-cieties. This may be related to ac-culturation and differences in nutri-ent intake, which usually lead to increased consumption of total fat, animal fat, animal protein, and sim-ple carbohydrates. Total and com-plex carbohydrate intake, on the other hand, decreases.[2,7]

Many people of Asian heritage adhere to yin-yang principles, which advocate dietary balance and mod-eration in eating. Overeating or obe-sity is not prevalent among many Chinese-Americans because of the belief that one should leave the table only 70% full. As a general rule, Asian Americans have good di-etary habits that should be rein-forced. Improvement in consuming calcium-containing foods is suggested.[2]

Blacks. Although black Americans are a heterogeneous group, several factors make it worthwhile to dis-cuss their diet separately. First, there are more low-income blacks, and low incomes are associated with less nutritious diets. Second, many black Americans are lactose intolerant, and their consumption of dairy foods is therefore lower. Third, dietary patterns are interrelated with culturally determined habits, obser-vation of ethnic holidays, and other cultural factors.

Although the food of blacks is not significantly different from that of other clients living in the same area, regional differences between the North and South are marked. South-ern diets are distinguishable be-cause they contain more corn, rice, pork, lard, legumes, and greens than Northern diets. Hot breads and fried foods are popular. Black Amer-icans may classify foods as heavy (cornbread, greens, legumes) or light (fruit, white bread). A balanced meal consists of a mixture of heavy and light foods. Some foods are also identified as strength foods, such as vegetables, meat, and milk.[1,2]

An important belief concerning the quality and character of the blood is useful for the nurse. Some blacks believe that a healthy body displays a balance of hot and cold. Blood is considered hot. High blood (excess blood in the body) can cause stroke and is believed to come from eating too much rich food or red meat, such as pork. The treatment is be-lieved to be dietary and involves use of astringent and acidic foods, such as vinegar, lemons, pickles, or epsom salts to open the pores and let excessive sweat escape. Some black Americans believe that low blood, a condition in which there is too little blood in the body, can be treated with diet. The dietary treat-ment consists of increased intake of liver, beets, rare meat, or milk. Note the emphasis on the color red and the bloodiness of the meat. The term *low blood* is sometimes con-fused with anemia, but biomedical and lay treatment may coincide, so adverse effects do not usually ensue.

Hispanic Americans. Although many cultures and subcultures are represented in this category, the di-etary beliefs and practices of Mexi-can-Americans will be discussed as an example of Hispanic dietary pat-terns. The staples of Mexican-Amer-ican diets feature beans and tortillas made from corn treated with lime (calcium carbonate). Other popular foods are eggs, chicken, lard, chili peppers, onions, tomatoes, squash, herb teas (especially mint and chamomile), sweetened packaged breakfast cereals, potatoes, bread, carbonated beverages, canned fruits, gelatin, ice cream, other sweets, and sugar. Although few fresh fruits are consumed, bananas and melons are popular. Milk is used primarily in hot beverages. Most foods are fried using lard, salt pork, and bacon fat. Large break-fasts are common.

In the Southwest, chili, chili con carne, enchiladas, tamales, tostadas, chicken mole, and nopalitos are favored by many Hispanics. Among Mexican-American migrant workers in California, favorite dishes include refried beans, tacos, tortillas, and, to a lesser extent, such middle-class American dishes as hamburgers, macaroni and cheese, and hot dogs. Compared with "typical Anglos," Mexican-Americans use more carbonated beverages, beer, and sweetened beverage mixes, and less milk, coffee, and tea.

The traditional Mexican-American diet has several desirable characteristics. The fiber content is high, and it contains a large amount of complex carbohydrates. The amount of animal fat is relatively low, and processed foods are used infrequently. Although Mexican-American diets are generally adequate for protein and energy, they often are low for vitamins A and C, iron, and calcium. The rate of obesity in Mexican Americans is two to four times the rate of white adults.[2] The prevalence of diabetes mellitus is twice as high in both men and women of Mexican heritage.[7] Paradoxically, Hispanic immigrants from Mexico have a better health profile than those who have been in the United States for a long time.[8]

Native Americans. With more than 500 tribes, American Indian and Alaska Native dietary practices vary widely. The contemporary American Indian diet combines indigenous natural foods with modern processed foods. In the Native American culture, food has great religious and social significance. Health is perceived as a state in which the entire being is in balance, whereas illness indicates disharmony or imbalance.

Traditional foods vary among tribes, but the basic Native American diet consists of corn, beans, and squash. For many tribes these three main staples are sacred. In geographic areas providing game and fish, these items are important food sources for many American Indians. Fruits, berries, roots, and wild greens are highly valued foods, but they are scarce in many areas, particularly large urban centers.

Approximately half of Native Americans live on reservations. When indigenous foods are unavailable on reservations, the daily diet consists of commodity foods provided by the U.S. Department of Agriculture and foods purchased at stores. Access to fresh fruits and vegetables is frequently problematic due to lack of availability or expense in areas in which these items are not locally grown.

Lack of refrigeration may limit some American Indians' consumption of fresh meat, milk, fruits, and vegetables. When relying on nonperishable foods for the bulk of the diet, there are often marginal or deficient states in key nutrients. Excessive amounts of refined sugar, cholesterol, fat, and calories are frequently consumed.

Food acceptance is often culturally related. Among Navajo, meat and blue cornmeal are considered strong foods, whereas milk is a weak food. Corn is a sacred food to many American Indian tribes and is used in ceremonies such as weddings. Dietary taboos against many foods exist among different tribes. For example, some Plains Indians place a taboo on the consumption of fish.

Poor nutrition is directly related to several leading causes of death. Heart disease and cirrhosis of the liver are common. The most significant nutrition-related health problem is obesity and obesity-related diabetes mellitus. Pima Indians have the highest reported incidence for non–insulin dependent diabetes mellitus, with a prevalence of nearly 50% in those older than 35 years. Low hemoglobin values are problematic, and mild thyroid deficiency is also frequent.[2,4]

Facilitating Dietary Change

When helping people to improve their nutrition practices, the nurse should remember that it is essential to understand and appreciate the culture and dietary practices of the group with which the client identifies. Eating is a personal matter carrying with it great cultural significance. Food patterns are generally deeply ingrained, contribute to psychological stability, and are hard to change.[2] People tend to change more outward aspects of their cultural background, such as clothing and language, earlier in their acculturation, whereas food habits persist for a much longer period of time. Each cultural food pattern has strengths and limitations. The positive characteristics have contrib-

uted to the group's survival over time. Most patterns reflect the environment in which the group originated and contain foodstuffs prevalent in the client's country of origin.

One of the few cultural universal truths concerning diet is that people never eat all that is edible in their environment. Culture determines what are acceptable and unacceptable foods. When counseling a client, the nurse should try to categorize nutrition practices as beneficial, neutral, or harmful to the client. Obviously, the ideal is to promote change only in those practices that are harmful to the client. Beneficial or neutral practices should be supported and encouraged. Nurses

should be aware of their own culturally based eating practices and attitudes and should be careful not to project those onto clients.

If it is necessary to change the diet for health or medical reasons, suggest minimal alterations to traditional foods. Recommending a diet that can be eaten by all members of the family increases the likelihood that the client will follow the regimen. The probability that the client will adhere to recommended dietary changes also increases when he or she has control over food choices, understands the meal plan, and feels responsible for following the suggestions.[2]

When suggesting dietary change, the nurse must consider the sym-

Continued on following page

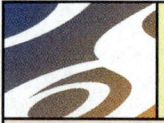

DIVERSITY IN HEALTHCARE *(Continued)*

bolic meaning of food to the individual. For example, *soul food* for many blacks grew out of the necessity of surviving as slaves and out of a need to express the group feeling of "soul." Soul food refers to collards, poke salad, and other greens and vegetables combined with fatback and cooked for long periods. Soul foods are usually well seasoned and economical.[2]

When the client is a recent immigrant to the United States, it may be necessary for the nurse to help with basic survival skills, such as buying, storing, and preparing foods in the new environment. Clients' food habits and beliefs should always be the basis on which to build or improve dietary practices. For example, the nurse might suggest to a febrile Hispanic client who adheres to the hot-cold theory that fluid intake could be improved by drinking sufficient quantities of herbal tea. Such a suggestion would match the client's belief system while achieving the goal of increasing fluid intake. The nurse should assure the client that Anglo-American foods are not necessarily better choices than their own culture's food. Likewise, the standard approach of three meals a day and four food groups should not be emphasized if it conflicts with the client's cultural dietary patterns. It is important to ask the client about possible food restrictions, taboos, or

intolerances, so that acceptable alternatives can be found without compromising nutrient intake.

In suggesting dietary changes, the nurse should be aware that most people not of Northern European descent may have some degree of intolerance to lactose, which is found in milk. Two-thirds of the world's population experiences lactose intolerance after early childhood due to reduced production of the enzyme lactase.[3,9] The majority of American blacks, Asians, Indians, Hispanics, and Middle Easterners are lactose deficient to some degree. Because the client may not be aware that he or she has lactose intolerance, it may be necessary for the nurse to inquire about the usual clinical manifestations of this condition. After drinking milk the person with lactose intolerance may have flatus, intestinal discomfort (such as cramping and abdominal pain), and, less frequently, vomiting and diarrhea. Many people simply say that milk "doesn't agree with them" or that they are allergic to milk. For lactose-intolerant clients, it is necessary to identify other culturally appropriate sources of calcium. For Asian American clients, the nurse might suggest calcium-rich foods such as leafy green vegetables, bok choy, tofu (soybean curd), and fish with edible bones. For Hispanic clients, the nurse might encourage the

consumption of corn tortillas (if the corn has been treated with lime which contains calcium carbonate), cheese, and *cafe con leche* (coffee with milk). Most people with lactose intolerance are able to tolerate fermented milk products such as yogurt, lactose-reduced milks, and sweet acidophilus milk to provide calcium.[1–3]

The nurse should recognize that food itself is only one part of eating. In some cultures, social contacts during meals are restricted to members of the immediate or extended family. The nurse should be aware of the individual's preference, particularly in situations fostering group dining, such as psychiatric/mental health institutions, extended-care facilities, and nursing homes, which sometimes encourage clients to eat in small groups. Traditional group nutrition education may also be inappropriate when it conflicts with cultural restrictions. In some Middle Eastern cultures, men and women eat meals separately, or women may be permitted to eat with their husbands but not with other males.

For members of many cultural groups, respect for authority and politeness in public may prevent clients from asking questions. Inviting the client to ask questions or to state any objections to the recommendations sometimes promotes communication. The nurse may indi-

Major Illnesses and Hospitalizations

The nurse asks the client about past problems with the GI system. Has the client been hospitalized or treated for peptic ulcer, anemia, hiatal hernia, jaundice, gallbladder disease, colitis, cancer, or a change in bowel habits? Has the client ever had surgery of the oral cavity, throat, stomach, abdomen, or rectal area? If so, determine dates and outcomes of the procedures. Ask whether the client has had diagnostic tests involving the GI system, such as barium swallow, upper GI studies, x-ray studies, or CT scan of the lower GI tract.

To continue the history, the nurse should note the client's general health status as well as previous GI disorders and surgery. The nurse should question whether the client currently has or previously has had a change in bowel habits, GI bleeding, jaundice, ulcers, colitis, or unexplained weight loss or gain.

Medications

Obtain detailed information about prescribed and over-the-counter medications, both currently used and taken previously. Does the client take antacids? If so, determine the type and the frequency of administration. Over-the-counter preparations for indigestion often contain sodium bicarbonate (baking soda), which is readily absorbed and may lead to metabolic alkalosis if ingested in sufficient quantities. Also, ask about the use of aspirin, aspirin compounds, and nonsteroidal anti-inflammatory drugs (NSAIDs), which may contribute to gastritis and gastric bleeding. Does the client take a vitamin or mineral supplement? Ask specifically about iron, because it can change the color and consistency of feces (black, tarry stools) and cause constipation. Does the client take laxatives or use enemas to aid elimination? Long-term use of laxatives and enemas can cause dependence.

cate that other alternatives are possible and that the advice is intended as a negotiable suggestion. If the recommendations are culturally unacceptable, the client may be polite and superficially compliant, but will ultimately disregard the suggestions. If the client is asked to keep a diary of foods eaten, the nurse may find excuses, such as forgetting, being offered as reasons for failing to follow instructions. Clients may resort to telling what they think the nurse wants or expects to hear.

It is sometimes difficult to determine how well the message has been understood by the client. Asking the client directly or through an interpreter to repeat the instructions, demonstrate the procedures, or summarize the main points of discussion will help provide feedback as to the success of communication efforts. Limiting discussion to the most relevant and understandable information and using culturally appropriate methods will enhance the nurse's ability to convey the message effectively. Teaching one concept at a time, limiting the length of time per session, and avoiding professional and technical jargon can help prevent the client from becoming overwhelmed with information.

The nurse should be aware that the degree of compliance in transcultural interchanges may be disappointingly less than expected. If a client's values are inconsistent with the underlying rationale for recommended change, the probability of noncompliance is high. Clients may agree to do something out of courtesy or fear, but fail to follow through with recommendations. Limited understanding of health issues may act as a disincentive for client compliance. It is especially difficult to motivate clients to undertake dietary change as a preventive measure for asymptomatic conditions. For example, the client with hypertension may perceive no need for a recommended low-sodium diet because he or she is experiencing no discomfort.

Having realistic expectations will give the nurse a sense of accomplishment and avoid feelings of frustration. Knowledge that an eating practice is harmful does not necessarily promote behavioral change, as is evident in people who are obese or who smoke. This is true regardless of the client's cultural background, educational level, socioeconomic status, or religious affiliation. The nurse must balance the clients' rights to determine their own future against the nurse's need to promote change. The goal should be to provide advice and recommendations in a positive and culturally appropriate manner that encourages learning and promotes the desired behavioral change.

---

[1] Andrews, M. M. (1995). Transcultural nursing care. In M. M. Andrews & J. S. Boyle (Eds.). *Transcultural concepts in nursing care* (pp. 49–96). Philadelphia: J. B. Lippincott.

[2] Davis, J. R., & Sherer, K. (1994). *Applied nutrition and diet therapy for nurses.* Philadelphia: W. B. Saunders.

[3] Bryant, C. A. (1985). The impact of kin, friend, and neighbor networks on infant feeding practices. *Social Science Medicine, 16,* 1757–1765.

[4] Indian Health Service. (1994). *Trends in Indian health—1994.* Rockville, MD: U.S. Department of Health and Human Services, U.S. Public Health Service.

[5] Andrews, M. M., & Hanson, P. A. (1995). Religion, culture and nursing. In M. M. Andrews & J. S. Boyle (Eds.). *Transcultural concepts in nursing care* (pp. 353–409). Philadelphia: J. B. Lippincott.

[6] Schwartz, E. (1995). Jewish Americans. In J. N. Giger & R. E. Davidhizer (Eds.). *Transcultural nursing: Assessment and intervention* (pp. 525–552). St. Louis: Mosby–Year Book.

[7] Bertorelli, A. M. (1990). Nutrition counseling: Meeting the needs of ethnic clients with diabetes. *Diabetes Educator, 11*(4), 284–285, 289.

[8] Marwich, C. (1991). HANES takes long look at Latino health. *JAMA, 265*(2), 177, 181.

[9] Overfield, T. (1985). *Biologic variation in health and illness.* Menlo Park, CA: Addison-Wesley.

Allergies

The nurse inquires about allergies to foods, taking care to distinguish between actual allergic response and client dislikes of certain foods. If the client reports food allergies, determine what GI manifestations result, such as cramping, flatulence, diarrhea, or other manifestations, such as hives or dyspnea.

Family Health History

A family history of certain GI problems may influence a client's current and past health problems. The nurse asks the client if any family members have had cancer, ulcers, or colitis. Many of these diseases are familial (e.g., ulcerative colitis and Crohn's disease), that is, they have a higher incidence within a family than would be expected by chance. Duodenal ulcers also occur more frequently in clients with blood group O, suggesting a possible genetic association.

Other disorders to inquire about include jaundice, alcoholism, hepatitis, cancer of the colon, intestinal polyps, obesity, peptic ulcers, and irritable bowel syndrome.

Psychosocial History

Sociologic and psychological factors, as well as the physical environment, can affect health.

Occupation

Ask the client about his or her occupation. Are substances present in the workplace that are toxic if ingested or absorbed, such as arsenic, mercury, or carbon tetrachloride? Does the client travel as part of the job, which can lead to exposure to unfamiliar foods, pathogens, or parasites? Does the client experience stress in the work-place?

Geographic Location

A history of travel outside of the United States should also be explored. Recent travel to foreign countries may be related to the onset of GI manifestations, such as diarrhea or nausea. Invasion by bacteria, helminths, and other parasites are the primary causes of such problems.

Nutrition

When assessing GI tract function, a diet history is an essential component of the health history. The client's dietary practices and nutritional status may contribute to GI disorders. These practices are influenced by the client's cultural and religious background, individual pref-erences, and physical and mental well-being. For exam-ple, foods with a high nitrosamine content (e.g., smoked and preserved meats) or a high fat content increase the risk of upper GI tract and colorectal cancer. Assess when and where meals are taken.

The nurse assesses the client's usual and current appe-tite and whether a change in appetite has occurred. The client should describe the usual foods and fluids, such as coffee, colas, and alcohol, that are typically consumed within a 24-hour period. The nurse can then evaluate, often with the assistance of a clinical dietician, the quality of the foods ingested and the client's understanding of a balanced diet.

The nurse should explore the relationship between food intake and possible GI manifestations. Gastric ulcer symptoms increase with food intake whereas duodenal ulcer manifestations decrease with food intake. Lactose intolerance causes abdominal bloating, diarrhea, and cramping, because of an insufficient amount of the en-zyme lactase. Lactase converts lactose, found in dairy products, into glucose and galactose. Other manifesta-tions, such as nausea and vomiting, difficulty swallowing, anorexia, early satiety, and diarrhea, should be noted.

Habits

Certain habits have a known effect on the GI system. Caffeine can cause gastritis and irritable bowel manifesta-tions. Alcohol can cause gastritis and eventual hepatic damage if it is used excessively. Nicotine irritates the GI mucosa and is linked to oral and esophageal cancers.

Ask the client whether aspects of the work or home environments are stress provoking, such as interpersonal relationships, job security, or financial concerns. Can the client relate GI manifestations, such as epigastric pain, nausea, diarrhea, or peptic ulcers, to stressful situations? Life-style habits also can affect elimination patterns. Ask whether the client has sufficient time the daily schedule to promote a regular pattern of bowel elimination.

Review of Systems

The nurse questions the client about other areas related to the GI system. Inquire about the condition of the oral cavity, such as the presence of dental caries, number and condition of teeth, condition of the gingivae, use of den-tures and their fit, problems of the oral cavity (e.g., le-sions, odor, excess salivation or dryness, sore tongue). Does the client have difficulty chewing or swallowing? Has there been any change in appetite or weight? If pain is reported with eating, is it related to specific foods or associated events? Do bowel habits, appetite changes, and other GI manifestations occur with hormonal changes during the menstrual cycle? Has the client had a change in bowel habits or stool characteristics? Are there prob-lems with hemorrhoids? Specifically, ask about problems of the hepatic and biliary systems, such as jaundice, pru-ritus, ascites, dark-colored urine, pale stools, or bleeding problems. (Detailed questions for the review of systems are found in Box 11–2.)

Physical Examination

Assessing the Oral Cavity

Begin the GI physical assessment with the oral cavity. Assessment of the oral cavity involves inspection and palpation. The nurse puts on gloves, faces the client, and begins by inspecting the lips. The lips are inspected for abnormal color, lesions, nodules, and symmetry.

Good illumination and instrumentation are essential in performing an assessment of the oral cavity. A headlight provides direct illumination and a head mirror provides indirect lighting of the mouth, both allowing the exami-ner's hands to be free to handle the equipment. A pen-light and tongue blade may also be used. Figure 59–1 presents and overview of assessment of the oral cavity, including terminology and normal findings.

After applying gloves, the examiner asks the client to remove any dentures or partial appliances so that all areas of the mouth can be visualized. The oral assessment be-gins at the left side of the client's mouth and continues in a clockwise fashion. The oral mucosa is inspected for redness, pallor, swelling, ulcers, or leukoplakia (a gray-white spot or patch). The gums are inspected for redness, pallor, recession, ulcers, and bleeding. Examine the teeth for evidence of dental caries and for missing or broken teeth. The tongue is inspected for color, ulcers, abnormal coatings, swelling, or a deviation to one side. Using the tongue blade or gauze as a retractor, the examiner moves the tongue to inspect the mucous membranes. The client is instructed to stick out the tongue and move it from side to side and upward and downward. This allows the examiner to observe the tongue for voluntary or involun-tary movement. Abnormal tongue movement may be due to infiltration of muscle or nerve by tumor or nerve en-trapment. While depressing the tongue, the examiner asks the client to say "aah." Examine the pharynx for any tonsil abnormalities, such as redness or swelling, lesions, ulcers, uvular deviations, and any unusual mouth odor.

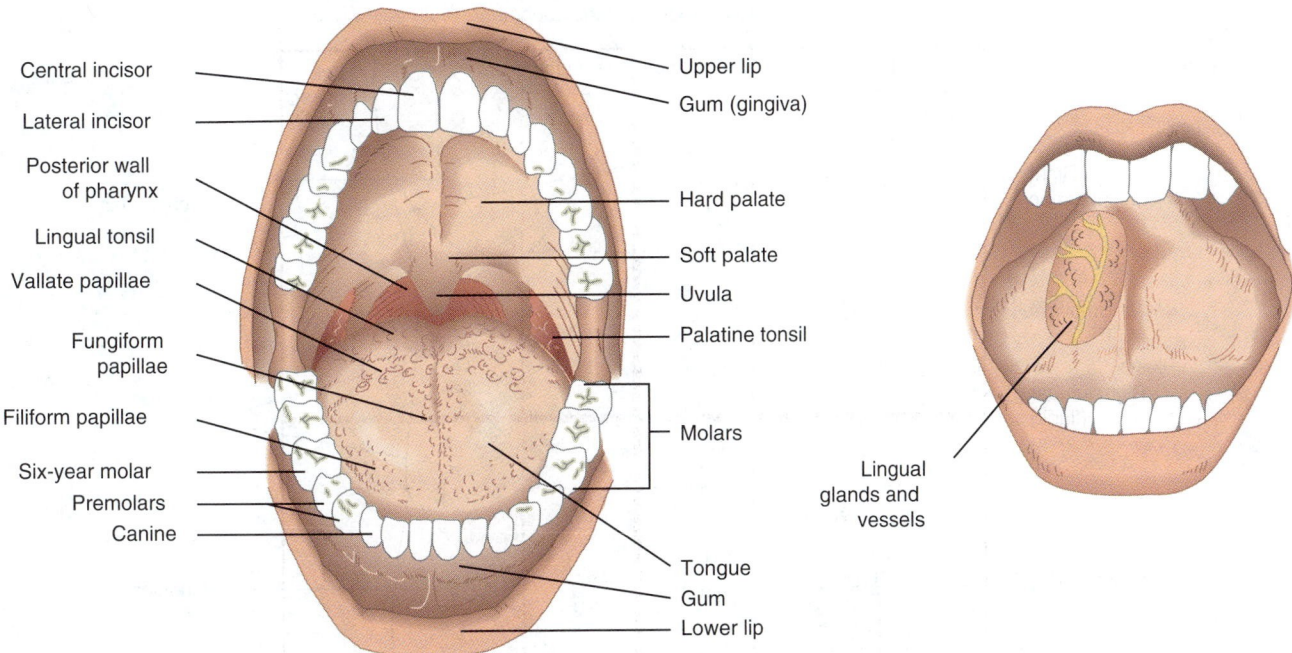

Figure 59–1. Assessment of the oral cavity: terminology and normal findings.

The lips, gingivae, buccal mucosa, and tongue are palpated, and the area is checked for any masses, swellings, or tenderness.

Ask the client to swallow. Is any difficulty noted with swallowing? Does the client experience frequent choking or other problems with swallowing?

Assessing the Abdomen

To assess the client's abdomen, have the client lie in a supine position with the arms at the sides. Bending the knees slightly helps to relax the abdominal muscles. Begin in the client's right lower quadrant and proceed in a clockwise manner. When assessing the abdomen, the nurse proceeds in the following sequence: inspection, auscultation, percussion, and palpation. This sequence varies from other body systems because in the GI system, auscultation is performed in the abdomen before percussion and palpation. This is because percussion and palpation can increase intestinal activity and, therefore, alter bowel sounds. You must be knowledgeable about the underlying structures of the abdomen for accurate assessment. Figure 59–2 shows the quadrant and anatomic regions of the abdomen and their underlying organs.

Inspection

Begin by inspecting the client's abdomen, noting the condition of the skin and the contour of the abdomen. The skin should be smooth and intact, with varying amounts of hair. Assess for the presence of rashes, discolorations, scars, petechiae, striae (stretch marks), and dilated veins. The contour of the abdomen is either flat, concave, rounded, or distended, depending on the client's body type. An irregular contour should be noted and could be due to a hernia, tumor, or previous surgery. The umbilicus is inspected for shape, position, and color. It should be concave, located at the midline, and the same color as the abdominal skin. The nurse also assesses for bulging flanks and glistening, taut skin, which are abnormal findings associated with ascites.

Abdominal movements are noted. Observe the abdomen for pulsation, especially by the abdominal aorta, and for peristaltic movement. Normally, peristaltic movements are not visible and should be reported. The rectal area is inspected after the entire abdominal examination is completed.

Assess for a separation of the rectus muscles (*diastasis recti*). Ask the client to either bear down and perform the Valsalva maneuver (if not contraindicated) or to attempt a situp or stomach curl. The increased intra-abdominal pressure enhances the separation of weakened rectus muscles at the midline, where a bulge appears. *Diastasis recti* results from obesity, pregnancy, or other conditions in which the abdominal muscles are subjected to sustained, increased intra-abdominal pressure.

Auscultation

Auscultation of the abdomen begins by listening with the diaphragm of the stethoscope, which provides information on bowel and vascular sounds. The stethoscope is lightly pressed on the abdominal wall in all four quadrants. Begin in the right lower quadrant at the ileocecal valve area, because bowel sounds are normally present there.[10] As air and fluid move through the GI tract, soft clicks and gurgles can be heard every 5 to 15 seconds. The frequency and character of bowel sounds should be noted, with a normal frequency rate of 5 to 35 bowel sounds, which occur irregularly, per minute. Borborygmi, or rapid, high-pitched, loud bowel sounds, represent hyperactive bowel,

Anatomic regions of the abdomen

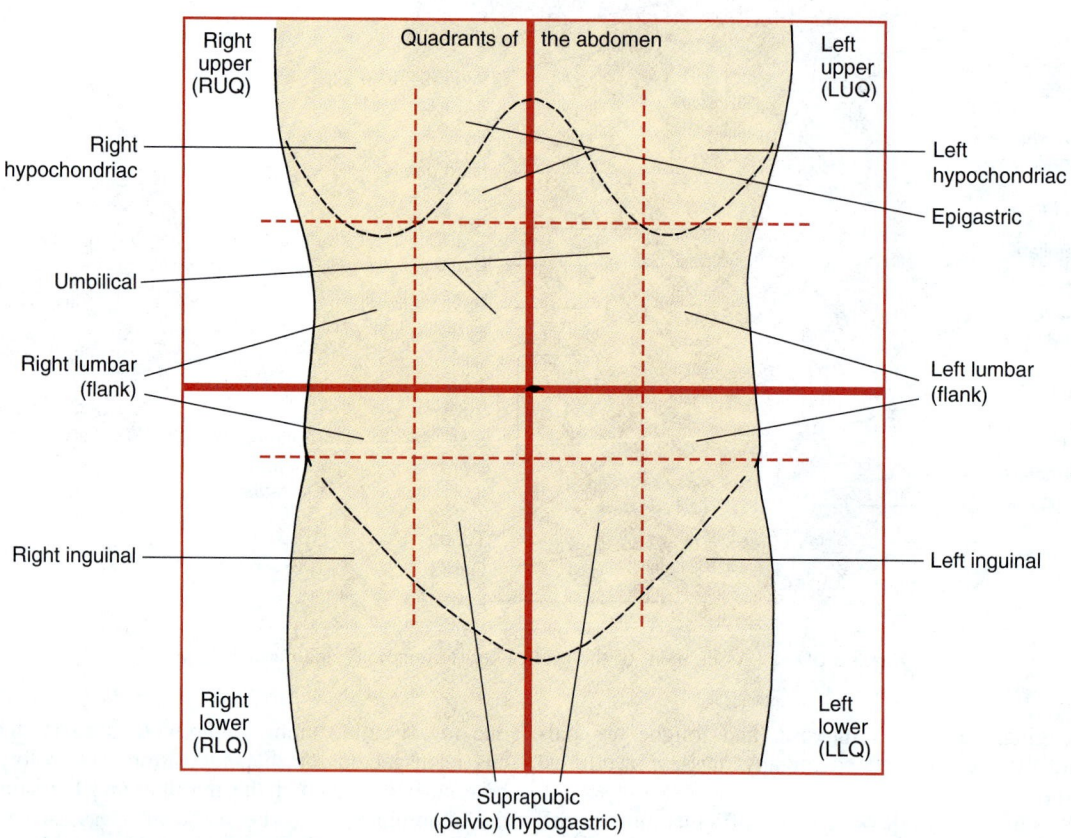

QUADRANTS OF THE ABDOMEN
AND THEIR UNDERLYING ORGANS*

Right Upper Quadrant (RUQ)
Adrenal gland (right)
Colon (hepatic flexure
  and portions
  of ascending and
  transverse)
Duodenum
Kidney (portion of
  right)
Liver (right lobe)
Gallbladder
Pancreas (head)
Pylorus

Left Upper Quadrant (LUQ)
Adrenal gland (left)
Colon (splenic flexure
  and portions
  of transverse and
  descending)
Kidney (portion of left)
Liver (left lobe)
Pancreas (body)
Spleen
Stomach

Right Lower Quadrant (RLQ)
Appendix
Bladder (if distended)
Cecum
Colon (portion of
  ascending)
Kidney (lower pole of
  right)
Ovary (right)
Salpinx (uterine tube;
  right)
Spermatic cord (right)
Ureter (right)
Uterus (if enlarged)

Left Lower Quadrant (LLQ)
Bladder (if distended)
Colon (sigmoid and
  portion of
  descending)
Kidney (lower pole of
  left)
Ovary (left)
Salpinx (uterine tube;
  left)
Spermatic cord (left)
Ureter (left)
Uterus (if enlarged)

*Small intestine loops in all quadrants.

ANATOMIC REGIONS OF THE ABDOMEN
AND THEIR UNDERLYING ORGANS

Right hypochondriac
Right lobe of
  liver
Gallbladder
Portion of
  duodenum
Hepatic
  flexure of
  colon
Portion of right
  kidney
Adrenal gland
  (right)

Epigastric
Pyloric end of
  stomach
Duodenum
Pancreas
Portion of
  liver

Left hypochondriac
Stomach
Spleen
Tail of
  pancreas
Splenic flexure
  of colon
Upper pole of
  left kidney
Adrenal gland
  (left)

Right lumbar
Ascending
  colon
Lower half of
  right kidney
Portion of
  duodenum
  and jejunum

Umbilical
Omentum
Mesentery
Lower
  duodenum
Jejunum and
  ileum

Left lumbar
Descending
  colon
Lower half of
  left kidney
Portions of
  jejunum and
  ileum

Right inguinal
Cecum
Appendix
Ileum (lower
  end)
Right ureter
Right
  spermatic
  cord
Right ovary

Suprapubic
Ileum
Bladder
Uterus (in
  pregnancy)

Left inguinal
Sigmoid colon
Left ureter
Left spermatic
  cord
Left ovary

Figure 59–2. Quadrants and anatomic regions of the abdomen and their underlying organs.

and they may occur normally in a hungry client or in a client with gastroenteritis. Hypoactive bowel sounds occur at a rate of one or fewer every minute, and they can be heard in clients with a paralytic ileus or after bowel surgery. To determine the absence of bowel sounds, the nurse must listen for a total of 5 minutes or at least 1 minute per quadrant. It is best to listen for 2 full minutes in the right lower quadrant before concluding that bowel sounds are absent.[16] Make sure the bladder is empty, because a full bladder can interfere with bowel sounds.

The nurse next uses the bell of the stethoscope to auscultate vascular sounds. Three abnormal sounds should be listened for: a bruit, a venous hum, or a friction rub. The nurse listens over the aorta, renal arteries, and iliac arteries. No bruits should be auscultated. A bruit heard over the aorta could indicate the presence of an aneurysm. A continuous venous hum heard in the periumbilical area can indicate engorged liver circulation. Listen for a friction rub, which sounds like two pieces of leather rubbing together, over the liver and spleen. If the sound is heard, it can indicate a hepatic tumor or splenic infarction.

Percussion

Abdominal percussion is used to determine the size and location of abdominal organs and to detect fluid, air, and masses. The nurse uses percussion in all four quadrants of the abdomen and compares sounds. Normally, percussion sounds over the abdomen are tympanic (high-pitched loud or musical over gas) or dull (thudlike sounds over fluid or solid organs). Percussion is used to determine the size and position of the liver and spleen (see Chapter 64 for a discussion of these assessments) and also can be used to assess the level of a distended bladder (see also Chapter 55). Abdominal percussion is contraindicated in

clients with suspected abdominal aneurysms and in those who have undergone abdominal organ transplants.

Palpation

To palpate the abdomen, the nurse starts by lightly depressing the abdomen (1 to 2 cm) in a systematic, quadrant-to-quadrant manner. The nurse assesses for masses, rebound tenderness, and areas of direct tenderness. Any areas of tenderness are cautiously examined last with deep palpation. Areas of involuntary abdominal rigidity and guarding are noted. Deep palpation is used next to determine the size and shape of abdominal organs and masses. Deep palpation should be performed cautiously and by a skilled nurse. Palpation of the kidneys is discussed in Chapter 55 and palpation of the liver and spleen in Chapter 64. Further discussion of palpation techniques is contained in Chapter 12.

Assessing the Anus and Rectum

Examination of the anus and rectum is potentially embarrassing and uncomfortable for the client. Agency policy and the nurse's skill level dictate the extent of rectal examination performed; nurses without advanced preparation may be limited to inspection of the perianal area. However, you should be familiar with rectal structures and expected physical findings when digitally assessing for fecal impaction or administering rectal medications (Fig. 59–3). The nurse uses a gentle approach and a matter-of-fact manner.

The client's position depends on the circumstances of the examination. A female client may be examined while in the lithotomy position immediately following assessment of the genitalia, in the Sim's position, or in a dorsal

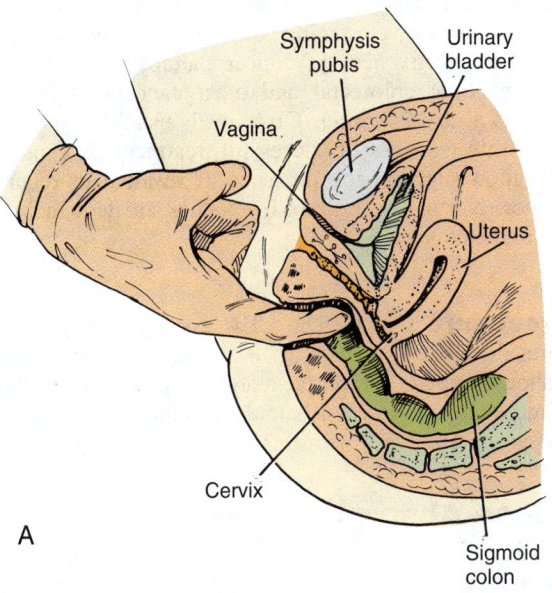
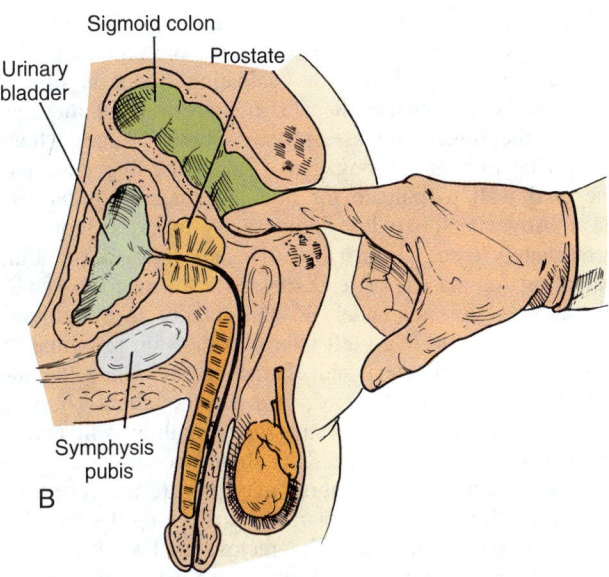

Figure 59–3. Palpation of the rectum in female (*A*) and male (*B*) clients.

recumbent position. A male client may be examined in the Sim's position or while standing and leaning across the examination table, a position which facilitates palpation of the prostate gland. Clients are draped accordingly. The nurse wears disposable gloves and uses water-soluble lubricant. A stool specimen is usually obtained at the end of the examination following removal of the finger from the rectum and is tested for occult blood (guaiac test). (This test is discussed later in the chapter.)

Inspection

Using the nondominant hand, the nurse gently spreads apart the buttocks to visualize the perianal area. Perianal skin is darker and coarser than the skin of the surrounding area and should be intact, moist, and without hair. The area should be free of excoriation, rashes, inflammation, ulceration, abscesses, lumps, fissures (cracks), fistulous openings, and hemorrhoids (dilated veins seen as reddened skin protrusions). The anus should be closed, without manifestations of rectal prolapse (protrusion of rectal mucosa through the anal opening).

Next, ask the client to bear down as if having a bowel movement. Look for the appearance of abnormalities such as rectal prolapse, internal hemorrhoids, polyps, and rectal fissures. The increased intra-abdominal pressure may cause abnormalities to become more prominent.

Palpation

The nurse lubricates the index finger of the dominant hand and places it over the client's anus. Instruct the client to bear down and, as the anal sphincter relaxes, insert the index finger slowly and gently into the anal canal, pointing the finger toward the umbilicus. If insertion is difficult or the nurse meets with resistance or rectal bleeding, stop the examination. Reassure the client that it is normal to feel like having a bowel movement while being examined digitally.

The anal canal extends toward the umbilicus approximately 3 cm (1¼ inch), where it joins the rectum at the anorectal junction. While the palpating finger is in the anal canal, instruct the client to tighten the anal muscles around the finger and assess anal sphincter tone, which should be firm and strong. Next, rotate the finger around the anal wall to palpate for nodules, masses, or tenderness. Advance the index finger to its fullest extent, approximately 6 to 10 cm (2 to 4 inches) into the rectum, palpating for masses or tenderness. Rectal mucosa should be smooth and nontender. If abnormality is noted, describe its location (e.g., left lateral wall, 1 cm proximal to internal anal sphincter) and characteristics. Once the index finger is fully inserted, instruct the client to bear down again and feel for a mass descending from above against the palpating finger. This should be absent.

In a female client, the nurse may palpate the cervix of the uterus through the rectovaginal wall along the anterior rectum (see Chapter 82). The rectovaginal wall is firm, smooth, and resilient. The nurse may mistake the cervix or a vaginal tampon for a rectal mass.

In a male client, the nurse may palpate the prostate gland through the anterior rectal wall. See Chapter 74 for a discussion of this part of the physical examination.

As the nurse withdraws the index finger from the client's rectum, he or she observes for the presence of stool on the glove. Feces, if present, is usually brown. Mucus, blood, or black, tan, gray, or tarry stool is abnormal. Test the stool for occult blood (described later in this chapter). If the nurse suspects that a sexually transmitted disease is present, a rectal culture is also obtained (see the discussion of collecting a stool specimen for culture later in this chapter). Wipe the perianal area clean and inform the client that the examination is completed.

Diagnostic Tests

Diagnostic measures are performed to locate the nature and level of the problem associated with diseases of the GI tract. The general methods of diagnosis include laboratory tests (Table 59–1), ultrasound, magnetic resonance imaging, radiographic tests, endoscopy, cytologic studies, and gastric analysis. Hematologic studies and electrolyte determinations indicate the general health status, but they do not give specific information about GI disorders.

Laboratory Tests

Carcinoembryonic Antigen

Procedure. Carcinoembryonic antigen (CEA) is a glycoprotein normally produced during the first or second trimester of fetal life. Normally, production is halted before birth. Increased CEA levels in clients other than neonates may indicate the presence of colorectal or other cancer. This test is not useful as a screening tool because increased CEA levels are also seen with cirrhosis, hepatic disease, and alcoholic pancreatitis, and they are also present in clients who smoke heavily. The test is used to assist in preoperative staging of colorectal cancer, to monitor the effectiveness of cancer therapy, and to test for recurrence of colorectal and other cancers. It is referred to as a *tumor marker*. CEA levels usually return to normal within 6 weeks of successful treatment. A continued elevation suggests the presence of residual or recurrent tumor. Normally, serum CEA values are less than 5 ng/ml in nonsmokers.

Preprocedure Care. The CEA assay requires venipuncture. In this test, as well as in all diagnostic tests, the nurse should explain the purpose and the procedure to the client and evaluate the client's understanding. No postprocedure care is necessary with this test.

D-Xylose Absorption Test

Procedure. Measurement of blood and urine levels of D-xylose, a monosaccharide absorbed in the small intestine, helps evaluate the absorption qualities of the small

Table 59–1. Laboratory Tests Used to Assess GI Function

Test	Normal Findings	Abnormal Findings
Complete Blood Count		
Red blood cells	4.2–5.4 million/mm³ (women) 4.5–6.2 million/mm³ (men)	Decreased values indicate possible anemia or hemorrhage
Hemoglobin	12–16 g/dl (women) 14–18 g/dl (men)	Increased values indicate possible hemoconcentration, caused by dehydration
Hematocrit	38%–46% (women) 42%–54% (men)	
Electrolytes		
Potassium	3.5–5.0 mg/L	Decreased values indicate possible GI suction, diarrhea, vomiting, intestinal fistulas
Calcium	8.0–10.5 mg/dl	Decreased values indicate possible malabsorption
Sodium	135–145 mg/L	Decreased values indicate possible malabsorption and diarrhea
CEA		
	<5 ng/ml (nonsmokers)	Increased values indicate possible colorectal cancer and inflammatory bowel disease.
D-Xylose Absorption		
	Blood levels peak (25–40 mg/dl) 2 hr after ingestion 80%–95% excreted in 5 hr	Decreased values indicate possible malabsorption
Fecal Analysis		
Stool for occult blood	Negative	Presence indicates possible peptic ulcer, cancer of the colon, ulcerative colitis
Stool for ova and parasites	Negative	Presence indicates infection
Stool cultures	No unusual growth	Presence of pathogens may indicate *Shigella, Salmonella, Staphylococcus aureus,* or *Bacillus cereus*
Stool for lipids	2 to 5 g/24 hr (normal diet)	Increased values indicate possible malabsorption syndrome and Crohn's disease

intestine and aids in the diagnosis of malabsorption. Decreased values of absorbed D-xylose in blood and urine indicate possible malabsorption in the small intestine. D-Xylose is given orally in water. All urine is then collected for a specified time, and blood is drawn 2 hours after D-xylose is given. The client is instructed to remain in bed during the test because activity alters the test results.

Preprocedure Care. The client receives nothing by mouth for 10 to 12 hours before the test. Before the administration of D-xylose, a blood sample and a first-voided morning urine specimen are collected.

Fecal Analysis

Stool examinations that may aid in the diagnosis of GI tract disorders include stool examination for occult blood, stool examination for ova and parasites, stool cultures, and stool analysis for lipids.

Stool Examination for Occult Blood

Procedure. Stool can be examined for occult blood to detect GI bleeding and to aid in the early diagnosis of colorectal cancer. The importance of this test is highlighted in the Nursing Research feature. The guaiac or orthotoluidine test is commonly used. The American Cancer Society recommends that the fecal occult blood test be combined with a digital rectal examination and flexible fiberoptic sigmoidoscopy for colorectal cancer screening of the average-risk client older than 50 years.[1, 18] A digital rectal examination should be done each year after the age of 40. A fecal occult blood test and a digital rectal examination should be done each year after the age of 50. In addition to these tests, the client should have a flexible sigmoidoscopy every 3 to 5 years. Clients with above-average risk for colorectal cancer should be evaluated with barium enema or colonoscopy as recommended by the physician.[1] The nurse or the client usually collects a total of three stool specimens (over 3 successive days). A

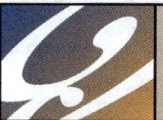

NURSING RESEARCH

Do Annual Tests for Fecal Occult Blood Really Make a Difference?

Mandel, J., et al. (1993). Reducing mortality from colorectal cancer by screening for occult blood. *New England Journal of Medicine, 328* (19), 1365–1371.

Mandel and colleagues completed the 13-year-long Minnesota Colon Control Study to evaluate the effectiveness of screening for fecal occult blood in reducing mortality from colorectal cancer. Participants (N = 46,551), aged 50 to 80, were randomly assigned to one of three groups: those who underwent annual occult blood screening, those who underwent biannual occult blood screening, and a control group that followed personal healthcare regimens. People with a history of colorectal cancer, familial polyposis, or chronic ulcerative colitis were excluded from the sample.

The incidence of colorectal cancer was found to be similar in all three groups. The cumulative annual mortality rate, however, was lower in the annually screened group (5.88 per 1,000) than in the biannually screened group (8.33 per 1,000) or the control group (8.83 per 1,000). Overall, cancer was detected at an earlier stage in the groups that underwent occult blood screening. Mortality at 13 years of follow-up was significantly lower in the annually screened group than in the control group.

Implications for Practice

Although tests for fecal occult blood do not reduce the incidence of colorectal cancer, they clearly increase the likelihood of early detection and cure. When working with clients over age 50, stress the importance of annual tests for fecal occult blood.

---

wooden applicator is used to apply the stool to one side of guaiac-treated paper. After the required solution is applied, the color is immediately noted. A positive result, which is blue, should be reported.

Preprocedure Care. If the orthotoluidine test is used, the client may be instructed to eat a high-fiber diet for 48 to 72 hours before the collection of the stool specimen. Red meats, poultry, fish, turnips, and horseradish should be avoided. The following medications should be withheld for 48 hours before the test: iron preparations, bromides, rauwolfia derivatives, steroids, indomethacin, and colchicine. Other tests for occult blood do not require dietary restrictions. There is no post-procedure care.

Stool Examination for Ova and Parasites

Procedure. Stool examination for ova and parasites is performed to detect intestinal infections caused by parasites and their ova (eggs). The nurse should collect the stool and send it immediately to the laboratory. The nurse should wear gloves when obtaining the specimen. Fresh, warm stool is required. If it cannot be examined within 30 minutes, the nurse should place the specimen in a preservative according to hospital protocol.

Preprocedure Care. The client should be instructed to avoid drugs such as castor oil, mineral oil, or antidiarrheal compounds, all of which may alter the feces. The client should be informed that the test usually re-

quires three stool specimens, one taken every other day or every third day. There is no post-procedure care.

Stool Cultures

Procedure. Stool cultures are performed to identify pathogenic organisms in the GI tract. If a stool culture shows no pathogens, detection of viruses can be performed by immunoassay or electron microscopy, which may help in the diagnosis of nonbacterial gastroenteritis. Stool should be collected using sterile technique and a sterile stool container and sent immediately to the laboratory. The nurse should wear gloves when obtaining the specimen. Fresh, warm stool is required. Storage in a refrigerator is contraindicated because the cool air retards bacterial growth. The stool may be collected for 3 consecutive days. Stool cultures can also be collected via sterile swabs. With the client in lithotomy position, insert the swab about 1 inch into the anal canal. Rotate the swab, moving it from side to side. Remove the swab and send it to the laboratory in the proper culture media.

Preprocedure Care. The nurse should report if the client is or has been taking any antibiotics recently. There is no post-procedure care.

Stool for Lipids

Procedure. Stool can also be examined for lipids. Normally, dietary lipids are almost completely absorbed in the small intestine. Excessive secretion of fecal fat (steatorrhea) may occur in various digestive and absorptive disorders, such as Crohn's disease. The nurse should collect a 72-hour stool specimen; the collected specimens should be stored on ice.

Preprocedure Care. The client should be instructed to eat a high-fat diet and to refrain from alcohol consumption for 3 days before the test and during the collection period. The client should avoid drugs that interfere with the test, such as mineral oil, neomycin, and potassium chloride. There is no post-procedure care.

Ultrasonography

Procedure. Ultrasonography is a noninvasive diagnostic procedure during which ultrasonic waves are directed into the deep structures of the body; their reflections (echoes) are recorded to produce an image of an organ or tissue.

Diagnosticians use ultrasonography on the GI system to identify pathophysiologic processes in the pancreas, liver, gallbladder, spleen, and retroperitoneal tissues. Ultrasound can identify fluid, masses (e.g., tumors), adipose tissue, abscesses, and hematomas. Ultrasound enhances the physical examination because palpable masses and areas of tenderness can be correlated with anatomic structures while the client is on the examining table. Gas in the abdomen may interfere with ultrasound waves.

Preprocedure Care. The client may be required to have nothing by mouth 8 to 12 hours before the procedure to reduce bowel gas. Reassure the client that the test is painless and safe. There are no specific post-procedure precautions or observations related to ultrasound.

Magnetic Resonance Imaging

Procedure. Magnetic resonance imaging (MRI) is a noninvasive test that uses application of an external magnetic field to visualize the soft tissues of the body. MRI can be used in addition to other GI diagnostic tests. MRI is used to study blood flow and to identify tumors, infections, and other abnormal tissue. The test is contraindicated in clients with pacemakers, aneurysm clips, automatic implantable cardiac defibrillators (AICDs), artificial joints, or orthopedic screws.

The client lies on a narrow table that slides into a magnetic body scanner. The client may feel claustrophobic inside of the tube and should be instructed that technicians are readily available in the next room. The client will hear a clanging noise during the procedure.

Preprocedure Care. The client may not receive anything by mouth for 6 hours before the procedure. The client should be instructed that the test requires lying still for the duration of the procedure, which can take from 60 to 90 minutes. All jewelry and metal appurtenances (e.g., glasses, partial dentures) should be removed. There is no post-procedure care.

Radiographic Tests

Flat Plate of the Abdomen

Procedure. A flat plate of the abdomen is an x-ray of the abdominal organs. This test can help to identify abnormalities such as tumors, obstructions, abnormal gas collections, and strictures.

Preprocedure Care. For this procedure, the client should be dressed in a hospital gown without any belts or jewelry. There is no post-procedure care.

Upper Gastrointestinal Series (Barium Swallow)

Procedure. An upper GI series permits radiologic visualization of the esophagus, stomach, duodenum, and jejunum. It can aid in the detection of strictures, ulcers, tumors, polyps, hiatal hernias, and motility problems.

The client drinks a radiopaque contrast medium (barium) while standing in front of a fluoroscopy tube. The client may be asked to assume other positions, such as lying on the x-ray table. This test is usually done after a barium enema or gallbladder radiographic series to prevent the swallowed barium from interfering with the other diagnostic images.

Preprocedure Care. The client is not allowed to have food or fluids for 6 to 8 hours before the test. The nurse should instruct the client about the procedure and about the barium preparation, including its thick consistency and chalky taste. The client is instructed that up to 16 oz of barium may need to be swallowed.

Postprocedure Care. A laxative is usually given to help expel the barium and to prevent a fecal impaction. The nurse should assess the abdomen for distention and bowel sounds. The nurse should also observe the stool to determine whether the barium has been completely eliminated. Initially, the client's stool is white in color, but it should return to its normal brown color within 72 hours. Constipation with a distended abdomen may indicate a barium impaction.

Because this procedure is most commonly done on an outpatient basis, the client should be instructed that the stool may appear white in color for up to 72 hours. If constipation and abdominal distention occur, the client should be instructed to call the physician immediately.

Lower Gastrointestinal Series (Barium Enema)

Procedure. A lower GI series is performed to visualize the position, movements, and filling of the colon. This test can aid in the detection of tumors, diverticuli, stenosis, obstructions, inflammation, ulcerative colitis, and polyps.

During a lower GI series, a radiopaque contrast medium (barium) is instilled via rectal catheter and radiographs are taken, with or without fluoroscopy. Air contrast studies can also be used for more detail. The client will be asked to assume several different positions to promote visualization during the 45- to 60-minute procedure. The procedure is often uncomfortable and can be very tiring, especially for elderly people. Clients often experience mild to severe abdominal cramps and the urge to defecate.

Preprocedure Care. In this procedure, adequate bowel preparation is essential and varies among institutions. Typical preparation for most adults includes placing the client on a low-residue or clear liquid (no milk products) diet for 2 days prior to the test. The client usually receives a potent laxative, such as magnesium citrate, for cleansing the bowel the day before the test. GoLYTELY or Colyte is often used in lieu of magnesium citrate, although this may vary throughout the country. The client receives nothing by mouth after midnight. The morning of the examination, a suppository or a cleansing enema may be administered. Ultrasound, abdominal scan, or colonoscopy, if indicated, should be performed first, because the barium interferes with these tests.

Postprocedure Care. A laxative or cleansing enema is often given after the test to empty the large bowel and to prevent barium impaction. The client is instructed that stools may be white for 24 to 72 hours following the examination and to increase the intake of liquids to prevent a fecal impaction. Any pain, bloating, absence of stool, or bleeding, should be reported to the physician.

Computed Tomography

Procedure. Tomography uses a beam of radiation to measure density differences in tissue. The data are processed by a computer and are reconstructed as cross-sections of the body. Computed tomography (CT) is used mainly to identify masses such as neoplasms, cysts, focal inflammatory lesions, and abscesses of the liver, pancreas, and pelvic areas. CT aids in evaluation of local tumor spread, especially if barium studies suggest the presence of tumor growth beyond the bowel wall (Fig. 59–4). Although CT has the advantage of providing a three-dimensional image, other diagnostic procedures are more valuable for most disorders of the gut. To distinguish normal bowel from abnormal intraperitoneal masses, dilute oral barium or other contrast media may be administered.

A radiation detector is used to visualize three-dimensional images of abdominal structures. This test may require the administration of a contrast material. The client will have to lie still and hold his or her breath when asked. Sedation with anti-anxiety agents may be ordered if the client cannot lie still or becomes claustrophobic. During the procedure, the client is instructed about a "clicking" sound as the scanner moves back and forth.

If contrast medium is used, the client should be taught that he or she may experience warmth, flushing of the face, a salty taste, and nausea. For the client with an allergy to iodine or contrast media, intravenous antihistamines, such as diphenhydramine hydrochloride (Benadryl), and corticosteroids, such as hydrocortisone sodium succinate (Solu-Cortef), should be ordered prior to administration of the contrast medium. Non-iodine contrast medium should be used when the client is allergic to iodine.

Preprocedure Care. The client usually receives nothing by mouth after midnight before the test. The client should be taught about this painless procedure. If contrast is to be used, the client should be asked about an allergy to iodine or shellfish. Non-iodine contrast medium is indicated if the client has an iodine allergy. No follow-up care is needed.

Endoscopy

Endoscopy is the direct visualization of the GI system by means of a lighted, flexible tube. It is more accurate than radiologic examination because the physician can directly observe sources of bleeding and surface lesions and determine the status of healing tissues.

Upper Gastrointestinal Endoscopy

Procedure. Upper GI tract endoscopy includes esophagoscopy, gastroscopy, and esophagogastroduodenoscopy (Fig. 59–5). These procedures are useful for examining clients with acute or chronic GI bleeding, pernicious anemia, esophageal injury, masses, strictures, dysphagia, substernal pain, and epigastric discomfort. Upper GI endoscopy should not be performed on clients with severe cardiovascular disease.

After the client is medicated, a flexible fiberoptic endoscopy tube is passed orally into the esophagus, stomach, pylorus, and duodenum. Some endoscopes are

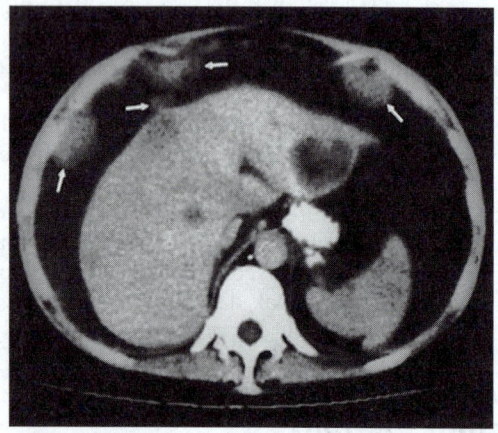

Figure 59–4. CT showing metastatic colon cancer. Scan of the upper abdomen shows ascites, peritoneal implants *(arrows)*, and hepatic metastases. The metastatic lesion in the left lobe of the liver has undergone partial necrosis. Its central necrotic cavity has a low density similar to that of the ascitic fluid. A thick, irregular margin of solid tumor tissue surrounds the cavity. (From Berk, J. E., et al. [1985]. *Bockus' gastroenterology* [4th ed.]. Philadelphia: W. B. Saunders.)

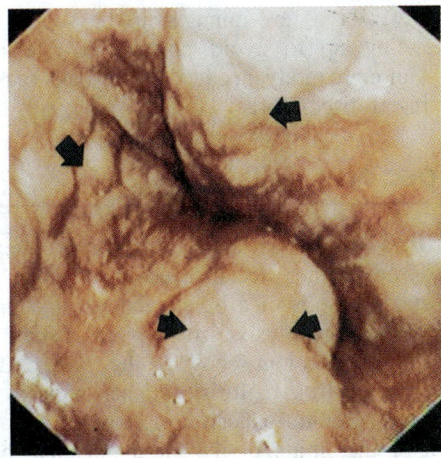

Figure 59–5. Endoscopic view of esophageal varices. Large dilated veins (*arrows*) course longitudinally down the distal esophagus. (From Wyngaarden, J. B., et al. [1996]. *Cecil textbook of medicine* [20th ed.]. Philadelphia: W. B. Saunders.)

equipped with a camera to enable the physician to obtain color photographs. Other endoscopic tubes have equipment for performing a biopsy or for securing cells for cytologic examination if cancer is suspected. Single polyps are sometimes removed via an endoscope.

Preprocedure Care. To prevent aspiration of the stomach contents into the lungs, the client receives nothing by mouth for 8 to 12 hours before the procedure. Outpatient clients may be instructed to take some regularly prescribed oral medications at home at 6:00 A.M. on the day of the procedure. The client may receive an anticholinergic medication to decrease oropharyngeal secretions and to prevent reflex bradycardia. Sedatives, narcotics, or tranquilizers such as diazepam (Valium), midazolam hydrochloride (Versed), or meperidine (Demerol) also may be given before the procedure to help relax the client. Antibiotic prophylaxis is necessary for the client with a history of cardiac valve disease or replacement. The client's dentures and any removable bridges should be taken out prior to the procedure to prevent dislodgement. The client's oral cavity also should be carefully assessed for the presence of infection or any lesions.

A local anesthetic is sprayed on the posterior pharynx to ease the discomfort and to prevent gagging when the tube is inserted. This anesthetic often tastes unpleasant and makes the tongue feel swollen. The client should not swallow saliva after the throat has been anesthetized. Saliva can drain from the side of the mouth when the client is placed in the left lateral decubitus (Sim's) position. The musculature of the tract tends to react with spasms and gagging if premedication is not used.

Endoscopic procedures require a signed consent. Provide complete preprocedure teaching because learning about the endoscopy enhances the client's cooperation. Despite the anesthesia, the client will experience some discomfort, nausea, and/or pressure. The client should be instructed to breathe through the nose and told that he or she will not be able to speak while the tube is in the GI tract. The client should also be told that the room will be dark and seem cool. Tell the client not to drive a motor vehicle for at least 12 hours after the test if sedation was used during the procedure.

Postprocedure Care. Vital signs are checked frequently as per agency protocol. The client is also placed on one side to prevent aspiration while the sedation and local anesthesia wear off. The client receives nothing by mouth until the gag reflex returns (2 to 4 hours). Test for return of the gag reflex by stroking the back of the throat with a tongue blade to see if the client gags. You also can ask the client to swallow and watch the throat for proper movement. Many endoscopic procedures are performed on an outpatient basis. The physician may order anesthetic throat lozenges or normal saline gargles for throat irritation or hoarseness once the gag reflex returns.

Assess the client after an endoscopy for signs of perforation, which include bleeding, fever, and dysphagia. The client with esophageal perforation has crepitus (crackling) in the neck from the leakage. Neck and throat pain, aggravated by swallowing or moving, may also occur. Midesophageal perforation can result in referred substernal or epigastric pain. Also, assess for cyanosis, pleural effusion, and back pain. Distal esophageal perforation may result in shoulder pain, dyspnea, or manifestations similar to those of perforated ulcer. Monitor the client for bradycardia and other arrhythmias secondary to sedatives and local anesthesia.

Lower Gastrointestinal Endoscopy (Colon Endoscopy)

Direct visualization of the bowel through a proctoscope, sigmoidoscope, or colonoscope is called colon endoscopy. This procedure is used when a client has a history of constipation, diarrhea, lower GI bleeding, or a strong family history of rectal or colon cancer. Colonic endoscopy is useful in diagnosing cancer, strictures, polyps, and ulcerative or inflammatory bowel lesions. Colon endoscopy is contraindicated in patients with inflammatory bowel disease, toxic megacolon, or strictures. This procedure sometimes is complicated by rectal bleeding and, rarely, bowel perforation. Antibiotic prophylaxis for all lower GI endoscopies is necessary for clients with cardiac valve disease or artificial valves.

Proctosigmoidoscopy

Procedure. Proctosigmoidoscopy is the endoscopic examination of the distal sigmoid colon, the rectum, and the anal canal. This test helps diagnose malignant and benign neoplasms and detects hemorrhoids, polyps, fissures, fistulas, and abscesses within the anal canal and rectum. Health professionals recommend this procedure for clients over 40 years on an annual or biennial basis, because the examination helps diagnose malignancy at an early stage.

A rigid proctoscope and a sigmoidoscope (rigid or flexible) are used to examine the bowel. Flexible fiberscopes decrease the possibility of perforation and permit examination above the rectosigmoid junction. The procedure involves three separate steps:

1. A digital examination, during which the examiner dilates the anal sphincter to detect an obstruction that might make the rest of the examination difficult.
2. Sigmoidoscopy, during which a 25- to 30-cm (10- to 12-inch) sigmoidoscope is inserted into the anus to visualize the distal sigmoid colon and rectum. A flexible sigmoidoscope also makes it possible to visualize the descending colon. The examiner may obtain specimens from suspicious-looking areas of the colon.
3. Proctoscopy, during which a 7-cm (2-inch) rigid proctoscope is inserted into the anus. This procedure helps the physician visualize the lower rectum and anal canal.

Preprocedure Care. To prepare the client for proctosigmoidoscopy, clearly explain the preparation for the procedure, the position for examination (knee chest or left lateral), and the discomfort that may accompany passage of the scope. For example, because the rectum is sensitive to temperature changes, the examining instrument will feel cool. Explain that the instrument will be advanced slowly.

When the entire colon is to be examined, the client usually

● Receives a clear liquid diet 24 hours before the test
● Takes a cathartic as ordered the night before the procedure
● Receives a cleansing enema the morning of the test to empty the bowel

Institutions employ various preparations for lower GI endoscopies. With one common preparation, the client drinks 1 gallon of Colyte or GoLYTELY at 7:00 P.M. (or earlier) the day before the test. The client may eat a regular lunch and clear liquid dinner before drinking an 8-oz glass of the solution every ten minutes. The solution has a metallic taste and is most palatable when it has been refrigerated. With another common preparation, the client limits the diet to clear liquids for 1 to 2 days before the procedure. On the evening before, the client drinks 1½ oz of Fleet Phospho-Soda, followed by 4 Dulcolax tablets 30 minutes later. The client is instructed to administer a Fleet enema in the morning before the procedure.

If bleeding or severe diarrhea is present, examination may be carried out without bowel preparation. To promote visualization, the client is placed in an inverted position (knee/chest), which allows the sigmoid colon to straighten. A left lateral Sim's position is suitable for clients who are aged, weak, or very ill.

Postprocedure Care. The client is observed for signs of perforation, such as bleeding, pain, and fever. Label and send any specimens obtained during the test to the laboratory immediately. Following the procedure, let the client rest for a few minutes in the supine position before standing up to avoid postural hypotension and fainting. Although rarely needed, a sitz bath may be ordered for rectal discomfort.

Colonoscopy

Procedure. If a client has a history of unexplained constipation or diarrhea, rectal bleeding, or lower abdominal pain, and if results of a barium enema and proctosigmoidoscopy are inconclusive, the physician may perform a colonoscopy. A colonoscopy is the preferred cancer screening method for high-risk clients with a positive family history of colon cancer. Colonoscopy provides visualization of the lining of the large intestine through a flexible endoscope, which is inserted rectally.

Preprocedure Care. For colonoscopy, the client is usually given intravenous (IV) sedation with Valium, Versed, Demerol, or Fentanyl, or a combination of these drugs, and is placed on the left side with the knees flexed. Once the lubricated colonoscope is inserted into the anus, a small amount of air is instilled to help the physician visualize the bowel lumen. When the colonoscope reaches the sigmoid junction, the client may be moved to the supine position, making it easier to advance the colonoscope past the splenic flexure. During the test, encourage the client to relax. Monitor vital signs throughout the procedure, watching for a vasovagal response leading to hypotension and bradycardia.

Postprocedure Care. The nurse monitors vital signs per protocol. The nurse should assess for signs of perforation, such as abdominal pain, bleeding, or fever. Some clients develop nausea before, during, or after the procedure, which may be treated with IV anti-emetics.

Exfoliative Cytologic Analysis

Procedure. Exfoliative cytologic analysis, developed by George Papanicolaou, is the study of cells that have sloughed off from a tissue. This procedure is used to distinguish between benign and malignant lesions. Malignant cells, which exfoliate more readily than normal cells, are collected by lavage and sent to the laboratory for analysis. Cells of the esophagus, stomach, small intestine, and colon can be examined. The contents of the stomach are examined for the presence of *Helicobacter pylori* bacteria, which can cause gastritis and peptic ulcer disease.

In this procedure, cells can be obtained from saline lavage through a nasogastric tube or from specimens obtained directly through an endoscopic procedure.

Preprocedure Care. A written consent is obtained. The client is placed on a liquid diet. For colon studies, laxatives and enemas are administered. The nurse should explain the procedure to the client.

Postprocedure Care. The client is allowed to rest and resume an appropriate diet. Follow-up care includes routine protocol per procedure used.

Gastric Analysis

Procedure. Gastric analysis is performed to measure secretions of hydrochloric acid and pepsin in the stomach. It can aid in the diagnosis of duodenal ulcer, Zollinger-Ellison syndrome, gastric carcinoma, and pernicious anemia. Two tests are performed in gastric analysis: (1) the basal cell secretion test and (2) the gastric acid stimulation test.

The client's nasogastric tube is attached to suction, and stomach contents are collected every 15 minutes for 1 hour. The nurse must properly label the specimens with the time and volume. If the basal secretion test suggests abnormal gastric secretion, a gastric acid stimulation test is usually performed immediately.

The gastric acid stimulation test measures the amount of gastric acid for 1 hour after subcutaneous injection of a drug that stimulates gastric acid secretion (e.g., pentagastrin, betazole). If results are abnormal, radiographic studies or endoscopy are usually performed to determine the cause.

A markedly increased level of gastric secretion may indicate Zollinger-Ellison syndrome, whereas moderately increased levels indicate a duodenal ulcer. Decreased levels of gastric secretion could indicate gastric ulcer or carcinoma.

Preprocedure Care. The client receives nothing by mouth for 12 hours before the test. A client who requires a coronary vasodilator may have an oral prescription temporarily changed to an ointment or sublingual preparation. A nasogastric tube is inserted, and any contents left in the stomach are removed. The client should avoid taking drugs that interfere with gastric acid levels (e.g., cholinergics, antacids).

Postprocedure Care. If the nasogastric tube is left in place, it should be clamped or attached to low intermittent suction if ordered. Drainage amount and color should be recorded.

Acid Perfusion Test (Bernstein Test)

Procedure. This test is performed to determine whether or not a client's chest pain is related to acid perfusion of the esophageal mucosa.

A nasogastric tube is inserted, and gastric contents are aspirated. Alternatively, 0.9% NaCl (normal saline) and 0.1% HCl are instilled into the lower esophagus. If the client does not experience pain, the test is considered negative. If pain occurs, 0.9% NaCl is administered until the pain ceases. To ensure that the pain is caused by acid perfusion, the 0.1% HCl is readministered. After the test, the nasogastric tube is withdrawn.

Preprocedure Care. The client should receive nothing by mouth the night before the test. The nurse should prepare the client for insertion of a nasogastric tube.

Postprocedure Care. After the procedure, the client may receive an antacid.

Conclusions

Once the nurse has a thorough knowledge of the structure and function of the GI system, the nurse must understand the diagnostic assessment of these organs. Systematic assessment of the client with possible disorders of the GI system can lead to prompt diagnosis and treatment. The nurse can facilitate this diagnostic process by adequately preparing the client for the diagnostic procedures and by assisting with or actually collecting assessment data.

Bibliography

1. American Cancer Society. (1996). *Cancer facts & figures*. Atlanta: Author.
2. Barkauskas, V., Stoltenberg-Allen, K., & Darling-Baumann, C. (1994). *Health and physical assessment*. St. Louis: Mosby–Year Book.
3. Chernecky, C., Krech, R., & Berger, B. (1993). *Laboratory tests and diagnostic procedures*. Philadelphia: W. B. Saunders.
4. Copstead, L. (1995). *Perspectives on pathophysiology*. Philadelphia: W. B. Saunders.
5. Dettenmeier, P. (1994). *X-ray assessment for nurses*. St. Louis: Mosby–Year Book.
6. Giger, J., & Davidhizar, R. (1995). *Transcultural nursing: Assessment and interventions* (2nd ed.). St. Louis: Mosby–Year Book.
7. Griffith, C. (1993). Colorectal cancer: Reducing mortality through early detection and treatment. *Physician Assistant, 17*, 25–34.
8. Guyton, A. C., & Hall, J. E. (1996). *Textbook of medical physiology* (9th ed.). Philadelphia: W. B. Saunders.
9. Heitkemper, M., et al. (1993). Women with gastrointestinal symptoms: Implications for nursing research. *Gastroenterology Nursing, 15*, 226–232.
10. Jarvis, C. (1995). *Physical examination and health assessment* (2nd ed.). Philadelphia: W. B. Saunders.
11. Kee, J. (1995). *Laboratory and diagnostic tests with nursing implications* (4th ed.). Norwalk, CT: Appleton & Lange.
12. Lang, C., & Ransohoff, D. (1994). Fecal occult blood screening for colorectal cancer. *JAMA, 271*(13), 1011–1013.
13. Laws, A. (1993). Does a history of sexual abuse in childhood play a role in women's medical problems? *Journal of Women's Health, 2*, 165–172.
14. Lehne, R. (1994). *Pharmacology for nursing care* (2nd ed.). Philadelphia: W. B. Saunders.
15. Mandel, J., et al. (1993). Reducing mortality from colorectal cancer by screening for fecal occult blood. *New England Journal of Medicine, 328*(19), 1365–1371.
16. Mayer, D. (1994). Commentary on social support and cancer screening among older black Americans. *Nursing Scan in Oncology, 3*(2), 10–11.
17. Mehler, E. (1994). Preparing your patient to use a fecal occult blood test. *Nursing, 24*(5), 32R.
18. Neugut, A. (1993). Colon cancer screening: Beyond reliance on fecal testing. *Consultant, 33*(10), 39–46.

19. Pagana, K., & Pagana, T. (1993). *Diagnostic testing and nursing implications: A case study approach* (4th ed.). St. Louis: Mosby–Year Book.

20. Pieper, B. (1992). A study of persons undergoing outpatient gastrointestinal radiography. *Journal of Enterostomal Therapy, 19,* 54–58.

21. Renkers, J. (1993). GI endoscopy: Managing the full scope of care. *Nursing, 23*(6), 50–55.

22. Sabiston, D. C., Jr. (Ed.). (1994). *Atlas of general surgery.* Philadelphia: W. B. Saunders.

23. Sabiston, D. C., Jr., & Lyerly, H. K. (Eds.). (1994). *Sabiston essentials of surgery* (2nd ed.). Philadelphia: W. B. Saunders.

24. Whitney, L. (1993). Acute abdominal pain: Revealing the source. *Nursing, 23*(9), 34–40.

25. Wyngaarden, J. B., & Smith, L. H. (Eds.). (1996). *Cecil textbook of medicine* (20th ed.). Philadelphia: W. B. Saunders.

Nursing Care of Clients with Ingestive Disorders

Jane Hokanson Hawks

The client with an ingestive disorder, regardless of the cause, may have a problem in the oral cavity or esophagus that leads to the identification of common nursing diagnoses such as *Altered Oral Mucous Membrane; Pain; Altered Nutrition: Less than Body Requirements; Impaired Verbal Communication;* or *Impaired Swallowing.* Usually the client will first experience pain in the mouth or esophagus or difficulty with swallowing. Shortly thereafter, oral communication and nutritional intake may be compromised. These complications may also result in the development of personal and family coping problems, as well as a lack of knowledge related to the treatment required for the disorder.

Dental Disorders

A person must have healthy teeth and gums for good general health. Health-care professionals (nurses, dental hygienists, dentists, dental physicians) strive to preserve healthy gums and natural teeth for as long as possible for these reasons:

- A person's natural teeth are almost always more functional in masticating food than a dental prosthesis.
- Effective mastication of food helps promote efficient digestion.
- Efficient digestion of food results in healthy gastrointestinal function and good general health.

The most frequent sources of tooth loss are dental decay and periodontal disease. Plaque is the major cause of both caries (decay) and periodontal disease.

Dental Plaque

Dental plaque is a soft mass of proliferating bacteria with a scattering of leukocytes, macrophages, and epithelial cells in a sticky polysaccharide-protein matrix that ad-

heres to the teeth. Food, especially carbohydrate, contributes to plaque formation. Bacterial enzymes liquefy food debris after a meal and use some of the carbohydrates, along with saliva, to form plaque. The sticky organic film begins to collect on the teeth within hours of eating or brushing. Plaque is transparent and colorless and escapes detection unless it (1) absorbs pigment from within the oral cavity or (2) is stained in the dental office by a disclosing solution. It can be removed only by mechanical cleaning.

Dental Caries

Development of dental caries (tooth decay) involves an erosive process that can cause progressive demineralization and destruction of the outer enamel of the tooth. If the condition is not treated, eventual damage to the pulp can occur. An estimated 90% to 99% of the U.S. population have experienced dental disorders.

Etiology and Risk Factors

Dental decay has many causes. Basically, decay depends on the following:

1. The resistance of the tooth enamel
2. The nature of the plaque (including its bacterial population)
3. The diet

Of these factors, dental plaque is probably the most important. The Risk Factors and Levels of Prevention feature lists other causes of dental caries.

Pathophysiology

Many dentists accept the theory that dental decay occurs when the acids produced by bacteria in the plaque begin to decalcify the inorganic tooth enamel when the pH is 5.6 or below. For decay to progress, both acid-producing cariogenic bacteria and carbohydrates must be present in

This chapter incorporates material written for the fourth edition by Shirley M. Ruder.

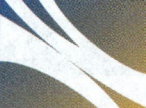

RISK FACTORS AND LEVELS OF PREVENTION

Dental Caries and Periodontal Disease

Risk Factors

Poor oral hygiene; lack of daily brushing and flossing; lack of regular dental visits; between-meals snacking

Levels of Prevention

Primary Prevention

- Encourage clients to brush and floss at least daily.
- Advise clients to maintain a healthy diet.
- Advise clients to drink fluoridated water.
- Encourage clients to limit between-meals snacking on high carbohydrate foods.

Secondary Prevention

- Teach clients with dental decay about the importance of daily brushing, flossing, and fluoride rinsing.
- Encourage clients to schedule dental visits every 6 months for regular cleaning and fluoride treatments.
- Recommend that children and adults have fluoride treatments.

Tertiary Prevention

- Encourage clients to schedule dental visits for regular cleaning and fluoride treatments, and for fillings, extractions, root canals, crowns, bridges, or dentures, as needed.
- Teach clients how to care for bridges and dentures.

the mouth. Any carbohydrate in the mouth will stimulate bacterial acid production, but sucrose stimulates the most acid. The longer carbohydrates remain in the mouth after ingestion, the longer it takes for the pH to return to normal levels. Therefore, increased frequency of food ingestion (particularly sticky substances such as caramels or honey) causes the acid level in the mouth to become elevated for longer periods of time, increasing the risk of cavity production.

Clinical Manifestations and Diagnostic Findings

The major manifestation of dental caries is pain in the affected tooth, especially when the tooth comes in contact with heat, cold, or certain foods. There may be no apparent manifestations. The dentist diagnoses caries through direct examination of the teeth and through x-ray studies.

Community and Self-Care

■ Medical Management

The best treatment for dental caries is prevention. Encourage clients in your care to brush and floss regularly, eat a diet low in simple carbohydrates, use fluoride, and schedule regular visits to the dentist for examination, cleaning, and treatment of dental caries.

Increasing the resistance of the enamel also helps prevent caries. The resistance of the enamel increases with the ingestion of fluoridated water during tooth formation and the continued use of fluoride throughout life. The daily use of fluoride rinses produces a more acid-resistant structure, enhances tooth mineralization, and interferes with bacterial growth. In addition, the dentist may apply topical fluoride to the teeth, especially in children.

■ Surgical Management

Treatment of dental caries may include the following:

1. Drilling out cavities and filling them with material to restore the tooth
2. Removal of the entire tooth (extraction) if the cavity cannot be filled
3. Preservation of the tooth by a root canal therapy (pulpectomy), followed by proper restoration

Any number of teeth can be removed because of disease. Teeth are usually replaced with some type of dental prosthesis (crowns, dentures, dental implants). If only one tooth or a few teeth are being removed, the procedure is usually performed with local anesthesia. Removing several teeth or having a full-mouth extraction may require sedation or general anesthesia. Potential complications include hemorrhage and abscess formation.

In root canal therapy, the entire pulp of the tooth is removed. The canal space within the roots is filled aseptically and sealed to prevent infection. Subsequent restoration of the tooth is essential to retain the tooth in a normal functional relation with the rest of the dentition. The tooth remains rooted in the gingiva and can still be used.

Periodontal Disease

Periodontal disease is defined as a spectrum of disorders of the gums ranging from gingivitis, in its least destructive form, to periodontitis, in its worst form. This is a very common problem and probably affects more than 90% of the population to some degree.

Etiology and Risk Factors

Plaque accumulating on the teeth is the major cause of both caries and periodontal disease. Once plaque has hardened to form calculus, it can be removed only by dental professionals with specialized instruments. The

Risk Factors and Levels of Prevention feature lists other causes of periodontal disease.

Pathophysiology

Plaque formation and subsequent bacterial colonization result in gingival inflammation (gingivitis) if the plaque is not removed by proper brushing and flossing. Pockets of inflammation form (Fig. 60–1) and gradually deepen. Eventually, inflammation causes destruction of the underlying tissues and separation of the gingiva from the tooth. In periodontitis, the inflammation extends from the gums into the alveolar bone and periodontal ligament, destroying the supporting structures of the teeth (Fig. 60–2). As a result, the teeth loosen and may require extraction.

Clinical Manifestations and Diagnostic Findings

The early form of periodontal disease is gingivitis. The late form of the disease is periodontitis or pyorrhea. Gingivitis is associated with gums that bleed from even minor trauma. Assessment usually reveals some alterations in the color of the gingiva, possibly swelling and ulceration, but rarely pain. In the late form of the disease, the dentist measures damage to the gums by determining the depth of gum recession.

Community and Self-Care

Most dental procedures are completed in an outpatient setting. To prepare the client for self-care at home, provide oral and written instructions on dental hygiene, manifestations of complications, how and when to notify healthcare personnel if complications arise, and instructions on a balanced diet. If the client has new dentures,

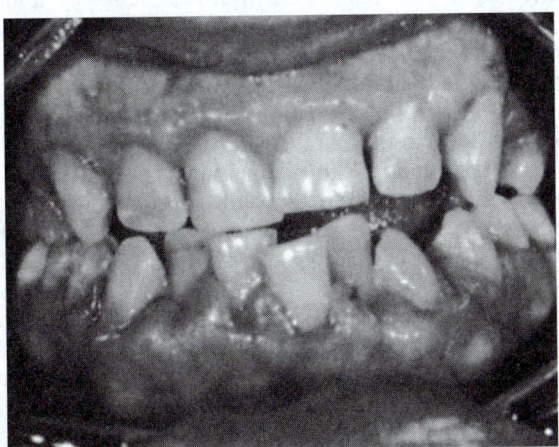

Figure 60–1. Gingivitis with erythema and inflammatory enlargement of the gingiva. (From Shklar, G. [1984]. The oral cavity, jaws, and salivary glands. In S. L. Robbins, et al. [Eds.], *Pathologic basis of disease* [3rd ed., p. 773]. Philadelphia: W. B. Saunders.)

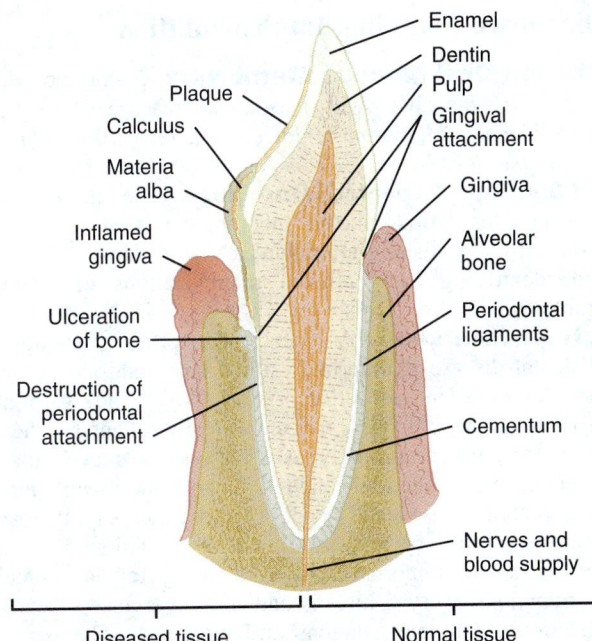

Figure 60–2. Periodontal disease. Normal tissues are shown on the right side, and tissues affected by periodontal disease are shown on the left side. Note the destruction of the alveolar bone and the periodontal fibers that normally hold the tooth in place.

the client should be able to demonstrate proper care of them.

■ Medical Management

Prevention is the most effective method of controlling periodontal disease. Plaque removal remains the best defense against gingivitis and, thus, periodontal disease. Simply rinsing the mouth does not remove plaque, because plaque cannot be removed without friction. Friction dislodges both plaque and other debris. Plaque can be decreased by thorough cleaning, cleaning after each meal, and cutting down on between-meal snacks, especially sticky, adherent foods. Good oral hygiene is based on toothbrushing, the use of dental floss, interdental cleaners, and water irrigation.

■ Nursing Management of the Medical Client

Assessment

Obtain a dental history from the client regarding dental problems, dental visits, and the client's current pattern of dental hygiene. Note the client's nutritional status, including eating habits and ability to chew, as well as the presence of dentures or dental appliances.

When examining the oral cavity, wear nonsterile gloves and use a tongue blade and flashlight. During inspection, note the general condition of the teeth and gingiva. Inspect for plaque buildup on the teeth and note any missing teeth or dental caries. The gingiva should be shiny, smooth, and a graduated red color. Note any edema or areas of tenderness.

Diagnosis, Planning, Implementation

Altered Oral Mucous Membrane. A common diagnosis for the client with periodontal disease is *Altered Oral Mucous Membrane related to dental disease and plaque buildup.*

Planning: Expected Outcomes. The client will prevent altered oral mucous membrane related to dental disease by establishing a regular pattern of dental hygiene and identifying early clinical manifestations of dental problems.

Implementation. As mentioned earlier, prevention of dental disease is of primary importance and should be the aim of client education. Assess the client's current dental hygiene practices, making sure the client brushes, rinses, and flosses properly. Also assess the client's diet, especially for refined and hidden sugars. The use of fluoride, both in rinses and added to the water supply, can also be helpful, barring any medical restrictions. Teach the client the importance of undergoing regular dental examinations every 6 months and the importance of early detection of minor irritations and infections. The dental hygienist may complete this teaching in outpatient settings.

Evaluation

The client's dental health should improve gradually with treatment and follow-up care.

■ Surgical Management

Surgical treatment of periodontal disease may include tooth extraction or root canal therapy as described under surgical management of dental caries.

■ Nursing Management of the Surgical Client

Assessment

Assessment of the client undergoing surgical management of periodontal disease is the same as that for the client undergoing medical management. Additionally, routine preoperative and postoperative assessments are necessary.

Diagnosis, Planning, Implementation

Hemorrhage. A common collaborative problem to address in the care of the surgical client is *Hemorrhage related to oral surgical procedure.*

Planning: Expected Outcomes. Hemorrhage will be prevented or detected and treated early after oral surgery, as evidenced by absence of bleeding.

Implementation. Postoperative care of a tooth extraction includes assessing the oral cavity for bleeding and monitoring vital signs (if the client stays in an inpatient facility or recovery area). A gauze pad is usually placed over the extraction site, and the client is instructed to bite down gently on the pad to maintain pressure. Ice also may be applied to the jaw over the site to decrease the blood flow and edema. Small amounts of bleeding

may be normal, but you should notify the dentist or physician or instruct the client to notify the dentist or physician if bleeding occurs for longer than 1 hour (see management of postextraction hemorrhage under Dental Emergencies).

The client usually requires analgesics to control pain. Instruct the client to eat soft foods and avoid hot or cold foods for several days. The client also should gently rinse the mouth with normal saline, but should avoid brushing any remaining teeth for 1 day.

Evaluation

The problem should resolve within a few days after the extraction. If the client continues to have pain or other problems, the client should return to the dentist for further evaluation.

■ Modifications for Elderly Clients

The elderly client may experience normal changes in the oral cavity as a result of aging. The oral mucosa is more susceptible to injury because of atrophy of the mucosa and a decrease in salivation. The teeth of the elderly are more prone to caries, and many clients have lost some or all of their teeth. There also may be a decrease in oral motor functions (chewing and swallowing). There is often an inability to perform normal hygiene practices resulting from a decrease in manual dexterity and strength.

The goal of dental care in the elderly is to retain permanent teeth as long as possible. Tooth loss is not a normal part of aging and is usually the result of periodontal disease or dental caries.

Dental Emergencies

A client who fractures a tooth must see a dentist immediately. Entry of bacteria into the canal of the tooth and the resulting infection may cause a dental abscess. An avulsed tooth is a tooth torn from the mouth by trauma. If it is found, reimplantation of the tooth should be attempted as soon as possible. It should be placed in a cool normal saline solution and reimplanted by the dentist or oral surgeon after the wound has been irrigated. Once the tooth has been reimplanted, wires or splints are used to stabilize it in place. Root canal therapy is required in cases of avulsion. Teeth that are embedded in the gum should be left alone but followed by a dentist. They usually return to normal position within 1 month.

Emergencies such as deep lacerations of the gums and fractures of the jaw must be treated by an oral surgeon. These lacerations bleed freely, because of the mouth's excellent blood supply. Application of local pressure to the site provides the best first-aid intervention. In any wound of this nature, prevent aspiration by carefully removing debris from the mouth. Either gently irrigate the mouth or allow the client to rinse the mouth.

Postextraction hemorrhage can be (1) primary, occurring within an hour or two of the extraction and usually caused by dislodging of the clot, or (2) secondary, probably caused by infection in the socket or a loose clot. Application of local pressure provides emergency intervention for both types of hemorrhage. Additional treatments include (1) applying a sterile gauze pad over the extraction site and (2) asking the client to bite down on the gauze to produce hemostasis. Sometimes biting down on a moistened tea bag is a successful home remedy. The pressure helps stop bleeding and the tannic acid in the tea helps promote hemostasis. If bleeding continues, instruct the client to contact or return to the dentist.

Oral Disorders

Stomatitis

Stomatitis is an inflammation of the oral cavity. It may be of infectious origin or a manifestation of a systemic condition. It may be caused by mechanical trauma such as injury or chemical trauma such as chemotherapy for cancer treatment. Jagged teeth, cheek-biting, and mouth-breathing may result in mechanical trauma. Certain foods and drinks and sensitivity to mouthwashes or dentrifrices may produce chemical trauma.

The inflammatory sloughing of tissue allows organisms to multiply; thus, stomatitis may lead to infection by viruses, bacteria, yeasts, or fungus.

Stomatitis is classified as primary or secondary depending on the cause. Primary stomatitis includes aphthous stomatitis (canker sore), herpes simplex, and Vincent's angina. Secondary stomatitis is caused when the client's resistance is lowered and an opportunistic infection results. Secondary stomatitis can be caused by a local or systemic disorder. Systemic disorders that can affect the oral mucous membranes include the following:

- Allergies
- Bone marrow disorders
- Nutritional disorders
- Disorders resulting from immunodeficiency or chemotherapy, radiation therapy, or immunosuppressive therapy

Aphthous Stomatitis (Canker Sores)

Canker sores are recurrent, small, ulcerated lesions of the soft tissues of the mouth, including the lips, tongue, and the inside of the cheeks. Canker sores can appear in all age groups, although young adult women are more frequently affected.

Etiology and Risk Factors

Although the cause of canker sores is unknown, possible causes include emotional stress, trauma, vitamin deficiency, food and drug allergies, endocrine imbalances, and viral infections. Prevention is almost impossible because the exact cause is unknown.

Pathophysiology

These lesions start as small, reddened areas that undergo central necrosis and ulceration. The lesions are not infective but are simply inflammatory, and they heal within 1 to 3 weeks without treatment.

Clinical Manifestations and Diagnostic Findings

Assessment usually reveals a well-circumscribed erythematous macule that undergoes necrosis (Fig. 60-3). Necrosis results in a well-defined pseudomembranous ulcer with an erythematous border. Lesions, although acutely painful, are not contagious and heal spontaneously within 1 to 3 weeks.

Management

Medical treatment with topical or systemic steroids may shorten the healing time. In addition, to suppress the recurrence of sores, suggest to clients prone to allergic reactions that they avoid tomatoes, chocolate, eggs, shell-

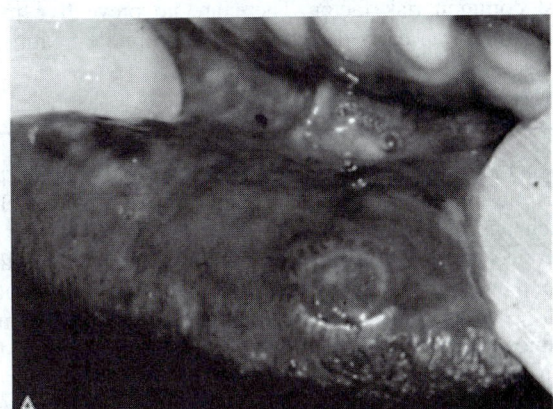
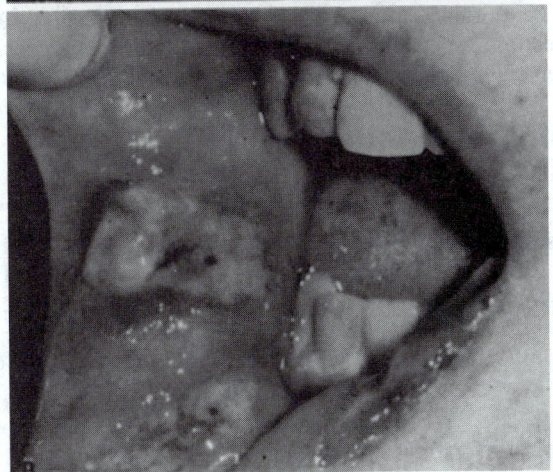

Figure 60-3. Aphthous stomatitis. *A*, A discrete round ulcer. *B*, Large necrotic lesions. (From Shklar, G. [1984]. The oral cavity, jaws, and salivary glands. In S. L. Robbins, et al. [Eds.], *Pathologic basis of disease* [3rd ed., p. 778]. Philadelphia: W. B. Saunders.)

fish, milk products, nuts, and citrus fruits. Some dentists report that the routine administration of systemic steroids may also prevent recurrence.

Herpes Simplex

Herpes simplex is a form of inflammation and ulceration caused by a viral infection. By the age of 5 years, 90% of the population has had an infection, usually asymptomatic, of primary herpes simplex. Secondary herpes is often seen in clients receiving immunosuppressants and in those with human immunodeficiency virus (HIV), or acquired immunodeficiency syndrome (AIDS).

Etiology and Risk Factors

Stomatitis caused by the *herpes simplex virus* (HSV) can occur as a primary or secondary infection. Primary HSV infection occurs as a result of the initial exposure to the virus and is often asymptomatic. Secondary HSV infection takes the form of *herpes labialis* (fever blister, cold sore). The current theory is that respiratory infections, sunlight, a fever, or emotional stress can reactivate the virus. Clients vary greatly in their susceptibility to secondary herpes simplex, but immunosuppression is the most common risk factor. There are no preventive measures other than early detection and appropriate treatment.

Pathophysiology

When the client is first infected with the primary herpes virus, lesions appear in the oral cavity. These vesicles, which appear throughout the oral cavity, rupture to form ulcerated areas that resemble canker sores and heal within several weeks. The client's tongue appears heavily coated with a characteristic white coating. The infection may produce manifestations of generalized infection in the client.

Secondary herpes is a recurrent infection that appears to lie dormant after the primary herpes infection. Any infection, especially upper respiratory infections, fever, or even sunlight can reactivate the virus.

Clinical Manifestations and Diagnostic Findings

Assessment reveals clear, vesicular lesions, most often appearing at the mucocutaneous junction of the lips (Fig. 60–4) and face. The lesions are contagious, last about 1 week, and heal without scarring. Later in the course of the infection, the tongue may appear coated, and the client may complain of a foul breath odor.

Management

General pain may be treated with analgesics. Unless the ulcer is secondarily infected, antimicrobial treatment does not affect the progress of the ulcer. Local ointments and anesthetics may soothe lesions. Clients who are immuno-

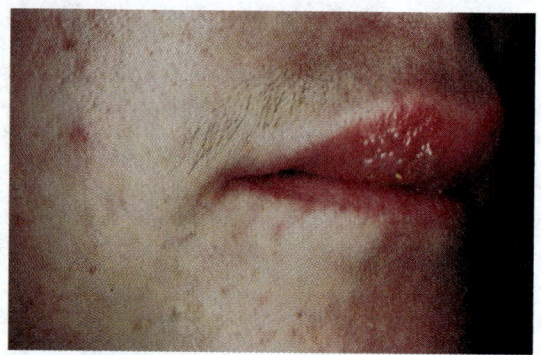

Figure 60–4. Herpes simplex of the lip. (From Hurwitz, S. [1993]. *Clinical pediatric dermatology* [2nd ed., p. 321]. Philadelphia: W. B. Saunders.)

compromised are started on intravenous acyclovir (Zovirax). Clients with competent immune systems also may be given acyclovir but in oral or topical forms.

Vincent's Angina (Necrotizing Ulcerative Gingivitis, Trench Mouth)

Vincent's angina is an acute bacterial infection of the gingiva. The incidence of Vincent's angina increases with age. This is probably related to the increased susceptibility to infections and changes in the oral cavity that occur with aging.

Etiology and Risk Factors

This acute inflammatory gum disease is caused by resident flora in the mouth, fusiform bacteria, and spirochetes. Precipitating factors include poor oral hygiene, nutritional deficiencies, lack of rest and sleep, local tissue damage, and debilitative diseases such as infectious mononucleosis, nonspecific viral infections, bacterial infections, blood dyscrasias, and diabetes mellitus. This condition is not contagious. Most of these factors are unavoidable and therefore unpreventable.

Pathophysiology

When systemic disease lowers one's resistance, susceptibility to one's own flora increases. The disease has a sudden onset and causes erythema and ulceration of the gingiva. The disease affects the entire oropharynx. Once the tonsils are removed, this disorder rarely recurs.

Clinical Manifestations and Diagnostic Findings

Assessment reveals ulcers covered with a pseudomembrane. A smear from an ulcer exudate identifies the causative organisms. Clients with Vincent's angina often have an elevated white blood cell (WBC) count. The client may complain of a foul taste, pain, a choking sensation, fever, thick secretions, anorexia, and occasionally, lymphadenopathy.

Management

Medical management consists of removing the devitalized tissue and correcting the underlying cause with rest, improved oral hygiene, a bland diet, and vitamins. Pain medications and saline, peroxide, or half-saline, half-peroxide mouthwashes promote comfort. The Nursing Research feature describes the effects of hydrogen peroxide rinses on the normal oral mucosa.

Candidiasis (Moniliasis)

Candidiasis (thrush) is caused by the organism *Candida albicans,* a yeastlike fungus, which is part of the normal flora of the oral cavity. Candidiasis of the oral cavity is commonly seen in clients who are immunosuppressed, such as those receiving chemotherapy or clients with HIV infection or AIDS. There is also a higher incidence in clients with diabetes mellitus and those who are pregnant; under stress; on high doses of, or prolonged, antibiotic therapy; or on prolonged periods of tube feeding.

Etiology and Risk Factors

When the client becomes immunosuppressed or has a decrease in some of the normal oral flora, an overgrowth of the normal flora *Candida* can occur. Critically ill clients with prolonged intubation often develop candidiasis. The major risk factors are immunosuppression and prolonged use of antibiotics that disrupts the normal flora. Clients with either risk factor should be monitored

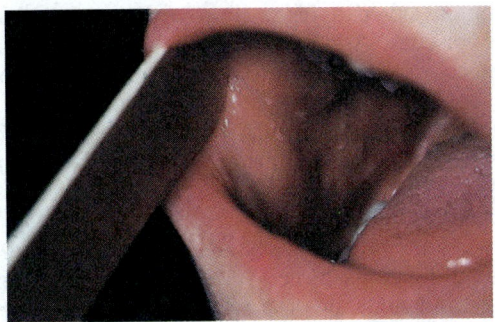

Figure 60–5. Oral candidiasis. Note the small white patches on the buccal mucosa. (From Moschella, S. L., & Hurley, H. J. [1992]. *Dermatology* [3rd ed., p. 231]. Philadelphia: W. B. Saunders.)

closely, and often prophylactic treatment is started for these high-risk clients.

Pathophysiology

Candidiasis is a secondary infection resulting from either an immunodeficiency or prolonged use of antibiotics. When the normal flora is disrupted, an overgrowth of the *Candida* organism may occur.

Clinical Manifestations and Diagnostic Findings

Assessment reveals white patches on the tongue, palate, and buccal mucosa (Fig. 60–5). These lesions adhere firmly to the tissues and are difficult to remove. The lesions are often referred to as milk curds because of their appearance. Clients often describe the lesions as dry and hot. Clients who have recurrent candidiasis infections should be examined for a possible systemic cause.

 ## Community and Self-Care

■ Medical Management

Medical management includes topical antifungal agents as well as other topical agents to alleviate the infection and provide pain relief. Analgesic medications, such as acetaminophen or aspirin, may also be administered to promote pain relief. Mouthwashes of half warm water or saline and half hydrogen peroxide are often ordered as part of an oral hygiene regimen. A bland, liquid, or puréed diet may be necessary. Prophylactic use of antifungal agents is indicated for high-risk clients.

■ Nursing Management of the Medical Client

Assessment

Clients with either risk factor should be monitored closely. Assess whether the client has pain, tenderness, or

---

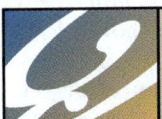

NURSING RESEARCH

Should Hydrogen Peroxide Rinses Be Used for Oral Care?

Tombes, M., & Gallucci, B. (1993). The effects of hydrogen peroxide rinses on the normal oral mucosa. *Nursing Research, 42* (6), 332–337.

This study examined the effects on the oral mucosa of hydrogen peroxide (quarter-strength and half-strength) mouth rinses in 35 randomly assigned volunteers. These rinses were associated with mucosal abnormalities and overwhelmingly negative subject reactions. However, subjects using the normal saline rinses had no significant changes.

Implications for Practice

These researchers do not recommend the use of hydrogen peroxide rinses for oral care. Rather, they recommend the use of normal saline rinses.

bleeding in any part of the oral cavity or has had any febrile episodes. Ask the client about a history of previous infection elsewhere in the body and the use of any medications such as antibiotics. Also ask the client about a history of treatment with radiation or chemotherapy, because both can affect the oral mucosa. Many times, prophylactic treatment for these high-risk clients may have been instituted.

To perform the oral assessment, have a tongue blade and good lighting. Inspect the oral cavity noting any areas of inflammation and whether vesicular eruptions, ulcers, white patches, or erythematous gingivae exist. The client should be examined by a dentist to rule out infection of dental origin.

Diagnosis, Planning, Implementation

Pain. A common nursing diagnosis for the client with candidiasis is *Pain related to altered oral mucous membrane and ulcerations.*

Planning: Expected Outcomes. The client's pain will be relieved or will be controlled as evidenced by the client expressing pain relief and demonstrating the ability to maintain normal nutrition.

Implementation. Assess for oral pain and administer analgesics, such as aspirin or acetaminophen, as ordered. Topical agents and topical mouth rinses often provide pain relief. Antifungal agents to rinse with and swallow are used to alleviate the infection. A change in diet to liquid or puréed foods often eases the discomfort of eating. The client should avoid spicy foods, citrus juice, and hot liquids.

Clients with painful lesions cannot tolerate commercial mouthwashes because of the high alcohol concentration in these products. A solution of warm water, half-strength hydrogen peroxide, or mouthwash formulas specific to many institutions are better tolerated and may promote healing.

The client should be given oral and written instructions regarding a dental hygiene regimen, diet, medications, and manifestations of complications. The client should demonstrate proper techniques of dental hygiene. Minimal home healthcare preparation is required unless the client requires alternative feeding routes. If the client is receiving tube feedings, referral to a home healthcare agency may be appropriate. If home care is not affordable, the client or significant other will need to be taught how to perform the tube feedings (discussed in Chapters 60 and 61). The client should be followed by a physician, a dentist, or a nurse to assess for recurrence.

Risk for Infection. The oral mucous membrane is impaired, so the nursing diagnosis of *Risk for Infection related to altered oral mucous membrane, ulcerations, and decreased resistance* is common in these clients.

Planning: Expected Outcomes. Infection will not develop or will be controlled, as evidenced by healing of lesions, absence of fever or elevated WBC count, and no evidence of secondary infection.

Implementation. If painful oral lesions are present, you may suggest modifications in the client's oral hy-

giene regimen. Gauze pads may replace toothbrushes, and oral rinses may be needed to clean the area of debris and promote healing. Oral pharyngeal cultures should be taken if infection is suspected. Antibiotics and antifungal agents may be used when positive cultures are found. Antifungal agents are frequently given as oral liquids to rinse and swallow.

Evaluation

The infection should clear up within a few days to a week in most clients. Assess the client for other risk factors if reinfection occurs.

Tumors of the Oral Cavity

Benign Tumors of the Oral Cavity

The most common benign tumors of the mouth are fibromas, lipomas, neurofibromas, and hemangiomas. As with benign tumors in other parts of the body, oral tumors cause problems primarily by occupying space and causing pressure. Benign tumors are usually excised if they cause functional or cosmetic problems.

Premalignant Tumors of the Oral Cavity

Leukoplakia. Leukoplakia is a potentially precancerous, yellow-white or gray-white lesion. It may occur in any region of the mouth. The size and shape of lesions vary, but they are usually elevated with a roughened or leathery surface and have clearly defined borders (Fig. 60–6). Leukoplakia is a common disorder of the oral mucous membranes, usually seen in persons in their 40s. Men are affected twice as often as women; however, the incidence is women is increasing.

Leukoplakia results from chronic irritation of the mucosa by physical, thermal, or chemical factors. Physical factors include poorly fitting dentures, broken teeth, cheek nibbling, and occlusion problems. Thermal and chemical

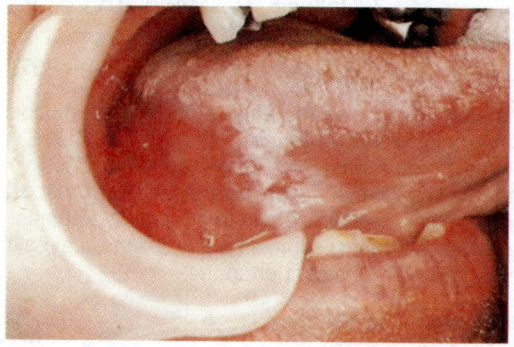

Figure 60–6. Leukoplakia of the lateral edge of the tongue. (From Sleisenger, M. H., & Fordtran, J. S. [1989]. *Gastrointestinal disease: Pathophysiology/diagnosis/management* [4th ed.]. Philadelphia: W. B. Saunders.)

factors arise from use of tobacco products, both inhaled and chewing products. Ingestion of excessively hot food and beverages also places the person at risk. It may also develop from systemic factors such as poor nutrition or syphilis.

Erythroplakia. Erythroplakia is a red, velvety-appearing patch that is often indicative of early squamous cell carcinoma. It occurs most frequently in persons in their 50s and 60s, with men and women equally affected. Risk factors are the same as those discussed for squamous cell carcinoma.

Malignant Tumors of the Oral Cavity

Cancers of the oral cavity account for less than 5% of total cases of body malignancies. Cancers in this area most frequently are seen in persons in their 40s and 50s, and in men more frequently than women. Cancers of the oral cavity are most often associated with alcohol consumption and tobacco use. With the increase of tobacco use in the younger age groups, especially the use of smokeless (chewing) tobacco, and use by women, the age and sex ratios are changing. The Risk Factors and Levels of Prevention feature lists overall risk factors for oral cancers.

Basal Cell Carcinoma. Basal cell carcinoma of the oral cavity occurs primarily on the lips. It starts as a small scab that develops into an ulcer with a characteristic pearly border. This cancer of the mouth accounts for about 4% of all cancers. Basal cell carcinoma is the second most common oral cancer.

Basal cell carcinoma primarily occurs as a result of excessive exposure to sunlight. It tends to occur more commonly in fair-skinned persons who are exposed to sunlight.

Squamous Cell Carcinoma. Squamous cell carcinoma is a malignant growth arising from tiny flat squamous cells that line mucous membranes. Squamous cell carcinoma is the leading type of oral cancer. Most tumors occur in clients older than 45 years of age. Common sites of squamous cell carcinoma include the lower lip and the tongue. Approximately 95% of cancers found on the tongue are squamous cell carcinomas. Malignancies of the tongue represent 1.0% to 1.5% of all malignancies in the United States.

The primary cause of squamous cell carcinoma is chronic irritation of the mucous lining of the mouth and oral cavity. The overuse of alcohol and tobacco is the primary cause of oral irritation. In combination, tobacco and alcohol are extremely destructive to the oral mucosa.

Squamous cell carcinoma develops from tiny cells that line the oral cavity. It can occur on the lips, buccal mucosa, tongue (Fig. 60–7), floor of the mouth, and tonsils. Squamous cell carcinoma is usually well differen-

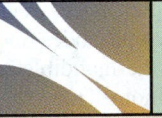

RISK FACTORS AND LEVELS OF PREVENTION

Oral Cancer

Risk Factors

Sunlight overexposure; tobacco (smoking and chewing); alcohol; poor oral hygiene with bacterial irritation; jagged teeth or improperly fitting dentures; hot or spicy foods or drinks; malnutrition; syphilis; cirrhosis of the liver; age over 45 years; family history of oral cancer

Levels of Prevention

Primary Prevention

● Teach clients to avoid excessive use of tobacco, alcohol, and hot and spicy foods and drinks.
● Encourage clients to maintain meticulous oral hygiene and a well-balanced diet.
● Encourage use of sunscreen during exposure to sunlight.

Secondary Prevention

● Screen smokers and drinkers of alcohol and teach them to stop smoking and to limit alcohol intake.
● Teach clients to limit intake of hot and spicy foods and drinks.
● Ensure that clients fix broken teeth and improperly fitting dentures.
● Teach persons at risk to observe for manifestations of oral cancer.

Tertiary Prevention

● Ensure that the client's tumor is excised and followed with chemotherapy and radiation as indicated.
● Provide nutritional support with tube feedings or feedings through a percutaneous endoscopic gastrostomy or gastrostomy tube.

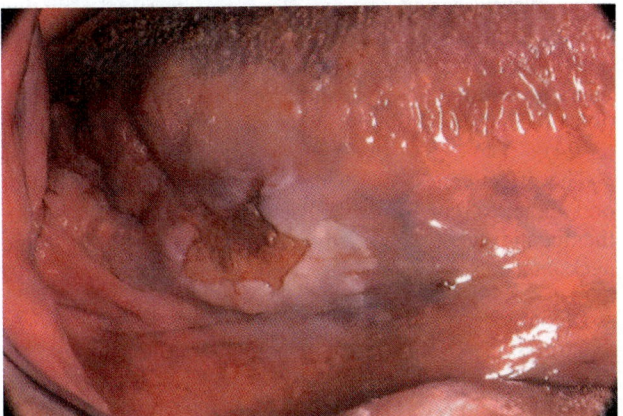

Figure 60–7. Oral squamous cell carcinoma. This is an ulcerated lesion with surrounding leukoplakia on the posterior lateral and ventral portions of the tongue. (From Neville, B. W., et al. [1995]. *Oral and maxillofacial pathology.* Philadelphia: W. B. Saunders.)

tiated and has a less than 10% metastasis rate. Cells metastasize by direct infiltration of local lymph nodes and can extend into the buccal fat and even to the mandible.

Manifestations of squamous cell carcinoma may include the presence of a sore or lesion in the oral cavity. Red-appearing (erythroplakia) squamous cell carcinomas may not be well delineated and often bleed easily. Because squamous cell carcinomas usually grow slowly, they may be large before manifestations are detected. Other manifestations can include a mild irritation of the tongue, sore throat, trouble with wearing dentures, or pain in the tongue or ear.

Only biopsy of lesions positively confirms a diagnosis of oral cancer. Cytologic examination of suspicious mucosa, while valuable in screening, unfortunately is not used widely enough to reduce the mortality rate. To be a valuable diagnostic aid, cytologic examination must be followed by biopsy when questionable cells are found. Biopsies may be performed with local or general anesthesia. To diagnose carcinoma at the base of the tongue, a laryngoscopic examination must be performed.

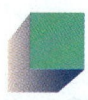

Acute and Subacute Care

■ Medical Management

The survival rate of oral cancer depends on the site and staging of the tumor (Table 60–1). Cancer of the lip has one of the highest cure rates of oral cancers. Squamous cell carcinoma of the tongue has the poorest prognosis because of the tongue's extensive vascular and lymphatic supply. Management of oral cancers includes radiation therapy, chemotherapy, and surgery, and again depends on the site and staging of the tumor.

Treatment of oral cancers with radiation can be given by external beam or interstitial radiation therapy. The external beam passes through the skin or mucous membrane to the tumor. Interstitial radiation (brachytherapy) involves implanting radioactive seeds into the tissue for a specific period of time. Because interstitial radiation affects local tissue, it is used for small lesions that have not infiltrated the surrounding tissue. The client with interstitial radiation is hospitalized and placed on radiation precautions while the materials are active (see Chapter 24).

The effectiveness of chemotherapy for the treatment of oral cancers remains to be determined. Several chemotherapeutic agents are used to treat clients with head and neck cancers:

Bleomycin
Cisplatin
Cyclophosphamide
Doxorubicin (Adriamycin)
5-Fluorouracil
Hydroxyurea
Methotrexate
Vincristine

Table 60–1. TNM Staging of Cancers of the Lip and Oral Cavity

Primary Tumor (T)

T_x	Primary tumor cannot be assessed
T_0	No evidence of primary tumor
T_{is}	Carcinoma in situ
T_1	Tumor 2 cm or less in greatest dimension
T_2	Tumor more than 2 cm but not more than 4 cm in greatest dimension
T_3	Tumor more than 4 cm in greatest dimension
T_4 (lip)	Tumor invades adjacent structures (e.g., through cortical bone, tongue, skin of neck)
T_4 (oral cavity)	Tumor invades adjacent structures (e.g., through cortical bone, into deep [extrinsic] muscle of tongue, maxillary sinus, skin)

Regional Lymph Nodes (N)

N_x	Regional lymph nodes cannot be assessed
N_0	No regional lymph node metastasis
N_1	Metastasis in a single ipsilateral lymph node, 3 cm or less in greatest dimension
N_2	Metastasis in a single ipsilateral lymph node, more than 3 cm but not more than 6 cm in greatest dimension; or in multiple ipsilateral lymph nodes, none more than 6 cm in greatest dimension; or in bilateral or contralateral lymph nodes, none more than 6 cm in greatest dimension
N_{2a}	Metastasis in a single ipsilateral lymph node more than 3 cm but not more than 6 cm in greatest dimension
N_{2b}	Metastasis in multiple ipsilateral lymph nodes, none more than 6 cm in greatest dimension
N_{2c}	Metastasis in bilateral or contralateral lymph nodes, none more than 6 cm in greatest dimension
N_3	Metastasis in a lymph node more than 6 cm in greatest dimension

Distant Metastasis (M)

M_x	Presence of distant metastasis cannot be assessed
M_0	No distant metastasis
M_1	Distant metastasis

Stage Grouping

Stage 0	T_{is}	N_0	M_0
Stage I	T_1	N_0	M_0
Stage II	T_2	N_0	M_0
Stage III	T_3	N_0	M_0
	T_1	N_1	M_0
	T_2	N_1	M_0
	T_3	N_1	M_0
Stage IV	T_4	N_0, N_1	M_0
	Any T	N_2, N_3	M_0
	Any T	Any N	M_1

■ Nursing Management of the Medical Client

Assessment

Carefully question the client about manifestations. A common finding is that of a painful ulcer. Also assess the client for difficulty in swallowing, white or red patches on the oral mucosa, bleeding in the mouth, lumps in the neck, pain referred to the ear, foul odor, and hoarseness. Question the client concerning the use of alcohol and tobacco, oral hygiene habits, and exposure to sun. Assess the rehabilitative needs of the client. Surgery can result in disfigurement and alterations in speech, and can cause the client to experience depression related to a change in body image.

Diagnosis, Planning, Implementation

Knowledge Deficit. A common nursing diagnosis for the client who is at risk of oral cancer is *Knowledge Deficit related to prevention and treatment of oral lesions.*

Planning: Expected Outcomes. The client will understand and comply with measures to maintain the oral mucosa as evidenced by statements of understanding of substances and activities to avoid and will be able to discuss the treatment regimen. There will be no evidence of lesions.

Implementation. Teach the client about the disease itself and treatment protocols. Because irritation is related to the development of leukoplakia, instruct the client to eschew tobacco, very hot drinks, and spicy foods. If dentures fit poorly, the client needs to consult with a dentist immediately for new ones. Give the client with poor nutrition guidelines for improving the diet. Supply pamphlets outlining the basic nutrients for good health, and refer the client to a dietitian as needed.

Again, the best intervention for oral cancer is prevention. Advise clients to

● Avoid chemical, physical, and thermal oral trauma.
● Perform careful, frequent oral hygiene, preferably three times daily.
● See a dentist if they have ill-fitting dentures.
● See a physician for any mouth lesion that does not heal in 2 to 3 weeks.

If the client is receiving radiation or chemotherapy, instruct the client about possible side effects of these forms of treatment. Provide the client with comfort measures to minimize the side effects, such as using antiemetics to prevent nausea and vomiting.

Altered Nutrition: Less than Body Requirements. Clients with oral cancers often have nutritional difficulties, so a usual nursing diagnosis is *Altered Nutrition: Less than Body Requirements, related to oral pain and difficulty eating and swallowing.*

Planning: Expected Outcomes. The client will maintain weight or show weight gain before surgery, as evidenced by an increase in intake, weight remaining stable, or weight gain of 1 lb per week preoperatively.

Implementation. The location, size, and pain associated with a tumor often interferes with the client's ability to eat. Small, frequent feedings often promote intake. Administering an analgesic 30 to 45 minutes prior to a meal often decreases pain associated with eating. Provide oral care before and after meals to remove oral odors and debris.

Unfortunately, treatments such as radiation alter salivation and taste perception. Xerostomia (dryness of the mouth) usually improves with the use of pilocarpine and artificial saliva. Suggest that the client chew sugarless gum or suck on sugarless candy drops to increase moisture. The client should perform frequent oral rinses with cool water to reduce dryness.

Evaluation

The best outcome would be that the client stopped the high-risk behavior and did not develop an oral cancer. If the cancer did develop, control of side effects and maintenance of nutrition would be the best outcome to evaluate.

■ Surgical Management

Surgical management of oral cancers can range from local excision of small tumors to extensive surgery for invasive tumors. Small tumors can be treated in outpatient facilities by local excision, radiation, or laser therapy. Small tumors of the floor of the mouth can be locally excised with or without removing a portion of the mandible. Small tumors in the anterior floor of the mouth can be excised and the area reconstructed with the use of a split-thickness skin graft. A thin layer of skin, usually from the anterior thigh, can line the surgical site, allowing the client to maintain good mobility and function of the tongue. Xeroform gauze is usually placed over the skin graft and sutured into place. This can restrict the tongue, causing aspiration of secretions. Because of this packing and as a result of postoperative edema, a tracheostomy tube is usually placed until edema subsides and the oral airway is patent. The client receives nothing by mouth (NPO) for 7 to 10 days after surgery to allow for healing. A feeding tube (nasogastric [NG], gastrostomy, or percutaneous endoscopic gastrostomy [PEG]) is used to provide nutrition until the client can resume oral feedings (see Chapter 61 for NG, gastrostomy, PEG, and percutaneous endoscopic jejunostomy tube feedings).

Invasive tumors require extensive surgical excision and usually involve removal of associated lymph nodes. Depending on the location, procedures may include a glossectomy (removal of the tongue), mandibulectomy (removal of the mandible), hemiglossectomy (removal of part of the tongue), or a radical neck dissection. A radical neck dissection is an extensive procedure that involves removal of all tissue under the skin, from the jaw down to the clavicle, and from the anterior border of the trapezius muscle to the midline. To remove the cervical lymph nodes in this procedure, the sternocleidomastoid muscle, the spinal accessory nerve, and the jugular vein have to be removed. A modified radical neck dissection involves removal of the lymph nodes only and is preferred with the disease is confined to mobile lymph nodes (see surgical management of cancer of the larynx). The Commando procedure is a very extensive oral operation in which part of the mandible is excised along with the oral lesion. This procedure is often combined with a radical neck dissection.

■ Nursing Management of the Surgical Client

Assessment

Assessment of the surgical client is similar to assessment of the medical client. The nurse should complete routine preoperative and postoperative assessments. Assessment of rehabilitative needs such as speech therapy and coping with disfigurement may also be required.

Diagnosis, Planning, Implementation

Knowledge Deficit. Many oral cancers require surgical intervention. Clients who are undergoing surgical treatment often experience *Knowledge Deficit related to surgical treatment of lesions.*

Planning: Expected Outcomes. The client will verbalize an understanding of and comply with surgical treatment measures.

Implementation. For the client scheduled for a surgical resection, ensure that the client understands the procedure to be performed and all its implications (such as a temporary or permanent tracheostomy). The client should receive adequate support before surgery to help the client cope with a possibly radically altered appearance. Instructions regarding postoperative procedures depend on the extent of the surgical resection. Instruct clients on the need for frequent assessment of vital signs, intravenous therapy, the availability of analgesics for pain, and oxygen therapy after surgery. Explain the purpose and care involved with a feeding tube.

Risk for Injury. Surgery for oral cancer involves many potential risks. *Risk for Injury related to surgical procedure, including hemorrhage, ineffective airway clearance, and possible wound infection* is an appropriate nursing diagnosis.

Planning: Expected Outcomes. The client will not develop injury, as evidenced by absence of excessive bleeding, maintenance of a patent airway, and wound healing without manifestations of infection.

Implementation. The extent of nursing care required by the client after surgery depends on the extent of the procedure. After local excisions, teach the client how to perform hygiene gently. If a dressing and packing are in place, monitor the amount of drainage. After the dressing and packing are removed, the client should rinse the oral cavity with a mild half-strength form of hydrogen peroxide and water or saline solution every 4 hours to remove debris and promote healing. If half-strength hydrogen peroxide and water is used, it should be followed by normal saline or water to prevent drying.

With more extensive surgery, the suture lines must be protected from trauma. Oral hygiene and oral suctioning are usually not implemented until healing has begun and the physician decides this type of cleaning can be performed.

Hemorrhage may occur at any time after surgery, especially with extensive resection of the tongue. Hemorrhage can be massive because of the large vessels that supply the mouth and oral area. Should bleeding occur, apply local pressure on the site until the bleeding stops spontaneously or stops with medical or surgical intervention. Surgical repair may be required. If an extensive resection was performed requiring skin grafts, monitor the site every 4 to 8 hours for drainage and for manifestations of infection.

The most critical postoperative intervention is to maintain a patent airway. If the surgical procedure has been extensive, there is usually a tracheostomy in place to help prevent respiratory difficulty from edema of the oral and pharyngeal structures. Clients at risk of ineffective airway clearance should be in semi- to high Fowler position after surgery to promote venous lymphatic drainage. The client may have a dusky appearance about the face from venous congestion. Pulse oximeter readings also should be used to determine whether or not the client is sufficiently oxygenated.

For the client with a tracheostomy, some blood-tinged mucus is normal in tracheal secretions for the first 48 hours after surgery. Bright-red bleeding from the tracheostomy tube or site is a manifestation of hemorrhage. Notify the physician immediately if this occurs.

Altered Nutrition: Less than Body Requirements. Often following surgical intervention for oral cancers, the client continues to have difficulties with nutrition. *Altered Nutrition: Less than Body Requirements, related to altered oral mucosa and surgical procedure* is an appropriate nursing diagnosis.

Planning: Expected Outcomes. The client will maintain or gain weight after surgery, as evidenced by a stabilization of weight and possibly a 1 lb per week weight gain.

Implementation. Immediately after surgery, monitor intravenous hydration. Assess bowel sounds every shift. The return of bowel sounds is often an indication to begin tube feedings. As outlined in Critical Monitoring, before adding each feeding to the feeding bag, assess the client for proper tube placement and retention of stomach contents. Administer nutritional supplements by pump or bolus feedings. In addition, the physician may order total parenteral nutrition (TPN) as the first line of nutritional management.

Once the edema has subsided, adequate healing has occurred, and the tracheostomy tube has been removed, the client may be restarted on oral feedings. The client should be cautioned about a decrease in sensation in the oral cavity after surgery. Swallowing should be carefully assessed before eating begins. Instruct the client to avoid

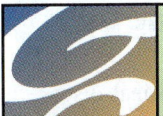

CRITICAL MONITORING

The Client with a Percutaneous Endoscopic Gastrostomy or Percutaneous Endoscopic Jejunostomy Tube

Interventions	Rationales
Weigh the client daily.	The client's weight gain or loss must be recorded.
Measure the length of the tube every 4 hours.	Measurement helps you to assess tube placement.
Aspirate the contents every 4 hours.	Aspiration helps you to assess the pH of stomach contents and determine if a residual amount exceeds 100 to 150 ml or more than 110% to 120% of the hourly rate. If this occurs, the feeding rate should be decreased or the feeding stopped for an hour.
Flush the tube with 50 to 100 ml of sterile saline or sterile water (or per institutional policy) after checking placement, administering medications, or giving a bolus feeding.	Flushing maintains patency of the tube and provides hydration.
Elevate the head of the bed at least 30 degrees during feedings and for 30 to 60 minutes after the tube feeding has been stopped.	Elevation prevents the client from aspirating tube feeding or stomach contents.
Monitor bowel sounds.	Monitoring helps you to assess for normal bowel activity.
Add blue food coloring to tube feedings.	Food coloring may indicate aspiration or a fistula.
Slow the tube feeding rate or decrease its strength.	Slowing the feeding rate controls diarrhea.
Refill the feeding bag every 4 hours. It should be rinsed and then refilled every 4 hours. (Never add to a solution that has been hanging several hours because of the risk of contamination.)	A solution that hangs for more than 4 hours can become sour or contaminated with bacteria.
Discard enteral feeding containers every 24 hours.	Discarding containers prevents contamination.
Rinse enteral feeding bags every 4 hours.	Rinsing feeding bags prevents contamination.
Keep the cuff of the endotracheal or tracheostomy tube inflated during feeding as appropriate.	Inflation prevents aspiration.

putting food directly on the surgical resection site. After meals, the client should always perform good oral hygiene.

On discharge, supply the client and family with complete instructions regarding diet, medications, manifestations of complications, and any treatments such as wound or tracheostomy care. Include information regarding how and when to contact healthcare providers. The client will need to be seen by the physician after discharge to ensure complete healing of any extensive surgical wounds. If the client has a tracheostomy, it may be permanent or may be closed at a later date. Clients who have undergone extensive surgery may need a referral to a home healthcare agency for possible assistance with respiratory support (home oxygen), suctioning, nutritional support, and wound care.

Impaired Verbal Communication.
When the client has a tracheostomy following surgery, a common diagnosis is *Impaired Verbal Communication related to the presence of tracheostomy.*

Planning: Expected Outcomes. The client will be able to communicate using alternative forms of communications, as evidence by the ability to communicate with staff and significant others.

Implementation. Help clients who cannot speak to express their needs, concerns, and feelings. Assess the client's literacy and then provide paper for the client to write on as a substitute for talking or provide the client with a picture board to use for communicating any needs. Ideally, this assessment and instruction are completed preoperatively. Check on the client frequently to reduce anxiety and loneliness. Also place the call light within easy reach and respond to the light promptly. If an intercom is used, it should be appropriately labeled regarding the client's limited ability to speak.

The client should be allowed to communicate by gestures or written notes if this approach puts the client at ease. Most important, your manner should communicate acceptance, compassion, and caring. It is common to treat clients who cannot talk as though they cannot hear or understand. Be alert to any tendency to treat these clients as though they were mentally incompetent or deaf. Help the client avoid social isolation by taking the client for walks and meeting others. Friendly social encounters and physical activity can help alleviate depression in this client.

Evaluation

The most favorable outcome is that the client heals within 6 weeks to 3 months depending on the extent of the radical surgery without complications. Another evaluation would be the client's ability to maintain an adequate intake of nutrients. If the client is able to self-feed via a tube until healing occurs and then to increase oral intake as able, nutritional status should remain adequate.

Disorders of the Salivary Glands

Inflammation

Parotitis, also known as surgical mumps, is inflammation of the parotid glands. It is the most common inflammatory condition affecting the salivary glands and probably results from inactivity of the glands caused by certain medications, such as diuretics, prolonged NG intubation, and lack of oral intake, such as that seen in postoperative clients. As secretions of the salivary gland diminish, oral bacteria have an opportunity to invade the gland and multiply. Interventions involve the following:

- Administering frequent oral hygiene to keep the bacterial count of the mouth low
- Keeping the client well hydrated
- Suggesting that the client use sugarless hard candies or chew sugarless gum to stimulate secretions of the glands

Calculi

Stones, or calculi, form in the salivary glands when the glands are inactive and the client has a metabolic condition favoring the precipitation of salts. A nidus or focus of origin is necessary for stimulating salt precipitation. Assessment reveals that irritation from the stones causes local inflammation, swelling, and pain when the gland is stimulated to secrete, as during chewing. Intervention requires local excision. Stones occur most commonly in the submaxillary glands, probably because of (1) the longer length of the duct and (2) production of viscous alkaline secretions.

Tumors

Most tumors in the salivary glands are benign. The most frequently seen malignant tumor is adenocarcinoma. Both types of tumors are characterized by enlargement of the gland. Pain occurs when expansion within the capsule of the gland creates pressure on sensory nerves. The treatment of choice for both benign and malignant tumors is usually surgical excision. If the tumor has recurred or is highly malignant, radiation therapy may also be used.

Disorders of the Esophagus

The most common manifestation of esophageal disease is dysphagia, difficulty with swallowing. Other manifestations include regurgitation, pain (which is probably linked with spasm), and heartburn.

Dysphagia

Dysphagia can be caused by any esophageal disorder. Specific causes include neuromotor malfunction, mechanical obstruction, cardiovascular abnormalities, and neurologic diseases.

Dysphagia Caused by Mechanical Obstructions

Mechanical obstructions causing dysphagia include congenital defects, carcinoma, and acquired conditions such as hiatal hernia. When an obstruction narrows the esophageal lumen, clients first experience dysphagia only with solid foods. Later, dysphagia becomes associated with semisolid foods and liquids. Finally, these clients are unable to swallow their own saliva. Obstructive disorders, particularly esophageal carcinoma, may be accompanied by weight loss and cachexia.

Dysphagia Caused by Cardiovascular Abnormalities

Dysphagia also may result from cardiovascular abnormalities, particularly in the elderly. Specific conditions that cause vascular dysphagia include an enlarged heart, an aortic aneurysm, and calcification of the descending aorta. Figure 60–8 shows the relationship of the heart and great arteries to the esophagus.

Dysphagia Caused by Neurologic Diseases

Dysphagia also may be caused by certain neurologic diseases such as cerebrovascular accident (CVA), multiple sclerosis, poliomyelitis, and amyotrophic lateral sclerosis. CVA is the most frequent cause of dysphagia.

Dysphagia from Other Causes

Dysphagia can be experienced after swallowing if food gets caught in the esophagus. Relief may be obtained by drinking liquids to force the impacted bolus through the narrow segment, or by retching to dislodge the food. Endoscopy is commonly used to remove food lodged in the esophagus if vomiting fails.

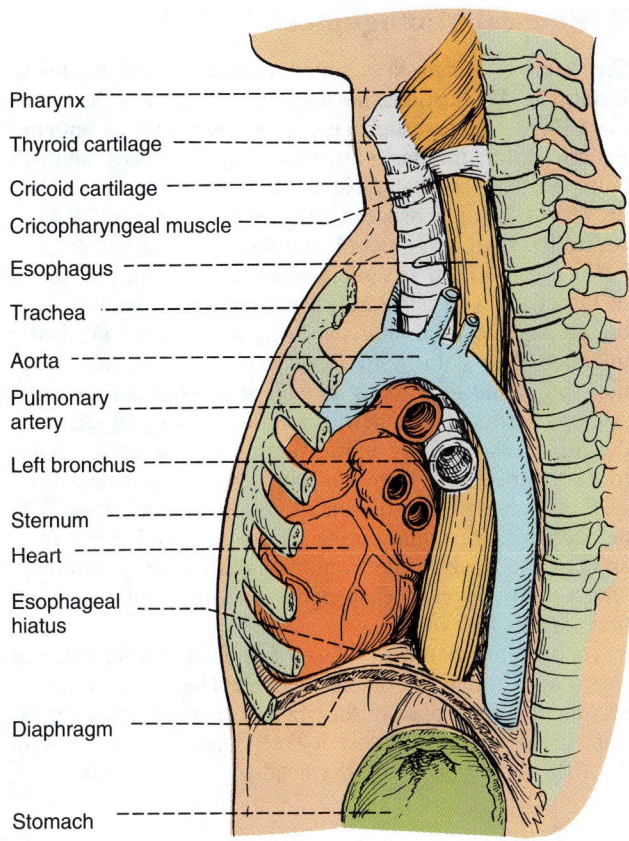

Pharynx

Thyroid cartilage

Cricoid cartilage

Cricopharyngeal muscle

Esophagus

Trachea

Aorta

Pulmonary artery

Left bronchus

Sternum

Heart

Esophageal hiatus

Diaphragm

Stomach

Figure 60–8. Relationship of the heart and great arteries to the esophagus.

Regurgitation

Regurgitation is the ejection of small amounts of chyme or gastric juice from the mouth without antecedent nausea. It is usually caused by an incompetent lower esophageal sphincter (LES). Regurgitation occurring immediately after swallowing results from structural or motor abnormality in the LES. Factors contributing to regurgitation include abnormal motor activity, increased abdominal pressure, and sphincter abnormality. Regurgitation occurs with pylorospasm, lesions proximal to the cardia, achalasia, hiatal hernia, reflux esophagitis, and esophageal ulcer or malignancy. Stooping or lying down facilitates the flow of gastric contents into the esophagus, thus exacerbating regurgitation.

Pain

Pain, which sometimes is constant or may occur only with swallowing, suggests diffuse esophageal spasm. Pain may result from alterations of the mucosa due to reflux disease, radiation, or viral infection. Pain that affects the esophageal mucosa and occurs with swallowing is called odynophagia. The client usually describes the pain as sharp, constricting, sticking, crushing, stabbing, or knife-like. Odynophagia is usually severe, quite distressing, and often associated with a deep and long-lasting pain. The

pain, located substernally, may radiate to the neck, back, upper thorax, and shoulder. Pain may occur throughout the day and can be confused with angina. Odynophagia can be triggered by a cold or carbonated beverage or solid food passing through the esophagus. The most common cause is the reflux of gastric contents into the esophagus.

Heartburn

Heartburn (pyrosis, indigestion, or dyspepsia) is another common manifestation of esophageal disease. Generally, it is a painful sensation of warmth and burning in the lower retrosternal midline. Clients may use the word "heartburn" to describe very different sensations. Therefore, it is essential to find out exactly what this term means to the client experiencing the manifestation. Heartburn usually means substernal, midline burning that tends to radiate, generally in waves, upward to the neck, resulting from abnormalities of the LES. Clients often describe this discomfort as cramping or knotting. Heartburn is often experienced with postural changes such as bending, stooping, or lifting, as well as when someone gulps food or liquids or ingests alcohol. Manifestations often are relieved by standing or eructating. Heartburn also arises in the presence of refluxed gastric or duodenal contents. Disorders most commonly associated with heartburn are reflux esophagitis, hiatal hernia, achalasia, and gastric stasis. Heartburn is common in persons with pyloric or duodenal ulcers and LES disorders.

Achalasia

Achalasia is a disorder characterized by progressively increasing dysphagia, with the client eventually having great difficulty swallowing and expressing the feeling that "something is stuck in the throat." Achalasia commonly occurs in persons in their 20s and 30s and appears with equal incidence in men and in women.

Etiology and Risk Factors

Achalasia is a chronic, progressive disease of unknown cause. Occasionally, the client can relate the onset to an episode of acute dysphagia, but usually achalasia has an obscure onset and is only noticed when the dysphagia becomes severe. Because achalasia is idiopathic, there are no identified risk factors. It is believed there may be a familial incidence of achalasia.

Pathophysiology

Achalasia is characterized by impaired motility of the lower two thirds of the esophagus. The LES fails to relax normally with swallowing. Inadequate functioning occurs because (1) nerve impulses are unable to pass through the esophagus or (2) sympathetic receptors are absent from the LES. There also may be degeneration of the ganglion cells or impairment of impulses from Auerbach's plexus (see Chapter 58). Impaired propulsion and a constricted LES result in accumulation of food and fluid within the lower esophagus. When hydrostatic pressure exceeds the force of resistance of the LES, the contents pass into the stomach. Complications of achalasia include reflux esophagitis with resultant ulceration (Fig. 60–9), which is discussed in the section on GERD. Aspiration of regurgitated esophageal contents may result in atelectasis and other pulmonary problems.

Clinical Manifestations and Diagnostic Findings

The initial manifestation of achalasia is dysphagia. It is difficult for food and fluid to pass through the LES. In the early stages of achalasia, the client may have substernal pain due to spasms of the esophagus or may be unable to eructate. The client may regurgitate undigested food eaten many hours earlier as well as large amounts of mucus that have been stimulated by esophageal irritation. As achalasia progresses, manifestations increase in frequency and severity. Upper respiratory infections, emotional disturbances, overeating, and pregnancy may aggravate the problem.

Diagnostic tests used to determine the presence of achalasia include the barium swallow, endoscopy, and manometry. The barium swallow is considered positive for achalasia if it reveals nonpropulsive waves and esophageal dilation. Also, barium may be retained. Endoscopy helps determine the status of the LES, dilation, and the presence of food. Manometry (measurement of pressure in the esophagus) confirms the diagnosis when there are elevated resting pressures in the LES, or slow, low-amplitude, or absent peristalsis.

Acute and Subacute Care

Management of the client with achalasia usually begins with medical treatment on an outpatient basis. Often, as the problem progresses, hospitalization is required for surgical procedures or for placement of a gastrostomy, PEG, or PEJ tube for nutritional support.

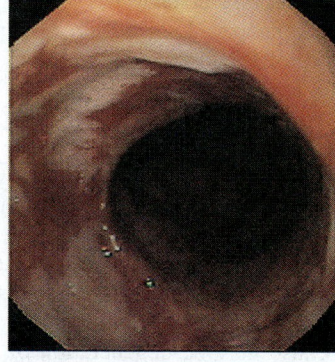

Figure 60–9. Endoscopic view of severe esophagitis.

■ Medical Management

Treatment of achalasia is aimed at relieving clinical manifestations. Medications have been investigated that relax the LES or lower esophageal pressures, such as anticholinergic drugs, nitrates, gastrointestinal hormones, and calcium channel blockers. None of these medications have proved to be of consistent value or effectiveness. Pain is controlled with non-narcotic and narcotic analgesics.

Changes in diet may often ease the pressure and reflux in the client with achalasia. Small, frequent feedings ease the passage of food, and semisoft, warm foods are better tolerated than cold, hard foods. The client should avoid hot, spicy, and iced foods as well as alcohol and tobacco. All foods should be chewed thoroughly to add saliva to the mixture, providing lubrication and allowing the bolus to pass more easily from the esophagus to the stomach.

The client should experiment with different positions to reduce pressure while eating. Some clients benefit from arching the back while swallowing. Restrictive clothing, which may increase esophageal pressure and regurgitation, should be avoided.

To prevent nocturnal reflux of food, the client should sleep with the head of the bed elevated. This may be accomplished by placing the client in a semi-Fowler position, using a wedge pillow to keep the head higher than the LES, or by elevating the head of the bed on 4- to 6-inch blocks.

■ Nursing Management of the Medical Client

Assessment

Obtain a history, noting the manifestations the client is experiencing, onset and duration of aggravating factors, and any methods the client uses for relief. Assess respiratory manifestations because the respiratory tract can be affected by reflux or regurgitation. Assess the client's nutritional status, noting any weight changes and the effects of esophageal manifestations on dietary habits.

Diagnosis, Planning, Implementation

Altered Nutrition: Less than Body Requirements. The client with achalasia experiences a great deal of difficulty swallowing, leading to the diagnosis of *Altered Nutrition: Less than Body Requirement, related to dysphagia.*

Planning: Expected Outcomes. The client will maintain an adequate nutritional intake, as evidenced by maintenance of ideal body weight or gaining back any weight lost at a rate of 1 lb per week.

Implementation. Consult with the client concerning dietary habits and daily intake of nutrients. Obtain a baseline weight and daily weights. Teach the client about changes in dietary habits that may relieve manifestations. A gastrostomy tube, PEG tube, or PEJ tube may be used to provide adequate nutritional support if dysphagia continues to be a problem (discussed under Surgical Management).

Pain. When the client experiences gastric reflux, the acid in the esophagus causes *Pain related to episodes of gastric reflux,* making pain an appropriate nursing diagnosis.

Planning: Expected Outcomes. The client will experience a decrease in pain or absence of pain, as evidenced by the client verbalizing a reduction in or absence of pain and ability to maintain oral intake.

Implementation. As stated, pain can be decreased or relieved through the use of medications (such as antacids and H_2-receptor antagonists), dietary changes, and repositioning. Assess the client every shift to determine whether medications, changes in diet, and positioning were effective in controlling or relieving pain.

Evaluation

The most appropriate outcome would be that the achalasia was controlled with medical treatment and the client's nutritional status was maintained.

■ Surgical Management

Surgical management of achalasia may involve dilating the lower esophageal sphincter (esophageal dilation) or enlarging the sphincter (esophagomyotomy). Esophageal dilation, or bougienage, forcefully dilates the LES (Fig. 60–10). This procedure, which is usually done on an outpatient basis, is used to help correct not only achalasia but esophageal spasms and strictures. Vigorous dilation has a 75% success rate. This procedure is performed with local anesthesia under radiologic guidance.

A more complex procedure, esophagomyotomy (Heller's procedure), may have to be performed. In this proce-

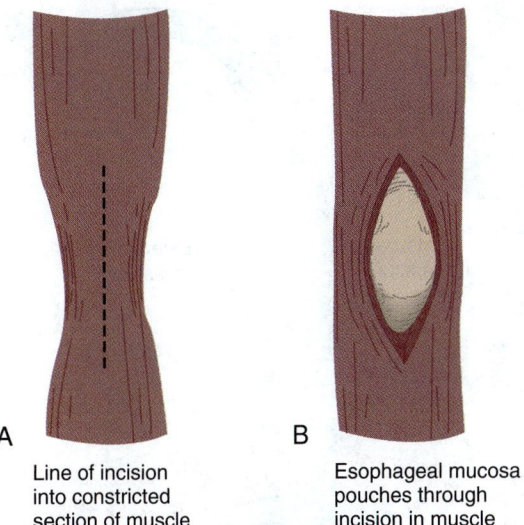

A — Line of incision into constricted section of muscle

B — Esophageal mucosa pouches through incision in muscle

Figure 60–11. Esophagomyotomy (Heller's procedure) is the surgical procedure of choice when a segment of esophagus narrows and causes functional obstruction.

dure, the surgeon enlarges the vestibule by incising the circular muscle fibers down to the mucosa (Fig. 60–11). Complications of esophagomyotomy include reflux esophagitis and restenosis.

If a client cannot swallow for long periods, a gastrostomy tube may be inserted. There are two methods of inserting a gastrostomy tube. The first involves making an incision in the wall of the abdomen and suturing the tube to the gastric wall. The second method is the PEG. Under local anesthesia, the physician inserts a cannula into the stomach through an abdominal incision. A suture is threaded through the cannula. A second physician uses an endoscope to pull the suture through the client's mouth. The PEG tube is attached and advanced down the esophagus, through the abdominal incision, where it is secured internally and externally by crossbars (Fig. 60–12). Some tubes have an internal balloon instead of an internal crossbar, while other tubes have internal and external crossbars and an internal balloon. Skin care around the percutaneous site is necessary postoperatively. The other procedure is the PEJ. Instead of inserting the tube in the stomach, it is inserted into the jejunum.

■ Nursing Management of the Surgical Client

Assessment

Obtain a history noting the onset and duration of manifestations the client is experiencing, aggravating factors, and any methods the client uses for relief. Again, the client's respiratory status and nutritional status should be assessed. In addition, routine preoperative and postoperative assessments are required.

Diagnosis, Planning, Implementation

Knowledge Deficit. In order to prepare the client for surgery, the nursing diagnosis *Knowledge Deficit re-*

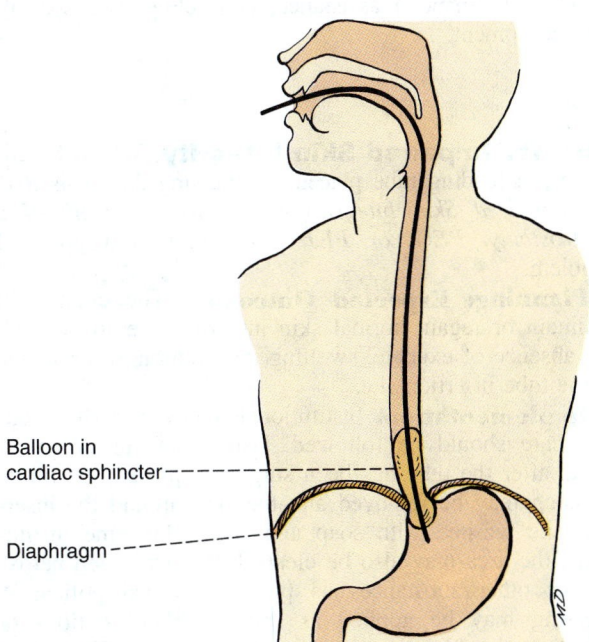

Balloon in cardiac sphincter

Diaphragm

Figure 60–10. Bougienage relieves dysphagia by dilating the lower esophageal sphincter.

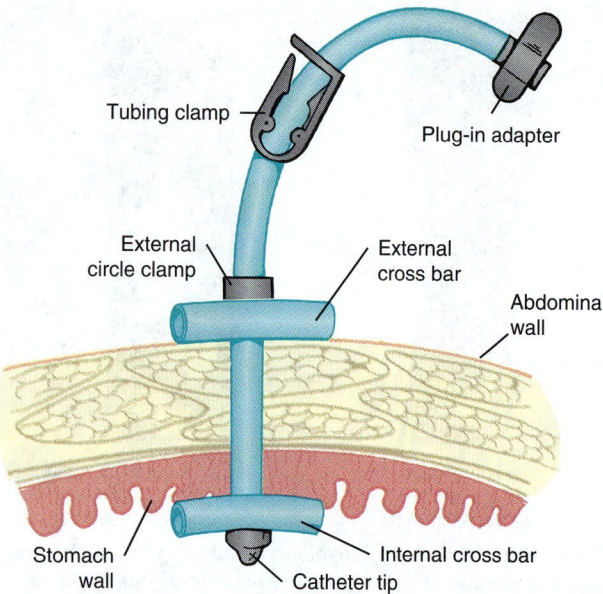

Figure 60–12. A percutaneous endoscopic gastrostomy tube in place for a client with achalasia.

lated to preoperative preparation and postoperative care is appropriate.

Planning: Expected Outcomes. The client will understand and be prepared for surgery, as evidenced by client questions and statements of understanding.

Implementation. Clients undergoing esophageal dilation should be told that they will be awake during the procedure. A local anesthetic is sprayed on the throat, and the client may receive an analgesic or tranquilizer. The client should take long slow breaths during passage of the bougies. As the bag is inflated, the client may feel a brief feeling of discomfort. Weighted bougies in increasing weight can also be used for dilation. Esophageal dilation is often performed on an outpatient basis.

Esophagomyotomy is a more complex procedure. The client will require a general anesthetic and remain hospitalized for more than 24 hours. Instruct the client undergoing an esophageal procedure about all the usual preoperative procedures, such as an NPO status after midnight, intravenous fluids, and preoperative medications. Also discuss pain control, drains, surgical dressings, and the presence of an NG tube, gastrostomy tube, PEG tube, or PEJ tube. The possibility of a thoracotomy approach being used to reach the esophagus requires instruction concerning chest tubes.

The client should receive written and oral instructions regarding diet, medications, and manifestations of respiratory complications related to esophageal reflux and aspiration.

Clients who have undergone an esophagomyotomy should be instructed to sleep with the head of the bed elevated and recognize manifestations of respiratory complications. Instruct the client in the manifestations of infection and esophageal perforation, and to notify the physician if any of these problems occur.

Altered Nutrition: Less than Body Requirements. For the client experiencing dysphagia, the nursing diagnosis *Altered Nutrition: Less than Body Requirements, related to dysphagia and placement of a gastrostomy, PEG, or PEJ tube* is appropriate.

Planning: Expected Outcomes. The client will maintain an adequate nutritional intake, as evidenced by maintenance of ideal body weight or gaining back any weight lost at a rate of 1 lb per week.

Implementation. A baseline weight and daily weights should be obtained. Follow institutional policy regarding care for the client with a gastrostomy, PEG, or PEJ tube. Typically, the client will be NPO for at least 24 hours before continuous or bolus tube feedings are begun. Nursing interventions include checking tube placement via measurement of the tube and checking pH of stomach contents and residual amounts every 4 hours. (This is not assessed via aspiration if the tube is placed in the jejunum, since these tubes are flushed, not aspirated.) If gastric return is greater than 100 ml, hold the feeding for 1 hour and repeat aspiration before continuing the feeding. After checking placement and administering bolus feedings or medications, the tube should be flushed with 50 to 100 ml of normal saline or water. The head of the bed should be kept elevated at least 30 degrees at all times for continuous feedings or for 1 hour after completion of intermittent bolus feedings. The enteral feeding bag and tubing should be changed every 24 hours and rinsed with water every 6 hours or following each intermittent feeding.

The client or significant others will require teaching if the feedings are required following discharge. Initially, home visits by a nurse may be necessary to assist the client with any home healthcare needs related to tube feedings, diet, medications, wound care, and to provide an ongoing evaluation of the client's condition. A referral to a social worker also might be needed to assist the client with financial assistance, counseling, and specialized equipment.

Risk for Impaired Skin Integrity. When the client has a feeding tube placed, the nursing diagnosis *Risk for Impaired Skin Integrity related to placement of a gastrostomy, PEG, or PEJ tube* identifies a potential problem.

Planning: Expected Outcomes. The client will maintain or regain normal skin integrity as evidenced by the absence of exudate, swelling, excoriation, or erythema at the tube insertion site.

Implementation. Institutional policy regarding routine care should be followed. Usually, about 12 to 24 hours after the tube has been surgically placed, the initial dressing may be removed and the skin around the insertion site washed with soap and water. In some institutions, the area may also be cleaned with hydrogen peroxide or other substances as per institutional policy. A dressing may be applied as needed. Manifestations of infection should be reported to the physician. The client or significant other must be taught about home care management.

Pneumothorax. A common collaborative problem in the postoperative client is *Pneumothorax related to surgical procedure and presence of chest tubes.*

Planning: Expected Outcomes. Injury will be prevented, as evidenced by absence of hemorrhage, no manifestations of perforation, normal temperature, and absence of manifestations of problems associated with the chest tubes, such as respiratory distress.

Implementation. After the performance of esophageal dilation, monitor the client for manifestations of perforation, such as elevated temperature, chest or shoulder pain, and subcutaneous emphysema. If any of these manifestations are noted, the nurse should notify the physician immediately. The client will require an x-ray study to determine whether or not air is in the mediastinum, indicating perforation.

After an esophagomyotomy, the client will have a thoracotomy incision and chest tubes in place. Maintain chest tube drainage, the NG or gastric drainage system, and manage the client's pain. (See Chapter 42 for care of the client with chest tubes.)

Evaluation

An appropriate outcome would be that the client maintained adequate nutrition and that the condition was reversed with surgery. The esophagus must heal completely before the client can return to eating the usual foods. An acceptable evaluation is that the client or significant others were able to continue tube feedings for at least 6 weeks after surgery.

■ Modifications for Elderly Clients

In older adults, an attempt is made to treat the client with more local measures (pain medications, positioning, and dietary modification) and, possibly, esophageal dilation.

Diffuse Esophageal Spasm

Diffuse esophageal spasm is a generalized neurogenic problem that interferes with esophageal motility. The client may experience chest pain (resembling that of angina pectoris), dysphagia, and odynophagia. Sometimes, this condition progresses to achalasia. Pain is sometimes relieved by sedatives, long-acting nitrates, and anticholinergics. Small, frequent feedings and a soft diet are recommended to decrease irritation and pressure. Esophageal dilation and esophagomyotomy may be required if the pain becomes severe.

Gastroesophageal Reflux Disease

Esophageal reflux is defined as the backward flow of gastric contents into the esophagus. *Gastroesophageal reflux disease (GERD)* is a term used to describe a syndrome resulting from esophageal reflux. Reflux exposes the esophageal mucosa to the gastric contents and gradually breaks down the esophageal mucosa. This condition,

sometimes referred to as *reflux esophagitis,* is often associated with a sliding hiatal hernia. However, reflux causing complications can occur without a hiatal hernia, and persons with a hiatal hernia may not have manifestations of reflux.

GERD can occur in any age group. It is estimated that 10% of the population has daily manifestations of GERD and as much as one-third of the population has monthly manifestations. Manifestations are often overlooked and attributed to stress.

Etiology and Risk Factors

The cause of GERD seems to be an inappropriate relaxation of the LES. The exact cause of the relaxation is unknown, but reflux occurs when there is

● An alteration in the innervation of the pressure zone in the region of the gastroesophageal sphincter
● Displacement of the angle of the gastroesophageal junction
● An incompetent LES

The Risk Factors and Levels of Prevention feature lists other potential causes of GERD.

Pathophysiology

Normally, a high-pressure zone exists in the region of the gastroesophageal sphincter. High pressure prevents reflux but permits the passage of food and liquids. When there is an alteration in this region, reflux occurs.

Reflux esophagitis also may occur with gastric or duodenal ulcer, after esophageal or gastric surgery, after prolonged vomiting, or after prolonged gastrointestinal intubation. The reflux most often consists of hydrochloric acid or gastric and duodenal contents containing bile acid and pancreatic juice. Frequent or prolonged reflux results in inflammation of the esophageal mucosa (esophagitis). The degree of reflux esophagitis present depends on the following:

1. Frequency of the reflux
2. Contents of the reflux
3. Buffering ability of the saliva and mucous secretion
4. Rate of gastric emptying

Clinical Manifestations and Diagnostic Findings

Clients with GERD may experience a sudden or gradual onset of manifestations. The client may complain of heartburn, odynophagia, dysphagia, acid regurgitation, water brash (the release of salty secretions in the mouth), or eructation. Pain in GERD is typically referred to as a burning sensation that moves up and down. If the condition is severe, the pain may radiate to the back, neck, or jaw. Pain usually occurs after meals and is relieved with antacids or fluids. Discomfort sometimes accompanies activities that increase intra-abdominal pressure, such as lifting or straining. The client may state that discomfort occurs when lying supine or when the stomach is dis-

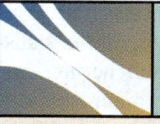

tended. Discomfort may be relieved by standing and walking. Dysphagia resulting from edema, spasm, or a narrowed lumen is intermittent and worse at the beginning of meals. Responses to pain-relieving measures (e.g., nitroglycerin) help to differentiate between esophagitis and problems of cardiac origin (e.g., angina pectoris).

Diagnosis rests on the demonstration of reflux. Barium swallow, esophageal manometry, esophagoscopy, esophageal biopsy, cytologic examination, analysis of gastric secretions, and acid perfusion tests confirm the diagnosis of GERD (see Chapter 59).

Acute and Subacute Care

Medical management is begun with clinic or office visits. However, surgical management will require the client to be hospitalized.

■ Medical Management

Pharmacologic Management

Antacids. Drug therapy for GERD usually starts with antacid therapy. Antacid therapy often provides prompt relief. Typically, the client takes 30 ml of antacid 1 hour before and 2 to 3 hours after each meal. Clients typically tolerate combination products such as calcium carbonate–magnesium carbonate (Mylanta) or magnesium hydroxide–aluminum hydroxide (Maalox). Aluminum hydroxide–magnesium carbonate (Gaviscon) is another excellent antacid because of its foaming action.

Histamine Receptor Antagonists. If manifestations are severe or persist, the client may be prescribed histamine receptor antagonists such as ranitidine (Zantac) or famotidine (Pepcid).

Other Medications. Bethanechol (Urecholine) may be added for clients with severe manifestations because it has been found to increase LES pressure and prevent reflux. Because bethanechol is a cholinergic drug, it is usually given with antacids and a histamine receptor antagonist because it can increase the secretion of gastric acid. It should be taken before meals.

Metoclopramide (Reglan) may be prescribed because it increases LES pressure by stimulating the smooth muscle of the gastrointestinal tract and increasing the rate of gastric emptying. This medication is taken before meals.

Cisapride (Propulsid) is prescribed for GERD because it has a triple mechanism:

1. It increases lower esophageal sphincter tone to reestablish the esophageal barrier.
2. It improves esophageal peristalsis to assist in clearance of acidic materials.
3. It promotes gastric emptying to reduce backpressure on the LES.

The drug is taken at least 15 minutes before meals and at bedtime.

Omeprazole (Prilosec), a proton pump inhibitor, suppresses secretion of gastric acid. It has been effective for short-term treatment of GERD. For persons with long-term therapy with nonsteroidal anti-inflammatory drugs (NSAIDs), misoprostol (Cytotec) has been useful for preventing gastric ulcer formation and, in some instances, GERD symptoms.

Anticholinergic drugs, calcium channel blockers, and theophylline should be avoided because they appear to decrease LES pressure or delay gastric emptying.

Dietary Management

In mild cases of GERD, diet changes may be sufficient to relieve manifestations. Instruct the client to follow this regimen:

- Restrict the diet to small, frequent feedings (four to six per day).
- Drink adequate fluids at meals to assist food passage.
- Eat slowly and chew thoroughly to add saliva to the food.

- Avoid extremely hot or cold foods, as well as spices, fats, alcohol, coffee, chocolate, and citrus juices.
- Avoid eating and drinking for 3 hours before retiring to prevent the common problem of nocturnal reflux.
- Elevate the head of the bed 6 to 8 inches to prevent nocturnal reflux.
- Lose weight if overweight to decrease the gastroesophageal pressure gradient.
- Avoid tobacco, salicylates, and phenylbutazone, which may aggravate esophagitis.

■ Nursing Management of the Medical Client

Assessment

Identify what manifestations the client has been experiencing. This assessment includes documenting when manifestations started, their frequency and severity, and the relationship of manifestations to food and various food products. Assist in maintaining the client's general appearance and nutritional status.

Diagnosis, Planning, Implementation

Pain. The client with GERD experiences reflux of acid into the esophagus leading to the nursing diagnosis of *Pain related to irritation of the esophagus caused by gastric reflux.*

Planning: Expected Outcomes. The client's pain will decrease or be absent, as evidenced by the client stating that the pain is decreased or absent.

Implementation. Instruct the client in the prescribed diet regimen and evaluate both the client's understanding and the effectiveness of the treatment. Administer medications ordered for the pain and document their effectiveness. Instruct the client in the prescribed medication regimen and evaluate the client's understanding of the treatment. Also help the client identify risk factors for GERD and instruct the client about life-style changes to reduce those risk factors.

■ Surgical Management

Surgery is the treatment for clients who do not respond to medical management. Any one of three different procedures may be used. They are (1) the Nissen fundoplication, (2) the Hill operation, or (3) the Belsey operation. The surgeon may use an open surgical approach or a laparoscopic approach to complete these procedures. Recovery is usually faster with the laparoscopic approach. The Nissen fundoplication is most frequently used and involves suture of the fundus around the esophagus (Fig. 60–13). An abdominal approach is usually used. An increase in pressure or volume in the stomach closes the cardia and blocks reflux into the esophagus. The surgery creates a valvelike substitute sphincter with inherent contractibility.

The Hill operation narrows the esophageal opening and anchors the stomach and distal esophagus to the median arcuate ligament (posterior gastropexy). This procedure reinforces the sphincter and recreates the gastroesophageal

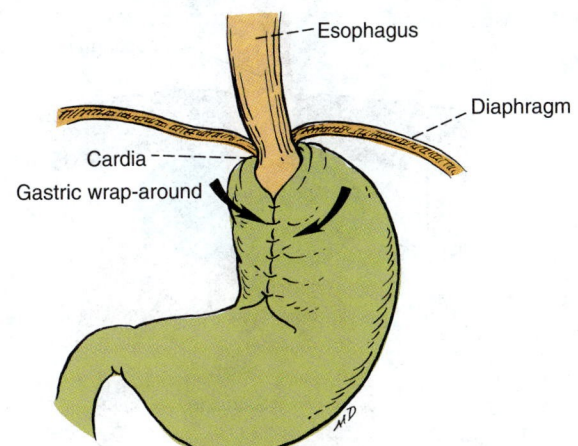

Figure 60–13. Nissen fundoplication for hiatal hernia. The gastric fundus is wrapped around the distal esophagus and sutured to itself.

valve. In the Hill procedure, there is a partial wraparound (180 degrees) of the stomach around the esophagus using an abdominal approach.

The Belsey (Mark IV) repair consists of plicating the anterior and lateral aspects of the stomach onto the distal esophagus. This creates the esophagogastric angle without opening the esophagus or the diaphragm. This procedure has a 280-degree esophageal wraparound and a thoracic approach.

Clients undergoing a surgical procedure are encouraged to follow the GERD antireflux medical regimen (medications, diet changes, life-style changes), because the recurrence rate is significant.

Clients with severe reflux may have an Angelchik prosthesis inserted. In this procedure, a laparotomy is performed and a synthetic C-shaped silicone prosthesis is tied around the distal esophagus (Fig. 60–14). The prosthesis anchors the LES in the abdomen and reinforces sphincter pressure. The success of this procedure is variable, depending on the severity of the problem. Clients with severe reflux may find this procedure unsuccessful.

■ Nursing Management of the Surgical Client

Assessment

The surgical client requires the same assessments as the medical client, as well as routine preoperative and postoperative assessments.

Diagnosis, Planning, Implementation

Risk for Injury. When the client has the GERD treated surgically, the nursing diagnosis *Risk for Injury related to surgical procedure and presence of chest tubes* is appropriate.

Planning: Expected Outcomes. Injury will be prevented, as evidenced by absence of hemorrhage, no manifestations of infection, normal temperature, and absence of manifestations of problems associated with the chest tubes such as respiratory distress.

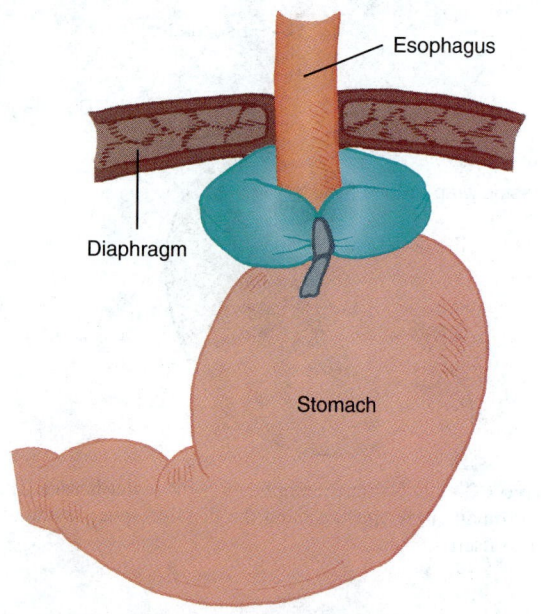

Figure 60–14. An Angelchik antireflux prosthesis in place.

Implementation. Preoperative care is basically the same as for other surgeries. Preoperative procedures include laboratory tests, preoperative medications, and an NPO status before surgery. Teach the client the importance of coughing and deep breathing after surgery to prevent respiratory complications. Clients will have an NG tube in place after surgery and the client should be taught the purpose and the nursing care associated with the NG tube.

If a thoracic approach is to be used, instruct the client on the purpose and care associated with chest tubes (see Chapter 42 for the care of the client with a chest tube). Postoperative breathing can be painful, so the client must cough and deep-breathe to avoid respiratory complications. With an abdominal incision, there is a greater chance of a wound infection. Assess the wound drainage for signs of infection.

The client will have an NG tube, and tube patency should be maintained to avoid stomach distention. Fluids are usually resumed after 24 hours and the diet is progressively advanced as tolerated as peristalsis returns. Small, frequent meals are provided to avoid overloading the stomach.

After fundoplication, the client could experience gas-bloat syndrome. This condition occurs if the wrap of the fundus is too tight, causing bloating and inability to eructate. Clients should avoid carbonated beverages, drinking with a straw, and gas-producing foods. Ambulation can assist peristalsis in removing air from the gastrointestinal tract. The condition is usually temporary. Instruct clients to report dysphagia, epigastric fullness, bloating, or excessive borborygmus to their physician.

Evaluation

If the medical treatment does not reverse the problem, then surgery is usually successful. The expected outcome

following surgery is complete recovery with normal nutrition.

Hiatal Hernia

A hiatal hernia, also referred to as a diaphragmatic hernia, is a condition in which the cardiac sphincter becomes enlarged, allowing a part of the stomach to pass into the thoracic cavity. There are two major types of hernias: (1) sliding hernias (type I) and (2) rolling or paraesophageal hernias (type II). In a sliding hernia, the upper stomach and the gastroesophageal junction are displaced upward into the thorax (Fig. 60–15). Sliding hernias account for approximately 90% of the total cases of esophageal hiatal hernias. With a rolling hernia, the gastroesophageal junction stays below the diaphragm, but all or part of the stomach pushes through into the thorax (Fig. 60–15).

The incidence of hiatal hernia is estimated as 5 per 1000 in the general population and may be as high as 60% in clients over 60 years of age. Females tend to be more often affected than males, and the incidence increases significantly with age. Sliding hiatal hernias may be noted in infants, but they usually do not produce manifestations until middle age. Rolling hiatal hernias are rarely noted in infants.

Etiology and Risk Factors

Hiatal hernias are related to muscle weakness in the esophageal hiatus, which loosens the esophageal supports and allows the lower portion of the stomach to rise into the thorax. As with other hernias, the muscle weakness is caused by a variety of conditions, such as aging, congenital muscle weakness, trauma, surgery, or anything that increases intra-abdominal pressure.

Risk factors for the development of hiatal hernias are any factors that lead to both weakness of the diaphragmatic muscle and increases in intra-abdominal pressure. The pressure may be increased by conditions such as obesity, pregnancy, or ascites.

Primary prevention of the hiatal hernia can be accomplished, or at least delayed, by losing weight and avoiding any activities that increase intra-abdominal pressure. Other than these measures, hiatal hernias are not preventable.

Pathophysiology

A hiatal hernia involves herniation of part of the stomach through a weakness in the diaphragm. The resulting regurgitation and motor dysfunction cause the major manifestations of hiatal hernia. With a sliding hernia, reflux appears to be caused by the exposure of the LES to the low pressure in the thorax. The major problem associated with a sliding hernia is the development of reflux.

With a rolling hernia, the LES remains below the diaphragm so reflux is not a problem. Complications of a

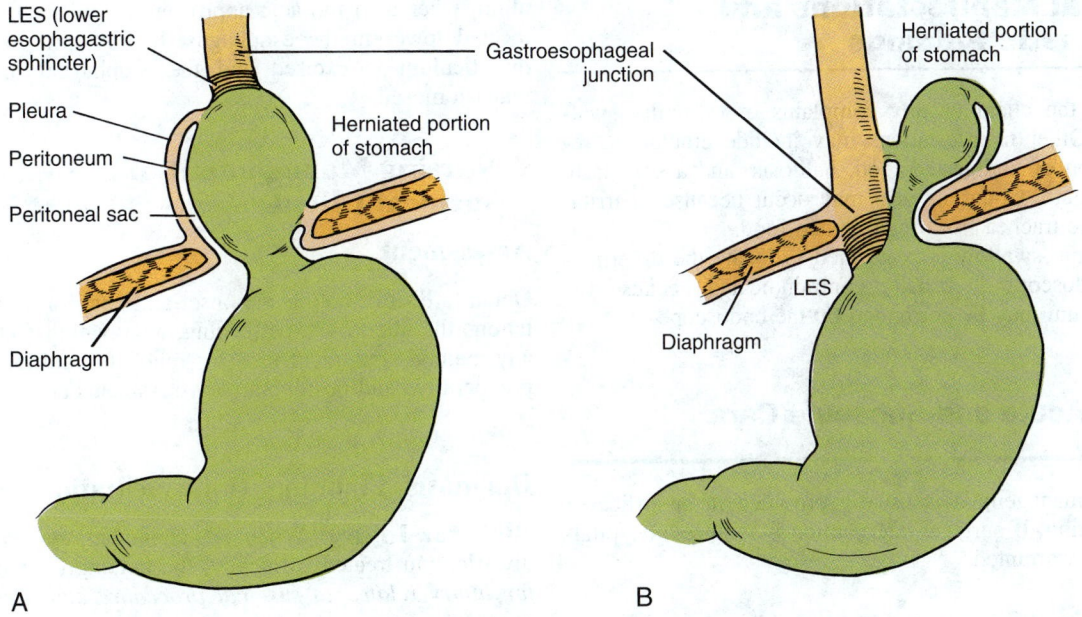

Figure 60–15. *A,* A sliding hiatal hernia. *B,* A rolling hiatal hernia.

rolling hiatal hernia include obstruction, strangulation, and the development of a volvulus.

Clinical Manifestations and Diagnostic Findings

Manifestations of hiatal hernia vary in kind and severity. In sliding hiatal hernias, clients may have heartburn 30 to 60 minutes after meals. In addition, reflux may result in substernal pain.

The client with a rolling hiatal hernia does not have manifestations of reflux. The client may complain of a feeling of fullness after eating or have difficulty breathing. Some clients experience chest pain similar to that of anginal pain. Pain is usually worse when the client assumes a recumbent position.

Hiatal hernias are diagnosed by a barium swallow, with fluoroscopy, showing the position of the stomach in relation to the diaphragm.

Management

The medical and surgical management for the client with a hiatal hernia is the same as that for the client with GERD.

The nursing care of the client with medical management of a hiatal hernia is the same as that for a client with GERD. As with GERD, the most common nursing diagnosis is *Pain related to irritation of the esophagus caused by gastric reflux.* The nursing care of the client with surgical management of a hiatal hernia is the same as that for the client with GERD. As with GERD, the most common collaborative problem is high risk of injury related to the surgical procedure and the presence of chest tubes.

Diverticula

Diverticula in the esophagus are saclike outpouchings in one or more layers of the esophagus. As food is ingested, it becomes trapped in a diverticulum and can later be regurgitated. The most common type of esophageal diverticulum is esophageal pulsion diverticulum (Zenker's diverticulum). Esophageal diverticula are considered rare. Zenker's diverticulum occurs three times more frequently in men than in women.

Etiology and Risk Factors

The cause of esophageal weakness could be a congenital defect, esophageal trauma, scar tissue, or inflammation. There are two categories of diverticula—(1) traction and (2) pulsion. In traction diverticula, the esophageal mucosa has pulled outward from the esophagus. Traction diverticula are most commonly found in the middle esophagus. In pulsion diverticula, the esophageal mucosa has pushed outward through a defect in the esophageal musculature. Pulsion diverticula are most commonly found in the upper esophagus. There is no means of prevention.

Pathophysiology

Diverticula in the esophagus are saclike outpouchings in one or more layers of the esophagus. They often develop in areas of muscle weakness that arise from esophageal trauma, congenital weakness of the esophageal wall, or scar tissue that forms from chronic inflammation of the esophagus. When food becomes trapped in a diverticulum, it may cause a local abscess. Infected diverticula place the client at risk for esophageal perforation because the mucosa is without the protection of the normal esophageal muscle layer.

Clinical Manifestations and Diagnostic Findings

Initially, the client usually complains of difficulty swallowing. Other manifestations may include eructation, regurgitation of undigested food, halitosis, and a sour taste in the mouth. Coughing also may occur because of irritation of the trachea from regurgitated food.

A barium swallow is performed to locate the diverticulum. Endoscopy is usually contraindicated because the diverticulum may be perforated by the endoscope.

Acute and Subacute Care

Medical management is usually provided in an office or clinic setting. If surgical intervention is required, hospitalization is warranted.

■ Medical Management

Medical management of manifestations of a diverticulum is achieved through dietary management and positioning. Small frequent feedings of semisoft foods often facilitate passage of food. The client should note what foods relieve or exacerbate the manifestations.

To prevent reflux of food, the client should have the head of the bed raised for 2 hours after meals. Nocturnal reflux can often be prevented by sleeping with the head of the bed elevated. The client also should avoid constrictive clothes and vigorous exercise after eating.

■ Nursing Management of the Medical Client

Assessment

Obtain a history from the client, noting the onset and duration of manifestations and whether or not they occur at mealtimes or at night. Assess the client's respiratory status because regurgitation can cause respiratory complications.

Diagnosis, Planning, Implementation

Pain. The client with difficulty swallowing often has the nursing diagnosis *Pain related to dysphagia.*

Planning: Expected Outcomes. The client will have a decrease in pain or an absence of pain, as evidenced by the client stating that the pain is decreased or absent, and by the client's ability to maintain oral intake.

Implementation. Teach the client the necessary changes in diet and how positioning can control manifestations. Encourage the client to try various foods and various positions to evaluate which are most effective.

■ Surgical Management

When manifestations become severe, surgery may be indicated. A cervical approach is used for Zenker's diverticulum, whereas a thoracic approach is used for diverticula located lower in the esophagus. In both procedures, the diverticulum is excised and the esophageal mucosa is reanastomosed.

■ Nursing Management of the Surgical Client

Assessment

Obtain a history noting the onset and duration of manifestations the client is experiencing, aggravating factors, and any methods the client uses for relief. In addition, routine preoperative and postoperative assessments are required.

Diagnosis, Planning, Implementation

Risk for Injury. When the client has the esophageal diverticulum treated surgically, the nursing diagnosis *Risk for Injury related to surgical procedure and presence of chest tubes* is appropriate.

Planning: Expected Outcomes. Injury will be prevented, as evidenced by absence of hemorrhage, no manifestations of infection, normal temperature, and absence of manifestations of problems associated with the chest tubes, such as respiratory distress.

Implementation. Discuss the normal preoperative routines. Tell the client that he or she will be NPO after surgery and an NG tube will be present until healing occurs. If a thoracic approach is used, preoperative and postoperative nursing care are similar to those for clients having thoracic surgery and chest tubes (see Chapter 42 for the care of the client after a thoracotomy and with chest tubes).

After surgery, the client's NG tube will be attached to low intermittent suction. Low intermittent suction is ordered by the physician to avoid trauma to the stomach lining. Assess the amount and color of the drainage during each shift. Check for continued bloody NG drainage as well as for manifestations of external bleeding. Do not irrigate or reposition the NG tube unless specifically ordered to do so by the physician. The Nursing Research feature describes the characteristics of feeding tube aspirates as a method of ascertaining tube location.

The client will receive intravenous fluids until tube feedings are begun. Once fluids and supplemental feedings are begun, record the client's response. Assess the client for manifestations of esophageal perforation, such as chest pain, elevated temperature, and subcutaneous emphysema.

Assess the client's pain and administer and evaluate prescribed analgesics. After surgery, the head of the bed should be elevated 30 degrees to reduce edema. Frequent practice of oral hygiene increases the client's comfort.

Following surgery, the client may be discharged with an NG or gastrostomy tube in place to allow for esophageal healing. The client should have written and verbal instructions about tube feedings, diet, and positioning. A visiting nurse should see the client at home to ensure that tube feedings are being tolerated well and continue visits until the feeding tube is removed.

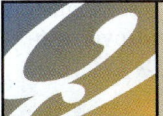

NURSING RESEARCH

What Does the Appearance of Aspirates from Feeding Tubes Indicate?

Metheny, N., et al. (1994). Visual characteristics of aspirates from feeding tubes as a method for predicting tube location. *Nursing Research, 43* (5), 282–287.

In this study, nurses classified feeding tube aspirates (N = 880) as being primarily clear or cloudy and as having one of six colors. Gastric aspirates were most frequently cloudy and green, tan or off-white, or bloody or brown. Intestinal fluids were primarily clear and yellow to bile-colored. In the absence of blood, pleural fluid was pale yellow and serous, and tracheobronchial secretions were usually tan or off-white mucus. However, respiratory aspirates often contained blood and therefore failed to have the expected characteristics of respiratory fluid. Staff nurses were able to characterize gastric and intestinal aspirates better than respiratory aspirates.

Implications for Practice

The appearance of aspirates is helpful in distinguishing between gastric and intestinal tube placement, but is of little value in ruling out respiratory tube placement.

Evaluation

An appropriate outcome for the client with a diverticulum is that the altered diet will control the problem. If surgery is required, the client should return to normal after healing occurs.

■ Modifications for Elderly Clients

Older adults are treated more conservatively, using diet and positioning rather than surgery. Surgery may entail too much risk for the older client.

Esophageal Neoplasms

Cancer of the esophagus takes the form of either squamous cell carcinoma or adenocarcinoma of the esophageal mucosa. In the United States, the incidence of squamous cell cancer of the esophagus is 4 per 100,000 males. The incidence is twice as high in males as in females, and it is higher in black, Japanese, and Chinese males than in white males. In northern China, the incidence in males is very high (130/100,000).[2] Adenocarcinoma of the esophagus occurs less often than squamous cell cancer and develops primarily in the distal esophagus. The Risk Factors and Levels of Prevention feature lists other contributing factors in esophageal cancer.

Etiology and Risk Factors

The cause of esophageal neoplasms is unknown, but researchers are studying environmental differences between locations with a low and a high incidence. In the Western world, evidence points to heavy smoking, nutritional deficiencies, and habitual ingestion of alcohol, hot foods, and hot drinks as underlying etiologic factors.

In other parts of the world, contaminants in the soil and food, high levels of nitrosamines, smoking opium, and nutritional deficiencies (especially of fruits and vegetables) have been linked to the condition. Chronic irritation from other esophageal problems such as achalasia, hiatal hernia, and stricture play a minor role in the development of esophageal cancer.

These are very preventable causes. Prevention particularly should be targeted toward the black male population in this country, because their risk is much higher. See the Risk Factors and Levels of Prevention feature.

Pathophysiology

Malignant tumors of the esophagus begin as slow-growing benign tissue changes. The majority of cancers are

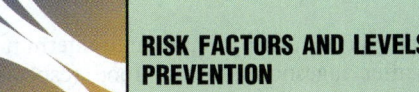

RISK FACTORS AND LEVELS OF PREVENTION

Esophageal Cancer

Risk Factors

Smoking of tobacco or opium; nutritional deficiencies; ingestion of hot foods and beverages; habitual ingestion of alcohol; nitrosamine ingestion; chronic irritation from gastroesophageal reflux disease (GERD), hiatal hernia, or achalasia

Levels of Prevention

Primary Prevention

- Encourage clients to limit smoking and chronic ingestion of alcohol, hot food and beverages, and nitrosamines.
- Encourage clients to consume a well-balanced diet.

Secondary Prevention

- Encourage clients to stop smoking.
- Advise clients to stop ingestion of alcohol, hot food and beverages, and food containing nitrosamines.
- Teach clients to follow life-style changes as recommended for GERD, hiatal hernia, and achalasia.

Tertiary Prevention

- Advise clients to seek and follow appropriate medical or surgical treatment for GERD, hiatal hernia, achalasia, alcoholism, and smoking abuse.

squamous epidermoid tumors that are commonly found in the middle or upper third of the esophagus. Because the esophagus has no serosal layer to limit its extension, it spreads rapidly. Esophageal tumors expand locally and very rapidly, and early spread to the lymph nodes is common. The rich lymphatic supply to the mucosa provides an excellent means for the tumor to metastasize widely. The tumors are typically intraluminal, ulcerating lesions that encircle the esophageal wall and extend upward and downward.

The disease is progressive and almost always fatal. As it progresses, most persons experience some pulmonary complications because of the formation of tracheo-esophageal fistulas that result in aspiration. If the condition is not treated, total esophageal obstruction is the inevitable outcome of the disease. Infiltration into blood vessels may predispose the client to hemorrhage.

Clinical Manifestations and Diagnostic Findings

Typically the first manifestations are dysphagia or odyno-phagia. Unfortunately, these manifestations are usually not apparent until the tumor involves the whole circumference of the esophagus. By the time the client becomes aware of a swallowing problem and seeks medical care, the tumor frequently has invaded the deeper layers of the esophagus and, sometimes, adjacent structures such as the bronchus.

At first, dysphagia is usually mild and intermittent, occurring only after ingestion of solid food (especially meat). Soon, dysphagia becomes constant, and manifestations of esophageal obstruction appear. These manifestations include an increase in salivation and mucus in the throat, nocturnal aspiration, regurgitation, and inability to swallow even liquids.

The diagnosis is confirmed by barium swallow, endoscopy, cytologic examination, and direct biopsy. Computed tomography (CT) scans provide an excellent definition of the size of the primary lesion and the extent of nodal involvement.

Acute and Subacute Care

■ Medical Management

Treatment of esophageal cancer depends on the location, size of the tumor, metastases, and the condition of the client. If the cancer is found in an early stage, the treatment is directed toward cure; however, it is usually detected in the late stages, when treatment becomes palliative and aimed specifically at allowing the client to continue eating.

Radiation Therapy. Radiation therapy is often used alone or in conjunction with surgery, either before or after surgery. Radiation provides palliation by reducing tumor size and slowing tumor growth. High-dose radia-

tion therapy may cause stenosis of the esophagus, so radiation treatments are usually administered over a 6- to 8-week period to minimize this effect.

Chemotherapy. Chemotherapy, combining several drugs, provides symptomatic relief. Chemotherapy combined with radiation and surgery is being studied.

Nutritional Management. Maintaining nutrition is a major goal for the client with esophageal cancer. In the beginning of the disease process, the client may be able to tolerate small, frequent feedings of soft or semisoft foods. As the disease progresses, feeding tubes may be needed. If necessary, a feeding gastrostomy or jejunostomy may be created. Short-term TPN may be used to improve the client's nutritional status before surgery. Proper positioning after meals is necessary in the client with frequent regurgitation, as well as in the client with a prosthesis. The head of the bed should always be elevated 30 degrees.

■ Nursing Management of the Medical Client

Assessment

Obtain data concerning the client's nutritional status. Most clients complain of dysphagia that is both persistent and progressive. The client initially may have difficulty swallowing solid foods and then progressively have difficulty swallowing soft foods and liquids.

A careful assessment of dysphagia is important. Other manifestations such as odynophagia, regurgitation, chronic cough, increased secretions, and hoarseness (due to involvement of the larynx) also are important to assess.

Diagnosis, Planning, Implementation

Altered Nutrition: Less than Body Requirements. Because of the progressively worsening dysphagia, the client with esophageal cancer exhibits the nursing diagnosis *Altered Nutrition: Less than Body Requirements, related to client's inability to swallow.*

Planning: Expected Outcomes. The client will maintain an adequate nutritional status, as evidenced by maintenance of stable body weight or slowed weight loss.

Implementation. Monitor the client's nutritional status throughout treatment, including daily weights, intake and output, and calories consumed. In the beginning, teach the client about diet changes that can make eating easier.

As the disease progresses, you may have to provide tube feedings. Assess the skin around the feeding tube for impairment of skin integrity caused by leakage of gastric juices. Wash the skin around the opening with a gentle soap and dry thoroughly twice daily or as needed. Apply protective ointments such as zinc oxide or karaya gum to the skin for further protection.

Risk for Impaired Swallowing. The client with esophageal cancer experiences increasing dysphagia which may lead to the diagnosis *Risk for Impaired Swallowing related to esophageal obstruction from tumor.*

Planning: Expected Outcomes. The client will not suffer from impaired swallowing, as evidenced by absence of choking and maintenance of a patent airway.

Implementation. Many problems arise when the client is unable to swallow. The client can easily choke on saliva and mucous secretions, and must spit frequently or drool. Constant wiping of saliva from the lips can cause irritation, cracking of the skin, and open lesions. Because it is impractical to collect this quantity of secretions in tissues, the client should carry a receptacle to receive the saliva. While hospitalized, clients are often taught to do self-suctioning. To prevent oral lesions and infections, and to provide comfort, the nurse should administer or assist with frequent oral care.

Risk for Ineffective Individual Coping. The client with cancer of the esophagus has many problems associated with both the disease itself and its treatment. This can lead to a nursing diagnosis of *Risk for Ineffective Individual Coping related to changes in body image and potentially terminal prognosis.*

Planning: Expected Outcomes. The client will effectively cope with the alterations in body image and potentially terminal prognosis, as evidenced by maintenance of activities and continued social interaction.

Implementation. In addition to meeting the client's physical needs, the nurse must provide emotional support. The gastrostomy tube may cause an alteration in body image and increased dependency. The drooling or need to spit constantly also may cause the client a great deal of emotional distress.

The poor prognosis of esophageal cancer necessitates psychological support and interventions aimed at helping the client and significant others prepare for the client's death.

■ Surgical Management

Esophageal dilation may be necessary throughout the course of the disease to treat strictures and tumor obstruction. The treatment should be performed by the physician as often as needed to relive dysphagia.

In advanced disease, a prosthesis may be inserted to bypass the tumor or to prevent aspiration in clients who develop fistulas. The prosthesis can maintain esophageal patency but can perforate the esophagus as the tumor size increases or become dislodged.

Surgery may be performed for cure or palliation, depending on the extent of the disease. There are three surgical procedures that can be performed. An esophagectomy is the removal of all or part of the esophagus. The resected esophagus is replaced with a Dacron graft. The esophagogastrostomy involves resecting the lower portion of the esophagus and anastomosing the remainder to the stomach, brought up into the thorax. The third procedure, esophagoenterostomy (also known as a colon interposition), involves resecting the esophagus and replacing it with a segment of the descending colon.

■ Nursing Management of the Surgical Client

Assessment

Obtain data concerning the client's nutritional status, ability to swallow, respiratory status, and ability to cope with the diagnosis. In addition, routine preoperative and postoperative assessments are required.

Diagnosis, Planning, Implementation

Risk for Injury. Surgery to treat esophageal cancer is often very extensive and usually requires a thoracic approach leading to the nursing diagnosis *Risk for Injury related to surgical procedure.*

Planning: Expected Outcomes. Injury will be prevented, as evidenced by absence of atelectasis, fever, wound infection, or problems associated with the chest tubes.

Implementation. Before surgery, clients usually require 2 to 3 weeks of nutritional support. Often, this support includes tube feedings or TPN. The client's weight and fluid and electrolyte status are monitored. Provide extensive instruction on postoperative respiratory care, including turning, coughing and deep-breathing, and chest physiotherapy. The client should be taught about all incisions, wound drainage tubes, feeding tubes, and chest tubes that may be present after surgery. Oral care should be performed four times a day to help prevent infection postoperatively. If an esophagoenterostomy is performed, a complete bowel preparation is performed before surgery.

After surgery, respiratory care is a high priority. The client may be placed on a ventilator (see Chapter 41 for care of a client receiving mechanical ventilation) in a critical care unit. Otherwise, the client must turn, cough, and deep-breathe every hour. Carefully assess the client's respiratory status and report any manifestations of atelectasis or pneumonia, and administer supplemental oxygen. Administer pain medication frequently, and assist the client in splinting the incision while coughing. Place the client in a semi-Fowler position to prevent reflux. Continually monitor the chest tube drainage for amount, color, and patency.

Assess the client's fluid and electrolyte status. Drainage from the NG, gastric, and all drainage tubes should be monitored at least every shift. The client will be NPO for 4 to 5 days until peristalsis returns. During the first 24 hours after surgery, NG or gastric drainage is bloody but should then change to a greenish-yellow color. If bloody drainage continues, it could indicate bleeding at the suture line and should be reported.

Leakage at the site of anastomosis may appear about 5 to 7 days after surgery. Assess the client for early manifestations of shock as well as manifestations of fever, fluid accumulation at the wound site, and manifestations of inflammation. Check all dressings for manifestations of bleeding, drainage, or separation of the suture lines.

The client should be started on small sips of water. If this intake is tolerated, the quantity is slowly increased. Supervise the client, making sure the client stays in an upright position, and monitor for manifestations of leakage at the anastomosis site. If this is tolerated, the client gradually progresses to pureed and semisolid foods. Teach the client the importance of small, frequent feedings and to always sit upright at meals and for 1 hour after meals to prevent overdistention of the stomach and reflux.

Upon discharge, the client and family should be given written and oral instructions concerning wound healing, nutritional support, respiratory care, and medications. Teach the client about possible wound and respiratory complications, manifestations that should be reported immediately, and how to contact appropriate members of the healthcare team.

Make appropriate referrals to community agencies. Most clients need a significant amount of assistance at home. Give the family information about services offered by the American Cancer Society and local hospice care if it becomes apparent that hospice care is necessary.

Evaluation

The poor prognosis means that successful control of symptoms may be the only reasonable outcome.

Vascular Disorders

The principal vascular disorder of the esophagus is varices. Because esophageal varices result from portal hypertension, this condition is discussed with liver disorders in Chapter 65.

Trauma

Major traumatic conditions of the esophagus include chemical burns, presence of foreign bodies, and injuries from external forces, such as endoscopic equipment. Chemical burns occur from the ingestion of acids or alkalis and sometimes from highly spiced foods. Thermal burns can result from drinking extremely hot liquids, accidental ingestion of foreign bodies that lodge in the natural narrow spots of the esophagus, and self-mutilation related to suicide attempts. Trauma can cause esophageal perforation with resultant contamination of the mediastinum and stricture formation as a complication of the healing process.

Treatment of esophageal strictures involves dilation of the esophagus or surgical excision of the diseased portion, and reanastomosis or interposition of a piece of gut from the stomach or colon (see under Esophageal Neoplasms).

Conclusions

Disorders of the mouth and esophagus range from fairly simple problems, such as dental caries, to complex and potentially lethal problems, such as cancer of the esophagus. Disorders throughout this oral-esophageal area, however, no matter how small, can interfere with the client's

nutritional intake. The nurse must always remember this fact when assessing and caring for clients with these disorders.

Thinking Critically

1. The client is a 72-year-old retired schoolteacher who lives with her 70-year-old sister. She is being evaluated for complaints of chest pain, which have become increasingly more frequent. Yesterday, while she was lifting flats of bedding plants to prepare for planting, she became dyspneic and collapsed. Her sister called the ambulance, and the client was admitted to a medical-surgical unit. This morning, she underwent an abdominal ultrasound prior to an upper GI series. The tests were followed by an ECG. When you last checked, she was sleeping soundly. Now her call light is on. As you enter the room, the client is gasping, clutching at her chest, and attempting to get out of bed, saying, "Please help me! I can't catch my breath!" What is your first priority?

Factors to Consider. Is the client experiencing symptoms of a cardiovascular problem or a gastrointestinal one? How could you tell the difference?

2. A 61-year-old woman is being treated as an outpatient for gastroesophageal reflux disease. She tells you that the doctor told her to take Maalox, but did not tell her how else to treat her condition. What would you teach her?

Factors to Consider. What life-style changes could help the client manage her condition?

3. An 18-year-old man is seen at a dental clinic following the blow of a soccer ball to the head. Several teeth were loosened by the impact. During the oral examination, you note that the gums are reddened and tender and bleed easily when probed with a tongue blade. The area under the left premolar is swollen, tender, and abscessed. The client pulls away and tells you to stop because it hurts too much to touch that tooth and states that "It's been hurting for the past several weeks." When questioned, the client states that he brushes his teeth once a day or every other day, has never flossed, and usually eats several candy bars a day. What nursing interventions are appropriate?

Factors to Consider. What might be the problem with the client's tooth? What could be the cause of his gingival problems?

Bibliography

1. Aliberti, L. (1993). Managing esophageal achalasia: Medical and nursing implications. *Gastroenterology Nursing, 16*(3), 126–130.
2. American Cancer Society. (1996). *Cancer facts and figures.* New York: Author.
3. Berry, S., et al. (1994). Intestinal placement of pH-sensing nasoin-

testinal feeding tubes. *JPEN: Journal of Parenteral and Enteral Nutrition, 18*(1), 67–70.

4. Bockus, S. (1993). When your patient needs tube feedings. *Nursing, 23*(7), 34–42.

5. Campbell, A., & Ferrara, B. (1993). Toupet partial fundoplication: Correcting, preventing gastroesophageal reflux. *AORN Journal, 57*(3), 671–679.

6. Chase, S. (1993). Antacids. *RN, 56*(8), 46–50.

7. Cheever, K. (1994). Fractured jaw: Your role after surgery. *Nursing, 24*(6), 32F.

8. Cole-Arvin, C., Notch, L., & Underhill, A. (1994). Identifying and managing dysphagia. *Nursing, 24*(1), 48–49.

9. Copstead, L. (1995). *Perspectives on pathophysiology.* Philadelphia: W. B. Saunders.

10. Eisenberg, P. (1994). Nasoenteral tubes. *RN, 57*(10), 62–70.

11. Eisenberg, P. (1994). Gastrostomy and jejunostomy tubes. *RN, 57*(11), 54–59.

12. Eisenberg, P. (1994). Feeding formulas. *RN, 57*(12), 46–53.

13. Georges, J., & Heitkemper, M. (1994). Dietary fiber and distressing gastrointestinal symptoms in midlife women. *Nursing Research, 43*(6), 357–361.

14. Good, M. (1995). A comparison of the effects of jaw relaxation and music on postoperative pain. *Nursing Research, 44*(1), 52–57.

15. Groenwald, S. L., et al. (Eds.) (1995). *Cancer nursing: Principles and practice* (3rd ed.). Boston: Jones & Bartlett.

16. Lee, N., Broome, A., & Pappas, T. (1994). Laparoscopic fundoplication: An alternate approach in the surgical treatment of esophageal reflux. *Today's OR Nurse, 16*(3), 44–45.

17. Lehne, R. (1994). *Pharmacology for nursing care* (2nd ed.). Philadelphia: W. B. Saunders.

18. Long, K., & Long, R. (1994). Treating gastroesophageal reflux disease. *Nurse Practitioner Forum, 5*(2), 63–64.

19. McCorkle R. (1996). *Cancer nursing: A comprehensive textbook.* (2nd ed.). Philadelphia; W. B. Saunders.

20. McGinnis, C., & Matson, S. (1994). How to manage patients with a Roux-en-Y jejunostomy. *American Journal of Nursing, 94*(2), 43–45.

21. Metheny, N., et al. (1993). Effectiveness of pH measurements in predicting feeding tube placement: An update. *Nursing Research, 42*(6), 314–331.

22. Metheny, N., et al. (1994). Visual characteristics of aspirates from feeding tubes as a method for predicting tube location. *Nursing Research, 43*(5), 282–287.

23. Miller, C. (1994). Alleviating the discomfort of gastroesophageal reflux disease. *Geriatric Nursing: American Journal of Care for the Aging, 15*(3), 171–172.

24. Miller, D., & Miller, H. (1995). Giving meds through the tube. *RN, 58*(1), 44–48.

25. Morton, L., & Fromkes, J. (1993). Gastroesophageal reflux disease: Diagnosis and medical therapy. *Geriatrics, 48*(3), 60–66.

26. Rakel, B., et al. (1994). Nasogastric and nasointestinal feeding tube placement: An integrative review of the literature. *AACN: Clinical Issues in Critical Care Nursing, 5*(2), 194–223.

27. Ricciardi, E., & Brown, D. (1994). Managing PEG tubes. *American Journal of Nursing, 94*(10), 29–31.

28. Robinson, M. (1994). Gastroesophageal reflux disease: Selecting optimal therapy. *Postgraduate Medicine, 95*(2), 88–102.

29. Rush, C. (1995). Gastrointestinal bleeding. *Nursing, 25,* 33.

30. Sabiston, D. (Ed.). (1994). *Atlas of general surgery.* Philadelphia: W. B. Saunders.

31. Sabiston, D., & Lyerly, H. (Eds.). (1994). *Essentials of surgery* (2nd ed.). Philadelphia: W. B. Saunders.

32. Saunderlin, G. (1993). Esophageal achalasia. *Gastroenterology Nursing, 15*(5), 191–196.

33. Shuster, M., & Mancino, J. (1994). Ensuring successful home tube feeding in the geriatric population. *Geriatric Nursing: American Journal of Care for the Aging, 15*(2), 67–84.

34. Sleisenger, M. H., & Fordtran, J. S. (Eds.). (1993). *Gastrointestinal disease: Pathophysiology/diagnosis/management* (5th ed.). Philadelphia: W. B. Saunders.

35. Spiro, H. (1994). Hiatal hernia and reflux esophagitis. *Hospital Practice, 29*(1), 51–66.

36. Swiech, K., Lancaster, D., & Sheehan, R. (1994). Use of a pressure gauge to differentiate gastric from pulmonary placement of nasoenteral feeding tubes. *Applied Nursing Research, 7*(4), 183–189.

37. Thompson, L. (1995). Taking a closer look at percutaneous endoscopic gastrostomy. *Nursing, 25*(4), 62–63.

38. Tombes, M., & Galucci, B. (1993). The effects of hydrogen peroxide rinses on normal oral mucosa. *Nursing Research, 42*(6), 332–337.

39. Whitney, L. (1993). Acute abdominal pain: Revealing the source. *Nursing, 23*(9), 34–41.

40. Whitney, L. (1994). Caring for a gastrostomy. *Nursing, 24*(8), 48–50.

41. Whitney, L. (1995). Vincent's angina, periodonitis, and stomatitis. *Nursing, 25,* 32.

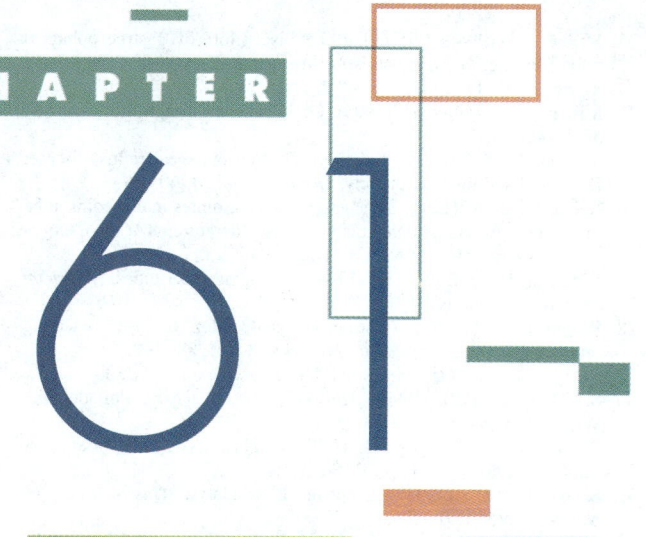

Nursing Care of Clients with Gastric Disorders

Jane Hokanson Hawks

The client with a gastric disorder usually has a problem with nutritional intake. As a result, the most common nursing diagnoses are altered nutrition (less than body requirements) and pain. With obesity and bulimia nervosa, the nursing diagnosis is altered nutrition (more than body requirements). Additional nursing diagnoses such as knowledge deficit related to dietary changes and pharmacologic management, fear, body image disturbance, and high risk for injury related to complications are also possible.

General Clinical Manifestations of Gastrointestinal Disorders

Manifestations of gastric dysfunction are caused by the following:

1. Excessive gastric secretions that erode stomach mucosa
2. Excessive motility
3. Retention of gastric contents

The most prominent manifestations are pain, acid eructation, anorexia, belching, nausea, vomiting, hemorrhaging, and diarrhea.

Pain

Pain is the most characteristic manifestation; it usually results from chemical irritation of nerve endings. Nerve irritation occurs when acid comes into contact with the eroded stomach mucosa. It also results from stretching and contracting of the stomach, caused in turn by increased motility and increased smooth muscle tension, as is found in an obstruction.

Anorexia

Anorexia, or loss of appetite, is often experienced by clients with malignancy or various other disorders. Hun-

This chapter incorporates material written for the fourth edition by Shirley M. Ruder.

ger is normally caused by several stimuli, including contraction of the empty stomach. When the stomach empties slowly or when gastric stasis occurs because of a gastric disorder, anorexia can result.

Nausea

Nausea is a result of conditions that increase tension on the walls of the stomach, duodenum, or lower end of the esophagus. Unpleasant stimuli or distention, gastritis, and carcinoma of the stomach can produce nausea. Vomiting may follow nausea or occur without it. Recall from Chapter 60 that vomiting is caused by stimulation of the emetic center. Vomiting is stimulated by the following:

- The chemoreceptor trigger zone (CTZ) in the fourth ventricle. The CTZ is stimulated by various drugs and body toxins. Conversely, medications of the phenothiazine derivative groups, such as chlorpromazine (Thorazine) and prochlorperazine (Compazine), depress vomiting caused by chemoreceptor stimulation. Serotonin antagonists, such as ondansetron (Zofran), block serotonin receptors in the vagus nerve and CTZ
- Nerve impulses, which can be excited by the following:

  Direct mechanical stimuli, as in increased intracranial pressure
  Chemical stimuli from bloodborne metabolites or toxic substances
  Sympathetic and parasympathetic afferent nerve impulses through the vagus, glossopharyngeal, vestibular, and splanchnic nerves; the most sensitive receptors are located in the proximal duodenum
- Unpleasant odors, subjects, and sights that stimulate higher-center impulses
- Distention of stomach or duodenum
- Decreased gastric motility
- Pain, because the pain centers are close to the vomiting centers in the medulla
- Increased intracranial pressure

Bleeding results from local trauma or irritations that cause erosion or ulceration of the GI tract mucosa. The disorders involved include stomach neoplasms, gastric ulcer, gastritis, anastomotic (marginal) ulcers, and duodenal ulcers. Duodenitis can also cause bleeding. Although bleeding may arise from numerous causes, up to three quarters of all cases of upper GI tract bleeding result from esophagogastric varices (venous), hemorrhagic gastritis (capillary), or peptic ulcer. Ulcers account for 80% of all upper GI tract hemorrhage.

Diarrhea

Diarrhea can be caused by increased peristalsis resulting from an increased gastrocolic reflex or from the effort of the stomach and intestines to eliminate a local irritant.

Belching and Flatulence

Swallowed air causes most belching and flatulence. It is easy to swallow air during eating and drinking, especially in the case of clients who ingest food rapidly. Frequently, clients attempt to belch to relieve a vague feeling of distress in the stomach caused by swallowed air. Attempting to belch with the mouth closed sometimes adds more air to the stomach than it removes.

Dyspepsia

Dyspepsia (indigestion) can be caused by such factors as strong emotions, GI tract disease, eating too rapidly, chewing inadequately, gas-forming foods (e.g., beans and cabbage), or food allergy.

Gastrointestinal Intubation

Gastric and intestinal tubes are inserted for several purposes: decompression, lavage, gastric analysis, and tube feedings. *Decompression* relieves the pressure caused by contents and gases that remain in the stomach or bowel because of some obstruction. Long intestinal tubes are sometimes used to dilate or release an obstruction. Postoperative decompression removes secretions that cannot pass through the GI tract because of edema and decreased gastric motility. Intubation helps prevent vomiting, distention, and obstruction.

Lavage is the irrigation or washing out of an organ. Gastric lavage washes out the stomach. It is used most frequently as an emergency treatment in poisoning. Lavage is also used for exfoliative cytology to determine the presence of abnormal cells.

Tube feeding or *gavage feeding*, referred to as *enteral nutrition*, is a method of giving clients fluids and nutrients via a tube when oral intake is inadequate or impossible.

Types of Tubes

Three types of tubes are used for decompression: (1) short nasogastric tubes are used for the stomach, (2) medium tubes extend into the duodenum or jejunum, and (3) long tubes are for the rest of the GI tract (Table 61–1).

Short Tubes

Short tubes include the Levin and Salem sump tubes. Short tubes are long enough to extend into the stomach but not into the bowel. These tubes are usually attached to suction. Occasionally, they may be used for enteral feedings over a short period. However, nasoduodenal tubes are preferred for feedings because of the high rate of aspiration pneumonia associated with nasogastric tube feedings.

■ Levin Tube

The Levin tube is an older, single-lumen tube used to remove fluid or gas or to obtain a specimen of gastric

Table 61–1. Gastric and Intestinal Tubes				
	Length	**Size (French)**	**Lumen**	**Other Characteristics**
Short Tubes				
Levin type (plastic or rubber)	125 cm (50″)	12, 16, 18	Single	
Salem sump	120 cm (48″)	12, 14, 16, 18	Double	Sump-type suction
Medium Tubes				
Dobhoff (nasoduodenal or nasojejunal)	160–175 cm (60–66″)	8, 10, 12	Single	Radiopaque, tungsten-weighted
Long Tubes				
Cantor	300 cm (10′)	16	Single	Mercury weighted
Harris	180 cm (6′)	14, 16	Single	Mercury weighted
Miller-Abbott	300 cm (10′)	12, 14, 16, 18	Double	Mercury weighted

contents. Because it only has one lumen, low intermittent suction is required to minimize the irritation of the gastric mucosa. Levin tubes may be made out of plastic, Silastic, or rubber.

■ Salem Sump Tube

The Salem sump tube is a double-lumen tube used to empty and decompress the stomach. Low continuous suction is used because the "pigtail" lumen on the Salem vents the tube and protects gastric mucosa from being sucked against the tube. The pigtail lumen should not be clamped or irrigated and should be kept higher than the client's stomach to prevent drainage.

Medium Tubes

Medium tubes include a variety of nasoduodenal (e.g., Dobhoff) tubes that extend into the duodenum and are designed for short-term feeding use. They are less likely to cause aspiration pneumonia because of their small size and weighted tip. Placement is verified via x-ray.

Long Tubes

The long tubes extend into the small bowel, sometimes for its entire length. They are between 1.8 and 3.0 m (6 and 10 ft) long and are used to prevent gas and fluid accumulation in the intestine, which is usually caused by intestinal obstruction. The more common long tubes are the Miller-Abbott, Cantor, and Harris tubes.

■ Miller-Abbott Tube

The Miller-Abbott tube is a double-lumen, 3 m (10 ft) tube. One lumen is used to introduce mercury or to inflate the balloon at the end of the tube, and the other is used for aspiration. Markings on the tube indicate how far the tube has been passed. Initial placement of this tube is usually completed by a physician, whereas you are responsible for advancing the tube as ordered.

■ Cantor Tube

The Cantor tube is used for aspirating intestinal contents and has only one lumen. It is 3 m (10 ft) long and is larger than the others. It has 4 to 5 ml of mercury in a bag at the end, which is wrapped about the tube before insertion. For intestinal intubation, the tube is threaded through the nose into the stomach and then through the pylorus, where peristaltic activity of the bowel carries it to the desired intestinal area.

■ Harris Tube

The Harris tube is a single-lumen, mercury-weighted tube, 1.8 m (6 ft) long. It has a metal tip that is introduced into the nostril after being lubricated. The weight of the mercury carries the tube by gravity. This tube is used for suction and irrigation.

Sometimes it is difficult to get intestinal tubes to pass through the pylorus. The client is instructed to lie on the right side. Once the tube has passed into the duodenum, it is advanced, as ordered, an additional 4.8 to 9.6 cm (2 to 4 inches) every hour or half-hour. Once the tube has reached the desired location, it is taped securely to prevent further advancement.

Other Tubes

For long-term enteral feedings, gastrostomy tubes (GT or G-tubes) or jejunostomy tubes (JT or J-tubes) are often placed surgically. The percutaneous gastrostomy (PEG), which is the most common, and the percutaneous jejunostomy (PEJ) were discussed in Chapter 60. The GT and JT can be inserted surgically or laparoscopically. These feeding tubes were also discussed in Chapter 60.

Inserting Gastrointestinal Tubes

Gastrointestinal tubes are generally inserted through the nose into the stomach or small intestine; they are rarely inserted through the mouth. Explain each step of the intubation procedure at the client's level of understanding. Assist the client to assume a high Fowler's position, which makes intubation easier. Measure the distance on the tube from the tip of the nose to the ear lobe, plus the distance from the ear lobe to the tip of the xiphoid process (called the NEX measurement). This approximates the distance that the tube must be passed to reach the stomach. Mark this distance on the tubing with adhesive. After measuring the tube, lubricate it and gently insert it through the nares and posterior nasal pharynx and into the oropharynx. Once the tube is in the oropharynx, instruct the client to swallow (sometimes the client is allowed to drink water at this point to help with tube passage). This measure is important because the sphincter at the proximal end of the esophagus remains closed except during swallowing. The larynx rises during swallowing, stretching the cricopharyngeal muscle and causing it to relax, thus reducing resistance to the tube. Swallowing also enables the tube to enter the esophagus rather than the trachea. After the tube passes the sphincter, advance it into the stomach.

To verify placement, perform at least two of the following activities:

1. Aspirate gastric contents
2. Instill air into the tube with a syringe and listen with a stethoscope for air passing into the stomach
3. Measure the pH of the aspirant
4. Check the x-ray of the tube with radiopaque lines

The Nursing Research feature describes the effectiveness of pH measurements in predicting feeding tube placements. The next Nursing Research feature addresses the use of a pressure gauge to differentiate gastric from pulmonary placement of nasoenteral feeding tubes. After confirming placement, secure the tube to the nose with hypoallergenic tape. (This procedure is used for short tubes only; medium tubes are checked with an x-ray, and long tubes need to be able to advance).

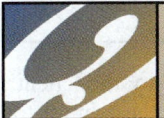

NURSING RESEARCH

Can the ph Value of Aspirated Fluid Indicate Feeding Tube Placement?

Metheny, N., et al. (1993). Effectiveness of pH measurements in predicting feeding tube placement: An update. *Nursing Research, 42*(6), 324–331.

Checking the pH of an aspirated fluid sample can help distinguish between gastric and intestinal placement of a feeding tube. A sample of 405 aspirates from nasogastric tubes and 389 aspirates from nasointestinal tubes was obtained. Eighty-five percent of the time, aspirate for nasogastric tubes had pH values ranging from 1 to 6. Eighty-seven percent of the time, nasointestinal aspirate had pH values greater than 6. These findings are consistent with the 1989 study by Metheny and co-workers.

Implications for Practice

The findings support the use of pH testing of tube feeding aspirate to determine placement of the tube. Values less than 6 suggest nasogastric placement while values greater than 6 suggest nasointestinal placement.

Suctioning Gastrointestinal Tubes

When suction is applied to a GI tube to remove accumulated gas and fluid, it is important to ensure that the GI mucosa is not traumatized. Excessive negative pressure causes the mucosa to be sucked into the openings on the tube, impairing the effectiveness of the suction and injuring the mucosa. Intermittent suction is commonly used to avoid this problem unless a double-lumen tube, such as the Salem sump, is used. Mucus tends to plug the openings of these tubes, so irrigate the openings as ordered to maintain or to check their patency (usually every 4 hours).

Nursing Management of Clients with Gastrointestinal Tubes

It is very important to maintain the client's comfort while the tube is in place. Some helpful nursing interventions include the following:

- Gently clean and lubricate external nares. They may become sore from crusted secretions around the tube. Always use a water-soluble lubricant.
- Tape the tube in a manner that prevents irritation to the nares.
- Administer frequent oral hygiene to remove debris, increase comfort, maintain a healthy oral cavity, and

stimulate saliva secretion. The client's mouth is usually dry because the absence of chewing prevents the normal stimulus to salivary secretions and because the presence of the tube causes mouth breathing.

- If possible, let the client chew gum or suck on sour candies or ice chips to help stimulate salivation. Excessive use will stimulate gastric secretions and cause electrolyte loss through the suction.
- Brush the client's teeth or assist the client to do so.
- Request an order for anesthetic mouth rinses or lozenges because clients frequently experience sore throats from the presence of the tube.

Placement of the tube in the throat may result in cricoid chondritis (irritation of the cricoid cartilage of the larynx) and laryngeal injuries. Presenting manifestations include the following:

Localized odynophagia
Pain radiating to the ears
Sore throat
Stridor
Bloody sputum
Mild hoarseness

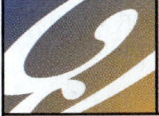

NURSING RESEARCH

Can a Pressure Gauge Help to Distinguish Gastric from Pulmonary Placement of Nasoenteral Tubes?

Swiech, K., Lancaster, D., & Sheehan, R. (1993). Use of a pressure gauge to differentiate gastric from pulmonary placement of nasoenteral feeding tubes. *Applied Nursing Research, 7*(4), 183–189.

The purpose of this study was to determine the reliability and validity of using a pressure gauge to differentiate gastric from pulmonary placement of nasoenteral tubes in 46 non-mechanically ventilated clients. It was anticipated that on inhalation, tubes properly placed in the gastric region would yield positive readings because of positive gastric pressures. Conversely, tubes inadvertently placed in the pulmonary system were expected to yield negative pressure readings because of the negative pulmonary pressures that exist on inhalation. Of the 46 subjects, 44 had positive gauge readings, and x-ray results showed that the nasoenteral tubes were in the gastric region. Two clients had negative gauge readings, and the x-rays showed that the nasoenteral tubes were in the pulmonary system.

Implications for Practice

The findings indicate that this method of assessing nasoenteral tube placement may be a safe, reliable, and cost-effective method of differentiating gastric from pulmonary tube placement.

Assess for these potential complications and report your findings immediately. The physician may order anesthetic lozenges or gargles to relieve the manifestations.

Frequently assess the material aspirated via the tube for color, odor, and quantity. Report any changes to the physician. It may be necessary to send samples of these secretions to the laboratory for analysis. Measure contents of the suction canisters to maintain an accurate record of GI losses. Metabolic alkalosis may result from a major loss of water and electrolytes. Monitor potassium levels, as potassium is one of the major electrolytes lost through suctioning.

Remember that the irrigating solution instilled into a GI tube is counted as intake, if is not removed when aspirating contents. Keep accurate records of how much is instilled and how much is aspirated from the tube during irrigations. Normal saline is often the irrigating solution of choice because water, a hypotonic solution, increases electrolyte loss through osmotic action if the tube is irrigated often.

Nutritional Support

Nutritional support is commonly required for clients with GI problems. Two types of nutritional support commonly used are enteral nutrition and parenteral nutrition.

Enteral Nutrition

Enteral nutrition contains nutrients (needed fats, carbohydrates, and proteins) that the client takes in via the GI tract. This nutrition can be supplemental to the general diet or can replace oral intake totally. In the case of clients with gastric and many GI tract disorders, this nutrition is often given through gastric or intestinal tubes, rather than orally.

GI feedings have physiologic and financial advantages over parenteral nutrition. They help to maintain GI structure (villi height and number) and the mucosal barrier. They also help to maintain GI motility that discourages bacterial overgrowth. Financially, enteral feedings are cheaper to administer. However, when the GI tract must rest because of illness or surgery, parenteral nutrition becomes the preferred choice for meeting nutritional needs.

Potential problems associated with enteral feedings, include the following:

Tube obstruction
Aspiration
Diarrhea
Distention
Constipation
Hyperglycemia
Hyperosmolar hyperglycemic nonketotic dehydration
Tube feedings syndrome
Hypercapnia
Electrolyte abnormalities

Routes and Formulas

Routes for tube feeding vary according to the client's condition. Several types of tubes exist for the administration of enteral feedings in clients who are unable to take them orally (e.g., nasogastric, gastrostomy, nasoduodenal, and jejunostomy tubes). Gastrostomy and jejunostomy tubes are preferred for long-term enteral feedings, whereas nasogastric and nasoduodenal tubes are common for short-term use.

Commercially prepared tube feedings as well as individually prepared formulas may be used to provide essential nutrients. The formulas differ in osmolality, digestibility, caloric density, lactose content, viscosity, fat content, fiber content, and expense. Many healthcare facilities mix their own tube feedings, which can then be tailored to suit the client. The physician, usually in consultation with the nutritionist, will determine the appropriate solution for each client. If diarrhea occurs, decreasing the concentration of the feeding and/or slowing the rate of administration usually controls the problem.

Methods of Administration

Tube feedings are administered either as a bolus feeding, as intermittent feedings, or by continuous infusion. The feeding can be administered by bolus push, gravity drainage, or infusion pump. The choice of the type of infusion and method of delivery depends on the disease and the client's ability to tolerate the feedings. Volumetric or peristaltic pumps are often employed to maintain a constant flow rate. Tubes smaller than 10F require a pump designed specifically for enteral feeding to maintain patency.

Continuous Feeding Method

The continuous feeding method is the method of choice for the critically ill and for clients fed via the small intestine. Continuous-drip feedings help to minimize cramping, nausea, and diarrhea. The rate of the continuous feedings is usually controlled with a feeding pump.

Intermittent Feeding Method

Intermittent feedings are given periodically; an administration set is used and the drip rate is adjusted to the client's tolerance. For example, a scheduled feeding of 400 ml is given over 30 minutes four to six times a day. Intermittent feedings are often the preferred method for clients on home tube-feeding regimens because they can be free of the feeding apparatus for part of the day and are able to engage in regular activities between feedings.

Bolus Feeding Method

For many years, the bolus method was the common procedure for tube feeding, and although it is theoretically obsolete, it is still occasionally practiced. To administer bolus feedings, pour a prescribed amount of room-temperature formula (usually 250 to 400 ml) slowly into the barrel of an Asepto syringe or funnel that is attached to the end of the feeding tube. The formula flows by gravity into the stomach or small intestine. This method is likely to cause nausea, vomiting, aspiration, diarrhea, or cramping, because large amounts of formula are given over a short period. The continuous or intermittent feeding methods are preferable.

Nursing Management of Clients Receiving Enteral Nutrition

Assessment

When administering tube feedings, review (1) the type of formula; (2) the time, frequency, and amount of feeding; and (3) the specific indications for the client. Most clients need a period of acclimatization to adjust to tube feeding, generally starting with a low rate and strength that is gradually increased until the desired amount of formula is being given.

Diagnosis, Planning, Implementation

Atelectasis, Pneumonia. Risks are associated with tube feedings. The most common potential complications are related to the collaborative problem *Atelectasis and Pneumonia related to aspiration of tube feeding.*

Planning: Expected Outcomes. You will prevent aspiration.

Implementation. The client should be sitting upright or have the head of the bed elevated at least 30 degrees. During the feedings, monitor for manifestations of intolerance, which include cramping, diarrhea, nausea, vomiting, aspiration, glycosuria, diaphoresis, and restlessness.

Before each tube feeding, explain the procedure to the client and significant others. Always check the placement of the tube. For gastric tubes, gently aspirate gastric contents with a syringe and measure the pH of the gastric contents. Antacids and gastric acid inhibitors can alter the pH. X-Ray confirmation is the most reliable way to ensure proper placement, but this method is impractical in most situations and is used almost exclusively to confirm initial tube placement. Injecting air into small-bore tubes is not always an accurate way to determine placement, because small-bore tubes can lodge in the bronchus without causing respiratory distress.

Check gastric residual volumes by aspirating stomach contents before each feeding, or every 4 to 8 hours. A residual volume greater than 100% to 120% of the previous hour's intake or greater than 100 to 150 ml indicates delayed gastric emptying. Notify the physician before giving additional formula. Re-instill the residual feeding to prevent excessive fluid and electrolyte losses unless the residual volume appears abnormal, e.g., contains coffee ground–like material, which is usually old blood. If this problem occurs, notify the physician.

To administer tube feedings, pour the formula into the bag attached to the feeding administration set. Prime the tubing prior to connecting the administration tubing to the feeding tube. This decreases air that can cause increased

gas. Start the feeding by releasing the clamp on the tubing or by turning on the pump. Assess the client's reaction to the feeding. If abdominal cramps develop, you may need to decrease the infusion rate. If the cramps continue, stop the infusion and notify the physician.

After the feeding, the client should remain in a sitting position or with the head of the bed elevated at least 30 degrees to promote gastric emptying and discourage regurgitation and aspiration. Make sure the client is comfortable and place the call light within easy reach. Chart the time of the feeding, amount of formula and water given, amount of residual volume, and the client's response to the feeding. Return to check on the client in 20 minutes, or sooner as needed.

The feeding tube should be flushed with 50 to 100 ml of water before and after intermittent feedings, every 4 hours during continuous feedings, and before and after any medications are administered via the feeding tube. If an obstruction occurs, try flushing the tube with water, saline, cranberry juice, or cola, after checking placement to be sure the tube is not in the lungs.

To minimize bacterial contamination, the feeding set should be changed every 24 hours. In addition, the bag should be rinsed every 4 hours, and no more than 4 hours worth of formula should be placed in the feeding set at one time.

Nursing management of the client receiving enteral feeding involves the same principles as does caring for someone with a nasal or oral tube. Possible complications include the following:

1. Vomiting and aspiration if the stomach is overfilled
2. Plugging of the tube
3. Dislocation of the tube into the trachea or lungs
4. Development of ulcerations and dried secretions in the nares
5. Tracheoesophageal fistula, which is a breakdown of the anterior esophageal wall, resulting from prolonged contact between the nasogastric tube and a tracheostomy tube, if present

With the development of soft, small-bore tubes, the last complication has become very rare. Suspect tracheoesophageal fistula when gastric contents appear in tracheal excretion. If it is not apparent, blue food coloring can be added to the feeding so that the coloring is apparent when the lungs are suctioned. Notify the physician, because this condition requires immediate intervention.

Risk for Fluid Volume Deficit. The client with a feeding tube is dependent on you for fluid intake and at risk for diarrhea. The potential nursing diagnosis is *Risk for Fluid Volume Deficit related to excess fluid loss or inadequate fluid intake.*

Planning: Expected Outcomes. The client will not develop a fluid volume deficit. He or she will have no manifestations of dehydration or diarrhea and will have an adequate intake of fluids.

Implementation. The client must be assessed for dehydration. Clients receiving tube feedings may lose fluids from excessive diarrhea, excessive protein intake, or osmotic diuresis. They also may not take in enough water. If the client continues to have problems with diarrhea, slow the rate and strength of the infusion or change to a more defined formula.

Carefully monitor for changes in skin turgor, vital signs, intake and output, mucous membrane moisture, level of consciousness, fever, and disorientation. The client's electrolyte and blood urea nitrogen (BUN) levels must be measured at regular intervals. Daily weights also should be obtained. Monitor for osmotic diuresis from high glucose load, especially if the infusion rate is increased. Keeping the formula at a constant infusion rate can also help ensure intake, as does routinely irrigating the tube with at least 50 ml of water every 4 hours. If sufficient water is not given, it will be taken from the tissues.

Constipation. Partly as a result of the fluid volume deficit, the nursing diagnosis *Constipation related to immobility and possible dehydration* is a common one.

Planning: Expected Outcomes. The client will not be constipated. He or she will have at least one bowel movement every other day with soft, formed stool.

Implementation. The client's dehydration status must be assessed to determine if dehydration is a possible cause of the constipation. Increasing the water intake may be a simple solution to this problem. The client should be encouraged to ambulate as much as possible to lessen the effect of immobility on bowel function. Assess bowel sounds for hypoactivity or absence of bowel sounds and notify the physician if these occur.

If constipation continues, a stool softener may need to be ordered. The contents of the formula of the feeding also could be changed to a fiber-enriched formula to improve defecation. Sometimes, simply allowing the client to use the toilet or a bedside commode can improve defecation.

Tube feedings should be discontinued if the client develops severe nausea, vomiting, increased abdominal girth, or epigastric and left upper quadrant pain, or if there is a large residual volume after feeding. It is important to stop the feedings because the client could vomit and aspirate the vomitus.

Diarrhea. Enteral feedings often alter bowel motility. Write the nursing diagnosis as *Diarrhea related to enteral feedings*.

Planning: Expected Outcomes. The client will not have diarrhea. The client will have at least one bowel movement every other day with soft, formed stool.

Implementation. Monitor the client for the presence of diarrhea. Possible causes of diarrhea include the following:

Bacterial contamination of the formula
Lactose intolerance
Osmotic action caused by hyperosmolar fluids
Fecal impaction
Concurrent drug therapy (especially antibiotics or elixirs containing sorbitol)
Low serum albumin level

Carefully assess bowel sounds for hyperactivity and notify the physician if hyperactive bowel sounds are heard.

The perianal skin should be carefully cleaned after each bowel movement and a skin barrier applied to prevent skin irritation. If diarrhea continues, carefully monitor the client for manifestations of fluid and electrolyte imbalances, especially hypokalemia.

Risk for Ineffective Management of Therapeutic Regimen (Individuals) and Risk for Ineffective Management of Therapeutic Regimen: Families. Clients are often discharged on tube feedings, so the nursing diagnosis is *Risk for Ineffective Management of Therapeutic Regimen (Individuals) or Risk for Ineffective Management of Therapeutic Regimen: Families related to tube feeding regimen for home feeding*.

Planning: Expected Outcomes. The client and significant others will understand how to self-administer tube feedings at home. They will be able to demonstrate correct procedures and explain possible problems and solutions.

Implementation. Some clients who require long-term enteral feeding are candidates for home enteral feeding programs. You or the dietician should assess the client's home environment and life-style before planning the program. Significant others should be included in teaching efforts. It is easy for the client to use prepared formulas rather than preparing them himself or herself. The use of prepared formulas also ensures that the client will receive all required nutrients. When chewing is important to the client's mental state, allow the client to chew food and spit it out.

Intermittent nocturnal feedings are the method of choice for home feedings so the client can be free of the equipment for at least part of the day. Clients need to sleep with the head of the bed elevated.

Be sure the client and significant others are taught proper storage of the formula, care of the administration apparatus, maintenance of tube patency, complications to monitor for, and when to notify the physician.

The Bridge to Home Healthcare provides suggestions for managing tube feedings at home.

Evaluation

The client should tolerate the enteral feedings without significant problems. If excessive side effects occur, the feedings should be adjusted to decrease these. The client and family should be able to learn to manage the feedings before discharge.

Parenteral Nutrition (Total Parenteral Nutrition or Hyperalimentation)

Many clients with GI tract disorders are unable to ingest, digest, or absorb sufficient nutrients to maintain a state of anabolism or positive nitrogen balance. These clients require total parenteral nutrition (TPN). One or more of the following criteria apply to these clients:

● Have debilitating diseases, such as malabsorption of the bowel
● Are unable to eat adequate amounts of nutrients

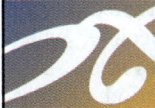

BRIDGE TO HOME HEALTHCARE

Managing Tube Feedings

Colette McVaney, R.N., B.S.N., *Visiting Nurse Association of Omaha, Omaha, Nebraska*

Knowing how to maintain patency of the feeding tube faciliates the transition from hospital to home care. Consistently flushing the tube before and after each feeding with water enhances the longevity of the tube. Although flushing the tube with carbonated beverages has been suggested, studies indicate few or no benefits as compared with flushing with water. Flush all types of feeding tubes with a 50 cc syringe; smaller syringes can create pressures high enough to rupture a tube.

Teach the patient and family to secure a nasogastric tube firmly to the nose or to either side of the face or to a position of comfort utilizing tape or a transparent occlusive dressing. When the patient has a percutaneous endoscopic gastrostomy or percutaneous endoscopic jejunostomy, observe daily for tube dislodgment, leaking, skin irritation and clinical manifestations of infection. Clean the site daily with hydrogen peroxide followed by normal saline rinse. Slide the external bridge away for cleaning and then reposition. No dressing is required. All caregivers need to use good handwriting technique.

Management of tube feedings varies with the type of infusion: continuous infusion with a pump, bolus infusion or infusion by gravity. Numerous commercial feedings are available to meet the individual's nutritional needs. When possible, refer patients receiving tube feedings to the agency's nutritionist for periodic evaluation. The physician and the nutritionist are responsible for assessing these needs. However, the client may tolerate one feeding better than another. Positioning the client at a 45-degree angle or greater helps him or her to tolerate the feedings. Changing the rate and frequency of infusion may decrease or eliminate nausea, diarrhea, and abdominal cramping.

Referral to a home care agency provides the family with an important resource. The family can contact the agency staff about difficulties such as cramping, nausea, diarrhea, or tube displacement. Successful tube feeding begins in the hospital and can continue at home with the cooperation of the client, family, home care nurse, nutritionist, and physician.

- Have gastric cancer or cancer cachexia
- Are undergoing chemotherapy or radiotherapy
- Have anorexia nervosa
- Have excessive metabolic needs (e.g., extensive burns or draining wounds)

TPN may also be used to rest the GI tract when a fistula or inflammatory bowel disease is present or after an intestinal obstruction is removed.

Routes and Formulas

TPN is most commonly administered through an indwelling subclavian catheter, which is inserted by the supraclavicular, intraclavicular, antecubital fossa, or internal jugular route into the superior vena cava (Fig. 61–1). A Hickman or Broviac catheter; tunneled, long-term central venous catheters; peripherally inserted central catheters (PICC); or subcutaneous ports can also be used. TPN is usually administered through a central line because it is a hypertonic solution that would rapidly inflame a peripheral vein. Most fat emulsions, however, are isotonic. Lower concentrations (less than 20%) of dextrose can be administered peripherally (peripheral parenteral nutrition), although fewer calories can be delivered.

When the GI tract cannot be used for alimentation, two types of solution are administered to provide nutritional support. Amino acid–dextrose solutions and fat emulsions combined with additives, such as electrolytes (sodium, potassium, chloride, calcium, magnesium, phosphate) and trace elements (zinc, copper, chromium, and manganese),

can maintain a positive nitrogen balance. Always check solutions for precipitate and hang lipid solutions higher than TPN. In some institutions, TPN and lipids are mixed in a 3 : 1 solution.

Complications

Complications that may occur during or after insertion of the catheter are caused by the following:

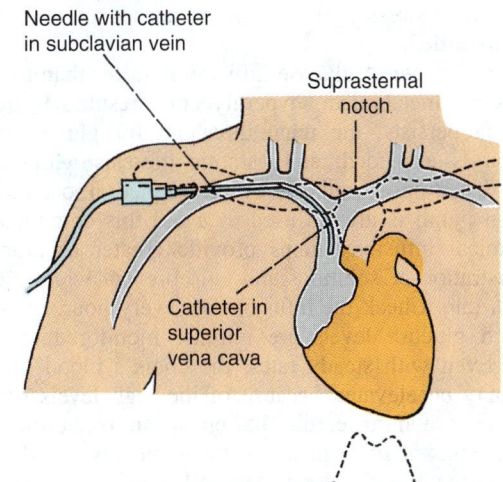

Figure 61–1. Insertion of catheter into superior vena cava via right subclavian vein. Once in place, this catheter may be used for total parenteral nutrition (TPN) administration.

1. Accidental perforation of the pleura leading to pneumothorax or hemothorax
2. Injury to the brachial plexus or the artery
3. Air embolism
4. Subclavian venous thrombosis

Other major complications of TPN therapy are infection, hyperglycemia, hypoglycemia, and other electrolyte imbalances.

Clients receiving TPN are very susceptible to infection, especially *Candida* septicemia. Concentrated glucose solutions provide a good medium for bacterial growth. Contamination of the catheter, solution, insertion site, tubing, or filters can lead to infection. Therefore, exercise stringent surgical asepsis in hanging TPN solutions, assisting with line insertion, or changing solutions or dressings.

Nursing Management of Clients Receiving Parenteral Nutrition

To minimize infection and sepsis, maintain strict aseptic technique during the insertion of the catheter, dressing changes, and changing bottles, filters, and intravenous tubing. Clinicians have developed rigid guidelines for accomplishing these duties, and they must be carefully followed. Procedures may vary in detail. To change the dressing, wear a mask and sterile gloves; apply an antiseptic solution, such as povidone-iodine, and an antibiotic ointment to the insertion site. After application of a dry, sterile dressing or transparent dressing, use tape to form an occlusive dressing that is impervious to air and small amounts of moisture.

A filter is commonly used in the intravenous tubing to trap bacteria and particles. The solution and administration equipment must be changed every 24 hours. Dressing changes are done every 48 to 72 hours on the basis of hospital policy, except right after placement of a tunneled catheter (in which case dressings are usually changed every 24 hours for the first 10 days). Povidone-iodine (Betadine) or an antibiotic ointment is often applied to the catheter insertion site with each dressing change, and an occlusive dressing is applied. Unused solution is always discarded.

When the rate of glucose infusion is faster than the rate of glucose metabolism, hyperglycemia results. If hyperglycemia persists, the renal threshold for glucose reabsorption is exceeded, and osmotic diuresis with subsequent dehydration and electrolyte depletion occurs. An infusion pump is always used to avoid this complication. Mechanical infusion pumps provide greater accuracy in administration of solutions and help prevent wide fluctuations in rate. Check the infusion rate every hour.

Blood glucose levels are initially monitored every 6 hours. Even with steady rates, the client's blood glucose level may be elevated because of the high levels of glucose being administered. The physician often orders a varying amount of regular insulin to be given, which is based on the client's blood glucose levels.

One of the body's major responses to high blood glucose levels, such as those found in clients receiving TPN, is increased insulin output from the pancreas. When a hypertonic glucose infusion is abruptly interrupted, insulin levels remain high while glucose levels decline, which results in rebound hypoglycemia. For this reason, TPN rates must be tapered off slowly over a period of days. Kinking of the tubing or catheter by position changes, occlusion of the catheter, failure of the mechanical pump, or allowing the infusion bottle to run dry can cause cessation of solution flow and subsequent hypoglycemia.

Venous thrombosis is another possible complication. It is characterized by neck vein distention (unilateral); unilateral edema of the arm, neck, or face; and shoulder pain. If this is suspected, notify the physician immediately.

Carefully check the flow rate of the pump for the TPN solution. Too rapid a flow of a solution can cause hyperglycemia. Too slow a flow fails to instill the needed nutrients. Do not increase the flow even if the infusion is behind schedule. In summary, when caring for clients receiving parenteral hyperalimentation, monitor vital signs and especially note an increase in temperature (a possible manifestation of infection). Monitor the intake and output, closely assessing for manifestations of dehydration or overhydration. Monitor nutritional status with daily weights and biochemical blood tests (e.g., BUN, creatinine, electrolytes, and minerals). Check the infusion site for manifestations of infection or inflammation. Use appropriate techniques to administer TPN, including the following:

● Always use an infusion pump.
● Always start TPN at a slow rate (usually 1 L given over 24 hours). In some institutions, 10% dextrose is given first. The rate is then advanced over 1 to 2 days until the rate that is desired to meet the client's nutritional requirements is met.
● Do not abruptly discontinue TPN. If TPN stops or the next bottle is unavailable, administer a 10% dextrose solution until the correct fluid can be obtained.
● Do not infuse any other solutions or medications via the TPN line (with the exception of intralipids).

The Nursing Research feature describes the caregiving experiences of family members of clients who are dependent on TPN at home.

Eating Disorders

Over the past several decades, eating disorders have become of increasing concern to nurses and other healthcare professionals. Anorexia nervosa and bulimia are now recognized as potentially life-threatening problems. Clients suffering from these disorders are frequently seen by medical-surgical nurses. You must understand these disorders to help clients recover.

Anorexia Nervosa

Anorexia nervosa is a loss of at least 15% to 25% of ideal body weight due to voluntary restriction of food intake. Clients with anorexia nervosa (usually young women) experience the following:

NURSING RESEARCH

How Does Caring for Clients who Are Dependent on Total Parenteral Nutrition Affect the Family?

Smith, C., et al. (1993). Responsibilities and reactions of family caregivers of patients dependent on total parenteral nutrition at home. *Public Health Nursing, 10*(2), 122–128.

A short, semi-structured interview based on the Roy adaptation model was used to gather data about the caregiving experiences of 20 relatives of adult TPN-dependent clients. Content analysis reflected frequently identified themes such as altered family responsibilities and negative and positive psychologic reactions to caregiving. The interviews suggested that caregivers master TPN technology but make little use of assistance from extended family or professionals. Although depression and fatigue were often reported, these family members felt capable and successful in their caregiving roles.

Implications for Practice

Families can be taught to care for clients with TPN at home.

1. Severe weight loss
2. Related physiologic changes associated with starvation, including cessation of menses
3. A complex of distorted mental perceptions, such as alterations in body image, weight phobia, and obsessive self-starvation associated with the fear of being fat

Since World War II, the incidence of anorexia nervosa has increased remarkably; the high-risk group consists of American girls between the ages of 12 and 18 years (estimated risk, 1 of 20).[20, 39] It most commonly occurs in females from the middle and upper classes in Western cultures. Males account for approximately 5% to 10% of the anorexia nervosa population. There is an increased incidence of anorexia nervosa in sports participants and in members of professions that require low body weight, such as gymnastics, wrestling, and ballet.

Etiology and Risk Factors

The cause of anorexia nervosa is not fully understood. It appears to be the result of many interacting cultural, social, familial, and psychological factors in a vulnerable client. As the Nursing Research feature suggests, sexual and physical abuse are contributing factors as well. The importance of each factor to a client can vary.

Young women with low self-esteem seem to be the highest risk group because they see thinness as a way to improve their self-confidence. American culture seems to worship thin fashion models, which encourages young girls to try to match this appearance.

Early recognition can lead to treatment before the client's life is in jeopardy. Although the disorder is psychological in origin and not responsive to education, instruction that centers around the avoidance of fad diets, proper nutrition, and ways to build self-confidence safely is valuable. Unfortunately, this disease is often denied by clients and families; therefore, preventive education is not possible.

Pathophysiology

The obvious pathologic changes associated with anorexia nervosa are physiologic, but the real disorder is psychological. The pathophysiologic changes include changes associated with the effects of starvation.

If not treated, this disorder can be fatal as a result of life-threatening fluid and electrolyte imbalances that are an offshoot of limited intake.

Clinical Manifestations and Diagnostic Findings

Clients are usually brought by family and friends for medical attention when weight loss is apparent. The client is usually younger than 25 years. Other manifestations, probably caused by the state of starvation, include the following:

Amenorrhea
Cachexia
Constipation
Fine hair covering the body (lanugo)

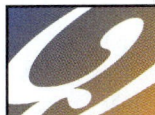

NURSING RESEARCH

Does Childhood Sexual Abuse Affect Women's Medical Problems Later in Life?

Laws, A. (1993). Does a history of sexual abuse in childhood play a role in women's medical problems? A review. *Journal of Women's Health, 2*(2), 165–172.

Although available literature is sparse and many studies lack methodologic rigor, data suggest that a history of sexual abuse in childhood is common in women with a history of chronic pain, functional bowel disorders, eating disorders, obesity, and alcohol abuse.

Implications for Practice

Healthcare providers should assess for a history of sexual abuse in clients with eating disorders and obesity.

Dry and sandpaper-like skin
Bradycardia
Periods of hyperactivity
Hypothermia
Hypotension

The blood pressure may be as low as 60/40 mm Hg. To induce weight loss, anorexics often subsist on fewer than 600 kcal/day; if they eat more, they often induce vomiting or use laxatives. Eventually, severe dieting causes extreme wasting and cachexia. The facial puffiness that is caused by parotid hypertrophy contrasts with the wasting of the rest of the body (Fig. 61–2).

Clients usually deny the existence of any problem, except a feeling of being fat. They seem to enjoy losing weight as evidence that they are achieving their goals. They often exhibit bizarre rituals associated with food, including hoarding food or handling it in ritualistic ways (such as lining up peas and then eating them one at a time). Other activities include excessive exercising and lack of sleep.

Clients often suffer from profound anemia diagnosed by a complete blood count. Electrolyte abnormalities such as hypokalemia, hypochloremic metabolic acidosis, metabolic alkalosis, or hypoglycemia, may be present. If the client is dehydrated, the BUN level may be elevated. Often serum cholesterol levels are elevated, although the reason for this is not fully understood. Other diagnostic tests may include a chest radiograph and electrocardiogram. Often, psychological testing is done by a psychiatrist as part of the diagnostic process.

Acute and Subacute Care

■ Medical Management

Nutritional rehabilitation and improvement of self-image are necessary for the client with anorexia. This is usually completed in an inpatient eating disorders unit and followed by lengthy outpatient care. Intervention must first focus on improving the state of nutrition so the client can undertake psychotherapy for the underlying problem. Eating is the preferred method of achieving weight gain, but sometimes the client refuses to comply. In this case, the physician may institute tube feedings or, in some cases, TPN supplementation. In addition, the client may receive a combined program of psychotherapy and behavior modification. Intervention is very lengthy and normally involves the client's significant others through family therapy.

■ Nursing Management of the Medical Client

Nursing management of the medical client with anorexia nervosa is discussed under the heading Nursing Management of Clients with Eating Disorders.

Figure 61–2. Physical signs of anorexia nervosa. The signs found in patients with bulimic complications are marked with an asterisk; those primarily due to starvation are without an asterisk. (From Andersen, A. E. [1985]. *Practical comprehensive treatment of anorexia nervosa and bulimia.* Baltimore: The Johns Hopkins University Press.)

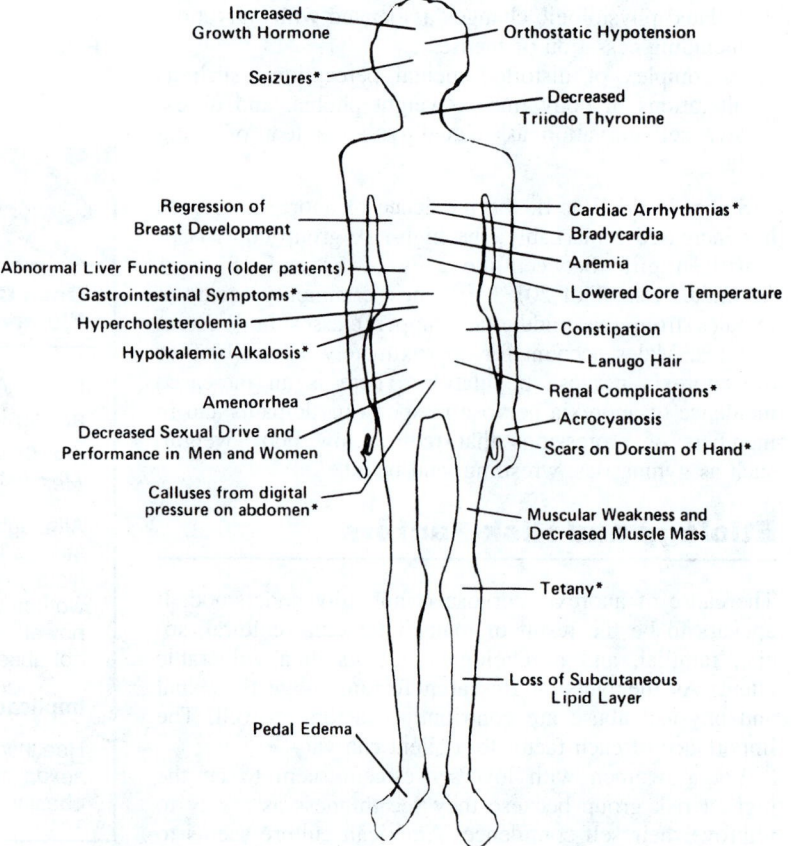

Bulimia Nervosa

Bulimia, also known as compulsive eating with self-induced vomiting, is another nutritional disorder. Bulimia can overlap with anorexia nervosa (i.e., anorectic clients may have episodes of bulimia). Bulimia is a common problem, especially among young women during late adolescence and young adulthood. Clients are typically of normal weight and from middle- to upper-class socioeconomic backgrounds. Most clients with bulimia maintain their weight, but they weigh less than the norm for their age and height. They are usually sociable and conforming, often appearing to be the ideal student, worker, or spouse.

Etiology and Risk Factors

As with anorexia nervosa, no one knows exactly what causes bulimia. One theory is that bulimia is a primary neurologic dysfunction, an electrical disorder, similar to epilepsy. Another is that the disorder is caused by a disturbance in the appetite/satiety center of the hypothalamus. Some researchers believe bulimia is learned behavior from dealing with stress and unpleasant feelings. Onset of the disorder can sometimes be traced to the young woman having been sexually or physically abused or on a strict weight loss diet.

The major factor, as with anorexia, is based on the societal ideal of the thin woman. Clients often have a history of poor family relations, low self-esteem, and poor impulse control.

Early recognition that the problem exists and quick intervention of mental healthcare providers to help the client come to terms with the behavior and to build self-confidence is very important. As with anorexia, the disease is often denied by clients and unrecognized by family members, so preventive education is not possible.

Pathophysiology

Clients often binge after some psychological-emotional factor such as depression, anxiety, anger, or even boredom. Bulimics ingest tremendous amounts of food during binges without extremes of hunger as the trigger. They may feel some hunger as a trigger; however, the intake of food is out of proportion to the hunger.

Bulimics often do experience weight gains on low-calorie diets and may have a history of being overweight. When they restrict their intake, they may have difficulty losing weight. They find that a large intake of food (sometimes thousands of calories at a sitting) followed by purging controls their weight.

Clients are aware that the eating pattern is abnormal and they fear they will lose complete control and be unable to stop eating at all. Other types of excessive behavior may be exhibited, such as alcohol or drug abuse or sexual promiscuity. The client has poor impulse control, resulting in overindulgence in many aspects of life.

Clinical Manifestations and Diagnostic Findings

Assessment reveals a history of repeated binge-eating episodes (rapid consumption of a large amount of food in 2 hours or less), with an awareness of abnormality and a fear of being unable to stop eating. Eating binges are followed by a depressed mood and self-deprecating thoughts. Manifestations of bulimia include consumption of high-calorie and easily ingested foods, inconspicuous eating, abdominal pain, excessive sleeping, self-induced vomiting, repeated attempts to lose weight, and frequent weight fluctuations of 10 lb or more.

Vomiting. Vomiting, the primary method of purging, decreases the physical pain of abdominal distention. Some clients use laxatives or severely restrictive diets after a bulimia episode. Amphetamines, diuretics, fasting, and excessive exercise may also be used to avoid gaining weight. Other psychological manifestations include impaired impulse control, fear of obesity, and low self-esteem. Bulimics, unlike clients with anorexia, report a strong appetite and usually binge several times a day. Binges occur most often in the late afternoon and evening and end with self-induced vomiting. Binges normally happen in secret. Clients with bulimia are aware that their eating is abnormal and may express concern about this behavior. Many clients with bulimia also abuse alcohol and drugs.

Depression. Depression marked by feelings of gloom, suicidal thoughts, irritability, and impaired concentration, are common. Clients with long-term bulimia also report loneliness, boredom, and anger. Except for frequent weight fluctuations, there are no known clinical manifestations of bulimia. Chronic vomiting, however, can lead to tooth damage (erosion of the enamel), irritation of the throat and esophagus, swelling of the salivary glands (caused by acidic reflux and constant stimulation), fluid and electrolyte imbalances, hair loss, and, occasionally, fistulas of the upper GI tract. Laxative abuse may further aggravate fluid and electrolyte imbalance and may cause rectal bleeding.

Acute and Subacute Care

■ **Medical Management**

Intervention for bulimia includes pharmacotherapy (serotonin blockers such as fluoxetine [Prozac]), aversion therapy, and psychotherapy. Sometimes a monoamine oxidase inhibitor medication (tranylcypromine sulfate) may be ordered to decrease the client's urge to binge. The most widely used modes of treatment are individual psychotherapy and self-help groups. Initially, this treatment is begun with the client admitted to an inpatient eating disorders unit and is followed with lengthy outpatient follow-up.

Treatment for bulimia has two goals: (1) to interrupt the binge/purge cycle by helping the client gain control of eating habits and (2) to change attitudes toward food, eating, body size, and self. Family therapy is also recommended to improve family interactions. Clients are encouraged to strengthen and explore relationships with family members.

■ Nursing Management of the Medical Client

Nursing management of the medical client with bulimia nervosa is discussed under the heading Nursing Management of Clients with Eating Disorders.

Obesity

Obesity is defined as weight 20% or greater than the desirable weight for adults of a given sex and height.

Obesity is caused by a caloric intake that exceeds energy expenditure. Many metabolic abnormalities are present in obese clients, but these are probably the result of obesity rather than the cause. When food intake equals metabolic needs, weight remains fairly constant throughout life. A weight gain sometimes accompanies aging because the client does not adjust food intake to lowered metabolism and diminished activity.

Atherosclerosis and its associated ischemic heart disease are caused by the altered metabolism of obesity. Hypertension and left ventricular hypertrophy occur because blood must be pumped through an enlarged vascular bed. Diabetes mellitus is four times more common in the obese client. Also, recent studies indicate a link between obesity and breast, endometrial, and ovarian cancer.

■ Medical Management

Activity increases both the energy output and the caloric deficit of a client after a weight loss diet. Thus, it is an excellent intervention. Any obese client on a calorie-restricted program should also have a planned, gradually increasing exercise program to help weight loss and muscle tone.

Most clients need the support and encouragement of others who understand the extreme difficulty of losing weight. The best intervention for obesity is appetite re-education, in which the client learns to eat and be satisfied with nutritious, well-balanced foods that are low in calories. Support groups such as TOPS (Take Off Pounds Sensibly), a nonprofit organization, and Weight Watchers help some clients. Overeater Anonymous groups use the Alcoholics Anonymous approach. Most of these groups teach nutrition as well as weight loss dieting. Because weight tends to be self-sustaining, vigilance and continued support are needed to maintain weight losses. No approach will work, however, unless the client is motivated to lose weight.

Obesity is controlled with dietary changes and exercise. A weight loss diet must provide fewer calories than the client's energy expenditure while consistently supplying the nutrients necessary for health.

■ Surgical Management

Morbidly obese clients who do not respond to dietary methods of weight loss may require surgical procedures to lose weight. Several surgical procedures can help the obese client. Many surgical approaches are designed to reduce the ability of the body to ingest or to absorb nutrients.

Food intake can be reduced by jaw wiring. Subcutaneous fat can be excised in a procedure called lipectomy. Both have advantages and disadvantages and do not always cause permanent weight reduction.

More permanent surgical approaches to weight loss have been undertaken. One approach, used in the past, involved severing the jejunum 14 inches from its beginning and anastomosing this end to the terminal ileum 4 inches above the ileocecal valve. This left the client with 18 inches of small bowel. This jejunal bypass surgical technique has been abandoned because of complications, especially hepatic failure.

The surgical procedure done currently is gastroplasty, or gastric stapling. The gastric stapling involves stapling the top part of the stomach, with creation of a small pouch to receive ingested food. A small opening left in the line of staples allows food to enter the rest of the stomach slowly. Depending on the size of the pouch created, the client can eat only about 30 ml of food every 5 minutes until satisfied. Before surgery, the client should receive psychiatric evaluation and begin participation in a support group. Because these clients are high surgical risks, an extensive preoperative assessment should be conducted. Postoperatively, special care must be taken with the nasogastric tube for preventing disruption of the suture line. Pulmonary complications often occur with gastric stapling.

Nursing Management of Clients with Eating Disorders

Assessment

A thorough history is necessary to differentiate the type of eating disorder from other illnesses. Carefully collect demographic data such as age and sex and get a thorough past medical history. Note the client's weight history, including the onset of the weight loss or weight gain and the reason for the change in weight. Information about the client's attitude and behavior related to food and weight are important. The client should describe his or her typical pattern of eating and be asked about the use of any appetite-suppressing medication, laxatives, and self-induced vomiting. Exercise patterns can also be important. Take a sexual history, including a menstrual history, and note whether amenorrhea is present.

Diagnosis, Planning, Implementation

Altered Nutrition: Less than Body Requirements. The client with anorexia often experiences *Al-*

tered *Nutrition: Less than Body Requirements related to inadequate food intake (anorexia nervosa).*

Planning: Expected Outcomes. The client will maintain body weight within normal limits, as evidenced by steady weight gain of 2 to 4 lb/week until ideal weight is reached.

Implementation. When caring for a client with anorexia nervosa, help the client select foods from all four food groups. The client is usually allowed to refuse a specific number of foods, such as two or three, so that some sense of control is felt. The client must eat only those foods provided by the dietary department and must eat all of the meal. Someone should remain with the client, talking, for at least 1 hour after meals to provide support and to prevent purging. Maintain an accurate calorie count on the client. The diet should allow the client to gain 2 to 4 lb/week. Weigh the client at regular intervals.

Help prevent the development of anorexia nervosa through education. By helping the public learn about the disease and its causes and manifestations, you can help prevent its development. Teach all clients a healthy, well-balanced diet. Speak out against fad diets and rapid weight loss approaches. If the client is overweight and seeking to lose weight, refer the client to a dietician and a support group and discourage fad diets.

Altered Nutrition: More than Body Requirements. Clients with bulimia nervosa and obesity often experience *Altered Nutrition: More than Body Requirements related to increased food intake (bulimia nervosa, obesity).*

Planning: Expected Outcomes. The client will maintain body weight within normal limits for client, as evidenced by steady weight loss of 1 to 2 lb/week until ideal weight is reached.

Implementation. Teach the client how to select a healthy diet with portions that are the correct size. Encourage clients to eat slowly and to develop a regular exercise pattern. Exercise is important, especially in bulimics and the obese, for it allows increased calorie intake.

Encourage the client to approach food, eating, and self-image in a new way. Help the client learn to eat a balanced diet from the four basic food groups. Help the client learn to choose proper foods in the right portions. Provide supervision and emotional support for the client to overcome stressful periods and break the cycle of binge/purge.

Dysrhythmias. Both anorexia and bulimia lead to altered fluid and electrolyte balance. The collaborative problem *Dysrhythmias related to alterations in rhythm secondary to hypokalemia (anorexia nervosa and bulimia)* is a common potential diagnosis.

Planning: Expected Outcomes. The client will maintain normal cardiac output, as evidenced by absence of cardiac dysrhythmias and adequate tissue perfusion.

Implementation. Monitor the client's serum potassium level at regular intervals. If the potassium level is low, administer potassium supplements as prescribed. If the potassium is at a dangerous level, intravenous replacement may be required. The client's potassium should return to normal once the diet is normalized and the condition controlled.

Body Image Disturbance. The client with an eating disorder often has a *Body Image Disturbance related to misconception of body size or negative feedings (all disorders).*

Planning: Expected Outcomes. The client will develop a more normal image of self, as evidenced by the client's statements concerning self and by client's ability to overcome the eating disorder.

Implementation. Recognize that clients suffering from eating disorders often have low self-esteem. These clients see the regulation of food and exercise of self-control in eating patterns and amounts as ways to prove themselves as being successful. It is important that the client's significant others help the client find other areas of self-regard unrelated to food.

Evaluation

If the client receives consistent and continued treatment, it is possible that the eating disorder can be overcome and the client can return to a normal weight.

Inflammatory and Neoplastic Disorders

Acute Gastritis

Gastritis is an inflammation of the gastric mucosa. Gastritis is classified as either acute or chronic. The incidence of gastritis is highest in the fifth and sixth decades of life; men are more frequently affected than are women. There is a greater incidence in clients who are heavy drinkers and smokers.

Etiology and Risk Factors

The acute form of gastritis may present with nausea and vomiting, epigastric discomfort or eructation, hemorrhage, malaise, and anorexia. It usually stems from the ingestion of a corrosive, erosive, or infectious substance. Aspirin and other nonsteroidal anti-inflammatory drugs, digitalis, chemotherapeutic drugs, steroids, acute alcoholism, and food poisoning (typically caused by *Staphylococcus* organisms) are common causes. In addition, food substances that can precipitate acute gastritis include excessive amounts of tea, coffee, mustard, paprika, cloves, and pepper. Foods with a rough texture or those eaten at an extremely high temperature can also damage the stomach mucosa. Ingestion of corrosive agents, such as lye or drain cleaner, also causes acute gastritis.

Disorders linked with acute gastritis include uremia, shock, central nervous system lesions, hepatic cirrhosis, portal hypertension, and prolonged emotional tension.

Acute gastritis is usually of short duration unless the gastric mucosa has suffered extensive damage. The Risk Factors and Levels of Prevention feature lists measures that the client can take to avoid gastritis.

Pathophysiology

The mucosal lining of the stomach normally protects it from the action of the gastric acid. This mucosal barrier is composed of prostaglandins. If this barrier is penetrated, gastritis occurs, with resultant injury to the mucosa. When hydrochloric acid comes into contact with the mucosa, injury to small vessels occurs with edema, hemorrhage, and possible ulcer formation. The damage associated with acute gastritis is usually limited.

Clinical Manifestations and Diagnostic Findings

Assessment typically reveals epigastric discomfort, abdominal tenderness, cramping, eructation, severe nausea and vomiting, and sometimes hematemesis. Sometimes GI bleeding is the only manifestation. When contaminated food is the cause of gastritis, the client usually develops diarrhea within 5 hours of ingestion of the offending substance.

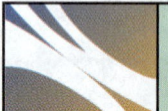

RISK FACTORS AND LEVELS OF PREVENTION

Acute Gastritis

Risk Factors

Consumption of alcohol, aspirin, NSAIDs, caffeine, nicotine, chemotherapeutic drugs, and spicy foods; other disorders such as uremia, shock, and cirrhosis; cancer treatments

Levels of Prevention

Primary Prevention

- Instruct the client to avoid irritants such as alcohol, aspirin, NSAIDs, caffeine, nicotine, and spicy foods.

Secondary Prevention

- Administer enteric-coated aspirin and other drugs if they must be taken on a regular basis.
- Administer histamine-receptor antagonists to decrease gastric acidity.
- Administer misoprostol (Cytotec) to protect against NSAIDs.

Tertiary Prevention

- Advise clients to treat medical disorders and follow orders for prescribed medications to minimize stomach irritation.

Diagnosis is based on a detailed history of food intake, medications taken, and any disorders related to gastritis. Also, the physician may perform a gastroscopic examination with a biopsy.

Acute and Subacute Care

Management of gastritis may begin in the inpatient or outpatient setting. For severe episodes and complications, hospitalization may be warranted, but it is rarely needed until chronic gastritis develops.

■ Medical Management

Intervention involves removing the cause or treating the condition symptomatically. Vomiting frequently responds to medications of the phenothiazine group; pain responds to antacids (which neutralize stomach acid) such as aluminum-magnesium combinations (Maalox) or H_2-receptor antagonists (which block the production of gastric acid) such as ranitidine hydrochloride (Zantac). If ingestion of nonsteroidal anti-inflammatory drugs (NSAIDs) is a problem, then misoprostol (Cytotec) may be prescribed to protect the stomach mucosa and suppress secretion of gastric acid. Initially, foods and fluids are withheld until nausea and vomiting subside. Once the client tolerates food, the diet includes decaffeinated tea, gelatin, toast, and simple, bland foods. The client should avoid spicy foods, caffeine, and large, heavy meals. In the continued absence of nausea, vomiting, and bloating, the client can slowly return to a normal diet.

■ Nursing Management of the Medical Client

Nursing management of the medical client with acute gastritis is described in the section on chronic gastritis.

Chronic Gastritis

This condition appears in three different forms:

- *Superficial gastritis,* which causes a reddened, edematous mucosa with hemorrhages and small erosions
- *Atrophic gastritis,* which occurs in all layers of the stomach, develops frequently in association with gastric ulcer and gastric cancer, and is invariably present in pernicious anemia; it is characterized by a decreased number of parietal and chief cells
- *Hypertrophic gastritis,* which produces a dull and nodular mucosa with irregular, thickened, or nodular rugae; hemorrhages occur frequently

Etiology and Risk Factors

Peptic ulcer disease, infection with *Helicobacter pylori* bacteria, or gastric surgery may lead to chronic gastritis. Other risk factors are similar to those for acute gastritis, such as consumption of alcohol, smoking, and ingestion of certain medications. Chronic gastritis is associated with atrophy of the gastrin glands. After gastric resection with a gastrojejunostomy, bile and bile acids may reflux into the remaining stomach, causing the condition. *H. pylori* infection can lead to chronic atrophic gastritis, which predisposes to the development of gastric cancer.[12] Age is also a risk factor; chronic gastritis is more common in older adults.

Pathophysiology

The initial pathophysiologic changes associated with chronic gastritis are the same as with acute gastritis. After being thickened and erythematous, the lining of the stomach becomes thin and atrophic. Continued deterioration and atrophy lead to loss of function of the parietal cells. When the acid secretion decreases, the source of the intrinsic factor is lost, which results in the inability to absorb vitamin B_{12}; this leads to the development of pernicious anemia.

Chronic gastritis usually heals without scarring but can cause hemorrhage and ulcer formation. The atrophic changes eventually result in minimal amount of acid being secreted into the stomach. This achlorhydria is a major risk factor for the development of gastric cancer.

Clinical Manifestations and Diagnostic Findings

Manifestations are vague and may be absent (because the problem is not an increase in hydrochloric acid). Assessment may reveal anorexia, a feeling of fullness, dyspepsia, belching, vague epigastric pain, nausea and vomiting, and intolerance of spicy or fatty foods.

Acute and Subacute Care

■ Medical Management

Intervention begins once the physician rules out cancer as a causative factor. Discomfort may lessen with a bland diet, small frequent meals, antacids, anticholinergics, sedatives, and avoidance of foods that cause manifestations. H_2-receptor antagonists such as famotidine (Pepcid), mucosal protectants such as sucralfate (Carafate), and NSAID protectors such as misoprostol (Cytotec) may also be prescribed. Sometimes the physician prescribes corticosteroids in the hope of inducing some parietal cell regeneration. Administer vitamin B_{12} if the client has pernicious anemia. If *H. pylori* bacteria are present, a combination of clarithromycin (Biaxin), metronidazole (Flagyl), and omeprazole (Prilosec) is administered to eliminate the bacteria. If one week of this regimen is unsuccessful in eliminating the bacteria, it may be repeated.

■ Nursing Management of the Medical Client

Assessment

When assessing the client with acute or chronic gastritis, carefully focus on risk factors. The client's diet, patterns of eating, use of prescription and over-the-counter drugs, and life-style, including alcohol consumption and cigarette smoking, are assessed.

Diagnosis, Planning, Implementation

Pain. The client with acute or chronic gastritis experiences *Pain related to irritation of the gastric mucosa.*

Planning: Expected Outcomes. The client will experience relief of discomfort by removing irritating agents, as evidenced by client's statement of pain relief.

Implementation. Focus on teaching the client about the causes of gastritis and foods that may aggravate the disease. Help the client assess factors that increase manifestations, such as stress or fatigue, and assist the client with techniques to reduce the discomfort.

Gaviscon, an antacid that produces a soothing foam, is the best antacid for gastritis. H_2-receptor antagonists (famotidine) and antisecretory agents that enhance mucosal defenses (misoprostol) may also provide pain relief.

On discharge, provide oral and written instructions about untoward manifestations, diet therapy, and prescribed medications. The client with chronic gastritis should be instructed to see the physician at regular intervals and be tested for the development of gastric cancer. This is particularly important for the client diagnosed with *H. pylori* infection and atrophic gastritis, because these are closely related to gastric cancer.

Altered Nutrition: Less than Body Requirements. A common diagnosis associated with clients with acute and chronic gastritis is *Altered Nutrition: Less than Body Requirements related to decreased appetite, nausea and vomiting, and pain.*

Planning: Expected Outcomes. The client will experience improved nutritional intake by eating a balanced diet, as evidenced by weight gain or cessation of weight loss.

Implementation. If the nausea and vomiting are severe, the client may be given nothing by mouth until these problems decrease in severity. Once the pain and nausea associated with gastritis have subsided, the client is usually willing to follow a prescribed, well-balanced diet. Help the client identify foods and beverages that stimulate the development of gastritis and encourage the client to avoid these agents.

Evaluation

Gastritis is usually controlled with medications and diet so the client's intake can be expected to return to normal. With chronic gastritis, continued use of medication and diet modification may be necessary for the treatment to be successful.

■ Surgical Management

If conservative measures have not controlled bleeding, surgery may be necessary. Subtotal gastrectomy, pyloroplasty, vagotomy, or total gastrectomy may be indicated with severe erosive gastritis. These procedures are discussed in the section on peptic ulcer disease.

Peptic Ulcer Disease

Peptic ulceration is a break in continuity of esophageal, gastric, or duodenal mucosa. It may occur in any part of the GI tract that comes into contact with gastric juices (hydrochloric acid and pepsin). The ulcer may be found in the esophagus, stomach, duodenum, or (after gastroenterostomy) jejunum.

The incidence of peptic ulcer disease occurs in approximately 10% of the population. Gastric ulcers are more likely to occur during the fifth and sixth decades of life; duodenal ulcers more commonly occur during the fourth and fifth decades for men. For women, the occurrence is about 10 years later in life. Men are more likely to develop both gastric and duodenal ulcers.

■ Duodenal Ulcers

Duodenal ulcers, which have a higher incidence than gastric ulcers, usually occur within 1.5 cm of the pylorus. They are usually characterized by high gastric acid secretion. Some are associated with normal gastric secretion associated with rapid emptying of the stomach. Hypersecretion of acid is attributed to a greater mass of parietal cells. Stimuli for acid secretion include protein-rich meals, calcium, and vagal stimulation. Clients with duodenal ulcers experience low pH levels in the duodenum for longer periods. They are sensitive to gastrin and secrete excess gastrin. Finally, clients with duodenal ulcers have more rapid gastric emptying. The combined effect of hypersecretion of acid and rapid emptying of food from the stomach reduces the buffering effect of food and results in a large acid load in the duodenum. Within the duodenum, inhibitory mechanisms and pancreatic secretion may be insufficient to control the acid load.

■ Gastric Ulcers

Gastric ulcers, which tend to heal within a few weeks, form within 1 inch of the pylorus of the stomach in an area where gastritis is common. Gastric ulcers are probably caused by a break in the "mucosal barrier." The barrier, which differs from the layer of glycoprotein mucus that overlies the gastric epithelium, normally allows hydrochloric acid to be secreted into the stomach without injury to the epithelial cells. An incompetent pylorus may decrease mucus production, the usual gastric defense. The reflux of bile acids through an incompetent pylorus into the stomach may break the mucosal barrier. Decreased blood flow to the gastric mucosa may also alter the de-

fensive barrier. Decreased blood flow may make the duodenum more susceptible to gastric acid and pepsin trauma. The recurrence rate in gastric ulcer is lower than in duodenal ulcer.

■ Stress (Stress-Erosive Gastritis) and Drug-Induced Ulcers

Besides peptic and gastric ulcers, acute gastric erosion, frequently called stress ulcers or stress-erosive gastritis, can occur after an acute medical crisis. Following are six major assaults that give rise to gastroduodenal ulcerations:

- Severe trauma or major illness
- Severe burns (sometimes called Curling's ulcers)
- Head injury or intracranial disease (frequently called Cushing's ulcers)
- Drug ingestion (e.g., aspirin, NSAIDs, and alcohol) that acts on the gastric mucosa (Fig. 61–3)
- Shock
- Sepsis

Etiology and Risk Factors

Peptic ulceration depends on the defensive resistance of the mucosa relative to the aggressive force of secretory activity. The defensive resistance of the mucosa depends on the following factors:

1. Mucosal integrity and regeneration
2. Presence of a protective mucus barrier
3. Adequate blood flow to the mucosa
4. Ability of the duodenal inhibitory mechanism to regulate secretion
5. Possibly the presence of adequate gastromucosal prostaglandins

The aggressive factors relate to the presence of *H. pylori* bacteria and the volume of hydrochloric acid and biliary acid. Ulceration occurs when aggressive factors exceed the defensive ones. The aggressive nature of the gastric juice may be the result of hypersecretion of gastric juices, increased stimulation of the vagus, decreased inhibition of gastric secretions, increased capacity or number of the parietal cells to secrete acid, or increased response of the parietal cells to stimulation. Certain medications

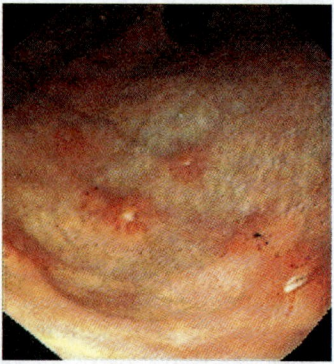

Figure 61–3. Gastric peptic ulceration caused by nonsteroidal anti-inflammatory drugs (NSAIDs).

increase the risk of ulcer formation (see Acute Gastritis), as do a variety of medical conditions, including Crohn's disease, Zollinger-Ellison syndrome, and hepatic and biliary disease. The Risk Factors and Levels of Prevention feature lists other factors that contribute to peptic ulcers.

Pathophysiology

Causation of more than 90% of all duodenal peptic ulcers and 70% of all gastric peptic ulcers has recently been attributed to *H. pylori*.[12] Eradication of the organism usually results in resolution of gastritis and subsequent ulcer healing. With multiple studies to support this data, many theories for peptic ulcer disease are being questioned.

In addition to *H. pylori*, two different mechanisms for the development of peptic ulcer disease in the stomach and duodenum have been proposed. In the stomach, it is thought that a breakdown in the normally protective epithelial lining occurs to cause gastric ulcers. Under normal circumstances, flow of hydrochloric acid from the lumen of the stomach is prevented by the presence of very tight, nonpermeable junctions between the epithelial cells and by the slightly alkaline layer of mucus that coats the surface of the gastric epithelium.

In the formation of a gastric peptic ulcer, this diffusion barrier may be interrupted by the chronic presence of such injurious substances as aspirin, NSAIDs, cortisone, adrenocorticotropic hormone (ACTH), caffeine, phenylbutazone (Butazolidin), alcohol, and chemotherapeutic agents. These substances may stimulate acid production, cause local mucosal damage, and/or suppress mucus secretion. The substances strip away the surface mucus and cause degeneration of the epithelial cell membranes, and massive diffusion of acid back into the gastric epithelial wall occurs.

The pathogenesis of duodenal peptic ulcers has a different proposed mechanism, as excess acid secretion is responsible for ulcer development. Activity of the vagus nerve is increased in persons with duodenal ulcers, particularly during a fasting state and at night. The vagus nerve stimulates the pyloric antrum cells to release gastrin, which in turn travels via the bloodstream and acts on the gastric parietal cells to stimulate the release of hydrochloric acid.

Another factor in peptic ulcer disease is the presence of emotional stress, which can cause an increase in gastric secretion, blood supply, and gastric motility by way of thalamus stimulation to the vagal nerves. Hormonal influence takes place via the hypothalamus through the pituitary adrenal route. When clients undergo stress reactions, the sympathetic nervous system causes the blood vessels in the duodenum to constrict, which makes the mucosa more vulnerable to trauma from gastric acid and pepsin secretion. On activation of the adrenal cortex, mucus production decreases, and gastric secretion increases. Together, these factors result in an increased vulnerability of the client to ulceration. Stress reactions thus cause an upset in the aggressive-defensive balance. Prolonged stress from burns, severe trauma, and other conditions can produce "stress ulcers," or stress erosive gastritis, within the GI tract.

Zollinger-Ellison syndrome is a condition characterized by abnormal secretion of gastrin by a rare islet cell tumor in the pancreas. Pathophysiologic changes associated with this syndrome include hypergastrinemia and diarrhea secondary to fat malabsorption from decreased duodenum-inactivating pancreatic lipase or from acid-induced injury of the villi. Besides gastric secretion, hyperplasia of the gastric mucosa is induced by the trophic effects of gastrin. Treatment of the Zollinger-Ellison syndrome is aimed at suppression of acid secretion.

Treated ulcers usually heal without difficulty. However, untreated ulcers or those not responding to treatment can result in perforation, hemorrhage, or obstruction, which may require surgical treatment. Some ulcers recur after healing, particularly if the risk factors associated with their development are not modified.

Critically ill clients are susceptible to stress ulcers. Gastric mucosal changes caused by stress develop within 72 hours in 78% of clients with greater than 35% burns. Stress ulcers manifest with superficial gastric erosions, often accompanied by painless massive gastric hemorrhage. The client characteristically has multiple lesions,

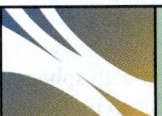

RISK FACTORS AND LEVELS OF PREVENTION

Peptic Ulcer Disease

Risk Factors

Infection with *Helicobacter pylori* bacteria; smoking (nicotine); steroids; aspirin; NSAIDs; caffeine; alcohol; stress; Crohn's disease, Zollinger-Ellison syndrome, and hepatic and biliary disease

Levels of Prevention

Primary Prevention

- Teach the client to avoid smoking; taking steroids, NSAIDs, and aspirin; ingesting caffeine and alcohol; and being subject to stress.

Secondary Prevention

- Treatment of *H. pylori* with clarithromycin (Biaxin), metronidazole (Flagyl), omeprazole (Prilosec).
- Administer misoprostol (Cytotec) to clients who are taking NSAIDs.
- Administer enteric-coated aspirin.
- Teach the client about stress management techniques.
- Administer histamine-receptor antagonists (to decrease stomach acidity) to clients at high risk for increased gastric acid secretion.

Tertiary Prevention

- Treat medical disorders that cause secondary peptic ulcer disease.
- Administer and ensure that the client complies with prescribed medication to minimize stomach irritation.

usually small and superficial, that do not extend through the muscularis mucosa. These lesions may give the appearance of "oozing blood." The mechanism causing stress ulcerations is unknown, but it probably involves ischemia. In the presence of acid, ischemia can produce erosive gastritis and ulcerations. Increased hydrogen ion back-diffusion and decreased mucosal perfusion may also contribute to stress ulcer formation. Low gastric pH (high acidity) is necessary for stress ulcer development.

Researchers continue to seek the precise mechanism by which stress ulcers occur. Few manifestations accompany stress ulcer. These ulcerations are typically painless unless perforation occurs; fortunately this is rare. Upper GI tract hemorrhage is the major manifestation of stress ulcer. About 10% of clients experience dyspepsia before hemorrhage, but typically there are no warning manifestations. Once stress ulcers cause profound hemorrhage, the mortality rate rises to about 50%.

Table 61–2 distinguishes the types of peptic ulcers.

Clinical Manifestations and Diagnostic Findings

Pain. The principal manifestation experienced by the client with ulcers is an aching, burning, cramplike, gnawing pain. The pain has a definite relationship to eating. With gastric ulcers, food may cause the pain, and vomiting may relieve it. Clients with duodenal ulcers have pain on an empty stomach, and discomfort may be relieved by the ingestion of food or antacids. Clients usually describe the pain as circumscribed in an area 2 to 10 cm in diameter, between the xiphoid cartilage and the umbilicus.

Gastric ulcer pain often occurs in the upper epigastrium, with localization to the left of the midline, whereas duodenal pain is in the right epigastrium. Ulcer pain also varies with the site, size, or penetration of the ulcer or the amount of surrounding fibrotic tissue.

In duodenal ulcers, steady pain near the midline of the back between the sixth and tenth thoracic vertebrae with radiation to the right upper quadrant may indicate perforation of the posterior duodenal wall. Fullness or hunger may also be present. Distention of the duodenal bulb produces epigastric pain, which may radiate to the back and thorax. Hydrochloric acid secretion may produce edema and inflammation, with resultant pain, or may activate motor changes, with increased spasm, intragastric pressure, and increased motility, also with resultant pain. In addition, ulcer pain tends to occur within distinct periods (periodicity).

The pain in both gastric and duodenal ulcers tends to recur daily for a while; it and all manifestations then disappear for months or years, to be followed eventually by another episode of pain.

Nausea and Vomiting. Clients with a duodenal ulcer usually have a normal appetite unless pyloric obstruction is present. Carcinoma, gastric ulcers, or gastritis may be associated with anorexia, weight loss, and dysphagia. Vomiting occurs more often with gastric ulcer than with uncomplicated duodenal ulcer. It also occurs more frequently when the ulcer is in the pylorus or antrum. Vomiting usually results from gastric stasis or pyloric obstruction. The client with a gastric ulcer or pyloric obstruction typically vomits undigested food. Severe retching and vomiting may suggest an esophageal tear.

Table 61–2. Classification of Peptic Ulcers

Assessment Data	Duodenal Ulcers	Gastric Ulcers
Location of ulcer	¼ to 1 inch from pylorus	Junction of fundus and pylorus, some in antrum
Acid secretion	Increased	Normal to decreased
Serum pepsinogen I	Increased	Normal

Serum gastrin
  Fasting
  Postprandial
	
	Normal
	Elevated
		
		Elevated

Blood group	Most frequently type O	No difference
Age at onset	25 to 50 years	Peaks at 45 to 54 years
Gender predominance	Men to women, 4:1	Men to women, 2:1
Associated gastritis	None	Common and increased
Pain	Occurs on empty stomach, 2 to 3 hr after meals or in middle of night; relieved by food and antacids	Variable pain pattern; may be made worse by food; antacids ineffective
Nutritional status	Usually well nourished	Probably malnourished
Malignancy potential	Rare, no increase in incidence	Occurs in approximately 10% of clients
Bleeding pattern	Melena more common than hematemesis	Hematemesis more common than melena
Recurrence	May occur as marginal ulcers after surgery	Recurrence unlikely after surgery

Bleeding. Clients with ulcers often bleed when the ulcer erodes through a blood vessel. Bleeding may occur as massive hemorrhage or may be occult from slow oozing. Approximately 25% of clients with gastric ulcers may experience bleeding.

Ulcers are diagnosed on the basis of manifestations, x-ray evidence, and endoscopy. The history and physical examination do not yield much significant data in an uncomplicated peptic ulcer. A complete blood count with decreased hematocrit and hemoglobin values may indicate bleeding. Stool for occult blood might also be positive, if bleeding is present.

The major diagnostic tests are an upper GI tract x-ray series and esophagogastroduodenoscopy (EGD). The EGD has several advantages. It allows the physician to take tissue specimens and to treat the ulcer with either multipolar electrocoagulation (MPEC) or heater-probe therapy (see Medical Management).

Acute and Subacute Care

■ Medical Management

The primary objective of intervention for peptic ulcer is to provide stomach rest. This may include such approaches as neutralizing or buffering hydrochloric acid, inhibiting acid secretion, decreasing the activity of pepsin and hydrochloric acid, and eradicating *H. pylori* from the GI tract. Specific measures include medications, physical and emotional rest, dietary management, and stress reduction.

Response to the therapeutic program varies with the client's perception of his or her health status and the degree to which life-style influences the ulcer disease. The following list enumerates the hallmarks of successful intervention:

1. The client experiences a decrease in pain with eventual elimination of all ulcer pain and related manifestations
2. The client eats a nutritionally sound diet and reports an increased tolerance to food
3. The client complies with the medication schedule
4. The client identifies stressors and and develops ways of dealing with or modifying them

Medications are prescribed for clients with peptic ulcer for four major reasons:

1. To eliminate *H. pylori* bacteria from the GI tract
2. To reduce secretions (hyposecretory drugs)
3. To neutralize acid (antacids)
4. To protect the mucosal barrier (mucosal barrier fortifiers) (Table 61–3)

Antibacterial Drugs

The antibacterial regimen used for treatment of *H. pylori* consists of clarithromycin (Biaxin), 250 mg bid, plus metronidazole (Flagyl), 250 mg qid, plus omeprazole (Prilosec), 20 mg bid. More than 90% of all clients are cured by following this protocol for 1 week. Fewer than

10% of clients require a second week of treatment or a variation of pharmacologic agents.

Hyposecretory Agents

Hyposecretory agents, which cause a reduction in acid secretions, include the following:

H$_2$-receptor antagonists
Prostaglandin analogs
Anticholinergics
Proton pump inhibitors
Antacids

H$_2$-Receptor Antagonists. H$_2$-receptor antagonists block histamine-stimulated gastric secretions (basal and stimulated) and are thus effective in the management of ulcer disease. Ranitidine hydrochloride (Zantac), one of the typical agents of the H$_2$-receptor antagonists, blocks the action of H$_2$-receptors and appears to inhibit gastrin release. It inhibits pepsin secretion and reduces the volume of gastric secretion. Maximal doses reduce food-stimulation secretion of acid by 75% to 85% in 3 hours. This medication appears to be effective in healing both gastric and duodenal ulcers. Ranitidine (Zantac) and famotidine (Pepcid) cause fewer complications than does the older agent cimetidine (Tagamet).

The client generally takes H$_2$-receptor antagonists every 6 hours for short-term management until the ulcer heals and manifestations subside, then once a day at bedtime. Although H$_2$-blockers are much more effective than are anticholinergic drugs alone, their effect is potentiated by anticholinergics. H$_2$-receptor antagonists do not appear to affect the rate of pepsin secretion or of gastric motility. The ulcer may recur after these medications have been discontinued, although rebound hyperacidity does not occur when they are stopped.

Prostaglandin Analogs. Prostaglandins are local tissue hormones that are formed from essential fatty acids. These hormones seem to be present in various forms in almost every tissue of the body. Two prostaglandins, E$_1$ and E$_2$, inhibit the secretion of gastric acid. Misoprostol is in this category.[25]

Anticholinergics. Excessive hydrochloric acid secretion and gastric motility can be partially prevented by decreasing vagal stimulation. Anticholinergics, as well as rest and sedation, accomplish this by blocking the action of acetylcholine on smooth muscles. This blockage decreases gastric motility and inhibits gastric secretion. Anticholinergics also delay gastric emptying time, thus prolonging the effect of foods and antacids. Reduced motility and consequent slowed gastric emptying cause a feeling of fullness. No proof exists that anticholinergics increase the rate of ulcer healing. However, they may enhance pain relief by relieving gastric distress caused by gastric spasm and hyperperistalsis.[25]

Anticholinergics are best given 1 hour after meals, when food-stimulated acid is at its peak. Their effects last 4 to 5 hours. Do not give anticholinergics to clients who are bleeding, because the stomach may become distended.

Table 61-3. Medications Commonly Used to Treat Peptic Ulcers

Medication	Action	Side Effects	Nursing Implications
Hyposecretory Agents			
Histamine (H₂)-Receptor Antagonists			
Cimetidine (Tagamet)	Same action as ranitidine	Fever, rash, headache, dizziness, somnolence, confusion (especially in elderly), hypotension, diarrhea, neutropenia, gynecomastia, and impotence	Monitor mental status of elderly; do not take antacids within 1 hr of cimetidine; take with meals and at bedtime; interacts with theophylline, phenytoin, warfarin, and beta-blockers; continue treatment for at least 8 wk to ensure healing
Ranitidine hydrochloride (Zantac)	Inhibits gastric acid secretion by blocking H₂-receptors on parietal cells	All side effects rare including nausea, constipation, bradycardia, increased liver enzymes, and headache	Give antacids at least 1 hr before or 2 hr after ranitidine; can be given in single bedtime dose; use cautiously in clients with liver or renal disorders; absorption not affected by food; interacts minimally with other drugs
Famotidine (Pepcid)	Same action as ranitidine	Headache, diarrhea, constipation, nausea, flatulence, increased blood urea nitrogen and creatinine, and rash	Do not take longer than 8 wk without physician's specific order; may be given with antacids; can be given in single bedtime dose; has no significant drug interactions
Nizatidine (Axid)	Same action as ranitidine	Diarrhea, rash bronchospasms, somnolence, joint pain, and sweating	Give as single bedtime dose or, if given twice a day, one dose at bedtime; assess for excessive drowsiness; monitor and record stools; do not give antacids within 1 hr of Axid; must be taken 4 to 8 wk for ulcer healing; notify physician if somnolence or rash develops
Prostaglandin Analogs			
Misoprostol (Cytotec)	Suppresses secretion of gastric acid and stimulates production of cytoprotective mucus	Diarrhea, nausea, abdominal discomfort, headache, and dizziness	Cannot be used in pregnancy because it stimulates uterine contractions; use for treatment in peptic ulcer disease currently under investigation; considered equivalent to cimetidine in ability to heal duodenal ulcers; useful in treating gastric ulcers also; recommended for clients on long-term aspirin or nonsteroidal anti-inflammatory drug therapy
Anticholinergics			
Dicyclomine hydrochloride (Bentyl)	Muscarinic antagonist; inhibits secretion of gastric acid in large doses	Headache, palpitations, dizziness, constipation, paralytic ileus, urinary hesitancy and retention, and dry mouth	Do not use in clients with obstructive uropathy, gastrointestinal obstruction, ulcerative colitis, unstable cardiovascular status, or toxic megacolon; use carefully in clients with narrow-angle glaucoma, hyperthyroidism, hiatal hernia, congestive heart failure, hepatic or renal disease; give ½ hr before meals and at bedtime; monitor vital signs and urine output; report blurred vision; maintain good fluid intake

Medication	Action	Side Effects	Nursing Implications
Hyposecretory Agents			
Antacids			
Aluminum hydroxide (Amphogel)	Buffers and neutralizes acid in gastrointestinal tract	Constipation, anorexia, intestinal obstruction, and hypophosphatemia	Give 1 to 2 hr after meals and at bedtime; do not give within 1 to 2 hr of H_2-receptor antagonists, enteric-coated drugs, or tetracycline; monitor and treat constipation; shake suspension well before use; follow tablets with water; contains salt, so contraindicated in large doses or long-term use with clients on sodium-restricted diets; used in clients with renal failure
Magnesium oxide (Mag-Ox)	Increases gastric pH to reduce pepsin activity; strengthens gastric mucosal barrier and esophageal sphincter tone	Diarrhea, nausea, and hypermagnesemia	Do not use in clients with renal disease; monitor for development of symptoms of hypermagnesemia; alter with aluminum or combination product if diarrhea occurs; do not give within 1 to 2 hr of H_2-receptor antagonists, tetracycline, or enteric-coated tablets
Aluminum-magnesium combinations (Riopan, Maalox, Mylanta, Gelusil)	Increases gastric pH to reduce pepsin activity; strengthens gastric mucosal barrier and esophageal sphincter tone	Mild constipation or diarrhea	Do not use in clients with renal disease; monitor bowel movements and signs of hypermagnesemia; Riopan low in sodium; do not give within 1 to 2 hr of H_2-receptor antagonists, tetracycline, or enteric-coated tablets
Calcium carbonate (Tums, Titralac)	Increases gastric pH to reduce pepsin activity; strengthens gastric mucosal barrier and esophageal sphincter tone	Constipation, gastric distention, rebound hyperacidity, hypercalcemia, and hypophosphatemia	Do not use in clients with renal disease; do not give with milk; monitor for symptoms of hypercalcemia and constipation; do not give within 1 to 2 hr of H_2-receptor antagonists, tetracycline, or enteric-coated tablets
Mucosal Barrier Fortifiers			
Sucralfate (Carafate)	In presence of mild acid condition, forms viscid and sticky gel and adheres to ulcer surface, forming a protective barrier	Dizziness, constipation, sleepiness, nausea, and gastric discomfort	Best on an empty stomach, 1 hr before meals and at bedtime; monitor for constipation; pain and ulcer symptoms may subside, urge client to take entire prescribed regimen; drug minimally absorbed, so few adverse reactions
Proton Pump Inhibitors			
Omeprazole (Prilosec)	Suppression of acid secretion by inhibiting H^+, K^+-ATPase (the enzyme that makes gastric acid	Headache, diarrhea, nausea, vomiting. Gastric cancer is a risk factor with long term use.	Usual dosage is 20 mg once a day for 4–8 wk; best taken in morning before breakfast.
Antibacterial Regimen to Eradicate H. pylori			
Clarithromycin (Biaxin); metronidazole (Flagyl); and omeprazole (Prilosec)	Eradicate *H. pylori* bacteria that cause peptic ulcer disease	Diarrhea, suprainfection with *Clostridium difficile*	Instruct client to take as ordered (usually twice daily for 7 days); monitor for diarrhea and signs of suprainfection; encourage client to take entire prescribed regimen

These agents are also contraindicated in clients who have pyloric obstruction, glaucoma, urinary retention, achalasia, or asthma. Dicyclomine hydrochloride (Bentyl) is a common anticholinergic used for clients with ulcers.

Unfortunately, anticholinergics suppress basal secretion more effectively than they suppress secretion in response to food. Also, to achieve sufficient suppression of secretion, the client must receive a large dose, which causes intolerable side effects: dry mouth, blurred vision, constipation, and sometimes urinary retention caused by bladder atony. For these reasons and because the H_2-receptor antagonists work better, anticholinergics are not used as frequently as they once were.

Proton Pump Inhibitors. Omeprazole (Prilosec) is a new anti-ulcer medication known as a proton pump inhibitor. The drug is the most effective agent available for suppressing secretion of gastric acid. Omeprazole undergoes conversion to its active form within parietal cells of the stomach. In active form, it causes irreversible inhibition of H+, K+-ATPase, the enzyme that generates gastric acid. Acid production decreases over 95% with one dose and will continue to decrease until several weeks after treatment has ceased.[25] The standard dosage is 20 mg once a day for 4 to 8 weeks.

Side effects from short-term therapy are minimal. Side effects include headache, diarrhea, nausea, and vomiting in less than 1% of clients taking the drug. With long-term therapy, there is concern about the risk of gastric cancer.

Antacids. The ideal antacid decreases acidity, is effective for a prolonged period, is pleasant to take orally, is not constipating or cathartic in nature, and is not absorbed, thereby eliminating systemic effects.

Calcium carbonate is a potent antacid but is constipating and triggers gastrin release, which causes a rebound acid secretion. Magnesium carbonate and magnesium oxide are also potent antacids but are also laxatives. They are sometimes prescribed to counteract the constipating effects of calcium carbonate. Frequently, the client takes these antacids alternately or balances dosages of each to produce a stool of the desired consistency.

Aluminum hydroxide, aluminum phosphate, and aluminum carbonate are less effective because they only partially neutralize the acid. Aluminum antacids can also be constipating. Sodium bicarbonate, a potent antacid, has a very brief effect and is absorbed systemically. Antacids that combine the effects of magnesium and either aluminum or calcium are on the market (e.g., Maalox and Mylanta).

Antacids are ordered to buffer gastric acid. They do not influence healing or prevent recurrence. They do, however, prevent the formation of pepsin, the protein-digesting enzyme. Antacids may also reduce the pyloroduodenal tone. For treatment of active peptic ulcer disease, sufficient antacid must be used to neutralize the hourly production of acid. Raising gastric pH from 1.3 to 2.3 produces 90% neutralization of gastric acid.

Generally, the goal of antacid therapy is to maintain a gastric pH of 3.0 to 3.5. For optimal effect, the client should take antacids about 1 hour after meals or feedings, at bedtime, and during periods of "rebound."

Some clinicians recommend that the antacid be mixed with water to ensure that it enters the stomach and does not simply coat the esophagus. Clients with esophageal reflux or hiatal hernia should take alginic acid, an additive present in Gaviscon. Alginic acid forms a viscous solution that floats to the top of the gastric contents and protects the esophageal mucosa. Table 61–4 summarizes manifestations to observe with antacids.

Mucosal Barrier Fortifiers

Mucosal barrier fortifiers are effective in (1) preventing hydrogen ion back-diffusion into the mucosa and (2) stimulating mucus production, which results in accelerated gastric ulcer healing.

Sucralfate (Carafate) is a sulfonated disaccharide that forms complexes with proteins at the base of a peptic ulcer. These complexes form a protective coat that prevents further digestive action of both acid and pepsin. Sucralfate does not inhibit acid secretion and has minimal acid-neutralizing ability. Instruct the client to take the recommended dosage of sucralfate 1 hour before each meal and at bedtime as needed for pain. Sucralfate should not be taken within 30 minutes of antacids.

Dietary Management

In uncomplicated ulcer disease, few physicians favor strict dietary changes. Evidence is scant to indicate that

Table 61–4. Precautions for Antacid Administration

Giving Antacids With	May Result In
Amphetamines or quinidine	Delayed drug elimination
Chlorpromazine and other phenothiazines	Decreased absorption with magnesium-aluminum
Diazepam (Valium)	Increased absorption rate
Dicumarol	Increased absorption with magnesium hydroxide
Digoxin (Lanoxin)	Decreased absorption (some antacids)
Enteric-coated tablets	Increased tablet dissolution and absorption rate
Iron salts	Decreased iron absorption: magnesium trisilicate or carbonates
Propranolol (Inderal)	Decreased drug absorption (aluminum hydroxide)
Tetracycline	Decreased absorption (especially with calcium, magnesium, and aluminum)

Adapted from Rosenberg, J. M., & Kirschenbaum, H. L. (1982). What to watch for with antacids. *Nursing Research, 31,* 54.

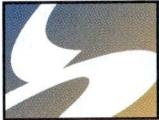

CASE MANAGEMENT

GI Hemorrhage
For Clinical Pathway, see Appendix D

Clinical Pathway from Birmingham Baptist Medical Center, Birmingham, Alabama
Information provided by Cindy Watson, B.S.N., M.Ed.

Development and Revision of Pathway

- DRG 174/174 (upper and lower GI hemorrhage) are high-volume, high-cost case types at our institution.
- The first task force met in October 1993. Two CareMaps were developed: one for upper GI bleed and one for lower GI bleed. These were implemented in April 1994. The two maps were combined into one CareMap in January 1995.
- Those involved in developing this pathway included the case manager, staff nurses, GI laboratory director, and physicians.
- A Continuous Quality Improvement team meets quarterly to review the data gathered from pathway use. These data drive pathway revision. For example, the data showed that there were very few upper GI bleed patients admitted and that intensive care was not utilized very often for the GI bleed patients. These data helped support the combining of the two pathways into one in January 1995.
- The pathway is revised as needed.

Use and Impact of Pathway

- All patients admitted with GI bleed are to be placed on this pathway. There is a uniform order set for GI bleed admissions. Variceal hemorrhage is excluded from this case type for data analysis purposes. However, most of those patients are placed on a pathway as well.
- Staff nurses and the case manager use the pathway every day.
- The pathway provides the nurses with the plan of care and allows them to focus on variations from that plan. They become very creative and professionally challenged when addressing variations in the expected plan and outcomes.
- Process improvements such as initial type and screen orders for blood have yielded cost savings. Overall savings are more apparent within medical subspecialties, such as gastroenterology. Overall, there has been a 3-day decrease in length of stay and a reduction of $1,000 variable cost per case.

---

diet treatment promotes or accelerates healing. Foods known to increase gastric acidity or cause discomfort should be avoided, such as coffee, alcohol, and milk.

Complications

Hemorrhage. Hemorrhage varies in degree from minimal, manifested by presence of occult blood in the stool (melena), to massive, manifested by vomitus containing bright red blood (hematemesis) (see Case Management feature). The usual manifestation of GI tract bleeding is either vomiting of coffee ground–type material or passing of tarry stools. Acid digestion of blood in the stomach results in a granular dark emesis, whereas digestion in the duodenum or below may result in a black stool. Hemorrhage tends to occur more often with gastric ulcers (Fig. 61–4), especially among the elderly.

Although the onset of hemorrhage may be associated with fatigue, nervous tension, upper respiratory tract infection, dietary indiscretion, alcoholism, or irritating drugs, there may be no known precipitating factor. Bleeding may manifest as either hematemesis or melena. Melena may occur with gastric ulcers but is more common with duodenal ulcers. Hematemesis usually indicates bleeding proximal to the ligament of Treitz at the duodenal level.

Manifestations depend on the severity of the hemorrhage. In mild bleeding (less than 500 ml), the client may experience only slight weakness and diaphoresis. Severe blood loss of more than 1 L per 24 hours may cause manifestations of shock, such as hypotension, weak thready pulse, chills, palpitations, and perspiration.

Intervention for massive bleeding aims to treat hypovolemic shock, prevent dehydration and electrolyte imbalance, and stop the bleeding. The client, who should be fasting, receives intravenous fluids until the bleeding sub-

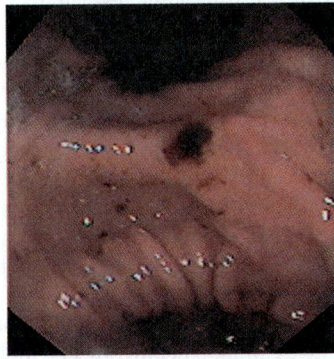

Figure 61–4. Bleeding ulcer on gastric mucosa.

sides. You or the physician may insert a nasogastric tube in the presence or absence of blood in the stomach to assess the rate of bleeding, to prevent gastric dilation, and to administer room temperature saline to remove blood from the stomach. The room temperature saline is cooler than the body temperature, which creates mild vasoconstriction. Cool saline lavage may also be instituted to promote gastric cooling, which although controversial, further curtails hemorrhage through its vasoconstrictive effect. Iced saline is rarely used today because it may lead to more mucosal damage by decreasing perfusion to the gastric mucosa and may cause a vagal response, decreasing systemic perfusion.

Arterial administration of vasopressin (via an infusion pump) can also successfully control acute hemorrhage. Vasopressin has few complications if given intravenously for less than 36 hours to control the bleeding.

Another approach to the control of bleeding is selective arterial embolization via angiography. The emboli may consist of autologous blood clots, with or without an absorbable gelatin sponge. A modified clot may be made with a mixture of the client's own blood, aminocaproic acid, and platelets. The client must remain on absolute bed rest for several days after bleeding has subsided. Rest decreases blood pressure and GI tract activity. When bleeding stops, the client is allowed bathroom privileges. If the individual requires narcotics, administer them with caution. Morphine sulfate can cause nausea and vomiting. However, it may calm the client who is extremely restless and apprehensive. A better alternative is to manage anxiety with non-narcotic alternatives.

During the first few days of hemorrhaging, gastric pH should be maintained between 5.5 and 7.0. To accomplish this, administer ranitidine intravenously every 4 hours for 4 days as prescribed. Monitor gastric pH at least each shift. Anticholinergics are not recommended for treatment of gastric hemorrhage. Administer antacids for 1 week to complement the ranitidine, but remember to give them 1 hour before or 2 hours after the ranitidine (Zantac) so the antacids do not interfere with its absorption. The client may require antacids every 30 minutes after starting intake of food or fluids. Antacids increase pH by direct hydrogen ion buffering.

If bleeding continues beyond 48 hours, recurs, or is associated with perforation or obstruction, surgery may be indicated. Increased surgical risk is associated with prolonged bleeding, multiple transfusions, debilitation, electrolyte imbalances, and increased age. Surgical procedures include partial gastric resection, excision of the ulcer, or vagotomy and pyloroplasty. Vagotomy and pyloroplasty with ligation of the eroded vessel may also be performed.

Blood volume depletion presents a major problem for the client with severe hemorrhage. For those who have suffered a massive upper GI tract hemorrhage, a primary objective of intervention is to replace blood volume. Restlessness and tachycardia are the earliest manifestations of hypovolemia. The client will also have a greatly decreased urine output, which should be monitored via a Foley catheter.

Two endoscopic procedures have been found to be safe and effective in treating bleeding ulcers: multipolar electrocoagulation (MPEC) and heater-probe therapy. In MPEC, a bipolar electric current cauterizes the bleeding lesion; in heater-probe therapy, direct heat cauterizes the lesion. Both procedures stop bleeding.

Perforation. Perforation is usually a surgical emergency. When the ulcer perforates, gastroduodenal contents empty through the anterior wall of the stomach into the peritoneal cavity, resulting in chemical peritonitis, bacterial septicemia, and hypovolemic shock. Peristalsis diminishes and paralytic ileus develops. Posterior perforation is not so clear, and often results in pancreatitis as the pancreas plugs the perforation (see manifestations of pancreatitis Chapter 66).

Perforation occurs most frequently with duodenal ulcers (Fig. 61–5). Perforation occurs when the ulcer erodes through the tunica muscularis. The client experiences sudden, sharp, severe pain beginning in the mid-epigastrium. As peritonitis develops, the pain spreads over the entire abdomen, which then becomes tender, hard, and rigid. (See discussion of peritonitis in Chapter 62.)

The degree of pain depends on the amount and type of contents that are spilled. Characteristically, the pain causes the client to bend over or draw the knees up to the abdomen in an effort to decrease the tension on the abdominal muscles. If the perforation occurs on the posterior gastric wall, however, it may erode through to adjacent organs and become sealed, causing few manifestations. Manifestations of pancreatitis usually develop when a perforation erodes into the pancreas.

If perforation occurs, the client needs immediate replacement of fluid, blood, and electrolytes and administration of antibiotics. Nasogastric suction should be instituted to drain gastric secretions and thus prevent further peritoneal spillage. A small perforation that closes immediately by adhering to the adjacent tissues usually causes only a small loss of gastric contents. In this instance, the client may recover without surgery. When surgery is necessary, the surgeon performs the following:

1. Evacuates the escaped gastric contents
2. Cleans the peritoneal cavity by flushing it out with normal saline or an antibiotic
3. Closes the perforation by patching it with a bit of omentum

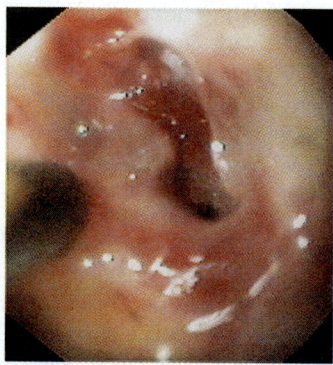
Figure 61–5. Perforation of a duodenal ulcer.

Vagotomy and hemigastrectomy or vagotomy and pyloroplasty can provide definitive control of both ulcer and its complications.

The Case Study describes the treatment of a client whose perforated ulcer was managed surgically.

After surgery, antibiotics are given to combat peritonitis. The nasogastric tube remains in the stomach until peristalsis returns. Postoperative complications include subphrenic abscess, hemorrhage, duodenal or gastric fistula, atelectasis, or pneumonia.

Obstruction. Long-standing ulcer disease causes scarring from repeated ulcerations and healing. Scarring at the pylorus frequently causes pyloric obstruction manifested most often by pain at night when the stomach cannot be emptied by peristalsis. Pyloric obstruction can also lead to vomiting. Surgery (pyloroplasty) is usually required to correct the problem.

■ Nursing Management of the Medical Client

Assessment

Nursing assessment involves gathering both psychosocial and pathophysiologic data concerning the client. To assess psychosocial aspects involving ulcer disease, ask the client about the following:

- Familial incidence of ulcer
- Ingestion of medications causing gastric irritation
- Cigarette smoking
- Alcohol intake
- Stressors
- Coping patterns

Questions about life-style, occupation, work, and leisure can yield valuable information. Physical assessment includes accurately observing and immediately reporting to the physician manifestations that help pinpoint the diagnosis or that might indicate the presence of a complication. Manifestations include pain, vomiting, and, occasionally, bleeding and changes in appetite. Always obtain a complete history of previous ulcer attacks, including frequency, duration, manifestations, and response to intervention.

Assessment also involves describing the bleeding, including hematemesis and melena. Note such factors as color, amount, consistency, and frequency. Bright red blood usually signifies new bleeding, whereas dark red blood indicates old bleeding. In severe bleeding, always maintain an accurate and up-to-date record of the client's hemoglobin, hematocrit, red blood cell count, and fluid intake and output.

Because of shock, the client may experience decreased renal blood flow, which causes a decrease in renal excretion and glomerular filtration rate. As the body absorbs the by-products of erythrocyte destruction and renal blood flow decreases, watch for an increase in BUN and ammonia levels. An elevated BUN level may follow dehydration resulting from vomiting. In addition, carefully assess the client for metabolic acidosis caused by vomiting.

Diagnosis, Planning, Implementation

Pain. One of the most common nursing diagnoses for the client with a peptic ulcer is *Pain related to gastric mucosal injury.*

Planning: Expected Outcomes. The client's pain will be relieved, as evidenced by healing of gastric or duodenal mucosal injury and the client's statement.

Implementation. Administer medications as ordered, for the following reasons:

1. To eliminate *H. pylori*
2. To neutralize gastric acids (antacids)
3. To reduce secretions (H_2 receptor antagonists, prostaglandin analogs, and proton pump inhibitors
4. To protect the gastric mucosa

Assess the effectiveness of the medication on the client's pain and notify the physician if the pain is not relieved by the medications.

Avoidance of strenuous physical activity decreases gastric secretions and peristalsis. Thus, a primary nursing goal is to promote recovery by helping the client achieve rest, both physically and mentally. Be alert for factors that interfere with the client's rest. Arrange the environment to encourage relaxation. If certain visitors or telephone calls agitate the client, discourage these visits or calls until the client improves.

Encourage clients who attempt to carry on their normal work routine (despite prescribed rest) to schedule physical and mental relaxation. Explore ways, with the client and significant others or co-workers, to reduce work responsibilities temporarily.

The diet must meet basic nutritional needs. Because an empty stomach stimulates gastric acid secretion, advise the client to eat small amounts at frequent, regular intervals. Discourage ingestion of alcohol, cola, tobacco, caffeine, milk, and foods that cause discomfort. The client may drink decaffeinated beverages.

During the acute phase, the client often requires a bland, nonirritating, and low-fiber diet. Significant others need to learn if there are any modifications in the client's diet. Have the dietician review the home diet with whoever will be cooking for the client.

Ineffective Management of Therapeutic Regimen (Individuals). For the client with an uncomplicated ulcer, most of the care must be done by the client at home. Write the nursing diagnosis as *Risk for Ineffective Management of Therapeutic Regimen (Individuals) related to cause of ulcer and measures to treat and prevent recurrence.*

Planning: Expected Outcomes. The client will understand and be able to discuss the cause of the ulcer and how to treat and prevent recurrence.

Implementation. Treatment for ulcer disease places the responsibility for self-care on the client. To maintain good self-care, the client must understand the pathophysiologic process underlying ulcer development and the rationale underlying intervention.

Perforated Ulcer Managed Surgically

Mr. Fong is a 50-year-old, divorced, second-generation Asian-American, who is the CEO of a local telecommunications firm. He has a history of peptic ulcer disease. Mr. Fong has been taking clarithromycin {Biaxin), 250 mg bid; metronidazole (Flagyl), 250 mg bid; and omeprazole (Prilosec), 20 mg bid, for 1 week. He reports that he has not been able to eat breakfast or lunch on a regular basis and has subsequently not taken the sucralfate as ordered. He arrived in the ER today per rescue squad with complaints of sudden onset of severe abdominal pain accompanied by emesis of bright-red blood at his office. Mr. Fong is admitted to your unit for preoperative diagnostic work-up and preoperative preparation.

Nursing Admission Assessment

Mr. Fong arrives on the unit accompanied by his girlfriend. He vomits bright-red blood upon admission and is unable to answer questions. He assumes the fetal position and clutches his abdomen.

Mr. Fong's girlfriend tells the nurse that she is not aware of any allergies. She states that he did take his medicine and ate breakfast this morning, but she is uncertain whether he ate lunch. Other pertinent preoperative assessment data include that Mr. Fong smokes two packs of cigarettes a day and drinks one or two alcoholic beverages every evening before dinner. He practices Buddhism.

In addition to his anti-ulcer medications, he has been taking ibuprofen-pseudoephedrine (Advil Cold & Sinus) three or four times a day for 5 days. Mr. Fong removed his partial bridge when he vomited the first time at the office. His contact lenses are still in place. Mr. Fong's girlfriend is concerned that his two teenage children will not arrive before their father goes to surgery.

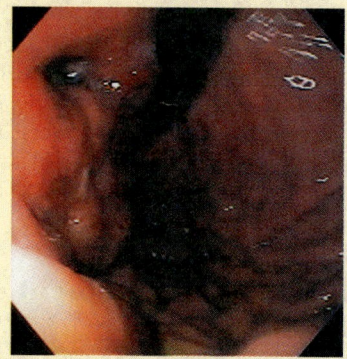

■ Endoscopic view of perforated peptic ulcer.

Nursing Physical Assessment

Height: 5′9″   Weight: 150 lb
(68.2 kg)

Vital Signs: BP = 90/50;
TPR = 99,120,22

LOC: Awake, restless, complaining of severe abdominal pain

EENT: Within normal limits

Cardiac: Tachycardia, regular rate and rhythm without gallop or murmur

Pulmonary: Lung sounds coarse and diminished bilaterally

Abdominal: Rigid, boardlike abdomen without bowel tones

Genitourinary: No urine output since admission; client denies urge to void

Peripheral pulses: 2/2 without edema

Mr. Fong's endoscopy revealed a perforated peptic ulcer and he was taken to the operating room for resection of the ulcer. He returns to your unit after 2 hours in the post-anesthesia care unit. Consider the postoperative orders and related

Emergency Room Diagnostic Test Results	
RBC	4.8 million/mm³ L
Hgb	13.5 g/dl
Hct	40%
WBC	8000/mm³
Sodium	140 mEq/L
Potassium	4 mEq/L
Chloride	101 mEq/L
Glucose	90 mg/dl
Prothrombin time (PT)	15 seconds
Partial thromboplastin time (PTT)	40 seconds
ECG	NSR
Chest x-ray	Within normal limits

nursing assessments and interventions expected in the care of Mr. Fong.

Mr. Fong is reluctant to take his pain medication because he is afraid of addiction. Two days postoperatively, he spikes a temperature of 101.6° F. On occasion, his cough is productive of thick, white sputum. His lungs remain coarse and diminished with scattered rhonchi and occasional wheezes bilaterally. A chest x-ray reveals bilateral atelectasis. Discuss how the nurse might have intervened to prevent this situation.

Mr. Fong's incision is clean, dry, and intact. His abdomen is tender, but soft. Bowel sounds remain absent and Mr. Fong denies flatus. NG intubation returns moderate amounts of green drainage. Consider the pathophysiology related to the continued absence of bowel tones.

Mr. Fong is 3 days postoperation and remains on an IV line and IV antibiotics. His hemoglobin is 7.6 g/dl and his hematocrit is 24%. He complains of being very thirsty and asks when he will be able to eat and drink. Discuss appropriate medical and nursing interventions.

Eight days postoperation, Mr. Fong is taking a soft diet and ambulating in the halls with good tolerance. He is scheduled for discharge in the morning.

Discharge Criteria

Average LOS (insurance certification): 8 days without complications; 14.2 days with complications; 5 to 6 days private insurance without complications

Complete discharge teaching (includes diet, medications, activity, stress management, and follow-up appointments)

Community referral: Smoking cessation program

Questions to Be Considered

1. Categorize Mr. Fong's surgeries according to the Categories of Surgical Procedures (Table 21–3). Define Mr. Fong's surgical procedures (refer to Table 21–2). Review the roles of the nurses on the perioperative team.
2. Compare and contrast local versus general anesthesia. Identify which type would be used for each of Mr. Fong's surgeries. Why?
3. Discuss the principles of surgical positioning. How would Mr. Fong be positioned for each of his surgical procedures? Include the rationale for your answer.
4. How is the routine preoperative abdominal surgery client prepared for surgery? Discuss how Mr. Fong's preparation was different and the related implications this would have for his recovery.
5. Explain informed consent. Describe the nurse's role in obtaining and completing informed consent forms.
6. Discuss the nurse's role in the promotion of wound healing. Include dietary management, wound care, positioning, rest, pain management, and pulmonary hygiene.
7. Discuss the psychosocial, spiritual, and cultural factors which may influence clients' attitudes about surgery and recovery. Apply these factors to Mr. Fong.
8. Compare and contrast the etiology, signs and symptoms, and management of peptic ulcer disease (gastric versus duodenal).

Initial Treatment Plan

Meds: Preoperative meds per anesthesia
IV: D5LR at 100 ml hr
Diet: NPO
Activity: Bedrest
Other: Surgical permit for upper gastrointestinal endoscopy with possible gastric or duodenal resection

Help the client with the following measures:

1. To understand the pathogenesis of the ulcer and the significance of the pain
2. To realize that healing takes place rapidly when the irritating effect is removed
3. To understand what caused the condition to develop and what must be done to lessen the stimulation
4. To discover which substances cause pain by stimulating secretion of gastric juices and eliminate them from the diet until the ulcer heals
5. To understand the importance of continuing the medical regimen, although pain is gone, until healing is completed
6. To recognize that once maintenance therapy stops, the ulcer may recur

Instruct the client to use acetaminophen instead of aspirin preparations when these are needed. Teach the client to examine the labels of all nonprescription medications, particularly cold remedies, for aspirin (acetylsalicylic acid), other salicylates, NSAIDs (such as ibuprofen and phenylbutazone), adrenocorticosteroids, and ACTH. These medications are ulcerogenic (ulcer causing), particularly when combined. If any of these medications must be taken, advise the client to check with the physician first, to eat between meals, and to use H_2-receptor antagonists or antacids.

Helping clients with ulcers cope with psychosocial problems is a vital part of intervention. Take the time to learn about their stressors. Discussing coping and relaxation techniques may enable clients to better deal with their problems.

Hemorrhage, Perforation, Pyloric Obstruction. The client with ulcer disease must be carefully monitored for the development of complications. Collaborative problems are *Hemorrhage, Perforation, or Pyloric Obstruction related to worsening of peptic ulcer disease and the development of complications.*

Planning: Expected Outcomes. The client will not suffer any complication or will have the complication diagnosed and treated early. There will be no hemorrhage, perforation, or obstruction, or early diagnosis and treatment of complications will ensure that injury does not occur.

Implementation. Monitor for the development of complications of ulcers including hemorrhage, perforation, or obstruction. Monitor vital manifestations closely for the development of manifestations of shock that might occur if bleeding is present. Document and report the occurrence of melena or hematemesis. If hemorrhage occurs, treat immediately to stop hemorrhage and prevent shock (see Chapter 22).

Monitor the client for the development of perforation. Assess the abdomen for pain, tenderness, or rigidity. Report suspected perforation to the physician immediately and prepare the client for possible surgery. The client should also be monitored for the development of gastric obstruction. If the client vomits, record the frequency and consistency (digested or undigested food or hematemesis) of the vomitus. If pyloric obstruction is present, the client

will require a nasogastric tube and administration of intravenous fluids until the problem is corrected surgically.

Evaluation

Medical management usually controls ulcer disease, often within a few weeks. Many clients must continue treatment to remain ulcer free.

■ Surgical Management

Surgery of the stomach is performed for the following reasons:

1. To reduce the stomach's acid-secreting ability
2. To remove a malignant or potentially malignant lesion
3. To treat a surgical emergency that develops as a complication of peptic ulcer disease
4. To treat clients who do not respond to medical intervention

Most chronic, recurring ulcers are eventually treated surgically. Surgery for prevention of ulcer recurrence is performed for the following reasons:

1. To facilitate enterogastric regurgitation of mucous secretions, bile, and pancreatic juice
2. To decrease the secretory capacity of the stomach by removing the parietal cells
3. To remove stimuli for hydrochloric acid secretion by cutting the vagus nerve
4. To eliminate the gastrin hormone mechanisms by antrectomy

If the physician suspects cancer in a gastric lesion, surgery is generally indicated. When an ulcer does not respond to intensive medical therapy and a definite diagnosis cannot be made by radiographic and endoscopic examination, surgery is performed to remove the lesion and to make certain it is not malignant.

Emergencies such as acute obstruction, perforation, and acute intractable hemorrhage are usually treated by immediate surgical intervention. Hemorrhage sometimes responds to medical management, but when medical approaches (such as cooling, vasoconstriction, and neutralization of acid) do not stop the bleeding, emergency surgery is required to save the client's life.

The surgical approaches to reducing the acidity of the stomach are (1) to sever nerves that stimulate the acid-secreting cells and (2) to remove the acid-secreting portions of the stomach.

Vagotomy

Vagotomy is performed to eliminate the acid-secreting stimulus to gastric cells. There are three types of vagotomy: (1) truncal, (2) selective, and (3) proximal (Fig. 61–6A). Truncal vagotomy involves completely cutting each vagus nerve. In selective vagotomy, the surgeon partially severs the nerves to preserve the hepatic and celiac branches. Proximal vagotomy also involves partial cutting, but in this instance, only the parietal cell mass is denervated; innervation of both the antrum and the pyloric sphincter is preserved. Cutting the vagal nerve fibers

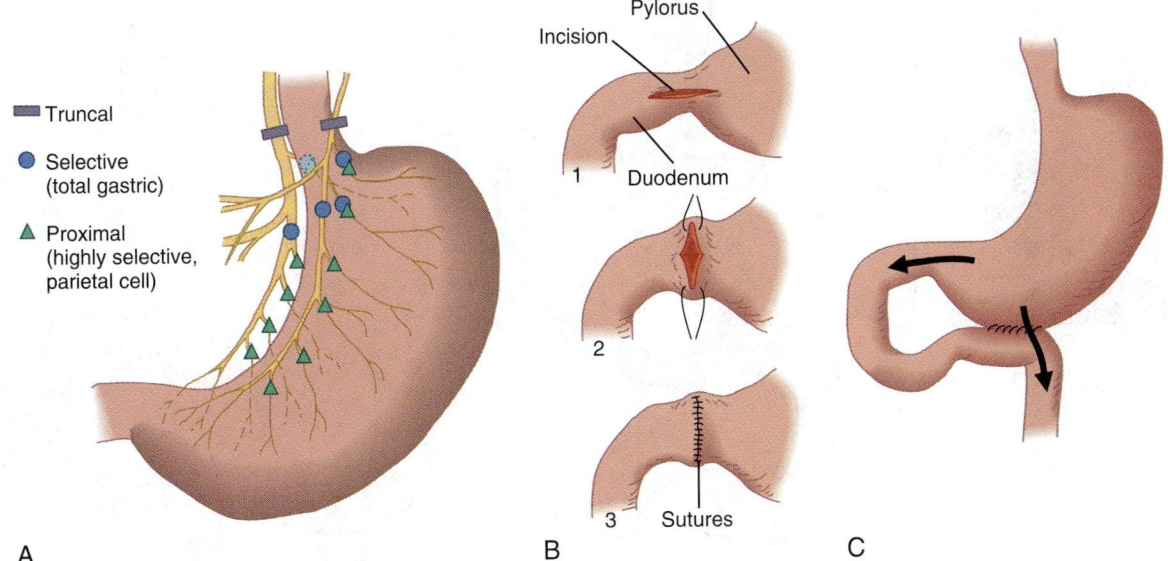

Figure 61–6. Vagotomy and drainage. *A*, Sites at which the three types of vagotomy are performed. *B*, Pyloroplasty provides a larger opening from stomach to duodenum to enhance emptying after vagotomy. *C*, Gastroenterostomy, another associated surgical procedure, creates a passage between the body of the stomach and the jejunum.

selectively avoids the problems of impaired emptying and diarrhea that follow the truncal vagotomy. It also eliminates the necessity for a drainage anastomosis to offset the gastric stasis. In addition, proximal vagotomy reduces acid secretion and preserves the function of the antrum.

Vagotomy with Pyloroplasty

Vagotomy with pyloroplasty involves cutting the right and left vagus nerves and widening the existing exit of the stomach at the pylorus. This procedure prevents stasis and enhances emptying, thereby preventing belching, weight loss, and feelings of fullness (Fig. 61–6*B*).

Gastroenterostomy

A simple gastroenterostomy (Fig. 61–6*C*) permits regurgitation of alkaline duodenal contents, thereby neutralizing gastric acid. In this procedure, a drain is made in the bottom of the stomach and sewn to an opening made in the jejunum. Because this neutralization interferes with the inhibition of gastrin release, a net increase in acid secretion may result. If the gastroenterostomy drains the stomach, it reduces motor activity in the pyloroduodenal area. Drainage also diverts acid away from the ulcerative area, which facilitates healing. A gastroenterostomy does not reduce the secretory capacity of the parietal cell mass, and the gastrin mechanism continues to function. Gastroenterostomy should be combined with vagotomy to reduce vagal influences.

Antrectomy

Antrectomy is performed to reduce the acid-secreting portions of the stomach. The procedure removes the entire antrum of the stomach; thus, the cells that secrete gastrin are excised. This delays or eliminates the gastric phase of digestion by withdrawing the source of stimulation for acid release and slows direct response to protein. The surgeon then anastomoses the remaining portion of the stomach to the duodenum. Antrectomy is often accompanied by vagotomy; thus, the cephalic and gastric phases of gastric secretion are eliminated and GI tract motor activity is decreased. It appears to prevent recurrence and is probably superior to more extensive procedures.

Subtotal Gastrectomy

Subtotal gastrectomy, a generic term referring to any surgery that involves partial removal of the stomach, may be accomplished by either a Billroth I or a Billroth II procedure (Fig. 61–7).

In a *Billroth I* procedure, the surgeon removes a part of the distal portion of the stomach, including the antrum. The remainder of the stomach is anastomosed to the duodenum. This combined procedure is more properly called *gastroduodenostomy*. It decreases the incidence of dumping syndrome that often occurs after a Billroth II procedure.

A *Billroth II* resection involves reanastomosis of the proximal remnant of the stomach to the proximal jejunum. Note that pancreatic secretions and bile continue to be secreted into the duodenum even after gastrectomy. Because these secretions are necessary for digestion, a route to the intestine must be preserved. Surgeons prefer the Billroth II technique for treatment of duodenal ulcer because recurrent ulceration develops less frequently with this procedure.

Total Gastrectomy

Total resection of the stomach is the principal intervention for extensive gastric cancer. This surgery involves removal of the stomach, with anastomosis of the esopha-

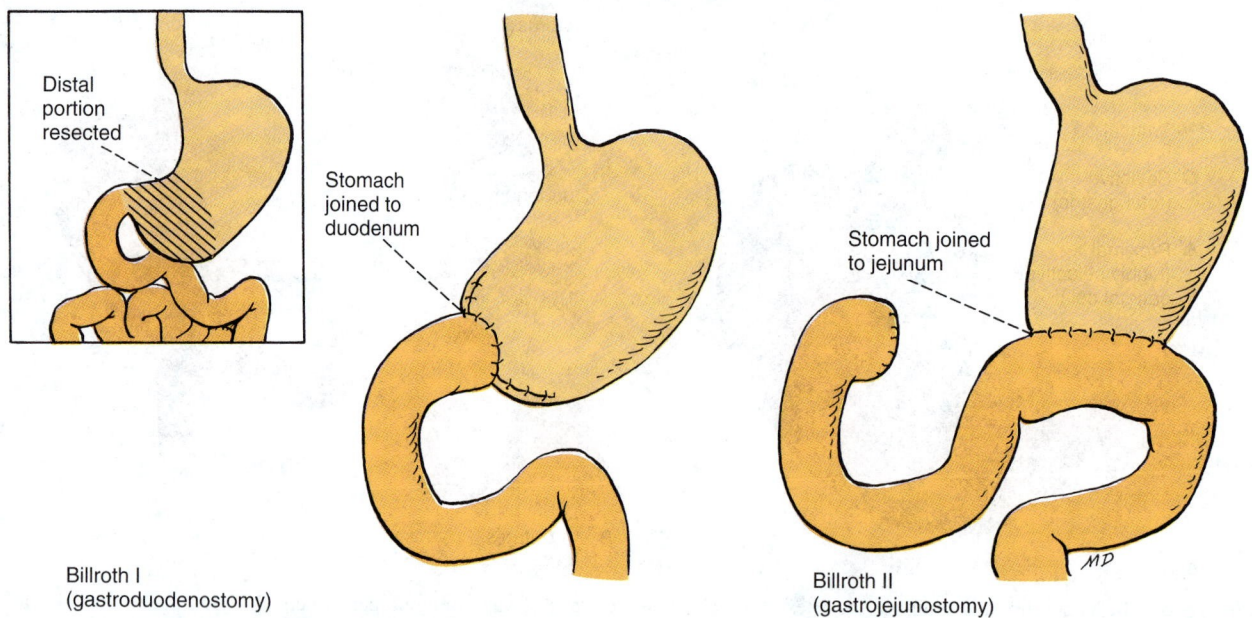

Distal
portion
resected

Stomach
joined to
duodenum

Stomach joined
to jejunum

Billroth I
(gastroduodenostomy)

Billroth II
(gastrojejunostomy)

Figure 61–7. Subtotal gastrectomy removes acid-secreting portions of the stomach. After removing the distal stomach *(inset),* a surgeon sutures the remaining portion of the stomach to the duodenum (Billroth I procedure) or to the proximal jejunum (Billroth II procedure).

gus to the jejunum, an esophagojejunostomy (Fig. 61–8). To perform total gastrectomy, the surgeon enters the chest; thus, the client returns to the recovery room with chest tubes.

Complications

Marginal Ulcers. A marginal ulcer can develop where gastric acids contact the operative site, either at the site of the anastomosis or in the jejunum. This ulceration may cause scarring and obstruction of the passages. Hemorrhage and perforation can also occur.

Hemorrhage. The reported incidence of hemorrhage after gastric surgery is 1% to 3%. It is usually caused by a splenic injury or slippage of a ligature. Assess the client postoperatively for manifestations of bleeding and intra-peritoneal hemorrhage.

Alkaline Reflux Gastritis. Alkaline reflux gastritis caused by duodenal contents occurs after gastric surgery in which the pylorus has been bypassed or removed. It also occurs after pyloroplasty and gastrojejunostomy. An associated vagotomy has usually been performed.

Acute Gastric Dilation. In the immediate postoperative period, distention of the stomach produces epigastric pain, tachycardia, and hypotension. The client complains of a feeling of fullness, hiccups, or gagging. This situation rapidly improves after insertion of a nasogastric tube or clearing of a plugged nasogastric tube. Report these manifestations to the physician immediately.

Nutritional Problems. Nutritional problems common after stomach removal include vitamin B_{12} and folic

acid deficiency, calcium metabolism disorders, and reduced absorption of calcium and vitamin D. Such problems result from (1) a shortage of intrinsic factor and (2) inadequate absorption because of rapid entry of food into the bowel. With the Billroth II gastric resection, there is a

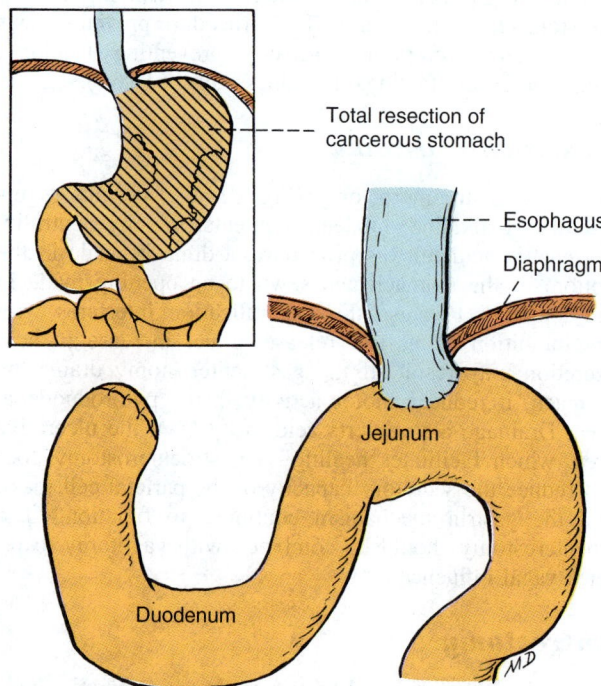

Total resection of
cancerous stomach

Esophagus

Diaphragm

Jejunum

Duodenum

Figure 61–8. Total gastrectomy *(inset)* with anastomosis of esophagus to jejunum (esophagojejunostomy), which is the principal intervention for extensive gastric cancer.

reduction in pancreatic juice and bile secretion because the usual stimulus of food passing through the duodenum is missing.

Dumping Syndrome. This postprandial problem occurs after gastrojejunostomy because ingested food rapidly enters the jejunum without proper mixing and without the normal duodenal digestive processing. It usually subsides in 6 to 12 months. Early manifestations, which occur 5 to 30 minutes after eating, involve the vasomotor disturbances of vertigo, tachycardia, syncope, sweating, pallor, palpitation, diarrhea, and nausea with the desire to lie down. The client's blood pressure and pulse may either rise or fall. Dumping syndrome is most common after the Billroth II procedure. Intestinal manifestations of dumping include epigastric fullness, distention, discomfort, abdominal cramping, nausea (with only occasional vomiting), and borborygmi (rumbling in the bowel). The client may experience tenesmus (ineffectual and painful straining to defecate). Pain is not present.

Early manifestations are probably caused by rapid movement of extracellular fluids into the bowel to convert the rapidly entering hypertonic bolus into an isotonic mixture. This rapid fluid shift decreases the circulating blood volume. A jejunum distended with food and fluid increases intestinal peristalsis and motility.

Late manifestations, which occur 2 to 3 hours after eating, are a result of (1) the rapid entry of high-carbohydrate food into the jejunum, (2) a rise in blood glucose level, and (3) excessive insulin.

Management of dumping syndrome involves decreasing the amount of food taken at one time and maintaining a high-protein, high-fat, low-carbohydrate, dry diet. Gastric emptying can be delayed by the following:

1. Eating in a recumbent or semirecumbent position
2. Lying down after meals
3. Increasing the fat content in the diet
4. Not taking fluids 1 hour before, with, or 2 hours after meals

The Client Education Guide provides a diet for clients with dumping syndrome.

The client may also be given sedatives and antispasmodic agents to delay gastric emptying. When manifestations persist, surgical intervention may include (1) reducing the size of the gastroenterostomy or (2) converting a Billroth II resection to a Billroth I by inserting a short segment of jejunum between the duodenal stump and the stomach.

Gastrojejunocolic Fistula. This postoperative complication follows recurrent peptic ulcer disease. The fistulas arise from perforation of a recurrent ulceration at the gastrojejunal anastomosis site. The perforation forms a fistula between the ulcer and adjacent bowel. Manifestations are variable but include fecal vomiting, diarrhea, weight loss, and anorexia. Belching of gas that has a fecal odor may also occur. The manifestations are caused by bacterial overgrowth in the small intestine.

Pyloric Obstruction. Pyloric obstruction, manifested by vomiting, occurs at the pylorus and is caused by

scarring, edema, inflammation, or a combination of these. When vomiting persists, the client is apt to develop alkalosis because large quantities of acid gastric juice are vomited (see Chapter 16). A client who vomits persistently is usually hospitalized to receive intravenous fluids fortified with electrolytes. Pyloroduodenal obstruction can cause gastric dilation, gastritis, and gastric stasis. These mechanisms create manifestations that gradually make it more difficult for the stomach to empty. Assess the client for feelings of fullness, distention, or nausea after eating, with a loss of appetite and weight loss.

Management of obstruction focuses on restoring fluid and electrolytes and decompressing the dilated stomach; if necessary, surgical intervention is instituted.

■ Nursing Management of the Surgical Client

Assessment

The client with surgical management of ulcer disease requires the same assessments by the nurse as the client being managed medically. In addition, routine preoperative and postoperative assessments are required (see Chapter 21).

Diagnosis, Planning, Implementation

Knowledge Deficit. An appropriate nursing diagnosis for the client undergoing surgery would be *Knowledge Deficit related to preoperative preparation, postoperative care, diet, and long-term prevention of recurrence.*

Planning: Expected Outcomes. The client will understand preoperative preparation, postoperative care, diet, and long-term prevention of recurrence, as evidenced by client's statements and no recurrence of ulcer disease.

Implementation. Surgical intervention for gastric and duodenal conditions may be either a planned procedure or an emergency. When emergency surgery is required (e.g., for acute obstruction, perforation, or hemorrhage), the client is very ill and is usually frightened. Provide calm, efficient, knowledgeable care and explain what is being done. Note and respond to the client's nonverbal behavior. Help significant others provide the client with empathy and emotional support.

When cancer is suspected, the client may want to talk about fears and concerns. Listen to the client carefully, respond to cues, and offer support and understanding. The client may wish to attend to personal matters before surgery (e.g., check a will, see a minister).

When elective surgery is done, the client will have an extensive series of preoperative examinations, such as a GI tract x-ray series, endoscopy, and perhaps acid-secretion studies (see Chapter 59). These may be done on an outpatient basis.

Preoperative teaching should include an explanation of what surgery generally involves. Explain that the client will have either a nasogastric tube or a gastrostomy tube and suction and that an intravenous infusion line will be placed in the hand or arm for fluids until the surgical site heals. Thoroughly demonstrate and discuss the importance of deep-breathing exercises or use of an incentive spirom-

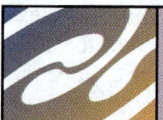

CLIENT EDUCATION GUIDE

Diet for Dumping Syndrome

Client Instructions in English (*Instrucciones para el cliente en inglés*)	Client Instructions in Spanish (*Instrucciones para el cliente en espanol*)
Eat five to six small meals every day.	Coma de 5 a 6 comidas pequeñas cada día.
Eat high-fat, high-protein, low-carbohydrate foods.	Coma alimentos altos en grasa y proteínas, pero bajos en carbohidratos.
Do not eat much roughage.	No coma muchos alimentos con substancias ásperas.
Avoid milk, sweets, and sugars.	Evite la leche, los dulces, y los alimentos con mucha azúcar.
Drink liquids between meals only (avoid liquids 1 hour before and after meals).	Beba líquidos sólo entre comidas (evite tomar líquidos 1 hora antes y después de las comidas).
Eat meat (beef, fish, pork, and poultry) and meat substitutes (cheese, peanut butter, and eggs); potatoes, rice, pasta, and starchy vegetables; white bread, rolls, muffins, cracker, and cereals; cooked vegetables; unsweetened cooked or canned fruits; dietetic drinks, jellies, and syrups; margarine, oils, butter, and salad dressings.	Carne (res, pescado, puerco, y pollo) y sustitutos de carne (queso, crema de cacahuate, y huevos); papas, arroz, pasta, y verduras que contengan carbohidratos; pan blanco, rollos, panecillos, galletas, y cereales; verduras cocidas; frutas cocidas sin azúcar o en conserva; bebidas dietéticas, jaleas, y almíbares; margarina, mantequilla, aceites, y aceites para ensalada (aderezos).
Eat the following foods with caution: Drink fluids 1 hour before and/or 2 hours after meals. Whole-grain breads, rolls, cereals, and pasta; foods made with milk; gas-producing vegetables (cabbage, onions, and broccoli); raw vegetables; fresh fruit; caffeinated beverages; mayonnaise; and salt.	Coma los siguientes alimentos con cuidado: Tome bebidas una hora antes y/o dos horas después de las comidas; panes integrales, panecillos, cereales, y pasta; comidas preparadas con leche; verduras que producen gas (repollo, cebolla, y brócoli); verduras crudas; frutas frescas; bebidas con cafeína; mayonesa; y sal.
Avoid spicy meats, soups, and potatoes; breads with frosting or jelly; sweetened fruit or fruit juice, cakes, pies, cookies; malts, milk shakes and milk products; carbonated beverages; alcoholic beverages; and spices, sugar, jelly, syrup, molasses, and honey.	Evite carnes con muchos condimentos, sopas, caldos, y papas; panes con capa de clara de huevos o jalea; fruta endulzada o jugo de fruta, pasteles, tartas, galletas; leche malteada, batido de leche, y productos lácteos; bebidas gaseosas; bebidas alcohólicas; y especias, azúcar, jalea, almíbar, melazas, miel.

eter. Warn clients that the high abdominal incision makes deep breathing very uncomfortable. The high incision also increases the risk of respiratory complications.

Postoperatively, some clients need help to reduce the number of stressors in their lives. Strategies for altering life-style may be an important part of the rehabilitation and recovery plan. When complications such as dumping syndrome occur, the client may feel disappointed. Many clients expect a rapid recovery and may be unprepared when complications do develop. Most clients can learn to control manifestations and lead a fairly normal life.

Postoperative Complications. After surgery, the client is prone to postoperative complications. The collaborative problem is *Postoperative Complications (immedi-*

ate and delayed) related to bleeding, distention, and atelectasis.

Planning: Expected Outcomes. The client will not suffer injury related to postoperative complications (immediate and delayed), as evidenced by decreasing bloody drainage from nasogastric tube, absence of abdominal distention, and normal breath sounds.

Implementation. Nursing care after gastric surgery is the same as postoperative care for any client recovering from major abdominal surgery. In addition to general postoperative care, the following functions should be performed:

- Check the drainage from the nasogastric tube
- Maintain nasogastric tube patency with saline irrigations as ordered

- Ensure that the tube is attached to suction, as ordered
- Assess the operative site for excessive drainage; too much fluid in the remaining gastric stump could cause increased pressure and injury
- Note the color and consistency of drainage from the operative site and report bleeding or hemorrhaging

Immediate complications after gastric surgery include gastric dilation, obstruction, hemorrhage, and disruption of the suture line. Also, observe for general surgical complications such as shock, hemorrhage, pulmonary problems, thrombosis, evisceration, infection (peritonitis), and paralytic ileus. Nausea and vomiting should not occur if the nasogastric tube is patent. Carefully measure and document intake (oral and intravenous) and output (urine, suction, and wound drainage).

The client will return from surgery with a nasogastric or gastrostomy tube for preventing the retention of gastric secretions. Carefully assess for abdominal distention. The nasogastric or gastrostomy tube should not be repositioned after gastric surgery because it is placed directly over the suture line. It should be irrigated gently with saline, *only* if specifically ordered.

The color of the drainage in the nasogastric tube may be bright during the early hours after surgery but should become dark red by the end of 24 hours. The drainage will have the appearance of coffee grounds several days after surgery.

Keep the client comfortable with liberal administration of pain medications. This helps the client to cooperate more fully during deep-breathing and coughing exercises. The Nursing Research feature compares the effects of jaw relaxation and music on postoperative abdominal pain. Give fluids by intravenous infusion as ordered until edema and swelling have diminished enough to allow fluids to pass the operative area (seen as a decrease in the gastric tube output and return of bowel sounds).

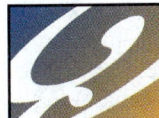

NURSING RESEARCH

Does Jaw Relaxation, Music, or Both, Relieve Pain After Surgery?

Good, M. (1995). A comparison of the effects of jaw relaxation and music on postoperative pain. *Nursing Research, 44*(1), 52–57.

This experimental study compared the effects of jaw relaxation and music, individually and combined, on sensory and affective pain following surgery. Eighty-four abdominal surgical clients were randomly assigned to four groups: jaw relaxation, taped music, a combination of jaw relaxation and taped music, and neither (control group). Interventions were taught preoperatively and used by subjects during the first ambulation after surgery. Indicators of the sensory component of pain were sensation and 24-hour narcotic intake. Indicators of the affective component of pain were distress and anxiety of pain. With preambulatory sensation, distress, narcotic intake, and preoperative anxiety as covariates, the four groups were compared using orthogonal a priori contrasts and analysis of covariance. The interventions were neither effective nor significantly different from one another during ambulation. However, after keeping the taped interventions for 2 postoperative days, 89% of experimental subjects reported them helpful for sensation and distress of pain.

Implications for Practice

Music and relaxation tapes are useful therapies in conjunction with analgesia for treatment of postoperative abdominal pain.

Altered Nutrition: Less than Body Requirements. After surgery the client is at *Risk for Altered Nutrition: Less than Body Requirements related to decreased nutrient absorption secondary to dumping syndrome.*

Planning: Expected Outcomes. The client will maintain adequate nutrition. He or she will be able to maintain weight at a normal level and with no evidence of dumping syndrome.

Implementation. When healing has occurred, clamp the tube and begin oral intake by giving the client clear water, usually 30 ml at a time. Aspirate the tube an hour or so later to see if the fluid has been retained. When GI function has returned (e.g., active bowel sounds, passage of flatus) and the client tolerates clear water, the nasogastric tube is usually removed and the diet progresses to soft foods; eventually, a regular diet of five or six small meals a day is given. The diet should not begin too early or progress too rapidly. At first, the client may experience discomfort if too much food is taken at one time.

Evaluation

Clients need to know that convalescence after gastric surgery tends to be slow. It may be 3 months before clients regain strength and even partial ability to eat in a more normal manner. It may take a year or so before they can eat three normal meals a day. Observe the client postoperatively for persistent gastric disturbances.

Gastric Cancer

Gastric cancer refers to the malignant neoplasms found in the stomach, usually adenocarcinoma, although there may be malignant lymphomas. For unknown reasons, the incidence of stomach cancer in the United States has diminished steadily during the last four decades. The incidence of gastric cancer in the United States has decreased from 25 per 100,000 to 4 per 100,000 during the past 40 years.[1] Despite the reduced incidence, gastric cancer is the sixth most common cause of death from cancer in the United

States. Although little is known of the cause, it is known that stomach cancer is twice as common in men as in women, more common in American whites, and more frequent in clients who have pernicious anemia. World-wide mortality rates vary greatly, possibly as a result of differences in diet, genetics, and soil composition.

Etiology and Risk Factors

Although no specific etiologic factors are associated with gastric cancer, several factors do seem to be associated with the development of the disease. It often develops in conjunction with chronic atrophic gastritis and affects individuals to whom the following characteristic apply:

1. Low socioeconomic status
2. Live in an urban area
3. Eat smoked fish
4. Are exposed to background radiation or trace metals in the soil

The presence of *H. pylori* in the stomach increases the incidence of gastric cancer. Other etiologic factors include achlorhydria and pernicious anemia. The changes in the mucosa may lead to an increase in the absorption of carcinogens from the diet, such as pickled foods, salted fish, and nitrates. Smoking also appears to be associated with an increased incidence of gastric cancer. There may also be a genetic factor because it does seem to run in families. Metal craftsmen, coal miners, bakers, and those working in dusty, smoky, and sulfur dioxide-containing environments are at greater risk. Wood or tobacco smoke, nitrite food preservatives, and overheated fat products may predispose clients to stomach cancer.

Avoidance of the carcinogenic agents is important, especially in clients with other risk factors such as chronic gastritis, *H. pylori* infection, and pernicious anemia. Cessation of smoking is a good primary preventive measure.

Pathophysiology

Gastric cancer most often arises from the mucous lining of the stomach. The majority of these cancers occur in the lesser curvature of the stomach in the pyloric and antral regions.

Most carcinomas of the stomach develop in its lower half. Prognosis is best for stomach cancer involving polypoid lesions; it is poor for ulcerating cancers and poorest for infiltrating forms. Stomach cancer spreads in the following ways:

1. By direct extension into the pancreas
2. Via the lymphatics
3. By hematogenous infiltration of the liver, lungs, and bones

The particular route depends on the location and the type of tumor. Some penetrate, some ulcerate, and some spread along the tissue planes (Table 61–5).

The disease is resectable in early stages before it has invaded the wall of the stomach. The 5-year survival rate is about 90% for local disease; this rate drops to less than 10% for stage III disease. In advanced gastric cancer, the

Table 61–5. TNM Classification for Gastric Carcinoma	
Primary Tumor (T)	
T_x	Primary tumor cannot be assessed
T_0	No evidence of primary tumor
T_{is}	Carcinoma in situ: intraepithelial tumor without invasion of lamina propria
T_1	Tumor invades lamina propria or submucosa
T_2	Tumor invades muscularis propria or subserosa
T_3	Tumor penetrates serosa (visceral peritoneum) without invasion of adjacent structures
T_4	Tumor invades adjacent structures
Lymph Node (N)	
N_x	Regional lymph node(s) cannot be assessed
N_0	No regional lymph node metastasis
N_1	Metastasis in perigastric lymph node(s) within 3 cm of edge of primary tumor
N_2	Metastasis in perigastric lymph node(s) more than 3 cm from edge of primary tumor, or in lymph nodes along left gastric, common hepatic, splenic, or celiac arteries
Distant Metastasis (M)	
M_x	Presence of distant metastasis cannot be assessed
M_0	No distant metastasis
M_1	Distant metastasis
Stage Grouping	
0	$T_{is}N_0M_0$
IA	$T_1N_0M_0$
IB	$T_1N_1M_0$
	$T_2N_0M_0$
II	$T_1N_2M_0$
	$T_2N_1M_0$
	$T_3N_0M_0$
IIIA	$T_2N_2M_0$
	$T_3N_1M_0$
	$T_4N_0M_0$
IIIB	$T_3N_2M_0$
	$T_4N_1M_0$
IV	$T_4N_2M_0$
	Any T, any N, M_1

survival rate is almost zero. Lesions higher in the stomach, especially around the cardia, have a poor prognosis because of the usual lateness of diagnosis.

Clinical Manifestations and Diagnostic Findings

Because the manifestations occur late in the course of the disease, stomach cancer is seldom diagnosed in an early stage. Furthermore, unless hemorrhage or perforation occurs, manifestations are vague and indefinite. The presence of a palpable mass, ascites, or bone pain from metastasis may be the first manifestation. Manifestations vary, depending on the location of the tumor in the stomach. If the neoplasm grows near the cardia, the client may experience dysphagia from early involvement of the esophagus. If the neoplasm is near the pylorus, manifestations may occur from obstruction.

Assessment reveals weight loss, a vague indigestion, anorexia, or a feeling of fullness or mild discomfort so insidious that the client does not recognize it as abnormal or seek medical assistance. Discomfort may be brought on or relieved by eating. Anemia from blood loss commonly occurs, and occult blood may be present in the stool. The presence of lactic acid and a high lactate dehydrogenase level in the gastric juice suggests carcinoma.

Gastric cancer is diagnosed by upper GI tract x-ray examination and gastroscopy. Gastroscopy allows the lesion to be viewed directly and permits cytologic brushing to facilitate the retrieval of cells for cytologic examination.

Acute and Subacute Care

■ Medical Management

Little effective medical treatment is available for gastric carcinoma. Clients may receive chemotherapy and radiation therapy, but the primary treatment for this condition is surgical resection.

At present, best results are achieved with multiple drug combinations. Those giving the best results are fluorouracil, mitomycin C, and doxorubicin (Adriamycin). Other combinations are currently being investigated in clinical trials. The combination of radiation and chemotherapy after surgery may be done.

TPN (hyperalimentation) is a method for providing nutrition to the client intravenously, thus bypassing the GI tract.

■ Surgical Management

Surgery is the only intervention that effectively treats stomach cancer. Unfortunately, because the diagnosis is usually late, surgery is more often palliative than curative. Gastrectomy, either partial or complete, depending on tumor location, is the usual procedure. Ideally, the surgeon removes all local growth and the associated lymph nodes. When an extensive tumor makes resection impractical or impossible and the pylorus is obstructed, the surgeon may perform a palliative gastroenterostomy (surgical creation of a passage between the stomach and small intestine). Chemotherapy and, less often, radiation may be used with surgery.

■ Nursing Management of the Surgical Client

Assessment

As mentioned, the manifestations associated with gastric cancer are usually vague. Clients may present with manifestations similar to those of ulcer disease, but frequently manifestations are not present until the tumor is advanced. Note on the client's history any risk or predisposing factors to the development of gastric carcinoma. These include a history of chronic gastritis, pernicious anemia, gastric surgery, or smoking. Also note in the client history if the client ingests large amounts of nitrates, smoked fish, salty foods, or pickled foods.

Diagnosis, Planning, Implementation

Pain. Both before and after surgery, a primary nursing diagnosis for the client is *Pain related to gastric erosion* and *Postoperative Pain related to high surgical incision.*

Planning: Expected Outcomes. The client will have pain controlled or experience a reduction in pain, as evidenced by client's statements.

Implementation. It is very important that the client receive pain relief. Pain that is not controlled can interfere with sleep and eating and contribute to overall physical and mental deterioration. See Chapter 17 for a detailed explanation of pain control. The client should have verbal and written instructions regarding medications, treatments, and follow-up care.

Altered Nutrition: Less than Body Requirements. After surgery, an important nursing diagnosis for the client with gastric cancer is *Altered Nutrition: Less than Body Requirements related to decreased appetite, pain, possible gastric obstruction, and nausea and vomiting.*

Planning: Expected Outcomes. The client will maintain nutritional intake to meet metabolic requirements, as evidenced by maintenance of normal body weight.

Implementation. Nutritional therapy is a very important aspect of management of the client with gastric cancer. TPN or jejunostomy tube feedings may be used postoperatively (or for clients with inoperable disease) to maintain the nutritional status.

Fear. Because of the uncertainty of the disease and its outcome, an appropriate nursing diagnosis for the client with gastric cancer is *Fear related to knowledge deficit, treatment, and life-threatening illness.*

Planning: Expected Outcomes. The client will have fear reduced or controlled, as evidenced by client's ability to understand and discuss disease and treatment options.

Implementation. The client needs an explanation of the disease and all treatment options. Reinforce information to the client as needed. The client also needs preoperative teaching concerning operative procedures (nothing by mouth; holding area; intravenous infusions). Information will help decrease the client's fear.

Postoperative complications include hemorrhage, obstruction, anemia, nutritional deficiency, dumping syndrome, duodenal stump leakage, gastric dilation, and delayed gastric emptying.

A home healthcare referral can assist the client with emotional support and treatments and provide an ongoing assessment of the client's condition. You might also refer the client to a dietitian, clergyman, and hospice team. Various community support groups are also available (e.g., I Can Cope).

Evaluation

The outcome of surgery for gastric cancer can leave the client with numerous problems. The prognosis for clients with gastric surgery is very poor, so the only appropriate outcome may be adequate control of manifestations and as good a quality of life as possible.

Congenital Disorders: Esophageal Atresia with Tracheoesophageal Fistula

Atresia of the esophagus with a fistula from the lower pouch and a blind upper pouch (type III) is described as the "classic picture" of the disease. There are six types of esophageal atresia; type III constitutes the largest percentage of cases. A wide variety and combination of treatment approaches may be employed, depending on the type of atresia and the condition of the infant who has been born with it. Ligation of the fistula usually takes place immediately. The esophagus is repaired at the same time if the infant's condition allows. If too wide a gap exists between the proximal and distal pouches in esophageal atresia without fistula, or if a leak occurs in the anastomosis, a reconstruction of the esophagus (colon transposition, colon transport, esophageal replacement) is performed.

The prognosis for complete recovery depends on many factors. The most common complication is stricture at the anastomosis site. Regularly scheduled dilation with Tucker dilators is necessary if stricture is present.

Conclusions

Gastric disorders are common; unless treated promptly and completely, they can continue to cause problems throughout the client's life. Help clients to learn a new way of eating to achieve and maintain health. This is a difficult task; however, unless the client modifies behavior—especially eating behaviors—many of the gastric disorders simply recur. The focus of nursing interventions will be education and modifications of the client's behavior to a healthier pattern.

Thinking Critically

1. You are caring for a client in a nursing home. The client has had a cardiovascular accident and is paralyzed, sometimes confused, and incontinent. She refuses to eat and drink after many episodes of coughing and choking at mealtimes. A small-bore feeding tube has been inserted. When you check the tube for the aspirate that indicates patency, you are unable to obtain any return aspirate. What nursing measures should be instituted to determine the problem? What is the priority nursing intervention?

Factors to Consider. What conditions contribute to the lack of aspirate return? What is your decision should the tube remain occluded?

2. You are assigned to care for two clients. One client is an elderly gentleman with a 6-month history of difficulty swallowing and weight loss of 25 lb. Esophageal cancer is suspected. The other client is a woman in her mid-30s with a diagnosis of Crohn's disease. She has been admitted with an exacerbation of the disease. How should nutritional needs be addressed for each client?

Factors to Consider. How should nutritional needs be met for the client with an upper gastrointestinal tract disorder? With a lower gastrointestinal tract disorder?

3. A young female executive comes to the health clinic with complaints of epigastric pain and malaise. She works under stress and smokes heavily. She is in a hurry and wants quick action. The physician recommends antacids for pain relief and an upper gastrointestinal x-ray film to rule out a duodenal ulcer. What further nursing assessment is required? What nursing interventions should you plan?

Factors to Consider. What places the client at risk for a duodenal ulcer? What teaching is required for medication and dietary management? How should changes in life-style be addressed?

Bibliography

1. American Cancer Society (1996). *Cancer facts and figures.* New York: Author.
2. McCorkle, R. (1996). *Cancer nursing: A comprehensive textbook.* (2nd ed.) Philadelphia: W. B. Saunders.
3. Berry, S., et al. (1994). Intestinal placement of pH-sensing nasointestinal feeding tubes. *JPEN: Journal of Parenteral and Enteral Nutrition, 18*(1), 67–70.
4. Bockus, S. (1993). Tube feedings. *Nursing, 23*(7), 34–42.
5. Cerda, J., et al. (1994). A revolution in peptic ulcer disease. *Patient Care, 28*(9), 18–28.
6. Chase, S. (1993). Antacids. *RN, 56*(8), 46–51.
7. Copstead, L. (1995). *Perspective on pathophysiology.* Philadelphia: W. B. Saunders.
8. Correa, P. (1991). Is gastric carcinoma an infectious disease? *New England Journal of Medicine, 325*(16), 1170–1171.
9. Eisenberg, P. (1994). Nasoenteral tubes. *RN, 57*(10), 62–69.

10. Eisenberg, P. (1994). Gastrostomy and jejunostomy tubes. *RN, 57*(11), 54–59.

11. Eisenberg, P. (1994). Feeding formulas. *RN, 57*(12), 46–53.

12. Fedotin, M. (1993). *Helicobacter pylori* and peptic ulcer disease: Reexamining the therapeutic approach. *Postgraduate Medicine, 94*(3), 38–45, 139–140.

13. Georges, J., & Heitkemper, M. (1994). Dietary fiber and distressing gastrointestinal symptoms in midlife women. *Nursing Research, 43*(6), 357–361.

14. Goldfinger, S. (1994). Peptic ulcer disease: Debugging the system . . . this study offered unprecedented evidence that ulcers can be cured with antibiotics. *Harvard Health Letter, 19*(8), 1–3.

15. Good, M. (1995). A comparison of the effects of jaw relaxation and music on postoperative pain. *Nursing Research, 44*(1), 52–57.

16. Goodman, T., & Simon, L. (1993). Minimizing the complications of NSAID therapy. *Journal of Musculoskeletal Medicine, 11*(2), 33–46.

17. Groenwald, S. L., et al. (1995). *Cancer nursing: Principles and practice* (3rd ed.). Boston: Jones and Bartlett.

18. Handerhan, B. (1993). Complications: Managing a perforated viscus. *Nursing, 23*(2), 92–95.

19. Harries, P. (1992). Facilitating change in anorexia nervosa: The role of occupational therapy. *British Journal of Occupational Therapy, 55*(9), 334–339.

20. Hoffman, L., & Halmi, K. (1993). Psychopharmacology in the treatment of anorexia nervosa and bulimia nervosa. *Psychiatric Clinics of North America, 16*(4), 767–778.

21. Jess, L. (1993). Acute abdominal pain. *Nursing, 23*(9), 34–41.

22. Keithley, J. (1993). The significance of enteral nutrition in the intensive care unit patient. *Critical Care Nursing Clinics of North America, 5*(1), 23–29.

23. Landau-West, D., Kohl, D., & Pasulka, P. (1993). Team treatment of eating disorders. *Nutrition in Clinical Practice, 8*(5), 220–225.

24. Laws, A. (1993). Does a history of sexual abuse in childhood play a role in women's medical problems? A review. *Journal of Women's Health, 2*(2), 165–172.

25. Lehne, R. (1994). *Pharmacology for nursing care* (2nd ed.). Philadelphia: W. B. Saunders.

26. Mamel, J. (1992). Clinical pharmacology of commonly used drugs in GI practice part 1. *Gastroenterology Nursing, 15*(3), 114–121.

27. Mamel, J. (1993). Clinical pharmacology of commonly used drugs in GI practice, part 2. *Gastroenterology Nursing, 15*(4), 156–162.

28. Mattox, T. (1993). Drug use evaluation approach to monitoring use of total parenteral nutrition: A review of criteria for use in cancer patients. *Nutrition in Clinical Practice, 8*(5), 233–237.

29. McGinnis, C., & Matson, S. (1994). How to manage patients with a Roux-en-Y jejunostomy. *AJN, 94*(2), 43–45.

30. Meades, S. (1993). Suggested community psychiatric nursing interventions with clients suffering from anorexia nervosa and bulimia nervosa. *Journal of Advanced Nursing, 18*(3), 364–370.

31. Metheny, N., et al. (1994). Visual characteristics of aspirates from feeding tubes as a method for predicting tube location. *Nursing Research, 43*(5), 282–287.

32. Metheny, N., et al. (1993). Effectiveness of pH measurements in predicting feeding tube placement: An update. *Nursing Research, 42*(6), 314–331.

33. Metheny, N., et al. (1993). How to aspirate fluid from small-bore feeding tubes. *AJN, 93*(5), 86–88.

34. Miller, D., & Miller, H. (1995). Giving meds through the tube. *RN, 58*(1), 44–48.

35. Olson, A. (1993). Women, obesity, and the results of medical management. *AWHONNS—Clinical Issues in Perinatal Women's Health Nursing, 4*(2), 220–226.

36. Osak, M. (1993). Nutrition and wound healing. *Plastic Surgical Nursing, 13*(1), 29–36.

37. Prevost, S., & Oberle, A. (1993). Stress ulceration in the critically ill patient. *Critical Care Nursing Clinics of North America, 5*(1), 163–169.

38. Rakel, B., et al. (1994). Nasogastric and nasointestinal feeding tube placement: An integrative review of the literature. *AACN: Clinical Issues in Critical Care Nursing, 5*(2), 194–223.

39. Rastam, M. (1994). Anorexia nervosa: Recent research findings and implications for clinical practice. *European Child and Adolescent Psychiatry, 3*(3), 197–207.

40. Rush, C. (1995). Action STAT! Gastrointestinal bleeding. *Nursing, 25*(8), 33.

41. Sabiston, D. (1994). *Atlas of general surgery.* Philadelphia: W. B. Saunders.

42. Sabiston, D., & Lyerly, H. (Eds.). (1994). *Essentials of surgery* (2nd ed.). Philadelphia: W. B. Saunders.

43. Sheldon, P., & Bender, M. (1994). High-technology in home care: An overview of intravenous therapy. *Nursing Clinics of North America, 29*(3), 507–519.

44. Smith, C., et al. (1993). Responsibilities and reactions of family caregivers of patients dependent on total parenteral nutrition at home. *Public Health Nursing, 10*(2), 122–128.

45. Surratt, S., et al. (1993). Troubleshooting a sump tube. *AJN, 93*(1), 42–47.

46. Swiech, K., Lancaster, D., & Sheehan, R. (1994). Use of a pressure gauge to differentiate gastric from pulmonary placement of nasoenteral feeding tubes. *Applied Nursing Research, 7*(4), 183–189.

47. Taylor, M. (1994). Total parenteral nutrition, part 1. *Nursing Standard, 8*(23), 25–28.

48. Taylor, M. (1994). Total parenteral nutrition, part 2. *Nursing Standard, 8*(24), 37–39.

49. Viall, C. (1994). Enteral feeding technology. *Nursing, 24*(8), 32J–32K.

50. Weber, M. (1995). Chemotherapy-induced nausea and vomiting. *AJN, 95*(4), 34–35.

51. White, J. (1993). Women and eating disorders. *AWHONNS—Clinical Issues in Perinatal Women's Health Nursing, 4*(2), 227–235.

52. Wilfley, D., & Grilo, C. (1994). Eating disorders: A women's health problem in primary care. *Nurse Practitioner Forum, 5*(1), 34–45.

53. Wyngaarden, J. B., et al. (1996). *Cecil Textbook of Medicine* (20th ed.). Philadelphia: W. B. Saunders.

54. Zaloga, G. (1993). Reagent testing: Bedside testing of gastrointestinal tract specimens. *Consultant, 33*(7), 80–82.

Nursing Care of Clients with Intestinal Disorders

Jane Hokanson Hawks

CHAPTER

62

The client with an intestinal disorder will usually have a problem with bowel elimination. Hence, the most common nursing diagnoses will be the following:

- Constipation
- Perceived Constipation
- Colonic Constipation
- Bowel Incontinence
- Diarrhea

Additional nursing diagnoses include:

- Altered Nutrition: Less than Body Requirements
- Pain
- Impaired Skin Integrity
- Fear
- Body Image Disturbance
- Knowledge Deficit related to dietary changes and pharmacologic management

General Clinical Manifestations

Manifestations of intestinal disorders vary according to which function (motility, digestion, or absorption) is disturbed and the cause of this disturbance. The major manifestations of dysfunction are:

- Hemorrhage
- Pain
- Tenderness
- Distention
- Vomiting
- Malabsorption
- Constipation
- Diarrhea
- Abdominal masses
- Abnormal fecal contents

Hemorrhage. Bleeding may be caused by trauma, ulceration, inflammation, or a growth that erodes through a

blood vessel (Fig. 62–1). The usual manifestation is blood in the stool (hematochezia) rather than in the vomitus (hematemesis). The amount of bleeding varies from a minute quantity that is invisible except by testing (occult blood) to large quantities that cause the stools to be bright red to tarry-black (melena). Because color comes from the digestive processes acting on the blood, the examiner can use the color change to determine the level of the bowel in which bleeding occurs. The rapidity with which the chyme passes through the bowel also affects stool color passed in a certain period and what color changes occur. For instance, slow bleeding from the duodenum may not increase peristalsis and may produce a tarry stool. If the rate of bleeding or of peristalsis increases, subsequent stools may become brighter in color.

Pain. Pain results from stimulation of nerve endings in the muscular or submucosal layers of bowel wall and from increased tension when the bowel is distended. Discomfort occurs in various places, including the involved portion of the bowel, another previously diseased area, or a nearby somatic portion of the body (referred pain). Previous surgical procedures also influence the site at which pain is felt.

Obstruction of blood supply to the intestine also can cause pain. Acute or partial occlusion of the mesenteric artery causes intermittent pain during digestion because of the increased need for blood at that time. This is sometimes called intestinal angina. Occlusion can occur in the major artery or one of the smaller branches.

Nausea and Vomiting. In intestinal disorders, nausea results from distention of the duodenum. If vomiting occurs and is fecal in nature, it originates from the bowel and is usually caused by a high small-intestinal obstruction.

Malabsorption. Malabsorption is a defect in the mechanism by which food is absorbed by the small intestinal mucosa. In the intestinal phase of absorption, the

---

This chapter incorporates material written for the fourth edition by Shirley M. Ruder and Esther Matassarin-Jacobs.

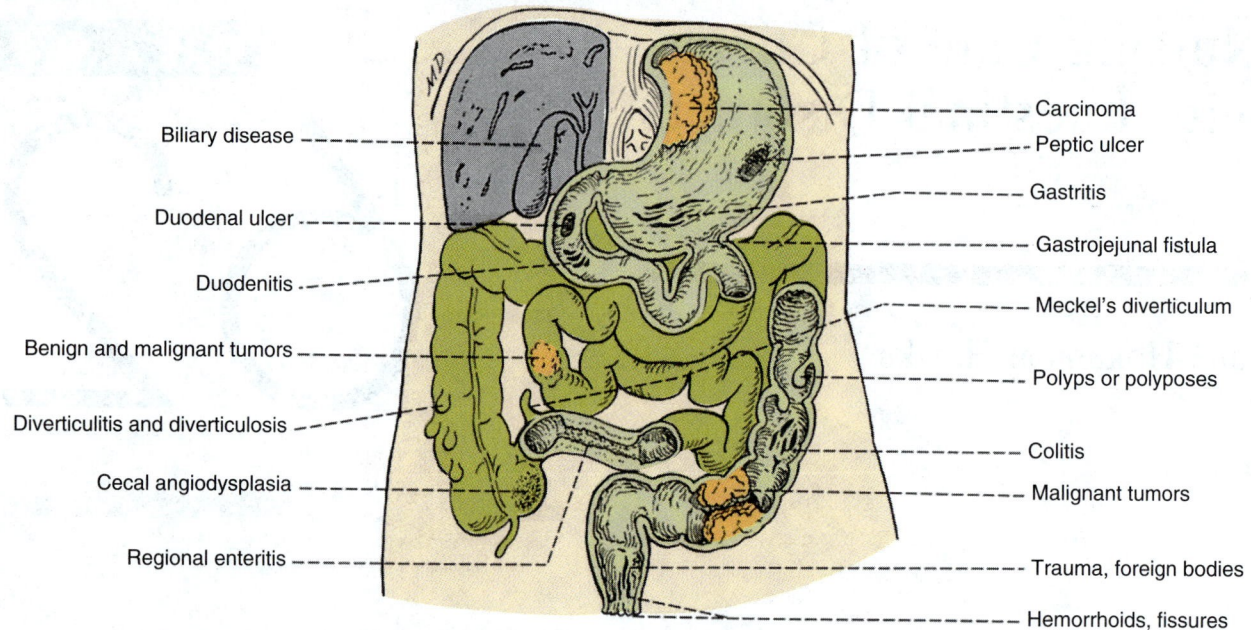

Figure 62–1. Causes of gastrointestinal bleeding.

intestinal villi secrete enzymes that stimulate intestinal motility and facilitate absorption. The active transport mechanism moves absorbed nutrients from the lumen of the small bowel to the intestinal submucosa and from the submucosa to the body's tissues by way of the circulatory and lymphatic system. Abnormalities may result from the following:

1. Loss of ileal function
2. Decreased production of pancreatic enzyme, especially inadequate secretion of lipase
3. Inflammation of the intestinal mucosa
4. Any surgical loss of absorptive mucosa, such as gastric, small bowel, or colon resection

Diarrhea. Rapid propulsion of intestinal contents through the small bowel usually results in diarrhea and may lead to a serious fluid volume deficit.

Constipation. Constipation, a very common manifestation, can be caused by inadequate fluid or bulk, mechanical blockage of the passage of intestinal contents (by a tumor), or slow peristalsis.

Abnormalities in Fecal Content. The presence of fats or other abnormal constituents, normally absorbed from the stool, indicates malabsorption. Other fecal abnormalities that may aid in diagnosis are bacteria, parasites, pus, blood, and abnormal quantities of mucus from the colon.

Disorders of the Large and Small Bowel

Inflammatory Disorders

Inflammation can occur in any portion of the bowel and can be caused by the following:

1. Organisms (any type)
2. Toxins produced by organisms
3. Infiltration of the bowel wall by granulomatous processes
4. Injury from radiation
5. Trauma
6. Medications

Infections and Infestations

Viral and Bacterial Infections: Gastroenteritis and Dysentery

Gastroenteritis is an inflammation of the stomach and intestinal tract that primarily affects the small bowel. It is associated with abdominal cramps, diarrhea, vomiting, and fever.

Viral gastroenteritis occurs throughout the world and is common. It often occurs in epidemic outbreaks.

Dysentery is an inflammatory condition affecting the colon. It is characterized by severe bloody diarrhea and abdominal cramping. Dysentery caused by *Escherichia coli* and *Shigella* occurs worldwide. *Shigella* infection occurs more frequently in children under 10 years of age and in homosexual populations.

Infection with *Clostridium difficile,* also known as pseudomembranous colitis, is a bacterial dysentery commonly seen in clients who have been receiving large doses of antibiotics or who have taken antibiotics for a long period of time. The condition is becoming increasingly common in the hospitalized population. The Nursing Research feature addresses the effect of *C. difficile* on hospitalized clients.

Another cause of dysentery is *Salmonella. Salmonella* is associated with ingestion of contaminated eggs or poultry, or other foods containing these contaminated products.

The cause of gastroenteritis is usually a virus or bacteria. The virus varies and is often referred to as the "flu." In staphylococcal food poisoning, the bacteria produce a toxin when infected foods are allowed to remain warm for a time before being eaten.

Amebic and bacterial organisms such as *Entamoeba histolytica, Shigella bacilli, Escherichia coli,* and *Salmonella* cause most dysentery. The organisms are transmitted by ingestion of contaminated foods and drinking water. Infected persons carry these organisms in the large bowel. Cholera also causes dysentery-like manifestations. *Clostridium difficile* occurs when the normal flora of the bowel is depressed by antibiotics. Spores are carried on healthcare workers' hands or contaminated equipment. The Risk Factors and Levels of Prevention feature lists

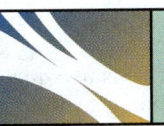

RISK FACTORS AND LEVELS OF PREVENTION

Gastroenteritis and Dysentery

Risk Factors

Viral: Overcrowding and confinement to the indoors

Bacterial: Improper handling and storage of foods, food handling by infected persons

Dysentery: Overcrowding, poor sanitary conditions, food remaining at a temperature high enough for organisms to incubate and colonize easily.

Levels of Prevention

Primary Prevention
● Instruct clients to avoid crowded conditions.
● Advise clients to obtain vaccinations against viral gastroenteritis.
● Encourage clients to follow proper food handling and storage techniques.
● Teach the importance of good hand-washing technique.
● Encourage cleanliness and proper sanitation.
● Caution clients to avoid the use of antibiotics over a long period of time.

Secondary Prevention

Assess clients who are on high or continued doses of antibiotics for signs of *C. difficile* infection.

● Tell clients to report signs and symptoms of infection secondary to antibiotic usage.
● Teach clients the proper methods for handling and storing food.

Tertiary Prevention

Promote bowel rest and replacement of fluids and electrolytes as needed to prevent complications.

● Instruct clients about their medication regimens as recommended.

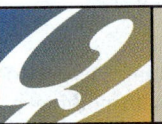

NURSING RESEARCH

How Does *Clostridium difficile* Affect Hospitalized Clients?

Yablon, S., Krotenberg, R., & Fruhmann, K. (1992). Diarrhea in hospitalized patients. *American Journal of Physical Medicine and Rehabilitation, 71*(2), 102–107.

This study examined the impact of *Clostridium difficile*–related disease in 33 rehabilitation hospital inpatients over a 13-month period. *Clostridium difficile* was determined to be the cause of diarrhea in 12 (36%) of the patients. Four patients were transferred to acute care because of the severeity of symptoms. A total of 120 therapy sessions were altered or cancelled because of the diarrhea.

Implications for Practice

A heightened awareness of this infection is indicated so that treatment may be initiated as soon as possible.

other factors that contribute to gastroenteritis and dysentery.

If *Staphylococcus* organisms multiply sufficiently, they can cause a violent gastroenteritis to develop in 2 to 4 hours. Bacterial or viral food poisoning usually develops within 16 hours after ingestion of contaminated food. Gastroenteritis is temporarily disabling, but the condition is of short duration and usually is not serious, except in infants, the very elderly, and weakened or debilitated persons. The last-named are at risk of life-threatening fluid and electrolyte imbalances.

Diarrhea associated with dysentery is caused, in part, by the inflammatory action of the organisms on the lining of the bowel. The organisms can invade and actually destroy the mucosal lining of the bowel, leading to fluid leaking into the bowel.

Endotoxins produced by the infective organisms stimulate the mucosal cells lining the bowel, leading to further diarrhea. These mucosal cells increase secretion of water and electrolytes into the intestinal lumen. The active secretion of chloride and bicarbonate ions in the small bowel leads to inhibition of sodium reabsorption. In order to balance the excess sodium, large amounts of protein-rich fluids are secreted into the bowel, overwhelming the large bowel's ability to reabsorb the fluid.

Dysentery can be fatal in debilitated, aged, and very young persons. Early detection and intervention with fluids and electrolytes are critical to prevent death or disability.

Assessment reveals possible vomiting, profuse diarrhea, and resultant severe fluid and electrolyte loss. Varying amounts of blood may be present in the stool, and the client may experience a mild-to-severe temperature elevation, depending on the causative organism.

Protozoal Infections: Amebiasis and Giardiasis

Amebiasis produces diarrhea when a protozoan *(Entamoeba histolytica)* invades the lining of the colon. Manifestations include rectal inflammation, blood, pus, and amebae in the stool. Metronidazole (Flagyl) is the drug of choice to treat this condition.

Giardiasis, a diarrheal illness, is caused by the protozoan *Giardia lamblia.* It generally spreads through the water system or spoiled food. Manifestations begin several weeks after exposure. Onset is abrupt with nausea, vomiting, excessive foul flatulence, and malabsorption, which causes weight loss. Most clients, however, are asymptomatic. Organisms infect the small intestinal mucosa and submucosa and are found in the stool. The medication of choice is tinidazole (Fasigyn). Other agents that may be used include metronidazole, quinacrine (Atabrine), and furazolidone (Furoxone). At present no agent is effective in preventing giardiasis.

Parasitic Infestations

The intestinal tract may be infested with any of several species of parasitic worms, including *Ascaris* (roundworms), *Enterobius* (pinworms), *Trichinella spiralis* (which causes trichinosis), and various species of tapeworms. These parasites are found worldwide and, often, in the poorer regions of the United States. Worm infestations can cause serious and even fatal disease if the parasites are not eradicated from the intestinal tract. Worms also may cause urinary tract infections or pruritus ani. Fortunately, most of these parasites are susceptible to medications such as mebendazole and pyrantel pamoate. Piperazine and quinacrine hydrochloride also may be used, but they produce more side effects. Treatment for all household members may reduce reinfection.

Schistosomiasis is caused by a blood fluke (a parasitic flatworm). It is prevalent worldwide. The cercariae of the parasite penetrate the skin, migrate to the liver via the lungs, and remain in intrahepatic portal venules until the worm matures. The mature worm, which does not multiply within humans, then moves into its final habitat. Depending on the species involved, the worm may settle in the veins of the large bowel, small bowel, or bladder, where it lays eggs. These eggs, which form pseudotubercles, are commonly found in the liver and veins of the abdomen and lungs but have been identified in every system of the body, including the nervous system. Some eggs are excreted in the urine or feces. Without adequate sewage disposal, the eggs may be deposited in water that contains a susceptible snail, thus continuing the cycle.

In humans, schistosomiasis may have no manifestations. It may be mild or severe, depending on the species of worm involved and the number present. The prognosis is usually good, although there is an increase in the incidence of bladder cancer in persons with this parasite. Schistosomes do not multiply within the body, but a large number may be present because of repeated infections. Their life span is probably about 3 to 5 years, but it may be as much as 30 years. Thousands of worms have been removed from a single client.

Schistosomiasis begins with dermatitis at the site of penetration, followed by a fever in 20 to 60 days, and later, by manifestations from the extrusion of eggs. Laboratory studies must examine the eggs or worms and identify the species before pharmacologic treatment can begin. Medications of choice include oxamniquine, metrifonate, praziquantel, and niridazole.

Acute and Subacute Care

■ Medical Management

Management of gastroenteritis includes resting the gastrointestinal tract and replacing fluids. Rest, with nothing by mouth (NPO) until the vomiting has stopped, is the best intervention. If the client has fluid depletion, an intravenous agent such as 0.45% sodium chloride (hypotonic) is administered. A potassium supplement may be ordered if the client's serum potassium level is low.

The client is started on small amounts of clear liquids, as tolerated. The client may be given an electrolyte replacement beverage. The diet is advanced after 24 hours, as tolerated. In gastroenteritis, the infecting agents need to be eliminated, so drugs that decrease intestinal motility are not administered.

If the infecting organism is *Shigella,* an anti-infective agent such as sulfamethoxazole with trimethoprim (Bactrim, Septra) is administered. In the case of prolonged diarrhea in which the stool is leukocyte-positive, antibiotics are given.

Antidiarrheals and antispasmodics may be given, but their use is controversial. Many of these medications slow intestinal motility, and they may actually increase the severity of the infection because these drugs keep the infection in contact with the bowel longer. The nonsystemic antidiarrheals, such as kaolin and pectin or bismuth subsalicylate (Pepto-Bismol), coat the intestinal mucosa, decrease intestinal secretions, and decrease the diarrhea. To be effective, these agents must be given frequently (every 30 minutes) in doses of 30 to 60 ml. However, antidiarrheal drugs are not given with *C. difficile* infection because the bacteria will multiply if gastrointestinal motility is slowed and the bacteria are retained.

■ Nursing Management of the Medical Client

Assessment

Most clients present with an acute onset of diarrhea. Carefully note a description of the diarrhea, including onset; number, color, and consistency of stools; and accompanying manifestations such as nausea and vomiting. Ask the client about recent foreign travel, eating habits, and antibiotic use.

Assess the client's abdomen. Examination may reveal hyperactive bowel sounds, distention, and tenderness. Dehydration and electrolyte imbalance may be present depending on the amount of fluids and electrolytes lost. Assess muscle weakness and fatigue due to hypokalemia. Metabolic alkalosis from bicarbonate loss is also a potential problem.

Diagnosis, Planning, Implementation

Diarrhea. The major manifestation of intestinal infections and infestations is diarrhea, so the primary nursing diagnosis for these clients would be *Diarrhea related to intestinal hypermotility secondary to irritation.*

Planning: Expected Outcomes. The client will have cessation of diarrhea, as evidenced by a decrease in the number of stools and the solid consistency of feces.

Implementation. Carefully examine all stool for blood and mucus, and record intake and output. Examine the client's anal area for irritation. After cleaning the area, apply a moisture barrier (e.g., petroleum jelly, zinc oxide).

Administer medications such as antibiotics and antiparasitics to treat the specific cause of the diarrhea. Antidiarrheals also may be ordered if the diarrhea is uncontrollable.

Provide written and oral instructions regarding diet and rest, as well as instructions about when and how to report any continued problems. Home healthcare needs are usually minimal unless the client is unable to prepare meals or obtain rest. The client must be reminded to wash his or her hands well and to maintain absolute cleanliness if other family members are sharing the bathroom.

Risk for Fluid Volume Deficit. Since diarrhea is one of the most common manifestations, the client is at risk for the nursing diagnosis *Risk for Fluid Volume Deficit related to gastrointestinal fluid and electrolyte losses.*

Planning: Expected Outcomes. The client will have return of normal fluid and electrolyte balance as evidenced by normal serum electrolytes and balanced intake and output.

Implementation. If the client shows manifestations of fluid and electrolyte imbalance, start intravenous fluids until oral fluids are tolerated. Then start clear liquids with electrolytes in small amounts until the client can tolerate a diet advanced to include toast and saltines. If this diet is tolerated, the diet is usually advanced to a bland diet, then to a general diet as tolerated.

Evaluation

Fluid volume deficit is usually a self-limiting problem and the major outcome is the control of fluid and electrolyte balance. If the problem does not resolve, further medical treatment is needed.

Appendicitis

Appendicitis is an inflammation of the vermiform appendix that develops most commonly in adolescents and young adults. It can occur at any age, but is rare in clients younger than 2 years of age and reaches a peak incidence in clients between 20 and 30 years old. It is not common in older adults, but when it does occur in this age group, rupture is more common.

Etiology and Risk Factors

Appendicitis can be caused by the following:

1. A fecalith (a fecal calculus or stone) that occludes the lumen of the appendix
2. Kinking of the appendix
3. Swelling of the bowel wall
4. Fibrous conditions in the bowel wall
5. External occlusion of the bowel by adhesions

There are no particular risk factors for appendicitis. It is not preventable, so early detection of the condition is important. Appendicitis is the most common cause of acute inflammation of the right lower quadrant of the abdomen.

Pathophysiology

When the appendix becomes obstructed, the intraluminal pressure increases, leading to decreased venous drainage, thrombosis, edema, and bacterial invasion of the bowel wall. With continued obstruction, perforation results.

After the initial obstruction, the appendix becomes increasingly hyperemic, warm, and covered with exudate progressing to gangrene and perforation.

Clinical Manifestations and Diagnostic Findings

The classic manifestations of appendicitis begin with acute abdominal pain, which comes in waves. At first, the pain may be perceived merely as discomfort that makes the client feel that passing flatus or having a bowel movement will bring relief. Unfortunately, many clients take a laxative during this period, which may lead to rupture of the appendix and peritonitis. The pain typically starts in the epigastrium or periumbilical region. It then shifts to the right lower quadrant as the inflammatory process spreads to involve the serosal layers of the bowel, thereby bringing the inflammatory process into contact with the peritoneum. The pain becomes steady rather than intermittent, and the client often guards the area by lying still and drawing the legs up to relieve tension on the abdominal muscles. Assessment also may reveal vomiting that begins after the pain starts, loss of appetite, low-grade fever, coated tongue, and bad breath.

Mild leukocytosis is usually present, with the white blood cell (WBC) count between 10,000 and 15,000/mm^3. Physical findings confirm the diagnosis. Pain at McBurney's point, which lies midway between the right anterior superior iliac crest and the umbilicus, may be diagnostic.

Acute and Subacute Care

■ Surgical Management

There is no medical treatment as such for appendicitis. Until surgery can be performed, intravenous fluids and antibiotics are administered.

Surgical intervention involves removing the appendix (appendectomy) within 24 to 48 hours of onset of the manifestations. The surgery can be performed through a small incision or laparoscopically. When the operation is performed in time, the mortality rate is less than 0.5%. Delay usually causes rupture of the organ and resultant peritonitis. Surgery is frequently delayed, however, because the diagnosis is difficult to make and clients often seek medical aid belatedly. Older clients may have very few manifestations and do not seek aid until after perforation has occurred.

Diagnosis also can be difficult in very young children. Numerous diseases mimic appendicitis:

- Mesenteric adenitis
- Ovarian cyst
- Cholelithiasis
- Renal or ureteral calculi
- Diverticulitis
- Meckel's diverticulum

The client may require antibiotics and surgical drainage if perforation occurs.

■ Nursing Management of the Surgical Client

Assessment

The client is usually admitted with severe abdominal pain. Carefully assess the pain, especially to determine its location. Also assess the client for rebound tenderness and the presence of peritonitis (see Peritonitis). Carefully assess the client's vital signs, fluid and electrolyte status, and laboratory data. The client with appendicitis should fast in preparation for surgery.

Diagnosis, Planning, Implementation

Pain. One of the most appropriate nursing diagnoses for the client with acute appendicitis is *Pain related to inflammation*.

Planning: Expected Outcomes. Client will verbalize decreased postoperative pain.

Implementation. The client's pain medication will be withheld until the diagnosis is confirmed. Sometimes, pain medication will not be given until the client is actually ready for surgery. Never give an enema or a laxative or apply heat to the abdomen of the client with appendicitis, because these actions could lead to perforation.

An abrupt change in the character of the pain preoperatively could indicate perforation. Postoperatively, pain control, as described in Chapters 17 and 20, should be practiced.

The client with uncomplicated appendicitis should be able to resume normal activity in 2 to 4 weeks. Discharge teaching and posthospital care for the client with an uncomplicated appendectomy are the same as for any client after surgery.

Risk for Fluid Volume Deficit. Another appropriate nursing diagnosis for the client with acute appendicitis is *Risk for Fluid Volume Deficit related to vomiting*.

Planning: Expected Outcomes. The client will maintain fluid and electrolyte balance as evidenced by balanced intake and output and electrolytes within normal limits.

Implementation. As soon as the client is admitted, intravenous fluids are started to maintain fluid balance, with electrolytes added as needed. If the client is vomiting, a nasogastric (NG) tube is inserted. Carefully measure intake and output and report discrepancies to the physician.

Risk for Infection. The diagnosis *Risk for Infection related to rupture of appendix* is common.

Planning: Expected Outcomes. The client will not develop an infection or will have rupture diagnosed early, as evidenced by removal of the appendix before rupture or prompt treatment of the rupture.

Implementation. Check the client's vital signs regularly, monitoring closely for an increase in temperature and a change in pulse and blood pressure, which may signify a ruptured appendix. The client's pain also should be closely monitored. If the pain becomes generalized throughout the abdomen and the abdomen becomes rigid and boardlike, rupture may have occurred.

If a rupture of the appendix is suspected, the manifestations should be reported to the physician immediately so the client can be prepared for surgery. Preoperative antibiotics are usually administered to reduce the infection.

After surgery, monitor vital signs, urine output, level of consciousness, and intravenous therapy, and assess the client's respiratory status and the surgical wound. The client may have a drain, and if the appendix ruptured, packing may be present. Assess the dressings, provide wound care, reposition the client, and adequately manage the client's pain.

If the client had a ruptured appendix with an infected wound, the client will have to be taught the proper way to care for the wound. Wound care usually includes irrigation of the wound with sterile saline and application of a sterile dressing at least several times a day. Assess the client's ability to function at home and to care for the wound. A home healthcare referral may be needed to assist the client with physical needs and to ensure that the wound is healing properly.

Evaluation

The usual outcome after an uncomplicated appendectomy is healing within a few weeks. If the appendix has ruptured, however, healing will take longer. With a ruptured appendix, healing cannot occur until the infection has cleared and the wound is clean. It may require a secondary closure after the wound is clean.

Peritonitis

Peritonitis is inflammation of the peritoneal membrane. The peritoneum is a semipermeable two-layered sac filled with approximately 1500 ml of fluid which covers all the organs in the abdominal cavity. Because it is well supplied with somatic nerves, stimulation of the parietal peritoneum that lines the abdominal and pelvic cavities causes sharp, well-localized pain. The visceral peritoneum is relatively insensitive. The incidence of peritonitis caused by perforation or rupture of abdominal viscus is hard to determine. Data usually relate to the underlying cause.

Etiology and Risk Factors

Peritonitis can be primary or secondary, or acute or chronic. The major sources of inflammation are from the gastrointestinal tract, from the external environment, and through the bloodstream. The peritoneum is able to produce an inflammatory reaction and wall off a localized process to combat an infection, if (1) the stimulus is not too massive or (2) the source of infection does not continue. For instance, a perforation (e.g., of a gastric ulcer) that continues to drain contaminants into the peritoneal cavity will overcome the ability of the peritoneum to localize and combat the inflammatory process.

Box 62–1 lists specific causes of peritonitis.

Normal bacterial flora of the intestine become a source of infection when they enter the sterile peritoneal cavity. The most common organism is *E. coli,* although streptococci, staphylococci, and pneumococci also may be involved.

There are no specific risk factors for peritonitis, because the condition is a result of another problem. The major preventive measure to consider with this disorder is early diagnosis of clients at risk of developing the condition secondary to one of its many causes. Early diagnosis and initiation of early treatment help to prevent spread of the infection.

Pathophysiology

Peritonitis creates severe systemic effects. Circulatory alterations, fluid shifts, and respiratory problems can cause critical fluid and electrolyte imbalances. The circulatory system undergoes great stress from several sources. The inflammatory response shunts extra blood to the inflamed area of the bowel to combat the infection. Peristaltic activity of the bowel ceases. Fluids and air are retained within its lumen, raising pressure and increasing fluid secretion into the bowel. Thus, the circulating blood volume diminishes.

The inflammatory process increases oxygen requirements at a time when the client's ability to ventilate has been reduced. The client has difficulty ventilating because of abdominal pain and increased abdominal pressure, which elevates the diaphragm.

Clinical Manifestations and Diagnostic Findings

Manifestations of peritonitis vary depending on the cause. Pain may be either localized or generalized. Well-localized pain that causes rigidity of abdominal muscles and

---

Box 62–1. Causes of Peritonitis

- Gangrenous cholecystitis
- Ruptured gallbladder
- Perforated carcinoma of the stomach
- Perforated gastric or duodenal ulcer
- Ruptured spleen
- Acute pancreatitis
- Penetrating wound of the gastrointestinal tract
- Ulcerative colitis
- Gangrenous obstruction of the small bowel due to (1) adhesions, (2) carcinoma, (3) volvulus, or (4) intussusception
- Perforation of Meckel's diverticulum
- Mesenteric thrombosis
- Perforation of a diverticulum
- Regional ileitis
- Appendicitis with perforation
- Ruptured retroperitoneal abscess
- Strangulated hernia
- Puerperal infection
- Salpingitis
- Septic abortion
- Ruptured urinary bladder
- Iatrogenic

pain that increases with any pressure or motion of the abdomen is characteristic of peritonitis. Also, the client usually experiences nausea, vomiting, and possibly a low-grade fever. Assessment reveals (1) absence of bowel sounds and (2) shallow respirations because the client is trying to avoid the pain caused by body movement.

The client with peritonitis commonly has an elevated WBC count (20,000/mm³) with a high neutrophil count. Abdominal x-rays studies are performed, which may show dilation and edema of the intestines, or free air or fluid in the abdominal cavity. If the client is vomiting, manifestations of altered fluid and electrolyte balance also may be present.

Acute and Subacute Care

■ Medical Management

If peritonitis is advanced and surgery is contraindicated because of shock and circulatory failure, oral fluids are prohibited and intravenous fluids are necessary for replacement of electrolyte and protein losses. Usually, a long intestinal tube is inserted through the nose into the intestine to reduce pressure within the bowel. Once the infection has become walled off and the client's condition improves, surgical drainage and repair can be attempted.

The other major treatment of peritonitis is intravenous antibiotic therapy with potent broad-spectrum agents.

■ Nursing Management of the Medical Client

See Chapter 61 for the nursing care of a client with an intestinal tube.

■ Surgical Management

Surgery may be performed to prevent peritonitis, such as with an appendectomy for an inflamed appendix or a colon resection for inflamed diverticulum. If the perforation is not prevented, then the major surgical intervention is incision and drainage of the abscess once it is walled off.

■ Nursing Management of the Surgical Client

Assessment

Obtain a thorough history including specific information about the client's pain. Assess the abdomen, noting the presence of bowel sounds. Palpate the abdomen, noting if the abdomen is firm, distended, or rigid. Note areas of tenderness. Also assess for the presence of rebound tenderness. The client may have a high fever, indicating peritonitis.

Diagnosis, Planning, Implementation

Septicemia. The client with peritonitis is at risk for the collaborative problem *Septicemia related to perforation and ischemia.*

Planning: Expected Outcomes. The client will not develop septicemia or other complications of peritonitis, or will have infection and complications adequately treated as evidenced by normal vital signs, no manifestations of inflammation, and absence of shock, renal failure, or adult respiratory distress syndrome (ARDS).

Implementation. Clients with peritonitis are acutely ill and are given broad-spectrum antibiotics immediately on admission to the hospital. Surgery is usually performed to repair the perforated organs as soon as clients are stable enough to withstand the stress of surgery. During surgery, any leakage can be cultured so specific antibiotic therapy can be implemented. The peritoneal cavity is usually thoroughly irrigated with an antibiotic solution during surgery to reduce the bacterial count. The wound is often packed open, or at least with drains, so infection can be treated.

Postoperatively, carefully monitor clients for the development of postoperative complications such as ARDS, sepsis, and shock. Closely monitor the client's vital signs. Immediately report any manifestations of sepsis, such as a drop or increase in temperature or drop in blood pressure. Upon discharge, provide the client with oral or written instructions regarding wound care, medications, activity restrictions, and follow-up visits.

Risk for Fluid Volume Deficit. The client with peritonitis is at risk for the nursing diagnosis *Risk for Fluid Volume Deficit related to vomiting.*

Planning: Expected Outcomes. The client will maintain normal fluid volume, as evidenced by adequate output, good skin turgor, and moist mucous membranes.

Implementation. Intravenous fluids are administered along with antibiotic therapy. In the client with peritonitis, maintain the NG tube (see Chapter 61). Also monitor the client's fluid balance by assessing vital signs, bowel sounds, urine output, skin turgor, intravenous fluid replacement, weight, and mucous membrane integrity.

Evaluation

Evaluate client outcomes based on the established plan. If the goals have not been achieved, the plan and interventions are revised to meet the client's needs.

Inflammatory Bowel Disease

Inflammatory bowel disease (IBD) includes two chronic inflammatory disorders: (1) Crohn's disease (regional enteritis) and (2) ulcerative colitis. Both diseases are characterized by periods of exacerbation and remission. These chronic, recurrent diseases predominantly affect younger people. Treatment is symptomatic and responses are often unpredictable. Frequently, clients with IBD require surgery, which may be followed by recurrence. Because of the similarities between Crohn's disease and ulcerative colitis, we compare and contrast these two conditions throughout the following discussion of IBD (Table 62–1).

Crohn's Disease. Crohn's disease is a chronic relapsing disease that may develop discontinuously in any segment of the alimentary tract. The most common location is the terminal ileum. Crohn's disease more characteristically involves the entire thickness of the bowel wall (transmural) but particularly the submucosa. The mortality rate is not high, but recurrences and complications can result in disability. Crohn's disease is more common in whites and among Jewish people. There is an increased incidence within families. It occurs at all ages but more often in the person's 20s. Both sexes are affected equally.[5,22]

Ulcerative Colitis. In contrast to Crohn's disease, which is transmural and segmental, ulcerative colitis is a disease that spans the entire length of the colon and involves only the mucosa and submucosa. The disease usually starts in the rectum and distal colon, and spreads upward beyond the rectosigmoid valve to involve most of the sigmoid and descending colon. Ulcerative colitis causes inflammation, thickening, congestion, edema, and minute lacerations that ooze blood and eventually develop

Table 62–1. Differentiation Between Crohn's Disease and Ulcerative Colitis

Characteristic	Regional Enteritis (Crohn's Disease)	Ulcerative Colitis
General Description		
Age at onset	Young	Young to middle age
Pathology and Anatomy		
Depth of involvement	Transmural (all layers of submucosa)	Mucosa and submucosa
Rectal involvement	50%	95%
Right colon involvement	Frequent	Occasional
Small bowel involvement	Involved, ileum narrow	Usually normal
Distribution of disease	Segmental	Continuous
Inflammatory mass	Chronic and extensive	Rare (crypt abscess)
Cobblestone-like mucosa and granuloma	Common	Absent
Mesentery lymph involvement	Edema and hyperplasia	Not involved
Toxic megacolon	Occasional	Occasional
Steatorrhea	Frequent	Absent
Malignancy results	Rare	After 10 years
Fibrous stricture	Common	Absent
Clinical Characteristics		
Course of disease	Slowly progressive	Remissions and relapses
Rectal bleeding	Occasional	Common (90%–100%)
Abdominal pain	Colicky (45%)	Predefecation (60%–70%)
Hematochezia	Unusual or absent	Almost always present
Diarrhea	Present (65%–85%)	Early and frequent (80%–95%)
Vomiting	Present (35%)	Present (15%)
Nutritional deficit	Common	Common
Weight loss	Present (60%–70%)	Present (10%)
Fever	Present (35%)	Present (10%)
Anal abscess	Common (75%)	Occasional (10%)
Fistula and anorectal fissure fistula	Common (80%)	Rare (10%–20%)
Systemic Manifestations		
Arthritis	20%	Uncommon (10%)
Peripheral sacrolitis	18%	18%–20%
Hepatobiliary involvement	Uncommon	15% cholestatic dysfunction 19%–38% fatty liver 30%–50% pericholangitis
Skin: erythema nodosum, pyoderma gangrenosum	Common	Present (5%–10%)
Nephrolithiasis	Occasional	Rare

into abscesses. The edema may lead to extreme friability of the mucosa, so bleeding occurs from any minor trauma. Ulcerative colitis is more common than Crohn's disease. It occurs at all ages, but has a higher incidence among young adults, women, and Jewish people. It has demonstrated a familial tendency.[5,22]

Etiology and Risk Factors

Crohn's Disease. The cause of Crohn's disease is unclear, although the literature suggests there is some genetic or hereditary basis. It is also considered an autoimmune disease. The only risk factors identified for Crohn's disease are genetic. There are no preventive measures that can be taken.

Ulcerative Colitis. Several theories have been advanced to explain the cause of ulcerative colitis. One theory is that the disease is of bacterial origin, because many clients have a history of bacterial infection before the onset of the condition. Researchers have also suspected an allergic reaction as a basis of the disease. Others believe that ulcerative colitis may be due to an altered immune status, because antibodies have been found in the colon. Still others suggest that destructive enzymes and a lack of protective substances in the bowel wall cause the inflammatory process. An emotional disturbance can precipitate an exacerbation or prolong an attack of the disorder, but it is not the primary cause. There are no preventable risk factors associated with ulcerative colitis. Once the client has the disease, controlling stress can help keep the disease in remission.

Pathophysiology

Crohn's Disease. Lesions typically develop in several separated segments of bowel. They are grossly visible and their color is dramatically different from that of normal tissue. Examination of the bowel tissue by endoscopy reveals edematous, heavy, reddish-purple areas. Granular spots also may be present. Enlarged lymph nodes appear in the submucosa, and Peyer's patches are seen in the intestinal mucous membrane. These areas undergo small superficial ulceration with granulomas and fissures. Fissures may completely penetrate the bowel wall, leading to fistulas and abscesses. Collections of lymphocytes throughout the mucosa, submucosa, and serosa are the only microscopic features of Crohn's disease. The small bowel wall becomes congested and thickened, and the lumen narrows.

Small-bowel–related complications of Crohn's disease include malabsorption, kidney stones, gallstones, and hydronephrosis. Anorectal problems include internal fistulas and abscesses. Nephrolithiasis, hydronephrosis, and growth retardation are other complications. Anal fissure is the most common lesion and is directly related to the severity of the diarrhea, which produces ulceration of the perianal skin. Pain commonly accompanies defecation. Perianal abscess may appear during the active phase of IBD. Pain is aggravated by walking, sitting, and defecation.

Assessment may reveal an area of induration, swelling, and redness. Internal fistulas characterize Crohn's disease of the ileum and right colon. Rectovaginal fistulas may occur in women. Incontinence is common as a result of breakdown in the relatively thin rectovaginal septum. Fistulas into the bladder precipitate recurrent urinary infections and, in some instances, even fecaluria. Treatment may include either drainage to control infection or excision.

Arthritis is a transient, acute, painful swelling present in 20% of clients with Crohn's disease. It may be polyarticular or monarticular. It most commonly affects the knees, ankles, and wrists. The client seldom suffers permanent limitation of motion.

Ulcerative Colitis. The appearance of the colon depends on the stage, activity, and severity of the disease. The most characteristic lesion of ulcerative colitis is an inflammatory infiltrate called crypt abscess. This abscess consists of polymorphonuclear leukocytes, lymphocytes, red blood cells, and cellular debris appearing at the base of the crypts of Lieberkühn. The crypt abscess secretions result in purulent discharge. The abscesses may become necrotic and may ulcerate.

Infections secondary to ulcerative colitis produce further inflammatory reactions in the mucosa and submucosa. When the inflammatory lesions heal, scarring and fibrosis, with narrowing, thickening, and shortening of the colon and loss of haustral folds, may follow.

Cancer of the colon is more common among clients with ulcerative colitis than among the general population. The incidence is greatly increased among those who develop ulcerative colitis before the age of 16 and those who have had the condition for more than 20 years.

Complications of ulcerative colitis vary with its severity and location. Ankylosing spondylitis and clubbing of the fingers are found in a few clients. Anemia and nutritional deficiency may occur, causing dry skin that lacks turgor. In addition, assessment reveals erythema, pustules, abscesses, and neurodermatitis.

Toxic megacolon is an extreme dilation of a segment of the diseased colon (often the transverse) that results in complete obstruction. Toxic megacolon usually occurs during an acute exacerbation, and it may follow hypokalemia, a barium enema, or the use of anticholinergics, narcotics, corticosteroids, or antibiotics. Bacterial overgrowth contributes to this complication.

Assessment reveals the following:

- Paralytic ileus
- Dehydration
- Fever
- Tachycardia
- Lethargy
- Leukocytosis
- Decreased serum protein and albumin levels
- Anxiety
- Prostration

In addition, perforation and peritonitis may complicate toxic megacolon.

Clinical Manifestations and Diagnostic Findings

Crohn's Disease. Crohn's disease may have acute manifestations, but the condition is usually slow and unaggressive. The client may be treated for mild and intermittent manifestations months before the diagnosis of Crohn's disease is made.

Assessment typically reveals abdominal pain, diarrhea, and weight loss due to nutritional deficits. The pain is usually intermittent. Terminal ileum involvement produces pain in the periumbilical region. The client experiences jejunal pain in the upper and left midabdomen. Pain of the ileum is intermittent and is felt in the lower right quadrant. A constant aching, soreness, or tenderness usually indicates advanced disease. The client may experience relief of discomfort after passing stool or flatus.

Diarrhea is usually less severe than that associated with ulcerative colitis. Stool consistency is typically soft or semiliquid. Malabsorption, associated with steatorrhea, may develop. If so, stools may be foul-smelling and fatty. Urgency to expel stools may awaken the person at night. In contrast to ulcerative colitis, the client rarely passes gross blood.

Passage of blood indicates ulceration. The client with severe steatorrhea, diarrhea, or long-standing enteritis may have associated nutritional deficits, weight loss, anorexia, pain, anemia, debility, fatigue, and metabolic disturbances. Nutritional deficits arise from the following:

1. A reduction in the intestinal absorptive surface
2. Impaired absorption of fat, vitamin B_{12}, folic acid, iron, calcium, and vitamins A, C, D, E, and K
3. Malabsorption of protein and carbohydrates

Alterations in bile salt and vitamin metabolism may result from surgery or mucosal defects. Metabolic requirements increase because of the inflammatory process and infection, decreased food intake, and nutrients lost in the feces because of rapid gastrointestinal transit time. Electrolytes lost from diarrhea include sodium, potassium, chloride, the trace elements (magnesium, zinc, copper), and minerals.

Nitrogen excretion remains normal if there is no loss of protein from the inflammatory exudate. The consequence of malnutrition may include the following:

● Loss of immunocompetence
● Decreased resistance to infection
● Diminished wound healing
● Diminished pancreatic enzyme output
● Impaired healing (fistula and surgical wounds)
● Decreased iron-binding capacity resulting from chronic infection or blood loss

Temperature elevation may occur with the following:

1. Acute inflammation
2. Associated fistulas, abscesses, or sinus tracts
3. Rheumatoid manifestations

Sudden, severe, right lower quadrant pain, leukocytosis, and tenderness accompany the elevated temperature. Nausea and vomiting are rare unless there is a small bowel obstruction.

Additional acute inflammatory manifestations include pain in the lower right quadrant, cramping, tenderness, flatulence, nausea, and diarrhea. Borborygmus (rumbling in the bowel) and increased peristalsis also may develop. Pain sometimes mimics acute appendicitis or bowel perforation, and manifestations may be confused with those of ulcerative colitis. If anal disease occurs, fissures, fistulas, skin tags, ulcers, and strictures may be present.

The client may experience periods of remission interrupted by exacerbations of active Crohn's disease. Because exacerbations often follow dietary indiscretions, emotional upsets, or illness, inquire into the client's life events at the time of the exacerbation.

Ulcerative Colitis. The predominant manifestation of ulcerative colitis is rectal bleeding. Clients often experience diarrhea, possibly 20 or more stools per day. The severity and frequency of diarrhea depend on the extent of involved colon. Severe diarrhea can cause a loss of 500 to 17,000 ml of water in 24 hours. Liquid stools occur with tenesmus and may contain blood, mucus, and pus. A sense of urgency and cramping abdominal pain may occur with the diarrhea. The client typically experiences colicky pain in the lower left quadrant.

Nausea, vomiting, anorexia, weight loss, and decreased serum potassium may occur with severe disease. In addition, the client loses plasma proteins, prothrombin, and fluids. The development of anemia depends on the degree of blood loss, severity of the illness, and dietary iron intake.

When the disease is acute, the client develops fever. Severe diarrhea or vomiting may cause metabolic acidosis. Physical findings include tenderness in the lower left quadrant, guarding, and (in severe ulcerative colitis) abdominal distention. Following remissions, ulcerative colitis may recur after bouts of emotional stress, dietary indiscretion, or the ingestion of irritants such as laxatives or antibiotics. Physical exertion, respiratory infections, and overfatigue also may cause an attack. As in Crohn's disease, ask about the client's life events prior to recurrences.

Crohn's disease and ulcerative colitis produce similar manifestations. Clients suffer from abdominal pain, fever, diarrhea, fluid imbalances, and weight loss. Remissions are followed by exacerbations of acute disease. Although bleeding is more common in ulcerative colitis, clients with severe Crohn's disease often experience bloody diarrhea.

Physical assessment may reveal certain characteristic manifestations. The general appearance of clients with IBD varies from reasonably healthy to wasted, drawn, and malnourished, with varying degrees of pallor. Some clients have fever and tachycardia. They usually report a steady and progressive weight loss. Inspection reveals a flat or concave shape of the abdomen, with visible peristaltic activity. Palpation of the abdomen reveals tenderness over the area of inflamed bowel. Increased bowel sounds are heard on auscultation. The rectal sphincter is found to be tight, the rectum empty, and the anal area irritated. Hemorrhoids and, in Crohn's disease, perianal abscess, fistula, or ulcers may be apparent.

Decreased levels of hematocrit and hemoglobin are usually noted. A barium enema study with air contrast is often performed to differentiate between ulcerative colitis and Crohn's disease. The client with suspected IBD routinely undergoes colonoscopy. Biopsy and cytologic studies also help distinguish between carcinoma, ulcerative colitis, and Crohn's disease.

Acute and Subacute Care

■ Medical Management

Pharmacologic Agents

Medical treatment, which primarily aims to control the manifestations, is similar for ulcerative colitis and for Crohn's disease. Because the inflammatory process in Crohn's disease involves deeper layers of the bowel wall and is more chronic, healing may occur more slowly than in ulcerative colitis. Thus, anti-inflammatory therapy, including steroids, is required for longer periods in Crohn's disease than in ulcerative colitis.

Fluids, electrolytes, and blood are replaced as needed to maintain the client's homeostasis. Physical activity should be kept to a minimum during the acute attack to decrease intestinal motility. The client with mild attacks

may work, but needs extra rest. The client with fever, toxemia, frequent bowel movements, bleeding, or pain sometimes requires bedrest. Failure of the inflamed colonic mucosa to reabsorb water and electrolytes, bile salts, and lactose interferes with control of diarrhea. The extent of large bowel involved in the disease influences the severity of diarrhea. The client should keep a record of the number of stools, their consistency and color, and the presence of blood.

Antidiarrheal Medications. Antidiarrheal preparations may provide symptomatic benefit (Table 62–2). Loperamide (Imodium) is superior to atropine-diphenoxylate (Lomotil) in controlling diarrhea of Crohn's disease, with fewer side effects. Opiates for diarrhea control may cause distention and megacolon. Hydrophilic mucilloids, such as psyllium or methylcellulose, may improve the consistency of stools and control incontinence. Antispasmodic medications such as belladonna extract, propantheline bromide, glycopyrrolate, or dicyclomine hydrochloride may reduce postprandial pain and diarrhea.

Diarrhea associated with IBD may be treated successfully by antimicrobial agents such as sulfasalazine (Azulfidine). The specific action is unknown, but the medication is retained by the connective tissue of the intestinal mucosa. Side effects include:

● Rash (most common)
● Headache
● Malaise

Table 62–2. Drugs Used in the Treatment of Diarrhea

Drug	Daily Dosage	Nursing Intervention
Diphenoxylate hydrochloride with atropine sulfate (Lomotil)	5 mg qid (altered doses for elderly are not specifically established)	1. Assess number of stools and consistency throughout treatment 2. Assess fluid and electrolyte balance 3. Assess for dry mouth, tachycardia, rash, and urinary retention 4. May be administered with food if gastrointestinal irritation occurs 5. Assess for abdominal distention, pain, and fever
Difenoxin hydrochloride with atropine sulfate (Motofen)	2 mg initially, then 1 mg after each loose stool	1. Assess number of stools 2. Assess for fluid and electrolyte balance 3. Assess for dry mouth, tachycardia, and urinary retention 4. Monitor for signs of addiction
Loperamide hydrochloride (Imodium)	4 mg initially, then 2 mg after each loose stool; maximum dose 16 mg/day	1. Assess number of stools 2. Assess for drowsiness, dry mouth, nausea and vomiting, constipation 3. Assess for abdominal distention, pain, and fever
Opium preparations (opium tincture, paregoric)	Paregoric: 5–10 ml, one to four times daily Tincture: 0.6 ml qid	1. Assess for nausea and vomiting 2. Dilute opium tincture in 15–30 ml of liquid 3. Assess for abdominal distention, pain, and fever 4. Monitor for signs of addiction

- Dizziness
- Aching
- Epigastric distress
- Lethargy
- Depression
- Nausea
- Vomiting

In an attempt to control diarrhea, tincture of opium and paregoric are sometimes given. Bowel rest and parenteral hyperalimentation may result in restored immunocompetence, greater resistance to infection, correction of nutritional deficiencies, and relief of edema and bowel inflammation.

Anti-inflammatory Medications.
Clients who fail to respond to general supportive measures may require anti-inflammatory medications. Adrenal steroids and corticotropin may be used with other therapy to reduce the body's response to inflammation. Steroids do not cure IBD, but by reducing inflammation, they may modify its course. The systemic effects of IBD also respond to steroids.

Antacids or histamine receptor antagonists should be given during steroid therapy to prevent gastric ulceration. Steroids reduce adrenal function and may impair resistance, causing defective healing of abscesses and fistulas. Remember that steroids may mask the manifestations of infection. They are not recommended for clients suffering from dehydration, potential perforation, or severe fluid and electrolyte imbalance. Steroids may be given intravenously, intramuscularly, rectally, or orally. Oral forms include hydrocortisone, prednisolone, and prednisone. Hydrocortisone also can be administered rectally as an enema or suppository. Corticosteroids interfere with intestinal absorption of calcium.

Immunosuppressive Agents.
6-Mercaptopurine, an immunosuppressive agent, is used when other treatment modalities fail and can be effective against chronic, unrelenting Crohn's disease and many of its complications. The medication should be used during the chronic phase. To be effective, therefore, the client must receive steroids or adrenocorticotropic hormone (ACTH) beforehand.

Other immunosuppressive agents are being explored as alternatives to steroids. Methotrexate (Folex) and cyclosporine (Sandimmune) are being administered to clients with Crohn's disease in experimental studies at this time. Transdermal nicotine is being explored as an alternative treatment for ulcerative colitis.

Anticholinergic Medications.
During acute exacerbations, the client is given anticholinergic medications to relieve abdominal cramps and help control diarrhea. Anticholinergics, antidiarrheal agents, and antispasmodics allow the colon to rest and decrease the gastrocolic reflex. Anticholinergics may decrease muscle spasm and discomfort, but have little effect on diarrhea. Withhold these medications if there are manifestations of obstruction. Treatment with these agents may cause further iatrogenic problems.

Anti-infective Medications.
Medications commonly used to prevent or control infections include the sulfonamides and antibiotics. If antibiotic therapy is effective, the client will experience a decrease in temperature, number of stools, and bleeding. Antibiotics may be given to control secondary bowel inflammation and infection. Sulfasalazine (Azulfidine) is the most commonly prescribed sulfonamide for management of both ulcerative colitis and Crohn's disease. Sulfasalazine can interfere with folate absorption and use.

Total Parenteral Nutrition

Total parenteral nutrition (TPN) is indicated for the client who (1) fails to respond to medical intervention, (2) is being prepared for surgery, or (3) has had an intestinal resection. This feeding method provides bowel rest by removing all stimulation of secretion and by decreasing fecal bulk. Weight gain, positive nitrogen balance, and a temporary remission of manifestations can occur. TPN appears to be more useful in Crohn's disease than in ulcerative colitis. When oral food and fluids are resumed, they should be chemically and mechanically nonirritating and high in calories, protein, and minerals. Exclude foods such as cocoa, chocolate, citrus juices, cold or carbonated drinks, nuts, seeds, popcorn, and alcohol.

Elemental diets provide nutritionally balanced meals. They are residue-free, low in fat, and digested mainly in the upper jejunum. Unfortunately, many of the enteral formulas are not very palatable, and client compliance often is low.

Anemia and vitamin B_{12} deficiency should be corrected nutritionally. Folate deficiency, which may be due to the therapeutic use of sulfasalazine, may be prevented by increasing dietary intake of folate, giving sulfasalazine between meals, or supplementing the intervention regimen with folic acid.

A diet high in protein and calories is given in an attempt to restore normal nutritional levels but is not always well tolerated. Anorexia and nausea and vomiting are often present and eating tends to increase diarrhea.

Complications

Nutritional deficiencies are the most common complications of IBD. These deficits derive from the following:

1. Decreased intake
2. Increased nutritional requirements
3. Increased losses
4. Side effects of certain medications

Diarrhea causes fluid and electrolyte losses with resultant muscle wasting and edema. Malabsorption due to bacterial overgrowth or mucosal involvement of the bowel may cause further problems. Deficiencies of all the fat-soluble vitamins, A, D, E, and K, and folate may develop. Vitamin K deficiency causes bleeding tendencies. Clients usually limit their dietary intake to control pain and diarrhea.

Therapeutic interventions such as special diets, antibiotic agents, and anti-inflammatory medications also may cause anorexia or stomatitis. Specific nutritional and metabolic problems caused by IBD include diminished absorption of vitamin B_{12} and trace metals, including zinc, calcium, and magnesium, and decreased reabsorption of bile salts.

Extraintestinal manifestations occur frequently in clients with IBD and complicate its management. Manifestations involve the joints (most common manifestation), skin, eyes, and mouth. The major skin manifestations are erythema nodosum and pyoderma gangrenosum. Local tissue involvement can cause rectal complications, such as anal fissures, and bowel complications, such as local abscesses, perforation, and stenosis from healing lesions. Infrequent nonspecific manifestations include osteoporosis, liver disease, peptic ulceration, and amyloidosis.

■ Nursing Management of the Medical Client

Assess the client's bowel elimination pattern, noting the number of stools, their color and consistency, as well as the presence of blood or steatorrhea. Also assess the client's abdomen. Note bowel sounds and the location of pain.

Diagnosis, Planning, Implementation

Diarrhea. One of the most common manifestations of inflammatory bowel disease is diarrhea, so one of the primary nursing diagnosis is *Diarrhea related to inflamed intestinal mucosa.*

Planning: Expected Outcomes. The client will experience a decrease in diarrhea, as evidenced by a decreased number of stools and a more solid consistency of stools.

Implementation. Antidiarrheal medications are commonly administered to control the client's diarrhea. See Table 62–2 for a summary of drugs commonly used to treat diarrhea. Closely monitor the number and consistency of stools.

Perianal excoriation often occurs with diarrhea. After every bowel movement, gently clean the skin with warm water, and apply a protective moisture barrier product.

Altered Nutrition: Less than Body Requirements.

The client with inflammatory bowel disease has many difficulties with nutrition, making *Altered Nutrition: Less than Body Requirements, related to diarrhea and malabsorption* a common nursing diagnosis.

Planning: Expected Outcomes. The client will increase nutritional intake to meet metabolic requirements, as evidenced by weight stabilization and, possibly, weight gain.

Implementation. Monitor the client's nutritional intake. The type of diet ordered depends on the condition of the client. If the client can tolerate food, encourage intake of fluids and food. Because eating stimulates the gastrocolic reflex and the urge to defecate, many people are afraid to eat. Small servings may allow the client to avoid this problem. Foods should be bland and easily digested to promote absorption during the short time the food remains in the bowel.

Clients with Crohn's disease are often on home TPN because they are unable to tolerate foods for long periods as a result of disease exacerbation. These clients also may have had multiple small bowel resections resulting in problems of malabsorption.

Pain. Another common nursing diagnosis for the client with inflammatory bowel disease is *Pain related to inflamed mucosa.*

Planning: Expected Outcomes. The client will experience a relief in abdominal pain, as evidenced by the client's statement of pain relief.

Implementation. Assess the client's pain and give pain medications as ordered. Note any changes in the client's complaints of pain, because they may indicate the development of complications. Narcotics are generally used sparingly so they do not mask manifestations. The client will need to be seen by the physician at regular intervals if the disease is being controlled medically.

Risk for Ineffective Individual Coping. Stress is associated with inflammatory bowel disease. Write the nursing diagnosis as *Risk for Ineffective Individual Coping related to stress of disease and exacerbations related to stress.*

Planning: Expected Outcomes. The client will cope effectively with the disease, as evidenced by fewer exacerbations and an improved coping style.

Implementation. Although emotional factors may not contribute to the cause of the disease, they do influence its course. The Nursing Research feature describes the effects of IBD on daily life. Prolonged stress often precedes the onset of IBD and exacerbations. Recommend that the client schedule a follow-up physical examination and colonoscopy every 1 to 2 years, depending on the duration of bowel disease manifestations and previous findings. Refer clients with IBD to the Crohn's and Colitis Foundation of America, 386 Park Ave. S., New York, NY 10016-7374, for support groups and information.

Because there is a high incidence of cancer with ulcerative colitis, a client who has had the disease for 5 years or more should also undergo a barium enema study and colonoscopy. Instruct the client to contact the physician at the first manifestation of IBD recurrence.

Evaluation

If the client does not respond to medical management for the treatment of IBD, as evidenced by the client achieving a remission, surgical intervention may be required.

■ Surgical Management

Surgery is commonly used to treat ulcerative colitis, but not Crohn's disease, except to treat complications. When medical management fails and the condition is intractable, surgical intervention is usually indicated for ulcerative colitis. Surgery may be indicated in both conditions for complications such as perforation, hemorrhage, obstruction, toxic megacolon, abscess, fistula, and intractability.

NURSING RESEARCH

How Does Inflammatory Bowel Disease Affect Daily Life?

Kinash, R., et al. (1993). Inflammatory bowel disease impact and patient characteristics. *Gastroenterology Nursing, 15*(4), 147–155.

This study describes the impact of inflammatory bowel disease on the daily life of 150 nonhospitalized adults and examines client characteristics and their relationship to the perceived impact. Most clients reported a low-to-moderate effect of the disease on daily life in self-report questionnaires and interviews. The greatest impact was reported in the areas of elimination, worry, recreation and leisure activities, sleep, and rest. Client characteristics that correlated positively with the impact variable were age (under 35 years), female sex, depressed mood, and an affective-oriented coping style.

Implications for Practice

Enhance client adaptation and satisfaction with life by focusing on client characteristics that are amenable to change and on areas of life where the impact of the disease is experienced most intensely.

Possible procedures that may be performed to treat ulcerative colitis include a total proctocolectomy with a permanent ileostomy, and restorative procedures such as an ileorectal anastomosis, an ileal pouch–anal anastomosis, and a Kock pouch.

Total Proctocolectomy

In a total proctocolectomy, the colon and rectum are removed and the anus closed. The terminal ileum is brought out through the abdominal wall and a permanent ileostomy formed (Fig. 62–2).

Ileorectal Anastomosis

Ileorectal anastomosis is another form of surgical management. The colon is resected, leaving a rectal stump. The terminal ileum is then anastomosed to this stump (Fig. 62–3). The client will have diarrhea postoperatively; however, in time, the stool usually becomes more solid.

Ileorectal anastomosis, an early alternative to total proctocolectomy, has several problems, however. The remaining rectum is often still affected by the disease, and further treatment, even eventual resection, is often required. There is also a significant incidence of rectal cancer among clients who have had this surgery. The newer procedures have essentially eliminated the need for this procedure because safer, more effective options are available.

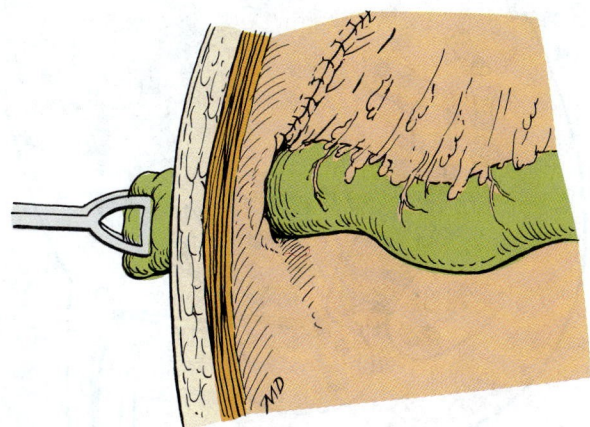

Figure 62–2. Ileum being drawn through the abdominal wall to form an ileostomy stoma.

Ileal Pouch–Anal Anastomosis

The ileal pouch–anal anastomosis (also known as the J pouch) prevents the need for an ostomy and preserves the rectal sphincter muscle. The rectal mucosa is excised and the colon removed. An ileoanal reservoir is then created in the anal canal, and a temporary loop ileostomy is formed. After healing has taken place, the ileostomy is reversed and stool drains into the reservoir, which is created by suturing two loops of bowel together (Fig. 62–4). This is often the preferred surgical procedure for clients with ulcerative colitis.

Continent Ileostomy, or Kock Pouch

A continent ileostomy, or Kock pouch, is a procedure in which a reservoir or pouch is constructed from a loop of ileum. This allows stool to be stored intra-abdominally

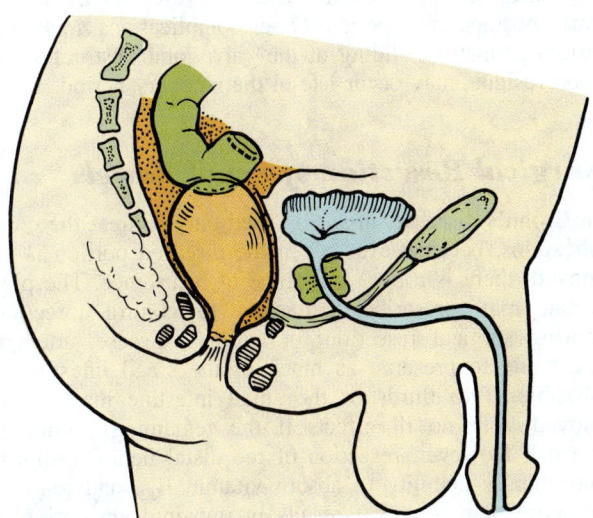

Figure 62–3. Ileorectal anastomosis following subtotal colectomy. This operation eliminates proctectomy with its attendant complications but does not provide definitive treatment for ulcerative colitis.

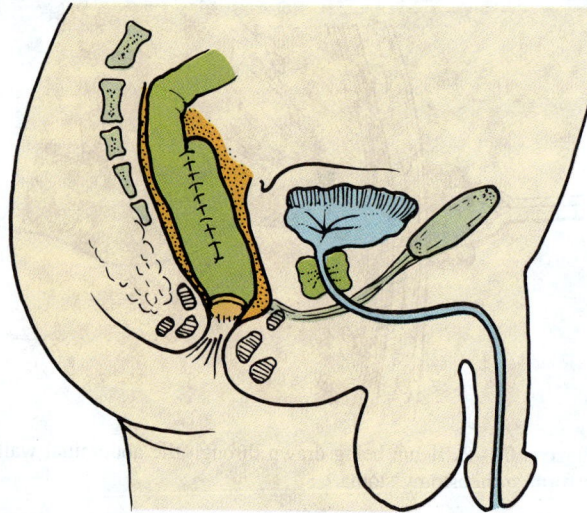

Figure 62–4. Ileal J pouch–anal anastomosis. The two-loop ileal pouch is simple to construct, provides adequate storage capacity, and is evacuated spontaneously and fully.

until it is drained through a nipple valve made from an intussuscepted portion of ileum (Fig. 62–5). The client has a flat stoma on the right side of the abdomen. This procedure is rarely done as a first choice by clients with ulcerative colitis because the ileal pouch–anal anastomosis is preferred. A continent ileostomy should not be done for Crohn's disease.

This continent ileostomy, or Kock pouch, has advantages because the client (1) does not need to wear an external pouch, (2) has minimal skin problems, and (3) usually has no leakage of stool or flatus. The client drains the pouch several times a day using a catheter, usually when a feeling of fullness occurs.

After the formation of the Kock pouch, suture line leakage with local or generalized peritonitis (the most frequent complication with the reservoir) occurs in the early postoperative period. Other complications, including fistula formation, sliding of the valve, and obstruction by food residue, may occur late in the recovery period.

Surgical Resection of Small Bowel

In Crohn's disease, surgery is used only to treat the complications, because even when the diseased portion is removed, there is a 50% incidence of recurrence. The physician may prescribe antibiotics to control infection. During surgical resection for Crohn's disease, attempts are made to preserve as much of the small intestine as possible. Two thirds of the small intestine may be removed with no ill effects if the remaining portion is normal. However, resection of the distal ileum results in the client's inability to absorb vitamin B_{12}, and removal of more than 6 to 8 ft results in impaired absorption of glucose, fat, and protein. If the colon is diseased, an ileotransverse colectomy (right colon and ileum), segmental colectomy, or total colectomy may be performed. A

total colectomy with ileorectal anastomosis may be the surgery of choice.

Complications

For 1 to 3 weeks after extensive small bowel resection, the client may be unable to tolerate oral intake and may have further losses in body protein or lean body mass. TPN is given until oral intake can be resumed. Diarrhea usually occurs during the first 6 weeks after surgery. Anemia (from iron deficiency, steatorrhea, or decreased protein absorption) also may ensue. Paralytic ileus is another possible complication.

■ Nursing Management of the Surgical Client

Assessment

Assessment of the surgical client is similar to assessment of the medical client. However, routine preoperative and postoperative assessments are also necessary.

Diagnosis, Planning, Implementation

Knowledge Deficit. The client who is to undergo surgical resection for inflammatory bowel disease has many learning needs. The nursing diagnosis is *Knowledge Deficit related to surgical procedure and possible ileostomy or other bowel resection.*

Planning: Expected Outcomes. The client will understand the surgical procedure and implications of bowel resection as evidenced by ability to describe the procedure and return to demonstrate ileostomy care.

Implementation. If the client is scheduled for an ileostomy, then ostomy surgery, a procedure that may provoke a life crisis, must be fully explained to the client. In some instances, a preoperative visit from a member of any ostomy association may be helpful. An enterostomal therapy nurse should assist with the preoperative preparation. Before surgery, the site of the ileostomy is selected, consideration being given to the location of the disease, body contours, convenience, and the type of clothing the client wears. If an ostomy pouch is indicated, the client may wear the pouch for 1 to 2 days before surgery to ensure comfort with the site selected. In order to provide assistance and support, assess the client's body image and feelings about loss of a major body part and wearing a pouch for a lifetime.

If the client is not having an ileoproctectomy, but one of the continence-sparing surgeries, extensive teaching is still required. The client needs to understand the type of bowel resection to be performed and the implications of this surgery. Some procedures may require a temporary ileostomy (ileal pouch–anal anastomosis), whereas others will require some altered elimination by the client (Kock pouch).

Postoperative care and care of the stoma or diversion should be reinforced before the client is discharged. The client with an ileostomy should be encouraged to join the

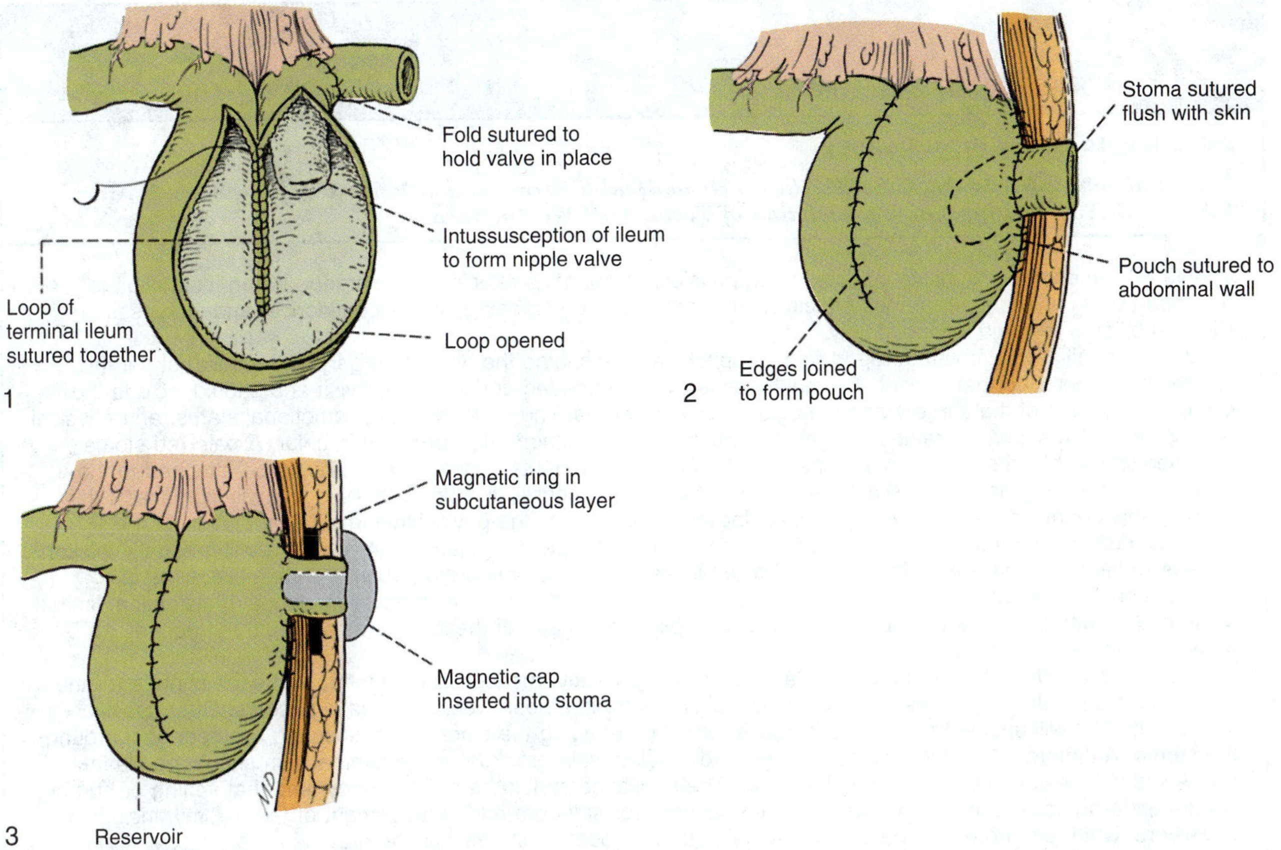

1   Loop of terminal ileum sutured together / Fold sutured to hold valve in place / Intussusception of ileum to form nipple valve / Loop opened

2   Stoma sutured flush with skin / Pouch sutured to abdominal wall / Edges joined to form pouch

3   Reservoir / Magnetic ring in subcutaneous layer / Magnetic cap inserted into stoma

Figure 62–5. Continent ileostomy (Kock pouch) with Maclet ring device. *1,* Loop of terminal ileum is sutured together and cut open. Using forceps, the surgeon intussuscepts the distal ileum to form a nipple valve. *2,* Free edges are sutured together to form the reservoir; the stoma is sutured flush with the skin, and the pouch is sutured to the abdominal wall. *3,* The magnetic ring is implanted in the subcutaneous layer and the stoma is closed with a magnetic cap.

United Ostomy Association. The Client Education Guide provides information about the equipment needed to care for an ileostomy. After a surgical resection, the client will need a follow-up appointment to ensure that healing has occurred. If the client experiences difficulty with self-care, a visiting nursing or enterostomal therapy nurse should visit the client at home to follow up on learning needs. The Bridge to Home Healthcare feature provides suggestions for making these visits useful.

Stomal Necrosis, Retraction, Prolapse, Stenosis, Obstruction.

The client undergoing stoma formation is prone to numerous complications. The collaborative problem is *Risk for Stomal Necrosis, Retraction, Prolapse, Stenosis, or Obstruction related to postoperative complications such as stomal cyanosis, distention, intestinal obstruction, and fluid and electrolyte imbalances.*

Planning: Expected Outcomes. The client will not suffer injury, as evidenced by minimal distention, rapid return of normal peristalsis, and absence of fluid and electrolyte imbalance.

Implementation. Monitor the stoma after surgery. Ensure that there is no pressure on the stoma that could

---

CLIENT EDUCATION GUIDE

Ostomy Supplies

Before you leave the hospital, find out where to purchase supplies for your ostomy. Obtain written instructions, including the brand name, order number, size of pouch, skin barrier, and pouch deodorants, as well as the name, address, and telephone number of a local medical supply facility. Ostomy supplies are very expensive; therefore, refer to *Ostomy Quarterly,* which lists mail-order houses that sell equipment at a discount. Talking with other ostomates at a local United Ostomy Association meeting may give you several money-saving ideas. United Ostomy Association's telephone number is 1–800–826–0826. *The Ostomy Book* by Barbara Dorr Mullen and Kerry Anne McGinn is an excellent publication written especially for clients and their families (Palo Alto, CA, Bull Publishing Co., 1992).

BRIDGE TO HOME HEALTHCARE

Adjusting to Life with an Ostomy

Mary Thomas, R.N., B.S.N., C.E.T.N. *Harris Home Health Services*, and **Jeanette Ghesquiere, R.N., B.S.N., C.E.T.N.** *Visiting Nurse Association of Texas*, **Fort Worth, Texas**

Clients will experience extensive emotional and physiologic changes after ostomy surgery. When instruction is provided to clients and their families effectively, it promotes understanding, instills confidence, and increases clients' ability to manage independently.

Before the initial visit, obtain a report from hospital staff describing the type of surgery and ostomy and if the ostomy is temporary or permanent. Thorough assessment is needed during the first visit and should include the client's knowledge of the surgery and the ostomy, his or her learning skills, dexterity, emotional status, and physical assessment. The stoma is created from mucosal tissue, which is normally beefy-red in color. A pale red stoma indicates limited blood supply. It will be moist with peristomal skin intact; outer edges should be attached to the skin. When cleaning the stoma, slight bleeding is normal. With aggressive cleaning, bleeding will increase. If this occurs, apply gentle pressure. Excessive bleeding is abnormal; call the physician immediately.

Expect daily output from the ostomy. Initially, the stool will be loose. Within 2 to 4 weeks, it will gradually thicken. Excessive flatus is common during the first 4 to 8 weeks. Teach ostomy clients about the manifestations of intestinal obstruction: nausea or vomiting, temperature of 101° F or more, severe abdominal pain, distention, limited or no output, and decreased bowel sounds. If clients experience any of these manifestations, they require immediate medical attention.

Instruct the client to change the ostomy appliance twice weekly, measuring the stoma with each change for the first 6 to 8 weeks. Inform clients that the stoma will shrink during those weeks as healing occurs. Offer specific instructions that will enable the client to increase skills in managing the ostomy and ensuring a proper seal around the stoma. An improper seal will cause leakage and result in skin breakdown. Peristomal skin should be clean and dry. Avoid lotions, creams, and harsh chemicals. The appliance should be changed any time that itching or burning occurs under the skin barrier. Provide written instructions for self-care and management of the ostomy, including the where, what, and how-to of purchasing supplies from a local retailer or mail-order house.

Diet and hydration are essential components of the teaching plan, because a significant amount of the bowel has been removed. Initially, the bowel will be swollen. Instruct the client to avoid foods high in fiber. These foods can lead to intestinal obstruction. Examples include corn, popcorn, mushrooms, peanuts, and Chinese foods. Within 4 to 8 weeks the bowel should return to normal size, allowing a slow return to a normal diet. Fluid intake should be increased to prevent constipation and dehydration. Increased intake is important for clients who have ileostomies because they are prone to experience alterations in potassium and sodium levels.

Community resource support groups are available to assist clients in coping with their diagnosis and changed body image. For information on local chapters in the client's area, call the United Ostomy Association at 1–800–826–0826, the American Cancer Society at 1–800–227–2345, or resources listed in your local telephone book. Contact the National Wound, Ostomy, and Continence Nurses Society at 1–714–476–0268 for information about enterostomal therapists (ETs) in your area. ET nurses provide ostomy clients with valuable instruction and support that helps them return to a normal life-style. ET nurses also have the skills to assist healthcare personnel manage complicated ostomies.

interfere with circulation. The color of the stoma should be assessed at frequent intervals. If the color becomes pale, dusky, or cyanotic, notify the physician immediately. If the blood supply to the stoma is compromised, the stoma may require surgical revision.

An NG, gastrostomy, or jejunostomy tube will be in place for several days after surgery to remove gases and fluids that would increase intestinal distention and put pressure on the suture line. The drainage must be accurately noted. The passage of flatus indicates return of peristalsis. As bowel sounds return, clamp the tube as prescribed and give the client ice chips and water. When the client has tolerated this for a minimum of 24 hours, the tube is usually removed and clear liquids are given.

Although most ileostomies are uneventful postoperatively, several complications can occur. The most com-mon is an intestinal obstruction that may be caused by obstruction of the lumen, adhesions, food, or stomal edema. Early manifestations include anorexia; abdominal cramps; no ileostomy drainage or a foul, brown, watery discharge in the pouch; or visible peristalsis. Other early postoperative complications include hemorrhage, hypoxia, and fluid and electrolyte imbalance. If there are severe or prolonged problems with absorption, an elemental diet or parenteral nutrition may be necessary.

Risk for Body Image Disturbance. The client with an ostomy has to face alterations in self-concept and body image. Write the nursing diagnosis as *Risk for Body Image Disturbance related to disturbance of life-style secondary to ostomy.*

Planning: Expected Outcomes. The client will experience a positive body image and self-concept, as evidenced by the client's statements and ability to care for his or her own ostomy without embarrassment.

Implementation. A few days after surgery, the client needs to begin to confront the stoma and to begin integrating its function and appearance into his or her body image. Help the client look at and touch the stoma as soon as possible. Always use proper terms for the stoma and equipment.

Clothing can be a concern for the client with an ostomy, and clothing options need to be discussed with the client. Discourage the client from wearing a tight waistband that might rub on the stoma. Encourage the client to try on various outfits to ensure that the stoma and pouch are not visible. A visit with another client with an ostomy, usually available through the local American Cancer Society chapter, often helps the client realize that the ostomy is easily hidden beneath clothing.

Encourage the client to verbalize feelings about the stoma and its appearance. The client may be very accepting of the stoma because the illness (ulcerative colitis) is now gone and the client's life may be more normal and productive than it had been with the disease. Young men and unmarried women may express the greatest concern about body image. It is also important to find out how family or significant others now view the client. Again, this might be a positive response, because the client may have been chronically ill prior to the surgery and now appears much healthier.

The client needs to be aware of the nearest ostomy supply center so equipment will be easy to obtain. Clients may want to join the local ostomy association or the United Ostomy Association for emotional support (see the Client Education Guide). This organization often helps clients regain self-esteem and improve their self-concept and body image. The successful rehabilitation of others helps clients believe that they, too, can return to a normal life-style.

Risk for Ineffective Management of Therapeutic Regimen (Individuals).

The client with a new stoma has much to learn about self-care. The nursing diagnosis is *Risk for Ineffective Management of Therapeutic Regimen (Individuals) related to ileostomy care, care following ileorectal anastomosis, care of an ileal pouch–anal anastomosis, or care of a continent ileostomy.*

Planning: Expected Outcomes. The client will understand proper care of (1) an ileostomy, (2) an ileorectal anastomosis, (3) an ileal pouch–anal anastomosis, or (4) a continent ileostomy, as evidenced by (1) ability to apply the appliance correctly, without leakage, and to empty the pouch appropriately; (2) absence of perianal breakdown; (3) absence of fecal leakage, or (4) ability to empty the reservoir correctly and absence of leakage.

Implementation. *Ileostomy.* The client must soon begin to master the skills needed to provide self-care. Consultation with an enterostomal therapy nurse, if available, may enhance teaching and care (see Management and Delegation feature). Initially, the client can sim-

ply observe the care of the stoma. Stoma care is the area of greatest concern to the client with an ileostomy. Begin by telling the client what the stoma looks like; that it extends ½ to ¾ inches beyond the abdominal wall, is 1 to 1½ inches in diameter, and is very red and swollen at first. Assure the client that permanent changes in stoma size usually occur within the first 3 to 4 months after surgery when the swelling subsides, with the stoma shrinking to a slightly smaller permanent size.

When changing the pouch, the client should learn to check the size and color of the stoma, assess the odor of the drainage, and observe for manifestations of irritation. When the ileostomy begins to function, the output is minimal. As the client takes in more food, the drainage becomes thicker in consistency and has a weak odor. The discharge is irritating to the skin because of the alkaline contents of the effluent. Because an ileostomy may drain continuously (drainage is related to eating patterns), a pouch must be worn continuously and the stoma must be covered with gauze when the pouch is being changed.

The pouch should be cut to fit the stoma, allowing only ¹⁄₁₆ inch of room around the stoma. If the pouch does not fit well, severe skin irritation can occur. Skin irritation can vary from redness to weeping dermatitis or ulceration. Irritation also can result from adhesives or frequent removal of the appliance. The skin should be washed and rinsed thoroughly between changes. With a two-piece setup, a pouch is snapped onto the faceplate which is applied to the skin. This allows for easy emptying of the pouch. The faceplate usually remains adherent to the skin for 5 to 7 days. It may need changing sooner if it becomes loose or if leakage occurs.

If skin irritation does occur, first check the fit of the pouch. The best initial treatment for this problem would be to reapply the ostomy appliance (one with a karaya gum or hydrocolloid skin barrier), ensuring a proper fit and seal. The skin barrier of the appliance is usually sufficient to protect and heal the skin. If this method does not work, other barriers must be used. A wide variety of skin care products are available. If the problems continue, consult an enterostomal therapy nurse for further assistance.

Skin infection also can occur. *Candida* is the most common cause. The peristomal skin takes on a rashlike appearance. An antifungal powder such as nystatin should be rubbed into the affected skin area. The barrier can then be applied over the powder.

The frequency with which the ileal pouch needs to be emptied varies with each client. It should be emptied when the pouch is approximately one-third to one-half full. Instruct the client to empty the pouch during times of low output, usually before meals, at bedtime, and on arising in the morning.

It is best to change the pouch when the ileostomy is the least active, usually first thing in the morning. When changing the pouch, all equipment should be ready before the old pouch is removed. Remove the old pouch carefully using a moist cloth. A piece of gauze may be held over the stoma until the new pouch is attached. Encourage the client to inspect and touch the stoma at this time. Remind the client with a new ileostomy to take ostomy supplies along when traveling. The client may want to

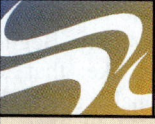

MANAGEMENT AND DELEGATION

Stoma Care and Application of Ostomy Appliances

The care of a mature stoma and the application of an ostomy appliance may be delegated to unlicensed assistive personnel. The assessment and care of a newly created ostomy should be performed only by a registered nurse. Prior to the delegation of stoma care and application of an ostomy appliance, consider the following:

- The age of the ostomy. Is this a postsurgical client with a new ostomy, or a client with an ostomy that is several weeks, months, or years old? For the client with a new ostomy, you or a trained ostomy nurse should provide care. For the client with a long-standing ostomy, you should assess the ostomy to ensure that the client is caring for it properly and that the stoma and surrounding skin are intact, prior to delegating care to assistive personnel.
- The client's need to learn self-care of the stoma and ostomy. You or a trained ostomy nurse should provide this instruction for a client needing to learn self-care.
- The client's acceptance of the ostomy, altered appearance, and bowel function. Clients having difficulty accepting their altered body image would benefit from having you or an ostomy nurse help them increase their acceptance and ability to cope with the new ostomy.
- The competency level of the unlicensed assistive personnel who will potentially perform this task.

The assistive personnel providing stoma care and applying ostomy appliances should be instructed to

- Provide privacy for the client.
- Place a waterproof pad around the ostomy or under the client, to protect the skin and bed linens.
- Empty the contents of the ostomy bag prior to removing the bag, noting the consistency, color, volume, and odor of the feces.
- Loosen the skin barrier with alcohol or another adhesive.
- Gently remove the barrier and bag while supporting the client's skin.
- Place a gauze pad or tissues over the exposed stoma to avoid soiling from leakage.
- Wash the skin around the stoma with warm water and a mild soap, and wash the stoma with clear water.
- Rinse the area with water and pat it dry.
- Note the color, moisture, and protrusion of the stoma and the condition of the surrounding skin.
- Create a circle 1/8-inch to 1/4-inch larger than the size of the stoma on the back of the appliance. A stoma-measuring guide may be helpful for this procedure.
- Prepare the barrier and appliance as a unit.
- Smooth the barrier to remove all air bubbles.
- Fill in irregular stoma borders with skin paste.
- Apply the unit, skin barrier, appliance, and bag around the stoma. Position the bag to hang in a dependent position. If the client is ambulatory, remember to position the bag for optimal drainage while the client is upright.
- Dispose of the soiled bag and appliance properly. Do this outside the client's room to prevent embarrassment over any odors.

Findings that are immediately reportable to you are black, tarry stools and overt signs of blood in the bag or bleeding from the stoma. Reddened, inflamed skin surrounding the stoma should also be brought to your attention. Information pertaining to the care and condition of the stoma should be recorded.

---

keep supplies handy in a shaving or cosmetic case instead of a suitcase.

Many different types of pouches are available (Fig. 62–6). Clients should try to find the best pouch for their needs. Small ileostomy drainage pouches are available for small adults and children. Foods such as eggs, fish, onions, cabbage, and some greens cause stool odor; therefore, deodorizing solutions and tablets may be placed in the pouch. Spinach, parsley, yogurt, and buttermilk reduce drainage odor.

The client also needs special instructions regarding prescription and over-the-counter medications. Enteric-coated tablets, such as iron preparations, vitamins, and hormones, multilayer tablets, time-release capsules, and gelatin capsules may not be absorbed in the small intestine.

The client should note if any medications are obvious in the pouch drainage. The physician will need to prescribe different medications or different forms of the medication.

The client who has had an ileostomy needs to pay close attention to fluid intake. It is very easy for this client to become dehydrated. The approximate output from an ileostomy is 1200 to 1500 ml/day. The client must monitor this output for any increase that could lead to severe fluid and electrolyte imbalance.

A low residue diet that is high in protein, carbohydrates, and calories is recommended after the surgery. Supplemental vitamins A, D, E, K, and B_{12} may be needed. Berries, whole-grain cereals, and raw fruits and vegetables can cause problems for clients with an ileostomy. Any foods that cause discomfort or diarrhea should

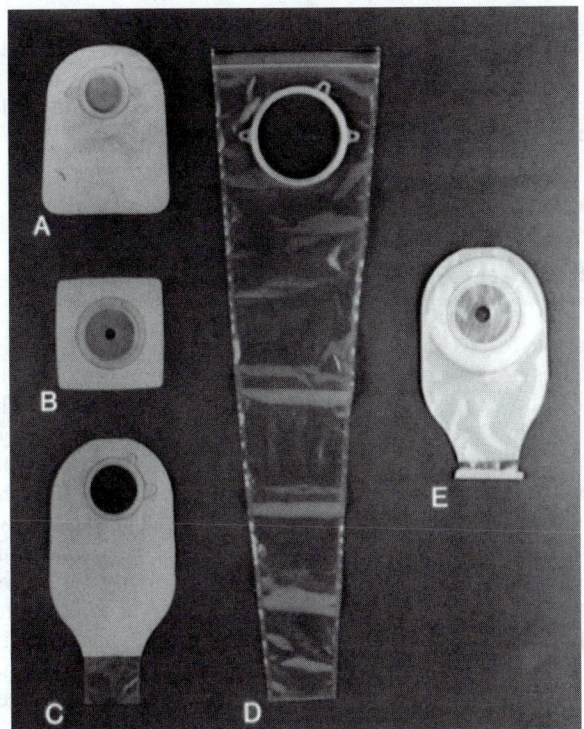

Figure 62–6. Colostomy and ileostomy pouches. *A,* Closed two-piece colostomy pouch. *B,* Skin barrier (second piece of two-piece pouches). *C,* Two-piece drainable colostomy and ileostomy pouch (transparent or flesh-colored). *D,* Colostomy irrigation sleeve. *E,* One-piece drainable colostomy and ileostomy pouch with clamp.

be omitted. Ingested foods will pass through the ileostomy within 4 to 6 hours. It is not advisable to eat a large meal close to bedtime.

Ileostomy clients must learn to chew their food well because the shortened bowel transit time means that poorly chewed food will be passed undigested. High fiber and high cellulose foods may absorb excessive moisture, leading to swelling and possibly constipation or even obstruction. Foods that should be avoided or limited, at least initially, include popcorn, peanuts, tough fibrous meats, skinned vegetables, rice, bran, and coconuts.

These clients often find, however, that their postoperative diet is less restrictive than the diet they followed with the disease. That diet was often very restricted preoperatively because so many foods increased the diarrhea and other manifestations. These clients often gain weight after surgery, sometimes to the point that they must begin to restrict their caloric intake.

Some clients with ileostomies tend to develop calcium oxalate, uric acid, or urinary calculi because of the increased amounts of fluid lost through the ileostomy leading to decreased urine output. Uric acid stones tend to form when urine volume is low and the urine is persistently acidic. Ingestion of sodium bicarbonate or potassium citrate will alkalinize the urine. Allopurinol may be used if uric acid levels remain elevated. Fluid intake should be at least 1500 ml/day.

Ileorectal Anastomosis. The client with an ileorectal anastomosis does not have to learn about stoma or

pouch care unless a temporary ileostomy is present. The major goal of teaching centers around the importance of defecating before the rectum becomes overly distended. Most clients find that they have four to five stools per day once their bodies have adjusted to the surgical alteration.

The feces in these clients are often described as pasty in consistency, and appear to contain fewer electrolytes than the drainage from a traditional ileostomy. It may take up to 1 year for the client's altered bowel to adapt.

Clients having the ileorectal anastomosis must understand the importance of follow-up meetings with the physician. They must understand that the remaining mucosa can become diseased with ulcerative colitis or Crohn's disease, requiring further resection and possibly formation of an ileostomy. They also need to know that they are at increased risk of development of rectal cancer. These clients have to receive regular proctoscopic examinations following their surgery.

The client should learn to avoid foods that may have caused diarrhea in the past. It is best to try new foods one at a time so their effect can be determined. The diet is usually not limited; however, it should include adequate fluids to avoid dehydration.

Ileal Pouch–Anal Anastomosis. The client with the ileal pouch–anal anastomosis also has no need to learn about stoma or pouch care unless a temporary ileostomy was created, which may often be the case. The client will learn to respond to the sensation to defecate so spillage does not occur. After the bowel adapts to the surgical alteration, the stool becomes more formed and many clients will have only five or six stools per day. The client should maintain an adequate fluid intake.

Continent Ileostomy, or Kock Pouch. During surgical formation of the Kock pouch, an evacuation catheter is inserted. A skin barrier and special gauze dressing are then applied. These hold the catheter in an upright position to avoid stress on a healing nipple valve. It is imperative to avoid distention of the ileostomy reservoir in the early postoperative period because of the pressure it would cause on the suture line. Thus, it is attached to straight drainage initially for several days. Then it is emptied every 2 hours for about 2 weeks.

Carefully observe for the start of ileal drainage, which usually starts 3 to 4 days postoperatively. About 2 weeks after surgery, the catheter is removed from the pouch. The marked catheter may then be used to drain the pouch. The intervals between drainings are gradually increased each week until the ileostomy is emptied four to six times per day and once or not at all at night.

To empty the reservoir, the client should sit up. The catheter is lubricated with a water-soluble lubricant and inserted into the stoma through the valve. Contents are allowed to drain by gravity through the catheter into the toilet, with complete drainage occurring in 3 to 5 minutes. A small gauze dressing is then applied over the stoma. The equipment is cleaned with mild soap and rinsed, and can be carried in a plastic case.

The reservoir volume continues to increase to a maximum of around 600 ml in 6 months. The client needs an oral intake of at least eight 8-oz glasses of fluid per day. No long-term restrictions are placed on physical activities.

Tell the client to wear a medical alert identification bracelet and carry a brief description of the pouch and drainage procedure in case of emergency.

The client needs to learn about dietary restrictions associated with a continent ileostomy. Foods that could cause a blockage of the valve and the stoma may need to be avoided. These foods include mushrooms and nuts. All foods need to be chewed thoroughly so partly digested food will not occlude the stoma.

Risk for Sexual Dysfunction. The client with an ileostomy does not have physiologic reasons for sexual dysfunction; however, psychological changes may occur. In this case, the nursing diagnosis is *Sexual Dysfunction related to concern about ileostomy and altered self-concept and body image.*

Planning: Expected Outcomes. The client will not develop a sexual dysfunction, as evidenced by ability to return to preillness sexual functioning and role.

Implementation. The ileostomy may cause concern about sexual activity and pregnancy. Encourage the client to express any such concerns and to discuss them with the sexual partner. Impotence is uncommon, and psychological reasons should be explored if it does occur. Pregnancy and normal vaginal delivery are possible. The United Ostomy Association has a wide variety of booklets available for clients with an ostomy. Titles include *Sex, Pregnancy and the Female Ostomate; Sex, Courtship and the Single Ostomate; Sex and the Male Ostomate;* and *Insight into the Emotional Aspects of Ileostomies and Colostomies.* The American Cancer Society has similar resources available.

The client and sexual partner should be encouraged to discuss sexuality and to verbalize any fears. Clients can be taught activities to lessen the intrusiveness of the pouch such as emptying it before intercourse, wearing a soft flannel pouch cover, and being open to using different positions for intercourse. If there are problems, a sexual therapist should be consulted for further information and assistance.

Evaluation

The client should be able to learn to care for the ostomy and to handle the altered elimination if teaching was adequate. If the client is unable to provide self-care within 6 weeks to 3 months of discharge, further teaching may be required.

■ Modifications for Elderly Clients

Crohn's disease and ulcerative colitis occur less often in the older age groups. The treatment, however, when it does occur in this age group, is the same as for the younger client.

If the aged client has an ileostomy or other diversion, teaching may take a little longer, but most older clients can learn to care for themselves without difficulty. If the client has an ileostomy, issues such as eyesight and dexterity are important. Sometimes the older client cannot

manipulate the clamp used to close the pouch. If the client is unable to manipulate the equipment, easier devices may be secured or a family member may have to assume that responsibility. Carefully assess the older client's ability to care for self and the appliance.

Neoplastic Disorders

Benign Tumors of the Bowel

Various kinds of benign tumors are found in the bowel. Polyps are the most commonly found benign tumor of the large bowel. A polyp is a lesion that projects into the lumen of the bowel. Some polyps have stems (pedunculated), whereas others do not (sessile). Polyps are usually benign lesions, but some types are precursors of cancer (i.e., premalignant tumors). Polyps are dangerous in two ways: (1) they can mask the presence of a malignant tumor and (2) they may serve as the focus for bowel obstruction or intussusception. Benign bowel tumors produce manifestations similar to those of malignant tumors. Some benign tumors bleed profusely and cause abdominal discomfort. Bleeding benign tumors are usually removed surgically.

Neoplastic Disorders of the Bowel

Cancer of the Small Bowel

Only about 1% of all gastrointestinal cancers involve tumors of the small bowel. The average age of onset is 53 to 58 years. Most tumors are in the ileum, with the remainder almost equally divided between the duodenum and jejunum. Manifestations are vague and nonspecific, and include:

- Weight loss
- Pain
- Anemia
- Nausea
- Vomiting
- Obstruction
- Palpable mass
- Hemorrhage

Surgery is the only intervention that offers hope of cure. Unfortunately, even with early diagnosis and bowel resection, only about 20% of clients survive 5 years. With late diagnosis, the 5-year survival rate decreases to about 5%.

Colon Cancer

Cancers of the colon are usually adenocarcinomas. In both sexes, colon and rectal cancer is the second most frequent cause of death from cancer in the United States, ranking just behind lung cancer.[1] It occurs with the same frequency in men and women. Most tumors are found in the distal portion of the large bowel, from the sigmoid colon to the anus. In recent years, the incidence of carcinoma of the right colon has increased, whereas that of the rectosigmoid area has decreased.

Even though early diagnosis reduces mortality, many clients still do not take advantage of screening techniques. Survival following diagnosis of colon cancer correlates with the stage of tumor invasion (Table 62–3).

Etiology and Risk Factors

The cause of colon cancer is not definitely known. There are identifiable predisposing factors, however. It does seem to be related to low residue, high fat diets and highly refined foods. There also seems to be a familial tendency for colon cancer. The risk of cancer increases with chronic ulcerative colitis, granulomas, and familial polyposis.

Epidemiologic studies indicate that diet may be a major factor in the development of cancer of the large bowel. Studies on bulk in stool and the rate of transit of fecal matter have so far given mixed results. Some researchers propose that metabolic and bacterial end products are carcinogenic and that constipation allows a longer contact with the bowel wall, thus increasing the probability of cancer developing. The Risk Factors and Levels of Prevention feature lists other factors that contribute to colon cancer.

Pathophysiology

Most malignant tumors (at least 50%) occur in the rectal area; another 20% to 30% are found in the sigmoid and

Table 62–3. TNM Classification of Colorectal Cancer			

Primary Tumor (T)

TX	Primary tumor cannot be assessed
T_0	No evidence of primary tumor
T_{is}	Carcinoma in situ
T1	Tumor invades submucosa
T2	Tumor invades muscularis propria
T3	Tumor invades through muscularis propria into subserosa, or into nonperitonealized pericolic or perirectal tissues
T4	Tumor perforates visceral peritoneum, or directly invades other organs or structures

Regional Lymph Nodes (N)

NX	Regional lymph nodes cannot be assessed
N_0	No regional lymph node metastasis
N1	Metastasis in one to three pericolic or perirectal lymph nodes
N2	Metastasis in four or more pericolic or perirectal lymph nodes
N3	Metastasis in any lymph node along course of a major vascular trunk

Distant Metastasis (M)

MX	Presence of distant metastasis cannot be assessed
M_0	No distant metastasis
M1	Distant metastasis

Stage Grouping[*]

0	T_{is}	N_0	M_0
I(A)	T1	N_0	M_0
	T2	N_0	M_0
II(B)	T3	N_0	M_0
	T4	N_0	M_0
III(C)	Any T	N1	M_0
	Any T	N2	M_0
	Any T	N3	M_0
IV(D)	Any T	Any N	M1

[*] Letters refer to Dukes' classification.

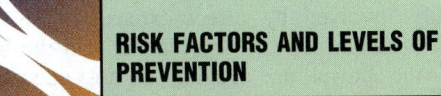

RISK FACTORS AND LEVELS OF PREVENTION

Colon Cancer

Risk Factors

Family history of colon cancer; previous colon cancer; age over 40 years; ulcerative colitis; high fat, low residue diet high in refined foods; familial polyposis; adenomatous polyps; living in a highly industrialized, urban society; slow bowel transit time

Levels of Prevention

Primary Prevention

Instruct clients to maintain a low-fat and high-fiber diet.

● Encourage clients to limit ingestion of refined foods.
● Tell clients to drink more fluids.

Secondary Prevention

Promote early detection through yearly digital rectal examinations for adults over 40.

● Monitor clients over age 50 with a stool guaiac test and yearly rectal examination
● Evaluate clients with flexible sigmoidoscopy every 3 to 5 years for persons at average risk. For persons at above-average risk, an evaluation with a barium enema or colonoscopy is recommended every 2 to 3 years.

Tertiary Prevention

Encourage use of bulk laxatives (Metamucil, etc.) for high-risk clients.

● Promote regular screening for persons with one or more risk factors.
● Encourage clients to follow a high fiber, low fat diet and to limit intake of refined foods.

descending colons. The remainder are found in the transverse and ascending colons, with twice as many found in the ascending colon as in the transverse colon.

Cancers of the colon almost always develop from adenomatous polyps. As this tumor becomes malignant, it increases in size within the lumen and begins to invade the bowel wall.

Colon cancer is staged using the TNM or Dukes' classification systems. The TNM system is presented in Table 62–3. Dukes' classification (A, B, C, D) correlates with the stage grouping (I, II, III, IV) and is the most commonly used system for colon cancer. The 5-year survival rates are as follows: Dukes' A, 80% to 90%; Dukes' B, about 60%; Dukes' C, 25% to 40%; Dukes' D, less than 5%.

Malignant bowel tumors spread (1) by direct extension to a nearby organ, as to the stomach from the transverse colon; (2) by lymphatic and hematogenous channels, usually to the liver; and (3) by seeding or implanting of cells into the peritoneal cavity.

The urinary bladder, ureters, and reproductive organs are frequently involved by direct extension. Also, the formation of a fistula between the bladder and the bowel or between the bowel and vagina is not uncommon. Blood-borne metastasis extends most frequently to the liver but also may involve the lungs, kidneys, and bones.

Clinical Manifestations and Diagnostic Findings

Manifestations of colon cancer include the following (Fig. 62–7):

- Rectal bleeding
- Changed bowel habits
- Tenesmus
- Intestinal obstruction
- Abdominal pain
- Weight loss
- Anorexia
- Nausea and vomiting
- Anemia
- Palpable mass

In general, tumors in the small bowel and right colon are more likely to cause abdominal pain, nausea, and vomiting. Because the large intestine distends, there are fewer early manifestations. Tumors in the left colon and rectum are more likely to cause passage of blood or mucus, an alteration in bowel habits, and a feeling that the bowel is not empty after defecation. Bleeding is the manifestation that often alerts the client to seek healthcare. When the tumor occludes the bowel, obstructive manifestations result.

Manifestations of carcinoma vary according to the area in which the tumor is found and the type of tumor involved. Tumors in the right colon are unlikely to cause obstruction because of its large lumen and the liquid quality of the feces. At this location, lesions often ulcerate, resulting in anemia. Anorexia, weight loss, weakness, and debility may be present at the time of diagnosis.

Lesions of the ascending and transverse colon often present with progressive obstruction. Tumors in the descending colon and rectum frequently cause obstructive manifestations but not weight loss, anemia, or dyspepsia. Most clients also report a change in bowel habits.

Early diagnosis improves the survival rate. American Cancer Society guidelines for early detection include a routine annual digital rectal examination beginning at age 40, an annual stool guaiac test and digital rectal examination at age 50, and a flexible sigmoidoscopy every 3 to 5 years, after two negative sigmoidoscopy examinations performed 1 year apart, after age 50.[1] High-risk clients

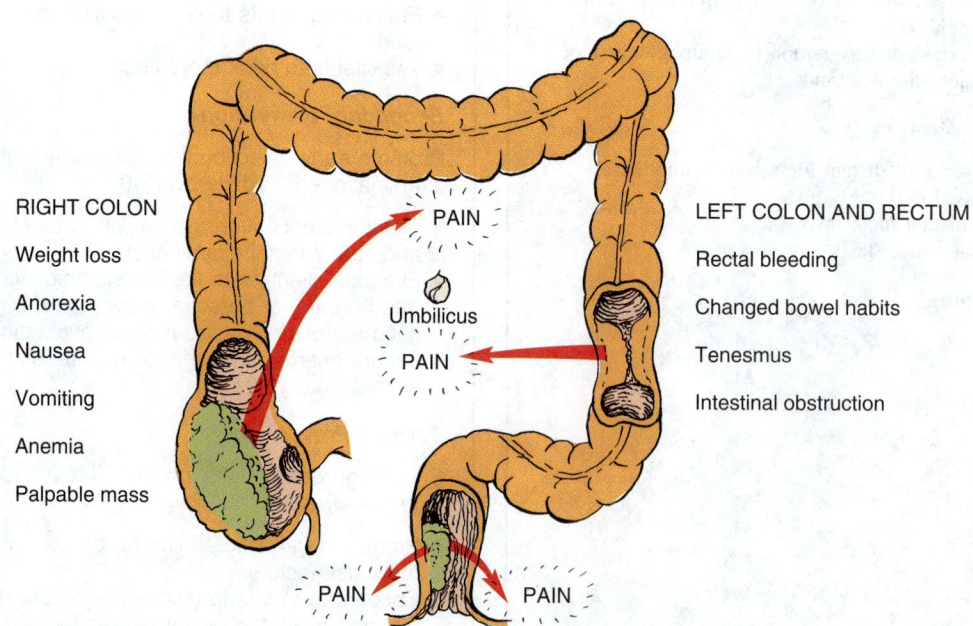

RIGHT COLON

Weight loss

Anorexia

Nausea

Vomiting

Anemia

Palpable mass

PAIN

Umbilicus

PAIN

LEFT COLON AND RECTUM

Rectal bleeding

Changed bowel habits

Tenesmus

Intestinal obstruction

PAIN   PAIN

Figure 62–7. Symptoms of carcinoma of the colon. Pain usually radiates toward the umbilicus or perianal area.

should have a barium enema or colonoscopy every 2 to 3 years. It is vital to explain to clients the necessity for early detection and the importance of reporting manifestations such as rectal bleeding and a change in bowel habits to their physician.

One third of malignant tumors of the distal colon and rectum can be felt with the examining finger. This makes digital rectal examination one of the more important diagnostic methods. A stool guaiac test is done to test for gastrointestinal bleeding. Carcinoembryonic antigen (CEA) may be elevated in colon cancer and aids in determining the progress of the disease. X-ray studies of the colon may show either a filling defect or a stricture. Ultrasound and computed tomography (CT) help establish tumor size and metastasis and identify more than one half of the tumors. Flexible fiberoptic scopes permit better visualization into the right colon, extend the diagnostic capabilities of the procedure, and allow biopsy (see Chapter 59).

Acute and Subacute Care

■ Medical Management

The primary treatment for colon cancer is surgery; however, medical treatment is used as an adjunct to improve survival in tumors that cannot be completely removed. Radiation therapy is often given before surgery in the hope that the malignant cells will not metastasize, and to reduce the size of the tumor and thus make it more resectable.

Local interventions at the tumor site after surgery include implantation of isotopes into the tumor area and electrocoagulation. Isotopes used include radium, cesium, and cobalt. Iridium has been used in the rectum.

Chemotherapy has had limited success, although 5-fluorouracil has produced some positive results. Recently, research has been conducted to improve this picture by using combinations of medications. Levamisol is the newest agent to be given with 5-fluorouracil. This combination has improved survival in Dukes' C tumors. Leucovorin also may be given with 5-fluorouracil, with or without levamisol to increase its effects. Chemotherapy may be used to reduce metastasis and control manifestations of metastasis. In clients with liver metastasis, intrahepatic arterial chemotherapy may be administered.

■ Nursing Management of the Medical Client

Care of the client undergoing medical treatment for colon cancer revolves around care of a client undergoing chemotherapy and occasionally radiation therapy. See Chapter 24 for further information on the care of these clients.

■ Surgical Management

Intervention depends on the type of tumor, its location and stage, and on the client's general condition (see Table 62–3). A variety of surgical procedures are performed to treat colorectal cancer (Figs. 62–8 and 62–9). All procedures entail colon resection. The tumor is removed with several inches of colon on either side of the tumor. An end-to-end anastomosis is performed, if possible.

Colostomy

A colostomy may have to be performed. This procedure involves creating an opening between the colon and abdominal wall, from which fecal contents will pass. A colostomy can be located in the ascending, transverse, descending, or sigmoid colon. A colostomy can be permanent or temporary. A temporary colostomy allows the bowel to rest and later may be reanastomosed. The temporary colostomy also can be used to treat inoperable bowel cancer, with the ostomy placed proximal to the

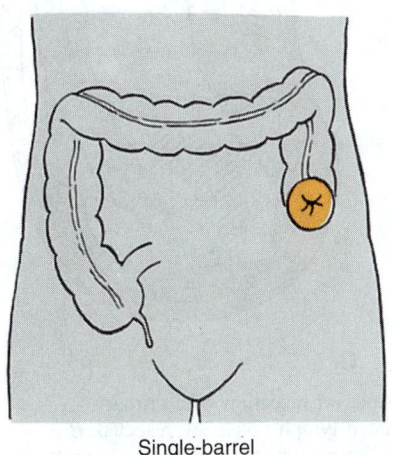
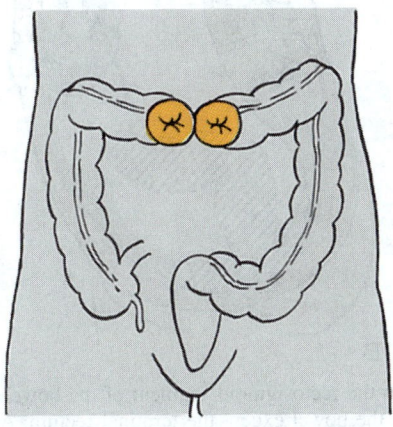
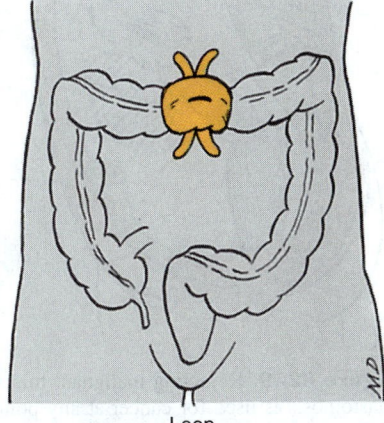

Single-barrel   Double-barrel   Loop

Figure 62–8. Types of colostomies. Single-barreled colostomies are usually permanent. Double-barred colostomies are usually temporary, and stomas may be adjacent or several inches apart. Loop colostomies are temporary and formed by bringing a loop of colon through the abdominal wall and supporting it with a plastic brace.

cancer. A temporary colostomy is made most commonly at the midpoint of the left colon or transverse colon, whereas a permanent colostomy is usually placed in the sigmoid colon. Because the main function of the large bowel is to absorb water, the colostomy is easier to manage nearer the sigmoid colon than in the transverse or right colon because the stool is formed.

A colostomy may also be single- or double-barreled. When only one loop end of bowel is opened onto the abdominal surface, it is called an end colostomy; the client has only one stoma. A double-barreled colostomy is one in which both loops, distal and proximal, are open on the abdominal wall. An end colostomy is permanent if the bowel distal to it has been resected. A double-barreled colostomy may be closed later depending on the disease present. A double-barreled colostomy can be two separate stomas, a loop with one stoma with two openings, or one stoma and a Hartmann's pouch (distal bowel closed off and placed left intra-abdominally).

Abdominal-Perineal Resection

Rectal tumors may require an abdominal-perineal resection, with the formation of a permanent or end colostomy. The affected colon and entire rectum is excised and the anus closed. Newer surgical techniques allow low sigmoid tumors to be removed while leaving the rectal sphincter intact. This allows normal bowel elimination to be maintained.

■ Nursing Management of the Surgical Client

Assessment

The client often presents with weight loss and a change in bowel habits. Obtain accurate descriptions of manifestations as well as an assessment of major risk factors, such as a family history of colon cancer, ulcerative coli-

tis, or familial polyposis. Assess the abdomen, noting any abnormalities, such as pain, distention, or masses.

Diagnosis, Planning, Implementation

Altered Nutrition: Less than Body Requirements.
Weight loss is a common manifestation of colon cancer. Therefore a common preoperative nursing diagnosis for the client with colon cancer is *Altered Nutrition: Less than Body Requirements, related to nausea and anorexia.*

Planning: Expected Outcomes. The client will attain an optimal level of nutrition, as evidenced by weight gain (or absence of weight loss), normal serum electrolytes, and normal protein levels.

Implementation. Preoperatively, a diet high in calories, protein, and carbohydrates but low in residue may be given to provide nutrition and reduce peristalsis. TPN may be required to provide the nutrients and vitamins the client requires.

Risk for Infection.
The client must have the bacteria level in the bowel lowered preoperatively to decrease the risk of infection. The nursing diagnosis is *Risk for Infection related to contamination from the bowel during surgery.*

Planning: Expected Outcomes. The client will not develop a postoperative wound infection or intra-abdominal infection, as evidenced by absence of fever or elevated WBC and good wound healing.

Implementation. Clients undergoing a bowel resection need a bowel preparation to minimize bacterial growth in the bowel and postoperative wound infection. This preparation usually includes the following:

- A low residue or liquid diet to reduce the fecal contents of the bowel
- Administration of cathartics orally such as polyethylene glycol–electrolyte solution (GoLYTELY) or other

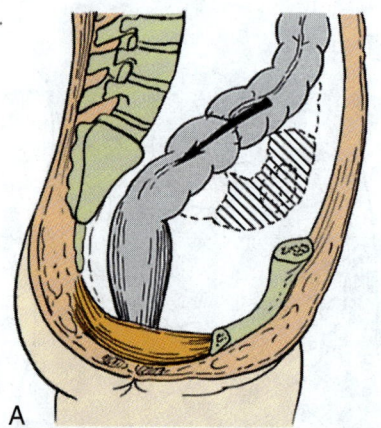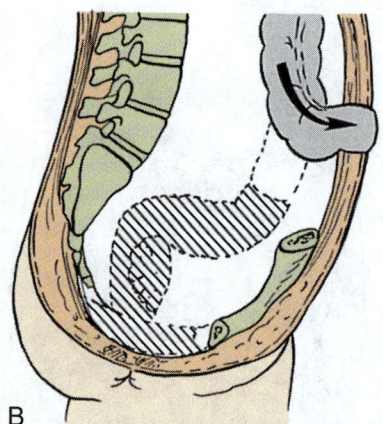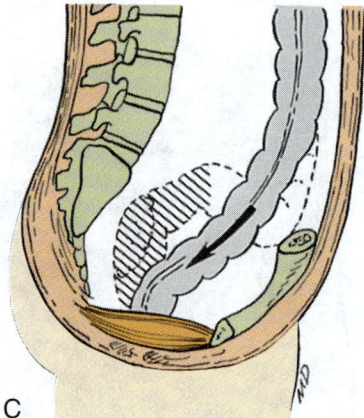

Figure 62–9. Resecting malignant tumors in the rectosigmoid segment of the bowel. *A,* Anterior resection with primary anastomosis is used for cancer at any point in the bowel except the terminal rectum. Associated lymph nodes are resected. *B,* Abdominoperineal (anteroposterior) resection with formation of permanent colostomy (Miles' operation) for cancer involving the anus and terminal portion of the rectum. *C,* Proctosigmoidectomy with pullthrough and preservation of external sphincter muscles is appropriate when the tumor is in the proximal rectum and unlikely to metastasize further.

agent, which is usually started at least 12 to 24 hours preoperatively
- Administration of antibiotics, such as sulfonamides and possibly neomycin and cephalexin, usually by mouth, for 12 to 48 hours preoperatively
- Administration of enemas to clean the bowel (the inside of the bowel lumen should be as clean and bacteria-free as possible)
- Blood transfusions to correct severe anemia

Anxiety. The client undergoing surgery for colon cancer will be prone to *Anxiety related to impending surgery and diagnosis of cancer.*

Planning: Expected Outcomes. The client will have lessened anxiety, as evidenced by the client's ability to understand preoperative teaching and respond appropriately.

Implementation. Identify the client's level of anxiety and provide supportive efforts. Explain all treatments and procedures fully. Clarify and reinforce the information provided by the physician. Encourage the client to ventilate his or her feelings and have time to meet with health team members to discuss treatments and prognosis. The client also needs to know the following:

- What to expect after the operation
- What measures are necessary to prevent complications, such as deep breathing and leg exercises
- The type of anesthetic to be used
- Whether an NG tube will be in place after surgery
- How treatment decisions will be made when the results of pathologic study are available

If a colostomy is necessary, an enterostomal therapy nurse should be asked to educate the client about the ostomy, answer questions, and advise on optimal placement of the stoma. If an enterostomal therapy nurse is not available, assume the responsibility for teaching the client about the stoma. The risk of sexual dysfunction should be explained to the client in a supportive atmosphere.

Risk for Injury. The postoperative client is at risk for the development of postoperative complications. The nursing diagnosis is *Risk for Injury related to postoperative complications, including infection, hemorrhage, wound disruption, thrombophlebitis, and abnormal stomal function.*

Planning: Expected Outcomes. The client will not develop an injury as evidenced by absence of manifestations of infection, bleeding, and evidence of wound disruption, thrombophlebitis, stomal ischemia, or bowel spillage.

Implementation. Immediate postoperative interventions are the same as those used for any major abdominal surgery. Additionally, if a colostomy was created, monitor the colostomy output and use special care to keep fecal contents from the colostomy (which contain bacteria) away from the surgical incision.

When creating a temporary loop colostomy, the surgeon brings a loop of bowel out through a wound that is separate from the surgical incision. To keep the loop from slipping back into the abdominal cavity, the surgeon places a rod or bridge beneath it. Although the surgeon usually opens the bowel with a cautery in surgery, he may wait 2 or 3 days postoperatively to open the bowel. Because there are no sensory nerve endings in the bowel wall, this procedure is essentially painless, except for some cramping. The surgeon usually indicates which is the proximal loop and which is the distal loop.

Assess for the return of peristalsis. Indications include passage of flatus and return of bowel sounds, which can be heard with a stethoscope. The client may remain on gastric suction until peristalsis returns. It usually takes several days before the client can receive food and fluids and, as the client tolerates food, he or she is slowly advanced to a regular diet.

Abdominal cramps commonly occur after surgery, as does distention of the bowel. Distention is uncomfortable and may cause pressure on suture lines. The insertion of a rectal tube for 20 to 30 minutes per physician order will help if the rectum contains gas.

Postoperatively, if an abdominal-perineal resection with creation of an end colostomy was performed, assess both the abdominal and the perineal wounds. The incision may be sutured completely closed. However, sometimes drains are left in the incision, which may be attached to a suction device such as a Hemovac. When suction is not used, a Penrose drain may be placed in the wound and you must change the dressing frequently or as ordered. A large amount of serous drainage can be expected from the perineal wound. It often takes several weeks to months for the wound to heal completely because of its size. Prepare the client to wear a rectal dressing throughout the healing period. The character, volume, and odor of the drainage should be assessed. If the drainage in any way suggests a developing infection, obtain a culture of the wound to identify the organism.

Occasionally, in the immediate postoperative period, sump drainage is placed in the perineal wound. This is also indicated if the wound becomes infected. The sump tube is attached to suction, allowing the wound to heal from its deepest portion without forming an abscess.

The perineal wound can be very painful, and the client should receive sufficient pain medication to control the pain. Once the packing is removed, the wound is irrigated and the client should take a sitz bath three to four times a day. The client will find a side-lying position much more comfortable.

Assess the client's stoma closely for the presence of stomal ischemia. The stoma should be red and moist. If it becomes dark or dusky, report this to the surgeon immediately. Clients may have a colostomy pouch over the stoma. Be sure that this pouch is not applying pressure to the stoma, interfering with its blood supply. When you change the pouch or empty it, prevent contamination of the surgical wound by fecal discharges. Monitor the return of bowel function by observing the type and quantity of discharges from the stoma.

The high lithotomy position associated with the abdominal-perineal resection is associated with an increased risk of development of postoperative phlebitis. To prevent this problem from developing, the client will often receive subcutaneous injections of heparin, usually 5000 units every 12 hours after surgery. Sequential pressure stockings or thigh-high antiemboli hose also must be worn. The client, with your help, also needs to perform leg exercises before and after surgery. Monitor the client for the development of manifestations of thrombophlebitis, such as redness, swelling, or the presence of Homan's sign.

Risk for Body Image Disturbance.
The client with an ostomy has to face alterations in self-concept and body image. Write the nursing diagnosis as *Risk for Body Image Disturbance related to life-style secondary to ostomy.*

Planning: Expected Outcomes. The client will adjust to changes in body image, as evidenced by the client's ability to identify and use effective coping methods in dealing with the disease and losses experienced.

Implementation. Provide emotional support while the client begins the process of adjusting to the colostomy. It is also important to provide extensive teaching regarding how to care for the colostomy.

A client's reactions to a new colostomy may range from apparently easy acceptance to total withdrawal from social contacts. How well clients adjust depends partly on their attitude toward excretory functions, previous knowledge about colostomies, and general ability to adjust to stressful situations.

Some clients refuse to look at the stoma and find it very difficult to accept its presence, whereas others begin to participate in stoma care almost immediately. Your reactions and manner toward the client and the care required can affect the client's adjustment. For some clients, the colostomy represents a "cure"; for others, it is palliation, as for those with extensive cancer.

Watson[46] has compared the phases of adjustment to an ostomy with the psychological phases experienced by a person in any crisis. The stages are the following:

1. Shock
2. Defensive retreat
3. Acknowledgment
4. Adaptation

Watson points out that during the first two stages, clients need a great deal of support, a realistic appraisal of their situation, and encouragement to participate in their own care. Clients must reach the acknowledgment phase before they are able to achieve any real rehabilitative gains. Once clients begin to care for their stoma with a degree of success, they are moving toward the final, or adaptive, level.

The client's significant others also must adjust to the colostomy. Help significant others by listening to their reactions and explaining the client's problems to them.

Continuing sexual relationships are one major concern for clients with colostomies and their significant others. There is no physical reason the client cannot enjoy normal sexual relations, although a small number of men become impotent after a radical perineal dissection. If this complication occurs, the physician may recommend a urology consultation to discuss treatment options for impotence. Psychological barriers may cause problems. With love, patience, understanding, and good hygienic practices, there should be no problem. However, it may take several months after surgery before a couple manage to reestablish a satisfactory sexual relationship. A referral to a social worker, counselor, psychiatric liaison, sex therapist, or registered nurse with a counseling background may be beneficial.

Risk for Ineffective Management of Therapeutic Regimen (Individuals).
The client with a colostomy needs to learn about self-care. The nursing diagnosis is *Risk for Ineffective Management of Therapeutic Regimen (Individuals) related to end colostomy care, irrigation, and possible complications associated with colostomies.*

Planning: Expected Outcomes. The client will understand care of the end colostomy, as evidenced by the client's ability to apply the pouch; care for peristomal skin; irrigate the colostomy, if applicable; and prevent or treat any associated problems.

Implementation. Carefully assess the client's physical condition and emotional and mental attitude toward the colostomy before attempting to teach ostomy self-care. Pace the teaching to the client's level of acceptance of the colostomy and his or her ability to manage it.

Teach the client how to correctly apply the pouch to the stoma. The client first should be taught to examine the stoma. A healthy stoma is red and slightly raised. The skin around the stoma (peristomal skin) should be clear, without evidence of irritation. The peristomal area should be cleaned well with a mild soap and water and dried well before the new pouch is applied. The skin should be treated with a skin barrier and the new pouch applied, cut about $\frac{1}{16}$ to $\frac{1}{8}$ inch larger than the stoma. The pouch should be changed about every 4 to 5 days or more often if leakage occurs. If a two-piece system is used, the faceplate may stay in place for 5 to 7 days unless leakage occurs. If it is changed after the bowel has been evacuated, there will be less risk of spillage during the change.

Teach the client how to empty the pouch when it is about one-half full. Show the client how to clean out the pouch when emptying it. The client should demonstrate the ability to empty and change the pouch independently before discharge. See the discussion of ileostomy care for further information.

The client must regularly clean the peristomal area to prevent irritation. The constant presence of moisture can lead to excoriation and can usually be prevented or healed with karaya gum or a light dusting of powder. Too much powder will prevent the pouch from sticking, however.

Clients with end colostomies can be taught to regulate the colostomy through regular irrigation. Clients who are physically, mentally, and emotionally capable should be encouraged to attempt irrigation and regulation, especially clients who had regular bowel habits before surgery and no other bowel disease. Although clients do not have to irrigate their colostomies, all clients who are able should be given the option of learning this technique. Some clients, in spite of irrigation, may never gain regularity. If they have not become regulated within 6 months, they probably will never be regulated.

Irrigation is taught in much the same way you would teach clients to self-administer an enema. The Client Education Guide lists the steps involved in colostomy irrigation. The best time for irrigation is when the client formerly had a daily bowel movement, because the bowel is already "trained" to evacuate at this time.

Clients find that by irrigating the bowel daily or every other day, the bowel evacuates after the irrigation and then does not empty until it is irrigated again.

If there is difficulty inserting the catheter, let a little solution flow in and rotate the catheter. If it will not go in, teach the client to apply gloves or a finger cot, lubricate the finger, and gently pass it into the stoma. This method will often dislodge any feces that may be near the stoma. If the client cannot pass a catheter and no obstruction is felt digitally, the client should notify the physician.

If cramping occurs, stop the solution temporarily, take a few deep breaths, and restart the solution slowly. Never use more than 1000 ml, irrigate more than once a day, or irrigate if diarrhea is present.

If there is no return after irrigation, the client should ambulate, gently massage the abdomen, and try drinking some warm water. If there is still no return, apply a pouch and try the irrigation again the next day. If there is no return, call the physician.

Diarrhea is a serious problem for clients with colostomies. Medications to slow the motility of the bowel should be prescribed by the physician. Two problems can result from diarrhea: (1) irritation of skin from digestive juices that have not been reabsorbed and (2) electrolyte imbalance when the condition persists. Encourage the client to drink water, broth, and plain tea; no solid food should be ingested until bowel motility returns to normal.

When hard stools are present, the client has difficulty evacuating the bowel and irrigating the colostomy. Fecal impactions also can occur. Sometimes the physician prescribes a stool softener such as docusate sodium (Colace). The client also needs to reevaluate the diet and increase the amount of fruit, vegetables, fiber, and water if constipation persists.

Flatus is an embarrassing problem because the client may have no control over its passage and no sensations to indicate when it is about to pass. Flatus can make clients avoid social situations. Clients can be taught how to muffle the passage of gas from their colostomies. Women may hold their purses or arms over the colostomy and men may hold their folded jackets or hats over the stoma to muffle the noise. Odor-proof pouches and those with charcoal filter discs are commonly available, but the most satisfactory way to control flatus is by diet. Because every client is different, clients have to learn by trial and error which foods cause gas. In general, nuts, cabbage, sauerkraut, broccoli, corn, cauliflower, and legumes are gas-forming foods. Swallowing air by eating too rapidly, chewing gum, or drinking carbonated beverages also cause intestinal gas.

Strictures of the stoma may occur after some surgeries because the rectus muscles of the abdominal wall tend to close over the artificial opening made through them. Some clients, especially those who do not irrigate, may be taught to dilate their stoma with a gloved, lubricated finger. This is usually not a problem in clients who irrigate because the irrigation nipple dilates the stoma.

In preparation for discharge, clients need support and knowledgeable advice as they learn to live with their colostomies. The enterostomal therapy nurse can help the client learn to manage and accept the ostomy, and to achieve a smooth transition from the healthcare facility to the home. Some cities have established ostomy rehabilitation clinics to help clients, and most large communities have an ostomy association that has contact with the American Cancer Society. These support groups are helpful because clients can share their ostomy concerns with others with similar problems. A home healthcare referral can add to the client's peace of mind, identify problems that might not otherwise be known, and ensure necessary follow-up care.

Before dismissal, advise clients that after major bowel surgery it may be several weeks before they regain their strength. Also tell them that when segments have been removed from the bowel, bowel habits may alter until the body adjusts to the situation. You may need to teach the client and significant others how to change dressings at home, because wounds may not be healed totally by the time the client is discharged. In general, teaching should include

- How to change dressings correctly
- Dietary or activity restrictions
- Manifestations of intestinal obstruction and perforation
- How to care for a colostomy, if applicable
- How and whom to notify if obstruction or perforation occurs

---

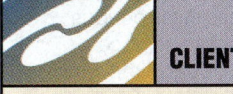

CLIENT EDUCATION GUIDE

Colostomy Irrigation

1. Assemble all the irrigation equipment and pouch, skin care products, and new colostomy pouch.
2. Remove and discard the old pouch.
3. Clean the peristomal skin.
4. Apply the irrigating sleeve and close off the distal end or place it in the toilet.
5. Using 500 to 1000 ml of warm tap water, suspend the solution container about 18 inches above the stoma. Clear the air from the irrigation tubing. Insert the lubricated cone (water-soluble lubricant) 2 to 4 inches into the stoma (NEVER FORCE THE CONE) and allow the solution to flow gently into the colon.
6. Once all solution has been instilled for 6 to 8 minutes, either allow most of the stool to pass into the toilet and then close off the pouch for another 30 to 45 minutes, or simply close off the end of the pouch until the bowel has evacuated.
7. Once the bowel has emptied, simply remove the sleeve, clean the stoma, and cover it with a small pouch or gauze pad.

Clients having problems with the colostomy should see an enterostomal therapy nurse. The client with an abdominal-perineal resection will need follow-up from the surgeon to ensure that the perineal wound is healing properly.

The Ethical Issues in Nursing feature, which deals with short-staffing, remarks on the individualized plans and hours of instruction required by the colostomy client.

Evaluation

The client should recover from surgery without complications and should be able to manage his or her colostomy within 6 weeks to 3 months. If the client is unable to accomplish self-care, the need for further teaching should be explored.

Other Disorders of the Large and Small Bowel

Herniations

A hernia is the abnormal protrusion of an organ, tissue, or part of an organ through the structure that normally contains it. Hernias most frequently occur in the abdominal cavity as a result of a congenital or acquired weakness of abdominal musculature. Hernias can occur at any age and in either sex. Indirect inguinal hernias are the most common type and typically occur in men. Direct hernias are found more commonly in older people. Incisional or ventral hernias occur most often in clients who had poor wound healing after surgery. Obese or pregnant clients are more likely to develop umbilical hernias.

Etiology and Risk Factors

Two factors must be present for a hernia to occur: (1) a defect in the integrity of the muscular wall and (2) increased intra-abdominal pressure.

Congenital muscle weakness is one risk factor combined with the factors that increase intra-abdominal pressure. The muscle weakness cannot be prevented, but exercises can be performed to strengthen weak muscles. Because obesity is one cause of increased intra-abdominal pressure, it can be prevented by weight control. Avoiding heavy lifting and straining also reduces intra-abdominal pressure. Early diagnosis is important to prevent incarceration and strangulation.

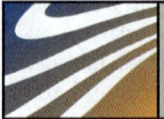

ETHICAL ISSUES IN NURSING

Short-Staffing

You are a nurse on a surgical unit with many clients with new colostomies. Your clients need to understand how their colostomy works, how to care for the skin surrounding the colostomy, what clothing is best to wear, how to select and use various appliances to maintain a secure and leak-free system, and what side effects to look for. Teaching these clients requires individualized plans and many hours of instruction, question-and-answer periods, and return demonstrations. Some nurses on your unit have left and administration has decided not to replace them. Since then, you have noticed that your unit is continuously left short-staffed. There is not enough time for adequate client teaching.

What ethical standards or principles guide you when you are faced with a chronic problem of understaffing on a nursing unit? All units occasionally face a problem with short-staffing. Many things can contribute to the problem: a flu outbreak among the nursing staff, several women out on maternity leave, or attendance at a nursing conference. These issues are temporary and usually can be resolved with a few telephone calls, one to the nurse-manager and a few to staff nurses requesting a few hours of overtime.

There is a difference when the staffing is chronically poor. If you constantly are unable to give high-quality nursing care, you must take action. Item 9 of the American Nurses Association (ANA) code states that "the nurse participates in the profession's efforts to establish and maintain conditions of employment conducive to high quality nursing care."

Staff nurses are obligated to provide nursing care that meets accepted standards. You are also obligated to correct the problem of short-staffing that interferes with providing nursing care that meets standards. This problem of staffing does not rest on your shoulders alone, however. While not abandoning your clients, inform those who can correct the problem. Supervisors, nurse-managers, physicians, and institution administration are obligated to correct the problem.

You must make a reasonable effort to ensure that safe, standard care is given. It may be possible to alter the assignments of other nurses temporarily to help alleviate the problem. Notifying the nursing supervisor may be necessary. If staffing is a chronic problem, the issue must be addressed by managers and administrators. Alternatives need to be identified and standards of care must be maintained. It may be possible to schedule nurses for unusual shifts to maximize the times clients are available for extended teaching sessions. An innovative volunteer program using former clients with colostomies as teachers may help. Whatever mechanisms are employed, standards must be maintained. As a last resort, the unit may need to be closed until adequate staff can be obtained.

Pathophysiology

Defects in the muscular wall may be congenital and due to weakened tissue or a wide space at the inguinal ligament, or may be caused by trauma. Intra-abdominal pressure most commonly increases as a result of pregnancy or obesity. Heavy lifting also causes increased pressure, as do coughing and traumatic injuries from blunt pressure. When two of these factors coexist with some tissue weakness, the person may develop a hernia. Increased pressure without a weakness is not likely to cause a hernia. Weakness, in addition to being present from birth, is acquired as part of the aging process. As clients age, muscular tissues become infiltrated and are replaced by adipose and connective tissues.

When the contents of the hernial sac can be re-placed into the abdominal cavity by manipulation, the hernia is said to be *reducible. Irreducible* and *incarcerated* are terms that refer to a hernia that cannot be reduced or re-placed by manipulation. When pressure from the hernial ring (the ring of muscular tissue through which the bowel protrudes) cuts off the blood supply to the herniated segment of bowel, the bowel becomes strangulated. Incarcerated hernias usually become strangulated. This situation is a surgical emergency because unless the bowel is released, it soon becomes gangrenous due to a lack of blood supply.

Hernias may penetrate through any defect in the abdominal wall, through the diaphragm, or through some internal structure within the abdominal cavity (Fig. 62–10). For the purposes of this discussion, only the more common types of hernias are covered. The most common hernias are the inguinal (both indirect and direct), femoral, umbilical, and incisional. (Hiatal hernia is discussed in Chapter 60).

Indirect Inguinal Hernia. This herniation occurs through the inguinal ring and follows the spermatic cord through the inguinal canal. It is more common in males than in females because of the space allowed for the testicles to descend. There is a high incidence of these hernias among infants and young persons. The incidence increases again among clients in their 50s, and then gradually decreases. These hernias can become extremely large and often descend into the scrotum.

Direct Inguinal Hernia. This hernia passes through the abdominal wall in an area of muscular weakness, not through a canal as do indirect inguinal and femoral hernias. It is more common in the elderly. Direct inguinal hernias gradually develop in an area that is weak due to congenital deficiency in the number of fibers it contains.

Femoral Hernia. A femoral hernia occurs through the femoral ring and is more common in females than in males. It begins as a plug of fat in the femoral canal that enlarges and gradually pulls the peritoneum, and almost inevitably the urinary bladder, into the sac. There is a high incidence of incarceration and strangulation with this type of hernia.

Umbilical Hernia. Umbilical herniation in the adult is more common in women and is due to increased abdominal pressure. It usually occurs in obese clients and in multiparous women.

Incisional or Ventral Hernia. This type of hernia occurs at the site of a previous surgical incision that has healed inadequately because of postoperative problems such as infection, inadequate nutrition, extreme distention, or obesity.

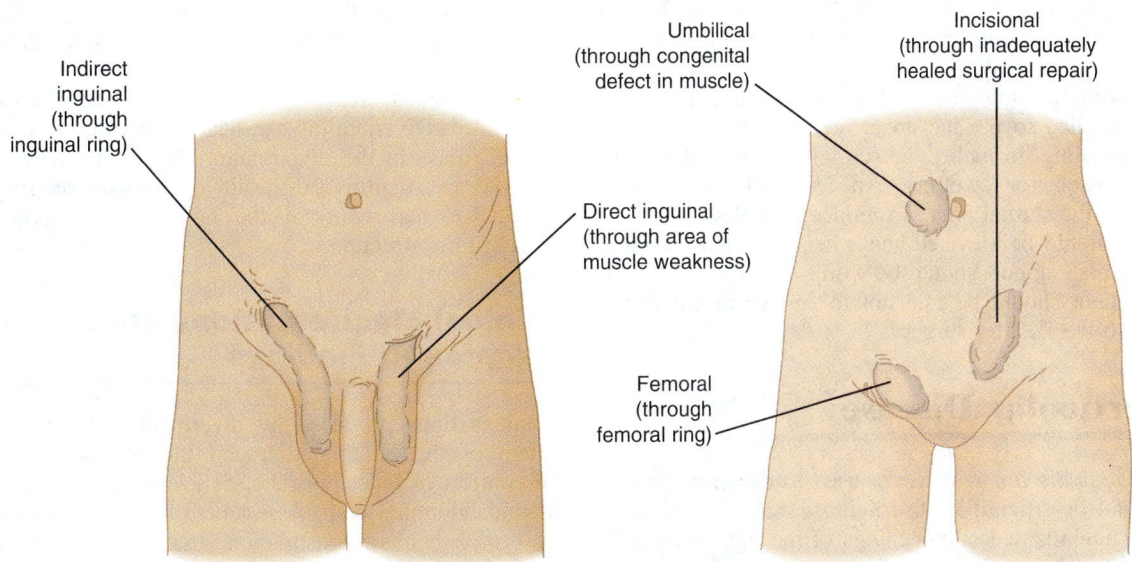

Figure 62–10. Common types of herniation.

Acute and Subacute Care

■ Medical Management

Hernias that are not strangulated or incarcerated can be mechanically reduced. A truss also can be used to keep the hernia reduced. A truss is a firm pad held in place by a belt. The pad is placed over the hernia after it has been reduced and left in place to prevent the hernia from recurring. The client is taught to apply the truss daily before arising. The client should carefully inspect the skin under the truss for any manifestation of breakdown.

■ Surgical Management

A hernia repair is performed using a small incision directly over the weakened area. The intestine is then returned to the perineal cavity, the hernia sac excised, and the muscle closed tightly over the area. Hernias in the inguinal region are usually repaired under spinal or local anesthesia. Most hernia repairs are now performed as outpatient procedures.

Some repairs are difficult because there is insufficient muscle mass to keep the intestines in place. In this case, steel mesh grafts are used to reinforce the area of herniation. Clients with difficult repairs are usually hospitalized for 1 to 2 days to receive prophylactic antibiotics.

■ Nursing Management of the Surgical Client

Make certain the client voids after surgery, because urinary retention is a common problem, especially in males. Return the client to a general diet as soon as the client tolerates food. When general anesthesia is used, postoperative progress is slower. Assure the client that during the immediate postoperative period the hernia will not recur. Some clients hesitate to become active because of this fear. Obese patients progress more slowly, heal more slowly, and may need more encouragement to participate in postoperative activities.

Following an inguinal hernia repair, an ice pack is usually applied to the incisional area to control pain and reduce swelling. In males, the scrotal area should be carefully assessed for swelling. An ice pack also can be applied to the scrotal area. To reduce scrotal swelling, the scrotum should be elevated and when the client is out of bed a scrotal support should be worn.

The client should be told not to engage in any lifting for 4 to 6 weeks after surgery.

Diverticular Disease

Diverticular disease is the term used to describe diverticulosis and diverticulitis. Diverticulosis refers to the presence of noninflamed outpouchings of the intestine. Diverticulitis is inflammation of a diverticulum. A diverticulum is a blind outpouching or herniation of intestinal mucosa through the muscular coat of the large intestine, usually the sigmoid colon.

Diverticular disease is common in men and women over 45 years of age and in the obese. It is present in approximately one third of the population over age 60 years. It is more common in the United States, the United Kingdom, Australia, and France.

Etiology and Risk Factors

Low fiber diets have been implicated in the development of diverticula, because these diets decrease bulk in the stool and predispose to constipation. In the presence of muscle weakness in the bowel, this increase in intraluminal pressure can lead to the formation of diverticula.

The causes of diverticulosis include atrophy or weakness of the bowel muscle, increased intraluminal pressure, obesity, and chronic constipation.

Diverticulitis occurs when undigested food blocks the diverticulum, leading to a decrease in the blood supply to the area and predisposing the bowel to invasion of bacteria into the diverticulum. The Risk Factors and Levels of Prevention feature lists contributing factors and preventive measures for diverticular disease.

Pathophysiology

Diverticula have narrow, flasklike necks, which communicate with the bowel lumen. Weak points in the bowel muscularis exist where branches of the blood vessels penetrate the colonic wall. These weak points create areas for bowel protrusion when there is increased intraluminal pressure.

Diverticula frequently develop in the sigmoid colon because of the high pressures in this area required to move the stool into the rectum.

Diverticulitis may be acute or chronic. If the diverticulum is not infected (diverticulosis), these lesions cause few problems. However, when fecaliths do not liquify and drain from the diverticulum, they may become trapped and cause irritation and inflammation (diverticulitis).

The inflamed area becomes congested with blood and may bleed. Diverticulitis can lead to perforation when the trapped mass in the diverticulum erodes the bowel wall. Chronic diverticulitis can result in increased scarring and, eventually, narrowing of the bowel lumen, potentially leading to obstruction.

Clinical Manifestations and Diagnostic Findings

Manifestations produced by diverticulitis depend on the extent of the inflammation and the site of occurrence. Discomfort includes episodic, dull, or steady left quadrant or midabdominal pain. Assessment also reveals alteration in bowel habits (constipation, diarrhea, or alternately, both), increased flatus, anorexia, and low-grade fever. The inflammatory process usually subsides within several

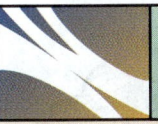

RISK FACTORS AND LEVELS OF PREVENTION

Diverticular Disease

Risk Factors

For diverticulosis: Chronic constipation, low fiber diet, obesity

For diverticulitis: Ingestion of indigestible fiber (e.g., corn, popcorn, and tomatoes or cucumbers with seeds) in clients with diverticulosis

Levels of Prevention

Primary Prevention

For diverticulosis:

- Instruct clients to maintain adequate bowel habits.
- Advise clients to consume a high fiber diet that helps prevent constipation.
- Encourage clients to lose weight if they are obese.

For diverticulitis:

- Encourage clients to avoid indigestible bulk to help prevent inflammation of the diverticula.

Secondary Prevention

For diverticulosis:

- Teach clients to avoid straining, coughing, lifting, and other factors that increase intra-abdominal pressure.
- Instruct clients to take bulk laxatives (Metamucil and other hydrophilic colloids).

For diverticulitis:

- Instruct clients to rest the colon by not taking anything by mouth until the pain subsides and fluids may be administered.

Tertiary Prevention

For diverticulosis and diverticulitis:

- Surgery to resect colon or ligate the sac may be required.
- Treatment prevention of complications such as hemorrhage, obstruction, abscesses, or perforation.

---

weeks. If the infection penetrates the pelvic floor or retroperitoneal tissues, abscesses may result. Extension of the inflammation to adjacent organs can lead to fistulas of the bladder or vagina and peritonitis. Repeated inflammation can result in narrowing of the bowel and obstruction.

Rectal bleeding occurs in about 15% of clients. Stools also may contain mucus. Urinary frequency can occur if the inflammation is in the proximity of the bladder. Straining, coughing, or lifting causes an increase in intra-abdominal pressure and manifestations. The clinician may palpate a tender mass on digital and rectal examinations.

Acute and Subacute Care

■ Medical Management

Asymptomatic diverticular disease requires no specific therapy other than modification of the diet. Mild disease can be treated by adherence to a high fiber diet and prevention of constipation with bran and bulk laxatives (hydrophilic colloids). Advise clients to notify the physician of any change in bowel movement pattern (constipation or diarrhea) or character (presence of mucus or blood), or if fever, abdominal pain, or urinary manifestations develop.

Diverticulitis may be treated conservatively with medical intervention by allowing the colon to rest. Clients with acute diverticulitis are on NPO status, may have an NG tube, and receive parenteral fluids until pain, inflammation, and temperature decrease. When the acute episode begins to subside, they can ingest oral liquids and, later, a progressively more inclusive diet.

■ Nursing Management of the Medical Client

Intervention also aims to control inflammation. Administer prescribed antibiotics and advise the client to:

1. Avoid activities that increase intra-abdominal pressure, such as bending, lifting, stooping, coughing, and vomiting
2. Drink at least eight glasses of water every day
3. Reduce weight if obese

■ Surgical Management

Surgery is indicated for clients who develop complications, such as hemorrhage, obstruction, abscesses, or perforation. Surgical procedures usually include ligation and removal of the sac or resection of involved bowel if there are complications. With abscess or obstruction, the surgeon performs a colon resection with a temporary colostomy, which is left in place until the client's condition improves. For some clients, the temporary colostomy alone allows the bowel to rest and heal.

■ Nursing Management of the Surgical Client

For information on the care of these clients see the discussion of colon resections.

Meckel's Diverticulum

Meckel's diverticulum is an outpouching of the bowel, a vestige of embryonic development found on the ileum within 10 cm of the cecum. The pouch may be lined with gastric mucosa or may contain pancreatic tissue. The gastric mucosal lining sometimes ulcerates and bleeds or perforates. In addition, the diverticulum may become inflamed and mimic appendicitis. Meckel's diverticulum is sometimes attached to the umbilicus by a fibrous band and may be the focus around which the bowel twists, causing obstruction. Treatment involves surgical excision of the diverticulum.

Obstruction

Partial or complete impairment of the forward flow of intestinal contents is known as an intestinal obstruction. Most obstructions occur in the small bowel, especially in the ileum, the narrowest segment. Obstructions of the small intestine are a common surgical emergency. Obstruction produces nausea, vomiting, dehydration, and severe pain. Intestinal obstruction has a high mortality rate if it is not diagnosed and treated within 24 hours.[34]

Etiology and Risk Factors

Obstruction of the small intestine may be caused by narrowing of the intestinal lumen due to inflammation, neoplasms, adhesions, hernia, volvulus, intussusception, food blockage, or compression from outside the intestine. Paralytic ileus, vascular problems such as mesenteric embolus or thrombus, or hypokalemia from diuretics or antihypertensive agents also may result in small bowel obstructions. Infections of the abdomen and sometimes of the thoracic cavity, such as lobar pneumonia, peritonitis, or pancreatitis, frequently produce an ileus of infectious origin.

Cancer accounts for approximately 80% of obstructions of the large intestine, with most occurring in the sigmoid colon. Other causes include diverticulitis and ulcerative colitis. Factors causing intestinal obstructions may be (1) mechanical, (2) neurogenic, or (3) vascular.

■ Mechanical Factors

Adhesions. Adhesions are probably the most common cause of obstruction in both the small and large intestine. Adhesions form after abdominal surgery, and for unknown reasons some clients develop massive adhesions. Irritants that remain in the abdomen following surgical procedures enhance the formation of adhesions. These fibrous bands of scar tissue can become looped over a portion of the bowel. These loops can then become either (1) the focus around which the bowel can twist (volvulus) (Fig. 62–11) or (2) the band that mechanically obstructs the bowel by external pressure. The presence of multiple adhesions increases the risk of obstruction.

Hernia. An incarcerated hernia may or may not cause obstruction, depending on the size of the hernial ring. However, the potential for obstruction is always present in any hernia. A strangulated hernia is always obstructed, because the bowel cannot function when its blood supply is cut off.

Volvulus. Volvulus is a twisting of the bowel that frequently occurs about a stationary focus (e.g., tumor or Meckel's diverticulum) in the abdominal cavity (see Fig.

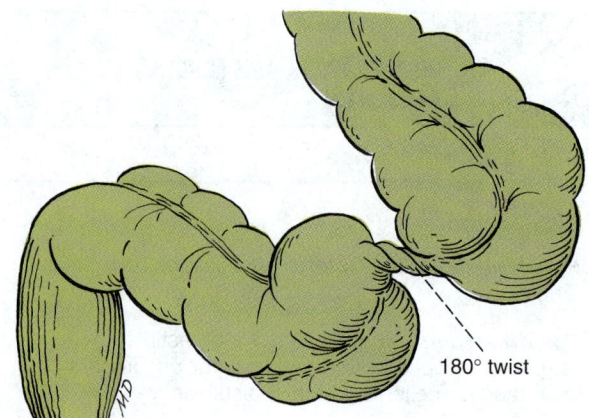

Figure 62–11. Volvulus. Intestine twists at least 180 degrees, causing obstruction and ischemia.

62–11). It can cause infarction of the bowel and can occur in either the large or small bowel. Volvulus can sometimes be corrected without surgical intervention. Successful decompression of the bowel with a long tube (Cantor or Miller-Abbott tube) releases pressure against the proximal end of the loop, thus allowing a small bowel volvulus to relax.

Intussusception. Intussusception, which sometimes complicates IBD, is a telescoping of the bowel (Fig. 62–12). The condition is often associated with tumor of the large bowel. Peristaltic action telescopes the proximal bowel into the bowel distal to it. Intramural lesions often cause intussusception.

Tumors. In the large bowel, tumors are the chief cause of obstruction. The process develops slowly and, because of the large lumen of the bowel, may become advanced before a fecal mass lodges at the constricted site and precipitates an acute obstructive process. In the small bowel, obstructive manifestations are frequently the first manifestation of a tumor. Even though the lumen of the small bowel is smaller, manifestations still do not occur early in the process because the intestinal contents are liquid.

■ Neurogenic Factors

An adynamic (or functional) obstruction, sometimes called a paralytic ileus, is caused by lack of peristaltic

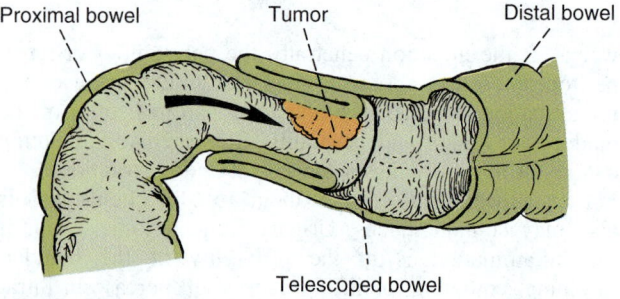

Figure 62–12. Intussusception. Portion of bowel telescopes into adjacent (usually distal) bowel.

activity. Paralytic ileus commonly occurs after abdominal surgery. The bowel ceases to function for a few hours to several days. Extensive surgical procedures in the bowel and in the retroperitoneal area may cause a postoperative neurogenic problem. Treatment involves aspiration of secretions by gastric suction until the bowel begins to function.

■ Vascular Factors

When the blood supply to any part of the body is interrupted, the part ceases to function and pain occurs. Blood is supplied to the bowel by way of the celiac and superior and inferior mesenteric arteries. These vessels have anastomotic intercommunications at the head of the pancreas and along the transverse bowel. Obstruction of blood flow can arise as a result of (1) complete occlusion (mesenteric infarction) or (2) partial occlusion (abdominal angina).

Complete Occlusion (Mesenteric Infarction).
Any occlusion of arterial blood supply to the bowel, as in mesenteric thrombosis, effectively stops bowel function. The usual cause is an embolus. The extent of the resulting manifestations is determined by the following:

1. The size of the vessel that is occluded
2. The length of bowel that is without a supply of blood
3. The rapidity with which the occlusion occurs

An acute occlusion, at its onset, causes intense abdominal pain, usually without manifestations of advanced intestinal obstruction. This is because the pain results from ischemic tissue rather than from obstruction. As the process advances, fever, leukocytosis, shock, and other manifestations of bowel gangrene develop. Acute mesenteric obstruction constitutes a surgical emergency and carries a high mortality rate (approximately 75%).

Surgical intervention must be initiated early. Sometimes, an embolectomy can restore circulation. The surgeon also must resect necrotic segments of the bowel.

Partial Occlusion (Abdominal Angina).
This condition usually results from atherosclerosis of the mesenteric arteries. It is a common, although often asymptomatic, problem. It is found at 33% of routine autopsies. Because there is an increased need for oxygenation during the digestive process, pain may develop 15 to 30 minutes after eating. Initially, pain may occur only after ingestion of a large meal. However, as the arterial process extends, it may occur even after a small meal, and eventually it becomes almost continuous.

Manifestations arise only when interruption of blood supply is sufficient to compromise bowel function. At this time, in addition to pain after eating, assessment reveals (1) a change in bowel habits, (2) nausea and vomiting, and (3) weight loss caused by restriction of intake by the client because of discomfort experienced when eating. Vascular or bypass grafts can sometimes improve the blood supply to the affected portion of the bowel.

Pathophysiology

Normally, 7 to 8 L of electrolyte-rich fluid are secreted by the bowel, and most of it is reabsorbed. When the bowel is obstructed, this fluid is partially retained within the bowel and partially eliminated by vomiting, causing severe reduction in circulating blood volume, resulting in hypotension, hypovolemic shock, and diminished renal and cerebral blood flow. Because fluid is lost but blood cells are not, the hematocrit and hemoglobin increase, thus increasing the potential for vascular occlusive disorders such as coronary, cerebral, and mesenteric thrombosis.

For instance, with the onset of an obstruction, fluids and air collect proximal to the site of the problem, causing distention. Manifestations occur sooner and are more intense in a small bowel blockage because the small bowel is narrower and normally more active. The large volume of secretions from the small bowel adds to the distention. The only significant secretion from the large bowel is mucus.

Distention causes a temporary increase in peristalsis as the bowel attempts to force the material through the obstructed area. Within a few hours, the increased peristalsis ends and the bowel becomes flaccid, thus reducing pressure within the lumen and slowing the process caused by the obstruction. Increased pressure within the bowel reduces its absorptive ability, which increases the fluid retention still further. Soon the intraluminal pressure reduces venous return, which increases venous pressure, congestion, and vessel fragility. This process, in turn, raises capillary permeability and allows plasma to extravasate into the bowel lumen and into the peritoneal cavity. The bowel wall becomes permeable to bacteria, and bowel organisms enter the peritoneal cavity. Increasing pressure in the bowel wall soon slows arterial blood flow, causing necrosis and, in some cases, toxemia and peritonitis.

Strangulation of the bowel results in decreased arterial blood supply. Necrosis and perforation may force the intestinal contents into the peritoneal cavity, causing peritonitis. Bacteria proliferate in the strangulated bowel and may form endotoxins. When the endotoxins are released into the peritoneal cavity or systemic circulation, there is rapid circulatory collapse with endotoxic shock, accounting for the high mortality rate associated with this condition. These complications are especially likely to occur in elderly persons, who tend to have atherosclerotic narrowing of these vessels, making thrombosis more likely.

Clinical Manifestations and Diagnostic Findings

Manifestations of intestinal obstruction depend on the following:

1. The level and length of bowel involved
2. The degree to which the obstruction interferes with blood supply
3. The completeness of the obstruction
4. The type of lesion producing the obstruction

Intestinal obstruction affects the bowel at local and systemic levels. Local changes in the bowel wall include congestion, fragility, reduced circulation, and increased pressure. Increased pressure leads to reverse peristalsis, producing vomiting that helps prevent overdistention of the bowel. These local effects result from (1) loss of fluids, electrolytes, and plasma; (2) bacterial proliferation; and (3) perforation. Systemic effects include a reduction in extracellular fluid and circulating blood volume, toxemia, and peritonitis.

The client with small bowel obstruction typically experiences abdominal pain in rhythmically recurring waves. The pain results from distention and the small intestine's peristaltic efforts to push its contents past the obstruction. Small intestinal pain is felt in the upper and midabdomen, whereas colonic pain is experienced in the lower abdomen. Soon after the small intestine becomes distended, you can see the peristaltic waves and hear accompanying high-pitched tinkling sounds. The client usually becomes nauseated and vomits, which brings some relief from the pain, provided the obstruction is high or proximal to the ileum.

If the obstruction is distal to the ileum, vomiting fails to empty the bowel completely, allowing the accumulation of fluids, residue, and gases. As the muscles become atonic, loops of small bowel dilate, compounding the problem of distention. Eventually, severe distention may raise the diaphragm, thereby inhibiting respirations. Hypoxia (due to inadequate respirations and decreased circulating blood volume and hypotension) often develops. Vomiting is more severe if the obstruction is located high in the small bowel. At first, vomitus is composed of semidigested food and chyme and later becomes watery and contains bile. Finally, the client vomits dark fecal material, the result of bacterial growth in the fluid that has stagnated in the obstructed bowel.

When the colon is obstructed, the competent ileocecal valve prevents regurgitation, and pressure within the lumen increases, resulting in distention. In some cases, the cecum may perforate. Obstruction of the colon results in altered bowel habits, lower abdominal pain, a desire to defecate, distention, and borborygmi. Vomiting is not a common manifestation because of the competent ileocecal valve. In the presence of an incompetent ileocecal valve, distention progresses to the small intestine. Vomiting that accompanies large intestine obstruction is a very late manifestation, and only occurs secondary to a distended small intestine.

Clients with vomiting may experience severe fluid and electrolyte imbalances. They lose not only water but also sodium, chloride, potassium, and bicarbonate. The result is an acute extracellular volume deficit (dehydration), which, in turn, lowers the circulating blood volume. Hydrogen ion imbalances frequently occur in intestinal obstructions, with metabolic acidosis being the most common problem.

Specific diagnostic tests include a plain film, which shows gas shadows; barium or radiopaque x-ray studies; and complete blood studies. Increased hemoglobin and hematocrit values may indicate dehydration. Leukocytosis may point to a strangulated bowel. A decrease in sodium, potassium, and chloride levels and a rise in nonprotein nitrogen and blood urea nitrogen (BUN) levels may indicate small bowel obstruction.

Acute and Subacute Care

■ Medical Management

The major treatment for an intestinal obstruction is the insertion of an intestinal tube (see the section on intestinal tubes in Chapter 61). Often, an intestinal tube both decompresses the bowel and breaks up the obstruction.

In adynamic ileus, the best intervention is rest and prevention of distention by gastric suction. Medications are not effective in stimulating bowel activity. The bowel will respond when it recovers completely from the effects of obstruction.

■ Nursing Management of the Medical Client

Assessment

Obtain a complete history of the onset of manifestations, eating patterns, food tolerance, vomiting episodes, stools (number per day and appearance), distention, and factors that increase or decrease pain.

During physical assessment, note the following:

● Abdominal distention
● The quality of bowel sounds
● The presence and extent of dehydration
● Muscle guarding or manifestations of abdominal pain.

A lack of bowel sounds indicates peritoneal irritation or adynamic ileus. Usually, in the case of bowel obstruction, auscultation reveals high-pitched peristaltic rushes with high, metallic tinkling sounds.

Diagnosis, Planning, Implementation

Fluid Volume Deficit. A priority nursing diagnosis for the client with an intestinal obstruction is *Fluid Volume Deficit related to vomiting, decreased intestinal reabsorption of fluid, and decreased intestinal secretions.*

Planning: Expected Outcomes. The client will maintain fluid balance, as evidenced by balanced intake and output, no manifestations of dehydration, and blood pressure within the client's normal range.

Implementation. Maintain good fluid balance in the client with an obstruction by carefully replacing fluids and electrolytes. Administer parenteral fluids with sodium chloride, bicarbonate, and potassium added as ordered.

Maintain an intestinal tube attached to suction to relieve the vomiting and distention (see the discussion of care of a client with intestinal tubes). If the obstruction is not mechanical, an intestinal tube can achieve decompression. If the obstruction is due to adhesions, hernia, or tumors, the tube stops at the point of obstruction and keeps the bowel decompressed above the obstruction.

Note the progress of an intestinal tube, the amount and type of drainage, and relief of distention and nausea.

Assess and measure drainage from the intestinal tube. Document color, odor, consistency, and volume. Inform the physician of blood levels of sodium, potassium, and bicarbonate, and the pH of the blood, all reflecting fluid and electrolyte balance.

For dismissal following medical resolution of the obstruction, the client needs to learn ways to prevent recurrence and maintain bowel elimination. The client needs to be seen at intervals after the obstruction is relieved to ensure that it has not recurred. The client's nutritional status also should be monitored to ensure that adequate nutrition is maintained.

Evaluation

Once the obstruction is relieved medically, the client should return to normal within a matter of days. If the obstruction cannot be relieved medically, surgery will need to be performed.

■ Surgical Management

If intestinal intubation does not relieve the obstruction, surgery is the only remaining option. The major objective in treating bowel obstruction is to relieve the cause and thus eliminate the problem. However, the cause is not always immediately obvious. Diagnosis of the cause of the acute abdominal condition may be difficult and must frequently be made during surgery. Document specific observations to aid in the diagnosis.

In most vascular and mechanically caused obstructions, surgical excision of the cause is the only intervention. Surgery relieves the obstruction and removes any ischemic bowel. Relieving the obstruction should reestablish bowel patency. The type of surgery depends on the location and type of obstruction. The surgeon may perform bowel resection, colostomy, or a bypass procedure.

■ Nursing Management of the Surgical Client

Assessment

Assessment of the surgical client is the same as assessment of the medical client. In addition, routine preoperative and postoperative assessments are required.

Diagnosis, Planning, Implementation

Risk for Altered Tissue Perfusion: Gastrointestinal. An appropriate nursing diagnosis for the client undergoing surgery for an intestinal obstruction is *Risk for Altered Tissue Perfusion: Gastrointestinal, related to intestinal obstruction.*

Planning: Expected Outcomes. The client will not develop an alteration in tissue perfusion to the bowel, as evidenced by the return of normal peristalsis and usual bowel elimination.

Implementation. The client will have the intestinal tube inserted to help relieve the obstruction. Recognize and immediately report to the physician manifestations

such as emesis, increasing distention and pain, and temperature elevation, all of which are manifestations of bowel strangulation.

If the blood supply becomes impaired, the client will require emergency surgery. The nurse must prepare the client for this procedure. Antibiotics are often given before surgery. Be careful about administering narcotics, because these medications may mask manifestations of increasing obstruction or impaired blood flow and some narcotics slow peristalsis.

The client with a bowel obstruction with impaired tissue perfusion requires an emergency bowel resection. (See the discussion of care of a client after a bowel resection with or without a colostomy.)

Prior to dismissal, the learning needs of the client are determined by the type of surgery required. The client with a temporary colostomy needs to learn to care for the colostomy. Without a colostomy, the client's learning needs are the same as for any client after a bowel resection.

Evaluation

Evaluate client outcomes based on the established care plan. If the goals were not achieved, revise the plan and interventions to meet the client's needs. The client should recover from surgery without complications.

Irritable Bowel Syndrome

Irritable bowel syndrome (IBS) is a functional disorder of motility in the small and large intestine. It develops without organic disease or anatomic abnormality. Other descriptive names for this condition are spastic colon, irritable colon, nervous indigestion, functional dyspepsia, pylorospasm, spastic colitis, intestinal neurosis, and laxative or cathartic "colitis." IBS is the most common gastrointestinal disorder in Western society, accounting for 50% of subspecialty referrals. It is more common in women than men and occurs during middle age.[22]

Etiology and Risk Factors

Several factors appear to be involved in the pathogenesis of IBS:

- Prediverticular disease characterized by increased width of the sigmoid circular muscles, increased segmentation, and nonpropulsive intraluminal pressures
- Psychological stress
- A low-residue diet
- Lactose intolerance

The Risk Factors and Levels of Prevention feature lists other factors that contribute to IBS as well as preventive measures.

Pathophysiology

IBS appears to be a disorder of gastrointestinal motility. Motility may be altered by any number of factors, including diet and emotions. The alteration in motility can

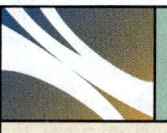

cause diarrhea, constipation, or alternating diarrhea and constipation. The structure of the bowel mucosa is not altered, although the disease continues whenever the client is exposed to the causative agents. Causative agents vary among clients; however, most clients can clearly identify them.

Clinical Manifestations and Diagnostic Findings

The client with IBS is usually found to have some combination of the following manifestations: abdominal pain, altered bowel function, constipation or diarrhea, hypersecretion of colonic mucus, dyspeptic manifestations (flatulence, nausea, anorexia), and some degree of anxiety or depression. Manifestations vary in intensity. Fiber, fruits, alcohol, and fatigue aggravate or precipitate manifestations.

Emotional disturbances affect the autonomic nervous system (ANS) and its innervation to the bowel. Disturbances of ANS function probably alter motor activity and transit time. Manifestations may mimic various organic and systemic diseases. Pain may be steady or intermittent, and there may be a dull deep discomfort with sharp cramps in the morning or after eating. The typical pattern consists of lower left quadrant abdominal pain and constipation or diarrhea. There may be tenderness over the sigmoid area.

Diarrhea tends to be the major problem but not usually at night. Nocturnal diarrhea tends to be associated with organic disease of the bowel. Examination of the stool reveals mucus but not blood. Eating may aggravate pain and defecation, and passing flatus or stool may provide temporary relief. Spastic contractions sometimes occur with stools that are small, dry, hard, and pelletlike. Other manifestations include abdominal disturbances such as nausea, distention, dyspepsia, eructation (belching), and borborygmus due to aerophagia and decreased gas motility. Anorexia, foul breath, sour stomach, flatulence, and cramps also may be present. Associated behavioral disturbances are anxiety, tension, nervousness, depression, sleep disturbances, weakness, or difficulty concentrating.

Because there are no confirmatory diagnostic tests for or histologic features of IBS, diagnosis generally is made by excluding other diseases. Diagnostic techniques, therefore, must eliminate the possibility that the client has organic gastrointestinal disease.

Clients over age 50 suspected of having IBS must be carefully evaluated to rule out malignancy or diverticular disease. When functional bowel disease develops, the client usually gives a history of nervousness and emotional disturbance. The client also may be bowel-conscious and a frequent user of cathartics and enemas. Palpation may demonstrate abdominal tenderness, particularly along the course of the colon.

Sigmoidoscopy or colonoscopy may reveal spasm and mucus in the colonic lumen. A barium enema is usually performed. A complete blood count and stool examination is needed to rule out the presence of occult blood, ova, parasites, and pathogenic bacteria.

Community and Self-Care

■ Medical Management

Treatment is palliative and supportive. Advise the client to limit responsibilities, seek rest, and adopt measures to reduce stress such as progressive relaxation, biofeedback, and a regular exercise routine. The client can control manifestations through diet, medication, and regular physical activity. The client must continue with routine follow-up assessment and care.

Sedative and antispasmodic medications may help the client feel more relaxed. Vegetable mucilages, such as psyllium hydrophilic mucilloid (Metamucil), can increase stool bulk.

A high fiber diet helps control IBS through the production of bulkier stools and reduction of tension in the walls of the sigmoid colon. Fiber helps manage both

NURSING RESEARCH

How Does Dietary Fiber Affect Gastrointestinal Symptoms?

Georges, J., & Heitkemper, M. (1994). Dietary fiber and distressing gastrointestinal symptoms in midlife women. *Nursing Research, 43*(6), 357–361.

In this descriptive study, 20 midlife women experiencing chronic distressing gastrointestinal symptoms recorded symptom severity in a diary over a 30-day period and dietary intake in a 9-day food record. A wide variability in symptom severity was noted. Significant negative relationships were present between dietary fiber intake and abdominal pain, awakening with abdominal pain, nausea, awakening with nausea, and awakening with rectal pain. No significant relationships were noted between amount of caffeine or alcohol intake and distressing gastrointestinal symptoms.

Implications for Practice

Women with GI manifestations should be encouraged to increase dietary fiber ingestion once physical abnormalities have been ruled out.

rhea to (1) limit foods that are gas-producing or irritating; (2) avoid caffeinated beverages, alcohol, and foods containing nondigestible carbohydrates, such as beans; and (3) eschew milk and milk products.

Acquired Megacolon

Acquired megacolon is a dilation of the colon above an area of obstruction. It may be secondary to any cause of severe constipation or obstruction (functional cause, rectal disease). In acquired megacolon, clients usually are incontinent of stool. Acquired megacolon usually occurs in the very young or very old. Treatment of acquired megacolon involves a retraining of bowel habits, behavior modification, removing impactions by using enemas or laxatives, and relief of any obstructions.

Disorders of the Anorectal Area

The major function of the rectum is to store feces until evacuation. When feces enter the rectum, peristalsis occurs. Many disorders in the rectal area result from constipation or failure to empty the rectum when peristalsis occurs.

At the mucocutaneous border of the anal canal, the mucous membrane changes to skin that has cutaneous somatic nerve endings. Because of this anatomic structure, lesions of the external anal canal are very painful. The two most common manifestations are bleeding and pain. Drainage of mucus and fecal matter and irritation of the skin by organisms can cause intense itching.

Hemorrhoids and skin tags may protrude from the anal opening, and there may be drainage of pus from abscesses. Bright-red blood per rectum usually indicates a lesion of the left colon or anorectal region. Blood on the toilet paper alone usually indicates perianal disease, whereas blood on the surface of a formed stool may suggest a polyp or carcinoma of the left colon or rectum. Blood mixed with the stool suggests inflammatory bowel disease or carcinoma of the proximal colon. Blood in the toilet bowl after the passage of formed stool suggests hemorrhoidal bleeding. All rectal bleeding must be evaluated by a physician.

Hemorrhoids are the most common source of bright-red blood in the stool. Carcinoma is the most serious source. Clinical features of rectal carcinoma often mimic those of hemorrhoids (sense of incomplete evacuation, stool caliber changes, and tenesmus). Carcinoma is suspected if there has been a change in bowel habits, loss of weight, or both.

constipation and diarrhea. In constipation, the softer, bulkier, and heavier stools produced by dietary fiber tend to decrease transit time. In diarrhea, the fiber diet helps absorb water, giving form to the stool and increasing transit time.

The Nursing Research feature describes the effects of dietary fiber on women with gastrointestinal manifestations.

Sources of fiber include unprocessed miller's bran, bran cereals, whole wheat, other whole grains such as brown rice, and fresh vegetables. Clients should drink six to eight glasses of water daily, because water helps regulate stool consistency and frequency. If diarrhea is a problem, the client needs to avoid foods that may cause diarrhea, such as cold drinks, and drink liquids between meals rather than at mealtime.

■ Nursing Management of the Medical Client

Reinforce the physician's explanation of the nature of the disorder, the intervention plan, and the prognosis. Make it clear to the client that the bowel responds to stress, foods, and medications. Emphasize the importance of regular hours, nourishing meals, and adequate sleep, exercise, and recreation. Help the client establish a regular bowel routine. Provide, as always, empathy and support.

Reinforce diet education. Advise the client with diar-

Hemorrhoids

Hemorrhoids are perianal varicose veins. Hemorrhoids may be internal or external (Fig. 62–13). Internal hemor-

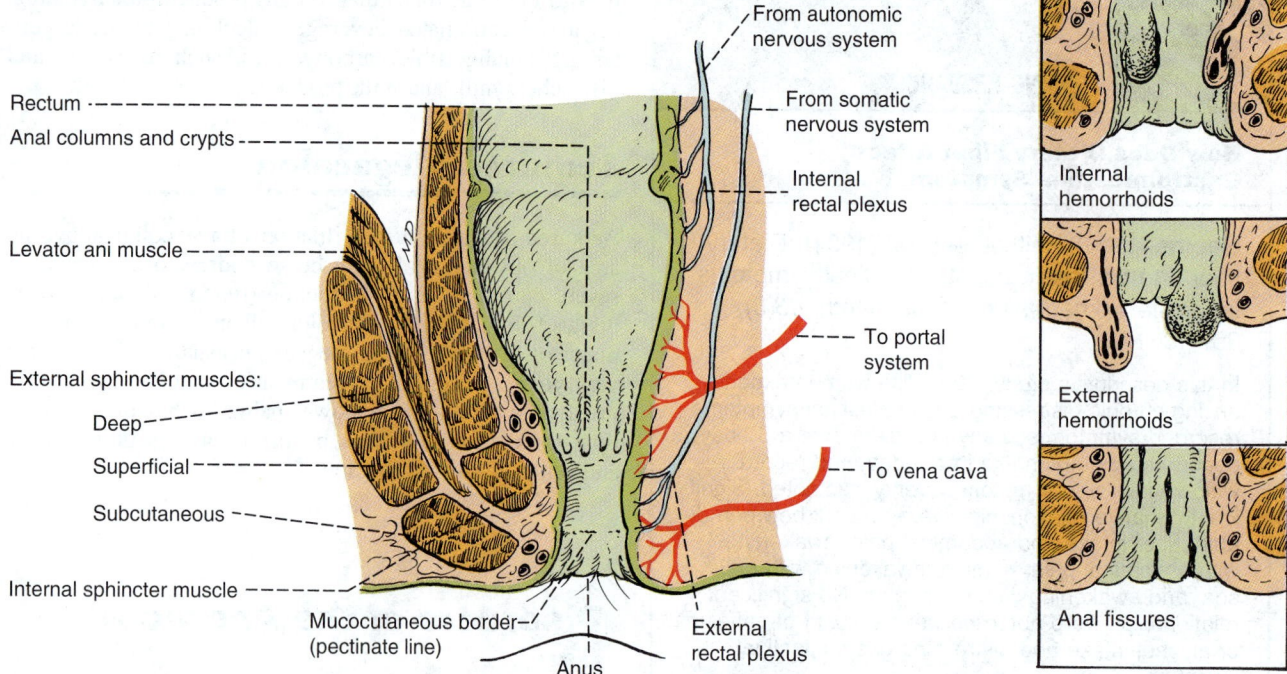

Figure 62–13. Structure of the anus and common disorders: internal hemorrhoids, external hemorrhoids, anal fissures.

rhoids are varicosities of the superior hemorrhoidal plexus occurring above the mucocutaneous border (pectinate line), are covered by mucous membrane, and are innervated by the autonomic nervous system.

External hemorrhoids are dilations of the inferior hemorrhoidal plexus that lie below the mucocutaneous junction and are covered by anal skin. As these vessels dilate, they stretch the overlying mucous membrane and skin and eventually protrude down the anal canal. This bulging plexus may be traumatized or pushed outside the anus by the passage of hard stool. Anal fissures are sometimes mistaken for hemorrhoids.

Hemorrhoids are a common disorder, affecting both men and women of any age, but the incidence is increased in people between 20 to 50 years old. Enlargement of hemorrhoids is caused by increased intra-abdominal pressure. Pregnancy, congestive heart failure, prolonged sitting or standing, and cirrhosis with portal hypertension also increase the incidence of hemorrhoids.

Etiology and Risk Factors

Both internal and external hemorrhoids may result from (1) the many anastomoses between the plexuses and (2) the lack of valves in the veins of the superior hemorrhoidal plexus, which leads into the portal vein. Internal hemorrhoids are frequently caused by portal hypertension. Any condition that increases constipation, intra-abdominal pressure, and hemorrhoidal venous pressure increases the risk of development of hemorrhoids. Some causes are constipation, diarrhea, prolonged straining, pregnancy, and obesity. Congestive heart failure also can cause hemorrhoids. Prevention of constipation through increased fiber

in the diet is an excellent measure to reduce the risk of hemorrhoid development.

Pathophysiology

Tenesmus increases intra-abdominal and hemorrhoidal venous pressures, leading to distention of the hemorrhoidal veins. When the rectal ampulla is filled with formed stool, venous obstruction is believed to occur. As a result of the repeated and prolonged increase in this pressure and the obstruction, permanent dilation of hemorrhoidal veins occurs. As a result of the distention, thrombosis and bleeding also may occur.

Clinical Manifestations and Diagnostic Findings

The major manifestation of external hemorrhoids is an enlarged mass at the anus. Internal hemorrhoids are characterized by bleeding and prolapse. Other manifestations include rectal itching and constipation. Pain may be present if there is associated thrombosis. The blood is bright red and may be seen in the stool or on the toilet tissue. A prolapse may occur in severe cases after exercise or after prolonged standing. Hemorrhoids may prolapse during defecation and spontaneously return, or the client may need to replace them manually. In some clients, hemorrhoids are prolapsed at all times.

External hemorrhoids are diagnosed by visual examination; internal hemorrhoids are diagnosed through history, digital palpation, and proctoscopy. Asking the client to strain during assessment causes the veins to enlarge, thus aiding diagnosis.

Community and Self-Care

■ Medical Management

Medical therapy is used only for small, uncomplicated hemorrhoids with mild manifestations. Treatment involves (1) reducing pressure by treating the constipation and (2) relieving pain by applying heat and astringent lotions. No other intervention is required.

Constipation unrelieved by diet may require use of a stool softener (docusate sodium) or a hydrophilic psyllium preparation. A topical anesthetic or steroid preparation such as lidocaine (Xylocaine) or steroid creams also reduces pain and itching.

Dietary changes used to treat constipation include increasing fluid and fiber in the diet. For pain, an initial application of cold packs, followed by warm sitz baths three to four times a day, should help.

Primary complications of hemorrhoids are bleeding, thrombosis, and hemorrhoidal strangulation. Severe bleeding from prolonged trauma to the vein during defecation can cause iron deficiency anemia. Blood oozes or may even spurt out following a bowel movement. Thrombosis within the hemorrhoids can occur at any time and is manifested by intense pain. Strangulated hemorrhoids, prolapsed hemorrhoids in which the blood supply is cut off by the anal sphincter, can result in thrombosis when blood within the hemorrhoid clots. Assessment reveals severe pain, extreme edema, and inflammation. Application of cold packs and elevation of the buttocks may allow the prolapsed hemorrhoid to reduce spontaneously.

■ Nursing Management of the Medical Client

The client should take measures to avoid constipation. The anal area is very painful, and the client may avoid defecating, resulting in hard stool or fecal impaction. Encourage the client to take bulk laxatives, stool softeners, or mineral oil as prescribed to promote stool passage. Monitor the stool for consistency and blood.

Counsel the client to eat fiber-containing foods and take ample fluids to prevent straining, and to avoid laxatives as far as possible. Remind the client not to sit on the toilet longer than necessary. This position impairs blood flow and puts added pressure on anal vessels. The use of witch hazel compresses are soothing to the mucosa.

■ Surgical Management

Several surgical procedures are used to treat hemorrhoids. These include sclerotherapy, rubber band ligation, cryosurgery, laser surgery, and hemorrhoidectomy.

Sclerotherapy is performed by the injection of a sclerosing agent between and around the veins. This produces an inflammatory reaction that leads to thrombosis and fibrosis. This procedure can be performed on an outpatient basis but requires one to four injections 5 to 7 days apart. The sclerosing agent can cause anal canal scarring.

A common procedure for internal hemorrhoids, ligation is performed in the physician's office. The client can usually carry on normal activities immediately after the treatment. Unfortunately, the procedure cannot be used for external hemorrhoids and may be only temporarily effective. The surgeon inserts a ligator, a small, double-lumen cylinder with a small rubber band on the inner layer, through an anoscope. The hemorrhoid is then grasped with forceps and pulled through the ligator. The rubber band is placed around the neck of the hemorrhoid. Although bleeding can occur, the most common problem is some pain during ligation. The client takes a bulk laxative after the procedure to avoid local trauma from a hard fecal mass. In 8 to 10 days, the rubber band cuts through the neck of tissue, and the tissue sloughs.

Cryosurgery, freezing of the hemorrhoids, is performed less commonly today. It is also an outpatient procedure. The freezing of the tissue leads to necrosis and sloughing of the hemorrhoids. The problems associated with this procedure are the prolonged periods of drainage, the amount of foul drainage, the presence of large residual skin tags, and possibly, incomplete destruction of the hemorrhoids.

Laser removal is the newest procedure. This also is performed on an outpatient basis. The hemorrhoid is burned off with the laser. There is minimal bleeding, although the procedure causes some pain.

With a hemorrhoidectomy, the vein is excised and the area is either left open to heal by granulation or closed with sutures. The open method is very painful but has a high rate of success. The suture method, although far less painful, is more likely to cause infection and result in poor healing.

Complications include infection, stricture formation as the lesion heals, and hemorrhage. Hemorrhage may occur immediately after surgery or about 10 days later as a result of sloughing of tissue. Also, bleeding may not be evident because it can occur into the rectum and not pass immediately.

■ Nursing Management of the Surgical Client

After the client has had a procedure to remove hemorrhoids, stress the importance of keeping the area clean and the stool soft but formed, to help prevent strictures. Encourage the client to wash the area after defecation and to pat it dry. Local moist heat, applied with a washcloth or piece of cotton to the anal opening for a few minutes, cleans, soothes, and promotes healing. Never apply heat in the immediate postoperative period because of the increased risk of hemorrhage. Most physicians prescribe sitz baths three or four times a day or as the client desires, beginning 12 hours after surgery.

Postoperative complications requiring nursing assessment include hemorrhage and urinary retention. The proximity of the bladder and tenderness in the area sometimes make urination difficult. Reestablishment of bowel habits is another potential postoperative problem. The client may need instruction on the relationship of proper diet and adequate fluid intake to bowel regularity, the physiology of defecation, and the importance of establishing a regular bowel routine.

After a hemorrhoidectomy, the client should take a warm sitz bath after each bowel movement or three to four times per day to relieve discomfort and spasm and to promote healing. Perianal irritation may be relieved with zinc oxide ointment. The most convenient perianal dressing is a sanitary napkin, although if there is no drainage, the client requires no dressing. The stools can be regulated by increasing dietary fiber intake, with the goal of one soft stool daily.

Postoperative pain can be controlled with parenteral and then oral analgesics. Warn the client to avoid vigorous perianal wiping during the immediate postoperative period. The client is usually given a stool softener and mineral oil to soften and lubricate the first stool. Warn clients that fainting can occur, from pain and vagal stimulation, during the first postoperative bowel movement. Clients should not be discharged until they have had a bowel movement.

Pilonidal Cyst

A pilonidal cyst occurs at the base of the sacrum, usually contains hair, and becomes infected, forming an abscess and then a sinus tract. It is most common in young adults, especially men. It may result from hairs that penetrate the skin and cause sinus tracts to form. Constant irritation (e.g., from clothing and perspiration from activity) can cause hairs to become embedded and then infected.

Acute pain and swelling result, followed by a discharge. Treatment involves surgical excision of the abscess. Healing is slow, and if the infectious process is not completely removed, the condition may recur. The client also may receive antibiotics.

Anal Fissure

An anal fissure is an ulceration or tear of the lining of the anal canal, usually on the posterior wall. An acute fissure occurs as a result of excessive tissue stretching and possibly from passage of a hard or large stool. The skin tear is tender and tends to reopen at subsequent defecation.

Chronic fissures are usually secondary to cryptitis (infectious material retained in the anal crypts). Sharp pain accompanies defecation, followed by burning. Severe muscle spasm of the sphincter usually accompanies chronic conditions. The client may try to avoid defecation, which aggravates the conditions.

If the acute lesion does not heal with local dilations, cleaning, and control of constipation, the tract can be excised surgically. A chronic fissure usually does not heal spontaneously and requires surgery.

Advise the client to (1) keep the stool soft with Metamucil, mineral oil, or docusate sodium, as prescribed; (2) have a bowel movement daily; and (3) clean the area after defecation, preferably with warm water. Sitz baths aid healing and may relieve pain. Suppositories with a local anesthetic may relieve constipation.

Anal Fistula

A fistula is a sinus tract that develops between two body cavities or between a body cavity and the surface of the body. A rectal fistula is a tract that leads from the anal canal to the skin outside the anus, or from an abscess to either the anal canal or the perianal area. It usually is preceded by an abscess. A fistula may heal over temporarily and then open and drain periodically.

This is a chronic condition for which surgery is the only cure. The surgeon excises the tract and cleans the area, leaving it open to heal by granulation. It may heal very slowly and be very painful. Advise the client to keep the area clean, especially after a bowel movement.

Anorectal Abscess

Anorectal abscesses form in several locations; Figure 62–14 illustrates the common ones. Most abscesses begin as cryptitis, with the formation of cysts that extend through the tubular ducts into the submucosal spaces. They also may originate from abrasions of the local tissues, with entry of a virulent organism. Anal intercourse may also cause a rectal abscess.

Treatment involves draining the abscess and surgical excision of any associated fistulas. It may take two stages of surgery to accomplish the needed resection.

Tumors

Carcinoma and melanoma can occur at the anus but are rare, constituting less than 5% of anorectal cancers. They spread by local extension into the perirectal spaces and then to the inguinal nodes. Some tumors are treated with radiation and chemotherapy, while others may require surgical excision. Surgical intervention involves excision of the anus with an abdominoperineal resection. Preoperative irradiation and chemotherapy are other modes of intervention for anal cancer. Regional intra-arterial infusion of 5-fluorouracil as palliative therapy can relieve pain and improve the quality of life for the client with rectal cancer.

Cancer of the anal canal or lower rectum can coexist with other rectal conditions, and the client may falsely attribute bleeding to a hemorrhoid instead of carcinoma. Anal cancers are more common in blacks and usually occur in clients with preexisting anal and perianal problems such as a fistula. Bleeding, pain, and tenesmus are characteristic manifestations. The client is usually aware of a lump near the anus that has bled and gradually becomes more and more painful, particularly during or just after a bowel movement. Many cancers are not diagnosed until they are large, and by then the prognosis is poor. A physician should investigate every case of rectal bleeding, even though it may be attributable to hemorrhoids or some other local rectal condition.

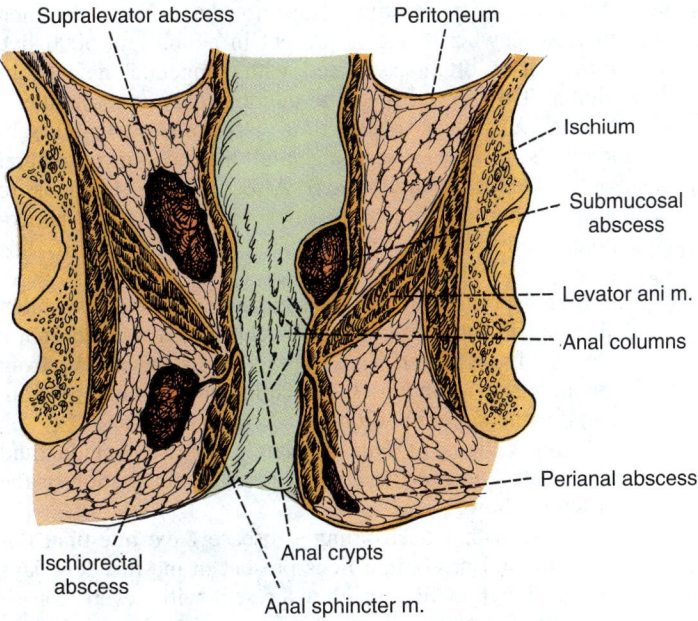

Supralevator abscess

Peritoneum

Ischium

Submucosal abscess

Levator ani m.

Anal columns

Perianal abscess

Ischiorectal abscess

Anal crypts

Anal sphincter m.

Figure 62–14. Abscesses of the anorectal area.

Blunt or Penetrating Trauma

Blunt or penetrating trauma to the abdomen refers to accidental or intentional trauma causing internal injuries. Most blunt abdominal trauma is caused by automobile steering wheel or pedestrian accidents, whereas most penetrating trauma is caused by gunshot wounds or stabbings.

Etiology and Risk Factors

Almost any kind of injury can cause blunt trauma to the abdomen. In automobile accidents, rapid, uncontrolled deceleration is the force that produces the trauma when the client's body hits the steering wheel or some other object. Penetrating trauma commonly results from gunshot wounds, which cause a great deal of internal damage. Stabbings are the next most common cause of penetrating abdominal wounds, although these wounds are less traumatic.

Trauma is the leading cause of death in adults under 40 and the fifth leading cause of death in all adults. Although not all of these cases of trauma are abdominal trauma, abdominal injuries are common with motor vehicle accidents. One method of prevention is wearing seat belts, which could decrease abdominal trauma in case of accidents.

Pathophysiology

Blunt trauma to the abdomen can cause shearing, crushing, or compressing forces that cause rupture of bowel and other abdominal structures.

Gunshot wounds can damage every structure in the abdomen. The gunshots may perforate the stomach or bowel, causing peritonitis and sepsis.

Stab wounds produce less trauma to internal abdominal structures because the abdominal organs have more time to shift out of the way of the penetrating instrument.

Clinical Manifestations and Diagnostic Findings

Assessment of the client first involves obtaining a thorough history of the accident so that the extent of blunt trauma can be estimated. For penetrating trauma, careful assessment of the position of entry and possibly exit wounds is vital.

The client may show manifestations of an acute abdomen with either type of trauma. With both injuries, either internal or external hemorrhage may occur. If the bowel is ruptured, manifestations of peritonitis are present. All abdominal drainage is closely assessed for the presence of bowel contents.

Abdominal lavage is commonly used to assess the presence of bleeding in all abdominal wounds. This involves instillation of a crystalloid solution into the peritoneal cavity followed by paracentesis (drainage of contents). Note and record the color and amount of the drainage.

A CT scan of the abdomen is now considered the base assessment of intra-abdominal injury. Angiography, intravenous pyelography, and other studies may be performed to assess different organs and the degree of trauma suffered.

 ## Acute and Subacute Care

■ Medical Management

If minimal blunt trauma was sustained without severe injury to any abdominal organs, then the client may simply be observed for problems once the diagnostic tests have been done. Penetrating trauma always requires some type of surgical intervention.

Pharmacologic Management

The client's pain is treated conservatively until the degree of trauma has been determined. If the bowel has been ruptured, large doses of intravenous antibiotics are given to control infection. If hemorrhage and shock are present, intravenous fluids, colloids, and vasopressors may be used.

Dietary Management

The client is NPO until the abdomen has been assessed and found to be intact.

Complications

The major complications of trauma are hemorrhage, shock, peritonitis, and sepsis.

■ Surgical Management

The treatment of choice for abdominal trauma with injury to the abdominal contents is an exploratory laparotomy. Depending on the injury, the surgery may be as simple as a closure of tears or as complex as a bowel resection and even a temporary colostomy.

■ Nursing Management of the Medical-Surgical Client

Careful assessment of the client's injury is vital. You often must prepare the client for immediate emergency surgery. Prepare the client as quickly as possible, knowing that postoperatively, much more teaching and support will be required.

Usually, once the injuries and repair have had sufficient time to heal and the infection has been adequately treated, the client will return to the hospital to have the temporary ostomy closed and the bowel returned to normal.

Prior to discharge, the client may need education regarding home healthcare, which may include ostomy care and extensive wound care. The client or significant others may have to learn to change dressings and to care for an open, draining wound. Follow-up care from a visiting nurse may also be required for the administration of antibiotics at home, further ostomy teaching, or wound care for an open draining wound.

Congenital Disorders

Hirschsprung's Disease

Hirschsprung's disease, or congenital megacolon, is hypertrophy of the colon due to absence of ganglion cells in the distal large intestine. This disorder is more common in male newborns and is present in about 1 in 5000 live births. It is often associated with congenital defects including Down syndrome and genitourinary abnormalities.

The functional obstruction associated with Hirschsprung's disease is a congenital absence of intramural neural plexus (aganglionosis). Affected bowel is unable to transmit normal peristaltic waves, resulting in a hypertrophied and dilated portion of intestine proximal to this area.

Hirschsprung's disease is characterized by a congenital absence of autonomic ganglion cells from the intramural plexus of the colon. The ganglion cells are absent from the anorectal junction, the rectum, and sometimes from parts of the sigmoid colon.

Complications of Hirschsprung's disease include fluid and electrolyte imbalances and possible perforation of the distended bowel.

Infants with Hirschsprung's disease have intestinal obstruction and meconium ileus present in the first few days of life. Later in life, children present with severe constipation and recurrent fecal impactions. Children with only a small segment of bowel involved may not demonstrate manifestations until after surgery.

In Hirschsprung's disease, digital examination shows the rectum to be empty. A barium enema study also confirms the absence of stool and usually shows a narrowed distal segment of bowel. A definitive diagnosis of Hirschsprung's disease is made from a full-thickness biopsy.

In Hirschsprung's disease, if obstruction is present, often a temporary colostomy is necessary. In some cases, a regular program of enemas can provide decompression. Several surgical procedures can be performed. Each of the major operations consists of dissecting the dilated bowel along with the portion of aganglionic bowel and then anastomosis. Later, most children achieve bowel control, but it is seldom completely normal. Anal dilation may be required.

Conclusions

Intestinal disorders are common and may cause problems for the client throughout life if they are not treated promptly and completely. Even with early treatment, many clients require ostomies for treatment of large and small bowel disorders. The resultant body image changes are the focus of nursing interventions to educate the client and facilitate modifications in behavior to promote health and adaptation to the changes.

Thinking Critically

1. **A young man is admitted with an exacerbation of inflammatory bowel disease. He reports frequent watery stools, general weakness, lack of appetite with a**

loss of 5 lb in a week, and cramping abdominal pain. What nursing history and physical assessment are required? How will his exacerbation be treated?

Factors to Consider. What are the clinical manifestations of inflammatory bowel disease? What are priority nursing interventions?

2. An elderly client has undergone a bowel resection with placement of a temporary transverse colostomy for treatment of colon cancer. He lives with his wife of 25 years. She is very interested in learning how to help her spouse manage care for the stoma and how to change the colostomy bags. What is your priority assessment? What teaching methods should you use to teach the client and his wife?

Factors to Consider. What is the appearance of a healthy stoma and healthy skin around the stoma? What dietary management is important?

3. A young man arrives in the emergency department in a highly anxious state. He has a history of numerous abdominal surgeries and now eliminates fecal material through a colostomy. He is handsome, appears very thin, and cannot sit still. He has a paper bag which he says contains a gun. He wants to shoot the doctor who did this to him. He wants to be admitted for a revision and asks that his bowel be "reconnected." What is your priority intervention? What psychosocial assessment should you pursue?

Factors to Consider. How is the client coping with his changed body function? What are relationships with others his age, especially women?

Bibliography

1. American Cancer Society. (1996). *Cancer facts and figures.* New York: Author.
2. Beitz, J. (1994). The ileoanal reservoir: An alternative to ileostomy. *Journal of WOCN, 21*(3), 120–125.
3. Copstead, L. (1995). *Perspectives on pathophysiology.* Philadelphia: W. B. Saunders.
4. Dancy, C., & Backhouse, S. (1993). Towards a better understanding of patients with irritable bowel syndrome. *Journal of Advanced Nursing, 18*(9), 1443–1450.
5. Doughty, D. (1994). What you need to know about inflammatory bowel disease. *American Journal of Nursing, 94*(7), 24–31.
6. Fitzsimmons, M., & Fales, L. (1993). Colon cancer prevention update. *Seminars in Oncology Nursing, 9*(3), 163–168.
7. Fulton, J. (1994). Chemotherapeutic treatment of colorectal cancer: Rationale, trends, and nursing care. *Journal of WOCN, 21*(1), 12–21.
8. Funovits, M., et al. (1993). Small intestine transplantation: A nursing perspective. *Critical Care Clinics of North America, 5*(1), 203–213.
9. Georges, J., & Heitkemper, M. (1994). Dietary fiber and distressing gastrointestinal symptoms in midlife women. *Nursing Research, 43*(6), 357–361.
10. Goldfinger, S. (1993). Irritable bowel syndrome: Hitting below the belt. *Harvard Health Letter, 18*(3), 1–3.
11. Griffith, C. (1993). Colorectal cancer: Reducing mortality through early detection and treatment. *Physician Assistant, 17*(1), 25–34.
12. Groenwald, S. L., et al. (1995). *Cancer nursing: Principles and practice* (3rd ed.). Boston: Jones & Bartlett.
13. Gurevich, I. (1994). Your patients don't need diarrhea, too! *RN, 57*(4), 52–55.
14. Guyton, A. C., & Hall, J. E. (1996). *Textbook of medical physiology* (9th ed.). Philadelphia: W. B. Saunders.
15. Hagel, M., McDonagh, J., & Rapp, C. (1994). Patients with long-term vascular access devices: Care and complications. *Orthopedic Nursing, 13*(5), 41–53.
16. Hampton, B., & Bryant, R. (Eds.) (1992). *Ostomies and continent diversions: Nursing management.* St. Louis: Mosby–Year Book.
17. Hanauer, S. (1993). Medical therapy of ulcerative colitis. *Lancet, 2,* 412–417.
18. Heitkemper, M., et al. (1993). Women with gastrointestinal symptoms: Implications for nursing research and practice. *Gastroenterology Nursing, 15*(6), 226–232.
19. Howard, J. (1993). Diarrhea: When is it important to investigate? *Medicine North America: The Add-On Journal of Continuing Medical Education, 16*(4), 299–304.
20. Jarrett, M., et al. (1994). Comparison of diet composition in women with and without functional bowel disorder. *Gastroenterology Nursing, 16*(6), 254–258.
21. Kelly, M. (1994). Patients' decision-making in major surgery: the case of total colectomy. *Journal of Advanced Nursing, 19*(6), 1168–1177.
22. Kinasch, R., et al. (1993). Inflammatory bowel disease impact and patient characteristics. *Gastroenterology Nursing, 15*(4), 147–155.
23. Kinash, R., et al. (1993). Coping patterns in patients with IBD. *Rehabilitation Nursing, 18*(1), 12–19, 67–68.
24. Kinzler, K., & Vogelstein, B. (1992). The colorectal cancer gene hunt: Current findings. *Hospital Practice, 27*(11), 51–58.
25. Krasner, D. (1993). Six steps to successful stoma care. *RN, 56*(7), 32–37.
26. Lang, C., & Ransohoff, D. (1994). Fecal occult blood screening for colorectal cancer. *JAMA, 271*(13), 1011–1013.
27. Lehne, R. (1994). *Pharmacology for nursing care* (2nd ed.). Philadelphia: W. B. Saunders.
28. Mandel, J., et al. (1993). Reducing mortality from colorectal cancer by screening for fecal occult blood. *New England Journal of Medicine, 328*(19), 1365–1371.
29. Marchiondo, K. (1994). When the Dx is diverticular disease. *RN, 57*(2), 42–46.
30. Mayer, D. (1994). Commentary on social support and cancer screening among older Black Americans. *ONS: Nursing Scan in Oncology, 3*(2), 10–11.
31. Mehler, E. (1994). Preparing your patient to use a fecal occult blood test. *Nursing, 24*(5), 32R.
32. Meissner, J. (1994). Caring for patients with ulcerative colitis. *Nursing, 24*(7), 54–55.
33. Metcalf, C. (1994). Effects of pregnancy on ulcerative colitis and Crohn's disease. *Professional Nurse, 9*(10), 685–688.
34. McConnell, E. (1994). Loosening the grip of intestinal obstruction. *Nursing, 24*(3), 34–41.
35. Neugut, A. (1993). Colon cancer screening: Beyond reliance on fecal testing. *Consultant, 33*(10), 39–46.
36. Paulford-Lecher, N. (1993). Teaching your patient stoma care. *Nursing, 23*(9), 47–49.
37. Phillips, S. (1995). Gut reaction . . . bowel disease. *Nursing Times, 91*(1), 44–45.
38. Pullan, R., et al. (1994). Transdermal nicotine for active ulcerative colitis. *New England Journal of Medicine, 330*(12), 811–815.
39. Quinless, F. (1994). When your patient undergoes bowel resection. *Nursing, 24*(2), 32c–32d.
40. Ripamonti, C. (1994). Management of bowel obstruction in advanced cancer patients. *Journal of Pain and Symptom Management, 9*(3), 193–200.
41. Sabiston, D. C., Jr. (1994). *Atlas of general surgery.* Philadelphia: W. B. Saunders.
42. Sabiston, D. C., Jr. & Lyerly, H. (Eds.). (1994). *Essentials of surgery* (2nd ed.). Philadelphia: W. B. Saunders.
43. Spollett, G. (1994). Nutritional management of common gastrointestinal problems. *Nurse Practitioner Forum, 5*(1), 24–27.
44. Tjandra, J., & Fazio, V. (1993). Current status of ileoanal reservoirs: 1992. *Journal of ET Nursing, 20*(2), 56–62.
45. Todd, D., & Dozois, R. (1993). Ileoanal reservoirs: Construction and management. *Journal of ET Nursing, 20*(1), 26–35.

46. Watson, P. (1985). Meeting the needs of patients undergoing ostomy surgery. *Journal of Enterostomal Therapy, 12,* 121–124.
47. Wilson, R. (1993). Patient teaching for an ileoanal reservoir. *Journal of ET Nursing, 20*(5), 199–203.
48. Witt, M. (1993). Current management of adults with colorectal cancer. *MEDSURG Nursing, 2*(2), 105–111.
49. Wyngaarden, J. B., et al. (1996). *Cecil textbook of Medicine* (20th ed.). Philadelphia: W. B. Saunders.
50. Yamaguchi, E., et al. (1994). Colonization pattern of vancomycin-resistant *Enterococcus faecium. American Journal of Infection Control, 22*(4), 202–206.

Liver, Biliary Tract, and Exocrine Pancreatic Disorders

Unit Editor: **BETTY BLAKE**

U N I T

13

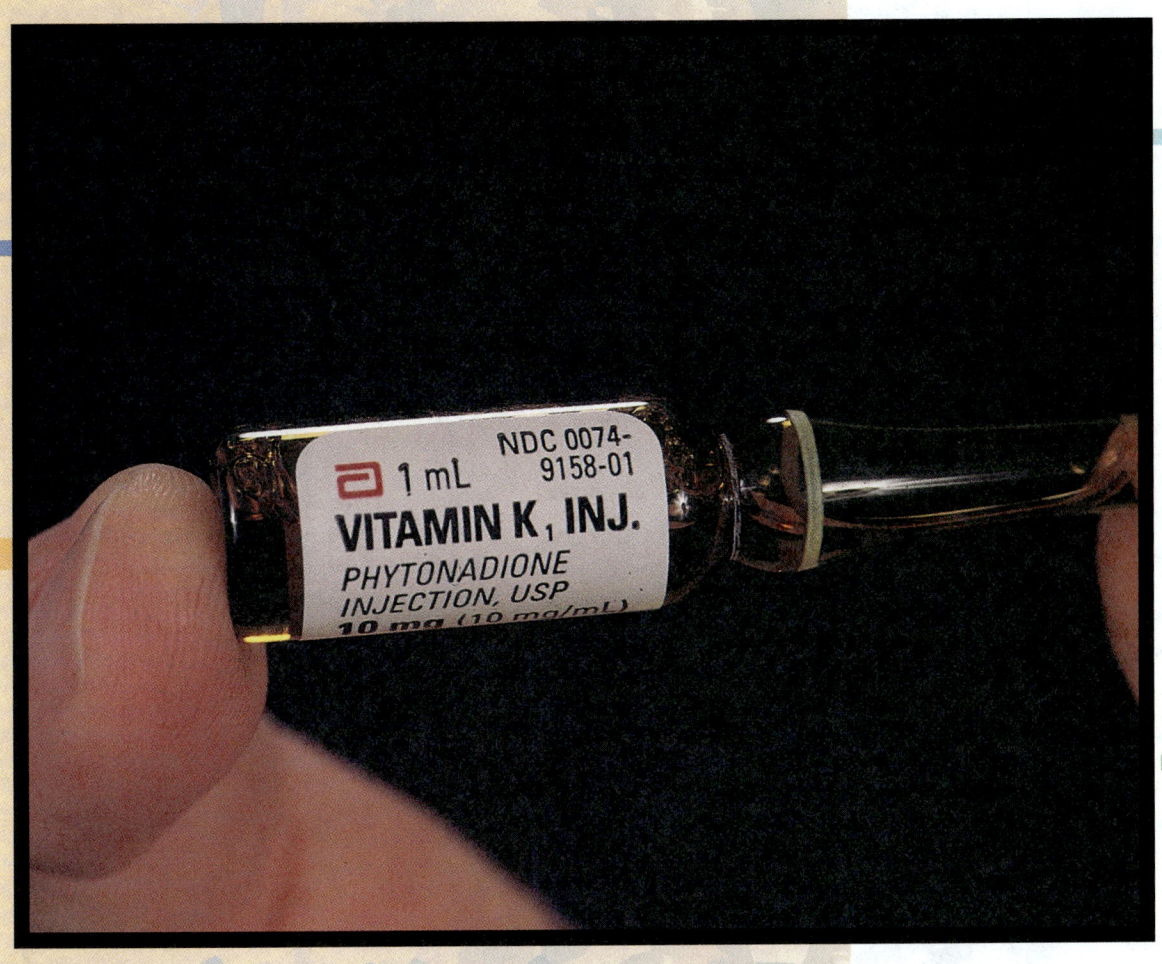

Structure and Function of the Liver, Biliary Tract, and Exocrine Pancreas

Esther Matassarin-Jacobs

Structure

Liver

The liver is the largest gland in the body, representing about 2.5% of body weight. It lies in the upper right quadrant of the abdomen, just below the diaphragm. The rib cage encloses the liver except for the lower margin (Fig. 63–1). The lungs extend over the liver's upper portion. The lower portion of the liver provides a roof for the stomach and intestines. A peritoneal covering blankets most of the liver and also the adjacent gallbladder (Fig. 63–2).

Note in Figure 63–2 that the liver divides at the falciform ligament into two major lobes, right and left. These two lobes, in turn, divide into superior and inferior portions of the posterior, anterior, medial, and lateral segments.

The hepatic artery supplies the liver with about one third of its blood, while the portal vein supplies the other two thirds. The hepatic artery carries oxygenated blood; the portal vein carries deoxygenated blood. The superior and inferior mesenteric veins and the splenic vein, which receive blood from the pancreas, spleen, stomach, intestines, and gallbladder, join to form the portal vein. The portal vein carries nutrients, metabolites, and toxins from the digestive organs to the liver for processing, detoxification, or assimilation. Agents such as prothrombin and fibrinogen (both vital to clotting) are added to the blood within the liver. The vasculature of the liver has been called the antechamber of the heart because it takes in all the gastrointestinal and splenic blood via the portal vein and returns it to the right side of the heart by way of the hepatic veins. Hence, any process impeding blood flow through the right atrium of the heart causes liver engorgement. Similarly, any process impeding blood flow through the liver causes engorgement of vessels draining the digestive organs.

This chapter incorporates material written for the fourth edition by Kris Strasburg.

Examine the hepatic portal system in Figure 63–3. In general, a portal circulation system is one in which blood from one or more organs circulates through another organ before returning to the heart.

The functional unit of the liver is the liver lobule, with the hepatocyte being the major cell. In the liver lobule, these cells are arranged hublike around a central vein. One side of the polyhedral hepatocyte faces the hepatic sinusoids, the capillary system of the liver. The other side faces the bile canaliculi. Incoming blood from the portal vein and the hepatic artery enters the sinusoids. As this blood passes through the liver lobules, many substances are exchanged between the blood and the hepatocytes. Lymphatic ducts drain waste products. Bile is formed in the hepatocytes, is secreted into the bile canaliculi, and then travels through bile ductules to the gallbladder. Endothelial and Kupffer's cells form the walls of the sinusoids. Kupffer's cells are an important part of the mononuclear phagocyte system (formerly called the reticuloendothelial system). The blood then courses into the central vein, the hepatic veins, and the inferior vena cava. The basic structure of a liver lobule is illustrated in Figure 63–4.

Biliary Tract

The gallbladder (Fig. 63–5) is a small, pear-shaped sac that can hold approximately 100 to 150 ml of bile. It receives its arterial blood supply from the cystic artery, which branches off the right hepatic artery. Venous blood is drained via the cystic veins. The celiac plexus, the vagus nerve, and the right phrenic nerve supply the gallbladder's innervation.

Bile is transported from the liver through the right and left hepatic ducts. The gallbladder serves as a reservoir for bile produced in the liver. Bile is necessary for the digestion of dietary fat. The gallbladder concentrates the bile, releases it into the cystic duct, which empties into the common bile duct, and finally into the small intestine

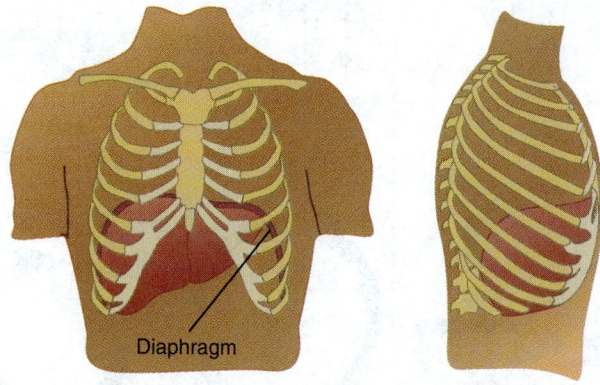

Figure 63–1. The liver, shown here from an anterior and right lateral view, is located just below the diaphragm.

(specifically the duodenum) (Fig. 63–6). When there is fat present in the intestine, a valve at the confluence of the common bile duct and the duodenum, called the sphincter of Oddi, opens to allow bile to flow into the intestinal tract. When there is no fat present, the sphincter remains closed and bile backs up into the gallbladder, where it is stored.

Figure 63–2. Segments of the right and left lobes of the liver. *A,* Anterior view. *B,* Inferior view.

Pancreas

The pancreas is a large, many-lobed gland that structurally resembles the salivary glands. It is located posterior to the greater curvature of the stomach. The head of the pancreas lies in the concavity of the duodenum, and its tail rests against the spleen (see Fig. 63–6). The liver lies above the pancreas, and the stomach passes close to the anterior surface. Major blood vessels, namely the aorta, inferior vena cava, and hepatic artery, are located very near the head of the pancreas and thus greatly complicate extensive surgery in this area.

The pancreas functions as (1) an endocrine gland, secreting insulin and glucagon directly into the bloodstream; and (2) as an exocrine gland, secreting multiple digestive enzymes into a system of ducts. These ducts flow into the duct of Wirsung and empty into the duodenum. The site where the duct of Wirsung joins the common bile duct and enters the duodenum is referred to as the ampulla of Vater (see Fig. 63–6). The sphincter of Oddi controls the release of both pancreatic juices and bile into the duodenum. The exocrine function of the pancreas is discussed in this unit. Endocrine function and disorders are discussed in Chapter 67.

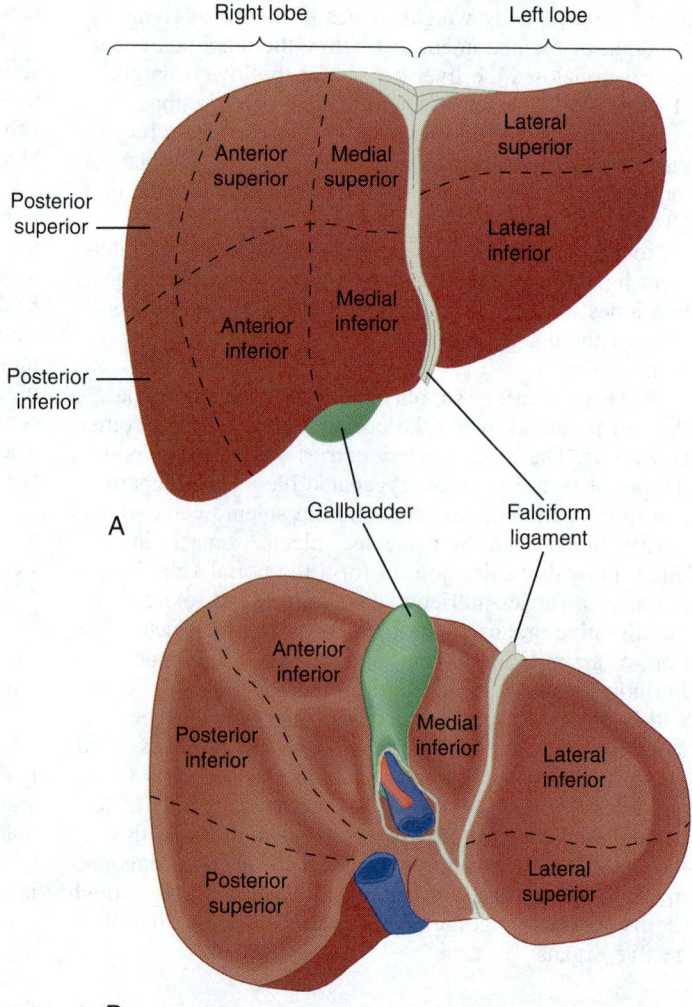

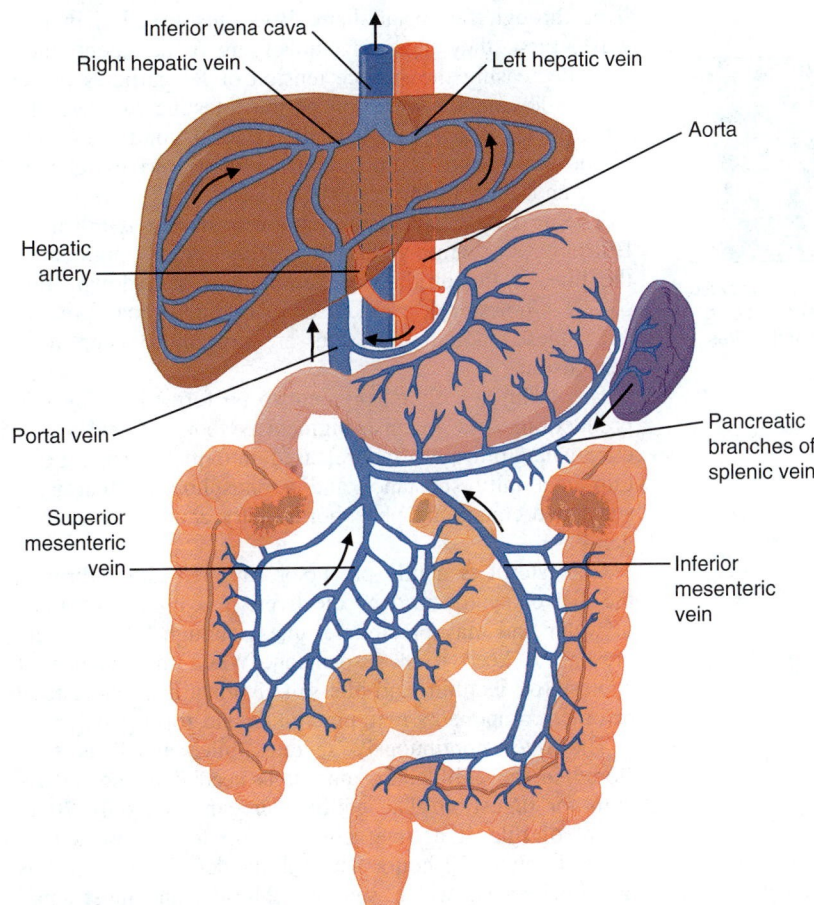

Figure 63–3. The hepatic portal system supplies the liver with blood from the digestive organs.

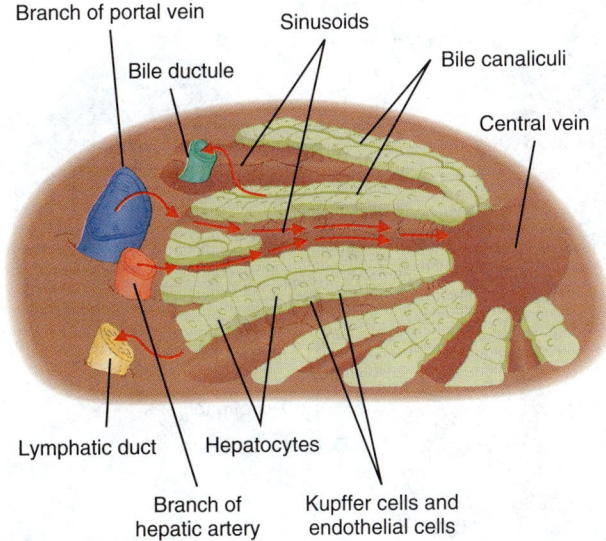

Figure 63–4. Diagram of a liver lobule. As blood from the portal vein and hepatic artery flows through the sinusoids toward the central vein, substances are exchanged between the blood and the hepatocytes. Lymphatic ducts drain the waste products. Bile produced in the hepatocytes is secreted into the bile canaliculi and travels through the bile ductules to the gallbladder.

Function

The liver, biliary system, and exocrine pancreas produce, detoxify, and store many substances in the body. The substances produced aid in the digestion, assimilation, and use of nutrients by the body.

Liver

■ **Bile Production**

The liver normally produces and secretes between 600 and 1200 ml of bile each day. The basic components of bile are water, bile salts, bilirubin, cholesterol, fatty acids, lecithin, sodium, potassium, calcium, chloride, and bicarbonate ion. Water is the most abundant component of bile, followed by bile salts. Because bile is concentrated in the gallbladder, this water and a large portion of the electrolytes (not calcium ions) are reabsorbed by the gallbladder mucosa.

Bile salts are produced by the liver in a quantity of about 0.5 g/day. The precursor of these bile salts is cholesterol, supplied either by the diet or synthesized by the

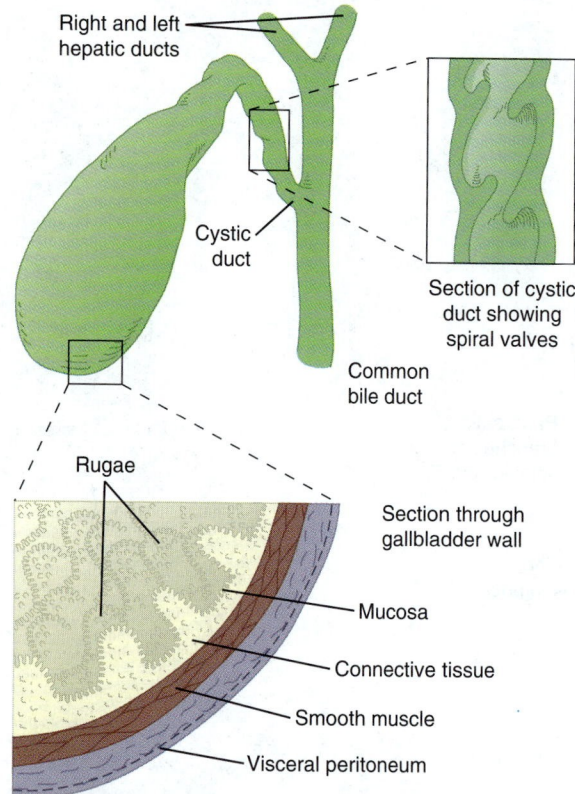

Figure 63–5. The gallbladder stores bile until needed to digest fat in the duodenum. *Insets* show a longitudinal section of spiral valves in the cystic duct and a section of the gallbladder wall.

liver through fat metabolism. Bile salts function in two ways. First, they have an emulsifying or detergent function, decreasing the surface tension of fat particles in the food, allowing the agitation of the intestine to break the fat globules into a much smaller size. Second, they help in the absorption of fatty acids, monoglycerides, cholesterol, and other lipids from the intestine.

The next most abundant component of bile is bilirubin. Bilirubin, an orange-yellow or greenish-yellow pigment in the bile, is the product of hemoglobin breakdown (Fig. 63–7). Cholesterol, a precursor of bile acid, may precipitate unless enough bile salts are present to keep it in suspension.

Biliverdin is the first pigment to be formed during bile production. This greenish pigment is soon reduced to unconjugated bilirubin and released into the plasma. Lecithin is a fatty substance and a phospholipid, that is, a substance containing phosphorus, fatty acids, and a nitrogen base.

Cholesterol is a bile precursor supplied either through the diet or synthesized by the liver. It is highly insoluble in water and may precipitate unless enough bile salts are present to keep it in suspension. When the balance of cholesterol, lecithin, and bile salts is disturbed, cholesterol or other components may precipitate and form gallstones.

The liver continuously secretes bile, which is then stored in the gallbladder until it is needed in the duodenum for digestion. The gallbladder can hold only 20 to 60 ml of bile at a time; however, up to 450 ml is produced in about 12 hours. The gallbladder can manage this amount because water, sodium, chloride, and most small

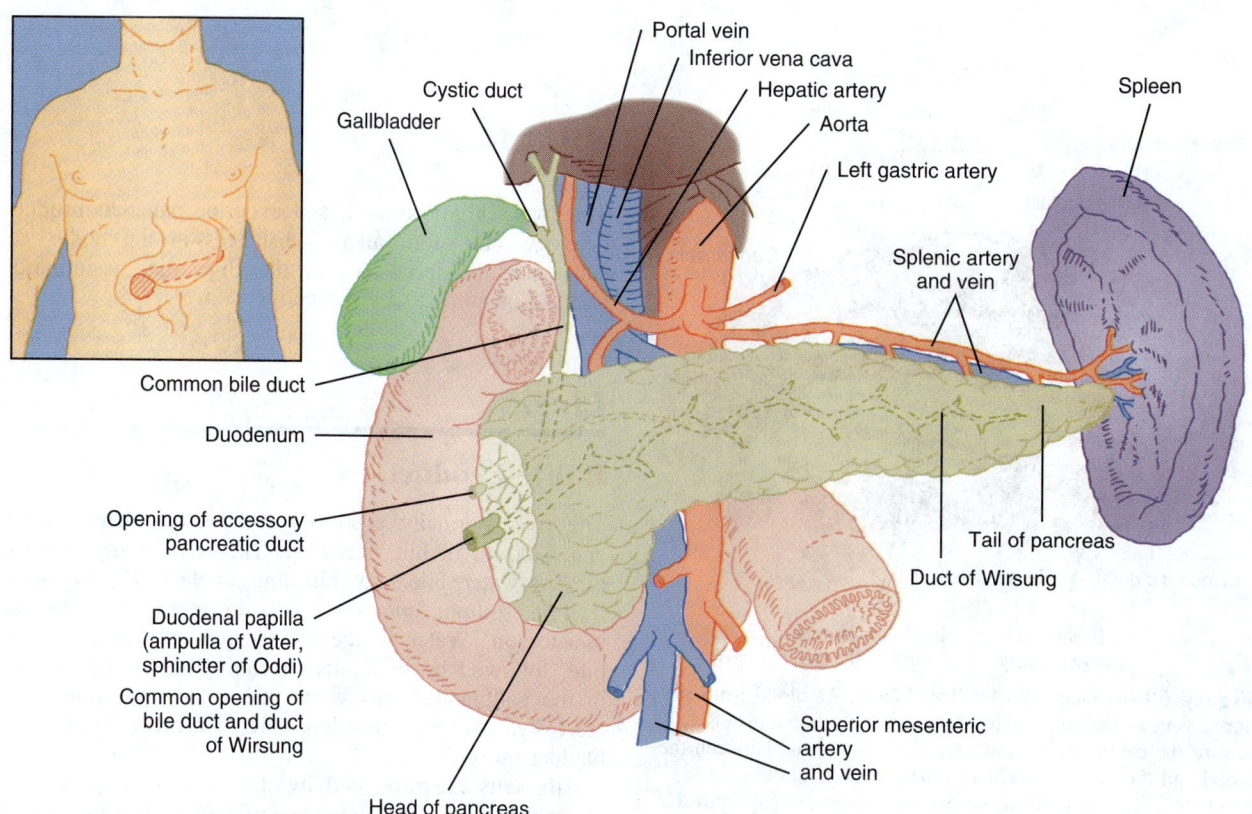

Figure 63–6. Pancreas and adjacent organs. *Inset* shows the anatomic location of the pancreas behind the stomach.

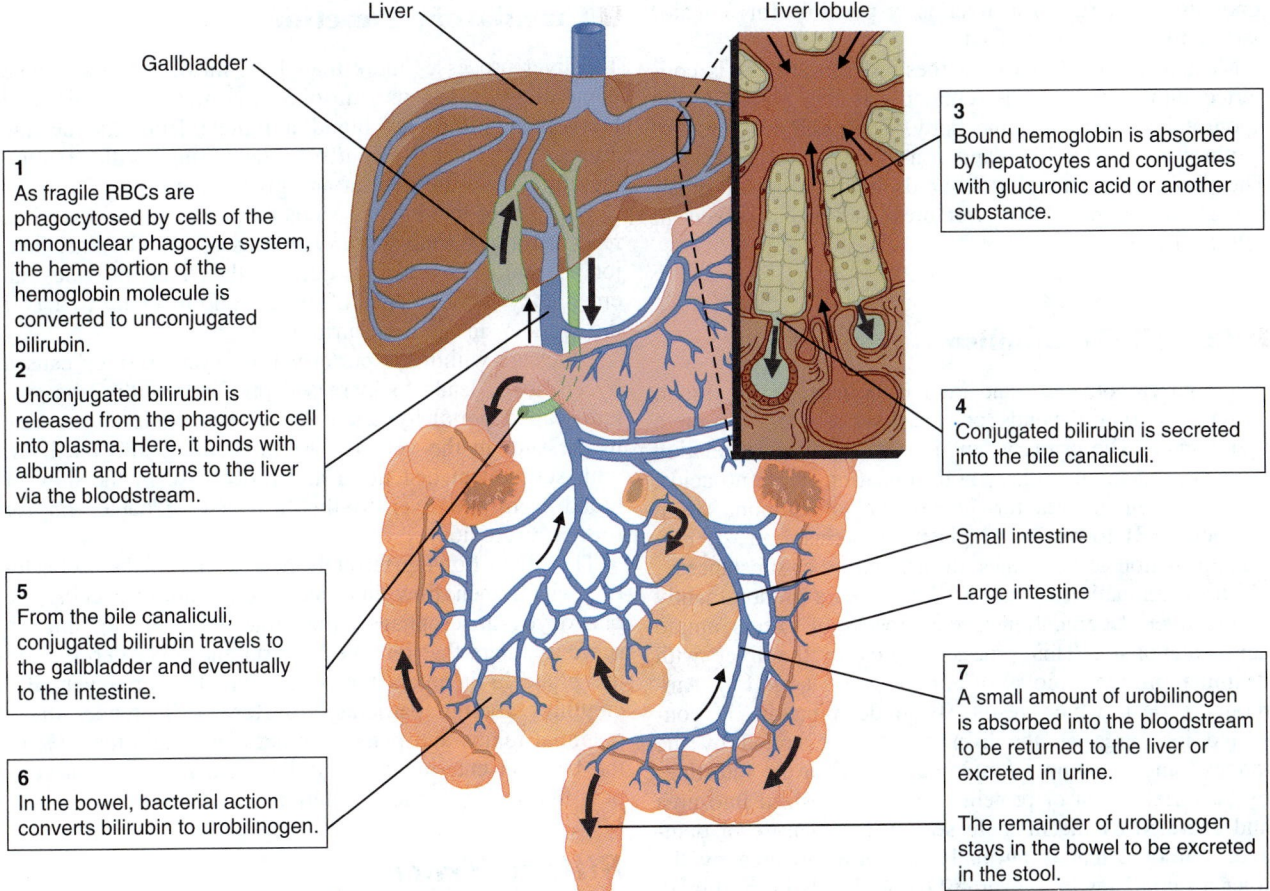

Liver

Gallbladder

Liver lobule

1
As fragile RBCs are phagocytosed by cells of the mononuclear phagocyte system, the heme portion of the hemoglobin molecule is converted to unconjugated bilirubin.

2
Unconjugated bilirubin is released from the phagocytic cell into plasma. Here, it binds with albumin and returns to the liver via the bloodstream.

3
Bound hemoglobin is absorbed by hepatocytes and conjugates with glucuronic acid or another substance.

4
Conjugated bilirubin is secreted into the bile canaliculi.

5
From the bile canaliculi, conjugated bilirubin travels to the gallbladder and eventually to the intestine.

6
In the bowel, bacterial action converts bilirubin to urobilinogen.

Small intestine

Large intestine

7
A small amount of urobilinogen is absorbed into the bloodstream to be returned to the liver or excreted in urine.

The remainder of urobilinogen stays in the bowel to be excreted in the stool.

Figure 63–7. Bile formation, metabolism, and excretion. *Inset* shows bile formation in the liver lobule. *Thin arrows* indicate the direction of blood flow; *fat arrows* indicate the direction of digestive system flow.

electrolytes are reabsorbed by the gallbladder mucosa. This process concentrates the bile from 5 to 20 times.

The gallbladder continues to store the bile until fatty foods enter the small intestine and stimulate the release of cholecystokinin. Cholecystokinin stimulates contractions of the gallbladder wall, and this process combined with simultaneous relaxation of the sphincter of Oddi allows the bile to flow into the duodenum and mix with the food. The gallbladder is also stimulated by cholinergic nerve fibers that also stimulate intestinal motility and secretion in other parts of the gastrointestinal tract. The gallbladder empties poorly in the absence of fatty foods but empties completely within 1 hour after a meal with adequate fat. Reabsorption of bile salts is almost total, and recycling occurs as they return to the liver.

The sphincter of Oddi must relax completely if adequate emptying is to occur. There are three mechanisms that help this occur: (1) cholecystokinin has a weak relaxant effect on the sphincter; (2) rhythmic contractions of the gallbladder wall transmit peristaltic waves down the common bile duct to the sphincter, leading to partial relaxations; and (3) relaxation phases of intestinal peristaltic waves cause the greatest relaxation of the sphincter and the intestinal wall.

■ Carbohydrate Metabolism

The major functions of the liver in relation to glucose metabolism are (1) *glycogenesis,* the conversion of glucose to glycogen, (2) *glycogenolysis,* the breakdown of glycogen to glucose, (3) storage of glycogen, (4) conversion of galactose and fructose to glucose, and (5) *gluconeogenesis,* the conversion of amino acids to glucose.

When glucose is not needed, the body stores it as glycogen. Later, if glucose is needed, the liver can break down glycogen to release glucose. If the blood sugar drops precipitously, gluconeogenesis occurs, which maintains a normal blood glucose.

■ Lipid (Fat) Metabolism

The major functions of the liver in relation to fat metabolism are (1) oxidation of fatty acids for energy, (2) formation of most lipoproteins, (3) synthesis of cholesterol and phospholipids, and (4) synthesis of fat from proteins and carbohydrates.

The liver provides energy from fats by splitting them into glycerol and fatty acids, followed by the oxidation of the fatty acids, leading to the release of tremendous amounts of energy. The liver is responsible for a major part of the metabolism of fats.

Most of the cholesterol synthesized in the liver is converted into bile salts; the remainder is transported in the lipoproteins throughout the body. Phospholipids are also synthesized in the liver and transported in lipoproteins. The cholesterol and phospholipids help form cell membranes and intracellular structures and are involved in cellular function.

■ Protein Metabolism

Although carbohydrate and fat metabolism are important, human survival depends on the liver's role in protein metabolism. The primary functions of the liver in relation to protein metabolism are (1) deamination of amino acids, (2) formation of urea for the removal of ammonia from the body, (3) formation of plasma proteins, and (4) biotransformation of hormones, drugs, and other substances.

The deamination of amino acids occurs predominantly in the liver. Degradation is the process of excess amino acid catabolism. This process begins in the liver with deamination, the removal of amino groups ($-NH_2$). Ammonia (NH^3), which results from deamination, is converted into urea by the liver and then excreted by the kidneys and intestines. Ammonia formed in the intestines by bacterial action or protein is also synthesized into urea and excreted by the liver. In severe liver disease or damage, ammonia that is normally converted to urea by the liver accumulates to dangerously high levels in the blood. As a result, a severe toxic state develops, called hepatic encephalopathy. This process can be slowed by the administration of medications such as neomycin, which destroys ammonia, producing bacteria in the gut, or lactulose, which binds ammonia and produces diarrhea, decreasing bowel transit time (see Chapter 65 for further discussion).

The liver also synthesizes plasma proteins, such as albumin, prothrombin, fibrinogen, and clotting proteins (factors V, VI, VII, IX, and X). Albumin is essential for maintaining plasma oncotic pressure, while the other proteins contribute to blood clotting (see Chapter 51). Plasma oncotic pressure prevents intravascular fluid from leaking out into the extravascular spaces, where it manifests as ascites and varying degrees of peripheral edema. Vitamin K, a fat-soluble vitamin, must be present for synthesis of several clotting proteins. Assimilation of vitamin K depends on the presence of bile in the intestine. Gamma globulins are the only plasma proteins not synthesized by the liver.

The liver primarily detoxifies and biotransforms hormones, drugs, and other chemicals. Some substances are deactivated by deamination, hydroxylation, oxidation, or reduction. Through conjugation, other substances become soluble in water, resulting in their excretion through the bile and, therefore, in feces or urine.

Clients with compromised liver function are at high risk of untoward reactions to many medications, all opiates, and many chemicals. The two major problems that result are prolonged action and increased potency of the substance.

■ Circulatory Function

The liver processes more than 1000 ml of blood a minute circulating through its sinusoids from the portal vein, and more than 350 ml of blood a minute from the hepatic artery. More than one fourth of the resting cardiac output, therefore, is in the liver at any given time.

Because of its size and sinusoid passages, the liver is a reservoir for storing large quantities of blood. When major systemic blood loss occurs, the liver provides an emergency blood supply of about 500 ml, or up to 1 L if the pressure in the right atrium is high.

Blockage within the portal venous system, often caused by cirrhosis, leads to increased pressures within the system, called portal hypertension. The result is an increase in pressure in the venous system draining into the liver, with subsequent distention and a decrease in the flow of blood from the liver to the heart (see Chapter 65 for further discussion).

The blood flowing through the intestine picks up bacteria, which then flow into the liver. Kupffer's cells, the phagocytic macrophages that line the hepatic sinuses, serve as filters that remove bacteria and other debris from the blood as it enters the liver from the portal vein. By engulfing foreign particles, Kupffer's cells render many potential toxins and pathogens harmless. Less than 1% of the bacteria entering the portal system from the intestine pass into the systemic circulation.

Biliary Tract

The bile ducts and gallbladder function as a collecting and concentrating system and as a reservoir for bile (see Fig. 63–7). Following surgical removal of the gallbladder, the bile ducts act as reservoirs and body processes proceed normally, but the ability to excrete large quantities of bile after ingestion of a fatty meal is lost. The function of the gallbladder was described in detail earlier in this chapter.

Pancreas

The pancreas normally produces 1200 to 1300 ml of pancreatic juice daily. Pancreatic juice is a clear alkaline solution carrying three major types of digestive enzymes.

1. Pancreatic amylase splits carbohydrates into dextrins and maltose.
2. Pancreatic lipase hydrolyzes fat to yield glycerol and fatty acids.
3. Pancreatic trypsin is one of a group of enzymes, including chymotrypsin and carboxypolypeptidase, that split proteins.

Trypsin is activated in the intestine, and, in turn, activates other proteolytic enzymes. The pancreas stores a special trypsin inhibitor to prevent autodigestion of pancreatic tissue. A dysfunction of the inhibitor may cause pancreatitis. The pancreatic juices, therefore, digest all three major types of food: proteins, carbohydrates, and fats. These enzymes are all secreted by the acini of the pancreatic glands. These juices also contain large quantities of bicarbonate ions that neutralize the acid chyme from the stomach present in the duodenum. The bicarbonate ions and water are secreted in large amounts mainly by the ductules and ducts leading from the acini. The amount of bicarbonate ion secreted here leads to amounts four to five times higher than that in the plasma.

Pancreatic secretion is stimulated by four basic factors: (1) acetylcholine, from the parasympathetic vagus nerve endings as well as other cholinergic nerves in the enteric nervous system; (2) gastrin, large quantities of which are secreted during the gastric phase of digestion; (3) cholecystokinin, secreted by the duodenum and upper jejunal mucosa when food enters the small intestine; and (4) secretin, secreted by the duodenal and jejunal mucosa when highly acidic food enters the small intestine.

The first three, acetylcholine, gastrin, and cholecystokinin, all stimulate the acinar cells more than the ductal cells. This causes large amounts of digestive juices to be secreted, but with little extra fluid in solution with these enzymes. These enzymes remain stored in the pancreas until they are washed into the duodenum by fluid secretion. Secretin, however, stimulates large amounts of bicarbonate ion to be secreted to neutralize acidic foods, but causes minimal secretion of the enzymes.

There are three phases of pancreatic secretion. The first is the cephalic phase. During this phase, the release of acetylcholine is stimulated by the same impulses that cause secretion in the stomach. The acetylcholine causes moderate amounts of pancreatic enzymes to be secreted, but little actually flows into the duodenum because little water and electrolytes are being secreted.

The gastric phase is characterized by further nervous stimulation of enzyme secretion. Also, the large amount of gastrin formed in the stomach stimulates more enzyme secretion. Because there is still little fluid, the enzymes remain in the gland.

During the intestinal phase, chyme enters the intestine, stimulating secretion and drastically increasing the amount of fluid in the pancreatic juice. Cholecystokinin also causes more enzymes to be secreted at the same time.

Secretin stimulates the production of copious amounts of bicarbonate ions without the stimulation of the acinar cells and, therefore, the enzymes. Secretin is released when the pH in the duodenum is less than 4.5, and release of secretin increases even more if the pH is below 3.0. This immediately results in large amounts of sodium bicarbonate in pancreatic juices being secreted and entering the duodenum. The acid from the stomach is immediately neutralized, stopping all peptic activity. This is a protective mechanism because the mucosa of the small bowel cannot tolerate the acidic pH of the gastric secretions.

Pancreatic enzymes work best in a neutral or slightly alkaline environment. Bicarbonate has a pH of about 8.0, raising the pH of the solution so that the pancreatic enzymes function efficiently.

The presence of food in the small intestine stimulates secretion of cholecystokinin. Cholecystokinin stimulates secretion of large amounts of pancreatic enzymes by the acinar cells.

Effects of Aging

With aging, liver, biliary system, and exocrine pancreatic functions all begin to deteriorate. In the liver, there is a decrease in the number and size of hepatic cells, leading to a decrease in both liver weight and mass. Fibrotic tissue also increases, leading to a decrease in protein synthesis, liver enzymes, and cholesterol synthesis.

The decrease in enzyme activity diminishes the liver's ability to detoxify drugs, increasing the risk of toxic levels of a variety of medications in the elderly.

The pancreas is also affected by the process of aging. There is calcification of the pancreatic vessels, and the size of the ducts change through distention and dilation. These changes lead to a decrease in the production of lipase, resulting in a decrease in fat absorption and digestion. The older person also may experience a decreased absorption of fat soluble vitamins and an increase of fat excreted through the feces (steatorrhea).

Conclusions

A thorough knowledge of the structure and function of the liver, biliary tract, and exocrine pancreas will help the nurse provide knowledgeable care to clients with disorders in these areas. In order to provide effective interventions, the nurse must understand the normal physiology of these organs.

Bibliography

1. Arias, I. M. (Ed.). (1994). *The liver: Biology and pathobiology* (3rd ed.). New York: Raven Press.
2. Bennett, J. C., & Plum, F. (Eds.). (1996). *Cecil textbook of medicine* (20th ed.). Philadelphia: W. B. Saunders.
3. Brown, R. E. (1994). *An introduction to neuroendocrinology.* New York: Cambridge University Press.
4. Christiansen, J. L., & Grzbouski, J. M. (1993). *Biology of aging.* St. Louis: Mosby–Year Book.
5. Cotran, R. S., Kumar, V., & Robbins, S. L. (1994). *Robbins pathologic basis of disease* (5th ed.). Philadelphia: W. B. Saunders.
6. DeGroot, L. J., Larsen, P. R., & Hennemann, G. (1996). *The thyroid and its diseases* (6th ed.). New York; Churchill Livingstone.
7. Gitlin, N., & Strauss, R. M. (1995). *Atlas of clinical hepatology.* Philadelphia: W. B. Saunders.
8. Gitnick, G. (Ed.). (1994). *Principles and practice of gastroenterology and hepatology* (2nd ed.). Norwalk, CT: Appleton & Lange.
9. Guyton, A. C. (1992). *Human physiology and mechanisms of disease* (5th ed.). Philadelphia: W. B. Saunders.
10. Guyton, A. C., & Hall, J. E. (1996). *Textbook of medical physiology,* (9th ed.). Philadelphia: W. B. Saunders.
11. Heatley, R. V. (Ed.). (1994). *Gastrointestinal and hepatic immunology.* New York: Cambridge University Press.
12. Kaplowitz, N. (Ed.). (1992). *Liver and biliary diseases.* Baltimore: Williams & Wilkins.
13. McCance, K. L., & Huether, S. E. (1994). *Pathophysiology: The biologic basis for disease in adults and children* (2nd ed.). St. Louis: Mosby–Year Book.
14. Melmed, S. (Ed.). (1995). *The pituitary.* Cambridge, MA: Blackwell Science.
15. Millward-Sadler, G. H., Wright, R., & Arthur, M. J. B. (Eds.).

(1992). *Wright's liver and biliary disease: Pathophysiology, diagnosis, and management* (3rd ed.). Philadelphia: W. B. Saunders.

16. Ming, S. C., & Goldman, H. (Eds.). (1992). *Pathology of the gastrointestinal tract.* Philadelphia: W. B. Saunders.

17. Pitt, H. A., Carr-Locke, D. L., & Ferrucci, J. T. (1995). *Hepatobiliary and pancreatic disease: The team approach to management.* Boston: Little, Brown.

18. Schaffer, E., & Thomson, A. B. (Eds). (1992). *Modern concepts in gastroenterology.* New York: Plenum Press.

19. Schiff, L., & Schiff, E. R. (1993). *Diseases of the liver.* Philadelphia: J. B. Lippincott.

20. Seeley, R., Stephens, T., & Tate, P. (1995). *Anatomy and physiology* (3rd ed.). St. Louis: Mosby–Year Book.

21. Sherlock, S., & Dooley, J. (1993). *Diseases of the liver and biliary system* (9th ed.). London: Blackwell Scientific.

22. Sleisenger, M. H., & Fordtran, J. S. (Eds.). (1993). *Gastrointestinal disease: Pathophysiology, diagnosis, management* (5th ed.). Philadelphia: W. B. Saunders.

23. Solomon, E. P. (1992). *Introduction to human anatomy and physiology.* Philadelphia: W. B. Saunders.

24. Tavoloni, N., & Berk, P. D. (Eds.). (1993). *Hepatic transport and bile secretion: Physiology and pathophysiology.* New York: Raven Press.

25. Thibodeau, G. A., & Patton, K. T. (1992). *Anatomy and physiology* (2nd ed.). St. Louis: Mosby–Year Book.

26. Thibodeau, G. A., & Patton, K. T. (1992). *The human body in health and disease.* St. Louis: Mosby–Year Book.

27. Zakim, D., & Boyer, T. D. (Eds.). (1990). *Hepatology* (2nd ed.). Philadelphia: W. B. Saunders.

Assessment of Clients with Liver, Biliary Tract, and Exocrine Pancreatic Disorders

Dianne Smolen

Individuals with hepatic, biliary tract, and exocrine pancreatic problems may have very specific complaints such as Fatigue, Altered Nutrition: Less than Body Requirements, Body Image Disturbance, or Impaired Skin Integrity. On the other hand, these same individuals may be bothered by vague, intermittent manifestations that are not localized. It becomes important, therefore, to carefully gather data and analyze the client's health history, presenting manifestations, nutritional status, life-style, and activities of daily living.

History

Assessment of clients with hepatic, biliary, and exocrine pancreatic disturbances includes an account of (1) the present illness, including the chief complaint; (2) the past medical history and family history, and (3) the psychosocial history and life-style patterns, including the environmental and occupational history.

During collection of historical data, help the client recall experiences and onset of manifestations by placing them in a time sequence. Linking events and disease manifestations helps establish the diagnosis and, in some cases, can even predict the course of the disease.

Chief Complaint

Thorough investigation of the client's chief complaint is necessary for accurate assessment. Similar to gastrointestinal manifestations, the manifestations of the hepatic, biliary, and pancreatic systems may be ambiguous and have puzzling causes. Explore each reported manifestation during the symptom analysis (see Chapter 11).

Common manifestations related to the hepatic, biliary, and pancreatic systems include problems associated with the gastrointestinal, neurologic, genitourinary, integumentary, or cardiovascular systems. Ask the client about the following manifestations:

Gastrointestinal

- Abdominal pain? Inquire about the site, type, predisposing factors, and frequency of pain. Right upper quadrant discomfort suggests gastrointestinal organ dysfunction. The distress may or may not be colicky.
- Nausea? Vomiting? Both of these manifestations occur in 70% of clients with pancreatitis.
- Anorexia? This manifestation is especially prevalent in liver disorders.
- Weight gain or loss?
- Chronic indigestion? This may be a manifestation of cholecystitis.
- Fatty food intolerance? This also may be diagnostic of cholecystitis.
- Excessive eructation?
- Disturbed bowel pattern? Constipation or diarrhea? (dark-colored, tarry stools)?
- Melena?
- Clay-colored stools? Acholic (without bilirubin) stools may occur briefly in viral hepatitis and are common in obstructive jaundice.
- Steatorrhea (bulky, foul-smelling, fatty stools)?

Neurologic

- Mild depression? This may be a manifestation of pancreatic cancer.
- A clouded sensorium?
- Irritability?
- Drowsiness? A change in mental status and neurologic manifestations can signal the development of hepatic encephalopathy.
- Pain? Pain, which may radiate to the back, can be a manifestation of a pancreatic, gallbladder, or biliary tract problem.

Genitourinary

- Dark-yellow or tea-colored urine? This indicates impaired excretion of bilirubin due to hepatocellular disease.

This chapter incorporates material written for the fourth edition by Kris Strasburg and Esther Matassarin-Jacobs.

Integumentary

- Jaundiced skin? Causes include viral hepatitis, cirrhosis, and drug-induced cholestasis or primary biliary cirrhosis.
- Unexplained puncture holes? May be the route of entry for hepatitis (types B or C) or other pathogens.
- Petechiae?
- Dilated abdominal veins? This may indicate hepatic cirrhosis.

Cardiovascular

- Nosebleeds or bruises easily?
- Hemorrhoids?
- Ascites (fluid accumulation in peritoneal cavity)?
- Edema of limbs?

All of these manifestations may be indicative of an hepatic disorder whereby fluid overload occurs related to the liver's improper functioning and metabolism of hormones such as aldosterone and antidiuretic hormone (ADH).

Other

- Yellow sclerae? This suggests biliary obstruction.
- Fever? This may indicate an acute gallbladder, pancreas, or liver problem.
- Intolerance to alcohol or medications?
- Fatigue? Malaise? These manifestations occur with hepatitis.

Past Health History

Major Illnesses and Hospitalizations

Ask the client to describe any past problems with jaundice, hepatitis, abdominal pain, gallbladder disease, anemia, or changes in bowel elimination such as diarrhea, clay-colored stools, or melena. Has the client ever been hospitalized for any of these problems or ever had surgery of the liver or gallbladder? Ask the client to recall if diagnostic procedures such as a gallbladder x-ray study, liver biopsy, or ultrasound examination of the gallbladder have ever been performed. Has the client ever received a transfusion of blood or blood products?

Procedures Causing Skin or Membrane Disruption

Has the client had recent blood tests, transfusions of blood products, dental procedures, ear piercing, tattooing, or any intravenous injection with a potentially contaminated needle? Such procedures are important to note in an assessment because breaks in the skin may be the route of entry for hepatitis virus (types B or C) or other pathogens.

Medications

Inquire specifically about medications the client currently is taking or has taken previously, including over-the-counter drugs. Many drugs and chemicals are potentially hepatotoxic such as alcohol, gold compounds, mercury, phosphorus, anabolic steroids, acetaminophen, isoniazid, halothane, sulfonamides, arsenic, thiazide diuretics, zidovudine (azidothymidine or AZT), and anticancer drugs such as methotrexate. Other medications to ask about are oral contraceptives, anesthetic agents, and antipsychotic agents.

Family Health History

The nurse asks the client if any family members have had cancer (especially of the bowel, liver, or pancreas), jaundice, bleeding disorders, hepatitis, nutritional deficiencies, alcoholism, obesity, pancreatic disease, or gallbladder disease. A history of these problems in family members increases the client's risk status for their occurrence.

Psychosocial History

Assessment of the client's psychosocial history and lifestyle patterns provide data about his or her physical and psychological status. Inquire about the client's occupation, environment, and habits.

Occupation and Environment

Ask about the client's occupation and work environment. Are there factors present that are known to cause liver damage? For example, heavy metals such as mercury and lead, anesthetic agents such as nitrous oxide, and chemicals such as carbon tetrachloride and certain pesticides are known hepatotoxins. Does the client engage in activities that increase the risk of exposure to substances causing hepatitis or pancreatitis? Ask about the following:

- Any close contact with hazardous waste
- Travel in areas where hepatitis or pancreatitis is endemic
- Eating raw or steamed shellfish (oysters, clams, scallops) from polluted water
- Swimming or bathing in polluted water
- Any known contact with hepatitis-infected animals or people
- Ingestion of mushrooms that were not purchased in a store

Habits

Ask the client about food intake, and use of alcohol and other recreational substances, such as use of illicit drugs. Eating patterns are important. Investigate the following:

- Food preferences

- Daily intake of proteins, carbohydrates, fats, and sodium
- Changes in eating patterns, including onset of changes
- Meal preparation—by whom, style of preparation
- Recent development of food intolerances

Carefully explore the client's use of alcohol and other mind-altering substances. Pay attention to alcohol use patterns, since alcoholism often accompanies liver and pancreatic disease causing fatty infiltration of the liver.

Be alert to whether the client provides confusing or conflicting data. Is the client's behavior altered in any way as the assessment proceeds? For example, does the client become angry, silent, or tearful? If significant others are present, do they corroborate the client's story? The client who does not acknowledge a substance abuse problem may not provide reliable information regarding usage. The client who takes illicit drugs may be unwilling to describe drug use patterns. If the client's history is suspected to be unreliable, ask significant others to provide additional information. (See Chapter 87 for a discussion of alcoholism and other drug use.)

Review of Systems

During the review of symptoms (ROS), the nurse includes questions about the gastrointestinal system, mental status, genitourinary system, integument, and cardiovascular system (see Current Illness and Chief Complaint). Specifically inquire about jaundice, pruritus (itching), abdominal swelling (edema or ascites), dark-colored urine, clay-colored stools, bleeding tendencies (purpura), spider angioma (spider nevi or telangiectasia), fatigue, and weight loss. Detailed questions for the ROS may be found in Box 11–2.

Physical Examination

Physical assessment for liver, biliary, or pancreatic dysfunction involves careful examination of the entire body.

General Health Status

Begin by assessing the client's general appearance and health status. Is there yellowing of the client's sclerae and integument? (See Chapter 65.) Does the client appear acutely or chronically ill? Is there a tense facial expression or fidgety movement indicating discomfort or pain?

Nutritional Status

Assess the client's nutritional status. Weigh the client and determine the amount of subcutaneous fat and muscular development. (Nutritional assessment is discussed in Chapter 11.) Obesity may accompany gallbladder disease. Malnutrition may exist in clients with a history of substance abuse or cirrhosis. Ascites may account for recent rapid onset of weight gain with accompanying loss of muscle mass.

Abdominal Assessment

Assessment of the abdomen includes inspection, auscultation, percussion, and palpation. Table 64–1 summarizes the key points of a physical examination for liver, biliary tract, and exocrine pancreatic disorders.

Inspection

Prior to examination, ask the client to point to any painful area and examine that section last. As stated earlier, hepatic and biliary pain is often located in the right upper quadrant. Pain that is dull and difficult to localize or describe may arise from an organ (viscera). Somatic pain is sharp, piercing, easy to localize, and arises from nerve endings in the peritoneum (Figure 64–1).

Inspect the abdomen for ascites (fluid-filled abdomen) and the prominent venous collateral networks common in cirrhosis. Characteristics of ascites include a distended abdomen with tight and glistening skin, bulging flanks, and prominent abdominal veins. Measure abdominal girth if ascites is present.

Auscultation

Auscultation for possible hepatic or biliary problems is performed by gently placing a warmed stethoscope on the client's right upper quadrant. With the client supine, note if a soft hum is heard during both the systolic and diastolic components of the heart beat. If present, it indicates increased collateral circulation between the portal and systemic venous systems, as might occur in hepatic cirrhosis. Also, listen for a friction rub. The presence of a friction rub, a grating sound heard with respiratory ventilation, indicates inflammation of the peritoneal surface of an organ, as from a liver tumor, chlamydial or gonococcal perihepatitis, or recent liver biopsy. If a systolic bruit accompanies a hepatic friction rub, carcinoma of the liver is suspected.

Percussion

Percuss the abdomen, especially the liver and spleen. Liver size is assessed by percussing the span of the liver at the right midclavicular line (RMCL) and the midsternal line (MSL). Begin by percussing in the RMCL either superior or inferior to the estimated borders of the liver. Superiorly, begin at the third intercostal space (ICS) over lung resonance and percuss down the thorax until the sound changes to dull. This level is marked on the skin with a pen. Inferiorly, start over a tympanic area and percuss upward until the sound changes to dull. This, too, is marked with the pen. At the MSL, percuss upward from above the umbilicus from tympany to dull and mark the change with the pen. Superiorly, percuss down the sternum until the percussion note changes. This, too, is marked. Measure the distance between each set of marks. At the RMCL, the liver span ranges from 6 to 12 cm (2½–5 inches) and at the MSL, it ranges from 4 to 8 cm

Table 64–1. Key Points of a Physical Examination: Hepatic, Biliary Tract and Exocrine Pancreatic Disorders

Steps	Normal or Common Findings	Significant or Abnormal Findings
Inspection		
Note:		
Color of skin	Same as or lighter than other areas	Redness, cyanosis, jaundice, lesions, ecchymosis, needlemarks, or hematomas
Eyes	White sclera	Sclera: yellow tint
Symmetry, contour, shape of abdomen	Flat, rounded abdomen	Distended, asymmetrical, masses
Surface of abdomen	Smooth	Tight, shiny; engorged, prominent veins, spider angiomas
Rectal area	No dilated veins (hemorrhoids)	Presence of distended veins (hemorrhoids)
General nutritional state Weigh Observe for ascites	Adequate for height and build	Obesity or malnutrition
Auscultation		
Place stethoscope (warmed) over right upper quadrant. Listen for vascular sounds or friction rubs.	No venous hums No friction rubs	Venous hum with both diastolic and systolic components
Percussion		
Abdomen: Note percussion sounds in four quadrants	Tympany over abdomen, bladder, intestines, aorta, and dull over liver, spleen, pancreas, kidneys, and uterus	Dullness over enlarged organs; indicates need for further assessment for ascites
Liver: Span. Percuss upward from below client's umbilicus on the right midclavicular line (MCL), until dullness is heard. Mark this point. Percuss downward from lung resonance in right MCL to dullness and measure distance between two marks.	Liver span is 6–12 cm. No tenderness	Liver span is greater than 12 cm
Note if tender, soft, or firm, smooth or nodular.	Slightly tender, soft, smooth surface	Nodular, more than slightly tender, hard
Spleen. Note size. Percuss downward in left posterior axillary line, beginning with lung resonance until dullness is heard.	Dullness between ribs 6 and 10	Dullness extends above sixth rib or covers large area—indicates enlargement
Palpation		
Use palmar surface of extended fingers		
Liver: Palpate lightly on right side and then palpate deeply	No tenderness, pain, masses	Tenderness, rigidity, nodules, enlarged
Spleen: Note: if spleen can be percussed, it is best not to palpate it. Palpate lightly on left side, distal to MCL.	No tenderness, pain, masses	Tenderness, rigidity, nodules, enlarged

| | Normal or | Significant or |
Steps	Common Findings	Abnormal Findings
Table 64–1. Key Points of a Physical Examination: Hepatic, Biliary Tract and Exocrine Pancreatic Disorders *(Continued)*		
Adaptations for Older Adults		
Inspection		
Contour	Sagging and rounded because of loss of muscle tone and accumulation of fat	
Palpation		
Note liver span and borders	Span may be shortened but border more easily palpated	Right upper quadrant or epigastric pain from the liver and biliary tract Epigastric pain from pancreas, stomach, or duodenum

(1½–3 inches). The lower border of the liver at the RMCL is usually at the right costal margin and the upper border is between the fifth and seventh ICSs. Liver size varies with body size. Measurements larger than the norms indicate liver enlargement. Ask the client to take a deep breath and hold it while you percuss the lower liver border in the RMCL again. Deep inspiration causes the liver to descend lower into the abdomen from the pressure of the diaphragm. The distance of liver descent is

marked and measured and ranges from 2 to 3 cm (about 1 inch). Use the marked level of liver descent as a guide for later palpation of the liver.

Spleen size may be determined by percussion, particularly if the spleen is enlarged. The spleen is located by percussion as a small area of dullness just posterior to the left midaxillary line (LMAL) between the 6th and 10th ribs. It normally has a span of approximately 7 cm (2½–3 inches). If the spleen enlarges, the area of dullness

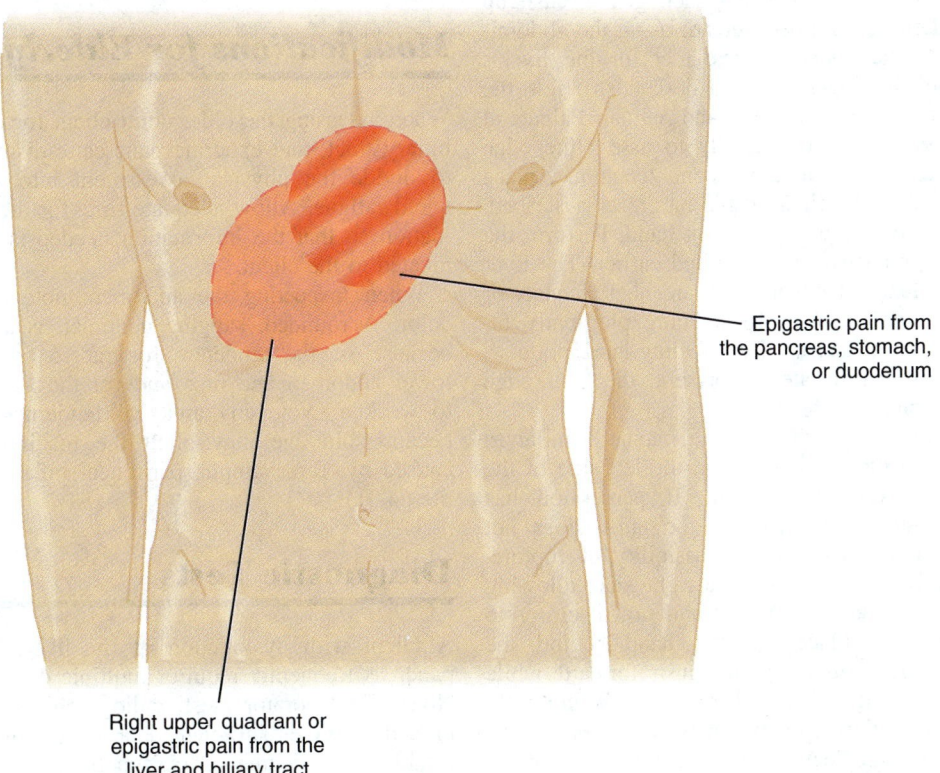

Epigastric pain from the pancreas, stomach, or duodenum

Right upper quadrant or epigastric pain from the liver and biliary tract

Figure 64–1. Location of abdominal pain with hepatic, biliary, or pancreatic disorders.

shifts inferiorly below the 10th rib and anteriorly toward or beyond the left anterior axillary line (LAAL).

Percussion also is used to assess the presence of ascites in the abdomen by observing for a fluid wave. The client is supine. Two nurses are needed to perform this assessment maneuver. One nurse places the edges of his or her hands on the client's abdominal midline to stabilize the abdominal wall. The second nurse places one hand on one side of the client's abdomen while briskly tapping the opposite side of the abdomen with the other hand. The second nurse feels for the movement of a fluid wave against the palpating hand opposite the side percussed.

Palpation

Perform light palpation initially to assess for muscle guarding or tenderness. Observe the client for facial grimaces, tensing, or other indications of discomfort. Next, perform deep palpation to evaluate tenderness, indicating possible inflammation. Light and deep palpation are discussed in Chapter 12. Because the peritoneum is often involved, evaluate for localized peritoneal irritation. Press the abdomen firmly at a point away from any tender area and then quickly remove the examining hand. Severe pain accompanies this maneuver when inflammation is present, indicating rebound tenderness. Perform liver palpation standing at the client's right side. Use one of two bimanual techniques. Place your left hand under the client's right posterior thorax over the 11th and 12th ribs and push the thorax upward. Place the right hand below the right costal margin at the previously marked level of liver descent as determined by percussion. The fingers point upward toward the costal margin. Then gently push up and in as the client takes a deep breath using the abdominal muscles. As the client inhales, feel for the liver's edge to slip over the finger tips as it descends. If felt, the liver's edge is firm, sharp, smooth, and regular. Palpate at several points medially and laterally to assess the edge along its inferior border. In the second technique, place the right hand below the right costal margin as described. Superimpose the left hand on the right hand. Perform the remainder of the maneuver as described earlier. The liver is difficult to palpate in clients who are obese, tense, or have taut abdominal muscles from being physically fit. Abnormal findings include the liver feeling hard, nodular, and tender. If extreme ascites is present, the liver edge will be nonpalpable.

Spleen palpation is performed in a manner similar to that for the liver, except it is done on the left side of the abdomen below the costal margin. If percussion has shown that the spleen is enlarged, the nurse does not usually palpate it because of the possibility of rupture. The client is asked to turn onto the right side, allowing gravity to bring the spleen forward and down, closer to the abdominal wall. Place the left hand behind the client's left posterior rib cage and push forward while palpating with the right hand. The spleen is normally nonpalpable. Congestion from portal hypertension results in enlargement of the spleen. This is a common finding in cirrhosis.

Blunt percussion (fist percussion) is performed to deter-

mine organ tenderness over the liver. This maneuver is performed after all other abdominal assessment techniques are completed to avoid producing discomfort should organ tenderness exist. When assessing for *liver tenderness,* use *only* indirect fist percussion over the costal margin at the RMCL to avoid trauma to the liver. This is also known as the liver tap. For comparison, perform indirect fist percussion over the left costal margin at the MCL (see Chapter 12 for a discussion of blunt percussion). Inform the client what is going to be done to avoid the reaction of surprise that may be misinterpreted as tenderness. The client's reaction to the blows is noted.

In addition to assessment of the abdomen, observe for systemic manifestations suggestive of hepatic, biliary, or pancreatic dysfunction. Such manifestations include jaundice; purpura; hair loss; weight loss; gynecomastia, which can develop from decreased metabolism of estrogen when the liver is dysfunctional; spider angiomas; and reddened palms (palmar erythema).

While taking the history and performing the physical assessment, continue assessment of the client's mental and neurologic status. Informally observe the client's verbal and nonverbal behavior. Note facial expressions at rest and while talking. Try to assess the client's mood. Is there evidence of anxiety, depression, apathy, anger, exhaustion, or hostility? If possible, question the client directly regarding his or her sensorium. Note the presence of confusion, disorientation, or lethargy. Question the client's use of alcohol and other substances. Since handwriting deteriorates with diminishing liver function, obtain a handwriting sample for subsequent comparison should the client develop progressive hepatocellular damage (see also Chapter 65).

Modifications for Elderly Clients

When assessing the older adult client for possible hepatic, biliary tract, and exocrine pancreatic disorders, remember to divide the physical assessment into several parts to avoid fatigue. Allow adequate time for the physical examination so that the information needed is clearly communicated to the client.

When inspecting the abdomen, note the contour and color. A rounded, sagging abdomen is a normal finding because of the tendency for fat to accumulate in the lower abdomen and hips and for the abdominal muscles to weaken. Note any areas of tenderness or discomfort because old age may blunt the manifestations of pain caused by, for example, peritoneal inflammation (see Table 64–1).

Diagnostic Tests

A client with dysfunction of the liver, biliary tract, or pancreas frequently requires multiple diagnostic measures. No single laboratory test, radiographic study, or surgical procedure yields sufficient data to confirm a diagnosis or establish the degree of malfunction. Afford the client a sense of self-worth and understanding during repeated diagnostic procedures. This helps gain the client's cooperation and also reduces the fatigue and anxiety that frequently accompany these work-ups.

Laboratory Studies

Familiarize yourself with common laboratory tests of liver, biliary, and pancreatic function. See Table 64–2 for a summary of these tests.

Immunologic Tests

Three types of immunologic tests may be used in diagnosing hepatobiliary disease. They include assays for globulins, mitochondrial antibody, and antinuclear and smooth muscle antibodies.[40]

■ Globulins

The concentration of serum globulins (as measured by serum protein electrophoresis or salt fractionation), while not diagnostic of liver disease per se, may be influenced by a wide variety of hepatic and extrahepatic factors and disease states. The cause of increased concentrations of serum globulins is thought to be related to the increased antibody production resulting from decreased removal of bacterial antigens from the portal blood or release of antigenic material from damaged liver cells. Elevated IgM concentrations are common in biliary cirrhosis and increases in globulin concentrations are commonly seen in cirrhosis and hepatitis.

■ Mitochondrial Antibodies

Antibodies directed against a component of the inner mitochondrial membrane appear in 90% of clients with primary biliary cirrhosis. Mitochondrial antibodies are also present in up to 25% of clients with chronic active hepatitis and postnecrotic cirrhosis. They are rarely present in extrahepatic biliary obstruction.

■ Antinuclear and Smooth Muscle Antibodies

Antinuclear and smooth muscle antibodies test positive in a variable percentage of patients with chronic active hepatitis. However, they are usually not present in association with hepatitis B or C. In addition, these antibodies also occur in a small number of clients with primary biliary cirrhosis.

Tests for Hepatitis Virus Infection

See Chapter 65 for information about these tests and their significance.

Ultrasonography

Ultrasonography uses high-frequency sound waves to examine the interior of the body. In abdominal ultrasonography, the examiner passes a transducer over the abdo-

men. Ultrasonography is noninvasive and generally accurate. Because it does not involve x-rays, it is safe for pregnant women. It lacks the ionizing radiation and the untoward side effects of radiologic procedures that use contrast media. (A discussion of radiologic techniques follows.) Because of the low risk involved, the health practitioner may recommend ultrasonography as the initial diagnostic study.

Ultrasonographic examination provides valuable diagnostic information for liver, pancreatic, and biliary tract conditions. It is a valuable diagnostic tool for the presence of gallstones or tumors as well as patency of vessels.

The technique proceeds rapidly and requires little or no preparation. Depending on the area to be examined, the client may or may not fast prior to the procedure. Reassure the client that the test is painless and safe. There are no specific precautions or observations following ultrasound.

Radiologic Studies

Many of the procedures used to diagnose disorders of the liver, pancreas, and biliary tract involve the use of x-rays. Plain x-ray films of the abdomen may show diaphragm elevation due to hepatic enlargement or calcification in the abdominal organs. Upper or lower gastrointestinal series using barium contrast medium also provide important information about the accessory organs of digestion, that is, the liver, gallbladder, and pancreas.

Radiologic studies using iodinated contrast media permit visualization of tubes and vessels. Before any of these procedures are performed, question the client about known hypersensitivity to iodine or seafood.

Oral Cholecystography (Gallbladder Series)

Cholecystography is an x-ray test for gallbladder or cystic duct disease. Oral cholecystography has been the standard examination for gallstones for almost 50 years. Although the use of oral cholecystography declined markedly with the advent of ultrasonography, the recent development of nonsurgical approaches to the treatment of cholelithiasis (e.g., lithotripsy and oral dissolution therapy) has led to a resurgence of interest in oral cholecystography.[18] While it is still clinically useful, it does predispose the client undergoing study to greater risks than does the similarly accurate cholecystosonography.

Procedure. During the test, radiography permits visualization of the gallbladder. When contraction of the gallbladder is desirable, the client consumes a high fat meal during the procedure. Following an oral cholecystogram, some people experience burning on urination due to the presence of the dye in the urine. Forcing fluids decreases this problem.

Poor or no visualization of the gallbladder indicates gallbladder disease, presumably because biliary obstruction prevents passage of the dye. Occasionally, stones

Table 64–2. Laboratory Tests of Liver, Biliary, and Pancreatic Function

Measurement	Normal Value*	Procedure	Interpretation
Biliary Excretion			

Serum bilirubin
  Direct (conjugated)
  Indirect (unconjugated)
  Total
	
	0.1–0.3 mg/100 ml
	0.2–0.8 mg/100 ml
	0.1–1.0 mg/100 ml
		Blood drawn without special preparation; protect sample from ultraviolet light or sunlight	Direct bilirubin increased with biliary obstruction, causing conjugated fraction to accumulate in plasma
			Indirect bilirubin increased with excessive erythrocyte hemolysis
			Total bilirubin measures direct and indirect levels together

Urine bilirubin	0	Urine collection (urine appears smoky or tea-colored); protect from light	Urine bilirubin measures conjugated bilirubin only; increased with biliary obstruction
Urine urobilinogen	0–1.0 Ehrlich units (EU)/24 hr or 0.5–4.0 EU/24 hr	2- or 24-hr afternoon collection placed in brown refrigerated bottle with sodium carbonate preservative	Urine urobilinogen decreased with biliary obstruction; increased with erythrocyte hemolysis
Fecal urobilinogen	75–275 EU/100 g	Entire stool specimen to laboratory	Fecal urobilinogen decreased with biliary obstruction; increased in erythrocyte hemolysis
Serum cholesterol	140–242 mg/100 ml	Blood drawn after low cholesterol diet for 12 hr	Cholesterol elevated when excretion blocked by bile duct obstruction, but reduced when severe liver damage reduces ability to synthesize it
Carbohydrate Metabolism			
Serum amylase Serum pancreatic isoamylase Urine amylase	80–150 Somogyi units/100 ml or 40–220 IU/L (depends on test used)	Blood drawn 1 to 2 hr after eating; preferably while no IV lines are infusing 2- or 24-hr urine collection with no preservative in bottle unless specified; 2- or 24-hr urine collection bottle must have a preservative Specimens collected for both *after voiding*	Pancreatic digestive enzyme released with breakdown of acinar cells; serum levels increase 2–3 hr after pain onset with pancreatitis and return to normal in 24–48 hr; elevations not directly correlated with severity; amylase test measures both pancreatic and salivary amylase; pancreatic isoamylase is a more specific test; urinary levels elevated longer with pancreatitis
Protein Metabolism			
Total protein Serum albumin Serum globulin Include α_1, α_2, β, γ	6–8.2 g/dl 3.5–5.0 g/dl 2.3–3.5 g/dl	Blood drawn without special preparation	Impaired protein synthesis or utilization caused by chronic liver disease, pancreatic insufficiency (albumin, α- and β-globulins); γ-globulins produced by B lymphocytes, not liver
A/G ratio (albumin/globulin)	1.0–2.0 g/dl	Blood drawn without special preparation	A decrease in the ratio may indicate chronic liver disease

Table 64–2. Laboratory Tests of Liver, Biliary, and Pancreatic Function (Continued)

Measurement	Normal Value*	Procedure	Interpretation
Protein Metabolism (Continued)			
Serum ammonia	0–150 μg N/dl	Blood drawn from person kept NPO except for water for 8–12 hr before the test Blood must be iced and tested immediately	Reduced synthesis of urea from body ammonia in severe hepatocellular damage produces elevated blood ammonia
Methemalbumin	Absent	Fluid from peritoneal or pleural tap analyzed	Product of hemoglobin digestion elevated when blood released into body fluids, as in hemorrhagic pancreatitis
Fat Metabolism			
Serum lipase	0–27 IU/dl	Blood drawn from fasting person	Pancreatic digestive enzyme is increased with acute pancreatitis and conditions leading to obstruction of ampulla of Vater
Metabolism of Foreign Substances			
Bromsulphalein (BSP) excretion	<5% retention in 1 hr	Control blood specimen (or sample) taken after fasting for 12 hr; BSP given, blood drawn at intervals	Dye retained with diminished hepatocellular ability to remove it from blood and excrete it; infrequently used
Serum Enzymes†			
Aspartate aminotransferase (AST)	0–41 IU/L	Blood drawn without special preparation	Serum AST, ALT, and LDH released from damaged liver, heart, kidney, and muscle cells; prolonged elevation in liver disease may be first indicator of chronic active hepatitis; a rapid drop may signal liver failure
Alanine aminotransferase (ALT)	0–41 IU/L (female values slightly lower than male values)		
Lactate dehydrogenase (LDH)	60–220 IU/L		
Alkaline phosphatase (ALP)	Male: 19–74 IU/L Female: 12–63 IU/L	Blood drawn without special preparation	Increase in biliary obstruction; produced by cells lining the biliary tract; this enzyme is also found in bone, intestine, and placenta
Serum 5′-nucleotidase	0.3–3.2 Bodansky units	Blood drawn without special preparation	Enzyme located mainly in liver and confirmation of liver disease occurs if ALP and this both elevated
Serum γ-glutamyltransferase (GGT)	<65 IU/L	Blood drawn without special preparation	Enzyme located in liver and kidney; elevation of GGT and ALP significant indication of liver disorders
Hepatitis Antigens and Antibodies			
	Negative for antigens Positive or negative for antibodies, depending on history	Blood drawn without special preparation	Antigens indicate hepatitis; antibodies indicate past or present hepatitis or immunization (hepatitis B)

Table continued on following page

Table 64-2. Laboratory Tests of Liver, Biliary, and Pancreatic Function (Continued)

Measurement	Normal Value*	Procedure	Interpretation
Hemostatic Function			
Prothrombin time (PT)	11.2–13.8 sec	Blood drawn without special preparation	Assesses function of extrinsic pathway in clotting process (factors I, II, V, VII, X) PT prolonged with (1) decreased synthesis of prothrombin due to liver cell damage or (2) decreased vitamin K absorption due to bile duct obstruction Vitamin K necessary for liver to synthesize prothrombin (factor II)
Platelets	250,000–500,000/mm³	Blood drawn without special preparation	May fall when spleen is enlarged in portal hypertension
Exocrine Pancreatic Function			
		Oral bentiromide given after overnight fast; urine is collected for 6 h	Pancreatic chymotrypsin splits bentiromide; para-aminobenzoic acid (PABA), a breakdown product, is excreted in urine; less PABA is excreted with pancreatic insufficiency
Antigens Associated with Cancer			
Alpha-fetoprotein (AFP)	<10 ng/mg	Blood drawn without special preparation	AFP is synthesized by fetus but not by healthy adult; AFP level >1000 ng/ml usually indicates hepatocellular carcinoma

* Normal values may differ significantly between laboratories.
† Trends in elevation are of particular importance in predicting the rapidity with which the liver is failing. If levels rise, fall, then rise again, liver failure may be occurring.

can be visualized as shadows within the opaque medium. The test results are accurate only when gastrointestinal and liver function allow absorption and conjugation of the dye.

Preprocedure Care. The evening before the examination, the client ingests a radiopaque dye determined by the fat content of the evening meal. If the client has a regular or low fat dinner, the client may receive ipodate sodium (Oragrafin). After a high fat dinner, the client must be given iopanoic acid (Telepaque). These dyes contain iodine. Carefully observe the client for allergic reactions even when the health history reveals no known allergies to iodine or seafood. Possible hypersensitive reactions include nausea and vomiting, diarrhea, abdominal pain, rash, and anaphylaxis. Diarrhea may result in nonvisualization of the gallbladder.

Conjugation of the dye occurs in the liver. Be aware

that these dyes are potentially toxic to the liver and kidneys. This is especially true in clients with preexisting hepatic or renal failure. Following excretion of the opaque medium into the bile, the gallbladder concentrates the contrast medium.

Postprocedure Care. The client can eat following the examination. There is no other specific care following the examination.

Cholangiography

A cholangiogram or cholangiopancreatograph allows visualization of the bile ducts. Following administration of an organic iodine dye (iodipamide meglumine, Cholografin Meglumine) x-ray filming begins.

Procedure. There are four types of cholangiography:

1. *Intravenous cholangiography* is used for common bile duct visualization. The radiopaque dye burns intensely upon injection.
2. *Percutaneous transhepatic cholangiography* involves injecting the dye directly into the ductal system, through the skin via a long, slender needle.
3. *Endoscopic retrograde cholangiography* (ERCP) involves passage of a side-viewing duodenoscope through the mouth to the papilla of Vater in the duodenum. The examiner passes a catheter into the common bile duct and, possibly, the pancreatic duct, that allows injection of contrast material into pancreatic and biliary systems.
4. *T-tube cholangiography* involves injecting dye into a preexisting bile drainage tube.

In all four types of cholangiography, failure of the opaque dye to pass through the bile ducts provides evidence of duct obstruction.

Preprocedure Care. Again, assess for iodine allergies. Possible allergic reactions include dyspnea, tachycardia, sweating, nausea, vomiting, and chills. Also, to prevent renal damage, instruct the client to drink ample amounts of fluid following administration of the dye. Or, if the client is unable to take adequate fluids orally, intravenous (IV) hydration with or without mannitol is frequently used.

Postprocedure Care. The client should be monitored for an allergic reaction for 24 hours following the procedure. Warn the client that there may be some discomfort with urination while the dye is excreted.

Angiography

Procedure. Angiography allows visualization of the hepatic, biliary, and pancreatic arterial vessels after administration of contrast medium. It is used to identify abnormalities of vascular structure and function, observe masses, and note bleeding sites in the pancreas, spleen, and portal system. Recall that angiography is also used in diagnosing disorders of the kidneys, lower extremities, and gastrointestinal tract. To inject the contrast media, the examiner usually introduces a needle into the femoral artery. Next, the needle is exchanged for a catheter, which is then passed into the celiac artery or one of its branches (superior mesenteric or hepatic). After contrast media injection, rapid sequence filming is done.

Preprocedure Care. Explain the purpose of the examination to the client. The client is usually NPO (nothing by mouth) for 6 to 8 hours before the test. Ask the client about any use of medications that might lead to bleeding, such as anticoagulants or nonsteroidal anti-inflammatory drugs (NSAIDs). These medications should be stopped up to a week prior to the test. Bleeding or clotting tests are usually ordered before the test. Remind the client that it will be necessary to lie very still during the examination. The client should be warned that there

may be a sensation of pressure during introduction of the catheter. Assess the pulses distal to the insertion site for comparison with pulses afterward.

Postprocedure Care. Following angiography, assess the needle insertion site for manifestations of bleeding, because with liver conditions, clients often have concurrent clotting disorders and this may lead to a hematoma. Assess the pulses below the level of catheter insertion.

Computed Tomography

Computed tomography (CT) is another radiologic technique used to diagnose and evaluate liver, biliary tract, and gallbladder disease, including distinguishing between obstructive and nonobstructive jaundice. A CT scan is performed by rotating a finely focused x-ray beam around the client. A computer then assembles data from the detector and provides an image. The constructed image yields a cross-sectional view (Fig. 64–2). Contrast media, when used, enhance the picture. Very dense structures, such as bone, appear white; less dense matter is gray; air is black. The client is instructed to fast, except for water, for 8 to 12 hours prior to the test.

Radionuclide Scanning

Radionuclide scanning, or scintigraphy, involves IV infusion of gamma-emitting isotopes. Following infusion, a scintillation detector is passed over the abdomen. This procedure investigates biliary duct patency and indicates whether a tumor or abscess is present in the liver, gallbladder, or pancreas. Useful isotopes include colloidal gold (^{198}Au), gallium (^{67}Ga), technetium (^{99}Tc), and sele-

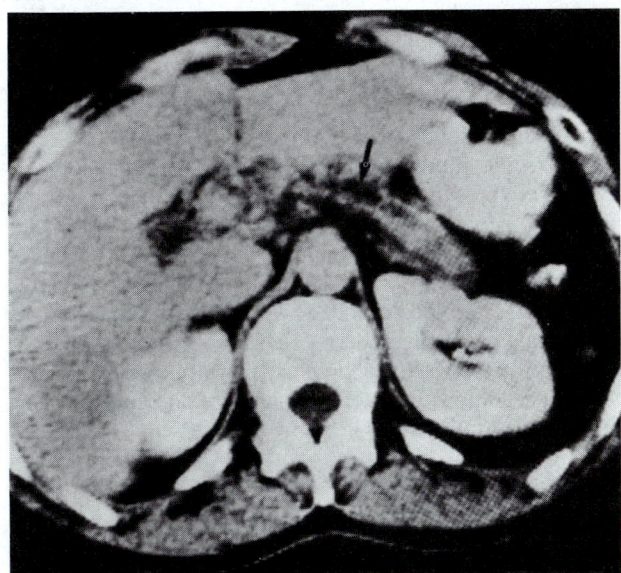

Figure 64–2. Computed tomographic scan of chronic pancreatitis. There is pancreatic atrophy and a dilated pancreatic duct *(arrow)* but no evidence of pancreatic calcification. (From Moss, A. A., et al. [1983]. *Computed tomography of the body.* Philadelphia: W. B. Saunders.)

nium (^{75}Se). ^{67}Ga accumulates in inflamed tissue. ^{99}Tc evaluates liver and biliary tract function. ^{75}Se is useful for identifying pancreatic abnormalities.

Paracentesis

Procedure. The purpose of paracentesis, or peritoneal tap, is to extract fluid accumulations in the peritoneum (ascites), to relieve intra-abdominal tension, which can impair the client's respiratory status, or to obtain the fluid to send for culture. Following cleaning of the skin and infiltration with a local anesthetic, the physician, using sterile technique, inserts a long aspirating needle with a syringe to collect a fluid specimen. To drain ascitic fluid (if desired), the physician inserts a trocar aseptically through a small stab wound below the umbilicus. This allows fluid (usually several liters) to drain slowly through a catheter into a collection bottle.

Preprocedure Care. The nurse actively participates in this procedure, which usually takes place at the bedside. Obtain written permission before the procedure begins and instruct the client regarding the procedure's purpose and the steps involved. Ask the client to void immediately prior to the procedure to decrease the risk of bladder puncture. Have the client sit upright on the edge of the bed, with the feet resting on a stool and the back well supported.

Postprocedure Care. The major complication of paracentesis is *hypovolemia* and shock secondary to fluid drainage from the peritoneum, and the resulting fluid shift from intravascular to interstitial space, as well as the sudden change in intra-abdominal pressure on the vessels. This fluid shift is exacerbated by hypoalbuminemia.

Assess vital signs and peripheral circulation every few minutes during and immediately following paracentesis. Observe for hypovolemic shock: pallor, tachycardia, decreased blood pressure, oliguria, and dyspnea.

Hepatic encephalopathy due to reduced tissue perfusion is another complication resulting from drainage of ascitic fluid. Ascitic fluid contains a high concentration of protein. Therefore, the physician may prescribe albumin infusions for 24 hours following paracentesis to compensate for protein losses. Potassium depletion may also occur following multiple paracentesis procedures. Infection, peritonitis, and bleeding due to vessel trauma occasionally complicate paracentesis.

Carefully assess for abdominal pain following paracentesis. In addition, monitor the puncture site for persistent leakage of ascitic drainage.

Peritoneoscopy

Procedure. Insertion of a peritoneoscope through an abdominal stab wound permits direct visualization of the liver and peritoneum. Visualization of structural changes aids in the diagnosis of cirrhosis and cancer. During peritoneoscopy, the examiner may take photographs and perform a biopsy.

Peritoneoscopy is relatively safe and simple. Contraindications include infections of the abdominal cavity, clotting disorders, or intestinal obstruction. In addition, the client must be able to cooperate throughout the procedure. Obesity and ascites interfere with test results.

Preprocedure Care. To prepare a client for peritoneoscopy:

1. Check that the written consent has been obtained.
2. Check the laboratory record to make certain the client has normal or adequate clotting factors. If not, inform the physician.
3. Check the client and healthcare record for contraindications to preprocedural medications.
4. Inquire whether the client is sensitive to local anesthetics.
5. Prepare the skin, and administer preprocedural medication when appropriate.
6. Instruct the client to take nothing by mouth and to empty the bowel and bladder just before the procedure begins.
7. Provide adequate teaching before and during the actual procedure.
8. Explain to the client that it may be difficult to breathe when air is placed in the abdominal cavity.
9. Instruct the client to elevate the abdominal wall by holding the breath to protect major organs during needle insertion.

Postprocedure Care. When peritoneoscopy includes liver biopsy, 24 hours of bedrest follows the procedure. If biopsy is not performed, the client resumes activity following recovery from the effects of the medication. Complications are uncommon and more often occur secondary to biopsy.

Possible postperitoneoscopy complications are pneumothorax, subcutaneous emphysema, air embolism, bile peritonitis, perforation of a hollow organ, and shoulder or abdominal pain.

Biopsy

Biopsy is the single most valuable diagnostic study because it is often the determining factor for final diagnosis. It involves removal of a sample of living tissue for analysis. Biopsies may be open or closed procedures. An open biopsy necessitates a general anesthetic and a major abdominal incision. A client may have an open biopsy at the time of a concurrent operative procedure. An advantage of the open biopsy is that the surgeon can observe the entire liver, identify grossly altered tissue, and remove the biopsy specimen for study.

A closed biopsy, or percutaneous liver biopsy, is the usual, current practice. It is performed under fluoroscopy and is a simpler procedure than open biopsy. It involves aspiration of a core of tissue via needle for histologic study. The conventional percutaneous liver biopsy is a blind procedure (Menghini's technique). The primary limitation of Menghini's technique is that the surgeon is unable to see where the needle is going. Nevertheless, this procedure may be appropriate for determining the cause of general hepatic disease (diffuse parenchymal involvement).

Contraindications to percutaneous liver biopsy are severe thrombocytopenia, local infection of the lung base, prolonged prothrombin time, peritonitis, massive ascites, an uncooperative client, and extrahepatic obstructive jaundice, especially with an enlarged gallbladder. The client with cancer or amyloidosis has an increased risk of postprocedure hemorrhage. Also, if the client is unable to remain still and cooperative during the procedure, the surgeon could accidentally puncture another organ.

Procedure. The liver biopsy procedure may be performed at the bedside, in a procedure room, or in a gastrointestinal unit using a local anesthetic. Check the client's chart for coagulation profile results as well as for a signed consent form. Sedation and analgesia, such as diazepam (Valium) or midazolam (Versed), may be given to help allay the client's fears and make him or her more comfortable. Place the client either in the supine position or in a left lateral position with the right arm elevated. Less frequently, you may ask the client to assume a prone position. During insertion of the needle, have the client exhale and then hold the breath on expiration for 5 to 10 seconds to avoid puncturing of the diaphragm (Fig. 64–3).

When the purpose of liver biopsy is to assess a focal lesion or abnormality, the blind procedure has definite limitations. The chance of inserting the needle into the wrong part of the liver and missing the lesion is great. With the use of concurrent ultrasonography, however, the physician is able to view the entire procedure and thus guide the needle. Guided biopsy allows better localization of a focal lesion or abnormality.

Fine-needle aspiration biopsy, often performed when a suspicious area of the liver is localized, helps diagnose malignancy. This approach is ideal when only a few cells are necessary for cytologic study. The risks of fine-needle aspiration biopsy are far less than a guided regular biopsy, because the tissue sample is much smaller. Also, this procedure greatly reduces any risk of tumor metastasis along the needle track.

There are few contraindications to the guided regular or fine-needle aspiration biopsy procedures. Clients with impaired coagulation associated with liver disease, however, may not be appropriate candidates for the closed procedure. When biopsy is indicated for these clients, a "plugged" biopsy procedure minimizes the risk of hemorrhage. This procedure allows injection of absorbable gelatin material on withdrawal of the biopsy needle. The gelatin material applies pressure to the bleeding site and closes the potential track. The client must be able to hold his or her breath for a period of up to 15 seconds.

Preprocedure Care. At least 2 weeks prior to having a liver biopsy, the client must refrain from ingesting aspirin, NSAIDs, or anticoagulants. In addition, blood clotting tests, i.e., prothrombin time, bleeding time, partial thromboplastin time and platelet count, and hematocrit are done in advance of the liver biopsy.

Before the liver biopsy begins, the client fasts for at least 6 hours. An explanation of the procedure is given, including its purpose, the insertion of an IV line during the procedure, and positioning during and after the procedure. When a client is given information about the procedure, the recovery period is smoother and less anxiety-producing. Emotional support is important to decrease apprehension and help a client feel more in control.

Postprocedure Care. Following percutaneous liver biopsy, perform the following nursing assessments and interventions:

1. Monitor vital signs every 15 minutes for 2 hours, every 30 minutes for 2 hours, and every 60 minutes for 4 hours.
2. Carefully assess for tachycardia and decreasing blood pressure, which may indicate hemorrhage.
3. Check the puncture site by monitoring the dressing, palpating the surrounding area for crepitus, and observing for hematoma formation.
4. Observe for pain in the right upper quadrant of the abdomen caused by a subcapsular accumulation of blood or bile, or at the right shoulder as a result of blood on the undersurface of the diaphragm.
5. Beginning 2 hours after the procedure, elevate the head of the bed 30 degrees. Two hours later, elevate it to 45 degrees. Maintain the client on bedrest for 24 hours following the procedure. The right side-lying position for the first 1 to 2 hours decreases the risk of hemorrhage and bile leakage.
6. Administer postprocedure medications on an individual basis, depending on the client's physical status.
7. Give vitamin K if prescribed.
8. Assess respiratory status for manifestations of dyspnea.

Inherent risks of the biopsy procedure include hemorrhage and puncture of adjacent organs or structures. Hem-

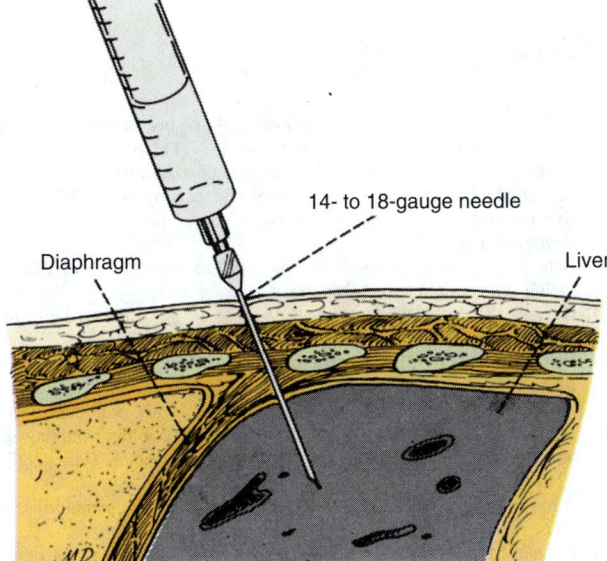

Figure 64–3. Percutaneous liver biopsy requires cooperation. The client must be able to lie quietly and hold his or her breath after exhaling.

14- to 18-gauge needle

Diaphragm

Liver

orrhage, the most serious complication, may result from penetration of the arterial tree or a distended vein radicle during the first 24 hours after the biopsy procedure. The risk of hemorrhage is increased if vascular channels are distended or if the client breathes during needle insertion into the liver. Puncture of a lung can cause pneumothorax. A large biopsy needle (14- to 18-gauge) can penetrate a dilated intrahepatic duct in a client with obstructive jaundice. Bile leakage and resultant peritonitis can develop. Bile peritonitis is treated with surgical decompression. Cross-contamination may occur following puncture of an adjacent organ. Clients with potentially effusive conditions (e.g., ascites, chronic lung disease) in addition to liver abnormality are at great risk of cross-contamination.

Portal Pressure Measurements

Measurements of portal pressure and flow help to (1) diagnose portal hypertension, (2) indicate the severity of portal hypertension, and (3) guide decisions as to appropriate intervention, which may include surgery. Also, the indirect calculation of sinusoid pressure helps determine the location of an obstruction in the liver and thus identify the underlying disorder. Normal portal pressure is 5 to 10 mm Hg. Portal hypertension is present when the wedged vein pressure is more than 5 mm Hg higher than the inferior vena cava pressure.[5]

Procedure. The major portal pressure measurements are the following:

- Wedged hepatic vein pressure (WHVP). In this procedure, portal pressure is obtained indirectly by percutaneous hepatic vein catheterization. The examiner uses either an arm vein or a femoral vein.
- Umbilical vein catheterization. This procedure allows direct measurement of portal pressure.
- Splenic pulp manometry. During manometry, the examiner places a needle between two of the lower ribs, inserting a manometer into the spleen.

Instruct the client to hold his or her breath during needle insertion and passage.

Preprocedure Care. Portal pressure measurements are minor surgical procedures that are performed in the operating room or a special studies laboratory. Often, the surgeon concurrently injects contrast media. These measures require standard preoperative and postoperative care.

Postprocedure Care. Carefully observe for bleeding or pneumothorax afterward. Carefully assess the incision site postoperatively for hematoma formation. Other care is the same as for the client following liver biopsy.

Analysis of Duodenal or Biliary Drainage

Duodenal and biliary drainage analysis assists in the diagnosis of cholelithiasis when the cholecystogram is inconclusive. Also, these procedures provide an alternative for clients allergic to iodine who cannot undergo cholecystography or cholangiography.

To prepare for the test, instruct the client to fast for 8 hours before the study. The study involves insertion of a single-lumen nasogastric tube into the stomach. The stomach contents are aspirated and the tube is slowly advanced until the aspirate changes to clear, golden, and alkaline. At this point, the tube is in the duodenum, and clear golden bile (called A bile) is collected.

The next step is to increase the flow of bile into the duodenum. Instillation of magnesium sulfate into the tube, or IV administration of secretin (sometimes followed by pancreozymin), stimulates bile flow. After administering these bile flow stimulants, it should be possible to aspirate 30 to 60 ml of concentrated bile (B bile) from the duodenum. Bile can also be collected through an endoscope.

Collected fluid is sent to the laboratory to be analyzed for volume and bicarbonate, enzyme, and bile content. Disproportions in the bile and pancreatic juice fractions indicate obstruction in the bile or pancreatic duct. The presence of cholesterol crystals indicates lithiasis.

Conclusions

Once a thorough knowledge of the structure and function of the liver, biliary tract, and exocrine pancreas is gained, the nurse must examine the diagnostic assessment of these organs. Systematic assessment of the client with possible disorders of the liver, biliary tract, or exocrine pancreas can lead to prompt diagnosis and treatment. You can facilitate this diagnostic process by adequately preparing the client for diagnostic procedures and by assisting with or actually collecting assessment data.

Bibliography

1. Balthazar, E. J. (1989). CT diagnosis and staging of acute pancreatitis. *Radiologic Clinics of North America, 27*(1), 19–37.
2. Barker, G. M., et al. (1994). The effects of azidothymidine therapy on pseudocholinesterase concentrations in asymptomatic HIV-positive patients. *Journal of the American Association of Nurse Anesthetists, 62*(4), 337–341.
3. Bates, B. (1995). *A guide to physical examination and history taking.* Philadelphia: J. B. Lippincott.
4. Bayless, T. M. (1989). *Current therapy in gastroenterology and liver disease* (Vol. 3, 3rd ed.). St. Louis: Mosby–Year Book.
5. Boyer, T. D. (1992). Cirrhosis of the liver and its major sequelae. In J. B. Wyngaarden, L. H. Smith, and J. C. Bennett (Eds.), *Cecil's textbook of medicine* (19th ed.). Philadelphia: W. B. Saunders.
6. Brown, A. (1991). Acute pancreatitis: Pathophysiology, nursing diagnosis and collaborative problems. *Focus on Critical Care, 18*(2), 121–130.
7. Burrell, L. (1993). *Adult nursing in hospital and community settings.* Norwalk, CT: Appleton & Lange.
8. Clouse, M. E. (1989). Current diagnostic imaging modalities of the liver. *Surgical Clinics of North America, 69*(2), 193–234.
9. Doughty, D. B., & Jackson, D. B. (1993). *Gastrointestinal disorders.* St. Louis: Mosby–Year Book.
10. Ebersol, P., & Hess, P. (1994). *Toward healthy aging: Human*

needs and nursing response (4th ed.). St. Louis: Mosby–Year Book.

11. Ferri, F. F. (1995). *The care of the medical patient* (3rd ed.). St. Louis: Mosby–Year Book.

12. For sharper diagnostic accuracy in identifying liver disease (1990). *Emergency Medicine, 22*(3), 127–130.

13. Friedman, L. S. (1995). Liver, biliary tract, pancreas. In L. M. Tierney, S. J. McPhee, & M. A. Papadakis (Eds.), *Current medical diagnosis and treatment* (34th ed.). Norwalk, CT: Appleton & Lange.

14. Guyton, A. C. (1991). *Textbook of medical physiology* (8th ed.). Philadelphia: W. B. Saunders.

15. Hogstal, M. O., & Keen-Payne, R. (1993). *Practical guide to health assessment.* Philadelphia: F. A. Davis.

16. Holland, P., & Hussain, I. (1989). Biliary lithotripsy: Nonsurgical treatment of gallstones. *Society of Gastrointestinal Assistants Journal, 3,* 158–162.

17. Hospitals must choose correct employee drug prophylaxis (1994). *Hospital Employee Health, 13*(6), 72–76.

18. Friedman, L., & Needleman, L. (1994). Hepato biliary imaging. In K. J. Isselbacher, et al. (Eds.), *Harrison's principles of internal medicine* (13th ed.). New York: McGraw-Hill.

19. Kee, J. L. (1995). *Laboratory and diagnostic tests with nursing implications* (4th ed.). Norwalk, CT: Appleton & Lange.

20. Kee, J. L., & Hayes, E. R. (1990). Assessment of patient laboratory data in the acutely ill. *Nursing Clinics of North America, 25*(4), 751–759.

21. Kohn, C. L., Brogenec, S., & Foster, P. F. (1993). Nutritional support for the patient with pancreatobiliary disease. *Critical Care Nursing Clinics of North America, 5*(1), 37–45.

22. Krech, R., & Walsh, D. (1991). Symptoms of pancreatic cancer. *Journal of Pain and Symptom Management, 6*(6), 360–367.

23. Lail, L. M., & Cotton, P. B. (1990). Risks of endoscopic retrograde cholangiopancreatography and therapeutic applications. *Gastroenterology Nursing, 13*(1), 239–245.

24. Li, C. P. K., & Ho-Tai, P. (1990). MR imaging of the liver: Technique considerations. *Applied Radiology, 18*(6), 10–15.

25. Melillo, K. D. (1993). Interpretation of abnormal laboratory values in older adults: Part I. *Journal of Gerontological Nursing, 19*(1), 39–40.

26. Melillo, K. D. (1993). Interpretation of abnormal laboratory values in older adults: Part II. *Journal of Gerontological Nursing, 19*(2), 35–40.

27. Melillo, K. D. (1993). Interpretation of laboratory values in older adults. *Nurse Practitioner, 18*(7), 59–67.

28. Mosley, J. W., et al. (1990). Non-A, non-B hepatitis and antibody to hepatitis C virus. *JAMA, 263,* 77–78.

29. Niedzwick, L., & Stringer, C. (1994). Liver biopsy and nursing intervention. *Gastroenterology Nursing, 17*(1), 17–19.

30. Podolsky, D. K., & Isselbacher, K. J. (1994). Diagnostic tests in liver disease. In K. J. Isselbacher, et al. (Eds.), *Harrison's principles of internal medicine* (13th ed.). New York: McGraw-Hill.

31. Rakel, R. E. (1990). *Conn's current therapy.* Philadelphia: W. B. Saunders.

32. Renkes, J. (1993). G.I. endoscopy. *Nursing 93, 13*(6), 50–55.

33. Sabiston, D. C., Jr. (1991). *Textbook of surgery: The biologic basis of modern surgical practice* (14th ed.). Philadelphia: W. B. Saunders.

34. Schiff, L., & Schiff, E. R. (1993). *Diseases of the liver* (7th ed.). Philadelphia: J. B. Lippincott.

35. Sleisenger, M. H., & Fordtran, J. S. (Eds.) (1989). *Gastrointestinal disease: Pathophysiology, diagnosis, and management* (4th ed.). Philadelphia: W. B. Saunders.

36. Swearingen, P. L. (1994). *Manual of medical-surgical nursing care* (3rd ed.). St. Louis: Mosby–Year Book.

37. Treseler, K. M. (1995). *Clinical laboratory and diagnostic tests* (3rd ed.) Norwalk, CT: Appleton & Lange.

38. van Sonnenberg, E., et al. (1989). Imaging and interventional radiology for pancreatitis and its complications. *Radiologic Clinics of North America, 27*(1), 65–72.

39. Versatile scavenging system to reduce occupational risk (1992). *Canadian Journal of Respiratory Therapy, 28,* 59–65.

40. Weisiger, R. A. (1992). Laboratory tests in liver disease. In J. B. Wyngaarden, L. H. Smith, & J. C. Bennett (Eds.), *Cecil's textbook of medicine* (19th ed.). Philadelphia: W. B. Saunders.

41. Zidovudine/acetaminophen interaction: Nurses' drug alert (1992). *American Journal of Nursing, 92*(11), 85.

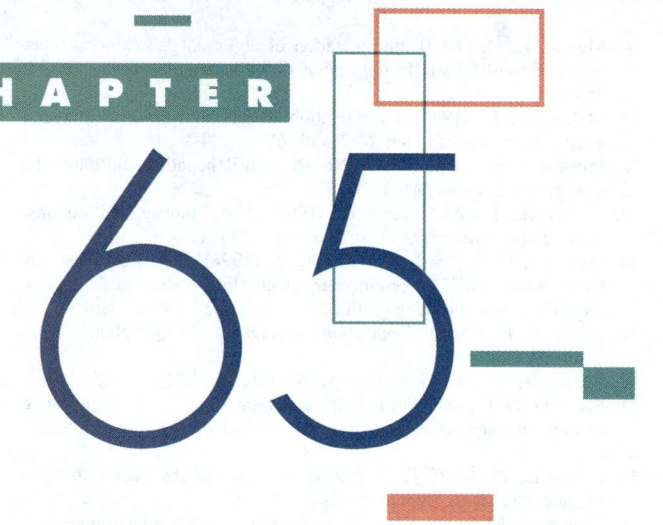

Nursing Care of Clients with Liver Disorders

Dianne Smolen

The liver plays a central role in many essential physiologic processes. It is the primary organ of lipid synthesis and functions to detoxify endogenous and exogenous substances such as hormones, drugs, and toxins. When there is alteration in the normal physiologic processes, numerous hepatic and extrahepatic manifestations of liver disease appear. Some of these manifestations are nonspecific to liver disease itself, whereas others are specific to liver disorders. Regardless of disease specificity, these hepatic and extrahepatic manifestations offer the initial clue to liver disease.

In this chapter we discuss the clinical features of liver diseases. In addition, we discuss their medical and surgical management and measures the nurse can take to assist clients with such nursing diagnoses as Impaired Skin Integrity, Fluid Volume Excess, Activity Intolerance related to fatigue, and Altered Nutrition: Less than Body Requirements.

Jaundice

Jaundice, or icterus, is the yellow pigmentation of the sclerae, skin, and deeper tissues caused by excessive accumulation of bile pigments in the blood. Bilirubin (bile pigment), a product of red blood cell breakdown, is deposited in the skin and excreted in the urine when present in the blood in excessive amounts (hyperbilirubinemia). This characteristic makes jaundice a valuable indicator of a variety of disorders involving either hemolysis or biliary obstruction. When there is an obstruction blocking the flow of bile into the intestine, jaundiced persons may have clay-colored stools due to lack of bilirubin and its

This chapter incorporates material written for the fourth edition by Esther Matassarin-Jacobs and Kris Strasburg.

metabolites in the intestine. For a description of normal bilirubin metabolism, see Figure 63–7.

Etiology and Risk Factors

Jaundice can be classified according to the location of the pathologic change. Jaundice may occur because of a problem (1) in the blood before reaching the liver (hemolytic jaundice), (2) within the liver itself (hepatocellular jaundice), or (3) after the bilirubin leaves the liver (obstructive jaundice). The pathologic causes underlying these three types of jaundice are outlined briefly here and in more detail in Table 65–1.

■ Hemolytic Jaundice

Hemolytic jaundice results from excessive red blood cell destruction. It may be due to transfusion reactions, hemolytic anemia, severe burns, or defective albumin binding. The liver normally compensates for the increased unconjugated bilirubin it receives by increasing its rate of bilirubin conjugation. The excess can then be excreted in the urine and feces. Hemolytic jaundice disappears once the rate of hemolysis slows.

■ Hepatocellular Jaundice

Hepatocellular jaundice is due to defective uptake, conjugation, or transport of bilirubin by the liver. Liver cell dysfunction or necrosis caused by hepatitis, for example, or defective bile transport in the bile canal and small bile duct can cause hyperbilirubinemia. Stagnation of bile in the hepatic cells or in the intrahepatic or extrahepatic bile ducts is called cholestasis. Unknown channels absorb the pooled bile components into the bloodstream. Although "obstructive jaundice" usually refers to jaundice caused by an obstruction such as a stone, hepatic cellular damage can also cause an obstruction sufficient to cause jaundice.

Table 65–1. Types of Jaundice (Icterus)

	Causes	Assessment	Conjugated (Direct) Bilirubin (0.1–0.3 mg/dl)	Unconjugated (Indirect) Bilirubin (0.2–0.8 mg/dl)	Total Bilirubin (0.1–1.0 mg/dl)	Urinary Bilirubin (0)	Urinary Urobilinogen (0–4 mg/day)	Fecal Urobilinogen (40–280 mg/day)	AST (5–40 Units/L)	ALT (5–35 Units/L)	PTT (30–40 sec)	PT (12–15 sec)
					Laboratory Tests (Reference Values)*							
Hemolytic jaundice	Excessive hemolysis caused by transfusion reactions, some types of anemia such as sickle cell anemia, hemolytic disease of newborn, severe burns, bacterial toxins, venoms, hypotonic parenteral solutions, etc. Defective albumin binding.	Liver function usually normal; compensates for ↑ bilirubin by ↑ metabolism of bilirubin.	Normal	↑	↑	None	↑	↑	Normal	Normal	Normal	Normal
Hepatocellular jaundice	Liver's inability to conjugate or transport bilirubin to canaliculi for excretion due to hepatitis, liver congestion, cirrhosis, metastatic cancer, prolonged use of medications metabolized by liver, etc.	Liver may be enlarged. Abdomen may be tender. May have bruising or bleeding due to vitamin K malabsorption.†	↑	↑	↑	↑	↑↓	↓	↑	↑	Prolonged	Prolonged
Obstructive jaundice	Blocked flow of bile into duodenum due to inflammation, scar tissue, stones, or tumors in liver, biliary, or pancreatic system.	↑ Level of unconjugated bilirubin if liver cell function is diminished. May have bruising or bleeding due to vitamin K malabsorption (bile is necessary for vitamin K absorption).† Abdomen may be tender. Stools are clay-colored (bile gives stool its dark color). Urine is brown to foamy (conjugated bilirubin is excreted in urine).	↑	Normal or ↑	↑	↑	↓	Absent or ↓	Normal or slightly ↑	Normaly or slightly ↑	Prolonged	Prolonged

AST, aspartate aminotransferase; ALT, alanine aminotransferase; PTT, partial thromboplastin time; PT, prothrombin time.
*Reference values vary among laboratories.
†Parenteral vitamin K will improve prothrombin time only if jaundice is due to posthepatic cause.
Source: From Friedman, L. S. (1995). Liver, biliary tract and pancreas. In L. M. Tierney, et al. (Eds.), *Medical diagnosis and treatment manual* (34 ed., p. 557). Norwalk, CT: Appleton & Lange.

■ Obstructive Jaundice

Obstructive jaundice results from impaired bilirubin transport and excretion in the biliary system. In this case, the problem arises from obstruction of an extrahepatic bile duct caused by occlusion of the common duct by gallstones.

Clinical Manifestations and Diagnostic Findings

Manifestations of jaundice include yellow sclerae, yellowish-orange skin, clay-colored feces, tea-colored urine, pruritus, fatigue, and anorexia. Table 65–1 presents the laboratory diagnostic tests that are used to identify the underlying cause and type of jaundice. The following diagnostic test results are consistent with jaundice:

- Increased levels of direct (conjugated) serum bilirubin (>0.4 mg/100 ml) when excretion is blocked
- Increased indirect (unconjugated) serum bilirubin values (>0.8 mg/100 ml) when excretion is blocked
- Absence of bilirubin in the urine (unconjugated bilirubin is water-soluble) or increased urinary bilirubin (due to high blood concentrations)
- Increased urinary urobilinogen (>4 mg/24 hr) depending on the liver's ability to absorb urobilinogen from the portal system
- Reduced fecal urobilinogen (<40 mg/24 hr) because it does not reach the intestine
- Increased alkaline phosphatase and cholesterol serum levels because they cannot be excreted into the bile as normal (due to liver cell damage)
- In extreme cases of fulminant liver failure, an unusually low cholesterol level, indicating the liver's inability to synthesize it
- Increased serum bile salts with consequent deposition in the skin, causing pruritus
- Prolonged prothrombin time (>40 seconds) due to reduced absorption of vitamin K

Acute and Subacute Care

■ Medical Management

Treatment of jaundice aims to resolve the underlying disease. See Chapter 53 for a discussion of interventions in hemolytic anemia (hemolytic jaundice). Time and rest compose the primary treatment of jaundice in hepatitis. Treatment of hepatocellular jaundice is discussed later. Treatment of obstructive jaundice includes dissolution therapy or surgical removal of the obstruction.

■ Nursing Management of the Medical Client

Assessment

The client should be closely observed for the development of jaundice. Often, the first manifestation the client notices is a change in taste, manifesting as a distaste for a food or drink the client liked, such as coffee. The sclerae should be checked daily for the development of yellow coloration. Pruritus is another early manifestation of developing jaundice.

Diagnosis, Planning, Implementation

Impaired Skin Integrity. The most common nursing diagnosis for the client with jaundice is *Impaired Skin Integrity related to pruritus.*
   Planning: Expected Outcomes. The client will have itching controlled, as evidenced by the client's state-

ments of relief, decreased dryness of skin, and a decrease in scratching by the client.
   Implementation. Pruritus, caused by an accumulation of bile salts in the skin, results from obstructed biliary excretion. Some clients experience only mild itching. Others suffer such extreme itching that they may tear at their skin or scratch in their sleep.
   Oral cholestyramine resin provides some relief by binding bile salts in the intestine so they can be excreted. Antihistamines also may relieve the itching, as might tepid water or emollient baths, avoiding alkaline soap, and frequent application of lotions. Phenobarbital has been effective in some cases because of its ability to enhance bile flow.
   Encourage the client to wear loose soft clothing; provide soft linens (cotton is best), and change soiled linen as soon as possible. Keep the room cool.

Body Image Disturbance. Clients with jaundice often experience problems related to the nursing diagnosis *Body Image Disturbance related to yellowing of skin and sclerae.*
   Planning: Expected Outcomes. The client will cope with body image disturbance, as evidenced by the client's not isolating himself or herself, verbalizing and demonstrating acceptance of appearance (grooming, dress, posture, eating patterns, and presentation of self), and initiating new, or reestablishing existing, support systems.
   Implementation. A highly visible manifestation of illness, jaundice may have a considerable emotional impact and may impair body image. Reassure the client that this is usually a temporary condition. Assist the client in personal hygiene. Encourage the client to express feelings about his or her self-image.

Knowledge Deficit. Clients with jaundice may experience the nursing diagnosis *Knowledge Deficit related to cause of jaundice.*
   Planning: Expected Outcomes. The client will understand the cause of jaundice, as evidenced by the client's statements and ability to define the illness.
   Implementation. Clients often wonder why they are jaundiced, how long the condition will last, and how to cope with the problem. Encourage the client to ask questions about his or her health, treatment, and progress. Jaundice usually begins to disappear within 4 to 6 weeks. The return of normal stool and urine color is an indication of resolution.

Evaluation

The jaundice should resolve with the treatment of whatever condition is causing it. As the jaundice lessens, the client's appetite, body image, and pruritus improves.

■ Surgical Management

Surgical exploration of the common bile duct (choledochostomy) enables the diagnostician to differentiate between choledocholithiasis (stone in the common bile duct) and tumor. If carcinoma (usually of the head of the pancreas) is discovered during exploration, the surgeon may perform a palliative anastomosis of the gallbladder to the jejunum to bypass the common bile duct. See Chapter 66 for more complete information on the surgical management of the client having a choledochostomy.

■ Nursing Management of the Surgical Client

See Chapter 66 for complete information on the nursing management of clients undergoing a choledochostomy.

Hepatitis

Simply stated, hepatitis is inflammation of the liver. This inflammation may be caused by a virus, bacteria, or toxic substance. Jaundice usually develops, and the liver is tender. Other systemic manifestations depend on the causative agent and the degree of organ disruption.

There are several different types of hepatitis. These include viral, toxic, chronic, and alcoholic hepatitis.

Viral Hepatitis

The development of serologic tests has made possible the identification of a growing number of specific viruses causing viral hepatitis. The more common of these are hepatitis A, hepatitis B, hepatitis C, hepatitis D (delta agent) and hepatitis E. Although the manifestations are similar, each of these conditions is caused by a different virus and differs in incubation period, mode of transmission, and severity (Table 65–2).

Hepatitis occurs worldwide.

Hepatitis A. Hepatitis A is endemic in some areas of the world, especially areas with poor sanitation. Epidemics do occur in countries with good sanitation, however.

Hepatitis B. Hepatitis B is found worldwide, even in remote areas. Its incidence increases in areas of high population density and poor hygiene.

Hepatitis C. The hepatitis C virus is responsible for over 90% of cases of post-transfusion hepatitis and many cases of sporadic hepatitis. Only 4% of cases of hepatitis are caused by hepatitis C; intravenous (IV) drug use accounts for 50% of the cases.[15]

Hepatitis D (Delta Agent). Hepatitis D is always found with hepatitis B. The delta agent is endemic in some areas, such as the Mediterranean countries, where up to 80% of hepatitis B carriers may be superinfected with it.[15]

Hepatitis E. Hepatitis E is an RNA virus distinct from hepatitis A and the enteroviruses. It is associated with hepatitis outbreaks in India, Burma, Afghanistan, Algeria, and Mexico.

Etiology and Risk Factors

Agents that may cause viral hepatitis include hepatitis A virus, hepatitis B virus, Epstein-Barr virus (which causes infectious mononucleosis), cytomegalovirus, rubella, herpes simplex, varicella virus, retrovirus, yellow fever virus, coxsackievirus, adenovirus, and Marburg virus.

Hepatitis A. Hepatitis A, also known as short-incubation hepatitis, infectious hepatitis, and MS-1 hepatitis, is caused by an RNA virus of the enterovirus family. Causes of epidemics include infected water, milk, or food, especially raw shellfish from contaminated waters.

People who work with animals imported from areas where hepatitis A is endemic are at increased risk, as are persons who eat raw or steamed shellfish. In the general population, those under 15 years of age are at most risk.

Hepatitis A is transmitted primarily by the fecal-oral route. It spreads from person to person by close contact or by the handling of feces-contaminated articles. Because the infected client's feces contain the virus before the onset of manifestations, the remaining household members are at risk. This problem also may spread in an institution such as a daycare center, prison, or facility for developmentally disabled people. Spread of the disease is enhanced by crowding and poor sanitation.

Hepatitis B. Healthcare workers are at high risk of hepatitis B because of their close contact with the blood of carriers. Clients who had multiple blood transfusions or dialysis are also vulnerable to this infection. Other high-risk populations are homosexually active males, morticians, persons who undergo tattooing, and parenteral drug abusers.

The major sources of this infection are carriers and clients with the acute process. Contact with the serum of an infected client is the major mode of transmission. The virus also may be transmitted by other body fluids, such as saliva and semen. Hepatitis B virus can survive on environmental surfaces for at least a week.

Hepatitis C. Hepatitis C is transmitted parenterally through the blood, by personal contact, and possibly by the fecal-oral route. In contrast to hepatitis A, but similar to hepatitis B, hepatitis C may be spread by carriers.

Because hepatitis C is also parenterally transmitted, the risk factors are similar to those for hepatitis B.

Hepatitis D (Delta Agent). Hepatitis D is transmitted only through blood contact, so it is seen most commonly in clients exposed to blood and blood products, such as IV drug users and hemophiliac individuals. The risk factors for hepatitis D are the same as for hepatitis B.

Hepatitis E. Hepatitis E is a waterborne virus that primarily affects young adults. It has a short incubation and there is no evidence that it becomes chronic.

The risk factors for hepatitis E include travel to countries that have a high incidence of hepatitis E and eating or drinking food or water contaminated with the virus.

Table 65–2. Comparison of Five Types of Viral Hepatitis

Factor	Hepatitis A	Hepatitis B	Hepatitis C	Hepatitis D (Delta Agent)	Hepatitis E
Incidence	Endemic in areas of poor sanitation. Common in fall and early winter	Worldwide, especially in drug addicts, homosexuals, people exposed to blood and blood products. Occurs all year	Posttransfusion, those working around blood and blood products. Occurs all year	Causes hepatitis only in association with hepatitis B and only in presence of HB$_S$Ag. Endemic in Mediterranean	Parts of Asia, Africa, and Mexico where there is poor sanitation
Incubation period	2–6 wk	6 wk–6 mo (12–14 wk avg.)	6–7 wk	Same as hepatitis B	2–9 wk
Risk factors	Close personal contact or by handling feces-contaminated wastes	Healthcare workers in contact with body secretions, blood, and blood products. Hemodialysis and posttransfusion clients. Homosexually active males and drug abusers	Similar to hepatitis B	Same as hepatitis B	Traveling or living in areas where incidence is high
Transmission	Infected feces, fecal-oral route. May be airborne if copious secretions. Shellfish from contaminated water. Also rarely parenteral	Parenteral, sexual contact, and fecal-oral route. Carrier state	Contact with blood and body fluids. Source of infection uncertain in many clients. Carrier state	Coinfects with hepatitis B, close perdsonal contact. Carrier state	Fecal-oral route, food- or water-borne. No carrier state
Severity	Mortality low. Rarely causes fulminating hepatic failure	More serious, may be fatal. Mortality rate 10–20%	Can lead to chronic hepatitis	Similar to hepatitis B. More severe if occurs with chronic active hepatitis B	Illness self-limiting. Mortality rate in pregnant women 10%–20%
Diagnostic tests	Anti-HAV. IgM positive in acute hepatitis; IgG positive after infection	HB$_S$Ag or anti-HB$_c$-IgM.	Anti-HCV or anti-HDV. Recombinant immunoblot assay	HDAg-positive	Anti-HEV.
Prophylaxis and active or passive immunity	Hygiene. Immune globulin (passive). Vaccine under development (active)	Hygiene, avoidance of risk factors. Immune globulin (passive). Hepatitis B vaccine (active)	Hygiene. Immune globulin (passive)	Hygiene. Hepatitis B vaccine (active)	Hygiene, sanitation. No immunity

anti-HAV, antibody to hepatitis A virus; anti-HB$_C$-IgM, antibody to hepatitis B–IgM; anti-HCV, antibody to hepatitis C virus; anti-HEV, antibody to hepatitis E virus; HB$_S$Ag, hepatitis B surface antigen.

Prevention

To a great extent, viral hepatitis can be prevented by proper controls within the home, community, and health-care facility setting. See the Risk Factors and Levels of Prevention feature for more information.

Hepatitis A

Personal Hygiene. Because transmission of hepatitis A and possibly hepatitis C is by the fecal-oral route, good personal hygiene is important. Strict isolation of clients is not necessary but hand washing after bowel movement is required. Food handlers, especially, must wash their hands thoroughly. In some facilities, the disease is present because residents are unable to care for themselves properly. Care providers must supervise hand washing by ambulatory residents. Personnel in daycare centers need to wash their hands carefully after changing diapers.

Water Supply. Treatment of municipal water supplies prevents transmission of hepatitis A virus. Private water

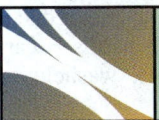

RISK FACTORS AND LEVELS OF PREVENTION

Hepatitis

Risk Factors

Hepatitis A. Individuals or populations who come in contact with contaminated food or water.

Hepatitis B. Homosexuals and intravenous drug users; clients and staff in hemodialysis units; physicians, nurses, dentists, and personnel working in clinical and pathology laboratories and blood banks; morticians; people who have tattoos.

Hepatitis C. Clients receiving blood transfusions; health professionals and laypersons who come in contact with blood and body fluids; handlers of primates (who are susceptible to infection).

Hepatitis D. Same as for hepatitis B.

Hepatitis E. Persons who live or travel in India, Burma, Afghanistan, Algeria, and Mexico.

Levels of Prevention

Primary Prevention

- Teach clients to pay strict attention to hygiene when preparing food, before leaving the toilet, and when in contact with people known to be exposed to hepatitis.
- Teach clients to avoid punctures by contaminated needles (or similar exposure to infective material).
- Encourage clients to avoid intimate sexual contact during the period of hepatitis B surface antigen (HB$_s$Ag) positivity.
- In the hospital, strict isolation may not be necessary if excreta, needles, and other medical supplies and utensils are carefully handled and discarded.

Secondary Prevention

- Advise clients to obtain passive immunization with immune globulin (within the first few days) if they have been in close contact with persons with hepatitis A.
- If clients travel in areas where public health and sanitation may be less than optimal, advise them to avoid drinking the water and eating fresh fruits, vegetables, and shellfish.
- Teach clients to request administration of a standard dose (0.02 ml/kg) of immune globulin before they embark on a trip.
- Administer hepatitis B vaccine to healthcare workers, clients, and individuals who come into contact with blood and body fluids.
- Administer hepatitis B immune globulin, which conveys passive immunity, after confirmed exposure to hepatitis B (i.e., needle puncture).
- Encourage clients to wear protective clothing and use good hand-washing technique when they are in contact with animals, especially primates.

Tertiary Prevention

- Teach all persons who come in contact with blood and body fluids the importance of basic public health and hygiene measures.
- Encourage clients to avoid strenuous activity and ingestion of excessive amounts of hepatotoxic agents (e.g., ethanol, acetaminophen).
- Instruct clients about possible infectivity to others.

supplies can be sources of contamination. Polluted fishing waters pose a threat. Shellfish that come from such waters are a major source of hepatitis A.

Restaurants. It is important for local health authorities to consistently and thoroughly inspect eating establishments. Serologic screening of food handlers for hepatitis A reduces its transmission. Because the disease can be transmitted via food, a person with active hepatitis A should not work in food services.

Animal Care. Isolating newly imported animals for a 2-month period would reduce the incidence of hepatitis A among people who handle them. If isolation is impossible, these persons need to wear protective clothing and use good hand-washing technique. If the risk of contamination is high, some physicians prescribe prophylactic standard immune globulin.

Active Immunization. An inactivated hepatitis A vaccine should be available commercially in the near future. It has proved effective in adults and children in clinical trials.

Passive Immunization. Again, physicians may prescribe standard immune globulin. Adverse effects of intramuscular injection include pain, tenderness, and at times hematoma formation. Immune globulin is helpful prophylaxis both before and after exposure. Immune globulin (gamma globulin, Gammar) is administered intramuscularly after exposure but not after the development of clinical manifestations. Clients who live in or visit high-risk areas can be protected for up to 3 months by immune globulin. The earlier in the incubation period that the prophylactic immune globulin is given, the greater the protection.

Hepatitis B

Control of Blood, Blood Products, and Skin-Piercing Instruments. Remember that hepatitis B is transmitted by the serum of the infected person. Therefore, blood, blood products, and instruments that pierce the skin and contact the vascular system are all potential sources of contamination. Some donor-related precautions that reduce the incidence of hepatitis B are the following:

1. Screening of donors' blood for hepatitis B virus surface antigen (HB_sAg), antibody to hepatitis B core antigen (anti-HB_c), antibodies to hepatitis C virus (anti-HCV), and elevated alanine aminotransferase (ALT), a "surrogate" marker of HCV[15]
2. Use of volunteer rather than paid donors
3. Registration of carriers
4. Sharing of accurate records between institutions
5. Testing of all pregnant women for HB_sAg. It is possible to reduce the transfusion recipient's exposure to hepatitis B by using blood products only when necessary, using only the necessary amount of blood or blood products, crosschecking laboratory data to re-

duce errors of reported results, avoiding commercially obtained blood, and encouraging clients who are having elective surgery to donate their own blood (autologous transfusions).

Many healthcare facilities use disposable equipment, especially needles and syringes, to reduce hepatitis transmission. Nondisposable equipment must be sterilized to prevent virus transmission. All healthcare workers, of course, follow the Centers for Disease Control universal precautions.

Personal Hygiene. Good personal hygiene reduces transmission. Clients with hepatitis B and hepatitis B carriers should not share razors, toothbrushes, washcloths, cigarettes, or other personal items.

Passive Immunization. Standard immune globulin may contain antibodies against hepatitis B. However, another preparation called *hepatitis B immune globulin* contains much higher levels of antibody. The vaccine is usually given in three doses. The second and third doses are given 1 month and 6 months after the initial dose. Physicians may prescribe hepatitis B immune globulin for postexposure prophylaxis when there has been percutaneous exposure to blood that contains HB_sAg.

Active Immunization. Hepatitis B vaccine may provide active immunization before exposure to hepatitis B virus. The injection is best given into the deltoid muscle. Authorities strongly recommend this killed virus vaccine for all persons in high-risk categories for hepatitis B, including not only healthcare workers but dialysis clients and attending personnel, clients requiring repeated transfusions, spouses of HB_sAg-positive persons, the sexually promiscuous (especially male homosexuals), prison workers, and handlers of primates. It may be used in conjunction with hepatitis B immune globulin after documented exposure to hepatitis B.

Hepatitis C

Recall that transmission of hepatitis C is similar to that of hepatitis B. Therefore, many of the same measures are useful in its prevention, although available evidence suggests that it is not as readily transmitted through sexual and household contacts as is hepatitis B. Physicians may prescribe standard immune globulin for postexposure passive immunization to hepatitis C. However, the role of this intervention as a preventive measure remains unclear, and at present, immune globulin is not officially recommended as prophylaxis. As with hepatitis A, there is no vaccine for active immunization against hepatitis C.

Hepatitis D (Delta Agent)

Because hepatitis D must coexist with hepatitis B, the hepatitis B vaccine can help prevent hepatitis D also. The precautions that help prevent hepatitis B also are useful in preventing delta hepatitis.

Hepatitis E

Since hepatitis E is responsible for waterborne hepatitis and is spread by the fecal-oral route in various parts of the world, attention to matters of personal hygiene and sanitation helps prevent the spread of this form of hepatitis, as it does with hepatitis A and hepatitis B.

Table 65–2 contains a summary of information on prophylaxis for the hepatitides.

Pathophysiology

The pathophysiology of viral hepatitis is similar regardless of the cause. Hepatocytes are damaged and become inflamed and necrosed by the body's immune response to the virus. This alters cellular function. The degree of functional impairment depends on the amount of hepatocellular damage. The endoplasmic reticulum (responsible for protein and steroid synthesis, glucuronide conjugation, and detoxification) is the first organelle to undergo change. Liver functions that depend on these processes are altered, the degree of impairment depending on the amount of damage to the endoplastic reticulum. Kupffer cells increase in size and number. Vascular and ductule tissues undergo inflammatory changes. The hepatocytes generally heal in 3 to 4 months.

Hepatitis A. Antibodies to hepatitis A virus (anti-HAV) appear early in the course of the illness. Both IgM and IgG anti-HAV are detectable in the serum soon after the onset of illness. IgM anti-HAV titers peak during the first week of the disease and usually disappear within 3 to 6 months. Detection of IgM anti-HAV is a valid test for demonstrating acute hepatitis. IgG anti-HAV peak titers occur after 1 month of the disease but may stay elevated for years; it is, therefore, an indicator of past infection.

Clients who are otherwise healthy usually recover from hepatitis A without major sequelae. Although hepatitis A has a low mortality rate, fulminant hepatitis A may result. The fulminant form resembles acute liver failure. It causes severe illness and even death.

Hepatitis B. The hepatitis B virus is a DNA virus that has an inner core and a surface envelope. The body forms antibodies to virus core antigen HB_cAg and HB_sAg. The presence of HB_sAg in the blood denotes (1) a previous or resolving infection with hepatitis B; (2) a continuing, chronic infection; or (3) immunization with immunoglobulin or hepatitis B vaccine.

Hepatitis C. The hepatitis C virus is a single-stranded RNA virus with properties similar to the virus that causes hepatitis B and hepatitis D. Hepatitis C virus is thought to be a pathogenic factor in conditions such as glomerulonephritis and autoimmune thyroiditis.

Hepatitis D (Delta Agent). Hepatitis D is a small defective RNA virus that causes hepatitis only in the presence of hepatitis B infection, and specifically only in the presence of HB_sAg.

Hepatitis E. The hepatitis E virus alters hepatocellular function in almost the same way as the other types of hepatitis viruses. It causes necrosis and liver cell damage.

Typically, persons with viral hepatitis completely recover from the illness in 3 to 16 weeks. Mortality from hepatitis A is low, except for the fulminant form. Persons with hepatitis B tend to develop more complications. One in 10 persons develops chronic active hepatitis as a result of hepatitis B, often leading to destruction of the liver. Cirrhosis may follow a severe case of hepatitis B or chronic active hepatitis. Primary hepatocellular carcinoma is a potential complication of chronic hepatitis.

Clinical Manifestations and Diagnostic Findings

Clients with viral hepatitis all experience liver inflammation and other sequelae that are similar. Hepatitis B and hepatitis D are usually the most severe, although they may be asymptomatic in some clients. The onset of manifestations varies from abrupt to insidious according to the incubation period and the degree of infectivity.

Manifestations of viral hepatitis are systemic and vary from client to client. Manifestations occurring during the earlier (prodromal) phase might include jaundice, lethargy, irritability, myalgia, arthralgia, anorexia, nausea, vomiting, abdominal pain, diarrhea or constipation, fever, and other flulike manifestations. Pruritus (itching) is typically mild and transient and may be more intense at its onset and termination. Jaundice may or may not be present, but when it is, it is first seen in the sclerae of the eyes and mucous membranes. Anicteric (without jaundice) hepatitis may or may not precede jaundice. Children with hepatitis are usually anicteric. Adults often note the appearance of darker urine and clay-colored stools a few days before clinical jaundice develops. The other manifestations often abate when jaundice appears, but they also may worsen.

If irritability and drowsiness become severe, assess for the possibility of hepatic encephalopathy. Deterioration of handwriting is an early manifestation of hepatic encephalopathy; thus, at each shift ask clients to write their name and observe their writing closely for changes. Asterixis, an abnormal muscle tremor sometimes called liver flap, may accompany encephalopathy. This manifestation is easily elicited by applying a blood pressure cuff and noting if the flapping is present when the cuff is released. Mild depression is not uncommon, because of (1) the nature of the illness (weakness, jaundice, itching, and nausea), (2) its length and cost, (3) confinement, and (4) forgetfulness and the inability to concentrate on completion of activities of daily living (ADLs).

Anemia may occur because of the decreased life span of erythrocytes. Erythrocyte destruction results from liver enzyme alterations. A transient hyperglycemia sometimes develops, and a client with diabetes may need to increase insulin dosage at this time. The liver is larger than normal with hepatitis and tender on palpation. Some people develop spider angiomas, palmar erythema, and gynecomastia, which disappear during the recovery period. A small percentage (5%–15%) of clients experience splenomegaly or enlargement of the posterior cervical lymph nodes. Occasionally, hepatitis B is accompanied by arthralgias, rash, vasculitis, or glomerulonephritis.

Major assessment findings and their pathophysiologic bases are summarized in Table 65–3.

Occasionally, the person develops cholestatic viral hepatitis syndrome. This uncommon disease process resembles mechanical obstruction. It is thus difficult to differentiate cholestatic viral hepatitis from biliary tract obstruction due to gallstones, strictures, and tumors. The cause and pathophysiology of this hepatitis variant are unclear. Cholestatic viral hepatitis syndrome causes jaundice, itching, and the typical flulike and gastrointestinal problems of hepatitis, but the manifestations often last longer and are more severe. Serum bilirubin reaches levels of 10 to 15 mg/100 ml. Diagnostic studies reveal elevations of serum lipoproteins, globulins, cholesterol, and alkaline phosphatase. Rarely, the liver progressively enlarges.

Other clients may manifest fulminant viral hepatitis. This life-threatening form resembles acute liver failure with manifestations of encephalopathy (increased excitability, insomnia, somnolence, and impaired mentation). The liver rapidly decreases in size. Other problems include gastrointestinal bleeding, disseminated intravascular coagulation, fever with leukocytosis and neutrophilia, hepatorenal problems of oliguria and azotemia, edema

Table 65–4. Serologic Tests for Viral Hepatitis

Hepatitis Type	Hepatitis A Antibody		HBsAg	HBsAb	HBcAb
	IgM	IgG			
Hepatitis A					
Acute	+	–	–	–	–
Immune	–	+	–	–	–
Hepatitis B					
Acute	–	–	+	–	+
Immune	–	–	–	+	+ or –
Chronic	–	–	+	+ or –	+ or –
Hepatitis C	Serologic markers in development				

HBcAb, hepatitis B core antibody; HBsAb, hepatitis B surface antibody; HBsAg, hepatitis B surface antigen.

and ascites, hypotension, respiratory failure, hypoglycemia, bacterial infection of the respiratory or urinary tract, or both, and thrombocytopenia and coagulopathy. The prognosis is poor, and death may occur before jaundice appears. A liver transplant may be performed to save the client's life.

Table 65–2 summarizes information on the modes of transmission and incubation periods of the hepatitides.

The serologic tests for viral hepatitis are presented in Table 65–4. Presence of HBsAg in the blood usually indicates that the person is infectious. Another antigen, HBeAg, is often associated with progression of acute hepatitis to chronic hepatitis and indicates a highly infectious state.

Levels of serum aminotransferases first rise and then begin to fall as bilirubin starts to increase. Levels that rise, peak, drop, and then rise again indicate severe liver damage and a poor prognosis. Jaundice may not be clinically recognizable until levels are about 3 mg/100 ml. Bilirubin that rises above 20 mg/100 ml and remains elevated for a long period may indicate severe liver necrosis, which has a poor prognosis. Mild prolongation of the prothrombin time sometimes occurs. The gamma globulin fraction and alkaline phosphatase are elevated in some clients. If hepatitis B is responsible, detection of HBsAg is possible even before the level of aspartate aminotransferase (AST) (formerly serum glutamic-oxaloacetic transaminase, SGOT) rises.

Acute and Subacute Care

■ Medical Management

The acute manifestations of hepatitis generally subside over 2 to 3 weeks. Complete clinical and laboratory re-

Table 65–3. Hepatitis Assessment Data

Assessment Data	Pathophysiologic Bases
Jaundice, clay-colored stools (no pigment); ↑ serum bilirubin; darkened urine (bilirubin and urobilin)	Impaired excretion of conjugated bilirubin Urobilin in blood excreted through kidneys instead of bowel
Pruritus	Bile salt accumulation in skin
Abdominal pain in right upper quadrant	Stretching of Glisson's capsule (surrounding liver) due to inflammation
Fever	Release of pyrogens in inflammatory process
Fatigue and weakness	Reduced energy metabolism by liver
Anorexia, nausea, vomiting	Changes in stomach or bowel
Bleeding tendencies	Reduced prothrombin synthesis by injured hepatic cells Reduced fat-soluble vitamin K absorption due to reduced bile in intestine
Anemia	Decreased red blood cell life due to liver enzyme alterations, hemorrhage

covery occurs in hepatitis A by 9 weeks and in hepatitis B and hepatitis C by 16 weeks. Less than 1% of clients with hepatitis develop severe complications.

Clients who have severe nausea and vomiting and have difficulty maintaining a fluid balance will need to be hospitalized if there is progressive deterioration.

General measures of treatment center around (1) pharmacotherapy, (2) dietary management, (3) management of activity level, (4) relief of pruritus, and (5) postexposure prophylaxis.

Clients are encouraged to monitor their activity level and avoid strenuous activity. If manifestations are severe, bedrest may be indicated with a gradual return to normal activity as manifestations subside. Management of pruritus may require emollients and lipid creams (e.g., Eucerin) to be prescribed. Corticosteroids have demonstrated no benefit in controlled studies of clients with viral hepatitis. Interferon-α, in preliminary trials, has proved to be of some benefit in acute hepatitis C, but further study is required.

Pharmacologic Treatment

Few medications are available for treating viral hepatitis. Antibiotics are not prescribed. Antiemetics control nausea and vomiting, but phenothiazines should not be used because they are biotransformed in the liver and therefore potentially toxic. Parenteral vitamin K may be given to clients with prolonged prothrombin time. Antihistamines may provide relief of pruritus but may cause excessive sedation.

Steroids. The corticosteroids are not necessary in uncomplicated cases of acute viral hepatitis, and authorities question their use in several cases. Corticosteroids may reduce the serum aminotransferase and bilirubin levels. However, they have no effect on liver necrosis or regeneration.

Estrogens. Estrogens can raise serum bilirubin levels. Therefore, clinicians need to evaluate the use of oral contraceptives during acute viral hepatitis.

Antilipemic Agents. The administration of an antilipemic cholestyramine, or urodiol, a gallstone-solubilizing agent, can relieve the pruritus associated with severe cholestatic liver disease. Cholestyramine acts by binding bile acids to form an insoluble complex that is excreted in the feces. Urodiol acts by inhibiting absorption of cholesterol.

Immune Globulin. Immune globulin, although not used to treat viral hepatitis, does provide prophylaxis for family and friends. If given early, standard immune globulin (proteins capable of acting as antibodies and formerly termed immune serum globulin) can prevent hepatitis A or mitigate the severity of manifestations. The hepatitis A virus does not remain in the blood long; therefore, there is no healthy carrier state for hepatitis A as there is for hepatitis B.

Vaccines. A vaccine is available to promote immunity to hepatitis B. It is administered prophylactically to persons such as healthcare workers who are considered at risk of developing hepatitis B. It is recommended that a person exposed to hepatitis B follow certain guidelines for receiving hepatitis B vaccine for prophylaxis, that is, proper sequencing of the injections.

Medications to Avoid. Clinicians administer very few medications to clients with hepatitis. Medications such as chlorpromazine, aspirin, acetaminophen, and a variety of sedatives are given as infrequently as possible because of their hepatotoxic properties.

Dietary Treatment

In general, a balanced diet high in carbohydrates and low in fat is recommended. Meals should be given in small portions and given four to six times daily. The client's food preferences should be accommodated. All alcoholic beverages are strictly forbidden.

Complications

Possible complications of hepatitis include fulminant hepatitis, chronic hepatitis, chronic persistent hepatitis, chronic active hepatitis, chronic carrier state, and aplastic anemia.

Fulminant Hepatitis. Fulminant hepatitis may occur in 1 to 2% of clients with hepatitis B and hepatitis C (rarely with hepatitis A). There is a progression of manifestations which include jaundice, hepatic encephalopathy, and ascites. The mortality rate varies with age but approaches 90% to 100%, especially in persons over 60 years old.

Chronic Hepatitis. Chronic hepatitis exists when liver inflammation continues beyond a period of 3 to 6 months. This disease may manifest as chronic persistent hepatitis (CPH) or chronic active hepatitis (CAH). Figure 65-1 compares biopsy findings in CPH and CAH.

Chronic Persistent Hepatitis. CPH may follow hepatitis B and hepatitis C. Most clients are asymptomatic although some may report fatigue, anorexia, and abdominal pain. Recurrent episodes are not acute in nature, and extrahepatic involvement seldom occurs. The clinical course is benign with fibrotic liver and cirrhosis developing only rarely. Clients with CPH generally have an excellent prognosis. Figure 65-2 illustrates common findings in CPH.

Chronic Active Hepatitis. CAH is demonstrated by elevated serum transaminase levels for more than 6 months. It is a complication of hepatitis B and hepatitis C. CAH causes a more severe illness than CPH. It leads to hepatic inflammation, hepatic necrosis, and progressive fibrosis with the client exhibiting manifestations of chronic liver disease such as splenomegaly and spider angiomas. These clients are also at risk of hepatocellular carcinoma.

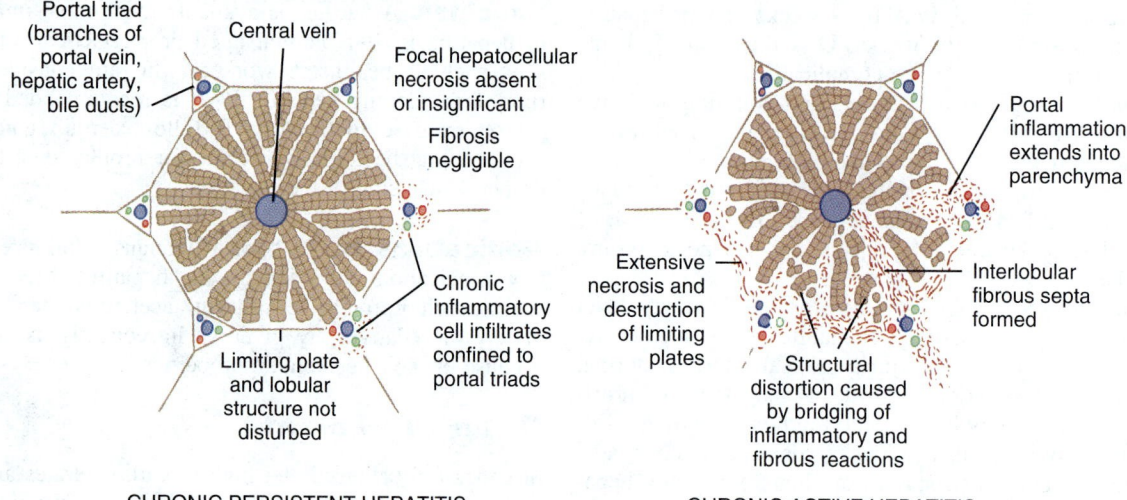

CHRONIC PERSISTENT HEPATITIS   CHRONIC ACTIVE HEPATITIS

Figure 65–1. Comparison of biopsy findings in chronic persistent hepatitis and chronic active hepatitis. Inflammation is confined to portal triads in chronic persistent hepatitis but extends into the parenchyma in chronic active hepatitis.

In most instances, CAH results from an autoimmune response or from the hepatitis B virus with or without superimposed hepatitis D infection. Autoimmune CAH is more common in females (Fig. 65–3), whereas hepatitis B CAH is more common in males. The pathogenesis in hepatitis B CAH indicates an autoimmune response with low-level anti-HB$_c$-IgM present in 70% of the clients.

Cytomegalovirus infection during an immunosuppressed state is another viral cause. CAH may also follow acute hepatitis C or post-transfusion hepatitis. When CAH presents in adolescents, it may arise from Wilson's disease, a hereditary disorder. In addition, methyldopa, dantrolene, nitrofurantoin, and isoniazid cause inflammatory changes consistent with CAH. Discontinuing the medication usually resolves the inflammatory process.

The onset of CAH is slow. Some clients report the manifestations of acute viral hepatitis, cirrhosis, or extrahepatic problems. Clients go to the acute care setting primarily for liver biopsy and the identification of extrahepatic sequelae, for example, thyroiditis, hemolytic anemia, amenorrhea, arthritis, urticaria, or glomerulonephritis.

There is no overall effective treatment for CAH. Some physicians may prescribe steroids, with or without azathioprine (Imuran), in the treatment of idiopathic CAH. This usually reduces manifestations, improves laboratory test results, suppresses the inflammatory response viewed on biopsy, and lowers the short-term and long-term morbidity and mortality.

With steroid therapy, fatigue and anorexia resolve in a few days or weeks. Laboratory values return to normal

PHYSICAL ASSESSMENT FINDINGS   LABORATORY FINDINGS

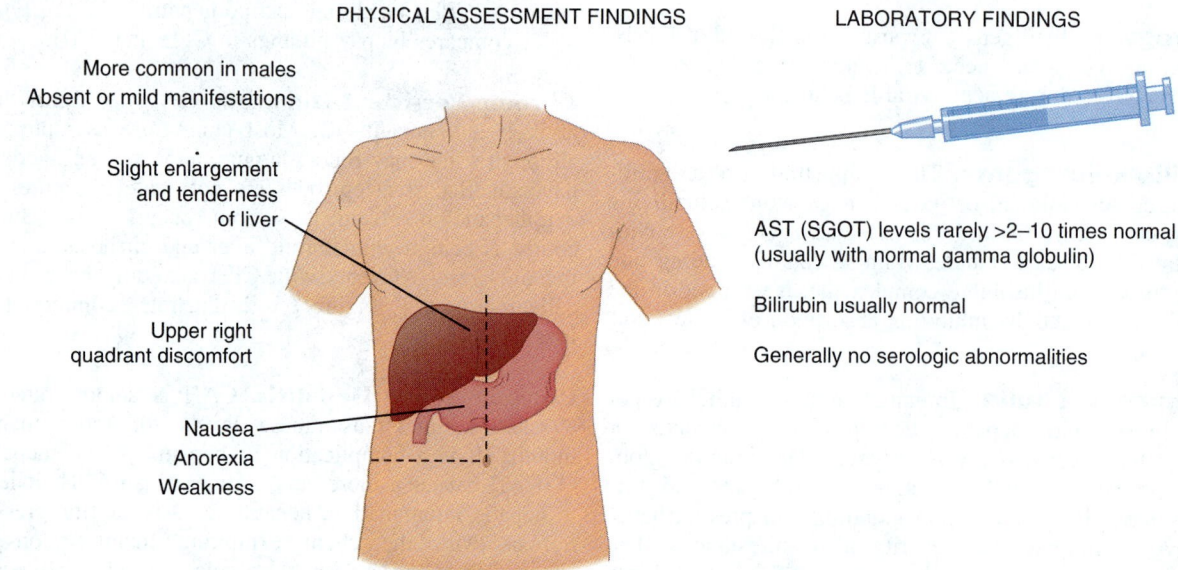

More common in males
Absent or mild manifestations

Slight enlargement
and tenderness
of liver

Upper right
quadrant discomfort

Nausea
Anorexia
Weakness

AST (SGOT) levels rarely >2–10 times normal
(usually with normal gamma globulin)

Bilirubin usually normal

Generally no serologic abnormalities

Figure 65–2. Chronic persistent hepatitis: common assessment findings. AST, aspartate amino transferase; SGOT, serum glutamic-oxaloacetic transaminase.

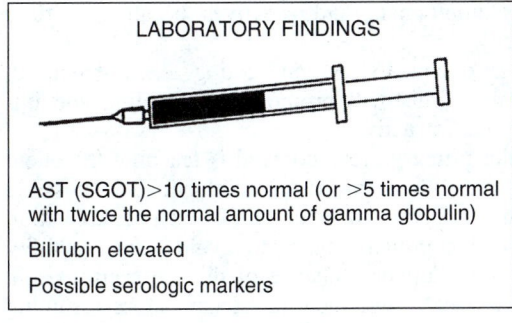

LABORATORY FINDINGS

AST (SGOT)>10 times normal (or >5 times normal with twice the normal amount of gamma globulin)

Bilirubin elevated

Possible serologic markers

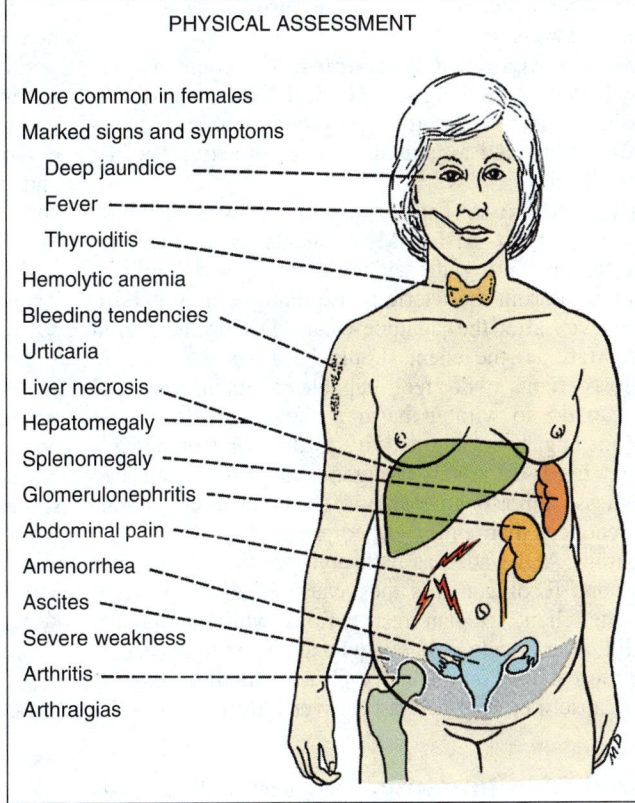

PHYSICAL ASSESSMENT

More common in females

Marked signs and symptoms

Deep jaundice

Fever

Thyroiditis

Hemolytic anemia

Bleeding tendencies

Urticaria

Liver necrosis

Hepatomegaly

Splenomegaly

Glomerulonephritis

Abdominal pain

Amenorrhea

Ascites

Severe weakness

Arthritis

Arthralgias

Figure 65–3. Chronic active hepatitis (idiopathic): common assessment findings. AST, aspartate aminotransferase; SGOT, serum glutamic-oxaloacetic transaminase.

within weeks or months. The physician reduces the dose of steroids in small increments to prevent a relapse and allow the adrenal glands time to resume normal secretion.

Clients being treated for CAH should be followed closely and have liver tests periodically. There is a need to monitor the possible side effects of drug treatments and perform liver biopsies every 6 months to 1 year. Untreated CAH has a high mortality rate. Death results from hepatic failure, bleeding varices, hepatic encephalopathy, or primary hepatocellular carcinoma.

Liver transplantation is a consideration for those persons with endstage liver disease that can no longer be medically managed.

Chronic Carrier State. In the United States, 0.1 to 0.5% of the population are in a chronic carrier state for hepatitis B.[10] A carrier state may also occur for hepatitis C in that blood donated by apparently healthy clients may transmit hepatitis C when transfused.

Aplastic Anemia. Aplastic anemia, although rare, has a high mortality rate when it occurs after acute viral hepatitis. No treatment has been demonstrated to be effective in reversing this condition.

Management of clients with complications is supportive and palliative. Therapy includes administration of (IV) fluids to provide hydration, correction of electrolyte abnormalities, administration of medications for relief of pain and nausea, and provision of adequate caloric intake.

Outcomes

Nearly all clients with acute viral hepatitis demonstrate normal results on liver function tests by 8 to 10 weeks. The clinical course, morbidity, and mortality of viral hepatitis, however, may vary considerably. In most cases, clients recover in 3 to 16 weeks with liver function tests demonstrating evidence of liver dysfunction for a longer time. Most clients recover completely with a mortality rate of less than 1%. The rate is reportedly higher in older people.[42]

■ Nursing Management of the Medical Client

Assessment

Always begin by questioning the client about possible exposure to risk factors to assess the type of hepatitis present. The presence of common manifestations, especially jaundice, is assessed, as are manifestations of progression of the disease, such as hepatic encephalopathy (see Hepatic Encephalopathy). Liver function studies are assessed and monitored to ascertain progression of the disease.

Diagnosis, Planning, Implementation

Fatigue. The client with hepatitis has tremendous metabolic demands leading to the nursing diagnosis *Fatigue* related to decreased metabolic energy production secondary to liver dysfunction.

Planning: Expected Outcomes. The client will relate the lessening of fatigue and the heightening of energy, as evidenced, respectively, by compliance with activity restrictions and a gradual increase in activity to the preillness level.

Implementation. Fatigue associated with hepatitis may interfere with ADLs. Most clients experience the greatest fatigue during the anicteric phase and begin to feel stronger during the icteric phase. Fatigue may persist, however, even after the jaundice clears. During the period of severe fatigue, the client should be advised to rest in bed. Most clients who feel capable of being up and around can do so without harm if they rest after meals and do not engage in any activity to the point of becoming overly tired. Because prolonged bedrest itself can lead to weakness, a reasonable activity level is more conducive to recovery than enforced bedrest.

Encourage ADLs such as bathroom privileges, personal hygiene, and feeding unless they cause excessive fatigue. Advise the client to plan rest periods while jaundiced, especially after meals. Clients who engage in excessive activity too early in the recovery phase sometimes experience a relapse, possibly leading to liver failure.

Impaired Skin Integrity. The client with hepatitis experiences jaundice leading to the nursing diagnosis *Impaired Tissue Integrity related to pruritus secondary to jaundice.*

Planning: Expected Outcomes. The client will have pruritus relieved, as evidenced by the client's statements of comfort and the absence of scratching.

Implementation. Clients with severe jaundice may suffer pruritus. See Jaundice for a discussion of nursing interventions for itching.

Evaluation

Since the clinical course of acute viral hepatitis varies considerably with each client, the nurse must carefully assess whether the goals have been met in the treatment of the client. Recovery without permanent liver damage is the most favorable outcome. Permanent damage may occur if the therapeutic regimen is not followed.

Community and Self-Care

■ Medical Management

Most clients recover from acute viral hepatitis, do not require hospitalization, and are appropriately managed at home. However, clinical and biochemical relapses may occur before full recovery. In addition, complications of acute viral hepatitis may develop and necessitate careful monitoring, especially in elderly clients.

There is no specific ongoing pharmacologic management of clients recovering from acute viral hepatitis. Advise the client to avoid alcohol and medications such as aspirin, acetaminophen, and sedatives because of their hepatotoxicity.

Encourage clients to continue eating a well-balanced, nutritional diet. This will promote liver healing and improve tolerance for activity.

One of the primary areas covered is teaching the client and significant others to avoid reinfection or possible spread of the infection to other family members. Caution the client and significant other to avoid sexual activity until there is no longer a chance of disease transmission. They should check with their physician before resuming sexual relations.

The client must understand the need for adequate rest so the liver can heal on its own. The client needs to be active enough to prevent complications of immobility but not so active as to risk relapse.

The client is expected to avoid reinfection or possible spread of the infection to other family members. The client is also expected to resume prehepatitis activities and not to develop complications.

■ Nursing Management of the Medical Client

Assessment

Assess the client's and family's ability to provide home and self-care. Their understanding of the disease and its implications are vital to successful management of the disease in the home setting.

Diagnosis, Planning, Implementation

Impaired Physical Mobility. An important factor for healing in the client with hepatitis is rest so that the liver can repair itself, which leads to an important nursing diagnosis, *Impaired Physical Mobility related to prolonged bedrest.*

Planning: Expected Outcomes. The client will regain mobility and not suffer from the complications of immobility, as evidenced by increasing mobility and the absence of complications.

Implementation. In very severe cases of hepatitis, the client may need to remain in bed for a prolonged period. In this case, you will need to intervene to prevent the complications of prolonged immobility, for example, pressure sores, contractures, anorexia, and depression. For detailed information on preventing problems due to immobility, see Chapter 74.

Altered Nutrition: Less than Body Requirements. In order for the liver to properly heal and regenerate, nutrition is important. Clients with hepatitis often have a decreased appetite, making the nursing diagnosis *Altered Nutrition: Less than Body Requirements related to anorexia, nausea, bile stasis, and altered absorption and metabolism* a common diagnosis.

Planning: Expected Outcomes. The client will maintain an intake of the required calories to maintain weight, as evidenced by no weight loss and possible weight gain.

Implementation. To help the client meet the nutritional requirements associated with hepatitis, the nurse needs to do the following:

- Provide a nutritious breakfast. Anorexia usually worsens during the day, so breakfast may be the best-tolerated meal.
- Encourage the client to avoid fatty food, which can induce nausea.
- In general, the diet should include the optimal amount of protein and carbohydrates to allow recovery of injured liver cells without overfeeding. If the client has no problem with protein metabolism, a normal intake is helpful for tissue repair. However, clients with very severe hepatitis who are in danger of developing hepatic encephalopathy require a diet low in protein (because of the buildup of ammonia in the blood). Alterations in fat metabolism differ according to the degree of interruption of bile production and excretion.
- Suggest multiple small meals. This allows the client with anorexia to ingest a diet of 2500 to 3000 calories more comfortably. Also, candy, juice, sweetened tea, and carbonated drinks can supply calories when nausea is a problem.
- Remind the client to avoid alcohol, because it is an extremely hepatotoxic agent.
- Tell the client that vitamin supplements are not generally necessary in uncomplicated hepatitis, provided the diet is adequate in nutrients. Vitamin K supplements, as ordered, may be administered if the prothrombin time is longer than normal.
- Clients who develop severe nausea and vomiting may obtain relief from antiemetics. However, before these medications are administered, their effect on liver function should be reviewed. Phenothiazines such as prochlorperazine (Compazine) are usually contraindicated. Clients who are unable to tolerate any oral intake may require IV nutrition.

Anxiety. It is often difficult to predict the outcome of hepatitis; therefore, the nursing diagnosis *Anxiety related to uncertainty of the effects of hepatitis* is a common diagnosis.

Planning: Expected Outcomes. The client will have a decrease in anxiety, as evidenced by the ability to discuss his or her feelings about the disease.

Implementation. Clients with hepatitis should be encouraged to express their feelings concerning the following:

1. Their illness
2. The duration and cost of the illness
3. Alterations in home life and in finances (especially for the parent of young children or for the sole breadwinner)
4. The effect of the illness on future health problems
5. The possibility of death if they are very ill.

Suggest psychosocial and financial counseling for the client who is disturbed. Teaching and subsequent understanding will greatly decrease anxiety.

Knowledge Deficit. In order for the client and significant others to manage hepatitis at home, the nursing diagnosis of *Knowledge Deficit related to cause of disease, modes of transmission, and its course* is a common diagnosis.

Planning: Expected Outcomes. The client will understand the disease and its treatment, as evidenced by the client's ability to state the causes of the disease and the rationales for treatment.

Implementation. Teaching for the client with hepatitis varies with the causative agent. In addition to teaching how to prevent recurrence and spread, instruct the client to return to former activity levels slowly in order to avoid a relapse. Instructions concerning the diet need to be clear.

Nursing intervention involves administering medications and supportive management. As stated previously, it is important to discontinue medications that may be causing inflammatory changes. Clients who cannot tolerate large doses of steroids may benefit from azathioprine and smaller steroid doses. Clinicians generally do not recommend steroid therapy for asymptomatic CAH, especially in elderly clients. In addition to pharmacologic intervention, bedrest is encouraged during the active phase of the disease. The client usually remains at home to convalesce. There may be periods of remission, but liver necrosis continues.

The client may need help at home after discharge because limits on activity will still have to be maintained. The client may need help with housework or shopping. The client needs to be seen at regular intervals after discharge to ensure that the liver is healing and no further damage has occurred.

Evaluation

Since hepatitis has no specific treatment, it is difficult to predict the exact course of the disease. With adequate rest and nutrition, the disease should resolve without complications.

■ Modifications for Elderly Clients

As clients age, the liver shrinks and consequently has less storage capacity. It also may have some age-related changes that place the elderly at higher risk of liver damage. Consequently, they are at greater risk of developing complications.

Toxic Hepatitis

Toxins and drugs may produce a wide variety of pathologic lesions in the liver. Some agents may cause toxic hepatitis, whereas others produce necrosis, cholestasis, or neoplasms. The extent and type of hepatitis produced by the toxin depends on the degree of exposure, the chemical properties of the hepatotoxin, and the genetic make-up of the individual. Most commonly, it is a toxic metabolite formed by the drug-metabolizing enzymes within the liver that is the causative agent. Table 65–5 lists some hepato-

Table 65–5. Substances Known to Be Hepatotoxic		
	Type of Liver Alteration	
	Hepatitis	*Cholestasis*
Dose-related	Acetaminophen	Oxymetholone
	Amanita phalloides (mushroom)	
	Aspirin	
	Benzene	
	Carbon tetrachloride	
	Chloroform	
	Methotrexate	
	Phosphorus	
	Tetracyclines	
Idiosyncratic	Halothane	Allopurinol
	Isoniazid	Anabolic steroids
	Methyldopa	Carbamazepine
	Nitrofurantoin	Chlordiazepoxide
	Oxacillin	Chlorpromazine
	Phenytoin	Chlorpropamide
	Quinidine	Diazepam
	Sulfasalazine	Erythromycin estolate
	Sulfa drugs	Flurazepam
	Sulfanilamides	Oral contraceptives
	Sulfonamides	Propylthiouracil
	Valproic acid	Thiazides

Source: Data from Di Marin, A. J. (1994). Gastrointestinal diseases. In A. R. Myers (Ed.), *Medicine,* (2nd. ed.; pp. 225–226). Philadelphia: Harwal.

toxic agents. Liver necrosis occurs within 2 or 3 days after acute exposure to a dose-related hepatotoxin. However, several weeks may pass before manifestations of idiosyncratic reactions appear. Persons with either process develop abnormal reactions to liver function tests.

People who are repeatedly exposed to hepatotoxins in minimal amounts but over long periods of time may develop chronic hepatitis or cirrhosis. Persons experiencing a hypersensitivity reaction may demonstrate eosinophilia, fever, arthralgia, and sometimes xanthomatosis (an excessive accumulation of lipids brought about by faulty lipid metabolism).

Nursing intervention consists of obtaining a detailed drug history and information about past exposure and the response to a suspect agent. This is followed by removal of the causative agent, rest, alleviation of side effects (e.g., cholestyramine for pruritus), and a high calorie diet with fats and protein, as tolerated. Protein intake may be restricted if there is evidence of impending hepatic encephalopathy. Steroids have not proved of value in treatment of drug-induced liver disease, although they may suppress the manifestations caused by the reaction of the toxic agent.

Renal failure sometimes appears as a complication of toxic hepatitis. Assessment and interventions for renal failure are discussed in Chapter 57.

Chronic Hepatitis

Chronic hepatitis was discussed earlier as a complication of acute hepatitis.

Alcoholic Hepatitis

Alcoholic hepatitis may be acute or chronic. It is caused by parenchymal necrosis resulting from heavy alcohol ingestion. Although sometimes reversible, this condition is the most frequent cause of cirrhosis. This fact is important because cirrhosis of the liver is a common cause of death among adults in the United States.

Clinical manifestations of alcoholic hepatitis usually develop following a bout of heavy drinking. Assessment reveals anorexia, nausea, abdominal pain, splenomegaly, hepatomegaly, jaundice, ascites, fever, and encephalopathy. Laboratory studies typically show anemia, leukocytosis, and an elevated serum bilirubin. Liver biopsy reveals a typically fatty-appearing liver.

Nursing intervention includes a high vitamin, high carbohydrate diet; folic acid and thiamine supplements; and parenteral fluids. Administration of liquid formulas may be useful in increasing caloric intake. Steroids sometimes have a beneficial effect, although their use remains controversial.

Hepatitis due to excessive alcohol intake has a poor prognosis, particularly if the client continues to use alcohol.

Cirrhosis

Cirrhosis of the liver is a chronic, progressive disease characterized by widespread fibrosis and nodule formation. Cirrhosis occurs when the normal flow of blood, bile, and hepatic metabolites is altered by fibrosis and changes in the hepatocytes, bile ductules, vascular channels, and reticular cells.

There are four major types of cirrhosis: Laënnec's (alcoholic, micronodular, and portal), postnecrotic (macronodular or toxin-induced), biliary, and cardiac (Table 65–6). The two major clinical problems in cirrhosis are (1) decreased liver function and (2) portal hypertension. The latter develops in severe cirrhosis.

The ninth leading cause of death in the United States in 1994 was cirrhosis with an age-adjusted death rate of 10.4 per 100,000. Of those, 45% were alcohol-related.[15] Men are more likely than women to develop alcoholic or Laënnec's cirrhosis. Cirrhosis is the fourth leading cause of death in persons between 35 and 54 years of age.

Worldwide, postnecrotic cirrhosis is the most common type of cirrhosis. It is also more common in women. Mortality is higher from all types of cirrhosis in men and nonwhites.

Etiology and Risk Factors

The causes of cirrhosis have not been clearly identified, although the relationship between cirrhosis and excessive alcohol ingestion is well established. Countries with the highest incidence of cirrhosis have the greatest per capita consumption of alcohol. Genetic predisposition with a familial tendency, as well as a hypersensitivity to alcohol, is seen in alcoholic cirrhosis.

The primary risk factor for cirrhosis is alcohol ingestion, especially in the absence of proper nutrition. Any client with a family history of alcoholism should avoid alcohol because of the increased risk. The Risk Factors and Levels of Prevention feature lists other factors that may contribute to cirrhosis.

Laënnec's or Micronodular Cirrhosis. This form of cirrhosis, as noted previously, is most commonly found in clients who chronically abuse alcohol. However, it is also found in nondrinkers. The quantity of alcohol that causes the diffuse scarring of micronodular cirrhosis varies from client to client. The amount of alcohol consumed daily appears to be a more important factor than the pattern (binge versus daily) of drinking or type of alcoholic beverage consumed. If the client is in a poor nutritional state, the damage is more likely and more severe.

Postnecrotic Cirrhosis. This type of cirrhosis usually follows acute viral hepatitis, although it may be due to exposure to industrial or chemical hepatotoxins such as carbon tetrachloride or arsenic.

Viral hepatitis is the primary risk factor for postnecrotic cirrhosis, and thus it is very important for the client with hepatitis to avoid other stressors and allow the liver to heal completely without further insult. Clients with hepatitis must avoid exposure to other hepatotoxins.

Avoidance of industrial or chemical compounds by working in well-ventilated areas and taking other safety measures reduces the risk from these toxins.

Biliary Cirrhosis. Biliary cirrhosis occurs secondary to chronic biliary inflammation or obstruction. Prompt treatment of biliary disorders helps reduce the risk of biliary cirrhosis.

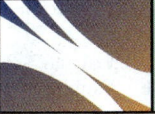

RISK FACTORS AND LEVELS OF PREVENTION

Cirrhosis

Risk Factors

Alcohol abuse; family history of alcoholism; biliary cirrhosis: primary—intrahepatic cholestasis (immune process suspected); secondary—obstruction of extrahepatic bile ducts; drugs (e.g. acetaminophen, methotrexate, methyldopa, isoniazid); chronic active hepatitis caused by hepatitis B or hepatitis C; hepatic congestion from severe right-sided, long-term heart failure; constrictive pericarditis; valvular disease; alpha$_1$-antitrypsin deficiency; infiltrative diseases (amyloidosis, hemochromatosis, glycogen storage diseases); Wilson's disease; nutritional: jejunal bypass

Levels of Prevention

Primary Prevention

- Urge clients to avoid alcohol ingestion.
- Advise clients to avoid travel to countries and areas where the incidence of hepatitis B, C, or E is high.
- Assist clients to learn how to maintain good nutritional status.
- Correct any mechanical obstruction to bile.
- Instruct clients to seek medical therapy for cardiovascular disorders.

Secondary Prevention

- Monitor clients for development of complications and deterioration in physical or mental status.
- Encourage clients to eat nourishing, well-balanced diets.
- Support client efforts to stop alcohol abuse.

Tertiary Prevention

- Teach clients the importance of compliance with treatment of cardiovascular disease.
- Teach clients about the dangers and risks of alcohol.
- Teach clients about the importance of avoiding alcohol if there is a family history of alcoholism.
- Show clients how to monitor for development of complications.
- Support clients in making life-style changes.

Table 65–6. Comparison of Postnecrotic, Biliary, Cardiac, and Laënnec's Cirrhosis

Definition	Etiology	Pathology	Assessment Data	Diagnosis and Prognosis	Intervention
Postnecrotic (macronodular) cirrhosis					
Most common worldwide form Massive loss of liver cells, with irregular patterns of regenerating cells	Postacute viral (types B and C) hepatitis Postintoxication with industrial chemicals Some infections and metabolic disorders	Liver small and nodular	Similar to Laënnec's except less muscle wasting and more jaundice	Needle biopsy of liver establishes pathologic processes Within 5 years 75% die of complications ↑ Serum aminotransferases ↑ Gamma globulins	Treat complications as needed
Biliary cirrhosis					
Bile flow is decreased with concurrent cell damage to hepatocytes around bile ductules	*Primary* Chronic stasis of bile in intrahepatic ducts Cause unknown Autoimmune process implicated *Secondary* Obstruction of bile ducts outside of liver	Early-stage biopsy reveals inflammatory process with necrosis of cells and ducts Hepatocytes are lost and scar tissue remains Endstage similar to postnecrotic	Generalized pruritus Dark urine Pale stools Jaundice Impaired bile flow Steatorrhea ↓ absorption of fat-soluble vitamins Elevated serum lipids ↑ Cholesterol deposits in subcutaneous tissues Signs of portal hypertension	Elevated serum bilirubin levels *Early:* 3–10 mg/100 ml *Late:* >50 mg/100 ml High elevations of alkaline phosphatase ↑ Gamma globulins ↑ Blood lipids Presence of lipoprotein X ↑ Serum bile salts Hypoprothrombinemia ↑ Antimitochondrial antibody in primary cases ↑ Serum copper in primary cases	*Primary* Treatment is symptomatic, e.g., high-calorie diet, lower intake of fats by 30–40 g/day if problems develop Cholestyramine for pruritus Supplement of fat-soluble vitamins *Secondary* Treatment to relieve mechanical obstruction

AST, aspartate aminotransferase; RUQ, right upper quadrant.
Data from Friedman, L. S. (1995). Liver, biliary tract and pancreas. In L. M. Tierney et al. (Eds.), *Medical diagnosis and treatment manual* (pp. 568–571). Norwalk, CT: Appleton & Lange; and Boyer, T. D. (1992). Cirrhosis of the liver and its major sequelae. In J. B. Wyngaarden, et al. (Eds.), *Cecil's textbook of medicine* (19th ed., p. 788). Philadelphia: W. B. Saunders.

Cardiac Cirrhosis. This type of cirrhosis is secondary to congestive heart failure with prolonged venous hepatic congestion. Adequate treatment of congestive heart failure can help prevent cardiac cirrhosis.

Pathophysiology

Cirrhosis is the final stage in many types of liver insults. The cirrhotic liver usually has a nodular consistency, with bands of fibrosis (scar tissue) and small areas of regenerating tissue. There is extensive destruction of hepatocytes. This alteration in the architecture of the liver alters flow in the vascular and lymphatic systems and bile duct channels. Periodic exacerbations are marked by bile stasis, precipitating jaundice.

Portal hypertension develops in severe cirrhosis. Recall that the portal vein receives blood from the intestines and spleen. Thus, an increase of pressure in the portal vein causes (1) a retrograde increase in pressure resistance and enlargement of the esophageal, umbilical, and superior rectus veins, which may result in bleeding varices; (2) ascites (the result of osmotic or hydrostatic shifts leading to fluid accumulation in the peritoneum); and (3) incomplete clearing of protein metabolic wastes, yielding an increase in ammonia, thus leading to hepatic encephalopathy.

Continuation of the process from unknown causes or

Definition	Etiology	Pathology	Assessment Data	Diagnosis and Prognosis	Intervention
Cardiac cirrhosis					
Chronic liver disease associated with severe right-sided long-term congestive heart failure (fairly rare)	Atrioventricular valve disease Prolonged constrictive pericarditis Decompensated cor pulmonale	*Early* Dark-colored liver enlarged by blood and edema fluid *Late* Liver capsule thickens and nodular scarring occurs	Slight jaundice, enlarged liver, and ascites in person with severe cardiac impairment over 10-year span RUQ pain during acute congestion Cachexia Fluid retention Circulatory problems	↑ Conjugated bilirubin in serum ↑ Sulfobromophthalein ↓ Albumin in serum ↑ Serum aminotransferases ↑ Alkaline phosphatase Liver biopsy *Prognosis* Depends on course of cardiac disease[26]	Cause of chronic congestive failure is treated if possible
Laënnec's cirrhosis					
Laënnec's cirrhosis (micronodular) Small nodules form as a result of persistence of some offending agent	Associated with alcohol absue	Scarring and collagen tissue deposits Regenerating nodules are very small Normal lobular structure is destroyed	May produce no symptoms for long periods Onset of symptoms may be insidious or abrupt *Early:* weakness, fatigue, weight loss *Later:* Anorexia, nausea, and vomiting Abdominal pain Ascites Menstrual irregularities Impotence Enlarged breasts in men Hematemesis Spider angiomas	Liver biopsy; history of alcohol abuse; high AST; high bilirubin (slight); anemia Prognosis depends on presence of complications and continued abuse of alcohol	Correction of vitamin and mineral deficiencies if any (e.g., folate, thiamine, pyridoxine, vitamin K, and minerals [magnesium and phosphate]; treat complications as needed (e.g., ferrous sulfate for anemia, IV vasopressin for esophageal varices, reduce or withhold dietary protein for hepatic encephalopathy or vitamin K for hemorrhagic tendency)

from alcohol abuse usually results in death from hepatic encephalopathy, bacterial (gram-negative) infection, peritonitis (bacterial), hepatoma (liver tumor), or complications of portal hypertension.

Clinical Manifestations and Diagnostic Findings

Table 65–7 gives the pathophysiologic bases for assessment data in advanced cirrhosis. Figure 65–4 illustrates the clinical characteristics of severe cirrhosis. Manifestations of cirrhosis diminish if the process is arrested at an early stage.

Cirrhosis is a disease that initially progresses slowly. Thus people with cirrhosis often discover the condition incidentally when seeking healthcare for other problems. In the early stages of cirrhosis, findings include hepatomegaly (enlarged liver), vascular changes, and abnormal laboratory tests. Palpation reveals a firm (scarred), lumpy (nodular), usually enlarged liver (although the liver becomes hard and shrunken in late cirrhosis).

In advanced cirrhosis, assessment reveals severe complications such as ascites, gastrointestinal bleeding from varices, or encephalopathy. Splenomegaly (enlarged spleen) indicates severe portal hypertension. Anemia, leukopenia, or thrombocytopenia may result from splenomegaly.

Laboratory results reveal impaired hepatocellular function: elevated liver serum enzymes (AST, ALT, and lactate dehydrogenase), hypoalbuminemia, anemia, and elevated prothrombin time. Liver biopsy provides definitive diagnosis and its sequelae.

Understanding Cirrhosis and Its Treatment

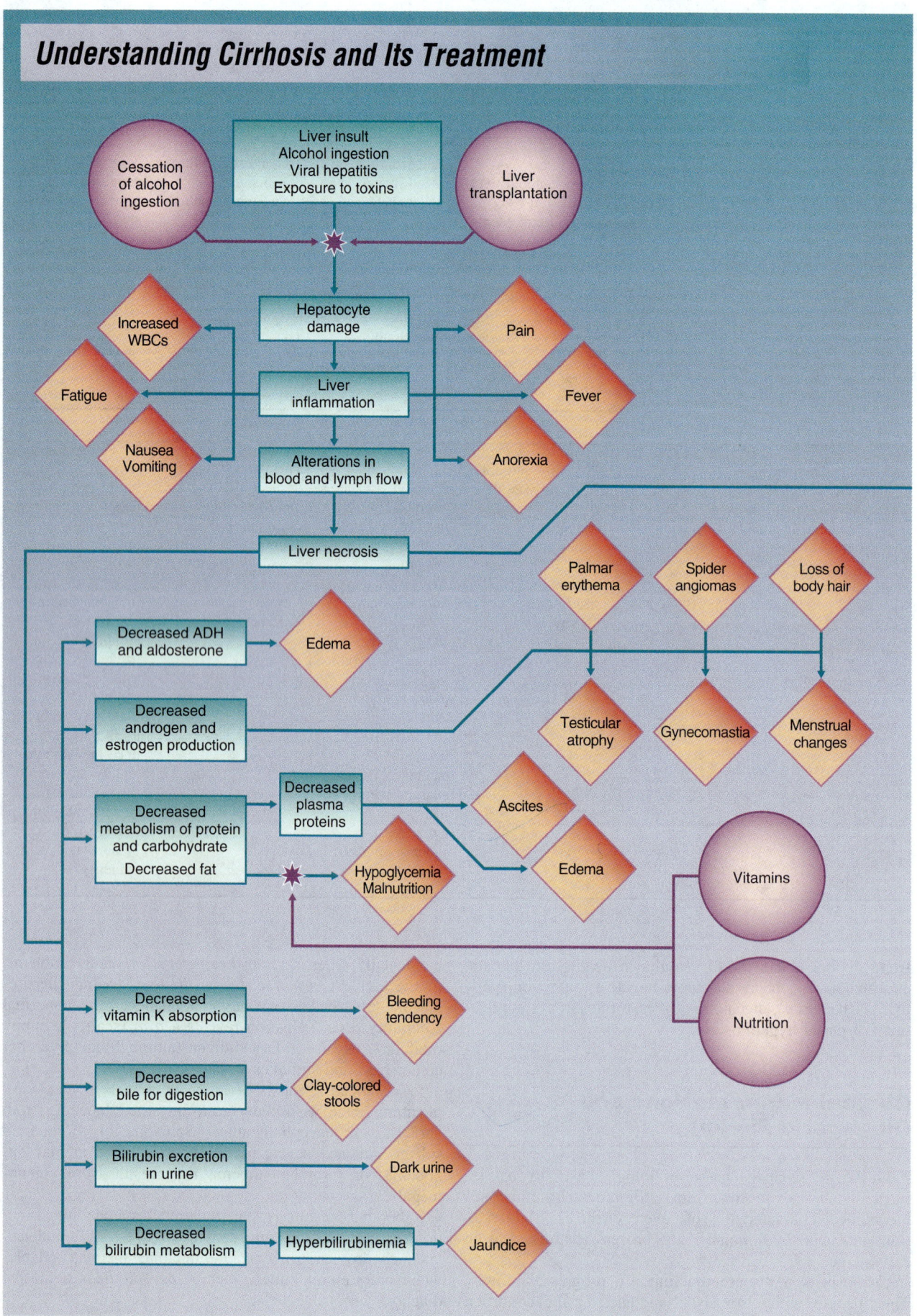

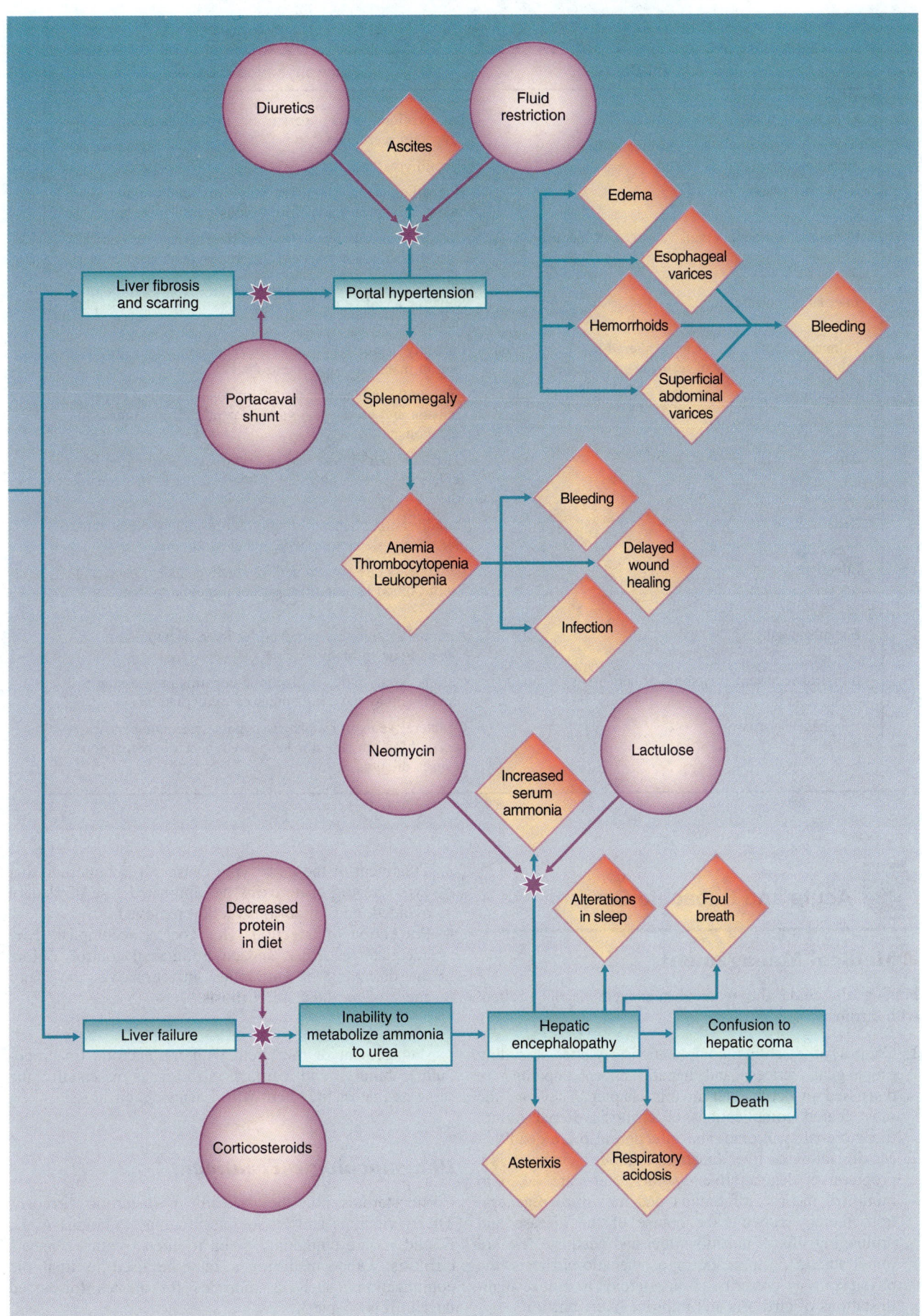

Table 65–7. Advanced Cirrhosis Assessment Data	
Assessment Data	**Pathophysiologic Bases**
Emaciation, ascites	Malnutrition, portal hypertension, hypoalbuminemia, and hyperaldosteronism
Splenomegaly	Portal hypertension
Lower leg edema	Hypoalbuminemia, hyperaldosteronism, and pressure of massive ascites obstructing venous return from legs
Prominent abdominal wall veins (caput medusae)	Collateral vessels bypass scarred liver to carry portal blood to superior vena cava; portal hypertension causes dilation
Internal hemorrhoids	Superior rectal veins dilate with pressure of portal hypertension
Palmar erythema, spider nevi, altered hair distribution; amenorrhea, atrophy of testicles, gynecomastia	Probably decreased hormone metabolism in liver, resulting in manifestations of estrogen excess
Bleeding tendency, especially gastrointestinal	Hypoprothrombinemia, thrombocytopenia; portal hypertension and esophageal varices; peptic ulcers common in alcoholism
Anemia	Gastrointestinal blood losses; erythrocyte destruction in enlarged spleen; folic acid deficiency due to inadequate diet
Renal failure	Rapidly failing hepatic function; occasionally precipitated by volume depletion; hepatorenal syndrome
Infections	Leukopenia due to enlarged, overactive spleen; bacteria in portal blood bypass liver, so not removed by Kupffer cells
Encephalopathy	Ammonia, no longer removed by liver, accumulates to levels toxic to brain
Initial or recurrent symptoms of hepatitis (jaundice)	Chronic viral, toxic, or alcoholic hepatitis progressing to cirrhosis may have inflammatory exacerbations
Esophageal varices	Collateral veins in esophagus bypass scarred liver to carry portal blood to superior vena cava; portal hypertension causes dilation

Acute and Subacute Care

■ Medical Management

Four goals guide the medical management of a client with cirrhosis:

1. Control of disabling complications. Ascites, bleeding esophageal varices, and hepatic encephalopathy are discussed in depth later in this chapter. They are the most feared complications of cirrhosis. Renal failure (hepatorenal syndrome) and infection also are deadly.
2. Maximization of liver function. Although cirrhosis is a progressive, degenerative disorder, steps are taken to minimize the risk of trauma and maximize regeneration, thereby slowing the course of the disease and prolonging life. A nutritious diet and adequate rest are important. In postnecrotic or posthepatic cirrhosis, the physician may prescribe corticosteroids to reduce manifestations of cirrhosis and improve liver function.

3. Treatment of the underlying causes. It is important that exposure to hepatotoxins be eliminated, use of alcohol avoided, and biliary obstruction removed.
4. Prevention of infection. This goal is accomplished by adequate rest, diet, and environmental control. Before the discovery of antibiotics, infection was the major cause of mortality in cirrhosis.

Management of the client with postnecrotic (macronodular), biliary, and cardiac cirrhosis is essentially the same as that of the client with Laënnec's cirrhosis.

Pharmacologic Treatment

Corticosteroids may be used for postnecrotic cirrhosis. The B vitamins and fat-soluble vitamins (vitamins A, D, E, and K) are commonly given to clients with Laënnec's cirrhosis. Other medications may be used to treat the complications, such as diuretics for ascites (discussed later in this chapter).

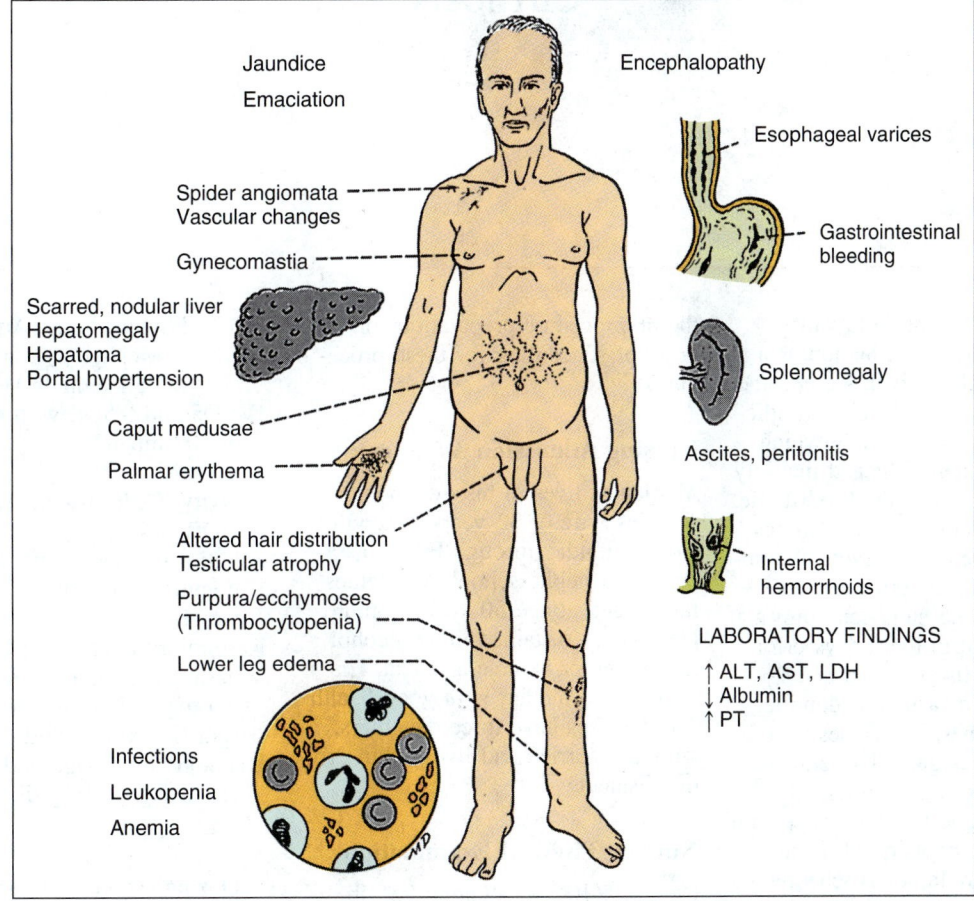

Figure 65–4. Liver cirrhosis: common assessment findings. ALT, alanine aminotransferase; AST, aspartate aminotransferase; LDH, lactate dehydrogenase; PT, prothrombin time.

Dietary Treatment

A nutritious diet is recommended for cirrhosis. The diet should be palatable with adequate calories and protein (75–100 g/day) unless hepatic encephalopathy is present. If there is fluid retention, restrict sodium. Fat intake need not be restricted.

■ Nursing Management of the Medical Client

Assessment

Because the manifestations of cirrhosis are sometimes vague and nonspecific, the client may not be aware of the disease's early manifestations. Assess the client closely for the presence of early manifestations, such as hepatomegaly, and carefully check the laboratory data for any indication of cirrhosis.

As the disease progresses, assess for manifestations of complications of cirrhosis, such as ascites, portal hypertension, or hepatic encephalopathy. These are discussed later.

When a client with cirrhosis is hospitalized, use laboratory data and the client's physical and psychosocial assessment data to guide care planning. Refer to the Case Study for further information about these tests.

Diagnosis, Planning, Implementation

Hemorrhage. Because of the increased risk of bleeding in the client with cirrhosis, the collaborative problem *Hemorrhage related to bleeding tendencies and varices* is an important problem.

Planning: Expected Outcomes. Hemorrhage will be prevented, as evidenced by absence of bleeding, normal vital signs, and urine output of at least 30 ml/hr.

Implementation. Monitor the client for bleeding gums, purpura, melena, hematuria, and hematemesis. Protect the client from physical injury from falls or abrasions and give injections to the client only when absolutely necessary, using only small-gauge needles. Be sure to apply gentle pressure after an injection.

Instruct the client to avoid vigorous nose blowing and straining with bowel movements. Sometimes stool softeners may be ordered. Advise the client to use a soft toothbrush and refrain from flossing until the bleeding has improved.

Cirrhosis

Mr. James is a 53-year-old white man on disability from his job as a warehouse forklift driver. He became unable to work after developing idiopathic peripheral neuropathy which resulted in frequent falls and inability to run the controls of the forklift. He uses a cane to ambulate. Mr. James is being admitted with severe abdominal pain and coffee-ground emesis. He reports that he had been vomiting bright-red blood in the 2 days prior to admission. His abdomen is distended, with a measured abdominal girth of 52 inches. Mr. James also states that he has gained several pounds and has had shortness of breath and fatigue for the past several weeks. He is a smoker, but denies alcohol use. Mr. James is scheduled for an upper gastrointestinal endoscopy and paracentesis followed by a CT scan of the abdomen. Review the preprocedure preparations and patient teaching required for these diagnostic tests. Also consider the influence of the preprocedure preparations on the order of scheduling for these procedures.

Nursing Admission Assessment

Mr. James lives in his own home with his wife of 32 years. His wife works Monday through Friday as a cook in a public school. Mr. James' father died at age 50 years of multiple injuries sustained in an alcohol-related motor vehicle accident. His 75-year-old mother is in good health. The Jameses have three daughters, who are married and live within driving distance.

Nursing Physical Examination

Height: 5'10"   Weight: 235 lb
                      (106.8 kg)
Vital signs: BP = 110/75; TPR =
                      100.3,95,25
LOC: Alert and cooperative
EENT: Moon-faced; sclerae are slightly icteric
Cardiac: Regular rate and rhythm with a grade I/VI systolic murmur
Pulmonary: Slight crackles in the bases bilaterally
Abdominal: Distended and taut; abdominal girth = 52 inches; fluid wave noted; bowel sounds high-pitched and hypoactive
Genitourinary: Voiding infrequently in small amounts; urine is dark amber
Peripheral Pulses: 3/3 with pitting pretibial and pedal edema
Skin: Bruising noted on extremities and abdomen

Initial Treatment Plan

Meds: Famotidine (Pepcid) 20 mg IV bid
      Buprenorphine (Buprenex) 0.3 mg IV q 4–6 h prn for pain

Phytonadione (Aqua-Mephyton) 2 mg IM qod
MVI 1 ampule IV qd
IV: D5 and 0.5NS with 40 mEq KCl at 100 ml/hr
Diet: NPO
Activity: Bedrest with BRP, elevate HOB
Additional assessments: Measure abdominal girth qd; I&O; daily weights
Respiratory treatments: O_2 2 L per nasal cannula, albuterol (Ventolin) 2.5 mg in 3 ml NS aerosol qid, spot O_2 oximetry qd.
Diagnostic tests: Hgb and Hct q 4 h; call if Hgb <10 g/dl, APTT daily

Oozing esophageal varices were discovered during Mr. James' endoscopy. The physician notes, as a probable cause, cirrhosis and portal hypertension. At the CT scan, the nurse tells Mr. James' daughter that liver disease is suspected. The daughter replies, "I'm not surprised. He's been drinking like a fish for years." Upon further inquiry, the daughter states that her father drinks both beer and hard liquor from morning until night while frequently skipping meals.

Mr. James' CT scan reveals a shrunken, cirrhotic liver, splenomegaly, and ascites. During the paracentesis, 60 ml of clear yellow fluid was aspirated. Initial results indicate the absence of abnormal or malignant cells and bacteria. Following diagnostic examinations, the physician discontinues the buprenorphine and orders acetaminophen (Tylenol) 650 mg q 4 h prn. Consider the rationale for this change.

In addition, the physician orders bumetanide (Bumex) 1 mg IV bid. A one-time dose of salt-poor albumin 25 g IV is also ordered. Consider the rationale of using these medications for treatment of ascites. Which of

Selected Admission Laboratory Values	
RBC	2.78 million/mm³
Hgb	11.0 g/dl
Hct	30.6%
WBC	12,300/mm³
Sodium	133 mEq/L
Potassium	3.1 mEq/L
Chloride	89 mEq/L
CO_2	32 mEq/L
Total protein	5.0 g/dl
Albumin	2.1 g/dl
Total bilirubin	1.5 mg/dl
Ammonia	79 µg/dl
AST	47 U/L
ALP	178 U/L
Hepatitis panel	Negative
APTT	62 seconds
Platelets	184,000/mm³
ANA	Negative

these orders should be implemented first? Why?

Mr. James' hemoglobin level remains stable, and no further bleeding is noted. He is started on an all-cooked, high carbohydrate, moderate protein (60–70 g/day) and low sodium (1–2 g/day) diet. He is to limit his intake of fluids to 1500 ml/day. The IV and IM vitamin K are discontinued. Vitamin K (phytonadione, Mephyton) 5 mg PO twice a week and a daily supplement of B vitamins are added to his medication orders. The famotidine is changed from the IV route to the PO route of administration. The bumetanide IV order is discontinued and replaced with an order for spironolactone (Aldactone) 25 mg bid and potassium (K-Dur) 20 mEq/day. Docusate (Colace) 100 mg/day is also ordered. Discharge is planned for tomorrow morning.

Discharge Criteria

Average LOS (insurance certification): 8.3 days

Initiate diet teaching, medication teaching, drug and alcohol incompatibilities, fluid restriction, report of bleeding tendencies, changes in mental status for client and significant others.

Complete community referrals for client and significant others.

What referrals would you make? Why?

Questions to Be Considered

1. Discuss the pathophysiologic changes that have led to Mr. James' ascites, peripheral edema, weight gain, bruising, and esophageal varices.

2. Discuss what further changes in Mr. James' diet and medications might be needed if certain laboratory values suggest progression of the disease process (e.g., serum ammonia levels, bleeding studies, liver enzymes, serum protein, bilirubin, etc.)

3. Mr. James' family decides to confront him about his alcohol consumption. Discuss the nurse's role in supporting the family's decision. Consider the ethical ramifications of your decision.

4. If Mr. James continues to abstain from alcohol, he is at risk of developing delirium tremens (DTs). What are the manifestations of this syndrome, and what treatments are indicated?

5. What is Mr. James' prognosis? Would he be eligible for a liver transplant? What factors would influence the transplant team's decision?

6. Had Mr. James' bleeding not been controlled, what medical and nursing interventions would have been indicated? Consider both medical and surgical management.

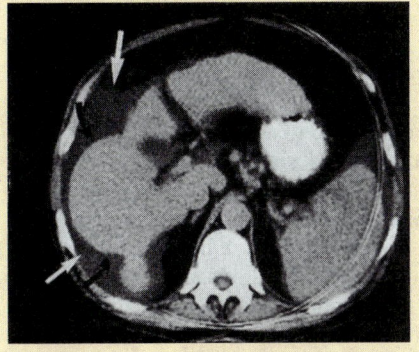

■ A CT scan of Mr. James' abdomen revealed a shrunken, cirrhotic liver, an enlarged spleen, and ascites *(white arrows)*. There is also a large regenerating nodule *(curved dark arrows)*.

Evaluation

Early in the disease the most favorable outcome is that manifestations may be managed if the client stops all alcohol intake and the intake of any substances toxic to the liver. If the desired outcomes are not achieved and the client develops disabling complications (such as hemorrhage), or liver function deteriorates, plans and interventions will need to be revised.

Community and Self-Care

■ Medical Management

A priority in the care of the client with cirrhosis is the need for the client to avoid the ingestion of hepatotoxins, especially alcohol. Other medications that should be avoided are also specified to the client. Table 65–8 lists drugs to restrict or avoid. The client should be encouraged to seek help (e.g., from Alcoholics Anonymous) with alcohol abstinence.

Significant others and the client are taught manifestations of progressive liver failure. The family should know what manifestations they need to report to the physician and when to seek immediate assistance, such as when bleeding from varices or a decrease in the level of consciousness occurs.

The home healthcare needs vary greatly among clients with cirrhosis. Those with milder disease may not need any assistance at home, whereas clients with encephalopathy may need extensive home care.

The client and significant others are taught the need for a nutritious diet. The diet should be rich in vitamins with adequate calories and protein (unless encephalopathy is present, in which case protein is limited). A list of foods

to be included in the diet is given to the client and family. If the client is experiencing edema, the client will probably be on a low sodium diet, possibly with fluid restrictions. If the client is on a thiazide diuretic, the diet should be high in potassium.

Major complications described later in this chapter may occur from liver disease. It is important to see the client at regular intervals to follow the progress of the disease. Periodic blood tests are performed to assess liver damage.

■ Nursing Management of the Medical Client

Assessment

Assess the client and significant others for their knowledge of the important aspects of self-care and continuing care. Cirrhosis, except in the late stages, is managed in the community rather than in the hospital.

Diagnosis, Planning, Implementation

Altered Nutrition: Less than Body Requirements. In order for the liver to regenerate, the client must have adequate levels of vital nutrients leading to the nursing diagnosis *Altered Nutrition: Less than Body Requirements, related to anorexia, impaired liver function, decreased absorption of fat-soluble vitamins, and diarrhea.*

Planning: Expected Outcomes. The client will take in adequate nutrition, as evidenced by no weight loss and no manifestations of malnutrition.

Implementation. The diet should provide ample protein to rebuild tissue, but not enough protein to precipitate hepatic encephalopathy. The diet should supply sufficient carbohydrates to maintain weight and spare protein. Fat restriction is not necessary. Total daily calories should range between 2000 and 3000. Place the client on daily weight, intake and output, and calorie counts to assess fluid and nutritional balance. Closely monitor the laboratory and nutritional panels for manifestations of improvement or further deterioration. If ammonia levels rise (normal levels are 70–200 μg/dl in whole blood and 56–150 μg/dl in plasma) protein and foods high in ammonia are restricted.

If the client has ascites or edema, sodium and possibly fluids should be restricted in the diet. Small frequent meals will make it easier for clients with anorexia to eat enough food. Adequate rest and a stable environmental temperature should be ensured to allow optimal use of calories. Administer prescribed medications such as antacids, antiemetics, antidiarrheals, or cathartics to decrease gastric distress, but avoid antiemetics such as phenothiazines.

The physician usually prescribes a maintenance multivitamin preparation and in severe malnutrition administers therapeutic levels of vitamins. Also, vitamins A, D, E, and K are supplied if fat absorption is present. The client with severe malabsorption may require IV vitamins with calcium gluconate supplementation. Encourage family or friends to provide desirable foods as permitted.

Table 65–8. Cirrhosis and Liver Failure	
Drugs to Restrict or Avoid	**Rationale**
Acetaminophen	Can cause fatal liver damage
Phenobarbital, phenytoin, Thorazine	Stimulates liver's major drug-metabolizing system; when liver diseased or damaged, drugs may not be metabolized properly and toxicity may occur; may also cause alteration in sensory perception and thought processes related to hepatic encephalopathy
Morphine, paraldehyde, codeine	Can cause spasms and pressure in the biliary tract, thus increasing discomfort
Alcohol	Stimulates liver's major drug metabolizing system; can damage liver further

Activity Intolerance. The client with cirrhosis often experiences severe fatigue leading to the nursing diagnosis *Activity Intolerance related to bedrest, lack of energy, and altered respiratory function (ascites).*

Planning: Expected Outcomes. The client will maintain a balance between rest and activity, as evidenced by the absence of fatigue and problems associated with immobility.

Implementation. Clinicians often prescribe rest for clients with cirrhosis, but how much rest is necessary is debated. During periods of acute malfunction, rest reduces metabolic demands on the liver and increases circulation. Long-term planning should include counseling the client to rest frequently and avoid unnecessary fatigue.

Risk for Injury. Because the liver is in a very precarious state, the nursing diagnosis *Risk for Injury related to continued intake of hepatotoxins* is a common one.

Planning: Expected Outcomes. The client will not suffer injury from continued intake of hepatotoxins, as evidenced by cessation of drinking and avoidance of all medications that might cause further damage.

Implementation. All known hepatotoxic medications (including alcohol) must be removed from therapeutic regimens. In addition, dosages of all drugs thought to be metabolized by the liver must be lowered. Administration of sedatives and opiates is to be avoided.

Knowledge Deficit. The client with cirrhosis must become involved in self-care if the treatment is to be at all successful. Therefore, *Knowledge Deficit related to* *disease and long-term treatment* is an important nursing diagnosis.

Planning: Expected Outcomes. The client with cirrhosis will understand the disease and the implications of long-term management, as evidenced by the client's statements.

Implementation. The client and significant others are provided with information in preparation for care at home. Clients with cirrhosis will live longer if they get adequate rest, abstain from alcohol, and eat nutritious meals.

Those clients with a history of alcohol abuse should be encouraged to seek assistance from support groups such as AA to stop drinking. Even if cirrhotic changes have begun in the liver, it is vital for the client to stop drinking before irreparable damage occurs. See Chapter 87 for further information on alcoholism. The Ethical Issues in Nursing feature also addresses care of the alcoholic client.

Evaluation

The outcome of cirrhosis depends on the client's ability to stop drinking early enough to prevent irreparable damage to the liver. If extensive damage has occurred, then recovery will not occur and the client will progress with manifestations of liver failure.

Complications of Cirrhosis

The clinical course of clients with advanced cirrhosis is often complicated by a number of sequelae. These in-

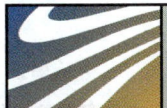

ETHICAL ISSUES IN NURSING

Do Nurses Have an Obligation to Care for a Client with a Life-Style Disease?

Cirrhosis of the liver can be a very serious and often deadly condition. Although cirrhosis may be caused by several different sources, alcohol abuse accounts for most cases. Cirrhosis can affect both men and women and does not discriminate by age. The endstages of liver cirrhosis are uncomfortable for the client and for those who care for him or her.

Healthcare workers who are not specialized in substance abuse often care for people who have abused alcohol or other substances. These clients appear in all nursing care settings—medical-surgical, intensive care, obstetric-gynecologic, and home healthcare. Because many nurses have not had formal training in the care of substance abusers, it is easy to misunderstand these clients. Caring for a person who has destroyed his or her liver through years of alcohol abuse is difficult, knowing that the problems were self-induced. When caregivers see these clients and their families go through such an emotional experience—all because the clients could not control their alcohol consumption—it is easy to judge the clients harshly. For example, if the client becomes demanding and requires more nursing time, it is easy to think unkindly of him or her. After all, had the client not abused himself or herself, the client would not be in this situation.

It is difficult not to prejudge persons with conditions brought about by substance abuse. Healthcare providers, although they do not approve of such abuse, have a responsibility to assist in the care of those who are in need. In the case of the alcoholic client with liver cirrhosis, you can refer the client and his or her family to a substance abuse center or other such service. Nurses who may care for substance abusers on an ongoing basis should receive special training in the care of such persons. It is natural to feel that those who abuse anything should more or less receive whatever comes from such activity; however, healthcare workers must look beyond the abusive personality and treat the person holistically.

clude portal hypertension, ascites, and hepatic encephalopathy.

Portal Hypertension

Portal hypertension occurs when there is a persistent increase in the pressure in the portal venous system as a result of increased resistance or obstruction of blood flow through the portal venous system.

Etiology and Risk Factors

Most cases of portal hypertension in the United States relate to cirrhosis. The portal vein is likely to be obstructed by a thrombus; a tumor is the next most common cause. Box 65–1 lists factors that may cause portal hypertension.

Pathophysiology

Recall that the normal flow to and from the liver depends on proper functioning of the portal vein (70% of inflow), the hepatic artery (30% of inflow), and the hepatic veins (outflow). Disease processes that damage or alter the flow of blood through the liver or its major vessels are responsible for the development of portal hypertension (see Box 65–1). The amount of liver dysfunction varies with the initial process, the length of the process, and individual differences. Portal hypertension may result from either increased blood flow in the portal vein or an increased resistance to flow within the portal venous system.

As noted in Chapter 63, normal portal pressure is 5 to 10 mm Hg. Portal hypertension exists when the pressure rises 5 mm Hg higher than the inferior vena cava pressure and collaterals form as a result of poor blood flow through major venous channels. The spleen and other organs that empty into the portal system also begin to undergo the effects of congestion. Eventually, clinical manifestations arise.

Clinical Manifestations and Diagnostic Findings

In clients with portal hypertension, assessment reveals slightly tortuous epigastric vessels that branch off the area of the umbilicus and lead toward the sternum and ribs (caput medusae); an enlarged, palpable spleen; internal hemorrhoids; bruits, which may be heard over the upper abdomen; and ascites, which typically appears when there is concurrent liver disease.

Direct measurement of portal pressure is possible only during laparotomy. The diagnosis of portal hypertension often relies on indirect measurements of portal pressure — liver scans, splenoportography, abdominal angiography, liver biopsy, and other laboratory data (see Chapter 64). Radiography and endoscopy procedures may be used to differentiate variceal hemorrhage from other types of gastrointestinal bleeding.

Box 65–1. Factors in the Pathogenesis of Portal Hypertension

Increased vascular resistance
  Intrahepatic
    Cirrhosis
    Infiltrations (e.g., tumors, sarcoidosis)
    Polycystic disease
    Schistosomiasis
    Noncirrhotic portal fibrosis (hepatic phlebosclerosis)
  Portal vein
    Thrombosis
    Tumor
    Infection (pyelophlebitis)
  Hepatic veins
    Thrombosis (Budd-Chiari syndrome)
    Veno-occlusive disease

Sustained high splanchnic inflow
  Splenomegaly
  Diffuse atrioventricular shunts(?)
  Major atrioventricular fistulas

Inadequate decompression via venous collaterals
  Esophageal
  Retroperitoneal
  Periumbilical
  Hemorrhoidal

From LaMont, J. T., & Isselbacher, K. J. (1977). Cirrhosis. In G. W. Thorn, et al. (Eds.), *Harrison's principles of internal medicine* (8th ed., p. 1611). New York: McGraw-Hill.

Emergency Care

■ Medical Management

One of the most serious disabling complications of portal hypertension is dilation of the superior rectal veins, abdominal wall veins, and esophagogastric veins. With conditions such as cirrhosis, portal pressure increases and causes esophageal veins to swell and distend. These swollen, dilated veins are called *varices*. Various factors can contribute to the rupturing of varices: portal pressure, increased intrathoracic pressure (coughing and straining at stools), irritation by food or alcohol, and erosion by gastric juices. The veins of the stomach and esophagus are most subject to rupture and when this occurs, it constitutes a medical emergency. Medical management of acute variceal bleeding involves vasoconstrictors (vasopressin [Pitressin] or somatostatin), beta-adrenergic blockers, balloon tamponade, sclerotherapy (endoscopic sclerosing of varices), or endoscopic ligation of varices.

Another mechanism that leads to hemorrhage involves the spleen. The splenic vein merges with the superior mesenteric vein to form the portal vein. When pressure increases in the portal system, damage to the spleen oc-

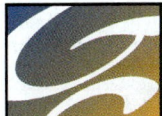

CRITICAL MONITORING

Esophageal Bleeding Secondary to Portal Hypertension

Blood pressure ≤ 90/60 mm Hg
Heart rate ≥ 100 BPM
Cool, clammy skin
Distal pulses <2+ on a 0–4+ scale
Slowed capillary refill (>2 seconds)
Diminished orientation to person, place, and time
Restlessness

curs. Damage to the spleen is not proportional to the increase in portal pressure. As the spleen enlarges, it tends to destroy blood cells, and especially platelets, which then increases the risk of hemorrhage and anemia.

Hepatic encephalopathy is an extremely dangerous complication of portal hypertension. This problem usually arises following a period of bleeding into the gastrointestinal tract. Digestion of this blood takes place in the intestines. Because blood is a protein, this process increases ammonia in the gut and bloodstream. In turn, the excessive ammonia disturbs brain function. The Critical Monitoring Feature lists assessment findings that mandate early intervention in esophageal bleeding secondary to portal hypertension. Hepatic encephalopathy is discussed later in this chapter.

Death often follows rupture of esophageal varices if the hemorrhage is not immediately controlled. To stop hemorrhage, health practitioners perform emergency measures: administration of vasopressin, balloon tamponade, injection sclerotherapy, endoscopic electrocautery, direct ligation of the bleeding varices, transhepatic embolization of the left gastric vein, or even urgent portocaval shunt surgery. Cold saline lavage is probably ineffective, but is done while waiting to transport the client to surgery or the gastrointestinal laboratory. Fluids, especially volume expanders and blood products, are administered to maintain volume.

Nonsurgical approaches to treat varices include endoscopic sclerotherapy and balloon tamponade.

Sclerotherapy

To perform sclerotherapy, the physician passes an endoscope into the esophagus and injects a sclerosing agent (e.g., morrhuate sodium) that flows into the varices. The sclerosing agent initially causes inflammation of the vein wall and then fibrosis. The physician may give repeated injections over a period of weeks until the varices are no longer prominent.

Balloon Tamponade

Applying pressure to ruptured varices via balloon tamponade may stop the hemorrhage. For this intervention,

the clinician inserts a Sengstaken-Blakemore or Minnesota tube into the stomach and inflates the esophageal and gastric balloons (Fig. 65–5). The pressure of the esophageal balloon against the varices may stop the bleeding. It is important to release this pressure periodically to prevent tissue necrosis. The esophageal balloon is not left inflated for more than 24 hours. Also, it is important to remove secretions and saliva that accumulate above the balloon to prevent aspiration. The Minnesota tube has a fourth port for aspiration of secretions above the esophageal balloon.

It is very important to ensure that the gastric balloon is inflated to prevent migration of the tube. You should also have scissors at the bedside so as to be able to remove the tube in an emergency.

Complications of balloon tamponade may occur in 15% or more of clients and include aspiration pneumonitis as well as esophageal rupture.

Vasopressin

When varices rupture, vasopressin 0.4 unit IV is routinely administered to stop variceal bleeding. Administration of vasopressin achieves temporary lowering of portal pressure. These agents reduce portal blood flow by constricting afferent arterioles. Direct infusion of vasopressin into the superior mesenteric artery is most effective. Serious side effects include hypothermia, myocardial and gastrointestinal tract ischemia, and acute renal failure. It is therefore, contraindicated in clients with a recent myocardial infarction. Vasopressin may be given in conjunction with nitroglycerin, which is administered IV, sublingually, or by patch to minimize vasoconstrictive side effects. Alternatively, somatostatin is at least as effective as vaso-

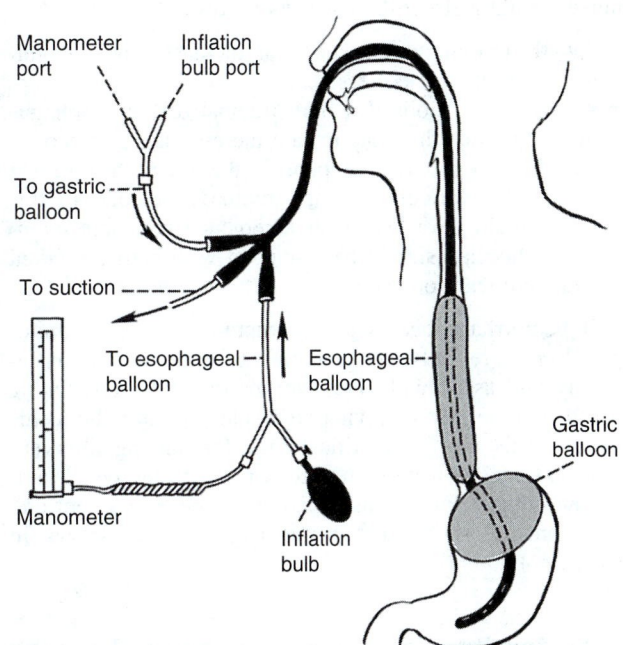

Figure 65–5. A Sengstaken-Blakemore tube may be used to control ruptured esophageal varices, a potential complication of portal hypertension.

pressin. Drug therapy may stop bleeding, but it has no effect on survival.

Beta-Adrenergic Blocking Agents

Beta-adrenergic blocking agents (e.g., propranolol, metoprolol [Lopressor] or atenonol) and their effectiveness in the management of acute variceal bleeding is limited because they reduce the heart rate (and hence the blood pressure) and mask the early manifestations of hypoglycemia. However, studies suggest they may reduce the risk of recurrent bleeding.

■ Nursing Management of the Medical Client

Assessment

The major assessment for the nurse to make is the presence of hemorrhage. The other important assessment is the client's condition after any intervention to treat the hemorrhage, such as the functioning of the Sengstaken-Blakemore tube. The client's vital signs are continuously assessed for any significant changes.

Diagnosis, Planning, Implementation

Hemorrhage. With the rupture of the varices, the collaborative problem that must be addressed immediately is *Hemorrhage related to portal hypertension, rupture of esophageal varices.*

Planning: Expected Outcomes. Hemorrhage will be controlled, as evidenced by the return of vital signs to normal and no further bleeding.

Implementation. The client can learn activities to help reduce the risk of rupture of esophageal varices. The nurse should instruct the client as follows:

- Avoid straining maneuvers that increase intra-abdominal or intrathoracic pressure.
- Avoid rough foods that may traumatize the esophagus or spicy foods that may irritate the esophageal mucosa.
- Develop an emergency plan if the client has severe esophageal varices that may rupture. Included in this plan should be a list of all emergency telephone numbers. The plan should be discussed with both the client and significant others.

If hemorrhage occurs due to ruptured varices, monitor blood pressure, pulse, respiration, and urine output continuously and assist with interventions to restore circulating blood volume. Monitor vital signs closely throughout this period. This is a very critical time for nursing intervention and can be a very stressful time for the client, family, and nurse. Further information on the assessment and treatment of shock and hemorrhage can be found in Chapter 22.

Risk for Impaired Gas Exchange. The client with ruptured varices is prone to many problems. A major potential problem is addressed in the nursing diagnosis *Risk for Impaired gas exchange related to decreased*

oxygen supply secondary to aspiration pneumonitis or obstruction occurring after balloon tamponade with the Sengstaken-Blakemore tube.

Planning: Expected Outcomes. The client will not suffer injury related to the Sengstaken-Blakemore tube, as evidenced by no respiratory distress, absence of aspiration, and no evidence of esophageal ischemia.

Implementation. It is important to remember that the pressure of the esophageal balloon on the esophagus not only stops hemorrhage but also may cause esophageal necrosis. As noted earlier, you must release the pressure on the esophagus periodically to prevent tissue damage. The physician should be consulted on how often to release balloon pressure, because practices vary widely.

Aspiration pneumonia is another complication of balloon tamponade. The inflated balloon in the esophagus prevents saliva and secretions from reaching the stomach. Ascertain if the tube used for tamponade has a suction port above the esophageal balloon. If not, insert a nasogastric tube to the upper balloon level or perform suctioning frequently to remove accumulating fluid.

Tubes inserted through the nose may cause erosion of the nares, especially if traction is applied to the tamponade (practices differ). To prevent this complication, clean and lubricate the external nares. Padding is provided if necessary.

The last complication of balloon tamponade is airway obstruction. This occurs when the gastric balloon deflates or breaks and traction on the tube pulls the esophageal balloon up into the oropharynx. Scissors should be kept at the bedside in case this emergency arises. Cut the tube and pull it out to restore airway patency. To prevent this complication, label each port of the tube to prevent accidental deflation of the gastric balloon.

Portal Systemic Encephalopathy. Because of the potential build-up of ammonia, the client with bleeding varices is likely to have the collaborative problem *Portal Systemic Encephalopathy related to increased risk of neurosensory changes secondary to hepatic coma occurring with gastrointestinal bleeding or accumulation of ammonia.*

Planning: Expected Outcomes. The client will be oriented to person, place, and time, and free of injuries that occur with neurosensory changes.

Implementation. Assess the client's level of consciousness and orientation on a regular basis (after performing a baseline assessment). Ask the client daily to write his or her name and assess for writing deterioration and possible rising ammonia levels. Also assess the client regularly for the development of asterixis. Monitor for gastrointestinal bleeding, including melena or hematemesis, because bleeding can precipitate hepatic coma. Report the bleeding promptly. Protect the client against injury by keeping the side rails up and the bed in the lowest position. Assist the client with ambulation as needed. Use caution when administering sedatives, antihistamines, and other agents that affect the central nervous system (CNS).

Evaluation

Although the acute episode of bleeding varices can usually be controlled, the development of varices is a sign of deterioration of the liver and increasing portal hypertension. The client will need a great deal of follow-up to prevent recurrence or further complications.

Acute and Subacute Care

■ Surgical Management

Overall, these clients are poor surgical risks because of their poor nutritional status, increased risk of infection, and deteriorating liver function. For bleeding esophageal varices the role of portosystemic shunt surgery after initial medical control of bleeding is uncertain. While shunts reduce the risk of recurrent hemorrhage, the overall mortality of clients undergoing such surgery is comparable with that of clients not operated on. This is because there is an increased incidence of encephalopathy when the shunted blood is not cleared of toxic substances, as well as on increased incidence of death from progressive liver failure. For these reasons, surgical creation of a portal shunt is reserved for clients who have not responded to other treatment, and who, despite periodic endoscopic sclerotherapy, continue to bleed.

Preoperative Management

Preoperative management of the client undergoing a portosystemic shunt includes an appraisal of the client's general physiologic condition and readiness for surgery. It also includes assessment of the client's neurologic, respiratory, and renal systems to establish a baseline. Blood and urine may be examined for the presence of infectious organisms and blood gas analysis done to assess general respiratory function.

Blood clotting mechanisms are analyzed, as well as the client's fluid, electrolyte, ammonia, protein, bilirubin, and enzyme levels. If the client has an inappropriate level of any one of these substances, measures are taken to correct the problem. If the hemoglobin and hematocrit are low, the client may receive a blood transfusion.

The client's general nutritional status is important and protein hydrolysates are administered by total parenteral nutrition (TPN) if indicated.

Surgical Procedure

There are several surgical approaches that reduce the danger of hemorrhage from varices caused by portal hypertension. Surgical approaches involve anastomosing the high-pressure portal system to the low-pressure systemic venous system. This creates a portosystemic shunt.

Surgical creation of a portosystemic shunt reduces portal hypertension by sending portal blood directly into the inferior vena cava, bypassing the liver (Fig. 65–6). Such a procedure lowers portal hypertension and thus the risk of rupturing esophageal varices.

Figure 65–6 illustrates some of the many portacaval shunt procedures possible. The goal of these procedures is threefold:

1. To reduce portal blood flow enough to prevent variceal hemorrhage
2. To preserve enough blood inflow to the liver to prevent hepatic encephalopathy and hepatic failure
3. To increase client comfort (this is a palliative procedure)

Achievement of these goals requires a delicate balance between the reduction of expendable blood flow and the preservation of essential blood flow.

A newer procedure is called the TIPS procedure—*t*ransjugular *i*ntrahepatic *p*ortosystemic *s*hunt. In this procedure, a stent is placed between the hepatic and portal vein. The goals of this shunting procedure are the same as for the other shunting procedures.

Postoperative Management

Management of the client after portacaval shunt procedures includes monitoring for the following:

- Presence of hemorrhage, hypovolemia, and oliguria
- Fluid and electrolyte imbalance (dilutional hyponatremia, ascites)
- Respiratory rate and rhythm (rales, atelectasis, labored breathing, pneumonia)
- Hypoalbuminemia
- Hypoglycemia
- Manifestations of infection (fever, increased white blood cells)
- Pain levels
- Mental status (alertness)

Complications

The major complications that can occur after a portocaval shunt procedure are bacteremia and disseminated intravascular coagulation (DIC), congestive heart failure, shunt clotting, and hepatic encephalopathy. Clients must be monitored closely to detect the onset of any of these complications and measures must be taken quickly if they manifest.

Outcomes

Clients who have portacaval shunts performed needed the surgery because other methods to control bleeding were unsuccessful. And, while the bleeding is stopped, the outcome of this surgery is an increased incidence of disabling encephalopathy and death from progressive liver disease.

■ Nursing Management of the Surgical Client

Assessment

After a portacaval shunt, assessment of the client's respiratory, neurologic, renal, and hemodynamic status is important. In addition, special attention is given to observa-

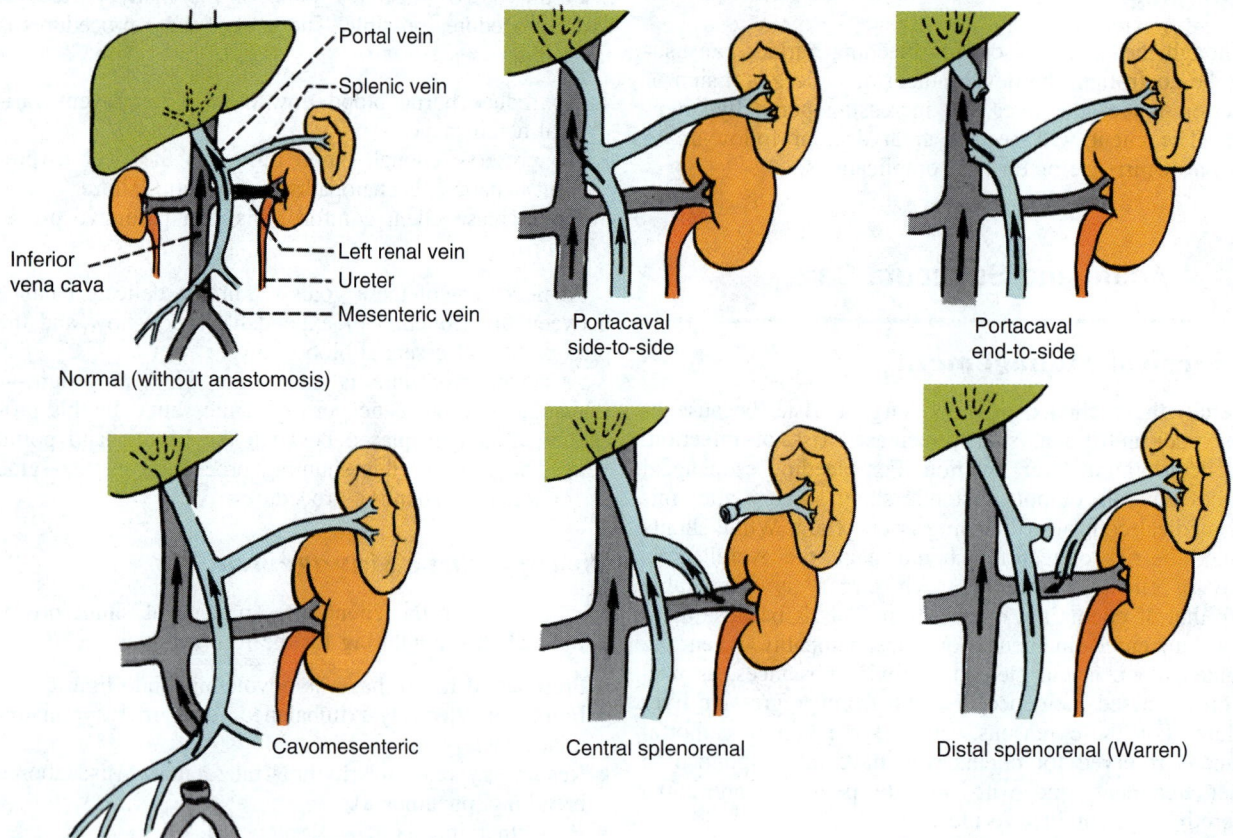

Labels in figure:
Portal vein
Splenic vein
Inferior vena cava
Left renal vein
Ureter
Mesenteric vein
Normal (without anastomosis)
Portacaval side-to-side
Portacaval end-to-side
Cavomesenteric
Central splenorenal
Distal splenorenal (Warren)

Figure 65–6. Some types of portacaval shunt procedures used to reduce portal hypertension.

tion of the operative site for any manifestations of shunt clotting such as pain, distention, or nausea.

Diagnosis, Planning, Implementation

Nursing diagnoses directed toward care of the client pre- and post-portacaval shunt surgery include hemorrhage, impaired gas exchange, and portal systemic encephalopathy and are discussed under Emergency Care. In addition, several other diagnoses are pertinent to the client undergoing liver surgery.

Ascites. The client with cirrhosis develops the collaborative problem *Ascites related to retention of fluids secondary to portal hypertension and liver failure.*

Planning: Expected Outcomes. A normovolemic state will be maintained, as evidenced by a stable or decreasing abdominal girth and a regular respiratory rate and rhythm.

Implementation. The client is assessed for retention of fluid that is likely to occur because of hemodynamic fluid shifts. Measure abdominal girth to obtain a baseline and then daily or every shift as appropriate for assessment of ascites. Also, monitor weight and intake and output. Output should not be less than intake. Assess the degree of edema from 1+ (barely noticeable) to 4+

(deep and pitting) and document. Be sure to check for clinical indicators of pulmonary edema, including dyspnea and orthopnea. See that appropriate pulmonary and respiratory therapy is initiated if the client has any respiratory involvement.

Risk for Altered Thought Processes. Hepatic encephalopathy is a risk after shunting procedures, leading to the nursing diagnosis *Risk for Altered Thought Processes related to development of hepatic encephalopathy secondary to shunt procedure.*

Planning: Expected Outcomes. Hepatic encephalopathy will be prevented or will be diagnosed early after shunt surgery, as evidenced by no decreased level of consciousness and no increase in blood ammonia level.

Implementation. When the client with portal hypertension undergoes portacaval shunt surgery, provide general postoperative care, as described in Chapter 21. In addition, assess the client for hepatic encephalopathy (see Clinical Manifestations and Diagnostic Findings under Hepatic Encephalopathy). If portal hypertension is due to liver disease, carefully monitor for postoperative hemorrhage, because bleeding tendencies often arise from liver cell malfunction. The shunt increases venous return to the heart, and because of this, cardiovascular function must be assessed carefully.

Recall that the client with portal hypertension often has ascites, hepatic encephalopathy, jaundice, bleeding tendencies, or alcoholism. Therefore, after surgery, carefully monitor laboratory data, including hemoglobin, hematocrit, prothrombin time, ammonia level, blood urea nitrogen (BUN), bilirubin, blood gases, and fluid and electrolyte levels.

If the hemoglobin and hematocrit are below normal, you may need to assist with administering a blood transfusion. If clotting time (prothrombin time) is not within normal limits, administer vitamin K. If the client is having difficulty breathing because of ascites, it becomes twice as important after surgery that you implement measures that improve respirations (turning, coughing, and deep-breathing; respiratory treatments; maintaining chest drainage system). Other areas where you may need to intervene for clients having a portocaval shunt include the following:

- Administering IV fluids plus blood or volume expanders such as dextran; maintaining patency and prescribed flow rates.
- Monitoring blood and urine values and noting any manifestations of infection (such as increased white blood cells and elevated erythrocyte sedimentation rate).
- Eliminating medications that sedate, depress the CNS, or that are known hepatotoxins (e.g., acetaminophen).
- Maintaining nutrition. While NPO (nothing by mouth, usually for several days postoperatively), administer TPN. When food intake begins, protein intake may be limited and advanced slowly as the client shows he or she can tolerate it (i.e., BUN, ammonia levels, and mental status remain within normal limits).
- Maintaining sterile technique when changing dressing(s).
- Maintaining patency if a gastrointestinal tube is in place.
- Assisting the client and family to cope with postoperative discomfort and with the chronicity issues of chronic liver disease and its sequelae.

When emergency shunt surgery is performed, there may be little time to give preoperative teaching and information to the client and significant others. Present careful explanations postoperatively to compensate for the lack of preoperative teaching.

Evaluation

Although these procedures may decrease the bleeding, the long-term prognosis for the client is poor. Clients often develop severe encephalopathy followed by coma and death.

Ascites

Etiology and Risk Factors

Ascites is the accumulation of fluid in the peritoneal cavity. It results from the interaction of several pathophysiologic changes. Portal hypertension, lowered plasma colloidal osmotic pressure, and sodium retention all contribute to this condition. Disease processes that lead to these events include cirrhosis of the liver, right-sided heart failure, tuberculous peritonitis, cancer, and complications of pancreatitis.

Pathophysiology

Any process that blocks the flow of blood through the liver sinusoids to the hepatic veins and vena cava causes an increase in hydrostatic pressure in the portal venous system. Most commonly, this problem develops in cirrhosis of the liver or right-sided heart failure. As portal pressure increases, plasma leaks directly from the liver capsule and the congested portal vein into the peritoneal cavity. Congestion of lymph channels occurs, leading to the leakage of more plasma into the peritoneal cavity. Loss of plasma proteins into ascitic fluid from the portal system reduces oncotic pressure in the vascular compartment. Reduction in oncotic pressure limits the vascular system's ability to hold onto or collect water.

In addition, hepatocellular damage reduces the liver's ability to synthesize normal amounts of albumin. Decreased albumin synthesis leads to hypoalbuminemia, which is exacerbated by leakage of protein into the peritoneal cavity. The circulating blood volume decreases from loss of colloid osmotic pressure. The secretion of aldosterone increases to stimulate the kidneys to retain sodium and water. As a result of hepatocellular damage, the liver is unable to inactivate aldosterone. Thus, sodium and water retention continue. More fluid is held, and the volume of ascites grows.

In summary, the three mechanisms that underlie ascites formation are as follows:

1. Portal hypertension results in increased plasma and lymphatic hydrostatic pressures causing lymphatic congestion leading to leakage of fluid into the peritoneal cavity.
2. Decreased albumin production in the liver results in decreased colloid osmotic pressure leading to leakage of fluid into the peritoneal cavity.
3. Decreased circulating volume leading to hyperaldosteronism results in renal sodium and water retention, further increasing fluid in the peritoneal cavity.

Clinical Manifestations and Diagnostic Findings

Ascitic fluid typically produces abdominal distention, bulging flanks, and a protruding (downward) umbilicus. Figure 65–7 depicts a client with ascites. Although large accumulations of ascitic fluid are obvious, small or moderate amounts may be more difficult to diagnose.

Diagnostic tests to confirm the presence of ascites include paracentesis, abdominal x-ray studies, ultrasonography, and computed tomographic (CT) scan. These tests may locate fluid in the peritoneal cavity. Paracentesis provides samples of fluid for analysis. Findings help de-

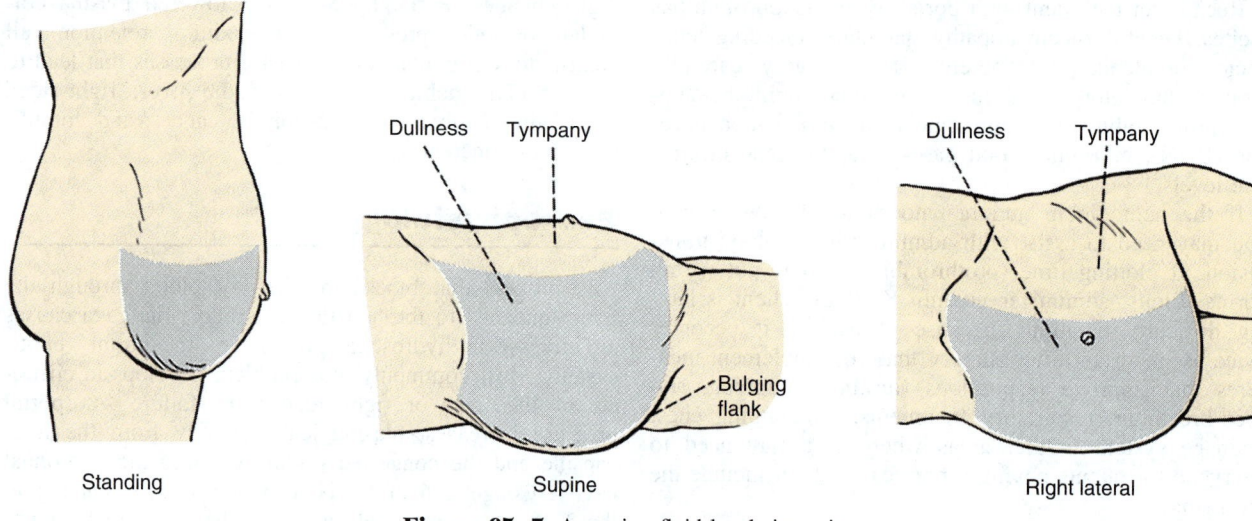

Figure 65–7. Assessing fluid levels in ascites.

termine the source of the ascites, such as the finding of malignant cells.

Acute and Subacute Care

■ Medical Management

The goal of intervention in ascites is to correct fluid and electrolyte imbalances by improving renal sodium excretion and restricting sodium and water intake. This involves discontinuing medications that inhibit prostaglandin synthesis (e.g., aspirin and indomethacin) and that thus impair renal sodium excretion.

Repeated large-volume paracenteses in combination with albumin (40 g) to maintain plasma volume are used to manage clients with ascites resulting from cirrhosis. However, repeated removal of fluid, protein, and electrolytes from the body causes severe disturbances of homeostasis. It is becoming more common to remove the least amount of fluid possible, such as 100 ml, to relieve manifestations such as shortness of breath.

Diuretic Therapy

Diuretics, especially spironolactone (Aldactone), are useful in reducing fluid retention. In addition, the physician may prescribe IV administration of albumin 10 g to replace each liter of ascitic fluid removed.

Dietary Treatment

The diet is a low sodium diet with restriction of fluids. Protein intake is moderate unless the client has manifestations of hepatic encephalopathy.

Complications

Complications of ascites include respiratory compromise and rupture of the umbilicus in cases of massive ascites. Infection can also occur and can be fatal. If these complications occur, monitor the client's respiratory status continuously as well as the blood pressure, temperature, pulse, respirations, and urine output.

■ Nursing Management of the Medical Client

Assessment

Some simple assessments that can be performed at the bedside are the following:

- Percussing the abdomen. If the client has ascites, the sound will be dull. (Abdominal assessment is discussed in Chapters 59 and 64).
- Measurement of circumference (abdominal girth).
- Turning the client laterally and percussing the abdomen (see Fig. 65–7). Because ascitic fluid flows to the lowest point in the abdomen, it will move downward when the client turns. This causes a shift in the area where dullness is heard.
- Tapping the abdomen to elicit a fluid wave.

The amount of distress that the ascites is causing also should be assessed. Ask whether the fluid is interfering with sleeping, eating, and breathing. Also assess for the presence of a hydrothorax or misplaced point of maximal impact (PMI).

Diagnosis, Planning, Implementation

Fluid Volume Excess and Fluid Volume Deficit. The client with ascites has a combination of volume problems leading to the nursing diagnosis *Fluid Volume Excess and Fluid Volume Deficit related to fluid shifts* *secondary to portal hypertension, hypoalbuminemia, and hyperaldosteronism.*

Planning: Expected Outcomes. A normal balance of fluid between the intracellular and extracellular spaces will be maintained, as evidenced by absence of hypovolemia, normal serum albumin, decreased abdominal girth, and normal blood pressure.

Implementation. The client is on a fluid restriction that must be strictly followed. To better space the fluids, give medications with meals, if possible, so these fluids can be used for medications. The abdominal girth should be measured daily and sometimes twice a day, and daily weights should be taken. Monitor intake and output daily. Output should be equal to or exceed intake. Aspirin should be avoided because it inhibits prostaglandin synthesis and, as noted previously, impairs sodium excretion by the kidney.

The client is monitored closely after a paracentesis. Check vital signs frequently to ensure that the client tolerated the procedure well and check the dressing carefully to ensure that excessive amounts of fluid are not lost. Sometimes a pouch is placed to collect leaking fluid. If too much fluid is lost, the physician may suture the site closed to prevent excess loss.

Ineffective Breathing Pattern. Ascites leads to many other problems making the nursing diagnosis *Ineffective Breathing Pattern related to increased intra-abdominal pressure on the diaphragm* a common diagnosis.

Planning: Expected Outcomes. The client will not suffer from an ineffective breathing pattern, as evidenced by the absence of shortness of breath and the presence of normal respiratory excursion.

Implementation. Position the client in the high Fowler position to facilitate breathing and monitor respiratory status for the development of atelectasis or pneumonia. Ask the client to cough and take a deep breath hourly to maintain adequate respiratory function. The client may need to use an incentive spirometer or receive ultrasonic treatments if the cough is ineffective.

Risk for Impaired Skin Integrity. The client with ascites may develop severe edema as well as other problems leading to the nursing diagnosis *Risk for Impaired Skin Integrity related to immobility, edema, and pressure from the abdomen.*

Planning: Expected Outcomes. The client will not develop impaired skin integrity, as evidenced by intact skin.

Implementation. Turn the client frequently, providing adequate support for the distended abdomen. If the client is on bedrest, a specialty mattress is used to prevent skin breakdown. Inspect the client's skin carefully daily and apply lotions and creams as necessary.

Knowledge Deficit. Once the acute problems associated with ascites are controlled, the client and significant others are faced with long-term control of the problem, leading to the nursing diagnosis *Knowledge Deficit related to ascites, treatment, and self-care following discharge.*

Planning: Expected Outcomes. The client will understand ascites, its treatment, and self-care following discharge, as evidenced by the client's statements and compliance with the treatment regimen and abstinence from alcohol.

Implementation. Discuss the causes of ascites with the client, making sure that the client understands ways to slow the recurrence. Ensure that the client understands the need for dietary modifications, fluid restrictions, and home healthcare needs. Help the client to understand that all alcohol intake must be stopped. Refer the client to AA for assistance with abstinence if necessary.

Evaluation

The client's ascites may be controlled to an extent, but, once cirrhosis is advanced, it is difficult to control. The most hopeful outcome is that the client stops drinking and further liver damage is prevented.

■ Surgical Management

The client with refractory and disabling chronic ascites may obtain relief from the insertion of a peritoneovenous shunt (e.g., LeVeen or Denver shunt). As Figure 65–8 shows, a properly functioning shunt moves fluid from the peritoneal (abdominal) cavity into the superior vena cava. Resolution of ascites may be dramatic after implantation of a peritoneovenous shunt. The shunt contains a one-way valve that prevents backflow of ascitic fluid.

Complications of shunt implantation include infection, hemodilution, DIC, congestive heart failure, and shunt clotting. For additional information, see the earlier discussion of surgical management of portal hypertension.

■ Nursing Management of the Surgical Client

Pre- and postoperative management of a client with ascites is similar to that of a client who has undergone surgery for portal hypertension and esophageal varices. See the discussion of nursing care of the client with surgical treatment of a hepatic problem.

Hepatic Encephalopathy

Etiology and Risk Factors

Hepatic encephalopathy comprises a spectrum of CNS disturbances. These disturbances may appear in conjunction with severe liver injury, liver failure, or portocaval shunt. The cause of this disorder is the liver's inability to metabolize ammonia to form urea, which is then excreted. Ammonia is a CNS depressant. Changes during the initial stages of hepatic encephalopathy include reduced mental

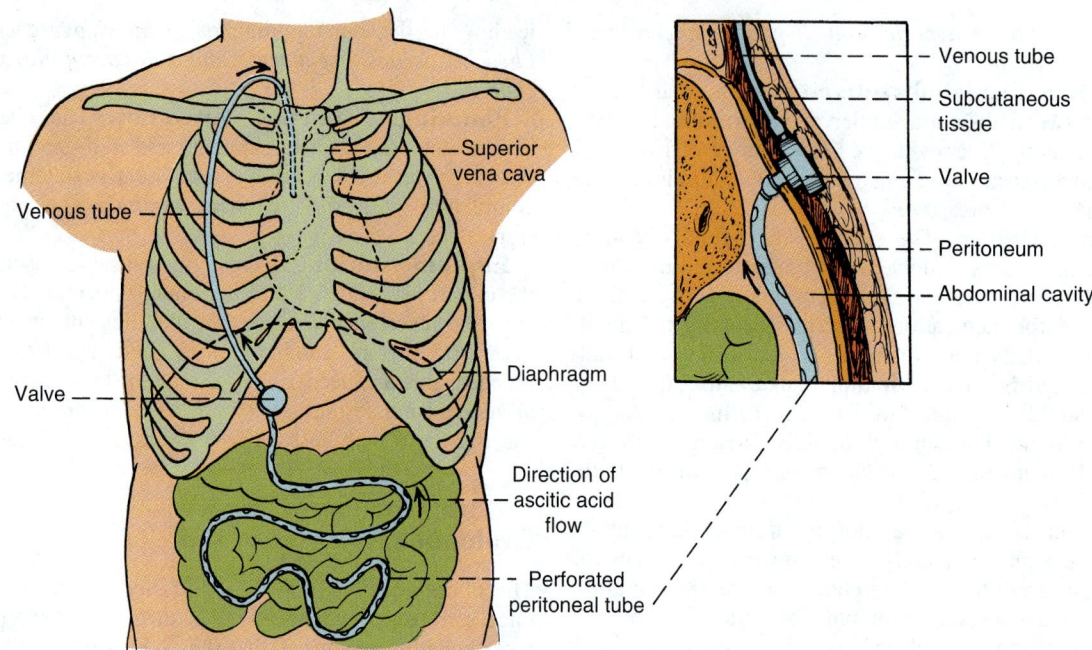

Figure 65–8. LeVeen peritoneovenous shunt for chronic ascites moves fluid from the peritoneal (abdominal) cavity into the superior vena cava.

alertness, confusion, and restlessness. Loss of consciousness, seizures, and irreversible coma occur in the terminal stage.

Pathophysiology

Hepatic encephalopathy is characterized by elevations of ammonia levels in the blood and cerebrospinal fluid. Ammonia is produced in the gastrointestinal tract when protein is broken down by bacteria, in the liver, and, in lesser amounts, by gastric juices and peripheral tissue metabolism. The kidneys are another source of ammonia in the presence of hypokalemia. More recently implicated as a cause of encephalopathy are false neurotransmitters, elevated levels of mercaptans (organic chemicals that contain the sulfhydryl radical, formed when the oxygen of an alcohol is replaced by sulfur), and fatty acids.

Normally, the liver converts ammonia into glutamine, which is stored in the liver and later converted to urea and excreted through the kidneys. Blood ammonia rises when the liver cells are unable to perform this conversion. Failure of the liver to perform this function may be due to liver cell damage and necrosis. It also may result from the shunting of blood from the portal system directly into the systemic venous circulation (bypassing the liver). In either case, as blood ammonia levels rise, many unusual compounds begin to form. Some of these (e.g., octopamine) apparently act as false neurotransmitters in the CNS. Ammonia also is a CNS toxin, with glial and nerve cells affected, leading to altered CNS metabolism and function.

Any process that increases protein in the intestine, such as increased dietary protein or gastrointestinal bleeding, causes elevated blood ammonia levels and possibly mani-

festations of hepatic encephalopathy in clients with hepatocellular failure or portal shunt (Box 65–2).

Clinical Manifestations and Diagnostic Findings

Manifestation of hepatic encephalopathy is primarily neurologic and progresses from mild mental confusion to deep coma. Hepatic encephalopathy impairs memory, attention, concentration, and rate of response. Sleep pattern reversal often occurs, with the client awake at night and sleepy during the day. Evaluate handwriting and speech for significant changes. Asterixis may be present. Some clients with hepatic encephalopathy develop hyperventilation with respiratory alkalosis because high ammonia levels stimulate the respiratory center. The presence of methylmercaptan causes a characteristic odor on the breath called fetor hepaticus.

Box 65–2. Hepatic Encephalopathy: Causes or Precipitating Factors

- Decrease in hepatocellular function
- Hypoxia
- Infection
- Diuretics (hypokalemia, alkalosis, and hypovolemia)
- Depressants (phenobarbital, narcotics, tranquilizers, and sedatives)
- Gastrointestinal bleeding
- Medications containing ammonium or amino compounds
- Paracentesis

Box 65–3. Stages of Hepatic Encephalopathy

Stage 1

Fatigue
Restlessness
Irritability
Decreased intellectual performance
Decreased attention span
Diminished short-term memory
Personality changes
Sleep pattern reversal

Stage 2

Deteriorated handwriting
Asterixis
Drowsiness
Confusion
Lethargy
Fetor hepaticus

Stage 3

Severe confusion
Unable to follow commands
Deep somnolence, but arousable

Stage 4

Coma
Unresponsive to painful stimuli
Possible decorticate or decerebrate posturing

As the client's condition deteriorates, characteristic delta waves appear on the electroencephalogram. As the syndrome progresses, the client's level of consciousness slowly diminishes, and confusion becomes more severe. However, the level of CNS depression commonly fluctuates.

Coma may eventually ensue, deepening until there is no pain response and the reflexes, including the corneal reflex, are completely absent. Box 65–3 lists the stages of hepatic encephalopathy.

Laboratory results show elevated blood ammonia and cerebrospinal fluid glutamine. Although these findings help to confirm the diagnosis of encephalopathy, they are not specific to encephalopathy.

Monitor serum ammonia levels, electrolytes, blood gases, and hepatic function tests (bilirubin, albumin, prothrombin, and enzymes) throughout the course. These findings help determine the degree of imbalance and the extent of hepatic injury and malfunction (see Chapter 64).

Acute and Subacute Care

■ Medical Management

The goals of intervention in clients with hepatic encephalopathy are (1) control or reduction of further degenerative processes, (2) correction or prevention of factors that may precipitate or aggravate encephalopathy, and (3) preservation of remaining physiologic functioning.

Seven principles guide intervention in hepatic encephalopathy:

1. Reduce protein in the intestine. Reducing dietary protein serves to reduce protein in the intestine. If no other precipitating factors are present, this alone may eliminate manifestations.
2. Prevent gastrointestinal bleeding, or, if it occurs, quickly remove the blood from the gastrointestinal tract with lactulose enemas. Gastrointestinal bleeding delivers a protein load to the gastrointestinal tract.
3. Reduce bacterial production of ammonia. Neomycin and lactulose are useful pharmacologic agents for this purpose.
4. Eliminate fluid and electrolyte imbalances, hypoxia, infection, and sedation.
5. Maintain safety and function in the unconscious client. The immobile client who lacks reflexes is vulnerable to numerous complications.
6. Prevent infection. Infection leads to increased tissue catabolism and increased protein load.
7. Remove drugs such as sedatives or those that are hepatotoxic.

Medications to Decrease Ammonia Levels

Neomycin and lactulose are given to reduce bacteria in the intestinal tract. Because neomycin is not absorbed into the circulation, it exerts a powerful effect on the intestinal bacteria responsible for ammonia production. Undesirable side effects result from the depletion of intestinal flora (e.g., diarrhea and vitamin K deficiency). Since neomycin is nephrotoxic, avoid its use in clients with renal insufficiency. Lactulose, which helps decrease blood ammonia levels by reducing absorption of ammonia, is given to clients to produce two to four stools a day. Antibiotics are administered to inhibit growth of gastrointestinal bacteria and magnesium sulfate or enemas are given after hemorrhage to clean out the intestines.

Low Protein Diet

Protein may be totally eliminated from the diet, with an intake of fruit juices and IV fluids, although this radical restriction leads to catabolism of the client's own protein stores. The usual protein restriction is 20 to 40 g/day. The client with chronic hepatic encephalopathy may need to adjust to a long-term, low protein diet (50–60 g/day), which can be difficult. These clients may tolerate vegetable and dairy protein better than meats. These proteins contain fewer amino acids that form ammonia than does meat. A diet high in vegetables and dairy products also helps prevent constipation which further reduces ammonia production.

Outcomes

Although intervention usually alleviates hepatic encephalopathy, the client may succumb to circulatory or respiratory complications, infection, or delirium and convulsions. Mortality is high among clients who progress into coma with hepatic failure. Health practitioners often use dramatic measures to reduce toxic levels of ammonia in the blood. Such measures include hemodialysis and exchange transfusions, which involve removal and replacement of approximately 80% of the client's blood. A liver transplant may be performed in cases of fulminant liver failure.

■ Nursing Management of the Medical Client

Assessment

When working with a client susceptible to hepatic encephalopathy, use interviewing and assessment techniques to evaluate psychophysiologic status. For example, has the client's normally neat handwriting become sloppy and difficult to read? Is speech slow and slurred? Observe the client for personality changes with labile feeling states and elicit flapping tremor (asterixis) by asking the client to dorsiflex the hand with the rest of the arm resting on the bed. The hand cannot be held steady.

The nurse who is with the client over time is often the best person to assess a change in level of mental functioning. Early detection of a depressed or confused level of consciousness greatly improves the client's chances of recovery. To make nursing progress notes relevant, describe behavior vividly and objectively ("States pigeons are pecking at his bedclothes") rather than offer interpretations that may have a different meaning for each reader ("Seems more confused"). As the client progresses into coma, make ongoing neurologic checks to determine the level of consciousness. See Unit 5 for neurologic assessment of comatose clients.

Diagnosis, Planning, Implementation

Risk for Ineffective Management of Therapeutic Regimen (Individuals) and Risk for Ineffective Management of Therapeutic Regimen: Families. The client and significant others are vital players in the control of encephalopathy, leading to the nursing diagnosis *Risk for Ineffective Management of Therapeutic Regimen (Individuals) and Risk for Ineffective Management of Therapeutic Regimen: Families, related to reduction in protein in the diet and long-term pharmacologic intervention with neomycin.*

Planning: Expected Outcomes. The client will understand and comply with the reduction in protein in the diet and long-term pharmacologic intervention with neomycin, as evidenced by the client's following a low-protein diet and stating reasons why neomycin should be taken.

Implementation. It is important that the client understand the importance of the protein-reduced diet in order to have the motivation to remain on this diet.

In addition to ensuring a low-protein diet, assess for manifestations of gastrointestinal bleeding, checking for bright blood in the stool or for black, tarry stools. As previously noted, bleeding results in protein accumulation in the gastrointestinal tract, which exacerbates hepatic encephalopathy. To reverse the progression of manifestations, constipation must be prevented. Administer cathartics and enemas to hasten the exit of protein material from the intestine.

Fluid Volume Deficit. The client often has difficulties with fluid volume leading to the diagnosis *Fluid Volume Deficit related to bleeding, decreased intake, and ascites.*

Planning: Expected Outcomes. The client will maintain a balanced fluid volume, as evidenced by normal blood pressure, absence of edema, absence of ascites, and balanced intake and output.

Implementation. Hypovolemia often precipitates hepatic encephalopathy by reducing hepatocellular perfusion. Fluid balance must be achieved, maintained, and monitored to prevent further hepatic injury and reduced renal perfusion. IV fluids are delivered evenly over time. Monitor vital signs and central venous pressure frequently. If necessary, measure urine output hourly.

Electrolyte and acid-base disturbances such as hypokalemia and alkalosis may precipitate hepatic encephalopathy or develop during its course. Laboratory tests indicate what replacement therapy is necessary.

Diarrhea. The client will need to learn to manage the side effects of medications leading to the nursing diagnosis *Diarrhea related to the laxative action of lactulose or neomycin sulfate.*

Planning: Expected Outcomes. The client will have diarrhea controlled, as evidenced by a decrease in the number of diarrheal stools.

Implementation. Intervention in severe hepatic encephalopathy commonly combines neomycin therapy with protein restriction and bowel cleansing. Administer the prescribed maintenance doses of neomycin and a low protein diet for clients with chronic hepatic encephalopathy. In addition, lactulose, a combination of galactose and fructose that passes through the intestine unchanged, is administered orally to decrease ammonia by trapping ammonium ions in the bowel. As noted earlier, the appropriate lactulose dosage causes two to four soft stool evacuations daily. If severe diarrhea occurs, the dosage is reduced to prevent further electrolyte imbalance.

Risk for Injury. Because of the multitude of problems faced by the client with encephalopathy, the nursing diagnosis *Risk for Injury related to loss of protective mechanisms secondary to hepatic coma* is a common problem.

Planning: Expected Outcomes. Injury or complications of immobility will be prevented or will be diagnosed early, as evidenced by the absence of problems related to immobility.

Implementation. Hypoxemia may precipitate hepatic encephalopathy by damaging the hepatic cell. To prevent and treat hypoxemia, attend to respiratory interventions (e.g., maintaining a patent airway).

Concurrent infection, with protein accumulating from tissue catabolism, requires rapid intervention. The client is particularly vulnerable to nosocomial infections. Wash your hands thoroughly and take other measures to prevent cross-contamination.

Be alert to possible harmful accumulations of ammonia due to diuretic therapy. Hypokalemia from the use of diuretics contributes to hepatic encephalopathy by increasing ammonia production in the kidney.

Finally, depressants may precipitate coma. Their use should be avoided. If agitation occurs in early encephalopathy, agents that are excreted partially through the kidney instead of the liver (e.g., phenobarbital) are administered. Phenobarbital should be administered with caution! Know which narcotics, tranquilizers, and sedatives are biotransformed by the liver. They are often contraindicated in clients with decreased hepatic function.

The immobile client who lacks protective reflexes such as the blink or gag reflex is vulnerable to numerous complications. Preventing complications requires intensive nursing intervention. These interventions are discussed further in Chapter 31 in the care of the client in a coma. Pneumonia and skin breakdown may be prevented by turning the client frequently and promoting lung aeration.

Physiologic agitation may appear as the body accumulates metabolic substances. Therefore, the client should be protected from self-injury, for example, by lowering the bed and padding the side rails. See Unit 5 for further discussion of the comatose client and the client with neurologic disturbances.

Evaluation

The prognosis for the client with hepatic encephalopathy is poor. Generally the best outcome that can be hoped for is maintenance with slowed deterioration.

Community and Self-Care

As the acute stages of cirrhosis subside, the ongoing care of the client with cirrhosis continues. If the client has been discharged, discharge teaching for the client with cirrhosis who has experienced complications is extensive. The family or significant others need to know how to reduce the incidence of complications from cirrhosis. Review the potential complications with the caregivers and how to prevent and treat them.

All medications, along with scheduled times of administration and their intended and adverse side effects, are reviewed.

Explain the importance of a well-balanced, nutritional diet to the client with specific information about limitations on dietary protein, sodium, and water. Family members and significant others need to be made aware of the need to encourage eating and still maintain food intake within prescribed limits.

The client's home may need to be altered to adjust for limitations in mobility. Safety precautions should be taken to help prevent injury to the client. The client's bedroom should be set up near the bathroom if the client is receiving diuretics.

The client's status needs to be followed closely. The client's caregivers need to be aware of any changes that require immediate medical attention. Diagnostic testing at regular intervals is continued to monitor the status of the liver.

Fatty Liver

Lipid infiltration is one of the more common metabolic diseases of the liver. These infiltrations cause liver enlargement and increased firmness and may result in decreased function. Liver biopsy establishes a definite diagnosis. Studies reveal that triglyceride is the major lipid, but small amounts of cholesterol and phospholipid also may have infiltrated the liver.

Major causes of lipid infiltrations include chronic alcoholism, protein malnutrition in early life, diabetes mellitus, obesity, Cushing's syndrome (natural or induced), jejunoileal bypass, prolonged IV hyperalimentation, chronic illnesses that involve impaired nutrition or malabsorption, some hepatotoxins (carbon tetrachloride and DDT), and Reye's syndrome in children.

Clients with moderate to severe lipid infiltration are frequently asymptomatic. However, clients with massive infiltration experience anorexia, abdominal pain, and sometimes jaundice. Laboratory studies demonstrate elevated serum alkaline phosphatase and bilirubin levels.

Recovery begins after the source of the problem is removed and metabolic balance and adequate nutrition are restored. Residual damage, if it occurs, usually follows persistent fatty infiltration and chronic alcoholism. Fat embolization may occur and can cause death.

Nursing intervention for clients with fatty infiltration of the liver includes the following:

1. Directing attention to correction of the cause (abstinence from alcohol, control of diabetes, weight loss, or correction of the intestinal absorptive defect)
2. Preparing the client for diagnostic procedures
3. Giving emotional support by allowing verbalization of concerns and fears
4. Giving supportive physical care including adequate nutritional intake
5. Designing teaching guidelines that promote proper diet and prevent a recurrence.

Liver Neoplasms

Tumors of the liver are either primary or metastatic. Primary liver tumors may arise from hepatocytes, connective tissue, blood vessels, or bile ducts. These tumors are either benign or malignant (Figure 65–9). Figure 65–10 presents a classification of the primary liver neoplasms.

Metastatic malignant tumors arise from the gastrointes-

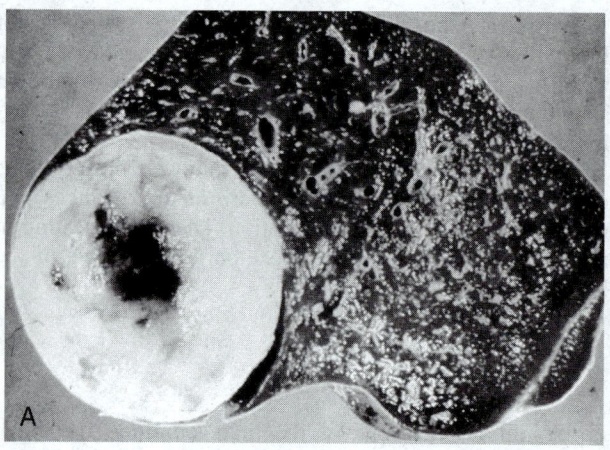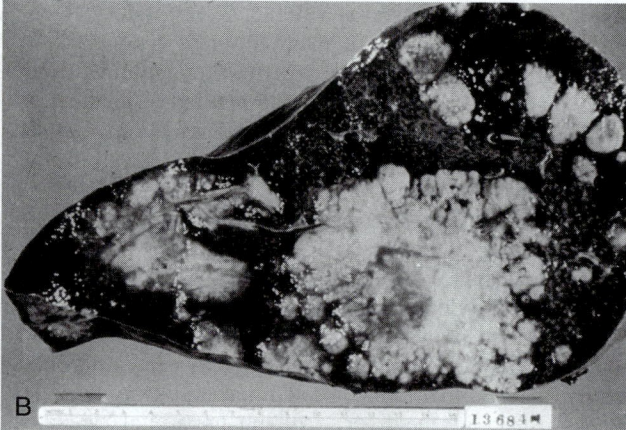

Figure 65–9. Benign liver tumor (*A*) and metastatic malignant liver tumor (*B*).

tinal tract (particularly the colon), the breasts, and the lungs.

■ Benign Hepatic Tumors

Hepatic adenomas are benign tumors of the liver occurring most commonly in women in their 20s and 30s. There has been an increased incidence of these tumors since the introduction of oral contraceptives. The fact that the tumors occur more commonly in women and in women who take oral contraceptives suggests a hormonal influence in their pathogenesis.

Although these tumors are classified as benign, they are nevertheless dangerous because of their vascularity. A benign adenoma may rupture, with consequent hemorrhage. Diagnosis is made by a combination of tests including sonography, CT scan, selective hepatic arteriography, and radionuclide scans. Liver biopsy is not suggested because the tumors are hypervascular.

Intervention for benign adenomas depends on its cause. Discontinuing oral contraceptives or androgens when a tumor appears to be hormone-dependent may correct the condition. Otherwise, treatment may include surgical excision of the involved liver segment. If acute hemorrhage calls for surgery, the surgeon may perform a hepatic lobectomy. Benign hepatic tumors have an excellent prognosis if they can be removed surgically before they rupture and cause death from hemorrhage.

ORIGIN	BENIGN	MALIGNANT
Hepatocytes	Adenoma	Hepatocellular carcinoma
Connective tissue	Fibroma	Sarcoma
Blood vessels	Hemangioma	Hemangioendothelioma
Bile ducts	Cholangioma	Carcinoma

Figure 65–10. Classification of primary liver neoplasms.

■ Malignant Hepatic Tumors

Primary Hepatocellular Carcinoma. Primary hepatocellular carcinoma (malignant hepatoma) is one of the most common tumors worldwide. It is four times more common in men than women. Etiologic factors that may contribute to hepatoma are hepatitis B, hepatitis C, cirrhosis, chronic liver disease, hemochromatosis, certain mycotoxins (aflatoxins), anabolic steroid use, and long-term androgen therapy.

Primary hepatocellular carcinoma is the main cause of death from cancer in many areas of the world, including sub-Saharan Africa and parts of Asia.

Following the diagnosis of liver cancer and if intervention fails to terminate the tumor process, the client usually dies of hepatic failure within 3 to 6 months. Surgical resection of the tumor is the only method of cure and may be attempted if the tumor is confined to one lobe. Many clients, however, do not have a resectable tumor because of underlying cirrhosis and involvement of both lobes.

Metastatic Hepatic Tumors. The liver is one of the common sites of metastasis for all cancers. In the United States, metastatic tumors of the liver are 20 times more common than primary liver tumors.

Etiology and Risk Factors

The liver is a common site of metastasis because of the liver's high rate of blood flow, its size, and portal drainage from the major abdominal organs. Tumors of the gastrointestinal tract, lung, and breast metastasize to the liver more frequently than do tumors of the prostate or thyroid.

Pathophysiology

Metastatic tumors spread to the liver by (1) direct extension from adjacent organs (stomach and gallbladder), (2) the hepatic arterial system, and (3) the portal venous system. Also, as a result of cell migration, the surface of the liver may become seeded with metastatic cells.

Unfortunately, these metastatic tumors may be far advanced before clinical manifestations or laboratory findings indicate their presence. For this reason, metastatic liver cancer carries a poor prognosis. Interventions with radiotherapy and chemotherapy may only be palliative.

Clinical Manifestations and Diagnostic Findings

Clients with primary (benign and malignant) and secondary (metastatic) tumors often present with similar manifestations. Early indicators of liver neoplasm are usually vague. Many clients with metastatic malignancy of the liver present with the following three types of manifestations: (1) manifestations that are specific only to the primary tumor, hepatic involvement being discovered incidentally in the course of a diagnostic evaluation; (2) nonspecific manifestations of anorexia, diaphoresis, fever, weight loss, and weakness; (3) manifestations of active liver disease such as abdominal pain, ascites, or hepatomegaly. Diagnostic studies and physical examination may reveal the following: elevated alkaline phosphatase, hepatomegaly, a liver mass, a friction rub or bruit over the liver, positive angiography, hypoproteinemia, blood-tinged ascites, decreased liver function, and reversal of the albumin-globulin ratio. Greatly elevated serum carcinoembryonic antigen (CEA) levels are often found when the metastases are from primary malignancies in the lung, breast, or gastrointestinal tract.

Some clients also may develop metabolic derangement such as polycythemia, blood sugar disorders, and high levels of calcium. Other clients may present with marked leukocytosis and anemia. Jaundice occurs more often when the bile ducts are the primary site or the tumor mass obstructs a major outflow duct. Other manifestations may be present, varying according to the concurrent pathologic condition. At times, the tumor process causes elevation of the diaphragm and some respiratory problems.

Although neoplasms of the liver create numerous clinical manifestations, many of these manifestations may not occur until the tumors have grown quite large. Malignant tumor cells may have replaced as much as 90% of normal liver tissue before liver insufficiency becomes clinically evident.

In primary hepatocellular cancers, diagnostic tests often reveal high levels of alpha-fetoprotein (AFP). This substance is sometimes present in clients who have metastatic tumors, but levels rarely match those found in clients with primary tumors.

A diagnosis of liver cancer is suggested by an elevated serum alkaline phosphatase level and by abnormal findings, obtained through ultrasound, CT, liver scan, or MRI. Cytologic examination of aspirated fluid can also be used to establish the diagnosis.

Liver biopsy is very helpful in diagnosis. The route of access may be percutaneous, direct via laparotomy, or through a peritoneoscope. Each method has its limitations.

Percutaneous procedures may cause seeding of tumor cells along the exit pathway. Laparotomy requires anesthesia and may be too dangerous. Peritoneoscopy may be impossible if there are extensive adhesions. Because all of these biopsy procedures require membrane puncture, be sure the client has an acceptable prothrombin time.

 ## Acute and Subacute Care

■ Medical Management

The treatment of liver cancer depends on the underlying tumor type. It is supportive and palliative. The long-term survival of clients with metastatic liver malignancies is dismal.

Chemotherapy

Regional perfusion of the liver directly into the hepatic artery to relieve pain or slow tumor growth may be useful. This may produce fewer side effects than systemic chemotherapy. Various chemotherapeutic agents have been used singly or in combination, systemically, with agents infused into the hepatic artery.

During surgery, the surgeon may implant a chemotherapy infusion pump. Such pumps, filled percutaneously, deliver medication continuously into the hepatic artery. In metastatic growths, the physician may prescribe systemic chemotherapy to reduce tumor size and pain.

Chemotherapeutic agents used to induce regression of primary and metastatic tumors of the liver include 5-fluorouracil (5-FU) and doxorubicin (Adriamycin) as single-dose therapy, and 5-FU with carmustine (BCNU), semustine (methyl CCNU), or streptozocin as combination therapy.

Radiation Therapy

Irradiation of liver tumors may provide temporary pain relief, but does not promote survival. Percutaneous biliary drainage or the internal placement of a biliary drain helps increase the passage of bile into the duodenum and decrease jaundice and discomfort.

Liver Transplant

Liver transplantation may be considered a therapeutic option in primary hepatocellular carcinoma, but recurrence of the tumor or metastases after transplantation limits the usefulness of this treatment.

Experimental Approaches

Some of the experimental approaches that are being evaluated for treatment of primary hepatic tumor include alcohol ablation via ultrasound-guided percutaneous injection, ultrasound-guided cryoablation, and gene therapy with retroviral vectors containing genes that express cytotoxic agents.

Complications

Tumor rupture, gastrointestinal hemorrhage from varices, progressive cachexia, and hepatic failure are the primary complications of hepatic tumors. Management of the client with these complications is supportive and palliative and will vary according to the client's overall condition and degree of liver impairment.

Outcomes

Prognosis is poor as most clients with hepatic carcinoma have a median survival of 3 to 6 months.

■ Nursing Management of the Medical Client

Nursing diagnoses and interventions for clients with liver neoplasms vary according to the amount of liver dysfunction and the treatment modalities. Plan to assess the client for metabolic malfunctions, bleeding problems, ascites, edema, inability to biotransform endogenous and exogenous (drug) wastes, hypoproteinemia, jaundice, and endocrine complications.

Take time to prepare the client in the diagnostic stage for the various procedures and assess carefully for postprocedure complications. In addition, assist the client and significant others to gain knowledge about the condition and offer the support necessary for them to cope with the uncertainty and fear associated with cancer. See Chapters 23 and 24 for detailed discussions of nursing care of clients with malignant tumors.

■ Surgical Management

For tumors that are small and confined to one liver segment or lobe, the surgeon may perform resection of the segment or lobe if the client is able to withstand the stress of surgery.

■ Nursing Management of the Surgical Client

Nursing management of the client pre- and postoperatively has many responsibilities. See the discussion of nursing management of the client who has undergone surgery for complications of portal hypertension.

Liver Transplantation

Liver transplantation is now considered a feasible form of intervention for a variety of endstage liver diseases. The number of liver transplants has continued to grow each year. In 1990, over 2500 people in the United States received liver transplants. Candidates for this procedure include clients with chronic liver disease. The following

are some of the most common conditions for which transplants are performed.

● Primary biliary cirrhosis (adult)
● Hepatitis—chronic or fulminant (usually adult)
● Sclerosing cholangitis (adult)
● Biliary atresia (pediatric)
● Alpha$_1$-antitrypsin deficiency (usually pediatric)
● Confined hepatic malignancy (adult or pediatric)
● Wilson's disease
● Budd-Chiari syndrome (hepatic vein obstruction)

Even though liver transplantation is indicated for clients whose chronic or acute liver disease is progressive, life-threatening, and unresponsive to medical therapy, the appropriate candidate for liver transplant is at lower risk (i.e., more likely to survive) if he or she is age 50 or younger; has lower bilirubin and albumin levels, decreased prothrombin time, and less edema; and is not suffering from life-threatening complications such as bleeding varices, severe hypertension or advanced cardiac disease, advanced catabolism, active alcoholism, or metastatic cancer.[15]

Clients with alcoholic cirrhosis, chronic viral hepatitis, and primary hepatocellular malignancies are more controversial liver transplant recipients. Clients with any one of these conditions are considered at high risk, but liver transplantation may be offered to carefully selected individuals. The alcoholic client, for example, must be willing to adhere to certain guidelines such as abstinence and a substance abuse treatment program in order to be eligible for a liver transplant. The client must be psychologically stable and have good support systems for the complex postoperative course.

Critical Care

■ Surgical Management

Preoperative Management

The client selected for liver transplantation must undergo a variety of tests including blood analysis, hepatic angiogram, abdominal CT scan, chest and hip x-ray, electrocardiogram (ECG), bone density studies, and nutritional assessment. The client may also have the opportunity to meet the transplant team. Matching donor and recipient organ size and blood and tissue type are important considerations in donor selection.

Surgical Procedure

Surgery generally lasts 8 hours but can last from 6 to 18 hours. The surgery may involve removal of the diseased liver *(orthotopic)* and insertion of the donor liver. Anastomoses of the vena cava, portal vein, hepatic artery, and bile duct are performed. A second approach is *heterotopic* where the diseased liver is left in during transplant. Orthotopic is by far the more common of the two. Because excessive bleeding may occur, large amounts of blood, blood products, and volume expanders are needed.

Postoperative Management

The major focus of care is to monitor for rejection, infection, and occlusion of vessels. The client needs to be in an intensive care unit with constant monitoring of the respiratory, cardiovascular, neurologic, fluid and electrolyte, and hemodynamic status. Liver function is also monitored through assessment of serum transaminases (ALT, AST), bilirubin, albumin, and clotting factors. Bedrest is necessary for several days and immunosuppressive therapy started before surgery must be continued on a regular schedule postoperatively. The Care Plan outlines nursing interventions and corresponding rationales for care of the client after a liver transplant.

Complications

Postoperative complications include infection, rejection, hemorrhage, atelectasis, failure of anastomosis, and acute renal failure. Rejection most commonly occurs between the 4th and 10th postoperative days. Manifestations of acute rejection include fever, tachycardia, right upper quadrant or flank pain, and increasing jaundice. Drugs such as azathioprine, an immunosuppressant, and steroids such as prednisone are used to stop the rejection; otherwise, rapid deterioration of liver function occurs. Cholangiocarcinoma is considered a contraindication in most cases because of the likelihood of recurrence of the tumor.

Outcomes

Teach the client and significant others about long-term, ongoing care. The Client Education Guide lists information that the client should know. As with other forms of transplant, immunosuppressive therapy (cyclosporine and newer experimental medications) prevents rejection of the transplanted liver.

■ Nursing Management of the Surgical Client

Preoperative Care

Assessment

Once the client has chosen transplantation as an alternative to care and is placed on the recipient waiting list, he or she will need to undergo an extensive physical and psychological evaluation. Focus on assessing the client's needs in relation to the amount of knowledge and information he or she has. Also, ascertain how the client and significant others are coping with the situation. In addition, the needs dictated by the extent of organ failure will guide care.

The specific nursing care needs of clients during the waiting period for a liver transplant depend on those mandated by the degree of endstage liver disease. Two needs of clients that guide nursing care include the following:

Diagnosis, Planning, Implementation

Knowledge Deficit. Because of the complexity of liver transplant and the complex regimen required after surgery, an appropriate nursing diagnosis for this client would be *Knowledge Deficit: Pretransplant recipient, related to transplantation process and care needed after transplant.*

Planning: Expected Outcomes. The client will become better informed about the transplantation process and the care needed after surgery, as evidenced by verbalization of specific information about the transplant procedure and description of pertinent care measures to be taken after surgery.

Implementation. Transplant recipients should be visited by the transplant team so that they can be given accurate information about the surgery. They also should have someone they can contact in case of an emergency or if they have a question. Clients need opportunities to meet the transplant team and ask them questions about the procedure. Care measures that will be administered post transplant need to be explained to the client, such as the kind and amount of medication that will be administered, the side effects of these drugs, and the need for

CLIENT EDUCATION GUIDE

Care After Liver Transplant

Know why each medication is important, when to take it, and what to do if you forget your medication and do not take it on time.

Although most clients do not go home with dietary restrictions, you may require a low sodium diet. Maintain a nutritious diet to help with healing.

Learn to manage fever, cough, malaise, nausea and vomiting, headache, and other untoward manifestations. Avoid self-medication with over-the-counter drugs and know when to call your physician.

Report any changes in liver function such as jaundice or changes in urine or stool to the physician. Any changes in liver function tests may indicate rejection.

Resume activities slowly. Although there are very few limitations on normal physical activities, the more vigorous ones, such as lifting or driving, may require your physician's permission.

Avoid crowds when taking large doses of immunosuppressants. Care for wounds and cuts, attend to mouth care and dental visits, and notify the transplant team if you are exposed to infectious disease.

You will need liver biopsies at months 3 and 6 and then yearly; frequent transplant clinic visits; routine checkups; regular cancer monitoring (Papanicolaou smear, breast or testicular examination, etc.); and regular dental visits.

CARE PLAN

Management of the Client After Liver Transplant

Nursing Diagnosis. Risk for Infection Related to Immunosuppression, poor nutritional status, loss of skin integrity, and presence of invasive lines.

Collaborative Problem. Organ Rejection; Occlusion of Vessels

Planning: Expected Outcomes. The client will demonstrate a reduced risk for infection as evidenced by no manifestations of rejection, maintaining a balanced nutritional state, maintaining skin integrity, and exhibiting no manifestations of inflammation at the IV insertion site.

Implementation: Nursing Intervention	Rationales
Observe for manifestations of respiratory compromise and readiness to wean from the ventilator.	Clients may be on a ventilator for 24 to 48 hours postoperatively. Incision under the diaphragm limits excursion because of pain and edema. Clients may have a chest tube in place.
Monitor fluid and electrolyte status, serum glucose, and pH.	Clients are always somewhat fluid-overloaded from receiving extensive volumes of blood products administered during the long surgical procedure. This overload could lead to pulmonary edema and congestive heart failure. Serum potassium will be decreased as a phenomenon of the transplant. Serum glucose will be increased as a normal event. pH will be normal to acidic.
Monitor for manifestations of bleeding and blood clotting factors.	Coagulopathy and thrombocytopenia may persist into the early postoperative period. The transplant procedure consists of several vascular anastomoses that may cause hemorrhage.
Monitor cardiovascular status, including blood pressure, pulse, central venous pressure, pulmonary artery pressures, ascites, and body temperature. Monitor for manifestations of infection.	Correlation of these factors can help diagnose early changes in cardiac and circulatory status. The highest rate of post-transplant nosocomial infections occurs in clients receiving liver transplants. Liver transplant clients are subject to systemic bacterial infection related to multiple invasive procedures; opportunistic bacterial, fungal, viral, and protozoal infections related to malnutrition and immunosuppression; and viral hepatitis from blood transfusions.
Follow immunosuppressive protocols.	The amount of immunosuppressant varies for each client. Maintaining proper levels of immunosuppressive drugs prevents rejection.
Monitor wound drains and bile drains for patency and bile characteristics (amount, color, consistency).	Obstruction of wound drains causes increased intra-abdominal pressure from accumulation of ascites and blood. Obstruction of bile flow can cause damage to the liver and biliary system.
Keep the client and significant others informed of changes and requirements.	The level of acuity may be alarming to both the client and significant others. The client will have difficulty expressing concerns because of grogginess and the presence of an endotracheal tube.
Teach the client and significant others about the procedures required postoperatively.	Both the client and significant others will require education about procedures such as cholangiography, liver biopsy, and abdominal ultrasound. Much of the teaching will have been done preoperatively unless the client required an emergency transplant as a result of fulminant liver failure.

Evaluation. The client does not develop manifestations of rejection or infection. The client should return to a relatively normal life after the transplant.

continuing care after the transplant. Clients need to know about the intensive care unit with its IV lines and monitoring devices, and the incision, and the dressings. The client needs to know that medications will be administered to control pain and nausea.

Ineffective Individual Coping. The client waiting for a liver transplant is under a great deal of stress leading to the nursing diagnosis *Ineffective Individual Coping related to situational crisis, threat of death, chronicity of illness, and change in the family role.*

Planning: Expected Outcomes. The client will cope with the anxiety of the waiting period as evidenced by being able to verbalize an understanding of how the transplant procedure may extend life and improve the quality of life for him or her and the family.

Implementation. The nurse will assist the client and significant others to learn new problem-solving strategies, as evidenced by helping them cope with any anxiety, depression, fear, anger, and uncertainty they may be experiencing. Offer encouragement and reassurance to the client and family and arrange family counseling or social work assistance if coping strategies that worked in the past work no longer. Offer support by being available for telephone calls, by coordinating support groups, and by calling families to let them know someone cares.

Evaluation

If the client is unable to verbalize specific pertinent information about liver transplant surgery and is unable to cope with the anxiety of surgery, then new plans and interventions are necessary to meet the client's preoperative needs.

Postoperative Care

Assessment

The nurse who works in the intensive care unit continually assesses the client's liver function and general physical status. The nurse must also assess the needs of the family and significant others who might have traveled long distances from home and are feeling powerless, stressed, and anxious. Soon after transplant the nursing staff need to formulate a plan of care appropriate to the postoperative needs of the client and family. Much of the care and many of the nursing diagnoses for a client who undergoes liver transplantation are the same as for a client after any other type of surgery.

Diagnosis, Planning, Implementation

Risk for Infection. Because of the immunosuppression required after the transplant, combined with the severity of the surgical procedure, a common nursing diagnosis for this client is *Risk for Infection related to impaired immune function, poor nutritional status, loss of skin integrity, and presence of invasive lines.*

Planning: Expected Outcomes. The client will demonstrate a reduced risk of infection as evidenced by no manifestations of rejection, maintaining a balanced nutritional state, maintaining skin integrity, and exhibiting no manifestations of inflammation at the IV insertion site.

Implementation. The client's temperature is monitored regularly and fever reported immediately. If fever is present, the source is sought from sputum, blood, urine, or wound drainage. Invasive lines, urinary catheters, and arterial lines should be removed as soon as possible to minimize the possibilities of infection. The general condition of the skin is assessed regularly and monitored for breaks or tears. Closely monitor the client during the

postoperative period. The Care Plan lists the postoperative nursing assessments and interventions and explains the rationale for each.

Rejection of Donor Tissue. One of the most critical problems associated with transplantation is possible rejection, making the collaborative problem *Rejection of Donor Tissue related to dysfunction of the transplanted organ or tissue* an important problem for the healthcare team to address.

Planning: Expected Outcomes. The client will not experience rejection of the transplanted liver, as evidenced by a lack of manifestations of organ failure.

Implementation. The nurse will assess the client for manifestations of organ failure, including increased serum enzymes; abnormal bilirubin, albumin, and clotting factors; increased temperature ($\geq 38°C$); tachycardia; malaise; hypertension; fluid retention; enlargement of the liver; and tenderness over the transplant site. Continue to administer immunosuppressive therapy (started before surgery) to prevent rejection and the reoccurrence of manifestations of organ failure. Administer nursing care based on the immunosuppressive therapy used.

Risk for Ineffective Management of Therapeutic Regimen (Individuals). The self-care regimen following liver transplantation is very complex for the client and significant others, leading to the nursing diagnosis *Risk for Ineffective Management of Therapeutic Regimen (Individuals), related to self-care (diet, physical activity) following transplant, medicines, manifestations of infection or rejection, follow-up care because of lack of previous exposure to information, and the large amount of information to comprehend.*

Planning: Expected Outcome. The client will discuss self-care involved in managing medications, diet, manifestations of rejection and infection, and physical activity and exercise.

Implementation. While the nurse is responsible for implementing the enormous physical care, the psychosocial needs of the client and significant others must also be met. Keep the client and significant others informed about the status of the transplanted organ. Allow them to express their concerns and fears and ask questions. Arrange short, frequent meetings between members of the healthcare team, transplant team, and the client and significant others to help clients and their significant others get answers to their many questions.

Explain why continuing the present medication regimen is important and why the client should never miss a dose. Also, explain the manifestations of infection and rejection if the client is not able to remember, needs a review, or did not receive complete information before surgery. Ask the client to repeat the information.

Evaluation

The client should recover from the liver transplant and be able to resume a normal life as long as medication and healthcare regimens are followed closely.

Liver Abscess

A liver abscess is a localized collection of pus and organisms within the parenchyma of the liver.

Liver abscess usually develops after one of the following three conditions:

1. *Bacterial cholangitis*, which results from obstruction of the bile ducts by stone or stricture
2. *Portal vein bacteremia*, which may develop following bowel inflammation or organ perforation
3. *Amebiasis* (infestation with amebae from tropical or subtropical areas)

Other predisposing factors are diabetes mellitus, infected hepatic cysts, metastatic liver tumors with secondary infection, and diverticulitis.

The client commonly reports right upper quadrant pain and abdominal and right shoulder pain. Assessment may also reveal liver enlargement, tenderness, nausea, vomiting, weight loss, anorexia, fever, and diaphoresis. At times, the client may develop a right pleural effusion. The liver's proximity to the base of the right lung contributes to this process.

Liver scans are extremely valuable in diagnosis. Other useful diagnostic measures include ultrasound, CT, and arteriography. Laboratory data reflect slight-to-marked elevations of aminotransferases, alkaline phosphatase, and bilirubin. High levels indicate the presence of concurrent obstruction. A positive blood culture occurs in some cases.

Intervention in hepatic abscess consists of (1) percutaneous drainage of the abscess with antimicrobial therapy, (2) surgical drainage of large abscesses with postoperative antimicrobial therapy, or (3) antimicrobial therapy without drainage for a few months. Any concurrent problem disposing the client to abscess requires attention as well. These clients are very ill. Early diagnosis and intervention reduce mortality from liver abscess to about 10%.

Abscesses due to amebic infestation (*Entamoeba histolytica*) are similar to other liver abscesses. The major difference in intervention is that physicians prescribe metronidazole (Flagyl) or chloroquine phosphate (Aralen Phosphate) instead of broad-spectrum antibiotics. It is important to dispose of feces carefully and to wash your hands to prevent transmission of this organism. Complications of an amebic abscess include rupture of the cyst into the pleural space, lung, bowel, and retroperitoneum.

When caring for the client with liver abscess, assess vital signs regularly. High temperature and rapid pulse may indicate the presence of general sepsis, a likely complication. Encourage movement, coughing, and deep-breathing to prevent or limit pulmonary complications related to hepatic abscess. Increase the client's fluid intake and provide skin care in the event of hyperpyrexia.

Help the client's significant others to accept the seriousness of the condition and provide a supportive environment that allows them to express their fears and concerns.

Hemochromatosis

Hemochromatosis is a disorder of iron metabolism. It is, however, often associated with portal hypertension and it causes hepatomegaly. Thus, we include it with liver disorders.

This process, which is relatively uncommon, affects men more often than women.

Primary hemochromatosis, a recessive inherited metabolic defect, causes increased iron absorption from the gastrointestinal tract. Secondary hemochromatosis is caused by alcoholism, excessive dietary intake of iron, or conditions that require repeated blood transfusions (e.g., chronic anemias).

Total body iron in most clients ranges from 2 to 5 g. Clients with hemochromatosis often have levels of 20 g or higher. The excess iron travels to parenchymal cells, where it is deposited as ferritin or hemosiderin. The liver and pancreas are most at risk. The heart, spleen, kidney, and skin undergo less damage. As these organs become fibrotic, loss of function occurs. As a result, the more common problems associated with hemochromatosis include diabetes, enlarged liver, cirrhosis, cardiac disease, increased skin pigmentation, and arthritis. A form of arthritis, pseudogout, in which calcium phosphate crystals accumulate in large joints, is also associated with hemochromatosis. It is the arthritis that often prompts clients to seek medical attention.

Diagnosis depends on the presence of (1) elevated plasma iron levels (above 150 μg/ml), (2) greater than 60% saturation of iron-binding protein (transferrin), and (3) manifestations of specific organ dysfunction. Liver biopsy provides the definitive diagnosis.

Intervention involves phlebotomy on a biweekly or weekly basis over a 1- or 2-year period (2 ml of blood = 1 mg Fe). Once the excess iron has been removed from the body, two or three maintenance phlebotomies per year keep body iron normal. If diagnosis of hemochromatosis occurs before cirrhosis develops, phlebotomy will reverse or prevent all the manifestations except arthropathy and hepatocellular carcinoma. Desferrioxamine mesylate, a chelating agent, also facilitates the removal of iron from the body.

When severe tissue damage with marked clinical manifestations occurs prior to diagnosis, the prognosis extends life from 1 to 8 years. The health practitioner manages the liver disease, cardiac disease, and diabetes, as necessary. Death usually follows cardiac failure, cirrhosis, hepatocellular carcinoma, hematemesis, or pneumonia.

Amyloidosis

Amyloid is a proteinaceous, starchlike substance that can infiltrate the liver and other organs. Accumulation of amyloid deposits causes tissues to cease functioning.

Clinicians may classify amyloidosis according to the type of protein that forms the amyloid deposits. The most common form of amyloidosis (primary amyloidosis) involves deposit of light-chain amyloid formed from immunoglobins. This abnormal protein material causes the most damage to tissues of cardiac, smooth muscle, skin, kidney, and liver origin. However, light-chain amyloid can accumulate in every organ except the CNS.

Amyloidosis due to deposition of protein A is associated with chronic inflammation in conditions such as tuberculosis, rheumatoid arthritis, ankylosing spondylitis, osteomyelitis, and bronchiectasis. Tissues most disturbed by this type of amyloidosis include those of the spleen, kidney, and liver.

Amyloidosis becomes a problem when it begins to interfere with organ function. Although many organs may be affected, the liver receives the greatest damage. Assessment reveals that hepatomegaly is the most noticeable effect of this pathologic process. Liver function remains relatively unaffected. Clinical jaundice rarely appears.

Liver biopsy provides excellent diagnostic data, but there is a high incidence of postbiopsy hemorrhage or liver rupture. Bleeding probably results from amyloid infiltration of the walls of small blood vessels. Clinicians find that gingival, skin, or rectal biopsy provides sufficient diagnostic data.

The physician may prescribe chemotherapy to treat light-chain amyloidosis and provide symptomatic relief. When kidney, heart, or gastrointestinal tract involvement occurs, the client usually experiences progressive deterioration. Assessment and interventions are designed for the specific organs involved. Death typically follows cardiac failure.

Intervention in amyloidosis associated with chronic inflammation consists of removing the primary cause and administering antimicrobial therapy to relieve chronic infection.

Congenital Conditions

Three congenital conditions affecting the liver are Wilson's disease, Caroli's syndrome, and congenital hepatic fibrosis.

Wilson's Disease

Wilson's disease leads to an accumulation of copper in the tissue of the liver, brain, and kidney. The primary manifestations of this disorder are abnormal liver function and neurologic changes. Hepatic manifestations may occur from early childhood to adulthood. This disease is usually chronic, but also may be acute. The acute form is often fatal unless a transplant can be performed. One of the hallmarks of this disease is the presence of Kayser-Fleischer rings encircling the cornea. These greenish-yellow–pigmented rings are due to copper deposits. Copper deposits also can be seen on liver biopsy. Penicillamine is the drug of choice to treat this problem.

Caroli's Syndrome

Caroli's syndrome is characterized by dilated bile ducts and cyst formations. The condition may be localized or

widespread. It usually presents soon after birth, but may not be diagnosed until early adulthood. Fever and bacterial cholangitis are usually the two manifestations that lead to diagnosis. Other manifestations may include right upper quadrant pain and jaundice, both of which may be caused by obstruction of the biliary tract by a cyst(s) or stone(s). Treatment consists of antibiotics, external biliary drainage, or even transplant.

Congenital Hepatic Fibrosis

Congenital hepatic fibrosis is characterized by portal hypertension caused by portal fibrosis. It usually presents as upper gastrointestinal bleeding from gastric or esophageal varices. Treatment ranges from blood transfusions and sclerotherapy to portacaval shunting (see Fig. 65–6).

Liver Trauma

Liver injury usually results from a penetrating injury or blunt trauma. Either may lead to laceration and hemorrhage.

Penetrating injuries are usually knife or missile wounds (gunshot). A knife wound generally is superficial and leaves a sharp clear edge, while missile wounds cause perforations through the liver tissue, that is, the entrance and exit points. The greater the velocity of the missile, the greater the damage. Often, a close-range missile injury is fatal because of the large amount of damage.

Blunt trauma (e.g., from a steering wheel or a fall) can have various effects, from small hematomas that remain under the liver capsule, to large, starlike lacerations from severe impact forces.

Intervention in hemorrhage constitutes the major immediate problem after injury. Monitor victims of trauma carefully for falling blood pressure and tachycardia which may indicate hemorrhage. The problem is more difficult when the liver's blood vessels or bile ducts are damaged as well. Later complications include bile peritonitis and abscess formation.

Intervention in liver injuries consists of control of the hemorrhage, debridement, and drainage. It may be necessary to remove liver lobes, but more often the major goal is to control hemorrhage. When a damaged blood supply causes sloughing of a hepatic segment, hemorrhage follows as a late problem.

Common postoperative problems include pulmonary infections and abscess formation. Clients are assessed postoperatively for manifestations of infection, for example, fever, chills, difficulty breathing, and so forth. Interventions to prevent pneumonia are performed. For information on preventing postoperative complications, review Chapter 21.

Conclusions

Hepatic disorders are complex and difficult for all involved. The nurse needs to have a thorough understanding of the liver and its functions to care for these clients. Many hepatic disorders are the result of the client's life-style, further complicating an already difficult problem. The nurse must therefore consider both the physiologic and psychosocial problems associated with many hepatic disorders. Helping the client make appropriate life-style changes is an important nursing function.

Thinking Critically

1. A 37-year-old man is admitted with a 10-day history of anorexia, fatigue, malaise, low-grade fever, dark urine, and upper abdominal discomfort. There is no history of jaundice, intravenous drug use, or blood transfusions. He is homosexual. Alcohol intake consists of several mixed drinks nightly and wine with dinner. The client's physical examination includes: temperature of 99.6° F, jaundice, blood pressure 150/80, and no spider nevi. The liver measures 12 cm in the mid-clavicular line and is moderately tender. The spleen is not palpable. Initial laboratory data: total bilirubin, 6.8 mg/dl (normal, 0.2–1.2 mg/dl); alkaline phosphatase, 240 units/L (normal, 20–90 units/L); aspartate aminotransferase (AST), 980 units/L (normal, 5–40); alanine aminotransferase (ALT), 1200 units/L (normal, 5–35 mU/mL). The white blood cell count is 5600/mm³ with a normal differential. What are the priorities for care in this situation? What interventions might be used?

Factors to Consider. Without further data, what would appear to be the major organ system(s) involved? What additional information do you, as his nurse, think it is necessary to obtain? If you are a student caring for this client and you inadvertently sustain a needle-stick from a syringe used to give an injection to this client, what action would you take?

2. A 48-year-old man presents to the emergency room. He felt well until 2 hours previously when he became nauseous and subsequently vomited a large amount of red blood and clots. He admits to a long history of heavy alcohol use and cigarette smoking. He takes no medications. Laboratory data: hemoglobin, 9.6 g/dl; hematocrit, 28.4%; platelet count, 92,000/mm³; prothrombin time, 16.5 seconds (normal, 11–15); alkaline phosphatase, 120 units/L (normal, 20–90); AST, 265 units/L; ALT, 112 units/L. What is likely to be a major underlying cause of this client's problem? Is it reversible? Can further damage be stopped? With the client vomiting blood, what should your priority interventions be?

Factors to Consider. What gastrointestinal disorders can be manifested in people who consume large quantities of alcohol? What risks does the client face in the present situation?

3. Your client is a 68-year-old man, diagnosed with cirrhosis, who is admitted for treatment of ascites and acute upper right abdominal pain. His abdomen is very large, and the ascitic fluid shifts whenever he moves from side to side. Diagnostic studies reveal that the cause of his pain is cholelithiasis, and surgery is scheduled. What are the client's priority needs on admission? What complications might he face following surgery?

Factors to Consider. What are the clinical manifestations of cirrhosis? Is the client with cirrhosis a good candidate for abdominal surgery?

Bibliography

1. American Cancer Society. (1996). *Cancer facts and figures.* New York: Author.
2. Bass, N. M. (1992). Toxic and drug-induced liver disease. In J. B. Wyngaarden, L. H. Smith, & J. C. Bennett (Eds.), *Cecil's handbook of medicine* (19th ed.). Philadelphia: W. B. Saunders.
3. Benning, C. R., & Smith, A. (1994). Psychosocial needs of family members of liver transplant patients. *Clinical Nurse Specialist, 8*(5), 280–288.
4. Boyer, T. D. (1992). Cirrhosis of the liver and its major sequelae. In J. B. Wyngaarden, L. H. Smith, & J. C. Bennett (Eds.), *Cecil's handbook of medicine* (19th ed.). Philadelphia: W. B. Saunders.
5. Bronsther, O., et al. (1994). Prioritization and organ distribution for liver transportation. *JAMA, 271*(2), 140–143.
6. Butler, R. (1994). Managing the complications of cirrhosis. *American Journal of Nursing, 94*(3), 46–49.
7. Caraceni, P., et al. (1994). When musculoskeletal, pulmonary, and cardiovascular findings herald hepatic dysfunction. *Consultant, 34*(3), 420–423.
8. Carpenito, L. J. (1995). *Handbook of nursing diagnosis* (6th ed.). Philadelphia: J. B. Lippincott.
9. Copstead, L. E. C. (1995). *Perspective on pathophysiology.* Philadelphia: W. B. Saunders.
10. Dienstag, J. (1994). Liver transplantation. In K. J. Isselbacher et al. (Eds.), *Harrison's principles of internal medicine* (13th ed.). New York: McGraw-Hill.
11. Di Marin, A. J. (1994). Gastrointestinal diseases. In A. R. Myers (Ed.). *Medicine* (2nd ed., pp. 225–226). Philadelphia: Harwal.
12. Doherty, M. M., & Carver, D. K. (1993). New relief for esophageal varices. *American Journal of Nursing, 93*(4), 58–63.
13. Felts, W. M., & Knight, S. M. (1992). The nature and prevention of viral hepatitis: What health educators should know. *Journal of Health Education, 23*(5), 267–274.
14. Ferri, F. F. (1995). *The care of the medical patient* (3rd ed.). St. Louis: Mosby–Year Book.
15. Friedman, L. S. (1995). In L. M. Tierney et al. (Eds.), *Medical diagnosis and treatment* (34th ed.). Norwalk, CT: Appleton & Lange.
16. Guyton, A. C. (1991). *Textbook of medical physiology* (8th ed.). Philadelphia: W. B. Saunders.
17. Hicks, F. D., Larson, J. L., & Ferrans, C. E. (1992). Quality of life after liver transplant. *Research in Nursing and Health, 15,* 111–119.
18. INH-associated hepatitis cases rare but potentially fatal (1993). *Hospital Infection Control, 20*(10), 143–144.
19. Isselbacher, K. J., & Dienstag, J. L. (1994). Tumors of the liver. In K. J. Isselbacher et al. (Eds), *Harrison's principles of internal medicine* (13th ed.). New York: McGraw-Hill.
20. Jackson, M., & Rymer, T. (1994). Viral hepatitis: Anatomy of a diagnosis. *American Journal of Nursing, 94*(1) 43–48.
21. Kerber, K. (1993). The adult with bleeding esophageal varices. *Critical Care Nursing Clinics of North America, 5*(1), 153–162.
22. Killeen, T. K. (1993). Alcoholism and liver transplantation: Ethical and nursing implications. *Perspectives in Psychiatric Care, 29*(1), 7–12.
23. Kimbrell, J. D. (1993). Acquired coagulopathies. *Critical Care Nursing Clinics of North America, 5*(3), 453–458.

24. Kucharshi, S. (1993). Fulminant hepatic failure. *Critical Care Nursing Clinics of North America, 5*(1), 141–152.

25. McLean, K., Kneteman, N., & Taylor, G. (1994). Comparative risk of bloodstream infection in organ transplant recipients. *Infection Control and Hospital Epidemiology, 15*(9), 582–584.

26. Myers, A. R. (Ed.). (1994). *Medicine.* Philadelphia: Harwal.

27. Nicholas, J. J., et al. (1994). The quality of life after orthotopic liver transplantation: An analysis of 166 cases. *Archives of Physical Medicine and Rehabilitation, 75,* 431–435.

28. O'Brien, E. (1992). Liver transplantation assessment. *The Lamp, 49*(5), 26–27.

29. Ockner, R. K. (1992). Acute viral hepatitis. In J. B. Wyngaarden, L. H. Smith, & J. C. Bennett (Eds.), *Cecil's handbook of medicine* (19th ed.). Philadelphia: W. B. Saunders.

30. Podolsky, D. K., & Isselbacher K. J. (1994). Alcohol related liver disease and cirrhosis. In K. J. Isselbacher et al. (Eds.), *Harrison's principles of internal medicine* (13th ed.). New York: McGraw-Hill.

31. Porth, C. M. (1994). *Pathophysiology* (4th ed.). Philadelphia: J. B. Lippincott.

32. Reishtein, J. (1993). Liver failure: Case study of a complex problem. *Critical Care Nurse, 26,* 36–47.

33. Rice, V. (1992). Fluid and electrolyte disorders in liver failure. *CINA Journal, 8*(1), 10–12.

34. Rosman, A. S., et al. (1993). Hepatitis C virus antibody in alcoholic patients. *Archives of Internal Medicine, 153,* 965–969.

35. Sabiston, D. C., Jr. (1991). *Textbook of surgery: The biologic basis of modern surgical practice* (14th ed.). Philadelphia: W. B. Saunders.

36. Scharschmidt, B. F. (1992). Acute and chronic hepatic failure. In J. B. Wyngaarden, L. H. Smith, & J. C. Bennett (Eds.), *Cecil's textbook of medicine* (19th ed.). Philadelphia: W. B. Saunders.

37. Scharschmidt, B. F. (1992). Bilirubin metabolism and hyperbilirubinemia. In J. B. Wyngaarden, L. H. Smith, & J. C. Bennett (Eds.), *Cecil's textbook of medicine* (19th ed.). Philadelphia: W. B. Saunders.

38. Siconolfi, L. (1995). Clarifying the complexity of liver function tests. *Nursing, 25*(5), 39–44.

39. Smith, S. L. (1993). The cutting edge in organ transplantation. *Critical Care Nurse, 26,* 29–30.

40. Smith, S. L., & Ciferni, M. L. (1992). Liver transplantation. *Critical Care Nursing Clinics of North America, 4*(1), 131–148.

41. Smith, S. L., Ciferni, M. L. (1993). Liver transplantation for acute hepatic failure: A review of clinical experience and management. *American Journal of Critical Care, 2*(2), 137–144.

42. Stein, R. (1993). The ABC's of hepatitis. *American Health, 12*(5), 65–69.

43. Tierney, L. M., et al. (Eds.). (1995). *Medical diagnosis and treatment* (34th ed.). Norwalk, CT: Appleton & Lange.

44. Wagener, M. W., & Yu, V. L. (1992). Bacteremia in transplant recipients: A prospective study of demographics, etiologic agents, risk factors, and outcomes. *American Journal of Infection Control, 20,* 239–247.

45. Werzberger, A., et al. (1992). A controlled trial of a formalininactivated hepatitis A vaccine in healthy children. *New England Journal of Medicine, 327*(7), 453–457.

46. Wilson, B. A., Shanson, M. T., & Strang, C. L. (1994). *Nurses Drug Guide.* Norwalk, CT: Appleton & Lange.

47. Wright, T. L. (1992). Parasitic, bacterial, fungal, and granulomatous liver disease. In J. B. Wyngaarden, L. H., Smith, & J. C. Bennett (Eds.), *Cecil's textbook of medicine* (19th ed.). Philadelphia: W. B. Saunders.

48. Wyngaarden, J. B., & Smith, L. H., Bennett, J. C. (Eds.). (1992). *Cecil textbook of medicine* (19th ed.). Philadelphia: W. B. Saunders.

49. Zaleznik, D. F. & Kasper, D. L. (1994). Intraabdominal infections and abscesses. In K. J. Isselbacher et al. (Eds.). *Harrison's principles of internal medicine* (13th ed.). New York: McGraw-Hill.

Case Study figure from Zakim, D., & Boyer, T. (1990). *Hepatology: A textbook of liver disease* (p. 670). Philadelphia: W. B. Saunders.

Nursing Care of Clients with Biliary Tract and Exocrine Pancreatic Disorders

Dianne Smolen

Disorders of the biliary tract and exocrine pancreas are discussed in this chapter. Some of the disorders are acute, while others are chronic. They may manifest with signs or symptoms that are similar to other conditions. The nurse plays an important role in assessing the client's manifestations, which, in turn, will lead to a definitive diagnosis and initiation of appropriate treatment.

Biliary Tract Disorders

Cholelithiasis (Gallstones)

The biliary tract is composed of the gallbladder, bile ducts, and the cystic duct. The cystic duct (from the gallbladder) joins with the hepatic duct (from the liver) to form the common bile duct (see Fig. 63–5). Recall from Chapter 63 that the function of the biliary tract is to transport bile (secreted by the liver) from the gallbladder (where it is stored) to the duodenum.

Disorders of the gallbladder and ducts are extremely common. In the United States alone, biliary tract disorders account for more than 500,000 hospitalizations annually. Disorders include cholelithiasis (gallstones), inflammatory conditions, infections, tumors, and congenital malformations.

The two most common conditions are cholelithiasis and associated cholecystitis (inflammation of the gallbladder). Approximately 98% of clients who present with symptomatic gallbladder disease have gallstones. Malignancies and congenital anomalies of the biliary tract are relatively uncommon.

Before beginning the discussion of biliary tract disorders, note the list of terms, presented in Table 66–1, that are used in association with these conditions.

It is estimated that 20 million people in the United States have gallstones, and that 475,000 cholecystectomies are performed every year. Studies show that the incidence of gallstones increases with age, as do the risks associated with cholelithiasis. Women account for nearly 70% of those treated for gallstones, although studies have suggested that the mortality rate is higher in men. Twice as many white Americans as black Americans are affected. The prevalence of this disease is much the same in Europe and Australia. Clients with diabetes mellitus and those with cirrhosis show an increased incidence of cholelithiasis.

Most of our present knowledge of cholesterol gallstones comes from the study of Pima Native American women in south-central Arizona, in whom the occurrence is 75% between the ages of 25 and 34 years old. Pigment stones are dominant in Asians and in black Americans.

Etiology and Risk Factors

The cause of gallstone disease is not well understood. Based on various theories, there are four possible explanations for stone formation.

First, bile may undergo a change in composition. Studies of subjects with cholesterol gallstones indicate that their bile is supersaturated with cholesterol but deficient in bile salts. The cholesterol saturation of bile seems to increase with age. Changes in bile composition, however, do not completely explain why gallstones form.

Second, gallbladder stasis may lead to bile stasis. Bile stasis may (1) change the composition of bile, (2) supersaturate bile with cholesterol, and (3) precipitate some bile constituents. Gallbladder stasis may result from decreased contractility of the gallbladder and spasm of the sphincter of Oddi. Total parenteral nutrition (TPN) without oral intake for longer than 1 month is associated with gallbladder sludge formation and cholelithiasis. Delayed emptying of the gallbladder may correlate with hormonal factors. This may explain why gallstones seem to be associated with pregnancy.

Third, infection may predispose a person to stone formation. Inflammatory debris can form a nidus (point of origin) for stone growth. The related tissue injury may

This chapter incorporates material written for the fourth edition by Cindy Kallsen.

Table 66–1. Biliary Tract Terminology	
Term	**Definition**
Chole-	Pertaining to bile
Cholang-	Pertaining to bile ducts
Cholangiography	X-ray study of bile ducts
Cholangitis	Inflammation of bile duct
Cholecyst-	Pertaining to gallbladder
Cholecystectomy	Removal of gallbladder
Cholecystitis	Inflammation of gallbladder
Cholecystography	X-ray study of gallbladder
Cholecystostomy	Incision and drainage of gallbladder
Choledocho-	Pertaining to common bile duct
Choledocholithiasis	Stones in common bile duct
Choledochostomy	Exploration of common bile duct
Cholelith-	Pertaining to gallstones
Cholelithiasis	Presence of gallstones
Cholescintography	Radionuclide imaging of biliary system

alter the composition of bile by increasing the reabsorption of bile salts and lecithin. Particular organisms may also play a part in stone formation by altering the composition of bile. For example, *Escherichia coli* increases the amount of bilirubin available for pigment stones and *Streptococcus faecalis* reduces bile salts.

Finally, genetics also seems to play some role in stone formation, as evidenced by its prevalence in Pima and Chippewa Native Americans.

Conditions that predispose clients to gallstone formation include those noted in Risk Factors and Levels of Prevention for cholelithiasis. Although obesity is a preventable risk factor, most risk factors are not. Maintaining a low fat diet and recommended weight helps prevent gallstone formation. Clients with risk factors should be aware of them.

Pathophysiology

Gallstones are generally divided into the following three groups: (1) cholesterol stones, (2) pigment stones, and (3) mixed stones. The incidence of a pure stone formation is rare, so stones are generally classified by the predominant substance.

Cholesterol stones are the most common; the incidence of cholesterol stones increases with age and is more common in women. The stones are usually smooth and whitish-yellow to tan. *Pigment stones* are present in about 30% of people with cholelithiasis in the United States. In these persons, the bile contains an excess of unconjugated bilirubin. Pigment stones are subdivided into black (associated with hemolysis and cirrhosis) and earthy calcium bilirubinate stones (associated with infection in the biliary system). *Mixed stones* may be a combination of cholesterol and pigment stones or either of these stones with some other substance. Calcium carbonate, phosphates,

bile salts, and palmitates make up the more common minor constituents of stones. Exactly why or how stones form is as yet unclear. It is known that most gallstones are formed in the gallbladder, but they may also form in the common duct or hepatic ducts of the liver. The actual incidence is not known, however, because some stones do not cause manifestations and pass through the ducts into the bowel unnoticed.

The pathologic findings are best interpreted from the clinical manifestations of the disease, which may be acute or chronic. Once a client becomes symptomatic, treatment and follow-up are essential to prevent progression to a more severe, and sometimes fatal, complication of gallbladder disease. Approximately one third of these complications are due to free perforation, which occurs when a gangrenous area becomes necrotic and bile breaks into the peritoneal cavity. Peritonitis with systemic distribution of pepsin has a mortality rate of approximately 20%. Pericholecystic abscess accounts for 50% of the complications and is the least severe, with a mortality rate of approximately 15%. Abscess formation occurs while the perforation is walled off by omentum or adjacent organs such as the colon, stomach, or duodenum.

Much less frequently (approximately 15% of clients), a fistula occurs when the gallbladder becomes attached to a portion of the gastrointestinal tract and perforates it. The duodenum is the most common site for this, followed by the colon. Occasionally, a stone is discharged into the small intestine. If the stone is large enough, it can obstruct the narrow terminal ileum, causing gallstone ileus.

Clinical Manifestations and Diagnostic Findings

Manifestations of biliary tract disorders are similar to those of a number of other conditions. Box 66–1 lists

RISK FACTORS AND LEVELS OF PREVENTION

Cholelithiasis (Gallstones)

Risk Factors

Diabetes, multiple pregnancies, vagotomy (interruption of vagus nerve innervating the fundus of the stomach), regional enteritis, ileal disease or resection (which results in bile salt depletion), long-term parenteral nutrition (which results in decreased gallbladder motility), cirrhosis of the liver, chronic hemolytic disorders (which result in increased bile pigments), obesity, exogenous estrogen administration, pancreatitis, caloric restriction with certain diets, clofibrate therapy (for treating hyperlipidemia), and cholestyramine therapy

Levels of Prevention

Primary Prevention

- Maintain a low fat, weight reduction diet.
- Consider birth control measures, if in high-risk category, to limit number of pregnancies.

Secondary Prevention

- Monitor clients carefully who are receiving total parenteral nutrition (TPN) for longer than 1 month.
- Encourage high-risk clients to see a physician regularly, especially if they have gastrointestinal complaints.
- Monitor high-risk patients for manifestations of infection of biliary tract including nausea, vomiting, anorexia, pain, and fever.

Tertiary Prevention

- Teach clients the importance of seeking regular medical checkups if manifestations of pain or gastrointestinal distress recur.
- Encourage clients to maintain low fat, weight reduction diet.
- Assist clients to seek birth control information if desired.

Box 66–1. Disorders with Manifestations Similar to Those of Chronic and Acute Cholecystitis

Chronic Cholecystitis

Angina pectoris
Chronic pancreatitis
Esophagitis
Hiatal hernia
Peptic ulcer
Pyelonephritis
Spastic colitis

Acute Cholecystitis

Acute appendicitis
Acute hepatitis
Acute myocardial infarction
Acute pancreatitis
Acute pyelonephritis
Intercostal neuritis
Intestinal obstruction
Perforated ulcer
Pleurisy
Renal calculus
Right lower lobe pneumonia

---

some of the more common diseases that must be differentiated from acute and chronic cholecystitis.

Less than half of persons with gallstones report any distress because gallstones cause no manifestations unless complications develop. The most specific and characteristic manifestation of gallstone disease is pain or biliary colic, which is caused by spasm of the biliary ducts as they try to dislodge stones. This pain usually follows the temporary obstruction of the gallbladder outlet. Characteristically, the pain starts in the upper midline area. It may radiate around to the back and right shoulder blade, although some complain that it passes straight through to the back and substernal areas.

The client is often restless, changing positions frequently to relieve the intensity of the pain. Pain may persist for only a few hours or several days and the interval between attacks is variable.

If the stone is blocking the cystic duct, the person may develop manifestations of acute cholecystitis (see Acute Cholecystitis). If the stone lodges in the common duct, gallstones may be complicated by cholangitis (inflammation of the bile ducts) and pancreatitis. *Jaundice* only appears when common duct obstruction is present.

Nausea and vomiting may occur; occasionally, self-induced vomiting alleviates the manifestations. Assessment may further reveal a history of flatulence, bloating, dyspepsia, eructation, intolerance for fatty foods, and vague upper abdominal sensations. Occasionally, clients who have these problems still have them after cholecystectomy.

Assessment of these clients becomes important in light of the fact that manifestations of biliary colic and coronary artery disease are remarkably similar. Considering the prevalence of both of these problems, accurate diagnosis is essential.

Many times, the diagnosis is made based on the manifestations alone. Physical findings are present only during an attack with pain, pain being the cardinal manifestation. The right upper quadrant or epigastric area is tender to palpation with voluntary muscle guarding, but manifestations of peritonitis are absent. The gallbladder is not palpable, and the temperature is normal.

Blood tests are unremarkable. Jaundice is not present unless there is common duct obstruction. For confirmation of the presence of gallstones, an abdominal ultrasound is very accurate and has advantages over oral cholecystography. Other tests may include computed tomography (CT), cholescintigraphy, cholangiography, and, rarely, biliary drainage examination.

Current trends, however, point to the use of endoscopic retrograde cholangiopancreatography (ERCP) and endoscopic retrograde catheterization of the gallbladder (ERCG) in diagnosis, especially for common duct stones. (See Chapter 64 for a discussion of these procedures.) Biliary ultrasonography (cholecystosonography) may be the initial study because it is accurate, safe, does not expose the client to ionizing radiation, and can be performed without preparation.

Acute and Subacute Care

■ Medical Management

For clients with symptomatic cholelithiasis, treatment is dictated by the frequency and severity of manifestations. It may mean hospitalization and (1) administration of parenteral analgesics for the discomfort of biliary colic (nitroglycerin may reduce colic as well); (2) insertion of a nasogastric tube for the symptomatic relief of vomiting or for those who have probable pancreatitis; (3) maintenance of fluid and electrolyte balance with intravenous fluids; and (4) monitoring for progression of abdominal complications, which may include bile duct obstruction, cholangitis, pancreatitis, acute calculous cholecystitis, and subsequent sepsis and death.

Endoscopy

Retrograde endoscopy for stone removal is an important nonsurgical alternative. To remove a gallstone from the common bile duct, the physician passes an endoscope orally into the duodenum, then passes a wire snare into the common bile duct through the ampulla of Vater, securing and removing the obstructing stone. The physician may elect to enlarge the ampulla of Vater by endoscopic papillotomy to allow passage of stones. If stones remain in the common bile duct after cholecystectomy and a T tube is still in place, the physician may pass a stone-retrieving basket or other device through the T tube tract to remove the stone.

Cholesterol-Dissolving Agents

An important nonsurgical intervention is the use of oral administration of agents for dissolving cholesterol gallstones. Chenodeoxycholic acid, or chenodiol, is not widely used because of its tendency to produce dose-related diarrhea. However, ursodeoxycholic acid (UDCA, ursodiol) has become widely used because it is effective and produces no side effects. Both drugs act by reducing the amount of cholesterol in bile; however, each drug uses a different mechanism. Oral chenodiol is contraindicated in clients with liver disease and in women of childbearing years because of its hepatotoxic effects on the developing fetus. There is evidence that the two drugs, administered together, produce a slightly better effect than when they are used individually. Of interest, diarrhea does not occur when the two drugs are combined.

Analgesics and Other Medications

Analgesics, usually meperidine (Demerol), may be administered intramuscular (IM) on a schedule or as needed for pain. Antacids are given to neutralize gastric hyperacidity and reduce associated pain, and antiemetics are given for nausea and vomiting. Antibiotics are administered to reduce the likelihood of infection.

Dietary Management

The client may be instructed to avoid foods that precipitate biliary colic. This could include eating a fatty meal, consumption of a large meal after fasting, or eating a normal meal. During an acute attack of biliary colic, the client remains NPO (nothing by mouth) with intravenous (IV) fluids administered to maintain hydration. The diet progresses according to the client's tolerance.

Complications

Complications arising from gallstone disease appear most commonly in clients who develop manifestations of biliary colic. The younger the age at initial diagnosis, the more likely the development of complications. People with diabetes mellitus and gallstones appear to be somewhat more susceptible to septic complications.

Outcomes

Because the gallbladder is left in place in all interventions except cholecystectomy, recurrence of stones is likely. Investigation continues on long-term prevention of the recurrence of gallstones.

■ Nursing Management of the Medical Client

Assessment

If the client is being admitted for evaluation and treatment of manifestations, the nurse's assessment should focus on collecting subjective and objective data, and noting the client's response to medications (i.e., analgesics). Assess the client's manifestations carefully to help determine the diagnosis. Also, assess the client's knowledge of the diagnostic process.

Closely monitor the client for manifestations of obstruction from the gallstones. Check vital signs at regular intervals to note inflammation associated with the stones.

Diagnosis, Planning, Implementation

Pain. Since one of the major manifestations of the disease is pain, *Pain related to biliary spasms* is the major nursing diagnosis.

Planning: Expected Outcomes. The client will demonstrate the absence of, or a decrease in, pain, as evidenced by the client verbalizing that pain is absent or decreased and that he or she is resting quietly.

Implementation. Administer pain medications as ordered and document and report the effectiveness of the medication. Meperidine is the drug most frequently ordered. Morphine is contraindicated because it may increase spasm of the sphincter of Oddi. Nitroglycerin may be ordered sublingually to relax smooth muscle and thereby decrease colic.

Other comforting measures may be helpful. Providing a quiet environment and using relaxation techniques such as a back rub or comfortable positioning may promote rest and enhance the effects of the analgesics.

Risk for Fluid Volume Deficit. Because of the associated gastrointestinal manifestations, write the nursing diagnosis as *Risk for Fluid Volume Deficit related to vomiting and nasogastric suctioning.*

Planning: Expected Outcomes. The client will maintain adequate hydration, as evidenced by normal skin turgor, moist oral mucous membranes, and urinary output equal to or greater than 30 ml/hr.

Implementation. If the client continues vomiting, obtain an order for a nasogastric tube with a suction attachment to relieve distention and vomiting. Suction also removes the gastric juices that stimulate cholecystokinin, which, in turn, causes painful contractions of the gallbladder. Nasogastric suction is usually maintained on a low intermittent setting.

Administer IV fluids as ordered. Assess and document intake and output, communicating discrepancies to the physician. Assess the client for manifestations of dehydration, such as dry mucous membranes, poor skin turgor, and urinary output less than 30 ml/hr. For a detailed discussion of fluid and electrolyte imbalances and nasogastric suction, see Chapters 15 and 61.

Knowledge Deficit. The client will have many learning needs, leading to the nursing diagnosis *Knowledge Deficit related to treatment modalities and diagnostic procedures.*

Planning: Expected Outcomes. The client will indicate understanding of therapeutics and diagnostics, as

evidenced by verbalizing understanding and manifesting a lower level of anxiety.

Implementation. The client who is in acute pain may have a short attention span. Give explanations that are simple and direct when the client is comfortable. Providing too much information when the client is in acute distress will only frustrate the client, and little will be understood or retained. Assessing the client's and significant others' level of understanding and their learning needs is helpful in giving them the information that is most pertinent to them. Provide simple and concise written information or films, as well as oral instruction if appropriate.

Risk for Injury. The client undergoing retrograde endoscopy will need the nursing diagnosis *Risk for Injury related to medication during retrograde endoscopy for stone removal.*

Planning: Expected Outcomes. The client will remain free from injury following retrograde endoscopy, as evidenced by the airway remaining patent without aspiration.

Implementation. Clients who undergo retrograde endoscopic papillotomy or stone removal will have a local anesthetic sprayed on the back of their throats. This intervention facilitates the passing of the endoscope. After the endoscopic papillotomy, carefully check for the return of the gag reflex below allowing oral intake. If these clients receive sedation, raise the side rails on the bed for their protection and keep the call light within reach.

Risk for Ineffective Management of Therapeutic Regimen (Individuals). The client and significant others will need to learn about the suggested therapeutic regimen leading to the nursing diagnosis *Risk for Ineffective Management of Therapeutic Regimen (Individuals) related to use of dissolution agents and prevention of further attacks.*

Planning: Expected Outcomes. The client will indicate an understanding of treatment and prevention of recurrence, as evidenced by his or her ability to verbalize indications for drugs and their side effects, dosage, and administration instructions, and ways to prevent recurrence.

Implementation. After assessing the level of understanding and learning needs, educate the client about the purpose of oral dissolution therapy, expected responses, and possible untoward reactions. Because the medication must be taken over a long period of time, help the client devise ways to remember to take the medication daily. For example, a pillbox that is divided into the days of the week clearly indicates if the client has missed a dose.

The client treated medically may be sent home with oral analgesics or other medications for comfort as well as an oral dissolution agent. Be sure the client and significant others are able to relate all necessary information to the nurse before discharge. Diet instructions may be necessary if ingestion of food precipitated the attack (i.e., if a fatty food caused the biliary colic, the client should receive information on a low fat diet).

The client should be given information on what to do should another attack occur. The client has probably been encouraged by the physician to consider elective cholecystectomy or other surgical intervention before the gallbladder disease progresses further. Written material on gallbladder disease should be provided at this time to aid in understanding and decision-making.

Evaluation

Most clients recover from acute cholecystitis without complications. Once the system is allowed to rest, the inflammation decreases and the client recovers. Clients do need to be monitored for the development of chronic cholecystitis.

■ Surgical Management

Whether to operate on a client with asymptomatic cholelithiasis (silent gallstones) is another area for debate. When is prophylactic gallbladder removal appropriate? The potential for serious complications (e.g., acute cholecystitis, choledocholithiasis, sepsis) can pose a significant risk. Elderly people and people with insulin-dependent diabetes have a high incidence of gallstones. Because such people are at high risk during acute biliary attacks and emergency procedures, surgeons may recommend that they undergo elective cholecystectomy to avoid later emergency surgery.

Other procedures that may be performed include extracorporeal shock wave lithotripsy, percutaneous cholecystolithotomy, and laparoscopic cholecystectomy.

Extracorporeal Shock Wave Lithotripsy

Extracorporeal shock wave lithotripsy may be used in a selected group of clients. These clients should have symptomatic cholelithiasis with fewer than four stones, each less than 3 cm in diameter. The surgical procedure is performed under general anesthesia. The client is placed in a large tub of water. Shock waves are directed at the stones as they are visualized on the TV screen. The shock waves are repeated until the stones are crushed. Contraindications to the procedure are the presence of common duct stones, recent acute cholecystitis, cholangitis, and pancreatitis.

Percutaneous Cholecystolithotomy

With a percutaneous cholecystolithotomy, surgeons extract stones using cystoscopes, stone baskets, and instruments designed for nephrolithotomy. Stones too large to extract manually can be fragmented using a lithotriptor or laser fiber. General anesthesia is not necessary for this procedure.

Research is currently taking place on the use of percutaneous insertion of a contact dissolution agent. With this procedure, a catheter is inserted into the gallbladder percutaneously and methyl *tert*-butyl ether (MTBE) is instilled directly into the gallbladder to dissolve cholesterol gallstones. When small amounts are infused and withdrawn four to six times per minute, stones dissolve in 1 to 3 days. Results from early treatments have been excellent.

Laparoscopic Cholecystectomy

Laparoscopic cholecystectomy has become the treatment of choice for symptomatic gallbladder disease. It is suitable for most clients, even those with acute cholecystitis, because there is minimal trauma to the abdominal wall. This makes it possible for clients to go home within 24 hours after the procedure and return to work within a few days instead of a few weeks, as is the case with a cholecystectomy.

Using general anesthesia, carbon dioxide is used to create pneumoperitoneum through a needle inserted near the umbilicus. Near the umbilicus, an endoscope is inserted through a small incision to view the gallbladder and determine the feasibility of success by this procedure. Three other small incisions are created: one for grasping the gallbladder, one for suction and irrigation, and another for dissection instruments and applying clips.

Cholecystectomy

Cholecystectomy consists of excising the gallbladder from the posterior liver wall and ligating the cystic duct, vein, and artery. The surgeon usually approaches the gallbladder through a right upper paramedian or upper midline incision. The common duct may be explored through this incision, if necessary. When stones are suspected in the common duct, operative cholangiography may be performed (if it had not been ordered preoperatively). The surgeon may dilate the common duct if it is not already dilated as a result of a pathologic process. This facilitates stone removal. The surgeon passes a thin instrument into the ducts to collect the stones, either whole or after crushing them.

Following exploration of the common duct, the surgeon usually inserts a T tube to ensure adequate bile drainage during duct healing (choledochostomy). The T tube also provides a route for postoperative cholangiography or stone dissolution, when appropriate.

Complications

Lithotripsy. Following lithotripsy, minor complications may include ecchymosis over the area of entry of the shock waves, gross or microscopic hematuria because of the proximity of the right kidney, and biliary pain when large fragments pass through the cystic duct.

Laparoscopic Cholecystectomy. Risks of laparoscopic cholecystectomy include hemorrhage, bile duct injury, and injury to other organs. However, the advantages of small scars and a short hospital stay have influenced the increased use of this procedure. Although the possible postoperative complications are the same as with traditional cholecystectomy, clients who undergo this procedure are at less risk because they are ambulatory sooner and usually require only oral analgesia. Because of the carbon dioxide pressing on the diaphragm, nausea, vomiting, and shoulder pain are more frequent if the client's head and torso are elevated too soon after surgery.

Cholecystectomy. Following cholecystectomy the client should be monitored for the usual postoperative complications such as hemorrhage, pneumonia, thrombophlebitis, urinary retention, and ileus. The risk of bile leakage into the abdominal cavity is more specific for surgeries involving the gallbladder. With hemorrhage and bile leakage, the client feels severe pain and tenderness in the right upper quadrant, abdominal girth increases, bile or blood may leak from the wound, blood pressure drops, and tachycardia develops.

Follow-up care is important. Overall, surgical procedures are successful in relieving the preoperative manifestations of gallstones. The most common cause of persistent postsurgery manifestations, especially after cholecystectomy, is an overlooked disorder such as esophagitis, peptic ulceration, pancreatitis, or irritable bowel syndrome.

■ Nursing Management of the Surgical Client

Preoperative Care

Preoperative care of the client facing gallbladder or biliary surgery is the same as that described in Chapter 21. In addition, preparation involves careful monitoring for early clinical findings that may indicate the onset of complications from infection or obstruction. For laparoscopic cholecystectomy, preoperative preparation involves the same measures taken for other clients going to surgery. They include NPO status after midnight, occasionally an enema to reduce colon mass and reduce the chance of incontinence contaminating the operative field, and sometimes an antibiotic.

Assessment

Generally, surgical management of cholelithiasis is elective and not performed in an emergency situation unless obstruction has occurred. Consequently, the client is typically knowledgeable about the procedure and the rationale for it. The client should be assessed, however, concerning knowledge of preoperative and postoperative care.

Diagnosis, Planning, Implementation

Knowledge Deficit. The preoperative client will have as a priority nursing diagnosis *Knowledge Deficit related to surgery and recovery.*

Planning: Expected Outcomes. The client will indicate an understanding of the procedure, as evidenced by ability to verbalize information regarding it, will demonstrate an ability to carry out coughing, deep-breathing, and leg exercises; and will have knowledge regarding the immediate postoperative course.

Implementation. Reinforce information given to the client regarding the surgical procedure. Determine the level of understanding and the learning needs of the client and significant other(s). Material should be provided, if available, that can be read or viewed at the client's own pace. Verbal instruction and a demonstration are necessary to ensure that the client can perform postoperative exercises (turning, coughing, deep-breathing, and wound splinting) properly as well as understand their importance.

The client also needs to have some knowledge of what to expect postoperatively (e.g., IV fluids; T tube placement and drainage, if applicable; and pain control and activity). Studies have shown that preoperative client education significantly reduces the risk of developing postoperative complications.

Anxiety. Because of the surgery and associated stress, a nursing diagnosis appropriate to these clients is *Anxiety related to the procedure and outcome.*

Planning: Expected Outcomes. The client will express and demonstrate feelings of comfort and show decreasing manifestations of anxiety, as evidenced by calmly discussing his or her apprehension, affirming that anxiety is decreasing, and ventilating feelings regarding the surgical procedure and diagnosis.

Implementation. Assess the client's level of anxiety by listening and observing. Reassure the client and acknowledge that the unknown is frightening. Thoroughly explain those things that may frighten the client, such as the diagnostic or preparatory procedures. Allow significant others to stay with the client as appropriate.

Postoperative Care

Respiratory status is carefully monitored after surgery of the gallbladder or biliary tract because of the potential for developing atelectasis and pneumonia. Drainage from any biliary tube needs to be monitored closely, as does drainage from the incision site, for amount, character, and color. Cardiovascular status is assessed carefully, as are manifestations of hemorrhage or shock. Hemorrhage, although rare, may occur if an inflamed gallbladder was adhered to the liver.

Analgesia for pain management is important and should be given on a regular basis to promote comfort and rest as well as to enhance the individual's ability to cough and deep-breathe.

Hydration and fluid balance must be maintained IV until the client is no longer NPO and receives fluids orally. When the client is allowed oral intake, the amount of fluid and food should be sufficient and well-balanced enough to maintain renal function (urine output no less than 50 ml/hr) and body weight (minimal loss of weight). Clients are generally allowed to progress to a regular diet, with fat content as tolerated.

Assessment

Postoperative assessment of the client is important. It includes careful monitoring of vital signs, breath and bowel sounds, and general level of responsiveness to check for complications such as hemorrhage, respiratory problems, or infection. In addition, intake is monitored to reflect renal function and output carefully measured including wound drainage, vomiting, or nasogastric suctioning.

The client's incision should be assessed for redness or swelling. The level of pain is monitored as are location, severity, and the effectiveness of any interventions. Following a laporoscopic cholecystectomy, a common postoperative pain pattern is referred pain to the shoulder. The shoulder pain occurs because of the CO_2 that was not released or absorbed by the body. CO_2 causes irritation of the purenic nerve and diaphragm and may decrease respiratory excursion.

Diagnosis, Planning, Implementation

Risk for Injury. The postoperative client is at risk for the development of many complications leading to the collaborative problem. Write the diagnosis *Risk for Injury related to postoperative complications of hemorrhage, infection, fluid and electrolyte imbalance, pulmonary changes (atelectasis, pneumonia), urinary retention, ileus, and decreased gastrointestinal motility.*

Planning: Expected Outcomes. The client will receive appropriate assessments and interventions for early detection and prevention of injury from postoperative complications, as evidenced by stable vital signs; normal pulmonary function; normal gastrointestinal function; laboratory values within normal limits; normal urinary function, which returns within 6 to 8 hours postoperatively; an intact incision that does not exhibit redness, odor, or purulent drainage; and no manifestations of thrombus or embolus.

Implementation. Take routine postoperative vital signs and assess for manifestations of shock, such as cyanosis, diaphoresis, cold clammy skin, decreased blood pressure, and increased pulse. As vital signs are checked, check dressings and drainage tubes at the same time for unusual amounts of bleeding or drainage. If any of the above-mentioned manifestations or changes occur, be sure to check vital signs frequently and notify the physician.

The client should change position at least every 2 hours. While the client is awake for turning, help him or her to cough and deep-breathe. Some hospitals use devices such as incentive spirometry to encourage lung expansion and spontaneous coughing. When using these devices, it is helpful to demonstrate their use prior to surgery.

Auscultate the lungs for rales, rhonchi, and diminished breath sounds every 4 hours for the first 24 hours and every 8 hours thereafter. If the client had a cholecystectomy, it will be even more difficult to take deep breaths and cough because of the location of the incision. Take extra care to ensure that the client is comfortable enough to breathe normally. Many physicians and nurses believe that smaller doses of narcotics given more frequently are beneficial. Splinting the incision helps as well.

Measure intake and output every 4 hours or more frequently, if ordered. Assess amounts for discrepancies. It is not unusual for new postoperative clients to be behind on fluids for the first few hours, so do not expect output to equal intake initially. Assess the client for edema along

with the lung sounds every 4 hours as another assurance that the client is tolerating the fluids that are being infused.

Unless the client is otherwise compromised (i.e., acutely ill at the time of surgery or has a history of other health problems such as heart disease or diabetes), laboratory work will probably not be ordered until the following day. These values should be monitored for indications of fluid and electrolyte imbalance (see Chapter 15).

Generally, the client voids within 6 to 8 hours after surgery. If not, assess the bladder for distention. It is normal for even an otherwise healthy client not to be able to void because of pain, discomfort, and position, nor to feel the need to void because of the effects of anesthesia and narcotics. The physician may order the client to be catheterized to empty the bladder initially. Also, the client may need an indwelling Foley catheter until fully ambulatory.

Occasionally, following surgery on the gallbladder, the client may return with a nasogastric tube to suction. Check the tube frequently to ensure that it is patent and that placement is correct for adequate drainage. A plugged or displaced tube not only causes distention, nausea, and vomiting but may place undue stress on the surgical site. Auscultate bowel sounds every 8 hours to note return of normal bowel activity. Depending on the surgery, the client may or may not be allowed oral intake before bowel sounds return.

For the more involved surgical procedure such as a cholecystectomy, clients are usually not allowed a normal diet until they have begun to pass flatus and bowel sounds are heard. After the client is allowed to have fluids or food, continue to assess the client for abdominal distention and normal bowel sounds to ensure that the intake is being tolerated. Early activity also helps the return of intestinal motility, so the client should be encouraged to begin progression of regular activities as soon as possible.

Many physicians order antiembolism stockings or some sort of sequential compression device to help prevent pooling of blood in the lower extremities and, thus, the development of thrombosis. However, the benefit of regular leg exercises should not be overlooked as a preventive measure. Even when the client is able to ambulate, leg exercises should continue. Also assess the lower extremities at least every 8 hours for redness, swelling, pain, and presence of Homans' sign.

If the dressings are to be changed by the nurse, the incision should be checked simultaneously for redness, swelling, drainage characteristics and amounts, and odor. If drains are present, such as a T tube, observe the drainage for its characteristics and amount. Check the client's temperature at least every 4 hours, or more frequently, if necessary. Keep the dressing and incision clean and dry because moisture enhances bacterial growth. Subjective complaints of increased pain may be the first manifestation that an infectious process is taking place. This is why it is important to document the location, type, and amount of pain routinely so that comparison can be made and a significant change in condition noted immediately. Many times it is the nurse's assessment that alerts the physician and facilitates the diagnosis of infection.

Pain. The client may be prone to problems related to the nursing diagnosis *Pain related to surgical procedure and incision.*

Planning: Expected Outcomes. The client will feel relief of pain, as evidenced by resting comfortably and quietly; blood pressure and heart rate will be within normal limits, and the client will be able to tolerate post-operative exercises and activities.

Implementation. Assess and document the level, location, and type of pain, as well as the client's response to pain medication. You may need to intervene and obtain new medication orders if the medication ordered is ineffective. It may be necessary to administer medication to coincide with activity to keep the client active. Non-pharmacologic measures are helpful as well. Providing a quiet environment (even limiting visitors, if necessary), changing the client's position, and rubbing the client's back are all important in relaxing the client and enhancing the effects of the pain medication. Be sure to assist the client in splinting the incision and instruct the client on the best way to get out of bed and to lie down.

Altered Oral Mucous Membrane. Another appropriate nursing diagnosis for this client is *Altered Oral Mucous Membrane related to NPO status, intubation, and nasogastric suctioning.*

Planning: Expected Outcomes. The client will have normal oral mucosa, as evidenced by an intact, moist oral cavity and verbalization of a reduction in, or absence of, discomfort.

Implementation. Offer oral care at least every 2 hours while the client is NPO. This may consist of rinsing the mouth with water, using mouthwash, swabbing with a moist swab, or assisting the client with brushing the teeth. Assess the oral mucous membranes at least every 8 hours for integrity, color, and moistness. While the client is NPO, it may be helpful to place a wet washcloth over the lips to humidify the air. Offering ice chips or sips of liquid as soon as allowed will provide much relief also.

Knowledge Deficit. Since the client will be faced with early discharge from the healthcare setting, the nursing diagnosis *Knowledge Deficit related to home health-care needs* is an important diagnosis to address.

Planning: Expected Outcomes. The client will verbalize and accurately demonstrate home healthcare needs and skills, as evidenced by ability to identify manifestations of infection; demonstrate wound care; name medications, their purpose, side effects, and administration instructions; and state activity and dietary restrictions.

Implementation. Educate the client about home healthcare as soon after surgery as possible to assess the client's learning potential and learning needs. Instruction should include wound care and dressing changes with return demonstration, as well as how to assess for manifestations of infection.

Be sure the client is knowledgeable about what manifestations should be reported to the physician and how to contact the physician. The client should be instructed to report jaundice, dark-colored urine, pale-colored stools, and pruritus. If the client is discharged with a drain or T tube in place, he or she should know the purpose of the tube, how to secure it, how to empty it, what amounts of drainage can be expected, and abnormal characteristics of drainage.

Explain and reinforce activity and dietary restrictions thoroughly. Instruct and question the client as to the medications he or she is being discharged with, the possible adverse effects, and the dosage and frequencies of the medications.

Evaluation

The client should heal without difficulty and be discharged within about 3 to 5 days after surgery (shorter with laparoscopic surgery).

■ Modifications for Elderly Clients

Gallstones in the older client may not cause pain, fever, or jaundice. Mental confusion, shakiness, and an elevated alkaline phosphatase may be the only manifestations of gallstones in the elderly. Nonsurgical decompression techniques may be preferred in high-risk elderly clients.

When the older client has a cholecystectomy, he or she is at greater risk of injury related to anesthesia, pain medications, and sometimes, the response to the trauma of surgery. Postoperative care should be modified to prevent injury. Especially in the immediate postoperative period, the side rails should be up, the bed in low position, and the call light within easy reach.

Depending on the older client's response to anesthesia and pain medication, frequent reorientation to the environment and circumstances may be necessary. Remind the older client how to summon help and why it is important to not get up alone. Be sure that all IV lines and drainage tubes are secure to prevent the client from inadvertently disconnecting or dislodging them.

In particular, older people have a tendency to become confused following surgery (especially at night), so be alert to this possibility. You may need to take precautions by having a physician order soft wrist or vest restraints or a device such as a bed check machine, which is placed under the client and sounds an alarm if it senses weight is no longer on it.

Acute Cholecystitis

Acute cholecystitis refers to acute inflammation of the gallbladder wall. There is an increased incidence of cholecystitis in clients who are overweight, especially those with sedentary life-styles. Certain ethnic groups, including Chinese, Jewish, and Italians, have a higher rate of the disease.

Etiology and Risk Factors

Obstruction of a cystic duct by a stone is the usual cause of acute cholecystitis. In 5% to 10% of clients, however, calculi obstructing the cystic duct are not found at surgery (acalculous cholecystitis). In over 50% of such cases, an underlying cause of the inflammation is not found.[14]

As noted in Risk Factors and Levels of Prevention for acute cholecystitis, the major preventable risk factors are sedentary life-style and obesity. If the client increases his or her level of activity and maintains a low fat diet, the risk of cholecystitis can be reduced.

Pathophysiology

Acute calculous cholecystitis, which appears to be caused by obstruction of the cystic duct, in turn causes distention of the gallbladder. Subsequently, (1) venous and lymphatic drainage is impaired, (2) proliferation of bacteria occurs, (3) localized cellular irritation or infiltration, or both, take place, and (4) areas of ischemia may develop. The inflamed gallbladder wall is edematous and thickened, and may have areas of gangrene or necrosis. *Empyema* is the term used to describe the gallbladder that contains pus, which is the equivalent of an intra-abdominal abscess and may be associated with severe sepsis. Recurrent episodes of acute cholecystitis cause fibrosis of the wall of the gallbladder.

Complications of untreated acute cholecystitis are usually associated with septic complications. Others are consequences of ischemia, inflammation, adhesions, and gangrene: perforation, pericholecystic abscess, and fistula.

Acalculous cholecystitis (cholecystitis without stones) is far less common than cholecystitis due to gallstones. It apparently can be triggered by (1) multiple blood transfusions, (2) gram-negative bacterial sepsis, or (3) tissue damage after burns, trauma, or extensive surgery. Other possible contributing factors include hyperalimentation, prolonged fasting, hypotension, anesthesia, narcotic analgesics, and mechanical ventilation with positive end-expiratory pressure. Clients with diabetes mellitus and systemic arteritis are also prone to this condition.

Clinical Manifestations and Diagnostic Findings

Inflammation of the gallbladder may be acute or chronic. The most common and reliable finding on physical examination is tenderness in the right upper quadrant, epigastrium, or both. Although persons with chronic and acute cholecystitis may complain of the same type of pain, the distinguishing factor is the severity and persistence of the pain. Chronic cholecystitis rarely lasts more than a few hours, whereas acute cholecystitis may last several days.

Pain in acute cholecystitis may be located in the epigastric, subscapular, or right upper quadrant regions. Sometimes, the pain is referred to the right scapula. The pain usually starts suddenly, increases steadily, and reaches a peak in about 30 minutes. During examination of the abdomen, extreme tenderness often causes the client to guard the upper right quadrant. When palpating the right subcostal area, ask the client to take a deep breath. If the client experiences extreme tenderness and stops breathing on inspiration, you have elicited Murphy's sign.

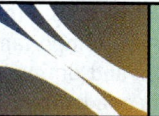

RISK FACTORS AND LEVELS OF PREVENTION

Acute Cholecystitis

Risk Factors

Obesity, sedentary life-style, and ethnic group such as Chinese, Jewish, Italian

Levels of Prevention

Primary Prevention

- Maintain a low fat, weight reduction diet.
- Establish an exercise and activity program.

Secondary Prevention

- Monitor high-risk clients for development of acute inflammation, as well as possible complications.
- Teach high-risk clients clinical manifestations of infection as well as manifestations of complications of untreated acute cholecystitis (gangrene, perforation, abscess, and fistula).
- Teach clients the benefits of exercise and healthy dietary habits.

Tertiary Prevention

- Encourage clients to maintain a low-fat, weight reduction diet.
- Support clients in establishing an exercise and activity program.
- Teach clients in high-risk ethnic groups the importance of regular checkups with a physician, especially if they have a history of gastrointestinal problems.

About 60% to 70% of clients with acute cholecystitis have experienced biliary colic episodes in the past.

In addition to pain, assessment of clients with acute cholecystitis reveals the following problems:

- Nausea and vomiting occur in 60% to 70% of clients.
- Approximately 80% of clients have an elevated temperature but this may be absent in the elderly, the immunocompromised, and those on steroidal therapy.
- Mild jaundice occurs in only 10% of cases.

See Table 66–2 for a summary of assessment data for cholecystitis and cholelithiasis.

Right upper quadrant tenderness, fever, and leukocytosis are highly suggestive of acute cholecystitis, particularly if other assessment data support this diagnosis.

The diagnostic examination for acute cholecystitis includes the following:

- Biliary ultrasonography is often the initial diagnostic procedure. Sonographic findings consistent with acute cholecystitis include (1) cholelithiasis, (2) focal tenderness over the gallbladder (sonographic Murphy's sign), (3) thickening of the gallbladder wall (greater than 3 mm), and (4) distention of the gallbladder lumen (greater than 5 cm).
- Aminotransferase, alkaline phosphatase, and bromosulfaphthalein values may be slightly abnormal.
- An abdominal x-ray study occasionally reveals the enlarged gallbladder. In 15% of cases, the gallstones contain enough calcium to be visible on film.
- Radionuclide imaging (cholescintigraphy) can provide additional information (when the diagnosis is clinically obscure) by pinpointing cystic duct obstruction. Confirmation is based on nonvisualization of the gallbladder.
- The white blood cell count is elevated in 85% of clients, with the exception of the elderly and those on steroid therapy.

See Chapter 64 for a discussion of other diagnostic techniques.

Acute and Subacute Care

■ Medical Management

Clients suspected of having acute cholecystitis may need to be hospitalized, and initial management should include administration of antibiotics effective against organisms found in the bile in approximately 80% of the cases. These organisms include both gram-positive and gram-negative aerobes and anaerobes: *Escherichia coli, Klebsiella aerogenes, Streptococcus faecalis, Clostridium welchii, Proteus* species, *Enterobacter* species, and anaerobic streptococci.

Antibiotics that are effective given singly include ampicillin, cephalosporin, or aminoglycosides. A combination of these drugs may be more effective in clients with diabetes mellitus or with debilitated conditions.

Further medical management is the same as for symptomatic cholelithiasis (see Cholelithiasis).

■ Nursing Management of the Medical Client

Assessment of these clients becomes extremely important because several other disease entities may produce the same manifestations (Box 66–1). Collect subjective and objective data and note the client's response to medications.

The nursing care plan is the same as for medical management of cholelithiasis except that it is certain these clients will receive a course of antibiotics. Observe the client for the development of complications, which may include increased pain in the right upper quadrant or jaundice (from an obstruction) and decreased or absent bowel sounds (from peritonitis). For additional information on nursing management, see Nursing Management of the Medical Client under Cholelithiasis.

Table 66–2. Cholecystitis and Cholelithiasis: Assessment Data

Assessment Data	Pathophysiologic Basis
Abdominal pain, most commonly right upper quadrant or epigastric; often radiates to back	In cholelithiasis, ductal spasm when a stone moves from gallbladder into ducts may cause waves of pain (biliary colic)
	In cholecystitis, pain may be steady (because of inflammation) and increases in severity with peritoneal extension
Nausea and vomiting	Distention of bile ducts initiates impulses to vomiting center
Fat intolerance	Contraction of inflamed gallbladder to release bile to digest fat often precipitates pain
Fever and leukocytosis	Response to inflammation
Jaundice	In cholelithiasis, obstruction to common bile duct causes increased serum bilirubin
	In cholecystitis, edema sometimes obstructs the duct enough to increase bilirubin levels

■ Surgical Management

Once the diagnosis of acute cholecystitis is made, the decision for early or delayed cholecystectomy depends on the risk factors. Delayed surgery is usually the correct decision in those clients who have unstable angina, significant carotid artery disease, congestive heart failure, cirrhosis, and other conditions that would increase their risk.

Cholecystectomy (surgical drainage of the gallbladder) for acute cholecystitis is more difficult than elective surgery because of the distended gallbladder. Usually, the gallbladder must be decompressed first to allow complete visualization of all surrounding structures and to avoid injury to the extrahepatic bile ducts.

Cholecystotomy is usually performed only when cholecystectomy is too dangerous, given all the risk factors. Although the procedure relieves the obstruction, the cure depends on the ability of the client's defense to resolve the inflammatory process. Treatment of complications of cholecystotomy is usually cholecystectomy.

■ Nursing Management of the Surgical Client

See the Nursing Management of the Surgical Client under Cholelithiasis.

Acute Acalculous Cholecystitis

Acute acalculous (absence of stones) cholecystitis accounts for approximately 4% to 8% of all cases of acute cholecystitis. Although it has not been proved, this condition is said to be increasing. It has a tendency to occur after or in association with other conditions, especially major trauma, burns, or surgery. Other preceding conditions include the postpartum period after a prolonged childbirth, bacterial sepsis, and debilitating systemic diseases such as cardiovascular disease, tuberculosis, and sarcoidosis. However, no apparent precipitating factor is present in as many as 50% of the clients.

The pathologic process does not differ from that of the calculous type except that the incidence of gangrene and perforation is higher. It is conjectural whether this is an inherent feature of the disease or the result of delayed diagnosis.

Recognition of the disease may be delayed when the client cannot communicate well because of concomitant disease or posttraumatic or postoperative states. The manifestations are the same as those of acute calculous cholecystitis—pain in the right upper quadrant, epigastrium, or both, and vomiting. However, although pain is the cardinal manifestation in the calculous type, it may be obscured or absent in acalculous cholecystitis because of narcotic administration, decreased level of consciousness, or abdominal pain from an incision or from another disease process. Significant physical findings are the same as those in acute calculous cholecystitis and the same diagnostic procedures are used.

The standard treatment is emergency cholecystectomy because of the increased risk of gangrene and perforation.

Chronic Cholecystitis

Chronic cholecystitis sometimes arises as a sequela to acute cholecystitis. Typically, however, it develops independently of acute cholecystitis. In addition, it is almost always associated with gallstones. Chronic cholecystitis principally affects middle-aged and older obese women. The female-to-male ratio is 3:1.

Assessment data for chronic cholecystitis are similar to those of acute cholecystitis with certain exceptions. In chronic states, (1) the pain is less severe, (2) the temperature is not as high, and (3) the leukocyte count is lower. Vague manifestations of dyspepsia, fat intolerance, heartburn, and flatulence accompany chronic cholecystitis. The client has usually experienced these manifestations for a long time as well as repeated attacks (mild or severe) of acute cholecystitis. Eventually, fibrous tissues begin to replace the normal muscle and mucosal tissues of the gallbladder. As a consequence, the gallbladder loses its ability to concentrate bile.

Diagnosis of chronic cholecystitis largely depends on ultrasonography. Other diagnostic procedures provide supplementary information. Diagnostic findings include (1) cholelithiasis, (2) gallbladder wall thickening (greater than 3 mm), and (3) delayed visualization or nonvisualization of the gallbladder on radionuclide scanning. Scarring from chronic inflammation may partially or completely obstruct the cystic duct and thus account for this delay in visualization or nonvisualization.

It may be difficult to differentiate chronic cholecystitis from other disorders. Conditions that produce manifestations similar to the manifestations of cholecystitis (acute and chronic) are listed in Box 66–1. The diagnostic process serves to rule out these conditions.

Conservative interventions include (1) a low fat diet, (2) weight reduction, and (3) administration of anticholinergics, sedatives, and antacids. When medical intervention is ineffective, cholecystectomy may be the treatment of choice. About 90% of clients obtain relief of manifestations after cholecystectomy. Ninety-five percent of the gallbladders removed contain stones.

Choledocholithiasis and Cholangitis

Choledocholithiasis is defined as stones in the common duct. Common bile duct calculi can arise from the gallbladder or hepatic ducts. Thus, common duct stones can occur in the absence of a gallbladder and are called primary common duct stones. Cholangitis is inflammation of the bile duct.

Common duct stones are found in 10% to 15% of clients with cholelithiasis. The incidence increases with age and the frequency of gallstones in the elderly population may be as high as 25%.[14] Frequently, inflammation or bacteria are present, and cholangitis may develop.

Etiology and Risk Factors

The cause is essentially the same as for cholelithiasis. This condition is sometimes combined with a narrowing of the papilla, which traps stones.

The risk factor for choledocholithiasis is that a small stone pass from the gallbladder and lodge in the common bile duct.

Pathophysiology

The pathophysiology is essentially the same as for cholelithiasis. The majority of bile duct stones are cholesterol or mixed stones. They form in the gallbladder and move into the biliary tree through the cystic duct.

Clinical Manifestations and Diagnostic Findings

Common duct calculi may be asymptomatic or cause biliary colic, bile duct obstruction, cholangitis, or pancreatitis. Early manifestations of choledocholithiasis are not easily distinguished from gallbladder colic or acute cholecystitis. Pain may be mild or severe and cannot be differentiated from gallbladder pain. Jaundice is intermittent if obstruction is intermittent but may be progressive if the stone becomes impacted.

Chills and fever, frequently recurring attacks of right upper quadrant severe pain, a history of jaundice, and mild elevation of serum bilirubin are manifestations of *cholangitis*. The white blood cell count is normal except when cholangitis is present. It is characteristic, however, to see an elevation of serum bilirubin and alkaline phosphatase, which results from obstruction. Serum amylase should always be measured to determine the presence of secondary pancreatitis.

Infrequently, manifestations of cholangitis are accompanied by shock and confusion, coma, or other central nervous system manifestations. This signals the presence of acute toxic cholangitis, a condition in which infected bile or pus is under pressure within the duct system. Emergency decompression of the duct system is necessary to prevent death.

To determine the diagnosis, ultrasonography, CT scan, and radionuclide imaging may be performed but are not reliable for the detection of common duct stones, although they can detect common duct dilation. Endoscopic retrograde cholangiography is indicated for those clients who have bile duct obstruction (as indicated by persistent jaundice) or bile duct dilation on ultrasonography. It allows visualization and endoscopic sphincterotomy when indicated.

Acute and Subacute Care

■ Medical Management

Medical management involves antibiotic therapy when cholangitis is present.

■ Surgical Management

Emergency intervention may be necessary but is rare unless severe ascending cholangitis is present. Usually, however, surgical management in some form is necessary for symptomatic choledocholithiasis.

Common duct stones in a client who has previously had a cholecystectomy is best treated by endoscopic sphincterotomy. The success rate is approximately 90%. Extracorporeal shock wave lithotripsy is used when stones are too large to extract via the endoscopic approach. Success can be achieved in 70% to 85% of these complicated cases. Most common duct stones are found and removed at the time of cholecystectomy.

Liver function should be thoroughly evaluated preoperatively by measuring the prothrombin time and if abnormal, restored to normal with administration of vitamin K. Antimicrobials should be given (e.g., mezlocillin IV along with either metronidazole or gentamicin IV).

Choledochostomy consists of opening the common duct surgically, removing stones, and inserting a T tube for drainage. Choledochostomy may be performed in conjunction with cholecystectomy. Otherwise, cholecystectomy may be necessary at a later date.

Postoperative antibiotics are not usually given after biliary tract surgery unless cultures of the bile obtained during the surgery are positive for organisms.

Surgical traumas or the presence of stones may result in ductal edema following choledochostomy. Inserting a T tube prevents bile from spilling into the peritoneal cavity and maintains patency of the duct (Fig. 66–1). T tubes may be attached to continuous gravity drainage or to collapsible bags in the dressing site.

Avoid tension on long tubing and obstruction by kinking. Carefully measure drainage from the T tube. The tube usually drains 300 to 500 ml in the first 24 hours. This amount decreases to less than 200 ml after 3 to 4 days. Record the volume and color of the drainage. To prevent excessive loss of bile, place the drainage bag for the T tube at the level of the abdomen rather than hanging the bag below the bed. At this height, bile flows into the bag only when pressure is high in the biliary tree.

Excessive T tube drainage may indicate obstruction. Occasionally, it signals development of a biliary fistula. Excessive bile losses may necessitate recycling the client's bile drainage. The bile may be returned to the client through a nasogastric tube or orally in a medium such as fruit juice.

Thick bile or bile containing blood clots may prevent drainage or cause inadequate amounts of drainage from the T tube. Without intervention, bile may begin to leak from the choledochotomy site instead of through the T tube. To prevent this problem, the physician may decide to irrigate the tube with sterile saline.

On rare occasions, tube dislodgment causes failure of the T tube to drain. The tube may dislodge from the common duct when the client moves from a supine to a sitting position. This complication may result from excessive tension during T tube insertion in surgery.

After a few days, the T tube will probably be clamped during meals to aid fat digestion. The tube remains in

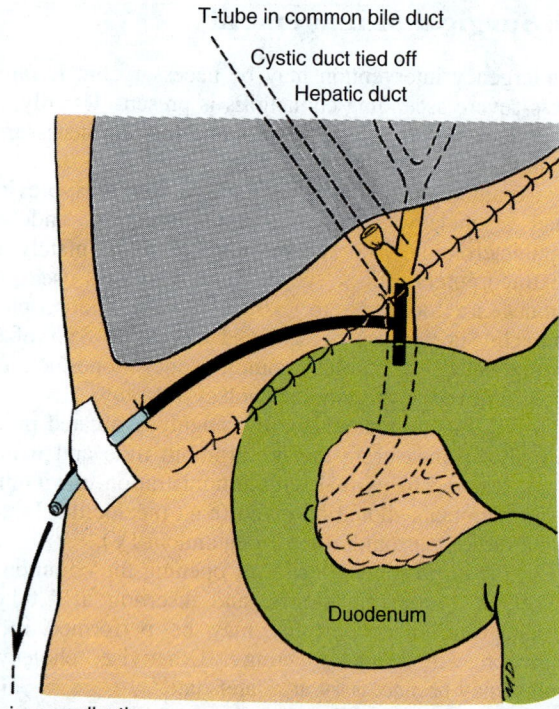

T-tube in common bile duct

Cystic duct tied off

Hepatic duct

Duodenum

To drainage collection

Figure 66–1. Tube placement. The surgeon ties off the cystic duct and sutures the T tube to the common bile duct, with the short arms of the T tube toward the hepatic duct and duodenum. The long arm of the T tube exits the body near the incision site. Skin suture and tape secure placement.

place for about 10 days. A T tube cholangiogram should be done on or about the seventh or eighth postoperative day to assess for bile duct obstruction. When the T tube cholangiogram indicates absence of obstruction, the surgeon may decide to remove the T tube. If a retained stone is discovered during cholangiography, the client may go home with the T tube in place. The surgeon may remove the stone through the T tube tract with a catheter at a later time.

■ Nursing Management of the Surgical Client

Nursing management is the same as for the client with a cholecystectomy.

Sclerosing Cholangitis

Sclerosing cholangitis is an inflammatory disease of the bile ducts that causes fibrosis and thickening of their walls and multiple short, concentric strictures. The disease is progressive and gradually causes cirrhosis, portal hypertension, and death from hepatic failure. It may also predispose the client to the development of cholangiocarcinoma. Some cases are associated with inflammatory bowel disease, 70% of which are ulcerative colitis. Sclerosing cholangitis and papillary stenosis are important complications of acquired immunodeficiency syndrome (AIDS). In addition, cytomegalovirus and cryptosporidia are observed frequently in such clients, indicating these

organisms may be involved in causing primary sclerosing cholangitis.

The cause has been linked to altered immunity, toxins, and infectious agents. Approximately two thirds of cases occur in clients under age 45. The male-to-female ratio is 3:2.

Usually, clients present with fatigue, anorexia, weight loss, jaundice, and pruritus. They sometimes complain of vague upper abdominal pain. The diagnosis is usually made by endoscopic retrograde cholangiography, clinical findings, and liver biopsy.

Medical management consists of corticosteroids and long-term antibiotic therapy when cholangitis is a recurrent problem. Immunosuppressants, bile acid–binding agents, colchicine, and penicillamine have been used. However, these agents do not alter the slow progressive course of the disease. Ursodiol, which improves primary biliary cirrhosis, is now being evaluated in the treatment of sclerosing cholangitis. Cholestyramine may help control the pruritus.

The success of surgical intervention is limited by the progressive nature of the disease and the recurrent cholangitis. Surgery is generally limited to procedures to open the ducts. Cholecystectomy should not be performed unless there is definite evidence of cholecystitis or cholelithiasis. Although surgical therapy may be life-saving in some circumstances, it has to be considered palliative in the overall context of the disease. The definitive management of these clients is liver transplantation, which is the procedure of choice. Survival rates with transplantation are 71% at 1 year and 57% at 3 years.

Carcinoma of the Gallbladder

Although cancer of the gallbladder is the most common malignant lesion of the biliary tract, it accounts for only 5% of all cancers at the time of autopsy. Of all clients who develop this malignancy, 91% are over the age of 50 and the incidence in women is four times that of men. However, the incidence of bile duct cancer is predominant in men. Native Americans, Hispanics, northeastern Europeans, Israelis, and Japanese immigrants to the United States are at greatest risk of developing cancer of the gallbladder. At least 70% of these clients have gallstones. Adenocarcinoma accounts for 82% of all cases.

The clinical presentation differs depending on the stage of the disease. There is no distinct pattern because the manifestations depend on the site of the lesion, its extent, and the presence or absence of preexisting biliary manifestations. Usually, however, the clinical manifestations are unrelenting right upper quadrant pain, weight loss, jaundice, and a palpable right upper quadrant mass.

At this point, treatment modalities and their effectiveness are widely debated. Treatment varies from radical resection, to palliative relief of duct obstruction, to chemotherapy or radiation. None have been found to increase survival.

The prognosis for cancer of the gallbladder is poor. About 88% of clients die within the first year, and only about 5% are alive at 5 years. The long-term survivors are generally those in whom the diagnosis of cancer had not been made prior to cholecystectomy and was determined by pathologic study.

Congenital Anomalies

Congenital anomalies of the gallbladder are very rare. Absence of the gallbladder seems to have a genetic link because several family members may be affected. Clients with no gallbladder may be asymptomatic, and the condition is discovered only incidentally.

Double and triple gallbladders are also rare, the latter being more so. Double gallbladders may share a common cystic duct and be completely separated, or they may be divided by a septum. An ectopic gallbladder is another rare occurrence.

Disorders of the Exocrine Pancreas

A client with a pancreatic disorder may have problems with both digestion and glucose use. Disorders of the pancreas fall into four groups: (1) inflammatory, (2) neoplastic, (3) traumatic, and (4) genetic. Box 66–2 lists pancreatic disorders under each category. The following sections include a discussion of exocrine illness. See Chapter 69 for hormonal disorders. Measures used to diagnose disorders of the pancreas include various laboratory and radiographic studies.

Acute Pancreatitis

Pancreatitis, or inflammation of the pancreas, may be acute or chronic. Acute pancreatitis is an inflammation of the pancreas that may result in autodigestion of the pancreas by its own enzymes. Acute pancreatitis is a fairly common but potentially lethal inflammatory process that results in varying degrees of pancreatic edema, fat necrosis, and hemorrhage. Typically, the manifestations of acute pancreatitis disappear once the causative factors are eliminated. Nine out of 10 people experience mild to moderate manifestations and improve with supportive care. Conversely, in 1 out of 10 clients, acute pancreatitis evolves into a severe life-threatening form. Studies have revealed that late complications of multisystem organ failure and pancreatic abscess contribute to most deaths. Pulmonary edema and congestion are also contributory factors.

Etiology and Risk Factors

In 90% of cases of acute pancreatitis, the cause is related to excessive alcohol intake or biliary tract disease. Alcohol abuse is the major cause of acute pancreatitis in urban areas of the United States. In other areas of the United States, Asia, and Europe, gallstone-associated pancreatitis is predominant. Although the exact mechanism of alcohol-related injury is unknown, the association is undeni-

---

Box 66–2. Classification of Pancreatic Disease

Inflammatory

Acute pancreatitis
Relapsing acute pancreatitis

In acute and relapsing acute pancreatitis, function and morphologic restoration may occur as causes (e.g., alcohol, gallstones) are eliminated.

Relapsing chronic pancreatitis
Chronic pancreatitis with acute exacerbations
Chronic pancreatitis

Permanent structural and functional damage has occurred; may be related to nutritional, metabolic, or endocrine factors.

Neoplastic

Parenchymal origin (acinar cells)

Adenoma
Acinar cell adenocarcinoma
Ductal origin
Cystadenoma
Adenocarcinoma

Islet cell origin

Insulinoma
Gastrin-producing tumor
Vasoactive intestinal peptide (VIP)–producing tumor
Glucagonoma

Other tumors derived from amine precursor uptake and decarboxylation (APUD) cells

Traumatic

Nonpenetrating or blunt trauma
Penetrating injuries

Genetic

Cystic fibrosis
Hereditary and familial pancreatitis

From Arvanitakis, C., & Cooke, A. R. (1978). Diagnostic tests and exocrine pancreatic function and disease. *Progress in Gastroenterology, 74,* 932.

---

able. Several theories exist regarding the effect of alcohol on the pancreas, but research continues. In gallstone-related pancreatitis, it is believed that gallstones migrating through the ampulla of Vater cause diversion of bile into the pancreatic duct and subsequent bile-induced pancreatic parenchymal injury. Other causes include the following:

- Hyperlipidemia, which may occur secondary to nephritis, castration, or exogenous estrogen administration, or as hereditary hyperlipidemia.
- Hypercalcemia arising as a result of hyperparathyroidism.
- Familial cases with no definite mechanism defined.

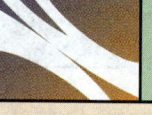

RISK FACTORS AND LEVELS OF PREVENTION

Acute Pancreatitis

Risk Factors

Alcohol abuse, cholecystitis, cholelithiasis, hyperlipidemia, hypercalcemia, pancreatic trauma, pancreatic ischemia, certain medications (estrogens, azathioprine), and any condition that causes pancreatic duct obstruction

Levels of Prevention

Primary Prevention

- Avoid alcohol.
- Avoid ingestion of large amounts of medications known to cause acute pancreatitis.
- Reduce dietary intake of fats (lipids) and calcium if blood levels run high.

Secondary Prevention

- Monitor lipid and calcium blood levels of high-risk clients.
- Teach clients risks associated with alcohol ingestion.
- Teach high-risk clients manifestations of infection.

Tertiary Prevention

- Encourage clients to enroll in an alcohol cessation program.
- Encourage clients to seek regular medical attention if in a high-risk group.

- Pancreatic trauma, such as penetrating or blunt external trauma, intraoperative manipulation, or ampullar manipulation and pancreatic ductal overdistention during ERCP.
- Pancreatic ischemia during episodes of hypotensive shock, cardiopulmonary bypass, visceral atheroembolism, or vasculitis.
- Drugs. Although azathioprine and estrogens have been directly linked with the disease, many other drugs are believed to have an association.
- Other general causes, such as pancreatic duct obstruction, duodenal obstruction, viral infection, scorpion venom, and idiopathic causes.

Alcohol abuse is a high-risk factor for the development of pancreatitis. Avoidance of alcohol is the best way to reduce the risk of the disease. The other major risk factors are cholecystitis and cholelithiasis. See Risk Factors and Levels of Prevention for acute pancreatitis.

Pathophysiology

The mechanism causing pancreatic damage remains unclear. The pathologic changes occurring in the pancreas may be due to premature activation of proteolytic and lipolytic pancreatic enzymes. These enzymes are normally activated in the duodenum. The pancreas normally releases protease in an inactive form (Table 66–3). Once in the intestine, the action of intestinal enterokinase converts pancreatic trypsinogen (one of the proteases) into trypsin. In pancreatitis, however, the activation of the proteases and lipases occurs prior to secretion into the intestine. This causes tissue damage in the pancreas.

Exactly how the enzymes become active in the pancreas is unknown, but they may be triggered by reflux of bile from the duodenum into the pancreatic duct or by pancreatic duct obstruction. The net effect of this enzymatic activation is autodigestion of the pancreas. Once pancreatic inflammation begins, a vicious circle continues the process of further tissue damage and enzyme activation. As the process becomes chronic, destruction of the pancreatic parenchyma occurs.

The clinical course in up to 90% of clients with acute pancreatitis follows a self-limited pattern. However, in

Table 66–3. Pancreatic Enzymes

Enzyme	Catalyzes Hydrolysis of:
Amylase	Carbohydrates into maltose and dextrins
Lipase	Fats into glycerol and fatty acids
Proteases	Proteins into peptides and amino acids
Trypsinogen Chymotrypsinogen Procarboxypeptidase Proaminopeptidase	Proteases are secreted in an inactive form; otherwise they would destroy pancreatic tissue. Once in the intestine, enterokinase acts on trypsinogen, coverting it to trypsin. Trypsin then acts on the other proteases to convert them to active enzymes

---

Box 66–3. Early Prognostic Signs of Acute Pancreatitis

At Admission

Age >55 years
WBC >16,000 cells/mm^3
Blood glucose >200 mg/dl
Serum LDH >350 units/L
Serum AST >250 units/L

During Initial 48 hours

Hematocrit falls >10 percentage points
BUN elevation >5 mg/dl
Serum calcium falls to <8 mg/dl
PaO$_2$ <60 mm Hg
Base deficit >4 mEq/L
Estimated fluid sequestration >6 L

AST, aspartate aminotransferase; BUN, blood urea nitrogen; LDH, lactic dehydrogenase; PaO$_2$, partial pressure of arterial oxygen; WBC, white blood cells.
Data from Ranson, J. H. C., et al. (1974). Prognostic signs and the role of operative management in acute pancreatitis. *Surgery, Gynecology and Obstetrics, 139,* 69.

10% to 15% of clients, a severe form of illness develops that requires a lengthy hospitalization, complications, and significant rates of morbidity and mortality. These clients present a major medical challenge by requiring an intensive care setting, hemodynamic monitoring, and frequent laboratory and radiographic evaluation.

One way to predict the severity of attack and overall prognosis is to use the predictive criteria identified by Ranson in 1974 (Box 66–3). Clients with two or fewer prognostic signs generally require only supportive care. Clients with three or four signs have a mortality rate of approximately 15%. If five or six prognostic signs are present, intensive care is required and the mortality rate reaches 50%. Clients with seven or more of these prognostic signs have an even higher mortality rate and truly test the limits of modern medicine.

Clinical Manifestations and Diagnostic Findings

Manifestations in clients presenting with acute pancreatitis vary from mild, nonspecific abdominal pain to profound shock with coma and death. The predominant clinical feature is abdominal pain, which normally begins in the midepigastrium and achieves maximal intensity several hours later. In most clients, the pain has a penetrating quality that radiates to the back. In clients with alcohol-associated pancreatitis, the pain often begins 12 to 48 hours after an episode of inebriation. Those with gallstone-associated pancreatitis typically experience pain after a large meal. Nausea and vomiting frequently accompany the pain.

Physical examination typically reveals fever, tachycardia, epigastric tenderness, and abdominal distention. Se-

vere hemorrhagic pancreatitis may produce two distinctive manifestations: Turner's sign (bluish discoloration of the left flank) and Cullen's sign (bluish discoloration of the periumbilical area). These signs, which occur in less than 3% of cases, are the result of blood-stained retroperitoneal fluid. Jaundice may be seen in clients with gallstone-associated pancreatitis but otherwise is uncommon in the initial phase of the disease.

Clients with severe pancreatitis may exhibit severe circulatory complications such as hypotension; pallor; cool, clammy skin; hypovolemia; hypoperfusion; and obtundation. As many as one third of clients have evidence of left pleural effusion or left hemidiaphragmatic elevation.

Other clinical findings include subcutaneous fat necrosis and cerebral abnormalities such as belligerence, confusion, psychosis, and coma. It is speculated that the cerebral abnormalities are caused by hyperosmolality, hypoperfusion and hypoxia, cerebral fat embolism, or disseminated intravascular coagulopathy. Transient hyperglycemia is found in 50% of clients, probably as a result of damage to the islets. All of the hormonal (endocrine) functions of the pancreas may be disrupted from tissue damage and the client may develop diabetes secondary to the disease. Hypocalcemia occurs in up to 30% of clients (Table 66–4).

Serum amylase is the most widely used test for the diagnosis of pancreatitis; however, the absence of an elevated serum amylase (hyperamylasemia) does not exclude the diagnosis. The absence of hyperamylasemia may reflect extensive pancreatic necrosis or failure of a chronically diseased gland. In most cases, hyperamylasemia is seen within 24 hours of the onset of manifestations and resolves within 7 days. If hyperamylasemia persists, it may indicate the development of complications.

The measurement of urinary amylase has been indicated as a sensitive index of the disease. Urinary amylase elevations persist for a longer period of time. Again, however, hyperamylasuria is not a true indicator of acute pancreatitis. Some support the use of the amylase-creatinine clearance ratio in the diagnosis. Unfortunately, acute pancreatitis may occur with a normal amylase-creatinine clearance ratio.

The elevation of serum lipase is a more accurate indicator of acute pancreatitis because lipase is solely of pancreatic origin. Also, the duration of hyperlipasemia often exceeds that of hyperamylasemia. However, hyperlipasemia may also be seen in perforated peptic ulcer, acute cholecystitis, and intestinal ischemia.

The serum lipase value is one of the most specific indicators of acute pancreatitis. Elevated serum lipase may be seen in clients with hereditary hyperlipidemia–associated pancreatitis or in alcohol-induced pancreatitis.

Additionally, a white blood cell count above 10,000 cells/mm^3 is common; also, hyperglycemia, mild azotemia, abnormal liver function tests, and hypocalcemia may be present.

Chest film findings are supportive but not specific for acute pancreatitis. They include left basilar atelectasis, elevated left hemidiaphragm, and left pleural effusion. These findings reflect the presence of a significant peridiaphragmatic retroperitoneal inflammatory process occurring in the region of the pancreas.

Table 66–4. Acute Pancreatitis: Assessment Data

Assessment Data	Pathophysiologic Basis
Extreme epigastric or umbilical pain, extending into back and flank	Edematous distention of pancreatic capsule; local peritonitis due to enzyme release into peritoneum; ductal spasm, or pancreatic autodigestion stimulated by increased enzyme secretion while eating
Persistent vomiting	Pain stimulates vomiting center; intestinal peristalsis reduced because of localized peritonitis
Abdominal distention, fever	Paralytic ileus of small bowel loop due to localized peritonitis
Shock and cardiac dysfunction	Release of pyrogens by tissue breakdown Hypovolemia caused by loss of fluid into the retroperitoneal space and decreased preload into the heart; release of kinins causes peripheral vasodilation and increased vascular permeability and toxemia
Hypocalcemia, usually mild, although tetany is possible	Calcium may be deposited in areas of fat necrosis; undigested intestinal fat traps calcium in feces
Impaired glucose tolerance	Some degree of islet involvement
Jaundice	Common bile duct obstruction by pancreatic edema
Pleural effusion	Spread of inflammation into surrounding tissues

Electrocardiographic findings may indicate ST-T wave changes. The changes are different from those of myocardial infarction.

Abdominal films may reveal nonspecific abnormalities: the presence of air in the duodenal loop indicating duodenal ileus; the sentinel loop sign, representing a dilated proximal jejunal loop; the colon cutoff sign, which is distention of the transverse colon; gallstones; or pancreatic calcifications.

Although no findings on upper GI series are specific for acute pancreatitis, the studies may reveal widening of the duodenal loop and anterior displacement of the stomach. Ultrasound can be used to detect pancreatic edema and acute peripancreatic fluid collections, but may be limited by the presence of air and fluid-filled loops of bowel.

Nearly all acute pancreatitis clients have some abnormality on CT scan. Pancreatic changes include parenchymal enlargement, edema, or necrosis. A CT scan is also helpful in identifying other structural changes that develop such as pancreatic pseudocyst, abscess, or phlegmon. A magnetic resonance imaging (MRI) study reveals the same information as CT.

Although endoscopic retrograde pancreatography has no role in the standard diagnostic evaluation of most clients with acute pancreatitis, it has proved helpful in some clients with recurrent pancreatitis by identifying correctable abnormalities (e.g., duct abnormalities).

Acute and Subacute Care

■ Medical Management

In many clients, acute pancreatitis is a mild disease that subsides automatically in a short time. With a pancreatic rest program of withholding food and fluid by mouth, keeping the client in bed, inserting a nasogastric tube, and giving pain medication, the client recovers without serious complications and further difficulty. At other times, as noted earlier, the client may be very ill and require care in the intensive care unit.

Acute pancreatitis is commonly associated with massive fluid isolation. Fluids can accumulate in the bowel secondary to ileus or in the peripancreatic region because of edema. Fluids also can be lost in the form of emesis. Therefore, an essential first step in the management of these clients is replacing lost body fluids, correcting hypovolemia, and restoring electrolyte balance. Normally, the success of fluid and electrolyte restoration is monitored by assessing the client's response by checking the heart rate, blood pressure, and urinary output. In clients with preexisting cardiac, pulmonary, or renal disease, or in clients with severe pancreatitis, invasive monitoring, including urinary catheterization, central venous pressure monitoring, or monitoring cardiac output and filling via a Swan-Ganz catheter, is indicated.

Those with severe hemorrhagic pancreatitis may require blood transfusions or transfusion of clotting factors to correct abnormal coagulation problems.

Often, a variety of electrolyte abnormalities are encountered. Clients with severe and persistent vomiting may require saline solutions containing potassium chloride. Serum calcium may be depressed secondary to hypoalbuminemia. Mild hyperglycemia is usually corrected with fluid volume replacement, but marked hyperglycemia or glycosuria requires careful insulin administration.

Treatment may involve attempts to suppress pancreatic exocrine function. Therapy to decrease these enzymes may include nasogastric suction, or administration of histamine H_2-receptor antagonists, antacids, anticholinergics, glucagon, calcitonin, somatostatin, and proglumide.

Analgesics

Pain is usually treated with narcotic analgesics, meperidine being the drug of choice. Morphine is contraindicated because it may cause spasm of the sphincter of Oddi, which could then potentiate ongoing pancreatic parenchymal injury.

Antibiotics

Antibiotics, in theory, are not necessary in most mild-to-moderate cases. However, prophylactic antibiotics may be ordered, particularly in the more severe cases of pancreatitis.

Dietary Management

Oral intake is prohibited initially but generally can be resumed once abdominal pain and tenderness have improved. Caution must be taken because premature return to oral intake has been associated with the development of pancreatic abscess and reactivation of inflammation. Clients with moderate to severe cases will need to be supported nutritionally by total parenteral nutrition (TPN). Administration of a carbohydrate- and amino acid–based solution along with lipids as a source of calories may be necessary.

Complications

Respiratory complications may require supportive measures such as oxygen administration and physical therapy, or the lesser supportive measures such as endotracheal intubation and positive pressure ventilation.

Outcomes

It may be necessary to perform peritoneal dialysis to rid the peritoneum of potentially toxic compounds commonly found in exudate from acute pancreatitis. Histamine, vasoactive kinins, elastase, prostaglandins, phospholipase A, trypsin, and chymotrypsin may mediate adverse systemic effects, such as hypotension, pulmonary failure, hepatic failure, and altered vascular permeability. This form of therapy is usually reserved for clients who show early clinical deterioration in spite of maximal intensive care support.

■ Nursing Management of the Medical Client

Assessment

Until a confirmed diagnosis is made, nursing should concentrate on treating the manifestations and preparing clients for diagnostic procedures. Assessing and documenting subjective and objective data may assist in making the diagnosis. Also, much of the nurse's role in these instances is educating the client and significant others regarding procedures and their rationale. Keep in mind that the degree of nursing intervention is directly related to the severity of the illness and the client's overall condition.

Most nursing interventions discussed in this section are an appropriate part of the medical management and surgical management of the client with pancreatitis. Refer to nursing management in both the medical management and surgical management sections for a complete understanding of the care required in acute pancreatitis.

Diagnosis, Planning, Implementation

Pain. A common nursing diagnosis for the client with pancreatitis is *Pain related to inflammation of the pancreas and surrounding tissue, biliary tract disease, obstruction of pancreatic ducts, and interruption of the blood supply.*

Planning: Expected Outcomes. The client will demonstrate an absence of, or a decrease in, pain, as evidenced by verbalizing this and resting quietly.

Implementation. The nurse should assess the location, severity, and character of the pain as well as the onset, duration, and precipitating or relieving factors. This assessment should be documented, and significant changes should be reported. Evaluate the client's response to pain and the therapies used to relieve discomfort.

Placing the client on NPO status not only rests the gastrointestinal tract but also decreases pancreatic stimulation. Keep in mind that even ice chips can stimulate enzymes and increase pain. Nasogastric suctioning removes hydrochloric acid (a powerful stimulant to the release of pancreatic enzymes) and helps decrease distention, thereby promoting comfort. Check the system frequently to ensure that nasogastric suction is functioning properly to avoid pooling and stimulation of enzyme secretion.

Be sure to administer pain medications in a timely manner. Remember that opiate narcotics may stimulate spasm of the ducts and increase pain. Meperidine is usually the drug of choice. Other drugs may be ordered (such as anticholinergics) to quiet the pancreas and decrease enzyme secretion.

Again, remember that nonpharmacologic measures are often helpful in relieving pain, relaxing the client, and enhancing the effects of narcotics. Positioning (a side-lying, knee-chest position with a pillow pressed against the abdomen or a sitting position with the trunk flexed may be helpful), back rubs, relaxation techniques, and a quiet environment all help promote comfort and rest.

Anxiety. Because of the uncertainty of the disease and the possibility of recurrence, an appropriate nursing diagnosis is *Anxiety related to change in health status, change in environment, and fear of pain returning.*

Planning: Expected Outcomes. The client will express and demonstrate decreasing manifestations of anxiety, as evidenced by calmly discussing his or her apprehensions, stating that anxiety and fear are decreasing, and displaying behavior associated with relaxation (e.g., resting quietly).

Implementation. Assess the client's level of anxiety by listening and observing. Reassure the client and acknowledge that the unknown is frightening. Explain procedures that may be frightening to the client. Remember that clients in pain or with acute anxiety may have a shortened attention span, so instruction should be simple and direct. Allow significant others to remain with the client as appropriate for added reassurance and comfort.

Hypovolemia and Electrolyte Imbalance.

A possible complication is *Hypovolemia and Electrolyte Imbalance related to vomiting, nasogastric suctioning, NPO status, shifting of body fluids, fever, and diaphoresis.*

Planning: Expected Outcomes. The client will receive appropriate assessments and interventions for early detection or prevention of fluid and electrolyte imbalance.

Implementation. Monitor vital signs for changes in pulse and blood pressure (fluid volume changes) and respiration (acid-base imbalance). If the client is in intensive care, hemodynamic monitoring should be assessed for changes in fluid and electrolyte status (see Chapter 15). Heart monitor rhythm changes may be the first indication of electrolyte imbalance. Check laboratory values for significant changes and observe for physical manifestations of hyperglycemia, hypocalcemia, and hypokalemia. Monitor the client's response to fluid administration and blood products by checking for edema, lung sounds, skin turgor, altered mucous membranes, and monitor intake and output. Significant changes should be reported promptly because these clients are at increased risk.

Ineffective Breathing Pattern.

The client with acute pancreatitis has the potential to develop many problems. One appropriate nursing diagnosis is *Ineffective Breathing Pattern related to abdominal distention or ascites, pain, or respiratory complications.*

Planning: Expected Outcomes. The client will maintain an effective breathing pattern, as evidenced by a respiratory rate within normal limits, relaxed respiratory effort, absence of cyanosis, and clear lungs.

Implementation. Assess the client's respiration for rate and effort. Assessment should include lung auscultation for decreased lung sounds (potential for atelectasis), rales or rhonchi (potential for pneumonia and pleural effusion), and cyanosis. Many times, these clients are on bedrest, which precludes the need for prophylactic nursing interventions of pulmonary hygiene (e.g., turning, coughing, deep breathing, and incentive spirometry). Keeping the client comfortable with analgesics enhances full inspiration and normal breathing patterns. Positioning, such as placing the client in the semi-Fowler or a side-lying position, may facilitate normal respiration.

Altered Nutrition: Less than Body Requirements.

Pancreatitis leads to many gastrointestinal manifestations making the nursing diagnosis *Altered Nutrition: Less than Body Requirements related to nausea and vomiting, NPO status, and nasogastric suctioning* a common nursing diagnosis for this client.

Planning: Expected Outcomes. The client will maintain adequate nutritional status, as evidenced by maintaining normal body weight, keeping blood sugar within normal limits, and finding no evidence of muscle wasting.

Implementation. Again, depending on the severity of illness, these clients may be NPO for an extended length of time. When extended fasting is necessary, nutrition is provided through hyperalimentation and lipids (see Chapter 60). Assess the overall nutritional status of the client by checking daily weights, tissue integrity, and the presence of adequate body fat and muscle mass.

You will recall that acute pancreatitis clients are allowed to have an oral diet when all abdominal pain and tenderness have resolved. However, if oral intake is resumed too soon, reexacerbation of manifestations may occur. Therefore, monitor the client's response to oral intake carefully and begin intake slowly with liquids before progressing to a normal diet. It may be necessary to administer antispasmodics, anticholinergics, and antacids to reduce gastric and pancreatic secretions. Also, if the pancreas has been severely damaged, it may be necessary to give replacement pancreatic enzymes to replace the enzyme deficit and aid in digestion. Monitor the effects of these drugs.

Knowledge Deficit.

Because of the complex nature of the disease and the importance of the client's understanding in lowering the risk of recurrence, the nursing diagnosis *Knowledge Deficit related to causes of pancreatitis, treatment, possible complications, and home healthcare* is important.

Planning: Expected Outcomes. The client and significant others will accurately verbalize home healthcare needs, as evidenced by ability to understand the diet; list medications, including indications, dosage, frequency, and side effects; and the manifestations of recurrence.

Implementation. Prepare clients for discharge by assessing their level of understanding and their learning needs. Also, discuss the medication regimen with the client, including the medication's purpose, dosage, frequency, and possible side effects and explain that an insulin supplement may be required because of pancreatic damage. Teaching should begin as soon as possible to ensure that the client and significant others are fully prepared to deal with glucose monitoring, diet, and insulin administration (see Chapter 69). Instruct the client about dietary restrictions, such as restrictions on alcohol, tea, coffee, spicy foods, and heavy meals, which stimulate pancreatic secretions and produce attacks of pancreatitis. Clients should understand the benefit of eating small, frequent meals high in protein, low in fat, and moderate to high in carbohydrates. Ensure that the client is aware of the manifestations of recurrence of pancreatitis and the importance of reporting these manifestations immediately. These manifestations include steatorrhea (fatty stools); severe back or epigastric pain; persistent gastritis, nausea, and vomiting; weight loss; elevated temperature; and manifestations of hyperglycemia.

Ineffective Individual Coping.

Although alcohol abuse is not the only cause of pancreatitis, it is a common cause leading to an important nursing diagnosis, *Ineffective Individual Coping related to alcohol abuse.*

Planning: Expected Outcomes. The client will learn to cope with life more effectively, as evidenced by admitting that alcohol is a problem, seeking help with abstinence, and seeking long-term support to develop more effective coping strategies.

Implementation. The client must be encouraged to face the problem that alcohol is causing. Spend time with the client and encourage him or her to talk about the problem. Recommend groups such as Alcoholics Anonymous and encourage the client to join such a program. Discuss supportive services available as necessary with the client and significant others.

The nurse also can help by working with significant others to better understand the client's problems with alcohol so that they can better help the client.

Evaluation

In the short term, the client should recover from acute pancreatitis without complications. Long-term recovery, however, often depends on the client's willingness and ability to alter his or her life-style.

■ Surgical Management

Operative intervention is indicated in four specific circumstances: (1) uncertainty of diagnosis, (2) treatment of pancreatic sepsis, (3) correction of associated biliary tract disease, and (4) progressive clinical deterioration despite optimal supportive care.

If it is necessary to facilitate drainage of the pancreatic duct, a procedure called longitudinal pancreaticojejunostomy Roux-en-Y (Puestow procedure) may be performed. This surgery, which relieves pain in most clients, involves opening the pancreatic duct and anastomosing it side to side to the proximal jejunum. If the client has extensive disease of the entire gland, a subtotal pancreatectomy may be performed. This surgery involves attaching a small remnant of the remaining head of the pancreas to the duodenum. A more extensive procedure, Whipple's operation (pancreaticoduodenectomy), may be necessary if the pancreatitis is confined to the head of the pancreas. The distal third of the stomach, the duodenum, common bile duct, gallbladder, and head of the pancreas are removed.

Complications

It has been previously discussed how difficult it may be to diagnose acute pancreatitis and to exclude other potentially fatal diagnoses. When such a condition exists, exploratory laparotomy is indicated to eliminate processes such as perforated viscus or acute mesenteric ischemia. Then, if uncomplicated acute pancreatitis is present, no manipulation is needed and the surgery is terminated. In presumed gallstone-associated pancreatitis, cholecystectomy and intraoperative cholangiography are favored. In clients with severe hemorrhagic pancreatitis with necrosis, debridement of necrotic tissue is performed and retroperitoneal drainage is established.

Ileus, abdominal distention and vomiting are possible postoperative complications and require nasogastric suction if they occur. Treatment of pancreatic abscess combines antibiotic therapy and surgical drainage. Operative

debridement is necessary to remove the thick, debris-filled, pastelike collections of infected necrotic material.

A serious complication of acute pancreatitis is adult respiratory distress syndrome (ARDS), which can occur within 3 to 7 days of the onset of pancreatitis and the administration of large volumes of fluid and colloids given to sustain blood pressure and adequate urine output. See the Critical Monitoring feature giving the assessment findings that mandate early intervention in ARDS secondary to acute pancreatitis.

Correction of Associated Biliary Tract Disease

Formerly, biliary tract surgery for gallstone-associated pancreatitis was deferred for up to 8 weeks. However, up to 50% of clients awaiting elective surgery had a recurrence of pancreatitis. Now, most surgeons proceed with surgery as soon as the initial manifestations of pancreatitis resolve.

If clients with severe pancreatitis do not respond to medical management, operative intervention may be indicated to debride necrosis, or again to exclude other possible diagnoses as causative factors.

■ Nursing Management of the Surgical Client

Preoperative Care

Preparing a client for pancreatic surgery is similar to preparing a client for biliary surgery. It requires close monitoring of the white blood cell count, hematocrit, serum electrolytes, serum calcium, serum creatinine, blood urea nitrogen (BUN), aspartate aminotransferase (AST) serum and lactic dehydrogenase (LDH), and arterial blood gases. Other measures may be necessary depending on the severity of the client's illness, such as insertion of a nasogastric tube, continued replacement of fluids, monitoring of central venous pressure, and blood cultures.

CRITICAL MONITORING

Manifestations of Adult Respiratory Distress Syndrome Secondary to Acute Pancreatitis

Acute respiratory distress: tachypnea, dyspnea, accessory muscle breathing, and cyanosis

Fever and dry cough that develop over a short time period

Fine crackles heard throughout lung fields on auscultation

Possible confusion and agitation

Hypoxemia with partial pressure of oxygen (PO_2) <50 mm Hg

Early—hypocapnia and respiratory alkalosis

Late—hypercapnia and respiratory acidosis

Preoperative nursing management of the client with acute pancreatitis is similar to nursing management discussed under Medical Management. Pay special attention to the nutritional status of the client, as well as the breathing pattern, fluid and electrolyte levels, anxiety level, and control of pain as the client is prepared for surgery.

Postoperative Care

Assessment

Following pancreatic surgery, it is necessary to (1) have a clear idea of the surgical procedure performed, its purpose, steps, and dangers; (2) be aware of the location and purpose of each drain inserted during surgery—if there are multiple drains, especially external drains, assess each for proper function; (3) continually assess tubes or drains that are in place for decompression; and (4) if a T tube or internal stent becomes nonfunctional, bring it to the surgeon's attention immediately to prevent leakage at the internal insertion site. Leakage may lead to peritonitis or fistula formation.

Following pancreatic excision, it is important to know how much pancreatic tissue was removed. When there is a decrease in endocrine tissue, control of blood sugar with insulin and diet becomes necessary. Exocrine loss does not pose immediate postoperative problems but will necessitate lifelong enzyme replacement when the client returns to oral ingestion.

Diagnosis, Planning, Implementation

See the nursing diagnoses discussed under Nursing Management of the Medical Client of acute pancreatitis relating to pain, fluid and electrolyte balance, breathing pattern, and nutrition. All are applicable in the postoperative situation. In addition, the following nursing diagnoses are specifically related to the postoperative period.

Risk for Injury. A common postoperative collaborative problem is *Risk for Injury related to malfunction of pancreatic drains or loss of endocrine and exocrine function secondary to removal of the pancreas.*

Planning: Expected Outcomes. The client will not experience injury, as evidenced by proper draining of pancreatic drains, and no manifestations of hypoglycemia or digestive disorders related to absence of exocrine enzymes.

Implementation. Assess for placement, location (internal or external), and proper function and patency of the drains. If the drains do not appear to be functioning, notify the physician immediately.

Assess the functional ability of remaining pancreatic tissue following excision of the pancreas, determining both endocrine and exocrine functioning and its long-term implications. If the client has lost all endocrine function, he or she will require insulin (see Chapter 69). Continue to monitor the client for manifestations of hypoglycemia and hyperglycemia.

With the loss of exocrine function, replacement of pancreatic enzyme function with medications such as pancre-

lipase (Pancrease) will be necessary. When the client begins to eat, watch for the development of diarrhea and steatorrhea, which indicate that insufficient pancreatic enzymes are present.

Risk for Ineffective Management of Therapeutic Regimen (Individuals). The client, following pancreatectomy, will have many and complex learning needs leading to the nursing diagnosis *Risk for Ineffective Management of Therapeutic Regimen (Individuals) related to care, postoperative nutritional needs, diabetic care, and pancreatic enzyme replacement.*

Planning: Expected Outcomes. The client will understand discharge instructions, as evidenced by the ability to describe and demonstrate appropriate wound care, diet, proper diabetes care, and correct administration and side effects of the medication regimen.

Implementation. Assess the knowledge of the client and significant others before providing appropriate learning guidelines prior to discharge. Provide instructions for wound care. The client will require changes in diet necessitated by the diabetes. Provide guidelines for nutritional needs and an appropriate low fat diet (see Chapter 69).

Provide the client with important information concerning diabetes, including information about hyperglycemia (polyuria, polydipsia, and polyphagia) and hypoglycemia (see Chapter 69).

Provide the client with information about medication (pancreatic enzymes), including action, side effects, and when to notify the physician.

Effective Management of Therapeutic Regimen: Individual. The client will need to control the alcohol problem and other potential problems associated with the disease. It is hoped that the nursing diagnosis *Effective Management of Therapeutic Regimen: Individual related to alcohol abuse, surgical procedure, severity of the pancreatitis, and need for follow-up care* will be a positive diagnosis.

Planning: Expected Outcomes. The client will discuss strategies to address the progression or complications of alcoholism and pancreatitis, which challenge his or her continued successful management.

Implementation. The client with loss of pancreatic endocrine function requires extensive education regarding diabetes and its care (see Chapter 69). All clients require instruction on good nutrition to maintain adequate output. The client will need to understand and follow a nutritious low fat diet.

Avoidance of alcohol is another area of postoperative education. The client needs to understand the problems that alcohol is creating and the importance of stopping drinking before irreversible damage is done.

Evaluation

The client may be seen by a visiting nurse after discharge to assess his or her ability to follow the postoperative regimen. The client will need to be seen at regular intervals to ensure that the postoperative regimen is being followed. The client's ability to abstain from alcohol should be carefully assessed and further counseling provided, if needed.

▪ Modifications for Elderly Clients

The older client may be less able to survive the life-threatening effects of pancreatitis. Treatment is the same, although surgery may not be performed unless the condition becomes life-threatening.

Chronic Pancreatitis

Chronic pancreatitis is a progressive, inflammatory, destructive disease of the pancreas. The incidence of chronic pancreatitis in the United States is approximately 4/100,000. Chronic pancreatitis involves progressive fibrosis and degeneration of the pancreas.

Pathophysiology

Characteristically, the pancreas is progressively destroyed by repeated flares of usually mild attacks of pancreatitis. After repeated attacks of acute pancreatitis, this inflammatory process results in scarring and calcification of pancreatic tissue and the damage is irreversible, affecting both endocrine and exocrine pancreatic functions. In the United States and other industrial countries, chronic alcoholism is the most frequent cause of chronic calcifying pancreatitis. Protein malnutrition is a cause of this disease in other parts of the world. Other causes include hyperparathyroidism, congenital anomalies, and pancreatic trauma.

Clinical Manifestations and Diagnostic Findings

In chronic pancreatitis, as in acute pancreatitis, dull pain alternates with severe pain, vomiting, fever, and jaundice. The client may experience some pain relief by sitting in bed with the knees flexed and pressing a pillow to the abdomen. The client generally experiences more pain when supine.

Because food may aggravate the pain, the client usually reduces food intake, resulting in weight loss. Reduction in digestive enzyme secretion eventually causes malnutrition and contributes to the weight loss.

Ultimately, because of involvement of islet tissue, the client develops hyperglycemia with manifestations of diabetes. Insulin-dependent diabetes mellitus occurs in up to one third of clients.

The client also suffers from (1) abdominal distention with flatus and cramps and (2) frequent passage of foul fatty stools (steatorrhea). Thus, the clinical group of manifestations that serves as a classic presentation of chronic pancreatitis is abdominal pain, weight loss, diabetes, and steatorrhea.

Additionally, many clients present with a history of narcotic analgesic abuse in an effort to control pain. Pain or digestive disturbance may motivate a person with chronic pancreatitis to seek help.

Because of a reduced amount of functioning tissue in chronic pancreatitis, pancreatic enzyme analysis may be normal. Blood studies may reveal a mild leukocytosis. X-ray studies may show reduced bowel motility, calcifications, and adhesions. Both ultrasonography and the more expensive CT study provide useful diagnostic data. Angiography indicates vascular changes. Cholangiography and cholecystography show biliary alterations, which may be either a cause or a consequence of the pancreatic disorder.

Pancreatitis frequently reveals bloody fluid that is high in amylase and methemalbumin from hemoglobin digestion. Other studies may be in order, especially when the diagnosis is obscure.

Acute and Subacute Care

▪ Medical Management

The three areas that are treated medically are (1) control of pain, (2) treatment of endocrine insufficiency, and (3) treatment of exocrine insufficiency.

The control of pain can be a major problem and is generally the sole indication for surgical intervention. For alcohol-related pancreatitis, total abstinence from alcohol is imperative and sometimes successful in itself for pain relief. Control of diet may reduce painful stimulation of pancreatitis enzyme secretion. Attempts to control pain pharmacologically should begin with non-narcotic analgesics and progress to narcotic analgesics, if needed.

Exogenous insulin therapy may be necessary because of destruction of islet tissue. Exocrine insufficiency is treated with exogenous pancreatic enzyme therapy. This therapy may include lipase, trypsin, or H_2-receptor antagonists.

▪ Surgical Management

The three major goals of surgical intervention for chronic pancreatitis are to (1) correct the primary tract disease (ampullar procedure), (2) relieve ductal obstruction (ductal drainage), and (3) relieve pain (ablative procedure). Several surgical approaches are available. The major operations are depicted in Figure 66–2.

The prognosis in chronic pancreatitis is good if acute attacks decrease in frequency. Replacement therapy for chronic fat indigestion permits a fairly normal life. If the client continues to drink alcohol, the prognosis is poor. Repeated attacks eventually cause death from shock or renal failure.

Pancreatic Pseudocysts

Pancreatic pseudocysts are localized collections of pancreatic secretions (high concentrations of amylase, lipase, and trypsin) in a cystic structure usually adjacent to the pancreas rather than within the parenchyma. Pseudocysts account for up to 75% of all cystic lesions of the pan-

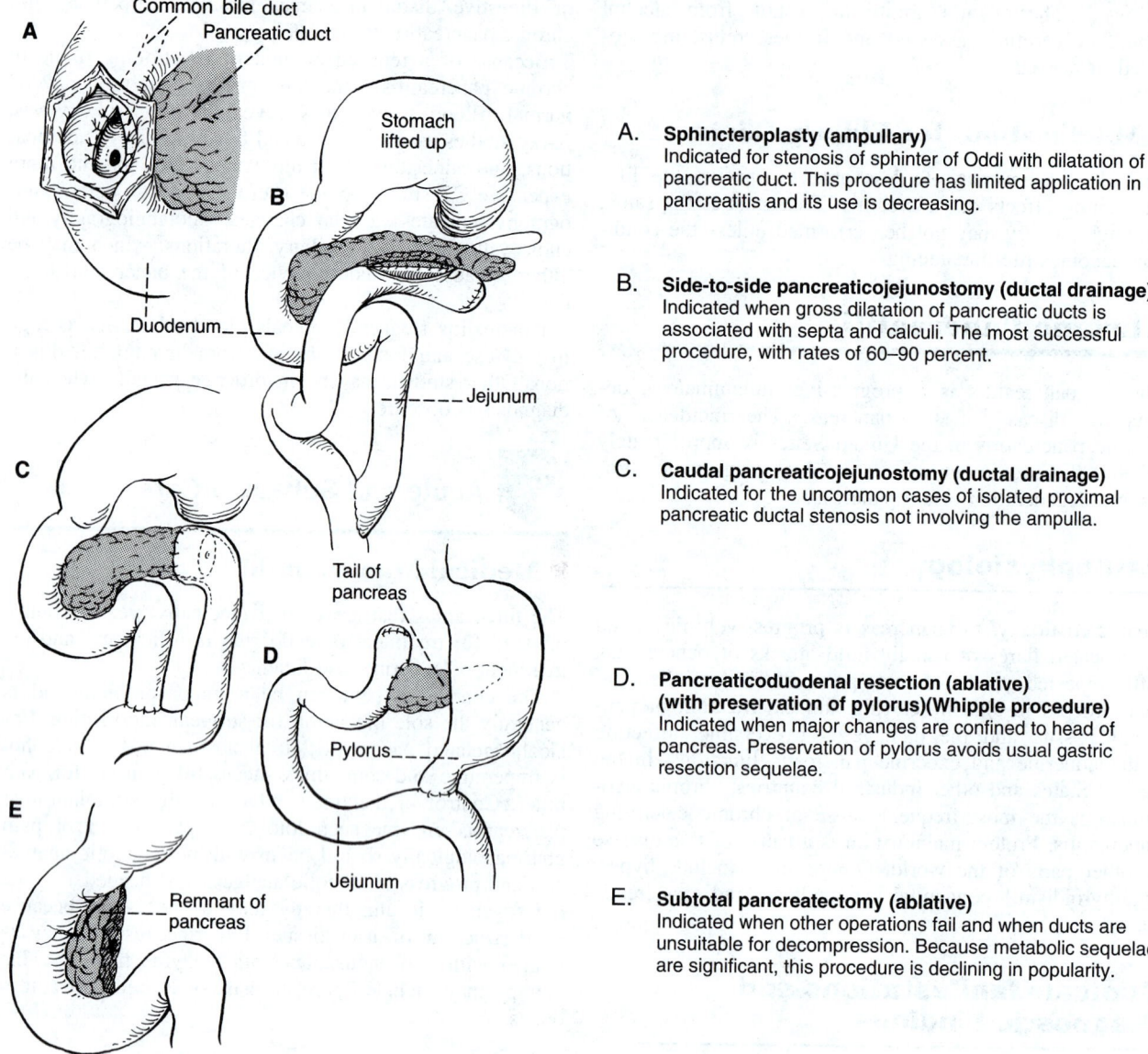

A. **Sphincteroplasty (ampullary)**
    Indicated for stenosis of sphinter of Oddi with dilatation of pancreatic duct. This procedure has limited application in pancreatitis and its use is decreasing.

B. **Side-to-side pancreaticojejunostomy (ductal drainage)**
    Indicated when gross dilatation of pancreatic ducts is associated with septa and calculi. The most successful procedure, with rates of 60–90 percent.

C. **Caudal pancreaticojejunostomy (ductal drainage)**
    Indicated for the uncommon cases of isolated proximal pancreatic ductal stenosis not involving the ampulla.

D. **Pancreaticoduodenal resection (ablative)**
    (with preservation of pylorus)(Whipple procedure)
    Indicated when major changes are confined to head of pancreas. Preservation of pylorus avoids usual gastric resection sequelae.

E. **Subtotal pancreatectomy (ablative)**
    Indicated when other operations fail and when ducts are unsuitable for decompression. Because metabolic sequelae are significant, this procedure is declining in popularity.

Figure 66–2. Operations for chronic pancreatitis and pancreatic cancer.

creas. Pancreatic pseudocysts develop in up to 10% of clients after an attack of acute alcoholic pancreatitis, but they may be associated with acute pancreatitis of other causes, chronic pancreatitis, trauma, and pancreatic neoplasm.

The most common clinical picture of a client with pancreatic pseudocyst involves abdominal pain, early satiety, nausea, and vomiting. Less common manifestations include pruritus, jaundice, sepsis, and hemorrhage. Essentially, diagnosis of pseudocyst is made through the same assessment as that used with pancreatitis.

Treatment is based on the presence or absence of manifestations, the client's age, and the size of the cyst. In about 25% of cases, the pseudocyst resolves spontaneously. Clients with this condition are followed with frequent ultrasound study to determine whether the cyst is decreasing in size. Persistent manifestations or pseudocyst-related complications require operative intervention.

Surgical procedures range from internal drainage of the pseudocyst (cystojejunostomy, cystogastrostomy, and cystoduodenostomy), pancreatic resection, distal pancreatectomy, and least often, percutaneous or endoscopic drainage.

Pancreatic Cancer

Cancer of the pancreas is the most common neoplasm of that organ. About 75% occur in the head and 25% in the body and tail of the pancreas. It is the fifth most common cause of cancer death, exceeded only by lung, colorectal, breast, and prostate cancer. Ninety percent of pancreatic cancer clients die within the first year of diagnosis. Cancer of the pancreas is more common in blacks than in whites, in smokers, and in males.

It appears to be linked to diabetes mellitus, use of alcohol, history of previous pancreatitis, smoking, and ingestion of a high fat diet.

Duct cell adenocarcinoma accounts for over 90% of cell types of malignant pancreatic exocrine tumors. Less common types of pancreatic exocrine cancer include cystadenocarcinoma and acinar cell carcinoma.

Periampullary adenocarcinomas originate in the region of the ampulla of Vater. Clients typically present with jaundice, significant unexplained weight loss, and abdominal pain. The majority of clients are managed operatively by either resection (about 30%) or palliative therapy to relieve manifestations such as jaundice.[41]

Carcinomas of the tail and body of the pancreas usually present with significant weight loss and abdominal pain. Because of their location, these tumors generally grow to a large size before manifestations occur and the diagnosis is made. Therefore, the resectability rate is low (less than 7%), and the prognosis is poor (5–6 month mean survival). The response to chemotherapy (fluorouracil) has been disappointing.

Cystadenocarcinoma of the pancreas is most frequently seen in women between the ages of 40 and 60 and accounts for less than 2% of all pancreatic exocrine neoplasms.

Acinar cell carcinoma of the pancreas is very rare, has no sex predominance, and is given the same surgical treatment as that used for ductal adenocarcinoma.

Surgical treatment is Whipple's operation, which involves a pancreatoduodenectomy with removal of the distal third of the stomach, pancreaticojejunostomy, gastrojejunostomy, and choledochojejunostomy (see Fig. 66–2). The nursing care for these clients is similar to that for Surgical Management of acute pancreatitis.

Pancreatic Transplantation

Transplantation of the pancreas was first developed in the mid-1960s. Advances in technique continue to be made. It is hoped that eventually pancreas transplantation will have an impact on the treatment of diabetes mellitus similar to that of kidney transplantation in the treatment of endstage renal disease.

Along with solving technological problems for advancement in technique, other problems are still being encountered that need resolving. They include organ donation and distribution and overcoming immunologic barriers.

■ Surgical Management

A candidate for a pancreas transplant, who is carefully assessed and evaluated, is most likely to have type II diabetes. Because there is a higher graft success rate in the population that receives a combined pancreas-renal transplant compared with a pancreas transplant alone, both transplants are often performed concurrently. Transplant procedures generally last from 4 to 6 hours.

Several surgical approaches are used with pancreas transplants. They include transplanting (1) a segmental portion, (2) an entire pancreas with or without all or part of the ampulla of Vater or part of the duodenum, or (3) isolated islet grafts. The primary concern when the entire pancreas is transplanted is management of the exocrine secretions from the pancreatic duct. When the entire pancreas is transplanted, it is placed in the lower pelvic cavity and the duct is connected to the urinary bladder to allow for drainage of the pancreatic enzymes. Urinary tests of the enzymes reveal the viability of the new pancreas. To help prevent complications such as thrombosis, the volume of blood flowing through the pancreas is kept at a high rate for 72 hours. Islet cell grafts are a specific approach to treatment but there are difficulties with isolating and preserving the grafts. They have been transplanted into sites such as the portal vein, renal capsule, and peritoneal cavity, among many other sites.

Graft rejection is a major complication. Immunosuppressants such as cyclosporine are used to lower the rate of rejection.

■ Nursing Management of the Surgical Client

The nursing management is similar to that of a client who has undergone liver transplantation. Hospitalization after transplant is usually 3 to 4 weeks. During that time, medication adjustments are made to achieve the appropriate dose of immunosuppressant for the individual client. Hemoglobin levels are monitored carefully, as is the blood sugar. The client will go off insulin and the need for strict adherence to a diet and constant monitoring of blood sugar will diminish.

Nursing diagnoses that apply to the patient after a pancreas transplant are similar to those noted for liver transplant except that clinical manifestations of rejection of a pancreas transplant differ. (A successful pancreatic transplantation is assessed by analyzing the blood glucose response and C-peptide levels. C-peptide levels are elevated and there is a normal blood sugar level 2 to 3 days postoperatively in a successful transplant.) Additional potential nursing diagnoses include the following:

- Altered Oral Mucous Membrane related to infection from immunosuppression
- Fluid Volume Excess or Deficit related to compromised organ function
- Impaired Gas Exchange related to ventilation-perfusion difficulty associated with fluid overload
- Activity Intolerance related to generalized weakness associated with the disease process, fluid and electrolyte imbalance, and poor nutrition
- Body Image Disturbance related to change in physical appearance and in role in the family and community

Pancreatic Trauma

The pancreas is injured in less than 2% of persons with abdominal trauma. Two thirds of pancreatic injuries are associated with penetrating abdominal trauma, and the rest are caused by blunt trauma. Clients with penetrating abdominal trauma show manifestations of hemorrhage, progressive peritonitis, and hypovolemia.

The presentation of blunt pancreatic trauma is varied. The majority of persons with blunt trauma have injuries to surrounding organs and vascular structures, and pancreatic trauma is discovered on treatment of these other injuries. In clients without injury to other areas, the only findings may be mild epigastric pain and tenderness; progressive deterioration will yield the diagnosis of pancreatic injury.

Treatment involves surgery to control hemorrhage, debride nonviable tissue, preserve viable tissue, and provide drainage of pancreatic secretions.

Cystic Fibrosis

Cystic fibrosis (CF) is a hereditary, chronic disease characterized by abnormal secretions of the exocrine glands. It is genetically transmitted as an autosomal recessive trait. Approximately 4% to 5% of the population are carriers, and the incidence in the United States is about 1 in every 1600 to 2000 white births.

Pancreatic exocrine function is affected by decreased lipase released into the bowel. This results in malabsorption of lipids and causes blockage of the pancreatic ducts by thick mucus. Pancreatic degeneration, fibrosis, and atrophy of tissues follow, with eventual development of fatty infiltration and loss of function. The intestines have thick, viscous mucus, which may cause a thick mass within the bowel. The lack of pancreatic enzymes causes steatorrhea.

Pulmonary complications are the most physically visible. These clients have obvious respiratory compromise, with frequent bronchopneumonia and chronic bronchitis.

Recent improvements in the management of infants and children with CF have led to a greater number of adults with CF. Typically, these persons have a small stature and appear somewhat emaciated. They are barrel-chested and have clubbed fingers.

Because the digestive problems encountered with CF are generally managed with diet and oral administration of pancreatic enzymes and fat-soluble vitamins, clients are hospitalized for treatment of respiratory complications rather than for intestinal problems. The current trend is to hospitalize the client routinely for thorough pulmonary hygiene with a full course of IV antibiotics (with emphasis on antifungals) and respiratory therapy.

Nursing diagnoses that may apply to people with CF include the following:

- Ineffective Airway Clearance related to thick, viscous, mucous secretions from the submucosal glands of the respiratory tract
- Altered Nutrition: Less than Body Requirements, related to lack of pancreatic enzymes
- Knowledge Deficit related to dietary management of CF

Interventions for clients with CF include:

- Prophylactic pulmonary support—expectorants, postural drainage, antibiotics, and exercise
- Administration of pancreatic enzymes

- Dietary management—high protein, high calorie, high salt, and low fat diet
- Replacement of fat-soluble vitamins

Conclusions

Biliary and exocrine pancreatic disorders are common but are extremely complex and diverse. The nurse needs a thorough understanding of biliary and pancreatic anatomy and physiology to understand these disorders. Some of these conditions are treated without further difficulty, such as cholecystitis, whereas others can become chronic and lead to a wide variety of other problems, such as pancreatitis. Teaching is vital to the care of these clients, and so the nurse must understand these conditions to initiate appropriate teaching plans.

Thinking Critically

1. A 40-year-old woman is admitted to the hospital complaining of colicky pain in the right upper abdominal quadrant. She states that the pain is worse when she eats fried foods. She also states that she has vomited on several occasions and it seems to relieve her manifestations. What are your priorities in assessing and caring for the client?

Factors to Consider. What types of diagnostic procedures should be scheduled? Why is an accurate assessment of the clinical manifestations important? What indications warrant insertion of a nasogastric tube?

2. You are assigned to care for a 32-year-old construction worker who has been admitted with severe upper abdominal pain radiating to his back and recurrent vomiting. This is his second admission for pancreatitis. He admits to drinking 1 pint of whiskey daily on the weekends and having several drinks nightly on weekdays. His alcohol intake has been greater in the past. Laboratory data include an amylase level of 750 units/L (normal 25–125 units); lipase, is 5.6 units/ml (normal, 10–140 units); aspartate aminotransferase (AST), 150 units/L (normal is 5–40 units) and alanine aminotransferase (ALT), 60 units (normal, 1–45 units). How do you feel about caring for this client?

Factors to Consider. Are you comfortable with the client's life-style? Do the biochemical studies support a diagnosis of pancreatitis? What do you need to consider if he complains of pain? What should you do if you discover he is allergic to meperidine?

3. A 73-year-old woman, comes to the emergency room with complaints of recurrent episodes of epigastric pain during the past 9 months. Chills, fever, and jaundice have occurred for the first time and have persisted for 4 days. Her white blood cell count is

normal. Serum bilirubin and alkaline phosphatase values are elevated. There is no history of alcoholism, blood transfusions, or hepatitis. The client takes no medications except an occasional "Bufferin for my arthritis." Her past medical history is unremarkable except for a cholecystectomy 10 years ago after an episode of cholecystitis. What are the priorities for care?

Factors to Consider. What are the client's clinical manifestations? Would surgical treatment alleviate the problem? What might cause stricture of the bile ducts?

Bibliography

1. Akiyama, H., et al. (1990). Percutaneous treatments for biliary diseases. *Radiology, 176,* 25.
2. Bartucci, M. R., Loughman, K. A., & Moir, E. J. (1992). Kidney-pancreas transplantation: A treatment option for ESRD and type I diabetes. *ANNA Journal, 19*(5), 467–474.
3. Bass, M. (1992). Pancreas transplantation: Detecting rejection and patient care. *ANNA Journal, 19*(5), 476–482.
4. Biorsch, G., et al. (1988). Clinical evaluation, ultrasound, cholescintography, and endoscopic retrograde cholangiography in cholestasis: A prospective comparative study. *Journal of Clinical Gerontology, 10,* 185.
5. Brodrick, R. L. (1991). Preventing complication in acute pancreatitis. *Dimensions of Critical Care Nursing, 10*(5), 262–270.
6. Cappell, M. S. (1991). Hepatobiliary manifestations of the acquired immune deficiency syndrome. *American Journal of Gastroenterology, 86,* 1.
7. Clearfield, H. R., & Borowsky, L. M. (1989). *Case studies in gastroenterology.* Baltimore: Williams & Wilkins.
8. Copstead, L. C. (1995). *Perspectives on pathophysiology.* Philadelphia: W. B. Saunders.
9. Cotton, P. B. (1990). Critical appraisal of therapeutic endoscopy in biliary tract disease. *Annual Review of Medicine, 41,* 211.
10. Ferri, F. F. (1995). *The care of the medical patient* (3rd ed.). St. Louis: Mosby–Year Book.
11. Fisher, R. L. (1989). Hepatobiliary abnormalities associated with total parenteral nutrition. *Gastroenterology Clinics of North America, 18,* 645.
12. Frey, C. F. (1993). Management of necrotizing pancreatitis. *Western Journal of Medicine, 159,* 675–680.
13. Friedman, L. S. (1995). Liver, biliary tract, and pancreas. In L. M. Tierney, et al. (Eds.), *Medical diagnosis and treatment* (34th ed.). Norwalk, CT: Appleton & Lange.
14. Greenberger, N. J., & Isselbacher, K. J. (1994). Diseases of the gallbladder and bile ducts. In K. J. Isselbacher, et al. (Eds.). *Harrison's principles of internal medicine* (13th ed.). New York: McGraw-Hill.
15. Guyton, A. C., & Hall, J. E. (1996). *Textbook of medical physiology* (9th ed.). Philadelphia: W. B. Saunders.
16. Hartshorn, J., Lamborn, M. & Noll, M. L. (1993). *Introduction to critical care nursing.* Philadelphia: W. B. Saunders.
17. Jones, W. G., Reilly, D. M., & Barie, P. S. (1991). Pancreatic injuries. *AORN Journal, 53*(4), 917–918.
18. Jurf, J. B., et al. (1990). Cholecystectomy made easier. *American Journal of Nursing, 90*(12), 38–39.
19. Jurkovich, G. I., et al. (1988). Cholecystectomy. Expected outcome in primary and secondary biliary disorders. *American Surgeon, 54,* 40.
20. Klar, E., et al. (1990). Pancreatic ischemia in experimental acute pancreatitis: Mechanism, significance, and therapy. *British Journal of Surgery, 11,* 1205.
21. Krumberger, J. M., (1993). Acute pancreatitis. *Critical Care Nursing Clinics of North America, 5*(1), 185–202.
22. Kulhman, J. E., et al. (1989). Complications of endoscopic retrograde sphincterotomy: Computed tomographic evaluation. *Gastrointestinal Radiology, 14,* 127.
23. Lee, S. P. (1990). Pathogenesis of biliary sludge. *Hematology, 12,* 2005.
24. Levitt, M. D. (1992). Pancreatitis. In J. B. Wyngaarden, et al. (Eds.), *Cecil textbook of medicine* (19th ed.). Philadelphia: W. B. Saunders.
25. McCance, K. L., & Huether, S. E. (1994). *Pathophysiology: The biologic basis for disease in adults and children* (2nd ed.). St. Louis: Mosby–Year Book.
26. McConnell, E. A. (1995). What's wrong with this patient? Investigating abdominal pain. *Nursing, 25*(5), 84–85.
27. McLaughlin, S. (1994) Pancreatic cancer and diabetes. *Diabetes Educator, 20*(1), 20–26.
28. Miller, F. J., & Rose, S. C. (1990). Intervention for gallbladder disease. *Cardiovascular and Interventional Radiology, 13,* 264.
29. Miyake, H., et al. (1989). Prognosis and prognostic factors in chronic pancreatitis. *Digestive Diseases and Sciences, 34,* 449.
30. Noone, J. (1995). Acute pancreatitis: An Orem approach to nursing assessment and care. *Critical Care Nurse, 15*(4), 27–37.
31. O'Hanlon-Nichols, T. (1995). Clinical snapshot. Protal hypertension. *American Journal of Nursing, 95*(11), 38.
32. Ohara, N., & Schaefer, J. (1990). Clinical significance of biliary sludge. *Journal of Clinical Gastroenterology, 12,* 291.
33. Pazdur, R. (1991). Pancreatic carcinoma: Evaluating patients for curative or palliative treatment. *Consultant, 31,* 57.
34. Peterson, T. (1995). Hepatitis C: A new enemy. *Nursing Times, 91*(36), 31–33.
35. Reber, H. A. (1990). The cause and management of the pain of chronic pancreatitis. *Gastroenterology Clinics of North America, 19,* 895.
36. Ritchie, A. C. (1990). *Boyd's textbook of pathology.* Philadelphia: Lea & Febiger.
37. Rogalla, C. J. (1991). Pancreatic duct calculi. *AORN Journal, 53*(6), 1506–1517.
38. Sabiston, D. C., Jr. (1991). *Textbook of surgery. The biological basis of modern surgical practice.* (14th ed.). Philadelphia: W. B. Saunders.
39. Smith, A., (1991). When the pancreas self-destructs. *American Journal of Nursing, 91*(9), 38–48.
40. Swearingen, P. L. (1994). *Manual of medical-surgical nursing care* (3rd ed.). St. Louis: Mosby–Year Book.
41. Tierney, L. M., et al. (Eds.). (1995). *Medical diagnosis and treatment* (34th ed.). Norwalk, CT: Appleton & Lange.
42. Trusler, L. A. (1992). Management of the patient receiving simultaneous kidney-pancreas transplantation. *Critical Care Nursing Clinics of North America, 4*(1), 89–95.
43. Ulander, K., et al. (1991). Needs and care of patients undergoing subtotal pancreatectomy for cancer. *Cancer Nursing, 14*(1), 27–34.
44. Urban, M. H. (1989). Endoscopic retrograde cholangiopancreatography. A diagnostic outpatient procedure. *AORN Journal, 50,* 572.
45. van Heerden, J. A., et al. (1991). Early experience with percutaneous cholecystolithotomy. *Mayo Clinic Procedures, 66,* 1005.
46. Zehrer, C. L., & Gross, C. R. (1994). Patient perceptions of benefits and concerns following pancreas transplantation. *Diabetes Educator, 20*(3), 216–220.

Metabolic Disorders

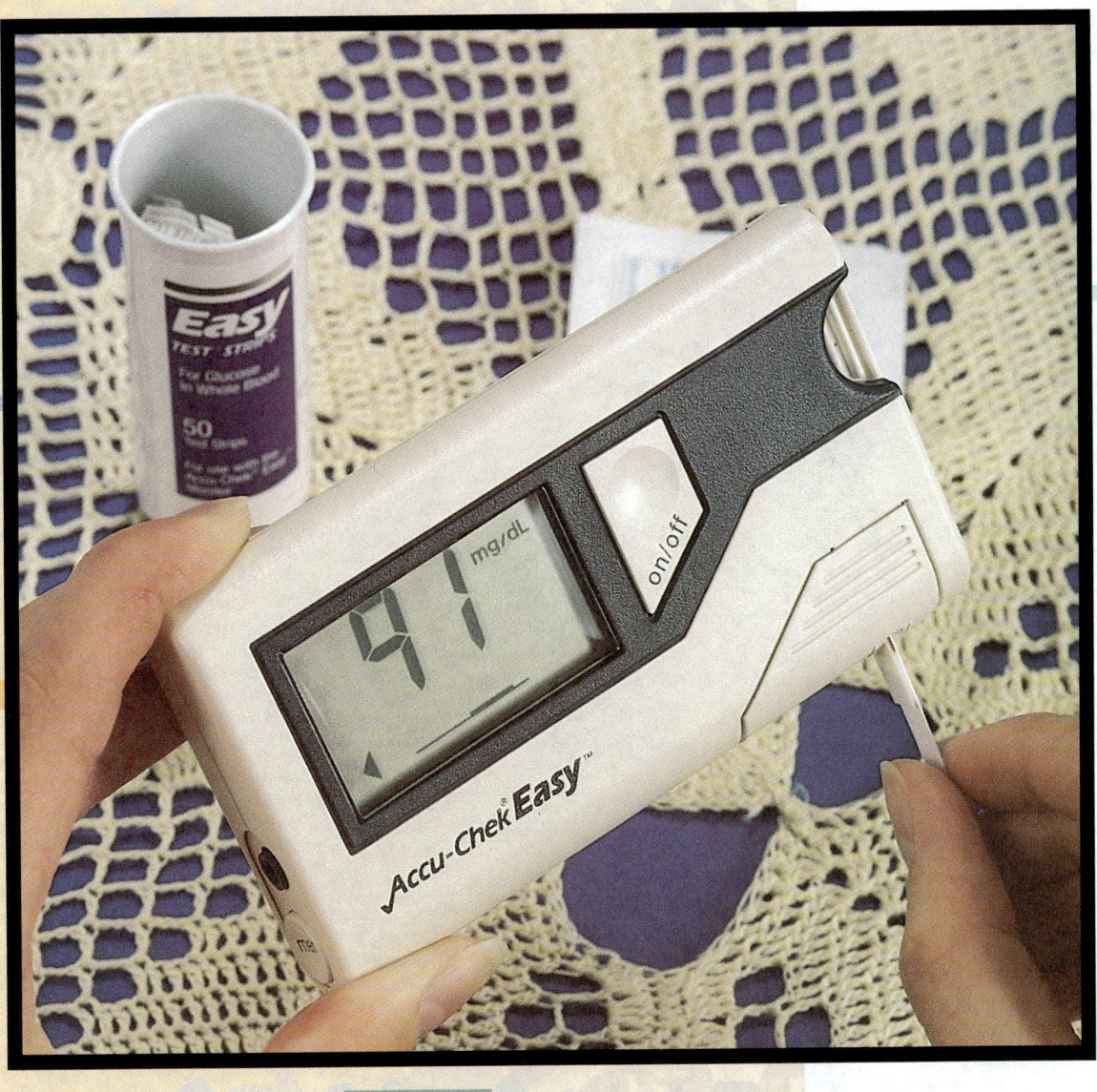

Structure and Function of the Endocrine System

Esther Matassarin-Jacobs

CHAPTER

67

The endocrine system often is considered one of the most complex systems in the human body. It is only in recent times that endocrine function has been understood and well defined. Prior to that time, the study of glands and hormones was considered to be more in the realm of ritual and magic than science and medicine. Endocrine disorders were not regarded as treatable physiologic problems. With the advent of endocrinology and the increased understanding of the system, nurses have found themselves deeply involved in the care of clients with endocrine disorders.

The nurse has a major role in the care of clients with endocrine disorders. The nurse is involved in assessment of these disorders, as well as the care of clients during treatment. Many of these disorders require minimal hospital care—during initial diagnosis and when severe complications occur. These clients remain at home, only seeking healthcare at periodic intervals. After extensive instruction, these disorders are usually controlled by the clients themselves.

This chapter covers the structure and function of the endocrine system as well as assessment of the system and all potential disorders. The remainder of this unit discusses specific disorders of the pituitary gland, endocrine pancrease, thyroid, parathyroid glands, adrenal glands, and gonads.

The Endocrine System

The endocrine system, in conjunction with the nervous system, controls and integrates body function. These two systems operate together to maintain homeostasis. Closely related in their functions, they are indistinguishable from one another in certain characteristics. For example, the adrenal medulla and the posterior pituitary glands are of neural origin. If they are destroyed or removed, the functions of these glands are partially taken over by the nervous system.

This chapter incorporates material written for the fourth edition by Diane Butts-Krakoff.

Although the communicative and integrative roles of the endocrine and nervous systems are similar, the precise ways in which each system functions differ. The nervous system sends its messages along nerve fibers, and neural responses are swift and selective. Also, neural effects usually are rapid in onset and of short duration. In contrast, the endocrine system sends its messages in the form of hormones via the bloodstream. Hormonal effects have a slower onset than neural effects but a longer duration of action. The actions of the endocrine system may be localized to one area, or generalized to all the cells of the body.

Structure

There are two type of glands: (1) exocrine and (2) endocrine. Exocrine glands release their secretions into ducts on body surfaces, such as the skin, or internal organs, like the lining of the intestinal tract. Exocrine glands include the liver, pancreas (an exocrine and endocrine gland), the breast, and lacrimal glands for tears. In contrast, endocrine glands release their secretions directly into the blood (Fig. 67–1). Endocrine glands include the following:

- Islets of Langerhans in the pancreas
- Gonads (ovaries and testes)
- Adrenal, pituitary, thyroid and parathyroid glands, and thymus

The endocrine glands are shown in Figure 67–2.

Hormones and Their Functions

The word *hormone* is derived from the Greek *hormon,* to set in motion or rouse. Hormones set into motion various processes that govern life. The endocrine system has five general functions:

1. Differentiation of the reproductive and central nervous systems in the developing fetus
2. Stimulation of sequential growth

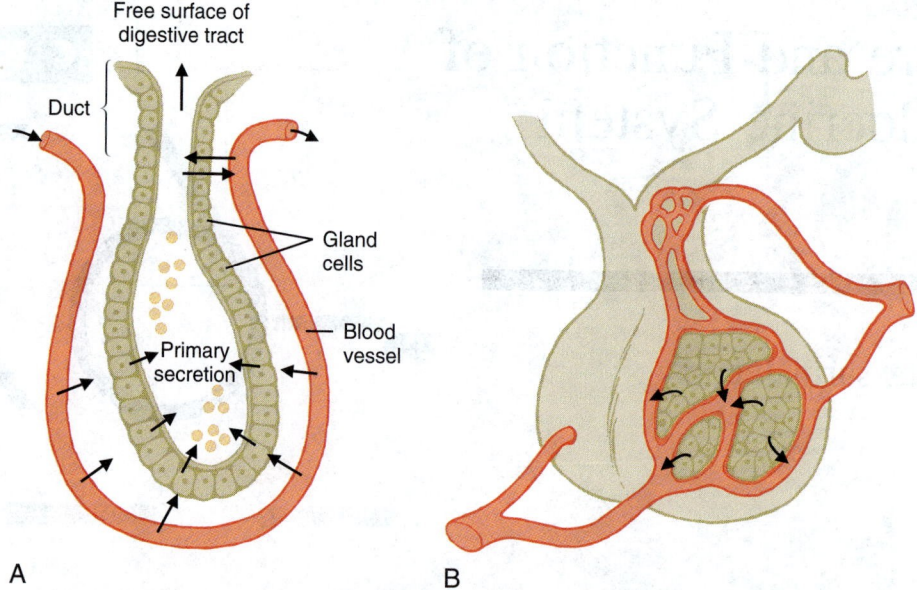

Figure 67–1. Differences between endocrine and exocrine gland function. *A,* Exocrine secretions pass through a duct to reach their final destination, which are free surfaces of the body (e.g., internal surfaces such as the lining of the gastrointestinal tract, or external surfaces such as the skin). *B,* Endocrine glands, on the other hand, are generally ductless. Hormones are released from the cells of the gland into the interstitial fluid, from which they may pass into the blood to circulate throughout the body.

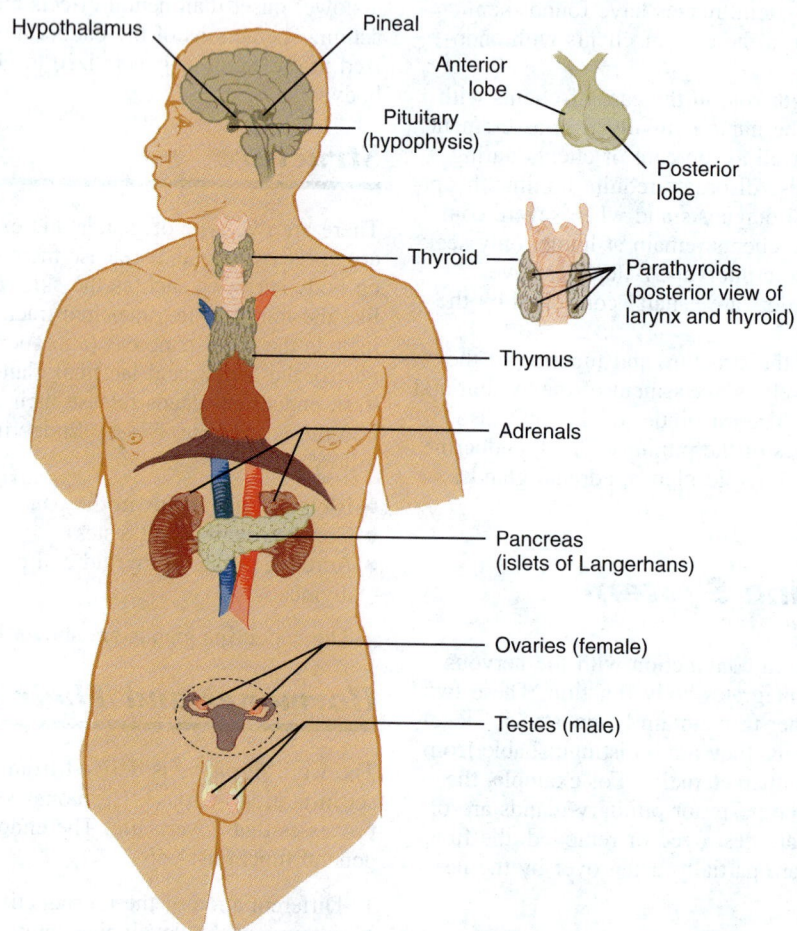

Figure 67–2. Organs of the endocrine system.

3. Coordination of the reproductive systems
4. Maintenance of optimal internal environment
5. Initiation of corrective and adaptive responses when emergency situations occur

The disorders that occur when the endocrine system is not functioning properly affect growth, reproduction, and adaptation to stress.

Classification

In terms of their chemical structure, hormones are classified as water-soluble or lipid-soluble. Water-soluble hormones include polypeptides (e.g., insulin, glucagon, adrenocorticotropic hormone [ACTH], gastrin) and catecholamines (e.g., dopamine, norepinephrine, epinephrine).

Lipid-soluble hormones include steroids (e.g., estrogen, progesterone, testosterone, glucocorticoids, aldosterone) and thyronines (e.g., thyroxine). Water-soluble hormones act via a second-messenger system, whereas steroid hormones are freely permeable to the cell membrane.

Characteristics

Although each hormone is unique in its own structure and function, all hormones have the following characteristics.

Hormones are secreted in one of three patterns. (1) *Diurnal* secretion is a pattern that rises and falls within a 24-hour period. Cortisol is as example of a diurnal hor-

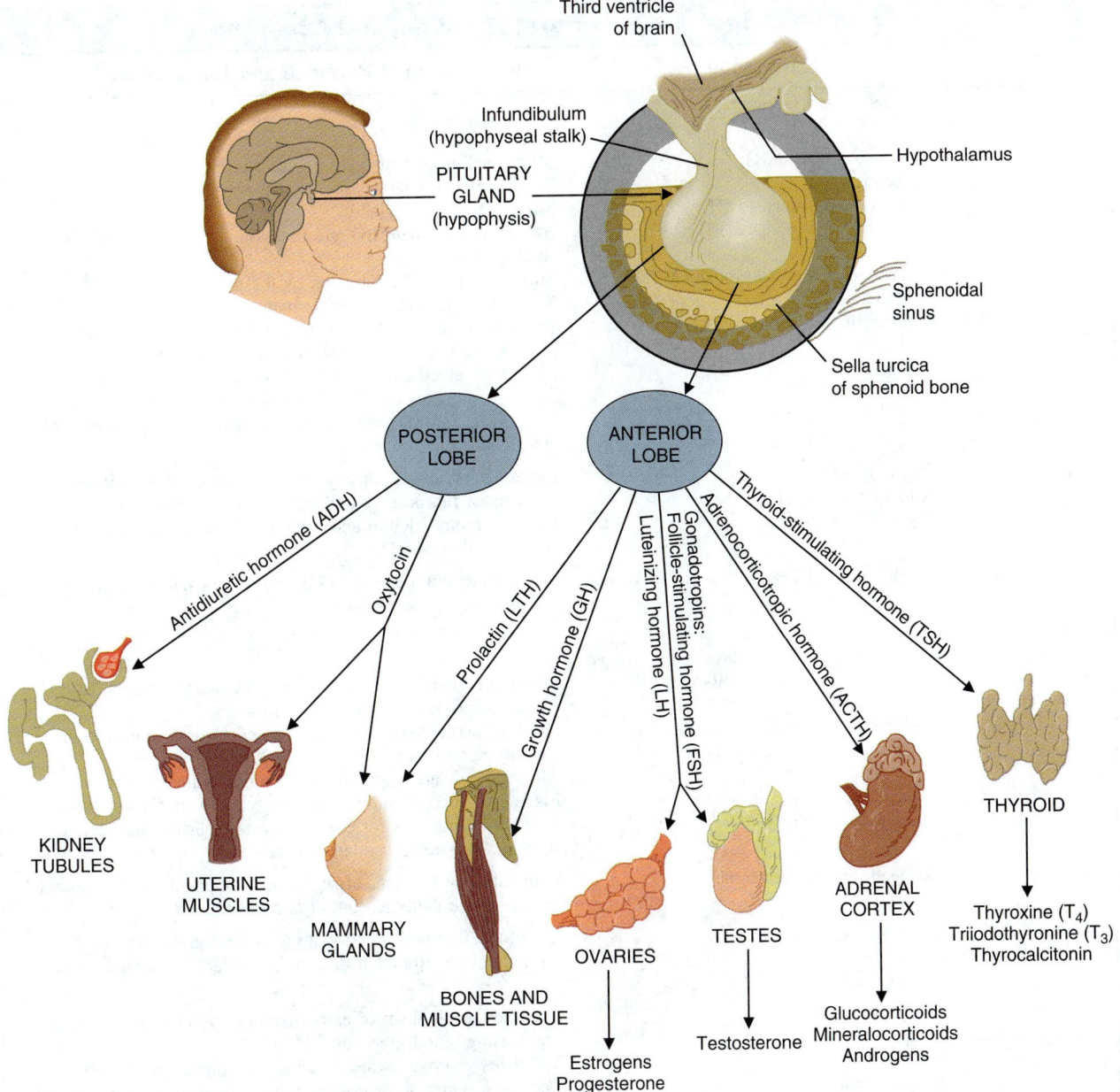

Figure 67–3. The pituitary gland is suspended from the hypothalamus by the infundibular or pituitary stalk. Shown here are hormones released by the pituitary gland and the target tissues on which they act.

mone. Cortisol levels rise in the morning and fall by evening. (2) *Pulsatile and cyclic* patterns of hormonal secretion rise and fall along another time frame, such as monthly. Estrogen is a cyclic hormone with peaks and troughs to produce a menstrual cycle. (3) The third type of hormonal secretion is *variable* and depends on levels of other substrates. Parathyroid hormone is secreted in response to serum calcium levels.

Hormones operate within a feedback system. Feedback loops can be positive or negative and allow the body to be maintained in an optimal environment. They control the rate of cellular activity. They do not initiate biochemical changes. Hormones affect only cells that contain appropriate receptors, which initiate a specific function. They have independent and interdependent functions. The

release of hormones from one gland often triggers the release of hormones from other glands. Hormones are constantly deactivated by the liver or other cellular mechanisms and are excreted by the kidney.

Regulation

■ Role of the Hypothalamus and Pituitary Glands

The two major endocrine glands are the hypothalamus and the pituitary. Endocrine activity is controlled directly or indirectly by the hypothalamus, which links the ner-

Table 67–1. Endocrine Structure, Function, and Assessment

Gland	Hormone	Action of Hormone and Target Gland
Pituitary		
Anterior lobe	Growth hormone (GH)	Stimulates growth of body tissues and bones
	Prolactin	Stimulates mammary tissue growth and lactation
	Thyrotropic hormone (TSH)	Stimulates thyroid gland
	Gonadotropic hormones (LH and FSH)	Affect growth, maturity, and functioning of primary and secondary sex organs
	Adrenocorticotropic hormone (ACTH)	Stimulates steroid production by the adrenal cortex
	Melanocyte-stimulating hormone (MSH)	May stimulate adrenal cortex; may affect pigmentation
Posterior lobe	Antidiuretic hormone (ADH, vasopressin)	Promotes reabsorption of water by the distal tubules and collecting ducts of the kidney, thus decreasing urine output
	Oxytocin	Stimulates ejection of milk from mammary alveoli into the ducts; stimulates uterine contractions; may possibly be involved in the transport of sperm in the reproductive tract of the female
Thyroid	Thyroxine (T_4)	Increases metabolic activity of almost all cells; stimulates most aspects of fat, protein, and carbohydrate metabolism
	Triiodothyronine (T_3)	
	Thyrocalcitonin (TCT)	Lowers serum calcium and elevates phosphate levels; opposite effect to that of PTH
Parathyroid	Parathormone (PTH)	Increases calcium levels and decreases phosphate levels; increases resorption of bone
Adrenal		
Cortex	Hormones divided into three main groups:	
	Glucocorticoids (primarily cortisol)	Promote carbohydrate, protein, and fat catabolism; increase tissue responsiveness to other hormones
	Mineralocorticoids (aldosterone)	Tend to increase sodium retention and potassium excretion
	Androgens (male hormones)	Govern certain secondary sex characteristics
		All corticoids are important for defense against stress or injury
Medulla	Epinephrine (Adrenalin) (80%)	Elevates blood pressure; converts glycogen to glucose when needed by muscles for energy; increases heart rate; increases cardiac contractility; dilates bronchioles
	Norepinephrine (20%)	
Ovaries	Estrogens and progesterone	Stimulate development of secondary sex characteristics; effect repair of the endometrium after menstruation
Testes	Testosterone	Essential to normal functioning of male reproductive organs; stimulates development of male secondary sex characteristics
Pancreas		
Islets of Langerhans	Insulin	Promotes metabolism of carbohydrates, protein, and fat, thus decreasing blood glucose levels
	Glucagon	Mobilizes glycogen stores, thus raising blood glucose levels
	Somatostatin	Decreases secretion of insulin, glucagon, growth hormone, and several gastrointestinal hormones (gastrin, secretin)

vous system to the endocrine system. In response to input from other areas of the brain and from other hormones in the blood, neurons in the hypothalamus secrete several releasing and inhibiting hormones. These hormones act on specific cells in the pituitary gland that regulate the production and secretion of pituitary hormones. The hypothalamus and pituitary gland are connected by a pedunculated infundibulum (Fig. 67–3).

The hormones secreted from each endocrine gland and the action of the hormones are listed in Table 67–1. Note that each of the hormones affects organs and tissues that are far removed from the location of their parent gland. For example, oxytocin, which is released from the posterior lobe of the pituitary gland, causes uterine contractions. The pituitary hormones that govern the secretion of hormones from other glands are called tropic hormones. Glands influenced by the hormones are called target glands (see Fig. 67–3).

The prostaglandins are a form of hormone, but their action is different from the other hormones. Rather than exerting a response in tissues far from their synthesizing tissues, prostaglandins appear to exert their effect in the tissue that synthesizes them. Prostaglandins inhibit gastric secretion, relax smooth muscle in the airway, increase urine flow, increase or decrease blood pressure, and stimulate uterine contraction.

■ Feedback Systems

Blood levels of hormones are also controlled by *negative feedback.* Once a hormone level is sufficient to produce its intended effect, further elevations in the hormone level are prevented by negative feedback. Rising levels of hormone negate the initial change that triggered the hormone release. For example, an increased secretion of ACTH from the anterior pituitary gland stimulates a rise in the release of cortisol from the adrenal cortex, causing a decrease in the release of more ACTH. Blood levels of substances other than hormones can also trigger hormone release and are controlled through a feedback system. The release of insulin from the islets of Langerhans in the pancreas is driven by blood glucose levels. A feedback system is shown in Figure 67–4.

■ Activation of Target Cells

Once the hormone reaches the target cell, it can influence how the cell functions in one of two methods: (1) through the use of intracellular mediators or (2) by activating the genes within the cell (Fig. 67–5). One intracellular mediator is cyclic adenosine monophosphate (cAMP), which is bound to the inner surface of the cell membrane. When the hormone attaches to the cell, the action of the cell is altered in some way. For example, when the pancreatic hormone glucagon binds to liver cells, elevated levels of AMP promote the breakdown of glycogen to glucose. When hormones activate cells by interacting with genes, the gene synthesizes messenger RNA (mRNA) and ultimately proteins (i.e., enzymes, steroids). These substances affect cellular reactions and processes.

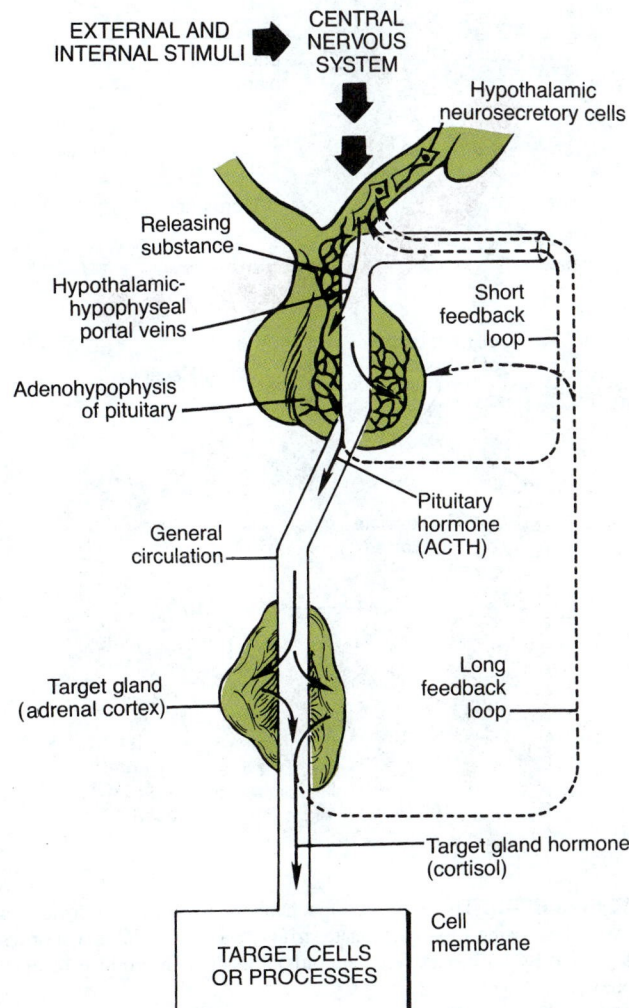

Figure 67–4. Regulation of hormone secretion by negative feedback. When the calcium level in the blood falls below normal, the parathyroid glands are stimulated to release more parathyroid hormone. This hormone acts to increase the calcium level in the blood, thus restoring homeostasis. If the calcium level exceeds normal, the parathyroid glands are inhibited and slow their release of hormone. This diagram has been simplified. Calcitonin, a hormone secreted by the thyroid gland, works antagonistically to parathyroid hormone and is important in lowering blood calcium concentration. (Modified from Spence, A. P., & Mason, E. B. [1987] *Human anatomy and physiology* [3rd ed., p. 485]. Menlo Park, CA: Benjamin-Cummings.)

The Endocrine Glands

Pituitary Structure and Function

The pituitary gland lies securely cradled within a small recess in the sphenoid bone called the sella turcica (see Fig. 67–3). About 70% of the gland is the anterior lobe, or adenohypophysis. The posterior lobe, or neurohypophysis, makes up the rest.

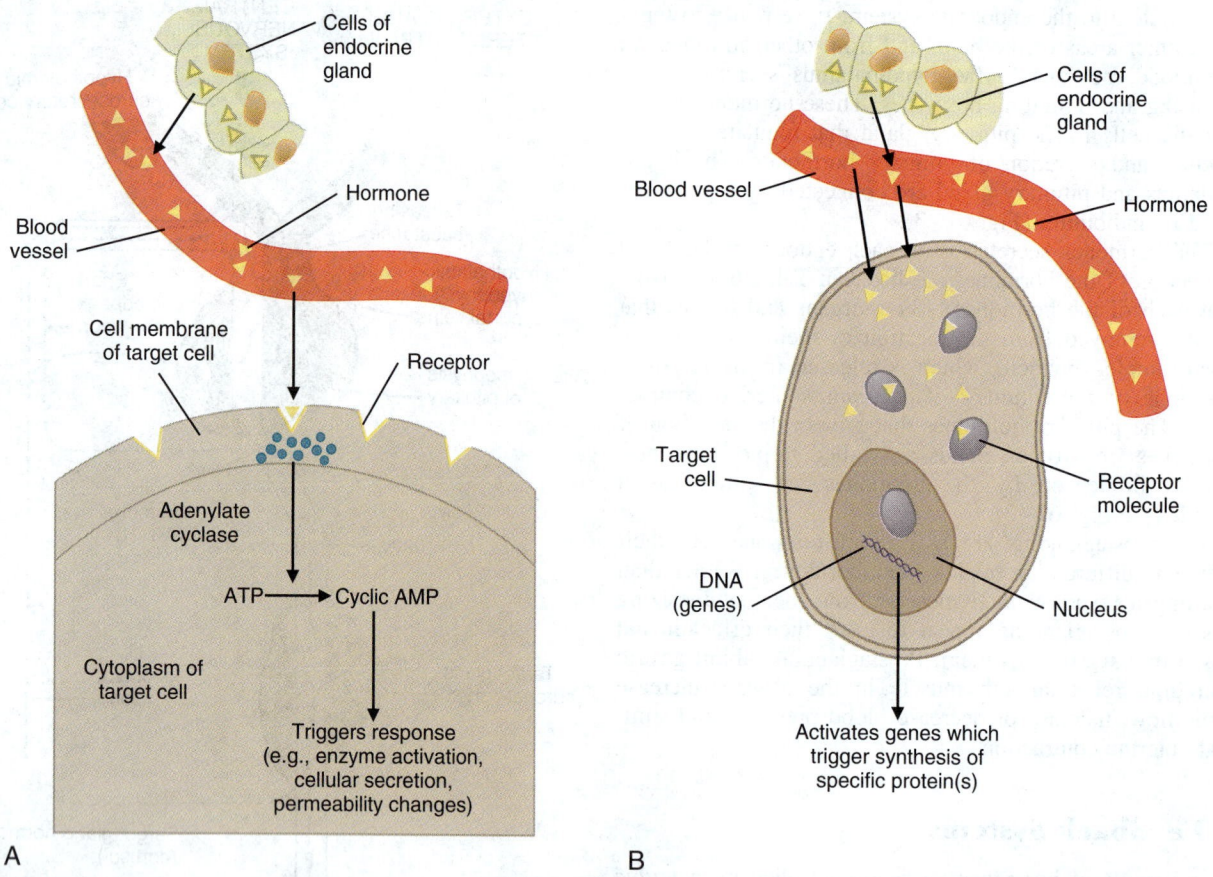

Figure 67–5. There are two mechanisms by which a hormone influences cellular function. *A,* Intracellular mediators, especially cyclic adenosine monophosphate, trigger various cellular responses, such as production of an enzyme. *B,* Genes can also be activated by hormones (e.g., steroids). Genes then produce messenger RNA, which triggers the production of proteins, such as enzymes.

Three basic cell types compose the adenohypophysis: (1) eosinophils, (2) basophils, and (3) chromophobes. The adenohypophysis synthesizes and releases six hormones (see Table 67–1): growth hormone (GH), ACTH, thyroid-stimulating hormone (TSH), prolactin (PRL), follicle-stimulating hormone (FSH), and luteinizing hormone (LH). Of these hormones, only GH and PRL act directly on the body's nonendocrine target tissues. The other four hormones stimulate the target glands governed by the pituitary (thyroid, adrenal cortex, testes, and ovaries), thereby indirectly influencing body structure and function (e.g., growth, intellectual and sexual development, and metabolism).

Target glands depend on stimulation from the anterior pituitary hormones to synthesize target gland hormones. If stimulation is excessive, the target gland becomes overactive; for example, too much ACTH from the pituitary stimulates the adrenal cortex to produce excessive amounts of cortisol, thereby causing hypertrophy and Cushing's disease. Conversely, inadequate pituitary production of a hormone causes the target gland to become hypoactive; for example, insufficient production of ACTH can cause secondary adrenocortical insufficiency.

The posterior lobe of the pituitary is called the neuro-

hypophysis because it is of neural (rather than glandular) origin. An extension of the hypothalamus, the posterior lobe stores and releases antidiuretic hormone (ADH) and oxytocin (a hormone that stimulates uterine and mammary gland contractions).

The production and release of anterior pituitary hormones is regulated by hypothalamic hormones. Note in Figure 67–3 that the hypothalamus lies above the pituitary gland and is connected to it by the hypophyseal (pituitary) stalk.

The hypothalamus continuously monitors information regarding the internal and external milieu via the central nervous system. These messages are transmitted to the pituitary gland by hypothalamic peptide hormones called releasing hormones. They travel within the portal blood that flows from the hypothalamus to the anterior pituitary, causing the release of hormones from the anterior pituitary gland.

The hypothalamus communicates with the posterior pituitary gland by way of nerve fibers in the hypophyseal stalk. Synthesis of the two posterior pituitary hormones occurs within the hypothalamus. The hormones then are transmitted to the posterior pituitary, where they are stored and released.

Thyroid and Parathyroid Structure and Function

■ Thyroid

The thyroid gland is located in the neck, just below the cricoid cartilage. It is shaped somewhat like the letter H. The right and left lateral lobes lie on either side of the trachea. The lobes are connected by a thin mass of tissue called the isthmus, which stretches over the surface of the trachea (Fig. 67–6). Each of the two lobes is composed of irregularly shaped lobules. These lobules, in turn, consist of a multitude of tiny sacs called follicles (Fig. 67–7) filled with a jelly-like, iodine-containing substance called colloid. The main component of colloid is thyroglobulin—the storage form of the hormone thyroxine.

Thyroxine is one of the three hormones secreted by the thyroid gland; triiodothyronine and thyrocalcitonin are the other two. The major role of thyroxine is to regulate body metabolism. Thyroxine also aids in the following:

- Regulation of growth and development (both physical and mental)
- Carbohydrate, fat, and protein metabolism
- Reproduction
- Resistance to infection

Thyroxine (T_4) ensures that oxygen consumption and heat production keep pace with the body's needs and activities. Too much thyroxine causes a dangerous increase in metabolism and a high rate of oxygen consumption. Conversely, too little results in a sluggish metabolism, a slowing of physical and mental function in the adult, and retardation of growth and development in the child.

Thyroxine production depends on (1) ingestion of sufficient protein and iodine and (2) the release of a vital anterior pituitary hormone called thyroid-stimulating hormone (TSH), thyrotropin, or thyrotropic hormone, TSH, as the name implies, stimulates the thyroid gland to pro-

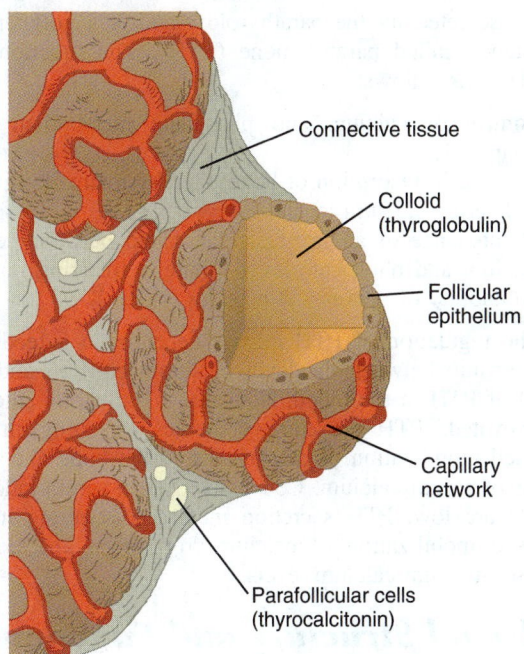

Figure 67–7. Microscopic view of the thyroid gland.

Connective tissue

Colloid (thyroglobulin)

Follicular epithelium

Capillary network

Parafollicular cells (thyrocalcitonin)

duce thyroxine. TSH release is controlled by a negative feedback system: low serum levels of thyroxine stimulate increased secretion of TSH, and high serum levels of thyroxine inhibit TSH secretion, thereby promoting a steady state of hormonal production and release.

Thyroxine production also depends on a number of environmental factors. Situations that speed thyroxine production are physiologic and psychological stress and prolonged exposure to cold. Factors that depress thyroxine secretion are excessive intake of dietary goitrogens (see later), ingestion of certain drugs (sulfonamides, salicylates, phenylbutazone, and para-aminosalicylic acid), and prolonged exposure to heat.

Thyroxine is stored as part of the thyroglobulin molecule in the thyroid follicles. Whenever the body's circulating thyroxine levels drop too low, thyroxine is released from thyroglobulin into the blood. Within the blood, thyroxine is bound to a plasma protein and is carried to organs and tissues in the form of protein-bound iodine.

Triiodothyronine (T_3), a second thyroid hormone, is much more potent than thyroxine. Thyroxine is converted to triiodothyronine by peripheral target tissues in the body.

Thyrocalcitonin (TCT), or calcitonin, the third thyroid hormone is a polypeptide produced by parafollicular cells located in the interstitial tissue between the follicles of the thyroid gland (see Fig. 67–7). Discovered during the 1960s, calcitonin is capable of lowering both plasma calcium and phosphate. Calcitonin acts in a manner opposite to that of parathormone. Its effect on maintaining calcium balance is minor compared with that of parathormone.

■ Parathyroid

The parathyroid glands are four small glands near to, attached to, or embedded in the thyroid gland. The hor-

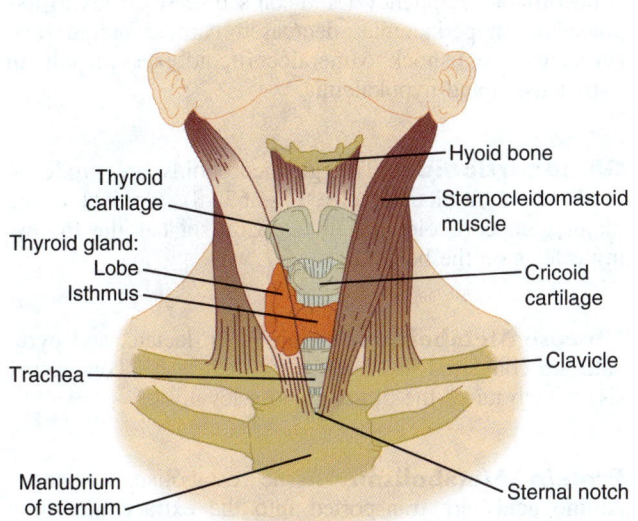

Hyoid bone

Sternocleidomastoid muscle

Thyroid cartilage

Thyroid gland:
Lobe
Isthmus

Cricoid cartilage

Trachea

Clavicle

Manubrium of sternum

Sternal notch

Figure 67–6. The thyroid gland.

mone secreted by the parathyroid gland is a polypeptide substance called parathormone (PTH). The functions of PTH are as follows:

- Control of calcium and phosphate metabolism (see Chapter 15)
- Increase in resorption of bone, thereby maintaining normal serum calcium levels
- Maintenance of an inverse relationship between serum calcium and phosphate levels, thereby fostering normal excitability of nerves and muscles

The regulation of PTH release depends on a feedback relationship between the level of serum calcium and the level of PTH in the blood. Note that when serum calcium is elevated, PTH secretion decreases, resulting in decreased mobilization of calcium ions from bone and lowering of serum calcium. Conversely, when serum calcium levels are low, PTH secretion increases, resulting in increased mobilization of calcium from bone and an increase in serum calcium levels.

Adrenal Structure and Function

The adrenal glands are small vital endocrine structures that rest upon the upper end of each kidney (Fig. 67–8). Each adrenal gland is composed of an inner core, the medulla, and an outer shell, the cortex. Both contribute to survival and well-being, but only the cortex is essential to life.

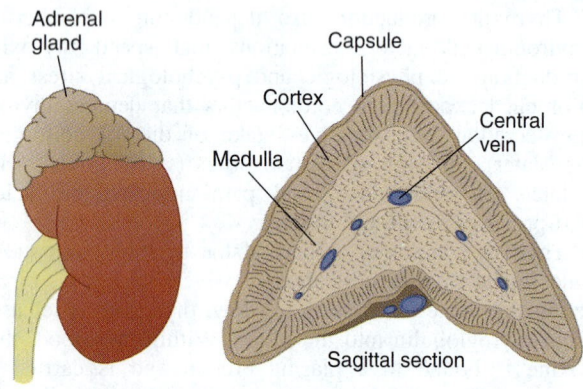

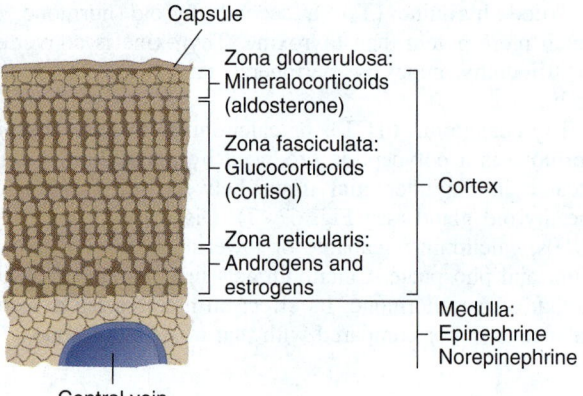

Figure 67–8. The adrenal glands rest upon the kidneys. A cortex surrounds the inner medulla and central vein. The cortex and medulla secrete specific hormones.

■ Adrenal Medulla

The adrenal medulla is a part of the sympathetic nervous system. It releases two potent hormones, epinephrine and norepinephrine. These hormones prepare an individual to meet and deal with threat and danger. During stressful situations, epinephrine acts (1) on the liver to convert glycogen into glucose, and (2) on the heart to increase cardiac output. It is the release of epinephrine that produces the cold sweat, pounding heart, deep rapid breathing, and a wide-eyed blank expression experienced in times of emergency. Norepinephrine produces extensive vascular constriction and a marked rise in blood pressure (BP) (see Table 67–1).

Overactivity of the adrenal medulla is usually caused by a catecholamine-producing tumor called a pheochromocytoma. This tumor is usually (but not always) found in the adrenal gland. Pheochromocytomas produce hypertension, hypermetabolism, and hyperglycemia. Surgical removal of the tumor is usually curative.

■ Adrenal Cortex

The adrenal cortex is essential to survival. Loss of adrenocortical hormones leads to death. The adrenal cortex synthesizes three classes of steroid hormones: (1) mineralocorticoids, (2) glucocorticoids, and (3) androgens. All are synthesized from cholesterol. As Boyd helpfully reminds us: "For persons with a desire to memorize things easily, the 3 functions [of the hormones of the adrenal cortex] may be represented by the letter S, as salt, sugar and sex. For the others, these categories are the mineralocorticoids, the glucocorticoids, and the androgenic hormones."[18]

Mineralocorticoids. The mineralocorticoids (primarily aldosterone in humans) are produced in the zona glomerulosa of the adrenal cortex (see Fig. 67–8). They regulate electrolyte balance by promoting sodium retention and potassium excretion. These physiologic activities, in turn, help sustain normal BP and cardiac output. Mineralocorticoid deficiency (Addison's disease) leads to hypotension, hyperkalemia, decreased cardiac output, and (in acute cases) shock. Mineralocorticoid excess results in hypertension and hypokalemia.

Glucocorticoids. The glucocorticoids are produced in the zona fasciculata (see Fig. 67–8). Cortisol is the major glucocorticoid in humans. Cortisol has the following effects on the body.

Glucose Metabolism. Amino acids, lactate, and pyruvate are converted in the liver to glucose (gluconeogenesis), which raises the blood glucose level.

Protein Metabolism. Tissue catabolism increases. Amino acids are transported into the extracellular fluid and to the liver, where they are converted to glucose. Tissue wasting is the result.

Fluid and Electrolyte Balance. Sodium retention and potassium excretion increase. Excessive glucocorticoid secretion results in hypervolemia and hypertension due to sodium and water retention. Note the similarity between these effects of the glucocorticoids and those of the mineralocorticoids.

Inflammation and Immunity. The glucocorticoids suppress the inflammatory response to tissue injury and the protective immune response to invasion by infectious agents. Recall from Chapter 2 that Selye called the glucocorticoids "anti-inflammatory corticoids." He believed that the principal action of glucocorticoids was to suppress inflammation in response to stress. In some cases, suppressing inflammation can be beneficial. For example, persons with arthritis (joint inflammation) obtain pain relief with cortisone injections. On the other hand, excessive glucocorticoids impede healing, decrease antibody formation, lower the number of circulating eosinophils and lymphocytes, and lower resistance to infection.

Stressors. Insufficient production of glucocorticoids (as noted in Addison's disease) decreases resistance to stress. Such individuals can die in shock following relatively minor trauma unless they quickly receive an injection of glucocorticoid (hydrocortisone).

Sex Hormones. The adrenal cortex secretes small amounts of sex steroids from the zona reticularis (see Fig. 67–8). Normally, the adrenals secrete few androgens and estrogens compared with the large amounts of sex hormones secreted by the gonads. Excess production of sex hormones by the adrenal gland, however, does cause symptoms. For example, excessive release of androgens causes virilism, whereas excessive release of estrogens (e.g., from an adrenal carcinoma) causes gynecomastia and sodium and water retention.

Pancreatic Structure and Function

The pancreas, a large fish-shaped organ that lies behind the stomach, is both an exocrine and an endocrine gland. The exocrine role of the pancreas is carried out by cells within the tubular and acinar units of the gland. These cells secrete hormones and digestive enzymes that catalyze the digestion of proteins, carbohydrates, and fats.

The endocrine functions of the pancreas are carried out by the islets of Langerhans. The islets, containing alpha, beta, and delta cells, are scattered throughout the pancreatic tissues. The islet cells are arranged in cords and are separated by a rich blood supply of capillaries. Insulin and glucagon, two hormones secreted by the islets, play a vital role in the control of carbohydrate metabolism. Insulin, synthesized by the beta cells, also helps control fat and protein metabolism. Insulin is a powerful hypoglycemic agent; insulin lowers blood sugar levels by promoting the passage of glucose into the cells. Conversely, glucagon, synthesized by alpha cells, is a hyperglycemic agent. It raises blood sugar by promoting the conversion of glycogen (the principal storage form of carbohydrate in mammals) to glucose within the liver. Somatostatin and gastrin are synthesized by the delta cells. Gastrin is used in the metabolism of foods, and somatostatin decreases the secretion of insulin, glucagon, growth hormone, gastrin, and secretin. Research is currently being conducted to explore the clinical usefulness of somatostatin.

Hormonal Factors Regulating Carbohydrate Metabolism

The hormones that regulate carbohydrate metabolism include the following: (1) insulin, (2) glucagon, (3) ACTH, (4) corticosteroids, (5) epinephrine, and (6) thyroid hormone.

Insulin and Glucagon

Insulin and glucagon are the two principal hormones controlling carbohydrate metabolism. Both hormones are small proteins. Insulin, the hypoglycemic factor, also helps regulate fat and protein metabolism. More specifically, insulin does the following:

● Stimulates the active transport of glucose into muscle and adipose tissue cells. For glucose to cross the cell membrane, insulin must connect with a receptor on the cell membrane. Some clients with diabetes mellitus have enough insulin but too few receptor sites, which thus reduces glucose transport into the cell. Others have inadequate insulin production from the pancreas. When insulin levels are inadequate, or insulin is unable to connect with a receptor, glucose remains outside the cells, raising the serum glucose levels above normal.
● Regulates the rate at which carbohydrates are used by cells for energy.
● Promotes the conversion of glucose to glycogen for storage and inhibits the conversion of glycogen to glucose.
● Promotes the conversion of fatty acids into fat, which can be stored as adipose tissue, and inhibits the breakdown of adipose tissue, the mobilization of fats, and the conversion of fat to ketone bodies.
● Stimulates protein synthesis within the tissues and inhibits the breakdown of protein into amino acids.

In sum, insulin actively promotes those processes that lower blood glucose levels (e.g., the transport of glucose into cells and the conversion of glucose to glycogen) and inhibits those processes that raise blood glucose levels (e.g., the conversion of glycogen and amino acids glucose). Insulin is, therefore, anabolic.

The amount of glucose in the blood regulates the rate of insulin secretion by the beta cells. As Figure 67–9 shows, when the blood glucose level rises, islet cells release insulin into the blood, allowing glucose transport into the cells and glucose conversion to glycogen. As the blood glucose level falls, insulin release from the islet cells slows until the blood glucose level drops slightly below normal. If food is consumed, the islet cells again release insulin.

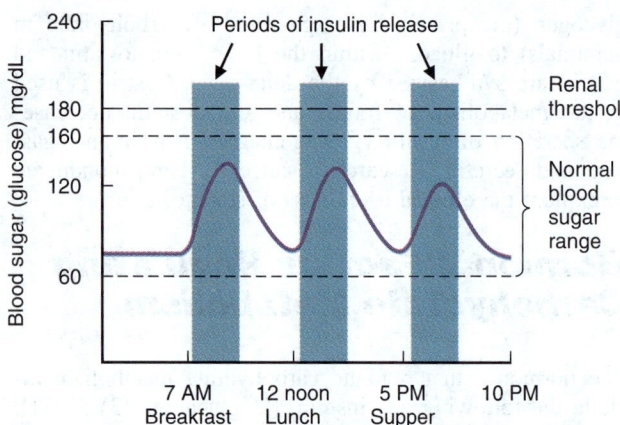

Figure 67–9. Insulin release and its effect on blood glucose levels following meals.

When there is a deficit of insulin, as with diabetes mellitus, the blood glucose level remains abnormally high. When there is an excess of insulin, as with an overdose of exogenous insulin, blood glucose levels may drop dangerously low, and insulin-induced hypoglycemia (insulin shock) develops.

In contrast to insulin, glucagon promotes a rise in blood glucose when glucose levels drop too low. Glucagon causes hyperglycemia by promoting the conversion of liver glycogen to glucose. Clients with diabetes mellitus often experience abnormalities in the secretion of both insulin and glucagon. Diseases involving only the alpha cells (glucagon secretion—either excess or deficiency) are rare.

What factors are necessary for the synthesis and release of insulin and glucagon? These essential hormones depend on the following three requirements:

1. A healthy pancreas with functioning alpha and beta cells.
2. A diet adequate in protein. Both insulin and glucagon are protein substances.
3. Normal potassium (K^+) levels. Insulin affects potassium mostly by inhibiting its leaving the cell.

When insulin or glucagon secretion is deficient, the person may receive the missing hormone by exogenous means. When injected, glucagon reverses hypoglycemia caused by excessive insulin. The person cannot take either of these hormones orally because they are inactivated within the gastrointestinal tract by proteolytic enzymes.

Other Hormonal Factors

Although insulin and glucagon play the predominant roles in carbohydrate regulation, the following hormones also influence blood glucose levels:

- ACTH and the glucocorticoids of the adrenal cortex raise serum glucose by increasing the formation of new glucose by the liver (gluconeogenesis) and decreasing the use of glucose in peripheral tissues. ACTH and the glucocorticoids also promote lipolysis and protein catabolism.

- Epinephrine, also released during stress, stimulates a rise in blood glucose by promoting the conversion of glycogen to glucose. Thyroid hormone stimulates almost all aspects of protein, fat, and carbohydrate metabolism.

Ovaries and Testes

The structure and function of the reproductive organs are described in Chapter 81.

Effects of Aging

The interaction of the endocrine system with the aging process has generated much study, but most data are inconclusive. The endocrine system has never been implicated as a cause of aging. There are changes in the endocrine glands and target organs that occur as a result of aging, however.

There may be a loss of self-regulation, leading to autoimmune or immunodeficiency disorders such as diabetes.

Theories of programmed change examine the genetic control of cell function. These theories suggest that cells are programmed to function only for a given time. The changes in the reproductive system, such as menopause, are an example of this theory.

As a result of changes with aging and disease, the target organs may lose their ability to respond to hormones. In addition, the hypothalamus and pituitary may be altered by changed levels of neurotransmitters.

Theories of stress and adaptation suggest that body structures wear out in time and are no longer able to adapt to stressors. This theory may help explain the inability of the elderly to respond to illness and stress.

Conclusions

The endocrine system works in unison with the nervous system to maintain homeostasis. There are two types of glands: (1) endocrine, which release hormones into the blood; and (2) exocrine, which release hormones into ducts. Endocrine glands include the pancreas, gonads, adrenal, thyroid, parathyroid, and thymus glands. Assessment of the client includes the usual history and physical examination. Blood levels of the various hormones can be determined.

Bibliography

1. American Association of Diabetes Educators. (1993). *Diabetes education: A core curriculum for health professionals.* Chicago: Author.
2. Bagdade, J. D. (1990). *Yearbook of endocrinology.* St. Louis: Mosby–Year Book.
3. Becker, K. L. (Ed.). (1990). *Principles and practice of endocrinology and metabolism.* Philadelphia: J. B. Lippincott.
4. Bennett, J. C., & Plum, F. (Eds.). (1996). *Cecil textbook of medicine* (20th ed.). Philadelphia: W. B. Saunders.

5. Braveman, L. E., & Utiger, R. D. (Eds.). (1991). *Werner and Ingbar's the thyroid* (6th ed.). Philadelphia: J. B. Lippincott.
6. Brown, J. C. (1993). An overview of gastrointestinal endocrine physiology. *Endocrinology and Metabolism Clinics of North America, 22*(4), 719–729.
7. Christiansen, J. L., & Grzbouski, J. M. (1993). *Biology of aging.* St. Louis: Mosby–Year Book.
8. Cotran, R. S., Kumar, V., & Robbins, S. L. (1994). *Robbins pathologic basis of disease* (5th ed.). Philadelphia: W. B. Saunders.
9. DeGroot, L. J. (Ed.). (1995). *Endocrinology* (3rd ed.). Philadelphia: W. B. Saunders.
10. Greenspan, F. S., & Baxter, J. D. (Eds.). (1994). *Basic and clinical endocrinology* (4th ed.). Norwalk, CT: Appleton & Lange.
11. Greer, M. A. (1990). *The thyroid gland.* New York: Raven Press.
12. Guyton, A. C. (1992). *Human physiology and mechanisms of disease* (5th ed.). Philadelphia: W. B. Saunders.
13. Guyton, A. C., & Hall, J. E. (1996). *Textbook of medical physiology* (9th ed.). Philadelphia: W. B. Saunders.
14. Kessler, C. A. (1992). An overview of endocrine function and dysfunction. *AACN Clinical Issues in Critical Care Nursing, 3*(2), 289–299.
15. Mazzaferri, E. L. (1993). *Advances in endocrinology and metabolism* (4th ed.). St. Louis: Mosby–Year Book.
16. McCance, K. L., & Huether, S. E. (1994). *Pathophysiology: The biologic basis for disease in adults and children* (2nd ed.). St. Louis: Mosby–Year Book.
17. Moore, W. T., & Eastman, R. C. (Eds.). (1990). *Diagnostic endocrinology.* Philadelphia: B. C. Decker.
18. Price, S., & Wilson, L. (1992). *Pathophysiology* (4th ed.). St. Louis: Mosby–Year Book.
19. Seeley, R., Stephens, T., & Tate, P. (1995). *Anatomy and physiology* (3rd ed.). St. Louis: Mosby–Year Book.
20. Solomon, E. P. (1992). *Introduction to human anatomy and physiology.* Philadelphia: W. B. Saunders.
21. Strauss, J. F., III. (1991). Steroid hormones: Synthesis, metabolism, and action in health and disease. *Endocrinology and Metabolism Clinics of North America 20*(4), 681–924.
22. Thibodeau, G. A., & Patton, K. T. (1992). *Anatomy and physiology* (2nd ed.). St. Louis: Mosby–Year Book
23. Thibodeau, G. A., & Patton, K. T. (1992). *The human body in health and disease.* St. Louis: Mosby–Year Book.
24. Toto, K. H. (1994). Endocrine physiology: A comprehensive review. *Critical Care Nursing Clinics of North America, 6*(4), 637–659.
25. Wilson, J. D., & Foster, D. W. (Eds.). (1992). *Williams textbook of endocrinology* (8th ed.). Philadelphia: W. B. Saunders.

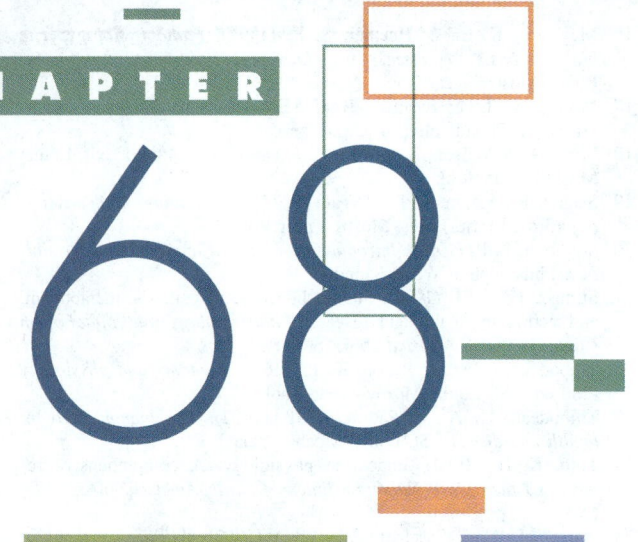

CHAPTER

68

Assessment of Clients with Endocrine Disorders

Carol Birch
Kerry H. Greear

Assessment of the endocrine system is often difficult because of the variety of manifestations that may occur. Each body system is affected by hormones; thus, clinical manifestations may be specific or nonspecific. Additionally, manifestations may be related to causes other than endocrine disorders. Thorough health history interviewing and physical examination assist in the diagnostic process.

History

Throughout the history interview, gather information about the client's present condition and previous medical history. Begin with the biographic data and proceed to the chief complaint, including a symptom analysis. Obtain the history for the presenting manifestations in chronologic order. Indicate onset, duration, intensity, and any alterations in growth patterns (weight and height changes in adulthood, hand, foot, or head size changes) (see Chapter 11). Collect additional subjective data about the client's past medical history, family history, psychosocial history, and life-style, and complete a review of systems (ROS).

Biographical and Demographic Data

Note the client's age, because the endocrine system is affected by the aging process. Fewer hormones may be produced, or their effect on the target organs may be diminished. For example, the incidence of diabetes mellitus increases with age.

Chief Complaint

The client's presenting manifestations may be specific or nonspecific. Common nonspecific manifestations include

This chapter incorporates material written for the fourth ediition by Diane Butts-Krakoff.

fatigue and depression, often accompanied by altered alertness, decreased energy, sleep pattern disturbances, weight changes, altered mood and affect, changes in the condition of the skin and hair, altered general appearance, and sexual dysfunction. Ask about the onset, duration, quality and characteristics, and severity of these manifestations, and about precipitating and relieving factors and associated manifestations. Some manifestations are specific for certain endocrine disorders, as the following examples illustrate.

Changes in Mental Status. The client may report increased nervousness, lability of mood, mental confusion, and depression. Extreme alterations in consciousness, such as coma, may occur in uncontrolled diabetes mellitus.

Changes in Vital Signs. Body temperature and pulse rate may be elevated due to hyperthyroidism. Kussmaul's respirations (deep rapid breathing) are a classic manifestation of diabetic ketoacidosis. Tumors of the adrenal glands, which cause increased secretion of epinephrine (e.g., pheochromocytoma), can result in hypertension. Insufficient levels of antidiuretic hormone (ADH) from the pituitary gland can cause dehydration, whereas oversecretion can cause excessive retention of body water.

Palpitations. Increased heart rate with sweating and flushing can occur in hyperthyroidism and also in pheochromocytoma.

Tremors. Uncontrolled tremors can be a possible indication of hyperthyroidism.

Fatigue. Fatigue may signify emotional stress or pathophysiologic changes.

Weakness. Weakness may be generalized or localized. Localized weakness often indicates a neurologic problem, which can be a complication of an endocrine disorder.

Changes in Appetite. The client may report polyphagia (excessive hunger) associated with diabetes mellitus or anorexia (lack of appetite).

Changes in Weight. Eating more but losing weight may indicate hyperthyroidism. Clients with hypothyroidism may gain weight.

Polydipsia and Polyuria. Abnormal thirst plus passage of large amounts of urine may indicate diabetes mellitus.

Changes in Bowel Habits. Frequent loose stools are a manifestation of hyperthyroidism, whereas constipation can indicate hypothyroidism.

Changes in the Reproductive Organs and Libido. Menstrual cycle irregularities (including amenorrhea), loss of libido, loss or premature development of secondary sex characteristics, impotence, and infertility are sexual changes characteristic of endocrine disorders.

Changes in Appearance. Acromegaly produces enlargement of the hands and feet and a coarsening of the facial features. Adrenocortical hyperfunction (Cushing's syndrome) is manifested in moon facies, thin extremities, and truncal obesity.

Growth Abnormalities. Growth may be delayed, stunted (dwarfism), excessive (gigantism), or inappropriate (acromegaly), especially growth of hands, feet, and head.

Skin and Tissue Changes. Hyperpigmentation occurs in chronic adrenocortical insufficiency (Addison's disease). Areas of hypopigmentation (vitiligo) may indicate other endocrine disorders. Delayed tissue healing and susceptibility to infection are associated with diabetes mellitus. Hard, nonpitting edema occurs in adult hypothyroidism (myxedema).

Changes in Hair. Excessive hair (hirsutism) in women may indicate ovarian or adrenocortical disorders. Axillary and pubic hair loss may indicate a pituitary disorder. Hair feels soft and silky in hyperthyroidism and coarse, dry, and brittle in hypothyroidism.

Changes in the Eyes. Exophthalmos (bulging eyes) is an important characteristic of hyperthyroidism. A pituitary tumor may cause partial or total loss of vision. Diabetes may cause temporary blurred vision or permanent blindness.

Bone and Joint Problems. Clients with hyperparathyroidism often develop bone pain, cysts, and fractures. Cushing's syndrome produces a rapid breakdown of bone.

Renal Colic and Urinary Stones. Renal problems, such as stone development, may follow the bone disorders found in hyperparathyroidism.

Tetany, Paresthesias, and Muscle Cramps. These manifestations may develop in clients with insufficient parathyroid hormone (PTH).

Past Health History

Explore the client's health history to determine the existence of previous endocrine disorders, abnormal patterns of growth and development, or head trauma, and to ascertain the general health status. Ask the client to identify *changes*, either general or specific, that have occurred in health status.

Growth and Development

Ask the client (or the client's family) whether any noticeable delays or accelerations in growth and development have occurred. For example, does the client have a history of being small or large for his or her chronologic age or genetic background? Ask about family members' growth patterns so that valid comparisons can be made. These questions should be asked with tact and understanding of their sensitive nature.

Ask about any changes in body size since physical maturation. Have any changes occurred in the size of the hands or feet or in the head circumference? For example, has the client had to buy shoes, gloves, rings, or hats in a larger size? Similarly, ask the client about changes in secondary sex characteristics, such as increased amounts of facial hair (in women) or decreased amounts (in men). For both men and women, ask about changes in pubic or axillary hair, such as in the amount and distribution. Does the female client have problems with menstruation, infertility, or pregnancy?

Major Illnesses and Hospitalizations

Ask the client to identify any history of head trauma, such as a forceful blow. Trauma can lead to hypopituitarism. Has the client been hospitalized for surgery to the head or neck? Does the client have a history of surgery, chemotherapy, or radiation therapy to the head or neck? Ask about related disorders, such as primary brain tumors, metastatic tumors, meningitis, brain infarctions, diabetes mellitus, diabetes insipidus, hypertension, and goiter.

Medications

Include all medications, past and current, in your history. Ask specifically about the use of hormones and steroids, including name, dose, and duration of use. Does the client have a history of using anabolic steroids? What over-the-counter medications are being used?

Family Health History

When assessing a client with an endocrine disorder, inquire into the family history. A number of endocrine disorders are inherited or associated with a familial trend.

Ask whether any family members have or have had problems similar to the client's. Disorders to inquire about include growth and development problems, obesity, goiter, hypothyroidism or hyperthyroidism, hypertension, low blood pressure (hypotension), diabetes mellitus, diabetes insipidus, autoimmune diseases (Addison's disease), and problems with the adrenal gland (e.g., pheochromocytoma).

Psychosocial History

Occupation and Environment

Inquire about the client's stress tolerance and coping patterns. Stressors can be either physiologic (illness) or emotional. Ask about job-related stressors, such as amount of time spent on the job both in the work setting and at home. Do strained interpersonal relationships at work contribute to increased stress levels? Does the client have opportunities to retreat from the workplace and to engage in recreational activities? Also ask about the home environment and family interpersonal relationships and obligations. What are the client's support systems? Does the client report effective current coping strategies? Ask family members to corroborate or to help identify behavior changes if possible.

Habits

Considering other aspects of life-style and coping, ask the client about such habits as smoking, exercise, diet, and sleep patterns. Ask the client to describe the usual patterns as well as any changes that may have occurred (see Chapter 11).

Review of Systems

A careful ROS is important if you suspect an endocrine problem. Review all body systems because endocrine disorders can affect multiple systems. Detailed questions for the ROS are found in Box 11–2.

Physical Examination

Physical examination of the endocrine system is integrated throughout the interaction with the client, beginning with the history interview. As the client responds to questions, observe the level of consciousness (orientation, alertness), memory, affect, and speech patterns. Note any anxiety or nervousness. Examine all body systems in a systematic manner from head-to-toe (see Chapter 12).

General Appearance

Observe the client's state of dress, growth and development, level of consciousness, orientation, and body size. Measure height and weight and compare to published norms. Observe extremities for proportionality to the rest of the body.

Vital Signs

Measure and assess vital signs. The temperature is elevated in hyperthyroidism or may be low normal or below normal in hypothyroidism. Observe respirations for altered rate and rhythm. Blood pressure changes include hypotension, hypertension, widening pulse pressure, and orthostatic changes with changes in the pulse rate.

Integument

Observe hair texture and distribution over body surfaces. Note brittleness of hair or alopecia. Inspect skin for color, pigmentation, striae, ecchymoses, or mottling. Palpate skin for texture, thickness, moisture, and diaphoresis. Inspect and palpate nails for color, texture, brittleness, presence of ridges, and peeling.

Head

Inspect head contour and shape. Note symmetry of facial features. Observe skin color for erythema or rash over the cheeks. Observe the client's facial expression for anxiety.

Eyes

Inspect and palpate the eyebrows, noting hair distribution. Observe eye position, symmetry, shape, and eyelid lag. Assess visual acuity, extraocular movements (EOMs), and visual fields. Inspect for lens opacity and eye edema.

Nose

Inspect mucosa for swelling and color. Listen for noisy or labored breathing.

Mouth

Note size and shape of the jaw. Inspect the oral mucosa color and the condition of the client's teeth. Note malocclusion. Observe tongue size and activity for fasciculations.

Neck

Listen to the client's voice for hoarseness or huskiness. Note clarity, pitch, and volume of speech. Ask the client

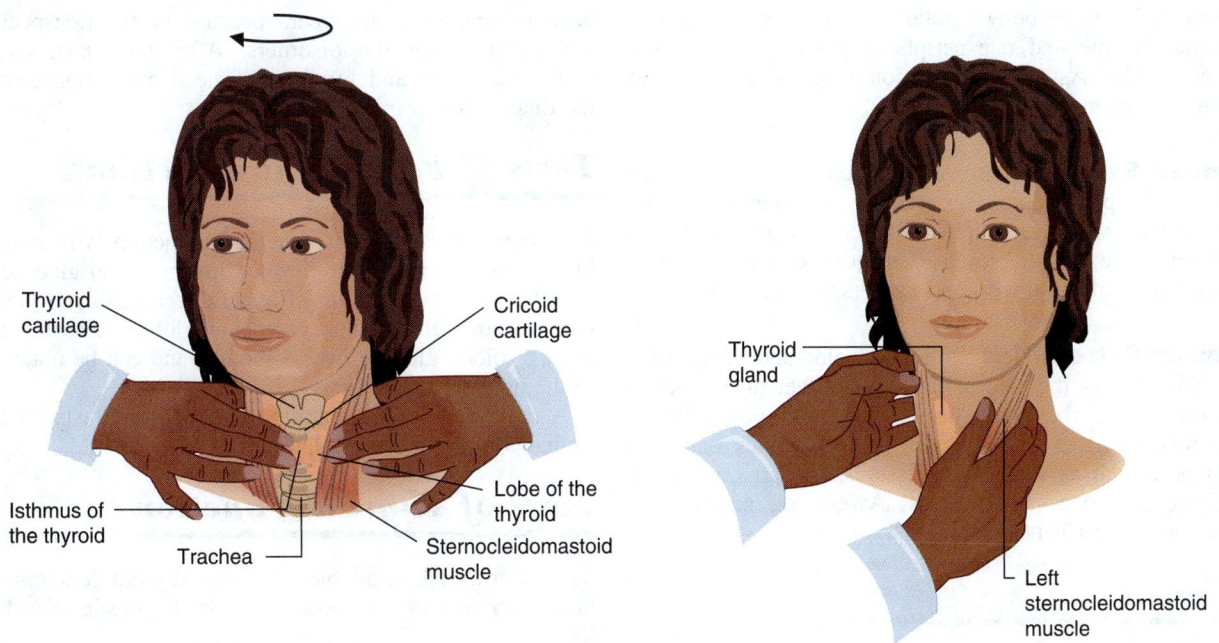

A Posterior approach   B Anterior approach

Figure 68–1. Palpation of the thyroid. *A,* Posterior approach. Stand behind the client. Ask the client to lower the chin to relax the neck muscles, and tilt the head slightly to the right. To examine the right lobe of the thyroid, use the fingers of your left hand to displace the trachea slightly to the right. This moves the thyroid laterally. You can then palpate the right lobe with the fingers of your right hand. Ask the client to swallow while you palpate; doing so causes the gland to rise in the neck. Repeat for the left lobe. Projection of the thyroid can be enhanced by having the client drink water. *B,* Anterior approach. Stand in front of the client. To palpate the thyroid gland's right lobe, flex the client's head toward the right to relax the neck muscles on that side. Use the fingers of your right hand to displace the trachea slightly to the client's right. Then ask the client to swallow while you palpate the right lobe of the thyroid with the fingers of your left hand. Repeat for the left lobe. You can also assess for thyroid enlargement by palpating deep on each side of the sternocleidomastoid muscle.

to swallow and observe for difficulty swallowing or pain; repeat this maneuver with the client's neck in a hyperextended position. Inspect the neck for symmetry, alignment, thickness or bulging over the thyroid gland, and examine the midline position of the trachea. Observe for scars related to thyroidectomy, trauma, or other neck surgery. Note presence of hyperpigmentation. Observe for forceful pulsations over the carotid arteries. Palpate the thyroid gland unless it is noticeably enlarged (vigorous palpation can stimulate release of thyroid hormone, which increases the risk of precipitating a thyroid crisis in a client with thyroid hyperplasia). If the thyroid gland is enlarged, auscultate the lobes for *bruits.*

The thyroid gland may be palpated using an anterior or posterior approach as described in Figure 68–1. In the anterior approach, gently run a finger down the anterior part of the neck, locating the thyroid and cricoid cartilages and the isthmus of the thyroid gland. The isthmus feels soft and compressible compared with the firmer cartilage ring just superior to it. Ask the client to swallow while you palpate the isthmus. It should rise in the neck and should not be enlarged. The thyroid gland is normally nonpalpable. If it is palpable, note the texture of the gland because it is usually smooth and firm, without lumps, roughness, hardness, asymmetry, or tenderness.

Palpate the back of the neck and over the area where the "buffalo hump" is found in clients with Cushing's disease.

Extremities

Examine the arms and legs for size, shape, and symmetry, and check their proportionality to the trunk. The distance from the symphysis pubis to the heel is usually

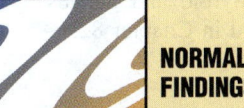

NORMAL PHYSICAL ASSESSMENT FINDINGS

Thyroid Gland

Inspection

The thyroid gland is not normally seen on inspection.

Palpation

Gland attached to trachea, can be felt to rise and fall with swallowing. Two irregular lobes to the gland with a connecting isthmus. Right lobe slightly larger than the left lobe. Texture rubbery without nodules. Nontender to palpation.

Auscultation

No bruits heard over either lobe.

about half of a body's total height. Note peripheral edema. Palpate and rate peripheral pulse amplitude (see Chapter 12). Assess deep tendon reflexes and observe their relaxation time (see Chapter 30).

Upper Extremities. Ask the client to extend the hands with palms down; observe for fine tremors. Inspect for thenar wasting, Dupuytren's contracture, and nail clubbing (see Chapter 39). Assess grip strength and muscle strength of the fingers and arms (see Chapter 73).

Lower Extremities. Note the color and distribution of hair. Assess the size of the client's feet in proportion to the rest of the body. Inspect for corns and calluses. Separate the toes and observe for deformities and skin changes, such as thickening, fissures, or nail thickening. Palpate and rate pedal pulses. Assess leg muscles for weakness (see Chapter 73).

Thorax

Inspect for gynecomastia in males. Auscultate for extra heart sounds, such as a systolic murmur (see Chapter 44).

Abdomen

Note areas of hyperpigmentation, such as in scars or striae. Observe the client for manifestations of pain during light palpation.

Genitalia

Observe the pattern of pubic hair distribution, particularly in female clients. A diamond-shaped (male) pattern is indicative of a masculinizing tumor. Note the size of the testes in male clients and the clitoris in female clients for comparison to expected norms.

The remainder of endocrine assessment consists of diagnostic studies, as the only endocrine glands accessible to physical examination are the thyroid and gonads. Assessment of the gonads is discussed in Chapter 82.

Diagnostic Tests

Tests of the endocrine system involve several general types of clinical evaluations. Blood levels of the various hormones are obtained through radioimmunoassay (RIA) and enzyme immunoassay (EIA). RIA is a technique in which antibodies to the hormone and radioisotope-tagged hormone are placed in a test tube with untagged hormone. The two types of hormones compete for sites on the antibodies. If most of the radioisotope-tagged hormone is bound to the antibody, the amount of untagged hormone is decreased. EIA is performed like RIA, except that enzymes are used instead of radioisotopes. This method allows hormones, such as thyroid hormone, to be tested in small amounts.

The client may have anxiety over the test and its possible results. Many clients with endocrine disorders have been misdiagnosed for years because of the nonspecific manifestations of the disorders. After the diagnosis is made, the client and family may need help coping with the diagnosis and ongoing care.

Tests of Pancreatic Function

Diagnostic assessment of pancreatic function is related to blood glucose levels. An elevated fasting blood glucose is usually the first indication of hyperglycemia. Glycosylated hemoglobin (Hb A_{1c}) or glycohemoglobin measures the average blood glucose over 3 months and can be obtained in the nonfasting state.

A more detailed presentation of diagnostic tests related to diabetes appears in Chapter 69.

Tests of Thyroid Function

Several tests are available to assess thyroid function. A brief overview of the most common diagnostic tests follows.

Serum Thyroxine and Triiodothyronine

Radioimmunoassay can measure serum concentrations of thyroxine (T_4) and triiodothyronine (T_3). T_4 is transported in the blood largely bound to thyroid-binding globulin; conditions that affect thyroid-binding globulin levels alter the serum T_4 concentration. Pregnancy and oral contraceptives both increase serum T_4. Phenytoin (Dilantin) may cause T_3 and T_4 readings to be low in euthyroid clients.

T_3 Resin Uptake

T_3 (like T_4) circulates in the bloodstream attached to plasma proteins and to erythrocytes. However, T_3 binds far more readily to plasma proteins than to erythrocytes. T_3 binds to erythrocytes only when plasma protein binding sites are limited.

If thyroid function is low or if serum protein levels are high, resin uptake of T_3 is depressed. On the other hand, if thyroid function is increased above normal or serum protein levels are low, resin uptake of T_3 is elevated. When compared with serum T_4 or T_3 levels, this test can detect abnormal plasma thyroid-binding globulin levels.

Radioiodine Uptake and Excretion Test

The body cannot distinguish between radiolabeled or "tagged" iodine and nonradiolabeled iodine. Consequently, the thyroid takes up radiolabeled iodine (^{131}I) and processes it just as it does regular iodine. Radioiodine is excreted in the urine just as is ordinary iodine. Thus, a scintillation scanner can measure the amount of radioactive iodine present in the thyroid after administration of a radioiodine preparation. The laboratory may measure the client's urine output of radioactive iodine following the test.

Many factors can distort findings. Before the procedure, therefore, question the client about the following, and inform the physician if the client answers "yes" to any of these questions:

- Have you taken any iodine-containing medications within the last 30 days? Any estrogens that can cause a false elevation?
- Have you undergone x-ray studies of the gallbladder, ureters, bronchi, fallopian tubes, or heart within the last 10 years?
- Within the last 2 weeks, have you principally eaten seafood? (Seafood is so rich in iodine that ^{131}I uptake could show a falsely low reading.)

Thyrotropin-Releasing Hormone Stimulation Test

Thyrotropin-releasing hormone (TRH) is released from the hypothalamus, and it normally stimulates release of thyroid-stimulating hormone (TSH) from the pituitary. During the TRH stimulation test, people with thyroid disorders are given TRH intravenously. A rise in TSH levels indicates that the pituitary is functioning normally. TSH levels do not rise in the presence of hyperthyroidism or if the pituitary cells that secrete TSH are diseased.

Serum Cholesterol

The serum cholesterol level may be elevated in primary hypothyroidism, which may explain why this condition is accompanied by a marked tendency toward atherosclerosis. Persons with hyperthyroidism usually have a lower serum cholesterol level. Serum cholesterol is not a specific test of thyroid function, however, because its levels are influenced by many other factors than thyroid hormone levels.

Antithyroid Antibody Tests

Many thyroid disorders are presumed to have an autoimmune basis, such as Hashimoto's thyroiditis, some types of myxedema, and Graves' disease (a form of hyperthyroidism). Serologic tests may be performed to determine if the client's blood contains antithyroid antibodies.

Basal Metabolic Rate

The basal metabolic rate (BMR) is estimated by measuring the amount of oxygen consumed by the body under basal conditions (a state of complete mental and physical relaxation). Test results can be altered by inadequate rest before the examination, anxiety and emotional stress, a noisy environment, and previous ingestion of medications that affect metabolism. The BMR, once the major test of thyroid function, has been largely replaced by newer, more sophisticated diagnostic techniques.

Achilles Tendon Reflexes

The Achilles tendon reflex test measures the amplitude and duration of the ankle jerk with a special instrument, which is used to tap the strong tendon at the back of the heel. People with hyperthyroidism may demonstrate a more rapid tendon reflex. Individuals with underactive thyroid glands or diabetes mellitus and pregnant women have slower reflexes and prolonged relaxation times.

Tests of Adrenal Function

Adrenal function tests are divided into medullary and cortical types. Adrenal hormones include cortisol, aldosterone, and adrenocorticotropic hormone (ACTH). Medullary hormones include the catecholamines.

Cortisone Suppression Test

Cortisol is secreted in a diurnal pattern, and levels are assessed at 8:00 AM and 8:00 PM. A cortisone suppression test is the suppression of the pituitary ACTH with dexamethasone. Normally, after administration of dexamethasone, 24-hour levels of ketosteroid in the urine drop 50%. Dexamethasone can also be given at midnight, and serum cortisol then assessed at 8:00 AM. In clients with increased adrenocortical stimulation, no decrease occurs in ketosteroid production in urine or in serum levels of cortisol.

Aldosterone Levels

Plasma levels of aldosterone, angiotensin II, and renin can be measured at any time. Plasma levels of aldosterone can be increased by giving potassium, restricting sodium, or having the client assume an upright position. Plasma levels of aldosterone can be decreased by infusing saline.

Serum Adrenocorticotropic Hormone

Serum levels of adrenocorticotropic hormone (ACTH) can be assessed after the infusion of synthetic ACTH. Urine levels of ketosteroid would be expected to rise to 25 mg in 24 hours; plasma levels of cortisol should rise to 10 to 40 μg/100 ml. Urine levels of ketosteroid can be measured with 24-hour urine specimens. Ketosteroids are metabolites of the hormones produced by the adrenal cortex. A preservative is required for the collection bottle, and if the client has an indwelling catheter, the urinary drainage bag is emptied frequently and the urine is refrigerated.

The adrenal cortex can be assessed for tumors by x-ray study, computed tomography (CT), and magnetic resonance imaging (MRI) scans.

Urinary Catecholamines

The function of the adrenal medulla can be assessed through urine levels of catecholamines and their metabolites (vanillylmandelic acid, or VMA). A 24-hour urine sample is collected and assayed. The adrenal medulla can be suppressed with the administration of ganglionic blocking agents, which normally decrease the urine levels of catecholamines. In clients with pheochromocytoma, a tumor of the adrenal medulla, ganglionic blocking agents have a negligible effect in controlling blood pressure. An older assessment test for pheochromocytoma, which involved blood pressure manipulation, is rarely performed today.

Tests of Pituitary Function

Imaging Studies

The structure of the pituitary gland can be assessed with skull x-ray study, CT, or MRI. Tumors of the pituitary may be visualized with these studies.

Hormone Assays

Hormonal disorders due to malfunction of the pituitary can lead to a wide variety of clinical manifestations, depending on which hormone is involved. Growth hormone and antidiuretic hormone are discussed here.

■ Growth Hormone Levels

Growth hormone (GH) is secreted in a diurnal pattern, and the level of growth hormone can be assayed. The blood sample is usually drawn in the morning to determine basal levels; usual levels are 3 g/ml. Growth hormone can be stimulated with administration of (1) levodopa (500 mg, orally), (2) insulin (0.1 units/kg, intravenously), or (3) bromocriptine (5 mg, orally). Following the stimulus, blood is drawn at intervals for up to 120 minutes. GH levels usually peak 60 minutes after stimulation.

■ Water Deprivation Test

An absence of antidiuretic hormone leads to diabetes insipidus. To diagnose diabetes insipidus, the client is given a water deprivation test. Water is withheld for 4 to 18 hours, and during this time the client's vital signs, urine output, and urine specific gravity are assessed hourly. Hypovolemic shock can develop from dehydration. A client without diabetes insipidus responds with decreased urine output and increased urine osmolarity. The client with diabetes insipidus is not able to respond and continues to produce high volumes of dilute urine (low osmolarity).

Conclusions

The endocrine system works in unison with the nervous system to maintain homeostasis. The endocrine system is composed of two types of glands: endocrine, which release hormones into the blood, and exocrine, which release hormones into ducts. Endocrine glands include the gonads, adrenal, thyroid, parathyroid, and thymus. The pancreas is both an endocrine and exocrine gland. Assessment of the client includes the usual history and physical examination. In addition, blood levels of the various hormones can be determined. Most important, your accurate and insightful assessment can help clients with endocrine disorders receive the correct diagnosis and timely treatment.

Bibliography

1. Bates, B. (1994). *A guide to physical examination* (5th ed.). Philadelphia: J. B. Lippincott.
2. Birch, C. (1997). Caring for people with endocrine disorders. In J. Luckmann (Ed.). *Saunders Manual of Nursing Care*. Philadelphia: W. B. Saunders.
3. Corbett, J. (1991). *Laboratory tests and diagnostic procedures with nursing diagnoses* (3rd ed.). Norwalk, CT: Appleton & Lange.
4. DeGowin, R. (1994). *DeGowin and DeGowin's diagnostic examination* (6th ed.). New York: McGraw-Hill.
5. Jarvis, C. (1996). *Physical examination and health assessment* (2nd ed.). Philadelphia: W. B. Saunders.
6. Kee, J. L. (1995). *Laboratory and diagnostic tests with nursing implications* (4th ed.). Norwalk, CT: Appleton & Lange.
7. McCance, K., & Huether, S. (1994). *Pathophysiology: The biological basis for disease in adults and children* (2nd ed.). St. Louis: Mosby–Year Book.
8. Price, S., & Wilson, L. (Eds.). (1994). *Pathophysiology* (4th ed.). St. Louis: Mosby–Year Book.
9. Sheldon, H. (1988). *Boyd's introduction to the study of disease* (10th ed.). Philadelphia: Lea & Febiger.
10. Wilson, J., & Foster, D. (1992). *Williams textbook of endocrinology* (8th ed.). Philadelphia: W. B. Saunders.

Nursing Care of Clients with Endocrine Disorders of the Pancreas

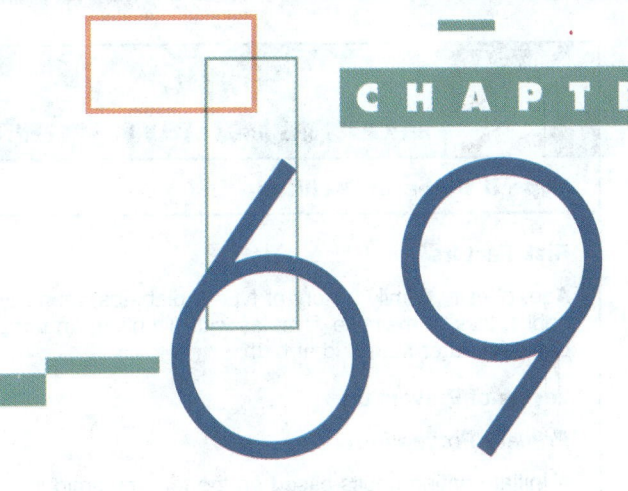

Carol Birch

Kerry H. Greear

Diabetes Mellitus

Diabetes mellitus is a syndrome caused by an imbalance between insulin supply and demand. It is characterized by hyperglycemia and associated with abnormal carbohydrate, fat, and protein metabolism. These metabolic abnormalities lead to the development of specific forms of renal, ocular, neurologic, and cardiovascular complications.

The overall term *diabetes mellitus* actually includes four subclasses: (1) type I (insulin-dependent diabetes mellitus, or IDDM), (2) type II (non–insulin-dependent diabetes, or NIDDM), (3) secondary diabetes mellitus, and (4) malnutrition-related diabetes mellitus. Besides diabetes mellitus, two other categories of abnormal glucose metabolism exist: (1) impaired glucose tolerance (IGT), and (2) gestational diabetes mellitus (GDM) (Box 69–1). This system for classification was developed by the National Diabetes Data Group of the National Institutes of Health with input from the World Health Organization.

Diabetes mellitus is a significant public health concern in the United States. Approximately 14 million Americans (one of every 20 people) have diabetes, but in about half that number the condition is undiagnosed. The economic costs of caring for people with diabetes accounted for $102.5 billion, close to one-seventh of total healthcare costs, in 1992.

Diabetes (and its complications) is the third leading cause of death from disease in the United States. Even when it does not kill, diabetes can cause major disabilities. For example, in the United States, diabetes mellitus is the single greatest contributor to blindness in adults, end-stage renal failure, and nontraumatic amputations. It is also a risk factor in coronary artery disease and stroke.

Type I diabetes mellitus accounts for approximately 10% of all known cases of diabetes mellitus in the United States. Annual incidence is 12 to 14 cases per 100,000 people younger than 20 years, with a prevalence of 1 case per 500 people younger than 16 years. It is one of the most common childhood diseases, being three to four times more common than chronic childhood diseases, such as cystic fibrosis, juvenile rheumatoid arthritis, or leukemia, and ten times more common than nephrotic syndrome or muscular dystrophy. Incidence is similar in males and females and lower in blacks, Hispanics, Asian Americans, and Native Americans than in whites. Delayed diagnosis is a serious problem. Approximately 40% of children with diabetes who are younger than 2 years old present to the healthcare provider in a coma; of these, approximately 5% die.

Type II diabetes mellitus accounts for approximately 85% to 90% of all known cases of diabetes mellitus in the United States. Approximately 7 million Americans have been diagnosed with this type of diabetes, but it is

> **Box 69–1. Types of Diabetes Mellitus and Other Categories of Abnormal Glucose Metabolism**
>
> Diabetes mellitus
> - Type I
> - Type II
> - Secondary and other types of diabetes
> - Malnutrition-related diabetes mellitus
> - Impaired glucose tolerance (IGT)
> - Gestational diabetes mellitus (GDM)
>
> ---
> Adapted from American Diabetes Association. (1994). *Medical management of non-insulin dependent (type II) diabetes* (3rd ed.). Alexandria, VA: Author.

This chapter incorporates material written for the fourth edition by Diane Butts-Krakoff and Joyce M. Black.

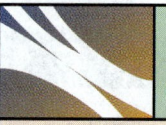

RISK FACTORS AND LEVELS OF PREVENTION

Type II Diabetes Mellitus

Risk Factors

Age, obesity, family history of type II diabetes, ethnicity, android (upper body or apple-type) fat distribution, dietary habits, lack of exercise, females with hirsutism and/or polycystic ovarian disease, gestational diabetes, and/or babies greater than 9 lb at birth

Levels of Prevention

Primary Prevention

- Initiate eating habits based on the food pyramid in school-age children.
- Promote avoidance of foods high in refined sugars and saturated fats.
- Encourage maintenance of ideal body weight starting in childhood.
- Teach the importance of regular exercise.
- Teach the importance of return to pre-pregnancy weight or ideal body weight postpartum.

Secondary Prevention

- Screen high-risk individuals: people with first-degree relatives with type II diabetes; obese individuals; members of high-risk races; people older than 40 years with any other risk factor; individuals with hypertension and/or hyperlipidemia; those with previous IGT: women with previous GDM or history of a baby weighing greater than 9 lb; and individuals with a history of recurrent infections.
- Perform periodic assessments to determine client's learning needs.
- Perform periodic examinations to assess glycemic control and screen for complications of diabetes.
- Utilize strategies shown to reduce complications of diabetes by teams made up of healthcare providers and individuals with diabetes.
- Prevent hypoglycemia or hyperglycemia with stress, illness, or exercise by closely monitoring blood glucose levels and taking early action.
- Perform daily foot care.

Tertiary Prevention

- Emphasize importance of controlling blood glucose levels to within as normal levels as possible.
- Teach diet and exercise programs to reduce obesity.
- Teach aggressive control of coexisting risk factors, such as hypertension and hyperlipidemia.
- No smoking.
- Teach avoidance of nephrotoxic drugs, such as NSAIDs (e.g., Motrin).
- Ensure yearly funduscopic examinations by an ophthalmologist and treatment as needed.
- Ensure prompt treatment of any foot abrasion or infection.
- Teach periodic visits to assess for learning needs.
- Teach routine follow-ups to assess for complications of diabetes.

estimated that an equal number of cases are undiagnosed. The prevalence is markedly increased in American Indians, blacks, and Hispanics, as well as in elderly and obese people (see Risk Factors and Levels of Prevention and Diversity in Healthcare features).

The number of people with secondary diabetes is small, but it will probably increase as people with pancreatic disease and endocrinopathies survive and as more people are treated with medications (such as glucocorticoids and thiazides) that can cause the disease.

Gestational diabetes occurs in approximately 4% of pregnant women, usually in the second or third trimester. After delivery, glucose tolerance in most clients returns to normal. However, type II diabetes develops in 40% to 60% of women with GDM within 5 to 15 years postpartum.

Etiology and Risk Factors

■ Type I Diabetes Mellitus (IDDM)

Predisposition to type I diabetes mellitus is inherited as a heterogeneous, multigenic trait. It carries a risk of 25% to 50% in identical twins, whereas siblings have a 6% risk and offspring a 5% risk. Despite this strong familial influence, 90% of individuals in whom type I diabetes develops do not have a first-degree relative with diabetes. An association also exists between type I diabetes and several human leukocyte antigens (HLAs). Environmental factors (such as viruses) appear to trigger an autoimmune process that destroys beta cells. Islet cell antibodies (ICAs) are present in increasing amounts over months to years as beta cells are destroyed. Fasting *hyperglycemia* (elevated

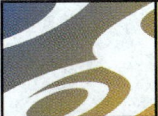

DIVERSITY IN HEALTHCARE

Diabetes in Native Americans

Approximately 1.5 million Native Americans live in the United States, including Inuits and Aleuts; many live on reservations. Diabetes was rarely diagnosed among Native Americans until the 1930s. Now, 60 years later, diabetes has become a major cause of morbidity and mortality among Native Americans, and the prevalence of diabetes is rising steadily in most tribes. Nearly all cases of diabetes diagnosed among Native Americans are type II diabetes mellitus.

To gain a more accurate picture of the prevalence of diabetes and impaired glucose tolerance in Native Americans, the Strong Heart Study[1] assessed the association of diabetes with four variables in Native Americans: age, obesity, family his-tory of diabetes, and amount of Native American ancestry.

The study sampled three large populations, one in Arizona (1,446 subjects), one in Oklahoma (1,449 subjects), and one in North and South Dakota (1,409 subjects). In all three populations, researchers found that diabetes was more prev-alent in Native American women than in Native American men. The Arizona population had the highest age-adjusted rates of diabetes: 65% in men and 72% in women. Diabe-tes rates in the populations studied in Oklahoma and North and South Dakota (38% in men and 42% in women, and 33% in men and 40% in women, respectively) were sev-eral times higher than those re-ported for the overall population of the United States. Interestingly, these diabetes rates were *lower* than in the overall population of Ari-zona.

Clearly, diabetes is an epidemic among Native Americans. Although standards of care and intervention for Native Americans with diabetes have been developed by the Indian Health Service, the findings of this study strongly suggest the need for diabetes prevention programs and periodic diabetes screenings for Na-tive Americans.

---

[1] Lee, E., et al. (1995). Diabetes and impaired glucose tolerance in three American Indian populations aged 45–74 years: The Strong Heart Study. *Diabetes Care, 18*(5), 599–610.

---

blood glucose level) occurs when 80% of 90% of beta-cell mass has been destroyed.

Identification of ICAs has made it possible to detect type I diabetes mellitus in its preclinical stage. Autoanti-bodies directed against insulin are found in 20% to 60% of clients with type I diabetes prior to initiation of exoge-nous insulin. The combination of high amounts of ICAs, insulin autoantibodies, and decreased first-phase insulin secretion (representing insulin stored within beta cells) is predictive of the onset of type I diabetes mellitus within 5 years.

■ Type II Diabetes Mellitus (NIDDM)

Type II diabetes mellitus also appears to be a heteroge-neous disorder involving both genetic and environmental factors. It is not associated with HLA tissue types, and circulating ICAs are rarely present. It is more common in identical twins (58% to 75% incidence). Obesity is a major risk factor; 85% of all clients with type II diabetes are obese. It is unclear whether impaired tissue (liver and muscle) sensitivity to insulin or impaired insulin secretion is the primary defect in this type of diabetes (see Risk Factors and Levels of Prevention).

Cases have been documented of families in which type II diabetes is present in all age groups and in which an autosomal dominant inheritance has been established. This form of diabetes is referred to as maturity-onset diabetes of the young (MODY).

Pathophysiology

■ Type I Diabetes Mellitus (IDDM)

Type I diabetes mellitus can be broken down into five stages of development:

Stage 1: Genetic predisposition
Stage 2: Environmental trigger
Stage 3: Active autoimmunity
Stage 4: Progressive beta-cell destruction
Stage 5: Overt diabetes mellitus

Type I diabetes mellitus does not develop in all indi-viduals with a genetic predisposition. Of the individuals with markers indicating genetic risk (DR3 or DR4 HLA markers), diabetes ultimately develops in fewer than 1%.

Environmental triggers have long been suspected in type I diabetes. Incidence is increased in both spring and fall and is coincidental with epidemics of various viral diseases. Active autoimmunity is directed against the beta cells of the pancreas and their products. ICAs and insulin antibodies serve to progressively decrease the effective circulating insulin level.

This slow, progressive insult to the beta cells and insu-lin molecules can result in an abrupt onset of manifesta-tions of diabetes. Hyperglycemia can be precipitated by acute illness or stress, which increases insulin demand beyond the reserves of the damaged beta-cell mass. When the acute illness or stress is resolved, the client may revert to a compensated state for a variable length of time until the diminishing beta-cell mass can no longer provide

Understanding Diabetes Mellitus and Its Treatment

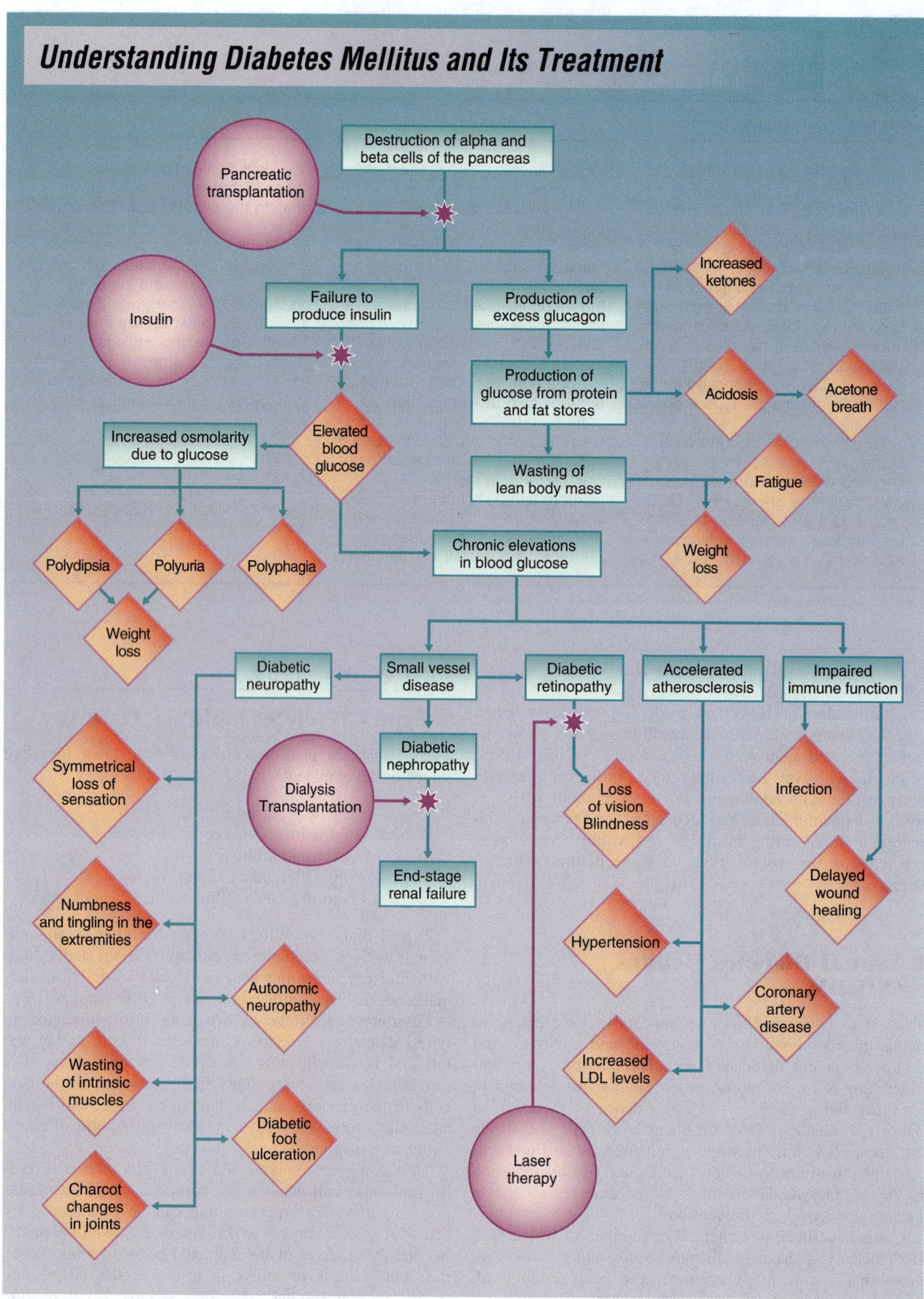

adequate amounts of insulin. This compensated state, referred to as the *honeymoon period*, typically lasts for 3 to 12 months.

The process ends when individuals do not produce enough insulin to sustain life. They become dependent on exogenous insulin administration to survive.

■ Type II Diabetes Mellitus (NIDDM)

The pathogenesis of type II diabetes mellitus differs significantly from type I. Limitation of beta-cell response to hyperglycemia appears to be a major factor in its development. Beta cells chronically exposed to hyperglycemia become progressively less efficient in response to further glucose elevations. This phenomenon, termed *desensitization*, is reversible with normalization of glucose levels. The ratio of proinsulin (a precursor to insulin) to insulin secreted also increases.

A second pathophysiologic process in type II diabetes mellitus is resistance to the biologic activity of insulin in both the liver and peripheral tissues. This is also known as *insulin resistance*. Clients with type II diabetes have a decreased sensitivity to glucose levels, which results in continued hepatic glucose production, even with high plasma glucose levels. This is coupled with an inability of the muscle and fat tissues to increase their glucose uptake. The mechanism causing peripheral insulin resistance is not clear; however, it appears to occur after insulin binds to a receptor on the cell surface (Fig. 69–1).

Insulin is a building (anabolic) hormone. Without insulin, three major metabolic problems occur: decreased glucose utilization, increased fat mobilization, and increased protein utilization.

Decreased Glucose Utilization

In diabetes, cells that require insulin as a carrier for glucose can take in only about 25% of the glucose they require for fuel. Nerve tissues, erythrocytes, and the cells of the intestines, liver, and kidney tubules do not require insulin for glucose transport, whereas the skeletal and cardiac muscles and adipose tissues do. Without adequate amounts of insulin, much of the ingested glucose cannot be utilized.

When adequate amounts of insulin are not present, blood glucose levels rise. This elevation continues because the liver is unable to store glucose as glycogen without sufficient insulin levels. In an attempt to restore balance and return blood glucose levels to normal, the kidney excretes the excess glucose. Glucose appears in the urine (*glucosuria*). Glucose excreted in the urine acts as an osmotic diuretic and causes excretion of increased amounts of water, resulting in fluid volume deficit.

Increased Fat Mobilization

Mainly in the type I diabetics, and occasionally in severely stressed type II diabetics, the body relies on fat stores for energy production when glucose is unavailable. Unfortunately, the process of fat metabolism leads to the formation of breakdown products called *ketones*. Ketones accumulate in the blood and are excreted through the kidneys and lungs. Ketone levels can be measured in the blood and urine and can serve as an indicator of uncontrolled diabetes. Ketones interfere with acid base balance by producing hydrogen ions. The pH can fall, and metabolic acidosis can develop (discussed later). In addition, when ketones are excreted, sodium is also eliminated, resulting in sodium depletion and further acidosis. The

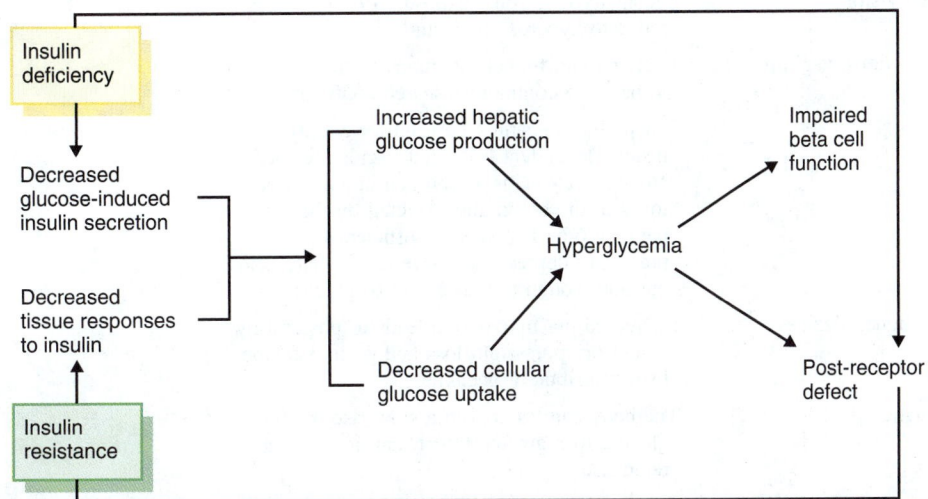

Figure 69–1. The relationship between insulin resistance and insulin secretion in type II diabetes mellitus. (Redrawn from American Diabetes Association [1994]. *Medical management of non-insulin dependent (type II) diabetes* [3rd ed.; p. 18]. Alexandria, VA: Author.)

excretion of ketones also increases osmotic pressure, leading to increased fluid loss. Also, when fats are the primary source of energy, body lipid levels can rise to five times normal, leading to increased atherosclerosis.

Increased Protein Utilization

Lack of insulin leads to protein wasting. In healthy individuals, proteins are constantly being broken down and rebuilt. In the type I diabetics, without insulin to stimulate protein synthesis, the balance is altered, which leads to increased catabolism. In this case, amino acids are converted to glucose in the liver, further elevating glucose levels. If untreated, the type I diabetic appears thin and emaciated.

The pathophysiologic processes of diabetes continue and lead to many acute and chronic complications. These are discussed later in the chapter.

Clinical Manifestations and Diagnostic Findings

Clients with type I diabetes mellitus usually present with cardinal manifestations (Tables 69–1 and 69–2) and sometimes already have complications such as ketoacidosis. Clients with type II diabetes mellitus may also develop the cardinal manifestations; however, because many of these clients are elderly, they may not recognize the abnormal thirst or frequent urination as being abnormal for their age. More commonly, they may only experience visual blurring, neuropathic changes such as tingling feet, or infections. Type II diabetes is commonly diagnosed when the client sees a healthcare provider for another problem.

Efforts to improve the management and prognosis of individuals with diagnosis must begin with prompt diagnosis and classification.

Table 69–1. Selected Clinical Manifestations of Diabetes Mellitus at Diagnosis

Clinical Manifestations	Pathophysiologic Bases	Type I Diabetes	Type II Diabetes
Cardinal manifestations			
Polyuria* (frequent urination)	Water not reabsorbed from renal tubules secondary to osmotic activity of glucose, leads to loss of water, glucose, and electrolytes	+ +	+
Polydipsia* (excessive thirst)	Dehydration secondary to polyuria causes thirst	+ +	+
Polyphagia* (excessive hunger)	Starvation secondary to tissue breakdown (catabolism) causes hunger	+ +	+
Weight loss*	Initial loss secondary to depletion of water, glycogen, and triglyceride stores; chronic loss secondary to decreased muscle mass as amino acids are diverted to form glucose and ketone bodies	+ +	−
Recurrent blurred vision	Secondary to chronic exposure of lenses and retina to hyperosmolar fluids	+	+ +
Pruritus, skin infections, vaginitis	Bacterial and fungal infections of the skin seem to be more common; research conflicting	+	+ +
Ketonuria	When glucose cannot be used for energy in insulin-dependent cells, fatty acids are used for energy; fatty acids are broken down into ketones in the blood and excreted by the kidneys; in type II diabetes, sufficient insulin is present to depress excessive use of fatty acids, but not enough to permit use of glucose	+ +	−
Weakness and fatigue, dizziness	Decreased plasma volume leads to postural hypotension; potassium loss and protein catabolism contribute to weakness	+ +	+
Often asymptomatic	The body can "adapt" to a slow rise in blood glucose to a greater extent than it can to a rapid rise	−	+ +

* Often referred to as *classic manifestations* of diabetes.
+, Sometimes seen; + +, usually seen; −, not usually seen.

Features	Type I	Type II
Synonyms	Insulin-dependent diabetes mellitus (IDDM), juvenile diabetes, labile or brittle diabetes	Non–insulin-dependent diabetes mellitus (NIDDM), adult or maturity-onset diabetes, mild diabetes
Age at onset	Usually occurs before age 30 years, but may occur at any age	Usually occurs after age 30 years, but can occur in children
Incidence	~10%	~85%–90%
Type of onset	Usually abrupt, with rapid onset of hyperglycemia	Insidious, may be asymptomatic or mildly asymptomatic; body adapts to slow onset of hyperglycemia
Endogenous insulin production	Little or none	Below normal, normal or above normal
Body weight at onset	Ideal body weight or thin	85% are obese; may be ideal body weight
Ketosis	Prone to ketosis, usually present at onset, frequently present during poor control	Resistant to ketosis, can occur with infection or stress
Manifestations	Polyuria, polydipsia, polyphagia, fatigue	Frequently none, may be mild manifestations of hyperglycemia
Dietary management	Essential	Essential
Exercise management	Essential	Essential
Exogenous insulin administration	Dependent on insulin for survival	20%–30% of clients may require insulin
Oral hypoglycemic agents (OHAs)	Not effective	Effective
Teaching needs	At diagnosis and ongoing	At diagnosis and ongoing

Because diabetes is a syndrome that affects multiple body systems, it is vital that diagnostic laboratory findings be correlated with the client's manifestations. The nurse plays an important role in diagnosis of diabetes mellitus. The nurse, as a member of the healthcare team, may perform the following:

● Set up screening clinics in the community (Box 69–2)
● Teach individuals and groups about risk factors and clinical manifestations of diabetes
● Teach clients about diagnostic testing techniques, including preparation, procedure, and follow-up

The nurse should be familiar with the following diagnostic/monitoring tests:

Random Blood Glucose. A blood sample for determination of glucose level may be drawn at any time and requires no preparation of the client. Results should be within normal limits for both nondiabetics and for diabetics with good control of blood glucose. Elevated levels of blood glucose may occur after meals, after stressful events, if the sample was drawn from above an intravenous (IV) site, or in cases of diabetes. See Table 69–3 for conditions and medications that can cause hyperglycemia (elevated blood glucose level) or hypoglycemia (decreased blood glucose level).

Fasting Blood Glucose. A fasting blood glucose sample (fasting blood sugar or FBS) is drawn when the client has not ingested any nutrients other than water for at least 3 hours. The FBS generally reflects glucose from hepatic production. If the client is receiving a dextrose IV solution, the results of the test must be analyzed with that variable in mind. In clients who are known to have diabetes, food and insulin are withheld until after the specimen is drawn. The FBS gives the best indication of overall glucose homeostasis. Critical values in adults are less than 60 mg/dl or more than 500 mg/dl.

Postprandial Blood Glucose. Postprandial blood glucose samples are drawn 2 hours after a standard meal and reflect the efficiency of insulin-mediated glucose uptake by peripheral tissues. Normally, the blood glucose should return to fasting levels within 2 hours. In the elderly, levels can rise by 5 to 10 mg/dl per decade after age 50 years due to the normal decline in glucose tolerance associated with aging. Smoking and drinking coffee can lead to falsely elevated values at 2 hours, whereas strenuous exercise can lead to falsely decreased values.

Self-Monitoring Blood Glucose. Development of devices that enable clients with diabetes to monitor their

Box 69-2. Guidelines for Screening in Clinics and the Community

Objective

To identify individuals with diabetes or diabetes risk factors through use of written or verbal questionnaires and measurement of glucose in blood samples. Individuals with risk factors and/or manifestations of diabetes should be referred to their healthcare provider for evaluation.

Screening

Measurement of plasma glucose levels should be limited to individuals identified as being at risk for having diabetes or for developing it in the future.

The screening test of choice is fasting blood glucose (FBS) FBS >115 mg/dl is an indication for further testing. Individuals with FBS ≤115 mg/dl should be retested in 3 years if they still have one or more diabetes risk factors.

Clients with random blood glucose test results ≥160 mg/dl should be referred to their healthcare provider for evaluation.

Minors and individuals with diagnosed diabetes should not be tested in a community screening program.

Follow-up

Community screening programs must have an established mechanism for referral. Written data must be given to the individual containing (1) individual's name, address, telephone number; (2) list of identified risk factors; (3) data on any tests performed (date, type, results, possibility of false-positive or false-negative results); and (4) a statement indicating need for follow-up with the healthcare provider and alternate resources for those without a provider.

Personnel conducting community screening programs must be adequately trained and able to demonstrate competency in knowledge of policies, procedures, and testing. OSHA guidelines must be followed.

----

* Glucose testing of pregnant women should not be performed in community screening programs. They should be referred to their healthcare provider for an oral glucose tolerance test.

Adapted from American Diabetes Association (1995). Screening for diabetes. *Diabetes Care, 18* (Suppl. 1), 5–7.

----

own blood glucose level has revolutionized diabetes care. These machines use reagent strips and/or a photometer and have a digital readout of blood glucose values. Some have memory chips. Self-monitoring of blood glucose (SMBG or glucose finger sticks) is recommended for all clients with diabetes, but it is required for people with type I diabetes, clients with insulin-requiring type II diabetes, highly motivated clients with type II diabetes, women with GDM, individuals utilizing an insulin pump, and clients whose diabetes is in poor control. These tests must be performed with extreme care and accuracy, because the results are utilized to adjust insulin, manage exercise, and monitor dietary management of diabetes. Most machines have a process to determine machine accuracy by use of control samples. This method of testing is not used to diagnose diabetes, but it is instrumental in managing diabetes.

Because SMBG utilizes whole blood and laboratories utilize serum or plasma for glucose determinations, the results of these monitoring methods are not equal. Whole blood glucose concentrations are approximately 12% to 15% lower than plasma concentrations because glucose is not distributed in hemoglobin. To compare SMBG results and laboratory levels of glucose, divide the serum or plasma level by 1.12, which represents the 12% difference between the two. The results of self-monitoring should fall within 15% to 20% of the laboratory results.

Glycosylated Hemoglobin (Hb A_{1c}). Glucose normally attaches itself to the hemoglobin molecule on a red blood cell. Once attached, it cannot dissociate. Therefore, the higher the blood glucose levels, the higher the levels of glycosylated hemoglobin (Hb A_{1c}). The results of this test show the average of the blood glucose levels over the previous 3 months, and it is therefore useful in the evaluation of long-term glycemic control. Hb A_{1c} samples can be drawn at any time during the day. Conditions that increase erythrocyte turnover, such as bleeding, pregnancy, or splenectomy, will lead to falsely low Hb A_{1c} concentrations. High aspirin doses, alcohol ingestion, uremia, elevated hemoglobin levels, and heparin therapy can cause falsely elevated levels of Hb A_{1c}. Normal values are 6% to 7%.

Glycosylated Albumin (Fructosamine). Glucose also attaches to proteins, primarily albumin. Fructosamine measures the average blood glucose over the previous 2 to 3 weeks. It is useful when short-term determinations of average blood glucose are desired. This test's role in clinical practice is not well defined.

Connecting Peptide (C-Peptide). When the proinsulin produced by the beta cells of the pancreas is broken apart by an enzyme, two products are formed: insulin and C-peptide. Since C-peptide and insulin are formed in equal amounts, this test indicates the amount of endogenous insulin production. Clients with type I diabetes usually have no or low concentrations of C-peptide. Clients with type II diabetes tend to have normal or elevated levels.

Oral Glucose Tolerance Test. The oral glucose tolerance test (OGTT) is often unnecessary for diagnosis of diabetes mellitus. Bedrest, infection, trauma, medications, and stress can alter the test results. It is not usually recommended in hospitalized clients. OGTT is unnecessary for diagnosing diabetes if the FBS is greater than 140 mg/dl.

The client needs to be on a diet that offers at least 150 g of carbohydrate per day for 3 days before the test. An FBS is drawn and then the client is given 75 g of glucose to drink. Blood samples are taken at intervals

Table 69–3. Selective Factors Contributing to Hypoglycemia and Hyperglycemia

	Predisposing Factors	Associated Medications
Hypoglycemia	Too much insulin Erratic absorption of insulin Sudden increase in activity Starvation Alcohol ingestion Age >60 years Acute illness Cerebral vascular accident Heart failure Decreased kidney function Gastric paresis Abnormal liver function Hypopituitarism Adrenocortical insufficiency	Insulin Salicylates/nonsteroidal anti-inflammatory drugs (NSAIDs) Sulfonamides Beta-blockers Sulfonylureas (oral hypoglycemia agents [OHAs]) Allopurinol Dicumerol Haloperidol Anticholinergic antagonists Monoamine oxidase inhibitors Para-amino benzoic acid Dextropropoxyphene Clofibrate Imipramine H_2-receptor antagonists
Hyperglycemia	Inadequate insulin Infection Inactivity Obesity IV dextrose Diabetes Emotional stress Physical stress Liver disease Hyperthyroidism Lack of OHA Decreased muscle mass Chronic pancreatitis	Diuretics, especially thiazides Beta-blockers Diphenylhydantoin Glucocorticoids Lithium Phenothiazines Progestins Levothyroxine NSAIDs Epinephrine Tricyclic antidepressants Oral contraceptives Rifampin Nicotinic acid Isoniazid

afterward (such as 1 and 2 hours). The client cannot consume any food or fluid, other than water, between the glucose load ingestion and the end of the test. Diagnosis of diabetes mellitus and IGT after the OGTT is dependent on fasting and follow-up glucose levels. See Table 69–4 for more information on these tests. The oral glucose load and levels diagnostic of diabetes are different for the pregnant client undergoing testing for GDM.

Urine Ketones (Ketonuria). Urine levels of ketones can be tested by clients, as well as in laboratories, by use of dip-strips. The presence of ketones indicates that the body is using fat as a major source of energy. Clients should test for urinary ketones when they are ill. The presence of nonfasting urinary ketones in a type II diabetic is major cause for concern.

Urine Protein (Proteinuria). A routine urinalysis tests the sample for protein. Proteinuria is a manifestation of nephropathy. Testing the urine for microalbuminuria shows early nephropathy, long before it would be displayed on a routine urinalysis.

Community and Self-Care

Diabetes mellitus is the prototype model for collaborative care, utilizing teams made up of the client, physician, nurse educator, nutritionist, social worker, pharmacist, counselor, pharmacist, exercise physiologist, and others (Fig. 69–2). The successful model recognizes the client as the primary provider of care. Living with a chronic illness requires the client to manage multiple dimensions of the condition, including manifestations of the disease, life-style changes, and the psychosocial aspects of chronic illness. A chronic care framework is more useful when working with diabetic clients.

In a chronic care model, the process of empowerment is valuable. Successful management of the chronic illness hinges on the healthcare team's integration of the client into the team. The team can collaborate to establish individualized goals, plans, and outcomes, which will assist the client to address the multiple dimensions of diabetes.

The coping tasks of chronicity identified by Miller[63] (Box 69–3) are utilized in the following model. The

Table 69–4 Diagnosis of Diabetes Mellitus and Impaired Glucose Tolerance (IGT) by Oral Glucose Tolerance Test

Test	Normal Results, mg/dl	IGT, mg/dl	Diabetes Mellitus, mg/dl
Fasting glucose (FBS)	≤115	<140	≥140 on 2 occasions
Serum blood glucose drawn ½ hour, 1 hour, or 1½ hours after 75-g glucose load	<140	140–199	≥200 on 2 occasions, after an FBS <140
Serum blood glucose drawn 2 hours after 75-g glucose load	<200	≥200	≥200

Adapted from American Diabetes Association. (1994). *Medical management of non-insulin dependent (type II) diabetes* (3rd ed.; pp. 7–9). Alexandria, VA: Author.

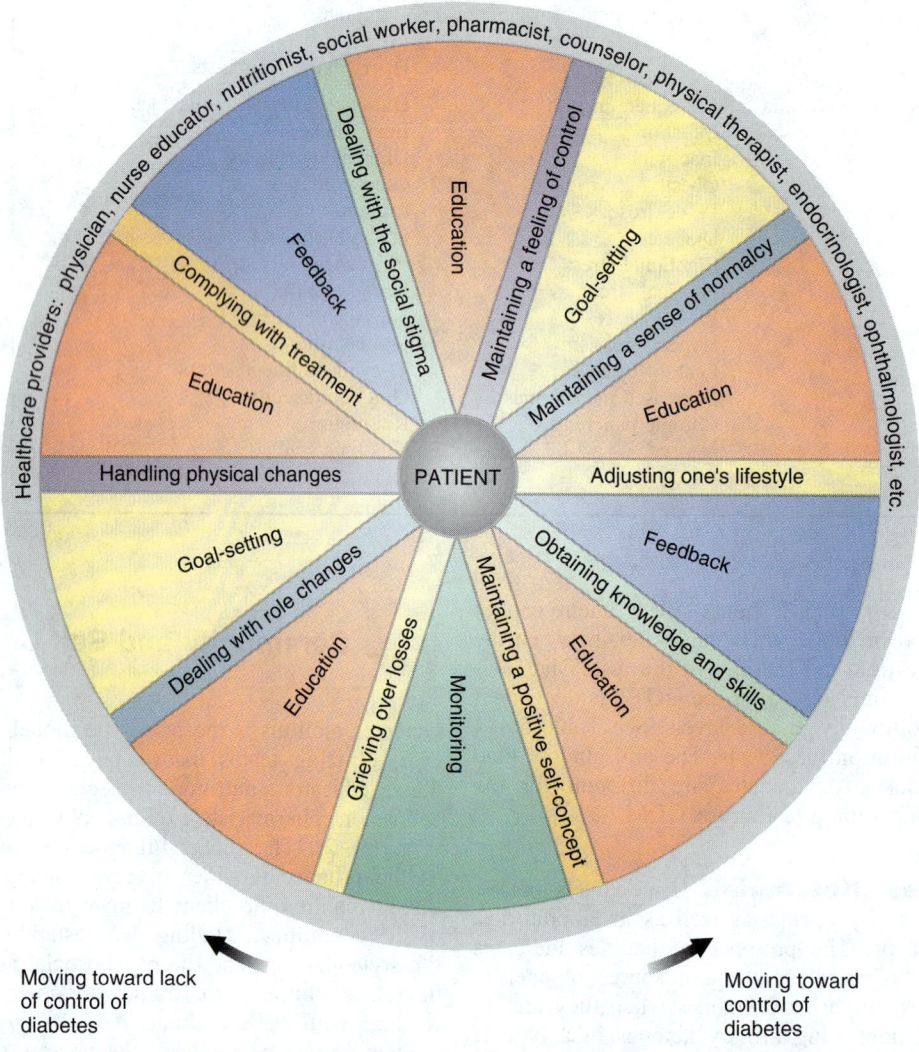

Figure 69–2. A collaborative model of diabetes management. In this model, the patient is viewed as the hub of the wheel to remind the team that the patient is the primary provider of care as well as the central component of the process of care. The coping tasks associated with the chronicity of the disease are viewed as the spokes of the wheel. These coping tasks are the link between the patient and the healthcare providers. Healthcare providers form the rim of the wheel. The rim is the same shape as the hub to reflect the commonality of patient and provider goals. Just as the wheel moves, so the direction of management may move or change: all components adjust and move together. (Redrawn with permission of Kerry H. Greear, M.S.N., R.N., C.N.P., Rapid City, SD.)

Box 69–3. Selected Coping Tasks of Clients Diagnosed with Diabetes Mellitus

- Maintaining sense of normalcy
- Modifying daily routine, adjusting life-style
- Obtaining knowledge and skill for continuing self-care
- Maintaining a positive concept of self
- Grieving over losses concomitant to chronic illness
- Dealing with role change
- Handling physical changes
- Complying with treatment regimens
- Dealing with social stigma of illness
- Maintaining feeling of being in control

Adapted from Miller, J. F. (1992). *Coping with chronic illness: Overcoming powerlessness* (2nd ed.). Philadelphia: F. A. Davis.

---

coping tasks, goal setting, education, monitoring, and feedback, by the healthcare team and the client, form the basis of the model.

■ Medical Management

Overall goals of care for clients with diabetes are (1) regulation of blood glucose and (2) prevention of acute and chronic complications. When diabetes is successfully managed, clients avoid the complications of hyperglycemia and hypoglycemia. Unfortunately, complications may develop in some clients with diabetes despite their vigorous efforts to carefully control the disease.

Diabetes management depends on the proper interaction of three factors: (1) physical activity, (2) diet, and, perhaps, (3) pharmacologic intervention with an oral hypoglycemic agent or insulin. Initial as well as ongoing client education is vital in assisting the client to manage this chronic condition. Interventions planned for the treatment of diabetes must be individualized; this means they must be based on the client's goals, age, life-style, nutritional needs, maturation, activity level, occupation, type of diabetes, and ability to independently perform the skills required by the management plan. Incorporation of psychosocial aspects into the overall plan is vital.

Initial goals for clients with newly diagnosed diabetes or clients in poor control of their diabetes should focus on the following:

1. Elimination of ketosis, if present
2. Attainment of desirable body weight
3. Prevention of manifestations of hyperglycemia
4. Maintenance of exercise tolerance
5. Maintenance of psychosocial well-being
6. Prevention of hypoglycemia

An overall goal is to learn to control the diabetes so it doesn't control the client.

Diabetes Control and Complications Trial

The Diabetes Control and Complications Trial (DCCT) showed that intensive control of blood glucose in clients with type I diabetes can prevent or ameliorate the complications of diabetes. It is believed that clients with type II diabetes would have similar benefits from normalization of glucose levels (see Nursing Research feature).

Physical Activity

A program of planned exercise is a critical part of the treatment plan for the client with diabetes. Exercise has the following effects on the body:

1. Lowers the blood glucose level by increasing carbohydrate metabolism
2. Facilitates weight reduction and proper weight maintenance
3. Increases insulin sensitivity
4. Increases high-density lipoprotein levels and decreases triglycerides levels
5. Decreases blood pressure
6. Decreases stress and tension

Components of Fitness. The three components of fitness are flexibility, muscle strength, and cardiovascular endurance. Aerobic exercise uses large muscles in repetitive motion, improves circulation, and strengthens the heart and lungs. Aerobic exercise also helps to lower blood glucose. Examples of aerobic exercise include jogging, bicycling, swimming, skiing, dancing, and walking.

Goals of Exercise. The goals of planned exercise are as follows:

- Exercise to 60% to 75% of the maximal heart rate for the client's age. This is determined by subtracting the present age from 220 and multiplying by 60% to 75%. Thus, a client 20 years old could exercise to a heart rate of 120 to 150 beats per minute, but a client 60 years old could exercise only to a heart rate of 96 to 120 beats per minute.
- Exercise for a period of 20 to 45 minutes at the desired heart rate.
- Exercise a minimum of three times a week.

Diabetic Dietary Management

Dietary management is an essential component of management of both types I and II diabetes mellitus. Approximately 30% of people with diabetes (type II) are treated with dietary measures only. Meal planning is intended to ensure a reasonably consistent food intake and a nutritionally adequate diet.

Some of the nutritional goals for adults with diabetes are (1) to maintain near-normal blood glucose levels by balancing food intake with exogenous or endogenous insulin levels and activity levels, (2) to achieve optimal

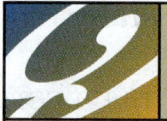

NURSING RESEARCH

How Do Conventional Therapy and Intensive Therapy Compare in the Effect on Clients with Diabetes?

The DCCT Research Group. (1993). The effect of intensive treatment of diabetes on the development and progression of long-term complications in insulin-dependent diabetes mellitus. *The New England Journal of Medicine, 329*(14), 977–985.

The Diabetes Control and Complications Trial (DCCT) was a multicenter, randomized, nearly 10-year clinical trial designed to compare intensive diabetes therapy with conventional diabetes therapy in regards to their effects on the development and progression of the early vascular and neurologic complications of type I diabetes mellitus.

The intensive therapy regimen was designed to achieve blood glucose levels as close to the normal range as possible by use of three or more insulin injections per day or treatment with an insulin pump. Conventional therapy consisted of one or two insulin injections per day.

Although retinopathy was the specific outcome studied, other adverse effects on renal, neurologic, and cardiovascular systems were also studied.

From 1983 through 1993 (with a range of 3 to 9 years and an average of 6.5 years), 1,441 clients at 29 centers were followed. Ages of the clients were 13 to 39 years at the beginning of the study. Major criteria for eligibility was insulin dependence (as noted by deficient C-peptide secretion) and absence of hypertension, hypercholesterolemia, and severe diabetic complications or medical conditions. Ninety-nine percent of the clients completed the study.

The following table compares the conventional therapy and intensive therapy regimens. Both groups had access to a diabetes treatment team and all necessary supplies.

Comparison of Clinical Groups in DCCT

	Conventional Therapy	Intensive Therapy
Insulin administration	One or two daily injections, including mixtures of rapid-acting and intermediate-acting insulins; daily adjustments were not made	Administration of insulin three or more times daily by injection or insulin per an insulin pump; dosage adjusted according to SMBG, dietary intake, and anticipated exercise
Goals	Absence of manifestations related to glycosuria or hypoglycemia; absence of ketonuria; maintenance of normal growth and development; ideal body weight; freedom from frequent or severe hypoglycemia	FBS, 70–120 mg/dl; postmeal blood glucose, <180 mg/dl; weekly 0300 blood glucose, >65 mg/dl; monthly Hb A_{1c}, <6%
Monitoring	Daily monitoring of urine or blood glucose; examinations every 3 months	SMBG at least 4 times daily; follow-up monthly and more frequently by telephone
Education	Regarding diet and exercise	Regarding diet, exercise, how to adjust insulin dosages

Implications for Practice

Intensive therapy delays the onset and slows the progression of chronic complications of diabetes by 35% to more than 70%. The risk of severe hypoglycemia was three times higher in the intensive therapy group. It was believed that risk of hypoglycemia was greatly outweighed by the reduction in microvascular and neurologic complications. On the basis of the results, it is recommended that most clients with type I diabetes mellitus be treated with closely monitored intensive regimens. Intensive therapy should be implemented with caution in clients with repeated severe hypoglycemia or unawareness of hypoglycemia. The risk benefit may be less favorable in children younger than 13 years and in clients with advanced complications, such as end-stage renal disease or cardiovascular or cerebrovascular disease. Clients beginning intensive therapy may be at risk for accelerated progression of retinopathy during the first year, with abnormalities usually disappearing by 18 months after starting therapy.

serum lipid levels, (3) to provide adequate calories for maintenance or attainment of reasonable weights and to meet increased metabolic needs when recovering from illness (reasonable weight is defined as the weight the individual and healthcare team acknowledge as achievable and maintainable both short and long term), (4) to prevent and treat acute and chronic complications of diabetes, and (5) to improve overall health.

Oral Hypoglycemic Agents

In clients with type II diabetes mellitus, pharmacologic intervention should be considered when the client cannot achieve normal or near-normal plasma glucose levels with nutrition and exercise therapies.

Oral hypoglycemic agents (OHAs) are often effective in clients with type II diabetes after nutrition and exercise therapy have failed. About 35% of clients with this type of diabetes take OHAs. The mechanism of action is complex; they work by stimulating the pancreas to release more endogenous insulin and to increase the number of insulin receptor sites throughout the body. They may also reduce hepatic production of glucose. These agents are not insulin, and they can only work if the pancreatic beta cells are able to produce insulin. They are not, therefore, used in type I diabetes. They are also contraindicated in pregnant and breastfeeding women, because they cross the placenta and are excreted in breast milk. Fever, traumatic injury, surgery, or other serious illness can increase blood glucose rapidly and render OHAs ineffective. When the condition is resolved, these clients can resume OHA therapy. Clients allergic to sulfa cannot take OHAs, and those with coronary artery disease, liver, or renal impairment should use them cautiously. Although most OHAs are classified as sulfonylureas and work the same way, they vary greatly in potency, duration of action, and dosage.

The client most likely to respond well to an OHA is one who develops diabetes after age 40, has had diabetes for less than 5 years, is of normal weight or obese, and has either never received insulin or has well-controlled diabetes with less than 40 units of insulin per day. Indications for these agents are random blood glucose level less than 300 mg/dl, fasting blood glucose level less than 250 mg/dl, and inadequate control after exercise and diet therapies.

First-generation sulfonylureas were discovered in the 1950s and second-generation drugs of this class were developed in the 1980s. They are outlined in Table 69–5. Note the smaller dosages of the newer agents that are required. Hypoglycemia is a potential side effect of all of these agents, and they may also cause gastrointestinal disturbances, hematologic reactions, cholestasis, rashes, and liver function changes. Risk factors for hypoglycemia during OHA treatment include advanced age, poor nutri-

Table 69-5. Oral Hypoglycemic Agents

Agent	Daily Dosage Range, mg	Duration of Action, hr	Frequency of Administration	Metabolism
First-Generation Sulfonylureas				
Tolbutamide (Orinase)	500–2,000	6–12	2–3 × day	By liver to inactive product
Chlorpropamide (Diabinese)	100–500	60	1 × day	70% by liver to active and inactive products, requires renal excretion
Tolazamide (Tolinase)	100	12–24	1–2 × day	By liver to active and inactive products, renal excretion
Second-Generation Sulfonylureas				
Glipizide (Glucotrol)	2.5–40	12–24	1–2 × day	By liver to inactive products
(Glucotrol XL)	5–60	24	1 × day	
Glyburide (Diabeta, Micronase)	1.25–12	16–24	1–2 × day	By liver to mostly inactive products
Glynase Pres Tabs	0.75–12	12–24	1–2 × day	
Biguanides				
Metformin (Glucophage)	500–2,550	(Unknown—half-life, 5.5)	1–3 × day	Excreted unchanged by kidneys
Precose (Acarbose)	75–100	4–6	3 × day with meals	Metabolized by the liver

tion, alcohol use, and hepatic or renal disease. Chlorpropamide, the longest-acting of these agents, is eliminated so slowly by the body that its effects can be seen for weeks. It can also cause hyponatremia in the elderly.

Second-generation sulfonylureas have fewer side effects, but they are more costly. No specific guidelines exist regarding which generation of drugs is better when everything is taken into account. In the absence of renal disease, tolazamide (Tolinase) may be a good choice. Whatever the choice of agent, the lowest recommended dose is prescribed with gradual increase every 1 to 2 weeks until adequate control or maximum dose is reached. If adequate control is not reached, the client may be a candidate for insulin therapy. Of all clients treated with sulfonylureas, approximately 60% to 75% will respond favorably. Primary treatment failures are diagnosed when an individual does not respond to a 1-month trial of an OHA at the maximum dose. Of clients who respond favorably in the initial months of treatment, 5% to 10% per year experience secondary treatment failures. Secondary failure may be the result of progression of diabetes or induced by treatable causes such as surgery, infection, or weight gain.

Drug interactions with sulfonylureas are frequent. Interactions can occur with agents that displace the OHA from plasma protein-binding sites (such as clofibrate, sulfonamides, and salicylates), compounds that alter hepatic enzyme activity (such as warfarin, levothyroxine, and alcohol), or medications that alter renal elimination (such as sulfonamides, salicylates, and allopurinol).

Metformin (Glucophage) is a guanidine derivative that decreases blood glucose levels in type II diabetic clients, primarily by an increase in glucose utilization. Because it does not stimulate insulin secretion, it is not associated with hypoglycemic reactions. It is used alone or with sulfonylureas to control hyperglycemia in clients who have primary or secondary failure with sulfonylureas alone. Metformin also decreases triglycerides and low-density lipoprotein (LDL) cholesterol levels. The major side effects are gastrointestinal, which include anorexia, nausea, abdominal discomfort, and diarrhea. Lactic acidosis is a rare complication. This drug should not be used in clients with kidney or liver disease, alcohol abuse, pregnancy, or cardiorespiratory insufficiency. As with sulfonylureas, metformin should be started at low doses, with gradual increases.

Precose (acarbose) is an oral agent released in 1996. It makes up another group of oral hypoglycemic agents for the patient with type II diabetes. Precose is an oligosaccharide (oral alpha-glucosidase inhibitor). It reversibly inhibits intestinal alpha-glucosidase enzymes thereby slowing carbohydrate digestion in the small intestine and delaying glucose absorption. Precose manages postprandial glucose peaks to improve glycemic control, reducing Hb A_{1c} (by 0.5 to 1.0 percentage points) levels to help prevent diabetes complications. Precose has no direct effects on fasting blood glucose levels.

Precose lowers blood glucose as an adjunct to diet. It may be prescribed alone or with a sulfonylurea when glycemic control cannot be achieved.

The recommended dosage of Precose is 25 mg TID to be taken with the first bite of the meal. Dosage may be adjusted at 4–8 week intervals. Maximum dose is 100 mg TID. Side effects related to dosages of 100 mg TID or greater include an increased risk of elevated transaminase levels. Liver toxicity is rare. Other side effects include intestinal distention, abdominal pain, diarrhea, and flatulence. These side effects are related to the mode of action and generally diminish after 4–8 weeks due to adaption of the small intestine enzyme activity.

Precose is contraindicated in clients with diabetic ketoacidosis, cirrhosis, inflammatory bowel disease, colonic ulceration or partial bowel obstruction. Precose is not recommended in clients with significant renal dysfunction (serum creatinine >2.0 mg/dl).

Client education topics must include hypoglycemia. Because Precose delays the absorption of multi-carbon carbohydrates, milk or glucose tablets must be used to treat hypoglycemia. Remember that Preocse has no effect on fasting blood glucose when used alone. It is imperative that Precose be taken with the first bite of a meal three times a day. It is important that patients continue to adhere to dietary instruction, a physical activity program, and regular testing of blood glucose. Certain drugs tend to produce hyperglycemia and may lead to loss of blood glucose control. These drugs include the thiazides and other diuretics, corticosteroids, phenothiazines, thyroid products, estrogens, oral contraceptives, phenytoin, nicotinic acid, sympathomimetics, calcium-channel blockers, and isoniazid. When such medications are administered to a client receiving Precose, the client should be closely observed for loss of blood glucose control.

Another OHA is being tested in clinical trials. Troglitazone, a member of the experimental class of drugs called *thiazolidinediones*, has decreased fasting and postprandial blood glucose levels, improved glucose tolerance, and increased insulin sensitivity. It also shows promise in preventing type II diabetes in obese clients.

Combination Therapy

In some clients with type II diabetes (mostly non-obese clients) who have primary failure to sulfonylurea agents, insulin therapy has been required to achieve metabolic control very early in their course of disease. In these clients, daily insulin dosage is markedly higher than in clients with type I diabetes. This is attributed to insulin resistance. Because sulfonylurea agents enhance the effect of endogenous insulin by reducing insulin resistance, it has been thought that combining insulin therapy with sulfonylureas may be effective. One regimen prescribed is an injection of an intermediate-acting insulin at bedtime with daytime coverage by a sulfonylurea (*b*edtime *i*nsulin with *d*aytime *s*ulfonylurea, or BIDS).

Insulin Therapy

Clients with type I diabetes mellitus do not produce enough insulin to sustain life. They depend on exogenous insulin administration on a daily basis. In contrast, clients with type II diabetes are not dependent on exogenous insulin for survival. They may need supplemental insulin for adequate glucose control, especially in times of stress or illness.

Insulin Types. Prior to 1991, insulin was classified by species (beef, pork, and human) and duration of action (short-, intermediate-, and long-acting). Since then, most clients are treated with human insulin (produced by recombinant DNA technology) which, in comparison to animal insulins, peak more precisely and predictably, have a shorter duration of action, have reduced antigenicity, and do not cause lipoatrophy or lipodystrophy at the injection site. Insulin works to lower blood glucose by (1) promoting the transport of glucose into cells, and (2) inhibiting conversion of glycogen and amino acids to glucose. See Table 69–6 for types of human insulin and comparative actions. Insulin types and species, injection technique, site of injection, number of insulin antibodies, and individual client response can all affect the onset, peak, and duration of action of the insulin. Insulin injected into the abdomen is absorbed fastest, followed by arm and leg, respectively.

The normal secretory pattern of endogenous insulins follows a basal level secretion with increased production in response to an incoming carbohydrate load. In clients with type I diabetes, the goal is to mimic this increase with injections of exogenous insulin.

Humalog, an insulin analog, was newly released in 1996. The action and potency of Humalog, as a hypoglycemic agent, is the same as human regular insulin, but the onset is immediate after subcutaneous injection and lasts for approximately 2 hours. Humalog should be taken immediately before eating.

Humalog is only approved, at this time, for subcutaneous or continuous insulin infusion pump use.

Humalog will provide many benefits in achieving glucose control and ultimately prevent or delay diabetes-related complications. A major point to remember and to emphasize to clients is that because it works so quickly, hypoglycemia can develop rapidly if adequate calories are not consumed immediately after injection.

Insulin Dosage. Insulin therapy should be individualized. For a client with newly diagnosed diabetes, a simple regimen with fixed doses may be used at first. The starting dose of insulin is 0.5 units/kg/day. Two-thirds of the dose is commonly given in the morning and one-third in the evening. The team works to adjust the numbers and timing of injections to smooth out normal patterns. Then the dose can be increased. Algorithms are detailed guidelines to help clients self-adjust the daily insulin dose, based on SMBG levels, food intake, exercise, and departures from normal routine (e.g., added stress or illness). These guidelines use a prospective (predictive) approach to blood glucose control.

Insulin dosage varies greatly. Two major considerations determine insulin dosage: (1) the client's requirements, and (2) the client's response to the insulin. After initial stabilization, the healthcare team assists clients to learn how to make adjustments in insulin doses, timing, food intake, and exercise. Unexplained fluctuations in blood glucose often occur. The team needs to help clients feel confident in their ability to control the diabetes.

Figure 69–3 shows various regimens for insulin delivery. The DCCT utilized a control group that used the standard twice-daily injections of regular plus NPH insulin. The experimental group utilized intensive treatment, which consisted of continuous subcutaneous insulin infusion (CSII, or insulin pump) or multi-dose treatment of three injections of regular insulin before meals and long-acting insulin at bedtime.

Insulin Pump Therapy. Small portable pumps for the continuous administration of regular insulin are sometimes used (Fig. 69–4). The small pump, worn externally, injects insulin subcutaneously into the abdomen through an indwelling needle site that is usually changed daily. Insulin is normally infused at a low, basal rate (i.e., a rate that matches the client's basal metabolic needs), with additional infusion of larger amounts (boluses) of insulin before meals.

			Action, hr*		
Action	**Preparation**	**Appearance**	*Onset*	*Peak*	*Duration*
Short-acting	Humalog (insulin lispro injection)	Clear	Immediate	.5–1.5	2–4
	Regular	Clear	½–1	2–3	3–6
Intermediate-acting	NPH	Cloudy	2–4	4–10	10–16
	Lente	Cloudy	3–4	4–12	12–18
	Premixed (70% NPH, 30% regular)	Cloudy	½–1	2 peaks: 3–4 and 8–12	16–24
Long-acting	Ultralente	Cloudy	6–10	None	18–20

Table 69–6. Types of Humulin Insulin and Comparative Actions

* Absorption rates may vary by 20% to 40% from day to day in any one client.
From American Diabetes Association. (1994). Medical management of insulin-dependent (type I) diabetes. (2nd ed.; p. 37). Alexandria, VA; Author.

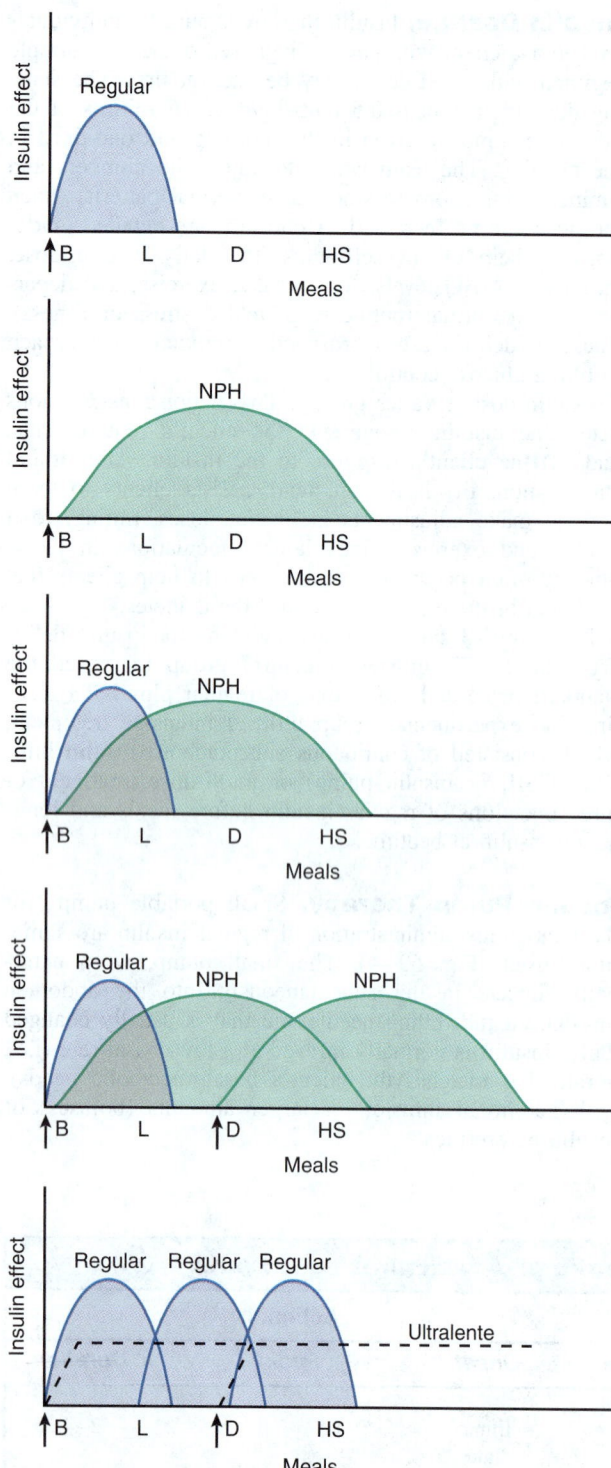

Figure 69–3. Insulin regimens. Only a few of a variety of possible regimens are shown here. Some clients require only one injection per day, whereas others may require split mixed doses (such as mixtures of NPH or Ultralente and regular insulin) or several doses of the same type of insulin (such as NPH insulin). Insulin regimens must be individualized for each client. B, breakfast; L, lunch; D, dinner; HS, bedtime.

Insulin pumps often improve blood glucose control by means of continuous subcutaneous insulin infusion. However, they do not have a built-in feedback mechanism for monitoring blood glucose levels. To benefit from an insulin pump, the client with diabetes must comply with dietary requirements and usually must deliver the correct premeal bolus of insulin. Clients must also monitor their blood glucose levels four to six times a day and make decisions regarding dosages by use of problem-solving skills.

Complications arising from use of insulin pumps include the following:

- Local infection at the injection site
- Hypoglycemia due to error in calculating insulin dosage or to pump malfunction
- Diabetic ketoacidosis due to injection of insufficient insulin for meeting regular or increased metabolic needs

For initiation of insulin pump therapy, the client must be supervised carefully in either an inpatient or an outpatient setting. During this time, the clinician adjusts the pump for basal and bolus doses before meals, according to the client's usual diet and exercise regimen and previous insulin requirements. Researchers are currently trying to produce an implantable pump that not only will administer insulin but also will monitor blood glucose levels much as a normal pancreas does.

Intensive Diabetes Therapy. Some clinicians and clients may decide to use an intensive diabetes therapy program rather than insulin pump therapy. In this therapy, the client must be willing to monitor blood glucose levels four to six times a day and take three to five insulin injections a day. Throughout the initiating period of the pump or intensive therapy, assess the client's knowledge concerning (1) the meal plan, (2) monitoring techniques, (3) management goals, and (4) manifestations of and intervention for hyperglycemia and hypoglycemia. The client also needs to be made aware of the extra financial and emotional burdens. The family and significant others need to be involved in the teaching process. Finally, the client needs to know that it cannot be guaranteed that either protocol will definitely prevent long-term complications.

■ Nursing Management of the Medical Client

Clients with newly diagnosed diabetes need extensive education for self-management. Long-term diabetics also need to have their management of diabetes reviewed. Many times, the nurse can discover errors in self-care or introduce them to newer technologies.

As in all chronic disorders, the client's physical condition, age, and basic personality must be considered when interventions are planned. For example, a client with IDDM may rebel if the diet and activities are too strictly controlled. Rebellion, in turn, may result in a self-destructive refusal to comply with any restrictions on diet or

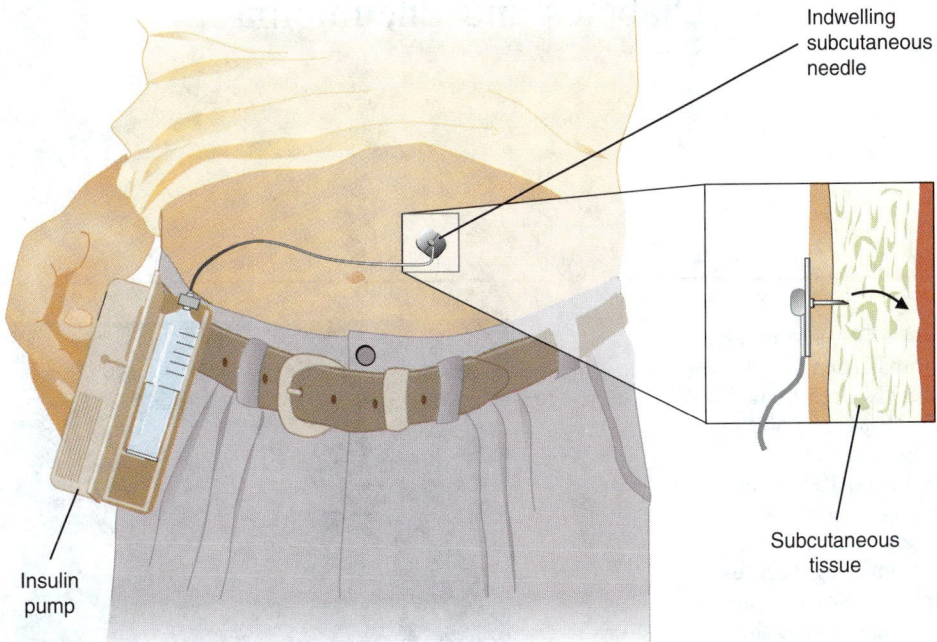

Figure 69–4. Insulin pumps are worn externally and connected to an indwelling subcutaneous needle, usually inserted in the abdomen.

activity. Another client may ritualize the diabetic regimen to the point that it totally dominates his or her life. An anxious client may worry so much about diabetes that the accumulated stress actually raises the blood glucose level.

Always investigate the client's habits and attitudes toward the illness before deciding on a plan of intervention and teaching. Tailor the plan as much as possible to the client's personality and life-style.

Diabetes education is often grouped into three main topic areas: (1) survival, (2) home care, and (3) improved life-style. Changes in life-style occur gradually over time and are dependent on the client's interest, willingness, and ability to make these changes. The healthcare team works together to develop an individualized plan of care. (See the Case Study for an example of such a plan of care.)

Generally, changes involve the following eight areas:

1. Healthy eating
2. Regular exercise
3. Taking any diabetes medications safely, regularly, and at specified times
4. Performing SMBG and urine ketone testing and utilizing the information
5. Performing routine foot care
6. Properly handling illness
7. Developing coping skills and a support system
8. Utilizing the healthcare system.

Despite the many behavior changes, most clients learn to successfully manage their diabetes.

Survival education is the critical information necessary to meet the immediate survival needs of the client. These vary widely from client to client. Insulin injection would

be a survival skill for a newly diagnosed type I client, but it is unlikely to be a necessary skill in a newly diagnosed client with type II diabetes. The simple mnemonic SUR-VIVE can be used to key into primary learning needs of the client:

S Simple pathophysiology (definition and general information on diabetes)
U Understand (relationship between food, stress, medicine, and blood glucose level)
R Regular exercise
V Variety of meal plans (basic nutrition principles)
I Insulin and/or OHA administration
V Value of normalizing blood glucose
E Educate entire family (emergency plans, identification alert, supplies)

When the client is comfortable with survival skills, he or she can progress to more in-depth information, such as treatment of hypoglycemia, monitoring, and management of insulin. Life-style improvement skills are higher-order skills and involve topics such as sick day management and adjusting medications, diet, or exercise based on SMBG.

Box 69–4 consists of teaching/learning guidelines for clients with diabetes.

Assessment

Clients with diabetes must be closely assessed for level of knowledge and ability to perform self-care. The type of diabetes, condition of the client, and plans for treatment are also important assessments to make.

Diabetes and Pneumonia

Ms. Washington is a 44-year-old black woman who has been sick for the past week. She has been treated with erythromycin (E-Mycin) 500 mg g 6 h and phenylpropanolamine-guaifensin (Entex LA) q 12 h as an outpatient after being seen in the clinic for a persistent cough, loss of voice, chest pain from coughing, fever, chills, and mild nausea without vomiting. She now reports that she has been coughing sputum that is brown to green, with small amounts of red blood present. Ms. Washington is also complaining of left shoulder pain of 3 days' duration, fatigue, sinus pressure, congestion, fullness in the ears, and postnasal drainage. She also reports frequent urination without dysuria or urgency and feeling thirsty all the time. Her history is significant for gestational diabetes 11 years ago, at which time she administered her own insulin injections. At this time, she is being admitted for failed treatment of pneumonia and control of new-onset diabetes. Consider whether Ms. Washington has type I or type II diabetes mellitus and the effect of that type of diabetes on her treatment plan and future complications.

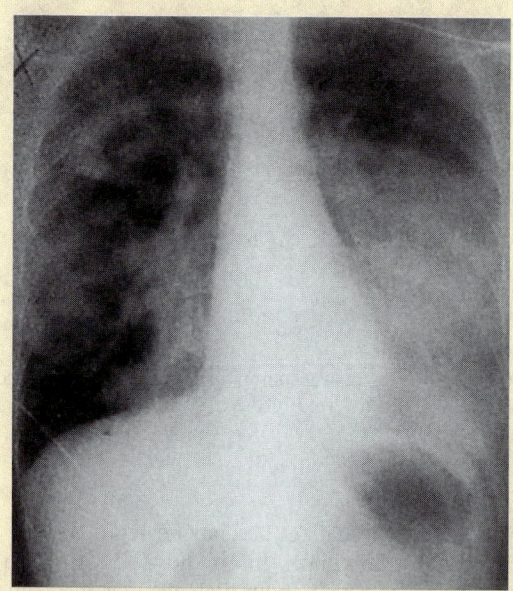

■ Ms. Washington's chest x-ray indicates the presence of thickened bronchioles with left lower lobe infiltrates. The cardiac silhouette is normal.

Admission Laboratory Values

RBC	3.7 million/mm³
Hgb	10.5 g/dl
Hct	31%
WBC	15,600/mm³
Neutrophils	81%
BUN	5 mg/dl
Creatinine	0.7 mg/dl
Cholesterol	176 mg/dl
Triglycerides	134 mg/dl
Potassium	5.3 mEq/L
Chloride	96 mEq/L
Sodium	139 mEq/L
Glucose	335 mg/dl

Nursing Admission Assessment

Ms. Washington is a single mother of an 11-year-old son. She works from 6 AM to 2 PM at McDonald's 6 days a week, where she stands at the counter. She reports that the benefits of the job are medical insurance and that she also receives free food for herself and discounted food for her son when he stops for breakfast on his way to school. Her father died of diabetes complicated by heart disease, and her mother died of diabetes complicated by CVA. She admits to smoking one pack of cigarettes a day for 20 years and denies use of alcohol. However, she reports drinking 1 gal of bottled fruit juice daily.

Nursing Physical Examination

Height: 5'7" Weight: 192 lb (87.3 kg).
Vital Signs: BP = 144/94;
TPR = 100.8, 78, 18

LOC: Alert and cooperative
EENT: Nasal mucosa unremarkable, yellow-green drainage on pharynx
Cardiac: Regular rate and rhythm without gallop or murmur
Pulmonary: Decreased breath sounds at bases, with the left greater than the right; wheezes and rhonchi noted at the left lower lobe; increased tactile fremitus
Abdominal: Soft and nontender with active bowel tones
Genitourinary: Reports vaginal itching and white "clumpy" discharge
Peripheral pulses: 3/3, without edema

Initial Treatment Plan

Meds: Cefazolin (Ancef) 1 g IV q 8 h
Triamcinolone acetonide (Kenaject-40) 40 mg IM now
Human insulin (Humulin)
NPH 20 U SQ AM, 10 U SQ PM, Sliding-scale insulin AC and HS: Humulin regular SQ

according to serum glucose level:

< 150 mg/dl 0 units
151–250 mg/dl 3 units
251–350 mg/dl 6 units
> 350 mg/dl Call

Saline flush IV lock bid and after meds

What effect, if any, would the admission medication orders have on Ms. Washington's blood glucose?

Diet: 1200 ADA; develop a sample 24-hour diet plan for Ms. Washington
Activity: As tolerated
Respiratory treatments: Albuterol (Ventolin) 2.5 mg in 3 ml NS aerosol qid; incentive spirometer Q 2 h while awake
Diagnostic tests: Blood sugars qid AC and HS; Repeat CBC, electrolytes, chest x-ray in AM

At 11:00 AM on day 2, Ms. Washington's serum glucose level is 265 mg/dl. How much insulin will she require?

Over the next 3 days, Ms. Washington's blood sugars stabilize. Her physician adds 10 U Humulin regular to her routine AM insulin dose and 5 U Humulin regular to her routine PM insulin dose and discontinues the orders for sliding-scale insulin. The physician writes an order for the client to continue monitoring blood sugars with a glucometer qid. Yesterday, her fluid intake was 1980 ml, and her urinary output was 1575 ml. She remains on her 1200 ADA diet, but says that she would like a Big Mac and French fries. Yesterday, the nurse discovered several candy bars in the drawer of Ms. Washington's bedside table.

Ms. Washington no longer complains of sinus pressure or postnasal drainage. Her cough remains produc-

tive of small amounts of white, thick sputum. Lung sounds remain diminished, but clear after coughing. She is able to raise her incentive spirometer measurement to 1500 ml. Her antibiotic has been changed to clarithromycin (Biaxin) 500 mg bid with food × 10 days. The physician has also ordered Miconazole (Monistat) vaginal cream daily. What instructions would you give Ms. Washington about administration of the vaginal cream?

Most recent laboratory values reveal a potassium of 4.0 mEq/L, chloride of 100 mEq/L, and sodium of 139 mEq/L. Her fasting blood sugar this AM was 95 mg/dl, and the WBC count was 10×10^9/L.

The physician is planning to discharge her tomorrow.

Discharge Criteria

Average LOS (insurance certification): 5.5 days

Initiate diabetes instruction for survival, home care, and improved lifestyle. Consider using the mnemonic SURVIVE to implement discharge teaching.

Complete community referrals. What referrals would you make? Why?

Questions to Be Considered

1. In the progress notes, Ms. Washington's physician reports a shift to the left in her WBC count. What does this mean? Discuss the relationship between diabetes mellitus and susceptibility to infection and response to treatment. What influence do infections exert over control of diabetes mellitus?
2. How would the physician's decision to prescribe mixed-dose insulin influence the triangle of control (diet, exercise, pharmacologic agents)? What are the benefits? What are the risks?

3. What influence did her socioeconomic status, race, and heredity have on Ms. Washington's development of diabetes mellitus? What continuing influence will these factors play in her regulation of the diabetes? What effect will her current employment likely have on Ms. Washington's compliance with, and ability to financially afford, diet, foot care, glucose monitoring, and exercise?
4. Based on the coping tasks presented by Miller (Box 69–3), identify specific behaviors that would convince a home health nurse that Ms. Washington is coping with her diabetes.
5. Describe the pathophysiologic basis for the change in Ms. Washington's potassium levels and her development of polyuria, polydipsia, polyphagia, and weight loss.
6. Ms. Washington's employer calls the nurses' station and asks, "Ms. Washington has informed me that she will be unable to return to work for 10 days. Is this true?" How would you respond? What are the ethical considerations you should make in formulating your response?
7. Ten days post discharge, Ms. Washington complains of fever, nausea, vomiting, and diarrhea. What directions would you give?

Box 69–4. Learning/Teaching Guidelines for Clients with Diabetes

I. Assess knowledge about diabetes mellitus, correct misinformation
II. Reteach or build on previously learned content to build baseline and confidence
III. General content for diabetic education includes:
   A. Basic anatomy and physiology of the pancreas
   B. Definition of diabetes and relationship to abnormal function of pancreas
   C. Manifestations of hyperglycemia
   D. Methods to control hyperglycemia:
      1. Diet must be individualized—refer to dietitian accordingly
      2. Exercise—client may need complete physical examination prior to exercise program to assess cardiac status, neuropathy, retinopathy, and nutritional needs (weight loss is commonly indicated)
      3. Oral hypoglycemic agents
      4. Insulin
      5. Recognize precipitating factors to development of hyperglycemia
   E. Insulin education: how/when/why/where to give insulin combinations
   F. Basic information about what diabetic client should do when ill and/or traveling
   G. When to call physician
   H. Daily blood glucose testing and recording
   I. Storing insulin and needles
   J. Needle disposal and universal precautions
   K. Using and recycling needles
   L. How to use a blood glucose monitor and test urine for ketones
   M. Complications of diabetes mellitus—definition, cause, manifestations, treatment
      1. Acute: Hypoglycemia, diabetic ketoacidosis, HHNK
      2. Chronic: Microvascular: retinopathy, nephropathy, neuropathy; macrovascular: cardiovascular, hypertension, peripheral vascular disease, infections
   N. Diabetics need routine physician follow-up to provide early diagnosis and treatment of acute and chronic complications, evaluation of present means of diabetic care, and treatment of co-existing medical disorders
   O. Identify available community and family resources
IV. Encourage client to keep written goals and diary outlining goals of weight, blood glucose, medicine administration, diet and exercise, and how he or she feels from day to day.

Adapted from Luckmann, J. (Ed.) (1995). *Saunders manual of nursing care.* Philadelphia: W. B. Saunders.

Diagnosis, Planning, Implementation

Altered Health Maintenance. The client with diabetes must be able to perform self-care to keep the condition well-controlled, leading to the nursing diagnosis *Altered Health Maintenance related to lack of knowledge about diabetes mellitus.*

Planning: Expected Outcomes. The client will relate the basic pathophysiologic mechanism of diabetes mellitus; explain the need for insulin, exercise, and diet in the treatment; and list the clinical manifestations of acute and chronic complications.

Implementation. The nurse or diabetes educator explains the basic pathophysiologic mechanism of diabetes to the client and family. Sometimes the information is given through classes or by videotape. The client should also be given some form of written information for reinforcement of the material. In addition, the nurse monitors for denial or anger about the diagnosis as part of a coping response.

Clients with diabetes must consult the clinician before starting an exercise program. Pre-exercise screening may include the following: history, physical examination, Hb A_{1c} assay, exercise stress test, foot evaluation, and blood glucose level. Many clients with diabetes may not be able to exercise intensely to a calculated heart rate because of pre-existing heart conditions, age, or joint problems. The client should be helped to choose an exercise regimen and to set reasonable goals, because any increase in activity level is beneficial. Walking is usually well tolerated. Using a stationary bicycle or swimming is possible for clients with foot problems. Clients with diabetes must start any new activity at a well-tolerated intensity level and duration, gradually (over a period of weeks or months) increasing the activity until they reach their exercise goals. They should include warm-up and cool-down periods before and after exercise. It is best to exercise at the same time of day, when possible. Because regular exercise is so important, have the client plan an alternative activity in case environmental or other factors make the usual exercise difficult. Unplanned exercise can be dangerous for clients taking insulin or oral hypoglycemic agents. During periods of exercise, the muscles are stimulated to take up glucose. Therefore, blood glucose levels can fall abruptly.

Clients should ensure they are adequately hydrated before starting exercise. They should eat 15 to 30 g of carbohydrate before exercise if the blood glucose level is less than 100 mg/dl and carry a carbohydrate snack as well as their diabetes identification. If blood glucose is 100 to 150 mg/dl, the client may exercise and have a snack later. If blood glucose is greater than 250 mg/dl and the client has not just eaten, ketone levels should be checked. Clients with glucose in this level should wait to exercise, because vigorous activity can raise blood glucose levels by releasing stored glycogen. Alcohol and beta-blockers should be avoided.

Risk for Ineffective Management of Therapeutic Regimen (Individuals).

The client with diabetes must understand and be able to self-monitor the glucose level, leading to a priority diagnosis of *Individual Risk for Ineffective Management of Therapeutic Regimen (Individuals) related to ability to test blood and urine.*

Planning: Expected Outcomes. The client will state personal goals for urine ketone and blood glucose testing parameters; demonstrate correct techniques for blood glucose tests (including timing of tests); demonstrate correct technique for urine ketone test (including timing of test) (type I diabetics only); test blood glucose at regular times, including during illnesses and when traveling; prick the side of the finger, where nerve endings are fewer and more blood is available; test urine for ketones when glucose is high (over 250 mg/dl) or during illnesses; keep a record of all tests performed and bring this record to regular, scheduled follow-up visits; and store testing materials away from heat, light, and moisture.

Implementation. All clients with newly diagnosed diabetes mellitus require teaching about urine and blood glucose monitoring. All clients with diabetes may require review or update of information for self-care.

Newer, easier, and more accurate blood glucose meters are constantly being made available. Only the basics are covered in this discussion, so the nurse must keep up-to-date on each meter's advantages and disadvantages.

Many different kinds of meters are available. Each client needs to be evaluated so that the proper meter is obtained. The client's ability to calibrate the meter and to visually interpret the digital reading needs to be considered. Some meters can be connected to a computer, which can convert blood glucose results into bar graphs or other printouts. Glucose meters are available for the visually impaired that give audio commands to use the device and to announce the blood glucose reading.

In addition to demonstrating the techniques of blood glucose self-monitoring, discuss the normal blood glucose range, goals for good control (individualized for each client), when to test, how to record test results, and what to do for abnormal results. Consult a diabetes educator for assistance in helping the client choose an optimal meter.

Some clients visually read blood glucose strips when they are not able or willing to purchase a meter. Make sure the client is not colorblind, or these results will be inaccurate. Compare the client's results with a blood glucose meter to check for accuracy.

Remember that with some meters and strips a 15% difference is seen between capillary blood and venous blood glucose levels. The capillary blood reading is lower. When insulin is being adjusted, make sure that this difference is accounted for. As long as the source of blood is consistent, no adjustment is required.

Both healthcare agencies and clients need to verify the accuracy of their blood glucose determinations. The Joint Commission on Accreditation of Healthcare Organizations (JCAHO) and other regulating bodies dictate the procedure and frequency for quality control of meters used in healthcare agencies. Many glucose meters are technique dependent. Because treatment is based on results, correct methods of use must be ensured. Clients can perform a self-test and simultaneously send a blood specimen to the laboratory to compare results. Manufacturers of meters also provide quality-control testing solutions, which clients should be instructed to use routinely (i.e., weekly). Quality control of glucose monitors is a constantly changing area; nurses and clients must keep up to date.

Urine testing for glucose is rarely done. Urine, however, can be tested for ketones (beta-hydroxybutyric acid, acetoacetic acid, and acetone). These substances appear in the urine of (1) clients who are fasting, (2) clients with IDDM who are insulin-deficient, and (3) clients with IDDM or NIDDM who have a secondary illness.

Ketones result from fat metabolism and are therefore present during fasting. In a client with diabetes, however, the presence of ketones may indicate a serious complication: diabetic ketoacidosis. Ketoacidosis is discussed further in the Acute Complications section of the chapter.

Knowledge Deficit.

For the diabetes to be under good control, the client must learn the necessary dietary principles, leading to the nursing diagnosis *Knowledge Deficit related to lack of knowledge about dietary management of diabetes.*

Planning: Expected Outcomes. The client will state the relationship of dietary management to blood glucose control; choose foods that meet caloric needs and offer a well-balanced diet; recognize the times at which it is necessary to substitute a food to maintain blood glucose control; discuss with the healthcare team difficulties seen in compliance with plans for diet; maintain blood glucose level within preset parameters; and maintain weight within preset parameters.

Implementation. A balanced nutritional plan is important for all clients, whether or not they have diabetes. Emphasize to the client and family that they are not eating a diabetic diet, but rather a balanced meal plan.

Adherence to nutrition principles is one of the most challenging aspects of diabetes management. It requires a team effort. For an effective plan, assessment of the individual's present eating patterns, knowledge of a healthy eating plan, and willingness and ability to modify patterns and nutritional needs is vital. Specific nutritional information should include the following:

● Appetite
● Food allergies
● Ethnic and cultural impact on food habits
● Ability to obtain (including financial ability) and prepare food
● Community resources currently used
● Amount and type of physical activity
● Chronic disease requiring dietary modification
● Gastrointestinal disease
● Vitamin, mineral, or food supplementation used

- Weight patterns
- Current eating patterns
- Dietary concerns of client
- Dental and oral health
- Medications with nutritional implications

The results of this assessment form a personal profile utilized to arrive at individualized goals.

The nurse, as a member of the healthcare team, must have a knowledge base of both nutritional assessment and appropriate interventions. The DCCT reaffirmed the importance of the team approach in successful diabetes management.

Basic nutritional assessment includes anthropometric measures, biochemical tests, physical assessment, and dietary evaluation. No single parameter can measure the client's nutritional status or determine problems or needs. Figure 69–5 shows how assessment fits into the total nutritional plan for the collaborative management of diabetes.

Following assessment, individualized goals are determined. Nutritional assessment and the client's understanding that optimal nutrition can lead to reduction of risk factors for chronic health problems and improve overall health constitute the starting point for goal selection.

For example, if the client has type II diabetes and is obese, teaching should emphasize that nutritional changes can assist in lowering blood glucose levels, decreasing lipid levels, and lowering blood pressure, as well as losing weight. Weight loss also appears to increase insulin sensitivity and to normalize liver glucose production. This client should understand that dietary treatment is the best and initial treatment. If nutritional status does not improve, glucose-lowering medications, insulin, lipid-lowering agents, and/or antihypertensives may be required.

A standard "diabetic diet" is no longer prescribed for all clients with diabetes; instead, many dietary options exist (Table 69–7). Basically, the client with diabetes should strive to follow the Dietary Guidelines for Americans (the Food Guide Pyramid) issued by the U.S. Department of Agriculture (USDA) and Health and Human Services in 1992 for current recommended nutritional guidelines.

Calories. Caloric restrictions, especially for people with lifelong obesity, may be perceived negatively. Obesity is a complex interaction between genetic and environmental factors. The most successful approach to weight reduction is unclear, but methods for the nurse to understand are caloric restriction, regular exercise, behavior modification, and peer/professional support. Moderate caloric reduction is described as a reduction of 250 to 500 calories per day below usual. Reduction of fat calories may be a good initial modification. Regular exercise (3 to 5 times/week) enhances weight loss and is a predictor for successful weight maintenance.

Protein. In general, individuals in the United States, with and without diabetes, consume more protein than is necessary to meet nutritional needs. Protein should be incorporated into the diet through a variety of foods. Very hypocaloric diets are often deficient in protein and may result in accelerated protein breakdown. High protein intake increases renal workload and glomerular filtration rate (GFR). Some studies in people with diabetes indicate that lowering protein intake may delay progression of nephropathy. At present, the lower end of the recommended scale (about 10% of daily calories) is sufficiently restricted and is recommended for clients with nephropathy.

A number of cases exist in which protein requirements vary from the adult recommended daily allowance

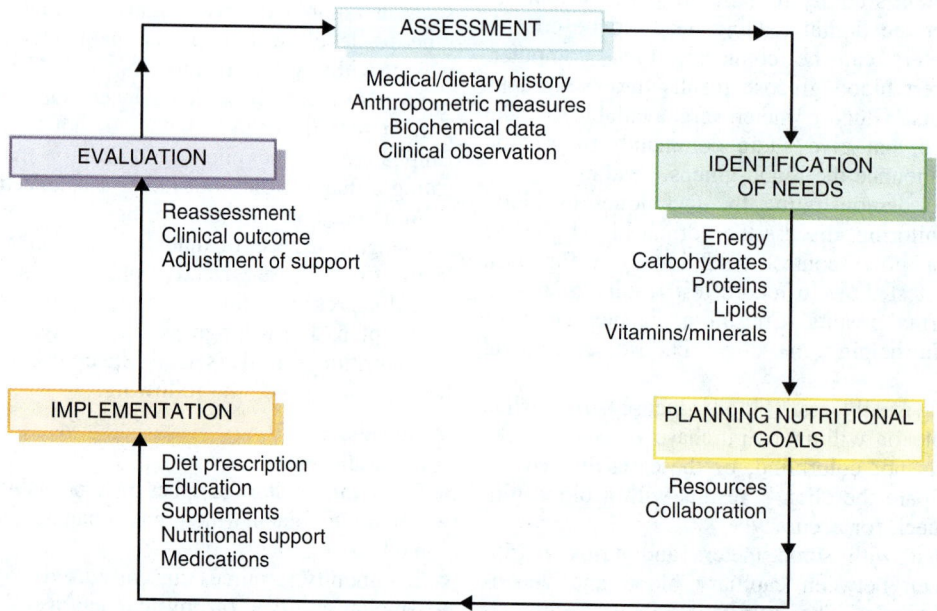

Figure 69–5. Assessment as part of the total nutritional plan for the collaborative management of diabetes. (Redrawn from Groth, K. [1995]. Nutritional alterations in critical illness. In L. C. Copstead [Ed.], *Perspectives on pathophysiology* [p. 1124]. Philadelphia: W. B. Saunders.)

Table 69–7. Currently Recommended Nutritional Guidelines for the Individual with Diabetes Mellitus	
Calories	Sufficient to achieve and maintain reasonable weight
Protein	Adequate to ensure maintenance of body protein stores; individuals with diabetes have the same protein requirements as nondiabetics; in general 10%–20% of the total daily calories should come from protein (equal to ~0.8 g/kg/day)
Fats	Less than 30% of calories should be from fat with less than 10% of that from saturated fat sources; if individualized risk factors indicate elevated VLDL and LDL, total calories from saturated fat may be reduced to 7%; cholesterol intake should be limited to 300 mg/day or less
Carbohydrates	50%–60% of total calories should be from carbohydrates; simple and complex sugars do not differ appreciably in their ability to worsen hyperglycemia
Fiber	Clients with diabetes are urged to consume 20–35 g of fiber per day, which is the same as the recommendation for all Americans

(RDA). This is true for infants, children, adolescents, and pregnant females.

Fat. The USDA national food consumption surveys reveal that the diets of most Americans are too high in fat. Approximately 36% of calories in the average adult diet come from fat, with approximately 13% from saturated fat. The general recommendation for the U.S. population is to decrease total dietary fat to 30% or less of total calories, with emphasis on reduction of saturated fat to less than 10%. This reduction is consistent with a diet to reduce cardiovascular disease. Clients with type II diabetes often have high triglycerides levels, high LDL and very-low-density lipoprotein (VLDL) levels, and low high-density lipoprotein (HDL) levels. This is a result of increased liver production of triglyceride-rich VLDLs, genetic predisposition, hyperinsulinemia, insulin resistance, or intra-abdominal fat accumulation. Limiting daily cholesterol intake to 300 mg is also recommended. All of these lipid-related dietary modifications are recommended for clients with diabetes as well as for all other Americans.

The guidelines further suggest that people with elevated LDL levels should reduce their intake of saturated fat to 7% of total calories and their intake of total cholesterol to less than 200 mg/day. Controversy continues about whether it is better to increase fiber and carbohydrates or to replace saturated fat with unsaturated fat.

Carbohydrates. For most of this century, the most widely held belief about dietary treatment of diabetes was that sugar should be avoided. Little or no scientific evidence supports this assumption. When fed as a single nutrient, sucrose produces a glycemic response similar to that of bread or pasta. In the United States, the average diet obtains almost half of total carbohydrate intake in the form of simple sugars. Clinical guidelines suggest that 50% to 60% of the diet should consist of carbohydrates, either in simple or complex form. An occasional high-sucrose dessert poses no problem for the client with diabetes when it is accounted for in the day's total caloric and carbohydrate plan. Because some desserts are also high in fat, however, they should be limited.

Fiber. Large amounts of fiber have an effect on serum lipid levels but probably an insignificant effect on glycemic control. The typical fiber intake in the United States is low (average, 10 to 12 g/day). Recommendations are to increase this to 20 to 35 g/day.

Sodium and Vitamins. Sodium has variable effects. Sodium intake recommendations for the client with diabetes are the same as for the general population: 2,400 to 3,000 mg/day. Most clients with diabetes do not appear to require routine vitamin and mineral supplementation. Research is continuing in the areas of magnesium and vitamin C and E supplementation.

Working as a team with the client database and a nutritionist, make a concrete medical nutrition therapy plan. The following are some helpful questions to ask clients:

What is your most important goal in managing your diabetes?
What are some changes you would like to make?
Of the changes we have talked about, what would you like to work on first?

Team members must remember their roles as providers of information and counselors. Most counseling on nutrition begins with basic overviews of nutrition, diabetes guidelines, and reading of labels. More in-depth counseling on meal planning and calorie counting, for example, can come later. Eating plans vary widely among individuals. Consistency within an eating style results in lower levels of glycosylated hemoglobins than does a haphazard eating style.

Type I Diabetic Diet Management. For the client with type I diabetes, meals should be adjusted to match insulin action. Breakfast should be eaten within 1 hour after the morning insulin dose and a carbohydrate should be eaten about 3 hours later; lunch should be eaten about 4 to 5 hours after the morning insulin dose. When multiple insulin injections are utilized, greater flexibility with meal timing is possible.

Because we can no longer rely on preprinted diet sheets and exchange lists of nutrients to give our clients, we need to rely more on our knowledge of nutrition, diabetes, behavior change, and education in working with clients. The following are examples of approaches used successfully to instruct clients with diabetes:

- Handouts available from government sources, such as the USDA's "The Food Guide Pyramid" and "Eating Right with the Dietary Guidelines". The USDHHS also has a publication called "Nutrition and Your Health: Dietary Guidelines for Americans," which uses the four basic food group approach.
- Individualized menus shaped between the client and dietitian.
- The exchange system, last revised in 1986, can help with uniform meal planning. It is available from the American Diabetes Association (ADA) in a simple pamphlet called "Healthy Food Choices," or in an expanded version called "Exchange Lists for Meal Planning."
- Counting components of the diet, such as counting calories and grams of fat.
- A point system that utilizes lists of foods with point values and a prescribed number of total points.
- The total available glucose (TAG) system, which looks at foods in terms of their metabolic effects. Highly motivated clients who desire flexibility may like this system.

A registered dietitian (preferably a certified diabetes educator) should always be consulted for initial evaluation and teaching of any client with a new diagnosis of diabetes. Each client should receive an individualized meal plan based on ethnic, religious, and cultural background; eating, cooking, and work habits; and food preferences.

All clients need to know the dietary basics, which include the following:

- Avoid adding sugar to foods (e.g., coffee, cereal)
- Avoid foods that are sweetened with sugar or honey (e.g., jellies, jams, cakes, ice cream)
- Check blood glucose levels regularly
- Keep periodic appointments with healthcare providers for evaluation of blood glucose control
- Be consistent regarding amount, distribution, and timing of nutrients
- Increase amount of carbohydrate in the meal before sustained exercise
- Limit intake of saturated fat and cholesterol

Risk for Ineffective Management of Therapeutic Regimen (Individuals).
The client must learn self-injection of insulin, leading to the nursing diagnosis *Individual Risk for Ineffective Management of Therapeutic Regimen (Individuals) related to knowledge of self-injection of insulin.*

Planning: Expected Outcomes.
The client will state that insulin lowers blood glucose; state the type or types of insulin prescribed and the onset, peak, and duration of each; take injections at regular times, 30 to 60 minutes before meals, every day, even when ill; wash hands before preparing insulin injection; demonstrate proper mixing of insulin; withdraw prescribed dosage, using sterile technique; when taking two types of insulin, withdraw the prescribed dosage of each insulin into one syringe without contaminating either bottle (regular insulin is drawn up first); demonstrate the correct technique of insulin injection; inject insulin into same site to be

able to safely rely on onset, peak, and duration; store at least one extra bottle of insulin in the refrigerator and not use insulin past the expiration date; purchase insulin syringes before all of the current supply has been used; wear a Medic-Alert bracelet or necklace, or carry an identification card; state manifestations and treatment of hypoglycemia; and always carry something for treatment of hypoglycemia.

Implementation.

Insulin Administration. When administered correctly, insulin acts as a life-saving medication for the insulin-dependent client. When administered incorrectly, insulin may cause complications ranging from tissue damage to lethal hypoglycemia (insulin shock). To administer insulin properly, the client must be familiar with insulin concentrations, syringes, storage, preparation for injection, and techniques for self-injection.

Insulin Concentrations. Insulin is prescribed in units. Thus, pharmaceutical companies prepare types of insulin (NPH, regular, Lente) in 10-ml glass vials that contain 100 units/ml. U-100 insulin contains 100 units of insulin per milliliter.

Insulin Syringes. The most commonly used syringe can deliver a maximum of 100 units in 1 cc. For smaller prescriptions, smaller syringes are available: for 50 units or less and for 30 units or less. Using a smaller syringe can enable the smaller insulin dosage to be more precise. Figure 69–6 shows three sizes of insulin syringes.

Insulin Storage. Vials of insulin not in use should be refrigerated. Avoid temperature extremes less than 36° F or greater than 86° F. Vials in use may be kept at room temperature. A slight loss of potency may occur after 30 days at room temperature. Mark the date on the vial when it was initially opened. The client should always have a spare vial on hand.

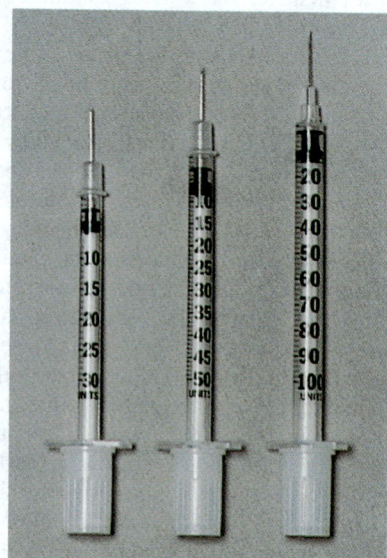

Figure 69–6. Examples of the sizes of insulin syringes that are available for precise measurement of insulin doses. (Courtesy of Becton Dickinson Consumer Products, Franklin Lakes, NJ.)

Insulin Preparation and Injection. Avoid excess agitation of bottle to prevent loss of potency, clumping, frosting, or precipitation. To minimize the discomfort associated with subcutaneous insulin injection, administer the insulin at room temperature. If alcohol is used to clean the site, wait until it has evaporated completely. Have the client try to relax. Penetrate the skin quickly. Do not change the direction of the needle once it has entered the subcutaneous tissue or while it is being withdrawn.

Prefilled Syringes. Prefilled syringes are chemically stable for up to 3 weeks when stored vertically, needle upward (so suspended particles don't clog the needle), in the refrigerator. The syringe should be gently rolled between the hands before administration. SMBG may need to be performed more frequently to check the effect of prefilling on glycemic control.

Mixing regular and NPH insulins in one syringe is acceptable and convenient. Premixed, fixed-proportion insulins are available commercially. These insulins are not suitable when daily variations in the dose or when short-acting insulin is required.

Site Selection and Rotation. Figure 69–7 illustrates the sites used for insulin injection. Insulin absorption varies from site to site. For avoidance of dramatic changes in daily insulin absorption, instruct the client to give injections in one area, about an inch apart, until the whole area has been used, then change to another site. Instruct the client to avoid sites above muscles that will be exercised heavily that day, because exercise increases the rate of absorption. The client who is taking two injections daily may use one site for the morning insulin and another site for the evening insulin. Some clinicians instruct their clients to use only the abdomen because of its more even and rapid absorption rate. Emphasize to the diabetic client the importance of adhering to a definite injection plan for avoiding tissue damage. Rotate injection sites in one area to decrease the variability of absorption.

Techniques for Self-Injection. The majority of clients who take insulin learn to give their own injections. It is primarily the nurse's responsibility to instruct clients with diabetes in the technique of preparing insulin and injecting themselves. The amount of teaching needed depends on the client's familiarity with insulin and the injection equipment. Teaching guidelines for clients with IDDM are discussed later in the chapter.

Equipment that the client must purchase for home use includes the following: (1) insulin of the type prescribed, (2) absorbent cotton, (3) approved syringes with needles, and (4) 70% ethyl or 91% isopropyl alcohol.

Although the prospect of daily injections for life is far from pleasant, the client's attitude toward this intervention may be largely influenced by the nurse. A matter-of-fact attitude helps the client understand and accept responsibility for self-care. Schedule a teaching/learning session for self-injection techniques. Some clients find it difficult to inject the needle into their own skin. For these clients, the nurse might select the site and inject the needle. Then, as the first step in self-injection, have the client push in the plunger and remove the needle. As the client gains confidence, self-injecting will be less traumatic. Jet injections can be used, which are pen-like devices. See the Client Education Guide for instructions on injections.

Evaluation

For a newly diagnosed diabetic, return demonstration should be expected for all activities with increasing proficiency over time. The client should not be expected to be able to accomplish complete self-care after a single teaching session. The amount of time required varies from client to client. Follow-up visits must be initiated to ensure that the client is following recommendations and has not developed problems with the therapeutic regimen. Over time, periodic repeat visits will help monitor the client's ability to perform self-care and anticipate any potential difficulties.

Before discharge, the client and family must have a basic understanding of diabetes and its management with blood glucose monitoring, insulin injections, nutrition, and exercise. Because diabetes is a chronic disorder, the client needs time to adapt to as well as to learn about the many changes that are occurring. Discussions should be held regarding the potential complications with any regimen (see Ethical Issues in Nursing). The client should be encouraged to anticipate a usual day at work, school, or home, and should be taught how and when insulin is to

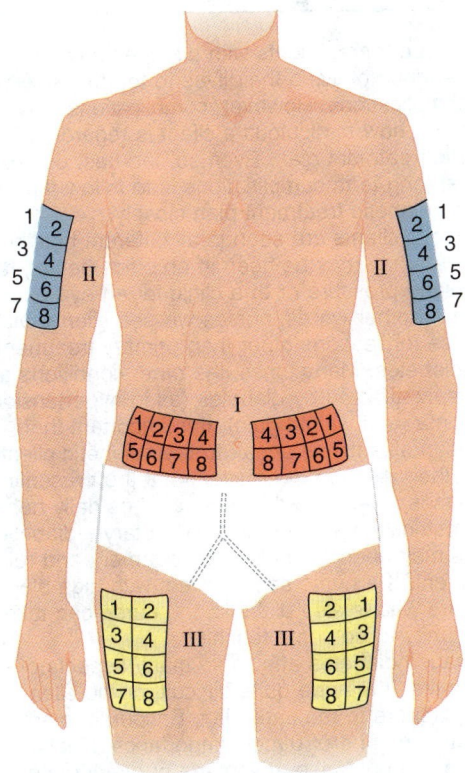

Figure 69–7. Sites used for insulin injection. The injection site can affect the onset, peak, and duration of action of the insulin. Insulin injected into the abdomen (area I) is absorbed fastest, followed by insulin injected into the arm (area II) and the leg (area III).

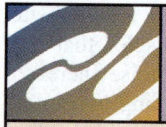

CLIENT EDUCATION GUIDE

Self-Injection of Insulin

Procedure

Wash hands.

Cleanse site (soap and water or 70% isopropyl alcohol).

Wipe top of insulin bottle with 70% isopropyl alcohol.

Roll bottle in palm of hands to resuspend (all but short-acting insulins).

Inject an amount of air that is equal to each dose into the bottle—short-acting last.

Insulin solution should be clear.

Aspirate prescribed amount of short-acting insulin into syringe first, intermediate- or long-acting insulin second.

Inspect syringe for air bubbles.

Pinch up and hold skinfold and inject at 90 degree angle.

If you are thin or have loose skin, inject insulin at 45 degree angle to avoid an intramuscular injection, which is absorbed faster.

Routine aspiration is not necessary.

Inject insulin.

If injection is painful or blood/serum oozes from site, apply pressure for 5 to 10 seconds.

Disposal

State laws require that needles and syringes be disposed as a single unit in a puncture-resistant container. It is unsafe to recap, bend, or break the needle.

Syringe Reuse

It is the manufacturer's intent and design that the insulin syringe and needle are to be disposed after one use. Research demonstrates that most people with diabetes reuse the needle and syringe until the needle becomes dull or bent or comes in contact with any surface other than skin. Most insulins have a bacteriostatic agent in them. If you reuse syringes and needles, the needle should be recapped after each use. Be aware that reusing may carry increased risk for infection, especially if you have poor personal hygiene, acute concurrent illness, or open wounds on hands. Discuss the practice of reuse with your practitioner before initiating (Can you safely recap the needle? Can you see clearly enough? How is your manual dexterity? Do you have a visible tremor?) Store syringes at room temperature. The potential benefit of using alcohol on the needle is unknown. It may remove the silicone coat on the needle and contribute to pain at the puncture site.

ally checked, as is the client's log of daily glucose levels and insulin. Female clients need to increase their insulin dose during menses.

The chronic changes that occur from diabetes are also assessed on an ongoing basis. The client's vision, kidney function, degree of neuropathy, hypertension, and skin condition are assessed.

If the client is elderly or debilitated, visiting nurses may be an excellent asset for the client. A referral to a visiting nurse organization or home health care agency should be initiated before discharge.

■ Modifications for Elderly Clients

Because nearly 20% of Americans age 65 or older have diabetes, the nurse must be aware of and understand the complications of diabetes in the elderly population.

Many changes that occur with normal aging affect glucose levels. Blood glucose levels increase with age; fasting levels increase about 1 mg/dl per decade and postprandial values by 6 to 13 mg/dl per decade. It is

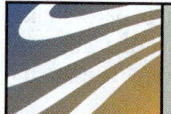

ETHICAL ISSUES IN NURSING

How Do Nurses Teach Compliance to Diabetic Clients?

With proper care, clients with diabetes have a very good chance of living their lives to the fullest with few complications. However, complications may arise no matter how meticulous a client is regarding the diabetic treatment plan. Even so, the best defense against long-term complications is to follow the prescribed diabetic treatment plan closely.

Diabetic clients are seen in all different healthcare settings. They may be seen in an office setting for high blood pressure or at a clinic for an eye examination. In other words, nurses will see clients with diabetes for reasons other than primary treatment of their diabetes. Many times, the other conditions are adversely affected by diabetes (as in hypertension, glaucoma, and weight gain). It is important that nurses in all settings speak to their diabetic clients about their disease (no matter what the presenting problem is). Because diabetes requires daily behavioral restrictions—predominantly dietary—diabetic clients may need a lot of encouragement and reinforcement. If a nurse sees a client with high blood pressure who is also diabetic, the nurse can take an opportunity to do some teaching.

Because diabetes affects so many aspects of the client's life, it may be quite difficult for the client to strictly adhere to the care plan. Encouragement and education can be of utmost importance. Healthcare providers should take advantage of every opportunity to assess their diabetic client's level of understanding and feelings about the disease. It is through this education that diabetic clients are given their best defense against the complications of their disease.

be given, how blood glucose is to be monitored, and what type of foods are to be eaten.

Diabetic clients need ongoing care for monitoring their self-care ability. Glycosylated hemoglobin levels are usu-

believed that peripheral receptor sites become less sensitive to insulin with time. A decline also takes place in glucose-regulating hormones (glucagon and epinephrine), and lean body mass. These may be accompanied by decreased physical activity and a poor diet. The elderly are more susceptible to severe hypoglycemia, which can lead to stroke, myocardial infarction, angina, or seizures. Diminished sensations may mask the manifestations of hyperglycemia. Accompanying changes in liver and kidney function and multi-drug regimens may exacerbate hypoglycemia.

In general, nutritional guidelines for elderly with diabetes are no different than those for elderly without diabetes. Elderly persons with diabetes are at increased risk for problems that can cause functional limitations. These include the following:

- Pain
- Incontinence of urine
- Decreased vision (retinopathy, glaucoma, cataracts)
- Decreased proprioception
- Postural hypotension

Mental status, functional abilities, and sensory function may interfere with the client's ability to understand and follow the treatment plan. In the elderly client, the risk of acute complications from hypoglycemia may outweigh the benefits of tight glucose control. The elderly client may enjoy good health and do very well on an individualized treatment plan. Working together to maximize health through improved diet and exercise may improve quality of life as well as glucose control.

Critical Care

■ Surgical Management

Some clients with type I are now receiving pancreas transplants. The first pancreas transplant was completed in 1966. Most (80%) pancreas transplants are now done concurrently with a kidney transplant. This is usually because the anti-rejection medications (i.e., cyclosporine) have such severe side effects, which include hyperglycemia and nephrotoxicity, that adequate renal function unaffected by nephropathy must be present. The client's own pancreas is left intact (98% of its function is exocrine in nature), and the new pancreas is usually anastomosed to the iliac artery and vein, where insulin can enter the systemic pathway. The exocrine secretions of the new pancreas drain into the bladder and are not absorbed. The client survival rate is 91% after transplant. Greater than 65% of clients receiving transplants no longer need insulin at 1 year afterward. Research is being conducted on the use of transplanted pancreatic islets rather than the entire pancreas.

Clients with type II diabetes do not benefit from pancreas transplants. Type II diabetes results from a failure of insulin action, which cannot be improved by adding a pancreas.

■ Nursing Management of the Surgical Client

The nursing care of the client undergoing a pancreas transplant is the same as that for any client undergoing major abdominal surgery. Care of the client following renal transplant is covered in Chapter 21. Postoperative care is directed not only at caring for the client's postsurgical needs but also at addressing the particular needs of a client who has undergone an organ transplant.

Acute Complications of Diabetes Mellitus

Hyperglycemia and Diabetic Ketoacidosis

Hyperglycemia results when glucose cannot be transported to the cells because of a lack of insulin. Without available carbohydrates for cellular fuel, the liver converts its glycogen stores back to glucose (glycogenolysis) and increases the biosynthesis of glucose (gluconeogenesis). Unfortunately, however, these responses aggravate the situation by raising the blood glucose level even higher.

In type I diabetes mellitus, as the need for cellular fuel grows more critical, the body begins to draw on its fat and protein stores for energy. Excessive amounts of fatty acids are mobilized from adipose tissue cells and transported to the liver. The liver, in turn, accelerates the rate at which it produces ketone bodies (ketogenesis) for catabolism by other body tissues, particularly muscle. As fat metabolism increases, the liver may produce too many ketone bodies. Ketone bodies accumulate in the blood (ketosis) and are excreted in the urine (ketonuria). Metabolic acidosis develops from the acidic (pH-lowering) effect of the ketones acetoacetate and beta-hydroxybutyrate. This condition is called *diabetic ketoacidosis*. Severe acidosis may cause the diabetic client to lose consciousness, a condition often called *diabetic coma*. Diabetic ketoacidosis is always a medical emergency and requires immediate medical attention.

Diabetic ketoacidosis is the most serious metabolic disturbance of type I diabetes and is a common cause of hospital admission. Diabetic ketoacidosis is identified in approximately 40% of clients with previously undiagnosed diabetes and is responsible for more than 160,000 hospital admissions each year. It occurs most frequently in teenagers and the elderly.

Etiology and Risk Factors

Diabetic ketoacidosis is primarily a complication of type I diabetes mellitus, although clients with NIDDM can also develop ketoacidosis during periods of extreme stress. A precipitating cause may be identified in 80% of clients. Causes of diabetic ketoacidosis commonly include (1) taking too little insulin; (2) omitting doses of insulin; (3) failing to meet an increased need for insulin due to surgery, trauma, pregnancy, stress, puberty, or infections;

and (4) developing insulin resistance as a result of the presence of insulin antibodies.

Pathophysiology

Diabetic ketoacidosis is marked by a relative or absolute lack of insulin. Insulin may be present, but not in sufficient amounts for the increased need of glucose due to the stressors present (e.g., infections).

When the body lacks insulin and cannot use carbohydrates for energy, it resorts to using fats and proteins. Excess counterregulatory hormones (e.g., glucagon, catecholamines, cortisol, and growth hormones) secondary to stress appear to play an important role in development of diabetic ketoacidosis. These hormones antagonize the effects of insulin and diabetic ketoacidosis by promoting hyperglycemia, osmotic diuresis, lipolysis with secondary hyperlipidemia, and acidosis. Figure 69–8 summarizes the pathophysiologic mechanism involved. The processes of catabolizing fats for fuel gives rise to three pathologic events: (1) ketosis and acidosis, (2) dehydration, and (3) electrolyte and acid-base imbalances.

Ketosis

We have already discussed the metabolic effect of lack of insulin on fat metabolism. In diabetic ketoacidosis, buffering by bicarbonate, which is excreted as carbon dioxide

and water, fails to compensate for ketosis. Respirations increase in rate and depth (Kussmaul's respirations) and the breath has a "fruity" or acetone-like odor.

The renal system then attempts to excrete enough ketone bodies to normalize pH. This excretion of ketones leads to osmotic diuresis and hemoconcentration. Hemoconcentration impedes blood circulation and leads to tissue anoxia and lactic acid production. This rise in lactic acid further acidifies blood pH. The rising tide of ketone bodies eventually overwhelms the body's defenses against hydrogen excess. With its buffer, respiratory, and renal defense systems depleted, the body finally succumbs to its acid overload, and diabetic coma can ensue.

Dehydration

Clients with ketoacidosis lose fluids from several sources. They excrete large amounts of urine in an attempt to eliminate excessive glucose and ketone bodies. Second, acidosis can cause severe nausea and vomiting, with resultant further losses of fluid and electrolytes (notably sodium and chloride). Finally, water is lost in the breath as the body attempts to rid itself of excess acetone and carbon dioxide. Typically, clients in diabetic coma lose an amount of water equivalent to 10% of body weight and approximately 40 g of sodium. Severe dehydration resulting from these fluid losses may be followed by hypovolemic shock and lactic acidosis.

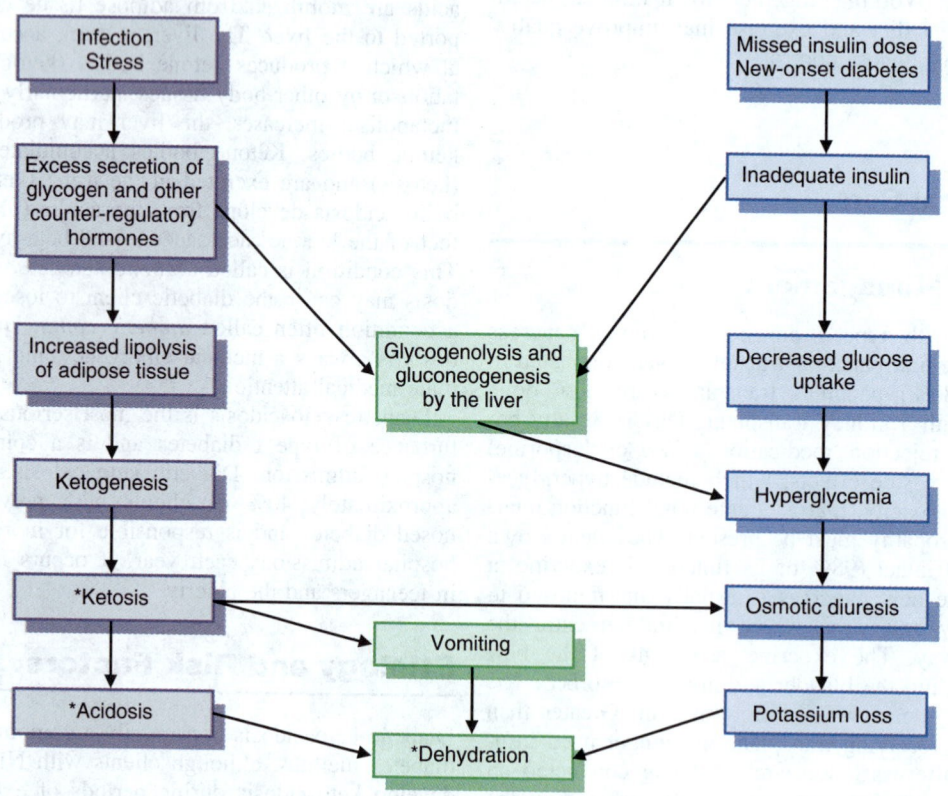

*Hallmarks of DKA

Figure 69–8. The pathophysiology of diabetic ketoacidosis. (Adapted from White, N. H., & Henry, D. N. [1992]. Special issues in diabetes management. In D. Haire-Joshu [Ed.], *Management of diabetes mellitus: Perspectives of care across the lifespan* [p. 250]. St Louis: Mosby–Year Book.)

Electrolyte Imbalance

As the pH of the blood decreases (acidosis), the accumulating hydrogen moves from the extracellular fluid to the intracellular fluid. Hydrogen moving into the cells promotes the movement of potassium out of the cells into the extracellular fluid, which results in severe intracellular potassium depletion. Initially, the intracellular potassium loss may go unrecognized because serum potassium levels are often normal or elevated. As the resulting osmotic diuresis continues, however, much potassium is excreted in the urine. If the client becomes severely dehydrated, hemoconcentration and oliguria may cause the serum potassium levels to rise still higher.

In addition to potassium losses, the client in metabolic acidosis loses excessive amounts of sodium, phosphate, chloride, and bicarbonate in the urine and vomitus.

Clinical Manifestations and Diagnostic Findings

Common presenting manifestations of the client in diabetic ketoacidosis are presented in Box 69–5.

Emergency Care

■ Management

Assessment priorities for the client with acute hyperglycemia are presented in Table 69–8. Management of diabetic ketoacidosis usually takes place in a hospital setting with care managed by the physician, nurse, and pharma-

cist. Dehydration resulting in hypovolemic shock, acute tubular necrosis, and uremia are major causes of death in cases of untreated diabetic ketoacidosis. Diabetic ketoacidosis is an emergency. Rapid medical care and nursing intervention are essential to correct the life-threatening abnormalities. Effective therapy is based on an understanding of metabolic changes that occur during diabetic ketoacidosis. Cornerstones of treatment are administration of fluids, insulin, and electrolytes.

Management goals in diabetic ketoacidosis are as follows:

1. Rehydration
2. Correction of electrolyte and acid/base imbalances
3. Shift from a state of fat catabolism to a state of carbohydrate catabolism by providing insulin
4. Identification and correction of those factors that precipitated the ketoacidosis. This must be done with great care. Fully correcting all biochemical abnormalities may take as long as 1 week after the client is able to eat solid food. A comprehensive flow sheet should be kept to follow intake, output, weight, fluids, electrolytes, insulin, and ketones (see Case Management).

Rehydration

Intravenous rehydration is required in for all clients who are vomiting, unable to drink, and have acidosis. Intravenous infusions of isotonic saline (0.9% sodium chloride) are started immediately. Usually, the client receives 1,000 ml of isotonic solution IV during the first hour (10 to 20 ml/kg), followed by an additional 2,000 to 8,000 ml of solution over the next 24 hours. Clients with compromised cardiovascular function may require slower IV fluid replacement (see the Critical Monitoring feature and Box 69–6).

A nasogastric tube may be necessary if the client is comatose or is vomiting and is likely to aspirate the vomitus. The client's mouth may be dry because of the nasogastric tube and as a result of dehydration. Frequent oral care is important.

Bowel sounds should be assessed frequently for changes. Once the client can tolerate fluids, fluid intake is encouraged. Drinking salted broth is beneficial to replenish needed sodium. Intake and output are recorded accurately. Most clients require a urinary catheter. Because clients with diabetes are more prone to infection, aseptic catheter care is essential.

Reversing Shock

If the client is in circulatory collapse, the physician may order blood, albumin, or other plasma volume expanders, such as dextran, to be administered alternately with normal saline solution. Also, the client may receive combinations of colloids and saline solution that raise the serum levels of both sodium chloride and plasma protein.

Restoring Potassium Balance

As a result of the lowered pH, potassium leaves the intracellular space in untreated ketoacidosis, and transient

---

Box 69–5. Common Presenting Signs and Symptoms in Diabetic Ketoacidosis

Signs

Tachycardia
Hypotension
Dehydration
Warm, dry skin
Hyperpnea or Kussmaul's respirations
Impaired level of consciousness or coma
Weight loss
Fruity odor of ketones on breath

Symptoms

Nausea and vomiting
Thirst and polyuria
Weakness and/or anorexia
Abdominal pain
Visual disturbances
Somnolence

Adapted from American Diabetes Association. (1944). *Medical management of insulin-dependent (type I) diabetes* (2nd ed.; p. 77). Alexandria, VA: Author.

Table 69–8. Assessment Findings for the Client with Acute Hyperglycemia

Problem	Key Assessments
Hyperglycemia	Finger stick and serum blood glucose levels and ketones Manifestations of hyperglycemia including polyuria, polyphagia, and polydipsia
Hyperosmolality	Serum osmolality, (BUN), and serum creatinine Manifestations of neurologic impairment including lethargy, disorientation, and behavioral changes
Dehydration	Flushed, dry skin, "tenting," dry mucous membranes Polyuria, oliguria, tachycardia, and hypotension
Electrolyte imbalances	Manifestations of imbalances: *Hyperkalemia:* Tachycardia, bradycardia, peaked T waves on ECG, ectopic beats, hypodtension, nausea, vomiting, diarrhea, hyperactive bowel sounds, paresthesias, muscle cramps *Hypokalemia:* Nausea, vomiting, diarrhea, ileus, muscle weakness and cramps, ectopic beats, hypotension, flattened T waves and U wave, fatigue, lethargy *Hyponatremia:* Nausea, vomiting, diarrhea, tachycardia, hypotension, lethargy, confusion, seizures, muscle weakness
Metabolic acidosis	Hypotension, arrhythmias, hyperventilation, lethargy, confusion, coma, headache, acetone breath
Hypoglycemia	Diaphoresis, tachycardia, palpitations, hunger, paresthesias, tremors, headache, confusion, slurred speech, blurred vision, shallow respirations
Fluid overload (may develop with insulin treatment for hyperglycemia)	Intake and output, jugular vein distension, dyspnea, pulmonary crackles, weight gain, bounding pulse, edema, confusion, increased blood pressure

Adapted from Reising, D. L. (1995). Acute hyperglycemia: Putting a lid on the crisis; and Acute hypoglycemia: Keeping the bottom from falling out. *Nursing 95, February*, 37, 39, 46.

hyperkalemia develops. The total body potassium level is depleted, despite a normal or elevated serum potassium level. Correct potassium replacement requires caution and timely action. Once intervention begins with fluids and insulin, dangerous hypokalemia may develop with weakness, extreme dyspnea, and even cardiac arrest. Hypokalemia occurs because potassium reenters the cells (along with glucose) with insulin administration, and potassium is excreted in the urine with rehydration and renal function restoration. General agreement exists on the following points of assessment and intervention:

- Frequently assess and measure urine output. Do not administer potassium to a client with low urine output; dangerous hyperkalemia may develop. Notify the physician promptly if the urine output falls dramatically or is less than 30 ml/hour.
- Assess the client continuously for manifestations of hyperkalemia (bradycardia, cardiac arrest, weakness, flaccid paralysis, oliguria) or hypokalemia (weakness, flaccid paralysis, paralytic ileus, cardiac arrest). Hyperkalemia may be present during the first 4 hours of intervention. Hypokalemia usually develops 4 to 24 hours after the initial intervention.
- Replace potassium carefully following protocols (see Box 69–7).
- Plan to begin potassium administration within 1 to 2 hours after starting insulin therapy and after adequate urine output is ensured.

- When the client has recovered sufficiently to resume eating and drinking, give foods and liquids that are high in potassium, such as orange juice or bananas.

Sodium chloride and phosphate levels also need to be closely monitored. Sodium is replaced by normal saline. Phosphate levels can vary the same as potassium does, and it can be replaced IV. Sometimes the physician will alternate potassium chloride with potassium phosphate in the IV fluid.

pH Correction/Insulin Administration

Clients presenting in diabetic ketoacidosis are usually suffering phosphate depletion from a combination of decreased food intake, excessive catabolism, and increased urinary excretion. As with administration of potassium, administration of insulin enhances movement of phosphate into cells, which further reduces plasma phosphate concentration. However, administering too much phosphate can induce hypocalcemia. Calcium levels should be checked before phosphate (as potassium phosphate) is given.

Clinicians usually administer sodium bicarbonate only to clients with a pH of 7.1 or less. Such replacement therapy partially corrects the metabolic acidosis. As the client's condition improves, normal body mechanisms restore the blood pH to normal.

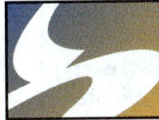

CASE MANAGEMENT

Diabetic Ketoacidosis

For Clinical Pathway, see Appendix D.

Clinical Pathway from Nashville Department of Veterans Affairs Medical Center
Nashville, Tennessee
Information provided by Wanda Shelton, M.S.N., R.N., and William Robertson, R.N.

Development and Revision of Pathway

- This diagnosis is one of the ten most frequent admitting diagnoses to the medical/coronary intensive care unit at the Nashville Department of Veterans Affairs Medical Center. By initially targeting the top ten diagnoses with the initial pathways, we covered approximately 86% of the admissions to the unit.
- Initially, a nursing task force reviewed data, drafted a pathway, and presented it to various disciplines involved in the care of the diabetic patient. Revisions were made to the draft, and brought to a multidisciplinary ICU Committee and to the ICU directors for approval.
- This particular pathway has been in use since April 1993. This does not include the initial development and validation period. That process took 6 to 9 months. April 1993 is the date when final approval was given for this pathway to be part of the permanent medical record.
- Aggregate variance analysis is done quarterly. Data from this analysis are evaluated to ensure appropriateness of the outcomes on the pathway. Task variance is done annually to ensure that the tasks on the pathway are current with physician and nursing practice standards. Variances indicate that the pathway needs revision.

Use and Impact of the Pathway

- This pathway is used only for the ICU portion of the patient's stay. Every patient who is admitted to the medical intensive care unit with diabetic ketoacidosis is placed on the pathway. Plans are under way for expanding pathways to include the entire hospital stay.
- Multidisciplinary patient care teams consisting of professional nurses, physicians, dietitians, and pharmacists use the pathway during daily rounds. MICU nurses use it to plan and manage care of the patient, and are always focused on the desired outcomes.
- Four major changes have occurred: (1) pathways have organized the care of diabetic ketoacidosis patients better than the previous methods; (2) the focus of care is now on outcomes/goals instead of tasks; (3) the pathway supports continuity of care among various providers; and (4) the pathway supports orientation of new staff to population-specific practice guidelines.
- We have not measured the impact of the pathway in actual dollars. However, we have demonstrated a decrease in the length of stay, increased patient and provider satisfaction, and decreased time in planning the care of these patients. All of these can be translated into cost savings.

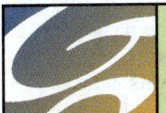

CRITICAL MONITORING

The Rehydration Process

- The best indication of degree of dehydration is weight loss, which may be determined if the client's baseline weight is known; loss may be 10% of total body weight
- Other clinical indices to monitor are tissue turgor, pulse, dryness of mucous membranes, levels of consciousness, thirst, hematocrit, and orthostatic hypotension
- Elderly clients and those with heart disease should have fluid replacement determined according to central venous pressure
- Too-aggressive fluid replacement (particularly with normal saline) may induce congestive heart failure; frequent auscultation of lungs is vital

Low-dosage insulin therapy (5 to 10 units/hour) will be ordered for the client in diabetic ketoacidosis. Although the blood glucose concentration is usually markedly elevated in diabetic ketoacidosis, a blood glucose level below 300 mg/dl does not exclude the diagnosis. The client in ketoacidosis may receive an initial IV bolus of regular insulin (0.15 units/kg) in the emergency room. Before starting an infusion of insulin, ask whether the client has already received insulin that day. Insulin should never be given subcutaneously to someone in diabetic ketoacidosis, because the subcutaneous tissues are dehydrated and poorly perfused with blood from dehydration and hypovolemic shock.

Traditionally, the hyperglycemia associated with diabetic ketoacidosis is treated with a bolus of regular insulin given IV. Then an "insulin drip" should be started. Either 0.9% normal saline (NS) or 0.45% NS, may be used, depending on the degree of dehydration and concurrent medical problems. Prepare the last amount of insulin in the smallest IV bag available (e.g., 100 units of regular

Box 69–6. Intravenous Fluid Replacement in Diabetic Ketoacidosis

Hour 1:

Provide 15–20 ml/kg of isotonic sodium chloride (0.9%) (normal saline) or full-strength Ringer's lactate (lactated Ringer's) solution

Hour 2:

Continue fluid as above at 15 ml/kg. If the client is hypernatremic, in congestive heart failure, or is a child, consider half-strength sodium chloride (0.45% normal saline)

Hour 3:

Reduce fluid intake to 7.5 ml/kg in adults. Fluid should be 0.45% normal saline.

Hour 4:

Adjust fluid intake to meet clinical need. Consider urine output rate in calculation.

When blood glucose approaches 300 mg/dl, change fluid to 5% dextrose in half-strength sodium chloride (D_5 0.45% normal saline). Continue IV fluids until client can ingest food and drink without vomiting.

From American Diabetes Association. (1994). *Medical management of (type I) insulin dependent diabetes* (2nd ed.). Alexandria, VA: Author.

---

insulin in 100 cc of IV fluid). This gives you a 1:1 ratio of regular insulin to IV fluid. Prime the IV tubing with the IV solution first, then add the regular insulin (insulin will adhere to the IV tubing). Label the IV bag very clearly with the dose and type of insulin added. The IV regular insulin must be administered very meticulously by a control pump and by frequent machine checks by the nurse.

After the bolus, infuse insulin at a rate of 0.1 unit/kg/hour. If no improvement in the acidosis occurs within 2 to 4 hours, the infusion rate should be doubled. Severe insulin resistance may be precipitated by severe stress. Glucose is normalized more quickly than acidosis.

Blood glucose levels need to be monitored every 30 minutes initially, preferably with a blood glucose meter. Rapid blood glucose test results allow the nurse to adjust the insulin infusion rapidly and correctly. When the blood glucose levels approach 250 mg/dl, the insulin infusion should be reduced and 5% dextrose added to the infusion so that the blood glucose level can be maintained at approximately 250 mg/dl for the first 12 to 24 hours. More rapid correction of hyperglycemia can lead to cerebral edema. Monitor the client's level of consciousness to closely assess for this uncommon complication. Blood glucose levels should be monitored every 1 to 2 hours after reaching 250 mg/dl, until they are stable.

As the client improves, decisions must be made about when to discontinue IV insulin and fluids and begin subcutaneous insulin administration. Normalization of the client's vital signs, correction of acidosis, and ability to take oral fluids are important considerations. Short-acting insulin is usually administered subcutaneously every 4 to 6 hours, with the first dose given 15 to 30 minutes prior to discontinuing IV insulin. The initial dose is approximately 0.2 units/kg. Subsequent doses are determined by blood glucose levels.

While correcting metabolic abnormalities, the cause of diabetic ketoacidosis must be pursued aggressively. Cultures of urine, throat, sputum, and blood; chest x-rays; and ECG may provide the source of stress.

Prior to discharge, the team reviews the situation that led to diabetic ketoacidosis and institutes teaching of risk factor reduction.

■ Prevention

Primary prevention of diabetic ketoacidosis is through client education. Preventing diabetic ketoacidosis is the long-term goal of good diabetes management. Clients and their families should understand enough about ketoacidosis to avoid what may cause it, to recognize its approach, to slow down or minimize its development, and to seek help fast if it begins to occur. To prevent diabetic ketoacidosis, clients with diabetes should learn to do the following:

- Take insulin in appropriate doses at appropriate times.
- Monitor blood glucose frequently (at least before each meal and at bedtime).
- Monitor urine ketone levels when blood glucose levels rise (above 250 mg/dl).
- Schedule regular appointments with the healthcare provider for regular review of blood glucose results,

Box 69–7. Potassium Replacement in Diabetic Ketoacidosis

In clients with adequate urine output, lead II of the 12-lead ECG may be used as a guide for plasma potassium (K^+) concentration. Flattening or inversion of the T wave with U wave and prolonged QT intervals indicate hypokalemia. Peaking of T waves, loss of P wave, and a disrupted QRS complex indicate hyperkalemia. Intravenous replacement of potassium is based on plasma K^+ concentration. If K^+ is:

<3 mEq/L, infuse ≥0.6 mEq/kg/hr
3–4 mEq/L, infuse 0.6 mEq/kg/hr
4–5 mEq/L, infuse 0.2–0.4 mEq/kg/hr
6 mEq/L, withold until K^+ is <6.0 mEq/L

Add K^+ to replacement fluid therapy. If concentration is 20–40 mEq/L and infusion into peripheral vein causes irritation, infuse into central vein.
Recheck plasma K^+ every 2 hours if plasma concentration is <4 or >6 mEq/L.

Adapted from American Diabetes Association. (1994). *Medical management of (type I) insulin dependent diabetes* (2nd ed.). Alexandria, VA: Author.

weight gains or losses, and general state of health and well-being.

● Recognize manifestations of infection (a major cause of diabetic ketoacidosis). The first manifestation of an infection in a foot or leg—or of an upper respiratory tract, urinary tract, or vaginal infection—should be reported immediately to the healthcare provider. Other stressors, such as family or emotional problems, can also precipitate diabetic ketoacidosis.

The client should call for assistance if any of the following develop:

● Anorexia, nausea, vomiting, or diarrhea
● Ketonuria persisting for more than 8 hours
● A febrile illness or infection
● Any manifestation of acidosis

Emphasize to the client that the greatest weapons against diabetic ketoacidosis are (1) regular, daily self-monitoring of blood glucose; (2) adherence to the diabetes management program; and (3) early recognition of and intervention in mild ketosis.

Hyperglycemic, Hyperosmolar, Nonketotic Coma

Hyperglycemic, hyperosmolar, nonketotic coma (HHNK) is another acute complication of diabetes. It is a variant of diabetic ketoacidosis. HHNK is characterized by extreme hyperglycemia (600 to 2,000 mg/dl), profound dehydration, mild or undetectable ketonuria, and the absence of acidosis. HHNK most commonly occurs in elderly clients with type II diabetes mellitus (see Box 69–8).

HHNK can be life-threatening. Mortality associated with HHNK is higher than with diabetic ketoacidosis (approximately 10% to 40%), primarily because clients are older and frequently have significant medical problems. HHNK sometimes occurs in people with undiagnosed diabetes and in those with diagnosed diabetes after a long period of uncontrolled hyperglycemia. The precipitating factors of HHNK may be the same as those precipitating diabetic ketoacidosis. There is almost always a precipitating factor.

The major difference between HHNK and diabetic ketoacidosis is the lack of ketonuria with HHNK. Because some residual ability remains to secrete insulin in type II diabetes mellitus, the mobilization of fats for energy is usually not present.

In the absence of adequate insulin, blood becomes concentrated with glucose. Glucose molecules are too large to pass into cells; therefore, osmosis of water occurs from the interstitial spaces and cells to dilute the glucose in the blood. Osmotic diuresis occurs. Eventually, the cells become dehydrated.

The client's fluid intake can initially balance the loss of fluid and glucose through the urine. The imbalance gradually becomes more severe as the client cannot match intake to output. In time, the client becomes obtunded and is unable to respond to thirst. At this point, the process is self-perpetuating.

The four major clinical features of HHNK syndrome are (1) severe hyperglycemia (600 to 2,000 mg/dl), (2) absence of or presence of slight ketosis, (3) profound dehydration (10% to 15% loss of body water), and (4) hyperosmolality of plasma and elevated blood urea nitrogen (BUN) level. Typically, the client experiences excessive thirst, altered level of consciousness (coma or confusion), and manifestations of dehydration.

The precipitating event should be determined and corrected as soon as possible, even while resuscitation is taking place. HHNK is treated with vigorous fluid replacement and administration of insulin and electrolytes. A common initial intervention is infusion of isotonic saline solution over a 2-hour period, followed by administration of hypotonic saline solution (0.45%). As in diabetic ketoacidosis, potassium, sodium, chloride, and phosphates are administered IV. Insulin is given via an

---

Box 69–8. Factors Associated with Nonketotic Hyperosmolar Coma (HHNK) Syndrome

Therapeutic Agents

▪ Glucocorticoids
▪ Diuretics
▪ Diphenylhydantoin
▪ Beta-adrenergic blocking agents
▪ L-Asparaginase
▪ Immunosuppressive agents
▪ Chlorpromazine
▪ Diazoxide

Therapeutic Procedures

▪ Peritoneal dialysis
▪ Hemodialysis
▪ Hyperalimentation
▪ Surgical stress

Chronic Illness

▪ Renal disease
▪ Heart disease
▪ Hypertension
▪ Previous stroke
▪ Alcoholism
▪ Psychiatric diagnosis
▪ Loss of thirst

Acute Illness

▪ Infection
▪ Gangrene
▪ Urinary tract infection
▪ Septicemia
▪ Burns
▪ Gastrointestinal bleeding
▪ Myocardial infarction
▪ Pancreatitis
▪ Cerebrovascular accident (Stroke)

From American Diabetes Association (1994). *Medical management of non-insulin dependent (type II) diabetes* (3rd ed.). Alexandria, VA: Author.

infusion pump, but usually at lower dosages, because the client is producing some insulin. Because of severe dehydration, plasma glucose levels fall rapidly with fluid administration. Dextrose is added to the IV fluid when the blood glucose level reaches about 250 mg/dl for preventing hypoglycemia. Because many clients in HHNK are elderly and have other cardiovascular or renal disorders, fluid volume and electrolyte changes must be carefully assessed, especially if acute or chronic renal failure complicates the course.

As the population ages, an increasing number of clients will experience HHNK, and nurses need to be alert for its manifestations. Before discharge, the nurse reviews the causes of HHNK with the client and family, including insulin injection (if necessary) and blood glucose testing techniques. The nurse helps the client understand how serious these acute complications are and how to prevent them in the future.

Hypoglycemia (Insulin Reaction)

Hypoglycemia is a common feature of type I diabetes mellitus and can also be seen in clients with type II diabetes treated with insulin and/or oral agents. The precise blood glucose level at which clients develop manifestations of hypoglycemia varies, but manifestations generally do not occur until the blood glucose level is less than 50 to 60 mg/dl.

Etiology and Risk Factors

Hypoglycemic reactions result from (1) an overdose of insulin or, less commonly, a sulfonylurea; (2) omitting a meal or eating less food than usual; (3) overexertion without additional carbohydrate compensation; (4) nutritional and fluid imbalances due to nausea and vomiting; and (5) alcohol intake.

Inadvertent or deliberate errors in insulin dose are a frequent cause of hypoglycemia. Other changes in the schedule of meals or insulin administration, vigorous unexpected exercise, or sleeping later than usual in the morning can also cause hypoglycemia. Alcohol, marijuana, or other drugs can mask a client's awareness of hypoglycemia in its earliest stages.

Hypoglycemia can also occur secondary to administration of an oral hypoglycemic agent (OHA). Most recorded cases have been in clients treated with chlorpropamide (Diabinese) which has a duration of action of 24 to 72 hours. Those at risk for hypoglycemia during OHA administration are clients older than 60 years; clients with poor nutritional intake; clients who use alcohol; clients with hepatic or renal dysfunction, or clients receiving multi-drug regimens. The hypoglycemic reactions can be severe and prolonged.

Pathophysiology

Normally, hypoglycemia triggers counterregulatory hormones, primarily glucagon and epinephrine, to promptly increase blood glucose levels by stimulating glucose release from the liver and inhibiting insulin secretion. Under usual conditions, this leads to normoglycemia.

In contrast, clients with type I diabetes have abnormalities in this feedback system. Typically, within the first 2 to 5 years of diabetes, the secretion of glucagon becomes deficient. Later, the secretion of epinephrine may become impaired secondary to subclinical neuropathy. The regulation of absorption of insulin from subcutaneous fat also becomes impaired. The combinations of these abnormalities make the client with type I diabetes susceptible to frequent development of hypoglycemia. In this respect, hypoglycemic shock is more dangerous than diabetic ketoacidosis. Approximately 10% of clients with type I diabetes suffer one severe reaction per year that requires emergency treatment. Untreated or prolonged hypoglycemia can cause permanent brain damage, memory loss, decreased learning ability, paralysis, and death.

Clinical Manifestations and Diagnostic Findings

Hypoglycemic manifestations are generally divided into two major categories: adrenergic and neuroglycopenic (Box 69–9). Adrenergic (autonomic) manifestations are those associated with rising epinephrine levels and are considered mild reactions. Cognitive deficits usually do not occur and clients are capable of self-treatment. Diaphoresis, although not mediated via adrenergic nerve endings, is usually considered along with the adrenergic manifestations of hypoglycemia. Adrenergic reactions usually occur during rapid decreases in blood glucose. They have been reported by clients with poorly controlled diabetes

---

Box 69–9. Manifestations of Hypoglycemia

Adrenergic (Increased Epinephrine)

- Shakiness
- Irritability
- Nervousness
- Tachycardia, palpitations
- Tremor
- Hunger
- Diaphoresis
- Pallor
- Paresthesias

Neuroglycopenic (Decreased Glucose to Brain)

- Headache
- Mental illness
- Inability to concentrate
- Slurred speech
- Blurred vision
- Confusion
- Irrational behavior
- Lethargy, severe
- Loss of consciousness
- Coma
- Seizure
- Death

when the fall in blood glucose level is rapid, even in the absence of hypoglycemia. These manifestations can also occur during other stressful or anxiety-provoking events. These "mild reactions" may produce only minimal disruptions of daily activities.

Moderate hypoglycemic reactions include neuroglycopenic reactions as well as adrenergic manifestations. Neuroglycopenic manifestations are those associated with lack of glucose availability to the brain and resultant decrease in cognitive functioning. These reactions typically produce longer-lasting and more severe manifestations than do mild reactions. Common manifestations are headache, irritability, drowsiness, weakness, and tremor. The client may need assistance in treatment. Severe hypoglycemic reactions render the client unable to self-treat. The client may be awake and alert, semicomatose, or comatose.

Hypoglycemia can occur at any time of day or night. It seems to occur most commonly (1) during exercise, (2) 8 to 24 hours after strenuous exercise, and (3) in the middle of the night. Occurrence of severe hypoglycemia appears to be more frequent in those suffering from hypoglycemic unawareness (discussed later in this section), defective glucose counterregulation (see earlier discussion), and autonomic neuropathy (see section on chronic complications of diabetes mellitus), as well as in those using intensive diabetes therapy.

The period during which the client is most likely to experience an insulin reaction depends on (1) the type of insulin given, (2) the client's response to that type of insulin, and (3) the timing of the insulin injection to food intake. When insulin is given in the morning, short-acting preparations tend to produce reactions before lunch; intermediate-acting insulins, 2 or 3 hours before dinner; and long-acting insulins, between 2:00 AM and breakfast. NPH or Lente insulin injected before dinner (5:00 PM) can cause hypoglycemia around 2:00 AM, when the normal blood glucose level is lowest because of the decrease in metabolism, and again at around 8:00 AM, when the insulin level peaks if breakfast is not eaten in time.

Acute and Subacute Care

■ Management

Management of hypoglycemia depends on the severity of the reaction (Table 69–9). For reversal of mild hypoglycemia, 10 to 15 g of simple carbohydrate works quickly to increase blood glucose levels and to stop manifestations of hypoglycemia. Reactions that occur during the night should be treated with a carbohydrate followed by a longer-acting mixture of carbohydrate and protein (e.g., 8 oz of milk). A blood glucose test (with a glucose meter) should be performed as soon as the manifestations are recognized. If a meter is not available, it is safer to assume and treat hypoglycemia. Blood glucose is retested in 15 to 30 minutes, and treatment is repeated if the level is not over 100 mg/dl. Moderate reactions may need two or more treatments with 10 to 15 g of carbohydrates (see Box 69–9).

Never force an unconscious or semiconscious client to drink liquids, because fluid may be aspirated into the lungs. The unconscious client with severe hypoglycemia needs glucagon or IV glucose immediately. Family members of clients with diabetes can administer glucagon at

Table 69–9. Interventions for Hypoglycemia	
Clinical Manifestations	**Interventions**
Mild hypoglycemia: Tremors Tachycardia Diaphoresis Paresthesias Excessive hunger Pallor Shakiness	10–15 g of carbohydrate (contained in following): 4 oz orange juice 6 oz regular soda 6–8 oz 2% milk 6–8 Life Savers candies 1 small (2-oz) tube of cake icing 4 tsp granulated sugar
Moderate hypoglycemia: manifestations listed above plus the following: Headache Mood swings Irritability Inability to concentrate Drowsiness Impaired judgment Slurred speech Double or blurred vision	20–30 g of carbohydrate Glucagon, 1 mg SC or IM
Severe hypoglycemia: Disorientation Seizures Unconsciousness	50% dextrose, 25 g IV Glucagon, 1 mg IM or IV

home in the event of a serious hypoglycemic reaction. Glucagon, administered intramuscularly or subcutaneously in the amount of 1 mg for adults, may eliminate the need for emergency department intervention. The pharmacy dispenses glucagon in the form of a powder with the diluent in a separate vial. Instruct the family how and when to mix and inject glucagon, and let them know that the client may experience nausea or vomiting on awakening. Even though glucagon is effective in the majority of clients, its effect is transient and slower than dextrose. Hypoglycemia often recurs. Medical assistance is advisable if hypoglycemia recurs, vomiting prevents oral intake, or status doesn't improve.

The client who experiences severe hypoglycemia in the hospital usually receives IV glucose (as 50% or 25% dextrose) in an amount of 10 to 25 g over 1 to 3 minutes. This is followed by an infusion of 5% dextrose at 5 to 10 g/hour until the client is fully recovered and is able to eat.

■ Prevention

Because insulin reactions are so common, newly diagnosed diabetic clients must understand the following:

1. Why reactions occur
2. When reactions are most likely to occur
3. The early clinical manifestations of hypoglycemia
4. The danger of severe or repeated reactions
5. The importance of early intervention
6. How to prevent insulin reactions

Whenever administration of insulin or an oral hypoglycemic agent is begun, the client must be taught to identify clinical manifestations and to manage hypoglycemia.

Once a client develops and then fully recovers from an episode of hypoglycemia, the nurse needs to thoroughly reassess the intervention program. In some cases, insulin reactions develop because the client carelessly prepares insulin dosages, fails to eat, or exercises excessively. Talk about dangers of repeated insulin reactions to the client who is careless in maintaining a normoglycemic balance. These dangers include loss of consciousness, trauma related to falling with loss of consciousness or injury to self from poor decision-making, seizures, loss of brain cells, and eventual death. Stress the importance of conscientious adherence to the therapeutic program.

In other cases, hypoglycemia develops because the prescribed insulin dosage is too large or the client's dietary intake is too small. Instruct the client to record the time and probable cause of any hypoglycemic episodes on the blood test record. The healthcare team can then evaluate the record together, making appropriate changes. Teach the client with type I diabetes to adjust diet and insulin by monitoring results. Finally, be certain that the client with diabetes obtains a diabetic identification tag or Medic-Alert bracelet and an identification card. Sometimes, clients who are suffering an insulin reaction behave as if they are intoxicated or mentally disturbed. By carrying proper identification, the client can avoid being arrested at a time when emergency care is desperately needed. Table 69–10 compares the data and interventions for diabetic ketoacidosis, HHNK, and hypoglycemia.

As for many chronic disorders, the client needs to develop a positive self-concept and a feeling of control. Help the client and significant others understand the complications associated with diabetes. Equally important, the nurse should assist the client to develop and maintain self-care skills that meet emotional and social needs as well as physical ones.

Other Hypoglycemic Disorders

Other manifestations of altered counterregulatory mechanisms in type I diabetes mellitus that the nurse should understand are: (1) hypoglycemic unawareness, (2) hypoglycemia with rebound hyperglycemia (Somogyi effect), and (3) dawn phenomenon.

Hypoglycemic Unawareness

Hypoglycemic unawareness refers to a syndrome in which people with diabetes are unaware they are hypoglycemic and therefore do not initiate treatment. In the Diabetes Control and Complications Trial (DCCT), about a third of all episodes of severe hypoglycemia seen in awake, intensively treated clients were not accompanied by sufficient manifestations so that clients could effectively prevent neuroglycopenia. In the past, this condition was incorrectly viewed as being rare and as only being associated with advanced neuropathy.

Repeated episodes of hypoglycemia seem to blunt the hormonal defense mechanisms that prevent hypoglycemia (blunted epinephrine response) and lower the level at which early hypoglycemic manifestations are perceived.

Theory speculates that beta-adrenergic blocking agents (such as propranolol) can cause hypoglycemic unawareness and can blunt adrenergic (epinephrine) effects in diabetics, because these effects are primarily mediated by beta-adrenergic receptors. Therefore, beta-blockers are contraindicated in clients with diabetes.

Clients with hypoglycemic unawareness (absence of manifestations of hypoglycemia when glucose level is <55 mg/dl) require consultation with an experienced physician. Increasing the frequency of SMBG, particularly before driving and after exercise, should be encouraged. Clients may wish to choose a slightly higher blood glucose target before meals and during the night. Self-management education and follow-up must be intensified for these clients. For clients with type I diabetes, maintaining good control is as much of a problem during the night as at any other time of day.

Hypoglycemia with Rebound Hyperglycemia (Somogyi Effect)

Hypoglycemia followed by "rebound" hyperglycemia, also known as the *Somogyi effect* or *Somogyi phenomenon*, may complicate diabetes management. This phenomenon has been implicated in the past as a common cause of fasting morning hyperglycemia. Studies have found it to be a rare occurrence. It usually results from excessive evening insulin dosing. The pathophysiology involves hy-

Table 69–10. Acute Complications of Diabetes

	Diabetic Ketoacidosis (DKA)	Hyperglycemia, Hyperosmolar, Nonketotic Coma (HHNK)	Hypoglycemia
Type of diabetes	Usually type I, may occur in type II	Type II	Type I or type II
Clinical manifestations	Warm/dry skin, nausea, vomiting, flushed appearance, dry mucous membranes, soft eyeballs, Kussmaul's respirations or tachypnea, abdominal pain, impaired consciousness, hypotension, tachycardia, acetone breath, acute weight loss Polyuria (early) Oliguria/anuria (late)	Same as DKA except Kussmaul's respirations and acetone breath usually not present Alterations in level of consciousness, severe dehydration Nausea and vomiting not present Tachypnea, shallow respirations	Mild reaction: tremors, palpitations, pallor, sweating, hunger Moderate reaction: headache, irritability, drowsiness, weakness, visual disturbances, decreased mental acuity Severe reaction: loss of consciousness, seizures
Precipitating factors	Undiagnosed diabetes Omission of insulin dose Puberty Infection Cardiovascular disorder Other physical or emotional stress, such as pregnancy or surgery Trauma	Undiagnosed diabetes Infection or other stress Medications: Dilantin, thiazide diuretics, steroids, chlorpromazine Dialysis GI bleed Hyperalimentation, MI Acute pancreatitis Central nervous system disorders Major burns rehydrated with high volumes of glucose	Delay or omission of meal Insulin overdosage Excessive exercise Improper timing of insulin and food
Onset of manifestations	Slow (hours to days) or quickly	Slow (hours to days)	Rapid (minutes to hours)
Laboratory findings:			
Plasma glucose	300–1,500 mg/dl	600–2,000 mg/dl	60 mg/dl or less
Serum sodium	Normal or decreased	Normal or increased	Normal
Serum potassium	Normal or elevated at first, then decreased	Same as DKA	Normal
BUN	Elevated	Elevated	Normal
Serum ketones	Elevated	Absent	Absent
White blood cells	Elevated	Elevated	Normal or elevated
Hematocrit	Elevated	Elevated	Normal
Urine glucose	Elevated	Elevated	Absent
Urine ketones	Elevated	Absent	Absent
Arterial blood gas	Metabolic acidosis with compensatory respiratory alkalosis	Normal (metabolic acidosis of shock is profound and prolonged)	Normal or slight respiratory acidosis
pH	Less than 7.3	Usually normal or slightly decreased	Normal
Osmolality	300–350 mOsm/L	Usually over 350 mOsm/L	Normal
Acute intervention	IV regular insulin IV fluids such as normal saline or half normal saline Potassium when urine output is adequate Sodium bicarbonate, rarely Phosphate, usually ECG Correct underlying problem	Correct underlying problem IV regular insulin IV fluids such as normal saline or half normal saline Potassium when urine output is adequate	Mild reaction: 10–15 g of simple carbohydrate Moderate reaction: one or more simple carbohydrate, glucagon may be needed, ½–1 mg Severe reaction: glucagon IM or SC, repeat × 1 in 10 minutes prn, may need IV glucose

Table continued on following page

	Diabetic Ketoacidosis (DKA)	Hyperglycemia, Hyperosmolar, Nonketotic Coma (HHNK)	Hypoglycemia
Table 69–10. Acute Complications of Diabetes *(Continued)*			
Preventive measures	Prompt medical attention when necessary Plan ahead for illness care Frequent SMBG when ill or during stressful events	Frequent SMBG when ill or during stressful events Prompt medical attention when necessary	Sleeping late should be planned in advance; if oversleeping >45 min is planned, changes in insulin or food intake may be necessary Have short-acting carbohydrate available when exercising or reduction of insulin dose before exercise Restricting alcohol intake Double-check insulin type and dosage prior to administration

→ → → Wearing ID alert band. Education for self-care. → → →

poglycemia leading to counterregulatory hormone secretion and resultant liver production of glucose. This increased glucose, along with insulin resistance secondary to increased hormone levels, could contribute to rebound hyperglycemia.

Nocturnal rebound hyperglycemia should be investigated by SMBG between 2:00 and 4:00 AM and again at 7:00 AM. If early morning levels are less than 50 to 60 mg/dl and those at 7:00 AM are greater than 180 to 200 mg/dl, rebound hyperglycemia may have occurred. Decreasing the intermediate insulin dose at suppertime, moving the intermediate insulin dose to bedtime, or increasing the size of the bedtime snack should prevent this phenomenon.

Dawn Phenomenon

The *dawn phenomenon* refers to an early morning (4 to 8 AM) rise in blood glucose level without preceding nocturnal hypoglycemia. Wearing off of insulin does not appear to be the sole cause of this phenomenon. It has been found in both type I and type II diabetes, and it probably occurs in people without diabetes. Growth hormone, increased insulin clearance, and diurnal variation in counterregulatory hormone levels seem to play a role.

The key clinical implication of dawn phenomenon is that attempts to normalize prebreakfast glucose levels often result in early morning hypoglycemia. Client SMBG and education regarding bedtime snacks, manifestations of nocturnal hypoglycemia, and importance of avoiding hypoglycemia are vital. Recent investigation has shown positive effects of the use of Ultralente instead of NPH insulin in the elimination of this phenomenon.

Chronic Complications of Diabetes Mellitus

Because people who have diabetes mellitus now live longer with the disease, their risk of developing chronic complications is greater. Chronic complications are the major causes of morbidity and mortality in clients with diabetes. These changes affect many body systems and can be devastating to clients and their families. These complications occur in clients with both type I and type II diabetes. Complications are classified as *macrovascular*, including coronary artery disease, cerebrovascular disease, hypertension, peripheral vascular disease, and infection; *microvascular*, including retinopathy and nephropathy; and *neuropathic*, including sensorimotor and autonomic dysfunction. See Box 69–10 for a list of chronic complications of diabetes.

Sustained increased glucose levels in the diabetic create an imbalance of substances used for making the matrix between cells. Enzyme systems normally convert glucose to other sugars, such as sorbitol and fructose to lower blood glucose. Sorbitol and fructose, as well as glucose, accumulate in the basement membrane of the cell and between the cells. Intracellular accumulations of sorbitol cause intracellular edema and affect function.

The microcirculation is affected by extracellular accumulation of glucose, sorbitol, and fructose. The thickened basement membrane increases the distance that nutrients and waste products must travel to and from the cell. As a result, the cells receive inadequate oxygen and nutrition and cannot rid themselves of waste. Unfortunately, the process starts as early as 2 years after the onset of diabetes.

Box 69–10. Chronic Complications of Diabetes Mellitus

Macrovascular complications

■ Coronary artery disease
■ Cerebrovascular disease
■ Hypertension
■ Peripheral vascular disease
■ Infection

Microvascular complications

■ Retinopathy
■ Nephropathy

Neuropathic complications

■ Sensorimotor neuropathy
■ Autonomic neuropathy
  Gastroparesis
  Neurogenic bladder
  Impotence

Mixed vascular and neuropathic diseases

■ Leg and foot ulcers

Clinicians often see clients with diabetes in the hospital with a myocardial infarction, with loss of cognitive and/or physical function as a result of a cerebral vascular accident, or with lower extremity amputation caused by peripheral vascular disease. Prevention of these all-too-common health problems should be a major focus of nurses working with clients with diabetes (see Table 69–11 for clinical manifestations, diagnosis, and interventions in macrovascular disease in diabetes.)

Macrovascular Complications

Coronary artery disease, cerebrovascular disease, and peripheral vascular disease are more common, tend to occur at an earlier age, and are more extensive and severe in people with diabetes (see Table 69–11). Macrovascular disease (disorder of large arteries) reflects atherosclerosis with deposits of lipids within the inner layer of vessel walls. The risk of developing macrovascular complications is higher in type I than in type II diabetes.

Macrovascular disease, especially coronary artery disease, is the most common cause of death in diabetics, accounting for 40% to 60% of all diabetics with macrovascular disease. The most common reasons for hospitalization in diabetics are for macrovascular complications. Diabetes is not only an independent risk factor for these complications, but it is also a major risk factor for development of hypertension and hyperlipidemia. Typically, VLDL and LDL levels are elevated and HDL levels are decreased. The most characteristic lipid abnormality in diabetes is an elevated triglyceride level. Therefore, the influence of diabetes in these diseases is multiplicative, not additive.

Data indicate that macrovascular disease has a tendency to occur years before the onset of clinical diabetes and to occur in people with impaired glucose tolerance at a similar rate as it does in those with type II diabetes. This phenomenon has been called *syndrome X* in the literature and further establishes the need for primary prevention. (See Box 69–11 for information on prevention of macrovascular complications.)

There is some speculation that type II diabetes may be one piece of a syndrome caused by insulin resistance. A well-established association has been demonstrated among hyperglycemia, hyperinsulinemia, dyslipidemia, and hypertension, which leads to coronary artery disease and stroke. The acronym CHAOS (coronary artery disease, hypertension, adult-onset diabetes, obesity, and stress) has been utilized to remind providers to look at the client's entire risk profile for cardiovascular disease when determining treatment for diabetes.

Successful weight reduction with a balanced diet improves lipid profiles, glucose intolerance, hypertension, and obesity; otherwise, successful treatment of macrovascular disease in the diabetic population parallels that in the non-diabetic population.

Coronary Artery Disease

Clients with diabetes are two to four times as likely as non-diabetics to die of coronary artery disease, and the relative risk factor for cardiovascular disease in women with type II diabetes is three to four times greater. Female sex does not protect the female diabetic from premature macrovascular disease. In many clients with diabetes, macrovascular events such as coronary artery disease are atypical or silent, and they often present as indigestion or unexplained congestive heart failure, dyspnea on exertion, or epigastric pain. Coronary artery disease is common in clients younger than 40 years if diabetes is of long duration. Clients with diabetes who have had a myocardial infarction (MI) have an increased chance of complications or of having a second infarction. Clients with diabetes who have an MI experience a higher incidence of congestive heart failure, shock, and arrhythmias. It has been suggested that insulin therapy in type II diabetes may actually increase atherosclerotic disease. It often leads to weight gain and increased blood pressure.

Cerebrovascular Disease

Prevention of cerebrovascular disease includes the same strategies as prevention of coronary artery disease: control of hypertension, lipids levels, and obesity; smoking cessation; exercise; and good nutritional practices.

Cerebrovascular disease, particularly atherothromboembolic infarctions manifested by transient ischemic attacks (TIAs) and cerebrovascular accidents (CVAs), are more common and severe in diabetes. The incidence is two to

Table 69–11. Macrovascular Disease in Diabetes: Clinical Manifestations, Diagnosis and Interventions

Clinical Manifestations	Diagnosis	Interventions
Cerebral Vascular Disease		
Atherothromboembolic infarctions *(transient ischemic attacks and cerebral vascular accidents)* are more severe, have higher mortality rate, have higher recurrence rate	History Manifestations Physical examinations CT scan MRI	Same as for nondiabetics plus: Improved glucose control, aspirin, Persantine, ticlopidine; ongoing education and support
Heart Disease (Coronary Heart Disease, CAD)		
Diabetics have a higher incidence of coronary artery changes that influence decreased oxygen and nutrients to myocardium. Clients have more *angina* and higher mortality with *myocardial infarction*. Manifestations are often "silent." Clients with a history of DM and MI have higher incidence of *congestive heart failure, shock* and *arrhythmias. Cardiomyopathy* may occur secondary to small vessel infarctions causing myocardial fibrosis and hypertrophy. Additional CAD manifestations: *Exertional weakness, peripheral edema, orthopnea, fatigue.* Features such as female sex, which normally protect one from premature heart disease, do not pertain to individuals with diabetes	History Manifestations Physical examination ECG Cardiac enzymes Cardiac catheterization Stress test Autopsy	Same as for non-diabetics with CVD plus: Improved glucose control, exercise, diet Hypertension control: Use of diuretics may worsen hyperglycemia if hypokalemia exists and may adversely affect lipid levels Beta-adrenergic blockers (may cause hypoglycemia), calcium-channel blockers, thrombolytic agents, aspirin, angioplasty, bypass surgery

three times greater in diabetic clients. The relative risk is higher in females, highest in the fifth and sixth decades of life, and much higher in clients with hypertension. In the United States, southeastern states are often referred to as the *stroke belt*, because of the sizable black population in that region with its increased prevalence of hypertension. Many clients presenting with CVAs have undiagnosed diabetes. In clients with diabetes, CVAs are more serious and have higher recurrence and mortality rates, especially in type II diabetics.

It is speculated that the increased prevalence of CVA in clients with diabetes may be related to the development of diabetic nephropathy and resultant proteinuria, hypertension, and platelet adhesiveness. Clients who present with CVA and high glucose levels have a much poorer prognosis than those with normoglycemia.

Studies have shown that ticlopidine, a platelet aggregation inhibitor, has been shown to be more effective than aspirin in lowering risk of cerebral infarction, especially in clients with diabetes. This drug may also cause increased cholesterol levels and neutropenia.

Hypertension

A 40% increased rate of hypertension has been noted in the diabetic population. Hypertension is a major risk factor for stroke and nephropathy. Inadequately treated hypertension augments the rate of development of nephropathy. Individualized pharmacologic treatment for hypertension greater than 140/90 mm Hg is suggested. Angiotensin-converting enzyme (ACE) inhibitors and calcium-channel blockers are the agents of choice for treatment. Beta-blockers and diuretics may increase glucose tolerance and lipid levels.

Peripheral Vascular Disease

In diabetes, incidence and prevalence of carotid bruits, intermittent claudication, absent pedal pulses, and ischemic gangrene are increased. More than 50% of nontraumatic lower limb amputations are associated with diabetic

Clinical Manifestations	Diagnosis	Interventions
Infection		
Diabetics have a higher incidence of *Pseudomonas external otitis* and *monilial skin infections,* common sites of infection in the diabetic include *urinary tract and skin*	History Manifestations Physical examination Laboratory data: serum—increased WBC and blood sugar; urine—increased WBCs	Improved glucose control; antibiotic, anti-fungals as required; follow-up with laboratory data; ongoing client education
Peripheral Vascular Disease (PVD)		
The presence of *carotid bruits, intermittent claudication, absent pedal pulses* and *ischemic gangrene* are increased in diabetes mellitus PVD and neuropathy augment the morbidity associated with trauma and infection in the lower extremity	History Manifestations Physical examinations Doppler studies Angiogram Neuropathy identification	Daily foot inspection aimed at prevention and early intervention; meticulous foot care, padded sport socks, well-fitting shoes; weight reduction; smoking cessation; safe exercise programs; ongoing education
Hypertension		
Usually asymptomatic	History Physical examinations Orthostatic blood pressures with pulse recordings Elevated BP readings at 2–3 recordings Urinalysis: 24-hour urine collection for protein, creatinine clearance and GFR Renal angiogram to evaluate for renal artery stenosis from atherosclerotic disease	Eliminate risk factors; educate client on this silent but deadly disease; diet education: low protein, low salt Pharmacological intervention dependent on blood pressure readings: diuretics, ACE inhibitors, calcium-channel blockers, alpha-blockers

changes such as sensory and autonomic neuropathy peripheral vascular disease, an increased risk and rate of infection, and poor healing. This chain of events, which may lead to amputation, is illustrated in Figure 69–9.

Infections

Clients with diabetes are susceptible to infections of many types. Infections, once they occur, are difficult to treat. Three factors that may contribute to the development of an infection include the following: (1) impaired polymorphonuclear leukocyte (PMN) function; (2) diabetic neuropathies; and (3) vascular insufficiency. Poor glycemic control augments these factors. Infected areas heal slowly because the damaged vascular system cannot carry sufficient oxygen, white blood cells, nutrients, and antibodies to the injured site. Infections increase the need for insulin and the possibility of ketoacidosis.

Urinary tract infections are the most common type of infections involving diabetic clients, particularly women. Factors that may influence urinary tract infections in diabetics include the inhibition of PMN activity while glycosuria is present. Glucosuria is associated with hyperglycemia. The development of a neurogenic bladder, which results in incomplete emptying and urinary retention, may also contribute to the risk of development of a urinary tract infection.

Diabetic foot infections are very common. Their occurrence is directly related to the three factors listed above plus hyperglycemia. Up to 40% of diabetics with foot infections may require amputation, and 5% to 10% will die despite amputation of the affected area. With proper education and early intervention, foot infections are usually eliminated in a timely manner.

The Care Plan provides instruction for the client with diabetes regarding prevention of foot infections. Effective foot care can be the initial break in the chain of events that leads to amputation (see Fig. 69–9) (see Bridge to Home Healthcare for more information).

Areas of the skin particularly subject to local infection by yeast organisms include the neck, axillae, and groin.

Box 69–11. Prevention of Macrovascular Complications in Clients with Diabetes

Primary Prevention

- Normalizing weight/reducing obesity
- Exercising
- Not smoking
- Normalizing lipid levels

Secondary Prevention

- Prompt recognition and treatment of hyperglycemia with exercise, food, and medication
- Aggressive treatment of hypertension, including regular blood pressure checks
- Screening high-risk clients (those with a family history of diabetes)

Tertiary Prevention

- Controlling angina
- Treating peripheral vascular disease
- SMBG to keep track of subjective and objective data
- Controlling risk factors for macrovascular disease
- Stressing medication compliance and follow-up
- Working closely with the client

In addition, obese women may develop raw infected areas beneath the breasts.

Microvascular Complications

Microangiopathy refers to the changes that occur in retinal and renal capillaries in diabetes. It has been made clear by the DCCT that consistent and tight glycemic control can prevent or stop microvascular changes (see the Nursing Research feature earlier in the chapter).

Diabetic Retinopathy

Diabetic retinopathy is the major cause of blindness among clients with diabetes. Approximately 80% of all clients with diabetes have some form of retinopathy 15 years after diagnosis.

Clients with type II diabetes develop retinopathy faster than do clients with type I diabetes. Manifestations may be evident 2 years after diagnosis. The client with type I diabetes may develop retinopathy 10 to 12 years after diagnosis.

Diabetes may be severely complicated by microangiopathy or vascular degeneration of the small vessels supplying the eyes and kidneys. The retina, which is the most essential structure of the eye, has the highest rate of

oxygen consumption of any tissue in the body. Consequently, if the retina is deprived of oxygen-carrying blood secondary to destruction of its capillaries, tissue anoxia develops swiftly.

Risk factors under investigation that may affect the development of retinopathy include chronic hyperglycemia, poor glycemic control, disease duration, hypertension, pregnancy, puberty, polyuria, and smoking (see Client Education Guide on p. 1999).

The three types of diabetic retinopathy are (1) nonproliferative (i.e., "background retinopathy"); (2) preproliferative; and (3) proliferative.

Nonproliferative diabetic retinopathy (NPDR) is the early phase of retinopathy. It is characterized by microaneurysms (outpouching) and intraretinal "dot and blot" hemorrhages. NPDR occurs in most clients with long-term diabetes, and in many cases it does not progress or affect visual acuity.

Preproliferative diabetic retinopathy involves further progression of the hemorrhages accompanied by decreasing visual acuity. It usually progresses to proliferative diabetic retinopathy.

Proliferative diabetic retinopathy is the final and most vision-threatening type. The weakened and damaged vessels (formed in response to ischemia) may rupture, causing retinal hemorrhage and exudates. It is the major cause of blindness in the United States.

Other Ocular Disorders

Blurred Vision. Blurred vision usually results from an abnormally elevated blood glucose level. Consequently, once the client's diabetes is under control, vision often clears. Clients should wait at least 6 weeks until blood glucose control is established before obtaining new prescription lenses.

Cataracts. A cataract is an opacity of the lens. Fortunately, surgical removal of the cataracts or use of glasses or implanted lenses helps restore vision in the majority of clients. Clients with diabetes are at higher risk of cataract formation and of glaucoma.

Clients who are visually impaired may continue to give their own insulin injections by using syringe magnifiers or other available devices. In some cases, the nurse may need to plan for a family member or home healthcare nurse to draw up the insulin for the client. Self-monitoring of blood glucose may be done with a special device that announces the result or with the help of another person. The Association for the Blind provides training that enables many visually impaired clients to maintain independence in daily living.

Nephropathy

Diabetic nephropathy is the single most common cause of endstage renal disease (ESRD). Approximately 35% to

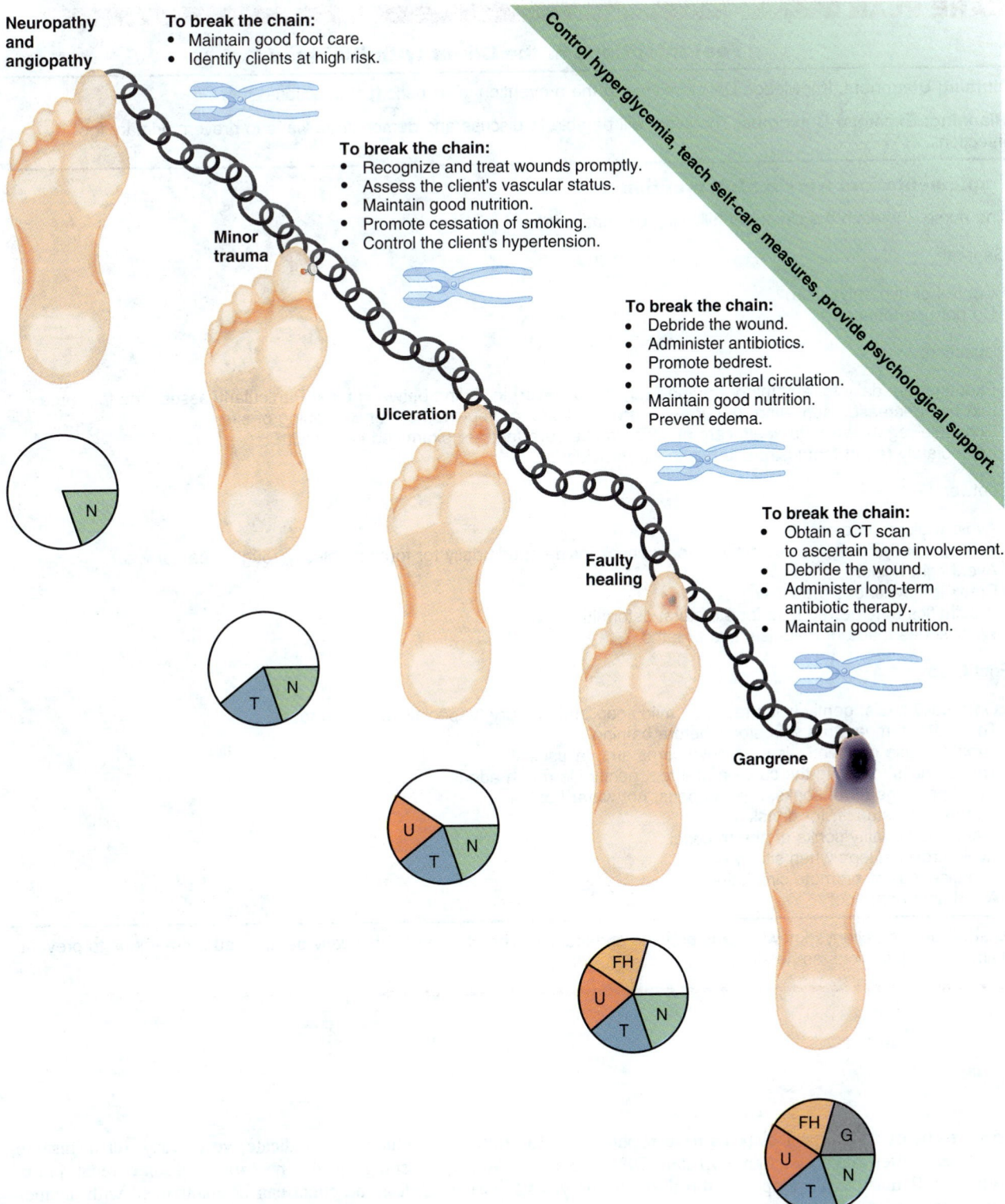

Neuropathy and angiopathy

To break the chain:
- Maintain good foot care.
- Identify clients at high risk.

Control hyperglycemia, teach self-care measures, provide psychological support.

To break the chain:
- Recognize and treat wounds promptly.
- Assess the client's vascular status.
- Maintain good nutrition.
- Promote cessation of smoking.
- Control the client's hypertension.

Minor trauma

To break the chain:
- Debride the wound.
- Administer antibiotics.
- Promote bedrest.
- Promote arterial circulation.
- Maintain good nutrition.
- Prevent edema.

Ulceration

To break the chain:
- Obtain a CT scan to ascertain bone involvement.
- Debride the wound.
- Administer long-term antibiotic therapy.
- Maintain good nutrition.

Faulty healing

Gangrene

Figure 69–9. Breaking the chain of events that leads to amputation in high-risk clients with diabetes mellitus. High-risk clients (those with neuropathy, vascular disease, structural deformities, abnormal gait, skin or nail deformities, or a history of previous diabetic ulcers or amputations) need frequent monitoring by the healthcare team. (Adapted from Pecoraro, R. E., & Burgess, E. M. [1992]. Pathways to diabetic limb amputation: Basis for prevention. *Diabetes Spectrum, 5*[6], 329–334.)

CARE PLAN

Foot Infections in the Client with Diabetes

Nursing Diagnosis. Knowledge Deficit related to the prevention of diabetic foot infections

Planning: Expected Outcomes. The client will be able to discuss and demonstrate ways to prevent primary foot infections.

Implementation: Nursing Intervention

The nurse will teach the client the following content areas:

General:

▪ Control of hyperglycemia
▪ Do not use tobacco

Inspection:

▪ Examine feet daily for any minor trauma (may need mirror) including between toes. Particularly assess the foot area that has decreased sensation, or current injury. Evaluate for improvement or worsening of site.
▪ Schedule regular visits to healthcare provider; make sure feet are examined each visit
▪ Immediately report foot lesions to healthcare provider

Footwear:

▪ Avoid walking barefoot
▪ Wear properly fitting, nonrestrictive shoes; check inside shoes daily for foreign objects, rough areas or wear
▪ Avoid tight hosiery
▪ Break in new shoes gradually
▪ Prosthetics may be required for structural deformities
▪ Wear shoes made of materials that breathe

Foot Care:

▪ On a daily basis, gently wash feet with mild soap and blot dry (especially between toes)
▪ Test water temperature with elbow before bathing
▪ Avoid the use of chemicals to remove corns and calluses
▪ Trim toenails following the curve of the toe, gently file rough edges
▪ Avoid prolonged foot soaks, heating pads, hot water bottles
▪ Use mild moisturizer for dry skin
▪ Wear good-quality socks of any material
▪ Avoid crossing legs when sitting
▪ Exercise legs to promote circulation
▪ Avoid going barefoot

Evaluation. The client's knowledge is ongoing and lifelong. The client will continually be updated on methods to prevent diabetic foot infections as needed.

45% of clients with type I diabetes have nephropathy 15 to 20 years after diagnosis. Approximately 20% of clients with type II diabetes develop nephropathy 5 to 10 years after diagnosis. Nephropathy, which is a consequence of microangiopathy, involves damage and eventual obliteration of the capillaries that supply the glomeruli of the kidney. Damage of the glomerular capillaries in turn leads to a complex of pathologic changes and manifestations (intercapillary glomerulosclerosis, nephrosis, gross albuminuria, and hypertension). Risk factors include poor glycemic control, duration of disease, and hypertension. Some clients now self-check microalbumin levels at home. This test can detect very small quantities of urinary albumin, which can indicate very early renal disease. With worsening of the nephrosis, chronic renal failure ensues. Unless the client can be maintained with hemodialysis or receives a renal transplant, uremia eventually causes death (see Chapter 57).

Clients with nephropathy monitor their blood glucose levels and blood pressure at home. ACE inhibitors can be used to decrease the microalbuminuria. Hypertension should be treated aggressively, as it can be the catalyst for the progression of nephropathy. Clients with nephropathy are taught to eat a low-protein diet and to avoid nephrotoxic drugs (e.g., gentamicin). If contrast dye is required for radiographic study, mannitol may be ordered,

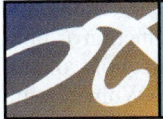

BRIDGE TO HOME HEALTHCARE

Diabetic Foot Care

Peg Neumann, R.N., M.P.H., *Visiting Nurse Association of Omaha, Omaha, Nebraska*

Normal foot care activities can be a real difficulty for the diabetic client. These clients may have diminished vision and difficulty reaching their feet because of the diabetes or other chronic diseases. Peripheral vascular complications, other circulatory complications, and the decrease of sensation and lack of healing in the extremities can combine to make even routine foot care a hazard. These problems are noted frequently by nurses during home and clinic visits, especially when clients are elderly.

The home healthcare nurse completes an initial assessment and evaluates the client's mobility, gait, hygiene, hydration, color, temperature, edema, pain, and sensation (or loss of sensation). Circulation is checked by palpating pedal pulses and the blanch/return time of nail beds. The nails are evaluated for thickness and discoloration due to possible fungal infection. The nurse needs to ask "Who has been cutting your toenails?" When the nurse plans to trim toenails for a diabetic client, check the physician's orders.

Toenails are easiest to cut after they are soaked in warm, soapy water or just after bathing. It is important to be able to see both sides of the cutting instrument before you cut, and then to protect your eyes from "flying" toenail pieces. Cut the nail to follow the curve of the toe; do not cut so straight across that edges are created that cause pressure on adjacent toes, and do not make such a rounded or short cut that tissue is left unprotected. File nails gently with an emery board to smooth the edges and prevent clothing snags and nail damage. If the nails have not been cut for an extended time, do not try to remove too much of the nail. Use a manicure stick to gently push the cuticle back. Tell the client that you will trim a portion of the nail today and will return in 1 or 2 weeks for further trimming. If the nails are so thick that they cannot be cut with a nipper or a clipper, or if they are so damaged by fungal infection that they cannot be cut, refer the client to a podiatrist.

Teach the client to inspect all foot surfaces daily. Use a mirror if needed. If red areas or ulcers are noted, the client should notify the nurse.

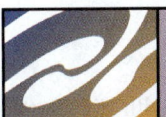

CLIENT EDUCATION GUIDE

Visual Complications of Diabetes

Diabetes can cause diabetic retinopathy, which can lead to vision loss.

There is a relationship between hyperglycemia and diabetic retinopathy. It is extremely important to normalize blood glucose levels.

Hypertension can worsen diabetic retinopathy. Its diagnosis and aggressive treatment are important.

If you have diabetic retinopathy, you should know that isometric exercises raise intraocular pressure and can aggravate proliferative retinopathy.

An ophthalmologist will be brought in to be part of your diabetes management team.

If you have any visual impairments, you can be referred to appropriate organizations for assistance.

If your vision is blurred while reading, you may have hyperglycemia or macular edema. Floaters may indicate hemorrhage, and flashing lights may indicate retinal detachment. If you experience any of these occurrences, you should report them.

Early laser photocoagulation therapy can reduce risk of vision loss.

Adapted from American Diabetes Association. Type II; and Herman, W. H. & Green, D. A. (1993). Microvascular complications of diabetes. In Haire-Joshu, D. (Ed.), *Management of diabetes mellitus: Perspectives of care across the life span.* St. Louis: Mosby–Year Book.

but the client must drink fluids after the test to clear the dye from the kidneys. Serum creatinine levels should be assessed before the administration of the contrast dye or other nephrotoxic agents.

Like diabetic retinopathy, diabetic nephropathy cannot be cured. However, prompt and adequate interventions for renal and bladder infections can prevent these causes of renal failure. Control of hypertension and tight glycemic control can contribute to a delay in the development of nephropathy or a decrease in its progression.

Unsuccessfully treated nephropathy progresses to end-stage renal disease. Treatment at this point includes hemodialysis, peritoneal dialysis, or a kidney transplant.

Neuropathy

Neuropathy is the most common chronic complication of diabetes. Nearly 60% of diabetics experience neuropathy. Even though nerve fibers do not have their own blood supply, they depend on the diffusion of nutrients and oxygen across the membrane. When axons and dendrites are not nourished, their transmission of impulses slows. In addition, sorbitol accumulates in nerve tissue, further diminishing both sensory and motor function. Both temporary and permanent neurologic problems may develop in clients with diabetes during the course of the illness. The neuropathy may be mild (causing minor inconveniences) or so severe that the quality of life is affected. Identified causes of diabetic neuropathy include vascular insufficiency, chronic elevations in blood glucose levels, hypertension, and cigarette smoking. Clients may present with mononeuropathy or polyneuropathy and may have sensory or motor impairment, depending on which nerves are involved.

Mononeuropathy. Mononeuropathy, or focal neuropathy, usually involves a single nerve or group of nerves. Mononeuropathies produce sharp, stabbing pains and are usually caused by an infarction of the blood supply. The muscles innervated by nerves affected by focal neuropathies are painful and are at risk for atrophy from disuse. Treatment may include surgical decompression for compression lesions.

Polyneuropathy. Polyneuropathy, or diffuse neuropathy, involves the sensory and autonomic nerves. Sensory neuropathy is the most common type of neuropathy. It is commonly assessed as bilateral, symmetrical, and affecting the lower extremities. The client describes tingling, numbness, burning, and mild to total sensory loss. This complication is a major factor in injuries to the lower extremities. Treatment includes foot care education to prevent trauma and ulcers. Painful neuropathy may be treated with tricyclic antidepressants, phenytoin, or carbamazepine. Polyneuropathy also may simply resolve spontaneously.

Autonomic Neuropathy. Autonomic neuropathy demonstrates itself in its effect in pupillary, cardiovascular, gastrointestinal and genitourinary functions.

Pupillary. Autonomic neuropathy of the pupil interferes with the pupil's ability to adapt to the dark. Pupil dilation is inadequate. Clients are at risk for accidents when driving at night. The environment should be well lighted at night.

Cardiovascular. Autonomic neuropathy of the cardiovascular system is evidenced by an abnormal response to exercise. A fixed heart rate may occur. Orthostatic hypotension may occur, which is dangerous. Resting tachycardia may occur.

Gastrointestinal. Autonomic neuropathy disorders frequently affect the GI tract. The client may experience dysphagia, abdominal pain, nausea, vomiting, malabsorption, postprandial hypoglycemia, diarrhea, constipation, or fecal incontinence. Gastroparesis (delayed stomach emptying) may give the client the feeling of stomach fullness. This may contribute to anorexia, decreased intake, weight loss, and labile blood glucose levels related to food malabsorption. Approximately 20% to 30% of diabetics have gastroparesis. Gastroparesis may be improved with metoclopramide, erythromycin, or clonidine.

Genitourinary. Bladder hypotonicity or neurogenic bladder is a frequent manifestation of autonomic neuropathy. Manifestations may include straining with urination, long periods of time between voiding, and decreased urinary stream. Urinary stasis may occur and develop into urinary tract infections. In the male client, autonomic neuropathy can contribute to erectile dysfunction (impotence) and retrograde ejaculation. Penile injections or implantable devices may improve function. Women with autonomic neuropathy may experience painful intercourse. Estrogen-containing lubricants can resolve this.

Special Situations in the Care of Clients with Diabetes

■ Management of the Diabetic Client Undergoing Surgery

Undergoing surgery is a stressful experience for anyone, but for the client with diabetes, surgery imposes several additional stressors. Surgery interrupts the client's usual therapeutic regimen; the diet must be temporarily changed, and the dosage of insulin or oral hypoglycemic agent readjusted; the stress of surgery raises serum glucose levels; the client is prone to infection; and the surgical incision itself becomes a new potential portal of entry for infectious agents. Furthermore, postoperative healing in these clients may be slow as a result of previously mentioned factors.

To offset these problems, clients with diabetes require special intervention, both preoperatively and postoperatively. Specific interventions vary, depending on whether the client has IDDM or NIDDM and whether the surgery is elective or emergent.

Preoperative Care

The goal of preoperative care for clients with diabetes is thorough regulation of blood glucose levels before surgery. Clients with IDDM need to be closely monitored for several days or even weeks before elective surgery to stabilize their condition and thereby decrease surgical risk. Sometimes a client with IDDM and poor glucose control requires emergency surgery. In this situation, the surgeon must make the critical decision between operating on a hypoglycemic or hyperglycemic client and postponing an emergency operation until the diabetes is controlled. In either case, the client needs constant monitoring of vital signs, frequent laboratory and bedside glucose meter studies, and vigilant nursing intervention.

In contrast, clients with well-controlled NIDDM usually undergo surgery with only slightly more risk than that of the general population. Typically, preoperative preparation for clients with diabetes includes the following:

● Preoperative laboratory tests, including (1) fasting and preprandial blood glucose levels; (2) glycosylated hemoglobin; (3) electrolytes, BUN, and creatinine; (4) complete blood count; (5) ECG and cardiac enzymes; and (6) chest radiograph
● Early morning scheduling of surgery so that the client's diet and insulin regimen undergo as little disruption as possible
● Omission of food, water, and oral hypoglycemic agents on the morning of surgery. One long-acting hypoglyce-

mic agent, chlorpropamide, should be discontinued 1 to 2 days before surgery because of its long half-life.

- Beginning an IV infusion of insulin for insulin-dependent or insulin-requiring clients. Glucose (5%) is usually also administered to prevent the possibility of hypoglycemia. If the surgery is relatively minor (e.g., cataract removal), the surgeon may order administration of a 5% dextrose solution infusion begun and of half the usual dose of intermediate-acting insulin. The anesthesiologist can monitor blood glucose levels in the operating room.

- A blood glucose determination performed and reported to the physician within 1 hour before the operation to ensure that the client (who has been NPO since midnight) will not develop hypoglycemia during surgery

Intraoperative Care

Once the client arrives in surgery, management again depends on the severity of the diabetes and the extent of the surgery. Regular insulin, based on the client's blood glucose levels and a sliding scale or an insulin protocol, can be given IV. Subcutaneous insulin should not be given intraoperatively because its absorption is affected by body temperature, circulatory blood volumes, and certain types of anesthetics.

Postoperative Care

After surgery, the goals of postoperative management are to stabilize the client's vital signs, correct fluid and electrolyte imbalances, reestablish control of the diabetes, prevent wound infection, and promote wound healing. The following are important postoperative interventions:

- Administer prescribed IV infusions and regular insulin until the client is able to take oral nourishment.

- Once the client is able to tolerate fluids, offer fluids that contain calories for prevention of hypoglycemia. Once the client can eat, food should be made available. Discuss the client's caloric level with a registered dietitian so that enough calories for postoperative wound healing are being provided.

- Obtain blood glucose level four to six times daily.

- Resume the client's prescribed preoperative insulin type (e.g., NPH, Lente) and dosage once blood glucose control is reestablished, foods are being consumed at adequate levels, and it has been reordered by the physician.

- Observe for manifestations of hypoglycemia after surgery. These may include a decrease in the blood pressure or an increase in the heart rate in a client who is still unresponsive from anesthesia.

- Avoid catheterization, if at all possible, to prevent bladder infections.

- Change wound dressings with meticulous sterile technique for prevention of wound infection.

- Observe for manifestations of skin breakdown and treat, especially if peripheral vascular disease or neuropathy is present.

- Assess the client's wound and incision frequently for manifestations of infection. Be alert for abnormal amounts of drainage or foul-smelling drainage.

■ Management of Diabetes when Sick

The Client Education Guide presents guidelines for the client to follow during illnesses.

■ Management of Diabetes when Traveling

All clients with diabetes face special challenges when they travel across different time zones since their mealtimes will be altered. Discuss with the client how to accommodate the diabetes regimen when traveling. Insulin therapy supplies and SMBG equipment should never be packed in checked baggage; it should be carried on board.

Conclusions

Diabetes mellitus is a chronic disease characterized by abnormalities in carbohydrate, fat, and protein metabolism. The two major categories of diabetes are (1) insulin-dependent diabetes mellitus (IDDM) and non–insulin-dependent diabetes mellitus (NIDDM). Meal planning, exercise, and medication are the main forms of treatment. Acute complications include hyperglycemia with diabetic ketoacidosis and hypoglycemia. Chronic complications are relentless and are a result of multiple effects in small and large vessels. Because diabetes is chronic, nursing management focuses on teaching the client and family how to manage the disorder on a day-to-day basis and how to assess for complications.

Thinking Critically

1. A client with type I IDDM takes 14 units of regular insulin and 32 units of NPH insulin SC at 7 AM and 5 PM every day. He is now hospitalized for pneumonia and nausea. It is 9:30 AM. On entering his room, you observe the client talking to his plants. What is your priority intervention? How will his confusion be resolved?

Factors to Consider. When does regular insulin peak? What might be the underlying cause of the client's confusion? How might you confirm the presence of hypoglycemia?

2. An elderly woman with type I IDDM calls the clinic and tells the nurse that she has the "flu." She tells the nurse that she usually takes Humulin N, 12 units, and Humulin R, 8 units, every morning. She did not take her insulin this morning because of vomiting, nausea, and an inability to eat. She tells the nurse she lives alone. What telephone advice is appropriate? How often should she monitor her blood glucose levels while she is ill?

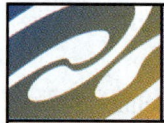

CLIENT EDUCATION GUIDE

Sick Day Management for Diabetes Mellitus*

You should have an individualized plan of care prescribed by the healthcare team to utilize during illness. Monitoring is an essential part of diabetes management, but this is even more vital during the stress of illness. Insulin requirements may be increased secondary to reduced activity and increased secretion of counterregulatory hormones. To prevent diabetic ketoacidosis, you should know the following:

SMBG: It is important to self-monitor blood glucose more frequently during illness, often every 2–4 hours. If premeal blood glucose values stay greater than 250 mg/dl, you should test for urine ketones and contact your healthcare provider.

Ketones: Urine ketones should be monitored when you feel sick and/or blood glucose is greater than 250 mg/dl. Test for ketones every 2–4 hours.

Insulin: Do not stop taking your insulin, even if you are vomiting and unable to eat. Additional regular insulin may be required, based on SMBG results.

Nutrition/Fluids: Adequate fluid intake and carbohydrates are essential during illness. Eating 10–15 g of carbohydrate every 1–2 hours and small quantities of fluid every 15–30 minutes is usually sufficient to prevent dehydration and ketoacidosis. Clear broth, tea, and ice chips are usually well tolerated. Examples of food and beverages containing about 15 g carbohydrate are as follows:

1 regular whole Popsicle
½ cup applesauce
½ cup regular soft drink
¾ cup ginger ale
½ cup orange or apple juice
1 cup Gatorade
½ cup regular gelatin

Notify your healthcare provider when you have any of the following manifestations:

- Illness that persists more than 24 hours
- Severe abdominal pain
- Fever over 100° F, oral
- Persistent diarrhea
- Vomiting with inability to take fluids greater for more than 4 hours
- Blood glucose levels difficult to control and/or moderate to large ketones in urine
- Shortness of breath or chest pain
- Acute visual loss
- Other unexplained manifestations

* Most applicable to clients with type I diabetes and those with type II diabetes receiving insulin therapy.

Factors to Consider. What learning needs does the client exhibit? When should the insulin be given? Is a clinic visit warranted?

3. The client is a 67-year-old woman who has a 25-year history of type I IDDM. She has been compliant over the years; with the advent of home glucose monitoring her blood sugar levels have been very well controlled. Her main problem is a significant history of hypertension, controlled with a daily antihypertensive. Lately, she finds that small cuts and bruises take longer than usual to heal. What are the chronic complications of diabetes mellitus? What teaching should you consider for this client?

Factors to Consider. What risks does this client face as a result of her long-term diabetic history? How would you approach teaching about complications?

Bibliography

1. Ahroni, J. H. (1993). Teaching foot care creatively and successfully. *The Diabetes Educator, 19*(4), 320–324.
2. American Diabetes Association. (1995). Continuous subcutaneous insulin infusion. *Diabetes Care, 18*(suppl. 1), 33.
3. American Diabetes Association (1995). Detection and management of lipid disorders in diabetes. *Diabetes Care, 18*(suppl. 1), 86–93.

4. American Diabetes Association (1993). Exercise and NIDDM. *Diabetes Care, 16*(suppl. 2), 54–57.

5. American Diabetes Association (1993). Foot care in patients with diabetes mellitus. *Diabetes Care, 16*(suppl. 2), 19–20.

6. American Diabetes Association (1993). Implications of the diabetes control and complications trial. *Diabetes Care, 6*(4), 225.

7. American Diabetes Association (1993). Implications of the diabetes control and complications trial. *Diabetes Care, 16*(11), 1517–1520.

8. American Diabetes Association (1993). Insulin administration. *Diabetes Care, 16*(suppl. 2), 31–34.

9. American Diabetes Association (1993). Magnesium supplementation in the treatment of diabetes. *Diabetes Care, 16*(suppl. 2), 79–81.

10. American Diabetes Association (1994). *Medical management of insulin-dependent (type I) diabetes* (2nd ed.). Alexandria, VA: Author.

11. American Diabetes Association (1994). *Medical management of non-insulin-dependent (type II) diabetes* (3rd ed.). Alexandria, VA: Author.

12. American Diabetes Association (1995). Nutrition recommendations and principles for people with diabetes mellitus. *Diabetes Care, 18*(suppl. 1), 16–19.

13. American Diabetes Association (1993). Prevention of type I diabetes mellitus. *Diabetes Care, 16*(suppl. 2), 14–15.

14. American Diabetes Association (1995). Screening for diabetes. *Diabetes Care, 18*(suppl. 1), 5–7.

15. American Diabetes Association (1993). Self-monitoring of blood glucose. *Diabetes Care, 16*(suppl. 2), 60–64.

16. American Diabetes Association (1995). Standards of medical care for patients with diabetes mellitus. *Diabetes Care, 18*(suppl. 1), 8–15.

17. Anderson, L. A., & Zimmerman, M. A. (1993). Patient and physician perceptions of their relationship and patient satisfaction: A study of chronic disease management. *Patient Education and Counseling, 20*(1), 27–36.

18. Arnold, M., et al. (1993). Guidelines vs practice in the delivery of diabetes nutrition care. *Journal of the American Dietetic Association, 93*(1), 34–39.

19. Auslander, W. (1992). Social contexts of management: Family and community environments. In D. Haire-Joshu (Ed.), *Management of diabetes mellitus: Perspectives of care across the life span* (pp 355–361). St. Louis: Mosby–Year Book.

20. Beaser, R. S. (1992). Fine-tuning insulin therapy. *Postgraduate Medicine, 91*(4), 323–330.

21. Beaser, R. S. (1995). Putting DCCT into practice. *Patient Care, 29*(6), 15–30.

22. Bell, D. S. H. (1994). Stroke in the diabetes patient. *Diabetes Care, 17*(3), 213–219.

23. Berne, R., & Levy, M. (1993). *Physiology* (3rd ed). St. Louis: Mosby–Year Book.

24. Bergenstal, R., & Rubenstein, A. (1995). Diabetes mellitus therapy. In L. J. De Groot (Ed.). *Endocrinology* (3rd ed.; pp. 1482–1505). Philadelphia: W. B. Saunders.

25. Bridges, R. M., & Deitch, E. A. (1994). Diabetic foot infections: Pathophysiology and treatment. *Surgical Clinics of North America, 74*(3), 537–555.

26. Brown, D. F., & Jackson, T. W. (1994). Diabetes: Tight control in a comprehensive treatment plan. *Geriatrics, 49*(6), 24–29, 33–36.

27. Brown, W. V. (1994). Lipoprotein disorders in diabetes mellitus. *Medical Clinics of North America, 78*(1), 143–155.

28. Coleman, W. C. (1992). Foot care and diabetes. In D. Haire-Joshu (Ed.), *Management of diabetes mellitus: Perspectives of care across the life span* (pp 215–248). St. Louis: Mosby–Year Book.

29. Collo, M. B., Johnson, J. L., & Kabadi, U. M. (1993). Combination sulfonylurea and insulin therapy in non-insulin dependent diabetes mellitus. *Nurse Practitioner, 18*(7), 40–48.

30. Coniff, R. F., et al. (1995). Multicenter, placebo-controlled trial comparing acarbose (BAY g 5421) with placebo, tolbutamide, and tolbutamide-plus-acarbose in non-insulin dependent diabetes mellitus. *American Journal of Medicine, 98*, 443–451.

31. Coniff, R. F., et al. (1995). Reduction of glycosylated hemoglobin and postprandial hyperglycemia by acarbose in patients with NIDDM. *Diabetes Care, 18*(6), 817–824.

32. Daly, A. (1994). Diabesity: The deadly pentad disease. *The Diabetes Educator, 10*(2), 156–162.

33. Davidson, M. B., et al. (1994) Real-world management of type II diabetes. *Patient Care, 28*(15), 68–86.

34. Dawson, L. Y. (1993). DCCT: Team approach takes center stage. *Diabetes Spectrum, 6*(4), 222–224.

35. DeFronzo, R. A., Goodman, A. M., & the Multicenter Metformin Study Group. (1995). Efficacy of metformin in patients with non-insulin dependent diabetes mellitus. *New England Journal of Medicine, 333*(9), 541–549.

36. Delahanty, L. (1992). Nutritional recommendations for cardiovascular complications of diabetes. *Nutrition Update, 18*(6), 543–544.

37. Diabetes Control and Complications Trial Research Group. (1993). The effect of intensive treatment of diabetes on the development and progression of long-term complications in insulin-dependent diabetes mellitus. *The New England Journal of Medicine, 329*(14), 977–985.

38. Etzwiler, D. D. (1994). Diabetes translation: A blueprint for the future. *Diabetes Care, 17*(suppl. 1), 1–4.

39. Fajans, S. (1995). Diabetes mellitus: Definition, classification, tests. In L. J. DeGroot (Ed.). *Endocrinology* (3rd ed.; pp. 1411–1422). Philadelphia: W. B. Saunders.

40. Farkas-Hirsch, R., & Hirsch, I. B. (1994). Continuous subcutaneous insulin infusion: A review of the past and its implementation for the future. *Diabetes Spectrum, 7*(2), 80–84, 136–138.

41. Foster, D. W., & McGarry, J. D. (1995). Diabetes mellitus: Acute complications, ketoacidosis, hyperosmolar coma, lactic acidosis. In J. L. DeGroot, (Ed.), *Endocrinology* (3rd ed.; pp. 1506–1521). Philadelphia: W. B. Saunders.

42. Franz, M. J., et al. (1994). Nutrition principles for the management of diabetes and related complications. *Diabetes Care, 17*(5), 490–511.

43. Friesen, J., et al. (1994). Diets for diabetes: More choices than ever. *Patient Care, 28*(15), 86–94.

44. Funnell, M. M., & Merritt, J. H. (1992). Diabetes and the older adult. In D. Haire-Joshu (Ed.), *Management of diabetes mellitus: Perspectives of care across the life span* (pp 505–564). St. Louis: Mosby–Year Book.

45. Garrison, M. W., & Campbell, R. K. (1993). Identifying and treating common and uncommon infections in the patient with diabetes. *The Diabetes Educator, 19*(6), 522–531.

46. Gates, G. (1994). Hyerlipidemias in diabetic patients: Is standard cholesterol treatment appropriate? *Postgraduate Medicine, 95*(2), 69–70, 77–84.

47. Gearhart, J. G., & Forbes, R. C. (1995). Initial management of the patient with newly diagnosed diabetes. *American Family Physician, 51*(8), 1953–1962.

48. Ginsberg, B. (1994). The role of technology in diabetes therapy. *Diabetes Care, 17*(suppl. 1), 50–55.

49. Glucophage (metformin hydrochloride tablets) package insert from Bristol-Myers Squibb.

50. Groth, K. (1995). Nutritional alterations in critical illness. In L.E.C. Copstead, (Ed.), *Perspectives in pathophysiology*. Philadelphia: W. B. Saunders.

51. Guyton, A. (1992) *Human physiology and mechanisms of disease* (5th ed.). Philadelphia: W. B. Saunders.

52. Haire-Joshu, D., & Funnell, M. M. (Eds.) (1993). Competencies in diabetes care for schools of nursing. *Diabetes Spectrum, 6*, 355–361.

53. Hanefeld, M. (1993). Acarbose efficacy review. *Practical Diabetes Supplement, 10*(6), S21–S27.

54. Harley, J. R. (1993). Preventing diabetic foot disease. *Nurse Practitioner, 18*(10), 37–44.

55. Hill, J., & Poirier, L. (1995). Helping patients manage their diabetes. *Patient Care, 29*(6), 97–120.

56. Howe, R. S., & Christman, C. (1991). Outpatient initiation of insulin: A nurse practitioner protocol. *Journal of the American Academy of Nurse Practitioners, 3*(1), 35–40.

57. Howey, D. C., et al. (1994). [Lys(B28) Pro(B29)] human insulin: A rapidly absorbed analogue of human insulin. *Diabetes, 43*, 396–402.

58. Hoyson, P. (1995) Diabetes 2000: Oral medications. *RN, 58*(5), 34–40.

59. Jasper, J. B., & Green, A. J. (1995). The neuropathies of diabetes. In L. J. DeGroot, (Ed.), *Endocrinology* (3rd ed.; pp. 1536–1568). Philadelphia: W. B. Saunders.

60. Katz, C. M. (1991). How efficient is sliding-scale insulin therapy? *Postgraduate Medicine, 89*(5), 46–57.

61. Kerr, C. P. (1995). Improving outcomes in diabetes: A review of the outpatient care of NIDDM patients. *The Journal of Family Practice, 40*(1), 63–73.

62. Kestel, F. (1994). Are you up to date on diabetes medications? *AJN, 94*(7), 48–52.

63. Kestel, F. (1993). Using blood glucose meters: What you and your patient need to know (part I). *Nursing 93, 23*(3), 34–41.

64. Klein, R. (1995). Diabetes mellitus: Late complications: Oculopathy. In L. J. DeGroot (Ed.). *Endocrinology* (3rd ed.; pp. 1522–1535). Philadelphia: W. B. Saunders.

65. Koda-Kimble, M. A. (1992). Diabetes Mellitus. In M. A. Koda-Kimble, & L. L. Young (Eds.). *Applied therapeutics: The clinical use of drugs* (5th ed.). Vancouver, BC: Applied Therapeutics.

66. Larsen, J., Duckworth, W., & Stratta, R. (1994). Pancreas transplantation for type I diabetes mellitus. *Postgraduate Medicine, 96*(3), 105–111.

67. Lehne, R. (1994). *Pharmacology for nursing care* (2nd ed.). Philadelphia: W. B. Saunders.

68. Lernmark, A. (1995). Insulin dependent (type I) diabetes: Etiology, pathogenesis, and natural history. In J. L. DeGroot (Ed.), *Endocrinology* (3rd ed.; pp. 1423–1435). Philadelphia: W. B. Saunders.

69. Miller, J. F. (1992). *Coping with chronic illness: Overcoming powerlessness* (2nd ed.). Philadelphia: F. A. Davis.

70. Olefsky, J. M. (1995). Diabetes mellitus (type II): Etiology and pathogenesis. In J. L. DeGroot (Ed.), *Endocrinology* (3rd ed.; pp. 1436–1463). Philadelphia: W. B. Saunders.

71. Orchard, T. J. (1994). From diagnosis and classification to complications and therapy. *Diabetes Care, 17*(4).

72. Pastors, J. G. (1992). Alternatives to the exchange system for teaching meal planning to persons with diabetes. *The Diabetes Educator, 18*(1), 57–63.

73. Pecoraro, R. E., Reiber, G. E., & Burgess, E. M. (1992). Pathways to diabetic limb amputation: Basis for prevention. *Diabetes Spectrum, 5*(6), 329–334.

74. Quinn, S. (1993). Diabetes and diet: We are still learning. *Medical Clinics of North America, 77*(4), 773–781.

75. Reising, D. L. (1995). Acute hyperglycemia: Putting a lid on the crisis. *Nursing 95, 25*(2), 33–40.

76. Reising, D. L. (1995). Acute hypoglycemia: Keeping the bottom from falling out. *Nursing 95, 25*(2), 41–48.

77. Skyler, J. S. (1991). Strategies in diabetes mellitus: Start of a new era. *Postgraduate Medicine, 89*(6), 45–63.

78. Spollett, G. R. (1993). Intensive insulin therapy in insulin dependent diabetes and combination therapy. *Nurse Practitioner, 18*(7), 27–38.

79. Strowig, S. (1995). Diabetes 2000: Insulin therapy. *RN, 58*(6), 30–36.

80. Thom, S. L. (1993). Nutritional management of diabetes. *Nursing Clinics of North America, 28*(1), 97–111.

81. Tinker, L. F., Heins, J. M., & Holter, H. J. (1994). Commentary and translation: 1994 nutrition recommendations for diabetes. *Diabetes Spectrum, 7*(4), 225–230.

82. Veves, A., et al. (1993). Painful neuropathy and foot ulceration in diabetic patients. *Diabetes Care, 18*(8), 1187–1189.

83. Vinicor, F. (1994). Is diabetes a public-health disorder? *Diabetes Care, 17*(suppl. 1), 22–27.

84. Wallberg-Henriksson, H. (1992). Exercise and diabetes mellitus. *Exercise Sport Scientific Review, 20*, 339.

85. Watson, J., & Jaffe, M. S. (1995). *Nurse's manual of laboratory and diagnostic tests* (2nd ed.). Philadelphia: F. A. Davis.

86. White, N. H., & Henry, D. N. (1992). Special issues in diabetes management. In D. Haire-Joshu (Ed.), *Management of diabetes mellitus: Perspectives of care across the life span* (pp. 249–309). St. Louis: Mosby–Year Book.

87. Woodworth, J., Howey, D., & Bowsher, R. (1993). [Lys (B28), Pro (B29)] human insulin (K): Dose-ranging versus Humulin R (H). *Diabetes, 42*(suppl 1), 54 A.

Nursing Care of Clients with Thyroid and Parathyroid Disorders

Carol Birch

Thyroid Disorders

Many terms to describe normal and abnormal states of thyroid function. *Euthyroid* signifies normal thyroid function and secretion. Thyroid abnormalities are basically of three types: (1) enlargement of the thyroid (*goiter*), (2) hyperfunction (*hyperthyroidism*), and (3) hypofunction (*hypothyroidism*). The last two conditions represent disorders of thyroid hormone secretion.

Enlargement of the thyroid gland may or may not be associated with abnormalities of hormone secretion. An enlarged thyroid may result from (1) lack of iodine, (2) inflammation, or (3) benign or malignant tumors. Enlargement may also appear in hyperthyroidism, especially Grave's disease.

Hypothyroidism

Hypothyroidism is a deficiency of thyroid hormone resulting in slowed body metabolism and heat production due to decreased oxygen consumption by the tissues; underactivity of the thyroid; and pronounced personality changes. The term hypothyroidism is not synonymous with myxedema.

Myxedema is a complication of hypothyroidism characterized by a generalized hypometabolic state. Myxedema coma is a life-threatening situation in which all body systems are severely compromised by the hypometabolic state.

The frequency of hypothyroidism depends on the population being studied. The incidence of overt hypothyroidism is 1 to 2/1000 in community surveys, and 5 to 20/1000 clients seeking medical care.

Hypothyroidism affects women more than men (about 4:1). Although hypothyroidism may be congenital (cretinism) and therefore present at birth, the highest incidence is in adults between 30 and 65 years of age. Approximately 95% of all persons with hypothyroidism have the primary form of the disease. Central hypothyroidism resulting from pituitary or hypothalamic disease accounts for less than 10% of the cases of hypothyroidism. Myxedema is most commonly identified in postmenopausal, hypothyroid women in their 60s.

Etiology and Risk Factors

There are several types of hypothyroidism: (1) primary, (2) secondary (pituitary disease), and (3) tertiary (hypothalamic disease).

Primary hypothyroidism may be caused by (1) congenital defects of the thyroid (cretinism), (2) defective hormone synthesis, (3) iodine deficiency (prenatal and postnatal), (4) antithyroid drugs, (5) surgery or radioactive therapy for hyperthyroidism, and (6) following chronic inflammatory (autoimmune) diseases such as Hashimoto's disease, amyloidosis, and sarcoidosis. Hashimoto's disease is the most common type of autoimmune hypothyroidism.

Secondary hypothyroidism develops when there is insufficient stimulation of the normal thyroid gland; consequently, thyroid-stimulating hormone (TSH) levels are increased. This may start as a malfunction of the pituitary or hypothalamus. It may also be caused by peripheral resistance to thyroid hormone.

Tertiary or *central hypothyroidism* can develop if the hypothalamus fails to produce thyroid-releasing hormone (TRH) and subsequently does not stimulate the pituitary to secrete TSH. This may be due to a tumor or other destructive lesion in the hypothalamic region.

There are two major forms of simple goiter: endemic and sporadic. Endemic goiter is principally caused by nutritional iodine deficiency. It tends to occur in "goiter belts," geographical areas characterized by soil and water deficient in iodine. Major goiter belts within the United States are the Midwest, Northwest, and Great Lakes region. Endemic goiter typically occurs in the winter and fall and is twice as prevalent in women as in men. Also, because the need for thyroid hormone is particularly great during growth spurts, pregnancy, and lactation, goiter commonly develops in adolescents, pregnant women, and nursing mothers living in iodine-deficient regions.

Sporadic goiter is not restricted to any geographical area. Major causes include the following:

● Genetic defects resulting in faulty iodine metabolism
● Ingestion of large amounts of nutritional goitrogens (goiter-producing agents that inhibit thyroxine [T_4] production) such as rutabagas, cabbage, soybeans, peanuts, peaches, peas, strawberries, spinach, and radishes, all of which contain goitrogenic glycosides
● Ingestion of medicinal goitrogens, for example, thioureas (propylthiouracil), thiocarbamides (aminothiazole, tolbutamide), and iodine in large doses. Some people take iodine-containing solutions as a tonic.

Subclinical hypothyroidism is defined as hypothyroidism that is diagnosed with a elevated TSH but normal to low-normal T_4. Manifestations resemble those of mild hypothyroidism with subtle cardiac defects, especially in clients with pre-existing cardiac disease. Subclinical hypothyroidism is found in from 20 to 120/1000 persons in the community. The causes are the same as those of primary hypothyroidism. Its prevalence increases with age. Low-dose levothyroxine sodium (Synthroid) is effective for relief of manifestations and improvement in cardiac function and the lipid profile. The Risk Factors and Levels of Prevention feature lists other risk factors for hypothyroidism.

Pathophysiology

The thyroid gland needs iodine to synthesize and secrete its thyroid hormones (THs): T_4, triiodothyronine (T_3) and thyrocalcitonin (calcitonin). Production of TH is dependent on the secretion of TSH from the anterior pituitary and the ingestion of adequate protein and iodine. The hypothalamus regulates the pituitary secretion of TSH via the negative feedback system.

If a person's diet lacks sufficient amounts of iodine or if the production of thyroid hormone is suppressed for any other reason, the thyroid enlarges in an attempt to compensate for hormonal deficiency. Under these circumstances, goiter is essentially an adaptation to a deficiency

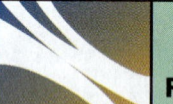

RISK FACTORS AND LEVELS OF PREVENTION

Hypothyroidism

Risk Factors

Most Common Factors. History of neck surgery or radioactive therapy for hyperthyroidism; radioiodine therapy for thyrotoxicosis and external radiotherapy; ingestion of large amounts of medicinal goitrogens: dopamine, glucocorticoids, adrenergic antagonists, propylthiouracil, methimazole, amiodarone, lithium, iodinated radiographic contrast agents, phenytoin, rifampin, carbamazepine; family history of thyroid disease.

Other Factors. Environment that is iodine-deficient in soil and water (primarily Third World); newborns; ingestion of large amounts of nutritional goitrogens: rutabagas, cabbage, soybeans, peanuts, cabbage, peas, strawberries, spinach; pregnant women, lactating mothers, adolescents with decreased thyroid hormones during times of growth spurts; elderly clients; clients with autoimmune disease; elderly men receiving aminoglutethimide (1000 mg/day or greater) for prostate cancer.

Levels of Prevention

Primary Prevention

Iodized salt and food additives have almost eliminated this problem in the United States. Educate clients at risk as to manifestations of hypothyroidism and benefits of early detection.

Secondary Prevention

Screen for early diagnosis at birth.
   Assess clients with risk factors and manifestations with physical examination and diagnostic thyroid function tests.

Tertiary Prevention

Administer hormonal supplements.
   Educate the client to enhance compliance and quality of life. Teach: purpose, side effects, frequency of hormonal supplement.
   Ensure that clients have follow-up visits with a physician to monitor medication and symptom relief.
   Encourage client to have regular thyroid function tests to evaluate serum thyroid-releasing hormone, thyroid-stimulating hormone, free thyroxine.

of TH. Enlargement of the gland will also occur in response to increased pituitary secretion of TSH. TSH stimulates the thyroid to secrete more T_4 when blood T_4 levels are low. Eventually, the gland may become so large that it compresses structures in the neck and chest, causing respiratory manifestations and dysphagia.

Decreased levels of TH lead to an overall slowing of the basal metabolic rate. This slowing of all body processes leads to achlorhydria (decreased secretion of hydrochloric acid in the stomach), decreased gastrointestinal tract motility, bradycardia, slowed neurologic functioning, and a decrease in heat production.

The most important changes caused by the reduced levels of TH are those affecting lipid metabolism. With the reduction in THs, there is a resultant increase in serum cholesterol and triglyceride levels and an increase in arteriosclerosis and coronary heart disease in clients suffering from hypothyroidism.

The THs also play a role in the production of red blood cells, so persons with hypothyroidism also show manifestations of anemia, with possible vitamin B_{12} and folate deficiency.

Myxedema, a mucinous edema, is caused by an accumulation of hydrophilic proteoglycans in the interstitial spaces. The reason for this problem remains unclear.

Clinical Manifestations and Diagnostic Findings

The manifestations of hypothyroidism depend on whether it is mild or complicated by myxedema or by myxedema coma.

Mild Hypothyroidism

Clients with mild hypothyroidism (the most common form) may be asymptomatic or may experience vague manifestations so ordinary as to escape detection. For example, clients may experience sensitivity to cold, lethargy, dry skin or hair, forgetfulness, depression, and some weight gain (Table 70–1).

The client's physical appearance changes. Often, obesity develops, features become coarse, hair becomes dry and sparse, and the skin feels dry, flaky, and inelastic. In addition, clients with hypothyroidism suffer from an intolerance to cold because of a decreased metabolic rate and a decreased basal body temperature. The client's ability to sweat also diminishes. Constipation and fecal impaction due to slowed peristaltic action and lack of normal physical activity constitute serious problems. Also, there is increased susceptibility to infection.

Vital sign changes may be minimal: the heart rate is normal or slow; blood pressure may be normal or a slight elevation of both systolic and diastolic pressures may exist; temperature may be normal to subnormal; respiration rate and rhythm may be affected by goiter size and degree of respiratory distress.

As the degree of hypothyroidism worsens, the thyroid may enlarge (goiter) in an attempt to produce enough T_4 (Fig. 70–1). Typically, clients seek medical advice when the goiter grows large enough to distort the appearance of the neck. They may also experience respiratory distress and dysphagia if the goiter is very large.

Myxedema

Myxedema may develop in clients with undiagnosed or undertreated hypothyroidism who experience stress. Stressors may include infection, drugs (phenothiazines, barbiturates, narcotics, anesthetics), respiratory failure, congestive heart failure, cerebral vascular accident, trauma, prolonged exposure to cold, metabolic disturbances, surgery, and seizures.

Myxedema is characterized by a dry, waxy type of swelling with abnormal deposits of mucin in the skin and other tissues. The edema is of the nonpitting type and is common in the pretibial and facial areas (Fig. 70–2).

Myxedema is most commonly diagnosed in hypothyroid women in their 60s. Untreated myxedema has been associated with severe atherosclerosis, and has been attributed to the increase in serum cholesterol concentrations, particularity low-density lipoprotein (LDL). TH replacement improves these changes.

Myxedema Coma

The major complication of hypothyroidism is myxedema coma. This is an extremely rare condition. Unrecognized and undiagnosed hypothyroidism may progress to myxedema coma, and may have a mortality rate approaching 100%.

Myxedema coma is characterized by a drastic decrease in the metabolic rate, hypoventilation leading to respiratory acidosis, hypothermia, and hypotension. Complicating factors include hyponatremia, hypercalcemia, secondary adrenal insufficiency, hypoglycemia, and water intoxication. It may be brought on by stress such as surgery, infection, or noncompliance with thyroid treatment.

Diagnostic tests for hypothyroidism confirm the clinical picture of hypometabolism and depressed thyroid activity (Table 70–2). The serum TSH level is elevated in hypothyroidism in an attempt to compensate for low levels of T_3 and T_4. Radioactive iodide uptake (RAIU) is decreased in hypothyroidism. A tracer dose of iodine 131 is given, and a thyroid scan is done 24 hours later to determine the uptake of ^{131}I by any nodules. "Hot nodules" absorb more isotope than normal tissue and are usually benign.

Clients with myxedema may also have hypercholesterolemia, hyperlipidemia, and proteinemia as a result of T_4 changes in the synthesis, mobilization, and degradation of serum lipids. Elevated lipid levels may be a contributing factor to the later development of cardiac problems. Dilutional hyponatremia may develop as a result of the marked impairment of water excretion related to decreased delivery of sodium and volume to the distal renal tubules as a result of decreased renal blood flow. Elevated creatine phosphokinase, aspartate aminotransferase, and lactate dehydrogenase may also develop secondary to altered metabolism.

Diagnosis of simple goiter is confirmed by history and laboratory tests. The client is often euthyroid; the manifestations and diagnostic manifestations of hypothyroid-

Table 70–1. Manifestations of Hypothyroidism and Hyperthyroidism

System	Hypothyroidism	Hyperthyroidism
Cardiovascular	$\downarrow$ HR + $\downarrow$ SV: $\downarrow$ CO $\downarrow$ Myocardial O_2 demand $\uparrow$ Peripheral vascular resistance Possible hypertension Hyperlipidemia Hypercholesterolemia Distant heart sounds	$\uparrow$ HR + $\uparrow$ SV: $\uparrow$ CO $\uparrow$ O_2 consumption Systolic BP $\uparrow$ 10–15 mm Hg Diastolic BP $\uparrow$ 10–15 mm Hg Palpitations Rapid, bounding pulse Possible congestive heart failure, edema
Hematologic	Normocytic, normochromic anemia Macrocytic anemia (pernicious) Easy bruising	No specific changes
Respiratory	Reduced hypoxic drive Hypercapnic ventilatory drive Respiratory muscle weakness Possible CO_2 retention on ABGs Dyspnea	$\uparrow$ Respiratory rate and depth Shortness of breath
Renal	Fluid retention $\downarrow$ Urinary output $\uparrow$ Total body water Dilutional hyponatremia $\downarrow$ Production of erythropoietin	Fluid retention $\downarrow$ Output
Gastrointestinal	$\downarrow$ Peristalsis Anorexia Possible weight gain Constipation $\downarrow$ Protein metabolism $\uparrow$ Serum lipids Delayed glucose uptake $\downarrow$ Glucose absorption	$\uparrow$ Peristalsis $\uparrow$ Appetite Weight loss Diarrhea $\uparrow$ Use of adipose and protein stores $\downarrow$ Serum lipids $\uparrow$ Gastrointestinal secretions Vomiting, abdominal pain
Musculoskeletal	Transient pain Muscle cramps and stiffness Slow movements $\uparrow$ Bone density $\downarrow$ Bone formation and resorption	Negative nitrogen balance Malnutrition Fatigue Muscle weakness Proximal muscle wasting Incoordination due to tremors
Integumentary	Dry, coarse, scaly skin Hair that falls out Thick, brittle nails Expressionless face Periorbital edema Thick, puffy skin: face and pretibial areas Cold intolerance	Profuse sweating Moist skin Flushed, warm skin Hair: fine, soft, straight, possible hair loss Heat intolerance
Endocrine	Normal to enlarged thyroid	Thyroid usually enlarged Bruit over thyroid
Neurologic	$\downarrow$ DTRs Muscle sluggishness Fatigue, somnolence Slow, deliberate speech Apathy, depression, paranoia Impaired short-term memory Lethargy	$\uparrow$ DTRs Fine tremors Nervousness, restlessness Emotional instability: anxiety, worry, paranoia
Reproductive	Females: menorrhagia, anovulation, irregular menses, decreased libido Males: decreased libido, impotence	Females: amenorrhea, irregular menses, $\downarrow$ fertility, $\uparrow$ tendency to spontaneous abortion Males: impotence, decreased libido $\downarrow$ Sexual development prepuberty
Other	Myxedema	Exophthalmos

ABGs, arterial blood gas analyses; BP, blood pressure; CO, cardiac output; CO_2, carbon dioxide; DTRs, deep tendon reflexes; HR, heart rate; O_2, oxygen; SV, stroke volume.

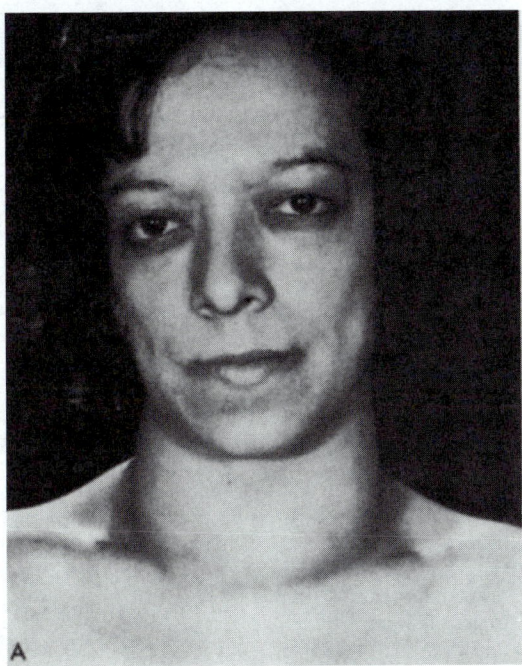
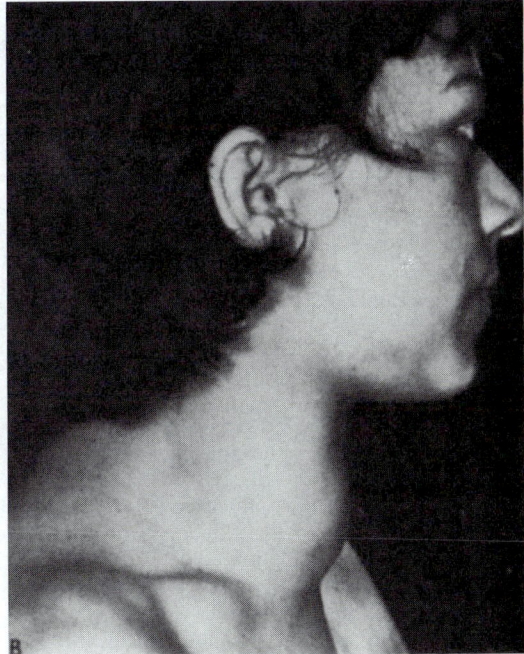

Figure 70–1. Massive thyroid enlargement caused by diffuse toxic goiter. *A,* Front view. *B,* Side view. (From Wilson, J. D., & Foster, D. W. [1992]. *Williams textbook of endocrinology* [8th ed.]. Philadelphia: W. B. Saunders.)

ism are seldom present because the gland enlarges enough to produce normal amounts of T_4. Needle biopsy of the goiter may be indicated to rule out malignancy.

Acute and Subacute Care

■ Medical Management

The goal of treatment of myxedema coma is to reverse the condition to save the client's life. Supportive measures are begun immediately, such as maintaining a patent airway, giving oxygen, and replacing fluids intravenously. The client is kept warm, and vital signs are closely monitored until the client begins to recover.

Levothyroxine sodium is given intravenously with glucose and corticosteroids. When administering TH to a client with myxedema heart disease, assess the client carefully for anginal pain, dyspnea, or orthopnea. The precipitating event causing the coma (surgery, infection, noncompliance) is evaluated and treated.

■ Nursing Management of the Medical Client

Assessment

Observe the client for the physical manifestations of myxedema, such as periorbital and facial edema, a blank facial expression, a thick tongue, and generalized slowing of all muscle movement.

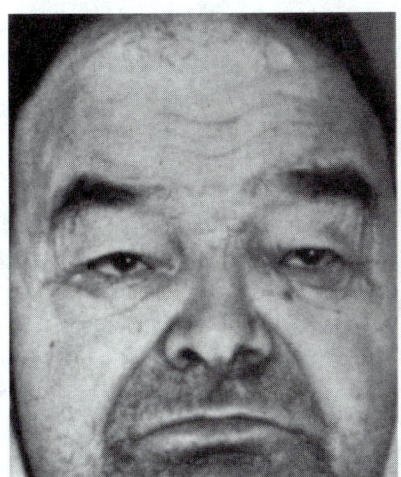
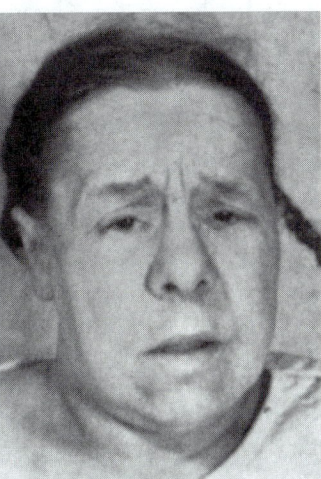

Figure 70–2. Typical facial appearance of myxedematous client. (From Wilson, J. D., & Foster, D. W. [1992]. *Williams textbook of endocrinology* [8th ed.]. Philadelphia: W. B. Saunders.)

Table 70–2. Diagnostic Tests for Thyroid Disorders*

Test	Description	Nursing Notes	Indications
Thyroid Function Tests			
Thyroid stimulating hormone (TSH) assay	TSH controls triiodothyronine (T_3) and thyroxine (T_4) release; TSH released from anterior pituitary	None	↑ : hypofunction of thyroid gland or anterior pituitary; primary hypothyroidism ↓ : pituitary disorders; hyperthyroidism; high dosages of dopamine or corticosteroids
Radioactive iodine uptake (RAIU)	Used to determine the metabolic activity of thyroid gland by measuring absorption of ^{131}I in thyroid	Client education: radioactive dose is small and harmless Contraindicated in pregnancy Drugs that may elevate results: barbiturates, estrogen, lithium, phenothiazines Seafood may elevate results Drugs that may decrease results: Lugol's solution, potassium iodide (SSKI), antithyroid, cortisone, aspirin, antihistamines 24-hr urine collection begins after oral tracer dose given. Thyroid scanned after 24 hr	↑ : hyperthyroidism, thyroiditis, liver cirrhosis; urine: hypothyroidism ↓ : hypothyroidism; urine: hyperthyroidism
Thyroid antibodies	Measures the presence of antibodies produced by body; may cause inflammation and destruction of thyroid gland	Note if client on oral contraceptives—these may elevate titers	↑ : thyroiditis
Free thyroxine (FT_4) concentration	FT_4 is metabolically active form of thyroxine	Results may be inaccurate with high estrogen levels or low serum protein levels	↑ : hyperthyroidism ↓ : hypothyroidism
Thyroxine (T_4)	A direct measurement of total amount of T_4 present in blood	Fasting is recommended Note on laboratory slip if client is taking thyroid supplements; levels can be increased by pregnancy or oral contraceptives	↑ : hyperthyroidism Normal– ↓ : hypothyroidism
Triiodothyronine (T_3) radioimmunoassay	Measures small amount of potent thyroid hormones; T_3 is active form of thyroid hormone	Same as T_4	↑ : hyperthyroidism, pregnancy, oral contraceptives Normal– ↓ : hypothyroidism, hypoprotein conditions

* The following drugs affect thyroid function test results: amiodarone HCl (Cordarone), corticosteroids, cough medicine (with iodine), dopamine HCl (Dopastat, Intropin), estrogens, lithium carbonate (Eskalith, Lithane, Lithobid), phenytoin (Dilantin), salicylates.
Adapted from Becker, K. L., et al. (1990). *Principles and practice of endocrinology and metabolism.* Philadelphia: J. B. Lippincott.

Test	Description	Nursing Notes	Indications
Thyroid Function Tests *Continued*			
T_3 resin uptake (T_3 RU)	Measures T_3 that is protein-bound	None	↑ : hyperthyroidism, low serum protein levels ↓ : high serum protein, hypothyroidism
Thyroid-binding globulins (TBGs)	Measures T_4 that is protein-bound	None	↑ : hyperthyroidism, low serum protein ↓ : high serum protein, hypothyroidism
Thyroid-releasing hormone (TRH)	TRH influences TSH release	None	↑ : hypothyroidism ↓ : hyperthyroidism
Diagnostic Imaging Studies			
Thyroid scan	Injection of radioactive isotopes used to identify thyroid gland	No preparation Radioactive iodine taken orally; dose is harmless Scanning done 24 hr later Be aware of contraindications such as potassium iodide, Lugol's solution, seafood intake, thyroid medications	Cold nodules: cancer Hot nodules: benign
Ultrasound	Identifies presence and size of gland location and nodules; differentiates solid tumors from fluid-filled cysts	No preparation necessary Remind client that he or she will not be radioactive Provide client education to alleviate anxiety	
Magnetic resonance imaging (MRI)	Used to visualize gland size, location, identify abnormalities	Test cannot be done in clients with metal implants (e.g., pacemakers, arthroplasties, skull plates) Assess for allergy to contrast media Inquire about claustrophobia	
Computed tomography (CT)	Identifies location and structure of gland	Client education Noninvasive Contrast media may be used; note allergy history	
Other Procedures Used to Diagnose Endocrine Disorders			
Fine-needle aspiration (FNA)	Provides sample of cells for histologic studies; usually used as thyroid biopsy	Client education for short, relatively pain-free procedure; observe site for swelling and bleeding	Benign or malignant

Diagnosis, Planning, Implementation

Risk for Heart Failure. The client with myxedema is prone to the development of severe arteriosclerotic heart disease and other cardiac abnormalities leading to the collaborative problem *Risk for Heart Failure related to sustained bradycardia, edema, and decreased urine output.*

Planning: Expected Outcomes. The client will maintain a normal cardiac output and will not develop heart failure, as evidenced by normal heart rate, evidence of normal perfusion, absence of edema, and urine output of at least 30 ml/hr.

Implementation. As the client is given the hormone replacement, the edema and puffiness will start to lessen. The nurse should continue to monitor intake and output, which becomes more balanced. Urinary output should increase significantly during thyroid therapy. Monitor the client's daily weight.

To help prevent further strain on the already overburdened heart, always help the client to turn so the client is not straining and placing an extra burden on the heart. If any new cardiac manifestations occur, notify the physician immediately. Do not give TH until the physician has reappraised the client's condition.

When administering thyroid preparations, assess the client carefully for manifestations of thyrotoxicosis (i.e., tachycardia, increased appetite, diarrhea, sweating, agitation, tremor, palpitations, shortness of breath). If any of these manifestations develop during thyroid therapy, notify the physician at once so the dosage can be reduced.

Hypothermia. The client with severe myxedema has a very low metabolic rate leading to an important nursing diagnosis of *Hypothermia related to slowed metabolic rate.*

Planning: Expected Outcomes. The client will not develop hypothermia, as evidenced by a normal body temperature.

Implementation. Provide the client with a comfortable, warm environment. Remember that hypothyroidism sharply increases sensitivity to cold. If necessary, supply extra clothing and warm blankets. Encourage the client to dress warmly and avoid extreme cold whenever possible.

Myxedema Coma. The client with acute hypothyroidism is prone to the development of coma leading to the collaborative problem *Myxedema coma related to hypersensitivity to anesthetics, sedatives, and narcotics secondary to decreased metabolic rate.*

Planning: Expected Outcomes. The client will not be given the usual doses of anesthetics, sedatives, and narcotics so that myxedema coma will not develop.

Implementation. The client should not receive sedatives unless it is absolutely necessary. If a sedative or narcotic must be given, administer no more than one-half to one-third the usual dose and then assess the client carefully for manifestations of respiratory depression or a decreased level of consciousness.

Risk for Impaired Skin Integrity. The client with myxedema is very prone to skin breakdown leading to the nursing diagnosis *Risk for Impaired Skin Integrity related to edema and dryness secondary to infiltration of fluid into interstitial spaces.*

Planning: Expected Outcomes. The client will have all skin remain intact, as evidenced by absence of injury and resolution of edema.

Implementation. Monitor the sacrum, coccyx, elbows, scapula, and other pressure points for manifestations of redness or tissue breakdown. Remember that edematous tissues are more prone to decubitus ulcer formation. Place the client on a strict turning schedule and on a pressure reduction mattress.

Evaluation

Evaluation outcomes are that the successful client shows no evidence of heart failure, edema, or skin impairment; temperature and urine output are normal for the client; and the client shows no further evidence of myxedema.

Community and Self-Care

■ Medical Management

Hypothyroidism

The goals of treatment of hypothyroidism are to correct TH deficiency, reverse manifestations, and prevent further cardiac and arterial damage.

For hypothyroidism to be reversed permanently, the client usually needs to take TH throughout life. Available thyroid medications include levothyroxine sodium, and desiccated thyroid, converted in the body to both T_4 and T_3 (Table 70–3). Levothyroxine sodium is the principal form of replacement therapy. Dosages vary with age, the severity of the hypothyroidism, general medical condition (particularly cardiovascular disorders), and client response to medical treatment. Clients with cardiac complications must be started on small doses of TH. Large doses could precipitate heart failure or myocardial infarction by increasing body metabolism, myocardial oxygen requirements, and consequently the workload of the heart.

Once clients have responded to TH therapy, they are placed on a lifetime maintenance dose of T_4 daily. Pharmacologic goitrogens are replaced with drugs that will not interfere with TH function. The drug of choice for thyroid replacement is levothyroxine sodium (see Table 70–3). Desiccated thyroid and liothyronine sodium (Cytomel), once commonly used in replacement therapy, are now used infrequently because of problems with fluctuating plasma levels and side effects. Dosage is based on the age of the client. Children and the elderly receive smaller doses.

Clients with hypothyroidism of long duration will notice an improvement of manifestations within 2 to 3 weeks of medication administration. Hoarseness, anemia,

Table 70–3. Medications Used to Treat Thyroid Disorders

Medication	Use	Usual Daily Dosage	Side Effects	Nursing Implications
Hyperthyroid Medications				
Propylthiouracil (PTU)	Antithyroid medication used to treat hyperthyroidism by inhibiting thyroid hormone synthesis. It slows T_4 clearance	100 mg PO tid 150 mg	Nausea, vomiting, diarrhea, loss of taste, skin changes, headache, dizziness, drowsiness, lymphadenopathy, hypersensitivity, agranulocytosis, hypothyroidism	Use carefully in combination with any drug that causes agranulocytosis; monitor blood counts; should not be used in the last trimester of pregnancy or during lactation; report any manifestations of infection; give every 8 hours around the clock; urge continued compliance because response is slow
Methimazole (Tapazole)	Antithyroid medication used to treat hyperthyroidism by inhibiting thyroid hormone synthesis	5–20 mg PO tid or 20–30 mg qd	Agranulocytosis, headache, drowsiness, diarrhea, nausea and vomiting, jaundice, urticaria, arthralgia, lymphadenopathy	Use carefully in pregnancy; monitor thyroid function closely; check CBC periodically; watch for signs of hypothyroidism, colds, other infections; stop drug if rash or lymphadenopathy occurs; give with meals to decrease GI effects; store in light-resistant containers
Saturated solution of potassium iodide (SSKI)	Antithyroid medication that blocks thyroid hormone production and release; used to treat hyperthyroidism prior to thyroidectomy	0.3–0.6 ml tid for 10–14 days before thyroidectomy (1 g potassium iodide per ml)	Diarrhea, nausea and vomiting, stomach pain, hypothyroidism, hypersensitivity, iodine poisoning, irregular heartbeat, productive cough	Use with caution in clients with TB, hyperkalemia, acute bronchitis, impaired renal function, or cardiac disease; safety not established in pregnancy, lactation, or childhood; give after meals with fruit juice; monitor potassium level; avoid sudden withdrawal; keep in light-protected bottle; avoid use of OTC drugs containing iodine; restrict iodine-rich foods and iodized salts; ensure preoperative compliance
Radioactive iodine (^{131}I)	Antithyroid medication that destroys thyroid tissue; used to treat hyperthyroidism; may be used to treat thyroid cancer	4–10 mCi PO for hyperthyroidism, 50–150 mCi for thyroid cancer	Feelings of fullness in neck, metallic taste, hypothyroidism, possible increased risk of leukemia later in life	Contraindicated in pregnancy and lactation for hyperthyroidism; stop all antithyroid medications 1 wk before giving ^{131}I; monitor thyroid function closely; give on empty stomach; institute radiation precautions on body secretions for 3 days after ingestion; teach client to avoid close, prolonged contact with children for 1 wk; should also sleep alone for 1 wk; client should not resume antithyroid medications for 6 wk

Table continued on following page

Table 70–3. Medications Used to Treat Thyroid Disorders *(Continued)*				
Medication	**Use**	**Usual Daily Dosage**	**Side Effects**	**Nursing Implications**
Hypothyroid Medications				
Levothyroxine sodium (Synthroid, Levothroid, Levoxine)	Thyroid replacement medication (T$_4$) used to treat hypothyroidism	Initial low dose daily increased until response to 100–200 mg/day in hypothyroidism (less in elderly clients); 0.2–0.5 mg IV in myxedema coma For myxedema, 5 μg/day increased to 50–100 μg/day maintenance dose; for thyroid hormone replacement, use 5 μg/day increasing to 12.5–25 μg/day PO	Rare hyperthyroidism, tremors, hunger, palpations, headache, nervousness, tachycardia, insomnia, heat intolerance, weight loss Manifestations of hyperthyroidism, diarrhea, abdominal cramps, vomiting, tachycardia, weight loss, heat intolerance	Use with caution in clients with acute MIs, hypertension, renal insufficiency, or diabetes and in elderly or pregnant clients; give a single dose in AM; watch for adverse effects early in treatment; do not use to treat depression or obesity; stress need for lifetime replacement; toxicity may last for weeks with overdosage; monitor for improvement of manifestations Dosage is monitored by serum free or total T$_4$ and thyrotropin levels Serum levels may be decreased when client is also taking aluminum hydroxide antacid Use with caution in clients with acute MIs, hypertension, renal insufficiency, or diabetes, and in elderly or pregnant clients; give a single dose in AM; watch for adverse effects early in treatment; smaller doses required for older clients; monitor pulse, blood pressure, and thyroid function

CBC, complete blood count; IV, intravenously; MIs, myocardial infarctions; PO, orally; qd, every day; T$_4$, thyroxine; tid, three times a day; GI, gastrointestinal; TB, tuberculosis; OTC, over the counter.

and changes in hair and skin may take many months to resolve.

Simple Goiter

The goals of treatment of simple goiter are to halt further enlargement of the thyroid gland and to promote regression of the gland.

Iodine. When enlargement is a compensatory reaction to iodine deficiency and consequent suppression of T$_4$ secretion, the client can be treated with preparations of iodine and TH. Iodine is administered in the form of either strong iodine solution (Lugol's solution) or saturated solution of potassium iodide (SSKI) drops. Iodine actually reduces the size and vascularity of the enlarged gland. However, the availability of iodized salt and thyroid hormones has made this replacement therapy with iodine obsolete in the United States.

Increased Iodine Diet. If the hypothyroidism and goiter are due to iodine deficiency, the client should be on a diet higher in iodine. This is accomplished simply by switching to iodized salt. Dietary goitrogens such as turnips, soybeans, rutabagas, and to a lesser degree, seafood, green leafy vegetables, carrots, and peanuts should also be avoided.

■ Nursing Management of the Medical Client

Assessment

Carefully assess the client for the presence of manifestations of hypothyroidism. Obtain a careful history; look for the manifestations that reflect a decrease in metabolic functions such as weight gain, excessive sleeping, and generalized fatigue. The Critical Monitoring feature lists other manifestations of decreased metabolic functions.

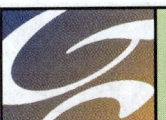

CRITICAL MONITORING

Hypothyroidism

Observations that should be monitored in a client who is hypothyroid or suspected of being hypothyroid. Serum laboratory tests confirm diagnosis.

Lethargy, depression
Sensitivity to cold, weight gain; Later, enlarged thyroid
Dry skin
Normal to subnormal temperature
Normal to slow pulse
Normal respiratory rate unless affected by goiter size
Normal to slight elevation of blood pressure
Augmentation of congestive heart failure

Also take a thorough diet history, looking particularly at the intake of iodine. Also question the client regarding the intake of goitrogenic substances and residence in a goiter belt.

Ask the client about other medical conditions that might be present, such as a previous history of hyperthyroidism treated with surgery or radioactive iodine, both of which predispose to hypothyroidism. Also investigate whether the client uses any medication that could lead to hypothyroidism; lithium, aminoglutethimide, sodium or potassium perchlorate, and cobalt can slow thyroid metabolism.

Diagnosis, Planning, Implementation

Altered Nutrition: More than Body Requirements.
The slowed metabolic rate make the client with hypothyroidism at risk for weight gain leading to the nursing diagnosis *Altered Nutrition: More than Body Requirements, related to slowed metabolic rate.*

Planning: Expected Outcomes. The client will return to normal weight, as evidenced by a loss of at least 2 lb per week.

Implementation. When thyroid medication is begun, the client's activity level and decreased edema often lead to significant initial weight loss without alteration in the diet. Typically, however, the appetite also increases as the medication begins to work. It is important, therefore, to provide low calorie diet education until the weight stabilizes at the ideal body weight. The client should develop more energy as the TH level returns to normal allowing the client to increase activity to help in weight loss.

Activity Intolerance.
The client with hypothyroidism often suffers from fatigue, making the nursing diagnosis *Activity Intolerance related to weakness and apathy secondary to decreased metabolic rate* a common nursing diagnosis.

Planning: Expected Outcomes. The client will develop increased tolerance to activity, as evidenced by a return to preillness activity levels.

Implementation. While the client is still suffering from hypothyroidism, energy levels will be decreased and the client will tire easily. Clients will usually decrease activity to compensate for the decreased energy they feel. Once TH replacement is begun, the client returns to a level of physical and mental activity that should gradually improve with hormone therapy.

Constipation.
The client with hypothyroidism has decreased gastrointestinal motility leading to the nursing diagnosis *Constipation related to decreased peristalsis secondary to slowed metabolic rate and activity intolerance.*

Planning: Expected Outcomes. The client will return to a normal preillness bowel pattern, as evidenced by a bowel movement at least every other day.

Implementation. Implement measures to prevent constipation and fecal impaction. As the hypothyroidism reverses and cardiac status improves, encourage more activity. Advise the client to drink six to eight glasses of water every day and to eat foods high in fiber such as fresh fruits, vegetables, and grains. If this is ineffective, a stool softener or cathartic may be indicated.

Risk for Ineffective Management of Therapeutic Regimen (Individuals).
Hypothyroidism is a lifelong disease which must be managed with the client's full participation leading to the diagnosis *Risk for Ineffective Management of Therapeutic Regimen (Individuals) related to pharmacologic regimen, nutrition, and follow-up care.*

Planning: Expected Outcomes. The client will understand the pharmacologic regimen, nutrition, and follow-up required for control of the condition, as evidenced by his or her statements and compliance with the therapeutic regimen.

Implementation. Once clients are mentally alert, evaluate their level of knowledge regarding the disorder and the importance of taking TH daily for life. Develop and implement a teaching plan based on each client's needs. Also, provide a written list (such as the one in the Client Education Guide) of the manifestations of thyroid deficiency or excess. Instruct the client and significant others to telephone the physician if those manifestations develop.

Endemic goiter can be prevented by the use of iodized salt. Adults require at least 50 μg of iodine per day. However, an adequate iodine intake guaranteed to prevent goiter is 200 to 300 μg/day. Iodized salt, used in the United States since 1924, contains 1 part iodine to 100,000 parts of salt. Thus, the average person, who ingests approximately 6.2 g of salt a day, is also taking 474 μg of iodine daily if the salt is iodized.

Many clients do not understand the need for iodized salt as a goiter preventive. Some believe that any additive to food or water is harmful and therefore do not use iodized salt. These two problems, plus the fact that many

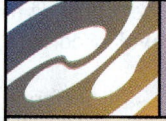

CLIENT EDUCATION GUIDE

Thyroid Supplements

The usual initial dosage in adults is 0.025 to 0.1 mg by mouth (PO) per day, increased by 0.05 to 0.1 mg PO every 1 to 4 weeks until the desired response is achieved. The maintenance dose is 0.1 to 0.4 mg/day.

Take the medication at the same time every day to maintain blood levels. Morning is preferred to prevent insomnia.

Side effects may occur relative to dosage and your sensitivity:

Central nervous system effects are nervousness, insomnia and tremor.
Cardiovascular manifestations may include tachycardia, palpitations, arrhythmias, angina pectoris, hypertension, and aggravation of pre-existing cardiac conditions such as congestive heart failure.
Gastrointestinal complaints may include an increase in appetite, nausea, diarrhea.

Other side effects resemble the symptoms of hyperthyroidism: headache, leg cramps, weight loss, heat intolerance, sweating, fever, and menstrual irregularities.

Do not take these drugs if you have had a heart attack, thyrotoxicosis, or untreated adrenal insufficiency.

Use these drugs with caution if you have angina pectoris, other cardiovascular disorders, renal insufficiency or failure, or poor circulation.

Notify your physician if you experience chest pain or manifestations of hyperthyroidism (may indicate overdose or manifestations of aggravated or difficult-to-control cardiac disease).

Notify your other physicians or healthcare providers, that you are using thyroid supplements. Thyroid hormones alter thyroid function test results. Thyroid supplements prolong prothrombin time. Therefore, if you are taking blood thinners, a smaller dose is required.

Notify your physician immediately if you are pregnant or plan to get pregnant so your dose can be adjusted accordingly.

---

modern foods are processed with cheaper noniodized salt, contribute to the potential for development of simple goiter. Nurses need to educate the public regarding the importance of iodized salt.

The discharge teaching centers around the need to understand and follow the medication regimen, the manifestations of hyperthyroidism and hypothyroidism, diet, and when to seek medical attention. Physical manifestations of hypothyroidism should decrease over a 3- to 12-week period as the TSH decreases. Impress on the client the need for iodized salt. The client should also be taught to eat a high fiber diet to prevent constipation. The client should be told to have TH levels checked at intervals until these levels are stabilized and then at regular intervals to be sure he or she is maintaining normal levels.

Evaluation

Once hypothyroidism has been diagnosed and replacement is begun, the condition reverses and the client can return to a normal level of hormone. After discharge, if the condition does not continue to reverse, the client will need to be assessed for compliance with the therapeutic regimen.

■ Modifications for Elderly Clients

Subclinical hypothyroidism is the combination of elevated TSH levels and normal T_3 and free T_4 levels without manifestations. Subclinical hypothyroidism occurs in up to 15% of postmenopausal women. The most common causes of subclinical hypothyroidism are, in order of frequency, autoimmune thyroiditis, Hashimoto's disease,

previous thyroid surgery or radioactive treatment, and noncompliance with prescribed T_4 replacements.

Medical treatment is not indicated for those clients who are without manifestations. Those clients with generalized complaints of hypothyroidism may benefit from small doses of T_4 which thus proves that their condition was symptomatic rather than subclinical. Remember, a principal hazard in giving T_4 to an elderly client is the development of ischemic heart disease, as evidenced by angina. Client response to therapy and serum levels must be observed closely.

The difficulty in diagnosing hypothyroidism in the elderly is that the manifestations are usually vague and generic to other disease processes. Hypothyroidism must be considered in the differential diagnosis of a variety of conditions affecting the elderly client.

Critical Care

Surgery is done for goiter that is very large, not responding to treatment, or putting too much pressure on other structures in the neck. Surgery is discussed in detail in the following section.

Hyperthyroidism

Hyperthyroidism is defined as excessive secretion of TH; thyrotoxicosis refers to the clinical manifestations that occur when the body tissues are stimulated by this increased TH.

Hyperthyroidism is a highly preventable endocrine disorder. Like most thyroid conditions, it is predominantly a disorder of women. It affects women four times as often as it does men, especially young women between the ages of 20 and 40 years.

Etiology and Risk Factors

Hyperthyroidism may be due to the overfunctioning of the entire gland or, less commonly, may be caused by single or multiple functioning adenomas of thyroid cancer. Also, overtreatment of myxedema with TH may result in hyperthyroidism. The most common form of hyperthyroidism is Graves' disease (toxic, diffuse goiter), which has three principal hallmarks: (1) hyperthyroidism, (2) thyroid gland enlargement (goiter), and (3) exophthalmos (abnormal protrusion of the eyes). Graves' disease is an autoimmune disorder mediated by IgG antibody that binds to and activates TSH receptors on the surface of the thyroid cells.

Other causes of hyperthyroidism may include toxic nodular goiter, toxic adenoma (benign), thyroid carcinoma, subacute and chronic thyroiditis, and ingestion of TH. The Risk Factors and Levels of Prevention feature lists other factors that may contribute to hyperthyroidism.

Pathophysiology

The pathophysiology behind the manifestations of Graves' hyperthyroid disease can be divided into two categories: (1) that secondary to excessive stimulation of the adrener-gic nervous system and (2) that due to excessive levels of circulating TH.

Hyperthyroidism is characterized by loss of the normal regulatory controls of TH secretion. Because the action of TH on the body is stimulatory, hypermetabolism results, with increased sympathetic nervous system activity. The excessive amounts of TH stimulate the cardiac system and increase the number of beta-adrenergic receptors. This leads to tachycardia and increased cardiac output, stroke volume, adrenergic responsiveness, and peripheral blood flow. Metabolism increases greatly, leading to a negative nitrogen balance, lipid depletion, and a resultant state of nutritional deficiency.

Hyperthyroidism also results in the alteration of secretion and metabolism of hypothalamic, pituitary, and gonadal hormones. If hyperthyroidism occurs before puberty, sexual development is delayed in both sexes, but after puberty it results in decreased libido in both men and women. After puberty, women will also exhibit menstrual irregularities and decreased fertility.

Clinical Manifestations and Diagnostic Findings

Because hyperthyroidism is caused by an excess secretion of TH, the clinical picture of Graves' disease is in many ways opposite to that of hypothyroidism. Assessment reveals a client who appears extremely agitated and irritable, with a hand tremor at rest. Despite a ravenous appetite, weight loss occurs as a result of the quickened metabolism. Because of the high levels of circulating TH, the client's body processes "speed up." As described in the Critical Monitoring feature, manifestations include

---

RISK FACTORS AND LEVELS OF PREVENTION

Hyperthyroidism

Risk Factors

Overtreatment of hypothyroidism, development of a "rebound effect" after radioiodine for partial thyroidectomy, history of posterior pituitary disease, hypothalamus disease, use of amiodarone hydrochloride as antiarrhythmic (atrial fibrillation)

Levels of Prevention

Primary Prevention

Provide education regarding manifestations of hyperthyroidism for those at risk.

Secondary Prevention

Provide prompt treatment and continued education about the disorder and medication to return the client to his or her usual quality of life.

Tertiary Prevention

Continue to provide education about the disorder and medication. Ensure that the client sees the physician yearly (or as needed) to monitor medication and thyroid levels.

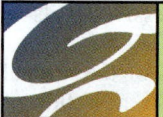

CRITICAL MONITORING

Hyperthyroidism

Observations that the nurse might make in a client who is suspected of, or diagnosed with, hyperthyroidism.

Anxiety, short attention span, irritability
Heat intolerance, unintentional weight loss
Warm, moist skin
Increased temperature
Increased pulse
Increased blood pressure
Fatigue and weakness
Augmentation of other disorders such as atrial fibrillation, congestive heart failure, angina, paranoia, and anxiety

loose bowel movements, heat intolerance, profuse diaphoresis, tachycardia, and incoordination due to tremor. Also, the skin becomes warm, smooth, and moist because of accelerated circulation to the tissues. The hair appears thin and soft.

Moreover, the client's emotions are adversely affected by the turbulent activity within the body. Moods may be cyclic, ranging from mild euphoria, to extreme hyperactivity, to delirium. The excessive hyperactivity in turn leads to extreme fatigue and depression, again followed by episodes of overactivity, and so forth. As a result of the client's chaotic emotional state, interpersonal relationships may deteriorate, further accentuating the emotional disturbance.

Goiter, the second characteristic of Graves' disease, is due to hyperplasia and hypertrophy of the thyroid cells. The gland may enlarge up to three to four times its normal size. Cellular overgrowth results in the release of excessive amounts of TH into the blood.

Exophthalmos is the third major manifestation of Graves' disease. The cause of the ophthalmologic changes in Graves' disease seems to be autoimmunity against retro-orbital tissues. The client who suffers from exophthalmos has protruding eyes and a fixed stare caused by the accumulation of fluid in the fat pads and muscles that lie behind the eyeballs (Fig. 70–3). Because the eyes are surrounded by unyielding bone, edema forces them forward out of their sockets, producing the typical facies of exophthalmos (see Fig. 70–3). In severe cases, clients may be unable to close their eyelids and must have their lids taped shut to protect the eyes. Without intervention, severe exophthalmos can progress to corneal ulceration or infection and loss of vision. In some cases, exophthalmos is not reversed by intervention. Exophthalmos may actually worsen with radioactive iodine (RAI) therapy for hyperthyroidism.

Graves' disease is diagnosed on the basis of (1) the client's often striking physical appearance (enlarged neck,

protruding eyes, agitated expression); (2) the manifestations of agitation, restlessness, and weight loss; and (3) laboratory findings. The serum TH levels are usually all elevated, although they occasionally may be within the normal range (so-called euthyroid Graves' disease). Serum cholesterol levels are usually depressed. See Table 70–2 for the usual laboratory findings.

Complications

The three major complications of Graves' disease are (1) exophthalmos, (2) heart disease, and (3) thyroid storm (thyroid crisis, thyrotoxicosis).

Exophthalmos. Exophthalmos develops as a result of proptosis, lid retraction, muscle swelling, and tissue edema from a prolonged hyperthyroid condition. Manifestations may include a gritty sensation in the eye, photophobia, lacrimation, inflammatory changes, and dyslogia.

Unlike the manifestations of goiter and hyperthyroidism, exophthalmos does not necessarily regress with therapy. Diuretics may alleviate some of the periorbital edema. Glucocorticoids such as prednisone are given in large doses to reduce inflammation of the periorbital tissues. Unfortunately, steroids produce many undesirable side effects, including acute psychoses. Estrogen therapy

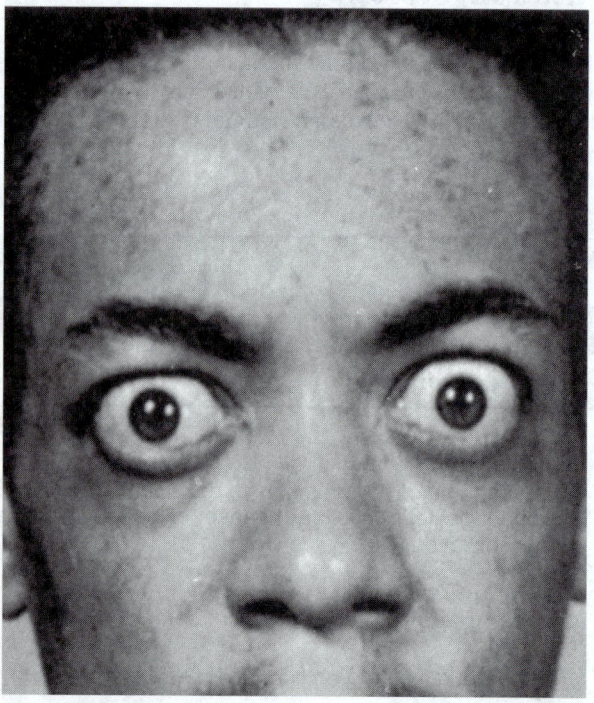

Figure 70–3. Extreme exophthalmos in hyperthyroidism. Because the eyes are surrounded by unyielding bone, fluid accumulation in the fat pads and muscles behind the eyeballs causes protruding eyes and a fixed stare in the client with exophthalmos. Without intervention, the client with severe exophthalmos may be unable to close the eyelids and may develop corneal ulceration or infection. Eventually, this can result in total loss of vision. (From Delp, M. H., & Manning, R. T. [1981]. *Major's physical diagnosis* [9th ed.]. Philadelphia: W. B. Saunders.)

is occasionally of value in postmenopausal women. Methylcellulose eye drops, ¼% four times daily, help reduce eye irritation. Radiation therapy to the retro-orbital tissues may help in severe cases. Surgical decompression of the orbits may be performed when all other measures fail to correct the exophthalmos. This procedure may save the client's vision when eye changes are severe.

A number of general nursing interventions also help to reduce eye discomfort and prevent corneal ulceration and infection. Instruct clients with exophthalmos to wear dark glasses. Warn them to avoid getting dust or dirt in their eyes. When they cannot close their eyelids easily or at all, have them wear a sleeping mask (available in drug stores) or lightly tape the eyes shut with nonallergic tape. Elevate the head of the bed at night and have the client restrict salt intake to relieve edema.

Heart Disease. Heart disease, the second complication of Graves' disease, poses a serious threat. Tachycardia almost always accompanies thyrotoxicosis, and atrial fibrillation may also appear. Congestive heart failure is found among older clients with long-standing thyrotoxicosis. Propranolol is the drug of choice, but is contraindicated if asthma or congestive heart failure are pre-existing conditions. The treatment of these cardiac complications is discussed in detail in Unit 8.

Thyroid Storm (Thyrotoxicosis). Thyroid storm (thyrotoxicosis) is a potentially fatal, acute episode of thyroid overactivity characterized by high fever, severe tachycardia, delirium, dehydration, and extreme irritability. It was once a commonly occurring crisis, but seldom develops today, thanks to modern intervention techniques. Factors that may precipitate thyroid storm include undiagnosed or untreated hyperthyroidism, infection, thyroid ablation, metabolic catastrophes, surgery, trauma, labor and delivery, myocardial infarction, pulmonary embolus, medication overdosage, or inadequate preparation of clients for thyroid surgery.

Clients with thyrotoxicosis may have an increase in clotting factor VIII. Despite this increase, the hyperthyroid client has an increased sensitivity to coumarin derivatives because of the accelerated metabolic clearance of the vitamin K–dependent clotting factors.

Thyroid storm is a clinical diagnosis; no laboratory tests serve to differentiate hyperthyroidism from thyroid storm in general.

Because it is an emergency, thyroid storm requires heroic intervention for control. The high fever is treated with hypothermic blankets; dehydration is reversed with intravenous fluids. Treatment of thyroid storm involves suppressing hormonal release, inhibiting hormonal synthesis, blocking conversion of T_4 to the more active T_3 and inhibiting the effects of TH on body tissues as well as treating the precipitating cause, if known. Blockade of TH release is usually achieved by the administration of iodides such as potassium iodide given orally. Sodium iodide may be given intravenously. Glucocorticoid, dexamethasone, and propylthiouracil are also commonly used oral drugs. Beta-blockers are given to decrease the effects of sympathetic nervous system stimulation and to treat tachycardia.

Acute and Subacute Care

■ Medical Management

The goals of care for clients with Graves' disease are to curtail the excessive secretion of TH and to prevent and treat complications. Choice of intervention is based on (1) age, (2) goiter size, and (3) whether other health problems exist.

The three major forms of therapy are (1) antithyroid medication, (2) radioiodine, and (3) surgery.

Antithyroid Medication Therapy

Antithyroid medication is recommended for clients under 18 years of age and for pregnant women. The major medications used to control hyperthyroidism include iodide, propylthiouracil, and methimazole (Tapazole) (see Table 70–3). Adrenergic blocking agents may also be administered as adjunctive therapy.

Propylthiouracil is the most commonly used antithyroid medication. It corrects hyperthyroidism by impairing TH synthesis. With the usual dosage regimen, propylthiouracil ameliorates Graves' disease within 4 to 8 weeks. However, several months may pass before manifestations completely abate. Once euthyroid, the client is given a maintenance dose of propylthiouracil, usually three times daily. Propylthiouracil, although an ideal medication in many ways, causes significant side effects in about 9% of clients using it.

The most serious toxic effect is agranulocytosis (see Chapter 53). A white blood cell (WBC) count should be obtained before initial administration of the medication. Instruct clients to report a sore throat, fever, or rash immediately to their physician so that further WBC tests can be performed and the client's condition evaluated. Less severe adverse reactions include mild allergies (rash and pruritus). Rarely, the client develops hepatitis or drug fever.

Methimazole acts to block the action of TH in the body. Unfortunately, methimazole also produces agranulocytosis in a small percentage of people.

Iodine therapy is prescribed for two reasons: (1) to reduce the vascularity of the thyroid gland before subtotal or total thyroidectomy and (2) to treat thyroid storm (see earlier). Iodine preparations temporarily act to prevent release of TH into the circulation by increasing the amount of TH stored within the gland. However, the stored TH is eventually released back into the circulation, once again producing hyperthyroidism. For this reason, iodine preparations are usually given only for a 10- to 14-day period before surgery. If iodine is given for a longer period or if it is given alone (i.e., not in combination with propylthiouracil), the thyroid gland may "escape" before thyroidectomy. "Escape of the thyroid" means that the iodine is no longer capable of maintaining

TH storage. As a result, TH floods the circulation, and hyperthyroidism returns in a more severe form than before.

The iodine medication of choice is potassium iodide. Lugol's solution is also used but is more expensive than potassium iodide and tends to inactivate antithyroid preparations within the bowel.

Adrenergic blocking agents are sometimes given as adjunctive therapy to control the activity of the sympathetic nervous system. There is now evidence that these agents are of great benefit to the "hyperthyroid heart," which has an increased sensitivity to catecholamines and an increased number of beta-adrenergic receptor sites. Therefore, these agents help lessen distressing manifestations such as palpitations and tachycardia. Tremor and nervousness may also be alleviated by adrenergic blocking agents. These medications include propranolol and reserpine.

Treatment of Graves' hyperthyroidism may require a long delay (weeks to months) between the start of therapy and substantial improvement or resolution of manifestations.

Radioiodine Therapy

Therapy with ^{131}I is principally prescribed for middle-aged and elderly clients. See the Case Study of hyperthyroidism and postmenopausal osteoporosis. This intervention offers many advantages: it is economical, is simple to administer, and can be prescribed on an outpatient basis. Radiotherapy is contraindicated in pregnant women and is rarely used in children.

The rationale behind ^{131}I therapy for Graves' disease is simple. The thyroid gland is unable to distinguish between regular iodine atoms and radioiodine atoms. Consequently, when the client receives a dose of ^{131}I, the thyroid gland picks up the radioiodine and concentrates it just as it would regular iodine. As a result, the cells that concentrate ^{131}I to make T_4 are destroyed by the local irradiation. Thus, TH secretion diminishes, and the manifestations of hyperthyroidism and goiter disappear. However, because radioiodine destroys thyroid cells, one of the major possible complications of ^{131}I therapy is myxedema. Therefore, assess for manifestations of hypothyroidism after ^{131}I therapy.

^{131}I is administered orally dissolved in water. Dosage is determined both by the size of the gland and by the thyroid's uptake of a tracer dose of radioiodine. After receiving the radioiodine, the client may go home unless the dosage is extremely large. In the latter case, the client must be placed in isolation for several days to prevent radioactive contamination. The manifestations of hyperthyroidism usually subside within 6 to 12 weeks after ^{131}I administration. Because of the delay in achieving a therapeutic response with ^{131}I, concurrent treatment with beta-adrenergic blockers may be desirable. Sometimes, resistant clients require a second or (in rare cases) a third dose of radioiodine. Once they become euthyroid, clients still need regular medical examinations, because hypothyroidism may develop several years after radiotherapy. Clients who become hypothyroid require lifelong hormone replacement with thyroid preparations.

Dietary Therapy

The client with hyperthyroidism needs a high calorie, high protein diet to compensate for the hypermetabolic state. A diet of 4000 to 5000 calories with high protein levels may be necessary to prevent the negative nitrogen balance and weight loss that occurs.

■ Nursing Management of the Medical Client

Assessment

Begin the assessment by obtaining a complete client history. By asking questions concerning weight, appetite, activity, heat intolerance, and bowel activity, you can assess for the presence of typical manifestations of hyperthyroidism.

Also question significant others about mood alterations experienced by the client. Mood swings, irritability, decreased attention span, and manic behavior may be experienced by the client with hyperthyroidism. Although the client may not be aware of some of the mood changes, the significant others can usually notice the changes.

Diagnosis, Planning, Implementation

Altered Nutrition: Less than Body Requirements. The client with hyperthyroidism is hypermetabolic, making the nursing diagnosis *Altered Nutrition: Less than Body Requirements related to accelerated metabolic rate* an important one.

Planning: Expected Outcomes. The client's weight loss will end, as evidenced by the client's ability to take in sufficient calories to return to ideal body weight.

Implementation. Provide the client with a well-balanced, high calorie diet. Clients with Graves' disease are usually extremely hungry because of the increased metabolism. Six full meals a day may be needed to satisfy their appetite. However, they may lose weight rapidly despite unusually large meals. Also, they usually are in a state of negative nitrogen balance. Therefore, encourage them to eat foods that are nutritious and contain ample amounts of protein, carbohydrates, fats, and minerals. Discourage eating of foods that increase peristalsis and thus result in diarrhea (e.g., highly seasoned, bulky, or fibrous foods). Clients should be weighed daily, and weight losses of more than 2 kg (4.4 lb) should be reported. If they continue to appear malnourished despite an ample diet, supplemental vitamins, particularly vitamin B complex, may be needed.

Activity Intolerance. Another nursing diagnosis related to the client's hypermetabolic state is *Activity Intolerance related to exhaustion secondary to accelerated metabolic rate.*

Planning: Expected Outcomes. The client will be able to engage in a normal level of activity, as evidenced by ability to maintain a proper balance of rest and activity to prevent exhaustion.

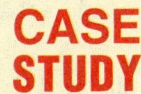

Hyperthyroidism and Postmenopausal Osteoporosis

Mrs. Gonzales is a 55-year-old Hispanic woman who presents at a free clinic for migrant farm workers. She is dressed in a lightweight sundress and sandals despite outdoor temperatures around 50° F. Mrs. Gonzales complains of pounding in her chest and shortness of breath without exertion. She relates that she has lost 20 lbs in the last 6 weeks even though she has been eating more than usual. A T_4 (thyroxine) level drawn in the clinic is twice the normal value. The nurse-practitioner has arranged for additional outpatient diagnostic studies.

Selected Outpatient Laboratory Values

RBC	3.8 million/mm³
Hgb	11.8 g/dl
Hct	35%
WBC	9000/mm³
Glucose	90 mg/dl
T_4	20 µg/dl
TSH	0 µIU/ml
^{131}I uptake	50% in 2 hours without evidence of malignancy
Calcium	10 mg/dl

Nursing Assessment

Mrs. Gonzales reports that she has worked in the fields all her life. She met her husband in California while they were picking grapes 40 years ago. They have three children who are married and also work in the fields. She does not get to see them often, however, because they cannot always get work in the same area. Mrs. Gonzales was born in Mexico. She speaks fluent Spanish and only a few words of English. She is concerned about how she and her husband will pay for her treatment.

Mrs. Gonzales reports that she went through "the change of life" 14 years ago. She cannot afford hormone replacement therapy. Mrs. Gonzales denies a family history of cancer, heart disease, or diabetes mellitus.

Nursing Physical Examination

Height: 5′5″ Weight: 105 lbs (47.7 kg)
Vital Signs: BP = 160/94; TPR = 99.6, 126, 24
LOC: Awake, alert, restless
EENT: PERLA, increased tears, photophobia, exophthalmos, goiter
Cardiac: Tachycardia, regular rate and rhythm, palpitations
Pulmonary: Lungs clear bilaterally
Abdominal: Soft, nontender, with hyperactive bowel sounds
Genitourinary: Within normal limits
Peripheral Pulses: 4/4, with slight pretibial and pedal edema

Initial Outpatient Treatment Plan

Meds: Propranolol (Inderal) 20 mg PO tid
Propylthiouracil (PTU) 100 mg PO tid
Artificial tears or other OTC eyedrops as needed
(Arrange for sample medications if possible)
Diet: As tolerated, no added salt
Activity: As tolerated; monitor heart rate; call if pulse >160 BPM at rest
Other: Call for difficulty swallowing or breathing, or other signs of enlarging goiter; return to clinic in 2 weeks

Based on the diagnostic work-up, Mrs. Gonzales will have radioactive iodine therapy. At her return visit, Mrs. Gonzales' T_4 is within normal limits. She reports that she has not had any more pounding in her chest. Her resting heart rate at the clinic is 84 BPM.

Review of her diet history reveals an average daily intake of approximately 2000 to 2500 calories consisting largely of tortillas, beans, and the foods currently being harvested in the fields. She reports that she does not drink milk or eat cheese because they cause bloating and diarrhea.

Mrs. Gonzales receives the prescribed dose of radioactive iodine orally and is instructed to return in 30 days for laboratory work and to call if any problems develop.

Discharge and Posttreatment Considerations

Average LOS (insurance certification): outpatient only
Complete posttreatment instruction
Coordinate health benefits with department of social services

Questions to Be Considered

1. What influence would Mrs. Gonzales' use of the Spanish language have on her treatment plan? Identify implications for formal nursing education preparation.
2. How might Mrs. Gonzales' care differ from that of a person with healthcare benefits? Discuss ethical considerations which may impact the allocation of scarce healthcare resources.
3. Compare and contrast the symptoms of menopause and hyperthyroidism. Discuss the implications for patient diagnosis and treatment.
4. Discuss the pathophysiology of the relationship between the pituitary gland and the thyroid gland. How is this manifested in Mrs. Gonzales' case?
5. Discuss the management of Mrs. Gonzales' diet before and after radioactive iodine treatment. Include cultural and economic factors in your discussion. In addition, consider the implications of Mrs. Gonzales being postmenopausal and lactose-intolerant.
6. Discuss the nursing implications and patient teaching aspects associated with Mrs. Gonzales' pre-radioactive iodine treatment prescription medications. Identify potential OTC drug contraindications in the pretreatment period. Discuss post-radioactive iodine treatment medication requirements and related patient teaching.

Implementation. Provide the client with an environment that is restful both mentally and physically. It is a challenge to help hyperthyroid clients relax. Assign these clients to a private room to promote rest and to prevent them from disturbing others through hyperactivity and restlessness.

Risk for Injury. There are many potential problems that can develop in the client with hyperthyroidism. Therefore, an important collaborative problem for this client is *Risk for Injury: corneal ulcerations, infection, and possible blindness related to inability to close the eyelids secondary to exophthalmos.*

　Planning: Expected Outcomes. The nurse will prevent corneal ulceration, infection, or blindness, as evidenced by no further development of exophthalmos.

　Implementation. The treatment should be started as soon as possible once the diagnosis is made so exophthalmos can be avoided, because the condition is irreversible. The client should use artificial tears and eye patches as needed to prevent irritation if the exophthalmos has already occurred. Once the treatment has begun, further exophthalmos should not develop.

Hyperthermia. The client with hyperthyroidism is in a hypermetabolic state leading to the nursing diagnosis *Hyperthermia related to accelerated metabolic rate.*

　Planning: Expected Outcomes. The client will not exhibit hyperthermia, as evidenced by return to normal body temperature.

　Implementation. Tell the client to stay in a cool environment. Remember that clients with Graves' disease suffer from heat intolerance. Use only a lightweight sheet for the top cover, and give them light loose pajamas. If the client is diaphoretic, the client may need to change the bed sheets and clothes frequently. Encourage the client not to overexert since this will raise the body temperature and metabolic rate.

Impaired Social Interaction. The client with hyperthyroidism suffers from hyperactivity. Therefore, an appropriate nursing diagnosis is *Impaired Social Interaction related to extreme agitation, hyperactivity, and mood swings.*

　Planning: Expected Outcomes. The client will not suffer from impaired social interaction, as evidenced by his or her ability to interact without difficulty without agitation, hyperactivity, or mood swings.

　Implementation. Explain to significant others that any bizarre, difficult behavior is likely to be temporary and should steadily improve with intervention. Maintain a quiet, understanding manner when caring for clients with Graves' disease. Accept their irritation and emotional outbursts as normal expressions of the disease.

　Incorporate occupational therapy into care planning. The occupational therapist may be able to provide clients with simple activities designed to distract them from focusing on the disorder (e.g., putting together a puzzle with large pieces, molding clay, watching television). For a very restless client, discuss with the physician the need for a sedative (such as diazepam [Valium]) or possibly one of the adrenergic blocking agents.

Evaluation

The client with Graves' disease should recover from the hyperthyroidism without difficulty once the medication regimen has begun.

■ Modifications for Elderly Clients

Hyperthyroidism in the elderly accounts for 10% to 15% of all thyrotoxic clients. Some clients present with typical manifestations of hyperthyroidism, especially when the diagnosis is Graves' disease. However, hyperthyroidism in the elderly is also notorious for presenting with atypical or minimal manifestations. It is often overlooked because the manifestations are not the usual ones. The manifestations are frequently attributed to aging. Weight loss, lack of eye findings, and normal-sized thyroid glands are frequently found on assessment. Many clients actually appear apathetic instead of hyperactive. Cardiovascular abnormalities such as congestive heart failure, atrial arrhythmias (usually digoxin-resistant), and various degrees of heart block may be caused by hyperthyroidism. If the cardiac condition is pre-existing, it may be aggregated by hyperthyroidism. A relative lack of tachycardia has been documented; approximately 40% of elderly clients have heart rates of less than 100 beats per minute.

　The diagnosis of hyperthyroidism is established by appropriate laboratory tests. It is usual to find an elevated T_4 and a suppressed TSH. Therapy for hyperthyroidism in the elderly is RAI.

Critical Care

■ Surgical Management

Surgery for hyperthyroidism has been performed since the early 1880s. Ideally, those selected are young and free from any condition that makes them poor operative risks (e.g., diabetes, heart disease, renal disease, drug allergies).

　A thyroidectomy (removal of the thyroid gland) may be total or partial. Total thyroidectomy is performed to remove thyroid cancer. Clients who undergo this operation must take TH on a permanent basis. Subtotal thyroidectomy is performed to correct hyperthyroidism and extreme cases of simple goiter. Approximately five sixths of the gland is removed, but because one sixth of the functioning gland is left intact, hormonal replacements may not be necessary. The parathyroid glands lie immediately posterior to the lobes of the thyroid and are often disturbed and sometimes inadvertently removed during surgery.

　Preoperative preparation for a subtotal thyroidectomy is extremely important. The client must be euthyroid before the operation, if possible. If the client is not euthyroid, the risk of thyroid storm occurring postoperatively is greatly increased. Therefore, preoperative care for clients with Graves' disease includes administration of (1) antithyroid drugs to suppress secretion of TH and (2) iodine preparations to reduce the size and vascularity of the organ, thereby diminishing the chance of hemorrhage (see Medical Management). Clients should be adequately rested, at optimal weight, and in good health before entering the operating room. Adequate preoperative preparation may take as long as 2 to 3 months.

Surgical treatment is effective in most people with Graves' disease. A small percentage remain hyperthyroid, and some develop hypothyroidism. Rarely, vocal cord paralysis or hypoparathyroidism may develop as a result of nerve damage or inadvertent removal of parathyroid gland tissue, respectively. Postoperative orders, rationale, and associated nursing interventions after thyroidectomy are presented in Table 70–4.

■ Nursing Management of the Surgical Client

Assessment

Assess the client for all the typical clinical manifestations associated with Graves' disease. Manifestations of the hypermetabolic state may be obvious with apparent weight loss, and exophthalmos may be readily apparent. Also question the client regarding visual difficulties, fatigue, weakness, tremors, or insomnia. See Critical Monitoring of Hyperthyroidism.

Diagnosis, Planning, Implementation

Risk for Thyroid Storm, Hypocalcemia, or Hemorrhage. The client undergoing a thyroidectomy should be euthyroid preoperatively. Thus the collaborative problem *Risk for Thyroid Storm, Hypocalcemia, or Hemorrhage related to surgical procedure and not being in a euthyroid state.*

Planning: Expected Outcomes. Thyroid storm, hypocalcemia, or hemorrhage will be prevented or will be detected early and the client protected from injury.

Implementation. Clients must be carefully prepared for a thyroidectomy for avoidance of complications (such as thyroid storm, hemorrhage). Outcomes of successful preparation of clients for thyroid surgery include the following.

- The client is euthyroid before entering the operating room. Tests of thyroid function must be within normal limits.
- Manifestations of thyrotoxicosis are greatly diminished or absent. The client appears rested and relaxed.
- Weight and nutritional status are normal, and any weight losses suffered earlier have been regained.
- Cardiac problems are under control, pulse rate is normal, and electrocardiographic tracings taken preoperatively show no dangerous arrhythmias.

For help in meeting these outcomes, the client undergoing a thyroidectomy is treated with antithyroid drugs, iodine preparations, bedrest, a nutritious diet, and supplemental vitamins. Thorough preparation may take months. However, once good health has been restored, the client can undergo surgery with confidence that the operation will be successful and the manifestations alleviated.

The immediate goals of postoperative care after thyroidectomy are to (1) maintain airway patency, (2) decrease the strain in the suture line, (3) relieve discomfort from the sore throat and tracheal irritation, (4) prevent pooling of respiratory secretions, and (5) prevent or relieve the complications of thyroidectomy.

Typical postoperative orders, their rationale, and important associated nursing interventions are outlined in Table 70–4. Assemble the equipment at the beside before the client returns from surgery (e.g., blood pressure cuff and stethoscope, additional pillows, oxygen, suction equipment, intubation supplies, and a tracheostomy set). Ampules of calcium gluconate should also be on hand in the medicine room or on the emergency cart.

Major complications after a thyroidectomy may include the following:

- Respiratory obstruction due to edema of the glottis, bilateral laryngeal nerve damage, or tracheal compression from hemorrhage
- Hemorrhage
- Weakness and hoarseness of the voice due to trauma or damage of one laryngeal nerve
- Hypocalcemia and tetany resulting from accidental removal of one or more parathyroid glands
- Thyroid storm (if the client is not euthyroid preoperatively)

Temporary hoarseness and voice weakness may occur if there has been unilateral injury to the recurrent laryngeal nerve during surgery. To assess the client's voice, ask What is your name? as soon as full recovery from anesthesia occurs. Have the client speak every 30 to 60 minutes thereafter, and carefully note any voice changes. If hoarseness or voice weakness is present, reassure the client that the problem will probably subside in a few days. Discourage unnecessary talking to minimize hoarseness.

Muscular twitching and hyperirritability of the nervous system may indicate hypocalcemic tetany. Hypocalcemia can develop after thyroidectomy if the parathyroid glands are accidentally removed during surgery. Manifestations may develop 1 to 7 days after surgery. If the client develops numbness and tingling around the mouth, finger tips or toes, muscle spasms, or twitching, call the physician immediately. Make sure calcium gluconate ampules are available at the bedside and the client has a patent intravenous line.

Risk for Ineffective Management of Therapeutic Regimen (Individuals). Hyperthyroidism is a chronic disease which must be managed with the client's full participation making the diagnosis *Risk for Ineffective Management of Therapeutic Regimen* (Individuals) *related to medications, eye care, and possible postoperative complications.*

Planning: Expected Outcomes. The client will understand eye care and possible postoperative complications, as evidenced by statements and ability to comply with the medication regimen.

Table 70–4. Postoperative Orders, Rationale, and Associated Nursing Interventions After Thyroidectomy

Postoperative Order	Rationale	Associated Nursing Interventions
Vital signs every 15 min until stable; then every 30 min for next 12 hr	After thyroidectomy, hemorrhage and respiratory obstruction may develop. Elevated pulse and hypotension indicate hemorrhage and shock. Dyspnea, stridulous respirations, and retraction of neck tissues indicate respiratory obstruction	Check dressing after checking vital signs. Observe for bleeding at front, sides, and back of neck. Examine back of neck and shoulders for bleeding because blood tends to drain posteriorly. Check dressing for tightness; uncomfortable tautness may indicate bleeding into tissues. Loosen dressing and call surgeon immediately
Semi-Fowler position when conscious unless client is hypotensive; support head and neck with pillows and sandbags; ambulate on day 2 as tolerated	Immobilization of head and neck is essential to prevent flexion and hyperextension of neck with resultant strain on suture line. Semi-Fowler position is used for comfort	Place sandbags on either side of head for immobilization and maintenance of good alignment. Warn client not to extend or hyperextend neck; reassure client that sandbags will prevent moving head too much. Gently rub back of neck to relieve tension. Support head and neck when moving or changing position
Fluids by mouth as tolerated; if nausea or vomiting, notify surgeon; soft diet on afternoon of day 2	Give intravenous fluids if nausea or vomiting. Otherwise, start oral fluids as soon as client is fully conscious	Maintain intake and output record for 2–3 days. Assess for difficulty swallowing. Normally this problem lasts for only 1–2 days postoperatively. Weigh client once a full diet is started; weight lost during early postoperative period should be regained
Meperidine (Demerol) or morphine sulfate every 3–4 hr as needed for pain in throat area	Meperidine and morphine sulfate are both used during early postoperative period to relieve pain and promote rest	Do not give narcotics if the client's respirations are below 12/min or he or she has respiratory congestion; consult physician for further orders

Implementation. Once the immediate postoperative period and its dangers have passed, turn your attention to teaching. Several important areas should be included in your teaching. First, teach the client how to support the weight of the head and neck when sitting up in bed. Show clients how to place their hands at the back of the head when flexing the neck or moving. Usually, they are able to perform this maneuver by the first postoperative day. Second, as the wound heals (around the second to fourth postoperative day), instruct the client in range-of-motion exercises for prevention of contracture. With the surgeon's permission, teach clients to flex the head forward and laterally, to hyperextend the neck, and to turn the head from side to side. Have them perform these exercises several times every day. Third, if a total thyroidectomy has been performed, give instruction concerning self-administration of thyroid medications, as outlined previously under Hypothyroidism. See the Client Education Guide on p. 2016.

Teach the client the medication regimen and the need for lifelong replacement therapy. Make an appointment for the clinic or physician's office after discharge. Serum thyroid levels are necessary to monitor treatment. Emphasize that the client who has had a thyroidectomy must see a physician at least twice yearly to avert possible complications (e.g., hypothyroidism, hypoparathyroidism, or recurrent hyperthyroidism) related to hormonal replacement.

For the postoperative thyroidectomy client, teach the client how to care for the incision once it has healed with the use of lanolin cream to soften the wound. This will help to lessen the scar.

As stated previously, the client needs to have the levels of TH measured at regular intervals until the replacement medication is adjusted to a maintenance dose. The client should then see the physician twice a year for examinations.

Evaluation

The client should be discharged within several days of surgery without difficulty. The wound should heal within about 6 weeks without infection.

Postoperative Order	Rationale	Associated Nursing Interventions
Cough and deep-breathe every half-hour; suction mouth and trachea if necessary	Pooling of mucous secretions in trachea, bronchi, and lungs will cause respiratory obstruction with resultant atelectasis and pneumonia. Secretions must be raised to prevent respiratory complications	Instruct client to cough and deep-breathe as taught during preoperative period. If client cannot raise secretions, gently suction mouth and trachea. Do not oversedate clients with profuse respiratory secretions; give narcotics judiciously
Have tracheostomy set, endotracheal tube, laryngoscope, and oxygen on hand	Acute respiratory obstruction due to hemorrhage, edema of glottis, laryngeal nerve damage, or tetany is an emergency. Equipment for establishing an airway and administering oxygen must be available for immediate use	Continuously assess for manifestations of airway obstruction, e.g., increasing restlessness, tachycardia, apprehension, cyanosis, stridulous respiration, and retraction of neck tissues. Report any of these manifestations to surgeon immediately
Continuous mist inhalation until chest clear	Humidification of air promotes easier breathing and helps to liquefy mucous secretions	Keep doors closed so that moist air is retained in room
Rectal temperature every 4 hr for 24 hr, then orally	One of the first manifestations of thyroid storm is an elevated temperature	Carefully assess for manifestations of thyroid storm: elevated temperature, extreme restlessness, agitation, and tachycardia. Report any elevation over 37.7° C (100° F) rectally or 37.2° C (99° F) orally
Assess client for hypocalcemia and monitor Ca^{2+}, Mg^{2+}, phosphorus	Inadvertent removal or devascularization of the parathyroid glands can cause postoperative hypoparathyroidism	Mild hypocalcemia can be asymptomatic. Severe hypocalcemia can produce circumoral paresthesias, positive Chvostek's or Trousseau's sign. Administer calcium supplements for hypocalcemic levels

Thyroiditis

Thyroiditis simply means inflammation of the thyroid gland. It appears in three basic forms: (1) acute suppurative, (2) subacute granulomatous (painful or de Quervain's thyroiditis) and subacute lymphocytic (silent or painless thyroiditis), and (3) chronic (Hashimoto's disease) thyroiditis.

Etiology and Risk Factors

Acute and subacute thyroiditis are uncommon disorders. Acute thyroiditis is more common in females, usually affecting women between the ages of 20 and 40 years, although it does occur in children and the elderly. The majority of clients have a pre-existing thyroid disorder. Eighty percent of the cases of subacute granulomatous thyroiditis are in women aged 40 to 50 years. There also appears to be a genetic predisposition to the subacute disease. Chronic thyroiditis or Hashimoto's disease is the

most common form of thyroiditis. Chronic thyroiditis is more common in women than in men and most commonly occurs in the 20s to 40s. The Risk Factors and Levels of Prevention feature lists other factors that may contribute to thyroiditis.

Acute suppurative thyroiditis is an uncommon inflammatory disease usually caused by bacterial invasion in the form of an abscess of the thyroid gland. *Streptococcus pyogenes, Staphylococcus aureus*, and *Pneumococcus pneumoniae* are the most common etiologic agents.

Subacute granulomatous thyroiditis is a self-limiting inflammatory condition. No etiologic agent has yet been identified, although it may be viral in origin and frequently follows a respiratory infection. Recently, autoimmune abnormalities have been described. There also appears to be a genetic predisposition to the development of both subacute granulomatous and lymphocytic thyroiditis.

Hashimoto's disease is a long-term inflammatory disorder. It is most commonly caused by autoimmune destruction of the thyroid gland. Genetic predisposition also plays a role in its causation.

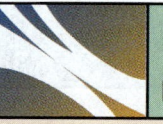

RISK FACTORS AND LEVELS OF PREVENTION

Thyroiditis

Risk Factors

Female sex, heredity, previous history of thyroid disease, previous thyroid or neck surgery, radioactive iodine treatment for hyperthyroidism, amiodarone treatment

Levels of Prevention

Primary Prevention

Educate clients at risk about manifestations of hyperthyroidism to promote early evaluation.

Secondary Prevention

Promote early identification and treatment to minimize potential morbidity of the disease process.

Tertiary Prevention

Educate the client regarding chronic effects of thyroiditis and lifelong medication dependency when hypothyroidism becomes chronic.

Pathophysiology

Acute thyroiditis is a state of acute infection and inflammation. Usually, one lobe of the thyroid is more affected than the other. Follicular destruction, cell infiltration, and colloid depletion occur. Microabscess formation is present.

Subacute thyroiditis has three phases. (1) It begins with a 3- to 4-week prodromal viral illness. Fever and malaise are experienced before the sudden onset of a tender goiter. The thyroid gland may enlarge two to three times its normal size. Mild hyperthyroidism may be present due to the sudden release of TH into the circulation. This occurs as a result of the inflammation and destruction of the thyroid gland. (2) In the second phase mild hypothyroidism develops due to incomplete recovery of the injured gland and exhaustion of stored THs. Relapse may occur. Hypothyroidism is rarely permanent. (3) The recovery phase may begin 2 to 4 months after onset.

Hashimoto's disease is manifested by an enlarged thyroid gland that may produce hypothyroid manifestations if the gland is destroyed by the autoimmune system. A euthyroid state may prevail if the gland is not destroyed.

Clinical Manifestations and Diagnostic Findings

Manifestations of acute thyroiditis include abrupt onset of unilateral anterior neck pain, with possible radiation to the ear or mandible on the affected side. Fever, diaphoresis, and other manifestations of bacterial toxicity may also be present.

Subacute granulomatous thyroiditis is usually painful, whereas subacute lymphocytic thyroiditis is usually painless. Assessment data may include characteristic anterior, unilateral neck pain that may occur with an abrupt onset, usually after a respiratory infection or viral episode. The Nursing Research feature discusses a study of *Pneumocystis carinii* thyroiditis in a client with acquired immunodeficiency syndrome (AIDS). Radiation to the ear on the ipsilateral side may occur. Manifestations of viral infection may be present that consist of myalgia, low-grade fever, lassitude, and sore throat. Approximately 50% of clients present with thyrotoxicosis.

Subacute lymphocytic thyroiditis is characterized by occasional hyperthyroidism and a painless goiter. The goiter is firm, diffuse, and mildly enlarged.

Manifestations of chronic thyroiditis include painless, asymmetrical enlargement of the gland, which in turn causes pressure on the surrounding structures and can lead to dysphagia and respiratory distress. Most clients are euthyroid; about 20% are hypothyroid, and less than 5% are hyperthyroid.

Diagnosis of thyroiditis may be made by evaluating serum T_3, free thyroxine (FT_4), RAIV, TSH, erythrocyte sedimentation rate (ESR), and thyroid antibodies. See Table 70–5 for the results of these tests. Clients with acute thyroiditis are typically euthyroid by laboratory tests.

For subacute granulomatous thyroiditis, laboratory findings reveal hyperthyroidism in approximately 50% of the clients. With subacute lymphocytic thyroiditis, laboratory diagnosis includes decreased RAIU, elevated T_3 and T_4, and frequently positive thyroid antibodies.

In chronic thyroiditis, immune antibodies are usually positive. The other thyroid function tests may be normal, increased, or decreased.

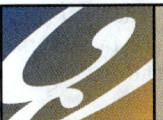

NURSING RESEARCH

Could Recent Development of Thyroid Swelling Be Related to AIDS Treatment?

Guttler, R., & Singer, P. (1993). AIDS treatment and *Pneumocystis carinii* thyroiditis. *Archives of Internal Medicine,* 153(3):393–396.

Opportunistic infections of the thyroid gland related to acquired immunodeficiency syndrome (AIDS) include cytomegalovirus, *Mycobacterium avium-intracellulare,* and *Pneumocystis carinii.* Inhaled pentamidine is commonly used as prophylaxis against *P. carinii* pneumonia. The recent emergence of *P. carinii* infection of the thyroid gland is likely related to the use of inhaled pentamidine prophylaxis, which appears to predispose to the development of extrapulmonary pneumocystosis.

Implications for Practice

A recently developed thyroid swelling should be evaluated by needle biopsy and smears so that appropriate therapy for *P. carinii* infection can be initiated promptly.

Acute and Subacute Care

■ Medical Management

Acute thyroiditis usually responds to parenteral antibiotic therapy. Treatment of subacute granulomatous thyroiditis is supportive. It may include salicylates, nonsteroidal anti-inflammatory agents, and oral glucocorticoids such as prednisone. The treatment goal in subacute lymphocytic thyroiditis is to provide relief of manifestations of hyperthyroidism with beta-adrenergic blocking agents. Antithyroid medications are not indicated.

The course of Hashimoto's disease varies. Some clients experience spontaneous remission, whereas others remain stable for years. In approximately one third of the cases, hypothyroidism develops as a result of gradual atrophy of the gland. Intervention is directed toward reducing the size of the gland and correcting any thyroid function abnormalities. Immunologic tests are not useful in monitoring these clients.

■ Surgical Management

Acute thyroiditis that does not respond to medical treatment may require incision and drainage of the affected gland. Depending on the size of the thyroid area to be incised and concurrent medical problems, the client may have the procedure done in the physician's office or as a short-stay procedure in the hospital. A fine-needle biopsy may be performed to rule out malignancy in chronic thyroiditis.

■ Nursing Management of the Medical-Surgical Client

Nursing care of clients with thyroiditis is usually supportive until the diagnosis is made. The care then, as with other thyroid disorders, revolves around helping the client learn correct medication administration. If surgery is necessary, care is the same as discussed earlier.

Discharge teaching is centered on making sure that clients understand their medication and how to take it. Clients should have their thyroid function monitored at regular intervals after discharge for the development of hyperthyroidism or hypothyroidism and for testing the effectiveness of medication.

Thyroid Cancer

The incidence of malignant tumors of the thyroid is rising. One reason may be the maturation of those people exposed to low-dose radiation early in life. They account for approximately 3 to 4 new cases per 100,000 popula-

Test	Chronic Hashimoto's or Lymphocytic Thyroiditis	Subacute Thyroiditis	Acute Thyroiditis
Serum triiodothyronine	↑ or ↓	↑ at first; ↓ later	Normal-low
Free thyroxine	↑ or ↓	↑ at first; ↓ later	Normal-low
Radioactive iodine uptake	Low or high-normal	Low	Low in about 40%
Thyroid-stimulating hormone	↑ or ↓	↓ at first; ↑ later	↓
Erythrocyte sedimentation rate	NA	↑↑	NA
Thyroid antibodies	↑	Not detected	NA

Table 70–5. Diagnostic Tests for Thyroiditis

NA, not applicable.
Adapted from Luckmann, J (Ed.) (1995). *Saunders manual of nursing care.* Philadelphia: W. B. Saunders.

tion per year in the United States. Thyroid cancer accounts for approximately 1% of cancer deaths. It has an incidence peak in the 60s but ranges from infancy to old age. Mortality is lowest in the young if the carcinoma is well differentiated. The ratio of females to males is 4:1. See Table 70–6 for the types of thyroid cancer.

Etiology and Risk Factors

Benign adenomas are usually not dangerous, although they rarely grow large enough to cause respiratory manifestations by pressing against the trachea. Occasionally, however, malignant transformation occurs, and the benign nodules become cancerous. Also, malignant transformation of benign nodules can apparently follow prolonged

stimulation of the thyroid gland by TSH. The Risk Factors and Levels of Prevention feature lists factors that may influence the development of thyroid cancer.

Pathophysiology

There are four major types of thyroid cancer: (1) papillary adenocarcinoma, (2) follicular adenocarcinoma, (3) medullary carcinoma, and (4) anaplastic carcinoma. Benign adenomas and malignant thyroid tumors constitute the third most common cause of thyroid enlargement (hypothyroidism and hyperthyroidism are the two most common causes). Like other benign tumors, most thyroid adenomas are usually well encapsulated and consequently do not spread or extend into other tissues. The incidence,

Table 70–6. Types of Thyroid Cancer: Incidence, Characteristics, Intervention, and Prognosis

Type	Incidence	Characteristics	Intervention	Prognosis
Papillary adeno-carcinoma	Constitutes 75% of thyroid cancers Affects clients in all age groups	Slow-growing firm tumor Palpable nodule Spreads to regional nodes in approximately 50% of cases Radiation-related thyroid cancer with 10- to 20-year latency period	Total or near-total thyroidectomy Others recommend lobectomy and isthmectomy	Excellent if cancer restricted to thyroid gland Lymph node metastasis is common Surgery usually curative
Follicular adeno-carcinoma	Constitutes 15% of thyroid cancers Mainly affects clients age 50 yr and older	Slow-growing nodule with about 15% metastasis to regional nodes at diagnosis Associated with radiation, iodine deficiency, endemic goiter, thyrotoxicosis	Total or near-total thyroidectomy Aggressive radioactive iodine therapy for metastases	Good but inferior to that of papillary adenocarcinoma 5-yr survival is 60%–90% Lymph node metastasis is uncommon Distant metastasis is common
Medullary thyroid carcinoma	Constitutes 5%–10% of thyroid cancers Mainly affects clients of all age groups Disease is familial in 20% of all clients	Growth rate is moderate Tends to secrete adrenocorticotropic hormone, serotonin Metastases to surrounding structures at diagnosis in 50% Associated with multiple endocrine neoplasia	Total or near-total thyroidectomy Radioactive iodine to ablate the gland	Lymph node and distant metastases are common 5-yr survival is 70%–80%
Anaplastic carcinoma (nondifferentiated)	Constitutes 5%–15% of thyroid cancers Mainly affects clients age 60–70 yr	Highly malignant Grows rapidly Local and widespread metastasis within 1 yr	Combination of thyroidectomy, external radiation therapy, chemotherapy, and tracheostomy as needed Aggressive therapy is palliative at best	Grave; mean survival, 6.2 mo; 10-yr survival, 1%

From Baker, K., & Feldman, J. (1993). Thyroid cancer: A review. *Oncology Nursing Forum, 20*(1), 95–104.

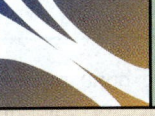

RISK FACTORS AND LEVELS OF PREVENTION

Thyroid Cancer

Risk Factors

Most Common Risk Factors. Previous radiation exposure to the head and neck; presence of thyroid nodule in client less than 20 or more than 60 years old

Other Risk Factors. Females have more nodules; males have higher incidence of malignancy; genetic factors: family history of thyroid cancer; family history of multiple endocrine neoplasia; previous history of thyroid cancer

Levels of Prevention

Primary Prevention

Assess the client's neck for a hard, irregular, painless nodule.
Shield the thyroid area if possible when radiation is done.

Secondary Prevention

Obtain thorough history, physical examination, thyroid function tests, or fine-needle aspiration as appropriate when nodule appears for early identification and treatment.

Tertiary Prevention

Ensure that clients have surgical intervention (partial or total thyroidectomy) after fine-needle biopsy results indicate questionable or malignant cell changes, or radiation treatment when indicated.

---

characteristics, intervention, and prognosis of each of these thyroid cancers are compared in Table 70–6.

Clinical Manifestations and Diagnostic Findings

The major manifestation of thyroid cancer is the appearance of a hard, irregular, painless nodule in an enlarged thyroid gland. The nodule itself is typically solitary, rapidly enlarging, and "cold" (i.e., it does not take up radioactive iodine) as opposed to benign adenomas, which may take up radioactive iodine. Also, if the tumor has metastasized, the client's lymph nodes are sometimes palpable. In long-standing cases, the client may suffer from respiratory difficulty and dysphagia, again due to the enlarged thyroid's pressing against neck structures. Thyroid cancer is diagnosed by fine-needle aspiration (FNA) biopsy.

Acute and Subacute Care

■ Medical Management

Chemotherapy, ^{131}I, external radiation, or TSH suppressive therapy may be used in metastasis. These have been discussed previously. Clients with a benign nodule usually undergo long-term suppression therapy with levothy-roxine. The goal is to suppress serum TSH without causing hyperthyroidism.

■ Surgical Management

Treatment usually includes removal of all or part of the thyroid. Neck resection may be done for metastases to the neck. Thyroid surgery is covered earlier in this chapter. As with a thyroidectomy for noncancerous lesions, the major complications postoperatively are respiratory distress, recurrent laryngeal damage, hemorrhage, and hypoparathyroidism.

■ Nursing Management of the Medical-Surgical Client

Nursing care of the client with thyroid cancer is similar to the care of any client undergoing a thyroidectomy. The client will also need the support and teaching a cancer client requires. If the client is to undergo chemotherapy, additional teaching is needed.

If the client has total thyroidectomy, replacement of TH is necessary. Discharge teaching is centered on making sure the client understands the medication and how to take it. There are no special home healthcare needs other than the needs of a client after thyroidectomy or the home healthcare needs of a client on chemotherapy or radiation therapy. The client should be checked at regular intervals for recurrence and should have thyroid function monitored.

Parathyroid Disorders

Hyperparathyroidism

Hyperparathyroidism is a disorder caused by overactivity of one or more of the parathyroid glands. Hyperparathyroidism is classified as primary, secondary, or tertiary. Hyperparathyroidism usually occurs in clients over the age of 60 years and affects females more than males by a ratio of 2:1. It is not related to age in clients with renal failure. The overall incidence of hyperparathyroidism is 27/100,000.

Etiology and Risk Factors

Primary hyperparathyroidism develops when the normal regulatory relationship between serum calcium levels and parathyroid hormone (PTH) secretion is interrupted. This occurs when either an adenoma or hyperplasia of the gland exists without an identifying injury.

Secondary hyperparathyroidism occurs when the glands are hyperplastic from malfunction of another organ system. This is usually the result of renal failure but may also occur with osteogenesis imperfecta, Paget's disease, multiple myeloma, and carcinoma with bone metastasis.

Tertiary hyperparathyroidism occurs when PTH production is irrepressible (autonomous) in clients with normal or low serum calcium levels. Risk factors are presented in the Risk Factors and Levels of Prevention feature.

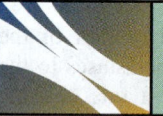

RISK FACTORS AND LEVELS OF PREVENTION

Hyperparathyroidism

Risk factors

Chronic renal failure, exposure to head and neck radiation and coexistence of Hashimoto's disease, history of neck exploration or thyroid surgery

Levels of Prevention

Primary Prevention

Educate clients at risk as to the manifestations of hyperparathyroidism.

Secondary Prevention

Seek early detection through evaluation of blood chemistry (Ca^{2+} levels, serum phosphate).

Tertiary Prevention

Educate clients about the disease process and medications prescribed for acute hypercalcemia; the surgical removal of parathyroid glands is definitive treatment.

Pathophysiology

The normal function of PTH is to increase bone resorption, thereby maintaining the proper balance of calcium and phosphorus ions within the blood (see Chapter 67). Excessive circulating PTH leads to bone damage, hypercalcemia, and kidney damage.

Primary Hyperparathyroidism

The severity of the hypercalcemia is reflective of the quantity of hyperfunctioning parathyroid tissue. The excessive quantities of PTH stimulate the transport of calcium into the blood from the intestine, kidneys and bone. Nephrolithiasis develops secondary to calcium phosphate kidney stones and the deposition of calcium in the soft tissues of the kidney. Pyelonephritis may complicate the nephrolithiasis. Bone resorption related to hypercalcemia may develop.

Myopathy is a common condition characterized by neuropathic atrophy and the development of proximal muscle weakness. Hypercalcemia can stimulate hypergastrinemia, abdominal pain, and peptic ulcer disease. Pancreatitis is also influenced by high calcium levels.

Secondary Hyperparathyroidism

Chronic renal failure (CRF) and hyperphosphatemia cause secondary hyperparathyroidism. As the glomerular filtration rate decreases in CRF, serum phosphorus rises. The increase in serum phosphorus causes the serum calcium level to fall. PTH secretion is stimulated. This increase decreases renal tubular absorption of phosphorus causing serum phosphorus levels to return to normal. As the glomerular filtration rate continues to decrease, PTH is secreted in increased amounts in order to decrease tubular reabsorption of phosphorus and maintain serum phosphorus at, or close to, normal limits.

Clinical Manifestations and Diagnostic Findings

Some clients with hyperparathyroidism may be entirely asymptomatic. Others suffer from a myriad of manifestations arising from the skeletal disease, renal involvement, gastrointestinal tract disorders, and neurologic abnormalities (Fig. 70–4 and the Clinical Monitoring feature).

Manifestations of bone disease range from backache, joint pain, and bone pain to pathologic fractures of the spine, ribs, and long bones. In long-standing cases, assessment reveals deformity and bending of the bones. Osteitis fibrosa with superperiosteal resorption or bone cysts, arthritis, or radiologic osteoporosis may be diagnosed.

Manifestations of renal involvement include (1) polyuria and polydipsia; (2) the appearance of sand, gravel, or stones within the urine; (3) azotemia; and (4) hypertension due to renal damage. Without intervention, renal insufficiency may progress to fatal renal hypertension and uremia.

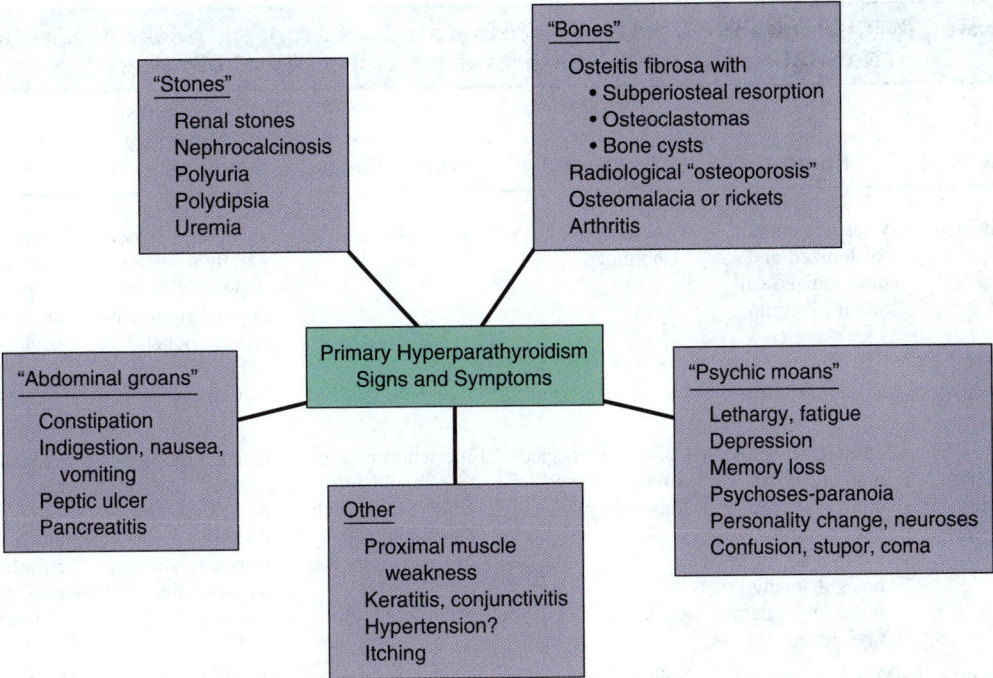

Figure 70–4. Signs and symptoms of primary hyperparathyroidism. (Adapted from Strewler, G. J., & Rosenblatt, M. (1995). Mineral metabolism. In P. Felig, J. D. Baxter, & L. A. Frohman [eds.], *Endocrinology and metabolism* [3rd ed., pp. 1407–1499]. New York: McGraw-Hill.)

Hypercalcemia mainly produces gastrointestinal tract manifestations (e.g., thirst, nausea, anorexia, constipation, ileus, and abdominal pain). Often, clients have a history of peptic ulcer or gastrointestinal tract bleeding. Assessment may also reveal psychiatric manifestations. Listlessness, depression, and paranoia are sometimes associated with high levels of serum calcium. Finally, calcium may form calcification within the eyes, impairing vision.

The major complications of hyperparathyroidism are the manifestations associated with hypercalcemia and those associated with treatment such as dehydration, hypocalcemia, and gastrointestinal tract manifestations.

The diagnosis of hyperparathyroidism mainly rests on laboratory and x-ray findings (Table 70–7). Serum calcium is elevated; serum phosphate is depressed; urine calcium and phosphorus are both high. In addition, alkaline phosphatase is elevated in the 25% of clients who have associated bone disease. Clients with skeletal damage have the following characteristic x-ray findings: diffuse demineralization of bones, bone cysts, subperiosteal bone resorption, and loss of the lamina dura surrounding the teeth. Ultrasound or magnetic resonance imaging (MRI) may be used for preoperative localization of the parathyroid glands.

 ## Community and Self-Care

■ Medical Management

The treatment of hyperparathyroidism includes (1) lowering severely elevated calcium levels, (2) increasing urinary calcium excretion with diuretics, and (3) long-term management of hypercalcemia with drugs to increase bone resorption of calcium.

Hydration and Calciuria

Serum calcium levels are lowered by hydration and calciuria. Hydration may be achieved with a normal saline

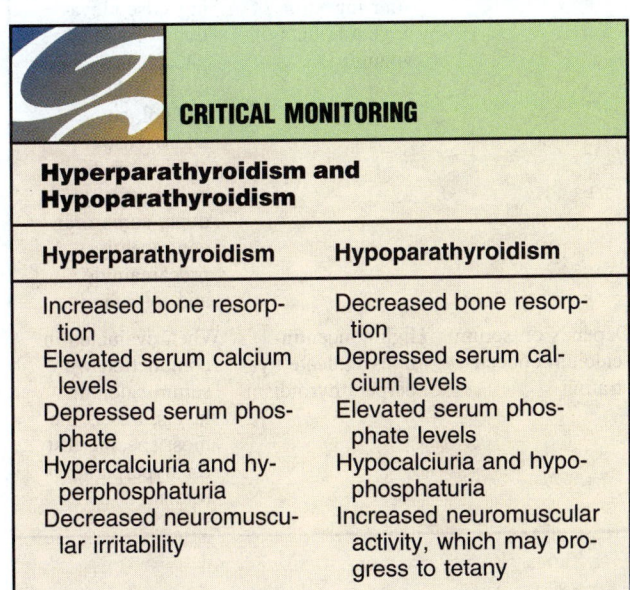

CRITICAL MONITORING	
Hyperparathyroidism and Hypoparathyroidism	
Hyperparathyroidism	**Hypoparathyroidism**
Increased bone resorption	Decreased bone resorption
Elevated serum calcium levels	Depressed serum calcium levels
Depressed serum phosphate	Elevated serum phosphate levels
Hypercalciuria and hyperphosphaturia	Hypocalciuria and hypophosphaturia
Decreased neuromuscular irritability	Increased neuromuscular activity, which may progress to tetany

Table 70–7. Diagnostic Tests of Parathyroid Function: Purpose, Procedure, Normal Range, and Interpretation of Abnormal Findings

Test	Purpose	Procedure	Normal Range	Interpretation of Abnormal Findings	Remarks
Total serum calcium	Measures amount of ionized and non-ionized calcium in serum	Venous blood to laboratory	4.8–5.2 mEq/L or 8–11 mg/dl	Elevated in hyperparathyroidism; depressed in hypoparathyroidism, tetany, rickets, nephrosis, and osteomalacia	Normally 50% of total serum calcium is ionized; amount of ionized calcium available decreases in alkalosis
Qualitative urinary calcium (Sulkowitch test)	Measures roughly amount of calcium in urine; used as quick method for diagnosis if tetany is due to hypoparathyroidism	Collect urine specimen and send to laboratory	Fine white precipitate should form when Sulkowitch reagent is added to urine specimen	Absence or decreased density of precipitate indicates low serum calcium and hypoparathyroidism	Medications that elevate serum calcium levels include vitamin D, parathyroid infection, and dihydrotachysterol
Quantitative urinary calcium (calcium deprivation test)	Measures exact amount of calcium in 24-hr urine specimen	Collect 24-hr urine specimen and send to laboratory	75–175 mg calcium per 24 hr	Elevated in hyperparathyroidism; depressed in hypoparathyroidism	Foods high in calcium include milk, cheese, molasses, turnip greens, and dandelion greens
Serum phosphorus	Measures amount of inorganic phosphorus in serum	Venous blood to laboratory	1.3–1.75 mEq/L (2.5–4.5 mg/dl) in adults	Depressed in hypoparathyroidism, uremia, and alkalosis; elevated in hyperparathyroidism, rickets, and osteomalacia	There is an inverse relationship between serum calcium and serum phosphorus
Serum alkaline phosphatase	Measures amount of alkaline phosphatase in serum; aids in diagnosing bone and liver disorders	Venous blood to laboratory	2.0–5.0 Bodansky units	Elevated in hyperparathyroidism, osteomalacia, rickets, healing fractures, and pregnancy and after ingestion of large amounts of vitamin D	Alkaline phosphatase is an enzyme normally present in small amounts in serum; some medications causing false elevations of alkaline phosphatase levels include allopurinol, some androgens, colchicine, erythromycin, methyldopa, some oral contraceptives, procainamide, and tolbutamide
PTH (parathyroid hormone) radioimmunoassay	Measures level of PTH in serum	Venous blood to laboratory	Depends on serum calcium concentration	High concentrations indicate hyperparathyroidism	When evaluated in conjunction with serum calcium levels, this is the most specific test for hyperparathyroidism

infusion. Normal saline is the fluid of choice because it both expands the volume and acts in the kidney to inhibit the resorption of calcium. Furosemide (Lasix), a loop diuretic, may also be used to promote calciuria after rehydration has occurred. Thiazide diuretics are not used since they promote calcium retention in the kidneys.

Antiresorption Agents

Drugs that inhibit bone resorption include plicamycin (Mithracin), gallium nitrate (Ganite), phosphates, and calcitonin. Plicamycin is a cancer chemotherapeutic agent that is very effective in lowering serum calcium levels. The hypocalcemic effect is seen after 24 hours and lasts for about 1 to 2 weeks. The dose is about one-tenth that used for cancer treatment, so the adverse effects are proportionally lower.

Gallium nitrate, a newer drug, is now being used more often because it has even fewer side effects. Glucocorticoids may be used to reduce hypercalcemia by decreasing gastrointestinal absorption of calcium. Etidronate (Didronel) or calcitonin may be used to decrease the release of calcium by bones. Drugs used to treat hypercalcemia are summarized in Table 70–8.

Low Calcium, Low Vitamin D Diet

The client with hypercalcemia should be on a low calcium, low vitamin D diet.

■ Nursing Management of the Medical Client

Assessment

There are no obvious manifestations of hyperparathyroidism and the resultant hypercalcemia. Elicit a good history from the client to see if any of the risk factors are present. The client may exhibit some psychological changes, such as lethargy, drowsiness, memory loss, and emotional lability, all manifestations seen in hypercalcemia.

Diagnosis, Planning, Implementation

Risk for Injury. The client with hyperparathyroidism is at great risk for injury leading to the nursing diagnosis *Risk for Injury related to demineralization of bones resulting in pathologic fractures.*

Planning: Expected Outcomes. The client will not suffer injury, as evidenced by absence of pathologic fractures or hypercalcemia.

Implementation. Protect the client from accidents. If bone involvement exists, the client may develop pathologic fractures from even small bumps or minor falls. Keep the client's bed in low position and use side rails. If the client is weak or has joint or skeletal disease, assist in ambulation.

If the client suffered from severe osteoporosis or pathologic fractures, some assistance may be required at home.

The client may need a visiting nurse to help assess the current home situation and make recommendations on how it could be made safer. The home will need to be cleared of articles such as throw rugs that might increase the risk of falling. The client may also need assistive devices such as a railing in the bathroom, a bedside commode, or a walker.

Altered Urinary Elimination. The development of urinary lithiasis in clients with hyperparathyroidism means that the nursing diagnosis *Altered Urinary Elimination related to renal involvement secondary to hypercalcemia and hyperphosphaturia* is appropriate.

Planning: Expected Outcomes. The client will return to a normal urinary output, as evidenced by no development of stones and urine output of 30 to 60 ml/hr.

Implementation. The client should take in at least 3000 ml of fluid a day. Dehydration is dangerous in clients with hyperparathyroidism because it increases the serum calcium level and promotes the formation of renal stones. Cranberry and prune juice may help make the urine more acidic. High urinary acidity helps prevent renal stone formation, because calcium is more soluble in an acidic urine than in an alkaline urine.

If the client has a kidney stone, strain all urine to detect gravel and stones. Save any specimens of abnormal urine for the physician to examine and for laboratory analysis. Also, observe the urine for blood and assess the client for renal colic (see Chapters 55 and 57).

Altered Nutrition: Less than Body Requirements. The client is likely to experience nutritional problems, making the nursing diagnosis *Altered Nutrition: Less than Body Requirements related to anorexia and nausea* an appropriate diagnosis.

Planning: Expected Outcomes. The client will have an adequate intake, as evidenced by absence of nausea and return to or maintenance of ideal body weight.

Implementation. Encourage a low calcium diet to correct hypercalcemia. Explain to the client that abstaining from milk and milk products may help alleviate some of the distressing gastrointestinal manifestations. The client who suffers from peptic ulcers will need to take antacids or histamine-receptor antagonists. Help the client develop a diet that is high enough in calories without dairy products. If necessary, have a dietitian see the client to help with meal planning.

Constipation. The client with hyperparathyroidism is prone to bowel problems leading to the nursing diagnosis *Constipation related to adverse effects of hypercalcemia on the gastrointestinal tract.*

Planning: Expected Outcomes. The client will maintain a normal bowel pattern, as evidenced by a daily bowel movement.

Implementation. Work to prevent constipation and fecal impaction resulting from hypercalcemia. Help the

Table 70–8. Drugs Used to Treat Hypercalcemia

Medication	Rationale	Dosage	Side Effects	Nursing Implications
Furosemide (Lasix)	Promotes renal excretion of calcium	Up to 100 mg IV	Volume depletion and dehydration, orthostatic hypotension, hypokalemia, hypochloremic alkalosis, hyperuricemia, dilutional hyponatremia, hypocalcemia, hypomagnesemia	Monitor intake and output carefully; monitor blood pressure and pulse; give with 0.9% sodium chloride; monitor serum electrolytes; watch calcium level closely
Plicamycin (Mithracin)	Chemotherapeutic agent that inhibits bone resorption and lowers serum calcium level	25 µg IV daily for 1–4 days	Thrombocytopenia, bleeding tendencies, nausea and vomiting, facial flushing, diarrhea; increased BUN and creatinine; decreased serum calcium, potassium, and phosphorus; anorexia	Therapeutic effect in hypercalcemia may not be seen for 24–48 hr and may last 3–15 days; monitor serum electrolytes, liver enzymes, and BUN and creatinine; monitor platelet count and watch for bleeding; watch for sudden drop in serum calcium; check closely for signs of hypocalcemia; give antiemetics before administration to reduce nausea
Etidronate disodium (Didronel)	Decreases release of calcium from bones	5 mg/kg PO daily as single dose 2 hr before meals, up to dose of 20 mg/kg	Diarrhea, nausea, bone pain, increased risk of fractures, elevated serum phosphate	Do not administer with food or antacids; monitor serum phosphate; tell client that onset of therapeutic effect may take several months; do not give for more than 6 mo continuously, stop, then restart after 3 mo; monitor renal function
Gallium nitrate (Ganite)	Inhibits bone resorption	100–200 mg/m² daily for 5 consecutive days	Increased BUN and creatinine, hypocalcemia, decreased serum bicarbonate, transient hypophosphatemia, anemia, hypotension, nausea and vomiting	Administer IV with 0.9% sodium chloride; monitor serum calcium, bicarbonate, and phosphate; check blood pressure at intervals; monitor renal function; check for signs of anemia
Calcitonin (Cibacalcin)	Used in secondary hyperparathyroidism; prescribed to decrease acidosis; acts as a phosphate-binding agent; nutritional supplement to the low-phosphate diet	0.5–1.0 mg SC daily or 2–3 times a week	Nausea and vomiting, urinary frequency, flushing of face and hands, hypocalcemia	Administer at bedtime to decrease nausea and vomiting; monitor for signs of hypocalcemia; treatment may last for 6 mo; monitor serum phosphate; warn client about transient facial flushing

BUN, blood urea nitrogen; IV, intravenously; PO, orally; SC, subcutaneously.

client to be as active as the extent of bone disease allows. Increase fluid intake and the amount of fiber in the diet. The client should drink at least six to eight glasses of water a day unless contraindicated. If constipation continues despite these measures, obtain an order for a stool softener or laxative.

Evaluation

Depending on the cause of the hypercalcemia, medical management may control primary hypercalcemia. If it does not, surgery may be required. If it is secondary to renal failure, the management will be more chronic in nature.

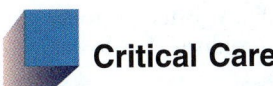

Critical Care

■ Surgical Management

Definitive treatment of primary hyperparathyroidism is surgical removal of the gland or glands causing hypersecretion of PTH. Usually, only the diseased parathyroid glands are resected. However, if all four glands are hyperplastic, three and one-half glands are removed. Fortunately, one half of a parathyroid gland is usually sufficient to maintain normal levels of circulating PTH.

Autotransplantation of the parathyroid glands is a useful modality for the management of clients with certain forms of hyperparathyroidism and radical neck surgery. After partial parathyroidectomy, it is possible to transplant the remaining healthy parathyroid tissue to a safer location, such as the brachioradialis muscle of the forearm. Reexploration of the neck in the future may cause laryngeal nerve damage and influence complications from the original surgery. Transplants take some time to come to full effect. Clients must be supplemented with calcium and vitamin D for prevention of hypoparathyroidism and hypocalcemia until the transplant matures.

If hyperparathyroidism is surgically treated early in its course, the chance of total recovery is good. Bone pain may disappear within 3 days after removal of parathyroid tissue, and bone lesions may heal completely. Unfortunately, serious renal disease may not be reversible by parathyroid surgery.

Complications

The complications of parathyroidectomy are similar to those of thyroidectomy and rarely occur. Hypocalcemia is a potentially life-threatening complication even if some parathyroid glands are left untouched because edema reduces their function. The client can also develop respiratory distress related to either hemorrhage or recurrent laryngeal nerve damage.

Outcomes

The cure rate for primary hyperparathyroidism after surgical removal is greater than 95%. This high success rate is directly related to the experience of the surgeon and adequate exploration of the neck.

■ Nursing Management of the Surgical Client

Assessment

The client undergoing surgery may have long-standing hyperparathyroidism and therefore should be assessed for the presence of complications of the disease. Renal function should be carefully assessed preoperatively.

Diagnosis, Planning, Implementation

Risk for Injury. The client undergoing surgery for hyperparathyroidism is at risk for a number of complications. Another important nursing diagnosis is *Risk for Injury related to preoperative drug sensitivities and postoperative complications.*

Planning: Expected Outcomes. The client will not suffer injury, as evidenced by no medication reactions preoperatively and the absence of respiratory distress, hemorrhage, and hypocalcemia after surgery.

Implementation. If the client is on digitalis, administer this medication with extreme caution. Clients with hypercalcemia are hypersensitive to digitalis and may quickly develop toxic manifestations.

During the postoperative period, new problems arise, some of which are the reverse of those found preoperatively. During the immediate postoperative period, nursing care is similar to that after thyroidectomy, that is, assess the client carefully for hemorrhage, airway obstruction, injury to the recurrent laryngeal nerve, and tetany. Also watch for manifestations of hormonal imbalance.

Mild tetany due to the fall in serum calcium is expected after removal of parathyroid tissue. Typically, the uncomfortable tingling of the hands and around the mouth that follows parathyroid resection is usually temporary. If it persists or is severe, however, calcium gluconate is administered intravenously.

Clients with bone disease require additional therapy after surgery. Removal of the parathyroid glands reduces bone resorption, and because bone rebuilding proceeds at a rapid rate, the client can develop the "hungry bones" syndrome. This is characterized by hypocalcemia and severe tetany resulting from the rapid utilization of calcium by the bones. For preventing low serum calcium levels due to bone recalcification, instruct these clients to eat foods high in calcium. Tetany is treated with injections of calcium gluconate. To maintain adequate calcium levels, oral calcium preparations are usually given for months until the skeletal tissues have been rebuilt. Finally, clients are encouraged to ambulate as soon as possible after surgery, because weightbearing speeds the recalcification process.

Evaluation

If the hypercalcemia was unrelieved by medical management, surgery is usually successful in relieving the condition. If a partial parathyroidectomy is unsuccessful, the client may need to have the remaining gland transplanted to the forearm to reduce absorption of the hormone. This usually eliminates the problem. As long as the client is followed in the immediate postoperative period, complications of hypocalcemia are usually controllable.

■ Modifications for Elderly Clients

Hyperparathyroidism in the elderly is an overlooked disease. It is estimated that 1/1000 men and 2/1000 women over the age of 60 years experience hyperparathyroidism. This disease often goes undiagnosed in the elderly because manifestations in the early stages are subtle and attributed to old age, depression, or anxiety. The manifestations only intensify as the level of serum calcium continues to rise and other physiologic and functional changes occur. Laboratory diagnosis is the same as for a younger client, but treatment may be complicated by medical problems and medication.

Hypoparathyroidism

Hyposecretion of the parathyroid glands produces a syndrome that is the reverse of hyperparathyroidism. That is, serum calcium levels are abnormally low, serum phosphate levels are abnormally high, and pronounced neuromuscular irritability (tetany) may develop.

Women are diagnosed with hypoparathyroidism more often than men. The incidence is related to thyroid surgery. The incidence of temporary hypoparathyroidism after total thyroidectomy ranges from 6.9% to 25%. The incidence after subtotal thyroidectomy is 1.6% to 9.0%.[13]

Etiology and Risk Factors

The causes of hypoparathyroidism are either iatrogenic or idiopathic. Iatrogenic causes include (1) accidental removal of the parathyroid glands during thyroidectomy, (2) infarction of the parathyroid glands resulting from an inadequate blood supply to the glands during surgery, and (3) strangulation of one or more of the glands by postoperative scar tissue. The Risk Factors and Levels of Prevention feature lists measures to prevent hypoparathyroidism.

Idiopathic hypoparathyroidism, like Graves' disease and Hashimoto's disease, may be an autoimmune disorder with a genetic basis. This type of hypoparathyroidism is far less common than the iatrogenic form. Pseudohypoparathyroidism (Albright's hereditary osteodystrophy) is an inherited form of hypoparathyroidism due to lack of end-organ responsiveness to PTH.

Pathophysiology

PTH normally acts to increase bone resorption, which in turn maintains proper serum calcium levels. The hormone also regulates phosphate clearance by the renal tubules, thereby maintaining the correct inverse balance between serum calcium and serum phosphate. Consequently, when parathyroid secretion is reduced, bone resorption slows, serum calcium levels fall, and severe neuromuscular irritability develops. Somewhat paradoxically, calcifications form in various organs (e.g., the eyes and basal ganglia). Also, without sufficient PTH, fewer phosphorus ions are secreted by the distal tubules of the kidney, renal excretion of phosphate falls, and serum phosphate levels rise.

The client may fully recover from the effects of hypoparathyroidism if the condition is diagnosed early, before the advent of serious complications. Unfortunately, cataracts and brain calcification, once formed, are irreversible.

Clinical Manifestations and Diagnostic Findings

The manifestations of hypoparathyroidism are mainly caused by low serum calcium levels. They are always more severe in clients who have an elevated serum pH (alkalosis) from any cause (e.g., ingesting antacids, hyperventilation). Manifestations worsen because when the pH of the blood rises, the amount of ionized calcium drops, although total serum calcium remains the same. With less ionized calcium available to the body, the manifestations resulting from hypocalcemia become more severe until the alkalosis is corrected.

Acute Hypoparathyroidism

Acute hypoparathyroidism is caused by accidental damage to parathyroid tissues during thyroidectomy. It is characterized by greatly increased neuromuscular irritability, which results in tetany. Clients with tetany experience painful muscle spasms, irritability, grimacing, tingling of fingers, laryngospasm, and arrhythmias. Assessment also reveals Chvostek's and Trousseau's signs. In some cases, tetany is so severe that a tracheostomy is required to correct acute respiratory obstruction secondary to laryngospasm.

Chronic Hypoparathyroidism

Chronic hypoparathyroidism is usually idiopathic. It causes lethargy; thin, patchy hair; brittle nails; dry, scaly skin; and personality changes. Ectopic calcification may appear in the eyes and basal ganglia. Thus, the client may develop cataracts and permanent brain damage accompanied by psychosis or convulsions. In addition, severe persistent hypocalcemia adversely affects the heart, causing arrhythmias and eventual cardiac failure.

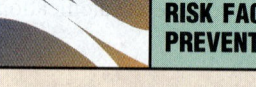

RISK FACTORS AND LEVELS OF PREVENTION

Hypoparathyroidism

Risk Factors

Thyroidectomy, partial (with inadvertent total) parathyroidectomy, postoperative neck exploration, status post neck radiation

Levels of Prevention

Primary Prevention

Educate the client regarding early detection of manifestations.

Secondary Prevention

Provide regular monitoring of parathyroid hormone, calcium, and phosphorus levels.
Provide client education.

Tertiary Prevention

Prevent tetany by administering calcium supplements for life.

The diagnosis of hypoparathyroidism is based on the following:

1. Physical examination findings related to hypocalcemia:
   - Presence of Chvostek's sign (spasms of facial muscles after a tap over the facial nerve, signifying facial hyperirritability)
   - Presence of Trousseau's sign (spasms of the wrist and hand after compression of the upper arm, as by a blood pressure cuff)
   - Hyperactive deep tendon reflexes (DTRs)
   - Circumoral paresthesia
   - Numbness and tingling of fingers
2. Laboratory findings of low calcium, low PTH, high phosphorus, decreased urine calcium
3. Radiographic studies of skull, computed tomography (CT) of the head, showing areas of calcification
4. Ophthalmic examination to reveal calcification of the lens that can lead to cataract formation.

Complications

If treatment is not begun rapidly in acute hypoparathyroidism, death can result from the respiratory obstruction secondary to tetany and laryngospasms.

In chronic hypoparathyroidism, the complications are calcifications in the eye and basal ganglia that can occur if treatment is delayed.

Acute and Subacute Care

■ Medical Management

Acute hypoparathyroidism (with its major manifestation of acute tetany) is a *life-threatening* disorder. The three goals of emergency care are to (1) elevate serum calcium levels as rapidly as possible, (2) prevent or treat convulsions, and (3) control laryngeal spasm and consequent respiratory obstruction.

The goal of intervention in clients with chronic hypoparathyroidism is to restore the serum calcium level to normal concentrations. This is done more gradually than with acute hypoparathyroidism.

Calcium Gluconate

In acute hypoparathyroidism, to elevate serum calcium levels quickly, the physician will prescribe 10% calcium gluconate solution in an intravenous infusion. While administering the calcium gluconate, instruct the client to inhale carbon dioxide by breathing into a paper bag. This causes a mild metabolic acidosis, which serves to elevate the amount of ionized calcium in the blood.

Oral Calcium Replacements

Once the condition has stabilized and the dangers of tetany have passed, the client is given oral calcium salts and vitamin D to maintain normal serum calcium levels. The goal of chronic hypoparathyroidism therapy is to keep the client asymptomatic with a serum calcium level of approximately 8.5 to 9.2 mg/dl.

The client is given oral calcium salts (either calcium gluconate, calcium lactate, or calcium carbonate) and vitamin D. Commercially available forms of vitamin D include ergocalciferol (vitamin D_2), and dihydrotachysterol (Hytakerol). Although ergocalciferol is a more reliable and less expensive drug than dihydrotachysterol or dihydroxycholecalciferol, all three forms of vitamin D are effective in correcting hypocalcemia. They are all obtainable as either tablets or oily liquids. Aluminum hydroxide gel (Amphojel) is also prescribed.

Parathyroid Hormone

The ideal treatment of this PTH-deficient condition is replacement of the absent hormone. A pure form of PTH has only recently been synthesized. See current journals for an update on pure PTH.

High Calcium, Low Phosphate Diet

The client with hypoparathyroidism should be on a diet high in calcium but low in phosphorus.

■ Nursing Management of the Medical Client

Assessment

Carefully assess the client at risk of acute hypoparathyroidism, such as the post-thyroidectomy client, for the development of hypocalcemia. Question the client about any manifestations of numbness and tingling around the mouth or in the finger tips or toes. Also check for a positive finding of Chvostek's or Trousseau's sign. It is also important to assess for any manifestation of respiratory distress secondary to laryngospasm.

In the client with chronic hypoparathyroidism, assess for the presence of obvious physical changes such as dry skin and hair. Also assess for the presence of a Parkinson's-like syndrome or the presence of cataracts. Also assess the teeth because pits may encircle the teeth, indicating enamel hypoplasia.

Diagnosis, Planning, Implementation

Muscle Tetany. The client with hypoparathyroidism is prone to hypocalcemia, which can lead to the collaborative problem *Muscle Tetany related to decreased serum calcium levels.*

Planning: Expected Outcomes. The client will not suffer any injury, as evidenced by calcium levels returning to the normal range, a normal respiratory rate, and blood gases within normal limits.

Implementation. When caring for clients with severe hypoparathyroidism, always be prepared for laryngeal spasm and respiratory obstruction. Have an endotracheal tube, laryngoscope, and tracheostomy set available when caring for clients with acute tetany.

When a client is at risk of sudden hypocalcemia, as after thyroidectomy, an ampule of intravenous calcium carbonate is usually kept at the client's bedside for immediate use if necessary. When the intravenous tubing is removed, it is sometimes capped so that rapid venous access is available. Sometimes clients are encouraged to take in a ready source of calcium carbonate such as Tums.

Risk for Ineffective Management of Therapeutic Regimen (Individuals).

Since hypoparathyroidism can be a chronic condition, the client must be able to provide self-care, making the nursing diagnosis *Risk for Ineffective Management of Therapeutic Regimen (Individuals) related to diet and medication regimen* an important diagnosis.

Planning: Expected Outcomes. The client will understand the diet and medication, as evidenced by the client's statements and ability to follow the diet and medication regimen.

Implementation. Teaching is important for the client with chronic hypoparathyroidism because this client will require lifelong medication and dietary modification.

When teaching the client about take-home medications, make sure the client knows that all forms of vitamin D, except dihydroxycholecalciferol, are slowly assimilated by the body. Therefore it may take a week or longer for the manifestations to improve.

Teach the client about a diet high in calcium but low in phosphorus. Remind the client to omit cheese and milk products from the diet, because these foods have a high phosphorus content. Tell the client that calcium supplements may be obtained in either tablet or solution form, depending on preference. Oral calcium administration is usually discontinued once the client responds successfully to vitamin D preparations.

Emphasize the importance of lifelong medical care for the client with chronic hypoparathyroidism. Instruct the client to have the serum calcium level checked by a physician at least three times a year. Normal blood serum calcium levels must be maintained to prevent complications. If hypercalcemia or hypocalcemia develop, the physician will need to adjust the treatment regimen to correct the imbalance.

Evaluation

If the hypocalcemia is transient secondary to a thyroidectomy, it usually resolves as edema decreases. If it is chronic, the client is usually able to manage the therapeutic regimen with minimal difficulty.

Conclusions

You must make careful assessments of clients with thyroid or parathyroid disorders. These disorders can be controlled and the manifestations reversed if they are diagnosed in a timely manner and prompt and proper treatment is begun. You are an important resource for these clients who require considerable education. You are also responsible for the close monitoring the client requires after surgery of either the thyroid or parathyroid gland. The client is particularly vulnerable during this postoperative period, and high-level nursing surveillance and intervention can mean the client recovers successfully.

Thinking Critically

1. A 64-year-old man comes to the clinic with a 6-month history of progressive fatigue, weakness, and dyspnea. On further questioning, you find that he has an unintentional weight loss of 30 lb despite an increased appetite.

Your physical examination reveals an alert and oriented man who looks his stated age. He is somewhat anxious. His attention span is short and you must repeat many questions. His heart rate is 118 beats per minute; blood pressure, 154/98 mm Hg; temperature, 101° F; the skin is warm and moist; deep tendon reflexes are hyperactive. What are priorities for care?

Factors to Consider. What additional subjective and objective data should you collect to confirm a diagnosis? What medication might he be started on after the diagnosis is made?

2. The client is a woman with a long history of chronic renal failure. She is on dialysis three times a week. She is currently hospitalized for a complicated pneumonia. Upon reviewing her laboratory values you note that her serum calcium level is 6.8 mg/dl. What are the implications for care?

Factors to Consider. What is the relationship of calcium metabolism to renal function? What are the dangers of a serum calcium at this level? What treatments should be initiated to treat this and what should be done to prevent recurrence?

3. A middle-aged woman comes to the clinic with symptoms of weight gain, lethargy, fatigue, and severe constipation. After diagnostic evaluation, the client is given Synthroid 0.1 mg, for hypothyroidism. What general information should you impart to the client about the hypothyroidism? About medication?

Factors to Consider. What should you teach about the expected therapeutic response to this medication? About side effects? How often are blood studies required for the client being treated with thyroid medications?

Bibliography

1. Angelucci, P. A. (1995). Caring for patients with hypothyroidism. *Nursing, 25*(5), 60–61.
2. Baker, K., & Feldman, J. (1993). Thyroid cancer: A review. *Oncology Nursing Forum, 20*(1), 95–104.
3. Baumann, D., & Wells, S. (1993). Parathyroid autotransplantation. *Surgery, 113*(2), 130–133.

4. Bemben, D., et al. (1994). Thyroid disease in the elderly. Part I. Prevalence of undiagnosed hypothyroidism. *Journal of Family Practice, 38*(6), 577–581.

5. Bemben, D., et al. (1994). Thyroid disease in the elderly. Part II. Predictability of subclinical hypothyroidism. *Journal of Family Practice, 38*(6), 583–588.

6. Bilezikian, J. P. (1994). Primary hyperparathyroidism: Another important metabolic bone disease women. *Journal of Women's Health, 3*(1), 21–32.

7. Burrow, G. N. (1995). The thyroid: Nodules and neoplasm. In P. Felig, J. D. Baxter, L. A. Frohman (Eds.), *Endocrinology and metabolism* (3rd ed., pp. 521–549). New York: McGraw-Hill.

8. Cannon, C. R. (1994). Hypothyroidism in head and neck cancer patients: Experimental and clinical observations. *Laryngoscope, 104*(11), 1–21.

9. Coffland, F. (1993). Thyroid induced cardiac disorders. *Critical Care Nurse, 13*(3), 25–50.

10. Corbett, J. V. (1992). *Laboratory tests and diagnostic procedures* (3rd ed.). Norwalk, CT: Appleton & Lange.

11. Cushing, G. W. (1993). Subclinical hypothyroidism. *Postgraduate Medicine, 94*(1), 95–107.

12. Figg, W. D., et al. (1994). *Archives of Internal Medicine, 154,* 1023–1025.

13. Fitzpatrick, L., & Arnold, A. (1995). Hypoparathyroidism. In P. Felig, J. D. Baxter, & L. A. Frohman (Eds.), *Endocrinology and metabolism* (3rd ed., pp. 1123–1135). New York: McGraw-Hill.

14. Frohman, L. A. (1995). Diseases of the anterior pituitary. In P. Felig, J. D. Baxter, & L. A. Frohman (Eds.), *Endocrinology and metabolism* (3rd ed., pp. 289–369). New York: McGraw-Hill.

15. Gagel, R., et al. (1993). Medullary thyroid carcinoma: Recent progress. *Journal of Endocrinology and Metabolism, 76*(4), 809–814.

16. Gharib, H. (1992). A strategy for the solitary thyroid nodule. *Hospital Practice, 27*(9A), 53–58.

17. Guttler, R., & Singer, P. (1993). *Pneumocystis carinii* thyroiditis. *Annals of Internal Medicine, 153*(3), 393–396.

18. Heitman, B., & Irizarry, A. (1995). Hypothyroidism: Common complaints, perplexing diagnosis. *Nurse Practitioner: American Journal of Primary Health Care, 20*(3), 54–60.

19. Helfand, M., & Crapo, L. M. (1990). Screening for thyroid disease. *Annals of Internal Medicine, 112*(11), 840.

20. Hershman, J., Ladenson, P., & Paulshock, B. (1992). A savvy approach to thyroid testing. *Patient Care, 26*(3), 134–137.

21. Hubener, J., Arnold, A., & Potts, J. (1995). Hyperparathyroidism. In L. DeGroot (Ed.), *Endocrinology* (3rd ed., pp. 1044–1060). Philadelphia: W. B. Saunders.

22. Isley, W. L. (1993). Thyroid dysfunction in the severely ill and elderly. *Postgraduate Medicine, 94*(3), 111–128.

23. Jossart, G. H. (1994). Well-differentiated thyroid cancer. *Current Problems in Surgery, 31*(12), 933–1012.

24. Kahky, M., & Weber, R. (1993). Complications of surgery of the thyroid and parathyroid glands. *Surgical Clinics of North America, 73*(2), 307–321.

25. Kaye, T. B. (1994). Thyroid function tests. *Postgraduate Medicine, 94*(1), 81–90.

26. Khanderia, U., Jaffee, C., & Theisen, V. (1993). Amiodarone-induced thyroid dysfunction. *Clinical Pharmacy, 12*(10), 774–778.

27. Kim, T. A. (1994). Primary hyperparathyroidism. *Orthopaedic Nursing, 13*(3), 17–27.

28. Kjellman, M., Sardelin, K., & Farnebo, L. (1994). Primary hypoparathyroidism—low surgical morbidity supports liberal attitude to operation. *Archives of Surgery, 129*(3), 237–240.

29. Kleerekoper, M., & Bilezikian, J. (1994). In search of a disease: Parathyroidectomy for nontraditional features of primary hyperparathyroidism. *American Journal of Medicine, 96*(2), 99–100.

30. Klein, I., Becker, O., & Levey, G. (1994). Treatment of hyperthyroid disease. *Annals of Internal Medicine, 121*(4), 281–288.

31. Kung, A. W. C., & Cheng, A. (1994). The incidence of ophthalmopathy after radioiodine therapy for Graves' disease: Prognostic factors and the role of methimazole. *Journal of Endocrinology and Metabolism, 79*(2), 542–545.

32. Lehne, R. (1994). *Pharmacology for nursing care* (2nd ed.). Philadelphia: W. B. Saunders.

33. Liel, Y., Sperber, A. D., & Shany, S. (1994). Nonspecific intestinal absorption of levothyroxine by aluminum hydroxide. *American Journal of Medicine, 97*(4), 363–365.

34. Makshagundam, S, & Barzel, U. (1993). Thyroid disease in the elderly. *Journal of the American Geriatric Society, 41*(12), 1361–1369.

35. Martinez, M., Derksen, D., & Kapsner, P. (1993). Making sense of hypothyroidism. *Postgraduate Medicine, 93*(6), 135–145.

36. McKenzie, J. M., & Zakarija, M. (1995). Hyperthyroidism. In L. DeGroot (Ed.), *Endocrinology* (3rd ed., pp. 676–711). Philadelphia: W. B. Saunders.

37. Miller, D. (1993). Endocrine angiography and venous sampling. *Radiologic Clinics of North America, 31*(5), 1051–1066.

38. Miller, W. L., & Tyrrell, J. B. (1995). Adrenal cortex. In P. Felig, J. D. Baxter, & L. A. Frohman (Eds.), *Endocrinology and metabolism* (3rd ed., pp. 521–549). New York: McGraw-Hill.

39. Molitch, M. E. (1995). Neuroendocrinology. In P. Felig, J. D. Baxter, & L. A. Frohman (Eds.), *Endocrinology and metabolism* (3rd ed., pp. 221–275). New York: McGraw-Hill.

40. Mundy, G. (1994). Evaluation and treatment of hypercalcemia. *Hospital Practice, 29*(6), 79–84.

41. O'Brien, T., et al. (1993). Hyperlipidemia in patients with primary and secondary hypothyroidism. *Mayo Clinic Proceedings, 68*(9), 860–866.

42. Olin, B. R. (Ed.) (1994). *Drug facts and comparisons* (48th ed.). St. Louis: Facts & Comparisons.

43. Pagana, K., & Pagana, T. (1993). *Diagnostic testing and nursing implications* (4th ed.). St. Louis: Mosby–Year Book.

44. Robertson, G. (1995). Posterior pituitary. In P. Felig, J. D. Baxter, & L. A. Frohman (Eds.), *Endocrinology and metabolism,* (3rd ed., pp. 385–423). New York: McGraw-Hill.

45. Sakiyama, R. (1993). Thyroiditis: A clinical review. *American Family Physician, 48*(4), 615–621.

46. Santen, R. J. (1995). The testes. In P. Felig, J. D. Baxter, & L. A. Frohman (Eds.), *Endocrinology and metabolism* (3rd ed., pp. 885–955). New York: McGraw-Hill.

47. Sawin, C., et al. (1994). Low serum thyropin concentrations as a risk factor for atrial fibrillation in older persons. *New England Journal of Medicine, 331*(19), 1249–1252.

48. Sessions, R., & Davidson, B. (1993). Thyroid cancer. *Medical Clinics of North America, 77*(3), 517–536.

49. Strewler, G. J., & Rosenblatt, M. (1995). Mineral metabolism. In P. Felig, J. D. Baxter, & L. A. Frohman (Eds.), *Endocrinology and metabolism* (3rd ed., pp, 1407–1499). New York: McGraw-Hill.

50. Toft, A. (1994). Thyroxine therapy. *New England Journal of Medicine, 331*(3), 174–179.

51. Tunbridge, W. M. G., & Caldwell, G. (1991). The epidemiology of thyroid diseases. In L. E. Braverman & R. O. Utiger (Eds.), *The thyroid: A fundamental and clinical text* (6th ed., 578–587). Philadelphia: J. B. Lippincott.

52. Utiger, R. (1995). Hypothyroidism. In L. DeGroot (Ed.), *Endocrinology* (3rd ed., pp. 753–768). Philadelphia: W. B. Saunders.

53. Utiger, R. D. (1995). The thyroid: Physiology, thyrotoxicosis, hypothyroidism and the painful thyroid. In P. Felig, J. D. Baxter, & L. A. Frohman (Eds.), *Endocrinology and Metabolism* (3rd ed., pp. 435–509). New York: McGraw-Hill.

54. Wartofsky, L. (1990). The thyroid gland. In K. L. Becher, et al. (Eds.), *Principles and practice of endocrinology and metabolism* (pp. 264–397). Philadelphia: J. B. Lippincott.

55. Wiseman, S., et al. (1993). The magnitude of hypercholesterolemia of hypothyroidism is associated with variation in the low density lipoprotein receptor gene. *Journal of Endocrinology and Metabolism, 77*(1), 108–111.

Nursing Care of Clients with Adrenal, Pituitary, and Gonadal Disorders

Carol Birch

Adrenocortical Disorders

Glandular hypofunction and hyperfunction characterize the major disorders of the adrenal cortex. Underactivity of the adrenal cortex results in a deficiency of glucocorticoids, mineralocorticoids, and adrenal androgens. The person with adrenal hypofunction is a prime candidate for experiencing powerlessness, injury, and knowledge deficit. Overactivity of the adrenal cortex results in excessive production of glucocorticoids, mineralocorticoids, and androgens or estrogens. The person experiencing adrenal hyperfunction will need to focus on preventing injury, acquiring effective coping mechanisms, and learning about the disease process.

Adrenal Insufficiency

Hypofunction of the adrenal cortex can originate from a disorder within the adrenal gland itself (primary adrenal insufficiency), or it may be due to hypofunction of the pituitary-hypothalamic unit (secondary adrenal insufficiency). Adrenocortical insufficiency can be either chronic or acute.

Chronic Primary Adrenal Insufficiency

Chronic primary adrenal insufficiency, or Addison's disease, is the result of idiopathic atrophy or destruction of the adrenal glands by an autoimmune process or other disease. Thomas Addison first described this disorder in 1849.

Etiology and Risk Factors

Primary adrenal insufficiency is rare. The incidence and prevalence in the United States are not known. It affects

This chapter incorporates material written for the fourth edition by Teresa Choate Loriaux.

persons of all ages and occurs in both sexes equally. As shown in the Risk Factors and Levels of Prevention feature for primary adrenal insufficiency, risk factors play an important role in identifying persons with adrenal insufficiency.

Primary adrenal insufficiency is caused by hypofunction of the adrenal glands. An autoimmune process accounts for 75% of primary adrenal insufficiency. Adrenal insufficiency is commonly seen in persons with acquired immunodeficiency syndrome (AIDS). Tuberculosis is the cause of about 20% of Addison's disease. Adrenal metastasis from the lung, breast, gastrointestinal tract, melanoma, or lymphoma may also cause primary adrenal insufficiency.

Secondary adrenal insufficiency is hypofunction of the pituitary-hypothalamic unit. The most common cause is chronic treatment with glucocorticoids for nonendocrine uses. Other causes include bilateral adrenalectomy, hemorrhagic infarction and necrosis of the adrenal gland, hypopituitarism resulting in decreased adrenocorticotropic (ACTH) secretion by the pituitary gland, pituitary tumor or infarction, and radiation.

Pathophysiology

Autoimmune-induced adrenal insufficiency is the most common cause of the disease. Lymphocytic infiltration of the adrenal cortex is the characteristic feature. Addison's disease is frequently accompanied by other immune disorders. Gradual destruction leads to chronic adrenal insufficiency. Continued loss of cortical tissue accompanies a deficiency of mineralocorticoids as well as glucocorticoids. Adrenocortical hypofunction results in decreased levels of mineralocorticoids (aldosterone), glucocorticoids (cortisol), and androgens (Fig. 71–1).

Clinical Manifestations and Diagnostic Findings

The onset of Addison's disease is usually insidious. The client experiences mild fatigue, languor, irritability, weight loss, nausea, vomiting, and postural hypotension

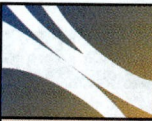

RISK FACTORS AND LEVELS OF PREVENTION

Primary Adrenal Insufficiency

Risk Factors

History of other endocrine disorders; taking glucocorticoids for longer than 3 weeks with sudden cessation; taking glucocorticoids more often than once every other day; adrenalectomy; tuberculosis

Levels of Prevention

Primary Prevention

- There is no primary prevention.

Secondary Prevention

- Assess and educate clients who are at risk for manifestations of adrenal insufficiency.
- Educate clients about supplemental steroids to prevent acute adrenal insufficiency.
- Teach clients about steroid use and dosages.
- Educate clients about the need for "sick days."

Tertiary Prevention

- Educate clients about physician follow-up for steroid levels.
- Educate clients about "sick day" care.

weeks or months before diagnosis of the disease. As the disorder progresses, manifestations intensify.

The development of clinical manifestations of adrenocortical insufficiency require the loss of over 90% of both adrenal cortices. Table 71–1 lists the clinical manifestations of adrenal insufficiency.

Diagnosis of Addison's disease depends primarily on blood and urine hormonal assays. Diagnostic tests of adrenalcortical function are presented in Table 71–2.

Primary adrenal insufficiency is characterized by a low cortisol production rate and a high plasma ACTH concentration. Secondary adrenal insufficiency is characterized by a low cortisol production rate and a low plasma ACTH concentration.

Other diagnostic tests may be ordered to evaluate the effects of hypofunction of the adrenals on the body: serum electrolytes (especially hyponatremia and hyperkalemia in primary adrenal insufficiency; hyponatremia alone in secondary disease); blood glucose; complete blood count (to assess for anemia); x-rays or computed tomography (CT) or magnetic resonance imaging (MRI) of the adrenals and pituitary.

Acute and Subacute Care

■ Medical Management

Addisonian crisis, or *acute adrenal insufficiency,* may occur when the client has been under stress without appro-

priate hormone replacement. Stressors include pregnancy, surgery, infection, states of dehydration or anorexia, fever, and emotional upheaval.

Manifestations are related to the degree of hormone deficiency and electrolyte imbalance. Manifestations may include sudden penetrating pain in the back, abdomen, or legs; depressed or changed mentation; volume depletion; hypotension; loss of consciousness; or shock.

The overall goal in treatment is to prevent the morbidity and mortality associated with the addisonian crisis. Untreated, addisonian crisis is fatal. The cause of the crisis must be determined and treated immediately. Hypotension and electrolyte imbalance need to be corrected quickly. Rapid rehydration is essential. An isotonic solution will usually correct the volume depletion, salt depletion, and hypotension. Hypoglycemia must be evaluated and corrected with intravenous (IV) glucose (D_5 solution IV or IV glucose push bolus). The client may also need oxygen, vasopressors, or volume expanders.

Hydrocortisone 100 mg is administered as an IV bolus, then 100 mg IV every 8 hours for 24 hours. The IV hydrocortisone is tapered as the client's status dictates. Oral hydrocortisone is initiated.

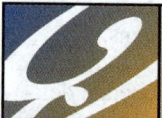

NURSING RESEARCH

Adrenal Insufficiency and AIDS

Freda, P., et al. (1994). Primary adrenal insufficiency in patients with the acquired immunodeficiency syndrome: A report of five cases. *Journal of Clinical Endocrinology and Metabolism, 79*(6), 1540–1545.

The most common cause of adrenal insufficiency is autoimmune disease. Pathologic abnormalities have been demonstrated in the adrenal glands of 50% to 78% of clients who are living with acquired immunodeficiency syndrome (AIDS). The human immunodeficiency virus (HIV) can directly infect the adrenocortical cells, but it is not known if HIV causes adrenal dysfunction in AIDS. Despite the high level of involvement of the adrenal glands by HIV, clinically significant adrenal insufficiency occurs in few clients.

AIDS is becoming a more common cause of adrenal insufficiency than autoimmune processes and tuberculosis.

Clients with AIDS are at risk of adrenal insufficiency because of peripheral resistance to glucocorticoids; tendency for the hypothalamic-pituitary-adrenal axis to be affected by infectious agents such as tuberculosis or toxoplasmosis; from drugs used to treat AIDS; and possible adrenal infiltration from opportunistic infections and viruses.

Implications for Practice

As the number of AIDS-infected people increases, we may see more adrenal insufficiency.

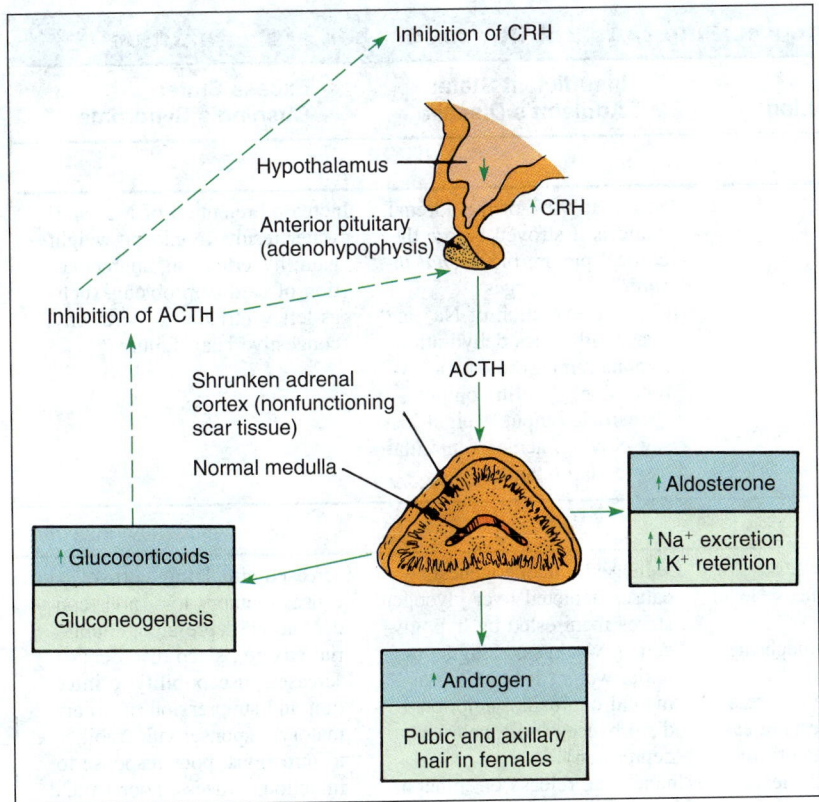

Figure 71–1. Effects of Addison's disease. *Dashed arrows* show feedback mechanisms.

Nursing Management of the Medical Client

Assessment

Monitor the client's vital signs closely while the disease is being diagnosed. Check the pulse carefully, at least every 4 hours. Take orthostatic blood pressure readings and pulses. Report drops in blood pressure or orthostatic changes.

As rehydration occurs and electrolyte imbalances are corrected, assess for manifestations of increased physical vitality and emotional well-being. Assess bony prominences for pressure sores in immobilized clients. With therapy, listlessness and exhaustion should gradually lessen and disappear.

Monitor for exposure to cold and infections. Immediately inform the physician if manifestations of infection develop, such as a sore throat or burning on urination. Remember, the client with Addison's disease cannot tolerate stress. Infection imposes additional stress on the body, and cortisol levels need to be higher during infectious illnesses.

Carefully assess for manifestations of sodium and potassium imbalance (see Chapter 15). Daily weights are indicated for objective measurement of fluid gain or loss. If steroid replacement therapy is inadequate, sodium loss and potassium retention continue uncorrected. If steroid dosage is too high, excessive amounts of sodium and water are retained and potassium excretion is high.

Diagnosis, Planning, Implementation

Addisonian Crisis. The client must engage in careful self-care or there will be an increased risk of the collaborative problem of *Addisonian Crisis related to adrenal insufficiency.*

Planning: Expected Outcomes. The client will not exhibit injury, as evidenced by the absence of hypotension, shock, or other manifestations of acute adrenal insufficiency.

Implementation. Closely monitor for manifestations of addisonian crisis, including:

1. Sudden profound weakness
2. Severe abdominal, back, and leg pain
3. Hyperpyrexia (although this may be suppressed by steroids) followed by hypothermia
4. Hypotension in association with high cardiac output, normal wedge pressure, and low systemic resistance
5. Coma
6. Renal shutdown and death

Addisonian crisis usually develops over a 24- to 48-hour period.

The development of an adrenal crisis constitutes a medical emergency that must be treated rapidly and vigorously. The three major goals of intervention are the following:

1. Reversal of shock
2. Restoration of blood circulation (the client usually suf-

Table 71–1. Adrenal Hormones: Function and Consequences of Dysfunction

Hormone	Usual Function	Insufficient State: Addison's Disease	Excess State: Cushing's Syndrome
Mineralocorticoids			
Aldosterone Stimulated by ACTH production Major control is renin-angiotensin system	Promotes retention of Na⁺ (and water) in kidney	More than 90% of the adrenal gland is destroyed before the clinical picture of *adrenal insufficiency* emerges. Increased excretion of Na⁺ and water influences dehydration, hyponatremia, orthostatic hypotension, ↓ urine output, ↓ cardiac output, weight loss, salt craving, acidosis, circulatory collapse, shock	Increased retention of Na⁺ and water results in edema, weight gain, hypertension, augmentation of cardiac problems such as left ventricular hypertrophy, congestive heart failure
Glucocorticoids			
Cortisol Regulated by ACTH release from anterior pituitary	Promotes gluconeogenesis Maintains plasma glucose level Promotes appetite Causes release of epinephrine from adrenal medulla Assists in adaptation to stress by ↑ gluconeogenesis releasing an anti-inflammatory response; augmenting release of catacholamines (epinephrine, norepinephrine) to increase blood pressure	Decreased gluconeogenesis causes depleted liver glycogen stores manifested by hypoglycemia, weakness, fatigue, anorexia, weight loss, vomiting, mental confusion, emotional disturbances (mild neurosis to depression) Inadequate release of epinephrine produces hypoglycemia, hypotension Lowers resistance to stress and produces a "hyperresponse" to stressors: hypoglycemia, hypotension, hyperthermia	Increased circulating cortisol causes memory loss, poor concentration, depression, euphoria, anxiety, sleep disorders Increased susceptibility to infection and suppression of inflammatory response: vulnerability to infections, poor response to infectious process, poor wound healing
ACTH release controls cortisol secretion	ACTH regulates melanocyte-stimulating hormone (MSH)	Stimulates an increase in MSH: increases skin and mucous membrane pigmentation, especially in fingers, toes, and sun-exposed body parts (skin appears bronzed)	No effect
Androgens			
Regulated by ACTH release from anterior pituitary		Females: Oligomenorrhea or amenorrhea, decrease in body hair Males: no manifestations in males because testes produce adequate quantities of sex hormone	Females: acne, thinning of scalp hair, excessive growth of body and facial hair in male pattern (hirsutism), menstrual irregularities, infertility common Males: decreased libido, impotence

fers from a deficit of at least 20% of extracellular fluid [ECF] volume)

3. Replenishment with essential steroids

Immediately on admission, a rapid infusion of 1000 ml of normal saline is administered with water-soluble glucocorticoid (hydrocortisone phosphate or hydrocortisone sodium succinate) added. The dosage of the prescribed glucocorticoid is gradually reduced. It is administered intramuscularly (IM) or IV every 8 hours on days 1 and 2 of the crisis and gradually reduced thereafter. Hypoglycemia is controlled by a glucose infusion, either an IV bolus or IV drip as part of rehydration. The precipitating event must be corrected.

Plasma, oxygen, and vasopressor medications may be indicated. Throughout the emergency period, do the following:

- Monitor blood pressure,
- Administer IV infusion and medications.
- Monitor hourly urine output and report oliguria (a manifestation of shock).
- Minimize exposure to emotional and physical stress.
- Observe for manifestations of glucocorticoid overdose and overhydration, such as generalized edema due to

Table 71–2. Diagnostic Tests of Adrenocortical Function

Test	Purpose	Nursing Notes	Interpretation
Cortisol level with dexamethasone suppression test	Evaluates function of adrenal cortex	Give dexamethasone before phlebotomy to suppress diurnal formation of ACTH Give 1 mg dexamethasone at 11 PM to suppress ACTH formation in time for 8 AM phlebotomy and later at 8 PM; estrogen therapy can falsely increase results	↑ Pituitary tumor, Cushing's syndrome or disease, hyperplasia of adrenal cortex (benign or malignant) ↓ Addison's disease
Cortisol plasma levels	Evaluates function of adrenal cortex	Plasma cortisol levels have diurnal effect: levels higher in AM than PM Fasting prephlebotomy 2 hours of supine activity are necessary before test because activity increases cortisol level Estrogens will increase level Aldactone (spironolactone) can cause false-positives	↑ Pregnancy, recent physical activity, obesity, Cushing's disease or syndrome ↓ Addison's disease
17-Hydroxysteroids (Porter-Silber reaction)	Measures metabolites of glucocorticoids and aldosterone	24-hour urine collection to be kept on ice Many drugs can invalidate results	↑ Cushing's disease or syndrome; ACTH administration; nonadrenal ACTH-producing tumor ↓ Addison's disease or exogenous steroid suppression
Cosyntropin test	Diagnoses adrenal insufficiency with ACTH stimulation	Give ACTH IV; 45 min later, obtain serum cortisol level	↑ Normal ↓ Dysfunction of hypothalamic-pituitary axis Secondary adrenal insufficiency
CT or MRI of adrenals	Identifies and locates adrenal glands	No preparation except client education	Small, atrophied glands = autoimmune adrenal insufficiency Bilateral enlarged glands = hemorrhage (with areas of high density), neoplasm
Rapid ACTH stimulation		Give cosyntropin IV; obtain plasma cortisol and aldosterone level at baseline + 30 minutes	↓ Cortisol and aldosterone = primary adrenal insufficiency
17-Ketosteroids	Measures steroid metabolites from adrenal cortex and testes (does not include testosterone)	24-hour urine test; keep collection cold; may need preservative Many drugs make test invalid	↑ Tumors of adrenal cortex or testes, Cushing's syndrome ↓ Hypofunction of adrenal, or in clients with removal of testes or ovaries
Aldosterone	Measures mineralocorticoid production	Client to be supine 2 hr before phlebotomy ↑ Aldosterone can cause ↑ extracellular fluid Oral contraceptive, sodium restriction, and potassium may ↑ level	↑ Primary or secondary hyperaldosteronism, severe liver dysfunction ↓ Addison's disease (may be undetectable or ↓ in Addison's)
Urinary cortisol level	Measures cortisol, not metabolites		↑ Adrenal hyperfunction, Cushing's syndrome ↓ Not necessarily adrenal hypofunction

Table continued on following page

Table 71–2. Diagnostic Tests of Adrenocortical Function (*Continued*)

Test	Purpose	Nursing Notes	Interpretation
Renin level	Measures renin, an enzyme produced by juxtaglomerular apparatus in response to decreased blood flow to kidneys	Client in supine position Results high in AM Note sodium content in diet on laboratory slip The following medications interfere with results: diuretics, estrogens, oral contraceptives, antihypertensives	↑ Hypertension, upright position with phlebotomy ↓ High sodium diet
Plasma ACTH or serum corticotropin	Tests anterior pituitary function as it may cause Cushing's syndrome, Addison's disease	Fasting sample Stress may artificially increase results	↑ Cushing's syndrome caused by bilateral adrenal hyperplasia or ectopic ACTH-producing tumors; Addison's disease (primary adrenal insufficiency) caused by adrenal gland failure, surgical removal of adrenals, adrenal suppression with long-term exogenous steroid supply ↓ Secondary adrenal insufficiency caused by hypopituitarism; cushingoid client may have adrenal adenoma as cause of hyperfunction
Captopril test	Rules out renal artery stenosis	Nuclear medicine captopril renal scan done first to evaluate resting glomerular filtration rule (GFR); captopril administered PO; GFR reevaluated after captopril	↓ GFR renal artery stenosis same ↑ GFR after captopril: negative for renal artery stenosis
Corticotropin-releasing hormone (CRH) stimulation	Measures CRH from hypothalamus to pituitary necessary to stimulate ACTH and cortisol release	Give CRH IV; measure plasma ACTH and cortisol at baseline and after 15, 30, and 60 min	↑ ACTH and cortisol indicate primary adrenal insufficiency ↓ ACTH and cortisol indicate pituitary or hypothalamic dysfunction, secondary adrenal insufficiency

fluid retention, hypertension, flaccid paralysis resulting from hypokalemia, psychosis, and loss of consciousness.

● Evaluate electrolytes for hyperkalemia, hyponatremia, and hypoglycemia and correlate these findings with client manifestations.

With rapid, efficient intervention, Addisonian crisis usually resolves within 12 hours. The client's condition stabilizes, and the convalescent period begins. When the client is able to tolerate food and fluids by mouth, steroid replacement can be administered orally.

After the immediate crisis is past, help the client prevent further development of adrenal insufficiency. Identification bracelets and emergency kits should be obtained for all clients with Addison's disease prior to their discharge from the hospital. Instruct clients to carry these items at all times. The client's name and diagnosis should appear on the identification bracelet, and a wallet card should state that the client receives daily hydrocortisone, and that the medication must be administered by injection in an emergency.

Dexamethasone can be kept in a prepared syringe in an emergency kit with sterile alcohol wipes for cleaning the injection site. The kit also should contain written information on the client's diagnosis, medication prescription, dosage schedules, and emergency phone numbers, including the physician's name and phone number.

Adrenal insufficiency is a potentially life-threatening condition, but when properly recognized and treated, it has little or no effect on life span. There are no dietary or activity restrictions.

Evaluation

Successful outcome of treatment is easily evaluated, usually within 12 hours of treatment. By this time the client should no longer exhibit any manifestations of addisonian crisis or would have died.

Community and Self-Care

■ Medical Management

Addison's disease was once fatal within months. Today, with the manufacture of synthetic corticosteroids (Table 71–3), clients with Addison's disease can live normal, active lives provided they receive adequate glucocorticoid replacement. Use corticosteroids with caution. Table 71–4 shows the adverse consequences of administering corticosteroids in selected disorders. Carefully assess clients for manifestations of hypercortisolism, which can result from excessive long-term cortisol therapy. Most clients receive glucocorticoid and minerocorticoid replacement.

Osteoporosis is a complication that may develop with excessive use of glucocorticosteroids. Closely observe clients with other medical problems that may be worsened with steroid usage (see Table 71–4).

■ Nursing Management of the Medical Client

Assessment

Carefully assess the client's ability to understand and perform self-care. The client will need extensive instruction in self-care activities to achieve independence.

Diagnosis, Planning, Implementation

Risk for Ineffective Management of Therapeutic Regimen (Individuals). The client with adrenal insufficiency must learn a complex self-care regimen. A common nursing diagnosis would therefore be *Risk for Ineffective Management of Therapeutic Regimen, related to insufficient knowledge of the disease, manifestations of complications, risks of crisis, overexertion, dietary management, identification, emergency kit, and pharmacologic management.*

   Planning: Expected Outcomes. The client will understand how to take steroids correctly, as evidenced by the client's statements and ability to comply with the therapeutic regimen.

   Implementation. Provide the client and significant others with written instructions for self-administration of steroids. (The client and significant others will have demonstrated their ability to prepare and administer injections.)

● Actions of prescribed hormones (hydrocortisone, fludrocortisone).
● Importance of taking medications daily, without fail, exactly as prescribed.
● Principles of self-administration of oral medications (e.g., check the label on the bottle before taking the medication; document when medications are taken and their side effects).
● Manifestations of over- and underdosage.
● Importance of hydrocortisone self-injection when unable to tolerate oral medication (because of nausea and vomiting) and during times of acute stress (motor vehicle accident, trauma) because the body is unable to compensate for its need for additional glucocorticoid coverage.
● Need for an IM self-injection kit to be available at all times.
● Need for a medical alert bracelet that carries the diagnosis and the need for cortisol replacement.
● Need for the client to contact a healthcare provider if questions arise after discharge from the medical center. Emphasize to clients who take glucocorticoids that they must call the physician to get a dosage increase when experiencing stressful situations (e.g., emotional upheavals, dental extractions, minor surgery, upper respiratory infections). The general rule is to double the glucocorticoid dosage for up to 1 week, depending on manifestations, then resume normal dosage. In addition, temporary mineralocorticoid dosage is reduced by 50% to avoid excessive salt retention and hypertension. Encourage clients to consult their physician for dose adjustment. The medication will need to be administered IM when nausea and vomiting prevent oral administration.

Finally, remind clients to adhere to semiannual appointments with their physician, even when they are in good health and the process of self-medication is proceeding smoothly. As in diabetes mellitus, the control of Addison's disease is a lifelong responsibility.

Evaluation

Appropriate outcomes for the client with Addison's disease would be that the client's weight remains stable, the vital signs remain within normal limits, cortisol levels remain within normal limits, and the client states that fatigue has decreased.

■ Modifications for Elderly Clients

Adrenal diseases are uncommon in older people. The effects of normal aging on the adrenals are unclear. It does appear, however, that ACTH and cortisol production remain constant throughout life. The elderly may be more sensitive to the side effects of steroid therapy because these problems (osteoporosis, hypertension, diabetes, etc.) may already exist in the client.

Secondary Adrenal Insufficiency

Secondary adrenal insufficiency is the result of a dysfunction in the hypothalamic-pituitary-adrenal (HPA) axis. Causes of secondary adrenocortical insufficiency include the following:

● Bilateral adrenalectomy.
● Hemorrhagic infarction and necrosis of the adrenal glands. Adrenal apoplexy can develop as a complica-

Table 71–3. Corticosteroids

Medication	Duration of Action	Indication	Mineralocorticoid/Glucocorticoid Activity	Side Effects (Relative to Dose and Duration)
Glucocorticoids				
Betamethasone (Celestone)	Long-acting	Chronic adrenocortical insufficiency, anti-inflammatory	Minor mineralocorticoid activity	*Fluid and electrolytes:* hypokalemia, hypocalcemia, congestive heart failure, hypertension
Cortisone (Cortone)	Short-acting	Inflammatory disorders, allergic disorders, Cushing's syndrome (suppression test), adrenocortical insufficiency	Minimal mineralocorticoid activity	*Musculoskeletal:* weakness, steroid psychosis, myopathy; aseptic necrosis of femoral and humeral heads; spontaneous fractures; osteoporosis
Dexamethasone (Decadron)	Long-acting	Adrenal hyperplasia, adrenal insufficiency with mineralocorticoid therapy; allergic states; addisonian crisis	Minimal mineralocorticoid activity	*Cardiovascular:* thromboembolism, arrhythmias related to hypokalemia; hypertension; myocardial rupture following recent infarction
Hydrocortisone (Hydrocortone, Synacort)	Short-acting	Chronic adrenal insufficiency, inflammatory disorders, allergic reactions, collagen disorders, nonsuppurative thyroiditis	Moderate mineralocorticoid activity	*Gastrointestinal:* pancreatitis, peptic ulcer, inflammatory bowel disease, ulcerative esophagitis
Methylprednisolone (Medrol)	Intermediate-acting	Immunosuppressant for transplant clients, adrenogenital syndrome, acute and chronic inflammatory diseases, allergic processes	Minimal mineralocorticoid activity	*Integument:* impaired wound healing, thin skin, petechiae, suppression of skin test reactions
Prednisolone (Delta-Cortef)	Intermediate-acting	Anti-inflammatory, immunosuppression	Minimal mineralocorticoid activity	*Neurologic:* convulsions, steroid psychosis
Prednisone (Deltasone, Orasone)	Intermediate-acting	Inflammatory conditions; immunosuppression	Minimal mineralocorticoid activity	*Endocrine:* amenorrhea, postmenopausal bleeding, development of cushingoid state, growth suppression in children, secondary development of insulin-resistant diabetes mellitus
Mineralocorticoids				
Desoxycorticosterone acetate (Doca acetate, Percorten acetate)		Addison's disease, salt-losing adrenogenital syndrome	No glucocorticoid activity	*Cardiovascular:* hypertension, fluid retention, weight gain, cardiomegaly *Endocrine:* drug-induced adrenal insufficiency
Fludrocortisone (Florinef)	Long-acting	Chronic adrenocortical insufficiency; salt-losing adrenogenital syndrome	Moderate glucocorticoid activity	*Integument:* bruising, diaphoresis *Other:* hypokalemia, allergic reaction

Table 71–4. Consequences of Corticosteroid Use in Selected Disorders*

Disorder	Consequence
Diabetes mellitus	Augments hyperglycemia
Inflammatory bowel disorders	Fluid retention may exacerbate peristalsis
Hypertension	Contributes to fluid retention
Congestive heart failure	Contributes to fluid retention
Renal insufficiency	Worsens fluid retention

* Corticosteroids are contraindicated in clients with viral, fungal, or tubercular infections.

tion of meningococcal septicemia or anticoagulant therapy.

● Hypopituitarism resulting in decreased secretion of ACTH by the pituitary gland, causing decreased secretion of cortisol and androgens by the adrenal gland (secondary adrenal insufficiency). Figure 71–2 illustrates the HPA axis.

● Suppression of hypothalamic-pituitary secretion of ACTH due to hypercortisolism caused by either (1) exogenous administration of corticosteroids, or (2) oversecretion of corticosteroids by an adrenal tumor. In both cases, the adrenal glands atrophy and become filled with lipids. Because the circulating levels of corticosteroids remain high, these clients do not develop manifestations of adrenocortical insufficiency unless steroid therapy is discontinued suddenly or the tumor is resected. Fortunately, if corticosteroid drug therapy is terminated by gradually reducing the dosage each day, adrenal gland function usually returns to normal.

Assessment reveals that clients with secondary adrenal insufficiency experience cortisol deficiency. Aldosterone continues to be secreted in sufficient amounts.

Treatment involves administering glucocorticoids, as in Addison's disease. Mineralocorticoid replacement is

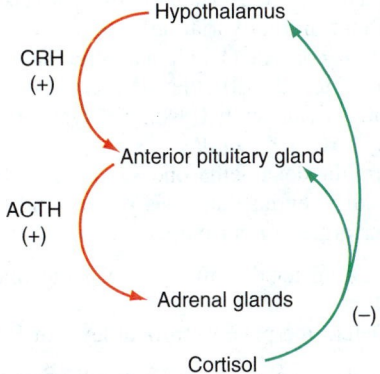

Figure 71–2. The hypothalamic-pituitary-adrenal (HPA) axis, demonstrating stimulation and feedback between the hypothalamus, anterior pituitary, and adrenal glands.

unnecessary. Instruct the client to wear an emergency identification bracelet and carry an emergency kit for hydrocortisone injection in case an adrenal crisis occurs.

Adrenocortical Hyperfunction

Hyperfunction of the adrenal cortex can result in excessive production of glucocorticoids, mineralocorticoids, and androgens. Major conditions of adrenocortical hyperfunction are:

● Hypercortisolism (glucocorticoid excess)
● Primary aldosteronism (aldosterone excess)

Hypercortisolism

Hypercortisolism, or Cushing's syndrome, was first described by Harvey Cushing in 1932. It results from overactivity of the adrenal gland, with consequent hypersecretion of glucocorticoids. Cushing's syndrome is relatively rare. The incidence is unknown. It occurs mainly in women, and the average age of onset is 20 to 40 years of age. It can, however, be seen up to age 60 years.

Etiology and Risk Factors

Iatrogenic hypercortisolism accounts for most hypercortisolism because of the frequent therapeutic use of high-dose glucocorticoids. Hypersecretion of cortisol can be caused by the following factors:

● A cortisol-secreting adrenal tumor. Adrenal tumors are responsible for approximately 30% of cases of Cushing's syndrome. Most (85%) are benign, but 15% are malignant.
● Adrenal hyperplasia is caused by overproduction of ACTH. The two sources of excessive ACTH secretion are:

> Pituitary hypersecretion and pituitary tumors cause approximately 70% of cases of Cushing's syndrome. These usually benign tumors are either small basophil adenomas or large chromophobe adenomas. Pituitary hypersecretion of ACTH resulting in glucocorticoid excess is called *Cushing's disease.*

> Ectopic secretion of ACTH (ectopic ACTH syndrome). ACTH-secreting tumors located outside the pituitary gland constitute a rare cause of Cushing's syndrome. Oat cell carcinoma of the lung, pancreatic islet cell carcinoma, and carcinoid tumors of the lung, gut, thymus, and ovary are the tumors that most frequently cause the ectopic ACTH syndrome (also known as *ACTH-dependent*).

Additionally, iatrogenic Cushing's syndrome, another form of the disorder, results from exogenous administration of synthetic glucocorticoids in supraphysiologic amounts. See the Risk Factors and Levels of Prevention feature for Cushing's syndrome.

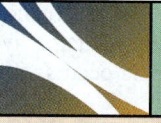

Pathophysiology

When Cushing's syndrome develops, the normal function of the glucocorticoids (see Chapter 67) becomes exaggerated and the classic picture of the syndrome emerges (Fig. 71–3). This exaggerated physiologic action of glucocorticoids appears as follows:

● Persistent hyperglycemia ("steroid diabetes").
● Protein tissue wasting, which results in:
    Weakness caused by muscle wasting
    Capillary fragility, resulting in ecchymosis.
    Osteoporosis caused by bone matrix wasting. Osteoporosis can become so severe that even mild trauma can cause fractures. Compression fractures can develop in the osteoporotic spine, leading to kyphosis and loss of height.
● Potassium depletion, leading to hypokalemia, arrhythmias, muscle weakness, and renal disorders.
● Sodium and water retention, which cause edema and hypertension.
● Hypertension, which eventually predisposes the client to left ventricular hypertrophy, congestive heart failure, and cerebrovascular accidents.
● Abnormal fat distribution (in conjunction with edema), results in a moon-shaped face, a dorsocervical fat pad on the neck (buffalo type), and truncal obesity with slender limbs. Also, pink and purple striae appear on the breasts, axillary areas, abdomen, and legs because

of thinning of the skin. Striking changes occur in appearance following both the development and cure of Cushing's syndrome. Old photographs can be useful in recognizing changes over time.

● Increased susceptibility to infection and lowered resistance to stress increase vulnerability to microorganisms of all types. Because of suppression of the inflammatory response, persons with Cushing's syndrome show few manifestations of infection. The client also demonstrates poor wound healing.
● Possible increased production of androgens can cause virilism in women. Manifestations of virilism include acne, thinning of scalp hair, and hirsutism (excessive bodily and facial hair in a male pattern).
● Mental changes include memory loss, poor concentration and cognition, euphoria, and depression. Some clients develop "steroid psychosis." Depression can predispose the client to suicidal thoughts.

Approximately 80% of the clients meet the criteria for a major affective disorder: 50% with unipolar depression, 30% with bipolar illness.

Clinical Manifestations and Diagnostic Findings

Figure 71–3 demonstrates the clinical picture of a client with Cushing's syndrome. The pathophysiology of the disease also provides a clear picture. Although clients have a classic "cushingoid" appearance, it is important to perform diagnostic studies (see Table 71–2).

Laboratory tests for Cushing's syndrome reflect hyperglycemia, fluid and electrolyte disturbances, and immunosuppressive responses that characterize excessive glucocorticoid secretion. Thus, in Cushing's syndrome, glucose tolerance decreases and glucosuria appears. The white blood cell count often rises above 10,000/mm³, but the total eosinophil count can drop below 50/mm³. Also, lymphocytes can fall below 20%. Both urinary 17-hydroxysteroids (17-HS) and blood cortisol are elevated.

Normally, plasma cortisol follows a diurnal pattern, rising in the early morning (10–25 μg/dl), gradually falling to less than 10 μg/dl in the evening, and approaching undetectable levels near midnight. Clients with Cushing's syndrome have elevated plasma cortisol levels throughout the day without diurnal variation.

Urinary free cortisol (UFC) measurement is used as a screening test to identify elevated urinary excretion of free cortisol. Clients with Cushing's syndrome will have UFC levels above 100 μg/day.

The overnight dexamethasone suppression test is often used in the differential diagnosis of Cushing's syndrome. It can be performed on an outpatient basis.

Day 1: Administer dexamethasone, 1 mg orally (PO) at 11 PM
Day 2: Determine plasma cortisol level at 8 AM

The normal range is below 5 μg/dl. Severe stress or depression can cause false-positive results (i.e., plasma cortisol greater than 5 μg/dl despite otherwise normal endocrine function). If dexamethasone fails to suppress the (HPA axis) (see Fig. 71–2) and the morning cortisol

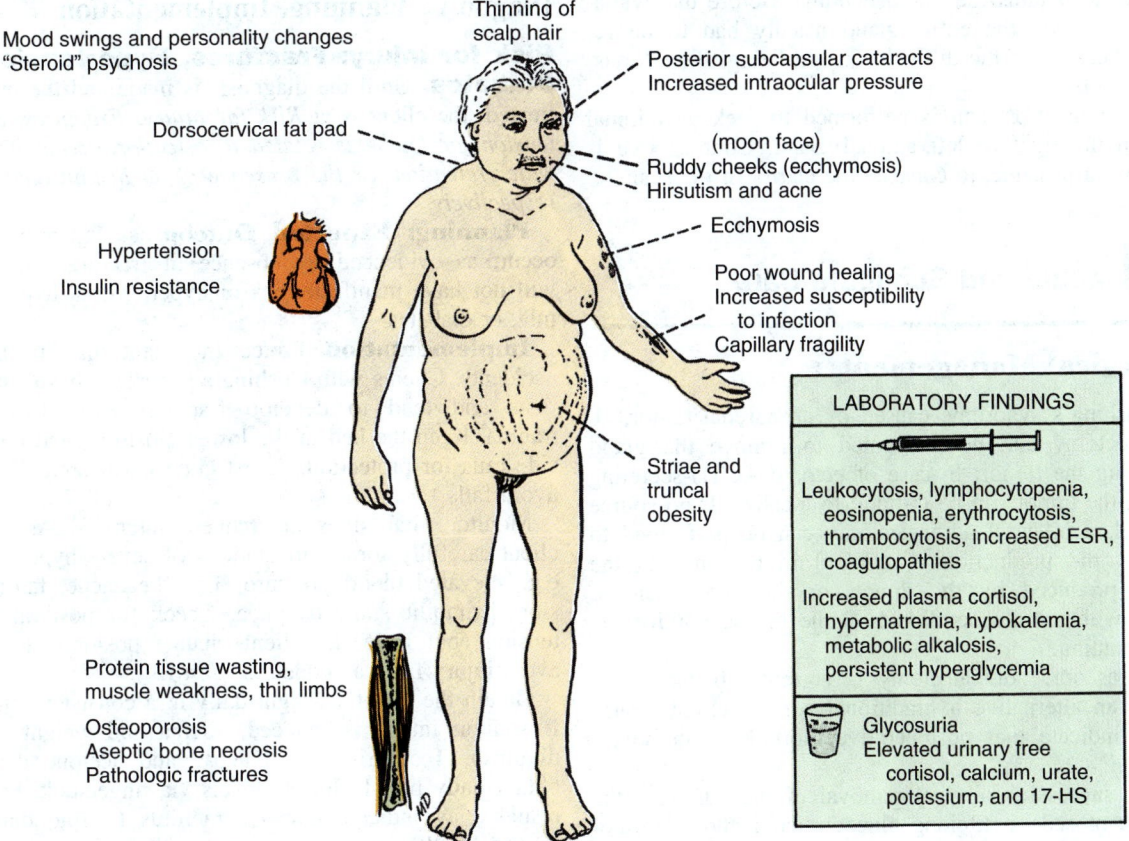

Mood swings and personality changes
"Steroid" psychosis

Thinning of
scalp hair

Posterior subcapsular cataracts
Increased intraocular pressure

Dorsocervical fat pad

(moon face)
Ruddy cheeks (ecchymosis)
Hirsutism and acne

Ecchymosis

Hypertension
Insulin resistance

Poor wound healing
Increased susceptibility
to infection
Capillary fragility

Striae and
truncal
obesity

Protein tissue wasting,
muscle weakness, thin limbs

Osteoporosis
Aseptic bone necrosis
Pathologic fractures

LABORATORY FINDINGS

Leukocytosis, lymphocytopenia,
eosinopenia, erythrocytosis,
thrombocytosis, increased ESR,
coagulopathies

Increased plasma cortisol,
hypernatremia, hypokalemia,
metabolic alkalosis,
persistent hyperglycemia

Glycosuria
Elevated urinary free
cortisol, calcium, urate,
potassium, and 17-HS

Figure 71–3. Assessment data for Cushing's syndrome. *Inset* refers to laboratory findings.

level is greater than 5 μg/dl, an abnormality of feedback is suggested that is compatible with Cushing's syndrome.

The standard dexamethasone suppression test (performed over 6 consecutive days) differentiates Cushing's disease (caused by pituitary oversecretion of ACTH) from other causes of Cushing's syndrome.

Days 1 to 6: Collect 24-hour urine for UFC.
Days 1 to 2: Obtain baseline value.
Days 3 to 4: Low-dose dexamethasone test: 0.5 mg PO q 6 h.
Days 5 to 6: High-dose dexamethasone test: 2 mg PO q 6 h.

The results show that suppression is interpreted as a fall in basal 17-HS of more than 50%. This is compatible with Cushing's disease and ectopic ACTH secretion.

Dexamethasone suppresses pituitary secretion of ACTH. Thus, by the second day of dexamethasone administration, levels of urinary 17-HS should be less than 2 mg in normal subjects. In the client with Cushing's disease (a pituitary disorder), levels of 17-HS drop due to a pathologic disruption in the HPA axis. ACTH-secreting pituitary adenomas are relatively resistant to dexamethasone. Cushing's syndrome and an ectopic ACTH-secreting tumor, on the other hand, usually do not respond to dexamethasone (i.e., levels of 17-HS do not decrease).

The plasma ACTH test demonstrates that low ACTH levels point toward an adrenal tumor as the cause of hypercortisolism. Overproduction of cortisol from the adrenal tumor provides negative feedback to the pituitary gland, which responds by reducing ACTH release. The high cortisol level also provides feedback to the hypothalamus, which reduces release of cortisol-releasing hormone (CRH).

The presence of an ectopic ACTH-producing tumor usually yields a normal or elevated ACTH level. ACTH production from the tumor is independent of pituitary production of ACTH. Thus, despite negative feedback to the hypothalamic-pituitary unit, ACTH levels remain high.

The inferior petrosal sinus sampling test (IPSS) is a radiologic test used to isolate the source of ACTH secretion (whether it is within the pituitary gland, and if so, where). The left and right petrosal sinuses carry blood from the pituitary gland to the jugular veins. Catheters are threaded into the inferior petrosal sinus via the femoral veins. By sampling ACTH levels drawn from the right and left petrosal sinuses, the side of the pituitary gland producing ACTH can be identified. If ACTH levels from the petrosal sinuses are greater than those from a peripheral site (the arm), a pituitary tumor is identified as the source of hypercortisolism. If central ACTH levels (petrosal) and peripheral ACTH levels (arm) are equivalent, an ectopic ACTH-secreting tumor is likely. The development of this test has allowed neurosurgeons to perform a hemi-hypophysectomy and remove only the half of the pituitary gland that contains the microadenoma. Before the availability of EPSS, the entire gland usually had to be removed because of the difficulty in localizing these "invisible" tumors.

An adrenal CT scan is performed to seek an adrenal mass in the right or left adrenal gland. Contrast dye is used, when possible, to enhance the clarity of the scan.

Acute and Subacute Care

■ Surgical Management

For Cushing's syndrome caused by an adrenal tumor, an adrenalectomy can be performed to remove the gland containing the tumor. In case of ectopic ACTH-secreting tumors, the tumor can be difficult to localize. If no source is found, a bilateral adrenalectomy can be performed to interrupt the production of cortisol in response to the ACTH produced by the tumor, or the client can be treated with antiglucocorticoids while the search for the tumor continues.

Laparoscopic adrenalectomy is currently being evaluated as an alternative to traditional adrenalectomy. Early studies indicate that postoperative morbidity can be reduced.[19,22]

After successful surgical removal of the adrenals, the client is placed on lifelong glucocorticoid and mineralocorticoid replacement. Most physical manifestations of Cushing's syndrome resolve after bilateral adrenalectomy.

The resection of most pituitary tumors causing Cushing's disease is performed via transsphenoidal hypophysectomy. Occasionally, large or anatomically complex tumors are excised via a transfrontal approach (see the discussion of hypophysectomy). A surgical cure rate of 85% to 90% has been documented. Because the HPA axis has been suppressed, adrenal insufficiency will develop postoperatively. The axis takes 12 to 24 months to recover. Replacement steroids are indicated during this time.

■ Nursing Management of the Surgical Client

Assessment

Begin by collecting a careful history from the client with potential Cushing's syndrome. The client may exhibit the characteristic clinical manifestations identified previously.

Support the client during the diagnostic phase of the disease. There is often a great deal of uncertainty at this point about the cause of the disorder. Explain to the client why these tests must be performed before treatment can be started.

During the preoperative phase, the client with Cushing's syndrome requires expert nursing assessment and care. The crucial problems of hypertension, edema, possible heart disease, diabetes mellitus, increased susceptibility to infection, decrease resistance to stress, and emotional lability must all be assessed and then brought under control prior to surgical treatment.

Diagnosis, Planning, Implementation

Risk for Injury: Fractures, Hypertension, or Diabetes. Until the diagnosis is made and the problem treated, the client is at *Risk for Injury: Fractures, Hypertension, or Diabetes related to osteoporosis, sodium and water retention, or the presence of an insulin antagonist, respectively.*

Planning: Expected Outcomes. Injury will not occur, as evidenced by absence of fracture. The client will not have manifestations of hypertension, hyperglycemia, or diabetes.

Implementation. Protect the client against falls and accidents. Clients with Cushing's syndrome have osteoporosis and tend to develop fractures even with mild trauma. Keep the bed in the lowest position, and raise the side rails for protection. Assist clients with ambulation to avoid falls.

Monitor vital signs at frequent intervals. Assess the client carefully for manifestations of severe hypertension, e.g., elevated blood pressure (BP), headache, failing vision, irritability, and dyspnea. Check for postural hypotension (but have the client change position slowly to avoid injury from a sudden drop in BP).

Obtain the client's weight daily in a consistent manner. If sodium intake is reduced, edema and weight should diminish. Test urine for glucose and acetone daily or obtain daily blood glucose levels via fingerstick. Positive results may indicate diabetes mellitus (steroid diabetes) caused by the insulin antagonist action of the excessive cortisol.

Knowledge Deficit. A typical nursing diagnosis for the client undergoing surgery to correct adrenocortical excess is *Knowledge Deficit related to the disease, surgery, and proper diet.*

Planning: Expected Outcomes. The client will understand the disease, the surgery planned, and the importance of a proper diet, as evidenced by statements of understanding and choice of a proper diet.

Implementation. It is important for clients to understand their condition and the proposed treatment. Give clients an opportunity to ask questions about the treatment and assess for their understanding of it.

Encourage a diet low in calories, carbohydrates, and sodium but with ample protein and potassium content. Such a diet promotes weight loss, reduction of edema and hypertension, control of hypokalemia, and rebuilding of wasted tissue. The client with diabetes mellitus or gastric ulcers requires a special diet (see Chapters 69 and 61, respectively).

Risk for Injury. After surgery, the client may have *Risk for Injury related to complications of the surgical procedure.*

Planning: Expected Outcomes. Injury will not occur or will be detected early, as evidenced by absence of shock, hemorrhage, infection, or addisonian crisis.

Implementation. On the morning of surgery, administer a glucocorticoid preparation IM or IV as prescribed. A water-soluble cortisol preparation (diluted in an IV infusion) may be given throughout the surgical procedure. Cortisol protects the client from development of acute adrenal insufficiency during adrenalectomy. Even if the surgeon plans to remove only one adrenal gland, temporary glucocorticoid support may be needed until the remaining adrenal gland begins to secrete sufficient amounts of cortisol. Because of the excessive secretion of cortisol by the tumorous gland, the healthy gland can atrophy and require time to readjust.

During the immediate postoperative phase, major goals are the following:

1. Prevention of shock
2. Prevention of infection
3. Maintenance of adequate cortisol levels
4. Control of pain and incisional discomfort.

Observe for manifestations of shock due to hemorrhage (hypotension, and rapid, weak pulse). Document vital signs every 15 minutes. Measure urine and record hourly output, observing for oliguria, a manifestation of shock and renal shutdown. Administer IV fluids, pressor amines, and corticosteroids as prescribed.

The manifestations of addisonian crisis resemble shock. Closely assess the client for the development of this complication, and administer IV cortisol in high doses until the manifestations subside. The client will continue to require increased amounts of steroids until the remaining adrenal returns to a normal level of functioning and the stress associated with the treatment subsides.

Encourage clients in coughing, turning, and deep-breathing to prevent respiratory infections. Employ meticulous sterile technique with wound care to prevent infection. Ileus is less common because the flank approach is usually used.

Risk for Ineffective Management of Therapeutic Regimen (Individuals). The client with a bilateral adrenalectomy will need to learn self-care. A typical nursing diagnosis would therefore be *Risk for Ineffective Management of Therapeutic Regimen (Individuals) related to self-administration of replacement hormones.*

Planning: Expected Outcomes. The client will understand self-administration of replacement hormones. The client will be able to repeat and comply with instructions and will not develop addisonian crisis or adrenal insufficiency.

Implementation. Following bilateral adrenalectomy, lifelong glucocorticoid replacement is essential. If only one adrenal gland has been removed, daily cortisol replacement continues until the remaining gland functions normally (usually 6–12 months later). Prior to discharge, the client and significant others need instruction on self-administration of replacement hormones (hydrocortisone). The client and significant others should successfully demonstrate the injection technique before discharge from the hospital.

Evaluation

If the surgical management of Cushing's disease is successful, the client will not develop injury secondary to the

surgery or develop addisonian crisis. If complications do occur, outcomes could be related to the successful management of the complications, such as control of hemorrhage, prevention of shock, and control of addisonian crisis.

Community and Self-Care

■ Medical Management

Radiation Therapy

Although surgery is the usual treatment for primary adrenal hyperplasia, other, palliative treatments are available (Table 71–5). Radiation therapy can be used to treat primary pituitary tumors and other ACTH-secreting adenomas. Radiation can be applied to the pituitary gland either internally or externally. Internally, the radiation is applied through a transsphenoidal implant. Radiation must be used with care because of the proximity of the optic nerve. Radiation is not always effective in even palliative treatment of tumors and may destroy normal tissue. For ACTH-secreting adenomas such as lung tumors, palliation is possible. Chapter 24 describes the care of the client undergoing radiation therapy.

Radiation therapy is commonly used concurrently with surgical or pharmacologic management to enhance its effectiveness and reduce long-term side effects.

Adrenal Blocking Agents

Medications that interfere with ACTH production or adrenal hormone synthesis are available. Mitotane (Lysodren) is a cytotoxic antihormonal agent that inhibits corticosteroid synthesis without destroying cortical cells. Aminoglutethimide (Cytadren) and trilostane (Modrastane) are other cytotoxic agents that block the synthesis of glucocorticoids and adrenal steroids.

ACTH-Reducing Agents

Cyproheptadine (Periactin), bromocryptine, or somatostatin is used to treat hypersecretion due to pituitary abnormalities causing in increased ACTH levels. This agent appears to interfere with ACTH production, thereby reducing the effect on the adrenals.

■ Nursing Management of the Medical Client

Assessment

Assess the client for ability to perform self-care and to manage the disease for the remainder of his or her life. The client's current level of knowledge must be assessed and a careful teaching plan developed.

Diagnosis, Planning, Implementation

Risk for Infection. The client on steroid replacement will be at *Risk for Infection related to lowered resistance to stress and compromised immune response.*

Table 71–5. Therapies for Cushing's Syndrome, Cushing's Disease, and Ectopic ACTH Syndrome

Condition	Responsible Lesion	Therapies	Remarks
Cushing's syndrome	Adrenal tumor (benign or malignant)	Adrenalectomy	Adrenalectomy for benign unilateral tumor; usually curative Bilateral adrenalectomy must be followed by lifelong administration of corticosteroids
	Adrenal carcinoma with widespread metastases	Surgery and chemotherapy (mitotane)	Chemotherapy largely unsuccessful
Cushing's disease	Pituitary tumor (or unidentified lesion) that secretes excessive amounts of ACTH	Microsurgical resection of pituitary adenoma	Pituitary surgery successful in 95% of cases
		Irradiation of pituitary gland	Irradiation successful in 75% of cases; therapeutic effects not apparent for months following initiation of therapy
		Total bilateral adrenalectomy (corrects adrenal hyperplasia due to excessive ACTH stimulation)	Total bilateral adrenalectomy must be followed by life-long replacement therapy with glucocorticoid and mineralocorticoid
Ectopic ACTH syndrome	Extra-adrenal malignant tumor	Surgical removal of ectopic malignant tumor; chemotherapy used to control hypercorticism and promote remission in clients with inoperable cancer	Surgery rarely successful because metastasis usually occurs before diagnosis; chemotherapy purely palliative

Planning: Expected Outcomes. Infection will not develop or will be detected early, as evidenced by absence of leukocytosis, fever, and other manifestations of infections.

Implementation. Protect clients from exposure to infectious organisms. Isolate clients from healthcare personnel and significant others with contagious disorders. Wash your hands meticulously before contact with client.

Because glycocorticoids suppress immune and inflammatory reactions, clients with Cushing's syndrome may experience only mild manifestations, even in the presence of a severe infection. The white blood cell count will not show significant elevation in immunosuppressed clients. A slight elevation in body temperature may indicate the presence of a severe infection.

Activity Intolerance. Clients receiving steroids may exhibit *Activity Intolerance related to fatigue and muscle weakness from protein wasting, persistent hyperglycemia (and possible diabetes mellitus), and potassium depletion.*

Planning: Expected Outcomes. The client will be able to balance rest and activity.

Implementation. Promote mental and physical rest for the client with Cushing's syndrome. Minimize stress and confusion so the client can achieve maximal periods of rest.

Risk for Impaired Skin Integrity. The client who is taking steroids is at *Risk for Impaired Skin Integrity related to tissue catabolism (thinning of skin), loss of connective tissue, and edema secondary to sodium and water retention.*

Planning: Expected Outcomes. The client will not develop impaired skin integrity, as evidenced by intact skin.

Implementation. Monitor the client's skin meticulously for the presence of breakdown. The client is extremely prone to breakdown from tissue catabolism. Avoid the use of tape or other irritants that may result in skin tearing or excoriation.

Altered Thought Processes. The client may exhibit *Altered Thought Processes (memory loss, cognitive impairment, mood swings, euphoria, or depression) related to increased levels of glucocorticoids and ACTH.*

Planning: Expected Outcomes. The client will not suffer from memory loss, cognitive impairment, or mood swings or these manifestations will be minimized.

Implementation. Anticipate clients' mood swings. Clients can become easily upset by changes in their appearance caused by the disease process. They also can become alarmed by the bizarre feelings and emotions they experience. Reassure the client that appearance and moods should gradually return to normal after the disorder is treated (see Fig. 71–3) unless the treatment requires steroid replacement. If clients have to receive steroid therapy, they will continue to experience some side effects.

Evaluation

Appropriate outcomes for the client would include the control of side effects from the steroid therapy. Since these cannot be completely avoided, the client's ability to control them would be an appropriate area to evaluate. Does the client know the manifestations of complications versus side effects?

■ Modifications for Elderly Clients

Elderly clients may exhibit excessive manifestations of Cushing's syndrome because these clients may already exhibit many of the characteristic manifestations, such as osteoporosis, hypertension, and diabetes. The client also is more prone to the side effects of steroid replacement therapy.

Primary Hyperaldosteronism

Aldosterone is the most powerful of the mineralocorticoids. Its primary role is to conserve sodium, and it also promotes potassium excretion.

The incidence of primary hyperaldosteronism in the hypertensive population is unknown. It is estimated to affect approximately 1%. It strikes females twice as often as males and appears most frequently in the middle-aged.

Etiology and Risk Factors

Primary hyperaldosteronism is the hypersecretion of aldosterone due to an adrenal lesion that is usually benign. The disease, which produces secondary hypertension and hypokalemia (in most) and hypernatremia, is also known as Conn's syndrome.

Secondary hyperaldosteronism is a consequence of a variety of conditions that cause an overproduction of aldosterone. These conditions may include sodium wasting renal disease, laxative or diuretic abuse, dehydration, cirrhosis with ascites, heart failure, and a decrease in intravascular volume. Hypertension is not a usual feature.

There are no particular risk factors for primary hyperaldosteronism. Risk factors for secondary hyperaldosteronism include chronic heart failure, cirrhosis with ascites, nephrotic syndrome, and hypertension caused by destructive renal artery disease. The preventive measures, therefore, are successful treatment and control of the causative disease process. The more successfully these factors are controlled, the less secondary hyperaldosteronism will be present.

Pathophysiology

Aldosterone affects the tubular reabsorption of sodium and water, and the excretion of potassium and hydrogen

ions in the renal tubular epithelial cells (Fig. 71–4). This leads to the development of hypernatremia, hypervolemia, hypokalemia, and metabolic alkalosis. With hypervolemia and hypernatremia, BP increases, often to very high levels, and renin production is suppressed. The hypertension can lead to cerebral infarcts and to renal damage.

Secondary hyperaldosteronism is due to continuous secretion of aldosterone secondary to high levels of angiotensin II, resulting, in turn, from high plasma renin activity. The decreased renal perfusion due to a variety of causes is the underlying mechanism.

Clinical Manifestations and Diagnostic Findings

Clients with primary hyperaldosteronism may be asymptomatic, but found to have hypertension, hypernatremia, and hypokalemia. Without intervention, they can develop all the complications of chronic hypertension, such as visual disturbances, heart failure, renal damage, and cerebrovascular accident.

Hypokalemia results from excessive urinary excretion of potassium ions (see Chapters 15 and 16). This problem, in turn, causes muscle weakness, paralysis, or cardiac arrhythmias, because K^+ loss reduces normal neuromuscular irritability. In addition, excessive excretion of K^+ results in polyuria. The large urinary output leads to polydipsia (excessive thirst). Finally, hypokalemia leads to metabolic alkalosis from (1) shifting of hydrogen ions into the cells in exchange for K^+ and (2) exchange of H^+ within the tubular cells for sodium ions from the tubular urine. Metabolic alkalosis causes a decrease in ionized calcium levels, which can result in tetany and respiratory suppression (see Chapters 15 and 16).

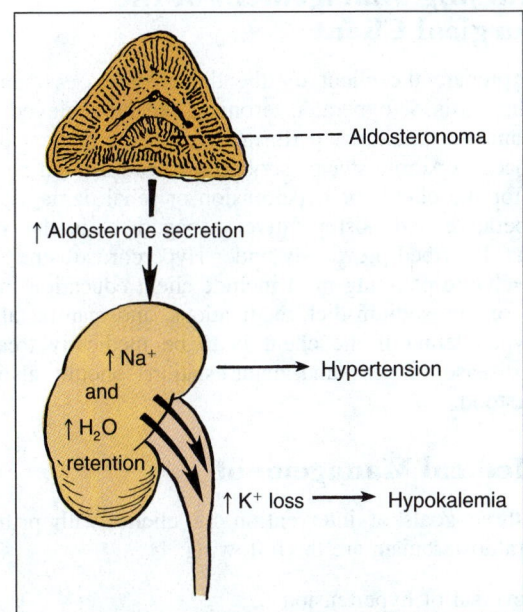

Figure 71–4. Effects of primary aldosteronism. Excessive aldosterone secretion causes increased Na^+ and water retention and increased excretion of K^+.

Despite sodium retention, clients with hyperaldosteronism rarely develop overt edema. Although ECF increases moderately, excessive water is normally excreted in the urine with potassium ions. Over time, the kidneys tend to adjust physiologically to excessive secretion of aldosterone, so water excretion reaches an equilibrium with sodium intake. The ability of the kidneys to eventually "escape" from the sodium- and water-retaining action of aldosterone is sometimes called the escape phenomenon.

Diagnosis of primary hyperaldosteronism is based on low serum potassium, alkalosis, and elevated urinary or plasma aldosterone with low plasma renin levels (elevated in secondary hyperaldosteronism). Additionally, radiographic studies may reveal cardiac hypertrophy resulting from chronic hypertension. Radionuclide scanning techniques using radiolabeled iodocholesterol allow visualization of the tumors.

Acute and Subacute Care

■ Surgical Management

Surgery is the treatment of choice for primary hyperaldosteronism. A unilateral or bilateral adrenalectomy must be performed. Clients undergoing a unilateral adrenalectomy may need temporary replacement of glucocorticoids, while those requiring bilateral adrenalectomies will need permanent replacement (see the discussion of Addison's disease). Clients usually receive glucocorticoids preoperatively to prevent adrenal hypofunction.

Surgical removal of the adrenals usually corrects the hypertension, hypokalemia, and hypernatremia.

■ Nursing Management of the Surgical Client

Help prepare the client for the diagnostic assessment so the diagnosis of hyperaldosteronism can be achieved rapidly and the treatment performed before permanent damage occurs. Administer prescribed medications and closely monitor the client for hypertension or renal damage. The preoperative and postoperative management is the same as that described previously under Hypercortisolism.

Discharge planning must include client education in the areas of low sodium diet, medications, and manifestations of hypokalemia if the client is to be medically treated. The disease process and manifestations should also be understood.

■ Medical Management

The three goals of intervention for clients with primary hyperaldosteronism are the following:

1. Reversal of hypertension
2. Correction of the hypokalemia
3. Prevention of kidney damage

In two thirds of the cases, removal of the aldosterone-secreting tumor completely resolves the hypertension.

Most clients have normal BP readings by the third postoperative month.

Unfortunately, the renal complications resulting from long-term hypertension tend to be progressive. Therefore, clients with primary hyperaldosteronism need to be diagnosed and treated early in the course of the disease.

If clients cannot be treated surgically, they are often given spironolactone (Aldactone) to increase sodium excretion and to treat the hypertension and hypokalemia. Hypertension may take 4 to 8 weeks to correct. The client's potassium level should be carefully monitored for the development of hyperkalemia, especially if the client has been receiving potassium supplements or has been on a high potassium diet (Box 71–1). Amiloride is the drug of choice for clients intolerant to spironolactone.

■ Nursing Management of the Medical Client

Assess the client's ability to manage the complex therapeutic regimen. Plan and implement a teaching program for self-care related to the medical management presented in the previous section.

Adrenomedullary Disorders

Two important tumors occur in the adrenal medulla: (1) pheochromocytoma, a tumor that results in hyperactivity of the gland, and (2) neuroblastoma, a malignant tumor made up of cells resembling a neuroblast. For a complete description of neuroblastoma, an important tumor in children, consult a pediatric textbook.

Pheochromocytoma

A pheochromocytoma is a catecholamine-secreting tumor of the chromaffin cells of the sympathetic nervous system usually found in the adrenal medulla.

Box 71–1. Complications of Spironolactone Administration

Spironolactone is the drug of choice for primary hyperaldosteronism. It effectively lowers blood pressure and improves hypokalemia. The administration of spironolactone is complicated by:

1. Side effects such as gastrointestinal discomfort, impotence, decreased libido, gynecomastia, and menstrual irregularities.
2. Increase in the half-life of digoxin. The client's digoxin dosage may be reduced based on serum levels.
3. Concomitant therapy with salicylates. Salicylates increase renal tubular excretion of canrenone, the major active metabolite of spironolactone, thus decreasing its effectiveness.

Pheochromocytomas are rare. Based on autopsy series, the incidence of pheochromocytoma is 0.1% of clients with diastolic hypertension. The condition is equally common in women and men. Although the disease can occur at any age, it is most common in middle age and rarely occurs after age 60.

Etiology and Risk Factors

The cause of pheochromocytomas is unknown. In some cases, pheochromocytomas appear to have a familial basis. They often occur in association with neuroectodermal diseases and with multiple endocrine neoplasia type IIA.

Pathophysiology

The pheochromocytoma, usually less than 200 g, is composed of chromaffin cells, so named (L. *affinis,* affinity) because they stain brownish-yellow with chromic salts. In 85% to 95% of cases, pheochromocytomas arise within the adrenal medulla. Occasionally, however, they develop from the chromaffin tissues found in the sympathetic paraganglia.

Pheochromocytomas are typically benign; less than 10% are malignant. Because of the excessive amounts of epinephrine and norepinephrine they secrete, they can produce severe manifestations and even death. Table 71–6 summarizes the effects of epinephrine and norepinephrine.

There are no known risk factors affecting the development of pheochromocytoma.

Once diagnosed, there are known risk factors that can influence the catecholamine release. Catecholamine release occurs in various frequencies and intensities. This is called a *paroxysm.* The Risk Factors and Levels of Prevention feature for pheochromocytoma lists factors causing a paroxysm. Without early intervention, the client is at risk of cerebral hemorrhage and cardiac failure. Fortunately, if pheochromocytomas are discovered early in their development, they can usually be removed surgically.

Clinical Manifestations and Diagnostic Findings

The client with pheochromocytoma may present with manifestations of diabetes mellitus (elevated blood glucose and glucosuria), hypertension (elevated BP, headaches), hyperthyroidism (increased metabolic rate, diaphoresis, agitation, rapid pulse, palpitations, emotional outbursts), and psychoneurosis (emotional instability).

Hypertension is the principal manifestation of pheochromocytoma, and can be persistent, fluctuating, intermittent, or paroxysmal. Typically, the client has episodes of high BP accompanied by pounding headaches. Other manifestations of sympathetic overactivity include sweating, apprehension, palpitations, nausea, and vomiting. Excessive release of catecholamine also results in excessive conversion of glycogen into glucose in the liver. Conse-

Table 71–6. The Effects of Epinephrine and Norepinephrine

Epinephrine	Norepinephrine
Cardiovascular System	
Constricts superficial blood vessels; in small doses, dilates muscle, brain, and coronary vessels, thus shunting blood supply to organs; essential for "fight or flight"	Constricts blood vessels (especially peripheral), causing increased peripheral resistance
Raises blood pressure	Raises blood pressure greatly
Increases cardiac output	Decreases cardiac output because of increased peripheral resistance
Increases pulse dramatically	Increases pulse moderately
Constricts spleen, shunting stored red blood cells into general circulation	
Increases coagulability of blood	
Respiratory System	
Increases rate and depth of respirations	
Dilates bronchi	
Nervous System	
Stimulates central nervous system, increasing alertness and producing a feeling of fright, excitation, and impending doom	
Dilates pupils	Dilates pupils
Inhibits gastrointestinal tract	Inhibits gastrointestinal tract
Metabolism	
Increases nonesterified fatty acid level of blood	Increases nonesterified fatty acid level of blood
Promotes conversion of glycogen to glucose	
Increases body metabolism	Increases body metabolism slightly

Data from Campese, V. M., & DeQuattro, V. (1989). Functional components of the sympathetic nervous system: Regulation of organ systems. In L. DeGroot (Ed.), *Endocrinology and metabolism* (2nd ed.). Philadelphia: W. B. Saunders.

quently, hyperglycemia and glucosuria occur during attacks. Such manifestations can develop spontaneously or be precipitated by emotional stress, physical exertion, or change in body position.

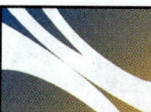

RISK FACTORS AND LEVELS OF PREVENTION

Pheochromocytoma

Risk Factors

Risk factors involved in stimulating a paroxysm in pheochromocytoma:

- Smoking
- Micturition
- Drugs that may influence catecholamine release: histamines, some anesthetics (halothane, thiopental, cyclopropane, methoxyflurane, fentanyl), atropine, opiates, steroids, glucagon
- Activities that might displace abdominal organs: bending, exercising, straining, vigorous palpation of the abdomen
- Pregnancy, especially the third trimester and labor

Levels of Prevention

Primary Prevention

- Advise clients to avoid the activities listed above.
- Tell clients that micturition should occur in small amounts, without urgency, avoiding a full bladder.
- Assist clients to stop the causative event if possible.

Secondary Prevention

- Monitor blood pressure regularly in at-risk clients.
- Ensure that clients take prescribed antihypertensives.

Tertiary Prevention

- Ensure that clients take prescribed medications to treat long-term effects of paroxysmal episodes.
- Educate clients about steroid replacement after adrenalectomy.

Acute attacks may be associated with profuse diaphoresis, dilated pupils, and cold extremities. Severe hypertension can precipitate a cerebrovascular accident or sudden blindness.

Because pheochromocytoma is curable, early and accurate diagnosis is essential. Current methods of diagnosis include the following:

1. History and physical examination. The client may describe symptomatic attacks over weeks, months, or even years. The BP may change with exertion or emotional upset. In long-standing cases, complications of intractable hypertension (e.g., visual disturbances), manifestations of heart disease (dyspnea, edema), and manifestations of kidney damage (albuminuria, proteinuria, and increased blood urea nitrogen) can coexist.
2. Chemical tests. Two hormonal assay tests are useful in diagnosing pheochromocytoma:
   a. Assay of urinary catecholamines and their metabolites (metanephrines and vanillylmandelic acid

[VMA]). Assays of catecholamines are performed on single-voided urine specimens, 2- to 4-hour specimens, and 24-hour urine specimens. The normal range of urinary catecholamines is up to 14 μg/100 ml of urine, with higher levels occurring in pheochromocytoma.

   b. Determinations of plasma catecholamine concentrations. Assays of urinary VMA levels are performed on 24-hour urine specimens only. Advise clients to avoid tea, chocolate, vanilla, and all fruits for at least 2 days before urine collection begins. Also, remind them not to take any medications for 2 to 3 days before the test. Normally, the amount of VMA is less than 7 mg/24 hours. Urinary VMA rises in clients with pheochromocytoma.
3. The laboratory also performs a direct assay of catecholamines (epinephrine and norepinephrine) in the blood. The normal range of catecholamines in the blood is epinephrine, 0.02 to 0.2 μg/L, and norepinephrine, 0.1 to 0.5 μg/L.
4. X-ray imaging. Various radiographic techniques can help confirm and identify adrenomedullary tumor location, such as CT and MRI.
5. Miscellaneous nonspecific laboratory tests. In the presence of pheochromocytoma, the basal metabolic rate increases, blood sugar rises to abnormal levels, and glycosuria can occur.

Acute and Subacute Care

■ Surgical Management

The primary treatment of a pheochromocytoma is surgical removal of one or both adrenal glands, depending on whether the tumor is unilateral or bilateral. The procedure is the same as that described for treatment of Cushing's syndrome.

Alpha-adrenergic blocking agents such as phentolamine (Regitine) can be used in an IV bolus or IV drip for hypertensive crisis. Oral phenoxybenzamine (Dibenzyline) is used at least 7 days preoperatively to control BP, reduce manifestations, and eliminate paroxysms prior to definitive treatment: surgical removal of the affected gland.

Surgical removal can cure most clients, provided the growth is discovered before cardiovascular damage becomes permanent. Some clients may be on less medication at discharge after surgery. The operation, however, is not without danger. There are two serious hazards. First, excessive discharge of pressor hormones during induction of anesthesia or manipulation of the tumor can cause extreme rises in BP and cardiac arrhythmias. Second, following resection of the tumor, BP can fall precipitously.

Lifelong steroid replacement must be initiated following a bilateral adrenalectomy.

Clients with pheochromocytoma may develop the following complications: hypertensive retinopathy, hypertensive nephropathy, myocarditis, increased platelet aggregation, cerebroaccidents, vascular and congestive heart failure. Death may occur from myocardial infarction, cerebrovascular accident, arrhythmias, irreversible shock, renal failure, or dissecting aortic aneurysm.

■ Nursing Management of the Surgical Client

Assessment

It is important to assess and control the client's BP preoperatively. Closely monitor the client for the development of stressful episodes before treatment has begun. It is also important to assess the client's neurologic status in case the client has a stroke from the extremely elevated BP.

Diagnosis, Planning, Implementation

Risk for Injury. The client with a pheochromocytoma is at great risk of injury preoperatively. Write the nursing diagnosis *Risk for Injury related to excessive release of epinephrine and norepinephrine preoperatively.*

   Planning: Expected Outcomes. Injury will not occur or will be detected early, as evidenced by the absence of hypertensive episodes and cardiovascular or cerebral damage.

   Implementation. During the preoperative phase, the goal of treatment is to prevent attacks of acute paroxysmal hypertension, thereby lowering the risk of further damage to the cardiovascular system. Important nursing interventions include the following:

1. Promoting rest and relief from stress
2. Administering prescribed sedatives
3. Providing a diet high in vitamins, minerals, and calories
4. Prohibiting beverages containing caffeine, such as coffee, tea, and colas
5. Monitoring vital signs

   In most cases, the physician will prescribe an alpha-adrenergic blocking agent such as phenoxybenzamine.

Risk for Injury. The client at is at increased risk of development of problems such as hypotension postoperatively. Write the nursing diagnosis as *Risk for Injury related to postoperative hypotension, hemorrhage, and shock.*

   Planning: Expected Outcomes. Injury will not occur or will be detected early, as evidenced by normotensive state and the absence of hemorrhage, shock, or addisonian crisis.

   Implementation. The first 24 to 48 hours after surgery is a critical period demanding vigilant nursing assessment and intervention. During the immediate postoperative period, observe for manifestations of shock and hemorrhage.

Following removal of the tumor, profound shock can develop as catecholamine levels drop. Hypotension can persist for 24 to 48 hours. Hemorrhage can occur because of the high vascularity of the adrenal glands. To prevent postoperative shock, do the following:

● Give IV fluids as prescribed, such as blood, plasma, dextran, or glucose in water to maintain blood volume.
● Administer IV pressors as prescribed at a rate sufficient to maintain BP within a safe range. Check BP as often as is necessary to titrate the medication.
● Carefully measure hourly urinary output. If the client voids less than 30 ml/hr, notify the physician. Oliguria can signify impending shock and consequent renal shutdown.
● Assess the client for manifestations of hemorrhage. Check the dressing every half-hour for bloody drainage. If the client is bleeding internally, an abdominal hematoma can develop, resulting in paralytic ileus. Manifestations of paralytic ileus include abdominal pain, distention, severe nausea, vomiting, and diminished or absent bowel sounds.
● If cortical tissue was resected during surgery, assess the client closely for manifestations of adrenal insufficiency (see the section on addisonian crisis). If both adrenal glands have been removed, the client must receive cortisol replacement for life.

Pain. Postoperatively, the client must be monitored for *Pain related to surgery, headache, and other manifestations of pheochromocytoma.*

   Planning: Expected Outcomes. The client will not suffer pain, as evidenced by the client's statements, normotensive state, and absence of painful expression.

   Implementation. When administering medication for incisional pain, monitor BP frequently. Remember that narcotics, particularly meperidine, produce hypotension as a side effect; however, withholding pain medication also can lead to hypotension (or even hypertension) and severe pain. It is important to control the pain so the client's level of stress will decrease.

Risk for Ineffective Management of Therapeutic Regimen (Individuals). Following a bilateral adrenalectomy, the client must learn self-care measures or he or she will be at *Risk for Ineffective Management of Therapeutic Regimen related to self-administration of corticosteroids.*

   Planning: Expected Outcomes. The client will understand self-administration of steroids. He or she will be able to explain administration of these drugs and comply with the medication regimen.

   Implementation. Once the critical postoperative period is over, most clients pass through an uneventful convalescence. Clients who will be self-administering corticosteroids need instruction concerning the administration and side effects (see the discussion of addison's disease).

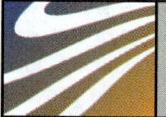

Evaluation

Successful outcome is evaluated by the client's ability to self-manage steroid replacement after surgery. Although side effects of steroids cannot be avoided, there are ways to minimize them and the client's ability to control these and avoid complications can be evaluated.

▪ Modifications for Elderly Clients

Elderly clients are more likely to suffer damage related to hypertensive episodes associated with the pheochromocytoma because their cardiovascular and cerebrovascular systems are likely to be weaker and prone to damage from the elevated pressure.

Anterior Pituitary Disorders

Disorders of the pituitary gland occur most frequently in the anterior lobe (Table 71–7; see also Fig. 70–2). Major causes of pituitary disease include the following:

1. Functioning tumors
2. Nonfunctioning tumors
3. Pituitary infarction
4. Genetic disorders
5. Trauma

The three principal pathologic consequences of pituitary disorders are:

1. Hyperpituitarism

Table 71–7. Pituitary Hormones

Name	Releasing Factor	Target Cells	Response	Increased Level	Decreased Level
Anterior Pituitary					
GH	GHRH	Bone, muscle	Stimulates growth; promotes active transport of amino acids into cell and influences lipid, CHO, and Ca^{2+} metabolism	Child: gigantism (before epiphyseal closure); child grows very tall. Adult: acromegaly (after epiphyseal closure); bones increase in thickness; increase in soft tissue growth	Child: dwarfism. Adult: lethargy, increased weight, loss of reproductive function, premature aging
ACTH	CRH	Adrenal cortex	Stimulates adrenal gland secretion of mineralocorticoids and glucocorticoids	Cushing's disease: increased amounts of cortisol and aldosterone	Addison's disease: decreased cortisol and aldosterone, increased MSH
TSH	TRH	Thyroid	Stimulates thyroid to increase secretion of thyroxine (controls rate of most chemical reactions in body)	Goiter; increased BMR; decreased weight; increased cardiac output, HR, and BP; increased cerebration; fine muscle tremors	Reduced thyroid activity; decreased BMR; increased weight; decreased cardiac output, HR, and BP; decreased cerebration; somnolence
Prolactin		Breast	Stimulates breast to lactate	Amenorrhea	Too little milk
FSH	LHRH	Ovaries, testes	Stimulates growth of ovaries and sperm		Late puberty
LH	LHRH	Ovaries, testes	Stimulates growth of follicles and increased secretion of estrogen and progesterone; increases testosterone secretion in the male	Excess testosterone, menstrual cycle disturbance	Amenorrhea; diminished progesterone and testosterone
Posterior Pituitary					
Oxytocin	Labor, sucking	Uterus, breasts	Stimulates uterus to contract at childbirth; stimulates lactation	Precipitates childbirth, excess milk	Prolonged childbirth, diminished milk
ADH (vasopressin)	Dehydration	Arterioles, distal renal tubule	Vasoconstricts arterioles to increase arterial pressure; increases water reabsorption in distal tubules, stimulates smooth muscle of gastrointestinal tract	Increased BP, decreased urinary output, edema	Diabetes insipidus, dilute urine, increased urinary volume

ACTH, adrenocorticotropic hormone; ADH, antidiuretic hormone; BMR, basal metabolic rate; CHO, carbohydrate; CRH, corticotropin-releasing hormone; FSH, follicle-stimulating hormone; GH, growth hormone; GHRH, growth hormone–releasing hormone; HR, heart rate; LH, luteinizing hormone; LHRH, luteinizing hormone–releasing hormone; MSH, melanocyte-stimulating hormone; TRH, thyrotropin-releasing hormone; TSH, thyroid-stimulating hormone.
Adapted from Davis, J., and Mason, C. (1979). *Neurologic critical care.* New York: Van Nostrand Reinhold.

2. Hypopituitarism
3. Local compression of brain tissue by expanding tumor masses.

Hyperpituitarism and Hyperprolactinemia

Etiology and Risk Factors

Hyperpituitarism is defined as oversecretion of one or more of the hormones secreted by the pituitary gland. It is primarily caused by a hormone-secreting pituitary tumor, typically a benign adenoma. Syndromes associated with hyperpituitarism are Cushing's syndrome, acromegaly, amenorrhea, galactorrhea, hyperthyroidism, and, rarely, hypergonadism in the male.

Pathophysiology

Prolactin (PRL) and growth hormone (GH) are the hormones most commonly overproduced by adenomas. They produce hyperprolactinemia and acromegaly (Fig. 71–5) respectively. The increased amounts of GH lead to rapid growth in all body tissues. This increased growth leads to gigantism if it occurs before closure of the epiphysis, and acromegaly if it occurs after epiphyseal closure.

Clinical Manifestations and Diagnostic Findings

Pituitary tumors produce both systemic effects and local manifestations. Systemic effects include the following:

1. Excessive or abnormal growth patterns due to overproduction of GH
2. Abnormal milk secretion (galactorrhea)
3. Overstimulation of one or more of the target glands, resulting in the release of excessive thyroid, sex, or adrenocortical hormones

Locally, pituitary tumors produce manifestations because the bony cranium that houses the tumor cannot expand to accommodate a growing mass. Local manifestations include visual field abnormalities resulting from pressure on the optic chiasm, headaches, and somnolence.

Table 71–8 for additional information related to hyperprolactinemia and acromegaly.

 Acute and Subacute Care

■ Surgical Management

The client with a pituitary tumor will need to have the tumor resected. There are a variety of approaches that can be used to remove a pituitary tumor. See Chapter 33 for specific information on hypophysectomy.

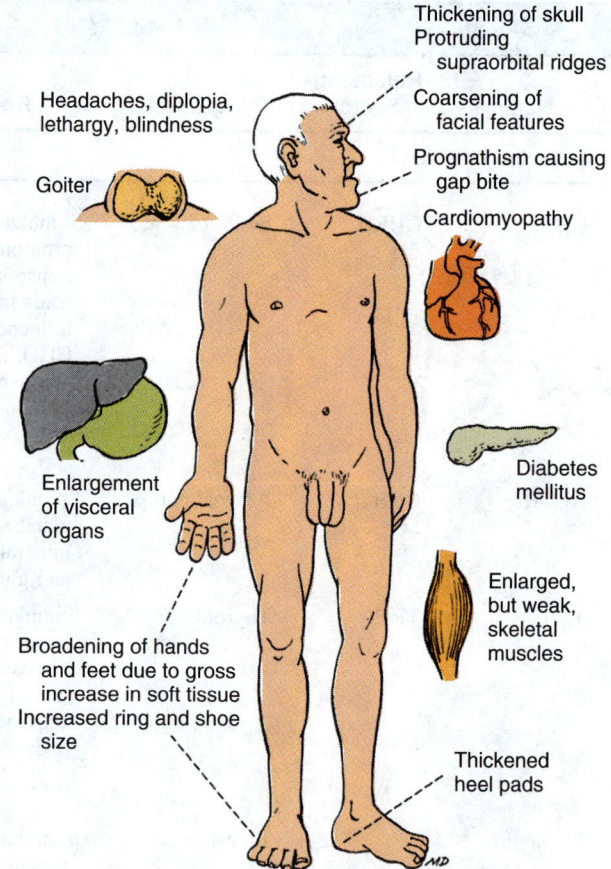

Figure 71–5. Assessment data for acromegaly.

Labels in figure:
- Headaches, diplopia, lethargy, blindness
- Goiter
- Thickening of skull
- Protruding supraorbital ridges
- Coarsening of facial features
- Prognathism causing gap bite
- Cardiomyopathy
- Diabetes mellitus
- Enlargement of visceral organs
- Enlarged, but weak, skeletal muscles
- Broadening of hands and feet due to gross increase in soft tissue Increased ring and shoe size
- Thickened heel pads

■ Nursing Management of the Surgical Client

Assessment

Most clients are frightened by the prospect of undergoing surgical removal of the pituitary gland. Provide the client and significant others with emotional support and comfort throughout the preoperative period. The initial manifestations are vague; therefore, clients will often have seen many physicians in the past and will have had multiple examinations and tests seeking a diagnosis. The client and family may be fearful, skeptical, or relieved with the final diagnosis of pituitary tumor. Assess the client's (1) reaction to the diagnosis, (2) expectations for the surgery, (3) educational needs related to the diagnosis and treatment plan, and (4) the available support network following discharge.

Your physical assessment of the client includes baseline vital signs and weight as well as neurologic assessment. The client should also have a preoperative eye examination by an ophthalmologist. These findings are essential to establish a baseline for postoperative comparison. To perform the neurologic assessment, check the following:

● Pupil equality and reactivity to light
● Handgrip for strength, equality, and ability to release on command

Table 71-8. Hyperprolactinemia and Acromegaly in Hyperpituitarism

	Hyperprolactinemia	Acromegaly
Hormone secreted	Excessive prolactin (PRL) causes prolactinoma	Excessive growth hormone (GH)
Risk factors	Hyperprolactinemia; estrogen therapy; oral contraceptive use; pregnancy may increase tumor size and dysfunction	None
Etiology	Pregnancy; hypothalamic-pituitary disorders; hypothyroidism; drug ingestion (estrogen or oral contraception)	Anterior pituitary adenoma; abnormal hypothalamic function (rare)
Pathophysiology	PRL-producing tumors deliver excess PRL systemically	GH-producing adenomas deliver excess GH systemically leading to rapid growth in other body tissues (with exception of the CNS) causing organomegaly; increase in tumor size within confined space can result in destruction of entire pituitary and cause hypopituitarism
Clinical manifestations related to hormone oversecretion	Abnormal lactation (galactorrhea) in nonlactating breast; amenorrhea; decreased vaginal lubrication; decreased libido in men; impotence; depression; anxiety; headache; visual loss	Local overgrowth of bone: skull and mandible; soft tissue overgrowth; lethargy; weight gain; paresthesias; glucose intolerance; coarse facial features; irregular or absent menses; enlargement of hands and feet over 1–10 yr; depression; headache; visual field impairment; osteoarthritis; paresthesias; impotence
Complications related to tumor growth	Headaches; visual disturbances affecting CN III, IV, VI; hypopituitarism; infertility; decreased bone growth	Hypopituitarism; neoplasms of gastrointestinal tract; increased mortality secondary to cardiovascular atherosclerosis, cerebral atherosclerosis, congestive heart failure, respiratory disease, hypertension, diabetes mellitus
Pharmacologic intervention	Bromocriptine is treatment of choice; bromocriptine can reduce PRL levels in 90% of clients; adverse reactions may contribute to noncompliance: nausea, headaches, dizziness, nasal stuffiness, hypotension, depression	Somatostatin analog octeotide is very effective in reducing GH levels; pharmacologic treatment may cause cholelithiasis; bromocriptine is effective in 60%–80% of clients
Surgical intervention	Transsphenoidal microsurgery; complications: residual tissue may produce elevated hormone levels, visual loss, diabetes insipidus, postoperative infection	Transsphenoidal microsurgery is treatment of choice; complications: same as in hyperprolactinemia
Radiation treatment	May decrease adenoma, but local complications are common because of tissue scarring and impairment of anterior pituitary function (hypopituitarism)	Produces slower decline of GH levels, implying higher morbidity related to atherosclerotic disease, respiratory disease, hypertension, diabetes mellitus, and gastrointestinal cancer; hypopituitarism
Diagnosis	Measurement of GH, ACTH, FSH, LH, PRL, testosterone, gonadotropins; thyroid function tests (T_3, T_4, FT_4, TSH); liver function tests (LDH, CPK, ASTT, alkaline phosphatase), coagulation studies; kidney function tests (serum creatinine, BUN, 24-hour urine collection for protein, creatinine clearance, GFR); urinalysis; pregnancy testing; CT or MRI for pituitary adenoma localization	Radioimmunoassay or enzyme-linked immunosorbent assay for GH level; serum GH level; insulin-like growth factor; CT scan or MRI for pituitary edema localization; oral glucose tolerance test may demonstrate hyperglycemia, — TT suppresses normal GH release 1–2 hr after ingestion; in acromegaly, GH level remains ↑

AST, aspartate aminotransferase; BUN, blood urea nitrogen; CPK, creatine phosphokinase; FT_4, free thyroxine; GFR, glomerular filtration rate; LDH, lactic dehydrogenase; T_3, triiodothyronine; T_4, thyroxine. For other abbreviations, see footnote to Table 71-7.

- Level of consciousness
- Orientation to time, place, person, and situation
- Appropriate response to stimuli
- Visual acuity and visual fields

Diagnosis, Planning, Implementation

Knowledge Deficit. Preoperatively, the client will need to be taught about the surgery and its implications.

A typical nursing diagnosis would be *Knowledge Deficit related to surgery and possible outcomes.*

Planning: Expected Outcomes. The client will understand the planned surgery and possible outcomes, as evidenced by the client's statements, questions, and ability to describe the procedure and outcomes.

Implementation. Explain the surgery to the client in detail, along with potential outcomes of surgical treatment. Use drawings of the brain to explain the transsphenoidal approach. Prepare the client for the presence of an indwelling urinary catheter, IV lines, and any other lines or monitors that may be needed after surgery. Tell the client that vital signs will be monitored closely following surgery.

Preoperative preparation also includes coaching the client in deep-breathing exercises and assisting in keeping records of intake and output.

Risk for Injury. A typical postoperative nursing diagnosis would be *Risk for Injury related to postoperative complications.*

Planning: Expected Outcomes. Injury will not occur from surgery, as evidenced by the absence of addisonian crisis, balanced intake and output, no manifestations of increased intracranial pressure, normal temperature, and absence of manifestations of cerebrospinal fluid (CSF) leakage or meningitis.

Implementation. Prior to surgery, the client usually receives an injection of IV cortisol. Glucocorticoids help the client to tolerate the stress of an operation that can result in loss of adrenocortical function.

Treatment following transfrontal hypophysectomy resembles that for any craniotomy (see Chapter 33). Immediately after surgery, assess for manifestations of cerebral edema and rising intracranial pressure (elevated BP, widened pulse pressure, low pulse rate, pupil changes, altered respiratory pattern).

The pituitary no longer produces tropic hormones; therefore, watch for manifestations of target gland defi-ciencies, such as adrenal insufficiency and hypothyroidism. In addition, diabetes insipidus can occur temporarily because of antidiuretic hormone (ADH) deficiency. This deficiency is related to surgical manipulation. Maintain strict documentation of intake and output. Notify the physician if urine output is greater than 200 ml/hr with a specific gravity of less than 1.005. The Critical Monitoring feature lists assessment findings that indicate an ADH imbalance.

Assess the client carefully for manifestations of meningitis, a potential complication of surgery. Report any temperature elevation, severe headache, irritability, or nuchal rigidity.

The client who has undergone transsphenoidal hypophysectomy requires frequent oral hygiene using a gauze sponge; the lips should be lubricated with petroleum jelly. The client should not brush his or her teeth for 2 weeks after surgery.

The nasal packing is usually removed in 2 to 5 days. After its removal, observe the client for rhinorrhea, which can indicate a CSF leak. Have the client report frequent postnasal drainage. Collect any serous drainage and test it for the presence of CSF (see Chapter 30) or send it to the laboratory for analysis. It is possible for the muscle or fat graft to dislodge, causing a CSF leak. Instruct the client to avoid sneezing, coughing, and bending over from the waist to avoid disrupting the graft.

Risk for Ineffective Management of Therapeutic Regimen (Individuals). Following a hypophysectomy, the client will have to take replacement hormones for life. The nursing diagnosis could be *Risk for Ineffective Management of Therapeutic Regimen related to self-administration of pituitary replacement hormones.*

Planning: Expected Outcomes. The client will understand self-administration of medication, as evidenced by the client's statements, ability to comply with the postoperative medication regimen, and absence of manifestations of hypopituitarism.

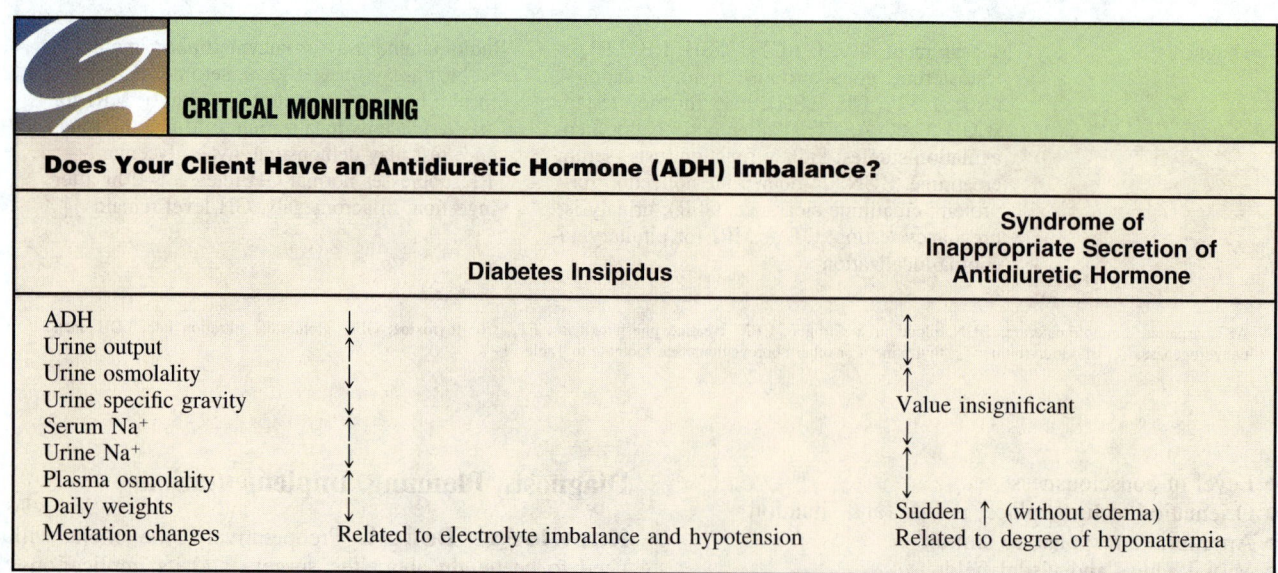

CRITICAL MONITORING

Does Your Client Have an Antidiuretic Hormone (ADH) Imbalance?

	Diabetes Insipidus		Syndrome of Inappropriate Secretion of Antidiuretic Hormone
ADH	↓		↑
Urine output	↑		↓
Urine osmolality	↓		↑
Urine specific gravity	↓		Value insignificant
Serum Na⁺	↑		↓
Urine Na⁺	↓		↑
Plasma osmolality	↑		
Daily weights	↓		Sudden ↑ (without edema)
Mentation changes	Related to electrolyte imbalance and hypotension		Related to degree of hyponatremia

Implementation. As stated earlier, people who have undergone complete hypophysectomy must take cortisone replacements for the rest of their lives. Instruct these clients to avoid gastric irritation by taking cortisone with milk, food, or an antacid. Advise clients to notify their physician if they develop gastritis, tarry stools, or frank blood in the stools.

Some clients also may require thyroid or sex hormone replacement. In addition, some will need vasopressin replacement to treat diabetes insipidus. Diabetes insipidus is usually transient following surgery, but can persist, indicating the need for chronic hormone replacement.

Evaluation

Appropriate outcomes following a hypophysectomy include the absence of postoperative complications and the client's ability to manage lifetime hormone replacement. If complications occur, appropriate outcomes would be that these are controlled without the client suffering permanent problems.

Sexual Disturbances

Excess secretion of gonadotropic hormones (luteinizing hormone [LH], follicle-stimulating hormone [FSH]) from pituitary tumors can produce sexual precocity in children. Excess PRL secretion can cause amenorrhea or galactorrhea (excessive flow of milk) in women. Physicians consider surgical removal to be the treatment of choice for radiologically demonstrable tumors.

Clients with increased PRL secretion and no radiologic or neurologic evidence of a pituitary tumor often respond to bromocriptine, an ergot-like compound. Clients with prolactinomas can be successfully treated with bromocriptine. Bromocriptine, a dopamine agonist, inhibits PRL secretion. Surgery is no longer the treatment of choice in most of these cases.

Hypopituitarism

In contrast to hyperpituitarism, hypopituitarism is a deficiency of one or more of the hormones produced by the anterior lobe of the pituitary. When both the anterior and posterior lobes fail to secrete hormones, the condition is called panhypopituitarism. Hypopituitarism and panhypopituitarism are rare disorders.

Etiology

The nine most important causes of hypopituitarism are known as the "nine I's":

*I*nvasive (most common)—pituitary tumors, central nervous system (CNS) tumors, carotid aneurysm

*I*nfarction—postpartum necrosis (Sheehan's syndrome), pituitary apoplexy

*I*nfiltrative—sarcoidosis, hemochromatosis

*I*njury—head trauma, child abuse

*I*mmunologic—lymphocytic hypophysitis

*I*atrogenic—surgery, radiation therapy

*I*nfectious—mycoses, tuberculosis, syphilis

*I*diopathic—familial

*I*solated—deficiency of an anterior pituitary hormone: growth hormone (GH), LH, FSH, thyroid-stimulating hormone (TSH), ACTH–lipotropic pituitary hormone (ACTH-LPH), PRL

Clinical Manifestations and Diagnostic Findings

The pituitary has enormous functional reserve; therefore, manifestations of hypopituitarism usually do not appear until 75% of the pituitary has been obliterated by tumors or thromboses. Manifestations depend on the age of onset as well as the hormones that are deficient.

The onset of hypopituitarism is usually gradual and the classic course of progressive hypopituitarism is an initial loss of GH and gonadotropic hormone, followed by deficiencies of TSH, then ACTH, and finally PRL.

Specific disorders resulting from pituitary hyposecretion include the following:

● Short stature. Severely stunted growth results from either (1) congenital lack of GH or (2) the development of space-occupying intracranial tumors, meningitis, or brain injury during early childhood.

● Sexual and reproductive disorders. Deficiencies of the gonadotropins (LH and FSH) can produce sterility, diminished sexual drive, and decreased secondary sex characteristics. Decreased FSH and LH lead to infertility and amenorrhea, diminished spermatogenesis, and testicular atrophy.

● Hypothyroidism. Because the synthesis of thyroid hormone depends on TSH, therapeutic ablation or pathologic destruction of the pituitary gland causes hypothyroidism unless the client receives thyroid hormone (see Chapter 70).

● Secondary adrenocortical insufficiency. Adrenal insufficiency can follow diminished synthesis of ACTH by the pituitary gland, which, in turn, causes diminished secretion of adrenocortical hormones by the adrenal cortex (see Fig. 71–2).

● PRL deficiency is symptomatic by absence of lactation in the postpartum woman.

Diagnosis of GH deficiency rests on the inability of stimulating agents such as levodopa, arginine, and insulin to increase plasma GH levels.

Measurement of ACTH levels can be performed to diagnose secondary adrenal insufficiency. Cortisol levels are low in both primary and secondary hypothyroidism; however, when it is a primary deficiency, ACTH levels are high. In the client with secondary hypopituitarism, ACTH levels are low.

Low serum thyroid hormone levels, together with low serum TSH levels, establish the diagnosis of hypothyroidism.

Sexual and reproductive disorders are diagnosed by

low levels of sex steroids and low levels of plasma FSH and LH.

Skull x-rays may reveal enlargement of the sella turcica, erosion of the sphenoid bone, or calcification of a suprasellar mass. CT scan or MRI may provide an enhanced view of an x-ray finding.

Management. Treatment of hypopituitarism involves (1) removal, if possible, of the causative factor (e.g., tumors) and (2) permanent replacement of the hormones secreted by the target organs.

Injections of human growth hormone (HGH) successfully treat GH deficiency. Previously, HGH was scarce and available for only a few clients, but HGH produced by recombinant DNA technology is now available.

Medications prescribed to replace hormones include the following:

1. Corticosteroids for correction of secondary adrenocortical insufficiency
2. Thyroid hormone for treatment of myxedema
3. Sex hormones to correct hypogonadism.

Assessment of the client with hypopituitarism revolves around assessment of the various target organs that are dependent on pituitary secretions. See the discussion of specific disorders such as Addison's disease or hypothyroidism for further information.

Nursing interventions also are directed at problems resulting from deficiency at the target organ. See the appropriate secretions for specific interventions.

Posterior Lobe (Neurohypophyseal) Disorders

Unlike the adenohypophysis, disease rarely destroys the neurohypophysis. Even if the posterior lobe becomes damaged or is surgically destroyed with the anterior lobe, hormonal deficiencies usually do not develop. This is because the hypothalamus continues to synthesize oxytocin and ADH. On the other hand, if the hypothalamus suffers damage, deficiencies of oxytocin and ADH develop even if the neurohypophysis is healthy and intact.

The major disorder of the posterior lobe is ADH deficiency (diabetes insipidus) (Fig. 71–6). Excessive ADH causes the syndrome of inappropriate secretion of ADH (SIADH), which can occur with lung cancer, head injuries, cranial surgery, pituitary tumors, encephalitis, poliomyelitis, and myxedema. Table 71–9 compares diabetes insipidus and SIADH.

Researchers have not documented oxytocin imbalances. For further information on oxytocin, consult an obstetrics textbook.

Gonadal Disorders

Testicular dysfunction can be primary, a disorder of testicular function, or secondary to a disorder of hypotha-

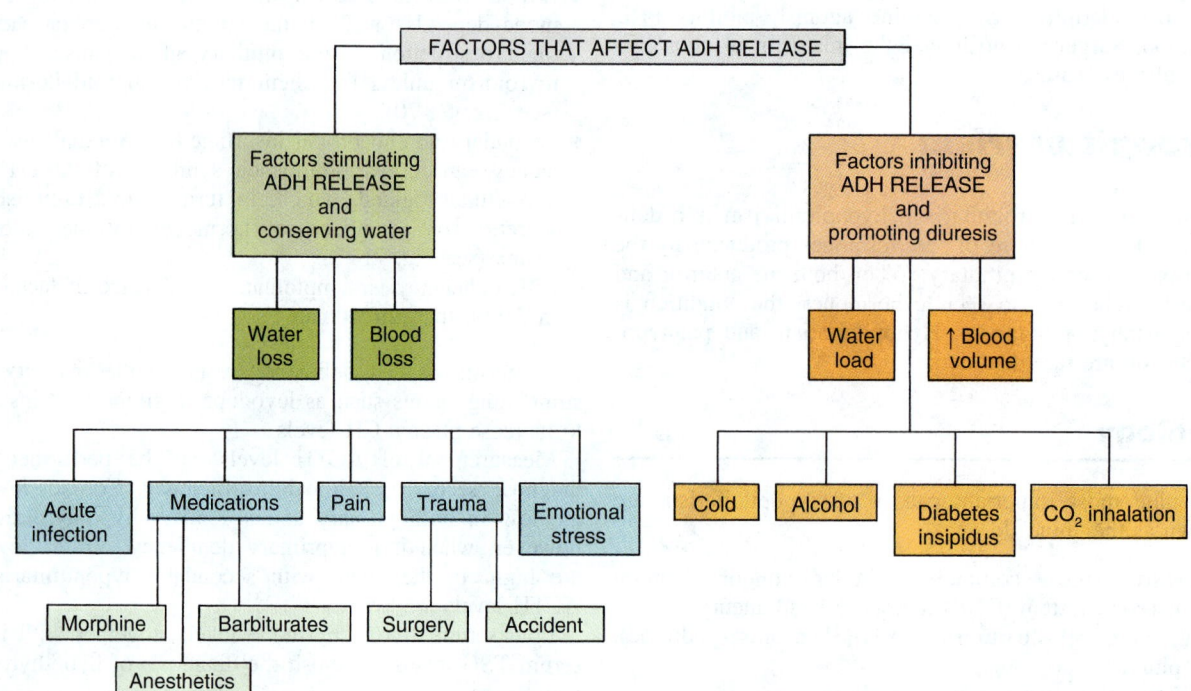

Figure 71–6. Factors that stimulate and inhibit the release of antidiuretic hormone.

Table 71-9. Comparison of Diabetes Insipidus and Syndrome of Inappropriate Secretion of Antidiuretic Hormone

	Diabetes Insipidus (DI)	Syndrome of Inappropriate Secretion of Antidiuretic Hormone (SIADH)
Definition	A deficiency of antidiuretic hormone (ADH, vasopressin) results in inability to conserve water	Excessive amounts of ADH secreted from posterior pituitary and other ectopic sources
Incidence	Unknown; DI idiopathic in about 30% of all clients with DI; tumors can be related to 25% of DI cases; head injury accounts for 16%; cranial surgery for 20% of DI cases	Approximately 80% of clients with small cell carcinoma have evidence of impaired ability to excrete water secondary to ectopic production of vasopressin
Etiology	Central CI or neurogenic DI: CNS interruption of anatomic integrity of posterior pituitary; localized or generalized edema from head trauma, vascular lesions, centrally acting drugs, or CNS infections may also cause central DI; ADH synthesis or release is affected; may be transient or permanent Complete DI occurs when there is disruption to hypophyseal tract and a complete absence of ADH Nephrogenic DI: rare hereditary disorder; acquired structural or functional change in kidney occurs; ADH produced normally, but distal and collecting tubules cannot respond Idiopathic DI	Ectopic production of vasopressin by malignancy is most common cause (degree of vasopressin impairment is relative to extent of malignant disease) see Risk factors below
Risk factors	Head injury, neurosurgery, hypothalamic tumors, pituitary tumors, brain infections or inflammation; drugs that inhibit vasopressin release: ethanol, glucocorticoids, adrenergic agents, phenytoin, narcotic antagonists, lithium	Vasopressin overuse (from DI); malignant conditions that may contain ectopic sources of vasopressin-like hormone: bronchogenic carcinoma; lymphoma of duodenum, brain, bladder; pancreatic cancer; prostatic cancer; increased intracranial pressure secondary to infectious processes or brain trauma; infectious processes—viral or bacterial pneumonia; drugs that may stimulate vasopressin release: vincristine, cyclophosphamide, thiazides, phenothiazines, carbamazepine, vinblastine, cisplatin, oxytocin; endocrine disorders: adrenal insufficiency, myxedema, anterior pituitary insufficiency; analgesics; vomiting
Pathophysiology normally ADH: increases kidneys' permeability to water to promote water reabsorption and decrease urine output; ADH is normally released in response to: ↑ serum osmolality and ↓ extracellular volume	With ADH deficiency: permeability of water is diminished resulting in excretion of large volumes of hypotonic fluid Three patterns may develop: (1) transient DI—abrupt onset within first few days after neurosurgery, resolves within several days; (2) permanent DI (prolonged DI)—abrupt and early onset, persists for several weeks or forever, usually occurs after damage to hypothalamus or neurohypophyseal stalk; (3) triphasic DI—immediate postinjury increase in urine volume with decrease in urine osmolality lasting 4–5 days; interphase occurs over next 5–7 days when urine volume; decreases to normal and is followed by a permanent phase of polyuria	Key features of ADH excess: (1) water retention, (2) hyponatremia, (3) hypo-osmolality; a continual release of ADH causes water retention from renal tubules and collecting ducts; extracellular fluid volume increases with dilutional hyponatremia; hyponatremia suppresses renin and aldosterone secretions causing a decrease in proximal tubule reabsorption of Na$^+$
Physical examination	Integumentary: dry, cool skin, dry mucous membranes Cardiovascular: tachycardia Physical manifestations related to specific electrolyte imbalance	Physical manifestations related to hyponatremia: decreased deep tendon reflexes, fatigue, headache, anorexia, nausea, decreased mental status, seizures, coma Physical manifestations related to fluid volume excess: weight gain without edema, jugular venous distention, tachycardia, tachypnea, rales

Table continued on following page

Table 71–9. Comparison of Diabetes Insipidus and Syndrome of Inappropriate Secretion of Antidiuretic Hormone (Continued)

	Diabetes Insipidus (DI)	Syndrome of Inappropriate Secretion of Antidiuretic Hormone (SIADH)
Clinical manifestations	Genitourinary: polyuria—a few liters to 18 L/day; clear urine; urinary frequency; nocturia Gastrointestinal: weight loss; polydipsia (if thirst mechanism intact) Integumentary: dry skin and mucous membranes Neurologic: mentation changes as electrolyte imbalance and hypotension worsen	Related to degree of hyponatremia: confusion, lethargy, irritability, seizures, coma Gastrointestinal: decreased motility with anorexia, nausea, vomiting; abrupt weight gain *without edema* of 5%–10%
Complications	Electrolyte imbalance; hypovolemia; hypotension; shock	Seizures; coma; permanent brain damage; disease processes already in progress may be complicated
Diagnosis	Urine: output—a few liters to 18 L/day; specific gravity 1.005; osmolality <200 mOsm/kg H_2O Plasma osmolality ↑ secondary to hypovolemia and dehydration Serum Na$^+$ ↑ secondary to hypovolemia and dehydration Serum osmolality >290 mOsm/kg H_2O Serum Na$^+$ ↓ secondary to volume depletion Water deprivation study: positive results Hypertonic saline test: positive for DI if there is little or no ↑ in plasma ADH levels	Serum Na$^+$ ↓; urine Na$^+$ ↑; blood urea nitrogen ↑; serum osmolality ↓; urine osmolality ↑; absence of hypotension, hypovolemia, or edematous states; water load test: positive for SIADH, abnormal water excretion; serum Na$^+$ remains ↓; serum osmolality remains ↓; urine osmolality remains ↑
Surgical management	Hypophysectomy to remove posterior pituitary tumor	None
Medical management	IV fluids; ADH replacement with DDAVP (desmopressin) IV, SQ, or intranasal; nasal solution bid is drug of choice; onset of action is 1 hr, 6–24 hours duration; pitressin tannate in oil is given IM; aqueous pitressin is used for acute, transient form of DI	Hypertonic IV fluids to correct hyponatremia; sodium restriction; diuretics to correct low plasma osmolality; monitor urine electrolyte loss; replace electrolyte loss; demeclocycline to facilitate free water clearance; treat the underlying cause
Nursing management	1. Know which clients are at risk 2. Monitor intake and output 3. Monitor for excessive thirst or urination 4. Assess serum and urine values: ↓ specific gravity, ↓ urine osmolality, ↑ serum osmolality, are early indicators of DI 5. Observe effects of DI on concurrent medical and surgical disorders 6. Client and family teaching	1. Know which clients are at risk 2. Monitor appropriate urine and serum laboratory tests 3. Assess for manifestations of hyponatremia by evaluating neurologic status 4. Monitor daily weights and intake and output 5. Observe for changes in concurrent disorders 6. Administer demeclocycline as ordered to interfere with ADH action; monitor for possible nephrotoxicity 7. Monitor for hypernatremia with fluid overcorrection 8. Client and family teaching
Prognosis	Excellent if there is compliance with vasopressin therapy	Dependent on cause and sodium level and serum osmolality; poor for client with bronchogenic carcinoma; seizures and coma contribute to chronic brain dysfunction

lamic-pituitary function. Primary testis dysfunction can involve the seminiferous tubules (germ cells or Sertoli's cells), Leydig's cells, or both. Germ cell abnormalities cause infertility by disrupting spermatogenesis.

Secondary sexual development and virilization are normal because testosterone production is not interrupted.

When Leydig cell function is impaired, testosterone production falls, and virilization is impaired.

Causes of primary hypogonadism include genetic defects, malnutrition, trauma, infection, renal failure, radiation, chemotherapy, and environmental toxins (e.g., lead, alcohol). The cause, however, is usually unknown. Klinefelter's syndrome, a chromosomal anomaly with a 47, XXY chromosome constitution, is an example of a genetic disorder causing primary testicular failure.

Secondary testicular dysfunction is frequently referred to as hypogonadotropic hypogonadism and results from inadequate secretion of gonadotropins. This complication leads to infertility and hypoandrogenism. The extent of LH and FSH deficiency and the age of onset determine clinical manifestations. Prepubertal hypogonadism leads to eunuchoid body proportions, small testes, and lack of virilization.

Examples of secondary hypogonadism include hypothalamic or pituitary tumors, trauma, degenerative lesions, and radiation. Kallmann's syndrome, a deficiency of gonadotropin-releasing hormone (GnRH) production by the hypothalamus, is an example of congenital secondary testicular dysfunction.

Persons with Kallmann's syndrome fail to mature normally because of gonadotropin deficiency. Midline defects such as cleft lip or palate, color blindness, anosmia, and ataxia are common findings in these persons.

Conclusions

Adrenal, pituitary, and gonadal disorders are not common, but are extremely complex and diverse. Obtain a thorough understanding of the adrenal, pituitary, and gonadal anatomy and physiology to help clients with these disorders. Most of these conditions (e.g., hypopituitarism) are acute and affect many body systems, whereas others become chronic and lead to a wide variety of other problems, such as Addison's disease. Teaching is vital to the care of these clients; understand these conditions so that appropriate teaching plans can be initiated.

Thinking Critically

1. The client is a woman with a 9-year history of Addison's disease. Normally, she takes her prescribed doses of a glucocorticoid (dexamethasone [Decadron]) and a mineralocorticoid (fludrocortisone [Florinef]) without fail. She is 29 years old and is otherwise in good health. The client stayed home from work today because she began to experience nausea, vomiting, diarrhea, and fever, with diaphoresis. Because of the nausea and vomiting, she did not take her medications. When her husband returned home at 5:30 PM, he found the client unconscious. What events led to the client's unconsciousness? How might missing her medications have affected the client?

Factors to Consider. What acute disorder do the nausea, vomiting, diarrhea, and fever suggest? What might be their impact on a person with Addison's disease?

2. A 50-year-old woman has been on glucocorticoids for 10 years for asthma. She is admitted to the hospital for sudden onset of severe low back pain. What factors may have contributed to her back pain?

Factors to Consider. What are the potential long-term effects of oral glucocorticoid therapy? What are their manifestations?

3. A 23-year-old man is admitted to your unit for a head injury related to an automobile accident. While doing your hourly checks, you note that his urine output has been 800 ml since the last check. Over the next 3 hours, the client excretes an additional 3000 ml of very clear urine. His BP has dropped, and his urine specific gravity is less than 1.005. What are your priorities for care?

Factors to Consider. Is the urine output within normal limits? How might his urine output be related to his head injury?

Bibliography

1. Ackermann, R. (1994). Adrenal disorders: Know when to act and what tests to give. *Geriatrics, 49*(7), 32–38.
2. Acromegaly Therapy Consensus Development Panel. (1994). Consensus statement: Benefits versus risks of medical therapy for acromegaly. *American Journal of Medicine, 97*(5), 468–473.
3. Anonymous. (1993). Headaches, diabetes insipidus and hyperprolactinemia in a woman with an enlarged pituitary gland. *American Journal of Medicine, 95*(3), 332–339.
4. Aron, D., & Tyrell, J. B. (1994). Glucocorticoids and Adrenal Androgens. In F. Greenspan & J. D. Baxter (Eds.), *Basic and clinical endocrinology* (4th ed., pp. 307–346). Norwalk, CT: Appleton & Lange.
5. Biglieri, E., Kater, C., & Ramsay, D. (1994). Endocrine hypertension. In F. Greenspan & J. Baxter (Eds.), *Basic and clinical endocrinology* (4th ed., pp. 347–369). Norwalk, CT: Appleton & Lange.
6. Birch, C. (1997). Caring for people with endocrine disorders. In J. Luckmann (Ed.), *Saunders manual of nursing care.* Philadelphia: W. B. Saunders.
7. Blevins, L., & Wand, G. (1992). Diabetes insipidus. *Critical Care Medicine, 20*(1), 69–79.
8. Blumenfeld, J. D., et al. (1994). Diagnosis and treatment of primary hyperaldosteronism. *Annals of Internal Medicine, 121*(11), 877–885.
9. Bryce, J. (1994). S.I.A.D.H.—Recognizing and treating syndrome of inappropriate antidiuretic hormone secretion. *Nursing, 24*(4), 33.
10. Chipps, E. (1992). Transsphenoidal surgery for pituitary tumors. *Critical Care Nurse, 12*(1), 30–39.
11. Cryer, P. (1995). Diseases of the sympathochromaffin system. In P. Felg, J. D. Baxter, & L. A. Frohman (Eds.), *Endocrinology and metabolism* (3rd ed., pp. 713–748). New York: McGraw Hill.
12. Edwards, C. (1995). Primary mineralocorticoid excess syndromes. In L. DeGroot (Ed.), *Endocrinology* (3rd ed., pp. 1775–1803). Philadelphia: W. B. Saunders.
13. Epstein, C. D. (1991). Fluid volume deficit for the adrenal crisis patient. *Dimensions of Critical Care Nursing, 10*(4), 210–217.
14. Ezzat, S., et al. (1994) Acromegaly—Clinical and biochemical features in 500 patients. *Medicine (Baltimore), 73*(5), 233–240.
15. Fazio, S., et al. (1994). Impaired cardiac performance is a distinct feature of uncomplicated acromegaly. *Journal of Clinical Endocrinology and Metabolism, 79*(2), 441–446.
16. Flogstad, A. K., et al. (1994). A comparison of octreotide, bromocriptine or a combination of both drugs in acromegaly. *Journal of Clinical Endocrinology and Metabolism, 79*(2), 461–465.
17. Freda, P., et al. (1994). Primary adrenal insufficiency in patients with the acquired immunodeficiency syndrome: A report of five cases. *Journal of Clinical Endocrinology and Metabolism, 79*(6), 1540–1545.

18. Giefer, C., & Cassemeyer, V. (1994). The syndrome of primary aldosteronism: A case study. *Medical Surgical Nursing, 3*(4), 277–284.

19. Go, H., et al. (1995). Laparoscopic adrenalectomy for Cushing's syndrome: Comparison with primary hyperaldosteronism. *Surgery, 117*(1), 11–17.

20. Goldfien, A. (1994). Adrenal medulla. In F. Greenspan & J. D. Baxter (Eds.), *Basic and clinical endocrinology* (4th ed, pp. 371–390). Norwalk, CT: Appleton & Lange.

21. Grinspoon, S. K., & Biller, B. (1994). Laboratory assessment of adrenal insufficiency. *Journal of Clinical Endocrinology and Metabolism, 7*(4), 923–931.

22. Guzaaoni, G., et al. (1994). Effectiveness and safety of laparoscopic adrenalectomy. *Journal of Urology, 152*(5), 1375–1378.

23. Handerhan, B. (1992). Recognizing adrenal crisis. *American Journal of Nursing, 22*(4), 33.

24. Jenkins, P. J., et al. (1995). The long term outcome after adrenalectomy and prophylactic pituitary radiotherapy in adrenocorticotropin-dependent Cushing's syndrome. *Journal of Clinical Endocrinology and Metabolism, 80*(1), 165–171.

25. Katz, E., & Adashi, E. (1990). Hyperprolactinemic disorders. *Clinical Obstetrics and Gynecology, 33*(3), 621–639.

26. Keiser, H. (1995). Pheochromocytoma and related tumors. In L. DeGroot (Ed.), *Endocrinology* (3rd ed., pp. 1853–1877). Philadelphia: W. B. Saunders.

27. Keljo, D. J., & Squires, R. H. Jr. (1996). Clinical problem-solving: Just in time. *New England Journal of Medicine, 334*(1), 46–48.

28. Lindaman, C. (1992) S.I.A.D.H.—is your patient at risk? *Nursing, 22*(6), 60–63.

29. Loriauz, D. L., & McDonald, W. J. (1995). Adrenal insufficiency. In L. DeGroot (Ed.), *Endocrinology,* 3rd ed., pp. 1731–1740). Philadelphia: W. B. Saunders.

30. Ludwig-Beymer, P., Huether, S., & Gray, D. P. (1993). Alterations of hormonal regulations. In K. McCance & S. Huether (Eds.), *Pathophysiology: The biologic basis for disease in adults and children* (2nd ed., pp. 656–707). St. Louis: Mosby–Year Book.

31. Miller, W., & Tyrell, J. B. (1995). The adrenal cortex. In P. Felig, J. D. Baxter, & L. A. Frohman (Eds.), *Endocrinology and metabolism* (pp. 555–711). New York: McGraw-Hill.

32. Nalbach, D., & Carson, M. (1991). Prolactinoma: A review and case study. *Critical Care Nurse, 11*(9), 48–49, 52–57.

33. Nieman, L., & Cutler, G. B. (1995). Cushing's syndrome. In L. DeGroot (Ed.), *Endocrinology* (3rd ed., pp. 1741–1769). Philadelphia: W. B. Saunders.

34. Norbiato, G., et al. (1992). Cortisol resistance in acquired immunodeficiency syndrome. *Journal of Clinical Endocrinology and Metabolism, 74*(3), 608–613.

35. Peterson, A., & Drass, J. (1993). How to keep adrenal insufficiency in check. *American Journal of Nursing, 93*(10), 36–39.

36. Schamess, A., Bernik, T., & Tenner, S. (1994). Refractory hypertension in Conn's syndrome. *Postgraduate Medicine, 95*(4), 199–206.

37. Shannon, M., Wilson, B. A., & Stang, C. (Eds.). (1995). *Govanni and Hayes Drugs and Nursing Implications* (8th ed.). Norwalk, CT: Appleton & Lange.

38. Shuey, K. (1994). Heart, lung and endocrine complications of solid tumors. *Seminars in Oncology Nursing, 10*(3), 177–188.

39. Siegel, R., & Melby, J. (1994). Fatigue: The role of adrenal insufficiency. *Hospital Practice, 29*(7), 59–71.

40. Sterns, R. (1991). The management of hyponatremic emergencies. *Critical Care Clinics, 7*(1), 127–142.

41. Stoffer, S. S. (1993). Addison's disease. *Postgraduate Medicine, 93*(4), 265–276.

42. Tyrell, J. B., Findling, J. W., & Aron, D. C. (1994). Hypothalamus and pituitary. In F. Greenspan, & J. D. Baxter (Eds.), *Basic and clinical endocrinology* (4th ed., pp. 64–127). Norwalk, CT: Appleton & Lange.

43. Weigel, R., et al. (1994). Surgical treatment of primary hyperaldosteronism. *Annals of Surgery, 219*(4), 347–352.

44. Werbel, S., & Ober, K. P. (1993). Acute adrenal insufficiency. *Endocrinology and Metabolic Clinics of North America, 22*(2), 303–328.

45. Werbel, S., & Ober, K. P. (1995). Pheochromocytoma. *Medical Clinics of North America, 79*(1), 131–153.

46. Yucha, C., & Suddaby, P. (1992). Assessing diabetes insipidus with the dehydration test. *Nursing, 22*(5), 32DD–32FF.

47. Zeiger, M. A., et al. (1993). Effective reversibility of the signs and symptoms of hypercortisolism by bilateral adrenalectomy. *Surgery, 114*(6), 1138–1143.

Musculoskeletal Disorders

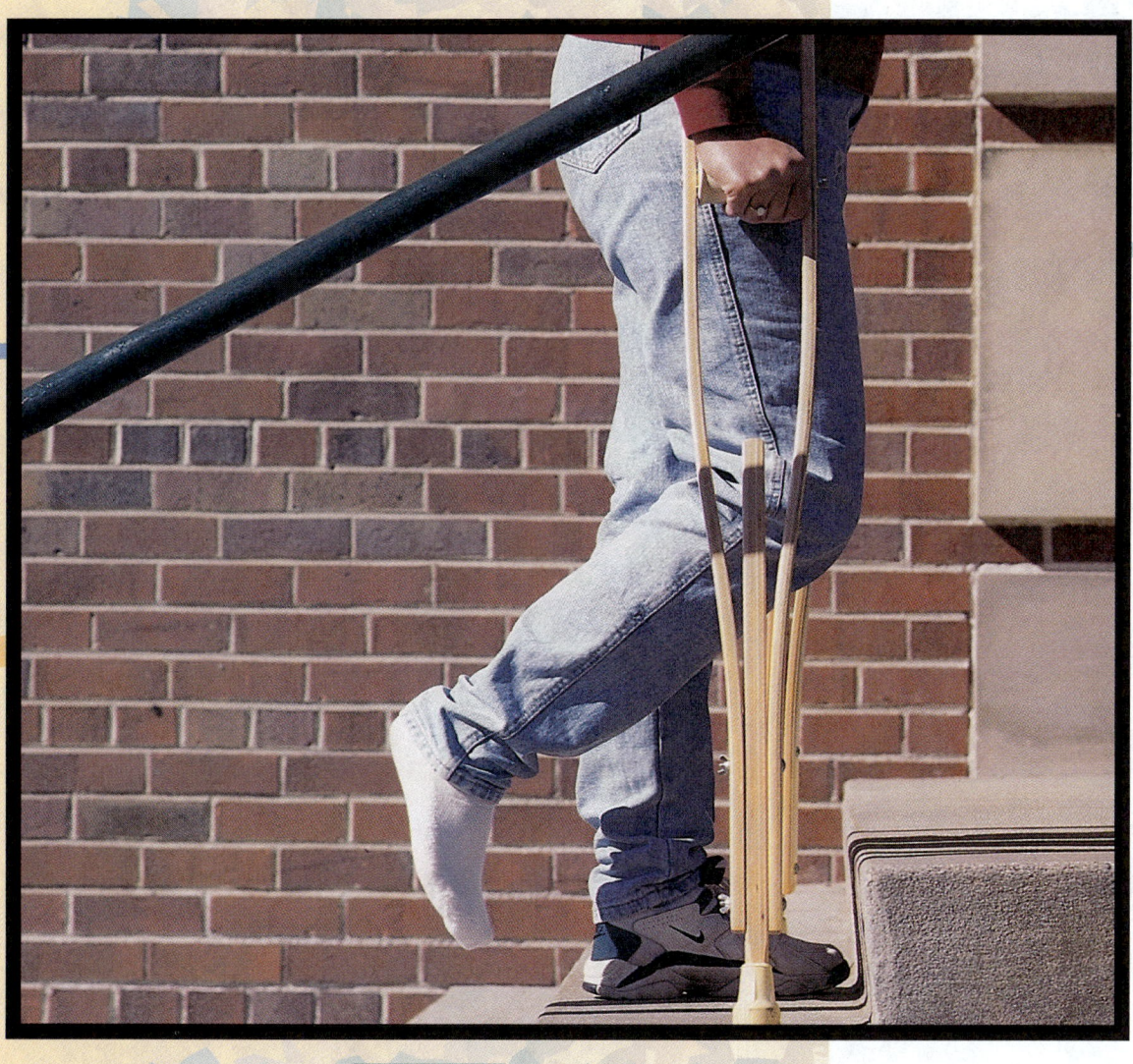

Structure and Function of the Musculoskeletal System

Joyce M. Black

Physiologically, the musculoskeletal system enables movement and position changes. The bony skeleton provides support and movable parts.

Muscles facilitate movement. Movement serves two general purposes. First, movement is necessary to perform normal activities of daily living. Second, movement in itself is a source of pleasure. Interest has increased in performing activities that contribute to physical fitness. This is partly because such activities promote physical health and also because they are enjoyable. People who participate in exercise programs describe feelings of well-being from regular physical activity.

Structure of the Skeletal System

The human skeleton is an endoskeleton (i.e., it lies *within* the soft tissues of the body). It is composed of living tissue that is capable of growth, adaptation, and repair.

The body contains 206 bones, which are divided into two major categories: the axial and appendicular skeletons. The axial skeleton comprises 80 bones, which include the skull, vertebral column, and thorax. The appendicular skeleton comprises 126 bones, which include the bones of the legs, arms, shoulders, and pelvis (Fig. 72–1). Our review will first examine the structure of the skeleton, then its functions. The same format is used for a discussion of muscles.

Bone Classification According to Shape

Long Bones. Most of the long bones are found in the upper and lower extremities. They are longer than they are wide (Fig. 72–2A). The humerus, radius, ulna, femur, tibia, fibula, and phalanges are the long bones.

Short Bones. Short bones (e.g., carpals, tarsals) do not have a long axis.

Flat Bones. Examples of flat bones are the ribs, skull, scapula, and portions of the pelvic girdle. Flat bones protect soft body parts or provide large surfaces for muscle attachments.

Irregular Bones. Irregular bones are of differing shapes, such as vertebrae, ear ossicles, mandible, and pelvis. Irregular bones are similar to other bones in structure and composition.

Structure of Bones

Gross Anatomy

A typical long bone has a shaft, called a *diaphysis*, and two ends called *proximal* and *distal epiphyses* (see Fig. 72–2). The diaphysis is a hollow cylinder of compact bone that surrounds a medullary cavity. The medullary cavity is a fat-storage site and is sometimes called the *yellow bone marrow cavity*. It is lined with a thin connective tissue layer called *endosteum*. The epiphyses are the ends of the bone from which bone grows. In children and young adults, the ends of the epiphyses are separated from the diaphyses by epiphyseal cartilage or plates. In adults, when bone growth is complete, the epiphyseal cartilage is replaced with bone, which joins it to the diaphysis. Fractures of the epiphyseal plates in children can lead to slow bone growth or limb shortening.

Bones are covered with a double layer of connective tissue called *periosteum* (see Fig. 72–2B). The outer layer of periosteum is well supplied with blood vessels and nerves, some of which enter the bone through Volkmann's canals (see Fig. 72–2C). The inner layer is anchored to the bone by bundles of collagen called *Sharpey's fibers*. There is no periosteum in joints, which are covered with articular cartilage.

This chapter incorporates material written for the fourth edition by Darrell A. Follman.

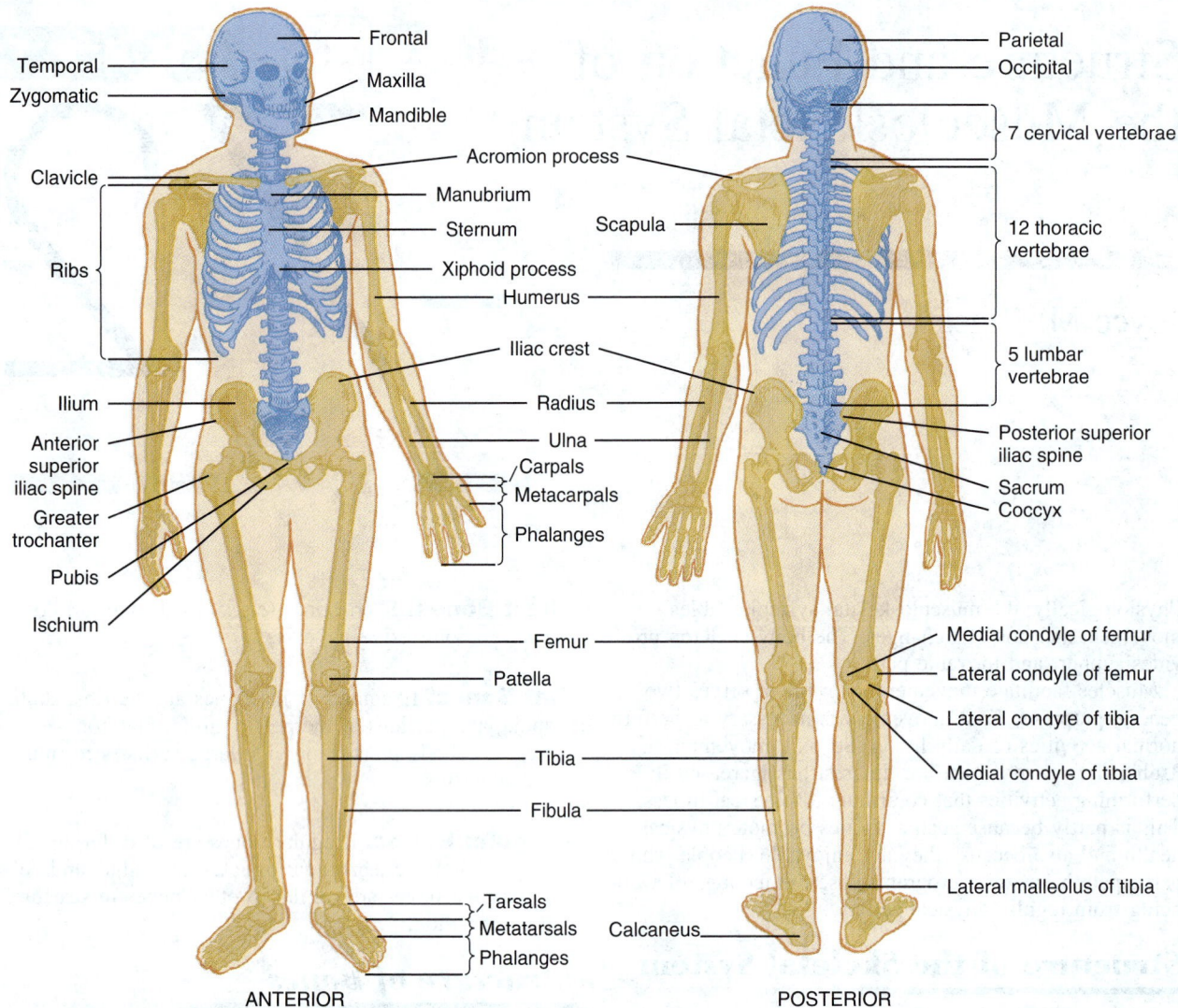

Figure 72-1. The human skeleton is composed of 206 bones. The axial skeleton is shown in blue, and the appendicular skeleton is shown in brown.

Microscopic Anatomy

When viewed through a microscope, compact bone is highly organized and solid. Compact bone is organized into structural units, called *haversian systems*. Each haversian unit contains a central canal, called the *haversian canal*; concentric layers of bone matrix, called *lamellae*; tiny spaces between the lamellae, called *lacunae*, which contain osteocytes; and small channels, called *canaliculi* (see Fig. 72–2D). Each haversian system looks like a separate cylinder, and together they resemble concentric rings. The large haversian canal runs through the center of long bones and contains blood vessels and nerves. The blood vessels transport nutrients to the bone and carry wastes away from the bone. Each haversian unit contains at least one capillary.

Spongy bone does not have the organizational structure of compact bone. The lamellae are not arranged in concentric circles. Rather, they are arranged in various directions that correspond with the lines of maximum pressure of tension placed on the bone. Spongy bone does have osteocytes embedded in lacunae, and lacunae intercommunicate via canaliculi. Blood reaches the osteocytes by passing through spaces in the bone marrow.

Composition of Bone

The organic framework is formed from collagen, which is similar to the collagen found in other connective tissues. Collagen provides bone with great tensile strength so that it can withstand stretching and twisting. The salts allow bone to withstand compression. The combination of collagen and salt makes bone exceptionally strong without being brittle. The composition of bone is analogous to that of reinforced concrete, which is used in construction. Steel rods provide tensile strength, and cement, sand, and gravel provide compression strength.

Bone contains three types of cells: (1) osteoblasts, (2) osteocytes, and (3) osteoclasts. Osteoblasts are bone-forming cells; they lay down new bone. Osteocytes are osteo-

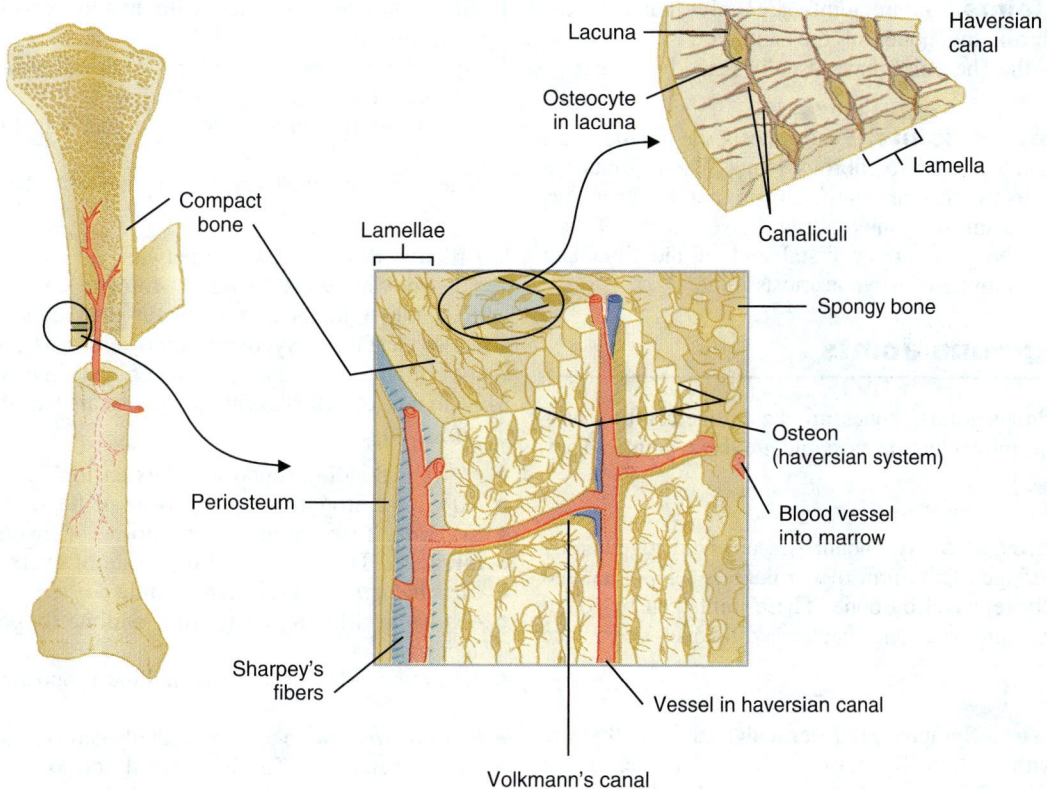

Figure 72-2. Structure of a long bone.

blasts that are found in the bone matrix. Osteoclasts are cells that resorb (remove) damaged or old bone cells during periods of growth or repair. Bone cells allow bone to grow, repair itself, and change shape. Even mature bone constantly changes, with new cells being formed and old cells being destroyed. The bone cells are surrounded by extracellular elements of tissue, called the *bone matrix*. The matrix contains collagen, fibers, proteins, carbohydrate-protein complexes, minerals, and ground substance. Ground substance is a gelatinous material that acts as a medium for the diffusion of nutrients, oxygen, and metabolic wastes between bone cells and blood vessels.

Function of the Skeletal System

Bones give form to the body: they support various tissues and organs and permit movement by providing attachments for tendons and ligaments. The skull and rib cage, for example, provide protection for the brain and special senses and lungs, respectively. Movement of the body is permitted by the articulation of joints and their attached muscles.

Bone houses the hematopoietic system, which manufactures blood cells. The marrow cavities within various bones serve as sites for blood cell formation. In adults, blood cells form in marrow cavities in the skull, vertebrae, ribs, sternum, shoulder, and pelvis. There are two types of bone marrow: yellow and red. The yellow marrow is found in the shafts of long bones and extends into the haversian systems. Yellow marrow is connective tissue that is composed of fat cells. Yellow marrow does not produce blood cells, except during times of increased blood cell need. Red marrow has the hematopoietic function (manufactures red and white blood cells). Red marrow is located in the cancellous bone spaces, found in flat bones. (See Chapter 51 for more information on blood cell production.)

Structure and Function of the Articular System

Articulations (joints) are places of union between two or more bones. Not all joints permit movement.

Types of Joints

Categorization of joints is according to degree of movement.

Fibrous Joints

Fibrous joints are articulations in which bones are held together by fibrous connective tissue. Very little material separates the ends of the bone, and little, if any, movement is possible. The edges of bone, called *sutures*, are grooves (also called *interdigitations*) that fit firmly together.

Suture Joints. Suture joints are only found in the skull. At birth, the bones of the skull are separated, to facilitate birth. The bones have usually fused by 2 years.

Syndesmosis Joints. Syndesmosis, or ligamentous, joints are another form of fibrous joints. These joints are held together by ligaments, which are not as strong as sutures. Syndesmosis joints allow "give" but not true movement. The joint at the distal end of the tibia and fibula is an example of a syndesmosis joint.

Cartilaginous Joints

In cartilaginous joints, bones are held together by cartilage. Slight movement is possible in these joints. They are of two types.

Synchondroses. Synchondroses are held together by hyaline cartilage. This form of cartilage is temporary and is eventually replaced by bone. These joints can be found between the epiphyses and diaphyses of bones and in the ribs.

Symphyses. Symphyses are articular surfaces that are covered with a thin layer of hyaline cartilage. Slight movement is allowed. Within the joint, the surfaces act as shock absorbers. The vertebrae are separated by symphyses.

Synovial Joints

Most of the joints in the body are synovial joints. They are freely movable, permitting position and motion changes. Synovial joints have four characteristics:

1. Bone surfaces are lined with hyaline cartilage called *articular cartilage*
2. Synovial membrane produces synovial fluid for joint lubrication and cartilage nourishment
3. Ligaments reinforce the capsule and help to limit motion
4. The joint is enclosed by an articular capsule (Fig. 72–3).

Articular discs are located between articular cartilage of some synovial joints to buffer forceful impact. Muscles help stabilize joints and maintain firm contact between articular surfaces. Synovial joints are classified by the shape of the articulating end of the involved bones. Movements of which synovial joints are capable include the following:

- *Flexion.* Bending (opposite of extension)
- *Extension.* Straightening (opposite of flexion)
- *Eversion.* Turning outward (opposite of inversion)
- *Inversion.* Turning inward (opposite of eversion)
- *Circumduction.* Moving in a circle
- *Abduction.* Moving away from midline (opposite of adduction)
- *Adduction.* Moving toward midline (opposite of abduction)
- *Internal rotation.* Turning medially on axis
- *External rotation.* Turning laterally on axis
- *Supination.* Facing upward, such as turning palm upward or forward (opposite of pronation)
- *Pronation.* Facing downward (e.g., turning palm downward or backward) (opposite of supination)
- *Protraction.* Drawing a body part, such as the mandible, forward (opposite of retraction)
- *Retraction.* Drawing a body part backward (opposite of protraction)

Various joint motions are shown in Chapter 73.

Figure 72-3. Structure of a synovial joint.

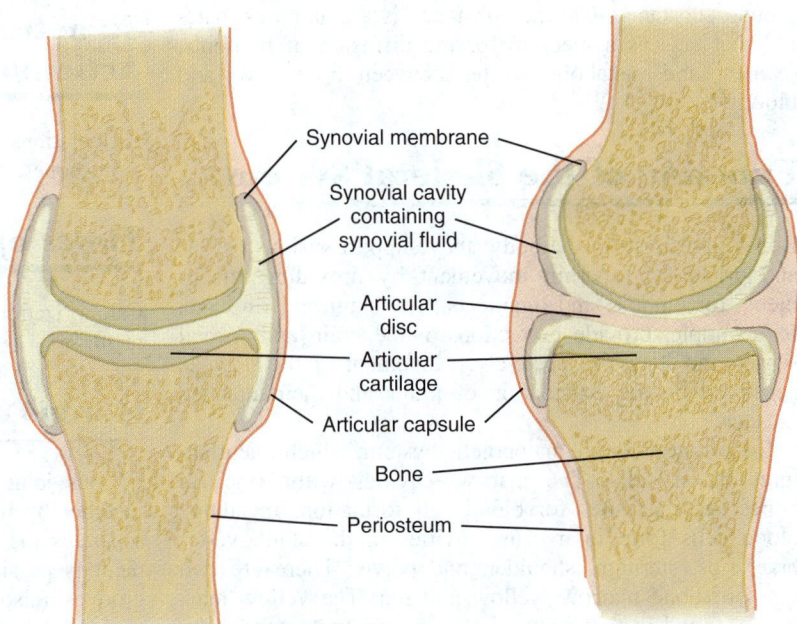

Synovial membrane

Synovial cavity containing synovial fluid

Articular disc

Articular cartilage

Articular capsule

Bone

Periosteum

Bursae and Tendon Sheaths

Synovial joints have two other structures that, although not actually a part of the joint, are associated with them. *Bursae* are small sacs lined with synovial membrane and filled with synovial fluid (Fig. 72–4). They act as cushions between structures. There are hundreds of bursae in the body. Some are subcutaneous, lying between bone and skin (e.g., the bursa between the olecranon process of the elbow and the skin). Most bursae lie between tendons and bones.

Tendon sheaths are cylindrical synovial discs similar to bursae. They are found where tendons cross joints and may be subject to constant friction. The sheath wraps around the tendon, forming a fluid-filled cushion for the tendon to slide through.

Ligaments

Ligaments connect bones at joints and provide stability during movement. Some ligaments, which are commonly injured, are briefly highlighted here.

In the shoulder joint, the head of the humerus is held in the shallow glenoid fossa of the scapula. It is loosely constructed and permits free movement, but it often dislocates. Two ligaments in the shoulder maintain joint stability: the coracohumeral ligament and the glenohumeral ligament.

The knee is a complicated joint and is prone to injury. The knee is a hinge joint, and it contains ligaments that restrict any other movements. The knee is stabilized medially by medial and collateral ligaments, which extend from the condyles of the femur to the tibia. The patellar ligament provides anterior strength. Additional knee stability is gained by the anterior and posterior cruciate ligaments. These ligaments extend diagonally from the superior surface of the tibia to the distal end of the femur, between the condyles (Fig. 72–5). When the knee is extended, the anterior cruciate ligament is taut, prevent-

ing overextension. When the knee is flexed, the posterior cruciate ligament becomes taut, preventing posterior slipping.

Structure and Function of the Muscular System

Muscles make up 40% to 50% of body weight. Muscles produce movement by contraction. Muscles also line tubes in the body to propel blood upward in the legs and excrete urine and feces. Muscles produce heat that is used to maintain body temperature. We will examine the structure of muscles and their function.

Types of Muscle

The body contains three types of muscles: skeletal, cardiac, and smooth muscle.

Gross Anatomy

■ Skeletal Muscle

Skeletal, or striated, muscle attaches to bones of the skeleton. The contraction of skeletal muscle exerts force on bones and moves them.

Skeletal muscle is voluntary muscle of the skeletal system. In most situations, however, the movement of skeletal muscle does not require conscious thought. (For example, you do not have to consciously think about moving your eyes or head to read this paragraph.)

When viewed through the microscope, muscle has transverse light and dark bands that give it a striped or *striated* appearance. Skeletal muscle is controlled by the somatic division of the peripheral nervous system.

Skeletal muscles are named according to (1) action (e.g., flexor, extensor); (2) shape (e.g., quadrilateral, pennate); (3) origin (i.e., stationary attachment of muscle to skeleton); (4) insertion (i.e., movable attachment of the

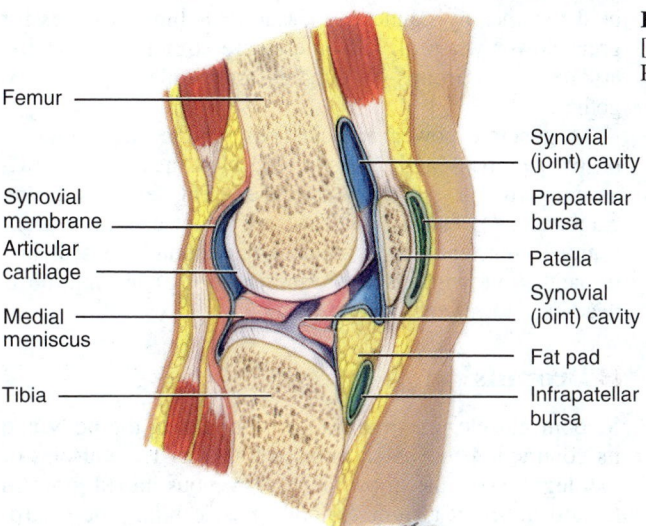

Figure 72-4. The bursa of the knee. (From Applegate, E. J. [1995]. *The anatomy and physiology learning system: Textbook.* Philadelphia: W. B. Saunders.)

Femur

Synovial membrane

Articular cartilage

Medial meniscus

Tibia

Synovial (joint) cavity

Prepatellar bursa

Patella

Synovial (joint) cavity

Fat pad

Infrapatellar bursa

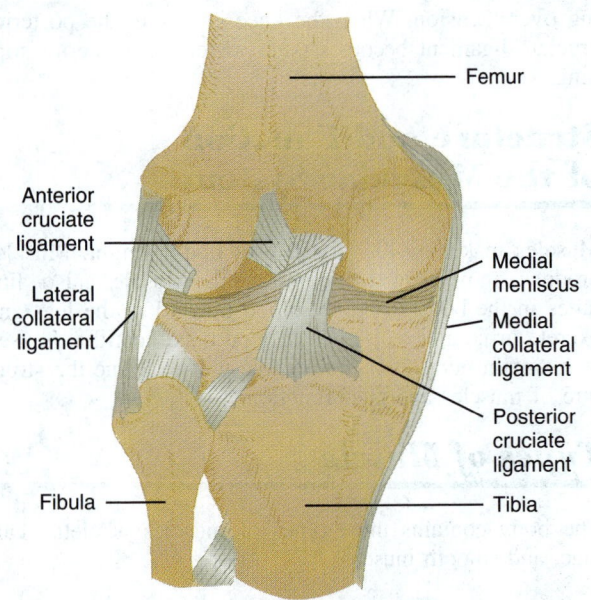

Femur

Anterior
cruciate
ligament

Lateral
collateral
ligament

Medial
meniscus

Medial
collateral
ligament

Posterior
cruciate
ligament

Fibula

Tibia

Figure 72-5. Ligaments provide stability for the knee. When the knee is extended, the taut anterior cruciate ligament prevents overextension. When the knee is flexed, the posterior cruciate ligament prevents the tibia from slipping posteriorly.

muscle); (5) number of divisions; (6) location; or (7) direction of fibers (i.e., transverse). Principal muscle groups are shown in Figure 72–6.

When viewed directly, skeletal muscle is composed of many individual muscle cells, called *muscle fibers*. These fibers are held together by thin sheets of fibrous connective tissue called *fascia*. Fascia also penetrates the muscle, separating it into bundles called *fasciculi*.

Skeletal muscle is attached to the bones of the skeleton by very thin extensions of fascia or by tendons. Tendons make a strong connection to bone.

■ Cardiac Muscle

Cardiac muscle, or myocardium, is involuntary muscle that occurs only in the heart. It is striated crosswise and lengthwise. Cardiac muscle is controlled by intrinsic factors (e.g., the amount of venous return to the right atrium), hormones, and signals from the autonomic nervous system. Cardiac muscle is discussed in Chapter 43.

■ Smooth Muscle

Smooth muscle is so named because it does not have the striations that are evident in skeletal muscle cells. This type of muscle is involuntary and nonstriated, and it is present in hollow structures (e.g., the digestive tract, blood vessels, and urinary bladder) and in other areas (e.g., the eye). The muscle is involuntary and controlled by the autonomic nervous system, hormones, and intrinsic factors in the muscle (e.g., food in the intestine).

Microscopic Anatomy

Under microscopic examination, muscle cells have many nuclei and are grouped into threadlike myofibrils. If you look closely at the myofibrils you can see alternating bands of light and dark, producing the visible striations. We can further divide the muscle cell into smaller segments, called *sarcomeres*. The sarcomere is the structure in the muscle where the actual contraction occurs. The sarcomeres are delimited by Z bands. Two bands are present in the sarcomere: a thick filament and a thin filament. The filaments are proteins that attach and cause the muscle to contract. Bands have also been labeled with letters, A or I, based on their appearance. The *sarcolemma* is the thin protective membrane that envelops every muscle fiber.

Functions of Muscle

■ Movement

Muscle contraction occurs when a stimulus excites an individual muscle fiber (see Fig. 72–7). The stimulus, a nerve impulse, releases stored acetylcholine from the end of the motor neuron. The acetylcholine crosses the neuromuscular junction and elicits an action potential (e.g., stimulatory electrical impulse). The action potential triggers the attachment of the thin and thick filaments in the sarcomere. Nerve fibers may supply more than 100 individual muscle cells. A continuous flow of stimuli maintains muscle tone (i.e., keeps muscles partially contracted, in a state of readiness for movement).

Muscle fibers relax between contractions because calcium ions that are released during the action potential are free only for a short time. Calcium quickly returns to storage in the sarcoplasmic reticulum in the muscle. If nerve impulses arrive in rapid succession so that calcium remains free, the muscle will continue to contract (called *spasm*).

Obviously, a single sarcomere does not have much power. Muscle fibers are arranged in bundles (fasciculi) held together by connective tissue. Bundling provides for great power when all sarcomeres are stimulated to action at one time. Groups of bundles are similarly bound together.

To generate power, muscle cells require large amounts of oxygen (O_2) and glucose. Muscles thus have a rich vascular (blood) supply. An oxygen debt develops during exercise if O_2 cannot be delivered to muscles in concentrations great enough to metabolize accumulations of lactic acid. Following exercise, increased O_2 consumption is necessary to relieve oxygen debt.

■ Propulsion

Smooth muscle lines the hollow conduits in the body and its contraction moves substances forward. The muscles of the legs assist the movement of venous blood upward toward the right atrium. Smooth muscle lining the gastro-

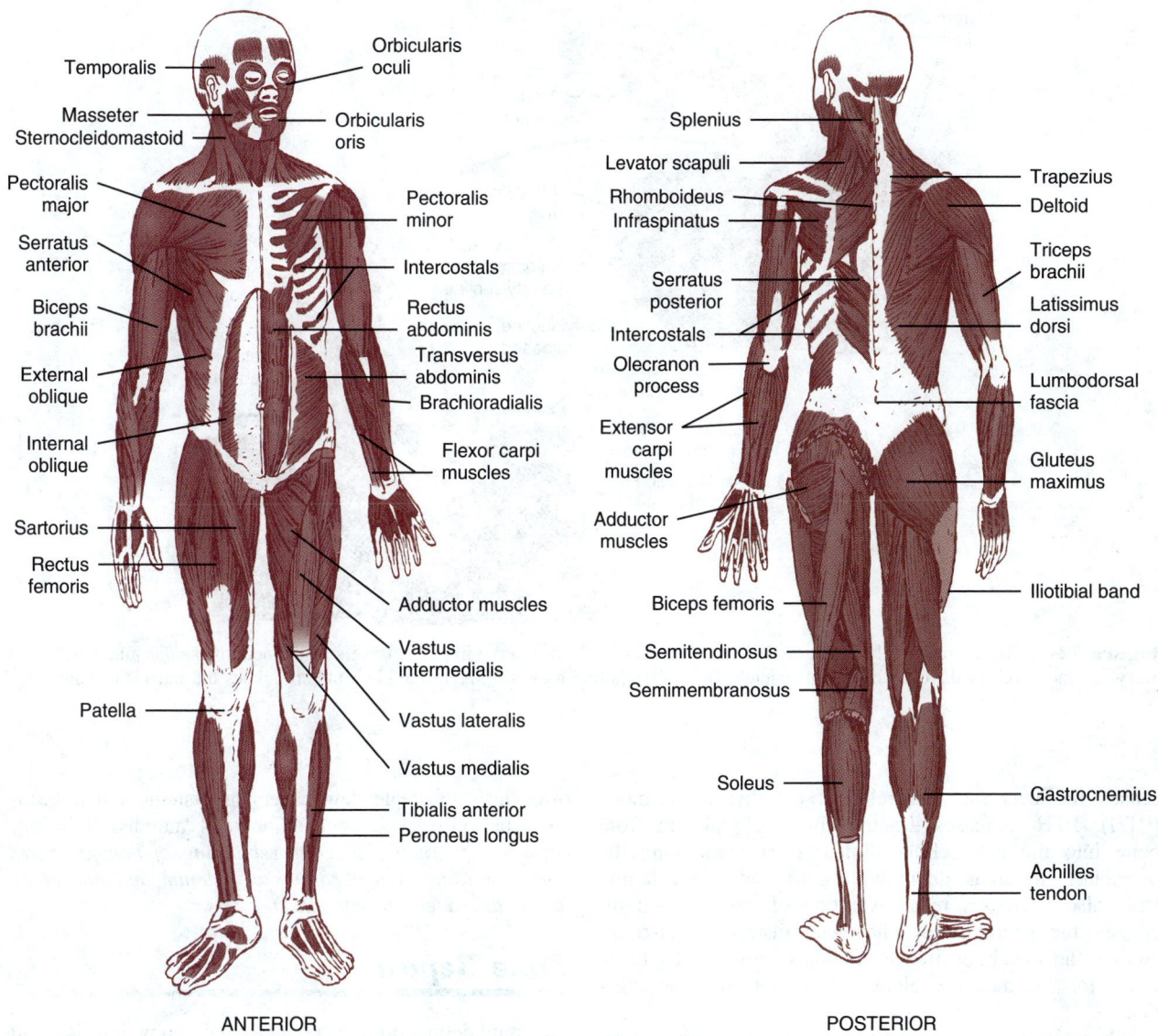

Figure 72-6. Principal muscle groups.

intestinal tract propels food through the tract during digestion. Finally, muscle in arterioles regulates arterial blood flow by causing vasodilation and vasoconstriction.

■ Heat Production

The activity of skeletal muscle produces body heat. Some of this heat can be used to maintain body temperature. During exercise, excess heat is released through sweating and vasodilation. When the body is cold, heat is generated by shivering.

Cartilage

Cartilage is a type of dense connective tissue that is prevalent throughout the musculoskeletal system. It can resist forces of tension and compression with considerable resilience. It is semiopaque (bluish white or gray) and has limited nerve and blood supply. Cartilage forms most of the skeleton of an embryo. Most of this cartilage gradually changes into bone by ossification. Three types of cartilage are found in the body: (1) hyaline cartilage, found in the respiratory tract, in developing bones, and at the ends of articulating bones; (2) fibrocartilage, found in certain ligaments and intervertebral discs; and (3) elastin cartilage, found in the nose and ears.

The Role of the Musculoskeletal System in Homeostasis

Bones also provide a crucial portion of mineral balance. Calcium, phosphorus, sodium, potassium, and other minerals are stored within the bones. These minerals can be mobilized and distributed as needed by other body systems. Bones store and release minerals for cellular metabolism. When blood levels of calcium fall, the parathyroid

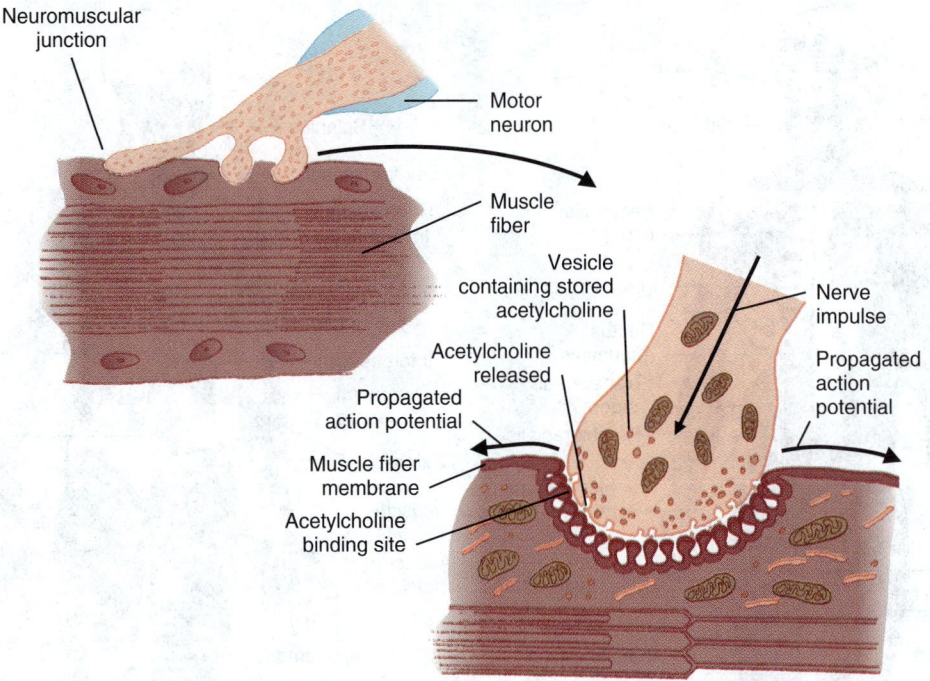

Figure 72-7. The neuromuscular junction. When a stimulus, such as a nerve impulse, travels to the neuromuscular junction, acetylcholine is released from storage in vesicles. The acetylcholine moves throught the cleft and stimulates the muscle to contract.

senses the decrease and releases parathyroid hormone (PTH). PTH increases the movement of calcium from bone into the extracellular fluids. PTH stimulating the osteoclasts to break down bone cells and free calcium. PTH also decreases renal excretion of calcium and increases the excretion of phosphate instead. It also increases the metabolic transformation of vitamin D_3 to its active form to increase calcium absorption from the intestine.

When serum calcium levels are high, calcitonin, a hormone from the thyroid gland, lowers plasma calcium. Calcitonin inhibits calcium removal from bone. Thus, the action of calcitonin is the opposite of the action of PTH.

Bone Remodeling

Throughout life the bone mass is continuously undergoing well-regulated processes of bone formation and bone resorption. The process of bone turnover is called *remodeling,* and it is one of the major mechanisms for maintaining calcium balance in the body. As much as 15% of the total bone mass normally turns over each year.

Remodeling is a three-phase process by which existing bone is resorbed and new bone is laid down to replace it. The cycle begins when a stimulus, such as a hormone, drug, or stressor, activates the bone cell precursors to become osteoclasts. In the second phase, osteoclasts gradually resorb the bone. They leave behind an elongated cavity, called a *resorption cavity.* The cavity matches the general structure of the haversian system or trabeculae. The third phase involves the laying down of new bone by the osteoblasts. The osteoblasts follow the path of the

osteoclasts to create new haversian systems and trabeculae. The entire process takes about 4 months. *It is very important to realize that the rebuilding of bone requires normal plasma concentrations of calcium and phosphate and is dependent on vitamin D.*

Bone Repair

The remodeling process repairs small bony injuries, but fractures and other wounds of bone heal in a different manner. Initially, the bone heals by forming a hematoma. The hematoma's fibrin provides a meshwork, which is the initial framework for healing. Granulation tissue is produced, called a *procallus.* Osteoblasts deposit disorganized clumps of bone matrix, or callus. The trabeculae and haversian systems follow. Finally, the bony edges are remodeled to the size and shape of the bone before injury.

Effects of Aging on the Musculoskeletal System

Aging affects bone, muscle, and tendons. Bone tissue is lost. The haversian systems in compact bone erode. The lacunae enlarge, and the outer surface becomes thin and porous. Eventually, the rate of loss exceeds the rate of growth. Cartilage becomes more rigid and fragile, and muscle bulk and strength decrease.[2] Skeletal muscle is replaced with fat. As muscle mass decreases, so does maximal strength, which can decline by 50% between 20 and 50 years. Several theories have been offered to explain these changes. Changes in activity, reduced circulation, cardiovascular disorders, and nutritional problems are often cited.

Disorders of the Musculoskeletal System

Musculoskeletal disorders are very common. Fractures, or broken bones, are due to forces applied to the bone that exceed its tensile or compressive strength. Osteoporosis is a condition of decreased calcium in bone that leads to weak and brittle bones. Disorders seen in the articular surfaces include rheumatoid arthritis and degenerative arthritis. The articular cartilage degenerates, leading to pain and decreased movement. Muscle disorders can be found in the muscle itself, such as muscular dystrophy, which is the progressive degeneration of muscle. Myasthenia gravis is loss of receptors on the muscle for acetylcholine, leading to profound muscle weakness.

Conclusions

The haversian system is the structural unit of bone. The major minerals in bone are calcium and phosphate, which are regulated by PTH and calcitonin. Bone is constantly remodeled, and every 4 months it has been completely replaced. Muscles provide movement, propel substances, and produce heat.

Bibliography

1. Berne, R., & Levy, M. (1993). *Physiology* (3rd ed.). St. Louis: Mosby–Year Book.
2. Guyton, A. (1995). *Textbook of medical physiology* (9th ed.). Philadelphia: W. B. Saunders.
3. Heveron, B., & Kaempffe, F. (1995). Tears of the rotator cuff. *Orthopaedic Nursing, 14*(6), 38–41.
4. McCance, K. L., & Huerther, S. E. (1994). *Pathophysiology* (2nd Ed.). St. Louis: Mosby–Year Book.
5. Mulvey, T. (1988). Anatomy and pathology of the shoulder complex. *Orthopaedic Nursing, 7*(3), 23–28.
6. Solomon, E. P., et al. (1990). *Human anatomy and physiology* (2nd ed.). Philadelphia: W. B. Saunders.
7. Spence, A., & and Mason, E. (1983). *Human anatomy and physiology* (2nd ed.). Menlo Park, CA: Benjamin Cummings.

Assessment of Clients with Musculoskeletal Disorders

Peggy Doheny
Carol Sedlak

Assessment of the client with musculoskeletal disorders involves gathering subjective data and historical data as well as conducting a physical assessment. The health history provides direction for further musculoskeletal system assessment. For example, the musculoskeletal physical examination can be either general (as in a screening examination) or local (for a specific problem or injury). Similarly, diagnostic tests can be either general or specific. These are helpful for making judgments about the client's musculoskeletal status based on data obtained from interviews, physical findings, and diagnostic tests.

Musculoskeletal assessment usually includes the client's functional abilities to perform activities of daily living (ADL) and to meet self-care needs. This also includes evaluating exercise habits and leisure activities that promote health. The focus of this chapter is on the assessment of the client's musculoskeletal system. Specifically, we address important historical and physical findings and laboratory and diagnostic tests pertinent to musculoskeletal assessment.

History

The musculoskeletal history includes the client's biographical and demographic data and chief complaint (including symptom analysis), including the past health history, family history, psychosocial history, and life-style data, and review of systems. Information is collected to help determine the nature and extent of the current disorder. If the client's chief complaint is related to trauma, the history interview is brief and focused on the cause of injury, or it may be deferred, depending on the extent of the injury. Once the client's condition is stable, a more complete history is obtained.

Biographical and Demographic Data

Personal information helps the nurse know the client as an individual. This enables individualized care planning.

For example, knowing where the client lives and the kind of transportation used helps the nurse understand the energy expenditure the client needs to keep an appointment. Identifying and getting to know significant others is essential in planning care. The client's age and sex may suggest possible causes of musculoskeletal manifestations. For example, 85% of people over age 70 have some osteoarthritis; osteoporosis occurs most often in postmenopausal women; Reiter's syndrome is most common in men between the ages of 20 and 40; osteogenic sarcoma is rare after age 40; and carpal tunnel syndrome occurs more often in women than in men.

Current Symptoms

Chief Complaint

The client is asked to describe the reason for seeking healthcare. Common clinical manifestations related to the musculoskeletal system include pain, tenderness, muscle tightness, muscle weakness, joint stiffness, cramps, muscle spasms, swelling, redness, deformity, reduced movement or joint range of motion (ROM), sensory changes, and other abnormal sensations. ADL may be affected. Ask the client and significant others to relate their perceptions of the problem and its cause. Their answers often provide not only information about areas for further assessment but also clues about personal fears and concerns.

Symptom Analysis

Conduct a symptom analysis for each manifestation the client reports (see Chapter 11). Examples of assessment questions for typical musculoskeletal manifestations follow.

Pain. Ask the client to point to the pain's exact location. Poorly localized pain is usually associated with problems in blood vessels, joints, fascia, or periosteum.

Ask the client to describe the pain. Is it an ache, a sharp pain, a throbbing? Throbbing pain is usually bone-related and aches are often muscular. Sharp pain is associated with fractures and bone infection. Ask the client to rate his or her pain on a scale of 0 to 10. Pain rating can be a reliable source of data to assess the intensity of pain. Does anything make the pain worse? Temperature changes? Movement? Lifting or carrying something heavy? Pain associated with movement is typical of joint problems. Degenerative hip conditions produce pain during weightbearing and during and after walking. Degenerative knee problems produce pain during and after walking. Vertebral disc herniation produces pain on bending or lifting and tends to radiate down one leg. Pain associated with osteoarthritis is worse in cold, damp weather. Is pain worse at any particular time of day? Does the pain wake the patient or prevent him or her from sleeping at night? Inflammation of bursae or tendons is worse at night. Degenerative joint pain is often worse at the end of a day. Ask the client if the pain is relieved with rest. Most musculoskeletal pain is helped by rest. Ask what medications help relieve the pain. Pain from inflammation is usually helped by aspirin or nonsteroidal anti-inflammatory drugs (NSAIDs). Narcotic analgesics are usually required for traumatic injury. Inquire if the patient has had any recent injuries. Sometimes a client does not relate a fall or other injury with current manifestations. Is the pain associated with chills, fever, rash, or a sore throat? Joint pain occurring 10 to 14 days after a sore throat may be from rheumatic fever.

Joint Stiffness. Ask the client to point to the joints that are stiff. Are the joints always stiff? How long does the stiffness last? Some conditions, such as ankylosing spondylitis, have remissions and exacerbations. Ask at what time of day is the stiffness worst? With degenerative joint disease, stiffness is often most severe in the morning after inactivity in bed. What relieves the stiffness? Temperature changes? Exercise? Coldness and lack of use generally increase joint stiffness. Heat may reduce muscle spasm. Heat applied to a recently injured joint may increase stiffness by increasing bleeding into and swelling of the joint. Does the joint lock? Does the client hear or feel bones rubbing together? Bone malalignment within a joint causes locking (joint cannot move). Crepitus (the sound of bone ends rubbing together) indicates fractures or joint destruction. Is there pain or weakness in muscles with certain movements? Weakness in muscles may be due to various neuromuscular disorders. If weakness is present, does it interfere with the client's usual activities?

Swelling. Ask the client how long he or she has had the swelling. Is there pain? Swelling and pain often accompany bone and muscle injury. With degenerative joint disease, swelling often does not develop for some time, maybe weeks, after pain is present or it may not develop at all. Is movement limited by the swelling? Limited movement is associated with soft tissue damage and swelling within a joint. Does rest give relief? Does ele-

vating the part give relief? Elevation reduces swelling in acute injuries. Ask the client if the body part was casted recently. Removing a cast can precipitate temporary swelling. A casted extremity may have muscle atrophy. Has the area been hot or red? Redness and heat indicate inflammation, infection, or recent injury; and are not usually present with degenerative conditions.

Deformity and Immobility. Has the deformity developed suddenly or gradually? A gradually developing mass may indicate a tumor. Is movement limited? Is movement limitation always present? Is it worse after activity? Does any particular body position make it worse or better? Immobility from degenerative joint disease varies with the severity of the condition. Ask how the deformity affects daily activities? Does the client use any supportive equipment such as crutches, a walker, or bandages? Use of such aids indicates the severity of the disability.

Sensory Changes. Does the client have a history of back pain or injury? If so, where is the pain located? Does the pain travel, for example, down the back of the leg? Does the client have problems walking? Any loss of feeling anywhere? Any tingling or burning sensation? Is loss of feeling associated with any pain? Pressure on nerves or blood vessels can occur from swelling, tumors, or fractures, causing loss of sensation. Sensory changes may be associated with pain in an arm or hand.

Past Health History

Ask the client about a number of past health problems because there are many diseases that can affect the musculoskeletal system. Both childhood and adult-onset disorders are explored because of the possible long-term effects.

Previous trauma, accidents, or surgery involving bones or joints are carefully assessed. The client may have sustained fractures, dislocations, strains, or sprains. Previous accidents leading to bony fracture may predispose the client to degenerative changes.

Childhood and Infectious Diseases

Some health conditions affect the musculoskeletal system either directly or indirectly. For example, diabetes may predispose the client to degenerative joint disease. Blood dyscrasias, such as hemophilia, may cause bleeding in joints that produces pain, swelling, tenderness, and deformity. Psoriasis may precede psoriatic arthritis. Trauma-producing cartilage damage may precipitate degenerative changes in a relatively young person. Ask about a history of tuberculosis, sickle cell anemia, poliomyelitis, inflammatory or degenerative arthritis, scurvy, rickets, osteomyelitis, soft tissue infection, fungus infection of bones or joints, and streptococcal and neuromuscular disorders.

Major Illnesses and Hospitalizations

In addition to diseases such as diabetes mellitus, tuberculosis, poliomyelitis, and arthritis, ask the client about hospitalizations related to musculoskeletal disorders, including trauma. If the client or significant others cannot remember details, ask for permission to obtain the medical records. Ask about past or present minor and major injuries, including the circumstances of the injury, the diagnosis of the injury, the treatment received, the duration of treatment, and any current problems resulting from the injury.

Musculoskeletal injury includes fractures, sprains, strains, and joint dislocations. Some injuries are minor and are treated on an ambulatory basis, whereas others are major and require prolonged hospitalization, surgery, or rest and immobilization. Ask whether the client has any residual impairment from the injury such as a need to use assistive devices, such as a cane, crutches, or walker. Also inquire whether there has been a need to change or adjust ADL because of lingering limitations.

Medications

Question the client carefully about past and present prescription and over-the-counter medications. Ask what the reasons are for taking each medication, and its dose, frequency, how long it was taken, and any observed side effects. Ask specifically about medication used for musculoskeletal problems, such as muscle relaxants, salicylates, NSAIDs, and steroids. Some medications affect the musculoskeletal system. For example, corticosteroids can precipitate necrosis of the head of the femur, leading to septic arthritis, and can also precipitate muscle weakness. High doses of anticoagulants can produce hemarthrosis (blood in joints); anticonvulsants may cause osteomalacia; phenothiazines may produce gait disturbances; potassium-depleting diuretics may produce cramps and muscle weakness; and amphetamines and caffeine cause generalized, increased motor activity. Use of NSAIDs for more than 4 weeks can lead to bleeding problems (especially gastrointestinal bleeding) due to decreased platelet aggregation. Renal and hepatic changes can also develop. Clients taking long-term NSAIDs need to have follow-up laboratory assessments to monitor the side effects of NSAIDs. Usually a complete blood count, urinalysis, liver enzymes, potassium, and creatinine are assessed. For the postmenopausal woman, inquire about use of hormonal replacement therapy with estrogen, which has been shown to modify the effects of osteoporosis.

Family Health History

Genetically related family history is important to identify musculoskeletal problems that have a familial predisposition, such as arthritis, osteoporosis, ankylosing spondylitis, gout, Heberden's nodes in osteoarthritis, muscular dystrophy, and scoliosis. Thirty percent of people with psoriatic arthritis have a family history of psoriasis.

Psychosocial History

The integrity of the musculoskeletal system allows people to function effortlessly. Yet there are many factors that can disrupt that integrity. Inquire about the client's daily activities and habits. When assessing clients with chronic illnesses and degenerative processes, ask if the disorder has affected the client's interactions with others and the client's view of himself or herself. Crippling illnesses often curtail social activity and lower self-esteem.

Occupation

Ask whether heavy lifting or strenuous activity is typical. This can cause muscle strain, degenerative vertebral disc problems, and other trauma. Low back pain can arise from jobs involving a lot of driving. Habitually carrying heavy objects, such as a mailbag, shoulder bag, attaché case, or other equipment, causes musculoskeletal problems by placing uneven pressure on the spinal column. Prolonged use of computers and keyboarding can cause orthopedic injuries (see Chapter 75 for discussion of repetitive strain injury).

Daily Activities

Are there any everyday activities that the client finds difficult or impossible, such as opening containers, pouring liquids, cutting up food; dressing; using zippers; fastening or unfastening buttons, snaps, or hooks; grooming; combing hair; applying make-up; running a bath and testing the water temperature; washing the hair; shaving; writing; getting out of the house; climbing stairs; or getting in and out of chairs or cars? Ask if there is anything in everyday life the client wants to do that manifestations prevent.

Try to ascertain the client's attention to safety. Ask about safety practices at work and at home. Does the client use the recommended equipment for recreational activities, such as correct shoes? Does the client use safety guards when using power tools? There is a high incidence of accidental injury among people who pay little attention to safety practices.

Exercise

Document details of the client's typical recreational activities and exercise pattern. Lack of exercise produces poor muscle tone, which leads to muscle strain. Sporadic exercise of poorly toned muscles causes muscle injury and spasm. In addition, the lack of warm-up exercises increases the likelihood of injury. Fractures and other trauma can arise from contact sports, such as football and hockey. Achilles tendon damage can arise from improperly landing on the heels while jogging. Pain in arm joints can arise from racket sports such as tennis and squash, which require a strong grasp, wrist extension, and forearm rotation. Ask about typical footwear. High-heeled shoes can shorten the Achilles tendons and pitch the center of gravity forward, leading to lordosis.

Nutrition

Dietary history is important to provide clues to musculo-skeletal problems. For example, obesity stresses weight-bearing joints and predisposes the client to ligamentous instability, particularly of the lower back. Poor calcium intake can precipitate fractures due to bone decalcifica-tion. Ask the client to list foods eaten on a typical day. Dietary history forms help with dietary assessment and teaching. Adequate dietary intake of vitamins A and D, calcium, and protein is important for musculoskeletal health. Ask about recent major weight changes. Excessive weight gain can place stress on the musculoskeletal system.

Habits and Safety

The client's habits and life-style can increase the risk of developing musculoskeletal disorders. Similarly, musculo-skeletal impairment affects the ability to perform ADL.

Review of Systems

Ask the client about problems such as muscle pain, spasm or tenderness; joint pain, stiffness, pain, swelling, or redness; weakness; limited movement; clumsiness; crepitus; backache; and changes in joints or bones. Each reported problem is investigated with a symptom analysis, as well as an inquiry about the effect the problem has had on the client's ability to perform ADL.

Assessment findings from other body systems some-times indicate musculoskeletal problems. Some examples are the following:

● Pain or burning when urinating is associated with Rei-ter's syndrome.
● Tachycardia and hypertension may accompany gout.
● Chronic diarrhea may occur when arthritis is associated with colitis or other gastrointestinal problems.
● Conjunctivitis may indicate Reiter's syndrome, and nongranulomatous uveitis may occur with ankylosing spondylitis.
● Skin changes may indicate musculoskeletal problems, for example, dry skin over the thumb and the first two fingers with carpal tunnel syndrome.
● Cramping leg pain on activity may signal intermittent claudication.
● Generalized muscle cramping may result from electro-lyte imbalances.
● Joint pain associated with recent chills, fever, or sore throat may be due to rheumatic fever.

Detailed questions for the review of systems (ROS) are found in Chapter 11, Box 11–2.

Physical Examination

Like other body system assessments, assessment of the musculoskeletal system proceeds in a systematic manner to avoid missing hidden problems. Use an examining room big enough for the client to move around in. Natu-

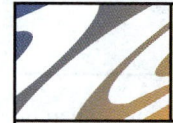

NORMAL PHYSICAL ASSESSMENT FINDINGS

Musculoskeletal System

Inspection

Joints in alignment; posture straight; gait smooth. Ex-tremities symmetrical and of equal length. Muscle groups symmetrical, without atrophy or fascicula-tions. Joints without erythema, swelling, or deformi-ties. Full range of motion (active and passive) in all major joints.

Palpation

Muscle groups firm, symmetrical, nontender; without masses or spasms. Joints stable and nontender; without heat, crepitus (palpable or audible), boggi-ness, or nodules. Muscle strength in all major mus-cle groups rated 5/5.

ral lighting is best for assessing skin color changes and swelling. Artificial light distorts some assessment find-ings. During musculoskeletal assessment, have the client sit, stand, and walk (unless any position is contraindicated by the client's condition).

The *musculoskeletal assessment* includes inspection and palpation of *muscle masses* for symmetry, involuntary movements, tenderness, tone, and strength; *joints* for sym-metry, crepitus, tenderness or pain, and ROM; and *bones* for deformity and leg length discrepancy. The nurse also tests the muscle-stretch or deep tendon reflexes (DTRs) using a percussion hammer.

General Musculoskeletal Examination

Using inspection and palpation, examine each body part. First, examine the body at rest. Then assess ROM and muscle strength (see discussion below).

When the client enters the examination room assess gait, body mobility, posture, general joint motion, and balance. While observing movement and gait, watch for gait patterns associated with specific disorders (see Chap-ter 30), objective evidence of discomfort, indications of joint stiffness or muscle weakness, lack of coordination, or deformities. Then have the client sit on the edge of the examination table. Look at the client's general appearance and body build. Examine the head, neck, shoulders, and upper extremities.

Have the client stand, and examine the chest, back, and ilium. Observe posture; body build; body contours; body alignment; and the cervical, thoracic, and lumbar spine. Also observe the relationships of various body parts to one another, for example, the relationship of feet to legs, legs to hips, and hips to pelvis (Fig. 73–1). Observe the client's stance and note any spinal deformities (Fig. 73–

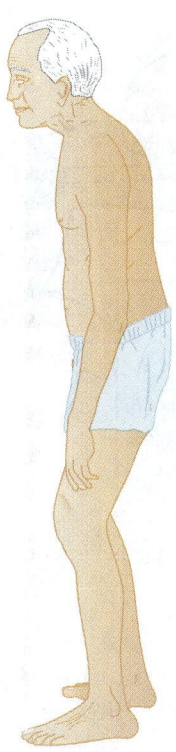

muscle tone (i.e., the state of tension in a muscle at rest, which is felt as firmness). Muscles should feel firm, smooth, and be bilaterally equal in size and nontender. A slight increase in mass, or *hypertrophy*, on the dominant side is normal, whereas *atrophy*, or decreased muscle size, on either side is abnormal. If muscle groups are noticeably asymmetrical in size, use a tape measure to assess limb circumference. Differences of 1 cm or less are considered within normal variation.

Assess *muscle strength* while putting the client's joints through active ROM. If a detailed assessment of muscle strength is necessary, each major muscle group can be assessed separately. Follow the guidelines in Table 73–1. (Note that the sternocleidomastoid and trapezius muscles are tested as part of the head and neck [i.e., cranial nerve] examination and are omitted from the table.) Test muscle strength by asking the client to repeat ROM while resistance is applied. Note the strength the client uses against the resistance. If there is weakness, decrease the resistance. Because the dominant arm is usually stronger, ask whether the client is right- or left-handed. Muscle

Figure 73–1. When performing a musculoskeletal assessment, have the client stand and walk, if possible. Observe the client's stance, joint mobility, and posture. If you were to assess this man only while he was reclining, you might not notice his posture, the curvature of his spine, and his limited range of motion.

2), such as (1) kyphosis, an abnormally increased roundness of the thoracic curve or "hump-back" look (Fig. 73–2A); (2) scoliosis, an obvious lateral deformity of the spine (Fig. 73–2B); or (3) lordosis, an, abnormal increase in the lumbar curve, or swayback (Fig. 73–2C). Other observable abnormalities include genu varum, or bowleg (Fig. 73–2D), and genu valgum, or knock-knee (Fig. 73–2E). The terms *varus(-um)* and *valgus(-um)* refer to the direction in which the apex of a deformity lies in relationship to the midline. With a varus deformity the apex of the deformity points toward the midline. With a valgus deformity it is bent or twisted away from the midline. In othropedics, these terms are often erroneously transposed, as in genu varum and valgum.

Last, have the client lie supine and examine the hips, knees, ankles, and feet for alignment, symmetry, or deformities. Determine leg length discrepancy by measuring from the anterior iliac spine to the medial malleolus. Measurements should be within 1 cm. If a discrepancy is noted, try to determine if it exists above or below the knee.

Muscles

Compare each muscle group with its contralateral side. Muscles should be free of *fasciculations* (fine muscle twitches) and smooth, without bulges or lumps. Palpate muscle groups gently, from proximal to distal, feeling the

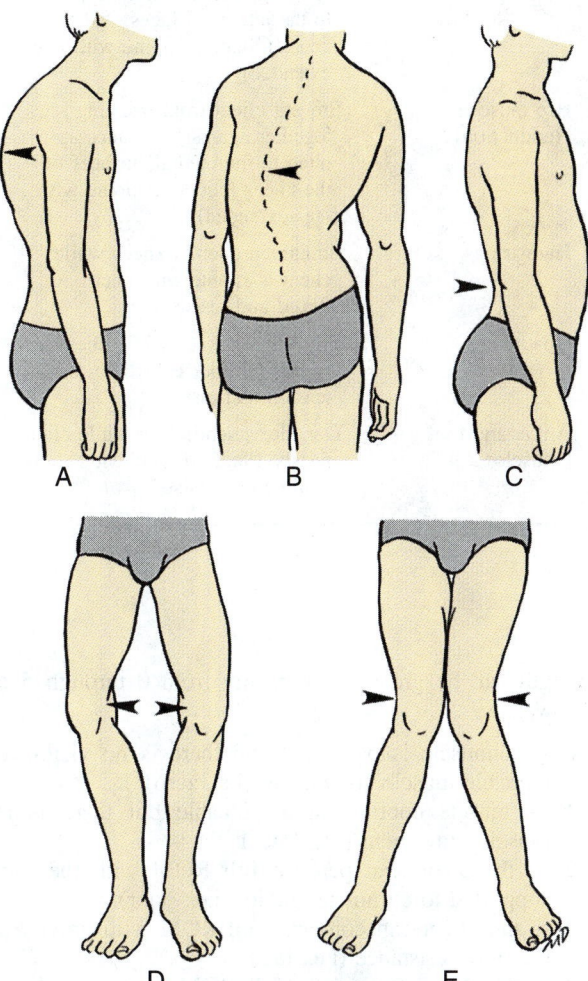

Figure 73–2. Musculoskeletal deformities observable during assessment. *A*, Kyphosis. *B*, Scoliosis. *C*, Lordosis. *D*, Genu varum. *E*, Genu valgum.

Table 73–1. Assessing Muscle Strength

Muscle Group	Technique
Deltoid	Push down client's arm while it is held up and client resists
Biceps	Hold client's arm in extension while it is fully extended and client flexes arm
Triceps	Keep client's arm in flexion while it is flexed and client extends arm
Wrist and finger muscles	Push client's fingers together while client spreads them and resists
Grip strength	Try to pull crossed index and middle fingers out from the client's grasp
Hip muscles	Hold down client's leg while it is fully extended and client lifts it off the table (client is supine)
Hip muscles (abduction)	Prevent client from spreading legs apart against resistance applied to the lateral surfaces of the knees (client is supine with legs extended)
Hip muscles (adduction)	Prevent client from bringing legs together against resistance applied to the medial surfaces of the knees (client is supine with legs extended)
Hamstrings	Straighten client's knees while client is supine with knees flexed and resists
Quadriceps	Flex client's knee while client is supine with knee partially in extension and resists
Ankle and foot muscles	Dorsiflex client's foot while client resists. Plantar flex client's foot while client resists

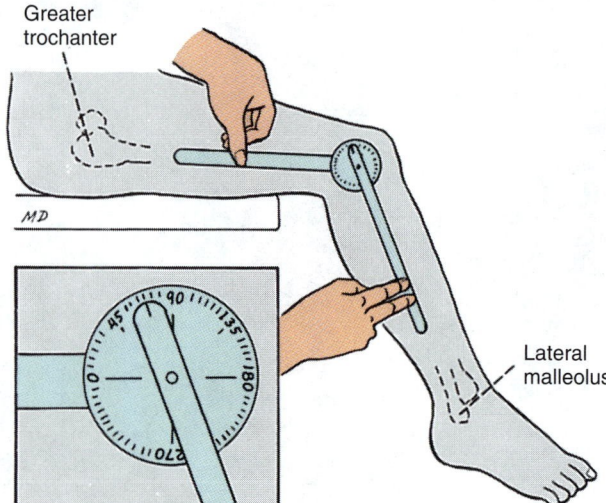

Figure 73–3. Use of a goniometer to measure joint range of motion.

The scale is included as part of the record to ensure understanding and consistency.

Joints and Bones

Inspect the joints and bones and compare findings bilaterally. They should be symmetrical and without redness, swelling, enlargement, or deformity. Each joint and bone is palpated for edema and tenderness, which should be absent. The joints also are palpated as they move for *crepitus* (grating sound or feeling), which is abnormal. Joints should feel smooth as they move, and nodules should not be present. ROM is the maximum amount of movement that a healthy joint is capable of. Measure ROM with a goniometer, which is based on the degrees of a circle (Fig. 73–3). This flexible, protractor type of instrument is placed on a joint to measure the angles created by joint movement. Figure 73–4 displays the joints that are assessed, and the types and degrees of ROM possible.

Special Tests of Joint Function

Some advanced practitioners use special assessments to determine if injury has occurred in the joints. Some of the more common tests are listed in Table 73–2; two of them are shown in Figure 73–5. These examinations are not usually included in the general orthopedic assessment and should be used only when the client's history indicates a possible injury and then only by persons trained to do these tests.

Neurovascular Assessment

A neurovascular assessment is essential for any client who has had a musculoskeletal injury because of the high risk of ischemia, deformity, or loss of function of an extremity.

strength can be graded numerically from 0 through 5 as follows:

0 = a muscle is paralyzed and there is no visible or palpable muscle contraction (i.e., zero).

1 = muscle contraction is palpable but there is no muscle movement (i.e., trace).

2 = the client can perform full ROM with the joint supported to eliminate gravity (i.e., poor).

3 = the client can complete full ROM with gravity as the only resistance (i.e., fair).

4 = the person completes full ROM against moderate resistance (i.e., good).

5 = the client completes full ROM against normal resistance and gravity (i.e., normal).

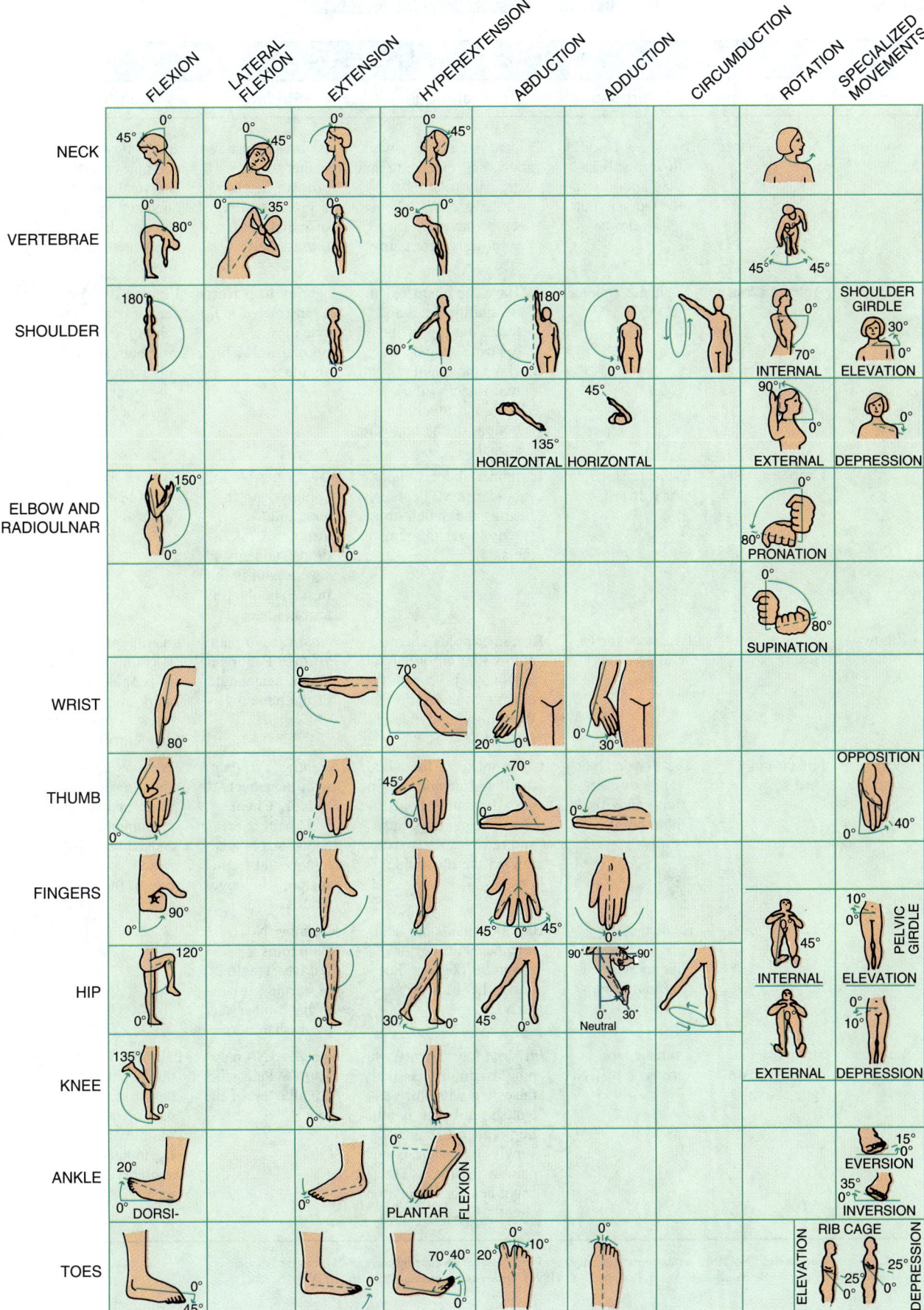

Figure 73–4. Joint range of motion (ROM). All joints are at 0 degrees when in their anatomic position. ROM begins at 0 degrees, as shown by the *solid lines.* Attainment of the average normal ROM is shown by *dotted lines* and the number of degrees in the angle formed by the two lines.

Table 73–2. Joint Function

Site	Test or Sign	Purpose	Technique	Findings	Comments
Shoulder	Adson's maneuver	Evaluates blood flow in subclavian artery; tests for thoracic outlet syndrome	Palpate radial artery while abducting, extending and externally rotating the arm; have client take a deep breath and turn head toward arm being tested	*Negative:* Pulse remains strong *Positive:* Marked decrease or loss of radial pulse during the test	Blood flow can be compromised by cervical rib, tumor, hematoma, or infection that has tightened neck muscles
	Apley's scratch test	Evaluates shoulder ROM	1. Have the client reach behind the head and touch the top of the opposite scapula 2. Have the client reach behind the back and touch the bottom of the opposite scapula	Inability to perform as instructed indicates less than normal ROM for shoulder	Limited ROM decreases functional ability; e.g., combing hair, pulling up a zipper, placing something in a back pocket
	Drop arm test	Evaluates for rotator cuff tear	Examiner abducts client's shoulder to 90 degrees. Instruct the patient to slowly lower the arms to the side	*Negative:* Able to comply with instructions *Positive:* Arm drops suddenly or severe pain is felt in the shoulder as arm is lowered	Positive test indicates tear in rotator cuff
Elbow	Tennis elbow test	Evaluates for lateral epicondylitis	Examiner holds client's elbow (thumb on lateral epicondyle). Pronate the client's forearm, flex the wrist fully, and extend the elbow	*Negative:* No pain *Positive:* Pain over lateral epicondyle of the humerus	Lateral epicondylitis is commonly seen in people who work at computers (word processing, data entry)
Wrist and hand	Finkelstein's test	Test for de Quervain's disease (tenosynovitis of the thumb)	Client makes a fist with the thumb inside the fingers. Examiner holds the client's forearm steady and deviates the wrist toward the ulnar side	*Negative:* No pain with maneuver *Positive:* Client feels pain over abductor pollicis longus and extensor pollicis longus tendons	Test may cause some discomfort in normal persons, so compare pain caused on "affected" side relative to the normal side
	Phalen's test	Evaluates for pressure on median nerve (carpal tunnel syndrome)	Backs of hands are held together with wrists flexed 90 degrees. Position is held for 60 seconds	*Negative:* No symptoms *Positive:* Tingling or burning in area of hand innervated by median nerve	
Lumbar spine	Straight leg raising (Lasègue's sign)	Evaluates for presence of HNP	*Involved leg:* Client is supine; examiner passively raises leg with knee extended until pain is felt. Leg is then extended slowly until there is no pain or tightness. The examiner dorsiflexes the client's foot	*Negative:* No pain *Positive:* Pain with dorsiflexion of the foot	Pain in posterior thigh indicates hamstring tightness Pain down entire leg indicates sciatic nerve involvement

ACL, anterior cruciate ligament; HNP, herniated nucleus pulposus; PCL, posterior cruciate ligament; ROM, range of motion.
Adapted from Maher, A. B., Salmond, S. W., & Pellino, T. A.: (1994). *Orthopaedic nursing*, Philadelphia: W. B. Saunders.

Site	Test or Sign	Purpose	Technique	Findings	Comments
Lumbar spine (continued)			*Uninvolved leg:* Client is supine and the leg raised as described above	*Positive:* Pain in opposite leg (not test leg) strongly suggests HNP	
Knee	Drawer test	Evaluates ligament stability in knee	*Anterior test:* Client lies on back, with knee flexed to 90 degrees and hip to 45 degrees. Hold the foot of the test leg in place. Draw the tibia forward on the femur. (Examiner's hands are around the tibia with the thumbs on the medial and lateral joint lines of the knee [see Fig. 73–5])	*Negative:* Movement 6 mm or less *Positive:* Movement more than 6 mm indicates tear in ACL	Ensure that PCL is not injured or anterior drawer test may be a false-positive. If PCL injury is suspected, check for posterior "sag" sign (gravity drawer test)
			Posterior test: Position patient as above. Tibia is pushed back on the femur	*Negative:* Tibia does not move back *Positive:* Feel and observe backward movement of the tibia. Indicates injury to PCL	
			Gravity test: (posterior sag sign): Patient lies supine with hips flexed to 45 degrees, and knees to 90 degrees	*Positive:* Tibia "sags" back on the femur. Indicates PCL is torn	With minimal swelling, the sag is very evident; there is obvious concavity distal to the patella
	Lachman's test	Evaluates injury to the ACL	Client lies supine, with knees between full extension and 30 degrees. One hand stabilizes the femur and the other hand moves the tibia forward (see Fig. 73–5B)	*Positive:* When tibia moves forward, infrapatellar tendon slope disappears	This test is the best indicator of ACL injury
	McMurray's test	Evaluates for medial and lateral meniscus injury	Client lies supine with injured leg fully flexed. Examiner cups heel with one hand and places the other hand on the knee (fingers on the medial joint line, thumb on the lateral joint line). Rotate the tibia medially, changing the degrees of flexion. Then rotate the tibia laterally, repeatedly changing the degrees of flexion	*Positive:* If a snap or click is heard, there is probably a meniscal tear	Evaluation of meniscal injuries is difficult and requires considerable experience. Because menisci have no blood or nervous supply, there may be no pain or swelling with injury

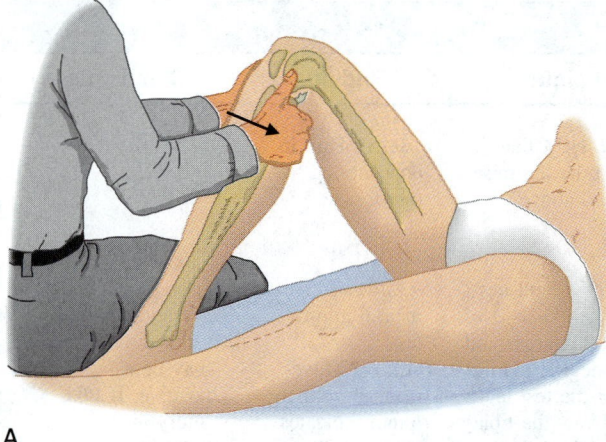

A

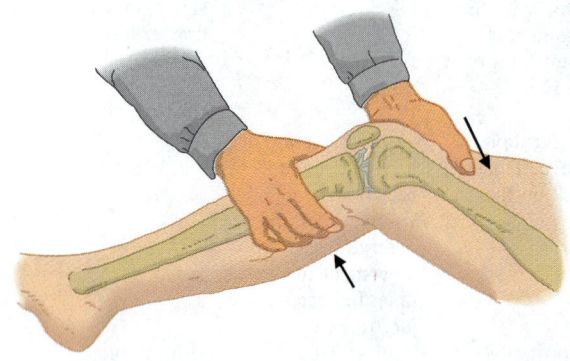

B

Figure 73–5. Special tests of joint function. *A*, The drawer test for instability of the knee ligaments. *B*, Lachman's test for anterior cruciate instability.

Components of Neurovascular Assessment

Components of a neurovascular assessment include checking for pain, pallor, temperature, pulses, capillary refill time, paresthesia, and mobility of the affected joints. The presence of pain using a client intensity rating scale of 0 to 10 can help determine if the pain is getting worse due to edema and compression on the nerves. Pallor, coolness, or cyanosis can indicate circulatory compromise in the extremity. Checking pulses and capillary refill bilaterally can assist in determining the adequacy of the blood supply to the small peripheral vessels. Capillary refill should occur in less than 2 to 3 seconds. Loss of sensation and motor function to an extremity can signal nerve injury.

Peripheral Nerve Assessment

Function in the major peripheral nerves is tested for sensation and motion. Have the client close the eyes when checking sensation. Light touch should be perceptible to the client if sensation is normal. If the client reports a

"pins-and-needles" sensation, further assessment is warranted. The client should be able to demonstrate active motion of a specific joint when requested to do so. If the client cannot move a joint and has pain when the joint is passively moved, suspect compartmental syndrome and perform further assessments, such as capillary refill, pulses, color, and warmth. Compartmental syndrome is discussed fully in Chapter 75. When casts prevent full neurovascular assessment, observation of edema, capillary refill, and joint movement can serve as a neurovascular assessment. Neurovascular assessment of the peroneal, tibial, radial, ulnar, and median nerves is shown in Figure 73–6.

Diagnostic Tests

Diagnostic tests are grouped according to tests that assess structure and tests that assess function. Tests can also be considered invasive or noninvasive. The following sections address x-ray studies, scans, computer imaging, arthroscopy, arthrocentesis, electromyography, and laboratory studies.

Noninvasive Tests of Structure

Radiography

Radiography (X-ray study) is the most widely used noninvasive musculoskeletal diagnostic procedure. X-ray examinations are important to (1) establish the presence of a musculoskeletal problem, (2) follow its progress, and (3) evaluate treatment effectiveness. A plain film is commonly obtained, usually an anteroposterior (AP) or lateral view, or both. Other common views include a notch (posterior or less commonly anterior) view of the knee in flexion, an oblique (45-degree angle) view, and a sunrise or patella view of the underside of the patella. The client is asked to remove any radiopaque objects that could appear on the x-ray film, such as jewelry. No additional preparation is needed except possibly analgesics for some clients. If possible, the client may be asked to assume various positions so that x-ray films may be taken from the most useful angles. This may be difficult or painful because x-ray tables are hard. Analgesia and other pain-relieving interventions may be needed after the x-ray.

■ Tomography

Tomograms (body section radiographs) are x-ray films showing details of structures otherwise hidden by overlying, radiopaque bone. This technique allows views of tissue at various planes as though slices had been made through the tissue. *Laminography* is sometimes used to locate bone destruction, small cavities, foreign bodies, and lesions overshadowed by other structures, and to evaluate whether a bone graft has united.

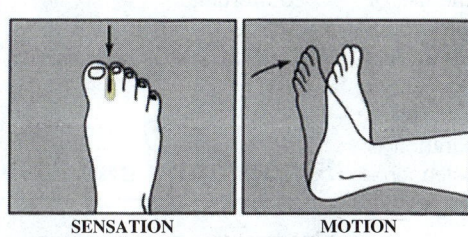

Peroneal Nerve

□ **SENSATION**
Prick the web space between the great toe and second toe

□ **MOTION**
Have patient dorsiflex ankle and extend toes at the metatarsal phalangeal joints

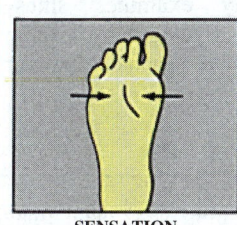
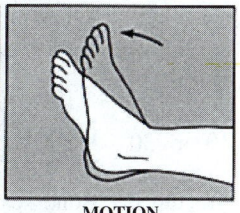

Tibial Nerve

□ **SENSATION**
Prick the medial and lateral surfaces of the sole of the foot

□ **MOTION**
Have patient plantar flex ankle and toes

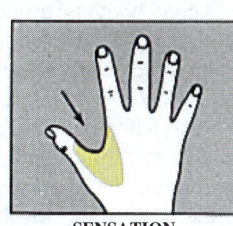
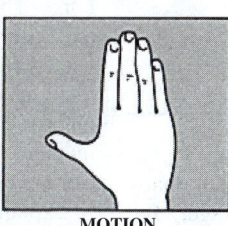

Radial Nerve

□ **SENSATION**
Prick the web space between the thumb and index finger

□ **MOTION**
Have patient hyperextend thumb then wrist and hyperextend the four fingers at the MCP joints

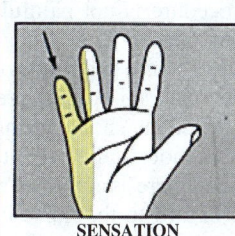
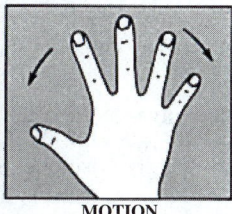

Ulnar Nerve

□ **SENSATION**
Prick the distal fat pad of the small finger

□ **MOTION**
Have patient Abduct all fingers

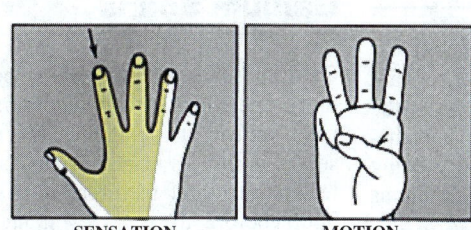

Median Nerve

□ **SENSATION**
Prick the distal surface of the index finger

□ **MOTION**
Have patient oppose thumb and small finger; note whether patient can flex wrist

Figure 73–6. Neurovascular assessment of the peroneal, tibial, radial, ulnar, and median nerves. (Modified from Stearns, G. M., & Brunner, N. A. [1987]. *Operative care* [Vol. 1, p. 89]. Rutherford, NJ: Howmedica.)

■ Fluoroscopy

Fluoroscopy is another type of radiologic test that provides a continuous picture of a structure. The images are viewed on a screen.

■ Dual-Energy X-Ray Absorptiometry

Methods used to measure bone density are performed to diagnose osteoporosis, because the condition is not evident on x-ray study until 30% to 50% of the bone mass is lost. One method of measuring bone mass is the use of dual-energy x-ray absorptiometry (DXA). This procedure uses an x-ray tube to generate dual-energy photons. The DXA has less radiation exposure and the test takes about 10 minutes. This test can detect osteoporosis in other sites, such as the wrist, spine, and hips. No preparation is required; the client may require teaching about osteoporosis once the findings are known.

■ Computed Tomography

Computed tomography (CT) scans use both x-rays and computers for three-dimensional physical assessment of various body areas. A contrast medium (iodine) is used and images appear on a computer screen in cross-sectional views. A complete examination takes 10 to 30 views or slides. CT scans are useful in assessing some bone and soft tissue tumors and some spinal fractures. Clients must remain still during the scan and the procedure can last between ½ and 1½ hours depending on the area scanned.

Magnetic Resonance Imaging

Magnetic resonance imaging (MRI) is a noninvasive imaging device that facilitates the early diagnosis of many conditions affecting tendons, ligaments, cartilage, and bone marrow. Preprocedure and postprocedure care is discussed in Chapter 13.

Invasive Tests of Structure

Other specialized radiographic procedures that are invasive allow more precise visualization and include arthrograms, sinography, and myelography.

Arthrography

An arthrogram is a radiographic examination of soft tissue joint structures. It is used to diagnose trauma to joint capsules or supporting ligaments, especially involving the shoulder, wrist, hip, ankle, or knee. Under local anesthesia, contrast or air is injected into the joint cavity using aseptic precautions. The joint is moved through ROM as a series of x-ray films is taken.

Prior to arthrography, the nurse should do the following:

1. Explain the procedure to the client and family and answer their questions.
2. Explain that the procedure may take up to an hour (follow-up x-rays are sometimes taken 30 minutes after the injection) and that the client will need to remain as still as possible except when asked to reposition.
3. Ask whether the client has any allergies, especially to local anesthetics, iodine, seafood, or contrast.

4. Suggest that the client void before the procedure to be comfortable.
5. Advise the client that the joint may be uncomfortable for 1 to 2 days afterward and to avoid strenuous exercise.

Sinography and Myelography

Sinography and myelography are similar to arthrography in that contrast is injected and x-ray films are taken. Sinography examines sinus tracks (deep draining wounds). Myelography examines the spinal canal and cord to detect herniated intervertebral discs.

Bone Scans

Bone scanning is skeletal imaging done after a radioisotope, which is taken up by bone, is injected intravenously (usually technetium Tc 99m). This substance migrates to bone. The whole body is usually scanned, although only an extremity may be scanned if a stress fracture is suspected (i.e., pinhole scan). Bone scanning is used to detect malignancies, osteomyelitis, osteoporosis, and some fractures (especially pathologic fractures). The isotope collects in these areas, indicating abnormal bone metabolism. The isotope does not collect in poorly perfused bone.

Explain the procedure to the client and family and answer their questions; the procedure takes about 1 hour, during which the client lies supine. Reassure the client that the procedure is not painful and there are no harmful effects from the isotopes. Suggest that the client urinate before the procedure for comfort.

After the scan, no special precautions are required except that the client should drink large amounts of water for 24 to 48 hours after the test to help eliminate the isotope. Since there is minimal radioactivity in the isotope there is no hazard to the nurse or others.

Gallium Scans

Gallium scans are similar to bone scans, but the test is more specific to bone disorders. Gallium is the isotope used, and it also migrates to brain, liver, and breast tissue. Gallium is taken up by bone more slowly than is technetium, and therefore it is given to the client 2 to 3 hours before the scan by a nuclear medicine technician. The scan requires 30 to 60 minutes to complete. Mild sedation may be needed for clients in pain or who are restless or elderly. No special follow-up care is required.

Indium Imaging

Indium imaging is the use of indium tagged to leukocytes to detect bone infection. The client's leukocytes are separated from a sample of blood and labeled (tagged) with indium. The tagged cells are reinjected. They accumulate in areas of bone infection and can be detected on scanning. No special preparation or follow-up care is necessary.

Biopsy

A biopsy is the removal and histologic examination of tissue for diagnostic purposes. Disorders such as infection and cancer of the bone and atrophy and inflammation of the muscle are detected. Bone or muscle may be biopsied during surgery or through a needle or bore not requiring a surgical incision. The latter are called aspiration, punch, or needle biopsies. Sometimes aspiration biopsy under radiographic control is performed, as into the spine. Bone biopsies are performed in the radiology department or an operating room under sterile conditions to prevent osteomyelitis. Local anesthesia is used. Bone or muscle biopsies take about 30 minutes.

Following the biopsy the nurse monitors the site for bleeding, swelling, and hematoma development. Because dressings usually surround the biopsy site, assessment is performed through analysis of the client's pain. Mild-to-moderate discomfort is usual; more severe levels of pain may signal complications. The biopsy site is elevated for 24 hours to reduce edema. Vital signs are monitored every 4 hours for 24 hours. A mild analgesic is usually required. Ongoing assessments of the site for signs of infection are performed by the nurse or client when discharged.

Arthroscopy

Arthroscopy (Fig. 73–7) is a common and very useful invasive type of diagnostic tool performed under local anesthesia in an ambulatory, same-day surgery facility.

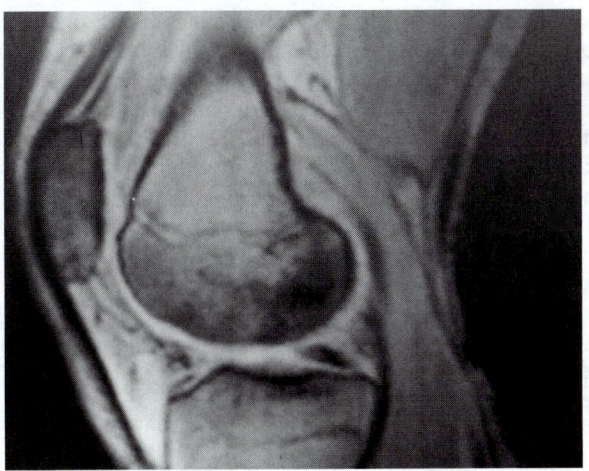

Figure 73–7. MRI of right knee.

An arthroscope is a small fiberoptic instrument that allows endoscopic examination of various joints, including the hip, knee, shoulder, elbow, and wrist, without making a large incision into the joint. Diagnoses made via arthroscopy are 98% accurate. Arthroscopy can be used for assessment or treatment. For example, biopsies can be taken, articular cartilage abnormalities can be assessed, or loose bodies can be removed and cartilage trimmed. The client is usually home and back to work sooner than if an arthrotomy (opening the joint) were performed. Arthroscopy is contraindicated in clients whose joint flexion is less than 50% (e.g., in fibrous ankylosis) or if skin or wound infection is present at the site. Complications are rare but include infection, hemarthrosis (blood in the joint), swelling, synovial rupture, joint injury, and thrombophlebitis.

Table 73–3. Synovial Fluid Analysis	
Tests	**Measurement and Norms**
Mucin clot test	The addition of 5% acetic acid to normal joint fluid results in a thick ropy clot that will not fragment when shaken. Fluid from an acutely inflamed joint results in a stringy loose clot
Viscosity	After taking normal synovial fluid between the thumb and index finger, a string of fluid 1 to 2 inches long will develop as the thumb and index finger are separated. Inflamed joints produce synovial fluid that is watery
Color, clarity, amount	Normal joint fluid varies from yellow to straw-colored, is clear, and is present in the joint in only minute quantities. Inflamed joints produce increased fluid that is turbid and gray in color
White blood cells	Normal synovial fluid has a low concentration, with predominately mononuclear cells. WBC $>2000/mm^3$ occurs in osteoarthritis; WBC $>100,000/mm^3$ with sepsis and polymyalgia rheumatica
Glucose	Blood and synovial fluid glucose levels need to be determined simultaneously in the fasting client. If the joint fluid glucose level is $<50\%$ of that of the blood, pyogenic infection should be suspected. However, greater differentials can occur with RA
Crystal studies	Presence of crystals in the synovial fluid indicates gout or pseudogout
Rheumatoid factor	RF may be found in synovial fluid before becoming evident in the blood. However, RF in synovial fluid is nonspecific, and cannot be relied on to provide meaningful support for a diagnosis of RA

RA, Rheumatoid arthritis; RF, rheumatoid factor; WBC, white blood cell.
From Schoen, D. (1988). Assessment for arthritis. *Orthopaedic Nursing, 7*(2), 31–39.

Instruct the client to fast from midnight the night before. Be sure the client and family know where the procedure will be performed and by whom and that appropriate consent forms are understood and signed. If a local anesthetic will be used, tell the client that there may be mild discomfort as it is administered and a thumping sensation may be felt as the arthroscope is inserted. Teach the client to watch for indications of postprocedure infection, such as temperature elevation or local inflammation at the incision site, and to report this promptly.

Ensure necessary pain relief after the procedure. Tell the client a normal diet may be resumed as soon as desired. Advise the client that unless surgical excision is performed and the surgeon gives specific instructions, walking is usually permitted after sensation has returned, but excessive exercise should be avoided for a few days.

Arthrocentesis

Joint aspiration, or arthrocentesis, is a method of aspirating synovial fluid, blood, or pus via a needle inserted into the joint cavity. It is used to diagnose rheumatoid arthritis and other inflammatory conditions or to remove fluid to relieve pain. The procedure is done under local anesthesia with aseptic precautions with or without fluoroscopy. Medication may be instilled into the joint if necessary, to alleviate inflammation in septic arthritis. Apply a compression bandage following arthrocentesis and rest the joint for 8 to 24 hours. (The results of synovial fluid analysis are summarized in Table 73–3).

Electromyography

Electromyography (EMG) is used to assess common complaints such as muscle weakness or altered gait, or lower motor neuron lesions. It measures the electrical potential associated with skeletal muscle contractions. Needles are inserted into muscles. Recordings of muscular electrical activity are then traced on an audiotransmitter, on an oscilloscope, and on recording paper. EMG helps diagnose neuromuscular conditions. A diagram of an EMG is shown in Chapter 30.

Explain the procedure to the client and family. Assure the client that the needle insertion is similar to a pinprick. Instruct the client not to take any stimulants or sedatives for 24 hours before procedure. Some clients who have nerve inflammation may have residual pain after electromyography. They may need a mild analgesic.

Laboratory Tests

Table 73–4 lists the most common laboratory tests for clients with musculoskeletal disorders. Chapter 13 includes laboratory tests specific for rheumatic problems.

Table 73–4. Common Laboratory Studies Used in Diagnosing Musculoskeletal Conditions

Test/Normal Value	Significance of Results
Antinuclear antibody (ANA) Normal: negative or at a titer ≤1:32	Positive tests are associated with systemic lupus erythematosus, rheumatoid arthritis, rheumatic fever, Raynaud's disease
C-Reactive protein (CRP) Normal: trace amounts	Positive in acute inflammation such as rheumatoid arthritis
Erythrocyte sedimentation rate (ESR) Normal: Westergren's method: males, 0–15 mm/hr females, 0–20 mm/hr Wintrobe's method: males, 0–9 mm/hr females, 0–15 mm/hr	Elevations common in arthritic conditions, infection, inflammation, cancer, cell or tissue destruction
Tests of Mineral Metabolism	
Calcium 8.0–10.5 mg/dl or 4.5–5.5 mEq/L	Decreased levels found in osteomalacia, osteoporosis. Increased levels found in bone tumors, Paget's disease, healing fractures
Alkaline phosphatase 30–90 units/L	Elevations found in bone cancer, osteoporosis, osteomalacia, Paget's disease
Phosphorus 2.5–4.0 mg/dl	Increased levels found in healing fractures, osteolytic metastatic tumor diseases
Muscle Enzymes	
Aldolase A 1.3–8.2 units/dl	Elevations in muscular dystrophy, dermatomyositis
Aspartate aminotransferase 10–50 units/L	Found in skeletal muscle, but primarily in heart and renal cells
Creatine kinase 15–150 units/L	Increased levels found in traumatic injuries, progressive muscular dystrophy, polymyositis
Lactate dehydrogenase (LDH$_4$, LDH$_5$) 60–150 units/L	Elevations in skeletal muscle necrosis, extensive cancer, progressive muscular dystrophy

Conclusions

The musculoskeletal system assessment begins with a complete history, including symptom analysis. Diagnostic studies commonly include x-ray study, and in recent years arthroscopy has been performed to diagnose and treat joint disorders at one procedure.

Bibliography

1. Bryan, V. (1990). Troubleshooting arthroscopic equipment. *Orthopaedic Nursing, 9*(1), 18–25.

2. Doheny, M., Linden, P., & Sedlak, C. (1995). Reducing orthopaedic hazards of the computer work environment. *Orthopaedic Nursing, 14*, 7–16.
3. Jarvis, C. (1996). *Physical examination and health assessment* (2nd ed.). Philadelphia, W. B. Saunders.
4. Long, J. S. (1996). Shoulder arthroscopy. *Orthopaedic Nursing, 15*(2), 21–32.
5. Maher, A. B., Salmond, S. W., & Pellino, T. A. (1994). *Orthopaedic nursing*. Philadelphia: W. B. Saunders.
6. Pavlik, M. (1991). Measuring bone mineral content. *Orthopaedic Nursing, 10*(2), 39–42.
7. Swartz, M. (1994). *Textbook of physical diagnosis* (2nd ed.). Philadelphia: W. B. Saunders.

74

Nursing Care of Clients with Musculoskeletal Disorders

Joan Lappe
Cleda L. Meyer

The musculoskeletal system is essential to humans if they are to perform activities of daily living. Although musculoskeletal disorders are not usually seen as life-threatening, disorders of the musculoskeletal system seriously affect the quality of life.

Metabolic Bone Disorders

Metabolic bone disorders result from inappropriate functioning of one or more metabolic processes. Manifestations are seen in both physical and chemical structure of the bone. Disorders that alter bony equilibrium and affect bone turnover can be due to estrogen deficiency, parathyroid gland abnormalities, vitamin deficiency, or malabsorption.

Osteoporosis

Osteoporosis was defined by the osteoporosis consensus development conference as a "systemic skeletal disease characterized by low bone mass and microarchitectural deterioration of bone tissue, with a consequent increase in bone fragility and susceptibility to fracture."[51] Fragility fractures are fractures that result from low trauma, such as bending over to pick up a newspaper, that would not cause fractures in healthy bone. Fragility fractures due to osteoporosis most commonly involve the hip, vertebrae, and radius (Colles' fracture). The term *osteopenia* refers to a reduction in the amount of bone per unit volume relative to that expected for the sex and age of the individual. Since many elderly persons have osteopenia but never develop a fracture, the World Health Organization has developed several general diagnostic categories to elaborate more specifically on the definition of osteoporosis.[29] The categories include the following:

This chapter incorporates material written for the fourth edition by Nina A. Rauscher, Helen A. Andrews, and Esther Matassarin-Jacobs.

1. Normal. A value for bone mineral density (BMD) or bone mineral content (BMC) that is not more than 1 SD below the young adult mean value (Fig. 74–1A).
2. Low bone mass or osteopenia. A value for BMD or BMC that lies between 1.0 and 2.5 SDs below the young adult mean value. Persons with those values include those in whom the prevention of bone loss would be most useful.
3. Osteoporosis. A value for BMD or BMC that is more than 2.5 SD below the young adult mean value (Fig. 74–1B).
4. Severe osteoporosis (or established osteoporosis). A value for BMD or BMC more than 2.5 SD below the young adult mean value *and* the presence of one or more fragility fractures.

Osteoporosis can be classified into primary and secondary forms. Primary osteoporosis refers to the occurrence of the condition among older persons in whom no secondary predisposing condition exists. This includes both postmenopausal osteoporosis and the osteoporosis of aging. Secondary osteoporosis results from an underlying condition, such as hyperparathyroidism, or an iatrogenic cause, such as long-term corticosteroid administration.

Etiology and Risk Factors

The cause of osteoporosis is unknown. Many factors, both genetic and environmental, are involved in the development of osteoporosis. The two most important risk factors are low peak bone mass and accelerated postmenopausal bone loss. (Peak bone mass is the maximum amount of bone that a person achieves.) Women have accelerated bone loss following menopause because of the loss of endogenous estrogen. Rapid bone loss also occurs in women who have early or surgically induced meno-

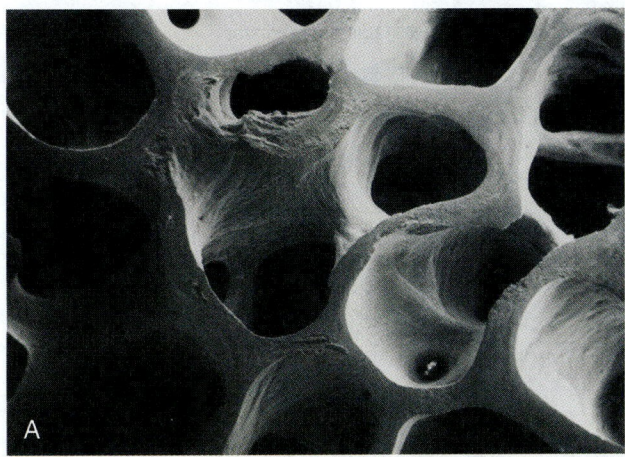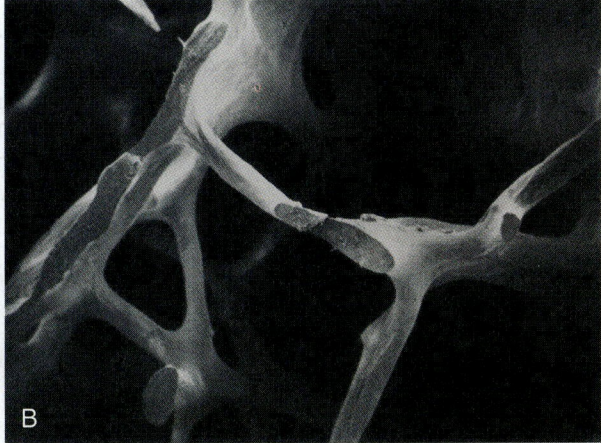

Figure 74–1. Electron micrographs of normal (*A*) and osteoporotic (*B*) bone. (Reproduced with permission from Dempster, D. W., et al. [1986]. *Journal of Bone and Mineral Research,* 1, 15–21.)

pause, in female athletes who cease to menstruate, and in women who have anorexia nervosa with amenorrhea. Both men and women experience age-related bone loss.

Evidence exists for a heredity predisposition to osteoporosis. It has been estimated that as much as 80% of the variance of peak bone mass is attributable to genetic influences. Women who have a family history of osteoporosis or postmenopausal dorsal kyphosis are at high risk of development of osteoporotic fractures. Other hereditary factors include northern European extraction, and blond hair and fair skin. Thin, small-framed women and men have a greater risk of fracture than persons with larger frames and more body weight.

Osteoporosis is a major public health problem in many countries, particularly in the United States and northern Europe. In the United States alone, osteoporosis affects 25 million people and is responsible for more than 1.3 million fractures each year, most of which occur in persons over 65 years old. Vertebral crush fractures are probably the most common type of osteoporotic fracture. One third of American women over 65 will eventually have a vertebral fracture. It is estimated that the female-to-male ratio of vertebral crush fractures is at least 10:1.[10] Hip fractures are one of the most important causes of death and disability among the elderly, primarily occurring in persons over 70 years of age. One third of the very old will experience a hip fracture. Fractures of the hip are two to three times more common in women than in men. The mortality rate of persons who have sustained hip fractures is 12% to 20% higher than in persons of similar age and sex who have not had a hip fracture. Among persons with hip fractures, 50% will need some help with activities of daily living and 15% to 25% will require placement in a long-term care institution.

Evidence exists that persons with one osteoporotic fracture are five times more likely to suffer another fracture than persons without a fracture. Osteoporotic fractures are more common in whites than in blacks, while persons of Asian extraction have a risk that falls between that of whites and blacks.

Pathophysiology

Bone is a dynamic tissue that undergoes continuous remodeling, the process by which old bone is replaced by new, with little or no net change in the mass or shape of the bone (Fig. 74–2). Bone remodeling serves two principal functions: (1) to replace old bone with new so that the biomechanical properties of the skeleton are not compromised by continuous use, and (2) to play a role in mineral homeostasis by transferring calcium and other ions into and out of the skeletal reservoir. The remodeling sequence starts with activation of *osteoclasts,* which resorb a small portion of bone over a relatively short period of time (as short as 7–10 days). Bone formation then takes place as *osteoblasts* form an organic matrix that is subsequently mineralized.

Although longitudinal growth usually is complete by about age 20, consolidation of bone continues so that peak bone mass is not attained until about 30 years of age. Although there is disagreement about exactly when bone loss naturally begins, it is well established that at the time of menopause women experience a marked acceleration in bone loss and may lose as much as 15% of their total mass within the first 5 years. The rate of loss then slows to a rate similar to that of men.

Peak bone mass and the subsequent rate and duration of bone loss are important determinants of whether skeletal integrity will be compromised to the degree that it eventually results in a low-trauma fracture. In addition, as bone tissue is lost, there are other alterations in the skeleton, such as changes in architecture, aging of the bone tissue, and accumulation of microdamage, that contribute to fracture risk. The supporting structures become so weak that even minimal stress can cause fractures. Spinal fractures occurring with osteoporosis are usually "compression fractures" which occur when one or more vertebrae collapse from carrying the weight of the upright body (see Fig. 74–1*A* and *B*).

Complications of osteoporotic vertebral fracture include loss of height and progressive dorsal kyphosis. The lower

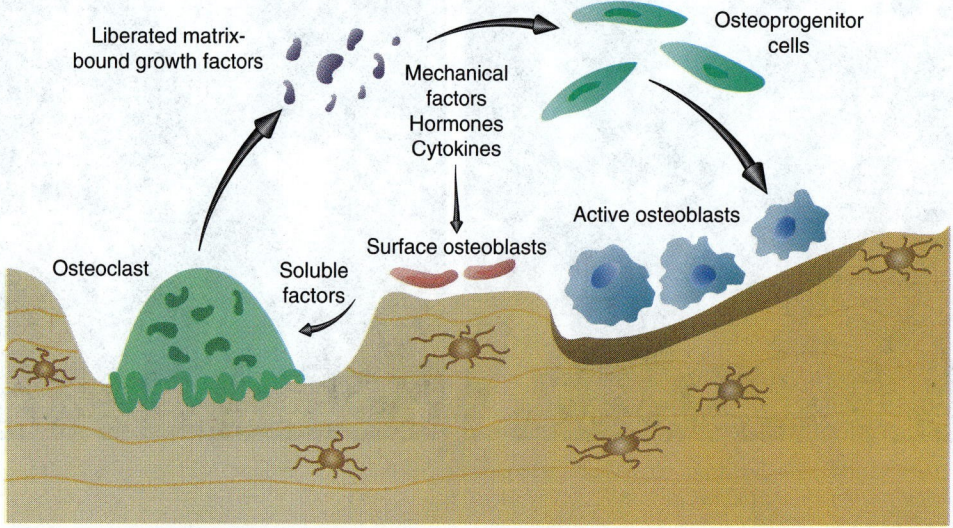

Figure 74–2. Bone remodeling is a process of bone resorption and bone formation. These two processes are controlled by systemic factors (the need for calcium) and local cytokines, some of which are found in the bone matrix. Cytokines are key in communication between the osteoblasts and the osteoclasts. (Modified from Cotran, R. S., Kumar, V., & Robbins, S. L. [1994]. *Robbins pathologic basis of disease* [5th ed., p. 1217]. Philadelphia: W. B. Saunders.)

ribs eventually rest on the iliac crests, and downward pressure on viscera causes abdominal distention and bloating. Respiration may also be impaired by restricted lung expansion. Self-esteem is affected by the obvious deformity and the difficulty in finding clothing that fits. Quality of life may be affected by chronic pain, and fear of subsequent fracture may cause people to reduce their activity.

Complications of hip fracture include death (12%–20% of persons who suffer a hip fracture die within the first year after the fracture) and disability. Many of these people require nursing home placement.

Clinical Manifestations and Diagnostic Findings

In many persons the diagnosis of osteoporosis is made after a fracture, often a vertebral compression fracture. Clinical manifestations of vertebral compression fracture include sudden onset of severe back pain that worsens on movement and is relieved by rest. This acute pain usually subsides within 2 to 6 weeks. The majority of compression fractures, however, are discovered accidentally on routine x-ray. Progressive vertebral deformities lead to shortened stature and marked kyphosis (Fig. 74–3). Impaired breathing, abdominal distention, and constipation may occur due to deformities of the spine. Bone loss can also occur in the mandible, which may lead to loss of teeth or poorly fitting dentures, as well as changes in the appearance of the client's face. The many changes in appearance can have a profound negative impact on the individual's self-esteem.

It is recommended that bone mass be assessed in clients at high risk of osteoporosis so that preventive interventions can be instituted before fractures occur. The position of the Scientific Advisory Board of the National Osteoporosis Foundation is that bone mass measurements should be performed in estrogen-deficient women. The diagnosis of low bone mass allows decisions about hormone replacement therapy (HRT). The best time to start HRT has not been clearly established. Based on the findings that women start to lose bone at least 1½ years before their last menses, bone mass measurements might best be done when women in their 40s or 50s start to skip menstrual periods. In addition, bone mass measurement is useful to determine the severity of osteoporosis in clients experiencing their first low-trauma fracture. Bone mass is commonly determined by dual-energy x-ray absorptiometry of the hip, spine, radius, and total body (Fig. 74–4). This technique has low risk and takes only a few minutes. Clinical evaluation should also include lateral radiographs of the thoracic and lumbar spine to determine the presence of compressed vertebrae, which may be asymptomatic.

Laboratory tests may be performed to rule out secondary osteoporosis or other metabolic bone diseases. These tests include blood count, urinalysis, multichannel screen, serum alkaline phosphatase, serum 25-hydroxyvitamin D, parathyroid hormone, ionized calcium, protein electrophoresis in urine and serum, and thyroid function.

Community and Self-Care

Preventive Measures

Once the clinical expression of osteoporosis has occurred, few therapeutic options are available. This emphasizes the

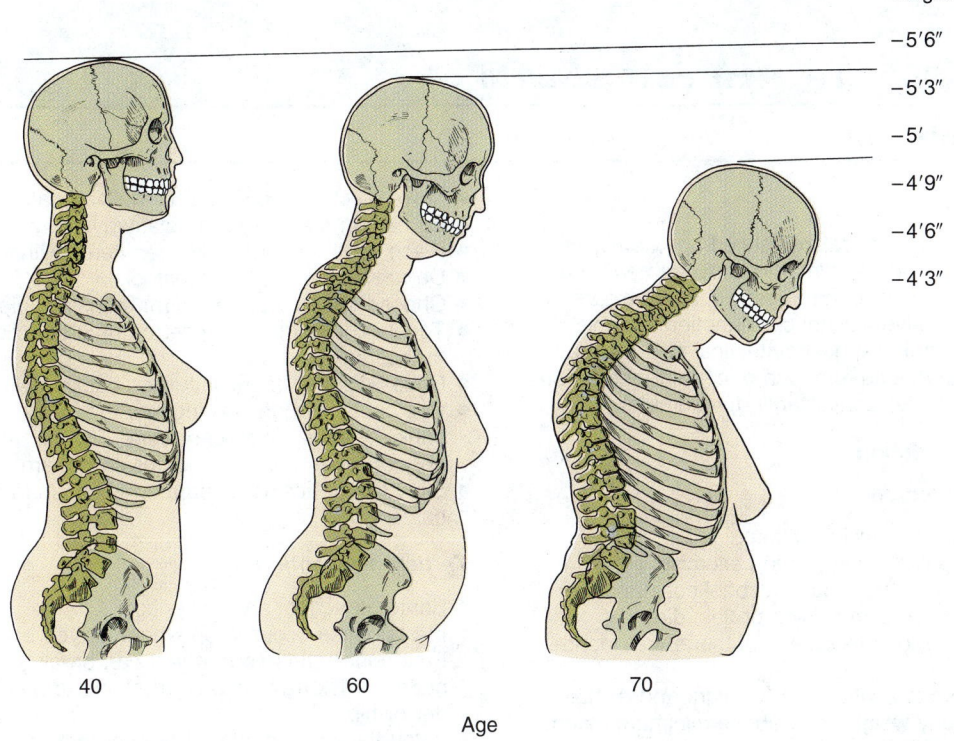

Figure 74–3. Osteoporotic changes: A normal spine at age 40, and osteoporotic changes at ages 60 and 70. These changes can cause a loss of height and result in dorsal kyphosis.

need for preventive measures, which can maximize peak bone mass and minimize the amount of bone loss that will occur. Strategies for preventing osteoporosis are most effective when started in childhood. This material is summarized in the Risk Factors and Levels of Prevention feature.

A well-balanced diet containing the recommended level of calcium is an important component of bone health (Box 74–1). The major sources of dietary calcium are dairy products. Calcium can also be obtained from calcium-fortified foods such as fortified orange juice. National surveys of dietary intake indicate that many Americans are not consuming enough calcium. As early as age 10, girls have calcium intake considerably below recommended levels.

Individuals who have difficulty digesting milk due to a lack of the enzyme lactase, which breaks down the milk sugar lactose, may be able to tolerate acidophilus milk, yogurt, and hard cheeses. Skim milk and low-fat yogurt can be recommended for persons who are trying to maintain low cholesterol diets.

Although dietary sources of calcium are preferred, research evidence supports recommending calcium supplementation for women with typically low calcium intake.

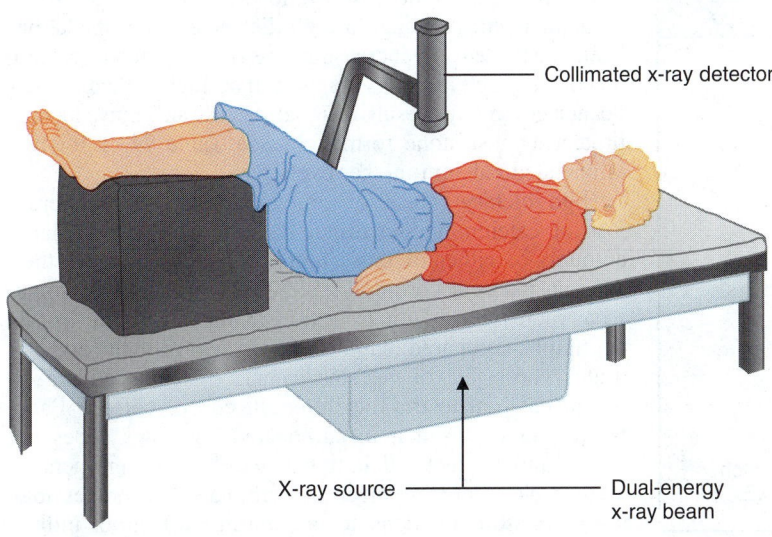

Figure 74–4. Dual-photon absorptiometry. (Adapted from an original illustration in *Clinical Symposia,* illustrated by Frank Netter, M.D., copyright by Ciba-Geigy Corporation.)

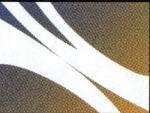

RISK FACTORS AND LEVELS OF PREVENTION

Osteoporosis

Risk Factors

Female, postmenopausal, advanced age, family history of osteoporosis, white, thin, and small-framed body build, sedentariness, calcium-deficient diet, cigarette smoking, excessive alcohol consumption, chronic illness (inflammatory arthritis, gastrointestinal disease, gastrointestinal surgery), long-term use of certain medications (corticosteroids, anticonvulsants, furosemide).

Levels of Prevention

Primary Prevention

- Achieve optimal calcium intake.
- Perform regular weightbearing exercise.
- Avoid smoking and regular alcohol consumption.
- Avoid a high sodium or high protein diet.
- Consider estrogen replacement therapy at menopause.
- Absorb adequate vitamin D (sunlight and diet).
- Maintain body weight at or above minimum recommended levels.

Secondary Prevention

- Same as primary prevention
- Teach clients how to provide an environment that protects against falls.
- Install phones in most rooms in the house.
- Install grab bars in bathtubs and showers.
- Apply nonskid strips on areas that get wet.
- Install a telephone and light switch near the bed.

- Move electrical cords out of walking paths.
- Be certain that carpet on stairways is not loose.
- Place commonly used kitchen items within reach.
- Do not use chairs as stepstools.
- Choose shoes that have firm, nonskid soles.
- Tennis shoes may provide too much traction and lead to tripping.
- Cover slippery floors with rugs backed with rubber.
- Use caution when walking into the lobby of a hotel, bank, hospital, or grocery store. Floors are often slippery or have a visually confusing pattern.
- Slow down; accidents happen when you do things in haste.

Tertiary Prevention

- Same as secondary prevention
- If a fall does occur, drop whatever you are doing. Free your hands so that you can break your fall. (It is better to risk fracturing a wrist than to break a shoulder or hip.)
- If you think you broke a bone, do not move and do not let others move you who are not medically trained.
- Arrange a signal. Use a professional alert system or use the telephone to call for help.
- If you think you are bruised and not seriously injured, try to get up into a chair. Do not put weight on the injured part. Apply ice to a bruise.
- Analyze what happened and identify what you can do to avoid a similar fall.

Box 74–1. Calcium Equivalents of Dietary Sources (300 mg)

1 cup of milk
1 carton of low fat yogurt with fruit
1¼ cup frozen yogurt
1 cup vanilla pudding
1 cup baked egg custard
1 oz Swiss cheese
1 slice cheese pizza (Pizza Hut)
½ cup ricotta cheese, part skim
1½ oz. cheddar cheese
2¼ cup cottage cheese
11 dried figs
4 cups broccoli
7 oz baked walleyed pike fillet
¾ cup whole dried almonds

Prepared by Patricia T. Packard, R.D., C.N., Creighton University Osteoporosis Research Center, Omaha, NE.

Calcium supplements vary in absorbability, some passing through the gastrointestinal tract intact. Tums and Os-Cal are known to be well absorbed. All calcium supplements should be taken with food to enhance absorbability. Chewing them rather than swallowing them whole also is recommended. Although a high dietary calcium intake has been suspected of increasing the risk of renal calculi, recent research findings suggest that high calcium diets do not commonly result in renal calculi and may, in fact, protect against stone formation. See Table 74–1 for recommended calcium intake levels.

High dietary intake of protein and sodium increases loss of calcium in the urine. Persons who take in large amounts of either of those nutrients should increase their calcium intake accordingly. Although caffeine does somewhat increase calcium excretion in the urine, the loss is negligible compared with the effects of protein and sodium. The effect of caffeine can be offset by adding 40 mg of calcium to the diet for each cup of coffee.[3] Phosphorus intake, as that in carbonated beverages, does not significantly affect calcium balance.[23] However, persons who drink a large number of carbonated beverages may not be consuming adequate calcium in the form of milk.

Table 74–1. Calcium Intake Levels Recommended by the National Institutes of Health Consensus Panel

Group	Calcium Intake (mg/day)
Infants	
Birth–6 mo	400
6 mo–1 yr	600
Children	
1–5 yr	800
6–10 yr	800–1200
11–24 yr	1200–1500
Adults	
Women 25–50 yr	1000
Postmenopausal women <65 yr	
Taking estrogen	1000
Not taking estrogen	1500
Women >65 yr	1500
Men <65 yr	1000
Men >65 yr	1500
Pregnancy	
400 mg + recommendation for age group	

Data from NIH Consensus Development Panel on Optimal Calcium Intake. (1994). Optimal calcium intake. *JAMA, 272,* 1942–1948.

Vitamin D plays a major role in both calcium absorption and bone metabolism. Vitamin D is made in the skin in the presence of sunlight or is obtained from food sources, primarily vitamin D–fortified milk. Although exposure to sunlight is necessary for cutaneous synthesis of vitamin D, prolonged exposure to sunlight does not necessarily increase the amount synthesized. An average of 15 minutes a day of sunlight exposure to hands, face, arms, and legs probably meets the requirements for most persons. While the use of sunscreen remains important to reduce photoaging and the risk of skin cancer, overuse of sunscreen is not advised. When sunscreen is applied so heavily that the skin receives no sunlight, vitamin D is not synthesized in the skin. Institutionalized, elderly, and other people who have limited sun exposure may need to supplement their diets with multiple vitamins containing vitamin D.

Clients of all ages should be encouraged to engage in regular weightbearing exercise, such as walking or running. Even in osteoporotic women, exercise programs have increased bone mass. Nonweightbearing exercise such as swimming and cycling has not demonstrated an effect on bone mass. Athletic women should be cautioned that exercising to the point of amenorrhea may be harmful to their bones. Frail, elderly people need to be assisted with some weightbearing, since immobility is known to result in bone loss.

Estrogen replacement therapy (ERT) has been proved effective in the prevention of postmenopausal osteoporosis. Estrogen maintains a positive calcium balance by decreasing the bone remodeling rate. ERT is most effective if started during the perimenopausal period, before rapid bone loss begins. However, there is evidence that ERT may be beneficial if started after menopause, even in women with established osteoporosis. The skeletal effects of estrogen are obtained with both oral and transdermal preparations. Rapid bone loss occurs if and when ERT is discontinued.

Estrogen is usually given in combination with progesterone in women with an intact uterus to prevent cancer of the uterus. Side effects of HRT include breast tenderness and vaginal bleeding. Administration of estrogen and progesterone continuously eliminates monthly bleeding in many women.

Home Care and Safety Measures

Clients with existing osteoporosis should be assessed for activity level and dietary adequacy, and appropriate teaching should be done to prevent further fractures. In addition, osteoporotic clients should be assessed for their risk of falling. Assessment includes visual acuity, medications that may cause dizziness or postural hypotension, and difficulties with balance or coordination. It is also important to assess the home environment for potential safety hazards. Evaluation of the home setting is performed via the admission assessment, discussions with the client, consultation with a specialist in social services, and home safety evaluation by a visiting nurse.

Discussion about fall prevention strategies is imperative. Clients who are prone to dizziness should be instructed to get up slowly from a lying position, sitting on the side of the bed first. They may need to have their eyeglass prescription updated to improve vision. An aid to ambulation, such as a cane or walker, may also be indicated to prevent falling. Alterations to the home may be recommended. Handrails in the bathroom, removal of scatter rugs, and increased lighting are some of the modifications that may be necessary.

Specific resources in the community that may be helpful to clients with osteoporosis include osteoporosis support groups and exercise programs. The National Osteoporosis Foundation, 2100 M St. N.W., Washington, DC 20037, is an excellent source of educational resources related to osteoporosis.

 ## Acute and Subacute Care

■ Medical Management

The goals of treatment of osteoporosis are to reduce bone loss and prevent further fracture. Furthermore, treatment is directed toward limiting pain and disability associated with existing fractures.

Pain Management

One of the most important interventions in the care of the patient with an osteoporotic fracture is pain management. Often clients present with back pain due to vertebral crush fracture syndrome. Strict bedrest lasting between 5 and 7 days has been found to be most effective in relieving pain and shortening the course of pain. The client should lie supine or in a side-lying position. After 5 to 7 days of bedrest, the client is instructed to gradually increase his or her activity.

Non-narcotic analgesics may be needed for 1 to 2 weeks to aid in relief of pain. If non-steroidal antiinflammatory medications are used, protect the client from gastric ulceration by administering medications with food or antacids.

Flexible corsets with Velcro adjustable fasteners may help to relieve back pain and fatigue. However, they will not correct the underlying problem of bone loss and spinal deformity. Corsets may be worn in bed but are most helpful if worn when the person is in the upright position.

Physical Therapy

Physical therapy is of utmost importance in the long-term treatment of back pain. Often chronic back pain is associated with decreased range of motion (ROM), weakness, muscle spasm, postural change, muscle tenderness, and decreased endurance. Physical therapy should be started during the period of bedrest with ROM exercises and mild resistive exercises of the extremities in bed. Heat or ice, ultrasound, and electrical stimulation may be used for pain relief. After acute pain subsides, patients should carry out exercises specifically prescribed for them, such as stretching and strengthening. Water aerobics may be initiated early in the treatment before the patient can tolerate weightbearing exercise. A long-term physical activity program should include weightbearing and aerobic exercise in addition to strengthening and flexibility exercise. Since osteoporotic clients are at risk of subsequent fractures, they should be taught how to move safely while maintaining or increasing physical activity.

Nutrition

Calcium nutrition is important in the management of osteoporosis. It reduces bone loss and the incidence of fractures. Calcium-rich foods and calcium supplements should be encouraged. Total calcium intake should be at least 1000 mg/day in women who are estrogen-replete and at least 1500 mg/day in those who are estrogen-deprived. Since diets low in calcium have been found to be low in other nutrients,[2] good general nutrition should be encouraged.

Pharmacologic Agents

Pharmacologic agents used for osteoporosis include calcitonin and estrogen. Calcitonin is a hormone that prevents bone loss by inhibiting bone resorption. In addition, it has analgesic effects, which may help to relieve pain associated with fractures. Calcitonin may cause nausea and flushing. The drug is administered daily by injection or nasal spray.

Estrogen replacement therapy has been found to be beneficial for postmenopausal women, even older women who did not start to take estrogen at menopause.[49]

Bisphosphonates, a class of antiresorptive drugs, are a new class of medication recently approved for treatment of osteoporosis. Alendronate (Fosamax) has been found to reduce the risk of fractured vertebrae by nearly half in postmenopausal women. The medication is safe and has few side effects. Alendronate should be taken with a full glass of water, and the client should be instructed to remain upright for an hour after taking it. If not taken according to directions, alendronate can cause gastrointestinal upset and pain.

■ Nursing Management of the Medical Client

Nursing management for the client with osteoporosis is detailed in the Care Plan.

Paget's Disease

Paget's disease, or osteitis deformans, is defined as a disorder of bone architecture characterized by an initial phase of increased rate of bone tissue breakdown by osteoclasts, followed by excessive abnormal bone formation by osteoblasts. New bone is not laid down according to the lines of stress, and this altered process leads to enlarged, distorted bones that are poorly mineralized. The diseased bone is structurally weak and prone to fractures. Paget's disease most frequently produces painful deformities of the femur, tibia, lower spine, pelvis, and cranium.

The cause of Paget's disease is unknown. One theory suggests that perhaps a slow virus with a long latent period causes Paget's disease. Although no definite hereditary pattern has been established, a familial clustering has been reported.

Paget's disease occurs worldwide, but it appears to afflict those of northwestern European extraction in North America. It is seen less frequently in Africa, Asia, and Scandinavia. In the United States, 2½ million people over the age of 40 are affected. It is more common in males than females.

Many people are diagnosed because they have experienced trauma, and their x-rays demonstrate the characteristic changes of the disease. Ten percent to 20% of persons with the disease are asymptomatic. Before clinical manifestations occur, x-rays show increased bone expansion and density. After clinical manifestations have developed, the bone shows a characteristic mosaic appearance (Fig. 74–5). A bone scan may be useful to determine whether a lesion in pagetoid bone is active or inactive. Computed tomography scans and magnetic resonance imaging are also used because they improve visualization of bone.

An increase in hydroxyproline during a 24-hour urine collection indicates osteoclastic activity. A normal or increased serum calcium, anemia, and increased alkaline phosphatase are indicative of the disease process.

In symptomatic Paget's disease, the most common presenting complaints include one or more of the following:

CARE PLAN

The Client with Osteoporosis

Nursing Diagnosis: Altered Nutrition: Less Than Body Requirements, related to calcium imbalance

Planning: Expected Outcomes. The client meets U.S. Recommended Daily Dietary Allowances requirements for calcium and vitamin D. The client describes foods high in calcium and types of calcium supplements. The client uses less caffeine and alcohol. The client discusses ways to avoid the effects of lactose intolerance (as needed).

Implementation: Nursing Intervention	Rationales
Teach the importance of diet to reduce the risk of further osteoporosis.	Dietary calcium is needed to maintain serum calcium levels, to maintain bone mass.
Refer to dietitian for consult.	Dietitians can offer assistance with food choices.
Encourage the client to eat foods high in calcium, such as plain yogurt, dairy products, seafood, sardines, green vegetables, calcium-fortified orange juice, and cereals.	These foods are excellent sources of calcium.
Provide current information about calcium supplements.	1000 to 1500 mg of calcium each day is easier to achieve with supplements.
Teach the need to reduce alcohol and caffeine intake.	Excessive alcohol and caffeine use increase bone resorption.
Teach ways to reduce risk of lactose intolerance, such as the use of acidophilus milk and commercially prepared lactase.	Lactose intolerance is caused by the inability to break down milk sugar lactose.

Evaluation: Changing nutritional habits takes time. Expect to have this as an active problem for many weeks. Encourage small improvements.

Nursing Diagnosis: Impaired Physical Activity related to osteoporosis

Planning: Expected Outcomes. The client complies with the physical mobility plan to level of independent activities of daily living (ADLs). The client uses assistive devices to perform independent ADL. The client identifies and avoids potential hazards, thereby avoiding falls and fractures resulting from minimal injury.

Implementation: Nursing Intervention	Rationales
Consult with physical therapist to develop an exercise program of weightbearing exercises and strengthening exercises such as walking, tennis, hiking, and ballroom dancing. Discuss the benefits of walking at least ½ mile three times a week. Teach the importance of exercise in prevention of osteoporosis.	Weightbearing exercises increase bone formation. Strengthening exercises increase muscle tone and circulation. National Institutes of Health (NIH) Consensus on Osteoporosis (1984) recommendations are walking, tennis, hiking, and ballroom dancing.
Assist with ADL allowing the client to remain independent.	Pain may limit the client's ability to perform ADL.
Evaluate the need for assistive devices for ADL and home use.	Devices may be needed for independent ADL.
Establish a hazard-free hospital environment:	A hazard-free environment will reduce the risk of falls.
● Provide adequate lighting	
● Adjust bed to lowest position with side rails up when client is in bed	
● Place necessary articles within client's reach.	
● Keep client area free of spills and clutter	

Evaluation: Increasing safe and weightbearing activities will require several weeks. The client will need to be pain free and develop muscle strength and flexibility before independence will be met.

Nursing Diagnosis: Pain related to fracture (vertebral, Colles' wrist, hip)

Planning: Expected Outcomes. The client experiences pain reduction or relief so the client may be independent.

Implementation: Nursing Intervention	Rationales
Assess pain medication needs. Plan medication schedule with the client.	The client may not be receiving adequate medication due to inadequate dosing, the need for around-the-clock administration, or iatrogenic causes.

Care Plan continued on following page

The Client with Osteoporosis (Continued)

Implementation: Nursing Intervention	Rationales
Administer non-narcotic analgesics.	Non-narcotic analgesics block production of chemical mediators of pain.
Monitor the effectiveness of analgesia.	Monitoring allows for revisions in the care plan.
Teach alternative modalities of pain relief, such as positioning, warm compresses, application of assistive devices, distraction, imagery, biofeedback, and hypnosis.	Alternative modalities have been found effective in reducing pain.

Evaluation: Pain relief should be accomplished within a few days when the client is immobile. Expect to revise plans to control pain once the client is mobile or exercising.

---

deep, aching bone pain, skeletal deformity (barrel-shaped chest or bowing of the tibia or femur, or kyphosis), changes in skin temperature, pathologic fractures through diseased bone, and symptoms related to nerve compression. Diseased bone pressing on the cranial nerves may result in vertigo, hearing loss with tinnitus, and blindness. Rheumatoid arthritis (RA), ankylosing spondylitis, and gout are commonly associated with Paget's disease.

Analgesics such as aspirin, indomethacin, or ibuprofen may relieve mild bone pain. Pain may also be relieved with heat therapy, massage, and bracing. Further orthopedic treatment may be indicated for severe disabling arthritis, severe bowing deformities of the femur or tibia, and pathologic fractures. Vigorous treatment of Paget's disease includes calcitonin and etidronate, both of which

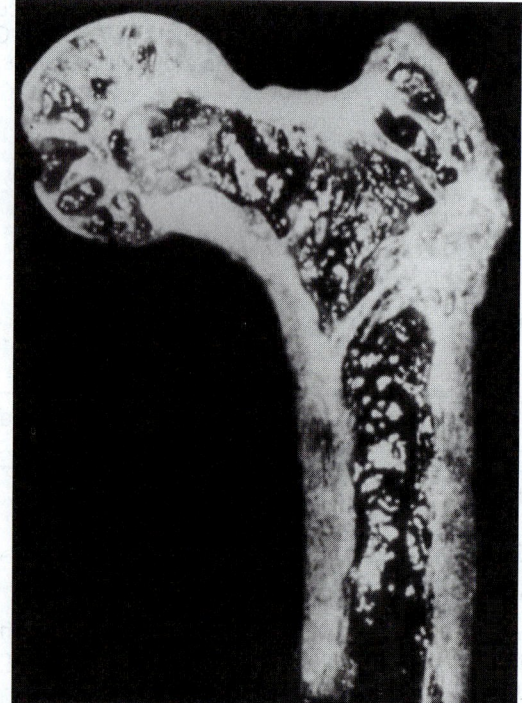

Figure 74–5. A pagetoid bone, demonstrating the characteristic mosaic pattern seen on x-rays. (From Merkow, R. L., & Lane, J. M. [1990]. Paget's disease of bone. *Orthopaedic Clinics of North America, 21*[1], 173.)

retard bone resorption. The antibiotic plicamycin (Mithracin) may be used to treat clients who are unresponsive to other treatments. Because plicamycin is cytotoxic it leads to several side effects, including hepatotoxicity, thrombocytopenia, nephrotoxicity, severe anorexia, nausea, and vomiting.

Osteomalacia

Osteomalacia is a disease in which the bone becomes abnormally soft because of a disturbed calcium and phosphorous balance secondary to vitamin D deficiency, resulting in marked deformities of the weightbearing bones and pathologic fractures.

Osteomalacia mainly affects women, and it is endemic in Asia. Occasionally, the disease can be found in strict vegetarians or in clients who have had gastrectomy. Primary hypoparathyroidism, renal tubular disorders, pancreatic insufficiency, hepatobiliary disease, and small intestine disease contribute to the incidence of osteomalacia. Women who have had multiple frequent pregnancies and who have breast-fed their children may have a higher incidence of the disease as well as persons on long-term anticonvulsants, tranquilizers, sedatives, muscle relaxants, or antidiuretics. Osteomalacia is similar to rickets, which occurs in children; therefore, the condition is called adult rickets.

Osteomalacia is always due to an inadequate concentration of calcium or phosphorus in the body fluids. Inadequate calcium or vitamin D in the diet may cause a decrease in the absorption of calcium from the intestine. Increased urinary excretion of calcium or the loss of calcium or phosphorus during pregnancy and lactation may cause osteomalacia.

Osteomalacia is characterized by widespread decalcification and softening of bones, especially in the spine, pelvis, and lower extremities. Bones become bent and flattened as they soften. In the spine, scoliotic and kyphotic deformities are present. Coxa vara deformity of the femoral neck due to pressure on the femoral neck is common.

Serum calcium and phosphorus levels are reduced, and the alkaline phosphatase level is moderately elevated. Urinary calcium and creatinine excretion levels are low.

X-rays indicate generalized demineralization with trabecular bone loss. Pseudofractures (Milkman's syndrome)

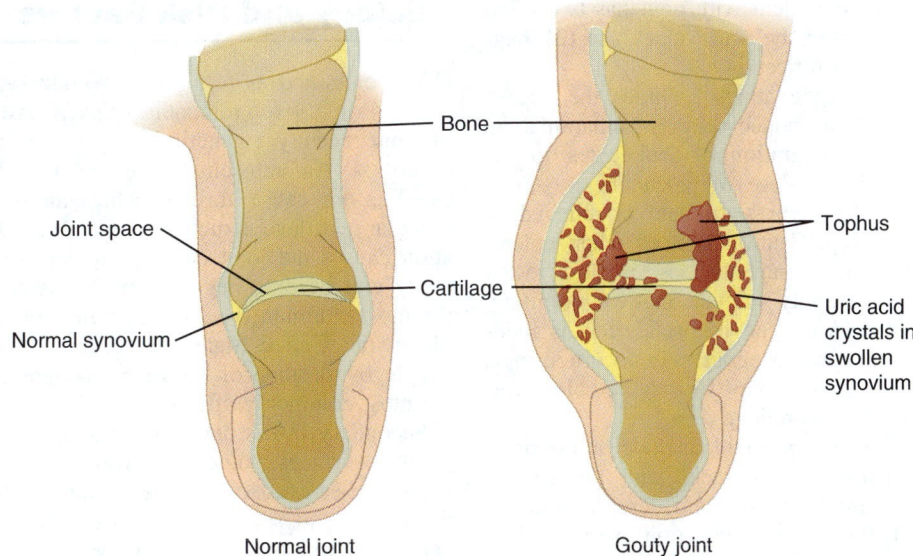

Figure 74–6. Comparison of a gouty joint and a normal joint.

and cyst formation are common. Compression fractures, and bowing and bending deformities of the long bones are often present. Biopsy may assist in diagnosis.

Intervention in osteomalacia includes vitamin D administered daily until signs of healing take place, when a daily low maintenance dose is continued. Adequate intake of calcium and phosphorous as well as protein should be ensured. Supplemental calcium in the form of lactate or gluconate is administered.

Gout and Gouty Arthritis

Gout is a metabolic bone disorder in which purine (protein) metabolism is altered and the by-product, uric acid, accumulates. Gout is classified as primary or secondary. Primary gout is caused by an inherited defect of purine metabolism leading to increased or decreased renal excretion. Primary gout accounts for 80% of all cases, of which 95% are males. The initial attack of gout occurs in the 30s or 40s.

Secondary gout is an acquired condition, following hematopoietic (multiple myeloma, polycythemia vera, and leukemia) or renal disorders. In hematopoietic disorders there is an increase in cell turnover and increased uric acid production. In addition, gout may develop from the rapid induction of chemotherapy or radiation therapy when there is massive destruction of cells. Renal disorders that decrease the excretion of uric acid may lead to gout. Hyperuricemia may also result from use of aspirin, thiazide, and mercurial diuretics, and some antituberculosis medications. Alcohol intoxication and starvation increase serum urate levels by inhibiting renal excretion due to lactic acidosis and ketosis, respectively. In addition, alcohol ingestion increases urate production by stimulating purine breakdown. Prolonged use of diuretics and other medications (levodopa, nicotinic acid, low-dose salicylates) also reduce excretion of uric acid and precipitate gout.

In the body, uric acid is made by the enzymatic break-

down of tissue and dietary purines. Hyperuricemia develops because of undersecretion or overproduction of uric acid. In addition to accumulating in the blood, uric acid accumulates in the synovial fluid, myocardium, kidneys, and ears. When uric acid levels reach a certain level, they crystallize and the crystals, called tophi, are deposited in connective tissue. Because the crystals are deposited in connective tissue, gout is classified as a form of arthritis (Fig. 74–6).

Clinical manifestations of gout develop in stages:

Stage I: Asymptomatic hyperuricemia.

Stage II: Acute attack with redness, swelling, and exquisite tenderness in one joint (toes, fingers, wrists, ankles, knees, or other joints). The great toe is the most common site. This first attack develops quickly, often overnight. Fever, tachycardia, malaise, and anorexia may be noted. The acute episode usually subsides within a week. As the edema subsides, pruritus and local desquamation (tissue loss) may be noted. Following the initial attack the affected joint returns to normal and the client may be asymptomatic for years. Eventually, other attacks occur.

Stage III: Asymptomatic hyperuricemia again. Laboratory and x-ray findings are unchanged from stage II.

Stage IV: Permanent changes in multiple joints with restrictions in movement. Tophi may be detected on the ears, hands, elbows, feet, and knees. Renal and cardiac disorders may also develop. The client may have uric acid renal stones, renal colic, and hypertension. Atherosclerosis occurs in about half of all clients.

Gout is diagnosed by the presence of persistent hyperuricemia (> 7.0 mg/dl) in addition to the clinical manifestations. The presence of uric acid in an aspirated sample of synovial fluid confirms the diagnosis.

The management of the client with gout has two components: (1) management of the acute attack and (2) long-term management of hyperuricemia.

Management of the acute attack includes the use of colchicine and NSAIDs to reduce pain and inflammation. Colchicine reduces the migration of leukocytes to the synovial fluids. The initial dose of colchicine is 0.6 to 1.0 mg followed by 0.5 mg/hr until pain is relieved or signs of toxicity develop. Caution is used when colchicine is given because the therapeutic dose is close to the toxic dose. Signs of toxicity include nausea, vomiting, and diarrhea. Other NSAIDs can be used, such as indomethacin. In resistant cases of gout, adrenocorticotropic hormone (ACTH) or steroids may be required. Ice over the inflamed joints may also relieve pain.

Medications to lower uric acid include allopurinol, which blocks formation of uric acid, and probenecid, which promotes resorption of uric acid deposits and excretion of uric acid. Long-term medication use is advised in clients who have more than two attacks of gout a year, secondary forms of gout, or persistent hyperuricemia. Salicylates (aspirin) antagonize the action of uricosuric agents and must not be used concurrently.

There are differing opinions on dietary treatment for gout. In the past, a low-purine diet was used, which eliminates many proteins from the diet. Some physicians have prescribed a decrease in red and organ meats; others prescribe no dietary changes at all.

Encourage ample fluid intake to promote excretion of uric acid. A moderate intake of distilled forms of alcohol does not seem to precipitate gouty attacks. Beer, ale, and wine may precipitate them. Excessive alcohol in any form should be avoided.

Encourage gradual weight loss after the initial attack. Weight loss alone may reduce the incidence of attacks and uric acid levels. A sudden loss of weight may precipitate an attack due to the destruction of cells.

Clients who can recognize early symptoms of gout can avert the attack in many cases by prompt use of colchicine or indomethacin. Long-term side effects (alopecia, bone marrow suppression, hepatic damage) from these agents, although rare, should be explained to the client.

Nursing management of the client with gout includes pain management. The client is usually placed at bedrest until pain subsides. Once ambulating, the client's need for crutches or a walker should be considered until gait is stable. Dietary restrictions, fluid requirements, and long-term self-management are taught to the client.

Connective Tissue Disorders

Osteoarthritis

Osteoarthritis (OA) is a noninflammatory joint disease, characterized by degeneration and loss of articular cartilage in synovial joints. OA was previously called degenerative joint disease (DJD), but the term DJD is generally considered inaccurate because there is no biochemical or metabolic degeneration.

Etiology and Risk Factors

OA is classified as primary or secondary, based upon its cause. Primary (or idiopathic) OA is associated with aging, but recently a genetic basis for the disorder has been described. An autosomal recessive trait has been implicated as one cause, through which the genes encoded for articular cartilage structure are altered. This gene alteration causes the joint cartilage to repair itself less effectively and become degraded more easily. Primary OA is the most common type, existing in about 60 million people in the United States. It occurs in about 50% of all people by the age of 16 years. Weightbearing joints are the most commonly affected.

Secondary OA is due to conditions that lead to damage to joint surfaces, sometimes from "wear and tear" of the joints. Other causes of OA are joint injury such as repetitive strain and sprains, joint dislocation, fractures, disorders that lead to abnormal movements (e.g., neurologic disease), and medications that stimulate the activity of collagen-digesting enzymes in the synovial membrane (e.g., steroids, colchicine).

Primary prevention of OA can be achieved with the reduction of injury seen in sports with the use of protective gear and warm-ups. Also, the reduction of repetitive motions, such as those in assembly-line work, decreases wear and tear on joints.

Pathophysiology

The pathophysiology of OA is the loss of articular cartilage due to enzymatic destruction (Fig. 74–7). Destruction begins in the matrix, leading to damage to proteoglycans and collagen. Layers of the cartilage loosen and

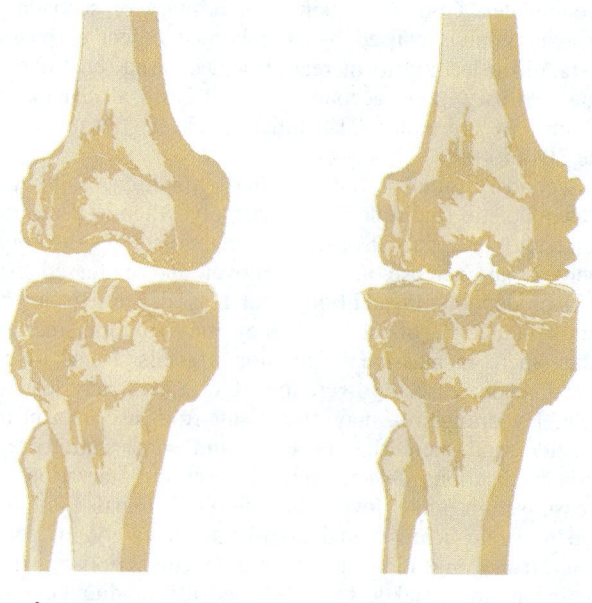

A　Normal　　　　　B　Degenerated

Figure 74–7. Pathologic changes seen in osteoarthritis. *A,* Normal bony surfaces for articulation are altered. *B,* There is loss of joint space and formation of osteophytes.

Table 74–2. Differential Diagnosis of Osteoarthritis and Rheumatoid Arthritis

	Osteoarthritis	Rheumatoid Arthritis
Pathologic changes	Cartilage degeneration, bone regeneration (spurs)	Inflammation of synovial membrane; bone destruction; damage to ligaments, tendons, cartilage, joint capsule
Joints affected	Hands, spine, knees, hips may be asymmetrical	Symmetrical (both sides): wrists, knees, knuckles
Features: symptoms	Localized pain and stiffness, Heberden's nodes, usually not much edema	Swelling, redness, warmth, pain, tenderness, nodules, fatigue, stiffness, muscle aches, fever
Other systems affected	None	Lungs, heart, skin
Prognosis: long-term	Less pain for some, more pain and disability for others; few severely disabled	Disease is less aggressive with time; deformity can often be prevented
Age: onset	Age 45–90. Most clients have some features with increasing age	Age 25–50
Sex	Males and females about equal	Females affected more often
Heredity	One form is familial	Familial tendency
Tests	X-rays	Rheumatoid factor (80%), blood test, x-rays, examination of joint fluid, Lyme titer
Treatment	Maintain activity level, exercise, joint protection, weight control, relaxation, heat, sometimes medication/surgery	Reduce inflammation, balanced exercise program, joint protection, weight control, relaxation, heat, medication/surgery

Modified from Maher, A., Salmond, S., & Pellino, T. (1994). *Orthopaedic nursing.* Philadelphia: W. B. Saunders.

eventually the subchondral bone becomes unprotected. In addition, cysts and fissures often develop in the bone. If the fluid content inside the cyst breaks open into the synovial space through the cartilage, further destruction of the joint occurs. When the cartilage is ruptured small pieces of bone that coat the surface may form abnormal bony growths in the joint space and surrounding bone. Osteophytes of new bone may break off and lodge in the synovial space, possibly leading to inflammation of the joint capsule.

Clinical Manifestations and Diagnostic Findings

It is important to differentiate OA from rheumatoid arthritis (RA) (see Table 74–2 and Chapter 28). RA is a systematic inflammatory joint disease with an autoimmune cause. Clients with RA tend to be young women. In contrast, clients with OA tend to be older men. RA begins in the smaller joints (e.g., hands and wrists); OA primarily affects weightbearing joints—the hips and knees. Laboratory studies in RA include elevated sedimentation rate and positive rheumatoid factor. There are no specific laboratory tests to confirm OA. Sometimes, the sedimentation rate is elevated if the client has synovitis. X-rays of OA show reduced joint space, and osteophytes may be visible.

Clinical manifestations of OA are aching pain, crepitus, and stiffness in involved large weightbearing joints. The client may also have enlarged joints, contractures, and muscle spasms. New bone growth in joints may lead to swelling, called Heberden's nodes (Fig. 74–8). When osteophytes lodge in the joint, swelling, called joint effusion, occurs.

Community and Self-Care

■ Medical Management

Medical management of the client with OA includes pain management, reduction of inflammation, and improvement of ROM and strength. Nonsteroidal anti-inflammatory drugs (NSAIDs) are used to reduce inflammation and pain. Narcotics are not used, because of the chronic nature of OA. In addition, local injections of steroids such as cortisone may be used for acute pain in a single joint. When joints become inflamed or acutely painful, they may be rested in splints that limit motion in the joint. Splints are not used for prolonged periods, because the joint tends to stiffen when immobilized and the client may have difficulty in regaining ROM. Skin traction or cervical collars may be used for OA of the vertebrae. Heat treatments can also be used to control pain and reduce inflammation. Other methods for pain control should also be used. There is no specific diet for OA, nor is there a diet that will "cure" OA. Obese clients are encouraged to lose weight and increase activity as allowed by their pain levels. Decreasing activity is not advised for any client with OA; the client should be taught to exercise daily despite mild discomfort. Im-

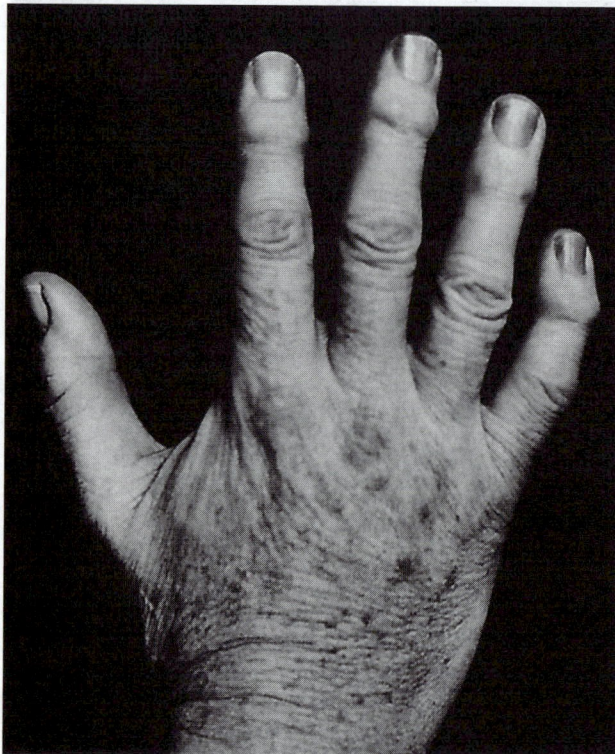

Figure 74–8. Heberden's nodes on the distal portions of the fingers in a client with osteoarthritis. (From Gartland, J. J. [1987]. *Fundamentals of orthopaedics* [4th ed., p. 125]. Philadelphia: W. B. Saunders.)

proved muscle tone and strength can relieve the chronic pain of OA. Low levels of exercise are as beneficial as high-intensity exercise.

■ Nursing Management of the Medical Client

Nursing management of the client with OA includes encouragement of activity. Walking, swimming, and water aerobics are some of the best activities. Ambulatory aids may be helpful by reducing the weight on involved joints. Weight reduction should be encouraged, if needed, because being closer to ideal body weight lessens strain on joints.

Pain should be managed with NSAIDs. Be certain to instruct clients to take NSAIDs with food, milk, or antacids to reduce the risk of gastric ulcerations. Ice or heat may be applied to the joints. Positions of comfort should be used only for short times. Discourage clients from propping a joint in flexion without stretching the joint. The continual use of flexion encourages contracture.

Promote self-care. Various devices can be purchased to facilitate self-care. Rubber grips can be used to open jars. Velcro closures can be placed on clothing rather than zippers or buttons. Front-closing garments and slip-on shoes should be worn.

Acute and Subacute Care: Osteotomy, Arthrodesis, and Total Hip Replacement

■ Surgical Management

Osteotomy

Osteotomy is the removal of a section of bone to realign a joint, and decrease joint strain. It is commonly performed for valgus (knock-knee) and varus (bowleg) deformities. After surgery, the leg is wrapped from toes to groin and elevated. Ambulation is allowed with toe-touch weightbearing.

Arthrodesis

Arthrodesis is fusion of a joint. This operation is reserved for joints that cannot be reconstructed. Initial immobility is provided with pins, braces, or casts.

Total Hip Replacement

Total hip replacement, or arthroplasty, is an operation to restore motion to the joint and function to the muscles, ligaments, and other soft tissue structures that control the joint. (See Chapter 28 for a discussion of shoulder, elbow and hand arthroplasty.)

Indications

Indications for surgery include a painful, disabling arthritic joint that is no longer responding to nonsurgical treatments. Severe hip pain can interfere with sleep, prevent walking, and impair or prevent sexual enjoyment. Usually, the subjective changes are the major driving force for surgery and not just changes of joint shape on x-ray. The prostheses used in arthroplasty were designed for older persons and for people with a relatively sedentary life-style. Young persons can have joint replacement surgery, but the failure rate (loosening of the prosthesis) is increased. Persons who are very active or heavy laborers are also not good candidates for arthroplasty. If both hips are involved, surgery is usually performed on the most severely affected hip. Several weeks later, when the client has recovered from the first operation, surgery is performed on the other hip. If the client is in excellent condition otherwise, both hips can be operated on together (although this is rare). A total hip replacement also may be performed for complications of femoral neck fractures, failure of previous reconstructive surgery (such as osteotomy and femoral head replacement), and complications of congenital hip disease.

Contraindications

Contraindications to hip arthroplasty include systemic infection, hip infection, diseases that are destroying bone, progressive neurologic diseases, and poor abductor muscle strength. In addition, the client's general health must be satisfactory to withstand anesthesia, blood loss, and surgical stress. Heart, lung, liver, and metabolic disorders are stabilized prior to surgery.

Techniques

The client lies in a lateral position for the surgery with the leg in a sling. A long incision is made along the lateral surface of the hip. The hip must be dislocated in order to replace the two surfaces. The two most common techniques for hip dislocation will be discussed. An established surgical technique is to temporarily remove the trochanter for exposure and then replace it following the arthroplasty. A newer technique is to place the incision more posterior and not remove the trochanter. As you will see later, the surgical approach is a very important aspect of postoperative care.

Once the hip is open the old femoral head is removed and the acetabulum is shaved to fit the new acetabular prosthesis. The prosthesis can be held in place with a glue (methyl methacrylate) or with cementless component. The cement can cause problems during insertion by causing nerve damage from heat and hypotension. The cement can also loosen in time. Newer implants are made with a porous metal coating and are inserted with a tight fit, known as a press fit. The implant is placed very snugly against the bone, and within about 6 weeks, new bone tissue grows between the pores and grafts to the new prosthesis. The bony growth serves as the fixation mechanism that holds the device in place. Issues of bony resorption are beginning to emerge. Therefore, further refinement in surgical techniques will continue to develop.

Sometimes, the greater trochanter with attachment of the abductor muscles is transferred distally on the femur to increase the efficiency of the abductor mechanism. When such a transfer is made, the greater trochanter is usually held in its new position by wires. The transfer must be protected until it heals in place (4–6 weeks). In this situation, progressive abduction exercises must be limited. Excessive exercise may cause nonunion or fracture of the osteotomy site.

Complications

Clients are at risk for many complications after total hip arthroplasty. Fortunately, most of them are rare. Nerve injury can develop after surgery due to peroneal nerve compression. Hemorrhage and hematomas can develop, especially in clients who have had major resections of tissue or revisional hip surgery. Infection is a serious concern, because osteomyelitis is very difficult to treat. Staples are used for wound closure because they are associated with a lower infection rate. Bladder infection is fairly common and may be iatrogenic or may have existed prior to surgery. In either case, the infection can spread into the wound and therefore should be treated promptly.

Thromboembolism is the most common and most serious complication after hip surgery. Embolism is responsible for more than 50% of the deaths after hip arthroplasty.

Leg length discrepancy can occur because leg length is difficult to determine accurately during surgery. Revisional surgery may be needed. Shoe elevators usually help.

Dislocation and subluxation is always a concern and several precautions are taken during and after surgery to prevent these problems. Clients at highest risk of dislocation and subluxation are those having a revision of a previous hip arthroplasty, who sustain some type of trauma (e.g., fall) after surgery, who have abductor weakness, or who accidentally place the hip in extremes of flexion, adduction, or internal rotation. Most dislocations occur within 6 weeks of surgery. The dislocation is usually precipitated by malposition when the client does not yet have muscle control or strength. Long-term complications include fractures, nonunion of bone, loosening of the femoral and acetabular components, and bone infection.

Outcomes

Total joint replacement results in immediate and substantial improvement in the client's pain, functional status, and overall health-related quality of life, which persist for years. Because of improvements in technology, more than 90% of all artificial joints never need revision.

■ Nursing Management of the Surgical Client: Total Hip Replacement

There is no universally accepted postoperative rehabilitation program after total hip arthroplasty. Although a pain-free hip can be obtained with limited efforts, a well-designed rehabilitation program will speed recovery of motion and function, diminish limping, and aid a return to independent living.

Preoperative Care

Assessment

The client's physical and psychological readiness for surgery is assessed. Many clients are admitted the same day as surgery, so most of the preoperative nursing assessment is completed by telephone interview. Ambulation is assessed, ideally by a physical therapist, and areas are identified that may need extra help postoperatively.

Diagnosis, Planning, Implementation

Knowledge Deficit. The common nursing diagnosis of knowledge deficit can be used to describe the client's previous inexperience with surgery in general, joint replacement surgery, or postoperative restrictions. The diagnosis can be written *Knowledge Deficit related to previous inexperience with surgery.*

Planning: Expected Outcomes. The client will understand the proposed surgery, postoperative restrictions, and rehabilitation, as evidenced by his or her statements and compliance with the postoperative regimen.

Implementation. Because of cost control measures,

most clients are admitted to a hospital room after the surgery, so the preoperative teaching is completed by nurses in the office setting and preoperative preparation room. In addition, the client is usually called the day prior to surgery to reinforce needed precautions (such as NPO [nothing by mouth], medications). The client and significant others are taught about the procedure and what the client can expect after surgery. Teach the client how to use crutches, a walker, or both. Encourage the client to practice using crutches or a walker. Assist the client to practice moving from bed to a chair or wheelchair without flexing the hip more than 90 degrees (limited flexion is needed after surgery to prevent dislocation of the prosthesis).

Physical therapists and nurses assess the client preoperatively and teach postoperative exercise. If the exercises are not understood preoperatively, the client may not be able to do them effectively after surgery, when pain and anxiety may be present. Exercises include quadriceps sets, gluteal sets, isometric hip extension and abduction exercises, as well as upper extremity strengthening exercises to prepare for crutch walking or use of a walker. Encourage the client to practice the exercises regularly.

Evaluation

Expect the client to be able to explain the operation and his or her role in recovery. Anxiety may interfere with learning. If you notice the client is quite anxious, try to lower anxiety prior to teaching.

Postoperative Care

Care of clients after total hip replacement does not differ significantly from the usual care given any postoperative client. (For a review of general postoperative care, see Chapter 21). The major difference is that the client cannot turn after a total hip replacement. Therefore, skin integrity is a concern, and pressure reduction mattresses are used, especially if the client is frail or malnourished. If female clients require urinary catheterization, they often cannot abduct and externally rotate the operative hip due to pain (and many times cannot move the nonoperative hip due to degenerative disease or RA). Therefore, extra assistance is usually needed to visualize the perineum.

Assessment

After total hip replacement, frequently assess neurovascular status. Check the color, warmth, movement, sensation, capillary refit, and pedal pulses in both feet according to hospital protocol. Monitor the client's position: The legs must remain abducted but not externally rotated.

The dressing applied immediately after surgery is usually heavy and bulky, and is left in place (but carefully assessed) until the surgeon removes it 2 to 3 days postoperatively. In addition, Hemovac drains are placed to drain excess blood fluid from the wound and to reduce dead space. Expect a moderate amount of bloody drainage for 48 hours. Drainage from the wound drains is usually less than 600 ml/24 hours or 200 ml/8 hours unless the client has been heavily hydrated with plasma expanders such as dextran. In this case, the amount of output from these drains can easily triple. Therefore, intake and output totals should be carefully calculated to assess fluid balance. After 48 hours, the wound is either re-covered with a light dressing or sometimes left open to the air. The wound is usually cleaned each shift according to the surgeon's orders.

Diagnosis, Planning, Implementation

Pain. Acute pain is a common and expected nursing diagnosis after any surgery. Joint replacement is no different. Write the diagnosis as *Pain related to local tissue trauma from surgical incision.*

Planning: Expected Outcomes. The client will be comfortable after surgery as evidenced by stating that the pain is tolerable, moving without grimacing, asking for fewer narcotics, or using narcotics of lesser strength.

Implementation. Immediately after surgery, pain is intense and usually requires injectable narcotics (intramuscular, patient-controlled analgesia [PCA], or epidural). As expected, pain is intensified with movement and decreases with inactivity. Clients often attempt to limit their activity and may refuse to get up to a bedside chair because they know it will hurt. It is important for the nurse to be empathic but to be reasonably insistent that the client ambulate, pointing out the serious complications of immobility in this group of clients. Medicate the client prior to any activity and monitor tolerance of the activity. Many clients can remain up in the bedside chair for only 15 to 20 minutes the first time (which is just long enough to make the bed).

Be certain to assess for complications of narcotic use. Respiratory depression is a concern, but not common. A very common problem is constipation, especially since the risk is increased with immobility and advanced age. Plan on administering laxatives and stool softeners and encourage the use of dietary fiber. Older persons worry about bowel function and it is important not to minimize their concerns. Many older persons routinely use some sort of bulk or fiber laxative at home. Therefore, the nurse is wise to plan ahead for these concerns.

It is important to consider that even though the arthroplasty will reduce pain in one joint, arthritis continues in all the other joints. Therefore, administer non-narcotic analgesics also to reduce generalized discomfort.

Impaired Physical Mobility. Several issues will influence the degree of immobility after joint replacement. These factors include pain, arthritis in other joints, and fear of movement. Write the diagnosis as *Impaired physical mobility related to pain or fear of movement.*

Planning: Expected Outcomes. The client will have improving physical mobility as evidenced by needing less assistance in transferring from the bed to a chair or wheelchair, rising from a sitting position to standing with less assistance, and using the walker or crutches safely.

Implementation. Since there is usually a lot of anxiety in moving orthopedic clients, a detailed discussion is provided on safe movement to and from the chair. This discussion is designed to help you move the client safely and to be aware of risk to your low back at the same time.

The client is usually assisted to a bedside chair the morning following surgery. Initially the client requires two persons to assist, one on each side. Use caution not to strain your back while helping the client to stand. Two important points are (1) to be close to the client while moving and (2) to avoid twisting motions. Slide the trapeze toward the foot of the bed first. This allows the client to assist with sitting up. Move the client to the edge of the bed, keeping the legs abducted. The client often needs help to pivot in bed to sit on the edge of the bed, due to weakness in hip abductors and upper arms. Once at the edge of the bed, position your foot to block the client's foot from slipping on the floor. Assist the client to a standing position by having the client push off with the hands from the bed. Support the client beneath the axillae. Remember to get close to the client to keep the center of gravity between you and your body. Do not let the client use the walker to pull himself or herself to a standing position. The walker will tip over. The walker should only be used once the client is standing. The amount of weightbearing on the operative leg is specified by the surgeon. It usually ranges from toe-touch to 25% weightbearing. The amount of pressure felt in the leg with these weight limits must be learned by the client. Once the client is standing, pause for a moment and have the client take some deep breaths. Ask about orthostatic hypotension (dizziness) before moving to reduce the risk of falls. Instruct the client to lift the walker first, then move the nonoperative leg, and finally the operative leg. Encourage the client to stand erect when using the walker, rather than stooped over looking at the floor. Once the client reaches the chair, he or she will be tired and want to drop quickly into the chair. Remind the client not to sit until he or she feels the back of the chair, and to use the arms of the chair to glide down into the seat. The leg may be elevated slightly for comfort.

Use a chair that has an elevated seat and arms. To see the amount of hip flexion needed for standing up from a chair, try standing up from a low chair without arms using only one of your legs. This amount of movement and stress could injure the hip. When moving from chair to bed, the client slides forward in the chair. This is to prevent excessive hip flexion. Again, the client pushes up from the chair using the arms of the chair and is assisted by two persons. The walker is then used, using the same ambulation process. Once in bed the client's leg is positioned in abduction.

Most clients are comfortable and alert enough the day after surgery to begin a program of bed exercises. Ankle pumps, quadriceps and gluteal isometrics, and gentle rotation exercises are begun. Straight leg raising, used after knee surgery, is not helpful after total hip arthroplasty. Physical therapy may be started as early as the second postoperative day. In addition to helping the client ambulate, physical therapy may include gentle, active, and assisted ROM exercises in sling suspension (within the pain-free range). Until discharge, the client continues exercises that increase ROM and strengthen hip muscles.

Progressive ambulation follows with crutches or a walker, and finally, a cane. If the client has upper extremity problems, like arthritis of the shoulders and hands, special types of walkers with arm platforms may be required for ambulation.

Risk for Compartment Syndrome and Nerve Injury.
Be aware of the collaborative problem of risk for compartment syndrome and nerve injury related to edema in the surgical site and external rotation placing direct pressure on the nerve.

Planning: Expected Outcomes. The nurse will monitor for signs of compartment syndrome. Do not allow the leg to rest in external rotation; pressure is applied to the peroneal nerve which runs close to the skin's surface behind the knee. If the nerve is injured due to ischemia from prolonged pressure, footdrop can result.

Implementation. Assess nerve function and circulation in the affected leg every 1 or 2 hours (or as directed by the physician) for the first day or so, then as often as the client's condition warrants. These assessments are called neurovascular assessments. They include assessment of bilateral pulses and quality, extremity skin color and temperature, capillary refill in the toes, sensation of the toes and feet, movement of toes, and dorsiplantar flexion of feet. Report any pallor, numbness, coolness, "needles and pins" sensation, or inability to move promptly.

Risk for Dislocation of the Prosthesis.
If the client had a standard surgical approach to total hip arthroplasty or had the trochanter repositioned, there is risk of dislocation because the hip is unstable while the trochanter heals again. To reduce the risk of dislocation, strain on the gluteals is minimized.

Planning: Expected Outcomes. The nurse will position the client to reduce risk of prosthesis dislocation and monitor for signs of dislocation.

Implementation
Proper Positioning. After total hip replacement, assess the client's position frequently while the client is in bed. Prevent external rotation or adduction of the affected leg and flexion of the hip of more than 90 degrees. The operative leg is placed at 15 degrees of abduction. Usually a triangular abduction pillow is used to maintain abduction and prevent extremes of flexion. Straps secure the limb to the pillow. The straps must be positioned carefully to avoid placing pressure on the peroneal nerve. Balanced suspension or traction may also be used to maintain abduction, but these interventions are uncommon. Keep the operative leg in an abducted position and in straight alignment. Use trochanter rolls to assist the weak leg to maintain straight alignment. Encourage and supervise prescribed exercises such as quadriceps sets. Muscle strengthening of the gluteal muscles helps prevent dislocation.

In addition, the client cannot turn to the side. Turning to the side either has the client lying on the incision or risking adduction of the leg if uppermost. Therefore, if an occupied bed must be made, it is made from top to bottom.

If the greater trochanter was transferred to the distal position on the femur to increase the efficiency of the abductor mechanism, progressive abduction exercises must be limited. Follow the surgeon's orders concerning movement and positioning.

Ambulation. The client is usually mobilized at the bedside on the first or second postoperative day. This may mean standing at the bedside briefly or being assisted to a chair. Be careful not to flex the hip joint greater than 90 degrees, and maintain abduction of the legs to prevent dislocation. Recall that one point of attachment for the gluteal muscles is the greater trochanter. Therefore, any movement that stretches the gluteal muscles (e.g., leaning forward to get up from a seated position) will increase the risk of injury. (Positions to avoid are shown in Figure 74–9).

Risk for Infection. Clients with joint replacement are at increased risk for serious infections, such as osteomyelitis, related to the use of implanted prostheses.

Planning: Expected Outcomes. The client will not develop an infection in the implanted prosthesis, as evidenced by a normal white blood cell (WBC) count, temperature, absence of purulent drainage, and no sign of inflammation.

Implementation. Prevention of infection is another priority in the client after hip replacement. These clients are at high risk of infection for several reasons. First, a foreign body has been implanted. Although the material used produces little inflammation, it is a potential source of infection because of the trauma of surgery. The client may also have been receiving anti-inflammatory agents, especially steroids or cytotoxic medications, which increase the risk of infection. This places the total joint replacement client at greater risk of infection.

Usually the client is started on prophylactic broad-spectrum antibiotics during surgery, and this therapy is continued for several days after surgery. If the client begins to exhibit any sign of infection in the operative site such as redness, fever, purulent drainage, or increasing incisional pain, any drainage is cultured and aggressive antibiotic therapy is begun.

Other preventive measures range from the use of staples for wound closure, because they are associated with a lower infection rate, and the use of strict aseptic technique when handling dressings or wound drains.

Risk for Thrombophlebitis. Thrombophlebitis is a common finding in persons who are immobile, have edema of the pelvic area, are of advanced age, have had previous problems with thrombophlebitis, are obese, have heart failure, or have had a transfusion. Choose the cause(s) that best describes your client; several of them may apply.

Planning: Expected Outcomes. The nurse will monitor for manifestations of thrombophlebitis and provide preventive care as prescribed.

Implementation. Assess the client twice daily for manifestations of thrombophlebitis. Manifestations of thrombophlebitis include pain and unilateral edema and

erythema in the leg. Homans' sign is usually positive, but it is important to recognize that a positive Homans' sign does not mean that the client has a blood clot. Other conditions, even things as simple as shin splints, can lead to a positive Homans' sign. In fact, many clients have blood clots but no manifestations.

To prevent the development of deep vein thrombosis (DVT), support stockings are applied to the client preoperatively and are maintained postoperatively. The stockings should be removed for about 1 hour twice daily. They can be washed, too, if needed. In addition, sequential compression devices can be used to promote venous return. Exercising the unaffected leg also helps prevent clot formation. Other preventive measures include aspirin, low-dose heparin, low-molecular-weight heparin, or warfarin, or a combination of these. All of these medications help to prevent thrombophlebitis without significantly increasing the risk of hemorrhage. Initially, a high-risk client is begun on injectable low-dose heparin and then switched to warfarin once oral intake is satisfactory. For 2 days, both heparin and warfarin are given. Warfarin has a slow onset and a long half-life; therefore, it is necessary to use both medications for a short time. The prothrombin time is monitored daily and the warfarin dose adjusted accordingly. Look for new orders each day.

To diagnose blood clots, venography or Doppler studies of the lower leg are commonly used. If the test is positive, that is, if blood clots are noted, continuous heparin is begun and the client is placed at bedrest with leg elevation. Frequent assessment for pulmonary embolism is needed. Recall that a thrombus can break off and move (called embolization). It commonly would travel to the lung and be called "pulmonary embolism, or PE." This is a lethal condition. To read more about DVT, thrombophlebitis, and PE, see Chapter 50.

Risk for Adrenal Insufficiency. Clients taking steroids to treat their arthritis are at risk for adrenocortical insufficiency, or addisonian crisis. When subjected to the stress of surgery, steroid-dependent clients may exhibit signs of adrenocortical insufficiency.

Planning: Expected Outcome. The nurse will monitor for manifestations of adrenocortical insufficiency. These manifestations include tachycardia, hypotension, diaphoresis, and a decreasing level of consciousness. This condition resembles hypovolemic shock, although in this case there is no bleeding and the client is not hypotensive. If there is abrupt cessation of adrenocorticoids, hypotension and diuresis can occur.

Implementation. Treatment of adrenocortical insufficiency or addisonian crisis is intravenous hydrocortisone administration, often in the form of Solu-Cortef. Once the client's level of steroids is increased, the clinical manifestations resolve very rapidly. Be aware of the possibility of this complication developing and be sure that the client receives increased steroid doses as prescribed, to prevent the crisis situation.

Evaluation

Progress toward goals is assessed every day. Clinical pathways are used by several facilities to guide care and

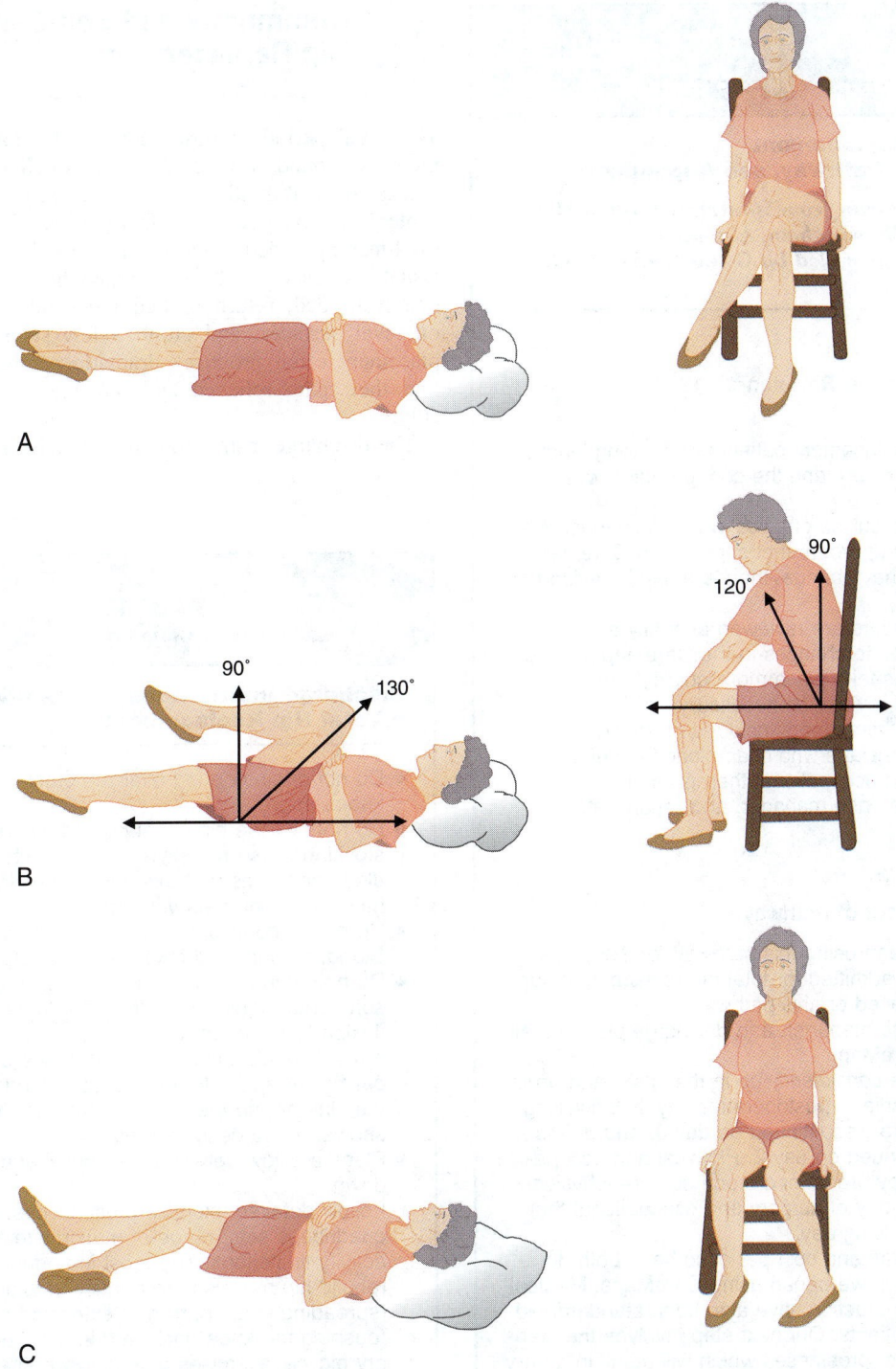

Figure 74–9. Positions to avoid after total hip replacement. It is essential that clients avoid positions that stretch the gluteal muscles. These positions include (*A*) crossing the operated leg across the midline of the body, (*B*) flexing the hip more than 90 degrees, and (*C*) rotating the leg externally. (Modified from Maher, A. B., Salmond, S. W., & Pellino, T. A. [1994]. *Orthopaedic nursing.* Philadelphia: W. B. Saunders.)

encourage progression. These plans also attempt to limit the number of tasks forgotten or overlooked, such as laboratory work. Discrepancies or deviations from the plan are usually recorded for later review.

Assess whether the outcomes have been met for the client who has had surgery. Because of controlled length of hospital stay, it is important to communicate with the extended care facility with respect to outcomes that are unmet.

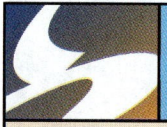

CASE MANAGEMENT

Total Hip Replacement
For Clinical Pathway, see Appendix D.

Clinical Pathway from Montclair Baptist Medical Center, Birmingham, Alabama
Information provided by Gwen Cooke, R.N., B.S.N., O.N.C.

Development and Revision of Pathway

- Total hip replacement patients had a long length of stay (10 days), and the cost per case was high.
- Revisions occur as practice patterns change. We have standing orders that support the CareMap and when they change, the CareMap is revised as necessary.
- Standing orders are reviewed annually and that usually leads to changes in the CareMap. If practice changes take place more quickly, the CareMap is revised as necessary.
- The development team included orthopedic nurses, physicians who championed CareMaps, physical and occupational therapists, the dietitian, the case manager, and rehabilitation staff.

Use and Impact of Pathway

- We have been using this pathway for 2½ years.
- All patients admitted for total hip replacement surgery are placed on this pathway.
- Nurses, case manager, and discharge planners all use the CareMap.
- Patients are *consistently* up in the chair, and up in the chair earlier—postoperative day 1. Indwelling catheters are discontinued on day 3, and drains are discontinued on day 2. Physical and occupational therapy are started much earlier—physical therapy the day of surgery and occupational therapy the following day.
- Length of stay and cost per case have both decreased since we began using CareMaps. Medical and nursing practice have also been standardized for these patients. Our next step involves the standardization of prostheses which will result in a very large cost savings for the institution and the payor. We are negotiating with three vendors (for prosthetic implants) to get a discounted price. We are also using Patient Demand Matching, a methodology whereby the type of hip prosthesis is determined by the characteristics of the patient and his or her life-style. An athlete, for example, would get a much more durable prosthesis designed to withstand vigorous exercise. A frail, elderly patient needs a much less expensive prosthesis. By understanding the patient's needs before surgery, we can reduce the cost of this procedure significantly.

Community and Self-Care: Total Hip Replacement

The usual period of hospitalization for total hip replacement is around 4 to 5 days. Most clients still require extensive rehabilitation, so they are sent to rehabilitation centers or extended-care facilities until they are able to function independently or with limited assistance. Usually clients can be discharged home when they can rise from bed, return to bed independently, walk alone on level surfaces, and climb a few steps. Total hip replacement often produces dramatic results. Clients often find their pain relieved and movement increased markedly.

The discharge instructions that the client and significant

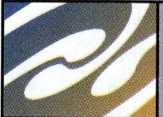

CLIENT EDUCATION GUIDE

Discharge Instructions for the Client After a Total Hip Replacement

- Do not cross one leg over the other—keep the knees apart.
- Do not flex the hip when putting on shoes and stockings. Use assistive devices such as long-handled shoehorns and extenders with clothespins, or have someone help you put them on.
- Do not sit continuously for longer than 1 hour. Stand, stretch, and take a few steps periodically.
- Do not sit in low, reclining, or rocking chairs. Low, soft seats require more than 90 degrees of hip flexion to stand up. Sit in a firm, high chair with arms. Use a raised toilet seat. Place a very secure bar beside the toilet to help you stand up. Bathe at the sink or use the shower. Put a lawn chair in the shower if you become tired.
- Place a pillow between the knees when lying down.
- Follow detailed exercise prescriptions, including quadriceps sets, range-of-motion exercises, and activity limitations. The most important exercises to rebuild hip muscles are abduction exercises (spreading legs apart) and extension exercises (pushing the knee backward into the bed). Stationary bicycle exercises may help when an adequate range of hip flexion is achieved.
- Avoid actions that place a strain on the hip joint, such as excessive bending, heavy lifting, jogging, and jumping.
- Use crutches or a walker for as long as prescribed.
- Climb stairs carefully.
- Wear support stockings on the unaffected leg and an Ace bandage on the affected leg until there is no swelling in the legs or feet and full activities are resumed.
- Do not drive a car for 6 weeks after surgery unless authorized by the physician.

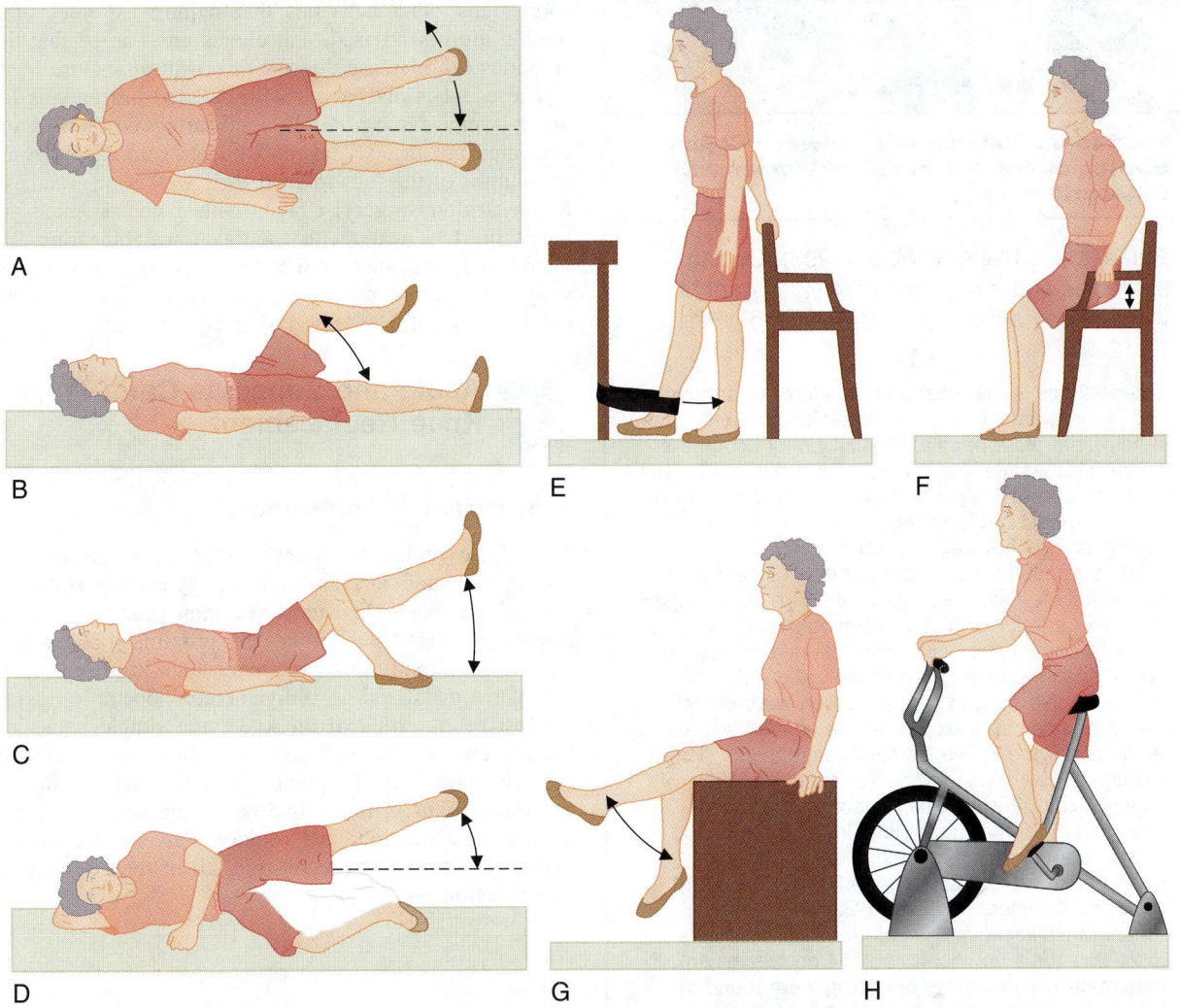

Figure 74–10. Exercises that may be used to increase strength and motion after total hip replacement. Each movement should be held for 3 to 6 seconds. The number of repetitions of each movement should be increased until each exercise is repeated 3 to 10 times to form a set. The client should repeat each set with the nonoperative leg. *A,* Leg spreader. While lying on a *firm* surface, the client gently moves each leg away from the body, holds them for 3 to 6 seconds, then returns them to midline. *B,* Bent knee raise. While lying on a flat surface, the client raises the hip with the knee bent to keep it parallel with the extended leg. *C,* Straight leg raise. The client lies on her back. Then the client tenses the muscles that go across the front of the knee. Keeping the other knee bent, the client raises her leg 1 or 2 ft, keeping the knee straight without arching her back. *D.* Side-lying leg raise. While lying on the unaffected side, the client bends the knee on that side and raises the affected leg, keeping the toes parallel to the floor. *E,* Standing leg extension. This exercise is used to strengthen the muscles in the back of the leg. The client secures an elastic belt or rubber tubing to the leg of a heavy, straight chair or table, then fastens it around the ankle, keeping it parallel to the floor. While holding onto a firm chair or other support, the client pulls the ankle back to midline. *F,* The client should raise herself gently out of a chair to increase the strength of the upper extremities. This exercise is good preparation for crutch-walking. *G,* The client should raise her leg from a sitting position to increase range of motion (ROM) and strengthen quadriceps tone. *H,* Stationary bicycling is one of the last exercises to be added to an exercise program following total hip replacement surgery. Stationary bicycling increases ROM, provides a warm-up before and after other exercises, and increases cardiovascular capacity.

others must receive are given in the Client Education Guide and in Figure 74–9. It is important for the client to know which activities are allowed and which may cause problems. The most important instruction is that the client not flex the hip greater than 90 degrees to prevent the hip from dislocating and to avoid extremes of internal rotation, adduction, and flexion of the hip. An elevated toilet seat is needed and one or two ordinary pillows between the knees when lying on the side. Showering is allowed once the wound is healed. Tub baths are allowed only if a stool is placed in the tub. A rubber mat and

handrails are needed. These devices should be installed before the client returns home from the hospital. Sexual activity can resume in the supine position. Exercises to be performed also should be included in the instructions (see Fig. 74–10). These restrictions continue for 6 months to 1 year after surgery. Clients should be reminded that this surgery does not cure their arthritis and that they will need to continue therapy for their disease. The client may require outpatient physical therapy or even a visiting therapist to maintain optimal function and to complete rehabilitation after total joint replacement surgery.

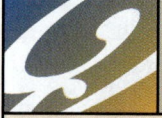

NURSING RESEARCH

What Is the Relationship Between Coping Strategies and the Health of Women with Osteoarthritis?

Burke, M., & Flaherty, M. J. (1993). Coping strategies and health status of elderly arthritic women. *Journal of Advanced Nursing, 18*(1), 7–12.

Osteoarthritis is the most common form of arthritis and is the greatest cause of disability and limitations in activity in older people. Disability may become so severe that women cannot manage a home. The use of housing for the aged is becoming more common and the impact of the social loss of a home on coping skills is not well understood.

The purpose of this study was to (1) investigate how elderly female residents in life-care communities cope with arthritis and (2) determine the relationship between coping strategies, physical health, psychological health, physical impairment, and pain.

A purposive sample of 130 women were drawn from a population of elderly, single women with osteoarthritis living in five life-care communities. Three instruments were used to collect data: the Ways of Coping Scale, the Arthritis Impact Measurement Scale, and the Musculoskeletal Impairment Index.

The mean age of the sample was 83.2 years. Mean health status scores were 3.3 on a scale of 0 to 10 with 0 indicating good health and 10 poor health. Musculoskeletal impairment mean score was 25.2 (18 equals no impairment, 54 equals maximum impairment). Three ways of coping were found in 90% of the sample and they were: "I maintained my pride and kept a stiff upper lip," "I prayed," and "I reminded myself how much worse things could be." These are considered self-controlling coping strategies.

Implications for Practice

The elderly bring a lifelong pattern of dealing with stress. These women may be reflecting either socially expected behavior or responding to the attitudes society has toward the aged. The use of positive reappraisal and spiritual dimensions are positive findings. Coping strategies are fundamental to an elderly person's ability to maintain independence in spite of physical and social losses.

There are some alterations that need to be made to the home. These alterations include devices such as ramps, good lighting, and modifications in floor plans that help the client maintain independence longer.

Clients with sedentary occupations can return to work after 6 to 8 weeks. At 3 months clients may return to work in occupations requiring limited lifting and bending. Manual labor is not encouraged after total hip arthroplasty. Limited athletic activity is permitted. Swimming, cycling, and golfing are acceptable. Jogging, racquet sports, and other activities that require extremes of hip motion are not advised, and clients are warned that these activities can increase the risk of prosthesis failure.

The client is discharged with detailed instructions for a home exercise program. Weightbearing is allowed on a cemented prosthesis, and most clients gain adequate muscle control of the legs to shed their walker or crutches by 6 weeks after surgery. Clients with a noncemented prosthesis need to walk with toe-touch weightbearing for 6 weeks and then another 6 weeks of crutch walking with weightbearing as tolerated. Stationary bicycle exercises can be helpful for at least 1 year after surgery.

Acute and Subacute Care: Total Knee Replacement

■ Surgical Management

Total knee replacement or arthroplasty is performed to relieve pain and increase function by adding stability to the arthritic knee. The most common procedures include resurfacing the distal femur, the proximal tibia, and the patella. Like total hip replacement, total knee replacement includes a metal and polyethylene component.

Most people think of the knee as a simple hinge joint, but actually it is an extremely complex joint with movement in three separate planes (Fig. 74–11). Flexion and extension occur in more than one plane and the knee has adduction, abduction, and rotation movements. Knee replacements attempt to reconstruct all of these motions for best function.

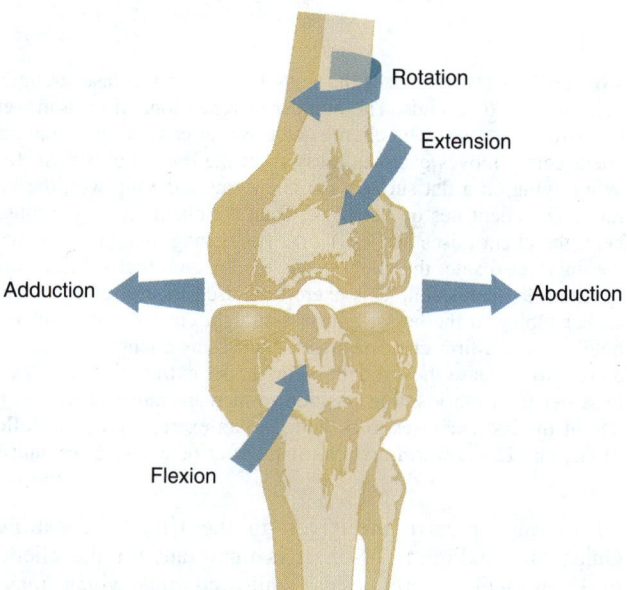

Figure 74–11. Movement of the knee occurs in three separate planes; the knee is not just a simple hinge joint. During normal gait, the knee moves through 70 degrees of flexion and extension, 10 degrees of abduction and adduction, and 10 to 15 degrees of internal and external rotation. (After Tooms, R. E. [1992]. Arthroplasty of the ankle and knee. In A. H. Chenshaw [Ed.]. *Campbell's operative orthopaedics* [8th ed., p. 391]. St. Louis: Mosby–Year Book.)

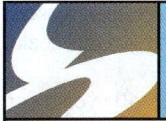

CASE MANAGEMENT

Total Knee Replacement
For Clinical Pathway, see Appendix D.

Clinical Pathway from Montclair Baptist Medical Center, Birmingham, Alabama
Information provided by **Gwen Cooke, R.N., B.S.N., O.N.C.**

Development and Revision of Pathway

- Total knee replacement patients had a long length of stay (9 days), and the cost was high.
- Revisions occur as practice patterns change. We have standing orders that support the CareMap and when they change, the CareMap is revised.
- Standing orders are reviewed annually and that usually leads to changes in the CareMap. If practice changes take place more quickly, the CareMap is revised as necessary.
- The development team included orthopedic nurses, physicians who championed CareMaps, physical and occupational therapists, the case manager, and rehabilitation staff.

Use and Impact of Pathway

- We have been using this pathway for 2½ years.
- All patients admitted for knee replacement surgery are placed on this pathway.
- Nurses, case manager, and discharge planners all use the CareMap.
- Patients are *consistently* up in the chair, and up in the chair earlier—the day of surgery or on postoperative day 1. Indwelling catheters and drains are discontinued on day 2. Physical therapy begins the day of surgery, occupational therapy begins the next day.
- Length of stay and cost per case have both decreased since we began using CareMaps. Medical and nursing practice have also been standardized for these patients. Our next step involves the standardization of prostheses which will result in a very large savings for the institution and the payor.

There are three types of knee prostheses: tricompartmental, bicompartmental, and unicompartmental. The tricompartmental prosthesis is the most commonly used. It contains implants to resurface the femur and tibia, and also resurfaces the patella (Fig. 74–12). A bicompartmental prosthesis is just the femoral and tibia components. It has been discarded because there was no patellar resurfacing and a high incidence of mechanical loosening. A unicompartmental device is used to replace the femoral and tibia surfaces of one side of the knee. This type of reconstruction is rare. The ideal prosthesis is yet to be designed.

Indications and Contraindications

The total knee arthroplasty is designed to relieve pain, provide motion with stability, and correct deformity.

Therefore it is used in persons with RA or degenerative joint disease of the knees. Because the durability of the prosthesis is not yet determined, the operation is best designed for older, sedentary persons and younger persons who have multiple joint problems. Total knee replacement is contraindicated in persons with severe osteoporosis, infection, or generally poor health.

Techniques

An incision is made along the superior surface of the leg, from about 4 to 5 inches above the patella to 2 to 3 inches below the patella. The bone is trimmed and the prosthesis is cemented or placed (if noncemented) into the bone. Varus and valgus deformities are also corrected. Flexion contractures can be corrected somewhat with bone resection, and, at times, with quadricepsplasty. Wound drains are placed and the knee is dressed in bulky compression dressings at about 35 degrees of flexion. Intravenous antibiotics are used prophylactically for 24 to 48 hours after surgery.

Complications

Possible postoperative complications include infection, thrombophlebitis, pulmonary embolism, peroneal nerve palsy, loosening of the prosthesis, and stress fracture of the tibia or fibula.

■ Nursing Management of the Surgical Client

Preoperative care is the same as for total hip replacement. Postoperative care is similar to that for total hip replacement, although there is more emphasis on active exercises because dislocation is not a problem in view of the anatomy of the knee. Antiembolism stockings and sequential compression devices are used to promote venous return and reduce the risk of DVT. Anticoagulants (see discussion under Total Hip Replacement) can also be used. It is common to have clients report pain with extension of the knee. This is due to flexion contracture of the knee that was present prior to surgery and usually from the client placing the knee in flexion to reduce pain. Keep the affected knee extended as much as possible, and use analgesics as needed.

The goal of knee rehabilitation is to obtain a maximal arc of comfortable joint motion with good quadriceps and hamstring control. After surgery, the client may be placed immediately in a continuous passive motion machine (CPM) or it can be started the morning after surgery (Fig. 74–13). The CPM should be used at all times except when not lying supine. The initial CPM setting is at 30 degrees of flexion and full extension. Then the degrees of flexion are slowly increased each day, until 90 degrees of flexion is reached. It is important for the CPM to be correctly applied to the client's leg with the knee gatch of the machine aligned with the knee. Quadriceps sets and ankle pumping exercises are started the first day.

To move the client to the chair from the bed, the client pivots in bed until sitting on the edge. Hold and slowly move the leg that was operated on. The client has little

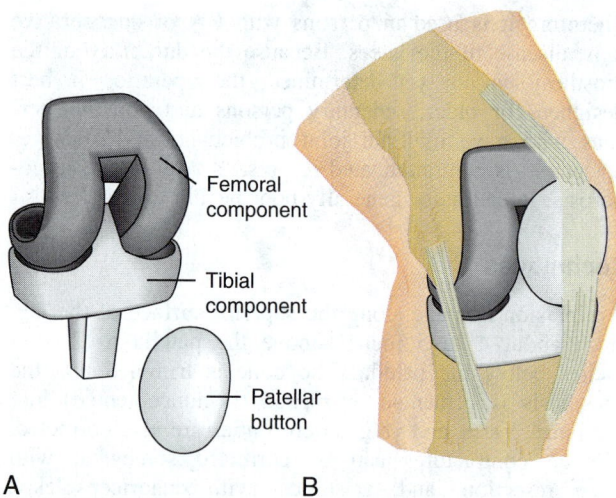

Figure 74–12. The tricompartmental knee prosthesis. *A,* Components of the prosthesis. *B,* The prosthesis in place.

control of this leg and often feels like he or she is going to fall. A walker is used for balance and weightbearing once standing. Weightbearing to pain tolerance is permitted with a cemented prosthesis. Only toe-touch weightbearing is allowed with noncemented prostheses. Record how much weightbearing was used and how it was tolerated (i.e., pain). Once in a chair the leg can be elevated if it aches, but letting the knee flex is beneficial. Crutch walking is permitted, rather than the walker, when the client can actively raise the leg from the bed indicating that he or she has control of the leg.

Curvatures of the Spine

The spine develops its characteristic curves during fetal development and early childhood. Abnormal spinal curves may develop due to defects in the bone, muscle, nerve, or other growth factors. They may also develop from tumors or injuries. Abnormal curves can occur in the thoracic spine, lumbar spine, or both sections.

Scoliosis

Scoliosis is defined as an abnormal lateral curvature of the spine. Adult scoliosis is a spinal curvature existing after skeletal maturity. A curve may present in any area of the spine—cervical, thoracic, thoracolumbar, or lumbar. There may be compensatory curves. The most common curve pattern is right thoracic, which produces a rib prominence.

The prevalence of scoliosis in the general population ranges from 2% to 4%. If the person has a positive family history for scoliosis, the risk of scoliosis is greater. Many adults with scoliosis have been diagnosed as children; have been observed for spinal curve progression; and have undergone exercise regimens, bracing, casting, and even some surgical intervention. Others have never

been formally diagnosed, and the curve has progressed, causing cardiopulmonary problems, resulting in the seeking out of medical care.

Adult scoliosis occurs in persons aged 40 years or older. Most cases are idiopathic and are defined as a structural spinal curvature of unknown cause, which arises during adolescence and persists into adulthood. Curves of less than 40 degrees, without symptoms, generally remain stable and do not require intervention. A progressive curve (>65 degrees) in the thoracic spine may be responsible for shortness of breath and fatigue. Other symptoms may include back pain, progressive spinal curvature accompanied by a reduction in height, cardiopulmonary failure, and cosmetic deformity. Evaluating the character, severity, and specific location of back pain helps determine whether or not the pain is caused by scoliosis. A progressive curve in the lumbar spine may be responsible for low back fatigue and pain. Back pain associated with scoliosis is usually located at the apex of the curve on either the convexity or the concavity. Early degenerative changes include spinal stenosis. If nerve root entrapment occurs, surgery is indicated.

Diagnosis is based on x-ray findings of a curvature of greater than 10 degrees, combined with structural changes in the spine, including vertebral rotation. Functional scoliosis occurs as a result of leg-length discrepancy or posture.

Surgical procedures for adults include the application of spinal instrumentation either through an anterior or posterior approach. These include the Cotrel-Dubousset instrumentation, the Harrington instrumentation, Harrington rods with spinous process wiring (Drummond or Wisconsin technique), Luque rods with sublaminar wires, Dwyer and Zielke instrumentations, as well as the creation of bone-grafted fusions (Fig. 74–14). The type of instrumentation used is based on the discretion of the surgeon. Other considerations include diagnosis, magnitude of the curve, flexibility of the curve, inherent strength of the bone, and the individual's ability to be immobilized postoperatively.

Nursing management focuses on education of the client on postoperative care, pain control, adequate fluid replacement, and progressive ambulation.[20] Refer to discus-

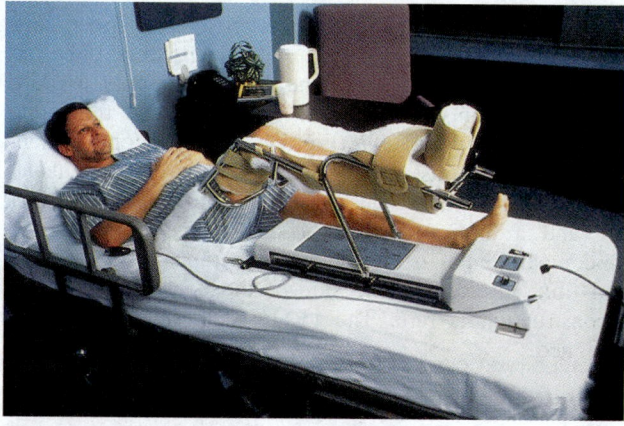

Figure 74–13. A continuous passive motion exerciser in use. (Courtesy of the Chattanooga Group, Inc., Hixson, TN.)

sion of nursing management of clients having lumbar fusion in Chapter 35 for more detail.

Kyphosis

Kyphosis, or "humpback," is excessive posterior curvature of the thoracic spine. Kyphosis can occur at all ages. It may be due to congenital anomaly, tuberculosis, or tumors, or it may be a compensatory mechanism for lumbar lordosis. Kyphosis is a classic sign of ankylosing spondylitis. When it occurs in women with osteoporosis, it is called a dowager's hump. The curvature can become so severe that functions of the lungs, heart, and gastrointestinal tract are altered. General management is with orthotic braces or corsets and exercise to strengthen muscles and ligaments. Osteoporotic women benefit from calcium and estrogen therapy. Spinal fusion with or without fixation rods may be required.

Lordosis

Lordosis is normal curvature of the lumbar spine. It can become exaggerated during pregnancy, with obesity, or in persons with large abdominal tumors. Structural changes in the spine do not occur in these instances, and once the problem is resolved, the condition resolves.

Hyperlordosis, or swayback, is fairly common in young children and in girls before puberty. It is thought to be due to rapid skeletal growth without appropriate growth of soft tissues such as fascia and muscles. This problem is self-correcting. Permanent hyperlordosis, which is rare, can occur due to degeneration of the intervertebral discs. Treatment includes bracing, spinal fusion, or osteotomy.

Bone Infections

Osteomyelitis

Osteomyelitis is a term used to describe any infection of the bone. Acute osteomyelitis responds to a 4- to 6-week course of intravenous antibiotics, whereas chronic osteomyelitis persists longer than 4 weeks and involves sequestered (necrotic bone that has separated from living tissue) areas of infection.

Osteomyelitis is generally bacterial in origin but may also be caused by viral or fungal infections. *Staphylococcus aureus* in the most common organism, but *Escherichia coli, Klebsiella, Proteus, Pseudomonas,* and *Salmonella* may also cause osteomyelitis. These organisms may be directly introduced into the bone, or they may be spread from adjacent soft tissue infection or travel through the blood to the infected site. The causative bacterial agent is able to multiply readily in bone because bone has a slow circulatory system.

Clinical manifestations of osteomyelitis include fever, usually above 101° F (38° C); localized pain or tenderness; erythema (redness); heat; and swelling around the affected bone.

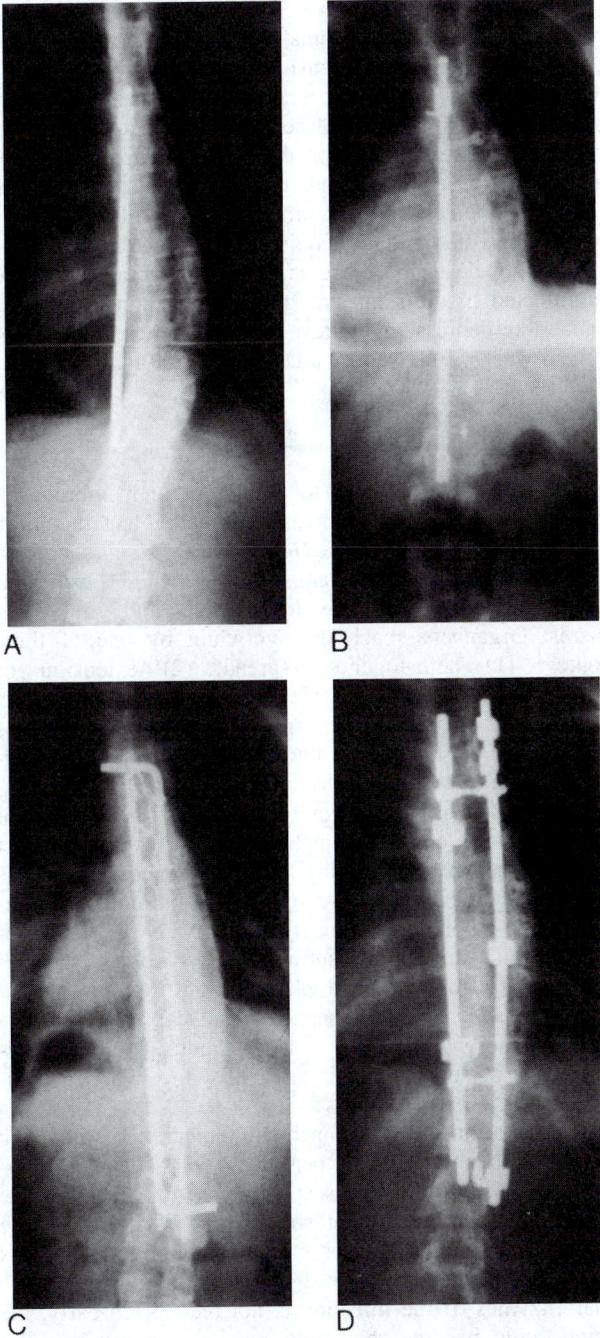

Figure 74–14. Radiographic appearance of instrumentation commonly used to correct scoliosis. *A,* A Harrington rod. *B,* A Harrington rod with spinous process wiring. *C,* Luque instrumentation. *D,* Cotrel-Dubousset instrumentation. (From Rodts, M. F. [1987]. Surgical intervention for adult scoliosis. *Orthopaedic Nursing, 6*[6], 12.)

Early diagnosis is important to prevent progression of the infection. Clinical manifestations are based on the area affected. Diagnostic tests include radionuclide bone scans, gallium scans, indium scans, computed tomography, and magnetic resonance imaging. In acute osteomyelitis, radiographic changes are usually not visible till 2 to 3 weeks after onset. Laboratory findings include an elevated WBC count, an elevated erythrocyte sedimentation rate (ESR), and if bacteremia is present, a positive blood culture for the organism causing the infection.

Needle aspiration or a percutaneous needle biopsy may assist with the diagnosis of acute osteomyelitis as well as relieve pressure from within the bone. Treatment requires administration of intravenous or intramuscular injection of one of the penicillin-type antibiotics for 4 to 6 weeks.

Chronic osteomyelitis requires sequestrectomy (surgical removal of dead bone) and saucerization (removal of scar or infected tissue, sequestra, and necrotic bone, leaving a saucerlike depression). Intravenous antibiotics are used for 4 to 6 weeks, followed by a course of oral antibiotics.

Septic Arthritis

Septic arthritis is invasion of the synovial membrane by pathogens. A variety of organisms may infect the joint, including *Staphylococcus, Gonococcus, Meningococcus,* and *Streptococcus* and gram-negative bacilli. Less common causes include tuberculosis fungal and viral organisms. Organisms reach the synovium by one of three routes: (1) hematogenous spread, (2) extension of adjacent musculoskeletal infection, and (3) from direct inoculation. Hematogenous spread, in which organisms reach the joint from a remote site, include upper respiratory infections, otitis media, and skin infections. Osteomyelitis adjacent to the joint may spread via the small capillaries that cross the epiphyseal (growth) plate. Direct inoculation can occur during invasive procedures such as arthroscopy or arthroplasty. Once the organism has invaded the joint, the synovial membrane swells and becomes infiltrated with neutrophils. Lysosomal enzymes are released from the neutrophils and destroy the articular cartilage, subchondral bone, and joint capsule. Cartilage can be readily digested in 3 to 24 hours. Clinical manifestations of septic arthritis are chills, fever, and a painful, tender joint.

Acute arthritis is a medical emergency requiring prompt treatment to avoid permanent joint damage. Management focuses on the use of cultures to find the exact organism and the original source of the infection. The joint fluid is aspirated for culture. Usually the joint is opened to drain the synovial fluid that is full of lysosomal enzymes. If the infection is not recognized early, the joint fluids become thick and need to be removed by continuous irrigation. Parenteral antibiotics are used for 2 to 3 weeks, followed by oral antibiotics. Acute septic arthritis can result in loss of joint function. Early use of active and passive range of motion exercises can reduce the risk of joint contractures and the loss of muscle strength. Chronic septic arthritis can also develop.

Bone Tumors

Primary Bone Tumors

Primary bone tumors (those originating in bone) may be benign or malignant. Benign tumors are characterized by their uniform density and well-defined margins. The most common benign bone tumor is a giant cell tumor (Fig. 74–15A). Malignant bone tumors are characterized by borders that extend into surrounding tissues. The most common malignant bone tumors are osteogenic sarcoma (Fig. 74–15B) and Ewing's sarcoma (Fig. 74–15C). Malignant bone tumors can also be metastatic from cancer elsewhere in the body. Primary bone tumors are described in Table 74–3.

The customary treatment of bone and soft tissue sarcomas has been amputation. Over the past two decades, much progress has been made in understanding the tumor, and in chemotherapy and radiation therapy, thereby enabling salvage of the limb. Research has shown that clients have the same disease-free survival rate with limb-sparing operations as those who have amputations.

Before surgery, the client undergoes chemotherapy and radiation therapy to reduce the tumor size and treat small metastases. During surgery, the tumor and a margin of normal bone are removed. The defect created by tumor removal is filled in with bone allograft. Bone grafts are usually from cadaveric donors. The recipients of bone allografts do not require immunosuppressive treatment because the bone is frozen after harvesting. Freezing diminishes the immune response of the bone tissue. The risk of contracting human immunodeficiency virus (HIV) is well over 1 in 1 million.[40] The bone graft is secured with metallic pastes and screws.

Prior to surgery, the healthcare team discusses the options with the client and family (many clients are adolescents or young adults). Autologous blood donations prior to surgery are not permitted for tumor resection; therefore, the family may wish to donate blood.

Following surgery, the limb is immobilized and elevated. Pain is usually severe and controlled with narcotic analgesics through epidural or PCA modes. Postoperative anemia may require transfusion. Complications of the surgery typify other orthopedic surgeries: infection, DVT, and nonunion of the bone grafts. Ambulation is begun the day after surgery, and the client is taught to walk with crutches.[34, 37]

Metastatic Bone Tumors

Skeletal metastases are the most common form of malignant bone tumor, and virtually every malignant tumor can metastasize to bone. Evidence suggests that distant metastases seem to develop from tumor seed cells that travel through the lymphatic system, blood vessels, and other surrounding tissues. Primary lesions of the prostate, breast, kidney, thyroid, and lung most commonly metastasize to bone. The femur, pelvis, ribs, and vertebrae are the most commonly affected bone sites. Pathologic fractures are common, especially in the acetabulum and proximal femur. Serum levels of alkaline phosphatase, calcium, and ESR may be elevated.

Pain may occur before changes are detectable on radiographic studies. Diagnosis may be made through x-rays, incisional biopsy, or frozen section. Many bone tumors produce typical patterns on radiographic studies. Whenever malignant lesions are suspected, anteroposterior and

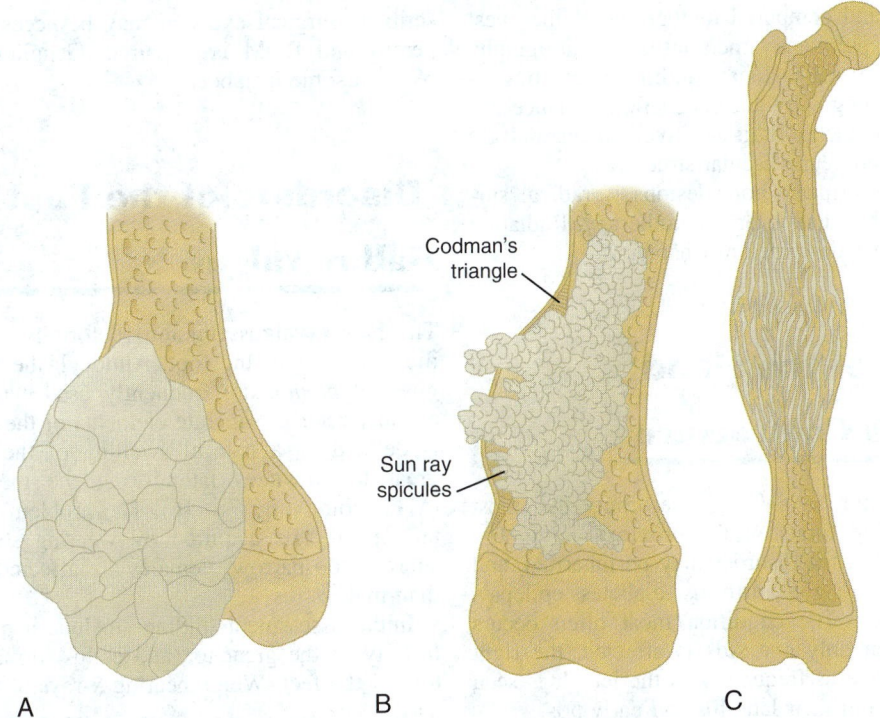

Figure 74–15. Bone tumors. *A,* A giant cell tumor. *B,* An osteogenic sarcoma. *C,* A malignant endothelioma (Ewing's sarcoma). (After Hughes, S. [1983]. *A short textbook of orthopedics and traumatology* [3rd ed.]. New York: ARCO.)

Table 74–3. Primary Bone Tumors

Classification/Name	Description
Benign chondrogenic Osteochondroma	Most common benign tumor. Commonly found in the femur and tibia; half of these clients are less than 20 yr old; tumor is usually solitary; about 10% of multiple osteochondromas develop into sarcomas
Chondroma	Common in mature cartilage in hands, feet, ribs, spine, sternum, or long bones; frequently leads to pathologic fractures.
Benign osteogenic Osteoid osteoma	Usually small tumors with clearly outlined area of reactive bone; common in the proximal femur, tibia, scaphoid bone, talus, or calcaneus; causes pain at night
Osteoblastoma	Rare tumor that evolves more rapidly and into a larger tumor than an osteoid osteoma; found in the vertebrae, distal femur, diaphysis of long bones, hands, and feet
Giant cell tumor	Aggressive and extensive lesion; rarely will recur and metastasize to the lung; commonly found in the distal femur, tibia, distal radius, sacrum, proximal humerus, and proximal fibula; produces pain, edema, and limitation in movement
Malignant osteogenic Osteogenic sarcoma	Most common primary malignant bone tumor; occurs in the metaphysis of long bones, at the sites of most rapid bone growth; common in the distal femur, proximal tibia, and proximal humerus; causes pain, swelling, and pathologic fracture; serum alkaline phosphatase is markedly elevated; prognosis improving with combination therapies, reaching 65% 5-yr survival; therapy includes chemotherapy and surgery
Ewing's sarcoma	Common in young adults and found in the pelvis and lower extremities; metastasizes quickly to the lungs and other bones; clinical manifestations include pain, edema, low-grade fever, leukocytosis, and anemia; improving prognosis with aggressive therapy; 65% 5-yr survival rate.
Chondrosarcoma	Common in the pelvis, ribs, proximal femur, and proximal humerus
Fibrosarcoma	Rare tumor of the femur and tibia

lateral chest films and computed tomograms of the chest are taken to detect pulmonary metastases. A scintigraphy (bone scan) is performed to locate additional osseous lesions. Computed tomography and magnetic resonance imaging are used to detect soft tissue involvement and the location of tumor and neurovascular structures.

The treatment of primary bone lesions is radical surgery, combined with radiation or chemotherapy. Radiation and chemotherapy are described in Chapter 24.

Disorders of the Hand

Dupuytren's Contracture

Dupuytren's contracture is a flexion deformity that most often affects the ring finger at the proximal joint. The cause is unknown, but the disorder may be inherited, and may also be seen with gout, arthritis, diabetes, epilepsy, and with alcoholism. The condition most often occurs bilaterally, but when only one side is affected, the right hand is involved twice as frequently as the left. It is seen most often in people in their late 40s and early 50s.

Initial assessment findings may reveal a bulky proliferation of tissue and contracting band palpated on the palmar crease opposite the ring or affected finger. Treatment includes finger-stretching exercises and surgical resection of the thickened palmar fascia.

Ganglion

A ganglion is the most common benign soft tissue mass in the hand, consisting of a round cystlike lesion overlying or adjacent to the wrist joint or tendon. The synovium surrounding the tendon degenerates, allowing the tendon sheath to buckle and weaken. The onset may be gradual or sudden, and it may follow trauma. Clinical manifestations include localized pain and a freely movable mass. Symptoms are exacerbated by dorsiflexion of the wrist. Treatment includes aspiration of the ganglion followed by injection of corticosteroid into the joint. NSAIDs are pre-

scribed. Surgical excision may be necessary if symptoms persist and ROM is impaired. Ganglion formation may recur in some instances.

Disorders of the Foot

Hallux Valgus

The hallux valgus (bunion) deformity is the most common disorder of the foot. Although the terms *hallux valgus* and *bunion* are frequently used synonymously, they actually refer to separate elements of the same disorder. It is defined as a painful swelling of the bursa when the great toe deviates laterally at the metatarsophalangeal (MTP) joint (Fig. 74–16). The problem may be congenital, or may be acquired by wearing shoes that are too short or too narrow. Females are affected more frequently than males.

Initial assessment findings include a painful valgus deformity of the great toe and callus formation on the bottom of the feet. Weightbearing x-rays of both feet may be used.

Treatment includes wearing open-toed shoes made of soft leather or sneakers. Metatarsal pads relieve some of the pressure from weightbearing. Intra-articular corticosteroid injections are given for acute bursitis, and analgesics are administered for pain. Simple bunionectomy involves osteotomy (bone resection) of the first metatarsal, removing the bony overgrowth and bursa (Fig. 74–16). Kirschner wires are inserted vertically through the toes and remain in place for 3 weeks postoperatively. Corks are placed on the tips of the wires for protection.

Hammer Toe

Hammer toe deformity is a flexion contracture of the proximal interphalangeal joint with extension or slight hyperextension of the distal interphalangeal joint (Fig. 74–17). Hammer toe deformity often accompanies hallux valgus. Clinical manifestations may include a family his-

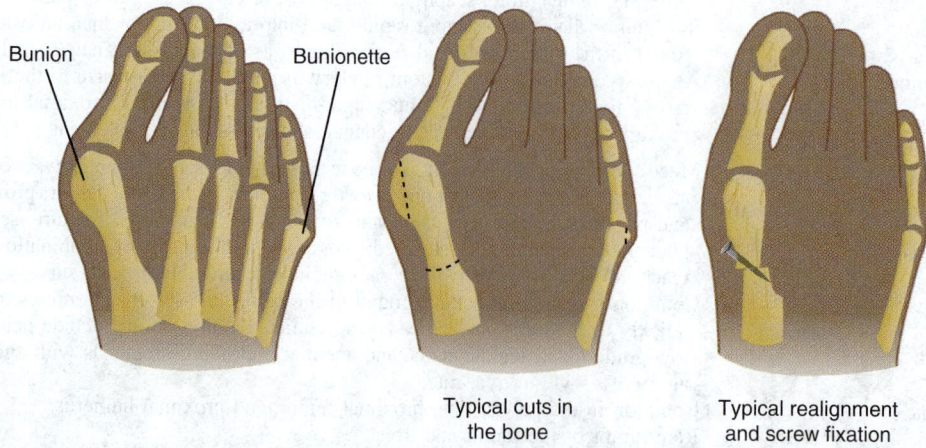

Bunion   Bunionette

Typical cuts in the bone

Typical realignment and screw fixation

Figure 74–16. ■ Bunions and their surgical correction.

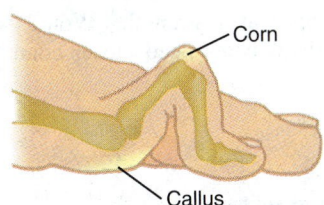

Figure 74–17. Hammer toe.

tory of hammer toe, RA, and clawfeet. Shoes may fit incorrectly, and there is often pain on walking, with alterations in stride length. Corns may be present on the dorsum of the toe. Treatment includes the use of pads to cushion the foot from the shoe, removal of corns, and passive stretching exercises. Surgical intervention involves osteotomy of the toe and resection of the proximal phalanx.

Morton's Neuroma (Plantar Neuroma)

Morton's neuroma, also known as a plantar neuroma or plantar digital neuritis, is the thickening of a nerve or the formation of a small tumor, secondary to pressure, in the area around the lateral branch of the medial plantar nerve. Pain is described as a severe, burning sensation, usually occurring in the web space between the third and fourth toes. Treatment is surgical excision of the neuroma. Palliative measures may include steroid injection and insertion of a metatarsal arch to relieve pressure.

Muscular Disorders: Muscular Dystrophy

Muscular dystrophy (MD) is a progressive, hereditary, degenerative disease of skeletal muscle. There are many forms of muscular dystrophy (Table 74–4), each with its own distinct characteristics and causes. All are progressive.

Three theories have evolved regarding the pathophysiology of muscular dystrophy. The membrane theory, which states that the cell membrane has been genetically altered, compromising the integrity of the cell and making it vulnerable to degeneration, is the most popular hypothesis. The neurogenic theory suggests a disturbance in nerve-muscle interaction. The vascular theory proposes that a lack of blood flow causes muscle and tissue degeneration.

Diagnosis of muscular dystrophy is often difficult, because the clinical manifestations are varied and similar to other muscular disorders such as myasthenia gravis or

Table 74–4. Clinical Features of Major Muscular Dystrophy (MD) Types

Clinical Features	Duchenne's MD	Limb Girdle MD	Becker's MD
Incidence	Most common	Not infrequent	Less common
Age at onset	Generally before age 3 yr	Usually by second decade	Majority between ages 5–15 yr
Inheritance	Sex-linked recessive gene, autosomal <10%	Usually autosomal recessive; may occur as autosomal dominant	Sex-linked recessive gene
Pattern of muscle involvement	Onset: selected symmetrical weakness of proximal pelvic muscles; 3–5 yrs later shoulder girdle muscles become involved	Proximal shoulder and pelvic girdle	Similar to Duchenne's MD
Late muscle involvement	All muscles, including facial, oculopharyngeal, and respiratory	Periphery; brachioradialis, hand and calf	Face is spared
Pseudohypertrophy	Calf muscles	Occurs in less than one third of cases	Calf muscles
Contractural deformities	Common	Late, milder than Duchenne's MD	Less common
Scoliosis/kyphoscoliosis	Common, late	Mild, late	Not severe
Heart involvement	Yes	Very rare	Late, uncommon
IQ	Decreased	Normal	Normal
Course	Steadily progressive	Much variation among clients but is slowly progressive	Slowly progressive

Modified from Doleysh, N., et al. (1991). Neuromuscular disorders. In S. W. Salmond, et al. (Eds), *Core curriculum for orthopaedic nursing* (2nd ed., p. 301). Pitman, NJ: National Association of Orthopaedic Nurses.

polymyositis. Muscle weakness is characteristic of all types. Elevated enzyme levels of creatine phosphokinase (CPK), abnormal muscle biopsy results, and an abnormal electromyogram (EMG) are found with muscular dystrophy.

Treatment includes corrective surgery for scoliosis or flexion contractures, long-leg braces, spinal braces, and exercise programs, including breathing exercises for respiratory decompensation. The prognosis of muscular dystrophy depends on the type and severity of the disease.

Conclusions

The focus of this chapter was on musculoskeletal disorders. These disorders include metabolic bone diseases, such as osteoporosis. Osteoarthritis is a common disorder. Its usual treatment is with joint replacement. Specialized nursing care is required after surgery to maximize outcomes. Bone tumors were also discussed. They can be benign or malignant primary lesions or metastatic tumors. Bone salvaging procedures are becoming more common in the management of these tumors.

Thinking Critically

1. A middle-aged client is concerned about bone loss resulting from osteoporosis. She tells you that her mother has severe osteoporosis, and she realizes her life-style and family history predispose her to osteoporosis. She asks you to suggest a life-style program for her and her daughters. How should you proceed?

Factors to Consider. What focused assessment should you complete? How should you complete teaching for the client and her daughters?

2. An elderly woman tells you her physician wants her to eat a diet high in calcium. He wants her to consume 1500 mg of calcium without taking enriched antacids or calcium supplements. This woman is lactose intolerant and has a hiatal hernia. She lives alone on a limited income. What problems might impair her compliance with the prescribed treatment regimen?

Factors to Consider. What dietary sources of calcium are appropriate for the lactose intolerant client? How does the presence of a hiatal hernia affect dietary intake?

3. You are seeing an elderly woman in her home with osteoarthritis to assist her in managing her diabetes. Over the past few months she has had increasing pain in her hips and knees. Her ability to walk has become limited. Several months later she is planning to have arthroplasty. How could she best be prepared for surgery?

Factors to Consider. Would it be advantageous to

improve her upper arm strength? Would weight control be helpful? Will diabetes need closer control during hospitalization?

Bibliography

1. Barden, R. M., & Sinkora, G. L. (1991). Bone stimulators for fusions and fractures. *Nursing Clinics of North America, 26*(1), 89–103.
2. Barger-Lux, J., et al. (1992). Nutritional correlates of low calcium intake. *Clinical and Applied Nutrition, 2,* 39–44.
3. Barger-Lux, M. & Heaney, R. (1994). Caffeine and the calcium economy revisited. *Osteoporosis International, 4,* 97–102.
4. Belinsky, J. B. (1993). Acetabular fracture: ORIF. . . .open reduction internal fixation. *Orthopaedic Nursing, 12,* 42–45, 48–50.
5. Bender, L. H. (1991). Osteogenesis imperfecta. *Orthopaedic Nursing, 10*(4), 23–31.
6. Boden, S. D., & Kaplan, F. S. (1990). Calcium homeostasis. *Orthopaedic Clinics of North America, 21*(1), 31–42.
7. Bridwell, K. H. (1988). Cotrel-Dubousset instrumentation. *Orthopaedic Nursing, 7*(1), 11–16.
8. Brosnan, H. (1991). Nursing management of the adolescent with idiopathic scoliosis. *Nursing Clinics of North America, 26*(1), 17–31.
9. Burns, S. (1996). Common foot problems. *Primary Care, 23*(2), 203–214.
10. Coe, F. L., & Favus, M. J. (1992). *Disorders of bone and mineral metabolism.* New York: Raven Press.
11. Dearborn, J., & Jergesen, H. (1996). The evaluation and initial management of arthritis. *Primary Care, 23*(2), 215–240.
12. Doheny, M. O., & Sedlak, C. A. (1987). Body image considerations for the adult scoliosis patient having spinal fusion surgery. *Orthopaedic Nursing, 6*(6), 18–22.
13. Doleysh, N., et al. (1991). Neuromuscular disorders. In S. W. Salmond et al. (Eds.), *Core curriculum for orthopaedic nursing* (2nd ed., pp. 299–303). Pitman, NJ: National Association of Orthopaedic Nurses.
14. Einhom, T. A., et al. (1990). Nutrition and bone. *Orthopaedic Clinics of North America, 21*(1), 43–50.
15. Ficner, H. B. (1993). Revision surgery in adult scoliosis patients. *Orthopaedic Nursing, 12,* 23–33.
16. Fueyo, L. (1991). Hand. In S. W. Salmond, et al. (Eds.), *Core curriculum for orthopaedic nursing* (2nd ed, pp. 239–250). Pitman, NJ: National Association of Orthopaedic Nurses.
17. Gagliardi, B. A. (1991). The impact of Duchenne muscular dystrophy on families. *Orthopaedic Nursing, 10*(5), 41–48.
18. Gertner, J. M., & Root, L. (1990). Osteogenesis imperfecta. *Orthopaedic Clinics of North America, 21*(1), 151–162.
19. Hahn, T. J. (1993). Metabolic bone disease. In W. Kelley, et al. (Eds.), *Textbook of rheumatology* (4th ed., pp. 1593–1628). Philadelphia: W. B. Saunders.
20. Hay, E. K. (1991). That old hip: The osteoporosis process. *Nursing Clinics of North America, 26*(1), 43–51.
21. Hunt, A. (1996). The relationship between height change and bone mineral density. *Orthopaedic Nursing, 15*(3), 57–66.
22. Kaiser, J. M., & Piasecki, P. A. (1991). Tumors. In S. W. Salmond, et al. (Eds.), *Core curriculum for orthopaedic nursing* (2nd ed, pp. 407–425). Pitman, NJ: National Association of Orthopaedic Nurses.
23. Kanis, J. A., et al. (1994). The diagnosis of osteoporosis. *Journal of Bone and Mineral Research, 9,* 1137–1141.
24. Kimmel, D. B., & Recker, R. R. (1994). Clinical assessment of bone strength. In R. Marcus (Ed.), *Osteoporosis* (pp. 49–68). Boston: Blackwell Scientific.
25. Lappe, J. M. (1994). Bone fragility: Assessment of risk and strategies for prevention. *Journal of Obstetrical, Gynecological, and Neonatal Nursing, 23,* 260–268.
26. Liscum, B. (1992). Osteoporosis: The silent disease. *Orthopaedic Nursing, 11*(4), 21–25.
27. Maier, T., & Pietrocarlo, T. (1991). The foot and footwear. *Nursing Clinics of North America, 26*(1), 223–231.

28. Martin, M. E. (1989). Oral antibiotics for the treatment of patients with chronic osteomyelitis. *Orthopaedic Nursing, 8*(3), 35–38.

29. Merkow, R. L., & Lane, J. M. (1990). Paget's disease of bone. *Orthopaedic Clinics of North America, 21*(1), 171–189.

30. Mitchell, N. R., et al. (1991). Infection. In S. W. Salmond, et al. (Eds.), *Core curriculum for orthopaedic nursing* (2nd ed, 251–263). Pitman, NJ: National Association of Orthopaedic Nurses.

31. Mooney, N. E. (1991). Pain management in the orthopaedic patient. *Nursing Clinics of North America, 26*(1), 81–84.

32. Mosher, C. M. (1991). The Papineau bone graft: A limb salvage technique. *Orthopaedic Nursing, 10*(3), 27–32.

33. National Osteoporosis Foundation. (1991). *Boning up on osteoporosis: A guide to prevention and treatment.* Farmington, CT. University of Connecticut Health Center.

34. NIH Consensus Development Panel on Optimal Calcium Intake. (1994). Optimal calcium intake. *JAMA, 272,* 1942–1948.

35. NIH Consensus Conference on Total Hip Replacement (1995). *JAMA, 273,* 1950–1956.

36. Nork, S., & Coughlin, R. (1996). How to examine a foot and what to do with a bunion. *Primary Care, 23*(2), 281–298.

37. Olson, B., Ustanko, L., & Warner, S. (1991). The patient in a halo brace: Striving for normalcy in body image and self-concept. *Orthopaedic Nursing, 10,* 44–50.

38. Pavlik, M. (1991). Measuring bone mineral content. *Orthopaedic Nursing, 10*(2), 39–43.

39. Piasecki, P. A. (1991). The nursing role in limb salvage surgery. *Nursing Clinics of North America, 26*(1), 33–41.

40. Prestwood, K., et al. (1994). The short term effects of conjugated estrogen on bone turnover in older women. *Journal of Clinical Endocrinology and Metabolism, 79,* 366–371.

41. Prior, J. C., et al. (1990). Spinal bone loss and ovulatory disturbances. *New England Journal of Medicine, 323*(18), 1221–1271.

42. Randall, R., Mann, J., & Johnston, J. (1996). Orthopedic soft-tissue tumors: Concepts for the primary care physician. *Primary Care, 23*(2), 241–262.

43. Recker, R. R., et al. (1995). Longitudinal studies of perimenopausal bone loss. *Journal of Bone and Mineral Research, 10 (Suppl. 1),* 146.

44. Recker, R., Dowd, R. et al. (1995). Patient care of osteoporosis. *Clinics in Geriatric Medicine, 11*(4), 625–640.

45. Recker, R. (1993). Clinical review 41: Current therapy for osteoporosis. *Journal of Clinical Endocrinology and Metabolism, 76,* 14–16.

46. Recker, R. R., et al. (1992). Bone gain in young women. *JAMA, 268,* 2403–2408.

47. Riggs, B., and Melton, L. (1992). The prevention and treatment of osteoporosis. *New England Journal of Medicine, 327,* 620–627.

48. Rodts, M. F., & Ruda, S. C. (1991). Spine. In S. W. Salmond et al. (Eds.), *Core curriculum for orthopaedic nursing* (2nd ed, pp. 357–361). Pitman, NJ: National Association of Orthopaedic Nurses.

49. Ross, P. D., et al. (1991). Evaluation of adverse health outcomes associated with vertebral fractures. *Osteoporosis International, 1,* 134–140.

50. Siris, E. (1995). Extensive personal experience: Paget's disease of bone. *Journal of Clinical Endocrinology and Metabolism, 80,* 335–338.

51. Tomaski, A. M., & Dobert, J. H. (1991). Metabolic bone disease. In S. W. Salmond, et al. (Eds.), *Core curriculum for orthopaedic nursing* (2nd ed., pp. 265–279). Pitman, NJ: National Association of Orthopaedic Nurses.

52. Urrows, S. T., et al. (1991). Profiles in osteoporosis. *American Journal of Nursing, 91*(12), 32–37.

53. Williams, M. A., Oberst, M. T., & Bjorklund, B. C. (1994). Post-hospital convalescence in older women with hip fracture. *Orthopaedic Nursing, 13,* 55–64.

Nursing Care of Clients with Musculoskeletal Trauma or Overuse

Joyce M. Black

Perhaps you have had a broken bone and can appreciate the pain such an injury causes. You can probably empathize with clients as they try to "live" in a cast. This chapter discusses various types of fractures and other musculoskeletal injuries, how they occur, techniques to manage them, and the nurse's role in their management.

Fractures

A fracture is a disruption of normal bone continuity that occurs when more stress is placed on a bone than the bone is able to absorb. Injury to surrounding soft tissue (skin, subcutaneous tissues, muscle, blood vessels, nerves, ligaments, and tendons) also often occurs. Although some fractures are life threatening (because of associated hemorrhage and shock), most are not.

About 25% of the population suffers some type of musculoskeletal injury yearly.[27] The injuries range from minor sprains to significant fractures, some of which result in major disability. Trauma remains the leading cause of death for persons between the ages of 1 and 44 years in the United States. Fractures constitute a high percentage of these injuries. Such injuries from motor vehicle accidents alone are estimated to cost more than $100 billion. About 90% of all fractures result in restrictions in activity or work disability days, and about 26% of clients with fractures require hospitalization.

This section discusses fractures in general. The classification of fractures, how they heal, and how they are managed are included, and traction and casts are examined in depth. The material that follows addresses various types of fractures and reviews their specialized management.

Classification

The more than 150 different types of fractures are classified in various ways: by fracture line, anatomic location, pattern of fracture, and appearance. Some of the more common types are described here and are shown in Figure 75–1. Compare and contrast the various types of fractures.

■ Classification by Communication with the Environment

The simplest method of describing a fracture is based on whether it is open to the environment (i.e., the bone protrudes through the skin) or closed (i.e., the skin is not broken).

Closed Fractures. A closed fracture is an uncomplicated fracture with intact skin over the fracture site (see Fig. 75–1A). In the past, these fractures were called *simple fractures*. The term "simple" can be misleading because the treatment is often as complex as for open fractures; therefore, this term is seldom used today.

Open Fractures. An open fracture is characterized by a break in the skin over the fracture site. The wound encompasses the skin (externally) and the fractured bone (internally). Because of the wound's communication with the external environment and extensive tissue damage, an open fracture always carries the potential for infection (see Fig. 75–1B). Open fractures are also called *compound fractures*. Open fractures are further divided into the following grades of severity:

Grade I: Wound smaller than 1 cm with minimal contamination
Grade II: Wound larger than 1 cm with moderate contamination and moderate soft tissue damage
Grade III: Wound larger than 6 to 8 cm with extensive soft tissue, nerve, and tendon damage and a high

This chapter incorporates material written for the fourth edition by Helen A. Andrews.

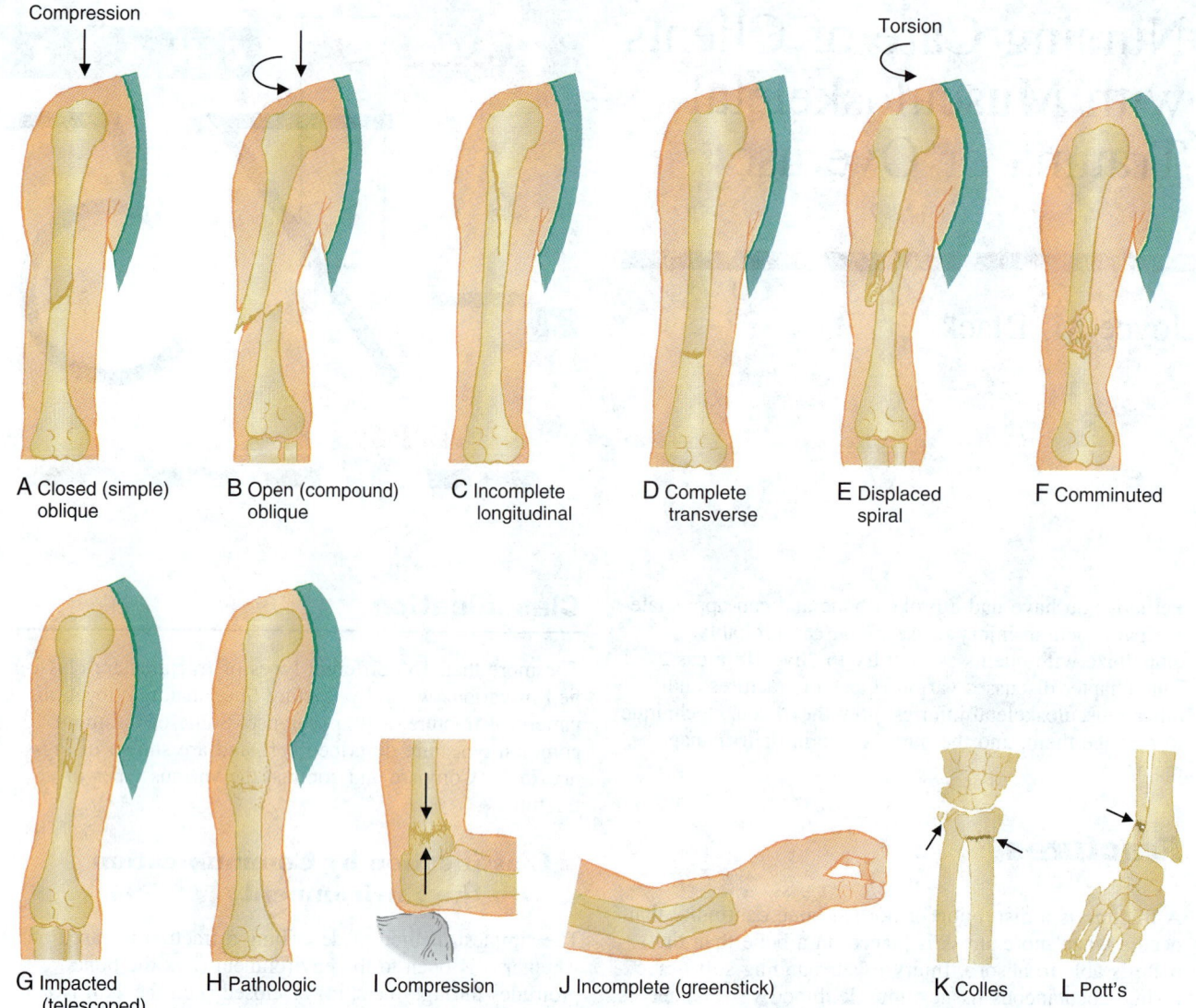

Figure 75–1. Common types of fractures.

degree of contamination. Some practitioners further subdivide this grade.

■ Classification by Fracture Pattern

The following terms describe fractures by the fracture line or the direction of the fracture:

Linear Fracture. The fracture line is intact. The line may be transverse or oblique. The fracture is the result of minor or moderate force applied directly to the bone.

Oblique Fracture. The fracture line occurs at an oblique angle (about a 45-degree angle) to the shaft (axis) of the bone (see Fig. 75–1A and B). Oblique fractures are usually produced by a twisting force.

Longitudinal Fracture. The fracture line extends longitudinally (see Fig. 75–1C).

Transverse Fracture. The fracture line is straight across the bone, that is, at a right angle to the bone's axis (see Fig. 75–1D). A transverse fracture is usually caused by an angulation force. Transverse fractures also occur in clients with bone disorders, such as Paget's disease, osteomalacia, and osteogenesis imperfecta.

Spiral Fracture. The fracture line forms a spiral encircling the bone (see Fig. 75–1E). Spiral fractures are usually caused by a twisting force with an upward thrust. They are usually the result of indirect forces. When seen in the upper extremities, spiral fractures may indicate abuse.

■ Classification by Type of Fracture

Avulsion Fracture. An avulsion fractures is one in which bone fragments are torn away from the body of the bone. Avulsion injuries occur when a direct force (pulling) is exerted on a bone with ligamentous resistance in the joint.

Compression Fracture. A compression fracture is produced by a compressive loading force applied to the long axis of the bone. Vertebral compression fractures are common in the elderly as a result of osteoporosis (see Fig. 75–1*J*). Gravity and body weight are the loading forces.

Comminuted Fracture. A comminuted fracture is produced by high-energy forces (e.g., motor vehicle accidents) that produce more than one fracture line, and bone fragments are crushed or broken into several pieces (see Fig. 75–1*F*). Severe soft tissue injury is frequently present as well. Many elderly clients suffer comminuted hip fractures during falls. A fall is seldom a high-energy force, but the bones are brittle and therefore break easily.

Greenstick Fracture. A greenstick fracture is one in which one side of the bone is broken and the other side is bent (like a stick of green wood). The cortex of the bone is buckled or cracked, but bone continuity is not completely disrupted. This type of fracture is also called an *incomplete fracture* (see Fig. 75–1*J*). These fractures usually occur in children, whose bones are still soft and pliable.

Impacted Fracture. An impacted fracture is one in which one end of the bone is impacted (driven) into the other end. (see Fig. 75–1*G*).

Pathologic Fracture. A pathologic fracture occurs when bone is weakened as a result of an underlying bone disorder, such as osteoporosis or tumor. Fractures usually occur with minimal trauma, or even with simple body movements, which would not damage normal bone (see Fig. 75–1*H*). With the prolonged survival of many patients with solid tumors, the incidence of bony metastasis is rising. Bony metastasis is seen in clients with cancer of the breast, prostate, thyroid, lung, and kidney. Pathologic fractures also occur with cancer of the bone.

Stress (Fatigue) Fracture. A stress fracture is a result of repeated stress on a bone, and there is usually no evidence of bone disease or trauma to explain the fracture. Muscles normally allow stress forces to be shunted away from the bone, but as muscles become fatigued, this protection is lost. Stress fractures are most commonly seen in marathon runners.

■ Classification by Eponym

Some fractures have been named by the physician who first described them:

Colles' Fracture. Colles' fracture is a common fracture in which the distal radius is fractured within 1 inch of the articular surface (see Fig. 75–1*K*).

Pott's Fracture. Pott's fracture occurs at the medial malleolus of the tibia and fibula and often is associated with rupture of the internal lateral ligament, chipping off of a piece of the medial malleolus, or both. The tibiofibular articulation is seriously disrupted (see Fig. 75–1*L*).

■ Classification by Appearance

This form of classification describes the appearance of the fracture and any bony fragments.

Burst Fracture. A burst fracture is one that results in multiple pieces of bone; although it is usually found at the ends of bone, it can occur in vertebrae.

Chip Fracture. A chip fracture is a small fracture in which a bony process near a joint is fragmented.

Complete Fracture. In a complete fracture, the fracture line extends through the entire bone substance, that is, the periosteum and cortex are disrupted on both sides of the bone (see Fig. 75–1*D*).

Displaced Fracture. In a displaced fracture, bone fragments are separated at the fracture line or the joint. These fractures may also be described according to the degree of displacement, such as minimal and complete (see Fig. 75–1*E*).

■ Classification by Point of Reference

The "rule of thirds" is used to classify fractures by a point of reference on the bone shaft. Fractures are termed *proximal third, midshaft,* and *distal third.* Fractures of the midshaft heal more slowly due to the decreased blood supply in that area.

■ Classification by Anatomic Location

Finally, fractures are also described by their anatomic location (e.g., the anatomic neck of the humerus or femur, or the surgical neck of the humerus or femur). A fracture involving a joint surface is called an *articular fracture.* A fracture near a joint but not entering the joint capsule is called an *extracapsular fracture. Intracapsular fractures* are fractures within a joint capsule.

Epiphyseal fractures involve the growth plate at the ends of long bones. These fractures may result in alterations in bone growth. (A complete discussion can be found in a pediatric nursing textbook.)

Any of the abovementioned terms used to describe fractures may be combined to provide a more complete description; for example, a client may have a "closed, completely displaced fracture of the distal third of the femur."

Etiology and Risk Factors

Bone fracture occurs when the bone is mechanically over-loaded. Factors that cause bone to fracture include the amount of force applied to the bone, the mechanical properties of the bone, and the amount of alteration in the bony structure from disorders such as osteoporosis or cancer. Direct force is the result of a moving object impacting the bone. Direct forces can include compression, torsion (twisting), or pulling. Indirect force can be caused by contracting muscles exerting a powerful pulling force on the bone. Other causes of fracture include stress or fatigue of the ligaments and pathologic disorders of the bone, which decrease the bone's ability to withstand mechanical stress.

The two types of bone materials also respond differently to stress and impact. Cortical bone is the compact outer layer of bone. Surprisingly, it is porous compared to trabecular bone. Even though cortical bone is more porous, it can bear a large amount of strain. Tendency to fracture cortical bone is influenced by the rate at which the bone is stressed and the orientation of the bone. Cortical bone can tolerate more stress along its axis (longitudinally) than across it.

Trabecular bone is the inner bone material. It is quite

RISK FACTORS AND LEVELS OF PREVENTION

Fractures

Risk Factors

Osteoporosis, cigarette smoking, falls, metastatic bony defects

Levels of Prevention

Primary Prevention

- Teach calcium supplementation for all women, especially those past menopause.
- Discourage cigarette smoking.
- Maintain safe environments, (good lighting, no scatter rugs) for elders.
- Keep hospital beds in a low position with side rails up when client is unattended.
- Encourage seatbelt use and use of protective gear for sports.
- Encourage early detection of breast and prostate cancers.

Secondary Prevention

- Teach prophylactic stabilization of impending fractures in persons with bony metastasis.

Tertiary Prevention

- Teach early management of fractures with stabilization.

---

dense and can tolerate more stress without fracturing. Trabecular bone has been described as being very similar to porous engineering materials that can be used to absorb energy on impact. On impact of stress the bone is elastic, but eventually the trabeculae fracture individually.

Risk factors and prevention of fractures are described in Risk Factors and Levels of Prevention.

Pathophysiology

At the time of fracture, muscles that were attached to the ends of the now fractured bone are no longer suspended across the length of the bone. The muscle can then spasm and pull the loose bony ends into various positions. Large muscle groups can create massive spasm and displace large bones, such as the femur. The distal portion of the fracture becomes displaced while the proximal portion remains in place. Displacement of the fracture ends and fragments of bone depend on the causative force and the degree of spasm in surrounding muscles. Displacement may occur sideways, at an angle (angulated), or as an overriding bone segment, and displaced segments may be rotated or offset.

When a bone is broken, the periosteum and blood vessels in the cortex, marrow, and surrounding soft tissue are disrupted. Bleeding occurs from the damaged ends of the bone and from nearby soft tissue (muscles). A hematoma forms in the medullary canal, between the fractured ends of the bone and beneath the periosteum. Bone tissue immediately adjacent to the fracture dies. This necrotic tissue stimulates an intense inflammatory response characterized by vasodilation, edema, pain, loss of function, exudation of plasma and leukocytes, and infiltration of other white blood cells. (Inflammation and wound healing are discussed more fully in Chapter 20). These initial steps build the foundation for bone healing.

■ Bone Healing

Bone is able to regenerate, unlike some other specialized body tissue. Fracture healing occurs by the formation of new bone tissue (to reunite bone fragments) rather than by the formation of nonspecialized fibrous scar tissue.

Healing time varies with the type of fracture and the type of bone. Impacted fractures require several weeks to heal, whereas displaced fractures may require months to years for complete healing.

The bones of the arm may heal in 3 months, whereas the tibia and femur require 6 months or longer. The greater the surface area of the fracture fragments, the more rapidly they heal (e.g., spiral fractures heal more rapidly than transverse fractures).

Most function returns in 6 months after bony union takes place, but complete function may not be regained for a year or more. In a year, a simple fracture resumes an almost normal appearance if the bone has been aligned correctly. Fracture healing occurs in the following five stages (Fig. 75–2).

Stage 1: Hematoma Formation. Within 72 hours, a blood clot forms at the fracture site. As the clot

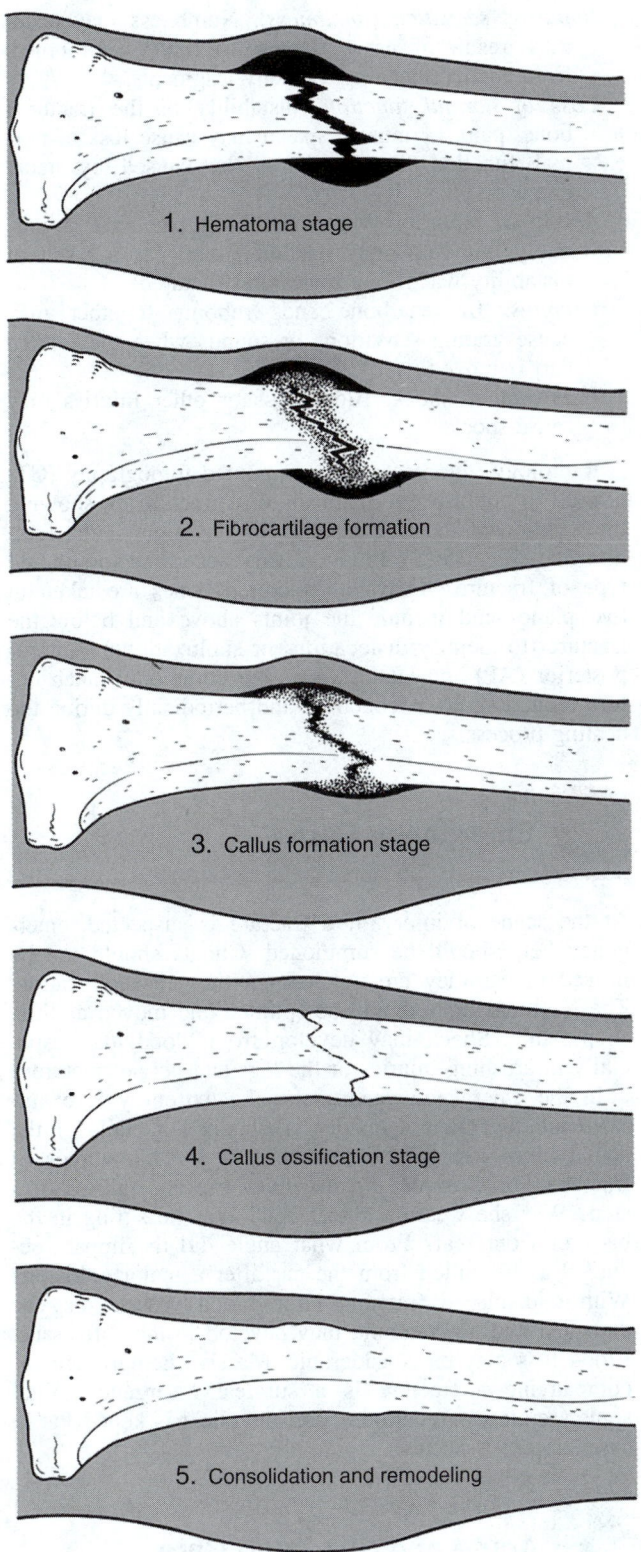

Figure 75–2. Stages of fracture healing.

coagulates, a loose, delicate mesh of fibrin forms around the fracture site. This fibrin mesh protectively encloses the damaged bone and acts as a scaffold for the ingrowth of capillary buds and fibroblasts. Blood supply increases

at the fractured bone ends. Unlike most hematomas, a hematoma that surrounds a fracture is not reabsorbed during healing. Instead, it undergoes changes and develops into granulation tissue.

Stage 2: Fibrocartilage Formation. This stage takes place over 3 days to 2 weeks. At the ends of periosteum, the endosteum and bone marrow supply the cells that proliferate and differentiate into fibrocartilage, hyaline cartilage, and fibrous connective tissues. Periosteal trauma serves as a catalyst for proliferation of osteoblasts. Osteogenesis is rapid, and bone formation, which is primarily dependent on blood supply to the area, occurs within a few days.

The periosteum is elevated away from the bone. After several days, the combination of periosteal elevation and granulation tissue forms a collar around the end of each fragment. The collars eventually advance, unite, and form a bridge across the fracture site.

Stage 3: Callus Formation. Three to 10 days after injury, the granulation tissue changes and a provisional callus (procallus) forms. Newly formed cartilage and bone matrix disperse through the soft tissue callus and increase in number until a provisional callus is established. The procallus is a large, loosely woven mass of bone and cartilage that is considerably wider than the normal bone's diameter. It secures the bone fragments but does not provide strength. A procallus extends some distance beyond the fracture line, serving as a temporary splint. In an uncomplicated fracture, the procallus usually reaches its maximal size in about 14 to 21 days after the injury. This mass is subsequently remodeled (see later discussion). Proper bony alignment is essential during this phase.

Stage 4: Ossification. A permanent callus of true, rigid bone eventually forms and closes the gap between the bones. Ossification first forms an external callus (between the periosteum and cortex), then an internal callus (medullary plug), and finally an intermediate callus (between the cortical fragments). During the third to tenth weeks of healing, the callus converts into bone, and healing can be confirmed by x-ray. This formation of bone firmly binds together the fractured ends and completes healing. Sometimes this stage is called the *union stage.*

Stage 5: Consolidation and Remodeling. At the same time that true bone is forming, the callus is remodeled by osteoblastic and osteoclastic activity. In effect, excess bone is chiseled away and absorbed from the callus. The amount and timing of bone remodeling is governed by the stresses imposed on the bone by muscles, weightbearing, and age. Children's bones remodel better than those of adults.

■ Factors Affecting Bone Healing

Because healing of fractures is a continuous sequential process, any interruption in the process may result in

Table 75–1. Factors Affecting Bone Healing	
Favorable	Location (distal or proximal shaft)
	Flat bones
	Minimal soft tissue damage
	Anatomic reduction
	Immobilization
	Weightbearing on long bones
Unfavorable	Wide separation of ends of fragments
	Distraction of fragments by traction
	Severe comminution
	Severe soft tissue damage
	Bone loss due to injury or surgical excision
	Motion/rotation at fracture site due to inadequate fixation
	Infection
	Impaired blood supply to one or more bone fragments
	Location (midshaft—decreased blood supply)

From Maher, A. B., Salmond, S. W., & Pellino, T. A. (1994). *Orthopaedic nursing.* Philadelphia: W. B. Saunders.

delayed healing. Factors affecting bone healing are shown in Table 75–1.

Clinical Manifestations and Diagnostic Findings

The clinical manifestations of fracture vary with site, severity, type of fracture, and amount of damage to other structures. Some fractures are immediately obvious and others produce few clinical manifestations, which would not be detected if x-ray films were not taken to assess the injury. See Table 75–2 for information about neurovascular assessments. Various combinations of the following clinical manifestations may be present:

Deformity. Strong muscle spasms may cause bone fragments to override; therefore alignment and contour changes occur, such as angulation, rotation, or limb shortening; bone depression; or altered curves in the injured site, especially when compared with the opposite side.

Swelling. Edema may appear rapidly from localization of serous fluid at the fracture site and extravasation of blood into adjacent tissues.

Bruising (ecchymosis). Bruising is a result of subcutaneous bleeding.

Muscle spasm. Involuntary muscle contraction may occur near the fracture.

Tenderness. Tenderness is present over the fracture site due to underlying injuries.

Pain. Immediate severe pain occurs at the time of injury. Following injury, pain may result from muscle spasm, overriding of the fractured ends of the bone, or damage to adjacent structures.

Impaired sensation (numbness). Numbness may occur as a result of nerve damage or nerve entrapment from edema, bleeding, or bony fragments.

Loss of normal function. Instability of the fractured bone, pain, or muscle spasm may cause loss of normal function. Paralysis may be caused by nerve damage.

Abnormal mobility. Movement of a part that is normally immobile may become mobile as a result of instability when long bones are fractured.

Crepitus. Broken bone ends rubbing together may cause grating sensations or sounds when the injured part is moved.

Hypovolemic shock. Blood loss or other injuries may cause shock.

Radiology, fluoroscopy, or computed tomography (CT) is used to confirm the diagnosis of a fracture by showing the location of the fracture and the direction of the fracture line (Fig. 75–3). Findings vary according to site and type of fracture. X-rays of fractured bones are taken in two planes and include the joints above and below the fracture (to identify dislocations or subluxations). Anteroposterior (AP) and lateral views are commonly taken before reduction, after reduction, and periodically during the healing process.

Emergency Care

At the scene of injury, if a fracture is suspected, emergency help should be summoned. Clients should not be moved unless they are not safe in the present location. The fractured limb should be splinted and moved as little as possible. Shock may develop from blood loss, especially in crushing injuries of the legs and pelvic fractures.

In the emergency department, the extremity is examined and the client's history is obtained. Details of the actual injury are helpful to determine the likely type of fracture. For example, did the client trip and fall off of a step? Was she wearing a seat belt? Was he sitting in the back or front seat? From what angle did the impact occur? Was he pulled from the car after a major collision? With a displaced fracture, large blood vessels may be damaged and a hematoma may develop in the soft tissue. Blood loss may be considerable. Massive hemorrhage accompanying a fracture is a surgical emergency. Vital signs are closely monitored, and the client is kept NPO in case surgery is needed.

Acute and Subacute Care

■ Medical Management

Primary goals of treatment of a fracture are preventing complications, returning an injured limb to maximal function, and achieving the best possible cosmetic result. When a fracture of an extremity divides a bone into two fragments, the fragments are referred to as the *proximal*

Table 75-2. Neurovascular Assessments

Parameter Being Assessed	Technique	Expected Finding
Color of affected extremity	Inspect the color of affected leg, foot, arm or hand; compare to opposite side	Color should be the same; it is normal to have some paleness (pallor) in injured tissues; if incisions are present, some redness (erythema) may be noted along incision lines
Temperature of affected extremity	Use dorsum (back) of your hand to assess temperature	Temperature should be the same in each extremity; report any coolness or heat in the extremity
Movement of affected extremity	Ask client to "move your toes/ fingers"	Movement should be the same on each side; if decreased movement is noted, determine if extremity normally moves (e.g., if the client has had a stroke, limited movement may have been present before); if client had surgery on toes or fingers, expect decreased movement due to pain and edema; look for even slight movement in the area
Sensation of affected extremity	Ask clients if they feel you touching their toes or fingers; ask specifically if they have "pins and needles" or if the extremity feels like it is "asleep"	Sensation should be the same on each side; any alterations in sensation should be reported
Capillary refill in nail beds	Compress nail bed and measure time needed for refill (return of color)	Should be 2–4 sec; slowing to 4–6 sec should be reported
Edema	Inspect for edema in both extremities	No edema should be present; if edema is noted in affected extremity consider if it is due to the trauma or surgery or thrombophlebitis; if present in both extremities, consider causes such as heart disease
Pain	Ask client to rate pain on scale of 0–10, with 0 being no pain and 10 being the worst pain they have ever felt	Pain is common in injured extremities; if no pain is reported, client may have recently had pain medication; uncontrollable pain usually signals compartment syndrome and should be reported
Pedal pulses	Palpate for pedal pulses on dorsum of foot	Pedal pulses should be present bilaterally; if absent, may be normal variation; absent pulses could also signal compression of vessels due to edema

(uncontrollable) fragment and the *distal* (controllable) fragment. The proximal fragment is the section of bone nearer the body. This fragment cannot be manipulated or moved when the fractured bones are being set (i.e., therapeutically correctly aligned) because of its muscle attachments and location. The distal fragment (farther away from the body) can be manipulated or moved to realign it with the proximal fragment.

Reducing Fractures

The first step in displaced fracture management is to reduce the fracture. Reduction is the process of manipulation of fractured bones to restore alignment and alleviate compression and stretching of nerves and vessels. Reduction is sometimes called *setting* a bone. Fracture reduction restores the injured bone to normal anatomic alignment, position, and length and brings the fractured fragments into close approximation. Fracture reduction is usually painful and requires local or general anesthesia.

Fortunately, not all fractures require reduction. For example, undisplaced fractures do not need reduction because the bone fragments are already correctly aligned. Splinting is used with such fractures to maintain alignment. A few fractures, such as distal phalanges, cannot be adequately splinted and are treated by resting the part until healing occurs.

There are three methods of fracture reduction, which can be used alone or in combination.

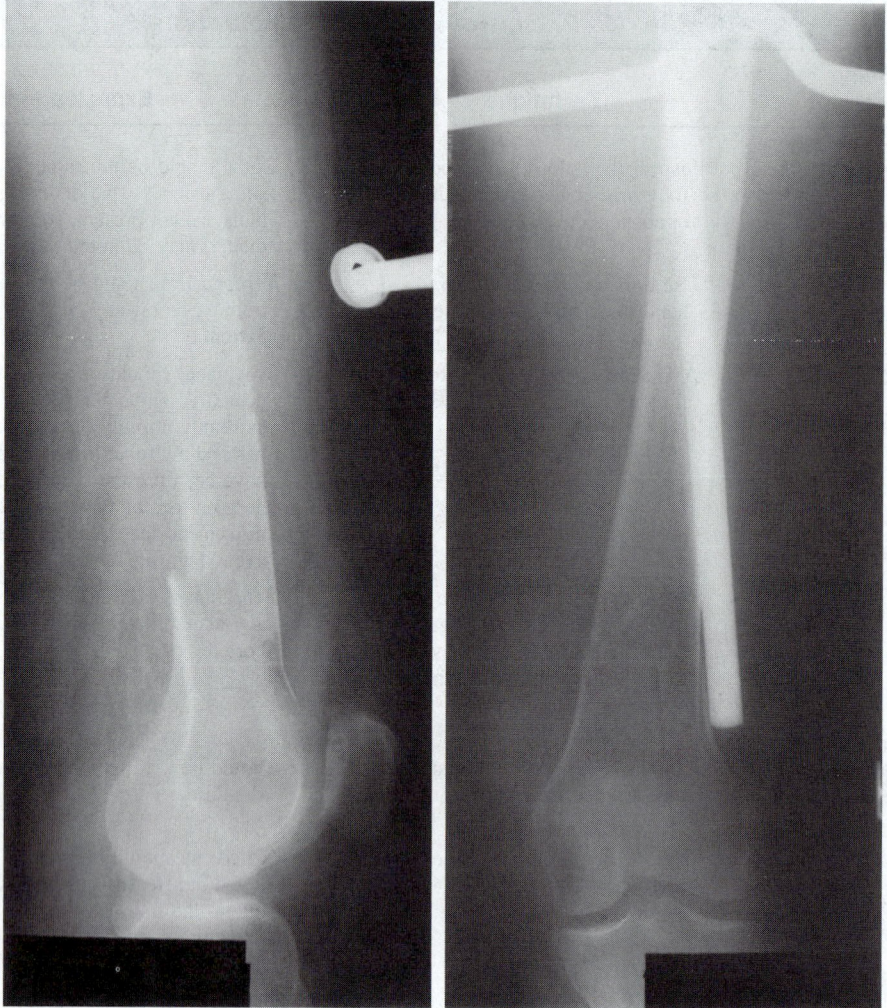

Figure 75–3. *A*, Fracture of the supracondylar femur. *B*, Reduction of the fracture with traction. The fracture was eventually pinned.

Closed Reduction

Closed reduction is a method of fracture realignment. A physician performs closed reduction by manually applying traction to move the ends of a bone together and restore alignment (Fig. 75–4). It should be performed as soon as possible after the injury to reduce the risk of loss of limb function, prevent or delay degeneration of the joint, and minimize the deforming effects of the injury. Closed reduction is performed under general anesthesia or local anesthesia, with or without sedation.

Four maneuvers are used for manual reduction. The first step is a longitudinal pull on the distal end of the fracture or extremity. This pull reverses the mechanism that produced the fracture and overcomes the initial muscle spasm, limb shortening, and overriding of bone fragments. The second step is disengagement of the bony ends of the fracture, which is sometimes done by rotating the distal portion. The third step is realignment of the

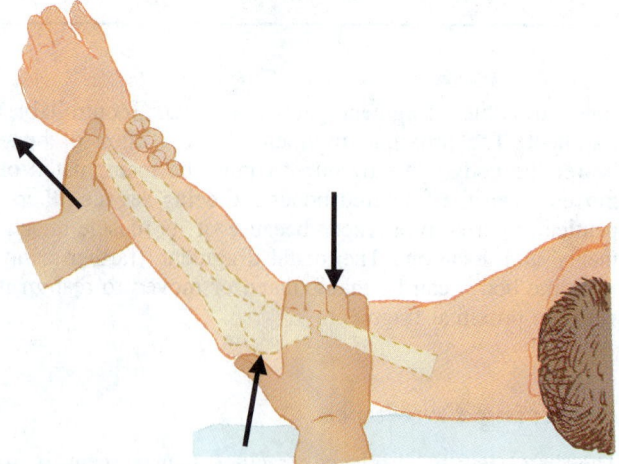

Figure 75–4. Closed reduction to realign a supracondylar fracture.

ends of the bone. This is a complex step, because several forces from various muscle groups are holding the bony fragments in various positions. Finally, the distraction force is released while alignment is maintained. After the distraction force is released, forces such as gravity, weightbearing, and muscle contraction begin again and can work to move the fragments once more. Following a closed reduction, x-ray films are taken and either a cast or traction is usually applied.

Open Reduction

In open reduction, an incision is made and the fracture is aligned during surgery under direct vision. At the time of surgery, various internal fixation devices may be applied to the fractured bone to maintain alignment (e.g., screws, plates, pins, wires, nails), or rods may be placed through bone fragments, fixed to the sides of the bone, or inserted directly into the bone's medullary cavity. For some fractures, open reduction is the treatment of choice, such as for compound fractures that are comminuted or accompanied by serious neurovascular injuries or for fractures with widely separated fragments or with soft tissue interposed between bone fragments. Open reduction is usually needed for fractures of the femur and fractured joints. Although internal fixation devices initially help immobilize a fracture and prevent deformity, they are not a substitute for bone healing. If proper bone healing does not occur, the metallic internal fixation devices succumb to stress and loosen or break. Examples of open reduction can be seen in the section on fractured hips.

Traction

Traction is accomplished by exerting a pull (on the head, body, or limbs) in two directions, that is, pull of traction and pull of countertraction. Traction may be applied (1) manually, by pulling on the body part with the hands (see earlier discussion); (2) mechanically, by exerting a pull on the body part with ropes and pulleys; (3) with devices inserted in casts (e.g., plaster traction); or (4) with braces (e.g., hyperextension braces). Traction for fracture management is most often produced by weights.

Advantages of traction include (1) a greater potential for exercising joints and muscles than is possible with casts and (2) elimination of the need for surgery and its risks. Major disadvantages of most types of traction are that prolonged hospitalization and bedrest are necessary.

The goal of traction is to return bone fragments to their normal position. Sometimes bones must be turned and pulled into alignment so that they can heal and the client can gain complete function and/or return to preinjury appearance and function. To return the bones to the proper position, various forces are applied. One force pulls the extremity distally (counteracting muscle spasms), and the countertraction pulls the opposite way. Countertraction may be produced with either the client's body weight or with other weights. The traction and countertraction must be of equal pulling force. A third force is created by the position of the limb (e.g., flexion of knee and hip). These forces combine to create the exact direction of pull along the long axis of the bone; this combination of forces is called the *vector of force*. It is imperative that the position of the pulleys and the angle of the splints not be readjusted without physician direction.

To reduce a fracture of a long bone, considerable pull is exerted on the distal fracture fragment to align it with the proximal fragment. The amount of traction needed to achieve alignment is usually intense, and it is applied for just a short time. Initially, many pounds of weight are needed to overcome the powerful muscle spasms. Once the spasms have stopped, the amount of weight is often lessened. Then when the fracture has been reduced, the amount of weight applied through the traction setup is the smallest amount required to maintain proper alignment and apposition of bone fragments.

When traction is properly applied in bed, the person is centered in the bed in a supine position and the affected part is held in alignment by a constant two-way pull. When applied to a long bone, the direction of traction is in line with the bone's long axis. When applied to the head or pelvis, the pull is in line with the spinal column. The bed is usually elevated under the part in traction to help with countertraction. For example, the foot of the bed may be elevated when traction is applied to lower extremities. If the bed is not elevated, the client tends to slide toward the weights, defeating the purpose of traction. With some types of traction, countertraction is applied with ropes, pulleys, and weights that pull in a direction opposite to the direction of the traction. These weights are usually attached behind the bed.

Methods of Applying Traction

Continuous Versus Intermittent Traction. Traction may be continuous (constant pull) or intermittent (periodic pull relieved by releasing the weights). Continuous traction typically is used to treat certain fractures or dislocations. Intermittent traction may be used to reduce flexion contractures. Prescriptions for intermittent traction state the precise length of time traction is to be applied.

Running Versus Suspension Traction. Running traction (straight traction) exerts a direct pull on the affected part without a splint to provide balanced support. It pulls in a single plane and may be unilateral or bilateral. Running traction may be applied to the skin (skin traction) or skeleton (skeletal traction). Buck's extension (see the section on skin traction) is an example.

Suspension traction (balanced traction) exerts a pull on the affected part and also supports the extremity in a splint, which is held in place by balanced weights attached to an overhead bar (Fig. 75–5A). Countertraction is supplied by a system of ropes, pulleys, and weights. With suspension traction, the pulling force remains the same even when the person moves, because countertraction takes up any slack caused by the movement. Thus, suspension traction allows more movement and activity than does running traction. This makes it easier to care for the client and improves the client's comfort.

Suspension traction may be applied to either the skele-

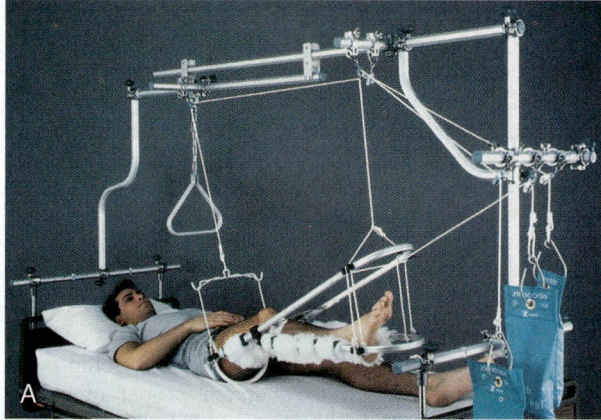

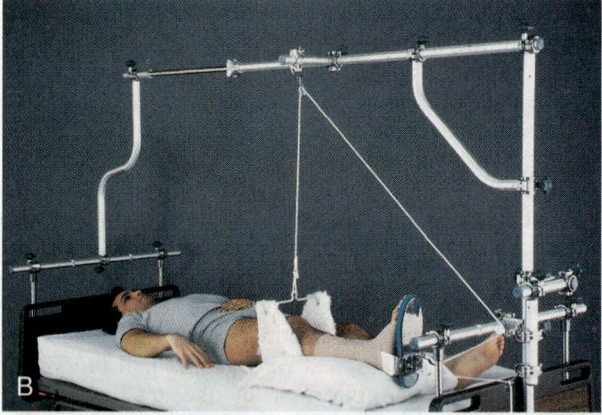

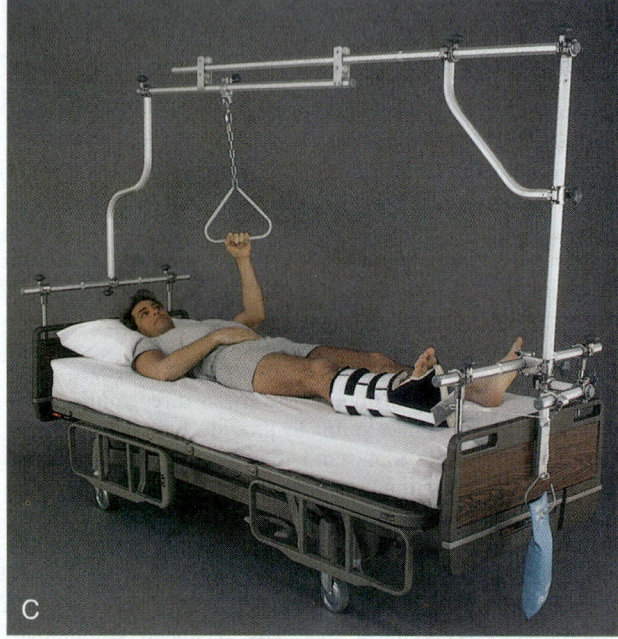

Figure 75–5. *A,* Balanced traction with a Thomas ring and a Pearson attachment. *B,* Russell's traction. *C,* Buck's traction. (Courtesy of Zimmer, Inc., Dover, OH.)

ton or skin and may use any type of splint. Examples of suspension traction are Russell's traction (see Fig. 75–5*B*) and a Thomas splint with a Pearson attachment. The traction must be continuous to be effective.

Skeletal Traction. Skeletal traction is accomplished by surgically inserting metal wires (Kirschner wires) or pins (Steinmann pins) through bones distal to the fracture site or by anchoring metal tongs (Gardner-Wells or Crutchfield tongs) in the skull. Kirschner wires and Steinmann pins are round stainless steel rods; they are typically inserted, with a hand drill, perpendicular to and completely through bone. A traction bow is attached to the wire or pin and the traction force is applied to the bow (also called spreader, stirrups, or calipers). The insertion site of pins, wires, or tongs determines the location at which traction force is applied.

Wires and pins are not inserted through joints. They are inserted so that they only penetrate skin, subcutaneous tissue, and bone. Joints, muscles, tendons, arteries, and nerves are avoided. Wires and pins are not inserted through skin that is infected, abraded, or affected by a rash. Inserting skeletal pins or wires is a sterile procedure performed under local or general anesthesia. Because the skin is opened for the placement of wires and pins, bone infection (osteomyelitis) is a potential (but rare) complication.

In the past, skeletal traction was used until bone healing took place. Now, its most common use is to reduce unstable fractures of long bones until the client is able to undergo more definitive surgical treatment, such as insertion of intramedullary nails and various plates.

Skin Traction. Skin traction applies traction to the underlying bones and other structures, such as muscles. It may be applied (1) with commercially prepared foam slings or (2) by encircling a body part with a halter, corset, or sling. Countertraction is provided by the person's weight when the bed is tilted away from the pull.

Removing Traction

When skeletal traction of a long bone is to be removed, the skin around the pin site is cleaned. A physician removes a wire by (1) depressing the skin around the wire end, (2) cutting the wire beneath the skin surface, and then (3) pulling the wire through from the opposite side. Cutting one end of the pin prevents the bone from being exposed to the contaminated end of the pin. The skin insertion and exit incisions are dressed with small sterile dressings. Clients are often placed in a cast to allow complete bone healing.

Types of Traction

Buck's Traction. Buck's traction is a form of skin traction exerted by a straight pull on one or both legs. It may be used to immobilize a limb for a short time (e.g., a fractured hip prior to internal surgical fixation) or to reduce muscle spasm. Other uses include treatment of arthritis, hip dislocation, hip tuberculosis, pelvic injuries, and fractures of the upper or lower leg. Buck's traction is applied by using a prefabricated boot. The boot should encase the lower leg to 1 to 2 inches below the knee, and the ankle movement should not be restricted. The traction should be continuous unless otherwise stated. If the weights must be removed, manual traction should be applied until the weights are replaced (see Fig. 75–5C).

Russell's Traction. Russell's traction is a modification of Buck's traction. Russell's traction adds a vertical pull by placing a sling under the leg above the knee. Russell's traction can be used to reduce or immobilize hip fractures or the shaft of the femur, especially in the adolescent. It also can be used for fractures of the tibial plateau in adults.

Cervical Traction. Cervical skin traction is used to hold the head in extension to treat muscle sprain, strain, and spasm. Cervical traction is usually applied with a head halter.

Cervical traction can also be skeletal traction used to stabilize fractures or dislocations of the cervical or upper thoracic spine. Two types of equipment are used for cervical traction: skull tongs and halo traction. Skull tongs (Gardner-Wells or Crutchfield) are a running traction with weight attached to the tongs, and the client is used as countertraction. The halo apparatus consists of a headpiece with four pins, two anterior and two posterior. Once the fracture is stable, the headpiece can be attached to a body jacket, called a *halo vest.*

Pelvic Traction. Pelvic traction is accomplished with a belt applied just above and encircling the iliac crests. The belt attaches to a spreader bar and pulley system. Traction is applied to the lumbar spine; up to 20 lb can be used. Some physicians order pillows beneath the legs; others want the foot of the bed to be elevated. If the backrest is excessively elevated, the client slides down in bed, creating an undesirable shearing force on the sacrum. The most desirable position is Williams's position (hips and knees each flexed 30 degrees). Pelvic traction should not increase a person's back or leg pain. If it does so, notify the physician. Pelvic traction is most often intermittent, but it can be continuous. Its use is uncommon because it has been shown to be of little value, and hospitalization is rarely used for low back strain.

Maintaining Vector of Force

The alignment of the bone is assessed daily; sometimes follow-up x-rays are used. Adjustments in angles of pull or weight may be needed.

Preventing Early Complications

Complications of fractures can be divided into early and late complications. Possible early complications of fractures include arterial damage, shock, nerve injury, compartment syndrome, Volkmann's ischemic contracture, fat embolism, deep vein thrombosis, pulmonary embolism, and infection.

Arterial Damage. Arterial damage may consist of contused, thrombosed, lacerated, severed, or spastic arteries. Arteries may be constricted by bandages or casts that are too tight. Indications of arterial damage include variable or absent pulse, swelling, pallor or patchy cyanosis distal to the fracture, continuing blood loss, pain, a large fracture hematoma, poor capillary return, poorly filled veins in a cold extremity, and paralysis or anesthesia distal to the fracture (in the absence of known neurologic injury). Promptly report and document assessment findings indicating arterial complications. Emergency intervention may include splitting or removing tight encircling casts or bandages, elevating or changing the position of the injured part, reducing fractures or dislocations, or surgery.

Shock. Hypovolemic shock is a potential problem because bony fragments can lacerate large vessels and cause bleeding. High-risk clients are those with femur and pelvic fractures. Even closed fractures can bleed.

Nerve Injury. Radial nerve injury is common with humeral fractures. Of course, bone fragments and edema can also injure nerves. Manifestations include paresthesia, paralysis, pallor, coolness of the extremity, increasing pain, and/or changes in the ability to move the extremity.

Compartment Syndrome. Compartment syndrome is a serious complication of fractures. Compartments are made up of muscles, bones, nerves, and blood vessels wrapped by a fibrous, inflexible membrane called fascia (Fig. 75–6A). The lower leg has four compartments: anterior, lateral, superficial and deep posterior. The arm has three compartments: superficial flexor, deep flexor, and extensor. The hand and foot also have compartments.

To understand compartment syndrome, it is important to realize that the fascia lining each compartment cannot expand. Therefore any increase in the compartment size due to bleeding or swelling will place pressure on pliable structures within the compartment, such as muscle, nerves, and blood vessels. Compartment syndrome can also develop if external pressure is applied, such as from a cast or a tight dressing.

Clinical manifestations of compartment syndrome are unrelenting ischemic pain that is not controllable with narcotic analgesics, pain with elevation due to decreased arterial inflow, and pain when the area is palpated or moved passively. Passive extension of the joint will cause pain in the compartment. In addition to pain, the client will have weak active movement, paresthesia (needles-and-pins sensation), diminished or absent pulses, coolness, or pallor of the affected extremity. The earliest sign of compartment syndrome is paresthesia. Pulselessness is a very late sign. If it is left untreated, in only 6 hours, compartment syndrome leads to a functionless extremity or requires amputation. Nursing assessment is critical and is described in the Critical Monitoring feature.

Compartment syndrome is managed by removing the cause of the compression. The cast or dressing is loosened or removed. If compartment syndrome is a result of edema or bleeding, a fasciotomy (incision into the fascia) is performed. Usually the incision is left open until the swelling decreases. For 2 to 3 days the area is loosely wrapped, and a skin graft may be performed eventually.

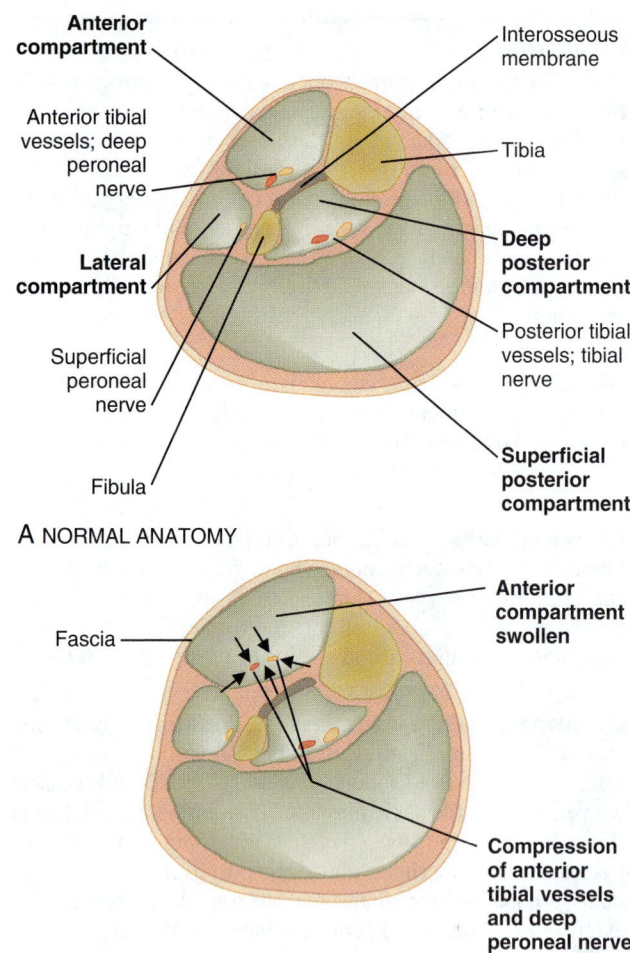

A NORMAL ANATOMY

B ANTERIOR COMPARTMENT SYNDROME

Figure 75–6. *A,* Compartments of the proximal third of the lower leg. The four compartments are (1) anterior, (2) lateral, (3) deep posterior, and (4) superficial posterior. *B,* Anterior compartment syndrome. As the compartment swells, it reaches a maximum size due to the inelastic fascia, which covers it. As edema continues, pressure is exerted on vessels and nerves within the compartment.

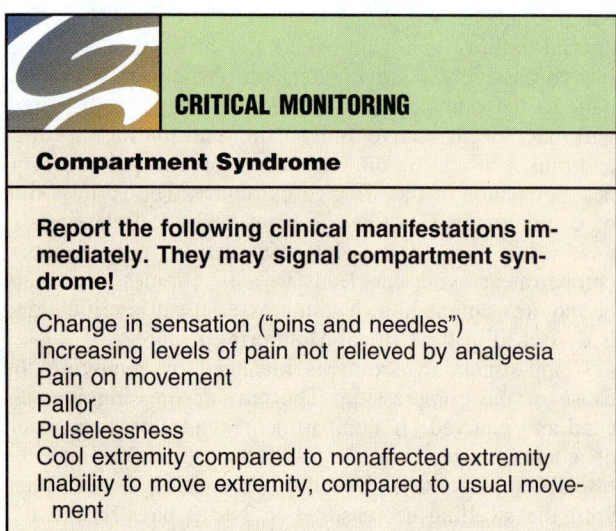

CRITICAL MONITORING

Compartment Syndrome

Report the following clinical manifestations immediately. They may signal compartment syndrome!

Change in sensation ("pins and needles")
Increasing levels of pain not relieved by analgesia
Pain on movement
Pallor
Pulselessness
Cool extremity compared to nonaffected extremity
Inability to move extremity, compared to usual movement

Volkmann's Ischemic Contracture. This serious and potentially crippling condition of the hand or forearm arises from a complication of a fracture around the elbow joint or forearm bones. It begins as a compartment syndrome that compromises arterial and venous circulation. If it is not relieved, pressure causes prolonged ischemia and muscle is gradually replaced by fibrous tissue that traps tendons and nerves. The typical end result is a permanent, stiff, claw-like deformity of the arm and hand. Numbness and paralysis are also often present. Volkmann's ischemic contracture most commonly arises after a supracondylar fracture of the humerus. It may also occur following other fractures of the elbow joint and forearm, crushing injuries of the forearm, and from tight bandages or casts. To avoid permanent deformity, compartment syndrome must be recognized and treated early.

Fat Embolism. Fat embolism is a relatively uncommon but potentially life-threatening complication of long-bone and pelvis fractures. Fat embolism syndrome occurs 24 to 48 hours after injury. The pathophysiology of fat embolism syndrome is similar to that of adult respiratory distress syndrome. The simplest explanation is that fat embolism develops when broken bones liberate fat from their marrow that embolizes to the lungs. Once fat droplets enter the circulation, they are too large to pass through pulmonary circulation. The emboli lodge in the capillaries and break down into fatty acids. Free fatty acids are toxic to lung parenchyma, capillary endothelium, and surfactant. The result is pulmonary hypertension and alterations in oxygen-carbon dioxide exchange.

The nurse must have a high index of suspicion for fat embolism syndrome. The classic picture of the client with fat embolism syndrome includes long bone fractures, altered mental status, tachypnea, tachycardia, hypoxemia, petechiae, and fever. Often it is difficult to distinguish fat embolism syndrome from pulmonary embolism. The distinguishing features are listed in Table 75–3.

Deep Vein Thrombosis and Pulmonary Embolism. Deep vein thrombosis (DVT) and pulmonary embolism (PE) are the most common causes of morbidity and mortality in orthopedic clients. Immobile clients with injuries of the pelvis and lower extremities are at highest risk. Clinical manifestations of DVT include unilateral leg edema, leg pain, and positive Homans' sign (not always a good indicator). Doppler studies may be used to determine if a clot is present. Clinical manifestations of PE are sudden dyspnea, tachypnea, chest pain, pallor, fright, and changes in mental status. DVT is fully discussed in Chapter 50 and PE is discussed in Chapter 41.

Infection. Infection following a fracture may be a result of contamination of an open fracture or it can be introduced at the time of surgery. *Pseudomonas* is a common infectious agent. Compound fractures may be complicated by tetanus or gas gangrene. Gas gangrene infections may develop in deep, grossly contaminated wounds. Gas gangrene is caused by anaerobic bacteria (various

Table 75–3. Comparison of Characteristics for Pulmonary Embolism and Fat Embolism Syndrome		
Characteristics	**Pulmonary Embolism**	**Fat Embolism Syndrome**
Pathophysiology and etiology	Local venous trauma Venous stasis Hypercoagulability	Fat globulin released from long bone or multiple fractures
Risk factors	Immobility Age > 40 History of heart disease, especially myocardial infarction or congestive heart failure Prior history of DVT or pulmonary embolus Surgery/trauma to hip, pelvis, or knee Obesity	Hypovolemia/shock Delayed immobilization or surgery Multiple fractures, especially long bones Joint replacement
Clinical manifestations*	Dyspnea Chest pain, worsened by deep breath Apprehension/anxiety Cough/hemoptysis Tachypnea > 30/min Localized rales Tachycardia > 140/min Low-grade fever Thrombophlebitis	Dyspnea Restless, agitated, confused, stuporous Tachypnea > 30/min Diffuse rales (late) Tachycardia > 140/min Fever > 103° F Petechial rash
Diagnostic assessment	ABGs (PaO$_2$ < 80 mm Hg)	Hypoxemia (PaO$_2$ < 60 mm Hg) Thrombocytopenia ↓ Hemoglobin Fat in urine and blood Increased sedimentation rate Increased levels of fibrin split products

Prevention	Early ambulation
	Leg elevation
	Elastic stockings
	Leg exercises
	Intermittent pneumatic compression
	Medications
	    Anticoagulants
	    Antiplatelet agents
		Immobilize fractures
		Adequate hydration
		O$_2$
		Corticosteroids

Management	Anticoagulation
	Surgical intervention
	    IVC interruption
	    Embolectomy
		O$_2$
		Fluid replacement
		Mechanical ventilation with PEEP
		Corticosteroids
		Maintain adequate hemoglobin

*Occur within 48 to 72 hours in venous thromboembolism. Occur within 24 to 48 hours in fat embolism. ABGs, arterial blood gases; DVT, deep vein thrombosis; IVC, inferior vena caval; PEEP, positive end expiratory pressure. Modified from Slye, D. (1991). Orthopedic complications. *Nursing Clinics of North America, 26*(1), 113–132.

species of *Clostridium*). These organisms produce a characteristic cellulitis in which gas is present under the skin. Assessment reveals (1) a precipitous drop in hemoglobin level, (2) an elevation in temperature, (3) a rapid pulse, (4) pain, (5) sudden local puffiness (with discoloration of tissues), and (6) thin, watery, extremely foul-smelling exudate. Crepitation may be felt on palpation of the skin as a result of the presence of gas bubbles in muscles and subcutaneous tissue. Treatment of gas gangrene involves opening the wound widely to admit air and permit drainage. Generous, multiple incisions are made through the

skin and fascia. Sutures and any gangrenous material are removed and the wound is irrigated. Anti-infective agents are administered. If massive gangrene develops, amputation is necessary.

Osteomyelitis is a severe bone infection. Organisms have direct access to bone in open fractures, but they can infect bone from other sources as well (e.g., sepsis, skin infections, cellulitis). Early osteomyelitis is readily treated if it is recognized. If it is not recognized early, osteomyelitis can become chronic and lead to leg-length discrepancy, deformity, or amputation.

■ Nursing Management of the Medical Client

Traction

When planning nursing intervention for people in traction, it is important to know (1) the nature of the injury, (2) the purpose of the traction, (3) how the traction device accomplishes its purpose, (4) which movements and positions are permitted, (5) potential complications associated with traction, and (6) appropriate intervention to prevent complications.

Care Before Traction Is Applied

Explain to the client and family the purposes of traction and the reasons why specific body positions must be maintained for long periods. Make sure they understand contraindicated movements or positions. Explain that moving into contraindicated positions defeats the purpose of traction and disrupts healing. Explain or demonstrate the use of the trapeze for independent movement. Explain that traction helps tight muscles to relax and that the client will probably feel more comfortable after a few hours. The physician tells the client how long traction is likely to be maintained. Techniques to perform self-care and to reduce boredom can also be described.

Before a pin is inserted, establish neurovascular baseline measurements for later comparison. Neurovascular assessment includes observation of color, warmth, movement, sensation, pedal pulses, and capillary refill.

Care After Traction Is Applied

Nursing care of a client in traction is presented in the Care Plan.

Care After Traction Is Removed

Immediately following traction removal, a client is often weak and unsteady. If a limb was immobilized, the muscle may display some atrophy. Orthostatic hypotension may occur if the client has been bedridden in a flat position for several days or more. To combat this problem, help the client very gradually resume a sitting (and later a standing) position. Elevate the head of the bed a little bit at a time to combat orthostatic hypotension. Raising the bed to a full sitting position may require several days. Have adequate help and provide careful physical support when a client first sits on the edge of the bed or gets out of bed. Safety precautions are imperative to prevent falls until the nurse is sure the client has secure balance, self-support, and strength.

Prepare the client for a lack of proprioceptor response (awareness of body position, movement, and posture) following traction removal. Explain that the client may feel faint or weak, and that joints may be stiff or unstable. Weakened limbs may require temporary support at their joints, and crutches may be needed for a while.

External Fixation

An external fixation device may be used as an alternative to either a cast or traction. An external fixator is a device consisting of pins that are placed through the skin into the fractured bone and connected to a rigid external frame. These devices are made of aluminum, titanium, or nylon. They are commonly used to treat massive open comminuted fractures with extensive soft tissue damage or neurovascular damage. Advantages of the external fixation system is that fractures can be adjusted in three dimensions. In addition, external fixation allows for fine adjustments and maintenance of limb length during and after its application. Some common external fixators are the Hoffmann, Anderson, Haynes, or Struder devices (Fig. 75–7). External fixators can be used on arms, legs, and, occasionally, fingers and/or the pelvis. Often, a cast is applied until healing is complete; this is especially common in fractures of the lower extremity.

Nursing care for the client with an external fixation device includes assessment of neurovascular compromise, assisting with impaired physical mobility, reducing the risk of infection, and assisting the client with self-care needs. Inspect exposed skin and pin sites twice daily for signs of infection. Slight redness and swelling at the site is normal. Infection is usually noted as marked redness and purulent drainage. Perform pin site care according to the institution's policy. Sometimes wound care is needed for open wounds, such as saline soaks. Usually, the client is ambulatory with a non-weightbearing gait. When the client is discharged, clothing will need to be specially fit. For example, a pant leg may need to be split up the inseam and then closed with ties or Velcro. Sweat pants or pants with snaps also work well. Women can wear full skirts. Underwear usually needs to be split down the sides and have Velcro closures attached to it. Clients with pelvic fixators need to reduce their intake of foods that increase intestinal gas, which leads to distension of the abdomen. Once the bone has healed, the external fixator is removed.

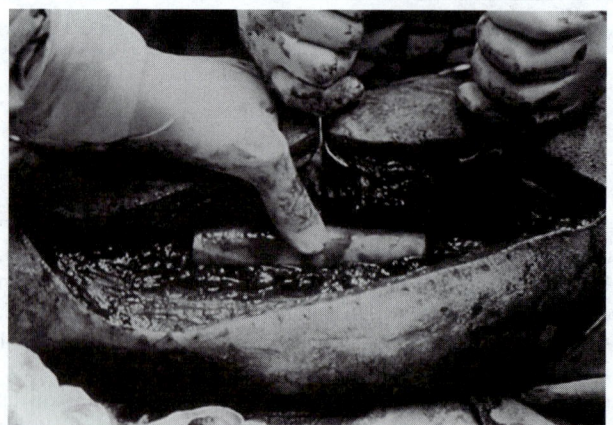

Figure 75–7. Bone grafting is sometimes used to correct fracture nonunion. Available bones are stored in a "bone bank" under refrigeration until they are required for a recipient.

CARE PLAN

The Client in Traction

Nursing Diagnosis. Risk for Impaired Skin Integrity related to inability to change position secondary to skeletal traction

Planning: Expected Outcomes. Client will retain intact skin, as evidenced by no reddened areas, no abrasions.

Implementation: Nursing Intervention	Rationales
Assess pressure points (sacrum, heels, skin under ropes and bones) every shift	These are common pressure points for clients in supine position
Provide skin care every shift by lifting client	Clients in traction cannot turn
Place therapeutic mattress on bed	Some mattresses (Geo-Matt) reduce surface pressure (eggcrate mattresses improve comfort only)

Evaluation. Expect the client's skin to remain intact with adequate pressure reduction interventions.

Nursing Diagnosis. Impaired Physical Mobility related to confinement in traction

Planning: Expected Outcomes. The client will not experience complications of immobility, as evidenced by maintaining preinjury ROM in noninvolved joints, not developing thrombophlebitis, having a bowel movement every other day, and maintaining clear lung sounds.

Implementation: Nursing Intervention	Rationales
Place all joints (except those immediately proximal and distal to fracture) through ROM every shift	ROM assists to maintain muscle tone
Assess lung sounds every shift	Immobility and use of analgesia may cause hypoventilation and atelectasis
Teach client to deep breathe and cough every shift	Deep breathing and coughing cause hyperventilation and clear secretions
Assess for clinical manifestations of thrombophlebitis: unilateral leg edema or pain; do not rely on Homans' sign as an indicator	The presence of Homans' sign is not an accurate indicator of thrombophlebitis; other signs are assessed
Monitor bowel movements	Constipation is a side effect of narcotic use and immobility
Encourage fluids and food containing fiber	Fiber and fluids assist to add bulk and soften stool, making its passage easier
Administer laxatives as needed	Laxatives irritate or stimulate the colon

Evaluation. After 3 to 5 days of immobility, clients may develop some of these complications. An aggressive prevention program should be effective.

Nursing Diagnosis: Risk for Injury related to traction

Planning: Expected Outcomes. The client will sustain no injury while in traction as evidenced by maintaining effective pulling force and desired vector of force.

Implementation: Nursing Intervention	Rationales
Ensure that weights hang freely from pulleys	If weights rest on the bed or floor, traction is not effective
Ensure that knots in the rope do not catch in the pulleys	Traction is not effective when knots catch in pulleys
Add and remove weights slowly with physician's order	Slow, steady pull reduces muscle spasms
Assess skin at pin site daily or bid for signs of infection	Infection can develop in pin sites
Pin site care per agency policy	Reduces risk of infection
Adjust the position of the bed per physician's orders	Provides countertraction

Evaluation. Expect the client to maintain adequate pulling forces via traction and with adequate nursing assessment and care.

Collaborative Problem. Risk for compartment syndrome and neurovascular compromise

Planning: Expected Outcomes. Clinical manifestations of compartment syndrome will be promptly recognized and reported.

Care Plan continued on following page

CARE PLAN

The Client in Traction *(Continued)*

Implementation: Nursing Intervention	Rationales
Monitor color, warmth, movement, and sensation of extremity distal to traction every shift Assess pedal (radial) pulse every shift Monitor reports of degree of pain and relief by analgesia Immediately inform physician of changes in skin color, pulses, skin temperature, motion, sensation or an increase in pain	Clinical manifestations of compartment syndrome include pallor, pulselessness, cool extremities, inability to move, loss of or change in sensation, and pain that is not relieved with usual analgesia Compartment syndrome demands immediate medical intervention

Evaluation. Risk of compartment syndrome exists until edema subsides (about 72 hours).

Nursing Diagnosis. Self Care Deficit related to inability to move in environment

Planning: Expected Outcomes. The client will participate in those self-care activities possible given sites of fractures.

Implementation: Nursing Intervention	Rationales
Place necessary equipment and supplies within easy reach	Facilitates maximal self-care and independence
Allow client to schedule procedures, such as bath or linen changes	Provides client some control
Medicate for pain prior to movement	Movement increases pain and spasm in fracture site

Evaluation. The client should be able to assist with his or her own feeding and bathing.

Nursing Diagnosis. Diversional Activity Deficit related to prolonged immobiity, inadequate environmental stimulation, or lack of variation

Planning: Expected Outcomes. The client will remain mentally and emotionally stable and demonstrate interest in surroundings.

Implementation: Nursing Intervention	Rationales
Plan varied activities of interest to the person to fill each day, such as reading, writing, listening to the radio, and watching television	Variety is a normal aspect of life
Be sure a telephone is convenient	Telephone can be used to maintain contact with significant others
Sit with, talk with, and touch the client as appropriate	Provides contact with nurses outside of usual activities (medications, cares)
Place the client's bed beside a window; keep the door open as possible	Allows passive interaction with outside
Provide accurate clock, current calendar and publications, clean eyeglasses and hearing aids, if worn by the client; obtain prism glasses if client is supine	Normal aids to orientation; prism glasses may help a person read more easily while lying flat
Have the radio and television clearly tuned, but do not leave them on continuously if the client cannot control them independently	Continuous noise can increase confusion

Evaluation. Problems with diversional activities develop after about 2 weeks, when pain is minimal and client must wait for bones to realign.

Community and Self-Care

■ Medical Management
Preventing Long-Term Complications

Joint Stiffness. Joint stiffness may follow edema, joint contracture, or muscle atrophy from prolonged immobilization. Joint stiffness is most common in the upper extremities (shoulder, elbow, finger).

Post-traumatic Arthritis. Post-traumatic arthritis is usually influenced by the severity of the initial injury and the initial bone reduction. Surgical joint replacement may eventually be needed.

Avascular Necrosis. Avascular necrosis is literally the death of bone tissue due to the absence of blood vessels supplying the tissues. *Aseptic necrosis* and *osteonecrosis* are other terms used to describe this problem. It most commonly occurs in femoral head and carpal fractures.

Reflex Sympathetic Dystrophy. *Reflex sympathetic dystrophy* (RSD) is a term applied to a variety of seemingly unrelated disorders having strikingly similar clinical manifestations and having the same pathophysiology. The term *reflex* indicates that the condition is a response to a stimulus that is traumatic, medical, infectious, or vascular; the term *sympathetic* indicates that the sympathetic nervous system is the neurologic pathway serving the development and maintenance of the syndrome; and the term *dystrophy* indicates that if this disorder is not treated it will result in permanent problems and trophic changes. RSD is defined as a syndrome of diffuse limb pain, often burning in nature, and usually following an injury or other noxious stimulus with variable sensory, motor, autonomic, and trophic changes. Examples of a few of the causes of RSD include sprains, dislocations, fractures, minor lacerations, burns, surgery on the hands, myocardial infarction, cerebral vascular accident, spinal cord disease, vascular disorders, and frostbite. Peculiar to RSD is the lack of correlation between the severity of the injury and the subsequent severity of RSD. In fact, severe trauma causing fractures of long bones and transection of nerves is less likely to develop into RSD than are minor injuries in areas richly supplied with nerves.

Regardless of the cause, the underlying pathophysiology is a prolonged normal sympathetic response to injury. Clinical manifestations occur in three phases:

1. Acute phase: Constant pain is present, usually of burning quality. The pain is aggravated by movement. Exaggerated sensation may be present in the knee area. The skin becomes smooth and taut with a decrease in normal skin wrinkles due to edema.

2. Dystrophic phase: Edema spreads, increasing the stiffness of joints and leading to muscular wasting. Pain remains the major manifestation and is still burning in nature. The skin is moist, cyanotic, and cold; hair is coarse. Manifestations of atrophy are present.

3. Atrophic phase: Pain is less prominent. Hair loss occurs in the extremity. The subcutaneous tissue and muscles are atrophied. All of the involved joints are characterized by extreme weakness and limited range of motion. Contractions of flexor tendons are present. Osteoporosis is evident. The client can develop depression and chronic pain syndromes. Anxiety increases over the chronicity of the problem, loss of work, and changes in social and family structures. Sleep is lost to pain and worry.

Management is based on the disease stage. In the acute phase, RSD can be completely reversed with sympathetic blockade. In the dystrophic phase, sympathetic blocks may still be used, although a larger series of blocks may be needed. In the atrophic phase, sympathetic blocks may still provide some relief, but the process can no longer be reversed. Physical therapy, psychological counseling, antidepressants for sleep, and nonsteroidal antiinflammatory drugs may be used. Nifedipine is being tried for its smooth muscle relaxation properties; this drug has not been fully studied, but it appears to be promising.

Malunion. Malunion is the healing of a fracture site in improper alignment. Malunion seen early in fracture healing can be corrected with adjustment of traction or reimmobilization. Malunion after healing is usually treated with surgery.

Delayed Union. Delayed union is the failure of a fracture to consolidate within 3 months to 1 year. Delayed union is usually due to a retardation of the healing process from previously discussed factors, such as decreased blood supply. Delayed union usually is correctable with additional time, correction of the cause, and the application of weightbearing to the fracture site.

Nonunion. Nonunion is the failure of a fracture site to consolidate and produce a complete, firm, and stable union after 4 to 6 months. Nonunion is characterized by excessive motion in the fracture site that leads to a false joint, or *pseudoarthrosis*. The risk factors for nonunion are the same as those presented earlier. Nonunion is commonly treated with bone grafts (Fig. 75–8), internal fixation, external fixation, electric bone stimulation, or combinations of these methods. Bone grafts can be from the client's own bone or cadaveric bone. The iliac crest is the most common donor site. When it is used as a donor site, expect the client to have more pain in the iliac donor site than in the surgical site. Psychological problems can develop in the client who uses cadaver bone due to worries

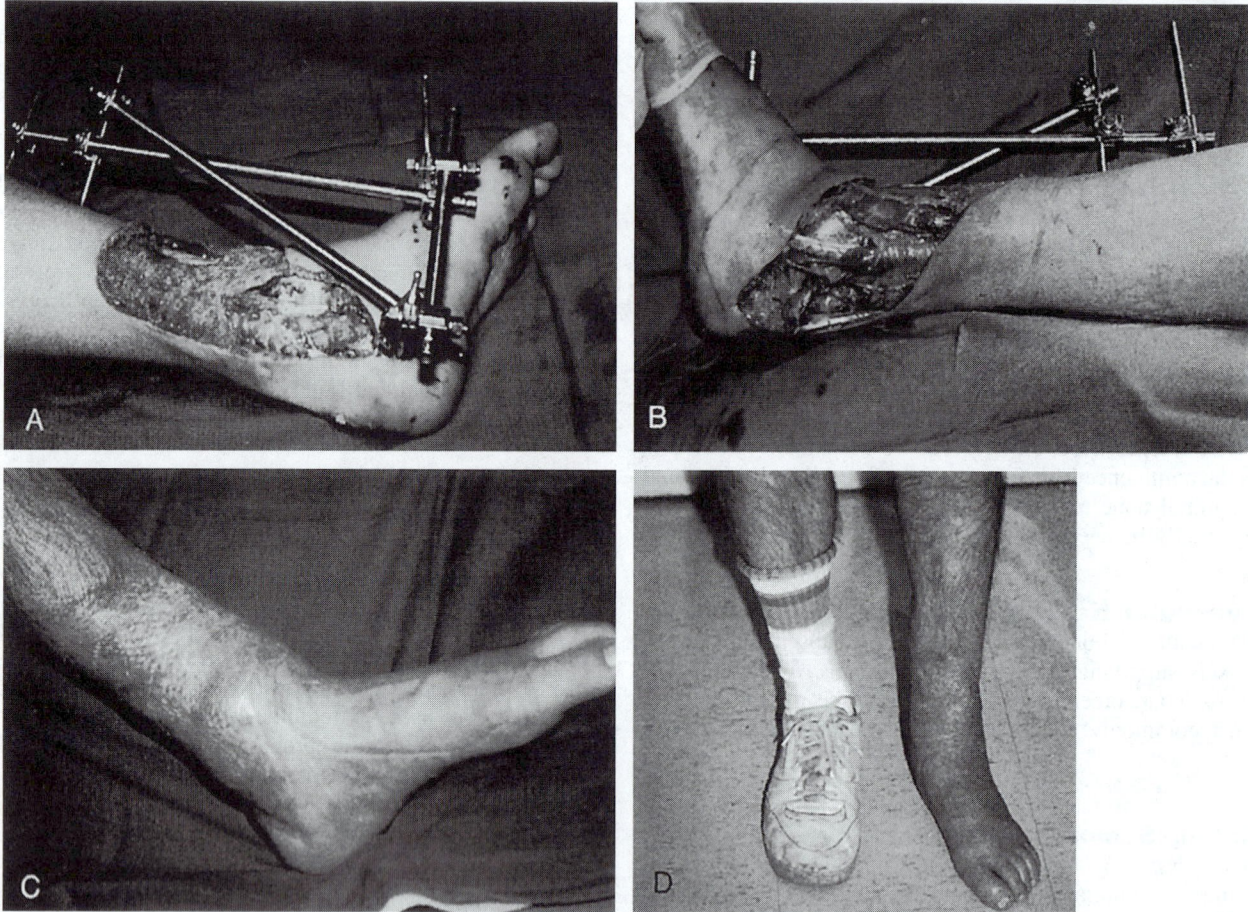

Figure 75–8. This client sustained severe fractures of the tibia and fibula. The fractures were managed with an external fixator device (*A* and *B*). The open wound was closed with a muscle flap and skin graft. *C* and *D,* the same client seen 8 months after surgery. He can stand with full weightbearing. (From Browner, B. D., et al. [Eds.]. [1992]. *Skeletal trauma: Fractures, dislocations, ligamentous injuries.* Philadelphia: W. B. Saunders.)

about transmission of hepatitis and human immunodeficiency virus (HIV).

Externally applied electrical current can stimulate bone growth. Direct-current stimulation via surgically implanted electrodes is the most common method of applying electrical stimulation. The system consists of a cathode, anode, and small current generator. The generator uses a lithium-iodine powder source with a life of 8 months. Nursing care after implantation is minimal, other than usual surgical recovery. Client education is important. While the electrical stimulation device is implanted, the client must not bear weight on the involved extremity for 6 to 8 weeks. Weightbearing on an unstable fracture prolongs healing time.

A surface form of electrical stimulation has also been developed, called capacitive-coupled simulation. The system consists of two small self-adhesive electrode pads placed on opposite sides of the fracture site and a 9-volt battery pack to provide power. This system cannot be used on clients with sensitivity to nickel, chromium, or stainless steel; clients with pacemakers; or clients with mental or physical conditions that preclude compliance. Clients need to be taught how to apply the device and to monitor for skin changes under the electrodes.

Casting

Casts are temporary devices of plaster or fiberglass that immobilize a body part, usually an extremity. However, clients can wear casts over the torso also. The purposes of a cast include (1) immobilization; (2) prevention or correction of deformity; (3) maintenance, support, and protection to realign bone; and (4) promotion of healing, which allows early weightbearing for ambulation. The types of casts are described in Table 75–4, and shown in Figure 75–9.

Applying a Cast

Casting Materials

Synthetic casting materials are made of fabric impregnated with high-density thermoplastic resin or fiberglass. These materials provide strong, lightweight casts that set in about 5 minutes. Synthetic casts come in a number of colors and patterns that can boost self-esteem in young or elderly clients. Synthetic casts maintain their shape and firmness even if they become wet. However, if a synthetic cast becomes wet, it must be thoroughly dried to

Table 75-4. Types of Casts

Name of the Cast	Description
Short arm	Used to treat stable metacarpal, carpal, distal radius, or humerus fractures or wrist sprains. Cast extends from the palm and thumb to midarm. May include a thumb spica for thumb fractures, or may be a hanging cast for humerus fractures.
Short leg	Used to treat fractures of the tibia, fibula, and ankle. Cast extends from the foot to below the knee. May be weightbearing or non-weightbearing.
Long leg	Used to treat unstable fractures of the femur, tibia, and/or fibula. Cast extends from foot to hip and holds the knee in flexion if fracture is unstable, to prevent weightbearing. If weightbearing is permitted, a cylinder cast is used.
Cast brace	Used to treat a stable distal femur fracture. Cast consists of two parts, above and below the knee, with a hinge at the knee to allow ROM.
Hip spica	Used to treat fractures of the hip and to immobilize the hip(s). Cast extends from midtrunk to foot or feet, hips abducted with an abductor bar. Opening made in cast for elimination of urine and feces. Fairly uncommon today.

prevent skin maceration. If there is no incision under the cast, a synthetic cast can be dried with a cast dryer or hair blow dryer on a low setting, although it takes several hours to dry.

Plaster of Paris (anhydrous calcium sulfate) bandages are individual rolls of precut crinoline, in various sizes, impregnated with plaster. The body part to be casted determines the amount of plaster to be used. Plaster casts take about 24 hours longer to dry than do synthetic casts. Plaster of Paris casts cannot get wet.

Casting Procedure

A cast may be applied in a physician's office, a clinic, an emergency room, in the operating room, or at a hospital bedside. In a hospital, the client is usually taken to an equipped cast room for cast application. Explain the procedure to the client and family. Skin preparation includes thoroughly cleaning the skin. Closely examine the skin while preparing it. Document the presence of any lesions, unremovable dirt, and foreign particles.

After the skin is prepared, it is covered with stockinette, web-roll, or padding. Make sure these coverings fit smoothly, without wrinkles. Wrinkles or uneven surface can abrade skin and lead to skin breakdown. Cut stockinette longer than the expected finished cast length, so that the excess portions can be pulled to cover exposed ends of the cast. When using the fiberglass material, the padding should be of a synthetic material. The padding may be applied more heavily over a bony prominence, but use caution because too much padding can cause pressure. When padding is applied, make sure it is smooth and even so that it does not cause pressure sores.

Plaster-filled bandages are submerged in a bucket of clean water, one at a time; the excess water is removed, and the bandage is applied to encircle the body part. Plaster bandages are applied in a wetter state than are synthetic bandages.

During cast application, support the extremity from underneath using the palms of the hands in such a way that pressure is not applied to any one area. Do not press fingertips into the cast or rest the cast on a hard or sharp surface. Doing so may cause flattening or indentations in the cast that might cause pressure problems. As soon as the casting procedure is complete, the client's skin is cleaned of excess casting material. An x-ray may be performed to verify correct bone alignment.

Never empty plaster-laden water into an ordinary sink because plaster sediment will solidify and plug the plumbing. If a sink with a plaster trap is not available, wait for sediment to settle into the bottom of the plastic-lined bucket, then drain the water from the top. Scrape the plaster sediment off the bottom of the pan and dispose of it in the garbage.

Drying a Cast

Synthetic casts are dry to the touch in a few minutes, but they take about 20 minutes to set completely. Synthetic casts dry with a thermal reaction and may feel hot. The client should be taught to expect the sensation of heat. Also, the surface is sticky and can cause skin irritation. Therefore handle synthetic casts only while wearing gloves. Plaster casts set rapidly but take several hours to dry completely (large casts may take several days). The water from a newly applied cast (green cast) eventually evaporates, leaving a mature cast of full strength.

Promote the circulation of warm, dry air around a damp cast to enhance moisture evaporation and to speed the drying process. Warn a person receiving a cast that heat (both plaster of Paris and fiberglass generate heat) is created during the cast's early setting (hardening) stages. The sensation of heat under a cast can be frightening if it is not understood. Allow the heat generated in a newly applied cast to dissipate into circulating air. Do not cover the cast while it is drying. It is usually helpful to put several layers of towels under the cast on the pillow to absorb the dampness from the cast. During the green period (while the cast is still damp), a casted person may feel cold and chill easily. Provide adequate covering while also allowing air to circulate around the cast. If the client has a large cast, avoid excessive chilling by covering some parts of the cast for a brief time and rotating the exposed portions.

Unless contraindicated, turn a client in a green cast periodically to expose more of the casted area to air.

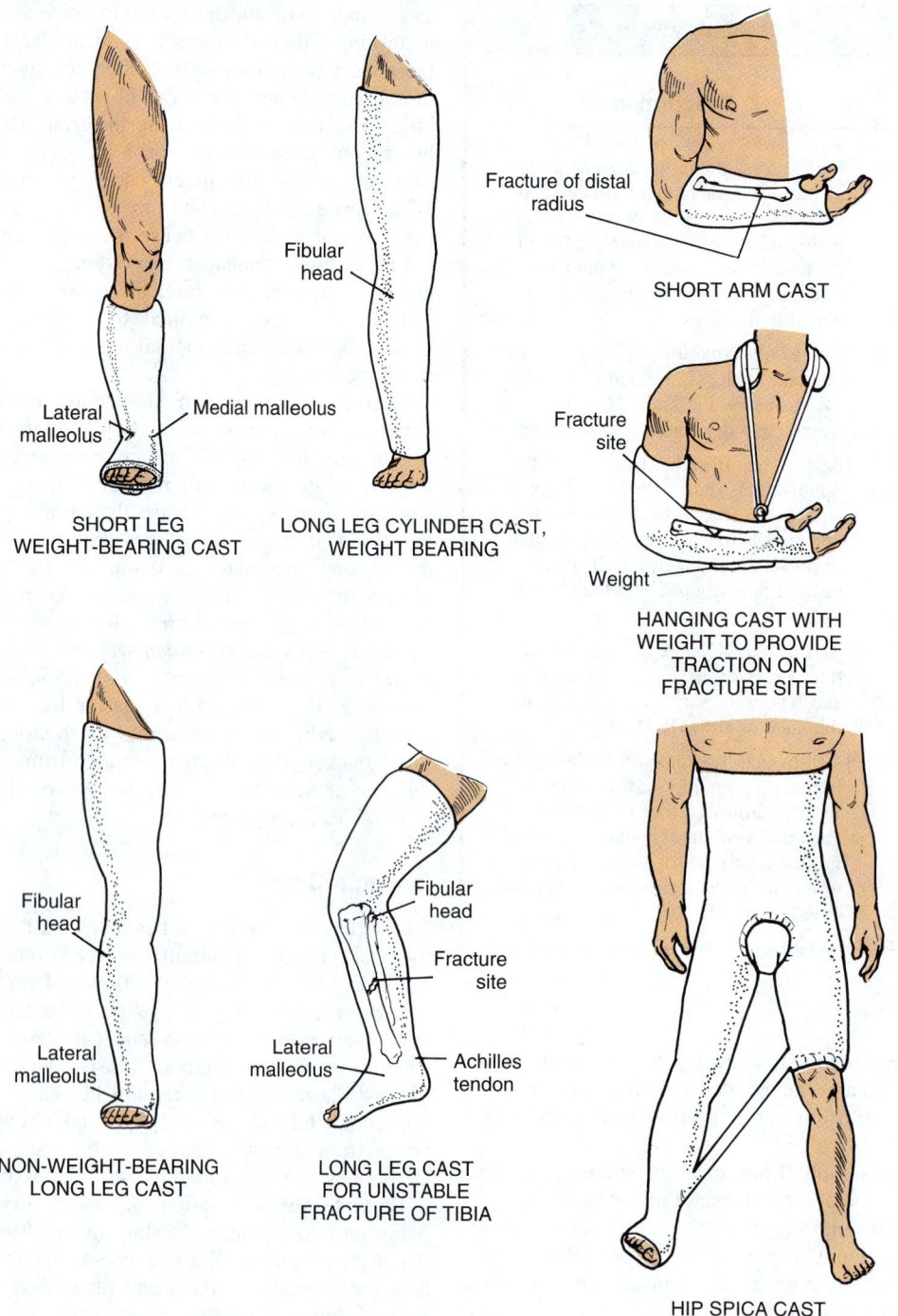

Figure 75–9. Common types of casts for extremity fractures.

Place new casts on pillows to protect them from pressure and flattening during drying. Occasionally, a cast dryer or a hair dryer on a low setting may be used to facilitate drying. However, never place a dryer too close to a cast or focus it on one spot. Rapid drying can burn skin under a cast or crack the cast. A wet plaster of Paris cast is musty smelling, dull on percussion, gray, and cold to the touch. A dry plaster cast is odorless, resonant on percussion, is white, and close to room temperature to the

touch. Wet, or green, fiberglass casts are a creamy color and feel hot to the touch. The surface also is sticky. The surface should not be touched without gloves until the cast is "dry" (about 20 minutes). A fiberglass cast should be handled as you would a plaster cast. Do not place a fiberglass cast over drainage-containing pads, such as incontinence pads, because paper and plastics will adhere and become a permanent part of the cast.

Once it is completely dry, a cast can be placed on a

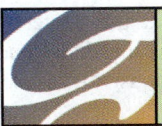

CRITICAL MONITORING

The Client in a Cast

Compartment Syndrome

- Pulselessness: slow nail bed capillary refill (greater than 3 sec)
- Skin pallor, blanching, cyanosis, or coolness
- Increasing pain, swelling, painful edema peripheral to cast, pain on passive motion
- Paresthesias (tingling, prickling), heightened sensitivity, numbness; hypesthesia (diminished sensitivity to touch); anesthesia (numbness)
- Motor paralysis of previously functioning muscles
- Hypesthesia (diminished sensitivity); anesthesia (numbness); paresthesias (tingling, prickling, heightened sensitivity, numbness)

Infection

- Musty, unpleasant odor over cast and/or at ends of cast
- Drainage through cast or cast opening
- Sudden unexplained body temperature elevation
- "Hot spot" felt on cast over lesion

Cast Syndrome

- Bloated feeling
- Prolonged nausea; repeated vomiting
- Abdominal distention; vague abdominal pain
- Shortness of breath

---

hard surface (e.g., a casted arm may rest on a table), but it is usually more comfortable to rest the casted area on pillows.

Windowing and Bivalving a Cast

Cutting windows in casts and bivalving casts are two techniques commonly used to relieve or prevent excessive pressure in casted body areas, or to provide access to or visualization of certain body parts. Windows may be cut (in dried casts) (1) to relieve pressure from abdominal distention (e.g., in a body cast or hip spica); (2) to prevent "cast syndrome"; (3) to assess a radial pulse (e.g., to check circulation in a casted arm); (4) to inspect areas of discomfort or areas of suspected tissue damage; and (5) to remove drains or care for wounds.

Bivalving a cast means splitting it along both sides (1) to allow tissue swelling, (2) to allow removal of half of it to facilitate care and taking of x-ray films, (3) to allow removal and reapplication while a client is learning to adjust to being without a cast, or (4) to make a half-cast for use as an intermittent splint (e.g., to prevent deformities). Once a cast is bivalved, either half can be removed easily without disturbing alignment. When reapplying a bivalved cast, the client's extremity should be handled carefully, with care taken not to pinch skin between the

two cast halves. When both halves of the cast are properly fitted, secure them with an elastic wrap.

Assessing for Complications of a Cast

Although casts are protective and therapeutic, they can also cause serious complications. The cast can cause pressure and constriction of the casted limb. The casted part can swell beneath the cast, leading to compartment syndrome (see earlier discussion). The cast can also rub on the skin and cause skin breakdown. Clinical manifestations of complications are found in the Critical Monitoring feature.

Cast syndrome is a serious complication that sometimes follows prolonged supine positioning, spinal surgery, or the use of a body cast. Cast syndrome is compression of the duodenum between the superior mesenteric artery anteriorly and the aorta and vertebral bodies posteriorly (Fig. 75–10). Clinical manifestations are nausea, abdominal pressure, vague abdominal pain, feelings of bloatedness, feelings of tightness, and inability to take a deep breath. Clients can develop complete gastrointestinal obstruction. Management includes cutting, windowing, or bivalving the cast, nasogastric intubation to decompress the intestine, intravenous fluids, and placing the client on

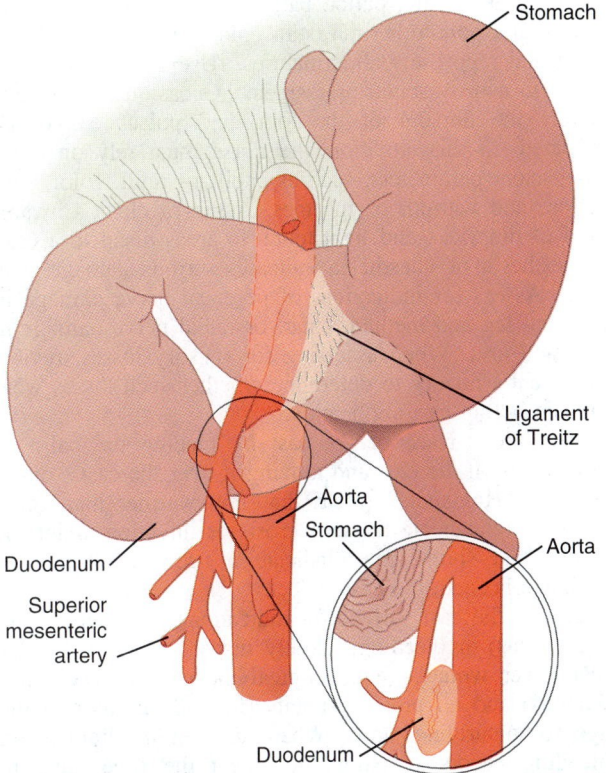

Figure 75–10. Cast syndrome is due to compression of the duodenum between the aorta and the superior mesenteric artery. The pressure is usually due to a tight body cast. (After Cohen, L. B., Field, S. P., & Sachar, D. B. [1985]. The superior mesenteric artery syndrome: The disease that isn't, or is it? *Journal of Clinical Gastroenterology, 7,* 113.)

NPO status (nothing by mouth). Antiemetics should be given sparingly to all persons in body casts because they can mask the manifestations of cast syndrome. Untreated cast syndrome can be fatal because it causes obstruction of the superior mesenteric vein, leading to gastrointestinal hemorrhage and necrosis. It can develop as late as several weeks or months after cast application. Thus, it is important to teach clients how to recognize the manifestations and to report abdominal pain and nausea.

■ Nursing Management of the Medical Client

Assessment

Thorough assessment and prompt intervention are essential to prevent cast-related complications. Establish an assessment pattern and always make observations sequentially. For example, in a casted extremity, assess the following:

1. Color
2. Movement of distal fingers or toes
3. Warmth
4. Sensation
5. Swelling
6. Pulses distal to cast

Another helpful way to remember some significant assessment findings with cast-related complications is the 6 Ps mnemonic: pain, pallor, paralysis, pulselessness, paresthesia, and poikilothermia (skin cold to the touch). Document and report any abnormalities. (Use Table 75–3 as a guide to neurovascular assessment). Occasionally, the cast covers the dorsum of the foot, and pulses cannot be palpated. In this situation, the nurse must rely on other assessment parameters, such as capillary refill, color, sensation, and warmth of the toes. Assess a client's awareness of pinpricks and light touch in areas distal to a cast. Hypesthesia or anesthesia indicates serious damage to a limb. Assess for indications of peroneal nerve damage in a casted leg and median, ulnar, or radial nerve damage in a casted arm. When assessing for sensory losses, review the client's history to determine whether such losses were present before cast application.

Feel the surface of the cast by placing the palm of your hand on the cast and moving it over the cast's entire surface. "Hot spots" (areas that feel warmer than other areas) may indicate tissue necrosis or infection under the cast. "Wet spots" may indicate a need for drying or drainage beneath the cast.

Assess the cast surface for indications of wound drainage (stains) or bleeding. Closely inspect areas of the cast that cover wounds (e.g., surgical incisions or accidental wounds) and all pressure points (for indications of damage to underlying skin). When an area of drainage or bleeding becomes visible, document the time, date its appearance, and describe the observation. Drainage on the surface of fiberglass casts may not appear at the area of the wound or incision. Because of the composition of the cast, the drainage may not wick outward; rather, it may wick to the dependent area if the cast is flat, or it may be found posterior and superior if the limb is elevated. The drainage may even seep out of the cast at the posterior and superior aspect of the elevated cast or the distal end of a dependent cast. Continued assessment is, of course, necessary.

Note odors indicative of tissue necrosis and infection. A cast often develops a sour smell after being worn a while, from perspiration and normal sloughing of outer skin layers. However, tissue necrosis emits an easily detectable, musty, strong, offensive odor. If the odor of mildew is present, especially with a fiberglass cast, the cast may have become wet at one time and not thoroughly dried. If this has occurred, the physician should be notified, and the cast will probably be changed.

Assess skin around cast edges for skin damage or swelling. Injury to an extremity and subsequent treatment (e.g., closed reduction, surgery) usually produces swelling, which progresses for the first 12 to 24 hours after injury or surgery. Swelling may be the greatest for the first 24 to 48 hours. Although mild swelling of exposed fingers and toes is not unusual, moderate or severe swelling associated with pain and discoloration is abnormal. When a casted part swells markedly, structures within the cast are constricted and compartment syndrome may result. Swelling may obstruct blood flow. The physician must be notified of these changes.

Intervention

Intervention to prevent or relieve excessive swelling typically includes (1) full-length elevation of the cast higher than the client's heart, (2) exercising the fingers or toes to stimulate circulation, and (3) placing ice bags around the cast. Pressure caused by swelling must be relieved by cutting the cast before irreversible damage occurs. Pressure (without swelling) by the edge of a cast against skin may be relieved by a position change or by loosely padding the uncomfortable area.

Positioning. A casted extremity should be elevated to minimize swelling and promote drainage. This procedure is especially important for the first 24 to 48 hours. Elevating a casted part stimulates circulation and reduces swelling (and thus pressure within the cast). Elevate casted extremities on pillows. A casted arm may be placed in a sling or arm immobilizer when the client is ambulatory. Support the entire arm, including the elbow, wrist, and hand (wristdrop leads to neurovascular complications), and keep the fingers higher than the elbow (to minimize swelling). If a sling or immobilization is not used, the person should be encouraged to exercise the uncasted joints, such as the shoulder or elbow, to prevent complications of disuse. Use a pillow to elevate the arm during sitting if this position is more comfortable.

Expose the buttocks of a client in a hip spica or body cast to prevent soiled or damp clothing during urination and to provide adequate skin care. Position the client carefully and comfortably on a fracture bedpan designed for use by clients wearing body casts or hip spica casts. Incontinence pads can be tucked into the edge of the cast to prevent soiling. Slightly raise the head of the bed to facilitate elimination and to prevent excrement from running under the cast. Raising head and shoulders slightly to use a bedpan is usually allowed unless the client is in shock, is hemorrhaging, or has a spinal injury. Damp, soiled casts become malodorous and may mold or break. Dampness also causes skin irritation and may increase the risk of infection if an open wound is present.

Frequent position changes are essential to prevent complications of immobility. A client with a cast often needs help to turn in bed. If possible, give the client turning instructions and encourage practice before the cast is applied. The nurse should always have adequate help to move and position a casted person. Roller boards and mechanical lifts can be used. Three or four people may be needed to turn a client who is in a body or hip spica cast. Wet casts are particularly heavy. Safe body mechanics should be used to prevent injury to the client or the nurse.

Foot drop may develop in a casted leg. The foot should be splinted or supported with 90 degrees of flexion in the ankle. Protect the toes of a casted foot from the pressure of bedclothing; stockings may provide warmth.

Ambulation. Clients in casts can often bear weight as soon as the cast is dry (Fig. 75–11). Synthetic casts can be walked on immediately after application. Plaster casts require 36 to 48 hours before weight can be borne. Weak, aged, and debilitated clients often find the weight of a cast difficult to deal with and may tire rapidly when

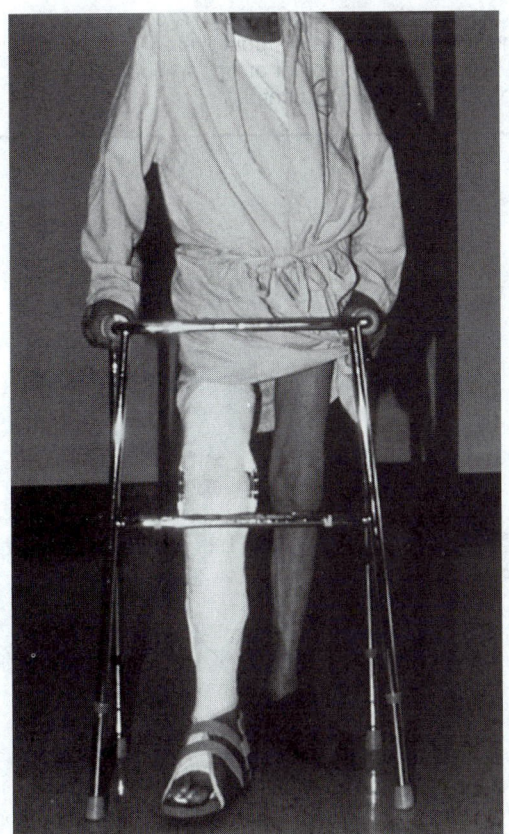

Figure 75–11. Older clients often feel more secure ambulating with the aid of a walker.

ambulating for the first few times. Observe them closely to prevent accidents. In addition, because a cast is heavy and inflexible, a client can easily lose his or her balance and fall. Safety straps should be used when assisting the client to stand for the first few times.

Instruct the client that more rest will be needed due to the need to heal the fracture and the extra energy used for ambulation. Pain may be experienced the first few times that a casted leg is lowered to a dependent position. Prepare the client for this pain. Explain that pain is not unusual and that it occurs as blood rushes into the leg. Initially, the nurse can assist the client to lower the leg for brief periods and gradually lengthen the time of dependence. Once the client's leg becomes accustomed to the increased blood, pain subsides.

Exercises. The nurse should instruct the client in exercises to stimulate circulation, increase venous return, enhance healing, and facilitate rehabilitation. Usually, exercises are prescribed for the joints above and below the cast. It usually is important to exercise the uncasted shoulder of a casted arm, because the shoulder joint can become stiff quickly (this is one reason a sling may be contraindicated). Also, the shoulder supports the weight of the arm cast. Teach the client not to hold the shoulder immobile but to periodically lift the casted arm up over the head and to move each finger frequently.

Isometric exercises do not actually move the limb or bend the joints, but they do contract the muscles. Isometric muscle exercises help maintain muscle strength and mass by combating weakness and disuse atrophy. The nurse should begin by teaching isometric exercises on unaffected limbs and then on casted areas. By practicing with the unaffected knee first, the client can see how the muscles contract without moving the limb. Teach a client with a casted knee to try to push down with the knee. This exercise (quadriceps setting) tightens leg muscles. To validate the instructions, the nurse can place a hand beneath the knee and ask the person to try to push the knee down onto the nurse's hand. In a casted arm, opening and closing the hand to make a fist provides isometric exercise for arm muscles.

A client confined to bed may need other exercises, such as gluteal setting, abdominal tightening, and deep breathing, to prevent complications and to strengthen muscles for future activities, such as crutch walking (see the Bridge to Home Healthcare). Teach the client full range-of-motion (ROM) exercises for uncasted structures and joints. Uncasted extremities need to be in optimal condition to perform the extra duties necessary to relieve the weight and work of casted areas. Encourage active exercise several times a day. Self-care activity provides significant indirect exercise.

Nutrition. Increased dietary fiber and fluids help clients with reduced mobility maintain normal bowel elimination. A person in a body cast or hip spica cast may need to avoid gas-forming foods to prevent abdominal distention. A general, well-balanced diet promotes wound healing. Elderly clients often need stool softeners because of decreased mobility.

Self-Care. The nurse should teach the client and significant others about skin care and how to prevent skin damage.

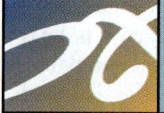

BRIDGE TO HOME HEALTHCARE

Managing Casts and Braces

Mary McQuin, B.S.P.T., *Visiting Nurse Association of Omaha, Omaha, Nebraska*

Common sense and ingenuity can help relieve the client's stress when an extremity is confined to a cast or brace.
   With leg braces, the bars parallel the shape of the leg, but do not touch the leg. Straps should maintain proper fit but never leave marks on the skin. Any strap that is too tight can cause swelling distal to that strap. If a short-leg brace has a T-strap on the lateral side of the shoe, it goes against the ankle and the cinch strap goes around the medial bar to prevent ankle inversion. Contact the orthotist for any needed adjustments. The plastic, custom-made braces encase the leg or ankle/foot nearly perfectly and have no T-strap. Put this brace into the shoe and let it act as a shoehorn when putting on the shoe. Bledsoe leg braces have foam sheets encasing the extremity; the hinge parallels the knee joint. If the foam feels itchy, cover with a towel, or dust lightly with medicated powder (kept away from incisions). Body braces should be applied over a cotton undershirt. Apply the brace while the client is in bed. Use a felt-tipped marker to label "top front." Pads go over bony prominences. Whenever a brace or cast exerts pressure or is too loose, use a towel, rolled washcloth, sponge, or cotton balls for padding. Mark the Velcro with a marker to indicate placement. If the client does not have enough pinch strength, poke a hole in the Velcro and run a string through it. Make a loop that the client can slip the fingers through to pull and release the closure. To allow braces to be worn under clothing or to facilitate dressing, wear larger sizes of clothes, open seams, or insert zippers or Velcro in the inner seams of pants legs.
   A cast should fit. Watch fingers and toes for discoloration or swelling; wiggling helps to maintain circulation and range of motion. Encourage "setting" exercises for the muscle under the cast. The cast supports the fracture/surgical site; actively moving the extremity helps to reduce swelling and pain. Initially, keep the extremity elevated on pillows, rolled blankets, or even balloons. To help reduce swelling or discomfort, a doubled zipper-fastener plastic bag of ice or wet towels frozen in bags can be placed on the cast. If swelling is severe, suspend the extremity from a vertical pole, such as an IV pole or coat rack. An elastic wrap, strips of sheet, or a towel can be used to keep the extremity in place and in good alignment. Even if it is casted, keep pressure off the heel. Cover sharp edges with moleskin. Use a washcloth over the rim of a long-leg cast to keep it clean. Never insert anything under a cast, as it may damage skin or the padding. Itching can sometimes be relieved by dribbling alcohol inside the cast.
   To keep the cast dry in the shower, wrap it in a plastic bag and secure the edges with tape. A commercial shower or lawn chair can be used. Provide a nonslip surface. If no shower is available, pour water over the client with a pitcher. While the client is using the toilet, prop the casted leg up on a foot stool or phone book. For dressing, reacher sticks or other assistive devices (barbecue tongs or forks) can be useful.

Removing the Cast

The length of time a client wears a cast varies with the type and extent of injury, disease, or surgery and the rate of healing. A cast is usually removed with an electric cast cutter, which resembles a small electric saw with a circular blade. Because of its appearance and noise, a cast cutter is often frightening. Show the client the cast cutter before using it and explain that it cannot cut skin because the blade does not whirl around and cut like a saw. Rather, it breaks the cast by oscillating or vibrating rapidly from side to side. When a cast cutter is used, the client may feel sensations of heat, vibrations, or pressure. Very rarely, a client suffers a burn from the cast cutter blades. A cast spreader may also be used to spread open a cut cast so that underlying padding material can be cut. Equipment used to remove casts is shown in Figure 75–12.
   Skin under a casted area often becomes very sensitive and is mottled and covered with yellow-brown scales or crusts of dead skin, oil, and exudate. Muscles under a cast may appear atrophied, and the extremity feels stiff and weak from inactivity. New aches and pains may

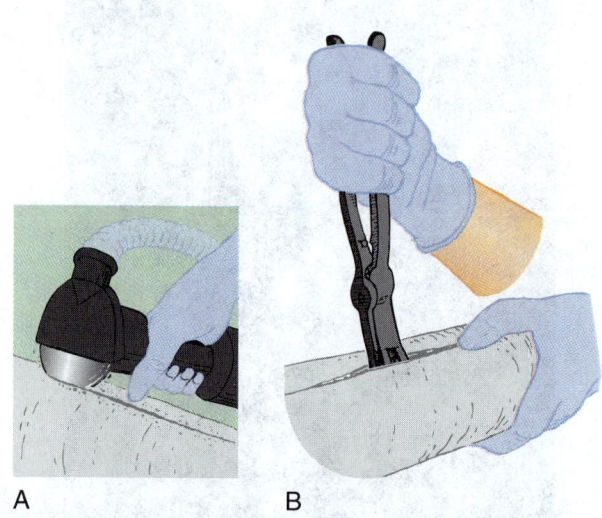

A   B

Figure 75–12. *A,* A cast saw, with its oscillating blade, "vibrates" plaster and synthetic cast material apart. The vibrating motion reduces the risk of cutting the client's skin. *B,* A cast spreader is a useful tool in performing cast removal. It is used to open a cast so that padding material can be cut out.

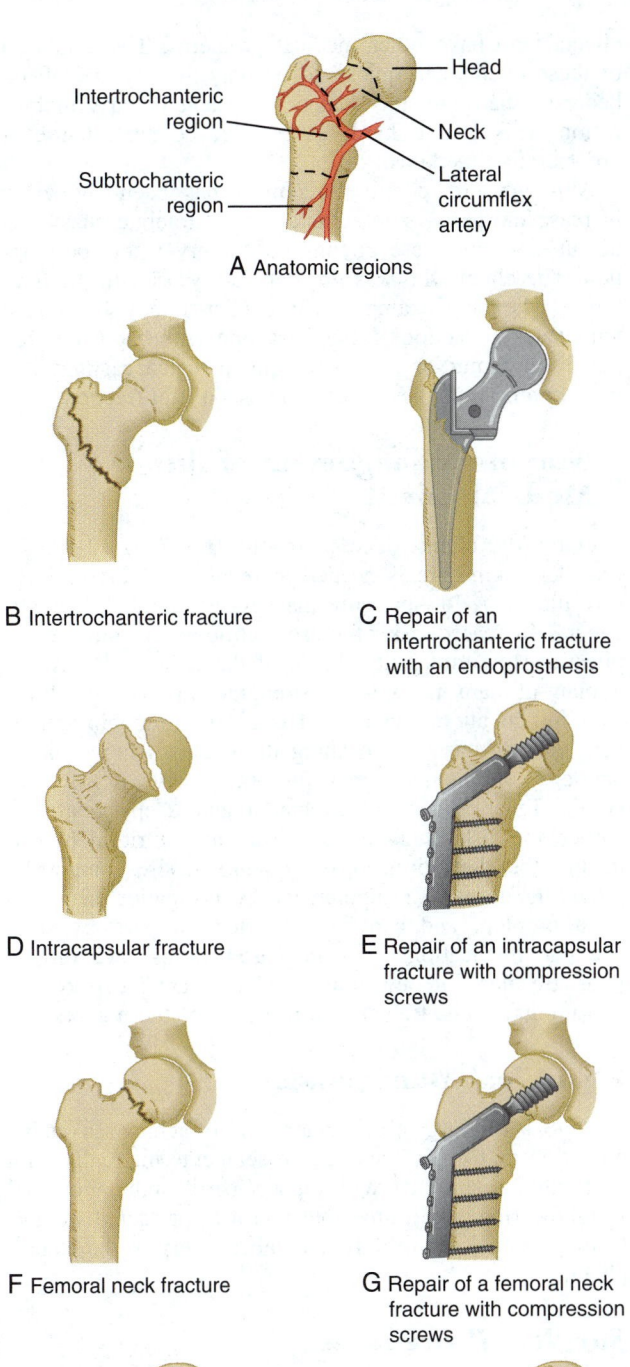

Figure 75-13. *A*, Anatomic regions of the proximal femur. Note the blood supply. *B*, Intertrochanteric fracture. *C*, Repair of an intertrochanteric fracture with an endoprosthesis. *D*, Intra-capsular fracture. *E*, Repair of an intracapsular fracture with screws. *F*, Femoral neck fracture. *G*, Repair of a femoral neck fracture with compression screws. *H*, Subtrochanteric fracture. *I*, Repair of a subtrochanteric fracture with compression screws.

appear with movement following cast removal, and muscles and tissues are subjected to new stresses and strains. The client's balance is altered, because removing a cast removes weight. The client needs to be prepared.

Gentle soaking and washing for a few days after a cast is removed returns skin to its normal appearance. Many clients want to vigorously scrub the skin, but this often causes irritation. After a gentle washing, dry the skin and lubricate it with cocoa butter, lanolin, or another emollient to promote softening. Because newly uncasted skin is sensitive and can burn easily, advise the person to prevent overexposure to the sun.

Following cast removal, swelling may develop for a while when the involved limb is dependent. Elevate the limb when the client is sitting or lying down. Swelling decreases with increased activity and improved muscle tone and circulation. Sometimes the physician recommends elastic bandages or stockings during ambulation to minimize swelling. Encourage ambulation, because intermittent weightbearing acts as an effective venous pump.

Rehabilitation

Rehabilitation is the restoration of the client to a preinjury or preoperative fitness level or to a greater level of fitness through a carefully planned program of exercises. Instructions are given by the physician according to the client's condition. A physical therapist often participates in rehabilitative care following cast removal. For example, a physical therapist may teach and supervise graded active exercises (to stimulate circulation and increase muscle strength) and joint ROM, and perform other prescribed activities such as whirlpool baths to force joints and muscles during recovery (by passive stretching exercises, resistive exercises, or forced movements). Placing excessive demands on stiff, weakened limbs may further impair motion by increasing fibrosis and excessively engorging the area with blood.

Intertrochanteric Hip Fractures

The proximal hip has been divided into four anatomic areas (Fig. 75-13A). Blood flow to the hip is an important influence on healing; you can see in the figure that some fractures can alter blood flow and thereby delay or prevent healing.

Each year more than 250,000 Americans suffer hip fractures; 90% of these fractures occur in clients older than 65 years. In addition to the $8.7 billion cost associated with the fractures, acute morbidity, long-term loss of function, substantial risk for institutionalization, and increased risk of death occur.[27] The incidence of these fractures is rising each year, paralleling the increased longevity of the world's population. Intertrochanteric fractures are the most common hip fracture (see Fig. 75–13*B*).

Etiology and Risk Factors

Hip fractures result from two major changes seen with aging: loss of postural stability and loss of bone mass. The most significant factor in the aged is the loss of postural stability and subsequent falls. Decreased bone mass does contribute to hip fractures, however. Bone mass decreases linearly with age. The combination of decreased bone mass and tendency toward falls explains why the incidence of hip fracture doubles every 5 years after the age of 50. Risk factors for osteoporosis are shown in Chapter 76.

Preinjury functional impairments are also common in the elderly who sustain hip fractures. One study revealed that before the fracture, clients had problems with ambulation in the community, using a bathtub, walking outdoors, and climbing stairs.[3]

Fall prevention programs are being developed in communities. These programs can be used to identify risk factors in the home. Some cities have used college students and community volunteers to fix identified problems with stairs and floors. These creative methods of risk reduction are excellent efforts on the part of many healthcare providers to help the aged.

Pathophysiology

The pathophysiology of fracture injury is discussed earlier in this chapter.

Clinical Manifestations and Diagnostic Findings

The vast majority of clients with intertrochanteric fractures are elderly. Women outnumber men by a 2:1 ratio, and most report a fall at home involving only a moderate amount of trauma, such as slipping out of a chair onto the floor. Immediately after the fall the client is unable to bear weight. Objective findings include a shortened, externally rotated hip and, sometimes, deformity along the lateral side of the hip if the fracture is displaced. Ecchymosis and tissue trauma from the fall may also be evident. Other sites of tissue trauma may also be present, such as forehead or hand lacerations.

Hip fracture is confirmed by anteroposterior x-ray. On occasion, the fractures may not be apparent on initial x-ray. Technetium bone scans or magnetic resonance imaging (MRI) may be needed to confirm the fracture.

Acute and Subacute Care

■ Medical Management

Intertrochanteric fractures are serious injuries. Extensive blood loss frequently occurs in older, more debilitated clients who have other medical problems. The condition of these clients can quickly deteriorate if they are left on bedrest. Therefore, the goal of treatment is early mobilization. This goal is hardly ever achieved through use of nonoperative methods.

Although nonoperative treatment has been shown to increase mortality, some clients cannot tolerate anesthesia or surgery. For these clients, no surgery is the best option. The client who was nonambulatory prior to the fracture is the best example. These clients may be treated with Buck's traction, skeletal traction with a pin through the distal femur or proximal tibia, or spica casting. The most common of these treatments is skeletal traction.

■ Nursing Management of the Medical Client

Plan for the client to be in traction for 8 to 12 weeks. Excellent skin care is needed to reduce the risk of pressure ulcers. A low-pressure mattress is essential. The client has increased risk of muscle atrophy and other complications of immobility. Physical therapists will develop a plan of care for muscle strengthening. Nurses direct attention to all of the other hazards of immobility. Prevent venous stasis by teaching the client to move his or her legs (or the nurse may preform passive ROM exercises). Teach the client to cough and deep breathe to reduce the risk of atelectasis. Maintain nutrition by adjusting the diet to meet the client's desires and/or by providing nutritional supplements. Constipation may also be a problem and can be prevented, in part, by stool softener medications and increased fluids and dietary fiber. Be alert for development of pressure ulcers on the sacrum and heels. Elevate the heels off of the mattress.

■ Surgical Management

The goal of surgical treatment is to achieve a stable reduction and to fix the fracture segments internally with a strong implant that will support early ambulation and weightbearing. The immediate return to protected weightbearing is critical to the functional recovery of the elderly client.

Surgical Procedures

Several devices are currently in use for the treatment of intertrochanteric hip fractures. They include a sliding hip screw, plates, intermedullary Ender pins, and intermedullary implants. Highly comminuted intertrochanteric fractures are managed with an endoprosthesis (see Fig. 75–13*C*).

Complications

Due in part to the age of the client and the presence of other medical problems, several complications can develop after surgery. Complications due to immobility are of the greatest concern. Intertrochanteric fractures are usually comminuted and the bone is more osteoporotic, leading to difficulty with good anatomic reduction of the fragments and fixation.

Deep Vein Thrombosis. The incidence of deep vein thrombosis in clients not receiving prophylaxis is reported to be 40% to 60% following hip surgery. Because approximately 20% of clients with deep vein thrombosis develop pulmonary emboli, the prevention of thrombosis is essential. Clients are assessed twice daily for unilateral leg pain, leg edema, and positive Homans' sign (pain with dorsiflexion of the foot). Measures to decrease the risk of deep vein thrombosis include the use of aspirin, heparin, enoxaparin sodium (Lovenox), warfarin, low molecular weight dextran, and external pneumatic compression devices. Leg exercises should be encouraged; ask the client to flex the feet and move the legs 10 times every hour. Antiembolism stockings are also commonly used. Many physicians order Doppler studies of the legs before discharge to determine if thrombi have developed.

Pressure Ulcers. Pressure ulcers occur in 20% to 70% of clients following hip fracture. It should be recognized that significant pressure has often been applied to the skin before the client is admitted to the nursing unit, from lying on a hard floor at home or on hard surfaces in ambulances, emergency departments, and x-ray departments. It is equally important to realize that clients with hip fractures often cannot turn due to pain or the location of the fracture. Therefore, many clients lie supine most of the time that they are in acute care. Prevention of ongoing ischemia is critical and can be accomplished by decreasing the risk of pressure through the use of pressure reduction (eggcrate or air) mattresses, excellent skin care, early ambulation, and elevation of the heels from the bed with rolled towels. Identification of high-risk clients can be made through the use of assessment tools such as the Braden tool, presented in Chapter 20.

Infection. Postoperative wound infection is possible, yet the incidence is declining because antibiotics are used before, during, and after surgery. When infection occurs, it can be superficial or deep. It may also develop because of persistent hematoma in the wound. To reduce the risk of hematoma, drains are used for 24 to 48 hours to divert blood. Drains are removed when drainage has decreased, usually in about 24 to 48 hours.

Acute Confusion. It has been reported that acute confusion develops in up to 51%[38] of older clients hospitalized for hip fractures. Postoperative confusion usually occurs in response to physiologic, psychological, or environmental changes. Physiologic changes include blood loss, previous strokes, hypotension, hypoxia, pain, urine elimination problems, urinary tract infections, malnutrition, and use of various medications. Psychological problems leading to confusion include stress due to pain or impending surgery, depression, and dementia. Environmental alterations include a change of environment, sleep deprivation, and social isolation. Early signs include forgetfulness, disorientation, fear, misperceptions, insomnia, daytime sleepiness, inattentiveness, and verbal reports of feeling "mixed-up" or "funny." Nursing interventions include accurate assessments of attention, memory, orientation, psychomotor behavior, sleep-wake cycle, and thinking. Management is directed at correcting the underlying problem.

Outcomes

Eventual recovery of clients after the repair of hip fractures is influenced by premorbid dementia, preoperative immobility, presence of intertrochanteric fracture, and advanced age.[1] Several large series report that of clients surviving 1 year after a fracture, only 50% achieve prefracture functional status.[25]

■ Nursing Management of the Surgical Client

Preoperative Care

Assessment

On admission, the client is usually weighed before being placed in bed. A complete assessment is performed, including the assessment of abrasions or other injuries from the fall.

While the client's condition is being stabilized for surgery, perhaps with blood transfusions or correction of underlying disorders such as heart failure, skin traction is commonly applied to the leg (e.g., Buck's traction). In general, the client is taken for surgical repair quickly, because placing an elderly person on bedrest increases the risks of immobility. In addition, delayed repair increases the risk of avascular necrosis.

Diagnostic tests may be used to assess the client's readiness for surgery and anesthesia. A complete blood count, prothrombin time, partial thromboplastin time, serum chemical analyses, urinalysis, chest x-ray, and ECG are the most common tests.

It is important to determine the client's level of preinjury function. Under the best circumstances, this is the level that most clients can expect to achieve after surgery. Unfortunately, it is more likely that some loss will occur in preinjury level of function. The client's social functioning appears to be a significant factor.[20] Preinjury social functioning not only determined the level achievable after surgery but also had an impact on the mortality rate after surgery. Recovery is also related to the client's social prior to surgery. Arm strength, mental status, ability to pull oneself to a sitting position, and serum albumin levels (as an indicator of nutritional status) also correlate to recovery. Sadly, only about 50% of clients return to preinjury functional levels after 1 year.

Diagnosis, Planning, Implementation

Risk for Impaired Skin Integrity. The prescribed limitations in movement and pain lead to the diagnosis of *Risk for Impaired Skin Integrity*. In addition, malnutrition, dehydration or frail skin increase the risk. The diagnostic statement may be *Risk for Impaired Skin Integrity related to prescribed complete bedrest, use of Buck's skin trac-*

tion and inability to purposefully move due to pain from fractured hip.

Planning: Expected Outcomes. The client will have reduced risk of impaired skin as evidenced by no reddened areas that do not blanch and no ulcerations on skin or under traction boot.

Implementation. Most clients with fractured hip are admitted through the emergency department. Plan on the client being immobile and place a pressure reduction mattress on the bed before the client arrives on the floor. The client can be turned slightly in Buck's traction for skin care and skin assessment. Skin care and assessment may be needed every 2 to 4 hours, depending on the client's condition.

Risk for Compartment Syndrome. Leg edema and bleeding within fascial compartments can lead to entrapment of nerves and vessels. This important diagnosis is stated as a collaborative problem, because nurses only monitor for its development and refer care to the physician. *It is stated as High Risk for Compartment Syndrome related to edema, tissue trauma, and bleeding within fascial compartments.*

Planning: Expected Outcomes. Clinical manifestations of compartment syndrome will be promptly recognized and addressed.

Implementation. The nurse monitors the color, capillary refill, warmth, movement, sensation, pedal pulses, and ability to dorsiflex and plantar flex the fractured leg using the nonfractured leg as a baseline. Clinical manifestations of compartment syndrome include pallor, pulselessness, paresthesia, pain, and paralysis of the leg. These findings must be reported to the physician immediately. Compartment syndrome was discussed more fully earlier in the chapter.

Pain. Tissue trauma and the fractured hip cause pain. This common diagnosis is stated as *Pain related to tissue trauma secondary to fractured hip.*

Planning: Expected Outcomes. The client will describe adequate pain relief, as evidenced by less facial grimacing and guarding with movement, ability to turn in bed or move in bed without reports of pain, and using decreasing amount of narcotics for pain relief.

Implementation. Most traumatic pain is managed with narcotic analgesics. Ice can be applied to the fracture site. Nonnarcotic analgesics, such as non-steroidal antiinflammatory drugs (NSAIDs) can also be given to control the acute pain, muscle spasms, and pain due to other chronic problems, such as arthritis.

Evaluation

The risk of compartment syndrome should subside within 24 to 48 hours. Risk of pressure ulcers remains as long as the client is at bedrest. Acute pain should subside once the fracture site has stabilized. Clients may have surgery within a few hours or days. Timing of surgery will adjust the goal attainment time frames.

Postoperative Care

Assessment

Routinely monitor vital signs, respiratory status, pain, blood loss through drains, and urine and bowel output. A urinary catheter may have been inserted prior to surgery.

Diagnosis, Planning, Implementation

Impaired Physical Mobility. Prescribed immobility and pain are the most common causes of immobility after hip surgery. The diagnostic statement would be written *Impaired Physical Mobility related to muscle weakness, pain, prescribed immobility.*

Planning: Expected Outcomes. The client will maintain adequate strength to regain physical mobility once able to ambulate, as evidenced by performing exercises while bedridden, transferring to the chair with decreasing need for assistance once ambulatory, and walking with a walker safely.

Implementation. The client is encouraged to perform various exercises for the upper and lower extremities. A trapeze is placed above the bed to facilitate upper arm and shoulder strength. Exercises such as quadriceps setting, gluteal setting, and leg movements up and down in bed maintain some muscle strength. Passive and active range of motion exercises should also be implemented.

When the client is allowed to be in the chair, the nurse assists the client to the edge of the bed while keeping the legs abducted. The client is assisted to stand by at least two nurses, and then to balance with the walker. The degree of weightbearing that the client can safely use must be reinforced as the client stands. Types of weightbearing are described in Table 75–5. If the client is unable to stand, a complete lift is usually performed to assist the client to the chair.

Table 75–5. Weightbearing Status

Non-weightbearing	The client does not bear weight on the affected extremity; the affected extremity should not touch the floor
Touch-down weight-bearing	The client's foot of the affected extremity may rest on the floor, but no weight is distributed through that extremity
Partial weightbearing	The client bears 30%–50% of his weight on the affected extremity
Weightbearing as tolerated	The client bears as much weight as he can tolerate on the affected extremity without undue strain or pain
Full weightbearing	The client bears weight fully on the affected extremity.

From Maher, A. B., Salmond, S. W., & Pellino, T. A. (1994). *Orthopaedic nursing.* Philadelphia: W. B. Saunders.

It is important to record the amount of assistance the client required for safe transfer to the chair. Use the guide listed in Table 75–6. You can also use these assessments to determine if your goal for increased mobility is being met. For example, if the client required maximal assistance by two nurses on the day after surgery, but by the next morning only needed one nurse's assistance, mobility has increased.

Physical therapists and occupational therapists aid the client's recovery. Physical therapists teach the client how to ambulate and strengthen muscles. Physical therapists also provide assistive devices for the client, such as elevated toilet seats, walkers, or crutches, and measure the client for the correct sitting height. The leg is measured from the back of the knee to the heel at the floor. Two to 3 inches are added to this length for the correct sitting height for chairs in the hospital and at home. Cushions can be added to raise the sitting height of chairs. These adjustments assist with moving from a sitting to a standing position.

Occupational therapists can instruct the client on how to get in and out of an automobile, how to use a tub bench for bathing, and how to use long-handled reachers, assistive devices, long-handled sponges, and sock aids.

Table 75–6. Transferring Techniques

Independent	The client is safe with transfers and requires no assistance
Standby assist of 1	The client is basically independent but may need verbal cues or observation if his judgment is questionable
Contact guard of 1	The client transfers well with hands on contact by physical therapist or nurse; this method is used if patient's judgment is questionable or for patients with slightly decreased balance
Minimal assistance of 1	The client requires minimal physical assistance from physical therapist or nurse to stand, sit, etc. (e.g., for lower extremity placement on footrest of wheelchair)
Maximal assistance of 1	The client requires maximal physical assistance by physical therapist or nurse to transfer (e.g., for extremity placement, trunk placement) and a lot of verbal cuing
Maximal assistance of 2	Same as for the previous example but requires two physical therapists or nurses; this necessitates good body mechanics and often calls for assistive devices (Hoyer lift, total lift)

From Maher, A. B., Salmond, S. W., & Pellino, T. A. (1994). *Orthopaedic nursing.* Philadelphia, W. B. Saunders.

Risk for Hip Dislocation. When the entire hip joint is replaced (arthroplasty) it can dislocate because the acetabular component does not enclose the femoral head as completely as does the bony acetabulum. Stress on the hip and surrounding muscles, such as gluteal stretching, can make the hip joint unstable. Gluteal stretching is most common when the hip is flexed, adducted, or when the client bends forward. Dislocation is not a common problem with endoprostheses. These devices, in contrast to total hip replacement, use the client's own acetabulum rather than an artificial acetabulum. They are therefore more stable.

Planning: Expected Outcomes. The client will be positioned so as to reduce the risk of hip dislocation.

Implementation. Handle the operated leg gently following hip surgery. Before moving the client, explain what is going to happen and how the client can help. An above-bed trapeze helps with moving. Teach the client how to use the trapeze. Avoid extremes of position following hip surgery. Keep the leg abducted (i.e., out to the side) at all times. Never adduct the leg past the body's midline (i.e., crossed over the other leg), or the head of the femur (or prosthesis) may dislocate out of the acetabulum. Place a pillow or A-frame abductor pillow between the client's legs to help maintain abduction and to remind the client not to cross the legs.

Avoid acute flexion of the operated hip. This can be caused by excessive elevation of the head of the bed. Check the physician's instructions about how high the head of the bed can be safely elevated. Some clients can have the head of the bed raised only 35 to 40 degrees. If the head of the bed can be somewhat elevated, instruct the client not to lean farther forward, because this practice further flexes the hip and may cause dislocation. Reduce the risk of clients bending forward by having self-care items in reach, such as the telephone, bed covers, and ice water.

Prevent external rotation of the leg on the operated side by placing a trochanter roll beside the external aspect of the thigh. Without this intervention, the operated leg may tend to lie slightly externally rotated when the person is supine. Elevate the heels as well.

Turn the client only with the physician's order following hip surgery. Several days following hip pinning, some clients are permitted to turn to the *nonoperative* side. When helping a client to turn following internal fixation, (1) avoid adduction of the operated leg and excessive movement, (2) prevent strain on the hip, and (3) keep the leg and hip in proper alignment. If the client is permitted to turn onto the operative side, roll the client gently toward you after placing pillows between the client's legs. The bed acts as a splint for the injured leg. If it is not possible to turn to either side, the client may be able to lift straight up off the bed by using a trapeze for back care and linen changes.

Commonly following an anterior surgical approach, the operated limb is positioned so it is internally rotated and in a neutral or an abducted position. The individual may be permitted to sit up unless the capsule has been removed. With a posterior approach the operated leg is positioned in slight abduction and external rotation (a change from "typical" positioning) and the client lies fairly flat.

Do not position the bed too low when a client is getting up after hip surgery. Less hip strain and bending occur if the bed is somewhat elevated. Be sure the bed is locked so it will not move while the client is getting up. For the same reasons, elevated toilet seats are needed following hip surgery once the client can go to the bathroom.

Usually when a client first gets up in a chair following hip surgery, the operated leg is kept extended, well supported, and elevated. Once the operated leg may be lowered, the client should sit with the hips even with the knees. Tell the client not to cross the legs but to keep both feet on the floor. The first few times the leg is lowered, assess for swelling and discoloration.

Pain. Tissue trauma of fractured hip and surgery leads to pain. This common diagnosis is stated as *Pain related to tissue trauma secondary to fractured hip and surgical incision.*

Planning: Expected Outcomes. The client will experience improved comfort, as evidenced by less facial grimacing and guarding with movement, ability to transfer to the chair or to ambulate without reports of pain, and use of a decreasing amount of narcotics for pain relief.

Implementation. Most surgical pain is managed with narcotic analgesics until the pain subsides somewhat. Morphine is commonly given by patient controlled analgesia (PCA) systems, although injections and epidural catheters for narcotic administration are also used for pain management. Usually within 3 to 4 days, less potent narcotics and non-narcotic analgesics are used for pain relief. Ice is also used to reduce sensation and edema. A client's discomfort from lying in one position (supine) can be decreased by placing a small, folded bath towel beneath the lumbar spine and by moving the legs slightly in bed.

Risk for Thrombophlebitis. The bedridden client with edema in the pelvic area from surgery is at very high risk of thrombus development, especially in the thigh and calf areas. The collaborative problem should read *Risk for Thrombophlebitis related to immobility and pelvic edema.*

Planning: Expected Outcomes. Clinical manifestations of thrombophlebitis will be promptly recognized and reported.

Implementation. Implementation of this problem was discussed under the section on complications.

Risk for Constipation. The side effects of narcotics and immobility lead to constipation. This common problem is stated as *Risk for Constipation related to side effects of narcotics and immobility.* Clients may also have a preexisting dependence on laxatives and this dependence could be another risk.

Planning: Expected Outcomes. The client will decrease risk of constipation by consuming high-fiber and bulk foods, adequate fluids, and having a bowel movement at least every 2 to 3 days.

Implementation. The nurse determines the client's usual defecation pattern and monitors for the return of bowel sounds after surgery. Once the client has resumed eating, foods with fiber, such as bran and prunes, should be encouraged. Some clients find that hot fluids, such as coffee, stimulate the bowels. Bowel programs should be instituted in the morning after breakfast because the gastrocolic reflex is strongest at that time. Docusate sodium (Colace) and other stool softeners are commonly prescribed. In addition, the client may require suppositories or enemas to maintain a normal bowel movement schedule. When possible, the client should be placed on a bedside commode to facilitate defecation. Many elderly clients monitor their bowel movements closely. The nurse is wise to consider their concerns and prevent constipation.

Evaluation

Care paths may be used to assess the degree of outcome attainment for clients with fractured hip repair. Expect pain to subside fairly soon. Many clients do not require injectable narcotics after 24 to 36 hours. Remember, though, that pain is an individual experience. Some of the expected outcomes for mobility may require extended periods of time to accomplish, depending on the status of the client before surgery. Most clients are transferred to subacute care for ongoing rehabilitation.

Because many clients with fractured hips are covered by Medicare, their hospital stay is very short and only a portion of rehabilitation can be accomplished in the hospital. Many clients benefit from transfer to an extended care facility, where they can complete their rehabilitation. Finding a location for ongoing rehabilitation is a collaborative effort among all members of the healthcare team, the client, and family. Family members need to be included in teaching and discharge planning. Subacute care focuses on improving muscle strength and self-care abilities.

Ochs[30] questions whether the clients see as much benefit when transferred to a community nursing home, where little rehabilitation is offered. Many clients remain as nursing home residents after a year because rehabilitation was incomplete and the client cannot maintain self-care.

Community and Self-Care

At the time of discharge to home, some clients may not be able to walk more than a few feet or transfer from bed to chair or wheelchair. In addition to ongoing rehabilitation, these clients need complete care to provide food, maintain hygiene, and address other needs of daily living. If the client is sent home, the nurse and social worker ascertain that the client's family can safely move the client and that other activities of daily living are provided for the client (see the Nursing Research feature).

Intracapsular Hip Fractures

The intracapsular area of the hip is the head of the femur. It is most commonly fractured in association with posterior hip dislocation. The fracture most commonly occurs due to motor vehicle accidents (see Fig. 75–13D). Significant force is required to fracture the head of the femur. Usually the force is also great enough to shear off bone against the acetabulum. The loss of bone leads to degenerative joint disease or avascular necrosis. Avascular necrosis is the death of bone tissue due to loss of blood supply. The vessels that feed the femoral head are commonly injured in the original trauma. The client may also develop joint fusion as a result of bone tissue overgrowth

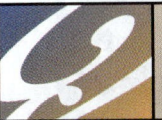

NURSING RESEARCH

How Do Older Clients with Hip Fractures Fare Once They Leave the Hospital?

Williams, M. A., Oberst, M. T., & Bjorkland, B. C. (1994). Posthospital convalescence in older women with hip fracture. *Orthopaedic Nursing.* *13*(4), 55–64.

Remarkably little is known about how clients with hip fractures fare during the early part of their convalescence after leaving the hospital. Recovery in hip fracture clients is generally measured by the assistance they require for activities of daily living. These data are usually compared to estimates of mobility prior to the fracture.

Before fracture, 90% of the women required no assistance with eating, dressing, care of appearance, getting in and out of bed, or using chairs. More than three quarters required no assistance with bathing, walking, or using stairs. After the fracture, the ability to eat and take care of one's appearance returned first. The ability to walk, use stairs, and bathe were very slow to return. The most rapid gain in functional ability was from weeks 2 to 8; after that, only small gains were noted. Perceived mobility correlated with assistance required for mobility. Mood states were initially depressed. Mood scores for persons going into nursing homes were lower than those persons discharged to home.

Implications for Practice

This study documents the long process of recovery of the ability to perform activities of daily living after hip fracture. The increasing number of these clients, as our population ages, makes these studies helpful for planing posthospital care and further legislative efforts to fund rehabilitation of these clients.

(called *heterotopic ossification*). Treatment is open reduction and internal fixation (ORIF) (see Fig. 75–13E). Sometimes an endoprosthesis is required.

Femoral Neck Fractures

Femoral neck fractures occur in persons who fall from significant heights or are involved in an automobile accident in which the knee strikes the dashboard (see Fig. 75–13F). Due to the nature of the trauma, several other problems are commonly seen in these clients. They often have head, chest, abdominal, or spinal injuries. Early care centers on protecting the limb to prevent further injury. The leg may be placed in Buck's traction with the knee flexed while the other life-threatening injuries are being managed. Four surgical procedures are common to repair femoral neck fractures (Fig. 75–13G): (1) insertion of a Knowles pin; (2) insertion of a Jewett nail; (3) insertion of a sliding nail or compression screw; and (4) hemiarthroplasty or total hip arthroplasty.

Following fixation with a Knowles pin, full weightbearing is not allowed because the pin does not pull the fracture fragments together (a process called *compression*). The Jewett nail also does not provide compression of the fragments, but it is a stronger device and the client can usually bear partial weight after surgery. The compression screw is the most commonly used device and has an advantage of drawing the fracture fragments together. The alignment of the fractures increases healing and allows for weightbearing. A hemiarthroplasty, with replacement of only the femoral component of the hip with a noncemented metallic prosthesis, can be performed. The use of noncemented prothesis is most commonly used in younger clients who have the capability of bone growth to "cement" the prothesis. Elderly persons tend to have osteoporosis with greater bone destruction than production; therefore, cemented prostheses are more common for elderly clients. A cemented prosthesis allows the client to perform full weightbearing. If the prosthesis is not cemented, the client is allowed only partial weightbearing for 3 to 7 days. Most hip fractures are not repaired with both a metal femoral prosthesis and a plastic acetabular prosthesis, which replaces the entire hip joint. If the client develops nonunion after hip fracture, a complete hip replacement can also be performed. Total hip arthroplasty is discussed in Chapter 76.

Subtrochanteric Femoral Fractures

Subtrochanteric fractures are located below the lesser trochanter of the femur (see Fig. 75–13H). They are also known as *extracapsular fractures*. Subtrochanteric fractures occur from low-energy trauma and frequently occur in osteopenic bone. These fractures have always been difficult to treat; loss of motion in the hip is common despite the best of care. Management is similar to other forms of hip fracture. The client can have surgical repair with nails or screws (see Fig. 75–13I). Nonoperative repair is also possible with traction and braces or casts.

Nursing management is the same as for other hip fractures.

Femoral Shaft Fractures

Femoral shaft fracture most often results from severe violence and occurs in young or middle-aged people. Fractures of the proximal femur are more common in the elderly. A fractured femur commonly causes marked displacement and deformity and extensive soft tissue damage with swelling. Blood loss at the time of injury is often considerable and the client can develop shock.

It is essential that the leg be protectively immobilized during transportation, such as with an air splint or Thomas splint. If the fracture is relatively simple and the client is in good general condition, with no skin damage, treatment may be by open reduction and internal fixation (ORIF) using intramedullary rod insertion (Fig. 75–14). This allows immediate ambulation (with guarded weightbearing). Fractures of the distal end of the femur may be reduced by continuous skeletal traction and manipulation or by internal fixation with rods, nails, plates, or screws. Care of the client in skeletal traction was discussed earlier in this chapter.

Condyle Fractures

The condyles are found at the distal end of the femur. Fractures of the condyles tend to occur in high-energy injuries in young clients. These fractures are often only one of several injuries sustained in motor vehicle accidents when the flexed knee strikes the dashboard. Previously, severe condylar fractures were managed with 6 to 12 weeks of traction followed by mobilization in a cast brace. Newer management of severe condylar fractures is open reduction and internal fixation with plates and screws and, for comminuted fractures, the use of bone grafting. Less severe types of condylar fractures still are appropriately treated with knee immobilizers and cast braces. Loss of knee motion is a common outcome and surgical revision surgery may be needed to improve alignment. If the client develops severe pain and disability with loss of function, the knee may require arthrodesis (fusion) or arthroplasty (joint replacement).

Pelvic Fractures

Pelvic fractures occur in nearly 30% of all multiple trauma injuries. Pelvic fractures are associated with injuries to the major arteries, lower urinary tract, uterus, testes, bowel and rectum, abdominal wall, and spine and spinal cord. Pelvic fractures can result in hemorrhage (the pelvis can hold as much as 4 L of blood), and usual clinical manifestations include hypotension, pain with pressure applied to the pelvis, and bleeding into the peritoneum or urinary tract.

Management of pelvic fractures depends on the severity of the fracture. Unstable, weightbearing pelvic fractures are treated with external fixation devices and through

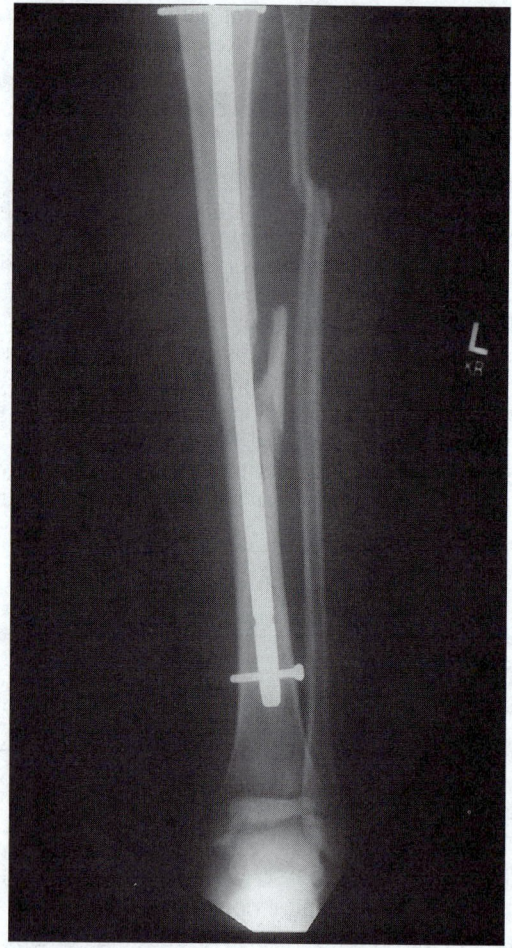

Figure 75–14. Open reduction and internal fixation with an intermedullary rod. Although this x-ray shows open reduction and internal fixation of a tibial fracture, the procedure is commonly used for femoral shaft fractures.

open reduction with internal fixation. Less severe fractures of non-weightbearing portions of the pelvis can be successfully treated with bedrest.

Nursing management centers around maintaining adequate circulation to the skin, because the client in traction can seldom turn. Low air-loss beds (e.g., KinAir) are beneficial. In addition, the client needs adequate pain control, assessment of neurovascular status, and assessment for complications such as thrombophlebitis and fat embolism.

Patellar Fractures

The patella (kneecap) can fracture during falls from heights, near falls, or direct blows. Manifestations include pain and a noticeable defect. Knee extension is often impossible due to pain and damage to extensor mechanisms. The patella can fracture in several patterns and management is based on the type of fracture. The bone fragments can be wired or, in cases of severe damage, the patella can be excised. Rupture of the extensor mechanisms of the knee is possible including the quadriceps tendon and the patellar tendon. Repair is needed. It is also possible to develop chronic ruptures, and for these problems, tendon lengthening or muscle transfer is required.

Tibial and Fibular Fractures

Tibial plateau fractures are usually due to forces that contact the lower leg from the sides (medial or lateral). The magnitude of the impact will determine the degree of bone damage. Fractures of the tibial shaft are among the most serious skeletal fractures. The fractures tend to be complex, and potential complications result from both the injury (compartment syndrome) and the treatment (infection from external fixation). Tibial shaft fractures often are due to crushing injury and are therefore contaminated.

Simple, nondisplaced fractures of the lower leg, tibia, and fibula are most commonly casted. Complex fractures may require traction or external fixation (see Fig. 75–8). In some clients, the fibula is sacrificed to serve as a bone donor for tibial fracture repair. Open fractures of the distal third of the leg are often slow to heal in many people as a result of diminished blood supply from atherosclerosis. Tibial fractures have a higher rate of nonunion.

Foot Fractures

Minimally displaced fractures of the foot are treated with open walking shoes, casts, or braces to reduce direct contact with the fracture site and to act as a splint. In fractures with significant displacement, open reduction and casting may be necessary. Pott's fracture occurs at the medial malleous of the tibia and fibula. Pott's fracture can occur from supination and eversion, pronation and abduction, or pronation and eversion. The mechanism of injury can produce a variety of fracture patterns. Open and closed reduction may be needed.

Upper Extremity Fractures

Fractures of the proximal humerus are common in the elderly. The fracture may be impacted or displaced. Impacted fractures are usually immobilized with a sling. Displaced fractures are treated by surgical open reduction and fixation with pins. Fractures of the dominant arm in elderly clients often make them dependent and immobile. The risk of falling is also increased because balance is reduced secondary to loss of the use of the arm.

Fractures of the shaft of the humerus are usually managed with traction via a hanging arm cast or a splint. Sometimes the fracture is surgically reduced and repaired with intermedullary rods or plates and screws. Nonunion is a common complication of humeral shaft fractures, and bone grafting may be required.

Fractures of the condyles of the humerus usually occur from a direct blow. These fractures can result in damage to the brachial or median nerves. The fracture is treated with ORIF, although skeletal traction and casts can be used.

Colles' fracture is a fracture of the distal radius resulting from a fall on an outstretched hand. It is most common in women. The distal radius has a large percentage of cancellous bone, the type that is most commonly affected by osteoporosis. These fractures can be treated by ORIF, splints, casts, or external fixation, depending on the severity of the injury.

The radius and ulna usually fracture together. The fracture may be treated with ORIF or casted. Closed reduction with casting is the most common form of treatment.

Fractures of the olecranon are common and usually result from a fall onto the elbow. Treatment includes closed reduction and long arm casting. Healing is slow. Once the cast is removed, range of motion in the elbow is very slow to return. Six weeks to 2 months is the usual length of time the cast is left on, and several months may be required for full return of function.

The most commonly fractured bone in the hand is the carpal scaphoid, and this injury most often occurs in young men. A fracture of one or more of the bones in the wrist and hand can occur. Closed reduction and casting is the usual treatment. Casts are usually worn for 6 to 12 weeks.

Fractures of the metacarpals and phalanges are seldom displaced. They are immobilized with splints for 10 days for phalangeal fractures, and 3 to 4 weeks for fractures of the metacarpals.

When managing clients with upper extremity fractures, the nurse assesses the client's radial and ulnar arteries as well as color, warmth, movement, sensation, and capillary refill in the fingers. The client's arm should be elevated on two pillows. During the night, the client needs frequent assessment to be certain the arm does not move into a dependent position. The arm can quickly swell and occlude arterial and nerve supply to the hand. Cast care should be taught to the client and family.

Sports Injuries

Overuse Syndromes

Overuse syndromes are common sports-related problems. They begin insidiously and although they are uncomfortable they do not completely stop a person's activity. Thus, the person may continue to exercise. However, continuing to exercise sets up a cycle that worsens the overuse syndrome. Overuse syndromes are related to specific athletic activities, such as excessive running. A gradual overload of stress produces microtrauma, causing inflammation and pain. Stopping the activity that is producing the syndrome usually corrects the problem. Intervention consists of resting the injured part, applying ice, and performing supervised gradual rehabilitative exercises of the part before returning to athletic activity.

The following people at greatest risk for overexercising and overuse injury:

1. Competitive athletes
2. First-time athletes
3. "Born again" athletes (i.e., people who were once very

active and begin to exercise again after a decade or so of sedentary living)
4. People recovering from injury

Some authorities suggest that exercising 5 days a week is beneficial and relatively safe, whereas exercising 6 or 7 days a week greatly increases the risk of injury, including overuse injury. Anatomic variants, for example, bone malalignment, also increase risk for overuse injury.

Overuse syndromes may be prevented by avoiding the following factors, which precipitate overuse injury:

- *Training errors,* such as progressing too fast or lack of conditioning
- *Improper technique,* such as elbow problems from poor tennis technique
- *Improper equipment,* such as incorrect shoes for the sport
- *Unsafe environmental factors,* such as a slippery surface

Prevention is the real key to these injuries. Stretching is extremely important before exercise requiring joint flexibility. Flexibility is determined mainly by muscles and much less by capsules and tendons. Stretching exercises affect muscles and are, therefore, important in increasing general flexibility. Stretching exercises also help maintain and increase ROM around a joint. They do not increase endurance or strength. Stretching exercises should be static (i.e., they should hold muscles in a stretched position for a few moments rather than repeatedly stretch and relax them). Static stretching (1) reduces the danger of overstretching or tissue damage, (2) causes less muscle soreness than a bouncing or ballistic stretch, and (3) relieves muscle soreness when it occurs. Box 75–1 summarizes some ways of preventing injuries in fitness programs.

Overuse syndromes can be grouped into four categories according to severity. In general, intervention depends on severity more than on the specific type of injury (Table 75–7). Management usually consists of rest, ice, and NSAIDs.

Some common overuse syndromes of the leg include the following:

- *Patellar tendinitis* ("jumper's knee"), which is caused by repetitive stress on the patellar tendon during jumping. The person experiences tenderness at the insertion of the patellar tendon on the tibia.
- *Plantar fasciitis,* which produces heel pain during or immediately after exercise and often on arising in the morning. It is caused by repetitive stress on the long plantar ligament that attaches to the plantar (sole) surface of the calcaneus (heel bone) with its fibers fanning out and attaching to the forefoot.
- *Lateral epicondylitis* (tennis elbow), which is caused by excessive irritation of the extensor carpi radialis brevis as it comes over the lateral epicondyle and radial head. It is common in tennis players, bowlers, and pitchers. Manifestations include pain just below the lateral epicondyle, inability to lift any object with the affected arm, and increased pain when the wrist is hyperextended while the elbow is straight.

Box 75–1. Preventing Injuries in Fitness Programs

Lack of fitness is one of the main causes of sport injury.

Warm-up and Stretching Exercises

Always warm up and stretch before strenuous exercises. To warm up means to begin and finish exercises gradually. Stretching exercises increase muscle flexibility.

Pacing

Build up an exercise program gradually. It takes at least 6 to 8 weeks to get into strong condition. Add small, gradual increments of exercise. Proceed gradually and do not overdo. Tired muscles are prone to injury.

Intensity

When preparing for a specific event, plan training programs accordingly (e.g., a marathon demands a more intense training program than does a 10K race).

Capacity Level

Exercise to the capacity of physiologic limits.

Strength

Build strength gradually to gain greater endurance, speed, and power.

Motivation

Success in an exercise program depends on individual motivation.

Relaxation

Relaxation exercises relieve fatigue and tension.

Routine

Regular exercise is more valuable and less likely to lead to injury than bursts of activity followed by long periods of inactivity.

- *Shin splints,* which occur in people who run vigorously. They usually result from overuse, improper footwear, failure to warm up, or running on hard surfaces. There is pain in the anterior portion of the lower leg. The pain results from the tendons tearing away from the tibia. If pain persists, stress fractures should be ruled out.
- *Stress fractures,* which are partial or complete fractures of bone that are due to recurrent submaximal trauma. They are common in, but not confined to, the lower limbs. Early stress fractures are difficult to identify on x-ray examination. Clinical manifestations include localized swelling and point tenderness across a bone. Most stress fractures are "hairline fractures" of the bone; therefore, it takes several weeks for new bone to be seen. Most stress fractures are preventable with proper preconditioning and preseason training.

Table 75–7. Grades of Overuse Injuries			
	Grade I	**Grade II**	**Grade III**	**Grade IV**
Assessment				
History	Hurts after, not during, activity	Hurts after and sometimes during activity	Hurts during and after activity	Hurts all the time
Physical examination	Generalized tenderness	Generalized tenderness over area	More localized tenderness	Localized tenderness
X-rays	Negative	Negative	Usually negative	May be positive
Bone scan	Negative	Negative	May be positive	Usually positive
Type of Tissue Injured	Soft tissue	Soft tissue	Soft, hard, or bony tissue	Hard or bony tissue
Management	Ice Treat underlying problem	Ice Correct underlying problem Anti-inflammatory medication, e.g., aspirin Decrease exercise 25% to 33%	Ice Correct underlying problem Anti-inflammatory medication, e.g., aspirin, NSAIDs; possibly prednisone Decrease exercise 50% to 75%	Ice Correct underlying problem Anti-inflammatory medication, e.g., aspirin, NSAIDs; possibly prednisone Stop exercising altogether

Adapted from The athlete's leg (1985). *Emergency Medicine, 17,* 83.

Strains

Strain is trauma to the body of a muscle or attachment of a tendon caused by overstretching, misuse, or overextension. Strains usually arise from twisting or wrenching movements. They may be acute (e.g., occur during unaccustomed vigorous exercise) or chronic (e.g., develop after repetitive muscle overuse). Strains may occur in any age group and in any body part that contains muscles and tendons.

There are three classifications of strains.

First-degree strain is identified by the gradual onset of muscle spasms, discomfort, and loss of ROM. No edema or ecchymosis is present. It involves pulling of the musculotendinous unit.

Second-degree strain is identified by extreme muscle spasms, pain, and edema, which develop immediately after injury. The area remains tender after acute symptoms subside. Ecchymoses develop within a few hours. This type of strain involves tearing or straining of the musculotendinous unit.

Third-degree strain is identified by severe muscle spasms, point tenderness, and edema at the rim of injury. A sensation of sudden tearing, or a snapping or burning sensation is felt. Very limited ROM results from spasms. This degree of injury usually represents a complete rupture of the musculotendinous unit.

X-ray examination is required to rule out the possibility of fracture. Acute strains require rest and, possibly, splint-ing. Elevate the injured part. Apply ice packs for the first 24 to 48 hours after injury to reduce swelling. Heat may be prescribed for comfort, to encourage reabsorption of blood and fluid, and to promote healing. Surgical repair may be necessary if rupture is present at the tendon-bone interface. During healing (4 to 6 weeks) movement of the injured part should be minimal. Activity should never be such that it produces symptoms, such as swelling or pain. After mature scar tissue has formed, the part can be gradually and progressively exercised. Avoid overactivity during rehabilitation.

Sprains

Ankle sprains are the most common injury resulting from recreational sports. A sprain is a ligament injury resulting from overstress causing damage to ligament fibers or their attachment. They commonly result from sudden injury or forced hyperextension. Sprains may be mild (grade 1), moderate (grade 2), or severe (grade 3). A mild sprain tears a few ligament fibers, but there is no loss of function and the ligament is not weakened. Therefore, protection of the ligament is not vital. A moderate sprain tears a portion of a ligament, producing some loss of function. Protection is vital to prevent further tearing. A severe sprain completely tears a ligament either from its attachment or within the ligament body itself. It is estimated that about 75% of sprains have complete ligament rupture. Complete rupture often requires surgical repair. Approximation of the ligament ends is important to ensure strength and stability of the ligament (Fig. 75–15).

Upper extremity sprains often result from overstressing a joint during sports activity, attempting to break a fall, or bracing the body against impact during a motor vehicle accident. Ankle sprains are often the result of missteps, motor vehicle accidents, or sports injuries. Cervical sprains most often result from whiplash injuries.

On physical examination, the severity of a sprain may not be apparent. With severe sprains the person may say the joint feels loose or like "something coming apart." The person may describe what feels like a snap, pop, or tearing. This usually indicates severe injury. The amount of swelling also indicates severity. Mild swelling (grade 1 sprains) results from microscopic ligament tearing, whereas severe swelling (grade 3 sprains) comes from bleeding into the tissues. Ecchymoses do not necessarily indicate either the severity or site of the injury. For example, gravity causes bruising in a part of the foot distal to a sprained ankle.

Following a sprain injury, tenderness to palpation develops, which is well localized at first and later becomes more diffuse. Other assessment findings include swelling, severe pain, discoloration, decreased motion (limited joint motion and function), and disability. Disability may not be very severe initially, but it may be extensive after 2 to 3 hours. X-ray studies may show soft tissue swelling but no evidence of bone or joint injury.

Immediate intervention includes elevating the injured joint and applying ice (see Management and Delegation). The joint may be immobilized by splinting, casting, or taping. Aircasts are also used for immobilization. Crutch walking without weightbearing is required. After about 3 days the client is reassessed. At that time, generally, a stirrup splint with pneumatic cushions (e.g., Aircast) is applied over a sock or over light, loose elastic wrap. The client is encouraged to bear weight progressively as tolerated and to discard the crutches as soon as comfort and security of walking permit. Immobilization may continue for 3 to 4 weeks. A mature scar forms in connective fibrous tissue in 4 to 6 weeks. Following complete healing, the person needs a carefully planned exercise program to avoid reinjury.

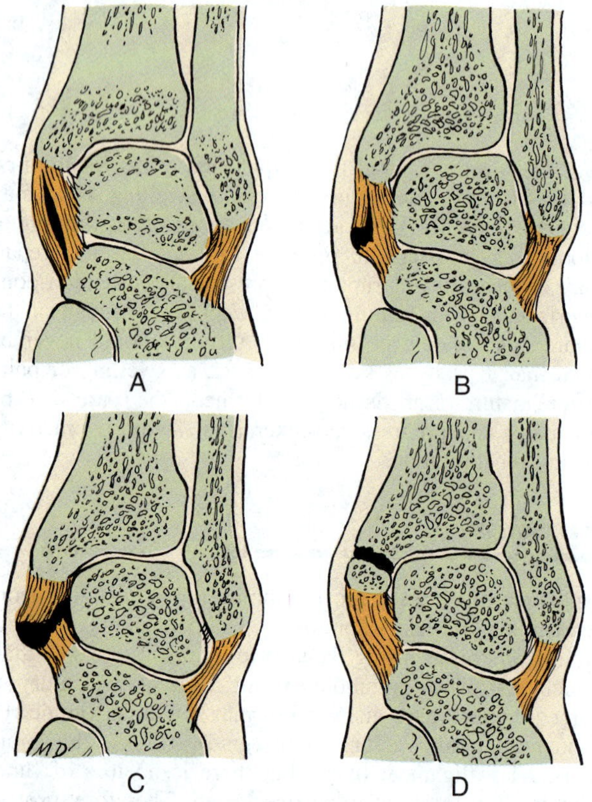

Dislocations and Subluxations

Dislocation and subluxation are both displacements of a joint from its normal position. Dislocation is the separation of both articulating surfaces. Subluxation occurs when the articulating surfaces lose partial contact. These injuries usually occur from direct or indirect pressure to the joint. For example, trying to break a fall down the stairs by holding onto a railing could dislocate the shoulder. A displaced bone may impede blood supply, tear ligaments, rupture blood vessels, damage nerves, and rupture muscle attachments. Dislocations and subluxations disrupt a joint by tearing the capsule and ligaments. They are often accompanied by a fracture of the joint surface.

Dislocations and subluxations may or may not produce visible deformity. Dislocation may alter the length of an affected extremity. Localized joint pain and loss of function may occur. A dislocation differs from a fracture in that it partially immobilizes a joint. (A fracture site typically has abnormal free movement.) X-ray films show the abnormality (i.e., complete or partial separation of the articulating surfaces). Some dislocations reduce themselves, leaving a sprain. Others require therapeutic reduction. Before treatment, assess and document the neurovascular status of parts distal to the injury. Once diagnosis is confirmed by x-ray examination, the dislocation or subluxation is reduced.

Figure 75–15. Various types of sprain (using the ankle as an example). *A,* Mild (grade 1) sprain. There is a small hematoma in a localized ligament area. A few fibers are separated. *B,* Moderate (grade 2) sprain. More severe fiber tearing than in *A.* No more than half of the fibers are torn. *C,* Severe (grade 3) sprain. Tearing is completely through the ligament. *D,* Sprain fracture. Ligament is completely torn off, and a fragment of bone is torn off also.

Rotator Cuff Tears

The rotator cuff is a complex of four muscles (supraspinatus, infraspinatus, teres minor, and subscapularis). These muscles stabilize the humeral head in the glenoid fossa. They also assist with abduction, forward elevation, and external rotation. The rotator cuff muscles can be injured during a fall or can degenerate. Clients report pain, weakness, and limited motion in the shoulder.

Treatment usually begins with conservative manage-

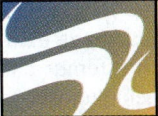

MANAGEMENT AND DELEGATION

Application of Heat and Cold

Heat is often applied to reduce swelling and inflammation. Heat can also be used to promote pain relief, increase circulation, promote healing, and reduce muscle spasms. Cold is often applied to reduce bleeding and inflammation. Cold can also be used to promote pain relief and prevent swelling.

Any equipment used to apply heat or cold may injure the client. Injury may result if the client is unable to perceive discomfort because of decreased peripheral circulation, decreased feeling, decreased sensorium, sedation, or agitation. The client may also be at risk if he or she cannot be left alone safely or if the client alters the controls of the heating pad or aquathermia pad.

The application of heat or cold to an inflamed or painful area that is closed may be delegated to unlicensed assistive personnel. A registered nurse should perform the application of heat or cold to an open wound, to an extremity of a diabetic client, or to a client with peripheral vascular disease. Prior to delegating the application of heat or cold, consider the following:

- What is the indication for the application of heat or cold? Check the physician's order. The order and indication may be sufficient to tell you whether you can delegate this task or not.
- What is the condition of the affected site? Assess for any areas of redness, swelling, breakdown, or scar tissue. It is important to know the baseline condition of the site prior to the application of heat or cold. There may be an indication to withhold this treatment or to confer with the physician about the order. You will also want to assess the condition of the site on completion of the treatment.
- What is the client's diagnosis? Is there any history of diabetes mellitus or impairment in sensorium or mentation? This may be an indication for you to perform this treatment yourself. If there is impairment of the client's mental or sensory status, it may be necessary for the unlicensed assistive personnel to remain with the client throughout the treatment.
- What is the competency level of the unlicensed assistive personnel who might perform this task?

The unlicensed assistive personnel providing the heat or cold application should be instructed to do the following:

- Wash their hands
- Assemble the necessary equipment. Instruct them as to which method of applying heat or cold is ordered.
- Check the temperature of the heat or cold device prior to applying it to the client's skin. A safe range for heat applications is 115° to 125° F for adults.
- Wrap any heat or cold application with a protective cover, such as a towel or flannel sleeve
- (If using a heating pad) start with the device on the lowest setting to initiate treatment
- Instruct the client not to adjust the heat setting
- Check the client's response immediately. If the device is too hot or cold, an adjustment is necessary. Double the protective layer between the device and the skin or allow the temperature of the device to moderate slightly.
- Check the client's skin after 5 minutes. If it is tolerated, leave the heat or cold in place for 20 minutes. If it is not tolerated, the heat or cold should be removed immediately, and you should be made aware of this. Assess the situation and notify the physician as appropriate.
- Remove the heat or cold application at 20 minutes and inform you that the treatment is complete

You are responsible to examine the affected area and reassess the client's skin at the completion of this treatment. You should document your findings and the client's response to treatment in the medical record. The unlicensed assistive personnel should immediately report any difficulty encountered during the course of treatment.

---

ment including rest, ice, antiinflammatory medications, and physical therapy. Surgery may be required to repair the rotator cuff. Postoperative management includes a short hospital stay, use of a shoulder immobilizer, and pain control. A program of exercise is taught to the client prior to discharge.

Prompt intervention is essential to prevent complications (i.e., ischemia or aseptic necrosis resulting from impaired blood supply to parts distal to the dislocation), and impaired nourishment of the articulating cartilage in the injured joint. Reduction is usually performed without surgery (closed reduction). Occasionally, surgery (open

reduction) is required (i.e., for knee injuries in which ligaments are completely ruptured). Closed manipulation is performed under general anesthesia. The physician pulls on the joint with a gradual steady pull and moves the bone back into correct alignment.

Following reduction of a dislocation or subluxation, the joint is immobilized by a splint or a cast. Immobilization may be needed for 3 to 6 weeks. Encourage prescribed active exercise of adjacent nonimmobilized joints. After immobilization is removed, encourage active motion of the injured part (i.e., voluntary muscle contraction). Passive stretching can be harmful.

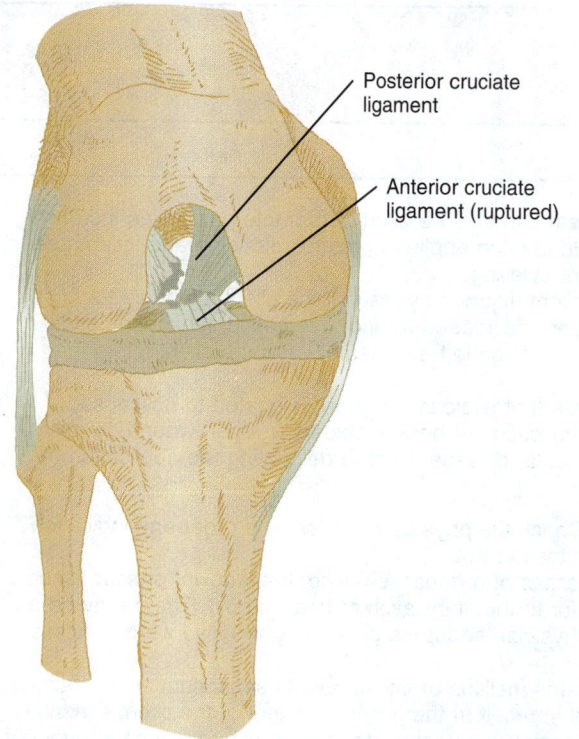

Posterior cruciate
ligament

Anterior cruciate
ligament (ruptured)

Figure 75–16. Anterior cruciate ligament injury, commonly caused by twisting of a hyperextended knee when landing after a jump shot in basketball.

Anterior Cruciate Ligament Injuries

The ligaments of the knee stabilize the joint and control motion. The anterior cruciate ligament (ACL) is the strongest and least compliant ligament within the knee. It functions primarily to prevent anterior displacement of the tibia on the femur as well as to control the rotary stability of the knee joint.

The anterior cruciate ligament is susceptible to injury and is the most frequently completely torn ligament of the knee (Fig. 75–16). Two basic mechanisms of injury exist. In the first type of injury, an excessive valgus force is applied to the knee. This type of force damages the medial collateral ligament (MCL) and the anterior cruciate ligament. "Clipping" in football is a common cause of this type of injury. The second type of injury to the anterior cruciate ligament occurs with hyperextension while the leg is internally rotated. This mechanism causes isolated anterior cruciate ligament rupture and more subtle manifestations. This type of injury commonly occurs during skiing, basketball, or gymnastics.

At the time of injury, a snapping sensation is felt and, at times, a popping noise is heard. Within hours, the knee becomes tense, swollen, stiff, and painful. If it is not treated, the knee will give way, leading to falls. The knee loses support during lateral pivots. The Lachman test results are positive, showing an anterior shift of the lateral

tibial plateau. The Lachman test is one of the most sensitive tests used to assess anterior cruciate ligament damage. The examiner holds the distal end of the femur and it is displaced posteriorly while the examiner attempts to pull the tibia forward. When the anterior cruciate ligament has been damaged, the tibia will travel forward. The drawer test for anterior cruciate ligament damage is not as reliable because the femur is held in a neutral position. False-negative results occur frequently using the drawer test.

Anterior cruciate ligament tears can be repaired within several weeks of injury and still allow the return of function and stability. Various devices, including autograft and artifical ligament materials, have been used for reconstruction. Reconstruction after the surgery requires an effective balance between mobilization and immobilization. Some clients are treated with continuous passive motion machines (CPM). The CPM is placed in the recovery room, where it provides support to the limb and puts the knee through preset degrees of passive ROM. The CPM is used at least 3 hours/day or until full ROM is achieved.

When the CPM is not used, the limb is placed in a long-leg limb brace set at 40 degrees flexion for 1 week. The client is taught to do isometric quadriceps setting, bent-knee leg raises, and foot exercises. Over the course of the next 4 to 6 weeks, progressive ROM exercises are added.

A newer form of reconstruction uses artificial grafts to reconstruct the anterior cruciate ligament. These clients can undergo rapid rehabilitation, obtaining full ROM in 3 to 4 days most of the time.

Meniscal Injuries

The meniscus is fibrous cartilage that lies on top of the tibia, between the tibia and the femur (Fig. 75–17) It acts as a shock absorber. It has very little blood supply and therefore heals very slowly, if at all, when torn. Manifestations of meniscal injury are popping or tearing sensations in the knee at the time of injury. The knee swells

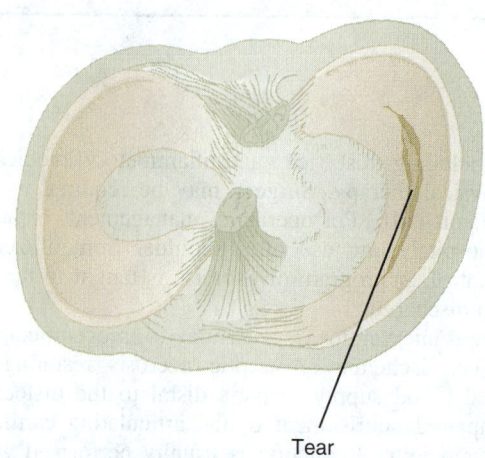

Tear

Figure 75–17. A tear of the meniscus of the knee.

over the next several hours. If the injury is severe, and the cartilage is torn, it can float or move within the knee joint and cause the knee to "lock" or "catch." Initial management is rest, elevation, ice, and pain medication. After the initial edema has subsided, quadriceps exercises are begun to strengthen the knee. If the knee continues to swell and hurt, surgery is considered. Arthroscopic surgery is most often required. If the pieces of cartilage remain in the knee, they can damage knee structures as they float and move. The arthroscope is inserted into the knee and the structures are either repaired or removed. Following surgery, the leg is elevated, ice compresses are applied, and pain is controlled. Rehabilitation included quadriceps strengthening and range of motion exercises. Activity is allowed once strength has returned.

Repetitive Motion Injuries

Repetitive motion injuries result from using the same muscle groups over and over without rest or stretch. Certain occupations create risk of very specific types of injuries. They are summarized in Table 75–8. Management usually centers around ergonomic positioning at workstations, proper work equipment, stretching of opposing muscle groups, and frequent breaks for stretching.

Remobilization After Traumatic Injury

Devices for remobilization include therapeutic exercise, continuous passive motion machines, passive and active ROM exercises, and active resistive ROM exercises. Therapeutic exercise increases joint ROM, muscle strength, and cardiovascular endurance. Before an exercise program begins, factors that limit exercise, such as pain and an inability to relax, must be known. Exercise should progress so that the client experiences only little muscle soreness. Pain in the exercising client may be due to chronic compartment syndrome.

Passive ROM exercises prevent joint contractures and maintain normal joint ROM. Passive ROM exercises can be performed by the therapist, nurse, or with equipment such as the CPM machine. Nursing considerations when using the CPM machine include assessing the client for proper fit of the device. It should fit so that it is not too tight in the groin yet is still able to bend at the knee. Because the client must be supine when using the machine, assess the skin of the sacrum and heels for signs of pressure. In addition, assess the groin for signs of irritation. The client should be taught about the purposes of the machine, to report any signs of pressure or irritation, and how to start and stop it.

Active ROM is the active contraction of muscle against the pull of gravity. Active ROM exercises are a part of gradual exercises that increase muscle strength and endurance. Examples include straight-leg raises and knee flexion and extension in a sitting position.

Active assistive ROM is the active contraction of muscle by the client against an external force applied by the therapist, a mechanical appliance, or the opposite extremity. Active assistive exercise is often the second step in a muscle reeducation and strengthening program. Examples of active assistive ROM include isotonic and isokinetic exercises. The best example of isotonic exercise is weight-lifting. An example of isokinetic exercise machines is the Cybex.

Ambulation is a three-dimensional activity involving the pelvis, legs, trunk, and upper extremities. Many factors can lead to difficulties in ambulation: disorders of the musculoskeletal system, nervous system, and cardiovascular system can all lead to abnormalities in gait. In addition, cognitive factors, balance, and coordination are also important for safe walking. Ambulation should be initiated as soon as possible after orthopedic surgery or immobility. Clients who have been bedridden for extended periods have muscle atrophy, weakness, decreased endurance, decreased cardiovascular fitness, and decreased joint flexibility, and they tend to develop orthostatic hypotension. See the earlier Nursing Research feature for a consideration of posthospital convalescence in clients with hip fractures.

A gradual progression of exercise is used to get these clients moving again. In bed, exercises should be used (e.g., ROM and active assisted ROM). The tilt table, a device that assists the client to an upright position, can be used for initial attempts at standing after long periods of bedrest.

Weightbearing status must be known before attempting to assist clients to ambulate safely. The degree of protective weightbearing is determined by the orthopedic physician. Types of weightbearing status are shown in Table 75–5. Ambulatory assistive devices, such as canes, walkers, and crutches, can be used. These devices are fully described in any basic nursing skills textbook.

Conclusions

Musculoskeletal trauma may range from simple strains and sprains to very complex, open, compound fractures that are life threatening. The nurse's role in the care of these clients is primarily to reduce the complications of immobility to promote early ambulation, and to teach the client how to prevent further injury.

Thinking Critically

1. A young man arrives in the emergency department holding his arm close to his body. The wrist is obviously misshapen, but swelling is minimal. He tells you he fell out of a tree while picking cherries and landed hard on his hand. It is painful for him to flex or twist his wrist from side to side. An x-ray of the wrist confirms a fracture. He is scheduled for a cast application. What intervention should be done immediately on arrival? What teaching should be completed about cast care?

Table 75–8. Repetitive Motion Injuries

Condition	Manifestations	Occupations at Risk	Usual Treatment
Neck			
Tension neck syndrome	Stiff, aching neck, headache	Typists, key punch operators, cashiers, and others who must maintain a restricted posture	Prevention is key: (1) pause frequently when typing or keying to stretch about 30 sec every 30 min; (2) place screen directly in front of typist, avoid twisting; (3) place material to be typed at eye level if possible; avoid having materials to be typed consistently on one side of typist; conservative*
Cervical syndrome	Pain on flexion or extension of the neck with radiation down the arm	Common in persons who assume awkward positions for a long time, such as painters, dentists	Conservative*, cervical collar, surgery
Shoulder			
Thoracic outlet syndrome	Numbness, pain, ischemia, and weakened pulse in upper extremity with hyperextension of the shoulder	Overhead assembly workers, automobile repair mechanics, letter carriers	Conservative,* transcutaneous nerve stimulation, surgery
Supraspinatus tendinitis	Pain on elevating arm above 70 degrees at the shoulder	Persons who must maintain abduction with elbow extended—painters, construction workers	Conservative,* physical therapy, steroid injections
Bicipital tendinitis	Pain over the bicipital tendon in bicipital groove	Window washers, construction workers, shipping clerks	Conservative,* physical therapy, steroid injections

*Conservative treatment consists of restriction of the harmful motion, splinting (if appropriate, and only for short periods of time or at night), application of ice or heat, mild analgesics and NSAIDs, and gentle stretching exercises.

Factors to Consider. How should you relieve the client's pain? What is involved in the healing process for a fracture? What complications might the client face because of the cast?

2. **A 48-year-old woman lost her footing while skiing. She arrives at the emergency department in obvious distress. Her leg is extremely painful and she will not allow anyone to touch the affected leg. Once clothing is removed, a noticeable lump is visible on the thigh, and medication is given to relieve the pain. After x-ray studies of the entire leg, she is told the femur is fractured. She is scheduled for application of a long-leg cast and admission to the orthopedic unit. What is your priority for care when she is admitted to your unit? What special complication is she at risk for?**

Factors to Consider. What are her immediate needs on arrival on the unit? What is the classic picture of the client with fat embolism syndrome?

3. **An elderly woman, age 80, has a history of thoracic and low back pain. X-rays reveal multiple compression fractures of the thoracic and lumbar area. Originally 5 feet tall, she has lost about 6 inches over the past 3 years. She calls the clinic to report onset of lumbar back pain after a fall in which she hit the end of a table as she landed on her back. How should you respond to her request for direction? What further assessments can be made over the telephone?**

Factors to Consider. How were the compression factors treated in the past? What in her nursing history might alert you to the ongoing problem with back pain?

Condition	Manifestations	Occupations at Risk	Usual Treatment
Elbow, Hand, and Wrist			
Lateral or medial epicondylitis (tennis elbow)	Local pain and pain on resisted hand motion	Repeated and forceful rotation of the forearm with the wrist bent; can be seen in bowlers, tennis players, and pitchers	Conservative,* steroid injections, surgery
deQuervain's tenosynovitis (inflammation of the extensor pollicus brevis tendons)	Gradual onset of pain, and sometimes swelling of the radial styloid; popping sensation on extension of the thumb	Middle-aged women and those subject to repetitive stress of the thumb	Conservative,* steroid injections, surgery
Carpal tunnel syndrome	Pain and paresthesias on percussion over the median nerve at the wrist (Tinel's sign) or with flexed wrists pressed together (positive Phalen's maneuver); night pain after 3–4 hr of sleep, morning stiffness, daytime numbness	Repetitive forced hand movements, keypunch operators, cashiers, typists, persons with degenerative joint disease	Prevention is key: (1) while typing pause frequently at least 30 seconds every 30 minutes; (2) adjust keyboard so the elbows are at 90 degree angle and wrists are straight; (3) do not rest wrists on a hard surface or restpad; wrists should "float" above keyboard; (4) use a light touch when striking the keys; conservative,* steroid injections, surgery
Ulnar nerve entrapment	Pain and paraesthesias on percussion of the ulnar nerve over the epicondyle (Tinel's sign); local swelling and tissue hypertrophy around elbow	Rheumatoid arthritis clients, occupational stress on elbow	Conservative,* surgery

Bibliography

1. Barangan, J. (1990). Factors that influence recovery from hip fracture during hospitalization. *Orthopaedic Nursing 9*(5), 19–29.
2. Barden, R. M. & Sinkora, G. (1991). Bone stimulators for fusions and fractures. *Nursing Clinics of North America, 26*(1), 89–103.
3. Bigos, S., Bowyer, O., Braen, G., et al. (1994). *Acute low back problems in adults. Clinical Practice Guideline No. 14.* AHCPR publication No. 95–0642. Rockville, MD: Agency for Health Care Polcy and Research, Public Health Service, U. S. Department of Health and Human Services.
4. Brown, F. (1996). Anterior cruciate ligament reconstruction as an outpatient procedure. *Orthopaedic Nursing, 15*(1), 15–20.
5. Commodore, D. B. (1995). Falls in the elderly population: A look at incidence, risks, healthcare costs and preventive strategies. *Rehabilitation Nursing, 20*(2), 84–89.
6. Currie, D. M., Gershkoff, A. M., & Cifu, D. X. (1993). Geriatric rehabilitation: Mid and late life effects of early-life disabilities. *Archives of Physical Medicine and Rehabilitation, 74,* S413–S416.
7. Doheny, M., Linden, P., & Sedlak, C. (1995). Reducing orthopaedic hazards of the computer work environment. *Orthopaedic Nursing, 14*(1), 7–15.
8. Farnworth, M. G., Kenny, P., & Shiell, A. (1994). The cost and effects of early discharge in the management of fractured hip. *Age and Aging, 23,* 190–194.
9. Folcik, M. (1991). Meniscal injuries. *Nursing Clinics of North America, 26*(1), 181–198.
10. Foreman, M. D. (1991). The cognitive in the hospitalized elderly: Incidence, onset, and associated factors. *Research in Nursing and Health, 12,* 21–29.
11. Funk, J., MacBrair, B., & Peterson, A. (1990). Tibial osteotomy. *Orthopaedic Nursing, 9*(2), 29–36.
12. Gelman, R., & Burns, S. (1996). Walking aches and running pains. *Primary Care, 23*(2), 263–280.
13. Greenspan, S. L., Myers, E. R., Maitland, L. A., et al. (1994). Fall severity and bone mineral density as risk factors for hip fracture in ambulatory elderly. *JAMA, 271*(2), 128–133.
14. Gross, R. (1991). Initial assessment and management of a patient with a gunshot wound to the femur. *Orthopaedic Nursing, 10*(6), 9–13.

15. Hansell, M. (1988). Fractures and the healing process. *Orthopaedic Nursing, 7*(1), 43–50.

16. Herron, D., & Nance, J. (1990). Emergency department nursing management of patients with orthopedic fractures from motor vehicle accidents. *Nursing Clinics of North America, 25*(1), 71–84.

17. Hereron, B., & Kaempffe, F. (1995). Tears of the rotator cuff. *Orthopaedic Nursing, 14*(6), 38–42.

18. Johnson, J., Barrett, A., Anderson, C., et. al., (1995). Roller traction: Mobilizing patients with acetabular fractures. *Orthopaedic Nursing, 14*(1) 21–24.

19. Johnson, L. (1989). Operative management of unstable pelvic fractures. *Orthopaedic Nursing, 8*(4), 21–26.

20. Jones-Walton, P. (1991). Clinical standards in skeletal traction pin site care. *Orthopaedic Nursing, 7*(4), 29–33.

21. Lyritis, G. P., & Johnell, O. (1993). Orthopaedic management of hip fracture. *Bone, 14*, S11–S17.

22. Maher, A., Salmond, S., & Pellino, T. (1994). *Orthopaedic nursing.* Philadelphia: W. B. Saunders.

23. Matthiesen, V., et al. (1994). Acute confusion: Nursing intervention in older adults. *Orthopaedic Nursing, 13*(2), 21–27, 29.

24. Miller, C. W. (1978). Survival and ambulation following hip fracture. *American Journal of Bone and Joint Surgery, 60,* 930–936.

25. Mims, B. (1989). Fat embolism syndrome: A variant of ARDS. *Orthopaedic Nursing, 8*(3), 22–27.

26. Mooney, N. (1991). Pain management in the orthopedic patient. *Nursing Clinics of North America, 26*(1), 73–88.

27. National Association of Orthopaedic Nurses. (1995). Telephone triage of upper extremity problems. *Orthopaedic Nursing, 14*(6), 31–36.

28. National Association of Orthopaedic Nurses (1990). *The impact of orthopaedic conditions on the health and economy of the United States.* Pitman, NJ: Author.

29. Nelson, L., et al. (1990). Improving pain management for hip fractured elderly. *Orthopaedic Nursing, 9*(3), 79–83.

30. Ochs, M. (1990). Surgical management of the hip in the elderly patient. *Clinics in Geriatric Medicine, 6*(3), 571–585.

31. Peters, V., & Ferkel, R. (1989). Arthroscopic surgery of the ankle. *Orthopaedic Nursing, 8*(5), 12–20.

32. Praemer, A. Furner, S., & Rice D. P. (1992). Costs of musculoskeletal conditions. In *Musculoskeletal conditions in the United States.* Park Ridge, IL: American Academy of Orthopaedic Surgeons.

33. Raj, P., et al. (1992). Reflex sympathetic dystrophy. In B. Browner, et al. (Eds.), *Skeletal trauma.* Philadelphia: W. B. Saunders.

34. Rorabek. C. H. (1992). Compartment syndrome. In B. Browner, et al. (Eds.), *Skeletal trauma.* Philadelphia: W. B. Saunders.

35. Ross, D. (1996). Chronic compartment syndrome. *Orthopaedic Nursing, 15*(3), 23–27.

36. Rousseau, P. (1993). Spontaneous fractures in the bedbound elderly. *Nursing Home Medicine, 1*(1), 17–19.

37. Rothenberg, J. (1991). Innovations in treating anterior cruciate ligament injury. *Orthopaedic Nursing, 10*(2), 17–26.

38. Ruda, S. C. (1991). Common ankle injuries in the athlete. *Nursing Clinics of North America, 26*(1), 167–180.

39. Scheck, R. K. (1992). Biology of fracture repair. In B. Browner, et al. (Eds.), *Skeletal trauma.* Philadelphia: W. B. Saunders.

40. Shea, K., & Folcik, M. (1989). Water sports injuries. *Orthopaedic Nursing, 8*(6), 11–17.

41. Sipos, D. A. (1995). Carpal tunnel syndrome. *Orthopaedic Nursing, 14*(1), 17–20.

42. Slye, D. (1991). Orthopedic complications: Compartment syndrome, fat embolism syndrome and venous thromboembolism. *Nursing Clinics of North America, 26*(1), 113–132.

43. Smrcina, C. (1991). Stress fractures in athletes. *Nursing Clinics of North America, 26*(1), 159–166.

44. Smrcina, C. (1988). Case study: Shoulder injury. *Orthopaedic Nursing, 7*(3), 57.

45. Strycula, L. (1994). Traction basics: Part I. *Orthopaedic Nursing, 13*(2), 71–74.

46. Strycula, L. (1994). Traction basics: Part II. *Orthopaedic Nursing, 13*(3), 55–59.

47. Strycula, L. (1994). Traction basics: Part III. *Orthopaedic Nursing, 13*(4), 34–44.

48. Strycula, L. (1994). Traction basics: Part IV. *Orthopaedic Nursing, 13*(5), 59–68.

49. Torburn, L. (1996). Basic protocols of rehabilitation for the ankle, knee, hip, and shoulder. *Primary Care, 23*(2), 389–403.

50. Verdon, M. (1996). Overuse syndromes of the hand and wrist. *Primary Care, 23*(2), 305–319.

51. Williams, M. A., Campbell, E. B., & Raynor, W. J. (1985). Predictors of acute confusion states in hospitalized elderly patients. *Research in Nursing and Health, 8,* 31–40.

52. Williams, M. A., Oberst, M. T., & Bjorkland, B. C. (1994). Posthospital convalescence in older women with hip fracture. *Orthopaedic Nursing, 13*(4), 55–64.

53. Wittington, C., & Carlson, C. (1991). Anterior cruciate ligament injuries: Evaluation, arthroscopic reconstruction and rehabilitation. *Nursing Clinics of North America, 26*(1), 149–158.

Integumentary Disorders

UNIT 16

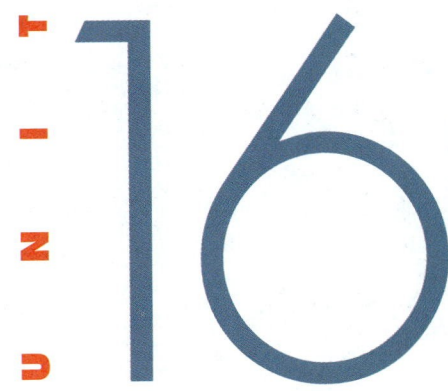

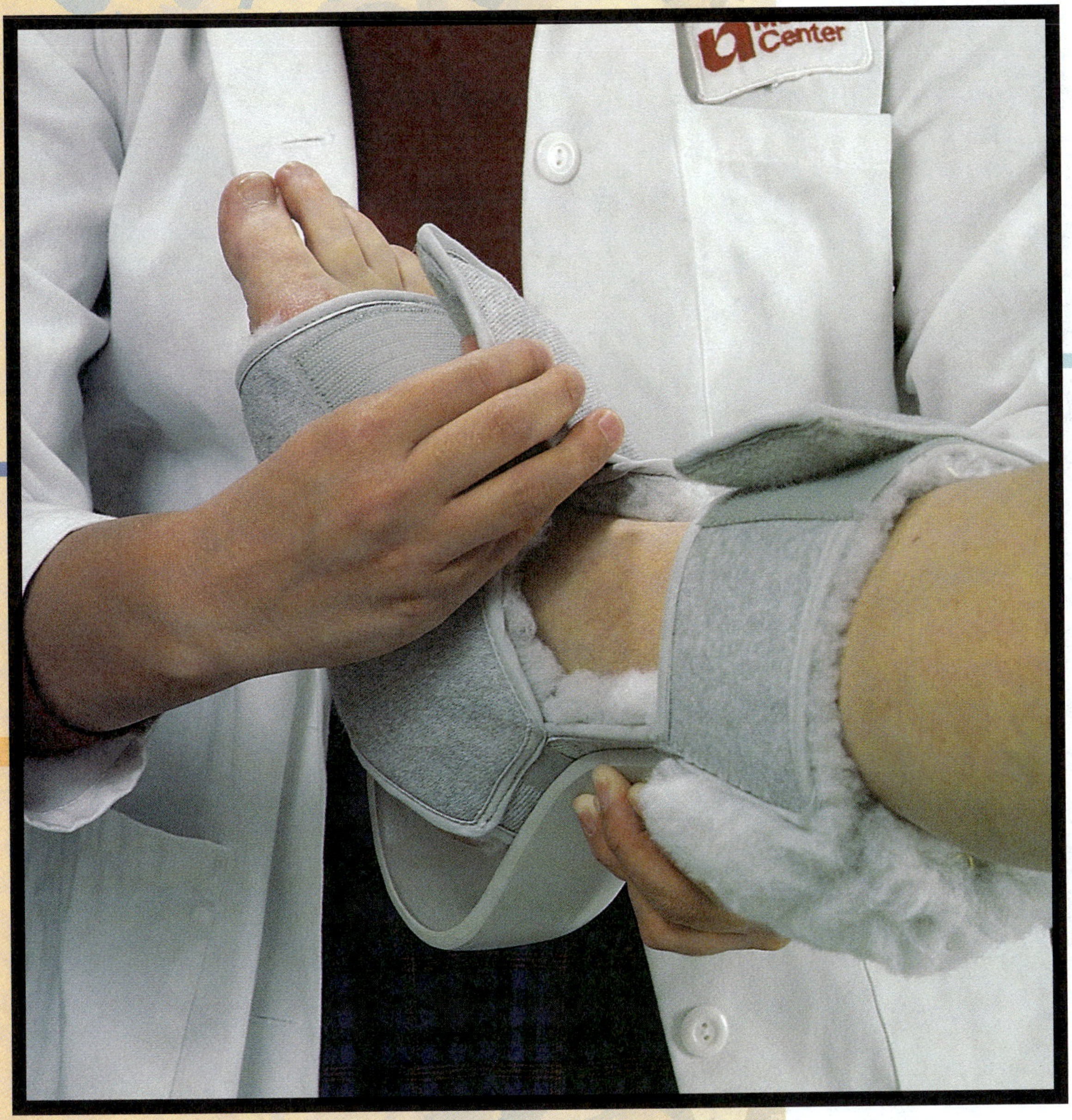

Structure and Function of the Integumentary System

Noreen Heer Nicol

Joyce M. Black

Skin, the largest and most visible organ of the body, plays a critical role in a person's physical and mental health. In both outpatient and inpatient practice settings, nurses have a unique opportunity to affect a client's dermatologic care significantly. Nurses have more prolonged contact with a client's skin than do most other healthcare professionals. Despite being the largest organ of the body, the skin is rarely taken as seriously as other organ systems such as the heart or the lung. The skin protects us from an array of natural and manmade attacks. Clients must appreciate the important role that the skin plays and should recognize that some skin conditions are indeed life-threatening. Forecasts indicate that by the year 2000, as many as 1 in 75 Americans will be afflicted by malignant melanoma, a life-threatening, often fatal skin cancer. Currently in the United States, one person dies every hour from skin cancer. Burn injury continues despite advances in fireproofing homes and clothes. Pressure ulcers, a serious alteration in skin integrity, lead to 60,000 deaths per year.

Skin is integral to self-image and self-esteem. Each client's unique appearance is established through the skin. The skin was once thought to reflect the "normal aging process" and how that aging process affected the genetic skin types we inherit. We now know it more likely reflects the cumulative amount of sun exposure over a lifetime. It is hoped that with education, untanned skin will once again be viewed as attractive and healthy. Likewise, cosmetic surgery should not be considered surgery for vanity, but surgery to enhance self-esteem.

Today's society has a long-standing prejudice against impaired skin that needs to be dispelled. Historically, skin diseases have been perceived as divine punishment for being spiritually and physically "unclean." Subtle punishment for skin diseases still exists because of ignorance. For example, a woman with atopic dermatitis may sit isolated and shunned in a waiting room because others view her scratching and eczematous lesions as contagious. A waitress is encouraged to work in the back of the kitchen so that customers will not notice the healed burn scars on her hands and body. Vitiligo, loss of pigment in the skin, is sometimes incorrectly labeled "white leprosy," and so on. Clients who have visible chronic skin problems often withdraw from social situations and have altered interpersonal relationships and increased social isolation. When these clients seek professional care for skin problems, psychosocial as well as physical concerns need to be met.

Structure of the Skin

Skin makes up 15% to 20% of body weight. Intact skin is always considered the body's primary defense system. It protects us from invasion by organisms, helps regulate body temperature, manufactures vitamins, and provides our external appearance. Skin has three primary layers— (1) epidermal (epidermis), (2) dermal (dermis), and (3) subcutaneous (subcutaneous fat) (Fig. 76–1)—as well as epidermal appendages (i.e., eccrine glands, apocrine glands, sebaceous glands, hair follicles, and nails).

Epidermis

The epidermis is the thin, stratified outer skin layer in direct contact with the external environment. The thickness of the epidermis ranges from 0.04 mm on the eyelids to 1.6 mm on the palms and soles. The epidermis consists of five layers and four cell types. Desmosomes, which are points of intercellular attachment that are critical for cell-to-cell adhesion, are also found in the epidermis (Fig. 76–2).

Keratinocytes

Keratinocytes are the principal cells of the epidermis. All five layers of epidermis consist of keratinocytes. Each layer of cells gradually differentiates into the next. The name of each layer, from inner- to outermost, reflects evolving differentiation: (1) stratum germinativum (basal

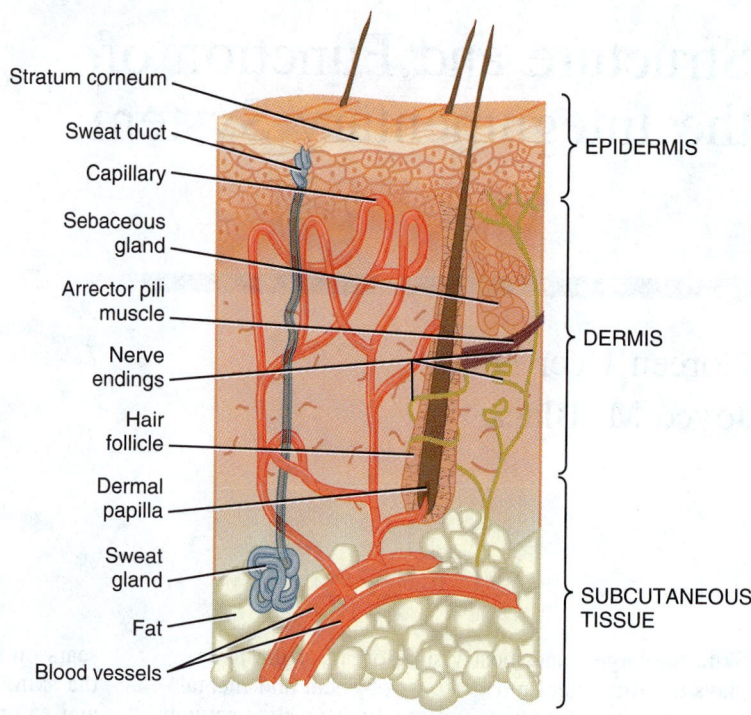

Figure 76–1. Structure of the skin.

cell layer), (2) stratum spinosum (prickle cells), (3) stratum granulosum (nucleated granular cells), (4) stratum lucidum (thin transparent layer), and (5) stratum corneum (the horny layer of dead keratinized cells). Keratinocytes produce keratin in a complex process as the cells begin in the basal cell layer, constantly change, and move upward through the epidermis. The entire process of differentiation from basal cell layer to horny cell layer requires 3 to 4 weeks. Thus, the epidermis constantly regenerates itself, providing a tough keratinized barrier.

Melanocytes

Melanocytes are epidermal pigment-producing cells that are intermittently found wedged between basal cells. Melanocytes produce melanosomes (pigment granules) that contain melanin (skin pigment). Skin color is produced by four pigments: (1) exogenously formed carotenoids (yellow), (2) melanin (brown), (3) oxygenated hemoglobin in capillaries (red), and (4) reduced hemoglobin in venules (blue). Melanin has the greatest role in skin color

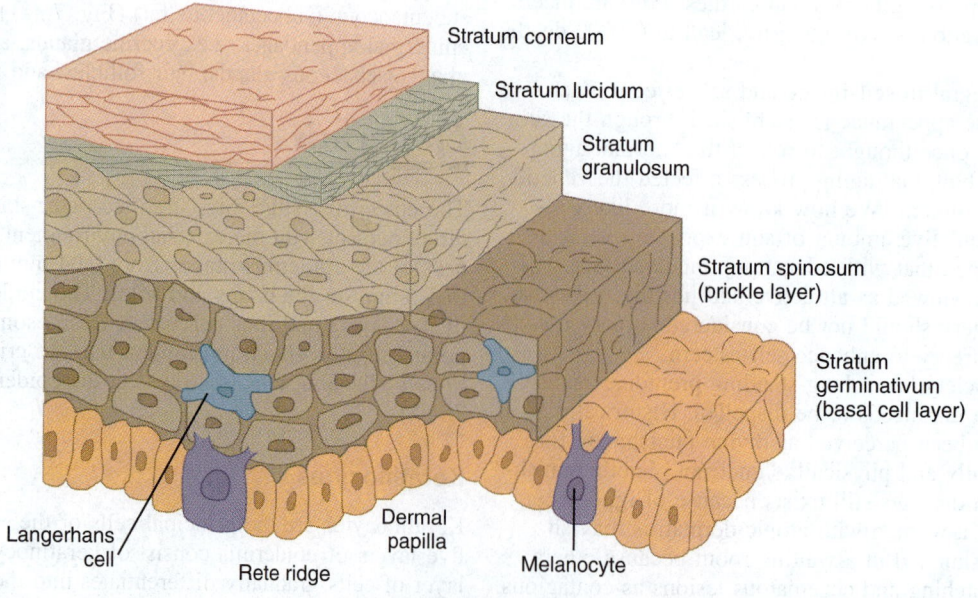

Figure 76–2. The epidermis.

and is produced in the epidermis and in corresponding layers of the hair follicle. Melanin is not produced in the dermis; however, it can be deposited in the dermis from the epidermis through various processes such as inflammation. Skin color differences result from the size and quantity of melanosomes as well as from the rate of melanin production. In blacks, there is an increase in the size and number of melanosomes—not melanocytes—as well as increased melanin production. The melanosomes in blacks are large, discrete, and dispersed. In whites, the melanosomes are small and aggregated and produce less melanin. Sun exposure initially increases the size and functional activity of both melanocytes and melanosomes. With chronic sun exposure, there is an increase in concentration of melanocytes as well as in size and functional activity.

Merkel Cells

Merkel cells are in the basal layer but can usually be located only by electron microscopy. They are thought to be touch receptors on palms, soles, and oral and genital epithelium, but are very scarce. A rare but highly malignant tumor called Merkel cell carcinoma develops from these cells.

Langerhans' Cells

Langerhans' cells are scattered among the keratinocytes located primarily in the epidermis; however, they can be seen in the dermis. These cells originate in the bone marrow and migrate to the epidermis. Langerhans' cells play a role in the cell-mediated immune responses of the skin through antigen presentation.

Epidermal Appendages

Epidermal appendages are downgrowths of epidermis into the dermis and consist of (1) eccrine glands, (2) apocrine units, (3) sebaceous glands, (4) hair, and (5) nails.

Eccrine Glands

Eccrine glands are sweat-producing glands that play an important role in thermoregulation; they are found throughout the skin except on the vermilion border (junction of the pink area of the lip with the surrounding skin) of the lip, ears, nail bed, glans penis, and labia minora. They are more numerous on the palms, soles, forehead, and axillae. Eccrine glands consist of two types of cells: (1) large, pale cells and (2) small, dark-staining cells. Sweat has the same composition as plasma in a less concentrated form. The main stimulus to eccrine gland secretion is heat. However, exercise and emotional stress also stimulate sweat production via cholinergic innervation. These glands exit the body independently of the hair shaft.

Apocrine Glands

The function of the apocrine glands, which occur primarily in the axillae, breast areolae, anogenital area, ear canals, and eyelids, is not known. It is theorized that these glands may be evolutionary remnants in humans and serve lower-order animals in sexual arousal. Mediated by adrenergic innervation, they secrete a milky substance that becomes odoriferous when altered by skin surface bacteria. These glands do not function until puberty and require a high output of sex hormone for activity.

Sebaceous Glands

Sebaceous glands are found throughout the skin except on the palms and soles. They are most abundant on the face, scalp, upper back, and chest. Sebaceous glands are associated with hair follicles that open onto the skin surface, where sebum is released. Sebum has a lubricating function and bactericidal activity. Sebum is a mixture of sebaceous gland–produced lipids and epidermal cell–derived lipids. Androgen is responsible for sebaceous gland development. In utero androgen causes neonatal acne. Sebum production is higher in males.

Hair and Hair Follicles

Hair is a nonviable protein end product found on all skin surfaces except the palms and soles. Each hair follicle functions as an independent unit and goes through intermittent stages of development. Hair develops from the mitotic activity of the hair bulb. Hair in different regions of the body spends different fractions of time in phases of growth. In a typical adult scalp, 85% to 90% of hairs are in an anagen (growth) phase. The remainder are in a telogen (rest) phase. About 50 to 100 hairs are lost each day. As a rule, the growing phase of hair on the eyebrows, trunk, and extremities does not exceed 6 months. Its resting phase is 3 to 4 months. Hair shape depends on what it looks like on cross-section. Straight hair has a round cross-section; curly hair has an oval or ribbonlike cross-section. Curved follicles also affect the curliness of hair. Melanocytes in the bulb determine hair color. Hair follicles usually occur with sebaceous glands, and together they form a pilosebaceous unit.

Nails

Nails are horny scales of epidermis. The nail matrix is the source of specialized, nonkeratinized cells that differentiate into keratinized cells, which make up the nail protein. The matrix for nail formation is located in the proximal nail bed. It grows forward from the nail fold to cover the nail bed. Fingernails grow about 0.1 mm/day. Their complete reproduction takes 100 to 150 days. Toenails grow one third as fast as fingernails do. A damaged nail matrix, which may result from trauma or aggressive manicuring, produces a distorted nail. Nails are also sensitive to physiologic changes (i.e., they grow more slowly in cold weather and during periods of illness). Nails and hair consist of keratinized and, therefore, "dead" cells. The ingestion of gelatin has not been shown to increase nail growth or strength.

Dermis

The dermis, a dense layer of tissue beneath the epidermis, gives the skin most of its substance and structure. It varies from 1 to 4 mm in thickness and is thickest over the back. The dermis contains fibroblasts, macrophages, mast cells, and lymphocytes, which promote wound healing. The skin's lymphatic, vascular, and nerve supplies, which maintain equilibrium in the skin, are in the dermis.

The dermis is divided into two parts: (1) papillary dermis and (2) reticular dermis. The papillary dermis, which contains increased amounts of collagen, blood vessels, sweat glands, and elastin, is in contact with the epidermis. The reticular dermis also has collagen but with increased amounts of mature elastic tissue.

The epidermis and dermis meet at the dermoepidermal junction. This area contains wavelike projections from the dermis called papillae. Papillae correspond to reciprocal structures in the epidermis. The subepidermal basement membrane zone is a semipermeable filter that permits fluid exchange of components such as nutrients, metabolites, and waste products.

Apart from sight and hearing, the major human sensory apparatus is in the skin. Sensory fibers responsible for pain, touch, and temperature form a complex network in the dermis. There are four primary types of sensation: pain, light touch, temperature (cold and warmth), and pressure. Pain may be caused by physical, chemical, or mechanical stimulation. Touch stimuli are received by hair follicles and the intervening skin. Itching arises from terminal nerve endings close to the skin surface; itching does not occur when the epidermis is absent. Temperature sense probably occurs through free sensory nerve endings in the epidermis.

The dermis also houses many other cells, vessels, and nerves. Table 76–1 lists the components of the dermis and their functions.

Subcutaneous Fat

The subcutaneous layer is a specialized layer of connective tissue. It is sometimes called the adipose layer because of its fat content. This layer is absent in some places such as the eyelids, scrotum, areola, and tibia. Age, heredity, and many other factors influence the thickness of the subcutaneous layer. Subcutaneous fat is generally thickest on the back and buttocks, giving shape and contour over bone. The primary functions of this layer are insulation from extremes of hot and cold, as a cushion to trauma, and as a source of energy and hormone metabolism.

Function of the Skin

The skin is a morphologically complex structure that serves several functions essential to life. The skin differs anatomically and physiologically in different areas of the body. Functions of the skin include protection, maintenance of homeostasis, thermoregulation, sensory reception, vitamin synthesis, and processing of antigenic sub-

Table 76–1. Skin Structure and Function

Structure	Normal Function
Epidermis	
Stratum corneum	Protection (from trauma, microbes)
	Barrier (prevents fluid, electrolyte, and chemical loss)
Keratinocytes (squamous cells)	Synthesis of keratin, 14-day migration through epidermis
Melanocytes	Melanosome production
	Synthesis of melanin (protection from sunburn, ultraviolet carcinogenesis)
	Determine skin color
Langerhans' cells	Antigen presentation
Basal cells	Epidermal reproduction (average of 457 hr between cell divisions), producing one basal cell and one squamous cell
Epidermal Appendages	
Eccrine unit	Thermoregulation by perspiration
Apocrine unit	Production of apocrine sweat (no known significance)
Sebaceous glands	Production of sebum (lipid mixture)
Hair follicles	Protection, cosmetic adornment
Nails	Protection and mechanical assistance
Dermis	
Collagen, reticulum, elastin	Major skin proteins; contribute to skin texture
Fibroblasts	Collagen synthesis; provide vital structural skin strength and wound healing
Macrophages	Phagocytosis of foreign substances and microbes; initiation of inflammation and repair
Mast cells	Provide histamine for vasodilation and chemotactic factors for inflammatory responses
Lymphatic glands	Removal of microbes and excess interstitial fluids
Blood vessels	Provide metabolic skin requirements, thermoregulation
Nerve fibers	Perception of heat and cold, pain, itching
Subcutaneous Adipose Tissue	Energy storage and balance, trauma absorption

stances. Table 76–1 summarizes major skin structures and functions.

Protection

The skin protects the body against many forms of trauma, including mechanical, thermal, chemical, and radiant. The intact tough epidermal layer is a mechanical barrier. Bacteria, foreign matter, other organisms, and chemicals penetrate it with difficulty. The oily and slightly acid secretions of its sebaceous glands protect the body further by limiting the growth of many organisms. The thickened skin of the palms and soles provides additional covering to absorb the constant use of or trauma to these areas.

Homeostasis

Skin forms a barrier that prevents excessive loss of water and electrolytes from the internal environment and also prevents the subcutaneous tissues from drying out. The effectiveness of this impermeable membrane is readily recognized when one observes the extreme loss of fluids that occurs with damage to the skin, as with burns and other injuries. Insensible loss of water and electrolytes occurs only through pores in this effective barrier.

Thermoregulation

The skin, under normal conditions, adjusts metabolic heat production to heat loss to maintain the thermal balance and the internal temperature of the body, which is approximately 37° C (98.6° F). The rate of heat loss depends primarily on the surface temperature of the skin, which is in turn a function of the skin's blood flow. The skin's blood flow varies in response to changes in the body's core temperature, as well as to changes in the temperature of the external environment. Generally, the vessels dilate during warm temperatures and constrict during cold. The hypothalamus is partly responsible for this control.

Sweating and subsequent cooling occurs from fluid evaporation from the skin. Sweating contributes significantly to the body's thermoregulation ability.

Sensory Reception

The primary function of the receptors in the skin is to sense temperature (hot and cold), pain, light touch, and pressure. Different nerve endings are responsible for responding to each type of stimulus, and they have varying concentrations over the body. For example, finger tips are more densely innervated than is the skin on the back.

Vitamin D Production

The epidermis is involved in synthesis of vitamin D. In the presence of sunlight or ultraviolet radiation, one of the sterols that is found on the malpighian cells is converted to form cholecalciferol (vitamin D_3). Vitamin D_3 assists in the absorption of calcium and phosphate from ingested foods.

Processing of Antigenic Substances

Cells in both the epidermis and dermis of the skin play an important role in the immune function of the body. Skin is now recognized not only as a physical barrier but as having an active role in immunologically mediated defense against various antigens. These specialized cells include Langerhans' cells and keratinocytes located in the epidermis, and lymphocytes located in the dermis. An antigen entering immunologically competent skin is likely to encounter a coordinated response of Langerhans' and T cells to neutralize its effect. An antigen entering diseased skin can induce and elicit immune responses. These reactions may be involved in the pathogenesis of many inflammatory skin diseases.

Cosmetic Adornment

Another function of skin, hair, and nails is to provide an outward appearance or "cosmetic adornment." The acceptance of the appearance of a person's skin, hair, and nails is critical to his or her psychosocial well-being. Depending on the situation and the person's perception, this can be a positive or negative experience. Skin disorders frequently are a high source of morbidity because we live in a beauty-conscious society. Healthcare providers must be acutely aware of the role that skin plays in a person's self-esteem and ability to function in relationships.

Effects of Aging on the Integumentary System

The skin undergoes numerous changes that one can see and feel throughout the life span. Many of these changes are natural, unchangeable, and harmless. Other changes may be bothersome or painful and often are treated in a variety of ways until there is acceptable resolution or acceptance of the condition. Other skin changes may go unnoticed and not be bothersome because they are slow-growing, such as senile keratosis.

Adolescence

During puberty, hormone secretion stimulates the maturation of hair follicles, sebaceous glands, and apocrine and eccrine units in certain body areas. Hair follicles on the face (males), pubic region, and axilla activate to produce coarse terminal hairs. Folliculitis (hair follicle inflammation) may occur on the thighs and buttocks. Sebaceous glands on the face, chest, and upper back become functional, and mild acne (inflammation of a pilosebaceous follicle) may occur. As the apocrine glands increase sweat production, perspiration and body odor become noticeable for the first time. These normal changes bother some teenagers. Skin irritation (excessive dryness) may result from excessive application of commercial skin products such as astringents or other products marketed for "oily" skin. Adolescents should be made aware that in many instances these over-the-counter products are often ineffective or more irritating than helpful.

Pigmented nevi, which may be flat or papular lesions, are other noticeable changes that occur during adolescence. The most common nevi are junctional, dermal, and compound nevi. These lesions are benign cluster melanocyte-like cells. The tendency to freckle is genetically inherited. These small, brown, macular lesions appear on sun-exposed areas and are promoted by sun exposure.

New nevi can appear after adolescence. Pigmented lesions that appear much later in life are called lentigo or senile lentigo. At any age, raised, pigmented lesions that bleed or change in color or size should be assessed by a physician. Such a lesion may simply be an irritated nevus requiring minor care or may have early malignant changes, for example, malignant melanoma (see Chapter 78 for discussion of malignant melanoma).

Adulthood

Temporary hormonal changes account for some of the adult skin changes. Pregnancy and birth control pills may change hormonal status and thus skin structures that are hormonally linked. Temporary changes in hair growth patterns and a temporary thinning of hair after pregnancy are common. Melasma is a condition of blotchy hyperpigmentation on the cheeks and forehead, the pathogenesis of which is unknown. Many etiologic factors have been implicated, such as pregnancy, oral contraceptives, and genetics. Melasma disappears after pregnancy, discontinuance of oral contraceptives, or correction of hormonal abnormalities. Hormonal and genetic changes also produce a recognizable male-pattern baldness (alopecia). Family history reveals a balding tendency that passes to subsequent generations. Excessive facial or body hair in women can be an androgen-related problem.

Heredity and exposure to environmental factors such as sun, tobacco, alcohol, and chemicals play a major role in many of the skin changes that occur in adults. Actinic keratosis (slightly raised, red, scaly papules), sebaceous cysts (enclosed cyst in the dermis), and acrochordons or "skin tags" (small flesh-colored papules) commonly occur singly or in combination. Some lesions (i.e., seborrheic keratosis and acrochordons) may be removed for cosmetic reasons, if desired, or if physically irritating. Actinic keratosis and sebaceous cysts need assessment and may be removed (see Chapter 78): actinic keratoses because of their premalignant status, and sebaceous cysts because of their infectious potential.

Older Adulthood

The skin of older people reflects the cumulative influence of environmental insults, decreased circulation, and di-

minished function of a variety of skin structures. As the stratum corneum becomes thinner, the skin reacts more readily to minor changes in humidity, temperature, and other irritants. Dry skin (xerosis) is a common problem due to a decrease in natural skin oils and sweat. Xerosis can range from mild flaking or roughness to severe cracking, itching, and scaling (see discussion of xerotic eczema, Chapter 78). Wrinkles appear with loss of elasticity and subcutaneous fat. Wrinkling is also caused by excessive sun exposure, the effects of gravity, and cigarette smoking. Epidermal thinning makes the skin more transparent in the elderly. Skin tears frequently result because of the epidermal thinning that occurs, especially in those elderly requiring routine use of oral corticosteroids for conditions such as asthma, chronic obstructive pulmonary disease, or connective tissue disease. Small, bright-red domes (cherry angiomas) are created by dilated blood vessels that form loops; these are harmless and often occur on the trunk. Seborrheic keratoses are raised black or brown spots or wartlike growths that look as though they have been pasted on the skin surface. These are common and also an inherited trait; they are not contagious or precancerous and are easily removed if cosmetically bothersome or physically irritating. Hair and nail growth is decreased. Hair loss is often noticeable on the trunk, pubic area, axillae, and limbs. Nails become brittle and may yellow and thicken. Loss of pigment causes gray hair.

Lentigines ("liver spots")—variously sized black or brown, flat lesions—are common. Lentigines may appear anywhere and have nothing to do with the liver. Those on the dorsum of the hand or on the face are probably promoted by prolonged sun exposure. The skin may also have a leathery or coarse appearance from excessive exposure to ultraviolet light. Because there is no known treatment for these lesions, protection from ultraviolet light is the only preventive measure.

Conclusions

The skin is the largest and most visible organ of the body. Anatomically, the skin is divided into three layers: the epidermis (outer layer), dermis (inner layer), and subcutaneous layer. The epidermis is further divided into five layers.

The skin serves many functions. It is the first line of defense against many forms of trauma. Skin maintains body temperature, prevents water loss, and provides sensations of hot, cold, pain, light touch, and pressure. Skin also produces vitamin D and recognizes antigens. Finally, healthy skin is aesthetically pleasing.

Aging is very evident in the skin. The older adult loses subcutaneous fat and elasticity. Wrinkles develop. Older adults can also develop lentigines, seborrheic keratoses, brittle nails, and gray hair due to normal changes in skin function.

Bibliography

1. Arnold, H. L., Odom, R. B., & James, W. D. (1990). *Andrew's diseases of the skin.* Philadelphia: W. B. Saunders.
2. Fitzpatrick, T. B., & Eisen, T. B. (1990). *Dermatology in general medicine.* New York: McGraw-Hill.
3. Jaubovic, H., & Ackerman, A. (1992). Structure and function of the skin. In S. Moschella & H. Hurley (Eds.), *Dermatology* (3rd ed.). Philadelphia: W. B. Saunders.
4. Nicol, N. H. (1994). Alteration of the integument in children. M. K. McCance & S. Huether (Eds.), *Pathophysiology—The biologic basis for disease in adults and children* (2nd ed.; pp. 1561–1577). St. Louis: Mosby–Year Book.
5. Nicol, N. H. (1994). Diseases of epidermal origin. In M. J. Hill (Ed.), *Skin disorders* (pp. 27–38). St. Louis: Mosby–Year Book.
6. Pogue, S. (1995). Vitamin D synthesis in the elderly. *Dermatology Nursing, 1*(2), 103–105.
7. Sams, V. M., & Lynch, P. J. (1990). *Principles and practice of dermatology.* New York: Churchill Livingstone.

CHAPTER 77

Assessment of Clients with Integumentary Disorders

Noreen Heer Nicol

A thorough health history assists in diagnosis of integumentary disorders, such as occupationally related contact dermatitis, or in revealing psychosocial aspects of disease processes. The medication history is important because side effects from certain medications can cause skin changes. The physical examination can confirm integumentary disorders as well as reveal disorders that the client may have omitted during the history.

History

The history includes asking questions about the current symptoms, past health history, medications, allergies, family health history, and psychosocial history, including occupational and travel history, and a review of systems.

Current Symptoms

Chief Complaint

The most common problems related to the integument are itching (pruritus), dryness, rashes, lesions, ecchymoses, lumps, and masses. The nurse asks about changes in the skin, hair, and nails that may be related to the chief complaint. Sample questions that attempt to elicit pertinent information related to the presenting dermatologic problem are listed in Table 77–1. Ask only one question at a time. Remember to pause after each question to give the client time to answer.

Symptom Analysis

A symptom analysis is completed, which includes definition of the problem, onset, location, duration, evolution of the lesion or eruption, aggravating and relieving factors,

medical intervention, self-treatment, and compliance/treatment factors. Sexual history may also be important if differential diagnosis includes a sexually transmitted disease (STD).

Past Health History

Various systemic diseases have cutaneous manifestations. It is important to find out whether the client has other systemic illness relevant to the skin, that is, immunologic, endocrine, collagen, vascular, renal, or hepatic conditions. Information on recent exposure to ticks, other insects, or infectious or childhood diseases is helpful, as is knowing the immunization status. Previous trauma and surgical intervention may give the explanation for unusual lesions or location. History of past allergic reactions to foods or medications is important for avoiding inadvertent reaction through readministration.

Medications

Prescription as well as over-the-counter medications that the client is currently taking or has recently finished should be noted. Sensitivity to antibiotics or other drugs in the form of a drug rash may not occur until the end of a routine course of the drug. Photosensitizing drugs (e.g., phenothiazides, tetracyclines, diuretics, sulfonamides) may cause a sunburn-like rash in areas of sun exposure. Topical preparations may include many preservatives or active ingredients that are known sensitizers. The most commonly encountered are neomycin, ethyl aminobenzoate (benzocaine), and diphenhydramine hydrochloride (Benadryl). Oral corticosteroids (e.g., prednisone), if used at high doses or routinely, can cause acne breakouts, thinning of skin, stretch marks, and many other systemic side effects.

Table 77–1. Dermatologic Assessment History: Sample Questions	
Information Needed	**Questions**
Chief complaint	"Please tell me what brings you here today."
Definition of problem (onset, location)	"Tell me more about the problem. Where did it start? Have you noticed this problem before?"
Duration	"When did it start? Does it come and go? Has it changed? Has it become better or worse?"
Accompanying symptoms	"Did you have any feelings—such as fatigue, nausea, skin tightness, skin burning—before this problem started? Does it itch?"
Evolution of lesion or eruption	"How does it feel now? Are you experiencing any discomfort? Do you feel tenderness, tightness? Does clothing irritate your skin? Do you have any problems sleeping? Does it limit any of your activities? Has it interfered with your normal daily routine?"
Aggravating and relieving factors	"Have you noticed whether the problem worsens after any of these activities: eating particular foods? Using cosmetics? Using soaps? Wearing clothing? Do changes in temperature or climate affect the problem? Does it worsen or improve with changes in season? Are you more comfortable when warm or when cool?"
Medical intervention	"Did you see a physician about this? Were you told what the problem was? Was any treatment recommended? Did it help?"
Self-treatment	"What have you tried to do on your own to get relief? What did you use? What over-the-counter or home remedies have you tried? What do you do yourself that helps the problem?"
Compliance and treatment factors	"How often were you able to apply or take prescribed medication? Were you able to complete prescribed treatment? How did you use the medication? (e.g., How did you apply it? How did you take it? For how long? Why did you stop?)"

Allergies

Ask the client about allergies to medications and foods (see previous discussion under Medications). Does the ingestion of certain foods cause itching, burning, or eruption of rashes? Fresh fruits that have been treated with pesticides or preservatives may also be problematic, as may prepared foods containing preservatives.

Inquire about substances that may cause local skin irritation or lesions on direct contact, such as textiles or metals. Wool is irritating to some people. Jewelry containing nickel may cause skin discoloration, irritation, rash, or other problems in people who are sensitive to this metal.

Family Health History

A family health history helps determine genetic predisposition to skin disorders as well as predisposition to parasitic or other conditions based on the family's life-style and living environment. Many dermatologic disorders or systemic disorders with a dermatologic presentation are passed on genetically to other family members. Genetically transmitted dermatologic conditions include alopecia (loss of patches of hair), ichthyosis, atopic dermatitis, and psoriasis. Systemic diseases with dermatologic manifestations include diabetes mellitus, blood dyscrasia, and collagen vascular diseases (lupus erythematosus).

Other diseases, such as scabies, are likely to be passed on to family members because of close and frequent exposure.

Psychosocial History

Psychosocial factors influencing the dermatologic disorders often play a large role, particularly in long-term and chronic processes. Skin disease can greatly affect life-style and self-image. Cultural and familial influences on how to care for a particular disorder may conflict with prescribed therapies. Misconceptions about skin problems (e.g., acne lesions can be scrubbed away) need to be determined and corrected. Visually or physically disabling chronic skin diseases have been associated with chronic unemployment, poor mental health, and even suicide. Sexual history should be assessed, as it can help alert or explain the presence of tissue trauma or lesions caused by sexually transmitted diseases.

Socioeconomic factors cannot be ignored. Compliance with outlined therapies and return for follow-up care are influenced by social expectations or financial ability to pay for medications or treatments. When recommending desired therapies or medications, consider the impact on the client's day-to-day routine, as well as what type of prescription insurance plan the client has. Many topical therapies, whether covered by insurance or not, are expensive, and expense is a factor that affects compliance.

Occupation and Travel

Occupational history is significant because a large number of skin problems are caused or worsened by exposure to irritants and chemicals in the home and work environment. It is important to understand what the client comes in contact with and to what extent. This could explain situations such as the chronic flaring of hand eczema whenever the client uses certain glues and glazes during a hobby project, the total body rash secondary to chemical mists penetrating nonprotective gear at the work site, or hand rash from latex glove allergies.[18, 20]

Travel history can be helpful. This is especially true if the travel included hiking or exposure to any variety of outdoor wonders that have resulted in dermatologic disorders such as poison ivy, poison sumac, and poison oak, or Lyme disease.

Habits

Inquire about the client's habits. Determine the frequency of hygiene practices, what products are used (e.g., soaps, lotions, abrasives), and whether cosmetics are used. Record products used, including brand names. Ask if there have been any changes in clothing or bedding and discuss how these items are cleaned. Review the client's diet history for intake of sufficient nutrients, such as water; protein; vitamins A, D, E, and C; and dietary fat. Also ask about exercise and sleep patterns, which affect circulation, nourishment, and repair of the skin. Does the client engage in recreational activities that involve prolonged exposure to the sun, unusual cold, or other conditions that may damage the integument? For example, does the client visit tanning salons often? More than 1 million persons/day use tanning salons, and federal regulation of salons is very limited. Nurses may want to advise clients that exposure leads to premature aging, increased risk of skin cancer development, risk of corneal burns if eye guards are not worn, exacerbation of photosensitivity diseases, and increased development of lentigines, or "liver spots."[17]

Review of Systems

A complete history of skin changes is important. The nurse specifically asks about past problems with unusual itching, dryness, lesions, rashes, lumps, ecchymoses, and masses. Has the client had problems with moles or other lesions, especially if they have undergone changes in size, shape, or color? A more complete list of questions for the review of systems appears in Table 11–4.

Physical Examination

Examination of the skin should be done as thoroughly as the examination of any other body organ. It cannot be done properly in the hall or at a quick glance, which is often asked of the dermatologist or the nurse. Inspection, palpation, and olfaction are used to assess hair, nails, and skin. Effective assessment requires knowledge, awareness,

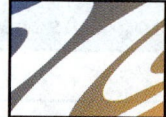

NORMAL PHYSICAL ASSESSMENT FINDINGS

Integumentary System

Inspection

Skin. Even skin tones, darker on exposed areas of face, neck, arms, and lower legs; lighter on trunk and back. Small tan freckles scattered over face and arms. Scars, striae absent.

Hair and Scalp. Hair evenly distributed over scalp. Clean, without nits or lice. No dandruff, scaling, or scalp lesions. Axillae and legs probably shaved; pubic hair distributed as inverted triangle from symphysis pubis to perineum (female). Pubic hair distributed in diamond pattern from below umbilicus to perineum (male).

Nails. Regular, smooth, oval shape. Pink nail beds. Cuticles manicured, clean. Nail bed angle <160° (no clubbing).

Palpation

Skin. Warm, well hydrated, smooth, elastic, nontender. No lesions, masses, or lumps.

Hair and Scalp. Hair non-oily, even-textured, resilient. Scalp smooth, intact, nontender.

Nails. Firm without tenderness or bogginess. Rapid blanch response.

---

and practice in describing skin of individuals of all ages and different life-styles and in recognizing normal and abnormal skin changes. The Normal Physical Assessment Findings feature describes normal conditions of the integumentary system.

Terminology

The terms used in dermatology have frequently been referred to as a foreign language and have been known to inhibit healthcare providers from using the correct terminology for skin disease. Use of standard terminology is important and often leads to differential diagnosis. The intent of this section is to clarify some of the commonly used dermatology terminology and to assist the nurse in recognizing and describing skin disorders. Table 77–2 is a glossary of commonly used dermatologic terms.

Types of Lesions

Examination and diagnosis of skin disorders are dependent on identifying skin lesions or changes. Two major types of lesions are distinguished: *primary* and *secondary* lesions.

Table 77–2. Glossary of Dermatologic Terms

Actinic	Pertaining to ultraviolet light (UVL)
Amelanotic	Without pigment
Circinate (pronounced *sir-sin-ate*)	Circular
Circumscribed	Limited to a certain area by sharply defined border
Coalesce	To merge one with another
Comedo	Plug in a skin duct containing keratin (open, blackhead; closed, whitehead)
Cytotoxic	Toxic to cells
Dermatome	Area of skin supplied by a single dorsal nerve root
Dermatophyte	Fungus that enters the skin's surface, causing infection
Desquamation	Scaling, peeling of epidermis
Discoid	Coinlike
Eczematous	General term for disease process characterized by scaling, weeping, crusting, and inflammation
Erythema	Redness
Exacerbation	Worsening of disease state
Exfoliative	Shedding of skin in fairly large quantities
Folliculitis	Hair follicle inflammation
Guttate	Small, water drop-sized lesions, usually widespread
Hives	Spontaneously occurring wheals
Hyperkeratosis	Thickening of stratum corneum, usually from repeated pressure or friction
Hyperpigmentation	Increased or excessive skin pigmentation (melanin) causing an area of skin to be darker than surrounding areas
Hypopigmentation	Decreased pigmentation
Indurated	Hard (tissue)
Intertrigo	Irritation of body areas with opposing skinfolds that are subject to friction
Lesion	Detectable change from normal skin structure
Maceration	Tissue softening or disintegration from excessive moisture
Milia	Small, white papules
Perioral	Around the mouth
Periungual	Under the nail plate
Pigmentation	Degree of skin or mucous membrane color
Plantar	Pertaining to sole of the foot
Polymorphic	Existing in many forms
Pruritus	Itching
Punctate	Pinpoint or dot-shaped
Sclerosis	Hardening or induration of skin
Sebum	Lipid excretion produced by sebaceous glands
Tautness	Degree of skin tightness
Texture	Tactile or visual skin characteristics, e.g., coarseness, dryness
Ultraviolet light (UVL)	Electromagnetic radiation from the sun (wavelengths 4–400 nm)
Urticaria	Wheals (hives)
Verruca	Lesion characterized by surface roughness, e.g., wart
Wheal	Lesion found in hives

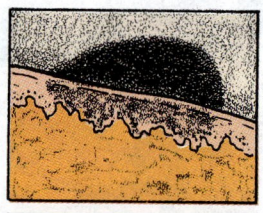

MACULE: Skin color change without elevation, i.e., flat (e.g., freckles or petechia). Described as a "patch" if greater than 1 cm (e.g., vitiligo).

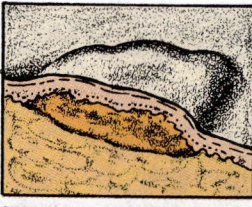

WHEAL (hive): Fleeting skin elevation that is irregularly shaped because of edema (e.g., mosquito bite or urticaria).

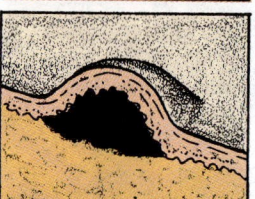

PAPULE: Elevated, solid lesion of less than 1 cm, varying in color (e.g., warts or elevated nevus).

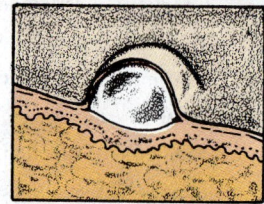

VESICLE (blister): Elevated, sharply defined lesion containing serous fluid. Usually less than 1 cm (e.g., blister, chickenpox, or herpes simplex).

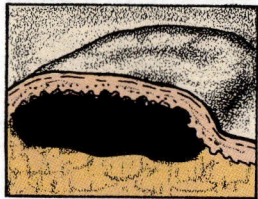

PLAQUE: Raised, flat lesion formed from merging papules or nodules.

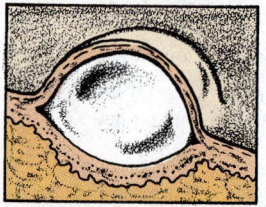

BULLA (plural, *bullae*): Large, elevated, fluid-filled lesion greater than 1 cm (e.g., second-degree burn).

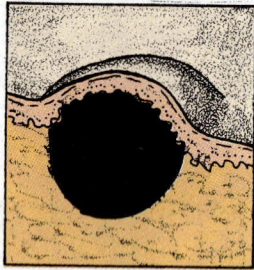

NODULE: Larger than a papule. Raised solid lesion extending deeper into the dermis.

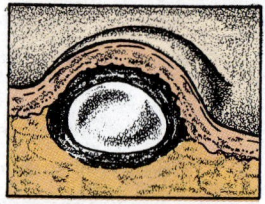

CYST: Elevated, thick-walled lesion containing fluid or semisolid matter.

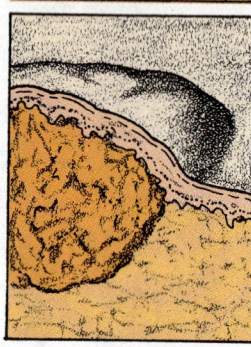

TUMOR: Larger than a nodule. Elevated firm lesion that may or may not be easily demarcated.

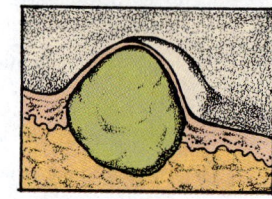

PUSTULE: Elevated lesion less than 1 cm containing purulent material. Lesions larger than 1 cm are described as boils, abscesses, or furuncles (e.g., acne, or impetigo).

Figure 77–1. Primary lesions: visually recognizable structural changes in the skin that have specific characteristics.

The primary lesion is the first lesion to appear on the skin and has a visually recognizable structure. Figure 77–1 describes 10 primary lesions: macule, papule, plaque, nodule, tumor, wheal, vesicle, bulla, cyst, and pustule. Frequently, the healthcare provider will not see a primary lesion and must depend on the client to "describe how it looked when it first appeared."

When changes occur in the primary lesion, it becomes a secondary lesion. These changes may be brought about by the client or the client's environment and often occur in the epidermal layer. These changes may result from many factors including scratching, rubbing, medication, natural disease progression, or processes of involution and healing. Figure 77–2 describes the following secondary lesions: scale, crust, erosion, deep ulcer, scar, lichenification, excoriation, fissure, and atrophy.

Examination Environment

A well-lit, private room with moderate temperature and neutral, white, or cream-colored walls is best for assessment. Excessive warmth can produce changes in skin color (e.g., redness) by causing vasodilation. Colored walls can affect normal skin hue (color). Ask the client to undress for a complete examination; provide a gown. Tell the client that all skin surfaces will be examined. Avoid unnecessary exposure as the examination proceeds.

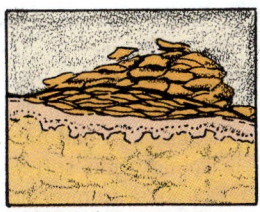

SCALE: Dried fragments of sloughed epidermal cells, irregular in shape and size and white, tan, yellow, or silver in color (e.g., dandruff, dry skin, or psoriasis).

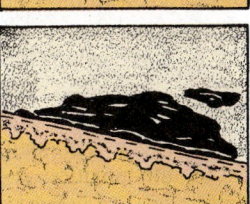

CRUST: Dried serum, sebum, blood, or pus on skin surface producing a temporary barrier to the environment (e.g., impetigo).

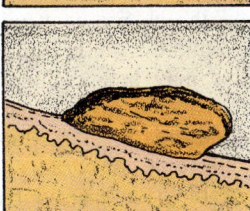

EROSION: A moist, demarcated, depressed area due to loss of partial- or full-thickness epidermis. Basal layer of epidermis remains intact (e.g., ruptured chickenpox vesicle).

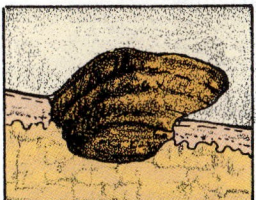

ULCER: Irregularly shaped, exudative, depressed lesion in which entire epidermis and upper layer of dermis are lost. Results from trauma and tissue destruction (e.g., stasis ulcer).

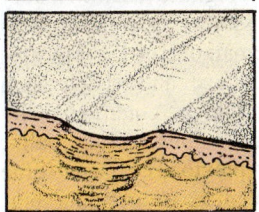

SCAR: Mark left on skin after healing. Replacement of destroyed tissue by fibrous tissue.

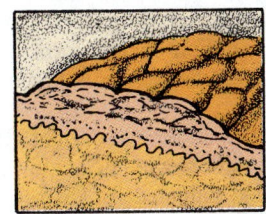

LICHENIFICATION: Epidermal thickening resulting in elevated plaque with accentuated skin markings. Usually results from repeated injury through rubbing or scratching (e.g., chronic atopic dermatitis).

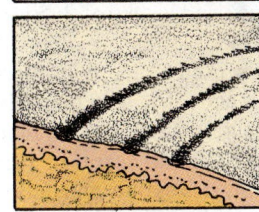

EXCORIATION: Superficial, linear abrasion of epidermis. Visible sign of itching caused by rubbing or scratching (e.g., atopic dermatitis).

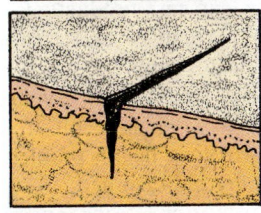

FISSURE: Deep linear split through epidermis into dermis (e.g., tinea pedis).

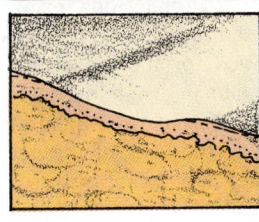

ATROPHY: Wasting of epidermis in which skin appears thin and transparent, or of dermis in which there is a depressed area (e.g., arterial insufficiency).

Figure 77–2. Secondary lesions: primary lesions that have changed because of the natural progression of the lesion or because of physical change (e.g., scratching, irritation, or secondary infection).

The examiner should have warm hands to avoid stimulation of the skin and to add to the overall comfort of the client.

Depth of Examination

Examination is systematic and as complete as appropriate. A total body skin examination includes hair, scalp, nails, mucous membranes, and the skin including the axilla, areas in skin folds, external genitalia, webs between toes and fingers, palms of hands, and soles of feet. Begin at the head and proceed to the toes. General changes can alter total body skin color (e.g., jaundice, cyanosis, pallor), thickness, turgor, temperature, and vascularity (e.g., purpura, petechiae). General findings such as these can suggest systemic disease and may require complete physical examination and appropriate work-up. The diagnosis of skin disease is accomplished by careful observation and work-up of individual lesions. This discussion is limited to assessment of hair, scalp, nails, and skin lesions.

Although you may examine the client's integument over the complete body surface at one time, this usually is not done in the screening examination. Rather, integument assessment is integrated throughout the physical examination as each body region is examined. However, for the purpose of discussion, assessment of the integument is presented as a separate body system. Significant or abnormal findings are commonly reported as part of each regional assessment, rather than separately.

Inspection and Palpation

Hair and Scalp

Hair distribution patterns are examined for symmetry and distribution according to age and sexual development.

Fine hair covers much of the body and is of the same color as scalp hair. Increased distribution occurs normally in the axillae and pubic areas. Excess body hair is known as *hirsutism.*

The hair and scalp are inspected under good light. If the nurse suspects lesions or infestation with lice, gloves are worn. The hair is inspected and palpated for distribution, thickness, texture, lubrication, and signs of infestation or infection. Natural hair color varies greatly (the nurse asks the client if hair dye is used because it alters texture). Hair should be resilient and distributed evenly over the scalp. Individual hair shaft diameter can range from thin and fine to thick and coarse; the shape of hair fibers can be straight, curly, or wavy. Texture and lubrication are affected by the type of hair care products used (e.g., harsh shampoo, curling irons, or hair dryers) as well as by a protein-deficient diet or health problems such as febrile illness, all of which tend to leave hair dry and brittle. Hair loss or thinning *(alopecia)* can result from genetic predisposition to baldness or to a health problem, such as recent chemotherapy or a thyroid disorder.

The *scalp* is inspected and palpated for lesions, excoriations (from scratching), lumps, or bruises, which should be absent. Hair shafts are examined for the presence of nits, which are the eggs of the human head louse *(Pediculus capitis)* and appear as particles of oval dandruff. The areas behind the ears and along the back of the neck are often where adult lice bite the scalp, which results in pustular lesions. It may be difficult to see adult lice on the scalp; they are very small (1 to 2 mm) with gray-white bodies.

If lesions are seen, the nurse describes them and asks the client about recent trauma or injury to the head. If the client has not already provided information during the health history interview, the nurse conducts a symptom analysis.

Nails

Inspect the client's nails for color, shape, texture, integrity, and thickness (Table 77–3). The nails reflect the client's overall health, indicating nutrition and respiratory status. The nail plate is usually transparent and colorless and, when viewed from the side, has a convex *shape.* The vascular bed underlying the nail plate gives the nail its color. In white clients, the *color* is pink, whereas it is darker in dark-skinned clients. A deficiency in hemoglobin is seen in the nail bed as pallor, and decreased arterial circulation appears as cyanosis. Perform a *blanch test* by palpating the nail beds to assess capillary refill. The nail bed is pressed firmly for 5 seconds, then quickly released while the rate of color return to the nail bed is observed. Color return should be immediate within 3 to 5 seconds in healthy individuals. Results of the blanch test should be documented as "rapid" or "sluggish" capillary refill. When palpated, the nail bed feels firm with no softness (i.e., bogginess) or tenderness.

Texture is smooth; healthy nails are of uniform thickness with no signs of dryness, softness, brittleness, splitting, peeling, ridges, or pitting. The *angle* formed between the nail plate and posterior nailfold is approximately 160 degrees without separation. Changes in nail shape and nail bed angle can indicate health problems. Clubbing of the nails is an increase of more than 160 degrees in the angle between the nail plate and nail base. The nail base of a clubbed nail is spongy and soft on palpation. These changes result from hypoxia (diminished tissue oxygenation). Nail clubbing commonly occurs in clients with congenital heart defects or chronic lung disease.

The tissue surrounding the nail should appear intact without signs of inflammation, jagged edges (hangnail), or dryness. Inferior or lateral nailfold inflammation is a sign of paronychia (i.e., nailfold infection). If these abnormalities are noted, the nurse asks the client about nail care habits such as biting or cutting cuticles. While examining the fingers and toes, the nurse may note common abnormalities such as calluses or corns. A *callus* is a flat, painless thickening of a circumscribed area of skin. Calluses usually occur on the hands and feet. A *corn* is a horny induration and thickening of the skin caused by friction and pressure and is often painful.

Skin

■ Color

Overall skin color is assessed during the health history interview. A more thorough assessment is conducted as the nurse proceeds through the remainder of the physical examination. Observe the client's face and visible skin surfaces for color tones, which should be congruent with the client's stated race. Abnormal findings include pallor (paleness), a flushed or ruddy complexion, cyanosis (blue cast), jaundice (yellow cast), and areas of irregular pigmentation. Normal variation occurs from one region of the body to another, particularly in those areas protected from the sun and exposure by clothing; these areas will be lighter. Overall color should be uniform. Skin tone may range over a variety of colors including light ivory to deep brown or blue-black, yellow to olive, or light pink to dark, ruddy pink.

Areas that are less pigmented reveal abnormal findings more readily than do more heavily pigmented surfaces. For example, *pallor* is best seen in the buccal (mouth) mucosa, especially in clients with dark skin. *Cyanosis* is evident more readily in less pigmented areas, such as the nail beds, lips, and palms. *Jaundice* sharply contrasts with the white of the sclera, especially in dark-skinned clients who have more carotene deposits. Jaundice is best assessed in dark-skinned clients by inspecting color changes in the hard palate (see Diversity in Healthcare).

Local areas of color change are examined closely. *Hyperpigmentation* describes areas of increased pigmentation; *hypopigmentation* describes areas of decreased pigmentation. Skin color also results from the circulation supply; an increased blood supply may indicate the redness of inflammation *(rubor),* whereas extreme pallor may be a result of anemia or impeded arterial circulation to the area.

Table 77–3. Assessing the Nails

Assessment Finding	Description	Causes
Normal nail	Nail shape is convex, and nailplate angle is approximately 160 degrees	
Beau's line	Horizontal depression in nail plate; depressions can occur singly or in multiples	Nail growth is disturbed temporarily; related to systemic illness (e.g., infection) or direct injury to the nail root
Splinter hemorrhages	Linear (vertical) red or brown streaks in the nail bed	Minor trauma to the nail bed; subacute bacterial endocarditis; trichinosis
Paronychia	Inflammation of the skinfold at the nail margin	Trauma; skin infection at the nail base
Spoon shape	Nail shape is concave as the nail curves upward from the nail bed	Use of strong detergents; iron deficiency anemia; syphilis
Clubbing	Increased angle between nail plate and nail base	Long-standing hypoxia

■ Moisture

Moisture refers to the skin's hydration level for both wetness and oiliness. Overall skin moisture in healthy individuals can be described as well-hydrated but should not be excessively moist. It often reflects ambient temperature and humidity levels. Moistness usually occurs in intertriginous areas (areas where skin touches skin), such as the axillae and groin. Skin that feels overly moist and cool (i.e., clammy) is abnormal. Skin that is overly dry, scaling, or cracked is also abnormal.

■ Temperature

Temperature is assessed with the dorsum of the hand. The skin should feel uniformly warm, because it reflects

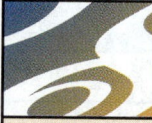

DIVERSITY IN HEALTHCARE

Biocultural Variations in the Integumentary System

To accurately and comprehensively assess the integumentary system of clients from various cultural backgrounds, the nurse must possess knowledge of biocultural variations. The nurse also must develop skill in assessing a wide range of color, temperature, and texture differences in the skin. Knowledge of normal biocultural differences and the ability to recognize the unique clinical manifestations of disease, especially in darkly pigmented clients, is important for providing safe and culturally competent nursing care.

In this box, the reader will learn to identify normal biocultural variations of the integumentary system prevalent in clients from diverse cultural backgrounds and recognize clinical manifestations of systemic and skin disorders with integumentary manifestations in clients from diverse cultures.

Normal Variations

The assessment of a client's integumentary system requires astute observational skills and the ability to recognize both subtle and overt changes in the color, temperature, and texture of skin. With repeated exposure to clients from culturally diverse backgrounds, the nurse's skill with these important assessments increases.

Melanin is responsible for the various skin colors and tones found in all people. Melanin protects the skin against harmful ultraviolet rays and provides a genetic advantage that accounts for the lower incidence of skin cancer among darkly pigmented black and Native American clients. Skin color occurs on a continuum, and color gradations are described by using a range of colors (e.g., ash, gray, light brown, medium brown, dark brown, yellow-brown, tan-brown). Intermarriage may result in a nearly endless combination of color gradations and a mixture or blending of other physical characteristics. It is important for the nurse to describe with accuracy the baseline skin color and to recognize variations that occur in the same individual.[1-6]

Variations in Pigmentation

Pigmentary disturbances are of great concern to clients of all races, but conditions of hypopigmentation and hyperpigmentation may be particularly disconcerting to people with darker pigmentation because pigmentary changes are more obvious and noticeable than in people with lighter skin. The following conditions of hypopigmentation and hyperpigmentation are examined: oral leukoedema, midline hypopigmentation, nail pigmentation, hormonal influences on sex organs, mongolian spots, and chronic low-grade trauma.

Oral leukoedema is characterized by the presence of pearly, whitish gray lesions of the mucosa of the mouth or tongue. The condition is present in 68% to 90% of blacks and 43% of whites, but it is rarely seen in the people of India. Oral leukoedema increases with age in all races and may be associated with oral hygiene and cigarette smoking.[1-4,6]

Midline hypopigmentation is a normal variant characterized by a faint or prominent line or band of macular hypopigmentation in the midsternal area (sometimes extending medially and laterally to the clavicles). Midline hypopigmentation may also appear in the form of discrete oval macules located primarily over the anterior chest and midsternal areas. The lesions also may extend upward to the neck and downward to the abdomen. Midline hypopigmentation occurs most commonly in black males and dark-skinned Latin Americans. It occurs in 70% of children, but this figure drops to less than 40% by the end of the third decade. The history, clinical appearance, age at onset, and lack of any associated symptoms distinguish it from other conditions such as vitiligo, tuberous sclerosis, nevus depigmentosus, and the depigmentation that often follows inflammation.[1-3,6]

Nail pigmentation appears as brown to black longitudinal bands or as diffuse pigmentation of the nail plate that results from increased melanocytosis in the nail matrix. The condition usually occurs bilaterally and increases in frequency with advancing age. The incidence in blacks exceeds 50% and may exceed 90% in heavily pigmented individuals. Care must be exercised to distinguish normal nail pigmentation from abnormal conditions, such as subungual nevi, malignant melanoma, changes secondary to chemicals, drugs, and radiation, and the pigmentation associated with Addison's disease and Peutz-Jeghers syndrome.[2,3,6]

Due to hormonal influences, the *sexual skin areas,* such as the nipples, areola, scrotum, and labia majora, are likely to be hyperpigmented. Among people of all races, in both adults and children, these areas are normally darker than are other parts of the skin. The difference is especially pronounced among clients of black and Asian descent. When assessing these skin surfaces on dark-skinned patients, observe carefully for erythema, rashes, and other abnormalities, because darker pigmentation may mask their presence.

Mongolian spots, irregular areas of deep blue pigmentation, are usually located in the sacral and gluteal areas, but they sometimes occur on the abdomen, thighs, shoulders, or arms. Mongolian spots are a normal variation in children of African, Asian, or Latin descent. By adulthood, the spots become lighter but are frequently still visible. Mongolian spots are present in 90% of blacks, 80% of Asians and Native Americans, and 9% of whites. Nurses unfamiliar with mongolian spots should be careful not to confuse them with bruises. Recognition of this normal variation is particularly important when dealing with children who might be erroneously identified as victims of child abuse.[1-6]

Finally, among the normal biocultural variations found in darkly pigmented clients is hyperpigmentation of the elbows and knees that is often associated with a roughened texture. Elbow and knee hyperpigmentation is seen primarily in black adults and appears to be a reaction to *chronic low-grade trauma.* If elbow and/or knee trauma is severe, gather further data concerning recent falls and accidents to distinguish the condition from more serious musculoskeletal or neurological conditions that may cause the client to lose balance, fall, and sustain injury; and to identify areas for client education

about safety (e.g., environmental hazards in the homes of the elderly, athletic injuries in young adults, and occupational injuries.)[6]

Abnormal Variations

Given that normal pigment distribution patterns in dark-skinned clients may mask some skin color changes associated with disease, nurses are

cautioned against the dangers of misinterpretation. The following symptoms of systemic and skin conditions that nurses sometimes find difficult to assess in dark-skinned clients will be examined: cyanosis, jaundice, pallor, erythema, petechiae, ecchymoses, keloids, pseudofolliculitis, post-inflammatory hypopigmentation and hyperpigmentation, and vitiligo.

Assessment of Cyanosis in Darkly Pigmented Patients

- Examine patient in favorable lighting conditions (e.g., use overbed light or natural sunlight)
- Be attentive to factors that may mask cyanosis by causing vasoconstriction:
    Environmental conditions (e.g., air conditioning, mist tents)
    Patient behaviors (e.g., smoking, medications causing vasoconstriction)
- Be aware that the region around the mouth is often darker in people of Mediterranean descent
- Examine the usual places in which cyanosis is found:
    Lips
    Nail beds
    Circumoral region
    Cheekbones
    Ear lobes
But be aware that darker skin may mask the underlying cyanosis
- When cyanosis is questionable, apply light pressure to create pallor. In cyanosis the tissue color returns slowly by spreading from the periphery to the center. Normally the color returns in less than 1 second, and it returns from below the pallid spot as well as from the periphery.
- Observe for other clinical manifestations of decreased oxygenation of the brain:
    Changes in level of consciousness
    Increased respiratory rate
    Use of accessory muscles of respiration
    Nasal flaring
    Positional changes and other manifestations of respiratory distress
- Cyanosis of an extremity may become more recognizable if the position of the extremity can be changed (from elevated to dependent or vice versa).

Symptoms of Systemic Disorders

Cyanosis is among the more difficult clinical signs to observe in darkly pigmented clients. Because peripheral vasoconstriction can prevent cyanosis even though serious anoxia is present, attention should be given to environmental conditions such as air conditioning, mist tents, and other factors that may lower the room temperature. It is also important to rule out vasoconstriction caused by hypovolemic shock by checking the capillary refill time, which is normally less than 3 sec-

onds. For the client to manifest clinical evidence of cyanosis, the blood must contain 5 g of reduced hemoglobin in 1.5 g of methemoglobin per 100 ml of blood.[1-3]

Dark-skinned Native American and black clients may not have bluish tones to their skin when it is cyanotic; rather, gray tones will be evident when assessing the palms of the hands, soles of the feet, mucous membranes, and sclera. Given that most conditions causing cyanosis also cause decreased oxygenation of the brain, other noncutaneous clinical symptoms, such as

changes in level of consciousness, will be evident. Cyanosis is usually accompanied by increased respiratory rate, use of accessory muscles of respiration, nasal flaring, and other manifestations of respiratory distress. Note that blanching of the skin and capillary refill time can also be helpful in assessment, as can monitoring of blood gas values and hemoglobin levels. Because the circumoral region is normally dark blue in persons of Mediterranean descent, the nurse should be especially observant for subtle color changes.[1-4]

Continued on following page

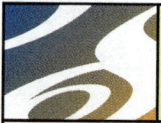

DIVERSITY IN HEALTHCARE *(Continued)*

Biocultural Variations in the Integumentary System

Cyanosis of an extremity may become more recognizable if the position of the extremity can be changed (e.g., from elevated to dependent). When cyanosis is questionable, apply light pressure to create pallor. In cyanosis, the tissue color returns slowly by spreading from the periphery to the center. Normally, the color returns in 1 to 3 seconds, and it appears to return from below the pallid spot and from the periphery.[1–3]

In both light- and dark-skinned patients, *jaundice* is best observed in the sclera. When assessing darkly pigmented clients, caution must be exercised to avoid confusing other forms of pigmentation with jaundice. Many darkly pigmented clients have heavy deposits of subconjunctival fat containing sufficient carotene to mimic jaundice. The fatty deposits become more dense as the distance from the cornea increases. The portion of the sclera that is revealed naturally by the palpebral fissure is the best place to accurately assess color. If the palate does not have heavy melanin pigmentation, jaundice can be detected there in the early stages (i.e., when serum bilirubin is 2 to 4 mg/100 ml). The absence of a yellowish tint to the palate when the sclera are yellow indicates carotene pigmentation of the sclera rather than jaundice. Light or clay-colored stools and dark golden urine often accompany jaundice in both light- and dark-skinned clients.[1–4,6]

Pallor in dark-skinned clients is observable by the absence of the underlying red tones that normally give brown or black skin its luster. The brown-skinned patient will manifest pallor with a more yellowish-brown color, and the black-skinned client will appear ashen or gray. Generalized pallor can be observed in the mucous membranes, lips, and nail beds, and care should be exercised to ensure that lipstick and nail polish have been completely removed. The palpebra conjunctiva and nail beds are preferred sites for assessing the pallor of anemia. When inspecting the conjunctiva, the nurse should lower the eyelid sufficiently to visualize the conjunctiva near the inner and outer canthi. The coloration is often lighter near the inner canthus.[1–3,6]

The pallor of impending shock is accompanied by other subtle manifestations, such as increasing pulse rate, oliguria, apprehension, and restlessness. Anemia, particularly chronic iron deficiency anemia, may be manifested by "spoon" nails, which are concave. A lemon-yellow tint to the face and slightly yellow sclera accompany pernicious anemia, which also is manifested by neurologic deficits and a red, painful tongue. Fatigue, exertional dyspnea, rapid pulse, dizziness, and impaired mental function accompany most severe anemias.[1–3,6]

Erythema is a form of macula characterized by diffuse redness over the skin; it is caused by capillary congestion. Capillary congestion is usually due to dilation of the superficial capillaries. The dilation usually is caused by a nervous mechanism within the body, inflammation, or some exposure to an external stimulus such as heat, sunlight, or cold. The degree of redness is determined by the quantity of blood present in the subpapillary plexus, whereas the warmth of the skin is related to the rate of blood flow through the arteries and veins. In assessing inflammation in dark-skinned clients, it is often necessary to palpate the skin for increased warmth, taut or tightly pulled surfaces that may be indicative of edema, and hardening of deep tissues or blood vessels. When assessing for joint inflammation in dark-skinned clients it is often useful to palpate the joints for warmth, because redness may not be readily apparent. For palpating, the dorsal surface of the fingers is the most sensitive to temperature sensations.[2,3]

The erythema associated with rashes is not always accompanied by noticeable increases in skin temperature. Macular, papular, and vesicular skin lesions are identified by a combination of palpation and inspection, combined with the client's description of symptoms. For example, clients with macular rashes usually complain of itching, and evidence of scratching will be apparent. When the skin is only moderately pigmented, a macular rash may become recognizable if the skin is gently stretched. Stretching the skin decreases the normal red tone, thus providing more contrast and making the macules appear brighter. Some disorders are characterized by generalized rashes that are seen in the mouth on inspection of the palate.[2,3]

The increased redness that accompanies *carbon monoxide poisoning* and the polycythemias can be observed in the lips of dark-skinned clients. Because lipstick masks the actual color of the lips, it should be removed before inspection.

In dark-skinned clients, *petechiae* are best visualized in the areas of lighter melanization, such as the abdomen, buttocks, and volar surface of the forearm. When the skin is black or very dark brown, petechiae cannot be seen in the skin. Most of the diseases that cause bleeding and microembolism formation, such as thrombocytopenia, subacute bacterial endocarditis, and other septicemias, are characterized by the presence of petechiae in the mucous membranes as well as on the skin. Thus, the nurse should inspect for petechiae in the mouth, particularly the buccal mucosa, and in the conjunctiva.[1–4,6]

Ecchymotic lesions caused by systemic disorders are found in the same locations as petechiae, although their larger size makes them more apparent on dark-skinned clients. When differentiating petechiae and ecchymoses from erythema in the mucous membrane, pressure on the tissue momentarily causes blanching of erythematous tissue, but not of petechial or ecchymotic tissue.[1–4,6]

Skin Conditions

Keloids are raised, firm, thickened, red scars that form at the site of a wound. Even relatively minor trauma, such as ear piercing, may result in keloid formation in individuals with the genetic predisposition, particularly black and Asian clients. The tissue response is out of proportion to the amount of scar tissue required for normal repair and healing, and the scar that results is excessively large. Keloids are sharply elevated and irregular and continue to enlarge following trauma. Keloids may be treated by local administration of corticosteroids, and large keloids may need excision followed by steroid injection. Laser therapy has been effective for some individuals.[1-4,6]

Pseudofolliculitis, more popularly known as "razor bumps" or "ingrown hairs," depending on their location, are caused by shaving. The sharp point of the hair, if shaved too closely, enters the skin and induces a foreign-body reaction. The symptoms include papules, pustules, and sometimes even keloids. Although the problem may occur among all races, particularly among people with very curly hair, it is more prevalent among blacks.[2,3]

Several common causes of *postinflammatory hypopigmentation and hyperpigmentation* are acne vulgaris, drug eruptions, dermatitis, impetigo, and tinea versicolor. The pigmentary changes are more noticeable in blacks than in whites.

Vitiligo is an abnormality of the pigment (lack of melanin formation) of unknown cause in which the melanocytes fail to function in some areas of the skin. Vitiligo is characterized by unpigmented skin patches and affects more than 2 million Americans, primarily those with dark skin. Clients with vitiligo also have a statistically higher than normal chance of developing pernicious anemia, diabetes mellitus, and hyperthyroidism. These factors are believed to reflect an underlying genetic abnormality.[1-4]

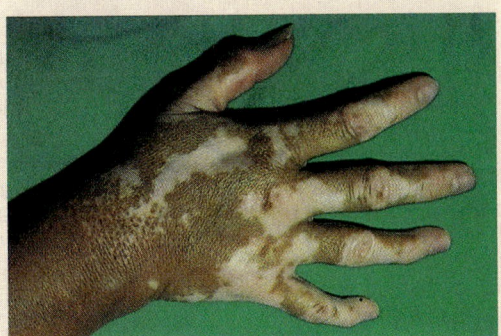

Vitiligo

Conclusions

A few concluding suggestions for better assessing darkly pigmented clients follow:

- When assessing individuals from culturally diverse backgrounds, observe the color, texture, and temperature of the skin and the client's overall behavior. Compare findings with baseline data to determine if, and when, change occurs.
- Be aware of the normal biocultural variations that may be associated with certain groups. For example, blacks commonly have brown freckle-like pigmentation of the gums, buccal mucosa, borders of the tongue, and nail beds; people of Mediterranean descent tend to have deep blue lips; some Asians have a natural yellow-olive color to the skin.
- Be sure that lighting, from either sunlight or artificial sources, is adequate. Flashlights and the soft illumination of many overbed lights provide insufficient light for identifying subtle color change.
- When possible, involve the client (and/or family) in assisting you to distinguish normal from abnormal skin changes. For example, you might remark, "You're looking a little ashen today. How does this compare to your usual skin color?"
- Provide an environment in which the temperature is conducive to physical examination, paying par-

ticular attention to excesses (i.e., too hot or too cold). Observe the location of air conditioning/ventilation ducts to determine their possible impact on the client. Lying on a cold table may cause blanching of the skin of the back, thus masking clinically significant pallor.
- Be aware that emotions, particularly anger and fear, can influence the client and may create temporary but misleading skin changes.
- Edema of the skin reduces the intensity of skin color by increasing the distance between the surface and the pigmented and vascular layers. Consequently, the darkly pigmented skin appears lighter in color. Edema also obscures the pathologic color changes associated with pallor, jaundice, and cyanosis.
- Color changes in both the adult and the child are best observed where pigmentation is most scarce, namely, the sclera, conjunctiva, nail beds, lips, buccal mucosa, tongue, palms, and soles.

The ability to identify normal biocultural variations in the integumentary system is important for the provision of culturally competent nursing care. The nurse must learn to integrate cultural knowledge and skill into the assessment, planning, implementation, and evaluation of nursing care for clients from diverse cultures.

Continued on following page

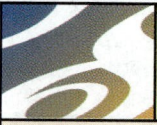

DIVERSITY IN HEALTHCARE *(Continued)*

Biocultural Variations in the Integumentary System

References

1 Andrews, M. M. (1995). Transcultural nursing care. In M. M. Andrews & J. S. Boyle (Eds.). *Transcultural concepts in nursing care* (pp. 49–96). Philadelphia: J. B. Lippincott.

2 Andrews, M. M. (1992). Skin, hair and nails: Transcultural considerations. In C. Jarvis (Ed.). *Physical examination and health assessment* (pp. 227–228). Philadelphia: W. B. Saunders.

3 Overfield, T. (1985). *Biologic variation in health and illness: Race, age and sex differences.* Menlo Park, CA: Addison-Wesley.

4 Giger, J. N., & Davidhizer, R. E. (1995). Biological variations. In J. N. Giger & R. E. Davidhizer (Eds.). *Transcultural nursing: Assessment and intervention* (pp. 127–161). St. Louis: Mosby–Year Book.

5 Leininger, M. M. (1995). Transcultural nursing perspectives; Basic concepts, principles, and culture care incidents. In M. M. Leininger (Ed.). *Transcultural nursing: Concepts, theories, research and practices* (pp. 57–92). New York: McGraw-Hill.

6 McLaurin, C. I. (1988). Cutaneous reaction patterns in blacks. *Dermatologic Clinics, 6*(3), 353–362.

circulation. Compare areas of hypothermia or hyperthermia with the same area on the opposite side.

■ Texture

Palpate texture by stroking the skin lightly with the finger tips. The skin should feel smooth, soft, and resilient. There should be no areas of lumps or unusual thickening or thinning (atrophy).

■ Turgor

Turgor is the skin's elasticity and is measured by the time it takes for the skin and underlying tissue to return to its original contour after being pinched up. Lightly pinch the skin over the forearm between the thumb and index finger, then release it. If the skin remains elevated (i.e., tented) for more than 3 seconds, turgor is decreased. Normal turgor is a return to baseline contour within 3 seconds when the skin is mobile and elastic. Turgor decreases with age as the skin loses elasticity. Assessment of turgor is shown in Chapter 12.

■ Edema

Palpate for edema, particularly if areas of taut, shiny skin are noted on inspection. Edema is the collection of fluid in underlying tissues that separate the skin's surface from pigmented and vascular layers, which results in a blanched appearance. It is an abnormal finding. Edematous areas are palpated for consistency, temperature, shape (i.e., extent), tenderness, and mobility. Press a finger firmly against the edematous area for 5 seconds to assess for *pitting edema,* that is, a residual indentation left by the finger's pressure when the fluid is displaced from the underlying tissue. The depth of pitting is expressed in millimeters or centimeters. Because of a variation in rating scales, it is more accurate for the nurse to state the depth of pitting rather than to rate it. Areas examined for

edema include over the sacrum (especially in bedridden clients), the feet, ankles, and over the tibia on the shins.

■ Tenderness

Tenderness is an abnormal finding and is elicited as the nurse palpates. No areas of tenderness should be found in a healthy, uninjured client.

■ Odor

The skin should be free of pungent odors. Odors, when noted, are usually present in the axillae and skinfolds or in open wounds and are related to the presence of bacteria on the skin, inadequate hygiene, or infection. Assessing odor in open wounds should be done following cleansing of the wound, as odor can be related to the drainage itself or related to the type of dressing used (e.g., hydrocolloid).

■ Lesions

Inspect the skin for detectable lesions. It is important to assess and describe the findings about any lesions in an orderly fashion: location; distribution; size; arrangement; color; configuration; secondary changes; and presence of drainage. Skin lesions are also palpated to determine the characteristics of contour (e.g., flat, raised, or depressed), size (using a measuring device), consistency (e.g., firm, soft), mobility, and tenderness. Lesions can be mobile or immobile (fixed to underlying tissue). Photographing lesions of concern is an excellent way to reliably document changes over time.

Location, Distribution, and Size. Location is described in reference to anatomic landmarks. Measure the lesions for size, because this helps to classify their type (e.g., macule, papule). If multiple lesions are present, the distribution pattern could be helpful in determining the

Table 77–4. Terminology for Skin Lesion Configuration and Distribution

	Description
Configuration*	
Annular	Ring-shaped
Iris	Concentric rings, "bull's eyes"
Gyrate	Spiral-shaped
Linear	Forming a line
Nummular	Coinlike
Polymorphous	Occurring in several forms
Punctate	Marked by points or dots
Serpiginous	Snakelike
Distribution†	
Solitary	Single lesion
Satellite	Single lesion occurring in close proximity to but separate from a large group of lesions
Grouped	Clustered
Confluent	Merged together
Diffuse	Widely distributed
Discrete	Separate from other lesions
Generalized	Diffusely distributed
Localized	Limited, clearly defined
Symmetrical	Bilaterally distributed
Asymmetrical	Unilaterally distributed
Zosteriform	Bandlike distribution of lesions along a dermatome

*Position of lesions relative to other lesions.
†Grouping, or pattern, of lesions over entire skin surface.

diagnosis. Extent of the presence of the lesions is noted. Lesions can be localized (confined to a specific area), regional, or generalized (present over a large surface). Compare sides bilaterally to determine if lesions are symmetrical or asymmetrical. Another commonly noted distribution is on sun-exposed areas. Certain diseases have a classic lesion distribution, such as herpes zoster (following along a nerve root dermatome). Table 77–4 gives other descriptions of common configurations and distributions. Figure 77–3 depicts the locations of common skin disorders found during physical examination.

Arrangement. The arrangement refers to the pattern of nearby lesions. Two of the typical patterns include "linear" and "satellite," which can also be helpful in confirming diagnosis. Linear lesions appear in a straight line (e.g., scabies). Satellite lesions appear as small peripheral lesions around a central larger lesion (e.g., diaper candidiasis).

Color. Skin lesions can assume a wide variety of colors; they may be flesh-colored, brown, red, yellow, tan, or blue. Color can be influenced by many factors, including the client's normal skin color, which may make accurate description difficult. Slight color changes can best be assessed in areas having the least amount of natural pigmentation and those with superficial capillary beds (i.e., buccal membrane of the mouth, mucosa, lips, nail beds, ocular conjunctiva, palms, and soles). These areas are especially important in assessing darkly pigmented skin.

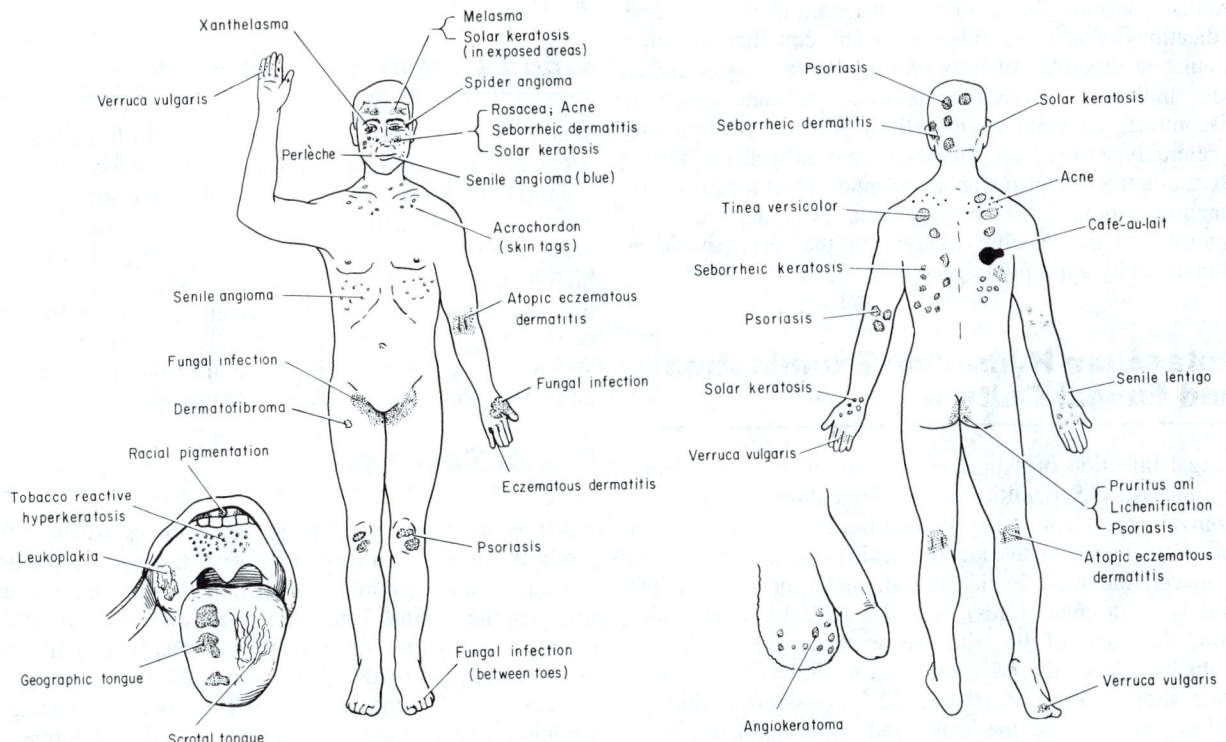

Figure 77–3. Common disorders encountered during physical examination of the skin. (From Fitzpatrick, T. B., et al. [1993]. *Dermatology in general medicine* [4th ed.]. New York: McGraw-Hill.)

Configuration. Configuration refers to the shape or the outline of the lesion. Most lesions are circular. The term *nummular* is used for a circular lesion when it is the diameter of a large coin (i.e., nummular eczema). *Annular* describes lesions found with an active ring-shaped border and some central clearing (e.g., granuloma annulare). Table 77–4 gives the description of other configurations that may be found during assessment.

Skin Self-Examination

Although it is key that all healthcare providers learn to do an accurate and complete assessment of the skin, it is probably more important to teach every individual from childhood how to do a skin self-examination. Routine self-examination greatly lowers individual risk from severe skin disorders, such as skin cancer. Using a full-length or hand mirror, individuals should be taught to examine their entire bodies to look for any changes in the skin. Danger signals in skin lesions to look for are listed in Box 78–1, in Chapter 78. Clients should be taught to visit their healthcare provider for further evaluation of any suspicious-looking lesions.

Diagnostic Tests

Before a diagnostic skin procedure (or treatment), the nurse should perform an assessment and document findings. Nursing intervention for diagnostic procedures includes explaining the procedure to the client and significant others and allowing them to ask questions and express concerns. Teach them appropriate wound care and indications of possible side effects and complications that should be reported, such as prolonged bleeding or infection (indicated by swelling, redness, drainage, increased discomfort, temperature elevation). Provide instructions (preferably written) for follow-up care as well as follow-up appointment and telephone number. Documentation of diagnostic procedures (exactly what was done and by whom) and the specific location of the lesion must be completed by appropriate personnel.

Potassium Hydroxide Examination and Fungal Culture

Fungal infection of skin, hair, or nails may be confirmed by microscopic identification and/or culture of scrapings from the area. Any scaly dermatitis may be scraped for this test. Typical sites are the scalp, intertriginous areas (between the toes, axillae, groin, under or between the breasts, abdominal folds), and the nailfold. Fine scales from the edge of the site are scraped with a No. 15 scalpel blade or the edge of a glass slide onto a second glass slide. A drop of 10% to 20% potassium hydroxide (KOH) is added to the scale, and a coverslip is placed over the specimen. Gentle pressure is applied to the coverslip to flatten the scales. The slide may be gently heated

to dissolve the keratin or the cells more quickly. The scrapings are examined under the microscope. For a culture, scrapings from a suspicious lesion are obtained and implanted onto the appropriate culture medium. For a nail culture, an altered, dystrophic nail is snipped and implanted into the medium. Debris from the nail's subungual area is less suitable for culturing.

Tzanck's Smear

Tzanck's smear is the microscopic assessment of fluids and cells from vesicles or bullae. The presence of multinucleated giant cells establishes a diagnosis of viral infection, such as herpes simplex or herpes zoster. An intact, recently evolved vesicle's top is removed and its base is scraped with a scalpel or small curet. The debris is smeared onto a slide, which is properly identified and sent for cytologic assessment.

Scabies Scraping

The test for scabies is most accurate when a papule that has not been scratched is chosen. The most difficult part of this procedure is finding the proper lesion from which to take the specimen, and it often requires preparation of several areas. When visible, a linear burrow is sampled to look for the mite or its eggs or feces. The best method is to shave off the top of the lesion with a No. 15 scalpel blade. The shavings are placed on a microscope slide, covered with immersion oil and a coverslip, and examined under low power on the microscope. Local anesthesia is not necessary, and fine bleeding should be expected. Some discomfort will occur when the lesion is opened.

Wood's Light Examination

Wood's light examination is assessment with a high-pressure mercury lamp that transmits long-wave ultraviolet light (UVA; 360 nm); it has several diagnostic uses. For example, it (1) detects superficial fungal and bacterial skin infections, (2) delineates pigmentary disorders by highlighting the degree of contrast between lesions and normal skin color, and (3) accentuates the contrast between hypopigmented and totally amelanotic areas. Wood's light ("black light") examination is done in a darkened room. The procedure is painless.

Patch Testing

Patch testing is done to attempt to identify substances that produce allergic skin responses. This testing is a painless procedure that requires a skilled evaluator to read and interpret the results. Patch testing is often done to differentiate between an *irritant* contact dermatitis and an *allergic* contact dermatitis. Small amounts of various substances or allergens are applied to the skin using a commercially prepared tape containing the allergens, or allergens are placed on aluminum discs placed on a special tape. The client and significant others need to understand that whereas potential allergic substances (allergens) can produce inflammatory skin reactions, compounds of low concentration are used to prevent possible excessive irritation. Patch testing should not be performed if acute dermatitis is present. The potential allergen could worsen the dermatitis. The tape must be worn for 48 hours without disturbing the patches; then it is removed. Interpretations are made at 48, 72, and/or 96 hours and sometimes at 1 week. An eczematous response at the test site with erythema, papules, or small vesicles indicates a positive reaction and confirms an allergic contact sensitivity to the substance on the disc.

Biopsy

Skin biopsy is the removal of a skin tissue specimen for histologic (cellular microscopic) assessment. There are three types: shave, dermal punch, and surgical excision. In all three procedures, local anesthesia is used, and small-gauge needles (26- to 30-gauge) are recommended to limit trauma to the skin. Clean or sterile technique as appropriate should be used in dealing with the biopsy site. Depending on size, location, and skill of the practitioner, a biopsy is usually a quick and almost painless procedure. The most common source of pain is the initial local anesthetic administration. The specimen is placed in a preservative such as formalin solution, properly identified, and sent for pathologic assessment.

Procedures

Shave Biopsy. A shave biopsy is performed to obtain tissue for analysis from possibly malignant epidermal growths, except potential melanoma (Fig. 77–4A). After skin cleansing and infiltration of local anesthesia, tissue is removed with a lateral motion by use of a scalpel with a No. 15 blade. Alternatively, a specimen can be obtained by snipping with curved tissue scissors. Tissue removed includes the epidermis and upper portions of the dermal layers. Hemostasis of the biopsy site is obtained by applying pressure, by using ferric subsulfate (Monsel's solu-

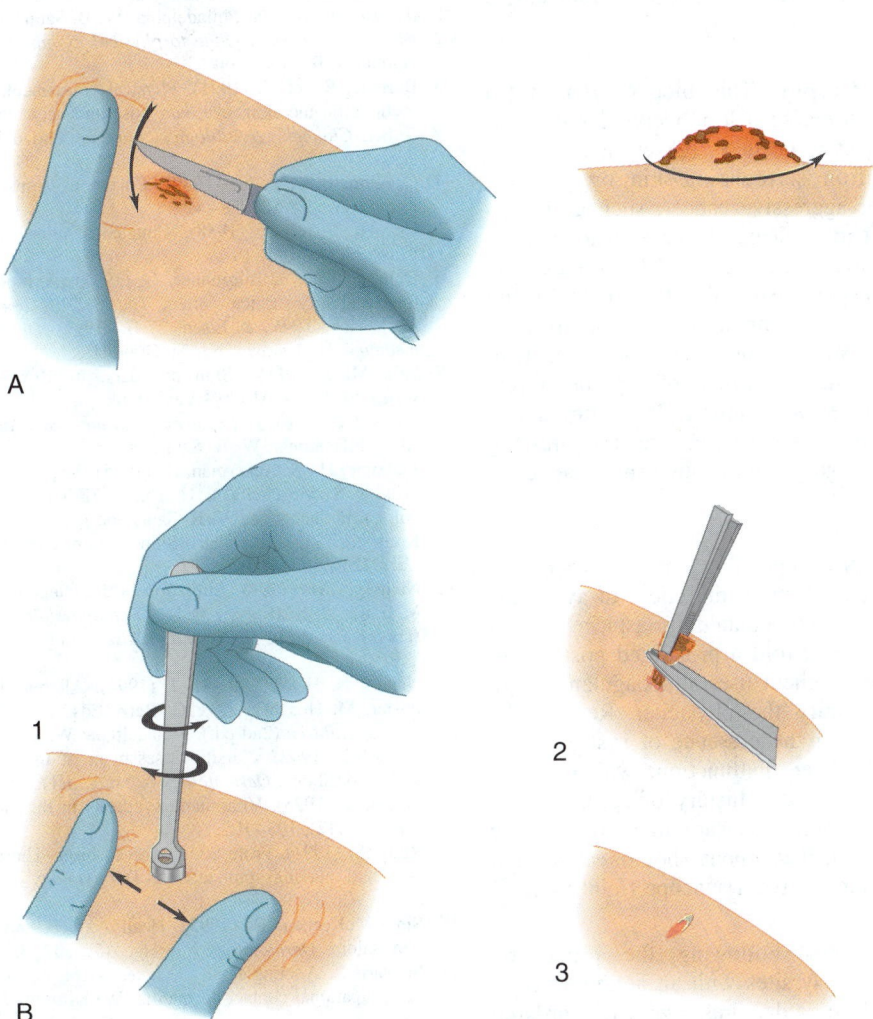

Figure 77–4. Skin biopsies. *A*, Shave biopsy: a tissue specimen is obtained by use of a scalpel (No. 15 blade) in a horizontal-lateral motion. *B*, Punch biopsy: a tissue specimen is obtained with the instrument pressed down firmly on the skin. The specimen is freed from surrounding tissue by a rotary back-and-forth cutting motion; the specimen base is severed with tissue scissors.

tion) or aluminum chloride solution, or by electrodesiccation (cautery).

Punch Biopsy. A dermal punch biopsy uses a circular instrument with a sharp cutting edge to remove a specimen of skin that includes epidermal, dermal, and subcutaneous tissue. This method is used for biopsy of a well-developed, mature lesion (Fig. 77–4*B*). An appropriate size of punch biopsy is chosen (from 2 to 6 mm). The skin site is cleaned, and a local anesthetic is injected. Skin surrounding the lesion is stretched taut and the punch is pressed firmly downward into the skin site. The instrument is rotated back-and-forth in a cutting motion that frees the lesion from surrounding tissue. The specimen is then gently grasped with a tissue forceps or needle, and its base is severed with scissors or a scalpel blade. Depending on the size of the biopsy, hemostasis can be achieved with pressure or application of ferric subsulfate (Monsel's solution) or aluminum chloride solution. The oval defect may be closed with a 4–0 or 5–0 silk or nylon suture to produce a linear scar. Sutures are removed after about 7 to 14 days (with facial biopsies, 3 to 5 days).

Surgical Excision Biopsy. This biopsy is used (1) when it is necessary to excise a lesion completely (e.g., when full skin thickness is needed), (2) when a lesion's borders are indistinct from surrounding skin, or (3) when there is a recurrent or aggressive cancer, such as malignant melanoma. The site is cleansed, the excisional lines are marked with a gentian violet pen, and local anesthetic is administered. The lesion is excised with a scalpel using one of a variety of surgical techniques; a commonly used one is an elliptical incision. Hemostasis is achieved with pressure and ligation (suturing closed) of superficial vessels. The incision is closed with sutures. The suture site is rinsed with saline-dampened gauze. A pressure dressing of sterile nonadhering gauze is applied and taped in place.

Preprocedure Care. Depending on the size of the excision, the nurse should instruct the client to avoid the use of aspirin and products containing aspirin for 48 hours before the biopsy to avoid a prolonged post-procedure bleeding time. If the client uses anticoagulants (e.g., heparin or warfarin), notify the physician. Review the client's medical history for the presence of systemic disease problems such as liver malfunction, which affects clotting time. If the client has a history of cardiac valve replacement, the nurse should be sure that prophylactic antibiotics are prescribed. The client should eat a light meal before the procedure to avoid syncope (fainting).

Postprocedure Care. Following the procedure, cover the majority of biopsy sites with an antibiotic ointment and a clean bandage or dry dressing, unless ordered otherwise. Many non-adhesive types of dressings are available and may be preferable for clients who have fragile or sensitive skin. Remind the client that follow-up assessment is necessary and plan a follow-up appointment for suture removal. Tell the client how and when biopsy results will be reported. Be aware that individuals will have different levels of anxiety about the biopsy results depending on the anticipated possible outcome (e.g., melanoma vs. wart).

Conclusions

Although the skin is the largest organ in the body, it is often taken for granted. The skin protects us from the sun and many dangerous elements, and helps fight diseases and infections. The top layers of healthy skin have the ability to regenerate and repair themselves every 3 to 4 weeks. Skin must be handled with care to maintain its many functions.

Bibliography

1. Arnold, H. L., Odom, R. B., & James, W. D. (1990). *Andrew's diseases of the skin.* Philadelphia: W. B. Saunders.
2. Bates, B. (1995). *A guide to physical examination.* (6th ed.). Philadelphia: J. B. Lippincott.
3. Burrage, R., et al. (1991). Physical assessment. An overview with sections on the skin, eye, ear, nose and neck. In W. Chenitz, et al. (Eds.), *Clinical gerontological nursing.* Philadelphia: W. B. Saunders.
4. Caughman, S., et al. (1989). Cutaneous signs of internal cancer. *Patient Care, 23*(2), 28–41.
5. Chapel, T., et al. (1988). Cutaneous signs of infection. *Patient Care, 22*(13), 185–197.
6. Dellasega, C., & Burgunder, C. (1991). Perioperative nursing care for the elderly surgical patient. *Todays OR Nurse, 13*(6), 12–17.
7. Fitzpatrick, T. B., & Eisen, T. B. (1992). *Dermatology in general medicine.* Hightstown, NJ: McGraw-Hill.
8. Hill, M. J. (1994). Skin disorders. In *Mosby's clinical nursing series.* St. Louis: Mosby–Year Book.
9. Jarvis, C. (1996). *Physical examination and health assessment* (2nd ed.). Philadelphia: W. B. Saunders.
10. Jaubovic, H., & Ackerman, A. (1985). Structure and function of the skin. In S. Moschella & H. Hurley (Eds.), *Dermatology* (2nd ed., vol. 1). Philadelphia: W. B. Saunders.
11. Kreisberg, S., et al. (1989). Skin signs of endocrine disease. *Patient Care, 23*(6), 73–86.
12. Nichol, N. H. (1994). Alteration in the integument in children. In J. McCance & S. Huetner (Eds.), *Pathophysiology—The biologic basics for disease in adults and children* (2nd ed.). St. Louis: Mosby–Year Book.
13. Nichol, N. H., & Hill, M. J. (1994). Altered skin integrity. In R. Foster, M. Hunsberger, & C. Betz (Eds.), *Family-centered nursing care of children* (2nd ed.). Philadelphia: W. B. Saunders.
14. Pogue, S. (1992). Nursing assessment of the elderly for dermatologic procedures. *Dermatology Nursing, 4*(1), 15–23.
15. Pogue, S. (1995). Vitamin D synthesis in the elderly. *Dermatology Nursing, 7*(2), 103–105.
16. Rudy, S. (1991). From conception to birth: The development of the skin and nursing implications. *Dermatology Nursing, 3*(6), 381–392.
17. Sinni-McKeehen, B. (1995). Health effects and regulation of tanning salons. *Dermatology Nursing, 7*(5), 307–312.
18. Stewart, L. A., Engleken, G. J., & Nicol, N. H. (1992). Essentials of occupational contact dermatitis. *Dermatology Nursing, 4*(3), 175–183.
19. Swartz, S. M., & Sherertz, E. F. (1993). The technique of patch testing: Role of the office staff. *Dermatology Nursing, 5*(2), 133–137, 144.
20. Truscott, W., & Roley, L. (1995). Glove-associated reactions: Addressing an increasing concern. *Dermatology Nursing, 7*(5), 283–292.

Nursing Care of Clients with Integumentary Disorders

Noreen Heer Nicol

General Principles of Dermatologic Nursing

Many effective treatments are available for skin problems. Some are specific to certain conditions. The following treatments are directed at skin cellular metabolism:

1. Altering skin temperature
2. Reducing or increasing blood flow
3. Adapting delivery of oxygen to and from skin tissue
4. Altering inflammatory responses
5. Adapting absorption of toxins and mediators.

Dermatologic therapies include the following:

1. Topical medications
2. Wound dressings
3. Soaks and wet wraps
4. Skin lubricants
5. Ultraviolet light (UVL) therapy.

Topical Medications

Topical Therapy

The skin's large surface area allows the absorption, penetration, and permeation of topically applied preparations. The factors that determine how well these processes occur include the patient's age, skin region, pathologic changes of the stratum corneum, cutaneous blood supply, and the vehicle of the topical medication. (The word *vehicle* is used here to mean the substance containing the medication or the form in which the medication is delivered.)

Topical therapy can be used to do the following:

1. Restore hydration
2. Alleviate symptoms
3. Reduce inflammation
4. Protect the skin
5. Reduce scale and callus

6. Cleanse and debride
7. Eradicate causative organisms.

Topical medications are chosen both for the action of the active ingredients (which are delivered directly to the skin surface) and for the vehicle. Topical medications have many different actions and cover a large spectrum of drug categories, including antibacterial, antifungal, antiparasitic and antipruritic (Table 78–1).

Topical Vehicles

Examples of various topical medication vehicles (Table 78–2) include ointments, creams, gels, aerosols, lotions, and powders. Ointments are more occlusive and therefore provide better delivery of the medication by preventing water loss from the skin. However, in some cases, especially periods of excessive heat or humidity, this occlusion may result in increased itching or skin infection; in these situations, creams may be better tolerated. Although creams spread more easily, they are less occlusive, and may produce increased drying in some persons. Sprays and lotions are available for use on the scalp and other hairy areas. The various ingredients used to formulate the different bases may be irritating to individuals, and care must be taken in recommending any product.

Both the active ingredient and the vehicle must be appropriate for the condition being treated. For acute dermatosis (i.e., weeping, blistering lesions), an aqueous (water-based) compound provides a drying effect. A greasy vehicle has the opposite effect: it promotes lubrication and occlusion and helps treat the dryness and scaling caused by chronic dermatosis. Differences in skin permeability also influence the effectiveness of topical medications. For example, absorption is increased in inflamed skin. Depending on the medication and the specific condition, topical medication may be applied to localized lesions or to larger skin surfaces. When increased absorption of the medication is needed, topical medication may be prescribed for application under an occlusive

Table 78–1. Dermatologic Topical Therapies

Category	Example	Action	Nursing Intervention
Acne products that are not purely anti-bacterials	Benzoyl peroxide (Benzagel, component of Benzamycin, Desquam, Panoxyl, Xerac) BP5, Xerac BP10)	Keratolytic Bacteriostatic Decreases production of irritant-free fatty acids in follicle	Applied once or twice a day after washing area Observe for dryness or redness
	Tretinoin (Retin-A)	Vitamin A acid Decreases cohesiveness of epithelial cells, causes desquamation	Applied once daily at bedtime, 20 min after washing area Instruct client to expect some redness and peeling within a week, lasting 3–4 wk Flare up of acne may occur in first 2–4 wks before improvement Clearing of acne requires 2–3 mo Avoid excessive sun exposure, and use sunscreen daily Keep agent away from eyes
Antibacterials	Bacitracin ointment Polysporin ointment	Increases cell wall permeability Interferes with metabolism	Clean skin of adherent crust and debris before application Apply 2–3 times daily, as prescribed
	Topical Erythromycin (T-Stat, Erycette, component of Benzamycin) Clindamycin (Cleocin-T) Mupirocin (Bactroban)	Anti-inflammatory	Observe for redness, itching, or burning
Antifungals	*Topical* Nystatin (Mycostatin) Clotrimazole (Lotrimin) Oxiconazole (Oxistat) Naftifine (Naftin)	Alters cell wall permeability	A 2- to 3-wk course of twice-daily application is necessary for adequate treatment Overapplication can irritate sensitive, damaged skin
Antimetabolites	5-Fluorouracil (Efudex, Fluoroplex)	Interferes with DNA synthesis Inhibits thymidylate synthetase activity Effective in treating large areas of sun-damaged skin having premalignant or malignant lesions, e.g., basal cell epithelioma	Apply medication with gloved hand, avoiding mucous membranes and eyes Teach the client expected response to the medication, e.g., a brisk inflammatory response with burning and itching Advise client to avoid sun exposure, which can increase the intensity of reaction
Scabicides Pediculicides	Lindane (for scabies and pediculosis) Pyrethrin (for scabies)	Absorbed through the exoskeleton of the arthropod, causing seizures and death of the organism	Be certain to treat webs of fingers and toes Avoid getting in eyes Observe for signs of re-infestation Observe for side effects (e.g., rash, redness, itching, burning, tingling) Full course of therapy needs to be completed Wash clothing in hot water or dry clean Seal clothing that cannot be washed or dry-cleaned in plastic for 30–35 days All sexual contacts must also be treated
Antipruritics	*Lotions/Pastes* Phenol (0.5%–2%) Menthol (0.1%–2%)	Antihistaminic effect, blocking histamine and serotonin effects	Apply frequently to reduce discomfort

Category	Example	Action	Nursing Intervention
	Camphor (1%–3%) Calamine lotion Baths, cornstarch Colloidal oatmeal (Aveeno)	Cool and soothe skin	Avoid the eyes If it contains anesthetic ingredient, apply as prescribed (2–4 times daily)
	Wet Dressings Potassium permanganate (1:4000–1:16,000) Aluminum acetate Burow solution (1:10–1:40) Boric acid (1 tbsp in 1 L of water) Normal saline (2 tsp salt in 1 L of water) Magnesium sulfate (8 tsp in 1 L of water)	Cool and soothe Some germicidal activity	Assess for contact sensitivity Use caution when entering and exiting tub; most solutions are slippery Protect linens from stains with wet dressings
Antiseptics	Chlorhexidine gluconate-alcohol (Hibiclens)	Effective against staphylococci, streptococci, and gram-positive bacteria	Use for irrigating and cleaning wounds, but not for packing, because it may cause dermatitis
	Acetic acid (0.25%) solution	Effective against *Pseudomonas*	Protect healthy skin with a layer of petrolatum, because it excoriates the skin
	Hydrogen peroxide (3%)	Destroys necrotic tissues	Use to irrigate and clean necrotic tissues from wounds Inhibits tissue formation, so avoid use in healing wounds
Corticosteroids (listed from lower to higher potency)	Hydrocortisone (Hytone) Desonide (DesOwen) Alclometasone (Aclovate) Triamcinolone (Kenalog) Fluocinolone (Synalar) Mometasone (Elocon) Halcinonide (Halog) Betamethasone (Diprosone) Diflorasone (Psorcon) Clobetasol (Ternovate)	Vasoconstrictive Antimitotic effect Anti-inflammatory *Note:* Potent corticosteroids should be avoided in treating face, neck, and intertriginous sites because increased side effects may occur	Apply in even amounts Monitor length of prescribed topical administration to avoid long-term side effects Use with care in clients with systemic bacterial, fungal, or viral infections May be applied to hydrated skin or with occlusive dressings to increase penetration
Dressings	Hydrocolloid gel (DuoDerm) Transparent film dressings (Tegasorb, Opsite) Zinc oxide in Unna boot	Create moist wound environment; provide bacterial barrier; encourage autolytic debridement; reduce pain; absorb wound exudate; provide cooling effect; become or are adhesive	All dressings should be used according to manufacturer's direction
Emollients, protectants	Petroleum jelly (Vaseline) Aquaphor ointment Eucerin creme Vanicream Neutrogena emulsion	Emollients provide a temporary barrier, protecting and softening skin Protectants cover skin and alleviate irritation	Apply evenly and smoothly; most useful when applied immediately after bathing Reapplication is required to provide protection when product has been absorbed or has worn off
Keratolytics	Salicylic acid (DuoFilm, Occlusal, component of Ionil shampoo, T/Sal shampoo, component of Meted shampoo, Keralyt gel) Lactic acid (Lacti Care lotion)	Soften keratin and loosen cornified epithelium of the stratum corneum Debride excessive scale Used in varying concentrations to treat conditions ranging from dry, ichthyotic scalps or skin to warts	Apply only to involved area; can produce irritation and erythema in normal skin If prescribed for scale debridement, discontinue as soon as scale disappears If erythema and irritation occur, seek physician's approval to reduce frequency of use

Table 78–1. Dermatologic Topical Therapies *(Continued)*

Table continued on following page

Table 78–1. Dermatologic Topical Therapies (Continued)

Category	Example	Action	Nursing Intervention
Sunscreens	Para-aminobenzoic acid (PABA) PABA esters Cinnamates Salicylates Anthranilates Benzophenone	Provide protection through absorption, reflection, and scattering of ultraviolet radiation	Apply liberally 30 min to 1 h before sun exposure Reapply after swimming or sweating or with prolonged ultraviolet exposure
Tars	*Coal Tar Products* PsoriGel T-Derm Estar gel	Keratolytic Keratoplastic Photosensitizing Antipruritic	May be applied locally to specific lesions or widely to skin Do not apply to face or intertriginous sites Explain drug's photosensitizing properties to client

Table 78–2. Topical Medication Vehicles

Category	Example	Action	Use	Nursing Implications
Powders	Talc, cornstarch	Leaves a film of powder May absorb fluid	Intertriginous dermatitis	Dry surface before applying to prevent caking; reapply often
Lotions Suspension-based	Calamine lotion	Leaves a thin film of powder as water evaporates	Pruritus	Shake lotions well before applying Observe for overdrying of skin Apply in long, even strokes along direction of hair growth
Solutions	Salicylic acid	Leaves a film of powder as alcohol base evaporates	Warts	Shake well before applying; observe for skin overdrying and dry, tight skin due to alcohol Apply as above
Aerosols	Triamcinolone acetonide aerosol	Leaves a thin film after alcohol evaporates	Pruritus, when direct application is painful	Shake well before applying; prevent inhalation by turning client's face to the side
Gels	Fluocinonide gel	Promotes drying of the skin	Eczema Pruritic rash	Observe for skin drying; avoid application to open skin areas (it burns)
Creams	Hydrocortisone cream	Leaves medication on skin after evaporation	Pruritus Eczema	Apply in thin layer along direction of hair growth Use during daytime Need to be reapplied often because perspiration or drainage may remove them
Ointments Water-in-oil	Eucerin	Lubricates skin	Xerosis Dermatitis	Removable with soap and water
Absorbent	Aquaphor	Lubricates skin	Xerosis, dermatitis	Difficult to remove; may feel greasy
Water-repellent	Petrolatum	Promotes absorption of water and medication	Xerosis, dermatitis	Retains heat, difficult to remove; observe for maceration; avoid use in hair-bearing areas

Table 78–3. Occlusive Dressings	
Purpose/Desired Effect	**Nursing Implications**
Produces airtight barrier, usually with plastic film Enhances absorption of topically applied medication (e.g., corticosteroids, keratolytics) by preventing evaporation Increases stratum corneum rehydration Softens hyperkeratotic areas by moisture retention	Clean skin site of debris and "old" medication before applying prescribed topical medication Apply topical medication while skin is still damp Apply plastic film (Saran wrap) snugly Use plastic bags for feet, polyethylene gloves for hands, plastic shower caps for scalp Press air out; seal borders with paper tape Leave dressing intact for 2–12 hr (as prescribed); then remove and gently clean the site Observe and document complications, e.g., maceration, oozing, signs of secondary fungal or bacterial infection, and folliculitis When occlusive dressings are used in conjunction with topical corticosteroids, frequent, prolonged use can result in permanent skin changes; these include striae, nonhealing ulcerations, telangiectases, erythema, and skin atrophy

dressing (Table 78–3). Ointments, creams, and gels have greatly increased absorption if they are applied to skin that is wet.

Topical Corticosteroids

Corticosteroids are among the most commonly used topical medications. Topical corticosteroids reduce inflammation by relieving itching, reducing blood flow by vasoconstriction, which reduces redness of the skin due to capillary dilation (erythema), and interfering with the action of many inflammatory cells. A large selection of topical steroids, ranging in potency from low to high, is available today. Low-potency topical steroids are now available in over-the-counter (e.g., hydrocortisone, 0.5% and 1.0%) and in prescription strength (e.g., desonide). Generally, low-potency steroids are safe to use for longer periods of time and even on thin-skinned areas like the face, groin, or underarms. Prolonged use should still be monitored. Medium- (e.g., triamcinolone or fluocinolone) to high-potency (e.g., halcinonide or fluocinonide) corticosteroids should be used with caution and for short periods of time and not on the face, groin, or underarms. High- or superhigh-potency (e.g., betamethasone dipropionate or clobetasol) steroids should be reserved for use on very acute or resistant dermatoses, areas with thick plaque such as psoriasis, or on areas with poor medication delivery, as in severe lower extremity stasis dermatitis where absorption is poor because of edema and poor blood supply. Clients should be told the strength of the topical steroid they are given and its potential side effects. The lowest-potency corticosteroid that is effective should be used. Side effects are more likely with prolonged use of medium- to high-potency topical corticosteroids. The most common side effect is skin atrophy, which presents as thin, shiny skin with increased prominence of blood vessels, which can be very fragile.

Clients must clearly understand how, when, and where to use topical steroids. Properly applying the medication

evenly and sparingly one or two times daily to the affected areas can eliminate many potential problems. It is rarely helpful to apply the topical corticosteroid more than twice a day. This increases the chance of side effects, makes the therapy more costly, and does not usually increase effectiveness. As the skin disorder improves, the frequency of use may be changed or a less potent topical corticosteroid prescribed. The condition can recur if treatment is stopped abruptly. When the skin disease disappears or comes under good control, a tar preparation, moisturizer, or other topical preparation may be substituted for the topical steroid.

Wound Dressings

Wound dressings allow control of the affected skin's environment and remain important in the treatment of wounds, ulcers, and recalcitrant dermatitis. Historically, the primary role of wound dressings has been protection. Today, their role is to create an environment that promotes healing (see Table 78–3). Dressings limit the exposure of injured skin to dirt, mechanical trauma, and irritants. Ulcers and denuded skin heal more quickly when kept damp by an occlusive or semiocclusive dressing because regenerating epithelium migrates more easily across a moist surface. These wounds are less painful when kept damp, and enhanced absorption of topical medications will occur.

The clinician is challenged to understand the properties of the hundreds of wound care dressings on the market. Wound dressing materials include film, hydrocolloid, hydrogel, foam, alginates, and gauze, among others. Opsite and Tegaderm are examples of transparent film dressings used for intravenous (IV) sites or superficial wounds with little drainage. The hydrocolloid dressings (e.g., Duo-Derm) are used for abrasions, blood donor sites, minor burns, or chronic wounds that have small-to-moderate amounts of drainage. Hydrogel dressings are calcium alginate dressings that are used to loosely pack a deeper wound that is heavily draining. Snug dressings, such as elastic wraps over the lower legs, effectively reduce edema and decrease healing time in stasis ulcers.

Finally, Unna boot, a dressing designed to be removed only by medical personnel at a later visit, can be extremely useful for treatment of stasis ulcers that have venous insufficiency or when there is a concern about client compliance, scratching, or even self-injury. Unna boot is a fixed, protective dressing that stimulates granulation tissue and restores epithelial growth. Dressings impregnated with zinc oxide paste, glycerin, and gelatin harden into a castlike dressing after application. Thus, the skin is protected from mechanical injury, and venous return is promoted. With use of warm water, the damaged skin surface is gently irrigated for removal of previous medication and debris. The damaged skin area is then measured and assessed. Prescribed topical agents (i.e., antibiotic ointments) may be applied. Next, starting at the dorsum of the foot, the dressing is applied. It is wrapped obliquely over the heel and up the calf. The greatest pressure is applied at the ankle and the lower third of the leg. The boot is completed just below the popliteal space. A layer of tube gauze is applied over the dressing. For additional support, an elastic bandage is secured appropriately with tape. Unna boot is removed weekly for assessing damaged skin and cleaning normal skin.

Ideally with all wound dressings, the area of damaged skin decreases, granulation tissue forms, and signs of inflammation are reduced. Treatment may continue for weeks until improvement occurs. It is important to instruct the client and family to keep the dressing intact and that they need to notify their healthcare provider if there is excessive drainage or localized pain (signs of infection). Routine follow-up is very important in wound care.

Soaks and Wet Wraps

Soaks can be done in a variety of ways and serve several purposes. Moisture softens dry epidermis and aids in removal of crusts. Removal of cellular skin debris promotes healing and improves absorption of topical medication. The risk of infection is reduced by the removal of necrotic tissue and occlusive crusts. Cooling also results from the gradual evaporation of water and acts as an antiinflammatory, thus relieving itching.

Soaks can be accomplished by either soaking the affected area or bathing for 15 to 20 minutes in warm—not hot—tap water. The agent added to the soaks is the least important aspect of this therapy. Addition of substances such as colloidal oatmeal (Aveeno) or starch to the bath water may be soothing to some people, but does nothing to increase water absorption. Coal tar preparations (Balnetar, T/Derm) have an anti-inflammatory effect and can be helpful in some eczematous and psoriatic conditions. Aluminum acetate (Burow solution), aluminum sulfate—calcium acetate (Dŏmeboro), and povidone-iodine (Betadine) are also effective antibacterial substances but additionally have drying effects. Bath oils are not recommended because they give the client a false sense of lubrication and make the bathtub very slippery. Clients leaving the bath should remove excess water by

gently patting with a soft towel. They should immediately apply the recommended occlusive substance. Immediate application of the occlusive substance to the damp skin is the most important detail, because if the skin is not occluded within 3 to 5 minutes, evaporation will begin to occur.

Wet wraps used immediately after soaking and occlusion can optimize hydration and topical therapy; this also promotes cooling of the skin. Wet wraps and occlusion can be done in a variety of ways. The location and severity of lesions often determine the choices. Total-body wet wraps can be accomplished by putting on wet pajamas or wet long underwear followed by dry pajamas or a dry or plastic sweat suit. The hands and feet can be covered by wet tube socks or wet cotton gloves followed by dry tube socks. Any extremity or the trunk can be covered by wet Kerlix gauze and occluded with elastic bandages or by pieces of tube socks, wet followed by dry. The face can be wrapped with two layers of wet Kerlix gauze followed by two layers of dry Kerlix gauze held in place with Spandex netting or other tubular dressings; holes are cut out for eyes, nose, and mouth. If the dressing becomes dry, it should be rewetted before removal because debridement by the wet-to-dry method produces tissue damage and pain. Gentle debridement usually still occurs if dressings are removed when damp.

Skin Lubricants

Agents to hydrate the skin play an important role in many xerotic, pruritic, and inflammatory skin disorders. Measures to prevent skin dryness include elimination of irritating or drying compounds, which may include soaps and solvents, and use of cleansing agents and moisturizers. Moisturizers may be classified as occlusive, emollient, and humectant.

Occlusive preparations are extremely effective when applied to damp skin because they prevent evaporative water loss and replace oils in the stratum corneum. The primary means of correcting dryness is to add water to the skin by bathing and then apply an occlusive substance to retain the absorbed water. To seal in the water, use occlusives such as white petrolatum (Vaseline) or petrolatum with mineral oil, wax, and wool wax alcohol (Aquaphor ointment). Occlusives are greasy and may be cosmetically undesirable to some.

Emollients contain fatty acids, oil, and other agents that soften and soothe the skin. Clients often prefer these cosmetically elegant products because they are formulated into lotions that can be poured from bottles and rubbed into the skin without leaving a greasy residue. Although the chemicals in these lotions provide benefit, the water loss continues. There are many emollients available in the form of lotions and creams. Lotions and creams may be irritating and drying because of the evaporative property of water and the substances used as preservatives, solubilizers, and fragrances. Lotions contain more water than creams do and thus evaporate more quickly.

If emollient products are not successful, it may be necessary to try more potent agents. Humectants are substances such as urea (Aquacare 10%, Carmol 20%) that attract and hold water, which results in transepidermal water migration. The alphahydroxy acids (AHAs) have again become very popular and effective additives; these hold moisture and reduce the rough scale that creates the sensation of dryness. The AHAs are naturally derived organic acids and include citric acid, glycolic acid, malic acid, and tartaric acid. Also popular with clients are additives such as aloe, vitamin E, jojoba, elastin, and collagen; however, no scientific evidence has shown that these have special, intrinsic properties beyond their minimal lubricating effects.

Ultraviolet Light Therapy

Artificially reproduced forms of ultraviolet light (UVL) are used therapeutically with topical or systemic photosensitizing drugs to cause desquamation (shedding or peeling of epidermis). UVL also temporarily suppresses mitosis of the basal cell layer by inhibiting DNA mitosis. Ultraviolet A (UVA) and ultraviolet B (UVB) are used to treat diseases responsive to UVL, such as psoriasis, vitiligo, cutaneous T-cell lymphoma, uremic pruritus, and chronic eczematous eruptions. Currently, three treatment modalities involve UVL: (1) UVA; (2) UVB, and Goeckerman and modified Goeckerman treatment; and (3) photochemotherapy or PUVA (psoralen plus UVA).

Every client must have a complete history and physical examination before initiation of any UVL therapy. Record the highlights of the client's history; take care to include the complete medication history because the client could be taking one or more of the many photosensitizing drugs (i.e., thiazide diuretics, tetracyclines). Clients should also be asked specifically about previous herpes simplex infections because these can be stimulated by UVL. Pretreatment assessment includes identifying solar-induced skin malignancies, cataracts, or lupus erythematosus. Clients with a history of basal cell or squamous cell epitheliomas are at risk of developing additional neoplastic changes with this treatment. Thus, potential benefit is weighed against potential risk. A complete ophthalmologic examination is important before treatment is started and yearly thereafter during long-term treatment. A history of cataract formation is a potential contraindication to PUVA therapy. Anyone showing early cataract changes needs extra photoprotective measures (e.g., the complete occlusion provided by goggles or PUVA glasses) and more frequent ophthalmologic assessments (every 3–6 months). The skin changes of clients with lupus erythematosus are aggravated by sun exposure, so phototherapy is contraindicated. Before therapy is initiated, an antinuclear antibody (ANA) test should rule out this condition when suspected.

Be aware that because treatments to the face and genitalia increase the risk of a cumulative effect of UVL, minimal exposure is indicated. Periodic assessments must be done throughout the course of therapy for signs of actinic damage (e.g., severe wrinkling, "tissue paper" transparency) or cutaneous malignancy. Post-therapy clients must be observed for potential side effects including dry skin, pruritus, and potential delayed (36–48 hours after exposure) phototoxic reaction (such as erythema,

vesicles, and pain). All phototherapy should be administered by qualified, and well-trained dermatologic staff.

Ultraviolet B Therapy

Ultraviolet B therapy requires no oral medications and is usually the first choice of UVL therapy before moving on to PUVA. Types of UVB therapy include plain UVB treatment, UVB with topical tar and topical anthralin (known as the Ingram method) or UVB with topical tar (referred to as the Goeckerman treatment or regimen).

One of the most common types of UVB therapy is the Goeckerman regimen and variants of it. This method uses the photosensitizing, keratoplastic, and antipruritic properties of topical tar preparations in conjunction with UVL in UVB wavelengths. It is often used to treat psoriasis vulgaris and atopic dermatitis. The procedure includes a therapeutic tar emulsion bath followed by an application of topical tar medication (e.g., crude coal tar in petrolatum). Several hours later, a specific dose of UVL is administered to the skin surface. If the client's condition is severe, hospitalization or daily care in an ambulatory or day-care setting may be necessary for this treatment. Outpatient phototherapy combined with treatment baths and tar applications at home can be helpful for those with less severe involvement.

Photochemotherapy

Photochemotherapy or PUVA combines oral or topical 8-methoxypsoralen with UVA. PUVA is used to treat severe, unresponsive forms of psoriaris, atopic dermatitis, cutaneous T-cell lymphoma, and alopecia areata or vitiligo. The potent systemic photosensitizing medications increase skin sensitivity to long wave UVL (UVA). In conjunction with exposure to artificially reproduced forms of UVA (PUVA therapy), these medications induce repigmentation (melanin production) in vitiligo and have an antimitotic effect in psoriasis and cutaneous T-cell lymphoma. Dosage is determined by body weight. The medication in taken orally with food to minimize nausea 1½ to 2 hours before UVL irradiation. Topical medication is used to treat localized sites and in clients in whom systemic administration is contraindicated (such as clients with liver or renal disease).

Clients taking these photosensitizing medications must protect the skin from ambient UVL irradiation before and for 8 hours after taking the medication. The client should (1) wear protective clothing, such as long sleeves, (2) apply sunscreen to exposed skin, (3) minimize natural skin exposure, and (4) wear dark-green or brown plastic sunglasses that are capable of screening both UVA and UVB to protect the eyes for 48 hours after taking the medication.

Combination Therapies

There are many combination therapies being used in phototherapy units across the United States. These include PUVA and various topical medications, PUVA and retinoid therapy (RE-PUVA), PUVA and methotrexate, PUVA and cyclosporine, PUVA and UVB, UVB and retinoids, and UVB and methotrexate. The indication for combination therapy is to accelerate clearing of lesions and reduce the total cumulative dose of UVL. These therapies should be done under protocol and by highly qualified dermatologic staff.

Psychosocial Aspects of Skin Disorders

Anger, frustration, and anxiety are commonly experienced by clients with skin disorders, which often exacerbates the condition. Clients with underlying skin disease are more likely to respond to stress, frustration, embarrassment, or any emotionally upsetting event with itching and scratching. Excitability and arousal of the central nervous system from an emotional upset can intensify the vasomotor and sweat responses in the skin and lead to the itch-scratch cycle (see Pruritus). In some instances, scratching is used as an expression of anger, because typically it will get an immediate response from those nearby. The added dimension of family hostility, rejection, and guilt can damage the family structure.

Learning about the acute or chronic nature of the given disorder, the exacerbating factors, and the management measures that can control it is important for both the client and family members. Maintaining a healthy outlook is important. Counseling and other psychosocial interventions are often very helpful in dealing with the frustrations of skin disease. It is especially helpful to adolescents and young adults, who may consider the lesions disfiguring or unattractive.

The client education needs of those affected by skin disease are vast. Healthcare providers need to consistently provide information that includes detailed skin care plans, general disease information, and availability of client-oriented support organizations as well as updates on encouraging research results. Most clients will forget or confuse the important skin care recommendations without written instructions. Clearly outlining the skin care recommendations to the client orally and in writing is essential for good outcomes. The Client Education Guide provides information about skin self-examination. Nurses play the major role in providing this important aspect of care. Adequate time and client teaching materials are needed to provide education effectively. Be resourceful in obtaining or writing educational materials and instruction sheets. Client education pamphlets are available through a variety of sources, including the many dermatologically oriented client support groups, professional dermatology agencies such as the Dermatology Nurses' Association, and the American Academy of Dermatology.

Common Skin Disorders

Pruritus

Pruritus (itching) is one of the most common manifestations of skin problems; it is a symptom, not a disease.

Pruritus has been defined as an unpleasant skin sensation, producing a strong desire to scratch, localized to or generalized over a body area. It can lead to damage if scratching injures the skin's protective barrier, possibly with resultant infection and scarring. Relieving this symptom, especially for chronically ill clients, is a nursing challenge because of its common occurrence and the major effect it may have on a person's quality of life.

Pruritus can be a secondary symptom of conditions ranging from dry skin to carcinoma. Systemic diseases that can cause generalized and severe pruritus include chickenpox, severe liver disease, diabetes mellitus, uremia due to chronic renal failure, drug hypersensitivities, intestinal parasites, and neoplastic conditions (i.e., leukemia and lymphoma).

Stimulation of itching can be initiated by almost any chemical or physical substance, especially if skin is damaged. Once the itch sensation is established, the client has an almost uncontrollable urge to scratch. Scratching leads to further skin damage and increased inflammation. Pruritus therefore increases, and so does the urge to scratch. Thus, the *itch-scratch-itch cycle* develops. In order to minimize skin trauma caused by scratching, fingernails should be kept short.

The client will usually volunteer subjective reports of the degree and location of itching. Listen carefully to the client's description of the severity and location of pruritus and seek information about how pruritus interferes with activities of daily living. Objective signs include excoriations or other secondary skin changes such as lichenification. Document all assessment findings.

Appropriate management of itching requires a complete assessment that attempts to discover the underlying cause and knowledge of appropriate therapeutic modalities for treatment.

Dry skin may either be the source of or contribute to pruritus, and it is often helpful to employ good hydration (see Xerotic Eczema) in addition to any other topical therapy. One bath or shower per day for 15 to 20 minutes with warm water and a mild soap should be immediately followed by the application of an emollient, with or without other topical medications, to prevent evaporation of water from the hydrated epidermis. Other topical medications often added to emollients to help alleviate itching include menthol (0.25%–0.5%), camphor (0.25%–0.50%), urea (10%–20%), and lactic acid (12%). Camphor and menthol produce a cooling effect. Topically applied antihistamines and anesthetics are relatively ineffective and are best avoided because they can be potent allergic sensitizers. This is especially true if these products are used on inflamed skin. Use of topical corticosteroids should be reserved for the treatment of a specific steroid-responsive dermatosis. Long-term application of topical steroids, especially on skin not affected with an eczematous condition, may result in thinning of the skin, striae, telangiectasias, and easy bruising.

Systemic antihistaminics may be prescribed. They are most helpful in disorders in which histamine is the principal mediator but may be of benefit through a sedative or even placebo effect. A trial of an H_1-blocker antihistaminic (hydroxyzine, diphenhydramine, chlorpheniramine) is appropriate either on a regular schedule or as indicated

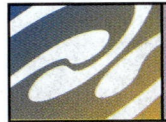

CLIENT EDUCATION GUIDE

Skin Self-Examination

You will need a bright light; a full-length mirror; a hand mirror; two chairs or stools; a blow dryer; body maps; a pencil. Examine your face, especially the nose, lips, mouth, and ears—front and back. Use one or both mirrors to get a clear view. Thoroughly inspect your scalp, using a blow dryer and mirror to expose each section to view. Get a friend or family member to help, if you can. Check your hands carefully: palms and backs, between the fingers and under the fingernails. Continue up the wrists to examine both the front and back of your forearms. Standing in front of the full-length mirror, begin at the elbows and scan all sides of your upper arms. Do not forget the underarms. Next focus on the neck, chest, and torso. Women should lift breasts to view the underside. With your back to the full-length mirror, use the hand mirror to inspect the back of your neck, shoulders, upper back, and any part of the back of your upper arms you could not view previously. Still using both mirrors, scan your lower back, buttocks, and backs of both legs. Sit down; prop each leg in turn on the other stool or chair. Use the hand mirror to examine the genitals. Check front and sides of both legs, thigh to shin; ankles, tops of feet, between toes, and under toenails. Examine soles of feet and heels.

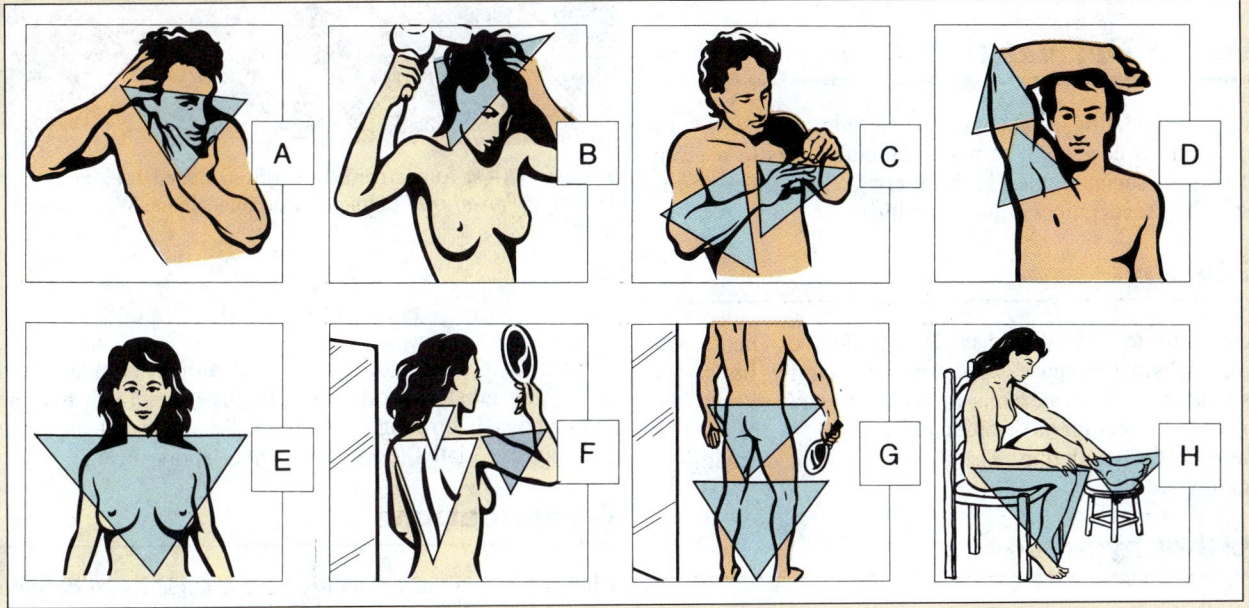

From The Skin Cancer Foundation (1992). *Skin cancer. If you can spot it, you can stop it.* New York: Author.

for itching. Tricyclic antidepressants (doxepin hydrochloride, amitriptyline hydrochloride) have a high binding capacity for histamine H_1 receptors and may be helpful to clients who would benefit from their antidepressant as well as antipruritic effect.

Elderly clients often have difficulty in following through with frequent bathing or showering because of decreased mobility. In this situation, when hydration cannot precede the application of moisturizers, more frequent application and use of more hydrating products may be needed. Additionally, the elderly may have difficulty applying the needed topicals properly, and assistive personnel may be required to offer the client proper therapy. Antihistaminics should be administered carefully with use of small doses initially because many elderly people have

a very low tolerance and may experience severe drowsiness, especially at the initiation of therapy.

Eczematous Disorders

Eczema is not a specific disease. Dermatitis and eczema are terms that may be used interchangeably to describe a group of disorders with a characteristic appearance. A few examples of eczema or dermatitis (and abbreviated definitions) include allergic contact dermatitis (eruptions from allergy to poison ivy, sumac, or oak or proven allergen); irritant dermatitis (eruption from direct contact with cosmetics, chemicals, dyes, or detergents); nummular eczema (appearance of coin-shaped, oozing, crusting patches); seborrheic dermatitis (yellowish-pink scaling of scalp, face, and trunk); stasis dermatitis (eruption resulting from peripheral venous disorders); and atopic dermatitis (characteristic distribution of eczema in persons with a family history of an allergic disorder). Eczema/dermatitis has three primary stages; eczema may manifest in any one of the three stages, or the three stages may coexist.

Acute dermatitis is characterized by extensive erosions with serous exudate or by intensely pruritic, erythematous papules and vesicles on a background of erythema. *Subacute dermatitis* is characterized by erythematous, excoriated, scaling papules or plaques that are either grouped or scattered over erythematous skin. Often, the scaling is so fine and diffuse that the skin acquires a silvery sheen. *Chronic dermatitis* is characterized by thickened skin and increased skin marking secondary to rubbing and scratching (lichenification); excoriated papules, fibrotic papules, and nodules (prurigo nodularis); and postinflammatory hyper- and hypopigmentation.

Atopic Dermatitis

Atopic dermatitis is a common, chronic, relapsing, pruritic type of eczema. The word "atopic" refers to a group of three associated allergic disorders: asthma, allergic rhinitis (hay fever), and atopic dermatitis.

Etiology

According to several studies, 75% to 80% of clients with atopic dermatitis have a personal or family history of asthma, hay fever, eczema, or food allergies. Atopic dermatitis is a common disorder affecting 0.5% to 1.0% of the world's population. The cause of atopic dermatitis is unknown.

Pathophysiology

Compared with normal skin, the dry skin of atopic dermatitis has a reduced water-binding capacity, a higher transepidermal water loss, and a decreased water content.[73] Water loss leads to further drying and cracking of the skin, which leads to more itching. Rubbing and scratching of itchy skin are responsible for many of the clinical changes seen in the skin.

Clinical Manifestations and Diagnostic Findings

Atopic dermatitis begins in many clients during infancy. The dermatitis is usually acute dermatitis, and the child has a red, oozing, crusting rash. As the child grows, the skin tends to show the chronic form of dermatitis, with thickened dry texture, brownish-gray color, and scales. The rash tends to become localized to the large folds of the extremities as the client becomes older. (Fig. 78–1). It is found mainly on elbow bends, backs of knees, the neck, eyelids, and the backs of hands and feet. Hand and foot dermatitis becomes a significant problem in some adults.

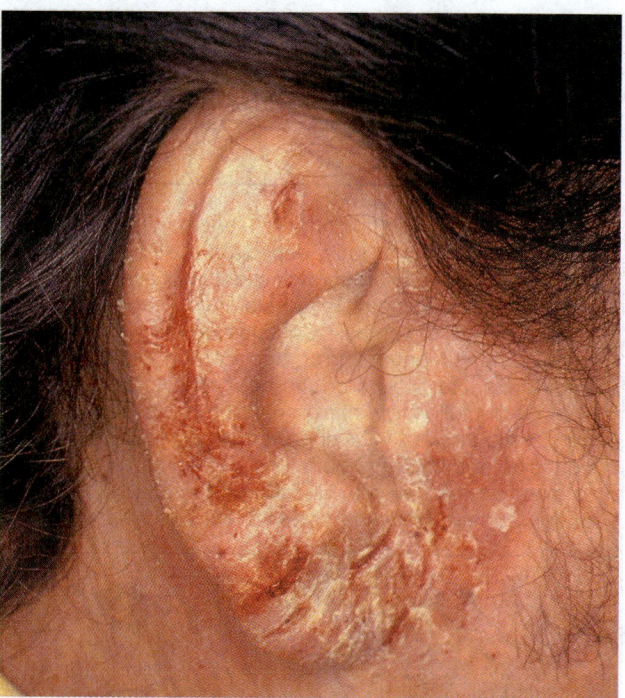

Figure 78–1. Atopic dermatitis. (From Callen J. P., et al. [1993]. *Color atlas of dermatology.* Philadelphia: W. B. Saunders.)

Pruritus is the major symptom of atopic dermatitis and causes the greatest morbidity. The urge to scratch may be mild and self-limiting, or it may be intense, leading to severely excoriated lesions, infection, and scarring.

Complications

Clients with atopic dermatitis have a tendency to develop viral, bacterial, and fungal skin infections. It is not clear whether these cutaneous infections arise secondary to a disruption of normal barrier function or reduced local immunity. The most common viral infection is herpes simplex, which tends to spread locally or become generalized. Honey-colored crusting, extensive serous weeping, folliculitis, pyoderma, and furunculosis indicate bacterial infection usually secondary to *Staphylococcus aureus* in clients with atopic dermatitis. Clients with atopic dermatitis are frequently heavily colonized with *S. aureus*. Superficial fungal infections may also appear more frequently.

Community and Self-Care

■ Medical Management

The goal of therapy is to break the inflammatory cycles that cause excess drying and cracking as well as the itching and scratching. Primary prevention begins with daily skin care that hydrates and lubricates the skin. The healthcare team's understanding of each client's disease pattern and the discovery and reduction of exacerbating factors are crucial to effective management of this chronic disorder. Other factors that must be considered include irritants, allergens, physical environment, and emotional stresses.

Hydration is the key to management but is often difficult to achieve. Soaks followed by application of occlusive substances is usually prescribed (see Soaks and Wet Wraps).

Allergens, food, and aeroallergens may be inciting factors in this disorder. Clients should avoid exposure to allergens to which there is both a positive test finding and for which a high degree of suspicion exists that dermatitis is precipitated by them. Stringent restrictions on clients are unjustified. Air conditioning may help reduce aeroallergen exposure at home and in the workplace. It is important to attempt to identify and eliminate triggers that cause the atopic dermatitis to flare. Many of these triggering factors are the same irritants that contribute to generalized pruritus (see Pruritus).

Dietary management of atopic dermatitis has continued to be a controversial subject. Food allergies in the causation of atopic dermatitis seem to be more significant in certain populations of young children and infants. The most common allergens that appear to be important are eggs, cow's milk, soy, wheat, nuts, and fish. Known allergens are avoided. Persons with food allergies must be taught to read labels and where to find cookbooks to assist in food preparation. Care must be taken to avoid malnutrition when any type of restrictive diet is used.

Occlusives, emollients, topical corticosteroids, and tar preparations can all be used topically in various combinations to control atopic dermatitis. Topical steroids are a very important component of therapy in treating eczema (see Topical Corticosteroids). These preparations are best absorbed into hydrated skin or by using wet wraps and occlusion. Topicals containing chemicals or drugs that could cause skin eruptions themselves are avoided.

Systemic medications may include antibiotics and antihistaminics. The use of a systemic corticosteroid is rarely warranted in atopic dermatitis. Some people view the systemic use of steroids as a "quick cure" and find them much easier to use than hydration and topical therapy. They should be avoided in this chronic non-life-threatening disorder. Although there may be dramatic improvement with their use, the recurrence of dermatitis after their discontinuation is equally dramatic. The side effects of long-term systemic steroid use are both unpleasant and dangerous.

If a short-term course of oral steroid therapy is given, it is important to taper the dosage as it is discontinued. Intensified skin care should also be instituted during the taper to suppress flaring of the dermatitis.

Recent research has suggested a variety of new therapeutic approaches. There are promising results with the use of the new immune response modifiers thymopentin and interferon-γ for therapy of severe atopic dermatitis as well as with etretinate and other experimental modalities. Clients with severe, recalcitrant disease should be made aware of research advances and encouraged to participate in trials, when possible, to give them a sense of hope.

■ Nursing Management of the Medical Client

The client with atopic dermatitis should be assessed for present bathing habits, use of moisturizers, present medication regimen, exposure to known allergens, environmental exposure and history of skin eruptions.

Nursing management of the client with atopic dermatitis is presented in the Care Plan.

■ Modifications for Elderly Clients

Dermatitis is a common skin disorder in the elderly. It may be caused by venous insufficiency, allergens, irritants, or underlying malignancy such as leukemia or lymphoma. Because elderly people often take many medications, dermatitis from drug-drug interaction is considered. The fragility of the skin as a result of the flattened epidermal-dermal junction and loss of dermis should be considered in planning any form of treatment.

Xerotic Eczema

Xerotic (dry) skin is dehydrated, and may present as erythematous, scaling, and finely cracked skin. Xerosis occurs in patches and may involve any skin surface. It is common in elderly people. If xerosis is severe, the skin is tight, itchy, and painful. Water loss causes xerotic chapping. The problem may be accentuated by use of drying skin cleansers, soaps, disinfectants, and solvents and infrequent use of moisturizers.

Environmental factors play a large role, especially those that increase water loss in the stratum corneum. Any factors that decrease the relative humidity exacerbate this condition, such as cold or dry winter air, especially in artificially heated rooms.

The treatment of xerotic skin consists primarily of use of hydration and moisturizers and avoidance of irritating factors. Teaching the client correct daily skin care is essential to treating this condition. See earlier discussion.

Stasis Dermatitis

Stasis dermatitis is the development of areas of very dry skin and sometimes shallow ulcers on the lower legs primarily due to venous insufficiency. The process of dermatitis begins with edema of the leg due to slowed venous return. The client commonly has a history of varicose veins or deep vein thrombosis. As the venous stasis continues, the tissue becomes hypoxic from inadequate blood supply. As the blood pools, hemoglobin is released from the red blood cell and is deposited in the tissues. This poorly nourished tissue begins to necrose. The clinical manifestations include itching, a feeling of heaviness in the legs, brown-stained skin, and open shallow lesions (Fig. 78–2). The lesions are very slow to heal because of the lack of oxygenated blood.

The legs need improved venous return. This can be accomplished with leg elevation, wearing support hose or elastic wraps daily, and refraining from crossing the legs. Clients should be instructed to raise the legs during the

CARE PLAN

The Client with Atopic Dermatitis

Nursing Diagnosis. Impaired Skin Integrity related to skin dryness

Planning: Expected Outcomes. The client will maintain skin that has good hydration and reduced inflammation, as evidenced by

■ Verbalizing increased skin comfort
■ Decreased flaking and scaling
■ Decreased redness
■ Decreased excoriations from scratching
■ Healing of previous areas of breakdown

Implementation: Nursing Intervention	Rationales
Bathe at least once every day for 15 to 20 minutes. Immediately upon leaving the bath, apply an appropriate emollient or prescribed topical. Bathe more often when clinical manifestations increase.	Soaking saturates the stratum corneum. Application of an occlusive moisturizer 2 to 4 minutes after the bath is critical for preventing evaporation of water from the hydrated epidermis.
Use warm water—not hot.	Hot water causes vasodilation, which increases pruritus.
Use superfatted soaps (i.e., Dove or Basis) or soaps for sensitive skin (i.e., Oil of Olay, Eucerin, Neutrogena, Aveeno, Oilatum, Cetaphil). Avoid bubble baths.	The use of drying soap may compound the problem. Superfatted soaps are less alkaline and less drying to the skin.
Apply occlusive topical emollient (i.e., Aquaphor ointment, Eucerin creme or lotion, Vanicream, Cetaphil cream or lotion, Moisturel lotion) or prescribed topical preparation two or three times per day.	Ointments and creams seal in water and thereby hydrate the skin. The particular emollient selected depends mostly on client preference and whether the ingredients in the base are irritants.

Evaluation. Outcomes should be met in 48–96 hours depending on severity of eczema, frequency of baths and adequate application of appropriate occlusive topical. Evaluate skin as often as possible.

Collaborative Problem. Alteration in Comfort related to pruritus

Planning: Expected Outcomes. The client will experience a decrease in pruritus, as evidenced by

■ Decrease in observed and reported scratching
■ Decreased excoriations from scratching
■ Decreased restlessness during sleep
■ Verbalizing increased skin comfort

Implementation: Nursing Intervention	Rationales
Explain the itching symptom as it relates to cause (i.e., dryness of the skin) and the principles of the selected therapy (i.e., hydration) and the itch-scratch-itch cycle.	Understanding the physiologic or psychological process and principles of itching and its treatment increases cooperation.
Wash all new clothes before wearing for removal of formaldehyde and other chemicals, and avoid use of fabric softeners.	Pruritus is often precipitated by irritant or allergic effects of certain chemicals or components of fabric softeners.
Change to a milder detergent and add a second rinse cycle to ensure removal of soap.	Residual laundry detergent in clothing may be irritating. The actual laundry soap that is used is not the key, but rather that all soap is rinsed out so that an irritant effect is avoided.
Wear open-weave, loose-fitting, cotton-blend clothing. Avoid overdressing, rough or wool fabrics, and tightly woven fabrics.	Light cotton-blend clothing allows air circulation and minimizes perspiration, which intensifies itching.
Work and sleep in comfortable surroundings with a fairly constant temperature (68–75° F) and humidity level (45–55%). Air conditioning in the home, particularly the bedroom, may be beneficial.	Extremes of temperature cause pruritus frequently secondary to vasodilation and increased cutaneous blood flow. In addition to providing a cooler environment, air conditioning will decrease aeroallergen exposure.

Continued on facing page

day, especially if they are employed at a job in which they stand still in one area for long periods of time (e.g., cashier). Additionally, it is beneficial to raise the foot of the bed with two-by-four blocks or books. When the client is up, walking instead of standing is encouraged to increase circulation. Stasis ulcers are treated with moisture-retentive dressings and gradient pressure wraps. Unna boots and skin grafts can be used.

The Client with Atopic Dermatitis *(Continued)*

Keep fingernails short, smooth, and clean.
Appropriate use of antihistamines may reduce itching to some degree.

Use sunscreen on a regular basis.
Immediately after swimming, take a shower or bath, washing with a mild soap from head to toe, and then apply an appropriate moisturizer.

Trimmed nails prevent damage and infection to the skin.
Histamine is one of the best-known itch mediators. The sedating antihistaminics also provide relief through tranquilizing effects.
Sunburn may cause flare of dermatitis.
Residual chlorine or bromine on the skin after swimming in a pool may be irritating.

Evaluation. Outcomes may not be achieved for days or weeks after eczema has been brought under control. Itching can become a learned behavior brought on by many things which may need to be modified through counseling, oral medications, and maintenance of good skin care.

Nursing Diagnosis. Risk for infection related to skin excoriation or decreased resistance to cutaneous viral, fungal and staphylococcal organisms

Planning: Expected Outcomes. The client will be free of infectious lesions, as evidenced by absence of pustules, exudate, or crusting

Implementation: Nursing Intervention

Explain to the client the signs of infection and be sure the client understands that the presence of these signs indicates need for medical intervention.
Ensure that the client understands the importance of not self-treating with leftover medication at home.

Emphasize that it is important to take the antibiotic on schedule over the entire course.

Rationales

Infections are a potentially serious complication of disorders of open skin.

Leftover medications may be outdated and may be inappropriate treatment. Medications can become contaminated and lead to infection or lose their potency.
The entire course of medication will completely eradicate the infectious organism.

Evaluation. Outcomes are usually achieved with 7 to 10 days of oral antibiotics. However, some clients require an extended course for complete clearing. Evaluation should be done at least in 7 days.

Nursing Diagnosis. Body Image Disturbance related to skin lesions and/or response of significant others to appearance

Planning: Expected Outcomes. The client will exhibit a positive self-concept, as evidenced by engaging in social activities, expressing feelings of importance and self-worth, enjoying interpersonal interactions

Implementation: Nursing Intervention

Encourage the client to teach others that eczema is not contagious unless severely infected.
Encourage the client and significant others to share feelings with one another and professional counselors, as needed, regarding the client's appearance and the chronic nature of eczema.
Reinforce the client's sense of identity and personal competence. Encourage self-management of eczema and understanding that controlling scratching will greatly reduce lesions.

Rationales

Eczema can be mistaken for impetigo or as an indication of uncleanliness, causing social isolation.
Unidentified fears and concerns may hinder interpersonal relationships.

Allowing the client to determine the need for various treatment modalities, such as when to initiate wet wraps or minor alterations in topical therapy, promotes a positive self-concept.

Evaluation. Outcomes are totally dependent on the degree of negative self-concept, chronicity of this process, and the degree to which eczema can be controlled. Depending on the age and motivation of the client, outcomes will be reached in weeks, months, years or unfortunately for a small few—never. Professional intervention should be facilitated early.

Contact Dermatitis

Contact dermatitis is an inflammatory response of the skin to chemical or physical allergens. *Irritant contact* *dermatitis* is due to exposure to a chemical or physical irritant such as cleaning products, fragrances, and topical skin care products. Clinical manifestations range from mild erythema to vesicles to ulceration (Fig. 78–3). *Allergic contact dermatitis* is a delayed hypersensitivity re-

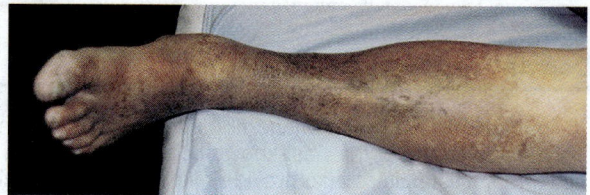

Figure 78–2. Stasis dermatitis. Note the dark, stained, shiny, and hairless quality of the leg.

action resulting from contact with an allergen. This reaction is an immune-mediated response by previously sensitized lymphocytes to a specific allergen. Common examples are poison ivy and nickel allergy. Clinical manifestations begin at the site of exposure with itching, stinging, erythema, and edema and may extend to more distant sites. Clients develop manifestations, possibly within an hour of contact or as late as 7 to 14 days after contact.

Management of contact dermatitis begins by determining the causative agent. Determining the agent usually begins by questioning the client about recent exposure to chemicals, metals, and the like. Patch testing is done to attempt to determine the specific agent. Pain and itching may be controlled with topical medication or wet dressings, as discussed earlier. Antihistaminics and steroids may be required. Each patch in a standardized test panel (T.R.U.E. test) contains a substance that is known to be a common cause of allergic contact dermatitis. When these tests provide a positive reaction, much can be done to teach the patient what to avoid (see Chapter 77).

Intertrigo

Intertrigo is superficial inflammatory dermatitis that occurs when two skin surfaces rub, which prevents adequate ventilation. Friction, heat, and moisture cause erythema and maceration, itching, and burning. Erosions and fissures with erythema and secondary bacterial or *Candida albicans* infection may occur. Whenever candidiasis presents, the healthcare provider must be careful to evaluate it completely. In an otherwise healthy person, it is a self-limiting disease that responds well to topical antifungal therapy. However, candidiasis can be the presenting sign of underlying systemic disease affecting the endocrine (e.g., diabetes) or immune (e.g., immunodeficiency syndromes) system. Intertrigo is common in hot, humid weather in neck creases, axillae, antecubital fossae, the perineum, finger and toe webs, abdominal skinfolds, and beneath the breasts, particularly those of obese clients. One of the most common causes of intertrigo is contamination with body fluids, as occurs in urinary incontinence.

The treatment of intertrigo is to eliminate maceration by promoting drying and to aerate the body skinfolds. For mobile clients, it is important to review environmental changes that promote drying of the body folds, such as loose-fitting cotton-blend clothing or periodic removal of clothing to dry off. Clients should be instructed to avoid

tight-fitting clothing such as jeans and activities that promote sweating. Care recommendations are very dependent on the degree of involvement and the overall condition of the skin. If the skin is still intact, recommendations include washing the area gently with tap water twice daily, rinsing, and drying the area, followed by liberal application of a talc-containing powder or a cellulose-containing powder (i.e., Zeasorb) for extra absorption. Never use cornstarch because it encourages *Candida albicans* overgrowth. If inflammation is present, low-potency topical corticosteroids in nonocclusive vehicles (i.e., hydrocortisone 1.0% or 2.5% cream or lotion) or combination steroid-antibiotic-antifungal (Vytone 1%) preparations may initially be helpful, but long-term use should be avoided. Apply cool, wet soaks with tap water or Burow solution three to four times daily for removal of exudate if secondary infection is present. In the event of fissuring, use of an antifungal-astringent-antiseptic drying dye preparation (Castaderm) to these areas once daily is effective but messy and may sting on application. Applying folded gauze or clean cotton handkerchiefs in skinfolds promotes healing by keeping skin surfaces apart.

Psoriasis Vulgaris

Psoriasis vulgaris is a chronic, recurrent, erythematous, inflammatory disorder involving keratin synthesis. Pruritus can be severe. Psoriasis occurs in both sexes, usually commencing in early adulthood. The Latin *vulgaris,* from *vulgus,* means "common." The cause of psoriasis vulgaris is unknown. However alterations in cyclic nucleotides, and possible immunologic abnormalities have been noted. Genetic predisposition is also possible.

Rapidly proliferating epidermal cells form small, scaly patches of skin that develop into erythematous, dry, scaling patches of various sizes. The course of psoriasis vulgaris is prolonged and unpredictable. Anxiety and stress often precede flares. Exacerbations and remissions are common. It usually recurs at intervals and lasts for in-

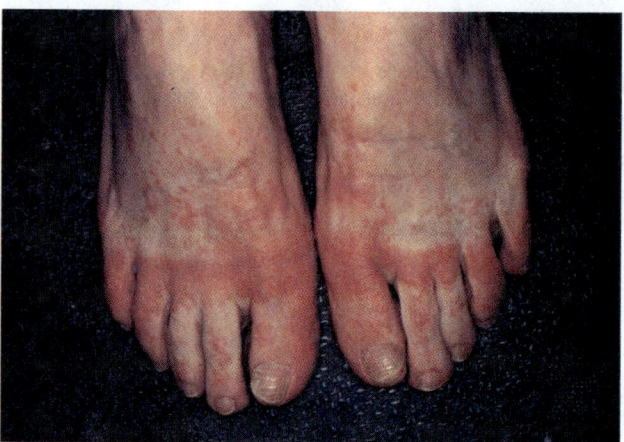

Figure 78–3. Contact dermatitis. (From Callen J. P., et al. [1993]. *Color atlas of dermatology.* Philadelphia: W. B. Saunders.)

creasingly longer periods. Spontaneous clearing is uncommon. Psoriatics have greater than normal colonization of *Staphylococcus* on plaques. Psoriatics who are human immunodeficiency virus (HIV)–positive are at high risk of infection from self-inoculation.

Psoriatic patches are covered with silvery white scales. The eruptions (usually symmetrical) commonly occur on the scalp, elbows, knees, and sacral regions (Fig. 78–4). Lesions may develop at the site of a previous injury, which is known as Koebner's phenomenon. A generalized eruption may occur with severe psoriasis vulgaris. A rare form of psoriasis (pustular psoriasis) produces generalized, sterile cutaneous pustules. Severe systemic involvement can be fatal. About 15% to 20% of clients with psoriasis have psoriatic arthritis, which primarily affects the distal joints and may be deforming. Nail dystrophies and pitting occur in about 30% to 50% of clients.

■ Medical Management

Mild psoriasis may be treated locally with natural sunlight or topical therapy, including tar preparations and topical corticosteroids (see Topical Corticosteroids) or intralesional corticosteroids. Injecting small, diluted amounts of corticosteroids (e.g., triamcinolone acetonide) into or just beneath a lesion gives a high drug concentration into the site. Potential localized side effects include atrophy, hypopigmentation, infection, and, rarely, ulceration. Keratolytic agents (e.g., salicylic acid) may remove scale and allow greater penetration of topical agents.

Anthralin is an effective topical therapy for psoriasis with widespread discrete lesions consisting primarily of thick plaques. There are varying methods of application. With all methods, it is important to apply medication only to the affected lesions, avoiding contact with normal surrounding skin. The client should wash hands immediately after application, leave medication on for the prescribed period of time, then remove it by showering or bathing. Anthralin products have the potential to stain

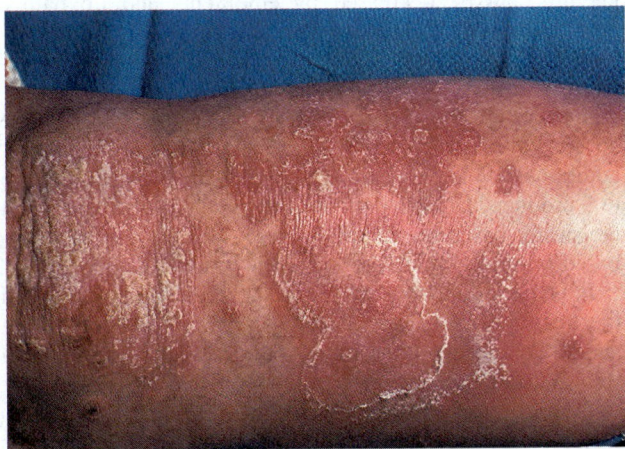

Figure 78–4. Psoriasis. (From Murphy, G. F., & Herzberg, A. J. [1996]. *Atlas of dermatopathology.* Philadelphia: W. B. Saunders.)

fabric, hair, skin, nails, furniture, and bathroom fixtures. For avoidance of excessive staining, it is recommended that medication be carefully applied and that as much medication as possible be removed with tissue or a previously stained towel before bathing.

Scalp care with psoriasis consists of removing scales and treating inflammation. Tar shampoos with keratolytic agents, followed by topical corticosteroid lotions, are useful. It is often necessary to use steroids under occlusion (under dressings) for percutaneous absorption to be enhanced; this can be accomplished on the scalp by using a plastic shower cap. There is no consistently effective treatment of psoriatic involvement of the nails. Usually, the scalp and nails improve with remission of psoriasis on the body surface.

Systemic treatment is sometimes prescribed for widespread psoriasis. The vitamin A derivative etretinate (Tegison) has been shown to be useful in pustular and erythrodermic psoriasis but not as useful in chronic plaque-type psoriasis. The mode of action may involve the correction of abnormal polyamine metabolism or leukocyte migration. The side effects of etretinate are similar to those of the oral retinoid isotretinoin (see Acne Vulgaris). Because of the teratogenicity of the drug and its extremely long half-life, its use in women of childbearing age is unwarranted. Widespread involvement may require whole-body irradiation with UVL (see earlier).

Antimetabolites (e.g., methotrexate) in small doses are useful for inhibiting DNA synthesis. Methotrexate is a folic acid antagonist used to treat psoriasis that is unresponsive to all topical therapies; it is reserved for the most severe cases. Methotrexate is potentially toxic to the renal, hepatic, and hematopoietic systems. Thus, baseline assessment (e.g., blood chemistry, complete blood count, and liver biopsy) is important before this medication is started. During treatment, periodic assessments are needed, including repeat liver biopsy. If any serious side effects develop, such as bone marrow depression (decreased white blood cell count and platelet count) or gastrointestinal tract bleeding, treatment is discontinued. For limiting potential liver damage, the client is advised not to consume alcohol throughout therapy. Because methotrexate may cause chromosomal abnormalities, effective birth control methods are important both for women and men before and during treatment. Nausea, the most common side effect, can be limited by taking methotrexate with food or taking prophylactic antiemetics.

■ Nursing Management of the Medical Client

Although the physician orders the medical regimen for the client the nurse and the physician collaborate in the ongoing assessment of the client's response to treatment and the development of new lesions.

The nurse's role in client care centers on teaching the client about the UVL treatments and medications. In addition, the nurse should assist the client in coping with an altered self-concept. The appearance of skin lesions may make the client feel "dirty" or untouchable. In addition, the smell of the tar preparations and the stain may add to the psychological reaction. The client is also at high risk of secondary infection in the open lesions. The client should be taught to keep the creams or ointments on and keep the areas clean and dry.

In order to keep psoriasis in remission, the client needs to control the causative factors. Adequate rest, nutrition, and exercise promote health. Stress should be minimized, and illness and infection treated early.

Acne Vulgaris

Acne is a common, self-limiting, multifactorial disorder. One of four clients affected has enough significant disease to seek professional treatment. Potential facial disfigurement is a major concern. Acne requires active treatment for control until it spontaneously resolves. The types of acne lesions are comedones (open and closed), pustules, papules, and nodules (Fig. 78–5). A closed comedone, or whitehead, is a noninflamed lesion that develops as the follicle enlarges with retention of horny cells. Open comedones, or blackheads, result from the continuing accumulation of horny cells and sebum, which dilate the follicles. Inflammation does not usually occur in comedones unless they are self-manipulated. Pustules and papules result as the inflammatory process progresses. Papules are at a deeper level in the dermis than pustules. Nodules result from total disintegration of a comedone and subsequent collapse of the follicle. Nodules are the hallmark of serious acne, and deep scarring may result.

The exact cause of acne is unknown. The principle factors are abnormal keratinization of the follicular epithelium, excessive sebum production, proliferation of *Propionibacterium acnes,* and inflammation secondary to the action of extracellular inflammatory products produced by *P. acnes.*

There is no scientific evidence that consumption of foods such as chocolate, nuts, or fatty foods affects acne. However, exacerbations coinciding with the menstrual cycle result from hormonal activity. Heat, humidity, and excessive perspiration also have a role in increased acne.

Treatment depends on the severity of acne. To prevent scarring, it is important to suppress inflammation. See Table 78–1 for a discussion of acne medications. Benzoyl peroxide (component of Desquam, Benzagel, Persa-Gel, Panoxyl) 5% and 10% has a potent antimicrobial effect. It will reduce the size and number of comedones present and may inhibit sebum secretion. Topical antibiotics (clindamycin and erythromycin) are also used. Tretinoin (Retin-A) has been found to be one of the most effective comedolytic agents, used alone or in combination with benzoyl peroxide. The irritant effects sometimes limit its usefulness. Clients should receive written instructions regarding use of tretinoin.

Failure of response to topicals indicates needed evaluation for addition of oral antibiotics (tetracycline or erythromycin). Tetracycline or erythromycin administered over an extended period (e.g., several months) suppresses *P. acnes* and decreases inflammation. Long-term systemic antibiotics can cause monilial vaginitis and gastrointestinal symptoms, and clients should be informed how to monitor for these and what interventions to take. Improvement may not be apparent for 4 to 6 weeks.

Hormone therapy may be indicated for severe cystic acne. Medication containing estrogens suppresses sebaceous gland activity. Estrogenic therapy requires treatment through a minimum of three to four menstrual cycles.

In severe cystic acne resistant to standard management, isotretinoin (Accutane) is used to inhibit inflammation. Dosage is determined by body weight and is taken in divided, daily doses for several months. The drug has many side effects and requires frequent follow-up visits and laboratory evaluations. Adverse effects include elevated triglycerides, skin dryness, cheilitis (lip inflammation), and eye discomfort (i.e., dryness, burning). Isotretinoin is a teratogen; thus, women of childbearing age should use an effective contraceptive for at least 1 month before starting this medication and should have a pregnancy screening test 2 weeks before treatment. This drug should not be used in women without strict and adequate contraception throughout the course of therapy and for a determined period after therapy. Reinforce the fact that close medical follow-up is needed and that dry skin and cheilitis can be decreased by emollients and lip balms. Vitamin A supplements are stopped during this treatment.

There is no convincing evidence that dietary management, abrasive scrubs, or oral vitamin A, has any beneficial effects in the management of acne. Some may notice an improvement in the summer months as a result of additional UVL exposure. Clients should be instructed to use products labeled noncomedogenic and cosmetics that are water-based to avoid contact with excessively oil-based products which are known to exacerbate acne.

It is important to explain the mechanism of acne and the treatment plan and to set goals of therapy. The client should understand that improvement is not usually seen for 4 to 8 weeks and therapy is usually required for months to years to achieve control. Assess the client's skin care practices. Reinforce compliance with topical or systemic therapy and appropriate skin-cleansing methods with special emphasis on not scrubbing the face and using only the agreed-upon topicals. Note areas of self-

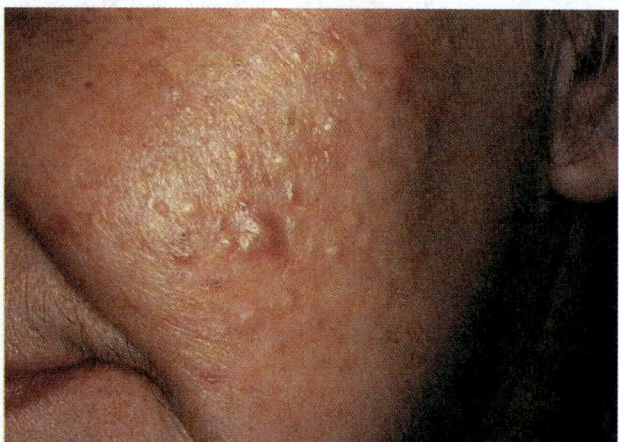

Figure 78–5. Acne. (From Callen J. P., et al. [1993]. *Color atlas of dermatology.* Philadelphia: W. B. Saunders.)

induced skin damage and emphasize to the client that he or she must not squeeze, prick, or pick at lesions.

Acne Rosacea

This chronic, inflammatory eruption, characterized by erythema, papules, pustules, and telangiectases, occurs on the face, especially the nose. Unlike acne vulgaris, comedones are generally not seen. Acne rosacea has an insidious onset, usually between ages 30 and 50 years, and affects women more frequently than men. It is more common in fair-skinned persons with a history of easy facial flushing. Precipitating factors that appear to make the flushing worse include tea, coffee, alcohol (especially wine), caffeine-containing products, sunlight, extremes of hot and cold, spicy foods, and emotional stress. Sebaceous hyperplasia of the nose (rhinophyma) is often associated with years of chronic acne rosacea. This results from chronic inflammation and increased connective tissues and may be mistaken for an indication of excessive alcohol consumption. Ocular changes such as eyelid inflammation and conjunctivitis may occur.

Avoidance of the stimuli that trigger acne rosacea may be sufficient for mild disorders. Clients should be instructed to avoid factors that provoke facial vasodilation, such as caffeine, excessive sunlight, alcohol (especially wine), temperature extremes, hot liquids and spicy foods. Systemic antibiotics used to be the mainstay of therapy. Antibiotics are given in small, usually tapered doses for long periods. Remind the client that improvement with systemic antibiotics will be gradual. Today, topical metronidazole (MetroGel) is the drug of choice for acne rosacea. A thin layer is applied twice daily with usually only minimal complaints by clients of dryness or burning. Relapse is common in clients who discontinue therapy.

Pressure Ulcers

A pressure ulcer is any lesion on the skin caused by unrelieved pressure resulting in damage of underlying tissue. Pressure ulcers occur commonly in areas subject to high pressure from body weight on bony prominences. Pressure ulcers have also been called bed sores and decubitus ulcers. The word *decubitus* comes from the Latin *decumbere,* to lie down. The ulcers were so named because they are common in bedridden clients.

Etiology and Risk Factors

Pressure ulcers develop when soft tissue (skin, subcutaneous tissue and muscle) are compressed between a bony prominence and a firm surface for a prolonged period of time. The period of time before breakdown varies among clients; very debilitated clients can have permanent tissue damage in less than 2 hours.

Malnutrition is a major risk factor. Malnourished clients have poor skin integrity and the skin is damaged easily. In addition, incontinence, immobility, and skin shearing can also lead to breakdown.

The incidence (number of new cases a year) of pressure ulcers in acute care facilities has ranged from 2.7% to 29.5%. The prevalence (number of cases at one point in time) in acute care settings ranges from 3.5% to 29.5%. Several groups are at increased risk, and therefore the incidence and prevalence are higher. Quadriplegic clients have a 60% prevalence, elderly persons with femoral fractures have a 66% prevalence, and clients in critical care have a 41% prevalence.

Prevention of pressure ulcers begins with identifying the client at risk. Risk factors for alteration in skin integrity can be determined by assessing sensory perception, moisture, activity, mobility, nutrition, and friction and sheer. The Braden Scale (Fig. 78–6) is an assessment tool that evaluates risk.

Pathophysiology

Continuous pressure on soft tissues between bony prominences and hard surfaces compresses capillaries and occludes the blood flow. If the pressure is relieved, a brief period of rebound capillary dilation (called reactive hyperemia) occurs and there is no tissue damage. If pressure is not relieved, microthrombi form in the capillary and completely occlude blood flow. A blister may form initially if there has been damage only to superficial tissues. Damage to underlying tissues creates a necrotic area of tissue. The necrotic tissue undergoes the process of inflammation as the body tries to rid it and ready the tissue for healing.

Clinical Manifestations and Diagnostic Findings

The clinical manifestations of pressure ulcers have been described in four stages (Fig. 78–7). Ulcers most commonly occur on the greater trochanter, heel, sacrum (Fig. 78–8), and ischial tuberosities.

The ulcer may or may not be covered with devitalized tissue. These tissues can be yellow, white, brown, or black. Ulcers covered with devitalized tissue cannot be staged accurately, until the necrotic tissue is excised.

Few additional diagnostic assessments are required for a diagnosis. Sometimes osteomyelitis is present in deep wounds. Bone scans are used for diagnosing this problem. Sinus tracts or tunneling can be diagnosed with a sinogram if needed. Sinography uses an injection of dye into a wound. If malnutrition is suspected as a cause, serum protein, albumin, or prealbumin may be used.

Acute and Subacute Care

■ Medical Management

The client with a pressure ulcer should have a complete history and physical examination. There are many causes of delayed healing, and in the case of pressure ulcers delayed healing is often the result of other health problems.

RISK PREDICTORS FOR SKIN BREAKDOWN

Patient's Name _____ Evaluator's Name _____ Date of Assessment

	1	2	3	4
SENSORY PERCEPTION ability to respond to discomfort	**1. Completely limited:** Unresponsive to painful stimuli, either because of state of unconsciousness or severe sensory impairment, which limits ability to feel pain over most of body surface	**2. Very limited:** Responds only to painful stimuli (but not verbal commands) by opening eyes or flexing extremities. Cannot communicate discomfort verbally, OR has a sensory impairment which limits the ability to feel pain or discomfort over one half of body surface	**3. Slightly limited:** Responds to verbal commands by opening eyes and obeying some commands, but cannot always communicate discomfort or need to be turned, OR has some sensory impairment which limits ability to feel pain or discomfort in one or two extremities.	**4. No impairment:** Responds to verbal commands by obeying. Can communicate needs accurately. Has no sensory deficit which would limit ability to feel pain or discomfort
MOISTURE degree to which skin is exposed to moisture	**1. Very Moist:** Skin is kept moist almost constantly by perspiration and urine. Dampness is detected every time patient is moved or turned. Linen must be changed more than one time each shift	**2. Occasionally Moist:** Skin is frequently, but not always kept moist, linen must be changed two to three times every 24 hours	**3. Rarely Moist:** Skin is rarely moist more than three to four times a week, but linen does require changing at that time	**4. Never Moist:** Perspiration and incontinence is never a problem, linen changed at routine intervals only
ACTIVITY degree of physical activity	**1. Bedfast:** Confined to bed	**2. Chairfast:** Ability to walk severely impaired or nonexistent and must be assisted into chair or wheelchair. Is confined to chair or wheelchair when not in bed	**3. Walks occasionally:** Walks occasionally during day, but for very short distances, with or without assistance. Spends majority of each shift in bed or chair	**4. Walks frequently:** Walks a moderate distance at least once every 1 to 2 hours during waking hours
MOBILITY ability to change and control body position	**1. Completely Immobile:** Unable to make even slight changes in position without assistance	**2. Very limited:** Makes occasional slight changes in position without help but unable to make frequent or significant changes in position independently	**3. Slightly limited:** Makes frequent though slight changes in position without assistance but unable to make or maintain major changes in position independently	**4. No limitations:** Makes major and frequent changes in position without assistance
NUTRITION usual food intake pattern	**1. Very Poor:** Never eats a complete meal. Rarely eats more than 1/3 of any food offered. Intake of protein is negligible. Takes even fluids poorly. Does not take a liquid dietary supplement, OR is NPO and/or maintained on clear liquids or IV for more than 5 days	**2. Probably Inadequate:** Rarely eats a complete meal and generally eats only about one half of any food offered. Protein intake is poor. Occasionally will take a liquid dietary supplement, OR receiving less than optimum amount of liquid diet or tube feeding	**3. Adequate:** Eats over half of most meals. Eats moderate amount of protein source one to two times daily. Occasionally will refuse a meal. Will usually take a dietary supplement if offered, OR is on a tube feeding or TPN regimen which probably meets most of nutritional needs	**4. Excellent:** Eats most of every meal. Never refuses a meal. Frequently eats between meals. Does not require a dietary supplementation
FRICTION AND SHEAR	**1. Problem:** Requires moderate to maximum assistance in moving. Complete lifting without sliding against sheets is impossible. Frequently slides down in bed or chair, requiring frequent repositioning with maximum assistance. Either spasticity, contractures or agitation leads to almost constant friction	**2. Potential Problem:** Moves feebly independently or requires minimum assistance. Skin probably slides against bedsheets or chair to some extent when movement occurs. Maintains relatively good position in chair or bed most of time but occasionally slides down	**3. No Apparent Problem:** Moves in bed and in chair independently and has sufficient muscle strength to lift up completely during move. Maintains good position in bed or chair at all times	

Key: 16, minimum risk; 13–14, moderate risk; 12 or less, high risk;
NPO, nothing by mouth; IV, intravenously; TPN, total parenteral nutrition.

Total _____ Score

Figure 78–6. The Braden Scale. (Courtesy of Barbara Braden and Nancy Bergstrom. Copyright 1988.)

Stage I

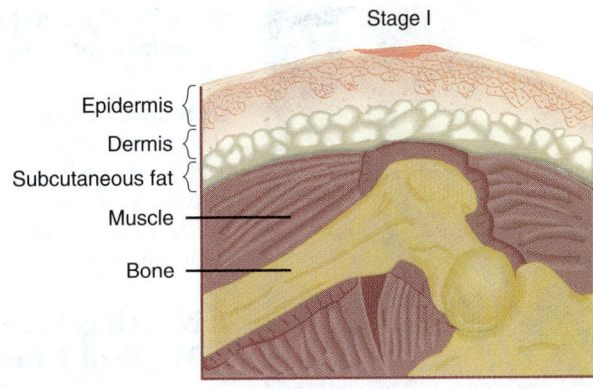

Epidermis
Dermis
Subcutaneous fat
Muscle
Bone

Non-blanching erythema of intact skin; the heralding lesion of skin ulceration

Stage II

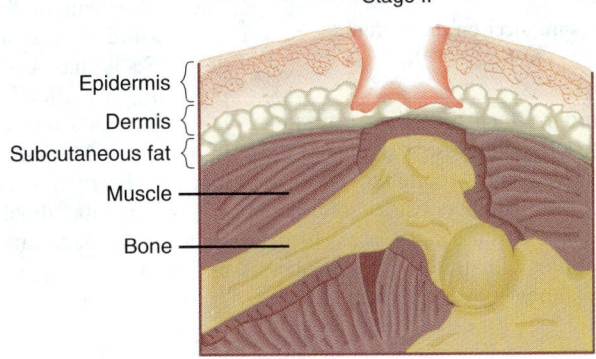

Epidermis
Dermis
Subcutaneous fat
Muscle
Bone

Partial-thickness skin loss involving epidermis and/or dermis. The ulcer is superficial and presents clinically as an abrasion, blister, or shallow crater.

Stage III

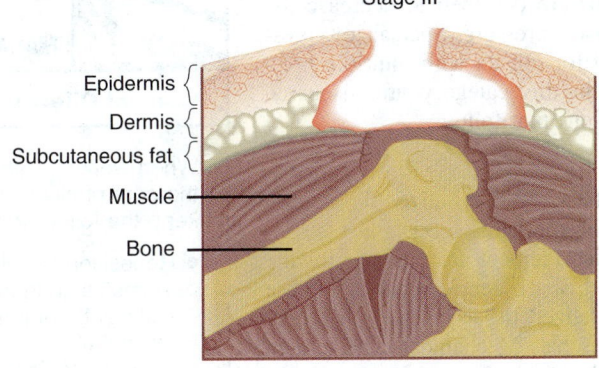

Epidermis
Dermis
Subcutaneous fat
Muscle
Bone

Full-thickness skin loss involving damage or necrosis of subcutaneous tissue, which may extend down to, but not through, the underlying fascia. The ulcer presents clinically as a deep crater with or without undermining of adjacent tissue.

Stage IV

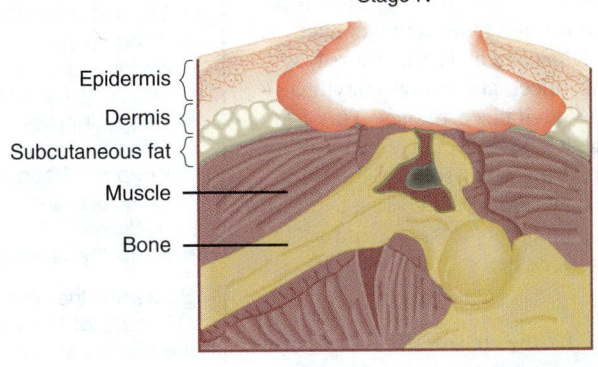

Epidermis
Dermis
Subcutaneous fat
Muscle
Bone

Full-thickness skin loss with extensive destruction, tissue necrosis, or damage to muscle, bone, or supporting structures (e.g., tendon, joint capsule, etc.)

Figure 78–7. The stages of pressure ulcers.

Managing Malnutrition. The association of malnutrition with pressure ulcer formation and delayed healing is quite clear. In fact, many clinicians believe that pressure ulcers are a serious indicator of malnutrition. If the client's albumin is less than 3.5 g/dl, the total lymphocyte count is less than 1800/mm³, the client is not eating or is at a body weight that is less than 80% of ideal body weight, consider nutritional supplementation. If the client

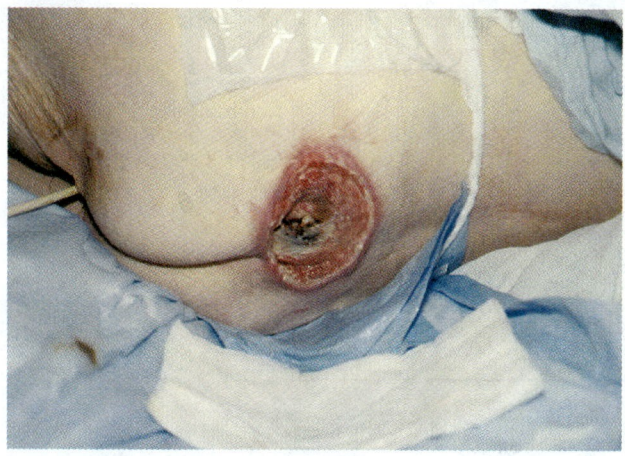

Figure 78–8. A pressure ulcer on the sacrum.

has no gastrointestinal disorders, feed the client oral supplements or by tube. Some clinicians use the phrase "If the gut works, use it" to sum up this recommendation. If the client has gastrointestinal problems, consider total parenteral nutrition. Of course, these more aggressive forms of feeding must be compatible with the client's wishes. Monitor nutritional status (as above) every 3 months.

Managing Tissue Loads. The term "tissue load" refers to the distribution of pressure, friction, and shear on the tissues. Interventions are designed to decrease tissue load and thereby decrease pressure. Special low-pressure beds may be required for clients with multiple pressure ulcers. Interventions in this category are discussed under nursing care, in sections that follow.

Providing Ulcer Care. Moist, devitalized tissue supports bacterial growth. Therefore, this tissue must be removed. Several forms of debridement are possible for the client with a pressure ulcer. Sharp debridement is the use of a scalpel to excise devitalized tissue (eschar). It works best for a thick, adherent eschar. Mechanical debridement is the use of wet-to-dry dressings, hydrotherapy, wound irrigation, and dextranomers to remove soft devitalized tissues. Enzymatic debridement is the use of topical debriding agents, such as collagenase, to remove necrotic tissues. Finally, autolytic debridement is the use of synthetic dressings to cover an ulcer and allow enzymes in the wound bed to digest the devitalized tissues. This form of debridement is the slowest and is usually reserved for clients who could not tolerate the other forms. Heel ulcers are not debrided unless they are clearly infected. All forms of debridement (except autolytic) are painful; the client should be given analgesics before beginning.

Monitoring Healing. If the ulcer does not heal within 2 weeks using adequate nutrition, pressure reduction, daily cleaning, and dressings, consider a 2-week trial of topical antibiotics. Swab cultures are not appropriate to diagnose infection in the ulcer. All pressure ulcers are colonized (covered with surface bacteria) and a swab cul-

ture will only detect surface colonization. Use a quantitative culture for suspicious infections.

Complications. Many complications have been associated with pressure ulcers. They include osteomyelitis, bacteremia and sepsis, and cellulitis. Amyloidosis, endocarditis, heterotopic bone formation, septic arthritis, and fistula from the ulcer to the perineum are rare but have been reported.

■ Nursing Management of the Medical Client

Assessment

The assessment of the client at high risk of development of pressure ulcers should include the risk factors. Braden's Scale has been developed to assist the nurse in predicting which clients are at greatest risk. In addition, laboratory data on hemoglobin, hematocrit, albumin, total protein, and lymphocytes should be assessed. It is important to realize that risk must be an ongoing assessment. Objective data about the pressure ulcer, size, depth, or stage of drainage, and condition of periulcer tissue should be noted.

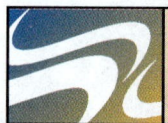

MANAGEMENT AND DELEGATION

Care of Clients with Pressure Ulcers

When working with unlicensed assistive personnel in the care of clients with pressure ulcers, help them to keep the following points in mind:

- Reposition the client *at least* every 2 hours. Even a small shift in the client's body weight may be sufficient, but it must be done every 2 hours at minimum.
- *Do not position the client on the ulcer.* If an ulcer is on the client's trunk, use a dynamic or overlay mattress. However, the use of these support surfaces does not eliminate the need for turning.
- If the client is wheelchair-bound, ensure that the padding provides adequate pressure relief by checking for "bottoming out."
- Keep all pressure off the client's heels. Use small pillows or foam to prevent direct contact.
- Keep the head of the bed at the lowest elevation to reduce shear and friction on the client's lower back.
- Keep the client's skin dry.

Be aware that even though you have delegated the skin care of this client, you are still accountable for the client's skin condition. Assess the client's entire skin surface every day. Ask for help in turning the client so that you can see the client's heels and sacrum. Use an assessment guide, such as the Braden Scale, to determine the risk of further ulceration.

Diagnosis, Planning, Implementation

Risk for Impaired Skin Integrity.
Clients who score between 12 and 16 on the Braden risk assessment are considered at risk. Scores below 12 are high-risk. This nursing diagnosis is written as *Risk for Impaired Skin Integrity related to malnutrition and unrelieved pressure.*

Planning: Expected Outcomes. The client will reduce the risk of impairment in skin integrity, as evidenced by no actual tissue breakdown and no persistent reddened areas.

Implementation. Preventive measures to reduce the risk of pressure ulcers cannot be overemphasized. In 1992, the U.S. Department of Health and Human Services developed guidelines for prediction and prevention of pressure ulcers in adults.[31] These guidelines are summarized here:

1. All clients at risk should have a systematic skin inspection at least once a day, paying particular attention to the bony prominences. Results of skin inspection should be documented.
2. Skin should be cleaned at the time of soiling and at routine intervals. The frequency of skin cleaning should be individualized according to need and client preference. Avoid hot water, and use a mild cleaning agent that minimizes irritation and dryness of the skin. During the cleaning process, take care to minimize the force and friction applied to the skin.
3. Minimize environmental factors leading to skin drying, such as low humidity (less than 40%) and exposure to cold. Dry skin should be treated with moisturizers.
4. Avoid massage over bony prominences. Current evidence suggests that massage over bony prominences may be harmful.
5. Minimize skin exposure to moisture due to incontinence, perspiration, or wound drainage. When these sources of moisture cannot be controlled, underpads or briefs can be used that are made of materials that absorb moisture and present a quick-drying surface to the skin. For information about assessing and managing urinary incontinence, see *Urinary Incontinence in Adults: Clinical Practice Guideline* (available from the Agency for Health Care Policy and Research [AHCPR]). Topical agents that act as barriers to moisture can also be used.
6. Skin injury due to friction and shear forces should be minimized through proper positioning, transferring, and turning techniques. In addition, friction injuries may be reduced by the use of lubricants (e.g., cornstarch and creams), protective films (e.g., as transparent film dressings and skin sealants), protective dressings (e.g., hydrocolloids), and protective padding.
7. When apparently well-nourished clients develop an inadequate dietary intake of protein or calories, caregivers should first attempt to discover the factors compromising intake and offer support with eating. Other nutritional supplements or support may be needed. If dietary intake remains inadequate and if consistent with overall goals of therapy, more aggressive nutritional intervention such as enteral or parenteral feedings should be considered.

   For nutritionally compromised clients, a plan of nutritional support or supplementation should be implemented that meets individual needs and is consistent with the overall goals of therapy.
8. If the potential exists for improving the client's mobility and activity status, rehabilitation efforts should be instituted if consistent with the overall goals of therapy. Maintaining current activity level, mobility, and range of motion is an appropriate goal for most clients.
9. Interventions and outcomes should be monitored and documented.
10. As the Nursing Research feature indicates, a client in bed who is assessed to be at risk of developing pressure ulcers should be repositioned at least every 2 hours if consistent with overall patient goals. A written schedule for systematically turning and repositioning the client should be used.
11. For clients in bed, pillows should be used to keep bony prominences (such as knees or ankles) from direct contact with one another.
12. Clients in bed who are completely immobile should have a care plan that includes the use of devices that totally relieve pressure on the heels, most commonly by raising the heels off the bed. Do not use doughnut-type devices; they are likely to cause pressure ulcers, not prevent them.
13. When the side-lying position is used in bed, avoid positioning directly on the trochanter.
14. Maintain the head of the bed at the lowest degree of elevation consistent with medical conditions and other restrictions. Limit the amount of time the head of the bed is elevated.
15. Use lifting devices such as a trapeze or bed linen to move (rather than drag) clients in bed who cannot assist during transfers and position changes.
16. Any client assessed to be at risk of developing pressure ulcers should be placed when lying in bed on a pressure-reducing device, such as a foam, static air, alternating air, gel, or water mattress.
17. Any person at risk of developing a pressure ulcer should avoid uninterrupted sitting in chair or wheelchair. The client should be repositioned, shifting the points under pressure at least every hour. Clients who are able should be taught to shift weight every 15 minutes.
18. For chair-bound clients, the use of a pressure-reducing device such as those made of foam, gel, air, or a combination of these is indicated. Do not use doughnut-type devices.
19. Positioning of chair-bound clients should include consideration of postural alignment, distribution of weight, balance, and stability, and pressure relief.
20. A written plan for the use of positioning devices and schedules may be helpful for chair-bound clients.*

---

*The clinical practice guide is available from the AHCPR at 1-800-358-9295.

NURSING RESEARCH

How Well Do Healthy Elderly Adults Tolerate an Every-2-Hour Turning Schedule?

Knox, D. M., Anderson, T. M., & Anderson, P. (1994). Effects of different turn intervals on skin of healthy older adults. *Advances in Wound Care, 7*(1), 48–56.

The 2-hour turning interval has been used without much scientific study as a nursing intervention for pressure ulcer formation. The purpose of this study was to compare the effects of 1-, 1½-, and 2-hour turning schedules on surface skin temperature, interface pressure, and skin color in healthy elderly adults.

In a convenience sample, 16 healthy adults were placed in beds and were turned every 2 hours, then every 1½ hours, and then every hour. The initial position was randomly assigned. Data collected included pain rating, interface pressure, temperature, blood pressure, and skin color changes.

The greatest increase in skin surface temperature was at the end of the 2-hour position in the trochanters. Mean interface pressures decreased at the end of 1½ hours and 2 hours; they increased at the end of 1 hour. These changes were not statistically significant. Skin redness increased according to the time; by 2 hours three subjects had severe redness. One subject had to terminate the study because of pain.

Implications for Practice

The traditional 2-hour turning schedule may not be frequent enough for the elderly debilitated client. The significance of skin temperature needs to be further studied, because plastic mattress covers and incontinence pads on hospital beds increase the skin temperature.

Evaluation

Outcomes should be met in 24 to 48 hours. Recall that skin can be impaired in just 2 hours. Therefore several hours are needed to determine if skin injury occurred prior to risk reduction measures.

Impaired Skin Integrity. Use this diagnosis to describe an actual pressure ulcer. State the diagnosis as *Impaired Skin Integrity related to pressure ulcer secondary to prolonged immobility, malnutrition, and unrelieved pressure.*

Planning: Expected Outcomes. The client will have healing of the ulcer, as evidenced by development of granulation tissue and decreasing ulcer size.

Implementation. Consistency among nurses is an important aspect in achieving wound healing. It is important to develop scientific protocols in ulcer care and use them. It is also important to give one protocol time to work before changing to another.

In 1994, the AHCPR established guidelines for pressure ulcer treatment.[7] The guidelines are summarized here. If you are caring for several clients with pressure ulcers, it would be wise to obtain the actual document. Wound care is discussed in Chapter 20. Pressure ulcer wound care does not differ.

1. Ensure adequate dietary intake to prevent malnutrition and delayed healing.
2. Assess nutritional status at least every 3 months in those clients at risk of malnutrition.
3. Provide oral supplementation, tube feeding, or hyperalimentation to place the client in positive nitrogen balance.
4. Supplement the diet with vitamins and minerals.
5. Assess and manage pain associated with the ulcer and its care.
6. Position the client to stay off of the ulcer.
7. Use positioning devices to hold the client in various positions. Do not use doughnut-type devices.
8. Establish a written turning schedule.
9. Maintain the head of the bed at the lowest elevation consistent with the client's other problems.
10. Use support surfaces for clients with multiple ulcers, those who are not able to keep off the ulcer surface. Begin with a dynamic surface or mattress overlay. Progress to low air loss beds or air-fluidized beds (Fig. 78–9) if the ulcer does not heal or if the client "bottoms out."
11. Check for bottoming out beneath the mattress (Fig. 78–10). Place your hand between the mattress and the bed. If you feel less than an inch of support the support surface is not adequate.
12. Prevent moisture from coming in contact with the client's skin.
13. Use support cushions for wheelchair-bound clients.
14. Teach wheelchair-bound clients to reposition themselves every 15 minutes.
15. Debride the ulcer of devitalized tissues.
16. Clean the wound with normal saline. Avoid antiseptics on the wound bed.
17. Use irrigation to clean the wound, Safe pressure ranges from 4 to 15 lb per square inch. A 35-ml syringe with a 19-gauge angiocatheter is a good device for irrigation.
18. Choose dressings that keep the wound bed moist and the surrounding skin dry.
19. Follow body substance isolation; use clean gloves and clean dressings for wound care.

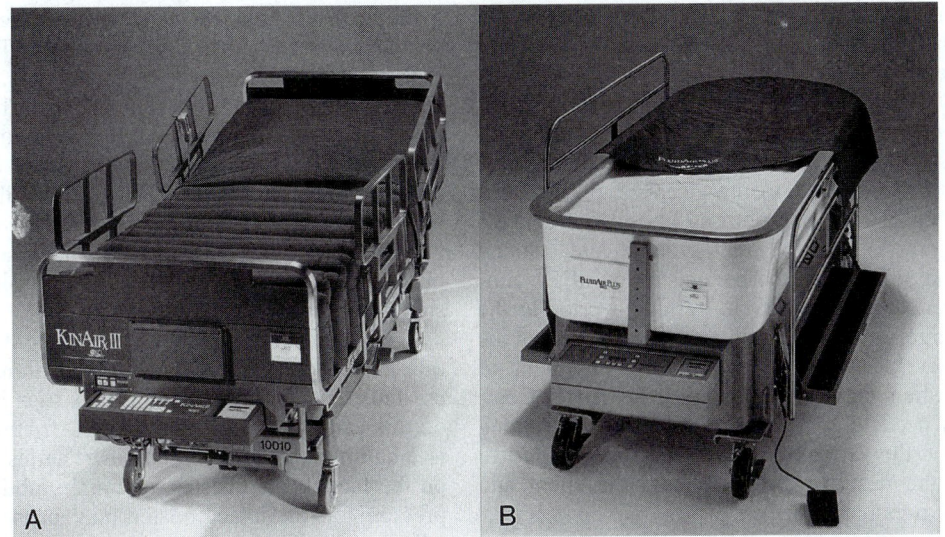

Figure 78–9. Pressure reduction surfaces. *A,* KinAir beds provide controlled air suspension to redistribute body weight away from bony prominences. *B,* FluidAir beds use air flow and bead fluidization. Both of these beds are covered with Gore-Tex fabric, which resists tearing. This fabric is also waterproof and acts as a barrier against bacteria. (Courtesy of Kinetic Concepts, Inc., San Antonio, TX.)

Evaluation

As the wound heals, the degree of goal attainment should be assessed every 3 to 4 days. Allow 2 weeks before changing the plan of care.

■ Surgical Management

Surgical repair is frequently performed on stage III and IV ulcers, on ulcers over 2 cm in diameter and in clients who can tolerate surgery. In stage III ulcers, undamaged tissue near the wound is rotated to cover the ulcer. In stage IV ulcers, musculocutaneous flaps are often used (see Chapter 80).

Community and Self-Care

Clients at high risk of pressure ulcers should be referred to home health agencies before discharge from acute case settings so that devices to reduce pressure can be obtained for home use. The family and client need to understand the importance of frequent turning. If the client is

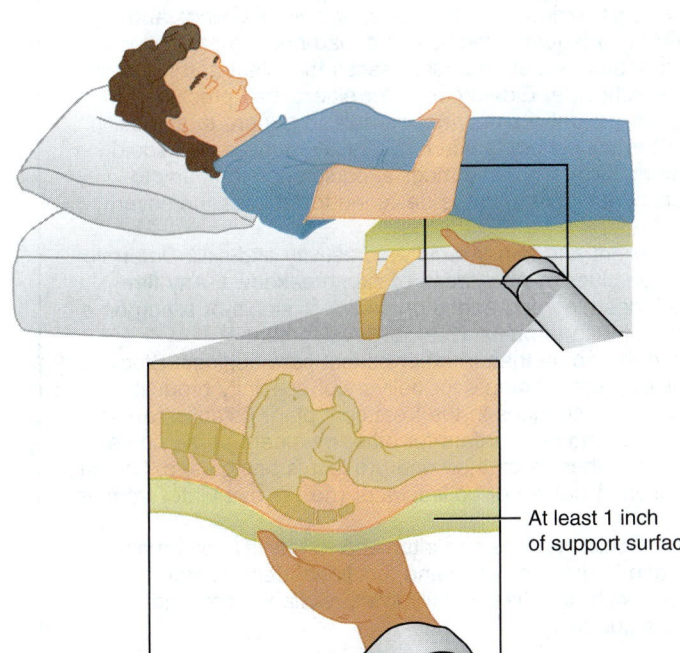

Figure 78–10. Assessing pressure relief. Slide your hand (palm up and fingers flat) under the support surface, just under the pressure point. Do not flex your fingers. With good support, there will be at least 1 inch of uncompressed support surface between your hand and the patient. (Modified from Gaymar Industries, Inc., Orchard Park, NY.)

At least 1 inch of support surface

wheelchair-bound and has arm function, he or she should be taught to lift the body with the arms off of the chair twice every hour for repositioning. Clients who are incontinent need to wear protective pads to absorb the urine or stool and be assessed often. The U.S. Department of Health and Human Services has developed a patient guide for preventing and treating pressure ulcers.[6,56]

If the client is going home with an unhealed ulcer, the client and family must be taught wound care, wound assessment, and sometimes, the administration of IV antibiotics. These interventions should be taught prior to the day of discharge, so that return demonstrations can be used to evaluate learning. In addition, procurement of equipment is often necessary, and this takes time. Community nurses need to be involved early in the planning of discharge of the client with an ulcer. The Bridge to Home Healthcare describes ways to help the client and family manage pressure ulcers.

Bullous Disorders: Pemphigus

Pemphigus is a chronic disorder that results in the development of blisters (called bullae). It is fairly uncommon in the general population but has an increased incidence in Jewish and Mediterranean peoples. There are several types of pemphigus: pemphigus vulgaris, pemphigus foliaceous, and pemphigus erythematosus. This discussion focuses on pemphigus vulgaris, the most common type.

Pemphigus is an autoimmune disease caused by circulating IgG autoantibodies. These autoantibodies react with the intracellular cement or the substance that holds epidermal cells together. The reaction causes intraepidermal blister (bulla) formation and acantholysis (loss of cohesion between epidermal cells).

Clinical manifestations include flaccid bullae that rupture easily, emitting a foul-smelling drainage and leaving crusted, denuded skin. Nikolsky's sign is when the epidermis can be rubbed off by slight friction or injury; this is a hallmark sign of pemphigus. The lesions are common on the face, back, chest, groin, and umbilicus. Even slight pressure on an intact blister may cause it to spread to adjacent skin.

Management includes large doses of steroids and immunosuppressives. Plasmapheresis has had some success with pemphigus. If the client has a large portion of denuded skin, management is similar to that for a burn client. The client is at increased risk of infection, fluid

---

BRIDGE TO HOME HEALTHCARE

Managing Pressure Ulcers

Bonnie Bolinger, R.N. C.E.T.N., *CAREONE, Tampa, Florida*, and Janice Cuzzell, M.A., R.N., *The Health Care Alternatives Group, Savannah, Georgia*

Providing home care for the client with pressure ulcers requires planning and preparation. Unlike the acute care environment, resources are often limited in the home. Wound care supplies and equipment may not be readily available. Physician communication is more difficult, sometimes delaying changes in the plan of care. Complex wound treatments, such as sharp debridement, may require patient transport to the hospital or a physician's office.

Assess the home for safety and functional capabilities such as refrigeration for some biologic dressings and compounded pharmaceutical solutions and supplies. Determine adequate electrical and load-bearing capacities for specialty beds. Procure whirlpool adaptations and safe and potable water sources. Assess the client and his or her caregiver's ability to care for wounds and maintain a turning schedule. Elders caring for elders may preclude an ideal turning schedule. Significant others with mobility or cognitive deficits may not be able to adhere to a specific regimen such as turning the client every 2 hours. A 2-hour turning schedule interrupts family routines and could lead to sleep deprivation for the caregiver. Make arrangements with a durable medical equipment company to provide pressure relief surfaces for bed and chair, or specialty equipment that is designed to address the severity or stage of the ulcer.

Adapting the home environment to meet the needs of the client and family requires creativity and skill. Determining where clients spend prolonged periods of time can provide clues to new areas of skin breakdown. Any firm, unyielding surface can produce an ulcer in unusual areas. Ridged, corded edges on chairs or stools or sitting on a firm toilet seat for extended periods can restrict blood flow and lead to pressure ulcer development.

Maintenance of equipment and supplies is more difficult in the home than in other patient care settings. Stock levels of skin and wound care supplies need to be determined. Arrangements for delivery of specialty products must be responsive to the written orders and not delay necessary changes in the treatment plan. Establish an intercommunication sheet in the home that flags a change in wound care orders for other members of the home care team. Leave specific directions for product use, especially when more than one product is being used. Normal saline can be made using this recipe: mix 8 tsp salt in 1 gallon of bottled or boiled water (do not use water from an outdoor well).

The home care team can address multidisciplinary needs. Social workers can intervene to identify community resources. Physical therapists and occupational therapists can address mobility and functional deficits. Home health aides provide additional full-body inspection and assist with activities of daily living. Collaboration and attention to detail will produce the desired result—an intact epidermis.

Text continued on p. 2222

Table 78-4. Common Skin Infections and Infestations

Name	Organism(s)	Clinical Manifestations	Management
Parasitic			
Scabies	*Sarcoptes scabiei*	Multiple straight or wavy thread-like lines beneath the skin, itching	Application of a scabicide with re-treatment of the residual eggs in 1 wk. All clothing and linen should be washed and dried in hot cycles or dry cleaned
Lice	*Pediculus humanus, Phthirus pubis*	Intense itching; scratch marks may be evident	Application of pediculicides. For head lice, the shampoo should be worked into dry hair until it is saturated. A fine-toothed comb should be used to remove the dead lice and nits. Brushes and combs should be washed in the pediculicide also. For body lice, a pediculicide lotion is applied to involved body areas. Clothing should be washed and dried in hot cycles or dry cleaned. Family members or close contacts should be treated, too
Bacterial			
Impetigo	Streptococcus A Staphylococci	Pruritic vesicle or pustule that breaks and leaves a thick honey-colored crust	Antibiotics until culture results available include erythromycin or dicloxacillin. Mupirocin preferable to oral antibiotics when lesions in small, localized area. Teach control of contagiousness; infection is contagious as long as skin lesions are present. Thorough hand washing, separate laundry for client's linens, separate washing of client's dishes
Folliculitis, furuncles, carbunicles	*Staphylococcus aureus*	White pustules on forehead, chest, upper back, neck, thighs, groin, and axillae. Furuncles are deeper inflamed nodules. Carbuncles are interconnected furuncles; often rupture expelling purulent, foul-smelling thick drainage	Localized folliculitis is treated with warm compresses, gentle washing and topical antibiotics. Furuncles are treated as folliculitis and are incised and drained (I&D) to avoid rupture. Carbuncles are treated with systemic antibiotics and I&D. Instruct client to use disposable razors to avoid reinfecting. Reduce spread of infection by careful hand washing and separate laundry of linens
Fungal			
Candidiasis	*Candida albicans*	Appearance depends on location. In the mouth, it is called thrush, and appears as white plaques with an underlying red base with fissures on corners of the mouth. Skin lesions are pruritic, red, and moist with eroded scales. Skin lesions are common to the axilla, gluteal, perianal, and interdigital folds. Vaginal thrush causes intense itching and a cheesy drainage.	Eliminate or control the predisposing factors such as antibiotics (which alter the flora), malnutrition, diabetes, immunosuppression, pregnancy, or use of birth control pills. Use topical antifungal powders and creams. Keep the skin dry, the environment cool
Tinea (several locations) Tinea corporis (on body) Tinea capitis (on scalp) Tinea cruris (jock itch) Tinea pedis (athlete's foot)	Variety of dermatophytes	Tinea capitis presents as patchy hair loss, inflammation, scales, and folliculitis. Tinea corporis appears as round red macules and papules with scales. They have advancing borders and healing centers. Tinea cruris appears as red lesions with raised borders. Tinea pedis causes scaling, maceration, pain, and vesicles.	Infection is controlled with antifungal solutions and creams. Acute lesions may require wet dressings, keratolytic agents, or both to remove the scales. Client is taught to reduce risk by thoroughly drying after a bath or shower, wearing absorbent underwear and socks, applying talc to intertriginous areas, and wearing open shoes during warm weather

Table continued on following page

Name	Organism(s)	Clinical Manifestations	Management
Viral			
Herpes simplex	Herpes simplex virus	Vesicles preceded by sensation of itching or burning. Clear exudate from vesicles, followed by crusting, common to the nose, lips, cheeks, ears, and genitalia.	No cure available. Treatment includes pain relief and topical anesthetics. Acyclovir, an antiviral drug, may decrease viral shedding and hasten healing. Avoiding the sun and using sunscreens reduce recurrent lesions on the lips. Reduce contagiousness by frequent hand washing, not picking at lesions, avoiding sexual intercourse and kissing while lesions are active, and not sharing lipsticks. Try to identify (and avoid or control) personal triggers for lesions
Warts	Human papillomavirus	Rough, fresh, or gray-colored skin protrusion	Numerous therapies, some over-the-counter. May require electrodesiccation or cryosurgery. Intralesional injections of cytotoxic drugs may also be used. No treatment also acceptable option.

Table 78–4. Common Skin Infections and Infestations (Continued)

and electrolyte imbalance, and stress response complications (i.e., stress ulcers, body system failure). In addition, nursing management focuses on self-concept and pain management. Potassium permanganate baths may be used to reduce the risk of infection, control the odor of the drainage, and ease the pain.

Infectious Disorders

Several organisms lead to skin infections and infestations. Common skin infections are described in Table 78–4. A few are discussed in detail here.

Erysipelas and Cellulitis

Erysipelas is an acute, superficial, rapidly spreading inflammation of the dermis and lymphatics. The usual causative agent is beta-hemolytic streptococcus group A. The organism enters tissue via an abrasion, bite, trauma, or wound. Fever and leukocytosis (elevated white blood cell count) are present. The skin is elevated, beginning with a small, bright-red area. The involved area spreads peripherally to become a plaque with sharp, indurated borders. Lesions are most common on the face and extremities. Recurrence in the same area is common, possibly because of underlying lymphatic obstruction.

Cellulitis is a skin infection into deeper dermis and subcutaneous fat which results in deep, red erythema without sharp borders that spreads widely through tissue spaces (see Fig. 78–11). The skin is erythematous, edematous, tender, and sometimes nodular. *Streptococcus pyogenes* is the usual cause of this infection; however, other pathogens may be responsible. Lymphangitis may occur; if cellulitis is untreated, gangrene, metastatic abscesses, and sepsis result.

Clients at increased risk of erysipelas and cellulitis include the elderly and clients with lowered resistance from diabetes, malnutrition, steroid therapy, and the presence of wounds or ulcers. Other predisposing factors include the presence of edema or other cutaneous inflammation or wounds (e.g., tinea, eczema, burns, trauma). There is a tendency for recurrence, especially at sites of lymphatic obstruction.

Erysipelas and cellulitis are treated by either oral or IV antibiotics which cover both *Streptococcus* and *Staphylococcus aureus*. Before antibiotics are administered, a culture and sensitivity test of the wound should be taken, although it is usually difficult to yield an organism on culture. Soaks may reduce edema and inflammation. The enzymes that facilitate a rapid spread of infection also seem to produce other significant manifestations such as high fever, tachycardia, confusion, and hypotension; appropriate interventions should be taken if these occur.

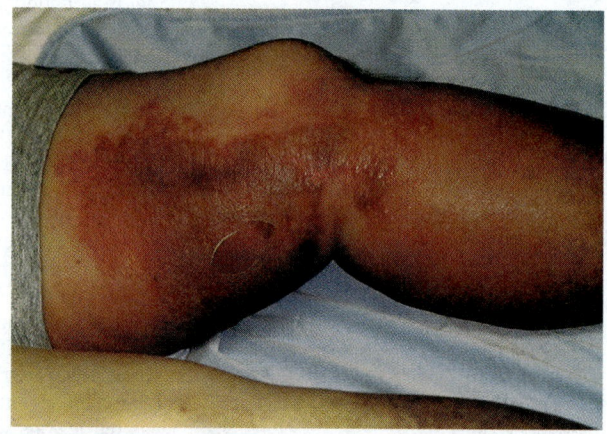

Figure 78–11. Cellulitis in a client with long-standing diabetes and stasis dermatitis.

Monitor the client's temperature and administer prescribed antipyretic medication. Prevent cross-contamination by teaching the client careful hand washing and careful disposal of linen, clothing, dressings, and so forth. Universal precautions should be used as appropriate. Close follow-up is necessary.

Herpes Zoster

Herpes zoster (Fig. 78–12), or shingles, is an infection caused by the reactivation of the varicella virus in clients who have had chickenpox. Although zoster is much less communicable than is varicella, persons who have not had chickenpox may develop it after exposure to a person with herpes zoster. An increased incidence of herpes zoster occurs in clients with lymphoma, leukemia, and acquired immunodeficiency syndrome (AIDS), probably because of their decreased immunologic response. Diagnostic tests may not be necessary because of the specific characteristics of herpes zoster; however, a Tzanck test will demonstrate multinucleated giant cells (see Chapter 77) and a viral culture is helpful.

The primary lesion of zoster is a vesicle. The classical presentation is grouped vesicles on an erythermatous base along a dermatome that appear 1 to 2 days after pain and itching at that site occasionally, only papules appear and not vesicles. Because they follow nerve pathways, the lesions do not cross the body's midline; however, rarely, the nerves of both sides may be involved. Herpes zoster lesions evolve into ulcers on the superficial mucous membrane (see Fig. 78–12)

The eruption clears in about 2 weeks unless the period between the pain and the eruption is longer than 2 days. In the latter situation, a prolonged convalescence may be expected. Residual pain, called postherpetic neuralgia, and itching are the major problems with herpes zoster. The pain may be constant or intermittent and vary from light burning to a deep visceral sensation. The duration of the pain can be weeks or months to years. Unfortunately, in the elderly, the pain generally lasts months to years. Another potential complication is herpes zoster involving the facial and acoustic nerves; involvement of the ophthalmic branch of the facial nerve requires close medical attention for avoidance of ocular complications.

Treatment for herpes zoster is antiviral medications like acyclovir (Zovirax) or given in a large dose orally or a smaller dose IV five times daily. Acyclovir when started early in the course of the disease, reduces acute pain as well as accelerates healing. Recent studies now suggest that early oral antiviral therapy will assist in reducing postherpetic neuralgia.[39] Analgesics and sedatives are prescribed for pain relief.

Topical therapy is primarily symptomatic: applications of cool compresses, use of cooling antipruritic preparations (see Table 78–1), and measures to prevent secondary infection. If pain is present, the client's normal pain tolerance and current pain level must be assessed. Systemic analgesics are usually required, and occasionally narcotics; however, in chronic pain, these may be addictive. Assess the effectiveness and side effects of prescribed analgesics. Because postherpetic neuralgia can last a long time, the client and significant others need continued intervention and support. Chronic pain management may include use of tricyclic antidepressants, phenothiazines, and other local physical modalities such as electrical stimulating units.

Nail Disorders

Disorders of the nail can be indicators of several dermatologic processes, such as an infection of the nail (e.g., paronychia), a fungal infection of the nail (e.g., onychomycosis), a dermatologic disease with prominent nail changes (e.g., psoriasis), or pigmentary abnormalities of the nail (e.g., melanoma).

Unguis incarnatus; (ingrown nail) is one of the most common nail conditions and is caused by improper nail trimming and by wearing tight or ill-fitting shoes. It primarily involves the great toes. A painful, warm inflammatory reaction results from excessive lateral growth of the nail into the nailfold. The nail acts as a foreign body, promoting granulation tissue. Decrease inflammation with warm soaks for 20 minutes several times a day. If the problem is minor, lifting the lateral portion of the nail by inserting a cotton wick prevents contact with the nailfold. Sometimes, the involved segment of the nailfold needs to be excised.

Paronychia, or infection around the nail, is characterized by red, shiny skin often associated with painful swelling. These infections frequently result from trauma, picking at the nail, or disorders such as dermatitis. Often these become secondarily infected with bacteria or fungus, which later involves the nail. As with ingrown toenail, warm soaks three or more times a day may reduce pressure and pain; however, incision and drainage of inflamed sites is frequently required. Appropriate cultures of the purulent material and the nail should be obtained. *Onychomycosis* is the term applied to any fungal infection of the nail, whether it is due to dermatophytes or candidiasis. Prescribed topical or systemic antibiotic or antifungal therapy, with emphasis on the need for compliance, is important for good outcome.

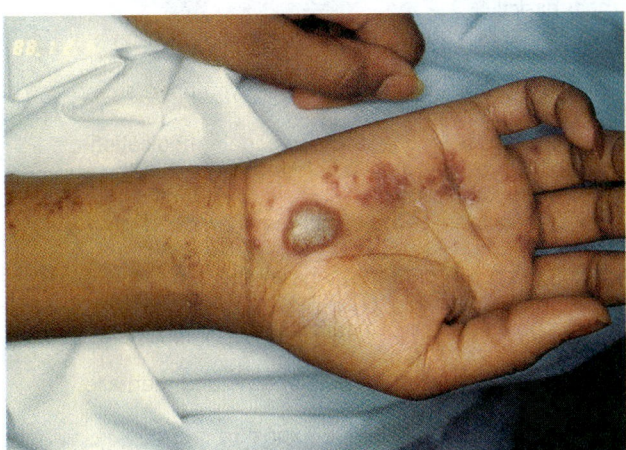

Figure 78–12. Herpes zoster. (From Callen J. P., et al. [1993]. *Color atlas of dermatology.* Philadelphia: W. B. Saunders.)

Clients should understand the importance of reducing trauma and irritation to involved nails by (1) trimming nails straight across to reduce further separation; (2) avoiding overmanicuring or self-induced trauma; (3) limiting chemical irritants such as soaps, cleansers, and nail products; and (4) keeping the nails dry.

Cancer of the Skin

Precursors to Cancer

Precursors to cancer of the skin include recurrent skin trauma and various skin lesions. In order to understand the role of prevention of skin cancer, they are discussed here.

Sunburn

Sunburn is an acute inflammatory skin response that occurs as a reaction to excessive exposure to sunlight. Dermatopathologic changes include the production of epidermal cells that have cytoplasmic and nuclear changes.

These changes are cumulative over the life span and lead to an increased incidence of skin cancer. *Photodamage* is a term used to describe repeated skin trauma from sun exposure.[51]

A first-degree sunburn produces mild, tender erythema followed by desquamation (peeling), which heals without scarring. Second-degree sunburn causes more extreme erythema and edema, and blistering results from damage to the epidermal cells. Deep sunburns are uncommon unless they are induced by artificial sources such as tanning lamps or booths. Deep sunburn produces burns (see Chapter 79).

Prevention is obviously the best therapy for sunburn. Client teaching emphasizing sun protection should never be omitted when caring for the sunburned client. The Client Education Guide lists specific precautions.

Treating sunburn involves decreasing inflammation and rehydrating the damaged skin. For localized, first-degree sunburn, apply cool tap water soaks for 20 minutes or until the skin is cool. This limits skin destruction, prevents edema, and potentially reduces blisters. Tepid tap water baths are indicated for large sunburned areas. After a bath or soak, apply water-based emollients, preferably refrigerated for an additional cooling effect. Emollients

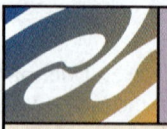

CLIENT EDUCATION GUIDE

Simple Guidelines to Help Protect You from the Damaging Rays of the Sun

1. Minimize sun exposure during the hours of 10 AM to 2 PM (11 AM to 3 PM daylight saving time), when the sun is strongest. Try to plan your outdoor activities for the early morning or late afternoon.
2. Wear a hat, long-sleeved shirt, and long pants when out in the sun. Choose tightly woven materials for greater protection from the sun's rays.
3. Apply a sunscreen before every exposure to the sun and reapply frequently and liberally, at least every 2 hours, as long as you stay in the sun. The sunscreen should always be reapplied after swimming or perspiring heavily, because products differ in their degrees of water resistance. Sunscreens with an SPF (sun protection factor) of 15 or more printed on the label are recommended.
4. Use a sunscreen during high-altitude activities such as mountain climbing and skiing. At high altitudes, where there is less atmosphere to absorb the sun's rays, your risk of burning is greater. The sun is also stronger near the equator, where the sun's rays strike the earth most directly.
5. Do not forget to use your sunscreen on overcast days. The sun's rays are as damaging to your skin on cloudy, hazy days as they are on sunny days.
6. Clients at high risk of skin cancer (outdoor workers, those who are fair-skinned, and those who have already had skin cancer) should apply sunscreens daily.
7. Photosensitivity—an increased sensitivity to sun exposure—is a possible side effect of certain medications, drugs and cosmetics, and birth control pills. Consult your physician or pharmacist before going out in the sun if you are using any such products. You may need to take extra precautions.
8. If you develop an allergic reaction to your sunscreen, change sunscreens. One of the many products on the market today should be right for you.
9. Beware of reflective surfaces! Sand, snow, concrete, and water can reflect more than half the sun's rays onto your skin. Sitting in the shade does not guarantee protection from sunburn.
10. Avoid tanning parlors. The ultraviolet light emitted by tanning booths causes sunburn and premature aging and increases your risk of developing skin cancer.
11. Keep young children out of the sun. Begin using sunscreens on children at 6 months of age, and then allow sun exposure with moderation.
12. Teach children sun protection early. Sun damage occurs with each unprotected sun exposure and accumulates over the course of a lifetime.

From The Skin Cancer Foundation, New York.

should also be applied throughout the day to soothe and relieve dryness. Lotions or foams containing camphor and menthol (e.g., Sarna) can also be beneficial. Avoid use of over-the-counter remedies containing local anesthetics (benzocaine, dibucaine [Nupercaine], or lidocaine [Xylocaine]) because they are rarely effective and have the potential of inducing contact sensitivity.

For second-degree sunburn, apply continuous cool, normal saline soaks or soaking baths to reduce oozing and edema. Aspirate very large blisters, and apply sterile dressings. Avoid debridement unless there is evidence of secondary bacterial infection. Silver sulfadiazine may be prescribed.

Prostaglandin inhibitors (aspirin) may be used to reduce erythema and inflammation in adults. Topical corticosteroids may be prescribed to be used sparingly in nonocclusive vehicles (i.e., lotion or gel) for their vasoconstrictive effects. Systemic corticosteroids are prescribed only for clients with very extensive, painful burns, but their use has declined because they seem to offer little efficacy in a reasonable dose range.

Actinic Keratosis

Actinic keratosis, the most common epithelial precancerous lesion in whites, is caused by sun exposure. It affects nearly 100% of the elderly white population. There is a small but definite risk of malignant degeneration and subsequent metastatic potential in neglected lesions.

Actinic keratosis most frequently occurs in areas of chronic, usually high-intensity sun exposure including face, tops of ears, back of the neck, forearms, and the back of the hand.

The clinical appearance of actinic keratoses can be quite varied. The typical lesion is an irregularly shaped, flat, slightly erythematous macule or papule with indistinct borders and an overlying hard keratotic scale or horn. In some cases, the erythema or horn may be absent. This scale can be periodically shed or peeled off, but then it regrows. The lesion varies in size from pinhead to several centimeters and is often more easily palpated than observed. Single lesions may be seen, but more often they appear in groups on a background of sun-damaged skin.[44]

■ Medical Management

Topical application of 5-fluorouracil (5-FU, Efudex), a topical antimetabolite, is presently one of the best approaches to treatment of widespread actinic damage with multiple lesions. The advantage of 5-FU is that large areas of widespread disease can be treated at the same time. Use of 5-FU not only removes the majority of premalignant and superficial malignant lesions that can be seen but also will uncover and destroy clinically undetectable lesions of this type. However, the major disadvantage is the therapeutic inflammatory response that often accompanies successful treatment. This response sequence is erythema usually followed by vesiculation, erosion, ulcerations, necrosis, and epithelialization.

The medication should be applied twice daily with a gloved hand, carefully avoiding eyes, nose, mouth, and scrotum. A porous gauze dressing may be applied over the medication for cosmetic reasons without increase in reaction. However, occlusive dressing should be avoided because of increased inflammatory response. Medication should be continued until the inflammatory response reaches the erosion, necrosis, and ulceration stage, at which time the medication should be stopped. The usual duration of therapy is 2 to 4 weeks; the client may experience extreme discomfort requiring pain medication by this point. At the time 5-FU is stopped, topical corticosteroid creams may be applied to reduce inflammation and provide the client with additional pain relief. Complete healing of the lesions may not be evident for 1 to 2 months after cessation of therapy.

■ Surgical Management

Cryotherapy. Cryotherapy using liquid nitrogen is the most common treatment for single or small numbers of actinic keratoses. Liquid nitrogen is usually applied with a cotton applicator or spraying device and requires no local anesthetic (Fig. 78–13A). The client does note a small amount of discomfort at the time of freezing, which may linger afterward. Application of a warm, damp washcloth intermittently to the site may bring relief. Freezing frequently results in inflammation with blister formation, and blister care should be reviewed with the client. Care must be taken to avoid overfreezing the site, which may result in scarring. Cryotherapy is cost-effective, easy to perform, and has minimal side effects.

Electrodesiccation and Curettage. Electrodesiccation produces superficial destruction through bursts of electrical current and is usually done under local anesthesia (Fig. 78–13B). The tissue is destroyed by mechanical disruption of cells and heat. The tissue is removed by scraping or scooping with a loop-shaped instrument called a curet (Fig. 78–13C). This method provides tissue for histologic diagnosis if needed. The wounds usually heal quickly with adequate wound care. Wound care should emphasize keeping the wound site moist with some nonsensitizing topical antibiotic ointment such as bacitracin.

Shave or Excisional Biopsy. Shave or excisional biopsy is indicated on lesions that are large or have other characteristics of a cutaneous malignancy (induration, erythema, erosion). It is often difficult to distinguish a large actinic keratosis from a squamous cell carcinoma without histologic diagnosis. Biopsy should also be done on lesions that persist after adequate treatment with 5-FU. Local anesthesia is given for a biopsy and allows electrodesiccation to be done painlessly after biopsy. Excisional biopsy requires primary closure of the site and may be a more extensive procedure than the lesion warrants; however, it ensures removal of the entire growth.

Skin Cancer

Skin cancer is the most common cancer in the United States and the number of new skin cancers and skin

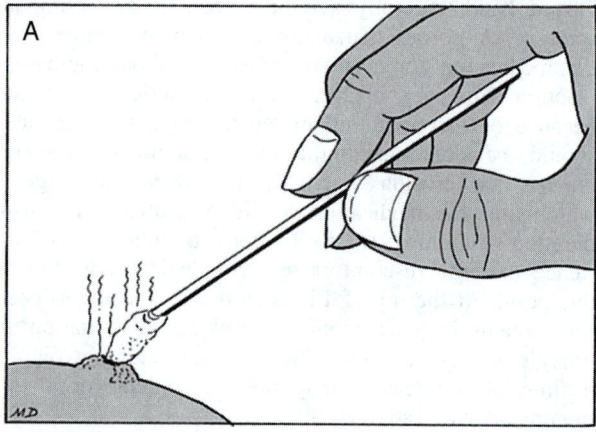

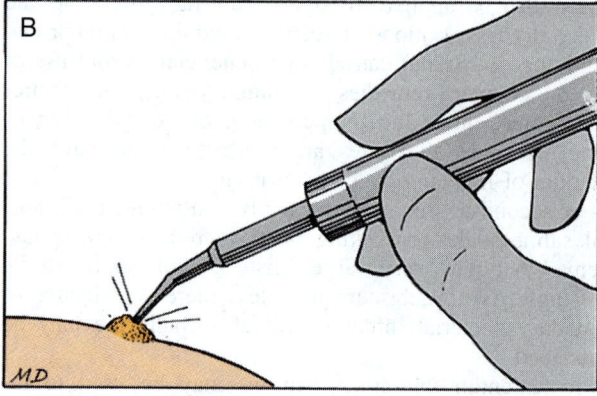

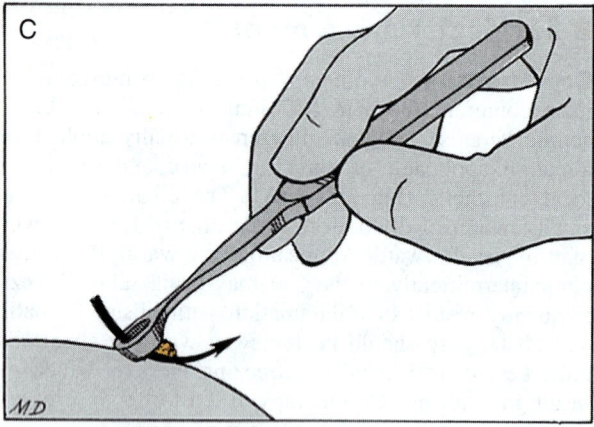

Figure 78–13. Methods for destroying skin lesions. *A,* Cryotherapy. Liquid nitrogen is applied with a saturated cotton-tipped applicator directly to the lesion or sprayed on. This causes tissue destruction by freezing. *B,* Electrodesiccation. Tissue is destroyed by heat from an electrical current; note gloved hand. *C,* Curettage. A curet (cutting instrument) removes tissue by scraping or scooping; note gloved hand.

cancer deaths are increasing at alarming rates. Skin cancer is a malignant condition caused by uncontrolled growth and spread of abnormal cells in a specific layer of the skin. The several different kinds of skin cancer are distinguished by the types of cells involved. Basal cell carcinoma, squamous cell carcinoma, and malignant melanoma are the three most common types of skin cancer. More than 90% of all skin cancers fall into the first two classifications. Both basal cell carcinoma and squamous cell carcinoma are slow-growing tumors that have a cure rate of 95% or greater with early treatment.

Etiology and Risk Factors

The cause of skin cancer is well-known. Prolonged or intermittent exposure to UVL radiation from the sun, especially when it results in sunburn and blistering, plays a key role in the induction of skin cancer, especially malignant melanoma. The majority of all non-melanoma skin cancers occur on parts of the body unprotected by clothing (face, neck, forearms, and backs of hands) and in persons who have received considerable exposure to sunlight. All persons are at risk of skin cancer regardless of skin tone and hair color, however, some persons are at much greater risk than others. In general, people with red, blond, or light-brown hair with light complexions or freckles, many of Celtic or Scandinavian origin, are most susceptible; blacks and Asians are least susceptible.

All persons should be taught to look at new moles or lesions and evaluate them for the danger signs. Danger signals in moles (pigmented nevi) are presented in Box 78–1. Suspicious lesions should be examined by a physician.

The history of a person's pattern of reaction to acute sun exposure is correlated with the his or her tendency to get actinic keratosis and skin cancer. Those who never

---

Box 78–1. Danger Signals Suggestive of Malignant Transformation of Moles

- *Change in color,* especially red, white, and blue, sudden darkening; mottled shades of brown or black
- *Change in diameter,* especially sudden increase
- *Change in outline,* especially development of irregular margins
- *Change in surface characteristics,* especially scaliness, erosion, oozing, crusting, bleeding, ulceration, development of a mushrooming mass on the surface of the lesion
- *Change in consistency,* especially softening or friability
- *Change in symptoms,* especially pruritus
- *Change in shape,* especially irregular elevation from a previously flat condition
- *Change in surrounding skin,* especially "leaking" of pigment from the lesion into surrounding skin or pigmented "satellite" lesions

tan and always burn after 1 to 2 hours of midday summer sun are most susceptible. Those who burn once or twice at the beginning of summer and then tan are somewhat less susceptible. Those who never burn and always tan are the least susceptible. The most severely affected persons usually have a history of long-term occupational (farmers, construction workers, surveyors, sailors) or recreational (swimmers, skiers, surfers, sunbathers) sun exposure.

Clinical Manifestations and Diagnostic Findings

■ Basal Cell Carcinoma

Basal cell carcinoma, the most common form of skin cancer, is a malignant epithelial tumor of the skin that arises from the basal cells contained in the epidermis.

The tumor is usually painless and slow-growing, generally appearing on sun-exposed skin, face, ears, head, neck, or hands. Occasionally, basal cell carcinoma may appear on the trunk, especially the upper back and chest. The majority are caused by chronic overexposure to UVL radiation, and only a few cases can be linked to arsenic, burns, scars, exposure to radiation, or genetic predisposition. Clinical and histologic findings are used to identify the tumor.

The most common clinical presentation of basal cell carcinoma is the nodular lesion (Fig. 78–14). This is a dome-shaped papule with a well-defined border with a classic "pearly" texture. Basal cell carcinoma has this flesh-colored "pearly" or shiny appearance because it does not keratinize. Telangiectatic vessels frequently overlie the lesion. As the lesion enlarges, the center may flatten or ulcerate; however, the border will still be raised and give a "rolled" appearance.

Basal cell carcinomas almost never metastasize. They can, however, be locally destructive and invasive through tissue. This is particularly true on the face, where a lesion can invade deep structures with resultant loss of an eye, ear, or nose. If untreated, the tumor can invade through

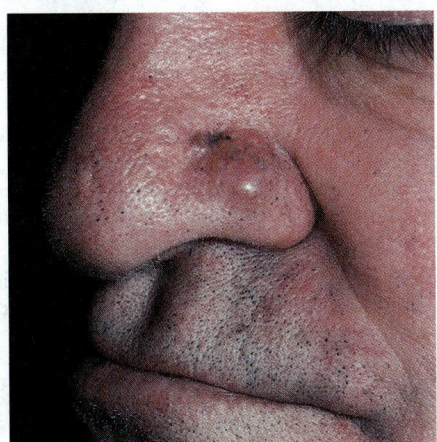

Figure 78–14. Basal cell carcinoma. (From Murphy, G. F., & Herzberg, A. J. [1996]. *Atlas of dermatopathology.* Philadelphia: W. B. Saunders.)

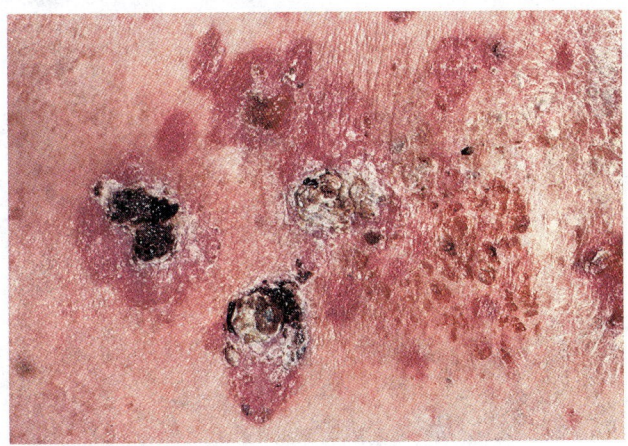

Figure 78–15. Squamous cell carcinoma. (From Murphy, G. F., & Herzberg, A. J. [1996]. *Atlas of dermatopathology.* Philadelphia: W. B. Saunders.)

bone and brain. However, if the tumor is identified and treated early, local excision or even nonexcisional destruction is usually curative.

Clients who have had one basal cell carcinoma are at greater risk of developing others. Recurrences of previously treated basal cell carcinomas are also possible but more unusual. The possible recurrence generally occurs within the first 2 years after removal or therapy.

■ Squamous Cell Carcinoma

Squamous cell carcinoma (Fig. 78–15) is the second most common skin cancer in whites. It is a tumor of the epidermal keratinocytes and rarely occurs in dark-skinned people. It is found on areas often exposed to the sun, typically the rim of the ear, the face, the lips and mouth, and the backs of the hands. Squamous cell carcinoma is more difficult to characterize than is basal cell carcinoma. These tumors are poorly marginated; the edge often blends into surrounding sun-damaged skin. Squamous cell carcinoma may present as an ulcer; a flat red area; cutaneous horn; indurated plaque; or hyperkeratotic papule or nodule. Often it presents as a red- to skin-colored papule surmounted by varying amounts of scale. These lesions grow more rapidly than does a basal cell carcinoma. These tumors are potentially dangerous because they may infiltrate surrounding structures, metastasize to lymph nodes, and be subsequently fatal.

■ Malignant Melanoma

Malignant melanoma (Figs. 78–16 and 78–17) is a cancer of melanocytes; it is the deadliest form of skin cancer. The incidence and death rate from melanoma are rising worldwide. In countries populated with fair-skinned whites, the incidence of melanoma and mortality have risen by 7% to 15% per year, more than doubling over the past decade. Whites have 10 times the incidence that blacks do.

UVL continues to be one of the most important causes of malignant melanoma. However, melanoma can appear

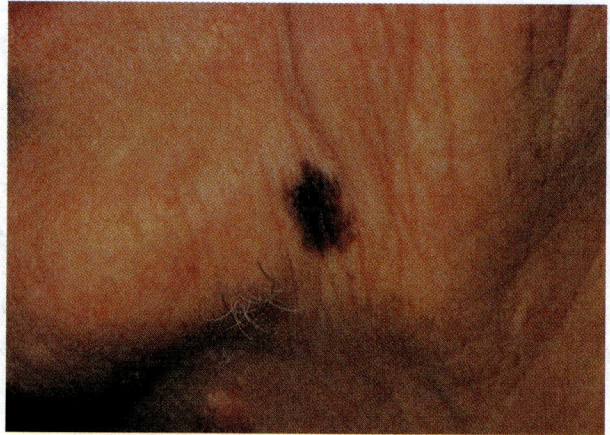

Figure 78–16. Superficial spreading melanoma.

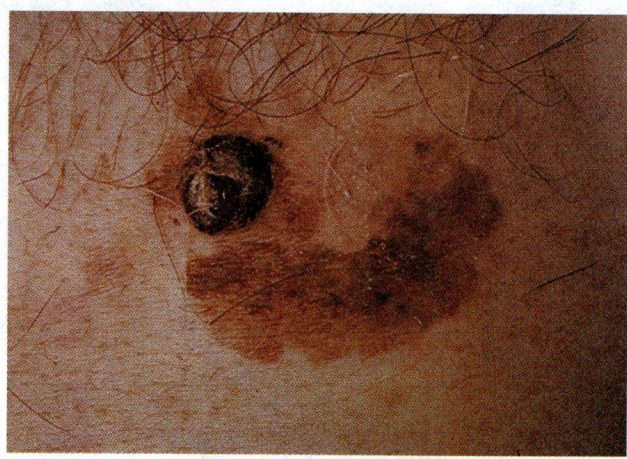

Figure 78–17. Nodular melanoma.

anywhere on the body, not just on sun-exposed areas. The majority of malignant melanomas appear to be associated with the intensity rather than the duration of sunlight exposure, in contrast to basal cell and squamous cell carcinomas. Melanoma tends to be observed more often in whites who have had a history of blistering sunburns or a family history of melanoma or atypical moles. The suspicion of melanoma is based on history as well as the clinical appearance. The cardinal clinical manifestation of melanoma is a change in a skin lesion observed over a period of months. If a lesion grows so fast that it doubles in size in 10 days, it is usually an inflammation. If a lesion changes so slowly that neither the client nor family is sure of a change, it is usually benign. Changes that may signal melanoma include doubling size in 3 to 8

months, change in diameter, bleeding, itching, ulceration, a change in color, or development of a palpable lymph node.

Melanomas usually have (1) various shades of brown, black, or blue within one lesion, (2) an irregular raised surface, (3) an irregular perimeter, (4) ulceration of the surface, and (5) crusting. Four types are presented in Table 78–5. The tumor can metastasize, usually to the brain, lungs, bones, liver, and skin, and is ultimately fatal. The prognosis of melanoma has become more predictable. Clinically, metastatic melanoma is universally fatal. Prognosis and mortality of melanoma that is not clinically metastatic at presentation depend critically on the depth of the lesion at the time of excision. The more superficial or "thin" the tumor, the better the prognosis.

Table 78–5. Types of Melanoma

Name	General Information	Clinical Manifestations
Superficial spreading melanoma (SSM)	The most common form of melanoma; slowly changing lesion with more rapid growth just before diagnosis	Deeply pigmented area contained within a brown nevus (freckle); usually flat and asymmetrical; as lesion grows, it can have variegations in color ranging from jet black to dark blue to pale gray or white; looks lacy, may have areas of no color within the lesions; usually 2 cm wide
Nodular melanoma (NM)	Second most common form of melanoma; more aggressive tumor and has a shorter clinical onset time than SSM	Common on the trunk, head, and neck; usually 1–2 cm in diameter; frequently begin in normal skin, rather than in a preexisting lesion; dark and more uniform in color; may resemble a blood blister or hemangioma; dome-shaped with sharp borders
Lentigo maligna melanoma (LMM)	Fairly uncommon tumor, typically appears on the face of white women; usually has been present for long period of time (5–15 yr)	Generally a large, flat lesion that looks like a stain on the skin; typically tan with various shades of brown; metastasis less common
Acral lentiginous melanoma (ALM)	Commonly occurs on palms and soles of feet; more common in dark-skinned persons, usually occurs in older people; evolves in short periods of time, a few months to years	Large lesion, about 3 cm in diameter; resemble LMM (a tan or brown flat lesion on the palm or sole); can be misdiagnosed as corns; ulceration is common; likely to metastasize

Management

■ Medical Management

Medical management begins by having a high index of suspicion for any type of skin cancer but specifically for melanoma. The need for early detection cannot be overemphasized in dealing with malignant melanoma. Any indication, whether it is a high-risk client or a suspicious lesion, is adequate reason for referral.

■ Surgical Management

Treatment of any and all skin cancers requires removal of the lesion. The tumor removed needs to have a specified margin free of tumor (differs depending on type of skin cancer) to guarantee full removal of the skin cancer.

A special surgical technique primarily used for the removal of skin malignancies such as basal cell and squamous cell carcinoma is Mohs' surgery. Mohs' surgery is also indicated for primary lesions in areas where preservation of normal skin is necessary (e.g., eyelids, pinna, nasolabial folds). The technique is based on a series of excisions. Careful microscopic tissue assessment "maps" the presence or absence of malignant cells within each specimen. The procedure may be lengthy. After all tumor tissue is removed, the wound is closed with sutures or with a flap (see Chapter 80) or allowed to close by secondary intention.

Basal cell and squamous cell carcinomas can also be excised and the area closed primarily or with a skin flap. The advantage of this technique is that it requires much less time, and the scar is controllable as a fine line. The tumor is completely excised with adequate margins of tumor-free tissue. If there is doubt about adequacy of margins, the specimen is sent for pathologic diagnosis (frozen section). Surgery can be combined with Mohs' technique.

The treatment of malignant melanoma is wide local excision. Surgical excision begins with a biopsy to determine the stage of the cancer. Biopsies are performed whenever the client cannot be assured that a lesion is benign. Excisional biopsy is the removal of the lesion and a narrow margin of normal-appearing tissue. This tissue is examined, and the melanoma is staged (Fig. 78–18).

Surgeons differ on the timing of the definitive surgery. Some surgeons excise the lesion after frozen-section examination while the client is still on the operating table. Other surgeons wait for the results of permanent section pathologic diagnosis and then proceed with definitive treatment. The final excision is usually completed within 1 week of biopsy. Nurses should be aware that although there is theoretical risk of tumor spread during biopsy, there is no convincing evidence that waiting 1 to even 6

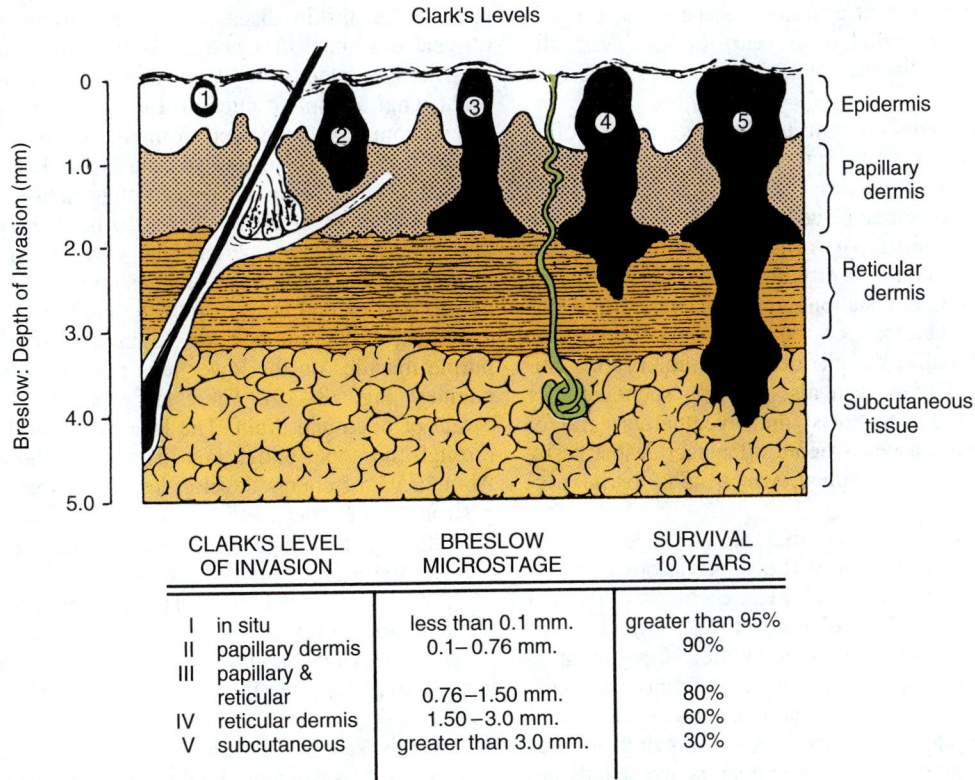

CLARK'S LEVEL OF INVASION		BRESLOW MICROSTAGE	SURVIVAL 10 YEARS
I	in situ	less than 0.1 mm.	greater than 95%
II	papillary dermis	0.1–0.76 mm.	90%
III	papillary & reticular	0.76–1.50 mm.	80%
IV	reticular dermis	1.50–3.0 mm.	60%
V	subcutaneous	greater than 3.0 mm.	30%

Figure 78–18. The combination of Clark's level of invasion and Breslow's depth of invasion allows prediction of 10-year survival in melanoma. (From Eisenbaum, S. L., & Black, J. M. [1988]. Melanoma. *Plastic Surgical Nursing, 8*[2], 42–47.)

weeks after biopsy jeopardizes the outcome. In fact, sometimes the delay gives the client time to prepare for surgery, both physically and psychologically.

Wide excision of the tumor with a 1- to 3-cm margin of normal-appearing skin is the treatment. The margin is based on the type of melanoma. The area is closed in surgery either primarily (skin edges sewn together) or with grafts or flaps.

Most clients with metastatic melanoma live less than 1 year.[4] There is no cure today for metastatic melanoma, but some therapies will improve the quality of life. A treatment plan is arranged on the basis of several factors: site of the tumor, number of metastases, rate of tumor growth, previous treatments, response to treatment, and the age, general health, and desires of the client.

Some treatments include surgery to remove metastatic lesions, radiation therapy, chemotherapy, and local hyperthermia. Of course, the client can opt for no further treatment.

Cutaneous T-Cell Lymphoma (Mycosis Fungoides)

Cutaneous T-cell lymphoma (CTCL), also known as mycosis fungoides, is a malignant disease involving the T helper cells. Malignant T cells in the blood migrate to the skin, where they have an affinity for the epidermis. The malignant cells continue to grow and change, eventually moving into the dermis. The cause is not known, and the course is unpredictable depending on the type of presentation. The three distinct presentations are patch, plaque, and tumor. Presentation of a tumor has the worst prognosis with a survival period of 3 years or less. Virtually every organ, especially the liver, spleen, and lungs, may be involved.

CTCL is extremely difficult to diagnose and is often misdiagnosed. In its early stages, CTCL can clinically mimic eczematous processes. The initial erythematous papules resemble eczematous conditions, including psoriasis and atopic dermatitis. The original eruptions of CTCL may be either transitory or prolonged and sometimes are pruritic. Clinical manifestations include eversion of the eyelids and hyperkeratosis of the palms and soles, often with fissuring. Finally, the plaques form tumors that ultimately ulcerate. Tumors can also develop spontaneously in previously unaffected areas, and eventual visceral or organ involvement ensues. Clients often feel desperate by the time diagnosis is confirmed, which adds to the psychological difficulties.

Control of pruritus is essential at all stages and is accomplished by rehydration of the skin, various dry skin therapy (see Xerotic Eczema), topical corticosteroids, and PUVA therapy (see Ultraviolet Light Therapy). Prevention of secondary infections is important. Nitrogen mustard and other chemotherapy agents are administered topically. They are applied daily and are often the initial treatment. Photophoresis, a treatment involving the removal of small amounts of blood that is irradiated and then returned to the body, is used frequently in more advanced stages. Total-body electron beam therapy with or without adjuvant chemotherapy is an aggressive approach often used. Unfortunately, even if these therapies succeed in clearing the skin, the disorder is still fatal because of systemic involvement.

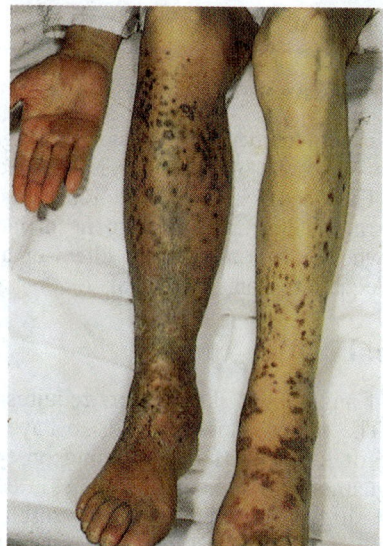

Figure 78–19. Kaposi's sarcoma.

Kaposi's Sarcoma

Kaposi's sarcoma is a vascular malignancy that presents as a skin disorder. It has a long history. Kaposi's sarcoma used to be a skin disease seen predominantly in 50- to 60-year-old men in Central or Eastern Europe. It was seen less frequently in blacks and the immunosuppressed (e.g., renal transplant clients). In the past 15 years, Kaposi's sarcoma has been seen in many clients with AIDS.

The cause of Kaposi's sarcoma is not known, although HIV and herpes virus have been suggested as cofactors in its development. It is considered to be due to a failure in the immune system, perhaps as a result of frequent or overwhelming infections. The lesions begin in the middermis and extend upward into the epidermis.

Kaposi's sarcoma lesions begin as red, dark-blue, or purple macules on the lower legs that coalesce into larger plaques (Fig. 78–19). These large plaques frequently ulcerate or open and drain. The lesions spread by metastasis through the upper body, then to the face and oral mucosa. About 75% of clients develop lesions of the lymph nodes, gastrointestinal tract, and lungs.[14] Clients also report pain and itching in the lesions; as Kaposi's sarcoma progresses, the legs become edematous.

Client history needs to be specific about sexual history when lesions of this type are present. All known risk factors for AIDS should be asked of the client such as homosexual activity, IV drug use, multiple sexual partners, etc.

Kaposi's sarcoma is diagnosed by skin biopsy, and a high index of suspicion should exist for those clients who are immunosuppressed. Local lesions can be excised or treated with intralesional chemotherapy. Systemic lesions are treated with a combination of interferon-α, cytotoxic agents, and radiation. General response to treatment is poor. A complete discussion of AIDS may be found in Chapter 27.

Nursing interventions include getting informed consent for HIV testing and addressing the client's questions and concerns. Patient education should include guidelines for safe sex and giving clients local and national patient resource groups' addresses and telephone numbers.

Conclusions

Skin disorders range from those that are a mere nuisance, such as dry skin, to life-threatening disorders, such as melanoma. Nurses frequently manage skin disorders independently, therefore, a thorough knowledge of the use of topical medications and therapies is critical. Because much of skin care is provided by the client or family, the nurse must use excellent teaching skills to convey needed self-care information.

Thinking Critically

1. You are caring for an elderly woman who has had a stroke that has left her with residual paralysis on the left side. She has also developed a pressure ulcer on the left trochanter, in part because she lies on her left side all the time. While caring for her on Monday, you convince her to sit in a chair and to lie on her right side. When you care for her again on Thursday, the ulcer is twice as large and deeper. She refuses to turn to the right and says "I like lying on my left side." What can you do to help this client?

Factors to Consider: What pressure reduction methods should be instituted? Is there any harm in lying on a pressure ulcer? Why might she be at increased risk because of malnutrition?

2. The client is a 72-year-old white man who had a large excisional biopsy on his forearm to rule out squamous cell carcinoma. The next day the client calls the office complaining of pain at the surgery site. What additional questions need to be asked, and what potential interventions might be necessary?

Factors to Consider: What signs and symptoms would indicate an infection is present? Is age a factor in wound healing?

3. The client is a healthy 41-year-old woman who presented to the clinic with a week-long history of intensely itchy, erythematous red lesions under her breasts. The rash appears to be spreading and some of the centers of the lesions developed tiny pustules. Additionally, the woman complains of a 12-lb weight loss over the past 6 months despite always feeling hungry and thirsty. She denies any medical problems or taking any current systemic or topical medications.

Factors to Consider: What diagnostic study can determine the cause of the problem? What endocrine disorder may be involved given the history of candidiasis, thirst, and weight loss?

Bibliography

1. Abel, E. A., et al. (1986). Drugs in exacerbation of psoriasis. *Journal of the American Academy of Dermatology, 15*(11), 1007–1022.
2. Alterescu, V. (1989). The financial cost of inpatient pressure ulcers to an acute care facility. *Decubitus, 2*(3), 14–23.
3. Arndt, K. W. (1989). *Manual of dermatological therapeutics* (4th ed:). Boston: Little, Brown.
4. Baumeister, L., & Nicol, N. H. (1994). Lupus and sun protection—what you need to know. *Pediatric Nursing, 20*(4), 371–375.
5. Bergstrom, N., et al. (1987). The Braden scale for predicting pressure sore risk. *Nursing Research, 36*(4), 205–210.
6. Bergstrom, N., et al. (1994). *Treatment of pressure ulcers clinical practice guideline*, No. 15. Rockville, MD. U.S. Department of Health and Human Services, Public Health Service, Agency for Health Care Policy and Research, AHCPR Publication No. 95-0652.
7. Black, J. (1991). Reconstructive surgery in the elderly. *Plastic Surgical Nursing, 11*(4), 151–162.
8. Black, J., & Black, S. (1987). Surgical management of pressure ulcers. *Nursing Clinics of North America, 22*(2), 429–438.
9. Braden, B., & Bergstrom, N. (1989). Clinical utility of the Braden scale for predicting pressure sore risk. *Decubitus, 2*(3), 44–51.
10. Braden, B., & Bryant, R. (1990). Innovations to prevent and treat pressure ulcers. *Geriatric Nursing, 4,* 182–186.
11. Clark, R. A. F., et al. (1990). Atopic dermatitis. In M. Sam & P. J. Lynch (Eds.), *Principles and practice of dermatology* (pp. 365–380). Philadelphia: W. B. Saunders.
12. Clark, R. A. F., et al. (1990). Current concepts in the management of the patient with atopic dermatitis. *Modern Medicine 58*(3), 78–94.
13. Cohen, I., et al. (Eds.) (1992). *Wound healing.* Philadelphia: W. B. Saunders.
14. Copper, D. (1990). Optimizing wound healing. *Nursing Clinics of North America, 25*(1), 165–180.
15. Curtis, A., et al. (1990). Hyperbaric oxygen therapy—An overview. *Plastic Surgical Nursing, 10*(2), 63–68.
16. Cuzzell, J., & Stotts, N. (1990). Trial and error yields to knowledge. *American Journal of Nursing, 90*(10), 53–61.
17. Dealey, C. (1991). The size of the pressure-sore problem in a teaching hospital. *Journal of Advanced Nursing, 16,* 663–670.
18. Deloach, E. D., et al. (1992). Osteomyelitis underlying severe pressure sores. *Contemporary Surgery, 40*(5), 25–32.
19. Dicken, C. H. (1984). Retinoids: a review. *Journal of the American Academy of Dermatology, 11*(10), 541–552.
20. Dermatology Nurses' Association. (1996). *Phototherapy administration guidelines for nurse phototherapists and phototechnicians.* Pitman, NJ: Author.
21. Drake, L. A., et al. (1990). Guidelines of care for acne vulgaris. *Journal of American Academy of Dermatology, 22,* 676–680.
22. Eisenbaum, S. L., & Black, J. M. (1988). Melanoma. *Plastic Surgical Nursing, 8*(2), 42–47.
23. Ellis, C. N., & Voorhees, J. J. (1987). Etretinate therapy. *Journal of the American Academy of Dermatology, 16*(1), 267–291.
24. Faller, N., & Lawrence, K. (1991). Nursing to promote healing. *Ostomy/Wound Management, 32*(1), 43–46, 48.
25. Farber, E. M., et al. (1983). Recent advances in the treatment of psoriasis. *Journal of the American Academy of Dermatology, 8*(3), 311–321.
26. Fitzpatrick, T. B., et al. (1990). *Dermatology in general medicine* (4th ed.), New York: McGraw-Hill.
27. French, E., & Sifner, K. (1991). A method for consistent documentation of pressure sores. *Rehabilitation Nursing, 16*(4), 204–207.
28. Glizzard, D. (1991). Understanding the pathophysiology of psoriasis. A nursing perspective. *Dermatology Nursing, 3*(5), 305–314.
29. Goodman, T., et al. (1990). Skin ulcers. *AORN Journal, 52*(1), 24–37.

30. Goss, R. (1992). Regeneration versus repair. In I. Cohen et al. (Eds.), *Wound healing.* Philadelphia: W. B. Saunders.

31. Green, E., & Kalz, J. (1991). Practice guidelines for management of pressure ulcers. *Decubitus, 4*(1), 36–42.

32. Huff, J. C., et al. (1993). Effect of oral acyclovir on pain resolution in herpes zoster: A reanalysis. *Journal of Medical Virology, 41*(Suppl. 1), 93–96.

33. Kaminski, M., & Devin, G. (1989). Nutritional management of decubitus ulcers in the elderly. *Decubitus, 2*(4), 20–30.

34. Keesling, B., & Friedman, S. (1987). Psychosocial factors in sunbathing and sunscreen use. *Health Psychology, 6*(5), 477–493.

35. Krasner, D. (1991). Resolving the dressing dilemma: Selecting wound dressings by category. *Ostomy/Wound Management, 35*(4), 62, 64–70.

36. Laudano, J. B., Leach, E. E., & Armstrong, R. B. (1990). Acne: Therapeutic perspectives with an emphasis on the role of isotretinoin. *Dermatology Nursing, 2*(6), 328–337.

37. Lawrence, W. (1992). Clinical management of nonhealing wounds. In I. Cohen, et al. (Eds.), *Wound healing.* Philadelphia: W. B. Saunders.

38. McCance, K., & Huether, S. (1994). *Pathophysiology* (2nd ed.). St. Louis: Mosby–Year Book.

39. Meehan, M. (1990). Multisite pressure ulcer prevalence study. *Decubitus, 3*(4), 14–17.

40. Menkes, A., et al. (1985). Psoriasis treatment with suberymemogenic ultraviolet B radiation and a coal tar extract. *Journal of the American Academy of Dermatology, 12*(1), 21–25.

41. Murphy, G. F., & Herzberg, A. J. (1996). *Atlas of dermatopathology.* Philadelphia: W. B. Saunders.

42. Nicol, N. H. (1987). Atopic dermatitis, the (wet) wrap-up. *American Journal of Nursing, 87*(12), 1560–1562.

43. Nicol, N. H. (1989). Early detection and prevention of skin cancer. *Dermatology Nursing, 1*(1), 11–20.

44. Nicol, N. H. (1989). Actinic keratosis: preventable and treatable like other precancerous and cancerous skin lesions. *Plastic Surgical Nursing, 9*(2), 49–55.

45. Nicol, N. H. (1989). What's new in sunscreens? Choices, choices, choices. *Pediatric Nursing, 15*(4), 417–418.

46. Nicol, N. H. (1990). Current considerations and management of atopic dermatitis. *Dermatology Nursing, 2*(3), 129–138.

47. Nicol, N. H. (1992). In S. Rudy (Ed.), *All about acne: A model workshop* (pp. 1–25). Pitman, NJ: Dermatology Nurses' Association.

48. Nicol, N. H. (1994). Alteration of the integument in children. In K. McCance & S. Huether (Eds.), *Pathophysiology—The biologic basis for disease in adults and children,* (2nd ed., pp. 1561–1577). St. Louis, Mosby–Year Book.

49. Nicol, N. H. (1994). Diseases of epidermal origin. In M. J. Hill (Ed.), *Skin Disorders,* (pp. 27–38). *Mosby's Clinical Nursing Series,* St. Louis, Mosby–Year Book.

50. Nicol, N. H., & Clark, R. A. F. (1988). Therapy of atopic dermatitis. In E. Farmer & T. Provost (Eds.), *Current therapy in dermatology*—2. Philadelphia: B. C. Decker.

51. Nicol, N. H., & Fenske, N. (1993). Focus on photodamage. *Dermatology Nursing, 5,* 263–277.

52. Nicol, N. H., & Hill, M. J. (1994). Altered skin integrity. In R. Foster, M. Hunsberger, & C. Betz (Eds.), *Family-Centered Nursing Care of Children,* (2nd ed., pp. 1645–1677). Philadelphia: W. B. Saunders.

53. Nicol, N. H., & Leung, D. Y. M. (1992). Management of the patient with atopic dermatitis. *American Journal of Asthma and Allergy for Pediatricians, 5,* 97–105.

54. Nicol, N. H., Ruszkowski, A. M. & Moore, J. A. (1995). Contact dermatitis and the role of patch testing in its diagnosis and management. *Dermatology Nursing,* (Suppl. Feb), 5–10.

55. Otson, B. (1989). Effects of massage for prevention of pressure ulcers. *Decubitus, 2*(4), 32–37.

56. Panel of the Prediction and Prevention of Pressure Ulcers in Adults (1992). *Pressure ulcers in adults: Prediction and prevention: Clinical practice guidelines.* AHCPR Publication No. 92-0050. Rockville, MD: Agency for Health Care Policy and Research, Public Health Service, U.S. Department of Health and Human Services.

57. Pochi, P. E., et al. (1991). Report on the Consensus Conference on Acne Classification. *Journal of American Academy of Dermatology, 24*(3), 495–500.

58. Provan, A., & Phillips, T. (1991). An overview of moist wound dressings: The under cover story. *Dermatology Nursing, 3*(6), 393–400.

59. Salasche, S. J. (1988). Actinic keratosis and keratoacanthoma. In E. Farmer & T. Provost (Eds.), *Current therapy in dermatology*—2 (pp. 74–76). Philadelphia: B. C. Decker.

60. Sams, V. M., & Lynch, P. J. (1990). *Principles and practice of dermatology.* New York: Churchill Livingstone.

61. Sater, B., et al. (1991). A protocol for the management of patients at high risk for pressure sores. In W. Chenitz, et al. (Eds.), *Clinical Gerontological Nursing.* Philadelphia: W. B. Saunders.

62. Scotto, J., & Fears, T. R. (1987). The association of solar ultraviolet and skin melanoma incidence among caucasians in the United States. *Cancer Investigation, 5*(4), 275–283.

63. Shelk, J. (1991). Phototherapy: A nursing overview. *Dermatology Nursing, 3*(6), 401–410.

64. Smith, A., & Malone, J. (1990). Preventing pressure ulcers in institutionalized elders: Assessing the effects of small unscheduled shifts in body position. *Decubitus, 3*(4), 20–24.

65. Sober, A. (1992). Management of rosacea. *Dermatology Nursing,* 1992, 4(6), 454–456.

66. Stern, R. S., et al. (1984). Isotretinoin and pregnancy. *Journal of the American Academy of Dermatology, 10*(5), 851–854.

67. Stern, R. S., et al. (1986). Risk reduction for nonmelanoma skin cancer with childhood sunscreen use. *Archives of Dermatology, 122*(5), 537–544.

68. Stern, R. S., et al. (1984). Topical versus systemic agent treatment for papulopustular acne. *Archives of Dermatology, 120*(12), 1571–1578.

69. Stewart, L. A., Engelken, G. J., & Nicol, N. H. (1992). Essentials of occupational contact dermatitis. *Dermatology Nursing, 4,* 175–183.

70. Stone, J. (1991). Pressure sores. In W. Chenitz, et al. (Eds.), *Clinical gerontological nursing.* Philadelphia: W.B. Saunders.

71. (1989). Sunlight, ultraviolet radiation, and the skin. *National Institutes of Health Consensus Development Conference Statement,* May 8–10, 7(8), 1–27.

72. Taylor, C. R., et al. (1990). Photoaging/photodamage and photoprotection. *Journal of The American Academy of Dermatology, 22*(1), 1–15.

73. Wemer, Y. (1986). The water content of the stratum corneum in patients with atopic dermatitis. *Acta Dermato-Venereologica* (Stockholm), 66, 282–284.

74. Wilkner, N. E., & Weston, W. L. (1988). Skin neoplasms. In R. W. Schrier (Ed.), *Medicine: Diagnosis and treatment* (pp. 513–530). Boston: Little, Brown.

75. Wiseman, D., et al. (1992). Wound dressings: Design and use. In I. Cohen, et al. (Eds.), *Wound healing.* Philadelphia: W. B. Saunders.

Nursing Care of Clients with Burns

CHAPTER 79

Gretchen J. Carrougher

Injuries that result from direct contact or exposure to any thermal, chemical, electrical, or radiation source are termed *burns*. Burn injuries occur when energy from a heat source is transferred to the tissues of the body. The depth of injury is related to temperature and the duration of exposure or contact.

Burn care has improved in recent decades, resulting in a lower mortality rate for victims of burn injuries.[32] Dedicated burn centers have been established with multidisciplinary burn team members who work together to care for the burn client and family. Advances in prehospital and inpatient care have contributed to survival. However, despite these advances, many people are still injured and die each year from burns. In the United States, approximately 1.4 million people seek medical attention every year for injuries caused by burns; of these, approximately 54,000 are hospitalized with severe injuries. Approximately 5,000 people die each year as a result of their burn injury.[9]

Etiology

Burn injuries are categorized according to the mechanism of injury.

Thermal Burns

Thermal burns are caused by exposure to or contact with flame, hot liquids, semiliquids (steam), semisolids (tar), or hot objects. Specific examples of thermal burns are those sustained in residential fires, explosive automobile accidents, scald injuries, clothing ignition, and ignition of poorly stored flammable liquids.

Chemical Burns

Chemical burns are caused by tissue contact with strong acids, alkalis, or organic compounds. The concentration, volume, and type of chemical, as well as the duration of contact, determine the severity of a chemical injury. Chemical burns can result from contact with certain household cleaning agents and various chemicals used in industry, agriculture, and the military. More than 25,000 products capable of causing chemical injuries have been identified.[25] Chemical injuries to the eyes and inhalation of chemical fumes are particularly serious.

Electrical Burns

Electrical burn injuries are caused by heat that is generated by the electrical energy as it passes through the body.[46] Electrical injuries can result from contact with exposed or faulty electrical wiring or high-voltage power lines. Individuals struck by lightning also sustain electrical injury.

The extent of the injury is influenced by the duration of contact, the intensity of the current (voltage), the type of current (direct or alternating), the pathway of the current, and the resistance of the tissues as the electric current passes through the body. Electrical contact with voltage greater than 40 is potentially dangerous; however, voltage greater than 1000 is considered to be high voltage and is associated with extensive tissue damage.

Radiation Burns

Radiation burns are the least common type of burn injury and are caused by exposure to a radioactive source. These types of injuries have been associated with nuclear radiation accidents, the use of ionizing radiation in industry, and from therapeutic radiation. A sunburn (solar radiation) from prolonged exposure to ultraviolet rays is also considered to be a type of radiation burn.

The amount of radioactive energy that an individual receives following exposure depends on the distance the person is from the source of the radiation, the strength of the radiation source, the duration of exposure, the extent of the body area exposed, and the amount of shielding between the source and the person.[4] An acute, localized radiation injury appears similar to a cutaneous thermal injury and is characterized by skin erythema, edema, and pain. In contrast, whole-body radiation causes systemic symptoms (radiation sickness) that are dose dependent.

Risk Factors

Data collected from the National Burn Information Exchange reveal that 75% of all burn injuries result from the actions of the victim, with many of these injuries occurring in the home environment. This section addresses risk factors in the adult; refer to a pediatric text for specific information about burns in children.

Contact with scalding liquids in either the kitchen or bathroom is often cited as a mechanism of injury.[15, 31, 96] Clients between the ages of 3 and 70 years with scald injuries often have mental or physical limitations.[77] Overturned coffee pots and cooking pans spilling hot liquid and grease, overheated foods, liquids cooked in microwave ovens, and hot tap water have been identified as specific causes.[30, 67] Because the severity of the burn is directly related to the temperature of the liquid and the duration of contact, efforts to reduce the incidence of scald injuries have included the recommendations of the Consumer Products Safety Commission and Underwriters Laboratory that the maximum temperature on the thermostats of hot water heaters be lowered and a warning label identifying the potential for injury be affixed to the water heater.[6] In addition, a relatively new thermostatic control system (anti-scald device) has been developed that, when installed at the faucet or shower head, shuts off the flow of water when the temperature rises above a predetermined temperature, typically 110° F (43.3° C).[102]

Everyday situations such as bathing and cooking may lead to a burn injury.[87, 96] Clothing ignition during routine meal preparation has also been cited, particularly in the elderly population.[60, 87, 95] Although this is a well-documented problem, no flammability standards exist for adult clothing manufacturers as they do for children's sleep-

wear manufacturers. See Box 79–1 for burn injury prevention recommendations in the home.

Residential fires are another common cause of burn injuries. Chimneys, vent flues, fixed heating units, fireplaces, central-heating systems, wood-burning stoves, ignition of wood-shingled roofs, cigarettes, and human error have all been implicated. Cigarette-related ignition of furniture and mattresses is the single leading cause of fire deaths, cited in 28% of fatal housefires.[1] Approximately 10% of residential fire deaths are attributed to children playing with matches or other ignition sources.[9]

Of primary importance in reducing injuries and deaths from residential fires is the presence of an operable smoke detector and fire extinguisher. It has been estimated that the risk of dying in a residential fire is reduced 50% when an operable smoke detector is in place.[36] Some suggest that insurance carriers should refuse to issue hazard insurance for residential properties if smoke detectors and fire extinguisher are not present on the premises.[91] See Box 79–2 for fire prevention recommendations in the home.

Pathophysiologic Response

The pathophysiologic changes that occur immediately following a cutaneous burn injury depend on the extent or size of the burn. For smaller burns, the body's response to injury is localized to the injured area. However, with more extensive burns (i.e., 25% or more of the total body surface area [TBSA]), the body's response to injury is systemic and proportional to the extent of the injury. Extensive burn injuries affect all major systems of the body. The systemic response to burn injury is typically biphasic, characterized by early hypofunction that is followed later by hyperfunction of each organ system.

Fluid and Electrolyte Balance

Immediately following a burn injury, vasoactive substances (catecholamines, histamine, serotonin, leukotrienes, kinins, and prostaglandins) are released from the injured tissues. These substances initiate changes in capillary integrity, allowing plasma to seep into surrounding tissues. Direct heat injury to vessels further increases capillary permeability, which permits sodium ions to enter the cell and potassium ions to exit. Overall, this creates an osmotic gradient, which leads to increases in intracellular and interstitial fluid and further depletes intravascular fluid volumes.[71] These substances exert their effect both locally (in the area of injury) and systemically. The burn-injured client's hemodynamic balance, metabolism, and immune status are altered.

Hyponatremia, hypernatremia, and hyperkalemia are common electrolyte abnormalities that affect the burn-injured client at different points in the recovery process. Extensive burns (greater than 25% TBSA) result in generalized body edema in both burned and nonburned tissues[26] and a decrease in circulating intravascular blood volume. Several studies have found that tissue water content doubles within 1 hour of injury. Hematocrit levels are elevated in the first 24 hours postinjury, demonstrating hemoconcentration from the loss of intravascular fluid. In addition, evaporative fluid losses through the burn wound are 4 to 20 times greater than normal[97] and remain elevated until complete wound closure is obtained. The result is a decrease in organ perfusion. If the intravascular space is not replenished with intravenous fluids, hypovolemic (burn) shock, and ultimately death, ensue for the victim of an extensive burn.

At approximately 18 to 36 hours after burn injury, capillary membrane integrity begins to normalize.[72] The initial rise in hematocrit seen early after injury falls to below normal by the third or fourth day postinjury due to red blood cell loss and damage at the time of injury. Over the ensuing days and weeks, the body begins to reabsorb the edema fluid, and the excess fluid is excreted via diuresis (Fig. 79–1).

Nervous System

The burn-injured client typically suffers no neurologic sequelae unless the injury was associated with neurologic trauma (e.g., fall, explosion), impaired perfusion to the brain, hypoxemia (e.g., closed-space fire), inhalation injury (e.g., exposure to asphyxiants or other toxic materials from the fire), electrical burn injury, or from the effects of drugs present in the body at the time of injury.

The client with a major burn injury is often awake and alert on admission to the hospital. If agitation develops in the immediate postburn period, the client may be suffering from hypovolemia or hypoxemia.

Cardiovascular System

Following a major burn injury, heart rate and peripheral vascular resistance increase in response to the release of catecholamines and to the relative hypovolemia, but initial cardiac output falls (hypofunction).[10] At approximately 24 hours after burn injury in persons receiving adequate fluid resuscitation, cardiac output returns to normal and then increases (2 to 2.5 times normal) to meet the hypermetabolic needs of the body (hyperfunction). This change in cardiac output occurs even before circulating intravascular volume levels are restored to normal.[10]

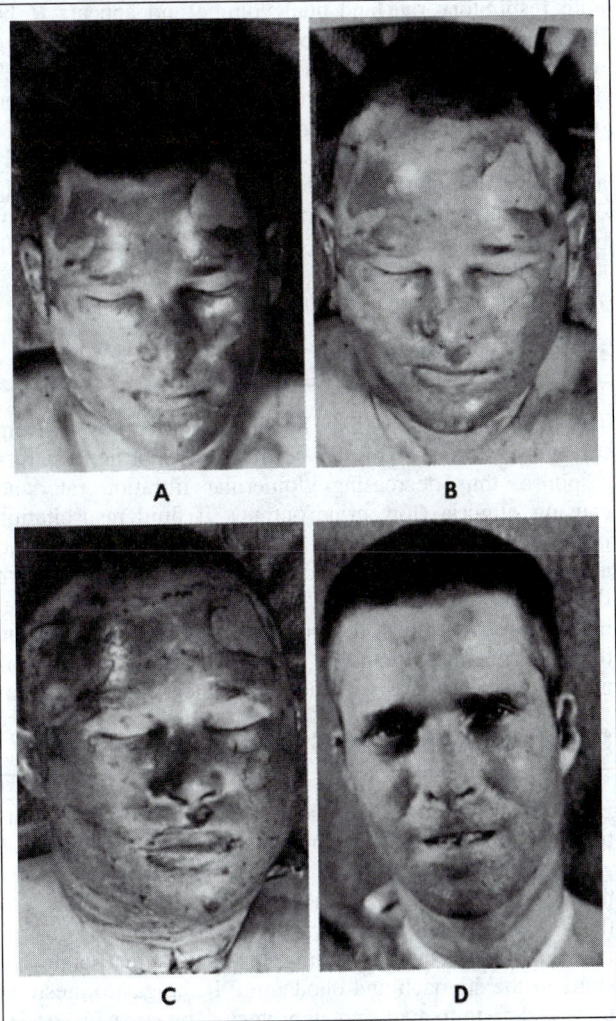

Figure 79–1. Facial edema at various times following a burn injury to the face and neck. Edema worsens over the first 24 to 48 hours following a burn. *A*, 3 hours after burn. *B*, 8 hours after burn. *C*, 24 hours after burn, when the edema has typically maximized. *D*, Complete healing after 40 days. (From Artz, C. P., et al. [1979]. *Burns: A team approach*. Philadelphia: W. B. Saunders.)

Arterial blood pressure is normal or slightly elevated unless severe hypovolemia exists.

Some research investigators have suggested that a myocardial depressant factor exists and circulates in the early postinjury period. Although a specific factor has yet to be identified, it may be the cause of unresponsiveness to fluid resuscitation in some clients with extensive burns.

Respiratory System

Without a concomitant inhalation injury, initial findings suggestive of pulmonary insufficiency are rare. Minute ventilation is often normal or slightly decreased early after a burn injury. Following fluid resuscitation, the client may exhibit a rise in minute ventilation (hyperventilation), especially if he or she is fearful, anxious, or in pain. This hyperventilation is the result of an increase in both respiratory rate and tidal volume and appears to be the result of the hypermetabolism that is seen after burn injury. It typically peaks in the second postinjury week and then gradually returns to normal as the burn wound heals or is closed by grafting.[84]

Pulmonary vascular resistance may increase slightly and lung compliance may decrease. The changes in lung compliance cause a proportionate increase in work of breathing. However, these changes are typically small, and in the absence of any pulmonary parenchymal (tissue) damage, they require no specialized treatment.

Urinary System

The body responds initially by shunting blood away from the kidneys as part of the normal neurohormonal stress response, thus decreasing glomerular filtration rate and causing oliguria (low urine output). If fluid resuscitation is delayed or inadequate, hypovolemia progresses and acute renal failure may occur. However, with adequate fluid resuscitation and a rise in cardiac output, renal blood flow will return to normal. Following resuscitation, the body begins to reabsorb the edema fluid and to eliminate it through diuresis. Urine output then increases.

Gastrointestinal System

Blood flow to the mesenteric bed is also diminished initially, leading to the development of intestinal ileus and gastrointestinal dysfunction in clients with burns greater than 25% TBSA.[83] With the reduction in blood flow to the gastric mucosa, ischemic changes to the upper gastrointestinal tract occur, resulting in small, superficial erosions to the stomach and duodenum. If the gastrointestinal tract is left untreated and unprotected by antacids or H_2 histamine receptor antagonists, the erosions can progress to ulcerations (called *Curling's ulcer* in burn clients) and gastrointestinal bleeding.

Following adequate fluid resuscitation, gastrointestinal motility returns, signaled by a return of bowel sounds, flatus, and stool production.

Immune System

Immune system function is depressed. Depression of lymphocyte activity, a decrease in immunoglobulin production, suppression of complement activity, and an alteration in neutrophil and macrophage functioning are evident following extensive burn injuries.[7, 39, 58, 75] In addition, the burn injury disrupts the body's primary barrier to infection. Together these changes result in some degree of immunosuppression, increasing the risk of infection and life-threatening sepsis.

Psychological Response

A myriad of psychological and emotional responses to burn injuries have been identified, ranging from fear to psychosis.[33] A victim's response is influenced by age, personality, cultural and ethnic background, extent and location of injury, and the resulting impact on body im-

age. In addition, separation from family and friends and the change in the client's normal role and responsibilities affect the reaction to burn trauma.

Four stages of psychosocial responses following burn trauma have been characterized by Lee: (1) impact, (2) retreat or withdrawal, (3) acknowledgment, and (4) the reconstructive period.[61]

The period of *impact* occurs immediately postinjury and is characterized by shock, disbelief, and feelings of being overwhelmed. The client and family may be aware of what is happening but may be coping with the situation poorly. Studies indicate that the families of critically ill patients have a need for assurance, proximity to the injured family member, and information. Specifically, families want to know how the family member is being treated, what is being done for him or her, specific facts about the client's progress, and why certain procedures are being done.[64]

Retreat is characterized by repression, withdrawal, denial, and suppression. Although seemingly destructive, these coping strategies may be protective in that they allow the client to maintain an intact psyche.

The third phase, *acknowledgment*, begins when the client accepts the injury and the resultant change in body image. Mourning of actual or perceived losses may be apparent. During this phase, clients may benefit from meeting with other burn-injured clients in one-to-one contact or group support meetings.

The final phase, *the reconstructive period*, begins when the client and family accept the limitations imposed by the injury and begin to plan realistically for the future. Client and family may benefit from job retraining.

Burn Pain

Considerable pain is associated with burn injuries. Burn victims typically describe two types of pain resulting from their injury: (1) background pain, and (2) procedural pain.

Background Pain. Background pain occurs while the client is at rest or is engaged in nonprocedural activities (e.g., when shifting position in bed or with chest wall movements that occur with a deep breath or cough). Background pain is described as continuous in nature and low in intensity, typically lasting the duration of the clinical course.[21]

Procedural Pain. Procedural pain is related to therapeutic measures commonly performed during burn care. About 52% of clients report moderate to severe pain during burn wound debridement,[28] and up to 84% of burned adults report intense pain levels during therapeutic procedures.[80] Procedural pain is described as acute and high in intensity.

Inhalation Injury

Exposure to asphyxiants and smoke commonly occurs with flame injuries, particularly if the victim was trapped in an enclosed, smoke-filled space (e.g., a residential fire). The incidence of inhalation injury has been estimated to be as great as 30% for persons injured in a fire.[74]

Clinical manifestations suggestive of inhalation injury include facial burns, erythema or swelling of the oropharynx or nasopharynx, singed nasal hairs, agitation or anxiety, tachypnea, flaring nostrils, stridor, wheezing, dyspnea, hoarse voice, carbonaceous (sooty) sputum, and cough. Fiberoptic bronchoscopy and xenon 133 lung scan can be used to confirm the diagnosis.[2, 24, 78]

The pulmonary pathophysiology that occurs with inhalation injury is multifactorial and relates to the severity and type of smoke or gases inhaled. Exposure to asphyxiants, smoke poisoning, and direct thermal or heat injury to lung tissue constitute the three facets of an inhalation injury. Each or all may coexist in the burn-injured client suffering from an inhalation injury.[41]

Asphyxiants

Exposure to asphyxiants is the most common cause of early mortality from inhalation injury.[29, 106] Carbon monoxide (CO), a common asphyxiant, is produced when organic substances (e.g., wood or coal) burn. It is a colorless, odorless, and tasteless gas that has an affinity for hemoglobin that is 200 times greater than that of oxygen. With inhalation of CO, the oxygen molecules are displaced and CO reversibly binds to hemoglobin to form carboxyhemoglobin (COHb). Tissue hypoxia occurs from an overall decrease in the blood's oxygen-delivering capability. COHb levels are easily monitored via blood serum levels in the clinical setting. Clinical manifestations of acute CO poisoning are related to the level of COHb saturation (Table 79–1).

Smoke Poisoning

Smoke poisoning results from the inhalation of the by-products of combustion: noxious chemicals and particulate matter. The pulmonary response includes a localized inflammatory reaction, a decrease in bronchial ciliary action, and a decrease in alveolar surfactant. Mucosal

edema occurs in the smaller airways, leading to audible wheezing on auscultation. After several hours, sloughing of the tracheobronchial epithelium may occur, and hemorrhagic tracheobronchitis may develop. Adult respiratory distress syndrome may follow.

Direct Thermal (Heat) Injury

Thermal burns to the lower airways of the pulmonary system are rare because of the protective reflex closure of the glottis and the ability of the respiratory tract to exchange heat effectively.[73] However, thermal burns to the lower airways can occur with the inhalation of steam or explosive gases or with aspiration of scalding liquids. Thermal burns to the upper airways (mouth, nasopharynx, pharynx, and larynx) are more common and generally appear erythematous and edematous with mucosal blisters or ulcerations. The mucosal edema can lead to upper airway obstruction, particularly during the first 24 to 48 hours after burn injury.

Classification of Burn Severity

The American Burn Association has published a severity classification schedule for burn injuries (Table 79–2). These guidelines are intended to assist the clinician in determining injury severity for the burn client. This classification schedule separates injuries into major, moderate, or minor categories. Clients with major burns are usually transferred to a specialized burn care facility after local emergency treatment has been provided. Clients with moderate burns can usually be treated on an inpatient basis at the receiving hospital. Clients with minor burns usually receive initial care in the emergency department and are then discharged for follow-up care on an outpatient basis.[5]

The severity of a burn injury is classified based on the risk of mortality and the risk of cosmetic or functional disability.[5] Factors that influence injury severity include the following:

- Burn depth
- Burn size (percentage of TBSA burned)
- Burn location
- Age of burn victim
- General health of burn victim
- Mechanism of injury

Burn Depth

Burn injuries are classified as a partial-thickness or full-thickness burn injury. Partial-thickness burn injuries are classified as first- and second-degree burns (Fig. 79–2). Full-thickness burn injuries are classified as third- and fourth-degree burns (Figs. 79–3 and 79–4). The appearance, sensation, and recovery course of these burns are compared in Figure 79–5.

Table 79–1. Clinical Manifestations of Carbon Monoxide (CO) Poisoning

CO Level (%)	Clinical Manifestations
5–10	Impaired visual acuity
11–20	Flushing, headache
21–30	Nausea, impaired dexterity
31–40	Vomiting, dizziness, syncope
41–50	Tachypnea, tachycardia
>50	Coma, death

Adapted from Cioffi, W. G., & Rue, L. W. (1991). Diagnosis and treatment of inhalation injuries. *Critical Care Clinics of North America, 3*(2): 195.

Table 79–2. American Burn Association Severity Classification for Burn Injuries

Major Burn Injury

25% TBSA burn in adults <40 yr
20% TBSA burn in adults >40 yr
20% TBSA burn in children <10 yr
                    or
Burns involving the face, eyes, ears, hands, feet, and perineum likely to result in functional or cosmetic disability
                    or
High-voltage electrical burn injury
                    or
All burn injuries with concomitant inhalation injury or major trauma

Moderate Burn Injury

15%–25% TBSA burn in adults <40 yr
10%–20% TBSA burn in adults >40 yr
10%–20% TBSA burn in children <10 yr
                    with
Less than 10% TBSA full-thickness burn without cosmetic or functional risk to burn involving the face, eyes, ears, hands, feet, or perineum

Minor Burn Injury

<15% TBSA burn in adults <40 yr
<10% TBSA burn in adults >40 yr
<10% TBSA burn in children <10 yr
                    with
<2% TBSA full-thickness burn and no cosmetic or functional risk to the face, eyes, ears, hands, feet, or perineum

TBSA, total body surface area.
Adapted from American Burn Association. (1984). Guidelines for service standards and severity classification in the treatment of burn injury. *American College of Surgeons Bulletin, 69*(10), 24–28.

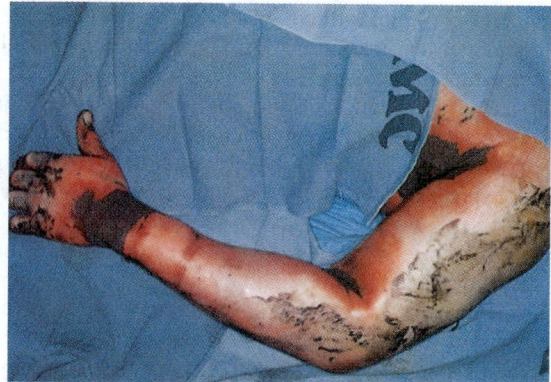

Figure 79–3. Full-thickness burn injury (third-degree burn).

Burn Size

The size of a burn (percentage of injured skin, excluding first-degree burns) is determined by one of two techniques: (1) the rule of 9s and (2) an age-specific burn diagram or chart. Burn size is expressed as a percentage of TBSA. The accuracy of the calculation varies with the method and the experience of the individual making the determination.[13, 38]

The rule of 9s was introduced in the late 1940s as a quick assessment tool for estimating burn size.[57, 66] The basis of this rule is that the body is divided into anatomic sections, each of which represents 9%, or a multiple of 9%, of the TBSA (Fig. 79–6). This method is easy,

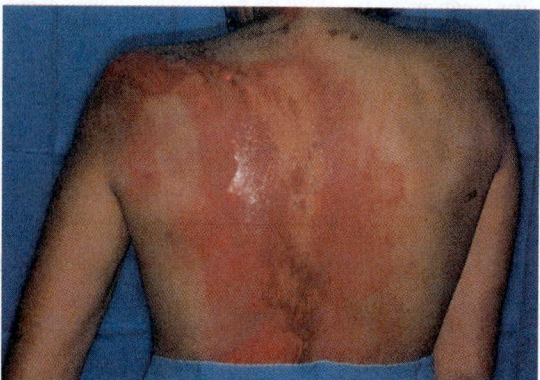

Figure 79–2. Partial-thickness burn injury (second-degree burn).

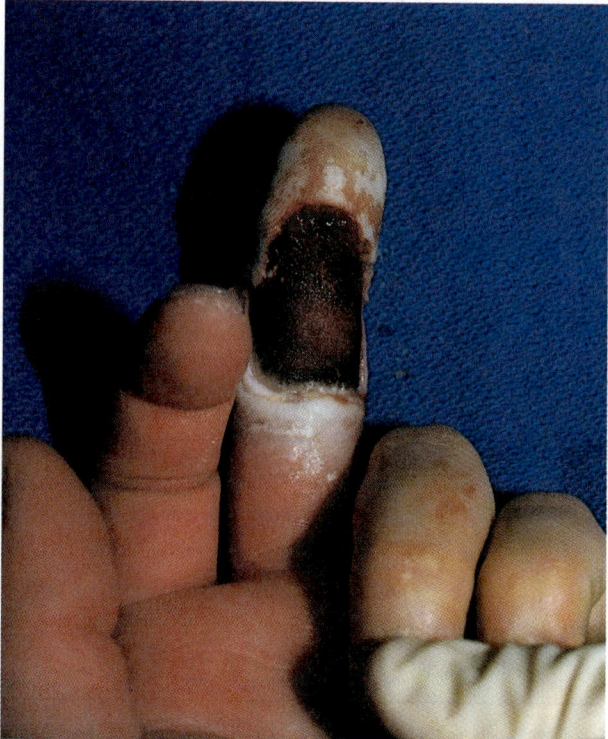

Figure 79–4. Full-thickness burn injury (fourth-degree burn).

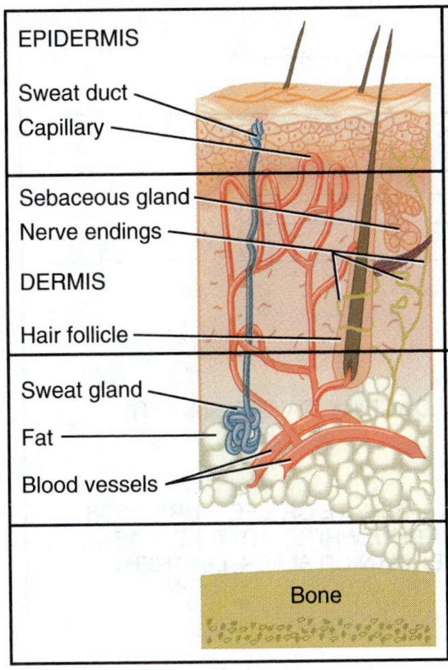
EPIDERMIS
Sweat duct
Capillary
Sebaceous gland
Nerve endings
DERMIS
Hair follicle
Sweat gland
Fat
Blood vessels
Bone

		WOUND APPEARANCE	WOUND SENSATION	COURSE OF HEALING
PARTIAL-THICKNESS BURN	1st-degree	Epidermis remains intact and without blisters. Erythema; skin blanches with pressure.	Painful	Discomfort lasts 48–72 hours. Desquamation in 3–7 days
PARTIAL-THICKNESS BURN	2nd-degree	Wet, shiny, weeping surface. Blisters. Wound blanches with pressure.	Painful. Very sensitive to touch, air currents	Superficial partial-thickness burn heals in < 21 days. Deep partial-thickness burn requires > 21 days for healing. Healing rates vary with burn depth and presence/absence of infection.
FULL-THICKNESS BURN	3rd-degree	Color variable (i.e., deep red, white, black, brown). Surface dry. Thrombosed vessels visible. No blanching	Insensate (↓ pinprick sensation)	Autografting required for healing
FULL-THICKNESS BURN	4th-degree	Color variable. Charring visible in deepest areas. Extremity movement limited	Insensate	Amputation of extremities likely. Autografting required for healing

Figure 79–5. Burn injury classification according to the depth of injury.

requiring no diagrams to determine the percentage of TBSA injured. Therefore, it has been used in emergency departments, where the initial triage occurs.

A burn diagram charts the percentages for body segments according to age and provides a more accurate estimate of burn size (Fig. 79–7).

Extent of burn injury is most accurate after initial debridement. Verify the TBSA after debridement.

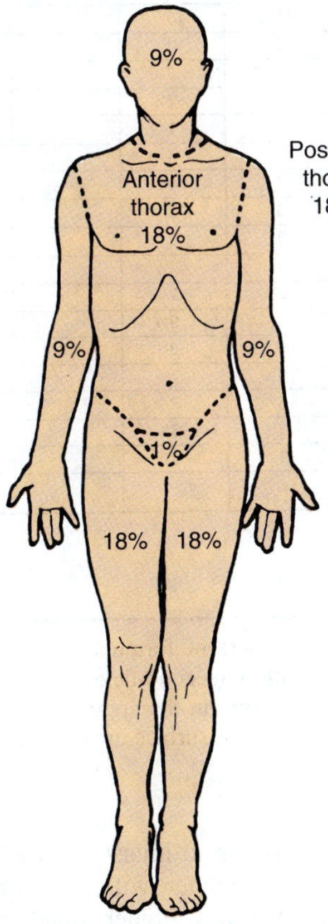
9%
Anterior thorax 18%
Posterior thorax 18%
9%
9%
1%
18%
18%

Figure 79–6. The *rule of 9s* provides a quick method for estimating the extent of a burn injury in the adult.

Burn Location

Burns of the head, neck, and chest frequently have associated pulmonary complications. Burns involving the face often have associated corneal abrasions. Burns of the ears are prone to auricular chondritis and are susceptible to infection and further loss of tissue. Burns of the hands and joints often require intense physical and occupational therapy and have implications for loss of work time and/or permanent physical and vocational disability. Burns involving the perineal area are prone to infection due to autocontamination by urine and feces. Circumferential burns of extremities may produce a tourniquet-like effect and lead to distal vascular compromise. Circumferential thorax burns may lead to inadequate chest wall expansion and pulmonary insufficiency.

Age

The client's age affects the severity and outcome of the burn. Mortality rates are higher for children younger than 4 years, particularly in the 0- to 1-year age group, and for clients older than 65 years.[15, 17, 47, 58, 66, 87]

High mortality and morbidity statistics in the elderly burn client result from the combination of functional impairments (slower reaction time, impaired judgment, and decreased mobility), living alone, environmental hazards, and significant preburn morbidity.[15, 47] Compounding this vulnerability to burn injury is the thinning of the skin and atrophy of skin appendages.

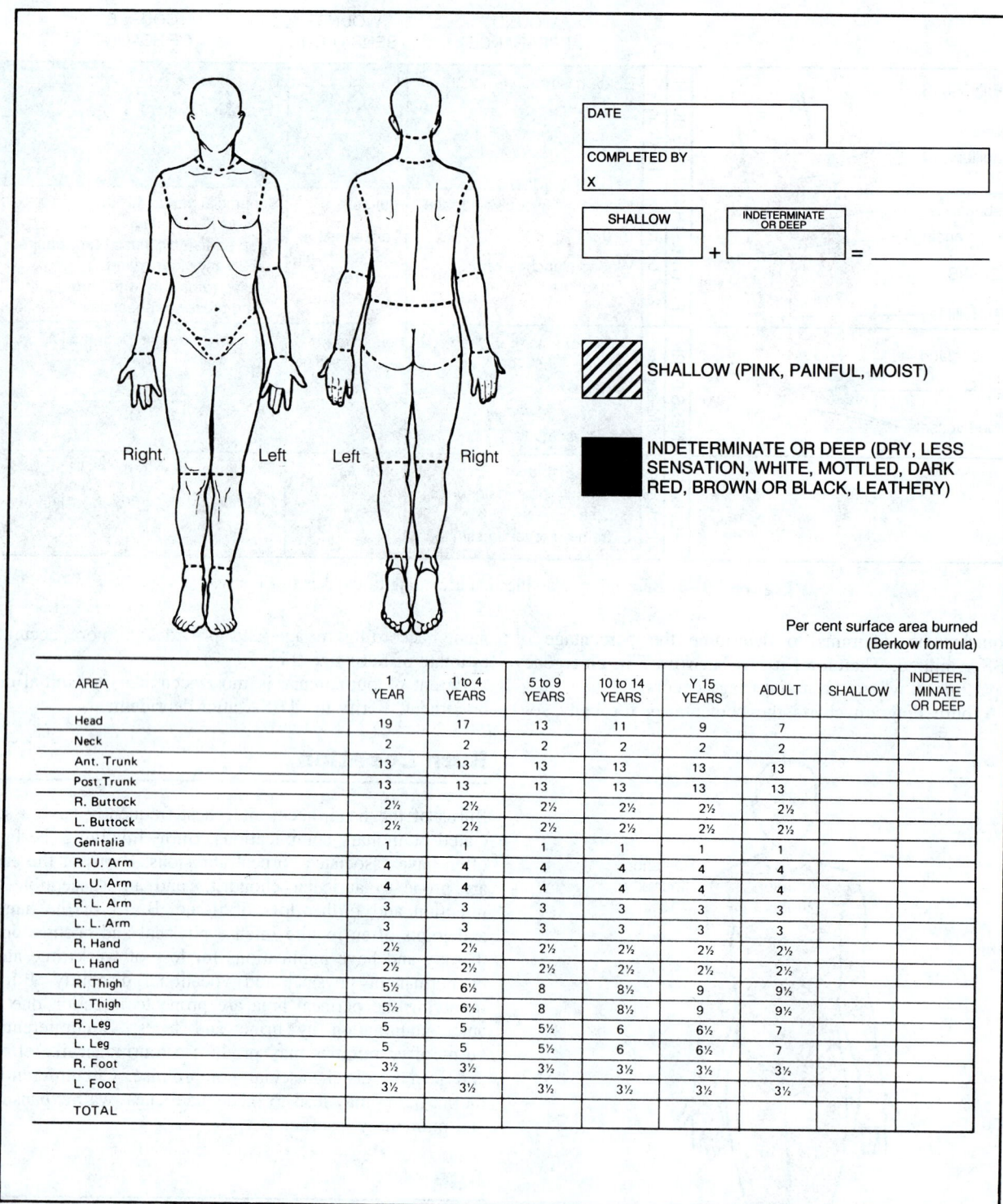

AREA	1 YEAR	1 to 4 YEARS	5 to 9 YEARS	10 to 14 YEARS	Y 15 YEARS	ADULT	SHALLOW	INDETER-MINATE OR DEEP
Head	19	17	13	11	9	7		
Neck	2	2	2	2	2	2		
Ant. Trunk	13	13	13	13	13	13		
Post. Trunk	13	13	13	13	13	13		
R. Buttock	2½	2½	2½	2½	2½	2½		
L. Buttock	2½	2½	2½	2½	2½	2½		
Genitalia	1	1	1	1	1	1		
R. U. Arm	4	4	4	4	4	4		
L. U. Arm	4	4	4	4	4	4		
R. L. Arm	3	3	3	3	3	3		
L. L. Arm	3	3	3	3	3	3		
R. Hand	2½	2½	2½	2½	2½	2½		
L. Hand	2½	2½	2½	2½	2½	2½		
R. Thigh	5½	6½	8	8½	9	9½		
L. Thigh	5½	6½	8	8½	9	9½		
R. Leg	5	5	5½	6	6½	7		
L. Leg	5	5	5½	6	6½	7		
R. Foot	3½	3½	3½	3½	3½	3½		
L. Foot	3½	3½	3½	3½	3½	3½		
TOTAL								

Figure 79–7. A sample chart for recording the extent and depth of a burn injury using the Berkow formula. To estimate burn extent using this chart, the nurse outlines the injured areas, excluding first-degree burns. Shallow (second-degree) burns are designated by parallel lines, and deeper (third- and fourth-degree) burns are designated by shading in the appropriate areas. The percentage of each injured anatomic area is then estimated using the age-specific table. Total body surface area (TBSA) burn is then calculated.

General Health

Debilitating cardiac, pulmonary, endocrine, and renal disease—specifically, diabetes, cardiopulmonary insufficiency, alcoholism, and renal failure—have been observed to in-fluence the client's response to injury and treatment.[47, 60, 83] The mortality rate for clients with preexisting cardiac disorders is 3.5 to 4 times higher than that for burn clients without cardiac disorders. Alcoholic clients with burns have a threefold increase in mortality rate over that of nonalcoholic clients with burns. In addition, alcoholic clients who survive the burn injury have longer hospital stays and more complications.[51, 54, 82] The increased morbidity among clients with burns who are alcoholics may be related to impaired immune function.[52] Obese clients with burns are also at increased risk due to cardiopulmonary complications.[85, 90]

Mechanism of Injury

The mechanism of injury is another factor used to determine the severity of injury. In general, special consideration is required for any electrical or chemical burn injury or any burn associated with an inhalation injury.

In electrical burn injuries, heat is generated as the electricity travels through the body, resulting in internal tissue damage. Cutaneous burn injuries may be negligible, but muscle and soft tissue damage may be extensive, particularly in high-voltage electrical injuries. The voltage, type of current (direct or alternating), contact site, and duration of contact are important considerations because they may affect morbidity. Alternating current (AC) is more dangerous than direct current (DC). It is often associated with cardiopulmonary arrest, ventricular fibrillation, tetanic muscle contractions, and long bone or vertebral compression fractures.[84] The risk of acute renal failure is greater in those with electrical injury, possibly due to the release of myoglobin from injured muscle tissue. Myoglobin precipitates in the renal tubules, causing renal damage, unless a brisk urine output is maintained.[84] In addition, victims of electrical injuries may have fallen from the point of electrical contact and sustained associated injuries. Cataract formation is also associated with high-voltage electrical injury, especially in cases in which contact points are on the head or neck.

In chemical burns, systemic toxic effects from cutaneous absorption of the offending agent may occur. Organ failure and even death have resulted from prolonged contact and absorption of different chemicals (e.g., hydrocarbons found in petroleum products).

Management

Minor Burns

Care of the client with minor burn injuries is frequently provided on an ambulatory or outpatient basis. In making the decision about whether to treat a client as an outpatient, the seriousness of the injury must first be assessed. As previously outlined (see Table 79–2), a minor burn injury in the adult is generally considered to be less than 15% TBSA (in clients younger than 40 years) or 10% TBSA (in clients older than 40 years) without a risk of cosmetic or functional impairment or disability.[5] In addition, consideration of the client's or caregiver's ability to perform wound care in the home environment is important.

Care of minor burn wounds includes (1) wound evaluation and initial care, (2) tetanus immunization, (3) pain management, and (4) education.

Wound Evaluation and Wound Care

An accurate history of the injury to include the date and time of the accident and the source of the burn (e.g., flame, hot liquid, chemical); an evaluation for any associated injuries is also necessary. All pertinent past medical history, to include drug allergies, medication history, and illnesses, should also be obtained.

Wound care for minor burns consists of cleansing, debridement, removal of any damaging agents (e.g., chemicals, tar), and application of an appropriate topical treatment. Burn wounds should be washed with a mild soap and rinsed thoroughly with warm water. If evaluation by a physician is delayed, the wounds may be covered with saline-soaked sponges to lesson the discomfort. Loose, nonviable tissue should be carefully trimmed away, and any hair should be shaved to within a 1-inch margin around the burn wound.

The removal of tar or asphalt is easily accomplished with the use of a citrus and petroleum product, Medisol (Orange-Sol, Inc.), or with mineral oil and a petroleum ointment, such as bacitracin (Fougera) or Neosporin (Burroughs Wellcome).

A minor chemical burn should be well irrigated with water for at least 20 minutes. Neutralizing agents are not recommended because the neutralizing reaction causes heat, which results in further tissue damage.

After the burn wound is cleansed and debrided, the size and depth of the injury should be carefully assessed and documented. Because minor burn wounds are not associated with an increase in susceptibility to infection, basic principles of wound healing are applied to these injuries. The wound should be kept clean and in a moist environment. Topical treatments for minor burn wounds can include twice-daily applications of a mild antimicrobial ointment (e.g., Bacitracin) or cream (e.g., silver sulfadiazine) and gauze dressing or a single application of a biosynthetic (e.g., Biobrane) or synthetic (e.g., Op-Site) product. Systemic antibiotics are rarely indicated.[99]

Pain Management

Pain management is often achieved with small doses of intravenous morphine sulfate or meperidine hydrochloride while the client is in the emergency department or burn clinic.[81] Oral analgesic agents are then prescribed for outpatient use.

Tetanus Immunization

The current protocol for tetanus immunization is the same for clients with minor burns as for clients with any other type of trauma. Clients who have been previously immunized against tetanus, but not within the past 5 years, should receive a tetanus toxoid booster. For clients who have not been immunized, tetanus human immune globulin and the first of a series of active immunizations with tetanus toxoid should be administered.[86, 99]

Education

While providing initial wound care, the nurse is responsible for teaching home wound care and the clinical manifestations of infection that necessitate further medical care. Other teaching needs include the need to perform active range-of-motion (ROM) exercises to maintain normal joint function and to decrease edema formation. The need for any follow-up evaluations or treatments should be confirmed with the client at this time.

Major Burns

The multiple organ system response that occurs following a major burn injury necessitates an interdisciplinary approach. The nurse, in consultation with other burn team members, is responsible for developing a plan of care that is based on assessment data reflecting the physical and psychosocial needs of the client and family or significant other.[11]

Nursing diagnoses, related goals, and interventions are presented in the Care Plan, and the phase(s) of recovery to which they are most applicable are specified. The clinical course of the burn client can be divided into three phases: the emergent (or resuscitative) phase, the acute phase, and the rehabilitation phase.[18, 81]

Emergency Care

The emergent phase begins at the time of injury with the prehospital care and concludes when capillary integrity is restored, typically at 48 to 72 hours following the injury. The primary goals during the emergent phase of recovery are directed toward sustaining life through prevention of hypovolemic (burn) shock and preservation of vital organ functioning. Ethical issues in treatment of massive burn is discussed in Ethical Issues in Nursing.

■ Prehospital Care

Prehospital care of the burn victim begins at the scene of the incident and concludes when institutional emergency medical care is obtained (Box 79–3). Prehospital care should begin with removing the victim from the source of the burn and/or eliminating the source of the heat. This action requires some consideration of the mechanism of injury so as to avoid further injury to the victim and/or injury to the rescuer.

■ Hospital Care

For clients with extensive burn wounds, initial care includes the following:

- Reevaluation of airway, breathing, and circulation (ABCs) and associated trauma
- Initiation of fluid resuscitation
- Placement of an indwelling urinary catheter
- Placement of a nasogastric tube
- Vital signs/baseline laboratory studies
- Pain management
- Tetanus immunization
- Data collection
- Wound care
- Psychological support
- Consideration for transport to a burn center

Airway/Breathing Assessment

With the exception of chemical burns, the burn wound should not take precedence over other life-threatening trauma or complications. For clients with chemical burns, wound irrigation should continue as the emergency medical team evaluates the victim. The adequacy of the airway and breathing should be reestablished and a re-evaluation for any associated trauma performed. The oropharynx is inspected for evidence of erythema, blisters, or ulcerations, and the need for endotracheal intubation is considered. If inhalation injury is suspected, administration of 100% oxygen via a tight-fitting non-rebreather face mask continues until carboxyhemoglobin levels fall below 15%.[78] Hyperbaric oxygen therapy has also been used for clients with high COHb levels and associated neurologic sequelae (see Chapter 20).

The head of the bed should be elevated to facilitate lung expansion if the client suffers no hemodynamic instability. If breathing appears to be compromised by tight circumferential trunk burns, bilateral escharotomies of the trunk may be necessary to relieve ventilatory compromise.

Intravenous Access

For adults with burn injuries affecting more than 15% TBSA, intravenous fluid resuscitation is generally required. Two peripheral large-bore intravenous (IV) lines placed through nonburned skin, proximal to any extremity burns, is preferred. IVs may be placed through burned skin if necessary; however, these lines should be secured with a suture. For clients with extensive burns or limited peripheral intravenous access sites, cannulation of a central vein (subclavian, internal or external jugular, or femoral) by a physician may be necessary.

TBSA Estimation

The percentage of burn injury is determined (see Fig. 79–7) and fluid resuscitation is initiated.

Fluid Resuscitation

Fluid resuscitation minimizes the deleterious effects of the fluid shifts. The goal of fluid resuscitation is to maintain vital organ perfusion while avoiding the complications of inadequate or excessive therapy.[78] Several formulas used to calculate fluid requirements are listed in Table 79–3. In the calculation of fluid infusion rates, the time of injury, and not the time at which fluid resuscitation was

Text continued on page 2249

CARE PLAN

The Burn-Injured Client

Nursing Diagnosis (E). Fluid Volume Deficit related to increased capillary leak and large fluid shift from intravascular to interstitial space.

Planning: Expected Outcomes. The client will have improved fluid balance, as evidenced by urine output of 30–50-ml/hour, clear sensorium, pulse rate <120 bpm without dysrhythmias, and blood pressure within expected range for age and medical history (pain control achieved).

Implementation: Nursing Intervention	Rationales
Assess for hypovolemia q 1 hour × 36 hours	Fluid shifts lead to hypovolemia
Obtain admission weight; weigh client daily	Weight is an accurate index of fluid balance
Monitor and document hourly intake and output	Urine output is a measure of effectiveness of fluid resuscitation
Administer intravenous (IV) fluid and electrolyte replacement per physician's order	IV fluids are used to restore fluid volume
Monitor serum electrolyte and hematocrit measurements	Hyponatremia, hyperkalemia and elevated hematocrit are common findings during the emergent phase

Evaluation. With adequate fluid resuscitation, expect fluid balance within 24 to 36 hours.

Collaborative Problem (E). Risk for paralytic ileus related to sympathetic nervous system response to injury.

Planning: Expected Outcomes. The nurse will monitor for normoactive bowel sounds, absence of abdominal distention, flatus production, and normal bowel movements.

Implementation: Nursing Intervention	Rationales
Assess need for placement of nasogastric (NG) tube	Ileus is common in burns >20% to 25% TBSA
Assess bowel function:	Bowel sounds indicate peristalsis is present
Auscultate bowel sounds q 4 hours	Abdominal distention indicates ileus
Observe for abdominal distention	Gastric output may require fluid replacement
Monitor gastric output and amount, color, presence of blood, and pH	Gastric ulcers are common following major burns

Evaluation. Expect bowel sounds to return once fluid volume is balanced.

Collaborative Problem (E). Risk for renal failure related to presence of hemochromagens in the urine due to deep burn and/or crush injury

Planning: Expected Outcomes. The nurse will monitor for visible urinary hemochromagens and adequate urine output of 75 to 100 ml/hour.

Implementation: Nursing Intervention	Rationales
Monitor and document hourly urine output and urine color	Urine is red or dark brown when hemochromagens are present
Ensure patency of urinary catheter	Catheter can become plugged with hemochromagens
Administer IV fluids per physician's order	Hemochromagens are flushed from the body
Send urine samples for urine myoglobin/hemoglobin levels per physician's order	This test provides quantitative information on risk of renal failure

Evaluation. Renal failure risk is a high-priority problem for first 24 to 36 hours. Once client has diuresis, the risk declines.

Nursing Diagnosis (E, A). Impaired Gas Exchange related to carbon monoxide poisoning, smoke poisoning, and heat damage to lungs

Planning: Expected Outcomes. Client will have improved gas exchange, as evidenced by unlabored respirations, 16 to 24/min; PaO_2, >90 mm Hg; $PaCO_2$, 35 to 45 mm Hg; SaO_2, >95%; and clear bilateral breath sounds.

Implementation: Nursing Intervention	Rationales
Assess for signs of respiratory distress as evidenced by restlessness, confusion, labored breathing, tachypnea, dyspnea, diminished and/or adventitious breath sounds, tachycardia, decrease in PaO_2 and SaO_2 levels, and cyanosis	Impaired gas exchange can lead to respiratory distress from hypoxemia

Care Plan continued on following page

CARE PLAN

The Burn-Injured Client *(Continued)*

Implementation: Nursing Intervention	Rationales
Monitor arterial blood gas and carboxyhemoglobin levels per physician's order	Data on effectiveness of respiration/oxygenation
Monitor SaO$_2$ levels continuously	SaO$_2$ levels provide noninvasive oxygenation data
Administer oxygen therapy as prescribed	Reduces hypoxemia
Instruct client on the use of incentive spirometer	Encourages deep breathing
Elevate head of bed	Facilitates lung expansion, reduces facial edema
Monitor need for endotracheal intubation	Intubation may be required to maintain oxygenation

Evaluation. Problems with gas exchange may require several days to resolve. If the client develops respiratory disease, it may be much longer.

Nursing Diagnosis (E, A). Ineffective Airway Clearance related to tracheal edema, airway epidermal sloughing, and depressed pulmonary ciliary action from inhalation injury

Planning: Expected Outcomes. Client will have effective airway clearance, as evidenced by clear bilateral breath sounds, clear to white pulmonary secretions, effective mobilization of pulmonary secretions, and unlabored respiration of 16 to 24/min.

Implementation: Nursing Intervention	Rationales
Have client turn, cough, and deep breathe q 1 to 2 hours × 24 hours, then q 2 to 4 hours while awake	Facilitates clearance of upper airways
Place oral suction device within client's reach for independent use	For removal of oral secretions and expectorated sputum
Perform endotracheal or nasotracheal suction prn, and monitor and document character of sputum	Suction removes secretions from upper airway. Sputum color, consistency, odor, and amount may indicate infection

Evaluation. If client is intubated, airway clearance problems remain well intubated and for several days after extubation.

Nursing Diagnosis. Altered Peripheral Tissue Perfusion related to constricting circumferential burns

Planning: Expected Outcomes. The client will have adequate peripheral perfusion, as evidenced by pulses present by palpation or Doppler, capillary refill of unburned skin <2 seconds, absence of numbness or tingling, and absence of increased pain with active ROM exercises.

Implementation: Nursing Intervention	Rationales
Remove all constricting jewelry and clothing	Constricting items may compromise circulation as edema ensues
Limit use of constricting blood pressure cuff in affected extremity	The constriction of the cuffs may reduce arterial inflow and venous return
Monitor arterial pulses by palpation or ultrasonic flow detector (Doppler) hourly for 48–72 hours	Pulses will diminish with circulation impairments
Assess capillary refill of unburned skin on affected extremity	Capillary refill will be prolonged with impaired circulation
Assess pain level with active ROM exercises	Ischemic tissues cause pain
Elevate affected extremities above the level of the heart	Reduces dependent edema formation
Encourage active ROM exercises	Promotes venous return and reduces muscle atrophy
Anticipate and prepare client for escharotomy	Escharotomy is used to restore circulation to compromised tissues

Post-escharotomy care:
  Assess adequacy of circulation:
  Check pulses
	These data indicate adequacy of perfusion

Note color, movement, and sensation of affected extremity	
Control post-escharotomy bleeding with pressure, electrocautery, or suturing of bleeding vessels	Viable tissue beneath eschar bleeds

Evaluation. Peripheral tissue perfusion should return to normal in 24 to 48 hours once the fluid shifts have stabilized.

Nursing Diagnosis (E, A). Hypothermia related to epithelial tissue loss and fluctuating ambient air temperature

Planning: Expected Outcomes. The client will remain normothermic, as evidenced by core body temperature between 99.6° and 101.0° F.

CARE PLAN

The Burn-Injured Client *(Continued)*

Implementation: Nursing Intervention	Rationales
Monitor the client's rectal or core temperature as indicated (hourly during the emergent phase and postsurgery)	Hypothermia may follow loss of skin as a thermal regulator and with some anesthetics
Limit the amount of body surface area exposed during wound care	Exposure leads to hypothermia; heat is lost in open wounds and after hydrotherapy by evaporation
Limit hydrotherapy treatment sessions to 30 min or less with water temperature 98° to 102.0° F	
Use external heat shields/radiant heat lamps	Provides an external source of heat
Keep procedure rooms and surgical suites warm	Heat is lost due to convection
If air-fluidized therapy bed is in use, monitor and maintain appropriate bed temperature and consider reducing the flow of fluidization if hypothermia develops	

Evaluation. The risk of hypothermia remains a problem as long as there is >15% to 20% ungrafted burn wound.

Collaborative Problem (E, A). Risk for stress ulcers related to neurohormonal stress response from the burn injury

Planning: Expected Outcomes. The nurse will monitor for gastrointestinal bleeding and will maintain gastric pH at greater than 5.

Implementation: Nursing Intervention	Rationales
Monitor and document gastric pH values and heme content q 2 hours while NG tube is in place	Acidic gastric secretions may lead to bleeding
Administer antacids and/or H$_2$ receptor antagonists per physician's order	These reduce gastric acid content
Monitor stools for occult blood	Stress ulcers cause bleeding, which may be excreted in stools

Evaluation. Stress ulceration can occur at any time following a burn injury.

Nursing Diagnosis (A). Altered Nutrition: Less Than Body Requirements related to increased metabolic needs for wound healing

Planning: Expected Outcomes. The client will have adequate nutrition, as evidenced by maintaining 85% to 90% of pre-burn weight and healing burn wounds, donor sites, and skin grafts.

Implementation: Nursing Intervention	Rationales
Obtain accurate pre-burn weight	Caloric needs are based on pre-burn weight
Consult dietitian	Dietitians perform nutritional assessments
Assess eating habits/patterns, food preferences, food allergies within 72 hours of admission	Assessment establishes a baseline
Record caloric intake (calorie counts)	Quantitative data on caloric intake is maintained
Weigh client daily to follow weight trends (except if operative procedure limits movement)	Weight should be stable if caloric needs are being met
Provide oral hygiene each shift and prn	Oral hygiene prevents stomatitis, enhances appetite
Provide an aesthetically pleasing environment	A pleasing environment is conducive to eating
Schedule treatments to provide for uninterrupted meal times	Interruptions may decrease calorie intake
Allow a period of rest prior to meal time if the client has endured a painful procedure or treatment	Pain decreases appetite
Provide aids and devices for eating utensils	Use of these devices facilitates self-care
Encourage family/significant other to bring favorite foods from home	Client may be willing to eat familiar foods
	Foods must be nutritionally sound
Provide nutritious supplements between meals	Caloric needs are often too high to be eaten in three meals
Provide positive reinforcement for eating	Anorexic clients may believe there is no benefit to eating
Consider other methods to meet caloric needs, such as tube feeding, total parenteral nutrition	Oral feeding may not provide adequate calories for healing

Evaluation. The client remains at nutritional risk until completely healed or grafted.

Care Plan continued on following page

CARE PLAN

The Burn-Injured Client *(Continued)*

Nursing Diagnosis. Risk for Infection related to loss of skin barrier, impaired immune response, presence of invasive catheters (indwelling urinary catheter and intravenous catheters), and invasive procedures (venous and arterial blood sampling and bronchoscopy)

Planning: Expected Outcomes. The client will have no burn wound microbial invasion, as evidenced by quantitative wound cultures <100,000 organisms; core body temperature at 99.6° to 101.0° F; no swelling, redness, or purulence will be present at invasive line insertion sites; and blood, urine, and sputum cultures will be negative.

Implementation: Nursing Intervention	Rationales
Administer tetanus prophylaxis prn	Anaerobic environment beneath eschar may allow tetanus organism to grow
Maintain infection control techniques	Good infection control techniques prevent cross-contamination
Instruct family/significant other on infection control measures	Informed family/significant other promotes compliance
Enforce strict handwashing	Clean hands minimize incidences of cross-contamination
Assess for clinical signs of infection: discoloration of wounds or drainage, odor, delayed healing; headache, chills, anorexia, nausea; change in vital signs; hyperglycemia and glycosuria; paralytic ileus, confusion, restlessness, hallucinations	Burn wound is open and client is immunocompromised; therefore, local wound infection or systemic infection is a risk
Before reapplying topical cream, cleanse and rinse the burn wound	Wound debris limits penetration of topical antimicrobial creams
Debride wound of loose, nonviable tissue	These tissues are a medium for bacterial growth
Shave or cut body hair in and around wound margins (exception: eyebrows and eyelashes)	Hair is contaminated and prevents cream adherence
Apply topical therapy (antimicrobial agent or temporary wound covering)	Topical therapy
Assess for signs of infection at catheter insertion site twice a day	

Evaluation. Infection remains an active problem as long as the client has open tissue, or invasive lines.

Nursing Diagnosis (E, A, R). Pain related to burn injury, exposed nerve endings, treatments, and anxiety

Planning: Expected Outcomes. The client will have more comfort as evidenced by verbalizing relief or control of pain/discomfort.

Implementation: Nursing Intervention	Rationales
Assess the client's response to pain with wound care, physical therapy, and at rest (background pain)	The client's response to pain at these points establishes a baseline
Medicate prior to painful procedures: 45 minutes for oral, 5 to 10 minutes for IV; do *NOT* administer intramuscular medications to clients with major burns during the emergent phase	Allow adequate time for onset of analgesia; intramuscular injections are not given because of erratic and diminished circulation, which impairs absorption
Explore relaxation techniques, music therapy, guided imagery, distraction, and hypnosis.	Nonpharmolocologic analgesics
Explain all procedures to the client and allow time for preparation	Explanations reduce anxiety
Talk to the client while providing care and performing procedures	Verbal contact promotes client's trust
Assess for the need of anxiolytic medications	Anxiety decreases pain threshold
Document the client's response to prescribed medications and nonpharmocologic treatments	Documentation is performed to evaluate effectiveness of interventions

Evaluation. Expect level of pain to decrease as burn wounds heal. Use of various pain relief measures may be needed for weeks to months.

Nursing Diagnosis (A, R). Self Care Deficit (Grooming, Bathing, Eating, Elimination) related to functional deficits resulting from the burn injury, pain, dressings, splints, and enforced immobility

Planning: Expected Outcomes. The client will have less self-care deficit and will demonstrate increased participation in self-care.

CARE PLAN

The Burn-Injured Client (Continued)

Implementations: Nursing Intervention	Rationales
Assess the client's ability to provide self-care	This assessment provides a baseline
Consult with occupational therapy regarding the need for assistive devices	Assistive devices can promote self-care
Encourage the client to participate in self-care tasks	Helps to motivate the client and overcome fear and dependency
Ensure that the client has adequate time to accomplish tasks	Adequate time for tasks helps establish self-control
Provide positive reinforcement when tasks are accomplished	Positive reinforcement promotes independence and motivation

Evaluation. Self Care Deficit may or may not resolve depending on the location and extent of burns and need for splints.

Nursing Diagnosis (E, A, R). Impaired Physical Mobility related to edema, pain dressings, splints, surgical procedures, and wound contractures

Planning: Expected Outcomes. The client will have improved physical mobility, as evidenced by returning to maximum activities of daily living with minimal disability and disfigurement.

Implementation: Nursing Intervention	Rationales
Assess ROM and muscle strength in burned areas prone to develop contractures every day and prn	This assessment determines baseline
Maintain burned areas in position of physiologic function within limits imposed by associated injuries, grafting, other therapeutic devices (see Table 79–7 for positioning recommendations)	The appropriate positions prevent/reduce contracture development
Explain rationale for activities and positioning to client and family; reinforce prn	Understanding improves compliance
Consult physical and occupational therapy for an individualized rehabilitation schedule; adjust schedule as needed	Will provide needed devices and teaching for ambulation and ROM
Wrap donor sites on burned legs and/or unburned legs with Ace bandage wraps (figure-8 technique) before placing in dependent position; as healing progresses, other elastic support bandages can be worn	Decreases capillary venous stasis, which impairs graft healing
Encourage active ROM q 2–4 hours while awake unless contraindicated because of a recent grafting procedure	Control postresuscitation edema and prevent muscle atrophy, tendon adherence, joint stiffness, and capsular shortening
Help client to ambulate to chair or to walking (unless contraindicated by a recent grafting procedure or other injuries)	Ambulation promotes muscle strength and cardiopulmonary reserve; after grafting, client remains on bedrest
Provide passive exercise and stretching if client is unable to actively participate (e.g., comatose or paralyzed)	Passive ROM maintains joint motion and muscle tone

Evaluation. Expect the client to begin ambulation early in the acute period. The problem should remain active until able to perform ADL and ambulate independently.

Nursing Diagnosis (A, R). Risk for Self Esteem Disturbance related to threatened or actual change in body image, physical loss, and loss of role responsibilities

Planning: Expected Outcomes. The client will develop improved self-esteem as evidenced by making social contact with others outside of immediate family, developing effective coping mechanisms through the stages of recovery, and verbalizing feelings about self-concept.

Implementation: Nursing Intervention	Rationales
Determine previous coping style	Previous coping styles will be tried by client
Provide an atmosphere of acceptance	New coping strategies cannot be learned during acute stress.
Explain projected appearance of burns and grafts during different phases of wound healing	This explanation provides information; may reduce misconceptions
Allow the client to progress at his or her own pace through stages of denial, grief, and acceptance of injury and recovery	Clients progress at varying rates depending on the degree of injury, perception of injury, support systems, and previous coping styles

Care Plan continued on following page

CARE PLAN

The Burn-Injured Client (*Continued*)

Implementation: Nursing Intervention	Rationales
Assess need for limit setting for maladaptive behavior; consult with burn team members to establish limits and treatment plan; explain and assist family/significant other to maintain same limits	Maladaptive behavior is harmful and is usually controlled by setting limits for all to follow
Promote client's self-confidence:	
Ensure continuity of care providers	Continuity of care providers promotes trust
Discuss all activities and procedures prior to initiation	Understanding reduces anxiety
Support client's role in care and treatment	Support motivates client; reduces fear
Keep client informed of progress	
Provide honest, positive reinforcement	Do not provide false hope of functional return if there is irreparable damage
Help family/significant other to interact with client	Family may be fearful and require guidance
Encourage interaction with others outside. Use family day passes	Encouragement facilitates societal reintegration
Help prepare client for social interactions after discharge by discussing potential situations and how client might deal with them	Such preparation provides rehearsal of events and reduces anxiety
Make home healthcare nurse or physical therapist referral as indicated	An appropriate referral will assess client's adjustment at home, ability to continue with needed therapy, further teaching, and care requirements

Evaluation. Self-esteem problems may resolve over months or years. This problem is followed up after discharge.

Nursing Diagnosis (E, A, R). Risk for Ineffective Family Coping related to the emergent and critical nature of the injury and separation from family/friends

Planning: Expected Outcomes. Family will have improved coping strategies, as evidenced by verbalizing goals of treatment regimen; emotional stressors, concerns, and behaviors; and understanding and knowledge of available support services.

Implementation: Nursing Intervention	Rationales
Prior to initial visit of family/significant other:	
Communicate extent of burn and changes in client's appearance	Preparation reduces fear
Provide family/significant other with information that meets their basic needs (information about lodging, location of cafeteria, parking)	Common needs of family members
Provide brief, simple explanations of procedures and equipment	Simple explanations are more readily retained
Determine how the client and family/significant other have coped with past stresses	Provides a baseline; previous coping methods will be used again
Allow for uninterrupted visitation during visiting hours if possible	Uninterrupted visits assist client to cope
Provide family/significant other with daily updates regarding changes in client's condition	A daily update maintains realistic perception of client's progress
Consult with psychologist, psychiatrist, social worker, or psychiatric clinical nurse specialist prn	These professionals may assist client to improve coping strategies
Encourage family/significant other attendance at support group meetings for family members	Provides support and helps to dispel misconceptions
For impending client transfer, provide family/significant other with support services to assist with travel	Support services during travel reduce anxiety during transition

Evaluation. Family coping issues will vary during the course of recovery. Early concerns with survival are replaced with worries over appearance and return to society. This problem may require long-term care to resolve.

E, emergent phase; A, acute phase; R, rehabilitation phase. Data from Dyer, C. & Roberts, D. (1990). Thermal trauma. *Nursing Clinics of North America 25*(1), 101–115; Burgess, M. D. (1991). Initial management of a patient with extensive burn injury. *Critical Care Nursing Clinics of North America, 3*(2), 175–177; Duncan, D. J., & Driscoll, D. M. (1991). Burn wound management. *Critical Care Nursing Clinics of North America, 3*(2), 202–204; Carlson, D. E., & Jordan, B. S. (1991). Implementing nutritional therapy in the thermally injured patient. *Critical Care Nursing Clinics of North America, 3*(2), 229–231.

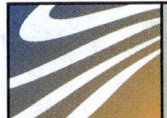

ETHICAL ISSUES IN NURSING

Should the Severely Burned Client Be Allowed to Refuse Treatment?

People who have sustained severe burns are perhaps the most fragile of all clients. The road to recovery is long and hard, and full recovery may never occur. In the most severe cases, the treatments may take months and induce intense pain. Even though months of whirlpool and debridement treatments may be undertaken, with the client experiencing severe pain with each treatment, death may be the end result. Even if death does not occur, return to a "normal" life may never happen.

Should the severely burned client be allowed to die without any medical intervention except pain management? Should a set of criteria be established to determine what treatment options are offered to the client? (These criteria would, of course, be based on the client's best interests, respect for the client's dignity as a person, and the availability of resources.) Should a client be allowed to refuse treatments, even if the chance of survival is good, simply because he or she believes that the quality of life after recovery will be unacceptably poor?

National statistics are available that are based on age, depth of burns, and degree of inhalation damage, among other factors, to assist caregivers in the burn unit in calculating the potential survival rate of a given burn client. The survival rate assists in the recommended treatment options, but clients may still choose death over treatment. Is a client in such a physical and mental state competent to make such a final decisions regarding survival? Undoubtedly, many challenges face both clients and caregivers in the burn unit setting. Each case should be evaluated individually, and caregivers should always be sensitive to the client and the client's family members. Many of the ethical questions regarding the care of burn clients are uncomfortable, and the answers are no less uncomfortable, if the questions can be answered at all.

initiated, serves as time zero. Therefore, if a burned client is delayed 2 hours in reaching an emergency department, he is 2 hours behind in fluid needs.

Although each formula is different, generally the first 24 hours after burn injury dictates the infusion of a balanced salt solution. The exact amount of fluid is based on the client's weight and the extent of injury. Other factors to be considered include the presence of an inhalation injury, a delay in initiation of resuscitation, or deep tissue damage. These factors tend to increase the amount of intravenous fluid required for adequate resuscitation above the calculated amount.[44] With the exception of the Evans and Brooke formulas, colloid-containing solutions are not given during this period due to the changes in capillary integrity that allow leakage of protein-rich fluid into the interstitial space, which increases edema formation. During the second 24 hours after burn injury, colloid-containing solutions are administered, along with 5% dextrose and water, in varying amounts.

It is important to remember that all resuscitation formulas serve only as guides and that they should be adjusted according to the client's physiologic response. Successful or adequate fluid resuscitation in the adult is signaled by stable vital signs, adequate urine output, palpable peripheral pulses, and clear sensorium (see Nursing Care Plan).

Assessment of Urine Output

An indwelling urethral catheter connected to a closed drainage system should be placed to measure hourly urine production. When hemodynamic monitoring is not used, urine output is the most readily available and reliable indicator for determining the adequacy of fluid resuscitation.[78, 83] For an adult, the hourly urine volume should be 30 to 50 ml. If hemochromogens (hemoglobin and myoglobin) are present in the urine, the hourly urine volume should be maintained at 75 to 100 ml for adults and 2 ml/kg for children weighing less than 30 kg. Urine hemochromogens are caused by the release of hemoglobin and myoglobin from damaged red blood cells and injured muscle. Hemochromogens cause the urine to become dark brown or red.

Insertion of a Nasogastric Tube

Many burn centers advocate the placement of a nasogastric tube for the unresponsive client and/or for clients

---

Box 79–3. Guidelines for Prehospital Care of Burn Victims

1. Remove the victim from the source of the burn:

   - Flame: Extinguish burning clothes
   - Chemical or scald: Remove saturated clothing
   - Chemical: Brush off any dry chemical and begin to copiously irrigate injured areas with water
   - Hot tar: Cool the tar with water
   - Electrical: Turn off electricity or remove the electrical source using a dry, nonconductive object (e.g., a piece of wood)

2. Assess the ABCs:

   - Establish airway
   - Ensure adequate breathing (100% oxygen via nonrebreather face mask for suspected inhalation injury)
   - Assess circulation

3. Assess for associated trauma
4. Conserve body heat
5. Consider need for IV fluid administration
6. Transport to hospital or burn unit

Data from Trunkey, D. D. (1983). Transporting the critically burned patient. In T. L. Wachtel, et al. (Eds.), *Current topics in burn care*. Rockville, MD: Aspen Publications.

Table 79–3. Fluid Resuscitation Formulas Used in Burn Care

Formula Name	First 24 Hours			Second 24 Hours		
	Electrolyte-Containing Solution	Colloid-Containing Solution	Dextrose in Water	Electrolyte-Containing Solution	Colloid-Containing Solution	Dextrose in Water
Evans	Normal saline 1 ml/kg/% burn	1 ml/kg/% burn	2000 ml	½ of first 24-hour requirement	½ of first 24-hour requirement	2000 ml
Brooke	Lactated Ringer's 1.5 ml/kg/% burn	0.5 ml/kg/% burn	2000 ml	½–¾ of first 24-hour requiremen	½–¾ of first 24-hour requirement	2000 ml
Modified Brooke	Lactated Ringer's 2 ml/kg/% burn	None	None	None	0.3–0.5 ml/kg/% burn	Titrate to maintain urine output
Parkland	Lactated Ringer's 4 ml/kg/% burn	None	None	None	0.3–0.5 ml/kg/% burn	Titrate to maintain urine output
Hypertonic saline solution	Fluid containing 250 mEq of sodium/L to maintain hourly urine output of 70 ml in adults	None	None	Same solution to maintain hourly urine output of 30 ml in adults	None	None

Adapted from Rue, L. W., & Cioffi, W. G., Jr. (1991). Resuscitation of thermally injured patients. *Critical Care Nursing Clinics of North America 3*(2), 185; and Wachtel, T. L., & Fortune, J. B. (1983). Fluid resuscitation for burn shock. In T. L. Wachtel et al. (Eds.), *Current topics in burn care* (p. 44). Rockville, MD: Aspen Publishers.

with burns of 20% to 25% or more TBSA, to prevent emesis and reduce the risk of aspiration.[81, 83] Gastrointestinal dysfunction results from the intestinal ileus that develops almost universally in clients during the early post–burn injury period. All oral fluids should be restricted at this time.

Management of Circumferential Burn Injuries

Circumferential burns of the extremities may compromise circulation. Elevating injured extremities above the level of the heart and active exercise help to reduce dependent edema formation. However, circulatory compromise may still occur. Therefore, frequent assessment of distal extremity perfusion is necessary. Doppler flowmeter assessment of the palmar arch vessels (upper extremity) and the posterior tibial artery (lower extremity) provides the most precise indication of peripheral perfusion and should be monitored regularly during the resuscitation period. The absence of flow or the progressive diminution of the Doppler flowmeter signal intensity is an indication that perfusion is impaired.[88]

An escharotomy is the appropriate treatment for circulatory compromise due to constricting, circumferential burns. A midlateral and/or midmedial incision of the involved extremity is made from the proximal to the distalmost extent of the full-thickness burn. The depth of the incision is limited to the eschar (Fig. 79–8). It is generally performed at the bedside without local or general anesthesia, because full-thickness burns are insensate. However, viable tissue beneath the escharotomy may bleed if cut, and the client may feel pain. Bleeding can be controlled with pressure, suture ligation, or electrocautery. Pain control is achieved with IV narcotic administration (see discussion on pain management). The burn wound with an escharotomy can be dressed with topical antimicrobial creams and gauze dressings.

If adequate tissue perfusion does not return following escharotomy, a fasciotomy may be necessary. This procedure, in which the fascia is incised, is performed in the operating room under general anesthesia. This procedure is usually necessary only in injuries caused by high-voltage electricity or those with concomitant crush injury.[88]

Vital Signs and Laboratory Studies

Vital signs provide baseline information as well as additional data for determining the adequacy of fluid resuscitation. Baseline laboratory studies should include blood glucose, blood urea nitrogen (BUN), creatinine, serum electrolytes, and hematocrit levels. Arterial blood gas and COHb levels should also be obtained, particularly if an inhalation injury is suspected. A chest x-ray study should be obtained for all clients with extensive burns or inhalation injury. Other laboratory tests, in addition to x-ray

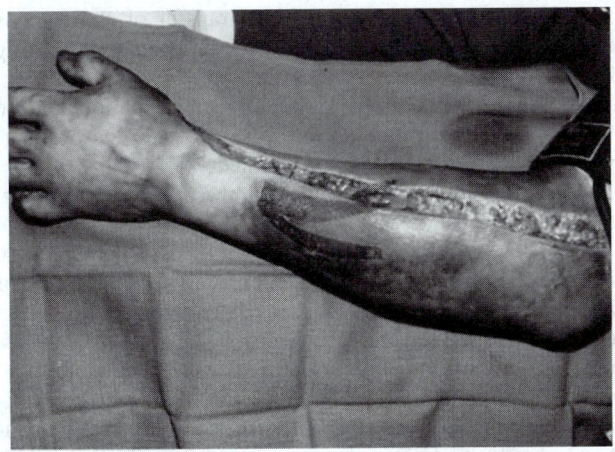

Figure 79–8. Escharotomy. Incision is made through the constricting burn eschar to permit expansion of the underlying subcutaneous tissues as edema forms.

studies to rule out fractures or associated trauma, should be obtained on an as-needed basis. Depending on the circumstances of the injury, an alcohol and/or drug screen may be indicated. Continuous electrocardiographic (ECG) monitoring should be initiated on all clients with major burn injuries, particularly those who have suffered a high-voltage electrical injury[83] or who have a history of cardiac ischemia or dysrhythmia.

Pain Management

Pain management is achieved through the administration of intravenous narcotic agents, typically morphine sulfate. In the adult, small doses are given intravenously and repeated in 5- to 10-minute intervals until pain appears to be under control. Extent of pain relief, blood pressure, pulse, respiratory rate, and state of consciousness should be assessed after each dose.

The intramuscular or subcutaneous routes are not used during this phase because absorption from the soft tissues is unreliable during the emergent period when hypovolemia and large fluid shifts occur. The oral route for pain medication administration is not used due to the likelihood of gastrointestinal dysfunction.

The effectiveness of pain management therapies should be evaluated. A variety of pain assessment techniques have been used with the burned adult. Pain assessment tools more commonly utilized during this phase are adjective and numeric scales, because they do not require a visual representation. With an adjective scale, the nurse asks the client to describe the level of pain (no pain, slight pain, moderate pain, or severe pain). With a numeric scale, the client is asked to rate the level of pain using a scale of zero to five or zero to ten. The nurse should instruct the client that the zero represents no pain and the highest number represents the worst pain possible. With this information, the nurse can compare the client's response before and after treatment and gain some idea of whether adequate pain control has been achieved.

Tetanus Immunization

Tetanus immunization for a client with a major burn is the same as for one with a minor burn (see earlier discussion).[97]

Data Collection

The client, people at the scene, and emergency medical personnel should be questioned regarding the incident.[18] Useful information includes the time of injury, the level of the client's consciousness at the scene, whether the injury occurred in an enclosed or open space, the presence of associated trauma, and the mechanism of injury. If the victim has suffered a chemical burn, knowledge of the offending agent, its concentration, duration of exposure, and whether irrigation was initiated at the scene is useful. For victims of electrical injuries, knowledge of the source, type of current, and the current voltage is useful in determining the extent of injury. Information concerning the client's past medical history as well as his or her general health should be obtained. Specifically, information regarding cardiac, pulmonary, endocrine, or renal disease should be obtained because it may have implications for treatment. Known allergies should also be identified, as should any current medication regimen.

Wound Care

Chemical Burns

Ideally, wound care for a chemical burn begins at the scene of the injury and includes prompt removal of all clothing (including undergarments, socks, and shoes), brushing off of any chemical powder from the skin (dry chemicals may be activated when mixed with water and cause greater injury), and continuous irrigation with copious amounts of water.

For chemical eye injuries, irrigate the eyes with a gentle stream of normal saline, flushing both the injured eye and the conjunctiva. It is recommended to irrigate the eyes from the inner canthus outward, to avoid washing any chemicals down the tear duct or toward to other eye.

Nonchemical Burns

If transfer to a burn center will be accomplished within 12 hours of injury, wound care should consist of covering the wound with sterile towels and placing clean, dry sheets and blankets over the client to maintain body heat. Clients with burns of the head and face should be positioned with the head elevated and all burned extremities elevated on pillows above the level of the heart. These measures help decrease formation of dependent edema. Unless transport time to the receiving medical facility is prolonged, debridement and application of topical antimicrobial agents is unnecessary. Definitive wound care begins following inpatient admission to the hospital.

Transport to a Burn Facility

Consideration of transfer to a specialized burn care facility is appropriate for all clients with major burn injuries (see Table 79–2). Prompt contact with the receiving burn center is important to facilitate a smooth transfer. All copies of medical records, which should include all fluids and medications given, hourly urine output values, and vital signs, must accompany the client.

Psychological Support

Both the client and family often perceive a real threat to survival during the emergent phase. This is commonly manifested as severe anxiety and fear. They may withdraw, have difficulty with concentration and in following simple instructions, or be uncooperative with treatment regimens.[92]

Nursing interventions employed during this phase of recovery should be designed to reduce the client's and family's anxiety, fear, and disorientation. The nurse can allay fears by talking in a soothing voice. Instructions and explanations should be simple and precede any painful procedure; they should be repeated as necessary. Orient the client frequently and allow him or her to verbalize fears.

To assist family members and significant others during this phase, the nurse should attempt to assess whether the family is equipped with the appropriate coping mechanisms and resources to meet their needs. Explanations need to be simple and repeated as necessary. Written materials, providing information concerning hospital resources (e.g., location of cafeteria, waiting rooms, chapel, public telephones) and policies (e.g., visiting hours, unit-specific policies) should be provided. Consultation with the psychiatric clinical nurse specialist, chaplain, or social worker can be helpful.[92]

Acute and Subacute Care

The acute phase of recovery following a major burn begins when the patient is hemodynamically stable, capillary integrity is restored, and diuresis has begun. This is generally considered to be at 48 to 72 hours after the time of injury.[81] Many of the same principles of care outlined in the emergent phase apply to the acute phase; however, more emphasis is placed on restorative therapies. The acute phase continues until wound closure is achieved.

Care of the burn-injured client during the acute phase focuses on the following:

- Infection control
- Wound care
- Wound closure
- Nutritional support
- Pain management
- Psychological support
- Physical therapy
- Control of scarring

■ Infection Control

The goals of infection control for the burn injured client are as follows: (1) to prevent transmission of exogenous microorganisms; (2) to control the transfer of endogenous microorganisms; and (3) to protect and support existing immunologic defenses.[102]

Sources of infection from autocontamination in the burn-injured client include the following: (1) the oropharynx, (2) fecal flora, and (3) unburned skin.

Sources of cross-contamination include the following: (1) staff, (2) visitors, and (3) the air.[83]

To prevent infection in the burn client, nursing care includes vigilant monitoring for clinical manifestations of impending infection and sepsis, maintenance of a clean environment to reduce the reservoir of microorganisms, use of aseptic technique for all invasive procedures and wound care, and timely administration of prescribed antimicrobial agents (systemic and topical). Universal precautions should be followed when caring for all clients with burn injuries; however, specific infection control practices and isolation techniques exist for all burn centers.[62] These practices include the use of gloves, caps, masks, shoe covers, scrub clothes, and plastic aprons. Strict handwashing is stressed to reduce the incidence of cross-contamination between clients and is the single most important means of preventing the spread of infection. Staff and visitors are generally prevented from client contact if they suffer from any skin, gastrointestinal, or respiratory tract infections. Refer to Box 79–4 for basic principles of infection control strategies.[102]

All visitors (this includes family members as well as healthcare providers from other departments) should be oriented to the infection control practices prior to their first contact with the burn injured client. At any one time, the number of visitors should be limited to ensure monitoring of compliance with infection control practices.

■ Wound Care

Care of the burn wound is ultimately aimed at promoting wound healing. Daily wound care involves cleansing, debridement of the eschar (devitalized tissue), and dressing of the burn wound.[94]

Box 79–4. Basic Principles of Infection Control

1. Thorough handwashing should be done before and after each contact with the burn-injured client
2. Protective garb (aprons or gowns) should be donned before each contact and promptly discarded after leaving the bedside or room
3. Gloves should be changed when they become contaminated with secretions or fluids from one anatomic site before contact with another site
4. Equipment, materials, and surfaces are considered contaminated for the individual client and should be properly decontaminated before use with another client

From Weber, J. M., & Tompkins, D. M. (1993). Improving survival: Infection control and burns. *AACN Clinical Issues in Critical Care Nursing* 4(2), 418–419.

Hydrotherapy

The wound is cleansed by the use of hydrotherapy. This is accomplished by immersion (Fig. 79–9, *A*), showering, or spraying (Fig. 79–9, *B*). A hydrotherapy session of 30 minutes or less is optimal for clients with acute burns.[93] Longer time periods may increase sodium loss (water is hypotonic) through the burn wound, heat loss, pain, and stress. During hydrotherapy, the wounds are gently washed using any one of a variety of solutions: dilute sodium hypochlorite,[35] dilute povidone–iodine,[20, 43, 49] and dilute chlorohexidine.[20, 99] Care should be taken to minimize bleeding and to maintain body temperature during this procedure. To prevent cross-contamination between clients, single-use, plastic hydrotherapy tub liners are available. Clients excluded from hydrotherapy are generally those who are hemodynamically unstable and those with new skin grafts.[20] If hydrotherapy is not used, wounds are washed and rinsed while the client is in bed, prior to the application of antimicrobial agents.

Debridement

Burn wound debridement involves the removal of the eschar. This serves to promote wound healing by preventing bacterial proliferation in and under the eschar.[35] Debridement of the burn wound is accomplished through mechanical, enzymatic, or surgical means.

Mechanical Debridement. Mechanical debridement can be accomplished with the careful use of scissors and forceps to lift and trim away loose eschar. Hydrotherapy softens and loosens eschar so it is more easily re-moved. Dressing changes are another effective means of mechanical debridement. This is accomplished by the use of wet-to-dry and wet-to-wet dressings. Mechanical debridement of the burn wound can be extremely painful; therefore, effective pain management is paramount.

Enzymatic Debridement. Enzymatic debridement involves the application of commercially prepared proteolytic and fibrinolytic topical enzymes to the burn wound eschar. These products selectively digest necrotic tissue, facilitating eschar removal. They require a moist environment to be effective and are applied directly to the burn wound. Pain and bleeding can be major problems associated with this treatment and should be checked for continuously throughout treatment. Enzymatic debridement agents are contraindicated for wounds communicating with major body cavities, exposed nerves, or nervous tissue and in fungating neoplastic ulcers.[14]

Surgical Debridement. Surgical debridement of the burn wound involves excision of the eschar and coverage of the wound. Early surgical excision begins during the first week after injury, once the client is hemodynamically stable. Advantages of early excision include early mobilization, reduction of pain (due to repeated dressing changes), early wound closure (reduces the potential for wound infection), and reduced length of hospitalization. A disadvantage to early excision is the risk of excising viable tissue that may heal with time.[42]

Two techniques of surgical debridement are currently used: tangential excision and fascial excision.[40] In tangential excision, very thin layers of eschar are sequentially

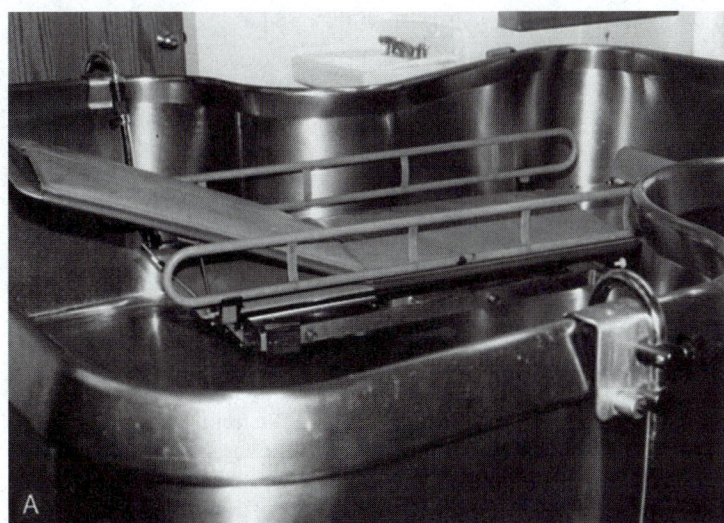
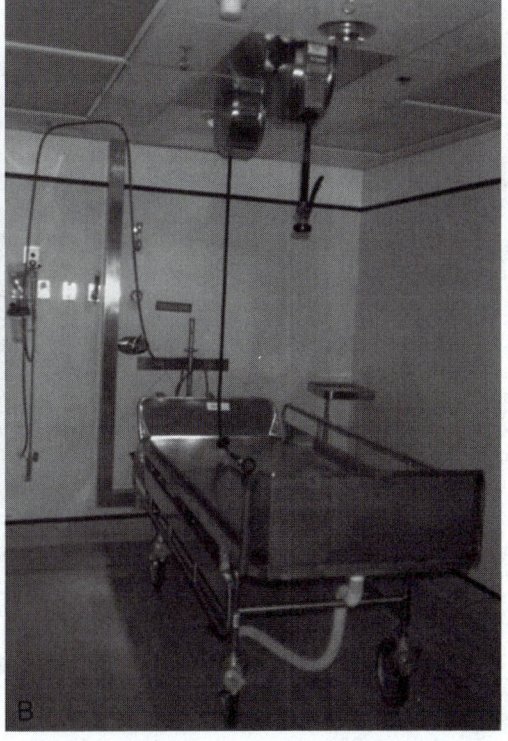
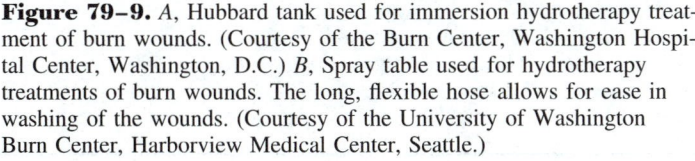

Figure 79–9. *A,* Hubbard tank used for immersion hydrotherapy treatment of burn wounds. (Courtesy of the Burn Center, Washington Hospital Center, Washington, D.C.) *B,* Spray table used for hydrotherapy treatments of burn wounds. The long, flexible hose allows for ease in washing of the wounds. (Courtesy of the University of Washington Burn Center, Harborview Medical Center, Seattle.)

shaved until viable tissue is reached. Fascial excision involves removing the burn tissue and underlying fat down to fascia. This technique is frequently used for very deep burns.

Application of Topical Antimicrobial Agents

Deep partial- or full-thickness burn wounds are treated initially with topical antimicrobial agents. These agents are applied once or twice daily following cleansing, debridement, and inspection of the wound. The nurse assesses for eschar separation, the presence of granulation tissue, and/or reepithelialization, and for signs of infection.[33] The most commonly used topical antimicrobial agents are listed in Table 79-4. Although no single agent is used universally, many burn centers choose silver sulfadiazine cream as the initial topical treatment.

Open Versus Closed Dressing Methods

Burn wounds are treated using either an open or closed dressing technique. For the open method, the antimicrobial cream is applied using a gloved hand (Fig. 79-10) and then left open to the air without gauze dressings. The cream is reapplied as needed, although formal reapplication occurs every 12 hours due to the duration of activity of the agent. The advantages of this method include increased visualization of the wound, greater freedom for mobility and joint motion, and simplicity in wound care.

Table 79-4. Topical Antimicrobial Agents Used in Burn Care

Agent	Antimicrobial Spectrum	Application	Side Effects	Nursing Considerations
Water-based creams				
1% Silver sulfadiazine	Broad spectrum, including some fungi and yeast	2× daily, 1/16-inch thickness Gauze dressing not required	Transient leukopenia typically appearing after 2 or 3 days of treatment Macular rash	Do not store in warm environment (e.g., warm client room)
Mafenide acetate	Broad spectrum, little antifungal activity	2× daily, 1/16-inch thickness Gauze dressing not required	Hyperchloremic metabolic acidosis from bicarbonate diuresis due to the inhibition of carbonic anhydrase Pain/burning sensation on application to superficial burns Maculopapular rash	Assess for side effects Assess adequacy of pain management; if pain and discomfort continue, consider other topical treatments Use cautiously in clients with acute renal failure
Solutions				
5% Mafenide acetate	Broad spectrum	Gauze dressing required and moistened with solution for application to the wound	Pain on application Pruritus Rash Fungal colonization	Remains investigational and requires informed consent Assess for side effects Assess adequacy of pain management
0.5% Silver nitrate	Broad spectrum, including *Candida* species	Multiple layers of gauze dressing required and moistened with solution for application to the wound	Hyponatremia Hypochloremia Hypokalemia Hypocalcemia	Check serum electrolytes daily Penetrates eschar poorly Remoisten dressings every 2 hours to avoid wound desiccation Protect the environment; stains everything a blackish-brown color
Petroleum-based ointments				
Polymyxin-B Neomycin sulfate Bacitracin	Gram-negative organisms Gram-positive and gram-negative organisms	Apply as needed in a thin layer; gauze dressing not utilized unless clothing protection is needed	Hypersensitivity (rash) Overgrowth of non-susceptible organisms including fungi	Assess for side effects

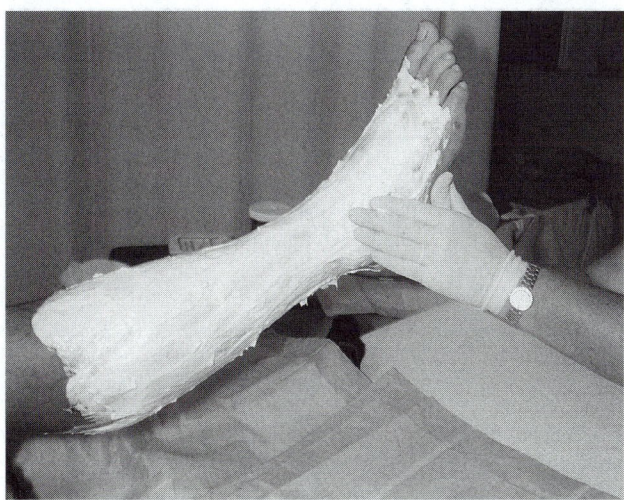

Figure 79–10. Silver sulfadiazine, a common antimicrobial cream used in burn care, is applied to the burn wound using a sterile, gloved hand. (Courtesy of the University of Washington Burn Center, Harborview Medical Center, Seattle.)

The disadvantages include an increased chance of hypothermia from exposure.

In the closed method of wound care, a gauze dressing is impregnated with antimicrobial cream and applied to the wound. For extremity injuries, to ensure that circulation is not compromised, the gauze should be wrapped from the distal portion of the extremity in a proximal direction. The advantages of the closed method are decreases in evaporative fluid and heat loss from the wound surface. In addition, gauze dressings may aid in debridement. The disadvantages of gauze dressings are mobility limitations and a potential decrease in effectiveness of ROM exercises. Wound assessment is also limited to the times at which dressing changes are performed.

■ Wound Closure

Temporary Wound Coverings

Temporary wound coverings are frequently used as a kind of wound "dressing." Table 79–5 outlines the most common biologic, biosynthetic, and synthetic wound coverings available. These products are temporary wound coverings, and each has specific indications. The character of the wound (depth of injury, amount of exudate, location of the wound on the body, and phase of recovery) and treatment goals are considered when choosing the most appropriate wound covering.

Autografts

Autografting is the surgical removal of a superficial layer of the client's own unburned skin, which is subsequently grafted to the excised burn wound. Because the epidermis is split rather than taken in full, these grafts are referred to as split-thickness grafts. This procedure is performed in the operating room while the client is under general anesthesia. Autografts can be applied either in a sheet (sheet graft) or in a meshed form (meshed graft). A sheet autograft is applied to the excised wound bed without altering in its integrity. Sheet autografts are often used to graft burns in visible areas. In contrast, a meshed autograft contains many little slits that allow for expansion of the donor skin. Meshing permits coverage of larger areas or irregularly shaped wounds and allows for drainage from a bleeding wound bed. When healed, the meshed pattern of the autograft remains visible. Therefore, meshed grafts are used on hidden body areas. When a thicker layer of skin is removed, consisting of the epidermis and the dermis, this is referred to as a full-thickness graft. For all autografts, the area of the body from which the skin was removed is referred to as the donor site (Fig. 79–11).

In addition to routine postoperative nursing care, care of the client after autografting includes the following:

● Assessment of bleeding from the graft site
● Proper positioning, elevation, and immobilization of the graft site
● Donor site care

Assessment of Bleeding

Bleeding beneath an autograft may prevent successful autograft adherence to the excised wound and may ultimately result in some degree of graft loss. This is particularly true for sheet autografts. Small amounts of blood or serum beneath sheet autografts can be removed by gently rolling (using a sterile cotton swab) the fluid a short distance to the periphery, where it can be absorbed with a sterile gauze pad. Rolling fluid over long distances, such as from the middle of the graft, is not recommended. The graft is lifted from its bed as the fluid is moved toward the edge. For large accumulations, aspiration of the blood and serum using a small-gauge needle (25 gauge) and syringe has been found to be effective.

Positioning and Immobilization

Autografts placed over joints or on lower extremities are often elevated and immobilized following surgery for 3 to 7 days. This period of immobilization allows the autograft time to adhere and attach to the wound bed. Immobilization can be accomplished in a variety of ways. Proper positioning, splinting, traction, and limb restraints have been used to prevent unwanted movement and shearing of autografts.

Donor Site Care

Various types of dressings are used to cover donor sites, depending on the size, location, and condition of adjacent skin or tissue. Nursing care depends on the type of dressing used. For example, a fine-mesh gauze dressing is allowed to dry, often assisted by radiant heat lamps. Once new epithelium forms beneath it, the gauze can be gently lifted and trimmed away. Removal of the gauze prior to this time will reinjure the donor site, causing pain and lengthening healing time. Donor sites treated with synthetic, semipermeable polyurethane film are often dressed with a compression bandage. This dressing, applied in the operating room, is left in place for one to several days to promote adherence of the polyurethane film to the donor

Table 79–5. Temporary Wound Coverings Used in Burn Care

Category/ Examples	Description	Indications	Nursing Considerations
Biologic			
Amnion	Amniotic membranes collected from human placentas	To protect partial-thickness burns To protect granulation tissue prior to autograft application	Cover dressing is changed every 48 hours with amnion.
Allograft homograft	Donated human cadaver skin harvested within 24 hours after death	To debride exudative wounds To cover excised wounds and test for receptivity prior to autograft application To cover and protect meshed autografts	Observe for wound exudate and signs of infection that may be indicative of a wound infection beneath the allograft/xenograft
Xenograft heterograft	Porcine skin is harvested after slaughter, then cryopreserved or lyophilized for storage	To promote healing of clean, superficial partial-thickness wounds	Xenograft over granulation tissue is changed every 2–5 days For superficial wounds, ensure that the wound is clean and well rinsed; apply xenograft with slight overlapping of edges to allow for shrinkage; trim away xenograft when skin beneath it has healed
Biosynthetic			
Biobrane (Winthrop Pharmaceuticals, New York)	Nylon fabric bonded to a silicone rubber membrane containing collagenous porcine peptides	Donor site dressing Protective cover over meshed autografts To promote healing of clean superficial partial-thickness wounds	Secure to the surrounding intact skin by staples, skin closure strips, tape, or sutures and then wrap with a gauze dressing; this outer dressing can be removed by 48 hours to check for adherence of the Biobrane; once adherence has occurred, the tape, sutures, and staples can be removed; the Biobrane can then be left exposed to the air New and healing donor sites of the legs require support during ambulation; the figure 8 Ace wrapping technique is recommended to minimize trauma to newly formed capillaries Assess for infection beneath the fabric and at wound periphery
Integra (Integra Life Sciences, Plainsboro, NJ)	Bilaminate substitute composed of collagen (dermal analog) and a Silastic covering (epidermal analog) The dermal analog is allowed to incorporate into the wound, becoming permanent	For application to excised wounds	The Silastic portion is removed after 2–3 days providing a wound bed for placement of a very thin split-thickness skin graft Assess for infection Protect the site from mechanical shearing forces
Calcium alginates (Curasorb, Kendall Co, Mansfield, Mass; Kalginate, DeRoyal Textiles, Camden, SC)	Dressing material derived from brown seaweeds (alginate) and calcium/sodium salts	Donor site dressing To promote healing of superficial partial-thickness wounds (contraindicated in full-thickness wounds)	To apply, irrigate wound with a physiologic solution, apply calcium alginate dressing to the wound, cover with an absorptive dressing The entire dressing should be changed when the outer dressing is saturated with drainage

Table 79–5. Temporary Wound Coverings Used in Burn Care *(Continued)*			
Category/ Examples	Description	Indications	Nursing Considerations
Transparent films (Bioclusive, Johnson & Johnson, Arlington, Texas; Op-Site)	Hypoallergenic film dressing that is occlusive, waterproof, and permeable to moisture vapor	Donor site dressing To promote healing of clean, small, superficial partial-thickness wounds	Use a margin of intact skin around the entire wound or donor site to adequately secure the dressing Assess for pooling exudate; if significant exudate forms that threatens the integrity of the closed dressing, drain the exudate aseptically with a small gauge needle and syringe; seal hole with a film patch
Non-adhering gauze (Aquaphor gauze, Beiersdorf Inc, Norwalk, Conn; Xeroform gauze)	Fine mesh gauze impregnated with ointment	Donor site dressing To cover meshed autografts To cover fragile, newly healed epithelium	Dressing material over donor site should remain intact until healed beneath (10–14 days) New and healing donor sites of the legs require support during ambulation; the figure-8 Ace wrapping technique is recommended to minimize trauma to newly formed capillaries

site and to reduce fluid accumulation. When the compression dressing is removed, the polyurethane film is left intact until new epithelium forms beneath it. For donor sites dressed with a specialized nylon fabric, staples, suture, or tape is used to keep the dressing in place. A compression dressing is applied in the operating room and left in place for at least 24 to 48 hours after surgery. At this time, the compression dressing can be removed and the donor site left open to the air. Staples and sutures should be removed by the third to fifth day after surgery. The nylon fabric remains adhered to the donor site and is peeled away once reepithelialization occurs beneath it (typically 10 to 14 days).

Despite the differences in dressings, the donor site wound requires the same meticulous care as other partial-thickness wounds, to expedite healing and prevent infection. If the donor site becomes infected, the dressing should be gently removed or soaked off. The wound can then be thoroughly cleaned and an antimicrobial agent

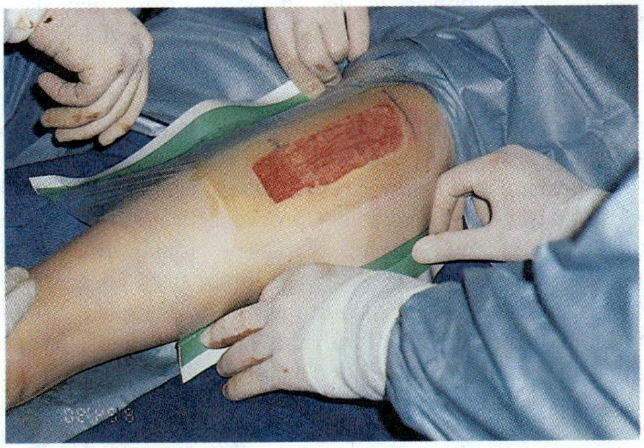

Figure 79–11. Harvesting donor skin from the lateral portion of the client's thigh.

applied. Once the donor site has healed, lubricating lotions can be applied to soften the area and reduce itching. Donor sites can be reused after they are healed.

Cultured Epithelial Autografts

Cultured epithelial autografting is a technique for wound closure of massive burn wounds. The process of autologous epithelial cell growth begins with taking a full-thickness skin biopsy from an uninjured body site. This biopsy is sent to a specialized laboratory for culturing and growth. Typically, in 3 to 4 weeks, several sheets of cultured epithelial autografts are ready for application. In the operating room, the cultured epithelial autograft sheets are carefully applied to an excised and nonbleeding wound bed and are secured in place with staples. Dressings are applied and moistened with an antibiotic solution shown to be nontoxic to the cultured epithelial autografts.

Reports demonstrating the successful use of cultured epithelial autografts in the treatment of massive burn wounds have been limited. Both early and late cultured epithelial autograft loss due to mechanical shearing, nutritional imbalance, infection, or an immune response have been reported.[76, 89, 93]

■ Nutritional Support

Maintenance of adequate nutrition during the acute phase is essential in promoting wound healing and preventing infection. Basal metabolic rates may be 40% to 100% higher than normal levels, depending on the extent of the burn.[48] This response is thought to be the result of a "resetting" of the hypothalamic-pituitary-adrenal axis, which leads to an increase in heat production.[16] Metabolic rates decrease as wound coverage is achieved. In addition, glucose metabolism is altered following a burn injury, resulting in hyperglycemia. Low levels of insulin

Table 79–6. Energy Calculation Formulas Used for the Burn-Injured Adult	
Author	**Formula for Daily Caloric Expenditure Estimate**
Curreri	(25 kcal/kg body weight) + (40 kcal × %TBSA burn)
Modified Harris-Benedict	RMR × activity factor × injury factor
USAISR	[Age- and sex-specific BMR × (0.89142 + 0.01335 × %TBSA burn) × m² × 24 × activity factor]

TBSA, total body surface area; RMR, resting metabolic rate; USAISR, United States Army Institute of Surgical Research; and BMR, basal metabolic rate.

during the emergent phase, inhibition of insulin activity by increased levels of circulating catecholamines, and increased gluconeogenesis during the acute phase have all been implicated in causing hyperglycemia in the burn client.

Aggressive nutritional support is required to meet the increased energy requirements necessary to promote healing and to prevent the untoward effects of catabolism. Several different formulas (Table 79–6) are currently used to estimate energy requirements by factoring several different indices: weight, sex, age, extent of burn, and activity or injury.[104]

Aggressive nutritional support is generally indicated for the burn client with any one of the following: 30% or greater TBSA burn, clinical course requiring multiple operations, need for mechanical ventilatory support, compromised mental status, and poor preinjury nutritional state.[19]

Methods for delivering nutritional support include oral diet, enteral tube feedings, peripheral parenteral nutrition, total parenteral nutrition, and a combination of these. The preferred feeding route is oral or enteral; however, the decision of how to best meet the nutritional needs should be individualized for all clients. Typically, parenteral nutrition is reserved for clients with a prolonged ileus or clients who fail to meet their nutritional needs by the enteral route.

During periods of immobility (e.g., following skin grafting to the hands) or when hand, wrist, or arm ROM is limited, assistive devices for eating are used to enable the client to feed himself or herself independently. Figure 79–12 illustrates several commonly utilized devices.

■ Pain Management

Physiologic factors that have an impact on pain include the depth of injury, extent of the burn, and stage of wound healing. Typically, partial-thickness burns and newly harvested donor sites are exquisitely painful due to stimulation of exposed nerve endings. In contrast, full-thickness burns are insensate because the superficial nerve endings have been destroyed. However, nerve endings located at a full-thickness burn wound's periphery can be extremely sensitive.

Psychological factors that influence the perception of pain include anxiety, fear, and ability to cope. Social factors include past experiences with pain, personality, family background, circumstances surrounding the injury, and separation from family and home. It is important to remember that the perception of pain and response to painful stimuli are individual and that the treatment plan should be individualized as well.

The most common approach to pain control is with the use of pharmacologic agents.[56, 79] Morphine sulfate, codeine, meperidine, fentanyl, hydromorphone, and methadone are opioid analgesics commonly used to control the pain associated with burn injuries and treatment. Other pharmacologic modalities used include patient-controlled analgesia (PCA); inhalation analgesics, such as nitrous oxide; oral analgesic pain cocktails; and narcotic agonist-antagonist agents.[68] Nonsteroidal anti-inflammatory agents (NSAIDs) are also prescribed for the treatment of mild to moderate pain.[56] When NSAIDs are used, extra precautions must be taken to avoid gastric ulceration.

Nonpharmacologic modalities used to treat burn-related pain include hypnosis, guided imagery, art and play therapy, relaxation techniques, distraction, biofeedback, and music therapy.[56, 68] These modalities have been found to be effective in decreasing anxiety and thereby decreasing the perception of pain. They are often used as adjuncts to the pharmacologic treatment of burn pain.

As previously mentioned, pain assessment is an integral part of any pain management program. In addition to the adjective and numeric pain scales (previously discussed), the visual analog scale (VAS) is often used to measure the sensory component of burn pain. The VAS is a 10-cm horizontal line, anchored with the words "no pain" on the left and "maximum pain" or "worst pain possible" on the right (Fig. 79–13). The VAS requires a visual representation of the scale so that the client can mark or point to the place on the scale that represents the level of pain.

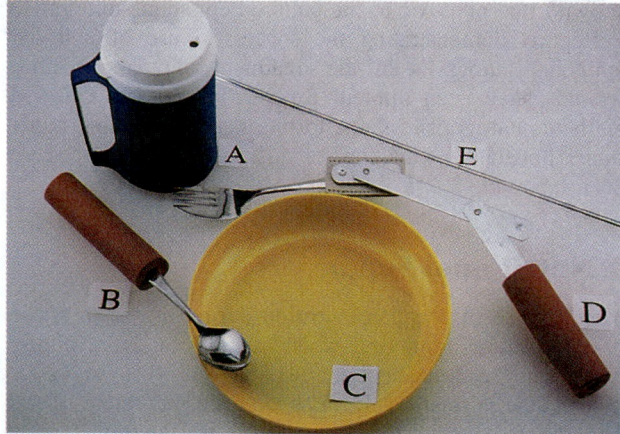

Figure 79–12. Mealtime assistive devices commonly used to increase client independence. Non-spill glass (*A*); large-handled spoon (*B*); plate with a lip and skid pad (*C*); long and large-handled fork (*D*); and long straw (*E*).

No pain

Worst pain
possible

Figure 79–13. Visual analog scale (VAS) used for pain assessment.

■ Psychological Support

The longest period of adjustment occurs during the acute phase.[70] The burned adult may demonstrate a variety of emotional and psychological responses. Anxiety and fearfulness continue related to potential disfigurement and perceived changes in role and identity. Depression, withdrawal, and regression may result.[100]

The client may begin discussing the burn injury or accident, recounting significant events[92] and searching for the meaning of what has happened.[100] Allowing expression of these worries and validating that they are "normal" is essential in providing support. Nurses need to actively listen and to allow the client to talk about the accident. Detailed and repetitious recounting of the injury is useful in desensitizing clients to the horror of what has happened and in decreasing nightmares.[100]

Reports of increased pain and the subsequent need for analgesia are common. The burned adult often voices a fear of inadequate pain relief, a sense of lack of control during painful procedures, and anxiety, all of which may lead to poor compliance and adherence to therapy.[92] Measures to reduce anxiety and promote a sense of personal control include client education, active listening by the staff, and client involvement in care.

Clients who have little information regarding what is to be done to them, how it may feel, and what resources or options exist to ease discomfort typically react with anxiety and a heightened pain response.[23] Providing preparatory information reassures the client that care and recovery are proceeding as planned and that nothing unusual is happening that could result in harm, thereby decreasing anxiety.[22] Educational measures that enhance the client's sense of personal control include education regarding various coping mechanisms and use of nonpharmacologic methods for pain control (e.g., controlled mental imagery, distraction, relaxation and breathing exercises). These interventions have been found to be effective in relieving pain-related distress and reducing use of analgesic medications.[103] Self-administered nitrous oxide and PCA are used in many burn centers for pain control, and they have been found to be valuable self-control modalities in pain management.

The healthcare team needs to demonstrate sensitivity toward the client through the practice of active listening. It is important that each member listen carefully and respond to the client's needs. Clients who feel that staff members are insensitive or too busy will believe that they have little control over their own pain relief.[23]

Many burn centers involve the client in their own care beginning soon after injury and find that this helps to reduce pain. Clients are encouraged to participate in wound care (e.g., bathing, simple debridement, dressing application) and physical therapy (e.g., active versus passive ROM exercises, application of splints and pressure garments). Negotiating therapy times with the client can result in better pain management and increased cooperation.

■ Physical Therapy

Maintenance of optimal physical functioning in the client with a burn injury is a challenge for the entire burn team. Nurses work closely with occupational and physical therapists to identify the rehabilitative needs of burn clients. An individualized program of splinting, positioning, exercise, ambulation, activities of daily living, and pressure therapy should be implemented early in the acute phase of recovery to maximize functional recovery and cosmetic outcome.

Wound contracture and hypertrophic scarring are two major problems for the burn client.[98] Wound contractures are typically more severe with extensive burns. Areas seemingly predisposed to contracture are the hands, head, neck, and axilla.[59] Measures used to prevent and treat wound contractures include therapeutic positioning, ROM exercises, splinting, and client/family education.[50, 98]

Therapeutic Positioning

Table 79–7 lists corrective and therapeutic techniques for positioning clients with specific areas of burn injury during periods of inactivity or immobilization. Allowing the burn client to assume a position of comfort most often contributes to contracture formation. Therefore, proper positioning should be maintained for the burn client while he or she is in and out of bed. These techniques place the affected area in a position that is in opposition to the anticipated contracture or deformity. For example to reduce risk of neck contractures, pillows are not allowed.

Exercise

Active ROM exercises are prescribed early in the acute phase of recovery to reduce edema and maintain strength and joint function. In addition, activities of daily living can be effective in maintaining function and ROM. Ambulation also maintains strength and ROM of the lower extremities and should begin as soon as the client is physiologically stable. Passive ROM and stretching exercises should be included as part of the daily treatment plan if the client is unable to perform active ROM exercises.[98]

Splinting

Splints are used to maintain proper joint position and to prevent or correct contractures. Two types of splints are

Table 79–7. Therapeutic Positioning for the Burn-Injured Client		
Burned Area	**Therapeutic Position**	**Positioning Techniques**
Neck		
Anterior	Extension	No pillow Small towel roll beneath shoulders to promote neck extension
Circumferential	Neutral toward extension	No pillow
Posterior or asymmetrical	Neutral	No pillow
Shoulder/axilla	Arm abduction to 90–110 degrees	Splinting Arms positioned away from the body and supported on arm troughs
Elbow	Arm extension	Elbow splint Elbows positioned in extension with slight bend at the elbow (no greater than 10 degrees of elbow flexion) Arms supported on arm troughs with the forearm in slight pronation
Hand		
Wrist	Wrist extension	Hand splint
MCP	MCP flexion at 90 degrees	Hand splint
PIP/DIP	PIP/DIP extension	Hand splint
Thumb	Thumb abduction	Hand splint with thumb abduction
Finger web spaces	Finger abduction	Web spacers of foam, silicone products, or custom-fitted pressure garments to decrease webbing formation
Hip	Hip extension	Supine with the head of bed flat and legs extended Trochanter roll to maintain neutral hip rotation (toes should be pointing toward the ceiling) Prone positioning
Knee	Knee extension	Supine with knees extended (toes should be pointing toward the ceiling) Prone positioning with feet extended over the end of the mattress Sitting in chair with legs extended and elevated Knee splint
Ankle	Neutral	Padded footboard Ankle positioning devices (avoid heel cord tightening)—provide heel protection to prevent pressure sore development

MCP, metacarpal interphalangeal joints; PIP/DIP, proximal/distal interphalangeal joints.

frequently used: static and dynamic. A static splint immobilizes the joint. Static splints do not replace exercise and are frequently applied for periods of immobilization, during sleeping hours, and in clients who cannot maintain proper positioning.[98] In contrast, dynamic splints exercise the affected joint. Care must be taken to ensure that all splints fit properly and do not apply excessive pressure that might lead to further tissue or nerve damage.

Education

Client and family education regarding correct positioning and the need for continued exercise is important. Written guides and handouts on positioning, splinting, and exercise routines can facilitate learning and cooperation.[50]

■ Control of Scarring

Hypertrophic scarring results from an overabundant deposition of collagen in the healed burn wound. The severity of hypertrophic scarring depends on several factors: burn depth, race, age, and type of autograft (sheet graft, meshed graft, cultured epithelial autograft).[55] The nonoperative method for minimizing hypertrophic scarring is pressure therapy.[98]

Several products are commercially available that provide continuous pressure over the healing burn wound. During the early acute stage of wound healing, elastic wraps and bandages can be used to apply continuous pressure to the healing skin while it is still fragile and vulnerable to mechanical shearing. Ultimately, custom-fit antiburn scar support garments (Fig. 79–14) can be or-

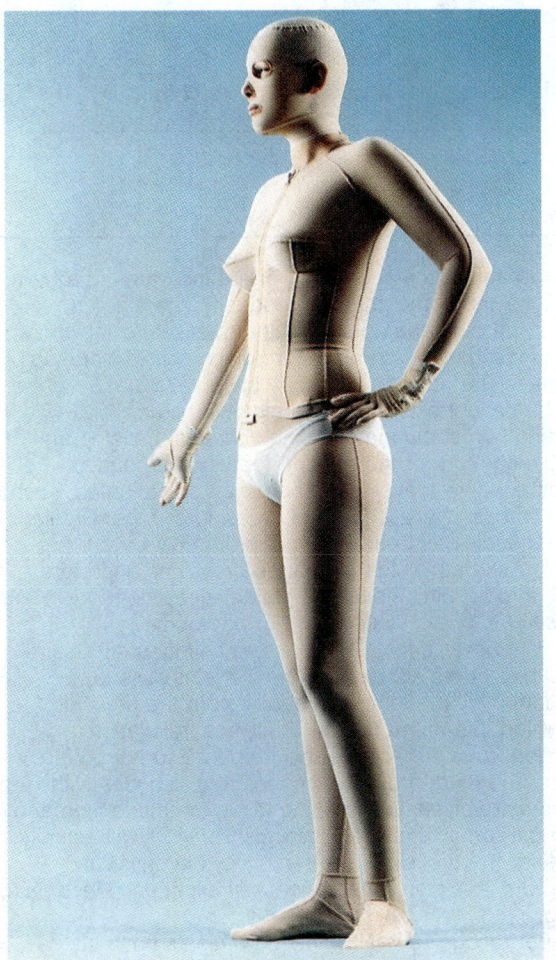

Figure 79–14. Client wearing custom-fitted anti-scar support garment. When worn 23 hours a day, this garment is effective in providing pressure therapy over healing burn wounds. Pressure therapy helps to minimize the development of hypertrophic scarring. (Courtesy of Medical Z Corporation, San Antonio.)

dered and worn 23 hours a day until the burn scar tissue has matured (typically 18 months to 2 years postinjury).

The term *keloid* is often misused to described hypertrophic scarring. By definition, a keloid is a sharply elevated, irregularly shaped, and enlarged mass of scar tissue that is caused by excessive amounts of collagen formation during connective tissue repair.[97] Keloids differ from hypertrophic scars in that they extend beyond the wound perimeter. They tend to occur in darkly pigmented individuals, may continue to grow years after the injury, and are more prone to recurrence, despite surgical excision.[12]

Community and Self-Care

The rehabilitation phase of recovery represents the final phase of burn care (see Bridge to Home Healthcare). Although this phase overlaps the acute care phase and lasts well beyond the acute inpatient hospitalization, the goals and principles of physical and psychological reha-

bilitation are similar to those described previously. Ultimately, a burn rehabilitation program is designed for the client to gain independence through achievement of maximal functional and emotional recovery. Measures to promote wound healing, prevent or minimize deformities and hypertrophic scarring, increase physical strength and function, promote emotional support, and provide education are part of the ongoing rehabilitation process.[98]

■ Education

Client and family education should focus on specific needs related to normal wound maturation, wound care, infection, nutritional needs and diet, physical therapy, exercise, and common emotional readjustment issues.

■ Wound Care Issues

Wound care issues of greatest concern during the rehabilitation period often relate to home care of healing wounds and fragile skin (this is especially true at time of discharge from the hospital) and to surgical options for treatment of wound contractures and hypertrophic scarring.

Prior to discharge from the hospital, the burned adult should be able to describe the normal process of wound healing with an emphasis on the special care and consideration of newly healed skin. Issues concerning care of dry skin, bathing/showering, sun and cold exposure, blisters, and itching should be reviewed thoroughly with the client (Box 79–5).

Surgical options for the treatment of wound contractures and scar include (1) split-thickness and full-thickness skin grafts, (2) skin flaps, (3) Z-plasty, and (4) tissue expansion. It is generally recommended that surgical release of contractures not be performed before 6 months postinjury or until the scar tissue has matured.[3, 45] These surgical options are discussed in depth in Chapter 80.

■ Emotional Support

Individuals during this phase of their recovery often voice excitement about leaving the hospital, yet some concern about returning to "life outside" is evident. Burn support groups utilizing group process are effective in assisting burned clients in reestablishing themselves in the outside world.[37] During therapy sessions, participants are encouraged to discuss their discharge concerns. Often, issues concerning poor body image (a deterrent to resocialization), interpersonal relationship problems, fear of returning home, finances, and career are revealed and discussed.[92] Staff intervention primarily consists of support[92] and education during this phase. Issues may develop when a home has been destroyed by fire (see Nursing Research feature).

Toxic Epidermal Necrolysis Syndrome

Toxic epidermal necrolysis syndrome (TEN) is a severe exfoliative dermatologic disease (Fig. 79–15). It is in-

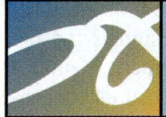

BRIDGE TO HOME HEALTHCARE

Burn Rehabilitation

Ruth Long, R. N., *Interim Healthcare, Auburn, California*

The transition from the critical care or rehabilitation unit of the hospital to home is an important milestone in a burn patient's recovery. The transition also presents many challenges for the home care team. Ideally, the team is multidisciplinary and includes the physician, nurse/case manager, physical therapist, and the medical social worker. If possible, make an appointment with the physician, nurses, and discharge planner before discharge to increase continuity of care. Find out how and where the patient was burned. The hospital staff may have valuable information to prepare for the patient's discharge, especially if the patient was burned in his own home.

On discharge, assess the patient and family's response to being home. During dressing changes, develop an environment to prevent infection and to provide the most possible comfort for the patient. Identify the needed dressing materials and a place to store them in the patient's home where they will not become contaminated, such as in a sealable plastic box or bag. Order supplies in quantities that can be used in one dressing change. Sterile dressings will not remain sterile until the next visit. Keep dressing supplies in one location, preferably covered. Storing the boxes that supplies come in helps keep them closed. Ask permission to change dressings and store supplies in one central location of the house, such as a spare bedroom. This helps the patient sleep better at night, since the pain from dressing changes is not associated with his or her "safe room" or bedroom.

Pain management is another great challenge. Not only does pain occur during the dressing changes, but also during the day and with physical therapy. The physical therapist and nurse should try to make joint visits during dressing changes. Team work will result in less pain for the patient. Call the family an hour before the dressing change to administer prescribed pain medication. Develop a comfortable milieu for the dressings: relaxation techniques, breathing exercises, and soft music will help the patient relax and control his response to pain. With the physician's approval, remove dressings gently in the shower. The extra moisture loosens and debrides with less pain. Cut the dressings off lengthwise in the direction of the extremities. Unwrapping takes too much time and causes anticipatory grief for the patient. Involve the patient with the removal of the dressings. Patients will actually experience less pain when they can control the pain stimulus. After the dressings are removed, the physical therapist can work with the patient to get more range of motion with less pain. The patient will experience less pain when two people support the extremities for wrapping or turning.

Post-traumatic stress is very real to patients, even if they do not recognize it. Not only do patients have stress related to the injury, but also to hospitalization and procedures such as ventilation, fluid resuscitation, painful dressing changes, and operations. Returning home to the place of injury or experiencing similar pain from dressing changes at home can emotionally scar the patient. Involve social workers for counseling, family adjustment, alternative pain management, and identification of post-traumatic stress.

---

cluded in this chapter because its pathophysiology and management are similar to those of burns. This syndrome is initially characterized by chills, fever, malaise, and myalgias followed by a body rash. Typically, the rash progresses to formation of vesicles and large confluent bullae that affect the epidermis and mucous membranes of the eyes, mouth, upper airways, and esophagus. Although the specific cause is unknown, TEN has been associated with the administration of various medications. Antibacterial agents, anticonvulsants, analgesics, and nonsteroidal anti-inflammatory agents have been implicated.[8, 34, 53, 105] Nondrug causes are uncommon, but they include viral, bacterial, and fungal infections and neoplastic disease.[8] This disorder, in which large areas of skin separate at the dermoepidermal junction, is similar to an extensive partial-thickness burn injury. Clients with TEN require specialized medical and nursing care (e.g., fluid resuscitation, daily wound care, nutritional support, physical and psychological therapy) similar to that routinely provided at most major burn centers. Medical and nursing treatment of the client with TEN is aimed at protecting the dermis and promoting reepithelialization. Early transfer and treatment to a burn center for the client with TEN is recommended to reduce morbidity and length of hospital stay.[53, 105]

Conclusions

Nursing care of the burn-injured client is both complex and challenging. The psychological and physical trauma sustained following a burn injury can be devastating for both the victim and the family or significant other. As a key member of the burn team, the nurse is responsible for an individualized plan of care that reflects the client's total condition as he or she progresses through the different phases of recovery. Priority issues and care change as the client moves from the critical emergent phase into, and ultimately through, the rehabilitative period. Therein lies the challenge to the burn care nurse.

Box 79–5. Skin Care after Hospitalization

Dry Skin/Itching

■ To prevent or treat dry skin, apply a thin layer of a moisturizer
■ Natural lubricants such as vitamin E or cocoa butter are commonly used to prevent excessive dry skin and itching
■ Products that contain perfume, alcohol, or lanolin should be avoided because they tend to irritate newly healed skin
■ If itching occurs, avoid scratching, as this may cause the skin to break open
■ A tepid bath followed by application of a moisturizer has been helpful in relieving itching
■ For severe itching, the client should contact his/her physician, who may prescribe a medication for relief

Bathing

■ Bathe as usual using a comfortable water temperature (newly healed skin is more sensitive to extreme water temperatures)
■ Wash using a mild soap, and rinse thoroughly
■ Ensure that all creams and loose skin particles are removed
■ Pat skin dry using a clean towel

Sun Exposure

■ Newly healed skin sunburns easily
■ Avoid direct sunlight by wearing light clothing and a large-brimmed hat
■ Apply sunscreen to any exposed areas and reapply as necessary to maintain adequate protection

Cold Exposure

■ Newly healed skin is more sensitive to the cold, which may cause slight tingling in the hands and feet
■ Wear warm clothing

Blisters

■ Blisters may develop in newly healed skin due to friction, mechanical trauma (bumping into objects), or from standing for prolonged periods without adequate support; avoiding these situations may decrease the incidence of blisters
■ Specific instructions on the care of blisters should be reviewed by the physician with the client prior to discharge

---

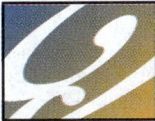

NURSING RESEARCH

How Do Victims of Home Fires React to Their Losses?

Stern, P. N., & Kerry, J. (1996). Restructuring life after home loss by fire. *IMAGE: Journal of Nursing Scholarship, 28* (1), 11–16.

Material possessions hold symbolic meaning for us. When our possessions are reduced to ashes and rubble by fire, part of our lives are destroyed as well. Home fires differ from other disasters in that they strike one household at a time. Community support for the victims is missing in these disasters, when compared to larger community problems, such as flooding.

The purpose of this study was to discover the experiences of home loss by fire. A ground theory method was used. The sample was victims of fire who had lost their dwelling to fire or had had damage so severe that they had been forced to vacate the premises. Fire victims were from North America, Europe, Southeast Asia, and Australia.

Fire victims described their loss as being akin to losing a family member. They spoke of feeling physically ill at the sight of their burned possessions. They went through a period of wandering aimlessly when purposeful action was almost impossible. Despite their helplessness, they were forced to take action to restore and restructure their homes. Victims also spoke of losing the fabric of their lives, the very structure to which they retreated to feel safe. The work of restoration was very difficult. The tools, records, photographs, and papers were all destroyed. While they were working through the losses, they needed a place to sleep, something to sleep on, and clothes to wear. In addition, if they were uninsured, they were not likely to ever recoup the financial loss. Furthermore, victims needed to keep working at their jobs to maintain employment.

Interactions with others included connected support with provision of home, clothes, and food. Sometimes, other people inflicted unintentional insults ("Aren't you lucky to be able to buy all new things?")

The victims restructured their lives with support from others. Their displays of grief were limited because extended grief responses were not socially acceptable. New rituals were developed, including using the fire as a benchmark for other life events, taking precautions, and becoming expert on fire prevention.

Implications for Practice

Nurses need to be aware of the tremendous impact fire has on life. Contacting community support agencies and providing needed support would be logical steps to assisting with the restructuring of lives destroyed by fire.

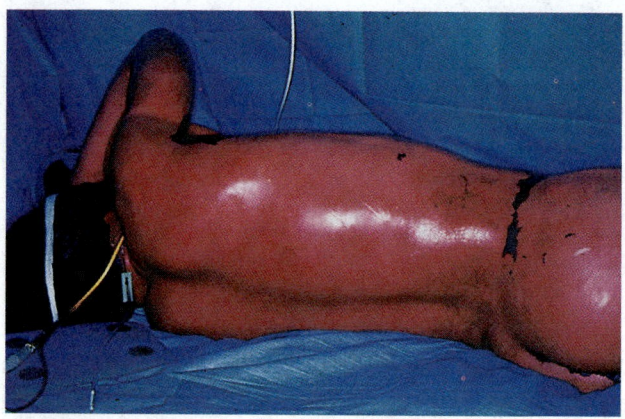

Figure 79–15. Client with toxic epidermal necrolysis syndrome (TEN).

Thinking Critically

1. The client is a 37-year-old man with a 45% TBSA flame burn sustained today at 8:00 AM. He was immediately taken to a nearby emergency department, where an IV line was placed and fluid resuscitation was started with lactated Ringer's solution, based on the Parkland formula. Following an evaluation that ruled out any concomitant life-threatening trauma, he was transferred to your burn center at 1:00 PM. Burn center admission data include the following:

Heart rate, 138 bpm; sinus tachycardia
Blood pressure, 162/100 mm Hg
Respiratory rate, 28 breaths/min, unlabored
Urine output 43 ml in the last 2 hours (urinary catheter in place); urine dark amber
Negative bowel sounds
Client is awake, alert, complaining of excessive thirst despite feelings of nausea; client vomited once in the ambulance en route to the burn center.
Admission weight, 72 kg
IV line was inadvertently pulled out during the transfer to the burn center; IV fluid intake 3 L since the time of injury

What priorities should be set for the client's care? What interventions should be undertaken?

Factors to Consider. What is the client's fluid volume status? What does the absence of bowel sounds tell you about his gastrointestinal status?

2. It is now 7 hours postinjury, and the client is complaining of pain in his right hand. The extent and depth of the client's burn injury are as follows: full-thickness circumferential burns to the right arm and forearm (palmar surface and fingers spared of injury); partial-thickness injury to the left forearm; full-thickness injury to the abdomen and chest; and partial-thickness burns to the buttock and right thigh; these total 45% TBSA. What assessments should you perform? What interventions should be undertaken?

Factors to Consider. What are the manifestations of tissue ischemia? How would you determine whether that is the client's problem? If it is, what should you do?

3. It is now 3 weeks since the client was injured. His wife has come to you with information that suggests that he is worried about never being able to work and support his family again (he is a farmer). She thinks that he is becoming depressed, and she feels helpless in this situation. What can you do to help both the client and his wife?

Factors to Consider. What professional resources might be helpful in addressing these concerns? What lay resources might be helpful? What factors related to the client's treatment might be contributing to his depression?

Bibliography

1. Achauer, B. M., & McGuire, A. (1989). Fire safe cigarettes—an update. *Journal of Burn Care and Rehabilitation, 10*(2), 173–174.
2. Agee, R. N., et al. (1976). Use of 133-xenon in early diagnosis of inhalation injury. *Journal of Trauma, 16*(3), 218–224.
3. Alexander, J. W., et al. (1981). Surgical correction of postburn flexion contractures of the fingers of children. *Plastic and Reconstructive Surgery, 68*(2), 218–226.
4. American Academy of Orthopaedic Surgeons. (1993). Burn injuries. In Heckman, J. D. (Ed.), *Emergency care and transportation of the sick and injured* (5th ed., revised). Rosemont, IL: Author.
5. American Burn Association. (1984). Guidelines for service standards and severity classification in the treatment of burn injury. *Bulletin of the American College of Surgeons, 69*(10), 24–28.
6. American National Standards Committee. (1981). *Standard Z21.10.1.* Washington, DC: Consumer Product Safety Commission.
7. Arturson, G., et al. (1969). Changes in immunoglobulin levels in severely burned patients. *Lancet, 1*(594), 546–548.
8. Avakian, R., et al. (1991). Toxic epidermal necrolysis: A review. *Journal of the American Academy of Dermatology, 25*(1, pt 1), 69–79.
9. Baker S. P., et al. (1992). *The injury fact book* (ed. 2; pp. 161–173). New York, Oxford University Press.
10. Baxter, C. R. (1974). Fluid volume and electrolyte changes in the early post-burned period. *Clinics in Plastic Surgery, 1*(4), 693–709.
11. Bayley, E. W., et al. (1990). Standards for burn nursing practice. *Journal of Burn Care and Rehabilitation, 10*(4), 362–374.
12. Bayley, E. W. (1990). Wound healing in the patient with burns. *Nursing Clinics of North America, 25*(1), 205–222.
13. Berry, C. C., et al. (1982). Differences in burn size estimates between community hospitals and a burn center. *Journal of Burn Care and Rehabilitation, 3*(3), 176–177.
14. Boots Pharmaceuticals. (1991). *Travase ointment—indications and usage* (product monograph). Lincolnshire, IL: Author.
15. Brodzka W., et al. (1985). Burns: Causes and risk factors. *Archives of Physical Medicine and Rehabilitation, 66*(11), 746–752.
16. Burdge, J. J., et al. (1986). Nutritional and metabolic consequences of thermal injury. *Clinics in Plastic Surgery, 13*(1), 49–55.
17. Burdge, J. J., et al. (1988). Surgical treatment of burns in elderly patients. *Journal of Trauma, 28*(2), 214–217.
18. Burgess, M. (1991). Initial management of a patient with extensive burn injury. *Critical Care Nursing Clinics of North America, 3*(2), 165–179.
19. Carlson, D. E., & Jordan, B. S. (1991). Implementing nutritional therapy in the thermally injured patient. *Critical Care Nursing Clinics of North America, 3*(2), 221–235.
20. Carrougher, G., & Marvin, J. (1989). Mechanical debridement: Views from University of Washington Burn Center at Harborview, Seattle, Washington (editorial). *Journal of Burn Care and Rehabilitation, 10*(3), 271–272.

21. Choiniere, M., et al. (1989). The pain of burns: Characteristics and correlates. *Journal of Trauma, 29*(11), 1531–1539.
22. Chapman, C. R. (1985). Psychological factors in postoperative pain and their treatment. In G. Smith & B. G. Covino (Eds.), *Acute pain* (pp. 22–41). London: Butterworths.
23. Chapman, C. R., & Turner, J. A. (1986). Psychological control of acute pain in medical settings. *Journal of Pain and Symptom Management, 1*(1), 9–20.
24. Cioffi, W. G., & Rue, L. W. (1991). Diagnosis and treatment of inhalation injuries. *Critical Care Nursing Clinics of North America, 3*(2), 191–198.
25. Curreri, P. W. (1979). Chemical burns. In C. P. Artz, et al. (Eds.), *Burns: A team approach* (pp. 363–369). Philadelphia: W. B. Saunders.
26. Demling, R. H., et al. (1984). Role of thermal injury-induced hypoproteinemia on edema formation in burned and non-burned tissue. *Surgery, 95*(2), 136–144.
27. Dyer, C., & Roberts, D. (1990). Thermal trauma. *Nursing Clinics of North America, 25*(1), 85–117.
28. Everett, J. J., et al. (1994). Pain assessment from patients with burns and their nurses. *Journal of Burn Care and Rehabilitation, 15*(2), 194–198.
29. Fein, A., et al. (1980). Pathophysiology and management of the complications resulting from fire and the inhaled products of combustion: Review of the literature. *Critical Care Medicine, 8*(2), 94–98.
30. Feldman, K. W., et al. (1978). Tap water scald burns in children. *Pediatrics, 62*(1), 1–7.
31. Feller, I., et al. (1982). Burn epidemiology: Focus on youngsters and the aged. *Journal of Burn Care and Rehabilitation, 3*(5), 285–288, 336.
32. Feller, I., et al. (1980). Improvements in burn care, 1965 to 1979. *Journal of the American Medical Association, 244*(18), 2074–2078.
33. Freeman, J. W. (1984). Nursing care of the patient with a burn injury. *Critical Care Nurse, 4*(6), 52–68.
34. Guillaume, J. C., et al. (1987). The culprit drugs in 87 cases of toxic epidermal necrolysis (Lyell syndrome). *Archives of Dermatology, 123*(9), 1166–1170.
35. Gordon, M. K. (1987). Burn wound care: Silver sulfadiazine application (editorial). *Journal of Burn Care and Rehabilitation, 8*(5), 429.
36. Hall, J. R., Jr. (1985). A decade of detectors: Measuring the effect. *Fire Journal, 79,* 37–43.
37. Hamill, W. T., et al. (1983). Stress management in burn cases. In T. L. Wachtel, et al. (Eds.), *Current topics in burn care.* Rockville, MD: Aspen Publications.
38. Hammond, J., & Ward, C. G. (1987). Transfers from emergency room to burn center: Errors in burn size estimate. *Journal of Trauma, 27*(10), 1161–1165.
39. Heideman, M., et al. (1978). Complement activation and hematologic hemodynamic and respiratory reactions early after soft tissue injury. *Journal of Trauma, 18*(10), 696–700.
40. Heimbach, D. M. (1987). Early excision and grafting. *Surgical Clinics of North America, 67*(1), 93–107.
41. Heimbach, D. M. (1983). Smoke inhalation: Current concepts (pp. 31–38). In T. L. Wachtel, et al. (Eds.), *Current topics in burn care.* Rockville, MD: Aspen Publications.
42. Heimbach, D. M. (1987). Early burn wound excision and grafting. In Boswick J. A. (Ed.), *The art and science of burn care.* Rockville, MD: Aspen Publications.
43. Helvig, B., & Curry, V. (1989). Mechanical debridement: Views from Shriners Hospitals for Crippled Children, Burn Unit, Galveston, Texas (editorial). *Journal of Burn Care and Rehabilitation, 10*(3), 272–273.
44. Herndon, D. N., et al. (1988). Inhalation injury in burned patients: Effects and treatment. *Burns, 14*(5), 349–356.
45. Huang, T. T., et al. (1978). Ten years experience in managing patients with burn contractures of axilla, elbow, wrist, and knee joints. *Plastic and Reconstructive Surgery, 61*(1), 70–76.
46. Hunt, J. L., et al. (1976). The pathophysiology of acute electric injuries. *Journal of Trauma, 16*(5), 335–340.
47. Hunt, J. L., & Purdue, G. F. (1992). The elderly burn patient. *The American Journal of Surgery, 164,* 472–476.
48. Ireton, C. S., et al. (1986). Evaluation of energy expenditures in burn patients. *Journal of the American Dietetic Association, 86*(3), 331–333.
49. Jarvis, R., & Weireter, L. J. (1989). Mechanical debridement: Views from Sentara Norfolk General Hospital, Norfolk, Virginia (editorial). *Journal of Burn Care and Rehabilitation, 10*(3), 273.
50. Johnson, C. L., & Cain, V. J. (1985). The rehab guide. *American Journal of Nursing, 85*(1), 48–50.
51. Jones, J. D., et al. (1989). Alcohol use and burn injury. *Journal of Burn Care and Rehabilitation, 12*(2), 148–152.
52. Kawakami, M., et al. (1991). Immune suppression after acute ethanol ingestion and thermal injury. *Journal of Surgical Research, 51*(3), 210–215.
53. Kelemen, J. J., et al. (1995). Burn center care for patients with toxic epidermal necrolysis. *Journal of the American College of Surgeons, 180*(3), 273–278.
54. Kelley, D., et al. (1992). Burns in alcohol and drug users result in longer treatment times with more complications. *Journal of Burn Care and Rehabilitation, 13*(2), 218–220.
55. Ketchum, L. D., et al. (1974). Hypertrophic scars and keloids. *Plastic and Reconstructive Surgery, 53*(2), 140–154.
56. Kibbee, E. (1984). Burn pain management. *Critical Care Quarterly, 7*(3), 54–62.
57. Knaysi, G. A., et al. (1968). The rule of nines: Its history and accuracy. *Plastic and Reconstructive Surgery, 41*(6), 560–563.
58. Kohn, J., & Cort, D. F. (1969). Immunoglobulins in burned patients. *Lancet, 1*(599), 836–837.
59. Kraemer, M. D., et al. (1988). Burn contractures: Incidence, predisposing factors, and results of surgical therapy. *Journal of Burn Care and Rehabilitation, 9*(3), 261–265.
60. Kravitz, M., et al. (1985). Thermal injury in the elderly: Incidence and cause. *Journal of Burn Care and Rehabilitation, 6*(6), 487–489.
61. Lee, J., (1970). Emotional reactions to trauma. *Nursing Clinics of North America, 5*(4), 577–587.
62. Lee, J. L., et al. (1985). Survey of isolation techniques (abstract). *Proceedings of the American Burn Association, 17,* 82.
63. Leonard, L. G., et al. (1982). Chemical burns: Effect of prompt first aid. *Journal of Trauma, 22*(5), 420–423.
64. Leske, J. S. (1991). Overview of family needs after critical illness: From assessment to intervention. *AACN Clinical Issues in Critical Care Nursing, 2*(2), 220–226.
65. Linn, B. S. (1980). Age differences in the severity and outcome of burns. *Journal of the American Geriatrics Society, 28*(3), 118–123.
66. Lund, C. C., & Browder, N. C. (1944). The estimation of areas of burn. *Surgery, Gynecology and Obstetrics, 79*(4), 352–358.
67. Maley, M. P. (1989). Scald burns associated with tap water. *Journal of Burn Care and Rehabilitation, 10*(2), 172–173.
68. Marvin, J. (1987). Pain management in the burn patient: Excerpts from a symposium on pain management at Harborview Hospital, Seattle, Washington, July 23, 1986. *Journal of Burn Care and Rehabilitation, 8*(4), 307–318.
69. Marvin, J. A., et al. (1991). Burn nursing delphi study: Setting research priorities. *Journal of Burn Care and Rehabilitation, 12*(2), 190–197.
70. Molter, N. C. (1993). When is the burn injury healed? Psychosocial implications of care. *AACN Clinical Issues in Critical Care Nursing, 4*(2), 424–432.
71. Monafo, W. W., Jr. (1971). *The treatment of burns: Principles and practices.* St. Louis: Warren H. Green.
72. Moncrief, J. A. (1979). Replacement therapy. In C. P. Artz, et al. (Eds.), *Burns: A team approach* (pp. 169–192). Philadelphia: W. B. Saunders.
73. Moritz, A. R., et al. (1945). The effects of inhaled heat on the air passages and lung: An experimental investigation. *American Journal of Pathology, 21*(2), 311–332.
74. Moylan, J. A., & Chan, C. (1978). Inhalation injury—an increasing problem. *Annals of Surgery, 188*(1), 34–37.
75. Munster, A. M., et al. (1970). The effect of thermal injury on serum immunoglobulins. *Annals of Surgery, 172*(6), 965–969.
76. Munster, A. M., et al. (1990). Cultured epidermis for the coverage of massive burn wounds—a single center experience. *Annals of Surgery, 211*(6), 676–679.
77. Murray, J. P. (1988). Study of the prevention of hot tap water burns. *Burns, 14,* 185–193.
78. Nebraska Burn Institute. (1994). *Advanced burn life support manual* (rev. ed.). Lincoln, NE: Author.
79. Perry, S. (1982). Management of pain during debridement: A survey of U.S. burn units. *Pain, 13*(3), 267–280.

80. Perry, S., et al. (1981). Assessment of pain by burn patients. *Journal of Burn Care and Rehabilitation, 2*(4), 322–326.
81. Philbin, P., & Marvin, J. A. (1982). Management of the pediatric patient with a major burn. *Journal of Burn Care and Rehabilitation, 3*(2), 118–125.
82. Powers, P. S., et al. (1994). Alcohol disorders among patients with burns: Crisis and opportunity. *Journal of Burn Care and Rehabilitation, 15*(4), 386–391.
83. Pruitt, B. A., Jr., & Goodwin, C. W., Jr. (1990). Burn injury. In E. E. Moore, et al. (Eds.), *Early care of the injured patient* (pp. 286–306). Philadelphia: Brian Decker.
84. Pruitt, B. A., Goodwin, C. W., & Cioffi, W. G. (1995). Thermal injury. In J. H. Davis, & G. F. Sheldon. (Eds.), *Clinical surgery.* St. Louis: Mosby–Year Book.
85. Purdue, G. F., et al. (1990). Obesity: A risk factor in the burn patient. *Journal of Burn Care and Rehabilitation, 11*(1), 32–34.
86. Robson, M. C., & Kucan, J. O. (1983). The burn wound. In T. L. Wachtel, et al. (Eds.), *Current topics in burn care* (pp. 55–63). Rockville, MD: Aspen Publications.
87. Rossignol, A. M., et al. (1985). Consumer products and hospitalized burn injuries among elderly Massachusetts residents. *Journal of the American Geriatrics Society, 33*(11), 768–772.
88. Rue, L. W., & Cioffi, W. G., Jr. (1991). Resuscitation of thermally injured patients. *Critical Care Nursing Clinics of North America, 3*(2), 181–189.
89. Rue, L. W., et al. (1993). Wound closure and outcome in extensively burned patients treated with cultured autologous keratinocytes. *Journal of Trauma, 34*(5), 662–668.
90. Sheridan, R. L., et al. (1992). Burns in morbidly obese patients. *Journal of Trauma, 33*(6), 818–820.
91. Silverstein, P., & Lack, B. (1987). Fire prevention in the United States—are the home fires still burning? *Surgical Clinics of North America, 67*(1), 1–14.
92. Summers, T. M. (1991). Psychosocial support of the burned patient. *Critical Care Nursing Clinics of North America, 3*(2), 237–244.
93. Teepe, R. G. C., et al. (1990). The use of cultured autologous epidermis in the treatment of extensive burn wounds. *Journal of Trauma, 30*(3), 269–275.
94. Thomson, P. D., et al. (1990). A survey of burn hydrotherapy in the United States. *Journal of Burn Care and Rehabilitation, 11*(2), 151–155.
95. Trunkey, D. D. (1983). Transporting the critically burned patient. In T. L. Wachtel, et al. (Eds.), *Current topics in burn care* (pp. 11–14). Rockville, MD: Aspen Publications.
96. Turner, D. G., et al. (1989). Cooking-related burn injuries in the elderly: Preventing the "granny gown" burn. *Journal of Burn Care and Rehabilitation, 10*(4), 356–359.
97. Wachtel, T. L., et al. (1983). Initial management of major burns. In T. L. Wachtel, et al. (Eds.). *Current topics in burn care.* (pp. 25–30) Rockville, MD: Aspen Publications.
98. Ward, R. S. (1991). The rehabilitation of burn patients. *Critical Reviews in Physical and Rehabilitation Medicine, 2*(3), 121–138.
99. Warden, G. D. (1987). Outpatient care of thermal injuries. *Surgical Clinics of North America, 67*(1), 147–157.
100. Watkins, P. N., et al. (1988). Psychological stages in adaptation following burn injury: A method for facilitating psychological recovery of burn victims. *Journal of Burn Care and Rehabilitation, 9*, 376–384.
101. Weaver, A. M., et al. (1993). Immersion scald burns: Strategies for prevention. *The Journal of Emergency Medicine, 11*(4), 397–402.
102. Weber, J. M., & Tompkins, D. M. (1993). Improving survival: Infection control and burns. *AACN Clinical Issues in Critical Care Nursing, 4*(2), 414–423.
103. Wernick, R. L., et al. (1981). Pain management in severely burned adults: A test of stress inoculation. *Journal of Behavioral Medicine, 4*, 103–109.
104. Williamson, J. (1989). Actual burn nutrition care practices—a national survey (part II). *Journal of Burn Care and Rehabilitation, 10*(2), 185–194.
105. Yarbrough D. R. (1996). Experience with toxic epidermal necrolysis treated in a burn center. *Journal of Burn Care and Rehabilitation, 17*(1), 30–33.
106. Zikria, B. A., et al. (1972). Smoke and carbon monoxide poisoning in fire victims. *Journal of Trauma, 12*, 641–645.

Nursing Care of Clients Undergoing Plastic Surgery

Joyce M. Black

Plastic surgery is the surgical subspecialty that concentrates on the restoration of function and form to body structures damaged by trauma, transformed by the aging process, changed by disease processes (such as skin cancer), and malformed as a result of congenital defects. Technology and plastic surgery techniques have improved rapidly. Plastic surgery is able to successfully address many problems (e.g., amputated digits, breast reconstruction following mastectomy, and distracting birthmarks) that could not be addressed just a few years ago.

Plastic surgery can be divided into two major areas: (1) aesthetic (cosmetic) surgery and (2) reconstructive surgery.

Aesthetic plastic surgery improves physical features that are already within "normal" range. Aesthetic surgery is performed for changes that result from aging, to alter inherited features, or because of a client's personal desire. Clients seeking aesthetic surgery are so dissatisfied with the appearance of one or more body parts that they are willing to undergo surgery. Because aesthetic surgery is considered "cosmetic" it is not covered by insurance, and clients pay out of pocket for procedures. Most clients are enthusiastic and happy because the surgery is a culmination of a personal desire that they have held for a long time. In contrast, other clients who are having aesthetic surgery may or may not have social support for their decision. The client may feel vain, embarrassed, or guilty about taking healthcare away from "people who really need it." Nurses need to be sensitive to these feelings in the client. Nurses also need to be comfortable with a person's normal desires to feel good about the way he or she looks.

Reconstructive surgery attempts to restore a more normal appearance to an abnormal or absent body part. The abnormality may be a result of injury or disease, it may be congenital, or it may be the cause of other medical problems. People undergoing reconstructive surgery are typically motivated to try to gain increased function of body parts and to improve their appearance. Although they may hope that plastic surgery will make them "normal," they usually know this may be unrealistic. Such clients are often struggling with diverse emotions: hope for a future without disease recurrence, eagerness to see final surgical results, hope that postoperative pain will be endurable, and weariness of the illness. The client having reconstructive surgery does have the advantage of social approval. Inasmuch as such a client is seen as a victim, society, as represented by either individuals or institutions, often provides treatment or makes appeals for payment of the operations.

Because of the significant impact of plastic surgical procedures on body image and self-esteem, psychological care is imperative. Throughout this chapter we address physical and psychological aspects of care. Plastic surgery is not only an operation on the skin, it reaches into the psyche of the individual.

Basic Principles of Plastic Surgery

Achieving Minimal Scarring

Minimal postoperative scarring is the hallmark of plastic surgery. It is very important to understand that no surgery can be done without creating a scar. Plastic surgery is conducted to minimize scars, so at times it seems like surgery can be done without scars. The quality of scarring is affected by many variables. The client's age, general health, skin type, and healing ability are important. Surgical technique and the quality of wound care also affect the healing process.

Skin Lines

Every individual has normal lines and skinfolds (Fig. 80-1). Incisions made perpendicular to these lines result in more obvious scars. Incisions made parallel to the lines heal camouflaged by natural skinfolds. Incisions can also

This chapter incorporates material written for the fourth edition by Terri Goodman.

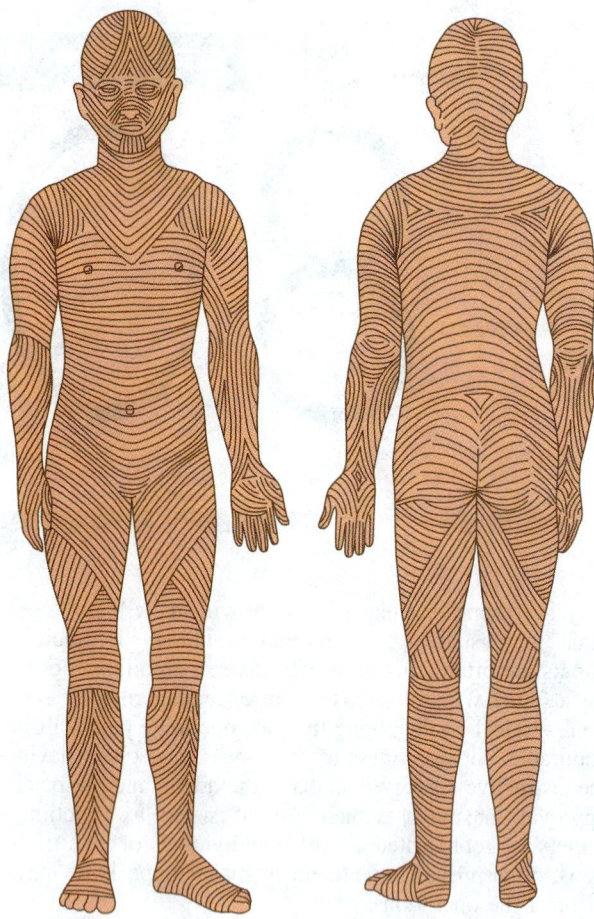

Figure 80–1. Langer's lines, which are important to consider in surgical incisions. To minimize scar formation, the surgeon makes incisions parallel to these lines rather than at right angles to them. Langer's lines are natural cleavage lines formed by the skin's fibrous tissue. Notice the lines in the palms of your hands.

be hidden in the scalp or by the eyebrow or concealed by clothing. A long incision parallel to these lines is less visible than a shorter incision placed at right angles. No amount of care in suturing can ensure an aesthetic scar if the incision is positioned at right angles or obliquely to the lines of minimal tension. Skinfolds and wrinkles become more pronounced with age, further obscuring incision lines.

Elliptical Incisions

When excising a lesion, the surgeon designs the incision lines to be longer than the lesion (Fig. 80–2). The resulting defect is elliptical, and the skin edges can be approximated easily. When the defect is round, tissues bunch at the ends of the incision, resulting in "dog ears."[21]

Suturing Techniques

To heal with minimal scarring, the edges of the skin incision must be approximated precisely, without undue tension. The suture lifts up the skin edges while it approximates them. Each suture puncture represents a miniature wound, and scar tissue forms at the site of each puncture. Suture lines must be kept clean, or stitch abscesses will develop and increase scarring. Sutures removed within 7 days leave no discernible suture marks or "tracks." Unfortunately, the skin on some areas of the body (e.g., the back) is thick and slower to heal and requires that sutures remain for a longer period of time. It is difficult to achieve fine scarring in these areas.

Other Variables

Blacks, people of Mediterranean origins, and other people with dark skin tend to develop more noticeable scars. Wounds located in such a way that the tissue moves as it heals (e.g., over joints) are also more prone to scarring. The skin of persons with malnutrition heals slowly, and the wounds may also develop more obvious scars.

Selecting Clients

The success of a plastic surgical procedure is determined by the degree to which it meets the client's expectations. A surgical procedure may produce excellent technical results, but the client will not consider it a success unless the results conform to expectations about a specific appearance or level of function. Therefore, it is essential that the surgeon and nurse understand what the client expects and that the client have a realistic view of what can and cannot be accomplished by surgery. The majority of plastic surgery procedures are not emergencies, and ample time is available to be certain the client is physically and psychologically prepared for surgery.

Because most procedures affect appearance, clients make a considerable emotional commitment when they elect to have plastic surgery. It is important to determine client characteristics that might indicate lack of satisfaction with a result. In addition to being in good physical health, the client must be psychologically healthy. Assessing the client's motivation is essential. Plastic surgery neither cures a person's underlying emotional problems nor alleviates major stress. An external change does not make a happy, well-adjusted person out of an individual

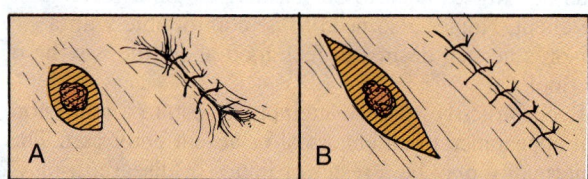

Figure 80–2. Elliptical excisions are used to reduce the scar. The *shaded area* shows the area of tissue removed with each lesion. *A,* If the ellipse is too short, puckers ("dog ears") form at the ends of the incision. This creates an unsightly scar. *B,* The correct length of elliptical incision for minimal scarring. (Redrawn from Grabb, W., & Smith, J. [1979]. *Plastic surgery* [3rd ed.]. Boston: Little, Brown.)

who is unhappy, poorly adjusted, or excessively stressed. Clients who expect plastic surgery to do so are poor candidates for plastic surgery. Nurses help to identify appropriate candidates for surgery. In most situations, the client feels that the physician is too busy and talks more openly to the nurse about the desires for the surgical outcome.

Understanding Motivations for Surgery

Many disorders can be corrected or improved with plastic surgery. Disorders range from life-threatening open fractures and gaping wounds to changes related to aging. The desire to be attractive or beautiful is a desire present in people of all cultures, but the perception of what is attractive varies. Adorning the body with paints or scars dates from ancient times to the present (e.g., lipstick, nail polish, tattoos). Some people decorate the body by wearing objects in their noses, ear lobes, or lips. Western society pressures people to continue to look young (perhaps by exercise) and to combat the normal physical changes of aging (perhaps by plastic surgery). For many years, people were limited to highlighting their positive features with make-up and clothing. Plastic surgery can correct their negative features.[41]

The importance of physical appearance varies among individuals; however it is an integral part of one's sense of self. The desire to want to physically resemble one's peers reasonably closely, e.g., to have acceptably "normal" facial features, is a normal desire. Clients' physical aspects are consistent with their idea of who they are as people. Trauma, disease states, congenital deformities, or multi-stage reconstruction procedures can result in alterations in appearance that have an impact on self-esteem and body image. Physical appearance carries significant meaning to overall quality of life for both males and females and should be considered throughout all phases of treatment.

A significant portion of any deformity rests in the client's perception of it. Perceptions develop in part from body image. Body image describes an individual's perception of his or her body—how the *person* thinks he or she looks, rather than an objective assessment of the person's characteristics. Body image is a factor in determining an individual's self-image, self-concept, and self-esteem. Individuals with a positive body image display more confidence and interact more easily with others. Body image changes continually, depending on individual expectations and feedback from others.

An individual with a physical deformity, real or perceived, can have a severely damaged body image. Even the usual processes of aging can be detrimental to body image. People's perception that they look like they're "getting old" can impair their level of confidence, affect their behavior, and interfere with their interactions in society. Body image is an important factor in the nursing assessment of the client having plastic surgery.

The client's ability to cope with a temporary or permanent, perceived or actual, disfigurement is also assessed. The nurse assesses the client's coping mechanisms. Some coping mechanisms may be effective; others may be ineffective. Men may have more difficulty expressing their feelings about their appearance than women. The nurse listens to the client, alert for positive and negative self-statements. The degree of anxiety and fear is noted. The nurse assesses the client's willingness or unwillingness to touch or look at involved body areas and the client's comfort in being near other people.

Techniques for working with clients who have alterations in body image are presented in Box 80–1.

Determining Realistic Expectations

A client who understands what is and is not a possible surgical outcome is said to have realistic expectations. Determining a client's expectations is a crucial first step before any surgery is performed. Most clients with conditions requiring plastic surgery have some degree of deformity. The deformity can be *actual,* that is, objectively observable by others (e.g., a missing breast or a deviated septum) or it can be *perceived,* that is, the client is aware of the deformity, but it may not be noticeable to others (e.g., fine facial wrinkling indicative of aging). It is important to clearly understand what the client sees and wants changed.

Clients with realistic expectations understand that facial rejuvenating surgery cannot stop the clock. A face lift cannot make a 65-year-old woman look like a 40-year-old. Realistic expectations are the realization that appearance will be improved, but aging continues.

Likewise, a face lift cannot get an unfaithful spouse to return home. As you might see, these expectations can be very private and may be hidden from the doctor and nurse during interviews. Clients with documented or suspected psychiatric illness may or may not be candidates for plastic surgery. A consultation with the psychiatrist or psychologist who is treating the client is necessary before any operation is undertaken.

The realistic client understands that plastic surgery does not occur as depicted in the movies: the bandages do not come off the next day, leaving the client perfectly healed and changed into a new person. Bruising can last for 2 weeks and swelling can persist for 6 months.

Realistic clients understand that they will have scars, but that the scars will be hidden in normal skin folds and will therefore be less noticeable. The nurse must help clients understand that any incision results in the formation of scar tissue. It is essential that the client have a realistic expectation of the location and extent of scarring that will result from the surgical procedure. The nurse must remind the patient that a scar matures over a long period of time. Some scars take as long as several years to achieve their final appearance.

Clients also need to understand that postoperative activities will need to be curtailed for a period. Clients who are very athletic and will not remain inactive during healing, or workaholics who will not take time off from work, present potential problems. Preoperative teaching includes helping the client develop realistic postoperative expectations. The client must understand how the surgery

Box 80–1. Supporting the Client Who Has a Changed Body Image

Many clients having plastic surgery experience some form of body image alteration. Clients may have body image changes before surgery due to disease or injury. They may also have problems after surgery from edema, bruising, or less than desired results. The nurse should anticipate these problems and work with the client as soon as possible to facilitate needed adjustments. You may want to work with the nursing diagnoses of *Risk for Body Image Disturbance* or *Self Esteem Disturbance related to perceived or actual disfigurement and changes in self-concept.* The expected outcome will need to be tailored to the client but may include improved self-image with incorporation of changed body part into body image as evidenced by effective coping and appropriate use of defense mechanisms, verbalizing feelings comfortably and appropriately, expressing satisfaction with changed body image, having the ability to openly verbalize feelings, making positive statements about self, having a normal level of anxiety and normal fears, comfortably looking at self in mirror and/or touching deformed body area, healed surgical site, or other scars, being able to be with others comfortably, and having no indications of depression.

Some interventions that you might find effective with clients who are experiencing body image disturbances include the following:

- Continue to assess apparent self-concept, coping methods, defense mechanisms, degree of anxiety, and fears frequently
- Assist client to explore and express feelings; do not use phrases such as "I know how you feel". These empty phrases build barriers to communication, whereas statements such as "you are angry" or "you seem depressed," for example, identify the feeling
- Be sensitive to client's feelings and needs
- Acknowledge client's feelings
- Present reality; building false hope is detrimental (reality need not be brutal, however)
- Healing is unpredictable; questions about healing should be referred to the surgeon
- Do not force the client to view or touch himself or herself; gently assist client to look at and touch deformity or healed surgical site (help incorporate it into client's self-concept and body image)
- Encourage client to begin meeting in public to begin desensitization to reactions of others, such as by taking walks in halls; desensitization begins in safe environments and proceeds to new situations, and the client is prepared for stares and remarks
- Discuss others' reaction to the client; support grief reactions
- If facial deformity is an issue, prepare visitors and family members before they see the client
- Look for vocal expression or hand gestures in cases of facial disfigurement; facial expression may be limited in clients with extensive facial scars or skin grafts
- Refer the client and family to local support groups, such as About Face
- Assist the client with techniques to camouflage scars; licensed aestheticians can assist with make-up choices and techniques

will affect usual routines. Thorough planning ensures minimum disruption in routines. Preoperative teaching must include information about restrictions on activity, the location and extent of scars, and the clinical manifestations of possible complications. Including family members in the teaching process promotes an effective support system for the client.

The ideal candidate has support from his or her family and significant others. Family members may react negatively, regarding the surgery as a waste of time, a waste of money, or an expression of vanity, placing the client at unnecessary risk during surgery. With short hospital stays, the family has taken over the caregiver role by providing postoperative care, which was in the past provided by nurses. The client may feel hesitant to rely on nonsupportive family members or may fear a negative postoperative result. The nurse has the unique opportunity to serve as the facilitator of positive interaction between the family and the client.[20]

Finally, the ideal candidate for surgery is healthy. Disorders such as hypertension and diabetes increase risk, but they do not prevent the client from having surgery. Alcohol and tobacco use should be stopped prior to surgery. Nutritional impairments are identified and corrected prior to surgery. Protein-carbohydrate malnutrition delays wound healing. Prior to a major operation, a complete blood cell count is taken, electrolyte levels are assessed, and a chest x-ray study and ECG (for clients older than 40 years) are performed. Other diagnostic assessments vary with specific procedures or with specific pre-existing medical problems.

Documentation Through Photography

Photographs are used extensively in plastic surgery. It is essential to document the client's condition prior to any surgical intervention. Once changes have been made in appearance, it is very difficult to remember the details of the original appearance. Photographic documentation provides an accurate record.

In office settings, nurses commonly photograph the client before and after surgery. By protecting the client's privacy and explaining the importance of photographic documentation, the nurse can make a photography session much less uncomfortable and embarrassing. The client must give written permission for photographs to be taken, especially if they are to be used for teaching purposes in addition to documentation for the medical record. Specific and standardized positions are used. Consistent positioning is critical to compare preoperative and postoperative views.[77]

Facial Rejuvenating Surgery

In childhood, skin is very elastic and is supported at maximum distention by adipose tissue (sometimes called "baby fat"). During aging, the skin loses elasticity and the subcutaneous fat diminishes and changes character. Skinfolds and wrinkles become increasingly noticeable. The tissue around the eyes and jowls sags, producing a drooping, tired, weary, or worried expression. The rate of skin change varies among individuals. Weight loss, sun exposure, genetic tendencies, and alcohol and tobacco use affect the speed and character of the changes.

Habitual exposure to the sun leads to several alterations in the skin. Many of the cutaneous changes once attributed to normal aging are in large measure due to chronic exposure to sunlight. Skin exposed to sunlight (natural sun and sun lamps) develops a chronic state of inflammation, which in its final stages leads to disintegration of the support matrix of elastin and collagen.

There is no ideal time to have surgery. Some people elect to have surgery very early to prolong a youthful appearance. Others wait until the effects of the aging process are pronounced. The client's physical and psychosocial health and support system determine the appropriateness of surgery. (See previous discussion about selection of a client for aesthetic surgery.)

Rhytidectomy

Rhytidectomy, also called *face lift*, removes the larger skin wrinkles and folds from the face and neck. The ideal candidate has large wrinkles or sagging facial skin. Fine circumoral wrinkles cannot be removed with face lift. Physical signs of aging occur throughout the body but are most obvious to others on the face. Rhytidectomy may restore a more youthful appearance to the face (maybe 5 to 10 years younger) by removing wrinkled skin from the forehead and along the eyes and mouth (Fig. 80–3). Rhytidectomy does not remove all of the wrinkles of the face. Clients may require acid peeling for fine wrinkles (see following discussion).[73, 76]

Prior to rhytidectomy, the person thoroughly shampoos the hair and washes the face. Men shave carefully. The nurse reconfirms that the client has maintained an NPO status (nothing by mouth) and has taken no medications containing aspirin.

Rhytidectomy is usually performed on an outpatient basis under general or local anesthesia with intravenous sedation. Incisions are made from the temple along the ear and out into the hair-bearing scalp behind the ear (Fig. 80–4). Through the incisions, excess facial skin is undermined and pulled back toward the ear. Undermining is a surgical technique in which the skin is separated from underlying structures. Most clients elect to have additional procedures done, such as tightening of the underlying fascia and/or facial suction lipectomy. Further adjuncts to face lift include brow lift, blepharoplasty, mentoplasty (chin revision), and, occasionally, rhinoplasty. On completion of the operation, facial compression dressings are applied.

Postoperatively, the client is placed in Fowler's position to reduce the risk of edema. Cold compresses can also be used to reduce swelling and bleeding. Suction drains are used to eliminate dead space and remove wound drainage. Drains are removed in 24 to 48 hours, when drainage has subsided. Facial movement (talking, and chewing) should be limited. Elevated blood pressure should be avoided by keeping the head elevated and resuming any prescribed antihypertensive medications. Coughing also increases blood pressure and should be avoided (by not operating on clients with colds) or treated if it occurs after surgery. Use antiemetics to reduce nausea and vomiting. Vomiting increases blood pressure and the risk of bleeding. Pain is minimal and can usually be managed with oral analgesics.

Complications of a face lift include hematoma, hair and skin loss, and nerve injury.[62] Hematomas are caused by small vessels that resume bleeding after the wound is closed. Large hematomas can cause tissue necrosis and must be surgically removed. Hematoma formation occurs

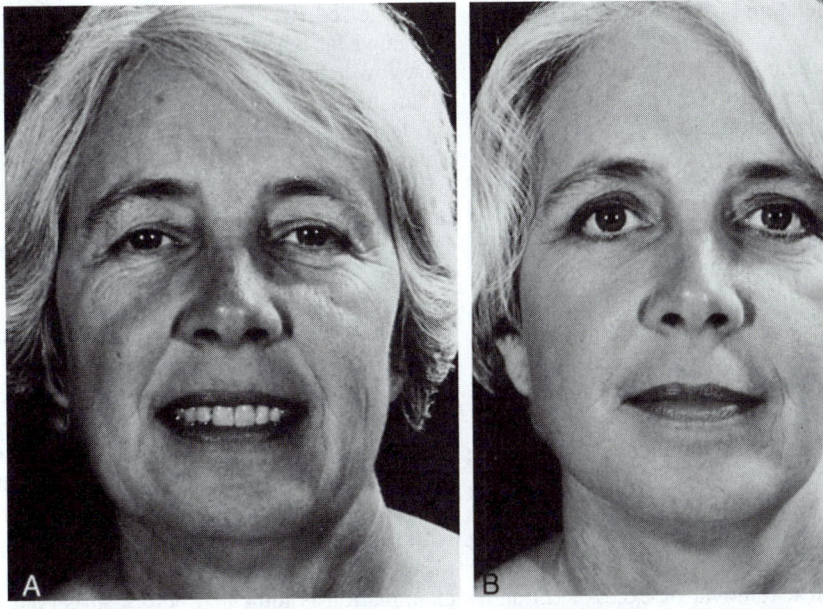

Figure 80–3. Before *(A)* and after *(B)* a face lift (rhytidectomy) and blepharoplasty.

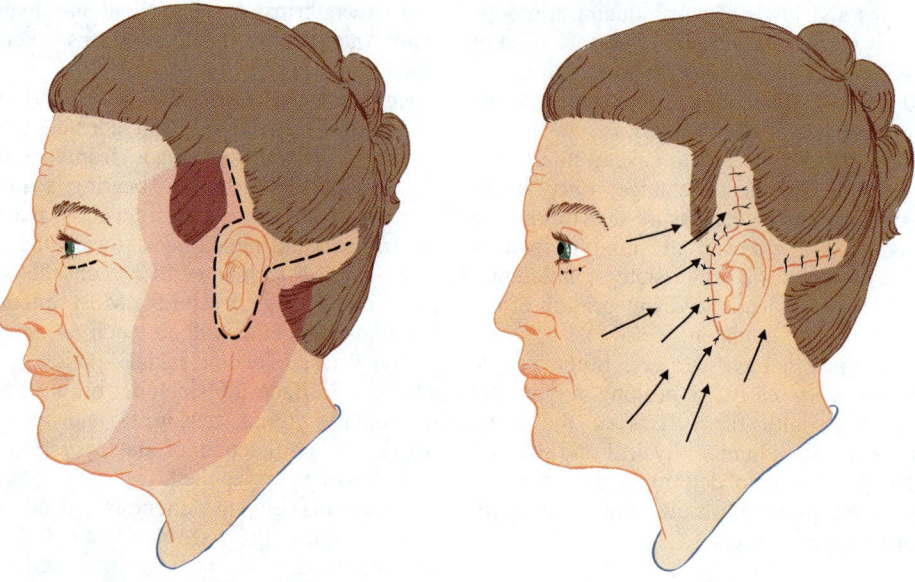

A Before face lift and blepharoplasty   **B** After face lift and blepharoplasty

Figure 80–4. Face lift (rhytidectomy) and blepharoplasty. Face lifts remove large wrinkles and folds of skin from the face and neck. *A,* The area in pink shows the amount of tissue that is undermined (lifted from the fascial connection) and moved during a face lift. The incision lines for the face lift go around the ear and into the hair-bearing scalp. Other incisions may also be used for face lifts. Note also the incision line beneath the eyelid for the blepharoplasty (to remove excess eyelid tissue). *B,* The postoperative near-final result, with tightened facial skin and neck folds.

most often in individuals who smoke or have pre-existing hypertension. Postoperative nausea and vomiting can also increase bleeding and hematoma formation. Hair loss is presumably due to altered circulation to hair follicles. The hair almost always grows back. Skin loss occasionally develops behind the ear, perhaps due to swelling or hematoma. Such a wound is allowed to heal by secondary intention and does not result in a very large scar. Nerve damage causing facial paralysis is a rare but devastating complication of facial surgery. Occasionally, facial paralysis results from nerve compression by a suture. When facial paralysis is observed, immediate surgical exploration to correct the problem and to prevent permanent damage is necessary.

The nurse assesses the client for complications, and the family and client are instructed to recognize the reportable changes in condition. Hematoma development is first noted as increasing facial asymmetry associated with pain or tightness on one side of the face. Increasing drainage and changes in facial sensation should also be reported.

Teach the client to keep the head of the bed elevated for 1 week to minimize edema and rest the face for 1 week to achieve fine scars (minimize talking and chewing by eating a soft diet). The surgeon usually removes dressings the morning after rhytidectomy. The face and hair may then be gently washed. Dandruff shampoo is avoided. The suture line should not be touched with creams or cosmetics until healing is complete.

Blepharoplasty

Blepharoplasty is the surgical removal of excess skin and periorbital fat from the upper or lower eyelid. The aging

process causes a loss of elasticity and relaxation of eyelid skin. Excess eyelid tissue in young and middle-aged people may be an inherited characteristic, an allergic reaction, or the result of cardiovascular or thyroid disease. Complete medical assessment is essential to rule out physical causes of excess eyelid skin. Most blepharoplasties are considered aesthetic operations, but if eyelid tissue obstructs vision, blepharoplasty is classified as being medically indicated.

Blepharoplasty is usually performed on an outpatient basis. General or local anesthesia with sedation can be used. Wide elliptical incisions are made on each eyelid. The excised wedge of excess tissue is lifted off and herniated fat is removed (Fig. 80–5).

A lower-lid blepharoplasty incision is placed an eighth of an inch below the edge of the eyelid. It begins near the tear duct and extends to the laugh lines on the eye's outer border. Extending the incision to the side of the eye prevents buckling of the tissues during healing. Sutures are removed on the third to fifth postoperative day. Rapid, uneventful recovery is typical. Blepharoplasty can be performed alone or with rhytidectomy (face lift). Complications from blepharoplasty are rare.

Because blepharoplasty clients are not hospitalized, preoperative nursing care is brief. The nurse confirms that the person has taken nothing by mouth since midnight. The presence of food or liquid in the stomach may necessitate postponing the operation. Preoperative near and distant vision is assessed in each eye by asking the person to read from a book and from something in the distance while one eye is covered. These baseline data are critical to assess postoperative visual changes. An ophthalmologic examination is indicated before surgery if vision problems are noted.

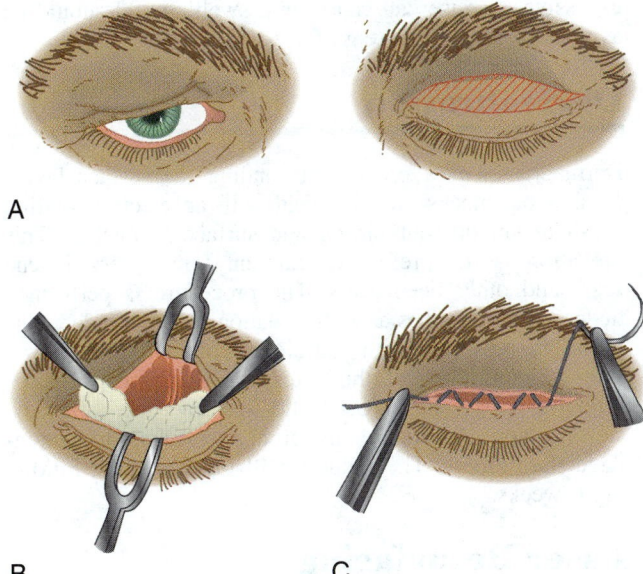

Figure 80–5. Blepharoplasty. An elliptical incision is made in the eyelid, and through it, excess tissue and fat are removed. *A*, The amount of tissue to be removed *(shaded area)* and the incision lines. *B*, The removal of herniated fat from beneath the skin and the muscles. *C*, Closure of the wound.

Following blepharoplasty, the head is elevated to reduce edema. Iced normal saline compresses are applied to the eyes as prescribed. Activity is limited for 1 week to reduce blood pressure elevations that often lead to increased edema and ecchymosis (bruising). Normally, severe pain is not experienced after blepharoplasty. An itching sensation, similar to having dry eyes, is usually experienced as a result of slight corneal swelling. This can be prevented with cold, wet dressings.

Postoperatively, the nurse teaches the client the following:

1. Immediately report to the surgeon changes in vision or eye pain not relieved by prescribed analgesia.
2. Apply cold compresses to the eyes as prescribed (typically for 24 to 48 hours after surgery). At home, clean washcloths soaked in ice water work well. The cloths should be damp and changed frequently. Freezing wet washcloths in plastic bags also works well.
3. Sleep on your back with your head elevated for the first 48 hours. Lying on one side causes facial edema on that side, which increases tension on the suture lines.
4. Use eyedrops during the day and eye ointment at night as directed to keep the corneas moist. In addition, use eye protection such as sunglasses. The blink reflex may be slower for a few days.
5. Avoid bending over from the waist for 48 hours.
6. Avoid vigorous activity for 1 month.
7. Bruising and swelling are common around the eyes for 7 to 10 days, so you may want to wear sunglasses. (The nurse will show the client how to apply and remove eyeglasses carefully to avoid bumping the incisions.)

Chemical Facial Peeling

Alpha-Hydroxy Peels

Alpha-hydroxy acids (AHAs) are a group of naturally occurring fruit acids that cause epidermolysis and detachment of keratinocytes of the superficial skin. AHAs can be used to remove acne scars, keratoses, warts, and superficial layers of skin. The best candidates for AHA peels are thin-skinned females with fair complexions and fine facial wrinkling. Trained nurses treat clients with AHA peels.

The skin is prepared for the peel with a 2-week skin-care regimen consisting of a facial wash and application of daytime treatment lotion and nighttime cream. The actual peel begins with the application of a prepeel solution. Skin that will not be peeled is protected. A thin layer of acid is applied to the face for a few minutes and then it is neutralized. Care after the peel includes application of skin moisturizers, gentle cleansing, use of sunscreen, and avoidance of abrasive agents.[59, 61]

Trichloracetic Acid Peels

Trichloracetic acid is generally used when a medium depth peel is required. TCA is indicated for clients with moderate actinic damage or for clients with pigment changes. TCA carries less risk than phenol peels (see following discussion) because systemic toxic effects are fewer, as are problems with hypopigmentation, and the ability to judge the depth of the peel while the chemical is still on the client's skin is enhanced.

The skin is prepared with a 2-week regimen of tretinoin (Retin-A) or glycolic acid in combination with a bleaching agent. If clients are taking estrogen, they should stop its use for 2 weeks prior to the peel. The actual peel begins with the application of a prepeel solution. The choice of skin preparation can affect the depth of the peel. Skin that will not be peeled is protected. TCA is applied to the face for a few minutes until the skin "frosts." It does not need to be neutralized. Care after the peel includes skin moisturizers, use of hydrocortisone to reduce edema and erythema, gentle cleansing, and use of sunscreen. The client often resumes the prepeel skin regimen after the peel. Hyperpigmentation is the most common complication.

Phenol Peels

The fine lines around the mouth and at the corners of the eyes can be treated with phenol peel. This process employs a caustic solution containing phenol that produces a controlled chemical burn of the top layers of skin. Chemical peel is best suited to fair-skinned people because individuals with darker skin tones may experience a change in skin color. Due to the advances with AHA peels, phenol peels are less common.

Before the procedure, the face is washed thoroughly and oil is removed with alcohol or a solvent. Intravenous sedation is usually required because the application of the solution causes a burning sensation until the anesthetic properties of the phenol take effect. Phenol is absorbed systemically, and during the procedure the client is monitored for dysrhythmias. The peeled area may be covered with several layers of waterproof adhesive tape to enhance penetration of the solution.

Considerable postoperative edema is common; this can be relieved by keeping the head elevated. If swelling interferes with vision, the client must have assistance to ensure safety. Talking should be limited and a liquid diet should be sipped through a straw for several days. Once the initial dressings are removed, antibiotic powder may be applied to form a crust, which must be kept dry for several days. With careful washing, the crusts will fall away as the tissue beneath heals. Peeled areas may remain hyperpigmented for some time. They should be protected with sunscreen for 1 year. Make-up cannot be worn until all areas have reepithelialized. When make-up is worn, it must be easily removable.[61]

Collagen Injection

Collagen is sometimes injected to fill in small wrinkles or depressed blemishes in the skin. The client's reaction to collagen is tested before treatment, because some people experience induration (hard, raised area) and swelling at the injection site. Clients with autoimmune disorders are not candidates for collagen injection.

Following collagen injections, the face should not be washed and face cream or make-up should not be applied for 3 to 4 hours. Normal skin care can then continue. Exposure to strong sunlight, alcohol consumption, and excessive exercise can cause mild swelling and should be avoided as prescribed (e.g., for a week).

Dermabrasion

Dermabrasion is a process of sanding the surface layers of skin on cheeks and forehead with an electric rotating brush to smooth out pitting and surface blemishes. This operation is the preferred treatment for depressed acne scars and other deep scars. The procedure is performed under local anesthesia with sedation. The abraded surfaces are covered with antibiotic ointment and gauze. Following removal of the gauze, the face weeps serous fluid for 5 to 7 days. Once the weeping stops and new skin has appeared, the client can apply makeup to camouflage the redness. The redness will fade over the following 6 weeks.

Laser Resurfacing

Laser treatment of skin wrinkles is becoming the preferred method of facial resurfacing. The wound produced is shallow because the energy is absorbed very superficially. An ultra-pulse laser is used.

Laser irradiations are quite painful. Some clients are able to tolerate the procedure with anesthesia provided with local sedation or through the use of topical anesthetics, such as eutectic mixture of local anesthetic (EMLA). The cream is applied for 1 to 2 hours and covered with an occlusive wrap (cellophane works well). Most clients need nerve blocks and local infiltration. The client should be told that the laser treatment will feel like multiple pin pricks or like a rubber band snapping against the skin.

At the conclusion, the client will have skin injury similar to a second-degree burn. Postoperative edema is significant, especially if the periorbital area has been treated. The edema can be reduced somewhat with ice packs and oral corticosteroids for 48 hours. Some clients also experience a burn sensation for 12 to 18 hours after treatment.

In 2 to 4 days, the residual tissue separates and sloughs off. Wound care after that time usually consists of hydrogel dressings. These dressings keep the wound bed moist and occluded, which promotes epithelialization and reduces pain. Hydrogel dressings are used for about 48 hours, after that time thin layers of antibacterial ointments or petrolatum are applied. Neither product is without problems—contact dermatitis can develop from antibacterials and acne-like lesions can develop from petrolatum.

The skin reepithelializes in about 5 to 10 days, depending on the depth of the injury. Varying degrees of erythema can remain, but clients can effectively cover the erythema with makeup that has a green foundation color. Milia can form and may require tretinoin (Retin-A), or they can be expressed. Sun-blocking agents are a must, as hyperpigmentation can develop.

Rhinoplasty

Rhinoplasty is the surgical correction of nasal deformities. Rhinoplasty is frequently performed as outpatient surgery with either local anesthesia and sedation or general anesthesia. Incisions are made inside the nose. Procedures are individualized and may include reshaping the bony dorsum of the nose, the tip of the nose, and/or the cartilage along the nares (nostrils). The nasal bones may be fractured to achieve the desired result. Following surgery, the inside of the nose may be packed and an external splint applied.

Preoperative nursing care focuses on teaching the client to breathe through the mouth after surgery and to not touch the nose. Postoperatively, assess for bleeding. While the client is sleepy from the anesthesia, excessive swallowing may be the only sign of bleeding. Examine the back of the throat with a flashlight to look for blood. Some bleeding is normal down the back of the throat and on the nasal packs and dressings. The nurse promptly reports excessive bleeding to the surgeon. The head of the bed is kept elevated to control postoperative edema. Nasal packing can be very uncomfortable. Pain management is important and can usually be achieved with oral analgesics (e.g., codeine or acetaminophen). Aspirin is avoided for 1 week before and 3 weeks after surgery.

In preparation for discharge, client education typically includes the following:

1. Sleep with the head of the bed elevated for 1 week.
2. Do not remove the external splints or nasal packing.
3. Do not blow the nose. Sneeze only through an open mouth.
4. Remain on a soft diet for 2 days.
5. After nasal packs are removed, avoid decongestant nasal sprays because they cause vasoconstriction and decrease the blood supply needed for healing.
6. After nasal packs and splints are removed, the nose will remain swollen and bruised for a while. Wait 12 months before judging the final results of the surgery.[70]

Body-Contouring Surgery (Lipectomy)

Generally, obesity is best treated by diet and exercise before any body contouring surgery is performed. An exception is some people who may become highly motivated to follow a weight-reducing diet after such surgery. Another exception is the presence of diet-resistant areas of fat. Fat distribution is based on sex, heredity, and corticosteroid use. It is generally accepted that rapid growth of fat cells occurs during childhood. It is also accepted that few new fat cells are made during adult life. If many fat cells were deposited during childhood, diet and exercise are not always effective for weight loss. Fat cells deposited during childhood are very resistant to decreasing and cannot be lost during dieting. Therefore, surgical removal is an option. As with all other surgery, careful preoperative assessment is necessary to try to identify realistic expectations. Body-contouring surgical procedures (lipectomy) remove excess fatty tissue, skin folds, or subcutaneous fat from various body parts, including the abdomen, thighs, arms, and buttocks.

Suction-Assisted Lipectomy

Suction-assisted lipectomy, or liposuction, is a technique used (1) to aspirate fatty tissue from areas of the body resistant to diet and exercise (lipodystrophy), (2) to contour flaps, and (3) to remove lipomas (benign fatty tumors). It is also used adjunctively with other plastic surgery procedures to create better contour and to enhance the aesthetic result. A blunt, hollow cannula is inserted through a very small incision (Fig. 80–6). The cannula, attached to a powerful suction machine, is passed back and forth through the subcutaneous tissue, sucking adipose tissue and creating a series of tunnels. The blunt tip pushes aside nerves and blood vessels. Precise surgical technique avoids ridges and dimpling on the surface as fatty tissue is suctioned away. Tumescent technique is the additional use of large volumes of dilute lidocaine and epinephrine. These medications promote vasoconstriction to minimize bleeding and provide postoperative analgesia. Compression dressings or elastic compression garments may be used to help collapse the tunnels and prevent fluid collection (hematoma and seroma), to maintain the desired body contour, and to promote healing. Complications of liposuction include hematoma, skin necrosis, infection, and undesirable scars or skin dimpling.

Following liposuction, clients rest for several hours. Because moderate to large quantities of tissue and fluid can be removed during liposuction, assess for hypovolemia and electrolyte imbalance (syncope, dizziness, and abnormal blood values). If drains are used, monitor the quantity and quality of drainage. Ice is effective in managing postoperative pain. Dressings usually remain in place for at least 24 hours. Nurses must ensure that dressings remain smooth and uniform or contour irregularities can result. Sometimes the client wears a compression garment for several weeks postoperatively to promote good healing.

Clients may gradually resume normal activity except for strenuous exercise. It may be 4 to 6 weeks before the client works up to the preoperative level of exercise. Resuming activity too rapidly may result in soreness and swelling. Bruising is common following liposuction and may take weeks to disappear completely.

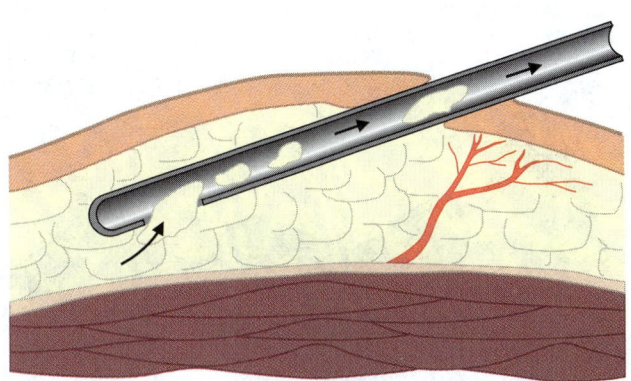

Figure 80–6. Suction-assisted lipectomy. To prevent extracting subdermal fat, the surgeon directs the opening of the suction cannula toward the muscle fascia.

Many clients expect the results of liposuction to be immediate. Usually up to 6 months is required for final results to be apparent after edema subsides and subcutaneous tissue heals. The nurse reinforces that results may not be apparent for 6 months following surgery. This period of time is required for complete resolution of edema and reconnection of soft tissues.

Abdominoplasty

Abdominoplasty is the removal of excess abdominal skin and fat and the repair and tightening of separated abdominal muscles. An incision is made across the lower abdomen, and tissue is undermined to the costal margin. The excess skin and fatty tissue are excised and recontoured. The umbilical stalk is detached and reattached once the overlying skin is in its proper position.

During abdominoplasty, the surgeon repairs diastasis (lateral separation of the rectus abdominis muscles, a benign condition occurring during pregnancy) and/or umbilical hernias. Indications for abdominoplasty include abdominal skin flaccidity (e.g., after multiple pregnancies and following major weight loss) and marked striae from pregnancy. An indwelling urinary catheter and surgical drains are inserted and compression stockings are applied in surgery.

Preoperative nursing care includes informing the client that drains and a urinary catheter will be in place after surgery, that a blood transfusion may be required, and that an intravenous infusion is continued until a diet is tolerated. After surgery, inspect the incision line for signs of pallor and/or lack of capillary refill. Taut skin can swell and impair capillary blood supply. Smoking is prohibited, because nicotine further restricts blood flow to the skin. Tension on the suture line needs to be minimized, to which end the client must lie in a contouring position (Fig. 80–7). The client also needs to walk in a "hunched-over" position until the swelling decreases and abdominal skin relaxes. The client is taught postoperative pain management techniques. Abdominoplasty is an abdominal operation and is uncomfortable. Adequate analgesia and other pain-relieving measures are essential.[17] Reinforce to unlicensed personnel that these clients require usual postoperative care (see Management and Delegation).

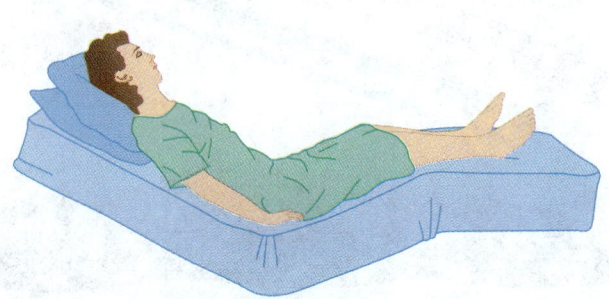

Figure 80–7. Position the client after abdominoplasty in a modified semi-Fowler's position, with the knees bent, to reduce strain on the incision line.

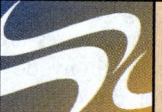

MANAGEMENT AND DELEGATION

Care of Clients Recovering from Plastic Surgery

When unlicensed assistive personnel are caring for clients after plastic surgery, reinforce the need for adequate pain management and routine postoperative care. It is not uncommon for people, including the client, to feel uncomfortable about asking for pain medications and for nursing assistance. Some people have the notion that surgery "for vanity" should hurt a little. This is a dangerous philosophy and should not be condoned. Any incision hurts, and these clients do not differ in their need for pain control. Likewise, routine vital signs, pulmonary care, monitoring intake and output, and encouraging ambulation are routine aspects of postoperative nursing care. Withholding care is not an acceptable manner of providing care.

Panniculectomy

Persons who have experienced major weight loss may develop excess loose skin and subcutaneous tissue over the abdomen, thighs, and arms. This tissue may hang in large folds, and laxity is greater in older people who have lost skin elasticity. Panniculectomy, the removal of excess drapes of tissue, usually requires more than one operation. The surgery is lengthy and there is risk of major blood loss. As much as 10 lb of redundant tissue has been surgically removed during one of these operations. Clearly this operation is not for the cure of the client's obesity, but it can offer some positive gains in self-esteem and reduction in health-related problems. Postoperative care is usually focused on reducing stress on the long suture lines. For example, place the client in Fowler's position after abdominal panniculectomy. Monitor the suture lines closely for signs of nonhealing. Fatty tissue is poorly perfused and the client may have pre-existing diet-induced malnutrition. During the healing phases, the client will need to consume adequate amounts of protein and carbohydrate to heal.

Reconstructive Plastic Surgery

One of the greatest challenges in plastic surgery is the reconstruction of deformities. The reconstructive "ladder," which is a guide to planning reconstruction (Fig. 80–8), asks the following questions:

- *What tissue is missing?* Is bone, muscle, subcutaneous tissue, or skin missing? If only skin is missing (e.g., burns), skin grafts are used for reconstruction. People with large pressure sores may be missing muscle, sub-

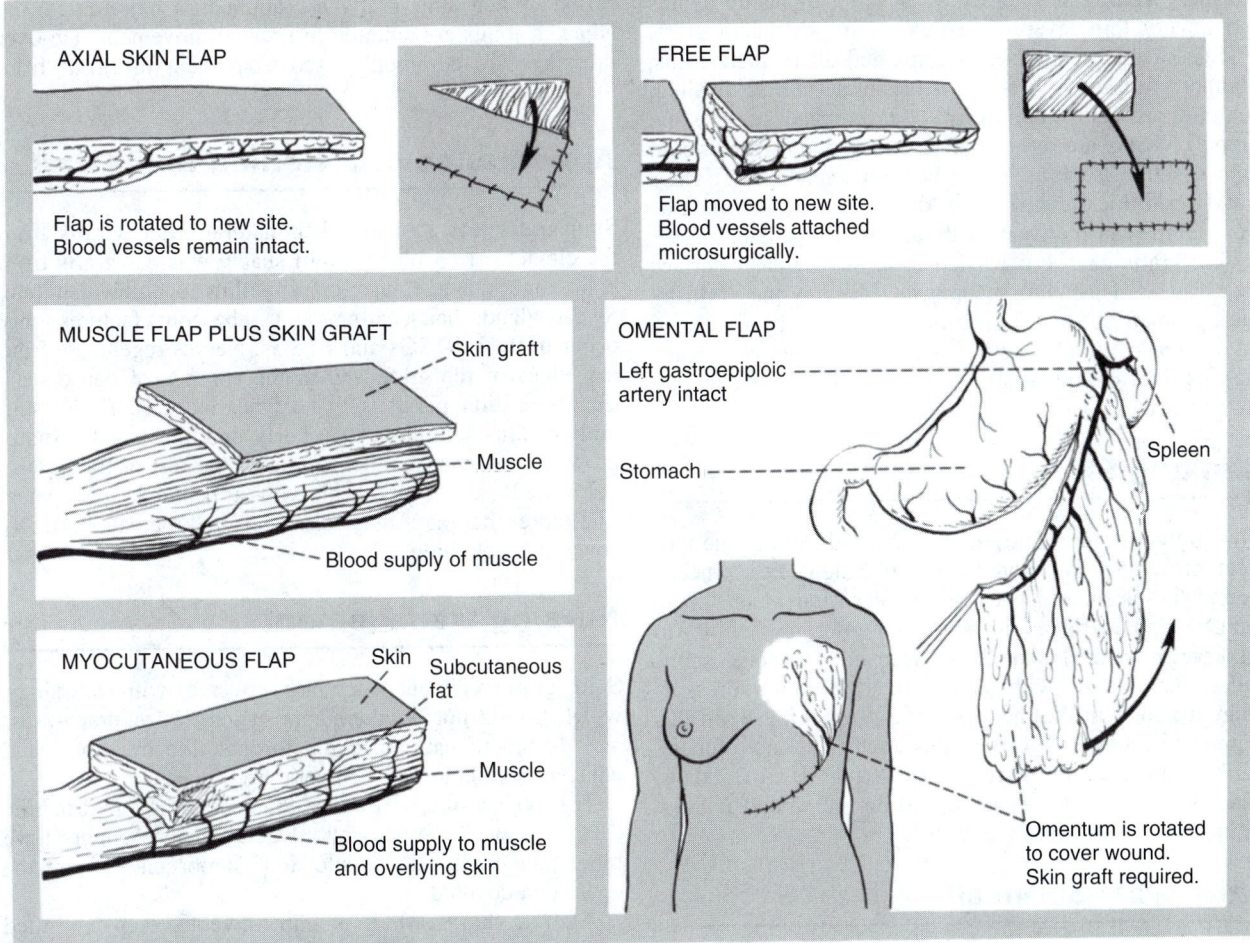

Figure 80–8. Common flaps.

cutaneous tissue, and skin, and a rotation flap containing all of these tissues may be used to repair the defect. Facial trauma may cause loss of bone as well as other tissues, and vascularized bone may be used in reconstruction.

- *Where is tissue available?* Some small defects have adequate tissue for repair nearby. This is ideal, because the tissue can be lifted from its base and rotated into the defect. Nearby tissue has the same color, thickness, and hair-bearing tendencies, contributing to a more natural appearance. If the tissue needed is not nearby, it may be moved from its location and attached to the defect by microscopic anastomosis (i.e., suturing small vessels and nerves with the aid of a microscope). Reconstruction with this technique is called *free flap reconstruction.*

- *What deficit might result from moving donor tissue?* Obviously, a person does not want a larger defect in the donor site than in the area being reconstructed! For example, a toe is often used to reconstruct a missing finger, but it is unlikely a person would give up a finger to rebuild a toe.

- *What is the simplest method to achieve the desired results?* The simplest method to close any wound is

simple suturing. More complex methods are used if adequate tissue is not available for primary closure or if a greater defect would result from simple suturing (e.g., a defect on the cheek might be closed by suturing, but it might pull the eyelid down into ectropion as it healed). Another method of closing a wound is to use a flap of nearby tissue and to rotate it onto the wound, maintaining the flap's own blood supply. Skin grafting is the third choice for reconstruction. The most complex form of wound closure is the free flap of skin, subcutaneous tissue, and, possibly, muscle or bone.

Reconstructive Modalities

Skin Grafts

A graft is tissue (e.g., skin, bone, nerve, or vessel) that is harvested without a blood supply from a donor site. It is transferred to a recipient site, where it develops a new blood supply. For the tissue to remain viable, or to *take,* a healthy vascular supply must be present at the recipient site.

Skin grafts are used extensively to resurface exposed surfaces. The grafts vary in thickness from very thin split-thickness skin grafts (STSGs), which contain epidermis and a very thin layer of dermis, to full-thickness grafts (FTSGs), which contain epidermis and all of the dermis. Thinner grafts are more likely to contract during healing, but they are also more likely to develop adequate blood supply. FTSGs are used in areas where contraction would limit function, such as on the hand or over joints. FTSGs leave a full-thickness defect in the donor site that must be closed, either primarily or with an STSG or a flap.

Skin grafts can be expanded to cover a greater surface area by use of meshing techniques. Meshing the graft, by cutting small slits in it, allows the skin to be expanded (like an accordian). Meshed skin grafts are used when there is little uninjured skin to use as a donor site (e.g., a major burn).

Banking Skin

Skin grafts can be removed or harvested during one surgical procedure and stored for application later, when a wound is clean or when an earlier graft has failed. Banked skin is folded in a dermis-to-dermis fashion, to preserve moisture, and it is wrapped in moist saline gauze. The gauze with skin is placed into a dressing impregnated with ointment (such as Vaseline gauze); this is put into a bottle, which creates an airtight environment. Banked skin can be stored at 4° C for 10 to 21 days. Later, the skin graft can be placed on the wound without the need for anesthesia.

Skin Graft Survival

A skin graft requires enough blood in its recipient site for survival. Capillary buds must revascularize the graft before the cells die. Blood supply that supports the growth of granulation tissue is usually adequate to support a skin graft. Good contact between the graft and the recipient bed is also critical. A thin fibrin network develops almost immediately after placement and serves as a temporary glue of sorts to hold the graft in place. Skin grafts require about 7 to 10 days to adhere and longer to mature.

Several factors reduce contact and thereby reduce skin graft survival. Collections of fluid between the graft and bed, improper tension on the graft, and movement of the graft on the bed are three common problems that lead to graft failure. Blood, serum, and purulent material may separate the graft from the bed. This collection prevents revascularization of the graft. A hematoma of only 0.5 mm delays the time for revascularization by 12 hours. A 5-mm thick hematoma delays revascularization by 120 hours. At body temperature, the skin graft cannot survive for the additional time, and necrosis begins.

Proper tension on the skin graft is critical once the skin graft has been sutured in place. If tension is insufficient, wrinkles develop that will never revascularize because they are not in contact with the recipient bed. Likewise, if the skin graft is too tight, it is stretched like a drumhead above the recesses of the wound, where the blood supply exists.

Movement between the graft and the bed will shear capillary buds from the bed, which prevents revasculari-

zation. When skin grafts are applied to extremities, the adjacent joints are splinted to prevent movement. Tie-over dressings are commonly used to prevent the graft from moving.

Appearance of a Healed Skin Graft

Skin grafts tend to carry their natural color. Grafts from the clavicle are a blush (pink) shade, whereas grafts from below the clavicle take on a yellow or brownish hue. Sweat gland, hair-bearing, and sebaceous features only occur in thick STSGs and FTSGs. Nerves regenerate from the edges of the graft, and in the absence of dense scarring, sensation parallels that of nearby skin. If the skin graft regains sensation, it is fairly durable. It will usually grow in a manner parallel to that of the rest of the body.

Meshed skin grafts heal with a pebbled appearance. Therefore they are only used on body areas normally covered by clothing.

Nursing Management

Skin graft recipient sites are covered with dressings, which should not be altered for at least 72 hours. Assess and document pain, bleeding through the dressings, and adjacent skin color and temperature.

The donor site is usually covered with a hydrophilic dressing, such as hydrocolloid gel. Because clients have more pain in the donor site, it is important to keep the open area covered.

After a skin graft, it is imperative to keep a grafted extremity elevated. If the graft is on the chest or back, be certain it is anchored well and that the client is positioned off of the grafted site. Avoid moving the grafted part. After the dressings are removed, continue to assess the skin graft for healing. The skin graft should become pink throughout (called a *take*). Blisters (small blebs of serum) can also shear the skin graft from the underlying wound. Document and report the presence of blisters to the surgeon. Blisters under a skin graft sometimes need to be drained. When prescribed, this is accomplished by inserting a small (25-gauge), sterile needle into the blister and letting the fluid run out onto a sterile dressing or a cotton tipped applicator. Rolling fluid to the edges of the skin graft is not advised, because it shears the graft from the capillaries in the bed en route. A standing order (prn) may be given for this intervention. Large accumulations may require surgical removal.

Flaps

Flaps are areas of tissue raised from one area of the body without being completely detached, so that the blood supply is intact; the flap is transferred (e.g., by rotation) to adjacent areas. Flaps of tissue can also be transferred to distant areas, where a blood supply is reestablished; these are called *free flaps* and are discussed in a later section. Local flaps are rotated or advanced to reconstruct an adjacent defect (see Fig. 80–8). An important consideration for flaps is the preservation of the nutrient blood vessels. These vessels are sometimes called the *pedicle*, because in the past, flaps were moved from site to site with a visible portion of tissue that "carried" the flap to the recipient site. This style of flap is now uncommon, but the term *pedicle* is still used. Flaps are commonly used to reconstruct defects following ablation for cancers or tissue loss from trauma. Flaps are also being used to heal extensive wounds from pressure ulcers and long-standing defects from osteomyelitis.

The skin of the flap, after transfer, maintains its original color and texture. This is why skin from the head and neck is used to reconstruct facial defects. If, for example, abdominal skin were used for facial reconstruction, it would be bulky and would increase in size if the patient gained weight, because the graft would respond just as if it were still in the abdomen.

Hair growth and sebaceous secretion remain the same as they were in the donor area. Sensation and sweating are lost immediately after transfer and usually return sometime between 6 weeks and 3 years later. These functions reappear as superficial nerves regrow into the tissues; therefore the sensation and sweating capacity match those of recipient site tissues.

Musculocutaneous Flaps

Flaps comprising both muscle and skin are called *musculocutaneous flaps*. They are commonly used to fill in defects where muscle is missing or where muscle may provide ample blood flow to heal osteomyelitis. These flaps are named by the muscle of origin. For example, large trochanteric pressure ulcers can be repaired with tensor fascia lata flaps, named for the tensor fascia lata muscle of the lateral thigh. Intrathoracic muscle flaps used for chest wall reconstruction include: serratus anterior, latissimus dorsi, and pectoralis muscles.

Tissue defects of the leg can also be treated with muscle flaps and skin grafting or musculocutaneous flaps. Currently, attempts are made to salvage all extremities unless nerve or vascular damage is irreparable, in which case amputation is preferred. It is common to treat less severe lower leg fractures with local rotation muscle flaps if possible. The use of these flaps has been overshadowed in recent years by the excitement over microvascular techniques, but definite indications exist for use of these local muscle flaps.

Care of the patient after a flap reconstruction centers on maintaining perfusion and reducing tissue injury to the flap. You may choose to design your nursing care under the nursing diagnosis of *Risk for Altered Peripheral Tissue Perfusion related to tissue transfer.*

For clients with this diagnosis, the expected outcome is that the client will maintain adequate peripheral tissue perfusion, as evidenced by usual color of skin, no pallor or cyanosis, warm and dry skin, blanching in 3 to 5 seconds, no edema or blebs, intact incisions, and controllable pain.

The flap is monitored for color, capillary refill, and dermal bleeding. Look for pallor, coolness, decreased capillary refill, or dark dermal blood on lancing (see Critical Monitoring feature) (lancing may not be allowed in

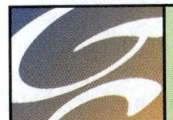

CRITICAL MONITORING

Musculocutaneous Reconstruction

Report the following findings immediately:

Development of coolness in the flap
Development of duskiness or pallor in the flap
Slowing of capillary refill in the flap
Loss of pulses (palpable or detected by Doppler) in the flap
Increasing pain in the flap

some settings). It takes a person with a fair amount of experience in clinical assessment of flaps to predict early flap demise using these subjective methods. Findings can vary because of oxygen content of the blood, capillary dilation, blood flow, and skin pigmentation. Therefore, in complex flaps, temperature and Doppler monitors and are used to monitor circulation. The extremity is usually elevated to improve venous return as long as elevation does not interfere with arterial flow.

Protecting the blood supply to a flap is a primary nursing responsibility. Nursing interventions are designed to avoid factors that can jeopardize blood flow. Position the client so that the flap is relaxed and elevated. Gravity promotes edema and venous congestion, both of which impede blood flow. Interventions to increase venous return include elevating the involved body part and applying elastic stockings or wraps as prescribed. Tension on the flap can stretch or kink the feeding blood vessels, reducing the flow of blood to the tissues. A blood clot can restrict blood flow. The first sign of compromised blood flow is pallor.

It is imperative to know the location of the pedicle that carries blood vessels to the flap. Most of the time the pedicle is buried, and little can be done to harm it. Some exceptions exist, though. When skin flaps are used, such as the deltopectoral flap, the pedicle is visible. Tracheostomy ties should not be tied tightly around the flap or circulation will be compromised to the distal portions. When the breast is reconstructed after mastectomy with a latissimus dorsi flap, the pedicle is located in the ipsilateral axilla. The client cannot lie on the ipsilateral side. Hydrate the client well, if prescribed, to help perfuse the flap. Maintain any postoperative splints to prevent tension on vessels. Limit the use of caffeine by the client and prohibit the use of nicotine by the client and by visitors.

Problems due to impaired arterial supply are apparent early after surgery. Altered perfusion due to venous obstruction may not be evident for a few hours.

Free Flaps

Free flaps are harvested from one area of the body to reconstruct a defect in a distant area. The donor tissue (skin, muscle, bone, or a combination of these) is detached from its blood supply at the donor site and reattached by microvascular anastomosis to arteries and veins at the recipient site. The development of microvascular techniques has made it possible to reconstruct defects that were previously untreatable.

The following list, while not exhaustive, includes the most common donor sites:

- Temporalis fascia, a thin conforming flap, is used to cover the dorsum of the foot or hand
- Radial forearm, a flap of skin and fascia, can be used for reconstruction of intraoral and extraoral defects; it can be combined with portions of the radius if bony reconstruction is needed
- Lateral forearm, a flap of skin and fascia, is used to cover body areas that demand thicker skin, such as weight-bearing surfaces
- Omentum, the fatty drape over the anterior abdomen, can be transplanted into spaces that require pliability, such as the frontal sinuses or chest wounds
- Latissimus dorsi, a large flap muscle with a skin segment, has a long pedicle and is useful for large bulky defects; it is called the "workhorse" for flap reconstruction and is common for facial, chest, and breast reconstruction
- Rectus abdominis, midline abdominal muscle and skin, has a long pedicle and is used for defects that require bulk
- Gracilis, a skin and muscle flap with a short pedicle, is used to reconstruct defects of the distal tibia, ankle, and heel, and for facial reanimation
- Serratus anterior, an easily sculpted flap, is used for provision of bulk and protection of lower extremity defects[2, 6]

Advantages to free flap reconstruction are numerous: it is a single operation, problems with immobility are lessened, new vascularization is provided to the area to aid in healing, mobilization of tissues is maximized, risk of flap loss is usually minimal, and the donor site is closed primarily. Disadvantages include a long operation (6 to 24 hours), two separate incisions, necessity for immediate reexploration of any vascular compromise, variable donor site morbidity, and need for sophisticated monitoring devices.

Prior to surgical reconstruction a flap can be prefabricated to build exactly what is needed for repair. Supplemental techniques, such as tissue expansion, may be used to augment the skin that is available for closure. Other advances have been made in the areas of bony and soft tissue reconstruction. Bone has traditionally been replaced with bone grafts or alloplastic materials. Recently, osteoinductive proteins capable of differentiating into bone were discovered.[8] These proteins have been combined with muscle flaps, and the tissue was transformed into useful bone. The future is bright for bone and joint reconstruction using these techniques.

Preoperative client characteristics to consider include health status and condition of potential donor tissue. Diabetes, cardiovascular, renal, and pulmonary disease do not present absolute contraindications, but these diseases do increase risk. The vessels used for a flap must not be in proximity to sites of previous trauma or radiation. Following trauma, widespread changes occur in the walls and perivascular tissues of the major vascular bundles. These changes have been labeled as post-traumatic vessel disease (PTVD). Vessels with PTVD are more difficult to dissect, are easily damaged, and have little resistance against clots. Donor sites are chosen using guidelines presented previously. The donor site pedicle is deliberately planned, so that the flap can comfortably reach the recipient site.

■ Free Flap Failure

When all goes well, one cannot argue with the obvious advantages of free flaps. The phantom called *free flap failure* looms large and leads to limited use of the procedure. Why do these flaps fail? A research study surveyed reconstructive surgeons who performed free flap grafts about flap failure. Thrombosis is the most common cause of failure. The rate of microvascular thrombosis is 3.7%; almost two-thirds of flaps with thrombosis were salvaged by timely revisions. It is suggested that the magnitude of the trauma is the most important factor related to the incidence of thrombosis. This conclusion is supported by the fact that none of 227 cases of head and neck or breast reconstruction using free flaps failed.[37]

■ Nursing Assessment

Following surgery, the free flap site is seldom dressed, so that clinical assessments can be performed. Several techniques have been developed in large clinical trials, but no consensus exists as to which is the best technique. The ideal monitoring system would provide a continuous recording of flap perfusion or flap metabolism. It should monitor both visible and buried tissues. Finally, the data should be easily interpreted by nursing personnel and junior medical staff.

Doppler Ultrasound. Surface Doppler ultrasound has become almost the standard method of assessment of arterial patency.[18] Doppler surface monitoring is used for free skin and muscle flaps, and reimplanted digits. Use of Doppler surface monitoring has some limitations, though. The axial artery must be located superficially, and sometimes venous obstruction still produces an arterial "hum." If venous obstruction is suspected, compression of the flap will produce a louder "hum." Implanted Doppler probes are also available and are in use in some centers.

Transcutaneous Oxygen. Determination of tissue oxygen tension would be the simplest technique for monitoring perfusion. Absolute PO_2 greater than 20 mm Hg seems to suggest adequate perfusion. Sudden falls of PO_2 below 20 mm Hg that do not respond to the administration of oxygen suggest arterial occlusion. As in other forms of monitoring, trends in data, rather than absolute values, should be monitored. Implantable probes have been developed for oxygen monitoring also.

Tissue pH. Measurement of tissue pH has been shown to be a more reliable index of perfusion than tissue oxygen. Arterial occlusion produces a rapid fall in tissue pH (0.66 pH units per hour in laboratory animals, compared with a fall of only 0.27 pH units per hour with venous occlusion).

Pulse Oximetry. Pulse oximetry is a good monitor for viability of digital free flaps or reimplanted digits. Digits will remain viable if the oxygen saturation remains above 95%. Loss of pulsatile flow is indicative of arterial occlusion; a decrease in saturation to 85% indicates venous obstruction.

Muscle Contractility. Ischemic muscles lose their contractility, and free muscle transfers can therefore be monitored by the continuing ability of the muscle to contract in response to electrical stimulation. Nerve stimulators are used to irritate the nerve every 15 minutes, and the response is recorded. A decrease in amplitude of the evoked potential is indicative of ischemia.

Photoplethysmography. Photoplethysmography is commonly used to monitor several types of free flaps, because it is noninvasive and reliable. Infrared light from a light-emitting diode will penetrate about 3 mm below the surface of the skin. Some of the light is reflected back to a photoelectric cell. Pulsatile changes in flow alter the proportion of light reflected back. Waveforms are monitored for changes. The waveforms can also be transmitted by telephone to remote stations for interpretation.

Clinical Assessment. Postoperative monitoring of free flaps used to be based solely on clinical assessment, which relied heavily on the experience of the nurse. In the past several years, the monitors just described have been used. It is interesting to note that some surgeons have abandoned external monitoring devices and are once more relying solely on the nurse's judgment. Most centers use a flow sheet to document color, texture, and temperature of the flap, Doppler pulses, and drainage from wound drains. Other postoperative care includes maintaining adequate hydration, keeping the client warm, managing pain and allowing only the appropriate activities. Clients may express some concern with the decision to salvage a body part and/or fear that the flap will fail and amputation will be required. The nurse needs to be supportive of the decision for surgery and allow time for expression of fears.

■ Long-Term Results

The ability to obtain soft-tissue coverage and limb salvage of a massively traumatized lower limb approaches 95%. Yet the true results are seen if the client can use the limb. A study was completed to examine the functional outcomes of 70 leg salvage procedures. The functional demands on the lower limb are great and include strength, stability, motion, and balance. Functional analysis of tibial shaft injuries revealed marked limitations in limb shortening, decreased ambulation, and mobility. Most clients require some sort of ambulatory-assist devices. Clients requiring free flaps or foot resurfacing did not have limb shortening, and all of them could wear shoes.

Implants

Implant material can be used to augment or replace tissue in all parts of the body. Facial structures (including the nose, chin, ears, orbital floor, and malar complex), breasts, bones and joints, and genitalia are often augmented or reconstructed with implant material. Polymers, such as medical-grade silicone, are used most frequently in plastic surgical procedures. Silicone prostheses can be very soft (breast prostheses), flexible (finger and toe joints), or rigid (bones and joints). Stainless steel, cobalt-chromium alloy (Vitallium), and titanium plates, screws, and wire are used to approximate, replace, and stabilize bone fragments (Fig. 80–9). Injectable collagen can be used to fill out skin depressions and fine wrinkles. Material for implants must be biocompatible and not rejected by body tissues. It must not cause severe foreign body reaction or infection. Implants must be noncarcinogenic, nontoxic, nonallergenic, and sterile.

Postoperatively, assessment and intervention focus on preventing displacement of the implant, ensuring adequate blood flow to the operative site, and preventing infection. Infection is a serious complication that could necessitate removal of the implant. Changes in temperature and local changes (e.g., drainage, increasing edema, hyperemia, and increasing skin temperature) may indicate a developing

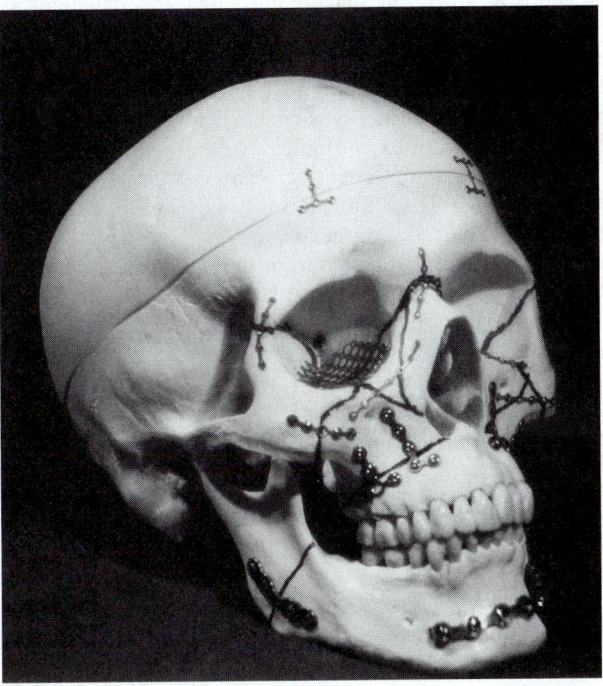

Figure 80–9. Titanium plates and screws used to treat facial fractures.

infection or implant rejection. Excellent wound care is imperative. The nurse must teach the client to recognize the clinical manifestations of infection so that treatment can be initiated quickly. Implants themselves are not painful, but the surgical procedure causes mild to moderate pain. Pain that is unrelieved with analgesics must be investigated.

Skin Expansion

Skin expansion is a technique used to increase the amount of local tissue available to reconstruct a defect. An inflatable silicone balloon is placed under the skin or muscle flap adjacent to a defect. The expander is inflated sequentially over several weeks or months to stretch the overlying tissue. When tissue is sufficient to resurface the adjacent defect, the balloon is removed and the flap is contoured (shaped) and advanced to cover the defect.

The process of skin expansion involves an extended period of time, commitment, and significant, although temporary, disfigurement. It is essential that the client be motivated, well prepared for the experience, and compliant. The client must be able to make additional trips to the physician's office where the expander will be inflated under sterile conditions. Each expander has an injection site into which a sterile needle is inserted percutaneously. Saline is injected slowly until the tissue is very tight over the expander. Sometimes a small amount of saline needs to be withdrawn to reduce discomfort. The tightness may be uncomfortable for several hours, but it subsides as the tissue begins to expand.

The nurse teaches the client to keep the incision and the injection site clean and dry to prevent infection. It is important that the client understand that pressure on the expander compromises blood flow and can cause tissue breakdown. Infection may require that the expander be removed altogether. If dehiscence of the incision line occurs, exposing the expander, the treatment need not necessarily be aborted. Fluid can be removed from the expander to relieve the tension. When the incision has healed sufficiently, expansion can begin again.

In most cases, the client can camouflage the expander with clothing. The clothing must be loose so that no pressure is placed on the expander. The client should sleep in a position that protects the expander from pressure. When the expander is placed in an exposed area, such as the neck or scalp, the client must be able to cope with the temporary physical inconvenience and insult to body image.

Nurses are instrumental in assisting the client in disguising the deformity caused by the expander. For example, when one breast is being expanded prior to reconstruction, the other breast will not match in size or shape. The nurse assists the client in padding the other side of the bra to reduce obvious asymmetry.

Lasers

The laser (acronym for *l*ight *a*mplification by *s*timulated *e*mission of *r*adiation) is a coagulating, vaporizing, and cutting instrument. A precise beam of laser light is directed onto tissue. The light is converted into heat energy that is absorbed by the cells. The heat vaporizes the cells. The advantages of laser surgery include precision and accuracy of cell destruction, reduced bleeding and swelling, and, sometimes, less postoperative pain. Operating time may be longer, but tissue damage is less, and the postoperative infection rate is lower.[75]

Laser light can be of different colors and wavelengths. Each is absorbed differently, depending on cell pigment and water content. The CO_2 laser is primarily a cutting and vaporizing tool. Its energy is absorbed by the water in cells, and therefore it penetrates tissue only superficially. The CO_2 laser is used primarily to excise or vaporize lesions such as warts, keloids, and vascular lesions. Argon, copper vapor, and pulsed-dye laser energy are preferentially absorbed by hemoglobin and are used primarily for coagulation. These types of lasers are used to treat birthmarks (e.g., port-wine stain), superficial vascular lesions, and pigmented lesions.

Laser energy generates intense heat and clients experience a burning sensation or a pin-pricking sensation. The tissue reaction can be similar to that of a second-degree burn with blistering. Ointment applied to the affected area for 2 to 4 weeks keeps the tissue moist until healing is complete. It is also essential that the area treated with laser energy be protected from sun exposure for several weeks.

Laser treatment to remove large pigmented lesions may require many operations. A single application may address only a small portion of the lesion, and the results are appreciated slowly as the site heals. Clients must be prepared for the length of time required and the inconvenience of multiple procedures.[75]

Craniofacial Surgery

Craniofacial surgery includes several techniques used for reconstruction of facial or skull deformities.[14] One approach for reconstructing facial bones is through a coronal incision (on the top of the skull). The skin and muscles over the forehead and face are lifted off the bones. Once the face is free of its soft tissue drape, bones are rearranged to correct congenital or acquired deformities. Bone grafts from the ribs, iliac crest, or skull may provide bone for reconstruction. Adults likely to undergo craniofacial surgery are those with facial fractures and facial skeletal tumors. Serious risks accompany the coronal approach to craniofacial surgery (e.g., death from increased intracranial pressure, blindness, brain damage, and infection, such as meningitis and osteomyelitis of the skull). Orthognathic surgery for jaw realignment is also considered craniofacial surgery.

Postoperative care following craniofacial surgery includes elevating the head of the bed to reduce edema. The client's head can and should be turned while being supported behind the coronal incision line. Care must be taken that no pressure is placed on areas of bone grafts. The client can lie supine or on the nonoperative side but not directly on the operated side of the head or cheek, because pressure on the bone grafts may dislodge them.

Neck flexion is permitted. Frequent neurologic assessment is important for increasing intracranial pressure (see Chapter 30) and intraocular pressure. Diplopia (double vision), which is usually the result of edema, is temporary, and it may be helped with alternating eye patches. Relatively mild doses of analgesics or narcotics may control discomfort. However, the donor sites for rib or iliac bone grafts are often very painful. Analgesics that contain aspirin are avoided because they increase risk of bleeding.

After orthognathic surgery, the client should be given pureed foods and liquids. The teeth are wired together to hold the bones in alignment. Care is the same as for the client with mandibular wiring after traumatic facial fractures (see later discussion).

Breast Surgery

Breast Augmentation

Clients seeking breast augmentation are often young women who have had chronic feelings of inadequacy and self-consciousness because of small or undeveloped breasts. Some clients are mature women who have developed postpartum breast atrophy.

In 1991, the use of implants for breast augmentation was placed under strict U.S. Food and Drug Administration (FDA) regulation. Current prostheses used for breast augmentation are durable, seamless, silicone rubber envelopes filled with saline. The prosthesis is inserted beneath existing breast tissue or the pectoralis muscle (called subpectoral placement) through an inframammary (under the breast), transaxillary (through the axilla), or periareolar (around the nipple) incision (Fig. 80–10). The implant can also be placed via endoscopic techniques.

Silicone-filled implants are currently being investigated by the FDA and are considered investigational.[71] The long-term risks of silicone filled implants are being studied. Although no scientific evidence currently exists to support a link between connective tissue disorders and silicone breast implants, silicone gel breast implants are available only from plastic surgeons involved in randomized clinical trials and for women who need breast reconstruction.

Thorough breast assessment is essential before breast augmentation to rule out breast cancer. Mammography is generally not done in women younger than 35, unless they have a positive family history of cancer or a suspicious lump.

Early complications of breast augmentation include changes in breast or nipple sensation, hematoma (collection of clotted blood), infection, or leakage from the prosthesis. The most frequent complication is capsule formation (fibrous sacs of scar tissue enclose the implant) followed by contracture of the scar. These complications cause excessive breast firmness and distortion of the breast into a hard, round ball. Possible causes of capsular contracture include infection, seroma (a collection of serosanguineous fluid), or hematoma. The basic problem in all of these cases is that the body's defense mechanisms respond to the prosthesis as a foreign body, and scar tissue forms around the prosthesis to wall it off.

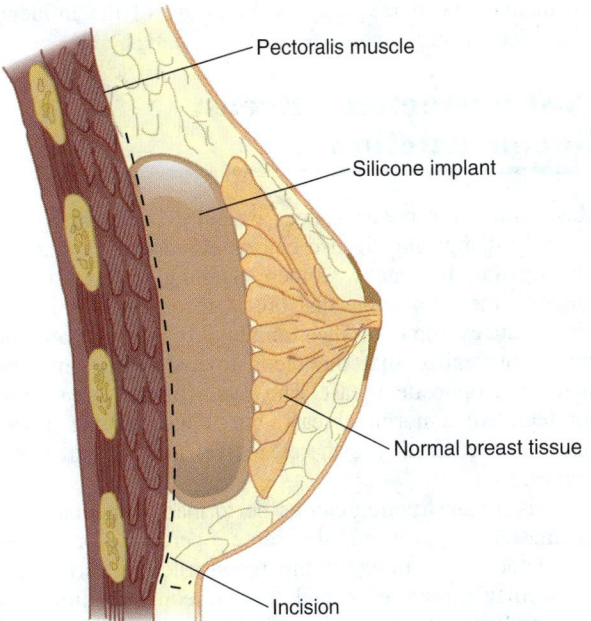

Figure 80–10. Augmentation mammaplasty is achieved by inserting a saline-filled implant beneath normal breast tissue (shown here) or beneath the pectoralis muscle. An inframammary approach is illustrated. Before beginning the retromammary dissection, the surgeon creates a subcutaneous flap. The incision is represented by a *dashed line*.

Capsules are usually treated with open (surgical) capsulotomy. Open capsulotomy, performed under general anesthesia, involves incising the capsule.

Breast massage maybe prescribed following breast augmentation with smooth-walled implants or after capsulotomy to reduce capsule formation. Breast massage typically begins postoperatively according to each surgeon's instructions. The nurse teaches the woman to push each breast up, to the side, and toward the middle of the chest, supporting the breast in each position for a count of ten. Women who have textured implants are usually not taught to do breast massage.

Discharge instructions usually include the following:

- To reduce edema, maintain a head-elevated position for a week when in bed.
- To reduce hematoma formation, get plenty of rest for a week (no excessive activity, take it easy)
- To avoid moving the pectoralis muscle and irritating the surgical site, do not raise the arms above the head for 3 weeks (e.g., while washing or brushing hair), do not play golf or tennis or swim for 6 weeks, sleep on the back and not on the stomach or sides, and be careful when closing car doors
- Because of their anticoagulant effect, do not use aspirin or aspirin-containing compounds
- Notify the physician if bleeding occurs or if a fever above 37.6° C (99.6° F) develops

The nurse caring for clients with breast implants must remain up-to-date by reading the scientific literature. Most women get their information on the implant issue from the media. The nurse needs to be aware of the influence of the media on women's fears and anxieties.[5, 29, 55]

Postmastectomy Breast Reconstruction

Mastectomy for breast cancer or other breast disease is not only disfiguring, it also causes emotional trauma (see Chapter 85). For many women planning to have a mastectomy, the knowledge that breast reconstruction is possible reduces some of their anxiety. It is important that the client realize that the reconstructed breast may not match the opposite breast. The reconstructed breast may not feel like a normal breast, but it has distinct advantages over external prostheses in feel and appearance in clothes.

Breast reconstruction can be performed immediately after mastectomy (during the same operation) or at any time later. The timing of the reconstruction varies with the woman's preference and the surgeon's opinion. The risks and complications are equal in immediate and delayed reconstruction. The psychosocial adjustment of the client must be addressed before surgery and throughout her surgical course. Concern also exists about the possibility that a woman might deny the seriousness of the cancer, which might reduce motivation for follow-up treatment with radiation therapy, if the breast is reconstructed immediately, although this has never been proven. The reconstructed breast does not reduce the effectiveness of radiation therapy, and may provide psychological strength for the woman to undergo radiation and chemotherapy.

Breast reconstruction is usually a collaborative effort among the general surgeon, the plastic surgeon, and the oncologist. A variety of reconstructive approaches, some of which follow, are available and depend on each client's needs and desires:

● Insertion of a tissue expander: A tissue expander is inserted under the chest muscles and expanded slowly over several weeks by adding fluid via percutaneous injection. After a few months, when the chest tissue has expanded, the expander is removed and an implant is inserted.

● Rotation of the latissimus dorsi muscle: This large, flat muscle is located in the back. The muscle and skin can be lifted up from the back, tunneled through the axilla, and formed into a breast mound on the chest. An implant may be inserted if needed. The incision is positioned so that it can be hidden under the brassiere. Functional loss of strength and shoulder abduction and loss of ability to pull may occur following latissimus dorsi breast reconstruction.

● Use of transrectus abdominal musculocutaneous (TRAM) flap: This form of breast reconstruction, which uses abdominal muscle and skin, does not usually require a prosthesis. The tissue can be rotated to the chest wall with the blood vessels intact, or the blood vessels can be reattached as a free flap through microsurgery. The donor site in the abdomen is closed as a modified abdominoplasty (Fig. 80–11). Although the contour of the abdomen is improved (flattened), the scar is usually visible. To undergo a TRAM flap, the woman must have sufficient redundant abdominal tissue. Previous abdominal surgery and smoking can be contraindications if the blood supply to the TRAM is impaired.

● Use of free flaps: Free flaps, including flaps from the gluteal area and TRAM, have also been used for reconstruction.

The breast reconstruction techniques just discussed rebuild the breast mound. Some women elect to also have the nipple-areola reconstructed. To achieve symmetry, nipple reconstruction should be delayed for several months following breast reconstruction. During the healing process, the contour of the reconstructed breast may change as the incisions heal and edema subsides. Nipples can be reconstructed with a variety of grafts, with a tattoo, or with a graft-tattoo combination (Fig. 80–12).

Figure 80–11. Breast reconstruction using transverse rectus abdominis myocutaneous flaps. *A*, Preoperative appearance. *B*, Postoperative appearance.

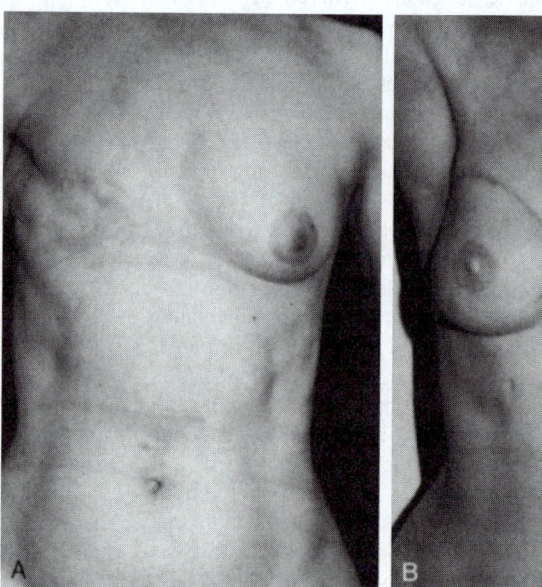

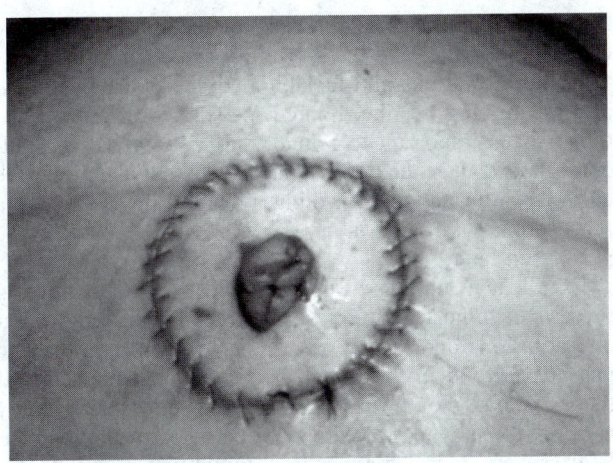

Figure 80–12. Nipple-areolar reconstruction. (From Hutcheson, H. A. [1989]. Nipple and areolar reconstruction. *Plastic Surgical Nursing,* 9[3], 105–110.)

Preoperative nursing care includes reinforcing the surgeon's discussion and teaching the client about the planned procedure and postoperative care. If surgery is being performed for known or suspected cancer, the nurse facilitates the expression of feelings (e.g., powerlessness, disbelief, anger, fear, or depression).

In addition to providing the postoperative nursing care required by any person having surgery (see Chapter 21), after reconstructive breast surgery the nurse assesses the flap or breast area, color, temperature, and capillary refill.

Pain management varies with type of surgery and the client's needs. Epidural analgesia has been used in breast reconstruction. When epidural analgesia is used, the nurse assesses the respiratory rate, degree of pain relief, and presence of numbness or paralysis in lower extremities every 2 hours. Caution must be used to protect the client from falling when ambulating. Narcotics can also be ad-

ministered via epidural routes, and they do not lead to numbness.

A woman with a recent subpectoral implant needs to know that initially the implant feels very firm and is higher on the chest than a normal breast. Over time, the muscle stretches, allowing the implant to drop and soften. Women with subpectoral implants do not wear bras, because the implant needs to move into the pocket created in the chest wall. Women having other types of surgery may or may not return from the operating room wearing a bra to support the breasts. A front-closing support bra, without wires, is preferred. Wearing a bra also helps some women feel more normal, encouraging a return to wellness.

Psychosocial readjustment to breast reconstruction, including incorporation of the reconstructed breast into the woman's body image, usually occurs 3 to 4 months after surgery. Following augmentation, most women incorporate a breast implant into their body image within weeks. They often report increased self-confidence, increased feelings of equality and self-worth, greater self-confidence, and improved sexual relationships.

Reduction Mammaplasty

Reduction mammaplasty surgically reduces the size of large, pendulous breasts. Women usually seek such surgery to reduce the physical and psychosocial discomforts of large breasts, for example, back pain, bra strap indentations in the shoulders, inability to wear normal clothing styles, intertriginous dermatitis (skin breakdown under large breasts), and being the subject of insensitive jokes or uncomfortable comments about breast size. These procedures may also be performed for men with gynecomastia (breast enlargement).

Many breast reduction techniques exist. Excess breast tissue is removed through incisions under the breast (Fig. 80–13). The nipple is transposed on a pedicle of tissue

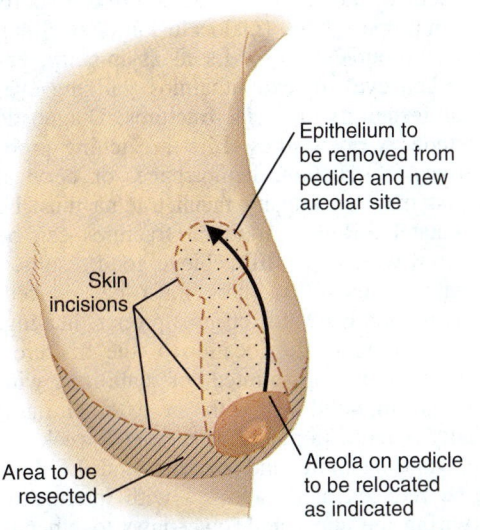

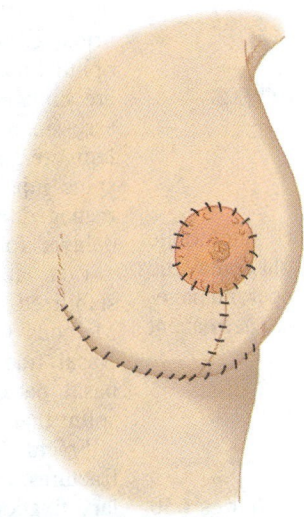

Figure 80–13. Reduction mammaplasty, in which breasts are surgically reduced. Excess breast tissue is removed, and the breast is recontoured. The nipple is relocated (e.g., moved higher) on a pedicle of tissue. The pedicle supplies the nipple with blood until new blood vessels form.

Epithelium to be removed from pedicle and new areolar site

Skin incisions

Area to be resected

Areola on pedicle to be relocated as indicated

PENDULOUS BREAST BEFORE SURGERY

SAME BREAST AFTER RECONTOURING

or grafted onto the newly formed breast. A possible complication is loss of blood supply to the nipple-areola complex. Altered sensation and the inability to perform breast-feeding are common adjustments after this procedure.

Assess the nipple-areolar complex after surgery, and report any duskiness or pallor. Manage pain with narcotics. Encourage ambulation and resume normal diet as soon as postoperative nausea subsides. The client will need to wear a bra after surgery, and she will require refitting due to the change in breast size. A front-opening bra is most comfortable to put on.[33]

Mastopexy

Mastopexy is the correction of mammary ptosis (drooping) to achieve an improved breast contour and position. Mastopexy may be performed with subcutaneous mastectomy or on normal breasts to improve contour and as part of a reduction mammaplasty. Postoperative care is similar to that for other types of breast surgery.

Subcutaneous Mastectomy

Some women develop premalignant lesions, have a high risk of breast cancer by family history, have had cancer in one breast, or have multiple suspicious breast nodules. These women may elect to undergo prophylactic mastectomy (a mastectomy done to prevent cancer) on one or both breasts. One alternative to simple prophylactic mastectomy is subcutaneous mastectomy, during which almost all of the breast tissue is removed, leaving only the nipple and areolar complex. An implant is inserted immediately, or tissue expanders may be used. This operation reduces the risk of later development of cancer in the operated breast. However, a few women develop tumors in the remaining bit of breast tissue within the nipple. Follow-up mammograms and breast self-examination are important to assist in the early detection of cancer. Postoperative care is similar to that for other types of breast surgery.

Repair of Traumatic Injuries

Facial Injuries

Injuries to the face are a common result of automobile accidents and physical violence. Although they may be serious, facial injuries are seldom fatal. Proper management helps to avoid sensory impairment and permanent disability and can minimize disfigurement.

Lacerations

Facial lacerations can range from very small injuries (.50 cm) that can be repaired under local anesthesia to extensive lacerations with soft tissue injury that require repair under general anesthesia. Prior to closure, wounds are cleansed of debris and devitalized tissue.

Facial lacerations and facial soft tissue injuries are usually distressing to the injured person and family. Although it is important to remain optimistic about the outcome and reduce anxiety, it is also essential to provide accurate information. Teaching includes the fact that a scar forms with any injury. Scar revision can also be performed later.

Excellent wound care, including cleansing and applying prescribed topical antibiotics, promotes the healing of facial abrasions and lacerations. A person who is NPO and has dried blood in the mouth needs frequent oral care. If the person's mouth has sutures, the mouth is simply rinsed with saline. Oral care *must* be performed, however. With severe facial trauma, soft toothbrushes suffice for oral care. Water Piks may further damage such injuries and their use is usually contraindicated. The nurse takes measures to prevent aspiration during oral care.

The nurse teaches the client and family to keep facial incision lines clean by applying a prescribed topical antibiotic. Skin incisions must not get wet (e.g., in the shower), because moisture allows bacteria to enter the wound along the sutures. Infected incisions tend to produce more scar tissue. (Wound care is also discussed in Chapter 20.)

Facial Fractures

Facial fractures can occur in the individual bones of the face: the nasal bones, orbit, malar prominence, mandible, or maxilla. Le Fort fractures are specific patterns of facial fractures (Fig. 80–14); they are classified as follows:

Le Fort I: Transverse fracture of the alveolar process separating the upper dental arch from the maxilla
Le Fort II: Fracture of the midface, maxilla, and orbits
Le Fort III: Fracture of the orbits that leads to craniofacial dissociation

The client with facial fractures has often been involved in an auto accident or an assault or has suffered a sports injury. Pain, improper bite (malocclusion), swelling, bruising, diplopia (double vision), facial asymmetry, enophthalmos (sunken eye), or exophthalmos (bulging eye) are clinical manifestations of facial fractures. Diagnostic assessment includes x-ray studies. Life-threatening problems (e.g., airway obstruction, hemorrhage, or cervical spine injury) that may accompany facial trauma must be managed immediately. Repair of facial fractures can be delayed for up to 3 weeks and still achieve good results.

Like all fractures, facial fractures must be reduced, stabilized, and immobilized to ensure proper healing. Methods vary according to the location of the fractures. Nasal fractures are reduced, splinted, or stabilized with nasal packing and immobilized with an external nasal splint that usually remains in place for at least 1 week.

Fractures of the mandible and maxilla and Le Fort fractures can be reduced and stabilized with intermaxillary fixation (wiring the upper and lower jaws together in occlusion) using arch bars. The jaws usually remain wired from 4 to 6 weeks. When small plates and screws are

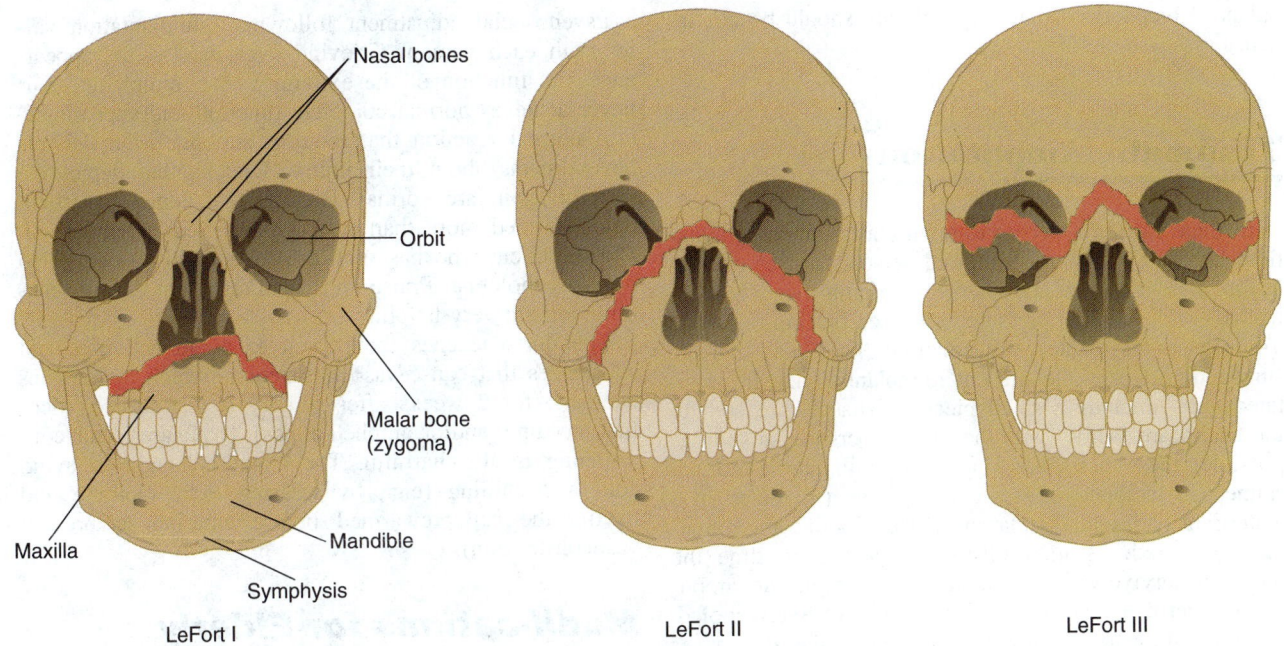

Figure 80–14. Le Fort fractures.

used to stabilize bone fragments, intermaxillary fixation may not be necessary.

Blowout fractures of the orbit can involve trapping of orbital structures between bone fragments, which may result in diplopia or enophthalmos. The integrity of the orbital floor is reestablished surgically and is stabilized with wire or small plates and screws. Implant material or bone graft might be used to complete the reconstruction. Malar (cheekbone) fractures may produce facial asymmetry. These fractures may also be stabilized with wire or small plates with screws. Malar implants may be necessary to reestablish facial symmetry.

The nurse assesses airway patency and breath sounds every 2 hours (more often if bleeding is present). Suction equipment is present at the bedside. The client is taught to breathe through the nose. Trying to open the mouth may dislocate the fracture. When the client has intermaxillary wiring, wire cutters should be in the client's possession at all times. If airway problems develop that cannot be managed with suction, the wires should be cut. The nurse and client need to be informed about which wires should be cut. Two wires are usually present on each side of the mouth, and they are the only wires that attach the top and bottom teeth. Do not try to cut off the bands attached to the teeth.

Facial edema and ecchymoses may be present. The head of the bed is elevated. Liquid tears may be needed if the client's ability to blink is decreased due to swelling, injury, or nerve damage.

The nurse assesses the client for diplopia and blurry vision. When these disorders are present, the nurse assists the client during ambulation to prevent injury.

The client remains on a liquefied diet until the wires are removed. Without adequate nutrition, clients can lose 10 to 20 lb during convalescence. The client is taught how to blenderize food and maintain adequate balances of carbohydrates, fat, protein, and calories. Milkshakes can be made with a wide variety of foods. High-calorie food supplements can augment the regular diet, and liquid multivitamins may be useful. Alcoholic and carbonated beverages can cause nausea and can fizz and foam in the back of the throat, leading to airway problems; they are to be avoided.

The nurse assesses the client for clear rhinorrhea or otorrhea. Rhinorrhea or otorrhea may indicate leaking cerebrospinal fluid (CSF), which must be reported to the physician. With CSF leakage, the potential exists for development of meningitis. To assess for rhinorrhea or otorrhea, the nurse observes the bed linens, because CSF dries in concentric, halo-like rings and does not crust.

Initially, the nurse and client must establish a means of communication. Although talking is possible through clenched teeth, hand signals or writing may be most effective initially. Trying to open the mouth may dislocate the fracture. Clients initially require reassurance that they will not choke or suffocate.

Oral hygiene aids in healing of oral wounds, prevents infection and destruction of teeth and gums, increases comfort, and enhances self-esteem. Rinsing the mouth with water or a mouthwash followed by a Water Pik on low pressure removes particles from the front of the mouth while the tissues are still tender. Once the initial swelling and tenderness subside, the teeth must be brushed and the mouth rinsed following every meal and at bedtime. Pieces of paraffin wax can be placed on the open ends of the wires if they irritate buccal surfaces.

Prior to discharge, the client and family need to be taught about the wires, diet, and oral care. Once the incisions have healed, the client can resume normal activities. However, while the jaws are wired, the client must carry a wire cutter and know which wires to cut. A well-balanced blenderized diet and oral care should be continued.

Traumatic Amputations

Immediate care of a person following a traumatic amputation, like that of any other injured person, focuses on lifesaving activities (see Chapter 89). Hemorrhage is controlled with direct pressure on the bleeding points. Tourniquets and cautery are not used. They may damage surrounding tissue and prevent reimplantation. All amputated parts, including small pieces of tissue, are sent to the healthcare facility with the injured person. As soon as possible, these parts are (1) rinsed with sterile normal saline, (2) wrapped in sterile wet gauze, (3) sealed in a watertight bag, and (4) placed on ice. Cooling the amputated part reduces metabolism, increasing the time the part can survive without blood. For example, an amputated finger can survive for 18 hours if effectively cooled. Although the part is rinsed with normal saline, it is never stored, left in normal saline or on dry ice, or frozen, which causes extensive cellular damage.

Reimplantation surgery is performed under regional block or general anesthesia. An operating microscope guides the surgical reattachment of arteries, veins, tendons, and nerves. With severe injuries, such an operation may take 12 to 18 hours. Following surgery, incisions are dressed, the extremity is immobilized with casts or splints, and the entire extremity is elevated.

Following reimplantation, a person requires careful, frequent nursing assessment (every 15 minutes) including documentation of the reimplanted part's color, temperature, and capillary refill. A reimplanted part may have blocked arterial or venous blood flow, which if it is not immediately corrected surgically will cause the part to die. Toes and fingertips are usually left uncovered for assessment. Doppler assessments help monitor pulses in the part. Temperature probes are often placed on the extremity. The surgeon usually states the ideal temperature range for reimplantations. A temperature decrease of 2° C or more in an hour or a decline to 32° C (89.6° F) demands immediate attention and is promptly reported to the surgeon. Aspirin is usually prescribed to reduce blood-clotting tendencies. A temperature at 34° to 36° C (93.2° to 96.5° F) is considered excellent for a reimplanted finger. Owing to lengthy anesthesia time (18 to 24 hours), nursing care also focuses on monitoring recovery from anesthesia.

An active rehabilitation program usually begins 2 weeks after injury and continues for months. Joint motion initially may be restricted by pins through joints and by bulky dressings. Because peripheral nerves take a long time to regenerate, protective sensation may be absent for months. The person must be careful to avoid injuring the part. Rehabilitation is accomplished through prescribed active and passive range-of-motion exercises several times each day. A final indication of the success of reimplantation is return of sensor-motor nerve function in the reimplanted part.

Psychosocial adjustment following reimplantation varies with each person. Grieving over the loss of appearance and function of the extremity (the reimplanted part never achieves normal complete function and appearance) is a normal reaction that requires support. Many clients have dreams about their injury. Dreams that depict the tragedy again are normal. Dreams that depict the client being harmed more than actually occurred are abnormal, and the client who has such dreams should be counseled by a psychologist. Praise and encouragement during rehabilitation are very helpful.

The nurse teaches the person to avoid activities and substances that cause vasoconstriction (which precipitates necrosis) for 2 weeks after surgery (e.g., tobacco, nicotine, cocaine, and/or amphetamines). Exposure to air conditioning is also harmful. The client is taught to avoid cold and chilling (e.g., by wearing extra clothing and having the car prewarmed before entering to prevent vasoconstriction).

Modifications for Elderly Clients

Many elderly clients have both aesthetic and reconstructive surgery. The nurse ascertains that the client understands the surgical plans, often by using education forms with large print. Many elderly clients routinely take anticoagulants and therefore tend to bleed more easily. Pressure dressings may be required for a longer period of time. Finally, some clients may resist not being independent with driving and self-care. Safety issues must be discussed. For example, the side effects of anesthetics and narcotics, as well as facial edema and sight-obscuring dressings, prohibit driving after facial surgery.[11, 35]

Conclusions

Effective nursing care makes a significant difference in postoperative outcomes for plastic surgery clients. Nursing care includes interventions to maintain both physiologic and psychological homeostasis. Successful plastic surgery procedures require a significant degree of client compliance with treatment protocols. With shortened hospital stays and an increased number of outpatient procedures, effective client teaching is imperative to ensure that the client has realistic expectations of surgery and has the ability to meet postoperative responsibilities.

Thinking Critically

1. You are caring for a woman who is scheduled to have a rhytidectomy. As you are reviewing her preoperative orders and education, she comments to you

that she hopes "this will work." You question her further on her comment, intending to review the actual operation and probable outcome of face lifts with her. She discloses that she believes that her restored youthful look will "keep" her new boyfriend interested in her during their planned vacation next week. How should you respond?

Factors to Consider. What are the elements of realistic expectations? How quickly do postoperative edema and ecchymosis resolve?

2. You are caring for a 50-year-old woman who had a right latissimus dorsi breast reconstruction this morning. You find her sleeping on her right side after surgery. Her Hemovac drain has not had any drainage for the past 4 hours. What nursing action should you take?

Factors to Consider. Where is the pedicle in a latissimus dorsi operation for breast reconstruction? What risk is present with the client lying on the Hemovac drain?

Bibliography

1. Ainslie, N., et al. (1996). Creating a realistic breast: The nipple-areola reconstruction. *Plastic Surgical Nursing, 16*(3), 156–165.
2. American Society of Plastic and Reconstructive Surgical Nurses. (1996). *Core curriculum for plastic and reconstructive surgical nursing* (2nd ed.). Pitman, NJ: Author.
3. Anderson, L. G., & Leroux, C. (1996). Routine surgery, routine patients? Never. *Plastic Surgical Nursing, 16*(1), 41–42.
4. Anderson, L. (1994). The plastic surgical nurse. *Nursing Clinics of North America, 29*(4), 817–825.
5. Anderson, R. C., & Larson, D. L. (1995). Patient concerns related to media coverage of silicone implants. *Plastic Surgical Nursing, 15*(2), 89–91.
6. Anderson, R. C., & Maksud, D. (1994). Psychological adjustments to reconstructive surgery. *Nursing Clinics of North America, 29*(4), 711–724.
7. Angell, M. (1996). Shattock lecture—Evaluating the health risks of breast implants: The interplay of medical science, the law, and public opinion. *New England Journal of Medicine, 334*(23), 1513–1518.
8. Black, J. (1996). Surgical options for wound healing. *Critical Care Nursing Clinics, 8*(2), 169–182.
9. Black, J. (1994). Surgical management of pressure ulcers. *Nursing Clinics of North America, 29*(4), 801–808.
10. Bondville, J. (1994). Pain-free harvesting of skin grafts with EMLA. *Plastic Surgical Nursing, 14*(4), 231–233.
11. Clamon, J., & Netscher, D. T. (1994). General principles of flap reconstruction: Goals for aesthetic and functional outcome. *Plastic Surgical Nursing, 14*(1), 9–14.
12. Clayton, B., et al. (1996). The TRAM flap in breast reconstruction. *Plastic Surgical Nursing, 16*(3), 133–138.
13. Francel T. (1992). Salvage of the massively traumatized lower extremity. *Clinics in Plastic Surgery 19*: 871–876.
14. Fowler, M. (1994). Body contouring surgery. *Nursing Clinics of North America, 29*(4), 753–761.
15. Furnas, H., & Rosen, J. (1991). Monitoring in microvascular surgery. *Annals of Plastic Surgery, 26*(3), 265–272.
16. Gayle, L., et al. (1991). Lower extremity replantation. *Clinics in Plastic Surgery, 18,* 437–447.
17. Gellis, M. B. (1996). Preoperative and postoperative instructions for liposuction of the jowl and chin. *Plastic Surgical Nursing, 16*(1), 57–58.
18. Gilboa, D., et al. (1990). Emotional and psychosocial adjustment of women to breast reconstruction and detection of subgroup(s) at risk for psychological morbidity. *Annals of Plastic Surgery, 25*(5), 397–401.
19. Gutek, E .P., Fowler, M. E., & Heeter, C. (1993). The forehead lift. *Plastic Surgical Nursing, 13*(4), 188–200.
20. Hart, D. (1996). Psychological outcomes of breast reconstruction. *Plastic Surgical Nursing, 16*(3), 167–171.
21. Hart, D. (1995). Women and saline breast implant surgery. *Plastic Surgical Nursing, 15*(3), 161–166.
22. Hinojosa, R. (1996). Anxiety of elective surgical patients' family members: Relationship between anxiety levels, family characteristics. *Plastic Surgical Nursing, 16*(1), 43–45.
23. Hinojosa, R. (1995). Postoperative nausea and vomiting: How nurses can help. *Plastic Surgical Nursing, 15*(2), 85–88.
24. Lusis, S. A. (1994). Nursing management of the elderly surgical patient. *Plastic Surgical Nursing, 14*(3), 139–146.
25. Khouri, R. K. (1992). Avoiding free flap failure. *Clinics in Plastic Surgery, 19,* 773–783.
26. Maksud, D., & Cogwell Anderson, R. (1995). Psychological dimensions of aesthetic surgery: Esssentials for nurses. *Plastic Surgical Nursing, 15*(3), 137–144.
27. Mangan, M. (1994). Current concepts in breast reconstruction. *Nursing Clinics of North America, 29*(4), 763–776.
28. McCain, L. (1995). A review of autoimmune disorders anecdotally linked to mammary implants. *Plastic Surgical Nursing, 15*(2), 68–77.
29. McCain, L., & Jones, G. (1995). Application of endoscopic techniques in aesthetic plastic surgery. *Plastic Surgical Nursing, 15*(3), 149–160.
30. McCain, L., & Jones, G. (1995). Endoscopic techniques in aesthetic plastic surgery. *Plastic Surgical Nursing, 15*(3), 145–148.
31. McCarthy, J. (1991). *Plastic surgery.* Philadelphia: W. B. Saunders.
32. Meland, N., & Weimar, R. (1991). Microsurgical reconstruction: Experience with free fascia flaps. *Annals of Plastic Surgery, 27*(1), 1–8.
33. Moncada, G. (1994). Traumatic injuries of the face and hands. *Nursing Clinics of North America, 29*(4), 777–789.
34. Monteiro, D. (1993). Surgical reconstruction of complex wounds. *Wounds, 5,* 129–134.
35. Netscher, D., & Clamon, J. (1994). Smoking: Adverse effects on outcomes for plastic surgical patients. *Plastic Surgical Nursing, 14*(4), 205–210.
36. Netscher, D. T., & Clamon, J. (1994). Methods of reconstruction. *Nursing Clinics of North America, 29*(4), 725–739.
37. Palcheff-Weimer, M., et al. (1993). The impact of the media on women with breast implants. *Plastic and Reconstructive Surgery, 92*(5), 778–775.
38. Pettis, D., & Vogt, P. (1992). Complications of suction-assisted lipectomy. *Plastic Surgical Nursing, 12*(4), 148–154.
39. Rubin, M. G. (1992). Trichloroacetic acid and other non-phenol peels. *Clinics in Plastic Surgery, 19*(2), 525–536.
40. Ryan, F., & La Fourcade, C. (1995). Skin care, chemical face peeling and skin rejuvenation. *Plastic Surgical Nursing, 15*(3), 167–171.
41. Salisbury, C., & Kaye, B. (1987). Complications following rhytidectomy. *Plastic Surgical Nursing, 7*(3), 76–83.
42. Simler, A. (1994). Endoscopic augmentation mammoplasty: The umbilical approach. *Plastic Surgical Nursing, 14*(3), 149–153.
43. Smith, J., & Aston, S. (1992). *Grabb and Smith's plastic surgery.* Boston: Little, Brown.
44. Spencer, K. (1996). Using the latissimus dorsi flap for breast reconstruction. *Plastic Surgical Nursing, 16*(3), 147–155.
45. Spencer, K. W. (1994). Selection and preoperative preparation of plastic surgery patients. *Nursing Clinics of North America, 29*(4), 697–710.
46. Springer, R. C. (1996). Rhytidectomy: From consultation to recovery. *Plastic Surgical Nursing, 16*(1), 27–30.
47. Tebbetts, J. B. (1992). Blepharoplasty: A refined technique emphasizing accuracy and control. *Clinics in Plastic Surgery, 19*(2), 329–350.
48. Vander Kam, V., & Achauer, B. (1995). Aesthetic rhinoplasty. *Plastic Surgical Nursing, 15*(3), 182–184.
49. Stombler, R. E. (1993). Breast implants and the FDA: Past, present and future. *Plastic Surgical Nursing, 13*(4), 185–187, 200.

50. Strzyzewski, N. M. (1995). The cycle of perioperative nursing care for plastic surgery patients. *Plastic Surgical Nursing, 15*(2), 78–81, 85.

51. Turpin, I. M. (1992). The modern rhytidectomy. *Clinics in Plastic Surgery, 19*(2), 383–400.

52. Vander Kam, V., & Achauer, B. (1993). Abdominoplasty. *Plastic Surgical Nursing, 13*(4), 217–220, 222.

53. Wentz, M. G. (1995). Clinical photography simplified: Developing a personal set of unformed view. *Plastic Surgical Nursing, 15*(4), 211–215.

54. Williams, L. (1994). Facial rejuvenation. *Nursing Clinics of North America, 29*(4), 741–752.

Reproductive Disorders

UNIT 17

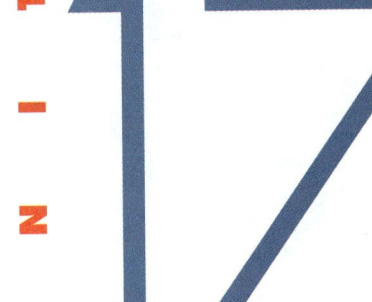

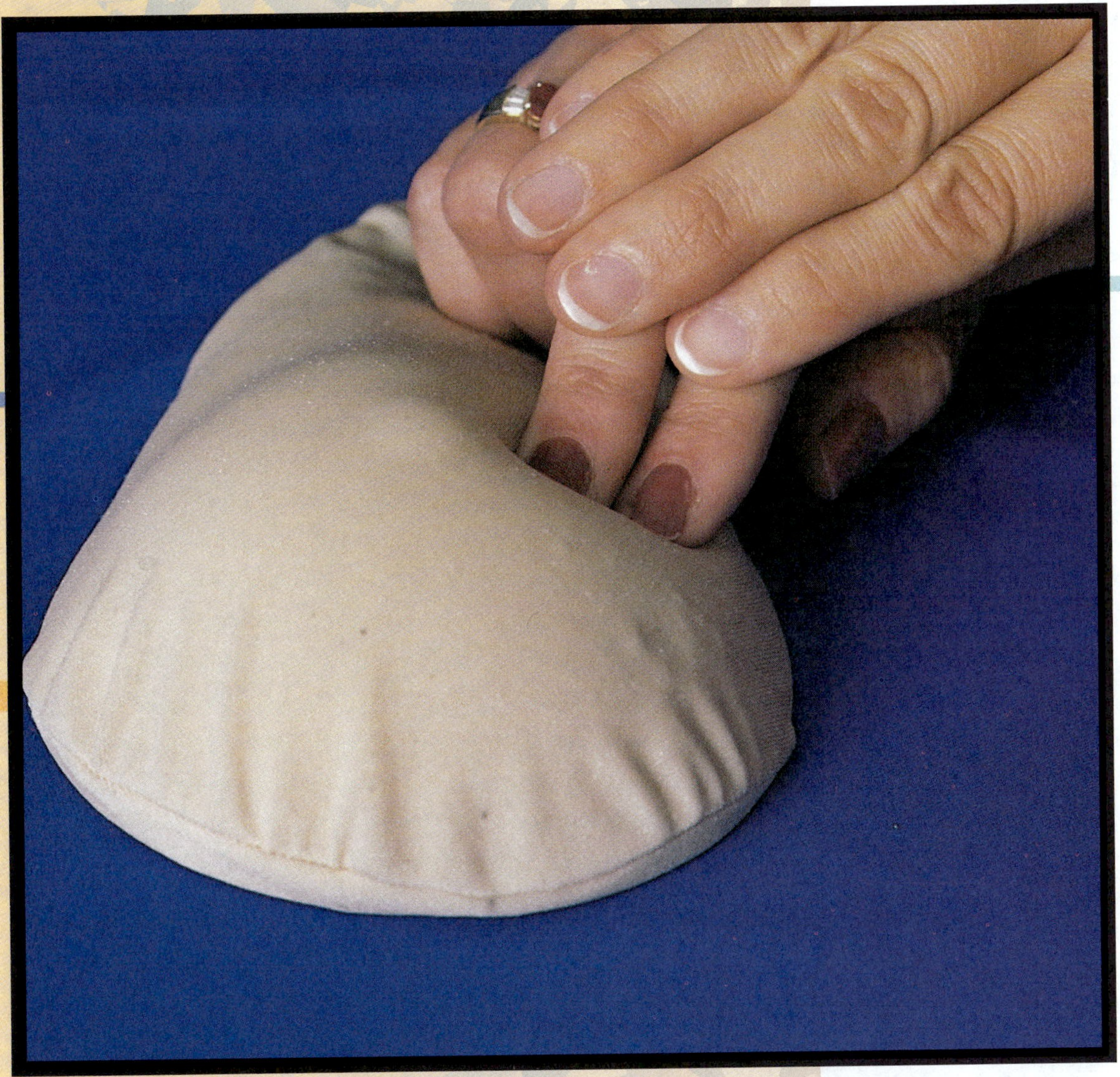

Structure and Function of the Reproductive System

Esther Matassarin-Jacobs

Gonadal Development

The gonads are the sex glands of the female (ovaries) and male (testes). Their primary function is to form the cells of human reproduction. The ovaries produce ova; the testes produce spermatozoa (sperm).

Gonadal development begins during the fifth week of fetal life. Gonadal differentiation occurs in the seventh and eighth weeks of gestation with the development of the testes in the male and the ovaries in the female. In the male, the wolffian ducts develop into the epididymis, vas deferens, and seminal vesicles. The müllerian ducts regress. In the female, the wolffian ducts regress and the müllerian ducts develop into fallopian tubes, uterus, and upper vagina. The external genitalia, the glans penis and scrotum, are complete in the male by 14 weeks of gestation. The clitoris, labia majora, and labia minora are complete in the female by 11 weeks of gestation.

Structure and Function of the Female Reproductive System

Female Reproductive Structure

The female reproductive organs (also called female genitalia, female genitals, or female organs of generation) consist of (1) externally (collectively termed the vulva or pudendum), the mons pubis (veneris), labia majora, labia minora, clitoris, fourchette, fossa navicularis, vestibule, vestibular bulb, Skene's ducts (glands), Bartholin's glands, vaginal opening (introitus), and, possibly, hymen, and (2) internally, two ovaries, two fallopian tubes, the uterus, and the vagina (Fig. 81–1).

This chapter incorporates material written for the fourth edition by Ann J. Clark and Lynne C. Carpenter.

External Female Genital Structures

The external female genital structures play a role in sexual stimulation and as a barrier to protect the body from foreign materials.

Mons Pubis (Veneris). This rounded pad of flesh lies over the symphysis pubis. It is covered with hair following puberty.

Labia Majora. These two elongated folds of tissue are separated by a cleft. Within the cleft, the vagina and urethra open. The labia majora connect anteriorly and posteriorly with commissures (the posterior one is not clearly defined).

Labia Minora. These are two small, thin, elongated folds of tissue. They lie, one on each side, between the labia majora and the vaginal opening, just inside and enclosing the vagina's vestibule. The labia minora each divide anteriorly, before uniting. They form the hoodlike prepuce of the clitoris and enclose the clitoris.

Clitoris. This small, elongated, highly sensitive erectile structure is located under the anterior labial commissure. It is partly hidden by the anterior portion of the labia minora. Usually covered by a prepuce, the clitoris is homologous to the male penis.

Fourchette. Located at the posterior commissure of the vagina, this tense band of mucous membrane connects the posterior end of the labia minora.

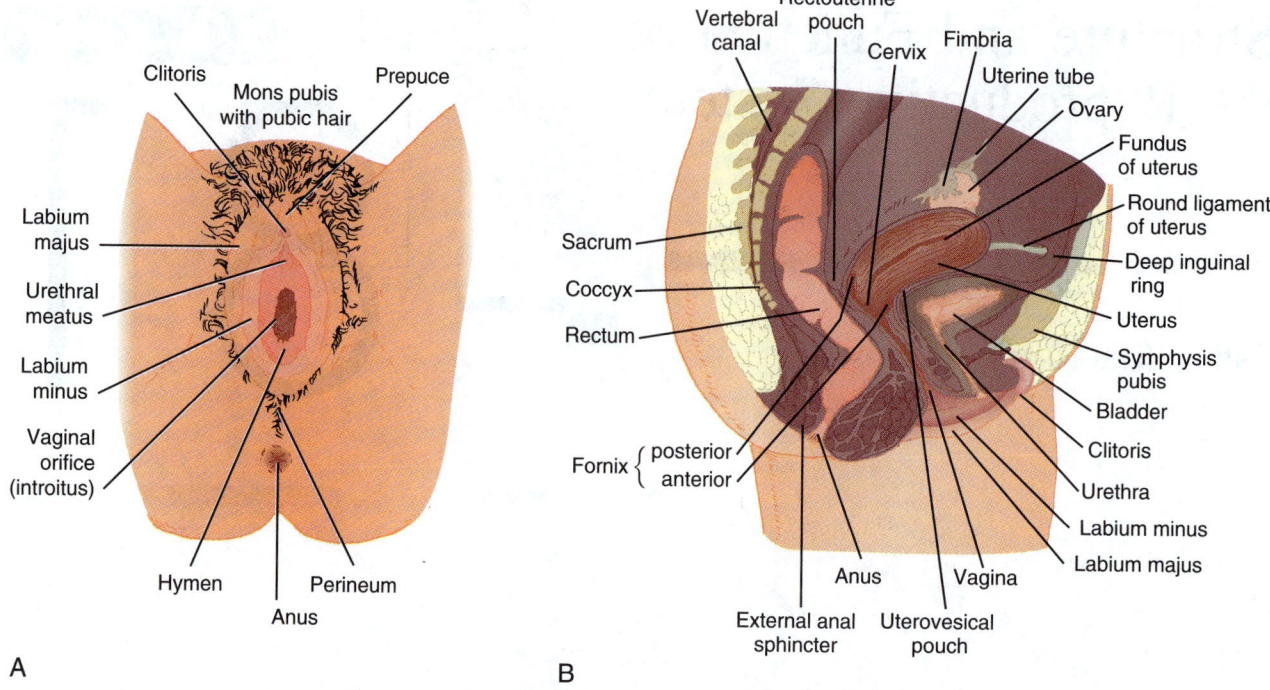

Figure 81–1. *A*, Anatomic landmarks of external female genitalia. *B*, Midsagittal section of the female pelvis.

Fossa Navicularis. This cul-de-sac, located anterior to the fourchette, separates the fourchette from the hymen. Following rupture of the hymen or parturition (childbirth), the fossa navicularis disappears.

Vestibule. The vestibule is an almond-shaped space between the labia minora. The clitoris is at the vestibule's anterior angle, and the fourchette is its posterior boundary. The vestibule's covering mucous membranes are delicate and pink. The four major structures opening into the vestibule are the (1) urethra, (2) vagina (posteriorly), and (3 and 4) two secretory ducts of Bartholin's glands (laterally). The perineum is posterior to the vestibule, between it and the anus.

Vestibular Bulbs. These two sacculated collections of veins (homologous to the male corpus spongiosum) lie on either side of the vagina.

Skene's Ducts (Glands, Tubules). The openings of these two glands lie on either side of the urethra's floor, just inside the urethral opening.

Bartholin's Glands (Vulvovaginal Glands). These two small mucoid-secreting glands (homologous to the male bulbourethral glands) lie on either side of the lower part of the vestibule, close to the vaginal orifice. During sexual excitement, Bartholin's glands cause secretion into the vestibule of the vagina.

Vaginal Opening (Introitus). The vagina is discussed later. The hymen, a fold of mucous membrane that

may or may not be present, partially covers the opening to the vagina. The hymen may be ruptured in various ways, for example, during exercise, sexual activity, surgery, vaginal examination, and insertion of tampons. In the past, the presence or absence of a hymen was used as proof of a woman's virginity or sexual activity. This unfortunate practice, based on ignorance and inaccurate folklore, has caused serious consequences. Pregnancy has been known to occur even with an undisturbed hymen. A ruptured or absent hymen does not necessarily indicate loss of virginity.

Perineum. The female perineum (perineal body) lies, externally, between the vulva and the anus. It is located between the thighs, below the pelvic diaphragm.

Internal Female Genital Structures

Ovaries

Ovaries are the female gonads, producing the female reproductive cell or germ cell (ovum, pleural ova) and hormones (estrogen and progesterone).

When a human ovum is fertilized by a human sperm, it can develop into a new human being.

Normally, there are two ovaries located in the pelvis, on either side of the uterus and below the fallopian (uterine) tubes (see Fig. 81–1). The ovaries are contained in the posterior surfaces of the broad ligaments. They are also supported by other ligaments connecting to the side of the pelvis (suspensory ligament) and to the uterus (utero-ovarian ligament). Each ovary is about the size, shape, and weight of an almond. Its surface is pale, and in young females, smooth. With age, the ovaries become pitted. When examined microscopically, each ovary (Fig. 81–2) consists of the following structures.

Germinal Epithelium.
The germinal epithelium is a single layer of cells (simple, cuboidal epithelium) covering the ovary's surface.

Tunica Albuginea.
The tunica albuginea is a capsule of dense, collagenous connective tissue beneath the germinal epithelium.

Stroma.
Stroma is the connective tissue beneath the tunica albginea. The stroma consists of a cortex (an outer, dense layer) and a medulla (an inner, loose layer).

Ovarian Follicles.
Ova in various stages of development with their surrounding tissue make up the ovarian follicles. Follicles, each containing a developing ovum, grow and mature in the stroma, close to an abundant blood and lymphatic supply. The cortex contains primary follicles (not yet growing) and mature or graafian follicles (ready to erupt and discharge mature ova). A mature follicle is an endocrine gland secreting estrogen hormones (see Estrogens). It consists of a mature ovum and its surrounding tissues.

At birth, there are several hundred thousand follicles. Each contains an oocyte (endstage ovum). They decrease in number as puberty approaches (the time when one first becomes functionally capable of reproduction) and gradually disappear around menopause.

Corpus Luteum.
The corpus luteum develops from a graafian follicle after ovulation (extrusion of a mature ovum). This glandular body produces the hormones progesterone and estrogen (see Estrogens and Progesterone).

Fallopian Tubes

Two fallopian tubes connect the uterus to the ovaries and are the usual site of fertilization. They convey either the fertilized or the unfertilized ovum to the uterus. Each fallopian tube is about 4 inches long. Although thin, the walls of the tubes have a serosal covering, a muscular layer, and a mucous lining. The mucous lining contains hairlike cilia that undulate, sweeping the ovum (along with muscular contractions) toward the uterus.

Supported by ligaments, each fallopian tube has four subdivisions: (1) the fimbriated end, nearest to the ovary, with small, fringed processes that cup over the ovary like a funnel; (2) the ampulla, the widest, longest part of the tube (where fertilization usually occurs); (3) the isthmus, a narrow, short, wavy portion of the tube adjacent to the uterus; and (4) the straight intramural (interstitial) portion, passing through the uterine wall.

Uterus

The uterus is a hollow, thick-walled, muscular organ (1–2 inches thick) that looks like an inverted pear. The organ is about 2 inches long, 2 inches wide at the widest part, and 1 inch wide at the narrowest point, that is, the cervix. The uterus is located in the pelvic cavity slightly below and between the fallopian tubes, almost at a right angle to the vagina (the passageway between the cervix and the vulva).

The normal uterus is movable in all directions. However, it maintains a normal position in the body cavity through the action of various ligaments and the pelvic floor. The right and left margins of the uterus are anchored by a pair of broad ligaments. A pair of uterosacral ligaments, on each side of the rectum, connect the uterus to the sacrum. The main ligaments that maintain the position of the uterus are the cardinal (lateral cervical) ligaments. If these ligaments are weak, the uterus is likely to drop into the vagina (prolapse). The cardinal ligaments run between the pelvic wall and the cervix and vagina. Round ligaments extend from the external genitalia to the uterus, just below the fallopian tubes.

The uterus is divided into three anatomic areas: (1) fundus, (2) corpus, and (3) cervix. The fundus (dome) is the area between the insertion of the two fallopian tubes. The corpus (body) of the uterus is the largest portion, separated from the cervix by a slight constriction (isth-

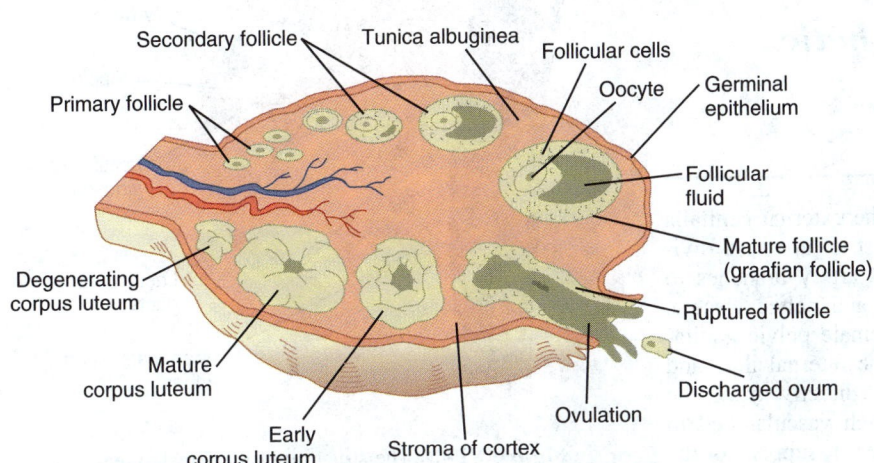

Secondary follicle — Tunica albuginea — Follicular cells — Oocyte — Germinal epithelium — Follicular fluid — Mature follicle (graafian follicle) — Ruptured follicle — Discharged ovum — Ovulation — Stroma of cortex — Early corpus luteum — Mature corpus luteum — Degenerating corpus luteum — Primary follicle

Figure 81–2. Histology of the ovary. Diagram of parts of an ovary in sectional view. The sequence of developmental stages that occur as part of the ovarian cycle begins with the primary follicle and ends with the degenerating corpus luteum.

mus). The cervix (neck) attaches to and projects into the vagina for a short distance. The cervical opening into the vagina is termed the external os. Its opening into the uterus is called the internal os or isthmus. The contents of the cervical canal include mucin-secreting glands. The cervix normally extends backward and downward. Usually, it forms almost a right angle with the vagina (angle of anteversion).

The body of the uterus is usually bent forward (anteflexion) over the urinary bladder. It is separated from the bladder by the uterovesical pouch. The rectum is behind the uterus. The posterior wall of the uterus is separated from the sigmoid colon above and behind the rectouterine pouch (cul-de-sac of Douglas). This cavity, an extension of the peritoneal cavity, usually contains coils of ileum.

The uterus has three functional layers: (1) the parametrium, the thin peritoneal and fascial covering of the uterus; (2) the myometrium (bulk of the uterus), a muscular layer composed of three layers, mainly of involuntary muscles; and (3) the endometrium, the mucous membrane lining the inner surface of the uterus. The superior two thirds of the endometrium responds cyclically to hormones. Menstrual flow results from shedding of the endometrial lining when the ovum is not fertilized. A fertilized ovum implants in the endometrium.

Vagina

This musculomembranous canal connects the uterus, through the cervical opening, with the external genitalia. The vagina has three layers: (1) epithelium, (2) fibrous connective tissue, and (3) a muscular layer. The vagina's upper third attaches to the cervix. At the level of attachment, there is a recess divided into an anterior part, a posterior part, and a lateral part.

The mucosa of the inner surface of the vaginal wall folds over in small ridges (rugae) extending laterally upward. This rugal pattern adds to the vagina's elasticity, making it very distensible. The rectum is posterior to its lower two thirds.

The vagina's smooth rugal pattern and elasticity diminish with age during the menopausal and postmenopausal years. The vagina can easily become infected from urethral or rectal secretions.

Pelvic Blood Supply, Innervation, and Lymphatic Drainage

Blood Supply

The most important blood supply to the external genitalia comes from the internal iliac (hypogastric) artery, a division of the common iliac artery. This artery branches to supply the pelvic floor, pelvic walls, and pelvic viscera. The principal vessels supplying the female pelvic genitalia are the (1) uterine arteries from the internal iliac and (2) the ovarian arteries which stem directly from the aorta. The uterine artery provides a rich vascular bed to the uterus, and anastomoses the arterial supply to the

vagina (vaginal arteries). The ovarian artery supplies blood to the ovaries, fallopian tubes, and body of the uterus. Venous drainage roughly parallels the arterial supply.

Innervation

Both the sympathetic and parasympathetic autonomic nervous systems innervate pelvic structures. The uterine myometrium is innervated only by the sympathetic nerve fibers. The perineum is supplied principally by the pudendal nerve.

Lymphatic Drainage

The pelvic lymphatics consist of a rich network of superficial and deep systems that roughly parallel the blood supply. There is an intermingling of the pelvic lymphatics and blood vessels. This is significant for the potential spread of cancer.

Breast Structure and Function

Breasts have an important role in our culture. Sexuality and femininity are associated with breasts. Because breasts are visible, their size and shape are often viewed as a measure of sexuality, femininity, and attractiveness. The physiologic function of female breasts is milk secretion to feed infants.

A breast (mamma) is a modified sebaceous gland and a skin appendage (Fig. 81–3). The female breast extends vertically from the second to sixth rib and horizontally from the sternum to the midaxillary line. It lies entirely

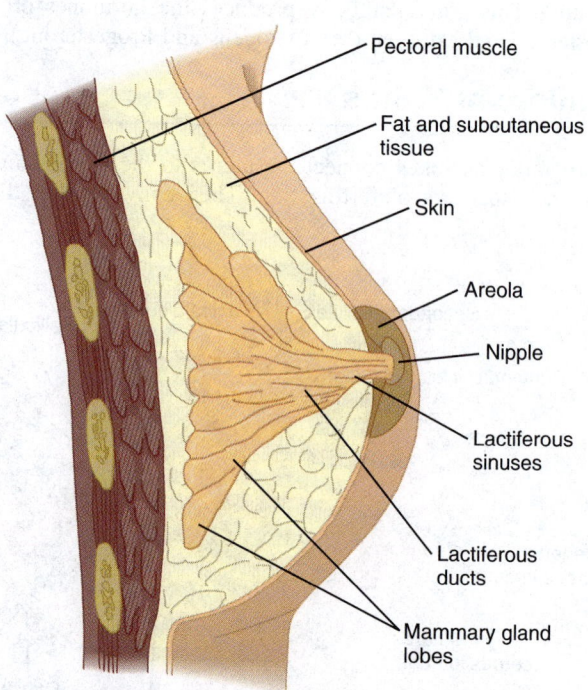

Figure 81–3. The structure of the female breast.

- Pectoral muscle
- Fat and subcutaneous tissue
- Skin
- Areola
- Nipple
- Lactiferous sinuses
- Lactiferous ducts
- Mammary gland lobes

within the superficial fascia of the anterior chest wall. The largest part of the breast rests on fascia of the pectoralis major and the remainder on fascia of the serratus anterior. An average nonlactating breast weighs between 150 and 250 g, and a lactating breast weighs 400 to 500 g.

The parenchyma of a breast consists of ductular, lobular, and acinar epithelial structures. The stroma of a breast is made of fibrous and fatty tissue. The central and upper portions are mostly glandular and the periphery is mostly fatty tissue. A breast consists of 12 to 20 lobes subdivided into lobules. These, in turn, are made up of acini. Breast lobes are arranged like the spokes of a wheel around the nipple. Each lobe is drained by a duct, 12 to 20 of which open on the nipple. Each duct opens independently on the surface of the nipple and has a dilated ampulla just before its opening. The largest amount of a breast's glandular tissue is located in its upper lateral quadrant. A projection of breast tissue extends from this quadrant into the axilla, that is, the tail of Spence. Because the upper quadrant and the tail of Spence contain the largest amount of breast tissue, this is the area where the majority of tumors occur (see Fig. 81–1).

A breast is fixed to the overlying skin and underlying pectoral fascia by fibrous bands (Cooper's ligaments). A fascial cleft on the breast's undersurface permits breast mobility. The nipple is located at the fourth intercostal space. Its base is surrounded by a circular pigmented area called the areola. The administration of estrogen increases pigmentation of the areola at any age. The areolar epithelium contains some small hairs and sebaceous glands, sweat glands, and accessory mammary glands. The sebaceous glands (Montgomery's glands) enlarge during pregnancy and lactation to lubricate the nipple.

The two main sources of the breast's blood supply are the lateral mammary artery and the lateral thoracic artery.

These arteries form an extensive network of anastomoses. The main veins follow the arterial pattern. Lymphatic pathways, in general, follow the pathways of the veins. There are three types of lymphatic drainage of the breast: (1) cutaneous or superficial lymphatic drainage from the skin; (2) areolar lymphatic drainage from the areola and nipple; and (3) glandular lymphatic drainage from deep glandular tissue (Fig. 81–4). The radical mastectomy, sometimes used to treat breast cancer, is based on lymphatic drainage pathways. In less radical surgery, axillary dissection determines the number of lymph nodes involved. This involvement is the best indicator of prognosis. The nerve supply is derived from the anterior and lateral branches of the fourth to sixth intercostal nerves.

Three types of physiologic changes affect the breast. The changes are related to (1) growth and development, (2) the menstrual cycle, and (3) pregnancy and lactation.

The hormones estrogen and progesterone act synergistically with the pituitary growth hormones prolactin and corticotropin to produce breast development and function. Estrogen is responsible for the growth of the breast and periductal stroma. Progesterone promotes the development of lobular and acinar structures. During the normal menstrual cycle, the cyclic secretion of these hormones is responsible for female breast structure. After menopause, the ovaries stop producing estrogen and progesterone. Estrogen is then produced by the adrenals through stimulation from the anterior pituitary. During this life stage, there is a continuous involution of the breast with loss of glandular elements and tissue atrophy.

During pregnancy, estrogen, progesterone, and pituitary hormones increase, increasing breast vascularity and the permeability and dilation of breast lymphatics. When pregnancy ends, prolactin initiates lactation. Prolactin and corticoptropin help maintain lactation. The "letting down" (flow) of milk is a complex response involving a mother's subjective response and the mechanical stimulation of

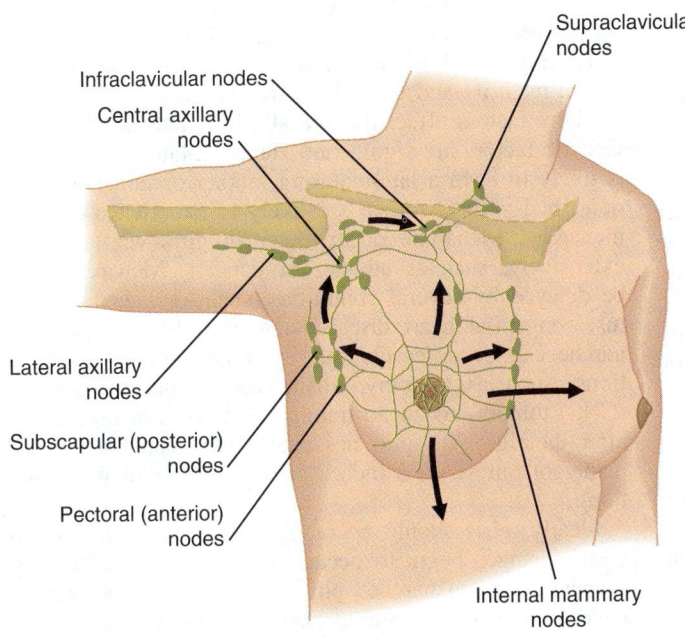

Figure 81–4. Routes of lymphatic drainage from the breast. These routes are very important routes of spread of breast cancer.

suckling. Suckling releases the pituitary hormone oxytocin into the bloodstream. This causes the mammary acini to contract and release milk into the duct system.

The male breast is similar to that of a preadolescent girl. It has a few ducts surrounded by connective tissue. Estrogen can cause a man's breast to enlarge (gynecomastia; see Chapter 83) due to growth of ducts and supporting tissue. Accumulation of fat in obese men can also make the breasts appear large.

Female Reproductive Function

Female Sexual Differentiation

The female reproductive system develops between week 5 and 18 of gestation. The wolffian ducts regress and the müllerian ducts develop into fallopian tubes, uterus, and upper vagina. The ovary secretes estradiol and progesterone. These sex steroids affect the growth, differentiation, and function of the female reproductive system.

Female Hormones

The ovaries manufacture hormones that (1) stimulate sexual desire; (2) interact with the hypothalamic-pituitary unit and the uterus for ovarian changes (follicular development, ovulation, corpus luteum formation), pregnancy (implantation of a fertilized ovum), or menstruation; and (3) have additional effects elsewhere in the body.

Estrogens

Estrogens (female sex hormones) produce cyclic changes in the uterine endothelium and vaginal epithelium. Estrogens are steroids secreted in both sexes by the adrenal cortex and in women by the ovary (main source) and placenta. Natural estrogens include estradiol, estrone, and estriol. When administered therapeutically, estrogens are usually given orally as a conjugate or as diethylstilbestrol (DES), a synthetic estrogenic substance.

Estrogens may be used therapeutically as a replacement hormone during menopause. They are administered, often alternating with progesterone, in the lowest effective dose (see Menopause).

The effects of hormones on menstruation are discussed later. The main effects of estrogenic stimulation on the body occur at puberty, and include breast growth (fatty tissue deposition, pigmentation), fat deposition in the vulva, pubic and axillary hair growth, bony pelvis growth and broadening, vaginal epithelial changes, and general growth.

Estrogens also influence the following:

- Positive nitrogen balance
- Calcium and phosphorus metabolism and calcium retention in bones
- Sodium chloride retention and, hence, sodium and water balance
- Control of blood proteins and lipids

- The vascular and skeletal systems
- Thyroid function, insulin production, and adrenal function.

It is not known precisely how these systems interact. Thus, it is controversial whether estrogen replacement should be given during menopause. Osteoporosis (increased bone porosity) is associated with estrogen deficiency in adult women.

Progesterone

Progesterone is a steroid hormone with varied functions. For example, it helps prepare the endometrium to receive and implant the fertilized ovum. After implantation, progesterone promotes development of the placenta (a spongy structure in the uterus that provides nourishment for a developing fetus) and the mammary glands.

Progesterone is used therapeutically to treat threatened abortion and menstrual problems, for example, dysmenorrhea or amenorrhea. It is obtained from the placenta and the corpus luteum.

Progesterone plays a minor role in sodium and water balance. It also influences nitrogen balance, breast function, and body temperature during the menstrual cycle.

Menarche

Menarche, the beginning of menstrual life, is a developmental milestone in a woman's life. The event is biologic, psychological, and social. A young woman experiencing menarche needs to understand what is happening to her. Psychosocial support and knowledge of how to take care of herself are essential.

Menarche is preceded by characteristic body changes occurring between ages 9 and 16. Breast development varies but takes about 4 to 5 years. The average age for menarche in the United States is now 12.8 years.

Dramatic changes in body image occur. Girls appear to act differently after menarche, and they see themselves differently. The body image is reorganized toward greater sexual maturity and feminine differentiation.

Many factors affect the age at which menarche occurs. Genetic factors are significant. Hence, a late-maturing girl is likely to have a late-maturing mother or father. Undernourished young women are likely to experience delayed menarche. Menarche occurs later in girls who exercise extensively, such as athletes or dancers. Menarche may be delayed by several conditions, such as diabetes mellitus, congenital heart disease, and ulcerative colitis. Menarche can occur earlier than average with other conditions, such as hypothyroidism, central nervous system (CNS) tumors, and head trauma. Girls start to menstruate after their growth spurt has peaked and usually increase in height only 2 to 3 inches after the onset of menstruation.

Ideally, girls should be taught about menarche as pubertal changes begin to occur. Girls who feel adequately prepared, for menarche, physically and psychosocially, have a more positive initial experience with menstruation.

Information about menstrual physiology, menstrual hygiene, and the personal experience is useful. Having appropriate sanitary products ready for use when menarche does occur is also helpful. The girl's mother or significant other female is critical to providing information and support. Some women need preparation for this role. Sex education also should be included in the preparation for menarche. Information should be provided about reproduction, and sexually active teenagers require contraceptive counseling.

Early menstrual cycles are often irregular and anovulatory (menstrual flow is not preceded by ovulation, production, and discharge of an ovum). Although regular menstrual cycles may not occur for several years, any individual cycle may be ovulatory and thus potentially fertile.

Menstrual Cycle

The menstrual cycle is a series of periodic, recurrent changes in the uterus, ovaries, cervix, and vagina (Fig. 81–5). The menstrual cycle consists of proliferative, secretory, and premenstrual phases and ends with menstruation. The proliferative phase ends with ovulation. Each phase is characterized by specific histologic changes in the endometrium.

The length of the menstrual cycle is calculated from the first day of menstruation (menstrual flow). This cycle is about 25 to 32 days but it can vary from month to month (even in the same woman).

The menstrual cycle depends on interactions between the CNS, anterior pituitary, ovaries, and uterus. Variations in the length of the proliferative phase typically cause variation in the length of the entire cycle. Environmental influences also may affect the menstrual cycle because the CNS adjusts the function of many glands in response to environmental stimuli. The menstrual pattern may be altered by climatic changes, emotionally traumatic experiences, stress, or acute or chronic illness.

Proliferative Phase

The proliferative phase of the menstrual cycle depends on the ratio of follicle-stimulating hormone (FSH) to luteinizing hormone (LH).

In the ovary, after menstrual flow has begun, primary follicles (containing oocytes, or primitive ova) and follicular cells begin to develop under the influence of FSH from the anterior pituitary gland (see Fig. 81–5). The thecal (stromal) cells surrounding ova produce estrogens. The level of estrogen produced by these cells begins to rise, which signals the pituitary to inhibit FSH production

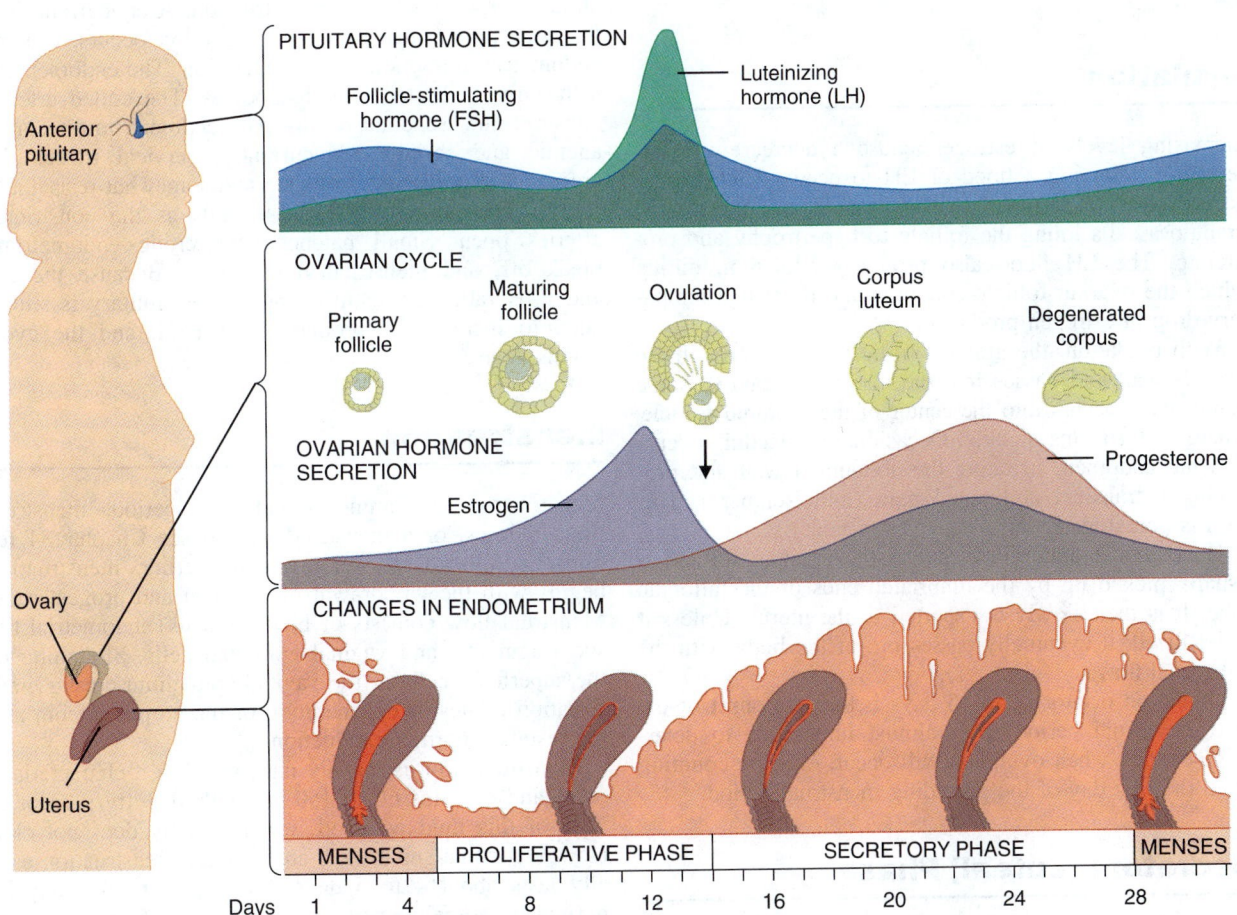

Figure 81–5. Menstrual (uterine) cycle. Note hormonal control of the menstrual cycle and the effects on ovaries *(center)* and endometrium *(bottom).*

and to stimulate secretion of LH. Then, acting together, the two pituitary hormones stimulate further estrogen production. Estrogens, in turn, further inhibit FSH release from the anterior pituitary. LH becomes dominant, stimulating further maturation of the follicle.

About 2 days before ovulation, one follicle (now called a graafian follicle) reaches full maturity. The remaining primary follicles degenerate, that is, follicle atresia takes place. The graafian follicle migrates to the ovary's cortex, where it ruptures through the ovary's wall (ovulation).

Meanwhile, in the uterus, related changes are occurring primarily in response to estrogen from the developing follicle. At the end of a menstrual flow, the uterine endometrium (containing surface epithelium, glands, connective tissue, spaces, and blood vessels) is very thin. Much of it has sloughed off during menstrual flow. Estrogen begins creating a new endometrial surface layer and restoring the uterine epithelium. It stimulates growth of glands and stroma. The epithelium becomes thicker and more vascular. Endometrial proliferation peaks about 2 days before ovulation.

The cervix also undergoes changes. The most important change is that mucous secretion greatly increases just before ovulation. The mucus is a clear fluid that is receptive to sperm.

Vaginal changes during the proliferation phase include proliferation and thickening of the vaginal epithelium due to estrogen. This change is greatest at the time of ovulation.

Ovulation

Increasing levels of estrogen cause a decrease in FSH secretion, allowing a flood of LH to occur. This process occurs over a 24-hour period, causing the thecal and granulosa cells lining the follicle to hypertrophy and proliferate. The LH flood also produces ovulation, during which the ovarian follicle collapses and there is a temporary drop in estrogen production.

With ovulation, the graafian follicle breaks through the ovary's wall and passes into the abdominal cavity. Some hemorrhage occurs into the center of the ruptured follicle, where a clot forms quickly. Occasionally, bleeding occurs into the abdomen, irritating the abdominal wall and producing a transient abdominal pain (mittelschmerz). This pain is occasionally mistaken for appendicitis.

Once in the abdominal cavity, the graafian follicle is usually picked up by the fimbriated ends of the fallopian tube. It is then slowly transported to the uterus. Unless it is fertilized, it eventually passes out of the body with the menstrual flow.

Ovulation occurs 12 to 15 days before the onset of the next menstrual period. It is almost impossible to determine exactly when ovulation will occur, even by counting from the first day of the preceding menstrual period.

Secretory (Luteal) Phase

During the secretory phase, which lasts 10 to 14 days, progesterone and estrogen promote the endometrium's se-

cretory activity. This is characterized by connective tissue hypertrophy. The arteries coil and become tortuous. The glands become larger and more tortuous, and abundantly secrete a substance containing glycogen. The endometrium becomes edematous, compact, and thickened, and is ready for implantation of a fertilized ovum. This development peaks 7 to 8 days after ovulation. This is the most favorable time for implantation.

In the ovary after ovulation, the corpus luteum (yellow body) develops within the ruptured ovarian follicle, as follows: the clot, which developed in response to hemorrhage when the follicle ruptured, is replaced with yellowish luteal cells containing lipids. These cells secrete progesterone and eventually form the corpus luteum. The corpus luteum is an endocrine body that secretes progesterone.

Formation of the corpus luteum occurs in response to stimulation from the LH flood. As the corpus luteum forms, increasing amounts of progesterone and some estrogen are produced. Full maturity of the corpus luteum occurs about 9 days after ovulation (Fig. 81–6). If implantation of a fertilized ovum (pregnancy) does not occur, the corpus luteum begins to degenerate.

Premenstrual (Ischemic) Phase

Degeneration (involution) of the corpus luteum occurs about 2 to 4 days before menstruation. A concurrent drop in progesterone and estrogen production occurs, causing endometrial retraction and degeneration. The endometrium is heavily infiltrated with leukocytes. The coiled arteries constrict and ischemia results. The endometrium becomes anemic and shrinks. Concurrently, cervical mucus decreases, becoming more opaque and somewhat resistant to sperm. The premenstrual phase ends as the constricted arteries open. Small patches of necrotic endometrium break off, and menstrual flow begins. Because the LH and FSH ratio has again changed, the pituitary is stimulated to increase its production of FSH, and the cycle begins again.

Menstruation

Menstruation is commonly called a period, menstrual flow, menses, or a menstrual period (see Chapter 84 for menstrual disorders). As discussed earlier, menstruation begins with the withdrawal of estrogen and progesterone. Menstrual flow consists of blood, mucus, endometrial tissue fragments, and vaginal epithelial cells. Sloughing of the superficial cells of the vaginal epithelium during menstruation relates to degeneration of the corpus luteum and the resultant hormone reduction.

Menstrual flow is usually dark red, has a characteristic odor, and contains 60 to 150 ml of fluid. Fifty percent to 75% of this fluid is blood, which usually does not clot. However, some small clots are normal. Menstruation usually lasts about 4 to 5 days, but 1 to 10 days may be normal for some women.

Discussion of methods of contraception (prevention of pregnancy) may be found in obstetrics nursing texts.

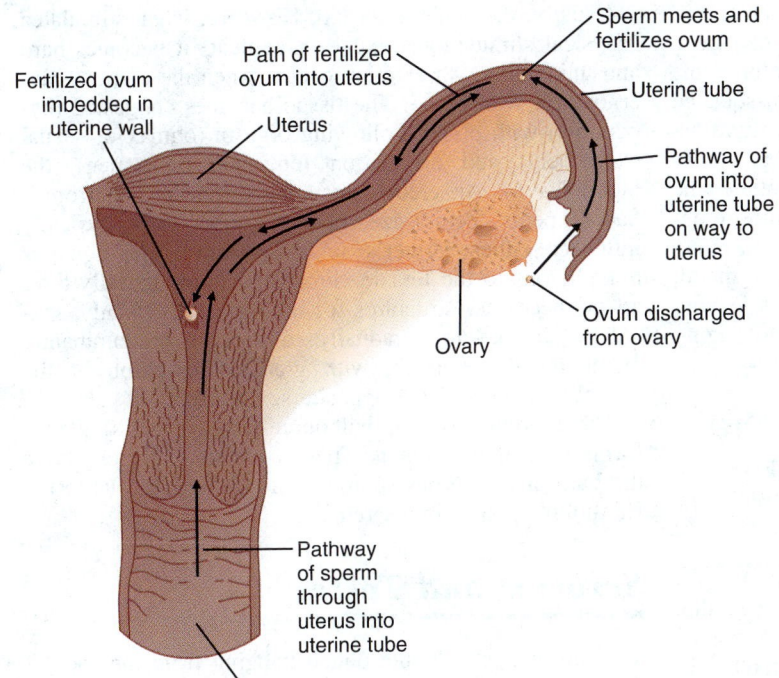

Figure 81–6. Pathways of sperm and ovum in the female reproductive organs. (Modified from Miller, B. F., & Keane, C. B. [1992]. *Encyclopedia and dictionary of medicine, nursing and allied health* [5th ed., p. 1085]. Philadelphia: W. B. Saunders.)

Menopause

Like menarche, menopause (permanent cessation of menstruation) is an important developmental event in a woman's life. Menopause produces physical changes, as well as having psychological and social implications for the woman.

Menopause is one of a complex sequence of biologic aging events of the climacteric or perimenopausal period. This period lasts about 15 to 20 years from, about age 40 to 60 years, during which time the body makes the transition from fertility to a nonreproductive status. The usual age at menopause is between 48 and 54 years, although it may occur as early as age 35. The average age at menopause appears to be increasing in industrialized countries.

The pattern of menstrual cessation varies. It may be abrupt but more often occurs over 1 to 2 years. Periodic menstrual flow gradually occurs less frequently, becoming irregular and less in amount. Anovulatory cycles are common during this time, and occasional episodes of profuse bleeding may be interspersed with episodes of scant bleeding. Menopause is said to have occurred when there have been no menstrual periods for 12 consecutive months. Any spontaneous uterine bleeding after this time is abnormal and requires investigation. Unplanned pregnancy may occur during the premenopausal period. Advise sexually active women to use contraception for at least 6 months after menses have ceased.

The cause of menopause is not known. However, certain predictable physiologic changes and experiences occur. Premenopausal ovaries contain abundant germinal structures in various stages of development. During the climacteric, a gradual decrease in the number of maturing ovarian follicles and a parallel decline in the production

of ovarian estrogen occur. Over time, as the ovaries become unresponsive to pituitary hormones, and toward the end of the climacteric, the ovaries atrophy. Other changes associated with menopause, such as hot flashes and vaginal atrophy, are related to decreased estrogen production.

Most women experience menopause without difficulty. The menopausal woman of today is younger-looking, active, and has more positive attitudes about menopause than in the past.[2, 24] The stereotype of the typical menopausal woman, a woman who is miserable with a varied range of symptoms for which she seeks medical assistance, has been disproved. Research shows that menopause itself does not cause poorer health or greater use of healthcare.[24] The perimenopause marks the beginning of the healthy aging process in women. However, some women do become distressed enough to require professional assistance.

Menstrual variation, such as irregular menses, skipped periods, and occasional scanty or moderately heavy menses, may happen a year or two before menopause occurs. Usually, these variations do not require any intervention.

Although further study is needed of the psychosexual changes associated with the perimenopausal period, it is likely that any changes that occur are the result of the complex interaction of anatomic, physiologic, psychological, and social factors. Vaginal lubrication may be reduced in the perimenopausal years, and this dryness may cause discomfort or bleeding with intercourse. Estrogen replacement therapy can usually relieve this discomfort. Some studies have reported lessened interest in sexual activity among menopausal women, but other authors claim freedom from pregnancy allows women to relax and enjoy intercourse more.

Menopause is not a disease. Most women pass through menopause with minimal or no problems. With increased life expectancy, the typical woman can spend over a third of her life in the postmenopausal years. This can be a time to set new goals. Nurses can help counter some misconceptions and negative connotations often associated with menopause by stressing the normal and positive aspects of the experience. The nurse should help to clarify misconceptions about menopause and differentiate the physiologic manifestations of menopause from midlife developmental changes. During the menopausal years, many women are faced with life situations that affect mood, such as growing older, adjusting to the children's leaving home, and accepting increased responsibility for aging parents.

Structure and Function of the Male Reproductive System

Male Reproductive Structure

The male reproductive organs (also called male genitalia, male genitals, or male organs of generation) consist of paired testicles (containing the seminiferous tubules, in which sperm is produced) lying within the scrotum, epididymides, seminal ducts, spermatic cords, seminal vesicles, ejaculatory ducts, bulbourethral (Cowper's) glands, the prostate gland, and the penis, through which traverses the urethra (Fig. 81–7).

The penis and scrotum are external, visible genitalia, whereas the other structures are internal. The male perineum is the external area between the scrotum and the anus.

Penis and Related Structures

The penis is both a sexual organ (organ of copulation) and an organ for urination. This cylindrical, pendulous structure suspends from its attachment to the pubic arch. The skin of the penis is dark, hairless, thin, and loose (permitting considerable distention).

Structurally, the penis consists mainly of erectile tissue, covered by skin, and is arranged into three columns. Two columns of erectile tissue (*corpora cavernosa*) form two lateral columns. The median column (*corpus spongiosum*) contains the urethra, which forms a passage for urine and semen. Each corpus is enclosed in a fascial sheath (*tunica albuginea*). All are surrounded by a thick fibrous envelope (*Buck's fascia*). The portion of the penis between its end or head and its attachment to the pubic bone is the shaft.

In males, the urethra's external opening (meatus or orifice) is in the glans (glans penis), the cone-shaped end or head of the penis. The glans is the conical expansion of the corpus spongiosum. The expanded posterior border of the glans is the corona. At its junction with the shaft is the coronal sulcus. A flap of movable skin (foreskin or prepuce) covers the glans. Smegma is a cheesy, thick, odoriferous secretion of sloughed-off epithelial cells that collects under the prepuce. (In females, smegma is the secretion of the apocrine glands of the clitoris, together with epithelial cells.)

Usually, the penis is flaccid. However, when stimulated (physical stimulation, sexual excitement) it becomes hard and unyielding. An erection occurs when the corpora cavernosa fill with blood. The tissue becomes congested (hyperemic) with blood. Following orgasm (climax of sexual excitement) and ejaculation (emission of semen), the blood leaves. An erect penis may differ in size from a flaccid penis. Penis size, however, does not physically influence either partner's sexual pleasure. The penis is homologous to the female clitoris. Embryos initially have all the necessary structures for both sexes. Normally, sexual organs develop gradually to become predominantly either female or male, with gradual involution of the sexual structures of the opposite sex.

The secretion of the bulbourethral (Cowper's) glands forms part of the semen. These two small glands above the bulb of the corpus spongiosum are homologous to the Bartholin's glands in the female.

Scrotum and Testes

The scrotum is a double pouch hanging from the root of the penis. Internally, beneath the scrotal skin, muscular contractile tissue (*tunica dartos*) separates the pouch's two halves. Externally, the scrotal skin is bisected in the middle by a *raphe* (ridge) where the two halves of the scrotum join. The raphe runs over the scrotum from the root of the penis to the anus.

Each half of the scrotum contains (1) a testicle with its epididymis and (2) part of a spermatic cord. The spermatic cord is held together by spermatic fascia. Each cord is made up of nerves, testicular vessels (spermatic artery, vein, lymph vessels), and the vas deferens. The vas deferens (ductus deferens, seminal duct) is the testicle's excretory duct. It is the continuation of the epididymis and is a tube of musculature about 46 cm (18 inches) long. The vas deferens conveys sperm from the testicle to the prostatic urethra, that is, from the epididymis to the ejaculatory duct. The ejaculatory duct then conveys semen to the urethra.

The scrotum's left side hangs lower than the right because the left spermatic cord suspends the testicles and extends from them into the inguinal ring. The cord goes through the inguinal canal, and the vas deferens continues into the abdominal cavity. It passes behind the bladder, anterior to the rectum, to join the duct of the seminal vesicle, becoming the ejaculatory duct. The spermatic cord is movable for protection from trauma and facilitates optimal spermatogenesis, that is, production of mature, functional sperm.

Testicles are the male gonads. They produce the male hormone (testosterone) and the male reproductive cells (sperm).

Testicles (testes) are smooth, solid, ovoid structures about 4.0 cm long and 2.0 to 2.5 cm wide. An inelastic, dense, fibrous *tunica albuginea* forms the outer coat of the testicle.

The epididymis is a small, oblong body resting on and beside the posterior surface of the testicle. Each epididymis consists of a convoluted tube 3.96 to 6.1 m (13–20 ft) long. The upper end of the testicle is capped by the

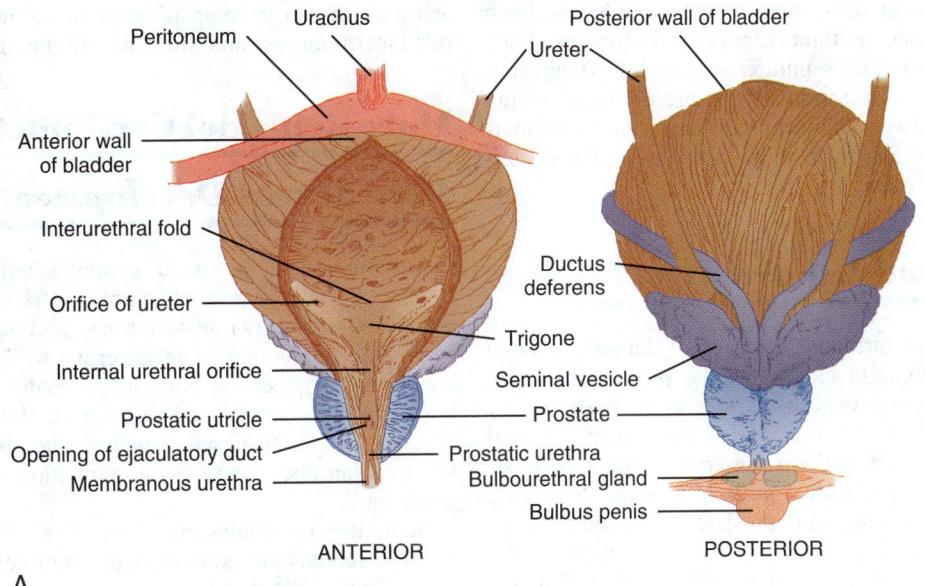

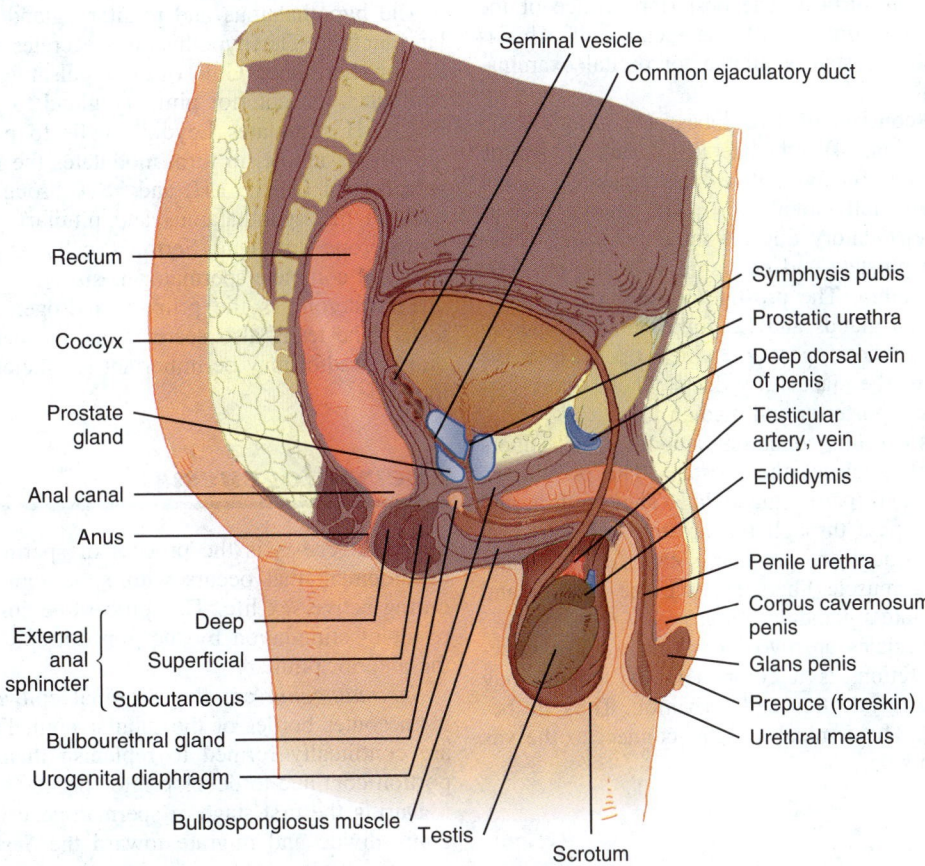

Figure 81–7. *A,* Internal and external aspects of the male urinary bladder and related structures. *B,* Midsagittal section of the male pelvis and external genitalia.

head of the epididymis. The body of the epididymis attaches to the posterior surface of the testicle. At the lower end of the testicle, the tail of the epididymis becomes continuous with the vas deferens which joins other ves-

sels to form the spermatic cord. The head of the epididymis contains 12 to 20 testicular efferent ducts.

Many lobules, separated by septa, divide a testicle. These lobules lead to straight ducts that join a plexus from which efferent ducts lead to the epididymis. Each lobule contains one to three seminiferous tubules. Each testicle has 600 to 1200 seminiferous tubules. Their combined length is almost a mile! Sperm are produced within these tubules. Between the seminiferous tubules are interstitial cells called *Leydig's cells,* the source of testosterone, the male hormone.

Prostate and Related Structures

The prostate gland surrounds the neck of the male urinary bladder and urethra. In childhood, the prostate is small, but with puberty, it grows to the size of a chestnut. The adult prostate gland (see Fig. 81–7) lies like a flattened cone in the pelvis, about 2 cm posterior to the symphysis pubis. A normal adult male's prostate weighs 15 to 20 g and is 4 to 6 cm long. The prostate is inverted, so its apex is inferior, and is suspended by the urogenital diaphragm. The base of the prostate is superior and at the bladder neck, anterior to the rectum. The bladder overlies the prostate's basal surface. The posterior surface of the prostate is in close contact with the rectal wall. This is the surface of the prostate available for digital examination.

The prostate consists of five lobes: (1) anterior, (2) posterior, (3) median, (4) right lateral, (5) and left lateral. A shallow, median furrow divides the prostate's lower part into right and left lateral lobes. The middle lobe is created by the ejaculatory ducts from either side. These ducts pierce the prostate and converge with the prostatic portion of the urethra. The prostate consists of (1) periurethral or internal glands and (2) follicle-like tubules in the prostate's peripheral portion, which opens into the urethra by way of the ejaculatory ducts. These ducts separate the prostate's posterior and median lobes.

A firm fibrous capsule, containing smooth muscle fibers in its inner layer, encloses the prostate. The prostate is partly muscular and partly glandular. The urethra and ejaculatory ducts pass through the prostate. The urethral portion passing through the prostate is called the prostatic urethra. Prostatic muscle fibers encircle the urethra and separate the prostate's glandular tissue.

The seminal vesicles are two 5-cm-long, saclike structures whose secretion, is a component of semen, may contribute to sperm nutrition and activation. They lie behind the bladder. The seminal vesicles connect to the vas deferens on each side.

Sperm

Sperm are mature male sex or germ cells that develop after puberty. Resembling tadpoles, sperm self-propel themselves by hairlike tails like flagella. A normal sperm (about 51 μm in length) has a flattened, broad, oval head with a nucleus. A middle piece or protoplasmic neck connects to the tail. During fertilization, the sperm's head pierces an ovum (female reproductive or germ cell). The sperm's tail is lost when fusion of two cells occurs. Sperm are produced in the seminiferous tubules of the testicles. Sperm develop in great quantities from spermatids (spermoblasts) and are stored in the vas deferens.

Male Reproductive Function

Male Sexual Development

Development of the male genitalia requires two hormones: (1) müllerian duct inhibitory factor, secreted Sertoli's cells, and (2) testosterone, secreted by Leydig's cells. The production of testosterone by Leydig's cells is supported by placental chorionic gonadotropin. Müllerian duct inhibitory factor mediates the involution of the müllerian duct. Testosterone supports the differentiation of the wolffian ducts and the differentiation of male external genitalia.

Seminiferous tubules constitute 90% of the mature testis. The tubules are composed of germ cells and Sertoli's cells. Germ cells develop into spermatozoa, and Sertoli's cells support spermatogenesis.

The hypothalamus and pituitary gland regulate testicular function. The hypothalamus secretes gonadotropin-releasing hormone (GnRH) in a pulsatile fashion. GnRH stimulates the anterior pituitary gland to produce LH and FSH. LH stimulates Leydig's cells to produce testosterone. Testosterone, in turn, modulates the regulation of the secretion of GnRH, LH, and FSH through negative feedback to the hypothalamus and pituitary gland. FSH and testosterone stimulate Sertoli's cells and germ cells to start and complete spermatogenesis.

Testosterone is the primary androgen secreted by the testis. The testis also secretes androstenedione and estradiol. Estradiol may be important for skeletal maturation in the male.

Spermatogenesis

Spermatogenesis is the process of sperm production and development that occurs within the seminiferous tubules during active sex life. This process begins at puberty as a result of stimulation by the gonadotropic hormones from the anterior pituitary.

Spermatogonia are the germinal epithelial cells found in the outer border of the tubular epithelium. These cells are continually formed to replenish themselves, while a portion continue to develop into sperm.

During the first stage of spermatogenesis, the spermatogonia divide and migrate toward the *Sertoli's cells.* The spermatogonia penetrate the membranes of Sertoli's cells and become enveloped within the cytoplasm of these cells. The spermatogonia continue this close relationship with Sertoli's cells throughout their development.

During the 24 days when it is in contact with Sertoli's cells, the spermatogonium changes and enlarges to form a primary spermatocyte. After this development, the spermatocyte splits into two secondary spermatocytes, each with only 23 chromosomes. After 2 to 3 days, the spermatocytes undergo a second division to form four spermatids, each with 23 chromosomes, half the original number. This means that the sperm that eventually fertilizes the female ovum contains half the genetic material, while the ovum contains the other half.

The period of spermatogenesis from germinal cell to sperm takes about 74 days. During this time, the spermatocytes lose some cytoplasm, the chromatin material of the head reorganizes to form a compact head, and the remaining cytoplasm and cell membranes collect at one end of the cell to form the tail of the sperm.

Hormonal Stimulation

Testosterone is essential to the growth and division of the germinal cells that form the sperm. LH stimulates Leydig's cells to secrete testosterone. FSH stimulates Sertoli's cells promoting spermatogenesis. Estrogens are formed from testosterone when Sertoli's cells are stimulated by FSH. Estrogen appears to be essential in spermatogenesis. Growth hormone promotes early division of spermatogonia.

Maturation in the Epididymis

After the sperm are formed in the seminiferous tubules, they spend several days passing through the epididymis. After the sperm have spent about 24 hours in the epididymis, they become motile. The sperm also become capable of fertilization, a process called maturation.

Sperm are stored in small amounts in the epididymis but are mainly stored in the vas deferens and the ampulla of the vas deferens. With low levels of sexual activity, the sperm can be stored there up to a month, maintaining their motility and fertility. When sexual activity is frequent, sperm may be stored only a few days.

Prostatic Fluid

The prostate secretes a milky fluid that forms part of the semen. This fluid aids the passage of sperm and helps keep them alive, supplying them with food, if needed. Prostatic secretion is manufactured in a network of branching glands embedded in muscle within the prostate. This muscle contracts during ejaculation, and prostatic secretions are ejected through the ejaculatory ducts into the urethra.

Semen

Semen (seminal fluid or ejaculate) is a viscid, thick, opalescent secretion discharged by males at the climax of sexual excitement or orgasm. It contains sperm and other secretions. About 10% of the semen is composed of sperm and fluid from the vas deferens, with about 60% made up of fluid from the seminal vesicles. The remaining 30% is composed of prostatic fluid and small amounts of mucoid secretion from the bulbourethral glands.

With sexual climax, the fluid and sperm are ejaculated through the urethra. Semen is slightly alkaline, with a pH

of about 7.5. The prostatic fluid contains a clotting enzyme, which causes the fibrinogen of the seminal vesicle fluid to form a weak coagulum that holds the semen near the uterine cervix. The coagulum dissolves in about 15 to 30 minutes, at which time the sperm becomes highly motile. The sperm can live within the vagina for 24 to 48 hours after ejaculation (see Fig. 81–6).

Conclusions

A thorough knowledge of the structure and function of the female and male reproductive systems is important if the nurse is to provide safe, effective care for clients with problems associated with the reproductive system. The nurse must be sensitive to the delicate nature of problems associated with this system, because many disorders affect sexuality.

Bibliography

1. Adashi, E. Y., & Leung, P. C. K. (Eds.). (1993). *The ovary.* New York: Raven Press.
2. Avis, N. E., & McKinley, S. M. (1991). A longitudinal analysis of women's attitudes toward the menopause: Results from the Massachusetts Women's Health Study. *Maturitas, 13,* 65–79.
3. Bates, G. W., & Boone, W. R. (1991). The female reproductive cycle: New variations on an old theme. *Current Opinion in Obstetrics and Gynecology, 3*(6), 838–843.
4. Bennett, J. C., & Plum, F. (Eds.). (1996). *Cecil textbook of medicine* (20th ed.). Philadelphia: W. B. Saunders.
5. Blackledge, G. R. P., Jordan, J. A., & Shingleton, H. M. (1991). *Textbook of gynecologic oncology.* Philadelphia: W. B. Saunders.
6. Buchsbaum, H. J., & Schmidt, J. D. (1993). *Gynecologic and obstetric urology* (3rd ed.). Philadelphia: W. B. Saunders.
7. Christiansen, J. L., & Grzbouski, J. M. (1993). *Biology of aging.* St. Louis: Mosby–Year Book.
8. Comhaire, F. H. (1993). Methods to evaluate reproductive health of the human male. *Reproductive Toxicology, 7*(Suppl. 1), 39–46.
9. Cotran, R. S., Kumar, V., & Robbins, S. L. (1994). *Robbins pathologic basis of disease* (5th ed.). Philadelphia: W. B. Saunders.
10. Copeland, L. J. (Ed.). (1993). *Textbook of gynecology.* Philadelphia: W. B. Saunders.
11. Ferin, M., Jewelewicz, R., & Warren, W. (1993). *The menstrual cycle: Physiology, reproductive disorders, and infertility.* New York: Oxford University Press.
12. Fogel, C. L., & Lauver, D. (Eds.). (1990). *Sexual health promotion.* Philadelphia: W. B. Saunders.
13. Gershenson, D. M., DeCherney, A. H., & Curry, S. L. (Eds.). (1993). *Operative gynecology.* Philadelphia: W. B. Saunders.
14. Guyton, A. C. (1992). *Human physiology and mechanisms of disease* (5th ed.). Philadelphia: W. B. Saunders.
15. Guyton, A. C., & Hall, J. E. (1996). *Textbook of medical physiology* (9th ed.). Philadelphia: W. B. Saunders.
16. Hacker, N. R., & Moore, J. G. (1992). *Essentials of obstetrics and gynecology.* Philadelphia: W. B. Saunders.
17. Hargrove, J. T., & Eisenberg, E. (1995). Menopause. *Medical Clinics of North America, 79*(6), 1337–1356.
18. Harlap, S. (1992). The benefits and risks of hormone replacement therapy: An epidemiologic overview. *American Journal of Obstetrics and Gynecology, 166*(6, pt. 2), 1986–1992.
19. Herbst, A. L., et al. (1992). *Comprehensive gynecology* (2nd ed.). St. Louis: Mosby–Year Book.
20. Jarvis, C. (1996). *Physical examination and health assessment* (2nd ed.). Philadelphia: W. B. Saunders.

21. Karlowicz, K. A. (Ed.). (1995). *Urologic nursing: Principles and practice.* Philadelphia: W. B. Saunders.

22. Knobil, E., & Neill, J. D. (Ed.). (1994). *The physiology of reproduction* (2nd ed.). New York: Raven Press.

23. McCance, K. L., & Huether, S. E. (1994). *Pathophysiology: The biologic basis for disease in adults and children* (2nd ed.). St. Louis: Mosby–Year Book.

24. McKinley, J. B., et al. (1987). Health status and utilization behavior associated with the menopause. *American Journal of Epidemiology, 125*(1), 110–121.

25. Prue, L. K. (1994). *Atlas of mammographic positioning.* Philadelphia: W. B. Saunders.

26. Seeley, R., Stephens, T., & Tate, P. (1995). *Anatomy and physiology* (3rd ed.). St. Louis: Mosby–Year Book.

27. Seidman, E. J. (Eds.). (1994). *Current urologic therapy.* Philadelphia: W. B. Saunders.

28. Smith, D. R. (1992). *General urology* (13th ed.). Los Altos, CA: Lange Medical.

29. Solomon, E. P. (1992). *Introduction to human anatomy and physiology.* Philadelphia: W. B. Saunders.

30. Tanagho, E. A., & McAninich, J. W. (1992). *Smith's general urology.* Norwalk, CT: Appleton & Lange.

31. Thibodeau, G. A., & Patton, K. T. (1992). *Anatomy and physiology* (2nd ed.). St. Louis: Mosby–Year Book.

32. Thibodeau, G. A., & Patton, K. T. (1992). *The human body in health and disease.* St. Louis: Mosby–Year Book.

33. Utian, W. H. (1991). Menopause: A proposed new functional definition. *Maturitas, 14*(1), 1–2.

34. Wagner, G. (1992). Aspects of genital physiology and pathology. *Seminars in Neurology, 12*(2), 87–97.

35. Walsh, P. C., et al. (1992). *Campbell's urology,* (6th ed.). Philadelphia: W. B. Saunders.

36. Yu, H. S. (1994). *Human reproductive biology.* Boca Raton, FL: CRC Press.

Assessment of Clients with Reproductive Disorders

Elizabeth Carlson

Esther Matassarin-Jacobs

Lynne C. Carpenter

Assessment of Clients with Gynecologic Disorders

In recent years there has been an increased emphasis on women's health concerns and on the importance of health promotion activities for women. Because many women receive most, if not all, of their primary healthcare from their obstetric and gynecologic healthcare provider, the scope of gynecologic care needs to broaden. Nurses participating in this area of healthcare must focus not only on the gynecologic condition of the woman but also on her total health maintenance needs. A thorough assessment includes the usual health history and physical examination, as well as a review of the woman's life-style, health habits, self-perception, body image, and developmental stage, with consideration of cultural, religious, socioeconomic, and educational factors. These factors influence the woman's health and health-seeking behaviors. A nonjudgmental attitude and respect for the woman's values will allow the nurse to provide more effective care. The woman's cultural or ethnic background, socioeconomic status, or sexual preference should not limit her access to, or quality of, healthcare.

Approach to Gynecologic Care

Women have the right to be informed and to participate actively in decisions about their health. A supportive, respectful attitude on the part of the nurse promotes the woman's participation in her care and ensures her comfort and cooperation. The nurse is also alert to sexist attitudes in the healthcare system, which may lead to women's health complaints being ignored or to unnecessary or inappropriate prescriptions being written. The nurse can be an advocate for the woman, positively influencing her perception of healthcare and the importance of health maintenance.

Providing privacy and creating an environment that is conducive to the expression of feelings allow a woman to express her concerns openly. It is important to assess the woman's understanding of healthcare information and to elicit her perception of her needs and problems. The nurse may need to repeat information, especially if the woman is anxious or stressed, for example, when information is received during a pelvic examination. Nurses can provide a sensitive, humane orientation to gynecologic healthcare. Through teaching and counseling, nurses provide valuable assistance with health maintenance for women.

The annual gynecologic examination provides opportunity for the nurse to discuss health maintenance activities with women. For example, a health visit for a Papanicolaou (Pap) smear is a good time to teach breast self-examination and to talk about risk factors associated with gynecologic cancer. It is also a good time to provide information about developmental changes such as adolescence, menarche, or menopause, and about menstrual hygiene and menstrual symptom management. Information on life-style factors that affect health maintenance, such as diet, exercise, adequate sleep and rest, stress management, cessation of smoking, and general risk factor identification, should also be discussed. If appropriate, the nurse provides the client with information about protection against sexually transmitted diseases (STDs).

After establishing rapport with the woman, the nurse performs a comprehensive gynecologic nursing assessment appropriate to the situation. (For a review of a comprehensive history and psychosocial assessment, see Chapter 11). A detailed history is followed by a systematic physical examination. The information obtained is the basis for nursing intervention.

History

The health history for the gynecologic system includes data related to the genital organs, the breasts, and other health information that relates to the reproductive system

This chapter incorporates material written for the fourth edition by Ann J. Clark.

and the woman's overall health status. It is preferable to obtain the history from the woman while she is still dressed and in a private area to maintain her level of comfort.

Chief Complaint

Ask the client to describe her reason for seeking gynecologic care. These data alert you to the possible nature of the client's problem, as well as to the level of the client's understanding of the problem. This information provides direction for the remainder of the health history interview as well as for health teaching. If the client has come for a specific problem rather than for a routine examination, ask the client to relate the history of the problem, including a symptom analysis (see Chapter 11).

Past Health History

The client's past health history has many components of significance for the reproductive system. These include childhood and infectious illnesses, major illness and hospitalizations, allergies, gynecologic history, family history, psychosocial history, and review of systems.

Childhood and Infectious Diseases

The most common childhood infectious illness to affect a woman of childbearing age is rubella. Ask the client if she has had rubella or been immunized against it. The woman who is contemplating pregnancy should have a rubella titer drawn to determine whether immunity exists because maternal rubella during the first trimester increases the risk to the fetus of congenital disorders. If the titer is negative (i.e. immunity is lacking), the woman is encouraged to receive an immunization. A woman who is already pregnant should not be immunized. After immunization, advise the client not to become pregnant for at least 3 months.

Major Illnesses and Hospitalizations

Ask the client about major illnesses such as diabetes, hypertension, thrombophlebitis, angina, anemia, thyroid disorders, cholecystitis, hepatitis, and migraine headaches. Diabetes is associated with increased morbidity and mortality in women who are pregnant or who take oral contraceptives. Pregnancy and oral contraceptive use are also linked with higher morbidity and mortality rates in women with a history of cardiovascular disease such as angina, hypertension, and thrombophlebitis. Anemia can result from menstrual disorders such as dysfunctional uterine bleeding, or it can be aggravated by normal menstruation, depending on the heaviness of flow. Endometrial implants (endometriosis) can cause painful menstruation and fertility problems so that the woman who wants

to become pregnant may need medication or surgery to reduce or remove the implants. Hypothyroidism and hyperthyroidism affect the menstrual cycle, as can other endocrine disorders. Renal and urinary tract disorders can interfere with sexual function.

Women with a history of migraine headaches or seizure disorders should avoid oral contraceptives because of the increased risk of migraines associated with their use. Cholecystitis may be aggravated by oral contraceptives; hepatitis and other liver disorders are a contraindication to estrogen because of its route of metabolism. The progesterones in oral contraceptives thicken respiratory secretions, which complicates the treatment of women with asthma or chronic obstructive respiratory disorders. Estrogens are generally contraindicated in women who have had breast cancer or cancers of the reproductive tract.

Ask the client about surgery involving the reproductive system. Specific surgical procedures include dilation and curettage (D & C), tubal ligation, cryosurgery or cryotherapy, cystocele and rectocele repair, hysterectomy, oophorectomy, and salpingectomy. Inquire about interruptions to pregnancies, such as planned or spontaneous abortions.

Medications

Ask the patient for a complete medication history. This includes prescription and over-the-counter medications as well as recreational or illegal substances that the woman takes. Contraceptive medications can include oral contraceptives, medroxyprogesterone (Depo-Provera) injections, and vaginal preparations. Ask about episodic medications, such as those used for menstrual and premenstrual discomforts (e.g., diuretics), and the clients use of herbal or other "natural" substances. Ask specifically about hormone replacement therapy (e.g., estrogen, progesterone, thyroid, corticosteroids). Recreational or illegal substances, such as alcohol, amphetamines, barbiturates, marijuana, and hallucinogens, may affect a person's sexual behavior and risk status for exposure to an STD.

Allergies

Ask the client about allergies to antibiotics, spermicides, and latex or rubber. Genitourinary infections are treated with antibiotics. Latex and rubber are used in contraceptive devices such as condoms and diaphragms, which are used in conjunction with spermicides. Allergies to these substances eliminate their use for contraception by these clients. Be alert and use vinyl gloves, instead of latex, during the physical examination.

Gynecologic History

The gynecologic history is discussed in the following paragraphs. For the menopausal or elderly woman or the woman who has had a hysterectomy, ask only the appropriate questions.

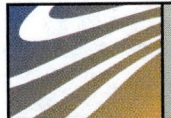

ETHICAL ISSUES IN NURSING

Should Pregnant Women Who Engage in Substance Abuse Be Held Liable for Damage to the Fetus?

The rights of procreation are continually challenged as technology allows more and more reproductive options. Much controversy exists around reproductive issues such as abortion, in vitro fertilization, surrogate motherhood, sperm banks, and genetic selection (to name a few). There is, however, controversy surrounding the right to reproduce that does not involve any modern technology. This controversy surrounds the responsibilities of the mother to her unborn baby.

Pregnant women who engage in substance abuse often are directly responsible for physical and mental handicaps that their babies are born with. These babies, who might otherwise have been healthy, will live their lives with disabilities that could have been prevented had their mothers not abused drugs or alcohol. Should such women be legally prosecuted for the harm they have inflicted on their children? Although a woman has a right to do with her own body what she wants, abusing toxic substances does not simply affect her body alone. Should a woman who gives birth to a baby addicted to cocaine and perhaps disabled for life be ordered by the courts not to procreate ever again? Is court-ordered sterilization ever ethically justified? Society has an obligation to help care for its members who are physically and mentally handicapped. Does society also have a responsibility to see that its members are not treated in such ways that intentional physical and mental handicaps result in order not to overburden the society? (Intentional means that had substance abuse not occurred, perhaps the handicaps might not have either.)

Nurses who care for babies and children who are handicapped from maternal substance abuse may develop negative feelings toward the parents of such babies and children. It is hard to see the innocent suffer, no matter what the cause. It is very important that caregivers in these situations express their concerns and emotions in an arena in which it is safe to do so, for instance, in team care conferences or informal sessions with a peer or social worker.

Breast History

Ask the client about breast pain or tenderness and its occurrence in relation to the menstrual cycle. Many women experience breast tenderness before menses onset as a result of hormonal changes. Inquire whether the woman has had or currently has breast lumps or masses. If a lump is present, ask the woman to describe its location, onset, and size, and whether it is painful. Determine if the lump has changed shape, size, consistency, or in the amount of tenderness since it was first noticed and if the lump changes with the menstrual cycle. Ask the woman the date of her last menstrual period in order to better evaluate a breast lump. The breasts become more firm and cystic during the luteal phase so that the best time to perform breast palpation is 7 to 10 days after onset of menses.

Ask about discharge from the nipple. Nipple discharge is abnormal in women who are not pregnant or lactating. If discharge is present, determine the color, consistency, amount, and odor.

Inquire about the practice of breast self-examination on a monthly basis. Ask not only about frequency of performance but also about technique to determine if the woman could benefit from a review of the procedure and supervised practice. Note whether the woman includes the axillary nodes as part of her self-examination. Last, ask if there is a history of breast cancer in blood-related female relatives, such as mother, sister(s), maternal grandmother, or maternal aunt(s). Incidence of breast cancer in these relatives increases a woman's risk of breast cancer.

Menstrual History

Ask the woman at what age she started menstruating. Ask the date of her last menstrual period; this is the first day of the most recent cycle. Ask the number of days per cycle and the regularity of her cycle. Have her describe the amount of flow by counting the number and type of pads or tampons used in 24 hours. Determine whether there are clots in the flow. Ask how long the menstrual period lasts. Ask if she experiences dysmenorrhea; if so, have her describe the pain, the duration, whether it occurs with every cycle, and what she uses for relief. Ask if she experiences midcycle bleeding, spotting, or pain. Are there any premenstrual manifestations? Does she have any menopausal manifestations, including menstrual cycle changes or manifestations of hormonal changes?

Contraceptive History

Document the woman's current contraceptive method (if any), her satisfaction with the method, duration of use, any contraceptive problems, and any desire to change methods. Ask about previous contraceptive methods, problems encountered, and reason for discontinuation. Ask if she wants any contraceptive information. For a woman of reproductive age, not sterilized, and heterosexually active, determine whether she wants to become pregnant.

Sexual History

Obtain a sexual history using a direct approach and terms the woman understands. The purpose of a sexual history is to identify sexual problems and give the woman an opportunity to ask questions or express concerns. Begin with general questions about whether the woman is satisfied and comfortable with her current sexual activity. A nonjudgmental approach is essential; make no assumptions about anything, including the sex or number of partners. Follow up on any concerns or issues she raises (Table 82–1). Of particular importance are difficulties or concerns she may have. Be alert for any risk-taking behaviors, including those putting her at risk of STDs. See Chapter 11 for further information on sexuality assessment.

Obstetric History

If the woman is in her childbearing years, ask if she thinks she may be pregnant. (Pregnancy may contraindicate mammography or other radiologic studies, as well as certain medications.) If the woman has been pregnant, obtain information about each pregnancy, including the delivery and postpartum period. Document details of any difficulties or complications (physical or psychosocial). Record any spontaneous or planned abortions. If the woman has never been pregnant, ask whether children were or are desired. If the woman has relinquished a child for adoption, explore her feelings about it. See Chapter 11 for detailed questions to assess the obstetric history.

Past Gynecologic and Genitourinary History

Ask about previous problems with genitourinary infections and vaginitis. Determine whether the woman has had a previous pelvic infection or STD and how it was treated (see Chapter 86 for more information on STDs). Were there any problems or complications as a result of this? Determine whether the woman experiences urinary incontinence and the circumstances when incontinence occurs (see Chapter 56 for a discussion of urinary incontinence).

Reproductive Health Practices

Seek information about menstrual, sexual, and gynecologic hygiene, including douching. Ask about the frequency of gynecologic examinations. If appropriate, ask if she protects herself against STDs and unwanted pregnancy.

Family Health History

A family history of diabetes, cardiovascular disease, or cancer of a reproductive organ may indicate that the woman is at a higher risk of developing those diseases. If the woman's mother received diethylstilbestrol (DES) during her pregnancy with the client, the woman may be at risk of cancer or structural and functional changes in the reproductive tract.

Psychosocial History

Occupation and Environment

Ask the woman about any exposures to toxins or radiation, including hazards encountered at work. Many substances can affect overall health status generally and reproductive function specifically.

Habits

Ask the client whether she smokes cigarettes. Smoking is associated with an increase in morbidity when used with oral contraceptives and also may be related to an earlier than normal onset of menopause. The use of alcohol and recreational drugs is also ascertained.

Domestic Violence

Asks if the woman is a victim of domestic violence. You should ask every client if there is violence in her life. It is important to explain to clients that the same question is asked of all women and that they are not being singled out because of race, nationality, or socioeconomic status. This is also a good time to educate women about options that exist for them should violence be or become a problem.

Psychosocial Factors

For many women, the genital organs and reproductive capacity have symbolic significance. Thus, problems in this area can affect a woman's sexuality and sense of femininity. Gynecologic problems may be associated with changes in a woman's self-concept, body image, personal identity, and role performance. Reproductive capabilities and the experience of sexuality and sexual activities may be affected. There may be psychological consequences for some women experiencing gynecologic disorders. For this reason, psychological assessment is especially important. A woman's outward reaction to gynecologic problems does not necessarily correlate with either her inner experience or the seriousness of the condition.

Sensitivity is vital in interviewing and examining a woman. Do not press the client for information that she appears hesitant to reveal. Remember that the woman herself may not understand her own responses. Empathic listening is supportive, often lessening the stress the woman feels.

Fear may be expressed because of a suspicion the woman holds of unhealthy changes in the genitals or of unwanted pregnancy. There may be anxiety and embarrassment in anticipation of a pelvic examination. Women may consider the pelvic examination unpleasant despite the insignificant risk of injury or physical pain. Other feelings that may be expressed include humiliation, guilt, or anger. In the event of deep, powerful feelings, women may avoid seeking gynecologic care. It has been suggested that intrusive gynecologic procedures may evoke

Table 82–1. Sexual Health Assessment

Sexual health assessment may include consideration of the client's current

- Knowledge about sexuality
- Attitudes about sexuality and toward sexual partner(s)
- Level of comfort and feelings of adequacy regarding own sexuality
- Concerns about sexuality of significant others
- Perception of own sex role and that of sexual partner(s)
- Sexual self-concept as a female or male
- Fears and anxiety about intimacy and other aspects of sexuality
- Self-perception of own body (body image)
- Ability to function sexually, e.g., to obtain an erection and control ejaculation, to please sexual partner, to achieve pain-free orgasm, to reproduce, to obtain adequate contraception, to obtain sufficient vaginal lubrication, to give and receive effective sexual stimulation and pleasure
- Typical sexual patterns and activities, e.g., partner choice (female, male, spouse, extramarital, multiple, single, same partner, different partners), frequency of sexual activity, type of sexual activity (vaginal, anal, oral, masturbation), partner satisfaction, self-satisfaction
- Level of interest in sexual activity (sex drive)
- Level of satisfaction regarding current sexual opportunity and activity
- Physical health problems affecting sexuality, e.g., menstrual problems, pregnancy, medication, surgery (colostomy, surgical amputation, recent heart surgery or brain surgery), paralysis, illness (hypertension, diabetes, recent myocardial infarction, "stroke"), injury (recent spinal cord injury, recent head injury, burns, traumatic amputations), sexually transmitted disease, genitourinary problems

Sexual History

There is no single approach to taking a sexual health history. Information obtained may relate to historical (past) information about the following:

Both Females and Males

- Pregnancies (information about unplanned pregnancies)
- Fertility management
- Genitourinary problems
- Sexually transmitted disease
- Sexual abuse, e.g., incest, rape, pedophilia, battering
- Relationship-partner history, e.g., number of sexual partners, sexual orientation (bisexual, homosexual, heterosexual)
- First experience of sexual activity
- Early sexual development and influences
- Adolescent sexual experiences
- Sexual techniques used, e.g., masturbation, intercourse (oral, vaginal, anal)
- Role models for sexuality, e.g., peers, parents, guardians, famous people, advertising models
- Spiritual-philosophical models influencing the client's sexuality

Females

History specific to menstruation, abortion, pregnancy

Males

History specific to impotence, noctural emissions

---

memories or strong reactions in women who have experienced childhood sexual abuse or sexual assault. The opportunity to express and discuss feelings with a nurse skilled in therapeutic communication may help these women cope more effectively and follow through with appropriate care. A therapeutic conversation can provide opportunities for clarifying a woman's misconceptions about her diagnosis, proposed treatment, and preventive care. Many women have never received accurate information about reproductive problems.

Review of Systems

Before the physical examination, review the physical health history, proceeding from head to toe. Areas of particular concern to the reproductive system for women include the cardiovascular system (hypertension, angina, myocardial infarction, and thrombophlebitis if oral contraceptives are taken concurrently); endocrine disorders such as hypo- and hyperthyroidism and disorders of the pitui-

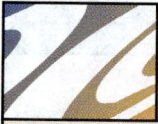

NORMAL PHYSICAL ASSESSMENT FINDINGS

Female Reproductive System

Inspection

Pubic hair distribution varies with stage of sexual development; clean, coarse. Labia majora covered with pubic hair in adult women; may gape open slightly. Labia minora pink, smooth. Clitoris midline, smooth. Urethral meatus pink, discharge absent. Vaginal orifice clean, without bulges. Vaginal walls intact, pink, glistening, rugae present; discharge, bulges, and masses absent. Cervix round with os round or oval in nulliparous women and slitlike in parous women; discharge absent.

Palpation

Pelvic floor musculature firm. Skene's glands without discharge or tenderness. Bartholin's glands without masses or tenderness. No bulges in vaginal wall with straining. Uterus anteverted, firm, smooth, mobile, nontender; without masses. Ovaries oval, firm, mobile, nontender.

---

tary gland; and liver disorders and cholecystitis. In addition, ask about problems involving the urinary tract and reproductive system such as urinary tract infection, urinary incontinence, vaginitis, and any bleeding disorders associated with menstruation (e.g., amenorrhea, dysmenorrhea, breakthrough bleeding, menorrhagia, postcoital bleeding). Detailed questions for the review of systems are found in Box 11–2.

Physical Examination

A standard gynecologic examination includes the following physical assessment and laboratory data:

- Vital signs (temperature, pulse, respiration, blood pressure)
- Height
- Weight
- Complete blood count
- Urinalysis
- Pelvic examination and Pap smear
- Physical assessment of heart, lungs, breasts and axillae, thyroid, and abdomen

See Chapter 44 for cardiac assessment, Chapter 39 for respiratory assessment, Chapter 68 for endocrine assessment, and Chapter 59 for assessment of the abdomen. Physical examination of the breasts and axillae and the reproductive organs follows. Unusual or abnormal findings obtained during the gynecologic history or physical examination require additional data. (See Chapter 12 for details of general physical assessment techniques.)

Examination of the Breasts and Axillae

The breast and axillae examination is an important part of the annual gynecologic examination. Good lighting is essential. Some examiners complete this portion of the examination before assessing the anterior lungs and heart. Because the breasts are sensitive and closely associated with sexuality, some nurses delay examining them until there has been more hands-on interaction with the client during the lungs and heart assessments. Others integrate the assessments so that the client is sitting for those portions of the heart, lungs, breasts, and axillae examination before being assisted to a supine position for the remaining portions. Any sequence is acceptable as long as the nurse is thorough, the client's privacy is maintained, and the client can tolerate the position changes. The nurse instructs the client in breast self-examination while performing it. See Chapter 84 for further information about breast self-examination.

The nurse asks the client when the last menstrual period began. Breasts are usually tender the week before onset of menses and least tender the week after. If the client reports that one breast is tender, the nurse begins palpation with the opposite breast. Thorough examination requires the client to have both breasts exposed for comparison.

Inspection

Breast inspection begins with the client seated with her arms at her sides. Then ask the client to raise her hands over her head. Finally, ask the client to press her hands firmly on her hips or together to tighten the pectoral muscles. Women with large or pendulous breasts are examined leaning forward at the waist and facing forward with the breasts hanging down (Fig. 82–1). The breasts are inspected for symmetry, size, shape, contour, and skin characteristics, including the vascular pattern, in all positions.

Breasts are symmetrical although it is not unusual for one breast to be slightly larger than the other. They should hang evenly between the third and fourth ribs with the nipples approximately level with the fourth intercostal space when the client sits with her arms at her sides. With aging and loss of tissue elasticity, the breasts hang lower, especially after pregnancy and breast-feeding. The contour is even, without manifestations of dimpling (retraction), masses, or surface flattening, which are abnormal. Skin color is the same as that of the abdomen. *Striae* (i.e., stretch marks from rapid skin stretching) may be present; recent striae are reddened, but they become paler with time. If venous patterns are noticeable, they should be symmetrical. There should be no local areas of hyperpigmentation or edema.

Ask the client to raise her arms over her head while you examine the lateral and undersurfaces of each breast. The contraction of the pectoral muscles will emphasize any manifestations of retraction or skin flattening. Areas of redness or excoriation may be noted in women with

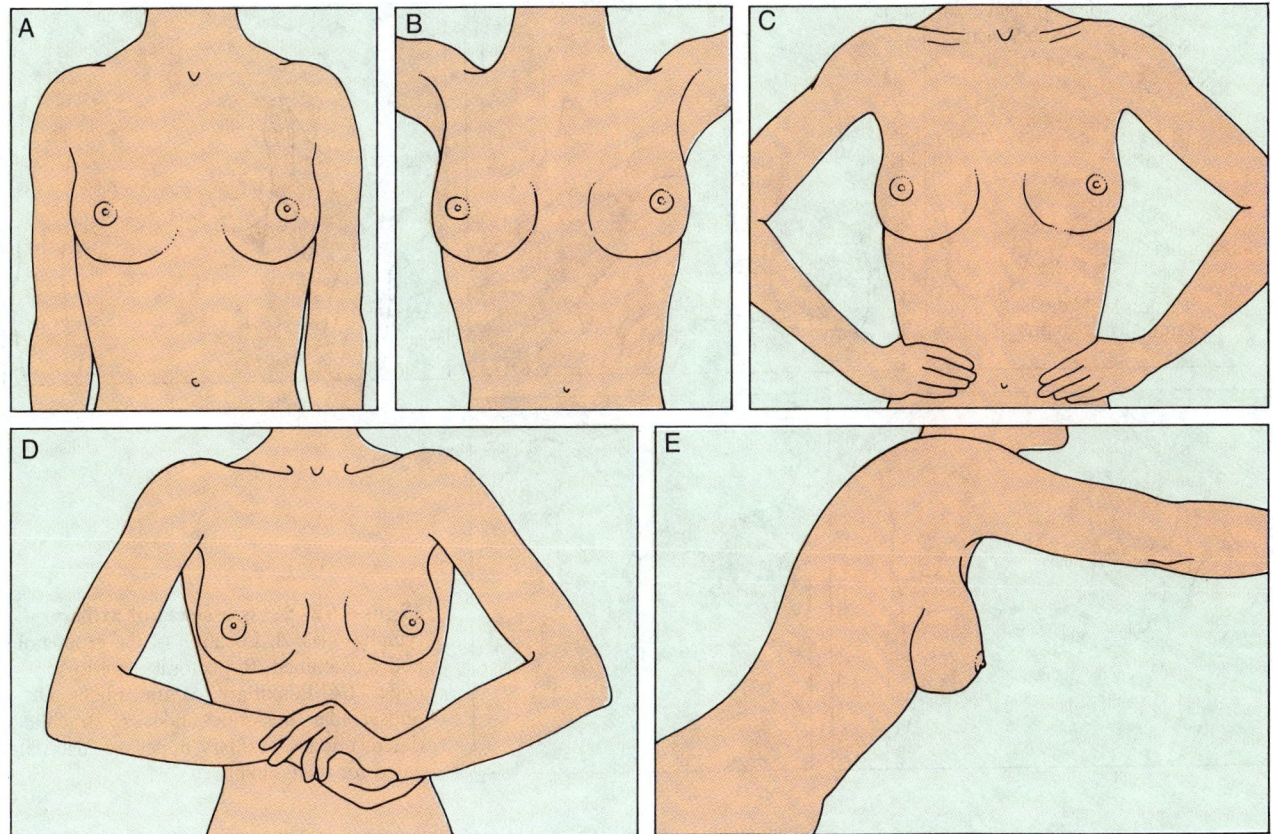

Figure 82–1. Positions for breast examination. *A*, Arms at sides. *B*, Hands raised over head. For tightening pectoral muscles, the examiner asks the client to press hands firmly on hips (*C*) or to press hands together (*D*). *E*, Breasts may also be examined with the woman leaning forward at the waist, allowing the breasts to hang down.

large breasts from brassiere rubbing or from underwires in poorly fitting brassieres. The breasts should elevate evenly so that the areolae remain at the same level. Then ask the client to put her hands on her hips and press inward firmly while you repeat the inspection for masses, retraction, or skin flattening.

The *areolae* and *nipples* are inspected for size, shape and contour, symmetry, surface characteristics, and masses or lesions. Areolae are pink in fair-skinned women and darker in dark-skinned women. Slight asymmetry is common, but the nipples should point in symmetrical directions. Masses or lesions are abnormal. There may be prominence of *Montgomery's tubercles* around the nipple, which is normal. The nipples are round or oval, equal in size, of the same color, soft, and smooth. If one or both nipples are inverted, ask whether this is a recent occurrence or has been present for a while and how long. Recent nipple inversion is abnormal, and the client is referred to the physician for follow-up. There should be no rashes, crusts, or discharge unless the client is in the late stages of pregnancy, when colostrum (a yellowish fluid) may leak from the nipples.

The *axillae* are inspected for rashes, masses, and areas of unusual pigmentation, which should be absent. Axillary hair is present unless the client removes it by shaving or with a depilatory.

Palpation

Palpation of axillae is done while the client is seated; breast palpation is facilitated with the client supine. Clients with large and pendulous breasts, with a history of breast masses or cancer, or who are at increased risk of breast cancer should have their breasts palpated in both positions.

Palpation of the axillae includes examination of five sets of *lymph nodes,* which are illustrated in Figure 82–2. Encourage the client to relax her arm, which assists in relaxing the muscles and eases palpation. Begin by palpating the edge of the pectoralis major muscle along the anterior axillary line, using a bimanual technique, if necessary, to examine the *pectoral (anterior) nodes.* Then reach high up into the axilla at the midaxillary line to palpate the *midaxillary (central) nodes* against the ribs and serratus anterior. Palpate the *subscapular (posterior) nodes* along the posterior axillary fold along the anterior edge of the latissimus dorsi. Palpate the *brachial (lateral) nodes* along the upper inner arm along the humerus. Last, palpate the *infraclavicular area.* The *supraclavicular nodes,* which receive lymphatic drainage from the breasts, are usually examined with the neck nodes. All the nodes should be nonpalpable, although the detection of one or

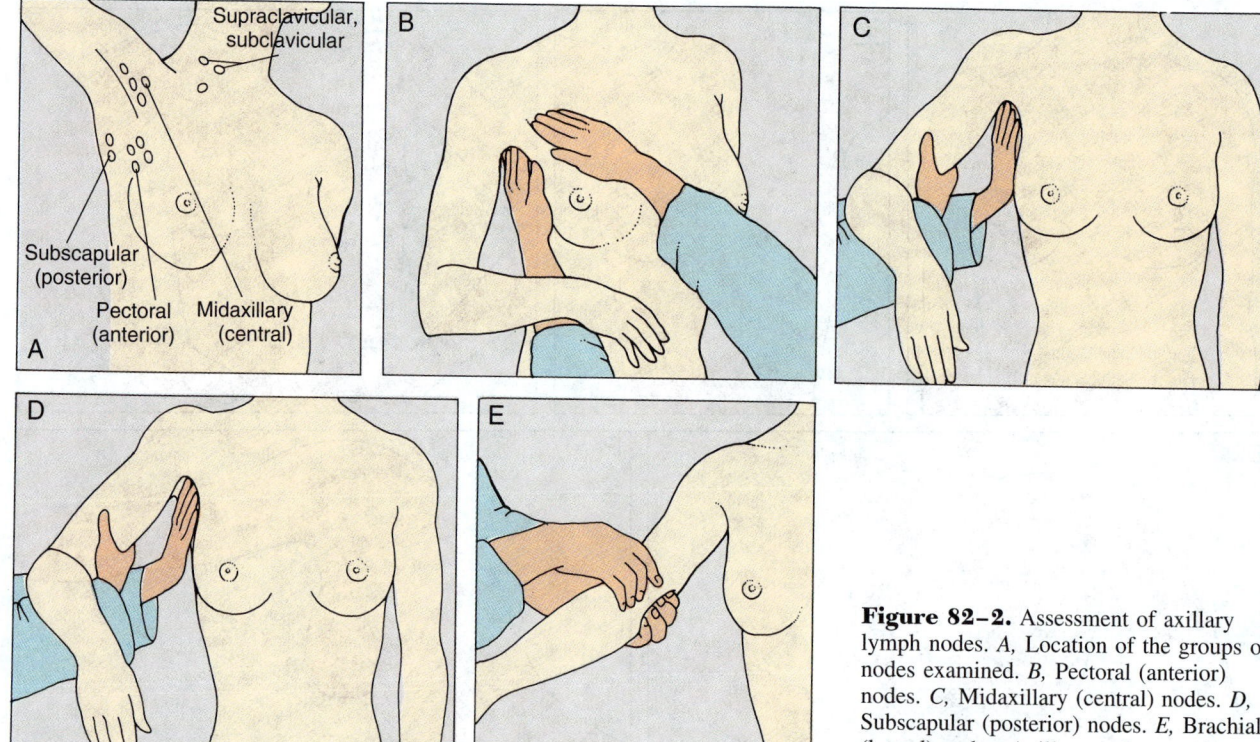

Figure 82–2. Assessment of axillary lymph nodes. *A,* Location of the groups of nodes examined. *B,* Pectoral (anterior) nodes. *C,* Midaxillary (central) nodes. *D,* Subscapular (posterior) nodes. *E,* Brachial (lateral) nodes. Axillary nodes are also palpated for male clients.

two small, nontender, mobile central nodes is often a normal finding. Abnormal findings include firm, fixed nodes that may or may not be tender. If nodes are palpated, note the number of nodes felt, their location, size, shape, mobility, tenderness, and consistency.

Breast palpation is conducted systematically so that all breast tissue, including the *tail of Spence* in the upper outer quadrant, is examined. Any one of several approaches may be used as long as each portion of the breasts, areolae, and nipples is palpated. The breast and areola may be palpated in concentric circles, in a wheel-and-spokes pattern, or back and forth from superior to inferior. When the client is sitting, you may prefer to use a bimanual technique, especially if the breasts are large. When supine, place a small folded towel under the client's shoulder to enhance breast flattening against the chest wall, and have her place her arm behind her head.

Slide your fingers along the tissue using a rotary motion to press the breast against the chest wall. Your fingers remain in contact with the skin surface. You will feel a firm, curved ridge along the inferior breast, which is the *inframammary ridge.* Breast consistency varies from firm and elastic in young women to stringy and nodular in older women. If the client reports a mass, begin palpation with the unaffected breast so that there is a basis for comparison. Pay particular attention to the upper outer quadrant and tail of Spence, where most of the glandular tissue is located and 50% of breast lesions are found. There should be no masses or local areas of warmth. If you feel a lump or mass, note its characteristics, including the exact location (and the position the client is in for the palpation) with the areola for a reference point, and its size, shape, contour, consistency, mo-

bility, tenderness, and discreteness. The breast can be visualized as having four quadrants plus the tail; the location of lesions can be diagrammed in the written record.

The areola and nipple are palpated gently. Compress the nipple between the thumb and index finger. There should be no discharge. Erection and wrinkling of the nipple with manipulation is normal.

Breast Self-Examination

Breast self-examination (BSE) is a technique that all women can use to assess their own breasts. The American Cancer Society (ACS) recommends that all women over the age of 20 perform monthly BSE.[2] Teaching the skills of BSE can be life-saving and is one of nursing's most important activities. With regular BSE, malignancy may be discovered early and treated. Regular monthly BSE is an essential health maintenance activity.

Women familiar with their breasts easily note the development of breast abnormalities early. Nurses have many opportunities to encourage and educate men and women about this important health maintenance procedure. Individualized instruction in BSE that guides the client in self-examination produces more thorough BSE performance than films, pamphlets, or posters. As with any teaching procedure, get a return demonstration and allow time for discussion and questions.

Emphasize to clients that the breasts easily lend themselves to self-examination by palpation and inspection in a mirror. Sexual partners may help perform breast examinations.

Techniques of BSE for a woman are described in Figure 82–3. As part of BSE instruction, educate the client about the risk factors for breast cancer (see Chapter 85). Each woman should be aware of her own risk factors. Emphasize the importance of obtaining professional con- sultation as soon as breast abnormalities are noted. It is important not to delay. Mention the following statistics: (1) 80% of breast lumps are not cancer[1,45]; (2) women who were taught and practiced BSE had tumors more

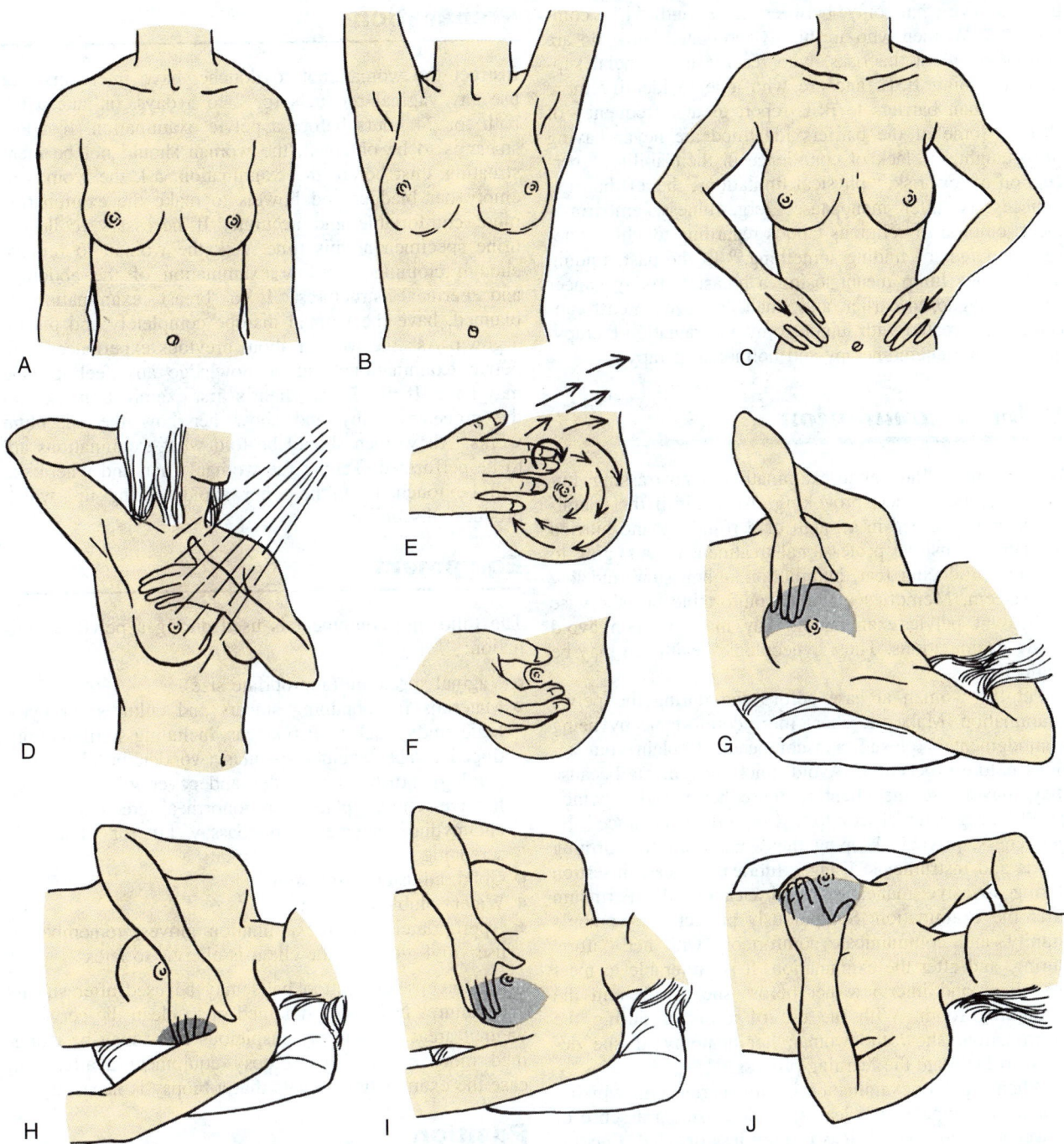

Figure 82–3. Self-examination of female breasts and axillae. Accomplished by observation and palpation. Various positions are assumed for observation while standing in front of a mirror. *A,* Arms relaxed at sides. Next, lean forward. *B,* Raise arms high overhead. Press arms behind head. *C,* Rest palms on hips and firmly press inward to flex chest muscles. *D,* In shower, examine breast contours. *E,* Method of palpating breast. With fingers flat, gently press with small circular motions around an imaginary clock face, that is, begin at 12 o'clock. Move an inch at a time toward the nipple. *F,* As a final step, squeeze the nipple gently between the thumb and index finger. Palpation of the breast is accomplished while lying down. *G,* Position to examine inner breast. *H,* Position to examine axilla. *I,* Position to examine outer breast. *J,* Entire process is repeated for opposite breast and axilla. (See text for discussion of technique and observations.)

amenable to treatment at diagnosis than women with breast cancer who did not perform BSE[49]; (3) one study showed that after 5 years, 75% of women who performed BSE were alive compared with only 57% of those who did not.[22] BSE definitely contributes to the early detection and improved survival of clients with breast cancer.

All women should do monthly BSE. However, studies have shown that only between 27% and 51% comply.[21,50,59] Women who are highly motivated and who are concerned about the risks, who receive more social support for doing BSE, and are who able to identify more benefits than barriers to BSE report greater frequency of BSE.[14] Some of the barriers identified are never having been taught,[27,42] lack of confidence in their ability,[26] perception of low risk,[50] physical limitations,[5] belief that it is unnecessary after menopause, forgetfulness, embarrassment, cultural or religious taboos regarding touching oneself, and fear of finding something.[60] In the past, finding a cancerous lump meant losing a breast.[26] Today cancer can be diagnosed earlier, and small, localized breast cancer can be treated with lumpectomy and radiation therapy, and possibly chemotherapy and hormonal therapy.

Pelvic Examination

Women often find pelvic examinations embarrassing, humiliating, and anxiety-provoking, especially if the examination is performed in a rough or perfunctory and hurried manner. Insensitive professional treatment is damaging to women, producing fear, humiliation, submission, and low self-esteem. Memories of an uncomfortable or otherwise unpleasant pelvic examination may make women avoid future examinations. Thus, gynecologic healthcare may be neglected.

Put the woman at ease before and during the pelvic examination. Make the client more comfortable by being nonjudgmental, relaxed, and competent. Explain your actions before proceeding. Avoid quick movements because they may cause the client to tense her muscles, which results in greater discomfort. Comfort is enhanced by gentleness, privacy, keeping the woman warm, warming hands and instruments, using a lubricant to ease insertion during invasive maneuvers, and cleaning the perineum after the examination. Scrupulously protect the woman's dignity, and communicate comfortably with her before, during, and after the examination. It is preferable to meet the client and interview her before she disrobes in the examining room. With the use of a mirror during the examination, show the woman her anatomy, if she desires, to facilitate the learning process.

When a pelvic examination is an experience in which a woman participates and learns, while retaining a sense of power and self-control, it is usually less dreaded. Encourage the woman to ask questions and express her concerns, feelings, and wishes. Some women are afraid the examiner will detect their sexual "secrets" from a pelvic examination. Make an effort to provide these clients with a sense of control over self-disclosure so they do not feel the nurse is prying or can "read their past."

Remain professional and avoid actions or remarks that may be misconstrued by the client as demeaning or sexu-ally provocative (e.g., using a firm touch instead of gentle stroking). Be aware that the client may become sexually stimulated and alter the sequence of the examination, if necessary, but continue in a professional manner. Some facilities mandate that a male examiner be accompanied by a woman assistant when examining a woman.

Preparation

Instruct the woman not to douche, have intercourse, or use any vaginal products for 2 to 3 days, or take a tub bath for 24 hours before a pelvic examination. If a Pap smear is to be obtained, the woman should not be menstruating. Just before the examination, ask the woman to empty her bladder and bowels to make the examination more comfortable and accurate. If necessary, collect a urine specimen at this time. Ask the woman to remove enough clothing to allow examination of the abdomen and perineal structures. If a breast examination is planned, have the woman disrobe completely and put on a gown. Ask the woman about previous experiences with pelvic examinations and acknowledge any feelings she may have. If this is the client's first examination, explain the procedure fully and show her how the speculum works. All women should be told what examinations are to be performed. Telling the woman when and where she will be touched can help her avoid tensing up, which produces discomfort.

Equipment

The following equipment is used during a pelvic examination:

- Vaginal speculum (appropriate size)
- Materials for obtaining smears and cultures for cytologic study, such as Pap smear, including sterile cotton-tipped swabs, vaginal spatulas (wooden or plastic) or cytology brush, glass slides and cover glass, cytology fixative, culture plates for gonorrhea screening, and a chlamydial enzyme immunoassay kit for chlamydia screening
- Good, adjustable light source
- Water-soluble lubricant
- Appropriately sized examination gloves; remember to use vinyl gloves if the client is allergic to latex

Long forceps and cotton balls may be used after smears and cultures have been obtained or to clean the cervix or vaginal areas so that any suspicious areas may be examined more easily. Have biopsy equipment available in case the examination reveals that a biopsy is necessary.

Position

The client is assisted in assuming a dorsal recumbent or lithotomy position and kept draped until the nurse is ready to proceed. In the lithotomy position, the woman's buttocks need to be flush with the end of the table. The client does not have to put her feet into stirrups if only the external genitalia are examined. Assist the client to flex and abduct her hips and knees with her arms at her sides or crossed over the chest. Adjust the height and distance of the stirrups from the examination table to match the woman's height. Being in a lithotomy position with one's perineum exposed is uncomfortable and embarrassing. Do not keep a woman exposed any longer than necessary. The client's head may be elevated on a small pillow for comfort. Clients who have lower back pain or a hip deformity may be unable to assume this position; an alternative position, such as Sims, will then be necessary (see Fig. 12–6), or have an assistant help the client abduct one or both legs. There must be an adjustable light source. Wear nonsterile, disposable examining gloves (latex unless the client has a latex allergy, in which case vinyl).

Technique

The nurse, with special preparation, may perform the complete pelvic examination. Two nurses should be present during a pelvic examination, and one should be a woman, to protect the examiner against accusations of sexual abuse. While the examiner is performing the examination, the second nurse offers the woman emotional support and gives aid during the examination. A consistent sequence should be followed during the pelvic examination. Consideration of the client's comfort is important at all times.

External Examination

Inspect the external genitalia and perineum (Fig. 82–4A). Assess secondary sexual characteristics (e.g., pubic hair distribution, developmental stage of external genitalia) during examination of the external genitalia and rectum because these areas are uncovered at this time. Before touching the client's perineum, place one hand on the client's thigh to avoid startling her. The *mons pubis* is a mound of tissue superior to the labia. In adults it is usually covered by *pubic hair* distributed as an inverse triangle over the mons, anterior perineum, and medial aspects of the upper thighs. The hair is inspected for nits and the skin for parasites, irritation, inflammation, edema, and lesions. There should be no offensive odor present. Any discharge should be scanty and clear.

Perineal skin is slightly darker than the rest of the body. The *labia majora* are symmetrical rounded, and full. If the client has had a previous vaginal delivery, the labia majora gape slightly and the *labia minora* are evident. After menopause, the labia majora slowly atrophy. They should be free of edema, inflammation, and lesions. The labia minora are thinner than the labia majora, and one side may be larger than the other. Gently separate the labia to inspect the vulva and remaining external structures. Place the thumb and index finger of your nondominant hand inside the labia minora and retract the tissues laterally. A firm hold is needed to avoid unnecessary manipulation of sensitive tissues.

Inspect the clitoris, urethral meatus, hymen (if present), and vaginal orifice (introitus); discharge, inflammation, edema, or lesions, should be absent. The *clitoris* is approximately 1 cm wide and 2 cm long and the same color

as the rest of the vulva. It can be the site of syphilitic chancres in young women, and the site of dry, scaly, nodular lesions that are malignant in older women. When examining the *introitus,* also inspect the *hymen,* which is just inside the introitus. The hymen may be prominent and restrict the vaginal opening in a virgin, or mostly absent in a sexually active client. *Bartholin's glands* are found near the posterior of the introitus and normally are not visualized or palpable. If inflammation and edema are present near the posterior introitus, palpate each gland between thumb and index finger. Insert the index finger into the introitus and rotate it laterally and posteriorly (see Fig. 82–4B). Palpate the gland against the thumb at the posterior aspect of the labia majora. Repeat the maneuver for the other side.

The *urethral meatus* is between the clitoris and introitus and can be difficult to locate, particularly in women who have had a vaginal delivery. It is a small slit just above the vaginal opening and the same color as surrounding tissues. In women who have had several vaginal deliveries, the opening may be located just inside the vaginal orifice. The meatus should be free of discharge, inflammation, or swelling. If these are present, palpate *Skene's glands* (paraurethral glands), which are at both sides of the urethral meatus (Fig. 82–4C). They are usually not visualized or palpable. Insert a gloved index finger palm up into the introitus and approximately 1 inch (2.5 cm) into the vagina. Then press gently upward to palpate the glands and note their characteristics. Draw the index finger along the vaginal wall as it is removed from the vagina so that any discharge is "milked" from the glands into the urethra and out the meatus. If a discharge is present, collect a specimen for culture and change gloves before proceeding further with the examination.

Vaginal Speculum Examination

Wearing gloves, insert a prewarmed vaginal speculum gently into the vagina (Fig. 82–5) *without* lubricants (lubricants interfere with the accuracy of various cytologic examinations, such as the Pap smear). An appropriately sized speculum is selected; specula differ in width and depth. Vaginal speculum insertion is easier and more comfortable for the woman if the speculum is warmed in warm water. If a lubricant is used, use a water-soluble lubricant. Place the index and middle fingers of your nondominant hand in the vaginal orifice and gently pull posteriorly. Insert the closed speculum at a 45-degree angle with the tip pointing downward into the vaginal orifice over your fingers (Fig. 82–5A). Withdraw the fingers while slowly rotating the speculum downward into the vagina until the handle is in a vertical position and insert the speculum to its base (see Fig. 82–5B). Open the blades to observe the vaginal walls and cervix (see Fig. 82–5C and D). Offer the woman a mirror if she wants to see her cervix.

Vaginal *mucous membranes* are moist and pink, without discharge. If a discharge is present, it should be thin and white to clear in color. Abnormal findings include dry or inflamed mucosa; a discharge that is thick, curdy, yellow, green, odorous, or profuse; ulcers; lesions;

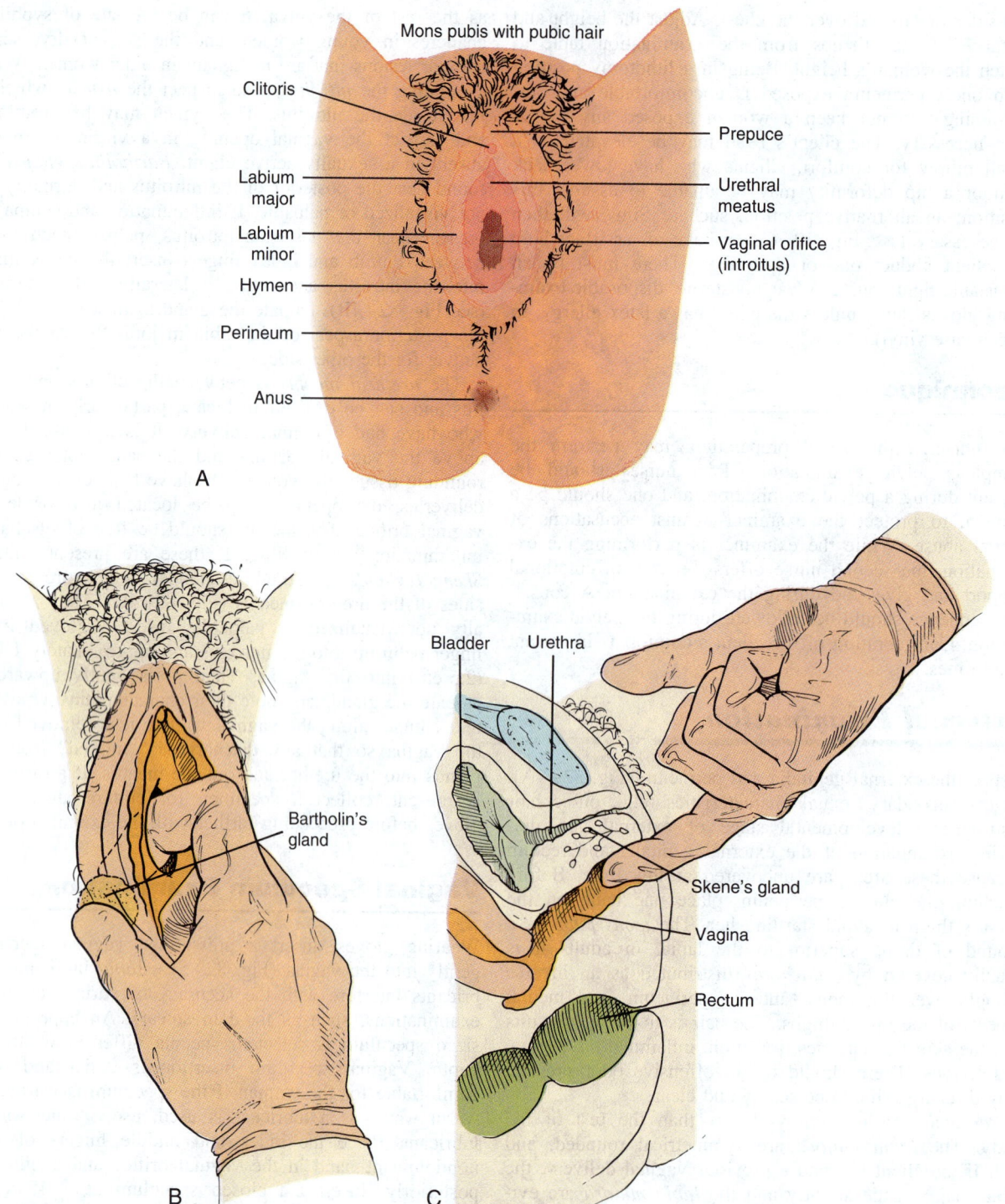

Figure 82–4. *A,* Anatomy of female perineum and external genitalia. *B,* Palpation of Bartholin's glands. *C,* Palpation of Skene's glands.

masses; and bulges of the vaginal wall (e.g., cystocele, rectocele).

The *cervical os* (see Fig. 82–5D) is usually round but may be irregularly shaped after pregnancy. It is pink and smooth; a discharge is usually present that varies from thin and clear to thick, white, and stringy, depending on the phase of the menstrual cycle. Abnormal findings include unusual color of the mucosa, abnormal consistency

of discharge, ulcerations, growths, masses, nodules, inflammation, and bleeding. If an abnormal discharge is present, a culture is obtained.

Before the speculum is removed from the vagina, a Pap smear and culture(s), if indicated, are obtained (see discussion of obtaining specimens later in this chapter). The speculum blades are left slightly open as they are withdrawn for visualizing the vaginal walls.

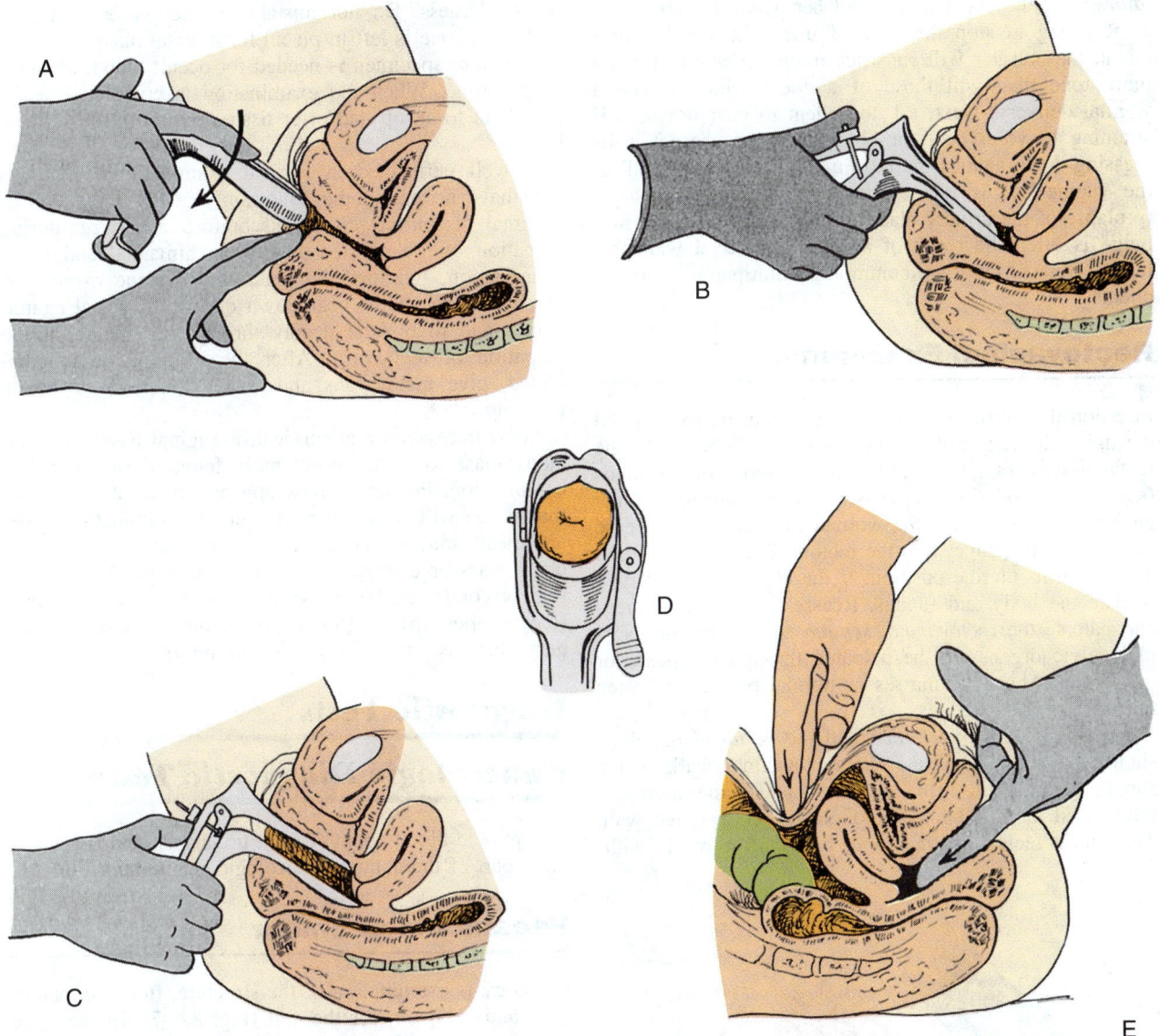

Figure 82–5. Pelvic examination and insertion of the vaginal speculum. *A,* The speculum blades are turned obliquely, and any pressure is directed downward onto the perineum. *B,* After full insertion, the blades are rotated to a horizontal position. *C,* Squeezing the speculum handles opens the blades. *D,* A full view of the cervix and cervical os. *E,* The bimanual examination. The abdominal hand presses the pelvic organs to be palpated toward the intravaginal hand.

Bimanual Examination

One or two fingers of the dominant hand are lubricated and inserted gently into the vagina, palm up, and the other hand is placed on the lower abdomen (see Fig. 82–5E). Palpate the pelvic contents between the fingers in the vagina and the hand on the abdomen. Locate and assess the *cervix.* Assess the size, shape, surface characteristics, consistency, position, mobility, and tenderness of the *uterine body* and *fundus.* Last, each of the *adnexal areas* (left and right) is palpated. Normal *ovaries* may or may not be palpated, and normal *fallopian tubes* are not palpable. Postmenopausal ovaries should not be palpable.

A normal cervix can be gently moved sideways without pain. The cervix should feel smooth and firm, located deep in the vagina on the anterior wall. It usually points

away from the fundus of the uterus, posteriorly. Abnormal findings include tenderness or pain with palpation, immobility, and an abnormal position.

The uterus is typically in an anterior position, but is retroverted or in midposition in 15% of women. It is normally firm, smooth, mobile, and nontender and is approximately 5.5 to 8.0 cm (2 ⅛–3 ⅛) in length. Abnormal findings include prolapse into the vagina, feeling hard or soft, being fixed in position, irregular contour, enlargement, or tenderness.

A normal ovary is 4 to 6 cm in diameter and feels smooth, firm, and oval. Slight tenderness on palpation is normal, but uncomfortable tenderness, pain, or masses are not.

Withdraw the hand, palm up, halfway from the vaginal orifice and assess the integrity of the *pelvic floor muscu-*

lature. Ask the client to contract her pelvic floor muscles as if trying to stop the flow of urine. In a nulliparous client, the muscles will constrict around your fingers with more tone than will those of a client who has had a vaginal delivery. Next, ask the client to bear down as if straining to void. Feel for bulging of the vaginal walls pressing down against the introitus. If the anterior wall of the vagina bulges, the client probably has a *cystocele* (prolapse of the urinary bladder). A posterior vaginal wall bulge is often the result of a *rectocele* (rectal wall prolapse). Both of these are common in multiparous or obese clients.

Rectovaginal Examination

Insertion the lubricated middle finger into the rectum and the index finger into the vagina (Fig. 82–6) be assess the rectal tissues for abnormalities, for example, hemorrhoids (see Chapter 62 for a discussion of examination of the anus and rectum). Ask the woman to bear down to ease insertion of the finger into the rectum. Rectal examination also confirms uterine position. If the uterus is retroverted, palpate the body and fundus. Reassess the adnexal areas and palpate the *rectovaginal septum* and *cul-de-sac*. Normal pelvic organs can be palpated through the posterior cul-de-sac. Abnormal masses or normal ovaries are often felt in the cul-de-sac.

Assess *anal sphincter tone* and the *rectal wall,* which should be smooth. Assess the rectovaginal wall, which should be smooth, firm, and resilient. If the uterus is retroverted, it may be felt through the rectovaginal wall. The cervix feels smooth, round, firm, and movable with-

out tenderness. Do not mistake the cervix or a vaginal tampon (if one is left in place) for a rectal mass.

If a stool specimen is needed for occult blood, obtain it at this time. When the examination is completed, assist the client to sit up and offer tissues or wipes for perineal hygiene.

If well performed, a vaginal examination in women who have no pathologic conditions usually causes no or minimal discomfort. Some discomfort may occur during palpation of the ovaries during the bimanual and rectal examination. Acknowledge this, and help the woman relax by asking her to bear down during the rectal examination and to breathe deeply through her mouth during palpation of the ovary. After the examination is completed, give instructions and conduct appropriate health teaching.

Sometimes abnormal cervical or vaginal tissue, a suspicious mass, or other problem is found during a pelvic examination. Perhaps colposcopy or biopsy of the abnormal tissue will be performed. Further examination under anesthesia may be necessary for exploration of a suspicious mass or unexplained tenderness. A pelvic examination is conducted before various other gynecologic tests (e.g., colposcopy, hysterosalpingogram) and before surgery (such as laparoscopy or laparotomy).

Diagnostic Tests

Gynecologic Diagnostic Tests

A complete blood count (CBC), urinalysis, and Pap smear are a part of the annual gynecologic examination.

Papanicolaou Smear

Cytology is examination of the structure, function, pathology, and chemistry of the cell (Fig. 82–7). In the gynecologic context, cytology refers to the Pap smear. The Pap smear identifies preinvasive and invasive cervical cancer.

Client Preparation. Tell the client that this test cannot be performed during menstruation. Also, tell the client not to douche for at least 24 hours prior to the test. The client needs to remove all clothing below the waist. The examination is performed with the client in the lithotomy position, using a speculum.

Procedure. A Pap test is based on the fact that cells (normal and abnormal) are shed from the lining of the uterus and cervix and pass into both uterine and cervical secretions. When a cytologic smear is made of these secretions and examined under a microscope, early cellular changes may be detected before disease becomes clinically apparent. The Pap test is up to 95% accurate in diagnosing early cervical carcinoma, provided, of course, that correct sampling and handling techniques are used. It is much less accurate (about 40%) in detecting endometrial carcinoma.

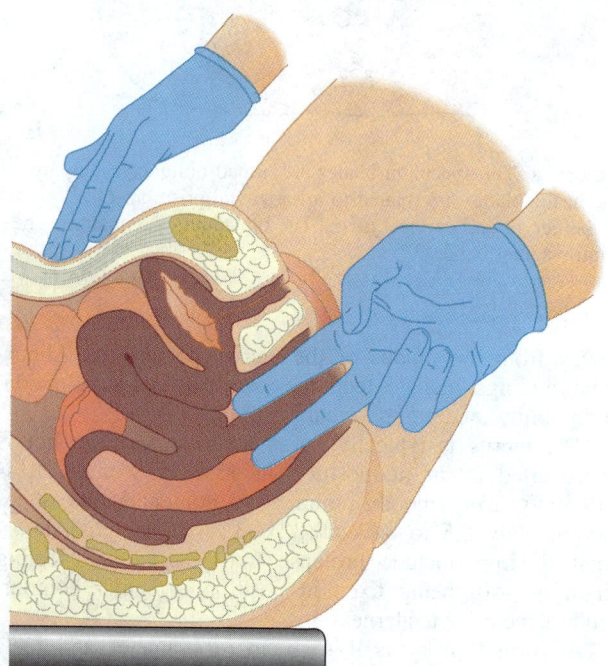

Figure 82–6. Rectovaginal examination. The examiner combines bimanual and rectal examination by inserting the index finger in the woman's vagina and the middle finger in the rectum.

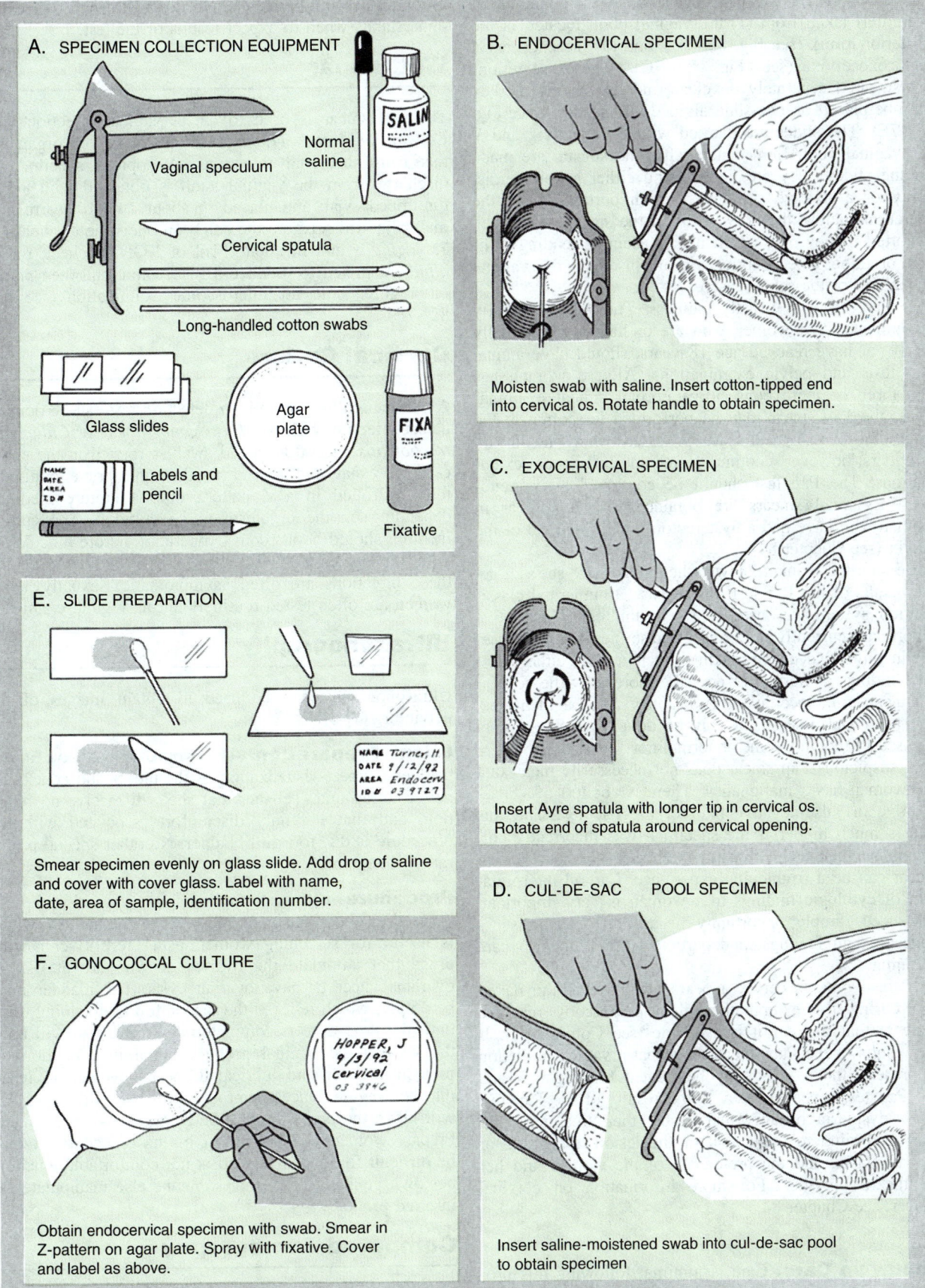

A. SPECIMEN COLLECTION EQUIPMENT

SALINE

Vaginal speculum

Normal saline

Cervical spatula

Long-handled cotton swabs

Glass slides

Agar plate

FIXA

Labels and pencil

Fixative

B. ENDOCERVICAL SPECIMEN

Moisten swab with saline. Insert cotton-tipped end into cervical os. Rotate handle to obtain specimen.

C. EXOCERVICAL SPECIMEN

Insert Ayre spatula with longer tip in cervical os. Rotate end of spatula around cervical opening.

E. SLIDE PREPARATION

NAME Turner, H
DATE 9/12/92
AREA Endocerv
ID # 03 9727

Smear specimen evenly on glass slide. Add drop of saline and cover with cover glass. Label with name, date, area of sample, identification number.

D. CUL-DE-SAC POOL SPECIMEN

F. GONOCOCCAL CULTURE

HOPPER, J
9/3/92
cervical
03 3846

Obtain endocervical specimen with swab. Smear in Z-pattern on agar plate. Spray with fixative. Cover and label as above.

Insert saline-moistened swab into cul-de-sac pool to obtain specimen

Figure 82–7. Collection of cervical cytology specimens.

Smears for the Pap test consist of a small amount of secretions taken from (1) the vaginal pool, located in the posterior fornix (see Fig. 82–7D), and (2) the endocervix and exocervix (see Fig. 82–7C). These secretions are smeared separately on clean and dry slides, or they may be placed on one slide divided into sections (see Fig. 82–7E). The slides are marked with *C* for cervix and *V* for vaginal pool. Immediately after the smears are made on the slides, they are fixed, using either a commercial spray or a fixative solution. It is important to fix the secretions before they dry. Cells in the specimen may be distorted if they dry, which makes accurate reading difficult or impossible. Lubricant is not used on the vaginal speculum for the same reason.

A Pap smear is usually painless. The ACS[2] currently recommends that women who are or have been sexually active, or have reached age 18 years, should have annual Pap tests and pelvic examinations. After a woman has had three or more consecutive normal annual examinations, the Pap smear may be performed less often at the discretion of her healthcare provider. Many healthcare providers, however, continue to recommend annual examinations. The Pap test should be continued after menopause. Vaginal smears are obtained for Pap smear in women who have had a hysterectomy with removal of the cervix (see Chapter 84).

Be sure the woman knows when and where she can get the results of her Pap test. In the past, a numerical classification system was used to report findings. Descriptive reports are currently preferred because they are more useful in clinical decision-making. Such reports either classify findings as normal or describe more fully the cellular changes seen. Specific infections may also be identified, and hormonal assessment may be done. A Pap test may be used to monitor some abnormalities.

A suspicious Pap smear does not necessarily mean that the woman has a malignancy. There is about a 5% false-positive or false-negative rate for the Pap test, and this rate is much higher if the specimen was incorrectly collected or handled. However, having an abnormal Pap smear can be a frightening experience. Careful interpretation of cytologic findings to a woman is very important. She needs ample opportunity to ask questions, discuss concerns and feelings, and participate in follow-up care planning.

If the woman's cervix appears abnormal to the naked eye during the examination, then colposcopy may be done at that time, if it is available (see Colposcopy). If the results of the Pap smear show that a vaginal infection is present, the woman may be treated for vaginitis and the Pap test repeated later. If the results of the Pap test show dysplasia or abnormal tissue, then treatment will vary according to the extent of the lesion, the grade of the dysplasia, and the preference of the woman and her healthcare provider. For more information on cervical cancer, see Chapter 84.

Follow-up Care. Care is minimal following this procedure. The client needs to be helped out of the stirrups and told not to get up too rapidly. Clean off any excess lubricant or allow the client to do so. Be sure the client understands when to expect results of the test.

Wet Smear

The wet smear is used to detect vaginal infection with *Candida albicans, Trichomonas vaginalis,* or organisms that cause bacterial infections. A copious specimen of discharge from the vaginal vault is obtained with a cotton-tipped swab and placed in about 1 ml of warm normal saline (to separate the cells) on one slide to check for *T. vaginalis* and in about 1 ml of KOH to check for *C. albicans,* mixed to produce a suspension, and then placed on a glass slide for microscopic examination (see Fig. 82–7E).

Cervical Culture

A cervical culture or antigen detection test can be done to detect infection with *Neisseria gonorrhoeae* or *Chlamydia trachomatis.* A cotton-tipped swab is rotated in the endocervical canal and placed in the appropriate culturette tube or rolled in a Z pattern onto a culture medium, depending on the organism to be cultured. The culture medium should be at room temperature before inoculation with the specimen (see Figs. 82–7B and F). Because these infections are often asymptomatic, sexually active women are often tested routinely during regular exams.

Ultrasonography

Ultrasonography can be used to obtain images of the pelvic organs.

Client Preparation. The woman must have a full bladder for best visualization of the uterus and adnexa by pelvic ultrasound. Tell her that she will receive no radiation, and that the only discomfort associated with the procedure is due to a full bladder. No other special preparation is required.

Procedure. Ultrasonography using a vaginal probe can be used to obtain an improved view of the adnexa, which is useful for screening women using fertility-enhancing drugs that stimulate the ovaries or who are at risk of ovarian cancer or have ovarian cysts. The bladder must be empty, which relieves the discomfort of retaining urine until the procedure is complete. The technician will hand the woman the vaginal probe covered in a condom or protective cover and lubricated for the woman to insert into her vagina. Once the probe is inserted, the technician will move the probe so that the best images are obtained. Prepare women for this aspect of the procedure. It may be difficult for a woman who is not comfortable touching her own genitalia or having someone else manipulate the inserted probe.

Computed Tomography

Client Preparation. There is no special preparation for computed tomography (CT) of the pelvis unless oral contrast medium is given; in that case the woman must be NPO (nothing by mouth) for at least 4 hours. She should remove all metal objects and empty her bladder prior to the test. Tell the woman she will hear a clicking noise from the machine and that she must remain motionless during the procedure. If she anticipates becoming anxious from being confined in the equipment, antianxiety medication prior to the procedure may help her. Tell her that the technician will be in the next room and can communicate with her by intercom.

Procedure. CT is a noninvasive diagnostic scanning technique that can be used to distinguish between benign and malignant lesions in the reproductive organs. It produces three-dimensional, cross-sectional images. It exposes the woman to radiation, but no more than that of a series of regular x-rays. Contraindications to CT include pregnancy, morbid obesity (over 300 lb), and allergy to iodine dye or shellfish if contrast medium will be used.

Magnetic Resonance Imaging

Client Preparation. There is no special preparation for magnetic resonance imaging (MRI). The woman will empty her bladder and remove all metal objects before the test. Tell the woman the machine will make a thumping sound periodically during the test. If she anticipates experiencing claustrophobia while being confined in the MRI apparatus, antianxiety medication or earphones may be helpful. The technician will be in the next room and able to talk with the woman by intercom.

Procedure. MRI is a noninvasive diagnostic procedure that uses a magnetic field and radiowaves to generate a multiplane, cross-sectional image of a body area. It can be used to detect primary and metastatic tumors of the reproductive organs. It does not use radiation or contrast medium, but is very expensive and not available at all facilities. Contraindications to this test include pregnancy, morbid obesity (over 300 lb), any implanted metal devices or fragments (including intrauterine devices, which would be drawn to the magnet), and inability to lie still within a confined space.

Endometrial Smear

An endometrial smear is made in a manner similar to a Pap smear (Fig. 82–8). The uterine lining is swabbed to obtain cells and secretions for examination. The test differs from a Pap test in that the cervix must be dilated under sterile conditions to obtain the specimen. The procedure is usually done during the first 12 hours after onset of menses, because the cervix is easier to enter at this time. Cervical dilation may cause cramping, which is usually relieved by analgesics and application of heat to the lower abdomen. The endometrial smear as a diagnostic test has been largely replaced by endometrial biopsy.

The American Cancer Society[2] recommends that women at high risk of developing endometrial cancer have an endometrial sample (biopsy or smear) taken at menopause. Subsequent samples are obtained according to level of risk.

Endometrial Biopsy

Client Preparation. The client needs to understand the purpose of the test and the procedure to be followed, including the use of an anesthetic block. A permit must be signed. Position the client as for a pelvic examination.

Procedure. A sample of endometrial tissue can be obtained for histologic study on an outpatient basis through the technique of endometrial biopsy. Endometrial tissue may be analyzed for menstrual disturbances, infertility, or endometrial cancer. The biopsy is performed after bimanual examination of the uterus. Because the biopsy may cause cramping, the woman may receive a paracervical block to relieve the discomfort. After dilating the cervix under sterile conditions, the healthcare provider passes a sounding instrument into the uterus to measure the depth of the uterine cavity. Then the healthcare provider inserts a cutting or aspirating instrument into the uterus and removes a small amount of tissue from the fundus for examination.

Follow-up Care. If cramping persists after the procedure, administer analgesics as ordered or apply heat to the lower abdomen.

Colposcopy

Client Preparation. Explain to the woman that the procedure is similar to a pelvic examination and that when the speculum is in place, a large microscope will be used to look at the cervix.

Procedure. Colposcopy involves using a magnifying instrument (colposcope) to examine the cervical epithelium, vagina, and vulva (Fig. 82–9). A colposcope is a stereoscopic binocular microscope, usually used with a magnification power of 15. Colposcopy is indicated for all women with Pap smears showing dysplasia and may be used to examine any suspicious lesion in the lower genital tract. In this office or clinic procedure, the woman is placed in the lithotomy position and her cervix is exposed with a vaginal speculum. A solution of 3% acetic acid (common household vinegar) is applied to remove mucus and cellular debris and to dehydrate slightly the cells on the cervix. The cervix and upper vagina are then inspected with the colposcope. Epithelial abnormalities can be detected as well as specific lesions. Biopsy is usually performed at the time of colposcopy if a suspicious lesion is present and can easily be done in the office or clinic without the use of anesthesia.

Use of colposcopy increases diagnostic accuracy and reduces the need for biopsy. The procedure is safe and painless and can be performed on pregnant women. (Cervical biopsy, however, is avoided on pregnant women.)

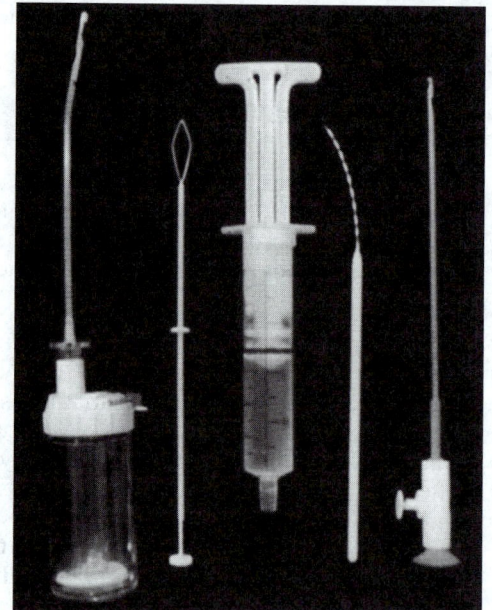

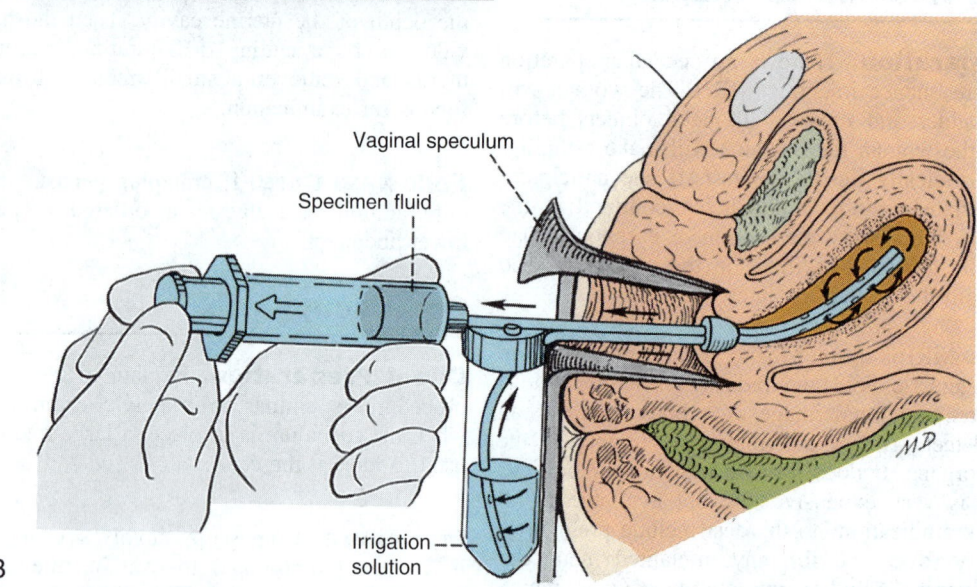

Figure 82–8. *A,* Endometrial sampling devices for uterine cancer screening. *Left to right:* Vakutage, Accurette, syringe for Karman cannula, Mi-Mark helix, and Karman cannula. *B,* Gravlee Jet Washer performing endometrial uterine lavage with sterile normal saline under negative pressure. Cells loosened by the "washing" are obtained for cytopathologic examination. *Arrows* indicate the flow of the irrigating solution and collection of the specimen. Fluid does not enter the fallopian tubes. A rubber plug at the cervical os helps create an airtight, negative pressure within the uterus. *Arrows* within the uterus show circulation of fluids within the uterus. (From Boone, M. I., et al. [1984]. Uterine cancer screening by the family physician. *American Family Physician, 30,* 157.)

Cervical Biopsy

Client Preparation. Explain the purpose of the test to the client. The test cannot be done while the client is menstruating and is best performed 1 week following the end of menses. The test is performed with the client in the same position as for a pelvic examination.

Procedure. Biopsies of suspicious cervical lesions identified with the naked eye or with colposcopic magni-

fication are usually performed in the outpatient setting with the use of little or no anesthesia. A solution of 3% acetic acid can be applied to the cervix to identify areas suspicious of dysplasia, metaplasia, or malignancy. These areas undergo a color change and appear white.

In an unusual situation, when colposcopy cannot identify an abnormal lesion on the cervix or vagina, Schiller's test may be performed. Schiller's iodine solution is applied to the vagina and cervix. Normal tissue takes up the stain and appears as a homogeneous mahogany-brown

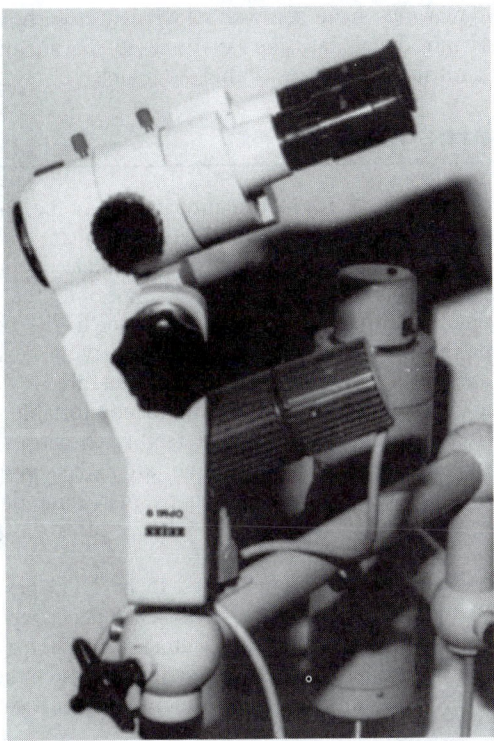

Figure 82–9. A colposcope, used to evaluate clients with an abnormal Papanicolaou smear and a grossly normal cervix. (From Hacker, N. F., & Moore, J. G. [1992]. *Essentials of obstetrics and gynecology* [2nd ed.]. Philadelphia: W. B. Saunders.)

color. Usually, abnormal tissue does not take stain as well and may appear light yellow instead. This is a positive finding and can indicate areas that need to be biopsied. A biopsy may be done when a cervical lesion is first noted or delayed until about 1 week after the menstrual period (when the cervix is least vascular). Multiple biopsies are usually obtained at specific sites with biopsy forceps (Fig. 82–10). Hemostasis is achieved with topical application of silver nitrate or Monsel's solution. The biopsies are usually somewhat painful. For ruling out disease in the endocervical canal, endocervical curettage may be performed.

Follow-up Care. Allow the woman to rest for a short time before discharge home. Instruct her to avoid activity for the next 24 hours. Although she may note a small amount of blood-tinged vaginal discharge, any excessive bleeding should be reported to the physician immediately. Advise her to abstain from vaginal sexual activity, avoid tampons, and avoid douching for several days to achieve hemostasis, lessen trauma, and promote healing.

Cold Conization

Today, colposcopy, biopsy, and endocervical curettage have largely replaced conization, but there are some circumstances in which it is indicated. When the lesion is in the endocervix or when the Pap smear suggests invasive carcinoma, conization may be done.

Client Preparation. Since this is a surgical procedure, the preparation is the same as for any client undergoing minor surgery. The client must sign a permit for the procedure. Mild sedation may be given prior to the start of the procedure if the client is very anxious.

Procedure. The goal of conization is to excise the cervical lesion entirely by cutting out a cone-shaped section of tissue with an adequate surgical margin. A cold knife blade is used to preserve histologic characteristics and avoid desiccation. Conization is usually performed in an outpatient room under general or spinal anesthesia. After excision of the specimen, curettage of the remaining endocervical canal is usually performed. The carbon dioxide laser can be used in place of the cold knife and is carried out the same way. Postoperative care is similar to that following D & C. Vaginal packing may be used to control bleeding for 24 to 48 hours.

Follow-up Care. Immediate complications include intraoperative or postoperative hemorrhage. Tell the woman that some vaginal discharge (often blood-tinged) usually occurs after 3 to 5 days and that her next two or three menstrual periods may be prolonged, heavier than usual, and possibly preceded by a dark-brown premenstrual discharge. Bleeding can occur about 1 week after surgery when the absorbable suture placed in the surgical bed reabsorbs. Complications are rare after conization but include infection, incompetent cervix, or cervical stenosis.

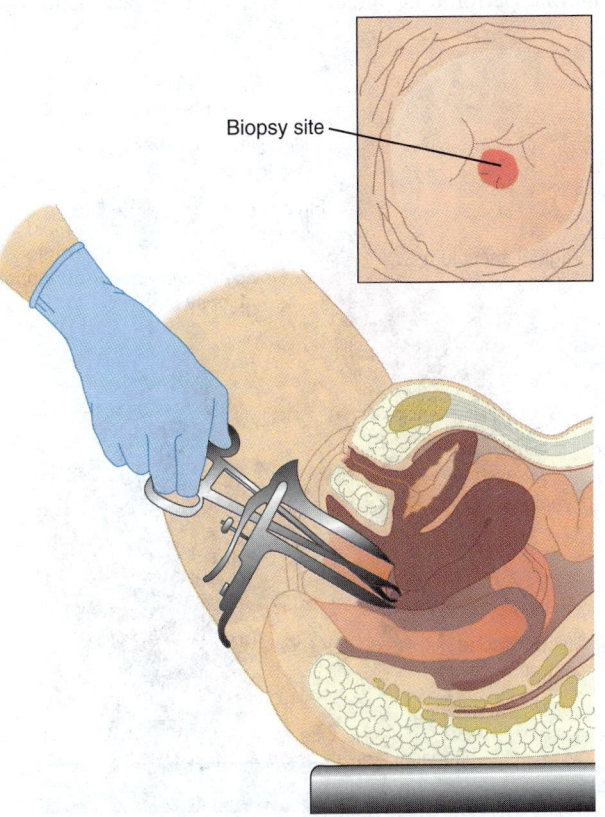

Biopsy site

Figure 82–10. Cervical biopsy.

Hysteroscopy

Client Preparation. Explain the procedure to the client. Position the client in the lithotomy position as for a pelvic examination.

Procedure. In this technique, the intrauterine cavity is directly viewed through an endoscope called a hysteroscope (Fig. 82–11). Hysteroscopes have a fiberoptic lighting system and use 5% glucose in water, highly viscous dextran solutions, or carbon dioxide as the uterine distending medium. After administration of an anesthetic, the hysteroscope is passed into the uterus via the vagina. The uterine cavity is distended and may be rinsed to clear away blood and secretory debris that would obstruct vision. In addition to direct visualization of the uterine cavity, directed biopsies and resections of endometrial abnormalities can be done. The hysteroscope can also be used to deliver a laser beam into the uterus for therapeutic procedures. Hysteroscopy may be used for (1) ruling out organic causes in abnormal uterine or postmenopausal bleeding, (2) examining suspected leiomyomas or polyps, (3) removing an intrauterine device with a missing string, (4) evaluating infertility, and (5) performing surgical techniques for uterine abnormalities. Hysteroscopy is contraindicated if the woman (1) has acute pelvic inflammatory disease, recurrent chronic upper genital tract infection, or recent uterine perforation; (2) has or is suspected of having cervical malignancy; or (3) is pregnant.

Follow-up Care. Complications include bleeding, uterine perforation, infection, and perhaps bowel injuries.

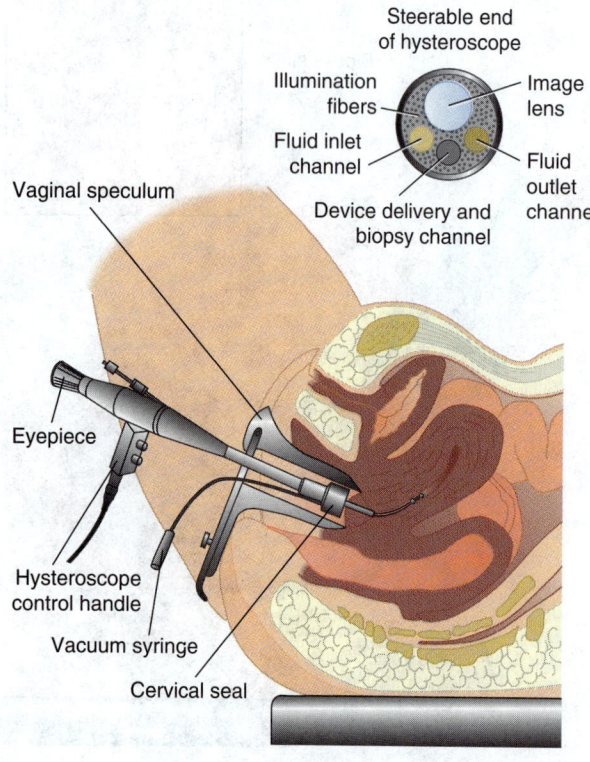

Steerable end
of hysteroscope

Illumination
fibers
Image
lens
Fluid inlet
channel
Fluid
outlet
channel
Device delivery and
biopsy channel

Vaginal speculum

Eyepiece

Hysteroscope
control handle

Vacuum syringe

Cervical seal

Figure 82–11. Hysteroscopy.

The woman may have some shoulder pain if carbon dioxide was introduced into the pelvic cavity during the procedure; it usually resolves within 24 hours.

Laparoscopy

Client Preparation. The preparation is the same as that for hysteroscopy. Preoperatively, a woman scheduled for a laparoscopy should be given a complete explanation of the procedure and how she can expect to feel afterward. She should have someone drive her to the hospital or clinic, because she may not feel like driving if she has local anesthesia and should not drive at all if she has general anesthesia. She will be more comfortable if she wears loose-fitting clothes to the facility, because it will be easier to prepare to go home after the procedure. Typically women having laparoscopy in a same-day surgery setting can go home 2 to 4 hours after the procedure.

The woman is usually instructed to be NPO past midnight on the day the laparoscopy is scheduled. Depending on the physician's preference, a cathartic or enema and a partial perineal shave might be required (usually they are not). Abdominal skin preparation (scrubbing and shaving) is done in the operating room.

Procedure. A laparoscope is a common diagnostic and therapeutic tool (Fig. 82–12). It is a telescope with an illuminated optical system that is inserted into the abdomen through a small incision near the umbilicus. Abdominal and pelvic organs can be visualized. Laparoscopy is a safe, convenient procedure that can be performed in hospitals, office, or clinics equipped for outpatient surgery. The postprocedure recovery period is short and the scar is small.

Laparoscopy may be performed (1) diagnostically, for conditions such as pelvic pain, pelvic masses, infertility, suspected ectopic pregnancy, and endometriosis; and (2) therapeutically, for procedures such as tubal ligation for contraceptive purposes and minor surgical procedures. The main contraindication to laparoscopy is serious cardiac or pulmonary disease. Previous lower abdominal surgery is not a contraindication, but should be considered.

Follow-up Care. Postoperatively, take vital signs every 15 minutes for the first hour, or until the woman is stable. If local anesthesia has been used, the woman can have fluids and a light snack as soon as she wants. After general anesthesia, the woman may have fluids and a light snack as soon as she is fully awake and has no nausea. Explain to the client that she may experience mild-to-moderate transient shoulder pain or a feeling of "bloatedness" as a result of the carbon dioxide or nitrous oxide used to distend the abdomen during the procedure (separating the organs and allowing better visualization). The discomfort usually lasts only a few hours and may be relieved by comfortable positioning or mild analgesics. The woman may also experience mild incisional pain or abdominal cramping for the first few hours or days after the procedure, which is usually relieved by rest. If she had general anesthesia, she might have a sore throat from

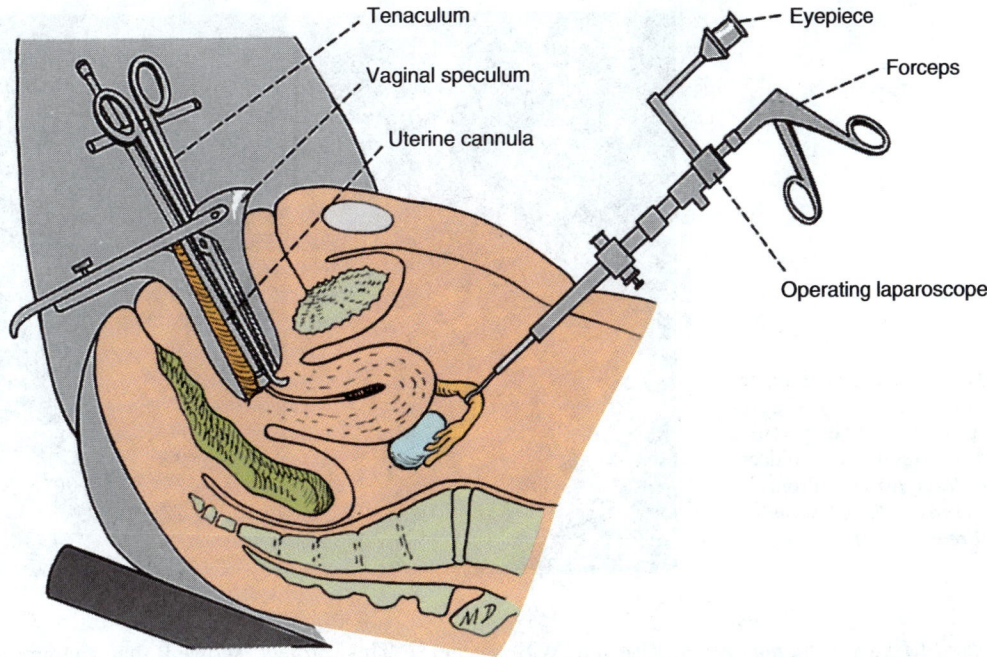

Figure 82–12. Laparoscopy.

intubation or a sore chest from insufflation. These manifestations usually disappear within 48 hours. Teach her how to keep the incision clean and dry. After it heals, the scar will be barely noticeable. Sexual intercourse can be resumed within a week or less.

Diagnostic Tests for the Breast

Breast Imaging Techniques

Various techniques have been tried in an effort to identify early-stage breast cancer in women accurately and safely when assessment indicates breast lesions. Such techniques are also important in finding an effective method to screen women without clinically apparent findings. At present, only mammography has been shown to be useful for widespread screening. Ineffective techniques include transillumination (also known as light-scanning and diaphanography) and thermography. While ultrasonography is not specific enough to identify lesions suspicious of cancer, it does differentiate cystic from solid lesions. CT scanning, MRI, and other tests are being investigated.

Mammography

A mammogram is a soft tissue radiographic breast examination used to detect small invasive and noninvasive tumors and benign lesions in the breast. Two common methods of obtaining mammograms are (1) film or screen mammography (Fig. 82–13) and (2) xeromammography (Fig. 82–14). The first method uses x-ray film. Xeromammography produces an electrostatic image on plastic-coated paper. Ductograms and pneumocystograms are specialized mammographic techniques. Each technique

has its own strengths and limitations and uses acceptably low radiation doses.

Client Preparation. Some common questions and possible answers about mammography include the following:

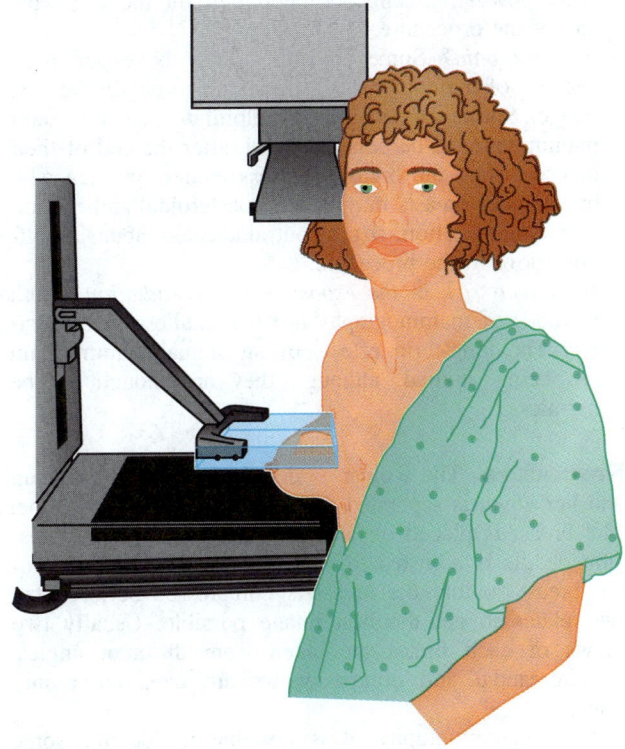

Figure 82–13. Mammography, a technique for x-raying the breast, is the most reliable mechanical method of detecting a breast cancer before it can be felt. It is also used to help diagnose breast cancer in women with symptoms.

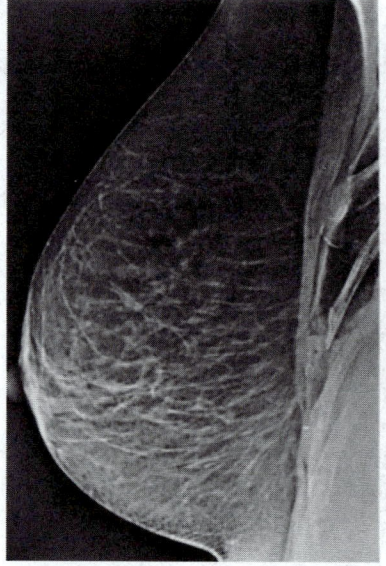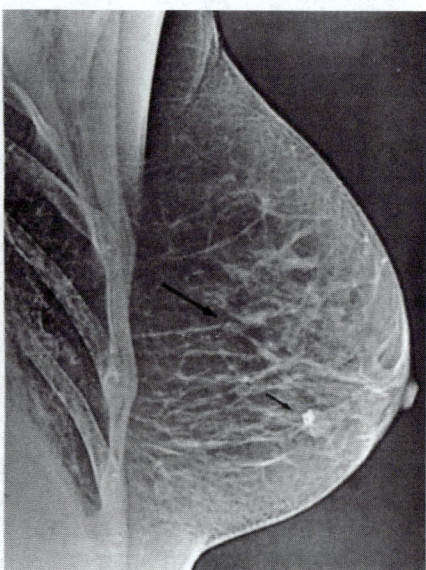

Figure 82–14. A xeromammogram, performed prior to a planned biopsy of a palpable mass that proved to be benign (*small arrow*), revealed the presence of a hidden cancerous lesion (*large arrow*). (From Lippman, M. E. [1987]. *Diagnosis and management of breast cancer.* Philadelphia: W. B. Saunders.)

- *How often should I have a mammogram?* Use the ACS or National Cancer Institute (NCI) guidelines for the age and risk group.
- *Cost?* Prices vary. Inquire at the facility where the mammogram will be performed. Tell the client it is worthwhile to compare prices.
- *Time involved?* About 15 to 30 minutes to complete the procedure. Results are usually available within 1 to 21 days, depending on the facility.
- *Preparation involved?* The woman should not wear any body powder, creams, or deodorant on the torso the day of the procedure.
- *Is there pain?* Some discomfort may be experienced because of the compression necessary to obtain the best image. Some women find it helpful to schedule their mammogram to be done the week after the end of their menses when the breasts are less tender. Women who have tender breasts may take a nonsteroidal anti-inflammatory medication, if not contraindicated, about a half-hour prior to the procedure.
- *Is there a risk in the exposure to the radiation?* Both methods of mammography use the smallest dose possible. The long-term effects of an annual mammogram are being studied, although they are thought to be harmless.

Procedure. The woman is disrobed from the waist up and her gown is separated to expose one breast at a time. The breast is placed on an x-ray plate and the compression paddle is adjusted to press against the other side of the breast so that the breast is compressed between the two plates to get the best image possible. Usually two views of each breast are taken from different angles. Cranial-caudal and oblique views are most commonly done.

With mammography, it is possible to identify some breast cancers before they reach a size that can be detected by palpation. The Breast Cancer Detection Demonstration Project (BCDDP) included 280,000 participants who were followed mammographically for at least 5

years.[61] This project showed that mammography alone detected 41.6% of the cancers—impressively high in the diagnosis of small cancers.

Current indications for mammography[20] include (1) diagnosis of potentially curable cancer, and follow-up after treatment, (2) questionable breast masses or other abnormal physical findings to help determine whether and where a biopsy should be performed, (3) detection of breast cancer when assessing a woman with metastatic cancer and the primary site is unknown, and (4) routine screening. There has been controversy about the age at which routine mammography in women should begin.[20] The ACS recommends a baseline mammogram for all women by age 40 and mammography screening of asymptomatic women aged 40 to 49 at intervals of 1 to 2 years and annually over age 50. The NCI recently dropped its recommendation to routinely screen women under the age of 50 years. Until there is further evidence, the decision when to begin mammography may be made on an individual basis, with the woman and her health-care provider together evaluating her risk for breast cancer as well as the possible risks and benefits of the screening test. A woman who is at high risk of breast cancer should follow the recommendations of her health-care provider.

Ductography

In a ductogram, a radiocontrast dye is injected through the areolar orifice of the duct. This is done to determine if there is a filling defect, duct ectasia, obstruction, or possible papilloma.

Pneumocystography

After aspiration of a nonpapable cyst under mammographic guidance, a pneumocystogram is done by injecting air to fill the cyst cavity and then performing another mammogram. The pneumocystogram helps visualize the walls of the cyst. A smooth wall usually indicates a simple cyst and may not require further evaluation or treatment. An irregular or thickened wall may indicate a complex cyst, hyperplasia, or other problem and a need for the cyst to be surgically removed.

Ultrasonography

Ultrasound of the breast involves scanning with an automated whole breast scanner and a handheld real-time sector scanner and is very useful in determining the consistency of breast masses. It differentiates cystic (fluid-filled) from solid lesions. It cannot differentiate solid benign from solid cancerous lesions. Ultrasound is useful in confirming the fluid consistency of cystic-appearing lesions seen on a mammogram. It is also useful in guiding fine-needle aspiration (FNA) of cysts and other breast masses. Ultrasonography requires no special preparation, is painless, and does not involve a radiation risk.

Laboratory Studies

No laboratory tests can screen for breast cancer. Some progress has been made in identifying biologic tumor markers for breast cancer that detect metastatic disease. Elevations in carcinoembryonic antigen (CEA), alkaline phosphatase, ferritin, and γ-glutamyltransferase seem to be associated with the recurrence of breast cancer. Other possible tumor markers that have been studied include C-reactive protein, acid glycoprotein, sialyltransferase, the urinary hydroxyproline–creatinine ratio, and gross cystic disease fluid protein.

Biopsy

Biopsy is essential to the diagnosis of breast cancer. No treatment should be undertaken without an unequivocal histologic diagnosis of cancer.

Client Preparation. The purpose of the biopsy should be completely explained to the client. Food and fluid restriction is necessary if intravenous (IV) sedation is to be used. Instruction should also include self-care activities following the procedure. Most women fear that the biopsy will result in cancer being found, so some clients may ask for information about what will happen if cancer is found (see Chapter 85).

Procedure. A core needle biopsy and FNA biopsy may be performed with local anesthesia during an office visit. A core needle biopsy is a simple procedure that takes just a few minutes. After the site is cleaned and prepared with povidone-iodine, a small core of tissue is obtained with a special needle, for example, a Vim-Silverman needle. The core of tissue removed is placed in formalin and sent to the pathologist for histologic diagnosis. Occasionally a suture is needed to close the skin.

FNA is a slightly different procedure. A needle and syringe are used to aspirate cells from a breast mass or fluid from a cyst. The cells are fixed on a slide (as in a Pap smear), and a cytologic diagnosis is made. Mammography is useful in guiding the needle for the FNA examination of nonpalpable lesions. FNA cytologic examination is useful for confirming the diagnosis of clinical and mammographic findings of fibroadenoma, a fibrocystic condition, intramammary lymph nodes, fat necrosis, subareolar papillomatosis, chronic subareolar abscess, and cancer. If the cytologic interpretation is that the specimen is acellular or has only blood and adipose cells present, then a biopsy or further evaluation is needed to rule out breast cancer. Both FNA and core needle biopsy take only a small amount of cells and tissue from a lesion. False-negative results are possible, so an open biopsy may still need to be performed.

Incisional or excisional open biopsies are usually performed in an operating room or a room equipped for minor operative procedures with local anesthetic or possibly with some IV sedation. About 35% of clients requiring an open biopsy for a breast lesion have a malignancy. Excisional biopsy removes the entire mass that was palpated. Incisional biopsy removes only a portion of the mass. In both cases the tissue removed is sent to the pathologist for histologic assessment. The incision is closed with sutures and a dressing (sometimes a pressure dressing) is placed over the site. Typically the dressing needs to stay in place for 24 to 48 hours before it is removed.

Percutaneous needle localization may be used to determine the area for an open biopsy if a mass is very small, for example, those detected by mammograms alone. Localization of the lesion is done in the radiology department by passing a thin needle into the suspicious area identified by mammography. The position of the lesion is confirmed with a repeat mammogram. The needle is secured in place with tape and the woman is taken to the operating room where an open biopsy is immediately performed. A frozen section examination is sometimes performed for rapid diagnosis.

Follow-up Care. After any biopsy instruct the woman to report any bleeding, swelling, or manifestations of infection. Normal activity is resumed as soon as possible. After an open biopsy vigorous activity should be avoided for 1 to 2 weeks. The woman may find that it is more comfortable to wear a supportive brassiere 24 hours a day until the site is healed so long as the wires and elastic do not rub on the incision.

Assessment of Men with Reproductive and Urinary Tract Disorders

Male reproductive and urinary tract problems are common and experienced by men of all ages. Assessing these disorders requires expertise on the part of the nurse. Expertise is required in both the history and psychosocial assessment, as well as in physical examination skills. The nurse must display sensitivity and tact when working with these clients because men are often uncomfortable discussing issues associated with these disorders.

History

A complete health history and physical examination are necessary for men experiencing reproductive problems. A sexual and reproductive history is important. History-taking provides an opportunity to (1) allow men to express sensitive concerns, (2) identify and dispel myths and misinformation held, (3) give health information, (4) offer referrals, and (5) facilitate further communication. Those aspects of history taking that address major risk factors pertinent to men's reproductive health are discussed here.

Chief Complaint

The client may present with problems related to the genitourinary or reproductive system or to sexuality. Areas in a chief complaint may include the following.

- Systemic disturbances, such as weight loss, fever, and malaise
- Voiding disturbances, such as frequency, polyuria, oliguria, nocturia, pyuria, enuresis, dysuria, urgency, or incontinence
- Disturbances in the character of urine, such as hematuria and pyuria
- Gastrointestinal disturbances, such as nausea, vomiting, anorexia, abdominal discomfort, constipation, or diarrhea
- Reproductive disturbances, infertility, history of STDs, genital lesions, or genital discharge in self and partner; genital trauma
- Sexual functioning, whether sexually active or celibate; changes in libido; changes in erectile ability; decreased ejaculatory ability; gynecomastia; effects of manifestations, disability, chronic disease, trauma, surgery, or treatment on sexual functioning

For each manifestation the client reports, the nurse conducts a symptom analysis (see Chapter 11).

Past Health History

Significant health history for the male reproductive system includes childhood and infectious diseases, immunizations, major illnesses and hospitalizations, medications, allergies, sexual and reproductive history, family history, psychosocial history, and review of systems.

Childhood and Infectious Diseases

The most significant childhood infectious illness to affect male fertility is mumps. Its occurrence in young men is associated with sterility. Ask the client whether he has ever had mumps or been immunized against it. The client also should be questioned about the presence of cryptorchidism at birth and the age at which the testicles descended or were brought down surgically.

Major Illnesses and Hospitalizations

Ask the client about major illnesses such as diabetes, hypertension, cerebrovascular accident (stroke), and myocardial infarction. Men who have diabetes frequently have problems with potency related to the accompanying neurologic and vascular changes. Hypertension and its serious complication of stroke can cause impotence due to physiologic or psychological factors. Impotence may also occur in men who have had myocardial infarctions because of a fear of precipitating another heart attack as a result of sexual excitement and activity. Be alert to the man's concerns and fears, remain nonjudgmental, and offer the support of counseling and referral to peer groups established for this purpose. Renal and urinary tract disorders can interfere with sexual functioning because of the close physiologic and anatomic relationships. Endocrine disorders can also interfere with sexual performance.

Ask the client about surgery involving the reproductive system. Specific surgical procedures include herniorrhaphy, vasectomy, prostatectomy, varicocelectomy, orchiopexy, and testicular torsion repair.

Medications

Obtain a complete medication history for prescription, over-the-counter, and recreational drugs. Some medications prescribed for hypertension may cause impotence (e.g., methyldopa, clonidine, guanethidine, and hydralazine). Tranquilizers can interfere with sexual performance. Recreational drugs that alter behavior can also affect physiologic reproductive function, for example, marijuana and hallucinogens.

Allergies

Ask the client about allergies to penicillin and sulfonamides or to rubber or latex. Male genitourinary disorders are often treated with these antibiotics, and latex and rubber are ingredients found in condoms as well as in the gloves commonly worn by the examiner during the physical examination. If the man is allergic to latex, wear vinyl gloves.

Sexual and Reproductive History

The sexual and reproductive history includes the following (see also Chapter 11 for further information on assessment of sexuality).

Breast History

Data should be collected about the breast and axillae for men, as well as women. Ask the client about breast pain or tenderness, masses, lumps, and nipple discharge. If any of these manifestations are present, perform an analysis of clinical manifestations (see Chapter 11). Ask whether the man or his sexual partner has noticed any changes in breast tissue, such as enlargement (*gynecomastia*). Gynecomastia can occur in obese or elderly men and as a side effect of some medications. Ask whether the client performs BSE, similar to that done by a woman. BSE should be performed on a regular, monthly basis following the same guidelines as those for a woman. If the client does not perform BSE, offer to teach him the technique (see the discussion on BSE earlier in this chapter).

Contraceptive History

Document the man's current contraceptive method (if any), his satisfaction with the method, the effect of contraception on sexual function, and any desire to change methods. Has the man used contraceptive methods previously, and if so, were there problems leading to their discontinuation?

Sexual History

Inquire about the client's patterns of sexual relationships. Can the man relate the total number of sexual partners he has had and the frequency of sexual activity? Multiple partners and contacts increase the client's risk of STD as well as human immunodeficiency virus (HIV) infection. Does the man use condoms during sexual intercourse? Does the client have homosexual or bisexual relationships, both of which increase the risk of HIV infection?

Does the client have any sexual concerns, such as an inability to attain or maintain an erection? If so, ask whether this is a problem that occurs frequently or occasionally. Is the client able to discuss sexual concerns with his partner? Have he and his partner developed ways to cope with or adjust to disturbances in sexual function? If sexual dysfunction exists, does the client want a referral to, or consultation with, a sex counselor?

Throughout the interview, ask questions directly. Instead of beginning questions with "why" (which puts the client on the spot to justify his behavior), phrase questions in such a way that it is assumed the client has performed in this way. This interview technique helps preserve the client's dignity and self-esteem instead of making him feel guilt or shame.

Past Genitourinary History

Ask about past problems with genitourinary infections, such as prostatitis. Determine whether the client has had a previous pelvic examination. Are there problems such as urinary incontinence or dribbling, hesitancy, weak urinary stream, or other manifestations? See Chapter 55 for an assessment of the urinary system.

Reproductive Health Practices

Inquire about sexual and reproductive hygiene. How often does the man examine his breasts and testes? Does he protect himself against STDs? See Chapter 11 for a discussion of health risk management.

Family Health History

Ask if there is a family history of infertility, diabetes, hypertension, cerebrovascular accidents, or endocrine disorders. Similar to women whose mothers took DES during pregnancy, men exposed to DES in utero are at increased risk of congenital anomalies, including structural defects of the genitourinary system and reduced semen levels.

Psychosocial History

Assess the following areas.

Occupation and Environment

Determine the type of work and recreational activities of the client to identify any exposure to chemicals, pesticides, heat, heavy metals, hormones, and radiation. These materials can directly affect the number and integrity of sperm and germinal tissue.

Habits

Assess the client's use of caffeine, alcohol, tobacco, and marijuana. These substances may affect the sperm count, contribute to impotence, or decrease the libido.

Psychosocial Factors

An overview of assessment areas pertinent to men with reproductive disturbances is presented here. When taking a nursing history from such men, consider the following factors. You will probably not be able to obtain detailed information in each of these areas, but the outline will signal areas that will help you to regard each man and his significant others as individuals and avoid stereotypic and possibly judgmental nursing care.

- *Self-concept.* How has the client's health affected how he feels about himself? How do his partner and significant others feel about him? What is his posture, dress, grooming? What is his emotional response? What is his mood? His tone?
- *Role relationships.* Who are the important people in this client's life? Who accompanied him to the health-care facility? Who is his most significant other? How is he able to carry out his various social roles (e.g., partner, husband, friend, father, worker)? How has his health affected his economic situation and his partner or significant others?
- *Communication.* How does the client communicate, both verbally and nonverbally, with you and his significant others? Does he maintain eye contact? Does he use gestures or touch? How does he speak (e.g., volume, tone, vocabulary, repetition)?
- *Value system.* What values, opinions, and beliefs does

the client hold? What is his predominant life-style? What is his cultural or subcultural background?

● *Coping with stress.* Who supports and nurtures the client? Does he experience intimacy with anyone? How connected is the client with significant others? What supports and resources does he have? How does he spend his leisure time? To what extent does he engage in physical activity or exercise?

● *Cognitive-perceptual.* How does the client use words? Can he read? What is his level of comprehension? What is his major source of reproductive health information?

Review of Systems

When conducting the review of systems, ask about diabetes, hypertension, stroke, myocardial infarction, angina, endocrine disorders, renal disorders, and urinary tract problems. Detailed questions for the review of systems may be found in Box 11–2.

Physical Examination

Skillful history-taking can help establish a therapeutic relationship that facilitates a successful physical examination. Many men find physical examination for problems of the reproductive system stressful and embarrassing. Genitals are viewed by many as private and even unclean.

Nurses can make a reproductive and sexual physical examination more comfortable for the man by sharing normal findings while proceeding. Explain each step carefully. Ways of increasing the client's comfort during the examination include maintaining eye contact, proceeding in an unhurried manner, and involving the client in self-examination.

Sometimes a man will have an erection during an examination. This possibility is lessened by a kind yet professional manner and a firm yet gentle touch. If the man does have an erection, explain that this is normal and has no sexual connotation.

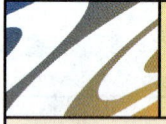

NORMAL PHYSICAL ASSESSMENT FINDINGS

Male Reproductive System

Inspection

Penis: Penis size and shape vary among normal adult men. Foreskin may or may not be present. If client circumcised, head of penis should be slightly rounded without discharge. For uncircumcised clients, smegma is a normal discharge that may appear under the foreskin. Normally the urinary meatus is seen at the tip of the head of the penis and is free of discharge or drainage.

Scrotum: Scrotal size and shape vary normally. The sac may hang below the penis or may be above the level of the penis. The left side of the scrotal sac is usually lower than the right. When exposed to cold, the scrotum contracts and appears much higher and smaller than when warm. The scrotal skin is thin and rugose. There is heavy hair surrounding the male genitalia, but usually only sparse hair on the scrotum itself. The scrotum can be transilluminated and should show no masses or areas of thickness.

Inguinal-Femoral Area: There should be no bulges noted over the inguinal or femoral area, either normally or with coughing or straining.

Palpation

Penis: No masses should be palpated along the penile shaft or head of the penis. There should be no tenderness even when the penis or head is gently squeezed.

Testicles: Two testicles are normally palpated in the scrotum. The testicles should be smooth and oval and similar in consistency. They should be mobile and equal in size. There may be slight tenderness when the testicles are palpated.

Epididymis: The epididymis should be easily palpated at the posterior portion of the scrotum. It may be found in the anterolateral or anterior area of the testes in a small percentage of men. There should be no tenderness.

Vas Deferens: The vas deferens should be palpated from the epididymis anteriorly. The vas feels cordlike and is mobile. It should be smooth, and nontender. No masses should be felt.

Inguinal Canal: The inguinal canal is palpated by invaginating the scrotal skin on both side. The spermatic cord is followed to the external inguinal ring, which is a triangular, slitlike opening. If large enough, the finger can be passed into the canal. There should be no bulge or mass in the canal either normally or when the client bears down or coughs.

Physical examination for reproductive problems focuses on findings that may be associated with reproductive or sexual problems. These may include the following:

- Inflammatory (e.g., enlarged, tender, movable, or fixed lymph nodes in the inguinal region)
- Endocrine and genetic (e.g., general body appearance for indications of conditions such as Cushing's syndrome or acromegaly; hair distribution; gynecomastia)
- Neurologic (e.g., gross neurologic examination of the lower extremities)
- Vascular (e.g., status of femoral and pedal pulses)
- Traumatic (e.g., hernia)

Follow an orderly sequence for the physical examination and teach the client how to do similar self-examinations regularly. The male breast and axillae are included here as part of the examination of the reproductive system.

Examination of the Breasts

It is important that the nurse examine the breasts of male clients. Although the incidence of breast cancer in men is low, it does occur because men have glandular tissue beneath each nipple. Likewise, the axillary nodes are examined.

Inspect and palpate the breasts and axillae while the man is sitting, following the same guidelines as discussed for the female breast examination. The male breast should be flat and symmetrical without nodules, edema, or ulceration. Enlargement (gynecomastia) may occur in obese or elderly men. Unilateral enlargement that persists past puberty is abnormal. Palpation reveals a small, flat disc of glandular tissue under the areola. There should be no masses or discharge. Axillary nodes should be nonpalpable (see Fig. 82–2).

Examination of the Genitals

Ensure that the client's urinary bladder is empty. The client may be supine or lying on his side with his legs spread slightly for the first portion of the genitalia examination but is asked to stand when the nurse assesses for inguinal herniation. An alternative position is to have the client stand for the entire examination of the genitalia while the nurse is seated on a stool. Because the male urethra is the common conduit for both urine and semen, examination of the male reproductive tract also includes assessment of the urinary system. Wear nonsterile, disposable examining gloves.

Inspect the external genitalia and perineum (Fig. 82–15), observing the *public hair* and *skin*. You must be familiar with normal growth and development of the male genitalia. Observe the client's general appearance and body build. Note the hair distribution. Pubic hair distribution in men is triangular with hair covering the symphysis pubis, base of the penis, and inner aspects of the thighs. Hair distribution may also spread toward the umbilicus in a diamond pattern. Hair is inspected for nits and the skin for parasites, rashes, excoriation, and lesions. Masses, lesions, edema, and offensive odors should be absent. *Scro-*

tal skin is darker than other skin surfaces and is loose and wrinkled.

The *penis* includes the penile shaft, prepuce (foreskin), glans, and urethral meatus (Fig. 82–16). Inspect and palpate these structures for lesions, nodules, swelling, inflammation, atrophy, and discharge. *Penile skin* in the unerect penis is wrinkled. The *foreskin,* if present, covers the glans. The foreskin is absent in a circumcised client. The nurse instructs the client to retract the foreskin to expose the *glans,* which is easily accomplished. You may note a small amount of cheesy, thick, white, odoriferous *smegma* between the glans and the foreskin, which is normal. If other discharge is noted, obtain a specimen for culture. The area between the glans and foreskin is a common site of venereal lesions. It is normally free of lesions; if any are present, palpate them for tenderness, size, shape, and consistency and change gloves before proceeding further.

Next, inspect the *urethral meatus,* which is located at the tip of the penis and looks like a slit. Malposition of the meatus on either the underside of the penile shaft (*hypospadias*) or upper side (*epispadias*) is usually a congenital condition. The normal meatus is pink and without ulcers, scars, inflammation, or discharge. Gently compress the glans between thumb and index finger to open the meatus and inspect for discharge. If the client reports a urethral discharge, ask the client to compress the penis from base to tip between his thumb and fingers in an attempt to express a discharge. If one is expressed, obtain a specimen for culture or microscopic examination. You may need to change gloves again before proceeding with the examination.

The *penile shaft* is gently palpated between the thumb and first two fingers. It is smooth and semifirm, and the skin should move easily over underlying structures. The normal penis is free of nodules, thickened or hard areas, and tenderness.

The *scrotum* is inspected and palpated for symmetry, size, shape, and swelling. The scrotum has a right and a left half, each containing a testis, epididymis, and vas deferens. The left testis hangs lower than the right. Scrotal size varies with ambient temperature; cold results in contraction, and warmth in relaxation. Ask the client to hold the penis to one side and then the other and to lift the scrotum up while she inspects it. The skin should be loose, without tension. The *testes* are ovoid, approximately 2 cm × 4 cm (⅘ inch × 1 ⅗ inches). On palpation, they are normally smooth, firm, and rubbery, without nodules, masses, or tenderness. Elderly clients have smaller, less firm testes. In younger, adolescent males, note if both testes are present in the scrotum. Testes may temporarily migrate as a result of being touched during examination or from exposure to cold air. They may be palpable later in the examination when the client is more relaxed. If a testis is not apparent, palpate the femoral and inguinal area. A client with an undescended testis is referred to the physician. A small (pea-sized), hard lump located on either the anterior or lateral aspect of a testis is suggestive of a malignancy, and the client is referred to the physician for follow-up. The testes are compared bilaterally and should be similar.

Palpate each *epididymis* between thumb and index fin-

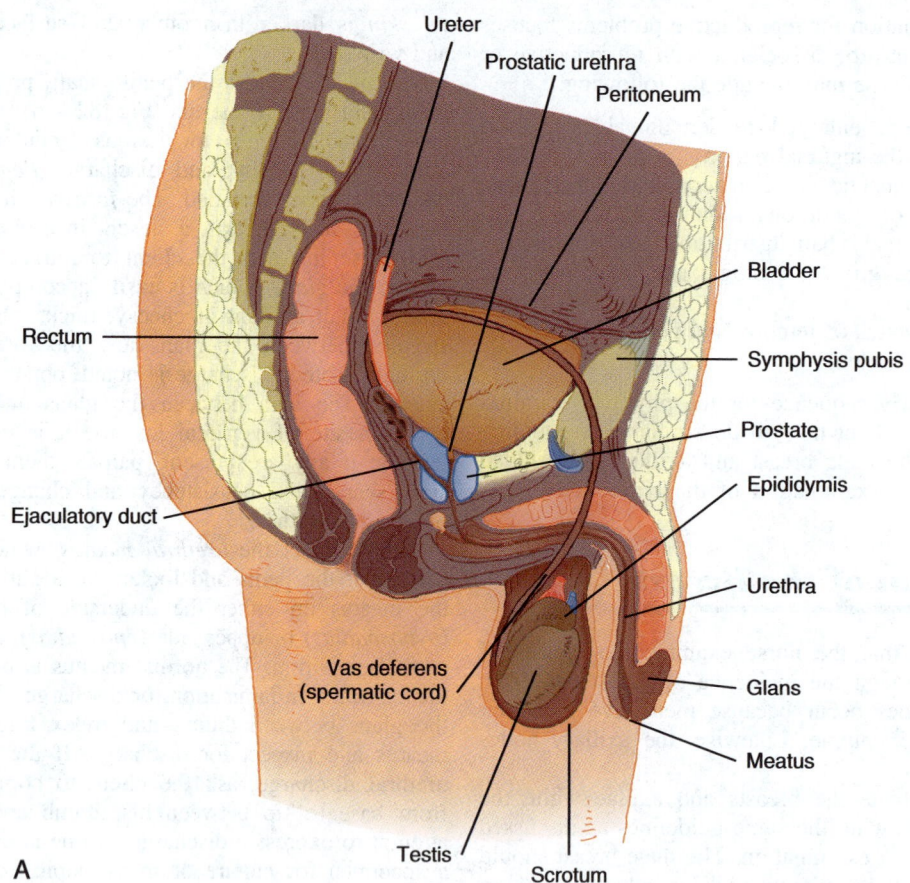

Ureter
Prostatic urethra
Peritoneum
Bladder
Symphysis pubis
Prostate
Epididymis
Urethra
Glans
Meatus
Rectum
Ejaculatory duct
Vas deferens
(spermatic cord)
Testis
Scrotum

A

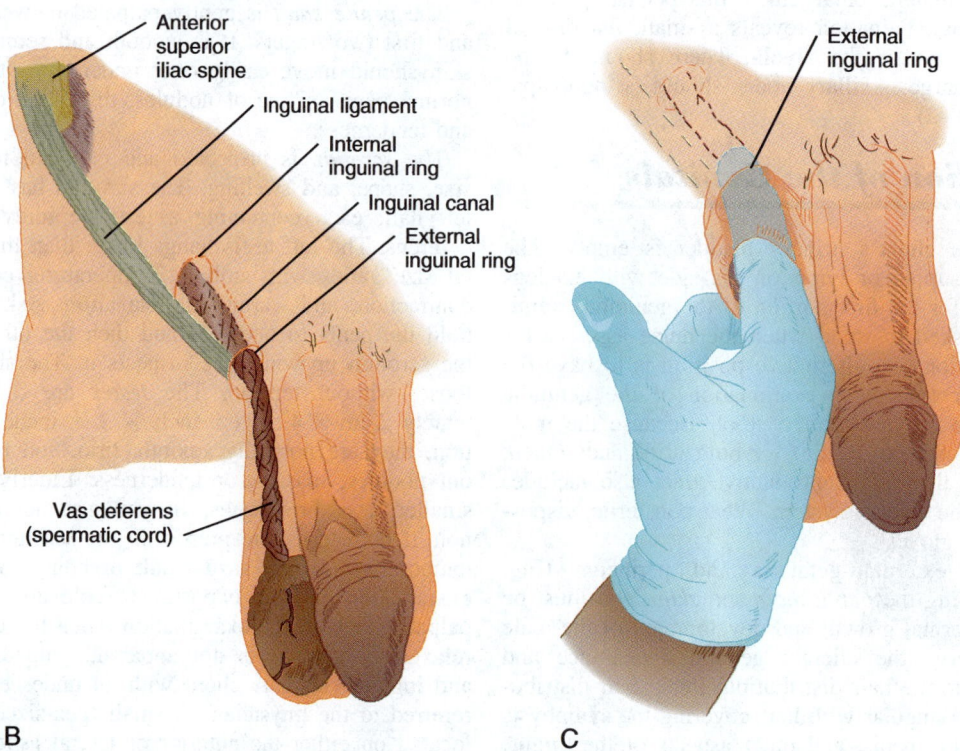

Anterior
superior
iliac spine
Inguinal ligament
Internal
inguinal ring
Inguinal canal
External
inguinal ring
Vas deferens
(spermatic cord)

External
inguinal ring

B

C

Figure 82–15. *A,* Male genitourinary anatomy. *B,* Anatomy of male inguinal structures. *C,* Palpation to detect an indirect hernia.

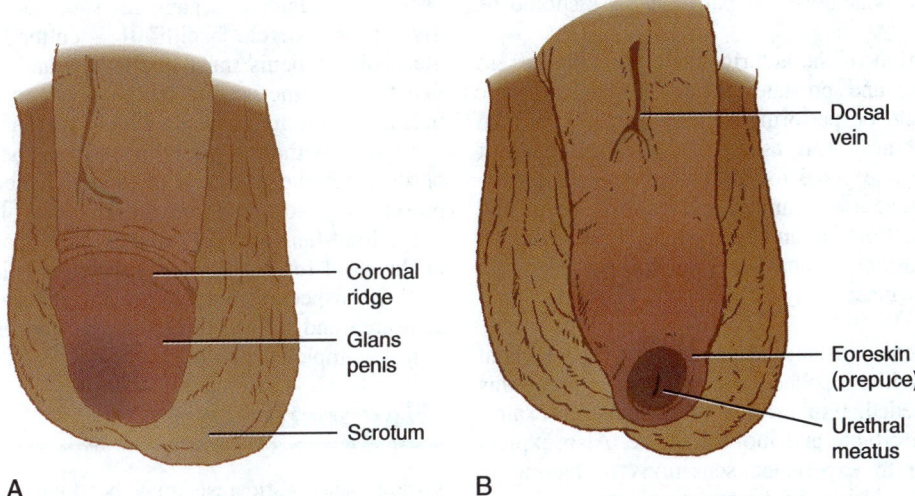

Figure 82–16. Appearance of a circumcised (*A*) and an uncircumcised (*B*) penis.

ger. The epididymis is located on the superior aspect of the testis and extends down the posterior surface. The epididymis feels soft, resilient, and tender. Swelling and hardness are abnormal. The *vas deferens* (spermatic cord) begins at the superior, lateral aspect of the testis. It is differentiated from the epididymis by its firmer, tubular feel. Compare your findings bilaterally. The vas deferens is palpated along its length toward the inguinal canal. Note any thickening or asymmetry, which is abnormal.

If you find swelling, nodules, or other abnormal results during the scrotal examination, perform *transillumination of the scrotum* (Fig. 82–17). Darken the room and shine

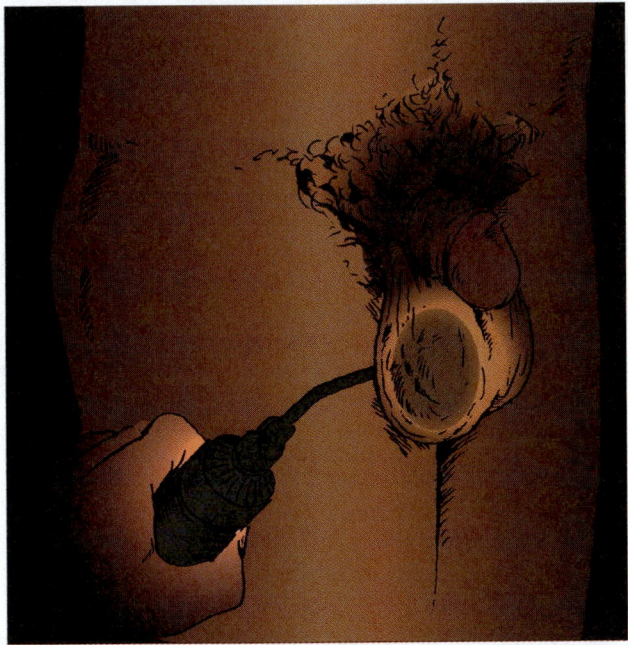

Figure 82–17. Transillumination of the scrotum. In a darkened room, place a strong, lighted flashlight or transilluminator next to the scrotum, as shown. Light normally passes through the scrotum (transillumination), but this does not occur with testicular tumor. A hydrocele will shine red.

a flashlight through the scrotum from behind the mass. A scrotum filled with serous fluid will transilluminate as a red glow. More solid lesions, such as a hematoma or mass, will not transilluminate and may be seen as a dark shadow. Record the characteristics of the abnormality, including whether it transilluminates.

Examination of the client for *inguinal herniation* is best performed while the client stands. A *hernia* is a prolapse or protrusion of a loop of intestine through the inguinal wall or canal. A *direct inguinal hernia* enters the inguinal canal behind the external ring because of a weakened abdominal wall; it does not pass through the inguinal canal. An *indirect inguinal hernia* enters the inguinal canal through the internal ring and can remain in the canal or pass down through the external ring and into the scrotum. A *femoral hernia* (more common in women) occurs inferiorly and more laterally than an inguinal hernia; it often has the appearance of an enlarged inguinal lymph node. Use the left index finger to palpate the client's right side and the right finger for the client's left side, with the client facing you.

Inspect the inguinal areas for bulges while the client stands quietly and again after he is instructed to bear down and strain as though attempting a bowel movement. Bulges should be absent. The presence of a *direct hernia* is assessed by gently inserting an index finger into the loose scrotal skin over the external inguinal ring; the finger does not enter to the external ring. Instruct the client to bear down while you feel for a bulge, which should be absent. To palpate for an *indirect hernia,* gently invaginate the scrotal skin with the index or little finger, following the vas deferens to where it passes into the external ring (see Fig. 82–15C). Asking the client to flex the knee on that same side may assist in relaxing the muscles so that the finger can be inserted through the external ring and into the inguinal canal. Advance the palpating finger as far as possible, and instruct the client to bear down while you feel for a tissue mass touching the finger. The mass retreats back up the canal when the client relaxes. Palpate the inguinal area directly for a *femoral hernia* while the client is relaxed and again after instructing him to bear down. A palpable mass should be absent.

After examination of the anterior male genitalia, assess the anus, rectum, and prostate gland. A rectal-prostatic examination should be performed during annually in men over 40 years of age. This assesses (1) for evidence of STD; (2) the prostate gland for alterations in size, consistency, and evidence of a tumor; and (3) for acute and chronic infection. Impress on the man the importance of regular rectal-prostatic examination as the best way to detect prostatic cancer early enough for effective treatment.

Just before rectal-prostatic examination, ask the client to empty his bladder. Collect a urine specimen at this time if one is needed. Explain that this makes the examination more comfortable and more accurate. Also explain that it is normal to experience sensations of having to urinate or defecate during the examination.

Two possible positions for the client during the rectal examination are (1) the knee-chest position with the buttocks elevated or (2) bending over from the hip with elbows placed either on the knees or on the examining table (see discussion of examination positions in Chapter 12). See Chapter 59 for a complete discussion of examination of the anus and rectum.

Wear a glove on the examining hand and apply water-soluble lubricant to the examining finger. To perform the examination, place the dominant hand on the client's hip to stabilize his position and to reassure him. Gently spread his buttocks with the nondominant hand. Observe the perineum and perianal areas for lesions, hemorrhoids, inflammation, or discoloration. Ask the client to bear down, explaining that this helps relax the anal sphincter and makes it easier to insert the examining finger. Insert the ball of the finger toward the anterior wall of the rectum. The normal prostate is located 2 to 5 cm beyond the anal sphincter along the anterior wall of the rectum. It is normally about 4 cm long and 5 cm wide (Fig. 82–18 A and B). The prostate is shaped like a doughnut wrapped around the neck of the urethra (Fig. 82–18 C). The posterior and lateral lobes only can be felt through the rectal wall (Fig. 82–18 D and E). The lateral lobes should be symmetrical. A normal prostate should feel smooth, rubbery, and firm, rather like the base of the thumb. In benign prostatic hypertrophy the prostate feels larger than normal, with a firmer consistency, like that of the chin. Tenderness and bogginess (like the cheek of the face) may indicate acute or chronic prostatitis. Carcinoma feels "stony hard" or like a "hard nodule," that is, a circumscribed area of induration. Any induration is abnormal. The seminal vesicles (superior and lateral to the prostate) are normally nonpalpable.

Prostatic massage may be indicated even when the client is asymptomatic, in order to diagnose prostatitis. Roll the pad of the index finger across the prostate, starting laterally and superiorly and moving toward the midline of the prostate (Fig. 82–18F). Then, strip (or "milk") the area of the seminal vesicles, starting laterally and superiorly, toward the midline (Fig. 82–18G). Send the resultant meatal secretions for microscopic examination. A large number of pus cells suggests prostatitis. Acid-fast organisms may be identified by staining. Cultures may be needed to identify organisms such as gonococci, chlamydia, or tubercle bacilli. If a culture is required, the glans of the penis must be cleaned and the bladder emptied to clean the urethra before prostatic massage. Collect meatal secretions in sterile culture media.

As you withdraw your finger from the client's rectum, observe for the presence of *stool* on the glove. Feces, if present, are normally brown. Mucus or blood and black, tarry, light-tan, or gray stool is abnormal. Test a sample of the stool for *occult blood*, which should be negative. If STD is suspected, obtain a rectal culture. Wipe the perianal area and inform the client that the physical examination is completed.

Diagnostic Tests

Various diagnostic tests may be done to assess for male reproductive disturbances. Men and their significant others are often anxious about diagnostic tests. Reduce anxiety by giving careful explanations before and during the tests. It is much less frightening if a client knows what to expect and is included in the process.

Learn the preparation necessary for each test. Sometimes sedation or pain relief is required. An informed consent authorization may be necessary. Physiologic preparations may be required (e.g., fasting, enema). During the test, keep the client informed about what is happening. Help him maintain the required positions. Observe him carefully during and after the test for adverse reactions, such as pain, excessive anxiety, pallor, or nausea.

Laboratory Tests

Blood Studies

■ Prostate-Specific Antigen

In the late 1980s a blood test was developed that has revolutionized screening for prostate cancer—the prostate-specific antigen (PSA), tested by immunoassay. PSA is a normal substance found in prostatic fluid that aids in the liquification of semen. PSA is found in the sera of men without prostate cancer, but, the normal levels are very low. The PSA level also increases with age. Some controversy exists over the normal level. It can be argued that of 4.0 ng/ml or higher may be normal only for men over the age 65 and a lower level is normal for younger men.[53] It should be remembered that prostatic massage or rectal examination within 48 hours of the examination can lead to elevated levels of PSA.

In order to further clarify the meaning of the PSA level, two newer tests have been added, the PSA density (PSAD) and the PSA velocity (PSAV). The former relates PSA level to prostate size while the latter looks at the rate of change in PSA level over time. The PSAD is combined with transrectal ultrasound to determine the volume of the prostate. Clients with PSAD levels less than 0.10 ng/ml are considered unlikely to have significant prostate cancer. As the levels rise, so does the likelihood that prostate cancer is present. Clients with a PSAV that rises more than 0.7 ng/ml/yr or that increases 20% or

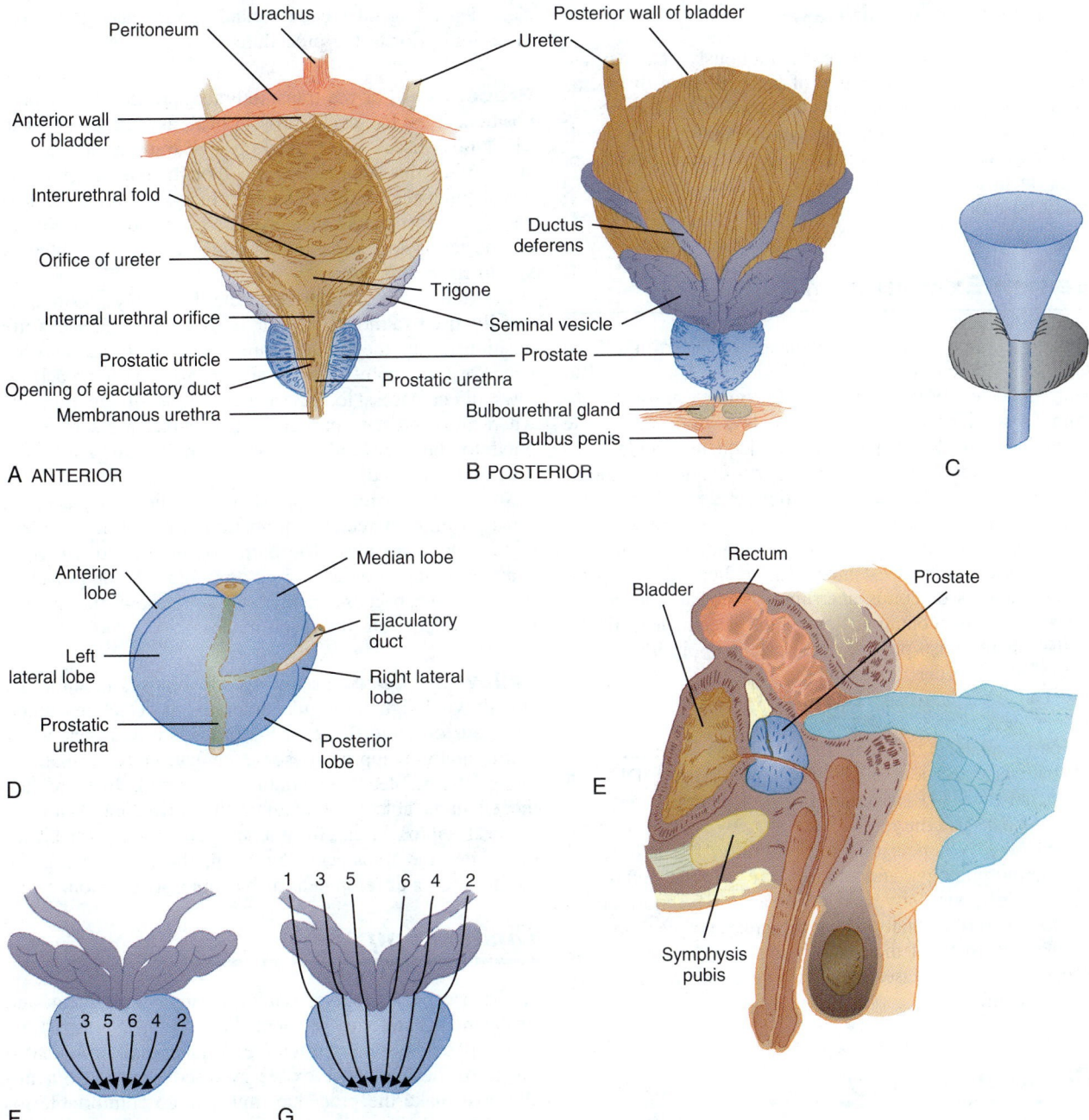

Figure 82–18. Rectal-prostatic assessment. *A* and *B*, Anterior and posterior views of the prostate gland. *C*, Diagrammatic representation of the anatomic position of the prostate gland. It surrounds the urethra rather like a doughnut wrapped around the outlet of a funnel. *D*, Posterior and lateral lobes of the prostate. *E*, Rectal examination. Insert a gloved index finger into the anus while the client is bearing down. Palpate all surfaces. *F*, Prostatic massage. Roll the pad of the index finger across the prostate, starting laterally and superiorly and moving toward the midline of the prostate. *G*, Seminal vesicles and prostatic massage. Use the same technique as for prostatic massage, but extend the finger higher over the area of the seminal vesicles.

more a year, are considered at high risk of having prostate cancer.

■ Serum Acid Phosphatase

Although acid phosphatase is contained in many tissues, the prostate value has been important for diagnosis. The development of the PSA assay, however, has decreased the importance of this test to the point that it may not be used in the future.[52] Part of the problem is that serum acid phosphatase is elevated after prostate cancer has spread beyond the gland. This makes it more accurate test for determining spread of prostate cancer rather than diagnosing the disease early.

Acid phosphatase levels can be abnormally elevated for 48 hours following prostatic massage or rectal examination or following administration of clofibrate. Alcohol, fluorides, oxalates, and phosphates can lead to artificially reduced levels of acid phosphatase.

■ Alkaline Phosphatase

Alkaline phosphatase is present ubiquitously. It is particularly associated with a variety of bone diseases. It is used as a diagnostic test in men with prostate cancer as a measure of possible bone metastasis. With higher levels in clients with known prostate cancer, the probability of bone metastasis is higher. Many medications can artificially raise or lower the level.

Semen Examination

Semen testing is done to evaluate for infertility. Two samples gathered at intervals of 2 to 4 weeks are used to accommodate normal variation. The client needs to abstain from ejaculation for 2 to 5 days prior to sample collection in order to produce an adequate sample. Prolonged abstinence may decrease sperm quality and motility, while more frequent ejaculations reduce sperm concentration and volume.

Masturbation into a clean, dry container in the laboratory or office is the best method of collecting the specimen. Condoms or coitus interruptus is not an appropriate method because contamination of the specimen is likely. If the client must provide the specimen outside of the laboratory or office, it should be kept at room temperature and brought to the laboratory within 30 minutes of collection.

Sperm analysis is done to (1) assess infertility, (2) evaluate effectiveness of a vasectomy, (3) test DNA in suspected rape, (4) prove sterility in a paternity suit, and (5) establish paternity. Only the first two areas are discussed here. When testing for infertility, the number of sperm, morphology, and motility are all assessed along with the pH, viscosity, and appearance. If abnormalities are found, further analysis for the presence of antibodies is also performed. If the test is being done to evaluate the effectiveness of a vasectomy, the presence or absence of sperm is sufficient.

Prostatic Biopsy

Following the finding of an abnormal PSA level, transrectal ultrasound, or digital rectal examination, a prostatic biopsy is done to test the suspicious area. The removal of a small amount of prostate tissue allows cytologic examination for the presence of prostate cancer.

Client Preparation. The tissue is be obtained transurethrally, transrectally, or perineally. It is important that the client understand the approach to be used and the preparation and procedure for it. Tell the client that he will be in the lithotomy position if a transurethral or perineal approach will be used and in Sims position if a transrectal approach is to be used.

Physical preparation oftens include enemas for the transrectal or perineal approach, either one enema or until clear depending on the physician's preference. The client must void prior to the procedure.

Procedure. For the transurethral approach, the client is positioned as for cystoscopy. Local anesthesia is used. The biopsy tissue is removed through transurethral endoscopy. With this approach, even though it is under direct visual guidance, malignant tissue may be missed. This is partly due to the fact that prostate cancer often begins in the posterior lobe, making it more difficult to obtain a specimen by this approach.

For the perineal approach, the lithotomy position is usually used, although it can be done from a jackknife position. After the perineal area is cleaned and anesthetized, one or more biopsies are taken. This approach allows direct access to the posterior lobe of the prostate, where most prostate cancers begin. Direct pressure is applied to the area and if there is no bleeding, a sterile dressing is applied.

With the transrectal approach, the client is placed in Sims position. A rectal examination is performed to identify any hard nodules. The biopsy is performed using the examiner's finger as a guide. Some think this approach is inappropriate because malignant cells from the nodule may be seeded into the rectal mucosa.

Follow-up Care. Following the biopsy, monitor the client's vital signs at regular intervals to detect any manifestations of hemorrhage. If the procedure was done using a transurethral approach, some hematuria is normal, although frank bleeding should be reported. Be sure that the client is able to void after the procedure. With the perineal approach, carefully assess the dressing for bleeding. After the transrectal approach, the client should be monitored for development of bleeding or infection.

Cystoscopy

A cystoscope is indispensable in both assessment and treatment of urologic problems. It is a metal instrument with optical systems providing a magnified illuminated image of the bladder. Flexible cystoscopes are also available and make the procedure much more comfortable for the client. Some indications for cystoscopy are the following:

- To determine the source of urinary bleeding
- To determine the cause of unexplained urinary manifestations
- To determine the source of pyuria
- To catheterize the ureters to localize the infection and for subsequent treatment
- To obtain biopsy specimens
- For follow-up examinations.

Cystoscopy may be done in a urologist's office or (if the client is symptomatic) in an operating room before surgery. Inspection of the bladder interior includes looking for trabeculation, diverticula, and bladder neck contracture and checking the size and contours of the prostatic lobes. Chapter 55 describes the procedure and client care in detail.

Computed Tomography

CT scans are used in the clinical staging of testicular tumors and prostate cancer. The client lies on an x-ray table, which moves him into various positions while scans are taken at various planes. If an injectable contrast medium is used, ask the client about any history of allergies. The procedure takes about 30 minutes.

Ultrasonography

Ultrasonic waves (sound waves too high in frequency for the human ear to hear) are "bounced off" tissue surfaces and produce an electronic image of body structures that can differentiate masses. This technique is used to visualize abnormalities of the prostate or scrotum. The procedure is done transrectally to help detect prostate lesions.

Prostatic ultrasonography is performed through a transrectal approach. The rectum needs to be free of feces prior to the test. The client is usually in a left lateral Sims position for the procedure. A rectal examination is performed followed by insertion of a well-lubricated transducer. A water-filled condom covers the probe to allow for the transmission of sound waves. The bladder also may be filled with fluid to improve the transmission of sound waves. The probe is moved along the prostate until adequate scanning has been accomplished. Some discomfort is associated with insertion and movement of the probe, but, once the examination is completed, there are no further effects.

Scrotal ultrasonography is performed to assess for testicular abnormalities. It is used to differentiate whether a mass is cystic, a solid tumor, or an abscess. It can also be used to diagnose epididymitis, hydrocele, spermatocele, scrotal hernia, or testicular torsion and associated infarction. The procedure is done with the client supine. The penis is gently taped to the lower abdomen to move it out of the way. The transducer is moved over the well-lubricated scrotum.

Magnetic Resonance Imaging

MRI provides three-dimensional images obtained by using field gradients in a magnetic field. MRI may be used to visualize pelvic structures, including the prostate, bladder, seminal vesicles, and penis. Metallic objects must be removed to prevent injuries. Clients with pacemakers, metal joint replacements, or surgical clips cannot undergo this study.

Urodynamic Assessment

Urodynamic studies measure (1) pressure (e.g., from the bladder or urethra), (2) urinary flow, and (3) striated muscle activity. Common tests use the uroflowmeter, cystometrography, electromyography, and urethral pressure profile. They are useful to determine the cause of frequency and decreased urinary stream in men (e.g., prostatic obstruction). Chapter 55 describes urodynamic testing in detail.

Client Preparation. Ask the client not to empty his bladder before the tests, because he will be asked to pass urine during the tests. Withhold sedatives, analgesics, and cholinergic or adrenergic drugs 6 to 8 hours before testing because these may interfere with bladder function.

Procedure. During the tests, the client is asked to void into a funnel or commode connected to a uroflowmeter, which measures voiding patterns (i.e., rate, time, volume, effort needed to initiate stream, strength and continuity of stream). During cystometrography, a urethral or suprapubic catheter is inserted and residual urine measured. Then, 30 ml of saline solution at room temperature is introduced into the bladder, followed by 30 ml of fluid at 110° to 115° F.

The client is asked to describe sensations as the bladder fills (e.g., need to void, nausea, flushing, discomfort, temperature). The bladder is drained, the catheter is connected to a cystometer, and normal saline or carbon dioxide is slowly introduced into the bladder. A transducer connected to the catheter records pressure changes in the bladder. The client is asked to report when he first feels the need to void, and then when he feels an urgent need to void. He voids when the bladder reaches its full capacity.

An electromyogram assesses sphincter activity during voiding. A needle electrode is inserted through the perineum into the external sphincter. Normally, sphincter activity ceases during voiding and resumes when the man voiding stops. The urethral pressure profile involves slowly withdrawing a catheter through the urethra. A transducer connected to the catheter measures the pressure as it is withdrawn.

Follow-up Care. These tests may be uncomfortable and embarrassing for the client. Document intake and output for 24 hours after the test. Document and report any hematuria.

Radioisotope Scans

Radioisotope scans may be used to assess testicular abnormalities (e.g., torsion, epididymitis, abscess, tumors, hydroceles, varicoceles, and spermatoceles). A radioactive substance is administered IV, and several scans are taken. Before a scan is taken, ask the client if he has any history of allergies.

Secretion Analysis

Body secretions from the throat, penis, and anus or lesions from the oral, pharyngeal, and perineal areas may be examined for microorganisms. A sterile applicator with a cotton tip is placed on or in the affected area and transferred to a sterile tube or slide. Be careful not to touch any other surface with the applicator.

Prevention of Male Reproductive Problems

Primary prevention (preventing a problem before it occurs) includes genetic counseling; immunization against infectious diseases; good nutrition; careful genital hygiene; the use of condoms to prevent STD; knowing one's partner; avoiding multiple sex partners; and avoiding sex (oral, anal, or genital) with a person who has genital lesions.

Secondary prevention (detecting and treating a problem early) includes activities such as screening (e.g., PSA levels in men over 50) and self-examination (see following).

Tertiary prevention (preventing complications and rehabilitation) is provided by most health professionals who provide care for clients experiencing acute and chronic diseases. For example, teaching men who have had a prostatectomy perineal exercises helps them regain urinary control.

Self-examination of the perineal and genital areas, including the penis, scrotum, and testes, is important. Avail yourself of opportunities to talk with men about this part of self-directed health care. Teach self-examination to all males past puberty. Such secondary prevention practices can be taught anywhere, including healthcare settings, schools and colleges, and workplace clinics. Self-examination can identify potential problems early when treatment is likely to be more successful; for example, testicular self-examination can detect testicular cancer while it is treatable.

Most men touch their genitals when urinating, bathing, and masturbating, but it may take a while for them to get used to touching their genitals for health assessment. It takes practice for a man to feel confident doing self-examinations. After a time, however, he will become familiar with his genital anatomy and able to identify abnormal changes. Explain the procedure carefully and provide opportunities for him to ask questions and express his concerns. Whenever possible, give the client literature to take home (the ACS publishes a useful pamphlet on testicular self-examination).

When teaching genital self-examination to men, instruct the client as follows:

- Develop the habit of doing self-examination once a month. Connect it in your mind with some other monthly event (e.g., paying bills, receiving the first paycheck of the month).
- Use a mirror to check inaccessible places (e.g., buttocks, perianal area, scrotum).
- Look for any changes from normal, such as swelling, lumps, tenderness, lesions, discoloration, asymmetry, or discharge.
- The best time to do a testicular self-examination is after a shower when you are warm, the scrotum is relaxed, and the testicles are easier to examine. When the testicles are cold, the scrotal skin contracts, making the testicles hard to feel. The left testicle is normally lower than the right because of a longer cord.
- The technique of testicular self-examination is as fol-

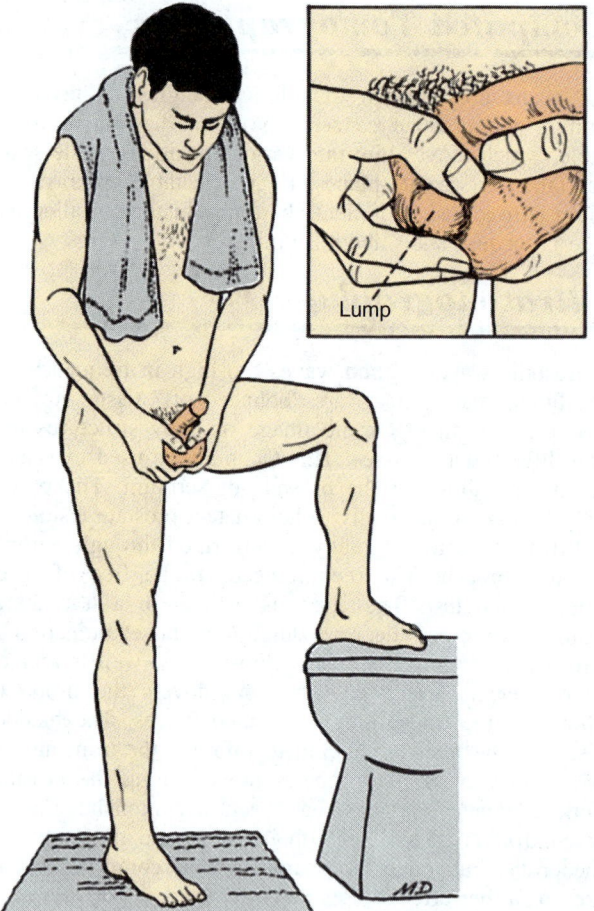

Figure 82–19. Testicular self-examination.

lows: hold the scrotum in the palms of your hands and examine each testicle with the thumbs and fingers of both hands. The index and middle fingers should be on the underside of each testicle with the thumbs on the top. Roll the testicles between your thumb and fingers (Fig. 82–19).

- A normal testicle is shaped like an egg and is about 4 cm (1 ⅗ inches) long. It feels firm but not hard (rather like an ear lobe), even rubbery, and quite smooth with no lumps.
- Examine the epididymides (behind the testicles). They should feel soft and may be spongy.
- Examine the spermatic cords, which ascend from the epididymides behind the testicles. They are normally firm, smooth, tubular structures.
- Do not hesitate to seek professional assessment and advice about anything unusual you find. It is better to learn that everything is all right rather than to wait too long.

Conclusions

It is very important to understand the proper assessment of the male and female reproductive systems. You must be aware not only of the physiology of this system but also of the psychological implications associated with reproductive disorders. Exhibit a concerned, caring attitude when assessing clients with reproductive disorders because disorders in this system are laden with psychosocial overtones. By assessing the client in a thorough but matter-of-fact manner, you can put the client at ease and perform a complete assessment.

Bibliography

1. American Cancer Society (1989). *Special touch: A personal plan of action for breast health* publication no. 87-1MM-Rev. 9/89-no. 2095-LE. Atlanta: Author.
2. American Cancer Society. (1992). *Guidelines for the cancer-related check-up.* Atlanta: Author.
3. American Cancer Society. (1995). *Cancer facts and figures, 1995* (publication no. 95-375M-no. 5008.95). Atlanta: Author.
4. Bates, B. (1995). *A guide to physical examination and history taking* (6th ed.). Philadelphia: J. B. Lippincott.
5. Baulch, T. S. et al. (1993). The relationship of visual acuity, tactile sensitivity, and mobility of the upper extremities to proficient breast self-examination in women 65 and older. *Oncology Nursing Forum, 19*(9), 1367–1372.
6. Benign Prostatic Hyperplasia Guideline Panel. (1994). *Benign prostatic hyperplasia: Clinical practice guideline.* AHCPR Publication no. 94-0583. Rockville, MD: Agency for Health Care Policy and Research, Public Health Service, U. S. Department of Health and Human Services.
7. Benign Prostatic Hyperplasia Guideline Panel. (1994). *Benign prostatic hyperplasia: Diagnosis and treatment.* AHCPR Publication no. 94-0582. Rockville, MD: Agency for Health Care Policy and Research, Public Health Service, U. S. Department of Health and Human Services.
8. Benign Prostatic Hyperplasia Guideline Panel. (1994). *Benign prostatic hyperplasia: Patient guide.* AHCPR Publication no. 94-0584. Rockville, MD: Agency for Health Care Policy and Research, Public Health Service, U. S. Department of Health and Human Services.
9. Betz, C. L., Hunsberger, M., & Wright, S. (1994). *Family-centered nursing care of children* (2nd ed.). Philadelphia: W. B. Saunders.
10. Bobak, I. M., & Jensen, M. D. (1993). *Maternity and gynecologic care* (5th ed.). St. Louis: Mosby–Year Book.
11. Bolander, V. R. (1994). *Sorensen and Luckmann's basic nursing: A psychophysiologic approach* (3rd ed.). Philadelphia: W. B. Saunders.
12. Bowers, A., & Thompson, J. (1992). *Clinical manual of health assessment* (4th ed.). St. Louis: Mosby–Year Book.
13. Campion, M. J., & Reid, R. (1990). Screening for gynecologic cancer. *Obstetrics and Gynecology Clinics of North America, 17*(4), 695–727.
14. Champion, V. L. (1991). The relationship of selected variables to breast cancer detection behaviors in women 35 and older. *Oncology Nursing Forum, 18*(4), 733–739.
15. Chernecky, C. C., Krech, R. L., & Berger, B. J. (1993). *Laboratory tests and diagnostic procedures.* Philadelphia: W. B. Saunders.
16. Dawson, N. A., & Vogelzang, N. (Eds.). (1994). *Prostate cancer.* New York: John Wiley & Sons.
17. Duffy, M. E. (1993). Determinants of health-promoting lifestyles in older persons. *Image: Journal of Nursing Scholarship, 25*(1), 23–28.
18. Feig, S. A. (1994). Mammographic screening of women 40 to 49 years. Is it justified? *Obstetrics and Gynecology Clinics of North America, 21*(4), 587–606.
19. Fogel, C. I., & Lauver, D. (1990). *Sexual health promotion.* Philadelphia: W. B. Saunders.
20. Frankl, G. (1988). Screening and detection of breast cancer. In M. E. Lippman, et al. (Eds.), *Diagnosis and management of breast cancer* (pp. 10–21). Philadelphia: W. B. Saunders.
21. Friedman, L. C., et al. (1994). Dispositional optimism, self-efficacy, and health beliefs as predictors of self-examination. *American Journal of Preventative Medicine, 10*(3), 130–135.
22. Fuller, J., & Schaller-Ayers, J. (1994). *Health assessment: A nursing approach* (2nd ed.). Philadelphia: J.B. Lippincott.
23. George, N., & Samntook, P. (1991). *Diagnostic picture tests in urology.* St. Louis: Mosby–Year Book.
24. Giger, J. N., & Davidhizar, R. E. (1995). *Transcultural nursing: Assessment and intervention* (2nd ed.). St. Louis: Mosby–Year Book.
25. Ginsberg, C. K. (1991). Exfoliative cytologic screening: The Papanicolaou test. *Journal of Obstetric, Gynecologic, and Neonatal Nursing, 20*, 39–46.
26. Glenn, B. L., & Moore, L. A. (1990). Relationship of self-concept, health locus of control, and perceived cancer treatment options to the practice of breast self-examination. *Cancer Nursing, 13*(6), 361–365.
27. Gonzalez, J. T. (1990). Factors relating to frequency of breast self-examination among low income Mexican American women: Implications for nursing practice. *Cancer Nursing, 13*(3), 134–142.
28. Gorrie, T. M., McKinney, E. S., & Nurray, S. S. (1994). *Foundations of maternal newborn nursing.* Philadelphia: W. B. Saunders.
29. Graham, S. (1994). Screening for prostate cancer. *Cancer, 74*(12), 3077–3079.
30. Gray, M. E. (1990). Factors related to practice of breast self-examination in rural women. *Cancer Nursing, 13*(2), 100–107.
31. Grimes, J., & Burns, E. (1996). *Health assessment in nursing practice* (4th ed.). Boston: Little, Brown.
32. Hacker, N. F., & Moore, J. G. (1992). *Essentials of obstetrics and gynecology* (2nd ed.). Philadelphia: W. B. Saunders.
33. Hamilton, P. M. (1993). *Basic maternity nursing* (7th ed.). St. Louis. Mosby–Year Book.
34. Hammerer, P. G., McNeal, J. E., & Stamey, T. A. (1995). Correlation between serum prostate specific antigen levels and the volume of the individual glandular zones of the human prostate. *Journal of Urology, 153*(1), 111–114.
35. Helvie, M. A., et al. (1990). Radiographic guided fine needle aspiration of non-palpable breast lesions. *Radiology, 174*(3141), 657–661.
36. Horton, J. A. (1992). *The women's health data book.* New York: Elsevier.
37. Jarvis, C. (1996). *Physical examination and health assessment* (2nd ed.). Philadelphia: W. B. Saunders.
38. Karlowicz, K. A. (Ed.). (1995). *Urologic nursing: Principles and practice.* Philadelphia: W. B. Saunders.
39. Kee, J. L. (1995). *Laboratory and diagnostic tests with nursing implications* (4th ed.). Norwalk, CT: Appleton & Lange.
40. Kenny, R. A. (1992). *Physiology of aging: A synopsis.* St. Louis: Mosby–Year Book.
41. Kirby, R., & Christmas, T. (1993). *Benign prostatic hypertrophy.* New York: Raven Press.
42. Kurtz, M. E., et al. (1993). Relationship of barriers and facilitators to breast self-examination, mammography, and clinical breast examination in a worksite population. *Cancer Nursing, 16*(4), 251–259.
43. Lauver, D., & Rubin, M. (1991). Women's concerns about abnormal Papanicolaou test results. *Journal of Obstetric, Gynecologic, and Neonatal Nursing, 20*, 154–159.
44. Lee, W. R., et al. (1995). Observations if pretreatment prostate-specific antigen doubling time in 107 patients referred for definitive radiotherapy. *International Journal of Radiation Oncology, Biology, and Physiology, 31*(1), 21–24.
45. Leitch, A. M., & Garvey, R. F. (1994). Breast cancer in a community hospital population: Impact of breast screening in stage of presentations. *Annals of Surgical Oncology, 1*(16), 516–520.
46. LeMone, P. (1993). Validation of the defining characteristics of altered sexuality patterns. *Nursing Diagnosis, 4*, 56–62.
47. Littrup, P. (1994). Prostate cancer screening. *Cancer, 74* (Suppl. 7), 2016–2022.
48. Littrup, P., & Goodman, A. C. (1994). Costs and benefits of prostate cancer screening: Investigators of the American Cancer Society–National Prostate Cancer Detection Project. *In Vivo, 8* (3), 423–427.
49. McCorkle, R., et al. (1996). *Cancer nursing: A comprehensive textbook.* Philadelphia: W. B. Saunders.
50. McMillan, S. C. (1990). Nurses' compliance with American Cancer

Society guidelines for cancer prevention and detection. *Oncology Nursing Forum, 17*(5), 721–736.

51. Mettlin, C., et al. (1993). Defining and updating the American Cancer Society guidelines for the cancer-related checkup: Prostate and endometrial cancers. *CA: A Cancer Journal for Clinicians, 43*(2), 42–46.

52. Mettlin, C., Jones, G. W., Murphy, G. P. (1993). Trends in prostate cancer care in the United States, 1974–1990: Observations from the patient care evaluation studies of the American College of Surgeons Commission on Cancer. *CA: A Cancer Journal for Clinicians, 43*(2), 83–91.

53. Mitchell, T. S. (1994). Screening for prostate cancer. *Urologic Nursing, 14*(1), 9–11.

54. Montie, J. E. (1994). Controversies in the early detection of prostate cancer. *In Vivo, 8*(3), 407–411.

55. Pleatman, M. A., & Cardona, R. R. (1990). Detection of breast cancer. *Obstetrics and Gynecology Clinics of North America, 17*(4), 729–740.

56. Pontie, J. E. (1994). Methods of early detection of prostate cancer: The role of prostatic specific antigen, transrectal ultrasound and digital rectal examination. *In Vivo, 8*(3), 413–414.

57. Quilligan, E. J., & Zuspan, F. P. (1994). *Current Therapy in Obstetrics and Gynecology* (4th ed.). Philadelphia: W. B. Saunders.

58. Reeder, S., Martin, L., & Koniak, D. (1992). *Maternity nursing* (17th ed.). Philadelphia: J. B. Lippincott.

59. Richardson, J. L., et al. (1987). Frequency and adequacy of breast cancer screening among elderly Hispanic women. *Preventive Medicine, 16*(6), 761–774.

60. Salazar, M. K. (1994). Breast self-examination beliefs: A descriptive study. *Public Health Nursing, 11*(1), 49–56.

61. Seidman, H., et al. (1987). Survival experience in the breast cancer detection demonstration project. *CA: A Cancer Journal for Clinicians, 37*(5), 258–291.

62. Shepard, E. D., & Shepard, C. A. (1990). *The complete guide to women's health* (2nd ed.). New York: Plume.

63. Smith, D. R. (1996). *General urology* (14th ed.). Los Altos, CA: Lange Medical.

64. Strasinger, S. K. (1994). *Urinalysis and body fluids.* Philadelphia: F. A. Davis.

65. Terris, M. K., et al. (1995). Prediction of prostate cancer volume using prostate-specific antigen levels, transrectal ultrasound, and systemic sextant biopsies. *Urology, 45*(1), 75–80.

66. Watson, J., & Jaffe, M. (1995). *Nurse's manual of laboratory and diagnostic tests* (2nd ed.). Philadelphia: F. A. Davis Co.

67. Yen, S. S. C., & Jaffe, R. (1991). *Reproductive endocrinology: Physiology, pathophysiology, and clinical management* (3rd ed.). Philadelphia: W. B. Saunders.

68. YoungKin, E. Q., & Davis, M. S. (1994). *Women's health.* Norwalk, CT: Appleton & Lange.

Nursing Care of Men with Reproductive Disorders

CHAPTER 83

Esther Matassarin-Jacobs

Today, men are showing more interest in being actively involved in health maintenance. This is evidenced by the increased interest shown by men in fitness and exercise, men's increased attainment of life-style factors related to fitness (such as stopping smoking), and men's increased participation in childbirth and parenting. As men learn to express their interest in general health maintenance, you can extend these interests to reproductive and urinary health maintenance. Men with health problems face both Altered Urinary Elimination and Risk for Sexual Dysfunction because their urinary and reproductive systems involve the same structures.

Psychosocial Factors Affecting Male Reproduction

When caring for men who are experiencing sexual, reproductive, or urinary problems, plan sensitive care to meet the psychosocial and physical needs of men who are undergoing very personal procedures. The urinary system and reproductive system are the same, so any problem in the urinary system may be seen as a threat to a man's reproductive system and sexuality. Men are often reluctant to ask for help because they see such problems as a potential threat to their sexuality and are embarrassed to talk about them.

Many stereotypes have been bandied about concerning men's reluctance to complain or to seek healthcare. Some are true, because men are less likely than women to seek healthcare, and some men do complain less. As the Ethical Issues in Nursing feature explains, however, urinary or reproductive problems and sexual preference are very personal, and the client may be very hesitant to talk about these problems.

Because men may be reluctant to ask for help, skillful therapeutic interaction is essential to help them express their concerns. Be very sensitive and give the client permission to talk about his problem. Be sensitive to the client's discomfort and attempt to put the client at ease.

Statements such as "Many men are concerned about how this problem will affect their sex lives," or "It is common to worry about how your partner might feel about this problem," and "What are some of your concerns?" may help the client begin to talk about his concerns.

Giving men permission to express their feelings and health-related concerns draws them and their significant others into the process of healthcare. Teaching men reproductive and urinary health maintenance and self-care contributes to their overall health.

Physical Factors Affecting Male Reproduction

Some men find reproductive assessment difficult and need considerable support. Some men simply refuse to participate, perhaps fearing abnormal results. Masturbation is necessary to obtain a semen sample, and some men find this difficult for personal, cultural, or religious reasons. Many men may not know what chemicals they have been exposed to at the work place. In the United States, not all states have right-to-know laws that require employers to inform workers of the following:

1. Any use of toxic agents
2. Possible harmful effects from toxic agents that are used
3. How to avoid exposure to toxic agents being used

Assessment of reproductive problems in men includes the following:

1. Careful reproductive history-taking of men at risk and of their partners, including exposure to hazards from occupations, hobbies, and environment
2. Sexual history of men at risk and of their partners
3. Careful history of other physiologic conditions, such as hypertension, diabetes, or prostate problems
4. Semen analysis

ETHICAL ISSUES IN NURSING

Should a Client's Sexual Life-Style Influence His Nursing Care?

Personal attitudes toward sexuality help make us who we are. Our sexuality is an important part of our personal identity and how we identify with others. Attitudes toward others who may not view sexuality in the same way influence our relationship with those people.

Homosexuality, especially among men, is a subject that produces various responses. AIDS has caused a negative reaction toward gay men because the first human immunodeficiency virus (HIV) outbreaks in North America and Europe were seen primarily in homosexual men. Although this virus now is seen in heterosexual as well as homosexual populations, a negative association with homosexuals remains.

Healthcare providers take care of many kinds of people who are certain to have different attitudes about sexuality. You may or may not be aware of the sexuality of your clients. Those who care for homosexual men need to confront their own feelings about providing such care, which may reflect social discomfort or the fear of contracting HIV. Although this fear is a reality for many healthcare professionals, all clients should be treated equally, with respect and dignity. Also, the use of universal precautions may alleviate some of the apprehensions associated with HIV. The sexuality of clients is just as private as the sexuality of caregivers, and the respect shown toward one's own private life-style should be shown equally to others, no matter what personal attitudes are held.

---

5. Hormone studies, for example, radioimmunoassay for follicle-stimulating hormone (FSH), luteinizing hormone (LH), and testosterone.

Environmental and Occupational Agents

The effects of a variety of chemical agents on the male reproductive system are well documented. In 1977, the toxicity of the pesticide dibromochloropropane (DBCP) was dramatically linked to adverse testicular effects in workers in a California plant manufacturing the chemical.[152] The workers suspected the problem when they realized as a group they had conceived few children. The following interesting findings were made: (1) low sperm counts correlating with the length of time men had worked in the plant and (2) higher than normal levels of FSH and LH. Some men's sperm counts improved after they were no longer exposed to the pesticide. DBCP has also been found in community water supplies in California and Arizona. It has since been banned from agricultural use in the United States except on Hawaiian pineapples (little residue having been found on pineapples).[34]

Other agents associated with adverse reproductive effects in men include the following:

1. Anesthetic gases used in operating rooms and dentists' offices
2. Carbon disulfide from rubber vulcanization
3. Estrogen during manufacturing
4. The pesticides ethylene dibromide and chlordecone (Kepone)
5. Inorganic lead from smelters, painting, and printing
6. Inorganic mercury from manufacturing and dental work

7. Microwaves leaking from machines
8. Neurotoxins from the manufacture of polyurethane foam
9. Ionizing radiation from x-rays and gamma-emitting radioisotopes
10. Uoulene diamine from chemical manufacturing
11. Waste water treatment at petroleum refineries
12. Cadmium contained in cigarettes

Reproductive effects of chemical exposure vary, including abnormal sperm counts, loss of motility, impotence, spontaneous abortion, birth defects, and decreased libido (sex drive).

Pharmacologic Agents

Whenever a man is taking any drug, the possibility of sexual or reproductive health effects should be considered during nursing assessment. When planning nursing care, always review the specific use and action of drugs being taken by clients. Ask a man the simple question "Have there been any changes in your sexual activity? Why?" because part of nursing history can reveal problems that may be corrected by medication changes.

Some drugs may actually enhance sexual and reproductive functioning, such as clomiphene citrate (Clomid), which increases the sperm count. Other drugs depress sexual and reproductive function, such as phenytoin (Dilantin), which decreases spermatogenesis. The effects of some drugs are variable, enhancing functioning in one man and depressing it in another. Drugs that delay ejaculation (alcohol, cocaine, and amphetamines) may improve sexual function in a man who ejaculates prematurely. However, overuse of such drugs may lead to other problems, such as erectile dysfunction. Many drugs (prescription, over-the-counter, and recreational) are known to have sexual and reproductive effects in males. Others may not have been identified yet.

Major sexual and reproductive effects of drugs on men include the following:

1. Decreased desire for sex (libido)
2. Decreased erectile ability (impotence)
3. Decreased ejaculatory ability
4. Decreased sperm quality
5. Gynecomastia

The following drugs may have one or more such effects:

- Antihypertensives may cause impotence, decreased libido, and ejaculatory difficulties. These drugs include:
  1. Diuretics such as spironolactone (Aldactone) and chlorthalidone (Hygroton)
  2. Metoprolol (Lopressor)
  3. Others, such as methyldopa (Aldomet) and clonidine (Catapres)
- Antipsychotics such as chlorpromazine (Thorazine) and thioridazine (Mellaril) may lead to impaired ejaculation, decreased libido, and priapism (prolonged, persistent erection without ejaculation)
- Tricyclic antidepressants, such as amitriptyline (Elavil) and imipramine (Tofranil), may lead to a decrease in libido and difficulty with erection, ejaculation, and orgasm
- Monamine oxidase inhibitor (MAO) antidepressants, such as phenelzine (Nardil) and tranylcypromine (Parnate), may lead to a decrease in libido.
- Hormones such as progestins, antiandrogens, and androgens, may lead to almost any of the problems already mentioned, including impotence and gynecomastia.
- Sedative-hypnotics and tranquilizers such as diazepam (Valium), chlordiazepoxide (Librium), and methaqualone (Quaalude); barbiturates such as secobarbital (Seconal) and pentobarbital (Nembutal); and ethyl alcohol may lead to a decrease in libido.
- Stimulants such as amphetamines (Adderall) and cocaine may lead to impotence and changes in libido.
- Chemotherapeutic agents, such as chlorambucil (Leukeran) and cyclophosphamide (Cytoxan), may lead to decreased sperm quality.
- Opiates such as morphine, heroin, and methadone (Dolophine) may lead to impotence.
- Steroids, especially anabolic steroids, may cause a decrease in libido.
- Recreational drugs such as marijuana, lysergic acid diethylamide (LSD), phencyclidine piperidine (PCP), and tobacco may lead to decreased libido and impotence.

Many other drugs have been found to affect sexual or reproductive function in men. These drugs include digoxin (Lanoxin), griseofulvin (Fulvicin), and cimetidine (Tagamet), which may cause gynecomastia; disopyramide phosphate (Norpace), disulfiram (Antabuse), and trimethoprim-sulfamethoxazole (Bactrim-Septra), which may cause impotence; and metronidazole (Flagyl), which may decrease libido.

Systemic Conditions

Sexual dysfunction and other reproductive problems may be associated with medical or surgical conditions, such as diabetes mellitus, renal disease, prostate surgery, and spinal injury. It is important to assess a man's previous level of sexual functioning. Be aware of the wide range of normal sexual and reproductive function to reassure clients about their normalcy. What may be normal for one man may be considered abnormal by another and, therefore, a cause for concern.

Vascular Conditions. Arteriosclerotic changes in the vascular system can lead to changes in blood flow to the penis. If these changes are severe enough, impotence may result. Hypertension itself or antihypertensive medications may lead to problems with potency. Strokes also may lead to impotence with related cerebral cortical output. In actuality, any vascular condition or treatment that alters blood flow may alter the blood flow to the penis.

Neurologic Conditions. Both the sympathetic and parasympathetic nervous systems are involved in achieving and maintaining an erection. Surgery of the prostate may lead to damage of the nerves responsible for erection. Many neurologic conditions, such as multiple sclerosis, Parkinson's disease, myasthenia gravis, amyotrophic lateral sclerosis, and spinal cord injuries, cause the client problems with sexual function, especially achieving and maintaining an erection.

Respiratory Conditions. Emphysema has been associated with sexual dysfunction in men. It is unclear, however, whether this is specifically caused by the disease, the medications often used to treat it, or simply the extreme fatigue associated with the hypoxemia.

Endocrine Conditions. Diabetes mellitus is one of the most common diseases leading to problems with sexual function. This is usually related to the altered blood supply from small-vessel disease associated with diabetes. Pituitary or gonadal problems associated with low levels of testosterone or high levels of prolactin lead to many sexual and reproductive disorders. Thyroid and adrenal disorders can also cause problems. Hypogonadism, either primary (a rare congenital problem) or secondary (as a result of mumps orchitis, chemotherapy, radiation, or surgical removal), lead to impotence and other sexual problems.

Genitourinary Conditions. Problems with the penis or testes can lead to difficulties with sexuality and reproduction. Conditions of the penis such as priapism, phimosis, or Peyronie's disease (all discussed later in this chapter) may cause erectile dysfunction. Testicular disorders such as varicocele, torsion, or hydrocele lead to decreased fertility. Prostate problems may also alter fertility because of alterations in prostatic fluid. Hypospadias and epispadias, depending on how far the meatal opening is from the glans, may cause impaired fertility related to problems with ejaculation.

Infertility

In 1982, one out of every eight couples in the United States were considered infertile (i.e., unprotected intercourse did not result in a pregnancy over a 12-month period). Requests for infertility services are increasing rapidly, now numbering in the millions.

Male infertility is extensive, occurring in 5% to 10% of married men. Ten percent to 15% of marriages are childless, and another 10% to 15% of married couples have fewer children than they would like. In 30% to 50% of such marriages, it is the man who is infertile. However, the two partners are best treated together. Minimal fertility in one partner can be offset by strong fertility in the other. However, if both partners are minimally fertile, infertility is more likely.

An awareness of these statistics alerts healthcare professionals to clients who may have concerns about infertility but who have difficulty expressing them.

Etiology and Risk Factors

Causes of male infertility include the following:

- *Pretesticular:* endocrinopathy and sexual dysfunction, such as excessive ejaculation frequency
- *Testicular:* varicocele (varicose testicular vein); failure of testicle to produce sperm because of effects of drugs, environmental factors, development of chromosomal abnormalities, mumps orchitis, or spinal cord injury
- *Post-testicular:* ejaculatory dysfunction or obstruction caused by trauma, infection, or surgery
- *Genitourinary:* infection
- *Immunologic:* sperm antibodies in one or both partners

Pathophysiology

The pathophysiologic mechanisms involved with infertility are different for the different etiologies. It is often related to the inability to produce normal sperm capable of reproduction. Men normally have about 425×10^6 sperm available for ejaculation. A sperm concentration of at least 20×10^6/ml, with a volume of 1.5 to 5.0 ml, must be available for reproduction. Sperm must also have adequate motility and normal morphology to be functional. Problems with either lead to infertility.

Motility is defined as the forward progressive movement of the sperm. Factors that decrease the motility of sperm include heat, cold, certain drugs (discussed earlier), bacteria, and the presence of antisperm antibodies. *Morphology* refers to the form and structure of the sperm. Unless more than 60% of the sperm have normal morphologic characteristics, infertility will result.

Other abnormalities include the viscosity of the sperm, which may indicate problems with the prostate. Inflammatory or immunologic processes may lead to decreased viscosity with clumping of sperm. Normal semen coagulate, then liquify. Abnormalities in the accessory glands may lead to problems with either coagulation or liquification.

A normal component of semen is fructose, which is androgen dependent and is produced in the seminal vesicles. Obstruction of the ejaculatory ducts or absence of the seminal vesicles or vas deferens results in an absence of fructose in the semen, which may increase infertility.

Clinical Manifestations and Diagnostic Findings

Both the man and his partner may need help and support to express concerns and fears about infertility. Failure to conceive may make severe demands on the couple, threatening their individual self-concepts, sex roles, relationship, and sexual interaction. Guilt and blame about previous sexual activity, sexually transmitted diseases (STDs), or abortion may come between them. Fear and anxiety may be lessened by taking an involved nursing history. This also provides you with the opportunity to give support, respond to questions, and explain diagnostic and treatment procedures.

Assessment of male infertility includes obtaining a detailed history (sexual, medical, and reproductive) and a thorough physical examination. Semen analysis includes the following:

1. Gross examination, noting volume, viscosity, and color
2. pH, concentration, motility, morphology, and sperm agglutination

Other, more specific tests of sperm function include the fructose concentration and the Sims-Huhner test to assess the penetration of cervical mucus by sperm. Additional tests are performed for azoospermia (absence of sperm in the semen) or oligozoospermia (less than the normal number of sperm in the semen). Other studies include tests for sperm antibodies in serum and chromosome karyotyping to detect genetic abnormalities.

Endocrinologic studies assess follicle stimulating hormone (FSH), luteinizing hormones (LH), prolactin, and serum testosterone levels, all of which can help to identify endocrinologic causes of infertility. For example, if FSH levels are high, spermatogenesis is probably arrested. If FSH is normal, azoospermia or oligozoospermia is probable because of obstruction in the post-testicular ducts, which may be corrected by microsurgery. A testicular biopsy provides further information about spermatogenesis.

A genitourinary source of infertility can be assessed through urinalysis, urine culture, serum creatinine assay, and examination of prostatic secretions.

Community and Self-Care

■ Medical Management

Pretesticular Causes. Treatment for pretesticular causes of male infertility varies. No treatment is available for primary testicular failure or hypogonadism. Testosterone may be prescribed to correct low testosterone levels.

This is accomplished through the use of a testosterone patch applied directly to the scrotum. Hyperprolactinemia may be treated by surgical removal of a pituitary tumor or by administration of bromocriptine (Parlodel).

Treatment of male sexual dysfunction is discussed in the Erectile Dysfunction section. For oligozoospermia caused by excessive frequency of ejaculation, recommend that the couple have intercourse only once every 36 hours during the woman's periovulatory period, because it takes 24 hours for a normal sperm count to be generated after ejaculation.

Testicular Causes. Treatment of testicular causes of male infertility also varies. Reduced spermatogenesis from testicular atrophy caused by infection may be treated by the following:

1. Avoiding factors that depress spermatogenesis, such as heat and use of drugs, alcohol, and marijuana
2. Keeping the testes cool by avoiding hot baths and tight clothing, or by using a commercially prepared, water-dampened scrotal cooling device (keeping the testes cool appears to improve the sperm count)
3. Good nutrition

Medications, such as human chorionic gonadotropin (hCG) or testosterone (Depo-Testosterone), are sometimes prescribed, with varying degrees of success. Varicocele is treated surgically.

Post-testicular Causes. Treatment for post-testicular causes of male infertility involves correcting ejaculatory abnormalities and obstruction. Ejaculatory abnormalities may be corrected by the split-ejaculate technique. The first half of the ejaculate contains more sperm than the second half. The first half may be used for artificial insemination or may be deposited in the vagina during intercourse, followed by withdrawal of the penis. Absence of ejaculation or retrograde (backward) ejaculation may be treated with drugs such as ephedrine, imipramine, or antihistamines. When the client experiences retrograde ejaculation, artificial insemination may be done using sperm from urine obtained by centrifuge. Obstructive infertility is treated by surgery.

Appropriate antimicrobial drugs are used to treat genitourinary infections. Immunologic causes of male infertility may be treated with steroids and artificial insemination of sperm that have been washed to remove antibodies contained in the sperm.

■ Nursing Management of the Medical Client

The client and his partner are often highly emotional during the diagnostic phase, and your sensitivity can ease this somewhat. Encourage the client and his partner to talk openly about their feelings. Be open to the emotions expressed, including anger and fear. Thorough and complete infertility assessment is expensive and is often ineffective. It is more effective to prevent infertility from developing. Clients who either want to conceive at present or may want to conceive in the future can try to prevent infertility in the following ways:

- Avoid excessive intake of alcohol
- Avoid tobacco, marijuana, and other recreational drugs
- Decrease exposure to occupational and environmental hazards, including toxic substances and radiation
- Keep the scrotum cool (e.g., avoid excessive heat, hot baths, and tight clothing)
- Avoid transmission of sexually transmitted organisms by limiting the number of sexual partners and by using condoms, diaphragms, contraceptive foam, and other spermicides, especially with new partners (STDs, particularly gonorrhea and infection by *Chlamydia trachomatis*, may account for up to 30% of cases of infertility in populations at high risk)
- Develop effective means of stress reduction
- Eat a well-balanced nutritious diet

An assessment begins with a thorough history and physical examination. The client needs to be prepared to undergo a variety of diagnostic tests, including sperm analysis. Be sure that the client understands the testing and the reasons for the various examinations.

Ensure that the client understands the medical regimen suggested and the importance of following it closely. If the treatment involves the use of testosterone patches, make sure the client understands their use and correct application. The Client Education Guide provides guidelines for application of these patches.

Referral for counseling or support groups, or both, for infertile couples may be appropriate. A nationally known support group in the United States is RESOLVE (Department P, Box 474, Belmont, MA 02178).

Erectile Dysfunction

Erectile dysfunction (impotence) was once thought to be entirely psychogenic in origin. We now know that about half of the cases have physiologic causes. The number is even higher in men older 50 than years.

Psychogenic Dysfunction. Indications of psychogenic erectile dysfunction include the following:

- Normal and sustained erection during foreplay, but loss of erection at the moment of intromission (penetration)
- Normal erection with some sexual partners but not with others
- Normal erection with masturbation but not with partners
- Sudden onset of total impotence in a man younger than 40 years
- Alternating periods of normal function and total impotence

Physiologic Dysfunction. Medications are one possible cause of erectile dysfunction (see preceding text). Other possible causes of physiologic dysfunction include the following:

- *Vascular:* arteriosclerotic changes, trauma to penile blood supply, hypertension, stroke, diabetes mellitus,

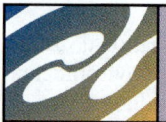

CLIENT EDUCATION GUIDE

Application of Testosterone Patches

Client Instructions in English (*Instrucciones para el cliente en inglés*)	Client Instructions in Spanish (*Instrucciones para el cliente en español*)
Clean and dry the scrotum carefully.	Limpie y seque cuidadosamente el escroto.
Shave the scrotum carefully, either with a safety razor without shaving cream or with an electric razor.	Rasure cuidadosamente el escroto con máquina de afeitar sin usar crema de afeitar, o máquina de afeitar eléctrica.
Before removing the patch from its plastic backing, heat it slightly with a hair dryer to help make it stick.	Antes de sacar el parche del refuerzo de plástico, caliéntelo ligeramente con una secadora de cabello para hacer que se pegue bien.
Apply the patch smoothly, holding it in place for a moment to help adherence.	Aplique suavemente el parche; sosténgalo por un momento para que se pegue bien.
Change the patch every 24 hours. It can be removed for bathing and then reapplied. Use the hair dryer to make it sticky again.	Cámbiese el parche cada 24 horas. Se lo puede quitar cuando se bañe y volvérselo a poner. Use la secadora de cabello para hacer adhesivo de nuevo.
Shave as often as needed to be sure the scrotum is kept free of hair. Hair will decrease the contact of the patch with the skin.	Aféitese tan a menudo como sea necesario para tener la seguridad de que el escroto está libre de pelo. El pelo disminuye el contacto del parche con la piel.
Notify the physician if a rash or any other problem develops.	Avisele al médico si le aparece un sarpullido (una erupción) o cualquier otro problema.
Have testosterone levels checked at intervals suggested by the physician.	Hágase controlar el nivel de la testosterona con la frecuencia que le recomiende el médico.

sickle cell anemia, leukemia, Hodgkin's disease, and aortic aneurysms
- *Neurologic:* interference with either sympathetic or parasympathetic innervation, degenerative diseases, and spinal cord injury
- *Genitourinary:* prostatitis, Peyronie's disease, and prolonged priapism
- *Endocrine:* hypopituitarism, hypogonadism, Cushing's syndrome, Addison's disease, hyperthyroidism, and extreme obesity leading to elevated estradiol levels and lower testosterone
- *Surgical:* bilateral orchiectomy, radical pelvic lymph node dissection, perineal prostatectomy, and some radical cystectomy procedures

Acute and Subacute Care

■ Surgical Management

Surgical treatment includes the use of penile prostheses, intracavernosal injections (using papaverine and prostaglandin E_1), and penile revascularization. Various penile prostheses are available. They comprise three basic types: semirigid, self-contained, and inflatable. Vacuum erection devices have also been in use for the last several years.

The original semirigid penile prosthesis (Small-Carrion) consists of a pair of plastic rods inserted within the corpus cavernosum (Fig. 83–1A). Silicone rods with a soft area at the scrotal junction are now available (Fig. 83–1B). The penis becomes permanently semirigid. Other semirigid prostheses include the Jonas malleable prosthesis, which has a silver wire center that allows the penis to be stabilized in a vertical or horizontal position, and the Finney prosthesis, which assumes a normal position when the client is standing, yet is firm enough for penetration.

Inflatable penile prostheses may be composed of the following:

1. Inflatable cylinders, with a pump placed within the scrotum and a reservoir in the abdomen (Fig. 83–1C),
2. A self-contained unit, with a pump and reservoir within the cylinder
3. A partially self-contained unit, with the pump in the cylinder and the reservoir in the scrotum

An erection is achieved through digital inflation of the cylinders, and the unit is deflated by a release valve at the side of the pump. The inflatable prosthesis is very

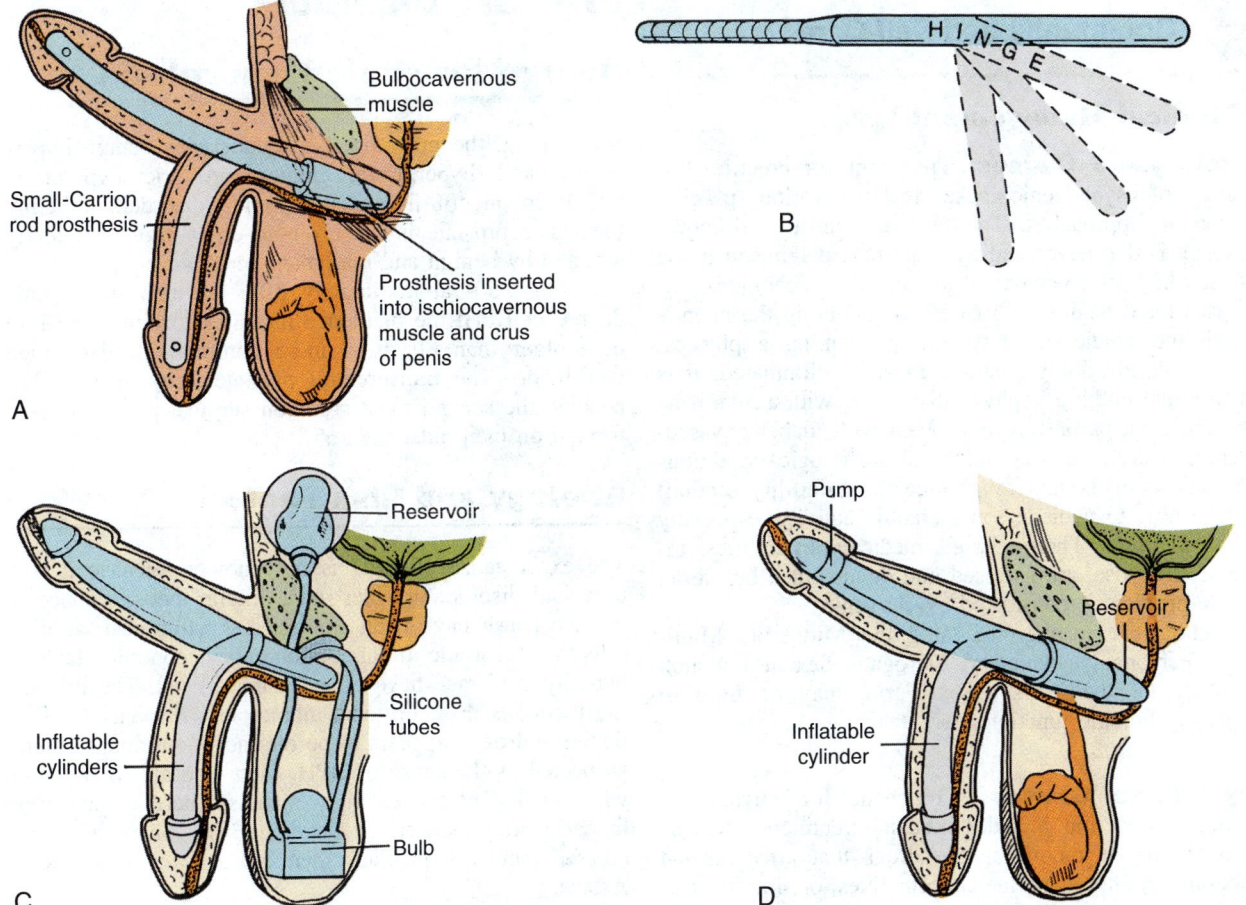

Figure 83–1. Penile prostheses. *A,* Small-Carrion prosthesis, consisting of plastic rods. *B,* Flexrod semirigid penile implant. *C,* Inflatable penile prosthesis. *D,* Self-contained penile prosthesis.

acceptable to the partner. The mechanical malfunction rate is at least 10% to 20%.

A newer variation of the semirigid model is the self-contained prosthesis (Fig. 83–1D). This prosthesis consists of a cylinder, a pump, and a reservoir filled with fluid. This prosthesis allows a more natural look in the relaxed state. It is inflated by pumping the prosthesis behind the head of the penis; fluid is then transferred from the reservoir near the rear of the device to the portion in the shaft, thereby producing an erection. A release valve can be pressed that allows the fluid to return to the reservoir. Semirigid prostheses can be implanted under local anesthesia and are successful in about 95% of cases. Semirigid penile prostheses are the most commonly used.

Penile revascularization may be used to correct vasculogenic erectile dysfunction. This surgical approach is still in its infancy. Microsurgical techniques are being tried to revascularize the dorsal or central penile arteries.

Intracorporeal injection therapy using papaverine and/or prostaglandin E₁ also may be used to achieve erection. This medication is administered by the client into the corporal bodies of the penis when erection is desired.

■ Nursing Management of the Surgical Client

Care of the client following implant of a penile prosthesis centers around teaching the client self-care of the prosthesis so that it will be used correctly. Physical care is the same as for any client undergoing surgery. Encourage the client to use pain medication after surgery before pain becomes severe. The genital area may be swollen and bruised after the procedure. The client will be told not to use the prosthesis (if an active prosthesis has been implanted) until complete healing has occurred.

The client who will use intracorporeal injections requires adequate teaching so that the procedure can be done independently. Teach the client the proper way to aspirate medication into the syringe and to clean the site of injection. For penile injections, the client should gently hold the penis against the thigh with one hand and inject the medication (papaverine or prostaglandin E₁) into the 3 or 9 o'clock position in the center of the penis. Try to rotate the sites between these two positions. Also teach the client proper disposal of the equipment.

Community and Self-Care

■ Medical Management

Psychogenic Causes. Treatment for erectile dysfunction of psychogenic causes includes various psychotherapeutic approaches. The best and most well-known approach is that developed by Masters and Johnson in the 1960s, which uses behavioral modification techniques.

Assessment begins with carefully gathering the client's sexual and medical history and performing a physical assessment. Physiologic causes must be eliminated. It is not true that nothing is physically wrong with a man if he can achieve a partial erection. Men with diabetic, vasculogenic, neurogenic, or endocrine pathologic conditions and men using certain drugs (see the Infertility section) may be able to achieve some erectile activity, especially in the morning. Therefore, all medical possibilities, including drug use, are assessed and documented before an erectile problem is considered psychogenic.

Psychometric testing, including the Minnesota Multiphasic Personality Inventory, Derogatis Sexual Function Inventory, or the Walker Sex Form, may be used to assess psychologic functioning.

Physiologic Causes. Treatment for physiologic erectile dysfunction includes medical treatment, such as discontinuing or modifying the drugs that affect sexual function, treating endocrine abnormalities, or simply treating the medical problem that is contributing to the dysfunction. If low levels of testosterone are discovered, replacement of the hormone may lead to improved functioning.

Physical examination includes complete blood count; urinalysis; examination of prostatic secretions; liver function studies; thyroid function tests; assessment for diabetes mellitus; and serum creatine, serum testosterone, LH, and prolactin assays.

■ Nursing Management of the Medical Client

Care of the client experiencing erectile dysfunction is similar to the care of the infertile client, as this is one cause of infertility. Use a sensitive, caring approach when working with these clients, because embarrassment may cause many men to avoid treatment. Care for erectile dysfunction of psychogenic origin may be long term and may require the client to undergo some form of counseling to resolve the disorder. Testing and diagnosis may be timely and discouraging for the client. Encourage the client to follow the suggested therapy.

When the cause of the dysfunction is physiologic, much of the initial care is centered around helping with the diagnostic process. Help the client understand the treatment of the primary medical or surgical problem that is causing the dysfunction. In many cases, erectile function will return once the primary condition is adequately treated.

Prostate Disorders

Benign Prostatic Hyperplasia

With aging, the prostatic tissue undergoes benign hypertrophy and hyperplasia. Benign prostatic hyperplasia (BPH) is one of the most common disorders affecting men. The prostate is the urologic organ most frequently affected by benign and malignant neoplasms.

By age 50, approximately 50% of men have some degree of BPH; the incidence increases to almost 90% in men older than 80. It is more common in black men worldwide. The transurethral prostatectomy (TURP) has become the second most common surgical procedure performed on men older than 65.[73]

Etiology and Risk Factors

The exact cause of BPH is not known. Because it is a universal disorder in older men, several theories concerning the cause have been examined. Factors such as diet, effects of chronic inflammation, socioeconomic factors, heredity, and race have all been considered. The prevailing theory is that hormonal alteration is responsible. Testicular androgen appears to be the most common hormone suspected as the cause of BPH. Men who are castrated or who develop permanent hypogonadism before puberty or in early adulthood rarely develop BPH. There is an increased incidence in black men and a lower incidence in Asians.

Aging is the major risk factor for the development of BPH with 80% of men over age 80 exhibiting some degree of BPH, so few primary preventions exist. Dietary factors have been examined with the conclusion that a diet high in yellow vegetables and other elements of Japanese diets appear to provide some protection against BPH. Early detection is the best secondary prevention available. Early detection can lead to early treatment, which can prevent complications related to urinary obstruction. Examination of the prostate by digital rectal examination annually for men older than 40 improves early detection.

Pathophysiology

Benign prostatic enlargement is an abnormal increase in number of normal cells (hyperplasia) in the prostate, rather than an increase in cell size (hypertrophy). Thus, although the disease was known as *benign prostatic hypertrophy*, *benign prostatic hyperplasia* is a more accurate name. With aging, the periurethral glands undergo hyperplasia. Gradually, they grow and compress surrounding normal prostatic tissue, pushing it toward the gland periphery, forming a false or surgical capsule. Tissue inside the capsule can be shelled out during surgery.

Many theories have been postulated concerning the pathophysiology of BPH. For BPH to occur, 5α-dihydrotestosterone (DHT) must be present and the client must be aging. DHT, the main prostatic androgen produced when testosterone is acted on by 5α-reductase, is a more

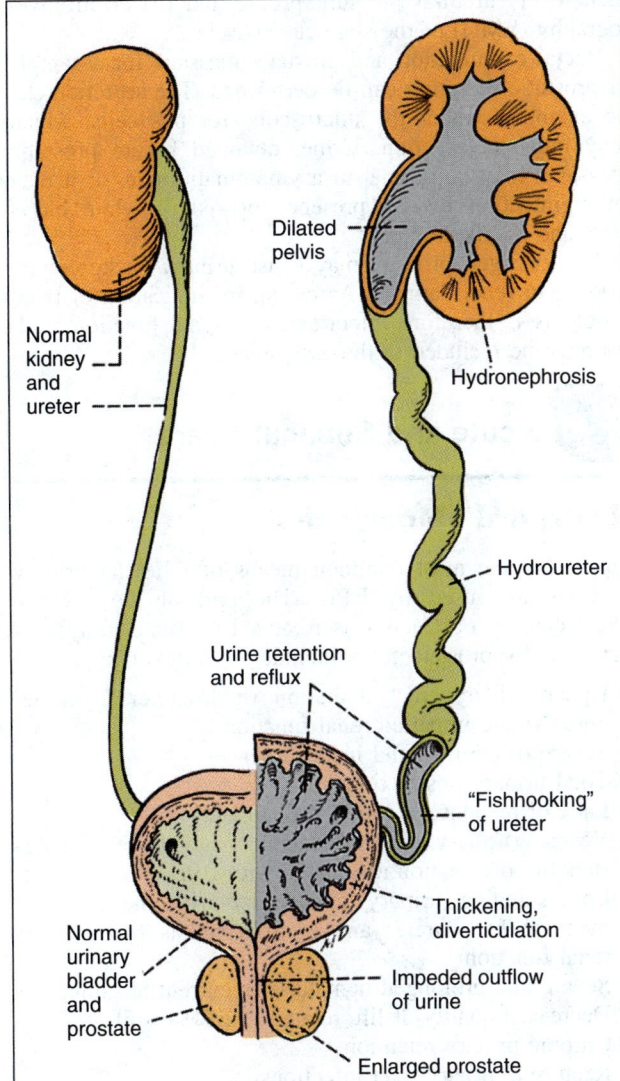

Figure 83–2. Complications of benign prostatic enlargement. *Left,* Normal kidney, ureter, bladder, and prostate. *Right,* Potential complications.

potent androgen within the prostate than testosterone itself. DHT, not testosterone, produces growth of prostatic tissue. The theory is that with BPH, increased levels of DHT combined with increased 5α-reductase activity lead to hyperplasia of prostatic tissue. Aging, on the other hand, lowers testosterone levels in relation to estrogen levels. Increased estrogen levels increase the longevity of prostatic cells, so cell death decreases. This leads to more cells being available to be acted on by the DHT, which leads to further hyperplasia.

Potential complications of prostatic enlargement (Fig. 83–2) include impeded urinary outflow and urinary reflux (backward flow) because of decompensation of the ureterovesical junction (see Bridge to Home Healthcare). Decompensation results from long-term elevated bladder pressure. Thickening, trabeculation (fibromuscular bands), and bladder wall diverticula may occur. Bladder diverticula may retain urine, causing infection and development of calculi. *Fishhooking* of the ureters is common (i.e.,

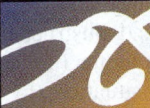

BRIDGE TO HOME HEALTHCARE

Intermittent Self-Catheterization for Men

Joyce Godin, *Godin Associates ET Nursing, LLC, Farmington, Connecticut*

Urinary retention is the inability to partially or completely empty the bladder. Retention may be caused by spinal cord injury, other neurologic diseases, or an enlarged prostate. When the bladder cannot be effectively emptied, it becomes overly distended and flaccid. Static urine becomes a medium for bacterial growth. Incontinence due to overflow voiding is frequently experienced.

Manual performance of a previously almost automatic function becomes necessary. Intermittent catheterization is an effective way to manage urinary retention, prevent overflow incontinence, and lessen incidence of urinary tract infections. To be successful, the client must be motivated to catheterize frequently enough to obtain 300 to 500 ml at each catheterization. Frequency is usually four to five times a day. As well as the ability to perform the procedure, the client also should have knowledge and understanding related to health and disease.

Clean catheterizarion is acceptable in the home setting. Care should be taken to ensure cleanliness of the equipment and the environment. Depending on client physical condition or limitations, catheterization may be performed sitting up in bed, on a chair, or on the toilet. Ambulatory men may prefer to stand. Supplies needed are as follows:

- Red rubber or clear vinyl 14F, 16 inch long, straight catheters
- Water soluble lubricant
- Soap and water, or cleansing towelettes, and paper towels
- Receptacle for urine
- Closed container, such as a resealable plastic bag or a plastic tube, for catheter storage

Procedure. Wash hands and penis. Lubricate tip of catheter. While holding penis at 45 degree angle from body, insert the catheter about 6 inches. Lower and direct the distal end of the catheter into toilet, urinal, or other receptacle. If no urine flows, insert catheter further until flow begins. When flow stops or slows, remove catheter slowly while turning it slightly. Wash and dry hands, penis, and catheter. Store catheter in closed container. If immediate catheter cleansing is not possible, place it in closed container for washing as soon as possible.

Men with incontinence related to radical prostatectomy rarely benefit from intermittent catheterization. Kegel exercises may be helpful to strengthen the sphincter muscle. Containment devices may be needed. If incontinence is intermittent or in volume of less than 90 ml, a drip collector that adheres to brief-type underpants is a good choice.

ureters loop downward like a fishhook as they enter the bladder). The ureters may be compressed and obstructed by the thickened bladder wall, causing hydroureter (ureter abnormally distended with urine). A similar situation (hydronephrosis) may develop in the kidneys, because urine flow is obstructed in the ureters and urine backs up. In this situation, the pelvis and renal calyces distend with urine and the renal parenchyma atrophies. Ultimately, prolonged urinary obstruction or reflux can cause renal insufficiency (see Fig. 83–2).

Clinical Manifestations and Diagnostic Findings

BPH usually develops slowly and may persist for a long time in a silent state without creating a major problem. As a man becomes older, he may assume that increasing frequency of urination is part of aging. Reduction in both the size and the force of the urinary stream is abnormal and should be assessed.

With developing BPH, the urinary stream first lacks force, then becomes weak and dribbling. A man feels unable to start voiding (hesitancy), and either strains to urinate or urinates more frequently. Often, terminal dribbling follows urination. There may be blood in the urine (a manifestation that is more common in benign hyperplasia than in cancer). The client also exhibits manifestations of frequency, urgency, nocturia, and urge incontinence.

As the prostate enlarges, a danger develops of complete urinary obstruction and retention. Retention may be precipitated by the following:

1. Chill
2. Alcoholic beverages
3. Infection
4. Delay in voiding
5. Bedrest

Some medications may also provoke retention, such as decongestants, anticholinergics, and antidepressants. Obstruction can be a painful emergency requiring catheterization. If retention is long-standing and large amounts of urine are removed, observe the person carefully for manifestations of shock. Table 83–1 (beginning on p. 2354) shows various types of urethral catheters.

BPH is assessed by the following measures:

1. A general physical examination, including rectal examination
2. Laboratory examination of blood, urine, and renal function
3. X-ray examination including intravenous pyelogram and cystography
4. Instrumental examination, including catheterization and cystoscopy

A prostate-specific antigen (PSA) test and a transrectal ultrasound may be done to rule out the presence of malignancy.

The client should be asked about the size and force of the urinary stream. Uroflowmetry may be performed. Straight catheterization after voiding assesses the amount of residual urine. Other studies used to assess obstruction include (1) urethral pressure profile and (2) electromyelography (EMG) of the sphincter muscles.

Rectal examination and prostatic massage for a sample of prostatic secretion can be performed. The secretion can be examined under the microscope for pus cells, which may indicate infection. Urine, obtained before prostatic massage, may be normal in asymptomatic men, or it may show infection by the presence of red or white blood cells and an alkaline pH.

The enlarged prostate may cause urinary backpressure, leading to renal damage. Assessing for indication of renal problems is therefore important, and renal function studies must be included in the assessment.

Acute and Subacute Care

■ Surgical Management

Surgery is the most common means of relieving urinary obstruction caused by BPH. The part of the prostate gland causing obstruction is removed (prostatectomy). Indications for prostatectomy include the following:

- Upper urinary tract dilatation (hydroureter, hydronephrosis) and impaired renal function
- Severe discomfort and inconvenience
- Total urinary obstruction
- Lack of response to medical treatment
- Vesical (urinary bladder) calculus, indicative of long-standing obstruction associated with BPH and infection
- Long-standing urinary obstruction with the development of hydroureter and hydronephrosis that impairs renal function
- Severe and prolonged hematuria (recurrent bleeding)
- Decreased quality of life related to BPH manifestations
- Chronic urinary retention
- Recurrent urinary tract infections

Preoperative Management

Preoperative care centers around establishing and maintaining urinary output and the prevention of complications. Clients who develop acute retention need to have urinary flow restored prior to surgery. This usually means that this client will require catheterization. The catheter will then be maintained until a more permanent solution can be attempted.

Procedures

Enlarged prostate tissue may be removed by various approaches (Fig. 83–3). These approaches include the following:

1. Transurethral resection of the prostate (TURP)
2. Suprapubic prostatectomy
3. Retropubic prostatectomy
4. Perineal prostatectomy

The method used depends on the size of the prostate and the general health of the client. The term *prostatectomy* is really a misnomer. The procedure is actually an adenectomy of new tissue growth, and the true prostate

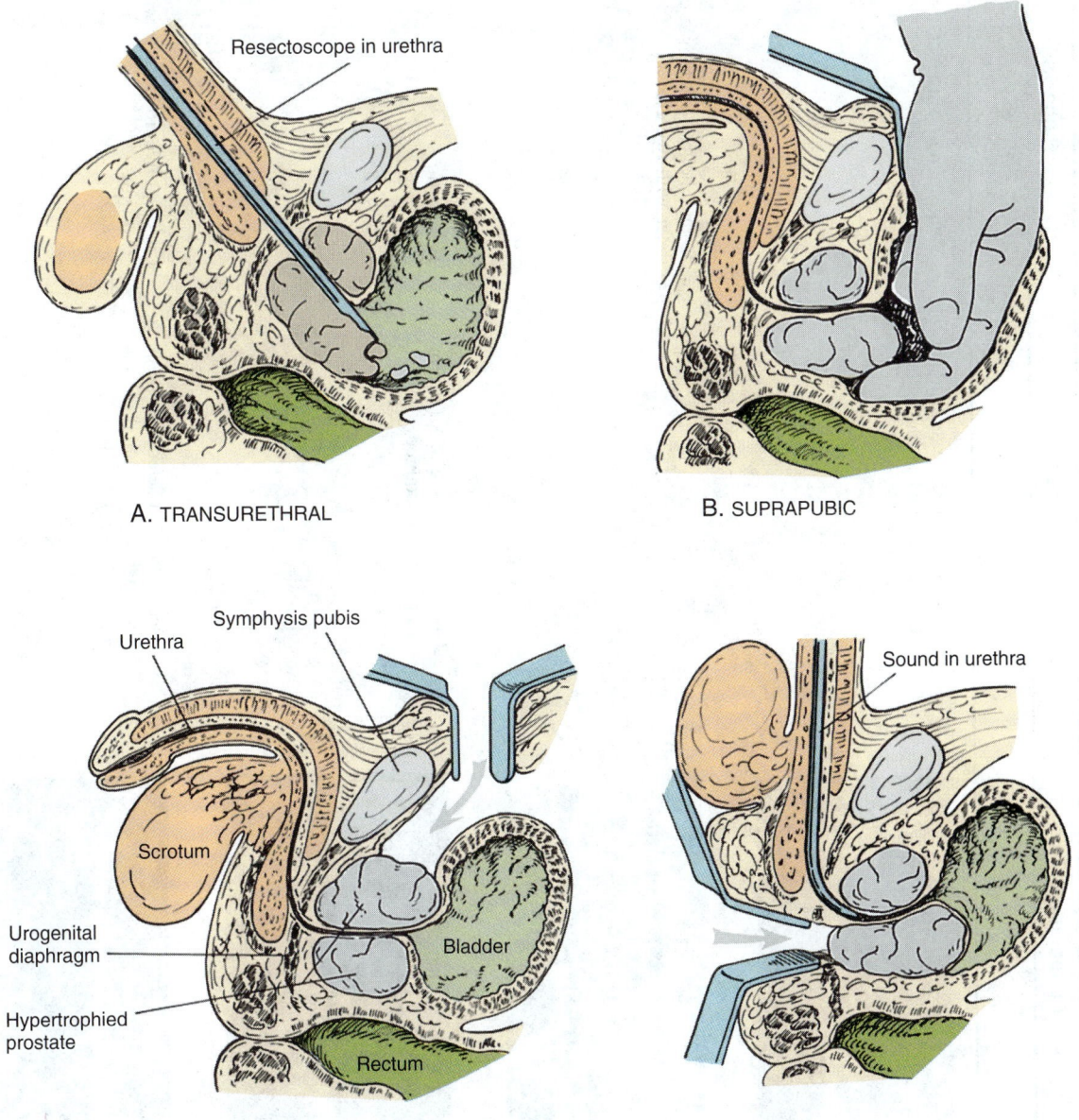

Figure 83–3. Surgical approaches to the prostate. *A,* Transurethral resection prostatectomy (TURP) is a closed method of treatment, that is, no incision is made, and the hyperplastic prostate tissue is removed through a resectoscope (like a cystoscope), which is inserted through the urethra. *B,* Suprapubic (transvesical) prostatectomy is an open method of treatment in which the hyperplastic prostatic tissue is enucleated through the anterior walls of the abdomen and bladder. *C,* Retropubic (extravesical) prostatectomy is an open method in which a low abdominal incision is made between the pubic arch and the bladder. *D,* Perineal prostatectomy is an open method involving an incision between the anus and the scrotum.

and fibrous capsule are not removed. The entire prostate is removed only during a radical prostatectomy, which is used only to treat some prostate cancers.

Transurethral Resection. Transurethral resection of the prostate (TURP) is the most widely used of all prostatic surgical techniques. TURP is especially suitable for men with relatively small prostatic enlargements or who are poor surgical risks. No incision is made. Repeated TURPs may be needed because of postoperative urethral strictures, bladder neck scarring, and continued hyperplasia of the remaining prostate tissue.

TURP is performed by inserting a resectoscope through the urethra (Fig. 83–3A). One of the two following types of resectoscope may be used:

1. A hot-loop resectoscope, which has a movable loop of wire that cuts tissue with a high-frequency current
2. A cold-punch resectoscope (rarely used), which punches out tissue, piece by piece, with a circular knife blade

In both cases, the surgeon is able to visualize the inside of the bladder by inserting a telescope through the resectoscope. Bleeding is controlled by cauterization. Irri-

Text continued on page 2358

Table 83–1. Urologic Instruments Most Commonly Encountered in a Clinical Setting

Name	Appearance	Purpose/Use	Remarks
Urinary Catheters			
1. Nélaton red rubber urethral catheter		One-time, immediate drainage of the bladder; used when indwelling catheter is not needed	Blunt, round-tip straight catheter with one eye
2. Robinson red rubber urethral catheter		Same as 1.	Round, hollow-tip straight catheter with two eyes
3. Councill red rubber urethral catheter (5-mL balloon)		Used when passage of a filiform or guide wire is required	Hole at tip
4. Tiemann coudé red rubber urethral catheter		Used when a catheter must be negotiated through a urethral, prostatic, or bladder neck blockage	Curved, olive-tip catheter with two eyes

5. Indwelling Foley urethral catheter	Used when a catheter must be retained in the bladder for continuous drainage	Various French sizes of catheters with 5- or 30-ml balloon
6. Three-way Foley urethral catheter	Used when irrigation of a retention catheter may be needed (e.g., after transurethral resection of the prostate)	Various French sizes of catheters with 5- or 30-ml balloon and a third port for irrigation
7. Coudé round-tip Foley urethral catheter	Used when retention catheter must be passed through urethral, prostatic, or bladder neck blockage	Curved tip; various French sizes of catheters with 5- or 30-mL balloon
8. Double-balloon Foley urethral catheter	Used when bladder drainage and pressure on a resected area must be accomplished simultaneously	
9. Malecot catheter	Sometimes used to drain and irrigate continent reservoirs; for temporary or continuous suprapubic drainage	Self-retaining winged catheter; design may have two or four wings; Stamey type used for suprapubic puncture

Table continued on following page

Table 83–1. Urologic Instruments Most Commonly Encountered in a Clinical Setting (*Continued*)

Name	Appearance	Purpose/Use	Remarks
Instruments Used for Urethral Dilation			
10. Otis bougie à boule		Catheterlike device used to dilate urethra; used to calibrate urethral passage	Olive tip; usually available in even sizes from 8–40 F
11. Walther sound. *A*, Dilator. *B*, Tapered dilator		Metal instrument used to dilate female urethra	Tapers toward handle
12. Béniqué sound		Used to dilate male urethra	Curve in tip is more pronounced than in other sounds
13. LeFort sound		Often used to dilate severe (usually trauma-induced) urethral strictures in males	Threaded tip for attachment of woven filiform

14. Catheter stylet or guide

Stiff wire inserted into a channel catheter to make it rigid for easier insertion into the urethra

Another type of guide is the filiform guide wire; has threads at the end to attach filiforms to aid in inserting a Councill catheter

15. Filiforms (A) and followers (B)

Used to establish access to the urinary bladder when urethral abnormalities exist or to dilate urethral strictures

Filiform is small and has different shaped tips; follower attaches to end of filiform once entry to bladder has been established; available in variety of French sizes

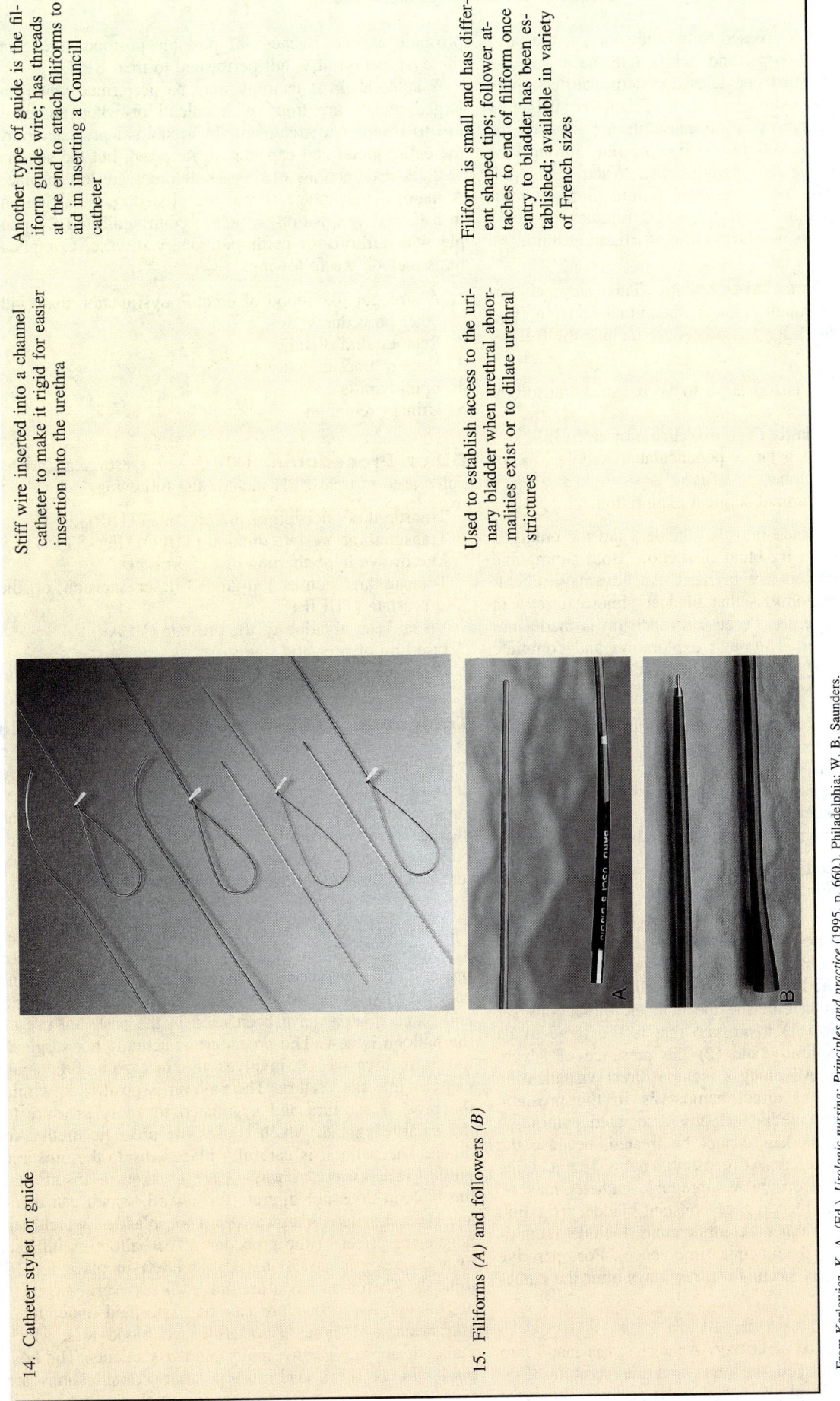

From Karlowicz, K. A. (Ed.). *Urologic nursing: Principles and practice* (1995, p. 660). Philadelphia: W. B. Saunders.

gating fluid can be passed into and out of the area through the resectoscope, and debris falls back into the bladder and is washed out. Closed-system, sterile gravity irrigation is used with a solution of isotonic irrigation fluid. Water is never used, because during surgery the client absorbs about 900 ml of irrigating fluid through the tissues and veins at the operative site. Water could precipitate hemolysis and acute renal failure. Surgery must be completed within about 60 to 90 minutes to avoid excessive blood loss and absorption of irrigating fluid.

Suprapubic Prostatectomy. This surgical approach is done through a lower abdominal incision (Fig. 83–3*B*). Indications for this procedure include the following:

1. A prostate that is too large to be resected transurethrally
2. Bladder abnormality (e.g., diverticula or calculi)
3. The presence of a large, pedunculated middle lobe or lateral prostatic lobes
4. A need for abdominal surgical exploration.

An incision is made into the bladder, and the enlarged tissue is enucleated by blunt dissection. Both suprapubic and urethral catheters are inserted. An advantage of suprapubic prostatectomy is that bladder abnormalities can be treated concurrently, because an incision is made into the urinary bladder. Thorough exploration and complete tissue removal are facilitated. Disadvantages include the following:

1. Difficulty in obtaining hemostasis (therefore, assess for shock and hemorrhage)
2. Bladder spasms
3. Urinary leakage into an abdominal wound around the suprapubic catheter
4. Relatively prolonged and uncomfortable convalescence

Incontinence sometimes occurs. A few men experience erectile dysfunction after this procedure.

Retropubic Prostatectomy. Retropubic prostatectomy is the most recently developed open method (Fig. 83–3*C*). A low abdominal incision facilitates approaching the prostate without entering the bladder. Indications for this procedure are (1) a prostate that is too large to be removed transurethrally and (2) the presence of severe urethral stricture. Advantages include direct visualization of the prostate and direct hemostasis in the prostatic fossa. A disadvantage is that any associated pathologic condition in the bladder cannot be treated, because the bladder is not entered. Also, osteitis pubis (pubic bone inflammation) may occur. A suprapubic catheter may be inserted to control bleeding, or constant bladder irrigation may be used. Infrequent complications include incontinence and erectile dysfunction (impotence). Postoperative urinary leakage may occur for a few days after the catheter is removed.

Perineal Prostatectomy. An incision is made into the perineum, between the anus and the scrotum (Fig. 83–3*D*). The perineal prostatectomy is performed to treat prostatic cancer. Because of possible postoperative erectile dysfunction, it is not performed to treat BPH.

A subtotal prostatectomy may be performed when enlarged glands are filled with calculi or when abscesses fail to respond to treatment. In a subtotal prostatectomy, the entire gland and capsule are removed, but the seminal vesicles and sections of the vas deferens are left in place. A major disadvantage is that the procedure is carried out in a lithotomy position, which is contraindicated for people with arthritis or cardiopulmonary disease. Complications include the following:

1. A stronger likelihood of erectile dysfunction than with other procedures
2. Rectourethral fistula
3. Urinary tract infections
4. Epididymitis
5. Urinary retention

Other Procedures. Other, newer, surgical procedures used to treat BPH include the following:

Transurethral incision of the prostate (TUIP)
Transurethral prostate dilation (TUPD) (Fig. 83–4)
Microwave hyperthermia of the prostate
Transurethral ultrasound-guided laser incision of the prostate (TULIP)
Visual laser ablation of the prostate (VLAP)
Insertion of prostatic stents
High-intensity focused ultrasound therapy

Transurethral Incision of the Prostate. The TUIP is an option for men with small prostates which cause outlet obstruction. This procedure has fewer postoperative complications and can be performed under local anesthesia for high-risk clients. Greater client satisfaction has also been reported with this procedure; many clients report no change in ejaculation, which makes this an excellent procedure for younger men with small glands.

Transurethral Balloon Dilation of the Prostate. Transurethral balloon dilation of the prostate is another procedure that has become increasingly popular. The concept of dilating the prostate is not new; sounds, bougies, and metal dilators have been used in the past, but use of the balloon is new. The procedure is actually not surgical, but it is invasive. It involves the insertion of a small catheter into the urethra. The balloon is positioned within the prostatic urethra and is inflated to apply pressure to the enlarged gland, which causes the prostatic urethra to dilate. The balloon is carefully placed inside the prostatic urethra in a variety of ways. Care is taken to ensure that the balloon does not migrate downward, which can damage the sphincter, or upward into the bladder, which can negate the effect of the procedure. The balloon is inflated to a diameter of a 75F to 90F and left in place for 15 minutes. The client has a urethral catheter overnight.

This surgical procedure can be performed under local anesthesia, and there is no associated blood loss, which makes it appropriate for many high-risk clients. The hospital stay is short, and postoperative complications are few. There are two major concerns with this procedure.

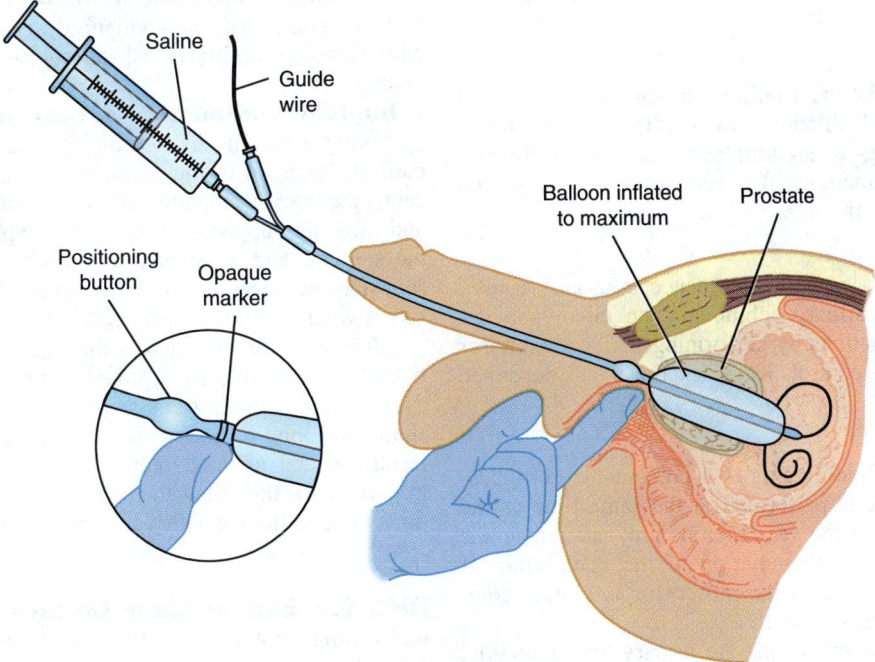

Figure 83–4. Balloon dilation of the prostate. (After Dowd, J. B., & Smith, J. J. [1990]. Balloon dilation of the prostate. *Urologic Clinics of North America, 17*[3], 673.)

First, because no tissue is removed, prostatic cancer could be missed. The other concern is the length of time for which the results of this procedure will be effective. Because it is such a recent innovation, clients have not been followed long enough to determine whether or not recurrence of the obstruction is common.

Hyperthermia. Microwave hyperthermia is one of the newest procedures being performed. Microwave hyperthermia is delivered via a rectal probe over a period of four to ten treatments. Each treatment lasts about 60 minutes and is performed without anesthesia on an outpatient basis. The treatment has shown some promising results, although the ultimate efficacy has not been shown.

Transurethral Ultrasound-Guided Laser Incision of the Prostate. TULIP is the newest treatment. It is similar to the TUIP, but a laser is used to make the incision. So far, few results are available, but data that are available look promising. The procedure causes minimal blood loss, it requires no irrigation, and the client does not need a catheter after surgery. This procedure is usually done in an ambulatory or outpatient setting.

Stents. The remaining new treatment is the insertion of a prostatic stent. This procedure is used for clients who are extremely poor operative risks. This hollow tube can be inserted through an endoscope into the prostatic urethra, where it holds the urethra open mechanically. It is safer than an indwelling urethral catheter because there is no risk of infection. The stent can be left in place for 4 to 6 weeks without problems. If left in place longer, epithelial cells will grow over the stent.

Ultrasound. An investigational treatment is the high-intensity focused ultrasound therapy. This treatment completely ablates the prostatic tissue. The ultrasound is delivered through a transrectal probe. The potential of this treatment is that it is much less invasive than many other procedures.

Postoperative Management

Monitoring fluid and electrolyte balance and renal function before, during, and after surgery is important. When constant bladder irrigation is used, fluid absorption (water intoxication or dilutional hyponatremia) during surgery can produce hypervolemia. Postoperative assessment includes observing for hypertension, bradycardia, weakness, and seizures.

Complications

The most common early complication of the open procedures and the TURP is postoperative bleeding. Other complications include the following:

1. Retrograde ejaculation (semen passing backward into the bladder instead of out through the penis) because of bladder neck surgical trauma
2. Urethral stricture
3. Bladder neck constriction
4. Urinary incontinence
5. Epididymitis

Retrograde Ejaculation. No treatment has been devised for retrograde ejaculation. Explain the condition to the client so he is not frightened by it. The condition results in sterility because the sperm are ejaculated into the bladder.

Urethral Stricture. Urethral stricture can be treated postoperatively with dilation with urethral sounds. If the stricture is severe, a urethroplasty can be performed. Bladder neck contractures, if severe, also can be treated with surgical reconstruction.

Incontinence. Urinary incontinence is usually caused by trauma to the urinary sphincter. The client can decrease the manifestations by performing perineal exercises to improve muscle control. Kegel exercises are described in Chapter 56.

Epididymitis. Epididymitis is a preventable complication if a vasectomy is performed at the same time as the prostatectomy. Tying the vas deferens prevents retrograde bacterial infection or inflammation of the epididymis. If the prostate is removed in its entirety or is almost completely removed, sterility results.

Other possible complications are urinary tract infection, obstruction, accidental displacement of the catheter, incontinence, impotence, and recurrence of manifestations.

Outcomes

Open prostatectomies appear to provide the best outcome as regards improvement of manifestations. These procedures also require the least follow-up treatment and provide the greatest increase in urine flow rate. The TUIP and TURP also produce significant improvement in manifestations. The TURP potentially requires more follow-up treatment than the other operations. All of the surgical procedures produce better long-term outcomes than do the medical treatments.[9]

■ Nursing Management of the Surgical Client

Assessment

Assess the client's ability to empty his bladder. The client's bladder should be palpated for distention. If the client is unable to void, the need for a urethral catheter should be assessed.

Careful preoperative assessment in both physical and psychosocial areas is important. The client's knowledge about the surgery and its outcome should be assessed. Because so many types of treatment are possible, the client may not understand the implications of the treatment he will be receiving.

Diagnosis, Planning, Implementation

Fear. Men often feel *Fear related to urinary problems, treatments, and threats to sexual functioning* because the urinary and reproductive systems are linked systems in the male. Prostate hyperplasia and treatment may lead to alterations in sexuality and reproduction.

Planning: Expected Outcomes. The client's fear will be controlled, as evidenced by his statements of understanding, ability to ask questions, and ability to rest quietly.

Implementation. Fear and anxiety may be lessened by taking a nursing history and giving appropriate explanations. Respond to the concerns of the client and significant others with empathic listening, accurate information, and ongoing support. Restating the explanations given by the surgeon and anesthetist when securing informed consent may be necessary, because stressed clients frequently forget what they have been told.

Informed consent requires that the man understand the risks (e.g., possible sexual dysfunction, including erectile dysfunction; retrograde ejaculation; and infertility) and short- and long-term benefits (e.g., relief of urinary manifestations and arrested reduction in renal function). It is important for the client to receive honest answers to questions concerning sexuality and reproduction.

Risk for Self Esteem Disturbance. The client undergoing treatment for BPH is at *Risk for Self Esteem Disturbance related to threats to sexuality from disease and treatment.*

Planning: Expected Outcomes. The client will not develop a disturbance in self-concept as evidenced by his willingness to discuss sexual issues.

Implementation. Most men undergoing prostatectomy are older than 50. The aging process compounds the psychosocial threat involved in intimate surgery. Such men may experience disturbing changes in self-concept, including body image, self-esteem, role performance, and personal identity. Sexual concerns may be a part of these changes.

It is usually helpful if the man and his significant other can talk about these concerns with a supportive person. They need reassurance that their concerns (including fears of being unable to perform sexually) are common to men who undergo major surgery. Recommendations for any restrictions on sexual intercourse and alternative sexual activity are best given in collaboration with the physician. Men who leave healthcare facilities with incontinence, weakness, pain, and indwelling catheters may have additional concerns and self-doubts.

Significant others also need support following prostatectomy. They may not understand what is happening and may be concerned about potential or actual changes in their relationship.

Hemorrhage. A common collaborative problem after all open prostatectomies is *Hemorrhage related to prostatectomy.*

Planning: Expected Outcomes. The client will not hemorrhage, as evidenced by absence of gross bleeding and maintenance of at least 30 ml of urine output per hour.

Implementation. Carry out the nursing assessment described in Chapters 21 and 22 to identify hemorrhage. In addition, observe the wound drains, wound packing, and catheter drainage for excessive bleeding. Wound drains may be in place after perineal, retropubic, or suprapubic prostatectomies. A suprapubic urinary catheter positioned directly into the bladder through the abdominal wall is in place after suprapubic prostatectomies. Sometimes, the balloon of the indwelling catheter (Foley type) is inflated with 30 ml or more of fluid, up to 100 ml (rather than the usual 5 ml) to promote hemostasis at the operative site within the prostatic capsule.

Some hematuria (blood in the urine) is usual for several days after surgery. However, frank bleeding, arterial or venous, may occur during the first day after surgery. Arterial bleeding is bright red, has numerous clots, and is viscous. Blood pressure may fall, and emergency surgical intervention may become necessary. Venous bleeding in the prostatic area may be controlled by increasing the pressure (adding fluid) in the balloon end of the urethral catheter, pulling the catheter tightly to move the balloon into the prostatic fossa, and taping the catheter to the thigh (called *applying traction*). Traction is left in place for 24 hours or more and is released by the physician when the bleeding has stopped. The physician also can remove fluid slowly from the balloon as the bleeding decreases.

Overdistention of the bladder must be avoided because it can precipitate secondary hemorrhage by placing undue strain on freshly coagulated blood vessels; it is therefore important to be sure that the Foley catheter is patent and draining.

Pain. A common nursing diagnosis for the client undergoing a prostatectomy is *Pain related to surgery and bladder spasms.*

Planning: Expected Outcomes. The client will have pain relieved or controlled, as evidenced by client's report.

Implementation. Pain control following surgery is discussed in Chapters 17 and 21. Additional pain can occur after prostatectomy if urinary drainage tubes become obstructed. The best intervention is to prevent catheters from becoming blocked. If a man experiences pain after a prostatectomy, first assess the drainage apparatus for patency. Relief of obstruction often alleviates pain without the need for analgesics. Clots are often the cause of the obstruction.

Bladder spasms also may occur because of bladder overdistention or irritation from an indwelling catheter balloon. Antispasmodic medications, such as belladonna and opium suppositories or propantheline bromide (Pro-Banthine), may be prescribed prophylactically to help prevent bladder spasms, especially in clients who require traction. They may cause complications, however. Clients with severe cardiac disease or glaucoma should not receive these agents. Antispasmodic drugs can cause constipation, and straining at stool can precipitate bleeding from the operative site, so stool softeners such as docusate sodium (Colace) are often given.

Risk for Injury. Postoperatively, catheters and drains are often in place. Write the nursing diagnosis as *Risk for Injury related to presence of urinary catheters, irrigation, or suprapubic drains.*

Planning: Expected Outcomes. The client will not develop an injury such as infection, catheter obstruction, water intoxication, or injury because of the catheter. White blood cell count will be normal, and wound healing and catheter drainage will be adequate. There will be no fever; hyponatremia, hypertension, or other manifestations of water intoxication; excessive bleeding or trauma from the catheter; urinary retention after catheter removal; or fistula formation from the suprapubic catheter.

Implementation. Indwelling catheters (urethral or suprapubic) are generally used to facilitate urinary drainage after all types of prostatectomies (see Table 83–1). Various types of catheter irrigation systems may be used with these catheters. Closed irrigation, referred to as a constant bladder irrigation (CBI) (Fig. 83–5), permits either constant or intermittent irrigation without the hazard of breaking aseptic technique. Isotonic irrigating fluid is used for intermittent irrigation, incorporating small amounts (usually 60 to 100 ml); for continuous irrigation, enough to maintain outflow of clear or slightly pink urine. The fluid must be isotonic, because water could lead to a depletion of electrolytes or to water intoxication (see Chapter 15).

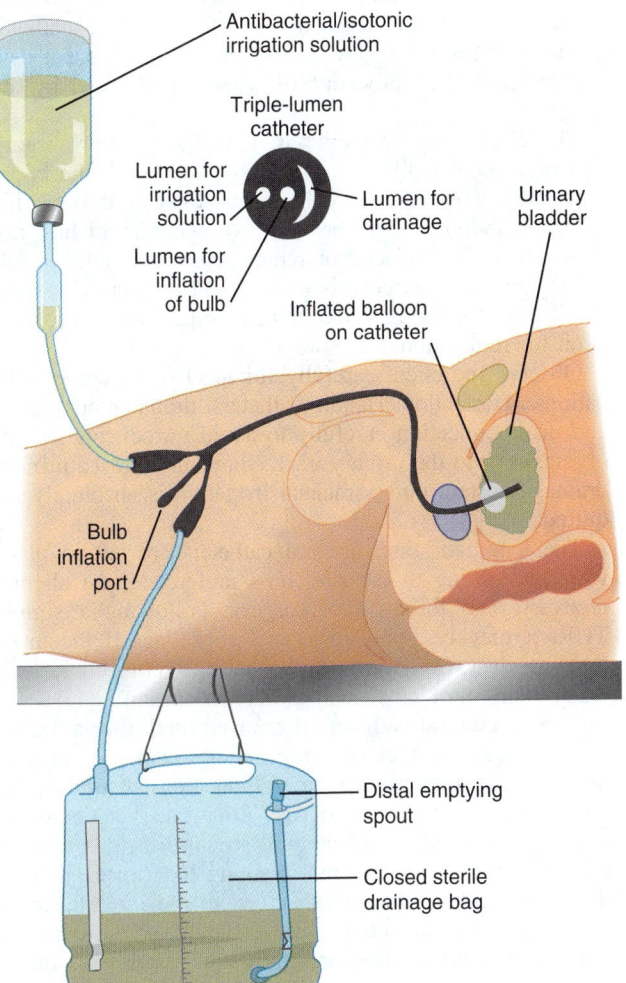

Figure 83–5. A closed bladder irrigation (CBI) system.

Frequently assess drainage from the catheter. Because the client usually receives intravenous fluid postoperatively, urinary catheters should be draining. Keep accurate records of intake and output, accounting for the amount instilled with the irrigation.

While a urinary catheter is in place, it must be kept patent (open, clear, and unobstructed). Urinary flow may become obstructed by blood clots, prostatic chips, mucous plugs, kinked tubing, or tube displacement. Frequently assess catheter patency to make sure it is draining.

The catheter may become blocked by clots or sediment, leading to complications such as infections, bladder distention, and painful bladder spasms. Some bladder spasms occur with bladder distention, whereas others are a response to irritation from the catheter balloon (from excessive fluid in the balloon to prevent bleeding).

It is important to prevent bladder overdistention, such as during irrigation or as a result of urinary obstruction. Bladder overdistention can cause hemorrhage by placing undue strain on freshly coagulated blood vessels. Assess the client for bladder overdistention by shutting off continuous irrigation and palpating the lower abdomen. If overdistention is present, catheter irrigation may clear clots or plugs and restore urinary drainage.

If there is resistance to the introduction of irrigating fluid into the catheter, or if there is no return of irrigating fluid through the tubing, *do not force the fluid*. If this occurs, contact the surgeon immediately. If a catheter cannot be cleared, it may have to be removed and a new one inserted. This procedure is usually performed by the surgeon.

The client may be confused immediately after surgery and may accidentally pull out the catheter. Tell the client repeatedly that he has a tube in his bladder through his penis or abdomen (whichever it is), and remind him not to touch it. A displaced or removed urinary catheter following prostatic surgery is painful and disrupts recovery. If the client does pull the catheter out, contact the surgeon for reinsertion.

Observe the client carefully for local or systemic indications of infection. Handle catheters, drainage apparatus, and urine collection carefully to avoid introducing microorganisms into the urinary tract. Maintain a closed urinary drainage system unless manual irrigation is absolutely required.

The length of time urethral catheters are left in place varies according to the surgeon's preference, the client's recovery, and the type of surgery. Following a simple TUR, it may be removed after 1 to 2 days if the urine remains clear. Sometimes the catheter is removed early if it is causing problems, such as bladder spasms.

After a urethral catheter is removed (and after a TUR), monitor the client closely for manifestations of urinary retention and urethral strictures. Indications of urinary retention include inability to pass urine and bladder overdistention. Indications of urethral stricture include a small urinary stream, dysuria, and straining to urinate. Talk to the client and significant others about the importance of urinating when the client first feels a desire to do so. Holding the urine may increase the possibility of retention.

Temporary urinary frequency or incontinence may oc-cur after the catheter is removed. Be understanding of the man's feelings and keep him dry without embarrassing him. Keep reminding him and his significant other that these problems are temporary, but that they may take some time to resolve. Urinary control usually returns quickly in young men, whereas in older men, a period of dribbling for up to 3 months is not unusual. Perineal exercises may reduce this problem (see next Nursing Implementation section). Additional surgery is sometimes required for persistent incontinence (see Chapter 56).

Wound drains are usually removed earlier than suprapubic drains. The suprapubic drain is left in place until urinary function has returned. Once the client is voiding well, the suprapubic drain can be removed. If it is removed before the client has returned to normal voiding, the wound may not heal properly, leading to fistula formation.

Ineffective Management of Therapeutic Regimen (Individuals).
The postoperative client has many learning needs in order to move to a state of self-care. The most appropriate diagnosis is therefore at *Risk for Ineffective Management of Therapeutic Regimen (Individuals) related to postoperative exercises and return of urinary function.*

Planning: Expected Outcomes. The client will understand postoperative exercises and return of urinary function, as evidenced by client's statements and increasing urinary continence.

Implementation. Throughout the postoperative period, tell the client about each procedure and expectation, such as not to strain at stool, and encourage his participation.

Catheters, Wound Drains, Urinary Drainage, and Irrigation. Provide information about related procedures. Answer questions patiently. Tell the client and significant other that it is important not to touch the equipment, pull out the tubes, or obstruct the drainage. Help the man learn ways of turning and getting out of bed without pulling on the catheter or kinking the drainage tubing. Remind the client not to lie on the tubing. Show the client and significant other how to make sure the tubing always remains above the level of the drainage bag, because if the tubing falls at or below the drainage bag the flow of urine may be impeded and actually pass back into the bladder.

Bloody urine is not unusual early in the postoperative period. For open prostatectomies, some wound drainage also may occur. The client who has had a suprapubic prostatectomy will have extensive drainage of urine from the suprapubic wound if a suprapubic catheter is not used.

Management of Common Sensations. Common sensations experienced by clients after a prostatectomy are that the ureteral catheter may cause bladder spasms and a sensation of needing to pass urine; following removal of a catheter, dribbling of urine and a sense of urgency may occur. Many men find it difficult to admit to discomfort or pain, such as from bladder spasms. Ask them frequently about this problem, and remind them of the importance of letting you know (see Chapter 17).

Self-Care Activities. Self-care activities include drinking increased amounts of fluids while a catheter is in place, performing bed exercises, incorporating early ambulation, and measuring fluid intake and urinary output. Prolonged sitting increases intra-abdominal pressure and may precipitate bleeding. Therefore, the man should avoid sitting except during meals. After he leaves the healthcare facility, driving an automobile or taking prolonged automobile rides should be avoided until at least 2 weeks after surgery, when the risk of bleeding lessens. Strenuous exercise is also contraindicated.

Advise the client not to strain during defecation for at least 6 weeks after surgery, because this can lead to bleeding from the operative site. Docusate sodium (Colace), prune juice, and milk of magnesia are usually satisfactory bowel stimulants during this time.

Perineal exercises help the client regain urinary sphincter control. From the second or third postoperative day, teach the client to breathe normally while contracting abdominal, gluteal, and perineal muscles 12 to 25 times/hour. A good way to describe this action is "Contract your muscles as if you have to pass urine urgently and there is no place to relieve yourself."

Another helpful exercise is to squeeze the rectal sphincter tensely while relaxing other body muscles. Teach the client to place his hands on his abdomen to assess abdominal tension. The abdomen should not be tense and a Valsalva maneuver should not occur when the exercise is performed correctly. During these exercises, it may help the man concentrate if he says aloud words such as relax and squeeze. Encourage the man to establish a planned schedule of exercising during waking hours and continue this routine until complete urinary control is achieved.

Post-discharge Care. The client is usually discharged 2 to 3 days or sooner after a TUR and a few days later for a suprapubic prostatectomy. It is a good idea not only to teach the client but also to provide him with written materials to refer to after discharge. Be sure he knows when and where to contact his surgeon next and how to get in touch with healthcare professionals if he has concerns before that time. Tell the client to be sure to report to the surgeon any bleeding, infection, or obstructed urine flow. However, give him support and permission to discuss any concern with a healthcare professional.

Advise the client to avoid strenuous activity for 4 to 6 weeks (e.g., mowing the lawn, lifting more than 20 lb). He will probably need extra rest while at the same time maintaining a balance of activity with ambulation. He may drive a car when given permission, usually after his first visit to the physician.

Advise the client to continue a high daily intake (at least 6 to 8 glasses/day) of nonalcoholic fluids to minimize clot formation. If he is discharged home with an indwelling catheter, provide him and his significant other with appropriate information about catheter insertion.

Sexual Dysfunction. The client will be at *Risk for Sexual Dysfunction related to removal of prostate, retrograde ejaculation, and sterility.*

Planning: Expected Outcomes. The client will not develop sexual dysfunction. He will be able to discuss fears and concerns with the staff.

Implementation. Retrograde ejaculation consists of the ejaculation of semen backward into the bladder rather than out through the urethra. The client experiences erection and orgasm, but normal ejaculation does not occur. Retrograde ejaculation may occur after a prostatectomy because when the prostatic capsule contracts, the semen passes more easily into the bladder rather than through the urethra. Semen passes into the bladder and mixes with the urine, producing cloudy urine. Advise the client to observe his urine for cloudiness and tell his physician if it occurs.

Erectile dysfunction (impotence) is a rare complication of prostatectomy and is more likely to occur after a perineal prostatectomy than after the other types. If this problem occurs, it is important to reinforce the man's masculine image. This is mainly achieved through supportive caring of the significant other. Educate the significant other to provide the necessary support.

Referral for sexual counseling may be helpful. The man needs to know that he can still please a partner and that lovemaking techniques other than intercourse may be necessary. The couple may need information about alternatives to intercourse, such as cuddling, stroking, or manual or oral stimulation to orgasm. Talking about options may enhance communications between the man and his partner. A penile implant may be considered (see the Erectile Dysfunction section).

Community and Self-Care

■ Medical Management

Several treatments can control benign prostatic hyperplasia. Prostatic massage, sexual intercourse, and hot sitz baths may relieve manifestations by releasing a small amount of prostatic fluid, which reduces the edema and therefore some of the problems associated with BPH. Urinary frequency then may be decreased, and stream flow increased. Mild or asymptomatic BPH may be associated with prostatitis, which causes increased prostatic swelling and worsening of manifestations. Antibiotics may relieve acute manifestations and possibly delay surgery.

Catheter insertion may be required to treat acute urinary retention. An indwelling catheter can be left in place until medical or surgical intervention decreases the acute retention. If the client is not a candidate for surgical intervention, long-term catheter use may be needed.

Definitive medical treatment is aimed at androgen deprivation (Table 83–2) to inhibit prostatic hyperplasia. This includes treatments such as prescribing estrogen, cyproterone acetate, or the nonsteroidal veterinary antiandrogen flutamide. The 5α-reductase inhibitor (Proscar) is also used without the side effects of estrogens or antitestosterones. It also lowers PSA levels, increases urinary flow, and decreases prostatic volume. Alpha-adrenergic blocking agents also decrease muscle tone and improve

Table 83–2. Medications Used to Treat Benign Prostatic Hyperplasia

Medications	Action
Testosterone-Ablating Agents	

Diethylstilbestrol (DES)
Flutamide (Eulexin)
Gonadotropin-releasing hormone analogs (GnRH)
   Nafarelin acetate (Synarel)
   Leuprolide (Lupron)
   Goserelin acetate (Zoladex)
Cyproterone acetate (Androcur)
	Testosterone-ablating agents decrease the amount of circulating testosterone levels leading to suppression of prostatic tissue growth; estrogens inhibit prostatic growth by suppressing release of luteinizing hormone–releasing agent; this leads to a decrease in testosterone; flutamide is an antiandrogen that competes with testosterone for androgen receptor sites; GnRH inhibits the release of pituitary gonadotropin; this prevents testosterone biosynthesis; cyproterone is a synthetic antiandrogen that acts as an androgen-receptor inhibitor

5α-Reductase Inhibitor	
Finasteride (Proscar)	A 5α-reductase inhibitor that blocks dihydrotestosterone without suppressing circulating testosterone; decreases prostatic tissue withour affecting potency or libido
Alpha-adrenergic Blocking Agents	
Phenoxybenzamine (Dibenzyline) Terazosin (Hytrin) Prazosin (Minipress)	Autonomic innervation of the bladder neck and prostatic smooth muscle is abundant; prostatic obstruction is caused in part by the neurogenic tone of the bladder neck and prostatic smooth muscle; these agents block the alpha-receptors, improving urination by decreasing outlet obstruction

voiding. Unfortunately, many clients still require surgical management.

■ Nursing Management of the Medical Client

Assessment

Men often have only a vague understanding about what an enlarged prostate is, and they may be afraid of the tests and results. Carefully explain each part of the assessment process. Show the client and significant other a picture of the reproductive organs and prostate and explain the effects of enlargement on urine excretion.

Ask the client to describe all urinary manifestations, including the pattern of urination, presence of urgency, frequency, decreased or altered urinary stream, hesitancy, and nocturia. Question the client about the presence of hematuria.

Diagnosis, Planning, Implementation

Altered Urinary Elimination. The client with BPH will usually experience manifestations such as frequency, urgency, hesitancy, change in stream, incontinence, retention, and nocturia. Write the nursing diagnosis as *Altered Urinary Elimination related to increasing urethral occlusion.*

Planning: Expected Outcomes. The client will not develop manifestations of BPH or those manifestations will decrease with treatment, as evidenced by ab-

sence of frequency, urgency, hesitancy, change in stream, incontinence, retention, or nocturia.

Implementation. The client may have urinary difficulties, such as obstruction, urinary retention, and diminished renal function. These problems may require early admission to the healthcare facility for treatment. An indwelling catheter may be inserted, or drainage achieved by cystostomy. Assess the client carefully for manifestations of shock caused by postobstructive diuresis.

Never force a urinary catheter. If it cannot be inserted with gentle pressure, contact a urologist. Emergency catheterization for complete bladder obstruction requires a urologist's skills and, possibly, special instruments, such as a stylet (thin wire) for insertion into the catheter lumen, metal catheters, or other firm, specially angled catheters (coudé).

Knowledge Deficit. The client suffering from BPH may experience *Knowledge Deficit related to lack of understanding of disease, manifestations, and medical treatments.*

Planning: Expected Outcomes. The client will understand disease, manifestations, and medical treatment as evidenced by client statements, increased fluid intake, and ability to follow medication regimen.

Implementation. It is important to maintain the client's fluid balance. Many clients limit their fluid intake to combat the manifestations of frequency and urgency they experience as a result of the prostatic enlargement. Clients increase their risk of urinary tract infection and even renal or cardiovascular dysfunction with this limited intake. The client should maintain, unless otherwise contraindicated, an intake of at least 2500 to 3000 ml/day to correct dehydration and azotemia (nitrogen waste products in the blood).

Some men find their manifestations considerably relieved by conservative interventions. The client can learn some techniques that will decrease his clinical manifestations and possible complications. Explain to the man that if his bladder is distended rapidly, it can increase his manifestations and precipitate acute retention; the hypertrophic muscle of the bladder can lose its tone if distended quickly. Advise the client to undertake the following:

1. Void whenever the urge to do so is felt; do not put it off
2. Avoid taking large quantities of fluid over a short period
3. Avoid alcohol, because its diuretic effect, with the volume of fluid, increases bladder distention

Alcohol ingestion is the most common precipitating factor for acute urinary retention.

Sympathomimetic drugs such as phenylpropanolamine and phenylephrine, found in common cold and cough remedies, worsen BPH. Warn the client not to take any of these medications.

Evaluation

The client should be able to manage the manifestations of the disease and take the medication appropriately. Clients should also continue to have follow-up to assess the usefulness of the medical treatment and to continue regular check-ups for prostate cancer.

Prostate Cancer

Prostate cancer is the most common cancer among men and the third leading cause of death among men in the United States. Most clients with clinically detectable prostate cancer are older than 50; therefore, the man's risk of prostatic cancer increases with each decade after age 50. Young men, however, appear to have more aggressive disease and are more likely to have metastasis at time of diagnosis.

Etiology and Risk Factors

The cause of prostate cancer is unknown, but epidemiologic studies suggest several associated factors. See Risk Factors and Levels of Prevention for specific risk factors associated with prostate cancer.

The condition tends to occur more in certain families. In the United States, black men are at greater risk than white men (it is not clear whether this is because of genetic or environmental factors, for example, income or exposure to occupational hazards).

Because the risk of prostatic cancer increases with age, it may be associated with the hormonal shifts associated with aging, such as lower amounts of androsterone and higher serum levels of estrogen and estradiol.

Differences in mortality rates in prostate cancer between Asians and whites have been associated with dietary differences. Japanese men have low rates of prostate cancer, yet those who migrate to the United States experience increasing rates, which suggests dietary habits as a possible factor. High fat consumption (typical of American diets) can alter cholesterol and steroid metabolism, which may increase the risk of cancer. Green and yellow vegetables (typical of Japanese diets) could have a protective effect against prostate cancer.

Occupational and environmental exposure to carcinogens may increase the risk of prostate cancer. A higher incidence is found in urban areas, which suggests that environmental exposure may be a factor. Occupations linked to higher rates of prostate cancer include (1) employment in fertilizer, textile, and rubber industries; and (2) work with batteries containing cadmium.

The observation by electron microscopy of virus particles in carcinomatous prostate tissue suggests that viruses may be associated with the disease. Gonorrhea is also associated with an increased incidence of prostate cancer, although it is assumed that people with gonorrhea may be exposed to a virus concurrently.

It is hoped that late prostatic cancer will become rare as increasing emphasis is placed on early diagnosis through routine rectal examinations, rectal ultrasound studies, measurement of prostate-specific antigen (PSA), and prompt intervention.

Pathophysiology

The appearance of prostate cancer is variable, which adds to the difficulty of diagnosis and staging and grading of the tumor. These tumors are usually adenocarcinomas. The tumor begins in the periphery of the posterior lobe of the gland, whereas BPH occurs centrally and is large by the time it restricts urination. The tumor may appear as normal prostate, which delays diagnosis. Typically, such lesions grow slowly and remain confined to the prostatic capsule, and if they occur late in life, the client may die of other causes. Sometimes, however, the tumor grows rapidly, and metastasis has occurred by the time a diagnosis is made, after which the client lives only a short time. Alternatively, the tumor may grow locally for a long time despite the potential for metastasis.

When the tumor spreads, it occurs mainly through direct extension to the bladder neck and seminal vesicles. Other spread occurs through lymphatic and hematogenous routes. Obturator and iliac nodes are commonly positive. With advanced disease, metastasis to the bone is common as is spread to the lungs and liver.

Clinical Manifestations and Diagnostic Findings

Unless BPH is present at the same time, manifestations of early prostatic cancer may be absent. The presenting findings are most often those of prostatitis, such as infection.

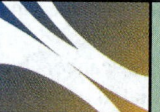

RISK FACTORS AND LEVELS OF PREVENTION

Prostate Cancer

Risk Factors

Genetic Tendency: Familial; blacks have higher rate than whites

Age: White men 65 years or older, high-risk or black men older than 40

Hormonal Factors: Men who had late puberty; men who have a high frequency of sexual experience, with high fertility; androgenic stimulation of the prostate over time

Dietary Factors: High intake of dietary fat

Chemical Exposure: Employment in fertilizer, textile, and rubber industries; work with batteries containing cadmium

Other: High levels of body fat; vasectomy done more than 20 years ago

Levels of Prevention

Primary Prevention

- Encourage clients to maintain a low-fat diet.
- Teach clients that a diet high in retinoids and carotenoids may reduce the risk of prostate cancer.
- Encourage chemoprevention with 5α-reductase inhibitor agents, such as finasteride.

Secondary Prevention

- Monitor men older than 50 with a yearly digital rectal examination combined with a PSA assay and transrectal ultrasound if indicated.
- Check PSA levels yearly for high-risk men and black men older than 40.
- Take biopsies of suspicious lesions.

Tertiary Prevention

- Suggest watchful waiting rather than aggressive treatment in selected clients.
- Teach perineal exercises to improve return of urinary control in post-TUR clients.
- Provide sexual counseling after radical perineal prostatectomy.

Obstruction is rare unless BPH is present, because the cancer is usually found in the periphery of the posterior lobe. Unfortunately, the tumor may escape detection until the disease is advanced. Also, 15% to 40% of men with prostate cancer present with late manifestations caused by metastasis, such as hip or back bone pain and possible sensory or motor changes from spinal cord compression. Rectal pressure or obstruction from local tumor growth may produce stool changes and painful defecation. Painful ejaculation also may be experienced. Late in the disease, thrombophlebitis and lower extremity lymphedema may occur as a result of the pelvic lymph node involvement.

Early diagnosis is essential. Diagnostic tests include the following:

Digital rectal examination
Laboratory tests, such as alkaline and acid phosphatase assays
Radiography

Rectal ultrasound
Computed tomographic (CT) scanning
Radionuclide imaging
Transrectal and percutaneous needle aspiration and biopsy
Assay of tumor markers, such as PSA

■ Digital Rectal Examination

Annual digital rectal examination is recommended for all men older than 40 because colon cancer and prostate cancer can be screened for at the same time. Examination every 6 months is recommended if (1) the client has a history of continuing urinary manifestations, especially if a blood relative has had prostate cancer, or (2) if he has BPH or has had subtotal prostatectomy. Even so, 10% to 20% of tumors are too small to be detected by rectal examination. A hard nodule in the prostate, particularly in the posterior lobe, of any man older than 50 years has about a 50% chance of being malignant.

■ Transrectal Ultrasound

Transrectal ultrasound is a newer modality used for early detection of prostate cancer. This simple diagnostic test is capable of discovering possibly twice as many prostate cancers as digital rectal examination. It is not used routinely, however. It is usually ordered if the PSA level is elevated or if abnormalities are felt on the digital rectal examination.

■ Tumor Markers

Tumor markers are another means of assessment. The serum level of acid phosphatase was the most important biochemical test in diagnosing prostate cancer. The newer and even more specific test is the PSA assay. The PSA test is particularly useful in monitoring clients with prostate cancer; an elevation of PSA signals that the tumor is growing. A combination of the digital rectal examination and transrectal ultrasound following an elevated PSA is considered the best screening for the disease.

Acid phosphatase is not usually a tumor-specific marker because it is produced in a number of body tissues. However, approximately 1000 times more acid phosphatase is present in the prostate than in any other body organ. High serum levels of prostatic acid phosphatase (PAP) are associated with metastatic prostate cancer. Determination of the PAP levels is useful in monitoring disease progression and in assessment of response to treatment. However, it is not as specific as the PSA and is considered much less useful today.

A new blood test called the reverse transcriptase–polymerase chain reaction (RT-PCR) can determine whether cells in circulation are producing PSA, a substance produced only by cancer cells. This test helps detect metastasis of prostate cancer and may lead to earlier treatment of the disease.

■ Other Tests

Laboratory tests screen for indications of bladder obstruction, tumor obstruction, or metastasis to areas such as the liver and bone marrow. These tests include complete blood cell count (CBC), SMA-12, blood urea nitrogen (BUN), creatinine, and liver function studies.

X-ray assessment includes chest radiography, intravenous pyelography (IVP), and lymphangiography, to screen for obstructive uropathy and metastases in the skeleton and lymph nodes.

Ultrasonography, CT scanning, and magnetic resonance imaging (MRI) assess for the local extent of the tumor. Although CT scanning does not differentiate cancer of the prostate from BPH, it is useful in assessing large tumors. Transrectal ultrasonography is useful in assessing the size and shape of the prostate, locating tumors within the capsule of the prostate, and monitoring tumor response to treatment.

Radionuclide imaging is used to detect bone lesions. Bone metastasis occurs in 75% to 85% of men with advanced prostatic cancer. Lesions may be detected by bone scans 6 months or more before abnormalities appear on a bone x-ray film.

■ Biopsy

Needle aspiration or biopsy is used to confirm suspected malignancy. Open perineal biopsy often is not performed because adverse effects, such as infection and trauma, are common. Tissue for histologic examination is obtained more readily by transperineal or transrectal needle biopsy. The transperineal approach avoids the risk of contaminating the prostate with fecal matter, but the transrectal approach is more accurate. A general anesthetic may be used and allows more accuracy because many samples may be taken with a small-bore needle.

After the needle biopsy, monitor the client for fever, urinary obstruction, hematuria, or rectal bleeding. Fine-needle aspiration of the prostate for cytologic analysis is usually performed without anesthesia. Percutaneous fine-needle aspiration may be used to determine metastatic sites, such as lymph nodes. Bone marrow aspiration is performed to confirm metastatic tumors, but it is positive only in widespread disease. Transurethral resection of the prostate is not recommended for biopsy, because tumors are usually located at the periphery of the prostate, particularly in the posterior lobe.

■ Staging and Grading of Tumors

Grading of prostatic cancer is intended to establish the activity or virulence of the disease. Staging is an attempt to define the extent to which the carcinoma has developed. Of the several methods of classification, no consensus presently exists for defining each stage. Box 83–1 outlines one classification.

Acute and Subacute Care

■ Medical Management

The treatment of prostatic cancer is controversial because of the varied biologic behavior of the disease and because staging methods do not accurately predict malignant potential. Various treatment combinations may be used, depending on the choices of the person and physician, and the stage that has been reached. For example, if the tumor is well differentiated and of low volume, TUR may be sufficient. Recent studies have questioned the use of aggressive therapy. Quality-of-life considerations are important and are now being considered when deciding treatment options. Recent studies have found that watchful waiting may be an appropriate option for many less aggressive prostate cancers.[149] However, if extensive metastases have developed by the time a diagnosis is made, palliative treatment may be all that is available.

Radiation Therapy

Radiation therapy includes the following:

1. Interstitial radiation
2. Combined interstitial and external-beam radiation
3. External-beam megavoltage radiation (see also Chapter 24)

Box 83-1. Staging and Grading of Tumors

Stage A: **Tumor microscopic (T_1N_0, M_0)**

A_1: Microscopic focus
A_2: Diffuse

Stage B: **Tumor macroscopic (T_{1-2}, N_0, M_0)**

B_1: One lobe involved, nodule ≤ 1.5 cm
B_2: Both lobes involved, nodule ≥ 1.5 cm

Stage C: **Tumor extracapsular (T_3, N_0, M_0)**

C_1: Localized, nodule ≤ 70 g
C_2: Pelvic sidewall fixation, nodule ≥ 70 g

Stage D: **Metastatic disease (T_4, N_{1-3+}, M_+)**

D_1: Confined to pelvis
D_2: Extrapelvic

Grading of the tumor is as follows (Gleason's score):

- *Grade I:* Well differentiated
- *Grade II:* Intermediate or moderately differentiated
- *Grade III:* Poorly differentiated

Interstitial radiation is used to control locally advanced tumors (usually stage B or C). Radioactive isotopes, such as iodine (^{125}I), are used to destroy tumors directly. One widely used technique is to perform a pelvic lymphadenectomy and to implant iodine seeds into the prostate with needles. The long half-life of these seeds allows delivery of an effective radiation dose for 1 year. Radiation falls off a short distance from the seeds, so normal tissue is protected. Complications include thrombophlebitis, lymphocele formation, edema, and obstructive problems during voiding.

Combined interstitial and external-beam radiation involves implanting gold in the prostate, followed by external-beam radiation. This approach is used for people with stage A_2, B, or C tumors. Gold is of higher energy than iodine and has a shorter half-life (2.7 days). Thus, an effective dose can be delivered in several weeks, followed by external-beam full pelvic radiation over several more weeks. Implanting gold alone would destroy surrounding tissue. Complications include edema of the penis and lower extremities, cystitis, and urethritis. A major advantage of interstitial therapy is preservation of erection for most men treated this way.

External-beam megavoltage radiation is used when tumors are confined to the prostate and surrounding tissue. A tumoricidal dose of 6500 to 7000 rad is usually applied at a rate of 175 to 200 rad daily to the prostate. Surrounding tissue is relatively spared. The result depends on the size and grade of the tumor.

Hormonal Therapy

Endocrine therapy is used based on an observation that prostate epithelial cells atrophy if they are deprived of androgens. Androgen is produced in the testicles and the adrenal gland. Endocrine therapy is used for the following functions:

1. To remove the source of androgen
2. To suppress pituitary gonadotropin
3. To interfere with androgen synthesis
4. To interfere with the action of androgen on the tissue

The first oral androgen blocker, flutamide (Eulexin), is one of the newest medications used to treat prostate cancer. The gonadotropin-releasing hormone (GnRH) analogs leuprolide (Lupron) and goserelin acetate (Zoladex) are also being used. These agents block the action or secretion of androgens, which stimulate tumor growth, without causing the side effects that estrogen does. Finasteride (Proscar) is also used.

Administration of estrogen (diethylstilbestrol [DES]) suppresses the release of pituitary gonadotropin and reduces serum testosterone levels. Side effects include cardiovascular manifestations and gynecomastia. Gynecomastia can be lessened by giving the client breast radiation before estrogen therapy.

Chemotherapy

Nonendocrine chemotherapy (either given singly or in combination) has been used with prostate cancers to treat or sometimes stabilize the disease. Examples of chemotherapeutic agents sometimes used are cyclophosphamide (Cytoxan), fluorouracil, estramustine phosphate (Emcyt), doxorubicin hydrochloride (Adriamycin), and mitomycin (Mutamycin), Taxol, and VP-16.

■ Nursing Management of the Medical Client

Many clients diagnosed with prostate cancer undergo what is now known as watchful waiting, that is, periodic but close observation. The side effects of treatment combined with the relatively long life expectancy of many men with prostate cancer make aggressive treatment an option for only certain clients. For many others, although they do have prostate cancer, no treatment may result in a life expectancy equal to or better than that of clients who are treated.[149] Help the client understand this option and the absolute need for careful follow-up.

Radiation Therapy

Nursing care of the client receiving radiation therapy is covered in Chapter 24. Teach these clients about the possibility of radiation cystitis or proctitis. The main care that clients must learn is the need to control diarrhea and to care for the perianal skin, which may become extremely excoriated. Antidiarrheals also may be used to help control the diarrhea and thereby keep the perianal skin free from irritation.

Hormonal Therapy

Hormonal therapy is often used for advanced disease, so care of these clients may involve care of a client with long-term disease that may become terminal. Drugs such as Proscar, however, are being used earlier in the disease with curative treatments. Help the client cope with the possible disease outcome. Many of the hormonal treatments produce chemical castration with the side effects of loss of secondary sexual characteristics and feminization. The client will need to cope with the alterations in sexuality. Help the client learn to cope with the impotence that may result along with the manifestations of feminization. Clients may refuse treatment because of the fear of impotence. These clients need a great deal of support to understand the options available.

■ Surgical Management

Transurethral Prostatectomy. Surgical approaches include transurethral prostatectomy (TURP), laser ablation, cryosurgical ablation, and radical prostatectomy (see Case Management feature). TURP may be used for well-differentiated tumors of low volume or to relieve obstruction in advanced disease. Repeated TURP is sometimes needed to maintain an adequate channel through the prostatic urethra. (See the discussion of TURP in the section on BPH.)

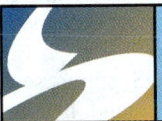

CASE MANAGEMENT

Transurethral Resection of the Prostate (TURP)
(For Clinical Pathway, see Appendix D.)

Clinical Pathway from Nashville Department of Veterans Affairs Medical Center, Nashville, Tennessee
Information provided by Jim Zeedar, R.N., and Ellen Moore, M.S.N., R.N.

Development and Revision of Pathway

- TURPs were (and continue to be) the highest-volume and most easily mapped genitourinary procedure being performed on the unit at the time pathways were initiated. It is also a diagnosis that works well in a pathway format. By choosing this diagnosis, we were able to use pathways on a large segment of our patient population while introducing the staff to a relatively variance-free pathway for initial training.
- This pathway was initiated in March 1993 and has been used steadily since its inception.
- Clinical leadership on the unit provided initial development of the TURP pathway. These included the nurse-manager and assistant manager, the surgical service attending physician, and the multidisciplinary service chiefs. Currently, the clinical staff is developing pathways with attending physician and service chief approval. The process remains nurse driven, beginning with the staff nurse and involving the appropriate clinical staff of each service involved in the client's care.
- All of our pathways are initially monitored for task and outcome variance to ensure reliability and validity. As practice changes, pathways are revised accordingly. The process is presently initiated by nursing service, as variance analysis is currently within this service's domain. Revisions are discussed and approved by the multidisciplinary development team and finally approved by the surgical task force oversight committee.
- All pathways are reviewed for 3 months when they are initiated. After the initial introduction and review period, the pathway is reviewed semi-annually to determine if revisions need to be made.

Use and Impact of the Pathway

- All clients undergoing the TURP procedure are admitted or transferred to our surgical unit and are placed on the pathway. If a client were to be admitted to another unit, the pathway would not be used at this time. Pathways are used only on specific units.
- The pathways are developed as a multidisciplinary tool, and all services are therefore encouraged to utilize the pathway. Nursing predominates in pathway utilization, especially with regard to documentation; however, other services are increasing their use of the pathway. The physician staff reviews the pathway daily for order entry, but they do not yet document directly on the pathway.
- The initiation of pathways has uniformly improved the quality and consistency of care provided on this unit by increasing the accountability of the nursing staff to move the client toward identified goals. Specific improvements noted with these pathways have been in early mobilization of clients, heightened attention to returning the patient to routine nutrition, and closer monitoring of hematuria and voiding patterns. Client education has also improved by standardizing the education expected and increasing the accountability for education.
- This pathway has impacted cost by decreasing the length of stay for TURP clients. This pathway immediately remedied a hesitancy to discharge on the weekends. By not holding clients unnecessarily over the weekend, the postoperative length of stay has decreased. Analysis of our multidisciplinary practices for TURP clients through pathway development and variance analysis has helped us improve the selection criteria for preoperative admission versus day-of-surgery admission, which also lowers the overall length of stay.

Laser Ablation. Laser ablation of the prostate (LAP) is a newer form of surgical treatment similar in procedure to the TURP. A laser fiber is introduced transurethrally to ablate the lateral lobes of the prostate. There is significantly less bleeding associated with the LAP than with the TURP, making it a safer procedure. The LAP so effectively controls bleeding that it has been used in clients who are receiving anticoagulant therapy. LAP does produce more edema than the traditional TURP, so clients may experience longer recovery of urinary flow.

Cryosurgical Ablation. Cryosurgical ablation of the prostate requires the insertion of cryoprobes, under guided transrectal ultrasound, into desired areas of the prostate to freeze and thereby destroy the tissue. This procedure produces less pain and less bleeding than traditional TURP and is much less invasive than open radical procedures. Because of the newness of the procedure, long-term statistics about success rates or long-term complications are not yet available. It is not always covered by insurance since it is not yet a proven treatment.

Radical Prostatectomy. Radical prostatectomy via a perineal (see Fig. 83–3D) or retropubic (see Fig. 83–3C) approach may be performed. Radical surgery involves removal of the following:

1. The entire prostate gland (rather than just enucleation)
2. The outer capsule
3. The seminal vesicles
4. Sections of the vas deferens
5. Possibly, portions of the bladder neck

This surgery may be recommended for men who fit the following criteria:

1. Have no other serious medical problems
2. Have a discrete tumor involving less than one lobe (i.e., stage B_1)
3. Have an expected survival of at least 10 to 15 years; it is sometimes used for men with stage B_2 or C tumors

Common side effects of radical prostatectomy are erectile dysfunction (in as many as 85% to 90% of clients or as low as 50% with nerve-sparing surgery) and incontinence (in 10% to 15% of clients). Both of these side effects are difficult for a man to experience and to discuss. Improved surgical techniques and advances in preventing and treating erectile dysfunction and incontinence help many men overcome these difficulties. For example, surgical techniques that carefully dissect around periprostatic autonomic nerves can avoid erectile dysfunction. Urinary incontinence usually occurs after postoperative removal of the catheter, but leakage generally subsides within 6 months in 85% to 90% of men. (For discussion of these problems, see the section on TURP.)

Artificial urinary sphincters (AUSs) have been surgically implanted for refractory urinary incontinence. An AUS is a fluid-filled system that consists of the following three parts:

1. A silicone rubber cuff that encircles the urethra
2. A pump that is implanted into the scrotum
3. A balloon that is inserted into the abdomen

The mechanism of an AUS functions as follows:

● When inflated with fluid, the cuff closes the urethra.
● The urethra is opened when the man manually squeezes the pump flat, moving fluid from the cuff into the balloon.
● When the man releases the pump, fluid moves from the balloon back into the cuff, closing the urethra.

The pump appears as a bulge in the scrotum just above the left testicle. It is seen on x-ray film because the fluid contains a small amount of dye.

Extensive postsurgical evaluation is necessary, including urodynamic testing, urethral pressure, cystography, IVP, and, sometimes, micturition studies. This procedure is recommended for people with a normal bladder and especially for those with incontinence following TURP. Initial postoperative pain is considerable. A Foley catheter is inserted during surgery and is removed in about 24 hours, when the swelling has subsided.

Once the physician has activated the AUS pump, several weeks after the swelling has subsided and healing has occurred, the client can learn to activate the pump. The client needs to pump the bulb only when feeling the sensation of a full bladder. Catheterization can be performed with the device in place, but the practice is not recommended.

Orchiectomy. Bilateral orchiectomy is the most effective way to remove the source of androgen. This surgical procedure removes the testicles, which lowers serum testosterone levels significantly.

■ Nursing Management of the Surgical Client

The physical nursing care for the client with prostatic cancer is essentially the same as that for a client with BPH and a TURP. The psychosocial and emotional care of these clients is very different because issues such as cancer and sexuality must be addressed (see Chapter 24). Aseptic technique is especially important after a perineal prostatectomy because of a high possibility of infection in a wound so close to the anal area. Meticulous aseptic technique is also necessary around the area of insertion of a suprapubic catheter.

Care for the client after laser ablation is simpler than for the TUR client, because bleeding is not a significant problem. A Foley catheter is present and requires the same nursing care as discussed under BPH. The client will probably go home with the catheter in place and will need teaching to maintain the system.

Following cryosurgical ablation, the client requires bladder retraining as for any prostatectomy. The client often has a suprapubic catheter in place rather than a Foley catheter. This allows the client to attempt voiding and to be able to drain any residual urine without recatheterization. Until the edema has subsided, the suprapubic catheter is left open to provide for urinary drainage. The catheter can then be clamped for 3 to 4 hours and the client can then try to void. Once adequate urinary control has been reestablished, the suprapubic catheter is removed. The client must also be taught to expect the

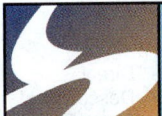

CASE MANAGEMENT

**Simple Orchiectomy (Prostatic Cancer)
For Clinical Pathway, see Appendix D.**

Clinical Pathway from Nashville Department of Veterans Affairs Medical Center, Nashville, Tennessee
Information provided by Jim Zeedar, R.N., and Ellen Moore, M.S.N., R.N.

Development and Revision of Pathway

- Orchiectomy is a short-stay procedure that was not performed frequently enough for the staff to remain highly proficient. By using pathways, a higher level of consistent care is ensured.
- This pathway was initiated in October 1994.
- Clinical leadership on the unit initially developed the simple orchiectomy pathway. This included the nurse-manager and assistant manager, the surgical service attending physician, and the multidisciplinary service chiefs. Currently, the clinical staff is developing pathways with attending physician and service chief approval. The process remains nurse driven, beginning with the staff nurse and involving the appropriate clinical staff of each service involved in the client's care.
- All of our pathways are initially monitored for task and outcome variance to ensure reliability and validity. As practice changes, pathways are revised accordingly. The process is presently initiated by nursing service as variance analysis is currently within this service's domain. Revisions are discussed and approved by the multidisciplinary development team and finally approved by the surgical task force oversight committee.
- All pathways are reviewed for 3 months when they are initiated. After the initial introduction and review period, the pathway is reviewed semi-annually to determine if revisions need to be made.

Use and Impact of the Pathway

- All clients admitted for this procedure are placed on the pathway. If a client were to be admitted to another unit, the pathway would not be used at this time. Pathways are used only on specific units.
- The pathways are developed as a multidisciplinary tool, and all services are therefore encouraged to utilize the pathway. Nursing predominates in pathway utilization, especially with regard to documentation; however, other services are increasing their use of the pathway. The physician staff reviews the pathway daily for order entry, but they do not yet document directly on the pathway.
- The initiation of pathways has uniformly improved the quality and consistency of care provided on this unit by increasing the accountability of the nursing staff to move the client toward identified goals. Specific improvements noted with these pathways have been in early mobilization of clients, heightened attention to returning the client to routine nutrition, and closer monitoring of hematuria and voiding patterns. Client education has also improved by standardizing the education expected and increasing the accountability for education.
- This pathway has had an impact on cost by decreasing the length of stay for clients undergoing simple orchiectomy. This pathway immediately remedied a hesitancy to discharge on the weekends. By not holding clients unnecessarily over the weekend, the postoperative length of stay has decreased. Analysis of our multidisciplinary practices for simple orchiectomy clients through pathway development and variance analysis has helped us to improve the selection criteria for preoperative admission versus day-of-surgery admission, which also lowers the overall length of stay.

prostatic tissue to slough off after the procedure. Fluid intake should be at least 6 to 8 glasses of fluid per day to help wash this tissue out. Also warn the client about potential swelling and bruising of the scrotum. The client may find that application of ice bags helps to relieve the pain. Also, swelling can be controlled through scrotal elevation with a Bellevue bridge (Fig. 83–6).

The client undergoing radical surgery, especially radical perineal prostatectomy, will have a dressing that necessitates nursing intervention. The surgeon may make the initial dressing change and delegate subsequent wound care to you. The man may be taught to change his own dressing. When a perineal incision is present, a double-tailed T-binder or mesh pants may be used to secure dressings. Cross the tails over the incisional area, and

position one tail on each side of the scrotum. Then, pull the tails up to the waistband and tie them securely. Some men find it more comfortable to wear a scrotal support to hold the dressing in place. Prevent wound trauma after perineal surgery by avoiding the use of enemas, rectal tubes, or rectal thermometers. Clean the wound thoroughly after each bowel movement. After perineal prostatectomy, a urethral catheter may be left in place for 12 to 14 days to allow for healing of the resected bladder neck and urethra.

Men with prostatic cancer and their significant others need ongoing sensitive support and accurate information to make the difficult decisions required of them. Their concerns are often considerable and may include the choices of available treatments, fear of death, anxiety about residual disability and illness, and the possible effects of the illness on people in their social network.

■ Modifications for Elderly Clients

Although prostate cancer occurs most commonly in men older than 50, treatment options will vary depending on the age of the client, the stage and grade of the cancer, and the wishes of the client. Hormonal manipulation appears to prolong survival significantly for the older client.

Prostatitis

Prostatitis (inflammation of the prostate gland) may be classified as (1) acute bacterial, (2) chronic bacterial, or (3) nonbacterial.

Acute bacterial prostatitis is usually caused by aerobic gram-negative rods, the coliforms (especially *Escherichia coli*), and *Pseudomonas*. Routes of infection (Fig. 83–7) include the following:

1. Urethral ascent
2. Descent from the urinary bladder or kidneys

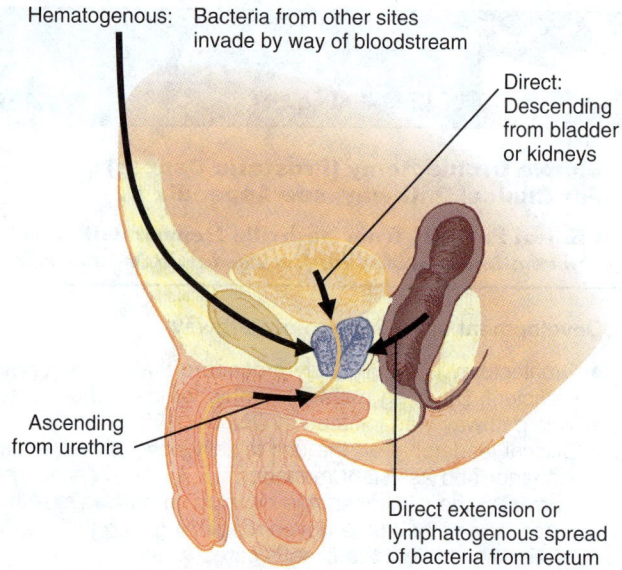

Figure 83–7. Postulated pathways of infection to the prostate gland.

3. Direct extension or lymphatogenous spread from the rectum
4. Hematogenous spread (via blood)

Assessment reveals chills and fever, low back and perineal pain, and urinary urgency, frequency, nocturia, and dysuria. Bladder outlet obstruction, myalgia (painful muscles), and arthralgia (painful joints) may occur. On examination (see Fig. 82–18), the prostate is extremely tender and swollen, yet it is firm, indurated, and warm to the touch. Acute cystitis (bladder inflammation) is common and is characterized by hematuria and cloudy, malodorous urine. Urine cultures identify the infecting organisms. Exudate from prostatic massage (see Chapter 82) can also identify the organism, but this is not usually performed because such massage is very painful for a client with prostatitis, and it can precipitate bacteremia. Transurethral instrumentation, including catheterization, is avoided during acute infection because it can push infection up into the bladder. Intervention includes rest, analgesics, stool softeners (constipation is painful with prostatitis), antimicrobial medication, sitz baths, and increased oral fluids. Occasionally the inflammation is so severe that the client cannot pass urine, and catheterization is needed. Hospitalization may be required for administration of parenteral antibiotics and supportive care.

Chronic bacterial prostatitis is a nonacute infection of the prostate gland. It is most commonly caused by the same organisms that cause acute bacterial prostatitis and has the same routes of infection. Some gram-positive bacteria, such as staphylococci and streptococci, have been thought to cause chronic bacterial prostatitis, but they rarely persist or lead to recurring infection. Chronic bacterial prostatitis is a less severe inflammation than the acute type. Some clients have no manifestations. A diagnosis may be made after finding bacteriuria (bacteria in the urine) on routine urinalysis. Other clients may experience the following symptoms:

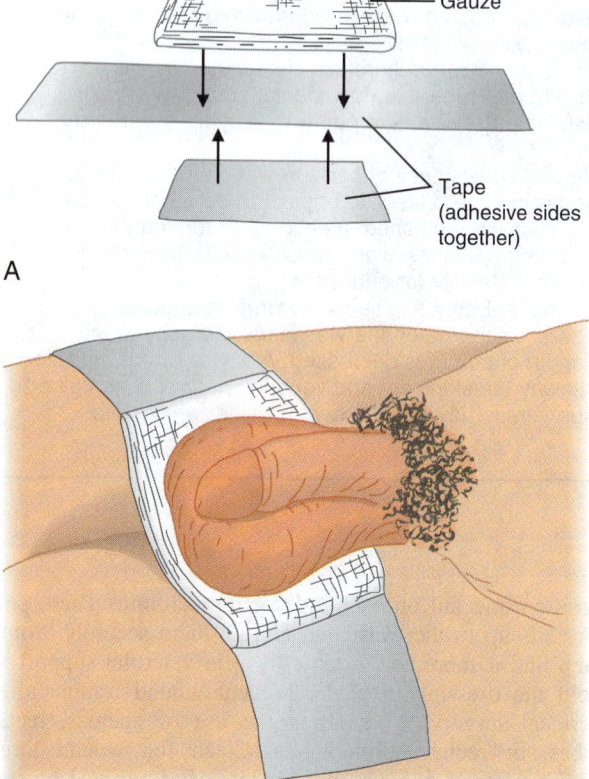

Figure 83–6. Scrotal support (Bellevue bridge type). *A,* Prepare the support by placing two pieces of tape with their adhesive edges together, the smaller piece in the center of the longer piece. This provides a "nonadhesive" segment between the client's legs. Place folded gauze on top of the support. *B,* Gently place the support under the scrotum, and attach the adhesive ends of the support to the thighs.

1. Voiding dysfunction, such as urgency, frequency, nocturia, and dysuria
2. Low back or perineal pain
3. Occasional myalgia (muscle aches) and arthralgia (painful joints)

On examination, the prostate may be normal or feel boggy or indurated. Inflammatory cells may be present in prostatic secretions. If the client has cystitis, organisms may be identified in urine specimens. If urine is not infected, organisms may be identified from mid-stream urine specimen, urethral specimens, and prostatic massage.

Treatment with antimicrobial agents is problematic because it is difficult to obtain therapeutic levels of drug in prostatic secretions during nonacute inflammations. Discomfort and pain may be relieved by sitz baths, anti-inflammatory agents, and anticholinergic drugs. Repeated prostatic massage and ejaculation may be helpful. Surgical intervention is rarely required. Long-term, low-dose antimicrobial drugs may control manifestations.

Nonbacterial prostatitis is the most common form of prostatitis. Its cause is unknown. It has the same manifestations as bacterial prostatitis, but no causative organism is found. On prostatic massage, abnormal numbers of inflammatory cells are noted in the prostatic fluid, but no infectious agent is found. Some experts believe that nonbacterial prostatitis may be caused by *Mycoplasma, Chlamydia,* or *Ureaplasma* species. Others suggest it may be an autoimmune disease.

Assessment findings of nonbacterial prostatitis are similar to those of bacterial prostatitis except that bacteria are not found in the urine or prostatic secretions. Diagnosis is made by systematically ruling out other types of prostatitis. This can be distressing for the client, because diagnosis and treatment are not specific. Intervention includes anti-inflammatory agents or short-term antimicrobial medication. Hot sitz baths and normal sexual activity are recommended. Dietary restrictions are not recommended unless the person finds them to be associated with manifestations. Opinions vary about the therapeutic benefits of prostatic massage.

Other Prostate Infections

Other prostate infections include the following:

1. Nonspecific granulomatous prostatitis in men prone to asthma or allergies
2. Prostatic abscess, caused primarily by *Escherichia coli*
3. Prostatic tuberculosis

Prostatodynia

Prostatodynia is a condition in which men experience manifestations similar to prostatitis, particularly prostatic and pelvic pain. There is no history of urinary tract infection and no apparent prostatic inflammation. Microscopic examination and culture of prostatic secretions are negative. Conditions associated with prostatodynia include the following:

- *Spasm* on voiding, detected by urodynamic testing, for which phenoxybenzamine hydrochloride (Dibenzyline) is usually prescribed
- *Tension myalgia* of the pelvic floor, treated by diathermy, physical therapy, and muscle relaxants
- *Emotional problems,* helped by counseling or psychiatric consultation

Testicular Disorders and Procedures

Testicular Cancer

Testicular cancer is the most common and serious solid tumor cancer in men between the ages of 15 and 35 years. Testicular cancer rarely occurs in men younger than 15 or older than 40. It is less common in black and Asian men. Two to three cases per 100,000 males are diagnosed in the United States each year.

Etiology and Risk Factors

The cause of testicular cancer is unknown. Exogenous estrogen and cryptorchidism are considered possible causes. The major risk factor for testicular cancer is cryptorchidism (undescended testicles). It is now recommended that any child born with an undescended testicle have an orchiopexy as soon as possible after birth. The longer the testicles are left undescended, the greater the risk of testicular cancer. Performing an orchiopexy, however, does not completely eliminate the risk of cancer.

The male offspring of women who used estrogen during the first trimester of pregnancy (called *DES sons*) or who were exposed to estrogen-progestin combinations frequently used in diagnostic tests to confirm pregnancy are at greater risk of developing testicular cancer.

As just noted, the term *DES sons* refer to men whose mothers took the drug diethylstilbestrol (DES), a synthetic estrogen, during pregnancy. Between 1940 and 1970, DES was given to pregnant women who had a high risk of spontaneous abortion. Vaginal cancer and other genital anomalies have been found in daughters of women who took DES. It is now being found that 30% to 70% of sons of such women have developed genital abnormalities, such as undescended testicles (increased risk of cancer), micropenis, meatal stenosis (narrowing of penile opening), varicocele, hypoplastic (underdeveloped) testicles, and epididymal cysts. DES sons also have an increased risk of infertility and abnormal semen.

The Risk Factors and Levels of Prevention feature and the Nursing Research feature explain that all men between the ages of 15 and 45 should practice testicular self-examination (TSE) on a regular monthly basis. Early detection can lead to early diagnosis and cure of this cancer. All young men over the age of 15 years should be taught how to perform monthly TSE and should be strongly encouraged to do this monthly (see Chapter 82 for TSE instructions).

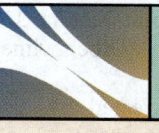

Testicular Cancer

Risk Factors

- Cryptorchidism (undescended testicles)
- Male offspring of women who took DES or oral contraceptives during the first trimester of pregnancy
- Family history of testicular cancer
- Higher rates in higher socioeconomic groups
- Lowest rate in black men

Levels of Prevention

Primary Prevention

- Ensure that children born with undescended testicles have an orchiopexy as soon as possible after birth.

Secondary Prevention

- Encourage all men from age 15 to 45 to practice monthly testicular self-examination.
- Teach high-risk men to have a yearly examination by a physician.

Tertiary Prevention

- Ensure that clients receive testicular implants following orchiectomy.
- Teach clients about sperm banking prior to treatment.

Pathophysiology

Most cases of testicular cancer (97%) are germinal cell tumors, such as seminoma (about 40% of all tumors), teratocarcinoma, embryonal carcinoma, or choriocarcinoma. Seminomas generally have a favorable prognosis (about a 90% 5-year survival rate) because they are usually localized and metastasize late. These tumors are usually treated with orchiectomy and radiation therapy. They are usually confined to the testes and retroperitoneal nodes.

Nonseminomatous germ cell tumors are not as sensitive to radiation therapy; however, with the advent of newer chemotherapy regimens following orchiectomy, the cure rate has risen to 95% overall, with 100% cure in stage I, 98% in stage II, and 80% in stage III.[59]

Nongerminal tumors make up the remainder of testicular cancers. These tumors arise from interstitial cells or cells that compose the fibrous or vascular networks. They are classified as either interstitial cell tumors or testicular adenomas and are usually benign.

The overall survival rate from all types of testicular cancer is about 89% in whites and 78% in blacks, although the occurrence rate is much lower in this group. This rate has increased dramatically in the last 10 years.

Metastasis occurs primarily through lymphatic spread. Drainage from the right testis is to the interaortal caval nodes, whereas the left drains to the preaortic nodes. Retroperineal nodes are commonly affected. Distant metastasis occurs most commonly to the lung and rarely to the liver, viscera, bone, or brain.

Clinical Manifestations and Diagnostic Findings

Most commonly, men with testicular tumors experience a painless enlargement, noted as heaviness, in the testicle (about 75% of cases). Some men describe it as a dragging sensation. Pain is rarely felt; however, the tumor is often found after an injury because the testicle is examined as a result of the injury. Hydrocele or hematocele may develop (Fig. 83–8). Some manifestations of testicular cancer resemble the manifestations of varicocele, and some are similar to the manifestations of prostatitis.

Assessment findings suggesting metastasis to the retroperitoneal lymph nodes include back pain, vague abdominal pain, nausea and vomiting, bowel and bladder changes, anorexia, and weight loss. If the lungs are involved, manifestations may include cough, dyspnea, and hemoptysis.

A thorough physical examination of the scrotum and testicles is the first diagnostic test performed. Unlike a simple hydrocele, a testicular tumor is not translucent on light examination.

A radical orchiectomy is the major diagnostic tool, because the entire testicle is removed for biopsy after a mass has been detected. Any testicular mass is considered malignant until proved otherwise. This approach is used because of the belief that a needle or open biopsy would lead to rapid spread, and because once the tumor has been shown to be a solid mass, its chance of being malignant is almost 100%.

Testicular tumors are staged as follows:

Stage I$_a$: tumor confined to testicle (T_1 N_0 M_0)
Stage I$_b$: metastasis to para-aortic or iliac nodes (T_1 N_1 M_0)
Stage II: tumor spread to retroperitoneal nodes but disease limited to below the diaphragm (T_{2-3}, N_2, M_0)
Stage III: tumor above the diaphragm or spread to body organs (usually the lungs) T_4, N_{3-4}, $M+$)

Other diagnostic tests used to determine the possible extent of the tumor include the following:

1. A chest x-ray study or CT of the lungs for lung metastasis
2. An abdominal and pelvic CT scan or MRI for retroperitoneal lymph node involvement
3. An IVP for urinary tract involvement
4. A lymphangiogram for retroperitoneal lymph node involvement (performed less frequently because CT and MRI are available)
5. Laboratory studies for serum alpha-fetoprotein (AFP), serum human serum gonadotropin-β subunit (hCG-β),

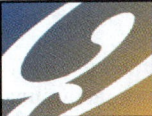

NURSING RESEARCH

Is Education about Testicular Self-Examination Effective?

Rudolf, V. M., & Quinn, L. M. (1988). The practice of TSE among college men: Effectiveness of an educational program. *Oncology Nursing Forum, 15* (1), 45–48.

Testicular cancer is the most common cancer in men aged 15 to 35. It is easily cured if detected early. Testicular self-examination (TSE) is an important tool for early detection, is done very easily, and yet is reported to be very rarely done by the men who would most benefit from it. This study replicated studies that demonstrate the lack of knowledge about testicular cancer. This study also looked at the effects of an educational program about testicular cancer and TSE. The program was presented to college men. The Health Belief Model was the theoretical framework for this study.

   A convenience sample of 64 college men enrolled in a physical education class at a private East Coast university were given a questionnaire on the Health Beliefs Survey for Testicular Cancer and Testicular Self-Examination. The group was white, of similar ages, and with similar low-risk factors.

   The results of the pretest showed that about half of the men had heard of testicular cancer and one-third stated they performed TSE. The scores on the seriousness and susceptibility subscales, however, showed little knowledge of testicular cancer among all subjects. After the education program, knowledge of testicular cancer did not increase significantly; however, the actual practice of TSE did increase significantly along with the subjects' knowledge of TSE and TSE technique.

   Several limitations of the study were described, including the lack of a randomized sample and the short length of time between the pre- and post-tests. Rudolph and Quinn also addressed the need for further education among college age men about the correct technique for TSE and the need to begin education about testicular cancer at the secondary school level. You can be instrumental in providing these educational programs to the groups that need them most.

Implications for Practice

It is apparent that knowledge of testicular cancer and TSE is not high among young men. This demonstrates the need for increased public awareness of this disease and the need for education of young men in the performance of TSE.

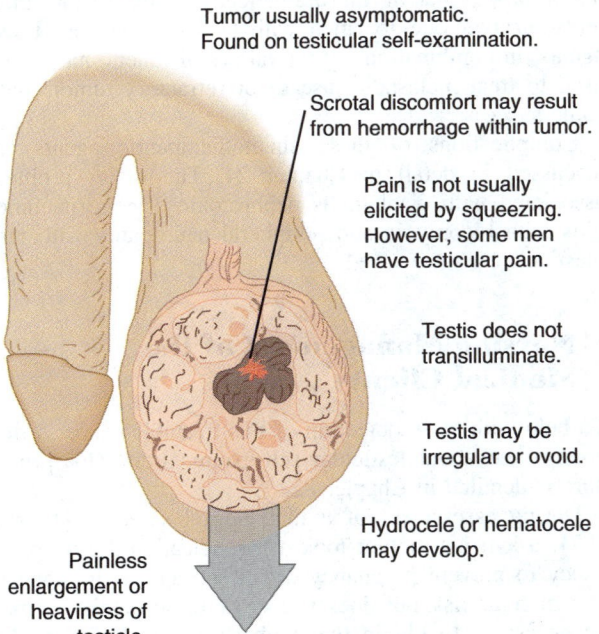

Tumor usually asymptomatic. Found on testicular self-examination.

Scrotal discomfort may result from hemorrhage within tumor.

Pain is not usually elicited by squeezing. However, some men have testicular pain.

Testis does not transilluminate.

Testis may be irregular or ovoid.

Hydrocele or hematocele may develop.

Painless enlargement or heaviness of testicle.

Figure 83–8. Some characteristics of tumors of the testes.

and lactic acid dehydrogenase (LDH) as tumor markers.

AFP levels are elevated only in nonseminomatous tumors. HCG-β is also elevated in nonseminomatous tumors, and hCG may be elevated in pure seminomas. Normally, hCG is present only in pregnant women. The elevation in men with testicular tumors also may lead to the development of gynecomastia. LDH levels may also be elevated.

Acute and Subacute Care

■ Surgical Management

Radical Orchiectomy. As discussed earlier, a radical orchiectomy is performed to diagnose testicular cancer, so it also is the primary treatment. A radical inguinal orchiectomy involves the removal of the testis, epididymis, and vas deferens. The spermatic cord is then ligated just inside the internal inguinal ring to prevent seeding of the cancer.

Retroperitoneal Lymph Node Dissection. The major surgical choice is whether or not to do a retroperitoneal lymph node dissection in addition to the radical orchiectomy. Because chemotherapy is so successful in treating even widespread disease, the use of this radical surgery has been questioned. It is major surgery with a significant mortality rate. Since the advent of the CT scan and MRI, the status of these nodes can be ascertained without surgery. Also, there is a high incidence of impotence after this surgery because many of the autonomic nerves necessary for ejaculation are located in this area. This is a significant concern given the ages of the clients. Many surgeons are opting simply for the radical orchiectomy and diagnostic studies of the retroperitoneal lymph nodes without surgical resection.

The group that supports the retroperitoneal node dissection believes that using this approach limits the amount of chemotherapy needed because the extent of the tumor spread can be removed. Also, with stage B_2 or higher tumors, retroperitoneal node dissection is often done after chemotherapy, when only a partial response is achieved.

The major complication of retroperitoneal node dissection is infertility due to retrograde ejaculation. If a bilateral orchiectomy is performed, both infertility and impotence occur.

Testicular Prostheses. The amputated testicle can be replaced with a testicular prosthesis. This reconstructive surgery is recommended to help the young man's self-esteem. There has recently been some controversy associated with the use of silicone implants. Although most of the publicity has been directed toward the dangers associated with breast implants, silicone-filled testicular implants were also removed from the market. Currently, only one prosthesis remains on the market. Although little evidence has emerged that testicular implants cause autoimmune disease, particularly because so few are performed as compared to breast implants, clients should be aware of the possible effects.

■ Nursing Management of the Surgical Client

Carefully assess the client's understanding of and readiness for surgery, because the time between finding a lump and undergoing a radical orchiectomy may be a few days at most. Today, this surgery is usually a same-day procedure with an overnight stay at most. The client will need to be taught how to monitor for the development of complications and self-care strategies. The scrotal area will be tender and slightly swollen after surgery. Ice bags should control the swelling. The client should watch for the development of excessive swelling or bruising, such as from hematoma formation. The client should be provided with complete written instructions and a follow-up appointment before discharge.

If the client undergoes a radical orchiectomy, hospitalization will be longer. Preoperatively, sperm banking should be discussed with the client, because fertility is often impaired postoperatively. The client may need

counseling from a reproductive specialist to understand all of the options available.

Postoperatively, the client must be monitored closely for possible problems associated with major abdominal surgery. The client will require adequate pain control, usually through the use of a patient-controlled analgesia (PCA) pump or epidural infusion to comply with vigorous coughing and deep breathing to prevent respiratory complications. The client may have a chest tube if the chest was entered during the dissection. Ambulation is begun the day after surgery and the client may be given low-dose heparin to help prevent postoperative phlebitis. Review postoperative care in Chapter 21. Before discharge, provide the client with written instructions to monitor for the development of postoperative problems. The client also may need to make follow-up appointments with an oncologist for further treatment.

■ Medical Management

The primary treatment for testicular cancer is surgical resection of the testicle. Radiation and chemotherapy also may be used.

Radiation Therapy. Seminomas are particularly radiosensitive. The perineum and pelvis and the mediastinal and supraclavicular nodes are also irradiated if the peritoneal nodes are positive. Side effects include common complications associated with pelvic radiation. Radiation is not used for nonseminomatous tumors because they are not very radiosensitive.

Chemotherapy. Chemotherapy is used for both seminomas and nonseminomatous tumors that show any sign of spread. The major agent used is cisplatin in combination with vinblastine and bleomycin. Cisplatin in combination with other agents dramatically increases the long-term survival rate for men with testicular cancer. These agents, in combination with a variety of others, have been used to treat metastatic disease or refractory tumors with some success.

Complications of these chemotherapeutic agents are discussed in detail in Chapter 24. The major problem associated with cisplatin is nephrotoxic effects (pneumonitis with bleomycin and peripheral neuropathy with vinblastine).

■ Nursing Management of the Medical Client

To help with early detection of this treatable cancer, teach young men about testicular self-examination. This procedure is detailed in Chapter 82.

During assessment of a man born between 1940 and 1971, ask if his mother took any medication during pregnancy to prevent pregnancy or miscarriage. If he appears at particular risk but does not know these details, it may be necessary to obtain the mother's medical history. Information and referral is available through DES Action,

Long Island Jewish-Hillside Medical Center, New Hyde Park, NY 11040.

Supportive nursing care is very important for these young men, both during diagnosis and treatment. Be very aware of the threat to sexuality that this condition and its treatment have on young men. Review Chapters 23 and 24 for the care of clients undergoing chemotherapy and radiation therapy.

Testicular Torsion

Testicular torsion (Fig. 83–9) occurs when a testicle is mobile and the spermatic cord twists, cutting off the blood supply. It is the most common testicular disorder in children. It can occur at any age but is most usual at puberty. Manifestations arise suddenly, with acute scrotal swelling and severe pain as blood supply to the testicles is interrupted. It does not appear to be associated with any particular physical activity or trauma.

If testicular torsion is suspected, a testicular scan and Doppler scan should be done to assess the blood supply. If the blood supply is increased, the manifestations may be caused by epididymitis, and if it is decreased, then they are probably caused by torsion.

Testicular torsion is an emergency requiring surgical intervention within 6 to 12 hours. The spermatic cord is untwisted and the testicle immobilized by suturing it to the scrotum (orchiopexy). Without prompt surgery, the testicle may atrophy or develop an abscess.

Orchitis

Orchitis is a rare, acute testicular inflammation. It may be associated with trauma or an infection elsewhere in the body, such as mumps, pneumonia, tuberculosis, and syphilis. Mumps orchitis, which occurs in 20% to 3% of men who develop mumps after puberty, is usually bilateral.

Assessment reveals edematous and extremely tender testicles, reddened scrotal skin, fever, and prostration. Treatment includes bedrest, scrotal support, local heat to the scrotum, and medication for pain relief and fever. The acute phase lasts about 1 week. Permanent sterility may occur if both testicles are affected, whereas decreased fertility may result if only one is affected.

Hydrocele, Hematocele, and Spermatocele

Hydrocele (see Fig. 83–9) is a painless collection of clear, yellow fluid anywhere along the spermatic cord. The soft intrascrotal mass is translucent to light (see Chapter 82). If complications develop, such as discomfort from enlargement or impaired circulation, aspiration or surgical drainage may be performed.

A hematocele is a collection of blood in the tunica vaginalis. A spermatocele is a dilatation, originating in the epididymis, containing a milky fluid and spermatozoa. Hematoceles are less likely to transilluminate on light examination than are hydroceles.

Varicocele

Varicocele (see Fig. 83–9C) is a dilation and varicosity of the pampiniform plexus (the network of veins supplying the testicles) within the scrotum. Ninety percent of varicoceles are left-sided. They occur in 15% to 20% of men between 15 and 25 years of age. The client may experience a pulling sensation, a dull ache, or scrotal pain. Pain may be relieved by masturbation or sexual intercourse.

On palpation, with the man standing, a varicocele feels like a mass of tortuous veins above and posterior to the testicle. When the man lies down, the mass abates. Although the condition is not clearly understood, varicocele is an important cause of male infertility. Treatment includes the use of a scrotal support, with surgery being performed only if complications occur, such as severe pain, or if the varicocele is thought to contribute to infertility.

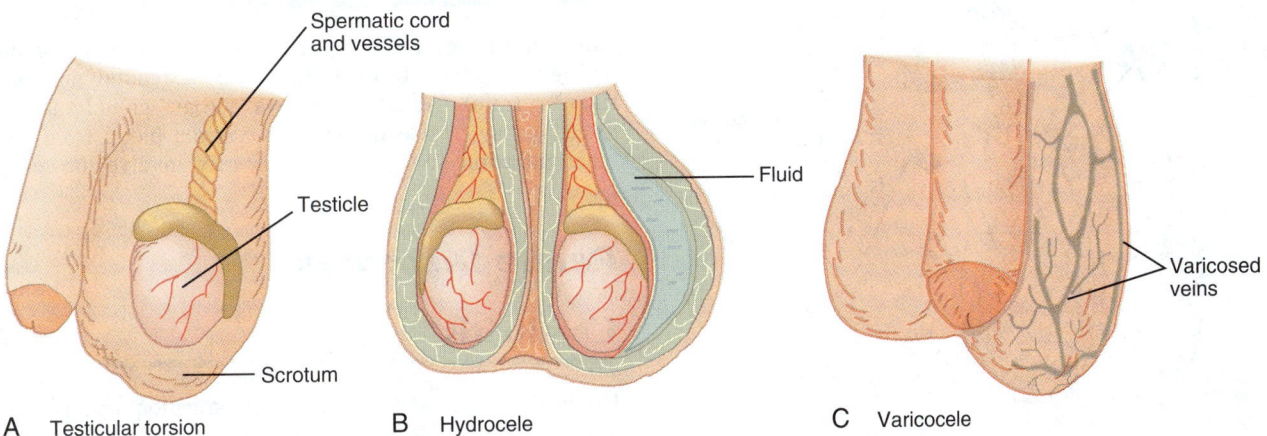

Figure 83–9. Disturbances of the testicles.

Vasectomy

A vasectomy is an elective surgical procedure performed as a permanent method of contraception (although sometimes a vasectomy can be surgically reversed). This procedure also is frequently performed after a prostatectomy to prevent retrograde epididymitis.

The surgery is usually performed under local anesthesia in the urologist's office or in an outpatient setting. The procedure, performed through a small incision in the scrotum, involves cutting out a segment of the vas deferens and folding and ligating the remaining ends (Fig. 83–10).

Postoperatively, slight pain and swelling are easily controlled with an ice bag and mild analgesia, such as acetaminophen. A scrotal support also increases client comfort. The client can resume sexual intercourse whenever he finds it comfortable, usually about 1 week after the procedure. The client must continue to practice other means of birth control until the follow-up semen analysis shows azoospermia, because live sperm are left in the ampulla of vas.

Undescended Testes

The most common congenital testicular condition is that of undescended testes (cryptorchidism) (Fig. 83–11). One (unilateral) or both (bilateral) testicles may be arrested in the abdomen, inguinal canal, low pelvis (intracanalicular), or high scrotum. Retractile testicle (descends into the scrotum but is occasionally pulled back into the inguinal canal), ectopic testicle (descends to the wrong area, e.g., perineum), and complete absence of a testicle may also occur. Undescended testicles occur in 1% of full-term male infants. If the condition is bilateral, the child should be assessed for intersexuality, especially if it is associated with other genital abnormalities.

Undescended testes are associated with infertility. The incidence of testicular cancer is high in men with undes-

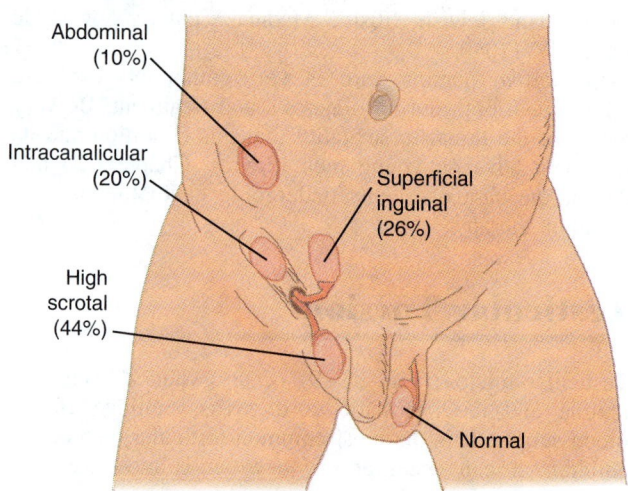

Figure 83–11. Undescended testis (cryptorchidism).

cended testes if the condition is not corrected before puberty. Treatment, which is surgical, is carried out when the child is between 1 and 2 years of age and certainly before age 6.

Eunuchoidism

Eunuchoidism is a congenital condition, characterized by the following signs:

Puberty does not occur
Genitals and prostate remain infantile
Voice is high pitched
Axillary and pubic hair are scanty
No beard hair develops
Skeletal proportions are abnormal

Medical advice should be sought if puberty is delayed and secondary sexual characteristics do not develop. Treatment with hormonal replacement may be possible.

Other Testicular Problems

Other testicular problems include tuberculosis spread through the blood from the lungs to the epididymis and testicles (rare). Actinomycosis (a chronic granulomatous disease) may invade the testicles via the blood from another infection site. Syphilis also may involve the testicles.

Penile Disorders

Urethritis

Urethritis is an acute urethral inflammation and is discussed under sexually transmitted diseases and urinary disorders (see Chapters 55 and 86).

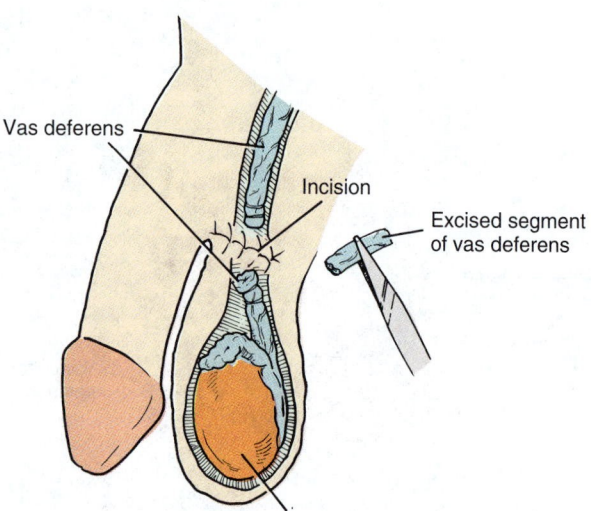

Figure 83–10. Vasectomy.

Urethral Stricture

Urethral stricture is caused by urethral scarring or narrowing. It may be congenital or caused by untreated or severe urethritis or urethral injury (including urologic instrumentation, e.g., cystoscopy). Manifestations are caused by obstruction: small-caliber urinary stream, hyperdistended bladder, infection, fever, and dysuria. Urethral strictures are released surgically by urethral dilation or urethroplasty. See Chapter 56 for further information.

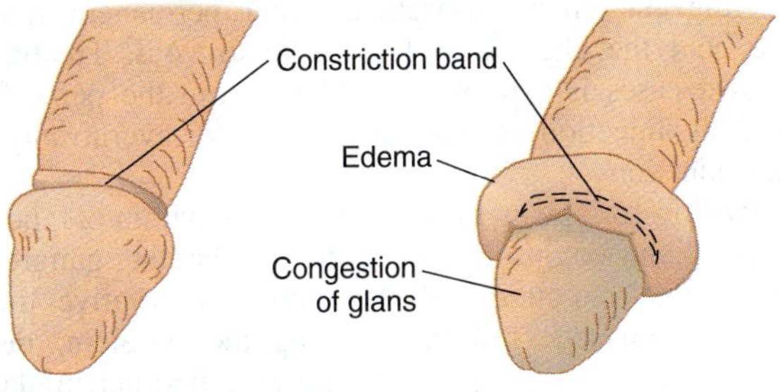

Phimosis

Phimosis occurs when the penile foreskin (prepuce) is constricted at the opening, making retraction difficult or impossible. It is caused by posthitis (preputial infection or inflammation), balanitis (inflammation or infection of the glans), or local trauma and inflammation. It is not usually painful, but it can lead to obstructive uropathy if it is severe enough. Prolonged phimosis, caused by the chronic inflammation and irritation, does predispose to penile cancer. Assessment reveals edema, erythema, tenderness, and purulent discharge. Intervention includes controlling infection with local treatment and broad-spectrum antimicrobial drugs.

Effective genital hygiene is essential to prevent acquired penile disorders. In uncircumcised males, the penis is cleaned by pulling the foreskin back gently and washing the area with a wash cloth (Fig. 83–12).

Routine circumcision has not been seen as medically necessary according to the American Academy of Pediat-

Figure 83–13. Paraphimosis.

rics and many other health professionals and health organizations. Circumcision may be indicated in clients with penile infection, phimosis, or paraphimosis. Circumcision should be done under general anesthesia. Potential risks include excessive bleeding, infection, and penile trauma. Recently, however, they have reconsidered this decision based on the fact that the rate of penile cancer is almost zero in circumcised men. It is now believed that this should be explained to parents who are making a decision. Some parents have religious or cultural reasons for circumcising their male children. Be sure uncircumcised men know how to retract the foreskin daily and clean the smegma from beneath it properly.

Paraphimosis

Paraphimosis (Fig. 83–13) occurs when a tight foreskin, once retracted, cannot be returned to its normal position. Paraphimosis sometimes occurs after rigorous cleaning, masturbation, sexual intercourse, catheter insertion, or cystoscopy if the foreskin is not returned to its normal position. Circulation is thus impeded, and the glans swells rapidly. It is painful and edema is commonly seen. The foreskin can be gently compressed either manually or with an elastic wrap. Manual reduction then may be attempted by gently pulling the foreskin. Surgical incision of the foreskin with local anesthesia may be necessary if the condition does not resolve.

Priapism

Priapism is a prolonged, persistent penile erection without sexual desire. It can last hours or even days and may be very painful. The condition is sometimes associated with leukemia or sickle cell anemia. Self-injection of medications (mainly papaverine) to treat impotence is the other common cause. It also may result from some medications, such as anticoagulants, alcohol, phenothiazines, alpha-adrenergic blockers, and marijuana.

Two major types of priapism have been defined using a physiology-based system. High-flow arterial priapism, the first, is less common, usually occurs after trauma, and is less painful. Low-flow veno-occlusive priapism, the second and more common form of the condition, is an emergency situation, and is extremely painful.

Low-flow priapism is considered an emergency situation because circulation to the penis is compromised, pre-

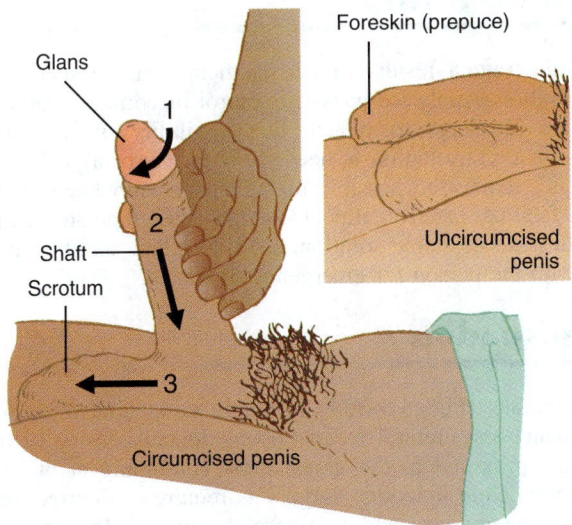

Figure 83–12. A circumcised and an uncircumcised penis. The foreskin of an uncircumcised penis should retract easily. During physical examination, ask the man to retract his foreskin himself. Effective genital hygiene is essential to prevent acquired penile problems. Many men have never been taught how to do this: *1,* Begin washing at the tip of the penis. For an uncircumcised penis, gently retract the foreskin and wash. *2,* Proceed down the penis shaft toward the body. *3,* Next wash the scrotum. Wash the anal area last.

disposing the client to ischemia and permanent impotence, and the client may be unable to void. Treatment for most cases is aspiration of blood from the penis followed by injection of phenylephrine intracavernosally in serial injections.

Low-flow priapism must be resolved within 24 hours or the client might develop penile ischemia, gangrene, fibrosis, and impotence. If the more conservative treatments are unsuccessful in resolving the problem, more invasive therapy is required to prevent permanent damage. Surgical treatment is designed to drain the congested blood from the corpora.

High-flow priapism often can be treated successfully with ice and compression. If this is not successful, the client may require selective embolization or ligation of the traumatized artery.

Be sensitive to the embarrassing nature of this problem. Men are often reluctant to admit that this problem has occurred and yet are often in severe pain. Be understanding and attempt to make the client comfortable while decreasing the client's embarrassment over this problem.

Penile Cancer

Penile cancer is a rare skin cancer occurring most often in older, uncircumcised men who have suffered chronic irritation and who have poor hygiene practices. Associated genital cancer sometimes develops in sexual partners (e.g., cervical cancer in females). Any dry, wartlike, painless growth on the penis or foreskin that fails to respond to antibiotics should be assessed for cancer. If an early diagnosis is made, excision and circumcision may be all that is necessary.

Many men find penile problems embarrassing and consequently do not seek medical attention for months. By this time, a lesion may be ulcerated, involve the foreskin and penile shaft, and have metastasized to the inguinal nodes. Penile shaft resection, and sometimes penile amputation and dissection of enlarged inguinal nodes, may be necessary.

Peyronie's Disease

Fibrous plaques develop near the dorsal midline of the penile shaft in middle-aged and older men. A high percentage of older men develop these plaques. Diagnosis is usually made only if you question the client about this during the history.

Assessment reveals penile curvature on erection, painful erection, and unsatisfactory vaginal penetration. Peyronie's disease is often associated with Dupuytren's contracture of the hand tendons. Surgical correction is often necessary, but other treatments are often tried, including waiting for spontaneous improvement.

Posthitis and Balanitis

Posthitis is foreskin inflammation. Balanitis is inflammation of the glans penis and the mucous membrane beneath it. This condition (Fig. 83–14) is caused by irritation and

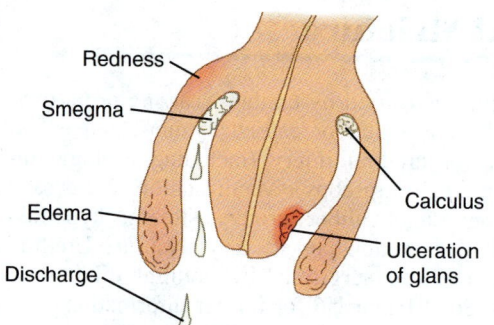

Figure 83–14. Posthitis and balanitis.

invasion of microorganisms. Good hygiene and thorough drying of the penis is recommended. Assessment for diabetes is important because diabetes predisposes the client to the development of secondary infection. Antibiotics help control local infection. Circumcision may be necessary.

Urinary Extravasation

Urinary extravasation is the escape of urine and other fluid into the perineum, scrotum, and penile tissue. It may be caused by trauma or may be secondary to urethral stricture. It is an emergency condition. Assessment reveals discoloration of the tissue, shock, and fever. Emergency intervention consists of alternative drainage of the bladder (urethral or suprapubic catheter) and drainage of the tissues with a Penrose drain.

Penile Injury

Penile trauma results in edema, hematoma, bruising, or laceration. Apply ice packs to control bleeding and appropriate dressings to reduce the possibility of infection. Urologic consultation is needed. With microsurgical techniques it may be possible to replant an amputated penis. To facilitate such treatment, dampen the amputated penis with a sterile saline solution, keep it chilled, and transport it with the person for emergency treatment.

Epispadias

Epispadias (Fig. 83–15A) is a rare congenital condition in which the urethral meatus opens dorsally on top of the penis, proximal to the glans, most commonly at the abdominopenile junction. Surgery is required to correct urinary incontinence and to return the urethra to a normal position in the penis. It is important to ask about this condition when taking the history.

Hypospadias

Hypospadias (Fig. 83–15B) is a congenital condition in which the urethral meatus opens on the ventral side of the penis. Common locations include the glans penis, penile

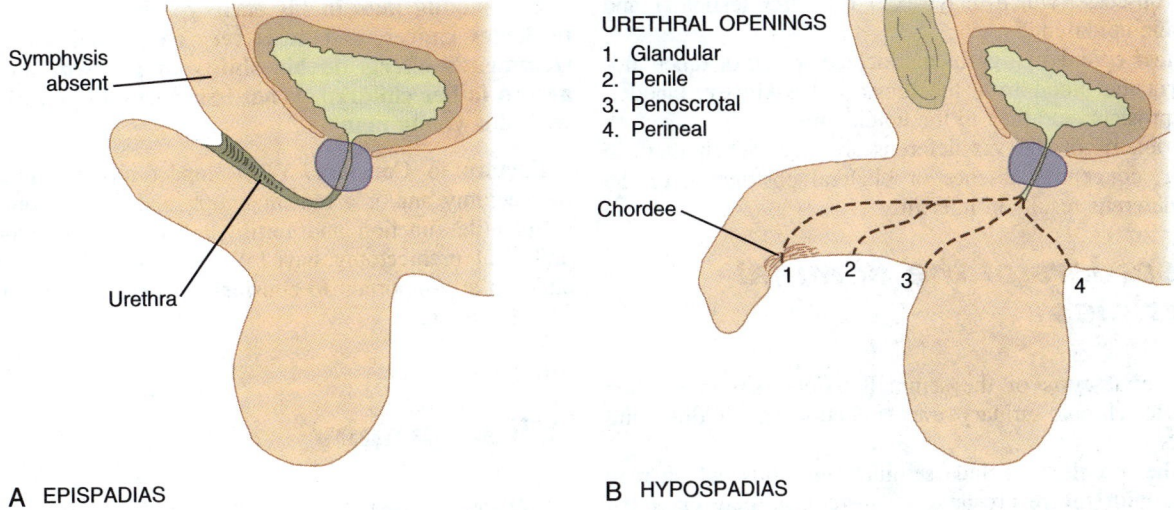

Figure 83–15. Epispadias and hypospadias.

shaft, penoscrotal junction, and perineum. Chordee (curvature of the penis) is often associated with hypospadias. Hypospadias occurs in about 1 in 300 live male births. Early assessment of internal reproductive organ development is necessary to confirm the child's sex. For psychological reasons, hypospadias should be repaired before the child starts school. It is important to ask about this condition when taking the history.

Scrotal Disorders

Infections

Scrotal skin is very thin and is in constant contact with clothes and the thighs. The scrotum's many rugae (folds) inhibit ventilation. It is, therefore, exposed to moisture and rubbing, and is prone to infection. Nonvenereal disorders, such as erysipelas, abscesses, fistulas, and gangrene, may occur. Parasites, such as scabies and lice, and many common skin diseases, such as fungal infections (*candidiasis,* also known as *jock itch*), contact dermatitis, drug eruptions, eczema, lichen planus, and psoriasis, may spread to the scrotum. Heat, friction, obesity, and tight clothing aggravate scrotal disorders. Medications (often topical) specific to the infection, good hygiene, and prompt intervention are essential.

Injuries

The most common scrotal injury is cutaneous tearing as a result of clothes being caught in machinery. Blunt or penetrating trauma also may occur. Saddle injuries also occur to the scrotum and perineum from accidents. First-aid intervention includes control of bleeding, by applying an ice pack, scrotal support (see Fig. 83–6), and rapid transportation of the client to a healthcare facility.

Edema

Scrotal edema may occur from infection, local irritation, and allergic reactions. It also can follow surgery, such as hernia repair or vasectomy. It also may be associated with systemic diseases, such as congestive heart failure. Scrotal support, such as a Bellevue bridge, increases comfort for the client (see Fig. 83–6).

Disorders of the Reproductive Ducts

The system of ducts through which spermatozoa pass from the testicles to the urethra includes the epididymis and the vas deferens.

Epididymitis is inflammation of the epididymis, most often caused by infection. Sometimes, however, it is caused by trauma or urinary reflux from the urethra through the vas deferens. Organisms can reach the epididymis via the blood or directly from the lower urinary tract or prostate. Epididymitis may be sexually transmitted, such as by infection with *Chlamydia trachomatis* and *Neisseria gonorrhoeae,* or nonsexually transmitted, such as by infection with *Enterobacteriaceae* or *Pseudomonas* species. Strain or pressure during voiding may force urine-containing pathogens from the urethra or prostate through the vas deferens to the epididymis.

Assessment reveals acute, painful scrotal swelling, often accompanied by nausea, vomiting, fever, and chills. It is important to distinguish acute epididymitis from testicular torsion. Intervention includes bedrest, scrotal elevation, ice packs, sitz baths, analgesics, and antibiotics. Also treat sexual partners for sexually transmitted forms of epididymitis. Nonsexually transmitted forms can be prevented by treating underlying causes of urinary tract infection and prostatitis. Complications include epididymal abscess (which may extend to the testicles) and chronic epididymitis.

Other epididymal problems include spread of tuberculosis via the blood from the lungs to the kidney, bladder, and prostate, and then to the epididymis.

Problems of the vas deferens are rare. When they do occur, congenital absence or bilateral obstruction of the vas deferens results in infertility.

Disorders of the Seminal Vesicles

Congenital cysts of the seminal vesicles are rare. They lead to chronic urinary tract infection in children and adults.

Other problems include seminal vesiculitis, which may occur with severe prostatitis. Tuberculosis may enter the genitourinary organs from the lungs via the blood. Infected urine passes through the prostatic urethra, invading the prostate and seminal vesicles. Intervention is the same as for prostatitis.

Conclusions

Male reproductive disorders can be complex problems for the client and the nurse. The client often finds that these disorders threaten sexuality and sexual function. These effects may be physiologic, but complex psychosocial problems also arise. You and the client may feel discomfort discussing issues of a sexual nature.

Prostate disorders are among the most common problems experienced by clients throughout their life. The nursing care associated with these problems can greatly influence the client's ability to adapt to the accompanying changes. Cancers of the male reproductive tract can be life threatening, but if they are detected early, they can be cured or at least controlled for long periods. You can play a major role in the early detection of these cancers. Teaching young men to perform TSE can increase the incidence of early diagnosis and treatment of testicular cancer.

Thinking Critically

1. Your client underwent a laser-assisted TURP yesterday. CBI is being used and his urine is dark to bright red with multiple clots. He is complaining of intense cramping pain in the lower abdomen. What further assessments should you make? What could be causing the cramping pain? What nursing action should you take?

Factors to Consider. Is the dark to bright red urinary output normal at this stage? What does the nature of the client's pain tell you about its likely cause?

2. A young man in his early 20s is diagnosed with testicular cancer, and he is very concerned about the treatment's effects on his ability to perform sexually and to father children. What issues should you discuss with this young man?

Factors to Consider. What impact might a bilateral orchiectomy and/or a radical lymph node dissection have on erectile function and fertility? What impact might a unilateral orchiectomy have? What options for fathering children are important to consider *before* the client undergoes treatment?

Bibliography

1. Adami, H. O., Baron, J. A., & Rothman, K. J. (1994). Ethics of prostate cancer screening trial. *Lancet, 343*(8903), 958–960.
2. Alpha Tocopherol, Beta Carotene Cancer Prevention Study Group. (1994). The effects of vitamin E and beta carotene on the incidence of lung cancer and other cancers in male smokers. *New England Journal of Medicine, 330*, 1029–1035.
3. Arcadi, J. A. (Dec. 1994). Transscrotal approach to testicular tumors: An anatomical approach. *Journal of Surgical Oncology, 57*(4), 261–265.
4. Austoker, J. (July 30, 1994). Screening for ovarian, prostatic, and testicular cancers. *British Medical Journal, 309*(6950), 315–320.
5. Baniel, J., et al. (1994). Complications of primary retroperitoneal lymph node dissection. *Journal of Urology, 152*(2 pt 1), 424–427.
6. Barry, M. J., et al. (Jan. 1995). Using repeated measures of symptom score, uroflowmetry and prostate specific antigen in the clinical management of prostate disease: Benign Prostatic Hyperplasia Treatment Outcomes Study Group. *Journal of Urology, 153*(1), 99–103.
7. Beach, P. R. (1994). Controversies of prostate cancer screening. *Journal of Urological Nursing, 13*(1), 650–655.
8. Beahrs, O. H., et al. (Eds.). (1992). *Manual for staging of cancer.* Philadelphia: J. B. Lippincott.
9. Benign Prostatic Hyperplasia Guideline Panel. (1994). *Benign prostatic hyperplasia: Clinical practice guideline.* Agency for Health Care Policy and Research publication No. 94–0583. Rockville, MD: U.S. Department of Health and Human Services.
10. Benign Prostatic Hyperplasia Guideline Panel. (1994). *Benign prostatic hyperplasia: Diagnosis and treatment.* Agency for Health Care Policy and Research publication No. 94–0582. Rockville, MD: U.S. Department of Health and Human Services.
11. Benign Prostatic Hyperplasia Guideline Panel. (1994). *Benign prostatic hyperplasia: Patient guide.* Agency for Health Care Policy and Research Publication No. 94–0584. Rockville, MD: U.S. Department of Health and Human Services.
12. Berger, N. S. (1993). Prostate cancer: Screening and early detection update. *Seminars in Oncology Nursing, 9*(3), 180–183.
13. Bhasin, S., deKretser, D. M., & Baker, H. W. (Dec. 1994). Clinical review 64: Pathophysiology and natural history of male infertility. *Journal of Clinical Endocrinology and Metabolism, 79*(6), 1525–1529.
14. Blaivas, J. F. (April 1, 1995). Urinary incontinence after radical prostatectomy. *Cancer Supplement, 75*(7), 1978–1982.
15. Bokemeyer, C., & Schmoll, H. J. (Jan. 1995). Treatment of testicular cancer and the development of secondary malignancies. *Journal of Clinical Oncology, 13*(1), 283–292.
16. Boring, C., Squires, T., & Heath, C. (1992). Cancer statistics for African-Americans. *CA—A Journal for Clinicians, 42*, 7–17.
17. Bowersox, J. (1993). Experts confer on vasectomy and prostate cancer risk. *Journal of the National Cancer Institute, 85*, 527–528.
18. Boyle, P. (1994). New insights into the epidemiology and natural history of benign prostatic hyperplasia. *Progress in Clinical and Biological Research, 386*, 3–18.
19. Brawer, M. K., & Ellis, W. J. (April 1, 1995). Chemoprevention in prostate cancer. *Cancer Supplement, 75*(7), 1783–1789.

20. Brenner, A. R., & Krenzer, M. E. (1995). Update on cryosurgical ablation for prostate cancer. *American Journal of Nursing, 95*(5), 44–48.

21. Bullman, T. A., Watanabe, K. K., & Kang, H. K. (Jan. 1994). Risk of testicular cancer associated with surrogate measures of Agent Orange exposure among Vietnam veterans on the Agent Orange Registry. *Annals of Epidemiology, 4*(1), 11–16.

22. Bullock, A. D., Basler, J. W., & Catalona, W. J. (1994). How to manage early prostate cancer. *Contemporary Oncology, 4*(1), 40–48.

23. Carapella, J. S. (1994). Radical prostatectomy: A case study. *Journal of Post Anesthesia Nursing, 9*(6), 344–349.

24. Cetinel, B., et al. (Nov. 1994). Update evaluation of benign prostatic hyperplasia: When should we offer prostatectomy? *British Journal of Urology, 74*(5), 566–571.

25. Chia, S. E., et al. (Sept.-Oct. 1994). Effect of cadmium and cigarette smoking on human semen quality. *International Journal of Fertility and Menopausal Studies, 39*(5), 292–298.

26. Chiou, R. K., et al. (June 1994). Randomized comparison of balloon dilation and transurethral incision for treatment of symptomatic benign prostatic hyperplasia. *Journal of Endocrinology, 8*(3), 221–224.

27. Comis, R. L. (Oct. 1994). Cisplatin: The future. *Seminars in Oncology, 21*(5 suppl 12), 109–113.

28. Crowe, H., & Costello, A. (June 1994). Laser ablation of the prostate: Nursing management. *Urologic Nursing, 14*(2), 38–40.

29. Dancer, S. E., & Logsdon, K. (Dec. 1994). Patient trajectory: Improving care for the radical retropubic patient. *Urologic Nursing, 14*(4), 151–172.

30. Dawson, N. A., & Vogelzang, N. (Eds.). (1994). *Prostate cancer.* New York: John Wiley & Sons.

31. Diamond, D. A., & Ransley, P. G. (Oct. 1994). Improved granuloplasty in epispadias repair: Technical aspects. *Journal of Urology, 152*(4), 1243–1245.

32. Dixon, C. M. (Aug. 1994). Right-angle free beam lasers for the treatment of benign prostatic hyperplasia. *Seminars in Urology, 12*(3), 165–169.

33. Donohue, J. P., et al. (1994). Stage I nonseminomatous germ-cell testicular cancer—Management options and risk-benefit considerations. *Worldwide Journal of Urology, 12*(4), 170–177.

34. Entrekin, N. M., & McMillan, S. C. (1993). Nurses' knowledge, beliefs, and practices related to cancer prevention and detection. *Cancer Nursing, 16*(6), 431–439.

35. Feldman, J. S. (1993). An alternative group approach: Using multidisciplinary expertise to support patients with prostate cancer and their families. *Journal of Psychosocial Oncology, 11*(2), 83–93.

36. Foster, R. S., et al. (1994). Stage II nonseminomatous germ-cell testicular tumors: The Indiana experience and risk-benefit analysis. *Worldwide Journal of Urology, 12*(3), 143–147.

37. Foster, R. S., et al. (1994). Fertility considerations in nerve-sparing retroperitoneal lymph-node dissection. *Worldwide Journal of Urology, 12*(3), 136–138.

38. Garner, C. (1994). Uses of GnRH agonists: Gonadotropin-releasing hormone. *Journal of Obstetric, Gynecologic, and Neonatal Nursing, 23*(7), 563–570.

39. Gilliland, F. D., & Key, C. R. (Jan. 1, 1995). Male genital cancer. *Cancer, 75*(1 suppl), 295–315.

40. Giovannucci, E. (April 1, 1995). Epidemiologic characteristics of prostate cancer. *Cancer Supplement, 75*(7), 1766–1777.

41. Giovannucci, E., et al. (Dec. 1, 1994). Obesity and benign prostatic hyperplasia. *American Journal of Epidemiology, 140*(11), 989–1002.

42. Giovannucci, E., et al. (1993). A prospective study of dietary fat and risk of prostate cancer. *Journal of the National Cancer Institute, 85*(19), 1571–1579.

43. Giwercman, A., et al. (1994). Current concepts of radiation treatment of carcinoma in situ of the testis. *Worldwide Journal of Urology, 12*(3), 125–130.

44. Gold, E. B., Lasley, B. L., & Schenker, M. B. (July-Sept 1994). Introduction: Rationale for an update. Reproductive hazards. *Occupational Medicine, 9*(3), 363–372.

45. Grace-Louthen, C. L. (1993). Commentary on treatment-related fatigue and serum interleukin-1 levels in patients during external beam irradiation for prostate cancer. *ONS Nursing Scan in Oncology, 2*(5), 9.

46. Graham, S. (Dec. 15, 1994). Screening for prostate cancer. *Cancer, 74*(12), 3077–3079.

47. Greco, K. E. (1993). Prostate cancer screening: Getting your patients to follow-up. *Urologic Nursing, 13*(3) 76–79.

48. Greco, K. E., & Kulawiak, L. (1994). Prostate cancer prevention: Risk reduction through life-style, diet, and chemoprevention. *Oncology Nursing Forum, 21*(9), 1504–1511.

49. Greenberg, D. B., et al. (1993). Treatment-related fatigue and serum interleukin-1 levels in patients during external beam irradiation for prostate cancer. *Journal of Pain and Symptom Management, 8*(4), 196–200.

50. Greenwald, P., Kramer., & Weed, D. (1993). Expanding horizons in breast and prostate cancer prevention and early detection. *Journal of Cancer Education, 8*(2), 91–107.

51. Gregoire, I. (March 1995). Pharmacologic erection program: An alternative solution for the man with erectile dysfunction. *Urologic Nursing, 15*(1), 10–13.

52. Grignon, D., & Sakr, W. (May-June 1994). Benign prostatic hyperplasia: It is a premalignant lesion? *In Vivo, 8*(3), 415–418.

53. Haas, G. P. (May-June, 1994). Epidemiology of early prostate cancer (introduction). *In Vivo, 8*(3), 403–405.

54. Haidl, G. (1994). New aspects of the aetiology of male fertility disorders. *Archives of Gynecology and Obstetrics, 255*(suppl 2), S301–308.

55. Hammerer, P. G., McNeal, J. E., & Stamey, T. A. (Jan. 1995). Correlation between serum prostate specific antigen levels and the volume of the individual glandular zones of the human prostate. *Journal of Urology, 153*(1), 111–114.

56. Harlan, L., et al. (Jan., 1995). Geographic, age, and racial variations in the treatment of local/regional carcinoma of the prostate. *Journal of Clinical Oncology, 13*(1), 93–100.

57. Hayes, R. B., et al. (Jan. 27, 1995). Prostate cancer risk in U.S. blacks and whites with a family history of cancer. *International Journal of Cancer, 60*(3), 361–364.

58. Held, J. L., et al. (1994). Cancer of the prostate: Treatment and nursing implications. *Oncology Nursing Forum, 21*(9), 1517–1529.

59. Hill, D. J. (1990). The patient with testicular cancer: Nursing management of chemotherapy. *Oncology Nursing Forum, 17*(2), 243—249.

60. Hobson, A. (1993). Commentary on a retrospective cohort study of vasectomy and prostate cancer in U.S. men. *Nursing Scan in Research, 6*(4), 2.

61. Holdcroft, C. (1993). Finasteride for benign prostatic hyperplasia. *Nurse Practitioner, 18*(3), 57–58.

62. Holmes, K., & MacInnes, P. (1993). A comparative study of nurse practitioners' perceptions of prostatectomy patients' sexual concerns vs. the stated sexual concerns of the prostatectomy patient. *Nursing Scan in Research, 6*(6), 6.

63. Horowich, A., & Bell, J. (March 1994). Mortality and cancer incidence following radiotherapy for seminoma of the testis. *Radiotherapeutic Oncology, 30*(3), 193–198.

64. Howards, S. S. (Feb. 2, 1995). Treatment of male infertility. *New England Journal of Medicine, 332*(5), 312–317.

65. Hutson, J. M., et al. (1994). Hormonal control of testicular descent and the cause of cryptorchidism. *Reproductive Fertility Development, 6*(2), 151–156.

66. Jardin, A., et al. (Nov. 1994). Long-term treatment of benign prostatic hyperplasia with alfuzosin: A 24–30 month survey, BPHALF Group. *British Journal of Urology, 74*(5), 579–584.

67. Karlowicz, KA (Ed.). (1995). *Urologic nursing: Principles and practice.* Philadelphia: W. B. Saunders.

68. Kass, E. J., & Reitelman, C. (Feb. 1995). Adolescent varicocele. *Urologic Clinics of North America, 22*(1), 151–159.

69. Keetch, D. W., & Andriole, G. L. (Jan. 1995). Medical therapy for benign prostatic hyperplasia. *American Journal of Roentgenology, 164*(1), 11–17.

70. Kenny, R. A. (1992). *Physiology of aging: A synopsis.* St. Louis: Mosby–Year Book.

71. Kingston, T. E., et al. (Jan. 1995). Further evaluation of transurethral laser ablation of the prostate in patients treated with anticoagulant therapy. *Australia and New Zealand Journal of Surgery, 65*(1), 40–43.

72. Kirby, R. (1994). BPH: When to rule out carcinoma of the prostate. *Progress in Clinical and Biological Research, 386*, 333–343.

73. Kirby, R., & Christmas, T. (1993). *Benign prostatic hypertrophy.* New York: Raven Press.

74. Klein, L. (1990). Current approaches to balloon dilatation of the prostate. *Astra Urologue, 20*(5), 1–7.

75. Kojima, M., & Babaian, R. J. (April 1, 1995). Algorithms for early detection of prostate cancer: Current state of the "art". *Cancer Supplement, 75*(7), 1860–1868.

76. Krainer, M., et al. (Jan. 15, 1995). Natural killer cell activity in long-term survivors of testicular cancer: Influence of cytostatic therapy and initial stage of disease. *Cancer, 75*(2), 539–544.

77. Kramer, B. S., et al. (1993). Prostate cancer screening: What we know and what we need to know. *Annals of Internal Medicine, 119*(9), 914–923.

78. Lassen, P. M., & Thompson, I. M. (March 1994). Treatment options for prostate cancer. *Urologic Nursing, 14*(1), 12–15.

79. Lee, W. R., et al. (Jan. 1, 1995). Observations if pretreatment prostate-specific antigen doubling time in 107 patients referred for definitive radiotherapy. *International Journal of Radiation Oncology, Biology, and Physiology, 31*(1), 21–24.

80. Little, J. S., et al. (1994). Unusual neoplasms detected in testicular cancer patients undergoing postchemotherapy retroperitoneal lymphadenectomy. *World Journal of Urology, 12*(4), 200–206.

81. Littrup, P. J. (Oct. 1, 1994). Prostate cancer screening. *Cancer Supplement, 74*(7), 2016–2022.

82. Littrup, P. J., & Goodman, A. C. (May-June 1994). Costs and benefits of prostate cancer screening: Investigators of the American Cancer Society–National Prostate Cancer Detection Project. *In Vivo, 8*(3), 423–427.

83. Littrup, P. J., & Goodman, A. C. (April 1, 1995). Economic considerations of prostate cancer: The role of detection specificity and biopsy reduction. *Cancer Supplement, 75*(7), 1987–1993.

84. Littrup, P. J., Goodman, A. C., & Mettlin, C. J. (1993). The benefit and cost of prostate cancer early detection. *CA—A Cancer Journal for Clinicians, 43*(3), 134–149.

85. Littrup, P. J., & Sparschu, R. (April 1, 1995). Transrectal ultrasound and prostate cancer risks: The "tailored" prostate biopsy. *Cancer Supplement, 75*(7), 1805–1813.

86. Litwin, M. S., et al. (Jan. 11, 1995). Quality-of-life outcomes in men treated for localized prostate cancer. *JAMA, 273*(2), 129–135.

87. Loescher, L. J. (1994). Prostate cancer: Controversies surrounding risk, screening, and management—introduction. *Oncology Nursing Forum, 21*(9), 1503–1504.

88. Long, K., & Long, R. (1994). Treating benign prostatic hyperplasia with medications. *Nurse Practitioner Forum, 5*(3), 126–127.

89. Lundsberg, L. S., Bracken, M. B., & Belanger, K. (Feb. 1995). Occupationally related magnetic field exposure and male subfertility. *Fertility and Sterility, 63*(2), 384–391.

90. Mahon, S. M., & Casperson, D. S. (1993). Focus on oncology: Mass screening for prostate cancer—a community hospital's experience. *Journal of Urological Nursing, 12*(1), 372–378.

91. Mahon, S. M., & Casperson, D. S. (1993). Focus on oncology: Vasectomy and the risk of prostate cancer. *Journal of Urological Nursing, 12*(4), 599–602.

92. Mainous, A. G., & Hagen, M. D. Public awareness of prostate cancer and the prostate-specific antigen test. *Cancer Practice, 2*(3), 217–221.

93. Malek, R. S., Barrett, D. M., & Dilworth, J. P. (Jan. 1995). Visual laser ablation of the prostate: A preliminary report. *Mayo Clinic Proceedings, 70*(1), 28–32.

94. Mason, M. (1993). *Male infertility: Men talking.* New York: Routledge.

95. Maxwell, M. B. (1993). Cancer of the prostate. *Seminars in Oncology Nursing, 9*(4), 237–251.

96. McKee, J. M. (1994). Cues to action in prostate cancer screening. *Oncology Nursing Forum, 21*(7), 1171–1176.

97. Mettlin, C., et al. (1993). Defining and updating the American Cancer Society guidelines for the cancer-related checkup: Prostate and endometrial cancers. *CA—A Journal for Clinicians, 43*, 42–46.

98. Mettlin, C., Jones, G. W., Murphy, G. P. (1993). Trends in prostate cancer care in the United States, 1974-1990: Observations from the patient care evaluation studies of the American College of Surgeons Commission on Cancer. *CA—A Journal for Clinicians, 43*, 83–91.

99. Miller, C. A. (1993). New medication for the treatment of benign prostatic hyperplasia. *Geriatric Nursing, 14*(2), 111–112.

100. Mitchell, T. S. (March 1994). Screening for prostate cancer. *Urologic Nursing, 14*(1), 9–11.

101. Moller, H., Knudsen, L. B., & Lynge, E. (July 30, 1994). Risk of testicular cancer after vasectomy: Cohort study of over 73,000 men. *British Medical Journal, 309*(6950), 295–299.

102. Monda, J. M., & Oesterling, J. E. (1994). Medical management of prostatic obstruction. *Journal of Urological Nursing, 13*(2), 717–738.

103. Montie, J. E. (May-June 1994). Controversies in the early detection of prostate cancer. *In Vivo, 8*(3), 407–411.

104. Montie, J. E. (Nov. 1994). Follow-up after radical orchiectomy for testicular cancer. *Urologic Clinics of North America, 21*(4), 757–760.

105. Moore, S., Shea, L., & Andriole, G. L. Evaluating and treating prostate cancer. *American Journal of Nursing, 94*(10), 16C–F.

106. Nacey, J. N., Meffan, P. J., & Delahunt, B. (Jan. 1995). The effect of finasteride on prostate volume, urinary flowrate and symptom score in men with benign prostatic hyperplasia. *Australia and New Zealand Journal of Surgery, 65*(1), 35–39.

107. Narayan, P., & Indudhara, R. (Nov. 1994). Pharmacotherapy for benign prostatic hyperplasia. *Western Journal of Medicine, 161*(5), 495–506.

108. Niehoff, M. L. (1994). Epidemiology and early detection of prostate cancer in the primary care setting. *Journal of the American Academy of Physician Assistants, 7*(3), 147–157.

109. Oesterling, J. E. (1994). The UroLume endoprosthesis: A summary of the European and North American experience. *Progress in Clinical and Biological Research, 386*, 561–575.

110. Oesterling, JE. (April 1, 1995). Prostate specific antigen: Its role in the diagnosis and staging of prostate cancer. *Cancer Supplement, 75*(7), 1795–1804.

111. Oesterling, J. E., et al. (1994). Endocrine therapies for BPH: Scientific rationale, clinical results, and patient selection. *Progress in Clinical and Biological Research, 386*, 231–250.

112. Ofman, U. S. (April 1, 1995). Sexual quality of life in men with prostate cancer. *Cancer Supplement, 75*(7), 1949–1953.

113. O'Hanlon-Nichols, T., Rosas, J., & Rogers, A. (1993). Subcutaneous abdominal implant: New treatment for prostate cancer. *Journal of Urological Nursing, 12*(1), 326–332.

114. Oliver, R. T. (May 1994). Testicular cancer. *Current Opinion in Oncology, 6*(3), 285–291.

115. Orihuela, E., et al. (Aug. 1994). Low-power laser radiation for the treatment of benign prostatic hyperplasia: Initial clinical experience. *Journal of Endocrinology, 8*(4), 301–304.

116. Overstreet, J. W. (July-Sept 1994). Clinical approach to male reproductive problems. *Occupational Medicine, 9*(3), 387–404.

117. Paschke, R., et al. (Sept 1994). Association of sperm antibodies with other autoantibodies in infertile men. *American Journal of Reproduction and Immunology, 32*(2), 88–94.

118. Pienta, K. J. (May-June 1994). The epidemiology of prostate cancer: Clues for chemoprevention. *In Vivo, 8*(3), 419–422.

119. Pienta, K. J., et al. (Jan. 1995). Effect of age and race on the survival of men with prostate cancer in the metropolitan Detroit tricounty area, 1973–1987. *Urology, 45*(1), 101–102.

120. Piente, K. J., & Esper, P. S. (1993). Is dietary fat a risk factor for prostate cancer? *Journal of the National Cancer Institute, 85*(19), 1538–1540.

121. Pontie, J. E. (May-June 1994). Methods of early detection of prostate cancer: The role of prostatic specific antigen, transrectal ultrasound and digital rectal examination. *In Vivo, 8*(3), 413–414.

122. Prostate cancer: Tracking down early metastasis. (1995). *Nursing 95, 25*(11), 64.

123. Razanauzskas, M., & Hoebler, L. (1994). Treating prostate cancer with cryosurgery. *Nursing 94, 24*(11), 66–68.

124. Reilly, N. J. (1994). The release of the clinical practice guideline: Benign prostatic hyperplasia: Diagnosis and treatment. *Urologic Nursing, 14*(2), 37.

125. Religo, W. M., & Larson, T. R. (1994). Microwave thermotherapy: New wave of treatment for benign prostatic hyperplasia. *Journal of the American Academy of Physician Assistants, 7*(4), 259–267.

126. Riehmann, M., & Bruskewitz, R. (1993). New options in benign prostatic hyperplasia. *Hospital Practice, 28*(2A), 17–18.

127. Rogers, E., et al. (Jan. 1995). Salvage radical prostatectomy: Outcome measured by serum prostate specific antigen levels. *Journal of Urology, 153*(1), 104–110.

128. Rosella, J. D. (Oct. 1994). Testicular cancer health education: An integrative review. *Journal of Advanced Nursing, 20*(4), 666–671.

129. Rosenberg, L., et al. (Sept 1, 1994). The relation of vasectomy to the risk of cancer. *American Journal of Epidemiology, 140*(5), 431–438.

130. Ross, R. K., et al. (April 1, 1995). Does the racial-ethnic variation in prostate cancer risk have a hormonal basis. *Cancer Supplement, 75*(7), 1778–1782.

131. Rozanski, T. A., & Bloom, D. A. (Feb. 1995). The undescended testis. Theory and management. *Urologic Clinics of North America, 22*(1), 107–118.

132. Ruckdeschel, J. C. (Oct. 1994). The future role of carboplatin. *Seminars in Oncology, 21*(5 suppl 12), 114–118.

133. Sanders, J. A., & Reese, J. H. (1994). The use of lasers as an alternative treatment for patients with benign prostatic hyperplasia: Transurethral ultrasound-guided laser-included prostatectomy. *Journal of Urological Nursing, 13*(1), 656–660.

134. Schroder, F. H. (Aug. 1994). 5-Alpha-reductase inhibitors and prostatic disease. *Clinical Endocrinology, 41*(2), 139–147.

135. Schulman, C. C., & Zlotta, A. R. (1994). Transurethral needle ablation (TUNA): Histopathological, radiological and clinical studies of a new office procedure for treatment of benign prostatic hyperplasia. *Progress in Clinical and Biological Research, 386*, 479–486.

136. Schulman, C. C., & Zlotta, A. R. (Jan. 1995). Transurethral needle ablation of the prostate for treatment of benign prostatic hyperplasia: Early clinical experience. *Urology, 45*(1), 28–33.

137. Seidmon, E. J., & Hanno, P. M. (1994). *Current urologic therapy 3.* Philadelphia: W.B. Saunders.

138. Small, E. J. (1993). Prostate cancer: Who to screen, and what the results mean. *Geriatrics, 48*(12), 35–38.

139. Smith, D. R. (1992). *General urology* (13th ed.). Los Altos, CA: Lange Medical.

140. Sommerfeld, H. J., et al. (April 1, 1995). Frontiers in prostate cancer: Telomeres and chaos. *Cancer Supplement, 75*(7), 2027–2035.

141. Sprouse, D. O. (April 1, 1995). Sexual rehabilitation of the prostate cancer patient. *Cancer Supplement, 75*(7), 1954–1956.

142. Stein, R., et al. (Nov. 1994). The fate of the adult exstrophy patient. *Journal of Urology, 152*(5 pt 1), 1413–1416.

143. Stepp, C. (1991). Balloon dilatation of the prostate: A historical review. *Urologic Nursing, 5*, 21–24.

144. Strasinger, S. K. (1994). *Urinalysis and body fluids.* Philadelphia: F. A. Davis.

145. Terris, M. K., et al. (Jan. 1995). Prediction of prostate cancer volume using prostate-specific antigen levels, transrectal ultrasound, and systemic sextant biopsies. *Urology, 45*(1) 75–80.

146. van Swol, C. F., et al. (1994). Optimization of laser prostatectomy. *Progress in Clinical and Biological Research, 386*, 511–519.

147. Waldman, A. R., & Osborne, D. M. (1994). Screening for prostate cancer. *Oncology Nursing Forum, 21*(9), 1512–1517.

148. Walsh, P., et al. (Eds.) (1992). *Campbell's Urology* (6th ed.). Philadelphia: W. B. Saunders.

149. Wasson, J. H., et al. (Jan. 12, 1995). A comparison of transurethral surgery with watchful waiting for moderate symptoms of benign prostatic hyperplasia: The Veterans Affairs Cooperative Study Group on Transurethral Resection of the Prostate. *New England Journal of Medicine, 332*(2), 75–79.

150. Waxman, E. S. (1993). Sexual dysfunction following treatment for prostate cancer: Nursing assessment and interventions. *Oncology Nursing Forum, 20*(10), 1567–1571.

151. Whorton, M. (1984). Environmental and occupational hazards. In J. Swanson & K. Forrest (Eds.), *Men's reproductive health.* New York: Springer.

152. Whorton, M., et al. (1977). Infertility in male pesticide workers. *Lancet, 2*, 1259.

153. Wilt, T. J., & Brawer, M. K. (April 1, 1995). The prostate cancer intervention versus observation trial (PIVOT): A randomized trial comparing radical prostatectomy versus expectant management for the treatment of clinically localized prostate cancer. *Cancer Supplement, 75*(7), 1963–1968.

154. Woodhouse, C. R. (Aug. 1994). The sexual and reproductive consequences of congenital genitourinary anomalies. *Journal of Urology, 152*(2 pt 2), 645–651.

155. Zimmern, P. E., & Leach, G. E. (1994) Nerve-sparing radical retropubic prostatectomy for localized prostate cancer: The pros and cons. *Cancer Supplement, 75*(7), 1944–1948.

84

Nursing Care of Women with Gynecologic Disorders

Elizabeth Carlson

The major themes that resound with almost all gynecologic disorders are sexuality (Altered Sexuality Patterns) and self-concept, including body image (Body Image Disturbance). Any disorder of the reproductive tract has the potential to cause actual or anticipated changes in sexual functioning or sexual identity. The disorder or its treatment may alter sexual functioning (i.e., by requiring temporary abstinence or the need to change the woman's usual positioning during vaginal intercourse). The disorders and their treatments have the potential to change the woman's perceived or actual body structure, which can lead to shame, embarrassment, and other negative responses.

To some women, alterations in sexuality and body image have a major effect on their femininity, or their feeling like a woman. Even in the 19th century, it was a commonly reported medical view that the reproductive organs dominated a woman's body. Some aspects of this view, which reduces women to the functioning of their body parts, persists in our culture today, which is why reproductive disorders can have such a far-reaching effect on women.

Menstrual Disorders

Women may experience some menstrual problems during their 30 or more years of menstruating. Women tend to readily seek professional help for obvious abnormalities such as excessive and irregular vaginal bleeding. However, they may not bring other menstrual problems to the attention of healthcare providers.

Women react to menstrual problems in differing, individual ways. Whereas some promptly seek healthcare, others may not for various reasons. For example, one

woman may hesitate and be unable to discuss menstruation because she views it as a personal, intimate problem that should be kept private. Another may have low self-esteem or have been told that such problems are to be expected, and will dismiss her own complaints as unimportant. Some women do not seek help because they feel that perhaps their problems will go away in time, whereas others question whether relief is really possible, or whether the treatment will be worse than the problem. Thus, many menstrual problems go undetected unless nurses are skillful and sensitive in assessment. Menstrual problems may be discovered by nurses when women are discussing unrelated concerns such as contraception needs. Some menstrual problems include dysmenorrhea, premenstrual syndrome, and abnormal uterine bleeding.

Dysmenorrhea

Until the early 1970s, dysmenorrhea (painful menstrual flow) was considered by many medical practitioners, as well as the lay public, to be mainly psychosomatic.[75] Women were told by everyone, including healthcare workers, that it was all in their heads or indicative of their inability to adjust to the feminine role. Thus, most women did not even consider asking for help with this problem. Today, however, dysmenorrhea is taken seriously as a health problem and new knowledge has provided the basis for useful therapies to relieve the discomfort.

Dysmenorrhea may be primary or secondary. Primary dysmenorrhea is believed to be caused by either a prostaglandin excess or an increased sensitivity to prostaglandins with no underlying pathologic pelvic disorders. Secondary dysmenorrhea begins with an underlying disease condition. The true incidence and prevalence of this condition are unknown, although most women are affected to some degree.[9] Ultimately, this discomfort has the potential to affect women's productivity and increase absentee-

This chapter incorporates material written for the fourth edition by Esther Matassarin-Jacobs and Ann J. Clark.

ism. Dysmenorrhea is a different entity than premenstrual syndrome (PMS) and requires different treatment modalities.[9] However, some women have manifestations of both.

Etiology and Risk Factors

There are a variety of causes of primary dysmenorrhea. These can be grouped into five factors:

1. Elevated uterine prostaglandins
2. Endocrine factors
3. Myometrial factors
4. Biochemical factors
5. Psychosocial factors

Each factor influences the system differently, although the outcome is the same: dysmenorrhea.

Secondary dysmenorrhea is suspected when (1) pain is concentrated in a specific area, or (2) pain is unilateral, or (3) its onset occurs after age 20. It may be caused by the following:

● Pelvic inflammatory disease (PID)
● Endometriosis
● Adenomyosis (invasion of uterine myometrium by endometrial tissue)
● Uterine prolapse
● Uterine myomas
● Polyps

Pathophysiology

It appears that prostaglandin synthesis at the time of menstruation produces strong myometrial contractions. The severe muscle spasms constrict blood vessels supplying the uterus, causing ischemia and pain. The excess prostaglandins in smooth muscle also help explain the presence of gastrointestinal manifestations, such as nausea and vomiting, and diarrhea or headache.

Clinical Manifestations and Diagnostic Findings

Primary dysmenorrhea characteristically begins 1 to 2 months after menarche in conjunction with ovulatory cycles. Generally, it increases in severity over several years until the woman is in her mid-20s and then begins to decline. Primary dysmenorrhea often decreases significantly after childbirth. It is often associated with prolonged menstrual flow and is more common in obese, sedentary women.

The discomfort of primary dysmenorrhea commonly begins 1 to 2 days before the onset of menstrual flow. The more severe discomfort is usually experienced during the first 24 hours of flow and typically subsides by the second day. Over half of the women experiencing dysmenorrhea also have systemic manifestations such as nausea and vomiting, diarrhea, syncope, headache, and leg pain.

Diagnosis is based on a thorough history, including what the woman has used for relief and what has helped.

A physical examination is done to rule out any underlying pathologic causes of dysmenorrhea.

Community and Self-Care

■ Medical Management

The current therapeutic approach to primary dysmenorrhea emphasizes prevention and education so that a women can participate in her own care. For women with mild manifestations who want to avoid medication, non-pharmacologic remedies might be effective. For example, biofeedback, therapeutic touch, or acupuncture might be helpful.

If contraception is desired as well as relief of dysmenorrhea, combination oral contraceptives may relieve menstrual pain. The resulting inhibition of ovulation results in decreased endometrial prostaglandin production and a concurrent reduction of uterine activity. For women with intrauterine devices (IUDs), removal of the device may lead to relief. An alternative form of contraception may be desired.

Exercise has also been used as a remedy for dysmenorrhea.[28] Exercise increases blood flows of beta endorphins, the body's endogenous opiates, making them available for pain relief. The exact mechanism responsible for relief is not known.

Prostaglandin synthesis inhibitors may provide relief via decreased prostaglandin activity, even in the presence of ovulatory cycles. Some commonly prescribed medications in this group are ibuprofen (Motrin), mefenamic acid (Ponstel), indomethacin (Indocin), and naproxen (Naprosyn). Ibuprofen (Advil, Nuprin) and naproxen sodium (Aleve) are available as nonprescription drugs in lower doses, which makes them easy to obtain.

These medications may have gastrointestinal side effects. Other possible side effects are sodium and water retention, skin rashes, and potential allergic reactions. For maximum effectiveness the medications should be administered either before or at the onset of menses. Sometimes, it is necessary to try several prostaglandin synthesis inhibitors until one with maximum effectiveness is found for the individual woman.

Treatment of secondary dysmenorrhea is directed toward the underlying cause. Antiprostaglandin agents may provide some relief.

■ Nursing Management of the Medical Client

Education and supportive reassurance are important nursing interventions for women with primary dysmenorrhea. Provide information about (1) the mechanisms involved in dysmenorrhea and (2) the actions and possible side effects of any prescribed medications. Assess the client's general health status. Encourage adequate nutrition and appropriate rest, sleep, and exercise. Assess stress, because stress may increase manifestations, and explore methods of stress management.

Premenstrual Syndrome

Premenstrual syndrome remained relatively obscure until recently, when extensive media coverage brought the syndrome to public attention. Despite its popularization, PMS is still not well understood. Much confusion surrounds its diagnosis, treatment, and management.

Various definitions of PMS appear in the literature. One is "any combination of emotional and physical features which occur cyclically in the female before menstruation and which regress or disappear during menstruation." [22] Premenstrual syndrome is somatic, not psychic, in origin, and it is a complex mechanism involving not only the endocrine system but both the autonomic and central nervous systems as well. A predominant alteration is the retention of body fluids.

The incidence of PMS is difficult to determine because of the variable manifestations and the lack of a clear understanding about the syndrome. PMS occurs mostly in the 30- to 40-year-old age group. Variable reports in the literature indicate that approximately 20% to 60% of all women experience some form of PMS. Probably only 20% to 40% of these women experience manifestations that disrupt their lives.

Etiology and Risk Factors

The cause of PMS is unclear; however, neuroendocrine mechanisms appear to be involved. It is not clear whether PMS is a single syndrome or a group of separate disorders.

Some theorized causes of PMS are the following:

- Estrogen-progesterone imbalance especially in estrogen excess and a progesterone deficiency, or estrogen deficiency at time of manifestations
- Estrogen, progesterone, and aldosterone interaction
- Excessive prolactin, hypothyroidism, or hypoglycemia
- Dietary factors such as vitamin B_6 and/or magnesium deficiency
- Life-style factors such as increased stress and poor diet

Clinical Manifestations and Diagnostic Findings

Typically, manifestations of PMS occur during the last few premenstrual days, and sudden relief of manifestations occurs with full menstrual flow. However, manifestations may begin with ovulation and may not be relieved until during or toward the end of menses. Characteristically, manifestations gradually worsen until menses begin.

Various manifestations are attributable to PMS, including altered emotional states, behavioral changes, somatic problems, altered appetite, and motor effects. Different sets of manifestations are experienced by individual women. Commonly, emotional manifestations may include tension, depression, irritability, hostility, insomnia, loneliness, crying easily, and indecision. Forgetfulness and mental confusion may occur. Psychosis and suicidal tendencies occur rarely. There is no evidence that the effects of PMS on women's productivity are any different from the effects of men's cyclicity on cognitive work. Somatic problems may include headache, breast tenderness and abdominal bloating, peripheral edema, joint pain and backache, hives, constipation, and exacerbation of preexisting conditions such as migraine and herpes.

Because PMS manifestations usually do not occur during the menstrual flow, women may not associate PMS with the menstrual cycle. Also, women may be reluctant to admit the apparent emotional changes. Such manifestations may be misdiagnosed as psychological or emotional problems.

To date, there are no objective methods of diagnosing PMS. Diagnosis is usually made by documenting the cyclic nature of the manifestations on a menstrual calendar. A diary of manifestations and menstrual periods is an essential part of assessing women suspected of having PMS.

A diagnosis of PMS requires a recurrence of manifestations for a minimum of three menstrual cycles. Diagnosis is made on the timing of manifestations rather than on the presence of particular manifestations.

Community and Self-Care

■ Medical Management

There is no known effective pharmacologic treatment for PMS. Treatment is directed toward relief of manifestations. What helps one woman may not be effective for another. A variety of therapies have been used.

Vitamins and Minerals

Daily intake of vitamin B_6 has improved some premenstrual manifestations. Other nonprescription drugs include calcium, vitamin A, magnesium, and trace elements. Essential fatty acid supplements are often recommended.

Medications for Symptomatic Relief

Prescription medications commonly include progesterone, oral spironolactone (Aldactone), oral bromocriptine (Parlodel), oral contraceptives, and tranquilizers. Spironolactone is a synthetic steroid aldosterone antagonist that inhibits the physiologic effect of aldosterone on the distal renal tubules. It is commonly used to treat the edema associated with excessive aldosterone secretion. Bromocriptine reduces serum prolactin concentrations by inhibiting prolactin release from the anterior pituitary. It has been used successfully in some cases of PMS. Sedatives and analgesics, including antiprostaglandins, are often used for relief.

■ Nursing Management of the Medical Client

Assessment

PMS is a significant problem for many women. Nurses are in a key position to help women identify and cope with PMS when it is present. There are typically several of the following manifestations present premenstrually: breast tenderness, fluid retention, abdominal bloating, craving for sweet or salty foods, acne, fatigue, dizziness or faintness, headache, and heart palpitations. The most bothersome manifestations, however, usually include mood swings, irritability, hostility, and depression and their effects on relationships, career, and other facets of life.

Diagnosis, Planning, Implementation

Knowledge Deficit. The client suffering from PMS has many learning needs making the nursing diagnosis *Knowledge Deficit related to syndrome and manifestation management* a common priority diagnosis.

Planning: Expected Outcomes. The client will understand PMS and the management of its manifestations, as evidenced by her statements, her ability to maintain a diary of manifestations and menstrual cycles, and her report of a decrease in manifestations.

Implementation. Educate the client about the need for keeping an accurate diary. Once the diagnosis of PMS is made, the woman needs information about the syndrome and reassurance that there is a physiologic basis for her manifestations, even though the mechanisms are not clearly understood. Women are often helped by the opportunity to talk about their feelings and experiences with PMS, especially because of the confusion and misconceptions surrounding the syndrome. Significant others also benefit from information and reassurance.

Altered Health Maintenance. The client with PMS often has poor health habits leading to the nursing diagnosis *Altered Health Maintenance related to poor health habits.*

Planning: Expected Outcomes. The client will improve her health habits, as evidenced by improved physical condition and decrease of PMS manifestations.

Implementation. Women who are in poor physical condition may be particularly susceptible to premenstrual difficulties. Thus the nursing assessment includes the woman's general life-style, sleep and dietary habits, and overall health maintenance.

Suggested dietary modifications include reducing salt and refined carbohydrate intake. Give careful attention to stress management and reduction (see Chapter 4). Adequate physical exercise and weight reduction (if necessary) are very important. It may also be helpful to reduce alcohol and caffeine intake, and stop or reduce smoking.

Risk for Ineffective Individual Coping. The client with PMS is often very upset by the manifestations of the condition, especially the psychosocial manifestations leading to the nursing diagnosis *Risk for Ineffective Individual Coping related to distress from manifestations of PMS.*

Planning: Expected Outcomes. The client will cope effectively with PMS and its manifestations, as evidenced by her statements and a decrease in manifestations.

Implementation. Another major nursing responsibility is assisting the woman and her significant others to cope with the manifestations of PMS. Make plans for coping with specific PMS manifestations on an individual basis, keeping in mind the woman's particular life-style and preferences. For example, a reallocation of responsibilities within the family might help to reduce the woman's stress. If she prefers to retain her current responsibilities, the nurse might help her learn how to manage them in ways that minimize stress. Support groups or educational sessions may be helpful as well. These sessions can serve as a forum for sharing information, providing mutual support, and discussing feelings. Nurses can help form such groups if none exist in the area. Self-help books can also be useful. Daily, vigorous exercise has been recommended to improve circulation (which might help some manifestations), reduce stress, and promote a sense of well-being.

Evaluation

A successful outcome would be the control of PMS manifestations. Many women find that with treatment, the manifestations can be controlled to some extent. If the treatment is not successful, psychosocial care of the client becomes even more important.

Abnormal Uterine Bleeding

Abnormal uterine bleeding encompasses a wide variety of menstrual disorders, such as lack of menstrual flow, irregular uterine bleeding, and excessive uterine bleeding. Changes in menstrual patterns can be frightening to the woman and if they are severe enough, manifestations can disrupt daily living. Sometimes, abnormal uterine bleeding indicates underlying disease conditions. The term *dysfunctional uterine bleeding* means abnormal uterine bleeding for which no organic cause can be found through the usual assessment techniques. Abnormal uterine bleeding always requires careful assessment by a qualified healthcare provider.

Amenorrhea

Amenorrhea means the absence of menses by age 16, which is primary amenorrhea, or the absence of menses for 6 months in a woman who previously had regular cyclic bleeding, or 12 months in a woman with a history of irregular bleeding, which is secondary amenorrhea. In the United States secondary amenorrhea affects about 4% of (nonpregnant) women.

Etiology and Risk Factors

There are many causes of amenorrhea (Fig. 84–1):

● Pregnancy and lactation
● Chromosomal abnormalities
● Structural genital malformations
● Hypothalamic dysfunction

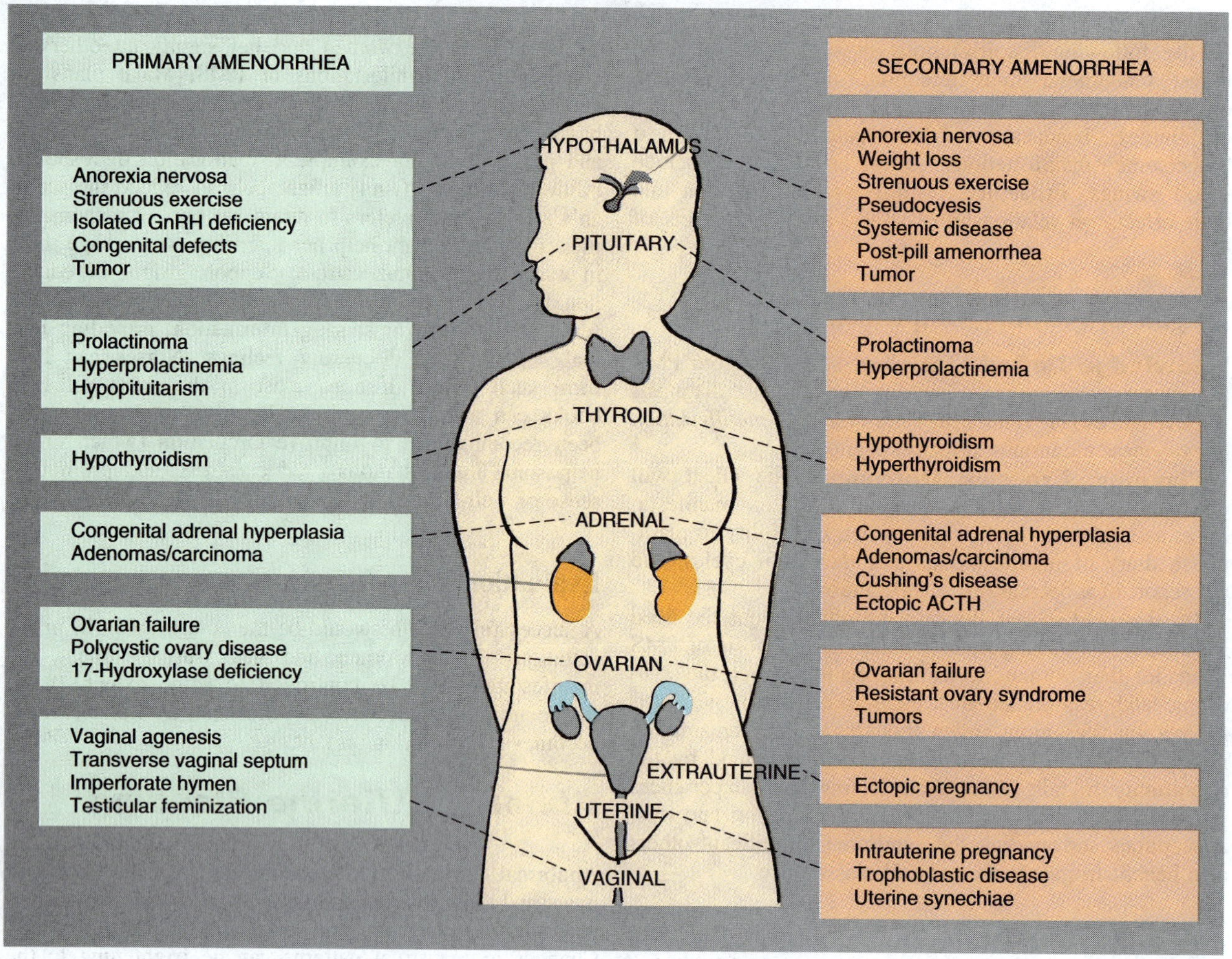

Figure 84–1. Causes of amenorrhea.

- Pituitary factors
- Ovarian factors
- Hypothyroidism and other endocrine factors
- Intense athletic training

These may be present alone or in combination.

Clinical Manifestations and Diagnostic Findings

The physical examination is usually normal. Manifestations, if any, are related to the cause of amenorrhea. Laboratory tests can be used to diagnose pregnancy or hormonal disorders.

Community and Self-Care

■ Medical Management

Treatment of amenorrhea depends in part on the woman's needs and wants. Particularly important are her wishes regarding childbearing.

If pregnancy is not wanted, medroxyprogesterone may be used to produce withdrawal bleeding. If pregnancy is wanted, ovulation induction with medications such as clomiphene citrate may be undertaken.

■ Nursing Management of the Medical Client

Absence of spontaneous menstrual flow before age 16 requires careful assessment, including history and physical examination. Pregnancy also must be ruled out for any woman of childbearing age experiencing secondary amenorrhea. Ask the woman about the presence of manifestations of pregnancy, such as breast tenderness, nausea, urinary frequency, weight gain, fatigue, or changes in food tolerance. Even if the woman has been consistently using birth control, pregnancy might have occurred.

Young girls may deny intercourse, meaning actual penetration, but may admit, on careful questioning, that sex play involving ejaculation between the thighs or near the introitus (opening into the vagina) did occur. Pregnancy can result from the migration of sperm in these situations. A pregnancy test is performed if there is any possibility that conception may have occurred. If the pregnancy test is positive, give the woman appropriate opportunity to discuss her wishes related to the pregnancy's continuation or termination.

Teaching opportunities are an important part of nursing care. Depending on the cause of amenorrhea, the woman may need help in gaining or losing weight, reducing energy drain from excessive physical activity, and stress reduction. Assess general health and help the woman plan and make changes as indicated.

Menorrhagia

The term *menorrhagia* means excessive vaginal bleeding at normal intervals and can cause women grave distress and inconvenience.

Etiology and Risk Factors

There are a number of causes of menorrhagia. These include:

1. Uterine fibroids and adenomyosis
2. Anatomic lesions
3. Spontaneous abortion
4. Inflammatory processes (e.g., endometritis and salpingitis)
5. Blood dyscrasias
6. Hypothyroidism
7. Intrauterine device (IUD) use
8. Endometrial carcinoma
9. Medications (e.g., anticoagulants)

Clinical Manifestations and Diagnostic Findings

Assessing the amount of blood loss can be difficult. Many women are unable to give a reliable history of blood loss. Ask women to compare the number of pads or tampons used during the abnormal period with the number used during a normal cycle. In a more controlled setting, it may help to weigh pads before and after use to estimate blood loss. Also, the usual tests to identify possible anemia may be performed. Diagnostic tests depend on the suspected cause.

Acute and Subacute Care

■ Surgical Management

Dilatation and curettage (D & C) may be performed for the abnormal bleeding, although this is currently believed to be unnecessary in most cases of menorrhagia. During dilation, the cervical opening is gradually enlarged using a dilator (Fig. 84–2). This is immediately followed by curettage (scraping the lining of the uterus with a curet).

Often, D & C is performed under light anesthesia as outpatient surgery.

Another surgical treatment is endometrial ablation, which is done on an outpatient basis. A laser fiber is used to destroy the endometrium by passing it through a hysteroscope. The destroyed tissues are then removed by irrigation of the uterus with saline. Sterility is likely, due to uterine scarring.

■ Nursing Management of the Surgical Client

Nursing management is the same for both procedures. Preoperatively, the woman restricts her food and fluid intake for anesthesia. The woman is placed in a lithotomy position for the procedure.

Postoperatively, the woman has a sterile perineal pad in place. The pad should be checked and changed frequently. The woman may have vaginal packing, which is usually removed within 24 hours.

During the first few hours, monitor the client closely for excessive vaginal bleeding. Also, assess her ability to urinate. Urination may be difficult, especially if vaginal packing is exerting pressure on the urethra. Report excess bleeding, inability to void, or excessive pain. The woman usually experiences only minimal uterine cramping postoperatively. Mild analgesics such as acetaminophen and codeine usually relieve any discomfort. Avoid aspirin for the first 24 to 48 hours to prevent excessive bleeding.

Follow-up instructions to the client include the following:

1. Avoid strenuous activity for about 1 week
2. Avoid douching and vaginal or rectal intercourse until the physician gives permission (usually about 1 week)
3. Expect a small amount of pinkish vaginal discharge, followed by a dark-red or dark-brown discharge during the healing process
4. Realize that subsequent menstrual periods may or may not be affected
5. Return for a follow-up appointment
6. Report any indication of complications to the surgeon. Following D & C, the next menses may not occur, may be on schedule, or may vary from the usual time of onset. Indications of possible complications include excessive bleeding, excessive pain, or an elevated temperature.

An important part of nursing care is to provide reassurance, because heavy vaginal bleeding can be very frightening.

■ Medical Management

If surgery is not done treatment may involve such medications as estrogens, progestins (alone or in combination with oral contraceptives), or antifibrinolytic agents, depending on factors thought to be associated with the cause.

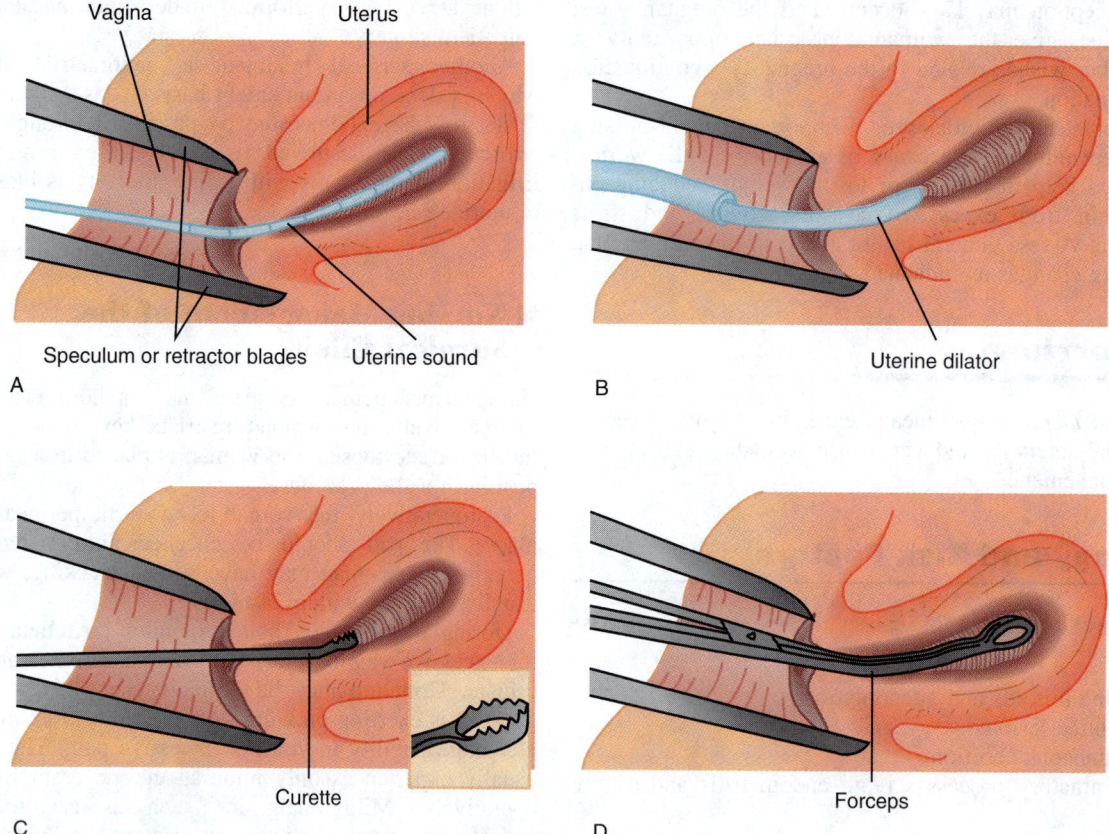

Vagina   Uterus

Speculum or retractor blades   Uterine sound

A

Uterine dilator

B

Curette

C

Forceps

D

Figure 84–2. Dilatation and curettage (D & C) of the uterus. *A,* The length and axis of the uterus is explored with a malleable uterine sound. *B,* A Kelly's speculum dilates the cervical os. Further gradual dilation is achieved with Hanks dilators in graduated sizes. *C,* The endocervical canal is curetted first; next, the uterine cavity. Tissue specimens are saved. *D,* Finally, the uterine cavity is explored with a polyforceps or common duct forceps.

Metrorrhagia

Metrorrhagia, or vaginal bleeding between menses, may occur as spotting or outright bleeding.

The possible causes of metrorrhagia include the following:

- Ectopic pregnancy
- Spotting with ovulation
- Cervical polyps
- Breakthrough bleeding with oral contraceptives
- Causes listed under menorrhagia

Pregnancy, as well as the presence of neoplasia, hormonal abnormalities, or physical abnormalities, needs to be ruled out or treated appropriately. Any anemia caused by excessive blood loss should be treated. For breakthrough bleeding in conjunction with oral contraceptives, the dosage of oral contraceptive can be adjusted or a different agent may be prescribed.

Menopause

Physiologic menopause is discussed in detail in Chapter 81.

Surgical Menopause

Menopause may be induced at any age by surgical removal of the ovaries, ablation with chemicals, or pelvic irradiation. Hysterectomy (removal of the uterus), not including removal of the ovaries, does not usually cause surgical menopause. However, some manifestations such as hot flashes have been reported following hysterectomy. In these instances, it is possible that blood vessels supplying the ovaries may have been injured, and the resulting loss of blood supply caused the ovaries to atrophy. Another possible cause of such manifestations could be the hormone imbalance produced by removal of the uterus and its loss as a hormone receptor.

Menopausal Difficulties

The most commonly reported menopausal difficulties are vasomotor instability, menstrual irregularities, and atrophic vaginitis. A wide variety of physical and psychosocial manifestations have been attributed to the perimenopausal period, but the only manifestations shown to be due to menopause itself and not the associated changes due to aging or stressful life events are vasomotor insta-bility, menstrual irregularities, and vaginal changes.

■ Vasomotor Instability

Manifestations of vasomotor instability, such as hot flashes, night sweats, and the occasional palpitations and dizziness associated with menopause, are probably caused by hormonal changes. Hot flashes are sudden involuntary waves of heat beginning in the upper chest or neck and proceeding up the face and head. These sensations last from a few seconds to an hour, and are aggravated by anything that increases heat production in the body. A hot flash may or may not be accompanied by a hot flush, which is a measurable change in skin temperature, a visi-ble pink to bright-red flush in skin color, and perspira-tion. A night sweat is a hot flash with or without a hot flush occurring in the night accompanied by perspiration, which can be profuse. Voda[73] describes the following types of hot flashes:

- Mild hot flash. A warm feeling, often so fleeting that it is barely noticeable. It may or may not be accompanied by dampness and slight skin flushing.
- Moderate hot flash. A warm to extremely warm feeling, longer and more noticeable than a mild hot flash. Often accompanied by sweat and sometimes skin flushing.
- Severe hot flash. An intense or extremely hot feeling. Usually accompanied by profuse and very uncomfort-able sweating or skin flushing. The thermal discomfort of a severe hot flash may cause a woman to stop her activity at the time of the hot flash and seek relief by the use of a fan, showering, removing or changing her clothes, or lying down. Other bodily sensations associ-ated with a severe hot flash are feelings of waves of heat, dizziness, a feeling of suffocation, inability to concentrate, and chest pain.

Generally, the subjective manifestation of the hot flash occurs about 45 seconds prior to the hot flush. The re-ported incidence of the hot flash varies for perimenopau-sal women from 68% to 92%, depending on the age group studied.[33] One study reported a prevalence rate of 88% for women experiencing natural menopause. How-ever, there is a great variance in both the quantitative and qualitative aspects of women's experiences of hot flashes. Women in other cultures do not all report experiencing hot flashes; they may not be a universal manifestation.

■ Atrophic Vaginitis and Other Changes

The vaginal mucous membrane is especially responsive to low estrogen levels. When these levels remain low both during and following menopause, vaginal walls become thinner and drier, and susceptibility to infection increases. These changes lead to an increase in vaginitis in meno-pausal women. Other manifestations may include vaginal irritation, burning, pruritus, leukorrhea, bleeding, and dys-pareunia (painful intercourse).

Vaginal epithelium loses its elasticity and subcutaneous fat after menopause. Pubic hair may become thinner. As the epidermal layer thins, the labia majora and minora flatten. The urethra may atrophy, and when this occurs, the incidence of cystitis and urethritis increase. The pubo-coccygeus muscles tend to lose their tone, and stress urinary incontinence also may occur. The effects of aging and previous childbearing also affect these changes.

Some women experience backache, joint pain, and other manifestations of osteoporosis. Osteoporosis is a skeletal disorder characterized by increased predisposition to bone collapse or fracture resulting from a reduced amount of bone mass. Estrogen seems to inhibit bone breakdown and loss. A decrease or absence of estrogen in conjunction with other risk factors may lead to osteoporo-sis (Chapter 75).

Many myths abound about depression occurring at the time of menopause but no relationship between depres-sion and menopause has been demonstrated. Women are no more prone to depression or emotional changes at menopause than at any other time in their lives. Psycho-social stress at the time of menopause, however, may affect menopausal manifestations. A woman's experience of menopause is affected not only by hormonal change but by her life circumstances and relationships.

Community and Self-Care

■ Medical Management

If vasomotor manifestations are severe, short-term treat-ment with hormone replacement therapy (HRT) may be used. Such therapy, lasting from a few months to 2 years, may relieve hot flashes. Generally, the therapy is discon-tinued gradually.

HRT (estrogen plus progesterone) may be part of the medical management of other perimenopausal manifesta-tions. Women must be informed of the advantages and potential dangers of HRT in order to make informed decisions about treatment. At this time there have been no studies of the benefits and risks of long-term use of HRT.

It is often difficult for women to decide about HRT because authorities differ markedly in their advice. HRT can alleviate vasomotor instability, vaginal and urinary tract atrophy, and dyspareunia.[44] It has also been studied as a preventive measure against osteoporosis and cardio-vascular disease, with some researchers claiming a protec-tive effect against breast cancer and others citing it as a risk factor for breast cancer development.[44]

In the mid- to late 1970s, evidence for an association between estrogen replacement therapy (ERT) and endo-metrial cancer was discovered. In subsequent years, this association has been studied extensively, and today estro-gen is given with a progestational agent to simulate the normal menstrual cycle. This provides a protective effect against endometrial cancer.[44] Unopposed ERT is, there-fore, no longer recommended for a woman with an intact uterus.

It is generally accepted that estrogens should not be given to women with the following:

1. Known or suspected breast or uterine cancer or any estrogen-dependent neoplasia (or a strong family history of the same)
2. Undiagnosed abnormal uterine bleeding
3. Previous or present thrombophlebitis
4. Acute liver or cerebrovascular disease
5. Risk factors such as obesity, varicosities, hypertension, and heavy smoking. (These risk factors become even more significant when they occur in combination.) Women with uterine fibromyomas, hyperlipidemia, severe varicose veins, chronic hepatic dysfunction, and diabetes mellitus require thorough assessment before estrogen is prescribed.

The use of ERT or HRT should be individualized according to the woman's needs, wishes, and individual manifestations and risks. The risk for women with fibrocystic breast disease is unclear, but careful assessment must be made. Risks should be assessed for endometrial cancer, osteoporosis, cardiovascular disease, and breast cancer. Both ERT and HRT are effective against perimenopausal hot flashes, atrophic vaginitis, and urinary tract changes. For relief of hot flashes, short-term therapy is usually effective with gradual withdrawal advised. Relief of urogenital problems may require long-term or even lifelong therapy.

Both ERT and HRT decrease the risk of developing osteoporosis. The optimal duration of therapy for osteoporosis prevention is not known, but it may be long-term to lifelong. Research is ongoing on the possible cardioprotective effects of ERT and HRT. Therapy for cardiovascular heart disease is lifelong.

At the present time, the risk from HRT for the development of breast cancer is unclear and further research is needed. If a woman opts for ERT or HRT, she should be carefully monitored for the development of breast cancer and receive breast examinations and mammography on a regular basis.

Estrogens used in replacement therapy are conjugated equine estrogens (Premarin), 0.625 mg; estrone sulfate, 0.625 mg to 1.25 mg; micronized 17-beta estradiol (Estrace), 1 to 2 mg; and transdermal 17-beta estradiol (Estraderm), 0.5 to 1.0 mg.[77]

Treatment regimens vary for estrogen-progesterone combinations. Estrogens may be used for 25 days each month or continually, whereas progesterones are generally prescribed for 10 to 14 days a month.[73] Low-dose continual progesterone therapy may be given along with continual ERT. The advantage of continued combined therapy is that withdrawal bleeding generally stops in about 6 months.

Side effects of progesterone therapy include bloating, depression, acne, breast tenderness, and premenstrual tension. However, side effects can generally be lessened by adjusting the dose or lengthening the duration of therapy. There have been, however, no studies of the benefits or risks associated with varying schedules for taking estrogens and progesterones together. Side effects may also be reduced by taking a natural form of progesterone rather than a synthetic progestin. Because of the side effects of progesterone, as well as the possibility that progesterones may unfavorably alter the high-density lipoprotein (HDL)–low-density lipoprotein (LDL) cholesterol ratio, unopposed estrogen has been recommended for women whose uterus has been surgically removed.

Transdermal estrogen patches are an alternative for women who cannot tolerate oral estrogens or for whom the hepatic effects of estrogen (increased secretion of renin substrate causing hypertension and increased clotting factors as a result of liver stimulation) are a problem.[43]

■ Nursing Management of the Medical Client

Many women require detailed information about what menopause is and what is happening to their bodies. Explain that hot flashes are a normal part of menopause. The nurse should provide practical suggestions for coping with hot flashes. The following information should be provided to women having difficulty with hot flashes:

- Dress in layers so that some clothing can easily be taken off and put back on as cooling commences.
- Avoid hot environments and keep the thermostat around 65° F or lower.
- Avoid getting excited, because emotional stress sometimes triggers hot flashes.
- Avoid highly seasoned, spicy foods, coffee, tea, and alcohol, if they trigger hot flashes. (Ask the client what spicy foods have this effect.)
- Keep a record or diary of when you experience hot flashes and try to identify common trigger(s) and work out ways of avoiding them.
- Learn to control your reactions to the hot flashes. (Voda[77] describes one woman's method of stopping hot flashes by imagining herself walking in snow and forcing herself to shiver.)
- Use cooling techniques, such as fans, showers, or applying cold cloths or ice cubes to various body parts.

The nursing role in working with menopausal women and their significant others involves providing support, education, and assistance in moving through this normal life experience as comfortably as possible. Accurate information about menopause and what to expect can be helpful and reassuring. Nurses need up-to-date information about menopause and its manifestations and their management, including HRT, in order to support women making important decisions.

Tailor assistance in coping with minor discomforts of menopause to the needs of the individual woman. The client may find the following self-care advice useful:

- *Vaginal dryness:* Intercourse and masturbation aid circulation and keep tissues flexible; use water-soluble vaginal lubricants as often as needed; use estrogen cream vaginally if needed.
- *Prevention of osteoporosis:* Take part in weightbearing exercises; increase calcium intake; stop smoking; reduce alcohol and caffeine intake.
- *Prevention of urinary tract infection:* Void frequently (every 2–3 hours); increase fluid intake; maintain good perineal hygiene; wear cotton underwear.

- *Pelvic relaxation:* Perform Kegel's exercises to increase muscle tone (see Chapter 56); lose weight if you are overweight.

Remind women experiencing menopause of the value of good health habits. Balanced nutrition and adequate sleep and rest are important. Exercising at least three times per week for 45 minutes will promote cardiovascular health. Nurses can be effective in assisting women to make menopause an affirmative experience.

Postmenopausal Bleeding

Postmenopausal bleeding, vaginal bleeding occurring after menopause, is a manifestation, not a diagnosis (Fig. 84–3). It requires careful assessment because it may be a manifestation of genital tract cancer. Other causes of postmenopausal bleeding include atrophic vaginitis, cervical polyps, fibroids, endometrial hyperplasia, and cervical erosion.

Pelvic Inflammatory Disease

Pelvic inflammatory disease (PID) refers to ascending pelvic infections, that is, those involving the upper genital tract (beyond the cervix).

Etiology and Risk Factors

Chlamydia trachomatis, gonococci, staphylococci, streptococci, and other pus-producing (pyogenic) organisms commonly cause PID. See the Risk Factors and Levels of Prevention feature for PID.

Pathophysiology

Once an infection is in the upper genital tract, it may travel along several routes (Fig. 84–4). Tuberculosis

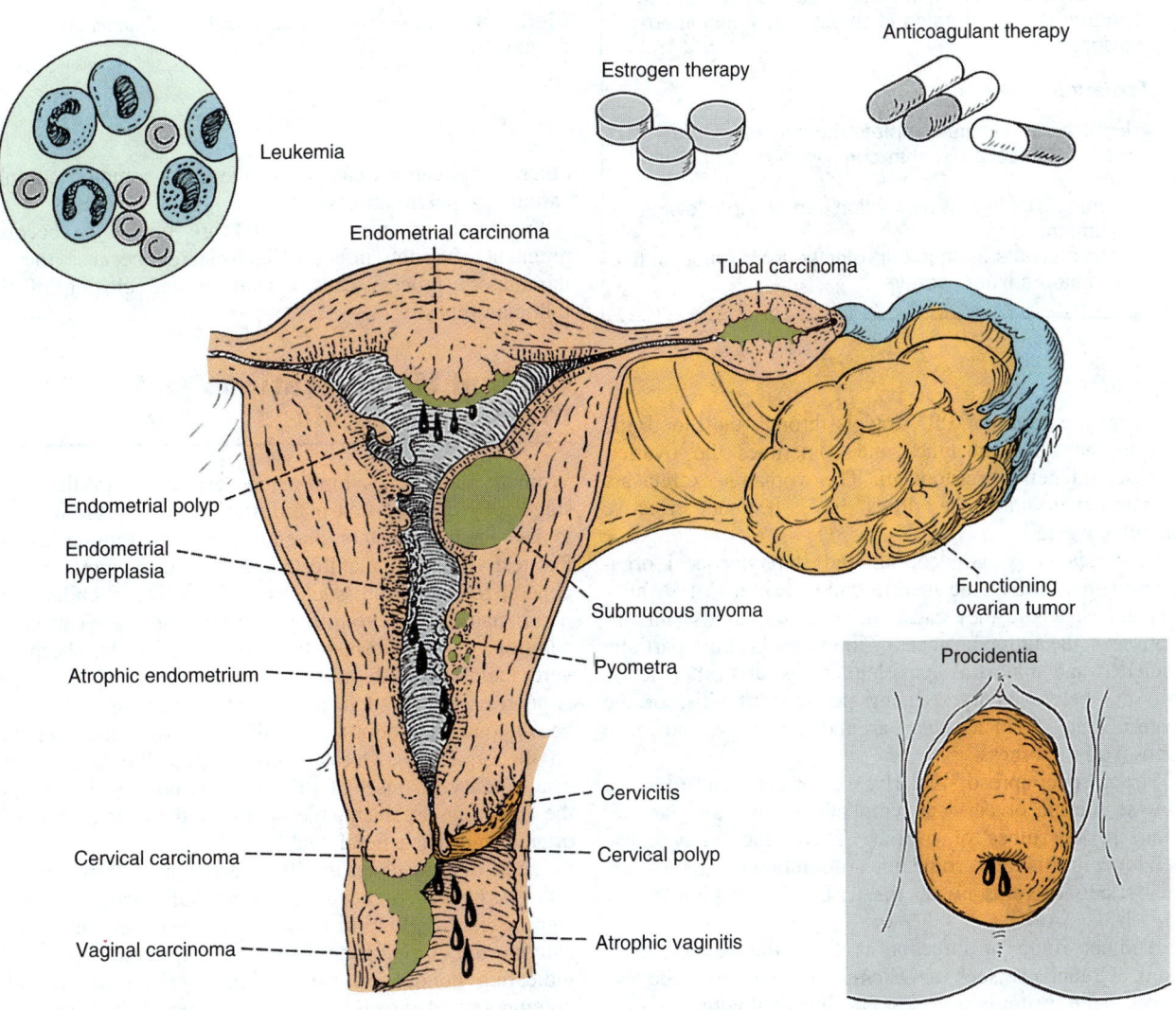

Figure 84–3. Causes of postmenopausal bleeding.

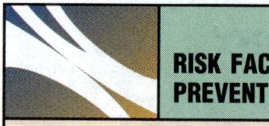

RISK FACTORS AND LEVELS OF PREVENTION

Pelvic Inflammatory Disease

Risk Factors

Chlamydia trachomatis, gonococci, staphylococci, streptococci, and other pus-producing organisms.

Levels of Prevention

Primary Prevention

- Educate clients to avoid unprotected intercourse.
- Advise clients to avoid multiple sexual partners.
- Advise clients to avoid the use of an IUD. If the client has an IUD, advise her to have no more than one sexual partner.
- Tell clients not to douche.

Secondary Prevention

- Tell clients to seek immediate treatment for any manifestations of a sexually transmitted disease.
- Tell clients to seek immediate treatment if a sexual partner is being treated for a sexually transmitted disease.

Tertiary Prevention

- Ensure that clients complete the course of treatment for infection so that complications do not develop.
- Remind clients that reinfection can occur following treatment.
- Advise clients to shun unprotected intercourse with untreated sexual partners.

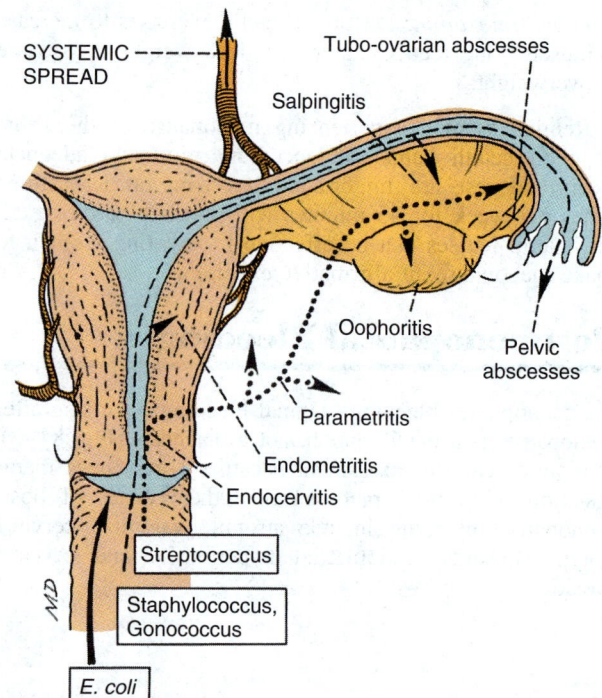

Figure 84–4. Routes of spread of pelvic inflammatory disease.

(TB), a rare cause of PID, travels through the blood and affects the fallopian tubes and sometimes the ovaries, uterus, and pelvic peritoneum. The woman's excreta are contaminated until the drugs have become effective (about 2 weeks).

C. trachomatis, gonococcal, and staphylococcal organisms spread along the uterine endometrium to the fallopian tubes, where they cause an acute salpingitis (inflammation of the fallopian tubes). The tubes become partially occluded and may drain pus, leukocytes, and other debris into the pelvic cavity, causing pelvic peritonitis, or the material may form a pocket around the ovary, causing a tubo-ovarian abscess.

Streptococci spread similarly, except they tend to travel via the uterine or cervical lymphatics across the parametrium to the tubes or ovaries. There, they may cause pelvic cellulitis and sometimes thrombophlebitis of the major pelvic veins, with the risk of development of emboli.

Another route of infection is from the pelvic cavity itself. Organisms such as *Escherichia coli* may be extruded from a ruptured viscus, causing peritonitis.

Complications may occur. Although septic shock and other complications can occur, the most common complication is a pelvic abscess.

Frequently, women with PID are unable to become pregnant after the infection has cleared because the inflammatory process causes scarring and closing of the fallopian tubes.

Clinical Manifestations and Diagnostic Findings

Women may be asymptomatic, especially in the early stages of PID. The first manifestation may be the inability to become pregnant or diagnosis through routine screening tests. Clinical manifestations include symptoms of a generalized infection, such as malaise, fever, chills, anorexia, nausea and vomiting, aching, and tachycardia. In addition, the woman usually experiences acute, sharp, severe aching on both sides of the abdomen or pelvis. Pain is aggravated by defecation and is accompanied by a heavy, purulent, odoriferous discharge (the odor depends on the organism). Occasionally, vaginal bleeding occurs. The rapidity of onset of PID depends on the virulence of the infecting organism, the status of the woman's pelvic organs, and her general health.

Other helpful clues to PID are obtained from the history. A history of acute lower genital tract infection is significant. It is helpful to know whether the pain accompanying the current illness began during menses (typically indicating gonococcal PID) or between menses (usually nongonococcal infections). Various other data, including a thorough sexual history, are important. Included is a his-

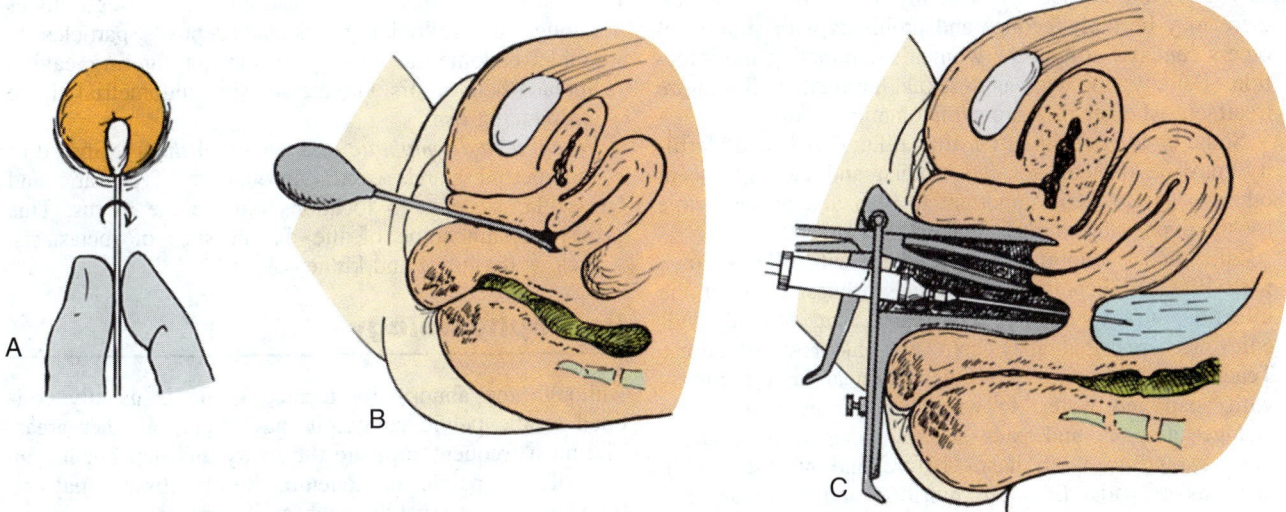

Figure 84–5. Some procedures used to diagnose pelvic inflammatory disease. *A,* Swabs may be obtained from the cervix, urethra, and rectum. *B,* The vaginal pool may be aspirated. *C,* Culdocentesis may be performed. Gram stains of cervical secretions show gram-negative intracellular diplococci. Cultures are placed on Thayer-Martin medium. Negative stains and cultures do not rule out gonococcal disease.

tory of contraceptive use, because the presence of an IUD correlates with a higher incidence of PID.

Manifestations of PID are combined with those of pulmonary TB (see Chapter 41) when TB is the cause of PID.

The usual laboratory tests for infection, including multiple cultures (Fig. 84–5), are performed. Some practitioners culture any evident drainage, and obtain specimens from various sites such as the cervix, vagina, and urethra. Additional cultures are helpful because it is not uncommon for several kinds of organisms to be involved or for organisms cultured from the cervix to differ from those found in the upper genital tract. When this occurs, several types of antibiotics may be necessary to treat the infection. Histologic examination of endometrial biopsy, ultrasonography of abscess, and laparoscopy may also be used in the diagnosis of PID, but are not as commonly used as cultures.

 Acute and Subacute Care

■ Medical Management

Most women are treated as outpatients, receiving antibiotics appropriate to the specific cause of the infection. Women with this condition are cautioned to avoid sexual activity, douches, and other activities that could worsen the infectious process. If the woman improves, she is usually evaluated in about a week to be sure the infection is gone. Advise the woman treated at home for PID to return for assessment if her condition deteriorates or her manifestations continue. Hospitalization may be necessary. A woman requiring hospitalization for PID is usually very ill.

PID caused by TB is treated with antitubercular medications (see Chapter 41). During hospitalization, appropriate antibiotics are given in maximal doses. The woman is placed in the semi-Fowler position to promote downward drainage. Pain management is important. Sitz baths or heat (applied periodically to the lower back or abdomen) may help relieve the pain. Analgesics are also used. Document the amount, color, odor, and appearance of the vaginal discharge. Make sure the client cleans the perineum frequently.

Other antibiotics are given as appropriate for the organisms cultured. See Chapter 86 for further information on the treatment of PID.

■ Surgical Management

Some abscesses are treated relatively easily; others require surgical intervention. Others may rupture, causing peritonitis. The type of surgical intervention and its timing (acute or after a cooling-off period) varies somewhat with the healthcare provider's philosophy and the presenting problem.

Treatment of some women with PID requires a laparotomy. While the infection is surgically removed, it may also be necessary to remove the uterus, ovaries, and tubes.

Surgery that is performed while PID is acute increases the woman's operative risk. This risk must be balanced against the risk of continuing unsuccessful medical therapy that can lead to chronic PID.

■ Nursing Management of the Medical/Surgical Client

Nursing care of women experiencing PID is directed toward providing health information and psychosocial support to the client and her significant others. Because

PID is often caused by sexually transmitted diseases, there may be guilt feelings and problems with significant others centered around the woman's contracting the infection. Usually, the woman's sexual partners will require treatment whether they are symptomatic or not.

Some women are infertile after PID. This loss of fertility may be difficult for the woman and her significant other to accept. It is important to plan and provide time for the expression of such feelings.

Education is important for the client with PID. Women with PID can benefit from factual discussion about the infection, how to identify recurrences, and general hygienic measures that may help prevent new infections. Teach the woman to wash her perineal area regularly with soap and water, to wipe from front to back, to change tampons and pads several times a day during menses, and to wash hands before and after changing tampons or pads. Balanced nutrition and adequate rest, sleep, and exercise can improve general health and reduce the risk of infection. Women need to know when they can resume sexual activity, how to ensure the safety of sexual encounters, and when other restrictions can be lifted.

Chronic Pelvic Inflammatory Disease

Chronic PID can occur if the acute phase of the illness does not respond to treatment or if treatment is inadequate. Clinical manifestations include chronic pelvic discomfort, menstrual disturbances or dysfunctional uterine bleeding, constipation, malaise, or periodic return of acute manifestations. Sterility, one of the more serious complications, results from destruction of part of the fallopian tubes and loss of their patency. Sterility is usually irreversible.

Treatment of chronic PID is aimed at removing the offending organism and improving the woman's general health. If treatment is unsuccessful, surgical removal of the pelvic organs may be necessary.

Uterine Disorders

Endometriosis

Endometriosis is an abnormal condition in which endometrial tissue (which normally lines the uterine cavity) is located in other sites. Endometriosis is found most commonly in premenopausal women aged 30 to late 40s. It rarely occurs in women younger than 20 years of age. Endometriosis appears to be hereditary, occurring more commonly in women whose mothers had the disorder. The highest incidence is in nulliparous white women.

Etiology and Risk Factors

The cause of endometriosis is unknown. Several theories have been proposed. Two theories are the following:

- *Implantation theory.* Menstrual flow regurgitates through the fallopian tubes and deposits particles of viable endometrial tissue outside the uterine cavity. Spread then occurs via metaplasia (endometrial tissue reproducing itself).
- *Vascular and lymphatic dissemination theory.* Spread of endometrial glands occurs through the lymphatic and vascular systems to locations outside the uterus. This may explain some of the distant sites of metastasis, such as the lungs and kidneys.

Pathophysiology

Although the abnormally located tissue is usually confined to the pelvic cavity, it may occur in other areas. The most frequent sites are the ovary and dependent portion of the pelvic peritoneum. Rarely, tissue may be found outside the pelvis, such as in surgical scars, lungs, and extremities. Possible sites of endometriosis are shown in Figure 84–6.

Regardless of the site, this misplaced endometrial tissue responds to hormonal stimulation and bleeds, producing a variety of manifestations. Scarring and inflammation occur at sites of endometriosis. Repeated episodes of interperitoneal bleeding (from hormonal stimulation of the endometrial tissue) cause adhesions. Eventually, one peritoneal surface may become fixed to another.

Infertility is a major complication of endometriosis. Usually the cause of infertility is unknown; sometimes, however, endometriosis produces tubal obstruction.

Endometrial tissue is hormone-dependent; therefore the tissue usually atrophies with the normal ovarian regression associated with menopause. It also regresses during pregnancy.

Clinical Manifestations and Diagnostic Findings

Manifestations of endometriosis relate more to the site than to the degree of disease present. Pain is the most characteristic manifestation of endometriosis. However, about one fourth of women with this condition are asymptomatic. Pain typically begins before the menstrual period, lasting for the duration of menstruation and sometimes for several days afterward. The intensity of pain is not correlated with the degree of endometriosis. Pain usually reaches its peak just before the onset of menstrual flow and during the first 1 or 2 days of the menstrual period. The pain may be located in a variety of areas, making the diagnosis more difficult. Unfortunately, some women with endometriosis are viewed as not having real pain and being neurotic.

Other manifestations of endometriosis include dyspareunia, menstrual irregularities, and infertility in the absence of tubal obstruction. When the condition occurs inside the ovary, it produces a chocolate cyst. Severe pain is associated with rupture of this cyst. Implants on the ureters may obstruct them, whereas those involving the rectum may be associated with bleeding, diarrhea, or obstruction. Bowel involvement can cause painful defecation.

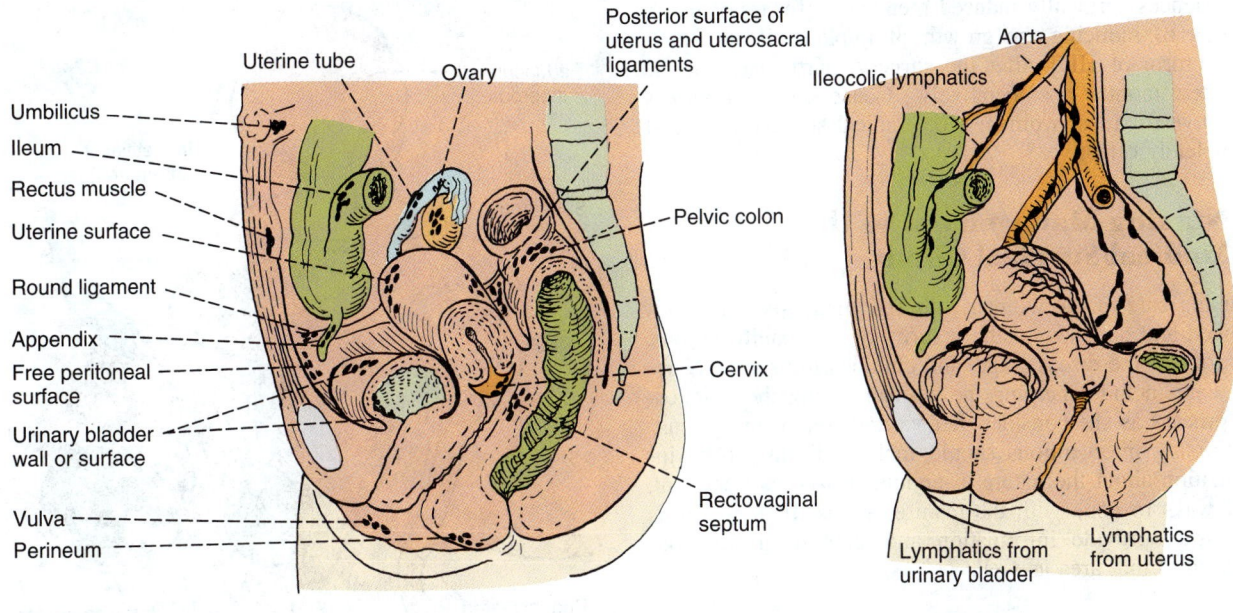

A. SITES OF ENDOMETRIOSIS

B. LYMPHATICS

Figure 84–6. Endometriosis. *A,* Sites of endometriosis. Those most frequently affected are the ovaries and the dependent pelvic peritoneum. However, as can be seen, many other sites can also be involved. *B,* Pelvic and lymph nodes are important.

Diagnosis is generally made by history, pelvic examination, and observation of lesions either by laparoscopic examination or pelvic surgery. Direct observation of lesions are necessary for a definitive diagnosis.

Community and Self-Care

■ Medical Management

Appropriate treatment of endometriosis depends on the woman's manifestations, age, parity, and extent of the disease. When the manifestations and extent of the disease are mild, the woman is given support, information about the disease, and some guidelines about ways to cope with the pain. Mild analgesics may be helpful. If manifestations become severe or the disease progresses, more treatment is generally necessary.

Medication may inhibit endometriosis enough to allow pregnancy, or at least relieve manifestations. Pharmacologic intervention includes inducing a pseudopregnancy with oral contraceptives, progesterone, or both. During the course of this treatment, progestins cause the ectopic endometrium to slough off. Thus, theoretically, the ectopic endometrial tissue no longer functions in abnormal sites. This type of treatment is not successful in all women.

The other hormonal treatment is to induce ovarian suppression or pseudomenopause. Danazol (Danocrine) is an antigonadotropin testosterone derivative that inhibits gonadotropin release and has other actions tending to cause the regression of endometriosis. The medication provides rapid and safe relief of manifestations, but it is very expensive, costing over $100 per month. It may cause side effects, such as acne, hirsutism, weight gain, decreased breast size, hot flashes, and vaginal dryness. Leuprolide (Lupron) is a synthetic analog of luteinizing hormone–releasing hormone that reduces endometrial pain and lesions. It can be given monthly as an intramuscular (IM) injection, which can cost $300 and up per injection, or daily as a subcutaneous injection that is self-administered, and is slightly less expensive. This medication also has associated menopausal side effects. Nafarelin (Synarel) acts as a synthetic analog of gonadotropin-releasing hormone (GnRH); because endometrial lesions are sensitive to ovarian hormones, it reduces the lesions. It is administered intranasally twice a day, is very expensive, and may cause menopausal side effects.

■ Surgical Management

Exploratory or therapeutic surgery directed at the endometriosis may make pregnancy possible. Conservative surgical intervention includes restoring normal anatomy and removing or destroying endometriotic foci. A carbon dioxide laser may be used to treat endometriosis by vaporizing adhesions and endometrial implants. Even if the client states that she does not want a future pregnancy, conservative surgery might be employed for a woman of childbearing age, in case she changes her mind.

More radical surgery involves removing the uterus, as many implants as possible, and possibly the ovaries. This surgery has wide-reaching consequences (i.e., for sexuality, cardiovascular health), so this surgery is generally only used when other measures have failed and the woman does not wish to retain her childbearing ability. This approach will cause surgically induced menopause and permanent sterility. (There is some controversy over whether a woman with a history of endometriosis who experiences surgically induced menopause for treatment is at risk of inducing the growth of implants if she takes some form of HRT after the surgery, particularly in the first few months postoperatively.) Conservative surgery is effective for most women. More radical surgery is almost completely effective.

■ Nursing Management of the Medical/Surgical Client

Nursing care of the woman with endometriosis is individualized and depends on the severity of her manifestations, severity of the disease, age, and childbearing status. Nursing care includes helping the woman during the diagnostic process as she considers her various treatment options.

Nursing interventions should include discussion of information about the nature of endometriosis, its treatment, and ways to cope with the manifestations. If infertility is an issue, provide information and support in decision-making in that area as well.

Benign Uterine Tumors (Leiomyomas)

Leiomyomas are the most common tumors of the female genital tract. They occur in more than 20% to 30% of all women during their menstrual years.[14] The incidence of leiomyomas in black women is two to three times greater than in white women.[32] Leiomyomas are more common in women approaching menopause.

Leiomyomas are known by various names (some not technically correct) related to the tissue involved (e.g., fibroids, fibromas, fibromyomas, fibroleiomyomas, myomas, and fiber balls). Leiomyomas are composed mainly of muscle and fibrous connective tissue.

Etiology and Risk Factors

The cause of leiomyomas is unknown. The growth of leiomyomas does seem to be related to estrogen stimulation because the fibroids often enlarge with pregnancy and decrease in size with menopause. Leiomyomas begin as a simple proliferation of smooth muscle cells. It has been theorized that this proliferation is stimulated by physical or mechanical means and may occur at points of maximal stress within the myometrium. With the multiple points of stress within the uterus due to contractions, there are often multiple fibroids (Fig. 84-7).

Pathophysiology

■ Classification

Leiomyomas may be classified according to their location. Those occurring in the uterine body are most common (see Fig. 84-7).

Intramural. Intramural lesions are found in the uterine wall, surrounded by myometrium. Clinical manifestations

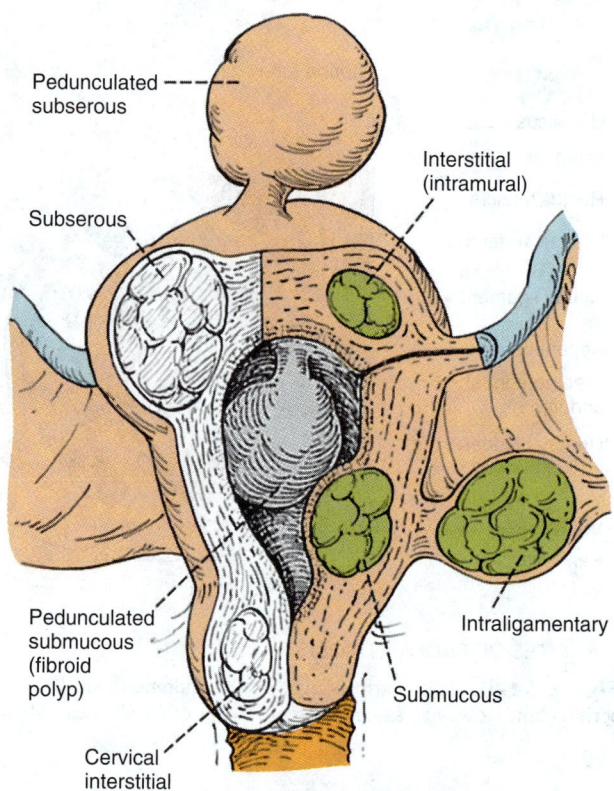

Figure 84-7. Some locations of leiomyomas (fibroids). Uterine leiomyomas, depending on their location and size, may interfere with sperm passage and implantation of a fertilized ovum.

may include increased uterine size, vaginal bleeding between menses, and dysmenorrhea.

Submucosal. Submucosal lesions occur directly under the endometrium, involving the endometrial cavity. The tumor may become pedunculated (grow on a stalk). Clinical manifestations may include prolonged vaginal bleeding, cramps, and the tumor may be seen protruding through the cervix.

Subserosal. Subserosal lesions are found on the outer surface (under the serosa) of the uterus. These tend to become pedunculated, to wander, and to be multiple and large. Clinical manifestations may include backache, constipation, and bladder problems.

Wandering or Parasitic. These lesions occur when a pedunculated leiomyoma twists on its pedicle and breaks off. It then attaches to other tissues, particularly the omentum.

Intraligamentary. Intraligamentary lesions are implants on the pelvic ligaments, and they may displace the uterus or involve the ureters.

Cervical. Cervical lesions occur infrequently and may obstruct the cervical canal.

■ Secondary Changes

Secondary changes can occur with all six categories of leiomyomas. These changes include the following:

- Hyaline degeneration, which occurs when the tumor outgrows the blood supply
- Cystic degeneration, which tends to follow hyaline degeneration, when the tumors become liquified and ultimately cystic
- Calcification, which is more common in large tumors
- Infection, which is more common in submucosal tumors
- Sarcomatous (malignant) degeneration, which is rare and is suspected with rapidly enlarging tumors, recurrent tumors, and when hemorrhage occurs with a known tumor
- Red (carneous) degeneration, which usually occurs during pregnancy with clinical manifestations of an acute abdomen (i.e., acute pain over the area of the leiomyoma, fever, tachycardia, nausea, vomiting, and abdominal rigidity)
- Acute torsion of the pedicle, which leads to acute disruption of the blood supply, with gangrenous changes and manifestations of acute abdomen
- Fatty degeneration, which is rare.

Clinical Manifestations and Diagnostic Findings

Frequently, leiomyomas are asymptomatic. Manifestations that do appear generally relate to tumor size, location, or number. Additionally, abnormal bleeding, often resulting in hypermenorrhea, may be present, and is related to the fibroid's hormone dependence.

Manifestations vary widely and occur in about half of women with leiomyomas. When they are present, they often relate to the size, location, and number of leiomyomas. The onset of manifestations most commonly occurs in the woman's late 40s and early 50s, just before menopause. Once menopause begins, manifestations often cease. It is rare for manifestations to begin after menopause, when leiomyomas tend to regress. If new manifestations develop during these years, other diagnoses, such as cancer, need to be ruled out.

The most common clinical manifestation of leiomyomas is abnormal uterine bleeding, which is excessive either in amount or duration. Frequently, it is accompanied by anemia and is associated with tiredness, weakness, and lethargy. Dysmenorrhea and a sensation of bearing down are often present. Urinary frequency is common when the tumor presses on the bladder. Urinary retention also may occur. Constipation, hydroureter, hydronephrosis, abdominal pain, and dyspareunia are less common manifestations.

Occasionally, the woman may have vaginal discharge. The discharge may be foul or water and blood-tinged. Abdominal pressure occurs if the leiomyoma is large enough to enlarge the abdomen. The tumor may be palpable. Also, the woman may have problems with sterility or a history of one or more spontaneous abortions.

A characteristic history, confirmed by abdominal and pelvic examination findings, usually establishes the diagnosis. Ultrasonography may indicate an abnormal uterine shape. Various disorders, such as cancer or a problem pregnancy, need to be ruled out before treatment is planned.

Acute and Subacute Care

■ Surgical Management

Asymptomatic women may require no treatment. However, when treatment is indicated, it typically consists of myomectomy (removal of a tumor without the removal of the uterus). Performing a myomectomy preserves the woman's reproductive organs and reproductive capability. Because of the many consequences of hysterectomy (removal of the uterus), it is preferable, if at all possible, to retain the uterus by performing a myomectomy. There are three types of hysterectomy that may be performed:

1. *Subtotal hysterectomy:* All of the uterus except the cervix is removed. (Rarely performed any longer, but if it is performed, remember that the woman still needs Papanicolaou [Pap] smears.)
2. *Total hysterectomy:* Removal of the uterus and cervix. The procedure can be performed either abdominally or vaginally.
3. *Total abdominal hysterectomy with bilateral salpingo-oophorectomy (TAH-BSO):* Removal of the uterus, cervix, fallopian tubes, and ovaries (Fig. 84–8).

A radical hysterectomy, which is performed only to treat cancer, is the same as a TAH-BSO plus removal of the lymph nodes, upper third of the vagina, and parametrium.

■ Nursing Management of the Surgical Client

Assessment

Many women may be asymptomatic; however, many will seek medical help because of some form of abnormal uterine bleeding. Obtain a thorough history from the client, especially concerning the time when the excessive bleeding occurs. Assess the woman's knowledge of her condition and the surgery, if one is planned. Pay particular attention to any question the woman has concerning sexuality after treatment.

Diagnosis, Planning, Implementation

Pain. Since pain is a common complaint in the woman with leiomyomas preoperatively, an appropriate nursing diagnosis for this client is *Pain related to dyspareunia and pelvic pain secondary to multiple or enlarged leiomyomas.*

Planning: Expected Outcomes. The client will have pain relieved or controlled, as evidenced by her statements of relief.

Implementation. The client can be taught ways to reduce pain associated with intercourse, such as assuming

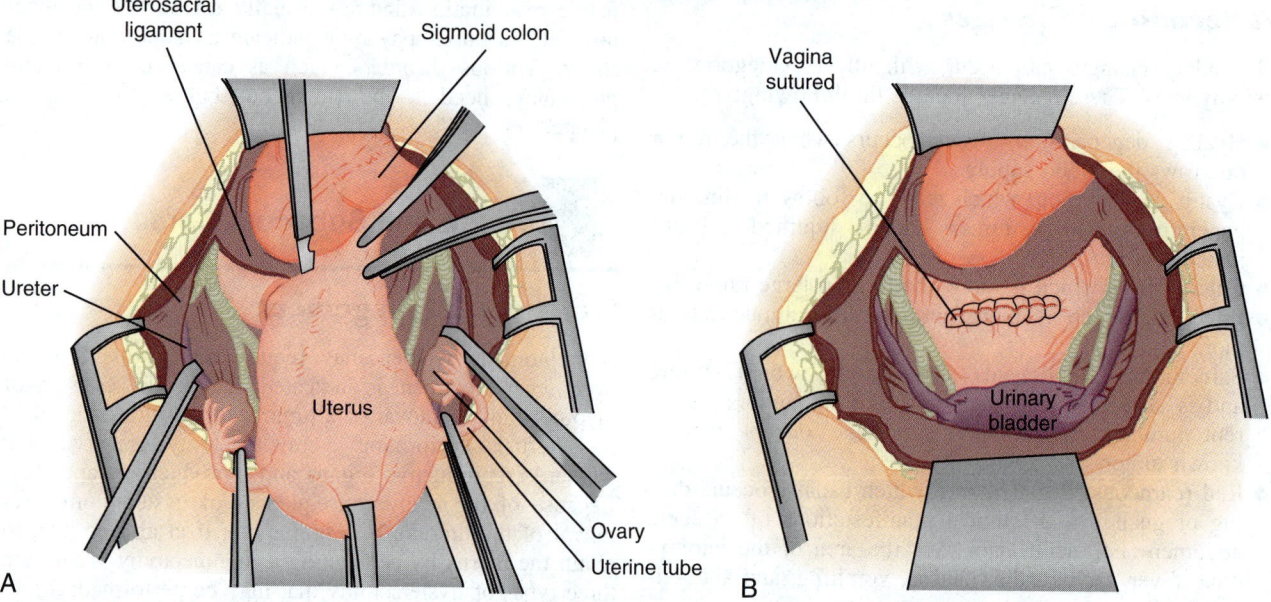

Figure 84–8. Total abdominal hysterectomy with salpingo-oophorectomy. *A,* The uterus with attached uterine tubes and ovaries is lifted out after it has been freed from the ligaments holding it. *B,* After the specimen has been removed en masse, the vagina is sutured closed.

positions in which leiomyomas are not pressed on during intercourse, and using water-soluble lubricants with intercourse.

Pain medications can be used for severe pain. Sometimes, sitz baths or the application of heat to the lower abdomen is helpful in relieving pain. See Chapter 17 for further methods of pain relief.

Knowledge Deficit. The client undergoing a hysterectomy will have many learning needs, making *Knowledge Deficit related to surgical procedure and possible outcomes of surgery* a priority nursing diagnosis.

Planning: Expected Outcomes. The client will understand surgery and outcomes, as evidenced by her statements.

Implementation. *Preoperative and Postoperative Teaching.* Frequently, a woman undergoing gynecologic surgery needs assistance in understanding her problem and the surgery being performed to correct it (see Ethical Issues in Nursing). She needs to understand her option and the difference between a myomectomy and a hysterectomy. She needs information as to what to expect postoperatively and how to care for herself.

If a woman is going to have a hysterectomy, she needs to understand that her reproductive capacity will be lost. If a woman is having her ovaries removed as well, a surgical menopause should be discussed with her. It is important to remember, however, that some women are relieved at the loss of the risk of unwanted pregnancy and the disappearance of severe manifestations.

It is particularly important for the woman to know that sexual intercourse will be perfectly normal following a hysterectomy, and her ability to achieve orgasm should not change. The woman should be told that once healing

has occurred, intercourse should be pain-free. Answer honestly any questions the woman has and encourage her to express her feelings and concerns about sexuality.

Discharge Teaching. Be sure the woman understands the type of surgery she had and what follow-up is needed. If she had a myomectomy, pregnancy is still an option, and she must continue to be followed with routine gynecologic examinations. If she has had a TAH-BSO, menopause and HRT should be discussed. Discharge teaching should also include the following instructions:

● Perform prescribed abdominal strengthening exercises so that the muscles affected by surgery can be restrengthened after the 2-month period is up.
● Avoid heavy lifting for about 2 months, to prevent straining the abdominal muscles that are healing.
● Avoid activities that increase pelvic congestion until the surgeon says they are safe. These activities include dancing, horseback riding, and prolonged standing. Optimal circulation is necessary to promote healing of pelvic tissues.
● Avoid vaginal and rectal sexual activities and douching until permitted by the surgeon, usually after about 6 weeks. Vaginal or rectal intercourse or douching could interfere with healing of the vaginal cuff or other healing tissues, and introduce infection.
● Report any fresh bleeding to the surgeon, and any abnormal (other than nonodorous, whitish, brownish, or yellowish liquid) vaginal discharge.
● Return for follow-up care as requested by the surgeon.

Risk for Dysfunctional Grieving. Many women experience grief over the loss of the female reproductive organs making *Risk for Dysfunctional Grieving related to loss of reproductive capacity and perceived loss*

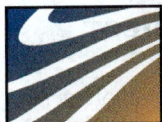

ETHICAL ISSUES IN NURSING

How Can Nurses Ensure That Patients Have Given Their Informed Consent?

Your client, Linda Anderson, has had some vaginal bleeding and is scheduled for a total abdominal hysterectomy. She is a 29-year-old unmarried woman who is an attorney in a large law firm. You are asked by the nurse-manager if she has consented to the procedure.

Linda has a right to informed consent. The medical and nursing staff are required to give each client adequate relevant information prior to interventions. This information is to enhance the client's ability to make decisions based on her own values and life plan.

There are five essential elements of informed consent: competence, disclosure, understanding, voluntariness, and authorization. Linda's specific surgery presents additional issues to consider such as consent to sterilization and the inability to conceive or continue a pregnancy.

In order to be considered competent, a client must be capable of making sound decisions. Linda must be able to autonomously authorize this surgery and be able to communicate her choices. These choices must be reasoned and congruous with her values. These choices should remain stable over time.

Currently, there is no assessment tool available to test a client's competence. Consequently, the determination of a person's competence can be difficult. A client may be competent to perform one task, but incompetent to perform another; therefore, it is beneficial to evaluate a client over time to ascertain the client's ability to make decisions about treatment options. When in doubt, a psychiatric consult is obtained.

Nurses informing clients about healthcare choices must disclose an adequate amount of information to the client. This information includes facts that the client typically considers important for consideration and information that the nurse thinks would be important for the client to consider. Disclosure of information is best accomplished when the client participates fully in a discussion, asking questions and obtaining clarification.

Linda must comprehend the risks and benefits of information to make an autonomous decision. She must understand enough information and appreciate the relevance of the information to her situation. Since Linda is to have a hysterectomy, she must clearly understand that she will no longer be able to participate in childbearing. Some clients may wish to harvest sperm or eggs and freeze them for later use.

Linda's decisions must be made independently, with no coercive influence from others. The healthcare professional's position, authority, and power should not unduly influence her decision.

Linda must actively approve the treatment plan. She must intentionally authorize the surgery.

These essential elements of informed consent are important for practice. Linda has a right to a consent process that is truly informed.

---

of femininity an appropriate nursing diagnosis for this client.

Planning: Expected Outcomes. The client will go through normal grieving over her loss after hysterectomy without developing dysfunctional grieving, as evidenced by her ability to express her feelings concerning the loss.

Implementation. When reproductive ability is lost, the client may well undergo a grief response. It is important to understand the grieving process and to be able to help the woman understand that what she is experiencing is normal. (Remember, however, that it is normal for some women to experience relief rather than grief.) The nurse should support normal grieving, including temporary denial, which is a part of the grieving process. If the client continues to experience grief beyond the normal degree, she may require counseling.

Risk for Infection. During surgery for a hysterectomy, the woman will have had a Foley catheter inserted leading to the nursing diagnosis *Risk for Infection related to surgical intervention and presence of a urinary catheter.*

Planning: Expected Outcomes. The client will not develop an infection or will have any infection diagnosed and treated immediately, as evidenced by normal urinary output without evidence of a urinary tract infection.

Implementation. The proximity of the bladder to the female reproductive organs increases the risk that urinary problems might occur postoperatively. These problems are even more likely to occur if a vaginal hysterectomy was performed, because of the pull on the musculature. A Foley catheter is usually inserted at the time of surgery to prevent bladder distention and injury during surgery. Sometimes it is left in place for 24 hours postoperatively. Potential problems that might occur postoperatively include urinary tract infection, difficulty urinating after the catheter is removed, and urinary retention.

When the Foley catheter is in place, instruct the woman to keep the urinary drainage catheter below the level of the bladder, to drink at least 2 to 4 L of liquid daily, and to report any urinary pain or discomfort. The nurse should check the urinary drainage system closely for leaks, provide complete perineal care every shift, and report any change in color or odor of the urine. It is normal for the urine to be slightly blood-tinged immediately postoperatively from the handling of the bladder during surgery. The color should return to normal after fluid intake increases.

Often a suprapubic catheter is also in place. This allows for removal of the Foley catheter first with the client being encouraged to void with the suprapubic catheter clamped. If the client becomes distended and is unable to void, the suprapubic catheter can be opened and drained without having to reinsert the catheter. This gives the client the opportunity to regain urinary control without recatheterization.

If a suprapubic catheter is not used, when the Foley catheter is removed observe for the first voiding, frequent voiding in small amounts, inability to void, or hematuria. If the woman experiences any of these manifestations, report it to the physician so that prompt treatment can begin.

Constipation. Because of bowel manipulation during surgery, the nursing diagnosis *Constipation related to bowel manipulation during surgery* is appropriate.

Planning: Expected Outcomes. The client will not become constipated and will have distention treated, as evidenced by return to a normal bowel pattern and absence of distention.

Implementation. Pain and discomfort following abdominal hysterectomy usually center around the incision and postoperative gas pains. After abdominal hysterectomy, gastrointestinal functioning returns slowly. Uncomfortable gas pains are often experienced during the early postoperative period. Early, frequent ambulation helps improve gastrointestinal function.

If gas pains persist, an enema may be prescribed to facilitate peristalsis and prevent constipation. Continue to encourage frequent ambulation to facilitate the return of normal gastrointestinal functioning. Six glasses of warm water a day also help peristalsis to return.

Evaluation

The client should recover from a hysterectomy without complications. She should return to normal activities within 6 weeks without permanent problems.

■ Medical Management

A plan of treatment for leiomyomas depends on manifestations, age, location and size of the tumors, onset of complications, and the woman's wish to become pregnant. In women who are not pregnant; do not have excessive bleeding or pressure on the bladder, bowel, or ureters; and do not have a rapidly growing tumor, leiomyomas can be assessed every 6 months by a practitioner. GnRH analogs, as discussed in the section on medical management of endometriosis, may be administered to reduce tumor size and inhibit their growth. Although malignant degeneration is rare, if the woman experiences a rapid increase in the size of the leiomyomas, more definitive therapy is considered.

Endometrial (Uterine) Cancer

Endometrial cancer is the second most common genital malignancy. It is estimated that 1 in 100 women in the United States will develop uterine cancer.[2]

Etiology and Risk Factors

Endometrial cancer is related to the hormone estrogen because estrogen is the primary stimulant of endometrial proliferation. The mechanism of malignant change has not been identified. See Risk Factors and Levels of Prevention feature for Endometrial Cancer for further information.

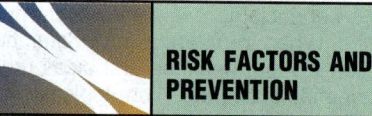

RISK FACTORS AND LEVELS OF PREVENTION

Endometrial Cancer

Risk Factors

- Exogenous estrogen replacement therapy for long periods without concomitant progesterone therapy
- Obesity (increased estrogen production and storage)
- History of pelvic radiation
- Hyperestrogenism: early menarche, late menopause, dysfunctional uterine bleeding, delayed onset of ovulation
- Old age
- Other reproductive cancer, including breast cancer
- History of infertility or habitual abortion
- Family history
- History of diabetes or hypertension
- White race
- Postmenopausal bleeding

Levels of Prevention

Primary Prevention

- Advise overweight clients to lose weight.
- Educate clients about the proper use of estrogens.
- Monitor clients for adequate control of diabetes and hypertension.

Secondary Prevention

- Advise women of menopause age or older to have a yearly pelvic examination and Pap smear (only effective in diagnosing endometrial cancer 50% of the time).
- Ensure that high-risk women have an endometrial tissue sample taken at menopause and at regular intervals.
- Assess any women experiencing postmenopausal bleeding.

Pathophysiology

The cell type in endometrial cancer is usually adenocarcinoma (involving the glands), a relatively slow-growing tumor that metastasizes late in its course. It tends to spread slowly to other organs. Most commonly, the carcinoma invades the uterus. From the uterus, it can spread to other peritoneal structures, including the lymphatics and blood vessels. It can then spread to the vagina, through the lymphatics to other areas, and occasionally to distant structures such as the brain and lungs.

Endometrial cancer may extensively invade the uterus, causing uterine enlargement. Extension of the cancerous process may occur along the endometrial surface to the cervix or fallopian tubes and ovaries. After invading the cervix, further spread resembles that of cervical cancer.

If cervical cancer is diagnosed early, its prognosis is relatively good. Once endometrial cancer has spread to the cervix, significantly invaded the myometrium, in-creased the size of the uterus, or spread outside the uterus, the prognosis is more serious.

Clinical Manifestations and Diagnostic Findings

Currently, there is no practical, accurate method of screening women for endometrial cancer. Thus, the cancer is usually discovered after the first manifestations appear. The most significant manifestation is some type of abnormal uterine bleeding, especially postmenopausal bleeding. This occurs relatively late in the disease. Other manifestations relate to invasion, metastasis to other organs, or both (Fig. 84–9).

A diagnosis of endometrial cancer is usually established by pelvic examination under anesthesia, followed immediately by D & C. D & C is used to obtain tissues for pathologic analysis. Women at high risk may have

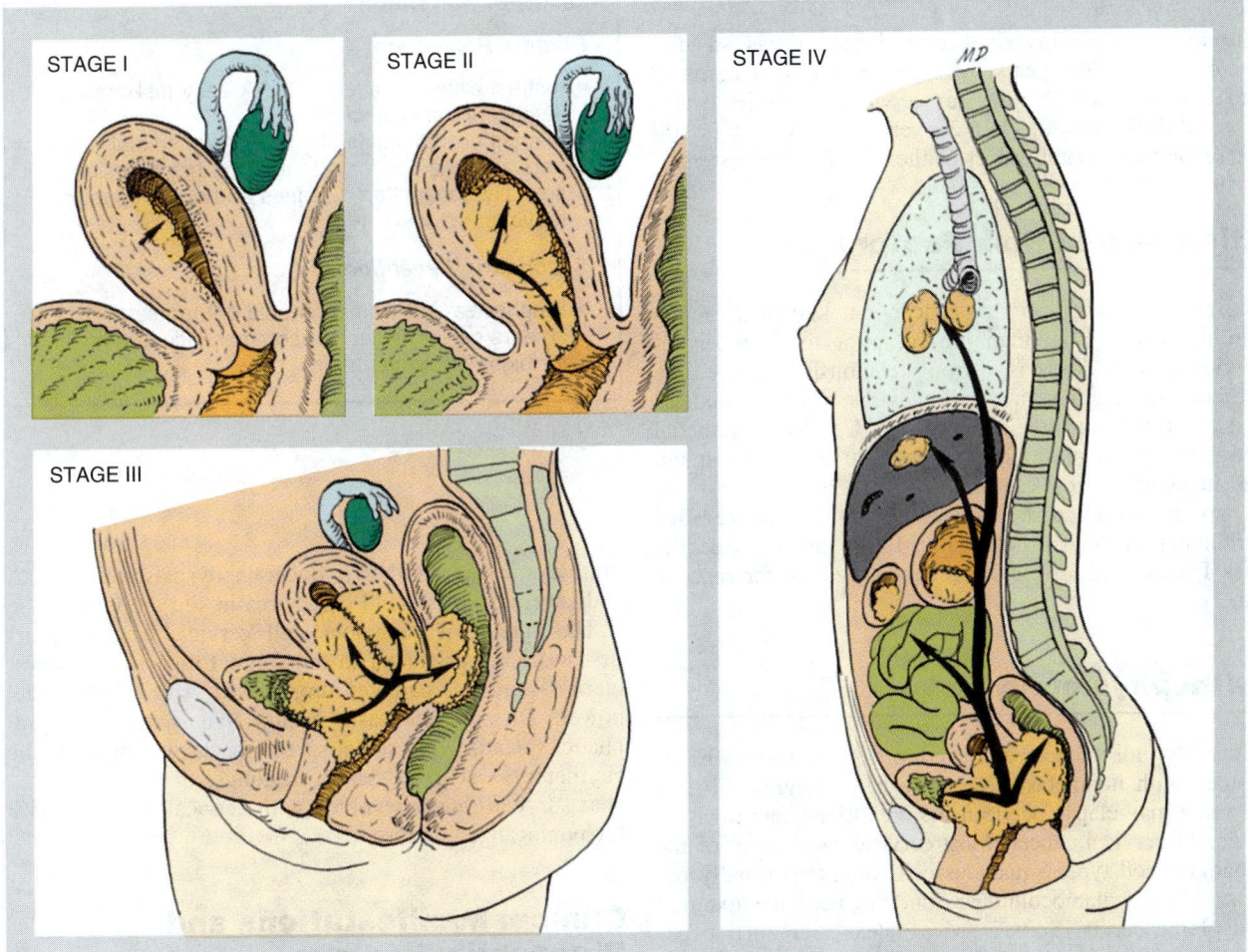

Figure 84–9. Staging uterine cancer. Stage 1: The tumor is confined to the uterine corpus. Stage 2: The cancer has invaded the cervix also. Stage 3: The cancer has spread beyond the uterus, but remains confined to the pelvis, such as in the bladder or rectum. Stage 4: Highest level of invasiveness as the cancer has spread beyond the pelvis, causing metastatic disease and large masses, such as in the liver or lungs.

periodic sampling via uterine washings. Occasionally, a hysterosalpingogram (an x-ray study using a contrast medium to show the uterus and fallopian tubes) or a hysteroscopy (use of an instrument to visualize uterine contents) is used to assist with the diagnosis.

Management

Precancerous endometrial changes may be treated with the hormone progesterone. Chemotherapy and hormonal therapy with estrogen and tamoxifen (Nolvadex) are used to treat late stages of endometrial cancer.

Endometrial cancer is generally treated with surgery, radiation, or a combination of both. Early endometrial cancer is surgically treated by a TAH-BSO. Surgery may be preceded or followed by irradiation, either external of internal.

See the sections on cervical cancer and uterine fibroids for nursing management.

Cervical Cancer

The incidence of invasive cervical cancer has steadily decreased over the years, whereas cervical carcinoma in situ has risen. Death rates for cervical cancer have also dropped 50% over the last 20 years; however, it is still the second most fatal cancer of the reproductive system.

Etiology and Risk Factors

The exact cause of cervical cancer is unknown, although chronic irritation is often present prior to diagnosis of cervical cancer. There is a strong relationship between the presence of the human papillomavirus types 16 and 18 and cervical intraepithelial neoplasia. Cervical intrathelial neoplasia has increasingly progressed to carcinoma in situ and invasive cervical cancer.

Pap smears are particularly important because cervical carcinoma in situ is potentially 100% curable. See the Risk Factors and Levels of Prevention feature for cervical cancer.

Pathophysiology

Potentially, all women with carcinoma in situ and 90% of women with nonmetastatic disease can be cured. Five to 10 years may elapse between the preinvasive and invasive stages of cervical cancer. Most cervical cancers are of the squamous cell type. Squamous cell carcinoma usually begins at the squamocolumnar junction near the external end of the cervix. Some cervical adenocarcinomas occur but are more difficult to diagnose. Adenocarcinoma generally involves the endocervical glands.

Cervical dysplasia, the earliest premalignant change noted in cervical epithelium, is now further divided into several levels of cervical intraepithelial neoplasia (CIN):

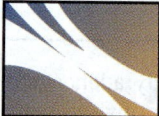

RISK FACTORS AND LEVELS OF PREVENTION

Cervical Cancer

Risk Factors

- Age: highest risk for carcinoma in situ is 25 to 40 years of age and highest risk for invasive cancer is age 40 to 60
- Black and Native American
- Prostitution
- Low socioeconomic class
- Multiparity
- Early age of first intercourse and frequent intercourse with multiple partners
- Early first pregnancy
- Postpartum lacerations
- Untreated chronic cervicitis
- Sexually transmitted disease
- Partner with history of penile or prostate cancer
- Infection with human papillomavirus

Levels of Prevention

Primary Prevention

- Instruct clients to avoid or seek early treatment of vaginal or cervical infection.
- Instruct clients to limit the number of sexual partners and use condoms to limit the transmission of sexually transmitted diseases and human papillomavirus.

Secondary Prevention

- Emphasize that women should get regular Pap smears per physician's recommendations (yearly for high-risk women).

mild dysplasia is CIN 1, moderate dysplasia is CIN 2, and severe dysplasia and carcinoma in situ are CIN 3.

The spread of squamous cell cervical cancer occurs first by direct extension to the vaginal mucosa, the lower uterine segment, parametrium, pelvic wall, bladder, and bowel. Distant metastasis occurs mainly through lymphatic spread, with some spread occurring through the circulatory system to the liver, lungs, or bones. The 5-year survival rate for women with cervical cancer is 65% for nonlocalized disease.

Clinical Manifestations and Diagnostic Findings

There are no early indications of carcinoma in situ or early cervical cancer. An abnormal Pap smear, however, is an indication for further assessment.

Late assessment findings include the presence of vaginal discharge and bleeding, especially after intercourse. Metrorrhagia (uterine bleeding between normal menses), postmenopausal bleeding, and polymenorrhea (increased frequency of menstrual bleeding) may be present. However, early bleeding also may occur as spotting or contact bleeding from cervical trauma secondary to sexual intercourse or douching. This early minimal bleeding increases in amount and duration as the cancer progresses. It usually indicates that the disease process involves the lymphatics.

Vaginal discharge, which is normally watery, becomes dark and foul-smelling as the disease advances. With infection of the neoplastic area, the discharge becomes more profuse and malodorous. Concurrent bleeding also adds to the unpleasantness of the condition.

Other assessment findings that develop as the disease progresses relate to the areas involved in the malignant process. These include pressure on the bowel, bladder, or both; bladder irritation; rectal discharge; manifestations of ureteral obstruction; and heavy, aching abdominal pain. Fistula formation may occur as the malignancy erodes through the walls of adjacent organs.

Pain is another late manifestation. It usually becomes a difficult problem with the onset of the cachexia (general wasting) that often accompanies the terminal stage of cancer.

The Pap smear is the primary diagnostic tool for cervical cancer. Further assessment of an abnormal Pap smear typically includes repeated cytologic and pelvic examinations. Also, colposcopic examination often helps locate lesions for biopsy. Biopsies are performed through a colposcope for better visualization. These biopsies are commonly performed as an office procedure and cause moderate discomfort to the client.

Less commonly, Schiller's test may be performed prior to biopsy. This test consists of cleaning the debris off the cervix and then painting the tissue with an iodine preparation. Abnormal tissue, which is glycogen-depleted, does not stain. The biopsy is then performed by removing a bit of tissue from various areas, including all areas that are not stained.

Occasionally, biopsies may be obtained by cold conization. This may be performed when colposcopic examination is not considered adequate. Cold conization involves obtaining a cone-shaped section of the cervix with a scalpel. This procedure provides more tissue for analysis, thus increasing the chances of identifying an area of invasive carcinoma, because invasive carcinoma and carcinoma in situ may coexist in the same woman. The procedure is particularly helpful if areas that are not readily visualized, such as the endocervical glands, are involved.

Sometimes, analysis of the tissue removed during a cold conization demonstrates that a wide area of normal tissue surrounds an excised malignancy. When this situation occurs, conization serves not only as the diagnostic procedure but may be the only treatment needed. This procedure allows the woman to maintain reproductive capacity, which may be an important consideration. Cautery or cryosurgery (freezing of the cervical tissues) may be performed instead of cold conization.

Acute and Subacute Care

■ Medical Management

Irradiation is used as primary therapy for early cervical cancer (see Chapter 24 for further information on radiation implants). It is usually curative, but it induces menopause.

Treatment of women with cervical cancer during pregnancy varies, depending on the stage of the cancer, the duration of the pregnancy, and the woman's wish for a child. A woman can usually complete the pregnancy if cervical intraepithelial neoplasia or carcinoma in situ is diagnosed. She may then be treated with conization 2 to 3 months post partum if further childbearing is wanted. However, if invasive cervical carcinoma is diagnosed in a pregnant woman, abortion is recommended up to 24 weeks in the pregnancy. After 24 weeks, therapy is delayed until the fetus is viable (28–32 weeks) and a cesarean section is performed. The woman may then be treated with either hysterectomy or irradiation in the postpartum period.

■ Nursing Management of the Medical Client

The care of a client with radiation implants is covered in Chapter 24.

Irradiation thins the vaginal epithelium and reduces vaginal lubrication. It may also cause vaginal adhesions and stenosis. Such changes can make vaginal sexual activities uncomfortable or painful. Vaginal penetration during the course of irradiation and the subsequent months minimizes the possibility of vaginal stenosis and contracture. Depending on personal preference, vaginal penetration and dilation can be accomplished with the woman's own fingers, a vaginal dilator, or her sexual partner's fingers or penis.

All women who have been treated conservatively for cervical cancer need information about recurrence. Encourage women who have been treated for cervical cancer to have frequent health examinations to diagnose a possible recurrence of the cancer early so it can be treated before it spreads too far. The client should have a pelvic examination and Pap smears scheduled at regular intervals as advised by the physician.

■ Surgical Management

Treatment ranges from cryosurgery, conization, or laser for local stage 0 tumors, to a radical hysterectomy for invasive cervical cancer.

Cryosurgery is the local freezing of abnormal cells and tissues with volatile gases such as nitrous gases (nitrous oxide, Freon, or carbon dioxide). Cell death results from dehydration and cell membrane destruction. Dead tissue then sloughs off.

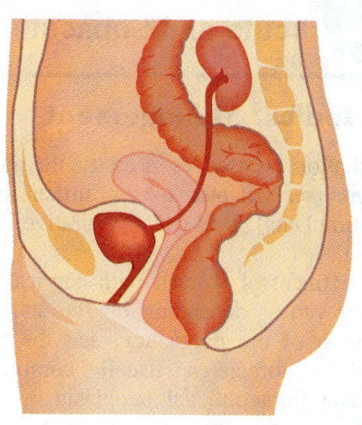

A   Normal anatomy

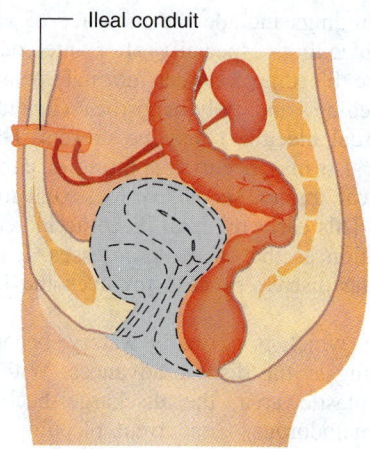

Ileal conduit

B   Anterior exenteration

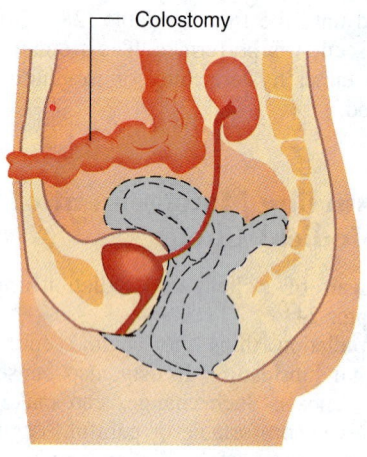

Colostomy

C   Posterior exenteration

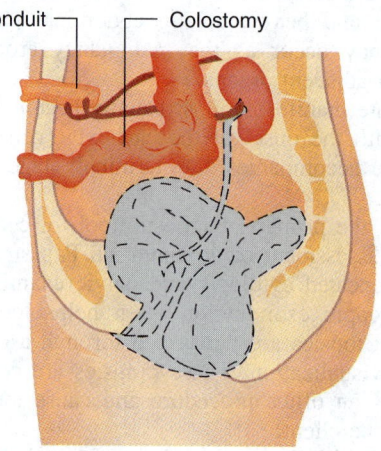

Ileal conduit   Colostomy

D   Total exenteration

Figure 84–10. Pelvic exenteration. *A*, Natural pelvic structures. *B*, Anterior exenteration—formation of the ileal conduit. *C*, Posterior exenteration—formation of colostomy. *D*, Total exenteration—formation of both ileal conduit and colostomy.

Conization is the removal of a small cone of tissue with a sharp instrument. Laser therapy also may be performed to remove abnormal tissue. There is usually minimal bleeding; however, the client may note a slight vaginal discharge.

A total abdominal hysterectomy can be used to treat carcinoma in situ in women who have finished childbearing or to treat invasive cancer. Pelvic exenteration (Fig. 84–10), an extremely radical procedure, is rarely performed. A total pelvic exenteration involves removal of all pelvic organs, including the uterus, tubes, ovaries, vagina, bladder, rectum, and colon. An ileal conduit and ileostomy are performed. With an anterior exenteration, the rectum and colon are left intact, but all other pelvic organs are removed and an ileal conduit is performed. In a posterior exenteration, the bladder is left intact, but the other pelvic organs are removed and an ileostomy is performed.

■ Nursing Management of the Surgical Client

Care of the client with a hysterectomy is discussed in the section on uterine fibroids. For women undergoing a pelvic exenteration, see Chapter 56 for care of the client with an ileal conduit and Chapter 62 for care of the client with a colostomy or ileostomy.

Nursing preparation of a woman for cryosurgery and laser therapy involves clarifying that this procedure is not actual surgery and an incision will not be made. Explain that the procedure is performed with a vaginal speculum in place, as during a routine pelvic examination. During treatment, a few women experience headaches, dizziness, flushing, and some cramping.

During the procedure, provide psychological support by (1) staying with the client; (2) informing her of what is to be done; (3) talking with her, listening to her, and facili-

tating her expression of concerns; (4) continuing to acknowledge her presence during the procedure rather than
excluding her; and (5) allowing her to retain as much
self-control as possible. For example, tell her what she
can do during the procedure to help it move along
quickly and smoothly. Also, discuss how she can help
manage postprocedure discomfort, such as performing
slow, deep breathing.

Assess the woman's discomfort during the procedure.
A mild analgesic may be prescribed for the pain following the procedure. Tell the client what to expect afterward. Mild pain may continue for several days. A clear,
watery discharge occurs. For about 14 days, this is followed by discharge containing debris (dead cells), which
may be malodorous. If the discharge continues longer
than 8 weeks, an infection is suspected.

Meticulous perineal hygiene minimizes the risk of infection and makes the client more comfortable. Healing
takes about 10 weeks. Showers or sponge baths should be
taken during this time; avoid tub or sitz baths.

Following a radical hysterectomy, the vagina is shortened and the trigone region of the bladder and the sigmoid colon may adhere to the vaginal apex. This may
cause dyspareunia felt deep in the pelvis. It is recommended that during penile penetration, the woman keep
her thighs adducted and use her thumb and index finger
at the vaginal opening to encircle the shaft of the penis,
providing some extra length to the vagina.

Some women with cervical cancer become terminally
ill despite vigorous treatment. When this situation occurs,
goals change and are directed toward physiologic and
psychosocial comfort. Pain relief (see Chapter 17) may be
accomplished through use of narcotic analgesics. Palliative irradiation also can be used as a pain relief measure
in many cases.

■ Modifications for Elderly Clients

Older clients may have cervical cancer treated by less
invasive methods. The older client undergoing internal
radiation treatments should be monitored closely following treatment for the development of fistulas.

Uterine Prolapse

Prolapse (descent, procidentia) of the uterus occurs in
three stages (Fig. 84–11):

- *First degree.* The uterus descends into the vaginal canal, and the cervix reaches but does not go through the
  introitus.
- *Second degree.* The body of the uterus is still within
  the vagina, but the cervix protrudes through the introitus.
- *Third degree.* The entire uterus and cervix protrude
  through the introitus, and the vaginal canal is inverted
  (turned inside out).

Risk factors for uterine prolapse include multiparity,
childbirth trauma, aging, and failure to maintain the perineal musculature. The occurrence of uterine prolapse has

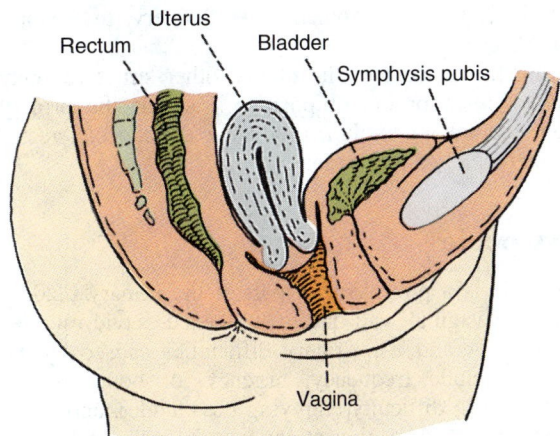

FIRST-DEGREE PROLAPSE

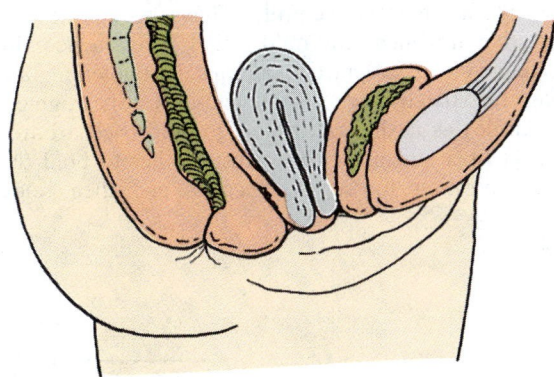

SECOND-DEGREE PROLAPSE

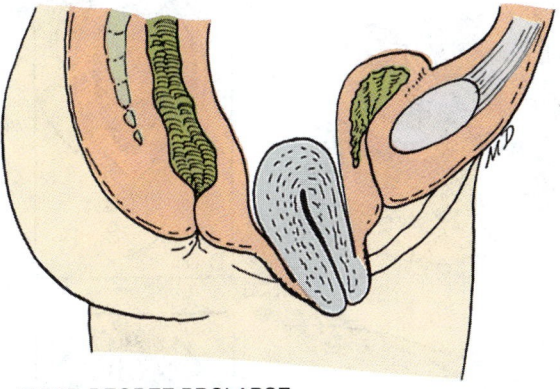

THIRD-DEGREE PROLAPSE

Figure 84–11. Uterine prolapse. White plastic cylinders,
placed at the ends of the applicator tandem and ovoids, keep the
radioactive implants properly positioned. The assembled device
is inserted as shown below. Cesium implants (at the tips of the
placement rod and wires) are inserted through the applicator and
left in place, close to the malignancy, for a prescribed length of
time.

decreased with improved obstetric care (e.g., less use of
forceps during delivery and better preparation of women
for labor). The nurse can help prevent prolapse by (1)
encouraging pregnant women to seek qualified obstetric

care and (2) teaching women, after delivery, to perform Kegel exercises.

During the descent of the uterus, other structures may be pulled down or out of position, such as the urinary bladder, rectum, or urethra, producing a cystocele, rectocele, enterocele, or urethrocele.

■ Cystocele

A cystocele is a protrusion of part of the urinary bladder through the vaginal wall due to weakened pelvic muscles (Fig. 84–12A and B). Urinary difficulties caused by the cystocele include frequency, urgency, or both; urinary tract infections; difficulty emptying the bladder; and stress incontinence. Mild manifestations may be relieved by pelvic (perineal) strengthening (Kegel) exercises. Kegel exercises may be prescribed to help a woman achieve pubococcygeal muscle control. This is a form of conservative treatment for mild stress incontinence. Instruct the woman to practice alternately tightening and relaxing her rectal and vaginal muscles. She tightens these muscles as if she were trying to hold back a bowel movement or a stream of urine. Instruct her to hold this tightened position for a few seconds and then relax.

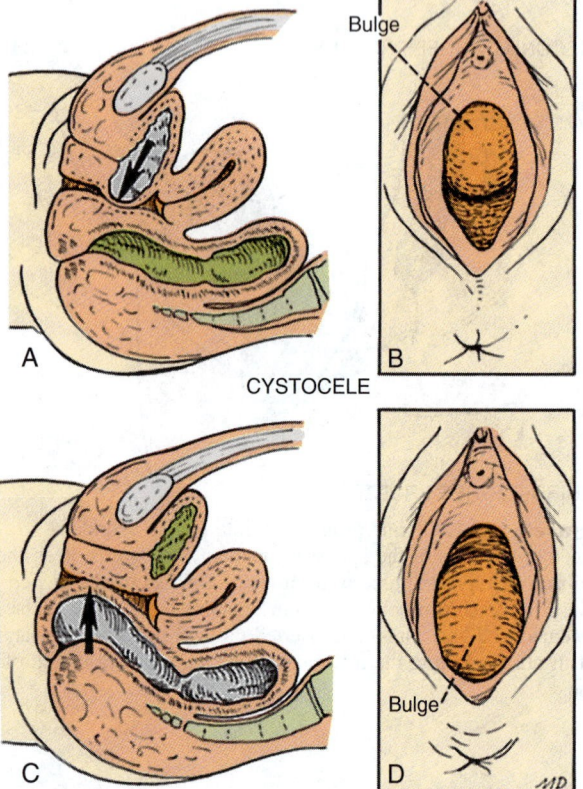

Figure 84–12. *A,* Cystocele. Note the bulging of the anterior vaginal wall. The urinary bladder is displaced downward. *B,* This pushes the anterior vaginal wall downward into the vagina. *C,* Rectocele. *D,* Note the bulging of the posterior vaginal wall.

These exercises can be performed frequently during the day, whenever the woman thinks of them. Or they may be performed a specified number of times (50–100) once or twice a day.

When manifestations are severe, a cystocele is corrected surgically by tightening the pelvic muscles to provide better bladder support. This type of vaginal surgery is known as anterior colporrhaphy or anterior repair. Nursing care is the same as for a vaginal hysterectomy (see the section on uterine prolapse).

■ Rectocele

A rectocele is the protrusion of a portion of the rectum through a weak place in the vaginal wall musculature (Fig. 84–12C and D). A rectocele produces constipation, heaviness, and hemorrhoids. Additionally, a rectocele may be associated with incomplete or complete tearing of the anal sphincter.

Surgical management is used to correct this problem by strengthening the weakened muscles. This is known as a posterior colporrhaphy or posterior repair. Occasionally, this procedure is performed with an anterior repair. It is then called an anteroposterior colporrhaphy or anteroposterior repair. A low residue diet and a cathartic are used before surgery to empty the bowel. Postoperatively, the client is given a low residue diet until healing occurs and then stool softeners to prevent straining. The client is warned to avoid constipation, which could cause recurrence.

■ Enterocele and Urethrocele

Other problems associated with uterine prolapse are enterocele (protrusion of a portion of the small intestine through the vaginal wall) and urethrocele (protrusion of a portion of the urethra through the vaginal wall). Because they result from weakened pelvic support, these conditions occur together, separately, or in conjunction with uterine prolapse. All these disorders cause pelvic pressure, backache, and other vague manifestations. Treatment is the same as for the cystocele and rectocele.

■ Complete Uterine Prolapse

Complete prolapse of the uterus usually develops gradually. When it is complete and also involves a cystocele, rectocele, and enterocele, the woman is said to have pelvic relaxation. When the cervix protrudes through the vaginal orifice, it is exposed and constantly irritated. Tissue changes occur, and malignant degeneration is possible. Also, the vaginal mucosa is subjected to drying, trauma, and irritation once it is exposed.

Clinical manifestations experienced by the woman with uterine prolapse do not necessarily correlate with the amount of prolapse present. However, most women with a significant degree of prolapse feel something is descending internally. Other findings include dyspareunia and vague abdominal problems, including feelings of pressure, dragging, heaviness, backaches, and bowel and bladder manifestations. Stress incontinence also may be present.

Acute and Subacute Care

■ Surgical Management

Treatment of prolapse depends on the extent of prolapse, the woman's age, and her wishes for childbearing. The most effective treatment is a vaginal hysterectomy, although a vaginal pessary may be used if surgery is not wanted. For a vaginal hysterectomy, an incision is made through the vaginal wall into the pelvic cavity. The uterus is removed from its supporting ligaments (broad, round, and uterosacral). The supporting ligaments are attached to the vaginal cuff to maintain the normal vaginal length. Special care is given to the Foley catheter to keep the bladder decompressed and pressure off the anterior vaginal muscles until adequate healing has occurred. When the catheter is removed, the woman must be taught to keep her bladder empty by voiding every 2 hours to help prevent recurrence.

■ Nursing Management of the Surgical Client

Postoperatively, the nurse should monitor the client closely for excessive vaginal bleeding. There is normally a small-to-moderate amount of pink, yellow, or brown serous drainage, or even a small amount of frank vaginal bleeding may occur. If heavy vaginal bleeding is accompanied by a rapidly distending, rigid abdomen, referred shoulder pain, and indications of shock, immediate surgery may be indicated. Other times of potential bleeding are the 4th, 9th, 14th, and 21st days following surgery as the sutures dissolve. If vaginal packing, a drain, or both are in place, the surgeon usually removes them after 24 to 48 hours. Often, postoperative sitz baths are prescribed, usually beginning on the first postoperative day.

■ Medical Management

Although it is used infrequently, a vaginal pessary may be prescribed as an alternative to surgery. This device is used to hold the uterus in the correct position. Pessaries come in different sizes and styles. After manually moving the uterus to a normal position, a pessary is inserted to keep it in place. A correctly inserted pessary cannot be felt and maintains the uterine position by holding the cervix posteriorly, which allows the uterus to fall forward. Before leaving the clinician's office, the woman should have a pelvic examination to ensure the pessary stays in place during bodily movements and that it does not interfere with urination.

■ Nursing Management of the Medical Client

A pessary irritates the vaginal mucosa. Therefore, instruct the client to douche twice a week with commercially prepared solutions of the proper pH or with vinegar, 1 tablespoon per pint of water, to remove vaginal debris. Follow-up care is important. Four to 6 weeks following insertion of the pessary, the woman needs professional reassessment. At that time, the clinician performs a pelvic examination to assess whether or not the pessary is irritating the tissues excessively. It may be changed or removed as indicated.

If it is left in place too long, a pessary may erode the cervix and adhere to the mucosa. Make sure the woman understands the need for frequent examinations. The pessary should be checked, removed, and cleaned every 3 to 4 months. Some women can be taught to do this themselves, but most women need assistance.

Polyps

Polyps are pedunculated tumors arising from the mucosa and extending into the opening of a body cavity. Genital polyps occur primarily in the uterus and cervix (Fig. 84–13). Uterine polyps may cause hypermenorrhea, intermenstrual bleeding, and postmenopausal bleeding. They occasionally undergo malignant changes, particularly in postmenopausal women. Cervical polyps may bleed following vaginal intercourse and are prone to infection.

If polyps are asymptomatic, they may simply be monitored. Since cervical polyps have a pedicle, they are easily removed by snipping or ligating them. This procedure is usually performed in the physician's office. Uterine polyps are not easily removed because of their location within the uterus. Uterine polyps do not usually require removal, but if removal is needed, it is usually performed by D & C.

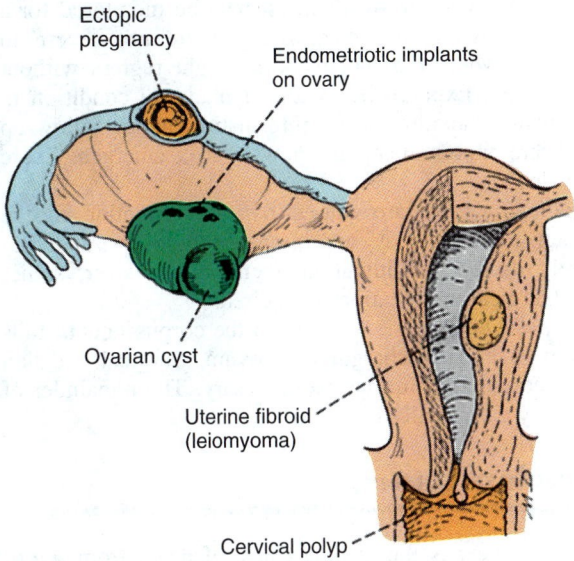

Figure 84–13. Common sites of some common benign gynecologic lesions.

Ovarian Disorders

Benign Ovarian Tumors

Benign ovarian tumors are either solid or cystic. Ovarian tumors are often asymptomatic until they are large enough to cause pressure. This makes early detection of malignancies difficult. Typical manifestations associated with pressure include constipation, urinary frequency, a full feeling in the abdomen, vague pelvic aching and sensations of heaviness, painful defecation, and dyspareunia. Acute pain may be experienced during menses. Often, the woman's abdominal girth increases and her clothes may not fit as well. Generally, the woman is unable to become pregnant.

Later manifestations include marked abdominal distention with dyspnea, peripheral edema, and anorexia. Pelvic pain may be present as a later manifestation if the ovarian tumor is growing rapidly. If the tumor produces hormones, there may be menstrual irregularities and masculinizing or feminizing effects.

Complications from ovarian tumors include (1) hemorrhage into a cyst, with rupture and possible infection; (2) torsion of a cystic pedicle; and (3) malignant changes.

Treatment depends on the type of tumor. Tumors are removed surgically, either through laparoscopy or open surgery, when they are bilateral, growing rapidly, or disrupt function of the pelvic organs or the ovary. Surgery may include removal of (1) only the tumor, (2) the tumor and the ovary or ovaries, or (3) the tumor, both ovaries and tubes, and the uterus. The type of nursing care needed depends on the specific type of surgery performed.

Ovarian cysts are physiologic tumors of ovaries. They are common and may or may not produce manifestations. When manifestations do occur, the women may experience pelvic pain that is often worse on one side, pressure in the lower abdomen, backache, and menstrual irregularities.

A woman with an ovarian cyst may be monitored for a month or two if her manifestations are not severe to determine whether or not the cyst might regress without intervention. Explain the treatment plan and condition to the client. She also needs information about follow-up healthcare appointments and how to seek emergency care if needed.

Follicular cysts are caused by fluid retention in the ovarian follicle. They are often symptomless and frequently disappear without intervention. However, sometimes surgical intervention is required.

Corpus luteum cysts form when the corpus luteum fails to regress after discharging the ovum. Surgical excision of the corpus luteum may be necessary. The remainder of the ovary can usually be saved.

Ovarian Cancer

Ovarian cancer is the leading cause of death from reproductive malignancies. The death rates have risen over time, probably due to lack of early detection methods.

Ovarian cancer ranks second to uterine cancer in incidence of female genital cancers. White women have a higher rate of ovarian cancer than black women.

Etiology and Risk Factors

The cause of ovarian cancer is unknown. A family history of ovarian cancer is one of the highest risk factors identified. An environmental link has been suggested, but there is no substantial evidence for this at present. Numerous other causes have been suggested and are currently under study. See Risk Factors and Levels of Prevention feature for ovarian cancer.

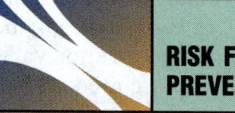

RISK FACTORS AND LEVELS OF PREVENTION

Ovarian Cancer

Risk Factors

- Age over 40 years
- Family history of ovarian cancer
- Nulliparity
- History of infertility
- History of heavy menstrual bleeding and dysmenorrhea
- North American or northern European descent
- Personal history of endometrial, colon, or breast cancer
- Obesity, especially with high intake of animal fats (under investigation)
- Use of ovulation-stimulating medications for infertility (under investigation)

Levels of Prevention

Primary Prevention

Tell clients that ovarian cancer may be prevented by anything that interrupts constant ovulatory cycles, such as:

- More than one full-term pregnancy
- Oral contraceptive use
- Breast-feeding
- Castration, bilateral oophorectomy

Secondary Prevention

- Encourage women to get a routine pelvic examination with bimanual rectovaginal examination.
- Determine CA-125 antigen levels in high-risk women.
- Obtain transvaginal ultrasound combined with bimanual pelvic examination, and Doppler studies for suspicious lesions.

Tertiary Prevention

- Obtain second-look surgery following chemotherapy.

Pathophysiology

Most ovarian cancers are epithelial tumors. However, some are adenocarcinomas. Ovarian cancer tends to grow and spread silently (without manifestations) until it causes pressure on adjacent organs or abdominal distention. When these pressure-related manifestations finally appear, the malignancy has usually spread to the fallopian tubes, uterus, and ligaments. Ovarian cancer often spreads to the other ovary and associated structures. The cancer may invade bowel surfaces, the omentum, liver, and other organs. When the pelvic blood vessels become involved, distant metastasis occurs. The usual routes of spread include lymphatic, hematogenous, local extension, and peritoneal seeding.

Ovarian cancer is the leading cause of death in women with genital cancer. Despite new treatment techniques, there has been no significant improvement in long-term survival rates for women with this disease.

Clinical Manifestations and Diagnostic Findings

Clinical manifestations of ovarian cancer include abdominal distention, urinary frequency and urgency, pleural effusion, malnutrition, pain from pressure caused by the growing tumor, and the effects of urinary or bowel obstruction, constipation, ascites with dyspnea, and ultimately, general severe pain. Indications of ovarian cancer do not typically occur until the malignancy is well established, which is often not until it has spread. Unfortunately, unless the malignancy is diagnosed early (e.g., when asymptomatic), most women eventually develop terminal cancer.

Palpation of the ovary in postmenopausal women should always be considered an abnormal finding and should be followed up.

Identification of a pelvic mass by palpation is usually the first assessment finding. However, detecting such a mass may be difficult in obese women or those who cannot relax during the examination. When an ovarian mass is suspected, a complete work-up is performed, including an intravenous pyelogram (IVP) and a barium enema. Ultrasonography may be performed to detect a mass. Generally, following the work-up, exploratory surgery is performed to look directly at the ovaries, and if the mass is malignant, it is resected.

Acute and Subacute Care

■ Surgical Management

The extent of an ovarian malignancy is determined by exploratory surgery. Ovarian cancer is usually treated aggressively. A young woman with a borderline malignancy may be treated conservatively with a TAH-BSO. However, generally, the surgery of choice is a TAH-BSO, partial or complete omentectomy, and removal of all visi-

ble tumor. The less residual tumor left, the better the prognosis.

Some women with ovarian cancer recover following treatment. Commonly, women who are clinically free of disease and who have received chemotherapy for 6 to 24 months have a second-look laparotomy to decide whether or not treatment should be continued. At this time, multiple biopsies are done to determine if any tumor is still present.

■ Medical Management

Adjuvant therapy varies with the stage of the disease. With stage I ovarian cancer, women typically receive irradiation or chemotherapy following surgery to destroy cancer cells that may have spread into the abdominal cavity. Intraperitoneal and systemic chemotherapy may be administered (see Chapter 24).

Women with stage II or later ovarian cancers typically receive the same treatment as those with stage I disease, with the inclusion of pelvic and, possibly, abdominal radiation. Intraperitoneal radioactive phosphorus is sometimes used.

■ Nursing Management of the Medical/Surgical Client

See the section on nursing care of the client with a TAH-BSO for care of the client with ovarian cancer.

Vaginal Disorders

Vaginal Discharge and Pruritus

The female reproductive tract maintains its integrity through various natural defense mechanisms. Inflammation and infection occur when organisms disrupt or overcome these natural defenses. The resulting manifestations, although usually not life-threatening, can be uncomfortable and annoying. Vaginal discharge and itching are among the most frequent problems women mention to healthcare providers.

All women have normal, nonbloody, asymptomatic vaginal discharge called *leukorrhea*. This discharge, secreted by the endocervical glands, is a clear exudate that keeps vaginal mucous membranes moist and clear. As this exudate passes through the vagina, it may become cloudy and acquire a slight odor as desquamated epithelial cells, leukocytes, and normal vaginal flora are added.

The amount of vaginal discharge often varies in relation to the menstrual cycle. It is greatest at ovulation and just before menses. Pregnancy, sexual stimulation, and oral contraceptives tend to increase the discharge. Some women view normal vaginal discharge and odor as offensive and to go great lengths to mitigate it. However, use of douches or vaginal deodorants may cause vaginal irritation and infection. The consensus in the medical literature is that periodic douching is unnecessary. There is some evidence that douching may actually be detrimental because it washes away normal protective mucus and bacterial flora of the vagina and may introduce other bacteria. Changes in the amount, color, character, or odor of vaginal discharges may indicate a problem.

The most common causes of vaginal discharge and irritation are vaginal infections; parasites, such as pinworms; sexually transmitted diseases (see Chapter 86); and mechanical or allergic irritants. An example of a mechanical irritant is a tampon left in place too long. Some forms of contraceptive creams or foams may be allergic irritants for some women.

Most inflammatory and infectious vaginal problems are accompanied by pathologic vaginal discharge, which may be copious, malodorous, and abnormal in color. The discharge frequently causes itching, irritation, and redness of the vulva and surrounding areas. It may be accompanied by burning and frequency of urination, anal discomfort, and pain in the lower abdominal region.

Vaginitis

Vaginitis is inflammation of the vagina, a common problem experienced by most women at some time in their life. Vaginitis has many causes and risk factors (see the Risk Factors and Levels of Prevention feature for vaginitis).

The vagina is a potential cavity with a normal protective population of flora, including various bacteria. The adult vagina is normally acidic because of lactic acid formed from the glycogen in desquamating vaginal epithelium. Normal vaginal function depends on a delicate balance between hormones and bacteria. Disturbance of this balance can precipitate infection.

Vaginitis is typically characterized by a change in vaginal discharge (i.e., it becomes profuse, odoriferous, and purulent).

Vaginitis is diagnosed on a pelvic examination. This examination may be painful because of the infection and must be performed as gently as possible. Some bleeding may occur during and after the examination. Tell the woman that pain and bleeding may occur, and provide her with a perineal pad.

Vaginitis can be a stubborn, discouraging problem. It requires early, vigorous treatment to avoid chronicity. Treatment is aimed at correcting the cause of the vaginitis. Attention must be given to the woman's overall health. See the Client Education Guide entitled "Preventing Vaginitis."

Atrophic Vaginitis

Atrophic vaginitis occurs in postmenopausal women. Atrophic, thin, vaginal mucosa and watery alkaline vaginal secretions provide an environment conducive to invasion by pyrogenic bacteria (as in simple vaginitis). Assessment findings include a discharge, which may be blood-flecked; a vaginal burning sensation; itching of the vagina and vulva; and dyspareunia. If secondary infection is present, vulval excoriation and burning with urination typically occur.

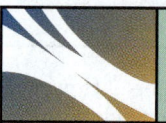

RISK FACTORS AND LEVELS OF PREVENTION

Vaginitis

Risk Factors

Any of the following can cause vaginitis:

- Change in normal vaginal flora
- Vaginal pH becomes more alkaline
- Virulent organisms invade the vagina

  These conditions can be caused by:

- Congestion of the pelvic organs
- Mechanical irritation
- Chemical irritation
- Vaginal infection
- Overmedication, especially with antibiotics
- Long-term steroid therapy
- Uncontrolled diabetes
- Acquired immunodeficiency syndrome

Levels of Prevention

Primary Prevention

- Ensure that clients' diabetes is well controlled.
- Advise clients to avoid douches and vaginal sprays.
- Advise clients to use adequate perineal hygiene.
- Advise clients to avoid long-term steroid and antibiotic use.
- Advise clients to avoid constricting clothing and synthetic underpants.

Secondary Prevention

- Instruct clients to seek early treatment for any change in vaginal drainage, especially malodorous or profuse vaginal drainage.
- Instruct clients to seek early treatment for any itching in the vaginal or perineal area.

Short-term use of estrogen cream is the usual medical treatment. If a secondary infection is present, additional therapy with an appropriate drug is added.

Vaginal Fistulas

Vaginal fistulas are abnormal tubelike passages from the vagina to the bladder (*vesicovaginal*), rectum (*rectovaginal*), or urethra (*urethrovaginal*) (Fig. 84–14). Fistulas are an extremely distressing and common problem in the genital and urinary tract.

Etiology and Risk Factors

Fistulas can be congenital or result from injury or surgery. About 10% of all fistulas occur in the female repro-

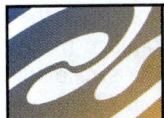

CLIENT EDUCATION GUIDE

Preventing Vaginitis

Client Instructions in English *(Instrucciones para el cliente en inglés)*	Client Instructions in Spanish *(Instrucciones para el cliente en español)*
Take care of yourself to prevent infection. Get enough rest, eat nutritious meals, and exercise at least three times a week.	Es importante que se cuide a sí misma para luchar contra una infección. Descanse bastante, coma alimentos nutritivos, y haga ejercicio por lo menos tres veces por semana.
After using the toilet, always wipe yourself from front to back to avoid spreading germs.	Limpiese siempre del frente hacia atrás después de usar el excusado (hacer del baño) para evitar la propagación de gérmenes.
Change tampons or sanitary pads at least four times a day during your menstrual period and wash your hands before and after each change.	Cambiese los tampones o toallas sanitarias por lo menos cuatro veces al día durante la menstruación (regla) y lavese las manos antes y después de cada cambio.
Avoid feminine hygiene sprays, which can be irritating. Soap and water are best for keeping yourself clean.	Evite el uso de aerosoles para la higiene femenina que pueden causar irritación. El agua y el jabón son mejores para guardarse limpia.
Avoid tight-fitting jeans, pants, pantyhose, non-cotton (e.g., nylon) underwear, or any garment restricting ventilation.	Evite usar pantalones de dril (jeans) o pantalones apretados, medias, calzones (nylon) o prendas interiores sin algodón, o cualquier prenda que restringe la ventilación.

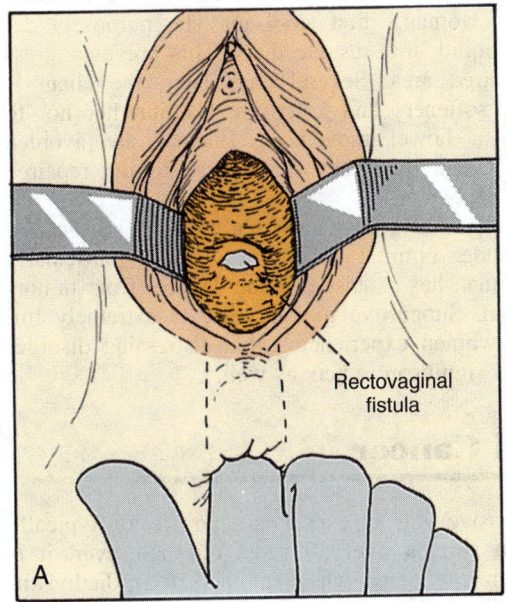

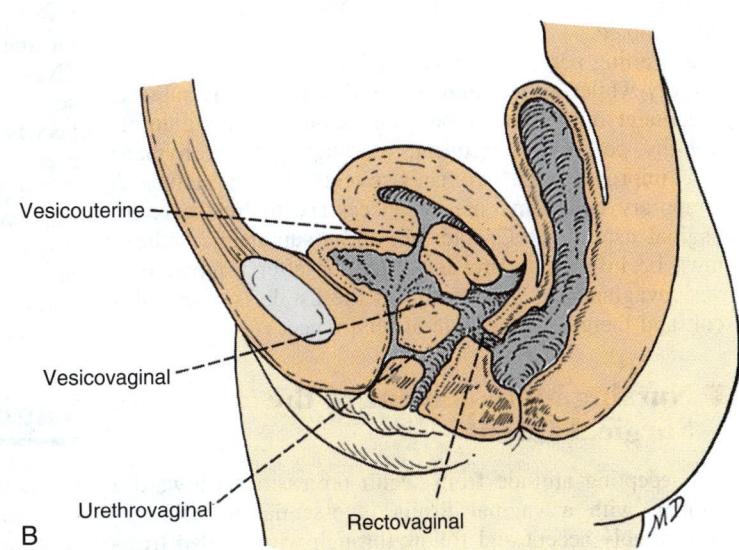

Figure 84–14. Vaginal fistulas. *A,* During examination, a rectovaginal fistula can be seen as the examiner's gloved finger (in the rectum) pushes upward toward the vagina. *B,* Locations of main types of vaginal fistulas.

ductive area. Vaginal fistulas may occur (1) as a result of the spread of a malignant lesion, (2) following irradiation for cancer, (3) as a result of venereal and other inflammatory disease (rare), and (4) after a prolonged, difficult labor and delivery.

Clinical Manifestations and Diagnostic Findings

Urine or flatus and feces leak into the vagina. Excoriation and irritation of vaginal and vulval tissues occur. Severe infection may occur. Rectovaginal fistulas may cause an offensive, particularly unpleasant odor. The woman experiences wetness and a sensation of feeling dirty.

In addition to producing unpleasant physical manifestations, vaginal fistulas produce severely distressing psychosocial problems. Women with vaginal fistulas often become social recluses, greatly disrupting their relationships with others and their social activities.

Women often do not seek professional healthcare until the problem becomes severe. Even then they may be embarrassed and reluctant to discuss it.

A fistulogram (injection of dye into the vagina) can be performed to assess the location and extent of the fistula.

Acute and Subacute Care

■ Surgical Management

The diagnosis and treatment of vaginal fistulas may be difficult. Treatment varies with the fistula's location, extent, and cause, and the woman's general condition. Small fistulas may heal spontaneously after 1 to 3 months; however, surgical excision is often needed. Surgery is not always successful. For this reason, it is important for the woman to be in optimal physical condition before surgery is attempted.

A waiting period of about 6 months is required prior to surgery while the inflammation and tissue edema subside. Treatment during this time focuses on preventing infection by performing frequent, thorough perineal hygiene and improving the woman's overall health status. A temporary colostomy may be necessary to treat a rectovaginal fistula (see Chapter 62) and a suprapubic catheter must be inserted to prevent distention after a repair of a vesicovaginal fistula. Excision of the fistula is often difficult and there is a high rate of recurrence.

■ Nursing Management of the Surgical Client

An accepting attitude from health professionals toward a woman with a vaginal fistula is essential to help her comfortably accept and follow through with needed treatments. During the time before surgery and again after surgery, the nurse helps the woman with a vaginal fistula to minimize the manifestations and care for herself.

Before surgery, some women inadvisably restrict their fluid intake in an attempt to decrease the drainage from a urinary fistula. This may actually increase the size of the fistula and increase the incidence of infection. Make sure the woman understands the importance of increasing her fluid intake to decrease the risk of infection. Perineal hygiene measures may include cleaning the perineum every 4 hours (with sterile materials after surgery), sitz baths, douches, and perineal pads (changed frequently). Deodorizing and comforting measures may include using vitamin A and D ointment, deodorant powders, and various types of prescribed weak acid or weak base irrigating solutions (depending on the urine pH). The solutions are poured over the perineum. Deodorizing douches also may be prescribed.

Caution a woman with a vaginal fistula to avoid using excessive pressure when douching because the water pressure may force the solution through the fistula tract, causing an infection.

Occasionally, an enema may be prescribed for a woman with a rectovaginal fistula to clean the bowel and temporarily decrease drainage. When an enema is done, a soft rubber catheter should be used. Gently insert the catheter above and away from the fistula tract.

Postoperatively, care is directed toward (1) avoiding stress on the repaired area and (2) preventing infection. A Foley or suprapubic catheter is used after a vesicovaginal or urethrovaginal fistulectomy to drain the urinary bladder. Careful attention is necessary to keep the catheter patent and draining. Also, provide and encourage enough fluid intake so that internal catheter irrigation is accomplished. The catheter is not routinely irrigated externally. If the catheter must be irrigated, use sterile solution and minimal pressure. Do not let the catheter become occluded because this pressure could reopen the fistula.

Rarely, women require an ileal conduit following fistula repair (see Chapter 56). After corrective bowel surgery, the woman's first stool may be purposely delayed with liquid, low residue diets. This prevents stress on the repaired area. Several days later, the client is given stool softeners and laxatives. Caution her not to strain with a bowel movement. Enemas are avoided because of the trauma they may cause to the repaired area.

Surgical repair of a vaginal fistula may not be successful, even under optimal conditions. This is particularly true if a woman has extensive tissue damage from tumors or irradiation. Supportive nursing care is extremely important for women experiencing this distressing disorder and for their significant others as well.

Vaginal Cancer

Primary invasive vaginal cancer is a rare lesion typically occurring in women over 50 years old. However, it is seen in younger women whose mothers took diethylstilbestrol (DES) during pregnancy. DES was widely prescribed in the United States from 1940 to 1960 for threatened miscarriage and other high-risk pregnancy problems.

Vaginal cancer in non-DES women is rare in black women and almost nonexistent in Jewish women.

Etiology and Risk Factors

The risk factor for vaginal cancer is maternal ingestion of DES (associated with clear cell vaginal cancer). Other potential causes of vaginal cancer include exposure to the drug in utero in girls and women between menarche and age 30 (adenocarcinoma), repeated pregnancies, the presence of syphilis, uterine prolapse, and pessary use. Leukoplakia and leukorrhea are often associated with vaginal cancer.

Pathophysiology

Primary in situ vaginal cancer also is rare, and when it occurs, it is usually part of an in situ vulval lesion. Secondary vaginal cancer is rare, but it may occur from trophoblastic disease.

The staging of vaginal cancer is similar to that used for other pelvic malignancies. The primary lesion and involvement of adjacent structures are considered. Primary invasive cancer tends to involve the anterior or posterior vaginal walls, or both. Complications may involve the urinary bladder or bowel, such as fistula formation.

Despite active treatment, the prognosis for vaginal cancer is generally poor. The overall cure rate reported by the American Cancer Society is about 35%. One-half of women with vaginal cancer die within 18 months of diagnosis.[2]

Low survival rates are due to (1) the rarity of the cancer (making it difficult to identify the best treatment), (2) the typically advanced stage of the cancer when diagnosed, and (3) the difficulty in treating this cancer with radiation or surgery because of the proximity of important structures.

Clinical Manifestations and Diagnostic Findings

Indications of vaginal cancer include foul vaginal discharge, painless vaginal bleeding, pruritus, pain (not associated with bleeding), and the presence of a vaginal mass or lesion. Urinary bladder manifestations such as pain and frequency may occur if a vaginal mass compresses the bladder.

Women exposed to DES in utero should receive careful examination of the cervix, along with cytologic examination of the cervix and any suspicious area in the vagina. Colposcopy may be used to identify areas to be biopsied. During pelvic examination, Lugol's solution may be applied to any vaginal areas that appear abnormal. Lack of staining identifies suspect areas. Unfortunately, the lesions of vaginal cancer are often well advanced before manifestations appear. Earlier lesions might be missed during pelvic examination.

Acute and Subacute Care

■ Medical Management

The usual treatment for vaginal cancer is either external or intravaginal radiation therapy or, less often, surgery. External radiation therapy is used for all stages of vaginal cancer. Internal radiation is generally used only in the earlier stages.

The difficulty of applying radiation to the vagina without harming adjacent tissues (i.e., bladder, rectum) has led some physicians to prefer surgical intervention.

■ Surgical Management

For earlier stages, radical hysterectomy, lymphadenectomy, and vaginectomy are performed. Vaginectomy refers to removal of the upper one third to one half of the vagina as part of the procedure in a radical hysterectomy. Pelvic exenteration (removal of pelvic organs, with an ileostomy and ileal conduit) is used in more advanced cancer when the bladder or rectum is involved. Pelvic exenteration is indicated when there are recurrent metastases.

■ Nursing Management of the Medical/Surgical Client

During assessment, ask young women born between 1940 and 1960 about medications their mothers may have taken during pregnancy. All whose mothers took DES when pregnant with them should have a gynecologic examination at least twice yearly beginning at menarche, or at age 14, whichever comes first.

Vaginal surgery may be anxiety-promoting and frightening to a woman. Ostomies (see Chapters 56 and 62) also may need to be performed, adding to the woman's fears and problems. Postoperatively, vaginal sexual activity is not possible unless vaginal reconstruction is performed.

Sexuality is an important nursing consideration in the care of women with vaginal cancer. Vaginal sex may be difficult after surgery or radiation therapy because of changes in the size and shape of the vagina. Assess the woman's previous sexual history and her self-esteem to identify possible problems. Create a therapeutic environment that allows the woman to feel comfortable discussing sexual concerns.

Discuss the potential impact of the disease process and treatment on sexuality, as appropriate. Potential problems include fatigue, pain, dyspareunia (secondary to radiation therapy), decreased libido, and altered body image (from surgery, radiation, or chemotherapy). If a partial vaginectomy (one-third to one-half removed) is performed, the woman can probably still enjoy normal vaginal sexual activity, using large amounts of lubricant and modified positioning, since vaginal tissue will stretch.

To cope with fatigue and pain, suggest that the woman schedule sexual activity after resting. Also, schedule pain medication so the peak of action coincides with sexual activity. A warm bath, back rub, positioning, or relaxation techniques might also help. Advise the client to use a water-soluble lubricant during intercourse and, perhaps, a vaginal dilator at other times to prevent vaginal fibrosis and tightening.

Vulvar Disorders

Vulvitis

Vulvitis (inflammation of the vulva) is caused by direct irritation of vulvar tissues or by direct extension of irritation from the vagina to the vulva. Itching and pruritus result. For information on the etiology of vulvitis, see the Risk Factors and Levels of Prevention feature for vulvitis.

Medical treatment is based on the specific cause of the condition. Itching (the most common manifestation) associated with vulvitis can be severe.

Antipruritics or antihistamines, such as hydrocortisone cream, diphenhydramine hydrochloride (Benadryl), or hydroxyzine hydrochloride (Atarax) may be given to relieve the itching, either locally or systemically.

Teach the client the following measures to relieve itching:

- Apply cold compresses
- Wear light, nonrestrictive clothing, including well-washed and well-rinsed cotton underpants (synthetic underpants tend to keep the vulvar area warm and moist)
- Avoid feminine hygiene sprays
- Apply prescribed hydrocortisone ointment or anesthetic sprays
- Keep the vulva clean and dry (e.g., clean after elimination—washing the vulva with soap and water, wiping with toilet tissue or a washcloth from front to back, rinsing and drying well, and applying cornstarch to maintain dryness)

Vulvar Cancer

Vulvar cancer is found mainly in women older than 50 years of age. It accounts for about 5% of female genital carcinoma.

Etiology and Risk Factors

Vulvar disorders such as leukoplakia, kraurosis, and diabetic vulvitis increase the risk of vulvar cancer. Sexually transmitted diseases, including the human papillomavirus, also increase the risk. See Risk Factors and Levels of Prevention feature for vulvar cancer.

Pathophysiology

Vulvar cancer arises from skin, urethra, glands, or subcutaneous tissues. Approximately 90% to 95% of vulvar cancers are squamous cell carcinoma. The rest are adenocarcinoma, Paget's disease, malignant melanoma, and sarcoma.

Vulvar cancer has a slow growth rate and remains localized for a long time. Most lesions are located in the labia, primarily the labia majora. Some are on the clitoris. Local spread may occur to the urethra, vagina, anus, and rectum. Lymphatic spread is to the inguinal femoral, pelvic, and finally, periaortic nodes. The usual causes of death from widespread vulvar cancer are distant metasta-

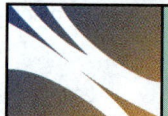

RISK FACTORS AND LEVELS OF PREVENTION

Vulvitis

Risk Factors

- Skin disorders
- Inflammatory problems
- Infection
- Vulvar kraurosis (dryness and atrophy of the vulva)
- Vulvar leukoplakia (atrophic disease of the older woman's external genitalia, with a white marble appearance of the skin, itching, and excoriation)
- Vulvovaginitis (inflammation of both vulva and vagina)
- Postmenopausal atrophy
- Irritation secondary to vaginitis
- Uncontrolled diabetes mellitus (with high amounts of sugar in the urine)
- Pediculosis or scabies
- Allergies
- Psychological problems
- Cancer
- Ulcerative glandular or skin lesions
- Systemic conditions
- Urinary incontinence
- Poor perineal hygiene

Levels of Prevention

Primary Prevention

- Encourage appropriate perineal hygiene, especially for women with incontinence, allergies, diabetes, and other irritants.
- Instruct clients to avoid use of feminine hygiene sprays.
- Help clients to maintain adequate health status (such as controlling diabetes).

Secondary Prevention

- Teach clients how to perform vulvar self-examination.
- Instruct clients to seek early and appropriate treatment of vulvar lesions.

Tertiary Prevention

- Provide sexual counseling for dysfunction associated with disease or treatment.

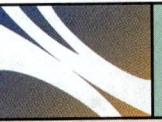

RISK FACTORS AND LEVELS OF PREVENTION

Vulvar Cancer

Risk Factors

Vulvar disorders such as leukoplakia, kraurosis, and diabetic vulvitis, and sexually transmitted diseases such as human papillomavirus infection.

Levels of Prevention

Primary Prevention

- Encourage early diagnosis and treatment of vulvar dystrophies (leukoplakia), kraurosis (vulvar and mucous membrane atrophy and dryness), and diabetic vulvitis.
- Teach clients how to prevent sexually transmitted disease, including human papillomavirus.

Secondary Prevention

- Ask clients about history of other primary malignancies (e.g., cervical cancer).
- Teach clients how to perform a regular vulvar self-examination using a mirror.

Tertiary Prevention

- Provide sexual counseling for clients after surgery.

---

sis, urethral obstruction, infection, uremia, hemorrhage, and general disability.

The prognosis is poor with vulvar invasive lesions. Five-year survival rates of clients with vulvectomy and lymphadenectomy are approximately 65%. Recurrence as well as distant metastasis may appear in the first 2 years. When lesions are diagnosed in an advanced stage with node involvement, the survival rate is only 8% to 10%.[2]

Clinical Manifestations and Diagnostic Findings

Leukoplakia vulvae is characterized by thickened gray patches of epithelium scattered over the vulva and perineum. Cracked areas in these patches provide an ideal medium for infection that can lead to ulceration and maceration. Eventually, these areas may become malignant.

Kraurosis also can become secondarily infected. It is characterized by a bright-red, smooth, almost transparent vulvar epithelium. Kraurosis is most common in postmenopausal women. With its progression, the vulvar tissues shrink and constrict the vaginal opening.

Both disorders cause itching and soreness or pain, or they may be asymptomatic. Both are diagnosed according to appearance.

Clinical manifestations of early vulvar cancer include pruritus, minimal vulval soreness, and tissue irritation with some bleeding. The potential seriousness of these relatively mild problems may not be appreciated by women or their healthcare providers because the manifestations are similar to those of nonmalignant vulvar lesions.

As the vulvar cancer progresses, clinical manifestations include vulvar edema and pelvic lymphadenopathy. Secondary infection may cause a foul-smelling discharge.

Diagnosis is made from biopsy of suspicious lesions.

Acute and Subacute Care

■ Medical Management

With leukoplakia, a biopsy to rule out cancer is indicated. In both disorders, infection is treated with an appropriate systemic antibiotic. Other manifestations are treated symptomatically.

Irradiation and chemotherapy are used less often than is surgical therapy. Irradiation is not generally used because the involved tissues do not tolerate it well. Chemotherapy is typically given unless metastasis has occurred. The agent of choice is then based on the extent of metastasis.

■ Nursing Management of the Medical Client

The nursing management of these clients is mainly supportive care throughout the diagnostic period. The itching can be treated symptomatically with antipruritic creams such as hydrocortisone.

■ Surgical Management

A vulvectomy is performed to remove abnormal tissue through procedures such as a skinning technique, local wide excision, or a simple or radical vulvectomy. A laser may be used in conjunction with these procedures to destroy specific abnormal tissue.

A simple vulvectomy involves removal of the labia majora and minora and possibly the glans clitoris. Occasionally, the perineal area is also removed, requiring plastic surgery to cover the vulvar area. However, extensive surgery is avoided if the woman's condition allows a simpler procedure.

A radical vulvectomy (Fig. 84–15) includes excision of tissue from the anus to a few centimeters below the symphysis pubis (skin, labia majora and minora, and clitoris). Bilateral dissection of groin lymph nodes also may be performed such as the superficial groin and deep inguinal, femoral, iliac, hypogastric, and obturator nodes.

■ Nursing Management of the Surgical Client

Assessment

For a woman experiencing vulvar surgery, psychosocial support is especially important and should begin preoperatively. Some problems the nurse might anticipate are

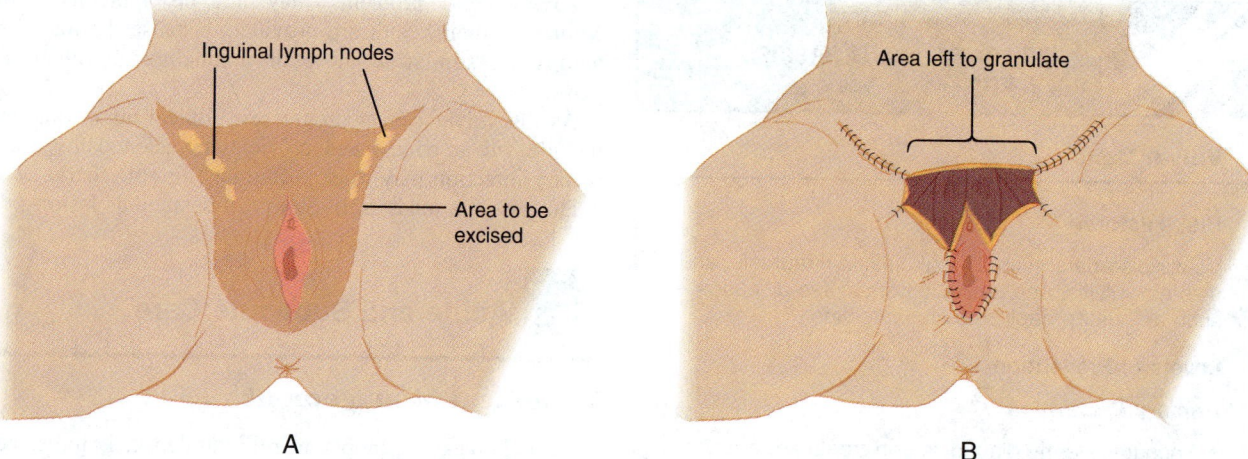

Figure 84–15. Radical vulvectomy. *A,* Area to be excised and line of incision *(dashed line).* The vulvar skin, underlying subcutaneous tissue and muscles, and regional lymph nodes are excised. If the anus is involved, the incision continues around it also. Inguinal and femoral lymph nodes are resected en bloc. *B,* Completed surgery. Perineal skin is approximated to the vagina, and a large area is left open to heal gradually by filling in with granulation tissue. A simple vulvectomy (not shown) does not remove the lymph nodes. Hence, the incision does not extend into the groin.

fear of disfigurement, grief over the loss of a body part, fear of death, and sexual concerns.

Preoperative preparation is similar to that for other gynecologic surgeries, but it will also include an enema, douche, and insertion of a Foley catheter.

Diagnosis, Planning, Implementation

Knowledge Deficit. The client who will undergo surgery to treat vulvar cancer will have many learning needs, leading to a priority nursing diagnosis of *Knowledge Deficit related to surgical procedure and outcomes of surgery.*

Planning: Expected Outcomes. The client will understand the surgical procedure and its outcomes, as evidenced by her ability to correctly explain the surgery and expected outcomes.

Implementation. Preoperative preparation is important for a woman scheduled for a vulvectomy so she (1) understands what the surgery entails, (2) knows what preoperative procedures will be performed, and (3) has an idea of what to expect in the postoperative period. See the Client Education Guide to postoperative radical vulvectomy instructions.

Potential Postoperative Complications: Hemorrhage, Thrombophlebitis, Infection, and Lymphedema. The client undergoing a radical vulvectomy is prone to many postoperative complications because of the extensive nature of the surgery. This leads to a number of important collaborative problems such as *Hemorrhage, Thrombophlebitis, Infection, and Lymphedema related to extensive surgery and dissection of groin lymph nodes.*

Planning: Expected Outcomes. The client will not suffer injury, as evidenced by absence of bleeding,

thrombophlebitis, infection, and absence of lower extremity lymphedema. Complications will be diagnosed early and normal wound healing will occur.

Implementation. In addition to routine postoperative care, Hemovacs or drains are present in the incision to remove drainage and reduce the risk of infection. Carefully monitor the amount of bleeding. A bed cradle is helpful in keeping bed linens away from the incision. The woman wears antiembolism or sequential compression stockings to prevent leg edema and thrombophlebitis. Also, it is important that she perform leg exercises to prevent circulatory problems. Low-dose heparin may be used prophylactically to reduce the risk of phlebitis.

Prevent infection in the incisional area through frequent dressing changes, perineal care (a Foley catheter is usually in place for 7–14 days or until adequate healing has occurred) or sitz baths after voiding and bowel movements, and meticulous wound care. Carefully monitor urination and bowel movements, with supportive care to prevent problems. Once healing has occurred, the woman may require reconstructive surgery.

Long-term physical complications of radical vulvectomy include edema of the lower extremities. Reduce lower extremity edema by applying support stockings or using sequential pressure devices. Keep the legs elevated as much as possible. Teach the client to avoid sitting with the legs dependent, standing, or crossing the legs.

Risk for Body Image Disturbance. The surgery for vulvar cancer is very extensive, removing the woman's external genitalia. This makes the nursing diagnosis *Risk for Body Image Disturbance related to radical surgery and loss of external genitalia* a high-priority diagnosis.

Planning: Expected Outcomes. The client will maintain a normal self-concept and body image, as evi-

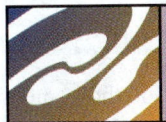

CLIENT EDUCATION GUIDE

Recovering from Radical Vulvectomy

Client Instructions in English (Instrucciones para el cliente en inglés)	Client Instructions in Spanish (Instrucciones para el cliente en español)
Avoid strenuous exercise involving the legs and pelvis.	Evite los ejercicios estrenuos de la pelvis y de las piernas.
Gradually resume normal physical activities.	Reanude gradualmente las actividades físicas normales.
Resume sexual activity, if desired, when the surgeon indicates. If intercourse is resumed, top or side positions are preferable to avoid direct pressure on the operative area. Water-soluble lubricants can be used for comfort.	Reanude la actividad sexual, si desea, cuando le indique el cirujano. Si las relaciones sexuales se reanudan, las posiciones por arriba o de lado son preferibles para evitar la presión directa en el area operada. Se pueden usar lubricantes solubles en agua para su comodidad.
Take showers rather than tub baths. Showers reduce the likelihood of postoperative wound infection. Gentle, thorough washing of the genital area is important. Wipe gently from front to back after bowel movements and urinating. Do not douche without permission from the surgeon.	Tome duchas en lugar de baños en la tina. Las duchas reducen la probabilidad de infección después de la operación. El aseo ligero pero completo del area genital es muy importante. Limpie suavemente del frente hacia atras después del movimiento del intestino (excremento) y de la orina. No se duche sin permiso del cirujano.
Notify the surgeon if any of the following problems occur:	Notifique al cirujano si cualquier problema de los siguientes occurre:
• Perineal pain unrelieved by prescribed medication	• Dolor en el perineo que no se mejora con el medicamento recetado
• Foul-smelling perineal discharge	• Desecho maloliente del perineo
• Heavy perineal bleeding or clots	• Sangrado pesado o coágulos
• Foul odor from the incision	• Mal olor de la incisión
• Change in color of the incision (especially manifestations of decreased circulation)	• Cambio en el color de la incisión (sobre todo, en los síntomas de circulación disminuida)
• Swelling of the groin or genital area	• Hinchazón de la ingle o del area genital
• Frequent urination, urinating in small amounts, or discomfort or burning on urination	• Orina con mucha frequencia, orina en cantidades pequeñas, o incomodidad o ardor cuando orina
• Temperature of 100° F (37.8° C) or higher	• Temperatura arriba de 100° F (37.8° C)
• Pain, tenderness, or redness in the calves.	• Dolor, sensibilidad, o rojez en al pantorrilla

denced by her ability to look at the wound and to express concerns about bodily alterations.

Implementation. Psychosocially, a vulvectomy may be a devastating experience for a woman because of its direct impact on the external genitalia. The surgery, especially a radical vulvectomy, may compromise the client's physical integrity and her sense of wholeness. Some important issues for a woman include (1) fear of recurrence and metastasis, (2) disfigurement, (3) concern over future sexual activity, and (4) fear of her partner's rejection.

Nursing care involves assisting the woman to redefine her self-image to include the physical changes of vulvectomy. Try to create an environment in which the woman is able to express her feelings. Provide her with an opportunity to mourn the loss affecting her sexuality. Encourage her to resume her normal activities as soon as possible to reinforce her feelings of self-worth.

The surgery can lead to stress in social relationships. The woman and her significant others may need help in coping with the aftermath of this radical surgery. Significant others may benefit from inclusion in sessions at which information and support are given to the client.

The impact of a vulvectomy on female sexuality has not been well described. The disfigurement of the surgery can lead to body image distortion that affects sexual functioning. Physical changes such as removal of the clitoris result in the woman's loss of the ability to experience orgasm. The woman may experience loss of sensation within the vagina. Also, introital stenosis may follow surgery, making intercourse painful or difficult and having a major impact on sexuality. If stenosis is present, it can be treated with vaginal dilators. If dilation is unsuccessful, plastic surgery should be considered.

Sexual counseling may be indicated for some women and their partners. The nurse can assist the client and her sexual partner by communicating openly with them, answering their questions, providing them with information about structural vulvar changes, and suggesting alternative forms of sexual arousal for the woman.

Lower extremity lymphedema can cause a change in clothing size and an upsetting change in appearance. In addition, some women have difficulty sitting for long periods. This makes activities such as long automobile trips difficult. Some women experience an unpredictable stream of urine following a radical vulvectomy. They must remove most of their clothing to avoid wetting themselves when voiding. Urinating into a funnel might be helpful.

Evaluation

This surgery requires a long recovery time. Many women develop wound infections and delayed wound healing leading to numerous problems. Delayed healing further impairs the woman's body image, leading to more difficulties. There are often prolonged urinary problems associated with the altered anatomy and poor healing. Given a long period of time, the woman can recover fully.

■ Modifications for Elderly Clients

An older woman is less likely to have radical excision because of the potential for poor wound healing. If she does have the radical surgery, the nurse needs to monitor her very closely for the development of complications.

Bartholinitis

Inflammation of Bartholin's glands can be caused by various organisms, including gonococci, streptococci, staphylococci, and *E. coli*. The infection involves the duct of the gland, producing edema and, eventually, obstruction. Because the inflamed gland cannot drain, it swells and an abscess forms. Cellulitis develops in the surrounding tissues, producing more pain and systemic manifestations. The abscess may rupture spontaneously or may require incision and drainage.

After the acute episode, occlusion of the duct by fibrosis and scarring causes retention of secretions and dilation of the duct. It then becomes a palpable, mobile cyst, which usually is not painful. Manifestations relate to the size of the cyst and include dyspareunia or pain on walking.

Systemic antibiotics specific for the causative organism are prescribed. Local heat with hot packs or sitz baths may help promote drainage. Surgery may be necessary, such as an incision and drainage or removal of the gland if cancer is suspected or for repeated infections with abscess formation.

Other Vulvar Disorders

Skin disorders of the vulva include many of those mentioned earlier, as well as chemical burns, irritation with harsh soaps, genital herpes (generally, herpes simplex virus type 2), psoriasis, folliculitis, and eczema. All are treated by removing the cause whenever possible and by the performance of meticulous perineal hygiene.

Both the itch mite *Sarcoptes scabiei* and the crab or pubic louse *Pthirus pubis* cause vulvar irritation. They are transmitted during sexual contact with an infected person, from infected bedding, or from toilets. Both the affected client and environment must be treated to get rid of the organisms and their eggs.

Other Gynecologic Disorders

Fallopian (Ovarian) Tube Cancer

The fallopian tubes are the least common gynecologic site of primary cancer. When it occurs, it most commonly affects women age 45 to 60. Secondary tubal carcinoma is more common. Generally it extends from ovarian or uterine sites. Infertility and nulliparity have been identified as high-risk factors.

Fallopian tube cancer is difficult to diagnose. Currently, there is no accurate, practical method for mass screening for this cancer. Both primary and secondary tubal cancers—like ovarian carcinoma—remain asymptomatic until late in the course of the malignancy. Fallopian tube cancer is relatively widespread. Its prognosis is poor. Late assessment findings include pain, abnormal uterine bleeding, and a watery vaginal discharge. Typically a mass can be palpated in the pelvis. Manifestations can vary, making it difficult to establish an accurate diagnosis.

Because of the late appearance of manifestations, treatment often begins late. The primary treatment is total abdominal hysterectomy and bilateral salpingo-oophorectomy. This is commonly followed by irradiation. Chemotherapy alone or in combination with irradiation may be given to women with widespread or recurrent disease.

Genital Tract Sarcomas

A very small percentage of genital tract malignancies in women are sarcomas, most commonly occurring in the uterus and ovaries. Uterine leiomyomas are one type of tumor that may undergo sarcomatous degeneration. However, this is rare in relation to the total incidence of leiomyomas in women.

Sarcomatous lesions tend to develop in younger women (20–30 years old) and grow rapidly. They metastasize, particularly to the lungs, and may result in death from pulmonary causes. Treatment usually includes wide excision of the involved area and normal surrounding tissue, at times followed by irradiation. The prognosis is poor.

Gestational Trophoblastic Disease

Gestational trophoblastic disease is a spectrum of neoplastic disorders. These disorders range from nonmalignant to highly malignant. The various disease forms are called hydatidiform mole, invasive mole (chorioadenoma destruens), and choriocarcinoma (chorionepithelioma). All share the following properties:

● They come from the trophoblast of human pregnancy (the trophoblast is a type of embryonic tissue through which the embryo receives nourishment from the mother).
● They represent invasion of the maternal host by fetal chorionic tissue (tissue of the human trophoblast).
● Fetal chorionic tissue produces a protein hormone called human chorionic gonadotropin (HCG). This hormone is produced in direct proportion to the amount of tumor present.
● Cure is possible with chemotherapy. These tumors can undergo spontaneous regression. However, this is rare for choriocarcinoma.

Hydatidiform Mole

Hydatidiform mole is relatively rare: about 1 in every 2000 to 2500 pregnancies. It occurs most often in women over age 40 and under 20. The risk increases after one mole has occurred. Hydatidiform mole is far more common in Asia (1 : 25 in Taiwan).

Indications of a hydatidiform mole include the following:

● Intermittent bleeding in the first trimester. Sometimes, this contains some characteristic grapelike tissue. Such tissue requires pathologic analysis.
● Excessively rapid uterine growth.
● Absence of fetal heart sounds, a fetal skeleton, and fetal movement.
● Spontaneous abortion at about 14 to 18 weeks' gestation.

There is a high correlation of hydatidiform mole with bilateral ovarian cysts, hyperemesis gravidarum, and eclampsia, particularly during the first trimester or early in the second trimester.

Medical diagnosis of a hydatidiform mole from a pathologic specimen. This is obtained either by spontaneous passage of tissue or by D & C. A persistently elevated HCG level in blood or urine is diagnostic. Also, it permits monitoring of the effects of treatment. If diagnosis is uncertain, ultrasonography, angiography of the uterine vessels, pelvic x-ray studies (showing absence of fetal outline), amniography, and serial HCG determinations help clarify the problem. Some of these activities must be used cautiously in case a viable fetus is present.

Hydatidiform moles are treated by evacuating the uterus. This may be performed by D & C, suction curettage, or hysterectomy. Follow-up care is of particular importance with hydatidiform moles and must be meticulous. HCG titer levels are checked frequently to make sure that metastatic invasion has not occurred.

Usually, HCG titers return to normal within a week of uterine evacuation. During early treatment, the titers are followed weekly, then every other week, and finally monthly for a year. In some centers, women are also treated with a course of chemotherapeutic agents to ensure that metastatic invasion has not occurred.

Invasive Mole and Choriocarcinoma

Invasive mole (chorioadenoma destruens) is a neoplasm of the chorion (gestational tissue) with grossly visible invasion of the uterine myometrium and, sometimes, of adjacent tissues. Metastases rarely occur, and the disease is often benign. About 15% of all molar pregnancies invade the myometrium. This disorder was previously treated by hysterectomy. However, chemotherapy is currently the treatment of choice. A precise diagnosis is difficult to obtain because tissue studies cannot be performed. Diagnosis is made by history and the clinical manifestations.

Choriocarcinoma is a malignant neoplasm of the chorion characterized by its tendency to metastasize early, rapidly, and widely. Choriocarcinoma tends to respond well to chemotherapy.

Choriocarcinoma is an extremely malignant, necrotic tumor. Its usual primary site is in the uterus. Choriocarcinoma develops later in about 3% of women having hydatidiform mole. Trophoblastic disease refers to invasive mole and choriocarcinoma. Its manifestations can imitate other conditions such as ectopic pregnancy or threatened abortion.

The primary site of choriocarcinoma may also occur in the ovaries (or in the testes in men). These forms of the disease are associated with a poor prognosis. They are not discussed here.

The clinical course of choriocarcinoma is capricious. Without intervention, it tends to progress rapidly, and is often fatal within 6 to 12 months. Metastases can occur to the lungs (most common), vagina, brain, or central nervous system (these respond poorly to treatment); liver (responds poorly); kidney; and spleen. A few women experience spontaneous remission without treatment.

Presenting assessment findings with choriocarcinoma may include heavy vaginal or abdominal bleeding or may relate to metastasis, such as pulmonary problems from metastasis to the lung. Death typically occurs from problems such as respiratory embarrassment or hemorrhage into the tumor.

Trophoblastic tumors are not radiosensitive. Methotrexate and actinomycin D are the drugs of choice in treating trophoblastic disease (invasive mole and choriocarcinoma). They are given in very large doses, with 1- to 2-week rest periods between courses of therapy. The response of the woman to treatment is measured by laboratory studies and serial HCG determinations. When the HCG titer level has returned to normal for about two courses of therapy, the treatment is stopped and the woman is followed closely.

Women with gestational trophoblastic disease (invasive mole or choriocarcinoma) require complex and expert nursing care. The disease process is confusing and frightening for the woman and her significant others. Because of the rapid progression of the disease, aggressive treatment must be begun quickly. There is generally little time to adapt to what is happening. Often, the woman becomes extremely ill because of the toxic effects of the medications used. Women and their significant others need support, reassurance, information, and meticulous nursing care.

When trophoblastic disease occurs, the pregnancy will be lost, adding additional stress to the woman and significant others. The woman probably has a knowledge deficit about the disease, and also experiences actual normal grieving. Assess the significance of the loss to the woman and her significant others. Then assess her well-being and coping responses and those of her significant others to identify any dysfunctional patterns or behavior. Provide

support by allowing the woman and her significant others to grieve, and by accepting and facilitating grief responses. Offer reassurance and provide information as the people involved become ready to learn more about what happened.

The prognosis of choriocarcinoma is directly related to the duration of illness and to the HCG titer level at the time of diagnosis. If the duration has been short and the titers are low, and if the woman's medication regimen is carefully managed, the prognosis may be excellent.

Conclusions

Female reproductive disorders can occur throughout the life span. These problems range from menstrual disorders to life-threatening malignancies. Primary and secondary prevention are particularly important for women with reproductive disorders, and the nurse can provide needed

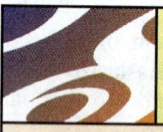

DIVERSITY IN HEALTHCARE

Women's Healthcare

From the moment of birth, cultural expectations for infant girls differ from those for boys. Parent-child relationships, social roles, childrearing practices, expected behaviors in health and illness, and expectations for survival differ markedly between the sexes. Anthropologists have noted that there are *asymmetries* in cultural roles for males and females, with wide variations being observed for different groups. For example, the temperamental attitudes traditionally regarded as feminine—passivity, responsiveness, and protectiveness of children—can be the masculine pattern in one group and outlawed for both sexes in another. The formerly accepted belief that certain behaviors are genetically sex-linked is no longer held by most social scientists. There are groups in which children of both sexes are more egotistic than boys in other cultures. The same sort of variability attaches to almost every kind of behavior.

Every known society recognizes and elaborates some differences between the sexes. Although there are groups in which men wear skirts and women wear slacks or trousers, there still remain characteristic tasks, manners, and responsibilities primarily associated with women or with men.

Cross-cultural studies of childbearing and childrearing reveal certain temperamental differences between the sexes. Differences in physical constitution, especially in endurance and strength, contribute to the characteristic differences in male and female activities, but there are individuals who fail to fit the norms. For example, during recent years American women have significantly extended the range of career opportunities open to them. Although it was formerly believed that women lacked the physical stamina necessary for traditionally male careers such as firefighters, police officers, surgeons, military aviators, and so on, women have demonstrated that some individuals can, and do, succeed in these fields. In some cases, legal action was needed before women were given the opportunity to demonstrate their capabilities. Similarly, laws were needed to force educational institutions to admit qualified women into certain disciplines. Gender issues have been an integral component of the ongoing dialogue among nurses, whose profession is comprised primarily of women.

Cultural expressions of sexual asymmetry may be associated with economics and occupations, but they are often found in other domains of activity as well. Although biology dictates that women will be mothers, the organization of families varies widely among cultural groups. In many traditional groups, a large part of a woman's adult life is spent giving birth to and raising children, which leads to a differentiation of domestic and public spheres of activity. Because women give birth and breast-feed children, the adult division of labor in all cultures reflects this biologic reality. Career-oriented women, for example, must make special child care arrangements, using spouse, extended family members, friends, day-care centers, or other supports to enable them to pursue career aspirations. Some employers provide maternity leave, and others offer both maternity and paternity leaves when a baby is born or adopted.

education so that women can become more aware of preventive measures. The physical care of these women is important; however, the psychosocial care of these clients is vital. (See Diversity in Healthcare for a discussion of cultural factors affecting women's health). The skillful and empathic nurse can assist the woman through what is often an extremely distressing diagnosis and treatment.

Nurses who need more information on reproductive issues should consult an obstetrics and gynecology text. Information on contraception, tubal ligation, abortion, and other issues can be found there.

Thinking Critically

1. The client, a 52-year-old woman, comes into the clinic stating, "I can't put up with it any longer!" Her last menstrual period was 4 months ago, she has had severe hot flashes and night sweats for almost 6 months with no abatement. Vaginal intercourse has become so painful that she and her husband have refrained from sexual activity for 3 months. She states that the night sweats are so bad that most nights she has been unable to get an uninterrupted night's sleep. What are your priorities for her care? What interventions might be used?

2. A 38-year-old woman enters the clinic with a complaint of acute, sharp, severe bilateral pelvic pain with a temperature of 102.2° F, a pulse rate of 100, a respiratory rate of 20, and chills. Her cervical culture shows gonococcal infection. She uses oral contraceptives for birth control. Besides teaching her about antibiotic medication, what is your priority in caring for her and what interventions are necessary?

3. The client, a 61-year-old woman, had a TAH-BSO 2 days ago for early endometrial cancer. Her Foley catheter was removed yesterday. Her temperature is 101.1° F, her pulse rate is 96, and her respira-

---

Culture also affects attitudes of healthcare providers toward lesbian and bisexual clients. Our society tends to assume women are heterosexual and base our care on this assumption. Lesbian women in our society are at higher risk for reproductive and breast cancers because of previous negative experiences with healthcare providers and fear of homophobic and/or hostile attitudes if the woman's sexual orientation is revealed.[12] Therefore, they are less likely to seek routine gynecologic examinations and screening tests.

Religion, Culture, and Women's Health

Many world religions provide guidelines or mandates related to women's reproductive functions. Religious tenets may require or encourage women to engage in certain practices during and after menstruation. For example, Jewish and Islamic laws encourage ritual bathing and indicate when sexual intercourse should occur in relationship to the menstrual cycle. Concepts such as "clean" and "unclean" are used to describe menstruation and activities appropriate for both sexes during the monthly period.

Contraception is perhaps the most frequent women's health issue discussed by members of religious groups. For example, many religions posit that one of the major purposes of marriage is procreation. For example, in the Torah Jews are admonished to be fruitful and multiply. It is considered a *mitzvah,* or good deed, to have at least two children. Since the holocaust of World War II, some Jewish couples believe that larger families should be encouraged to replace those who were lost. Birth control is, however, permissible in traditional and liberal homes. Although Hasidic and Orthodox Jews rarely employ vasectomy, contraception by either partner is acceptable in most Jewish congregations. The Church of Jesus Christ of Latter-Day Saints (Mormons) encourages married couples to raise large families and provides a theological rationale for its importance. Mormons have the highest birth rate of any religious group in the United States. In the Roman Catholic tradition, the conjugal act should be one that is love-giving and potentially life-giving. Only natural means of contraception, such as abstinence, the temperature method, and the ovulation method, are acceptable. Antiovulants may be used therapeutically to assist in regulating the menstrual cycle, but not for contraceptive purposes. For the Baha'ist, begetting children is considered the highest physical fruit of existence. The Baha'i teachings imply that birth control constitutes a real danger to the foundations of social life. Because Jewish, Mormon, Baha'i, and Catholic religious beliefs hold that life begins at conception, the use of intrauterine devices and abortion for contraceptive purposes is prohibited. Sterilization is opposed by many religions because it is viewed as a form of bodily mutilation and interferes with the natural reproductive capabilities of the woman's body.

Continued on following page

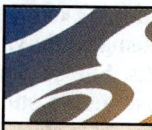

DIVERSITY IN HEALTHCARE *(Continued)*

Women's Healthcare

Abortion, artificial insemination, sterility and genetic testing, and other procedures are frequently the topic of religious doctrine and interpretive religious writings. The reader is encouraged to contact religious representatives from religious groups for the official position on these and to refer to selected nursing resources for further information. It is important for the nurse to ask the client about her religious health-related beliefs and practices as part of the initial and ongoing assessment. Despite the official position of religious leaders, individuals vary widely in their personal interpretations. The nurse must also allow for change over time. For example, despite the official Roman Catholic opposition to many contraceptive methods, the majority of Catholic couples in the United States report that they use oral contraceptives. Some Catholics have changed their attitudes toward abortion since the legalization of abortion with Roe v Wade decision by the Supreme Court. Nurses might find it useful to ask the woman if she would like to include others in her decision-making about procedures. For example, a rabbi, priest, elder, bishop, or other religious representative may be helpful to the client in examining the religious, moral, and ethical aspects of decision-making.

Throughout history, certain religious images and symbols have been used uncritically to legitimate the dominance of men over women. Nurses may care for women who have been victimized by a pattern of male domination that is culturally bound and perpetuated by certain religious imagery. Nurses should be aware that religious sex-role imagery can exert a powerful influence in the woman's life and may determine her treatment choices.

Menstruation

Each woman holds culturally defined and learned sets of beliefs about her bodily functions. Attitudes toward menstruation are often culturally based, and the adolescent girl may be taught a variety of folk beliefs and practices at the time of puberty. Among Mexican Americans, menstruation is often considered an unpleasant but natural condition requiring circumspect behavior. For example, menstruating females are not permitted to walk barefooted, wash their hair, or take showers or baths. Some Mexican Americans believe that sour or iced foods cause menstrual blood to coagulate, and some Puerto Rican women have been taught that drinking lemon or pineapple juice will increase menstrual cramping. The nurse should be aware of these beliefs and respect the cultural practices. By encouraging sponge baths and the frequent changing of tampons or pads, the nurse can promote hygienic habits during menstruation without becoming judgmental about cultural beliefs.

Some Arab women who practice Islam, such Palestinian, Lebanese, Jordanian, Saudi Arabian, and other Near or Middle Eastern women, and some African women, have ethnoreligious prohibitions and duties during and after menstruation. In Islam, blood is considered to be unclean *(najis)*. The blood of menstruation, as well as the blood lost during childbirth, renders the woman impure or potentially polluting. In Islamic legal language, the term used for menstruation is *hayz,* and the menstruating woman is called *ha'iz.*

Because one must be in a pure state in order to pray, the *ha'iz* are forbidden to perform certain acts of worship such as touching the Qur'an (Koran), entering a mosque, praying, and participating in certain feasts. During the menstrual period, sexual intercourse is forbidden for both men and women. When the menstrual flow stops, the woman performs *ghusl,* a ritual washing to purify herself.

Navajo attitudes toward menstruation are traditionally expressed in two customs. The first in the life of a girl is the puberty ceremony, the *kinaalda,* which announces the achievement of menarche. While in the past fertility was the goal of the ceremony, today the most common reason given for the *kinaalda* is educational. It equips the girl with the knowledge to participate in society as an adult female. Despite celebration of the first two menses, during subsequent menses Navajo women are constrained by taboos. Menstruating women may not look at sand paintings, enter a ceremonial hogan, be a patient, attend or lead a sing, or join in the dancing that occurs at certain ceremonies. Restrictions on work and physical activity vary widely according to the degree of acculturation. Certain taboos related to the disposal of the dangerous menstrual fluid and the proper disposal of pads. Attitudes toward intercourse during menstruation are variable.

Infertility

In many cultures of the world, fertility is still considered the primary function of women. Fertility is linked to their social status and reproductive ability. Infertile women are confronted with a twofold problem: They cannot fulfill their culturally sanctioned role, and they do not receive support from family or society. Failure to fulfill their reproductive role and satisfy familial and societal expectations within the culture may lead to personal and social crises.

Blenner[2] studied the approach used by healthcare providers in the treatment of infertile clients from diverse cultural backgrounds. Findings from in-depth interviews with healthcare providers in Southern California revealed three types of providers: (1) the culturally unaware, (2) the culturally nontolerant, and (3) the culturally sensitive. Culturally unaware providers failed to recognize different cultural needs and treated all clients in the same way, an approach that led to noncompliance. For example, at the time of the pelvic examination, a healthcare provider caused bleeding in an Orthodox Jewish woman. Because Jewish law requires ritualistic purification and abstinence from intercourse for 8 days after vaginal bleeding occurs, the couple was unable to have intercourse during the woman's most fertile period of the cycle in that month. Culturally nontolerant providers recognized diverse needs, but they were unwilling to tolerate cultural conflicts in treatment or to change treatment protocols. This often resulted in providers terminating treatment or making referrals to another provider. Culturally sensitive providers acquired information on cultural beliefs, worked within clients' limitations, and adapted tests and treatment protocols to meet clients' needs. For example, two women from Middle Eastern cultures (in which tampons are not worn) reported embarrassment over the transvaginal probe used for sonography. Given that full bladder transabdominal sonograms provide the necessary data without vaginal entry, the healthcare provider modified the diagnostic testing in a culturally appropriate manner at their next visit.

Menopause

Despite the current emphasis on aging, feminism, and women's health, the experiential reality of menopausal women from various cultures has not been studied sufficiently. The woman's perception of menopause and the self-care practices that she is likely to use are influenced by cultural factors. Few studies have placed menopause within the cultural context of other life experiences occurring during midlife. Buck and Gottlieb[3] studied eight menopausal Mohawk women to determine the meaning of menopause to them. The results revealed four major issues experienced in midlife that are related to the concept of time: (1) it is time for me, (2) being where I should be, (3) time for myself, and (4) my time is spent meaningfully. Women fell into two categories. Those "in synchrony" viewed their lives as following expected time pathways. Those "out of synchrony" identified aspects of their lives as problematic. Those in the latter category either demonstrated an action orientation aimed at remedying the situation or reported feeling "stuck."

Treatment of menopause as an estrogen-deficiency disease medicalizes the experience. Hormone replacement therapy's benefits and risks are also unknown. The Women's Health Initiative is studying their use over a 10-year period. Lichtman recommends weighing many factors in counseling women on HRT, including severity of symptoms and the woman's risk factors for cardiovascular disease and osteoporosis.

Cancer

Disparity exists between the scientific advances made for white women compared with those for their black, Hispanic, Asian, and Native American counterparts. Studies have documented the complex relationships among biologic, behavioral, and sociocultural factors that affect cancer incidence, treatment, and outcomes.[11] The following discussion of breast and cervical cancer screening and prevention programs is intended to identify the culture-specific needs of women from diverse groups.

Cancer Screening

Although screening tests for the early detection of various types of cancers are available, there are differences in the extent to which they are used by women from diverse cultures. National, state, and local programs aimed at increasing cancer screening for women from diverse cultural backgrounds have had limited success in reaching target populations.

Breast Cancer. Cancer mortality rates among black, Asian, Hispanic, Asian, and Native American women have been studied by the U.S. Department of Health and Human Services for the purpose of reducing the excess incidence found among minority women. There has been little change in 5-year survival rates for breast cancer during the past 20 years. Although the incidence of breast cancer is lower among black women, the death rate from this disease is higher for black women than for their white counterparts. Breast cancer is the leading cause of cancer mortality among black women, with elderly black women being particularly vulnerable. While white women have a 75% survival rate, their black counterparts have a 62% survival rate.

Factors that prevent black women from using breast cancer screening include cost, accessibility, availability, lack of knowledge, healthcare provider variables, and lack of community involvement. Programs for breast cancer screening that address cultural factors are successful in achieving their goals, while others fail. Although costly, mobile mammography units that visit ethnic neighborhoods on a regular basis have been effective in increasing the number of black women who are screened for breast cancer. Advertising in the media and church bulletins has also been beneficial. The involvement of black churches in promoting participation in breast cancer screening programs has increased the number of black women who are screened, especially the older adult population. The use of parish nurses and other grassroots community-based healthcare providers has significantly improved participation in screening programs by black women.

Continued on following page

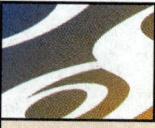

DIVERSITY IN HEALTHCARE *(Continued)*

Women's Healthcare

Cervical Cancer. Black women have the highest rate of screening for cervical cancer, which has significantly reduced the death rate of black women from this type of neoplasm. The decline in death rates from cervical cancer has been widely attributed to the use of Papanicolaou (Pap) smears for early detection. Pap smear screening rates, beliefs about appropriate screening intervals, and factors affecting screening were examined in a nationwide study. Results indicate that through age 69, black women are screened at similar or higher rates than whites.

A videotape and brochure about the importance of the Pap smear have been developed by the Aleutian Islands Association and the Alaska Area Native Health Service. The 12-minute videotape portrays Alaska native women (Eskimos, Indians, and Aleuts) engaging in healthy life-styles and discussing cervical cancer and Pap tests. Older female relatives share their stories and experiences with Pap tests and cervical cancer with a young woman celebrating her 18th birthday. The brochure discusses the Pap test, normal and abnormal results, and follow-up for abnormal results. The brochure is illustrated by an Alaskan artist.

Hispanics, particularly those speaking only or mostly Spanish, are least likely to have received a Pap smear within the last 3 years. Overall, the most frequently reported reason for not having had a recent Pap smear was procrastinating or not believing it was necessary.

Although Pap smear screening is relatively common, there are subgroups that remain resistant to it. Research indicates that Spanish-speaking women under age 39 are least likely to participate in Pap testing. Cubans are much less likely to be compliant than Puerto Ricans or Mexicans. Nurses need to consider cultural reasons for the lower participation rate by Hispanic women. For example, disrobing and submitting to a pelvic examination is regarded by some Hispanic women as immodest and improper. Some Hispanic women will allow female healthcare providers to conduct examinations of the genitalia, but refuse to be examined by a male. Educational programs should focus on unscreened women who underestimate its importance, procrastinate, or fail to receive advice from their healthcare provider stressing the benefits of early detection. Grassroots support from women in the Hispanic community who undergo regular Pap testing should be solicited to encourage other women to be tested as well.

Immigrants

Since 1975 nearly 1 million refugees have entered the United States. Although the majority come from Southeast Asia, there have been large waves of immigrants from Mexico, Central America, and Eastern Europe (Russia and Bosnia and Herzegovina). Adding a new dimension to American society, these new arrivals have challenged the healthcare system. A frustrating aspect for nurses is the radically different worldview of these multiple cultural groups. Perceptual differences include varying definitions of kinds and causes of diseases; behaviors to avoid when ill; appropriate kinds of treatment; patterns of accessing care and selecting care providers, including tradi-

---

tory rate is 16. **Her blood pressure is 128/74. She complains of flank pain and urinary hesitancy. Her urine output for the past 4 hours is 120 ml, which is the total from three separate voidings. Her urine is cloudy and has a slightly foul odor. What is your priority and what interventions are needed?**

Bibliography

1. Alexander, L. L. (1994). *New dimensions in women's health.* Boston: Jones & Bartlett.
2. American Cancer Society. (1995). *Cancer facts and figures.* New York: Author.
3. Avis, N. E., & McKinlay, S. M. (1995). The Massachusetts Women's Health Study: An epidemiologic investigation of the menopause. *Journal of the American Medical Women's Association, 50*(2), 45–49.
4. Baird, S. B., et al. (1991). *Cancer nursing: A comprehensive text.* Philadelphia: W. B. Saunders.
5. Barder, D. J., et al. (1995). Weight gain in infancy and cancer of the ovary. *Lancet, 345*(8957), 1087–1088.
6. Betz, C. L., Hunsberger, M., & Wright, S. (1994). *Family-centered nursing care of children,* (2nd ed.). Philadelphia: W. B. Saunders.
7. Biley, A. (1995). Making sense of diagnosing and treating endometriosis. *Nursing Times, 91*(9), 32–34.
8. Bobak, I. M., & Jensen, M. D. (1993). *Maternity and gynecologic care* (5th ed.). St. Louis: Mosby–Year Book.
9. Booten, D. A., & Seideman, R. Y. (1989). Relationship between premenstrual syndrome and dysmenorrhea. *AAOHN Journal, 37*(8), 308–315.
10. Brucks, J. A. (1992). Ovarian cancer: The most lethal gynecologic malignancy. *Nursing Clinics of North America, 27*(4), 835–845.
11. Callahan, J. C. (Ed.). (1993). *Menopause: A midlife passage.* Bloomington: Indiana University Press.
12. Carol, R. (Ed.). (1994). *Alternatives for women with endometriosis: A guide by women for women.* Chicago: Third Side Press.
13. Chang, J., et al. (1995). A matched control study of familial epithelial ovarian cancer: Patient characteristics, response to chemotherapy and outcome. *Annals of Oncology, 6*(1), 80–82.
14. Cherry, S. H., & Runowicz, C. D. (1994). *The menopause book: A guide to health and well-being for women after forty.* New York: Macmillan.
15. Chinn, P. L. (Ed.). (1994). *Developing nursing perspective in women's health.* Gaithersburg, MD: Aspen.
16. Choi, M. W. (1995). The menopausal transition: Change, loss, and adaptation. *Holistic Nursing Practice, 9*(3), 53–62.
17. Christiansen, C. (1995). What should be done at the time of menopause? *American Journal of Medicine, 98*(2A) 56S–59S.
18. Cunningham, G., et al. (1993). *Williams obstetrics* (19th ed.). Norwalk, CT: Appleton & Lange.

tional healers; and patterns of decision-making within the family. A study by Frye[8] reveals that Cambodian refugee women conceptualize equilibrium as important in their health. Unfortunately, few healthcare providers understand the concept of balance (hot and cold and Yin and Yang) and equilibrium that is so essential for healing among Cambodian and other Asian women refugees. Health-related behaviors are congruent with the traditional health structure, but blending of traditional and biomedical healing practices is prevalent in many cultures. The need for language and cultural comfort was the primary theme identified in the study by those seeking to access care and care providers.

Bibliography

1. Adebajo, C. O. (1992). Female circumcision and other dangerous practices. In M. N. Kisekka (Ed.), *Women's health issues in Nigeria* (pp. 1–12). Zaria: Tamaza.
2. Blenner, J. L. (1991). Health care providers' treatment approaches to culturally diverse infertile clients. *Journal of Transcultural Nursing, 2*(2), 24–31.
3. Buck, M. M., & Gottlieb, L. N. (1991). The meaning of time: Mohawk women at midlife. *Health Care for Women International, 12*(1), 41–50.
4. Douglas, C. J., Kalman, C. M., & Kalman, T. P. (1985). Homophobia among physicians and nurses: An empirical study. *Hospital and Community Psychiatry, 36,* 1309–1311.
5. Eliason, M. J. (1993). Cultural diversity in nursing care: The lesbian, gay or bisexual client. *Journal of Transcultural Nursing, 5*(1), 14–20.
6. Eliason, M. J., & Macy, M. N. (1992). A classroom activity to introduce cultural diversity. *Nurse Educator, 17,* 32–36.
7. Eliason, M. J., & Randall, C. E. (1991). Lesbian phobia in nursing students. *Western Journal of Nursing Research, 13*(3), 363–374.
8. Frye, B. A. (1991). Cultural themes in health care decision making among Cambodian refugee women. *Journal of Community Health Nursing, 8*(1), 30–44.
9. Griffin, F. N. (1994). Perceptions of African American women regarding health. *Journal of Cultural Diversity, 1*(2), 32–35.
10. Indian Health Service (1995). Pap test videotape and brochure available. *IHS Provider, 20*(5), 71.
11. Kagawa-Singer, M. (1995). Socioeconomic and cultural influences on cancer care of women. *Seminars in Oncology Nursing, 11*(2), 109–119.
12. Rankow, E. T. (1995). Breast and cervical cancer among lesbians. *Women's Health Issues, 5,* 123–129.
13. Smith, E. M., Johnson, S. R., & Guenther, S. M. (1985). Health care attitudes and experiences during gynecologic care among lesbians and bisexuals. *American Journal of Public Health, 75,* 1085–1087.
14. Stephany, T. M. (1992). Promoting mental health: Lesbian nurse support. *Journal of Psychosocial Nursing, 30,* 35–38.

19. Delgado, G., Potkul, R. K., & Dolan, J. R. (1995). Retroperitoneal radical hysterectomy. *Gynecologic Oncology, 56*(2), 191–194.
20. DeMonico, S. O., Brown, C. S., & Ling, F. W. (1994). Premenstrual syndrome. *Current Opinion in Obstetrics and Gynecology, 6*(6), 499–502.
21. Edge, V. (1994). *Women's health care.* St. Louis: Mosby–Year Book.
22. Ensign, J. E., et al. (1988). Premenstrual syndrome. *AORN Journal, 47*(4), 962–971.
23. Eschenbach, D. A., & Mead, P. B. (1992). Vaginitis: Varying management approaches. *Contemporary Obstetrics and Gynecology, 37,* 25.
24. Eskin, B. A. (Ed.). (1994). *The menopause: Comprehensive management* (3rd ed.). New York: McGraw-Hill.
25. Flay, L. D., & Matthews, J. H. (1995). The effects of radiotherapy and surgery on the sexual function of women treated for cervical cancer. *International Journal of Radiation Oncology, Biology, Physics, 31*(2), 399–404.
26. Fogel, C.I., & Woods, N.F. (Eds.). (1995). *Women's health care: A comprehensive handbook.* Thousand Oaks, CA: Sage Publications.
27. Freeman, H. P., Muth, B. J., & Kerner, J. F. (1995). Expanding access to cancer screening and clinical follow-up among the medically underserved. *Cancer Practice, 3*(1), 19–30.
28. Gannon, L. (1988). The potential role of exercise in the alleviation of menstrual disorders and menopausal symptoms: A theoretical synthesis of recent research. *Women & Health, 14*(2), 105–127.
29. Gershenson, D. M., DeCherney, A. H., & Curry, S. L. (Eds.) (1993). *Operative gynecology.* Philadelphia: W. B. Saunders.
30. Gorrie, T. M., McKinney, E. S., & Murray, S. S. (1994). *Foundations of maternal newborn nursing.* Philadelphia: W. B. Saunders.
31. Hacker, N. F., & Moore, J. G. (1992). *Essentials of obstetrics and gynecology* (2nd ed.). Philadelphia: W. B. Saunders.
32. Hamilton, P. M. (1993). *Basic maternity nursing* (7th ed.). St. Louis: Mosby–Year Book.
33. Harper, D. C. (1990). Perimenopause and aging. In R. Lichtman & S. Papera (Eds.), *Gynecology: Well woman care* (pp. 405–424). East Norwalk, CT: Appleton & Lange.
34. Hartage, P., & Devesa, S. (1995). Ovarian cancer, ovulation and side of origin. *British Journal of Cancer, 71*(3), 642–643.
35. Herbst, A. L., et al. (1992). *Comprehensive gynecology* (2nd ed.). St. Louis: Mosby–Year Book.
36. Hoffman, M. S., & Spellacy, W. N. (1995). *The difficult vaginal hysterectomy: A surgical atlas.* New York: Springer-Verlag.
37. Horton, J. A. (Ed.). (1995). *The women's health data book: A profile of women's health in the United States* (2nd ed.). New York: Elsevier.
38. Kenney, J. W., & Reuss, H. (1994). Human papillomavirus as expressed in cervical neoplasia: Evolving diagnostic and treatment modalities. *Health Care for Women International, 15*(4), 287–296.
39. Kerber, R. A., & Slattery, M. L. (1995). The impact of family history in ovarian cancer risk. The Utah Population Database. *Archives of Internal Medicine, 155*(9), 905–912.
40. Landau, C. (1994). *The complete book of menopause: Every woman's guide to good health.* New York: G. P. Putnam's.
41. Leuning, C. (1995). Women and health: Power through perseverance. *Holistic Nursing Practice, 8*(4), 1–11.

42. Lewis, L. L. (1995). One year in the life of a woman with premenstrual syndrome: A case study. *Nursing Research, 44*(2), 111–116.

43. Lichtman, R. (1996). Perimenopausal and postmenopausal hormone replacement therapy: I. An update of the literature on benefits and risks. *Journal of Nurse-Midwifery, 41*(1), 3–28.

44. Lichtman, R. C. (1991). Perimenopausal hormone replacement therapy. Reviews of the literature. *Journal of Nurse Midwifery, 36*(1), 30–48.

45. Lichtman, R. C., & Papera, S. (Eds.). (1990). *Gynecology: Well-woman care.* Norwalk, CT: Appleton & Lange.

46. Lobo, R. A. (Ed.). (1994). *Treatment of the postmenopausal woman: Basic and clinical aspects.* New York: Raven Press.

47. Magos, A. L., et al. (1995). Transvaginal endoscopic oophorectomy. *American Journal of Obstetrics and Gynecology, 172*(1, Pt.1), 123–124.

48. Mamsen, A., et al. (1995). The possible role of ultrasound in early cervical cancer. *Gynecologic Oncology, 56*(2), 187–190.

49. Miller, A. B. (1995). An epidemiological perspective on cancer screening. *Clinical Biochemistry, 28*(1), 41–48.

50. Munhall, P. L. (Ed.). (1994). *In women's experience.* New York: National League for Nursing.

51. Nezhat, F., et al. (1995). Complications and results of 361 hysterectomies performed at laparoscopy. *Journal of the American College of Surgeons, 180*(3), 307–316.

52. Ornitz, A. W., & Brown, M. A. (1993). Family coping and premenstrual symptomology. *Journal of Obstetric, Gynecologic and Neonatal Nursing, 22,* 49–55.

53. Ovarian cancer: Screening, treatment, and followup (April 5–7, 1994). *NIH Consensus Statement, 12*(3), 1–30.

54. Paul, H. (1994). Ten trends in women's health. *Healthcare Forum Journal, 37*(1), 19–21, 23.

55. *The PDR family guide to women's health and prescription drugs.* (1994). Montvale, NJ: Medical Economics Data.

56. Power, E. J. (1993). Pap smears, elderly women and Medicare. *Cancer Investigations, 11*(2), 164–168.

57. Rayome, R. G., King, C., & King, T. (1995). Patient with nocturnal enuresis and stress incontinence after previous hysterectomy and radiation therapy for cervical cancer. *Journal of Wound, Ostomy, and Continence Nursing, 22*(1), 64–67.

58. Reeder, S., Martin, L., & Koniak, D. (1992). *Maternity nursing* (17th ed.). Philadelphia: J. B. Lippincott.

59. Rodriguez, C., et al. (1995). Estrogen replacement therapy and fatal ovarian cancer. *American Journal of Epidemiology, 141*(9), 828–835.

60. Reid, R., Absten, G. T. (1995). Lasers in gynecology: Why pragmatic surgeons have not abandoned this valuable technology. *Lasers in Surgery & Medicine 17*(3), 201–301.

61. Rosser, S. V. (1994). *Women's health—missing from US medicine.* Bloomington: Indiana University Press.

62. Scarabelli, C., et al. (1995). Systemic pelvic and para-aortic lymphadenectomy during cytoreductive surgery in advanced ovarian cancer: Potential benefit on survival. *Gynecologic Oncology, 56*(3), 328–337.

63. Schnare, S. (1993). Hormone therapy. *Contemporary OB/GYN-NP, 1*(3), 3–5.

64. Seltzer, V., & Pearse, W. H. (Eds.). (1995). *Women's primary health care.* New York: McGraw-Hill.

65. Severino, S. K., & Moline, M. L. (1995). Premenstrual syndrome: Identification and management. *Drugs, 49*(1), 71–82.

66. Slade, M. (1994). Managing menopause. *American Health: Fitness of Body & Mind, 13*(10), 66–69.

67. Soper, D. E. (1994). Pelvic inflammatory disease. *Infectious Disease Clinics of North America, 8*(4), 821–840.

68. Star, W. L., Lommel, L. L., & Shannon, M. T. (Eds.). (1995). *Women's primary health care: Protocols for practice.* Washington, DC: American Nurses Publication.

69. Strausz, I. K. (1993). *You don't need a hysterectomy: New and effective ways of avoiding major surgery.* Reading, MA: Addison-Wesley.

70. Sullivan, N. (1990). Dysmenorrhea. In R. Lichtman & S. Papera (Eds.), *Gynecology: Well woman care* (pp. 345–353). East Norwalk, CT: Appleton & Lange.

71. Taylor, D. (1996). The perimenstrual symptom management program: Elements of effective treatment. *Capsules and Comments in Perinatal and Women's Health Nursing 2*(2), 140–146.

72. Teaff, N. L., & Wiley, K. W. (1995). *Perimenopause: Preparing for the change: A guide to the early stages of menopause and beyond.* Rocklin, CA: Prima.

73. Voda, A. M. (1994). Risks and benefits associated with hormonal and surgical therapies for healthy midlife women. *Western Journal of Nursing Research, 16*(5), 507–523.

74. Whipple, B. (1995). Four common questions about women's health: What you and your patients need to know about PMS, drug testing in women, eating disorders, and urinary incontinence. *American Journal of Nursing, 95*(2), 16A-B,16D.

75. Williamson, M. L., (1992). Sexual adjustment after hysterectomy. *Journal of Obstetric, Gynecologic, and Neonatal Nursing, 21,* 42–47.

76. Wright, S., et al. (1995). Short-term Lupron or danazol therapy for pelvic endometriosis. *Fertility and Sterility, 63*(3), 504–507.

77. Youngkin, E. Q., & Davis, M. S. (Eds.). (1994). *Women's health: A primary care clinical guide.* Norwalk, CT: Appleton & Lange.

Nursing Care of Clients with Breast Disorders

Lynne C. Carpenter

One of eight women will develop breast cancer in her lifetime.[2] Because breast cancer is such a feared disease, a woman who finds a breast lump or problem will probably first suspect cancer, and then worry about losing her breast and about dying, all within seconds after the discovery of the breast problem. Therefore, in addition to caring for women with breast disorders, nurses have an important role in teaching women about normal breasts; common benign breast problems; breast self-examination and mammography; and risk factors for, incidence of, and treatments for breast cancer.

Public Attitudes and Knowledge About Breast Lesions

The fear of breast cancer is common. Women and men who develop a breast problem become anxious about whether they have cancer. Thus, assessment not only is directed at differentiating between malignant and nonmalignant lesions but also focuses on gathering information about concerns of the client and significant others and their coping strategies. Such assessment forms the basis of subsequent nursing and medical intervention.

Many misconceptions exist about breast cancer. In a 1981 National Cancer Institute study, half of those surveyed were incorrect in thinking that a breast injury could cause cancer. Many did not know that nipple changes can be a manifestation of breast cancer. Also, many did not know about diagnostic procedures for breast cancer or treatment options other than surgery.[53] However, despite such misconceptions, public awareness about breast cancer has grown. In the past, the subject was often avoided, or information, often inaccurate, was secretly and fearfully shared. Now breast cancer is openly discussed and information about it frequently is presented in mass media. Controversies continue to arise over the cause of breast cancer, diagnostic methods, and treatment options. These controversies are reported in the popular press.

Facts about the disease, treatment, and prognosis need to be clarified.

Nurses have an educational role concerning breast lesions. By allowing clients to talk about breast cancer, correcting misinformation, and supplying accurate facts when possible, nurses can reduce associated fear, anxiety, and misinformation. Women may then seek earlier assessment, diagnosis, and effective treatment. Factual answers to questions are not always available. However, by maintaining a comfortable therapeutic relationship, nurses can support clients and their families.

Nurses need to provide current information about breast cancer. Controversies do exist, however. One current controversy involves risk factors. Which factors are important, and who is at greatest risk for developing breast cancer? Also, there are various opinions about the use of mammography in screening for breast cancer. Is mammography safe, and if so, which women should have it? Other controversies involve treatment selection. Four major methods of treatment are surgery, radiation therapy, hormonal therapy, and chemotherapy with cytotoxic agents. A newer treatment, high-dose chemotherapy and an autologous bone marrow transplant, is also available. Nurses are often involved in supporting clients as they make difficult decisions.

Breast Cancer

Breast cancer refers to a group of malignant diseases that commonly occur in the female breast and infrequently in the male breast. In 1995, it was estimated that 183,400 new breast cancers would occur in the United States and that about 46,240 deaths would occur from breast cancer.[146] One in every eight women is expected to develop breast cancer. Because of improvements in early detection and treatment, the 5-year survival rate for breast cancer has improved. This has helped stabilize (although not actually decrease) the mortality rates from breast cancer over the past 50 years despite an increasing incidence of breast cancer. Breast cancer, however, is the leading cause of cancer deaths in women between the ages of 14 and 54 years.[146] Lung cancer is now the leading cause of cancer deaths in all women; breast cancer is second.

Breast cancer in men is rare. In 1995, 1400 new male breast cancer diagnoses were made and 240 deaths occurred.[146] Breast cancer is often diagnosed in a more advanced stage in men than in women.

Etiology and Risk Factors

The cause of breast cancer has not been definitely established; genetic predisposition and hormonal factors may be involved. Recently the BRCA-1 gene on chromosome 17 has been cloned. Women and men who are carriers of this gene are at a significantly higher risk for breast, ovarian, and prostate cancer. Some women who are carriers are having prophylactic mastectomies to prevent breast cancer. Research is being done to identify other genes as well.[10] Other factors have been associated with a significantly increased risk of breast cancer.[11, 71, 133] However, many women diagnosed with breast cancer have no risk factors.

Risk factors related to ovarian function suggest a hormonal influence. Artificial menopause before the age of 35 years reduces the risk of breast cancer to one third of that experienced by women who undergo natural menopause.[46] Hormonal and other factors associated with a moderate risk include (1) early menarche, (2) late menopause, (3) nulliparity, (4) exogenous estrogen given for menopause manifestations (contraceptives do not seem to produce higher risk), and (5) history of cancer of the uterus, ovary, or colon.

Risk factors under study as possible causes of increased incidence of breast cancer include (1) oral contraceptives, (2) exogenous hormones, (3) above-average weight and height (especially in postmenopausal women), (4) diet high in total fat, (5) alcohol consumption, (6) ovarian-pituitary dysfunction, (7) genetic factors, (8) benign breast disease, and (9) radiation exposure.[73, 80, 124]

Factors that may lower a woman's risk of breast cancer include (1) late menarche, (2) early menopause, (3) premenopausal oophorectomy, (4) maintaining a normal or lighter-than-average weight after menopause, and (5) Asia (Japan especially) or Africa as place of birth.

For the best prognosis, it is extremely important for breast cancer to be detected early, before metastases occur. Breast self-examination, mammography, and a thorough breast examination by a clinician are important in early detection.

One of the nurse's roles, therefore, is to encourage all women to practice breast self-examination and to follow the screening advice of the American Cancer Society (Box 85–1). Nurses also have a role in identifying women at risk for developing breast cancer and convincing them of the necessity for appropriate, careful assessment. Unfortunately, little can be done in the way of primary prevention to reduce most risk factors for breast cancer. Exceptions are maintaining normal or lighter than average body weight and reducing dietary fat (e.g., meat, dairy products). Growing evidence suggests that dietary

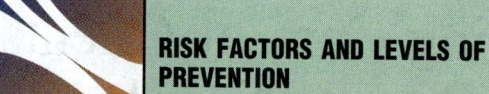

RISK FACTORS AND LEVELS OF PREVENTION

Breast Cancer

Risk Factors

- Gender: 99 : 1, women > men
- Age: Risk increases with age
- Place of birth: North America; Northern Europe
- Socioeconomic status: High
- Age at first full-term pregnancy: older than 30 years
- Menstrual history: Early menarche; late menopause
- Health history: Mammographic pattern of dysplastic parenchyma; past diagnosis of atypism, hyperplasia, or other benign proliferative disease in breast biopsy; large dose of radiation therapy to the chest; previous history of cancer in one breast
- Family history: Mother or sister with history of breast cancer; any first-degree relative with breast cancer; BRCA-1 gene carrier

Levels of Prevention

Primary Prevention

- Eat low-fat, high-fiber diet
- Maintain weight within 20% recommended body weight

Secondary Prevention

- Perform monthly breast self-examination
- Clinical examination yearly by healthcare provider
- Mammograms as appropriate for age
- Consultation with clinician about personal risk

Tertiary Prevention

- Breast reconstruction
- Arm exercises after surgery
- Exercises and positioning to prevent lymphedema

fat promotes carcinogenesis because of its effect on hormone activity.

Consideration of how women can prevent and detect early manifestations of any breast disease should be the

Box 85–1. Important Factors for Successful Breast Self-Examination

Examine the breasts at the same time each month
Examine the breasts in a consistent pattern
Examine all surfaces: the breast, tail of Spence, and axilla
Examine all depths of the tissue: use pads of fingers and press deeply
Check for discharge, inspect the breasts visually, and palpate for changes
Report any changes to the physician

primary focus of home healthcare nursing. First, women need education about their level of risk. Women at high risk include those older than 55 years, never married, older than 30 years at first pregnancy, or with a family history of breast cancer, especially if they are carriers of the BRCA-1 gene.

Women can make changes in their life-style to lower their risk of developing breast disease. Monthly breast self-examinations are essential. Most lumps are found by women themselves. The earlier breast cancer is detected, the greater the chance of cure. Besides breast self-examination, an examination by a physician should be done every 3 years for women 20 to 40 years of age and every year for women over 40 years.

Diet is another area in which women can make sufficient changes for preventing disease. A low-fat diet can play an important part in prevention. Decreasing fat intake to 20% of dietary calories is an admirable goal. Alcohol intake increases risk in relation to the amount of alcohol consumed.

Certain foods are helpful in decreasing risk. Cruciferous vegetables (broccoli, cabbage, cauliflower) help convert estrogen to a form less likely to cause cancer. Vitamin A (beta-carotene foods, orange and dark green vegetables) inhibits abnormal cell growth. Soybeans suppress estrogen production.

Women should be informed about and encouraged to have mammograms. Mammograms can detect very small tumors long before they might otherwise be found by manual breast examination (Fig. 85–1). The recommendations for mammograms are as follows: obtain a baseline at 40 years of age unless high-risk factors exist; repeat every 1 to 2 years at ages 40 to 50 years and yearly after age 50 years.

The American Cancer Society is an excellent source for further information about the prevention, detection, and treatment of breast cancer. Call 1–800–ACS–2345.

Pathophysiology

Various histopathologic types of breast cancer exist with various prognoses.[46] These include intraductal carcinoma, infiltrating ductal carcinoma, medullary carcinoma, muci-

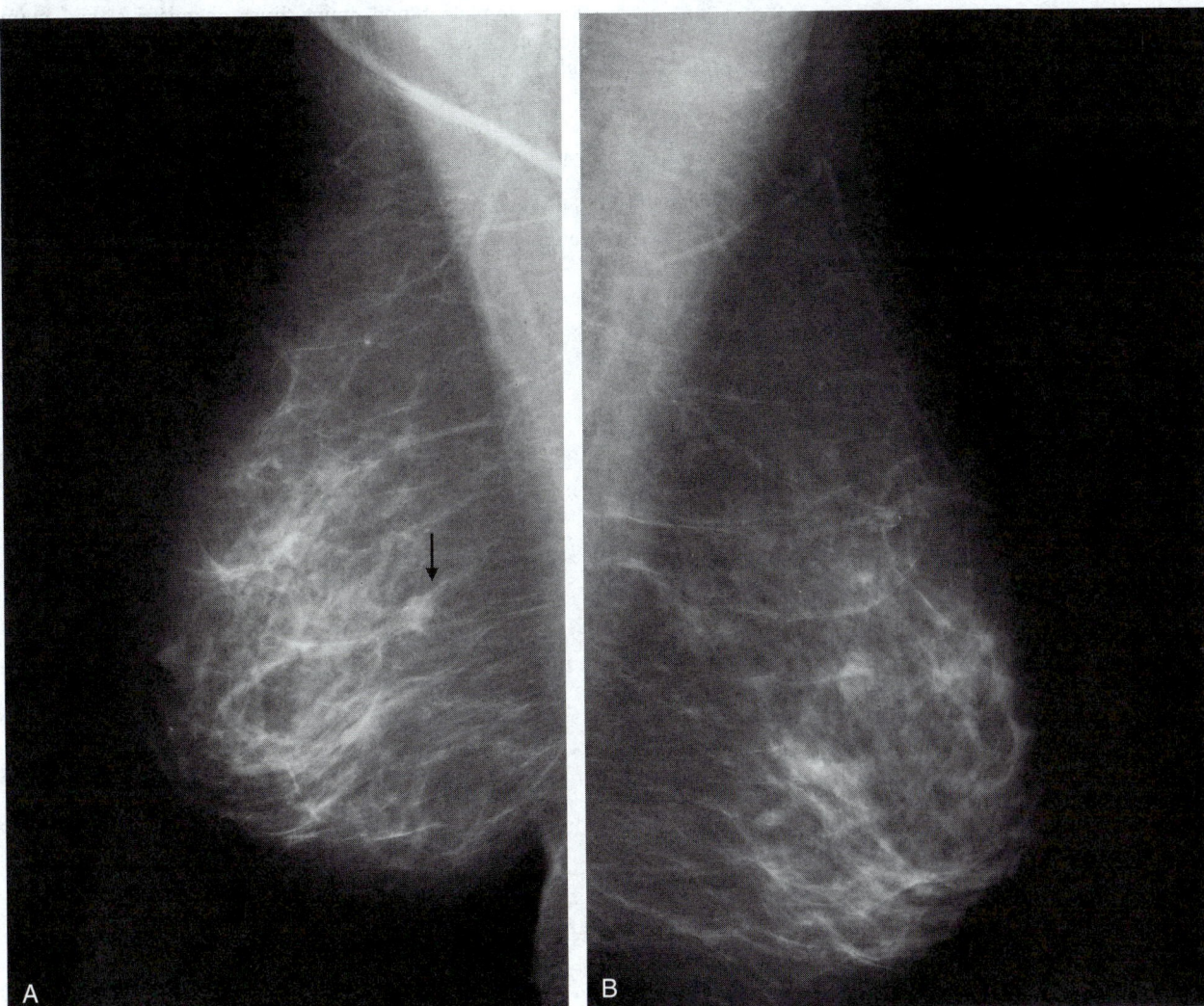

Figure 85–1. *A,* Screening mammogram (right mediolateral oblique view) of a 56-year-old woman with a strong family history of breast cancer detected a small, irregular, nonpalpable mass (*arrow*), which was highly suspicious for malignancy. *B,* The left mediolateral oblique view of the same patient shows a normal breast.

nous or colloid carcinoma, tubular carcinoma, lobular carcinoma in situ, infiltrating lobular carcinoma, inflammatory breast cancer, and Paget's disease.

Intraductal Carcinoma.

Intraductal carcinoma, also known as *ductal carcinoma in situ*, is a precancerous marker lesion that indicates a higher risk for invasive ductal breast cancer.[62] It arises from the ductal epithelium and is confined to the ducts. Axillary metastases are uncommon. Prognosis is excellent. If left untreated, intraductal carcinoma will develop into invasive ductal carcinoma.

Infiltrating Ductal Carcinoma.

Infiltrating ductal carcinoma (no other specification recognized) is found in 70% to 80% of breast cancers. It is palpated as a stony-hard lump. Frequently, metastasis to axillary lymph nodes occurs. Infiltrating ductal carcinoma has the poorest prognosis of the ductal carcinomas.

Medullary Carcinoma.

Medullary carcinoma is found in 5% to 7% of breast cancers. Frequently, it reaches large size. However, the prognosis is better than for many types of breast cancer.

Mucinous (Colloid) Carcinoma.

Mucinous carcinoma, found in 3% of breast cancers, frequently occurs with other types of breast cancer. It is slow-growing and can become quite large. Prognosis is good when the breast cancer is predominantly mucinous.

Tubular Carcinoma.

Tubular carcinoma frequently occurs with other types of breast cancer. Axillary metastases are uncommon. Prognosis is better than for infiltrating ductal carcinoma.

Lobular Carcinoma In Situ.

Lobular carcinoma in situ is a precancerous marker lesion that indicates a higher risk for invasive breast cancer. It arises from the mammary lobules and is usually a microscopic incidental finding with removal of a benign breast lesion. Checkups every 6 months without treatment may be indicated, or bilateral mastectomies may be performed because of the bilaterality of lobular carcinoma in situ that may or may not develop into infiltrating lobular breast cancer.[63]

Infiltrating Lobular Carcinoma.

Infiltrating lobular carcinoma is found in 5% to 10% of breast cancers. It usually presents as an area of ill-defined thickening rather than a lump. Multicentricity or involvement of the opposite breast may be found. Frequently, metastasis occurs to axillary lymph nodes.

Inflammatory Breast Cancer.

Inflammatory breast cancer is characterized by skin redness and induration. Edema, redness, warmth, and induration are frequent associated findings. Frequently, palpable axillary and supraclavicular nodes and distant metastases are involved. Prognosis is poor.[52]

Paget's Disease.

Paget's disease is found in 1% to 4% of breast cancers. A special classification characterizes Paget's disease, which includes a relatively long history of crusting and scaling skin changes in the nipple with burning, itching, or bleeding.

Clinical Manifestations and Diagnostic Findings

The nurse should be alert to assessment findings indicating breast cancer, although detection may be difficult. Initially, breast cancer typically appears as a unilateral single mass or thickening, most often in a breast's upper outer quadrant (Fig. 85–2). The mass is usually painless, nontender, hard, irregular in shape, and nonmobile. Nipple discharge and retraction, edema with *peau d'orange* skin, and dimpling may be present. A palpable mass, which is found by the client, is the presenting feature in 64% to 70% of cases of breast cancer[39]; 4% to 30% of lesions are found by mammography.

Pretreatment assessment varies. Chest x-ray examination, complete blood count, liver chemistries, and mammography of the opposite breast are frequently done. Other studies are in question, however. Bone scans or liver scans can give false-positive results and yield little useful information in asymptomatic clients. Some physicians believe scans should be used only for clients with stage III disease or abnormal liver chemistries. Others believe that a baseline study, especially a bone scan, is valuable for later comparison.

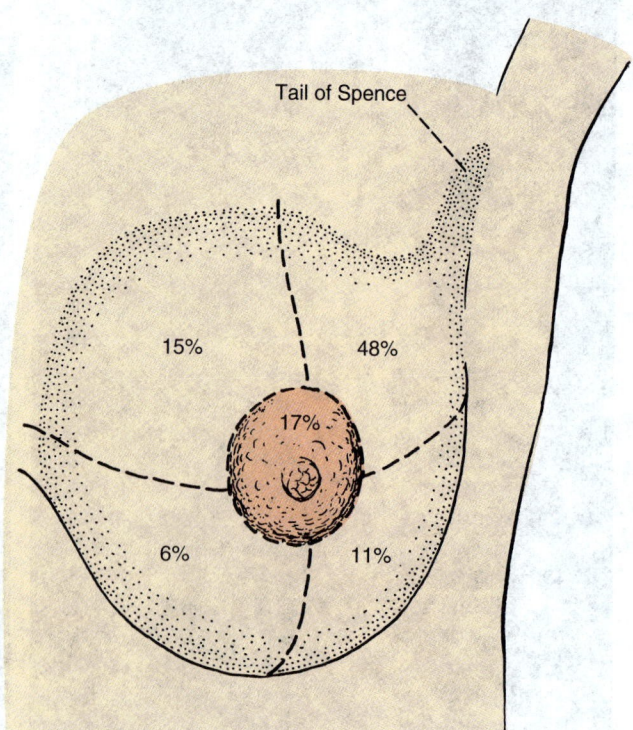

Figure 85–2. Frequency of occurrence of breast cancer according to location. Note that the highest occurrence is in the upper outer quadrant and the tail of Spence.

Tumor markers (substances produced either by the tumor itself or by the body in response to tumor tissue) may be present in the serum of a client with breast cancer. The tumor markers—carcinoembryonic antigen (CEA) and CA 15-3—are easy to obtain and correlate with changing disease status. Trying to identify these markers and to follow them after diagnosis is recommended.

Numerous staging systems (see Chapter 24) have been developed for cancer. The staging of a cancer is based on (1) the size of the primary lesion, (2) the extent of the cancer's spread to regional lymph nodes, and (3) the presence or absence of metastases. Staging provides prognostic information; Figure 85-3 illustrates the clinical staging of breast cancer. The commonly used TNM staging system (Table 85-1) groups breast cancer according to the characteristics of the primary tumor (T), regional lymph nodes (N), and distant metastases (M).[9] With breast cancer, subgroup assignments are made according to tumor size, tumor attachment to underlying structure, and other characteristics (e.g., edema).

Several other parameters are useful in determining the prognosis for women with breast cancer and deciding on its treatment.[29, 44, 46, 100, 132] These include histology, multicentricity, estrogen-progesterone receptor status of the tumor, and the immunocompetence of the woman. If cancer is found in two or more locations (multicentric) in the breast, the woman will probably not be a candidate for lumpectomy or quandrantectomy. If the tumor is estrogen-progesterone receptor-positive, she will probably receive antiestrogen hormonal therapy.

Tests of the proliferative activity of the tumor are gaining popularity. *Ploidy* refers to the degree of multiplication of chromosome sets. *Diploid* or *euploid* indicates an exact multiple of the haploid number of chromosome. *Aneuploid* indicates a deviation from an exact multiple of the haploid number *and a poorer prognosis. The S phase index* identifies the percentage of tumor cells in S phase of the cell growth cycle. The higher the percentage of cells in S phase, the more aggressive the cancer. The labeling index measures the uptake of thymidine, which is used primarily in DNA synthesis or in the S phase of the cell growth cycle.

Studies are also looking at the role of oncogenes in

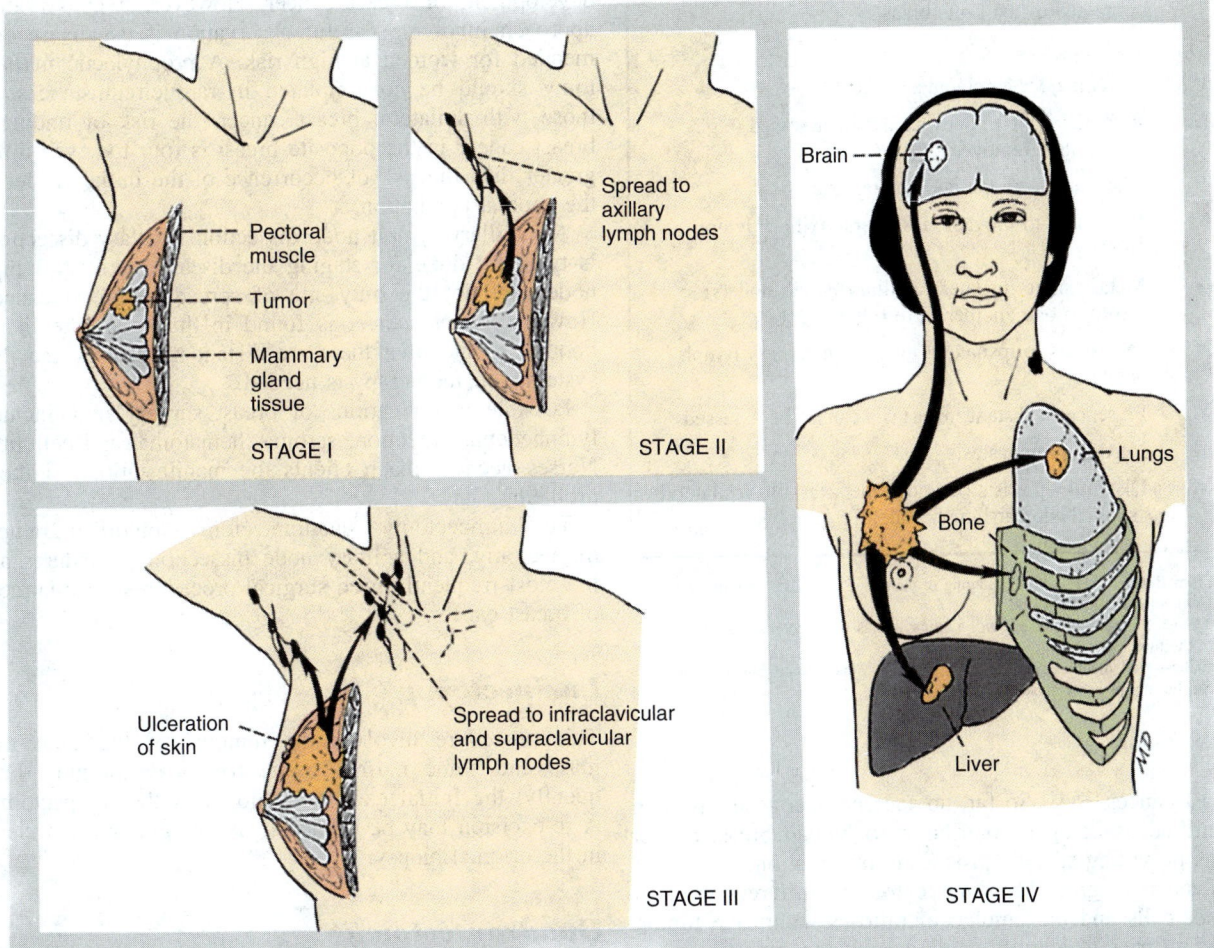

Figure 85-3. Clinical staging of breast cancer. Stage I: tumor less than 2 cm and confined to the breast. Stage II: tumor up to 5 cm, or axillary lymph nodes contain early metastasis. Stage III: tumor larger than 5 cm, or extends to the chest wall or skin, or involvement of the infraclavicular or supraclavicular lymph nodes. Stage IV: distant metastasis such as to the brain, bone, or liver.

Table 85–1. Staging of Breast Cancer, American Joint Committee on Cancer and International Union Against Cancer

T_X	Primary tumor cannot be assessed
T_0	No evidence of primary tumor
T_{is}	Carcinoma in situ: intraductal carcinoma, lobular carcinoma in situ, or Paget's disease* of the nipple with no tumor
T_1	Tumor 2 cm or less in greatest dimension
T_{1a}	0.5 cm or less in greatest dimension
T_{1b}	More than 0.5 cm but not more than 1 cm in greatest dimension
T_{1c}	More than 1 cm but not more than 2 cm in greatest dimension
T_2	Tumor more than 2 cm but not more than 5 cm in greatest dimension
T_3	Tumor more than 5 cm in greatest dimension
T_4	Tumor of any size with direct extension to chest wall† or skin
T_{4a}	Extension to chest wall
T_{4b}	Edema (including *peau d'orange*) or ulceration of the skin of the breast or satellite skin nodules confined to the same breast
T_{4c}	Both (T_{4a} and T_{4b})
T_{4d}	Inflammatory carcinoma
N_X	Regional lymph nodes cannot be assessed (e.g., previously removed)
N_0	No regional lymph node metastasis
N_1	Metastasis to movable ipsilateral axillary lymph node(s)
N_2	Metastasis to ipsilateral axillary lymph node(s) fixed to one another or to other structures
N_3	Metastasis to ipsilateral internal mammary lymph node(s)
M_X	Presence of distant metastasis cannot be assessed
M_0	No distant metastasis
M_1	Distant metastasis (includes metastasis to ipsilateral supraclavicular lymph node[s])

From Beahrs, O. H. (1991). Staging of cancer. *CA: A Cancer Journal for Clinicians, 41*(2), 122–124.
* Paget's disease associated with a tumor is classified according to the size of the tumor.
† Chest wall includes ribs, intercostal muscles, and serratus anterior muscle, but not pectoral muscle.

breast cancer.[135, 148] So far, no specific oncogene has been identified as being a contributor to human breast cancer or as providing specific prognostic information.

Cancer is graded on the cytologic differentiation of tumor cells and the number of mitoses within the tumor. Grading tries to identify some degree of a tumor's malignancy or to estimate its aggressiveness. Low histologic grade indicates that the cancer is well differentiated and carries a better prognosis than a higher-grade tumor.

Acute and Subacute Care

■ Surgical Management

Surgery is important in the diagnosis and treatment of most breast cancers.[90] Some breast surgical procedures are very disfiguring (e.g., radical mastectomy and modified radical mastectomy). However, less extensive procedures may be used (e.g., lumpectomy and quadrantectomy).

From the initial surgical procedure to diagnose breast cancer, a portion of the tissue is sent for estrogen and progesterone receptor assay. If high levels of estrogen or progesterone receptors are present, then a woman may need hormonal therapy. (See preceding discussion of hormonal therapy.)

Occasionally, a mastectomy is performed to prevent breast cancer in women who are at high risk for breast cancer. When a mastectomy is done to prevent breast cancer, it is called a *prophylactic mastectomy*. Reconstructive surgery (see Chapter 80) may be performed at the same time or delayed. Prophylactic mastectomy is controversial. The goal is to decrease the likelihood of development of breast cancer. However, a conservative approach involving careful observation is usually recommended for women at high risk. A prophylactic mastectomy should be contemplated in rare circumstances. In those with unilateral breast cancer, the risk of finding a breast cancer in the opposite breast is four to seven times greater than the risk of occurrence of the initial cancer in the general population.

An axillary lymph node dissection (axillary dissection) is typically done for staging the disease. Axillary lymph nodes are not the only site of spread of breast cancer. However, when cancer is found in the nodes the likelihood is greater that there are distant metastases and that systemic chemotherapy is needed.

Possible complications of breast surgery may include lymphedema, infection, seroma, hematoma, and cellulitis. Nurses need to teach clients the manifestations of these problems.

The lumpectomy, quadrantectomy, modified radical mastectomy, and axillary node dissection procedures are the most frequently used surgical procedures for treatment of breast cancer.[86, 119]

Lumpectomy

This procedure involves the removal of the cancerous mass and some normal tissue for clean margins. Frequently, the initial excisional biopsy is the lumpectomy. A re-excision may be needed if the margins are not clean in the original biopsy.

Quadrantectomy

This procedure removes the quadrant of the breast in which the cancer is located. A greater portion of normal tissue surrounding the cancer is removed with some of

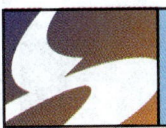

CASE MANAGEMENT

Breast: Mastectomy

For Clinical Pathway, see Appendix D.
Clinical Pathway from Birmingham Baptist Medical Center, Birmingham, Alabama
Information provided by Carol Murphy, R.N., O.C.N.

Development and Revision of Pathway

- This pathway was initiated to minimize hospital stay and to assist with coordinating breast care across the continuum from prediagnosis through outpatient treatment following surgery.
- The pathway was initiated in February 1994.
- The team that developed the pathway included registered nurses, a clinical pharmacist, a chaplain, a dietitian, and physicians. Consulting members included social service staff, rehabilitation staff, operating room scrub and circulating nurses, recovery room nurses, and nurses from the outpatient cancer center.
- We hold quarterly continuous process improvement meetings with a multidisciplinary group whose members are involved with the care of the mastectomy patient. Everyone on the team has an opportunity to recommend changes in the pathway.
- Maps are reviewed at least twice a year, but no more than quarterly, for possible revision.

Use and Impact of Pathway

- Patients who undergo mastectomy are placed on this pathway unless they are having breast reconstruction as part of the mastectomy procedure. A woman undergoing reconstruction at the time of mastectomy has a different postoperative recovery period and should be placed on a pathway that specifically addresses her care related to the reconstructive surgery.
- The nursing staff uses the pathway daily to guide care. More physicians are reviewing the pathway on daily rounds as well.
- There have been many positive changes in nursing practice since we initiated this pathway. Preoperative and postoperative education are started earlier; documentation of patient education has improved; and staff nurses have assumed responsibility for patient education rather than relying only on the clinical nurse specialist. The clinical nurse specialist has become a resource for the staff nurses as they take on more responsibility for education.
- The length of stay for breast surgery patients has steadily declined, from 4 days to 2.3 days. The variable cost has decreased from $1500 per case to $1370 per case in less than 2 years.

the overlying skin and underlying muscular fascia, to provide a wide margin of cancer-free tissue.

Modified Radical Mastectomy

This procedure involves the en bloc removal of the breast, axillary lymph nodes, and overlying skin. This is the most commonly performed mastectomy.

Axillary Node Dissection

This procedure removes ipsilateral lymph nodes. It is part of the lumpectomy, modified radical mastectomy, and the standard mastectomy. An axillary node dissection may be the only additional surgical procedure needed by a woman who has had an excisional biopsy for diagnosis and removal of a small breast cancer with clean margins. The axillary dissection is not usually done to treat the disease, but it determines the disease stage and the need for chemotherapy.

Total (Simple) Mastectomy

This procedure involves resection of breast tissue and some skin from the clavicle to the costal margin and from the midline to the latissimus dorsi. The axillary tail and pectoral fascia are also removed. Axillary nodes are not removed. This procedure is rarely used to treat diagnosed breast cancer. More frequently, bilateral simple mastectomies or total mastectomies are done to prevent breast cancer in women who are at high risk for having the disease.

Standard Radical Mastectomy

This procedure involves the en bloc removal of the breast, overlying skin, pectoral muscles, and axillary nodes. It removes the local lesion and the axillary nodes with a wide "safety margin" of surrounding tissue. Dissatisfaction with treatment results and morbidity has caused the number of radical mastectomies performed for primary breast cancer to decline sharply.

Extended Radical Mastectomy

This procedure involves the removal of the internal mammary nodes in addition to the structures removed during the standard radical mastectomy. This procedure currently has few advocates because it does not seem to be significantly more effective than is irradiation in preventing recurrence from internal mammary metastases.

Surgical Hormonal Manipulation

A bilateral oophorectomy has been used for more than 80 years as a form of hormonal therapy in premenopausal women with advanced breast cancer. Radiation to the ovaries may also be used to achieve castration (stopping the function of the ovaries), but it may take up to 2 months for the therapy to be effective.

In castrated or postmenopausal women, other surgical procedures, such as bilateral adrenalectomy or hypophysectomy (removal of the anterior pituitary), can be used

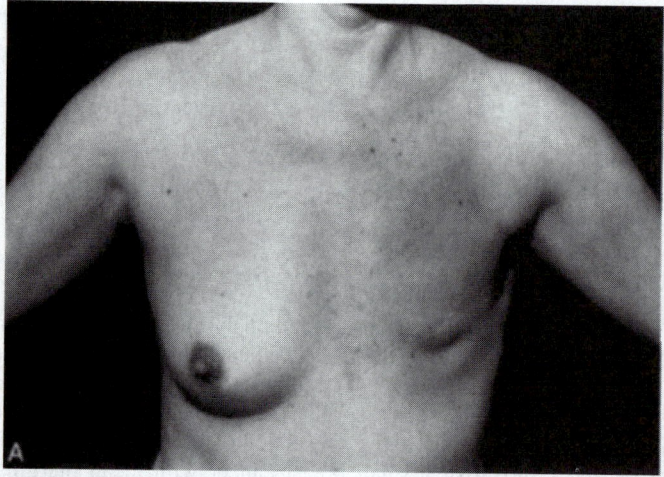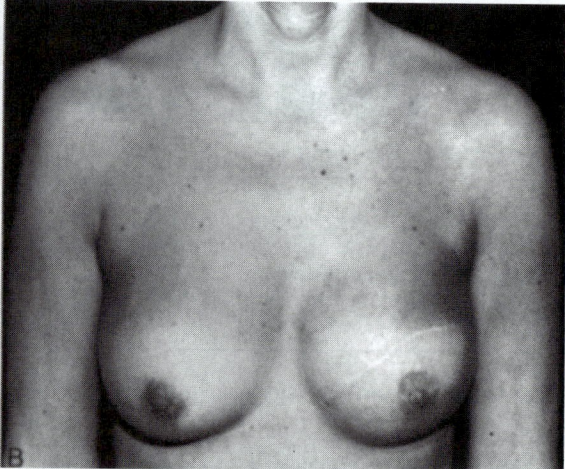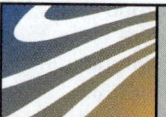

Figure 85–4. An ideal result of reconstructive surgery using a latissimus dorsi myocutaneous flap and an implant. *A,* Preoperative appearance. *B,* Postoperative appearance. A subpectoral implant was used in the right breast for symmetry. (From Bland, K. I., & Copeland, E. M. (Eds.) [1991]. *The breast: Comprehensive management of benign and malignant disease.* Philadelphia: W. B. Saunders.)

to further decrease the remaining low level of estrogen. If an adrenalectomy is used, daily cortisone replacement is required to prevent adrenal crisis and fludrocortisone acetate (Florinef) is required to replace the adrenal salt-regulating hormone, aldosterone. Hypophysectomy also requires daily replacement of cortisone, thyroid hormone, and, if necessary, posterior pituitary hormones (e.g., vasopressin or antidiuretic hormone).

Daily replacement therapy after bilateral adrenalectomy or hypophysectomy is required for life. A medical identification bracelet should be worn at all times after such surgery. A card indicating the type and dose of necessary replacement medications should also be carried.

Breast Reconstruction

Breast reconstruction is an option for women who have had a mastectomy.[16, 17, 70, 145] Consideration needs to be given to a woman's overall health and ability to tolerate a prolonged operation, the stage of disease, the need for radiation therapy or chemotherapy, and the woman's expectations (Fig. 85–4).

New techniques provide the woman with choices for the type and timing of reconstruction. Breast reconstruction can be done by use of tissue expanders, implants (see Ethical Issues in Nursing), latissimus dorsi muscle flap, transverse rectus abdominis muscle flap, or gluteus maximus muscle flap.[33, 66, 84, 100, 113, 127] The nurse needs to know about each of these procedures to answer the client's questions (see Chapter 21). A woman may choose to delay reconstruction until after radiation or chemotherapy is complete, or she may choose immediate reconstruction, to be done at the same time as the mastectomy, so she isn't missing a breast when she regains consciousness.

Breast reconstruction can help restore the woman's balance, symmetry, and body image. The nurse can help the woman while she is deciding about reconstructive surgery, while preparing for reconstructive surgery, and while recovering from the surgery (see Chapter 21).

Knowing about reconstruction and whether it is an option for her may help a woman with breast cancer cope with the need for a mastectomy. The nurse can provide information about reconstruction.

ETHICAL ISSUES IN NURSING

Are Silicone Implants a Safe Alternative for Breast Reconstruction?

For many women with breast cancer, breast implants allow both physical and mental treatment for the disfigurement that may result from surgery. For other women who simply wish to enhance their breasts, implants produce desired esthetic effects. Silicone breast implants have been in use since 1902, and millions of women throughout the world have undergone breast augmentation. No matter what opinions are held about breast implants, it is generally accepted that women have a right to such a procedure if they so choose.

Does this right to choose silicone breast implants imply a duty of the implant manufacturers to produce a safe product? It has been proposed but never proven that silicone leakage from breast implants causes various systemic side effects, some of which may be very serious. If this is true, does the Food and Drug Administration have an obligation to ban such implants to protect certain members of society from harm? Should a woman have the right to have silicone breast augmentation if she is adequately informed of the possible side effects that may occur should such implants rupture or leak silicone?

If silicone is the problem, perhaps saline implants may be the solution. Women could still choose to have augmentations but not have to worry about the possible side effects that silicone may cause. Autonomy would be preserved and beneficence fostered.

■ Nursing Management of the Surgical Client

Preoperative Care

Assessment

The assessment of the woman should begin with assessment of the breasts, identification of the woman's risk factors, a description of the lump or lesion, and current fears or concerns. It is also important to find out how the client discovered the lump.

The preoperative period before breast surgery for cancer or possible cancer is a very stressful time. Many fears surface, and the lives of the client and significant others are disrupted. A contradiction exists because usually the client feels well despite impending surgery. The preoperative period may also be stressful for health professionals. Nurses need an opportunity to explore their personal feelings about breast cancer before they can satisfactorily help others.

Nurses providing preoperative care assess the woman's and significant others' reactions to the frightening experience. The woman and significant others need an opportu-nity to talk about the surgery and feel that someone cares about them. Nursing assessment focuses on the woman's knowledge level, coping ability, self-concept, and sexual concerns. It helps to include the sexual partner in assessment and planning. Nurses need to be knowledgeable about all aspects of care and the therapeutic plan for each client so that they can accurately answer questions (see Nursing Care Plan).

Diagnosis, Planning, Implementation

Knowledge Deficit. The nursing diagnosis may be expressed as *Knowledge Deficit related to available options of treatment and surgery* (if chosen).

Planning: Expected Outcomes. The client will understand the available treatment options and surgery (if chosen), as evidenced by the client's questions and statements concerning options and the client's ability to explain her choice.

Implementation. The woman should receive information about recommendations and treatment options before surgery or treatment is initiated. The nurse can help women understand treatment options.[86, 139, 142] Because the typical hospital stay for a modified radical mastectomy or lumpectomy and axillary node dissection surgery is 1 to 3 days, preoperative teaching is done on an outpatient basis. The nurse needs to consider postoperative teaching along with preoperative care.

Nursing assessment provides data about knowledge deficits for use in formulating a teaching plan. This includes preoperative activities, explanations of surgery, postoperative care, discharge planning, and ways in which the client can participate. The woman's anxiety level may be so high that new information cannot be remembered, so it is important to provide written as well as verbal instructions. It is important to evaluate learning and to repeat information as often as necessary.

Risk for Ineffective Individual Coping and Risk for Ineffective Family Coping. The nursing diagnosis may be expressed as *Ineffective Individual Coping, and Ineffective Family Coping related to diagnosis of cancer and surgical changes in breast.*

Planning: Expected Outcomes. The client will cope with the diagnosis of cancer and surgical changes in the breast, as evidenced by client's statement of acceptance and decisions about treatment; the family will also cope effectively, as evidenced by support given to the client.

Implementation. Preoperatively or before any treatment, assess the client's and significant others' coping ability and concerns. Do not rush the assessment. Identify the coping mechanisms usually used by the client and significant others. Are there any potentially disabling coping patterns? Use this information as the basis of support. The woman may fear pain, mutilation, death, loss of control, and the hospital environment. Use these findings to establish a plan of care to help the client use positive growth-producing coping and to avoid disabling coping.[69]

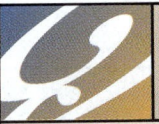

NURSING RESEARCH

Does Ability to Concentrate Differ Between Women Who Have Undergone Mastectomy versus Breast-Conserving Surgery?

Cimprich, B. (1992). Attentional fatigue following breast cancer surgery. *Research in Nursing and Health, 15*(3), 199–207.

A study was conducted on women who had surgery for early stage (I or II) breast cancer to determine their ability to direct attention (concentrate) during the early phase of their illness. This is important, because the ability to concentrate or direct attention is critical in listening to explanations of treatment options and self-care patient education.

This study compares the attentional deficits of women who had either mastectomy or breast-conserving surgery. It was found that women in the two different surgical groups did not differ significantly in attentional capacity and functioning. Also, it was found that attentional functioning decreased as time passed after surgery.

Implications for Practice

The findings support the need for nurses to assess the patient's ability to concentrate before initiating patient teaching and to include written materials that can be referred to later, along with verbal instructions. Interventions to help restore attentional capacity are needed by all women, regardless of type of surgery.

CARE PLAN

The Woman with a Modified Radical Mastectomy

Nursing Diagnosis. Ineffective Individual Coping related to mastectomy and diagnosis of breast cancer

Planning: Expected Outcomes. The client will begin to adapt to her emotional stressors, will use her resources to improve her coping, and will identify potentially disabling coping. Effective coping is identified, supported, and strengthened.

Implementation: Nursing Intervention	Rationales
Assess the client's stressors, resources, supports, and problem-solving skills.	There is a lot of hope for women with breast cancer.
Determine coping strategies that have been useful for the client in the past and reinforce them.	Productive coping strategies are reinforced.
Emphasize that periods of depression, anger, and the like are normal; describe the benefits of emotional release of feelings and tensions; provide opportunity for talking.	Clients have less anxiety when they know that their response is normal.
Encourage asking questions and seeking information.	Promotes autonomy.
Allow time for the client to verbalize fears and anxieties (do not appear to be in a hurry).	Reduces anxiety.
Reinforce positive self-care behavior and each step in getting well.	Ineffective coping may lead to lack of adherence to treatment regimens.
At the time of diagnosis or of the appointment for preoperative history and physical examination, refer the client to the American Cancer Society's Reach for Recovery program or the YWCA's Encore program.	Community support programs can provide ongoing help.
Refer the client to other professionals (social worker, psychologist, family counselor) and community support groups for emotional and psychosocial counseling as needed.	Ineffective coping may lead to prolonged depression or other psychiatric, social, or emotional disorders.

Nursing Diagnosis. Impaired Skin Integrity related to mastectomy and the placement of drains

Planning: Expected Outcomes. The client will exhibit healing of the incision, as evidenced by the absence of drainage, sutures, and infection. The client will demonstrate appropriate care of the incision at discharge. The client will identify potential complications and appropriate manifestations to report to the physician or nurse.

Implementation: Nursing Intervention	Rationales
Assess the dressing for bleeding or drainage.	Early detection of bleeding promotes early treatment.
Empty the drain. Measure and record the drainage every shift. Note the color and consistency of the drainage.	Wound drainage is normally sanguineous at first.
After dressing changes, observe the incision for healing; there should be no indications of infection, hematoma formation, erythema, induration, tenderness, or purulent drainage.	Previous radiation or chemotherapy can retard wound healing.
Begin teaching wound care at the first dressing change; prepare the client to look at the incision at the first dressing change by describing the incision to her.	These interventions support body image changes.
Teach the manifestations of infection, hematoma, or recurrence of breast cancer in the incision (a growing lump).	Assists the woman to be independent in self-care.
Discuss that it is normal to have decreased sensation in the surgical area or to have phantom breast pain.	Knowing normal changes after surgery reduces anxiety.
Instruct the client that after the incision heals she may massage the area with cocoa butter to keep the skin soft and increase healing; tell her that redness and swelling will fade with time.	Complaint scar tissue pulls less with movement, thereby reducing scar; redness and edema fade over weeks as healing ensues.

Nursing Diagnosis. Impaired Physical Mobility related to modified radical mastectomy

Planning: Expected Outcomes. The client will demonstrate knowledge related to potential mobility problems. The client will progress toward full range of motion (ROM); full ROM of hand, arm, and shoulder will return by 2 to 3 months postoperatively. The client identifies potential complications and manifestations of edema to report to the healthcare team.

CARE PLAN

The Woman with a Modified Radical Mastectomy *(Continued)*

Implementation: Nursing Intervention	Rationales
At the time of the preoperative history and physical examination, send a referral to physical therapy to see the client on postoperative day 1 or 2.	It is possible to regain full ROM.
Assess for manifestations of infection or impairment of circulation.	Removal of axillary lymph structures can lead to edema.
Instruct the client to keep the arm elevated on a pillow when she is lying down or sitting.	Promotes venous and lymph return.
After the client's anesthesia wears off, begin helping her to ambulate and instruct her to begin flexion and extension of the fingers, wrist, and lower arm.	Using the arm improves circulation.
Instruct the client to begin performing her ADLs (including dressing herself) with the arm on the operative side.	Promotes arm mobility and self-care.
Instruct the client to limit upper arm ROM to the level of the shoulder only.	Reduces pull on the incision.
After the axillary drain is removed, begin progressive full ROM of the upper arm.	If radiation therapy is needed, the woman will need to have her arm above her head to keep it safely out of the treatment field.
Instruct the client to use pain medication as needed to allow exercise without hindrance from pain.	
Teach ROM exercises to use at home after the drain is removed.	Full ROM returns in time after edema subsides.
Instruct the client to avoid infection and trauma to the operative site and left arm; teach hand care; the client must follow this for the rest of her life.	Because the lymph nodes have been removed, the woman is more vulnerable to trauma, edema, and infection.

Evaluation. The client will understand and undergo modified radical mastectomy with no significant problems. The affected arm should remain mobile without swelling or limitations. The wound will heal without complications

Evaluation

A positive outcome would be that the client was adequately prepared for surgery and its outcomes. Recovery from the surgical procedure is usually uncomplicated. Delayed grieving for the loss is not uncommon even months after the surgery.

Postoperative Care

Assessment

Postoperative assessments should also include the client's psychological reaction to the surgery. Other important assessments include the wound, drains, presence of lymphedema, clinical manifestations of infection, and pain.

Diagnosis, Planning, Implementation

Body Image Disturbance. A nursing diagnosis of *Body Image Disturbance related to impending changes in breast and sexuality* may be appropriate.

Planning: Expected Outcomes. The client will develop a positive body image, as evidenced by wearing usual make-up, own nightgown, and other feminine attire after breast surgery.

Implementation. If the assessment reveals problems with body image or sexuality, the nurse may choose to include other healthcare professionals (e.g., social worker,

sex therapist) in the plan of care for addressing these needs adequately. It may be helpful for someone who has had a similar surgery to talk with the woman preoperatively or postoperatively.

Women who undergo surgery for breast cancer experience a sense of loss; changes in their routine life, social interactions, self-concept, and body image; and fear of death.[69, 82] These women may benefit from opportunities to interact with nurses in ways in which they feel comfortable expressing their fears and problems.

Recovery during the postoperative period after mastectomy takes a lot of energy. A client's usual coping strategies may not be effective. Not everyone perceives or handles stress in the same way. Displacement, projection, denial, hope, prayer, meditation, stoicism, fatalism, or any combination of these reactions may occur. Clients who have surgically lost a breast may adapt in the same way they would to any loss. Phantom breast manifestations in the missing breast are not uncommon.[79]

Effective postoperative care is essential for successful psychosocial and physical rehabilitation. During the 1- to 3-day hospital stay, the focus of nursing care is toward recovery from surgery and anesthesia and aimed at discharge planning for self-care postoperative management. The client's self-image improves with self-care activities.

Losing a breast or having breast cancer may not exert its full impact until the client goes home. Many clients are surprised by events such as the amount of pain and discomfort, marked fatigue, slow incision healing, arm

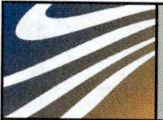

ETHICAL ISSUES IN NURSING

Communication Problem or Ethical Dilemma?

Sarah Smith, a 92-year-old woman, is admitted with a small lump in her breast. The surgeon has scheduled her for a mastectomy. The nurse who is caring for this client preoperatively feels that this is an inappropriate operation. She wonders if an ethics consultation should be called.

Nurses who practice in medical-surgical settings often encounter situations that require the understanding of ethical principles and the ability to use ethical decision-making skills. Nursing involves doing good for the client, but it is sometimes difficult to decide what nursing actions are "good" or best for the client. Situations can arise that the nurse may identify as an ethical dilemma. An ethical dilemma is a problem in which none of the solutions is satisfactory. The emergence of an ethical dilemma involving the care of a client is stressful for all concerned.

Frequently, however, the problem that initially seems like an ethical dilemma is actually a problem of communication. Clients can express ideas about treatment goals differently to nurses and physicians. Problems can also arise when a client's preferences are understood differently by different members of the healthcare team. It is also possible that what is said to a client and what is heard by the client are not the same. Misunderstandings between the client and the healthcare team can lead to many problems. To complicate the equation even further, problems can also arise when the client's goals are clear but communication of these goals between physicians and nurses or other members of the healthcare team is poor.

It is therefore essential that nurses gather all of the facts about a situation and be sure of the client's goals before identifying a problem as an ethical dilemma. If the client's goals are understood similarly by the healthcare team, then communication has been good. But if there still remains a problem of what is the "right" thing to do, the nurse may indeed be faced with an ethical dilemma requiring further analysis.

In this case, when the nurse questions the surgeon, she is surprised by the surgeon's answer. The surgeon states that he, too, was initially against this surgery. But the client, Ms. Smith, is completely alert and oriented, lives independently, and has always been in charge of her life, and she is the one who requested the surgery to remove the cancerous lesion. Ms. Smith insisted that she did not wish to spend her limited remaining years worrying about the cancer growing inside her. When the nurse understood that this surgery was the patient's preference and that she had a good rationale, the nurse was satisfied that no ethical dilemma existed.

swelling, and feelings of jitteriness. Ordinary things, such as finding a comfortable position in bed, may be difficult and painful. The woman has to decide whether to hide the incision from significant others or let it be seen. The defect may be camouflaged for a woman by an appropriately fitted brassiere or a special bathing suit or evening dress, but doubts and fears about her attractiveness may affect even the most secure woman.[65, 122]

Body image is further altered by weight gain and alopecia. If a woman wishes, a suitable wig can be obtained before hair is lost. Fatigue, decreased libido, and periods of depression are common in women receiving chemotherapy and radiation therapy. It may help a woman to talk with others who face the same problems. Breast cancer support groups may also be beneficial.

As time passes, a reorganization and restructuring of the lives of the woman and significant others takes place. During this time, the woman resumes her role in society. Significant changes in this role may be necessary. Women cope differently; feelings of sexual inadequacy, poor body image, and loss of a sense of femininity are common. The woman needs to share her concerns. Nurses are often able to offer such support. Nurses can offer understanding and facilitate communication between the client and significant others. Certain events, such as fitting the permanent prosthesis, can cause a breakdown in denial that a woman may have been using after a mastectomy. A new lump or any new problem may precipitate aspects of the grieving

process (e.g., anger, depression, and regression). Fear of metastases or recurrence of cancer may cause new manifestations to become magnified and every new pain to cause new anxiety.

Breast cancer support groups often provide a place for talking about shared and individual problems.[120] Women encountering similar problems and finding solutions may effectively help each other. It often helps to realize that one is not alone in feelings and problems. Find out details about such support groups in the community and share this information as appropriate.

Risk for Impaired Skin Integrity. The nursing diagnosis may be expressed as *Risk for Impaired Skin Integrity related to surgery or radiation therapy.*

Planning: Expected Outcomes. The client will not develop impairments in skin integrity after surgery or radiation therapy, as evidenced by healing skin without redness, infection, hematoma formation, or breakdown.

Implementation. Postoperatively, a pressure dressing is usually used initially. A drain, connected to gentle suction, prevents blood or serum collection in the operative space after a modified radical mastectomy or axillary node dissection. The nurse needs to instruct the woman about emptying the drain and recording the amount of drainage; the physician is notified if the drain becomes plugged, is dislodged, or shows manifestations of infection, or if frank bleeding develops.

When the dressing is changed, gently encourage the woman to look at the incision. Seeing the incision for the first time is often a difficult experience. A matter-of-fact approach by the nurse can help. Future dressing changes can be used to teach methods of cleaning the incision at home and watching for manifestations of infection.

During radiation therapy, scaling, flaking, dryness, itching, erythema, hair loss, rash, or dry desquamation of the involved skin may occur. Careful treatment of the skin is important in minimizing the skin effects of radiation therapy.[43, 83] Nurses need to teach women how to care for their skin (see Chapter 24).

Risk for Injury. The nursing diagnosis may be expressed as *Risk for Injury related to increased risk of infection and lymphedema secondary to axillary node dissection.*

Planning: Expected Outcomes. The client will not experience injury, as evidenced by absence of infection or lymphedema.

Implementation. Arm edema (e.g., lymphedema) was a common complication after the standard radical mastectomy. However, with less extensive surgery, it occurs less frequently. Arm edema (on the operative side) can occur immediately postoperatively, or secondary edema may occur months or years after surgery.[36, 54, 142] In the immediate postoperative period, encourage arm exercises; elevate the arm to promote lymphatic drainage and prevent infection. Wearing an elastic bandage or a custom-fitted pressure-gradient elastic sleeve may also be helpful. Place a sign on the woman's bed warning that no blood pressure readings, injections, intravenous lines, or blood sampling should be performed on the arm on the operative side. These procedures can cause circulatory impairment or infection.

After the woman leaves the hospital, burns, cuts, and abrasions are the most frequent sources of infection. After axillary node dissection, secondary edema from infection in the arm may cause some permanent edema. Also, postoperative radiation to the axilla often increases the frequency and degree of arm edema. Explain that the client is vulnerable to secondary edema in the arm on the operative side for the rest of her life and that any trauma to the arm may lead to edema and infection.

The client should be warned of the possible occurrence of numbness, which many women notice after a mastectomy. This sensation is often described as a feeling that a rubber band has been placed around the arm. This sensation resolves in time, and normal sensation gradually returns.

Knowledge Deficit. The nursing diagnosis may be written as *Knowledge Deficit related to postoperative arm exercises, postoperative care, and care of the breast prosthesis.*

Planning: Expected Outcomes. The client will understand postoperative arm exercises, postoperative care, and care of the breast prosthesis as evidenced by

return demonstration of arm exercises and care and client's statements concerning further treatment.

Implementation. Plan interventions for restoring strength and full hand, arm, and shoulder range of motion. Sometimes a surgeon attempts to enhance mobility by placing the arm on the operative side at a right angle to the chest wall immediately postoperatively.

Early limited postoperative arm exercises are important and usually started within 24 hours after surgery. Teach the client to perform hand and wrist movements and to flex and extend the elbow hourly. Encourage self-care activities (e.g., feeding, combing hair, washing face) and other activities that use the arm, with care taken not to abduct the arm or raise the arm or elbow above shoulder height until the drains are removed.

When wound healing is well established and axillary drains are removed, begin abduction and external rotation of the upper arm, including pendulum swings to improve shoulder function, forward and lateral elevation of the arms, overhead pulley suspension to obtain full elevation, and wall climbing and rope running (Fig. 85–5). Exercises may need to be approved by the physician. Arrangements for a physical therapist to assist with range of motion and strengthening exercises may need to be made at the time surgery is planned because the short hospital stay may allow time to do this postoperatively. It is important for the nurse to provide written and verbal instructions about arm precautions after axillary node dissection (see Fig. 85–5 and Client Education Guide).

The Reach for Recovery program of the American Cancer Society is a rehabilitation program for women who have had breast surgery. This program is designed to help women meet common psychosocial, physical, and cosmetic needs. With authorization of the physician, volunteers from this program visit the hospital or the home and give the woman information and help, including the following:

● A Reach for Recovery kit, ball, book, rope, and temporary soft cotton prosthesis (for women who have had a mastectomy)
● Postoperative axillary node dissection exercises
● Discussion of brassiere comfort, various breast prostheses, clothing adjustments, and personal problems as appropriate

Women who have had a mastectomy may wear a temporary lightweight prosthesis immediately after the sutures and drains are removed. This may help the woman's adjustment to the loss of her breast. A soft, cotton breast form may be supplied by the Reach for Recovery visitor; cotton padding inserted into a pocket sewn into a lightweight brassiere is also a good temporary substitute. A permanent prosthesis should not be purchased until the wound has healed completely, because the incision site may change. Prostheses are expensive. They may be purchased in foundation departments in most large stores or at medical-surgical supply stores that sell durable medical equipment. Most of these stores have fitters to help women obtain the right fit. It would be helpful for the nurse to learn about suppliers in the local area so she can provide a name to the client. Most private and govern-

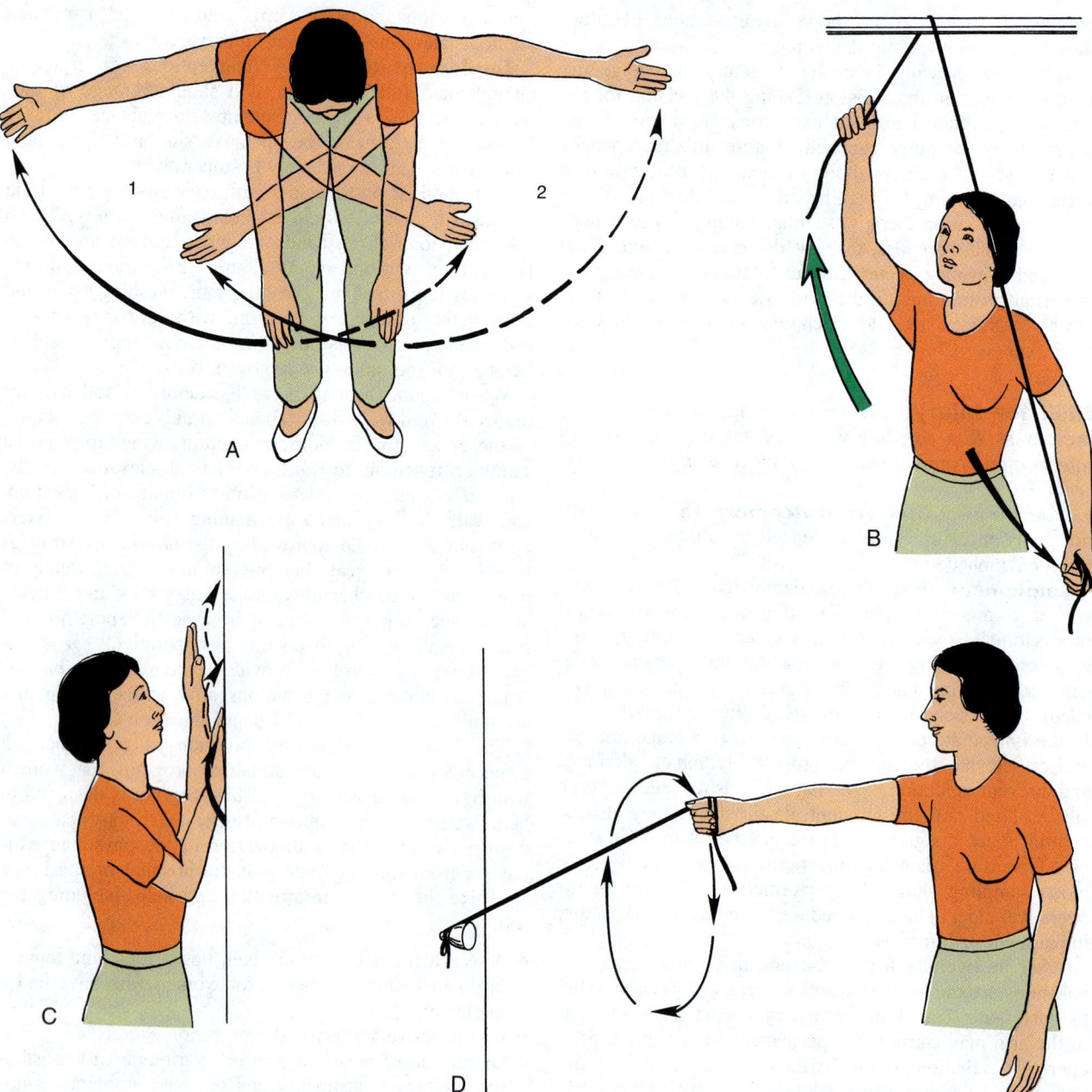

Figure 85–5. Postmastectomy exercises. *A*, Arm swings. The client stands with feet 8 inches apart and bends forward from the waist, allowing the arms to hang toward the floor. She then swings both arms up to her sides to reach shoulder level. Next, she swings her arms back to the center, then crosses her arms at the center. Throughout this exercise, the client should not bend her elbows. If possible, she should do this and the other exercises in front of a mirror to ensure even posture and correct motion. *B*, Pulley motion. Using the operated arm, the client tosses a 6-foot rope over a shower curtain rod (or over the top of a door that has a nail in the top to hold the rope in place for the exercise). She grasps one end of the rope in each hand, then slowly raises the operated arm as far as comfortable by pulling down on the rope on the opposite side. The client should keep the raised arm close to her head. Then the client reverses this motion to raise the unoperated arm by lowering the operated arm, and repeats the entire sequence. *C*, Hand wall climbing. The client stands facing a wall with the toes 6 to 12 inches from the wall. She then bends her elbows and places her palms against the wall at shoulder level. Then, she gradually moves both hands up the wall in a parallel path until incisional pulling or pain occurs. (The client should mark that spot on the wall to measure her progress.) She then walks her hands down the wall to shoulder level. The client should move closer to the wall as the height of her reach improves. *D*, Rope turning. The client ties a rope to a door handle, then holds the rope in the hand of her operated side. She backs away from the door until the arm is extended away from her body, parallel to floor. She then swings the rope in as wide a circle as possible, increasing the size of the circle as mobility returns.

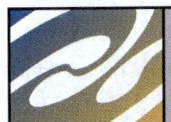

CLIENT EDUCATION GUIDE

Arm Care After Axillary Lymph Node Dissection

Because you have had an axillary node dissection, the affected arm may swell and is less able to fight infection. Use your arm normally following these recommendations.

Avoid burns while cooking or smoking
Wear a long-length oven mitt
Do not reach into a hot oven with this arm
Do not hold a cigarette in the affected hand
Avoid sunburn and insect bites
Wear long-sleeve shirts and gloves
Use sunscreen
Use insect repellent to avoid bites and stings
Avoid cuts, pinpricks, and scratches
Wear gloves when gardening
Do not work near thorny plants or dig with your hands
Use a thimble when sewing
Use an electric razor with a narrow head for underarm shaving to reduce the risk of nicks or scratches
Never cut or pick at cuticles; use hand cream or lotion
Wash cuts promptly; treat them with antibacterial medication and cover them with sterile dressing, and check often for redness, soreness, pus, or other manifestations of infection
Avoid strong detergents, harsh chemicals, and abrasive compounds
Wear protective gloves while doing dishes and cleaning
Avoid other trauma
Have all injections, vaccinations, blood samples, and blood pressure tests done on the other arm whenever possible
Wear a Medic Alert identification tag that cautions against test injections or blood pressure readings on the affected arm
Carry your handbag and other heavy objects on the other arm
Wear watch or jewelry loosely, if at all, on the operated arm
Avoid elastic cuffs on blouses and nightgowns
Use a lanolin hand cream a few times each day
Wear an elastic sleeve if recommended by your physician
Contact your physician if the arm or hand becomes red, is swollen, or feels hot; in the meantime, try to keep your arm over your head and periodically pump your fist

---

Adapted from National Cancer Institute (1987). *After breast cancer: A guide to followup care* (NIH publication No. 87–2400). Washington, DC: Author.

---

ment insurance plans pay for at least the first prosthesis and brassiere.

Community and Self-Care

■ Medical Management

Public knowledge is increasing about treatment options for breast cancer. Historically, breast cancer identified on a frozen section was immediately treated with a Halsted radical mastectomy at the time of the biopsy. Typically, the woman and her family did not know she had cancer or that her breast was to be removed until after the surgery was over. Now women and their families want to be informed about treatment options and included in treatment decision-making before it is initiated.[75] Nurses must be knowledgeable about recent advances in treatment as well as about treatment controversies to support women and their significant others as they make decisions.[74, 109] It is important for the nurse to know that a woman diagnosed with early-stage breast cancer may live a long, healthy life and also keep her breast.

Because of greater understanding of tumor biology, it is now recognized that breast cancer requires multimodality therapy.[22, 23, 47, 59, 138] Historically, it was believed that cancer spread locally to the lymph nodes in an orderly, defined manner. If this were true, radical mastectomy should eliminate the disease. It is now known that breast cancer does not spread in an orderly manner and that cancer cells metastasize through the bloodstream to other organs such as bone, lung, brain, and liver. Because of this, less radical surgical procedures are used in combination with radiation therapy, hormonal therapy, or chemotherapy.[72, 102] In 1988, 62% of breast cancer clients had mastectomies, 9% had no surgical procedure, and 25% had only partial mastectomies.[103] Now various treatment combinations are used to cure breast cancer through local, regional, or systemic treatments. Women who have early small breast cancers may be best served by first having a mastectomy or lumpectomy to be followed by radiation therapy, chemotherapy, or hormonal therapy as indicated. Women with locally advanced stage II breast cancer may be better served by having hormonally synchronized chemotherapy to shrink the breast cancer lesion before surgery and radiation therapy. Local and regional treatment involves treating the breast and chest wall. Mastectomy or adjuvant radiation therapy in combination with a lumpectomy or a quadrantectomy is used for local control of stage I or II breast cancer. Adjuvant (given after surgery) or neoadjuvant (given before surgery) chemotherapy or hormonal therapy may be given to reduce the risk of recurrence. Chemotherapy and hormonal therapy treat potential or known metastatic disease for systemic control. Hormonal therapy is used to treat women with estrogen and progesterone receptor-positive breast cancer. Chemotherapy is used to treat women with positive lymph nodes (stage II), locally advanced cancer (stage III), metastatic breast cancer (stage IV), and even some women with lymph node–negative (stage I) disease.

Multimodal Therapy

To provide multimodality therapy, a multidisciplinary evaluation is needed to determine the best course of treatment. A few major cancer treatment centers provide a consultation appointment at which surgical oncologists, medical oncologists, radiation oncologists, plastic surgeons, gynecologists, pathologists, mammographic radiology specialists, specialized nurses, and social workers are all available at one appointment to evaluate the woman and her disease and to recommend the best treatment combination.[6, 15, 43, 60] In many communities, the team consultation during one appointment may not be feasible. However, before any treatment is initiated, it is best for the woman to be evaluated for the need for each treatment modality and to determine the best therapeutic plan. This multidisciplinary evaluation before treatment is still possible in most communities through a series of appointments to specialists so long as the primary healthcare provider coordinates all appointments to occur in a timely manner and oversees the sequencing of treatment and follow-up. The nurse is important in facilitating the multidisciplinary process in both the major treatment centers and in other settings. Whatever the setting, the nurse has a major role in helping the woman through all phases of diagnosis and treatment.

Most breast cancer treatment is done on an outpatient basis. Mastectomy and other breast procedures that include axillary lymph node dissection typically involve only a 2- to 3-day hospital stay. To have continuity of care for the woman undergoing multimodality therapy, the nurses in the various treatment disciplines need to collaborate and share assessment information, nursing care plans, and reports on the woman's progress.

Women with breast cancer at any stage fear disfigurement and death. Much has been written about the psychosocial impact of breast cancer.[25] Some women choose to have reconstructive surgery to rebuild their breasts and create new nipples. Breast reconstruction helps some women adjust to the loss of their breast.

With more women receiving breast-conserving procedures, it is important for nurses and health professionals to consider the impact of these therapies. It has been shown that the women who have breast-conserving surgical procedures feel better about the appearance of their nude body than do women who have had mastectomy. However, the psychological impact of having breast cancer has not been eliminated.[118, 121, 132, 141] A woman who has had a lumpectomy and radiation therapy will still have scars and other physical changes that will remind her that she has had breast cancer. Because she has kept her breast, she may worry about recurrence or wonder if she should have had a mastectomy. Daily radiation treatments for several weeks may delay resumption of her normal pattern of daily activities. Also, the woman will have to cope with the side effects of radiation therapy. Some of the common complaints are tenderness, change in the texture of the breast, and arm or hand numbness.[14, 55]

Radiation Therapy

Radiation therapy (see Chapter 24) is used in breast cancer treatment as follows:

- The breast and the underlying chest wall are irradiated for local control in stage I or II breast cancer after lumpectomy or quadrantectomy.
- Women who are poor surgical candidates because of health problems, such as heart disease, typically receive radiation therapy to their breast.
- The chest wall is irradiated if it is involved or for local control after mastectomy with positive margins.
- The axilla is irradiated in women at high risk for axillary metastases who are poor surgical candidates for axillary dissection or have gross disease that was not surgically excised.
- The supraclavicular region is irradiated if positive axillary nodes are found.
- Additional areas are irradiated for management of metastatic disease of the brain, bone, or skin.

Radiation in combination with lumpectomy or quadrantectomy is an accepted treatment for early stage (e.g., stage I or II) breast cancer.[104, 111, 168] An axillary dissection is usually done for staging purposes. Eligibility for these treatment choices are as follows: (1) lesions less than 5 cm, (2) no large or fixed axillary nodes, (3) no demonstrable disease, (4) clear surgical margins, and (5) breasts that can be easily evaluated mammographically. Lumpectomy and quadrantectomy with dissection of axillary lymph nodes (for staging) and radiation to the breast area have produced good results. The survival rates and incidence of local and distant recurrence are equal to those with mastectomy.[46] Radiation therapy can be administered through an external beam and via iridium implants.

External beam radiation is administered by a cobalt machine or linear accelerator; it is given on an outpatient basis 5 days a week, with approximately 5000 rad given over 5 weeks.[72] Regional lymph nodes may be treated if they were not removed.

A concentrated boost of radiation is given to the small area where the tumor is located. A radiation boost to only the small area involved reduces the risk of side effects while treating the area of highest risk of disease. After more than 5000 rad is given to the entire breast, the incidence of side effects increases. However, if the total radiation dose is too low, the risk of recurrence increases. The boost of radiation can be given with several additional linear accelerator treatments by electron beam therapy or via an interstitial iridium implant.

Interstitial implant therapy using iridium (^{192}Ir) is an in-hospital procedure. The insertion of the iridium implant may be done with local anesthesia. Stainless steel guide needles are threaded through the tumor area at 1-cm intervals. Flexible plastic tubes are inserted in the guide needles. The guide needles are then removed, leaving the tubing in place. Strands of radioactive iridium seeds are threaded through each tube (Fig. 85–6). The seeds, at 1-cm intervals, form a grid with those above and below to cover the tissues evenly with radiation. At the end of the insertion procedure, a button is attached, and the ends are

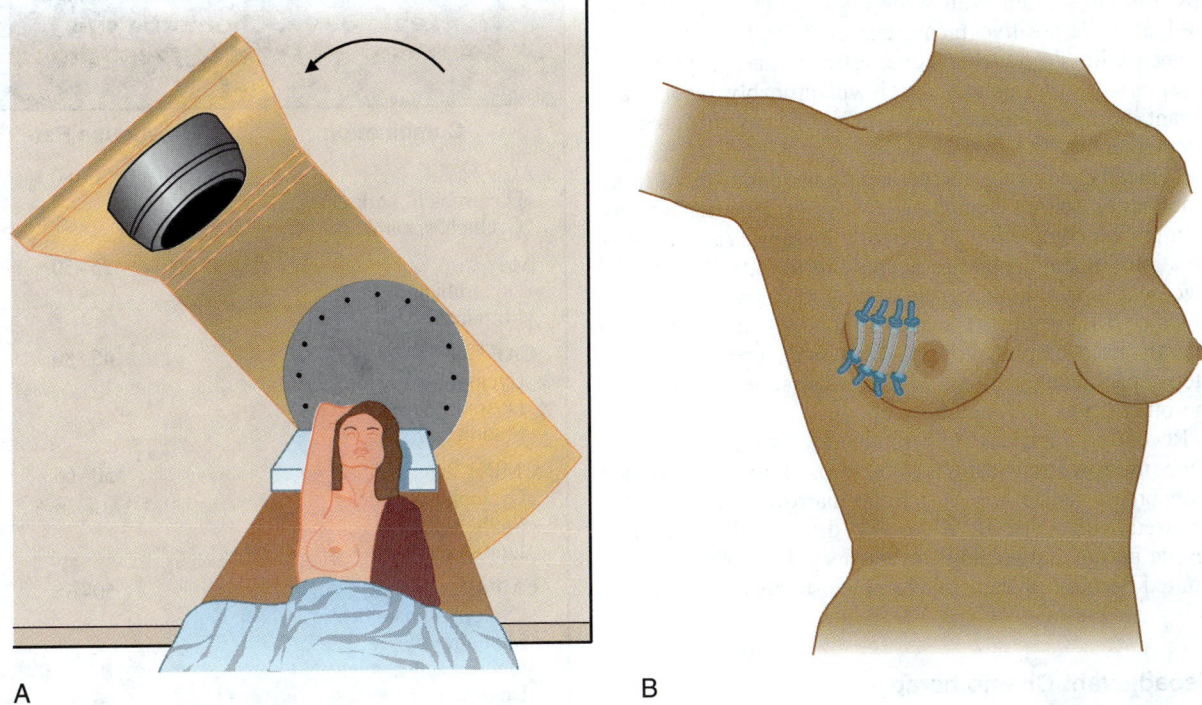

Figure 85–6. Radiation therapy is given via an external beam or iridium implants.

crimped and then cut to prevent the seeds from falling out. An x-ray film confirms the implant's location. The length of time that the implant must remain in place is usually 2 or 3 days. The procedure is mildly uncomfortable. The woman is able to be up and about in her room. Radiation precautions related to time, distance, and shielding are maintained.

Radiation therapy, in combination with lumpectomy or quadrantectomy, effectively treats early stage breast cancer and avoids the psychosocial trauma of mastectomy. It is surprising to some healthcare professionals that this treatment modality is not used more frequently. Let us consider three objections to the use of radiation for treatment of breast cancer. The first is concern that undetected cancer may remain after the identified tumor is removed by the excisional biopsy. However, several studies show that survival and local control are equal to those achieved with mastectomy.[67, 104, 111] A second objection is the concern that radiation might induce new cancers in the remaining breast or adjacent tissue. However, radiation has been used for more than 30 years, and thus far the incidence of secondary malignancies attributable to radiation therapy for breast cancer is small.[38, 110] The third objection is the thought that the breast may not be cosmetically pleasing after radiation because of fibrosis or pigment changes. However, in most cases, the skin changes are minimal.

Side effects from radiation to the breast include the following:

- Temporary skin changes (common) (e.g., itchy, dry, tender, red, swollen, or dry desquamation)
- Fatigue
- Dry throat (rare); this occurs in the later weeks of treatment as a result of radiation's effect on pharyngeal

mucosa if the supraclavicular area is irradiated; although often described as a "lump in the throat," it should not interfere with eating
- Pneumonitis (rare); this is indicated by dry cough and dyspnea and is due to inflammatory changes in the irradiated underlying lung
- Arm edema (rare); this may occur after axillary irradiation
- Increased susceptibility to rib fracture; this may occur in the irradiated field

Radiation therapy can be a long, difficult process for the client being treated. It is emotionally taxing to receive treatments daily for 5 to 7 weeks. Nursing support is needed during this period. Women receiving radiation therapy have many of the same fears as do those who are having mastectomy: fear of death, fear of mutilation, and feelings of sexual inadequacy. These are compounded by the stress of daily treatments and the fatigue that occurs with radiation therapy.

Chemotherapy

Adjuvant Chemotherapy

Adjuvant chemotherapy is given after surgical removal of any measurable cancer. The goal of adjuvant chemotherapy is to prolong disease-free survival while helping the client maintain a high quality of life. Before 1988, premenopausal women with breast cancer in the lymph nodes commonly received chemotherapy. It was felt that women with node-negative breast cancer and postmenopausal women with positive lymph nodes would not benefit from chemotherapy. In 1988, a clinical alert was issued from the National Cancer Institute recommending consideration of adjuvant chemotherapy or hormonal therapy for all women with node-negative breast cancer as well as node-positive breast cancer.[89, 147] Premenopausal women with T_1, node-negative, estrogen and progesterone receptor–positive breast cancer will probably receive adjuvant hormonal therapy and may or may not receive chemotherapy.[46, 48]

Typically, adjuvant chemotherapy is administered in an ambulatory setting beginning a few weeks after surgery or after the completion of radiation therapy. Various combinations of antineoplastic agents are used.[19, 41, 73, 137, 147] Cyclophosphamide (Cytoxan), methotrexate, and fluorouracil (CMF regimen) make up one of the most frequently used combinations. Doxorubicin, prednisone, thiotepa, paclitaxel, tamoxifen, and vincristine are some of the other drugs that may be used.

Recently, high-dose chemotherapy with autologous bone marrow transplant has been used to treat women with breast cancer.[1, 21, 32, 79] Bone marrow transplant may be used with stage II, III, or IV disease. Bone marrow rescue permits larger doses of agents, which otherwise are limited because of their severe myelosuppressive toxicity.

Neoadjuvant Chemotherapy

Neoadjuvant chemotherapy is given to treat locally advanced breast cancer (stage III) before surgical removal of the cancer. The goal of neoadjuvant chemotherapy is to evaluate the response of the measurable cancer to treatment.

Women with a breast cancer tumor greater than 5 cm in the breast or axilla may receive neoadjuvant chemotherapy and hormonal therapy before surgery or radiation therapy.[128, 130, 140] The goal is to shrink the local disease and reduce the risk of systemic spread. Recently, hormonal synchronization with combination chemotherapy has been under investigation. Because it is known that certain cell cycle-specific chemotherapies (e.g., methotrexate and fluorouracil) are more effective on growing cells, estrogen is given to stimulate cell growth to maximize cell kill. In one study,[140] doxorubicin and cyclophosphamide are given on day 1 of the cycle. On days 6, 7, and 8, estrogen is given. The cell cycle–specific chemotherapies methotrexate and fluorouracil are given on day 8. On days 9 through 14, tamoxifen is given. A new treatment cycle of the same drugs begins on day 22. The women receive 17 cycles of this chemotherapy. Surgery and radiation therapy usually take place (1) after disease is stable, (2) when there is no palpable tumor, (3) when the disease has progressed, or (4) around the ninth cycle.

Systemic Therapy for Metastatic Breast Cancer

When the cancer has spread outside the breast and the ipsilateral axillary regions, systemic therapy is necessary. Some of the antineoplastic agents used to treat metastatic breast cancer include cisplatin, cyclophosphamide, doxorubicin, fluorouracil, methotrexate, mitomycin, paclitaxel, thiotepa, vinblastine, and vincristine. No one combination offers a clear advantage. Table 85–2 lists the commonly used combinations of drugs.

Table 85–2. Chemotherapy Combinations Used to Treat Breast Cancer

Combination	Response Rate (%)
AC Doxorubicin (Adriamycin) Cyclophosphamide	50–80
AM Doxorubicin Mitomycin	25–50
CAF Cyclophosphamide Doxorubicin Fluorouracil	45–80
CMF Cyclophosphamide Methotrexate Fluorouracil	50–65
CMFA Cyclophosphamide Methotrexate Fluorouracil Doxorubicin	50–65
CMFP Cyclophosphamide Methotrexate Fluorouracil Prednisone	50–60
CMFVP Cyclophosphamide Methotrexate Fluorouracil Vincristine Prednisone	50–60
VAC Vincristine Doxorubicin Cyclophosphamide	50

Adapted from Harness, J. K., et al. (1988). *Breast cancer collaborative management*. Chelsea MI: Lewis Publishers.

Side Effects of Chemotherapy

Common side effects for most antineoplastic chemotherapy combinations include varying degrees of alopecia (hair loss); constipation; depression of red blood cells, white blood cells, and platelets; diarrhea; fatigue; menopausal manifestations; nausea; peripheral neuropathy; photosensitivity; sterility; stomatitis; vaginal dryness; vomiting; and weight gain.[24, 37, 45, 73, 93] Several of the agents have their own specific toxic side effects (see Chapter 24). In addition to these side effects, receiving chemotherapy may reduce the woman's social, household, and work-related activities; cause problems in marital, sexual, and family life; and cause a financial burden that can change the woman's quality of life.[144] Understanding this can help the nurse plan and provide appropriate support for women receiving chemotherapy.

Hormonal Therapy

Some breast cancers respond to hormonal therapy because they contain high levels of receptor proteins that are specific for certain steroids. These receptor proteins are capable of binding estrogen, progesterone, androgen, and corticosteroids. It is standard practice for breast biopsy tissue that is diagnosed as cancer to be sent for estrogen and progesterone receptor assay.[46] Estrogen and progesterone receptor assay involves the laboratory examination of 100 to 200 mg of cancerous breast tissue. The breast cancer tissue is considered estrogen receptor–positive or progesterone receptor–positive if the assay results indicate that 10 femtomole (fmol) or more of the receptors are present.[129] Generally, if the results are less than 10 fmol, the tissue is considered estrogen receptor–negative or progesterone receptor–negative.

It is important to know the estrogen status of breast tumors because estrogen receptor–positive tumors are associated with slower growth rates, less aggressive behavior, and longer survival. Both estrogen receptor–positive and progesterone receptor–positive results predict tumors that will respond well to hormonal manipulation. Hormonal therapy may successfully treat metastases to bone, lymph nodes, skin, remaining breast tissue, and lung. It is rarely successful in treating brain or liver metastases. Various medical and surgical methods have been used with varying degrees of success (Table 85–3).

Tamoxifen is the antiestrogen commonly used.[51, 68] Other antiestrogens are under investigation. Tamoxifen is administered orally in the treatment of estrogen receptor–positive breast cancer. It is often prescribed for years. It has relatively few side effects, most of which are fairly well tolerated by most women. Side effects may include hot flashes, vaginal dryness, nausea, vomiting, hypercalcemia, or a flare response (a transient flare of breast cancer manifestations). These side effects often decrease after a few weeks. The nurse needs to help the woman cope with side effects, particularly menopause-type side effects (e.g., hot flashes and vaginal dryness).

Estrogen has been used since 1950 to treat breast cancer in postmenopausal women.[46] The antitumor effect may take several weeks to occur. Side effects commonly include anorexia, nausea, vomiting, sodium and fluid retention, increased libido, withdrawal bleeding, and hypercalcemia. Rarely, a flare response of the disease with increased bone pain may occur. This usually indicates a good response to therapy.

Androgens are usually less effective than estrogen, but they may be superior for bone metastases. Side effects include virilization and increased libido. Progesterone, in large doses, is also used for those who have previously responded to other additive hormones.

Aminoglutethimide may be prescribed to inhibit adrenal steroid production in metastatic breast cancer. This therapy is superior to adrenalectomy. It avoids the need for lifelong replacement therapy, which must be continued after adrenalectomy or hypophysectomy. When aminoglutethimide is used, adrenal suppression leads to a reflex rise in adrenocorticotropic hormone, which can overcome the effect of aminoglutethimide. Therefore, suppressive doses of corticosteroids must be given. However, corticosteroids need to be continued only as long as the aminoglutethimide is used. Possible side effects of aminoglutethimide include lethargy, dizziness, visual blurring, and rash. These effects are dose-dependent and transient.

■ Nursing Management of the Medical Client

Assessment

The nurse has an important role in caring for women with breast cancer and their families. The nurse needs to consider the emotional, social, cognitive, spiritual, and

Table 85–3. Effectiveness of Endocrine Therapy for Metastatic Breast Cancer

	% Responding to Therapy	
	Receptor-Positive	*Receptor-Negative*
Tamoxifen	54	9
Estrogen	57	9
Androgen	43	8
Progestins	35	8
Aminoglutethimide	54	6
Oophorectomy	33	6
Adrenalectomy	46	10
Hypophysectomy	?	?
(36% response rate receptor status unknown)		

Adapted from DeVita, V. T., et al. (1989). *Cancer: Principles and practice of oncology* (3rd ed.). Philadelphia: J. B. Lippincott.

physical factors involved, whatever the treatment combination.

Diagnosis, Planning, Implementation

Knowledge Deficit. The nursing diagnosis may be expressed as *Knowledge Deficit related to chemotherapy and radiation therapy.*

Planning: Expected Outcomes. The client will understand chemotherapy and radiation therapy as evidenced by client's statements concerning further treatment and possible problems associated with therapy.

Implementation. Teaching is a major role for the nurse who is caring for clients receiving radiation therapy. Many clients have misconceptions about radiation. Through assessment, the nurse identifies misconceptions and develops a teaching plan to clarify misunderstandings and meet the woman's needs.[26, 87] The booklet *Radiation Therapy and You*[94] may help the client and is free of charge from the National Cancer Institute by calling 1–800–4–CANCER. See Chapter 24 for further information on radiation therapy.

Nurses are responsible for educating women receiving chemotherapy. This includes teaching them the names of medications being received, how the medications are administered, expected side effects, side effect management, preventive measures, and complications that must be reported to the physician or nurse (e.g., infection, fever, bruising, bleeding, or mouth sores). For example, adequate fluid intake is required with cyclophosphamide therapy to prevent hemorrhagic cystitis. For more information, see Chapter 24.

Altered Nutrition: Less than Body Requirements. The nursing diagnosis may be expressed as *Altered Nutrition: Less than Body Requirements related to nausea, vomiting, and stomatitis secondary to chemotherapy.*

Planning: Expected Outcomes. The client will take in adequate nutrition, as evidenced by absence of nausea and vomiting, control of stomatitis, intake of adequate calories daily, and no loss of weight.

Implementation. Nausea, vomiting, anorexia, stomatitis, and taste change are common side effects of chemotherapy. Yet an adequate nutritional intake is essential for providing strength and well-being. Stomatitis may make eating and drinking extremely difficult. Careful oral hygiene and topical analgesics may help. Adequate dosage and timing of antiemetics can control nausea and vomiting. The client may need to try different foods to find appealing ones. Emphasize the importance of good nutrition by helping the woman find high-calorie and high-protein foods that can be tolerated. Monitor weight and dietary patterns. Meeting nutritional needs can be difficult and must be individualized.

Knowledge Deficit. The nursing diagnosis may be expressed as *Knowledge Deficit related to discharge needs and follow-up care.*

Planning: Expected Outcomes. The client will understand discharge needs and follow-up care as evidenced by the client's ability to describe the care and potential needs.

Implementation. The nurse should also talk to the client about the development of fatigue so that the woman realizes that this is a common occurrence with chemotherapy or radiation therapy. The woman needs to balance activities with periods of rest so she does not become overtired. Reassure the woman that this feeling will gradually fade.

The client and significant others should be told about delayed grieving, which commonly occurs in women 2 to 3 months after mastectomy. This is a normal phenomenon for which the client and significant others should be prepared.

There is usually no need to provide specific home healthcare for the woman after breast cancer and treatment. The major need after discharge, as previously discussed, is for the woman to know how, where, and when to obtain a permanent prosthesis. Encourage the client to continue support groups such as Encore, Reach for Recovery, or Y-ME, as appropriate.

After surgery or radiation, clients with breast cancer need some professional attention for life. Health follow-ups initially are required every 3 to 4 months and later every 6 to 12 months. The risk of recurrence as well as the possibility of developing a second cancer in the remaining breast is high. Monthly breast self-examination and an annual mammogram and breast physical examination are advisable. Metastases may appear 15 years or more after removal of the primary tumor.

Evaluation

To adequately evaluate the outcome of care, the nurse must carefully assess the client's level of knowledge and understanding of continuing care. Acceptance of the change in body image can be evaluated by the woman's ability to look at her mastectomy and to discuss the future in terms of a permanent prosthesis. The presence of lymphedema does not mean the client is not using appropriate preventive measures; it can occur despite preventive measures. If the client is not meeting the expected outcomes, the plan of care should be reevaluated and appropriate changes made.

■ Modifications for Elderly Clients

The care of older women with breast cancer is similar to the care of younger women. The only difference might be in the extent of treatment.[7, 91] If the older woman is not in good health generally, radiation therapy and hormonal manipulation may be all that is recommended.

Metastatic Breast Cancer

Metastatic breast cancer is a chronic disease.[46, 73, 106] Metastases have been known to occur up to 25 years after the initial diagnosis of breast cancer. Alternatively, breast cancer can be a rapidly progressive terminal disease.

Knowledge of the usual metastatic patterns with breast cancer and common complications can aid early recognition and effective treatment. Metastases usually develop in one or more of the following sites: lymph nodes, skin, remaining breast tissue, bones, lung, pleura, peritoneum, liver, and central nervous system. Women with metastases to the liver or central nervous system have a poorer prognosis.

Treatment of metastatic disease may involve radiation therapy, hormonal manipulation, chemotherapy, or possibly surgery.[136] A combination of treatments is usually employed. Excellent palliation can be achieved for metastatic breast cancer, which offers longer survival for this disease than for many other types of cancers.

Hypercalcemia is a common complication of metastatic breast cancer. It may be due to bone involvement or hormonal therapy. Prompt treatment includes hydration and diuretics. Mithramycin or a newer drug, gallium citrate, is initiated for severe hypercalcemia.

Spinal cord compression, usually from extradural metastases, is a complication requiring prompt diagnosis and intervention for prevention of paraplegia. Assessment findings such as back pain, leg weakness, and sphincter disturbances indicate possible spinal cord compression. Treatment involves radiation therapy or surgery, often followed by chemotherapy.

Nursing care of women with metastatic breast cancer involves helping them manage the complications caused by the disease and the side effects caused by treatment. Providing support for the women and significant others is equally important. Physical manifestations may be difficult to manage.

Currently women with metastatic disease are treated using autologous bone marrow transplantation and high-dose chemotherapy.[1, 32] This procedure involves having the woman donate her own bone marrow, either through bone marrow aspiration or through peripheral stem cell pheresis. The client is then given very high dose chemotherapy followed by reinfusion of her own marrow or stem cells after the chemotherapy has destroyed her own marrow. Further information on bone marrow transplantation can be found in Chapters 24 and 27.

Previously established coping mechanisms may falter during this period, as hope dwindles and energy is spent coping with pain, physical problems, and fears. Unresolved issues may resurface. In addition to providing physical care, assist the woman and significant others to reestablish effective coping mechanisms. Women with breast cancer need a strong support system and people with whom they can comfortably and helpfully discuss their problems. Nurses can help provide this support where it is lacking. Nurses need to identify and reinforce beneficial coping to help the woman with advanced breast cancer live a meaningful life.[5, 30]

Breast Cancer in Men

Breast cancer in men is rare.[31, 40, 50] The incidence is 1% of that of women. The average age at occurrence is about 60 years (10 years older than the average for women). Factors associated with an increased risk of breast cancer in men include high estrogen levels, obesity, testicular abnormalities or injury, Klinefelter's syndrome, exposure to ionizing radiation, increased prolactin level, use of phenothiazines, and having a first-degree male or female relative with breast cancer.

Assessment findings indicating male breast cancer include a painless lump beneath the areola or, more often, nipple discharge, retraction, crusting, or ulceration. Staging is the same as for women. Biopsy is necessary for diagnosis of male breast cancer. It is as important to test for estrogen receptors in men as it is in women.

Initial treatment consists of a radical or modified radical mastectomy. Postoperative radiation is frequently used. The pattern of metastasis is similar to that in the female, with soft tissue, bone, and visceral site involvement occurring frequently. Hormonal therapy is very important in the treatment of metastasis, because estrogen receptors have been found in 84% of the tumors.

Tamoxifen and an orchiectomy are the primary hormonal therapies used to treat disseminated male breast cancer. Tamoxifen has provided a response rate of 71% in estrogen receptor–positive male breast cancer. Orchiectomy provides a mean response rate of 55% in men of all ages. Other hormonal manipulations are used in men as in women.

Chemotherapy should be administered for the same indications and with use of the same dose schedules as for women with metastatic disease. Adjuvant chemotherapy may also be useful in those with stage II disease, but experience with this therapy is lacking at present.

Benign Breast Disease

Fibrocystic Breasts

Ninety percent of all women have cysts. Fibrocystic breasts are not a disease per se although the label *fibrocystic breast disease* is often given to the condition (Box 85–2). Fibrocystic breasts are the most frequently occurring condition of the female breast.[35, 64, 83, 141] The exact cause is unknown, although some evidence indicates hormonal imbalance may be associated with it. The fibrocystic condition typically improves during pregnancy and lactation. It occurs during the reproductive years and disappears with menopause.

Typical fibrocystic lesions are fluid-filled cysts that are round, well circumscribed, and movable. Depending on the amount of fluid in the cyst, it may feel soft or hard.

Assessment findings may include nodularity and tenderness. Pain occurs, and the cysts frequently increase in size premenstrually. Cysts are generally aspirated rather than biopsied surgically. However, if there is any question, a biopsy is done. A biopsy is necessary if the cyst keeps recurring after being aspirated.

Once the diagnosis is confirmed, treatment is symptomatic.[105, 116] Conservative measures include breast support with a firm brassiere, local applications of heat or ice, mild analgesics, or the occasional use of diuretics. Recently, it has been found that reducing methylxanthines (e.g., caffeine and theophylline medications) is associated with reduction of manifestations.

Box 85–2. Causes of Breast Masses for Three Age Groups

Under 35 years
Fibrocystic condition
Fibroadenoma
Mastitis
Traumatic fat necrosis
Carcinoma of breast

Between 35 and 50 years
Fibrocystic condition
Carcinoma
Fibroadenoma
Traumatic fat necrosis
Mastitis
Papilloma

Over 50 years
Carcinoma
Fibrocystic breast
Fat necrosis
Paget's disease of breast
Acute mastitis
Papilloma

Data from Robbins, S. L., et al. (1984). *Pathologic basis of disease* (3rd ed., p. 1190). Philadelphia: W. B. Saunders.

Medications have been used with some success in treating fibrocystic breasts. Large doses of vitamin E relieve manifestations in some women but may raise cholesterol levels. Danazol, a synthetic androgen, may be used continuously for 3 to 6 months and repeated if manifestations recur. Side effects include menstrual irregularities, fluid retention, acne, muscle cramps, or possible hepatic dysfunction. Danazol should be used only for severe fibrocystic breasts.

Hyperplasia and Atypical Hyperplasia

Ductal hyperplasia is found in 20% of all breast biopsy specimens.[131] Atypical lobular hyperplasia is found in 1% of breast biopsy specimens. Hyperplasia and atypical hyperplasia can be diagnosed only by pathologic examination of breast tissue from a biopsy. Finding hyperplasia or atypical hyperplasia indicates that a woman is at increased risk for breast cancer.

Fibroadenoma

Fibroadenoma is a common breast tumor that usually occurs in young women, most frequently between the ages of 15 and 30 years.[127, 131] This tumor is usually a nontender, round, firm, or rubbery mass 1 to 3 cm in diameter. Movability of the adenoma in the breast tissues is one of its most distinctive characteristics. Excision is the only effective treatment.

Papilloma

Intraductal papillomas are lesions growing in the terminal portion of a duct (solitary) or throughout the duct system of a sector of breast (multiple or intraductal). Papillomas typically occur in women in their 40s. A ductogram may help in locating the papilloma.

Solitary intraductal papillomas are usually not precancerous. Multiple papillomas may occasionally be cancerous. Intraductal papilloma is usually indicated by a serous, serosanguineous, or bloody discharge from the nipple. Often, no mass is palpable, although a small soft tumor in a central or periareolar portion of the breast is usually present. It is necessary to excise the lesion and have the tissue examined to determine whether it is benign or malignant.

Duct Ectasia

Duct ectasia, a disease of ducts in the subareolar zone, occurs in aging breasts, usually in perimenopausal or postmenopausal women. Manifestations may include a palpable dilated duct; a thick, sticky nipple discharge; and burning pain, itching, and inflammation. There appears to be no association with cancer. However, biopsy is performed because on physical examination it is difficult to differentiate duct ectasia from cancer. Recommended treatment is excision of the ducts.

Fissure of the Nipple

A nipple fissure is a painful longitudinal ulcer in the nipple that occurs in nursing mothers because of irritation from the infant's sucking. Nurses can teach women prenatally to condition their nipples by washing, drying, and massaging to help decrease the incidence of this problem. Teach nursing mothers to wash their hands before feeding the baby, to wash and dry their nipples after breastfeeding, and to avoid astringent soaps or perfumed creams on the nipples. Lanolin-based, bland creams may relieve sore nipples. Drying the nipples and exposing them to a heat lamp is also helpful. Frequent breastfeeding helps reduce engorgement and decrease vigorous sucking. Refer to your maternity nursing textbook for further information.

Lactation Mastitis

Lactation mastitis, a localized, indurated, painful area, may develop when bacteria enter the breast through a cracked nipple.[34, 49, 123] Bacteria may be carried by a nursing mother's hands or by an infant with an oral, eye, or skin infection. Infection of the milk provides a medium for bacterial growth; continued breast-feeding or the manual expression of milk helps to empty the breast. Antibiotics are also prescribed.

Breast Abscess

Breast abscesses[58] frequently occur during lactation when bacteria enter through a cracked nipple. Subareolar abscess is a low-grade subareolar infection in young nonlactating women. Skin over the abscess is red and edematous. Pain, chills, and fever may occur. Antibiotics, analgesics, and warm, moist compresses are used. Weaning may be necessary for resolution of a breast abscess in a lactating woman.

Mastodynia and Mastalgia

Mastodynia and *mastalgia*[85, 131] refer to breast pain. Breast pain is the most common breast complaint. Pain is not usually associated with breast cancer. Many women have cyclic premenstrual mastodynia. Women with cyclic premenstrual mastodynia usually have lumpy breasts (nodularity) and pain for the week before menses. After any other problems have been ruled out, treatment is symptomatic. Wearing a well-fitting brassiere for support, particularly during jogging and other bouncing exercise, may be helpful. Decreasing salt and caffeine intake may also be helpful.

Gynecomastia

Gynecomastia,[12, 18] hypertrophy of one or both male breasts, is common at puberty and in older men. It occurs 60% to 70% of the time at puberty and typically resolves spontaneously in 1 to 2 years. The hormonal mechanism causing gynecomastia is not well understood, although some suggest it is due to increased estrogen. Careful assessment and follow-up are required to rule out causes such as tumors, thyroid or hepatic problems, or Klinefelter's syndrome.

Reassure the man that the condition is temporary. If the gynecomastia causes severe psychosocial trauma, reduction mammaplasty or medications such as an antiestrogen (e.g., tamoxifen) or a synthetic androgen (e.g., danazol) may be prescribed.

Men aged 50 to 70 years occasionally develop gynecomastia that usually regresses spontaneously after a few months to a year. This is not associated with endocrine abnormality. Because cancer is more common in this age group, any lesions found may require biopsy for differentiation from cancer. Certain medications (Box 85–3) can cause gynecomastia in any age group.

Mammaplasty

Women who are uncomfortable with the appearance of their breasts often have a poor body image. Some women who have small breasts seek surgical procedures to enlarge their breasts, such as augmentation mammaplasty. Augmentation mammaplasty has been a popular cosmetic procedure that uses implants or myocutaneous tissue to either (1) enlarge underdeveloped breasts or (2) reconstruct breasts after removal of benign or malignant lesions.

Breasts change over time. With advanced aging, the breasts atrophy and lose some glandular tissue. Some women have large, heavy breasts that are uncomfortable. Breast reduction surgery, or reduction mammaplasty, may benefit them. Reduction mammaplasty may help alleviate neck pain, backaches, possible curvature of the spine, and painful brassiere strap irritation.

Augmentation mammaplasty and reduction mammaplasty are discussed in Chapter 80. Women having such surgery believe it increases their attractiveness. There has been some controversy about the safety of silicone and polyurethane implants.[4, 107] In 1992, the Food and Drug Administration restricted use of these implants because of problems with rupture of the implants, leakage of silicone, and resultant health problems. Nurses can help women understand the facts about the risks and benefits of mammaplasty.

Box 85–3. Drugs Associated with Gynecomastia

Amiodarone	Digitalis	Methotrexate
Anabolic steroids	Domperidone	Methyldopa
Bumetanide	Estrogens	Nifedipine
Busulfan	Ethionamide	Nitrosoureas
Cannabis	Flutamide	Oral contraceptives
Cimetidine	Furosemide	Phenytoin
Clomiphene citrate	Heroin	Reserpine
Cyproterone acetate	Human chorionic gonadotropin	Spironolactone
D-Penicillamine	Isoniazid	Sulindac
Diazepam	Ketoconazole	Theophylline
Diethylpropion hydrochloride	Marijuana	Tricyclic antidepressants
Diethylstilbestrol	Medroxyprogesterone acetate	Verapamil
		Vincristine

Adapted from Bland, K. I., & Page, E. M. (1991). *The breast: Comprehensive management of benign and malignant disease.* Philadelphia: W. B. Saunders.

Conclusions

Diseases of the breast are usually benign conditions that occur throughout the life cycle. Breast cancer, however, has greatly increased in incidence over the last 30 years. The nurse has a vital role in teaching clients early detection methods so that breast cancer can be detected at a curable stage.

All diseases of the breast potentially pose problems in body image and sexuality. Even benign fibrocystic disease can cause breast tenderness and possibly interfere with sexual functioning. Breast cancer and the possibility of a mastectomy as treatment can be extremely threatening to a woman's body image. The nurse can help the client cope with these potential threats and successfully adapt to any changes that occur.

Thinking Critically

1. The pathology report of your client's breast biopsy reads "8 mm invasive ductal carcinoma, invasive carcinoma to the margins, estrogen and progesterone receptor–positive." The client is considering further treatment and asks you what her options are. How would you respond?

Factors to Consider. What treatment options might the client have? What interventions might be required?

2. Your client has come to surgery clinic 10 days postoperatively following a modified radical mastectomy. The breast incision line is clear and intact. Her J-P drain is sutured in place in the axilla. The skin around the drain is clear and intact. Drainage is serosanguineous, and the client has recorded 25 ml and 20 ml of drainage per 24 hours for the last 2 days. The client looks at the incision and the drain and asks questions while you examine her incision and drainage site. She asks when the drain will come out, when she can drive her car, when she can shower and resume her normal activities, and when can she be fitted for a prosthesis. What would you tell her? What else should you assess? What medical and nursing care does this client need during this appointment? What other teaching needs does she have?

Factors to Consider. Think about what structures are removed as part of the modified radial mastectomy. What are their functions and what does that imply about the client's self-care needs? Consider the client's needs in this immediate postoperative period, in a few months, and over the long term.

3. Two years ago your client was treated for stage II cancer of the right breast that was treated with a quadrantectomy (margins negative), axillary lymph node dissection (8 of 19 nodes positive), radiation therapy of the chest and axilla, and six courses of CAF (Cytoxan, Adriamycin, and fluorouracil) chemother-apy. **Today, she presents with pain, tingling, and swelling of her right hand and arm. She states that while she noticed intermittent problems with slight swelling over the past 6 months, it has become severe over the past 2 weeks and is affecting her ability to work as a court stenographer. What further information should you assess? What are your priority interventions?**

Factors to Consider. What do pain, tingling, and swelling of the hand and arm suggest in a client who has undergone lymph node dissection?

Bibliography

1. Affronti, M. L., et al. (1990). Autologous bone marrow transplant for the treatment of advanced breast cancer. *Innovations in Oncology Nursing, 6*(4), 2–6, 19–21.
2. American Cancer Society. (1995). *Cancer facts & figures* (publication No. 95–375M–No. 5008.95–LE). Atlanta: Author.
3. American Cancer Society. (1989). *Special touch: A personal plan of action for breast health* (publication No. 87–1MM–Rev. 9/89–No. 2423–LE). Atlanta: Author.
4. Angell, M. (1994). Do breast implants cause systemic disease? Science in the courtroom. *New England Journal of Medicine, 330*(24), 1748–1749.
5. Arathuzik, D. (1991). Pain experience for metastatic breast cancer patients: Unraveling the mystery. *Cancer Nursing, 14*(1), 41–48.
6. August, D. A., et al. (1993). Benefits of a multidisciplinary approach to breast care. *Journal of Surgical Oncology, 53*(3), 161–167.
7. August, D. A., et al. (1995). Age-related differences in breast cancer treatment. *Annals of Surgical Oncology, 1*(1), 45–52.
8. Baird, S. B., et al. (1991). *Cancer nursing: A comprehensive textbook.* Philadelphia: W. B. Saunders.
9. Beahrs, O. H. (1991). Staging of cancer. *CA: A Cancer Journal for Clinicians, 41*(2), 121–125.
10. Biesecker, B. B., et al. (1993). Genetic counseling for families with inherited susceptibility to breast and ovarian cancer. *JAMA, 269*(15), 1970–1974.
11. Bilimoria, M. M., & Morrow, M. (1995). The woman at increased risk for breast cancer: Evaluation and management strategies. *CA: A Cancer Journal for Clinicians, 45*(5), 263–278.
12. Bland, K. I., & Page, D. L. (1991). Gynecomastia. In K. I. Bland & E. M. Copeland (Eds.), *The breast: Comprehensive management of benign and malignant diseases* (pp. 135–168). Philadelphia: W. B. Saunders.
13. Blesch, K. S., et al. (1991). Correlates of fatigue in people with breast cancer or lung cancer. *Oncology Nursing Forum, 18*(1), 81–87.
14. Bodner, S., & Flynn, K. T. (1987). Symptom distress of women treated with conservative surgery and primary radiation for carcinoma of the breast (abstract 234). *Oncology Nursing Forum, 14*(suppl.), 140.
15. Bord, M. A., & Carpenter, L. C. (1990). A coordinated approach to comprehensive breast care. *Innovations in Oncology Nursing, 6*(2), 13–19.
16. Bostwick, J. (1995). Reconstruction following mastectomy. *CA: A Cancer Journal for Clinicians, 45*(5), 289–304.
17. Bostwick, J. (1990). Reconstruction after mastectomy. *Surgical Clinics of North America, 70*(5), 1125–1140.
18. Braustein, G. D.(1993). Diagnosis and treatment of gynecomastia. *Hospital Practice, 28*(10A), 37–46.
19. Breitmeyer, J. B., & Henderson, I. C. (1990). Adjuvant chemotherapy of breast cancer. *Surgical Clinics of North America, 70*(5), 1081–1113.
20. Brinker, N., & Harris, C. M. (1990). *The race is run one step at a time.* New York: Simon & Schuster.

21. Burns, J. M., et al. (1995). Critical pathway for administering high-dose chemotherapy followed by peripheral blood stem cell rescue in the outpatient setting. *Oncology Nursing Forum, 22*(8), 1219–1224.

22. Buzdar, A. U. (1994). Breast cancer: Diagnostic strategies—therapeutic tactics. *Consultant, 34*(4), 606–608, 611–612.

23. Cady, B., & Stone, M. D. (1990). Selection of breast-preservation therapy for primary invasion breast carcinoma. *Surgical Clinics of North America, 70*(5), 1047–1059.

24. Camp-Sorrell, D. (1991). Controlling adverse effects of chemotherapy. *Nursing 91, 12*(4), 34–41.

25. Carlsson, M., & Hamrin, E. (1994). Psychological and psychosocial aspects of breast cancer and breast cancer treatment: A literature review. *Cancer Nursing, 17*(5), 418–428.

26. Cawley, M., et al. (1990). Informational and psychosocial needs of women choosing conservative surgery/primary radiation for early stage breast cancer. *Cancer Nursing, 13*(2), 90–94.

27. Cimprich, B. (1992). Attentional fatigue following breast cancer surgery. *Research in Nursing and Health, 15*(3), 199–207.

28. Cody, R. L., & Wicha, M. S. (1988). Contemporary chemotherapy. In J. K. Harness, et al. (Eds.), *Breast cancer: Collaborative management* (pp. 157–177). Chelsea, MI: Lewis Publishers.

29. Collins-Hattery, A. M., & Blumberg, B. D. (1991). S Phase index and ploidy prognostic markers in node negative breast cancer: Information for nurses. *Oncology Nursing Forum, 18*(1), 59–62.

30. Coward, D. D. (1991). Self-transcendence and emotional well-being in women with advanced breast cancer. *Oncology Nursing Forum, 18*(5), 857–863.

31. Crichlow, R. W., & Galt, S. W. (1990). Male breast cancer. *Surgical Clinics of North America, 70*(5), 1165–1178.

32. Crouch, M. A. (1994). Current concepts in autologous bone marrow transplant. *Seminars in Oncology Nursing, 10*(1), 12–19.

33. d'Angelo, T. M., & Gorrell, C. R. (1989). Breast reconstruction using tissue expanders. *Oncology Nursing Forum, 16*(1), 23–27.

34. Dahlen, H. (1993). Lactation mastitis. *Nursing Times, 89*(36), 38–40.

35. Deckers, P. J., & Ricci, A. Jr. (1992). Pain and lumps in the female breast. *Hospital Practice, 27*(2A), 67–73, 77–78, 87–90.

36. Dennis, B. (1993). Acquired lymphedema: A chart review of nine women's responses to intervention. *American Journal of Occupational Therapy, 47*(10), 891–899.

37. Dodd, M. J. (1993). Side effects of cancer chemotherapy. *Annual Review of Nursing Research, 11*, 77–103.

38. Doherty, M. A., et al. (1993). Multiple primary tumours in patients treated with radiotherapy for breast cancer. *Radiotherapy and Oncology, 26*(2), 125–131.

39. Donegan, W. L. (1992). Evaluation of a palpable breast mass. *New England Journal of Medicine, 327*(13), 937–942.

40. Donegan, W. L. (1991). Cancer of the breast in men. *CA: A Cancer Journal for Clinicians, 41*(6), 339–354.

41. Dorr, F. A., & Friedman, M. A. (1991). The role of chemotherapy in the management of primary breast cancer. *CA: A Cancer Journal for Clinicians, 41*(4), 231–241.

42. Dunne-Daly, C. F. (1995). Skin and wound care in radiation oncology. *Cancer Nursing, 18*(2), 144–160.

43. Durant, J. R. (1990). How to organize a multidisciplinary clinic for the management of breast cancer. *Surgical Clinics of North America, 70*(4), 977–983.

44. Elledge, R. M., et al. (1992). Prognostic factors in breast cancer. *Seminars in Oncology, 19*(3), 244–253.

45. Fieler, V. K., et al. (1995). Patients' use of prevention behaviors in managing side effects related to chemotherapy. *Oncology Nursing Forum, 22*(4), 713–716.

46. Fisher, B., et al. (1993). Neoplasms of the breast. In J. F. Holland, et al. (Eds.), *Cancer Medicine* (3rd ed.; pp. 1706–1774). Philadelphia: Lea & Febiger.

47. Fisher, B. (1991). Biological perspective of breast cancer: Contributions of the national surgical adjuvant breast and bowel project clinical trials. *CA: A Cancer Journal for Clinicians, 41*(2), 97–111.

48. Fisher, B., et al. (1989). A randomized clinical trial evaluation of sequential methotrexate and fluorouracil in the treatment of patients with node-negative breast cancer who have estrogen-receptor-negative tumors. *New England Journal of Medicine, 320*(8), 473–478.

49. Foxman, B., et al. (1994). Breast feeding practice and lactation mastitis. *Social Science and Medicine, 38*(5), 755–761.

50. Franciosa, D., & Shaw, S. J. L. (1994). Breast cancer and benign breast disease in men. *Nurse Practitioner Forum, 5*(1), 56–58.

51. Gibson, D. F. C., & Jordan, V. C. (1990). Adjuvant antiestrogen therapy for breast cancer: Past, present, and future. *Surgical Clinics of North America, 70*(5), 1103–1113.

52. Glass, J. L., & Frazee, R. C. (1995). Inflammatory breast cancer. *American Surgeon, 61*(2), 121–124.

53. Gordon, R. S. (1981). Survey finds U.S. women knowledgeable about breast cancer. *JAMA, 245*(9), 918.

54. Granda, C. (1994). Nursing management of patients with lymphedema associated with breast cancer therapy. *Cancer Nursing, 17*(3), 229–235.

55. Graydon, J. E. (1994). Women with breast cancer: Their quality of life following a course of radiation therapy. *Journal of Advanced Nursing, 19*(4), 617–622.

56. Grindel, C. G., et al. (1989). Food intake of women with breast cancer during their first six months of chemotherapy. *Oncology Nursing Forum, 16*(3), 401–407.

57. Grooff, P. N., et al. (1993). Lobular carcinoma in situ: What clinicians need to know. *Hospital Practice, 28*(6), 122, 125, 129–130.

58. Grundfest-Broniatowski, S., & Bauer, T. W. (1988). Benign breast disease. In S. Grundfest-Broniatowski & C. B. Esselstyn (Eds.), *Controversies in breast disease: Diagnosis and management* (pp. 3–42). New York: Marcel Dekker.

59. Harness, J. K. (1988). Organizing for collaborative management: What are the options? In J. K. Harness, et al. (Eds.), *Breast cancer: Collaborative management* (pp. 3–9). Chelsea, MI: Lewis Publishers.

60. Harness, J. K., et al. (1987). Developing a comprehensive breast center. *American Surgeon, 53*(8), 419–423.

61. Helvie, M. A., et al. (1990). Radiographic guided fine needle aspiration of non-palpable breast lesions. *Radiology, 174*(3141), 657–661.

62. Henderson, I. C. (1987). Adjuvant chemotherapy and endocrine therapy in patients with operable breast cancer. *Principles and Practice of Oncology Update, 1*(3), 1–14.

63. Hetelekidis, S., et al. (1995). Management of ductal carcinoma in situ. *CA: A Cancer Journal for Clinicians, 45*(4), 244–253.

64. Hockenberger S. J. (1993). Fibrocystic breast disease: Every woman is at risk. *Plastic Surgical Nursing, 13*(1), 37–40.

65. Hughes, K. K. (1993). Psychosocial and functional status of breast cancer patients: The influence of diagnosis and treatment choice. *Cancer Nursing, 16*(3), 222–229.

66. Hutcheson, H. A. (1986). TAIF: New option for breast reconstruction. *Nursing 86, 16*(2), 52–53.

67. Jacobson, J. A., et al. (1995). Ten-year results of a comparison of conservation with mastectomy in the treatment of stage I and II breast cancer. *New England Journal of Medicine, 332*(14), 907–911.

68. Jordan, V. C. (1993). Targeted hormone therapy for breast cancer. *Hospital Practice, 28*(3), 55–62.

69. Kahane, D. H. (1993). The management of the psychosocial impact of breast cancer. *Nurse Practitioner Forum, 4*(2), 105–109.

70. Kalinowski, B. H. (1990). Options and decisions: Reconstructive surgery: Rehabilitation after mastectomy. *Innovations in Oncology Nursing, 6*(1), 2–9.

71. Kelsey, J. L., & Gammon, M. D. (1991). The epidemiology of breast cancer. *CA: A Cancer Journal for Clinicians, 41*(3), 146–165.

72. Kinne, D. W. (1991). Surgical management of primary breast cancer. *CA: A Cancer Journal for Clinicians, 41*(2), 71–84.

73. Knobf, M. T. (1991). Breast cancer. In S. B. Baird, et al. (Eds.), *Cancer nursing: A comprehensive textbook* (pp. 425–451). Philadelphia: W. B. Saunders.

74. Knobf, M. T. (1990). Early-stage breast cancer: The options. *American Journal of Nursing, 90*(11), 28–30.

75. Kuhrik, N. S., et al. (1994). Evaluating women with fibrocystic breast condition. *American Journal of Nursing, 94*(7), 16A–D.

76. Kushner, R. (1984). *Alternatives.* Cambridge, MA: The Kensington Press.

77. Leis, H. P. (1991). Prognostic parameters for breast cancer. In K. I. Bland & E. M. Copeland (Eds.), *The breast: Comprehensive*

management of benign and malignant disease (pp. 331–350). Philadelphia: W. B. Saunders.

78. Lierman, L. M. (1988). Phantom breast experiences after mastectomy. *Oncology Nursing Forum, 15*(1), 41–44.

79. Lin, E. M., et al. (1993). Autologous bone marrow transplantation: A review of the principles and complications. *Cancer Nursing, 16*(3), 204–213.

80. Lindsey, A. M., et al. (1987). Endocrine mechanism and obesity: Influences in breast cancer. *Oncology Nursing Forum, 14*(2), 47–51.

81. Lippman, M. E., et al. (Eds.). (1988). *Diagnosis and management of breast cancer.* Philadelphia: W. B. Saunders.

82. Loveys, B. J., & Klaich, K. (1991). Breast cancer: Demands of illness. *Oncology Nursing Forum, 18*(1), 75–80.

83. Mack, E. (1990). Most breast lumps aren't cancer! *RN, 53*(12), 20–23.

84. Mangan, M. A. (1994). Current concepts in breast reconstruction. *Nursing Clinics of North America, 29*(4), 763–776.

85. Mansel, R. E. (1988). Diagnosis and treatment of mastalgia. In S. Grundfest-Broniatowski & C. B. Esselstyn (Eds.), *Controversies in breast disease: Diagnosis and management* (pp. 63–77). New York: Marcel Dekker.

86. Marchant, D. J. (1994). Invasive breast cancer: Surgical treatment alternatives, *Obstetrics and Gynecology Clinics of North America, 21*(4), 659–679.

87. Mast, D. E., & Mood, D. W. (1990). Preparing patients with breast cancer for brachytherapy. *Oncology Nursing Forum, 17*(2), 267–270.

88. McGowan, K. L. (1989). Radiation therapy: Saving your patient's skin. *RN, 52*(6), 24–27.

89. McGuire, W. L. (1988). Clinical alert from the National Cancer Institute (editorial). *Breast Cancer Research and Treatment, 12*(1), 3–5.

90. Moore, M. P., & Kinne, D. W. (1995). The surgical management of the primary invasive breast cancer. *CA: A Cancer Journal for Clinicians, 45*(5), 279–288.

91. Morrow, M. (1990). Management of nonpalpable breast lesions. *Principles and Practice of Oncology Updates, 4*(1), 1–11.

92. Muss, H. B. (1993). How to treat the older woman with breast cancer. *Contemporary Oncology, 3*(5), 27–29, 33–34, 37–39.

93. Nail, L. M., et al. (1991). Use and perceived efficacy of self-care activities in patients receiving chemotherapy. *Oncology Nursing Forum, 18*(5), 883–887.

94. National Cancer Institute. (1995). *Radiation therapy and you* (NIH publication No. 92–2227). Washington, DC: Author.

95. National Cancer Institute. (1994). *Advanced cancer: Living each day* (NIH publication No. 94–856). Washington, DC: Author.

96. National Cancer Institute. (1994). *What you need to know about breast cancer* (NIH publication No. 94–1556). Washington, DC: Author.

97. National Cancer Institute. (1993). *Chemotherapy and you* (NIH publication No. 94–1136). Washington, DC: Author.

98. National Cancer Institute. (1993). *Taking time: Support for people with cancer and the people who care about them* (NIH publication No. 94–2059). Washington, DC: Author.

99. National Cancer Institute. (1993). *When cancer recurs: Meeting the challenge again* (NIH publication No. 93–2709). Washington, DC: Author.

100. Ojeda-Fournier, H., & Evans, G. R. D. (1994). Rehabilitation after mastectomy: The role of breast reconstruction. *Physician Assistant, 18*(11), 39–40, 43–44, 46–47.

101. Osborne, C. K. (1990). Prognostic factors in breast cancer. *Principles and Practice of Oncology Update, 4*(3), 1–11.

102. Osbourne, M. P., & Borgen, P. I. (1990). Role of mastectomy in breast cancer. *Surgical Clinics of North America, 70*(5), 1023–1046.

103. Osteen, R. T., et al. (1992). Regional differences in surgical management of breast cancer. *CA: A Journal for Clinicians, 42*(1), 39–43.

104. Osteen, R. T., & Smith, B. L. (1990). Results of conservative surgery and radiation therapy for breast cancer. *Surgical Clinics of North America, 70*(5), 1005–1021.

105. Page, D. L., & Simpson, J. F. (1991). Benign, high-risk, and premaligant lesions of the mamma. In K. I. Bland & E. M. Copeland (Eds.), *The breast: Comprehensive management of benign*

and malignant diseases* (pp. 113–134). Philadelphia: W. B. Saunders.

106. Palmer, G. A. (1993). Breast cancer: Diagnosis and treatment. *Nurse Practitioner Forum, 4*(2), 100–104.

107. Pennisi, V. R. (1990). Long-term use of polyurethane breast prostheses: A 14-year experience. *Plastic and Reconstructive Surgery, 86*(2), 368–371.

108. Pfeiffer, C. H., & Mulliken, J. B. (Eds.) (1984). *Caring for the patient with breast cancer: An interdisciplinary/multidisciplinary approach.* Reston, VA: Reston Publishing.

109. Pierce, P. F. (1993). Deciding on breast cancer treatment: A description of decision behavior. *Nursing Research, 42*(1), 22–28.

110. Pierce, S. M., et al. (1992). Long-term radiation complications following conservative surgery (CS) and radiation therapy (RT) in patients with early stage breast cancer. *International Journal of Radiation Oncology, Biology, Physics, 23*(5), 915–923.

111. Pierce, S. M., & Harris, J. R. (1991). Role of radiation therapy in the management of primary breast cancer. *CA: A Cancer Journal for Clinicians, 41*(2), 85–96.

112. Piper, B., et al. (1989). Fatigue patterns over time in woman receiving CMF chemotherapy for breast cancer (abstract 355). *Oncology Nursing Forum, 16*(suppl.), 217.

113. Priestly, M. (1992). Breast reconstruction following mastectomy. *British Journal of Nursing, 1*(3), 118–121.

114. Rebner, M., et al. (1989). Breast microcalcifications after lumpectomy and radiation therapy. *Radiology, 170*(3), 691–693.

115. Robbins, S. L., et al. (1984). *Pathologic basis of disease* (3rd ed.). Philadelphia: W. B. Saunders.

116. Rogers, K., & Coup, A. J. (1990). *Surgical pathology of the breast.* London: Wright.

117. Russell, L. C. (1989). Caffeine restriction as the initial treatment for breast pain. *Nurse Practitioner, 140*(3), 36–40.

118. Rust, D., & Kloppenborg, E. (1990). Don't underestimate the lumpectomy patient's needs. *RN, 53*(3), 58–64.

119. Saleh, K. L. (1992). Practical points in the care of the patients post-breast surgery. *Journal of Post Anesthesia Nursing, 7*(3), 176–178.

120. Samarel, N., & Fawcett, J. (1992). Enhancing adaptation to breast cancer: The addition of coaching to support groups. *Oncology Nursing Forum, 19*(4), 591–596.

121. Schag, C. A., et al. (1993). Characteristics of women at risk for psychosocial distress in the year after breast cancer. *Journal of Clinical Oncology, 11*(4), 783–93.

122. Schain, W. S., et al. (1994). Mastectomy versus conservative surgery and radiation therapy: Psychosocial consequences. *Cancer, 73*(4), 1221–1228.

123. Scheiderman, H. (1994). What's your diagnosis? . . . Answer: Acute mastitis. *Consultant, 34*(12), 1711–1712.

124. Schottenfeld, D. (1988). Epidemiology of the breast. In J. K. Harness, et al. (Eds.), *Breast cancer: Collaborative management* (pp. 55–68). Chelsea, MI: Lewis Publishers.

125. Schover, L. R. (1991). The impact of breast cancer on sexuality, body image, and intimate relationships. *CA: A Cancer Journal for Clinicians, 41*(2), 112–120.

126. Schumann, D. (1994). Health risks for women with breast implants. *Nurse Practitioner, 19*(7), 19–20, 23–25, 29–30.

127. Schydlower, M. (1982). Breast masses in adolescents. *American Family Physician, 25*(2), 141–145.

128. Semiglazov, V. F., et al. (1994). Primary (neoadjuvant chemotherapy and radiotherapy compared with primary radiotherapy alone in stage IIb-IIIa breast cancer. *Annals of Oncology, 5*(7), 591–595.

129. Sheth, S. P., & Allegra, A. C. (1991). Endocrine therapy of breast cancer. In K. I. Bland & E. M. Copeland (Eds.), *The breast: Comprehensive management of benign and malignant diseases* (pp. 937–947). Philadelphia: W. B. Saunders.

130. Sorace, R. A., & Lippman, M. E. (1988). Locally advanced breast cancer. In M. E. Lippman, et al. (Eds.), *Diagnosis and management of breast cancer* (pp. 272–295). Philadelphia: W. B. Saunders.

131. Souba, W. W. (1991). Evaluation and treatment of benign breast disorders. In K. I. Bland & E. M. Copeland (Eds.), *The breast: Comprehensive management of benign and malignant diseases* (pp. 715–729). Philadelphia: W. B. Saunders.

132. Spindler, J. (1991). Seeing through the mask of cancer. *Nursing 91, 12*(5), 37–40.

133. Stefanek, M. E. (1990). Counseling women at high risk for breast cancer. *Oncology, 4*(1), 27–37.

134. Sunderland, M. C., & McGuire, W. L. (1990). Prognostic indicators in invasive breast cancer. *Surgical Clinics of North America, 70*(5), 989–1004.

135. Taylor, D. L. (1995). Physiology insight: Close-up on oncogenes . . . How mutant genes trigger cancer. *Nursing, 25*(6), 57.

136. Vogel, C. L. (1991). Treatment of metastatic breast cancer. *Seminars in Oncology Nursing, 7*(3), 194–199.

137. Walters, P. (1990). Chemo: A nurse's guide to action, administration, and side effects. *RN, 53*(2), 52–67.

138. Waltman, N. (1994). Treatment options for the patient with breast cancer. *Plastic Surgical Nursing, 14*(1), 15–26.

139. Ward, S., & Griffin, J. (1990). Developing a test of knowledge of surgical options for breast cancer. *Cancer Nursing, 13*(3), 191–196.

140. Weber, B. L., et al. (1992). *High-response rate and breast conservation in locally advanced breast carcinoma (LABC) using combined modality therapy with hormonal synchronization* (meeting abstract). Proceedings of the Annual Meeting of the American Society of Clinical Oncology, 11, p. A127.

141. Wellisch, D. K., et al. (1989). Psychosocial outcomes of breast cancer therapies: Lumpectomy versus mastectomy. *Psychosomatics, 30*(4), 365–373.

142. Whitman, M. (1994). Breast surgery: Helping patients choose. *Nursing, 24*(8), 25.

143. Whitman, M., & McDaniel, R. W. (1993). Preventing lymphedema, an unwelcome sequel to breast cancer, *Nursing, 23*(12), 36–39.

144. Wilson, S., & Morse, J. M. (1991). Living with a wife undergoing chemotherapy. *IMAGE: Journal for Nursing Scholarship, 23*(2), 78–84.

145. Winer, E. P., et al. (1993). Silicone controversy: A survey of women with breast cancer and silicone implants. *Journal of the National Cancer Institute, 85*(17), 1407–1411.

146. Wingo, P. A., et al. (1995). Cancer statistics, 1995. *CA: A Cancer Journal for Clinicians, 45*(1), 8–30.

147. Wolmark, N. (1989). 1989: The year of adjuvant therapy in node-negative breast cancer. *Principles and Practice of Oncology Updates, 3*(12), 1–10.

148. Yarbro, J. W. (1992). Oncogenes and cancer suppressor genes. *Seminars in Oncology Nursing, 8*(1), 30–39.

Nursing Care of Clients with Sexually Transmitted Diseases

Patricia E. Downing

Sexually Transmitted Diseases: An Overview

The term *sexually transmitted diseases* (STDs) refers to a broad group of conditions that are usually or can be transmitted by genital, oral, or anal sexual contact. STD has replaced the older term *venereal disease* (VD), which was narrowly defined as a disease transmitted only by sexual intercourse. The newer term STD better reflects the broad spectrum of organisms and diseases now recognized as being sexually transmitted (Box 86–1). In addition to the five classic venereal diseases (gonorrhea, syphilis, chancroid, lymphogranuloma venereum, and granuloma inguinale), sexually transmitted diseases include infectious diseases such as chlamydial infections, genital herpes, genital warts, trichomoniasis, acquired immunodeficiency syndrome (AIDS), and some enteric and ectoparasitic infections. The number of diseases in this category increases as new agents are implicated in the sexual transmission of disease.

STDs share several characteristics:

- Despite their biologic differences, STDs are transmitted by sexual activity between opposite or same sex partners (not only vaginal/penile sex, but also oral and anal sex).
- Having one STD confers no immunity to future reinfection with that STD or to other STDs.
- All sexual partners of the infected client need to be assessed for treatment.
- STDs frequently coexist in the same client (e.g., a client may have both *Chlamydia* infection and gonorrhea).

The last fact may be responsible for some treatment failures. Current treatment guidelines for STDs are available in the United States from the division of STD, Centers for Disease Control and Prevention (CDC), Atlanta.

STDs represent a very serious public health problem. These diseases occur worldwide, have been recognized since the beginning of recorded history, affect all age groups and socioeconomic strata, and are associated with substantial morbidity and, in some cases, mortality. Although most are well understood and are relatively easily identified, the incidence of STDs continues to increase. Thus, the scope of the health problem they create is increasing rather than decreasing.

Except for the common cold and influenza, STDs are the most prevalent communicable diseases in the United States. Every year, STDs are diagnosed in more than 12 million people in this country. Out of these 12 million people, 25% (3 million) are adolescents. Most sources describe STD rates as epidemic. Whereas AIDS is probably the best publicized and most dangerous, the most common STDs are *Chlamydia*, gonorrhea, genital herpes, venereal warts, and syphilis.

Official national STD incidence statistics are published routinely by the CDC and by local health authorities, but the actual incidence of STDs is unknown. Accurate statistics are difficult to compile for a number of different reasons. Statistics are only as good as the accuracy of case reporting, and reporting is not mandatory for all STDs. In fact, STD case reporting is required by all states primarily only for AIDS, hepatitis B, and the five classic STDs (gonorrhea, syphilis, chancroid, lymphogranuloma venereum, and granuloma inguinale). Rates for other STDs, such as genital herpes and genital warts, are based on estimates derived from local studies and physician reports. These estimates are thought to be low. Even rates developed from mandatory case reporting are believed to be low because of underreporting. Nearly 1 million new cases of gonorrhea, for example, are reported to public health officials yearly, but it is generally believed that at least another million cases go unreported.

Anyone who engages in intimate physical contact can contract and transmit an STD. The age-specific rates for STDs are highest for sexually active adolescents and young adults, but all age groups are at risk. No age group is safe. The fetus and neonate can be infected perinatally across the placenta and during vaginal birth. Infants and

Box 86–1. Sexually Transmitted Diseases

STDs Caused by Bacteria

Gonorrhea
Chlamydial infection
Syphilis
Bacterial vaginosis
Nongonococcal urethritis
Chancroid
Lymphogranuloma venereum
Granuloma inguinale
Sexually transmitted enteric infections

STDs Caused by Viruses

Acquired immunodeficiency syndrome (AIDS)
Genital herpes
Genital warts
Hepatitis B

STDs Caused by Protozoa

Trichomoniasis

STDs Caused by Fungi

Vulvovaginal candidiasis

STDs Caused by Ectoparasites

Scabies
Pediculosis pubis

children can be infected through child abuse or incest. The elderly can be infected or experience residual sequelae from infections transmitted earlier in their lives. Risk factors for STDs are listed in Risk Factors and Levels of Prevention.

The increase in the estimated incidence of STDs worldwide is due to many factors. Among bacterial STDs (especially gonorrhea and chancroid) antibiotic-resistant strains have become widely disseminated. The incidence of gonorrhea, for example, once thought to be under control, has increased since the evolution of penicillinase-producing *Neisseria gonorrhoeae*. Also, many societies with increased mobility, sexual freedom, unemployment, and drug abuse have become more permissive. The use of intrauterine devices and oral contraceptives may be related to transmission of STDs because they may lower the female's resistance to infection. Lack of knowledge also plays a role in the incidence of STDs. It is sometimes difficult for people to get accurate information about sexual activities and to decide if and how such activities fit their chosen life-style. Controversy over sex education in schools continues. Only recently have the media and concerned organizations begun to present accurate information about sex and STDs in a manner designed to appeal to young people.

Although STDs can be passed nonsexually, most of the diseases, as the term STD implies, are transmitted sexually. This is because the causative organisms thrive in a

warm, dark, moist environment and survive only very briefly outside that environment. Transmission therefore requires some mode of close intimate contact. It follows logically that prevention and control must concentrate on breaking the chain of sexual transmission. According to the CDC, the prevention of STDs should focus primarily on changing high-risk sexual behaviors. Health promotion interventions for STDs are listed in Risk Factors and Levels of Prevention.

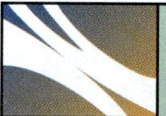

RISK FACTORS AND LEVELS OF PREVENTION

Sexually Transmitted Diseases

Risk Factors

High Risk

Having multiple sex partners; engaging in unsafe, unprotected sex practices; abusing drugs; being an adolescent or young adult; being medically underserved; having low socioeconomic status; belonging to a racial or ethnic minority; having a history of prior STDs; having a history of current STDs; failing to comply with treatment for an STD

Low or No Risk

Practicing sexual abstinence; being in mutually monogamous relationship

Levels of Prevention

Primary Prevention

Provide health education about STDs; promote comprehensive sex education classes in schools; provide risk reduction counseling; respond to the health-seeking behaviors of clients; promote "safe sex" practices (e.g., condom use); teach clients about good genital hygiene; advise clients to get hepatitis B vaccinations; engage and participate in research for the prevention of STDs.

Secondary Prevention

Conduct screening tests for asymptomatic high-risk groups; be alert for STDs in asymptomatic infected people; provide effective diagnosis and prompt treatment of infected people; conduct follow-up evaluations after the completion of treatment for STDs; promptly report STDs to the Health Department; identify all sexual contacts of people infected with STDs; counsel and treat all sexual contacts of people infected with STDs.

Tertiary Prevention

Advise clients about the surgical correction of the sequelae of STDs (e.g., tuboplasty); advise clients about rehabilitation from the effects of STDs.

Table 86–1. Management of Common Sexually Transmitted Diseases

Condition (Causative Organism)	Diagnostic Methods	Manifestations	Treatment of Choice*	Mandatory Reporting	Sexual Partner Treatment†
Gonorrhea *(Neisseria gonorrhoeae)*	Smear culture	Incubation period: 3–8 days Female: asymptomatic or • Thick, purulent vaginal discharge • Genital irritation • Dysuria, urinary frequency • Pharyngeal infection • Conjunctivitis • Late: pelvic pain (PID) Male: asymptomatic or • Urethral discharge • Dysuria, urinary frequency • Pharyngeal infection • Conjunctivitis • Late: scrotal pain (epididymitis) • Perineal pain (prostatitis) Disseminated infection, either sex: • Bacteremia • Arthritis-dermatitis syndrome	Ceftriaxone IM once or Cefixime PO once or Ciprofloxacin PO once or Ofloxacin PO once *plus* Doxycycline PO for 7 days Ceftriaxone IM or IV every 24 hours, continued for 24–48 hours after improvement begins	Yes	All contacts within the preceding 30 days should be examined, cultured, and treated presumptively
Chlamydial infections *(Chlamydia trachomatis)*	Culture Antigen-antibody tests Enzyme immunoassay (ELISA) Monoclonal antibody test	Incubation period: 7–21 days Female: asymptomatic or • Mucopurulent vaginal discharge • Dysuria • Abnormal vaginal bleeding • Pelvic pain (PID) Male: asymptomatic or • Mild dysuria • White or clear urethral discharge • Testicle pain (epididymitis)	Doxycycline PO for 7 days or Azithromycin PO once	Yes*	All contacts within 30 days should be examined and treated
Syphilis *(Treponema pallidum)*	Dark-field microscopy (chancre, granulomata lata) Serologic antibody tests (STS) • Nonspecific, e.g., VDRL • Specific, e.g., FTA-ABS	Incubation period: 10–90 days Primary stage • Painless chancre at site of exposure • Regional lymphadenopathy Second stage • Maculopapular rash • Generalized lymphadenopathy • Mucous patches • Condylomata lata • Fever, malaise	Primary, secondary, and early latent syphilis: benzathine penicillin G IM single dose	Yes	All contacts with early syphilis (primary, secondary, or latent syphilis of 1 year's duration) should be evaluated and treated All contacts within 90 days should be treated presumptively

Table continued on following page

Table 86–1. Management of Common Sexually Transmitted Diseases *(Continued)*

Condition (Causative Organism)	Diagnostic Methods	Manifestations	Treatment of Choice*	Mandatory Reporting	Sexual Partner Treatment†
	Cerebrospinal fluid (late syphilis)	• Alopecia Latent stage • Asymptomatic Late stage • Cardiovascular changes, e.g., aortic aneurysm • Central nervous system changes, e.g., paresis, tabes dorsalis, dementia	Late latent and late syphilis: benzathine penicillin G IM weekly for 3 weeks Neurosyphilis: aqueous penicillin IV every 4 hours for 10–14 days		

Genital herpes
Herpes simplex virus (HSV) type I or II, primarily type II
	Culture
	Pap smear
		Incubation period: 3–7 days
		Acute phase
		• Paresthesia/burning at site of exposure
		• Painful genital vesicles that ulcerate
		• Fever, chills, muscle aches
		Latent phase
		• Asymptomatic
			No cure
			Acute episodes:
			  Acyclovir PO for 5–10 days
			Severe episodes:
			  Acyclovir IV every 8 hours for 5–7 days
			Recurrent episodes:
			  Suppressive therapy—acyclovir daily for 4 months to 5 years
				No	All contacts of clients with active lesions should be evaluated and, if symptomatic, treated

Genital warts Human papillomavirus (HPV)	Pap smear Colposcopy Biopsy	Incubation period: 1–2 months Single or multiple painless genital or anorectal warts	No cure Topical podophyllin or Topical trichloroacetic acid (TCA) or Cryotherapy or electrocautery or CO_2 laser or surgical excision	No	All contacts should be evaluated and, if symptomatic, treated

* Not mandatory in all states in the United States.
† *CDC 1993 sexually transmitted diseases treatment guidelines.*
IM, intramuscularly; IV, intravenously; PID, pelvic inflammatory disease; PO, orally.

Community and Self-Care

■ Medical Management

Most commonly, STDs are treated with the anti-infective agent specific to the causative organism. Table 86–1 discusses the management of each STD; specific information on each STD is given later in the chapter.

■ Nursing Management of the Medical Client

Assessment

Assessment of the client with a sexually transmitted disease includes the identification of the manifestations of the STD, a careful physical assessment, and a complete sexual history. (See Chapters 11 and 82 for detailed descriptions of the physical assessment of the male and female reproductive systems.) Remember that perhaps as many as 60% to 80% of STDs are asymptomatic. High-risk clients should be assessed for possible STDs regardless of whether physical manifestations of STDs are present at the time of a visit to a healthcare provider.

The sexual history obtained from a client includes sexual orientation, sexual activities, number of sexual partners, previous STD infections, exposure to STDs, use of contraceptives, and manifestation history. (See Table 82–1 for an outline of a comprehensive sexual history.) Remember that sex partners may include persons of the same sex as the client.

Nurses need to be well informed about the variety of sexual activities, their effect on the transmission of STDs, and the common manifestations to assess. It is necessary for a health professional to separate a personal view of morality from appropriate nursing activities. At times, this is difficult for some nurses.

There is a social stigma associated with STDs (see Ethical Issues in Nursing). Many clients are ashamed of having an STD and try to keep the diagnosis secret. Many associate STDs with low social status and immorality, and many have misconceptions and fears about the dangers of STD.

Other social problems may surface with the discovery of an STD. For example, newly infected clients may be angry at the responsible sexual partners or may be hesitant to identify or inform their sexual partners about the STD. When a marital or committed relationship is involved, further problems, such as worry about infidelity or potential infertility, may develop.

Treatment can be sought in various facilities, including health department STD clinics, physician offices, Planned Parenthood, and community-based clinics. Such clinics deal with STDs frequently and often have staff especially sensitive to the needs of clients with STDs. Strict confidentiality is essential. This is especially, but not exclusively, important to gay men and lesbians, who may be at risk of discrimination if their sexual orientation is disclosed. To provide confidentiality, some clinics use a code rather than the term "homosexual" or "bisexual" to record sexual orientation in the client's record.

Diagnosis, Planning, and Implementation

Knowledge Deficit. The client with an STD probably has many learning needs, which makes *Knowledge Deficit related to lack of understanding of the causes, treatments, and prevention of STDs* the priority nursing diagnosis.

Planning: Expected Outcomes. The client will understand the cause, treatment, and prevention of specific STD, as evidenced by client's statements, avoidance of STDs, successful treatment of STD, and, if possible, no recurrence of STD.

Implementation. Provide information about the transmission, prevention, and treatment of STDs. When caring for clients with STDs, nurses obtain privileged/private information and provide instruction about these diseases (see the Client Education Guide on p. 2465). Both activities require sensitivity and skillful interaction.

Myths about STDs abound and need to be corrected. Many women and men, for example, erroneously believe that hormonal oral contraceptives protect them against STDs. These clients need to be informed about the inability of hormonal contraception methods to prevent STDs. Although dual use may be viewed as more difficult, condom use in conjunction with non–barrier contraceptive methods must be promoted. Also, some men erroneously think that the routine urine tests they undergo for certain sports are a check for STDs, and that a negative test indicates they are free of STDs. These clients need to know that sports urine examinations test for drugs *only*.

Supply accurate, factual STD information to help the client avoid reinfection of self or infection of others (see the Client Education Guide on p. 2465). Include the following topics in teaching sessions about STDs:

- Name, nature, and seriousness of the condition
- Mode of transmission
- Actions to take to prevent the spread of infection to others
- Incubation periods

ETHICAL ISSUES IN NURSING

Does the Right to Privacy of Clients with STDs Supersede the Right-to-Know of Potentially Infected Partners?

Sexually transmitted diseases (STDs) are a very serious public health problem. These diseases may predispose people to various cancers and may cause sterility and even death. Because of the seriousness of these diseases, the laws of some states in the United States require health professionals to report clients who test positive for syphilis, gonorrhea, or chlamydial infection to the Department of Public Health. The Department of Health then initiates follow-up of those clients. Follow-up includes notification of the sexual partners of the infected client so that treatment may be initiated for them as well.

The practice of reporting sexual contacts of people infected with STDs raises several ethical questions involving the right to privacy. Does a Public Health Department have the right to know the identities of the sexual partners of those with STDs, even if it is in the best interests of the public at large? Should the infected client alone be responsible for disclosing such information to his or her partners? Do partners of infected clients have a right to be told of their partner's infection, so that they may seek treatment?

Healthcare workers who care for people with STDs have an obligation to protect the privacy of their clients as well as an obligation to assist those who have potentially been infected. As a nurse, you must inform your infected clients of the public health guidelines that you must follow. Information given to public health departments should be as honest and concise as possible. Clients do have a right to privacy, but this privacy must be altered when the rights of others to information affecting their own health are involved.

BRIDGE TO HOME HEALTHCARE

Teaching About Sexually Transmitted Diseases

Sandra Elsea, R.N., M.N., *Visiting Nurse Association of Omaha, Omaha, Nebraska*

When you are caring for a client with a sexually transmitted disease (STD), it is important that you take a nonjudgmental approach. STDs affect the client not only physically but also emotionally. The diagnosis of an STD interferes with the client's sense of sexuality, which is a very personal, sensitive part of the identity. Nursing interventions related to assisting clients with STDs encompass three major areas: casefinding, education, and follow-up.

People who have contracted an STD need educational materials and teaching. Include in those instructions information about the specific infection that the person has contracted: the mode of transmission, the importance of compliance with the full course of treatment, and the potential short- and long-term consequences of noncompliance with the recommendations for treatment and follow-up.

Do not assume that the client has a basic understanding of anatomy and physiology. Selecting appropriate language and using teaching methods with which the client can identify are more likely to result in the desired changes in behavior patterns.

The concept of "safer sex" is a major teaching objective. Teaching about "safer" sexual practices must include the use of condoms, avoiding sexual contact with people who have many different sexual partners and with people who use illicit drugs, and avoiding sexual practices that cause bruising or damage the skin. Also teach other preventive behaviors, such as daily bathing with a mild soap, maintaining the normal vaginal flora by avoiding the use of feminine hygiene sprays, avoiding the use of tight synthetic clothing, and avoiding unnecessary douching.

It is important that the client understand the importance of honest disclosure and responsible behavior in relation to the diagnosis and treatment of STDs. Reporting of sexual contacts and accepting responsibility for treatment and follow-up are important concepts to communicate to the client. These behaviors are critical if the outcome of an STD is to be positive for the client, and in many cases they are critical if the outcome is to be positive for those who are close to the client.

- Manifestations of infection
- Asymptomatic problems
- When and how to seek treatment
- Treatment methods
- Importance of follow-up care (when and how to obtain it)
- Consequences of not completing treatment
- Risk and consequences of recurrent infections.

The latex condom (*rubber*) is the most effective mechanical barrier to STD infection. Use of the latex condom should be promoted for sexually active people who are at risk for STDs. Sexually active males and females must be taught to use condoms properly, effectively, and consistently. Condom failure is primarily due to improper or inconsistent use, rather than to product defect. The Client Education Guide on pp. 2466–2467 provides instructions for correct condom use.

In the United States and other countries, a variety of community and national programs are available in which healthcare professionals collaborate with laypersons. Nurses play a pivotal role by identifying community resources available to their clients. Most public health agencies have STD prevention and treatment programs that are open to the public. Clients can also obtain information anonymously from the National STD Hotline (1–800–227–8922) or the National AIDS Hotline (1–800–342–AIDS).

Anxiety. The client with an STD often experiences a great deal of fear and uncertainty, which makes *Anxiety related to uncertainty of condition and social stigma* an important nursing diagnosis.

Planning: Expected Outcomes. The client will have a decrease in anxiety, as evidenced by a realistic understanding of disease, seeking treatment, and showing an acceptance of the condition.

Implementation. Learning of an STD can threaten a client's self-concept and pose potential physical problems, such as possible infertility or damage to a fetus. Feelings of guilt, apprehension, and rejection by others may be expressed. The nurse should work with the client to reduce anxiety by being warm and supportive, facilitating the expression of feelings, and encouraging effective coping strategies. The client needs to be kept informed about what is happening and what to expect.

A nonjudgmental attitude is essential for providing quality care for a client with an STD. It is important that personnel examine their own attitudes toward sexuality and sexual behavior. Although one's own moral values are important in guiding personal behavior, prejudicial attitudes may interfere with therapeutic professional relationships. Bias and prejudice can be communicated in both obvious and subtle ways that make the affected client feel uncomfortable, judged, and discounted. A prejudiced health professional cannot provide comprehensive healthcare.

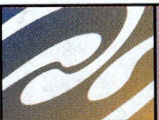

CLIENT EDUCATION GUIDE

Sexually Transmitted Diseases

Client Instructions in English *(Instrucciones para el cliente en inglés)*	Client Instructions in Spanish *(Instrucciones para el cliente en español)*
Treatment will not protect you from getting this disease again. Having had a sexually transmitted disease also doesn't give you immunity. You can get the same disease again, or you can get another sexually transmitted disease, if you don't take precautions.	El tratamiento no le asegura protección si contrae esta enfermedad otra vez. El haber tenido esta enfermedad transmitida sexualmente no le da inmunidad. Puede contraer la misma infección otra vez, o contraer otra enfermedad transmitida sexualmente, si no toma precauciones.
It is best to wait until your test results show that your infection is cured before you resume sexual activity. If you wait, you will not be in danger of spreading the infection to your sex partners, or possibly of getting the disease again yourself. If you feel that you can't wait, be sure to use barrier protection, such as a condom.	Es mejor esperar hasta que los resultados de los exámines indiquen que ya se ha curado de la infección, antes de volver a tener relaciones sexuales. Si espera no estará a riesgo de pasarle la infección a su compañero(a) sexual, o de contraer la infección otra vez. Si cree que no puede esperar para tener sexo, entonces asegurese y use protección tal como el condón.
We would like to see you again on [appointment date] to be sure that your infection is cured.	Por favor regrese el [día de la cita], para revisarlo y asegurarnos de que se ha curado.
For women: When you have your routine gynecologic examination, ask your doctor to check for sexually transmitted diseases. You may have a sexually transmitted disease even if you don't have any symptoms.	*Para mujeres:* Cuando le hagan su examen ginecológico, pidale al doctor que la examine para ver si tiene señas de infecciones sexuales. Puede tener una enfermedad infecciosa que se le ha ya transmitido sexualmente, aunque no tenga síntomas.
For men: If your symptoms come back, see your doctor for treatment right away.	*Para hombres:* Si vuelve a tener síntomas, vea al doctor para que le dé tratamiento inmediatamente.

The nurse needs to be very skillful in interpersonal communication to help clients seeking counsel or treatment for STD. Such clients need encouragement, support, and accurate information. Moralistic, judgmental attitudes do not change others' sexual behavior. Instead, they may deter clients from seeking adequate care. An accepting professional attitude may ensure treatment and prevent the transmission of disease to sexual partners or to infants, prenatally and postnatally.

Evaluation

If the client receives adequate treatment, most STDs can be cured or controlled within a short time.

Gonorrhea

Gonorrhea (lay terms: *clap, white, drips, strain, dose*) can be divided into two categories: local and disseminated infection (see Table 86–1).

● *Local infection* can involve the mucosal surfaces of the cervix, urethra, and rectum; vestibular glands; pharynx; or conjunctiva.
● *Systemic infection (disseminated gonococcal infection)*

involves bacteremia with polyarthritis, dermatitis, endocarditis, and meningitis. Systemic infection is more common in women than in men.

Etiology and Risk Factors

Since 1975, the overall number of reported cases of gonorrhea has declined. Despite this, gonorrhea continues to be one of the most prevalent STDs in the United States. In addition, it is widely believed that gonorrhea is underreported, and that the actual number of cases is much greater than those reported. Incidence varies with age and may be increasing rather than decreasing in adolescents. Teenagers and young adults are at highest risk. Most gonorrhea occurs in persons aged 15 to 29 years, with the highest rate in those aged 20 to 24 years.

Pathophysiology

Gonorrhea is caused by the gram-negative diplococcus *Neisseria gonorrhoeae*. The incubation period is variable, usually 3 to 8 days, sometimes longer. The causative organism does not survive long outside the body. Gonorrheal infection, therefore, is almost always transmitted by

CLIENT EDUCATION GUIDE

How to Use a Condom

Client Instructions in English *(Instrucciones para el cliente en inglés)*	Client Instructions in Spanish *(Instrucciones para el cliente en español)*
Before Intercourse	**Antes de Tener Relaciones Sexuales**
Discuss condom use with your sexual partner *before* you begin to have sex.	Discuta el uso del condón con su compañero(a) *antes de* empezar la relación sexual.
Decide that you will have sex *only* when you use a condom.	Haga la decisión de tener sexo *solamente* cuando use un condón.
Before you have sex, practice using a condom.	Antes del sexo, practique como usar el condón.
Keep condoms in a handy place.	Guarde los condones en un lugar conveniente.
To Use a Male Condom	**Uso de un Condón Masculino**
Use a *new latex* condom *each time* you have sex. Put the condom on before your genitals touch your partner's genitals. Do not use natural membrane condoms.	Use un condón *de látex nuevo cada vez que tenga* relaciones sexuales. Pongase el condón antes de que sus genitales toquen a su compañera(o). No use condónes hechos con membranas naturales.
Place a spermicide containing nonoxynol 9 inside the condom, unless you or your partner is allergic to it. These spermicides are available in your drug store without a prescription.	Ponga un espermaticida que contenga Nonoxinol 9 dentro del condón, a menos que su compañera(o) sea alérgico(a) a éste. Puede conseguir estos espermaticidas en la farmacia. No necesita receta.
Place the rolled up condom on the head of the erect penis.	Ponga el condón en la "cabeza" del pene cuando esté erecto.
Pinch the end of condom to create a little space to catch what you ejaculate.	Apriete la punta del condón para formar un área que recoja el semen (el líquido de la eyaculación).
Unroll the condom until your fingers reach the base of the penis. The condom should unroll easily. If it doesn't, replace it with a new one.	Desenrolle el condón hasta que los dedos lleguen a la base del pene. El condón debe desenrrollarse fácilmente. Si no se desenrolla bien, use otro condón nuevo.

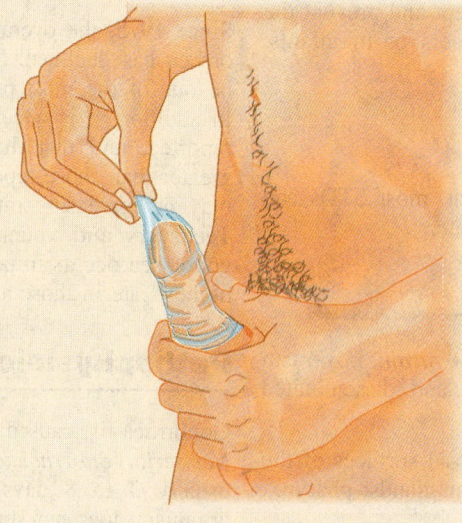

Client Instructions in English *(Instrucciones para el cliente en inglés)*	Client Instructions in Spanish *(Instrucciones para el cliente en español)*
Right after ejaculation, hold the condom firmly at the base of the penis and withdraw the penis before the erection goes away.	Inmediatamente después de la eyaculación, sujete firmemente el condón en la base del pene y saque el pene antes que termine la erección.
Throw the condom away in a safe place. Never reuse a condom.	Tire el condón en un lugar seguro. Nunca vuelva a usar el mismo condón.
If you use a lubricant, use only a water-soluble lubricant. Never use oil-based lubricants such as petroleum jelly, baby oil, cooking oil, or shortening.	Si usa lubricante, use sólo un lubricante que sea soluble en agua. Nunca use lubricante con aceite tal como vaselina, aceite para bebé, aceite para cocinar, o manteca.

To Use a Female Condom	**Uso de un Condón Femenino**
Squeeze the inner ring of the pouch between your fingers and insert it into the vagina.	Apriete entre los dedos el anillo interno de la bolsita y póngaselo en la vagina.
Advance the inner ring until the ring is just behind the pubic bone.	Avance el anillo interno hasta que sienta que llega al hueso de la pelvis.

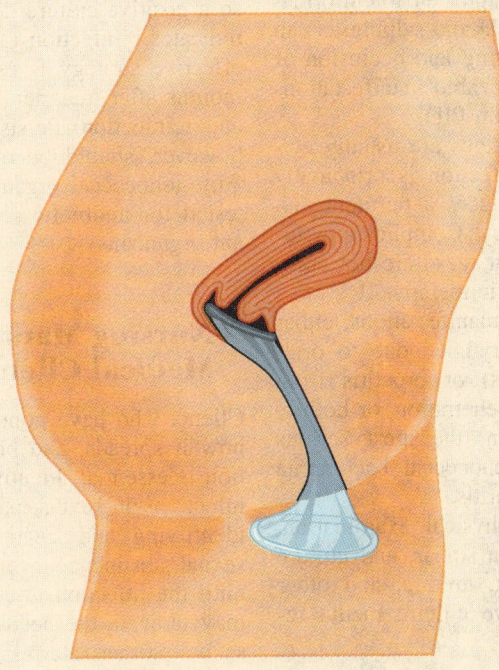

Leave one inch (2.25 cm) of the pouch's open end (the outer ring) outside the vagina.	Deje una pulgada (2.25 cm) de la bolsita afuera de la vagina.
Immediately after ejaculation, twist the outer ring and gently pull out the pouch.	Immediatamente después de la eyaculación, tuerza el anillo externo y saque (retire) suavemente la bolsita.
Throw the condom away. Never reuse a condom.	Tire el condón en un lugar seguro. Nunca vuelva a usar el mismo condón.

Adapted from The American College of Obstetricians and Gynecologists (1995). *ACOG patient education: Gonorrhea and Chlamydia* (pamphlet AP071). Washington, DC: Author.

direct sexual contact. The few rare exceptions to sexual transmission are (1) infection in children, who can develop gonorrhea from close contact with their mother's infected areas (vaginal or other mucous membranes), and (2) infection of medical personnel with lacerations, who can develop gonorrhea from contact with infected discharges. No lasting immunity prevents reinfection.

Clinical Manifestations and Diagnostic Findings

The endocervical canal is the primary site of gonorrheal infection in women. In the majority of women, the urethra is also infected. Infection can also involve the vestibular glands and anus. The vagina is resistant to the infection in adulthood, though before puberty it is not. The disease may be asymptomatic in women. In fact a large carrier population exists (i.e., people who carry the organism and have no manifestations, but who can transmit the disease). When symptomatic, manifestations may include heavy, yellow-green, purulent vaginal discharge; cervical erythema; a red, swollen, sore vulva; abnormal menstrual bleeding; dysuria; and urinary frequency.

The most common complication of gonorrhea in women is salpingitis (inflammation of fallopian tubes), which can progress to the serious complication of pelvic inflammatory disease (PID). (See Chapter 84 for information on PID and salpingitis.) Both PID and salpingitis can produce infertility secondary to scarring and occlusion of the fallopian tubes. The first recognizable manifestations of gonorrhea in women may arise from PID.

In men with gonorrhea, manifestations are usually evident earlier than in women. The infection is principally one of the anterior urethra that produces a purulent discharge, dysuria, and urinary frequency. Complications include epididymitis and prostatitis, but these are not common with early and complete antibiotic therapy.

In addition to the gender-specific manifestations, either sex may have conjunctivitis or pharyngitis due to oral-genital contact (fellatio, cunnilingus) or proctitis from anal contact (oral-anal contact, anal penetration, or both).

Disseminated gonococcal infection, the most serious form of gonorrhea, results from gonococcal bacteremia and is often manifested by septic arthritis.

Diagnosis is made by history, physical examination, identification of the gonococcus on a smear, and culture of the exudate from the endocervix, urethra, and other infected areas. Culture with selective culture media remains the cornerstone of diagnosis.

Community and Self-Care

■ Medical Management

When gonorrhea is first detected, all clients should be screened for syphilis by a serologic test and should be offered confidential testing and counseling for HIV infection. People with HIV infection and gonococcal infection should receive the same treatment as people not infected with HIV.

Gonorrhea is treated aggressively with antibiotics. Penicillin was once the treatment of choice, but therapy is now complicated by the development of penicillin-resistant organisms. The recommended regimen for uncomplicated gonorrhea is a single intramuscular dose of ceftriaxone (Rocephin), or a single oral dose of cefixime (Suprax), ciprofloxacin (Cipro), or ofloxacin (Floxin). Any of these single doses is followed by oral doxycycline (Vibramycin) for 7 days. Doxycycline is added for the presumptive treatment of co-infection with *Chlamydia trachomatis,* because chlamydial infections commonly co-exist with gonorrheal infections. For clients who cannot tolerate ceftriaxone sodium, a single intramuscular injection of spectinomycin (Trobicin) plus oral doxycycline can be used.

For clients with disseminated gonococcal infection, the recommended regimen is hospitalization and administration of ceftriaxone, given intramuscularly or intravenously every 24 hours and continued 24 to 48 hours after improvement begins. This is followed by cefixime or ciprofloxacin, given orally for a full week.

After completion of therapy for uncomplicated gonorrhea, a follow-up examination and culture may be done 4 to 7 days post-therapy. Treatment failure following combined ceftriaxone-doxycycline therapy, however, is rare, so a positive culture done immediately after therapy often indicates reinfection rather than treatment failure. A more effective strategy is reexamination with a culture 1 to 2 months after treatment. This detects both treatment failure and reinfection. Persistent manifestations after treatment, however, should be evaluated with a follow-up culture. Any gonococcal organisms shown on reculture should be tested for antibiotic sensitivity to identify possible resistant organisms.

■ Nursing Management of the Medical Client

Clients who have gonorrhea must understand the disease, how it spreads, and how it is treated. Self-care information is essential. Identify the possibility of reinfection and infection of sexual partners. Discuss the importance of identifying and treating all sexual partners. Encourage sexual abstinence or use of a male or female condom until the infection is cured. Recurrence due to reinfection may indicate the need for improved client education and sexual partner referral.

Warn pregnant female clients of the danger of infecting their newborns during delivery. Advise these women to refrain from sexual activity until their condition is cured. Oral sexual activity should be avoided if there is a pharyngeal infection. Clients receiving treatment for gonorrhea must understand the importance of taking the *complete* course of prescribed medications and of returning for follow-up evaluation after completing the medication.

Treatment for gonorrhea is subject to change as organisms become more resistant. Many clients are not aware that the regimen of antibiotics used to treat gonorrhea is usually much different from that used for most other infections, and some mistakenly think that an antibiotic taken for some other problem (e.g., a respiratory infection) will also "cure" gonorrhea. Public education is an essential part of the fight against STDs.

Sexual contact investigation is essential for the prevention and control of gonorrhea. All sex partners exposed to gonorrhea within the preceding 30 days should be examined, cultured, and treated presumptively. Reporting sexual contacts can be difficult and frightening for an infected client. Ask for contact information in a positive, nonthreatening, sensitive way during the initial treatment visit. However, this is best asked after the treatment is administered, to keep the client from becoming anxious and possibly avoiding necessary care.

Chlamydial Infections

Chlamydia is the nation's most common bacterial sexually transmitted disease (see Table 86-1). The number of new cases per year is estimated to be at least 3 to 4 million, three times that of gonorrhea. Unlike gonorrhea, however, no comprehensive national surveillance system for *Chlamydia* is fully functional, so the exact incidence is unknown.

Etiology and Risk Factors

The causative organism, *Chlamydia trachomatis,* is a nonmotile, gram-negative bacterium. This organism is the most common cause of what was previously diagnosed as nonspecific vaginitis in females, and nonspecific urethritis (NSU) or nongonococcal urethritis (NGU) in males. The incubation period is 7 to 21 days.

C. trachomatis is always transmitted by intimate sexual contact, never by casual contact. Women usually acquire the infection during intercourse with an infected male. Homosexual males can also transmit the infection through oral-anal contact or anal penetration. The infection does not cross the placenta, but passage through the birth canal of an infected woman can cause conjunctivitis and pneumonia in newborns.

Pathophysiology

Chlamydial infection is known as "the great sterilizer." Undetected and untreated cases can progress to serious, irreversible consequences. *C. trachomatis* causes an inflammation that leads to scarring and ulceration of involved tissue. In men, the infection can cause a stricture of the urethra or extend to the epididymis. The ensuing epididymitis can produce sterility. In women, the infection can extend to the endometrium and salpinx; the major consequence is salpingitis with subsequent infertility or high risk of ectopic pregnancy. Secondary extension to the female peritoneum can cause a PID very similar to that resulting from gonorrhea. (See Chapter 84 for a discussion of PID.) A serious systemic complication, more

common in males, is Reiter's syndrome, which consists of urethritis, polyarthritis, and conjunctivitis.

Clinical Manifestations and Diagnostic Findings

Chlamydial infections primarily affect the cervix, urethra, and rectum. In most cases, the infection is asymptomatic for an extended period. When present, manifestations closely resemble those of gonorrhea, but they are less severe.

In women, the primary site of infection is the endocervix. The organism produces an edematous cervix that causes a yellow, mucopurulent vaginal discharge. This discharge may be accompanied by spotting at menstrual midcycle or with sexual intercourse. *C. trachomatis* also causes urethritis with dysuria and frequency in women. Bartholin duct involvement also produces purulent discharge.

In males, the chief manifestation is urethritis with dysuria and a clear to mucopurulent discharge. In both sexes, proctitis and pharyngitis may develop with rectal and orogenital contact.

Because there are few or no manifestations, the diagnosis of chlamydial infection is difficult and often missed. Clients tend not to seek medical treatment. Manifestations are often nonspecific and are virtually indistinguishable clinically from those of gonorrhea. For this reason, and because these two infections often coexist, it is recommended that diagnostic tests for both be done when either condition is suspected. Presumptive treatment for *Chlamydia* in clients being treated for gonorrhea is appropriate, particularly when no diagnostic test for *Chlamydia* is performed.

The definitive test for the fast and accurate diagnosis of *Chlamydia* has yet to be developed. The best and most sensitive diagnostic test for chlamydial infections is the tissue culture of cellular material from the urethra, endocervix, or rectum. This test, however, is expensive and is not widely available.

Rapid nonculture detection tests done on urogenital secretions are readily available. These tests include direct fluorescent antibody (DFA) microscopy to detect elementary bodies, and enzyme-linked immunosorbent assay (ELISA) or monoclonal antigen-antibody tests to detect *C. trachomatis* antigens. Although less accurate than a culture, these tests have the advantage of being more convenient, rapid, and less expensive than a culture. For men who refuse to allow the insertion of a cotton applicator 2 to 4 cm into the urethra to obtain an adequate urethral specimen, the ELISA test can be used to detect *C. trachomatis* antigen in the initial 10 to 20 ml of voided urine.

These rapid tests are recommended for the screening of asymptomatic high-risk clients in whom chlamydial infections would otherwise go undetected. Priority groups for testing are high-risk pregnant women, adolescents, and women with multiple sex partners. The Papanicolaou (Pap) smear has no diagnostic value in the diagnosis or screening of chlamydial infection.

Community and Self-Care

■ Medical Management

All sexual contacts within 30 days before diagnosis should be examined and treated. In clinical settings in which testing for chlamydial infection is not available, treatment is often prescribed on the basis of clinical diagnosis only or as co-treatment for gonorrhea.

Doxycycline given orally for 7 days or one dose of azithromycin (Zithromax) is the treatment of choice for chlamydial infection. To increase the absorption and efficacy of the antibiotic, clients should be instructed to take the medications 1 to 2 hours after meals and to avoid iron, dairy products, and antacids. If salpingitis and other serious sequelae are to be prevented, it is imperative that treatment be started early and that the entire course of antibiotics be completed. Antichlamydial therapy is almost always effective. To confirm a cure, a repeat culture should be done 4 to 7 days after treatment whenever possible.

■ Nursing Management of the Medical Client

Clients should be instructed about the sexual mode of transmission of chlamydial infections. The increased risk of infection with multiple sex partners should be stressed. Clients should also be informed of the serious danger of sterility, particularly for the female. Infected clients should avoid all sexual activity (intercourse, oral-genital contact, oral-anal contact, or anal penetration) until cured, and condoms should be used thereafter for prevention of reinfection.

Syphilis

Syphilis (lay terms: *bad blood, lues, pox,* and *syph*) is a systemic, highly infectious disease caused by the delicate motile spirochete *Treponema pallidum* (see Table 86–1). The incubation period varies from 10 to 90 days, averaging 20 to 30 days. Although currently less common than gonorrhea, syphilis can progress to irreversible blindness, mental illness, paralysis, heart disease, and death.

Etiology and Risk Factors

Syphilis became less prevalent after the advent of penicillin, but it has not been eradicated. In fact, the incidence has been rising since about 1960. It is the third most commonly reported communicable disease in the United States. Adolescents, young adults, and homosexual males are at greatest risk.

Pathophysiology

Although *T. pallidum* cannot survive long outside the body, syphilis is highly infectious. Sexual transmission of *T. pallidum* occurs only when the mucocutaneous lesions of primary and secondary syphilis are present. The organism enters the body through intact mucous membranes or abraded skin, almost exclusively by direct sexual contact (acquired syphilis). After entry, the organisms multiply locally and disseminate systemically through the bloodstream and lymphatics. The infection can also be passed transplacentally from an untreated pregnant woman to her fetus during any stage of the disease (congenital syphilis). Rarely, syphilis has been contracted through nonsexual personal contact, accidental inoculation, or blood transfusion from a syphilitic donor.

Clinical Manifestations and Diagnostic Findings

Syphilis is characterized by well-defined sequential stages that occur over a period of years: primary, secondary, latent (early latent and late latent), and late or tertiary. The manifestations vary with each stage.

■ Primary Stage

Primary syphilis has two principal manifestations: the appearance of a chancre and regional lymphadenopathy. Typically, a chancre is an oval ulcer with a raised firm border that does not bleed readily and is painless unless infected.

The chancre develops at the site of inoculation, usually the genitalia, anus, or mouth. Most commonly, a single chancre occurs about 4 weeks after initial infection. Chancres in women are often not noticed. Lymphadenopathy occurs as lymph glands near the chancre become enlarged. Nodes are painless, firm, and discrete. If untreated, a chancre heals spontaneously in 4 to 6 weeks, leaving a thin, atrophic scar.

■ Secondary Stage

If untreated, secondary syphilis develops 6 to 8 weeks after infection. Indications of the second stage include the following:

- *Generalized rash.* Typically a maculopapular and non-pruritic rash appears on the palms of the hands and soles of the feet (few other diseases cause a rash in these locations).
- *Generalized nontender discrete lymphadenopathy*
- *Mucous patches.* Gray, superficial patches occur on the mucous membranes in the mouth and may be accompanied by a sore throat.
- *Condylomata lata.* These are broad-based, flat papules that can usually be easily distinguished from the typical narrow-based, pedunculated growth of condylomata acuminata (genital warts). They may develop in warm, moist body areas—most commonly on the labia or anus or at the corners of the mouth. Condylomata lata are highly contagious.
- *General flulike manifestations.* These include nausea; anorexia; constipation; headache; muscle, joint, and bone pain; and a chronically elevated temperature.
- *Patchy hair loss* from eyebrows and scalp (alopecia).

Secondary stage manifestations usually disappear after 2 to 6 weeks. A latency period then begins.

■ Latent Stage

The latent stage of syphilis typically has no manifestations. Latent syphilis is defined as those periods after infection with *T. pallidum* when clients are seroreactive but show no other evidence of disease. The disease during this stage is noninfectious except via blood transfusion or transplacental spread. The disease is not transmitted by sexual contact during the latent phase unless a rare recurrence of the secondary syphilitic mucocutaneous skin lesions takes place during early latent syphilis. Serologic tests for syphilis in all prospective blood donors is essential. Latent stage syphilis usually occurs about 2 years after the primary lesion and can last as long as 50 years. In about two thirds of infected clients, the disease remains in this stage, without causing further problems.

■ Tertiary Stage

If untreated, in 1 to 35 years about a third of infected clients develop devastating, irreversible complications, such as chronic bone and joint inflammation, cardiovascular problems (e.g., valvular involvement, aneurysms), granulomatous lesions (gummas) on any part of the body, and central nervous system problems (including mental illness, slurred speech, ataxic gait, paralysis, judgment loss, and senility). This late, or tertiary, stage is not infectious, but it may be terminal if untreated. (Chapter 30 discusses central nervous system manifestations.)

The diagnosis of syphilis is based on health assessment and various laboratory studies. The laboratory tests are both direct and indirect. A direct test identifies the causative organism. Indirect tests merely identify antibodies of the causative agent. *T. pallidum* cannot be cultured.

Primary or secondary stage lesions can be scraped and the causative organism identified directly with a dark-field microscope technique or silver salt staining. Dark-field examination must be done by an expert, because other spirochetes that closely resemble *T. pallidum* are present in oral and genital mucosa. This test confirms a diagnosis of syphilis in the primary stage (when other tests are generally negative) and secondary stage.

Serologic tests for syphilis are indirect tests that detect antibodies. These antibodies are not present in the serum until 4 weeks *after* the appearance of the chancre. Such tests include the VDRL (Venereal Disease Research Laboratory) and fluorescent treponemal antibody absorption (FTA-ABS) tests.

The VDRL test for nonspecific antibodies is the most commonly used screening test for syphilis. It is negative in the early primary stage before antibodies to *T. pallidum* are formed and are present in the circulation. It may be falsely positive if performed during the early stages of several common viral illnesses (e.g., mumps, measles, hepatitis, chickenpox, infectious mononucleosis). Results are given as nonreactive, borderline, weakly reactive, or reactive. Reactive and weakly reactive results are considered to be positive.

The FTA-ABS serologic test is more specific in that it measures antibodies specific to *T. pallidum.* It is used when the VDRL is positive, but the diagnosis of syphilis is still not certain. A false-positive result is possible in clients with infectious mononucleosis and lupus erythematosus. The FTA-ABS test usually becomes positive 3 to 4 weeks after the infection. Once positive, treponemal antibody tests usually remain positive for life, regardless of treatment or cure. In late neurosyphilis, cerebrospinal fluid may be examined for characteristic findings.

Syphilis often coexists with other infections. The CDC recommends that all clients with syphilis be counseled on the risks of *human immunodeficiency virus* (HIV) infection (AIDS) and be encouraged to undergo HIV testing. Clients with late manifestations of AIDS may fail to have positive serology test results.

Community and Self-Care

■ Medical Management

Parenteral penicillin remains the treatment of choice for all stages of syphilis. All stages of syphilis respond to penicillin therapy, but the structural changes present in late syphilis are irreversible despite successful treatment. The dosage schedule and length of therapy are determined by the stage of the disease and current guidelines for treatment. For primary, secondary, and early latent syphilis, the treatment of choice is benzathine penicillin G, given intramuscularly in one dose. For nonpregnant clients who are allergic to penicillin, oral doxycycline or tetracycline for 2 weeks may be given, but they are not as effective as penicillin.

Treatment failure can occur with any given regimen. Compliance is often a problem. Clients should be reexamined clinically and serologically at 3 and 6 months following treatment. No definitive criteria for cure exist. With successful treatment, ideally, no evidence of disease should be present, and serial serologic test titers should decline.

■ Nursing Management of the Medical Client

A client with syphilis needs healthcare information and psychosocial support. Nurses must provide clients with accurate information about transmission, early detection, treatment, follow-up, reinfection, sequelae, proper hygiene, and safe sexual habits. The nurse should individualize health teaching to meet the client's particular needs and psychosocial situation. A diagnosis of syphilis can be frightening and difficult to accept.

Clients with primary or secondary syphilis should abstain from sexual contact for at least 1 month after treatment. All sexual contacts must be identified and treated. Most practitioners treat contacts as if they have primary syphilis, whether or not infection is evident. When an infected, untreated woman has been in the asymptomatic latent stage for at least a year, she is not considered infectious unless she becomes pregnant. Then she can infect her fetus. Adequate treatment is curative, but reinfection is possible and can be detected by clinical reexaminations and monitoring serologic titers. An infection does not confer lasting immunity.

Genital Herpes

Genital herpes is a recurrent, systemic viral infection (see Table 86–1). Although recognized for centuries, genital herpes has received renewed attention because of its epidemic incidence. Now one of the most common STDs, it is the most common cause of genital ulceration. Its peak incidence occurs in the adolescent and young adult.

Etiology and Risk Factors

Caused by herpes simplex virus (HSV) type II, the infection is closely related to other herpes infections such as the classic cold sore caused by HSV type I. Type I herpes is mainly nongenital, occurring above the waist (often on the lips or nose). Type II herpes occurs primarily below the waist as a sexually transmitted genital infection. It is, however, possible for HSV type I to cause genital infections and for HSV type II to cause oral lesions.

Pathophysiology

The HSV organism is present in the exudate of the lesion. The disease can be transmitted while a lesion is present and for 10 days after a lesion has healed. Genital herpes is usually transmitted by direct contact with the exudate during sexual activity, but transmission is possible by fomites, such as towels used by an infected person. Many cases of genital herpes are acquired from persons who do not know they have an infection or who are asymptomatic at the time of sexual contact. In addition, newborns can be infected during vaginal delivery when active genital lesions are present. Birth by cesarean section prevents infection of the fetus under these conditions.

Clinical Manifestations and Diagnostic Findings

Manifestations of genital herpes usually occur 3 to 7 days after contact. Initially, a burning sensation or paresthesia is noted at the site of inoculation. Next, numerous small vesicles with an erythematous border form painful, shallow ulcers that then crust and heal with a scar in about 2 to 4 weeks.

The major problem of HSV infections is recurrence. About half to three quarters of infected clients have a recurrent infection within 1 year of the first episode. The herpes virus is believed to lie dormant in the body, probably in the trigeminal ganglion (HSV-I) and sacral ganglion (HSV-II), until it is activated and another episode of genital herpes, with the characteristic lesion, occurs. Certain situations such as stress, infection, trauma, menses, or sexual activity seem to trigger recurrent episodes.

Characteristically, recurrent genital herpes causes local, but not systemic manifestations. Prodromal sensations of burning or paresthesias may be experienced before the vesicles erupt. The vesicles tend to reappear at the site of previous infection, but recurrent infections can involve new sites. Manifestations are similar to those associated with primary infection, although they are usually less severe. Vesicles rupture in 24 to 48 hours, and the syndrome generally lasts 7 to 10 days.

Potential complications of HSV infections include aseptic meningitis and transverse myelitis. Women are at risk for spontaneous abortions, and some evidence has suggested that HSV-II predisposes to carcinoma of the cervix.

A diagnosis of genital herpes can often be made by the presence of vesicles. The diagnosis is confirmed by a viral culture, direct immunofluorescence staining, or antigen detection testing of the vesicular exudate. A Pap smear can be done in women. The presence in the Pap smear of multinucleated giant cells, with or without inclusion bodies, is characteristic of a herpes infection.

Community and Self-Care

■ Medical Management

Palliative measures include keeping the involved area clean and dry, wearing loose-fitting nonsynthetic undergarments, and using sitz baths, cool applications, and analgesic medications, such as aspirin, for pain relief.

Genital herpes is a chronic disease. It has no cure. The recommended treatment for an acute primary or recurrent infection is acyclovir (Zovirax), an antiviral agent taken orally for 5 to 10 days. For clients who experience frequent recurrences (six or more episodes in 1 year) daily suppressive therapy is used. Acyclovir taken daily for 4 months to 3 years has been shown to prevent or reduce the frequency and/or severity of recurrence in the vast majority of clients. After 1 year, the acyclovir should be discontinued to assess the need for continued suppressive therapy. If genital herpes recurs, the daily therapy is resumed.

■ Nursing Management of the Medical Client

When the vesicles of active genital herpes rupture, they release a highly contagious exudate. Therefore, clients as well as healthcare personnel must observe strict medical asepsis. For avoiding autoinoculation from the genital area to other body sites, clients should be advised to wash their hands thoroughly after any contact with the herpetic lesions. HSV infections of the eye are particularly serious. Infected clients should have separate towels and other personal items and should be instructed to avoid touching their eyes. Sexual contact should be avoided during initial and recurrent infections. The use of condoms during latent periods is encouraged because of the possible risk of transmission even when manifestations are not present. Women should be told to have annual pelvic examinations and Pap smears because of the association of HSV with cervical cancer.

Many clients find that coping with genital herpes is emotionally difficult. Tremendous psychosocial stress may develop because the infection cannot be cured and recurrence cannot be predicted. Its reappearance can significantly affect sexual activity. The pain caused by these lesions is especially problematic. Psychosocial support includes providing clients with accurate information about the infection. Support groups may be helpful in dealing with feelings of anger, guilt, and shame that are common in these clients.

Genital Warts (Condylomata Acuminata)

Genital warts, the fourth most common STD, are venereal warts caused by the human papillomavirus (HPV); they are usually transmitted by sexual contact (see Table 86–1).

Genital warts are benign growths that typically occur in multiple, painless clusters on the vulva, vagina, cervix, perineum, anorectal area, urethral meatus, or glans penis 1 to 2 months after exposure. Oral, pharyngeal, and laryngeal lesions can also occur. HPV can cause laryngeal papillomatosis in infants born to mothers with vaginal warts.

Diagnosis is typically made by observation of the warts. Subclinical warts can be identified by Pap smear and colposcopy of the cervix and vagina. Biopsy of lesions may be done to differentiate venereal warts from carcinoma or condylomata lata lesions of the secondary stage of syphilis.

■ Medical Management

There is no cure for genital warts. A wide variety of chemical, mechanical, and ablative techniques are used for visible lesions, but no specific antiviral therapy for the papillomavirus is available. Treatment varies somewhat by site and severity and is also guided by client preference. Treatment is more successful if the warts are small and have been present for less than a year.

Topical Therapy

The most common pharmacologic treatment is podophyllin in compound tincture of benzoin or trichloroacetic acid (TCA) applied topically to the warts *only*. Topical treatments are repeated every week until all of the lesions have disappeared and the skin is healed. Podophyllin is contraindicated during pregnancy because of its abortifacient properties.

Topical podofilox is the only agent approved for self-application by clients at home. For safe application the client must be able to see and reach the warts easily. Podofilox, like podophyllin, is contraindicated during pregnancy because of potential myelotoxic and neurotoxic effects. If warts persist after topical keratolytic treatment

is completed, other modes of therapy should be considered.

Other Treatments

Warts can also be treated with cryotherapy with liquid nitrogen or a cryoprobe. For extensive warts, carbon dioxide lasers, electrocautery, and simple surgical excision can be used. The antiviral drug interferon has also been used, but this therapy is expensive and is associated with a high frequency of adverse side effects. Again, remember that genital warts are not cured, and recurrence is very common.

■ Nursing Management of the Medical Client

The nurse needs to inform clients with genital warts that no cure exists. Treatment ameliorates the manifestations of the warts, but no treatment has been shown to eradicate the papillomavirus. Clients must be warned that they are at increased risk for genital malignancy. HPV infections are strongly associated with cancer of the cervix and vulva in women and squamous cell carcinoma of the penis in men. All women with genital warts should have a Pap smear at *least* every year and, when indicated, cervical colposcopy and biopsy. The detection and treatment of subclinical HPV infection in men may be important for the prevention of genital carcinoma in women.

Acquired Immunodeficiency Syndrome

AIDS is a viral STD that has reached worldwide epidemic proportions in the past decade. Unknown until 1981, AIDS has emerged as a major STD.

HIV infection has had an impact on the transmission of STDs, and vice versa. People with AIDS are more susceptible to other STDs. These coexistent STDs require more aggressive therapy and tend to recur. Conversely, people infected with an STD, especially those with genital ulcerations (e.g., syphilis, herpes, and chancroid), are more susceptible to AIDS. On the positive side, national campaigns to prevent and control the transmission of the HIV have had a beneficial effect on the incidence of some STDs (e.g., reduced incidence of hepatitis B in the homosexual population).

AIDS is discussed in detail in Chapter 27.

Trichomoniasis

Trichomoniasis is a protozoal infection causing vulvovaginitis. It is one of the three most common types of vaginitis (i.e., trichonomiasis, bacterial vaginitis, and vulvovaginal candidiasis). Although not life-threatening, trichomoniasis has a very high incidence worldwide and remains a major health problem.

Trichomoniasis is caused by the anaerobic, flagellated, parasitic protozoan *Trichomonas vaginalis*. The organism is almost always transmitted sexually. *T. vaginalis* prefers an alkaline environment (pH 6 to 7), and alterations in the vaginal flora make a woman more susceptible to infection. Trichomoniasis can be very resistant to treatment. Recurrence is very common.

Manifestations may be minor, especially in an infected male. In a female, manifestations include a copious, malodorous, yellow-green vaginal discharge. This is irritating to the vulva and causes severe itching, burning, and excoriation and maceration of the vulvar tissues. Occasionally, the cervix is covered with punctate hemorrhages ("strawberry cervix"). The vaginal mucosa appears reddened and slightly edematous. Some women experience dyspareunia (pain during vaginal sexual activity). The organism does not affect the uterus or fallopian tubes.

If trichomoniasis extends to the urethra, urinary frequency and burning with urination may occur. This is the most common manifestation in a male. Anal involvement may also occur, either asymptomatically or with a slight discharge. Bladder and anal involvement are more common when the infection has become chronic.

A diagnosis of trichomoniasis can be established immediately in the healthcare facility by obtaining a fresh, warm, wet mount and identifying the highly motile trichomonad under the microscope. Cultures can be obtained to establish the diagnosis, but they are rarely necessary.

A wet mount is obtained by placing a drop of vaginal exudate on a glass slide, mixing in a drop of saline, and covering it with a cover slide. The vaginal speculum used to obtain the exudate must be inserted without lubrication to avoid destroying the organism. If possible, instruct the woman not to douche before the vaginal examination. Reassurance and a calm attitude can help allay the woman's anxiety and minimize any discomfort with the examination.

■ Medical Management

The preferred treatment for trichomoniasis is a single oral dose of metronidazole (Flagyl). Trichomoniasis is almost always transmitted sexually from one partner to another, which makes simultaneous treatment of all partners absolutely necessary for a cure. Advise clients taking metronidazole not to drink alcoholic beverages so that side effects of nausea, vomiting, and headaches are prevented. Flagyl should not be taken during the first trimester of pregnancy because it may adversely affect fetal development. *T. vaginalis* does not affect the fetus.

Single-dose metronidazole therapy is usually curative, but recurrence is common. Clients should be instructed to seek prompt treatment if manifestations return. Metronidazole may be given in a 7-day regimen for recurrent infection.

■ Nursing Management of the Medical Client

Clients with trichomoniasis should refrain from sexual intercourse while the infection remains active. If this is not possible, use of a male or female condom is recommended until a cure is effected. Emphasize to the client the importance of good perineal hygiene. Treatment for a recurrent infection should be continued through the wom-

an's menstrual period, because the vagina is more alkaline during this time of the cycle, and a flare-up is likely to occur. After therapy has been completed, clients are evaluated and treated again if necessary.

Bacterial Vaginosis

Bacterial vaginosis, the term now used for what was once called nonspecific or *Gardnerella* vaginitis, is a very common condition in adult women.

Like vulvovaginal *Candida* (yeast) infections, the bacteria causing bacterial vaginosis are found in the normal vagina. The infection is thought to be caused by the overgrowth of a number of different organisms, including *Gardnerella vaginalis* and vaginal anaerobes, which occurs when the normal flora and pH of the vagina are altered.

The vulvovaginitis produced by bacterial vaginosis is mild or asymptomatic. The main manifestation is a mild to moderate malodorous vaginal discharge. The discharge is usually thin, watery, grayish white in color and tends to adhere to the vaginal wall. The malodor is described as "fishy," and it is often more noticeable after sexual intercourse. Manifestations are almost always confined to the vulvovaginal area. Mild vaginal burning and irritation may occur, but redness and pruritus are not common.

Bacterial vaginosis is evaluated mainly by physical examination of the vagina, microscopic examination of the discharge, and determination of its pH. Diagnosis is made on the basis of the presence of at least three of four of the following manifestations:

● Homogeneous gray or white discharge that is adherent to the vaginal wall
● Vaginal fluid pH of >4.5 (normal pH, 4.0 to 4.5)
● Positive "whiff" test—fishy odor elicited when potassium hydroxide (KOH) is added to the vaginal fluid
● Clue cells (desquamated vaginal epithelial cells characteristically stippled by the adherence of coccobacilli to their surfaces) seen either on saline wet mount or on Gram stain of vaginal fluid

■ Medical Management

The recommended treatment for bacterial vaginosis in nonpregnant women is metronidazole (Flagyl), given orally for 7 days. Single-dose regimens can be used to improve compliance, but they are less effective than the 7-day regimen.

■ Nursing Management of the Medical Client

Clients receiving metronidazole (Flagyl) should be cautioned to abstain from alcohol consumption during and for 24 hours after the medication is taken to prevent intense nausea, vomiting, and headache. Bacterial vaginosis is not necessarily transmitted sexually, though its occurrence is associated with sexual activity. Treatment of male partners is recommended only with recurrent or resistant infection. Even so, treatment of the male has not been shown to be highly beneficial for either partner. Clients are advised to avoid sexual intercourse during treatment, and condom use is recommended to prevent recurrence, which is common.

Vulvovaginal Candidiasis

Though occasionally transmitted sexually, candidiasis (yeast infection) of the vagina and vulva is generally not considered an STD. (See Chapter 84 for discussion of vulvovaginal candidiasis.)

Chancroid

Chancroid is a highly contagious infection caused by the gram-negative *Hemophilus ducreyi* bacillus. The initial papules/pustules produce multiple, painful, irregular, and deep genital ulcers, often accompanied by tender inguinal lymphadenopathy. Although chancroid is more common in the tropics, the incidence is endemic in many areas of the United States. Chancroid is well established as a co-factor for HIV transmission. There is a high rate of HIV infection in clients with chancroid in the United States and other countries.

Definitive diagnosis requires the culture of *H. ducreyi*. However, it is difficult to isolate the organism, and culture of *H. ducreyi* is not offered by all laboratories. Thus, a probable diagnosis may be made if the client has one or more painful genital ulcers without clinical and/or serologic evidence of syphilis or genital herpes. Sexual contacts within 10 days of the onset of manifestations should be examined and treated. Infected clients should also be tested for HIV and syphilis.

Recommended treatment is oral azithromycin or ceftriaxone given intramuscularly in a single dose, or erythromycin given orally for 7 days.

Lymphogranuloma Venereum

Lymphogranuloma venereum is a systemic infection common in the tropics but rare in the United States. The infection is caused by certain strains of *C. trachomatis*. The primary lesion is a small, painless papule on the glans penis or the vaginal mucosa that heals spontaneously and may go unnoticed.

Markedly tender, enlarged, and inflamed inguinal lymph nodes (buboes), which are usually unilateral and appear 2 to 6 weeks after the primary lesion, are the most common clinical manifestations. Eventually, draining ulcerations, scarring, lymphatic obstruction, and marked external genital deformity may occur. Rectal fibrosis and strictures are late sequelae.

Definitive diagnosis is made on the basis of a culture positive for *C. trachomatis.* Recommended therapy is doxycycline, given orally for 21 days. Orally administered erythromycin or sulfisoxazole (Gantrisin) are alternatives.

Granuloma Inguinale

Granuloma inguinale (donovanosis), a chronic infection that occurs most often in tropical regions and rarely in the United States, is caused by the small gram-negative bacillus *Calymmatobacterium granulomatis*.

Granuloma inguinale is characterized by genital and perianal papular lesions. These become painless, gradually enlarging, ulcerating granulomatous lesions that cause tissue destruction that is difficult to differentiate from cancer. Diagnosis is made by microscopic identification of Donovan bodies (inclusion bodies of the causative organism) in a smear taken from edge scrapings of the lesion.

Granuloma inguinale is treated with antibiotics such as tetracycline or streptomycin. Penicillin is not effective.

Hepatitis B

Hepatitis B is a reportable STD. Sexual contact is the most frequently reported mode of transmission of the hepatitis B virus (HBV) although bloodborne and perinatal transmission also can occur. Clients at high risk for sexually transmitted hepatitis B are heterosexuals with multiple partners, sex partners of intravenous drug users, and homosexual males. Sexually transmitted hepatitis B has decreased dramatically in the homosexual population. This is thought to be most likely the result of the modification of high-risk sexual behavior in this group to prevent AIDS. This is the only STD for which there is a vaccine.

See Chapter 65 for further discussion of hepatitis B.

Pediculosis Pubis and Scabies

Cutaneous infestation with pubic lice (pediculosis pubis) or mites (scabies) results either from close physical contact or contact with contaminated objects, such as linens and clothing. Because sexual transmission is possible, these conditions are included in STDs.

For further discussion of these ectoparasitic infections, see Chapter 78.

Sexually Transmitted Enteric Infections

Dysenteries and hepatitis caused by enteric pathogens are typically acquired from food or water contaminated with fecal matter. Since the mid-1970s, it has been recognized that these pathogens can also be transmitted by oral and anal sexual contact. Sexually transmitted enteric infections include shigellosis, salmonellosis, amebiasis, giardiasis, and hepatitis A. Homosexual males are at highest risk for these infections.

See Chapter 62 for discussion of dysentery, and Chapter 65 for discussion of hepatitis A.

Conclusions

Sexually transmitted diseases are more prevalent now than ever before. This phenomenon is attributable to many factors. The improper and indiscriminate use of antibiotics has produced a number of resistant organisms. Sexual activity, especially among adolescents and young adults, has increased. Many STDs are asymptomatic and go undetected. The economic cost of STDs increases as the number of cases increases. Nurses have an ever-increasing responsibility and role in the prevention, early detection, and treatment of these diseases.

Thinking Critically

1. A 20-year-old unmarried man comes to a walk-in STD clinic with a purulent urethral discharge. His diagnosis is uncomplicated gonorrhea. The client has no known allergies. He is sexually active with multiple partners. He gives a temporary address. What are the priorities of care? What are the priority interventions?

Factors to Consider: In planning for this client, consider the fact that gonorrhea is the most commonly reported STD in the United States. What impact would the client's status as a walk-in client have on your planning? What impact would the fact that the client gave only a temporary address have on your planning? What diseases are likely to coexist with gonorrhea?

2. Your client is a 65-year-old widowed woman who comes for treatment of acute, symptomatic genital herpes. Her sexual contact is a male friend who told her when their sexual relationship began a few months ago that he had a history of genital herpes, but that because he had no active lesions, there was no risk of her becoming infected. She is humiliated at having developed herpes, and tells you she feels dirty and contaminated. What are the goals of care? What interventions might be used?

Factors to Consider: How accurate is the client's knowledge about the transmission of genital herpes? What are the client's psychosocial needs?

3. A 25-year-old monogamous woman seeks outpatient treatment for the irritating, malodorous vaginal discharge of trichomoniasis. She has had trichomoniasis before, and metronidazole (Flagyl) was prescribed. What interventions should the care of this client include?

Factors to Consider: Knowing that metronidazole is usually curative, consider what might have caused the client's recurrence.

Bibliography

1. American College of Obstetricians and Gynecologists. *ACOG guide to preconception care* (1990). Washington, DC: Author.
2. Andreoli, T. E., et al. (1993). *Cecil essentials of medicine.* Philadelphia: W. B. Saunders.
3. Benenson, A. S. (Ed.). (1990). *Control of communicable diseases in man.* Washington, DC: American Public Health Association.
4. Brodman, M., et al. (1993). *Straight talk about sexually transmitted diseases.* New York: Facts on File.
5. Carlin, F. (1994). STD–Sexually transmitted diseases (non HIV). *SCCMA-The Bulletin,* March-April, p. 7.
6. Cates, W., Jr., et al. (1990). Sexually transmitted diseases: Overview of the situation. *Primary Care, 17,* 1.
7. Centers for Disease Control and Prevention (1993). *Division of STD/HIV prevention 1992 annual report.* Atlanta: US Dept of Health and Human Services.
8. Centers for Disease Control and Prevention (1990). Management of genital infection caused by human papillomavirus. *Reviews of Infectious Diseases, 12,* S621-632.
9. Centers for Disease Control and Prevention (1991). *Sexually transmitted diseases, clinical practice guidelines.* Atlanta: US Dept of Health and Human Services.
10. Centers for Disease Control and Prevention (1993). 1993 Sexually transmitted diseases treatment guidelines. *Morbidity and Mortality Weekly Report, 42* (No. RR–14).
11. Center for Disease Control and Prevention (1993). Surveillance for gonorrhea and primary and secondary syphilis among adolescents, United States 1981–1991. *Morbidity and Mortality Weekly Report, 42*(No. RR12), 1.
12. Centers for Disease Control and Prevention (1993). Update: Barrier protection against HIV infection and other sexually transmitted diseases. *Morbidity and Mortality Weekly Report, 42,* 589.
13. Condom availability for adolescents. (1995). *ACOG Committee Opinion, 154,* 1.
14. Custodio, D. E., et al. (1991). Sexually transmitted diseases. *Topics in Emergency Medicine, 13,* 66.
15. Durbin, M., et al. (1993). Multiple sex partners among junior high school students. *Journal of Adolescent Health, 14,* 202.
16. Featherston, W. E. (1990). Sexual identity and practices relating to the spread of sexually transmitted diseases. *Primary Care, 17,* 29.
17. Genital human papillomavirus infections. (1994). *ACOG Technical Bulletin, No. 193.*
18. Gonorrhea and chlamydial infections. (1994). *ACOG Technical Bulletin, No. 190.*
19. Grimes, D. (1991). *Infectious diseases.* St Louis: Mosby–Year Book.
20. Holmes, K. K., et al. (Eds.) (1990). *Sexually transmitted diseases.* New York: McGraw-Hill.
21. Hook, E. W., et al. (1992). Acquired syphilis in adults. *New England Journal of Medicine, 326,* 1060.
22. McIlhaney, J. S. (1991) *Safe sex.* Grand Rapids, MI: Baker Book House.
23. Melvin, S. Y. (1990). Syphilis: Resurgence of an old disease. *Primary Care, 17,* 47.
24. Nettina, S. L., et al. (1990). Diagnosis and management of sexually transmitted genital lesions. *Nurse Practitioner, 15,* 34.
25. Noller, K. L. (1992). Talking to the HPV-infected patient. *OB/GYN Clinical Alert, 9,* 39.
26. Nourse, A. E. (1992). *Sexually transmitted diseases.* New York: Franklin Watts.
27. Pagana, K. D., et al. (1992). *Mosby's diagnostic and laboratory test reference.* St. Louis: Mosby–Year Book.
28. *1995 Physicians General Rx.* (1995). Riverside, CT: Denniston Publishing Inc.
29. Progress toward achieving the 1990 objectives for the nation for sexually transmitted diseases. (1990) *Morbidity and Mortality Weekly Report, 39,* 53.
30. Talashek, M. L., et al. (1990). Sexually transmitted diseases in the elderly: Issues and recommendations. *Journal of Gerontological Nursing, 16,* 33.

Multisystem Disorders

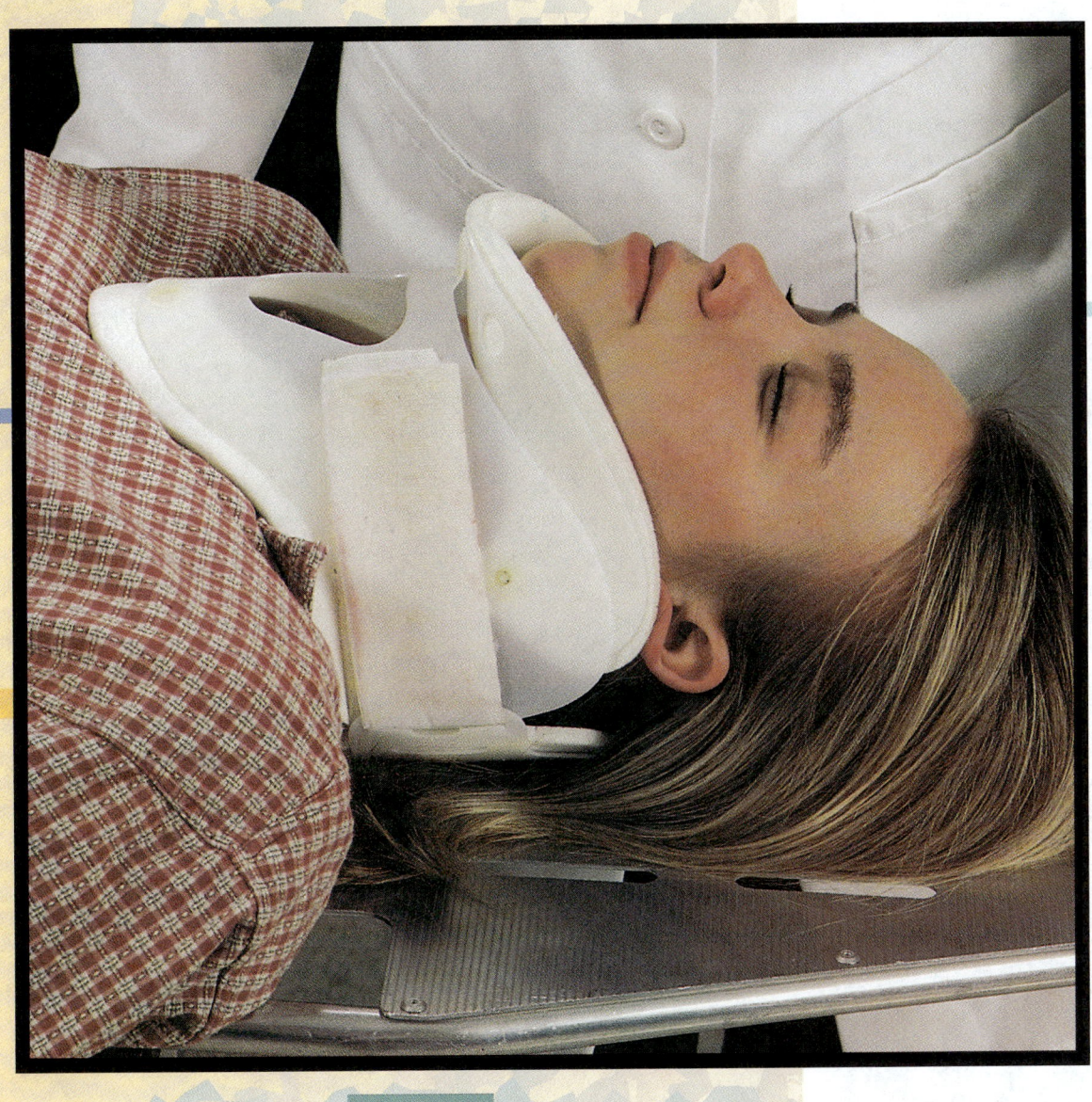

Substance Abuse

Linda Carman Copel

As the client passed through the hospital door, it was the beginning—the first step of many on the journey back from the world of drugs and alcohol. No longer need this person be entangled in the cycle of pain, ineffective coping with addictive substances, more pain, and more drugs. The client, struggling to think clearly, had the following thoughts: "I must be dying. My body hurts. Where am I? What is going on here? How did this happen? I can't stand it. What are they doing to me? They can't help me. I can't help me. No one can help me. My life has always been a mess. There is nothing I can do."

Clients with psychoactive substance abuse disorders struggle with an inability to problem-solve. They are unable to use adaptive behaviors to handle life stresses, traumas, and demands. Ineffective coping, defensive coping, denial, poor nutrition, risk of injury, and a risk for infection are a few of the nursing diagnoses specific to the assessment data obtained from these clients.

Nurses are challenged by the myriad of physical and emotional health problems faced by clients with addiction. Their health histories and at-risk behaviors culminate in problems ranging from liver and cardiovascular disease to depression and the possibility of being human immunodeficiency virus (HIV)–positive. The client's physical condition is further compromised by nutritional deficits and fluid and electrolyte imbalances. In addition, many clients suffer from injuries, either self-inflicted trauma or violence at the hands of others. Often, multiple injuries in various stages of healing are evident upon examination. Underlying the physical problems are the emotional wounds from both past and present life situations. Without effective coping skills clients have a strong tendency to repeat their self-destructive pattern of behavior over and over. The inability to perceive reality accurately and develop and maintain supportive relationships hinders successful life-style changes. Accelerating bouts of depression and feelings of powerlessness continue, perpetuating a sense of incompetence. A pervasive sense of failure overwhelms many of the clients.

Studies show consistently that substance-abusing clients need both medical and psychiatric nursing care to achieve their highest level of functioning and to maintain sobriety. Nurses have the challenge of not only dealing with the addicted client's many physiologic problems but also with the effects and withdrawal symptoms of the drugs involved. Even as you seek to assess and diagnose the physiologic effects of abused substances, clients typically offer defensiveness and denial. These clients' lack of responsibility for their personal behavior and a constant blaming and manipulating of others are typical characteristics that require your attention and intervention along with the physiologic issues. As much as any client population, this one challenges the entire healthcare team to provide holistic treatment for physical, emotional, and spiritual needs.

Frameworks for Explaining Addictive Behaviors

Over the last 100 years, clinicians and researchers have attempted to develop and refine the knowledge base on substance-abusing individuals. Early studies of alcoholism noted generational patterns of alcoholism in families. Based on this observation, the theory arose that alcoholism may have a genetic component. However, there is no evidence to support this supposition with other commonly abused drugs.[15,36,37,41,52]

Various explanations of the causes of substance abuse have focused on three conceptual frameworks:

1. Biologic
2. Psychological
3. Sociocultural

However, there is no one identifiable cause of substance use. Rather, typically, a combination of factors coalesce to produce drug use patterns. A person may be at risk of developing substance abuse because of a complex combination of biologic, psychological, and sociocultural varia-

---

This chapter incorporates material written for the fourth edition by Carol Ren Kneisl.

bles. All aspects of the client's background must be considered when initiating treatment. In addition to what the client brings to the treatment setting, the theoretical approach the team uses to view the underlying dynamics of substance abuse will influence the process of recovery.

Biologic Framework

The biologic theory, or disease concept, of substance abuse views addiction as a physiologic condition that can be diagnosed and treated. The emphasis is on physiologic causes, such as genetic predisposition, defects in metabolism, neurobiologic abnormalities, or abnormal levels of chemicals in the body.[35] Historically, studies attempting to link genetic transmission of alcoholism have been unable to find a target gene.

Present research focuses on examining the inherited biochemical abnormalities that may predispose an individual to developing alcoholism.[4] It is now believed that alcohol dependence is a combination of interwoven social and psychological variables in people who are physiologically vulnerable.[33] For example, people of East Asian ancestry tend to experience a physical reaction to alcohol characterized by tachycardia, a sensation of warmth and flushing, and generalized discomfort. The response is believed to be related to the lack of activation of the enzyme aldehyde dehydrogenase, resulting in the accumulation of acetaldehyde, a toxic product of alcohol metabolism.[4,49] This physiology may be the reason that Asian-Americans tend to have the lowest rate of alcohol consumption and associated substance use problems compared to other racial groups.[49] Hence, an examination of biologic differences associated with the use of alcohol warrants continued investigation.

Psychological Framework

Psychological theories attempt to explain the variables that may predispose an individual to substance use. According to the psychoanalytic model, the person is viewed as being fixated at the oral stage of development, seeking gratification of needs through behaviors such as drinking. With the psychodynamic approach, a person experiences both interpersonal and intrapersonal difficulties which provide the foundation for the addiction.

Behavioral theories regard addiction as a learned behavior that can be unlearned in a manner similar to changing negative habits or dysfunctional behaviors. A family systems approach emphasizes that relationships, roles, and unhealthy communication patterns among family members contribute to addictive behaviors; this dysfunctional life-style is transmitted to future generations.[11]

For years researchers and clinicians have sought without success to discover an addictive personality type. Some common characteristics noted in clients who abuse substances are low self-esteem, low frustration tolerance, inability to cope with physical and emotional pain, depression, lack of healthy relationships, and involvement in high-risk behaviors. Proponents of the psychological theories believe that individuals engage in substance use in an attempt to feel better about themselves and to meet their emotional needs. Thus, the use of a psychoactive substance becomes reinforced and eventually evolves into an addiction.

Sociocultural Framework

The sociocultural theories view substance use from the perspective of cultural and social norms within various groups in society. The issue of whether to use drugs, what type of drugs to use, and how and when to use them are determined by factors in a person's background. Such factors may include values, belief systems, spiritual orientation, ethnicity, sex, family standards, or the contemporary social environment. The relationships between any or all of these variables can contribute to a person's susceptibility to drug use and potential for addiction treatment and ongoing recovery.

Definitions and Terminology of Substance Abuse

According to the *Diagnostic and Statistical Manual of Mental Disorders (DSM-IV)*,[2] the substance-related disorders comprise the range of substance use from taking a drug of abuse, to the adverse effects of any medication, to exposure to toxic substances. The DSM-IV lists 11 types of substances commonly abused: alcohol, amphetamines, caffeine, cannabis, cocaine, hallucinogens, inhalants, nicotine, opioids, phencyclidine (PCP), and the group "sedatives, hypnotics, or anxiolytics."[2] In addition, it is appropriate to include polysubstance dependence and other substance-related disorders, particularly toxins or prescribed and over-the-counter medications.[2]

To understand and assess substance abuse it is essential to become familiar with the associated terminology. Table 87–1 lists and defines these substance abuse terms. In working with clients who are actively using substances, the nurse must also have knowledge about the types of drugs commonly used, the major routes of administration, and the effects. Drug effects are listed in Table 87–2, in order from the least severe to the most severe clinical manifestations. The order and severity of manifestations are influenced by the size of the dose and the length of time the drug has been used.

General Assessment for Substance Abuse

The purposes of a drug and alcohol assessment are to (1) determine if substance abuse exists, (2) evaluate the relationship between substance abuse and other healthcare problems, and (3) implement effective health promotion and health restoration interventions. All clients must be assessed for the use and misuse of chemical substances. Clients who struggle with addiction are found at all stages of life and therefore in all clinical specialties. It is a common occurance for a client who abuses drugs to be hospitalized for an injury, illness, or surgical procedure. The nurse-generalist must identify clients with actual or

Table 87-1. Substance Abuse Terms and Their Definitions

Term	Definition
Psychoactive substance	A substance that affects a person's mood or behavior
Substance abuse	Continued use of a psychoactive substance despite the occurrence of physical, psychological, social, or occupational problems
Substance dependence	A range of physiologic, behavioral, and cognitive symptoms indicating that a person persists in using the substance, ignoring serious substance-related problems
Physiologic dependence	The body's physical adaptation to a drug, whereby withdrawal symptoms will occur if the drug is not used
Psychological dependence	The emotional need or craving for a drug either for its effect or to prevent the occurrence of withdrawal symptoms
Addiction	A compulsion, loss of control, and progressive pattern of drug use, characterized by behavioral changes, impaired thinking, unkept promises to stop usage, obsession with the drug, neglect of personal needs, decreased tolerance, and physiologic deterioration
Polysubstance abuse	Concurrent use of multiple drugs
Intoxication	An altered physiologic state resulting from the use of a psychoactive drug
Overdose	Accidental or deliberate consumption of a drug in a dose larger than is ordinarily used, resulting in serious toxic reaction or death
Tolerance	State resulting from metabolic changes in cell functions, whereby the tissue reaction to a drug declines and the person needs to take increasing amounts to achieve the same effect
Cross-tolerance	State whereby the effect of a drug is decreased and greater amounts are required to achieve the desired effect because the person has become tolerant to a similar drug
Predisposition	Any factor that increases the likelihood of an event occurring
Potentiation	The ability of one drug to increase the activity of another drug when taken at the same time
Drug misuse	Any use of a drug that deviates from medical or socially acceptable use
Dual diagnosis	The coexistence of a major psychiatric illness and a psychoactive substance abuse disorder
Blackout	An acute situation in which a person experiences a period of memory loss for activities as a direct result of using drugs or alcohol
Withdrawal	Discontinuation of a substance by a person who is dependent on it
Detoxification	The process of withdrawing a person from an addictive substance in a safe manner
Toxic dose	The amount of a drug that produces a poisonous effect
Recidivism	The tendency to relapse into a former pattern of substance use and associated behaviors
Recovery	Return to a normal state of health whereby the person does not engage in problematic behavior, and continues to meet life's challenges and personal goals
Sobriety	Complete abstinence from drugs while developing a satisfactory life-style
Abstinence	Voluntarily refraining from activities or use of substances that cause problems in the physiologic, psychological, social, intellectual, and spiritual arenas of a person's life

Table 87–2. Characteristic Effects of Abuse of Major Substances

Drug Classification and Street Names	Route of Administration	Effects*
Alcohol	Oral	Relaxation and sedation Decreased inhibition Lack of coordination Unsteady gait Slurred speech Nausea and vomiting Transient visual, tactile, or auditory hallucinations Anxiety Psychomotor agitation High risk of permanent liver or brain damage
Amphetamines Dexedrine Methamphetamine "Ice" "Uppers" "Crank" "Speed"	Oral, injected, smoked	Grandiosity Hypervigilance Hypertension or hypotension Tachycardia or bradycardia Mydriasis (dilated pupils) Euphoria Appetite suppression Personality changes Antisocial behavior Psychosis similar to paranoid schizophrenia
Caffeine	Oral	Stimulation of senses Alertness and enhanced performance Anxiety and restlessness Flushed face Talkativeness Tremors or muscle twitching Tachycardia or cardiac arrhythmias Insomnia Irritation of the stomach
Cannabis Marijuana "Grass" "Pot" "Hash" "Weed"	Smoked, oral	Mild intoxication Increased appetite Dry mouth Lack of coordination Impaired judgment and memory Sexual arousal Tachycardia Visual hallucinations
Cocaine "Coke" "Crack" "Snow" "Blow" "Lady" "Powder"	Oral, injected, inhaled	Talkativeness Grandiosity Hypervigilance Anxiety Impaired judgment Tachycardia or bradycardia Hypertension or hypotension Mydriasis Muscle twitching Respiratory depression Hallucination, paranoid delusions, or paranoia Formication (sensation of insects crawling on the skin) Personality changes Antisocial behavior Euphoria followed by depression and feeling letdown

Table 87–2. Characteristic Effects of Abuse of Major Substances *(Continued)*

Drug Classification and Street Names	Route of Administration	Effects*
Hallucinogens Lysergic acid diethylamide (LSD) "Acid" Peyote Psilocybin Mescaline	Oral, inhaled	Intensified perceptions and feelings Synesthesia (seeing sound or hearing colors) Visual, auditory, or tactile hallucinations Fear of losing one's mind Mydriasis Tachycardia Palpitations Blurred vision Dizziness, weakness, and tremors Altered perceptions (flashbacks) Impaired judgment and bizarre behavior Mood swings and psychotic-like symptoms
Inhalants Spray can propellants Paint Paint thinner Glue Gasoline Cleaning fluid	Inhaled	Euphoria and giddiness Headache Dizziness, fatigue, or drowsiness Nystagmus (involuntary rapid eye movements) Unsteady gait or tremors Slurred speech Blurred vision or diplopia (double vision) Damage to major organs: lungs, liver, and kidneys Cardiac arrest
Nicotine	Inhaled, oral	Tachycardia Vasoconstriction Irritation of oral mucosa Persistent cough Damaged alveoli and bronchioli Emphysema High risk of oral, laryngeal, or lung cancer
Opioids Morphine Codeine Methadone Dilaudid Heroin "Smack" "Horse"	Oral, injected, inhaled	Immediate euphoria followed by dysphoria Psychomotor retardation or agitation Slurred speech Impaired judgment and memory Sedation and respiratory depression Constricted pupils Decreased sexual and aggressive drives
Phencyclidine (PCP) "Angel dust" "Hog"	Oral, injected, inhaled	Grandiosity and illusions of strength Impulsiveness Psychomotor agitation Assaultive behavior Decreased sensory awareness Hypertension and tachycardia Unsteady gait and lack of coordination Nystagmus Mood swings and paranoia
Sedatives, hypnotics, and anxiolytics Benzodiazepine (e.g., diazepam (Valium), alprazolam (Xanax), chlordiazepoxide (Librium) Secobarbital (Seconal) Pentobarbital (Nembutal) Methaqualone (Quaalude)	Oral, injected	Incoordination and unsteady gait Slurred speech Nystagmus Sedation Inappropriate sexual behavior and aggressive drives Impaired judgment Mood swings

*Drug effects are arranged in order of appearance, with prolonged use or a high dose of the drug associated with appearance of the later effects.
From Copel, L. C. (1996). *Nurses; clinical guide to psychiatric/mental health nursing.* Springhouse, PA: Springhouse.

potential substance problems (see Bridge to Home Healthcare) and institute a collaborative team approach to provide healthcare (see Ethical Issues in Nursing).

Influencing the ability of nurses to provide care are their personal thoughts and feelings about substance abuse and the people who become addicts. Self-awareness about substance use and abuse is essential if the nurse is to establish a therapeutic relationship and provide treatment. The Seaman-Mannello Scale, a Likert-type scale that assesses nurses' attitudes toward alcohol and alcoholism, and the National Council on Alcoholism and Drug Dependence Scale are two instruments that can provide the nurse with insight about personal values and beliefs about substances.[32] Nurses can also examine their personal attitudes and their own use of drugs and alcohol by considering the questions of how, when, where, and under what conditions they use them. Individual beliefs about drug and alcohol use come from the nurse's family background and previous knowledge about and experience with addicted people. This information allows nurses to anticipate their response patterns toward this group of clients. If nurses know their feelings and beliefs, they will be able to recognize a judgmental attitude, rejecting behaviors, or enabling behaviors. This knowledge can prevent the nurse from being drawn into power struggles regarding the client's manipulative behavior.

In addition to self-assessment measures for nurses, there are instruments to use with clients for the purpose of gaining information about their drug and alcohol use. Examples of these instruments are listed in Box 87–1. Note that to effectively use a tool as a piece of the assessment process, the nurse must have thorough knowledge of how to score the instrument and how to correctly interpret the findings.

Interviewing the substance abuse client presents a nursing challenge because of the client's tendency to deny or minimize the problem. A comprehensive assessment includes the client's history and physical examination. Here is where use of the previously mentioned screening tools can be helpful. Laboratory studies are done that address cardiac, liver, kidney, and respiratory functioning, as well as urine toxicology. A thorough mental status assessment is a requisite part of the examination. The major components of this assessment are listed in Table 87–3. Attention is paid to the psychosocial evaluation, especially the components that address difficulties in family, occupational, social, or leisure functioning. Some clinicians recommend that after the history and physical examination are completed, the healthcare provider should do a specific drug and alcohol history that asks about drug usage for the 11 major psychoactive substances, plus other prescription and over-the-counter substances.[12] Components of a drug and alcohol history are listed in Box 87–2.

Although all clients need to be assessed for substance abuse, of special concern are those who by virtue of lifestyle or social conditions may be at increased risk of abuse. Adolescents, women (particularly pregnant women), racial and ethnic minorities, homosexual women and men, clients with HIV infection or acquired immunodeficiency syndrome (AIDS), homeless people, older adults, and healthcare professionals are identified as popu-

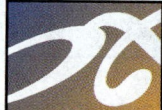

BRIDGE TO HOME HEALTHCARE

Detecting Substance Abuse

Jane Allen Augsten, R.N., B.S.N., *Bergan Home Health Care, Omaha, Nebraska*

Clinical manifestations of substance abuse can appear in a myriad of ways, including physiologic, social, and behavioral changes. When substance abuse is suspected, the community health nurse is an essential team member working with the family, physician, clinic and school nurses, and other concerned health providers. Together, this team can identify the missing pieces of the puzzle that the substance abuser presents.

Regardless of the client's age, social, economic, professional, or educational status, substance abuse can be a problem that eventually leads to changes in the client's behavior and life-style. Be alert to these changes, both overt and covert, in the home setting. It is very important for the nurse to trust his or her senses and instincts in gathering information, because substance abusers often use denial and concealment because of fear of detection.

However, in the comfort of the home, defenses may be lessened. Carefully listening to conversations and observing the environment and family interactions can reveal diminishing income. As substance abuse increases, less money is available for basic needs such as food, house and car payments, and rent. Conversely, a sudden increase in income or goods could be related to selling drugs.

The nurse's sense of smell can help detect the use of drugs and alcohol. The pungent odor of marijuana lingers in a home long after its use. Likewise, tell-tale alcohol breath is difficult to disguise. Using your vision to simply observe is one of the least intrusive means of detecting substance abuse. Noticing a pattern of increased visitors and observing drug paraphernalia or accumulated liquor and alcohol containers alerts the nurse to possible substance abuse.

Last, but equally important, instinct and intervention are useful tools for detection. The nurse needs to recognize behavior changes. Examples include (1) school children who arrive late, are frequently absent, or are inadequately dressed; (2) missed appointments with teachers, physicians, and clinics; and (3) at-risk adults who are noncompliant with medications, begin falling or burning themselves, or show a change in general appearance. Isolated instances can emerge into disruptive patterns that complete the pieces of the substance abuse puzzle.

You have a distinct advantage to see, hear, and observe suspected substance abusers in their home setting. In this way, the nurse offers valuable insight to the healthcare team from the time the family is admitted to service until dismissal.

ETHICAL ISSUES IN NURSING

What Considerations Should Be Made for Substance Abusers Who Are Being Treated for Other Medical Problems?

Substance abuse is a problem that touches all cultures throughout the world. Its effects are seen in the young and the old, and its addiction has no mercy. Because the abuse of chemical substances leads to health problems, healthcare workers see these clients often—perhaps not primarily because of their substance abuse but because their abuse plays a part in their illness. How ethical is the treatment rendered to those who are substance abusers?

For instance, the alcoholic client who is admitted for a surgical procedure requires special attention. He or she was told to not drink for several days prior to surgery, but the reality is that he or she drank up to the night before. Postoperatively, the client begins to develop DTs and must be aggressively restrained. The challenges facing the nursing staff caring for a postoperative client with DTs are great. Client safety is a serious matter, as are wound healing and adequate nutrition. The client may be treated to reduce symptoms. In other cases, the client may be simply left to detoxify "cold turkey."

What is the ethical thing to do in the treatment of substance abusers who are being treated for other medical problems? Nurses deal with these kinds of situations every day. Should clients who are known substance abusers be admitted to the hospital several days prior to a surgical procedure to rid their systems of substances that could adversely affect the outcome of their surgery? If so, what are the financial constraints of such a policy? Should all substance abuse clients be required to seek counseling for their abuse as a prerequisite to receiving other forms of healthcare?

As previously stated, nurses see substance abuse clients in all areas of practice and for all kinds of health problems. Although healthcare may not be contingent on treatment of their substance abuse, nurses can assist such clients by providing information on such treatment programs in their areas.

---

lations that require special prevention, treatment, and education about substance abuse.[3,6] Extra attention must be given to clients with chronic physical or mental illnesses. Self-medication can occur in vulnerable populations as a coping strategy to relieve physical and emotional pain associated with a chronic illness. Often, after obtaining a comprehensive assessment, the nurse may discover that a client struggles with polysubstance abuse. Such clients require specialized care during the withdrawal process, based on the particular combination of drugs used.

Assessment and Management of Substance-Abusing Clients

The immediate result of overconsumption of any psychoactive substance is acute intoxication. Nurses in an emergency department or a medical-surgical setting may care for clients suffering from trauma as a direct result of acute intoxication. In addition to treating the client's injuries, the nursing care of intoxication consists of monitoring vital signs, especially respiratory status, since respiratory depression or arrest can occur. The nurse must be vigilant for symptoms of shock, cardiac arrhythmias, electrolyte imbalances, or subdural hematomas. Typically, intravenous fluids are given to prevent dehydration. Note that some people become intoxicated but do not seek medical intervention because no injuries or emergencies bring them to healthcare facilities.

When there is a sharp reduction or cessation in the use of a psychoactive substance, the process of withdrawal occurs. Depending on the specific drug, withdrawal may begin within 8 to 12 hours or be delayed for 1 to 3 days. Prompt recognition of withdrawal symptoms can promote client safety and prevent complications. Factors that influ-

---

Box 87–1. Examples of Substance Use Screening Tools

For Use with Adults

- Michigan Alcoholism Screening Test (MAST)[42]
- Short Michigan Alcoholism Screening Test (SMAST)[38]
- Addiction Severity Index[27]
- The CAGE Questions[9]
- T-ACE (a modified version of the CAGE used with pregnant women)[48]
- Alcohol Use Disorders Identification Test (AUDIT)[10]
- Alcohol Dependence Scale[46]
- Self-Administered Alcoholism Screening Test (SAAST)[50]
- Alcohol Use Inventory[18]

For Use with Adolescents

- Guided Rational Adolescent Substance Abuse Profile (GRASP)[1]
- Problem Severity Scales for Assessment of Alcohol and Drug Abuse[17]

ence the withdrawal process include the specific drug(s) used, the dose taken, the method of intake, the time of last use, and the length of time the drug has been used. The nurse must also consider the overall health of the client, particularly the functioning of the kidneys, lungs, and liver, the principal organs that metabolize and excrete drugs. An overview of common withdrawal symptoms for alcohol and other substances appears in Table 87–4.

Box 87–2. Components of a Drug and Alcohol History*

- How often the drug was used (past and recent use)
- Age at first use
- Duration of use
- Age at last use
- Method of use
- Quantity used
- Initial and current reaction(s) to the drug
- How the drug was obtained or the use of the drug supported
- What has been done to reduce drug use
- Client's perception of use of the drug as a problem
- Use of drug related to any health problems

Table 87–3. Components of the Mental Status Assessment

General appearance	Appearance versus stated age Grooming and hygiene Posture, gait, and station Interaction during the interview Facial expressions Orientation or level of consciousness
Motor behavior	Restlessness Agitation Lethargy Tremors
Speech	Clarity and coherence of speech Rate of speech Volume and intonation Barriers to communication, such as confusion or delusions Vocabulary appropriate to socioeconomic background
Affect	Flat or labile
Mood	Euphoric, anxious, fearful
Thought processes	Thoughts presented as normal, concrete, scattered, or illogical Delusions—a false belief that is firmly maintained despite evidence to the contrary
Perception	Awareness of self and environment Illusions—misinterpretation of external stimuli Hallucinations—sensory experiences with no external stimuli present
Memory	Memory for remote, recent, and immediate past General knowledge level Ability to calculate Ability to think abstractly Insight Judgment or problem-solving ability

Alcohol

Ethyl alcohol, or ethanol, a central nervous system (CNS) depressant, is found in alcoholic beverages. The ingested alcohol is absorbed directly into the bloodstream from the stomach and proximal part of the small intestine. Since alcohol is water-soluble, it circulates easily throughout the body and readily passes through the blood-brain barrier. Approximately 95% of alcohol is metabolized in the liver, with the remaining 5% being excreted through the lungs, kidneys, and skin.[30] The body's metabolism for oxidizing alcohol is accomplished through the liver enzyme alcohol dehydrogenase. This process breaks down the alcohol to acetaldehyde, which is further broken down to acetic acid, which then goes through the citric acid cycle to become carbon dioxide and water. From this chemical process it is evident that alcohol can affect every aspect of the body. A growing number of young people may be using drugs to enhance alcohol's effect, as discussed in Diversity in Healthcare.

A blood alcohol level (BAL) is a test used to measure the concentration of alcohol in a person's blood. The purpose of the test is to detect and estimate the level of alcohol in the brain. The legal intoxication level in most states is 100 mg/dl (0.10%), with a few states using 0.08%.

Although some studies suggest that small amounts of alcohol can be harmless or even healthful, large amounts produce a predictable series of deleterious effects. After drinking one or two alcoholic beverages, one experiences a depression of the inhibitory regions of the brain that manage judgment, self-control, speech, and motor coordination. Alcohol is classified as a CNS depressant that affects all levels of the brain, starting with the reticular activating system and the cerebral cortex. Alcohol suppresses the inhibitory neurotransmitter gamma-aminobutyric acid (GABA). When the release of GABA is decreased, the initial results are an excitement or euphoric response. With acute alcohol intoxication, the alcohol continues to accumulate in the brain, and depression of the cerebral cortex, cerebellum, and midbrain occurs. In severe brain depression, disruption of the spinal reflexes,

Table 87–4. Common Withdrawal Symptoms Associated with Psychoactive Drugs

Drug Classification	Major Withdrawal Symptoms
Alcohol	Nausea and vomiting Tremors and weakness Sweating Tachycardia Hypertension Delusions Agitated behavior Hallucinations and nocturnal illusions
Amphetamines	Dysphoria Disorientation Fatigue and depression with suicidal potential Disturbed sleep and unpleasant dreams Hallucinations or delusions
Caffeine	Irritability and nervousness Inability to concentrate Headache Tremors Lethargy
Cannabis	No acute withdrawal symptoms; other symptoms appear over varying time periods following withdrawal Amotivational syndrome (inability to concentrate or complete tasks) Chronic respiratory problems Memory and learning difficulty Suppressed prolactin and testosterone levels
Cocaine	Severe craving for drug Severe depression ("postcoke blues") Fatigue Psychomotor agitation or retardation Anxiety Insomnia or hypersomnia Increased appetite
Hallucinogens	Symptoms appear over varying time periods following withdrawal Apprehension, fear, or panic Hyperactivity Sweating Tachycardia Altered perceptions (flashbacks) Perceptual distortions, especially hallucinations
Inhalants	Symptoms appear over varying time periods following withdrawal CNS damage (cerebral atrophy or peripheral neuropathies) Acute or chronic renal failure Bone marrow depression Cardiac arrhythmias Respiratory damage (lung or sinus damage, pneumonitis, emphysema, respiratory depression) Liver disease (hepatitis, cirrhosis)
Nicotine	Irritability and nervousness Headache Inability to concentrate Craving for cigarettes Fatigue and dizziness Tremors and palpitations

Table 87–4. Common Withdrawal Symptoms Associated with Psychoactive Drugs (Continued)	
Drug Classification	**Major Withdrawal Symptoms**
Opioids	Dysphoria Anxiety Insomnia Increased respirations and yawning Sweating Lacrimation and rhinorrhea (nasal discharge) Tremors and muscle twitching Mydriasis (dilated pupils) Piloerection (erection of the hair) Nausea, abdominal cramps, and vomiting
Phencyclidine (PCP)	Symptoms may appear over varying time periods following withdrawal Anxiety Withdrawn, catatonic state Hypertension Seizures Bizarre behavior and speech associated with temporary psychosis
Sedatives, hypnotics, and anxiolytics	Anxiety Sweating Tachycardia Tremors Nausea and vomiting Insomnia and disturbing dreams Transient visual, auditory, or tactile hallucinations Seizures

From Copel, L. C. (1996). *Nurses' clinical guide to psychiatric/mental health nursing.* Springhouse, PA: Springhouse.

respiratory system, cardiac functioning, or temperature regulation occurs. At this point the intoxicated person may become unconscious, and without treatment death may occur.

Early clinical manifestations of alcohol withdrawal, such as tremors, anorexia, anxiety, restlessness, and insomnia, tend to occur within 6 to 8 hours after ingesting the last drink. During the next 2 to 3 days, the client may further experience disorientation, nightmares, abdominal pain, nausea, and diaphoresis, and elevated temperature, pulse, and blood pressure. Visual and auditory hallucinations may also occur. *Delirium tremens* (DTs) is the term used to denote severe withdrawal or life-threatening complications of alcohol withdrawal. With DTs the client is at risk for cardiac arrhythmias, hypertension, increased respirations, profuse sweating, delusions, and hallucinations.

Many clients are prescribed medications to decrease the withdrawal symptoms and prevent DTs from occurring. The benzodiazepines are commonly used because they cause less respiratory depression and hypertension. Typically, the physician orders either a long-acting benzodiazepine, such as diazepam (Valium) or chlordiazepoxide (Librium), or a short-acting benzodiazepine, such as lorazepam (Ativan) or oxazepam (Serax). The long-acting benzodiazepines are often used to facilitate the withdrawal process. For clients who have severe liver dysfunction or a high degree of cognitive impairment, the short-acting benzodiazepines are used. There are also

nonpharmacologic approaches to treating withdrawal. The social model, or the non-medicinal treatment model, incorporates the use of an extensive physical examination followed by close medical supervision while in therapy. Several research studies have shown that approximately 75% of the clients enrolled in these programs improve.[31,54]

The major nursing interventions for a client experiencing withdrawal center around the continuous monitoring of manifestations and promoting a safe, calm, and comfortable environment. During the withdrawal period, clients need reassurance and support, because they may feel they will not survive the ordeal of detoxication. In the immediate period after the withdrawal syndrome has ceased, the nurse can refer the client for further assessment and treatment of addiction or its complications. At this time, especially after what the client has been through, it is essential for the nurse to address with the client the relationship between drug use and the concomitant acute or chronic physical health problems. Common medical consequences of alcohol abuse are identified in Table 87–5.

Amphetamines

Amphetamines have been used to treat narcolepsy and attention deficit hyperactivity disorder (ADHD). People

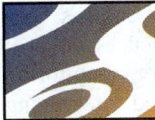

DIVERSITY IN HEALTHCARE

Flunitrazepam (Rohypnol) Use in Young Adults

A sleeping medication from the benzodiazepine family named flunitrazepam (Rohypnol, also known as "roachies," "ribs," "roofies," or "rope") has been increasingly used by young adults, particularly college students. Although the drug is marketed in other countries, it is not legally available in the United States. However, Rohypnol can be obtained from illicit drug dealers who smuggle the substance in from Mexico and Colombia. Worldwide, there is concern expressed about the expanding use of Rohypnol, especially the nasal method of abuse, known as snorting.[5]

A major concern about Rohypnol is its use in conjunction with alcohol. The combination of these two drugs causes CNS depression, which has been reported in some cases to be lethal.[47] For a person who uses Rohypnol only, the usual effects are lack of motor coordination and impairment of thought processes. Under the influence of Rohypnol, people tend to lose their ability to make judgments, resulting in a variety of risky behaviors. When alcohol and Rohypnol are used concurrently, the effects are intensified. Young adults have indicated that they take the drug when drinking beer to enhance the effects of the alcohol. Clients from an outpatient community mental health clinic who used alcohol and Rohypnol together reported that under the influence of these drugs, they engaged in criminal activities, such as breaking and entering. There are also clinical reports of becoming the victim of rape or gang rape after using this drug.[28] Persons under the influence of alcohol and Rohypnol have experienced blackouts lasting from 6 to 24 hours.

Physical and psychological dependence can occur with Rohypnol, just as it occurs with other benzodiazepines. Withdrawal symptoms usually occur 2 to 10 days after discontinuing the drug.[25] When a patient withdraws from Rohypnol, medical management and supportive care is mandated. Special monitoring must be provided for symptoms that indicate simultaneous withdrawal from alcohol and Rohypnol.

Healthcare professionals who treat clients withdrawing from Rohypnol administer phenobarbital orally or intramuscularly to assist the client through the withdrawal process. According to Smith and colleagues,[47] the dosage of phenobarbital used for the treatment of withdrawal is 30 mg for each 1 mg of Rohypnol taken. If the client has been using both alcohol and Rohypnol, the nurse must also be vigilant for symptoms of alcohol withdrawal. It is likely that clients withdrawing from both substances will receive both phenobarbital and either chlordiazepoxide (Librium) or diazepam (Valium). In the case of Rohypnol overdose, a specific benzodiazepine antagonist called flumazenil (Romazicon) is used.[21]

Although Rohypnol appears to be a new illegal drug, it has been used on the streets for years. Throughout the world, benzodiazepines, particularly flunitrazepam (Rohypnol), clorazepate (Tranxene), and diazepam (Valium), have been used by heroin addicts to enhance the highs obtained from the opiates. Today, Rohypnol is also used to extend poor-quality heroin.

The dangers of Rohypnol have been minimized in our society because people view this drug as just another type of diazepam. What people fail to realize is that although Rohypnol is in the benzodiazepine family, it is at least 10 times more potent than diazepam. Since Rohypnol is an inexpensive drug, costing only several dollars per pill, it can be easily purchased by young people. It has been postulated by practitioners in the field of addiction treatment that Rohypnol will become a drug of choice for high-school and college-age youth; it is further believed that Rohypnol could be "the Quaalude of the next generation."[45]

---

often use them illegally to remain awake and alert, increase their ability to perform physical tasks, or produce a state of euphoria (a "high"). The abuse of amphetamines has been noted by the National Institute on Drug Abuse to be most commonly found in the 18- to 34-year-old age group.[34] The pattern of abuse tends to be daily chronic use or periodic binge use that ends with the user overwhelmed by exhaustion ("crashing").

Amphetamines stimulate the CNS and accelerate the activity of the heart and brain. The mode of action for amphetamines is to block the reuptake of dopamine and norepinephrine by interfering with the transport protein, ultimately causing dopamine and norepinephrine to accumulate at the synapses.[14] Amphetamines are metabolized by the liver enzymes and excreted in the urine. In some cases, after continual drug use, half of the drug may be excreted from the body unchanged.[6]

When a client is intoxicated with amphetamines the clinical findings may include cardiac arrhythmias, hypertension, fever, labile emotions, paranoia, delusions, panic reactions, or psychosis. Client management centers on frequent assessment of vital signs and basic body functioning, as well as providing safe, supportive care. Closely monitor the client for changes in cardiac or neurologic status, since myocardial infarction and cerebral hemorrhage have occurred from amphetamine use. Often, antipsychotics are used to decrease the CNS stimulation, or else sedatives are given. In some instances, intravenous amino acids are given to speed up the detoxification process of stimulant drugs.[7]

Frequently, amphetamines cause psychological dependence, with craving behavior being very common. Abrupt cessation of the drug can precipitate anxiety, agitation, severe depression, hyperphagia, and hypersomnolence. An

Table 87–5. Medical Consequences of Alcohol Abuse

Body System	Consequences
Cardiac	Arrhythmias Hypertension Cardiomyopathy Congestive heart failure Beriberi heart disease
Gastrointestinal	Gastritis Gastric or duodenal ulcers Perforated gastrointestinal ulcers Esophageal varices Pancreatitis Interference with absorption of vitamin B_{12}, thiamine, and folic acid Malabsorption syndrome Alteration in nutrition, with potential for malnutrition Wernicke-Korsakoff syndrome Enlarged or fatty liver Liver enzyme changes Cirrhosis Alcoholic hepatitis Portal hypertension Ascites Hepatic encephalopathy
Hematopoietic	Anemia Thrombocytopenia Leukopenia Capillary fragility Spider nevi Palmar erythema
Neurologic	Peripheral neuropathy Brain atrophy
Musculoskeletal	Myopathy Decreased bone density with risk of fracture Fractured bones related to trauma
Immune	Depressed immune system Increased susceptibility to infections
Respiratory	Altered respirations Chronic obstructive pulmonary disease Pneumonia Tuberculosis
Endocrine	Testicular atrophy Gynecomastia Irregular menses Decreased libido Hypoglycemia Alcoholic ketoacidosis

amphetamine psychosis may occur if the client has continuously used high doses. Nursing care focuses on providing rest, orienting the client as necessary, monitoring for both physical and emotional changes, and intervening to prevent complications of the drug's adverse effects or withdrawal symptoms.

Caffeine

In the United States, caffeine—a CNS stimulant—is the most commonly used psychoactive substance. Products that contain caffeine include coffee, tea, chocolate, cola beverages, and both prescription and nonprescription medications. People rely on caffeine to promote wakefulness, elevate their sense of well-being, decrease fatigue, and facilitate motor activity. The mode of action within the body is stimulation of the CNS, thereby exciting the respiratory system and increasing body metabolism.[6] Caffeine is absorbed from the gastrointestinal tract, broken down in the liver, and excreted in the urine. The intake of a large quantity of caffeine can cause intoxication, manifested by cardiac arrhythmias, sleep disturbances, mood changes, increased production of urine, gastrointestinal discomfort, and anxiety, especially panic attacks. Caffeinism and caffeine withdrawal syndrome are seen only with long-term use of caffeine, usually a documented intake of greater than 500 mg/day.[41]

The nursing care of these clients begins with recognition of the clinical manifestations of excessive caffeine use and withdrawal. Monitoring the manifestations presented and observing for additional problems, such as whether the caffeine is exacerbating known health problems, is appropriate nursing management.

Cannabis

Cannabis derivatives or marijuana is the most widely used illegal drug in the United States, with over 55% of young adults reporting personal use of the substance.[19] The mode of action of marijuana is not clearly understood, and researchers continue to try to identify the mechanism that accounts for its effects on the CNS and cardiovascular system.[6,26] Tetrahydrocannabinol (THC) has been identified as the active ingredient in marijuana and the agent responsible for the psychological effects. The amount of marijuana that crosses the blood-brain barrier depends on the method of intake used. THC is absorbed in fatty tissues, primarily the brain and testes, and slowly released back into the bloodstream, where it is eventually excreted in urine and feces.[41]

Clients who use marijuana experience manifestations of intoxication. These symptoms are euphoria, mood changes, memory impairment, tremors, decreased body temperature, dry mouth, lack of coordination, elevated blood pressure and heart rate, and injected conjunctivae (bloodshot eyes). It has been noted that the CNS, cardiac, immune, and reproductive systems are affected by the use of marijuana. Long-term use also influences respiratory functioning, and the marijuana residues in the lungs are considered more carcinogenic than tobacco residues.

Withdrawal from marijuana is typically an uncomfortable, but not life-threatening, process. Nursing care includes monitoring the physical and emotional response of the client to the drug. It is often helpful for a nurse, family member, or friend to stay with the client, provide reassurance, and talk the client through the anxiety. Usually the client is not hospitalized unless preexisting medical conditions or the coexistence of another psychoactive substance complicates the withdrawal process. For most clients the initial effects of the drug dissipate within 4 to 6 hours; however, the effects of drug intoxication may last as long as 5 days.[23]

Cocaine

Cocaine is a narcotic obtained from the leaves of the coca plant, originally used by the Indians of the Andes to alleviate feelings of hunger and fatigue and promote endurance. Today cocaine is readily available on the illicit market in the form of cocaine hydrochloride, which is soluble in water and used intravenously, inhaled (snorted), or as "crack," a form of concentrated (freebase) cocaine that is smoked.

Cocaine stimulates the CNS and blocks the conduction of peripheral nerve impulses. Continued use of cocaine will increase the amount of dopamine present in the synapses of nerve cells by preventing dopamine reuptake. Cocaine also acts to decrease the breakdown of dopamine and other catecholamines, thereby increasing the level of catecholamine activity at the nerve cell synapses.[39] Cocaine is metabolized in the liver and excreted in the urine. Evidence of cocaine use can be extracted from a urine sample for up to approximately 72 hours after use.

In assessing for the effects of cocaine, remember that cocaine stimulates the CNS and the cardiovascular system. Cocaine abuse has led to myocardial infarctions in young, presumably healthy individuals. An overdose of cocaine causes tremors, seizures, and delirium. Death can also occur from cardiac or respiratory failure. Intervention is based on treating these identified problems and acting to prevent cardiac and respiratory complications. Often cocaine intoxication is not seen in medical-surgical settings, since the half-life of cocaine is approximately 60 minutes.[13] Nursing management of a cocaine overdose focuses on preventing or handling cardiovascular collapse, respiratory distress, delirium, and hyperthermia. Withdrawal from chronic use of cocaine (called "bingeing") results in an exhausted state known as "crashing." Here the client experiences a profound sense of depression, has memories of the cocaine-induced feelings of euphoria, and has cravings for the drug. Often, the client is hospitalized if there is severe depression with suicidal risk, if coexisting medical problems necessitate intense monitoring or treatment, or if there are medical problems directly related to complications of intravenous use. Besides providing the physical care required for the cocaine-dependent client, the nurse makes the client aware of the need to develop effective coping skills.

Hallucinogens

Hallucinogens, also known as psychedelic drugs, are both natural and synthetic substances that produce illusions, delusions, hallucinations, and alterations in thoughts, perceptions, and feelings. It has long been known that the effects of hallucinogens differ among individuals and are therefore unpredictable. An individual's personality may influence the particular reaction that occurs after use of a hallucinogen. Characteristic of lysergic acid diethylamide (LSD) and other psychedelic drugs is the subjective sensation of heightened awareness, the ability to look inward, and a feeling of oneness with the universe.

The mechanism of action of hallucinogens is unknown. Hallucinogens are usually ingested, then absorbed from the gastrointestinal tract, metabolized in the liver, and excreted in the bile and feces.[6] The length of action of most hallucinogens is between 6 and 12 hours.[41] The effects of hallucinogens are similar to other stimulants in that the user experiences euphoria, dilated pupils, anxiety, and increased respirations, blood pressure, and heart rate. Panic attacks occur while in a state of intoxication, accompanied by feelings of paranoia, confusion, hallucinations, possible dissociation, and loss of contact with reality. The resulting inability to perceive the environment accurately, impaired judgment, and the feeling of having special powers make the person prone to dangerous activities. Suicide, homicide, and other acts of violence have been reported in persons under the influence of hallucinogenic drugs. Some users also experience flashbacks. During a period of intoxication, or because of a flashback experience or the reliving of a "bad trip," a person may be brought to a healthcare setting. The nurse must carefully assess the client for both physiologic and psychological problems. Nursing care focuses on attending to the panic that the client is experiencing, as well as providing for client safety and creating a nonstimulating environment. It is important that someone stay with the client until the effects of the hallucinogen have worn off. In the case of a severe overdose, be prepared to intervene for possible seizures, extremely high temperatures, and cardiac distress.[41] Withdrawal symptoms may occur over a period of time, so be vigilant for possible neurologic abnormalities and psychiatric concerns.

Inhalants

Inhalants are chemicals that give off fumes or vapors that readily pass through the blood-brain barrier to produce an alteration in consciousness. Commonly used inhalants are solvents (glue, gasoline, nail polish remover, lighter fluid, paint thinner), aerosols (hair spray, insecticides), and anesthetics used for recreational purposes (nitrous oxide, chloroform, ether). The probable mechanism of action is that these volatile substances alter the biologic membranes of the cells of the CNS and affect the metabolism of neurotransmitters in the brain.[41] Inhalants are metabolized in the liver and kidneys. Low doses of inhalants cause initial CNS excitement within minutes of use. Immediately after inhaling a volatile substance through the nose or mouth (also known as "huffing"), the user experiences a high accompanied by feelings of giddiness and euphoria. There is a decrease in inhibitions, and a slowing of the heart rate, respiratory rate, and overall mental activity. With inhalant intoxication the client manifests many physical symptoms, such as delirium, cardiac arrhythmias, irritation of the mucous membranes of the nose and mouth, cough, and depression of brain waves. Depending on the substance inhaled, the effects may last from a few minutes to several hours.[41] Continuous use of volatile substances results in brain, lung, liver, kidney, and bone marrow damage. Withdrawal symptoms associated with inhalants vary with the specific substance used. Sudden death related to the use of inhalants can occur from life-threatening arrhythmias and hypoxia. Nursing care concentrates on prompt intervention when emergency situations occur, such as seizures, loss of consciousness, or respiratory arrest. Effective management of the client's acute and chronic physiologic problems remains your primary goal.

Nicotine

Smoking is an addictive habit practiced throughout the world. It is the leading cause of preventable death in the United States. Nicotine is absorbed through the lungs and within seconds it crosses the blood-brain barrier and acts to stimulate the CNS. It is metabolized in the liver and excreted in the urine. It is known to adversely affect the cardiovascular, respiratory, and gastrointestinal systems. An overdose of nicotine is not a common occurrence. If intoxication should develop, administration of oxygen and the treatment of symptoms are the nurse's priorities. Nicotine withdrawal occurs within 24 hours of smoking cessation. The withdrawal symptoms are uncomfortable, and the nurse can support the client through this process and assist with developing effective strategies for dealing with the manifestations.

Opioids

Opioids comprise drugs produced from opium along with manufactured or semisynthetic narcotics. In the human body there are natural opiates that facilitate feelings of well-being. Chemicals known as endorphins are neurotransmitters that connect with opiate receptors in the brain. When a person uses opiates or other narcotics, there is an interference created in the natural opioid system and a disruption of the functions of the neurotransmitters in the brain.[14] Opioids are metabolized in the liver and excreted in the bile and urine.

An opioid overdose constitutes a life-threatening situation due to seizures, shock, respiratory depression, or cardiac arrhythmias. The client is usually in an unconscious or lethargic state, and without appropriate medical treatment may die. The nurse assesses and intervenes with the healthcare team to provide the required emergency care. Establishing an airway, monitoring cardiac functioning and treating arrhythmias, maintaining hydration, and administering a narcotic antagonist such as naloxone (Narcan) are the nursing care priorities. Hospitalization, with close monitoring of all body systems, is instituted for at least a 24-hour period. For the client experiencing opioid withdrawal, focus on assessing and intervening for a variety of physiologic, psychological, and behavioral symptoms; these tend to occur within 72 hours of last drug use. Nursing care consists of constant monitoring of withdrawal symptoms, along with providing rest, nutrition, and a comfortable environment. The initiation of a methadone program is used to prevent severe withdrawal symptoms. Often clients are referred to residential treatment programs to learn how to develop new, drug-free lifestyles.

Phencyclidine (PCP)

Phencyclidine is a synthetic drug that has stimulant, depressant, and hallucinogenic properties.[6] PCP has been shown to not only increase the production of dopamine but also block its reuptake, thus causing an increase in blood pressure and heart and respiratory rates. It also increases acetylcholine in the CNS, thereby generating cholinergic effects manifested as diaphoresis, drooling, and pupillary constriction. Serotonin is also believed to be altered by the presence of PCP, resulting in a lack of coordination, slurred speech, and nystagmus.[19] PCP is metabolized in the liver and excreted in the urine. Intoxication from PCP lasts up to 6 hours, and the effects of the drug are unpredictable. A person may experience euphoria, disorientation, or the racing or slowing of thoughts. In emergency departments the client may be confused, hostile, violent, paranoid, or panicked. Nursing assessment of PCP intoxication often reveals severe cardiac or respiratory distress which can lead to cardiac arrest. Clients under the influence of PCP can be in a psychotic-like state, have nystagmus, abnormal muscle movements, and severe hypertension. Nursing care concentrates on the assessment of subtle changes in vital signs and level of consciousness, gastric lavage if PCP has been ingested, and acidification of the urine.[41] In PCP withdrawal, the nurse will see variable presentations of symptoms, particularly abnormal muscle movements. Careful monitoring of the client's physical and mental condition is warranted to minimize health problems.

Sedatives, Hypnotics, and Anxiolytics

Drugs in the group "sedatives, hypnotics, and anxiolytics" are considered to be CNS depressants. These medications are directly absorbed from the gastrointestinal tract into the bloodstream, where they enter the brain, are metabolized in the liver, and eliminated via the kidneys. In cases of overdose, the nurse sees decreased CNS functioning, along with the slowing of the cardiac and respiratory systems. Monitoring of vital signs and the initiation of emergency procedures are done based on the clinical symptoms and medical problems presented. An overdose of any of these depressant drugs constitutes a medical emergency, with some clients requiring hospitalization in an intensive care unit. Nursing care focuses on mainte-

Table 87–6. Health Consequences of Commonly Abused Drugs	
Drug Category	**Health Problem**
Amphetamines	Hypertension Excoriations from scratching at nonexistent "bugs" under the skin Cardiac arrhythmias Seizures Paranoid psychosis
Caffeine	Hypertension Arrhythmias Angina Peptic ulcers Tremors Insomnia
Cannabis	Irritation of lung tissue Chronic sinusitis Chronic pharyngitis Lowered testosterone level
Cocaine	Damaged nasal septum Aspiration Bronchitis Hypertension Stroke or stroke-like symptoms Endocarditis Hepatitis Pulmonary emboli Skin ulcers or abscesses Acquired immunodeficiency syndrome (AIDS) Seizures Myocardial infarction Respiratory failure
Hallucinogens	Hypertension Cardiac arrhythmias Flashbacks
Inhalants	Lung damage Hepatitis with possible liver failure Kidney failure Bone marrow depression with possible aplastic anemia Cardiac arrhythmias Respiratory arrest Muscle weakness Gastrointestinal distress Peripheral neuropathy Brain damage
Nicotine	Lung cancer Oral cavity cancer Cancer of the larynx Myocardial infarction Cerebrovascular accidents Angina Chronic obstructive pulmonary disease Bronchitis Gastric ulcers
Opioids	Pneumonia Lung abscess

Table 87–6. Health Consequences of Commonly Abused Drugs *(Continued)*	
Drug Category	**Health Problem**
Opioids *Cont.*	Atelectasis Pulmonary fibrosis Tuberculosis Bacterial endocarditis Cardiac arrhythmias Anemia Viral hepatitis (types A and B) Osteomyelitis Myositis ossificans (drug user's elbow) Phlebitis Hypergammaglobulinemia Splenomegaly Arthritis Lymphadenopathy Nephritis or kidney failure AIDS Eye-ground abnormalities from adulterants in street drugs
Phencyclidine (PCP)	Confusion and severe agitation, which precipitates accidents Hypertension Impaired immune functioning Hallucinations Seizures
Sedatives, hypnotics, and anxiolytics	Mental slowness, poor judgment, and difficulty thinking Impaired motor performance Abrupt withdrawal similar to alcohol withdrawal Seizures

nance of adequate respiratory and cardiovascular status, hydration, and possible gastric lavage if the drugs were taken within the last 4 to 6 hours.[41] In withdrawal situations, the nurse promotes safety and rest, while treating a variety of both physical and emotional manifestations. Nursing care priorities are awareness of the possibility of delirium, seizures, fever, and changes in cardiac and respiratory status, as well as the interaction between adverse effects of the drug and preexisting medical problems. Table 87–6 summarizes common health problems observed in clients who abuse drugs other than alcohol.

Nursing Care of Substance-Abusing Clients

The nurse plays a vital role in the care of the client experiencing intoxication and withdrawal. Nurses also meet basic needs, develop a therapeutic relationship, and teach both the client and family about addiction and its impact on the entire family. Nursing strategies for meeting actual or potential health problems are implemented for nursing diagnoses generated from assessment data.

Nursing diagnoses commonly applied to the substance abuse population are listed in Box 87–3.

Education is an essential component of care if the client is to look at the need for personal life-style change. The main components of a drug education plan for clients and families are outlined in Box 87–4. Sometimes clients who abuse alcohol are referred for various treatment options and given disulfiram (Antabuse) to deter their drinking. Clients on Antabuse must be carefully instructed about the drug. Information to include in a teaching plan is provided in Box 87–5.

Substance abuse has a major impact on family members. The family often tries to deal with the substance-abusing member by altering his or her behavior and compensating for the addict's unfilled responsibilities. Often the family inadvertently isolates itself from others as it focuses most of its energy on the member who is addicted. Personal needs of the caregiver and of other adults and children go unmet. Family members are strongly affected by the addiction and must be involved in the recovery process. A caring, supportive, and educative response from the nurse conveys that the family's concerns are understood and will be included in the treatment program.

Box 87–3. Common Nursing Diagnoses for Clients Who Abuse Substances

- Acute confusion
- Anxiety
- Communication, impaired verbal
- Denial, ineffective
- Family processes, altered
- Fatigue
- Fear
- Grieving, dysfunctional
- Hopelessness
- Individual coping, ineffective
- Infection, risk of
- Injury, risk of
- Knowledge deficit (specify)
- Noncompliance (specify)
- Nutrition, altered: less than body requirements
- Pain
- Parenting, altered
- Personal identity disturbance
- Poisoning, risk of
- Powerlessness
- Role performance, altered
- Self-care deficit (bathing, hygiene, dressing, grooming, feeding, toileting)
- Self-esteem, chronic low
- Sensory and perceptual alterations (specify) (visual, auditory, kinesthetic, gustatory, tactile, olfactory)
- Sexuality patterns, altered
- Skin integrity, risk of impaired
- Sleep pattern disturbance
- Social interaction, impaired
- Social isolation
- Spiritual distress
- Thought processes, altered
- Trauma, risk of
- Violence, risk of, self-directed or directed at others

Box 87–4. Components of a Client and Family Education Plan

- Concept of addiction
- Physical health problems associated with addiction
- Nutritional status
- Feelings and behaviors of all family members associated with addiction
- Areas of life affected by substance use: family, social, spiritual, sexual, occupational, financial, legal, and leisure
- Roles family members play in addiction
- Treatment options and treatment process
- Aftercare and self-help support groups or 12-step groups
- Community resources
- Skill building in the areas of communication, expression of feelings, socialization, and coping strategies
- Impact of both addiction and the recovery process on the roles and responsibilities of all family members
- Client confidentiality and right to privacy protected under the 1975 Federal Drug and Alcohol Abuse Act

Drug and Alcohol Intervention

Confrontation on Drug Abuse

In medical-surgical settings, nurses and other members of the healthcare team may receive a request for assistance from family members, who believe that the client needs to obtain drug and alcohol treatment. To confront the client about drug abuse, a carefully orchestrated format, called a therapeutic intervention, can be implemented.[55] The overall purpose of a therapeutic intervention is to confront the client with his or her drug use and mandate that the client participate in drug and alcohol treatment. This intervention must be planned in advance and executed under the guidance of a healthcare provider who has a drug and alcohol counseling background. In preparation for the intervention, all participants compose a list of situations in which they have personal knowledge about the client's drug and alcohol behaviors.

The basic format of the therapeutic intervention is to gather a group of family and friends together who realistically bring the client face to face with the addiction problem. In an objective and nonjudgmental manner these individuals state their concerns about the client, their observations about the client's substance abuse behavior, and overall caring about the person's well-being. A plan for obtaining help from these significant people is presented to the client. This plan includes treatment recommendations and may contain a reservation for a particular treatment facility. It is believed that this loving and open confrontation will break through the abuser's denial and defensiveness. The client's family and friends must also state the consequences that will immediately ensue if help is refused.

Treatment Options

After completing a comprehensive health history and providing healthcare for the client, the nurse is in an optimal position to recommend a treatment modality that corresponds to the needs of the client and family members. Activities that nurses would be involved in range from primary prevention (education), to secondary prevention (outpatient services), to tertiary prevention (inpatient or outpatient detoxification and rehabilitation). The common interventions for all three levels of care are listed in Table 87–7. A list of community resources that can provide education and support to substance-abusing clients and their families appears in Box 87–6.

Prevention of Relapse

It is common for clients in the recovery process to be at risk of relapse or a return to substance abuse. Nurses anticipate the possibility of relapse, and prepare clients with strategies that may prevent it from occurring. Relapse needs to be viewed as a potential part of the illness process, much like the potential course of any other

Box 87–5. Information on Disulfiram to Include in a Teaching Plan

- Inform the client that disulfiram (Antabuse) is not a cure for alcoholism; it only discourages drinking.
- Before initiating Antabuse, ask if the client has had any allergic reactions to substances such as sulfites, preservatives, or dyes.
- Ask if the client has a history of seizures; severe mental illness, particularly psychosis; serious cardiac disease; kidney disease; diabetes mellitus; hypothyroidism; or skin allergies.
- Ask if the client is taking anticoagulants (increases their effect), isoniazid (INH) (increases CNS effects), metronidazole (Flagyl) (may increase toxicity), or phenytoin (Dilantin) (may increase toxicity).
- Instruct client not to ingest any alcohol or use any products containing alcohol within 12 hours before taking Antabuse, while taking Antabuse, and for at least 14 days after discontinuing Antabuse.
- Explain to the client that it is necessary to read the labels on all products, because alcohol is found in many foods, medicines, and personal hygiene products. Examples of these products are sauces, vinegars, cough syrups, tonics, elixirs, mouthwash, colognes, and after-shave lotions.

- Tell the client not to inhale chemicals that may contain alcohol, such as paints, varnish, or shellac.
- Encourage the client not to use alcohol-containing products that are applied topically. Alcohol absorbed through the skin can cause redness, itching, headache, and nausea.
- Identify common side effects, such as headache, fatigue, a metallic or garlic-like aftertaste, or skin rash that the client may experience during the first 2 weeks of taking Antabuse. Inform the client that these symptoms resolve as the body adjusts to the medication.
- If the client ingests alcohol while on Antabuse, the following symptoms can occur: blurred vision, chest pain, confusion, dizziness or fainting, palpitations, flushing, diaphoresis, nausea, vomiting, headache, and dyspnea. These symptoms last as long as alcohol is in the body. If the client drinks a large amount of alcohol, more serious symptoms, such as seizures, myocardial infarction, unconsciousness, or death may occur.
- Instruct the client to carry a card specifying that he or she is taking Antabuse, listing symptoms that occur if he or she ingests alcohol, and stating whom to contact in case of an emergency.

chronic illness. Seeing relapse as client failure sets the client up for defeat instead of recovery. *Relapse* is an all-encompassing term used to describe a person who slips back into substance use after a period of abstinence. This regression can occur at any point in time, and may be defined as one-time use, brief intermittent use, or daily long-term use.

Physiologic, emotional, and social variables all contribute to relapse. Clients must be taught ways to assess their strengths and identify situations that can distract them from their recovery. It is common for factors such as peer pressure, stress, and negative feelings to trigger a relapse. Some relapse prevention strategies to include in educational programs are listed in Box 87–7.

Table 87–7. Levels of Treatment Strategies

Level of Prevention	Activities	Resources
Primary prevention	Education to prevent substance abuse Risk factor identification Life-style guidance	School programs Community programs Health promotion activities
Secondary prevention (outpatient)	Assessment and intervention of early physical and emotional issues and problems Educational interventions Pharmacologic interventions Self-management strategies Support and self-help groups Psychotherapy	Medical facilities as appropriate Individual, family, or group therapy Psychoeducational groups Self-help groups (e.g., AA, NA, CA, Al-Anon, Alateen, Naranon, ACOA)*
Tertiary prevention (inpatient or out-patient)	Interventions to monitor withdrawal and prevent or treat complications Focusing on relapse prevention Determining plan for aftercare and methods of obtaining support Individual, family, or group therapy	Medical services, such as detoxification Aftercare, such as partial programs, supervised living, or halfway house Individual, family, or group therapy Psychoeducational groups Self-help groups (e.g., AA, NA, CA, Al-Anon, Alateen, Naranon, ACOA)*

*See Box 87–6, Resources.

Box 87–6. Resources

- Alcoholics Anonymous (look in the local telephone directory or call New York, NY: 212-686-1100 for information throughout the United States)
- Al-Anon (look in the local telephone directory or call New York, NY: 212-254-7230 for information throughout the United States)
- National Alcohol Hotline 24-hour HelpLine: 1-800-ALCOHOL
- Adult Children of Alcoholics (look in the local telephone directory or call Torrance, CA: 213-534-1815 for information)
- Children of Alcoholics Foundation, Inc. (call New York, NY: 212-351-2680 for information)
- BACCHUS (Boast Alcohol Consciousness Concerning the Health of University Students) (call Denver, CO: 303-871-3068 for information)
- MADD (Mothers Against Drunken Driving) (call Austin, TX: 817-268-6233 for information)
- Narcotics Anonymous (look in the local telephone directory or call Van Nuys, CA: 818-780-3951 for information)
- Cocaine Anonymous (call Los Angeles, CA: 800-347-8998 or 213-559-5833 for information)
- National Cocaine Hotline: 1-800-COCAINE
- National Clearinghouse for Alcohol and Drug Information (call Rockville, MD: 301-468-2600 for information)
- National Asian Pacific American Families Against Drug Abuse (call Bethesda, MD: 301-530-0945 for information)

Surgery and Substance Abuse

Clients who abuse substances often experience accidents, injuries, or illnesses that require surgical intervention. In fact, many injuries seen by nurses in emergency departments are directly related to drug and alcohol use. A nurse must be skillful in observing for subtle changes and perform frequent assessments in order to intervene immediately and prevent the escalation of manifestations. Usually the traumatized client requires immediate surgery; hence, a thorough drug and alcohol assessment may not be done. It is a challenge for the nurse to differentiate between medical problems, psychiatric disorders, and substance abuse disorders in a timely manner.

Box 87–7. Strategies to Prevent Relapse

- Assess and build on the client's coping skills.
- Take opportunities, such as role-playing, that help the client practice coping methods.
- Assist the client in identifying personal risks of relapse.
- Identify people, places, and things that can interfere with maintaining sobriety and encourage the client to minimize contact with these obstacles and develop ways to handle them.
- Change environmental variables where possible.
- Discuss the concept of craving, how to identify it, what may trigger it, and how to handle it.
- Focus on the client's physiologic feelings and sensations, and develop methods to handle them.
- Teach strategies that promote a healthy life-style, such as exercise, nutrition, stress management, and relaxation techniques.
- Encourage participation in support groups or self-help groups.
- Recommend group or individual therapy if the client has family-of-origin problems, struggles with daily functioning, or mental illness.

If a client is addicted to CNS depressant drugs, a larger amount of an anesthetic may be needed to produce the desired effects. This situation occurs because the client will have a higher tolerance to the anesthetic drug. For clients with liver impairment and overall poor health, anesthetics cannot be properly metabolized, and the effect of sedation will be prolonged. While undergoing surgery, the addicted client is at risk of cardiac arrhythmias, respiratory depression, hemorrhage, and depletion of catecholamines. In the postoperative period, these clients are prone to cardiac, respiratory, urinary, hemorrhagic, and wound complications. The experience of pain may be intensified, since the client often has tolerance to the pain medication. Carefully assess whether the client requires increased doses of medication for pain relief and needs to be slowly weaned from the medication during the recovery process. Some addicted clients may experience drug withdrawal postoperatively, because withdrawal has been delayed by the use of anesthetics.

The Impaired Healthcare Professional

Healthcare professionals can become addicted to drugs and alcohol just like other members of society. Research on the prevalence of substance abuse among nurses has revealed no difference between nurses and non-nurses. Further, the prevalence of substance abuse among health professionals overall does not differ from that in the general population.[53] Many addicted healthcare professionals first started using drugs and alcohol in response to physical illness and pain, emotional difficulties, and work pressures.[24] The requirements of the role of professional nurse make it a very stressful occupation. On a daily basis the nurse is faced with the responsibility of coordinating and directly providing care for patients who are in pain and crisis. The pressure of handling resources; making decisions; interfacing with both medical and non-medical personnel; working long hours, often with inadequate staff;

Box 87–8. Signs of a Chemically Impaired Colleague

- Alcohol on breath
- Mood changes or confusion
- Difficulty making judgments and impaired memory
- Red eyes with flushed face
- Unsteady gait
- Tremors or impaired eye-hand coordination
- Irritability or hyperactivity
- Lethargy or dozing on breaks
- Disheveled appearance
- Wearing long sleeves or a sweater constantly, even in hot weather
- Incorrect drug counts
- Accidents, spillages, or drugs frequently being wasted
- Frequently found in the bathroom, nurses' lounge, or off the unit
- Recurrent unfinished assignments or patient care mistakes

---

and being responsible for the daily operation of the medical-surgical unit places overwhelming demands on the nurse. In addition, nurses have access to narcotics and operate on the premise that medications are a useful vehicle for relieving pain and altering states of feelings. Specialized knowledge about drugs and experience with administering them and watching their efficacy may lead health providers to view drugs as a "pharmacologic coping method."[51] It is a method that can ultimately backfire.

The signs of a chemically impaired colleague are subtle and easily overlooked by peers and supervisors. Even other healthcare professionals may deny and avoid the problem rather than confront the individual suspected of being chemically dependent. It is essential that all nurses be aware of signs of chemical dependence in peers. Box 87–8 outlines some signs that indicate a colleague could be chemically impaired. Document questionable or problematic incidents, and be willing to participate in an intervention if deemed appropriate. Remember that a peer who suffers from addiction is unable to meet the requirements of your state nurse practice act. Some states have a law that mandates reporting of an impaired colleague. As with clients, steps must be taken to assist the impaired nurse to obtain treatment (see Ethical Issues in Nursing for a discussion of the issues involved). The use of an employee assistance program (EAP) or peer support or assistance groups from the state nurses' association are two mechanisms that can facilitate referrals to treatment and assist with the recovery process. Although peer assistance programs vary from state to state, most programs offer support, referral services, monitoring during recovery, and educational programs targeted to the healthcare professional.

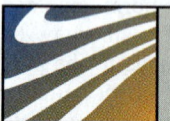

ETHICAL ISSUES IN NURSING

What Ethical Issues Surround Your Relationship to an Impaired Nurse?

You suspect that Sandy, a nurse coworker, is abusing narcotics. You decide to confront her. Sandy confides in you that she is addicted to cocaine. What is your moral responsibility?

The addicted nurse presents an unfortunate situation for all involved. You face an ethical dilemma. Should you break Sandy's trust in your friendship by telling the nurse-manager that Sandy is abusing drugs? Or should you not tell the nurse-manager and risk the harm that may come to clients in your unit if Sandy continues to deliver nursing care while under the influence of narcotics?

You can support your decision to tell the nurse-manager with the principle of beneficence to the clients on the unit. The third item in the ANA Code for Nurses supports you in safeguarding clients when healthcare and safety are affected by the incompetent, unethical, or illegal practice of others. On the other hand, you could support your decision to not tell the nurse manager by calling on principles of trust, privacy, and friendship. What should you do?

We value friendships and relationships. We have all confided in another person something that we would not want the world to know. Good working relationships are important to good nursing care. But concern for client safety in this situation should take precedence over trust and privacy issues. The clients on this nursing unit could be in real danger if Sandy's narcotic addiction continues. As a professional, your first duty is to your clients. You must ensure safe, competent nursing care. While concern for client safety is paramount, it does not have to be at the exclusion of concern for a friend.

If Sandy continues to abuse drugs while practicing nursing, she will undoubtedly make mistakes. These mistakes, besides the possibility of injuring clients, will also damage Sandy's reputation as a good nurse. Therefore, concern for Sandy's health can also motivate you to tell the nurse-manager about Sandy's addiction. Sandy needs help in recognizing the seriousness of her situation and an opportunity to get help.

You should discuss with Sandy your intentions to tell the nurse-manager and give Sandy time to think about her situation. By allowing about a week for Sandy to think about her situation, you are acknowledging the high value you place on Sandy's friendship and trust while still actively protecting client safety.

Conclusions

Substance abuse remains a major health issue, affecting individuals, families, and communities. Yet, despite this reality, many clients with substance abuse disorders are not diagnosed, and therefore do not obtain treatment. A lack of knowledge about addiction can perpetuate stigmatization of the client. The challenge for nurses is to become informed about both the effects of drugs and appropriate strategies for treatment. Keen assessment skills, decision-making skills, and compassion are the prerequisites for comprehensive nursing care of the myriad of physiologic and psychological needs presented by these clients.

Nurses play a vital role in developing and implementing drug and alcohol prevention strategies. Teaching people how to use effective coping strategies, ways to handle crises, and how to develop support systems are the primary steps that must be incorporated into the care. As for nurses, the importance of spending time cultivating relationships and allowing one's self to engage in leisure activities will decrease feelings of frustration, hopelessness, and burnout.

Thinking Critically

1. A group of young college-age students celebrated the end of the semester with a week-long party. Alcoholic beverages were plentiful; food was not a primary priority. A young couple brought their friend to the emergency department. They report their suspicions that she may have a drinking problem (e.g., erratic behavior, presence of alcoholic beverages in the dormitory room, smell of alcohol on her breath). They were unable to awaken her for any length of time and are worried that she drank too much. She has not had a drink for about 6 hours. What assessment is required? What nursing actions are appropriate?

Factors to Consider. How likely is it for the client to experience delirium tremens (DTs)? How will the client be treated?

2. You are a registered nurse in the local "Driving Under the Influence of Alcohol" (DUI) teaching program. Your topic is "Alcohol and the Human Body." The audience is made up of clients mandated by the court to attend. After the presentation, which focuses on the complications associated with long-term drinking, there is a question-and-answer period. The clients ask, "If alcoholism is a disease, why are we treated as criminals?" "I didn't drink so much, why did they pull me over?" What might these questions indicate?

Factors to Consider. Is alcoholism a disease of addiction? What psychologic factor is evident in such questions?

Bibliography

1. Addiction Research Corporation. (1986). *GRASP: Guide's rational adolescent substance abuse profile.* Piscataway, NJ: Rutgers University Center of Alcohol Studies.
2. American Psychiatric Association. (1994). *Diagnostic and statistical manual of mental disorders* (4th ed.). Washington, DC: American Psychiatric Association.
3. Bennett, E. G., & Woolf, D. (1991). *Substance abuse* (2nd ed.). Albany, NY: Delmar.
4. Blum, K., et al. (1990). Allelic association of human dopamine D2 receptor gene in alcoholism. *Journal of the American Medical Association, 15*(263), 2055–2060.
5. Bond, A., et al. (1994). Systemic absorption and abuse liability of snorted flunitrazepam. *Addiction, 89*(7), 821–830.
6. Burns, E. M., Thompson, A., & Ciccone, J. K. (1993). *An addictions curriculum for nurses and other helping professionals* (vol 2). New York: Springer-Verlag.
7. Cocaine withdrawal. (1987). *Emergency Medicine, 19*(8), 65.
8. Copel, L. C. (1996). *Nurses' clinical guide to psychiatric/mental health nursing.* Springhouse, PA: Springhouse.
9. Ewing, J. A. (1984). CAGE. *Journal of the American Medical Association, 252*(14), 1906.
10. Fleming, M. F., & Barry, K. L. (1992). *Addictive disorders.* St. Louis: Mosby–Year Book.
11. Freeman, E. M. (Ed.). (1993). *Substance abuse treatment: A family systems perspective.* Newbury, CA: Sage.
12. Galanter, M., & Kleber, H. D. (1994). *Textbook of substance abuse treatment.* Washington, DC: American Psychiatric Press.
13. Gold, M. S., & Gianini, A. J. (1989). Cocaine and cocaine addiction. In A. J. Gianini & A. E. Slaby (Eds.), *Drugs of abuse* (pp. 83–96). Oradell, NJ: Medical Economics Books.
14. Goldstein, A. (1994). *Addiction: From biology to drug policy.* New York: W. H. Freeman.
15. Goodwin, D. W. (1985). Alcoholism and genetics: The sins of the fathers. *Archives of General Psychiatry, 42,* 57–61.
16. Green, P. (1989). The chemically dependent nurse. *Nursing Clinics of North America, 24*(1), 81–94.
17. Henly, G. A., & Winters, K. C. (1988). Development of problem severity scales for the assessment of adolescent alcohol and drug abuse. *International Journal of the Addictions, 23,* 65–85.
18. Horn, J. L., et al. (1984). *Alcohol use questionnaire (AUQ).* Toronto, Ont.: Addiction Research Foundation.
19. Jaffe, J. H. (1990). Drug addiction and drug abuse. In A. G. Gilman, A. S. Nies, & L. P. Taylor (Eds.), *Goodman and Gilman's: The pharmacological basis of therapeutics* (pp. 522–573). New York: Macmillan.
20. Jefferson, L. V. (1995). Chemically mediated responses and substance-related disorders. In G. W. Stuart & S. J. Sundeen (Eds.), *Principles and practices of psychiatric nursing* (pp. 569–605). St. Louis: Mosby–Year Book.
21. Keller, C. M. (1994). Flumazenil: A new benzodiazepine-specific antagonist. *Journal of the American Academy of Physicians Assistants, 7*(8), 595–598.
22. Kim, M. J., McFarland, G. K., & McLane, A. M. (1993). *Pocket guide to nursing diagnoses.* St. Louis: Mosby–Year Book.
23. Klahr, A. L., Roehrich, H. G., & Miller, N. S. (1989). Marijuana. In A. J. Gianini & A. E. Slaby (Eds.), *Drugs of abuse* (pp. 97–126). Oradell, NJ: Medical Economics Books.
24. Lachman, V. D. (1988). The chemically dependent nurse. *Holistic Nursing Practice, 2*(4), 34–45.
25. Lader, M. (1994). Anxiolytic drugs: Dependence, addiction, and abuse. *European Neuropsychopharmacology, 4*(2), 85–91.
26. Marx, J. (1990). Marijuana receptor gene cloned. *Science, 249,* 624–626.
27. McLellan, A. T., et al. (1992). The fifth edition of the addiction severity index. *Journal of Substance Abuse Treatment, 9*(3), 199–213.
28. Monheit, D., & Cursillo, R. (October 19, 1995). Personal communication.
29. Murphy, S. A. (1988). Addiction nursing: An agenda for the 1990s. *Issues in Mental Health Nursing, 9*(2), 115–126.

30. Nace, E. P., & Isbell, P. I. (1991). Alcohol. In R. J. Frances & S. I. Miller (Eds.), *Clinical textbook of addictive disorders* (pp. 43–68). New York: Guildford Press.

31. Naranjo, C. A., Sellers, E. M., & Chater, M. (1983). Nonpharmacologic intervention in acute alcohol withdrawal. *Clinical Pharmacology and Therapeutics, 34,* 814–819.

32. National Institute on Alcohol Abuse and Alcoholism. (1984). *Alcohol abuse curriculum guide for nurse practitioner faculty* (vol. 3). DHHS Publication No. ADM 84-1313. Rockville, MD: Health Professions Education Curriculum Resources Series.

33. National Institute on Alcohol Abuse and Alcoholism. (1990). *Seventh special report to the U.S. Congress on alcohol and health: From the secretary of health and human services.* DHHS Publication No. ADM 90-1656. Rockville, MD: U.S. Department of Health and Human Services.

34. National Institute on Drug Abuse. (1991). *National household survey on drug abuse: Population estimates 1991.* DHHS Publication No. ADM 92-1887. Rockville, MD: U.S. Department of Health and Human Services, National Institute of Drug Abuse.

35. Naegle, M. A. (1988). Theoretical perspectives on the etiology of substance abuse. *Holistic Nursing Practice, 2*(4), 1–13.

36. Peele, S. (1986). The implications and limitations of genetic models of alcoholism and other addictions. *Journal of Studies on Alcohol, 47,* 63–73.

37. Peele, S. (Ed.). (1988). *Visions of addiction: Major contemporary perspectives on addiction and alcoholism.* Lexington, MA: Lexington Books.

38. Pokorney, A. D., Miller, B. A., & Kaplan, H. B. (1992). The brief MAST: A shortened version of the Michigan Alcoholism Screening Test. *American Journal of Psychiatry, 129,* 342–348.

39. Ritz, M. C., et al. (1987). Cocaine receptors on dopamine transporters are related to self-administration of cocaine. *Science, 237,* 1219–1223.

40. Schuckit, M. A. (1986). Alcohol and alcoholism. In E. Braunwald, K. J. Isselbacher, & R. G. Petersdorf (Eds.), *Harrison's principles of internal medicine* (11th ed.). New York: McGraw-Hill.

41. Schuckit, M. A. (1989). *Drug and alcohol abuse.* New York: Plenum Medical Book Co.

42. Selzer, M. L. (1971). The Michigan Alcoholism Screening test: The quest for a new diagnostic instrument. *American Journal of Psychiatry, 127,* 1653–1658.

43. Selzer, M., Vinokur, A., & van Roojan, L. (1975). A self-administered short alcohol screening test (SMAST). *Journal of Studies on Alcoholism, 36*(1), 86.

44. Shaw, J. M., Kleeson, G. S., & Sellers, E. M. (1981). Development of optimal treatment tactics for alcohol withdrawal: Assessment and effectiveness of supportive care. *Journal of Clinical Psychopharmacology, 1,* 382–389.

45. Skerjl, R. (November 11, 1995). Personal communication.

46. Skinner, H. A., & Horn, J. L. (1984). *Alcohol Dependence Scale (ADS): User's guide.* Toronto, Ont.: Addiction Research Foundation.

47. Smith, D. E., Wesson, D. R., & Calhoun, S. R. (1995). *Rohypnol (flunitrazepam) fact sheet.* (Available from the Haight-Ashbury Free Clinics, Inc., 409 Clayton Street, San Francisco, CA 94117.)

48. Sokol, R. J., Martier, S. S., & Ager, J. W. (1989). The T-ACE questions: Practical prenatal detection of risk-drinking. *American Journal of Obstetrics and Gynecology, 160,* 863–870.

49. Sue, D. (1987). Use and abuse of alcohol by Asian Americans. *Journal of Psychoactive Drugs, 19,* 57.

50. Swenson, W., & Morse, R. (1973). The use of self-administered alcoholism screening test (SAAST) in a medical center. *Mayo Clinic Proceedings, 50,* 204–208.

51. Sullivan, E. J. (1991). Impaired health care professionals. In G. Bennett & D. S. Woolf (Eds.). *Substance abuse: Pharmacologic, developmental, and clinical perspectives* (2nd. ed., pp. 293–304). Albany, NY: Delmar Publishers.

52. Tarter, R. E., Alterman, A. I., & Edwards, K. L. (1985). Vulnerability to alcoholism in men: A behavioral-genetic perspective. *Journal of Studies on Alcohol, 46,* 329–356.

53. Trinkoff, A. M., Eaton, W. W., & Anthony, J. C. (1991). The prevalence of substance abuse among registered nurses. *Nursing Research, 40*(3), 172–175.

54. Whitfield, C. L., Thompson, G., & Lamb, A. (1978). Detoxication of 1,024 alcoholic patients without psychoactive drugs. *Journal of the American Medical Association, 17*(239), 1409–1411.

55. Williams, E. (1989). Strategies for intervention. *Nursing Clinics of North America, 24*(1), 109–120.

Basic Concepts of Emergency Care

Linda Lorraine Armstrong Lazure
Jean Elizabeth DeMartinis

CHAPTER 88

An emergency is any sudden illness or injury that is perceived to be a crisis threatening the physical or psychological well-being of a person or group. This serious situation may be the result of an accident, a medical condition, or a natural disaster that requires immediate intervention. The emergency continues until the condition is stable or no longer threatens the client's well-being. Emergency situations can occur anywhere, such as the community, emergency department, and even on nursing units. Therefore, it is important for all nurses to have the basic knowledge and skills needed for rapid assessment, intervention, and safe management of emergencies.

Improvements in prehospital care, in emergency medical systems, and in transport to regional trauma systems, together with advances in medical and nursing management of clients in emergency situations, have led to increased survival.[4, 29] Quick and competent emergency care is the key to rapid stability, prevention of complications, and early recovery.

Emergency nursing requires a broad knowledge base to provide safe and competent care to clients with a variety of conditions. Nurses must make rapid and sound assessments regarding clients' physiologic responses and psychosocial behaviors. They must be adept in crisis intervention, communication, triage, trauma care, and be able to provide care in uncontrolled or unpredictable environments.

More than 80% of clients who seek emergency care do not have life-threatening problems. These clients are often diagnosed, treated, and then discharged from further care in the emergency department. Therefore, teaching clients about their diagnosis and treatment during the discharge process is a major nursing role. Many emergency departments provide written instructions as well as verbal teaching. Clients and/or family members should know what has been done, what follow-up care is necessary, and what should be done if the condition worsens. Never assume a client or family member will remember verbal instructions. Write everything down.

For many, the emergency department may be the usual source of healthcare, and emergency nurses may be the only contact the client has with the healthcare system. Nurses must be aware of clients who frequently return to the emergency department. These clients may have special health needs, have exacerbations of chronic conditions, be victims of abuse, have no primary healthcare provider, or have little or no health insurance. Research has shown that clients use emergency departments because they perceive their symptoms as serious, and emergency departments are viewed as faster and more convenient than clinics.[2] Until permanent solutions to overcrowding are found, it is important that healthcare professionals be nonjudgmental and do not refuse care to any client.[3, 18]

Recently, private insurance companies and managed care consortiums have imposed stringent criteria regarding payment for emergency department visits. Clients may be required to call their physicians for approval of the visit before arriving at the emergency department to ensure payment of the incurred expenses.

Ethical and Legal Considerations

Consent to Treatment

Informed consent to treatment means that clients are apprised of all treatments and procedures and agree to these before implementation. So the client understands the implications of any treatments, the information must be presented in a language in which the client is fluent and at an appropriate level. In general, clients should be informed each time a procedure is done for them.[7] By being informed, clients also have the right to refuse any treatments or procedures before they are implemented.

This chapter incorporates material written for the fourth edition by Lisa L. Strohmyer.

However, informed consent is valid only if the client is of "adult years and sound mind." Not all adult clients are capable of giving informed consent. Clients with emergencies may be hypoxic or intoxicated or have an altered level of consciousness.[8, 25]

When a client is unable to give consent or is unconscious, emergency treatment can be provided under the emergency doctrine. As the Ethical Issues in Nursing feature explains, this doctrine implies that the client would have consented to treatment if able, because the alternative would have been death or disability. The emergency doctrine removes the need for obtaining informed consent before emergency treatment and care are initiated.

Right to Privacy and Confidentiality

All clients have a right to privacy, and clients with emergencies are no different. This right includes the need for consent to use names and photographs of the client, not allowing unauthorized persons into the client's hospital area, and not disclosing private facts to the public or falsely representing the client to the public. Information about the client's condition, treatments, and outcomes is to be respected and handled with discretion. Any communication about the client's condition, treatments, and documentation are confidential and disclosed only with the client's permission.

Mandatory Reporting

Mandatory reporting laws require hospitals, nurses, and physicians to notify the appropriate local, state, or federal agency when certain conditions or incidents occur. These include child, spouse, or elder abuse; motor vehicle crashes; injuries resulting from violence; attempted suicides; animal bites; overdoses; and poisonings. Certain communicable disorders, such as meningitis, sexually transmitted diseases, and food poisonings, are also reportable to the state health department. When injuries are suspected or identified, the nurse must notify the physician in charge of the care and other individuals identified by hospital policy. The appropriate agency must be notified and a report filed.

Physical Evidence and Chain of Custody

Meticulous documentation and handling of evidence are of particular concern in situations in which injury resulted from a violent crime, such as a shooting or sexual assault. All evidence discovered during the examination is recorded. Documentation of samples includes the bodily location from which the sample was obtained and when and to whom it was delivered.

Evidence should be maintained in its original condition. Clothing is stored in a paper bag instead of plastic to prevent decomposition. If clothing needs to be cut off the client, special attention is taken not to destroy evidence inadvertently.

ETHICAL ISSUES IN NURSING

Are Emergency Personnel Obliged to Honor Clients' Advance Directives?

During emergency situations, clients and their significant others parallel the healthcare team's treatment goal, that is, survival. Once this goal is achieved, the true reality of each situation is often painful and tentative at best. How should a client whose condition may be reduced to a persistent vegetative state be treated medically? Can family members who feel their loved one would not want to continue living in such a physical state decide to discontinue treatment?

It is universally accepted that emergency care workers have a duty to assist those in need in whatever capacity is appropriate for stabilizing the condition. However, several well-known court cases have spawned legislation regarding the client's right to direct the care for certain treatments or situations. The Patient Self-Determination Act (PSDA) was enacted as part of the Omnibus Budget Reconciliation Act (OBRM) of 1990. It mandated that all adult clients entering hospitals, home health agencies, skilled nursing facilities, and hospice programs be provided, on admission, written information about clients' rights to accept or refuse medical or surgical treatment and the right to formulate advance directives. As defined in this law, "advance directives" are written instructions (a living will or directions obtained from a durable power of attorney for health care) recognized under state law relative to the provision of care when an individual is incapacitated. The law was intended to increase people's awareness of organ/tissue donation and their rights to make decisions about life-sustaining measures.

What about emergency cases for which such information may not be available? In the absence of an advance directive, emergency clients will be treated in the same fashion, that is, an attempt will be made to stabilize their condition. After the condition is stabilized and a definitive diagnosis is made, an advance directive is useful in guiding care decisions. When clients seek help from emergency personnel, the personnel assume an obligation to assist them. All personnel who work in such settings need to be familiar with the institutional and state policies on advance directives.

Bullets

Bullets removed from a client's body or recovered from clothing are handled with great care. When a bullet is removed, the physician usually makes a mark on the bottom of the bullet. This identifying mark may be referred to later during an investigation or trial. The bullet is then placed in a sealed bag, labeled, and given to proper authorities. The bag is sealed so that removal of the seal will be obvious. If a bullet is kept in the emergency department for any reason, it is kept in a locked, secure place. All persons having access to the bullet must sign for it; thus, a chain of custody is maintained. This information is included on the medical record.

Specimens

Specimens obtained for legal purposes, as opposed to clinical purposes, include blood samples for determination of blood alcohol levels and items obtained during the examination of an alleged sexual assault victim. When a blood alcohol determination is desired by either the client or legal authorities, the client's written permission must be obtained before the specimen is drawn. No client may be forced into having a blood sample drawn. In many instances, police officers have a kit with the necessary equipment for drawing the specimen. Isopropyl alcohol or any antiseptic solution containing alcohol must not be used as a skin preparation before a blood alcohol specimen is drawn. These agents may falsely elevate the blood alcohol level and render the test invalid. The nurse must know the laws within the state that identify who may draw blood for alcohol level determinations.

Once the specimen is drawn, it is handed to a police officer, who signs a document that indicates that the specimen has been received. The tube is sealed, and an identifying mark is placed on the seal. The chain of custody is similar to that for bullets. Documentation of the procedure on the client's clinical record, along with the nurse's signature and the name and badge number of the officer, is important.

Laws Governing Client Transfer

Federal laws, the 1986 Consolidated Omnibus Budget Reconciliation Act (COBRA) and 1990 Omnibus Budget Reconciliation Act (OBRA), have been passed in response to inappropriate client transfers and denial of care. Provisions of the COBRA/OBRA legislation require treatment for all clients with emergency conditions and pregnant women with active contractions, regardless of ability to pay. This includes an appropriate medical screening examination, necessary stabilizing treatments, and appropriate transfer to another facility with consent, if indicated. It is important for emergency nurses to be aware of the hospital guidelines and transfer protocols. Nurses can be active client advocates and ensure that clients receive necessary emergency treatments. Failure to comply with COBRA/OBRA legislation may result in substantial fines and penalties.[3, 27, 29]

Emergency Nursing Care

The Emergency Nurses Association defines emergency nursing care as the "assessment, diagnosis and treatment of perceived, actual or potential, sudden or urgent, physical or psychosocial problems that are primarily episodic or acute. These may require minimal care or life-support measures, client and significant other education, appropriate referral and knowledge of legal limitations."[11]

Initial Nursing Assessment

On first being confronted with a seriously ill or injured client, gain as much information as quickly as possible. The initial impression is important for early identification and intervention of life-threatening clinical manifestations (Box 88–1). Historical information provides clues to the urgency of the situation and treatment priorities. Client management consists of a brief history and primary assessment, resuscitation of vital functions, a thorough secondary assessment, and definitive care. Age and cultural differences should be considered when approaching and examining clients.

The history provides clues to the priority assessments and interventions. A history should include information about when and where the emergency occurred, what has been done, and whether the client has any known health problems, such as hypertension or diabetes. One way to remember the required information is through the mnemonic AMPLE:

A—Allergies
M—Medications currently prescribed or being used
P—Past medical and surgical history
L—Last meal
E—Events preceding the emergency and any care rendered

Another mnemonic, PQRST, may also aid in remembering the essential elements of the health history as it relates to the clinical manifestations of the presenting problem.[5, 14]

P—Problem, pain; provocation of current illness
Q—Quality
R—Region, radiates
S—Signs, symptoms; severity
T—Time of onset, duration

Box 88–1. Assessment Findings Implying a High Priority for Care

Significant alteration in vital signs (e.g., hypotension or hypertension, hypothermia or hyperthermia, cardiac dysrhythmias, respiratory distress)
Altered level of consciousness
Chest pain, especially in clients older than 35 years
Severe pain
Bleeding not controlled by direct pressure
Conditions that will worsen from delay in treatment (e.g., chemical burns, drug or toxic substance ingestion, allergic reaction, impaled objects)
Sudden vision loss
Dangerous, aberrant, or disruptive behavior
Psychologically devastating conditions (e.g., sexual assault, death or near-death of a loved one)
Elderly or very young client
Symptom that is vague but causes the triage officer (emergency assessor) concern

Table 88–1. Triage Categories

Category	Definition	Emergency Examples
Emergent	Life-threatening emergency Usually involves the ABCs The client may die without immediate intervention	Airway obstruction, cardiac arrest, chest pain with dyspnea or cyanosis, shock, coma, open chest wounds, sudden vision loss, psychologically devastating conditions, cerebrovascular accident, sudden paralysis
Urgent	Emergencies that require intervention within a few hours	Intraperitoneal bleeding, severe pain, persistent nausea, vomiting, diarrhea, or sudden changes in speech
Nonurgent	Not life-threatening Interventions may be delayed beyond a few hours	Soft tissue injuries, surface trauma, extremity fractures without circulatory compromise

Establishing Priorities: Triage

The goal of emergency care is prompt, effective resuscitation and stabilization of critically ill or injured clients. The process of determining priorities of client care, directing the client to the most appropriate care source, and providing prompt and timely emergency care is called *triage*.

Triage ensures that clients who require immediate attention for life-threatening emergencies receive it. Although triage categories may vary, three common categories are emergent, urgent, and nonurgent (Table 88–1). Because a complete assessment is difficult to do, it is wise to err on the side of assigning a higher triage priority than a lower one. Clients may have other injuries that were not initially assessed. It is important to reassess those waiting for care and to change priorities as needed.

The use of experienced emergency nurses in triage provides safe, efficient, and cost-effective care. An effective triage nurse possesses three critical qualities: expert assessment skills, nonjudgmental communication and interviewing techniques, and organizational skills to regulate control of traffic flow into the treatment areas.[25, 28]

Many clients enter the emergency department in a state of crisis. Therefore, the triage nurse must be knowledgeable about common responses to crises and be able to react quickly and in a calm manner. The ability of the triage nurse to assess, intervene, and communicate effectively helps to establish rapport and trust with the client and significant others.

Telephone triage occurs when a client calls the emergency department for help with a crisis, in an emergency situation, or for healthcare advice. Despite the advent of crisis lines and emergency 911 numbers, many callers contact the emergency department first. This places nurses who perform telephone triage in a "first-responder" position. Many physician's offices and health maintenance organizations (HMOs) have been practicing telephone triage. Ideally, telephone triage should be conducted with safeguards for proper documentation, training, standards, protocols, and adequate staff. Specially trained emergency department RNs should be responsible for telephone triage and can be assisted by sophisticated computer soft-

ware packages. Telephone triage incorporates eight important points, enumerated in Box 88–2.

Documentation

Documentation of assessments, interventions, and client responses is essential. Because time is often limited, preprinted flow sheets that contain key assessment and intervention areas are frequently used. During life-threatening

---

Box 88–2. Telephone Triage

Telephone triage includes the following eight important points:

1. With all crisis levels, when possible, stay on the line with the caller while contacting 911. A model telephone triage system includes a crisis team interface, standard documentation forms, conference call capabilities, direct lines, and call tracing capabilities.
2. Beware of caller noncompliance. The nurse could use one of two strategies, depending on the severity of the call: dial 911 directly, or make a verbal contract with the caller to an agreed-on course of action.
3. Develop crisis intervention "crash cards." These would contain developed action protocols or treatments modeled after medical dispatcher instructions.
4. Develop protocols for a suicide in progress or suicidal threats.
5. In a crisis, expect impaired judgment. The nurse needs to remain calm and coach the caller in first aid or actions that the caller can perform, such as opening the door for arriving paramedics.
6. Believe it when the caller says it is an emergency.
7. Get complete information. Preprinted checklists can help accomplish the baseline data collection.
8. Always err on the side of caution.

Data from Wheeler S. Q. (1989). ED telephone triage: Lessons learned form unusual calls. *Journal of Emergency Nursing, 15*(6), 401–407; and Tipsord-Klinkhammer, B., & Noska, A. R. (1966). Telephone triage: An ED alternative? *The Nursing Spectrum, 9*(6),4.

situations, critical data may be recorded on a communication board mounted on the treatment room wall, so that all members of the team are able to visualize important data rapidly. Information typically written on the communication board may include initial and subsequent vital signs, coma score, trauma score, laboratory and other diagnostic studies ordered/completed, team members, intravenous fluids/blood administered, urine output, and whether significant others were notified or present. Ideally, one person is responsible for documentation.

Computer use can simplify obtaining data about the client's history, including previous hospital admissions and treatment regimens. Various software programs can be used to supplement diagnostic and treatment protocols.

Discharge teaching sheets can be generated and individualized quickly and completely.

Priority Nursing Interventions

Airway Patency

Airway obstruction commonly is caused by the tongue and foreign bodies, such as food (e.g., "a cafe coronary"), teeth, bone fragments, or blood clots. In a conscious client, assist the client to remove the obstruction by initiating an abdominal thrust. Figure 88–1 illustrates thrust techniques for unconscious clients.

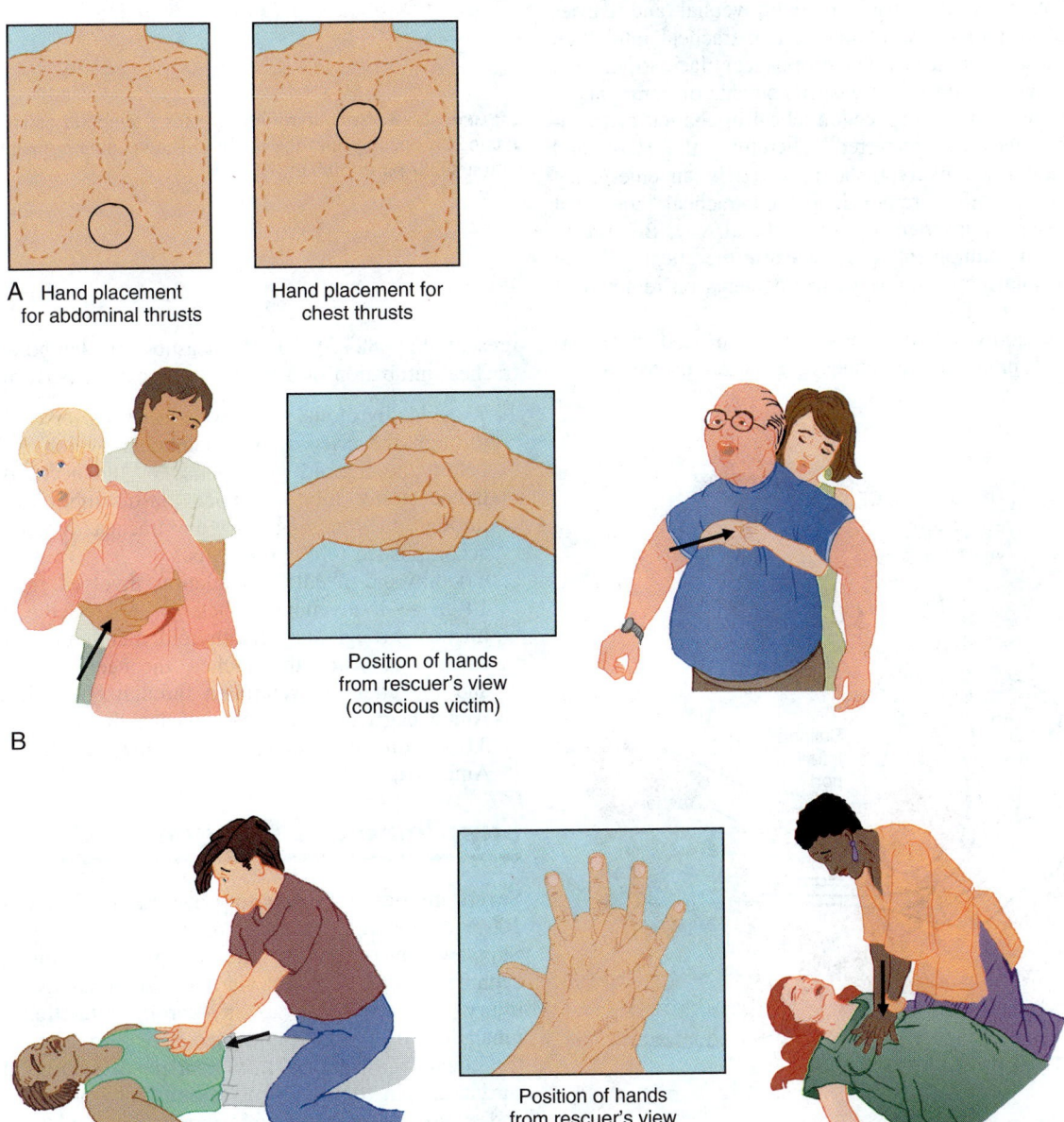

A Hand placement for abdominal thrusts

Hand placement for chest thrusts

B

Position of hands from rescuer's view (conscious victim)

C

Position of hands from rescuer's view (unconscious victim)

Figure 88–1. The Heimlich maneuver, which is used for removal of foreign bodies that are blocking the upper airway. Vigorous upward chest or abdominal thrusts produce a rush of air that expels the foreign body. The abdominal thrust is the original Heimlich maneuver. The chest thrust is an adaptation that is useful for obese or pregnant victims. Use four quick thrusts in the positions shown. *A,* Hand placement. *B,* The Heimlich maneuver for conscious victims. *C,* The Heimlich maneuver for unconscious victims.

If the airway is open but the client is not breathing, begin rescue breathing (see cardiopulmonary resuscitation [CPR], Chapter 45). Watch for the chest to rise and fall, which indicates that the airway is open. Various artificial airways are used when the airway is not patent or is inadequate (see Chapter 41). A nasopharyngeal airway can be inserted if the client is semiconscious; an oropharyngeal airway is used if the client is unconscious and without a gag reflex. Additional airway adjuncts for unconscious clients older than 15 years include an esophageal obturator airway (EOA) (Fig. 88–2) and an esophageal gastric tube airway (EGTA), which is a modification of the EOA with a port for a nasogastric tube. These two airways are used as temporary measures until endotracheal intubation or tracheotomy can be performed. The use of esophageal airways is controversial and carries potential complications of inadvertent tracheal intubation with subsequent asphyxia, esophageal laceration, and vomiting and aspiration of gastric contents on removal.

In the hospital setting, endotracheal intubation or tracheostomy tubes are preferred. Therefore, the EOA and EGTA are more likely to be removed in an emergency department.[5] Before removal, an endotracheal tube must be successfully inserted to protect the airway. Be sure to have suction equipment ready, because the client is likely to vomit and may aspirate gastric contents on removal of the EOA or EGTA.

Two cricothyroidotomy procedures are used when endotracheal intubation is impossible or an obstruction is

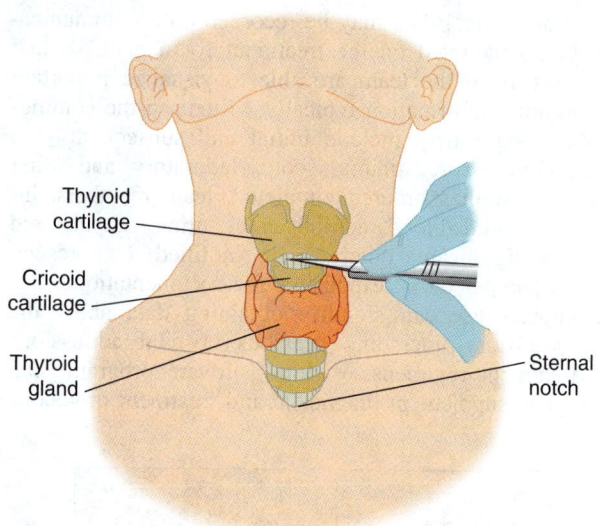

Figure 88–3. Cricothyrotomy creates a temporary airway by making an opening into the trachea. The opening is maintained with a small plastic tube.

present (Fig. 88–3).[16] Both measures are temporary until tracheal intubation or a tracheotomy can be performed:

1. A cricothyrotomy involves a transverse incision through the cricothyroid membrane, which is located below the thyroid prominence of the neck. A small tracheostomy tube or other plastic tube is inserted through the opening into the trachea. Ventilation is accomplished through the tube.
2. Cricothyroid needle cannulation involves inserting a 14-gauge intravenous catheter with a needle into the trachea through the cricothyroid membrane. Once the catheter is inside the trachea, the needle is removed, and the client is ventilated through the catheter. An Ambu bag can be used by placing the adaptor from a 3.0 endotracheal tube between the catheter and the Ambu bag.

Supplemental Oxygen

Severe injuries and respiratory distress indicate a need for 100% oxygen for treatment of any resultant hypoxemia. Supplemental oxygen is initiated up to 5 L/min by nasal cannula or 6 to 10 L/min via mask in situations of severe injury or stress, such as myocardial infarction, smoke inhalation, or shock. Supplemental oxygen is provided if the client has chest pain, clinical manifestations of poor cardiac output (decreased pulse and blood pressure), signs and symptoms of hypoxemia (confusion, anxiety, or restlessness), profuse bleeding, or nausea. Although noninvasive oxygen monitoring, such as pulse oximetry, is widely used, it should be remembered that accuracy decreases in the presence of widespread peripheral vasoconstriction, severe blood and fluid loss, and increased amounts of carboxyhemoglobin.[16]

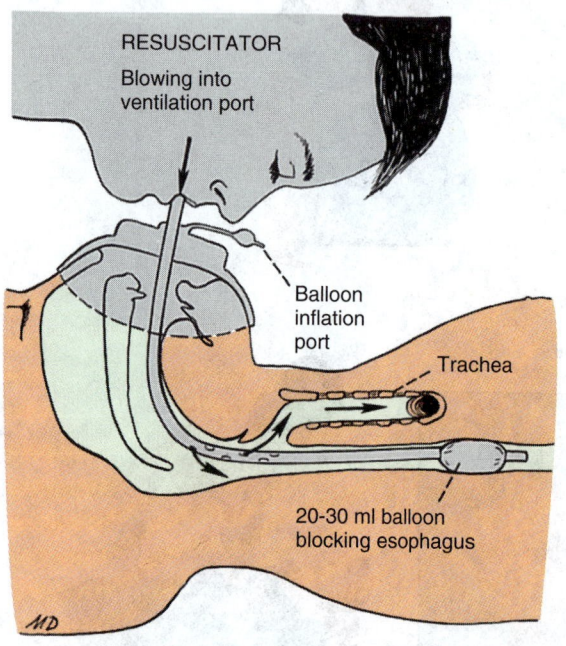

Figure 88–2. The esophageal obturator airway, a ventilatory device used for resuscitation in emergencies. The face mask anchors the airway and seals off the client's mouth and nose. The lungs are ventilated via openings in the flexible tube at the level of the pharynx. The risk of aspiration of gastric contents is minimized by the inflated balloon at the distal end of the tube, which blocks the esophagus.

Spinal Precautions and Immobilization

In a client with a decreased level of consciousness and a history of traumatic injury (or in whom a potential for traumatic injury is suspected), the spinal column is immobilized to prevent neurologic injury. The ideal precaution for spinal immobilization includes a cervical collar, two rolled towels or intravenous bags, or a head immobilizer placed on each side of the head and taped securely across the forehead onto a long backboard (Fig. 88–4).[19, 30]

Cardiopulmonary Resuscitation

If the client is not breathing and has no pulse, begin CPR (see Chapter 45). CPR aids in perfusing the tissues. Keep in mind that the client needs to have enough blood volume to circulate with CPR. If the client is bleeding profusely, large-bore intravenous lines need to be inserted immediately to restore intravascular fluid volume with fluids or blood products. Remember not to hyperextend the neck if a cervical spinal injury is suspected.[2]

Brief Neurologic Examination

After the *a*irway, *b*reathing, and *c*irculation (ABCs) are stabilized, conduct a brief neurologic assessment. Observe the client's general appearance, mental status, and orientation. Make note of any eye opening, verbal, and motor responses to verbal, tactile, and noxious stimuli. Observe for any posturing and spastic or flaccid extremities. Assess for abnormal breath or body odors (e.g., alcohol, gasoline, chemicals, urine, or feces), facial expressions, tremors, asymmetry, or obvious deformities.[7, 13, 19, 29]

One of the most common clinical manifestations of an emergency is pain. Acute pain may result from soft tissue injury, ischemia, or peripheral nerve damage, such as in a crush injury or compartment syndrome. Perform a symptom analysis. The mnemonic PQRST, presented earlier, may be used to elicit a more complete picture of the client's perception of the pain experience. Because pain is a subjective response, therapy must be individualized.[24, 32]

Any loss of sensation should be further assessed. It may be the result of spinal cord injury and spinal shock, cerebral hemorrhage, or neurovascular compromise.

Secondary Nursing Assessment

The secondary assessment involves a complete head-to-toe assessment guided by the client's chief complaint.[5] Objective physical assessments are performed (Fig. 88–5), concentrating on areas relating to the client's chief complaint. Keep in mind that not all of the assessment procedures are performed on every client with an emergency, but these are a guideline for establishing priorities. For instance, in a client with a migraine headache, an abdominal assessment is inappropriate. However, if the client complains of vague shoulder pain, an abdominal

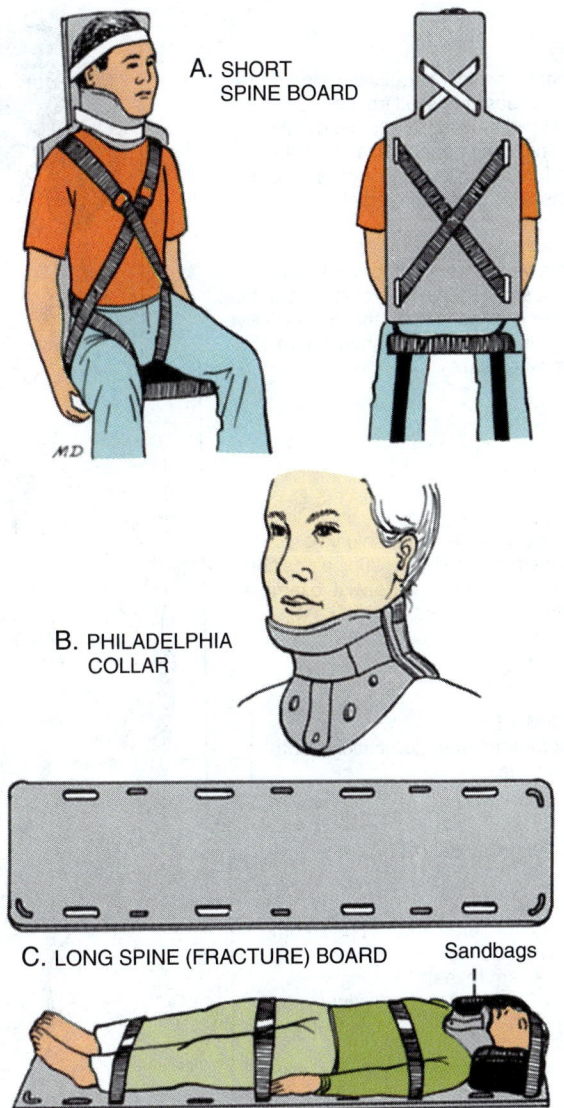

Figure 88–4. Spine immobilization devices. *A,* The short spine board is applied to a client who is seated (e.g., in an automobile) and is applied, along with a cervical collar, before extrication from the vehicle. *B,* The Philadelphia collar is a two-piece, hard, molded plastic device that can be applied without manipulating the neck and provides good immobilization of the cervical spine. *C,* The long spine (fracture) board is made of wood and contains cut-out sections along the sides for securing restraining straps and for lifting the injured client.

assessment is appropriate for ruling out referred pain, such as occurs with gallbladder disease.

Discharge Teaching

Because of the short time of the interaction, teaching conducted by emergency nurses must be specific to the client's most pressing problems. Emphasis is placed on return demonstration or verbal understanding. Information includes recognizing the most likely or significant complication, how and when to obtain follow-up care, and what to do if complications occur. A discharge instruction

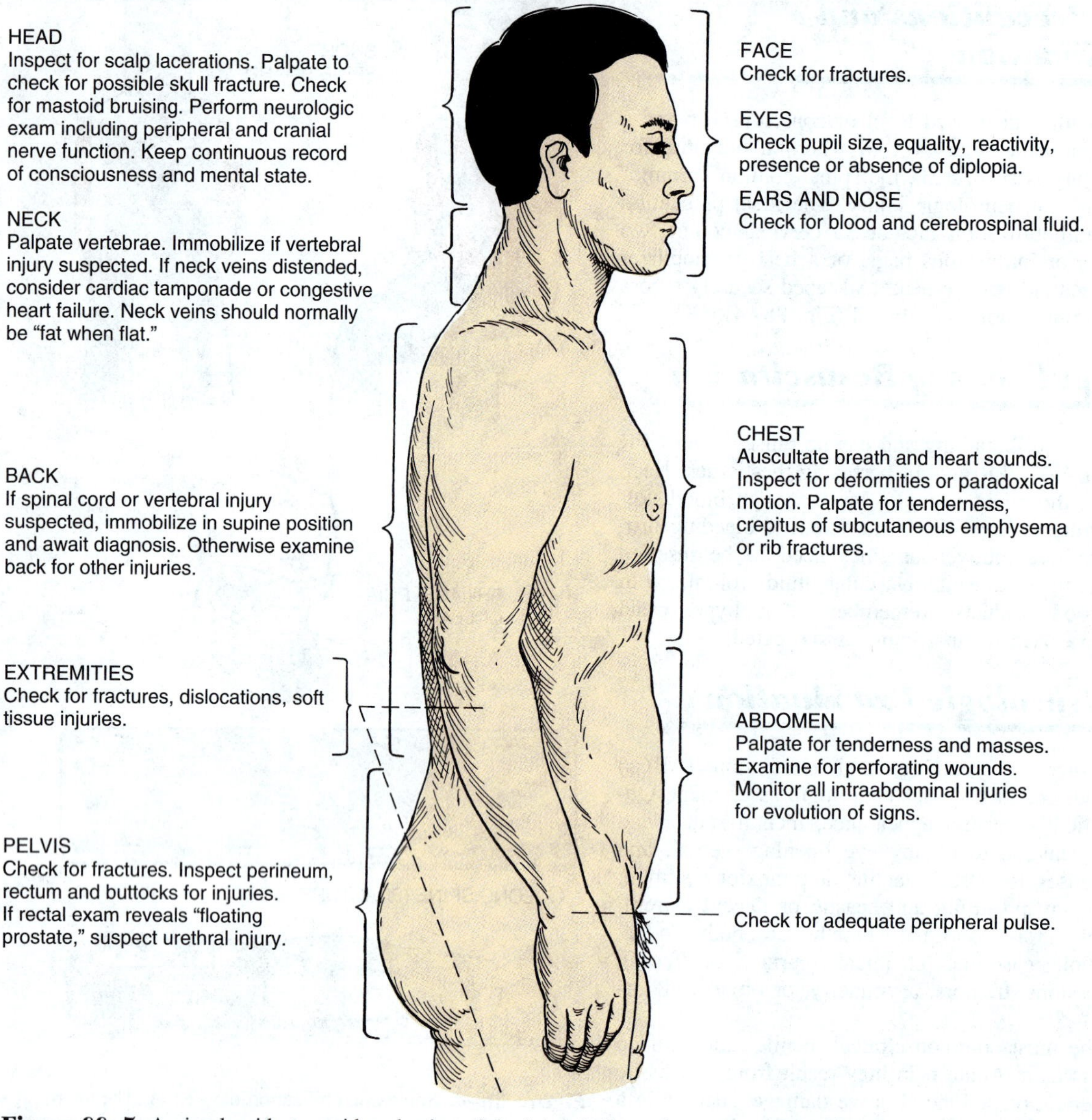

HEAD
Inspect for scalp lacerations. Palpate to check for possible skull fracture. Check for mastoid bruising. Perform neurologic exam including peripheral and cranial nerve function. Keep continuous record of consciousness and mental state.

NECK
Palpate vertebrae. Immobilize if vertebral injury suspected. If neck veins distended, consider cardiac tamponade or congestive heart failure. Neck veins should normally be "fat when flat."

BACK
If spinal cord or vertebral injury suspected, immobilize in supine position and await diagnosis. Otherwise examine back for other injuries.

EXTREMITIES
Check for fractures, dislocations, soft tissue injuries.

PELVIS
Check for fractures. Inspect perineum, rectum and buttocks for injuries. If rectal exam reveals "floating prostate," suspect urethral injury.

FACE
Check for fractures.

EYES
Check pupil size, equality, reactivity, presence or absence of diplopia.

EARS AND NOSE
Check for blood and cerebrospinal fluid.

CHEST
Auscultate breath and heart sounds. Inspect for deformities or paradoxical motion. Palpate for tenderness, crepitus of subcutaneous emphysema or rib fractures.

ABDOMEN
Palpate for tenderness and masses. Examine for perforating wounds. Monitor all intraabdominal injuries for evolution of signs.

Check for adequate peripheral pulse.

Figure 88–5. A visual guide to rapid evaluation of the injured client after the immediate treatment priorities have been covered. After the initial examination, monitor the client's state of consciousness and vital signs frequently while x-rays are taken and laboratory studies are performed.

sheet reinforcing this information is given to the client or significant other at discharge, and teaching is documented on the emergency record.[6]

Psychosocial Needs in Emergencies

The psychosocial needs of clients and significant others vary widely during an emergency. A number of factors influence reactions to emergencies. Some of these factors include little or no time to prepare; little experience with the type of stressor; little or no guidance available for assuming an expected role; loss of control and feelings of helplessness; the amount of time spent in crisis and its on-again, off-again nature; the disruption to client and family roles, responsibilities, and routines; and the perceived danger to and emotional impact on the client and family.

Client reactions are unique. Common defense mechanisms and coping strategies include denial, regression, distraction, and rationalization. Some clients are anxious, fearful, and, occasionally, angry. Others experience loss of control, loss of individuality, and possible loss of dignity. Remember, all behavior is purposeful, and defense mechanisms help maintain psychological integrity. The mechanisms and strategies used are usually based on past experiences and previous coping styles.

Some behavioral responses may be related to the physiologic process of the emergency and should be considered. For example, anoxia can cause agitation, restlessness, and irritability. In addition, cognitive impairment

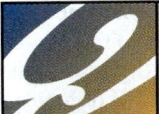

NURSING RESEARCH

How Should Violent Behavior in the Emergency Department Be Handled?

Emergency Nurses Association. (1994). *Prevalence of violence in emergency departments: Report by the ENA*. Park Ridge, IL: Author.

Societal violence has reached epidemic proportions and violence in the workplace is becoming more common. The emergency department, once thought of as only the endpoint for such violent acts, has been the locale for such assaults, particularly directed at healthcare workers. Previous studies have also speculated that such violence may be underreported because of a belief that such violence comes with the chaotic nature of emergency nursing or that reporting is too much of a bother.

The Emergency Nurses Association conducted a national survey to define violence within the workplace, identify factors contributing to that violence, and identify measures to prevent such violence and foster a safe work environment. Of the 4,600 surveys sent to emergency department nurse managers, 1,400 responded (30.4% return). Violence in the workplace was defined as follows:

- Verbal assaults, which included abusive language, profanity, stalking threats, obscene telephone calls, and threats of future injury
- Physical assault with weapons, such as guns, knives, homemade weapons, and tear gas spray
- Physical assault without weapons, including hitting, spitting, biting, kicking, pinching, and pulling hair

Based on the study definitions, 97% of the 1,400 respondents reported that emergency department staff were exposed to verbal abuse more that 20 times per year. Exposure to physical assault without weapons was reported by 87% of the respondents to occur one to five times per year, whereas 24% were exposed to physical assault with weapons one to five times per year.

Common contributing factors to the violence against emergency department staff included alcohol abuse, drug abuse, anger or high stress, open access to the emergency department, and psychiatric illness. These were consistent with previous research findings. Additional factors contributing to the emergency department violence were prolonged waiting times, gang-related activities, trauma, and staff-staff conflicts.

Although 97% of the managers indicated that they would report these violent incidents to appropriate personnel, 3% would not because violence was considered part of the job or the incident was not important enough to report. Safety measures to protect personnel had been initiated by 73% of the respondents' hospitals. Hospital security staff responded 42% of the time to restrain clients or visitors one to five times a month. However, 31% of the security officers had no formal training in handling a violent client, and only 19% had some form of self-defense training.

Implications for Practice

Emergency department nurses are exposed to a serious amount of verbal assault and violence. Both verbal and physical assault without weapons were considered common occurrences, and physical assault with weapons occurred with enough frequency to warrant concern for staff safety. Safety measures such as panic buttons, visitor control policies, locked entry mechanisms, video cameras, full-time security personnel, and protective glass are just a few of the physical structure changes taking place in emergency departments. Educational programs need to be developed to help staff identify, prevent, and address violent situations. Self-defense classes and appropriate techniques for "taking down" violent clients need to be taught to all personnel dealing with emergency clients and visitors.

---

and behavioral changes may result from head injury, trauma, substance ingestion, and metabolic disorders. Carefully assess behaviors and reactions, but always keep in mind the potential for physiologic effects.[24] The Nursing Research feature explores the problem of violent reactions in the emergency department.

The needs of significant others require special attention in emergency settings. Unless they accompanied the client to the emergency department, they may be notified by telephone. Advising significant others of the client's presence in the emergency setting by telephone requires tact and sensitivity. Exercise caution as you discuss the urgency of the situation. It is important to advise significant others to have someone else bring them to the hospital (Box 88–3).

Communicate to team members and make a note on the medical record about when significant others have been notified or whether they are present. It is important that the nurse providing the care periodically gives the significant others clear explanations regarding the client's condition, treatment, and progress using easily understood language. Significant others need to have opportunities to visit the client as appropriate. Before they visit, prepare significant others about the client's condition and appearance. Be sure to include the presence of tubes, equipment, bandages, and other devices. This is particularly important when there is disfigurement or loss of ability to communicate.

A private waiting area may help significant others cope with an emergency. The area should have a telephone,

Box 88–3. Summoning Family Members to Come to the Emergency Department

Giving the news of a client's death or critical condition over the telephone is difficult for staff (and for the person receiving the news). The following points help ensure that necessary information is given and obtained:

- Pre-establish definitions for *serious, critical, guarded,* and other terms, so all staff use the same terms. Use the same term consistently during conversation with family.
- Pre-establish a standardized format or protocol for making telephone notation.
- If you are providing care to the client, take a few moments to deal with your own feelings before making the call.
- Notify family members as soon as possible so they can begin anticipatory grieving.
- State your name, position, and work area and give institutional information.
- Do not give the bad news first; rather, present the facts chronologically. Begin with the onset of injury or illness, location of occurrence, prehospital treatment, treatment efforts rendered in the emergency department, and the client's response to treatment. By presenting the circumstances clearly, it is usually not necessary to say that a client has died. The family member usually asks. If you are asked directly if the client is dead, be honest. If the client is still alive, ask the family member if she or he understands the gravity of the prognosis.
- Clarify the client's condition if, in fact, it appears that survival is likely. Family members (in a state of emotional shock) may not process information well and may assume that the client is in worse condition than is the case.
- Present information in a factual way, asking for periodic feedback to make sure you are being understood.
- Prevent reckless driving by family members on their way to the hospital. Ask if you should notify someone else to bring them or anyone else to the hospital to serve as support. Ask the person you speak with to write down the instructions you give to reach the hospital and emergency department. Finally, ask the person to drive safely.
- If the family is coming, ask how soon they will be arriving and give them instructions about where to park. Give your name so they can ask for you on arrival. Notify the front desk personnel of the family's impending arrival.
- If death has already occurred, ask if the family members are coming to the emergency department or whether they would like to see their loved one. If they are not coming to the emergency department, discuss administrative details, such as funeral arrangements, medical examiner's cases, autopsy, handling of valuables, and the like. Ask about any special wishes regarding religious ceremonies, organ donation, or other arrangements.
- At the end of your call, repeat your name and telephone number. Ask the person you talk with to write it down so that any additional questions can be discussed. If death has occurred, encourage family members to call with any concerns. Unresolved issues or concerns impede the normal grieving process.

food, assorted beverages, comfortable chairs, current magazines, and nearby toilet facilities. A map on the wall showing the waiting area in relationship to the rest of the hospital helps orient people and provides direction (e.g., to the cafeteria).

Death and Dying in Emergency Settings

Unexpected death in the emergency department presents different problems to significant others and healthcare givers than expected death from a prolonged illness. There is often little time to interact with the dying client or to provide grief and loss counseling. Significant others may be overwhelmed by the suddenness of the event and feel there is not enough time to resolve "unfinished business" with the dying person.

Because there may not be much time before death actually takes place, make sure the dying client and significant others have ample opportunity to be together. Delay, if possible, procedures that will disrupt communication between the dying client and significant others, such as endotracheal intubation.

Allowing significant others to be present during resuscitation is not necessarily disruptive, as traditionally thought, and it can help survivors move through grief work in a less traumatic way. It can lessen their doubts about the loved one receiving the best care and it can involve them in decisions regarding termination of protracted and futile resuscitation measures.

Religious support can be extremely important for the client and significant others, and you should have a clear understanding of how to access that support.

The client's condition should be communicated to significant others periodically with clearly stated, factual information.

When telling the family about a death, use the following guidelines[1, 9, 20–22]:

- Designate a support person to stay with the family.
- Be aware of your appearance. Make sure your professional title and hospital affiliation are on your name badge and that your uniform is clean.
- Do not respond quickly to questions such as "Is he dead?" Get a sense of the environment. Sit down and introduce yourself. Make eye contact and use the client's name.
- Briefly relate the circumstances preceding the death. Explain what was done in the emergency department in terms that the family can understand. Then tell the family that resuscitation was not successful and the client is dead. If you use other terms such as "He is gone," you may have to reexplain or clarify. Remain silent after these statements so that the family has time to react to the news.
- Talk to the family about the events. Reassure them the client was not in pain (unless this is obviously not so).
- Avoid clichés.
- Express your sorrow for their loss, and scan the group for those who need further support.

- Encourage family members to view the body, particularly in instances of sudden death or trauma.
- Because preservation of legal evidence is often important in sudden death, advise significant others beforehand of the various tubes and devices present.
- Determine the client's wishes concerning organ donation. Required request laws (federal and state) facilitate this question because all hospitalized clients are asked about organ donation. Do not press for organ donation. The family may need to view the body and make arrangements for burial first.
- Assess the family's knowledge and level of understanding by using the open-ended statement, "Tell me what you know about the situation so far."
- A follow-up telephone call or visit may be beneficial in answering the questions or concerns of the significant others.
- Referral to a support group that assists survivors is often helpful. The healthcare facility or community social service agency can provide a list of the support groups in each area.
- Answer any questions about autopsy.

The Nursing Research feature suggests that such guidelines should be incorporated into basic and continuing education programs.

Organ Donation

The significant growth and development in the field of transplantation may be attributed, in part, to increased awareness on the part of public and healthcare professionals regarding organ donation, procurement, and transplantation. The emergency department nurse must be knowledgeable in identification of potential donors, the mechanisms and methods for procurement, and clinical care of the potential donor.[18]

Asking a family about organ/tissue donation may be difficult for all concerned. The nurse caring for the client may include the topic with the other death decisions (funeral home and autopsy) that must be made before leaving the emergency department. An organ/tissue procurement agency representative may be the best person to conduct the extensive interview in a sympathetic, yet professional, manner. According to the Uniform Anatomical Gift Act (UAGA 1968; revised version adopted 1987), family members who have the right to give consent if the deceased client has not made a decision about donation prior to death include (in order of legal priority): (1) spouse; (2) adult children; (3) parents; (4) adult siblings; (5) grandparents; (6) legal guardian.

Appendix A summarizes religious beliefs and practices affecting healthcare in general. Table 88–2 explains the religious and cultural beliefs related to death, organ/tissue donation, and transplantation. It should be remembered that this information is general and that individual differences do exist within religious and cultural groups.

Table 88–3 details which organs/tissues can be donated according to donor characteristics. General organ/tissue donor criteria include (1) known cause of death; (2) no history of a significant disease process in the

NURSING RESEARCH

How Should the Family Be Told of the Client's Death?

McQuay, L. E., et al. (1995). "Death-telling" research project. *Critical Care Nursing Clinics of North America, 7*(3), 549–555.

The way in which families are informed of a sudden death in the emergency department can have a profound effect on the grief response and subsequent bereavement process. Compassionate and humane "death-telling" techniques may not be taught in either medical or nursing schools.

The goal of this three-phase study was to educate medical residents about death-telling. In phase I, a videotape that had been developed for the study was used to illustrate grief reactions and various death-telling techniques. A 21-point evaluation checklist was developed and later used to analyze 42 death-telling events over a 6-month period. It was concluded that the physicians were not meeting many of the families' needs, and the process of tissue donation and autopsy were poorly managed. During phase II of the project, 45 medical residents were randomly assigned to four groups to test, via a role-playing exercise evaluated by the 21-point measurement tool, various methods of knowledge acquisition about death-telling. Group 1 had no instruction; group 2 received lecture only; group 3 viewed the videotape; and group 4 received the lecture and viewed the videotape. A telephone survey was conducted, during phase III, of 35 family members of sudden death victims.

Although specific comparisons between the groups were not reported, the researchers did provide feedback from both family members (phase III) and observers (phase II). Initially, the physician mentioned organ/tissue donation only 7% of the time before the educational sessions and almost 50% following the program. Families reported that information updates were inadequate (89%) and only 24% of the physicians used the word "dead," even after the educational program.

Implications for Practice

Although the physician has been the traditional "death-teller," the professional staff closest to the family may be the more appropriate team member to disclose the news. Therefore, more education about death-telling should be incorporated into basic and continuing education programs.

specific organ/tissue; (3) no untreated sepsis. Additional organ donor criteria are (1) brain death; (2) no history of extracranial malignancy; (3) relative hemodynamic stability; (4) blood group compatability; (5) newborn donors must be full-term (> 2000 g). It should be remembered

Table 88–2. Religious and Cultural Customs and Beliefs Related to Death and Organ Donation/Transplantation

Religious (or Cultural) Group	Death	Organ Donation/Transplantation
Religious Group		
Adventist	Dead are asleep until return of Jesus Christ	Individual and family may receive or donate organs
Baha'i	No official rituals	Both permitted
Baptist	Desire clergy present	Both approved if donor not endangered
Buddhist	"Last rite" chanting may be practiced at bedside	Matter of individual conscience
Church of Christ	No official rituals	No official position
Church of God	"Home-going ritual"	No conflict
Church of Jesus Christ of Latter Day Saints (Mormons)	Proper to bury dead in ground; cremation is discouraged	Personal choice; reflection encouraged
Eastern Orthodox Church	"Last rites"; cremation discouraged	No conflict; both are permitted
Episcopalian	"Last rites" not mandatory; desirable— Litany at the Time of Death read	No conflict if donor is not violated
Friends (Quakers)	Do not believe in life after this life	Both are permitted
Grace Brethren	No "last rites"; burial or cremation permitted	No conflict; they encourage both
Greek Orthodox	"Last rites"	Organ transplantation has always been acceptable
Hindu	Certain prescribed rites followed by priest; bodies cremated	No conflict
Islamic (Muslim, Moslem)	Patient must confess sins and beg forgiveness before death; family present	Organ donation provided that donors consent in advance in writing; not stored in organ banks
Jehovah's Witness	No official "last rites"	Do not encourage organ donation; a matter for the individual conscience; all organs drained of blood before transplantation
Judaism	Relatives and close friends remain with the deceased; no cremation	Donation or transplantation of organs requires rabbinical consultation
Lutheran	"Last rites" are optional	Both are acceptable and encouraged
Mennonite	No formal prescribed action	No conflict; both acceptable
Methodist, United	Believe in divine punishment after death; good rewarded, evil punished	Encourages both
Pentecostal (Assembly of God, Foursquare Church)	No official "last rites"	No official position
Presbyterian	Read scripture and pray	Encourage and endorse organ donation
Roman Catholic	"Last rites"	Transplantation and organ donation permissible
Russian Orthodox	Do not believe in autopsies, embalming, or cremation	Donation/transplantation of kidneys, eyes and tissues permitted; heart donation/transplantation not allowed
Cultural Group		
African-American	Funeral attendance symbolizes respect; "sticking together"; cultural rituals and quick "pulling together" by the family facilitates this process	No conflict with organ donation/transplantation
American Indian	Burial practices vary among tribal groups	Information not available
Black Muslim	Carefully prescribed procedure for washing and shrouding and funeral rites	Will accept a transplant if needed to live

Table 88–2. Religious and Cultural Customs and Beliefs Related to Death and Organ Donation/Transplantation *(Continued)*

Religious (or Cultural) Group	Death	Organ Donation/Transplantation
Chinese-American	Chinese have an aversion to death and to anything concerning it; funeral rituals crucial to the well-being of descendants	Information not available
Hispanics (Puerto Rican, Mexican, Latino)	Spirit of the dying person needs reassurance from the living; a wake held 1 day prior to funeral; use of funeral home popular; "Luto" (or mourning) is marked by wearing black and subdued behavior	No conflicts; whole family participates in the decision
Japanese-American	Among Buddhists death is considered a passage; rituals: body of a dead loved one is prepared by close family member, a bath of warm water, purification rites before the body is wrapped in a white kimono	Organ donation a matter of individual conscience
Southeast Asian Americans (Vietnamese, Cambodian, Laotian, Hmong)	Oldest male makes decisions; death of an infant is deeply mourned; expressions of grief vary	Information not available
West Indian (Haitian, Jamaican, Dominican Republican)	Death arrangements are usually made by the male kinsman of the deceased; death caused by angry voodoo spirits can give rise to conflicting feelings of guilt and anger	Permitted according to the specific religious beliefs of the individual

Data from McQuay, J. E. (1994). Cross-cultural customs and beliefs related to health crises, death, and organ donation/transplantation: A guide to assist health care professionals understand different responses and provide cross-cultural assistance. *Critical Care Nursing Clinics of North America, 7*(3): 581–594, an appendix adapted from Turner, J. W. (1987). Appendix: Attitudes and requirements of various religious groups. In DeGroot, K. D., & Damato, M. B. *Critical care skills* (pp. 389–395). Norwalk, CT: Appleton & Lange.

that the only absolute restriction against seeking organ/tissue procurement is a documented case of HIV infection. If the potential donor had any other infection, the local organ/tissue donation service should be consulted before assuming that the organs/tissues can't be used.

Medical Examiner's/Coroner's Jurisdiction

A medical examiner (or coroner), who is a physician with special training in forensic pathology, is concerned with determining the manner and cause of death in a given instance. In the United States, the following types of deaths are reported to the medical examiner's office:

1. Suspected suicides or homicides
2. Deaths in which the deceased has not been attended by a physician within 24 hours before death
3. Deaths with suspicious circumstances
4. Deaths caused by accidents
5. Deaths after surgery
6. Deaths associated with firearms or weapons
7. Deaths occurring as a result of crime
8. Stillbirths
9. Deaths resulting from drugs

10. Deaths possibly associated with hazards to public safety (infectious diseases that may cause epidemics).[14]

When notified of a death, the medical examiner may accept or decline jurisdiction for determining the manner and cause of death. If jurisdiction is accepted, the medical examiner may conduct an autopsy or other investigation or grant the hospital permission to perform an autopsy. Permission from significant others for postmortem examination in these circumstances is not required.

When the medical examiner plans to conduct the autopsy, it is important that all evidence be preserved. Therefore, all tubes, instruments, and devices are left in place, especially intravenous catheters. The deceased is not washed, nails are not cleaned, and any body fluids on the deceased at the time of death are left undisturbed, as is clothing. Clothing that had been removed during emergency treatment of the deceased is carefully placed in a paper bag so that decomposition does not obscure any evidence. When removing clothing during emergency treatment, do not cut through bullet holes, stab wound tears, or other tears. Do not wash the clothing. All valuables and clothing must be inventoried with the medical examiner's staff. Only they may release these items to significant others. Refer to the discussions of specimen

Table 88–3. Organ and Tissue Donor Review Chart

	Kidney	Heart	Liver	Pancreas	Heart for Valves	Bone	Skin	Eye	Ear
Age (years)	0–65	2–50	1 mo.–65	1–65	0–55	16–55	14–75	0–100+	8–100+
Cardiac arrest resuscitated	Prob. OK	No	Prob. OK	Prob. OK	OK	Heart-beating cadaver not mandatory	Heart-beating cadaver not mandatory	Heart-beating cadaver not mandatory	Heart-beating cadaver not mandatory
Chest/abdominal trauma	Important	Extremely important	Extremely important	Important	Little importance	Little importance	Little importance	Not important	Not important
No active systemic infections	Mandatory	Mandatory	Mandatory	Mandatory	Mandatory	Mandatory	Mandatory	N/A	Mandatory
No presence or history of communicable disease	Mandatory	Mandatory	Mandatory	Mandatory	Mandatory	Mandatory	Mandatory	Mandatory	Mandatory
Hypotension	Sensitive	Very sensitive	Very sensitive	Sensitive	N/A	N/A	N/A	N/A	N/A
Vasopressor (i.e., dopamine sensitive)	Yes	Very	Very	Yes	N/A	N/A	N/A	N/A	N/A
Weight important	No	Yes	Yes	No	No	No	>100 lb	N/A	N/A
Body build important	No	Yes	Yes	No	No	No	No	No	No
Blood type	Mandatory	Mandatory	Mandatory	Mandatory	N/A	N/A	N/A	N/A	N/A
Additional physician consults required	Usually not	Yes	Possibly	Usually not	No	No	No	No	No
Additional laboratory data needed	Yes, kidney specific	Yes, heart specific	Yes, liver specific	Yes, pancreas specific	No	No	No	No	No
Time needed to set up additional teams	No	Yes	Yes	Yes	No	No	Possible	No	No
Tissue may be retrieved after cardiac death	No	No	No	No	Yes, up to 12 hr after death; the whole heart is retrieved in the OR	Yes, up to 24 hr in the OR under sterile conditions	Yes, up to 36 hr if refrigerated	Yes, up to 6 hr; place ice packs on the eyes after closing them	Yes, up to 48 hr; may be procured following embalming

From Gill, A. G. (1993). Organ donation. In R. L. Boggs & M. Wooldridge-King (Eds.), AACN procedure manual for critical care (3rd ed.). Philadelphia: W. B. Saunders.

collection and chain of custody earlier in this chapter. A copy of the medical record is given to the medical examiner's staff. The record must be detailed, with special attention given to injuries and marks noted on arrival of the deceased, and a description of and location of tubes, surgical incisions, venipunctures, and other therapeutic interventions.

Conclusions

Emergency nurses must be experienced in communication, assessment, and psychomotor skills. Initial assessment, or triage, is used to prescribe a level of care for best outcomes. Priority nursing interventions include the ABCs. An emergency doctrine prevails and allows treatment of clients who are unable to give consent. When clients die suddenly, the family requires skilled and compassionate care.

Thinking Critically

1. A 23-year-old man walks into your emergency department. He tells you that he was in a motor vehicle accident about 4 hours ago. The police were at the scene, but he refused to be transported to the emergency department because he felt fine, and he went home. At home, however, the client started to experience worsening shoulder and posterior neck pain. His mother urged him to come to the emergency department. He tells you that he has "numbness" in his fingers and a "tingling" feeling in his right elbow. If you were the triage nurse, what potential problems would you consider that this client might have? Would you classify the client as emergent, urgent, or nonurgent? What measures should you take to ensure the client's safety?

Factors to Consider. What injuries sustained in a motor vehicle accident might account for the client's symptoms?

2. A 35-year-old man was brought in to your emergency department by the city police, who were arresting him for drunk and disorderly conduct. He was involved in a barroom brawl, during which he acquired several small lacerations about the face and arms from broken glass, a hit to the head, and kicks to his ribs. He is conscious, verbally abusive, and threatening to fight his way out of the emergency department because he wants "to go home and be left alone." He has twice threatened you with bodily harm if you persist in preventing him from leaving. How would you proceed with this case?

Factors to Consider. Whom should you call? Would it be appropriate to sedate this client? What should you do if the client actually harms you physically?

Bibliography

1. Allen, P. L. (1994). Overview of the organ donation process. *Critical Care Nursing Clinics of North America, 6*(3), 553–565.
2. American Heart Association (1994). *Textbook of advanced cardiac life support.* Dallas: Author.
3. American Hospital Association (1990). Emergency transfer (client dumping): Provisions of budget bill. *Washington Watch, 11,* 9–10.
4. Beaver, B. M. (1990). Care of the multiple trauma victim: The first hour. *Nursing Clinics of North America, 25*(1), 11–21.
5. Blair, F. A., & Hall, M. M. (1994). The nursing process: Assessment and priority setting. In A. R. Klein, et al. (Eds.), *Emergency nursing core curriculum* (4th ed.). Philadelphia: W. B. Saunders.
6. Bracken, L. J., & Rossier-Martinez, R. (1994). Education. In A. R. Klein, et al. (Eds.), *Emergency nursing core curriculum* (4th ed.). Philadelphia: W. B. Saunders.
7. Cardona, V. D., & Von Rueden, K. T. (1994). Nursing practice through the trauma cycles. In V. D. Cardona, et al. (Eds.), *Trauma nursing: From resuscitation through rehabilitation* (2nd ed.). Philadelphia: W. B. Saunders.
8. Chave, W. (1994). Legal concerns in trauma nursing. In V. D. Cardona, et al. (Eds.), *Trauma nursing: From resuscitation through rehabilitation* (2nd ed.). Philadelphia: W. B. Saunders.
9. Coolican, M. B. (1994). Families facing sudden death of a loved one. *Critical Care Nursing Clinics of North America, 6*(3) 607–612.
10. Donovan, M. R., & Matson, T. A. (Eds.). (1994). *Outpatient case management: Strategies for a new reality.* Chicago: American Hospital Publishing.
11. Emergency Nurses Association (1995). In J. Dains, et al. (Eds.), *Standards of emergency nursing practice* (3rd ed.). St. Louis: Mosby–Year Book.
12. Fadale, J. (1990). Overcrowding, comfort, consideration, convenience. *Journal of Emergency Nursing, 16*(3), 132–133.
13. Halpern, J. S. (1989). Mechanisms and patterns of trauma. *Journal of Emergency Nursing, 15*(5), 380–388.
14. Halpern, J. S. (1994). Clinical notebook: Mnemonics used for client assessment. *Journal of Emergency Nursing, 20*(3), 219–220.
15. Heffernan, L. (1996). Legal, economic, and religious issues. In F. Chabalewski (Ed.), *United Network for Organ Sharing Donation and Transplantation: Nursing curriculum.* Washington, D.C.: U.S. Department of Health and Human Services, Health Resources & Services Administration.
16. Hurn, P. D., & Hartsock, R. L. (1994). Thoracic injuries. In V. D. Cardona, et al. (Eds.), *Trauma nursing: From resuscitation through rehabilitation* (2nd ed.). Philadelphia: W. B. Saunders.
17. Kollef, M., & Goodenberger, D. (1995). Critical care and medical emergencies. In G. A. Ewald & C. R. McKenzie (Eds.), *Manual of medical therapeutics* (28th ed.). Boston: Little, Brown.
18. Lenehan, G. P. (1989). ED gridlock and blaming the victim. *Journal of Emergency Nursing, 15*(3), 211–213.
19. Lower, J. (1994). Neurological emergencies. In A. R. Klein, et al. (Eds.), *Emergency nursing core curriculum* (4th ed.). Philadelphia: W. B. Saunders.
20. McQuay, J. E. (1995). Support of families who had a loved one suffer a sudden injury, illness, or death. *Critical Care Nursing Clinics of North America, 7*(3), 541–547.
21. McQuay, J. E. (1995). Cross-cultural customs and beliefs related to health crises, death, and organ donation/transplantation: A guide to assist health care professionals understand different responses and provide cross-cultural assistance. *Critical Care Nursing Clinics of North America, 7*(3), 581–594.
22. McQuay, J. E., et al. (1995). "Death-telling" research project. *Critical Care Nursing Clinics of North America, 7*(3), 549–555.
23. Park, A. H. (1996). Nursing care of the potential donor. In F. Chabalewski (Ed.), *United Network for Organ Sharing Donation and Transplantation: Nursing curriculum.* Washington, D.C.: U.S. Department of Health and Human Services, Health Resources & Services Administration.
24. Puntillo, K., & Tesler, M. D. (1993). Pain. In V. Carrieri-Kohlman, A. M. Lindsey, & C. M. West (Eds.), *Pathophysiological phenomena in nursing* (2nd ed.). Philadelphia: W. B. Saunders.
25. Ramler, C. (1990). Triage. In S. Kitt & J. Kaiser (Eds.), *Emergency*

nursing: A physiologic and clinical perspective. Philadelphia: W. B. Saunders.

26. Scanlon, A. M. (1994). Psychosocial responses of the human spirit: The journey of trauma. In V. D. Cardona, et al. (Eds.), *Trauma nursing: From resuscitation through rehabilitation* (2nd ed.). Philadelphia: W. B. Saunders.

27. Southard, P. A. (1994). Legal issues. In A. R. Klein, et al. (Eds.), *Emergency nursing core curriculum* (4th ed.). Philadelphia: W. B. Saunders.

28. Tipsord-Klinkhammer, B., & Noska, A. R. (1996). Telephone triage: An ED alternative? *The Nursing Spectrum, 9*(6), 4.

29. Veise-Berry, S., & Beachley, V. (1994). Evolution of the trauma cycle. In V. D. Cardona et al. (Eds.), *Trauma nursing: From resuscitation through rehabilitation* (2nd ed.). Philadelphia, W. B. Saunders.

30. Walleck, C. A. (1994). Central nervous system II: Spinal cord injury. In V. D. Cardona, et al. (Eds.), *Trauma nursing: From resuscitation through rehabilitation* (2nd ed.). Philadelphia: W. B. Saunders.

31. Wheeler, S. Q. (1989). ED telephone triage: Lessons learned from unusual calls. *Journal of Emergency Nursing, 15*(6), 401–407.

32. Whelan, A. J. (1995). Patient care internal medicine. In G. A. Ewald & C.R. McKenzie (Eds.), *Manual of medical therapeutics* (28th ed.). Boston: Little, Brown.

Nursing Care of Clients with Medical-Surgical Emergencies

Linda Lorraine Armstrong Lazure
Jean Elizabeth DeMartinis

Emergency department (ED) clients present problems that range from minor to catastrophic. This wide variation in severity is compounded by the large number of possible situations that may be encountered, ranging from minor lacerations to traumatic death. The ED nurse must not only be familiar with these problems but must also be able to individualize the immediate care and discharge teaching. The following overview of common selected emergencies, their management, and priority discharge teaching needs provides a framework for basing nursing interventions in the ED. Two overriding tenets should guide the nurse's care: (1) the "ABCs" (i.e., *A*irway, *B*reathing, *B*leeding, *C*irculation, *C*ervical spine, and *C*onsciousness level) as a guide to clinical decision making, and (2) a caring, client-centered focus. The focus of this chapter is on identifying general principles, priorities, and management of common emergencies encountered by adult clients.

Altered Level of Consciousness

An altered level of consciousness may range from restlessness and disorientation to unconsciousness. The causes of an altered level of consciousness include hypoxic, metabolic, and pathologic conditions of the brain. The mnemonic device "vowel [*a, e, i, o, u*] tipps" is a helpful guide to determining the cause of unconsciousness. *a*, alcohol; *e*, epilepsy; *i*, insulin; *o*, opiates; *u*, urates; *t*, trauma; *i*, infection; *p*, psychogenic; *p*, poison; *s*, shock.

Obtain key historical information from significant others or prehospital personnel. Include any history of trauma; chronic health problems (e.g., diabetes, hypertension, heart or renal disease); use of prescription, over-the-counter, or street drugs or home remedies; alcohol use; mental health history; general health status; activities when the client was last seen or communicated with; temperature of environment in which the client was found; and clues that may help to determine cause (e.g., medication bottles, incontinence, medical alert tag or card).

Assess the color of the skin, the respiratory pattern, pupillary reaction, motor function, odors, nuchal rigidity, and posturing. Institute measures to stabilize the ABCs. Monitor vital signs and assess neurologic status. Calculate and document the Glasgow Coma Scale score (see Chapter 31), pupillary responses, and reflexes. Insert an intravenous (IV) line and draw blood for laboratory work (complete blood count [CBC]), glucose, calcium, electrolytes, creatinine, magnesium, drug screen, and alcohol level).

Because the history may be inadequate for determining whether thiamine deficiency is probable, thiamine (vitamin B) 100 mg IV may be routinely administered prophylactically. Administer IV dextrose if the client has a history of hypoglycemia or a low serum glucose. Glucose paste may also be applied sublingually, or intramuscular glucagon may be administered to raise the blood sugar. IV dextrose for all clients with an altered level of consciousness is controversial.

Naloxone (Narcan) 2 mg IV may be administered if a narcotic overdose is suspected, and it can be repeated. Use caution, however, because if the drug that is reversed by naloxone has a longer half-life, the effect of the drug may last longer than the effect of naloxone, and the client may lapse back into unconsciousness. Thus, observation for several hours is usually indicated for recurrence of clinical manifestations in these clients.

Ongoing nursing management includes safety measures. Manage airways and secretions for prevention of aspiration. Position the client on the side while maintaining spine immobilization, and suction as needed. Protect the eyes from drying by applying artificial tears and taping the eyelids shut (use cellophane rather than adhesive tape). Be sure to check the eyes for contact lenses and

This chapter incorporates material written for the fourth edition by Lisa L. Strohmyer.

remove if present. Be alert to the possibility of an eye prosthesis. Prevent skin necrosis by position changes and skin care. Protect from falls by raising the side rails and locking them. Minimize the potential for increased intracranial pressure by positioning the head in neutral alignment, hyperventilating with 100% oxygen before suctioning, suctioning for short periods of time, and avoiding the use of restraints if possible.

Prepare for and assist with diagnostic studies (e.g., computed tomography [CT] scans or magnetic resonance imaging). If toxic ingestion is suspected, institute gastric lavage (see Poisoning and Overdose) with an endotracheal tube in place. Provide continuous psychosocial support for both the client and significant others. Remember, the extent of hearing is unknown, so refrain from discussing the client's condition at the bedside.[19,31]

Multiple Trauma

Multiple trauma includes injury to more than one body system. There are many different scoring systems used to categorize and determine severity of injury. One of these is the Champion Trauma Score (Table 89–1). Points are assigned on the basis of the client's responses, and a total score is obtained. Optimally, a client with a Champion Trauma Score of less than 12 should be transferred to a tertiary trauma system. The Champion Trauma Score correlates highly with mortality. Another measure of injury severity is the Revised Trauma Score (RTS) (Table 89–2).

The *mechanism of injury* is a term used to describe how an injury occurred. For example, knowing if a person in a motor vehicle accident was struck head-on or from the side helps predict the likely injuries. Knowing the mechanism of injury helps in estimating the amount of force applied and provides insight into the pattern of injury. Box 89–1 lists questions to be asked to determine the mechanism of injury.

In addition to the mechanism of injury, the type and extent of injury also involve environmental conditions (weather, geographical location) and the characteristics of the client such as age, gender, nutrition, underlying disease processes, and any conditions altering cognitive function and judgment (alcohol, drug use, or fatigue).

The history and mechanism of injury constitute vital information and must be obtained promptly. This information helps guide assessment and intervention. Experienced emergency nurses can often anticipate common associated injuries most likely to be present on the basis of accurate information about the mechanism of injury. In addition, injuries should be matched with the reported mechanism. Clients and significant others may deny or falsify the history of injury for various reasons.

Two common differentiations of the mechanism of injury are penetrating and blunt (nonpenetrating) injuries. We examine these more closely.

Penetrating Injuries

Penetrating injuries cause a break in the integrity of the skin. The severity of penetrating injuries depends on two

Table 89–1. Champion Trauma Score

Glasgow Coma Scale (GCS)

Eye-opening response	Spontaneous	4
	To voice	3
	To pain	2
	None	1
Best verbal response	Oriented	5
	Confused	4
	Inappropriate words	3
	Incomprehensible sounds	2
	None	1
Best motor response	Obeys command	6
	Localizes pain	5
	Withdraws (pain)	4
	Flexion (pain)	3
	Extension (pain)	2
	None	1
Total	Apply this score to GCS portion of Trauma Score	3–15

Trauma Score

GCS (total points from above)	14–15	5
	11–13	4
	8–10	3
	5–7	2
	3–4	1
Respiratory rate	10–24/min	4
	25–35/min	3
	36/min or greater	2
	1–9/min	1
	None	0
Respiratory expansion	Normal	1
	Retractive/none	0
Systolic blood pressure	90 mm Hg or greater	4
	70–89 mm Hg	3
	50–69 mm Hg	2
	0–49 mm Hg	1
	No pulse	0
Capillary refill	Normal	2
	Delayed	1
	None	0
Total trauma score		1–16

Trauma score	16	15	14	13	12	11	10	9	8	7	6	5	4	3	2	1
Percentage survival	99	98	96	93	87	76	60	42	26	15	8	4	2	1	0	0

From Moore, E. F., et al. (1990). *Early care of the injured patient.* Philadelphia: B. C. Decker.

factors: (1) the anatomic location of the injury and (2) the amount of energy transferred to the body. The amount of energy transferred is determined by the force of the penetrating object at the time of impact. Because, in general, stab wounds are inflicted with less force than gunshot wounds, the client has a better prognosis than he or she

Table 89–2. Calculation of Revised Trauma Score (RTS) Based on Three Components

A. If Glasgow Coma Scale (GCS) score is:	Coded Value is:
13–15	4
9–12	3
6–8	2
4–5	1
3	0
B. If respiratory rate (RR) is:	
10–29	4
> 29	3
6–9	2
1–5	1
0	0
C. If systolic blood pressure (SBP) is:	
> 89	4
76–79	3
50–75	2
1–49	1
0	0

Each of these scores is then used in the equation: RTS = $0.9368 \times (GCS) + 0.7326 \times (SBP) + 0.2908 \times (RR)$

From DeKeyser, F. G. (1994). Trauma nursing research: A description and means of evaluation. *Critical Care Nursing Clinics of North America*, 6(3), 441–449.

Box 89–1. Questions to Be Asked of Clients with Various Traumatic Injuries

Motor Vehicle Crashes

Were you the driver or passenger?
Were you wearing a seatbelt or shoulder harness (or both)?
Did you hit the steering wheel or the dashboard? If so, with what part of your body?
Did you lose consciousness? If so, for how long?
How fast was the vehicle going?
What did the vehicle hit?
Did the vehicle hit a moving object or a nonmoving object? (Paramedics may assist by describing the condition of the car.)
Where is your pain?
How far were you thrown?
What is the condition of the other passengers?

Blunt Trauma from Falls

How far did you fall?
What precipitated the fall?
What did you land on?
Where is your pain?
Did you lose consciousness?

Gunshot Wounds

How long ago did the incident occur?
How many shots did you hear?
What type of gun was it?
From what direction do you think the bullet entered you?
Where is your pain?

Penetrating Wounds or Stab Wounds

How long ago did it happen?
How many times were you stabbed?
How long was the knife?
How far in did it go?
From what direction were you stabbed?
Where is your pain?

From Kih, S., et al. (1995). *Emergency nursing*. Philadelphia: W. B. Saunders.

would have were the gunshot injury in the same location. Remember to consider potential injuries to underlying organs and tissues. For instance, if an injury resulted from a stab wound, consider the length of the object and the direction of the wound for an idea of additional injuries. A thoracic wound may involve an interruption in the heart, lungs, tracheobronchial tree, great vessels, or even diaphragm, depending on whether the injured client was inspiring (diaphragm down) or expiring (diaphragm up) at the time of injury. Because of the location of the diaphragm, a diagnostic peritoneal lavage is often performed for evaluation of possible abdominal injury by penetrating wounds below the nipple line.[19,29] Predicted injuries from penetrating trauma are shown in Table 89–3.

Blunt Injuries

Blunt (nonpenetrating) injuries result in significant injuries that may be more difficult to detect. These injuries involve direct, indirect, and acceleration-deceleration forces. For instance, in a motor vehicle crash, the driver (traveling at the speed of the car) strikes the steering wheel. The force of the impact is exerted through the chest structures and may result in broken ribs, cardiac or pulmonary contusions, pneumothorax, or a ruptured aorta. Or the client's head may hit the windshield, which causes frontal lobe damage to the brain; then as the head falls backward, damage to the occipital lobe can occur. Solid organs (liver, spleen) are more likely to be crushed or compressed. Hollow, air-filled organs (lung, intestines)

are more likely to burst when compressed or subject to blast forces. Predicted injuries from blunt trauma are shown in Table 89–4.

Primary Assessment and Priority Interventions

With a multiply injured client, time is vital. Determine priorities by the ABCs, and implement the general interventions immediately. If spinal trauma is suspected, further neck injury is prevented by neck immobilization through the use of a cervical collar and backboard. Keep in mind that the airway may be obstructed by either positioning or by the tongue, blood, or loose teeth. Ensure an adequate airway and ventilate with 100% oxygen as needed.

Table 89–3. Predicted Injuries from Penetrating Trauma			
Type of Event	**Position or Location**	**Mechanism**	**Predicted Injury**
Gunshot wound	Victim may be shot close up or at a distance; victim may be leaving or running from assailant; victim may have been facing assailant	Should be an entrance wound but may not have an exit wound; caliber and velocity of weapon are directly related to extent of injury; damage is not only caused by the bullet itself but by the vibrating effect of the missile and the speed at which it travels	Severe blood loss; major organ penetration and damage depend on entrance and exit sites and associated organs
Stab wound	Victim may have been stabbed in back, abdomen, or chest from the front; object used to stab the victim may still be in place	Tissue damage at site and organs depends on length and width of object; location affects severity of injuries	Severe blood loss; mild to severe chest injuries such as pneumothorax, hemothorax, myocardial or aortic laceration; abdominal injuries or peripheral sites of injury
Impaled by other objects	Victim falls on object or during motor vehicle accident; object is impaled into victim, such as steering-wheel column	Tissue damage at site of object and organs that it impales depends on length, width, and location	Severe chest, head, and abdominal injuries; severe blood loss

Modified from Beaver, B. M. (1990). Care of the multiple trauma victim: The first hour. *Nursing Clinics of North America, 25*(1), 11–21.

Initiate two large-bore IV lines for rapid infusion of fluids. Draw blood while inserting an IV line. Prepare for possible blood transfusions by drawing a type and cross-match (T&C).

Control external bleeding by direct pressure, pressure dressing, or rapid fluid replacement if the client is hypotensive (crystalloid or colloid). The client may be in cardiac arrest from shock, chest injuries, or respiratory failure. Start cardiopulmonary resuscitation (CPR) immediately if no respirations or pulse is present. Remember, if the client has lost fluid volume, CPR will not be fully effective until fluid volume is restored. Consider use of a pneumatic antishock garment (PASG) (see Chapter 22).

Obtain a full set of vital signs and repeat at least every 15 minutes until the client is stabilized. Perform a brief neurologic and mental status examination. Calculate the Glasgow Coma Scale and trauma scores. Initiate a flow sheet for documentation of assessments, interventions, and client responses. Do the following:

1. Undress the client completely (by cutting off clothes, if necessary).
2. Cover the client with a sheet or blanket.
3. Remove any helmet carefully to avoid neck flexion.
4. Spread the helmet open.
5. Apply manual traction to the head.
6. "Walk off" the helmet while maintaining traction.
7. Push the helmet off the head.
8. After the helmet is off, lower the client's head and ask whether the client notices a change such as numbness, tingling, or a change in perceived level of pain. Ensure that the client's clothes or valuables are safeguarded, and use the proper chain of custody, especially if

criminal or suspicious acts are associated with the trauma.

Obtain a urinalysis after inserting a urinary catheter, and monitor urine output every 15 to 30 minutes. (Blood noted at the urinary meatus may mean a ruptured bladder or injury to the urethra so the catheter should not be inserted.) Urine output is a key indicator of adequate perfusion and should be monitored with fluid replacement. At least 0.5 to 1.0 ml/min, or 30 to 60 ml/hr of urine should be produced.[2,13,19,27]

Secondary Assessment and Interventions

Proceed with a complete head-to-toe examination. Remember the possibility of associated injuries, and keep in mind the various internal structures potentially affected by the known injury pattern.

Insert a nasogastric tube, if indicated. Test the gastric aspirant for blood and connect to suction. Keep the client NPO (nothing by mouth). Nasogastric tubes are not inserted if a basilar skull fracture is suspected because of possible insertion into the cranium; instead, an orogastric tube may be used to decompress the stomach. Battle's sign, a bruising over the mastoid bone, and blood in the ear canal are signs of a basilar skull fracture. If blood or clear fluid is coming out of the nose or ears, note if it leaves a yellow "halo" around the coagulated blood on the bed sheets, which may indicate a cerebrospinal fluid leak.

X-rays of the cervical spine, or chest and CT scans or magnetic resonance imaging, are often used to diagnose

Table 89–4. Predicted Injuries from Blunt Trauma

Type of Event	Position or Location	Mechanism	Predicted Injury
Automobile accident	*Driver* (with 3-point seatbelt)	Body travels forward, striking head on windshield, rear-view mirror, or hood of car; chest may hit steering wheel; knees may hit dashboard	Lacerations, bruises on head and face, abdominal injury from lap belt; possible broken clavicle or first rib; acceleration-deceleration injuries
	Driver (with lap belt only)	Same mechanism but more severe	Abdominal and bladder injuries, cervical spine injury, lumbar spine injuries, facial injury, major chest trauma, head injury, and pelvic fracture; acceleration-deceleration injuries
	Driver (unrestrained)	Same mechanism but much more severe	Severe head and neck and chest injuries; femur fracture, other fractures; acceleration-deceleration injuries
	Passenger (front) (3-point restraint)	Body travels forward, striking windshield or dashboard, or is pushed to one side	Lacerations and bruises of face, head, chest; abdominal injuries from lap belt; acceleration-deceleration injuries
	Passenger (lap belt only)	Same	Facial fractures, head injury, cervical spine injury, abdominal injury, bladder injury, lumbar spine or pelvic fractures; acceleration-deceleration injuries
	Any passenger (unrestrained)	Thrown through the windshield or other window or lands on the floorboard or front seat	Severe head injuries, femur fracture, knee fracture or other injury; other system injuries, other fractures; acceleration-deceleration injuries
Pedestrian accident	*Pedestrian* struck by car while walking or standing		
Motorcycle accident	*Motorcyclist* hit by vehicle; motorcyclist impacting with immovable object	Victim is thrown into objects, such as car, tree, etc.; may be run over by vehicle; helmet may protect from head injuries	Major head, chest, and abdominal injuries; fractures of lower and upper extremities; crush injuries; neck and spinal injuries
Fall or jump greater than 10 ft	Victim may: 1. Land on feet or heels or head and outstretched hands 2. Land on back and head 3. Land on buttocks or in sitting position	Depends on the distance of the fall and how victim landed	Heel and ankle fractures, knee fractures, wrist or upper extremity fractures, compression; fractures of vertebrae, lumbar spine fractures, hip fractures, major organ injuries, head and neck injuries, aortic tear
Altercation or beating	Victim standing or lying down; hit with blunt object	Hit in head, abdomen, kicked in kidneys, abdomen, bladder	Head injuries, lacerations, bruises, major organ injuries, i.e., kidney, spleen, and liver
	Child abuse	Hit anywhere on body	Fractures

Modified from Beaver, B. M. (1990). Care of the multiple trauma victim: The first hour. *Nursing Clinics of North America, 25*(1), 11–21.

injuries. If a portable x-ray machine is not available, coordinate x-ray studies so the client makes only one trip to the radiology department. Accompany unstable patients to x-ray.

Administer a tetanus booster if wounds are present. Splint fractures, apply ice, and elevate the area. Clean and dress wounds. Wounds are repaired only after the client is stabilized or in the operating room.

Provide emotional support to the client and significant others. Allowing the family into the room during resuscitation remains controversial. If appropriate, and the family chooses to observe, a support person should be designated to be with them to explain what is happening. Only one or two family members should be in the room at one time and they may leave at any time. This arrangement may actually be beneficial when families are asked whether resuscitation efforts should be continued. If the family is not in the room, they should receive frequent factual updates regarding the client's condition.

Pain medication is commonly not given initially for clients with multiple trauma and cardiovascular instability. Medication may mask the identification of significant injuries and interfere with accurate neurologic assessments. Self-administered nitrous oxide and oxygen may help clients with significant amounts of pain or those undergoing painful procedures. If narcotics are given, they are administered in small IV doses.

Elderly clients with traumatic injuries have special needs. The body's compensatory mechanisms may be delayed, and chronic health problems and medications may contribute to complications. For instance, a client with a heart condition who is taking a beta-blocker does not present with tachycardia in the presence of shock. The elderly may also be predisposed to adverse drug reactions because of their higher rate of drug use and physical factors, such as altered drug absorption, distribution, metabolism, and excretion. Also, abuse of the elderly is an increasing problem that may appear as multiple trauma.[5,26]

Respiratory Emergencies: Near Drowning

Clients who initially survive suffocation after submersion in a water or fluid medium are diagnosed as near drowning. Another term, *immersion syndrome,* is used by some clinicians to describe near drowning.

Freshwater drowning (i.e., swimming pool) is more common than saltwater drowning. Alcohol or drug ingestion, overestimation of swimming skills, hypothermia, hyperventilation, and hypoglycemia are risk factors.

Both freshwater and saltwater wash out alveolar surfactant. Freshwater also changes the surface tension of surfactant. The loss of surfactant leads to alveolar collapse, intrapulmonary shunting, and hypoxemia. Poor perfusion and hypoxemia result in acidosis and eventual pulmonary edema.

Near drowning compromises the respiratory system and leads to hypoxia, hypercapnia, cardiac arrest, and severe alterations in fluid-electrolyte balance. Bronchospasm, from aspirating water into the lungs, causes most drowning deaths. Cerebral edema from metabolic derangement is a major cause of death.

Obtain a history of the submersion. Include the length of submersion, temperature of the water, any associated injuries, and type of water.

Begin assessment and interventions with the ABCs. Note any respiratory efforts and adventitious sounds. Open the airway while maintaining spinal immobility. Assess the level of consciousness. Look for signs of hypoxia, such as confusion, irritability, lethargy, or unconsciousness. Obtain a complete set of vital signs. Additional injuries may be present in a client with near drowning. These include associated trauma, spinal cord injury from diving, air embolism from scuba diving, and seizures.

For respiratory insufficiency, intubate and ventilate with 100% oxygen and 5 to 10 cm of positive end-expiratory pressure (PEEP) to prevent the alveoli from collapsing. If the client is breathing, provide respiratory support with a non-rebreather mask.

Remove the client's wet clothing, and wrap the client in a warm blanket. Core rewarming may be indicated if the client is hypothermic. Rewarm the client slowly to avoid a rapid influx of metabolites (lactic acid) that may be trapped in the cold extremities.

Once the vital functions are stabilized, correct any acid-base or electrolyte abnormalities. Diagnostic studies include ABGs, CBC, electrolytes, appropriate toxicology studies if alcohol or drug ingestion is suspected, and a chest x-ray. Clients have a high risk of developing pulmonary edema, even several hours after the incident. Care must be taken to monitor the neurologic status. A deteriorating level of consciousness may indicate cerebral edema, severe acidosis, or increased hypoxia.[6]

Chest Trauma

The chest is a large, exposed portion of the body that is very vulnerable to impact injuries. Because it houses the heart, lungs, and great vessels, chest trauma frequently produces life-threatening disruptions. Injury to the thoracic cage and its contents can restrict the heart's ability to pump blood or the lungs' ability to exchange air and oxygenate blood. Major dangers associated with chest injuries are internal bleeding and punctured organs. Chest injuries can range from relatively minor bumps and scrapes to severe crushing or penetrating trauma.

Chest injuries may be penetrating or nonpenetrating (blunt).

- Penetrating chest injuries may cause an open chest wound, permitting atmospheric air into the pleural space and disrupting the normal ventilation mechanism. Penetrating chest injuries may seriously damage the lungs, heart, and other thoracic structures.
- Nonpenetrating (blunt) injuries are most commonly deceleration injuries associated with motor vehicle crashes. Blunt chest trauma may also result from falls or blows to the chest.

Initial assessment is directed toward identifying and treating immediate life-threatening conditions. Any client with chest trauma should be considered to have a serious injury until it is proved otherwise. Airway patency, adequacy of breathing, and circulatory sufficiency (i.e., presence of shock) are always of primary concern.

Once initial emergencies have been addressed, the client is assessed more thoroughly (Box 89–2). A medical history helps identify any pre-existing conditions that may

Box 89-2. Assessment of and Therapeutic Intervention for the Chest Trauma Victim

Maintain airway, breathing, and circulation

Obtain a quick history

What happened?
What was the mechanism of injury?
How long ago did it happen?
Where is the pain? Does it radiate?
Is there anything that makes the pain better or worse?
What does the pain feel like?
How severe is the pain on a scale of 1 to 10?
Is there any medical history?

Perform a quick (1-minute) evaluation

Check for shortness of breath and cyanosis.
Check vital signs.
Check skin color and temperature.
Check wound size and location.
Check for paradoxical chest movement.
Check for distended neck veins.
Check for tracheal deviation.
Listen for respiratory stridor.
Listen for bilateral breath sounds.
Look for epigastric and supraclavicular indrawing.
Give rough estimate of tidal volume.
Assess intercostal muscle use.
Assess accessory muscle use.
Check for subcutaneous emphysema.
Listen for sucking chest wounds.
Listen to heart sounds.

Provide therapeutic intervention

Maintain airway.
Ensure adequate air movement.
Administer oxygen.
Cover any open chest wound.
Control flail segment.
Insert needles or chest tube into anterior chest wall of affected side if tension pneumothorax is present.
Initiate a large bore intravenous line (two or more lines if possible, but do not delay transport to do this).
Do pericardiocentesis, if indicated.
Get chest x-ray film if more than three ribs are fractured, because victim is considered multitraumatized and the search for associated injuries must go on. It is essential at this time to obtain a cross-table lateral cervical spine x-ray film for detection of cervical spine injury before any other diagnostic tests are initiated or the victim is moved.
Frequently recheck vital signs.
Monitor for dysrhythmias.

From Sheehy, S. B. (1985). *Emergency nursing: Principles and practice.* St. Louis: Mosby-Year Book.

---

injuries. A chest film and electrocardiogram (ECG) are obtained for detecting possible pulmonary or cardiac impairment.[19,23,29]

Management

Ventilation-perfusion imbalances may result from atelectasis, hemopneumothorax, flail chest, aspiration, or pulmonary contusion. Oxygen or mechanical ventilation may be required. General respiratory status (e.g., rate and depth of respirations, chest movement, spontaneous vital volumes) and ABGs should be monitored closely. Deterioration may indicate previously undetected injury or late-developing complications.

Therapeutic measures such as thoracentesis, chest tube insertion, bronchoscopic aspiration, or thoracotomy (Chapters 39 and 41) may be indicated. Maintain effective functioning of any equipment used (e.g., chest drainage system). Help the client and significant others understand these procedures and the rationale for their use. Clients with chest injuries may experience significant hypovolemia. Fluid replacement is with blood and blood products, if indicated, or with crystalloid IV solutions (e.g., lactated Ringer's solution, normal saline). Monitor continually for signs of shock. Shock often results from hypovolemia, but in the chest-injured client it may also be caused by cardiac tamponade, cardiac contusion, flail chest, or tension pneumothorax. Central vascular pressure readings (central venous pressure [CVP] or pulmonary artery pressure) require careful interpretation. Once the cause of shock is determined, rapid treatment is crucial (see Chapter 22).

Excessive blood loss may further compromise the client's oxygenation. External bleeding should be carefully assessed, and blood loss should be estimated. Internal bleeding may result from injuries to the thoracic or abdominal viscera, torn muscles, or fractures. Considerable bleeding (i.e., 2 L or more) into the pleural space may occur. This is usually detected quickly. Bleeding into areas such as the chest wall (e.g., from torn intercostal muscles) is more difficult to assess. A liter of blood can accumulate between the chest wall muscles without producing much swelling.

A chest-injured person may require large quantities of blood replacement. Until the results of typing and crossmatching are available, the client is given O-negative blood. The volume of blood replacement is determined through assessment of clinical findings, hemodynamic measurements, and laboratory results (e.g., hemoglobin and hematocrit). When possible, surgery is delayed until the blood volume is restored.

Pain associated with chest injuries may cause the client to breathe rapidly and shallowly, which leads to atelectasis and pooling of tracheobronchial secretions. Analgesics minimize pain and permit periods of rest and relaxation. They also allow the client to cough and take deeper breaths. Narcotics are most effective if given IV. Intercostal nerve blocks or epidural analgesia may be used in clients with underlying health problems. Splinting the chest may also be helpful.

further complicate the injury. A thorough physical examination should be performed, with care being taken not to focus only on obvious injuries. Information about the accident (obtained from the injured client or witnesses) assists in the diagnosis of regional as well as anatomic

Complications

Severe chest trauma may produce numerous complications, including the following:

- Pneumothorax
- Tension pneumothorax and mediastinal shift
- Open pneumothorax and mediastinal flutter
- Hemothorax
- Fractured ribs
- Fractured sternum
- Flail chest

■ Pneumothorax

Pneumothorax is the presence of air in the pleural space that prohibits complete lung expansion. Air may escape into the pleural space from a puncture or tear in an internal respiratory structure (e.g., bronchus, bronchioles, alveoli). This form of pneumothorax is called closed or spontaneous pneumothorax (Fig. 89–1A). Fractured ribs commonly lead to closed pneumothorax. Air may enter the pleural space directly through a hole in the chest wall (open pneumothorax) or diaphragm.

Clinical manifestations of moderate pneumothorax include tachypnea; dyspnea; sudden sharp pain on the affected side with chest movement, breathing, or coughing; asymmetrical chest expansion; diminished or absent breath sounds on the affected side; hyperresonance (tympany) to percussion on the affected side; restlessness, anxiety; and tachycardia.

Clinical manifestations of severe pneumothorax include all the preceding and distended neck veins; PMI shift (point of maximal impulse of heart beat); subcutaneous emphysema; decreased tactile and vocal fremitus; tracheal deviation toward the unaffected side; and progressive cyanosis.

Chest films may reveal a slight tracheal shift away from the affected side and retraction of the lung back from the parietal pleura. (Remember, in pneumothorax, the collection of air is between the visceral and parietal pleura.) On chest x-ray, pneumothorax is expressed as a percentage. For example, a client may have a complete 100% to a partial 10% pneumothorax. The use of percentages allows for evaluation of progress on repeat x-rays. If pneumothorax is suspected (but respiratory distress is too severe to permit x-ray confirmation), the physician may insert an 18-gauge needle (emergency thoracentesis) into the second or third intercostal space in the midclavicular line. Aspiration demonstrates whether free air is present in the pleural space.

However, most physicians prefer to insert a chest tube immediately into the pleural space via the fourth intercostal space at the mid- or anterior axillary line. The chest catheter is connected to closed chest drainage. (Management of closed chest drainage is discussed in Chapter 42). The catheter permits the continuous escape of air and blood from the pleural space. Thus, it helps the lung expand by reestablishing subatmospheric pressure (i.e., negative pressure) in the pleural space (necessary for normal ventilation). Sometimes thoracotomy is done to ex-

plore the chest surgically and repair the site of origin of the pneumo- or hemothorax.

Open Pneumothorax and Mediastinal Flutter

An open pneumothorax occurs with sucking chest wounds. With this type of wound, a traumatic opening in the chest wall is large enough for air to move freely in and out of the chest cavity during ventilation (Fig. 89–1B). This abnormal movement of air through the chest wound produces a slurping or sucking noise that is audible in a quiet environment.

Open sucking chest wounds may result from accidental injuries or surgical trauma. For example, if a chest drainage catheter is accidentally pulled out of a chest, the remaining puncture incision in the chest wall may become a sucking wound.

When an open sucking chest wound is detected, emergency intervention includes immediately covering the wound securely with anything available. An airtight covering usually prevents tension pneumothorax and preserves ventilation of the opposite lung. Do not waste time looking for a sterile gauze petrolatum dressing (the ideal covering for such a wound) if it is not immediately available. Immediately cover it with whatever is at hand (e.g., a towel) until someone can bring a sterile petrolatum dressing. When possible, fix the temporary dressing firmly in place with several strips of wide tape.

If the client is conscious and cooperative, ask the client to take a very deep breath and then attempt to blow it out while keeping mouth and nose closed. This pushing effort against a closed glottis helps push air out through the chest wound and reexpand the lung. When the client does this, apply the dressing before the client can inhale again.

Stay with the chest-injured client after a dressing has been applied to a sucking wound. Assess carefully for indications of tension pneumothorax and mediastinal shift. This may develop if the air leak is in the lung or a bronchus, which permits air to escape into the pleural space. In such a situation, closing the chest wall wound with an airtight dressing prevents the outflow of escaping air. Thus, an open pneumothorax has been accidentally converted into a tension pneumothorax. If the client appears to be developing tension pneumothorax after sealing of the wound, immediately unplug the seal to allow the air to escape.

Although it is dangerous to have air moving in and out of the pleural space with each respiration (open pneumothorax), it is far more dangerous when air moves only into the pleural space and cannot move back out (tension pneumothorax). Closed chest drainage will be necessary to (1) remove the air from the pleural space and (2) allow the lung to reexpand if collapsed.

In addition to dyspnea and collapse of the lung on the affected side, the client with an open pneumothorax may experience mediastinal flutter. This complication results from air rushing in and out of the thoracic cavity on the affected side. With inspiration, the mediastinal structures (heart, trachea, esophagus) and collapsed lung are pushed toward the unaffected side. Then, with expiration, these

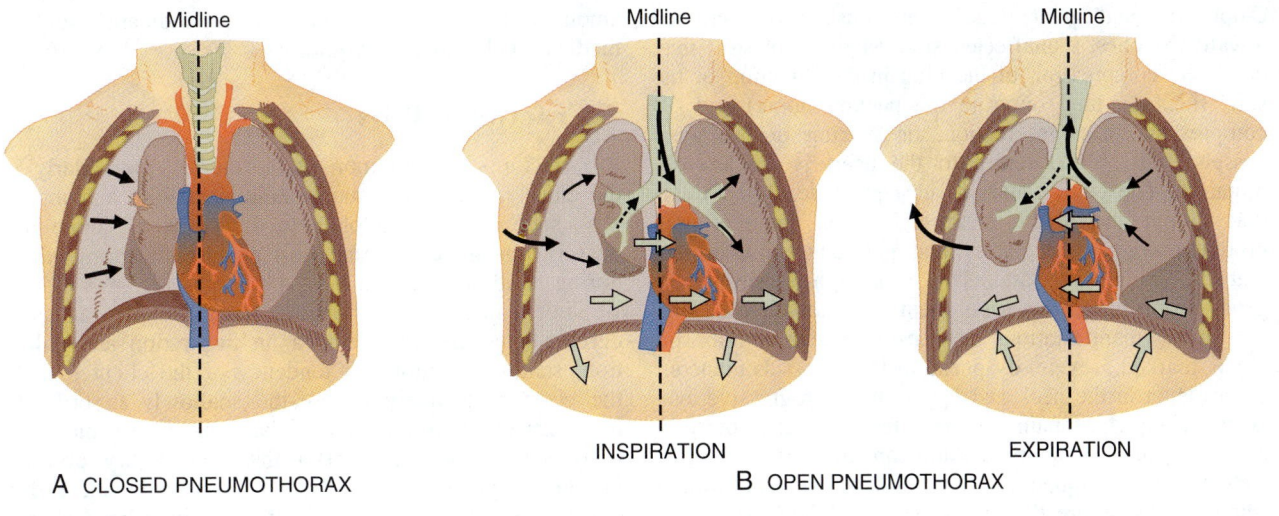

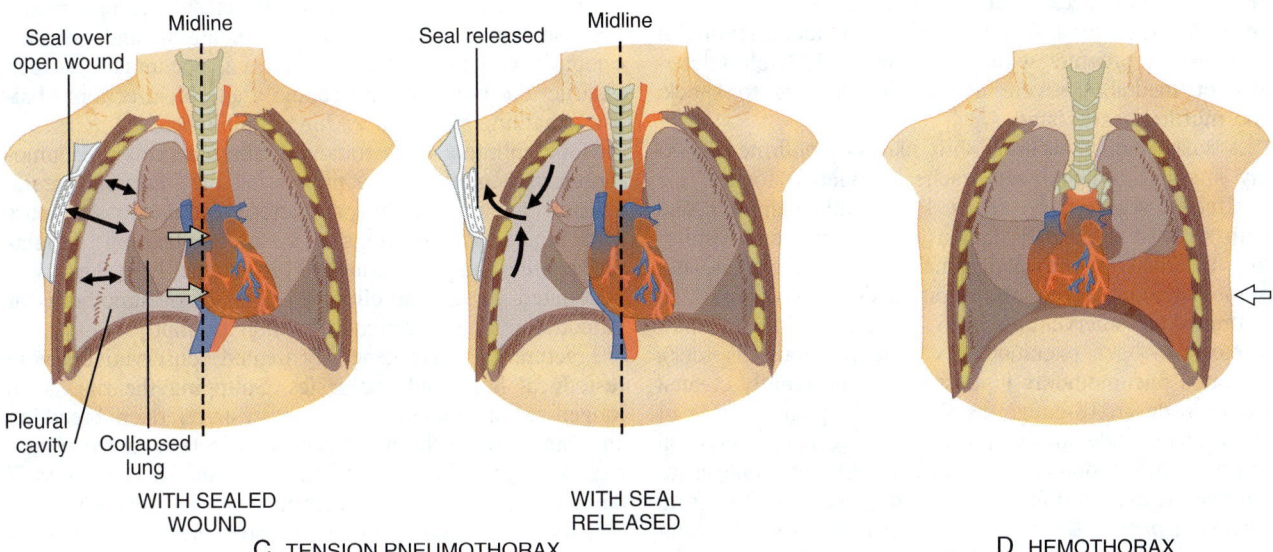

Figure 89–1. *A,* Pneumothorax. Lung collapses as air gathers in the pleural space. *B,* Open pneumothorax (sucking chest wound). *Solid arrows* indicate air movement; *open arrows,* structural movement. A chest wall wound connects the pleural space with atmospheric air. During inspiration, atmospheric air is sucked into the pleural space through the chest wall wound. Positive pressure in the pleural space collapses the lung on the affected side and pushes the mediastinal contents toward the unaffected side. This reduces the volume of air in the unaffected side considerably. During expiration, air escapes through the chest wall wound, lessening positive pressure in the affected side and allowing the mediastinal contents to swing back toward the affected side. Movement of mediastinal structures from side to side is called mediastinal flutter. *C,* Tension pneumothorax. *Left,* If an open pneumothorax is covered (e.g., with a dressing), it forms a seal, and tension pneumothorax with a mediastinal shift develops. A tear in lung structure continues to allow air into the pleural space. As positive pressure builds in the pleural space, the affected lung collapses, and the mediastinal contents shift to the unaffected side. *Right,* Tension pneumothorax is corrected by removing the seal (e.g., dressing), allowing air trapped in the pleural space to escape. *D,* Massive hemothorax (*arrow*) below the left lung, causing collapse of lung tissue.

structures move back toward the affected side. Fluttering, back-and-forth movements of these vital mediastinal structures produce severe cardiopulmonary embarrassment, which is fatal if not treated promptly.

Tension Pneumothorax and Mediastinal Shift

Tension pneumothorax (Fig. 89–1C) is a serious type of pneumothorax in which air enters the pleural space with

each inspiration, becomes trapped there, and is not expelled during expiration (i.e., one-way valve effect). Pressure builds in the chest as the accumulation of air in the pleural space increases. Tension pneumothorax most commonly occurs with blunt traumatic injuries and is frequently associated with flail chest injuries.

If untreated, tension pneumothorax collapses the lung on the affected side as intrapleural pressure or tension increases. It may then cause a mediastinal shift. This means the contents of the mediastinum (heart, trachea, esophagus, and great vessels) are pushed or "shifted" toward the chest's unaffected side. Mediastinal shift may cause (1) compression of the lung in the direction of the shift (i.e., the lung opposite the pneumothorax) and (2) compression, traction, torsion, or kinking of the great vessels; thus, blood return to the heart is dangerously impaired. The latter causes a subsequent decrease in cardiac output and blood pressure. Tension pneumothorax produces serious circulatory and pulmonary impairment that can be rapidly fatal. This is a high-priority emergency requiring prompt assessment and intervention.

Clinical manifestations of tension pneumothorax include marked, severe dyspnea; tachypnea; subcutaneous emphysema in the neck and upper chest; progressive cyanosis; acute chest pain on the affected side; hyperresonance (tympany) to percussion on the affected side; tachycardia; asymmetrical chest wall movement; diminished or absent breath sounds on the affected side; and extreme restlessness and agitation. Other clinical manifestations include neck vein distention; laryngeal and tracheal deviation or shift to the unaffected side; a feeling of tightness or pressure within the chest; a PMI shift laterally or medially; severe hypotension leading to shock; and muffled heart sounds.

A suspected mediastinal shift may be confirmed by x-ray study. Laryngeal and tracheal deviation toward the unaffected side can be detected by gentle palpation and with x-ray study. ABGs demonstrate hypoxia and respiratory alkalosis. When mediastinal shift is severe and not immediately corrected, respiratory acidosis may ensue.

Immediate intervention is to convert tension pneumothorax into open pneumothorax (a less serious disorder). An open pneumothorax is most easily and rapidly created by inserting an 18-gauge needle into the pleural space of the affected side at the level of the second intercostal space at the midclavicular line. Prompt thoracentesis to remove air may be life-saving. As trapped air rushes from a tension pneumothorax, the tension is relieved, the lung reexpands, and, if mediastinal shift is present, it corrects itself. After emergency treatment, a chest catheter is used to promote lung expansion.

■ Hemothorax

Hemothorax may be present in clients with chest injuries. A small amount of blood (less than 300 ml) in the pleural space may cause no symptoms and may not require intervention (blood will be reabsorbed spontaneously). Severe hemothorax (1400–2500 ml) may be life-threatening because of resultant hypovolemia and tension (Fig. 89–1D). Clinical manifestations include dullness to percussion on the affected side, tachycardia, hypotension, and shock.

A chest film confirms a diagnosis of hemothorax. If the client is in severe distress, the physician may aspirate blood from the pleural space by inserting a 16-gauge needle into the fifth or sixth intercostal space at the midaxillary line. To drain intrathoracic accumulations of blood, the physician inserts a large-caliber (36F or larger) chest catheter, which is then connected to a drainage system. An initial drainage of 500 to 1000 ml is considered moderate and may not require additional treatment. An initial drainage of 1500 ml or more or continued large amounts of drainage (200 ml/hr) is an indication for immediate exploratory thoracotomy.

■ Fractured Ribs

Rib fractures are common chest injuries, particularly in the elderly. They are usually associated with a blunt injury, such as a fall, a blow to the chest, or (more frequently) the impact of the chest against a steering wheel during rapid deceleration.

Clinical manifestations include localized pain and tenderness over the fracture area on inspiration and palpation; shallow respirations; tendency of the client to hold the chest protectively or breathe shallowly in order to minimize chest movements; bruising or surface markings (may or may not be present) at the site of injury; protruding bone splinters if the fracture is compound; and a clicking sensation during inspiration if costochondral separation or dislocation is present.

Fractured ribs predispose to atelectasis and pneumonia because the pain causes shallow breathing and prevents effective coughing. Thus, secretions accumulate, which obstruct the bronchi and become a site of infection. Shallow breathing also reduces lung compliance.

Bone splinters from fractured ribs may cause pneumothorax or hemothorax by puncturing the lung and pleura. Chest films are carefully reviewed for 24 to 48 hours after injury for indications of these complications. Bright-red sputum may be coughed up if the lung has been penetrated. Assess the client for signs of pneumothorax or hemothorax and report such findings promptly.

Fractured ribs are generally treated conservatively with rest, local heat, and analgesics. Strapping the ribs is no longer recommended because it restricts deep breathing and can increase the incidence of atelectasis and pneumonia. The pain from fractured ribs usually lasts 5 to 7 days. Complete healing occurs in approximately 6 weeks.

If pain is severe enough to impair ventilation significantly, a local anesthetic may be injected at the fracture site itself. Intercostal nerve blocks may also be used. A client with an underlying chest or heart disease (e.g., chronic obstructive pulmonary disease, congestive heart failure) may benefit particularly from this type of pain management. A chest film should be taken after this procedure to ensure that pneumothorax has not occurred. Adequate pain control and splinting of the chest during coughing and deep breathing help the client with rib fractures to carry out these painful but vital activities more comfortably. Hospitalization may be required, especially in the elderly, whose vital capacity may be significantly compromised.

■ Fractured Sternum

Sternal fractures usually result from blunt deceleration injuries, such as impact from the steering wheel. They are usually accompanied by other major injuries, such as flail chest; pulmonary and myocardial contusions; ruptured aorta, trachea, bronchus, or esophagus; and hemothorax or pneumothorax. Clinical manifestations include sharp, stabbing pain; swelling and discoloration over the fracture site; and crepitus. The main priority is to control associated injuries. A client with a nondisplaced fracture may need analgesics or intercostal nerve blocks for pain relief. Severe sternal fractures may require surgical fixation.

■ Flail Chest

Severe chest injuries that compress the rib cage often produce a crushed chest in which the ribs are pushed in on lung tissue. By definition, a flail chest consists of fractures of two or more adjacent ribs on the same side, and possibly the sternum, with each bone fractured into two or more segments (Fig. 89–2). The flail segment most commonly involves the lateral side of the chest. It is common for a fractured rib end to tear the pleura and lung surface, thereby producing hemopneumothorax. It is also common for a crushed chest to have a flail segment. Pulmonary edema, pneumonitis, and atelectasis often develop rapidly when the chest is crushed, because fluids tend to increase and collect at the injured site.

The "flail" segment no longer has bony or cartilaginous connections with the rest of the rib cage. Lacking attachment to the thoracic skeleton, the flail section "floats," moving independently of the chest wall during ventilation. This disrupts the normal bellows action of the thorax by causing paradoxical motion.

During paradoxical motion, the flail portion of the chest and its underlying lung tissue are (1) "sucked in" with inspiration, instead of expanding outward as normal, and (2) "blown out" with expiration, instead of collapsing normally inward. This alteration in normal chest wall mechanics diminishes the client's ability to achieve an adequate tidal volume and produce an adequate cough. Hypoventilation and hypoxemia may result, which leads to respiratory failure. Furthermore, mediastinal structures tend to swing back and forth (mediastinal flutter) with significant paradoxical motion. These swings may seriously affect circulatory dynamics, producing elevated venous pressure, impaired filling of the right side of the heart, and decreased arterial pressure.

In addition, pulmonary contusion occurs. This produces an accumulation of fluid in the affected alveoli, which leads to intrapulmonary shunting and further hypoxia. The full effects of pulmonary contusion may not be manifested until the height of the body's inflammatory response in 24 to 48 hours.

The client with a flail chest will experience emotional and physical distress while trying to breathe in spite of excruciating pain. The client is typically cyanotic and severely dyspneic. Respirations are usually rapid, shallow, and grunting. Paradoxical movement of the chest wall is usually obvious. Hypercapnia and hypoxia worsen as the effort necessary to breathe further depletes the already diminished oxygen supply. Frequent assessment of blood gases is needed to monitor respiratory effectiveness and detect acidosis. A variety of factors may produce metabolic and respiratory acidosis in chest-injured clients.

Treatment is usually with intubation and mechanical ventilation. These actions (1) restore adequate ventilation, thus reducing hypoxia and hypercapnia; (2) decrease paradoxical motion by using positive pressure to stabilize the chest wall internally; (3) relieve pain by decreasing movement of the fractured ribs; and (4) provide an avenue for removal of secretions. Internal stabilization with continuous ventilation may require 21 days or more. Muscle relaxants or musculoskeletal paralyzing agents may be administered to reduce the risk of separation of the healing costochondral junctions.

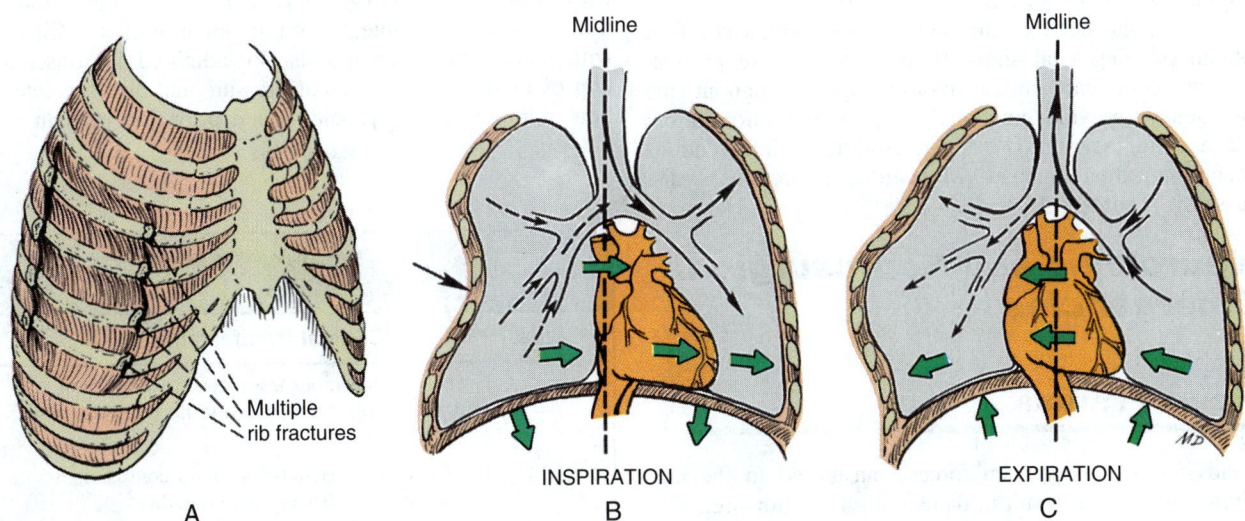

Figure 89–2. Flail chest. *Solid arrows* indicate air movement; *open arrows*, structural movement. *A,* A flail chest consists of fractured rib segments that are unattached (free-floating) to the rest of the chest wall. *B,* On inspiration, the flail segment of ribs is sucked inward. The affected lung and mediastinal structures shift to the unaffected side. This compromises the amount of inspired air in the unaffected lung. *C,* On expiration, the flail segment of ribs bellows outward. The affected lung and mediastinal structures shift to the affected side. Some air within the lungs is shunted back and forth between the lungs instead of passing through the upper airway.

Chest Pain

Chest pain is one of the most common complaints of clients entering an ED. A client with chest pain presents a diagnostic and management challenge. Effective triage is essential for early detection of and intervention in life-threatening conditions. Clients with chest pain are triaged as emergent until the cause is found. There are several causes of chest pain (see Table 44–1). Because the pain experience is subjective, careful assessment of the pain is important. Perform a complete symptom analysis.

Proceed with an objective assessment in the ABC order. Compare breath sounds bilaterally for the presence of any rales or wheezing. Listen to the heart sounds. Listen for a friction rub (possible pericarditis) or murmurs (valvular disease or endocarditis). Assess for the presence of adrenergic (elevated blood pressure, tachycardia, diaphoresis, dilated pupils, and anxiety) or cholinergic influences (bradycardia, nausea, and vomiting). Assess for distension of neck veins, which may be a clue to impaired venous return to the heart. Determine the level of consciousness. This may be diminished because of hypoxia. Obtain a full set of vital signs.

Provide supplemental oxygen via mask or nasal prongs. Apply a cardiac monitor for monitoring the heart rate and rhythm. A rapid way to do this is to apply the defibrillator pads for a quick look after explaining to the client that this is done to determine the heart rate and rhythm. If cardiac origin is suspected, obtain a 12-lead ECG. Secure IV access via a saline lock or begin an infusion of 5% dextrose with a microdrip or infusion pump at a keep-open rate. Treat any present dysrhythmias (see Chapter 46). Nitroglycerin is commonly used to treat angina or ischemic pain; this may be sublingual, IV, or dermal. Be sure to monitor blood pressure after the dose because it may cause hypotension. For severe pain, morphine 2 to 4 mg IV is administered. Be sure to assess respirations, vital signs, and pain control.

Position the head of the bed for the client's comfort. Obtain ongoing vital signs. If dysrhythmias are present, provide continual cardiac monitoring. Throughout the emergency, provide emotional support and information; use a calm, reassuring manner. Additional interventions depend on the diagnosis. Myocardial infarction is discussed in Chapter 44.

Neurologic and Neurosurgical Emergencies

Head Trauma

Head injuries result from forces transmitted to the cranium. Injuries can result in damage to the following:

1. The skull without brain injury
2. The brain without skull damage
3. The skull and brain

The brain and skull may be damaged by indirect trauma or direct trauma. Indirect injury occurs with a shearing motion, as in rear-impact collisions when the head is snapped backward and then forward, causing bruising that results in concussion. Direct trauma results from a force applied directly to the head. These are further divided into open and closed injuries. An open injury occurs when the client is hit with an object like a baseball bat or a bullet. Indirect or blunt trauma occurs most often in motor vehicle accidents, motorcycle collisions, and aggravated assaults when the head is struck by a stable object.

Care of clients with severe head injury is discussed fully in Chapter 34. We focus our discussion on head injuries that are often treated and released in the ED.

Concussions

A *concussion* is defined as a transient episode of neurologic dysfunction that occurs after blunt trauma. The injury is usually the result of a blow to the head, a fall, or a motor vehicle accident. The temporary loss of function may be caused by temporary ischemia or neuronal depolarization after acetylcholine release.

Concussions are classified into four grades based on the clinical manifestations (Table 89–5). Clinical manifestations of concussion are confusion, dizziness, amnesia, and may or may not include a loss of consciousness. Other manifestations can include changes in vital signs or respiratory patterns, diplopia, nausea, vomiting, and often headache. The Glasgow Coma Score is usually normal. There are three types of amnesia that can occur after concussion:

1. Anterograde: no memory of the events after the injury. There are often problems learning new material.
2. Retrograde: no memory of events prior to the trauma.
3. A combination of both types.

Management is usually directed at detecting more serious head injuries, and providing pain relief. Most clients with mild concussion (grade I) will be discharged home, if they have a reliable person to monitor them. Clients with more severe concussions are admitted for observation of increasing intracranial pressure and also for detection of more serious problems and provision of pain relief.

Table 89–5. Classification of Concussions	
Grade	**Clinical Manifestations**
I	No loss of consciousness, transient confusion (few minutes), rapid return to normal functioning, no amnesia.
II	Brief loss of consciousness, mild confusion, some amnesia, usually anterograde.
III	Loss of consciousness for less than 6 hrs, profound confusion, anterograde and retrograde amnesia.
IV	Loss of consciousness over 6 hrs, confusion, anterograde and retrograde amnesia.

Be sure to include the following teaching and learning points in the discharge instructions for clients with head injuries and their significant others.

- Wake the client every 2 hours (for the next 8 hours) and check level of consciousness and orientation.
- Give only liquids initially for the first 8 hours, then progress to a regular diet.
- Give acetaminophen for headache. If a stronger medication is required, contact a physician. (*Note:* Emphasize this, because clients may have narcotics from previous illnesses and must understand that narcotics are contraindicated in head injury.)
- Notify a physician or return to the ED if any of the following occur: one or both pupils become dilated and nonreactive; the level of consciousness decreases; irritability or confusion occurs; inability to use an arm or leg develops; seizure is experienced; or there is continued vomiting.
- Provide written as well as oral instruction, and include an appropriate telephone number for additional questions once the client returns home.

Skull Fractures

The type of skull fracture will depend upon the velocity and type of object striking the head. A low-velocity impact tends to produce a linear skull fracture without bony displacement or neurologic changes. Linear skull fractures of the temporal bone can lead to epidural hematoma. Management is observation and can usually be done at home, if the client has a reliable observer.

Basilar skull fractures occur from blunt trauma, such as a fall. These fractures are not always apparent in skull x-rays or CT scans. Diagnosis is usually made by clinical manifestations of raccoon eyes (periorbital ecchymosis), Battle's sign (ecchymosis of the mastoid area), hemotympanium, and cerebrospinal fluid rhinorrhea or otorrhea. Hearing loss and facial nerve palsy may develop, but are later signs. The client is admitted for observation of increasing intracranial pressure (ICP) and bleeding. Usual changes noted with elevations in ICP may not develop (i.e., changes in motor function) because pressure develops below the motor strip. Look for irritability and pain due to changes in vital signs (such as bradycardia) as a result of increased ICP. Antibiotics are used to reduce the risk of meningitis.

Depressed skull fractures are a cause for concern. The cranium is displaced into the brain. If the scalp is lacerated, there is communication between the outside environment and the brain. There is also increased risk of bleeding from the bony fragments lacerating blood vessels. Surgery is usually indicated to remove bone fragments and repair the dura.

Penetrating skull fractures and head injuries are often fatal. These injuries include gunshot wounds, stab wounds, and falls onto sharp objects that impale the skull. Any client admitted with a history of head trauma should undergo full assessment, even if the client does not look ill. Surgery may be required for clients with penetrating head wounds to debride damaged tissues. If the client has a massive, nonsurvivable head wound, it is usually not treated with surgery. Instead, the client is evaluated for potential organ donation.

Spinal Injuries

All persons who sustain traumatic injury are at risk of spinal cord injury. These injuries result in loss of motor or sensory function that may be permanent. See Chapter 35 for further discussion of spinal injuries.[45]

Assess and maintain the ABCs. Remember to suspect a cervical spine injury in all unconscious trauma victims and with injuries above the clavicle. Immobilize the spine by applying a hard cervical extrication collar or Philadelphia collar and placing the client on a long spine board.

Respiratory insufficiency may be present, especially with a cervical spine injury, because the phrenic nerve (controls the diaphragm during respiration) exits the spinal column between C3 and C4. Keep in mind the risk of hypotension related to neurogenic shock.

Clients with spinal cord injuries may be fully conscious and aware of motor and sensory losses. Fear and anxiety are often present. Be sure to communicate with the client and provide information about any treatments and procedures. Remain calm and reassure the client. Provide comfort measures, and maintain the client's dignity.

Abdominal Emergencies

Acute Abdominal Pain

Abdominal pain is common; its causes are numerous. Serious abdominal emergencies requiring immediate assessment and management must be identified. The term *acute abdomen* is used to describe sudden onset of abdominal pain. Common causes of acute abdomen are shown in Figure 89–3.

Include the following specific historical information:

- Assess the pain for location, quality, and duration and ask if it radiates. Determine if there is a history of injury.
- Is there a history of nausea, vomiting, or loss of appetite? What is the amount and character of the emesis, if present?
- When was the last bowel movement? Was it normal? What was the character of the stool? When did the client last eat? What did the client eat?
- What medication or remedies have been used in an attempt to relieve the pain?
- Determine the menstrual history in all sexually active females of childbearing age.

Assess the abdomen in order of inspection, auscultation, percussion, and palpation. Assess the client's position. Often a client lying with flexed knees has an inflammatory process (peritonitis), whereas a restless client unable to find a comfortable position may have a colic-type pain (ureteral calculi). Assess for distention, masses, umbilical protrusion, and discoloration around the flank or umbilicus. Look for evidence of blunt or penetrating trauma. Auscultate for bowel sounds.

Priorities of care focus on maintaining the ABCs. Be

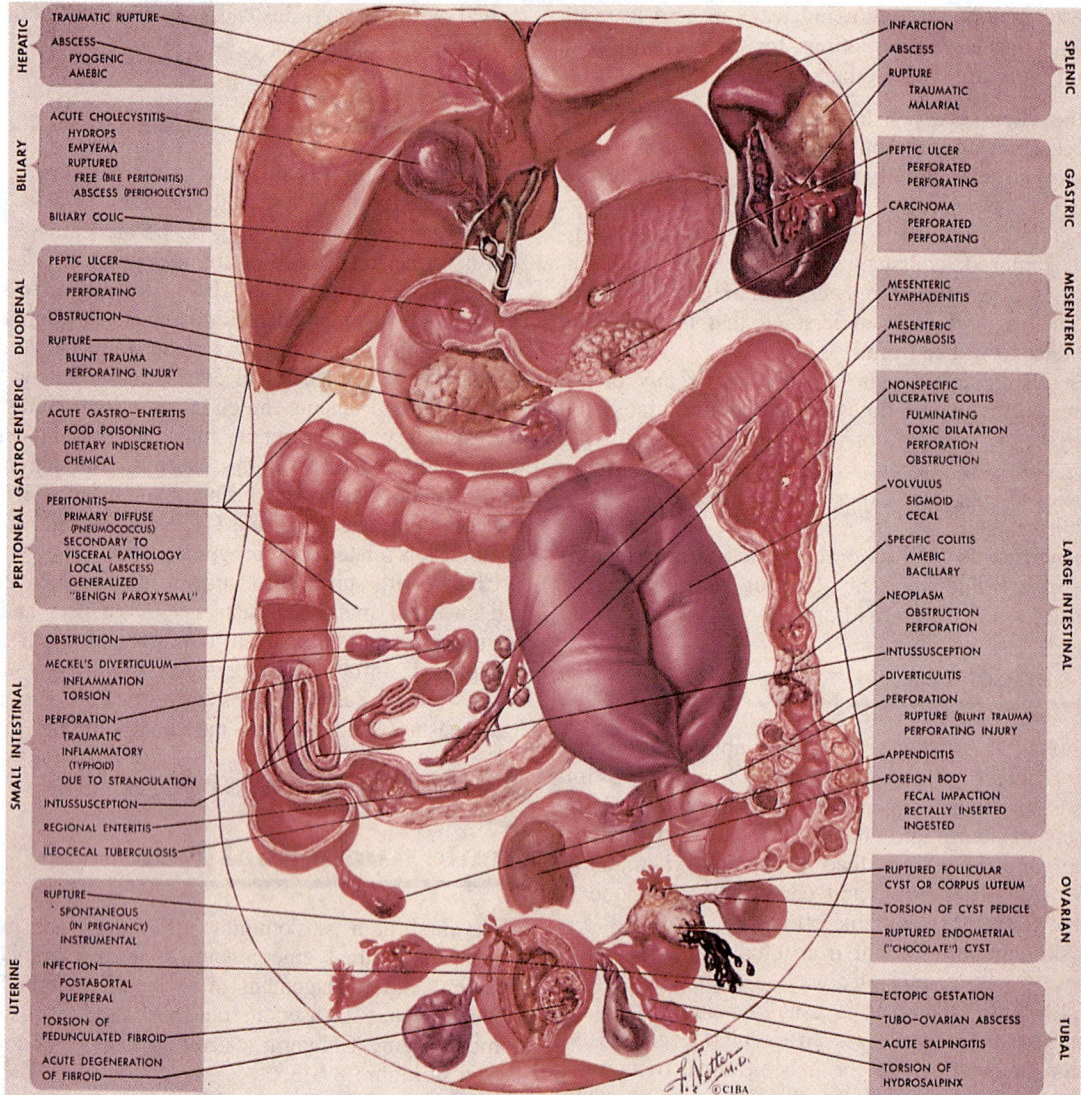

Figure 89–3. Differential diagnosis of acute abdominal pain. (© Copyright 1996. CIBA-GEIGY Corporation. Reprinted with permission from the Ciba Collection illustrated by Frank Netter, M.D. All rights reserved.)

sure to monitor vital signs for changes. Initiate IV access as needed for hydration and infuse lactated Ringer's solution or normal saline until hypotension or orthostasis is resolved. Keep the client NPO until the cause of the abdominal pain is identified.

Gastrointestinal Bleeding

The causes of gastrointestinal bleeding are many. The three major causes of upper gastrointestinal bleeding are peptic ulcer disease, gastritis, and esophageal varices. Massive gastrointestinal bleeding can also occur from hematologic disorders that decrease platelet numbers or function. Lower gastrointestinal bleeding is most often caused by hemorrhoids and polyps of the colon. The clients can appear perfectly normal or be in frank shock.

Immediate interventions focus on cardiovascular stabi-

lization, identification of the source of bleeding, and attempts to stop the bleeding. Additionally, psychosocial support for the client and significant others is important. Massive bleeding is frightening, and many procedures that may be uncomfortable are carried out rapidly in the initial phase of care.

Upper gastrointestinal bleeding is a common reason for ED visits.

Upper GI bleeding is often treated with a nasogastric tube to evacuate contents and lavage the stomach. Controversy exists about the temperature of the water for lavage. Some believe that cold water interferes with coagulation, whereas others support the use of cold water to cause vasoconstriction. Lavage should continue until the returning fluid is clear. Endoscopy is used to identify the source of the bleeding.

If the client has bleeding esophageal varices, bleeding is controlled by applying pressure to the lower esophagus.

A balloon is inserted and dilated to control bleeding; the process is called *tamponade*.

Abdominal Injuries

Abdominal injuries provide a challenge to healthcare providers. The manifestations of abdominal injuries are often subtle and require astute assessment and intervention. The mechanism of injury, knowledge of abdominal structures, and an index of suspicion provide clues for rapid detection and management of clients with abdominal injuries. Missed abdominal injuries are an all-too-frequent cause of preventable death following blunt trauma.

Abdominal injuries, caused by blunt or penetrating trauma, may result in significant organ injury and shock. Low-velocity trauma (e.g., fist) usually results in single-organ injury. High-velocity trauma (e.g., motor vehicle crash) often produces multiple-organ involvement. Once the mechanism of injury is identified, keep in mind the potential of associated injuries to underlying organs and tissues. Blunt trauma is more likely to cause injury to the solid organs (spleen, liver, pancreas, kidneys).

Penetrating abdominal injuries are often caused by gunshot or stab wounds. The underlying injuries will depend on the mechanism of injury, trajectory, and location. Infection (peritonitis) is a common complication of penetrating abdominal trauma, especially if the bowel is ruptured. Hemorrhage and shock may develop if major blood vessels, liver, and spleen are injured. The client with a penetrating abdominal injury requires surgical exploration.

Clinical manifestations include abdominal pain, distention, rigidity, nausea, vomiting, altered or absent bowel sounds, hypotension, and shock. Assess for any open wounds. If open wounds are present, evisceration may occur. Exposure of abdominal contents to air may dry them out and lead to necrosis. If an open wound is found, cover it with a warm, moist, sterile towel.

The spleen is the abdominal organ most commonly injured by blunt trauma. Splenic injury can also be associated with left upper quadrant injuries, left lower rib fractures, or left pneumothorax. Be sure to watch for shock and support the circulatory status.

Liver injury may result from abdominal trauma and should be suspected with right lower rib fractures. The liver is highly vascular, and injury may result in shock and bleeding disorders (clotting factors such as fibrinogen and prothrombin are synthesized in the liver). Surgical repair through hemostatic agents and repair of blood vessels may be indicated.[3,11]

Manage and support the ABCs. Provide supplemental oxygen. Initiate one to two large-bore IV lines and begin fluid support. Obtain serial vital signs. Insert a urinary catheter if there is no blood at the meatus and obtain urinalysis and specific gravity. Insert a nasogastric tube, test the aspirate for blood, and connect to suction to decompress the stomach. Obtain abdominal x-ray studies (flat plate, upright, and lateral decubitus views). Prepare the client for an IV pyelogram if hematuria is present. An ultrasonogram or CT scan of the abdomen may be performed if the client is stable. A culdocentesis may be done on females.

A diagnostic peritoneal lavage is performed by a physician to determine the presence of blood in the abdominal cavity (Fig. 89–4). The area below the umbilicus is anesthetized, and a large angiocatheter or peritoneal dialysis catheter is inserted into the abdomen. A syringe is attached to the catheter, and an attempt is made to aspirate blood. One liter of normal saline is infused into the abdomen and drained by gravity. The fluid is evaluated for gross blood and sent to the laboratory for evaluation. If the finding is positive, surgery is required.

Many clients with blunt abdominal trauma are assessed and discharged from the ED. However, some injuries (delayed rupture of the spleen) may not become apparent for several hours or days. Therefore, it is important to emphasize the need for repeat evaluation, particularly if the following symptoms occur:

- Increased localized or generalized abdominal pain
- Shoulder pain unrelated to shoulder trauma (Kehr's sign, suggestive of diaphragm irritation due to fluid or blood in the abdominal cavity)
- Malaise, lethargy, or dizziness suggestive of slow blood loss

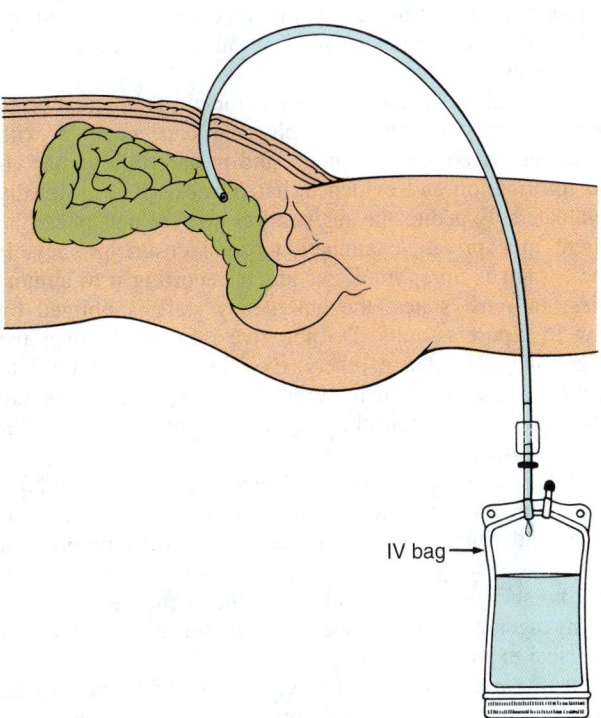

IV bag →

INTERPRETATION OF RESULTS

Positive result	Free-flowing blood on aspiration Grossly bloody lavage return >100,000 RBC/mm³ >500 WBC/mm³ Exit of lavage fluid from urinary or thoracic catheters
Equivocal result	50,000–100,000 RBC/mm³ 100–500 WBC/mm³
Negative result	<50,000 RBC/mm³ <100 WBC/mm³

Figure 89–4. Diagnostic peritoneal lavage.

- Fever of unexplained origin
- Nausea or vomiting, particularly if there is persistent hematemesis or melena

Alleged Sexual Assault

Healthcare providers are required to use the term "alleged sexual assault" when caring for clients who may be victims of rape. Rape is a legal term. Although people who experience sexual assault may be male, most are female. Victims of sexual assault should be advised that health professionals are required to use the term "sexual assault" rather than "rape." Otherwise, they may understandably become infuriated by the staff's seeming insensitivity and lack of understanding.

Sexual assault victims often experience both acute and long-term physical and psychological trauma. This results from the assault itself and the events that follow the assault. The psychological trauma, known as *rape-trauma syndrome,* may last only a few days to weeks or may last many years.[22, 32]

Lengthy legal proceedings, public humiliation, and destruction of social relationships prolong recovery. Although sexual assault victims may not be physiologically compromised on arrival in the emergency care setting, they are psychologically fragile and should be afforded the highest triage priority.

The goal of emergency care for these clients is to provide sensitive, thorough physical care coupled with empathic psychosocial support and to carefully gather vital information and evidence that in most cases is legally evaluated. Expedite the registration process and place the client in a private examination room; ensure privacy. If the assault is unreported, encourage reporting it to authorities. In most states, the emergency staff is obliged by law to report assaults. Do not give information over the telephone to media or others. Explain to the client not to wash, gargle, or douche until necessary specimens are obtained. Provide the client an opportunity to bathe after the examination.

Obtain a detailed history and physical examination after explaining the need for detail. Take the history immediately and only once. Sexual assault victims report that giving a history is almost as traumatic as the assault. Record the history in detail, using the client's own words. Many agencies have a special form for this history and physical examination.

Begin assessments and interventions with the ABCs. Some clients have massive trauma with loss of consciousness. For others, the physical result of the sexual assault may not be obvious. Consider possible sexual assault in unconscious clients with traumatic injury when the history is unknown or suspicious. Some common signs include ecchymotic areas, especially of the face or neck, and multiple contusions or lacerations. Assess for trauma to the larynx and fracture (with or without dislocation) of the mandible. Record extent, location, and treatment of all injuries. Pictures may be included. Some victims may not have any visible injuries, but this should not negate the client's claim of assault. In females, a gynecologic exami-nation should be carried out only once, preferably by a practitioner experienced in caring for these clients who will be available for court trial.[36,37]

Note the condition of the client's clothing. Clothes may be stained, torn, or disheveled. However, they may be used as court evidence. Be sure to handle them carefully. Clothes are often taken by the police as evidence, so make arrangements for clean clothes to be brought to the client. Place clothes in a paper bag.

Obtain specimens for laboratory study. These include cultures for chlamydia and gonorrhea; hanging drop analysis and smears for the presence of sperm and their motility; acid phosphatase in vaginal secretions; police laboratory analysis of foreign pubic hairs in which hairs obtained by combing through the client's hair and plucking pubic hair from several sites are compared; and serologic fluorescent treponemal antibody studies. A human immunodeficiency virus (HIV) screen, such as the enzyme-linked immunoassay (ELISA) to detect antibodies to HIV, may also be done. The client may be counseled to repeat the HIV screen 3 to 6 months later because a negative antibody test does not conclusively exclude the possibility of HIV infection. Specimen collection and chain-of-custody principles should be followed. Antibiotics may given to prevent or treat sexually transmitted diseases.[9] Medications for prevention of pregnancy may be given.

Emotional responses may vary. Keep in mind the use of defense mechanisms that preserve psychosocial integrity. Do not assume that a lack of concern or relative calm means that the assault did not occur or that the client is handling it well. Feelings of guilt, humiliation (especially after meeting with police), and fear may inhibit many victims from expressing their feelings. Provide psychosocial support and clear, understandable explanations. Obtain the client's permission to contact sexual assault counselors if they are available and it has not already been done. Suggest that someone stay with the client for several days after the event for support.

Discharge teaching includes the following:

1. Schedule follow-up care in 4 to 6 weeks for test results, pregnancy test, and psychosocial support.
2. Provide the name and number of someone to contact if the client is unwilling or unable to use counseling resources at the time of emergency treatment.
3. Discuss some emotional responses to this type of trauma (rape-trauma syndrome).
4. Stress the importance of pregnancy prevention drug treatment.
5. Advise that menses should start within 7 days after completion of treatment; if this does not occur, dilation and curettage is arranged.

Be sure to document the history, assessments, interventions, and discharge teaching carefully. These hospital records are often placed in a "security file" because of their possible use in court. Only the medical records department should release records and information and only to authorities with proper credentials.

Ocular Emergencies

Ocular emergencies, involving the eye and surrounding structures, range from mild corneal abrasions to avulsion of the eye. High triage priorities include retinal detachment or hemorrhage, cloudy cornea, irregular corneal light reflex, "ciliary flush" (red ring of dilated deep vessels at the corneal-scleral junction), blurred or decreased vision, pain, or photophobia. Immediate referral to an ophthalmologist is necessary.[19,24]

Chemical Eye Burns

Take the history. The conjunctiva is often reddened, and there is severe pain. Copious tearing may be present unless deeper structures are involved. Be sure to determine what measures, if any, have been taken to relieve the pain or remove the chemical.

Reassure the client and explain all procedures. Immediately irrigate the eye copiously with normal saline, water, or other mild solution. The eye's pH may be frequently tested and used to guide irrigation. Irrigation may continue until the pH is in the 6 to 7 range. Often it is necessary to use a short-acting local anesthetic to irrigate the eye adequately. Evert the upper lid to observe for and remove chemical particles (especially important with alkali burns). Alkali burns may need continuous irrigation for several hours, and special irrigation devices are available. Other chemical burns should be irrigated for at least 20 minutes. Antibiotic drops, ointments, or irrigants may be used. Pain is often due to blepharospasm, and a mydriatic (homatropine, cyclopentolate [Cyclogyl]) may relieve the pain. Patch both eyes if necessary to immobilize the affected eye. If the burn is significant, the client is usually referred to an ophthalmologist or admitted.

Ocular Foreign Bodies

Ocular foreign bodies include surface, embedded, and impaled objects. The client will complain of "something in the eye" or pain with blinking. Often the history is compatible with a foreign body. Pain and tearing may be present.

Be sure to remove any contact lenses, and place in sterile saline solution. Contact lenses may become dislodged, which makes removal by the client difficult. The lenses are often found under the upper eyelid.

Surface foreign bodies may be removed by simple saline irrigation administered by nursing staff. Anesthetizing the eye may be necessary prior to irrigation. Embedded or impaled objects are left intact until they are removed by an ophthalmologist. Stabilize the object by applying dressings (moistened with normal saline) around the base of the object and securing the object to the head. Avoid exerting pressure on the globe, and immobilize the head. Do not attempt to stop bleeding from the eye or eyelids with direct pressure. This can cause further injury. Foreign bodies made of metal may quickly begin to rust and a ring may be noticed around the object. Wood particles must also be removed quickly by an ophthalmologist.

Following eye irrigation, the eye is stained. Corneal abrasion, if present, is treated with antibacterial eye drops or ointment and patching of the eye. Follow-up care in 24 hours is indicated. Assessment of visual acuity should be completed and recorded before discharge. If one eye is patched, the client should be warned not to drive because of the loss of depth perception.

Ocular Avulsions

Avulsion of the eye from its socket may result from either blunt or penetrating trauma. The eye will be extruded from the orbit with obvious deformity and pain. However, even with rapid and expert care, the probability of preserving vision in the affected eye is slim.

Protect the eye from drying by gently applying sterile dressings moistened with warm saline. Apply an eye protector (cone, shield, paper cup) and secure it gently to the head with Kling or Kerlix gauze. Patch the unaffected eye, and immobilize the head. Provide reassurance, but do not give false hopes about saving the eye. Obtain a prompt referral to an ophthalmologist. Prepare the client for surgery and keep the client NPO.

Musculoskeletal Emergencies

Musculoskeletal emergencies include fractures, amputations, joint dislocations, muscle strains, and ligament and tendon damage. These disorders are discussed in Chapter 75.

Traumatic Amputations

Traumatic amputations involve obvious total or partial severing of an extremity or digit. The severity of bleeding depends on the extent of trauma to surrounding tissues. A crush injury and complete amputation may not bleed profusely because of muscle spasms in the arterial walls. However, a partially severed limb may require a tourniquet to control bleeding.

Hypotension, shock, and tachycardia may be present if the client sustained significant blood loss. Maintain and support the ABCs. Initiate IV and fluid resuscitation. Control hemorrhage by direct pressure with use of a clean, sterile dressing if possible. Draw blood for laboratory studies (CBC, T&C). Prepare the client for surgery.

The amputated part, including detached teeth, should accompany the client to the hospital because replantation with microsurgery is sometimes possible. Wrap the amputated part in saline-soaked gauze and place it in a plastic bag or container. Place the container on ice. Do not place the amputated part directly on ice. Do not use dry ice or freeze or totally submerge the tissue. In addition, the part should not be cleaned, disinfected, debrided, or perfused before transportation.

Soft Tissue Emergencies

Damage to the skin and soft tissues is a common emergency. The types of soft tissue injury are contusions, abrasions, puncture wounds, lacerations, and avulsions.

Always assess and maintain the ABCs. Assess the wound for location, size, depth, and degree of contamination; assess for associated injuries, amount of tissue loss, and viability of wound edges and of amputated tissue. Determine the history and mechanism of injury. Include information about where the injury occurred, the length of time since the injury, and allergies. Obtain an immunization history and the need for a tetanus booster. Assess the range of motion, perfusion, and sensation distal to the wound.

Stop bleeding by direct pressure or application of a pressure dressing. These wounds should be considered contaminated. Clean the area around the wound and copiously irrigate with normal saline. A high-pressure device (8 psi) made of a 30-ml syringe with an 18-gauge plastic catheter attached can clean the wound with only minimal damage to healthy tissue. Mechanical scrubbing is not advised unless the amount of debris in the wound is overwhelming. Scrubbing damages healthy tissue, prolongs wound healing, and increases inflammation. The area around the wound may need to be shaved. Do not shave eyebrows; they are used for landmarks to repair extensive facial lacerations.

Because of potential exposure to anaerobic organisms, tetanus prophylaxis is given. For wound management, the need for active immunization depends on the client's immunization history and the condition of the wound. The recommendations for tetanus prophylaxis are outlined in Table 89–6.

Td (tetanus and diphtheria toxoid) is the preferred preparation for active tetanus immunization in adults. If passive immunization is needed, human tetanus immune globulin (TIG) is given. The recommended dose of TIG for wounds of average severity is 250 units intramuscularly. When TIG and Td are given concurrently, separate syringes and separate sites should be used.[34,42]

Anesthesia may be needed to clean the wound properly. Lidocaine 1% without epinephrine is used on fingers, toes, the tip of the nose, and ears and in elderly clients with thin skin. Lidocaine with epinephrine is used in other areas to minimize bleeding or prolong anesthesia.

The wound may be closed noninvasively (e.g., with adhesive paper strips). The wound edges are pulled together and maintained with the tape.

Wounds that require suturing include those with gaping wound edges; with visible subcutaneous or deeper structures; and those located over joints, where joint movement opens the wound edges. Although minor suturing is a fairly simple skill, the consequences of an inappropriately sutured wound may lead to poor wound healing, scarring, and infection. Nurses who have received specialized training may suture uncomplicated lacerations.

After wound closure, gently remove any prep solution or old blood and apply a dressing. Begin with gauze dressings to absorb drainage. Then apply a layer to provide slight pressure. A woven roll of gauze (Kling or

Table 89–6. Summary of Recommendations of Advisory Committee on Immunization Practices for Tetanus Prophylaxis in Routine Wound Management—United States, 1991

History of Adsorbed Tetanus Toxoid (Doses)	Clean, Minor Wounds		All Other Wounds*	
	Td†	TIG	Td†	TIG
Unknown or <3	Yes	No	Yes	Yes
≥3‡	No§	No	No¶	No

* Such as, but not limited to, wounds contaminated with dirt, feces, soil, saliva; puncture wounds; avulsions; and wounds resulting from missiles, crushing, burns, and frostbite.
† For children <7 years old, DTP (DT, if pertussis vaccine is contraindicated) is preferred to tetanus toxoid alone. For persons ≥7 years of age, Td is preferred to tetanus toxoid alone. Diphtheria and tetanus toxoids and acellular pertussis vaccine (DTaP) may be used instead of DTP for the fourth and fifth doses.
‡ If only three doses of *fluid* toxoid have been received, then a fourth dose of toxoid, preferably an adsorbed toxoid, should be given.
§ Yes, if more than 10 years since last dose.
¶ Yes, if more than 5 years since last dose. (More frequent boosters are not needed and can accentuate side effects.)
DT, diphtheria-tetanus; DTP, diphtheria-tetanus-pertussis; Td, tetanus-diphtheria toxoid; TIG, tetanus immune globulin.
From Prevots, R., et al. (1992). Tetanus surveillance—United States, 1989–1990. *Morbidity and Mortality Weekly Report, 41* (SS-8), 1–9.
From: Kitt, S., et al. (1995). *Emergency Nursing*. Philadelphia: W. B. Saunders Co. Used with permission.

Kerlix) may be held in place by either adhesive tape or an elastic net. Avoid placing adhesive tape over the wound area; occlusive tape may foster moisture accumulation and maceration of wound edges. A thin film of antibiotic ointment may be applied directly to the wound to minimize crusting and promote a thinner scar. A transparent dressing may be used in wounds not expected to swell or that have large amounts of drainage.[34] The Client Education Guide provides discharge teaching for care of sutured lacerations.

Heat Emergencies

Exposure to increased environmental temperature may lead to heat emergencies.[29] As the temperature increases, the sweat glands attempt to cool the body through diaphoresis (sweating). As the temperature continues to increase, the body compensates with profuse sweating. Unless fluids and salts are replaced, hypotension, dehydration, sodium depletion, and electrolyte imbalances may occur from excess fluid loss through perspiration.

Clients who are very young, elderly, or certain medications are at greater risk of developing heat emergencies. Some medications reduce the ability to sweat; these include antihistaminics, beta-blockers, anticholinergics, and phenothiazines. Other medications, such as amphetamines and neuroleptics, increase heat production. Be sure to assess the client's history for cardiac, pulmonary, or renal

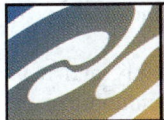

CLIENT EDUCATION GUIDE

Care of Sutured Lacerations

1. Keep the wound and dressing clean. You may shower. Do not expose the wound to moisture for prolonged periods of time.
2. Keep the area elevated. Mild swelling is expected. You may apply ice.
3. *Wet dressing:* If the dressing gets wet, remove it, blot the wound dry with a sterile gauze pad, and reapply a sterile dressing. Repeat this procedure every day until the stitches are removed, unless instructed otherwise.
4. *Dressing changes:* Remove the dressing after 2 days and reapply a sterile dressing. Repeat this procedure every day until the stitches are removed, unless instructed otherwise.
5. *Signs of infection:* If any of the following signs of infection appear, contact a physician immediately:
   a. Wound becomes red, swollen, tender, or warm.
   b. Wound begins to drain or fester.
   c. Red streaks appear around the wound.
   d. Tender lumps appear in the groin or under the arm.
   e. Chills or fever occur.
6. *Infection check:* Because of the nature of your injury, the possibility of infection is increased. Please return to be checked in _____ days.
7. *Stitch Removal:* The physician suggests that the stitches be removed in about _____ days.
8. *Tetanus immunization:* For your records, you/your child received the following:
   a. Tetanus toxoid _____
   b. DT (diphtheria-tetanus) _____
   c. DPT (diphtheria-pertussis-tetanus) _____
   d. Other _____

diseases and drug regimens. At discharge, these clients need to learn about the side effects of drug regimens and ways to avoid or reduce exposure to extremes in temperature. The elderly often are unable to afford air conditioning and are frequent victims of heat exhaustion. In the summer of 1995, several hundred impoverished elderly people died in Chicago from heat stroke.

Heat cramps are muscle spasms of arms, legs, and occasionally the abdomen related to sodium depletion from excessive perspiration. Remove the client from the hot environment and administer oral fluids containing salt.

Heat exhaustion results from dehydration. Manifestations include hypotension, headache, dizziness, faintness, anorexia, nausea, prostration, weakness, and collapse. The skin may be cool and clammy. Vital signs vary, depending on the extent of volume depletion. Remove the client from the heat. Administer oral or IV fluids as needed.

Heat stroke is an emergency and requires immediate treatment for survival. There are two forms of heat stroke: (1) classic heat stroke and (2) exertional heat stroke.

Classic heat stroke is seen most commonly in the poor, the elderly, the chronically ill, people with heart disease, the obese, and alcoholics. Hot, humid weather lasting 3 days or more increases the risk of heat stroke in these people. The stress of heat increases the demand on the heart.

Exertional heat stroke is more common in laborers, farmers, military recruits, athletes (especially football players and long-distance runners), and people who work in boiler rooms or foundries. Symptoms of their form of heat stroke are similar to classic heat stroke except this group sweats. They tend to develop lactic acidosis and have more severe bleeding problems.

Rapidly reduce body temperature (immerse or sponge with cool water). A hypothermia blanket may be used. Start an IV line and provide cardiovascular support. Apply a cardiac monitor and obtain frequent vital signs. Administer chlorpromazine or diazepam to reduce shivering. Provide supplemental oxygen. Insert a urinary catheter unless recovery is prompt. Admit the client to the hospital.

Cold Emergencies

Hypothermia

Hypothermia[27,29] is defined as a lowered core body temperature, usually below 34.4° C (94° F). It may occur in divers, people exposed to cold weather, and near drowning victims. Some clients appear dead yet have a feeble pulse. Pupils may be fixed and dilated. Manifestations depend on the client's core temperature:

- 34.4° C (94° F), amnesia or sluggishness
- 32.2° C (90° F), cardiac dysrhythmias, especially premature ventricular contractions
- 30° C (86° F), loss of muscle coordination, possible unconsciousness
- 25° C (77° F), cardiac arrest

Support the ABCs. Endotracheal intubation may be indicated. Initiate CPR when indicated. Be aware that often there is a great deal of water on the floor during immediate resuscitation of a client with profound hypothermia. Use a battery-powered defibrillator, rather than one connected to a higher voltage wall outlet, to protect the staff from electrical hazard.

Insert an esophageal thermometer or rectal thermometer probe. Start IV and CVP lines if hypothermia is severe. Monitor cardiac rhythm and obtain a 12-lead ECG. Insert a urinary catheter and monitor output every 30 minutes.

Core rewarming is performed by use of heated oxygen, and gastric, urinary bladder, and peritoneal lavage with heated fluids. Do not apply external heat to a profoundly hypothermic client. It causes vasodilation and further cardiovascular collapse. Peripheral rewarming is usually delayed until the core temperature has been raised. Resuscitation is not usually successful until adequate core rewarming has been achieved and efforts should not be abandoned until rewarming is accomplished. If necessary, the client may be transferred to the operating room for rewarming with a bypass machine.[26,27]

Frostbite

Frostbite is damage to tissues and blood vessels as a result of prolonged exposure to cold. Fingers, toes, nose, and ears are often affected. There may be initial numbness, paresthesia, and pallor of the affected part. Often, severe pain, swelling, erythema, and blistering (similar to a second-degree, partial-thickness burn) occur once the client is in a warm environment. Necrosis and gangrene may develop in severe cases.

Handle the tissues gently. Rewarm the affected part with tepid water (about 105° F). Do not massage the client; this may result in further tissue damage. Do not debride blisters. Apply bulky dressings to permit drainage and provide protection.

Bites

Snake Bites

Four poisonous snakes are found in the United States. Three of these are pit vipers (rattlesnakes, copperheads, and cottonmouths), and the other is the coral snake. Since exotic snakes are kept in zoos and by some individuals, the possibility always exists that a victim of a non-native snake bite could present in the emergency department.

Not all who are bitten are envenomated. Snakes can regulate the amount of venom actually injected. Therefore, treatment is based on clinical manifestations.

The "slash-and-suck" treatment of snake bites unfortunately only removes a small amount of venom. There are pumps that can be applied to the wound prior to reaching the hospital. Do *not* apply ice to the wound. Treatment is based on manifestations. When there is only local pain, edema, and ecchymosis, and coagulation studies are normal, the client is observed for 6 to 8 hours.

When there is moderate to severe pain, edema, and ecchymosis, results of coagulation studies are mildly to severely abnormal, or the client is unstable, antivenin is used. The use of antivenin is not without potentially serious complications. Antivenins are derived from horse serum and can prompt an allergic reaction. Skin testing is performed prior to use of the antivenin.

Pit viper venom primarily produces proteolytic (tissue damage) and hemotoxic effects. Envenomated pit viper bites are usually painful and are oozing blood from visible fang marks. The area becomes edematous and erythematous. Compartment syndrome and blistering may develop.

Elapid bites (those from coral snakes and cobras) may result in little or no pain at the bite site. Venom causes neurotoxic effects ranging from ptosis and dysphagia to respiratory paralysis.

The fear and anxiety that coexist with snake bites can lead to strong autonomic and vagal responses, such as nausea, vomiting, or diarrhea. It is important that these manifestations not be confused with systemic findings of envenomation.

Maintain and support the ABCs. Act calmly and reassure the client. Position the client at rest, immobilize the involved part, and place it at heart level. Apply a constricting band above the site to minimize lymphatic and superficial venous return. It should not be tighter than a watchband. Start one or two large-bore IV lines and infuse Ringer's lactate.

Administer antivenin by IV drip within 1 hour. Dosages range from 5 to 30 vials, depending on the degree of envenomation and the client's age and size. Monitor very closely for allergic response and bleeding.

Prevention is the best therapy. Advise the client to wear high leather boots and thick trousers when walking through areas known for snakes. Heavy gloves should be worn when climbing in rocky areas.

Animal Bites

Animal bites may result in puncture wounds, lacerations, and avulsions, especially if the client pulled away from the animal while its teeth were clenched in his or her tissue. There is a potential for infection from bacteria normally residing in the animal's mouth (e.g., *Pasteurella multocida*). Be sure to assess the possibility of rabies from the biting animal. Rabies is an infectious virus that affects the CNS, especially the brain. The incidence of rabies in domesticated animals is very low in the United States, but the disease is almost always fatal.

Obtain the history of the bite. Include the type of animal, owner of the animal, description of the incident (provoked or unprovoked), location of the animal, and the animal's immunization history and state of health. Assess the type of wound (e.g., stab, tear) and amount of tissue damage. Be sure to include a neurovascular and musculoskeletal assessment.

Carefully clean, irrigate, and debride the wound. Sutures may be needed for closure. Assess for possible associated fractures, especially of the hand or head. Apply a bulky, fluffy, and absorbent dressing. Place fingers in the position of function. Administer tetanus prophylaxis and antibiotics as prescribed. Rabies prophylaxis is used if the animal cannot be found and kept for observation, in areas where rabies is endemic, or if there is a high index of suspicion for rabies. Report the incident to public health officials, animal control services, or police. Be sure to provide psychosocial support for the client and significant others. The experience of being bitten by a domestic animal, particularly a family pet, can be devastating.

Human Bites

Human bites may be self-induced (tongue laceration), result from dental abrasions (usually superficial at the metacarpophalangeal joint incurred during a fist fight if the client's knuckles hit the opponent's teeth), or be penetrating bites causing puncture wounds and tissue loss. Human bites can cause severe necrotizing infections and require vigorous intervention.

Determine the history of the bite. Assess the neurovascular and musculoskeletal function carefully. Increased pain over the site may indicate a fracture. Fractures and tendon lacerations, especially of the hand, are common. Obtain x-ray studies if indicated.

Carefully clean and vigorously irrigate the wound. Open and debride puncture wounds. Wounds are usually not sutured unless they are large or located on the face. Loosely placed sutures or adhesive strips may be used. Administer broad-spectrum antibiotics and tetanus prophylaxis. The client with severe human bites may be admitted for at least 24-hour observation.

Insect Bites and Stings

Reactions to the secretion of insect venom into the skin from either a bite or a sting will cause varying degrees of reaction in the client. Insect stings from honeybees, bumblebees, wasps, hornets, and yellow jackets imbed a firm, sharp stinger into the skin from which the venom is secreted. The venoms are proteins with enzymatic activity that may cause local and/or systemic reactions. Reactions are generally classified as allergic or toxic. Within 2 to 60 minutes after the sting, a red papule or wheal may appear. Local symptoms include swelling, warmth, and itching at the site. Systemic reactions may include shortness of breath, nausea and vomiting, diarrhea, headaches, and joint aches. If the reaction is severe enough, anaphylaxis may occur (see Chapter 22).

A bite by either a brown recluse or black widow spider may cause severe reactions. Since one bite by a brown recluse can be more serious than several bites by a black widow, an accurate diagnosis is essential. From a brown recluse bite, the client will report a sharp pain at the instant of the bite with subsequent redness and swelling. More severe reactions occur in fatty areas, and tissue necrosis may begin within 4 hours. A distinctive blue-gray halo appears around the bite site, followed by a vesicular or pustular lesion. The center of the lesion seems to sink and necrose, leaving a deep ulcer that takes months to heal.

General interventions for insect bites and stings are aimed at treating systemic or local reactions, removing the venom effect, or breaking down the protein. Local reactions are treated with ice at the site, antihistamines, and nonsteroidal anti-inflammatory agents. The protein bonds in the venom may be broken down by proteolytic agents such as household meat tenderizer. A paste is made by adding a few drops of water to the powder and applying it to the site. Systemic reactions are treated with a variety of agents depending on the nature of the symptoms.[36]

Poisoning and Overdose

Accidental or intentional poisonings (overdoses) requiring emergency care occur frequently.[20,28,29] Nearly all poisonings are unintentional and 80% occur in the home. Substances most frequently involved include medications, cleansers, and personal care products. Substances most frequently associated with fatalities are carbon monoxide, analgesics, antidepressants, sedatives and hypnotics, and stimulants and street drugs. Phone inquiries are often received by ED staff regarding poisonings. It is important that nurses responsible for emergency care be knowledgeable about the management and complications of poisoning and overdoses. Various resources are available (poison control centers, poison index, and toxicology tests). Approximately 3.2 million poisonings are handled by U.S. poison centers or U.S. healthcare facilities. An emergency nurse needs a working knowledge of agents commonly used or abused, especially currently popular street drugs. Table 89–7 lists substances most often ingested by clients seen by poison-control centers and EDs.

Obtain an accurate history. Include the following questions:

1. Was the substance inhaled, injected, ingested, sniffed, or confined to skin surfaces?
2. How long ago was the event, and what was the amount?
3. In what kind of environment was the client found?
4. Were there any associated incidents (fire, trauma, near drowning)?
5. Is there a history of prescribed medications? Allergies? Medical problems?
6. What is the state of physical and mental health?

Keep in mind that despite careful fact-finding and detailed questioning, a history of the nature and amount of the toxic substance and the time since ingestion may be grossly inaccurate. Clients who have ingested toxic substances may exaggerate or minimize the conditions of an overdose in order to achieve other goals. The history is considered in planning the care. However, reliance on physical examination is also important.

Table 89–7. Poisonous Substances Most Frequently Ingested by Clients

Exposures

AAPCC	DAWN
Analgesics (10.5%)	Cocaine
Cleaning substances (10%)	Alcohol in combination
	Heroin, morphine
Cosmetics (8.1%)	Marijuana, hashish
Plants (6.9%)	Phencyclidine (PCP)
Cough and cold preparations (5.6%)	combinations

Deaths

AAPCC	DAWN
Antidepressants	Cocaine
Analgesics	Alcohol in combination
Stimulants and street drugs	Heroin, morphine
Sedatives, hypnotics	Codeine
Cardiovascular drugs	Diazepam

AAPCC = American Association of Poison Control Centers; DAWN = Drug Abuse Warning Network.
Modified from Koda-Kimble, M. A., et al. (1992). *Handbook of applied therapeutics.* (2nd ed.). Vancouver, WA: Applied Therapeutics.

The acronym *SIRES* is an aid to remembering the essentials of care in cases of poisoning:

Stabilize the client.
Identify the toxic substance.
Reverse its effect.
Eliminate the substance from the body.
Support the client and significant others (physically and psychosocially).

Stabilize the ABCs. Perform a rapid physical examination. Start IV lines, and obtain appropriate laboratory studies including a toxicology screen. Initiate a cardiac monitor, and obtain an ECG.

Select an appropriate means of reversing or eliminating the toxic substance. Home-remedy methods of inducing emesis (such as manual stimulation of the posterior pharynx, drinking saltwater or mustard water, or eating raw eggs) may be listed in first-aid books or on container labels. These measures are often unsafe and ineffective. The safest and most effective method of inducing emesis is administration of syrup of ipecac.

Syrup of ipecac is safe and effective when used in properly selected clients (Box 89–3). The dose is 15 to 30 ml (age 1–10 years, 15 ml; over 10 years, 30 ml), administered orally, preceded or followed by several hundred milliliters of warm water or other solution (juice). Emesis usually occurs within 15 to 20 minutes. However, a second dose can be given 20 minutes after the first dose. Do not give more than two doses. It is important that enough oral fluid be given to prevent retching and possible esophageal tears. Save emesis for possible toxicologic analysis. Note the presence or absence of pill particles.

Gastric lavage may be indicated. However, it is believed to be less effective than emesis in removing ingested substances from the stomach. Thus, it is reserved for use in clients with CNS depression, those with diminished or absent gag reflex, or those unable to cooperate with emetic therapy. Remember that gastric lavage is not a deterrent to future overdose attempts and should not be used as a punitive measure.

Gastric lavage involves inserting a large-bore (30F–36F, in adults) Ewald tube through the nose or mouth

Table 89–8. Antidotes Commonly Used in Managing Poisoned or Overdosed Clients

Substance	Antidote
Cholinesterase inhibitors, e.g., organophosphate insecticides, nerve gases, carbamates	Atropine Pralidoxine (2–PAM)
Iron	Deferoxamine
Insulin	Dextrose 50%
Mercury, arsenic, lead, other heavy metals	Dimercaprol, disodium edetate, penicillamine
Methanol, ethylene glycol	Ethanol
Lead	Ethylenediaminetetraacetic acid (EDTA)
Acetaminophen	Acetylcysteine (Mucomyst)
Narcotics and narcotic derivatives, opiates	Naloxone (Narcan)
Cyanide	Amyl nitrite, sodium nitrite, sodium thiosulfate
Carbon monoxide	Oxygen
Atropine, scopolamine, tricyclic antidepressants	Physostigmine (Antilirium)
Anticoagulants, e.g., warfarin (Coumadin), salicylates	Vitamin K

Data from Koda-Kimble, M. A., et al. (1992). *Handbook of applied therapeutics* (2nd ed.). Vancouver, WA: Applied Therapeutics.

Box 89–3. Cautions in the Use of Ipecac

- Use only syrup of ipecac, not ipecac fluid extract.
- Always ensure an intact gag reflex before giving ipecac. Do not assume a physician has done this.
- Ipecac may be ineffective in inducing emesis after ingestion of substances with antiemetic properties.
- Ipecac in large doses may be cardiotoxic. Lavage may be necessary if emesis does not occur.
- Frequently reassess the client. The client may become obtunded when the emesis occurs, and aspiration may result.
- Ipecac is most effective when adequate amounts of oral fluids are administered.

and then washing out the stomach contents with normal saline. The volume of each run of fluid instilled into the stomach varies, depending on the age and tolerance of the client (250–500 ml in adults). Avoid volumes in excess of 500 ml, because large volumes may foster passage of substances into the duodenum. Lavage is carried out until the fluid return is clear.

Absorptives are also used. Activated charcoal powder, usually mixed with water, is administered in doses of 25 to 50 g (0.5–1.0 g/kg) to absorb any remaining particles of toxic substance. This may be administered orally or inserted through a Ewald tube. Because it is black and does not easily mix in water, activated charcoal may be mixed with cherry syrup, sorbitol, or similar substances to make it more palatable.

Antidotes or antagonists may be used in selected cases for management or diagnosis of the toxin (Table 89–8). Remember that although an antidote may produce significant results initially, the half-life of the toxic substance may be longer than the antidote. For instance, naloxone (Narcan) is a potent narcotic antagonist used in opiate overdoses. Even though the client may initially respond rapidly, as the naloxone wears off the client may become obtunded. Clients receiving antidotes or antagonists must be observed for several hours before being discharged.

Other measures, depending on the client's condition, include diuresis, fluid loading, cooling or warming, anticonvulsive therapy, antidysrhythmic therapy, hemodialysis, hemoperfusion, or exchange transfusions. Nursing care involves assessing the client and the responses, carrying out therapies, and providing supportive care. Remember that an accidental or intentional poisoning may be reported to a poison control facility or additional agency.

For the client who intentionally overdoses, empathy and understanding are necessary. Vindictive or hostile attitudes are destructive and maximize feelings of guilt and low self-esteem. If the client is awake, one way to foster communication is to say, "It must have been hard for you to decide to do this." The client may then feel able to talk about problems and may be more receptive to counseling. Remember the suicide attempt may be repeated while the client is receiving care for the overdose. Be sure to implement suicide precautions, particularly if the client expresses a desire to harm himself or herself again.

A psychiatric evaluation is indicated for all clients who intentionally overdose or whose intentions seem unclear. The evaluation should occur before discharge, and plans for follow-up care should be well established. Investigate and use available support systems. Someone should stay with the client for the next several days. Provide a telephone number for the crisis team or clinic and written instructions for follow-up care.

Domestic Violence

Domestic violence is an increasingly serious problem.[8,19,23,38] This problem affects all ethnic, cultural, and religious groups across all sociologic levels. Especially vulnerable are pregnant women, adolescents, and the elderly. Three to 4 million women in the United States have been reported to be abused by their partners each year. It has been estimated that 22% to 35% of women who visit EDs present with manifestations related to ongoing abuse. From 4% to 14% of geriatric trauma has been reported to be due to violent assaults. Unfortunately, less than 10% have been documented on ED records as victims of domestic violence. Lack of public and professional awareness has allowed the problem of abuse to remain hidden. The importance of accurate assessment and identification by the ED nurse cannot be overemphasized.[19,22]

Most victims have back and neck injuries, CNS and sensory deficits, headaches, and other musculoskeletal injuries. Bruises and wounds in various states of healing indicate previous injury. Cigarette burns, penetrating injuries, and sexual abuse may also be encountered. In the elderly, neglect is more prevalent.

Separate all suspected victims from their partners or significant others until the battering has been ruled out. The batterer may be very protective and not want close examination of the family member. Obtain history and physical assessment data from the victim. When necessary, diagnostic tests specific to sexual assault may be done and photographs may be taken. Once the crime is validated, the appropriate civil authorities must be called.

The victim may need to be referred and transported to a shelter. Discharge planning is vital since many of the victims feel compelled to return to the abusive environment.[7,22,32]

Conclusions

Emergency care is very challenging and rewarding. By knowing and using the principles of emergency care, nurses can function effectively, regardless of the environment in which the care is delivered. Because of the variety of emergency problems encountered, nurses need to be responsible and accountable for updating their knowledge and skills. Besides mastering technical skills, nurses provide psychosocial care to clients and significant others. As a specialty, emergency nursing provides stimulating professional opportunities. Emergency nurses are active in health promotion, prevention, education, research, and emergency care. Emergency nurses are on the forefront of providing competent and professional care to a variety of clients and significant others.

Thinking Critically

1. A 60-year-old man has come in to your emergency department with a complaint of headache. He stated that he never had headaches until about 2 weeks ago when he began awakening in the mornings with head pain. The headache would go away each day after he had been up and around for a few hours and had taken aspirin. However, in the last few days, neither aspirin nor acetaminophen has helped and the headache has become nearly continuous. His wife states that his speech and balance have been off a little. He wonders if there can be any connection between his headaches and a recent fall he took in the garage or to his blood pressure being up some. Describe how you would proceed with the evaluation of this client. What further information should you elicit from him? What is your assessment priority? What triage classification would be best for this client? What interventions should you anticipate?

Factors to Consider. What diagnostic assessments should you anticipate? What should you include in your physical examination and nursing history?

2. The client is a 28-year-old woman who entered your emergency department with the complaint of continuous abdominal pain for the last two days. She states that she had been awakened in the night with sudden onset of severe pain in her right lower quadrant 2 days ago. The pain is sharp, radiates to her groin, and then goes pretty much everywhere and has actually "doubled her over" twice since it began. She states that she has taken ibuprofen 600 mg twice with little relief. The pain was dulled but did not go

away. Describe how you would proceed with the evaluation of this client. What triage classification would be best for this client? What would you include in your nursing history and physical assessment? What interventions should you anticipate?

Factors to Consider. What medical diagnoses do the clinical manifestations mimic? What diagnostic studies should you anticipate?

3. The client is a 70-year-old man who has been brought to your emergency department by ambulance. His wife states that he has become increasingly confused over the past few months. Within the past few days he has become worse, is hard to awaken in the mornings, and is "sleepy" all day. This progressed until today when she couldn't keep him awake at all, so she called an ambulance and had him brought in. He has a long history of HTN, CAD, DM, and depression. Ambulance records show evidence that the client is difficult to arouse, but upon aggressive stimulation he kind of "wakes up" and will follow basic commands. His vital signs are stable but his pulse is slow and irregular and his blood pressure is now lower than his "norm." His wife has brought his medications with her in a large paper bag. What is your priority assessment? What should you include in your physical assessment? What interventions should you anticipate?

Factors to Consider. What body systems should you assess? What diagnostic studies should you anticipate?

Bibliography

1. Allen, R. J., & Graber, M. A. (1994). Pulmonary medicine. In M. A. Graber, R. J. Allen, & R. T. Levy (Eds.), *The family practice handbook*. St. Louis: Mosby–Year Book.
2. American Heart Association (1994). *Textbook of advanced cardiac life support* (3rd ed.). Dallas: Author.
3. Bastnagel Mason, P. J. (1994). Abdominal injuries. In V. D. Cardona, et al. (Eds.), *Trauma nursing: From resuscitation through rehabilitation* (2nd ed.). Philadelphia: W. B. Saunders.
4. Beaver, B. M. (1990). Care of the multiple trauma victim. The first hour. *Nursing Clinics of North America, 25*(1), 11–21.
5. Bobb, J. (1994). Trauma in the elderly. In V. D. Cardona et al. (Eds.), *Trauma nursing: From resuscitation through rehabilitation* (2nd ed.). Philadelphia: W. B. Saunders.
6. Bryant, K. K., & Hammond, L. L. (1994). Environmental emergencies. In A. R. Klein et al. (Eds.), *Emergency nursing core curriculum.* (4th ed.) Philadelphia: W. B. Saunders.
7. Campbell, J. C., et al. (1994). Battered women's experiences in the emergency department. *Journal of Emergency Nursing, 20*(4), 280–288.
8. Cardona, V., & Von Rueden, K. T. (1994). Nursing practice through the trauma cycles. In V. D. Cardona et al. (Eds.), *Trauma nursing: From resuscitation through rehabilitation* (2nd ed.). Philadelphia: W. B. Saunders.
9. Centers for Disease Control and Prevention. (1993). 1993 Sexually transmitted diseases treatment guidelines. *MMWR, 42,* 1–102.
10. Coolican, M. B. (1994). Families: Facing the sudden death of a loved one. *Critical Care Nursing Clinics of North America, 6*(3), 607–612.
11. Cummings, S. P., & Cummings, P. H. (1994). Abdominal emergen-

cies. In A. R. Klein et al. (Eds.), *Emergency nursing core curriculum* (4th ed.). Philadelphia: W. B. Saunders.
12. DeKeyser, F. G. (1994). Trauma nursing research. A description and means of evaluation. *Critical Care Nursing Clinics of North America, 6*(3), 441–449.
13. Emergency Nurses Association (1995). *Standards of emergency nursing practice* (2nd ed.). St. Louis: Mosby–Year Book.
14. Fackler, C. (1994). Genitourinary and gynecological emergencies. In A. R. Klein et al. (Eds.), *Emergency nursing core curriculum* (4th ed.). Philadelphia: W. B. Saunders.
15. Faylor, J., & Royer, C. (1991). Intraosseous infusion for emergency intravascular access. *Trauma Talk Newsletter* (fall), Omaha: Saint Joseph Hospital at Creighton University Medical Center.
16. Flynn, M. B. (1994). Wound management of the traumatically injured patient. *Critical Care Nursing Clinics of North America, 6*(3), 491–499.
17. Gill, B. A. (1993). Organ donation. In R. L. Boggs & M. Wooldridge-King (Eds.), *AACN manual for critical care* (3rd ed.). Philadelphia: W. B. Saunders.
18. Gin, N., et al. (1991). Prevalence of domestic violence among patients in three ambulatory care internal medicine clinics. *Journal of General Internal Medicine, 6,* 317–322.
19. Graber, M. A. (1994). Emergency medicine. In M. A. Graber, R. J. Allen, & R. T. Levy (Eds.), *The family practice handbook*. St. Louis: Mosby–Year Book.
20. Halpern, J. (1989). Mechanisms and patterns of trauma. *Journal of Emergency Nursing, 15*(5), 380–388.
21. Halpern, J. (1994). Orthopedic emergencies. In A. R. Klein et al. (Eds.), *Emergency nursing core curriculum.* (4th ed.) Philadelphia: W. B. Saunders.
22. Henderson, A. D., & Erickson, J. R. (1994). Enhancing nurses' effectiveness with abused women, *Journal of Psychosocial Nursing, 32*(6), 11–15.
23. Hurn, P. D., & Hartsock, R. L. (1994). Thoracic injuries. In V. D. Cardona et al. (Eds.), *Trauma nursing: From resuscitation through rehabilitation.* (2nd ed.) Philadelphia: W. B. Saunders.
24. Jarvis, C. (1996). *Physical examination and health assessment* (2nd ed.). Philadelphia: W. B. Saunders.
25. Judkins, D., & Iserson, K. (1991). Rapid admixture blood warming. *Journal of Emergency Nursing, 17*(3), 146–151.
26. Koda-Kimble, M. A., et al. (1992). *Handbook of applied therapeutics* (2nd ed.). Vancouver, WA: Applied Therapeutics.
27. Kollef, M., & Goodenberger, D. (1995). Critical care and medical emergencies. In G. A. Ewald & C. R. McKenzie (Eds.), *Manual of medical therapeutics* (28th ed.). Boston: Little, Brown.
28. Lee, G. (1994). Dental, ear, nose, and throat emergencies. In A. R. Klein et al. (Eds.), *Emergency nursing core curriculum* (4th ed.). Philadelphia: W. B. Saunders.
29. LoCicero, J., & Mattox, K. (1989). Epidemiology of chest trauma. *Surgical Clinics of North America, 69*(1), 15–19.
30. McQuillan, K. (1994). Initial management of traumatic shock. In V. D. Cardona et al. (Eds.), *Trauma nursing: From resuscitation through rehabilitation* (2nd ed.). Philadelphia: W. B. Saunders.
31. Mitchell, P. H. (1994). Central nervous system I: Closed head injuries. In V. D. Cardona et al. (Eds.), *Trauma nursing: From resuscitation through rehabilitation* (2nd ed.). Philadelphia: W. B. Saunders.
32. Ozmar, B. (1994). Encountering victims of interpersonal violence. Implication for critical care nursing. *Critical Care Nursing Clinics of North America, 6*(3), 515–523.
33. Schuller, D. (1995). Pulmonary diseases. In G. A. Ewald & C. R. McKenzie (Eds.), *Manual of medical therapeutics* (28th ed.). Boston: Little, Brown.
34. Snell, G. (1994). Laceration repair. In J. L. Pfenninger & G. C. Fowler (Eds.), *Procedures for primary care physicians*. St. Louis: Mosby–Year Book.
35. Strange, J. M. & Kelly, P. M. (1994). Musculoskeletal injuries. In V. D. Cardona et al. (Eds.), *Trauma nursing: From resuscitation through rehabilitation* (2nd ed.). Philadelphia: W. B. Saunders.
36. Uphold, C. R., & Graham, M. V. (1994). *Clinical guidelines in family practice* (2nd ed.). Gainesville, Fla: Barmarrae Books.
37. U.S. Department of Health and Human Services. (1994). *Clinician's handbook of preventive services: Put prevention into practice*. Washington, DC: Public Health Service, Office of Disease Prevention and Health Promotion.

38. U.S. Preventive Services Task Force. (1996). *Guide to clinical preventive services* (2nd ed.). Baltimore: Williams & Wilkins.

39. Vary, T. C., & Kearney, M. T. L. (1994). Pathophysiology of traumatic shock and multiple organ system failure. In V. D. Cardona et al. (Eds.), *Trauma nursing from resuscitation through rehabilitation* (2nd ed.) Philadelphia: W. B. Saunders.

40. Von Rueden, K. T., & Dunham, C. M. (1994). Sequelae of massive fluid resuscitation in trauma patients. *Critical Care Nursing Clinics of North America, 6*(3), 463–472.

41. Walleck, C. A. (1994). Central nervous system II: Spinal cord injury. In V. D. Cardona et al. (Eds.), *Trauma nursing: From resuscitation through rehabilitation* (2nd ed.). Philadelphia: W. B. Saunders.

42. Weigelt, J. A., & Klein, J. D. (1994). Mechanism of injury. In V. D. Cardona et al. (Eds.) *Trauma nursing: From resuscitation through rehabilitation* (2nd ed.). Philadelphia: W. B. Saunders.

43. Whitney, J. D. (1994). Wound healing. In V. D. Cardona et al. (Eds.), *Trauma nursing: From resuscitation through rehabilitation* (2nd ed.). Philadelphia: W. B. Saunders.

Appendixes
A–D

Religious Beliefs and Practices Affecting Healthcare

APPENDIX A

Religious Group	Beliefs and Practices
WESTERN RELIGIONS	

Judaism
Orthodox and some Conservative Jewish groups

Care of women: A woman is considered to be in a ritual state of impurity whenever blood is coming from her uterus, such as during menstrual periods and after the birth of a child. During this time, her husband will not have physical contact with her. When this time is completed, she will bathe herself in a pool called a *mikvah.* Nurses need to be aware of this practice and be sensitive to the husband and wife because the husband will not touch his wife. He cannot assist her in moving in the bed, so the nurse will have to do this. An Orthodox Jewish man will not touch any women other than his wife, daughters, and mother.

Dietary rules: (1) Kosher dietary laws include the following: No mixing of milk and meat at a meal; no consumption of food or any derivative thereof from animals not slaughtered in accordance with Jewish law; use of separate cooking utensils for milk and milk products; if a client requires milk and meat products for a meal, the dairy foods should be served first, followed later by the meat. (2) During Yom Kippur (Day of Atonement), a 24-hour fast is required, but exceptions are made for those who cannot fast because of medical reasons. (3) During Passover, no leavened products are eaten. (4) May say benediction of thanksgiving before meals and grace at the end of the meal. Time and a quiet environment should be provided for this.

Sabbath: Observed from sunset Friday until sunset Saturday. Orthodox law prohibits riding in a car, smoking, turning lights on and off, handling money, and using television and telephone. Nurses need to be aware of this when caring for observant Jews at home and in the hospital. Medical or surgical treatments should be postponed if possible.

Death: Judaism defines death as occurring when respiration and circulation are irreversibly stopped and no movement is apparent. (1) Euthanasia is strictly forbidden by Orthodox Jews, who advocate the strict use of life-support measures. (2) Prior to death, Jewish faith indicates that visiting of the person by family and friends is a religious duty. The Torah and Psalms may be read and prayers recited. A witness needs to be present when a person prays for health so that if death occurs God will protect the family and the spirit will be committed to God. Extraneous talking and conversation about death are not encouraged unless initiated by the client or visitors. In Judaism, the belief is that people should have someone with them when the soul leaves the body, so family and/or friends should be allowed to stay with clients. After death, the body should not be left alone until buried, usually within 24 hours. (3) When death occurs, the body should be untouched for 8 to 30 minutes. Medical personnel should not touch or wash the body but allow only an Orthodox person or the Jewish Burial Society to care for the body. Handling of a corpse on the Sabbath is forbidden to Jewish persons. If need be, the nursing staff may provide routine care of the body, wearing gloves. Water in the room should be emptied, and the family may request that mirrors be covered to symbolize that a death has occurred. (4) Orthodox Jews and some Conservative Jews do not approve of autopsies. If an autopsy must be done, all body parts must remain with the body. (5) For

Religious Group	Beliefs and Practices
WESTERN RELIGIONS (*Continued*)	
	Orthodox Jews, the body must be buried within 24 hours. No flowers are permitted. A fetus must be buried. (6) A 7-day mourning period is required by the immediate family. They must stay at home except for Sabbath worship. (7) Organs or other body parts such as amputated limbs must be made available for burial for Orthodox Jews, because they believe that all of the body must be returned to earth. *Birth control and abortion:* Artificial methods of birth control are not encouraged. Vasectomy is not allowed. Abortion may be performed only to save the mother's life. *Organ transplant:* Donor organ transplants generally are not permitted by Orthodox Jews but may be allowed with rabbinical consent. *Shaving:* The beard is regarded as a mark of piety among observant Jews. For the very Orthodox, shaving should not be done with a razor but with scissors or electric razor, because a blade should not contact the skin. *Head covering:* Orthodox men wear skull caps at all times, and women cover their hair after marriage. Some Orthodox women wear wigs as a mark of piety. Conservative Jews cover their heads only during acts of worship and prayer. *Prayer:* Praying directly to God, including a prayer of confession, is required for Orthodox Jews. Nurses should provide quiet time for prayer.
Reform Jews	*Care of women:* Reform Jews do not observe the rules against touching. *Dietary rules:* Reform Jews usually do not observe kosher dietary restriction. *Sabbath:* Usually worship in temples on Friday evenings. No strict rules. *Death:* Advocate use of life support without heroic measures. Allow for cremation but suggest that ashes be buried in a Jewish cemetery. *Organ transplant:* Donation or transplantation of organs allowed with permission of a rabbi. *Head covering:* Generally pray without wearing skull caps.
Christianity Roman Catholic	*Holy Eucharist:* For clients and healthcare providers who are to receive communion, abstinence from solid food and alcohol is required for 15 minutes (if possible) prior to reception of the consecrated wafer. Medicine, water, and nonalcoholic drinks are permitted at any time. If a client is in danger of death, the fast is waived because the reception of the Eucharist at this time is very important. *Anointing of the sick:* The priest uses oil to anoint the forehead and hands and, if desired, the affected area. The rite may be performed on any who are ill and desire it. Clients receiving the sacrament seek complete healing, and strength to endure suffering. Prior to 1963, this sacrament was given only to clients at time of imminent death, so the nurse must be sensitive to the meaning this has for the client. If possible, the nurse calls a priest before the client is unconscious but may also call when there is sudden death, because the sacrament may also be given shortly after death. The nurse records on the care plan that this sacrament has been administered. *Dietary habits:* Obligatory fasting is excused during hospitalization. However, if there are no health restrictions, some Catholics may still observe the following guidelines: (1) Anyone 14 years or older must abstain from eating meat on Ash Wednesday and all Fridays during Lent. Some older Catholics may still abstain from meat on all Fridays of the year. (2) In addition to abstinence from meat, persons 21 to 59 years of age must limit themselves to one full meal and two light meals on Ash Wednesday and Good Friday. (3) Eastern Rite Catholics are stricter about fasting and fast more frequently than Western Rite Catholics, so it is important for the nurse to know if a client is Eastern or Western. *Death:* Each Roman Catholic should participate in the anointing of the sick as well as the Eucharist and penance before death. The body should not be shrouded until after these sacraments are performed. All body parts that retain human quality must be appropriately buried or cremated.

Appendix continued on following page

Religious Group	Beliefs and Practices
WESTERN RELIGIONS (*Continued*)	

	Birth control: Prohibited except for abstinence or natural family planning. Referral to a priest for questions about this can be of great help. Nurses can teach the techniques of natural family planning if they are familiar with them; otherwise, this should be referred to the physician or to a support group of the church that instructs couples in this method of birth control. Sterilization is prohibited unless there is an overriding medical reason.
	Organ donation: Donation and transplantation of organs are acceptable as long as the donor is not harmed and is not deprived of life.
	Religious objects: Rosary prayers are said using rosary beads. Medals bearing the images of saints, relics, statues, and scapulars are important objects that may be pinned to a hospital gown or pillow or be at the bedside. Extreme care should be taken not to lose these objects, because they have special meaning to the client.
Eastern Orthodox	*Holy Eucharist:* The priest is notified if the client desires this sacrament.
	Anointing of the sick: The priest conducts this in the hospital room.
	Dietary habits: Fasting from meat and dairy products is required on Wednesday and Friday during Lent and on other holy days. Hospital clients are exempt if fasting is detrimental to health.
	Special days: Christmas is celebrated on January 7 and New Year's Day on January 14. This is important to the care of a client who is hospitalized on these days.
	Death: Last rites are obligatory. This is handled by an ordained priest who is notified by the nurse while the client is conscious. The Russian Orthodox Church does not encourage autopsy or organ donation. Euthanasia, even for the terminally ill, is discouraged, as is cremation.
	Birth control: This, as well as abortion, is not permitted.
Protestant	*Holy Communion:* Notify clergy if the client desires.
Assemblies of God (Pentecostal)	*Anointing of the sick:* Members believe in divine healing through prayer and the laying on of hands. Clergy is notified if client or family desires this.
	Dietary habits: Abstinence from alcohol, tobacco, and all illegal drugs is strongly encouraged.
	Death: No special practices.
	Other practices: Faith in God and in the healthcare providers is encouraged. Members pray for divine intervention in health matters. Nurses should encourage and allow time for prayer. Members may speak in "tongues" during prayer.
Baptist (over 27 different groups in the United States)	*Holy Communion:* Clergy should be notified if the client desires.
	Dietary habits: Total abstinence from alcohol is expected.
	Death: No general service is provided, but the clergy does minister through counseling, prayer, and Scripture as requested by the client or family, and the client is encouraged to believe in Jesus Christ as Savior and Lord.
	Other practices: The Bible is held to be the word of God, so the nurse should either allow quiet time for Scripture reading or offer to read to the client.
Christian Church (Disciples of Christ)	*Holy Communion:* Open communion is celebrated each Sunday and is a central part of worship services. The nurse notifies the clergy if the client desires it, or the clergy may suggest it.
	Death: No special practices.
	Other practices: Church elders as well as clergy may be notified to assist with meeting the client's spiritual needs.
Church of the Brethren	*Holy Communion:* Usually received within church, but clergy will give it in the hospital when requested.

Religious Group	Beliefs and Practices
WESTERN RELIGIONS *(Continued)*	

	Anointing of the sick: Practices for physical healing as well as spiritual uplift and held in high regard by the church. The clergy is notified if the client or family desire. *Death:* The clergy is notified for counsel and prayer.
Church of the Nazarene	*Holy Communion:* Pastor will administer if the client wishes. *Dietary habits:* The use of alcohol and tobacco is forbidden. *Death:* Cremation is permitted, and term stillborn infants are buried. *Other practices:* Believe in divine healing but not to the exclusion of medical treatment. Clients may desire quiet time for prayer.
Episcopal (Anglican)	*Holy Communion:* The priest is notified if the client wishes to receive this sacrament. *Anointing of the sick:* Priest may administer this rite when death is imminent, but it is not considered mandatory. *Dietary habits:* Some clients may abstain from meat on Fridays. Others may fast before receiving the Eucharist, but fasting is not mandatory. *Death:* No special practices. *Other practices:* Confession of sins to a priest is optional: if the client desires this, the clergy should be notified.
Lutheran (18 different branches)	*Holy Communion:* Notify the clergy if the client desires this sacrament. Clergy may also inquire about the client's desire. *Anointing of the sick:* The client may request an anointing and blessing from the minister when the prognosis is poor. *Death:* A service of Commendation of the Dying is used at the client's or family's request.
Mennonite (12 different groups)	*Holy Communion:* Served twice a year, with foot washing as part of ceremony. *Dietary habits:* Abstinence from alcohol is urged for all. *Death:* Prayer is important at time of crisis, so contacting a minister is important. *Other practices:* Women may wear head coverings during hospitalization. Anointing with oil is administered in harmony with James 5:14 when requested.
Methodist (over 20 different groups)	*Holy Communion:* Notify the clergy if a client requests it prior to surgery or another health crisis. *Anointing of the sick:* If requested, the clergy will come to pray and sprinkle the client with olive oil. *Death:* Scripture reading and prayer are important at this time. *Other practices:* Donation of one's body or part of the body at death is encouraged.
Presbyterian (10 different groups)	*Holy Communion:* Given when appropriate and convenient, at the hospitalized client's request. *Death:* Notify a local pastor or elder for prayer and Scripture reading if desired by the family or client.
Quaker (Friends)	*Holy Communion:* Because Friends have no creed, there is a diversity of personal beliefs, one of which is that outward sacraments are usually not necessary because there is the ministry of the Spirit inwardly in such areas as baptism and communion. *Death:* Believe that the present life is part of God's kingdom and generally have no ceremony as a rite of passage from this life to the next. Personal beliefs and wishes need to be ascertained, and the nurse can then act on the client's wishes.
Salvation Army	*Holy Communion:* No particular ceremony. *Death:* Notify the local officer in charge of the Army Corps for any soldier (member) who needs assistance. *Other practices:* The Bible is seen as the only rule for one's faith, so the Scriptures should be made available to a client. The Army has many of

Appendix continued on following page

Religious Group	Beliefs and Practices

WESTERN RELIGIONS *(Continued)*

	its own social welfare centers, with hospitals and homes where unwed mothers are cared for and outpatient services provided. No medical or surgical procedures are opposed, except for abortion on demand.
Seventh-Day Adventist	*Holy Communion:* Although this is not required of hospitalized clients, the clergy are notified if the client desires.
	Anointing of the sick: The clergy are contacted for prayer and anointing with oil.
	Dietary habits: Because the body is viewed as the temple of the Holy Spirit, healthy living is essential. Therefore, the use of alcohol, tobacco, coffee, and tea and the promiscuous use of drugs are prohibited. Some are vegetarians, and most avoid pork.
	Special days: The Sabbath is observed on Saturday.
	Death: No special procedures.
	Other related practices: Use of hypnotism is opposed by some. Persons of homosexual or lesbian orientation are ministered to in the hope of correction of these practices, which are believed to be wrong. A Bible should always be available for Scripture reading.
United Church of Christ	*Holy Communion:* Clergy are notified if the client desires to receive this sacrament.
	Death: If the client desires counsel or prayer, notify the clergy.
Other Christian Science	*Dietary habits:* Because alcohol and tobacco are considered drugs, they are not used. Coffee and tea are often declined.
	Death: Autopsy is usually declined unless required by law. Donation of organs is unlikely, but is an individual decision.
	Other practices: Do not normally seek medical care, because they approach healthcare in a different, primarily spiritual, framework. They commonly utilize the services of a surgeon to set a bone but decline drugs and, in general, other medical or surgical procedures. Hypnotism and psychotherapy are also declined. Family planning is left to the family. They seek exemption from vaccinations but obey legal requirements (e.g., report infectious diseases and obey public health quarantines). Nonmedical care facilities are maintained for those needing nursing assistance in the course of a healing. *The Christian Science Journal* lists available Christian Science nurses. When a Christian Science believer is in the hospital, the nurse should allow and encourage time for prayer and study. Clients may request that a Christian Science practitioner be notified to come.
Jehovah's Witnesses	*Dietary habits:* Use of alcohol and tobacco is discouraged, because these harm the physical body.
	Death: Autopsy is a private matter to be decided by the persons involved. Burial and cremation are acceptable.
	Birth control and abortion: Use of birth control is a personal decision. Abortion is opposed based on Exodus 21:22–23.
	Organ transplants: Use of organ transplant is a private decision and if used must be cleansed with a nonblood solution.
	Blood transfusions: Blood transfusions violate God's laws and are therefore not allowed. Clients do respect physicians and will accept alternatives to blood transfusions. These might include use of nonblood plasma expanders, careful surgical techniques to decrease blood loss, use of autologous transfusions, and autotransfusion through use of a heart-lung machine. Nurses should check unconscious patients for medic alert cards that state that the person does not want a transfusion. Since Jehovah's Witnesses are prepared to die rather than break God's law, nurses need to be sensitive to the spiritual as well as the physical needs of the client.
The Church of Jesus Christ of Latter-Day Saints	*Holy Communion:* A hospitalized client may desire to have a member of the church priesthood administer this sacrament.

Religious Group	Beliefs and Practices
WESTERN RELIGIONS *(Continued)*	

	Anointing of the sick: Mormons frequently are anointed and given a blessing by laying on of hands before going to the hospital and after admission. *Dietary habits:* Abstinence from the use of tobacco; beverages with caffeine such as cola, coffee, and tea; alcohol and other substances considered injurious. Mormons eat meat but encourage the intake of fruits, grains, and herbs. *Death:* Prefer burial of the body. A church elder should be notified to assist the family. If need be, the elder will assist the funeral director in dressing the body in special clothes and will give other help as needed. *Birth control and abortion:* Abortion is opposed except when the life of the mother is in danger. Only natural means of birth control are recommended. Artificial means can be used when the health of the woman is at stake (including emotional health). *Personal care:* Cleanliness is very important to Mormons. A sacred undergarment may be worn at all times by Mormons and should only be removed in emergency situations. *Other practices:* Allowing quiet time for prayer and the reading of the sacred writings is important. The church maintains a welfare system to assist those in need. Families are of great importance, so visiting should be encouraged.
Unitarian Universalist Association	*Death:* Cremation is often preferred to burial. *Other practices:* Use of birth control is advocated as part of responsible parenting. Strong support for a woman's right to choice regarding abortion is maintained. Unitarian Universalists advocate donation of body parts for research and transplants.
Unification Church	*Baptism:* No baptism. *Special days:* Sunday mornings are used to honor Reverend and Mrs. Moon as the true parents, and members get up at 5:00 A.M., bow before a picture of the Moons three times, and vow to do what is needed to help the Reverend accomplish his mission on earth. *Death:* Believe that after death one's place of destiny will depend on his or her spirit's quality of life and goodness while on earth. In the afterlife, one will have the same aspirations and feelings as before earth. Hell is not a concern, because it will not be a place as heaven grows in size. Persons who leave the Unification Church are warned that Satan may try to possess them. *Other practices:* All marriages must be solemnized by Reverend Moon in order to be part of the perfect family and have salvation. The church supplies its faithful members with life's necessities. Members may use occult practices to have spiritual and psychic experiences.
Islam	*Dietary habits:* No pork is allowed, nor alcoholic beverages. All halal (permissible) meat must be blessed and killed in a special way. This is called *zabihah* (correctly slaughtered). *Death:* Prior to death, family members ask to be present so that they can read the Koran and pray with the client. An Imam may come if requested by the client or family but is not required. Clients must face Mecca and confess their sins and beg forgiveness in the presence of their family. If the family is unavailable, any practicing Muslim can provide support to the client. After death, Muslims prefer that the family wash, prepare, and place the body in a position facing Mecca. If necessary, the healthcare providers may perform these procedures as long as they wear gloves. Burial is performed as soon as possible. Cremation is forbidden. Autopsy is also prohibited except for legal reasons, and then no body part is to be removed. Donation of body parts or organs is not allowed, because according to culturally developed law, persons do not own their body. *Abortion and birth control:* Abortion is forbidden, and many conservative Muslims do not encourage the use of contraceptives because this inter-

Appendix continued on following page

Religious Group	Beliefs and Practices

WESTERN RELIGIONS (Continued)

	feres with God's purpose. Others feel that a woman should only have as many children as her husband can afford. Contraception is permitted by Islamic law. *Personal devotions:* At prayer time, washing is required, even by those who are sick. A client on bedrest may require assistance with this task before prayer. Provision of privacy is important during prayer. *Religious objects:* The Koran must not be touched by anyone ritually unclean, and nothing should be placed on top of it. Some Muslims wear *taviz,* a black string on which words of the Koran are attached. These should not be removed and must remain dry. Certain items of jewelry, such as bangles, may have religious significance and should not be removed unnecessarily. *Care of women:* Because women are not allowed to sign consent forms or make a decision regarding family planning, the husband needs to be present. Women are very modest and frequently wear clothes that cover all of the body. During a medical examination, the woman's modesty should be respected as much as possible. Muslim women prefer female doctors. For 40 days after giving birth and also during menstruation, a woman is exempt from prayer because this is a time of cleansing for her.
American Muslim Mission	*Dietary habits:* In addition to refusing pork, many will not eat traditional black American foods, such as corn bread and collard greens. *Death:* The family is contacted before any care of the deceased is performed. There are special procedures for washing and shrouding the body. *Other practices:* Quiet time is necessary to permit prayer. Members are encouraged to use black physicians for healthcare. Because these clients do not smoke, their request for a nonsmoking roommate should be honored.

EASTERN RELIGIONS

Hinduism	*Dietary habits:* Some sects are vegetarian, believing meats and intoxicants to be too stimulating to the senses. *Belief about illness:* View illnesses as a result of misuse of the body or a consequence of sins committed in a previous life. They do not oppose medical treatment, but view its effect as transitory. Believe that praying for health is the lowest form of prayer. *Death:* See death as a union with Brahman (God) achieved through prayers, ritual, purity, self-control, detachment, truth, nonviolence, charity, and compassion toward all creatures. Following death, one will be reborn (reincarnated) into a future life based on the behavior in this life. The record of behavior is called *karma.* Eventually, the process of rebirth stops which is called *moksha.* A priest may be called at the time of death, and may tie a thread around neck or waist as a blessing. The family washes the body, and it is cremated. *Other practices:* Offer daily worship at a shrine in the home. Daily offering to god, and morning and evening rites. Society is organized into castes, or strata. People are born into a caste, and the caste shapes one's entire life. Hindus practice a discipline of the mind and body, called yoga, to reach God. In the highest state, a meditating yogi does not see, hear, taste, feel, or smell. Beyond good and evil, time and space, he is one with God.
Buddhism	*Death:* Believe that salvation depends on one's own right living. Believe in reincarnation. Can speed the process toward Nirvana, the goal of all humanity's striving, through acts of merit. Meditation, worship, and prayer are some of the acts of merit. Buddhists may drive themselves into more and more ritual or contemplation in the hope that their last moments of consciousness may be filled with thoughts worthy enough to

Religious Group	Beliefs and Practices
EASTERN RELIGIONS *(Continued)*	
Taoism/Confucianism	elevate them to a higher existence. Last rites of chanting may be performed at bedside. *Renunciation:* The most important Buddhist feasts. Young boys are taught to despise the world's vanity and the boy spends a night in a nearby monastery. *General beliefs:* Founded on ethical principles of Confucius. God is not clearly defined as in other religions. Taoism is a mixture of magic and religion. Believe that humans and nature are inseparable, and that if heaven is upset, earth does not prosper. This relationship is described as yin and yang, which are two interplaying forces. When yin and yang are in balance, good occurs. *Death:* The dead are remembered in all festivals. The fate of the dead in the afterworld depends not only on the life they led but also on being properly honored after death. Otherwise they may become demons. Graves are mounds like those dedicated to the gifts of the soil. Graves and houses must be in harmony with the universe, otherwise evil will befall the occupants.

Modified from Carson, V. B. (1989). *Spiritual dimensions of nursing practice.* Philadelphia: W. B. Saunders.

A Health History Format That Integrates the Assessment of Functional Health Patterns

Functional Health Pattern	Assessment
Health perception–health management	Quality of usual and current health rated on a scale of 1 to 10 Self-rating of the importance of health on a scale of 1 to 10 Perceived ability to control and manage health Resources used in health management including primary healthcare provider Self-care measures to maintain or prevent disruption of health status Health habits (e.g., seatbelt use, diet, alcohol consumption, tobacco use) Complete description of present health problem (i.e., chief complaint) Expectations for outcome of current health problem Expectations for care givers Previous illnesses or hospitalizations, reaction to these events, and their outcomes Developmental history, including childhood illnesses and immunizations Ability to manage and comply with recommended treatment of health problems Current medications, including over-the-counter and recreational (street) drugs Allergies Environmental factors affecting health (e.g., occupation, home, leisure) Socioeconomic factors affecting health (e.g., financial concerns, healthcare insurance, living conditions) Knowledge and use of community resources to manage health Family history
Nutritional-metabolic	Recall of usual food and fluid intake for the past 24 hours Comparison of the 24-hour recall diet to typical pattern of diet intake Quality of appetite Dietary restrictions (medical order) Food preferences and dislikes Use of food supplements (e.g., vitamins) Knowledge level of dietary recommendations (e.g., food guide pyramid, recommended dietary allowances, special dietary guidelines) Past alterations in dietary habits (e.g., bulimia nervosa, anorexia nervosa) Usual weight Minimum and maximum weight range Recent weight gain or loss (how much? time span? intentional?) Social significance of food Who shops for food items? Who usually prepares meals? Religious or cultural beliefs affecting diet or meal preparation Ability to swallow and chew Are there any feeding problems?
Elimination Bowel	Usual bowel habits, including frequency, time of day, color, consistency, assistive devices used (e.g., laxatives, suppositories, enemas), constipation, diarrhea Change in bowel habits; describe
Bladder	Usual frequency, amount, color of voiding Assistive devices used (e.g., self-catheterization) Problems with frequency, urgency, burning, retention, incontinence, dribbling, dysuria, polyuria, nocturia
Skin	Condition, color, temperature, turgor, lesions, edema, pruritus
Activity-exercise	Description of usual daily activities Weekend schedule, if different from daily

Functional Health Pattern	Assessment
Activity-exercise (Continued)	Occupation-related activities
	Leisure activities including hobbies
	Description of exercise regimen
	Limitation in ambulation, bathing, dressing, toileting, and feeding
	Dyspnea with exertion
	Fatigue
Sleep-rest	Usual sleep habits including bedtime, hours of sleep obtained, wake-up time
	Problems falling asleep or staying asleep
	Sleep aids used, including medications, food, beverages, and sexual intercourse
	Rating of quality of sleep obtained (does client feel rested?)
	Periods of decreased wakefulness during the day
	Naps or rest periods
Cognitive-perceptual	Ability to understand
	Educational level obtained
	Self-rating of intelligence level
	Ability to communicate with others
	Ability to make decisions and the relative ease or difficulty experienced with decision making
	Ability to see, hear, feel, taste, smell
	Compensations made for sensory deficits and their effectiveness
	Problems with vertigo, heat or cold intolerance
	Pain (including a symptom analysis)
	Desire to learn
Self-perception–self-concept	Description of self, including strengths and weaknesses
	Major concerns
	Health goals
	Body image and feelings about self
	Level of satisfaction with current age
	Perceived developmental level
	Emotional status
	Effect of illness on self-perception
	Personal factors contributing to illness, recovery, health maintenance
Role relationship	Language, quality of speech and relevancy
	Ability to express self
	Family life, including family members and their relationships to client
	Roles client and family members fill
	Interpersonal relationships within family
	Support systems within family, including person client feels closest to
	Family-related problems including living arrangements, parenting, marital problems, abuse
	Occupation and job-related role expectations
	Problems at work
	Societal relationships beyond family or work
	Most important person to client
	Type of neighborhood or community in which client lives
	Participation in social groups (e.g., church, clubs)
	Perceived contributions to society
Sexuality-reproductive	Level of satisfaction with role as male or female
	Anticipated changes related to health problem (e.g., fertility, libido, impotence, pregnancy, contraception, menstruation)
	Sexual activity, including how long client has been sexually active, number of partners, use of contraceptives
	Known exposure to venereal diseases, including HIV
	Level of satisfaction with intercourse
	Problems with intercourse (e.g., premature ejaculation, impotence, pain, bleeding)
Female	Menstrual history including age at menarche, description of typical cycle, last menstrual period, age at menopause, or symptoms of menopause
	Obstetric history including number of pregnancies, number of births, problems during pregnancy or labor and delivery

Appendix continues on following page

Functional Health Pattern	Assessment
Female *Continued*	Practice of breast self-examination, knowledge of technique, compliance
	Last Pap test and results, frequency of pelvic examinations and Pap tests
Male	Circumcision
	Age at climacteric and description of symptoms experienced
	Practice of testicular self-examination, knowledge of technique, compliance
	Prostate examination, prostate-specific antigen test and results
Coping-stress tolerance	Coping strategies used and their effectiveness
	Personal loss or major changes in past year
	Comfort and security needs
	Most stressful event in life and reaction to it
	Use of stress management techniques and their effectiveness (e.g., eating, sleeping, self-medication, counseling, exercise, biofeedback)
	Effect of stress on life-style and ability to function, including decision making
Value-belief	Most important value to client
	Sources of strength and hope
	Importance of religion, type, and frequency of worship
	Life goals
	Values influencing decision making and ability to resolve moral questions
	Recent changes in values or beliefs
	Conflict in values or beliefs with those of significant others
	Spirituality needs, particularly during time of illness or hospitalization

Laboratory Values of Clinical Importance in Medical-Surgical Nursing

Reference laboratory values can provide guidelines for the clinician to use when assessing clients with a wide variety of problems. It should be remembered that the laboratory values given here are for reference only, and are not absolute normal values. The nurse also should remember that there is no sharp dividing line between normal and abnormal. Clients with only slightly elevated values may have apparent disease whereas those with more elevated values may not. Trends in laboratory values are often much more valuable than the single value.

When analyzing laboratory values, consider the following questions:

- Is the value an expected abnormal finding? For example, creatinine is normally elevated in clients with renal failure.
- Is the value an unexpected abnormal finding? For example, elevated blood glucose levels in a client without diabetes may signal a disease.
- Is the value an unexpected normal finding? For example, a client with angina and probable myocardial infarction would be expected to have elevated isoenzymes. Normal levels may mean the client has another cause of chest pain.
- Is the value an expected normal finding? For example, a healthy client should have a normal CBC.

Using the analytic technique, the nurse is guided on when to call the physician. Remember that the laboratory only reports findings; nurses help interpret their significance.

This section provides a summary of the common laboratory diagnostic studies for use as a quick reference. A complete explanation of the diagnostic study and its meaning is covered in the appropriate section (such as liver function studies in Chapter 64). This section simply provides a handy way to check the normal values for the most common diagnostic studies. For details concerning the meaning of the value, see the appropriate section in the text.

The following abbreviations are used throughout the laboratory studies:

g = gram
kg = kilogram
mg = milligram (10^{-3})
μg = microgram (10^{-6})
ng = nanogram (10^{-9})
pg = picogram (10^{-12})
L = liter
ml = milliliter
dl = deciliter (100 ml)
fL = femtoliter
mm = millimeter
mm^3 = cubic millimeter
U = unit
mU = milliunits
μU = microunits
mOsm = milliosmole
mol = mole
μmol = micromole
nmol = nanomole
pmol = picomole
fmol = femtomole (10^{-15})
mEq = milliequivalent
μm = micron

Reference Values in Hematology (For some procedures the reference values may vary, depending on the method used)

Test	Conventional Units	SI Units
Acid hemolysis test (Ham)	No hemolysis	No hemolysis
Alkaline phosphatase, leukocyte	Total score 14 to 100	Total score 14 to 100
Cell counts		
Erythrocytes		
Males	4.6 to 6.2 million/mm^3	4.6 to 6.2×10^{12}/L
Females	4.2 to 5.4 million/mm^3	4.2 to 5.2×10^{12}/L
Children (varies with age)	4.5 to 5.1 million/mm^3	4.5 to 5.1×10^{12}/L
Leukocytes, total	4500 to 11,000/mm^3	4.5 to 11.0×10^9/L

Table continued on following page

Reference Values in Hematology (For some procedures the reference values may vary, depending on the method used) *(Continued)*

Test		Conventional Units	SI Units
Leukocytes, differential	**Percentage**	**Absolute**	**Absolute**
Myelocytes	0	0/mm³	O/L
Band neutrophils	3 to 5	150 to 400/mm³	150 to 400 × 10⁶/L
Segmented neutrophils	54 to 62	3000 to 5800/mm³	3000 to 5800 × 10⁶/L
Lymphocytes	25 to 33	1500 to 3000/mm³	1500 to 3000 × 10⁶/L
Monocytes	3 to 7	300 to 500/mm³	300 to 500 × 10⁶/L
Eosinophils	1 to 3	50 to 250/mm³	50 to 250 × 10⁶/L
Basophils	0 to 0.75	15 to 50/mm³	15 to 50 × 10⁶/L
Platelets		150,000 to 350,000/mm³	150 to 350 × 10⁹/L
Reticulocytes		25,000 to 75,000/mm³	25 to 75 × 10⁹/L
		0.5% to 1.5% of erythrocytes	
Coagulation tests			
Bleeding time (template)		2.75 to 8.0 min	2.75 to 8.0 min
Coagulation time (glass tubes)		5 to 15 min	5 to 15 min
Factor VIII and other coagulation factors		50% to 150% of normal	0.5 to 1.5 of normal
Fibrin split products (Thrombo-Welco test)		<10 µg/ml	<10 mg/L
Fibrinogen		200 to 400 mg/dl	2.0 to 4.0 g/L
Partial thromboplastic time (PTT)		20 to 35 sec	20 to 35 sec
Prothrombin time (PT)		12.0 to 14.0 sec	12.0 to 14.0 sec
Coombs' test			
Direct		Negative	Negative
Indirect		Negative	Negative
Corpuscular values of erythrocytes			
Mean corpuscular hemoglobin (MCH)		26 to 34 pg	0.40 to 0.53 fmol
Mean corpuscular volume (MCV)		80 to 96 µm³	80 to 96 fL
Mean corpuscular hemoglobin concentration (MCHC)		32% to 36%	0.32% to 0.36%
Haptoglobin		26 to 185 mg/dl	260 to 1850 mg/L
Hematocrit			
Males		40 to 54 ml/dl	0.40 to 0.54 volume fraction
Females		37 to 47 ml/dl	0.37 to 0.47 volume fraction
Newborns		49 to 54 ml/dl	0.49 to 0.54 volume fraction
Children (varies with age)		35 to 49 ml/dl	0.35 to 0.49 volume fraction
Hemoglobin			
Males		14.0 to 18.0 g/dl	2.17 to 2.79 mmol/L
Females		12.0 to 16.0 g/dl	1.86 to 2.48 mmol/L
Newborns		16.5 to 19.5 g/dl	2.56 to 3.02 mmol/L
Children (varies with age)		11.2 to 16.5 g/dl	1.74 to 2.56 mmol/L
Hemoglobin, fetal		<1.0% of total	<0.01% of total
Hemoglobin A_{1C}		3% to 5% of total	0.03% to 0.05% of total
Hemoglobin A_2		1.5% to 3.0% of total	0.015% to 0.03% of total
Hemoglobin, plasma		0 to 5.0 mg/dl	0 to 0.8 µmol/L
Methemoglobin		30 to 130 mg/dl	4.7 to 20 µmol/L
Sedimentation rate (ESR)			
Wintrobe			
Males		0 to 5 mm/hr	0 to 5 mm/hr
Females		0 to 15 mm/hr	0 to 15 mm/hr
Westergren			
Males		0 to 15 mm/hr	0 to 15 mm/hr
Females		0 to 20 mm/hr	0 to 20 mm/hr

Reference Values for Blood, Plasma, and Serum (For some procedures the reference values may vary, depending on the method used)

Test	Conventional Units	SI Units
Acetoacetate plus acetone		
Qualitative	Negative	Negative
Quantitative	0.3 to 2.0 mg/dl	3 to 20 mg/L
Acid phosphatase, serum (thymolphthalein monophosphate substrate)	0.11 to 0.60 U/L	0.11 to 0.60 U/L
Adrenocorticotropin, plasma (ACTH)		
6:00 AM	10 to 80 pg/ml	10 to 80 ng/L
6:00 PM	<50 pg/ml	<50 ng/L
Alanine aminotransferase, serum (ALT, SGPT)	7 to 35 U/L	7 to 35 U/L
Albumin, serum	3.5 to 5.5 g/dl	35 to 55 g/L
Aldolase, serum	1.5 to 12.0 U/L	1.5 to 12.0 U/L
Aldosterone, plasma		
Supine	3 to 10 ng/dl	0.08 to 0.30 nmol/L
Standing		
Males	6 to 22 ng/dl	0.17 to 0.61 nmol/L
Females	5 to 30 ng/dl	0.14 to 0.83 nmol/L
Alkaline phosphatase, serum (ALP)	20 to 90 U/L (30° C)	20 to 90 U/L (30° C)
Ammonia nitrogen, plasma	15 to 49 μg/dl	11 to 35 μmol/L
Amylase, serum	25 to 125 U/L	25 to 125 U/L
Anion gap	8 to 16 mEq/L	8 to 16 mmol/L
Ascorbic acid, blood	0.4 to 1.5 mg/dl	23 to 85 μmol/L
Aspartate aminotransferase, serum (AST, SGOT)	7 to 40 U/L	7 to 40 U/L
Base excess, blood	0 ± 2 mEq/L	0 ± 2 mmol/L
Bicarbonate		
Venous plasma	23 to 29 mEq/L	23 to 29 mmol/L
Arterial blood	18 to 23 mEq/L	18 to 23 mmol/L
Bile acids, serum	0.3 to 3.0 mg/dl	3 to 30 mg/L
Bilirubin, serum		
Conjugated	0.1 to 0.4 mg/dl	1.7 to 6.8 μmol/L
Unconjugated	0.2 to 0.7 mg/dl	3.4 to 12 μmol/L
Total	0.3 to 1.1 mg/dl	5.1 to 19 μmol/L
Calcium, serum	9.0 to 11.0 mg/dl	2.25 to 2.75 mmol/L
Calcium, ionized, serum	4.25 to 5.25 mg/dl	1.05 to 1.30 mmol/L
Carbon dioxide, total, serum or plasma	24 to 30 mEq/L	24 to 30 mmol/L
Carbon dioxide tension, blood PCO_2	35 to 45 mm Hg	35 to 45 mm Hg
β-Carotene serum	40 to 200 μg/dl	0.74 to 3.72 μmol/L
Catecholamines, plasma		
Epinephrine	15 to 55 pg/ml	82 to 300 pmol/L
Norpinephrine	65 to 400 pg/ml	384 to 2364 pmol/L
Ceruloplasmin, serum	23 to 44 mg/dl	230 to 440 mg/L
Chloride, serum or plasma	96 to 106 mEq/L	96 to 106 mmol/L
Cholesterol, serum or EDTA plasma		
Desirable range	<200 mg/dl	<5.18 mmol/L
LDL Cholesterol	60 to 180 mgdl	600 to 1800 mg/L
HDL Cholesterol	30 to 80 mg/dl	300 to 800 mg/L
Copper		
Males	70 to 140 μg/dl	11 to 22 μmol/L
Females	85 to 155 μg/dl	13 to 24 μmol/L
Cortisol, plasma		
8:00 AM	6 to 23 μg/dl	170 to 635 nmol/L
4:00 PM	3 to 15 μg/dl	82 to 413 nmol/L

Table continued on following page

Reference Values for Blood, Plasma, and Serum (For some procedures the reference values may vary, depending on the method used) *(Continued)*

Test	Conventional Units	SI Units
Cortisol, plasma *(Continued)*		
10:00 PM	<50% of 8 AM value	<0.5% of 8 AM value
Creatine, serum	0.2 to 0.8 mg/dl	15 to 61 μmol/L
Creatine kinase, serum (CK, CPK)		
Males	55 to 170 U/L	55 to 170 U/L
Females	30 to 135 U/L	30 to 135 U/L
Creatine kinase MB isozyme, serum	0.0 to 4.7 ng/ml	0.0 to 4.7 μg/L
Creatinine, serum	0.6 to 1.2 mg/dl	53 to 108 μmol/L
Ferritin, serum	20 to 200 ng/ml	20 to 200 μg/L
Fibrinogen, plasma	200 to 400 mg/dl	2.0 to 4.0 g/L
Folate		
Serum	1.8 to 9.0 ng/ml	4.1 to 20.4 nmol/L
Erythrocytes	150 to 450 ng/ml	340 to 1020 nmol/L
Follicle-stimulating hormine, plasma (FSH)		
Males	4 to 25 mU/ml	4 to 25 U/L
Females	4 to 30 mU/ml	4 to 30 U/L
Postmenopausal	40 to 250 mU/ml	40 to 250 U/L
γ-Glutamyltransferase, serum		
Males	5 to 38 U/L	5 to 38 U/L
Females	5 to 29 U/L	5 to 29 U/L
Gastrin, serum	0 to 200 pg/ml	0 to 200 ng/L
Glucose (fasting), plasma or serum	70 to 115 mg/dl	3.89 to 6.38 mmol/L
Growth hormone, plasma (HGH)	0 to 10 ng/ml	0 to 10 μg/L
Haptoglobin, serum	26 to 185 mg/dl	260 to 1850 mg/L
Immunoglobulins, serum		
IgG	550 to 1900 mg/dl	5.5 to 19.0 g/L
IgA	60 to 333 mg/dl	0.60 to 3.3 g/L
IgM	45 to 145 mg/dl	0.45 to 1.5 g/L
IgD	0.5 to 3.0 mg/dl	5 to 30 mg/L
IgE	<500 ng/ml	<500 μg/L
Insulin (fasting), plasma	5 to 25 μU/ml	36 to 179 pmol/L
Iron, serum	75 to 175 ng/dl	13 to 31 μmol/L
Iron-binding capacity, serum		
Total	250 to 410 μg/dl	45 to 73 μmol/L
Saturation	20% to 55%	0.20 to 0.55
Lactate		
Venous blood	4.5 to 19.8 mg/dl	0.50 to 2.2 mmol/L
Arterial blood	4.5 to 14.4 mg/dl	0.50 to 1.6 mmol/L
Lactate dehydrogenase, serum (LD, LDH)	100 to 190 U/L	100 to 190 U/L
Lipase, serum	10 to 140 U/L	10 to 140 U/L
Lipids, total, serum	450 to 850 mg/dl	4.5 to 8.5 g/L
Luteinizing hormone, serum (LH)		
Males	6 to 18 mU/ml	6 to 18 U/L
Females		
Premenopausal	5 to 22 mU/ml	5 to 22 U/L
Midcycle	3 × baseline	3 × baseline
Postmenopausal	>30 mU/ml	>30 U/L

Test	Conventional Units	SI Units
Magnesium, serum	1.8 to 3.0 mg/dl	0.75 to 1.25 mmol/L
Osmolality	286 to 295 mOsm/kg H_2O	2.85 to 295 mOsm/kg H_2O
Oxygen blood		
Capacity (varies with hemoglobin)	16 to 24 vol%	7.14 to 10.7 mmol/L
Content, arterial	15 to 23 vol%	6.69 to 10.3 mmol/L
Saturation, arterial	94% to 100%	0.94 to 1.00
Tension, Po_2	75 to 100 mm Hg	75 to 100 mm Hg
P_{50}	26 to 27 mm Hg	26 to 27 mm Hg
pH, arterial blood	7.35 to 7.45	7.35 to 7.45
Phenylalanine, serum	<3 mg/dl	<0.18 mmol/L
Phosphate, inorganic, serum	3.0 to 4.5 mg/dl	1.0 to 1.5 mmol/L
Potassium, serum or plasma	3.5 to 5.0 mEq/l	3.5 to 5.0 mmol/L
Prolactin, serum		
Males	1 to 20 ng/ml	1 to 20 μg/L
Females	1 to 25 ng/ml	1 to 25 μg/L
Protein, serum		
Total	6.0 to 8.0 g/dl	60 to 80 g/L
Albumin	3.5 to 5.5 g/dl	35 to 55 g/L
α_1-Globulin	0.2 to 0.4 g/dl	2 to 4 g/L
α_2-Globulin	0.5 to 0.9 g/dl	5 to 9 g/L
β-Globulin	0.6 to 1.1 g/dl	6 to 11 g/L
γ-Globulin	0.7 to 1.7 g/dl	7 to 17 g/L
Pyruvate, blood	0.3 to 0.9 mg/dl	0.03 to 0.10 mmol/L
Sodium, serum or plasma	136 to 145 mEq/L	136 to 145 mmol/L
Testosterone, plasma		
Males	275 to 875 ng/dl	9.0 to 10.0 nmol/L
Females	23 to 75 ng/dl	0.8 to 2.6 nmol/L
Pregnant	38 to 190 ng/dl	1.3 to 6.6 nmol/L
Thyroid-stimulating hormone, serum (TSH)	0 to 7 μU/ml	0 to 7 mU/L
Thyroxine, free, serum (FT_4)	1.0 to 2.1 ng/dl	13 to 27 pmol/L
Thyroxine, serum (T_4)	4.4 to 9.9 μg/dl	57 to 128 nmol/L
Triglycerides, serum	40 to 150 mg/dl	0.4 to 1.5 g/L
Triiodothyronine, serum (T_3)	150 to 250 ng/dl	2.3 to 3.9 nmol/L
Triiodothyronine uptake, resin (T_3RU)	25% to 38% uptake	0.25 to 0.38 uptake
Urate		
Males	2.5 to 8.0 mg/dl	0.15 to 0.48 mmol/L
Females	1.5 to 7.0 mg/dl	0.09 to 0.42 mmol/L
Urea, serum or plasma	24 to 49 mg/dl	4.0 to 8.2 mmol/L
Urea nitrogen, serum or plasma	11 to 23 mg/dl	3.9 to 8.2 mmol/L
Viscosity, serum	1.4 to 1.8 × water	1.4 to 1.8 × water
Vitamin A, serum	20 to 80 μg/dl	0.70 to 2.80 μmol/L
Vitamin B_{12}, serum	180 to 900 pg/ml	133 to 664 pmol/L

Reference Values for Urine (For some procedures the reference values may vary, depending on the method used)

Test	Conventional Units	SI Units
Acetone and acetoacetate, qualitative	Negative	Negative
Albumin		
Qualitative	Negative	Negative
Quantitative	10 to 100 mg/24 hr	10 to 100 mg/24 hr
Aldosterone	3 to 20 μg/24 hr	8.3 to 55 nmol/24 hr
δ-Aminolevulinic acid	1.3 to 7.0 mg/24 hr	10 to 53 μmol/24 hr
Amylase	3 to 20 U/hr	3 to 20 U/hr
Amylase/creatinine clearance ratio	1% to 4%	0.01% to 0.04%
Bilirubin, qualitative	Negative	Negative
Calcium (usual diet)	<250 mg/24 hr	<6.3 mmol/24 hr
Catecholamines		
Epinephrine	<10 μg/24 hr	<55 nmol/24 hr
Norepinephrine	<100 μg/24 hr	<590 nmol/24 hr
Total free catecholamines	4 to 126 μg/24 hr	24 to 745 nmol/24 hr
Total metanephrines	0.1 to 1.6 mg/24 hr	0.5 to 8.1 μmol/24 hr
Chloride (varies with intake)	110 to 250 mEq/24 hr	110 to 250 nmol/24 hr
Copper	0 to 50 μg/24 hr	0 to 0.80 μmol/24 hr
Cortisol, free	10 to 100 μg/24 hr	27.6 to 276 nmol/24 hr
Creatinine	15 to 25 mg/kg body weight/24 hr	0.13 to 0.22 mmol/kg body weight/24 hr
Creatinine clearance (corrected to 1.73 m^2 body surface area)		
Males	110 to 150 ml/min	110 to 150 ml/min
Females	105 to 132 ml/min	105 to 132 ml/min
Dehydroepiandrosterone		
Males	0.2 to 2.0 mg/24 hr	0.7 to 6.9 μmol/24 hr
Females	0.2 to 1.8 mg/24 hr	0.7 to 6.2 μmol/24 hr
Estrogens, total		
Males	4 to 25 μg/24 hr	14 to 90 nmol/24 hr
Females	5 to 100 μg/24 hr	18 to 360 nmol/24 hr
Glucose (as reducing substance)	<250 mg/24 hr	<250 mg/24 hr
Hemoglobin and myoglobin, qualitative	Negative	Negative
17-Hydroxycorticosteroids		
Males	3 to 9 mg/24 hr	8.3 to 25 μmol/24 hr
Females	2 to 8 mg/24 hr	5.5 to 22 μmol/24 hr

Test	Conventional Units	SI Units
5-Hydroxyindoleacetic acid		
Qualitative	Negative	Negative
Quantitative	<9 mg/24 hr	<47 μmol/24 hr
17-Ketosteroids		
Males	6 to 18 mg/24 hr	21 to 62 μmol/24 hr
Females	4 to 13 mg/24 hr	14 to 45 μmol/24 hr
Magnesium	6.0 to 8.5 mEq/24 hr	3.0 to 4.2 mmol/24 hr
Metanephrines (see Catecholamines)		
Osmolality	38 to 1,400 mOsm/kg H_2O	38 to 1,400 mOsm/kg H_2O
pH	4.6 to 8.0	4.6 to 8.0
Phenylpyruvic acid, qualitative	Negative	Negative
Phosphate	0.9 to 1.3 g/24 hr	29 to 42 mmol/24 hr
Porphobilinogen		
Qualitative	Negative	Negative
Quantitative	<2.0 mg/24 hr	<9 μmol/24 hr
Porphyrins		
Coproporphyrin	50 to 250 μg/24 hr	77 to 380 nmol/24 hr
Uroporphyrin	10 to 30 μg/24 hr	12 to 36 nmol/24 hr
Potassium	25 to 100 mEq/24 hr	25 to 100 mmol/24 hr
Pregnanediol		
Males	0.4 to 1.4 mg/24 hr	1.2 to 4.4 μmol/24 hr
Females		
Proliferative phase	0.5 to 1.5 mg/24 hr	1.6 to 4.7 μmol/24 hr
Luteal phase	2.0 to 7.0 mg/24 hr	6.2 to 22 μmol/24 hr
Postmenopausal	0.2 to 1.0 mg/24 hr	0.6 to 3.1 μmol/24 hr
Pregnanetriol	<2.5 mg/24 hr	<7.4 μmol/24 hr
Protein		
Qualitative	Negative	Negative
Quantitative	10 to 150 mg/24 hr	10 to 150 mg/24 hr
Sodium	130 to 260 mEq/24 hr	130 to 260 mmol/24 hr
Specific gravity	1.003 to 1.030	1.003 to 1.030
Urate	200 to 500 mg/24 hr	1.2 to 3.0 mmol/24 hr
Urobilinogen	<4.0 mg/24 hr	<6.8 μmol/24 hr
Vanillylmandelic acid (VMA) (4-hydroxy-3-methoxymandelic acid)	1 to 8 mg/24 hr	5 to 40 μmol/24 hr

Reference Values for Therapeutic Drug Monitoring

	Therapeutic Range	Toxic Levels	Proprietary Names
Antibiotics			
Amikacin, serum	25 to 30 μg/ml	Peak > 35 μg/ml Trough > 5 to 7 μg/ml	Amikin
Chloramphenicol, serum	10 to 20 μg/ml	>25 μg/ml	Chloromycetin
Gentamicin, serum	5 to 10 μg/ml	Peak > 12 μg/ml Trough > 2 μg/ml	Garamycin
Tobramycin, serum	5 to 10 μg/ml	Peak > 12 μg/ml Trough > 2 μg/ml	Nebcin
Anticonvulsants			
Carbamazepine, serum	5 to 12 μg/ml	>12 μg/ml	Tegretol
Ethosuximide, serum	40 to 100 μg/ml	>100 μg/ml	Zarontin
Phenobarbital, serum	10 to 30 μg/ml	Vary widely because of developed tolerance	Luminal
Phenytoin, serum	10 to 20 μg/ml	>20 μg/ml	Dilantin
Primidone, serum	5 to 20 μg/ml	>15 μg/ml	Mysoline
Valproic acid, serum	50 to 100 μg/ml	>100 μg/ml	Depakene
Analgesics			
Acetaminophen, serum	10 to 20 μg/ml	>250 μg/ml	Tylenol Datril
Salicylate, serum	100 to 250 μg/ml	>300 μg/ml	
Bronchodilator			
Theophylline, serum (aminophylline)	10 to 20 μg/ml	>20 μg/ml	Theo-Dur
Cardiovascular Drugs			
Digitoxin, serum (specimen must be obtained 12 to 24 hr after last dose)	15 to 25 ng/ml	>25 ng/ml	Crystodigin
Digoxin, serum (specimen must be obtained 12 to 24 hr after last dose)	0.8 to 2.0 ng/ml	>2.4 ng/ml	Lanoxin
Disopyramide, serum	2 to 5 μg/ml	>5 μg/ml	Norpase
Lidocaine, serum	1.5 to 5.0 μg/ml	>6 to 8 μg/ml	Xylocaine
Procainamide, serum (measured as procainamide + N-acetyl procainamide)	4 to 10 μg/ml 10 to 30 μg/ml	>16 μg/ml >30 μg/ml	Pronestyl
Propranolol, serum	50 to 100 ng/ml	Variable	Inderal
Quinidine, serum	2 to 5 μg/ml	>10 μg/ml	Cardioquin Quinaglute Quinidex Quinora
Psychopharmacologic Drugs			
Amitriptyline, serum (measured as amitriptyline + nortriptyline)	120 to 150 ng/ml	>500 ng/ml	Amitril Elavil Endep Limbitrol Triavil
Desipramine, serum (measured as desipramine + imipramine)	150 to 300 ng/ml	>500 ng/ml	Norpramin Pertofrane
Imipramine, serum (measured as imipramine + desipramine)	150 to 300 ng/ml	500 ng/ml	Antipress Janimine Tofranil
Lithium, serum (obtain specimen 12 hr after last dose)	0.8 to 1.2 mEq/L	>2.0 mEq/L	Lithobid
Nortriptyline, serum	50 to 150 ng/ml	500 ng/ml	Aventyl Pamelor

Reference Values in Toxicology

	Conventional Units	SI Units
Arsenic, blood	3.5 to 7.2 μg/dl	0.47 to 0.96 μmol/L
Arsenic, urine	<100 μg/24 hr	<1.3 μmol/24 hr
Bromides, serum	0 Toxic above 17 mEq/L	0 Toxic above 17 mmol/L
Carboxyhemoglobin, blood Symptoms occur	<5% saturation >20% saturation	<0.05 saturation >0.20 saturation
Ethanol, blood	<0.05 mg/dl <0.005%	<1.0 mmol/L
Marked intoxication	300 to 400 mg/dl 0.3% to 0.4%	65 to 87 mmol/L
Alcoholic stupor	400 to 500 mg/dl 0.4% to 0.5%	87 to 109 mmol/L
Coma	>500 mg/dl >0.5%	>109 mmol/L
Lead, blood	0 to 40 μg/dl	0 to 2 μmol/L
Lead, urine	<100 μg/24 hr	<0.48 μmol/24 hr
Mercury, urine	<100 μg/24 hr	<50 nmol/24 hr

Reference Values for Cerebrospinal Fluid

	Conventional Units	SI Units
Cells	<5/mm^3 All mononuclear	<5 $\times$ 10^6/L All mononuclear
Electrophoresis	Predominantly albumin	Predominantly albumin
Glucose	50 to 75 mg/dl (20 mg/dl less than serum)	2.8 to 4.2 mmol/L (1.1 mmol/L less than serum)

IgG
   Children <14 yr
   Adults
	<8% of total protein
	 <14% of total protein
		<0.08 of total protein
		 <0.14 of total protein

IgG index $\dfrac{\text{CSF/serum IgG ratio}}{\text{CSF/serum albumin ratio}}$	0.3 to 0.6	0.3 to 0.6
Oligoclonal banding on electrophoresis	Absent	Absent
Pressure	70 to 180 mm H$_2$O	70 to 180 mm H$_2$O
Protein, total	15 to 45 mg/dl	150 to 450 mg/L

Reference Values for Feces

	Conventional Units	SI Units
Bulk	100 to 200 g/24 hr	100 to 200 g/24 hr
Dry matter	23 to 32 g/24 hr	23 to 32 g/24 hr
Fat, total	<6.0 g/24 hr	<6.0 g/24 hr
Nitrogen, total	<2.0 g/24 hr	<2.0 g/24 hr
Water	Approximately 65%	Approximately 0.65

Reference Values for Semen Analysis		
	Conventional Units	**SI Units**
Volume	2 to 5 ml	2 to 5 ml
Liquefaction	Complete in 15 min	Complete in 15 min
Leukocytes	Occasional or absent	Occasional or absent
Count	60 to 150 million/ml	60 to 150×10^6/ml
Motility	>80% motile	>0.80 motile
Morphology	80% to 90% normal forms	0.80 to 0.90 normal forms
Fructose	>150 mg/dl	>8.33 mmol/L

Reference Values for Assessment of Gastrointestinal Function		
Test	**Normal Range**	**Significance of Abnormal Findings**
Complete blood count		

Red blood cells	4.2 to 5.4 million/mm³ (women)
	4.5 to 6.2 million/mm³ (men)
		Decreased values indicate possible:
		  Anemia
		  Hemorrhage

Hemoglobin	12 to 16 g/dl (women) 14 to 18 g/dl (men)	Increased values indicate possible: Hemoconcentration caused by dehydration
Hematocrit	38% to 46% (women) 42% to 54% (men)	
Electrolytes		

Potassium	3.5 to 5.0 mg/L	Decreased values indicate possible:
		  Gastrointestinal suction
		  Diarrhea
		  Vomiting
		  Intestinal fistulas

Calcium	8.0 to 10.5 mg/dl	Decreased values indicate possible: Malabsorption

Sodium	135 to 145 mg/L	Decreased values indicate possible:
		  Malabsorption
		  Diarrhea

D-Xylose	Blood levels peak (25 to 40 mg/dl)
	  2 hr after ingestion
	80% to 95% excreted in 5 hr
		Decreased values indicate possible:
		  Malabsorption

Carcinoembryonic antigen	Less than 5 ng/ml (non-smokers)	Increased values indicate possible:
		  Colorectal cancer
		  Inflammatory bowel disease

Fecal analysis		

Stool for occult blood	Negative	Presence indicates possible:
		  Peptic ulcer
		  Cancer of the colon
		  Ulcerative colitis

Stool for ova and parasites	Negative	Presence indicates: Infection

Stool cultures	No unusual growth	Presence of pathogens may indicate:
		  Shigella
		  Salmonella
		  Staphylococcus aureus
		  Bacillus cereus

Stool for lipids	2 to 5 g/24 hr (normal diet)	Increased values indicate possible:
		  Malabsorption syndrome
		  Crohn's disease

Reference Values for Tumor Markers

Test	Reference Value	Conditions in Which Levels Are Elevated
α-Fetoprotein (AFP)	<10 ng/ml	Lung, nonseminomatous testicular, pancreatic, colon, and stomach cancers, and choriocarcinoma
CA–125	<35 units	Ovarian cancer
Calcitonin	<100 pg/ml	Medullary thyroid, small cell lung, and breast cancers, and carcinoid
Carcinoembryonic antigen (CEA)	0 to 2.5 ng/ml non-smokers <3.0 ng/ml smokers	Colorectal, breast, lung, stomach, pancreatic, and prostate cancers
Estrogen receptors	Negative <10 fmol/mg	Breast cancer
Human chorionic gonadotropin (HCG)	0 to 5 IU/L	Choriocarcinoma, germ cell testicular, lung, liver, stomach, pancreatic, endometrial, and liver cancers
Progesterone receptor assay	Negative <10 fmol/mg	Breast cancer
Prostatic acid phosphatase	0.26 to 0.83 U/L	Metastatic prostate cancer
Prostate-specific antigen (PSA)	0 to 4 ng/ml	Prostate cancer
CA–19-9		Pancreatic and colon cancer
CA–15-3		Breast cancer

Modified from Conn, R. B. (1991). *Current diagnosis 8* (8th ed., pp. 1307–1312). Philadelphia, W. B. Saunders.

Appendix D1: CVA/TIA

✝ **MONTCLAIR**
BAPTIST MEDICAL CENTER

COORDINATED CareMap®
CASE TYPE—CVA/TIA
DRG - 14/15   ALOS - 6 DAYS

(Addressograph)

_____

ROOM NO: _____   AGE: _____   DIABETIC: YES _____ NO _____

PHYSICIAN(S): _____ CONSULTING PHYSICIAN: _____

DIAGNOSIS: _____ OTHER DIAGNOSIS: _____

CASE COORDINATOR: _____

ALLERGIES: _____

_____

_____

FAMILY PHONE NUMBERS: (_____) _____   RELATIONSHIP: _____

(_____) _____   RELATIONSHIP: _____

(_____) _____   RELATIONSHIP: _____

11-7			7-3			3-11		
SIGNATURE	INITIAL	DATE	SIGNATURE	INITIAL	DATE	SIGNATURE	INITIAL	DATE

COORDINATED CareMap® — CVA/TIA

M-93-5376 REV. 12/21/93 P

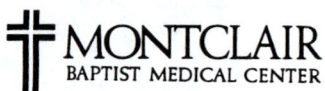
MONTCLAIR
BAPTIST MEDICAL CENTER

COORDINATED CareMap®
CASE TYPE – CVA/TIA

CVA LOS – 6 DAYS
TIA LOS – 2 DAYS

Key: Highlight completed task and goals.
Address variances in nurses' focus notes and circle variances on map.
Once variances completed - highlight and date.
Draw black line through non-applicable tasks/goals.

PAGE 2

	DAY 1 Date _____ RN Init. _____	DAY 2 Date _____ RN Init. _____	DAY 3 Date _____ RN Init. _____
ACTIVITY High risk for skin breakdown r/t ↓ mobility High risk for thrombus formation &/or PTE r/t ↓ mobility High risk for physical impairments r/t ↓ mobility, motor skills (balance, coordination, musculoskeletal contracture, foot drop, self-feeding, BR activities)	Assess skin q shift →→→→→→→→→→→→ Establish skin care regimen Consult ET nurse prn Turn/Reposition q 2° Check for incontinence q 2° **GOAL:** No redness or skin breakdown BR ROM qs Ted Hose: remove @ HS, replace @ 6A Consult PT/OT for Day 2	→→→→→→→→→→→→→→→→→→→→ Implement skin care regimen →→→→→→→ →→→→→→→→→→→→→→→→→→→→ **GOAL:** No redness or skin breakdown OOB to chair today BSC or BRP Ted Hose: remove @ HS, replace @ 6A PT/OT visit (establish position plan as indicated)	→→→→→→→→→→→→→→→→→→→→ →→→→→→→→→→→→→→→→→→→→ **GOAL:** No redness or skin brkdwn. Follow PT position plan as indicated OOB to chair TID →→→→→→→→→→→→→→→→→→→→ Ted Hose: rem. @ HS, rep. @ 6A **GOAL:** No evidence of contractures, swelling or ↑ warmth of extremities
D/C PLANNING	DCP Assessment DCP Consult		**GOAL:** Dschg. TIA pt. c̄ resolution of symp. and completion of dx testing **GOAL:** Discharge needs identified & documented by DPCN Consult PMRU for Evaluation
ELIMINATION Risk for bowel elimination impairment r/t constipation High risk for bladder elimination impairment r/t incontinence/retention Risk for intake/output imbalance	Assess for BM q s Insert foley or place condom c̄ incontinence or retention Monitor I/O qs	Assess need for LOC D/C Foley **GOAL:** Pt. has BM, Establishes pre-CVA voiding pattern/continent maintains balance i & O, U/O > 30cc/hr, adequate hydration.	Assess need for LOC →→→→→→→→→→→→→→→→→→→→
NUTRITION High risk for deficient oral intake	Document % intake Full liquid diet Elevate HOB 70-90°during meals Follow speech swallowing guidelines (as indic.)	→→→→→→→→→→→→→→→→→→→→ Regular as tol. c̄ no swallowing diff. →→→→→→→→→→→→→→→→→→→→ →→→→→→→→→→→→→→→→→→→→ Assess need for dietary consult **GOAL:** Dietary intake > 50% po, albumin > 3.0, no swallowing difficulties.	→→→→→→→→→→→→→→→→→→→→ →→→→→→→→→→→→→→→→→→→→ →→→→→→→→→→→→→→→→→→→→
PSYCHOSOCIAL/SPIRITUAL Risk for coping difficulties r/t emotional lability, altered body image, cognitive impairments Potential Pt./Family Faith Crisis	Assess need for Chaplain Consult q d **GOAL:** Pt./Family verbalize thoughts/feelings re: spirituality	**GOAL:** Pt./Family verbalize thoughts/feelings re: illness	**GOAL:** Pt./Family verbalize thoughts/feelings re: illness
NEURO-CARDIOPULMONARY High risk for development of or ↑ ICP, sensory, motor &/or visual deficits High risk for hemodynamic instability r/t arrythmias High risk for resp. distress r/t oxygenation, airway maintenance, breathing patterns High risk for aspiration r/t ↑ secretions &/or swallowing difficulties.	Neuro checks q 2° x 4, then q 4° VS q 2° x 4, then q 4° Cardiac Monitor O₂ Saturation (spot check) →→→→→→→→→ O₂ @ 2-4 L/NC or mask →→→→→→→→→→→ Assess breath sounds & character q 8° Clear airway secretions prn Speech Consult **GOAL:** Pt. experiences no swallowing difficulties, or pocketing of food. Maintain patent airway, clear, even bilateral breath sounds.	Neuro checks q 4° VS q 4° →→→→→→→→→→→→→→→→→→→→ →→→→→→→→→→→→→→→→→→→→ →→→→→→→→→→→→→→→→→→→→ →→→→→→→→→→→→→→→→→→→→ **GOAL:** Swallowing s̄ S & S of aspiration, adequate hemodynamic status c̄ no major ↓ or ↑ of BP (maintain loose control) HR 60-100 RR 12-24 BS < 200 for DM	Neuro checks q 8° VS q 8° D/C cardiac monitor D/O O2 **GOAL:** Oxygenation >90, no symptomatic arrythmias x 48h →→→→→→→→→→→→→→→→→→→→
SAFETY High risk for injury r/t possible seizures, falls, one-sided neglect	Seizure precautions Assess for motor sensory & cognitive deficit qs HOB ↑15° Assess need for restraints, siderails ↑ x 4 flat call light Call light within reach Bed in lowest position Room free of clutter **GOAL:** Pt. free from injury	→→→→→→→→→→→→→→→→→→→→ →→→→→→→→→→→→→→→→→→→→ →→→→→→→→→→→→→→→→→→→→ →→→→→→→→→→→→→→→→→→→→ →→→→→→→→→→→→→→→→→→→→ **GOAL:** Pt. free from injury	→→→→→→→→→→→→→→→→→→→→ →→→→→→→→→→→→→→→→→→→→ →→→→→→→→→→→→→→→→→→→→ →→→→→→→→→→→→→→→→→→→→ **GOAL:** Pt. free from injury
TEST/PROCEDURES NOTE ER CVA/TIA CARE MAP	**GOAL:** Pt./Family verbalizes understanding of test/procedures PT, PTT EKG PBS c̄ Diabetics CBC, S7, CT Scan	S-18, Carotid Doppler, Echo	**GOAL:** Pt./Family verbalizes understanding of test/procedures
MEDICATIONS Risk for drug induced CNS changes High risk for major bleeding/bruising r/t anticoag./antiplatelet meds Knowledge deficit r/t needs for med counsel.	IV @ KVO Assess for adverse drug reactions (ADR) **GOAL:** Pt. s̄ S&S of sedation, confusion, AMS, major bleeding, bruising, thrombocytopenia, neutropenia	→→→→→→→→→→→→→→→→→→→→	SL IV D/C IVF Begin med counseling per educational needs
TEACHING Knowledge deficit r/t medications, self-care, etc.	Assess for knowledge deficit	Assess need for education channel programs: • Overweight • Diet Management • High Blood Pressure Compliance	Begin education re: • S & S of recurrent stroke • Skin care regimen • Positioning/Transfer • ADL assistive measures • Risk factors • Swallowing Precaut.
COMMUNICATIONS Risk for speech &/or cognitive impairment r/t cerebral injury			**GOAL:** Oriented to person, place, environment & situation. **GOAL:** Comprehension of yes/no questions, ↑ auditory comprehension of one-part commands.

COORDINATED CareMap® — CVA/TIA

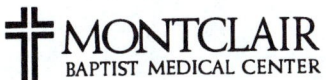

COORDINATED CareMap®
CASE TYPE—CVA/TIA

Key: Highlight completed task and goals.
Address variances in nurses' focus notes and circle variances on map.
Once variances completed - highlight and date.
Draw black line through non-applicable tasks/goals.

(Addressograph)

PAGE 3

DAY 4 Date _____	DAY 5 Date _____	DAY 6 Date _____	DAY 7 Date _____
RN Init. _____	RN Init. _____	RN Init. _____	RN Init. _____
→→→→→→→→→→→→→→→→→ →→→→→→→→→→→→→→→→ **GOAL:** No redness or skin brkdwn.	→→→→→→→→→→→→→→→→ →→→→→→→→→→→→→→→→ **GOAL:** No redness or skin brkdwn.	→→→→→→→→→→→→→→→→ →→→→→→→→→→→→→→→→ **GOAL:** No redness or skin brkdwn, Pt./Family verbalize understanding & demonstrate skin care regimen.	**GOAL:** No redness or skin brkdwn.
→→→→→→→→→→→→→→→→ →→→→→→→→→→→→→→→→ Ted Hose: rem. @ HS, rep. @ 6A	→→→→→→→→→→→→→→→→ →→→→→→→→→→→→→→→→ Ted Hose: rem. @ HS, rep. @ 6A	→→→→→→→→→→→→→→→→ →→→→→→→→→→→→→→→→ Ted Hose: rem. @ HS, rep. @ 6A	**GOAL:** Pt./Family demonstrates proper positioning, ROM &/or transfer skills
		GOAL: Arrangements complete for equipment, supplies &/or community resources.	**GOAL:** Pt./Family verbalize under-standing of f/u care: • MD visit • Outpatient PT/OT • _____ • _____
Assess need for bladder training	→→→→→→→→→→→→→→→→	Reinforce bladder training regimen c̄ Pt./Fam as indicated→→→→→→→	**GOAL:** Pt./Family verbalizes understanding of bladder training regimen
→→→→→→→→→→→→→→→→ →→→→→→→→→→→→→→→→ →→→→→→→→→→→→→→→→	→→→→→→→→→→→→→→→→ →→→→→→→→→→→→→→→→ →→→→→→→→→→→→→→→→	**GOAL:** Meets established nutritional needs (oral & oral plus tube feedings) →→→→→→→→→→→→→→→→	
GOAL: Pt./Family verbalize thoughts/feelings re: illness	Assess for signs of depression **GOAL:** Pt./Family verbalize thoughts/feelings re: illness **GOAL:** Pt./Family aware of prognosis	→→→→→→→→→→→→→→→→ **GOAL:** Pt./Family verbalize thoughts/feelings re: illness	
Neuro checks q 8° VS q 8°	Neuro checks q 8° VS q 8°	Neuro checks q 8° VS q 8°	**GOAL:** No evidence of ↑ neuro deficit
→→→→→→→→→→→→→→→→	→→→→→→→→→→→→→→→→	→→→→→→→→→→→→→→→→ **GOAL:** Oral skills appropriate for deglutition. Adequate hemodynamic status maintained.	
→→→→→→→→→→→→→→→→ →→→→→→→→→→→→→→→→ →→→→→→→→→→→→→→→→ →→→→→→→→→→→→→→→→ **GOAL:** Pt. free from injury	→→→→→→→→→→→→→→→→ →→→→→→→→→→→→→→→→ →→→→→→→→→→→→→→→→ →→→→→→→→→→→→→→→→ **GOAL:** Pt. free from injury	→→→→→→→→→→→→→→→→ →→→→→→→→→→→→→→→→ →→→→→→→→→→→→→→→→ →→→→→→→→→→→→→→→→ **GOAL:** Pt. free from injury	→→→→→→→→→→→→→→→→ →→→→→→→→→→→→→→→→ **GOAL:** Pt. free from injury
		GOAL: PT adjusted for correct range. CBC @ baseline c̄ no S&S of ADR	**GOAL:** Pt.\Family verbalizes understanding of home meds
Continue/Reinforce Teaching	→→→→→→→→→→→→→→→→	→→→→→→→→→→→→→→→→	**GOAL:** Pt./Fam. verbalizes understanding of topics.
			GOAL: Responds to yes/no questions verbally and non-verbally. **GOAL:** Appropriate reasoning/decisions for performance of ADL's & provision for personal safety

COORDINATED CareMap® — CVA/TIA

M-93-5376 REV. 12/30/93 P

Appendix D2: Lumbar Laminectomy

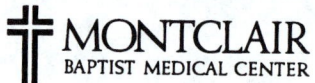
MONTCLAIR
BAPTIST MEDICAL CENTER

COORDINATED CareMap®
LUMBAR LAMINECTOMY/MICRODISCECTOMY
Key: Highlight completed task.
Address variances in nurses' focus notes and circle in red

	PRE-OP	P. O. D. OF SURGERY
	Date/Int. _____	Date/Int. _____
NEUROMUSCULAR High risk for altered sensory-motor function. Neurovascular Checks	On Admission	**Goal: Sensory-motor function at pre-op level or increased N - D - E** **Goal: No S & S deep vein thrombosis N - D - E**
ACTIVITY Impaired physical mobility Risk for Self-Care Deficit: Bathing, Toileting, dressing	Up Ad Lib	**Goal: Up to BR c assist w/in 8 hrs. after arrival to floor** Maintain normal curves of back in assisting c movement N - D - E **Goal: Compliance c activity restriction, no bending, twisting or lifting. N - D - E**
PAIN		**Goal: Pain controlled c I.M. pain meds. N - D - E**
PULMONARY Risk for respiratory insufficiency and retained secretions R/T surgery	Assess BBS on Adm.	**Goal: Bilateral breath sounds at pre-op baseline N - D - E** Assess BBS q shift N - D - E Cough and deep breathe q 2 hr x 12 hrs., then q 4 hr N - D - E **Goal: No S & S pulmonary embolism N - D - E**
INTEGUMENTARY High risk for impaired wound healing and infection Wound Care VS	q 8 Hr.	Assess Lumbar dressing q 2 hr. x 12 hrs., then q 4 hr. N - D - E q 15 min. x 4, q 30 min. X 2, q 1 hr x 2, then q 4 hr. N - D - E

FLUID BALANCE, NUTRITION, ELIMINATION   IV Fluids   Diet
   Elimination
   Lab Tests
	NPO p MN
	
	 CBC, U/A
	 Age > 40, EKG on record within last 30 days
	 CXR w/in past 6 mos.
		Goal: Absence of N & V N - D - E
		 D/C I.V. when tolerating p.o. fluids N - D - E
		
		 Reg. Diet (Begin c 1st scheduled meal)
		 Encourage p.o. fluids N - D - E

RISK FOR KNOWLEDGE DEFICIT OF EXPECTED PROGRESSION OF CARE IN HOSPITAL AND AT HOME   Pre-op Care
   Post-op Care
   Body Mechanics
   Wound Care
	Goal: Verbalizes use of patient/family map Review patient/family map
	
	 Goal: Verbalizes Intro to post-op exercises and body mechanics Body mechanics/ADL
		Reinforce T, C, DB (NSG) N - D - E
		
		 Reinforce maintenance of neutral body position/ body mechanics/ post-op exercises (NSG) N - D - E
		
		 VARIANCES
		 _____
		 _____
		 _____
		 _____
		 _____
		 _____

COORDINATED CareMap® — LUMBAR LAMINECTOMY/MICRODISCECTOMY

M-93-5071 REV. 2/21/94 P

✝ MONTCLAIR
BAPTIST MEDICAL CENTER

COORDINATED CareMap®
LUMBAR LAMINECTOMY/MICRODISCECTOMY
Key: Highlight completed task.
Address variances in nurses' focus notes and circle in red

(Addressograph)

P.O.D. 1	P.O.D. 2
Date/Int. _____	Date/Int. _____
Goal:Sensory-motor function at pre-op level or increased N - D - E	**Goal:Sensory-motor function at pre-op level or increased N - D - E**
Goal: No S & S deep vein thrombosis N - D - E	**Goal: No S & S deep vein thrombosis N - D - E**
Ambulate w/Assist N - D - E Maintain normal curves of back in assisting c movement N - D - E Bath per Dr.'s order **Goal: Compliance c activity restriction, no bending, twisting or lifting. N - D - E**	**Goal: Independent ambulation** Up Ad Lib Maintain normal curves of back in assisting c movement N - D - E **Goal: Compliance c activity restriction, no bending, twisting or lifting. N - D - E**
Encourage move to P.O. PRN pain meds	**Goal: Pain controlled c P.O. meds.**
Assess BBS q shift while awake N - D - E	Assess BBS q shift while awake N - D - E
Goal: No S & S pulmonary embolism N - D - E	**Goal: No S & S pulmonary embolism N - D - E**
	Goal: Temp < 99° F N - D - E
Goal: Wound edges approximated w/o redness or purulent drainage N - D - E	**Goal: Wound edges approximated w/o redness or purulent drainage N - D - E**
Assess Lumbar dressing q 8 hr. while awake N - D - E Dressing change per Dr.'s orders N - D - E q 4 hr. while awake N - D - E	Remove Lumbar dressing q 8 hr. on discharge N - D - E
	Goal: BM before D/C
Assess need for laxative	
Reinforce T, C, DB (NSG) N - D - E	Reinforce T, C, DB (NSG) N - D - E
	Goal: Verbalizes and demonstrates appropriate body mechanics and ADL's
Reinforce maintenance of neutral body position/ body mechanics/post-op exercises (NSG) N - D - E	
Provide wound care instruction	**Goal: Verbalizes correct steps for wound care and S & S of infection**
VARIANCES _____ _____ _____ _____ _____ _____	VARIANCES _____ _____ _____ _____ _____ _____

COORDINATED CareMap® — LUMBAR LAMINECTOMY/MICRODISCECTOMY

Adapted from CareMap® System, The Center for Case Management

M-93-5071 REV. 2/21/94 P

Appendix D3: COPD

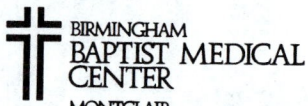

BIRMINGHAM BAPTIST MEDICAL CENTER MONTCLAIR

Coordinated CareMap®
CASE TYPE – COPD/ASTHMA
Key: *Highlight completed tasks and goals in yellow.*
Address variances in nurse's notes and circle in red.

(Addressograph)

PATIENT PROBLEM	1-4 HOURS/DIRECT ADMISSION ONLY Date/Init. _____	DAY 1 Date/Init. _____
PULMONARY Risk for pulmonary function altered.	GOAL: Stable pulmonary function AEB: • RR 18-25 • Effective airway clearance • no change in mental status/LOC • using diaphragmatic muscles for breathing • no restlessness/anxiety • ABX & Theo. IV given within 45 mins. of admission. Vital signs. O₂ - nasal/mask. UDN c bronchodilator. MDI Antibiotic IV within 45 min. of admission. Theophyllin IV within 45 min. of admission. Steroid IV within 45 min. of admission. IV fluids/saline lock. Pharmacy to assess drug orders. Assess drug allergies and notify pharmacy.	GOAL: Stable pulmonary function AEB: • RR 18-25 • effective airway clearance • no change in mental status/LOC • using diaphragmatic muscles for breathing • no restlessness/anxiety Vital signs q 8 hrs. Assess breath sounds q shift. D - E - N O₂ - nasal/mask. UDN c bronchodilator. MDI IV Fluids.
TESTS High risk for anxiety R/T tests, procedures, and hospitalization.	GOAL: Labwork/Tests completed within 45 min. of admission. Sputum C&S (collect within 45 min. of adm. Document attempts) If unable, RT to induce. S7 CBC CXR ABG (collect within 45 min. of adm.) Theophyllin level U/A PBS (if indicated) EKG	GOAL: Labwork/Tests within expected limits. Assess sputum report for acceptability. Notify MD to reorder if unacceptable.
ACTIVITY Risk for activity intolerance. Risk for mobility impairment R/T illness.	Assess for skin breakdown and document.	GOAL: Tolerates activity progression AEB: • stable HR, B/P, and RR • performs self care with assistance • feeds self Assist with personal care daily. Active ROM q 2 hrs. Initiate skin care protocol.
GASTROINTESTINAL Risk for nutrition alteration < body requirements. Risk for bowel function altered.	GOAL: Stable GI function AEB: • active bowel sounds • abdomen nondistended GI assessment.	GOAL: Stable GI function AEB: • active bowel sounds • abdomen nondistended • normal bowel pattern GI assessment q 8 hrs. D - E - N GOAL: Nutritional intake meets body requirements AEB: • dietary intake > 50% per meal • po intake ≥ 2000cc/day Assess po intake (I&O q 8 hr). Assess need for supplemental intake q 8 hrs. D - E - N
TEACHING Knowledge deficit R/T disease process, medication, and preventative measures.		GOAL: Pt./Family participates in identifying learning needs AEB: • verbalizes understanding of plan of care • demonstrates ability to follow instructions Assess knowledge of disease process. COPD Patient Booklet. Asthma Patient Booklet. Teach purse-lip breathing. Assess special needs.
DISCHARGE PLANNING Risk for self-care deficit. Risk for home maintenance management impaired.	GOAL: Pt./Family participates in identification of discharge needs: • pt./family verbalize needs • pt./family acknowledge D/C process Notify Case Manager ext. 5528. DCP assessment.	GOAL: Pt./Family participates in identification of discharge needs: • pt./family verbalize needs • pt./family acknowledge D/C process Discharge planning nurse to see if indicated.
PSYCHOSOCIAL/SPIRITUAL Risk for coping ineffective family. Risk for coping ineffective individual.		GOAL: Demonstrates adequate coping, AEB: • verbalization of fears and anxieties • demonstrates compliance with care • participates in care Allow time to verbalize concerns. Pastoral care prn. Assess response to care/treatment. Assess support system.

Coordinated CareMap® – COPD/ASTHMA

M-93-5047 (B) REV. 2/28/95 P

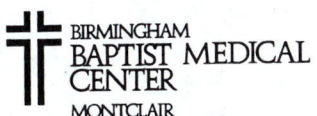

BIRMINGHAM
BAPTIST MEDICAL
CENTER
MONTCLAIR

Coordinated CareMap®
CASE TYPE – COPD/ASTHMA
Key: *Highlight completed tasks and goals in yellow.*
Address variances in nurse's notes and circle in red.

(Addressograph)

DAY 2	DAY 3	DAY 4
Date/Init. _____	Date/Init. _____	Date/Init. _____
GOAL: Stable pulmonary function AEB: • RR 18-25 • effective airway clearance • no change in mental status/LOC • using diaphragmatic muscles for breathing • no restlessness/anxiety Vital signs q 8 hrs. Assess breath sounds q shift. D - E - N O₂ - nasal/mask. UDN c̄ bronchodilator. MDI IV Fluids. Pharmacy for medication review.	**GOAL: Stable pulmonary function AEB:** • RR 18-25 • effective airway clearance • no change in mental status/LOC • using diaphragmatic muscles for breathing • no restlessness/anxiety • VS WNL's • SAO₂ ≥ 92% • breath sounds clear • weaning steroids Vital signs q 8 hrs. Assess breath sounds q shift. D - E - N O₂ - wean O₂. MDI Pulse Ox. x 1 (If on O₂). Call MD if < 90%. Change to po antibiotics. Change IV to saline lock. Assess need to change IV site.	**GOAL: Stable pulmonary function AEB:** • RR 18-25 • effective airway clearance • no change in mental status/LOC • using diaphragmatic muscles for breathing • no restlessness/anxiety • VS WNL's • SAO₂ ≥ 92% • breath sounds clear • weaning steroids Vital signs q 8 hrs. Assess breath sounds q shift. D - E - N D/C O₂. D/C UDN. MDI Change to po theophyllin. Change to po steroids. IV site care. Pharmacy to assess discharge meds.
GOAL: Labwork/Tests within expected limits Theophyllin level CBC Survey 6 (repeat if abnormal previously) Assess preliminary sputum results. PBS (if indicated).	**GOAL: Labwork/Tests WNL AEB:** • Thephyllin level WNL • CBC WNL • Survey 6 WNL (if ordered) • PBS WNL (if ordered) PBS (if indicated).	
GOAL: Tolerates activity progression AEB: • stable HR, B/P, and RR • performs self care • tolerates chair 1 hour TID OOB in chair TID. Up in chair with meals. Skin care protocol.	**GOAL: Tolerates activity progression AEB:** • stable HR, B/P, and RR • performs self care • tolerates ambulation TID Ambulate with assistance BID. Up in chair with meals. Skin care protocol.	**GOAL: Tolerates activity progression AEB:** • stable HR, B/P, and RR • performs self care • tolerates ambulation Ambulates independently QID. Skin care protocol.
GOAL: Stable GI function AEB: • active bowel sounds • abdomen nondistended • normal bowel pattern GI assessment q 8 hrs. D - E - N	**GOAL: Stable GI function AEB:** • active bowel sounds • abdomen nondistended • normal bowel pattern GI assessment q 8 hrs. D - E - N	**GOAL: Stable GI function AEB:** • active bowel sounds • abdomen nondistended • normal bowel pattern GI assessment q 8 hrs. D - E - N
GOAL: Nutritional intake meets body requirements AEB: • dietary intake > 50% per meal • po intake ≥ 2000cc/day Assess po intake. Assess need for supplemental intake q 8 hrs. D - E - N	**GOAL: Nutritional intake meets body requirements AEB:** • dietary intake > 50% per meal • po intake ≥ 2000cc/day Assess po intake. Assess need for supplemental intake q 8 hrs. D - E - N	**GOAL: Nutritional intake meets body requirements AEB:** • dietary intake > 50% per meal • po intake ≥ 2000cc/day Assess po intake. Assess need for supplemental intake q 8 hrs. D - E - N
GOAL: Identified learning needs met AEB: • verbalizes understanding of plan of care • demonstrates ability to follow instructions • verbalizes special needs Smoking cessation information as appropriate. Assess knowledge of disease process. Encourage questions Teach: progression of activity, pulmonary care and equipment needs.	**GOAL: Identified learning needs met AEB:** • verbalizes understanding of progression of care • demonstrates ability to follow instructions • verbalizes special needs Assess: knowledge of measures to prevent infection and symptoms to report to physician at home. Teach: progression of activity, pulmonary care and equipment needs.	**GOAL: Identified learning needs met AEB:** • verbalizes understanding of progression of care at home Reinforce prior instructions prn. Discharge instructions: - COPD booklet - Asthma booklet - Medications - Pulmonary care - Purse-lip breathing
GOAL: Pt./Family participates in identification of discharge needs: • pt./family verbalize needs • pt./family acknowledge D/C process • pt./family participates in decision making. Discharge planning nurse to see if indicated.	**GOAL: Pt./Family participates in identification of discharge needs:** • pt./family verbalize needs • pt./family acknowledge D/C process • pt./family participates in decision making. Assess and arrange for home health care and equipment needs. Assess need for SNU. Assess need for pulmonary rehab.	**GOAL: Pt./Family participates in identification of discharge needs:** • pt./family verbalize needs • pt./family acknowledge D/C process • pt./family participates in decision making. Discharge plans completed.
GOAL: Demonstrates adequate coping, AEB: • verbalization of fears and anxieties • demonstrates compliance with care • participates in care Allow time to verbalize concerns. Pastoral care prn. Assess response to care/treatment. Assess support system.	**GOAL: Demonstrates adequate coping, AEB:** • verbalization of fears and anxieties • demonstrates compliance with care • participates in care Allow time to verbalize concerns. Pastoral care prn. Assess response to care/treatment. Assess support system.	**GOAL: Demonstrates adequate coping, AEB:** • verbalization of fears and anxieties • demonstrates compliance with care • participates in care Allow time to verbalize concerns. Pastoral care prn. Assess response to care/treatment. Assess support system.

Coordinated CareMap® – COPD/ASTHMA

M-93-5047 (B) REV. 2/28/95 P

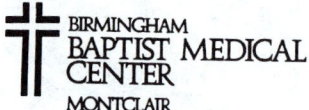

BIRMINGHAM
BAPTIST MEDICAL
CENTER
MONTCLAIR

Coordinated CareMap®
CASE TYPE – COPD/ASTHMA
Key: *Highlight completed tasks and goals in yellow.*
Address variances in nurse's notes and circle in red.

(Addressograph)

PATIENT PROBLEM	DAY 5
	Date/Init. _____
PULMONARY Risk for pulmonary function altered.	**GOAL: Stable pulmonary function AEB:** • RR 18-25 • effective airway clearance • no change in mental status/LOC • using diaphragmatic muscles for breathing • no restlessness/anxiety • VS WNL's • SAO₂ ≥ 92% • breath sounds clear • weaning steroids Vital signs q 8 hrs. Assess breath sounds q shift. D - E - N MDI D/C saline lock. Review pulmonary discharge instructions.
TESTS High risk for anxiety R/T tests, procedures, and hospitalization.	PBS (if indicated).
ACTIVITY Risk for activity intolerance. Risk for mobility impairment R/T illness.	**GOAL: Tolerates activity progression AEB:** • stable HR, B/P, and RR • performs personal care • increased activity time • independent ambulation Up ad lib. Skin care protocol.
GASTROINTESTINAL Risk for nutrition alteration < body requirements. Risk for bowel function altered.	**GOAL: Stable GI function AEB:** • active bowel sounds • abdomen nondistended • normal bowel pattern GI assessment q 8 hrs. D - E - N **GOAL: Nutritional intake meets body requirements AEB:** • dietary intake > 50% per meal • po intake ≥ 2000cc/day Assess po intake. Assess need for supplemental intake q 8 hrs. D - E - N
TEACHING Knowledge deficit R/T disease process, medication, and preventative measures.	**GOAL: Identified learning needs met:** • verbalizes understanding of progression of care at home Reinforce prior instructions. Review discharge instructions: - COPD booklet - Asthma booklet - Medications - Pulmonary care - Purse-lip breathing
DISCHARGE PLANNING Risk for self-care deficit. Risk for home maintenence management impaired.	**GOAL: Identified discharge needs met:** • pt./family describes home plan of care • pt./family demonstrates ability to manage home care Review home plan of care. Review discharge medications and instructions.
PSYCHOSOCIAL/SPIRITUAL Risk for coping ineffective family. Risk for coping ineffective individual.	

Adapted from CareMap® System, The Center for Case Management

M-93-5047 (F) REV. 2/28/95 P

Appendix D4: Pneumonia

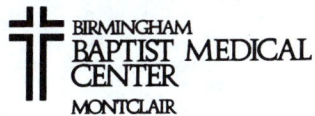

BIRMINGHAM
BAPTIST MEDICAL
CENTER
MONTCLAIR

Coordinated CareMap®
CASE TYPE – PNEUMONIA
Key: Highlight completed tasks and goals in yellow.
Address variances in nurse's notes and circle in red.

PATIENT PROBLEM	DIRECT ADMISSION ONLY/1-4 HOURS Date/Init. _____	DAY 1 Date/Init. _____
PULMONARY Risk for pulmonary function altered.	**GOAL: Stable pulmonary function AEB:** • unlabored respirations • Using diaphragmatic muscles for breathing • RR 18-25 • effective airway clearance • no restlessness/anxiety • no change in mental status/LOC • Antibiotic administered within 4 hours of admission Vital signs Assess cough & sputum production UDN c bronchodilator Begin 1st antibiotic within 4 hours of admission IV fluids/saline lock Pharmacy to assess drug orders Assess drug allergies and notify pharmacy	**GOAL: Stable pulmonary function AEB:** • unlabored respirations • Using diaphragmatic muscles for breathing • RR 18-25 • effective airway clearance • no restlessness/anxiety Vital signs q 4 hours Assess breath sounds q shift. D-E-N O2 – nasal/mask UDN c bronchodilator IV fluids
TESTS High risk for anxiety R/T tests, procedures, and hospitalization.	**GOAL: Labwork/Tests w/i expected limits, sputum specimen collected w/i 2 hours of admission** Sputum C & S, gram stain (collect within 2 hours) If unable to collect sputum, document attempts and RT to induce CBC • S7 • U/A • EKG • CXR Consult MD for the following: ABG, Serum Mycoplasm, Legionella studies, blood cultures x 2, albumin	**GOAL: Labwork/Tests w/i expected limits; acceptable sputum specimen** Assess sputum for acceptability Notify MD to reorder if unacceptable Notify MD if unable to obtain sputum
ACTIVITY Risk for activity intolerance. Risk for mobility impairment.	Assess for skin breakdown and document	**GOAL: Tolerates activity progression AEB:** • Stable HR, B/P and RR • Performs personal care with assist. • Feeds self Assist with personal care daily Encourage active ROM q 2 hours Initiate skin care protocol
GASTROINTESTINAL Risk for nutrition alt. < body requirements. Risk for bowel function altered.	**GOAL: Stable GI function AEB:** • Active bowel sounds • Abd. nondistended GI assessment	**GOAL: Stable GI function AEB:** • Active bowel sounds • Abd. nondistended • Normal bowel pattern GI assessment q 8 hours. D-E-N **GOAL: Nutritional intake meets body requirements AEB:** • Dietary intake > 50% per meal • PO intake ≥ 2000 cc/day Assess need for supplemental intake q 8 hrs. D-E-N I&O q shift. D-E-N
TEACHING Knowledge deficit R/T disease process, medication and preventive measures.		**GOAL: Pt./Family participates in identifying learning needs AEB:** • Verbalizes understanding of plan of care • Demonstrates ability to follow instruction Assess knowledge of disease process Pneumonia Booklet Assess special needs
DISCHARGE PLANNING Risk for self-care deficit. Risk for home maintenance management impaired.	**GOAL: Pt./Family participates in identification of discharge needs:** • Pt./Family verbalize needs • Pt./Family acknowledge D/C process Notify Case Manager ext. 5528 DCP Assessment	**GOAL: Pt./Family participates in identification of discharge needs:** • Pt./Family verbalize needs • Pt./Family acknowledge D/C process Discharge planning nurse to see if indicated
PSYCHOSOCIAL/SPIRITUAL Risk of coping ineffective family. Risk for coping ineffective individual.		**GOAL: Demonstrates adequate coping AEB:** • Verbalization of fears and anxieties • Demonstrates compliance with care • Participates in care Allow time to verbalize concerns Pastoral care prn Assess response to care/treatment Assess support system

Coordinated CareMap® – PNEUMONIA

M-94-5022 (B) REV. 2/28/95 P

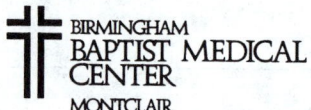

BIRMINGHAM
BAPTIST MEDICAL CENTER
MONTCLAIR

Coordinated CareMap®
CASE TYPE – PNEUMONIA
Key: *Highlight completed tasks and goals in yellow.*
Address variances in nurse's notes and circle in red.

(Addressograph)

DAY 2	DAY 3
Date/Init. _____	Date/Init. _____
GOAL: Stable pulmonary function AEB: • **unlabored respirations** • **RR 18-25** • **effective airway clearance** • **Using diaphragmatic muscles for breathing** • **no restlessness/anxiety** Vital signs q 4 hours Assess breath sounds q shift. D-E-N O2 – nasal/mask UDN c bronchodilator MDI IV fluids Pharmacy for medication review	**GOAL: Stable pulmonary function AEB:** • **unlabored respirations** • **RR 18-25** • **effective airway clearance** • **VS WNLs** • **SAO2 > 92%** • **secretions clear** • **Using diaphragmatic muscles for breathing** • **no restlessness/anxiety** • **Afebrile** • **Breath sounds clear** • **respirations noiseless** Vital signs q 8 hours Assess breath sounds q shift. D-E-N O2 – Wean O2 Assess need to D/C UDN MDI Pulse Ox - x 1 (If on O2). If < 90% report to MD Evaluate change to po antibiotics Assess need to change IV site
Assess preliminary sputum results	**GOAL: Labwork/Tests WNL AEB:** Assess sputum sensitivity report CBC S6 (report if abnormal previously) Identify causative organism
GOAL: Tolerates activity progression AEB: • **Stable HR, B/P and RR** • **Tolerates chair 1 hour TID** • **Performs personal care** OOB in chair TID Up in chair with meals Skin care protocol	**GOAL: Tolerates activity progression AEB:** • **Stable HR, B/P and RR** • **Tolerates ambulation** • **Performs personal care** Ambulate with assistance BID Up in chair with meals Skin care protocol
GOAL: Stable GI function AEB: • **Active bowel sounds** • **Normal bowel pattern** • **Abd. nondistended** GI assessment q 8 hours. D-E-N **GOAL: Nutritional intake meets body requirements AEB:** • **Dietary intake > 50% per meal** • **PO intake ≥ 2000 cc/day** I&O q shift Assess need for supplemental intake q 8 hrs. D-E-N	**GOAL: Stable GI function AEB:** • **Active bowel sounds** • **Normal bowel pattern** • **Abd. nondistended** GI assessment q 8 hours. D-E-N **GOAL: Nutritional intake meets body requirements AEB:** • **Dietary intake > 50% per meal** • **PO intake ≥ 2000 cc/day** I&O q shift Assess need for supplemental intake q 8 hrs. D-E-N

GOAL: Identified learning needs met AEB:
• **Verbalizes understanding of plan of care**
• **Demonstrates ability to follow instruction**
Smoking cessation info. as appropriate
Assess knowledge of disease process
Teach: progression of activity
     pulmonary care and equipment needs
	GOAL: Identified learning needs met AEB:
	• **Verbalizes understanding of plan of care**
	Assess knowledge measures to prevent infection and symptoms to report to MD
	Teach: progression of activity
	     pulmonary care and equipment needs

GOAL: Pt./Family participates in identification of discharge needs: • **Pt./Family verbalize needs** • **Pt./Family acknowledge D/C process** • **Pt./Family participates in decision making** Discharge planning nurse to see if indicated	**GOAL: Pt./Family participates in identification of discharge needs:** • **Pt./Family verbalize needs** • **Pt./Family acknowledge D/C process** • **Pt./Family participates in decision making** Assess and arrange for home health care and equipment needs Assess need for SNU
GOAL: Demonstrates adequate coping AEB: • **Verbalization of fears and anxieties** • **Demonstrates compliance with care** • **Participates in care** Allow time to verbalize concerns Pastoral care prn Assess response to care/treatment Assess support system	**GOAL: Demonstrates adequate coping AEB:** • **Verbalization of fears and anxieties** • **Demonstrates compliance with care** • **Participates in care** Allow time to verbalize concerns Pastoral care prn Assess response to care/treatment Assess support system

Coordinated CareMap® – PNEUMONIA

M-94-5022 (B) REV. 2/28/95 P

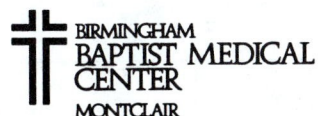
BIRMINGHAM
BAPTIST MEDICAL
CENTER
MONTCLAIR

Coordinated CareMap®
CASE TYPE – PNEUMONIA
Key: *Highlight completed tasks and goals in yellow.*
Address variances in nurse's notes and circle in red.

DAY 4	DAY 5
Date/Init. _____	Date/Init. _____

DAY 4	DAY 5
GOAL: Stable pulmonary function AEB: • **uniabored respirations** • **Using diaphragmatic muscles for breathing** • **RR 18-25** • **no restlessness/anxiety** • **effective airway clearance** • **Afebrile** • **VS WNLs** • **secretions clear** • **Breath sounds clear** • **respirations noiseless** Vital signs q 8 hours Assess breath sounds q shift. D-E-N D/C O2 D/C UDN MDI Convert to po antibiotics Change to saline lock IV site care Pharmacy to assess discharge meds.	**GOAL: Stable pulmonary function AEB:** • **uniabored respirations** • **Using diaphragmatic muscles for breathing** • **RR 18-25** • **no restlessness/anxiety** • **effective airway clearance** • **Afebrile** • **VS WNLs** • **secretions clear** • **Breath sounds clear** • **respirations noiseless** Vital signs q 8 hours Assess breath sounds q shift. D-E-N D/C saline lock
GOAL: Tolerates activity progression AEB: • **Stable HR, B/P and RR** • **Performs personal care** • **Tolerates ambulation** Ambulate independently Skin care protocol	**GOAL: Tolerates activity progression AEB:** • **Stable HR, B/P and RR** • **Performs personal care** • **Independent ambulation** Up ad lib
GOAL: Stable GI function AEB: • **Active bowel sounds** • **Abd. nondistended** • **Normal bowel pattern** GI assessment q 8 hours. D-E-N **GOAL: Nutritional intake meets body requirements AEB:** • **Dietary intake > 50% per meal** • **PO intake ≥ 2000 cc/day** I&O q shift Assess need for supplemental intake q 8 hrs. D-E-N	

GOAL: Identified learning needs met AEB:
• **Verbalizes understanding of progression of care at home**
Reinforce prior instructions prn
Discharge instructions
   • Pneumonia booklet
   • Medications
   • Pulmonary Care
	GOAL: Identified learning needs met AEB:
	• **Verbalizes understanding of progression of care at home**
	Reinforce prior instructions prn
	Review discharge instructions
	   • Pneumonia booklet
	   • Medications
	   • Pulmonary Care

GOAL: Pt./Family participates in identification of discharge needs: • **Pt./Family verbalize needs** • **Pt./Family acknowledge D/C process** • **Pt./Family participates in decision making**	**GOAL: Identified discharge needs met:** • **Pt./Family describe home plan of care** • **Pt./Family demonstrates ability to manage home care** Review home plan of care Review discharge medications and instructions
GOAL: Demonstrates adequate coping AEB: • **Verbalization of fears and anxieties** • **Demonstrates compliance with care** • **Participates in care** Allow time to verbalize concerns Pastoral care prn Assess response to care/treatment Assess support system	

Adapted from CareMap® System, The Center for Case Management

M-94-5022 (F) REV. 2/28/95   P

Appendix D5: CAG/PTCA

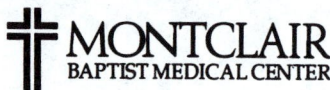

COORDINATED CARE MAP
CASE TYPE—PRE CAG/PTCA / DCA / LASER
Key: Highlight completed task and goals.
Address variances in nurses' focus notes and circle variances on map.
Once variances completed - highlight and date.
Draw black line through non-applicable tasks/goals.

PAGE 2

	DAY 1 – PRE-PROCEDURE DATE/RN INT. _____	CATH LAB DATE/INT. _____
CARDIOVASCULAR *High risk for:* *Alt. in tissue perfusion.* *Bleeding and hematoma.* *Dysrhythmia.* *Chest pain R/T CAD.* *Retroperitoneal bleed R/T procedure.*	VS per protocol Monitor cardiac rhythm-report any changes. Assess and record pedal pulses. Instruct pt. to notify nurse of chest pain. Grade CP on scale of 1-10. Treat CP per protocol. **GOAL:** Hemodynamically stable. CP relieved.	Continuous monitoring of HR, BP, O2 Sat. Sedate to maintain ↓ anxiety but able to follow commands. Assess groin for hematoma or bleeding. Assess DP pulses. **GOAL:** Hemodynamically stable post procedure. No hematoma. Baseline pulses present. **CAG ONLY:** _____ Fr. removed @ _____ by _____ . _____ Fr. removed @ _____ by _____ . Pressure held _____ min.
GI/NUTRITION *Alteration in food tolerance R/T contrast dye.* *Alteration in intake R/T supine position.* *Dehydration R/T procedure.*	NPO	
RENAL/FLUID BALANCE *High risk for:* *Alt in renal function* *UTI R/T indwelling catheter*	Assess BUN, Cr. – Notify MD if abnormal prior to procedure. Insert foley catheter if female (PTCA only). Have pt. void prior to procedure. **GOAL:** BUN, Cr, WNL	
TESTS	EKG PT (notify if > 16) CBC S6 (treat K+ < 4.0 per protocol) Type & Screen (PTCA only)	
INTEGUMENTARY *High risk for:* *Infection R/T invasive procedure and I.V.*	Prep both groins. Report temp > 101. **GOAL:** Temp. < 101.	
ACTIVITY *High risk for:* *Activity restriction R/T procedure.* *Musculoskeletal pain* *R/T activity restriction.*	Up ad lib Assess for hx of arthritis or back problems.	
PSYCHOSOCIAL/SPIRITUAL *High risk for:* *Fear & anxiety R/T procedure & CAD.*	Assess need to verbalize. Allow pt. & family time to verbalize. Assess support system. **GOAL:** Pt./Family verbalizes feelings.	
PT./FAMILY TEACHING **Discharge Planning** *High risk for:* *Knowledge deficit R/T procedure & plan of care.*	Provide unit & room orientation. Heart Smart Book - review invasive procedure section and pt./family care map. View Channel 3 program - Heart Cath and/or PTCA. **GOAL:** Pt. verbalizes understanding of important aspects of cath. and/or PTCA procedure, i.e. purpose, expected outcomes, activity limitations.	Explain each phase of the procedure. Explain typical sensations pt. may experience such as pressure, "hot flush" and/or chest tightness. **GOAL:** Pt. verbalizes understanding of important aspects of cath. and/or PTCA procedure.
CONSULTS	Identify need for consults, i.e. chaplain, DC planner, dietician. Make appropriate referrals. **GOAL:** Pt./family participate in ID of need for consults.	

COORDINATED CARE MAP — CAG / PTCA / DCA / LASER

✝ MONTCLAIR
BAPTIST MEDICAL CENTER
COORDINATED CARE MAP
CASE TYPE—POST PTCA / DCA / LASER
Key: *Highlight completed task and goals.*
Address variances in nurses' focus notes and circle variances on map.
Once variances completed - highlight and date.
Draw black line through non-applicable tasks/goals.

PAGE 3

(Addressograph)

DAY 1–POST PTCA WITH SHEATH	DAY 2–Post PTCA (SHEATH REMOVAL)	DAY 3
DATE/RN INT. _____	DATE/RN INT. _____	DATE/RN INT. _____
Check site, VS, pulse q 15 x 4, q 30 x 2, q 1 x 3 then per protocol. **GOAL: Baseline DP pulses present, no hematoma, HCT > 30.** Monitor rhythm & observe for S/S reocclusion. For severe back pain assess for retroperitoneal bleed. **GOAL: No CP, ST ↑, N/V, or retroperitoneal bleed. HD stable.** Lesion site(s)_____ _____	# _____ Fr. sheath removed @ _____ by _____ . Pressure held _____ min. ⟩Cath Lab **GOAL: No hematoma p̄ sheath removed. Baseline pulses present.** →→→→→→→→→→→→→→→→→→→→ →→→→→→→→→→→→→→→→→→→→ **AFTER SHEATH REMOVED:** Check site, VS, pulse q 15 x 2, q 30 x 2, then per protocol. **DO NOT TURN X 4 HRS.** Sandbag x 2 hrs. **GOAL: Baseline DP pulses present, no hematoma, HCT > 30.** **GOAL: No CP, ST ↑, N/V, or retroperitoneal bleed. HD stable.**	VS per protocol. D/C Telemetry at discharge. **GOAL: No chest pain. Stable rhythm.**
AHA Phase I No caffeine Encourage liquids (2000cc/24°) **GOAL: Tolerates diet and liquids without N/V.**	→→→→→→→→→→→→→→→→→→→→ →→→→→→→→→→→→→→→→→→→→ →→→→→→→→→→→→→→→→→→→→ **GOAL: Tolerates diet and liquids without N/V**	→→→→→→→→→→→→→→→→→→→→ →→→→→→→→→→→→→→→→→→→→ **GOAL: Dietry intake ≥75% of meal without N/V.**
I & O q shift Foley PRN (male) **GOAL: UO ≥ 30cc/hr. or 240cc/8 hrs.**	→→→→→→→→→→→→→→→→→→→→ **GOAL: UO > 30 cc/hr or 240cc/8 hr.** **BUN, Cr, WNL.**	→→→→→→→→→→→→→→→→→→→→ D/C foley when BR complete **GOAL: No S & S of UTI** **BUN, Cr, WNL.**
EKG – on return to CCU. ACT q 6° while on heparin Cardiac profile now & q 8 hrs. x 2.	EKG ACT q 1° p̄ heparin DC'd until < 150 (Notify cath. lab to DC sheath when ACT <150) S6 Hct	**GOAL: Lab values WNL.**
Assess groin site for redness, swelling, or discharge q 4°. Assess IV site for redness swelling, or discharge q 4°. Report temp >101. **GOAL: No S/S of infection at groin or IV site. Temp. <101.**	→→→→→→→→→→→→→→→→→→→→ →→→→→→→→→→→→→→→→→→→→ →→→→→→→→→→→→→→→→→→→→ **GOAL: No S/S of infection at groin or IV site. Temp. <101.**	→→→→→→→→→→→→→→→→→→→→ →→→→→→→→→→→→→→→→→→→→ →→→→→→→→→→→→→→→→→→→→ **GOAL: No S/S of infection at groin or IV site. Temp. <101.**
Bedrest w/affected leg straight. HOB ↑ ≤ 30° or 45° w/sheath obturator. **GOAL: Compliance with activity restrictions. Back pain/musculoskeletal pain relieved.**	Bedrest until _____ . Keep affected leg straight for 4 hrs. p̄ sheath removal. May ↑ HOB 30°. **GOAL: Able to tolerate activity level 4-6 after BR complete. Back pain/musculoskeletal pain relieved.**	Progressive ambulation to level 7. **GOAL: Increased activity w/o CP or SOB.**
Answer or seek answers to Pt./Family questions. Assess feelings re procedure and treatment plan. **GOAL: Pt./Family verbalizes ↓ anxiety and fear.**	→→→→→→→→→→→→→→→→→→→→ →→→→→→→→→→→→→→→→→→→→	Assess response to recommended lifestyle modification. →→→→→→→→→→→→→→→→→→→→ **GOAL: Pt./Family verbalizes ↓ anxiety and fears.**
Stress importance of keeping affected leg straight & still, and avoidance of lifting head off pillow. Heart Smart Book - review Heart Facts section. **GOAL: Pt. verbalizes basic understanding of CV anatomy in relation to his/her CAD.**	Explain groin anesthesia/sheath removal procedure. Heart Smart Book - review Heart & Circulatory Problems, and Healthy Lifestyles sections. View channel 3 program - I Am Joe's Heart, Learning to Relax, and Towards a Healthy Heart. **GOAL: Pt. verbalizes understanding of groin anesthesia/ sheath removal. Pt. verbalizes understanding of risk factors, angina, and chest pain management.**	Heart Smart Book - review Heart Medications section. Review home medication regime. Instruct pt. not to lift heavy objects or strain hard for a few days and to follow home walk program. **IF AMI RETURN TO AMI CARE MAP DAY 5.** **GOAL: Pt. verbalizes understanding of home meds and DC plans. Pt. verbalizes understanding of home walk instructions.**
Consult Cardiac Rehab — Home Walk program.		**GOAL: Pt./family verbalizes needs met through referrals.**

COORDINATED CARE MAP — CAG / PTCA / DCA / LASER

M-93-5312 REV. 9/20/93 P

COORDINATED CARE MAP
CASE TYPE—POST CAG
Key: *Highlight completed task and goals.*
Address variances in nurses' focus notes and circle variances on map.
Once variances completed - highlight and date.
Draw black line through non-applicable tasks/goals.

PAGE 4

	POST CATH
	DATE/RN INT. _____
CARDIOVASCULAR *High risk for:* *Alt. in tissue perfusion.* *Bleeding and hematoma.* *Dysrhythmia.* *Chest pain R/T CAD.* *Retroperitoneal bleed R/T procedure.*	Monitor rhythm. Check cath site, VS, pulses, q 15 x 4, q 30 x 2, q 1 x 2, then per protocol. Treat chest pain per protocol. Grade CP on scale of 1-10. **GOAL:** Hemodynamically stable. Baseline pulses present. Chest pain relieved.
GI/NUTRITION *Alteration in food tolerance R/T contrast dye.* *Alteration in intake R/T supine position.* *Dehydration R/T procedure.*	AHA Phase I No caffeine Encourage fluids **GOAL:** Tolerates diet w/o N & V with intake ≥ 50%. Fluid intake 2000cc/24°.
RENAL/FLUID BALANCE *High risk for:* *Alt in renal function* *UTI R/T indwelling catheter*	I & O x 24° Assess ability to void Foley PRN **GOAL:** UO ≥ 240cc/8 hours.
TESTS	
INTEGUMENTARY *High risk for:* *Infection R/T invasive procedure and I.V.*	Assess IV site for redness, swelling or discharge q 4°. Assess groin site for redness, swelling or discharge q 4°. **GOAL:** No S/S of infection at IV or groin site. Temp. <101.
ACTIVITY *High risk for:* *Activity restriction R/T procedure.* *Musculoskeletal pain* *R/T activity restriction.*	Bedrest until _____ Keep affected leg straight while on BR. HOB ≤ 30° while on BR. Progressive activity p bedrest complete. **GOAL:** Compliance with activity restriction while on bedrest then able to tolerate progressive ambulation. Back pain/musculoskeletal pain relieved.
PSYCHOSOCIAL/SPIRITUAL *High risk for:* *Fear & anxiety R/T procedure & CAD.*	Answer or seek answers to pt./family questions. Assess feelings re procedure and treatment plan. **GOAL:** Pt. verbalizes decreased anxiety and fear.
PT./FAMILY TEACHING **Discharge Planning** *High risk for:* *Knowledge deficit R/T procedure & plan of care.*	Discuss procedure and outcome: **RESULTS:** Normal _____ Heart Smart Book-review Healthy Lifestyle section. Discuss follow-up diagnostic plan. **Medical Tx** _____ Heart Smart Book - review CV anatomy, Healthy Lifestyle and medications section. View channel 3 programs on CAD. **Transfer to:** PTCA Care Map _____ , AMI Care Map _____ , CHF Care Map _____ , CABG Care Map _____ (If CTS consult notify CV Surgical Case Coordinator (5258). **GOAL:** Pt. verbalizes understanding of cath. results and plan of care. Pt. verbalizes understanding of risk factors, lifestyle modifications, and medications.
CONSULTS	**GOAL:** Pt./family verbalizes needs met through referrals.

COORDINATED CARE MAP — POST CAG

Appendix D6: CABG

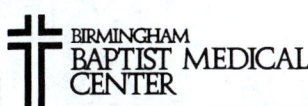

BIRMINGHAM BAPTIST MEDICAL CENTER MONTCLAIR

Coordinated CareMap®
OPEN HEART SURGERY – CABG & VALVE
Key: *Highlight completed tasks and goals.*
Circle variances and focus.
Date and highlight variances once completed.

(Addressograph)

PAGE 2	PRE-OP DATE	DAY OF SURGERY (Acutal P.O.D.: _____)	P.O.D. 1 (Acutal P.O.D.: _____)	P.O.D. 2 (Acutal P.O.D.: _____)
	Date/Init. _____	Date/Init. _____	Date/Init. _____	Date/Init. _____
CARDIOVASCULAR High risk for decreased cardiac output or altered hemodynamics	GOAL: Stable CV function with SBP > 90 < 150. HR 60-100. Vital Signs QID	OUTCOME: GOAL: Hemodynamic parameters within normal limits for patient within 16 hours after arrival in OHICU (CI, SVR, LA, PAP, BP) NSR with rare ectopy. Vital Signs every 30 minutes Continuous ECG monitoring RA LA ART PA Pacing wires present	GOAL: Stable CV with SBP > 90 < 150. HR 60-110 NSR with rare ectopy. Vital Signs every 2 hours Telemetry continues D/C RA, D/C LA, D/C ART, D/C PA Pacing wires present	GOAL: Stable CV with SBP > 90 < 150. HR 60-110 NSR with rare ectopy. Vital Signs every 4 hours Telemetry continues Pacing wires present
PULMONARY High risk for respiratory insufficiency, retained secretions, and inadequate oxygenation.	GOAL: Clear airways with SPO2 > 90. SPO2 check	GOAL: Extubated and with normal breathing patterns within 6 hrs. after arrival in OHICU. ABG's and SPO2 per protocol Suction PRN Extubated @ ____ Nasal O2 @ ____ GOAL: Oriented x 3, normal thought process Vibropercussion q 2 hrs. while awake.	GOAL: Clear airway and adequate oxygenation, SPO2 > 90. ↓ nasal O2, maintain SPO2 ≥ 90 May use O2 PRN Incentive Spirometry + CPT q 2° while awake, cough and deep breathe q 2°.	GOAL: Off nasal O2, with minimal resp. effort, SaO2 > 90. D/C nasal O2 if Sat > 90. I/S q 2-4° w.a. Cough and deep breathe q 4° SPO2 q 8 hrs. x 3
ELIMINATION GASTROINTESTINAL NUTRITION High risk for altered bowel function and nutrition	GOAL: Stable digestive process and normal nutritional state. NPO after midnight	GOAL: NGT patent, no N and V. NGT - Gravity NPO until extubated then ice chips D/C NGT post extubation	GOAL: BS present, no N and V. Ice chips to clear liquids then progress as tolerated to full liquid then Phase I AHA diet or _____ ADA	GOAL: Absence of N and V Assess need for supplemental intake Phase I AHA diet or _____ ADA
PSYCHO-SOCIAL/ SPIRITUAL Coping difficulties related to surgery and recommended lifestyle change	GOAL: Effective coping pattern 1. Assess support system and need to verbalize. 2. Consider allowing time to listen. 3. Consult Pastoral Care if requested.	1. Assess response to recommended treatment and allow time to listen. 2. Answer to seek answers to patient/family questions. 3. Pastoral Care if requested.	1. Assess response to recommended treatment and allow time to listen. 2. Pastoral Care if requested.	GOAL: Pt./Family will verbalize emotions/concerns to nurse 1. Assess response to recommended treatment and allow time to listen. 2. Pastoral Care if requested.
ALTERED FLUID BALANCE High risk for hypovolemia		GOAL: Normal LAP/PAD and U/O > 20 cc/hr, CTD < 200/hr I & O hourly Pre-Op Weight: _____ lbs. Foley Catheter care Chest tube care	I & O q 2 hr. Daily weights – bedtime Foley Catheter care GOAL: CTD < 200/shift, U/O > 30/hr Chest tube care	GOAL: Normal bladder function I & O q shift Daily weights – bedtime D/C foley D/C chest tube
ACTIVTY High risk for decreased mobility	Up ad lib	GOAL: Absence of motor deficits Passive ROM Bedrest Dangle x 2 after extubation ↑ HOB 20° Turn q 2 hrs. if stable	GOAL: Tolerates activity progression Transfer to OHIS or OHPC Ambulate in room tid for one minute Feeds self - in chair for all meals Dangle with assistance	GOAL: Tolerates activity progression HOB as desired, ↑ FOB-CABG Ambulate in room TID for 1-2 min. Feeds self - in chair for all meals Ambulate in hall BID Bath w/assistance
SKIN/WOUND High risk for impaired skin integrity/wound healing and infection	Chin to toe prep Hibiclens bath GOAL: Absence of skin abrasions	GOAL: Dressings dry and intact. All incisions covered: Chest, leg, RA/LA sites, chest tubes, peripheral IV, triple lumen.	GOAL: Incisions dry and intact Incisions covered: RA/LA wires, chest tubes, chest. Leg incisions open to air. Incision care BID. Triple lumen remains	GOAL: Absence of purulent drainage. Clean chest incision when tubes out. Gauze dressing if needed. Incision care BID. Triple lumen dressing care.
PAIN MANAGEMENT		GOAL: Pain controlled with IV pain meds.	GOAL: Pain controlled with IV pain meds.	GOAL: Pain controlled with po pain meds.
KNOWLEDGE DEFICIT of expected progression of care in hospital and at home	GOAL: Verbalizes and understands surgery prep, I/S, immediate post-op expectations. Film _____ Booklet _____ Patient CareMap® _____	Reinforce I/S, weaning, extubation, coughing and deep breathing, equipment. Topics reinforced GOAL: Verbalized understanding of above	Teaching/Understands 1. Progression of activity 2. Routine care, Meds, Equipment 3. Begin D/C instructions w/family 4. Evaluate D/C needs 5. Review patient CareMap	Reinforce teaching: Activity O2, medications, diet. Review plan of care GOAL: Verbalizes understanding Review patient CareMap
LAB WORK/ TESTS	EKG, CBC TYPE/CROSS S-27 HCT/HGB U/A PT/PTT GOAL: Labwork WNL	GOAL: Labwork WNL HCT/HGB } On Admit K+ CXR ACT BS if diabetic	GOAL: Labwork WNL HGB/HCT } at 0500 K+ PT if valve - consult pharmacy	GOAL: Labwork WNL HGB/HCT } at 0500 K+
CONSULTATION	Consult Case Manager	Evaluate need for discharge planning	Consult Cardiac Rehab Consult pharmacy if valve	

Coordinated CareMap® – OPEN HEART SURGERY (CABG & VALVE)

M-93-5455 (B) REV. 1/24/95 P

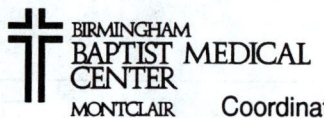

BIRMINGHAM BAPTIST MEDICAL CENTER
MONTCLAIR

Coordinated CareMap®
CABG
Expected discharge 106, 107 – POD 5

PAGE 3

(Addressograph)

P.O.D. 3	P.O.D. 4	P.O.D. 5	P.O.D. 6	P.O.D. 7
(Acutal P.O.D.: _____)	(Acutal P.O.D.: _____)	(Acutal P.O.D.: _____)	(Acutal P.O.D.: _____)	(Acutal P.O.D.: _____)
Date/Init. _____	Date/Init. _____	Date/Init. _____	Date/Init. _____	Date/Init. _____
GOAL: Stable CV function with SBP > 90 < 150. NSR with rare ectopy. Vital Signs QID Telemetry continues Pacing wires present	**GOAL: Stable CV function with SBP > 90 < 150. NSR with rare ectopy.** Vital Signs QID D/C Telemetry 2 hrs. after wires removed **GOAL: Normal sinus rhythm with occasional to no PVC/PAC's.** D/C wires if rhythm stable for previous 24 hrs.	**GOAL: Stable CV function with SBP > 90 < 150. NSR with rare ectopy.** Vital Signs QID		
GOAL: Clear breath sounds and effective airway clearance. Off of Nasal O2. I/S q 4° while awake. Cough and deep breathe q 4°	**GOAL: Clear breath sounds and effective airway clearance.** I/S QID QID	**GOAL: Lungs clear to auscultation and by CXR** I/S QID QID		
Assess need for PRN laxative. **GOAL: Tolerates diet > 50% no N and V.** Phase I AHA diet or _____ ADA diet	Bowel movement **GOAL: Resume normal pre-op bowel pattern. Absence of N & V.** Tolerates Diet Phase I AHA diet or _____ ADA diet	**GOAL: Tolerates diet with normal GI processes.** Phase I AHA diet or _____ ADA diet		
GOAL: Effective coping patterns 1. Assess response to recommended treatment and allow time to listen. 2. Answer or seek answers to patient/family questions. 3. Pastoral Care if needed.	**GOAL: Effective coping patterns** 1. Assess response to recommended treatment and allow time to listen. 2. Answer or seek answers to patient/family questions. 3. Pastoral Care if needed.	**GOAL: Pt./Family compliant with place of care.** 1. Assess response to recommended treatment and allow time to listen. 2. Answer or seek answers to patient/family questions. 3. Pastoral Care if needed.		
GOAL: Minimal edema, normal voiding. Daily weights	**GOAL: Post-op weight within 5 lbs. pre-op weight. Hct > 21** Daily weights	**GOAL: Post-op weight stable.** Weight _____ lbs. Daily weights		
GOAL: Tolerates activity progression HOB as desired, ↑ FOB Walk in hall w/assist 2-4 min. TID. Feeds self - in chair for all meals. Up in chair 1 hr. TID Performs own personal care	**GOAL: Independent ambulation** HOB as desired, ↑ FOB Walk in hall 5 min. QID In chair for all meals. Up in chair 1 hr. QID Performs own personal care	**GOAL: Tolerates progression of independent activity.** HOB as desired, ↑ FOB Walk in hall independently 5 min. QID In chair for all meals. Up in chair 1 hr. QID Performs own personal care		
GOAL: Temp < 101. Invasive line sites w/o redness or purulent drainage. All incisions open to air Incision care BID Triple lumen remains	**GOAL: Temp < 101. Incisions w/o purulent drainage.** D/C triple lumen 2 hr. after wires removed. All incisions open to air Incision care BID	**GOAL: No inflammation or purulent drainage from incisions. Temp. < 100°F.** D/C incision care.		
Pain meds prn	Pain meds prn	Pain meds prn		
Reinforce instructions on activity, telemetry, diet, meds, I/S **GOAL: Verbalizes understanding of above.** Review patient map	Receives instructions for: Diet ____ Stress ____ Cardiac Rehab/Home Activity ____ Receives Booklet ____ **GOAL: Verbalizes understanding of above.**	**GOAL: Understands discharge instructions.** Reinforce discharge instructions verbalizes understanding medication supplements provided Review discharge CareMap		
Resume home diabetic regimen	**GOAL: Labwork** CBC S-6 } in AM ECG } in PM CXR	**GOAL: CBC, S-6 WNL**		
Continue to evaluate discharge planning needs.	Cardiac Rehab Evaluation Home Walk Instructions	Home Walk Instructions		

Coordinated CareMap® – OPEN HEART SURGERY-CABG

M-93-5455 (B) REV. 1/24/95 P

✝ BIRMINGHAM
BAPTIST MEDICAL
CENTER
MONTCLAIR   Coordinated CareMap®
OPEN HEART SURGERY – VALVE
Expected Discharge - POD 7

Page 4   (Addressograph)

P.O.D. 3	P.O.D. 4	P.O.D. 5	P.O.D. 6	P.O.D. 7
(Acutal P.O.D.: _____)	(Acutal P.O.D.: _____)	(Acutal P.O.D.: _____)	(Acutal P.O.D.: _____)	(Acutal P.O.D.: _____)
Date/Init. _____	Date/Init. _____	Date/Init. _____	Date/Init. _____	Date/Init. _____
GOAL: Stable CV function with SBP > 90 < 150. NSR with rare ectopy or controlled A-Fib. Vital Signs QID Telemetry continues Pacing wires present	**GOAL: Stable CV function with SBP > 90 < 150. NSR with rare ectopy or controlled A-Fib.** Vital Signs QID D/C telemetry 2 hrs. after wires removed D/C wires if rhythm stable for pervious 24 hours	**GOAL: Stable CV function with SBP > 90 < 150. NSR with rare ectopy or controlled A-Fib.** Vital Signs QID	**GOAL: Stable CV function with SBP > 90 < 150. NSR with rare ectopy or controlled A-Fib.** Vital Signs QID	**GOAL: Stable CV function with SBP > 90 < 150. NSR with rare ectopy or controlled A-Fib.** Vital Signs QID
GOAL: Clear breath sounds and effective airway clearance. Off of Nasal O2. I/S q 2-4° while awake. Turn, cough and deep breathe q 4°	**GOAL: Clear breath sounds and effective airway clearance.** I/S q 2-4° while awake. Turn, cough and deep breathe q 4°	**GOAL: Clear breath sounds and effective airway clearance.** I/S QID QID	**GOAL: Lungs clear to ausculation and by CXR.** I/S QID QID	I/S QID QID
Assess need for PRN laxative. **GOAL: Tolerates diet > 50% no N and V.** Phase I AHA diet or _____ ADA diet	Bowel movement **GOAL: Tolerates > 50% diet, normal GI process.** Phase I AHA diet or _____ ADA diet	**GOAL: Tolerates > 50% diet, no N and V.** Phase I AHA diet or _____ ADA diet	**GOAL: Resume normal pre-op bowel pattern. Tolerates diet.** Phase I AHA diet or _____ ADA diet	 Phase I AHA diet or _____ ADA diet
GOAL: Effective coping patterns 1. Assess response to treatment and allow time to listen. 2. Answer or seek answers to patient/ family questions.	**GOAL: Effective coping patterns** 1. Assess response to treatment and allow time to listen. 2. Answer or seek answers to patient/ family questions.	**GOAL: Effective coping patterns** 1. Assess response to treatment and allow time to listen. 2. Answer or seek answers to patient/ family questions.	**GOAL: Family and Pt. compliant with Plan of Care.** 1. Assess response to treatment and allow time to listen. 2. Answer or seek answers to patient/ family questions.	**GOAL: Family and Pt. compliant with Plan of Care.** 1. Assess response to treatment and allow time to listen. 2. Answer or seek answers to patient family questions.
GOAL: Minimal edema, normal voiding. Daily weights	**GOAL: Absence of weight gain.** Daily weights	**GOAL: Post-op weight within 5 lbs. of pre-op weight. Lab work normal.** Daily weights	**GOAL: Post-op weight stable.** Weight _____ lbs.	
GOAL: Tolerates activity progression Walk in hall w/assist 2-4 min. TID. Feeds self - in chair for all meals. Up in chair 1 hr. TID Performs own personal care	**GOAL: Independent ambulation.** Walk in hall 2-5 min. QID In chair for all meals. Up in chair 1 hr. QID Performs own personal care	**GOAL: Tolerates progression of independent activity.** Walk in hall independently 5 min. QID In chair for all meals. Up in chair 1 hr. QID Performs own personal care	**GOAL: Tolerates progression of independent activity.** Walk in hall independently 5 min. QID In chair for all meals. Up in chair 1 hr. QID Performs own personal care	**GOAL: Tolerates progression of independent activity.** Walk in hall independently 5 min. QID In chair for all meals. Up in chair 1 hr. QID Performs own personal care
GOAL: Temp < 101. Invasive line sites w/o redness or purulent drainage. All incisions open to air Incision care BID Triple lumen remains	**GOAL: Temp < 101. No purulent drainage.** All incisions open to air D/C Triple Lumen	**GOAL: Temp < 101. No purulent drainage.** D/C incision care.	**GOAL: No inflammation or purulent drainage from incisions. Temp. <100°F.**	
Pain meds prn **GOAL: Pain controlled**	Pain meds prn	Pain meds prn	Pain meds prn	Pain meds prn
Reinforce instructions on activity, telemetry, VS, diet, Coumadin, I/S Review Patient Map **GOAL: Verbalizes understanding of above instructions.**	Reinforce instructions on activity, telemetry, VS, diet, Coumadin, I/S Review Patient Map **GOAL: Verbalizes understanding of above instructions.**	Receives instructions for: Diet _____ Stress _____ Cardiac Rehab _____ Coumadin _____ Receives Booklet _____ Review Patient Map	Receives instructions for: Diet _____ Stress _____ Cardiac Rehab _____ Coumadin _____ Receives Booklet _____ Review Patient Map	**GOAL: Understands discharge instructions.** Reinforce discharge instructions Medication supplements Discharge CareMap
Resume home diabetic regimen Daily PT	CBC S-6 } in AM ECG CXR } in PM Daily PT	**GOAL: CBC, S-6 WNL** **GOAL: PT regulated for INR. 2.5-3.5** Daily PT	**GOAL: PT regulated with INR. 2.5-3.5** Daily PT	**GOAL: Protime regulated with INR. 2.5-3.5** Daily PT
Pharmacy	Cardiac Rehab Eval. Home Walk Inst. Pharmacy	Pharmacy	Pharmacy	

Coordinated CareMap® – OPEN HEART SURGERY-VALVE   M-93-5455 (F) REV. 1/24/95 P

Appendix D7: Pacemaker

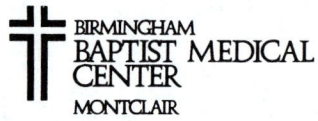
BIRMINGHAM
BAPTIST MEDICAL CENTER
MONTCLAIR

Coordinated CareMap®
CASE TYPE – PACEMAKER
Key: Highlight completed tasks and goals.
Circle variances and address in notes.
Date and highlight variances once completed.

PATIENT PROBLEM	PRE-PROCEDURE Date/Init. _____	DAY OF PROCEDURE Date/Init. _____
CARDIOVASCULAR Risk for altered hemodynamics.	GOAL: Stable CV function AEB SBP > 90, DBP > 50. Vital Signs QID.	GOAL: Stable CV function AEB SBP > 90, DBP > 50, pacing with appropriate capture & sensing. Vital signs q 15 min. x 1 hr., q 1 hr. x 4 hrs., then QID. Telemetry continuous.
PULMONARY Risk for altered pulmonary function.	GOAL: Stable pulmonary status AEB unlabored respirations, clear breath sounds, RR 15-25. Assess pulmonary status q shift.	GOAL: Stable pulmonary status AEB unlabored respirations, clear breath sounds, RR 15-25. Assess pulmonary status q shift.
GASTROINTESTINAL Risk for nausea & vomiting.	GOAL: Stable digestive processes AEB no nausea or vomiting. NPO after clear liquid breakfast.	GOAL: Stable digestive processes AEB no nausea or vomiting. AHA Phase I.
SKIN/WOUND Risk for altered skin integrity and infection.	GOAL: Maintain skin integrity AEB absence of skin abrasions, temp < 101° F Prep right & left side of chest and neck. **Antibiotic IV on call to cath lab.**	GOAL: Absence of signs and symptoms of infection AEB pacemaker drsg dry & intact, temp. < 101° F. Assess pacemaker site q shift.
FLUID BALANCE Risk for altered fluid balance.	GOAL: Maintain fluid balance AEB Urine output > 240cc q 8 hrs. I&O q shift. Void prior to procedure. Saline lock.	GOAL: Maintain fluid balance AEB Urine output > 240cc q 8 hrs. I&O q shift. D/C IV fluids when pt. is tolerating po fluids.
ACTIVITY Risk for impaired activity progression.	GOAL: Tolerates activity AEB independent ambulation. Up ad lib.	GOAL: Tolerates activity progression post procedure AEB ability to ambulate with assistance. Bedrest x 2 hrs., then up with assistance. Elevate HOB 30° or as desired.
PAIN MANAGEMENT Risk for altered comfort level.		GOAL: Effective coping with pain AEB pain controlled by medication. Assess pain level with vital signs.
PSYCHOSOCIAL/SPIRITUAL Risk for ineffective coping.	GOAL: Effective coping patterns AEB patient/family participation in plan of care. Assess response to plan of care q shift. Encourage verbalization. Assess need for pastoral care consult.	GOAL: Effective coping patterns AEB patient/family participation in plan of care. Assess response to plan of care q shift. Encourage verbalization. Assess need for pastoral care consult.
TEACHING Risk for knowledge deficit.	GOAL: Pt./family participate in identification of learning needs AEB verbalizing understanding of procedure, pre & post procedure care, plan of care. Video. AHA booklet. Pt./family map. Notify Patient Educator, Ext. 5533	GOAL: Identified learning needs met AEB pt./family verbalize understanding of use of transmitter, pacemaker follow up, signs and symptoms to report, how to check pulse. Pt./family map. Transmitter and pacemaker follow up teaching.
DISCHARGE PLANNING Risk for impaired home management.	GOAL: Pt./family participate in identification of D/C needs AEB verbalization of needs. Initial D/C assessment. Consult Case Manager, Ext. 1611.	GOAL: Pt./family participate in identification of D/C needs AEB verbalization of needs. Assess D/C needs q day.
TESTS/PROCEDURES	GOAL: Lab values WNL. CBC, UA, PT (if pt. on coumadin, notify MD if pt. > 14 seconds) S6 (treat K+ per protocol). EKG	

Coordinated CareMap® – PACEMAKER

M-95-5029 (B) REV. 4/17/95 P

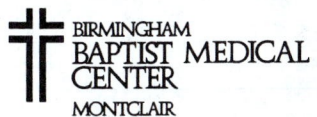
BIRMINGHAM
BAPTIST MEDICAL
CENTER
MONTCLAIR

Coordinated CareMap®
CASE TYPE – PACEMAKER

(Addressograph)

POST PROCEDURE

Date/Init. _____

GOAL: Stable CV function AEB SBP > 90, DBP > 50, pacing with appropriate capture & sensing.

Vital signs QID.
Telemetry continuous.

GOAL: Stable pulmonary status AEB unlabored respirations, clear breath sounds, RR 15-25.

Assess pulmonary status q shift.

GOAL: Nutrition intake meets body requirements AEB food intake > 50%, no nausea or vomiting.
AHA Phase I.

GOAL: Absence of signs and symptoms of infection AEB pacemaker site dry & intact, temp. < 101° F.

Remove pacemaker drsg.
Assess pacemaker site q shift.

GOAL: Maintain fluid balance AEB Urine output > 240cc q 8 hrs.
I&O q shift.
D/C saline lock.

GOAL: Tolerates activity progression AEB independent ambulation.

Up ad lib.

GOAL: Effective coping with pain AEB pain controlled by po medication.

Assess pain level with vital signs.

GOAL: Effective coping patterns AEB patient/family participation in plan of care.
Assess response to plan of care q shift.
Encourage verbalization.
Assess need for pastoral care consult.

GOAL: Identified learning needs met AEB pt./family verbalize understanding of use of transmitter, pacemaker follow up, signs and symptoms to report, how to check pulse.

Notify Patient Educator, Ext. 5533
Pt./family map.
Transmit baseline pacemaker EKG to follow-up clinic.

GOAL: Identified D/C needs met AEB pt./family verbalize ability to manage home care.

Review home plan of care.

Coordinated CareMap® – PACEMAKER

M-95-5029 (B) REV. 4/17/95   P

Adapted from CareMap® System, The Center for Case Management

Appendix D8: GI Hemorrhage

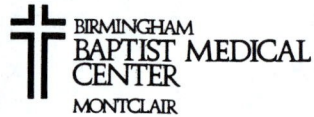

BIRMINGHAM
BAPTIST MEDICAL
CENTER
MONTCLAIR

Coordinated CareMap®
CASE TYPE – GI HEMORRHAGE
Key: Highlight completed task.
Address variances in nurses' focus notes and circle in red.
Once variances completed - highlight and date.

PAGE 2

CATEGORY	DAY # 1 DATE/INT. _____	DAY # 2 DATE/INT. _____
TEST/PROCEDURES Risk of increased instability of condition R/T delay in tests/procedures.	**GOAL: Tolerates test/procedures; EGD/colonoscopy completed.** T & S PT/PTT CBC Hct q 6 hrs. Renal Profile Upper Endoscopy Colonoscopy Prep as ordered	**GOAL: Labwork/tests WNL; Hct stable, no hematemesis, melana or rectal bleeding** Hct q 8 hrs.
MEDICATIONS/TREATMENTS Risk of recurrance of GI Bleed R/T irritation/ulceration of site.	**GOAL: Exhibits appropriate therapeutic response to medicinals; no adverse drug/blood reactions** IV H₂ blockers Transfuse per MD orders IV Fluids	**GOAL: Exhibits appropriate therapeutic response to medicinals; no adverse drug/blood reactions** IV H₂ blockers IV Fluids
GI Risk for altered bowel function.	**GOAL: Stable GI function; no active bleeding; NG tube patent.** NG Tube Document color, amount, character of aspirate, emesis, stool. Collect specimens as ordered.	**GOAL: Stable GI function; no active bleeding.** D/C NGT Collect specimens as ordered.
NUTRITION Risk for altered nutrition - less than body requirements.	**GOAL: Stable digestive processes; no vomitting, diarrhea.** NPO	**GOAL: Stable digestive processes; tolerates p.o. intake; no vomiting, diarrhea.** Clear liquids, advance as tolerated.
ACTIVITY Risk for activity intolerance R/T weakness.	**GOAL: Compliant with activity restriction** Bedrest	**GOAL: Tolerates activity progression** Chair t.i.d.
CARDIOVASCULAR Risk for fluid volume deficit R/T GI blood loss.	**GOAL: Stable CV function; adequate fluid balance, stable LOC, skin w/d, UOP > 60cc/h, VS WNL - (SBP > 90, HR 60-100).** VS q 4 hrs. I&O q shift Foley	**GOAL: Stable CV function; adequate fluid balance, stable LOC, skin w/d, UOP > 60cc/h, VS WNL - (SBP > 90, HR 60-100).** VS q 8 hrs. I&O q shift D/C Foley
PSYCHOSOCIAL/SPIRITUAL Risk for ineffective coping R/T illness, bleeding.	**GOAL: Effective coping patterns; pt./family verbalize thoughts & feelings re: illness & demonstrate compliance c care** Allow pt./family to verbalize thoughts, feelings re: illness & assess response to care & treatment	**GOAL: Effective coping patterns; pt./family verbalize thoughts & feelings re: illness & demonstrate compliance c care** Allow pt./family to verbalize thoughts, feelings re: illness & assess response to care & treatment
TEACHING Knowledge deficit R/T illness, procedures, preventative measures.	**GOAL: Pt./family participate in identification of learning needs; pt./family verbalize understanding of procedure, prep, & post procedure care.** Assess knowledge deficit & begin teaching as indicated: • procedures • treatments • medications	**GOAL: Identified learning needs met; pt./family verbalize understanding of progression of care.** Continue teaching: • diet • medications • activity • assessment & preventative measures.
DISCHARGE PLANNING	**GOAL: DCP needs identified & addressed.** DCP assessment Consult case manager to evaluate discharge needs.	**GOAL: DCP needs identified & addressed; DCP assessment completed.**

Coordinated CareMap® – GI HEMORRHAGE

BIRMINGHAM BAPTIST MEDICAL CENTER
MONTCLAIR

Coordinated CareMap®
CASE TYPE – GI HEMORRHAGE
Key: Highlight completed task.
Address variances in nurses' focus notes and circle in red.
Once variances completed - highlight and date.

(Addressograph)

PAGE 3

DAY # 3	DAY # 4
DATE/INT. _____	DATE/INT. _____
GOAL: Labwork/tests WNL; Hct WNL or baseline x 48 hrs.; no hematemesis, melana or rectal bleeding Hct q a.m.	**GOAL: Labwork/tests WNL**
GOAL: Exhibits appropriate therapeutic response to medicinals; no adverse drug/blood reactions Δ to p.o. meds D/C IVF Δ IV to SL	**GOAL: Exhibits appropriate therapeutic response to medicinals; no adverse drug/blood reactions** D/C SL
GOAL: Stable GI function; normal bowel pattern.	**GOAL: Stable GI function; normal bowel pattern; benign abdomen.**
GOAL: Stable digestive processes; p.o. intake ≥ 50% of meals; no nausea, vomitting, diarrhea. Advance diet as tolerated.	**GOAL: Stable digestive processes; tolerates 100% of meals; nutritional intake meets body requirements.** Diet as tolerated.
GOAL: Tolerates activity progression Up in room	**GOAL: Pt./family/S.O. able to manage care** Up ad lib
GOAL: Stable CV function; adequate fluid balance, stable LOC, skin w/d, UOP > 60cc/h, VS WNL - (SBP > 90, HR 60-100). VS q 8 hrs. I&O q shift	**GOAL: Stable CV function; adequate fluid balance, stable LOC, skin w/d, UOP > 60cc/h, VS WNL - (SBP > 90, HR 60-100).** VS q 8 hrs. I&O q shift
GOAL: Effective coping patterns; pt./family verbalize thoughts & feelings re: illness & demonstrate compliance c̄ care Allow pt./family to verbalize thoughts, feelings re: illness & assess response to care & treatment	**GOAL: Effective coping patterns; pt./family verbalize thoughts & feelings re: illness & demonstrate compliance c̄ care** Allow pt./family to verbalize thoughts, feelings re: illness & assess response to care & treatment
GOAL: Identified learning needs met; pt./family verbalize understanding of progression of care. Continue/reinforce teaching	**GOAL: Identified learning needs met; pt./family verbalize understanding of:** • _____ • _____ • _____ • _____
GOAL: DCP plans completed, needs identified, arrangements completed.	**GOAL: DCP plans completed, needs identified, arrangements completed.**

Coordinated CareMap® – GI HEMORRHAGE

M-94-5278 (B) REV. 1/6/95   P

Adapted from the Center for Case Management, Inc.

Appendix D9: Diabetic Ketoacidosis

Standard Form 507		c43—16—81472p–3 GPO

CLINICAL RECORD	**Report on**	COLLABORATIVE PLAN OF CARE: DIABETIC
	or	
	Continuation of S.F.	KETOACIDOSIS ALOS: 3DAYS
	(Strike out one line) (Specify type of examination or data)	

Admission Date & Time _____	DAY 1 ____	DAY 2 *(Sign and date)* ____	DAY 3 ____
OUTCOME	Hemodynamically stable B/P > 90 sys., UOP > 30 cc/hr Temp. < 100.5 ⟶		
	Serum glucose ≤ 300 with insulin infusion	Glucose ≤ 250 with SQ daily and sliding scale insulin	
	Electrolytes and acid/base balance WNL ⟶		
		Absence or decrease in nausea/vomiting. Tolerates liquid diet. Absence of s/s of hypoglycemia	
OUTCOME MET	YES NO ____	YES NO ____	YES NO ____
SIGNATURE			
CONSULTS	Pulmonary Endocrinology	Dietary Social Service	Diabetic Educator (if newly diagnosed)
TESTS	Renal I, II Glucose every 4 hrs x 24 hours then every 6 hours Twice daily Mag, PO^4 CBC with diff, platelets ABG's every 6 hours x 24 hours, then twice daily Serum ketones Lactic acid Urine, sputum and blood cultures U/A Chest x-ray, abdominal films EKG		
ACTIVITIES	Bedrest with BSC		

(Continue on reverse side)

PATIENT'S IDENTIFICATION *(For typed or written entries give: Name—last, first, middle; grade; date; hospital or medical facility)*

REGISTER NO.   WARD NO.

PAGE 1 OF 2

REPORT ON _____ or CONTINUATION OF ___

STANDARD FORM 507

General Services Administration and Interagency Committee on Medical Records
FIRMR (41 CFR) 201-45.505
October 1975   507-107

Standard Form 507   c43—16—81472p—3   GPO

CLINICAL RECORD	Report on	COLLABORATIVE PLAN OF CARE: DIABETIC
	or	
	Continuation of S.F.	KETOACIDOSIS ALOS: 3DAYS

(Strike out one line) (Specify type of examination or data)

(Sign and date)

TREATMENTS
Accuchecks hourly X 24 hours, then every 4 hours X 24, then every 6 hours
Continuous cardiac monitoring per SOC
SaO_2 monitoring continuously
Daily weights
Hourly intake and output
Arterial line (for blood draws)   d/c A-Line

MEDICATIONS
IVFs of normal saline (NS) or $\frac{1}{2}$ NS for hydration
Insulin infusion as ordered ————————→ Change insulin to SQ
                                                                                          with supplemental sliding scale

Supplemental K^+ and Mg^+ as ordered
Antibiotics
Antiemetics as ordered

NUTRITION   NPO   Clear Liquids   ADA Diet

TEACHING   Explain treatments   Assess patient/family
                        and procedure   knowledge r/t diabetes
                                                          Reinforce current knowledge
                                                          if adequate.
                                                          Referral to Diabetes Educator
                                                          for additional learning needs.

DISCHARGE PLANNING   Transfer to Ward

Admission Date_____Admission Time_____Discharge Date_____Discharge Time_____LOS_____

Documentation of review of Care Map for individual shifts will be made on the ICU Flowsheet.

Author:

Physician Reviewer:

Multidisciplinary Review Group: MICU Committee
DOF: April, 1993   *(Continue on reverse side)*

Appendix D10: Total Hip Replacement

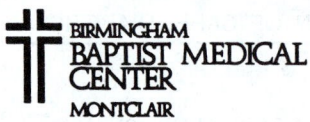

BIRMINGHAM
BAPTIST MEDICAL
CENTER
MONTCLAIR

Coordinated CareMap®
CASE TYPE – TOTAL HIP REPLACEMENT
Key: Highlight completed task.
Address variances in nurses' focus notes and circle in red.
Once variances completed - highlight and date.

PAGE 2

PATIENT PROBLEM	PRE-OP	IMMEDIATE POST-OP
	DATE/INT. _____	DATE/INT. _____
PAIN Pain R/T degenerative joint disease & surgery	GOAL: Understands pain management options (PAT) PAT discusses pain management options. Instruct pt. & family that pain is managed, but not eliminated PAT Anesthesia consults, EMA	GOAL: Pain controlled at level < 7. D-E-N Epidural or PCA for pain. D-E-N
MUSCULOSKELETAL Limited mobility & impaired ADL's R/T disease process. Potential for hip dislocation	GOAL: Understands mobility restrictions & activity progression. PAT Pt. oriented care map.	Begin Rehab Protocol exercises.
CIRCULATORY Potential for DVT, PE & fat emboli R/T surgery & imposed immobility Increased risk for blood loss	GOAL: No s/s of anemia. Pt. taking Trinsicon, as ordered. PAT Identify risk of DVT. PAT CBC. PAT Type & screen for 3 u PRBC. PAT EKG, if over 40 years old & not done in past 30 days. PAT Assess cardiac status & record. EMA	GOAL: Absence of cardiac arrhythmia. D-E-N Continuous cardiac monitoring. D-E-N GOAL: Maintain SBP > 90, DBP > 50, HR > 50. D-E-N VS q 15 min. x 4, q 30 min. x 4, q hr. until stable then q 4 hr. D-E-N. GOAL: Pedal pulses 2+ and capillary refill < 3 sec. in operative leg. D-E-N Assess pedal pulses q 2 hr. D-E-N Assess capillary refill q 2 hr. D-E-N Assess temp. of extremities q 2 hr. D-E-N GOAL: No evidence of DVT, P.E. or fat emboli. D-E-N Athrombic device on D-E-N Assess calf q shift. D-E-N GOAL: Hct ≥ 30 Hct
NEUROLOGY Potential for neurological deficits to operative leg R/T surgery.	Assess neurological status & record. EMA	GOAL: No evidence of parasthesias or foot drop in operative leg. D-E-N Assess sensation in operative leg q 2 hr. D-E-N Assess Plantar/Dorsiflexion in operative leg q 2 hr. D-E-N
PULMONARY Mod. risk for ineffective respirations R/T surgery & immobility	Assess pulmonary status & record. EMA	GOAL: Adequate oxygenation AEB: clear breath sounds & resp. > 12 & < 26. D-E-N Assess for normal breathing patterns & central cyanosis q 4 hr. D-E-N Ausculate breath sounds q 4 hr. D-E-N I/S q 2 hr. D-E-N CDB q 2 hr. D-E-N
INTEGUMENTARY Potential for infection R/T operative site, drains & IV site. Potential for alteration in skin integrity R/T imposed immobility & surgery.	Assess condition of skin and record. EMA	GOAL: Drsg. dry & intact s fresh drainage soaking through. D-E-N Incision & drain site covered. D-E-N GOAL: IV site s redness or swelling. D-E-N Assess IV site q shift. D-E-N GOAL: Drain < 200cc/shift. D-E-N Drain intact. D-E-N GOAL: Absence of prolonged reddened areas. Skin intact. D-E-N Turn q 2 hr. D-E-N
NUTRITION ELIMINATION Potential for constipation R/T immobility & pain meds. Potential for loss of appetite R/T inactivity & pain. Potential for altered fluid balance R/T surgery.	Assess GI status & record. EMA	GOAL: Maintain adequate fluid balance. D-E-N IVF's infusing. D-E-N I & O q shift. D-E-N GOAL: Tolerates liquids. D-E-N GOAL: UOP ≥ 240cc/shift. D-E-N Monitor foley drainage q shift. D-E-N
PSYCHOSOCIAL Anxiety R/T unknown surgery, temp, lifestyle changes & potential lack of a support system. Temporary loss of independence R/T surgery & lifestyle changes.	Complete discharge planning assessment	
KNOWLEDGE DEFICIT Knowledge deficit R/T surgery, post recovery activity, temporary lifestyle changes & dietary resources to aid in healing.	GOAL: Pt. verbalizes understanding of present meds & is compliant c regimen. PAT GOAL: Pt. & family verbalizes understanding of surgical process & post-op care. PAT, EMA GOAL: Pt. & family verbalizes understanding of importance of diet healing. PAT Give pt. oriented care map. PAT	GOAL: Pt. & family verbalizes understanding of hip precautions. Instruct pt. to maintain abduction of legs. < 60° of hip flexion & to avoid internal rotation of surgical leg. Teach pt. to use I/S

M-94-5275-1 (B) REV. 3/20/95 P

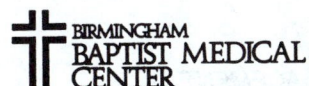

BIRMINGHAM BAPTIST MEDICAL CENTER

Coordinated CareMap®
CASE TYPE – TOTAL HIP REPLACEMENT
Key: Highlight completed task.
Address variances in nurses' focus notes and circle in red.
Once variances completed - highlight and date.

PAGE 3

(Addressograph)

	POD 1	POD 2	POD 3	POD 4
	DATE/INT.	DATE/INT.	DATE/INT.	DATE/INT.
PAIN	GOAL: Pt. verbalizes a decrease in pain to level 5-6. D-E-N Epidural or PCA for pain. D-E-N	GOAL: Pt. verbalizes pain at level 5-6. D-E-N Epidural or PCA for pain. D-E-N	GOAL: Pt. verbalizes a decrease in pain to level ≤ 5. D-E-N D/C Epidural or PCA Begin po pain meds. D-E-N	GOAL: Pt. verbalizes pain at level ≤ 5. D-E-N PO pain meds. D-E-N
MUSCULOSKELETAL		Consult OT for ADL/Home eval. & treatment Chair BID am/pm PT BID am/pm Fall precautions	Consult OT for ADL/Home eval. & treatment Chair BID am/pm PT BID am/pm Fall precautions	Consult OT for ADL/Home eval. & treatment Chair BID am/pm PT BID am/pm Fall precautions
CIRCULATORY	GOAL: Absence of cardiac arrhythmia. D-E-N D/C Telemetry GOAL: Maintain SBP > 90, DBP > 50, HR > 50. D-E-N VS q 4 hr. D-E-N GOAL: Pedal pulses 2+ and capillary refill < 3 sec. in operative leg. D-E-N Assess pedal pulses q 4 hr. D-E-N Assess capillary refill q 4 hr. D-E-N Assess temp. of extremities q 4 hr. D-E-N GOAL: No evidence of DVT, P.E. or fat emboli. D-E-N Athrombic device on D-E-N Assess calf q shift. D-E-N GOAL: Hct ≥ 30 Hct	GOAL: Maintain SBP > 90, DBP > 50, HR > 50. D-E-N VS q 4 hr. D-E-N GOAL: Pedal pulses 2+ and capillary refill < 3 sec. in operative leg. D-E-N Assess pedal pulses q shift. D-E-N Assess capillary refill q shift. D-E-N Assess temp. of extremities q shift. D-E-N GOAL: No evidence of DVT, P.E. or fat emboli. D-E-N Athrombic device on while in bed. D-E-N Assess calf q shift. D-E-N GOAL: Hct ≥ 30 Hct	GOAL: Pt. returns to pre-admission VS status. D-E-N VS q 4 hr. D-E-N GOAL: Pedal pulses 2+ and capillary refill < 3 sec. in operative leg. D-E-N Assess pedal pulses q shift. D-E-N Assess capillary refill q shift. D-E-N Assess temp. of extremities q shift. D-E-N GOAL: No evidence of DVT, P.E. or fat emboli. D-E-N Athrombic device on while in bed. D-E-N Assess calf q shift. D-E-N GOAL: Hct maintaining or increasing. Hct	GOAL: Pt. returns to pre-admission VS status. D-E-N VS q shift. D-E-N GOAL: Pedal pulses 2+ and capillary refill < 3 sec. in operative leg. D-E-N Assess pedal pulses q shift. D-E-N Assess capillary refill q shift. D-E-N Assess temp. of extremities q shift. D-E-N GOAL: No evidence of DVT, P.E. or fat emboli. D-E-N D/C athrombic device Assess calf q shift. D-E-N
NEUROLOGY	GOAL: No evidence of paresthesias or foot drop in operative leg. D-E-N Assess sensation in operative leg q 4 hr. D-E-N Assess Plantar/Dorsiflexion in operative leg q 4 hr. D-E-N	GOAL: No evidence of paresthesias or foot drop in operative leg. D-E-N Assess sensation in operative leg q shift. D-E-N Assess Plantar/Dorsiflexion in operative leg q shift. D-E-N	GOAL: No evidence of paresthesias or foot drop in operative leg. D-E-N Assess sensation in operative leg q shift. D-E-N Assess Plantar/Dorsiflexion in operative leg q shift. D-E-N	GOAL: No evidence of paresthesias or foot drop in operative leg. D-E-N Assess sensation in operative leg q shift. D-E-N Assess Plantar/Dorsiflexion in operative leg q shift. D-E-N
PULMONARY	GOAL: Adequate oxygenation AEB: clear breath sounds & resp. > 12 & < 26. D-E-N Assess for normal breathing patterns q shift. D-E-N Ausculate breath sounds q shift. D-E-N I/S q 2 hr. D-E-N CDB q 2 hr. D-E-N GOAL: Temp < 101.5 D-E-N Monitor temp q 4 hr. D-E-N	GOAL: Adequate oxygenation AEB: clear breath sounds & resp. > 12 & < 26. D-E-N Assess for normal breathing patterns q shift. D-E-N Ausculate breath sounds q shift. D-E-N I/S q 2 hr. D-E-N CDB q 2 hr. D-E-N GOAL: Temp < 101.5 D-E-N Monitor temp q 4 hr. D-E-N	GOAL: Lungs return to pre-surgical status. Assess for normal breathing patterns q shift. D-E-N Ausculate breath sounds q shift. D-E-N I/S q 2 hr. D-E-N GOAL: Temp < 100.5. D-E-N Monitor temp q 4 hr. D-E-N	GOAL: Lungs return to pre-surgical status. D-E-N Assess for normal breathing patterns q shift. D-E-N Ausculate breath sounds q shift. D-E-N I/S q 2 hrs. D-E-N GOAL: Temp < 100. D-E-N Monitor temp q shift. D-E-N
INTEGUMENTARY	GOAL: Drsg. dry & intact s fresh drainage soaking through. D-E-N Incision & drain site covered. D-E-N GOAL: IV site s redness or swelling. D-E-N IV site care daily GOAL: Drain < 200cc/shift. D-E-N Drain intact. D-E-N GOAL: Absence of prolonged reddened areas. Skin intact. D-E-N Turn q 2 hr. D-E-N	GOAL: Wound s redness, purulent drainage or excessive edema. D-E-N If drain d/c'd change drsg. c sterile technique. GOAL: IV site s redness or swelling. D-E-N IV site care daily GOAL: Drain < 150cc/shift. D-E-N D/C drain. GOAL: Absence of prolonged reddened areas. Skin intact. D-E-N Turn q 2 hr. D-E-N	GOAL: Wound s redness, purulent drainage or excessive edema. D-E-N Change drsg. daily c sterile technique. D/C IVF's if PCA/epidural d/c'd GOAL: Drain < 50cc/shift. D-E-N Monitor & inform MD when goal is achieved to GOAL: Absence of prolonged reddened areas. Skin intact. D-E-N Turn q 2 hr. while in bed. D-E-N	GOAL: Wound s redness, purulent drainage or excessive edema. D-E-N Change drsg. daily c sterile technique. GOAL: Absence of prolonged reddened areas. Skin intact. D-E-N Turn q 2 hr. while in bed. D-E-N
NUTRITION ELIMINATION	GOAL: Maintain adequate fluid balance. D-E-N IVF's infusing. D-E-N I & O q shift. D-E-N GOAL: Returns to pre-surgical diet. D-E-N GOAL: UOP ≥ 240cc/shift. D-E-N Monitor foley drainage q shift. D-E-N	GOAL: Maintain adequate fluid balance. D-E-N D/C IVF's. I & O q shift. D-E-N GOAL: Returns to pre-surgical diet. D-E-N GOAL: UOP ≥ 240cc/shift. D-E-N Monitor foley drainage q shift. D-E-N	GOAL: Maintain adequate fluid balance. D-E-N D/C I & O GOAL: Returns to pre-surgical diet. D-E-N GOAL: Pt. has BM LOC prn D/C foley	GOAL: Returns to pre-surgical diet. D-E-N GOAL: Returns to pre-surgical bowel patterns.
PSYCHO-SOCIAL	GOAL: Pt. will verbalize anxiety R/T hosp. stay. Consult Chaplain, prn.	GOAL: Begin home care/community resource arrangements. Consult DPN Assess pt. explain options & initiate post-op placement. DPN		GOAL: Pt. verbalizes readiness to transfer to rehab unit. D/C to PMRU, if applicable. (Have up by 12 noon.)
KNOWLEDGE DEFICIT	Reinforce use of I/S	GOAL: Pt. verbalizes understanding of the need to maintain hip precautions during ADL's & transfers. Instruct pt. in ADL's & home care. OT Instruct pt. in transfers & ambulation. PT Reinforce use of I/S.	GOAL: Pt. verbalizes understanding of po method of pain control. Instruct on po pain control, includes S.E.	

M-94-5275-2 (F) REV. 3/20/95 P

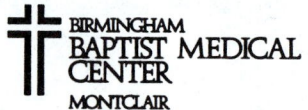

BIRMINGHAM
BAPTIST MEDICAL
CENTER
MONTCLAIR

Coordinated CareMap®
CASE TYPE – TOTAL HIP REPLACEMENT
Key: Highlight completed task.
Address variances in nurses' focus notes and circle in red.
Once variances completed - highlight and date.

PAGE 4

	POD 5	POD 6	POD 7	POD 8
	DATE/INT. _____	DATE/INT. _____	DATE/INT. _____	DATE/INT. _____
PAIN	GOAL: Pt. verbalizes pain at level ≤ 5.D-E-N	GOAL: Pt. verbalizes pain at level ≤ 5.D-E-N	GOAL: Pt. verbalizes pain at level ≤ 4.D-E-N	GOAL: Pt. verbalizes pain at level ≤ 4.D-E-N
	PO pain meds. D-E-N	PO pain meds. D-E-N	PO pain meds. D-E-N	PO pain meds. D-E-N
MUSCULOSKELETAL	Consult OT for ADL/Home eval. & treatment Chair BID am/pm PT BID am/pm Fall precautions	Consult OT for ADL/Home eval. & treatment Chair BID am/pm PT BID am/pm Fall precautions	Independent c ADL's Chair BID am/pm PT BID am/pm Fall precautions	Chair BID am/pm PT BID am/pm Fall precautions
CIRCULATORY	GOAL: Pt. returns to pre-admission VS status. D-E-N VS q shift. D-E-N GOAL: Pedal pulses 2+ and capillary refill < 3 sec. in operative leg. D-E-N Assess pedal pulses q shift. D-E-N Assess capillary refill q shift. D-E-N Assess temp. of extremities q shift. D-E-N GOAL: No evidence of DVT, P.E. or fat emboli. D-E-N Assess calf q shift. D-E-N	GOAL: Pt. returns to pre-admission VS status. D-E-N VS q shift. D-E-N GOAL: Pedal pulses 2+ and capillary refill < 3 sec. in operative leg. D-E-N Assess pedal pulses q shift. D-E-N Assess capillary refill q shift. D-E-N Assess temp. of extremities q shift. D-E-N GOAL: No evidence of DVT, P.E. or fat emboli. D-E-N Assess calf q shift. D-E-N	GOAL: Pt. returns to pre-admission VS status. D-E-N VS q shift. D-E-N GOAL: Pedal pulses 2+ and capillary refill < 3 sec. in operative leg. D-E-N Assess pedal pulses q shift. D-E-N Assess capillary refill q shift. D-E-N Assess temp. of extremities q shift. D-E-N GOAL: No evidence of DVT, P.E. or fat emboli. D-E-N Assess calf q shift. D-E-N	GOAL: Pt. returns to pre-admission VS status. D-E-N VS q shift. D-E-N GOAL: Pedal pulses 2+ and capillary refill < 3 sec. in operative leg. D-E-N Assess pedal pulses q shift. D-E-N Assess capillary refill q shift. D-E-N Assess temp. of extremities q shift. D-E-N GOAL: No evidence of DVT, P.E. or fat emboli. D-E-N Assess calf q shift. D-E-N
NEUROLOGY	GOAL: No evidence of parasthesias or foot drop in operative leg. D-E-N Assess sensation in operative leg q shift. D-E-N Assess Plantar/Dorsiflexion in operative leg q shift. D-E-N	GOAL: No evidence of parasthesias or foot drop in operative leg. D-E-N Assess sensation in operative leg q shift. D-E-N Assess Plantar/Dorsiflexion in operative leg q shift. D-E-N	GOAL: No evidence of parasthesias or foot drop in operative leg. D-E-N Assess sensation in operative leg q shift. D-E-N Assess Plantar/Dorsiflexion in operative leg q shift. D-E-N	GOAL: No evidence of parasthesias or foot drop in operative leg. D-E-N Assess sensation in operative leg q shift. D-E-N Assess Plantar/Dorsiflexion in operative leg q shift. D-E-N
PULMONARY	GOAL: Lungs return to pre-surgical status. D-E-N Assess for normal breathing patterns q shift. D-E-N Ausculate breath sounds q shift. D-E-N I/S q 2 hr. w.a. D-E-N GOAL: Temp < 100. D-E-N Temp q shift. D-E-N	GOAL: Lungs return to pre-surgical status. D-E-N Assess for normal breathing patterns q shift. D-E-N Ausculate breath sounds q shift. D-E-N I/S q 2 hr. w.a. D-E-N GOAL: Temp < 100. D-E-N Temp q shift. D-E-N	GOAL: Lungs return to pre-surgical status. D-E-N Assess for normal breathing patterns q shift. D-E-N Ausculate breath sounds q shift. D-E-N I/S q 2 hr. w.a. D-E-N GOAL: Temp < 100. D-E-N Temp q shift. D-E-N	GOAL: Lungs return to pre-surgical status. D-E-N Assess for normal breathing patterns q shift. D-E-N Ausculate breath sounds q shift. D-E-N I/S q 2 hr. w.a. D-E-N GOAL: Temp < 100. D-E-N Temp q shift. D-E-N
INTEGUMENTARY	GOAL: Wound s redness, purulent drainage or excessive edema. D-E-N Change drsg. daily c sterile technique. GOAL: Absence of prolonged reddened areas. Skin intact. D-E-N Turn q 2 hr. while in bed. D-E-N	GOAL: Wound s redness, purulent drainage or excessive edema. D-E-N Change drsg. daily c sterile technique. GOAL: Absence of prolonged reddened areas. Skin intact. D-E-N Turn q 2 hr. while in bed. D-E-N	GOAL: Wound s redness, purulent drainage or excessive edema. D-E-N Change drsg. daily c sterile technique. GOAL: Absence of prolonged reddened areas. Skin intact. D-E-N Turn q 2 hr. while in bed. D-E-N	GOAL: Wound s redness, purulent drainage or excessive edema. D-E-N Change drsg. daily c sterile technique. GOAL: Absence of prolonged reddened areas. Skin intact. D-E-N Turn q 2 hr. while in bed. D-E-N
NUTRITION ELIMINATION	GOAL: Returns to pre-surgical diet. D-E GOAL: Returns to pre-surgical bowel patterns.	GOAL: Returns to pre-surgical diet. D-E GOAL: Returns to pre-surgical bowel patterns.	GOAL: Returns to pre-surgical diet. D-E GOAL: Returns to pre-surgical bowel patterns.	GOAL: Returns to pre-surgical diet. D-E GOAL: Returns to pre-surgical bowel patterns.
PSYCHO-SOCIAL				GOAL: Pt. verbalizes readiness to go home.
KNOWLEDGE DEFICIT	GOAL: Family/S.O. involved in pt.'s care Family/S.O. to go to P.T. c pt. for home care instructions.			GOAL: Pt. verbalizes understanding of D/C instructions.

Adapted from the Center for Case Management, Inc.

M-94-5275-2 (B) REV. 3/20/95 P

Appendix D11: Total Knee Replacement

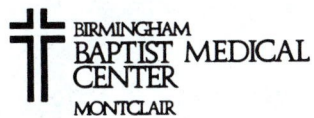

BIRMINGHAM BAPTIST MEDICAL CENTER MONTCLAIR

Coordinated CareMap®
CASE TYPE – TOTAL KNEE REPLACEMENT
Key: Highlight completed task.
Address variances in nurses' focus notes and circle in red.
Once variances completed - highlight and date.

PAGE 2

PATIENT PROBLEM	PRE-OP	IMMEDIATE POST-OP
	DATE/INT. _____	DATE/INT. _____
PAIN Pain R/T degenerative joint disease & surgery	**GOAL: Understands pain management options (PAT)** PAT discusses pain management options. Instruct pt. & family that pain is managed, but not eliminated PAT Anesthesia consult, EMA	**GOAL: Pain controlled at level < 7. D-E-N** Epidural or PCA for pain. D-E-N
MUSCULOSKELETAL Limited mobility & impaired ADL's R/T disease process.	**GOAL: Understands mobility restrictions & activity progression. PAT**	**GOAL: Pt. tol. CPM c̄ only minimal discomfort. PT** CPM at _____ degrees. **GOAL: Pt. tol. BS, supine TKR exercises c̄ assistance. PT.**
CIRCULATORY Potential for DVT, PE & fat emboli R/T surgery & imposed immobility Increased risk for blood loss	**GOAL: No s/s of anemia. Pt. taking Trinsicon, as ordered. PAT** Identify risk of DVT. PAT CBC. PAT Type & screen for 3 u. PRBC. PAT EKG, if over 40 years old & not done in past 30 days. PAT Assess cardiac status & record. EMA	**GOAL: Absence of cardiac arrhythmia. D-E-N** Continuous cardiac monitoring. OR-PACU D-E-N **GOAL: Maintain SBP > 90, DBP > 50, HR > 50. D-E-N** VS q 15 min. x 4, q 30 min. x 4, q hr. until stable then q 4 hr. D-E-N. **GOAL: Pedal pulses 2+ and capillary refill < 3 sec. in operative leg. D-E-N** Assess pedal pulses q 2 hr. D-E-N Assess capillary refill q 2 hr. D-E-N Assess temp. of extremities q 2 hr. D-E-N **GOAL: No evidence of DVT, P.E. or fat emboli. D-E-N** Athrombic device on D-E-N **GOAL: Hct ≥ 30** Hct
NEUROLOGY Potential for neurological deficits to operative leg R/T surgery.	Assess neurological status & record. EMA	**GOAL: No evidence of paresthesias or foot drop in operative leg. D-E-N** Assess sensation in operative leg q 2 hr. D-E-N Assess Plantar/Dorsiflexion in operative leg q 2 hr. D-E-N
PULMONARY Mod. risk for ineffective respirations R/T surgery & immobility.	Assess pulmonary status & record. EMA	**GOAL: Adequate oxygenation AEB: clear breath sounds & resp. > 12 & < 26. D-E-N** Assess for normal breathing patterns & central cyanosis q 4 hr. D-E-N Ausculate breath sounds q 4 hr. D-E-N I/S q 2 hr. D-E-N CDB q 2 hr. D-E-N
INTEGUMENTARY Potential for infection R/T operative site, drains & IV site. Potential for alteration in skin integrity R/T imposed immobility & surgery.	Assess condition of skin and record. EMA	**GOAL: Drsg. dry & intact s̄ fresh drainage soaking through. D-E-N** Incision & drain site covered. D-E-N **GOAL: Absence of prolonged reddened areas.** **Skin intact. D-E-N** Turn q 2 hr. D-E-N **GOAL: IV site s̄ redness or swelling. D-E-N** Assess IV site q shift. D-E-N **GOAL: Drain < 200 cc/shift. D-E-N** Drain intact. D-E-N
NUTRITIONAL ELIMINATION Potential for constipation R/T immobility & pain meds. Potential for loss of appetite R/T inactivity & pain. Potential altered fluid balance R/T surgery.	Assess GI status & record. EMA	**GOAL: Maintain adequate fluid balance. D-E-N** IVF's infusing. D-E-N I & O q shift. D-E-N **GOAL: Tolerates liquids. D-E-N** **GOAL: UOP ≥ 240cc/shift. D-E-N** Monitor foley drainage q shift. D-E-N
PSYCHOSOCIAL Anxiety R/T unknown surgery, temp. lifestyle changes & potential lack of a support system. Temporary loss of independence R/T surgery & lifestyle changes.	Complete discharge planning assessment	
KNOWLEDGE DEFICIT Knowledge deficit R/T surgery, post recovery activity, temporary lifestyle changes & dietary resources to aid in healing.	**GOAL: Pt. verbalizes understanding of present meds & is compliant c̄ regimen. PAT** **GOAL: Pt. & family verbalizes understanding of importance of diet healing. PAT, EMA** Give pt-oriented care map. PAT	**GOAL: Pt. & family verbalizes understanding of CPM.** Instruct pt. on purpose of CPM & proper positioning of leg in CPM. Teach pt. to use I/S.

M-94-5276-1 (B) REV. 12/8/94 P

BIRMINGHAM BAPTIST MEDICAL CENTER
MONTCLAIR   Coordinated CareMap®

CASE TYPE – TOTAL KNEE REPLACEMENT
Key: Highlight completed task.
Address variances in nurses' focus notes and circle in red.
Once variances completed - highlight and date.

PAGE 3

(Addressograph)

	POD 1	POD 2	POD 3	POD 4
	DATE/INT. ___	DATE/INT. ___	DATE/INT. ___	DATE/INT. ___
PAIN	GOAL: Pt. verbalizes a decrease in pain to level 5-6. D-E-N Epidural or PCA for pain. D-E-N	GOAL: Pt. verbalizes pain at level 5-6. D-E-N Epidural or PCA for pain. D-E-N	GOAL: Pt. verbalizes a decrease in pain to level ≤ 5. D-E-N D/C Epidural or PCA Begin po pain meds. D-E-N	GOAL: Pt. verbalizes pain at level ≤ 5. D-E-N PO pain meds. D-E-N
MUSCULOSKELETAL	GOAL: Pt. tol. CPM c̄ 5-10° advancement daily. PT AM/PT PM CPM at ___ degrees. GOAL: Pt. able to perform supine TKR exercises c̄ assistance. PT AM/PT PM GOAL: Pt. tol. dangling on BS & transfer to chair c̄ max. asst. of 2 while maintaining proper wt. bearing status. PT AM/PT PM GOAL: Pt. tol. amb. c̄ asst. device & c̄ max. asst. of 2 while maintaining proper wt. bearing status. PT AM/PT PM	GOAL: Pt. tol. CPM c̄ 5-10° advancement daily. PT AM/PT PM CPM at ___ degrees. GOAL: Pt. able to perform supine & sitting TKR exercises c̄ asst. & 0-60° ROM actively. PT AM/PT PM GOAL: Pt. able to transfer to chair c̄ mod. asst. of 1 while maintaining proper wt. bearing status. PT AM/PT PM GOAL: Pt. tol. amb. c̄ asst. device c̄ mod. asst. of 1 while maintaining proper wt. bearing status. PT AM/PT PM Chair BID AM/PM P.T. BID AM/PM	GOAL: Pt. tol. CPM c̄ 5-10° advancement daily. PT AM/PT PM CPM at ___ degrees. GOAL: Pt. able to perform supine & sitting TKR exercises c̄ asst. & 0-60° ROM actively. PT A</PT PM GOAL: Pt. able to transfer to chair c̄ mod. asst. of 1 while maintaining proper wt. bearing status. PT AM/PT PM GOAL: Pt. tol. amb. c̄ asst. device c̄ mod. asst. of 1 while maintaining proper wt. bearing status. PT AM/PT PM Chair BID AM/PM P.T. BID AM/PM	GOAL: Pt. tol. CPM c̄ 5-10° advancement daily. PT AM/PT PM CPM at ___ degrees. GOAL: Pt. able to perform all TKR exercises c̄ verbal cues & 0-85° ROM activity. PT AM/PT PM GOAL: Pt. able to transfer to chair c̄ min. asst. of 1 while maintaining proper wt. bearing status. PT AM/PT PM GOAL: Pt. tol amb. c̄ asst. device c̄ min. asst. → verbal cues while maintaining proper wt. bearing status. PT AM/PT PM Chair BID AM/PM P.T. BID AM/PM
CIRCULATORY	GOAL: Absence of cardiac arrhythmia. D-E-N D/C telemetry GOAL: Maintain SBP > 90, DBP > 50, HR > 50. D-E-N VS q 4 hr. D-E-N GOAL: Pedal pulses 2+ and capillary refill < 3 sec. in operative leg. D-E-N Assess pedal pulses q 4 hr. D-E-N Assess capillary refill q 4 hr. D-E-N Assess temp. of extremities q 4 hr. D-E-N GOAL: No evidence of DVT, P.E. or fat emboli. D-E-N Athrombic device on D-E-N GOAL: Hct ≥ 30 Hct	GOAL: Maintain SBP > 90, DBP > 50, HR > 50. D-E-N VS q 4 hr. D-E-N GOAL: Pedal pulses 2+ and capillary refill < 3 sec. in operative leg. D-E-N Assess pedal pulses q shift. D-E-N Assess capillary refill q shift. D-E-N Assess temp. of extremities q shift. D-E-N GOAL: No evidence of DVT, P.E. or fat emboli. D-E-N Athrombic device on while in bed. D-E-N GOAL: Hct ≥ 30 Hct	GOAL: Pt. returns to pre-admission VS status. D-E-N VS q 4 hr. D-E-N GOAL: Pedal pulses 2+ and capillary refill < 3 sec. in operative leg. D-E-N Assess pedal pulses q shift. D-E-N Assess capillary refill q shift. D-E-N Assess temp. of extremities q shift. D-E-N GOAL: No evidence of DVT, P.E. or fat emboli. D-E-N Athrombic device on while in bed. D-E-N GOAL: Hct maintaining or increasing. Hct	GOAL: Pt. returns to pre-admission VS status. D-E-N VS q shift. D-E-N GOAL: Pedal pulses 2+ and capillary refill < 3 sec. in operative leg. D-E-N Assess pedal pulses q shift. D-E-N Assess capillary refill q shift. D-E-N Assess temp. of extremities q shift. D-E-N GOAL: No evidence of DVT, P.E. or fat emboli. D-E-N D/C athrombic device
NEUROLOGY	GOAL: No evidence of parasthesias or foot drop in operative leg. D-E-N Assess sensation in operative leg q 4 hr. D-E-N Assess Plantar/Dorsiflexion in operative leg q 4 hr. D-E-N	GOAL: No evidence of parasthesias or foot drop in operative leg. D-E-N Assess sensation in operative leg q shift. D-E-N Assess Plantar/Dorsiflexion in operative leg q shift. D-E-N	GOAL: No evidence of parasthesias or foot drop in operative leg. D-E-N Assess sensation in operative leg q shift. D-E-N Assess Plantar/Dorsiflexion in operative leg q shift. D-E-N	GOAL: No evidence of parasthesias or foot drop in operative leg. D-E-N Assess sensation in operative leg q shift. D-E-N Assess Plantar/Dorsiflexion in operative leg q shift. D-E-N
PULMONARY	GOAL: Adequate oxygenation AEB: clear breath sounds & resp. > 12 & < 26. D-E-N Assess for normal breathing patterns q shift. D-E-N Ausculate breath sounds q shift. D-E-N I/S q 2 hr. D-E-N CDB q 2 hr. D-E-N GOAL: Temp < 101.5 D-E-N Monitor temp q 4 hr. D-E-N	GOAL: Adequate oxygenation AEB: clear breath sounds & resp. > 12 & < 26. D-E-N Assess for normal breathing patterns q shift. D-E-N Ausculate breath sounds q shift. D-E-N I/S q 2 hr. D-E-N CDB q 2 hr. D-E-N GOAL: Temp < 101.5 D-E-N Monitor temp q 4 hr. D-E-N	GOAL: Lungs return to pre-surgical status. D-E-N Assess for normal breathing patterns q shift. D-E-N Ausculate breath sounds q shift. D-E-N I/S q 2 hr. D-E-N GOAL: Temp < 100. D-E-N Monitor temp q 4 hr. D-E-N	GOAL: Lungs return to pre-surgical status. D-E-N Assess for normal breathing patterns q shift. D-E-N Ausculate breath sounds q shift. D-E-N I/S q 2 hr. D-E-N GOAL: Temp < 100. D-E-N Monitor temp q shift. D-E-N
INTEGUMENTARY	GOAL: Drsg. dry & intact s̄ fresh drainage soaking through. D-E-N Incision & drain site covered. D-E-N GOAL: Absence of prolonged reddened areas. Skin intact. D-E-N Turn q 2 hr. D-E-N GOAL: IV site s̄ redness or swelling. D-E-N IV site care daily. GOAL: Drain < 200cc/shift. D-E-N Drain intact. D-E-N	GOAL: Wound s̄ redness, purulent drainage or excessive edema. D-E-N If drain d/c'd change drsg. c̄ sterile technique. GOAL: Absence of prolonged reddened areas. Skin intact. D-E-N Turn q 2 hr. D-E-N GOAL: IV site s̄ redness or swelling. D-E-N IV site care daily. GOAL: Drain < 50cc/shift. D-E-N Mon. & inform M.D. when goal achvd. to D/C drain.	GOAL: Wound s̄ redness, purulent drainage or excessive edema. D-E-N Change drsg. daily c̄ sterile technique. GOAL: Absence of prolonged reddened areas. Skin intact. D-E-N Turn q 2 hr. while in bed. D-E-N D/C IVF's if PCA/epidural D/cd.	GOAL: Wound s̄ redness, purulent drainage or excessive edema. D-E-N Change drsg. daily c̄ sterile technique. GOAL: Absence of prolonged reddened areas. Skin intact. D-E-N Turn q 2 hr. D-E-N
NUTRITION ELIMINATION	GOAL: Maintain adequate fluid balance. D-E-N IVF's infusing. D-E-N I & O q shift. D-E-N GOAL: Returns to pre-surgical diet. D-E-N GOAL: UOP ≥ 240cc/shift. D-E-N Monitor foley drainage q shift. D-E-N	GOAL: Maintain adequate fluid balance. D-E-N D/C IVF's. I & O q shift. D-E-N GOAL: Returns to pre-surgical diet. D-E-N GOAL: UOP ≥ 240cc/shift. D-E-N D/C foley	GOAL: Maintain adequate fluid balance. D-E-N D/C I/O GOAL: Returns to pre-surgical diet. D-E-N GOAL: Pt. has BM LOC PRN	GOAL: Returns to pre-surgical diet. D-E-N GOAL: Returns to pre-surgical bowel patterns.
PSYCHO-SOCIAL	GOAL: Pt. will verbalize anxiety R/T hosp. stay. Consult Chaplain, prn.	GOAL: Begin home care/community resource arrangements. Consult DPN Assess pt., explain options & initiate post-op placement. DPN		GOAL: Pt. verbalizes readiness to transfer to rehab unit. D/C to PMRU, if applicable. (Have up by 12 noon)
KNOWLEDGE DEFICIT	Reinforce use of I/S	GOAL: Pt. verbalizes understanding of the need to maintain hip precautions during ADL's & transfers. Instruct pt. in ADL's & home care. OT Instruct pt. in transfers & ambulation. PT Reinforce use of I/S	GOAL: Pt. verbalizes understanding of po method of pain control. Instruct on po pain control, includes S.E.	

M-94-5276-2 (F) REV. 12/8/94   P

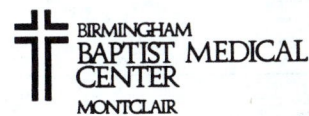

BIRMINGHAM BAPTIST MEDICAL CENTER
MONTCLAIR

Coordinated CareMap®
CASE TYPE – TOTAL KNEE REPLACEMENT
Key: *Highlight completed task.*
Address variances in nurses' focus notes and circle in red.
Once variances completed - highlight and date.

PAGE 4

	POD 5	POD 6	POD 7	POD 8
	DATE/INT. ____	DATE/INT. ____	DATE/INT. ____	DATE/INT. ____
PAIN	GOAL: Pt. verbalizes pain at level ≤ 5. D-E-N	GOAL: Pt. verbalizes pain at level ≤ 5. D-E-N	GOAL: Pt. verbalizes pain at level ≤ 4. D-E-N	GOAL: Pt. verbalizes pain at level ≤ 4. D-E-N
	PO pain meds. D-E-N	PO pain meds. D-E-N	PO pain meds. D-E-N	PO pain meds. D-E-N
MUSCULOSKELETAL	GOAL: Pt. tol.CPM c 5-10° advancement daily. PT AM/PT PM CPM at ___ degrees. GOAL: I c all TKR exercises & 0-90° ROM actively. PT AM/PT PM GOAL: I c all transfers while maintaining proper wt. bearing status. PT AM/PT PM GOAL: I c amb. c asst. device while maintaining proper wt. bearing status. PT AM/PT PM	GOAL: Pt. tol.CPM c 5-10° advancement daily. PT AM/PT PM CPM at ___ degrees. GOAL: I c all TKR exercises & 0-90° ROM actively. PT AM/PT PM GOAL: I c all transfers while maintaining proper wt. bearing status. PT AM/PT PM GOAL: I c amb. c asst. device while maintaining proper wt. bearing status. PT AM/PT PM	GOAL: Pt. tol.CPM c 5-10° advancement daily. PT AM/PT PM CPM at ___ degrees. GOAL: I c all TKR exercises & 0-90° ROM actively. PT AM/PT PM GOAL: I c all transfers while maintaining proper wt. bearing status. PT AM/PT PM GOAL: I c amb. c asst. device while maintaining proper wt. bearing status. PT AM/PT PM	GOAL: Pt. tol.CPM c 5-10° advancement daily. PT AM/PT PM CPM at ___ degrees. GOAL: I c all TKR exercises & 0-90° ROM actively. PT AM/PT PM GOAL: I c all transfers while maintaining proper wt. bearing status. PT AM/PT PM GOAL: I c amb. c asst. device while maintaining proper wt. bearing status. PT AM/PT PM
	Chair BID AM/PM P.T. BID AM/PM	Chair BID AM/PM P.T. BID AM/PM	Chair BID AM/PM P.T. BID AM/PM	Chair BID AM/PM P.T. BID AM/PM
CIRCULATORY	GOAL: Pt. returns to pre-surgical VS status. D-E-N VS q shift. D-E-N GOAL: Pedal pulses 2+ and capillary refill < 3 sec. in operative leg. D-E-N Assess pedal pulses q shift. D-E-N Assess capillary refill q shift. D-E-N Assess temp. of extremities q shift. D-E-N GOAL: No evidence of DVT, P.E. or fat emboli. D-E-N Assess calf q shift. D-E-N	GOAL: Pt. returns to pre-surgical VS status. D-E-N VS q shift. D-E-N GOAL: Pedal pulses 2+ and capillary refill < 3 sec. in operative leg. D-E-N Assess pedal pulses q shift. D-E-N Assess capillary refill q shift. D-E-N Assess temp. of extremities q shift. D-E-N GOAL: No evidence of DVT, P.E. or fat emboli. D-E-N Assess calf q shift. D-E-N	GOAL: Pt. returns to pre-surgical VS status. D-E-N VS q shift. D-E-N GOAL: Pedal pulses 2+ and capillary refill < 3 sec. in operative leg. D-E-N Assess pedal pulses q shift. D-E-N Assess capillary refill q shift. D-E-N Assess temp. of extremities q shift. D-E-N GOAL: No evidence of DVT, P.E. or fat emboli. D-E-N Assess calf q shift. D-E-N	GOAL: Pt. returns to pre-surgical VS status. D-E-N VS q shift. D-E-N GOAL: Pedal pulses 2+ and capillary refill < 3 sec. in operative leg. D-E-N Assess pedal pulses q shift. D-E-N Assess capillary refill q shift. D-E-N Assess temp. of extremities q shift. D-E-N GOAL: No evidence of DVT, P.E. or fat emboli. D-E-N Assess calf q shift. D-E-N
NEUROLOGY	GOAL: No evidence of parasthesias or foot drop in operative leg. D-E-N Assess sensation in operative leg q shift. D-E-N Assess Plantar/Dorsiflexion in operative leg q shift. D-E-N	GOAL: No evidence of parasthesias or foot drop in operative leg. D-E-N Assess sensation in operative leg q shift. D-E-N Assess Plantar/Dorsiflexion in operative leg q shift. D-E-N	GOAL: No evidence of parasthesias or foot drop in operative leg. D-E-N Assess sensation in operative leg q shift. D-E-N Assess Plantar/Dorsiflexion in operative leg q shift. D-E-N	GOAL: No evidence of parasthesias or foot drop in operative leg. D-E-N Assess sensation in operative leg q shift. D-E-N Assess Plantar/Dorsiflexion in operative leg q shift. D-E-N
PULMONARY	GOAL: Lungs return to pre-surgical status. D-E-N Assess for normal breathing patterns q shift. D-E-N Ausculate breath sounds q shift. D-E-N I/S q 2 hr., w.a. D-E-N GOAL: Temp < 100. D-E-N Temp q shift. D-E-N	GOAL: Lungs return to pre-surgical status. D-E-N Assess for normal breathing patterns q shift. D-E-N Ausculate breath sounds q shift. D-E-N I/S q 2 hr., w.a. D-E-N GOAL: Temp < 100. D-E-N Temp q shift. D-E-N	GOAL: Lungs return to pre-surgical status. D-E-N Assess for normal breathing patterns q shift. D-E-N Ausculate breath sounds q shift. D-E-N I/S q 2 hr., w.a. D-E-N GOAL: Temp < 100. D-E-N Temp q shift. D-E-N	GOAL: Lungs return to pre-surgical status. D-E-N Assess for normal breathing patterns q shift. D-E-N Ausculate breath sounds q shift. D-E-N I/S q 2 hr., w.a. D-E-N GOAL: Temp < 100. D-E-N Temp q shift. D-E-N
INTEGUMENTARY	GOAL: Wound s redness, purulent drainage or excessive edema. D-E-N Change drsg. daily c sterile technique. GOAL: Absence of prolonged reddened areas. Skin intact. D-E-N Turn q 2 hr. while in bed. D-E-N	GOAL: Wound s redness, purulent drainage or excessive edema. D-E-N Change drsg. daily c sterile technique. GOAL: Absence of prolonged reddened areas. Skin intact. D-E-N Turn q 2 hr. while in bed. D-E-N	GOAL: Wound s redness, purulent drainage or excessive edema. D-E-N Change drsg. daily c sterile technique. GOAL: Absence of prolonged reddened areas. Skin intact. D-E-N Turn q 2 hr. while in bed. D-E-N	GOAL: Wound s redness, purulent drainage or excessive edema. D-E-N Change drsg. daily c sterile technique. GOAL: Absence of prolonged reddened areas. Skin intact. D-E-N Turn q 2 hr. while in bed. D-E-N
NUTRITION ELIMINATION	GOAL: Returns to pre-surgical diet. D-E GOAL: Returns to pre-surgical bowel patterns.	GOAL: Returns to pre-surgical diet. D-E GOAL: Returns to pre-surgical bowel patterns.	GOAL: Returns to pre-surgical diet. D-E GOAL: Returns to pre-surgical bowel patterns.	GOAL: Returns to pre-surgical diet. D-E GOAL: Returns to pre-surgical bowel patterns.
PSYCHO-SOCIAL				GOAL: Pt. verbalizes readiness to go home.
KNOWLEDGE DEFICIT	GOAL: Family/S.O. involved in pt.'s care Family/S.O. to go to P.T. c pt. for home care instructions. Family/S.O. to go to P.T. c pt. for home care instructions.			GOAL: Pt. verbalizes understanding of D/C instructions.

Adapted from CareMap® System, The Center for Case Management

M-94-5276-2 (B) REV. 12/8/94   P

Appendix D12: TURP

CARE MAP

TURP

EST. LOS 4 DAYS

DAY # 1   **HOSP. DAY # ____**   **POST OP. DAY # ____**

DATE: ___/___/___

GOALS: VERBALIZES PRE/POST-OP ROUTINES

CONSULTS	**DIET**	**ACTIVITY**	**TEST**
ANESTHESIA ____	REGULAR ____	AD LIB ____	RENAL I&II + GLU ____
SOCIAL SERVICE ____	NPO AFTER MN ____		CBC W/DIFF ____
			PT & PTT ____
			T&H ____
			U/A URINE C&S ____
MEDS	**EQUIPMENT**		EKG ____
	VOLUREX ____		CXR ____

TREATMENTS	**D/C PLAN**	**TEACHING**
VS Q SHIFT ____	ASSESSMENT ____	VOLUREX ____
ADMISSION ASSESS PER STANDARD ____		TCH PLAN:PREOP SURG ____
THERAPY		FOLEY CATH/OHI ____

ADDITIONAL NARRATIVE _____

_____

_____

_____

_____

_____

NAME	INITIAL	NAME	INITIAL

CARE MAP

TURP

EST. LOS 4 DAYS

DAY # 2 DAY OF SURGERY　　　　　HOSP. DAY # ____　　　　　POST OP. DAY # ____

DATE: ___/___/___

GOALS: VERBALIZES SATISFACTORY COMFORT
　　　　　STABLE HEMODYNAMICS

CONSULTS	DIET	ACTIVITY	TEST
	CL. LIQ ADV. TO REG. IF TOL. ____	BEDREST 6–8HR ____	
		THEN OOB WITH ASSISTANCE ____	

MEDS　　　　　　　　　　　**EQUIPMENT**

IV　　　　　　　　____　　　VOLUREX ____

ANTIBIOTICS　　　____　　　OHI　　　____

ANTISPASMODICS　____

PAIN MEDS　　　　____

STOOL SOFTENER ____

TREATMENTS　　　　　　　**D/C PLAN**　　　　　　　**TEACHING**

VS Q4H　　　　　　　____

OHI TO KEEP URINE
　　PINK　　　　　　____

HAND IRRIGATE
　　FOLEY PRN　　____

VOLUREX Q4H　　____

THERAPY

ADDITIONAL NARRATIVE _____

_____

_____

_____

NAME	INITIAL	NAME	INITIAL

CARE MAP

TURP

EST. LOS 4 DAYS

DAY # 3   **HOSP. DAY # ____**   **POST OP. DAY # ____**

DATE: ___/___/___

GOALS: RESOLVE ACUTE HEMATURIA
INDEPENDENT AMBULATION

CONSULTS	**DIET**	**ACTIVITY**	**TEST**
	REGULAR ____	AMBULATE IN HALL ____	CBC ____
			RENAL1&11+GLU ____

MEDS   **EQUIPMENT**

PAIN MEDS   ____   VOLUREX ____

ANTIBIOTICS   ____   OHI   ____

ANTISPASMODICS ____

STOOL SOFTENER ____

TREATMENTS   **D/C PLAN**   **TEACHING**

VS Q SHIFT   ____   MEDS   ____

CLAMP OHI PER HO ____   ACTIVITY RESTRICTIONS ____

OHI PRN HEMATURIA ____

VOLUREX Q4H
HEP LOC. IV   ____

THERAPY

ADDITIONAL NARRATIVE _____

_____

_____

_____

_____

_____

NAME	INITIAL	NAME	INITIAL

CARE MAP

TURP

EST. LOS 4 DAYS

DAY # 4   **HOSP. DAY #** ____   **POST OP. DAY #** ____

DATE: ___/___/___

GOALS: VOIDING INDEPENDENTLY W/O SIGNS OR SYMPTOMS OF INFECTION OR RETENTION

CONSULTS	**DIET**	**ACTIVITY**	**TEST**
	REGULAR ____	AD LIB ____	

MEDS   **EQUIPMENT**

PAIN MEDS ____

ANTIBIOTICS ____

STOOL SOFTENER ____

TREATMENTS	**D/C PLAN**	**TEACHING**
D/C FOLEY PER HO ____	DISCHARGE ____	S/SX INFECTION ____
SERIAL URINES ____		ACTIVITY RESTRICTIONS ____
VS Q SHIFT ____		RECURRENT HEMATURIA ____
D/C HEP LOC. ____		

THERAPY

ADDITIONAL NARRATIVE _____

_____

_____

_____

_____

_____

_____

NAME	INITIAL	NAME	INITIAL

Appendix C13: Orchiectomy

CRITICAL PATH

SIMPLE ORCHIECTOMY
PROSTATIC CA

EST. LOS 3 DAYS

DAY # 1   **HOSP. DAY # ____**   **POST OP. DAY # ____**

DATE: ___/___/___

GOALS: Verbalizes pre & post op routines. ____

CONSULTS	**DIET**	**ACTIVITY**	**TEST**
ANESTHESIA ____	REGULAR ____	AD LIB ____	CBC/DIFF
	NPO @ MN ____		RENAL 1
			GLUCOSE
			PT/PTT
			U/A
MEDS	**EQUIPMENT**	**THERAPY**	CXR
			EKG

TREATMENTS	**D/C PLAN**	**TEACHING**	
ADM. ASSESS ____		S/SX INFECTION ____	
VS Q SHIFT ____		REQUESTING PAIN MEDS ____	
ASSESS PAIN STATUS ____			
ASSESS VOIDING ____			

ADDITIONAL NARRATIVE _____

_____

_____

_____

_____

_____

NAME	INITIAL	NAME	INITIAL

CRITICAL PATH

SIMPLE ORCHIECTOMY
PROSTATIC CA

EST. LOS 3 DAYS

DAY # Day of Surgery   HOSP. DAY # ____   POST OP. DAY # ____

DATE: ___/___/___

GOALS: STABILIZE HEMODYNAMICS ____

VERBALIZES SATISFACTORY COMFORT ____

CONSULTS	DIET	ACTIVITY	TEST
	CL. LIQ ____	OOB W/ ASST. ____	
	ADV. TO REG. ____		

MEDS	EQUIPMENT	THERAPY
PAIN MEDS ____		
ANTIBIOTICS ____		

TREATMENTS	D/C PLAN	TEACHING
VS Q4H ____		
ASSESS WD. DRAINAGE ____		
ASSESS VOIDING ____		

ADDITIONAL NARRATIVE _____

_____

_____

_____

_____

_____

_____

NAME	INITIAL	NAME	INITIAL

CRITICAL PATH

SIMPLE ORCHIECTOMY
PROSTATIC CA

EST. LOS 3 DAYS

DAY # 3   **HOSP. DAY #** _____   **POST OP. DAY #** _____

DATE: ___/___/___

GOALS: Verbalizes discharge instructions. _____

CONSULTS	DIET	ACTIVITY	TEST
	REGULAR _____	AD LIB _____	

MEDS	EQUIPMENT	THERAPY
Pain meds _____		

TREATMENTS	D/C PLAN	TEACHING
VS Q SHIFT _____	D/C TO HOME _____	REVIEW S/SX INFECTION _____
APPLY DRY DRESSING _____		TEACH D/C MEDS _____
		NO STRENUOUS ACT./ LIFTING FOR 2 WEEKS _____
		SHOWERS ONLY x 1 WEEK _____

ADDITIONAL NARRATIVE _____

_____

_____

_____

_____

_____

_____

NAME	INITIAL	NAME	INITIAL

Appendix C14: Mastectomy

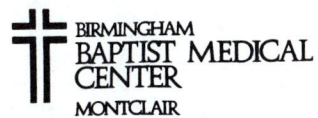 **BIRMINGHAM BAPTIST MEDICAL CENTER** MONTCLAIR

Coordinated CareMap®
CASE TYPE – MASTECTOMY
DRG – 257, 258
Key: *Highlight completed tasks.*
Address variances in nurses' focus notes in red.

PATIENT PROBLEM	PAT — Date/Init.	EMA — Date/Init.
CARDIO-PULMONARY Altered hemodynamics R/T surgery	**GOAL: NSR on EKG** Assess C/P status EKG, if > 40 yrs. & not done in past 30 days. CBC Survey 27 Chest X-ray	**GOAL: NSR on EKG** Assess C/P status EKG, if > 40 yrs. & not done in past 30 days.
Increased risk for atelectasis R/T surgery.	**GOAL: Verbalizes understanding of post-op pulmonary toilet regimen.** Instruct re T, C, DB	Instruct re T, C, DB
Increased risk for DVT & PTE.	**GOAL: Verbalizes understanding of TED stockings & SCD.** Instruct re TEDS & SCD.	**GOAL: Maintains adequate venous return.** Apply TEDS. Apply SCD per MD order.
FLUID BALANCE Risk for altered fluid balance/diet.	**GOAL: Verbalizes understanding pre-op NPO instructions.** Instruct re NPO. **GOAL: Verbalizes understanding post-op diet progression.** Instruct re post-op diet regimen.	**GOAL: Compliance c NPO pre-op status** NPO
PAIN Alteration in comfort R/T surgery.	**GOAL: Verbalizes understanding of pain management.** Discuss pain management vs. absence of pain.	**GOAL: Verbalizes understanding of pain management.** Discuss pain management vs. absence of pain.
INTEGUMENTARY Potential for infection at op site and/or drain site.	**GOAL: Verbalizes understanding of incision location & purpose of drains.** Instruct re surgical incision & post-op drains.	**GOAL: Verbalizes understanding of incision location & purpose of drains.** Reinforce pre-op instruction.
ACTIVITY Alteration in mobility R/T surgical procedure. Self-care deficit R/T decreased mobility & pain c movement.	**GOAL: Verbalizes understanding of post-op activity progression & restrictions.** Instruct re plan of post-op activity/mobility restrictions c progression.	
PSYCHOSOCIAL/SPIRITUAL Fear R/T Cancer dx & future implications. Fear R/T change in sexual self concept.	**GOAL: Verbally acknowledges feelings of anxiety R/T surgery.** Encourage expression of feelings. Assess pt./family support system. Discuss available inpt. support services, i.e. social service, pastoral care.	**GOAL: Verbally acknowledges feelings of anxiety R/T surgery.** Encourage expression of feelings. Pastoral care visit.
KNOWLEDGE DEFICIT R/T surgical procedure R/T pre-op preparation	**GOAL: Verbalizes understanding of EMA admitting process & surgical procedure.** Instruct re admission process & pre-op procedures. Instruct re use of home meds.	**GOAL: Verbalizes understanding of EMA admitting process & surgical procedure.** Reinforce instructions.
R/T acquisition of prosthesis	**GOAL: Verbalize understanding of plan for prosthesis acquisition.** Notify Reach for Recovery. Instruct re available resources i.e. financial	
R/T discharge/home care	Notify Breast Care Team.	

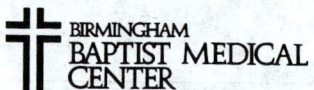

BIRMINGHAM BAPTIST MEDICAL CENTER
MONTCLAIR

Coordinated CareMap®
CASE TYPE – MASTECTOMY
DRG – 257, 258
Key: Highlight completed tasks.
Address variances in nurses' focus notes in red.

(Addressograph)

DAY OF SURGERY	POD 1	POD 2
Date/Init. _____	Date/Init. _____	Date/Init. _____
GOAL: SBP > 90, DBP > 50, HR > 50, R > 12. VS q 15 min. x 4 q 30 min. x 2, q 1 h x 4, q 4 h. D-E-N	**GOAL: SBP > 90, DBP > 50, HR > 50, R > 12.** VS q 4 h. D-E-N	**GOAL: SBP > 90, DBP > 50, HR > 50, R > 12.** VS q 8 h. D-E-N
GOAL: Clear bilateral lung sounds. Auscultate lungs q 8 hr. D-E-N Assist c T, C, DB q 2 hr x 4, D-E-N	**GOAL: Clear bilateral lung sounds.** Auscultate lungs q 8 hr. D-E-N	
GOAL: No s/s of DVT or PTE. Apply TEDS. D-E-N Apply SCD per MD order. D-E-N Assess L.E. for temp redness & calf tenderness q 8 hr. D-E-N Dangle & OOB with help 4-6 hrs. post-op. D-E-N	**GOAL: No s/s of DVT or PTE.** Remove TEDS for bath then reapply. Maintain SCD when in bed. D-E-N **GOAL: Independent ambulation q.i.d.** Assist with first walk in hall then amb. q.i.d. D-E-N	**GOAL: No s/s of DVT or PTE.** Remove TEDS for bath then reapply. D/C SCD. **GOAL: Compliance with ambulation.** Up ad lib. Assess compliance. D-E-N
GOAL: Tolerates 500cc p.o. q 8 hrs. post-op s N & V. Sips of clear liquid. Advance diet as tol. Measure & record amt. q 8 hrs: Heplock IV or maintain IV KVO if PCA. D-E-N **GOAL: Voids freely, UOP = 250cc q 8 h x 24 hr** Measure & record UOP q 8 hr. D-E-N	**GOAL: Tolerates regular diet.** Regular diet. Record % taken. D-E Encourages 6-8 glasses fluids per 24 hr. D-E-N **GOAL: Voids freely, UOP = 250cc q 8 h x 24 hr.** Measure & record UOP q 8 hr. D-E-N	**GOAL: Tolerates regular diet.** Regular diet. Record % taken. D-E Encourages 6-8 glasses fluids per 24 hr. **GOAL: Voids freely, UOP = 250cc q 8 h x 24 hr.** Measure & record UOP q 8 hr. D-E-N
GOAL: Pain controlled at level < 7. Assess pain level q 4 hr. D-E-N Reinforce instructions R/T PCA pump mgt. if ordered. Elevate arm on operative side on 1-2 pillows. D-E-N	**GOAL: Pain controlled c p.o. meds & s adverse drug reactions.** Assess pain level q 4 hr. D-E-N Offer p.o. analgesics prn. D/C PCA pump if ordered. Elevate arm on operative side on 1-2 pillows. D-E-N	**GOAL: Pain controlled c p.o. meds & s adverse drug reactions.** Assess pain level q 4 hr. D-E-N Offer p.o. analgesics prn. Elevate arm on operative side on 1-2 pillows. D-E-N
GOAL: Dressing dry & intact. Assess dressing q 4 hr. Reinforce prn. D-E-N	**GOAL: Dressing dry & intact.** Assess dressing q 4 hr. Reinforce prn. D-E-N	**GOAL: Wound s s/s of infection.** Dressing change per MD.
GOAL: Drains patent & compressed. Assess drains for patency and compression q 2 hr. x 4 D-E-N Measure & record drainage q 8 hr. & prn. D-E-N	**GOAL: Drains patent & compressed.** Assess drains for patency and compression q 2 hr. x 4 D-E-N Measure & record drainage q 8 hr. & prn. D-E-N	**GOAL: Drains patent & compressed.** Measure and record drainage q 8 hr. & prn. D-E-N **GOAL: Describe s/s of infection.** Instruct re s/s of infection c patient & significant other.
GOAL: Compliant c activity restrictions. Encourage arm activity within levels of comfort or as ordered per MD. D-E-N	**GOAL: Compliant c post mastectomy exercise regimen.** Instruct re limitations & restrictions. **GOAL: Participates in self-care activities.** Assess need for assistance c bath.	**GOAL: Compliant c post mastectomy exercise regimen.** Reinforce instructions. **GOAL: Perform ADL c minimal assistance.** Assess need for assistance c bath.
GOAL: Verbalizes thoughts/feelings re surgery & future implications. Encourage expression of thoughts & feelings. D-E-N Assess need for inpt. support services. D-E-N	**GOAL: Verbalizes thoughts/feelings re surgery & future implications.** Encourage expression of thoughts & feelings. D-E-N Assess need for inpt. support services. D-E-N	**GOAL: Verbalizes thoughts/feelings re surgery & future implications.** Encourage expression of thoughts & feelings. D-E-N Assess need for inpt. support services. D-E-N **GOAL: Verbalizes feelings of self-worth.** Actively listen. Provide positive reinforcement. D-E-N Instruct re post-op support services.
GOAL: Decreased anxiety R/T post-op process & procedures. Reinforce pre-op teachings. D-E-N Instruct re post-op process. D-E-N Notify surgical CNS. D-E-N Notify Case Coordinator. D-E-N	**GOAL: Verbalizes understanding of post-op drain management.** Instruct & demonstrate drain management.	**GOAL: Patient or significant other demonstrates ability to manage drain.** Reinforce instructions of POD 1. D-E-N Provide measuring cup. Observe technique.
	GOAL: Verbalize understanding of BSE post-op. Instruct re BSE of operative site.	**GOAL: Verbalize understanding of plan for medical follow-up.** Review discharge instructions.

Coordinated CareMap® – MASTECTOMY
Adapted from CareMap® System, The Center for Case Management

M-94-5279 (B) REV. 12/9/94 P

Discussion of "Thinking Critically" Exercises

Chapter 15

1. Because the client has a suspected influenza virus, a private room should be assigned and strict isolation should be initiated until the diagnosis is ruled out. Although a thorough nursing history is important, priority assessments include checking the level of consciousness and cardiac function, because brain and cardiac changes will indicate the seriousness of the fluid and electrolyte losses and direct the nature and speed of intervention. Interventions should focus on replacement and prevention of further fluid and electrolyte losses. Ensure that the intravenous line is patent and flowing at the prescribed rate. An antiemetic should be given intravenously for the most immediate effect. Give an acetaminophen suppository to decrease fever and prevent secondary fluid loss from diaphoresis. If diarrhea persists, give an antidiarrheal medication as soon as the client can retain clear liquids. An intravenous antibiotic may also be prescribed. Consult the physician for any of the above prescriptions as necessary. Continue to monitor the client's response to treatment. If the client's level of consciousness or dysrhythmia worsens, consult the physician immediately. More aggressive fluid and electrolyte replacement with cardiac monitoring may be necessary.

2. The client who has a third-space fluid shift must be monitored closely for presence of hypovolemia and hypervolemia. When fluids shift from the vascular space to the interstitial space, the client may become hypovolemic; when the fluid shifts back to the vascular space, the client may become hypervolemic. Thus, intravenous administration must be closely monitored. Vital signs, skin checks for dehydration and edema, level-of-consciousness monitoring, and the hematocrit levels in relation to the hemoglobin levels must be monitored. Assess breath sounds and urine output. The frequency of these assessments is dictated by the physical condition and mental status of the client and are performed hourly to every 4 to 8 hours.

Chapter 16

1. "Eyeballing" the pH reveals acidemia, and the low HCO_3^- indicates metabolic acidosis. The degree of decrease in the PCO_2 is consistent with partial compensation. The client's diabetes and recent diarrhea could both be contributory to metabolic acidosis, but the type of diabetes must be considered. Calculation of the anion gap would also be helpful. Considering her loss of intestinal fluid over the past week as well as the effects of hydrogen ion imbalance on other cations, electrolytes should be monitored carefully. Closely monitor electrolytes for which imbal-

ances may result in life-threatening complications.

2. The pH represents alkalemia, and the low PCO_2 is consistent with respiratory alkalosis. The client's rapid pulse and diaphoresis might suggest gastrointestinal bleeding—a risk given his history—but assessment of blood pressure and hydration status would tend to refute this as the immediate problem. Also, blood loss would promote metabolic *acidosis*, inconsistent with the pH. The circumstances surrounding the episode suggest an anxiety-induced imbalance. The nurse should consider intervening immediately (if emergency department protocol permits) to increase the client's PCO_2 and relieve symptoms. Educational intervention or referral aimed at reducing the risk of recurrent anxiety should also be considered.

3. The slightly acidemic pH and elevated PCO_2 indicate respiratory acidosis that is fully compensated. Given the client's history, it is likely that this is a chronic condition, but this could be confirmed with use of an acid-base map and access to prior ABG analyses. Whether the lung fluid represents congestive heart failure or pneumonia, the client is at risk for worsening respiratory status. You must carefully monitor his oxygenation status, and if oxygen therapy is started, you must closely monitor his ventilatory response. Cardiac failure and chronic respiratory failure often coexist, and diuretic therapy instituted for congestive heart failure could further complicate the electrolyte and acid-base picture. Serum potassium could be elevated or decreased, and serum values may not be representative of total body potassium. Monitoring of the electrocardiogram would be helpful in detecting cardiac effects of potassium imbalance.

Chapter 17

1. A thorough pain history along with neurologic checks should be completed. Be sure to include a history of migraine headaches and any neurologic or sensory disturbances that will help differentiate between a chronic and an acute disorder. Until an acute event such as a cerebral hemorrhage or a brain tumor is ruled out, nursing interventions should be directed at providing comfort measures and expediting any diagnostic tests that are ordered.

2. The client and family are taught the complications of opiate analgesia (respiratory depression, circulatory depression, constipation, paresthesia, and physical dependence and addiction). They should be able to assess the client for any complications while understanding the effect the medication may have on an elderly person. A member of a pain

management team, the nurse, the client, and family may work together to manage pain in a satisfactory manner in collaboration with the physician. Consideration is given to the client's wishes when developing a dosing schedule such as may be ordered for breakthrough pain. Although the caregiver has a record of when the medication was administered, the family may not always be aware of the most recent time of medication administration. The nurse should check for client response to pain (effectiveness, associated side effects, complications). The family may also be taught response time of the medication as well as the expected and unexpected side effects and what to do should the side effects occur. It would be helpful to teach the family about pain assessment, especially if some medications are ordered as needed.

Chapter 18

1. The first step is to find out what product the client has been using from the health food store. You will also want to know how much she has been taking, for how long, and in what quantity. The next step is to find the answer to her question. It will be important to consider the mechanism of action, side effects and contraindications for the prescribed medication and for the herbal remedy, as well as the client's beliefs about their effectiveness. You could refer the question back to the person who gave her the prescription. It may be useful to consult a pharmacist, a specialist in alternative therapies, or the research literature about the respective substances. You and the client will need to decide together how to approach the problem and what role, if any, you will take in that decision. Whatever the eventual strategy, the important considerations here are safety and empowerment toward self-care management.

2. The elderly client would most likely develop sensory deprivation related to his physical illness and environmental limitations. There is a remote possibility that the younger man could develop sensory overload, depending on the nature of the head injury. The nurse should assess both clients for behavioral changes, physical changes, and changes in sleep patterns. Because prevention is important, the nurse should adjust the environment to provide stimulation (for sensory deprivation) or decrease stimulation (for sensory overload). For example, the elderly client should be encouraged to look outside as much as possible, and his family and friends should be encouraged to visit. Family and friends should also be encouraged to communicate with a client who has had a stroke. The client might also be moved to a room closer to the nurses' station where the extra activity

can stimulate his environment. If sensory overload occurs in the younger client, the number of visitors at a time should be limited. The duration and loudness of the radio and television should be monitored.

3. A thorough sleep assessment should be completed and compared to the sleep pattern disturbance present before the pregnancy began. The nurse should explore the possibility of a dependency on sleep medication with the client and try to determine what helps or hinders sleep. Perhaps the same problems are persisting and are compounded by the needs of the two babies. The mother's lack of sleep may interfere with her ability to care for the children and assume her previous role (e.g., wife, mother to other children, caretaker, professional, student). The mother may not have confidence in her ability to care for a family, may have unfulfilled needs and wants, and may simply not know how to handle the situation without the use of medication. After a discussion of sleep routines and any necessary teaching, the client should be asked to return for an evaluation. If the sleep disturbance persists, the client should be referred to the appropriate healthcare provider, such as a sleep clinic, for further evaluation.

Chapter 20

1. Red, lumpy tissue is granulation tissue and indicates that the ulcer is healing. The wound should be covered with a moisture-retentive dressing, such as a hydrocolloid dressing. Use of the wet-to-dry dressings should be stopped.

2. Because emergency surgery was required, there was no time to adequately prepare the client for the prolonged period of not eating after surgery. Because he was malnourished before the operation, he is at increased risk of delayed healing as a result of decreased protein calorie intake and increased risk of infection. Without increased nutritional support healing will not occur. The physician needs to be approached about hyperalimentation until the client's gastrointestinal function has returned.

In addition, 3 L of intravenous (IV) fluids per day may place him into fluid overload. Lung sounds, heart sounds, and urine output will need to be closely monitored. The IV potassium will be required until he is taking oral feedings (or placed on hyperalimentation). His IV site will need to be assessed often; IV potassium is an irritant and the IV site can quickly develop phlebitis.

Ideal body weight for a 5'5" man is around 130 lb. He is markedly underweight. He also more than likely does not have a layer of fat over his bony prominences and is at high risk for pressure ulcer formation. He will need a pressure-reduction mattress and frequent turning to reduce his risk of pressure ulcers. Long-term dietary management will be needed. You may want to contact social services and/or investigate shelters and soup kitchens in his area.

Chapter 21

1. The client should be taught how to cough, deep breathe, and turn and move the extremities. Ask for a quick demonstration at this time and remind the client to hold a pillow (to act as a splint) against the incision when coughing. The client will be concerned about pain after the surgery and will also want to know about length of stay. Without complications, the client will most likely be discharged the following day. Teach about the availability of pain medication as needed, and that the client should ask for medication should pain occur. Preoperative measures include documentation of vital signs, results of completed blood studies, record of medication administered preoperatively, presence of an intravenous line, time of last voiding, shave preparation (this may also be completed in the operating room), the presence of capped teeth or dentures, the presence of a hearing aid, and other information deemed necessary by the institution. To accomplish this in a short time, a team approach to care is practiced.

2. Common problems in the older adult, such as diabetes mellitus, anemia, malnutrition, dehydration, and atherosclerosis, may have an impact on the course of recovery and should be considered when planning care. Generally, the immune system does not function effectively, so the client may be at risk for a wound infection. Fluid and electrolyte imbalances occur frequently in older adults, so intravenous fluids and electrolyte replacement therapy are initiated and followed by oral hydration. The gastrointestinal system of older adults may be sluggish, and the effects of the general anesthesia may result in constipation. The effects of the anesthesia may also produce weakness, and the client may not have strength to cough, deep breathe, and move the extremities in bed as often as possible. You should be alert to possible complications through ongoing assessment of the client's progress. Older persons may deny that pain is present or may not feel pain as acutely as a younger person. You should perform ongoing pain assessments so that medication therapy can be initiated in a timely manner. Age-related changes in body functioning should be considered during all stages of the nursing process, especially when caring for elderly or compromised clients.

Chapter 22

1. In considering this problem, the priority assessments are airway and breathing. The client has a gunshot wound to the chest and may have a pneumothorax, hemothorax, or both; he will need supportive interventions such as oxygen supplementation and chest tube placement. The next priority is cardiovascular status. He has probably experienced profound hemorrhage and will need rapid fluid replacement. To accomplish rapid fluid resuscitation, a peripheral intravenous line using a 14- or 16-gauge needle or a central line will be placed for administration of isotonic solutions, plasma expanders, and blood. Continuous assessment of respiratory and cardiovascular status is imperative for this client. Prepare for surgical intervention to repair the damage from the gunshot wound and stop the bleeding.

2. Initial admission information from the client's family suggests problems with oxygenation and perfusion. To evaluate what might be happening to him, a thorough assessment of respiratory and cardiovascular status should be performed. Consideration should also be given to the fact that he had abdominal surgery during which the abdominal cavity was exposed to the contents of the colon. In addition to the bacterial exposure that occurred during surgery, the client's age suggests decreased immune system functioning, which indicates increased risk for infection. Performing blood cultures may help to determine the presence of systemic bacteremia. The nurse should anticipate the need for cardiac monitoring, oxygen saturation monitoring, and the provision of supplemental oxygen.

3. Priority assessments always begin with the ABCs. Once the nurse has determined that the client's airway is open and that supplemental oxygen has been provided, detailed assessment of his cardiovascular status should be made. If a Swan-Ganz catheter is not already in place, one will be inserted to allow evaluation of cardiac output and other hemodynamic parameters. Considering the client's cardiac history, fluid resuscitation would not be the first intervention. His cardiovascular status is not a result of hypovolemia, but rather a result of failure of the heart's pumping ability. Interventions that would be most helpful at this point are those that support cardiac function and maintain cardiovascular stability: vasoactive drugs such as dopamine and dobutamine, strict maintenance of fluid and electrolyte balance, and cautious administration of IV fluids balanced with administration of diuretics and electrolyte replacement.

Chapter 24

1. You can develop a tool (brief checklist with space for more focused data) to help focus assessment on factors such as smoking; sunlight exposure; ionizing radiation exposure; nutrition and diet; alcohol consumption; use of smokeless tobacco; estrogen intake; and occupational hazards. Presence of these factors indicates that you should conduct an expanded life-style assessment. An in-depth assessment on any one (or a combination) of these factors will dictate the course of teaching. You should teach the client how to avoid factors involved with the development of cancer and you should support choices made to change life-style behaviors. Plan to use teaching aids such as video presentations, computer-assisted instruction, and handouts. Group teaching sessions can be planned for evening presentations. The client may need referral to agencies that specialize in specific areas, such as non-smoking seminars and dietary counseling. Follow-up visits would be helpful in monitoring the client's progress in achieving behavioral change.

2. The client is in the age-range for the development of testicular cancer. His friend should come in for a physical examination and diagnostic testing. You should ask if the friend does testicular self-examination on a monthly basis and ask if the friend is seeking medical help for the problem. Inform the client that blood studies for tumor markers (α-fetoprotein and human chorionic gonadotropin) would be done. Other studies also would be performed. The friend would be referred to a specialist for management of care. A young man with possible testicular cancer would have concerns such as prognosis, treatment, how the disease would affect marriage

and fathering children, possible changes in life-style, and effect on self-image and self-concept. Until a diagnosis is made, answer in general terms as best you can, and recommend that the friend seek help as soon as possible.

Chapter 27

1. Diagnosis of *Pneumocystis carinii* infection is made by examination of bronchial secretions or lung tissue. This is accomplished by bronchoscopy, transbrachial lung biopsy, or sputum induction. The client will be treated for 3 weeks with trimethoprim-sulfamethoxazole (Bactrim or Septra), parenteral pentamidine, or dapsone-trimethoprim. Any client with a CD4+ cell count lower than 200 would be treated prophylactically. It is important that the client completes the CD4+ cell count as scheduled. The systemic candidiasis is treated with antifungal agents, such as ketoconazole and fluconazole.

You should conduct an in-depth nursing history and a physical examination of the skin and mucosa (oral, vaginal, and rectal mucosa are frequently affected) and gastrointestinal function (lack of appetite and weight loss). Be alert to signs of impending opportunistic infections (e.g., fever, weight loss, anorexia, sweating). A general assessment of vital signs, lung sounds, and bowel sounds should be completed. It is important to explore sexual activity and provide teaching about safe sex if high-risk behaviors are a factor. Universal precautions are maintained and explained to the client and significant others.

2. The following criteria fit the client: end-stage disease is present in a transplantable organ; conventional therapy has failed to treat the condition successfully; and further progression of problems associated with the diseased organ may be fatal. The client cannot have a malignancy or irreversible infection and must be well enough to survive the transplantation surgery. When the client arrives at the designated hospital, she will begin learning about the transplant procedure, postoperative course, post-transplantation self-care requirements, and the medication regimen. She will be taught preoperatively about coughing and deep breathing and moving and turning after the surgery. She will be monitored closely in an intensive care unit after the surgery.

Psychological care and support are important throughout the process of candidate selection and transplantation. There are many ups and downs, and the wait may become unbearable. The client will be evaluated on her ability to comply with post-transplantation self-care. She must be willing to comply with treatment and deemed able to do so before being placed on the list. Her life will be different following the successful transplantation in that dialysis will be discontinued. Remember that over time the client has developed a support system in the dialysis staff and may feel abandoned even while she is happy that the transplantation was a success. She may be able to return to work (if she was not working because of weakness and scheduling of dialysis treatments), so her self-concept will change. Plan for time preoperatively and postoperatively to discuss feelings and plans for life after a transplant.

3. You may choose to have the clients introduce one another, using first names only. Because it is a small group, it would be helpful to place the clients in a circle while you present the information. Use visual aids, such as large signs listing the major topics. A handout may be used. Remember that we are a visual society and learn from seeing; thus, you may want to make use of an informational videotape followed by a question-and-answer period. Focus on general information, such as transmission and prevention. You should indicate the greatest areas of viral concentration in the body (blood, semen, cerebrospinal fluid, and cervical-vaginal secretions). Relate this to how the virus is transmitted (direct contact with any of the fluids mentioned). Discuss the risks of unprotected sex and multiple sex partners. The clinic may offer free condoms. Discuss the risk associated with using shared needles and the relationship to HIV infection. Teach avoidance of contact with blood and other body fluids (as much as possible, given their homeless status) and to try to wash the hands as frequently as possible if such contact is made.

Provide ample time for questions such as "I'm pregnant; can my baby get AIDS?" "What's the difference between HIV and AIDS?" "Where can I get tested?" "What should I do if my partner won't use protection?" Offer time for individual counseling should any of the clients indicate it is needed. You can also ask the clients about information that they would like to have presented at another session.

Chapter 28

1. You should find out when she has been taking her prednisone because it should be taken with food to decrease gastric irritation. You will also want to determine if she has had any nausea, vomiting, or diarrhea (manifestations of gastrointestinal [GI] bleeding). Advise her to stop taking ibuprofen because it further irritates the GI mucosa. You will want to see her in the clinic today to assess for actual bleeding, reassess her hemoglobin, and assess for occult blood in stool. She should be taught again about timing of medications.

2. You should pay particular attention to completing a thorough joint assessment (e.g., pain, range of motion, presence of inflammation, strength) in addition to an assessment that will help plan care postoperatively (e.g., general health, allergies, medication history). The client may have an unrealistic understanding of her postoperative abilities or she may be in denial regarding a change in life-style. She may be an excellent candidate for rehabilitation services and may be able to adapt her skills to another job.

Chapter 31

1. The priority for treatment of a person suffering from a neurologic trauma is airway. Even if no current alterations are noted in the client's airway, the nurse should always treat him as if he has sustained a cervical injury. A cervical collar should be placed and left on until the x-rays rule out cervical injury. It is possible that the neck could have been twisted during the fall. The Glasgow Coma Scale (e.g., best eye opening, best motor response, best verbal response) plus assessment

of the pupillary response to direct and indirect light gives a quick indication of his neurologic baseline. Inspecting and palpating the head and scalp for depressions, bone instability, crepitus, lacerations, penetrating injuries, or clear or amber-colored drainage from the nose or ears may indicate a basilar skull fracture. Bruising behind the ears ("battle sign") or around the eyes ("raccoon sign") lends a high suspicion for a skull fracture or an extradural hematoma. Drainage from the ears or nose may be the result of cerebrospinal fluid leakage secondary to meningeal tearing. Injury to the temporal fossa is the most common site for an extradural hematoma secondary to damage to the middle meningeal artery or vein. This type of hematoma can cause medial shifting and result in uncal and hippocampal herniation. The nurse needs to question the client and/or his wife about other signs and symptoms, such as a temporary loss of consciousness. Persons with temporal extradural hematomas often lose consciousness for a short period of time, but if the internal bleeding stops, they become lucid. A headache of increasing severity in addition to other manifestations, such as vomiting, change in level of consciousness, and seizure, usually indicate an enlargement of the hematoma. Rapid loss of consciousness, ipsilateral (same-sided) pupillary dilation, and contralateral (opposite-sided) hemiparesis indicate herniation, which is a serious complication. The nurse must anticipate these changes and obtain a baseline assessment very quickly. If a physician is not present, one should be notified as soon as the client arrives or before arrival, if notified by the squad team. In this way, you can prevent delay in obtaining a CT scan or an MRI, which may be essential to diagnosing an extradural hematoma. This condition is often considered a medical emergency and is treated by surgical ligation of the bleeding vessels with removal of the hematoma. Prognosis is good if the surgical repair is done before bilateral pupillary dilation occurs.

2. Several involuntary eye movements can develop after head injury. Oculovestibular assessment can help clarify whether the client's brain is functioning. Some medications (for example, barbiturates) can produce effects that mimic brain death; thus, medication use must be taken into account when evaluating for brain death. The client's mother is understandably anxious and may not be able to accurately process information about her son's condition. You should plan for extra time to support the mother and family members. A pastoral referral may also be helpful.

Chapter 32

1. The client is experiencing signs of acute decreased cerebral perfusion. Cerebral perfusion is the first priority, which includes managing airway, oxygenation, and blood pressure. Assess the airway for patency and suction if necessary, remembering to hyperoxygenate before, between, and after suctioning. Ensure that the oxygen delivery system is functional and set appropriately. Ensure that his head is in anatomic position and that the headrest is elevated to 30 degrees. Administer the prn antihypertensive, sublingually if ordered. Oxygenation, increasing venous jugular

return, and lowering blood pressure must be done quickly to promote improved cerebral perfusion. Proceed with a full neurologic assessment, watching for localizing signs of neurologic compromise. Avoid unnecessary nursing interventions, such as replacement of the nasogastric tube, which would only increase the intracranial pressure further. Perform the assessment quickly and notify the physician for further direction. The suddenness of the change is significant. It is usually indicative of an embolus or ruptured aneurysm.

2. The Glasgow Coma Scale is a well-documented, reliable tool for measuring levels of intracranial pressure. However, subtle signs of a change in intracranial pressure are not always revealed by the Glasgow Coma Scale. The finding that this client was slower to respond, combined with the changes in her pupillary reactions, was very significant. (Even the "slowness to respond" is a significant change in and of itself.) The physician ordered a CT scan, which confirmed an increase in cerebral edema. By the time she returned from the radiology department the client was oriented to name only, and her right pupil was not only sluggish but also larger than the left pupil. The physician ordered intravenous steroids and intravenous osmotic diuretics to decrease the edema. Because of prompt recognition that the "critical monitoring" goes beyond monitoring results of the Glasgow Coma Scale, the client's level of consciousness was quickly restored to normal without any irreversible effects.

Chapter 33

1. Airway management and protecting the client are the top two priorities. Manage these priorities simultaneously by taking the pillow or a blanket and placing it between the client and the rail while turning the client to his or her side. Turning the client on his or her side prevents airway obstruction from the tongue and decreases the risk for aspiration. You can also call for help, "I need help in here," while turning and protecting the client. Other interventions include staying with the client during the entire seizure and observing the characteristics of the seizure. Suctioning may be necessary.

Once the seizure is over, assess the client's vital signs and provide oral care if the client bit his or her tongue, or perineal care if incontinence occurred. Having a seizure is a very frightening experience; provide emotional support for the client and family. The amnesia of the actual seizure is common. If this is his or her first seizure, explain that this is a common consequence of a seizure. If the client has had seizures before, he or she will usually be aware that a seizure has occurred because of tongue biting, incontinence, or lethargy that occurs in the post-ictal phase. Teach the client and family about seizure precautions. See the Risk Factors and Levels of Prevention feature for seizure precautions.

2. The multidisciplinary rehabilitation team will meet to discuss plans for treatment, expected progression, and tentative discharge for the client. The client will be treated medically and receive referral for nutrition therapy. She will receive physical therapy, occupational therapy, and will be referred to other services as needed. You will be responsible for physical care and psychological support as well as teaching about how to prevent complications related to the impaired ability to move normally. Remember to assess the client's learning needs and design teaching that will enhance the client's compliance. You should include the family in the teaching, especially those family members who will be responsible for care after discharge.

3. Because increased intracranial pressure is a major complication of intracranial surgery, you should assess for a decreased level of consciousness with associated headaches, visual and speech disturbances, muscle weakness and paralysis, pupil changes, respiratory changes, seizures, and vomiting. General interventions include observation for serous drainage from the ears or nose, seizures, and possibility of meningeal infection (2 to 3 days postoperatively). You should also administer osmotic diuretic therapy and steroids and monitor for neurologic changes and respiratory status. Keeping the head of the bed elevated is imperative. In addition, you should use nursing interventions that prevent the complications of surgery performed under general anesthesia.

Chapter 34

1. Generalized weakness, fever, and chills suggest the presence of infection. Because of this client's neurogenic bladder, one of your first concerns should be the possibility of a urinary tract infection as a cause of this client's manifestations. You should teach the client again about maintaining a 2000 ml/24 hour routine. He should attempt to void every 3 hours. Review with the client and family the procedure for intermittent self-catheterization.

2. Confusion and paranoia are not typical manifestations of Parkinson's disease. This client may be having some side effects from dopaminergic agents, which are prescribed for Parkinson's disease. Confusion can develop when these drugs have been used for several years. When planning the care of this client, it is important to determine how likely it is that he will injure himself or others. To begin that determination, you will need to find out whether this is the first time the client has experienced these manifestations.

3. The client's difficult breathing is very likely related to her weakness and fatigue. You will need to consider whether she is at risk for respiratory compromise and whether you need to prepare for respiratory support. The weakness itself may result from either myasthenic crisis or cholinergic crisis. It is also possible that the addition of other medications may have increased the client's myasthenic symptoms.

Chapter 35

1. A cervical collar would have been placed on the client's neck at the accident scene. This may have been replaced by a hard cervical collar in the emergency department. Nevertheless, anticipate cord trauma whenever a client has head injury. Even if the airway is compromised, maintain cervical cord alignment. Only a jaw thrust maneuver is to be used for airway resuscitation. Anticipate that swelling will occur at least two levels above and below the actual cord injury as part of the normal response to trauma. The physician will prescribe medications, such as high doses of steroids, to decrease cord swelling. When the injury is at a high thoracic level, anticipate cervical cord involvement. A tracheostomy tray must be kept at the client's bedside at all times in case the injury ascends to the fourth cervical cord level, where the phrenic nerve, which innervates the diaphragm, is located. Notify the physician, even in the middle of the night, of the slightest change in data indicating ascending cord dysfunction. Use Table 35–2 to review the signs of ascending loss. Remember that the spinal cord is like the brain in that it does not tolerate prolonged ischemia. Ischemia will lead to death of tissue and permanent dysfunction from the level of the cord injury downward. Through astute assessments, you can play a key role in preventing or minimizing permanent cord injury.

2. In examining this problem, the first priority should be to maintain the client's neck in alignment. Keeping him calm is a second priority. You could consider giving him a sedative, but consider its onset time. Also consider what other sources, such as awakening in unfamiliar surroundings, might be contributing to his increased restlessness. Methods to consider for calming the client down and maintaining spinal alignment include orienting him to the room, asking about his concerns, and checking bladder distention. Regardless of the method chosen, he must be aided in remaining in bed with the traction in place and spine in alignment.

3. The first priority is to determine the extent of vascular insufficiency. Methods to consider for assessing vascular sufficiency include checking and comparing pedal pulses, capillary refill time, and ability to discriminate soft and hard touch. The next priority is relieving the client's headache. During the first 48 postoperative hours, you should check (every 2 to 4 hours) the client's motor abilities and sensation in the extremities. In addition to the usual postoperative care, the client should be turned using the log-rolling technique. Changes in assessment should be reported to the surgeon and monitored closely.

Chapter 36

1. The first question to ask is whether the client has taken anything for discomfort. If not (some people are reluctant to take medication of any kind), suggest that the client take acetaminophen (either plain or with codeine) and call back within an hour. If the pain is unrelieved or worse, and if the nausea persists, it is imperative that the client not wait until morning to be evaluated. Unrelieved pain and nausea indicate that the client's intraocular pressure may be elevated. You should suggest that the client's wife call a relative or friend to provide transportation.

2. Although it is understandable that the client is drowsy from anesthesia, it is very important to assess her visual acuity as ordered. Any sudden vision loss in the early postoperative period indicates pressure on the optic nerve. The pressure may be due to edema or hemorrhage. Check the bulb to be sure that the drain is patent. You can expect a small amount of serosanguineous drainage (10 to 30 ml). Carefully remove the tape on

the incisional dressing at the temple and observe for signs of swelling and ecchymosis. Stimulate your client by raising the head of the bed to a full, upright, sitting position and explain why reading the vision card is so important. Get another nurse to gently hold the eyelids open with cotton applicator sticks or gloved fingers. Hold the vision card 14 inches from the client's face and encourage her to read the smallest line she can see. Notify the surgeon immediately if the client's acuity is not within the parameters specified by the surgeon. Sudden vision loss may indicate a need to reoperate to relieve a hematoma that is pressing on the optic nerve.

Chapter 37

1. You should complete a thorough nursing history and physical assessment with emphasis on the function of the ear and hearing problems. Investigate the client's ability to provide care for himself or herself following surgery. If the type of surgery is known, you can provide verbal and written instructions for postoperative home care. The client should be taught about prescribed positioning, how to blow the nose properly, and how to sneeze and cough so that tympanic pressure is maintained. The client should also be alerted to hearing changes that may include decreased hearing in the affected ear (due to packing), cracking or popping in the ear, minor earache and discomfort in the cheek and jaw, and swelling of the ear. Other instructions, such as changing the cotton packing or restrictions on lifting, are specific to the practitioner and to the client's life-style.

2. You should proceed with a more thorough history of the ear infections and complete an examination of the ear and hearing ability. Recurrent ear infections can affect overall hearing, and along with the presbycusis, the client is at risk for hearing loss. You should teach about the hearing loss associated with aging and that there is no medical or surgical treatment for this condition. Emphasize the importance of completing a prescribed course of medication and explain how antibiotics target the bacteria causing the infection. Demonstrate how to instill eardrops and ensure that the client has the ability to self-administer the drops.

Chapter 40

1. The first step in evaluating the client with a tracheostomy who has difficulty breathing is to determine if the airway is obstructed. Feel for the movement of air through the tracheostomy tube to determine tube displacement or obstruction by secretions. Remove and clean the inner cannula or discard the disposable inner cannula to remove crusted secretions. Suction the tracheostomy to remove excess secretions. Assess the client's vital signs and check the oxygen saturation using a pulse oximeter. If the client has normal oxygen saturation levels yet continues to experience difficulty, provide reassurance and support. Remember that pain and anxiety can also result in the complaint of "trouble breathing." Do not medicate for pain or anxiety before evaluating the client. Some analgesics and antianxiety medications can depress respiration and result in increased difficulty in breathing. Document any changes

and notify the physician if the problem is not resolved.

2. When the entire larynx is removed, the client has a permanent tracheostomy, and therefore the esophagus and trachea are anatomically separated. This separation prevents aspiration of stomach contents during vomiting, but it does not reduce the risk of strain on the suture line or burning the GI tract with stomach contents. The nausea is likely due to side effects of anesthesia or the analgesics the client is receiving. Monitor for nausea after the next dose of narcotics to determine if the drug is the culprit. The client should be treated with an antiemetic. He should not be fed by nasogastric feeding until bowel function has returned, as evidenced by bowel sounds, feelings of hunger, and passage of flatus.

3. When first discovering a client with a nosebleed, you should pinch the anterior portion of the nose for 5 to 10 minutes. Most common nosebleeds occur on the anterior septum. Apply ice compresses to promote vasoconstriction. Instruct the client to lean forward to prevent any blood from draining into the throat. If these measures do not stop the bleeding, nasal packing and/or a posterior packing may be required. Monitor the client's vital signs and prepare the client for evaluation of the bleeding site and insertion of packing. Remember to provide emotional support as the client may become very anxious if the bleeding does not stop with simple measures.

Chapter 41

1. The first priority is to help the client regain her normal breathing pattern. Ask her to sit straight up and assist her in removing any clothing that is heavy or constricting. A respiratory therapist may be called to administer a nebulizer treatment. Ask questions that will require only a nod of the head for a response. Assess the lungs fields for crackles and wheezing. Provide a basin and tissue for use when coughing. A chest x-ray may be ordered. If the breathing does not improve, intravenous aminophylline may be initiated. Ask the client to drink water to help break up the mucous secretions. The client should be monitored frequently to determine the progress of treatment. Once the breathing is eased, you should plan to talk with the client about triggers that can cause an acute episode similar to the one she has experienced. Emphasize that she cannot tolerate physical exercise at the level she expects and that the cold air may have caused airway spasms. The client may need support in approaching her spouse to reduce his smoking and in asking him to smoke outdoors instead of inside the home. Review how she self-administers the inhalers for correctness of administration. If breathing improves, she may be observed in the clinic for a period of time. The intravenous line will be removed before discharge. If the shortness of breath and wheezing persist, she is a candidate for an acute care admission.

2. Chest pain is an emergency; you should assess this client immediately. She has been bedridden for 2 to 3 days, which increases her risk of pneumonia, atelectasis, and pulmonary embolism. Obtain a set of vital signs,

check oxygen saturation, listen to lung sounds, and ask the client to describe the pain. Apply low flow oxygen. Pneumonia would lead to fever, tachycardia, decreased oxygen saturation, pain with inspiration, yellow sputum, and crackles. Pulmonary embolus would lead to anxiety, decreased oxygen saturation, pain with inspiration, frothy or blood-tinged sputum, and crackles. Her pelvic surgery and immobility make pulmonary embolus the most likely problem. The physician needs to be notified immediately.

3. Your first intervention is to complete an assessment of lung sounds to verify presence or absence of crackles and to obtain a set of vital signs. Stay with the client to help allay her fears. Administer oxygen at a low flow rate. Arterial blood gas analyses are completed. Arterial hypoxemia (low PO_2) and hypocapnia (low PCO_2) may be present. A "stat" chest x-ray will rule out other possible diagnoses. Although a ventilation/perfusion scan may be ordered, a pulmonary angiogram offers the most effective means of diagnosing pulmonary emboli. The most successful method of treatment consists of quick recognition of the condition and prompt, aggressive treatment. The client will be treated with anticoagulants and fibrinolytic therapy. Oxygen is administered and the client may be placed on a ventilator. If oxygen is used, elevate the head of the bed to reduce dyspnea. Morphine is used to relieve chest pain and allay apprehension and anxiety. The client with an acute pulmonary embolus will be transferred to the pulmonary intensive care unit where his or her condition can be monitored more closely.

Chapter 42

1. In this situation, the first priority is to avoid any further compromise to the client than has already occurred. Your best intervention would be to reestablish water seal drainage, either by reconnecting the system or by submerging the end of the tube in a sterile fluid. If neither of these options is possible, it is better to leave the tube open temporarily (sustaining or extending the open pneumothorax initiated by the disconnection) than to clamp off the tube (possibly producing a closed, tension pneumothorax). Simultaneously, the client should be watched closely for signs of acute respiratory distress; if they develop, the physician should be notified immediately.

2. Your first priority is to respond promptly and try to determine what the problem is. The alarm indicates that the pressure required to deliver the preset tidal volume is exceeding the limit set (usually 10 to 15 cm H_2O above the inspiratory pressure required to ventilate the client). Thus, something is blocking airflow delivery. Check the visible possibilities first. Assess the client—he may still be coughing in response to suctioning or may be biting on the endotracheal tube, or more secretions may have been loosened, necessitating additional suctioning. Next, check the machine—is the tubing kinked or has water condensed in it? The priority is to reestablish adequate ventilation as quickly as possible. If you cannot rapidly identify and correct the problem, take the client off the machine and ventilate with a manual resuscitation bag. Stay with the client and continue

ventilating until a respiratory therapist can check the machine. If no apparent causes are visible, there may be an "internal" problem; for example, bronchospasm in response to suctioning may be causing increased airway resistance; the client may have developed a pneumothorax; or the endotracheal tube may have slipped out of position. Notify the physician for further direction.

3. After making the client comfortable and completing a history and physical examination, you should prepare the client for the procedure. Teach the client about the purpose of the thoracentesis (drainage of air or fluid), use of fluid in the diagnostic process, positioning, importance of not moving during the procedure (moving can cause the needle to pierce the pleural space and injure the visceral pleura or lung parenchyma), and care after completion. A thoracentesis tray should be placed in the room along with any other equipment deemed necessary by the physician.

Chapter 45

1. When you make this home visit, your first priority should be to assess the client's cardiopulmonary status prior to initiating the dobutamine therapy. This includes assessing heart and lung sounds, vital signs, and body weight. You need to consider how the client's blood pressure and heart rate will respond to the dobutamine therapy and you will need to monitor the blood pressure and heart rate periodically during the procedure. Your next priority should be to assess the client's understanding of insulin-dependent diabetes, glucose monitoring, and insulin administration. You should check the glucose level and may need to clarify misconceptions and reinforce discharge teaching.

2. Pain control is of primary importance. Continued pain is a symptom of myocardial ischemia. Pain also places more stress on the already damaged heart. The client should also receive oxygen and electrocardiographic monitoring should be instituted. Anticoagulants and stool softeners are also given to prevent further complications. The first 6 hours are crucial. To be effective, thrombolytic agents must be given within the first 3 to 6 hours following onset of chest pain.

3. Complications in the elderly include dysrhythmias related to aged sinoatrial node cells, drug toxic effects related to impaired hepatic and renal perfusion, multiple drug-drug interaction, and decreased physical stamina. During the surgery, a saphenous vein from the leg is harvested and used to bypass the blockage in the coronary vessel. It remains a common surgery because it alleviates the angina in clients who are refractory to medical treatment.

Chapter 46

1. This rhythm is sinus tachycardia or supraventricular tachycardia. The rate is 140 beats per minute. Although some tachycardia is normal with increased activity, the heart rate should not increase to this level. You should assess for tolerance of the rhythm by assessing for manifestations of decreased cardiac output. If the client cannot tolerate the rhythm, he should be returned to his room by

wheelchair, placed on bedrest, and reassessed often.

2. In addition to doing a complete neurologic examination, you need to assess the client's heart rate and rhythm and auscultate the heart and lungs. It is possible that pacemaker malfunction could be causing these syncopal episodes. If this is the case, the low heart rates may also result in congestive heart failure. Once you have confirmed the presence of a pacemaker, you must determine when the pacemaker was inserted, how long it has been since it was checked, and the type, model, and mode of the pacemaker. This information is necessary to evaluate functioning and to check the pacemaker. The physician may decide to reprogram the pacemaker.

Chapter 47

1. The fact that the client hit the steering wheel with his chest should alert you to take his vital signs and complete a more thorough cardiac assessment that includes observation for hypotension, dyspnea, and tachycardia as well as jugular vein distention, cyanosis of lips and nails, muffled heart sounds, diaphoresis, and paradoxical pulse. The client needs immediate intervention. The procedure of choice is pericardiocentesis, performed by the physician in which fluid or air is removed from the pericardial sac.

2. Helping to position your client for maximal ease of breathing might help; have him sit upright, with arms resting on pillows, to allow maximal chest expansion, and use of supplemental oxygen. Nursing actions that may help him include talking to him about completing advance directives. Advance directives will direct his healthcare when he is no longer able to make his own decisions. He could specify on his Living Will that he does not wish to be placed on a ventilator. Discussing advance directives with his family and his physician could help improve his psychological state by increasing his feeling of control.

3. The client's previous mitral valve prolapse placed him at risk for infective endocarditis. The newly transplanted kidney and subsequent medication regimen to counter rejection places this client at a high risk for infective endocarditis. Prophylactic antibiotic treatment to prevent endocarditis is extremely important for this client and will require the client's utmost attention. The nurse must coordinate the educational objectives with the physician and ensure the client's understanding regarding prophylactic therapy. A learning needs assessment of the client and his spouse should be completed prior to the teaching sessions.

Chapter 50

1. Many possibilities could explain the continued elevation in blood pressure. He could be anxious. He may have started the medications, then developed side effects and quit taking them; he could also have developed some other problems, such as renal disease. Begin unraveling this problem by asking him about his compliance with the medications. You may have to open the discussion by addressing common side effects, such as fatigue and impotence, to get the client to be honest.

2. The client's venous stasis ulcers are worsened by his chronic standing. The wounds need to be debrided before they will heal; whirlpool baths, enzymatic agents, or wet-to-dry dressings will all work well. His homeless state makes it very unlikely that he can care for the ulcers effectively. As long as he maintains this life, the ulcers will not stay healed. He needs to elevate his legs to decrease edema (which is almost impossible). Consider finding him placement in a shelter if he is willing.

Chapter 53

1. Her history of gastric resection and lack of follow-up care (because of the move) have put her at risk for developing pernicious anemia because of malabsorption of vitamin B_{12} from lack of intrinsic factor. The client exhibits manifestations of poor tissue perfusion (shortness of breath, fatigue) caused by a lack of oxygen carrying capacity of the RBCs. Hence, you would first assess for manifestations of pernicious anemia. It would be important to draw a CBC. Be alert to abnormally low amounts of RBCs (<3 million/mm³), elevated MCV and MCHC, and lower values of WBCs and MCH. Unconjugated bilirubin also may be elevated, as would LDH. Teach the client the need for life-long vitamin B_{12} maintenance through monthly injections. You may be involved in teaching a family member to administer the injections or in arranging for home health services to do this. You also would teach the client about other medications (such as folic acid) and proper nutrition.

2. The client's chemotherapy will cause a reduction in all of his blood cells, including thrombocytes. His bleeding gums are probably related to reduced platelets. You would ask him to return to the clinic so that his CBC could be evaluated. Based on the results, further interventions could be planned. Of particular interest would be the RBC, WBC, and platelet counts. You would instruct the client on thrombocytopenic precautions, such as avoiding activities that could cause bruising, using only electric razors, and using soft foam toothbrushes. In addition, you should evaluate him for anemia (weakness, shortness of breath) and neutropenia (elevated temperature, other manifestations of infection).

3. Hypercalcemia develops in 30% of all newly diagnosed clients with multiple myeloma because of the bone destruction caused by the rapidly dividing plasma cells. Hypercalcemia raises action potentials in nerve cells, thus requiring a larger-than-normal stimulus for excitation. Hence, manifestations of lethargy, paralytic ileus, and vomiting are common. The priority assessment for this client is her airway. Given her lethargic condition, ensure that her airway is and remains patent. This is especially important given her episodes of vomiting. She should be positioned with the head of the bed up and with her head turned to the side. She should be monitored constantly, and suction equipment should be available. A serum calcium level should be drawn, and you should anticipate the administration of intravenous saline and furosemide (Lasix) to increase the excretion of calcium. A Foley catheter may be inserted.

Intake and output should be strictly monitored. An antiemetic may be required.

Chapter 56

1. The probable cause of the client's problem is a urinary tract infection; however, to thoroughly assess the problem, you must look for other manifestations, such as urgency and frequency. A urine culture and sensitivity is needed to accurately diagnose the problem and identify the exact organism for correct antibiotic therapy. She should learn about the medications and the importance of completing the entire course of treatment. She should be questioned about her current hygiene practices, such as bathing, use of bubble bath, and manner of cleansing after urinating or having a bowel movement. You should discuss proper hygiene that can be used to help prevent further infections, such as showering, use of cotton underwear, increasing her fluid intake to at least 3 L/day, and voiding immediately after intercourse. Your teaching will help the client to avoid further infections, which is important because of the long-term problems that can result from recurrent infections.

2. The client appears to be experiencing several problems. First the amount of urine from the catheter is decreased. This problem could be related to a drop in fluid volume, an occlusion of the catheter, or a problem with the new pouch. The nurse will need to make further assessments to identify the cause of the problem. Some areas to assess include estimated blood loss during surgery, urine output since surgery, total output from all sources, blood pressure, and fluid intake. To assess for patency, the catheter should be gently irrigated by the surgeon. The second problem is the potentially impaired blood flow to the stoma. The stoma must be assessed carefully and if circulation is impaired (blue, pale, or dusky stoma), the surgeon must be notified immediately. You can assess the client to be sure that nothing is tight around the stoma or possibly impinging on its blood supply. Review the Critical Monitoring feature for more ideas concerning this problem.

Chapter 57

1. The client may be suffering from acute pyelonephritis secondary to cystitis. Cystitis is common in newly married women. She must have a urinalysis and should be assessed for pain and tenderness over the kidney area (CVA tenderness). She might also be passing a renal stone; however, if the urine contains many WBCs and some RBCs, she probably has an infection. A flat plate x-ray of the abdomen along with serum electrolytes and uric acid assays could be done to rule out calculi. Think about what teaching would be required if the client has pyelonephritis secondary to cystitis. Antibiotics would be given after a culture and sensitivity and must be taken for a full 10 to 14 days, with a follow-up culture to be sure the bacteria have been eradicated.

2. Your priority is to establish that the client has adequate renal function in his remaining kidney. Diagnostic tests, including creatinine, BUN, electrolytes, and an intravenous pyelogram, will be needed to adequately assess renal function. Remember that diabe-

tes may have affected his kidneys. The client is not going to be able to pass a large calculus independently. Think about the surgical procedures that may be required. They range from lithotripsy to open surgery. Remember that his diabetes may cause problems for him postoperatively.

3. Your first suspicion should be hypovolemia. Review his intake. He may also be experiencing some sort of pump failure. You would need to look at his BUN and creatinine. Review laboratory study values for renal failure. Compare the treatment you would institute if it is a volume problem versus a pump problem. Think about a volume depletion problem versus an inability to circulate existing volume and, possibly, a fluid overload problem.

Chapter 60

1. Your first priority is to get the client back in bed, with the head of the bed elevated to promote respiration. Next, obtain her vital signs and try to calm her. Administer oxygen and notify the physician. Once they are available, the test results will most likely determine whether symptoms are due to a hiatal hernia or angina. In the meantime, an immediate ECG and chest x-ray with a portable x-ray machine might be helpful. Changes in the ECG suggestive of cardiac ischemia point to a cardiac problem. If the problem is a hiatal hernia, the chest x-ray may show part or all of the stomach above the diaphragm. If the physician has ordered oral viscous lidocaine, you might also administer it to determine whether it relieves the client's pain. If the pain is unrelieved, it is most likely cardiac in origin.

2. Teach the client to limit her intake of caffeine, nicotine, fat, spicy foods, and alcohol; eat six small meals a day; reduce weight if needed; avoid lifting, straining, and bending; avoid restrictive, tight-fitting clothing; sleep with the head of the bed elevated; avoid lying down for at least 1 hour after eating; and take prescription or over-the-counter antacids as ordered by the physician. Specific teaching related to the medications ordered is warranted.

3. The client's gingival problems most likely result from poor dental hygiene. Teach him about brushing and flossing his teeth at least twice a day, and preferably after each meal and at bedtime. Additional teaching should focus on scheduling routine dental visits, limiting high-carbohydrate snacks, and use of fluoride rinses. One of the client's teeth appears to be abscessed. He will probably undergo a pulpectomy and incision and drainage of the abscessed tooth in an outpatient setting. The pulpectomy is the treatment of choice because it will allow the young man to preserve his tooth while removing the diseased pulp of the tooth.

Chapter 61

1. Usually, aspirate cannot be obtained because the ports of the tube are not positioned in a pocket of fluid or because the tube is blocked. If aspirate cannot be obtained, first try to push air (30 to 60 ml), using a large syringe, into the tube. This will move the tube away from the gastrointestinal mucosal folds. If the client belches immediately fol-

lowing air insufflation, the tube's ports are probably in the esophagus. If this occurs, advance the tube and check its position again.

Next, pull back on the plunger of the large syringe. If aspirate is obtained, observe the color and measure the volume and pH; then immediately flush the tube with water or saline to prevent clogging. If you are still unable to aspirate fluid, push air into the tube again and pull back on the plunger.

If these steps do not work, place another 20 ml of air into the tube with a large syringe. Then remove the large syringe and attach a 10- or 12-ml syringe to the feeding tube and attempt to aspirate fluid with the smaller syringe. Use of the smaller syringe to aspirate will result in less negative pressure to collapse the tube. Repeat this step if necessary. However, after inflating the tube with the large syringe, reattach the smaller syringe and leave it for 15 minutes before attempting to aspirate again. If you are unsuccessful, this step may be repeated again with an extension of the waiting time to 30 minutes.

If none of these steps works, try changing the client's position (e.g., from side to side). If the tube is in the duodenum, placement on the right side may be helpful. If the tube is in the fundus of the stomach, a supine position may be helpful.

If you are unable to inject air *and* aspirate contents, the tube may be clogged or knotted. Do not use great force. The decision to remove the tube should be made. This decision may be based on agency policy. You should notify the physician and prepare for reinsertion if the tube has been removed. (Adapted from Metheny, N., et al. (1993). How to aspirate fluid from small-bore feeding tubes. *American Journal of Nursing*, (5), 86–88.)

2. For achalasia, esophageal cancer, and oral cancer, keep the rest of the gastrointestinal tract operational and functioning as normally as possible. The same is true for the client who has difficulty swallowing following a cerebrovascular accident. Hence, for these situations, enteral feedings with the insertion of a feeding tube, or perhaps a G-tube or J-tube, would promote the client's nutritional status by using the rest of the gastrointestinal tract. For long-term purposes, this avenue would be the least expensive and would minimize risks such as infection.

With acute pancreatitis and bowel obstruction, the gut must be rested. Therefore, parenteral nutrition would be the first choice. In an exacerbation of Crohn's disease and with short-bowel syndrome, parenteral nutrition would also be the first choice because nutrients may not be absorbed via the short-bowel and inflamed gut associated with Crohn's disease.

3. The nurse must assess for a smoking history; use of steroids; aspirin, caffeine, and alcohol; and stress. A thorough pain assessment is also required. Plan to teach that antacids neutralize gastric acid and increase gastric pH. They should be taken 1 to 2 hours after meals. Some side effects may include constipation, diarrhea, anorexia, and electrolyte imbalances. Advise the client with a duodenal ulcer to avoid spicy foods, alcohol, milk, and caffeine, as well as any other foods that cause distress. Plan for time to discuss life-style with the client. The client should relate the causes of duodenal ulcer

and identify from her own experience the behaviors that place her at risk for ulcer disease. Suggest small but consistent changes in behavior rather than the massive changes in diet and life-style, which could contribute to more stress. Offer support and encouragement when the client suggests changes in behaviors that will enhance healing. A referral to a nonsmokers' support group may prove helpful.

Chapter 62

1. A thorough nursing history of bowel elimination patterns is warranted, noting the number, color, and consistency of stools. Ask if the client noticed any blood or fat globules in the stool. Focus on the changes of the past 5 to 7 days. Ask about his history of weight gain and loss and secure a thorough assessment of pain. Note any changes in pain status because they may indicate the possibility of complications. If the client eliminates stool at the time of the examination, check for occult blood and observe for color and consistency. Weigh the client, who will be placed on NPO status. Check for skin turgor as an indicator of dehydration. Complete an abdominal assessment that includes inspection for distention, auscultation for bowel sounds, and palpation.

To stabilize the client's condition, the immediate problems should be addressed. The diarrhea will be controlled by the administration of antidiarrheal medications. Observe the perianal area for skin excoriation and provide care for skin that is irritated. Until the diarrhea resolves, the client will need fluid replacement and maintenance. When oral intake is permitted, encourage intake of fluids and foods. Suggest small servings of bland food so the intestinal tract is not irritated and can begin to heal. Administer medication ordered for pain relief. Plan for time to listen to the client and address his coping behaviors. He may need referral to a local support group so that he can learn to cope with his disease more effectively.

2. You should assess the partners for their ability and willingness to learn. In particular, explore the reasons why the client is not participating in his care. Observe for depression and denial in the client. Your teaching-learning assessment will help you to plan discharge teaching for both. Plan to pace the teaching so that they are not overwhelmed. Show the stoma to the client and spouse and explain what is normal and what changes require physician notification. It would be helpful to show how to remove and apply a colostomy bag on an abdominal model made for this purpose. Encourage the client to inspect the stoma and surrounding skin and to empty, remove, and change the colostomy bag. If the spouse observes, suggest she offer praise and encouragement to increase her husband's self-concept and acceptance of the change in body function. The client is taught to avoid foods that cause gas, such as nuts, cabbage, corn, and legumes. Drinking carbonated beverages can cause flatus. The stoma and surrounding skin should be cleansed and the pouch changed about every 4 to 5 days. When leakage occurs, the pouch should be changed. Refer him to an enterostomal therapist if there are pouch problems. If the client

is having difficulty accepting the colostomy, he should be referred to a local support group.

3. Your priority intervention is to help the client to calm down. At the same time, you must convince him to relinquish the paper bag in the interest of safety. Speak in a calm manner and encourage him to express his concerns. Plan to listen and do not rush. Determine his acceptance of the bowel diversion and ask how he sees himself as a person and a man. Ask what triggered these feelings. Explore his relationships with others. Did he give up a job he liked? Refrain from certain sports? Fear a sexual relationship? Fear rejection because of the colostomy? Fear that others would know or find out about his colostomy? Whether the anxiety and ineffective coping have been building over time or this is a relatively recent occurrence, you must refer the client to professional personnel equipped to respond to a crisis such as this. The surgeon may also be notified of the client's presence in the emergency department and may choose to talk with the client and listen to his concerns.

Chapter 65

1. With an alkaline phosphatase value that is twice normal, which indicates a significant degree of cholestasis, and AST and ALT both well over 10 times normal, there is indication of major liver injury. A diagnosis of acute viral hepatitis B was made from a positive HB$_s$Ag test and positive IgM anti-HBc serologic studies, so you would have needed initial serologic tests. You would also ask the client about medications that he might have been taking (because of their hepatotoxic effects), about any bleeding problems, and whether he has had pruritus. You would need to inquire about whether he and/or his sexual partner had received hepatitis B (HB) vaccine and advise them that they should receive the vaccine if they have not. With tact and diplomacy, you would need to remind this client that he should modify sexual behavior. In thinking about the priorities for care, you might consider that management of fatigue secondary to liver dysfunction is important. Also, teaching the client about the causes of hepatitis and modes of transmission would be critical. Clients are at high risk for impaired skin integrity related to pruritus, so you should keep the client's skin moist and the environment cool. The client must be encouraged not to scratch his skin and to keep his nails short and smooth. If you are "stuck" with a bloody HB-infected needle and have been immunized, you should be tested for anti-HB$_s$. If an inadequate antibody is found, one dose (0.06 ml/kg) of hepatitis B immune globulin (HBIG) should be given immediately, as should an HB vaccine booster dose. If you have not been immunized, you should be given one dose of HBIG immediately and an HB vaccine series should be initiated.

2. This client was found to be suffering from alcoholic cirrhosis and esophageal varices (Laënnec's cirrhosis). Although the liver is protected from further damage by cessation of alcohol intake, changes in liver structure are irreversible.

With a client who is vomiting blood, the first priority is to monitor vital signs, stabilize

the client hemodynamically, and establish a patent airway. You may be required to clear the stomach and note the amount of blood loss. If a nasogastric tube is inserted, use great care, because the varices could rupture. You may also need to prepare the client for a blood transfusion if the hemoglobin and hematocrit indicate the need. A definitive diagnosis of the etiology must be established before treatment can begin. In this case, we know the source of the bleeding. A Sengstaken-Blakemore tube may be inserted to help stop the esophageal bleeding. This tube can stop bleeding esophageal varices, but it does have its drawbacks. The gastric balloon may rupture and allow the esophageal balloon to pull up and occlude the larynx. If this occurs, the tube should be cut with scissors to decompress the balloons. Also, when the balloon is inserted, great care must be taken to ensure proper placement so that the gastric balloon is not in the esophagus when it is inflated. This could be devastating.

3. In addition to the ascites, the client may exhibit malnutrition, edema of the lower extremities, jaundice, gastrointestinal bleeding tendencies, palmar erythema, and an enlarged liver and spleen. These manifestations are usually found in clients with advanced cirrhosis. Your client's priority is comfort. Raise the head of the bed to enhance breathing and administer medication to relieve the abdominal pain. In certain instances, paracentesis may be considered. Follow with an in-depth assessment to establish baseline information. You should explore cardiac, renal, and nutritional dysfunctions. The client's condition would need to be stabilized as soon as possible so that surgery could be performed.

Your client would be a candidate for surgery and is subject to all complications associated with receiving general anesthesia. Healing would be a problem, as the pressure of the ascitic fluid may be forced through the wound incision made for the cholecystectomy. The client may be sluggish in his response to requests for coughing and deep breathing and moving and turning. He might need extra encouragement and praise to use the incentive spirometer and extra assistance in moving and turning. It would also be important to maintain adequate nutrition for healing as well as proper body functioning. Remember that there may be sodium and fluid restrictions to consider.

Chapter 66

1. The client is having pain, which by itself would make her very uncomfortable; however, she is also nauseated and vomiting. Your first priority is to give her an antiemetic, administer pain medication, and assess the need for insertion of a nasogastric tube. If you observe abdominal distention and continued nausea and vomiting, it is likely that nasogastric suction is needed. Next, she is most likely dehydrated. She is not able to keep oral fluids down, so you will need to replace fluids intravenously.

Diagnostic procedures that could be scheduled might include a biliary ultrasound, endoscopic retrograde cholangiopancreatography or endoscopic retrograde catheterization of the gallbladder.

It is important to carefully assess clients with these symptoms because even though your client has the typical manifestations of acute cholecystitis, there are multiple serious conditions that present with similar manifestations (e.g., biliary colic and acute myocardial infarction).

2. Caring for a client who admits to drinking as your client does will require you to be flexible and sensitive. You will need to encourage the client to face his alcohol problem and to seek assistance. You will also need to examine your own feelings about caring for clients who have alcohol abuse problems and seek ways that will help you meet the responsibility of caring for these individuals.

The biochemical studies in general support a diagnosis of pancreatitis. The serum amylase level may be elevated for many reasons (vomiting, morphine, intestinal obstruction, and azotemia [high level of nitrogen in blood]). However, elevations of five or more times the upper limit of normal are usually due to pancreatitis.

For complaints of pain from pancreatitis, opiate narcotics such as morphine are contraindicated because they cause pain from spasm of the sphincter of Oddi. Generally, meperidine (Demerol) is ordered. However, since your client reports that he is allergic to meperidine, you should call the physician for another pain medication.

3. The priorities for your client's care consist of the obvious need for relieving her pain and making her as comfortable as possible during the episodes of fever and chills. You may need to give an antipyretic and place blankets over her when she is having chills. If she spikes a temperature over 101° F, you may need to call the physician for another, or a different, antipyretic. You also need to consider that she may need surgery and you need to assist in her preparation. You should allay some of her anxiety and let her express her thoughts and fears.

The client's manifestations are highly suggestive of choledocholithiasis. During the initial assessment, the client is asked whether a tube drained bile into a bag for 7 to 10 days following the surgery, indicating that a bile duct exploration was performed. Previous common bile duct manipulation is a common cause of bile duct stricture and later development of choledocholithiasis.

Chapter 69

1. Remember that regular insulin peaks about 2 hours after injection. Because the client appears confused, your first priority is to quickly assess for hypoglycemia. Assess for tachypnea, hunger, and orientation. Next, check his blood glucose with the glucometer on your unit to confirm his hypoglycemia. Administer additional carbohydrates to quickly increase his blood sugar. This simple form of carbohydrate will take about 20 to 30 minutes to increase his blood sugar. Assess blood sugar, vital signs, and other manifestations for resolution of the hypoglycemia in 20 to 30 minutes. Next, try to find out why the client became hypoglycemic: What was his prebreakfast blood sugar? Did he eat his entire breakfast? Did he receive his usual morning insulin dose? Analyze your data and notify his physician. A change in insulin dosage may be

indicated. Pay close attention to dietary intake and future blood glucose levels. Remember to document all of your data and interventions in the client record.

2. The nurse should tell the client never to omit her insulin. Infection is a stressor that causes a release of epinephrine, which causes glycogen to be converted to glucose and thus raises the blood glucose level. The client should be taught to take liquids or semisolids (e.g., broth, sherbet, ices) every hour and keep a record of all intake (food and fluid) in the event a clinic visit becomes necessary. If she is still unable to eat after substituting liquids for four or five meals, she should notify her physician. The client should ask a friend or relative to stay with her. You should also tell her to test her blood glucose every 3 to 4 hours until she returns to her usual state of health.

3. Many body systems are affected by long-standing diabetes because the cell is unable to receive nutrition and rid itself of waste because of the thickened membrane. Chronic complications include the neuropathies (especially peripheral neuropathy), the ocular disorders (blurred vision, diabetic neuropathy, and cataracts), kidney disorders (diabetic nephropathy and pyelonephritis), and infections. Diabetics are prone to infections and are noted for an impaired healing response to injury, whether from an infection or trauma. Your client needs a thorough assessment focused on the development of new complications. The client should be taught (or retaught) about the observations necessary to detect onset of complications. You should ask the client to tell you what she knows about complications of diabetes and how to prevent them. For example, with the change in healing ability, you might focus on teaching about skin inspection and foot care. Nutrition and control of the hypertension should also be reviewed.

Chapter 70

1. The client's current history and physical examination suggest hyperthyroidism. Although the immediate findings are not life-threatening, he is in need of palliative treatment to prevent complications. Your collaborative efforts with the physician may include the following: low dose oxygen supplement to reduce oxygen need, heart rate, and respiratory rate and a beta-blocker to reduce heart rate and increase systolic time. Respiratory rate and blood pressure will also be reduced by the actions of a beta-blocker. Depending on the level of anxiety he is experiencing, a mild sedative may be prescribed. Teach the client about the laboratory work being ordered (triiodothyronine, thyroxin, and thyroid-stimulating hormone). Present a calm, slightly cool environment for your client, who is probably experiencing heat intolerance. Investigate his history further for cardiac disorders that may be augmented by hyperthyroidism.

2. The client has secondary hyperparathyroidism. Remember that chronic renal failure influences hyperphosphatemia. This combination causes hyperparathyroidism. As the glomeruler filtration rate (GFR) decreases, the serum phosphate level increases and serum calcium levels fall. Via the negative feedback

system, secretion of parathyroid hormone is stimulated to decrease phosphorus absorption in the renal tubules.

Calcium carbonate (Os-Cal) will probably be prescribed for this client. This will reduce her phosphorus absorption and provide a calcium supplement. A vitamin D_3 supplement such as calcitriol (Rocaltrol) will be prescribed to further facilitate calcium absorption. The goal will be to get the phosphorus level to as normal a level as possible.

3. The client should be taught about the basic function of the thyroid gland and how it relates to the changes she has experienced. Teach about the major side effects such as anxiety, insomnia, tremors, and irritability; tachycardia, palpitations, angina, and arrhythmias; nausea and diarrhea; menstrual irregularities; sweating and heat intolerance; and weight loss. Therapeutic response is evaluated on the absence of weight loss; diuresis; vital signs within normal limits; absence of constipation; increased appetite; warm, moist skin; increased energy; and an increased sense of well-being. You should tell the client at what point the changes are abnormal and should be reported to the physician. Blood studies are usually done according to the practitioner's protocol, generally every 6 months or when indicated by a change in usual body functioning.

Chapter 71

1. The client most likely experienced an exacerbation of her Addison's disease, triggered by an acute bout of influenza. The nausea, vomiting, diarrhea, and fever with diaphoresis that accompany influenza can spell disaster in clients with Addison's disease. The diarrhea and diaphoresis probably caused her to lose a great deal of fluid. Because she did not take her fludrocortisone acetate (Florinef Acetate) today, her aldosterone deficiency promoted an increase in sodium excretion. Remember that the mineralocorticoid aldosterone normally conserves sodium (and consequently water) and promotes the excretion of potassium. Missing the fludrocortisone dose would have caused the water excretion to increase. These losses were worsened by the fluid loss from vomiting, diarrhea, and diaphoresis.

The client probably became severely dehydrated and passed out from dehydration and hypotension. She also experienced glucocorticoid deficiency because she did not take her morning dexamethasone (Decadron). When a client becomes glucocorticoid-deficient, gluconeogenesis decreases, with resultant hypoglycemia and deficiency of glycogen in the liver.

2. The long-term use of glucocorticoids may have promoted protein tissue wasting. This results in muscle wasting (in the lower back) and osteoporosis. It is not uncommon for clients on long-term therapy with glucocorticoids to experience sudden and severe back pain with minimal movement or minimal trauma. Even fractures of the vertebrae can occur easily.

3. Your client probably has diabetes insipidus related to his head injury. Your first priority is to call the physician. Present your objective data (increased urine output, clear urine, decreased specific gravity, decreased blood pressure), which suggest diabetes insip-

idus. The next priority would be to have the laboratory perform any tests ordered to support the diagnosis of diabetes insipidus. Expect the physician to order tests of serum urine osmolality and serum and urine electrolytes. Expect to participate in a water deprivation study or hypertonic saline test. Give intravenous fluids as aggressively as permissible, given the client's overall condition. A vasopressin replacement should produce quick results and decreased urine output. Monitor electrolytes until they stabilize under the influence of vasopressin.

Chapter 74

1. You should complete a focused assessment on nutrition as well as life-style for both the mother and daughters. The daughters should be included in any discussion of nutrition and life-style, given the family predisposition to osteoporosis. They should be taught how exercise and diet affect bone loss. Their diet should include calcium-rich, low-fat foods. Teach them how overconsumption of alcohol, cigarettes, and coffee can increase bone loss. Teach that exercise should be moderate, consistent, and most important, weightbearing. Each family member should be able to choose the exercise that best fits her life-style, so long as it meets the previously mentioned criteria. Perhaps you can suggest that each individual take responsibility for planning a week's menus that would include calcium-rich foods.

2. Cheese, yogurt, and acidophilus milk are recommended for clients who are lactose intolerant. Remember to suggest sources of vitamin D and the need for daily exposure to sunshine. The client's hiatal hernia limits intake of foods high in fat and sugar as well as spicy foods. You might suggest a consultation with a nutritionist so that the client can learn to select calcium-rich foods that are within her budget.

3. Your first priority is to gather a more in-depth assessment of pain, numbness, tingling, and other physical changes associated with carpal tunnel syndrome. Determine if the problem is unilateral or bilateral and how long it has persisted before treatment was sought. Focus on how many hours a day the repetitive use of the hands occurs. Medical treatment includes the use of nonsteroidal anti-inflammatory medications, application of a wrist splint during working hours, and possible steroid injections. The client may be counseled to arrange the work schedule so that keyboarding chores are interspersed with other duties to provide rest. Ergonomically, the company may provide a padded rest below the keyboard and a newer type of keyboard that allows a more natural hand position. The client may need to decrease his after-work time on the computer to provide rest. If such measures are not effective, he may be sent for a consultation for surgery.

Chapter 75

1. Provide support for the affected extremity by placing the forearm on a padded board and securing it with soft cotton gauze before the client goes to the radiology department. This measure, along with supporting the arm so it does not dangle, may alleviate the pain of the moment. Complete a more focused

assessment regarding a history of previous fractures and healing. Ask about diet and life-style, especially his occupation. The client should be told that heat may be generated during the drying process, which occurs over a short period of time. While it is drying, the cast should be handled gently so that impressions that could cause circulation problems under the cast do not occur. A wet cast has an odor; it is odorless when dry. The client should be taught not to place objects inside the cast and to observe for swelling of the fingers of the affected hand. The edges of the cast may be protected with small strips of bandages applied around top and bottom edges. The client may be given a prescription for pain in case it is needed. He should elevate the arm on pillows when he is sleeping. If he notices an odor coming from the cast, has excessive pain, or observes gross swelling of the fingers (they may also tingle and make the cast feel tight), he should notify the physician as soon as possible. He may or may not be able to return to work, depending on his occupation.

2. When the client arrives on the unit, you should provide elevation for the casted extremity and provide comfort measures, including analgesic medications to ease the pain. Complete a basic but thorough admission assessment. You should be aware of the changes associated with fat embolus, because this complication usually occurs in the first 24 to 48 hours after injury, and this client is at risk. Be particularly observant for altered mental status, tachypnea, tachycardia, hypoxemia, petechiae, and fever.

3. Before any advice is given, you should complete a more focused assessment to be certain that the client has not injured herself more and to discern if there is a positive history for osteoporosis. The concern is for a fractured hip. If possible, the client should be directed to the nearest emergency department for further evaluation. Her personal physician may also choose to take this call; the client might then be advised to remain on bedrest for a number of weeks (with bathroom privileges). She may need physical therapy to resume walking or she may be taught to use a walker with wheels for ambulation. Her ability to lift objects may be restricted for weeks to months, until healing occurs. The physician may also order calcium injections for a period of time (administered by a home health nurse). More recently, calcium in nasal spray form has been introduced and may be indicated in this case because it can be self-administered.

Chapter 78

1. Consider options to relieve the pressure despite the client's desire to lie on her left side. Low-pressure mattresses may help, but the ideal is to not have her lie on the ulcer at all. The ulcer developed as a result of unrelieved pressure, and it will not heal with continued pressure. You will also need to examine the reasons she has not been sitting up in the chair and how you might make her comfortable on the right side. Her chair will also need a cushion. Finally, examine her nutritional status. Even though it appears that this pressure ulcer developed overnight, tissue

damage has actually been occurring for many days.

2. Skin of the elderly is more fragile and has the potential to break down and to develop infection surrounding an incision site with sutures. Symptoms to ask about include tenderness and erythema at the site and whether it has clear borders, drainage, edema, and if the client is febrile. Additionally, there should be clarification of how the wound care is being done. Ask the client to return to the office for evaluation depending on results of the telephone triage process. Potential interventions include systemic antibiotics and a change in the wound care recommendations utilizing a dressing to absorb drainage if it is present.

3. This woman needs to be evaluated and looked at for several differential diagnoses related to the rash, which after KOH testing proves to be candidiasis. Provide comprehensive teaching related to how to relieve the discomfort. These measures are similar to those used in relieving intertrigo. In addition, teach the client to use antifungal medications properly. Additionally, the weight loss, thirst, and candidial infection indicate presenting signs of diabetes for this otherwise seemingly healthy woman. Diabetes education needs to be addressed comprehensively. The candidiasis may not resolve until the diabetes is under control.

Chapter 79

1. The client is suffering from hypovolemia. Therefore, one of the first priorities in this case is to re-establish a patent intravenous (IV) line for fluid administration. Perform a calculation of the client's fluid resuscitation needs using one of the established resuscitation formulas. Then adjust the rate based on the client's response. The following is a calculation of his fluid resuscitation needs based on the Parkland formula: 4 ml of lactated Ringer's solution $\times$ 45% TBSA burn $\times$ 72 kg = 12,960 ml of lactated Ringer's solution to be given in the first 24-hour period following injury.

Half of the total calculated fluid needs (6,480 ml) should be delivered in the first 8 hours after injury. Because it is now 5 hours after injury and the client has already received 3,000 ml of IV fluid, his IV rate should be set at 1,160 ml/hour. At this hourly rate, he should receive the remainder of the fluid required for the first 8 hours (3,480 ml) by 4:00 PM. The remaining half of the total calculated fluid needs (6,480 ml, or 405 ml/hour) are to be delivered IV over the next 16 hours (4:00 PM to 8:00 AM).

Another concern is the client's gastrointestinal status and the potential harm that he would suffer if he were to aspirate vomitus. The client has developed an ileus.

Actions include treatment of hypovolemia with IV fluids (in progress) and evacuation of gastric contents. Place a vented nasogastric tube and attach it to low, continuous suction. Assess vital signs at least hourly until the fluid status stabilizes.

2. The client may be developing tissue ischemia in his right hand from constricting burn eschar. Assessment parameters to be monitored include the following: Doppler flow checks of the vessels of the palmar arch

and the radial and ulnar arteries; capillary refill checks of the unburned fingers; pain sensation and level present at rest and with active range of motion; and evidence of swelling. Comparing the right and left hands will help determine whether tissue ischemia is actually developing. If the data support tissue ischemia, communication with the physician must be immediate so that the appropriate treatment (an escharotomy) can be performed in a timely manner. Interventions include elevation of the extremities to reduce the formation of dependent edema, judicious use of pain medication, removal of constricting dressings or blood pressure cuffs (if applicable), continued monitoring, and client/family education.

3. Emotional and psychological support of the burn-injured client must be individualized, based on assessment data. Talking with the client to determine his concerns is a good first step and will help to establish a baseline from which you can develop a plan of action. Consulting with specialists, such as psychiatric clinical nurse specialists, psychologists, or psychiatrists, is often helpful. If physically able, the couple may benefit from participation in a support group, where client and family concerns are discussed in a supportive environment with people who have similar problems and needs. Demonstrate support and concern with continued active listening. Investigate whether poor pain control or excessive anxiety may be present and compounding the client's concerns. Continue to evaluate the problem and alter the plan of care as needed.

Chapter 80

1. People who have plastic surgery to make other people happy (in this case a boyfriend) are usually sorely disappointed. If her boyfriend does not stay "interested," the client may not have the psychological stamina to accept other possible causes, such as personality differences or incompatibility. In addition, she will still be bruised and swollen next week. Because persons with unrealistic expectations are not good surgical candidates, the surgeon planning to do this woman's operation should be notified.

2. The client needs to be turned to a supine position and/or onto the other side. She is lying on the pedicle of the flap, which supplies blood to the transferred skin and muscle. The pedicle is in the axilla and on the ribs. The muscle is moved from the back to the chest. She is also lying on the drainage tubing, which is increasing her risk of hematoma, a common cause of flap failure.

Chapter 83

1. The client's pain is most likely due to bladder spasms. Postoperative bladder spasms may be caused by a variety of problems, such as heavy clots, too rapid flow of the continuous bladder irrigation (CBI), a large-ballooned Foley catheter, traction on the catheter, or bladder distention. When dealing with bladder spasms, begin by checking the actual flow through the catheter. Also, at 1 day after the procedure, the urine should be pink—not dark or bright red. Increase the CBI and note the output. If the catheter appears to be draining slowly, you may need to irrigate it manually.

2. It is impossible to predict with absolute certainty what effects treatment will have on the client's ability to perform sexually and to father children. If the client has a bilateral orchiectomy, he will be infertile and may be impotent. If he has a unilateral orchiectomy, the outcome will depend on whether he has a retroperitoneal lymph node dissection. The node dissection carries with it a high risk of impotence. The effect of chemotherapy on fertility is unknown, as are the long-term genetic effects of chemotherapy in men. Second primary tumors are known to occur following treatment for testicular cancer. Sperm banking can always be offered as an option.

Chapter 84

1. It appears that the client is perimenopausal, because she has classic manifestations of menopause but has not been without menses for 12 months. It might be useful to know what her FSH level is, to confirm this. Because her manifestations are disruptive to her life, relief is the priority. You can discuss her options as far as treatment of her disruptive manifestations, including methods to help lessen the discomfort of hot flashes and using vaginal lubricants, changing sexual position, and increasing foreplay as well as frequency of vaginal intercourse when it becomes more comfortable.

Another option might be the use of short-term hormone-replacement therapy. You can present this as an option that might be especially useful for her night sweats, which are interrupting her sleep. You need to obtain a good history from her to evaluate any contraindications and you must present both the benefits and risks of such a treatment. Provide a supportive, nonjudgmental atmosphere in which she can ask questions and express feelings and concerns.

2. Obtaining a sexual history is necessary to assess the client's risk for sexually transmitted diseases and to develop a plan for prevention. It is also important to assess her level of understanding of the transmission of sexually transmitted diseases and to use this assessment as the basis of your teaching plan. (She may not know, for example, that oral contraceptives protect against pregnancy but not against infection.) Assessment of her perineal hygiene, which may include the use of douches, should also be done. To prevent recurrence, teaching should include information about modes of transmission and methods to reduce transmission; identification of symptomatic and asymptomatic clients; information about how infected clients are diagnosed and treated; and evaluation, treatment, and counseling of all sex partners of the infected client.

3. The client has all the manifestations of urinary tract infection (UTI), which may be related to iatrogenic infection from the Foley catheter insertion, maintenance, or the surgery. The manifestations must be reported to the physician right away so the problem can be diagnosed and treated as soon as possible. Once diagnosis is made and treatment is begun, client teaching about the treatment (including the antibiotic given) and prevention of UTI is necessary. Explain the risk factors related to the recurrence of UTI. You should teach the client about maintaining a high

fluid intake, voiding immediately after sexual intercourse, avoiding the use of tampons, using good perineal hygiene, and wearing cotton underwear. Remember to teach about the signs and symptoms of UTI.

Chapter 85

1. At this point, you do not have all of the information necessary for staging and treatment planning. The client should be given all information about options, including modified radical mastectomy. A lumpectomy may be performed if the tumor is limited to one area. Tamoxifen and other chemotherapy should also be discussed, as should lymph node dissection.

2. With a modified radical mastectomy, the breast itself is removed along with the nipple and the local and axillary lymph nodes. The main structures to worry about for long-term care are the lymph nodes. Their removal predisposes the client to the development of lymphedema. In the immediate postoperative period, it is important to prevent swelling in the affected extremity and to begin exercises from the elbow down. Movement at the level of the shoulder will be delayed until healing occurs at the level of the shoulder.

Answer all of the client's questions concerning activity based on your knowledge of the healing process. Encourage her regarding care of the drain and the incision if healing seems normal. Assess for the presence of lymphedema and provide appropriate information.

3. This swelling most likely represents lymphedema. Assess the degree of swelling by comparing size. Assess for the presence of edema elsewhere in the body in case the problem is unrelated to the surgery. A top priority is to reduce the swelling in the arm. Check the circulation in this arm to be sure that the swelling has not impaired it. Once the immediate problem has resolved, teach the client how to prevent the problem in the future.

Chapter 86

1. Because of the widespread incidence of gonorrhea, the priority goal is to prevent the transmission of the disease from this client to others. Because the client came to the clinic as a walk-in, and because he gave only a temporary address, this may be your only opportunity to see him. You want your interventions to be as complete as possible. Your first intervention would be to administer the antibiotic of choice for the gonococcal infection and the presumed co-infection of *Chlamydia* as ordered. Use single-dose regimens if there is a concern about compliance. Next, you want to give the client information about the prevention and treatment of gonorrhea and other STDs (such as how the diseases are transmitted and "safe sex"). Finally, guaranteeing confidentiality, you would obtain information about the client's sexual contacts. You would obtain this information last, after you have administered antibiotics, to reduce the chance of having the client refuse treatment.

2. The client's problems are her lack of knowledge about genital herpes, her considerable psychological distress over contracting the condition, and her need for treatment. One goal might be to provide accurate infor-

mation about infection with genital herpes simplex virus. You would emphasize that there is no known cure and that transmission of the virus is possible during asymptomatic periods as well as symptomatic periods. Another goal might be to relieve the client's emotional distress by encouraging her to express her feelings. You could suggest that she contact a support group. If the distress is extreme, you could refer her to a sexual counselor. Of course, interventions for this client would also include the treatment of this acute episode of genital herpes. Recommended treatment is acyclovir (Zovirax) orally for 5 to 10 days. The area should be kept clean and dry. Sitz baths, cool applications, and analgesics may be helpful.

3. You might begin by trying to determine whether there was a problem of noncompliance with the previous drug regimen. Did the previous healthcare provider forget to warn the client not to drink alcoholic beverages when taking metronidazole? If so, did nausea and vomiting resulting from the combination of metronidazole and alcohol cause the client to stop taking the drug too soon? Perhaps the client did not understand that simultaneous treatment of her and her husband was absolutely necessary to effect a cure. Did she know to avoid sex until she and her husband were cured? If, as is likely, the client did not take her previous course of treatment properly, a likely course of treatment for the current infection is a repeat course of metronidazole therapy. You will want to ensure that the client fully understands how to take the drug and that her husband is also treated. Because metronidazole is contraindicated during the first trimester of pregnancy and because the client is of childbearing age, be sure to ask about the possibility of pregnancy before beginning therapy with metronidazole.

Chapter 87

1. Complete a physical assessment with vital signs, level of consciousness and response to pain, and lung sounds. Remember that most information needed for an accurate appraisal of the continuing problem is contained in a nursing history. The history must be deferred until the patient regains consciousness. Try to elicit more information from her friends as to type of alcohol ingested, length of time the drinking problem has existed, and particular changes in behavior that others have noticed (e.g., drinking from a flask, drinking rather than eating). Agency protocol would require a blood alcohol level be drawn. An intravenous line should be started for fluid replacement. Determine the client's level of consciousness. You should observe for early signs of delirium tremens: anxiety, anorexia, insomnia, and tremors. She may become hyperalert, irritable, have jerky movements, and startle easily. The symptoms develop within a few hours of stopping drinking and peak at about 24 hours. Pulse and blood pressure are typically elevated and diaphoresis may occur. During the first 48 hours of withdrawal, seizures may occur; you should maintain seizure precautions during this time. The client will most likely be admitted to an observation unit until her condition stabilizes. She may receive a psychiatric consultation and be referred to

Alcoholics Anonymous (AA) for continuing help with her problem.

2. Although alcoholism is a disease of addiction, the client still makes a choice to drink or not to drink. If the choice is to drink, the client needs to know the consequences: physical, psychosocial, financial, and marital. When the client is ready to admit to the problem, he or she will be open to suggestions of attending AA meetings and becoming abstinent.

Denial is very much in evidence if clients are not ready to accept responsibility for their actions. Remember that any addiction requires self-disclosure and acceptance of the disease, intense therapy (counseling sessions, daily AA meetings, admission to an alcohol rehabilitation center, employee assistance program), and ongoing support. Until the client experiences the stages of loss and grief, he or she will not be ready to accept a diagnosis of alcoholism and voluntarily change the alcoholic life-style.

Chapter 88

1. This client may have a cervical spine fracture and his status would be classified as urgent. Safety measures would include immediate application of a cervical collar, immobilization of the head and neck on a stretcher, and cross-table lateral x-rays. Advise the client to keep his head perfectly still. Do not leave him alone. The client should undergo a complete neurologic examination but a full range-of-motion examination should not be performed until a cervical fracture has been ruled out.

2. Your first priority is to insist that the police officers who brought the client stay in the room with you and the client. Second, have someone alert your emergency department manager and hospital security personnel. Next, try to calm the client by talking calmly and quietly. Try to get him to stay long enough to be assessed and treated. If he continues to be combative and abusive, he will need to be restrained so that he can undergo the necessary assessments and treatments. He should not be sedated, because he has a head injury, is intoxicated, and may vomit. Do not get into a shouting match with the client. If at any time and in any way the client causes you physical harm, you must complete a special report form and report the incident to your manager.

Chapter 89

1. Your priority in this case is to treat the client in need of emergency care, because you must rule out evidence of cerebral bleeding as soon as possible. Even though he is still conscious and has entered your department in no acute distress, he has progressed from a potentially urgent case to an emergent case because he has told you he sustained a fall (potential head injury), has taken aspirin (known anticoagulant properties), and may have hypertension. At this point you do not yet know if his blood pressure problem has been diagnosed and is being treated or if it is something he just noticed. He may be having a stroke. You need to proceed by getting his vital signs immediately while asking questions of him or his wife about the following: his headache, his blood pressure, his fall, how

much aspirin has he taken, and when he or his wife first noticed his speech and balance problems. The priority for your physical assessment, once you have the vital signs, is to perform a thorough neurologic examination to rule in or out your hypotheses regarding his condition. You must anticipate that he will most likely be admitted for a more complete work-up and that blood chemistries, clotting studies, and a CT scan of the head will be first on the list. You will stabilize the client, assist in collecting specimens, and accompanying him to the radiology department. You will keep him quiet, confine him to the gurney, and keep the head of the bed elevated 30 degrees. He and his wife must be kept informed and reassured.

2. The client is exhibiting signs of an "acute abdomen." Several possible etiologies, which are potentially life-threatening, can cause the same symptoms. Therefore, you should consider her an emergent case and begin your assessments immediately. She has stated that her pain starts in the RLQ and radiates to her groin, and that it has been intense. You need to find out more information that can help you rule in or out potential differential diagnoses of pelvic inflammatory disease, appendicitis, right ovarian cyst (possibly ruptured), ectopic pregnancy, or renal stones. After getting the vital signs, your first priority is to use your PQRST mnemonic to more fully assess her pain (direct and rebound pain), while performing a complete abdominal examination. You need to find out when her LMP was, if she is sexually active, if she has ever been pregnant before, if there is anything that precipitates her pain, if she had a fever, if she had any similar problems before, if she had nausea or vomiting, bleeding, dizziness or lightheadedness on standing, or progressive distention. You will want to draw blood ordered for a human chorionic gonadotropin pregnancy test and blood chemistries and obtain urine for analysis. You must anticipate that the client will be admitted for a more complete work-up. Keep her on bed rest. Your interventions will become specific once you have responses to your intense inquiry and have finished the physical examination. You may be ordered to secure an IV access, initiate IV fluids, keep her NPO, and prepare her for further diagnostic evaluation. You will continue to monitor her response to treatment. If her level of pain increases sharply and her vital signs show evidence of shock, immediate medical and nursing intervention is required.

3. The client's case would normally be considered urgent, but her increasing dyspnea is a red flag to a potential respiratory crisis and should alert you to consider her case emergent. Your first priority in this case is to stabilize her condition by following the principles of the ABCs. Obtain vital signs—including auscultation of lung sounds for crackles and wheezes—and peak flow readings and possibly ABGs immediately. According to the findings, priority interventions could include oxygen therapy, pulse oximetry, bronchodilator therapy, and a chest x-ray. She may have developed a pulmonary contusion, pneumothorax, or hemothorax from her fall on the curb and/or she may have developed adult-onset asthma precipitated by her increased exertion from her intense training. You must

question her more once she is breathing more easily regarding her fall and her breathing since then. You will want to know if she has ever had asthma or any other breathing problem. Metered-dose inhalation treatment may be all that is ordered, with detailed discharge teaching regarding inhalation therapy and how to recognize and control environmental and psychological asthma triggers. However, if her condition continues to worsen and your respiratory assessment shows evidence of a possible localized problem near where she injured herself when she fell, or if x-ray results show signs of contusion or collapse, immediate medical (e.g., chest tube insertion, anti-inflammatory agent administration) and nursing intervention (IV access, fluid administration, continued frequent vital signs) will be required. She will be admitted when stable.

4. Your first priority is to assess the ABCs. While taking the client's vital signs, oxygen therapy may be initiated at 2 to 4 L/minute per nasal cannula. Oxygen alone may help arouse him. Blood should be drawn for an immediate spot blood glucose to check for diabetic ketoacidosis versus insulin shock and a specimen should be sent for chemistry analysis, drug levels, and a lipid profile. A catheter may need to be inserted if he is not awake enough to give you a urine specimen. Because he has coronary artery disease, hypertension, and an irregular pulse, a 12-lead ECG may be helpful to determine if there is cardiac ischemia or injury. If blood glucose is normal, you may proceed with further inquiry of his wife. Ask her about his medications and how he has been taking them, how his diet has been, if he has ever had a problem like this before, and if he ever had a stroke

or recent chest pain. He may be suffering from medication reaction or overdose from any one or a combination of his medications if he is taking several—which seems likely if his wife has them in a large paper bag! You will need to record all of his medications. Your priority system assessments include cardiovascular, respiratory, and neurologic function, while keeping him on bedrest with the head of the bed elevated 30 degrees. Other interventions will follow initial laboratory and examination findings. Drug antagonists, IV glucose or insulin, CT of the head, and other IV fluids to prevent hypovolemia, are all interventions that may be ordered according to initial findings. It is likely that the client will be admitted for observation.

Index

Note: Page numbers in *italics* refer to illustrations; page numbers followed by t refer to tables; page numbers followed by b refer to boxes.

A

A beta fibers, in pain transmission, 344
A delta fibers, in pain transduction/transmission, 343, 344
A Patient's Bill of Rights, 41, 47
AA (anesthesiologist's assistant), 468
AAACN (American Academy of Ambulatory Care Nursing), 139
AAAHC (Accreditation Association for Ambulatory Health Care), 139
AAI (atrial demand) pacemaker, 1320b
Abdomen, assessment of, in cardiovascular disorders, 1217
  in regional examination, 219t–221t
  emergencies of, 2529–2532
  flat plate of, 1713
  injuries of, *2531,* 2531–2532
  physical examination of, 1707–1709, *1708,* 1845–1848, *1847*
    in endocrine disorders, 1952
    normal findings in, 1699b
  trauma to, 1829–1830
    clinical manifestations of, 1829
    diagnostic findings in, 1829
    etiology of, 1829
    management of, complications of, 1830
      medical, 1829–1830
      nursing, 1830
      surgical, 1830
    pathophysiology of, 1829
    risk factors for, 1829
Abdominal angina, and small intestinal obstruction, 1821
Abdominal aortic aneurysm, 1425–1428, *1426*
  management of, community/self care in, 1428
    medical, 1426
    surgical, 1426–1427
      complications of, 1427
      nursing care in, 1427–1428
    rupture of, 1426
Abdominal distention, in acute pancreatitis, 1923, 1924t
  postoperative, 490
Abdominal films, diagnostic, 250
Abdominal muscles, weak, and urinary incontinence, 1605
Abdominal pain, 356
  acute, 2529–2530, *2530*
  in rheumatic fever, 1328
Abdominal reflex, 726, 729t
  assessment of, in regional examination, 221t
Abdominal wall, veins of, in cirrhosis, 1878t
Abdominal-perineal resection, for colon cancer, 1812, *1812*
  nursing care after, 1813–1814

Abdominoplasty, 2276, *2276*
Abducens nerve, assessment of, *719,* 720
ABGs. See *Arterial blood gases (ABGs).*
ABI (ankle-brachial index), 1383
Ablation therapy, for dysrhythmias, 1314
ABMT (autologous bone marrow transplantation), for cancer, 585
ABO blood group system, 1455, 1455t
  in blood component compatibility, 1521t
  in spontaneous abortion, 1456b
Abortion, religious beliefs about, 2545–2551
  spontaneous, ABO incompatibility in, 1456b
Above-knee prosthesis, *1422*
Abscess(es), anorectal, 1828, *1829*
  brain, 857–858, *858*
    clinical manifestations of, 858
  breast, 2453
  crypt, in ulcerative colitis, 1796
  liver, 1902
  lung, 1138–1139
  perinephric, 1674
  peritonsillar, 1080
  renal, 1673–1674
  subdiaphragmatic, 1168
Absence (petit mal) seizures, in epilepsy, 837
Absolute neutrophil count (ANC), during chemotherapy, 582
Absorptiometry, x-ray, dual-energy, in osteoporosis, 2100, *2101*
  of musculoskeletal disorders, 2093–2094
Absorption, 274b
  in gastrointestinal tract, 1685
  in large intestine, 1696
  in small intestine, 1693–1694
Abstinence, definition of, 2481t
Abstract reasoning/thinking, assessment of, 195
  changes in, cerebrovascular accident and, 792
Abuse, of elderly, 89–90, 90b
  detection of, 90b
AC (doxorubicin [Adriamycin], cyclophosphamide), for breast cancer, 2448t
Acalculous cholecystitis, 1916
  acute, 1918
Acarbose (Precose), for diabetes mellitus, 1967t, 1968
Accidents, screening for, 208t
  vehicle, blunt trauma in, 2521t
Accommodation, 937
  testing of, 720, 944–945
    in increased intracranial pressure, 782
Accreditation, of ambulatory care settings, 138–139

Accreditation Association for Ambulatory Health Care (AAAHC), 139
Accupril (quinapril), 1396t
Accutane (isotretinoin), for acne vulgaris, 2212
ACE (angiotensin-converting enzyme) inhibitors, 1396t
  for heart failure, 1286
    with extracellular fluid volume excess, 288
Acebutolol (Sectral), 1395t
  for angina pectoris, 1257t
Acetaminophen (Tylenol), antidote to, 2538t
  avoidance of, in cirrhosis, 1882t
  in pain control, 375t
  therapeutic monitoring of, reference values for, 2562
Acetazolamide (Diamox), for glaucoma, client teaching about, 957t
  side effects of, 839t
Acetic acid solution, 2199t
  for open wounds, 445t
Acetylcholine, in muscle contraction, 2078, *2080*
  in pancreatic secretion, 1841
  in sleep, 398
Acetylsalicylic acid, for angina pectoris, 1257t
Achalasia, 1733–1737
  clinical manifestations of, 1734
  diagnostic findings in, 1734
  etiology of, 1733
  management of, in elderly, 1737
    medical, 1734
    nursing, 1734–1735
    surgical, 1735, *1735, 1736*
      nursing care in, 1735–1737
  pathophysiology of, 1733–1734, *1734*
  risk factors for, 1733
Achilles tendon reflex, 729t
  in thyroid function testing, 1953
Acid(s), fixed, regulation of, 329–331, *330, 331*
  volatile, regulation of, lungs in, 328–329, *329*
Acid perfusion test, 1717
Acid phosphatase, reference values for, in cancer, 557t
  serum, in male reproductive disorders, 2337
Acid-ash diet, for urinary tract infections, 1574, 1577t
Acid-base balance, compensation in, 332, *333*
  correction in, 332–333
  disorders of, 328–340
    clinical manifestations of, 337–338
    complex, 336
    critical monitoring in, 337b

Acid-base balance (Continued)
  diagnostic findings in, 337–338
  in coma, 752
  management of, 338–340
    medical, 338
    nursing, 338–340, 338b
  metabolic acidosis in, 335t, 336
  metabolic alkalosis in, 335t, 336
  prevention of, 336–337
  respiratory acidosis in, 333–335, 334t
  respiratory alkalosis in, 333–335, 334t
  triple, 336
  in shock, 504–506, 506
  regulation of, 328–333
    chemical buffer systems in, 331–332
    kidneys in, 329–331, 330, 331
    lungs in, 328–329, 329, 1033, 1057
    systems for, interaction of, 332, 332–333, 333
Acid-base map, 333
Acidemia, 333
Acid-fast bacilli (AFB) smear, in tuberculosis diagnosis, 1142
Acidification, of urine, for urinary tract infection, 1574
Acidosis, kidneys in, 1543
  lactic, in shock, 503, 506
  metabolic. See Metabolic acidosis.
  respiratory, 333–335, 334t
    critical monitoring in, 337b
    etiology of, 333–335, 334t
    postoperative, causes of, 488
Acinar cell carcinoma, of pancreas, 1931
ACL (anterior cruciate ligament), injuries of, 2166, 2166
Aclovate (alclometasone), topical, 2199t
Acne, medications for, 2198t
Acne rosacea, 2213
Acne vulgaris, 2212, 2212–2213
Acoustic nerve, assessment of, 719, 721
Acoustic neuroma, 845, 1002–1003
  and hearing impairment, 994
Acquired immunodeficiency syndrome (AIDS), 2473
  diagnostic tests for, 611
  infectious agent in, 416t
  management of, in elderly, 635–636
    medical, 627–631
    nursing, 631–635, 632b
    surgical, 636
  neoplasms in, 630–631
  nursing diagnoses in, 632b
  ocular manifestations of, 977
  opportunistic infections in, 627–630
  toxoplasmosis in, 860
Acral lentiginous melanoma (ALM), 2228t
Acromegaly, in hyperpituitarism, 2062, 2062, 2063t
ACS (American Cancer Society), 564b
  guidelines of, for cancer screening, 552, 553t
ACTH. See Adrenocorticotropic hormone (ACTH).
Actin filaments, 1196, 1196, 1197
Actinic, definition of, 2183t
Actinic keratosis, 2225
Action potential, of cardiac cells, 294, 1195, 1195

Action potential (Continued)
  of electrolytes, 293–294, 294, 295
Activated clotting time, in hemorrhage, 1467t
Activities of daily living (ADLs), in elderly, 87
  in spinal cord injury, 907
  pain effect on, 363, 365b
Activity, diversional, deficit in, in fracture, 2144
  impaired, in osteoporosis, 2105
  pattern of, 206
  physical, after myocardial infarction, program for, 1264–1266, 1265b
  postoperative, promotion of, 492
Activity intolerance, in cardiomyopathy, 1344
  in chronic arterial occlusion, 1409–1412, 1412
  in chronic obstructive pulmonary disease, 1120–1121
  in cirrhosis, 1883
  in heart failure, 1288
  in hypercortisolism, 2054
  in hyperthyroidism, 2020–2022
  in hypothyroidism, 2015
  in multiple sclerosis, 876
  in myocardial infarction, 1273–1275
  in pneumonia, 1137–1138
  in rheumatic fever, 1330
Activity tolerance, measurement of, perceived exertion scale in, 1126
Acupressure, in pain control, 349b, 371
Acupuncture, for pain, 349b, 388–389
  in anesthesia, 476–477
Acute abdomen, 2529–2530, 2530
Acute arterial occlusion, 1424
Acute bacterial endocarditis, 1331
Acute care, 120–132
  for elderly, 96
  future of, 131–132
  hospitals in, 120–121, 121b, 122b
  legal issues in, 130
  performance improvement in, 130–131, 130b, 131b
    clinical indicators of, 130, 130b
    qualities in, 131b
  quality, delivery of, 125–131, 127b, 128t, 130b, 131b
  regulatory requirements in, 129–130
  risk management in, 131, 132b
Acute hemolytic transfusion reaction, 1529t
Acute lymphocytic leukemia (ALL), 1487, 1488
  classification of, 1488t
  management of, medical, 1489–1490
Acute nonlymphocytic leukemia (ANLL), 1487
  management of, medical, 1490
  pathophysiology of, 1488
Acute pain, 351–352, 352
Acute renal failure (ARF), 1636–1641
  client education in, 1641b
  clinical manifestations of, 1638–1639
  diagnostic findings in, 1638–1639
  etiology of, 1636–1637, 1637
  management of, in elderly, 1641
    medical, 1639–1640

Acute renal failure (ARF) (Continued)
  nursing, 1640–1641, 1641b
  nonoliguric, 1638
  oliguric, 1638–1639
  pathophysiology of, 1637–1638
  risk factors for, 1636–1637
Acute respiratory failure, 1169–1170, 1170b
  causes of, 1170b
Acute tubular necrosis (ATN), in shock, 510
  nephrotoxins and, 1627, 1627b
Acutrim (phenylpropanolamine hydrochloride), for urinary incontinence, 1611t
Acyclovir (Zovirax), for genital herpes, 2472
  for herpes simplex virus encephalitis, 859
  for herpes zoster, 2223
AD. See Alzheimer's disease (AD).
ADA (Americans with Disabilities Act), 111b, 129
  ambulatory care standards of, 138
Adaptation, of receptors, in nerve impulse conduction, 690
  to chronic conditions. See Chronic conditions, adaptation to.
Adaptic gauze, indications for, 443t
ADC (AIDS dementia complex), 631
Addiction, definition of, 2481t
  to opioid analgesics, 377
Addictive behavior, framework for, 2479–2480
  biologic, 2480
  psychological, 2480
  sociocultural, 2480
Addis concentration test, 1561
Addisonian crisis, 2042
  after total hip replacement, 2114
  in postanesthesia care unit, 483
  nursing care in, 2043–2047
Addison's disease, 2041–2047
  clinical manifestations of, 2041–2042
  etiology of, 2041
  hormonal dysfunction in, 2044t
  in acquired immunodeficiency syndrome, nursing research on, 2042b
  management of, in elderly, 2047
    medical, 2042, 2047, 2048t, 2049t
    nursing, 2043–2047
  pathophysiology of, 2041, 2043
  prevention of, 2042b
  risk factors for, 2041, 2042b
ADEA (Age Discrimination and Employment Act), 129
Adenocarcinoma, of kidney, 1671
  of lung, 1153t
  of pancreas, 1931
  of thyroid, 2028t
Adenocard (adenosine), for dysrhythmia, 1308t
Adenohypophysis, disorders of, 2060–2066
  and sexual disturbances, 2065
  structure/function of, 1941–1942
Adenoids, 1023
Adenoma, hepatic, 1896, 1896
  pituitary, 846
Adenosine (Adenocard), for dysrhythmia, 1308t
Adenosine triphosphate (ATP), in shock, 503

Adenotonsillectomy, 1079
  indications for, 1079
ADH. See *Antidiuretic hormone (ADH)*.
Adhesions, and small intestinal obstruction, 1820, *1820*
Adipose tissue, measurement of, 237, *240*
Adjustment, impaired, in vertigo, 1014
Adjuvant chemotherapy, for breast cancer, 2447–2448
ADLs (activities of daily living), in elderly, 87
  in spinal cord injury, 907
  pain effect on, 363, 365b
Admission, to hospital, methods of, 121, 121b
Adnexal areas, examination of, 2319
Adnexal disease, red eye in, 942b
Adolescence, integumentary system changes in, 2177–2178
Adrenal blocking agents, for hypercortisolism, 2053
Adrenal cortex, disorders of, 2041–2056
  function of, *1944*, 1944–1945
    diagnostic tests of, 2045t–2046t
  hyperfunction of, 2049–2056
  structure of, *1944*, 1944–1945
Adrenal cortical compounds, for chemotherapy, classification of, 577t
Adrenal cortical steroid inhibitors, for chemotherapy, classification of, 577t
Adrenal glands, disorders of, 2041–2069
  function of, *1944*, 1944–1945
    tests of, 1953–1954
  hormones of, 1940t
    dysfunction of, 2044t
    function of, 2044t
  in hypertension, 1389
  in shock, 508
  structure of, *1944*, 1944–1945
Adrenal insufficiency, 2041–2049
  acute, 2042
  after total hip replacement, 2114
  in acquired immunodeficiency syndrome, nursing research on, 2042b
  primary, chronic. See *Addison's disease*.
  secondary, 2047–2049, *2049*
Adrenal medulla, disorders of, 2056–2060
  structure/function of, 1944
Adrenalectomy, for breast cancer, 2437–2438, 2449, 2449t
  for hypercortisolism, 2052, 2054t
  for pheochromocytoma, 2058–2059
  for primary hyperaldosteronism, 2056
Adrenergic antagonists, peripheral-acting, 1397t
Adrenergic blocking agents, for hyperthyroidism, 2020
  for shock, 515
Adrenergic fibers, 703
Adrenocorticotropic hormone (ACTH), 2061t
  actions of, 1940t
  deficiency of, in hypopituitarism, 2065
  dysfunction of, 2044t
  for multiple sclerosis, 874
  function of, 2044t
  in Addison's disease, 2042
  in carbohydrate metabolism, 1946

Adrenocorticotropic hormone (ACTH) *(Continued)*
  in secondary adrenal insufficiency, 2049
  measurement of, in adrenal function testing, 1953
  overproduction of, in hypercortisolism, 2049
  plasma level of, 2046t
  reference values for, in cancer, 557t
Adriamycin (doxorubicin), cyclophosphamide (AC), for breast cancer, 2448t
Adriamycin (doxorubicin), mitomycin (AM), for breast cancer, 2448t
Adson's maneuver, 2090t
Adult(s), immunization of, recommendations for, 422t
  integumentary system changes in, 2178
  older. See *Elderly*.
Adult Children of Alcoholics, 2497b
Adult day care, for elderly, 99
Adult respiratory distress syndrome (ARDS), 1170–1184
  clinical manifestations of, 1171–1172
  diagnostic findings in, 1171–1172, *1172*
  etiology of, 1170, 1170b
  in acute pancreatitis, critical monitoring in, 1927b
  management of, *1171*
    medical, 1172, 1172b
    nursing, 1172–1184
  pathophysiology of, 1170–1171
  risk factors for, 1170
Adult-onset medullary cystic disease, 1679
Advanced directives, 47
  for elderly, 102
  in dementia of Alzheimer's type, 870
  in emergency patient, ethical issues in, 2502b
  in terminal cancer, 567
Advanced-practice nurses (APNs), 12–14, 136
Adventitious breath sounds, 1046, 1048t
Advil (ibuprofen), for rheumatoid arthritis, 664t
  in pain control, 375t
Advocacy, ambulatory care nurse in, 141b, 142
  in client confusion, ethical issues in, 768b
  of elderly client, 101b
AEDs (automated external defibrillators), 1312
Aerosols, 2200t
  for hypersensitivity, 641
Aerotitis media, 1009
AFB (acid-fast bacilli) smear, in tuberculosis diagnosis, 1142
Affect, assessment of, 195, 710t, 716–717
AFP (alpha-fetoprotein), in cancer diagnosis, 558t
  in hepatobiliary assessment, 1852t
Afterload, 1200, *1201*
  in heart failure, increase in, 1277, 1277t
  reduction of, 1285–1286
Afterloading, in radiation therapy, 573
Age, advanced, in postoperative wound infection, 490
  assessment of, 233–234
    preoperative, 453

Age *(Continued)*
  in burn severity classification, 2239
  in cancer, 540
  in coronary artery disease, 1238
  in hypertension, 1388
  in immunity, 604–605
  in pain response, 346–350
  of clients, variations in, 14–16
Age Discrimination and Employment Act (ADEA), 129
Ageism, 88
Agency for Health Care Policy and Research (AHCPR), guidelines of, for acute pain management, 352
  for cancer pain management, 358–359
AGF (angiogenesis factor), in wound healing, 429
Aging, 81–102. See also *Elderly*.
  and sexuality changes, 77t
  cultural aspects of, 83–84
  in illness, 34
  of biliary tract, 1841
  of cell, 267–268, 268t
  of endocrine system, 1946
  of gastrointestinal tract, 1696
  of heart, 1204
  of hematologic system, 1459
  of integumentary system, 2177–2178
  of liver, 1841
  of lymphatic system, 1376
  of musculoskeletal system, 2080–2081
  of nervous system, 705–707
  of pancreas, 1841
  of respiratory system, 1034
  of urinary tract, 1545
  of vascular system, 1376
  physiologic changes of, 268t
  study of, 81–82
Agnosia, assessment of, 711t
  cerebrovascular accident and, 790–791
Agranulocytosis, 1497–1498
  clinical manifestations of, 1498
  diagnostic findings in, 1498
  etiology of, 1497
  management of, medical, 1498
    nursing, 1498
  pathophysiology of, 1497
  risk factors for, 1497
Agraphesthesia, 724
AHA (American Hospital Association), 4, 175b
AHAs (alphahydroxy acids), 2203
AHCPR (Agency for Health Care Policy and Research), guidelines of, for acute pain management, 352
  for cancer pain management, 358–359
AHF (antihemophilic factor), 1517
AICD (automatic implantable cardioverter-defibrillator), 1312–1313
AIDS. See *Acquired immunodeficiency syndrome (AIDS)*.
AIDS Action Council, 619b
AIDS dementia complex (ADC), 631
AIDS retinopathy, 977
Air conduction, testing of, 720, 721
Air conduction hearing loss, 994b
Air plethysmography (APG), in peripheral vascular assessment, 1384

Airborne particles, health risks of, 204t
Airborne precautions, 424
Airway(s), 1021–1026
  artificial, for respiratory complications, in
    postanesthesia care unit, 482, 482
  assessment of, in major burns, 2242
  clearance of, ineffective, 1180
    after brain tumor surgery, 854
    after cardiac surgery, 1014
    after partial laryngectomy, 1089–1090
    after spinal cord injury, 899–900, 907
    after thoracic surgery, 1160
    in asthma, 1110
    in burns, 2244
    in chronic obstructive pulmonary dis-
      ease, 1120
    in head trauma, 827
    in pneumonia, 1136–1137
    with tracheostomy, 1072–1074, 1074
  lower, disorders of, 1105–1131
    function of, 1025, 1025–1026, 1026t
    structure of, 1024, 1025
    thermal burns of, 2237
  maintenance of, after oral cancer surgery,
    1730
    in postanesthesia care unit, 482, 482
    in unconscious patient, 751
    postoperative, 485–487, 487
  obstruction of, after laryngeal surgery,
    1088
    in atelectasis, 1134b
    tracheostomy tubes and, 1070
  patency of, maintenance of, in emergency
    nursing care, 2505, 2505–2506, 2506
  suctioning of, in increased intracranial
    pressure, 783
  trauma to, endotracheal tube suctioning
    and, 1175t
  upper, disorders of, 1067–1103
    hemorrhagic, 1076–1082
    infectious, 1076–1082
    inflammatory, 1076–1082
    neoplastic, 1082–1100
    function of, 1023–1024
    obstructions of, 1100–1102
    structure of, 1021–1023, 1022–1024
Airway resistance, 1027
AJCC (American Joint Committee on Cancer), cancer performance status scale of,
  560, 560t
Akinesia, 723b
Alanine aminotransferase (ALT), in hepatobiliary assessment, 1851t
  reference values for, in cancer, 557t
  testing of, before blood transfusion, 1524t
Al-Anon, 2497b
Alarms, in electrocardiography, setting of,
  1222
  of ventilators, 1186
Albright's hereditary osteodystrophy, 2036
Albumin, administration of, for shock, 519
  decreased, in ascites, 1889
  effect of, on calcium level, 314
  functions of, 1447, 1448t
  glycosylated, in diabetes mellitus, 1962
  in acid-base balance, 331
  serum, in hepatobiliary assessment, 1850t
  transfusion of, 1520t

Albumin/globulin ratio, in hepatobiliary assessment, 1850t
Albuterol, for hyperkalemia, 312
Alclometasone (Aclovate), topical, 2199t
Alcohol, 35
  abuse of, 2486–2488
    effects of, 2482t
    in acute pancreatitis, 1921–1922, 1922b
    in cirrhosis, 1873
    in Native Americans, 198t
    management of, 201t
    medical consequences of, 2490t
  avoidance of, in cirrhosis, 1882t
  complications of, intraoperative, 457
  consumption of, in epilepsy, 842
    in respiratory disorders, 1039
  effects of, cardiovascular, 1210
    perioperative, 457
  restriction of, for hypertension, 1393
  withdrawal from, symptoms of, 2487t
Alcoholic hepatitis, 1872
Alcoholics Anonymous, 2497b
Alcoholism, hypomagnesemia in, 323
  prevention of, 201t
Aldactone (spironolactone), 1394t
  characteristics of, 1285t
  complications of, 2056b
  for hyperaldosteronism, 2056, 2056b
  for premenstrual syndrome, 2388
Aldolase A, tests of, in musculoskeletal disorders, 2096t
Aldomet (methyldopa), 1396t
  in surgical client, 458t
  urine color with, 1557t
Aldosterone, dysfunction of, 2044t
  function of, 2044t
  in fluid balance regulation, 275, 276,
    277
  in hypertension, 1389
  in hypokalemia, 305
  measurement of, 2045t
    in adrenal function testing, 1953
Alendronate (Fosamax), for osteoporosis,
  2104
ALG (antilymphocyte globulin), for renal
  graft rejection, 1662
  in organ transplantation, 644t
Algiderm, indications for, 443t
Algor mortis, 271
Alkalemia, 333
Alkaline phosphatase (ALP), in cancer, reference values for, 557t
  in hepatobiliary assessment, 1851t
  in male reproductive disorders, 2338
  in musculoskeletal disorders, 2096t
  serum, in parathyroid disorders, 2032t
Alkaline reflux gastritis, in peptic ulcer disease, 1778
Alkalosis, contraction, 336
  hypokalemia in, 305
  kidneys in, 1543
  metabolic, 335t, 336
    critical monitoring in, 337b
    etiology of, 335t, 336
    posthypercapneic, 336
  respiratory, 333–335, 334t
    critical monitoring in, 337b
    etiology of, 334t, 335

Alkylating agents, for chemotherapy, classification of, 577t
ALL (acute lymphocytic leukemia), 1487,
  1488
  classification of, 1488t
  management of, medical, 1489–1490
Allen's test, in arterial blood gas analysis,
  339, 1056, 1057
  in peripheral vascular assessment, 1382
Allergen, in hypersensitivity, 636
Allergic alveolitis, 1150
Allergic reactions, and distributive shock,
  500
  prevention of, 200t
  to intravenous pyelography, 1563
  to medications, clinical manifestations of,
    640t
Allergic rhinitis, 1080
Allergic transfusion reaction, 1529t
Allergy(ies). See also Hypersensitivity.
  atopic, 638–639
  history of, in ear disorders, 986
    in eye disorders, 942
    in gastrointestinal disorders, 1705
    in gynecologic disorders, 2308
    in hematologic disorders, 1462
    in immune disorders, 608
    in integumentary system disorders, 2181
    in male reproductive disorders, 2330
    in respiratory disorders, 1039
    in urinary tract disorders, 1550
  testing for, in immune disorders, 612
  to analgesia, 379
  to contrast agents, 252b
Allogeneic donor, preparation of, for bone
  marrow transplantation, 1495–1496
Allogeneic transplants, 642
Allograft homograft, in burn wound cover-
  ing, 2256t
Allopurinol (Zyloprim), for renal calculi,
  1667
ALM (acral lentiginous melanoma), 2228t
Alopecia, 2186
  chemotherapy and, 583
ALP. See Alkaline phosphatase (ALP).
Alpha₁-receptor blockers, 1395t
Alpha₂ agonists, centrally acting, 1396t–
  1397t
Alpha-adrenergic receptors, in cardiac regu-
  lation, 1203
Alpha-beta blockers, 1395t
Alpha-delta activity, 405
Alpha-fetoprotein (AFP), in cancer diagno-
  sis, 558t
  in hepatobiliary assessment, 1852t
Alphahydroxy acid peels, 2273
Alphahydroxy acids (AHAs), 2203
ALS (amyotrophic lateral sclerosis), 886–
  888
  bulbar, 887
ALS Society of America, 887b
ALT (alanine aminotransferase), in hepato-
  biliary assessment, 1851t
  reference values for, in cancer, 557t
  testing of, before blood transfusion, 1524t
Altace (ramipril), 1396t
Altercation, blunt trauma in, 2521t
Altered family processes, 57

Aluminum acetate, topical, 2199t
Aluminum hydroxide (Amphojel), for peptic ulcer disease, 1769t
Aluminum intoxication, hemodialysis and, 1654
Alveolar lavage, 1062
Alveolar macrophages, 1026
Alveolar pneumonia, 1135
Alveolar pressure, 1030
Alveolar unit, 1028, *1029*
Alveolar ventilation, $PaCO_2$ in, 1056–1057
Alveoli, structure of, 1028–1029, *1029*
Alveolitis, allergic, 1150
Alzheimer's disease (AD), 863–872
  caregiver respite in, 870b
  client education in, 867b
  clinical manifestations of, 864–865, 864b
  diagnostic findings in, 864–865
  etiology of, 863
  home safety in, 868b
  management of, community/self care in, 865–872
    medical, 865, 866t
    nursing, 865–872, 867b, 868b, 870b, 871t–872t
  pathophysiology of, 863–864, *864*
  risk factors for, 863
  sleep disorders in, 404
AM (doxorubicin [Adriamycin], mitomycin), for breast cancer, 2448t
Amantadine (Symmetrel), for Parkinson's disease, 880t
Amaurosis, 951
Ambulation, after musculoskeletal trauma, 2167
  after spinal cord injury, 905–907
  after total hip replacement, 2114
  for urinary calculi, 1596–1597
  postoperative, preoperative preparation for, 461
  with cast, 2151, *2151*
Ambulatory care, 135–143
  definition of, 136b
  settings for, 137–139, 138b, 139b
    accreditation of, 138–139
    certification of, 138–139, 139b
    controls/standards for, 138
    features of, 137
  terminology in, 136b
Ambulatory care nursing, 12
  definition of, 136b
  development of, 135–137, 136b
  medical model of, 139–140
  nursing model of, 140
  roles of, 140–143, 141b
    in clinical practice, 140–142
    in quality improvement, 142–143
    in research, 142–143
  scope of, 139–143
  studies of, 137
Ambulatory Care Nursing Administration and Practice Standards, 136–137, 136b
Amebiasis, 1790
  and liver abscess, 1902
Amelanotic, definition of, 2183t
Amenorrhea, 2389–2391, *2390*
  clinical manifestations of, 2390
  diagnostic findings in, 2390

Amenorrhea *(Continued)*
  etiology of, 2389–2390, *2390*
  in cirrhosis, 1878t
  management of, community/self care in, 2390–2391
    medical, 2390
    nursing, 2390–2391
Americaine (benzocaine), 473t
American Academy of Ambulatory Care Nursing (AAACN), 139
American Association of Homes for the Aging, 97b
American Association of Retired Persons, 97b
American Cancer Society (ACS), 564b
  guidelines of, for cancer screening, 552, 553t
American Hospital Association (AHA), 4, 175b
American Indian Health Care Association, 619b
American Joint Committee on Cancer (AJCC), cancer performance status scale of, 560, 560t
American Muslim Mission, beliefs/practices of, 2550
The American Parkinson's Disease Association, 887b
American Society of Anesthesiology's physical status classification, 469
American Spinal Injury Association (ASIA) Impairment Scale, 893
Americans with Disabilities Act (ADA), 111b, 129
  ambulatory care standards of, 138
Amicar (aminocaproic acid), for disseminated intravascular coagulation, 1512
Amikacin, therapeutic monitoring of, reference values for, 2562
Amiloride (Midamor), 1394t
Amino acids, deamination of, liver in, 1840
Aminocaproic acid (Amicar), for disseminated intravascular coagulation, 1512
Aminoglutethimide (Cytadren), for breast cancer, 2449, 2449t
  for hypercortisolism, 2053
Aminoglycoside antibiotics, ototoxic, 986b
Aminophylline, for asthma, 1110–1111
  therapeutic monitoring of, reference values for, 2562
Amiodarone (Cordarone), for dysrhythmia, 1308t
Amitriptyline (Elavil), in pain control, 374
  therapeutic monitoring of, reference values for, 2562
  urine color with, 1557t
Amlodipine (Norvasc), 1396t
Ammonia, in hepatic encephalopathy, 1892, 1893
  removal of, liver in, 1840
  serum, in hepatobiliary assessment, 1851t
Ammonia buffer system, 330, *330*
Amnesia, after concussion, 2528
Amniocentesis, schedule for, 208t
Amnion, in burn wound covering, 2256t
Amphetamines, abuse of, 2488–2490
  effects of, 2482t
  health consequences of, 2493t

Amphetamines *(Continued)*
  withdrawal from, symptoms of, 2487t
Amphojel (aluminum hydroxide), for peptic ulcer disease, 1769t
AMPLE, in emergency nursing assessment, 2503
Ampulla, in balance, 984
Amputation, 1415–1424
  care in, postoperative, 1420–1424
    preoperative, 1419–1420
  closed (flap), 1418, *1418*
  considerations in, 1418
  for thromboangiitis obliterans, 1431
  in diabetes mellitus, avoidance of, *1997*
  level of, 1418, *1419, 1420*
  open (guillotine), 1418, *1418*
  rehabilitation after, potential for, 1418
  traumatic, 2288, 2533
Amsler grid, 947
Amylase, in acute pancreatitis, 1923
  pancreatic, 1692t, 1840, 1922b
  serum, in hepatobiliary assessment, 1850t
  urine, in hepatobiliary assessment, 1850t
Amyloidosis, 1902–1903
Amyotrophic lateral sclerosis (ALS), 886–888
  bulbar, 887
ANA Code for Nurses, 41, 41b
ANA Standards of Nursing Practice, 41
Anaerobic bacterial pneumonia, 1136t
Anal fissure, 1828
Anal fistula, 1828
Anal reflex, 727, 729t
Anal sphincter, female, examination of, 2320
  tone of, assessment of, 1554
Analgesia, 724
  adjuvant, 377–378
  administration of, methods of, 382–386, *383, 384,* 385t
    principles of, 379–382
  effectiveness of, factors in, 378–379
  epidural, *383,* 383–384
  for intracranial hemorrhage, 815
  for otitis externa, 1005
  for pulmonary embolism, 1129
  in elderly, 391–392, 392t
  in pain control, 372–386, *373*
  intraspinal, *383,* 383–384
  mechanisms of, 373–374, 373t
  non-opioid, 374
  nurse-administered (demand), 382
  opioid (narcotic), 374–377, 375t, 376b
  oral, administration of, equianalgesic chart for, 375t
  patient-controlled. See *Patient-controlled analgesia (PCA).*
  potency of, oral, 379, 380t–381t
    relative, 378–379
  spinal, *383,* 383–384
  subcutaneous, continuous, 383
  time action of, 379
  transdermal, 382–383
  types of, 374–378
Analgesia system, 344
Analgesics, for acute pancreatitis, 1924–1925
  for cholelithiasis, 1910

Analgesics (Continued)
  for urinary tract infections, 1576t
  nephrotoxicity of, 1627
  therapeutic monitoring of, reference values
    for, 2562
Anaphylactic (type I) hypersensitivity, 638–
    639, 638t, 639t, 640t
Anaphylactic shock, 486t, 638
  causes of, 639t
  clinical manifestations of, 512–513
  definition of, 497
  etiology of, 500
  management of, 524t
  prevention of, 501b
  skin testing and, 637
Anaphylactic transfusion reaction, 1529t
Anaphylactoid purpura, 1508
Anaphylaxis, causes of, 639t
  chemical mediators of, 638t
Anaplastic, definition of, 534t
Anaplastic carcinoma, of thyroid, 2028t
Anaprox (naproxen), for rheumatoid arthri-
    tis, 664t
  in pain control, 375t
ANAs (antinuclear antibodies), in hepatobil-
    iary disease, 1849
  in musculoskeletal disorders, 2096t
  in systemic lupus erythematosus, 675
Anasarca, 286
  in right ventricular failure, 1282
Anatomical dead space, 1024
ANC (absolute neutrophil count), during
    chemotherapy, 582
Androcur (cyproterone acetate), for benign
    prostatic hyperplasia, 2364t
Androgens, actions of, 1940t
  dysfunction of, 2044t
  for breast cancer, 2449, 2449t
  for chemotherapy, classification of, 577t
  function of, 2044t
Anectine (succinylcholine chloride), 472t
Anemia, 1458, 1469–1485
  acquired, 1471–1481
    classification of, 1470b
  and heart failure, 1278
  aplastic. See Aplastic anemia.
  bone marrow failure and, 1477–1478
  chemotherapy and, 582
  classification of, 1470b
  clinical manifestations of, 1470–1471
  congenital, 1481–1485
    classification of, 1470b
  diagnostic findings in, 1470–1471
  etiology of, 1469
  folic acid deficiency in, 1474, 1476–
    1477
  hemolytic. See Hemolytic anemia.
  hemorrhagic, 1481
    classification of, 1470b
  in chronic renal failure, 1645
  in cirrhosis, 1878t
  in viral hepatitis, 1865, 1866t
  iron deficiency. See Iron deficiency ane-
    mia.
  management of, community/self care in,
    1471
    medical, 1471
    nursing, 1471

Anemia (Continued)
  megaloblastic, 1474–1477
  normocytic, 1477
  pathophysiology of, 1469–1470, 1470b
  pernicious. See Pernicious anemia.
  risk factors for, 1469
  screening for, 208t
  secondary, 1481
  sickle cell. See Sickle cell anemia.
  vitamin B_{12} deficiency in, 1474, 1476
Anesthesia, 468–477, 724
  American Society of Anesthesiology's
    physical status classification in, 469
  caudal, 476
  choice of, variables in, 468
  epidural, 475
  field block, 474
  general. See General anesthesia.
  inhalation, 471, 471–472
  intravenous, 471
  intravenous regional (extremity) block,
    476
  local, 474
    agents for, 473t–474t
    in pain control, 372
  monitored, 476
  nephrotoxicity of, 1627, 1627b
  neuroleptic (balanced), 471
  nurse, 467–468
  peripheral nerve block, 474–475
  preoperative preparation for, 463–464
  providers of, 467–468
  rectal, 472
  regional, 468t, 472–476, 473t–474t, 475,
    476t
    characteristics of, 468
    types of, 474–476, 475, 476t
  spinal, 475, 475
    benefits of, 475
    complications of, 476t
    positioning for, 475, 475
  topical, 474
    agents for, 473t–474t
    in pain control, 372
  types of, 468t
Anesthesiologist, role of, 466
Anesthesiologist's assistant (AA), 468
Aneurysm(s), 1425–1428
  aortic, abdominal. See Abdominal aortic
    aneurysm.
  dissecting, chest pain in, assessment of,
    1208t
  thoracic, 1429–1430
  arteriovenous, head trauma and, 826
  classification of, 1425, 1425
  intracranial, 812, 812
    diagnosis of, 814, 814
    rupture of, 813
      and cerebrovascular accident, 785
  mycotic, 786
  peripheral, 1430
Aneurysm clipping, for intracranial hemor-
    rhage, 815–816
Aneurysm precautions, 815
Angelchik prosthesis, for gastroesophageal
    reflux disease, 1739, 1740
Anger, in dementia of Alzheimer's type,
    pharmacologic treatment of, 866t

Angina, abdominal, and small intestinal ob-
    struction, 1821
  Vincent's. See Vincent's angina.
Angina decubitus, 1254
Angina pectoris, 1251–1258
  chest pain in, assessment of, 1208t
  clinical manifestations of, 1253–1254
  diagnostic findings in, 1253–1254
  etiology of, 1251
  intractable, 1254
  management of, community/self care in,
    1255–1258
    emergency, 1254–1255, 1256t–1257t
    outcomes of, 1255
  nocturnal, 1254
    sleep disorders in, 405
  pathophysiology of, 1251–1253, 1253b
  postinfarction, 1254
  risk factors in, 1251
  stable, 1253
  unstable, 1253
  variant, 1254
Angiocardiography, types of, 1232, 1232t
Angiogenesis, in wound healing, 432
Angiogenesis factor (AGF), in wound heal-
    ing, 429
Angiography, 254
  cerebral, in neurologic assessment, 736–
    738, 737
  complications of, 1385
  contrast, in peripheral vascular assessment,
    1384–1385, 1385
  coronary, in angina pectoris, 1254
  digital venous, 736–737
  fluorescein, 951–952, 952
  in cancer diagnosis, 556
  in cardiovascular assessment, 1232, 1232t
  in hepatobiliary disease, 1853
  in intracranial aneurysm diagnosis, 814,
    814
  in pulmonary embolism diagnosis, 1128,
    1128
  interventional, 736
  nursing care after, 254, 1385
  preprocedure care in, 254
  procedure for, 254, 254
  pulmonary, 1062
  renal, 1564–1565
Angioplasty, balloon, 1413
  laser-assisted, 1413
  transluminal, percutaneous, 1245, 1245,
    1247b, 1413
Angioscopy, in peripheral vascular assess-
    ment, 1386
Angiotensin, in shock, 507
Angiotensin-converting enzyme (ACE) in-
    hibitors, 1396t
  for heart failure, 1286
    with extracellular fluid volume excess,
      288
Angle structures, of eye, 937, 938
Angle-closure glaucoma, 952, 953. See also
    Glaucoma.
  red eye in, 942b
Anglicans, beliefs/practices of, 2547
Animal bites, 2536
Animals, care of, in hepatitis A prevention,
    1864

Anion gap, in metabolic acidosis, 336
Anions, 293
Anisocoria, 720
Anisocytes, 1466t
Ankle(s), muscles of, strength of, assessment of, 2088t
range of motion of, *2089*
sprains of, 2163–2164, *2164*
Ankle jerk, *726,* 727, 729t
Ankle-brachial index (ABI), 1383
Ankylosing spondylitis (AS), 678, *679*
ANLL (acute nonlymphocytic leukemia), *1487*
management of, medical, 1490
pathophysiology of, 1488
Anorectal abscess, 1828, *1829*
Anorectum, disorders of, 1825–1828
tumors of, 1828
Anorexia, in gastrointestinal disorders, 1748
in rheumatic fever, 1328
in right ventricular failure, 1282
in viral hepatitis, 1865, 1866t
Anorexia nervosa, 1756–1758
clinical manifestations of, 1757–1758, *1758*
diagnostic findings in, 1757–1758
etiology of, 1757
management of, medical, 1758
nursing, 1758
pathophysiology of, 1757
risk factors for, 1757
Anosmia, 719, 1050
ANPs (atrial natriuretic peptides), in fluid balance regulation, 277
in sodium regulation, 295
ANS (autonomic nervous system), 701
disorders of, assessment of, 728–730
in cardiac regulation, 1202–1203
structure/function of, 703–704, *704*
Antabuse (disulfiram), education about, 2496b
Antacids, administration of, precautions for, 1770, 1770t
for gastroesophageal reflux disease, 1738
for peptic ulcer disease, 1769t, 1770
Anterior cerebral artery, cerebrovascular accident of, clinical manifestations of, 788t
Anterior chamber, of eye, examination of, 944
Anterior chamber reaction, 950
Anterior cord syndrome, 895, *896*
Anterior cruciate ligament (ACL), injuries of, 2166, *2166*
Anteroinferior cerebellum, cerebrovascular accident of, clinical manifestations of, 788t
Anteroposterior (AP) chest x-ray, 1060
Anteroposterior repair, for rectocele, 2410
Anthralin, for psoriasis, 2211
Anthranilates, topical, 2200t
Anthraquinone laxatives, urine color with, 1557t
Antiandrogens, for chemotherapy, classification of, 577t
Antibacterial drugs, for peptic ulcer disease, 1767, 1769t
topical, 2198t
Antibiotics, antitumor, classification of, 577t

Antibiotics *(Continued)*
complications of, intraoperative, 457
for acute cholecystitis, 1917
for acute pancreatitis, 1925
for agranulocytosis, 1498
for chronic obstructive pulmonary disease, 1111t
for cystic fibrosis, 1149
for glomerulonephritis, 1631
for increased intracranial pressure, 775
for inflammatory bowel disease, 1799
for multiple organ system failure, 530
for otitis externa, *1004,* 1004–1005
for shock, 520
for urinary tract infections, 1574, 1576t–1577t
nephrotoxicity of, 1627, 1627b
ototoxic, 986b
resistance to, 421b
therapeutic monitoring of, reference values for, 2562
Antibody(ies). See also *Immunoglobulin(s).*
antinuclear, in hepatobiliary disease, 1849
in musculoskeletal disorders, 2096t
in systemic lupus erythematosus, 675
creation of, B cells in, 599, *600*
in immunity, 601–602, *602*
mitochondrial, in hepatobiliary disease, 1849
smooth muscle, in hepatobiliary disease, 1849
thyroid, testing of, 2010t
Antibody-mediated immunity, *1454*
Anticalcium agents, for multiple myeloma, 1499
Anticancer medications, in postoperative wound infection, 490
Anticholinergics, for inflammatory bowel disease, 1799
for Parkinson's disease, 878
for peptic ulcer disease, 1767–1770, 1768t
Anticipatory grieving, after spinal cord injury, 910
in glaucoma, 956
Anticoagulants, antidote to, 2538t
complications of, intraoperative, 457
for cerebrovascular accident, 793
for pulmonary embolism, 1128
for venous thrombosis, 1434
monitoring of, 1435
in hemostasis, 1458
Anticonvulsants, for epilepsy, 839t
in pain control, 377
prophylactic, after intracranial surgery, 852
therapeutic monitoring of, reference values for, 2562
Antidepressants, in pain control, 377
tricyclic, antidote to, 2538t
effect of, on male reproductive system, 2345
in pain control, 374
Antidiarrheal medications, for inflammatory bowel disease, 1798–1799, 1798t
Antidiuretic hormone (ADH), 2061t
actions of, 1940t
imbalance of, critical monitoring in, 2064b
in blood flow regulation, 1374

Antidiuretic hormone (ADH) *(Continued)*
in cardiac regulation, 1203
in fluid and electrolyte balance, *275,* 275–277, 1542
in shock, 508, *508*
release of, factors in, 2066, *2066*
Antidotes, to poisons, 2538t
Antidysrhythmics, 1314
Antiembolism stockings, 461
Antiestrogens, for chemotherapy, classification of, 577t
Antifungals, topical, 2198t
Antigen(s), exposure to, 598
histocompatibility, 1456
processing/presentation of, 599
skin in, 2177
sequestered, release of, in autoimmunity, *654,* 655
transport of, to peripheral lymphoid tissues, 598, *599*
Antigen skin testing, in cancer diagnosis, 559
Antigenic determinants, 653
Antigenicity, 414
Antigen-presenting cells (APCs), in immune response, 598–599
Anti-HBc, testing of, before blood transfusion, 1524t
Anti-HCV, testing of, before blood transfusion, 1524t
Antihemophilic factor (AHF), 1517
Antihemophilic globulin, 1516t
Antihistamines, for chronic obstructive pulmonary disease, 1111t
for hypersensitivity, 641
for pruritus, 2204
Anti-HIV, testing of, before blood transfusion, 1524t
Anti-HTLV-1, testing of, before blood transfusion, 1524t
Antihypertensives, 1394t–1397t
effect of, on male reproductive system, 2345
for chronic renal failure, 1654
for increased intracranial pressure, 775
Anti-inflammatory medications, for inflammatory bowel disease, 1799
for rheumatoid arthritis, 662–665, 664t
Antilipemic agents, for viral hepatitis, 1867
Antilymphocyte globulin (ALG), for renal graft rejection, 1662
in organ transplantation, 644t
Antimetabolites, for chemotherapy, classification of, 577t
topical, 2198t
Antimicrobials, topical, for burns, 2254, 2254t
Antineoplastic agents, side effects of, 581b
Antinuclear antibodies (ANAs), in hepatobiliary disease, 1849
in musculoskeletal disorders, 2096t
in systemic lupus erythematosus, 675
Anti-parkinsonian drugs, intraoperative complications of, 457
Antiplatelet therapy, for angina pectoris, 1255, 1257t
for cerebrovascular accident, 793
Antipruritics, topical, 2198t–2199t

Antipsychotics, effect of, on male reproductive system, 2345

Antiresorption agents, for hyperparathyroidism, 2033

Antiretroviral therapy, in human immunodeficiency virus infection, 623–624

Anti-scar support garment, 2260–2261, *2261*

Antiseptics, 2199t

Antispasmodics, for intracranial hemorrhage, 814

for urinary tract infections, 1576t

Antithrombin III, for disseminated intravascular coagulation, 1512

Antithymocyte globulin (ATG), for renal graft rejection, 1662

in organ transplantation, 644t

Antithyroid antibody tests, 1953

Antithyroid medications, for hyperthyroidism, 2019–2020

Antituberculosis agents, 1144t–1145t

Antitumor antibiotics, classification of, 577t

Antral irrigation, for sinusitis, 1077

Antrectomy, for peptic ulcer disease, 1777

Anuria, 1548, 1554

in shock, 521

Anus, female, assessment of, 224t

male, assessment of, 223t

physical examination of, *1709,* 1709–1710

normal findings in, 1699b

structure of, 1695

Anxiety, alleviation of, in pain management, 366

brain tumors and, 851

cancer and, 541

chest pain in, assessment of, 1209t

in acute pancreatitis, 1925–1926

in acute renal failure, 1641

in cholelithiasis, 1913

in chronic obstructive pulmonary disease, 1121

in colon cancer, 1813

in dementia of Alzheimer's type, pharmacologic treatment of, 866t

in dysrhythmias, 1322–1323

in heart failure, 1288–1289

in intervertebral disc surgery, 922

in myocardial infarction, 1272

in pain response, 350

in sexually transmitted diseases, 2464–2465

in urinary tract disorders, 1551

in viral hepatitis, 1871

mechanical ventilation and, care plan for, 1180

with tracheostomy, 1075–1076

Anxiolytics, abuse of, 2492–2494

effects of, 2483t

health consequences of, 2494t

withdrawal from, symptoms of, 2488t

AOO (atrial fixed-rate) pacemaker, 1320b

Aorta, assessment of, in regional examination, 220t

Aortic aneurysm, abdominal. See *Abdominal aortic aneurysm.*

dissecting, chest pain in, assessment of, 1208t

thoracic, 1429–1430

Aortic bodies, in blood flow regulation, 1374

Aortic dissection, 1428–1429

classification of, 1428–1429

clinical manifestations of, 1429

complications of, 1429

etiology of, 1428–1429

management of, 1429

nursing, 1429

Aortic regurgitation, *1345*

clinical manifestations of, 1348

management of, medical, 1349

surgical, 1349

pathophysiology of, 1348

Aortic stenosis, *1345*

clinical manifestations of, 1348

management of, medical, 1348–1349

surgical, 1349

pathophysiology of, 1348

Aortic valve, 1193

disease of, 1347–1349

clinical manifestations of, 1348

diagnostic findings in, 1348

etiology of, 1348

management of, medical, 1348–1349

surgical, 1349

pathophysiology of, 1348

risk factors for, 1348

Aortoiliac disorders, 1407

AP (anteroposterior) chest x-ray, 1060

Apache II criteria, modified, for multiple organ system failure diagnosis, 529t

APCs (antigen-presenting cells), in immune response, 598–599

APD (automated peritoneal dialysis), 1649

APG (air plethysmography), in peripheral vascular assessment, 1384

Aphakia, management of, 960

Aphasia, 690

assessment of, 711t

cerebrovascular accident and, 789

ineffective coping in, 806

management of, 805

types of, 789

Apheresis, for chronic myelogenous leukemia, 1491

Aphthous stomatitis, *1723,* 1723–1724

clinical manifestations of, 1723, *1723*

diagnostic findings in, 1723

etiology of, 1723

management of, 1723–1724

pathophysiology of, 1723

risk factors for, 1723

Apical impulse, 1213

Aplastic anemia, 1477–1478

clinical manifestations of, 1477–1478

diagnostic findings in, 1477–1478

etiology of, 1477

hepatitis and, 1869

management of, medical, 1478

nursing, 1478

pathophysiology of, 1477

risk factors for, 1477

Apley's scratch test, 2090t

Apnea, *238*

Apneustic respiration, *238*

APNs (advanced-practice nurses), 12–14, 136

Apocrine glands, 2175, 2176t

Appearance, abnormal, in eye disorders, symptom analysis in, 941

in endocrine disorders, 1949, 1950

Appendicitis, 1791–1793

clinical manifestations of, 1791–1792

diagnostic findings in, 1791–1792

etiology of, 1791

management of, surgical, 1792

nursing care in, 1792–1793

pathophysiology of, 1791

risk factors for, 1791

Appetite, changes in, in endocrine disorders, 1949

Applanation tonometer, 949, *949*

Apraxia, 723

cerebrovascular accident and, 787

Apresoline (hydralazine), 1397t

for heart failure, 1286

for hypertensive emergency, 1405t

Aquaphor, 2200t

Aquaphor gauze, for burns, 2257t

Aquaphor ointment, 2199t

Aquatag (benzthiazide), 1394t

Aqueduct of Sylvius, 698, *698*

Aqueous humor, 937, *938*

Arab-Americans, pain response in, 347b

Arachnoid, 697, *697*

Arbovirus encephalitis, 859

Arcuate arteries, 1537

Arcus senilis, 940, 944

ARDS. See *Adult respiratory distress syndrome (ARDS).*

Aredia (pamidronate sodium), for multiple myeloma, 1499

Areflexia, post-traumatic, 895

Areolae, inspection of, 2313

ARF. See *Acute renal failure (ARF).*

Arfonad (trimethaphan), for hypertensive emergency, 1405t

Argyll Robertson pupil, 928–929

Arm(s), edema of, after mastectomy, 2443

exercises of, after lung cancer surgery, *1158*

Arousal, assessment of, 710t

from sleep, physiology of, 398–400, *399*

Arousal disorders, sleep-related, 403

Artane (trihexyphenidyl), for Parkinson's disease, 880t

Arterial blood gases (ABGs), analysis of, 247–248, 338–339, 338b, 1055–1057, *1056*

errors in, sources of, 339, 340t

in asthma, 1108t

in shock, 514

Arterial bypass, 1414, *1414*

complications of, 1415

nursing care in, 1415, 1416–1417

plan for, 1416–1417

Arterial embolization, for bleeding ulcer, 1772

Arterial lines, 1263b

Arterial pressure, 1201–1202, *1202*

Arterial steal, 1407

Arterial thoracic outlet syndrome, 1430

Arteriography. See also *Angiography.*

of ear, 991

Arterioles, structure of, 1371, *1371*

Arteriosclerosis, 1376

Arteriovenous aneurysm, head trauma and, 826

Arteriovenous fistula, internal, for hemodialysis, 1651–1652, *1652*

Arteriovenous graft, internal, for hemodialysis, 1652

Arteriovenous malformations (AVMs), 816

Arteriovenous shunt, external, for hemodialysis, 1651, *1652*

Arteritis, cranial, 680–681
  giant cell, 681

Artery(ies). See also names of specific arteries.
  damage to, fractures and, 2139
  disorders of, 1405–1432
    symptoms of, 1377–1378, 1379t
  embolism vs. thrombosis of, 1424
  insufficiency of, signs of, 1378
  large, blood flow through, 1372–1374
  occlusion of, acute, 1424
    chronic. See *Chronic arterial occlusion.*
  structure of, 1369, *1371*
  types of, 1369
  ulcers of, 1424
  wall of, layers of, 1241, *1242*

Arthritis, gouty, *2107,* 2107–2108
  in Crohn's disease, 1796
  in rheumatic fever, 1328
  post-traumatic, in fracture, prevention of, 2145
  rheumatoid. See *Rheumatoid arthritis (RA).*
  secondary, 681
  septic, 2122

Arthritis Self-Management Program, 175b

Arthrocentesis, 2096

Arthrodesis, 2110
  for rheumatoid arthritis, 672

Arthrography, 2094

Arthroplasty, for rheumatoid arthritis, 672–674, *673*

Arthroscopy, 255–256, *2095,* 2095–2096
  procedure for, 255–256

Arthus reaction, 639

Articular cartilage, 2076, *2076*

Articular fracture, 2131

Articular system, structure/function of, 2075–2077, *2076–2078*

Artificial heart, 1354

Artificial urinary sphincter (AUS), for urinary incontinence, after radical prostatectomy, 2370

Arytenoidectomy, 1101

AS (ankylosing spondylitis), 678, *679*

Asbestos, exposure to, and cancer, 540

A-scan ultrasonography, of eyes, 951, *951*

Ascending pathways, of spinal cord, structure/function of, 694–696, 696t

Ascites, 289, 1889–1891
  clinical manifestations of, 1889–1890, *1890*
  complications of, 1890
  diagnostic findings in, 1889–1890, *1890*
  etiology of, 1889
  in cirrhosis, 1878t
  in hepatobiliary disease, 1845
  in portal hypertension, 1888

Ascites *(Continued)*
  management of, medical, 1890
    nursing, 1890–1891
    surgical, 1891, *1892*
  pathophysiology of, 1889
  percussion in, 1848
  risk factors for, 1889

Asepsis, failure of, in postoperative wound infection, 491
  surgical, 478

ASIA (American Spinal Injury Association) Impairment Scale, 893

Asians, ancient, healthcare in, history of, 18–19
  dietary practices of, 1702b
  human immunodeficiency virus infection in, 617b–618b
  skin examination in, 2188b

Aspartate aminotransferase (AST), in hepatobiliary assessment, 1851t
  in musculoskeletal disorders, 2096t
  in myocardial infarction, 1261, *1262*
  reference values for, in cancer, 557t

Asphyxiants, exposure to, in burns, 2237, 2237t

Aspiration, fine-needle, in cancer diagnosis, 558
  in thyroid disorders, 2011t
  of liver, 1855
    contraindications to, 1855
  in Parkinson's disease, prevention of, client education about, 882b
  of bone marrow, 1466–1468
    in leukemia, 1489
  of chest lesions, 1064–1065
  of joint, 2096
  risk for, after partial laryngectomy, 1089, *1090*
    after spinal cord injury, 898, 900
    in cerebrovascular accident, 799
    in consciousness disorders, 755–757
    with tracheostomy, 1074–1075

Aspirin, for angina pectoris, 1255, 1257t
  for cerebrovascular accident, 793
  for rheumatoid arthritis, 663, 664t
  in pain control, 375t
  in surgical client, 458t

Assault, in emergency department, handling of, 2509b

Assemblies of God, beliefs/practices of, 2546

Assertiveness training, in Wallingford Wellness Project, 175

Assessment, in cross-cultural nursing, 63–65, 64b
  health risk appraisal in, 65
  history in, 63–65, 64b
  physical assessment in, 65
  in diagnostic testing, 242
  in family nursing, 55, *55,* 56b–57b
    guidelines for, 55, 56b–57b
  in sexual health promotion, 76–77
  in spiritual care, 68, 72, 72b
  in therapeutic family communication, 58
  preoperative, 453–461, 453t, 454t, 458t, 460b

Assist/control ventilation, 1177, 1178t

Assisted-living facilities, for elderly, 100

Assistive listening devices, 997

AST (aspartate aminotransferase), in hepatobiliary assessment, 1851t
  in musculoskeletal disorders, 2096t
  in myocardial infarction, 1261, *1262*
  reference values for, in cancer, 557t

Astereognosis, 724

Asthma, 1105–1111
  adult, action plan for, 1109t
  case management in, 1124b
  client education in, 1112b–1113b
  clinical manifestations of, 1105–1106
  clinical pathway for, 2572–2574
  critical monitoring in, 1110b
  diagnostic findings in, 1105–1106, 1108t, *1109*
  dyspnea in, nursing research on, 1108b
  etiology of, 1105
  management of, community/self care in, 1110–1111, *1111,* 1111t
    emergency, 1106–1107
    medical, 1107, *1107*
    nursing, 1108–1110
  occupational, 1150, 1151t
  pathophysiology of, 1105
  prevention of, 200t, 1106b
  risk factors for, 1105, 1106b
  sleep disorders in, 405

Astigmatism, *975,* 976

Astrocytes, 687, *688*

Astrocytoma, 844, *846*

Asymmetrical septal hypertrophy, 1341

Asystole, ventricular, *1309,* 1310

Atelectasis, 1133, 1134b
  causes of, 1134b
  during enteral nutrition, 1753
  endotracheal tube suctioning and, 1175t
  postoperative, 486

Atenolol (Tenormin), 1395t
  for angina pectoris, 1257t
  for dysrhythmia, 1308t

ATG (antithymocyte globulin), for renal graft rejection, 1662
  in organ transplantation, 644t

Atherectomy, coronary, directional, 1245–1246, *1246*
  peripheral, 1413

Atherogenesis, response-to-injury theory of, 1243, *1243*

Atheroma, 810

Atherosclerosis, in chronic renal failure, 1645
  in coronary artery disease, 1238

Atherosclerotic parkinsonism, 878

Athetosis, 723b

ATN (acute tubular necrosis), in shock, 510
  nephrotoxins and, 1627, 1627b

Atonic seizures, in epilepsy, 838

Atopic allergies, 638–639

Atopic dermatitis. See *Dermatitis, atopic.*

Atopy, 636

ATP (adenosine triphosphate), in shock, 503

Atrial demand (AAI) pacemaker, 1320b

Atrial dysrhythmias, 1297–1302, *1299, 1300*

Atrial fibrillation, *1300,* 1301–1302

Atrial fixed-rate (AOO) pacemaker, 1320b

Atrial flutter, *1300,* 1301

Atrial gallop, 1216
Atrial kick, 1297
Atrial natriuretic peptides (ANPs), in fluid
    balance regulation, 277
  in sodium regulation, 295
Atrial synchronous ventricular (VDD) pace-
    maker, 1320b
Atrioventricular (AV) block, first-degree,
    1303, 1303–1304
  second-degree, 1303, 1304
  third-degree, 1303, 1304
Atrioventricular interval, 1319
Atrioventricular junctional dysrhythmias,
    1302, 1302–1304, 1303
Atrioventricular (AV) node, 1198
Atrioventricular (AV) valves, 1193, 1194
Atrium, left, 1191, 1193
  right, 1191, 1193
Atrophic vaginitis, 2414
  in menopause, 2393
Atrophy, 2185
  of muscles, 2087
    inspection of, in peripheral vascular as-
      sessment, 1380
Atropine, antidote to, 2538t
  for asthma, 1106
  for shock, 521
Atropine sulfate, preoperative, 465t
Attention, disorder of, 765
Attention span, assessment of, 195
Attitudes, assessment of, culture in, 193t
Audiometric tests, 991, 992
Audiometry, impedance, 991
  schedule for, 207t
Auditory acuity, testing of, 721, 988–989,
    990
Auditory brain stem response test, 991
Auerbach's plexus, 1689–1690
Augmentation mammaplasty, 2283, 2283–
    2284
Aura, before seizures, 836
  definition of, 835b
Auranofin (Ridaura), for rheumatoid arthri-
    tis, 664t
Auricle, structure of, 980, 981
AUS (artificial urinary sphincter), for uri-
    nary incontinence, after radical prostatec-
    tomy, 2370
Auscultation, 230, 230–231
  of abdomen, 1707–1709, 1845, 1846t
    in cardiovascular assessment, 1217
  of cardiovascular system, normal findings
    in, 1206b
  of gastrointestinal tract, normal findings
    in, 1699b
  of heart sounds, 1214–1217, 1215
  of hematologic system, 1463b
  of hepatobiliary system, 1846t
  of neurologic system, 718
    normal findings in, 717b
  of peripheral vascular system, 1378b,
    1382–1383
  of respiratory system, 1045, 1045–1047,
    1047, 1047t
    normal findings in, 1042b
  of thyroid gland, 1951b
  of urinary tract, 1556b
  sounds in, 230–231

Auscultatory gap, 237
Autoantibodies, in systemic lupus erythema-
    tosus, 675
Autochthonous flora, in pathogen resistance,
    594
Autogenic training, in pain control, 349b,
    369
Autografts, epithelial, cultured, for burns,
    2257
  for burns, 2255–2257, 2257
Autoimmune disorders, 653
  and hemolytic anemia, 1480
  testing for, in immune system assessment,
    612
Autoimmunity, 653–655, 654
  helper T cell tolerance in, loss of, 654,
    654–655
  theories of, 654, 654
Autologous bone marrow transplantation
    (ABMT), for cancer, 585
Autologous transplants, 642
Autolytic wound debridement, 441
Automated external defibrillators (AEDs),
    1312
Automated peritoneal dialysis (APD), 1649
Automatic implantable cardioverter-defibril-
    lator (AICD), 1312–1313
Automatic language, 792
Automaticity, disturbances in, and dysrhyth-
    mias, 1295–1297
  atrial, 1297–1299
  atrioventricular, 1302, 1302–1303
  ventricular, 1305–1310
  of heart, 1196
Automation, in American healthcare system,
    62
Automatisms, during seizures, 837
Automobile accident, blunt trauma in, 2521t
Autonomic dysreflexia, critical monitoring
    in, 909, 909b
  in neurogenic bladder dysfunction, 1617
  in spinal cord injury, 894–895, 909, 909b
Autonomic nervous system (ANS), 701
  disorders of, assessment of, 728–730
  in cardiac regulation, 1202–1203
  structure/function of, 703–704, 704
Autonomic neuropathy, diabetic, 2000
Autonomous neurogenic bladder, 1615,
    1616
Autonomy, in decision-making, in chronic
    conditions, 118b
  in ethics, 40
  of clients, ethical issues in, 47
  of elderly, 102
Autopsy, value of, 271b
Autoregulation, in increased intracranial
    pressure, 772
Autotransfusion, for shock, 519
Autotransplantation, of kidney, for renal cal-
    culi, 1669
  of parathyroid glands, 2035
AV (atrioventricular) block, first-degree,
    1303, 1303–1304
  second-degree, 1303, 1304
  third-degree, 1303, 1304
AV (atrioventricular) node, 1198
AV sequential fixed-rate (DOO) pacemaker,
    1320b

AV sequential (DVI) pacemaker, 1320b
AV synchronous (VAT) pacemaker, 1320b
AV (atrioventricular) valves, 1193, 1194
Avascular necrosis, in fracture, prevention
    of, 2145
Aveeno Bath (colloidal oatmeal bath), 2199t
AVMs (arteriovenous malformations), 816
Avulsion fracture, 2130–2131
Axid (nizatidine), for peptic ulcer disease,
    1768t
Axillae, assessment of, in health history,
    184b
  in regional examination, 219t
  physical examination of, 2312–2316,
    2313–2315
Axillary lymph nodes, assessment of, 610
Axillary node dissection, arm care after,
    2443, 2445b
  for breast cancer, 2437
  injury risk after, 2443
Axillofemoral grafting, 1414, 1414
Axons, 685–686, 686
Azathioprine (Imuran), after heart transplan-
    tation, 1353, 1354b
  for multiple sclerosis, 874
  for myasthenia gravis, 885
  for renal graft rejection, 1662
  for rheumatoid arthritis, 664t
  in organ transplantation, 644t
Azithromycin (Zithromax), for chlamydial
    infection, 2470
AZT (zidovudine), for human immunodefi-
    ciency virus infection, 624
Azulfidine (sulfasalazine), for diarrhea, in
    inflammatory bowel disease, 1798–1799
  for rheumatoid arthritis, 664t
  urine color with, 1557t

B

B cells, 1452
  assay of, in immune disorder assessment,
    611
  in immune response, 599, 600
  T cell interaction with, in autoimmunity,
    654, 655
Babinski's reflex, 727, 728, 729t
BACCHUS (Boost Alcohol Consciousness
    Concerning the Health of University Stu-
    dents), 2497b
Bacille Calmette-Guérin (BCG), for bladder
    cancer, 1584
  for interstitial cystitis, 1580
Bacitracin, for open wounds, 445t
Bacitracin ointment, 2198t
Back, lower, care of, client education in,
    918b
  neurologic assessment of, 718
    normal findings in, 717b
Back brace, after intervertebral disc surgery,
    924
  for spinal cord injury, 900, 902
Back pain, 356–357
Back strain, and intervertebral disc hernia-
    tion, 917
Baclofen (Lioresal), in pain control, 374,
    378
Bacteremia, 244

Bacteremia (Continued)
  nosocomial, 418t, 419
  portal vein, and liver abscess, 1902
Bacteria, and cell damage, 270
  in urine, 1559
Bacterial meningitis. See Meningitis, bacterial.
Bacterial vaginosis, 2474–2475
Bacteriuria, 1559
  asymptomatic, treatment of, 1574
  screening for, 208t
Bactrim (trimethoprim-sulfamethoxazole),
  for urinary tract infections, 1575t
  in Pneumocystis carinii pneumonia prophylaxis, 625
Bactroban (mupirocin), topical, 2198t
Badge, film, in radiation therapy safety, 573
Baerveldt seton, for glaucoma, 957
BAL (blood alcohol level), 2486
Balance, assessment of, 236
  in regional examination, 222t
  disorders of, 1010–1016
    central, 1011
    clinical manifestations of, 1011–1012, 1012t
    diagnostic findings in, 1011–1012, 1012t
    etiology of, 1010–1011
    management of, medical, 1012–1013
      nursing, 1013–1016, 1013b, 1014b–1015b
      surgical, 1015–1016
    pathophysiology of, 1011
    peripheral, 1010–1011
    risk factors for, 1010–1011, 1051b
  inner ear in, 984
Balanced (neuroleptic) anesthesia, 471
Balanitis, 2380, 2380
Ballismus, 723b
Balloon angioplasty, 1413
  laser-assisted, 1413
Balloon dilation, transurethral, of prostate,
  for benign prostatic hyperplasia, 2358–2359, 2359
Balloon tamponade, for bleeding esophageal
  varices, 1885, 1885
  complications of, 1886
Band neutrophils, in differential count, interpretation of, 436t
Baptists, beliefs/practices of, 2546
Barbiturates, allergic reaction to, clinical
  manifestations of, 640t
  for increased intracranial pressure, 775
Bard absorption dressing, indications for, 443t
Barium enema (lower gastrointestinal series), 251, 1713–1714
Barium swallow (upper gastrointestinal series), 250–251, 1713
Baroreceptors, in blood flow regulation, 1373
  in cardiac regulation, 1203
  in fluid balance regulation, 277
  in hypertension, 1389
  in shock, 502
Barotrauma, 1009
Barrel chest, 1040, 1043
Barriers, in infection control, 423
Barthel index, in chronic conditions, 115t

Bartholinitis, 2422
Bartholin's glands, 2294
  examination of, 2317, 2318
Basal cell carcinoma, 2227, 2227
  of oral cavity, 1727
Basal cell secretion test, 1717
Basal cells, structure/function of, 2176t
Basal ganglia, structure/function of, 691, 692
Basal metabolic rate (BMR), estimation of,
  in thyroid function testing, 1953
  in burns, 2257–2258, 2258t
Base excess, 338b
Basilar artery, 699, 700
Basophils, functions of, 1448t
  in blood dyscrasias, 1465t
  in hematopoiesis, 1451
  in wound healing, 429
  reference values for, in cancer, 557t
Bath, colloidal oatmeal, 2199t
  cornstarch, 2199t
Bathing, after burn injury, 2263b
BCG (bacille Calmette-Guérin), for bladder
  cancer, 1584
  for interstitial cystitis, 1580
Beating, blunt trauma in, 2521t
Beau's line, 2187t
Becker's muscular dystrophy, 2125t
Beclomethasone dipropionate (Beconase),
  indications for, 641
Beconase (beclomethasone dipropionate), indications for, 641
Bed, FluidAir, 2219
  KinAir, 2219
  Roto-Rest, 759
    after spinal cord injury, 908
  swing, 122
  transfer from, in cerebrovascular accident, 801
Bedrest, for intervertebral disc herniation, 920
  promotion of, for venous thrombosis, 1435
Bedtime insulin with daytime sulfonylurea
  (BIDS), for diabetes mellitus, 1968
Bed-wetting, 403
Behavior, addictive, framework for, 2479–2480
  altered, head trauma and, 826
  assessment of, 190, 233–236
  emotion-focused, 110
  health seeking, in chronic arterial occlusion, 1412
  nonverbal, 190
  patterns of, in stress response, 28
  problem-focused, 110
  type A, in coronary artery disease, 1241
  verbal, 190
  violent, in emergency department, nursing
    research on, 2509b
Behavior modification, for urinary incontinence, 1610, 1611–1612
  in pain management, 369–370
Belching, in gastrointestinal disorders, 1749
Beliefs, assessment of, 191t, 196
  culture in, 193t
  pattern of, 211
  religious, healthcare effects of, 2544–2551
Bellevue bridge, 2371, 2372

Bell's palsy, 930, 930–931
Below-knee prosthesis, 1422
Belsey operation, for gastroesophageal reflux disease, 1739
Benadryl (diphenhydramine), for Parkinson's disease, 880t
  for shock, 520
  in pain control, 374
Benazepril (Lotensin), 1396t
Bence Jones protein, 1558
Bendroflumethiazide (Naturetin), 1394t
Beneficence, in decision-making, in chronic
  conditions, 118b
  in ethics, 40
Benign, definition of, 533
Benign paroxysmal positional vertigo
  (BPPV), 1010–1011
Benign prostatic hyperplasia (BPH), 2350–2365
  and urinary tract infection, 1578
  clinical manifestations of, 2352
  complications of, 2351, 2351–2352
  diagnostic findings in, 2352
  etiology of, 2350
  management of, community/self care in,
    2363–2365, 2364t
    medical, 2363–2364, 2364t
    nursing, 2364–2365
    surgical, 2352–2360, 2353
      complications of, 2359–2360
      nursing care in, 2360–2363
      outcomes in, 2360
  pathophysiology of, 2350–2352, 2351
  preoperative, 456
  risk factors for, 2350
Béniqué sound, 2356t
Benson's relaxation response, in pain control, 349b
Bentyl (dicyclomine hydrochloride), for
  peptic ulcer disease, 1768t, 1770
Benzagel (benzoyl peroxide), 2198t
Benzocaine (Americaine), 473t
Benzodiazepines, for alcohol withdrawal, 2488
Benzophenone, topical, 2200t
Benzoyl peroxide (Benzagel), 2198t
Benzthiazide (Exna, Aquatag), 1394t
Benztropine (Cogentin), for Parkinson's disease, 880t
Bepridil, for angina pectoris, 1256t
Bereaveness, cultural issues in, 70b–71b
Berger's disease, 1634
Berkow formula, in burn severity classification, 2240
Bernard and Cannon's theory, of homeostasis, 21
Bernstein test, 1717
Beta-adrenergic blocking agents, 1395t
  for angina pectoris, 1254–1255, 1257t
  for asthma, 1106
  for bleeding esophageal varices, 1886
  for congestive heart failure, with extracellular fluid volume excess, 288
  for dysrhythmia, 1308t
  with intrinsic sympathomimetic activity, 1395t
Beta-adrenergic receptors, in cardiac regulation, 1203

Betadine (povidone-iodine), for open wounds, 445t
Betamethasone (Celestone, Diprosone), 2048t
  topical, 2199t
Betaseron (interferon beta-1b), for multiple sclerosis, 874
Betaxolol (Kerlone), 1395t
Bethanechol (Urecholine), for gastroesophageal reflux disease, 1738
  for urinary tract infections, 1576t
Biaxin (clarithromycin), for peptic ulcer disease, 1767, 1769t
  in *Mycobacterium avium-intracellulare* complex prophylaxis, 625
Bicarbonate, assessment of, in arterial blood gas analysis, 338b
  distribution of, 293t
  plasma, in serum pH regulation, 332
Bicarbonate buffer system, 329, *330*
Biceps, strength of, assessment of, 2088t
Biceps jerk, *726, 727,* 729t
Bicipital tendinitis, 2168t
Bicycle ergometry, in cardiovascular assessment, 1225
BIDS (bedtime insulin with daytime sulfonylurea), for diabetes mellitus, 1968
Bier block, 476
Bigeminal pulse, 1212
Biguanides, for diabetes mellitus, 1967t
Bilateral pneumonia, 1135
Bile, excretion of, laboratory tests for, 1850t
  production of, liver in, 1837–1839, *1839*
  storage of, gallbladder in, 1835–1836, *1838,* 1838–1839
Bile salts, 1837–1838
Biliary cirrhosis, 1873, 1874t–1875t
Biliary drainage, analysis of, 1856
Biliary tract, age-related changes in, 1841
  disorders of, 1907–1932
    assessment of, 1843–1856
      diagnostic tests in, 1848–1856
      history in, 1843–1856
      physical examination in, 1845–1848, 1846t–1847t, *1847*
  structure/function of, 1835–1841, *1837*
  terminology of, 1908t
Bilirubin, in bile, 1838, *1839*
  in urine, 1558
    in hepatobiliary assessment, 1850t
  level of, in jaundice, 1859t, 1860
  serum, in hepatobiliary assessment, 1850t
Bilirubinuria, 1558
Biliverdin, in bile, 1838
Billroth I procedure, for peptic ulcer disease, 1777, *1778*
Billroth II procedure, for peptic ulcer disease, 1777, *1778*
Bimanual examination, of female reproductive system, *2319,* 2319–2320
Biobrane, in burn wound covering, 2256t
Bioclusive, for burns, 2257t
  indications for, 443t
BioDyne, *759*
Biofeedback, for urinary incontinence, 1610, 1611
  in pain control, 349b, 370

Biologic response modifiers, for cancer, 585–587
Biomedical model, of illness, 20–21
Biopsy, excisional, for actinic keratosis, 2225
  in cancer diagnosis, 569
  in cancer diagnosis, 558–559
    cervical, 2407
    prostate, 2367
  in hepatobiliary disease, 1854–1856, *1855*
  in respiratory assessment, 1064–1065
  incisional, in cancer diagnosis, 568–569
  needle, in cancer diagnosis, 568
  of breasts, 2329
  of cervix, 2324–2325, *2325*
  of endometrium, 2323
  of kidneys, 1568–1569, *1569*
  of lymph nodes, in Hodgkin's disease, 1501
  of musculoskeletal system, 2095
    in neurologic disorders, 741
  of prostate, 2338
  of skin, *2195,* 2195–2196
  shave, for actinic keratosis, 2225
  types of, 257
Biotransformation, liver in, 1840
Biot's respiration, *238*
Birth control, religious beliefs about, 2545–2551
Birth defects, prevention of, 204t
  screening for, 208t
Bisoprolol (Zebeta), 1395t
Bisphosphonates, for osteoporosis, 2104
Bites, 2536–2537
Björk-Shiley tilting disc valve, *1352*
Black widow spider bite, 2537
Black wounds, management of, 439, *439*
Blackhead, 2212
Blackout, definition of, 2481t
Blacks, dietary practices of, 1702b
  human immunodeficiency virus infection in, 616b–617b
  hypertension in, 198t, 1389
  skin examination in, 2188b–2189b
  urban, attitudes of, toward death and dying, 71b
Bladder, anatomy of, *1538,* 1538–1539, *1539*
  congenital anomalies of, 1620
  control of, in spinal cord injury, 901–902
  disorders of, 1571–1621
  distention of, after intervertebral disc surgery, 924
    after prostatectomy, 2362
    after spinal cord injury, 908
    and urinary tract infection, 1572
  diverticula of, and urinary retention, 1601
  dysfunction of, in multiple sclerosis, 874
  exstrophy of, 1620
  function of, 1544–1545
    assessment of, 713t
  neurogenic. See *Neurogenic bladder dysfunction.*
  physical examination of, 1553
  spasms of, after prostatectomy, 2361
  trauma to, 1619–1620
Bladder cancer, 1582–1595
  clinical manifestations of, 1583

Bladder cancer *(Continued)*
  diagnostic findings in, 1583
  etiology of, 1582
  management of, in elderly, 1594–1595
    medical, 1583–1584
      complications of, 1584
      outcome of, 1584
    nursing, 1584–1585
    surgical, 1585–1588, *1586, 1587*
      care after, 1587
      complications of, 1587–1588
      nursing care in, 1588–1595, 1589b, 1590b, 1591b, *1592,* 1593b
      outcome of, 1588
  pathophysiology of, 1582–1583
  prevention of, 1582b
  risk factors for, 542b, 1582, 1582b
  staging of, 1582–1583, *1583*
  survival in, 538t
Bladder decompression drainage, 1603
Bladder neck, repair of, for urinary retention, 1603
  stricture of, and urinary incontinence, 1605
Bladder neck support prosthesis, for urinary incontinence, 1609
Bladder pain, 1548–1549
Bladder training, after spinal cord injury, 911
  for urinary incontinence, 1610
  in neurogenic bladder dysfunction, 1617
Blanch test, 1043, 2186
Blast crisis, 1488, *1489*
Bleeding. See also *Hemorrhage.*
  after arterial bypass, 1415
  after prostatectomy, 2361
  assessment of, in burn autografting, 2255
  disorders of, assessment of, 1461–1462
  esophageal, in portal hypertension, critical monitoring in, 1885, 1885b
  gastrointestinal. See *Gastrointestinal bleeding.*
  in cervical cancer, 2407
  in cirrhosis, 1878t
  in peptic ulcer disease, 1767
  in viral hepatitis, 1865, 1866t
  postmenopausal, 2395, *2395*
  uterine, abnormal, 2389–2395
Bleeding precautions, in leukemia, 1493
Bleeding time, in hemorrhage, 1467t
Blended family, 53
Blepharitis, 973
Blepharoplasty, *2272, 2272*–2273, *2273*
  client education in, 2273
Blepharospasm, in Parkinson's disease, 878
Blindness, central area, assessment of, 947
  glaucoma and, 956
Blinking, disorders of, 974
  examination of, 944
Blisters, *2184*
  after burn injury, 2263b
Blocadren (timolol), 1395t
  for angina pectoris, 1257t
Blood, acceptability of, confirmation of, before blood transfusion, 1525
  administration of, for shock, 519
  buffer systems of, in pH regulation, 331–332

Blood (Continued)
  characteristics of, 1447
  control of, in hepatitis B prevention, 1864
  dyscrasias of, complete blood count in, 1465t
  functions of, 1448t
  in human immunodeficiency virus infection transmission, 615
  loss of, in hypovolemic shock, management of, 522t
    postoperative, prevention of, 487
  occult, stool examination for, 1711–1712, 1711t, 1712b
    nursing research on, 1712b
  reference values for, 2557–2559
  release of, from blood bank, 1525
  testing of, delegation of, 244b
  whole, transfusion of, 1520t–1523t
Blood alcohol level (BAL), 2486
Blood cells, formation of. See Hematopoiesis.
Blood chemistry, in urinary tract assessment, 1562
Blood coagulation tests, in cardiovascular assessment, 1219–1220
Blood components, tranfusion of, 1520t–1523t
  during chemotherapy, 582
Blood cultures, 244
Blood flow, local factors in, 1375
  renal, in glomerular filtration rate, 1541
  through large arteries, 1372–1374
  through tissues, 1374–1376
    resistance to, 1375
    velocity of, 1374
Blood glucose. See Glucose, blood.
Blood glucose meters, 1975
Blood groups, 1455–1456, 1455t
  in diverse cultures, 1456b
Blood pressure, capillary, changes in, in shock, 509–510
  classification of, 1391, 1391t
  determinants of, 1202, 1202
  high. See Hypertension.
  improvement of, modified Trendelenburg's position for, nursing research on, 518b
  limb, assessment of, 1383
  management of, in cerebrovascular accident, 796
  measurement of, 237, 1399
    after cardiac surgery, 1357
    delegation of, 234b
    first-occasion, follow-up for, 1391, 1391t
    in cardiovascular assessment, 1211, 1211–1212
    in intracranial hemorrhage, 815
    in shock, 525
    schedule for, 209t
  paradoxical, measurement of, 1211–1212
  postural, measurement of, 1211, 1211
  regulation of, 1202–1204
    factors in, 1373–1374
    kidneys in, 1543
    renin-angiotensin-aldosterone system in, 1390, 1390
Blood products, control of, in hepatitis B prevention, 1864

Blood salvage, for autologous transfusion, 1518
Blood smear, stained, in sickle cell anemia diagnosis, 1514
Blood studies, 245–248
  arterial sampling in, 247–248
  in cancer diagnosis, 556
  in ear disorders, 992
  in male reproductive disorders, 2336–2338
  microcapillary collection in, 246–247
  results of, analysis of, 248
  serial port sampling in, 247
  venipuncture in, 246, 246t, 248
Blood supply, occlusion of, and small intestinal obstruction, 1821
  to central nervous system, 699, 700
  to esophagus, 1687
  to heart, 1194, 1194–1195
  to large intestine, 1695
  to pelvis, 2296
  to small intestine, 1692–1693
  to stomach, 1689
Blood transfusion, 1518–1530
  autologous, 1518
  complications of, delayed, 1527–1530
  directed donation in, 1518
  equipment/devices for, 1525
  for anemia, 1471
    pernicious, 1476
  in Jehovah's Witnesses, ethical issues in, 1519b
  initiation of, 1525–1527
  monitoring during, 1527, 1528b, 1529t
  preparation for, 1518–1525
    assessment in, 1518
    blood release request in, 1525
    client teaching in, 1518–1519
    informed consent in, 1518–1519
    pretransfusion testing in, 1519–1524, 1524t
    venous access in, 1524–1525
Blood typing, 1455–1456, 1455t
Blood urea nitrogen (BUN), measurement of, in cardiovascular assessment, 1220
  in urinary tract assessment, 1562
  preoperative, 453t
Blood vessels, changes in, in hypertension, 1390
  disorders of, and male reproductive disorders, 2345
  function of, 1372–1376
  in hemostasis, 1457
  pulmonary, disorders of, 1105–1131
  renal, abnormalities of, 1676–1677
  skin, structure/function of, 2176t
  structure of, 1369–1372, 1373, 1374
Blood viscosity, 1375
Blood volume, decreased, in ascites, 1889
Blood warmers, for blood transfusion, 1526–1527
Blood-brain barrier, 699
Blue Cross/Blue Shield, 5b
  history of, 6
Blunt percussion, in hepatobiliary assessment, 1848
Blunt trauma, 2519, 2521t
  to chest, 2522

BMC (bone mineral content), in osteoporosis, 2098
BMD (bone mineral density), in osteoporosis, 2098
BMR (basal metabolic rate), estimation of, in thyroid function testing, 1953
  in burns, 2257–2258, 2258t
BMT. See Bone marrow transplantation (BMT).
Board-and-care homes, for elderly, 100
Body box, in lung volume measurement, 1051, 1054
Body build, assessment of, 234
Body frame, size of, assessment of, 237, 239b
Body image, assessment of, 191t
  changed, nursing care in, 2270b
  disturbance of, after arterial bypass, 1417
    after vulvectomy, 2420–2422
    in bladder cancer, 1588–1589
    in breast cancer, 2441–2442
    in colon cancer, 1814
    in eating disorders, 1761
    in inflammatory bowel disease, 1804–1805
    in jaundice, 1860
    in leukemia, 1493
    in rheumatoid arthritis, management of, 669–670
    in urinary tract disorders, 1552
  positive, postoperative, promotion of, 492
Body odor, assessment of, 235
Body plethysmography, 1051, 1054
Body substance isolation (BSI), 423
Body-contouring surgery, 2275–2276
Bone(s), classification of, 2073, 2075
  composition of, 2074–2075
  cortical, 2132
  demineralization of, in chronic renal failure, 1646
  disease of, in hyperparathyroidism, 2035
  disorders of, in endocrine disorders, 1949
    metabolic, 2098–2108
  infections of, 2121–2122
  of dying patient, donation of, guidelines for, 2514t
  physical examination of, 2088
  remodeling of, 2080, 2099, 2100
  repair of, 2080
  structure of, 2073–2075, 2075
  trabecular, 2132
  tumors of, 2122–2124
    metastatic, 2122–2124
    primary, 2122, 2123, 2123t
Bone conduction, testing of, 720, 721
Bone conduction hearing loss, 994b
Bone growth, abnormal, in spinal cord injury, 904
Bone healing, 2132–2134, 2133, 2134t
  factors in, 2133–2134, 2134t
Bone marrow, 565, 595
  allogeneic, 1495
  aspiration of, in hematologic system assessment, 1466–1468
    in leukemia, 1489
  autologous, 1495
  collection of, for bone marrow transplantation, 1496, 1496

Bone marrow (Continued)
  failure of, and anemia, 1477–1478
  functions of, 595
  in immunity, 597
  sources of, for bone marrow transplantation, 1495
  structure/features of, 1449
  syngeneic, 1495
  tests of, in immune disorder assessment, 611
Bone marrow transplantation (BMT), 584–585, 1495–1497
  allogeneic, 585, 1496–1497
    bone marrow infusion in, 1496–1497
    recipient preparation for, 1496
  autologous, 585
    in metastatic breast cancer, 2451
  complications of, 585, 649t
  criteria for, 646
  for chronic leukemia, 1492
  graft-versus-host disease after, 1497
  harvesting in, 1495–1496, 1496
    allogeneic donor preparation in, 1495–1496
    histocompatibility testing in, 1495
    marrow collection in, 1496, 1496
    peripheral stem cell collection in, 1496
  indications for, 1495
  process of, 585
  syngeneic, 585
  types of, 585
Bone matrix, 2075
Bone mineral content (BMC), in osteoporosis, 2098
Bone mineral density (BMD), in osteoporosis, 2098
Bone pain, 355
Bone scans, 2094
Bony orbit, structure of, 935
Boost Alcohol Consciousness Concerning the Health of University Students (BACCHUS), 2497b
Borborygmi, 1707
Boric acid, topical, 2199t
Borrelia burgdorferi, 416t
Bougienage, for achalasia, 1735, 1735, 1736
Boutonnière deformity, in rheumatoid arthritis, 659, 659, 674
Bowel cancer, screening for, 209t
Bowel elimination, in cancer, 587b
Bowel function, assessment of, 713t
Bowel habits, changes in, in endocrine disorders, 1949
Bowel incontinence, after spinal cord injury, 908
Bowel retraining, after spinal cord injury, 911
Bowel sounds, auscultation of, 1707–1709
Bowels, control of, in spinal cord injury, 901–902
  ischemia of, in abdominal aortic aneurysm, 1428
Bowleg, 2087, 2087
BPH. See Benign prostatic hyperplasia (BPH).
BPPV (benign paroxysmal positional vertigo), 1010–1011

Brace(s), after cerebrovascular accident, 800
  back, after intervertebral disc surgery, 924
    for spinal cord injury, 900, 902
  management of, home healthcare in, 2152b
Brachial lymph nodes, palpation of, 2313, 2314
Brachial plexus, postoperative compromise of, critical monitoring of, 673b
Brachial plexus block, 384, 384
Brachioradialis reflex, 729t
Brachytherapy, 570
Braden Scale, 2213, 2214
Bradycardia, 236
  sinus, 1200, 1298–1299, 1299
Bradykinesia, 723b
  in Parkinson's disease, 878
    client education about, 881b
Bradykinin, in anaphylaxis, 638t
  in blood pressure regulation, 1204, 1375
  in shock, 507
  in wound healing, 430
Bradypnea, 238
Brain, cancer of, survival in, 538t
  edema of, 774
  in illness, 26–27
  injury to, secondary, 830, 830–831
    traumatic, 820–831. See also Head trauma.
  structure/function of, 659–661, 690–693
  surgery of, stereotactic, in pain control, 387
Brain abscess, 857–858, 858
  clinical manifestations of, 858
Brain death, criteria for, 271, 750–751
Brain stem, contusion of, clinical manifestations of, 824, 824
  structure/function of, 693, 693, 694t
  tumor of, clinical manifestations of, 847t
Brain stem response test, auditory, 991
Brain swelling, 774
Brain tumors, 843–856
  clinical manifestations of, 846–847, 847t
  diagnostic findings in, 846–847
  etiology of, 845
  management of, community/self care in, 855–856
    medical, 847–848
    nursing, 848
    surgical, 849, 849–851, 850
      complications of, 850–851
      nursing care in, 851–855, 852b
  metastatic, 845
  nursing research on, 852b
  pathophysiology of, 845
  risk factors for, 845
  sites of, 846
  types of, 844, 844–845, 845
Brawny edema, 1380
BRCA-1 gene, in breast cancer, 2432, 2433
Breast(s), abscess of, 2453
  disease of, benign, 2451–2453
  female, assessment of, in health history, 184b
    in regional examination, 219t
    diagnostic tests for, 2327, 2327–2329
    disorders of, 2431–2454

Breast(s) (Continued)
  lesions of, misconceptions about, 2431
  physical examination of, 2312–2316, 2313–2315
  structure/function of, 2296, 2296–2298, 2297
  surgery of, 2283–2286
  male, examination of, 2333
Breast augmentation, 2283, 2283–2284
  discharge instructions after, 2283
Breast cancer, 2431–2451
  clinical manifestations of, 2434, 2434–2436
  cultural beliefs about, 2427b
  diagnostic findings in, 2434–2436, 2435
  etiology of, 2432–2433
  in men, 2451
  management of, 199t
    community/self care in, 2445–2449
    in elderly, 2450
    medical, 2445–2449
    nursing, 2449–2450
    surgical, 2436–2438, 2437b, 2438
      nursing care in, 2439–2445, 2439b
  metastatic, 2450–2451
    systemic chemotherapy for, 2448, 2448t
  pathophysiology of, 2433–2434
  prevention of, 201t, 2432b
  risk factors for, 542b, 2432–2433, 2432b
  screening for, 209t
  staging of, 2435, 2435, 2436t
  survival in, 538t
  types of, 2434
Breast history, female, 2309
  male, 2330–2331
Breast reconstruction, after mastectomy, 2284, 2284–2285, 2285, 2438, 2438, 2438b
  silicone implants for, ethical issues in, 2438b
Breast reduction, 2285, 2285–2286
Breast self-examination (BSE), 2314–2316, 2315
  schedule for, 209t
  success of, factors in, 2432b
Breast-conserving surgery, concentration ability after, nursing research on, 2439b
Breath odor, assessment of, 235
Breath sounds, adventitious, 1046, 1048t
  normal, 1046, 1047t
  location of, 1047
Breathing, assessment of, in major burns, 2242
  pattern of, in consciousness disorders, 745, 747
    ineffective, in acute pancreatitis, 1926
      in ascites, 1891
      in asthma, 1109–1110
      in dialysis, 1658
      in pneumonia, 1137
      mechanical ventilation and, 1180
  rescue, with tracheostomy tube, 1071–1072
  rhythmic, in pain control, 370
Breslow's depth of invasion, in skin cancer, 2229
Bretylium (Bretylol), for dysrhythmia, 1308t
  for shock, 521

Bretylol (bretylium), for dysrhythmia, 1308t
  for shock, 521
Bricker's procedure, for bladder cancer, 1585
Broca's aphasia, 789
Bromocriptine (Parlodel), for Parkinson's disease, 880t
  for premenstrual syndrome, 2388
Bromsulphalein (BSP) excretion, in hepatobiliary assessment, 1851t
Bronchial breath sounds, 1046, 1047t
Bronchiectasis, 1125–1126
Bronchioles, structure of, 1024, *1025, 1029*
Bronchitis, obstructive, chronic, clinical manifestations of, 1114, *1116,* 1116b, 1118t
  pathophysiology of, 1111–1113
Bronchodilators, for chronic obstructive pulmonary disease, 1111t
  therapeutic monitoring of, reference values for, 2562
Bronchogenic carcinoma, 551
Bronchophony, 1046
Bronchopleural fistula, 1167
Bronchopneumonia, *1138*
Bronchopulmonary segments, 1028
Bronchoscopy, 256, *1061,* 1061–1062
  care in, postprocedure, 256
    preprocedure, 256
  procedure for, 256
  uses of, diagnostic, 256
    therapeutic, 256
Bronchospasm, endotracheal tube suctioning and, 1175t
  prevention of, 200t
Bronchovesicular breath sounds, 1046, 1047t
Bronchus, cancer of, survival in, 538t
  structure of, 1024, *1025*
Brooke formula, for fluid resuscitation, in burns, 2250t
Brown recluse spider bite, 2537
Brown-Séquard syndrome, 895, *896*
Brudzinski's sign, 828
  in bacterial meningitis, 856, *857*
Bruising, in fracture, 2134
Bruit, auscultation of, 1382–1383
  in gastrointestinal tract assessment, 1709
  in thyroid examination, 1951
  of carotid arteries, 1213
Brunner's glands, 1693
Bruxism, sleep, 403
B-scan ultrasonography, of eyes, 951
BSE (breast self-examination), 2314–2316, *2315*
  schedule for, 209t
  success of, factors in, 2432b
BSI (body substance isolation), 423
BSP (bromsulphalein) excretion, in hepatobiliary assessment, 1851t
Bubbling, in suction control bottle, of closed chest drainage system, 1164
  in water-seal compartment, of closed chest drainage system, 1163–1164
Buck's fascia, 2302
Buck's traction, *2138,* 2138–2139
Buddhism, beliefs/practices of, 2550–2551
  about death and dying, 69b

Buerger-Allen exercises, 1412, *1412*
Buerger's disease. See *Thromboangiitis obliterans.*
Buffer systems, blood, in pH regulation, 331–332
  urinary, 329–330, *330, 331*
Buffering reactions, 331
Bulbar cavernous urethra, 1545
Bulbar disorders, 861
Bulimia nervosa, 1759–1760
  clinical manifestations of, 1759
  diagnostic findings in, 1759
  etiology of, 1759
  management of, medical, 1759–1760
    nursing, 1760
  pathophysiology of, 1759
  risk factors for, 1759
Bulla, *2184*
Bullectomy, for chronic obstructive pulmonary disease, 1119
Bullets, handling of, 2502–2503
Bullous disorders, 2220–2222
Bumetanide (Bumex), 1394t
  characteristics of, 1285t
Bumex (bumetanide), 1394t
  characteristics of, 1285t
BUN (blood urea nitrogen), measurement of, in cardiovascular assessment, 1220
  in urinary tract assessment, 1562
  preoperative, 453t
Bundle branch block, 1310
Bundle of His, 1198
Bunions, 2124, *2124*
Bupivacaine (Marcaine, Sensorcaine), 473t
  in pain control, 372
Bupivacaine hydrochloride (Marcaine HCl), 473t
Buprenex (buprenorphine), administration of, 380t
Buprenorphine (Buprenex), administration of, 380t
Burn(s), 2233–2264
  and hypovolemic shock, 498
  chemical, 2233
    of eyes, 2533
  circumferential, management of, 2250, *2251*
  electrical, 2233
    injury mechanism in, 2241
  etiology of, 2233–2234
  inhalation injury in, 2236–2237, 2237t
  major, management of, acute/subacute care in, 2252–2261
    emergency, 2242–2252
    in hospital, 2242–2252
    prehospital, 2242, 2249b
  management of, community/self care in, 2261
  minor, management of, 2241–2242
  nursing care plan in, 2243–2248
  of esophagus, 1746
  pain of, 2236
  pathophysiologic response to, 2234–2236, *2235*
  prevention of, 2234, 2234b
  psychological response to, 2236
  radiation, 2233–2234

Burn(s) *(Continued)*
  rehabilitation of, home healthcare in, 2262b
  risk factors for, 2234, 2234b
  severity of, classification of, 2237–2241, *2238–2240,* 2238t
    age in, 2239
    depth in, 2237, *2238, 2239*
    general health in, 2240–2241
    injury mechanism in, 2241
    location in, 2239
    size in, 2238–2239, *2239*
  thermal, 2233
    of lower airways, 2237
  treatment refusal in, ethical issues in, 2249b
Burn facility, transport to, 2251–2252
Burow solution, 2199t
Bursae, 2077, *2077*
Burst fracture, 2131
Business/industry, in healthcare system, 4
Busulfan (Myleran), for chronic myelogenous leukemia, 1491
Butorphanol (Stadol), administration of, 380t
Butterfly needle, for venipuncture, 246, *248*

C

C & S (culture and sensitivity), 243
C fibers, in pain transduction/transmission, 343–344
CA (carbonic anhydrase), in volatile acid regulation, 328
CA-15-3, in breast cancer, 2435
  in cancer diagnosis, 558t
CA-19-9, in cancer diagnosis, 558t
CA-125, in cancer diagnosis, 558t
CABG. See *Coronary artery bypass graft (CABG).*
CAD. See *Coronary artery disease (CAD).*
CAF (cyclophosphamide, doxorubicin [Adriamycin], fluorouracil), for breast cancer, 2448t
Caffeine, abuse of, 2490
  effects of, 2482t
  health consequences of, 2493t
  cardiovascular effects of, 1210
  restriction of, for hypertension, 1393
  withdrawal from, symptoms of, 2487t
CAH (chronic active hepatitis), 1867–1869, *1868, 1869*
CAL (chronic airflow limitation), 1021. See also *Chronic obstructive pulmonary disease (COPD).*
Calamine lotion, 2199t, 2200t
Calan (verapamil), 1396t
  for angina pectoris, 1256t
  for dysrhythmia, 1308t
  for urinary incontinence, 1611t
Calcification, in chronic renal failure, 1646
Calcitonin (Cibacalcin), actions of, 1943
  for hypercalcemia, 321, 2034t
  for osteoporosis, 2104
  in cancer diagnosis, 558t
  reference values for, in cancer, 557t
Calcium, 1516t

Calcium (Continued)
  dietary, recommendations for, 2103t
    sources of, 318b, 2102b
  distribution of, 293t
  for shock, 521
  functions of, 314
  imbalances of, 314–322. See also Hyper-
    calcemia; Hypocalcemia.
  in cardiac action potential, 1195, 1195
  in muscle movement, 2078
  in neurotransmitter release, 687
  in osteoporosis prevention, 2101–2102,
    2102b, 2103t, 2104
  inadequate, management of, 200t
  ionized, 314
  measurement of, in cardiovascular assess-
    ment, 1220
    in gastrointestinal tract assessment,
      1711t
  metabolism of, tests of, in musculoskeletal
    disorders, 2096t
  plasma, range for, 296b
  preparations of, for chronic renal failure,
    1654
  reference values for, in cancer, 557t
  regulation of, parathyroid hormone in,
    314–315, 315
  replacement of, for hypocalcemia, 318
    for hypoparathyroidism, 2037
  serum, total, in parathyroid disorders,
    2032t
  supplementation of, for hypertension, 1393
    in chronic renal failure, 1655
  urinary, qualitative, in parathyroid disor-
    ders, 2032t
    quantitative, in parathyroid disorders,
      2032t
Calcium alginates, for burns, 2256t
  in wound management, indications for,
    443t
Calcium antagonists, 1396t
Calcium carbonate (Tums, Titralac), for
  peptic ulcer disease, 1769t, 1770
Calcium channel blockers, for angina pectoris, 1255, 1256t
  for dysrhythmia, 1308t
Calcium gluconate, for hyperkalemia, 312
  for hypoparathyroidism, 2037
Calcium renal calculi, 1666
Calciuria, in hyperparathyroidism, 2031–
  2033
Calculations, assessment of, 195
Calculus(i), renal. See Renal calculi.
  salivary gland, 1732
  urinary. See Urinary calculi.
Caldwell-Luc procedure, 1078
Calicectasis, in urinary reflux, 1599
Callus, 2186
  formation of, in bone healing, 2133, 2133
Caloric testing, in consciousness disorders,
  750, 750
  in neurologic assessment, 740
Calorie-restriction diet, client education in,
  1403b
Calories, expenditure of, in burns, 2257–
  2258, 2258t
  guidelines for, in diabetes mellitus, 1976,
    1977t

Calories (Continued)
  in wound healing, 434t
  reduction of, for hypertension, 1401–
    1402, 1403b
Calymmatobacterium granulomatis, and
  granuloma inguinale, 2475
cAMP (cyclic adenosine monophosphate),
  hormone activation by, 1941, 1942
Camphor lotion, 2199t
Canaliculi, 2074, 2075
Canalplasty, for otitis externa, 1005
Cancer, 533–561. See also specific organ
  involved.
  assessment of, 544–560
  clinical manifestations of, 554
  coping with, enabling/hindering factors in,
    563, 563b
    strategies for, 563, 563b
  definition of, 533
  diagnosis of, 552–560
    angiography in, 556
    antigen skin testing in, 559
    biopsy in, 558–559
    blood studies in, 556, 557t–558t
    computed tomography in, 556
    coping with, home healthcare in, 587b
    cytologic examination in, 556–558
    direct visualization in, 559
    history in, 554
    lymphangiography in, 556
    magnetic resonance imaging in, 559
    mammography in, 556
    physical examination in, 554
    positron emission tomography in, 555
    psychosocial issues in, 552–554, 554b,
      562–564
    radiography in, 555–556
    radioisotope scans in, 555
    ultrasonography in, 559
  epidemiology of, 534
  ethical issues in, 588b
  etiology of, 539–540
  grading of, 559–560, 560t
  impact of, 541–544
    financial, 542–544
    physical, 541
    psychosocial, 541
  incidence of, 534–535, 535
  information about, resources for, 564,
    564b
  mortality of, 535, 536
  nursing care in, 568–587
    challenge of, 533–534
  nutrition in, 35
  pain of, 358–359
    nerve block for, 385
  pathogenesis of, 537–539
  patient needs in, 564, 564b
  physical performance rating in, 560, 560t
  predisposing factors in, 540–541
  prevention of, 203t, 204t, 542b–543b,
    544–560, 551, 551–552, 552b, 553t
    genetic testing in, 551–552, 552b
    risk analysis/modification in, 551, 551
    screening in, 552, 552b, 553t
  psychosocial aspects of, 562
  recurrent, palliation of, 566
  research into, 544

Cancer (Continued)
  clinical trials in, 544
    ethical issues in, 544
  risk factors for, 542b
  screening for, ethical issues in, 554b
  second malignancies in, 587–588
  sexuality in, 78
  staging of, 559–560, 560t
  survivorship of, 535, 537, 564–566, 565b
  terminal, 566–568, 567b
    nursing care in, 567–568
  terminology of, 533, 534t
  treatment of, 562–588
    at home, 565b
    biologic response modifiers in, 585–587
    bone marrow transplantation in, 584–
      585
    chemotherapy in, 573–584. See also
      Chemotherapy.
    goals of, 568
    psychosocial aspects of, 562–564, 563b,
      564b
    radiation therapy in, 570–573. See also
      Radiation therapy (RT).
    surgery in, 568–570
      curative, 569
      diagnostic, 568–569
      exploratory, 569
      palliative, 569
      preventive, 570
      reconstructive, 569–570
    termination of, ethical issues in, 567b
  trends in, 535–537, 538t
  warning signals of, 552, 552b
Candida albicans, 417t
  and urinary tract infection, 1571
Candidiasis, 2221t
  in acquired immunodeficiency syndrome,
    628
  infectious agent in, 417t
  oral, 1725, 1725–1726
    clinical manifestations of, 1725, 1725
    diagnostic findings in, 1725
    etiology of, 1725
    management of, community/self care in,
      1725–1726
      medical, 1725
      nursing, 1725–1726
    pathophysiology of, 1725
    risk factors for, 1725
  renal, 1673
  scrotal, 2381
  vulvovaginal, 2475
Canker sores. See Aphthous stomatitis.
Cannabis, abuse of, 2490–2491
  effects of, 2482t
  health consequences of, 2493t
  withdrawal from, symptoms of, 2487t
Canthus, ocular, 936, 937
Cantor tube, 1749t, 1750
Capacitance vessels, 1371
CAPD (continuous ambulatory peritoneal
  dialysis), 1648–1649
Capillaries, dilation of, in wound healing,
  428, 429
  structure of, 1371, 1371
Capillary blood pressure, changes in, in
  shock, 509–510

Capillary exchange, 1375
Capillary fragility test, in hemorrhage, 1467t
Capillary pressure, 1202
Capillary refill, 1043
  inspection of, in peripheral vascular assessment, 1380
Capitation, 5b, 9
Caplan's syndrome, in rheumatoid arthritis, 659
Capnography, 1055
Capoten (captopril), 1396t
  in surgical client, 458t
Capreomycin, for tuberculosis, 1145t
Capsaicin, in pain control, 378
Captopril (Capoten), 1396t
  in surgical client, 458t
Captopril test, 2046t
Caput medusae, in cirrhosis, 1878t
Carafate (sucralfate), for peptic ulcer disease, 1769t, 1770
Carbamazepine (Tegretol), for dementia of Alzheimer's type, 866t
  for trigeminal neuralgia, 930
  in pain control, 374
  side effects of, 839t
  therapeutic monitoring of, reference values for, 2562
Carbaminohemoglobin, 329
Carbidopa-levodopa (Sinemet), for Parkinson's disease, 878–879, 880t
Carbohydrates, for hypoglycemia, 1989
  in diabetes mellitus, guidelines for, 1977, 1977t
  inadequate intake of, cellular effects of, 270
  metabolism of, hormones in, 1945–1946, 1946
    laboratory tests for, 1850t
    liver in, 1839
Carbon dioxide, excessive, in shock, 507
  in volatile acid regulation, 328–329, 329
  partial pressures of, 1032t
  transport of, in gas exchange, 1032
Carbon monoxide, antidote to, 2538t
  in coronary artery disease, 1240
Carbon monoxide poisoning, 269
  in burns, 2237, 2237t
  skin changes in, biocultural variations in, 2190b
Carbonic anhydrase (CA), in volatile acid regulation, 328
Carbonic anhydrase inhibitors, for glaucoma, client teaching about, 957t
Carbuncles, 2221t
Carcinoembryonic antigen (CEA), in cancer, 558t
  of breast, 2435
  measurement of, in gastrointestinal tract assessment, 1710, 1711t
Carcinogenesis, stages of, 539
Carcinogens, chemical, 539
  physical, 539–540
Carcinoma, definition of, 534t
Carcinoma in situ, 550
Cardene (nicardipine), 1396t
  for angina pectoris, 1256t
Cardiac catheterization, 1230–1232
  care after, 1232

Cardiac catheterization (Continued)
  complications of, 1231–1232
  family needs in, nursing research on, 1248b
  in cardiomyopathy, 1340t
  left-sided, 1231
  preparation for, 1231–1232
  right-sided, 1231
Cardiac cirrhosis, 1874, 1874t–1875t
  in right ventricular failure, 1282
Cardiac conduction system, 1197–1198, 1198
Cardiac cycle, 1198–1199, 1199
Cardiac death, sudden, in coronary artery disease, 1244
Cardiac enzymes, in cardiovascular assessment, 1219
Cardiac function, postoperative, maintenance of, 487
  regulation of, 1202–1204
Cardiac index, 1199–1200
Cardiac muscle, 2078
Cardiac output, 1199–1200
  calculation of, 1200, 1200b
  changes in, causes of, 1235, 1235t
  decreased, after cardiac surgery, 1012, 1013b
    in cardiomyopathy, 1343–1344
    in dysrhythmias, 1321–1322
    in heart failure, 1287
    in myocardial infarction, 1270–1271
  improvement of, modified Trendelenburg's position for, nursing research on, 518b
  in blood pressure, 1202
  measurement of, 1235
    in shock, 526
Cardiac pressures, 1200, 1201
Cardiac standstill, 1309, 1310
Cardiac surgery. See Heart, surgery of.
Cardiac tamponade, 1337, 1337–1338, 1337b
  after cardiac surgery, 1014
  critical monitoring in, 1337b
Cardiac valves. See Valve(s), cardiac.
Cardiogenic shock, after myocardial infarction, 1266
  clinical manifestations of, 512
  etiology of, 497, 499–500
  management of, 523t
  prevention of, 501b
  risk factors for, 499–500
  tachycardia and heart failure with, case study of, 1268–1269
Cardiomyopathy, 1338–1350
  dilated (congestive). See Dilated cardiomyopathy.
  hypertrophic. See Hypertrophic cardiomyopathy.
  management of, community/self care in, 1342
    medical, 1341–1342
    nursing, 1342
    surgical, 1342
  nursing care plan in, 1343–1344
  prevention of, 1339b
  restrictive, 1338, 1338, 1340t
  risk factors for, 1339b
  types of, 1338, 1338, 1340t

Cardiomyoplasty, for heart failure, 1290
Cardiopulmonary bypass, during open heart surgery, 1354–1355, 1355
Cardiopulmonary resuscitation (CPR), in emergency nursing care, 2507
  television portrayal of, nursing research on, 1313b
Cardiopulmonary support, for pulmonary embolism, 1129
Cardiorespiratory endurance, in fitness, 174b
Cardiotonic medications, for shock, 521
Cardiovascular drugs, therapeutic monitoring of, reference values for, 2562
Cardiovascular system, abnormalities of, and dysphagia, 1732, 1733
  age-related changes in, 268t
    physical changes with, 454t
  autonomic neuropathy of, diabetes mellitus and, 2000
  complications of, after renal transplantation, 1663
    in postanesthesia care unit, 483
  disorders of, and sleep disorders, 404
    assessment of, 1205–1237
      diagnostic tests in, 1217–1237
      history in, 1205–1211
      in urinary tract assessment, 1554–1555
      physical examination in, 1211–1217
        normal findings in, 1206b
      postoperative, 484
      preoperative, 455
    hypertensive, 1390
    prevention of, 200t, 202t
    renal disorders in, 1626
    risk factors for, 167t
  epinephrine effects on, 2057t
  in alcohol abuse, 2490t
  in anemia, 1470
  in burns, 2235
  in chronic renal failure, 1645
  in extracellular fluid volume excess, 287t
  in hematologic disorders, 1463
  in hepatobiliary disease, 1844
  in hypercalcemia, 321t
  in hyperkalemia, 312t
  in hypernatremia, 303t
  in hypocalcemia, 317t
  in hypokalemia, 309t
  in hyponatremia, 299b
  in shock, 506–507
  in thyroid disorders, 2008t
  norepinephrine effects on, 2057t
Cardioversion, 1313–1314
Carditis, in rheumatic fever, 1328
Cardizem (diltiazem), 1396t
  for angina pectoris, 1256t
Cardura (doxazosin), 1395t
Care, acute. See Acute care.
  coordination of, ambulatory care nurse in, 141b, 142
  direct, provision of, hospital nurse in, 123
  early-morning, on day of surgery, 464
  emotional, intraoperative, 477
  interdependent, 123
  outpatient, 137
  perioperative, recipients of, 451
  physical, provision of, in pain management, 367–368

Care *(Continued)*
  plan of, definition of, 136b
  quality, provision of, 126
    right to, 126
    staffing for, 126
  subacute, 121–123
    chronic, 123
    general, 123
    transitional, 123
      long-term, 123
Care plan. See *Nursing care plan.*
Caregiver role strain, in dementia of Alzheimer's type, 869–872, 870b, 871t–872t
Carina, 1024
Caroli's syndrome, 1903
Carotid artery(ies), examination of, in cardiovascular assessment, 1213
  rupture of, after laryngeal surgery, 1088
Carotid bodies, in blood flow regulation, 1374
Carotid endarterectomy, complications of, 811
  for transient ischemic attacks, 810–811, *811*
    nursing care in, 811–812
  outcomes in, 810
Carotid vessels, assessment of, in regional examination, 219t
Carotid–cavernous sinus fistula, 816–817
Carpal scaphoid, fracture of, 2161
Carpal tunnel syndrome (CTS), *927*, 927–928, 928b, 2169t
  surgery for, home care after, 928b
Carpentier-Edwards prosthetic valve, *1352*
Carteolol (Cartrol), 1395t
Cartesian dualism, 27
Cartilage, 2079
  hyaline, 2076
  laryngeal, 1023, *1024*
Cartilaginous joints, 2076
Cartrol (Carteolol), 1395t
Case fatality rate, 414
Case management, explanation of, 13b
  in cerebrovascular accident, 784b
  in chronic obstructive pulmonary disease, 1124b
  in diabetic ketoacidosis, 1985b
  in elder care, 98–99
  in gastrointestinal hemorrhage, 1771b
  in lumbar laminectomy, 922b
  in mastectomy, 2437b
  in orchiectomy, 2371b
  in pacemakers, 1315b
  in percutaneous transluminal coronary angioplasty, 1247
  in pneumonia, 1139b
  in total hip replacement, 2116b
  in total knee replacement, 2119b
  in transient ischemic attacks, 784b
  in transurethral resection of the prostate, 2369b
  nurse in, 125
Case managers, nurse, 13
Case study, of cardiogenic shock, tachycardia, and heart failure, 1268–1269
  of cirrhosis, 1880–1881
  of diabetes, with pneumonia, 1972–1973

Case study *(Continued)*
  of hyperthyroidism, with postmenopausal osteoporosis, 2021
  of meningioma, fractured hip, and possible cerebrovascular accident, *794,* 794–795
  of perforated ulcer managed surgically, 1774–1775
Cast(s), 2146–2150
  application of, 2146–2147
  bivalving of, 2149
  complications of, assessment for, *2149,* 2149–2150, 2149b
  critical monitoring in, 2149b
  drying of, 2147–2149
  in urine, 1559
  management of, home healthcare in, 2152b
    nursing care in, 2150–2153
  rehabilitation after, 2153
  removal of, *2152,* 2152–2153
  types of, 2146–2147, 2147t, *2148*
  windowing of, 2149
Cast brace, 2137t, *2148*
Cast syndrome, monitoring for, *2149,* 2149–2150, 2149b
Cataplexy, 400
Catapres (clonidine), 1396t
Cataracts, 958–961
  age-related, 958
  clinical manifestations of, 959, *959*
  diabetes mellitus and, 1996
  diagnostic findings in, 959, *959*
  etiology of, 958
  formation of, 939–940
  management of, 199t
    community/self care in, 961
    surgical, *959,* 959–960
      complications of, 960
      nursing care after, 960–961
      nursing research on, 960b
      outcome in, 960
  pathophysiology of, 958–959
  removal of, care after, client education in, 961b
  risk factors for, 958
Catarrhal exudate, 435t
Catecholamines, assay of, in pheochromocytoma, 2058
  in hypertension, 1389
  release of, in shock, 507
  urinary, measurement of, in adrenal function testing, 1954
Catheter(s), evacuation, for continent ileostomy, 1807
  for peritoneal dialysis, 1649, *1650*
    complications of, 1650
  for total parenteral nutrition, insertion of, 1755, *1755*
  Groshong, *579*
  Hickman, *579*
  in hemodynamic monitoring, in shock, 526
  in urinary output monitoring, in shock, 526
  retention, for urinary retention, 1602–1603, 1602b
    complications of, 1602–1603
  Swan-Ganz, in hemodynamic monitoring, in shock, 526

Catheter(s) *(Continued)*
  positioning of, *1234*
  quadruple-lumen, *1234*
  ureteral, blockage of, in bladder cancer, 1590
    care of, 1597–1598
  urethral, 2354t–2357t
    after prostatectomy, care of, 2362
  urinary, insertion of, at home, 1602b
Catheter stylet/guide, 2357t
Catheterization, after prostatectomy, *2361,* 2361–2362
  after spinal cord injury, 901–902, 908
    in home care, 911
  after vaginal fistula repair, 2416
  cardiac. See *Cardiac catheterization.*
  clean vs. sterile, 1618
  during hysterectomy, and infection, 2403–2404
  for urine specimen collection, 245, 1555–1556
  intermittent, in neurogenic bladder dysfunction, 1618
    in multiple sclerosis, 875
  of urinary reservoir, 1594
  umbilical vein, 1856
  urethral, and urinary tract infection, 418, 1572
Cations, 293
Cat's eye reflex, 970
Cauda equina, 701
Cauda equina syndrome, 895, *896*
Caudal anesthesia, 476
Cauliflower ear, 1007
Causalgia, 353, 357
Cavernous sinus thrombosis, 816
CBC. See *Complete blood count (CBC).*
CBI (closed bladder irrigation) system, after prostatectomy, 2361, *2361*
CCK (cholecystokinin), 1691t
  in pancreatic secretion, 1841
  release of, 1839
CCPD (continuous cycling peritoneal dialysis), 1649
CCUs (critical care units), sleep patterns in, nursing research on, 407b
CD4 cell count, in human immunodeficiency virus infection, 623
  in immune disorder assessment, 611
CD4+ cells, in human immunodeficiency virus infection, 620–621
CDC National AIDS Clearinghouse, 619b
CDs (cluster designations), *597*
CEA (carcinoembryonic antigen), in cancer, 558t
  of breast, 2435
  measurement of, in gastrointestinal tract assessment, 1710, 1711t
Cecum, structure of, 1694
Celestone (betamethasone), 2048t
Cell(s), 261–271. See also particular types of cells.
  aging, 267–268, 268t
  alterations in, precancerous, 267, *267*
  assessment of, in neurologic assessment, 741
  atrophy of, 267, *267*

Cell(s) *(Continued)*
cancer, appearance of, 546
division/differentiation of, 546
growth of, 545, *546*
normal cells vs., 547t
connective tissue, 265
death of, 270–271
endoplasmic reticulum of, 265–266
epithelial, 265
function of, 261
alterations in, 266–271
genetic disorders of, 266–267
Golgi apparatus of, 266
growth of, disturbances of, 267, *267*
neoplastic, 267
hypertrophy of, 267, *267*
in shock, *506*
infiltration of, 267
injury to, bacterial, 270
chemical, 269
electrical, 269
hypoxic, 269
mechanical, 270
mechanisms of, 269–270
nutritional, 270
radiation, 269
thermal, 269
viral, 270
lysosomes of, 266
microfilaments of, 266
microtubules of, 266
mitochondria of, 265
muscle, 265
necrosis of, 270–271
nerve, 265
normal, cancer cells vs., 547t
characteristics of, 544–545, *545*
nucleus of, 264–265
organelles of, 262–266, *264*
organs of, 266
replication of, 261–262, *263*
structure of, 261, *262*
alterations in, 266–271
tissues of, 266
transformation/derangement of, in cancer, 537–539
types of, 261
Cell cycle, 544–545, *545*
Cell membrane, 262–264, *264*
in active transport, 263
in bulk transport, 263–264
in diffusion, 263
in intercellular communication, 264
Cell-mediated immunity (CMI), 595, 602, *603, 1453*
Cell-mediated/delayed (type IV) hypersensitivity, 638t, 640–641
Cellulitis, *2222,* 2222–2223
Celontin (methsuximide), side effects of, 839t
Central area blindness, assessment of, 947
Central auditory dysfunction, 994
Central cord syndrome, 895, *896*
Central hearing loss, 994b
Central lobe, 691, *692*
Central nervous system (CNS), divisions of, 690–701
in ventilation, 1030, *1031*

Central nervous system (CNS) *(Continued)*
structures of, nutritional, 697–701, *698, 700, 701*
protective, *697,* 697–701, *698, 700, 701*
Central pain, 356–357
Central sleep apnea syndrome, 402
Central transtentorial herniation, 773, *773*
Central venous pressure (CVP), 1233–1234
measurement of, 1212–1213, *1213*
in shock, 514, 525
in fluid replacement evaluation, 520
indications for, 1236t
monitoring of, after cardiac surgery, 1357
Centrilobular emphysema, 1114, *1114*
Cephalexin monohydrate (Keflex), for urinary tract infections, 1577t
Cerebellar herniation, 774
Cerebellar medulloblastoma, *846*
Cerebellum, cerebrovascular accident of, clinical manifestations of, 788t
structure/function of, 693, *693*
tumor of, clinical manifestations of, 847t
Cerebral angiography, in neurologic assessment, 736–738, *737*
Cerebral contusion, clinical manifestations of, 824
Cerebral cortex, 690, *692*
lesions of, and pain, 357
Cerebral disorders, 834–862
Cerebral edema, 774
head trauma and, 825
Cerebral hemispheres, 690
Cerebral hypoxia, in left ventricular failure, 1281
Cerebral perfusion pressure (CPP), 771
measurement of, 778
Cerebral perfusion studies, 738
Cerebral sinuses, lesions of, 816–817
Cerebral tissue perfusion, altered, after cardiac surgery, 925
in brain tumors, 848, 853–854
in cerebrovascular accident, 797–798, 799
in head trauma, 827–828
in increased intracranial pressure, 782–783
studies of, 738
Cerebral veins, 699, *700*
lesions of, 816–817
Cerebrospinal fluid (CSF), composition of, 698t
in ear, testing for, 993
leakage of, after intracranial surgery, 850
structure/function of, 698–699, 698t
values for, abnormal, significance of, 735t
normal, 735t
reference, 2563
Cerebrovascular accident (CVA), 784–808
case management in, 784b
clinical manifestations of, 787–792, 787t, 788t
clinical pathway for, 2567–2569
complications of, 799
diabetes mellitus and, 1993–1994, 1994t
diagnostic findings in, 787–792
effect of, on marriage, nursing research on, 790b
etiology of, 784–786, *785*

Cerebrovascular accident (CVA) *(Continued)*
management of, community/self care in, 807–808
dietary, 796, 796t
emergency, 792
in elderly, 807
medical, 793–797, 796t, 798–799
nursing, 797–798, 799–807, *801,* 804b
occupational therapy in, 798
pharmacologic, 793
physical therapy in, 798
speech therapy in, 798
supportive, 796–797
surgical, 807
meningioma and fractured hip with, case study of, *794,* 794–795
outcomes in, 799
pathophysiology of, 786–787
risk factors for, 784–786, 786b
swallowing difficulties in, home management of, 804b
Cerebrovascular disorders, 771–832
diabetes mellitus and, 1993–1994, 1994t
diagnostic tests for, 733
Cerebrum, structure/function of, 690–691, *691, 692*
Certificate of need (CON) review, 7–8
Certification, of ambulatory care settings, 4–5, 139b
Cerumen, 981
impaction of, 1006–1007
production of, external ear in, 982
Cervical biopsy, 2324–2325, *2325*
Cervical cancer, 2406–2409
clinical manifestations of, 2406–2407
cultural beliefs about, 2428b
diagnostic findings in, 2406–2407
etiology of, 2406
management of, in elderly, 2409
in pregnancy, 2407
medical, 2407
nursing, 2407
surgical, 2407–2408, *2408*
nursing care in, 2408–2409
pathophysiology of, 2406
prevention of, 203t, 2406b
risk factors for, 542b, 2406, 2406b
screening for, 209t
survival in, 538t
Cervical chordotomy, percutaneous, for pain, 386, *387*
Cervical collar, 925, *925*
Cervical culture, 2322
Cervical fusion, 924–925, *925*
home care after, 926b
Cervical intraepithelial neoplasia (CIN), 2406
in acquired immunodeficiency syndrome, 631
Cervical lymph node dissection, for laryngeal cancer, 1088
Cervical os, examination of, 2318, *2319*
Cervical spine, disorders of, 924–925, *925*
fracture of, 891, *893*
injury to, and quadriplegia, 893
emergency management of, 896–898, 897, *897*
laminectomy of, home care after, 926b

Cervical spine (Continued)
  surgery of, care after, 925
Cervical syndrome, 2168t
Cervical traction, 2139
Cervix, cytologic studies of, specimen collection for, 2321
  examination of, 2319
CF (cystic fibrosis), 1148–1149, 1932
  treatment of, 1149
Chalazion, 972–973, 974
Champion Trauma Score, 2518, 2518t
Chancre, in syphilis, 2470
Chancroid, 2475
Chaotic family, 54
Charcot's joint, 929
Chemical ablation, of dysrhythmias, 1314
Chemical burns, 2233
  of eyes, 2533
  wound care in, 2251
Chemical facial peeling, 2273–2274
Chemical fumes, health risks of, 204t
Chemical injury, of cells, 269
Chemicals, and hemolytic anemia, 1479
  endogenous, in pain modulation, 344–345
  in blood flow regulation, 1374
  ototoxic, 986b
Chemonucleolysis, for intervertebral disc herniation, 920
Chemoreceptor trigger zone (CTZ), 1748
Chemoreceptors, in cardiac regulation, 1203
  in shock, 502
Chemosis, carotid–cavernous sinus fistula and, 816–817
Chemotaxis, in wound healing, 430
Chemotherapy, 573–584
  adjuvant, for breast cancer, 2447–2448
  administration of, 576–580, 578b, 579, 580
    routes of, 578–579, 579, 580
      alternative, 579, 580
      intravenous, 578–579, 579
  classification of, 576, 577b
  client/family education about, 584, 584b
  clinical trials in, 573–575
  drug development in, 573–575
  effects of, on male reproductive system, 2345
    toxic, 580–584, 581b
      risk factors for, 581b
  extravasation of, management of, 576
  for bladder cancer, 1584
  for brain tumors, 848
  for breast cancer, 2447–2449
    metastatic, 2448, 2448t
    side effects of, 2448
  for colon cancer, 1811
  for esophageal cancer, 1744
  for Hodgkin's disease, 1502, 1503t
  for hypercortisolism, 2054t
  for laryngeal cancer, 1086
  for leukemia, acute, 1490–1491
    complications of, 1490–1491
    chronic, 1492
  for liver cancer, 1897
  for lung cancer, 1154
  for multiple myeloma, 1499
  for oral cancer, 1728
  for prostate cancer, 2368

Chemotherapy (Continued)
  for renal cancer, 1673
  for testicular cancer, 2376
  hypersensitivity reaction to, 578, 578b
  intravesical, nursing care in, 1585
  mechanism of, 575–576, 576t
  neoadjuvant, for breast cancer, 2448
  nursing management of, 584, 584b
  objective of, 575, 575b
  outpatient, 579–580
  safety precautions in, 576
  tumor response to, 575b
Chenodeoxycholic acid, for cholelithiasis, 1910
Chenodiol, for cholelithiasis, 1910
Chest, deformities of, 1040–1042, 1043
  examination of, in cardiovascular assessment, 1213–1217, 1214, 1215
  flail, 2527, 2527
  inspection of, in respiratory assessment, 1040–1042, 1043
  lesions of, aspiration of, 1064–1065
  movement of, inspection of, 1042
  trauma to, 2522–2527, 2523b
    complications of, 2524–2527, 2525, 2527
    management of, 2523
Chest drainage, assessment of, after cardiac surgery, 1358–1359
  after lung cancer surgery, 1163
  closed. See Closed chest drainage.
Chest pain, 2528
  assessment of, 1037, 1205–1206, 1208t–1209t
  in pericarditis, 1336
  pleuritic, 1166
Chest tubes, after lung cancer surgery, 1156–1157
  clamping of, 1165
  removal of, 1165–1166
  suctioning of, 1164
Chest wall, changes in, in chronic obstructive pulmonary disease, 1117
  configuration of, 1040, 1043
  palpation of, 1043–1044
Chest x-ray, 1058–1060, 1059
  diagnostic, 250
  in cardiomyopathy, 1340t
  in cardiovascular assessment, 1227
  preoperative, 453t
  procedure for, 1059–1060
Chewing, 1685–1686
Chewing reflex, 728
Cheyne-Stokes respiration, 238
  assessment of, in cardiovascular assessment, 1217
  in left ventricular failure, 1281
CHF (congestive heart failure). See also Heart failure.
  corticosteroids in, consequences of, 2049t
  extracellular fluid volume excess in, management of, 288
Chief complaint, 187
  in cardiovascular disease, 1205–1207
  in ear disorders, 985
  in endocrine disorders, 1948–1949
  in eye disorders, 941
  in gastrointestinal disorders, 1698–1699

Chief complaint (Continued)
  in gynecologic disorders, 2308
  in hematologic disorders, 1461
  in hepatobiliary disease, 1843–1844
  in immune disorders, 607
  in integumentary system disorders, 2180, 2181t
  in male reproductive disorders, 2330
  in musculoskeletal disorders, 2083
  in neurologic disorders, 709
  in respiratory disorders, 1035–1037, 1036, 1037t
  upper, 1047–1048
  in urinary tract disorders, 1547
Childhood diseases, history of, in cardiovascular disorders, 1207
  in ear disorders, 985–986
  in eye disorders, 942
  in gynecologic disorders, 2308
  in immune disorders, 608
  in musculoskeletal disorders, 2084
  in neurologic disorders, 714
  in respiratory disorders, 1038
  in urinary tract disorders, 1550
Children of Alcoholics Foundation, Inc., 2497b
Chinese, ancient, healthcare beliefs of, 19
  attitudes of, toward death and dying, 70b
  health/illness beliefs of, 61
  pain response in, 347b
Chip fracture, 2131
Chlamydia trachomatis, 417t
Chlamydial infections, 2469–2470
  clinical manifestations of, 2469
  diagnostic findings in, 2469
  etiology of, 2469
  infectious agent in, 417t
  management of, 2461t
    community/self care in, 2470
    medical, 2470
    nursing, 2470
  pathophysiology of, 2469
  risk factors for, 2469
  testing for, schedule for, 210t
Chlorambucil (Leukeran), for chronic lymphocytic leukemia, 1492
  for rheumatoid arthritis, 664t
Chloramphenicol, therapeutic monitoring of, reference values for, 2562
Chlorhexidine gluconate–alcohol (Hibiclens), 2199t
Chloride, concentration of, 294, 294t
  distribution of, 293t
  imbalances of, 295
  in acid-base balance, 331
  plasma, range for, 296b
  serum, preoperative evaluation of, 453t
Chloride shift, 328
Chloroprocaine hydrochloride (Nesacaine), 473t
Chloroquine, urine color with, 1557t
Chlorothiazide (Diuril), 1394t
  characteristics of, 1285t
Chlorpropamide (Diabinese), for diabetes mellitus, 1967t
  in surgical client, 458t
Chlorthalidone (Hygroton), 1394t
  characteristics of, 1285t

"Choked disc," 846
Cholangiography, 1852–1853
  intravenous, 1853
  retrograde, endoscopic, 1853
  transhepatic, percutaneous, 1853
  T-tube, 1853
Cholangitis, 1918–1920
  bacterial, and liver abscess, 1902
  clinical manifestations of, 1919
  diagnostic findings in, 1919
  etiology of, 1919
  management of, medical, 1919
    surgical, 1919–1920, *1920*
  pathophysiology of, 1919
  risk factors for, 1919
  sclerosing, 1920
Cholecystectomy, for acute cholecystitis,
    1918
  for cholelithiasis, 1912
    complications of, 1913
  laparoscopic, for cholelithiasis, 1912
    complications of, 1912–1913
Cholecystitis, acalculous, 1916
  acute, 1918
  acute, 1915–1918
    clinical manifestations of, 1916–1917
    diagnostic findings in, 1916–1917, 1917t
    etiology of, 1915–1916
    management of, medical, 1917
      nursing, 1917
      surgical, 1918
    pathophysiology of, 1916
    prevention of, 1916b
    risk factors for, 1915–1916, 1916b
  chronic, 1918
Cholecystography, oral, 1849–1852
Cholecystokinin (CCK), 1691t
  in pancreatic secretion, 1841
  release of, 1839
Cholecystolithotomy, percutaneous, for cho-
    lelithiasis, 1912
Choledocholithiasis, 1918–1920
  clinical manifestations of, 1919
  diagnostic findings in, 1919
  etiology of, 1919
  management of, medical, 1919
    surgical, 1919–1920, *1920*
  pathophysiology of, 1919
  risk factors for, 1919
Choledochostomy, for choledocholithiasis,
    1919
  in jaundice, 1860
Cholelithiasis, 1907–1915
  assessment data in, 1917t
  clinical manifestations of, 1908–1910,
    1909b
  diagnostic findings in, 1908–1910, 1909b
  differential diagnosis of, 1909b
  etiology of, 1907–1908
  in hemolytic anemia, 1479t
  management of, in elderly, 1915
    medical, 1910
      complications of, 1910
      outcomes in, 1910
    nursing, 1910–1912
    surgical, 1912
      complications of, 1912–1913
      nursing care in, 1913–1915

Cholelithiasis *(Continued)*
  pathophysiology of, 1908
  prevention of, 1909b
  risk factors for, 1907–1908, 1909b
Cholera, infectious agent in, 416t
Cholestatic viral hepatitis syndrome, 1866
Cholesteatoma, 1009
Cholesterol, 35
  in bile, 1838
  serum, elevation of, in coronary artery dis-
    ease, 1241
    in hepatobiliary assessment, 1850t
    in thyroid function testing, 1953
    reduction of, for hypertension, 1401,
      1402b, 1408
  testing of, schedule for, 209t
Cholesterol gallstones, 1908
Cholesterol-dissolving agents, for cholelithi-
    asis, 1910
Cholestyramine, for viral hepatitis, 1867
Cholinergic crisis, in myasthenia gravis,
    885, 886b
Cholinergic fibers, 703
Cholinergics, for urinary retention, 1601
  for urinary tract infections, 1576t
Cholinesterase inhibitors, antidotes to, 2538t
Chondritis, cricoid, manifestations of, 1751
Chondroma, 2123t
Chondrosarcoma, 2123t
Chordae tendineae, 1193
Chordotomy, cervical, percutaneous, 386,
    387
  for pain, 386, *387*
Chore services, for elderly, 99
Chorea, 723b
  in rheumatic fever, 1328
Chorioadenoma destruens, 2423–2424
Choriocarcinoma, 2423–2424
Choroid, structure of, 937, *938*
Choroid plexus, 698
Christian Church, beliefs/practices of, 2546
Christian Scientists, beliefs/practices of,
    68b, 2548
Christmas disease, 1515t
Christmas factor, 1516t
Chromaffin cells, in pheochromocytoma,
    2057
Chromosomes, analysis of, in neurologic as-
    sessment, 741
  replication of, 264
Chronic active hepatitis (CAH), 1867–1869,
    1868, 1869
Chronic airflow limitation (CAL), 1021. See
    also *Chronic obstructive pulmonary dis-
    ease (COPD).*
Chronic arterial occlusion, 1405–1424
  clinical manifestations of, 1406–1407
  diagnostic findings in, 1406–1407
  etiology of, 1405
  management of, community/self care in,
    1407–1408
    in elderly, 1412
    medical, 1407–1408
    nursing, 1408–1412, *1412*
    surgical, 1412–1414, *1414*
      nursing care in, 1415–1424
  pathophysiology of, 1405–1406, *1406*
  risk factors for, 1405

Chronic arterial occlusion *(Continued)*
  sites of, 1406, *1406*
Chronic conditions, 105–119
  adaptation to, 106–112
    physical, promotion of, 117
    physiologic, 108, 109t
      challenges in, 108
    psychological, 108–111, 110b, 117
      challenges in, 110–111, 110b
      coping in, 110
      phases of, 109–110
      promotion of, 117
    social, 111–112, 111b
      challenges in, 112
      communication in, 111–112
      family in, 112
      promotion of, 117–118
      social change in, 112
  definition of, 105
  management of, 112–118
    case management in, 113
    funding issues in, 112–113
    home healthcare in, 113
    hospice care in, 113
    long-term care facilities in, 113
    nurse-managed clinics in, 113
    nursing, 113–118
      adaptation in, 117–118
      adjusting to changes in, 117
      assessment in, 114, 115t
      client education in, 116–117
      clinical manifestation control in, 117
      diagnosis in, 116
      evaluation in, 118
      implementation in, 116
      planning in, 116
      time restructuring in, 117
    rehabilitation centers in, 113
  manifestations of, 114
  risk factors for, 106, 106t
  sexuality in, 78
  stages of, 105–106, 106t
    chronic, 106
    diagnostic, 106, 107t
    prediagnostic, 105–106
    terminal, 106
Chronic hepatitis, 1867–1869, *1868, 1869*
Chronic lymphocytic leukemia (CLL), *1487*
  management of, medical, 1491–1492
  pathophysiology of, 1488
Chronic myelogenous leukemia (CML),
    1487
  management of, medical, 1491, *1491*
  pathophysiology of, 1488
Chronic obstructive pulmonary disease
    (COPD), 1111–1124
  case management in, 1124b
  clinical manifestations of, 1114–1115,
    1115–1117, 1116b
  clinical pathway for, 2572–2574
  complications of, 1115
  dyspnea in, assessment of, nursing re-
    search on, 1037b
  etiology of, 1111
  management of, community/self care in,
    1124
    critical, 1115
    in elderly, 1123

Chronic obstructive pulmonary disease (COPD) *(Continued)*
  medical, 1115–1119, 1119t
  nursing, 1119
  pharmacologic, 1111t
  surgical, 1119–1123, *1123*
  nursing care plan for, 1120–1123
  oxygen conservation in, home healthcare in, 1125b
  pathophysiology of, 1111–1114, *1114*
  quality of life in, nursing research on, 1127b
  risk factors for, 1111
Chronic pain, 352
  management of, 368
  nerve blocks in, 385t
Chronic pain syndrome, characteristics of, 353
Chronic persistent hepatitis (CPH), 1867, *1868*
Chronic primary adrenal insufficiency. See *Addison's disease.*
Chronic renal failure (CRF), 1641–1665
  and hyperparathyroidism, 2030
  assessment of, 1644–1647
  client education in, 1657b
  clinical manifestations of, 1644–1647
  diagnostic findings in, 1647
  etiology of, 1641
  management of, *1642–1643*
    dialysis in. See *Dialysis; Hemodialysis.*
    dietary, 1655
    medical, 1647–1655
    nursing, 1655–1660
  pathophysiology of, 1641–1644
  risk factors for, 1641
Chronic venous insufficiency, 1436
Chronobiology, of sleep, 397
Chronopharmacology, 397
The Church of Jesus Christ of Latter-Day Saints, beliefs/practices of, 2548–2549
Church of the Brethren, beliefs/practices of, 2546–2547
Church of the Nazarene, beliefs/practices of, 2547
Churning, haustral, 1695
Chvostek's sign, in hypocalcemia, 318, *319*
  in hypoparathyroidism, 2037
Chylomicrons, 35
Chyme, 1690
Chymopapain, for intervertebral disc herniation, 920
Chymotrypsinogen, pancreatic, 1922b
Cibacalcin. See *Calcitonin (Cibacalcin).*
Cicatricial ectropion, 974
Cigarette smoking, cardiovascular effects of, 1210
  in bladder cancer, 1582
  in coronary artery disease, 1238–1239
Cilia, of respiratory tract, 1025, *1025*
Ciliary body, structure of, 937, *938*
Cimetidine (Tagamet), for interstitial cystitis, 1580
  for peptic ulcer disease, 1767, 1768t
  for shock, 520
  preoperative, 465t
CIN (cervical intraepithelial neoplasia), 2406

CIN (cervical intraepithelial neoplasia) *(Continued)*
  in acquired immunodeficiency syndrome, 631
Cineangiography, 1232
Cingulate herniation, *773, 774*
Cingulotomy, for pain, 386, *387*
Cinnamates, 2200t
Cinobac (cinoxacin), for urinary tract infections, 1575t
Cinoxacin (Cinobac), for urinary tract infections, 1575t
Cipro (ciprofloxacin), for urinary tract infections, 1576t
Ciprofloxacin (Cipro), for urinary tract infections, 1576t
Circadian rhythms, 397
  in sleep disorders, 403
Circinate, definition of, 2183t
Circulating nurse, role of, 466
Circulation, assisted, 1354
  for shock, 516–518, *517,* 518b
  cardiac, *1193*
  collateral, in coronary artery disease, 1242–1243
  disorders of, ocular manifestations of, 977
  in metastasis, 548
  liver in, 1840
  maintenance of, in unconscious patient, 751
  of kidneys, 1537
  systemic, in shock, 502–503
Circulatory depression, opioid analgesics in, 377
Circulatory overload, in transfusion reaction, 1529t
Circumflex artery, 1194, *1194*
  lesion of, electrocardiographic changes in, 1225t
Circumscribed, definition of, 2183t
Cirrhosis, 1872–1884
  and liver failure, 1882t
  biliary, 1873, 1874t–1875t
  cardiac, 1874, 1874t–1875t
    in right ventricular failure, 1282
  case study of, 1880–1881
  clinical manifestations of, 1875, 1878t
  complications of, 1883–1895
  diagnostic findings in, 1875, *1879*
  etiology of, 1873–1874
  Laënnec's, 1873, 1874t–1875t
  management of, *1876–1877*
    dietary, 1879
    medical, 1878–1879, 1882
    nursing, 1879–1883
    pharmacologic, 1878
  pathophysiology of, 1874–1875
  postnecrotic, 1873, 1874t–1875t
  prevention of, 201t, 1873b
  risk factors for, 1873–1874, 1873b
Cisapride (Propulsid), for gastroesophageal reflux disease, 1738
Cisterna magna, *698, 699*
Cisternal puncture, in neurologic assessment, 736
Citizen vs. non-citizen care, ethical issues in, 915b
Civil Rights Act of 1964, 129

CJD (Creutzfeldt-Jakob disease), 872–873
CK (creatine kinase), in myocardial infarction, 1261, *1262*
  measurement of, in cardiovascular assessment, 1219
  in musculoskeletal disorders, 2096t
Clarithromycin (Biaxin), for peptic ulcer disease, 1767, 1769t
  in *Mycobacterium avium-intracellulare* complex prophylaxis, 625
Clark's classification, of cancer, 560
  of skin, *2229*
Claudication, intermittent, 1377
  in chronic arterial occlusion, 1406
Claudication distance, 1378
Clean-catch urine specimen, 1555
Cleanliness, in American healthcare system, 62
Clearance studies, renal, *1560,* 1560–1561
Cleocin T (clindamycin), topical, 2198t
Click, ejection, 1216
Client(s), critically ill, family needs of, nursing research on, 58b
  dignity of, protection of, ethical issues in, 467b
  "do not resuscitate," surgery in, ethical issues in, 460b
  motivation of, in health promotion, 170
  nurse relationship with, ethical issues in, 46
  perioperative, stress in, 451, 451t
  preparation of, for health history interview, 186
    for physical examination, 231–233, *232*
    draping in, 231
    positioning in, 231, *232*
    psychological, 231–233
    on day of surgery, 464–465, 465t
  role of, in home healthcare, 149
  transport of, from operating room, 480
    to surgery, 465
  underinsured, care of, ethical issues in, 9b
  variations in, 14–16
Client advocacy, of elderly, ethical issues in, 101b
Client education, after total hip replacement, 2116b
  for blood transfusion, 1518–1519
  in Alzheimer's disease, 867b
  in arm care, after axillary node dissection, 2443, 2445b
  in asthma, 1112b–1113b
  in blepharoplasty, 2273
  in calorie-restriction diet, 1403b
  in cataract postsurgical care, 961b
  in cerebrovascular accident, in bed-wheelchair transfer, *801*
  in chemotherapy, 584, 584b
  in chronic conditions, 116–117
  in colostomy irrigation, 1815b
  in condom use, 2466b–2467b
  in consciousness disorders, 762b
  in diabetes mellitus, in macrovascular complication prevention, 1996b
    in visual complication prevention, 1999b
  in dumping syndrome diet, 1780b
  in ear infection, 1008b
  in foot care, 1410b–1411b

Client education *(Continued)*
in halo vest use, 906b
in head trauma, 829b
in home care, after carpal tunnel release, 928b
after cervical laminectomy/fusion, 926b
in infective endocarditis, 1334b
in insulin self-injection, 1980b
in irradiated skin care, 571b
in liver transplantation, 1899b
in low back care, 918b
in low-fat, low-cholesterol diet, 1402b
in low-sodium diet, 1400b–1401b
in migraine headaches, 818b
in obstructive sleep apnea syndrome, 402b
in ocular prosthesis management, 972b–973b
in ostomy supplies, 1803b
in pain control, 361
in Parkinson's disease, 881b–882b
in permanent pacemaker, 1322b
in pulmonary tuberculosis, 1146b
in radical neck surgery exercises, 1096b–1098b
in radical vulvectomy, 2421b
in renal failure, acute, 1641b
chronic, 1657b
in rhinoplasty, 2275
in sexually transmitted diseases, 2465b
in shock, 527b
in skin self-examination, 2205b
in status epilepticus, 840b
in stress testing, 1226b
in stump/prosthesis care, 1423b
in substance abuse, 2495b
in sunburn prevention, 2224b
in sutured laceration care, 2535b
in swallowing, after partial laryngectomy, 1091b
in testosterone patch application, 2348b
in thyroid supplements, 2016b
in topical pain relievers, 668b
in tracheoesophageal puncture care, 1094b
in transcutaneous electrical nerve stimulation units, 389b
in transient ischemic attacks, 808b
in urinary calculus prevention, 1598b
in urinary diversion care, 1593b
in vaginitis prevention, 2415b
Clindamycin (Cleocin T), topical, 2198t
Clinic, nurse-managed, in chronic conditions, 113
Clinical indicators, in performance improvement, 130, 130b
Clinical nurse specialists (CNSs), 12–13
Clinical pathway, for asthma, 2572–2574
for cardiac valve surgery, 2583
for cerebrovascular accident, 2567–2569
for chronic obstructive pulmonary disease, 2572–2574
for coronary artery bypass grafting, 2578–2582
for diabetic ketoacidosis, 2588–2589
for directional coronary atherectomy, 2578–2579
for gastrointestinal bleeding, 2586–2587
for lumbar laminectomy, 2570–2571

Clinical pathway *(Continued)*
for mastectomy, 2603–2604
for microdiscectomy, 2570–2571
for orchiectomy, 2600–2602
for pacemaker, 2584–2585
for percutaneous transluminal coronary angioplasty, 2578–2579
for pneumonia, 2575–2577
for total hip replacement, 2590–2592
for total knee replacement, 2593–2595
for transient ischemic attack, 2567–2569
for transurethral resection of the prostate, 2596–2599
Clinical technicians, 125
Clinical unit, postoperative nursing in, 484–492, 486t, *487, 489, 491*
Clinically significant electrolyte abnormalities (CSEA), indicators of, 296b
Clinoril (sulindac), for rheumatoid arthritis, 664t
Clitoris, 2293, *2294*
examination of, 2317
CLL (chronic lymphocytic leukemia), *1487*
management of, medical, 1491–1492
pathophysiology of, 1488
Clobetasol (Temovate), topical, 2199t
Clonazepam (Klonopin), side effects of, 839t
Clonic phase, of tonic-clonic seizure, 837, *837*
Clonidine (Catapres), 1396t
Clonus, 728
Closed bladder irrigation (CBI) system, after prostatectomy, 2361, *2361*
Closed chest drainage, activity with, 1165
after lung cancer surgery, 1157, 1163, *1163*
promotion of, 1164–1165, *1165*
removal of, 1165–1166
suction in, 1164
apparatus for, assessment of, 1164
tubing of, clamping of, 1165
water seal of, assessment of, 1163–1164
Closed circuit helium method, of lung volume measurement, 1051
Closed fracture, 2129, *2130*
Closed reduction, of fractures, *2136,* 2136–2137
Clostridium difficile, in hospitalized clients, nursing research on, 1789b
Clostridium tetani, 857
Clot retraction, in hemorrhage, 1467t
Clotrimazole (Lotrimin), topical, 2198t
Clotting factors, disorders of, 1506–1512
Clozapine, for dementia of Alzheimer's type, 866t
Clubbing, 1042–1043, *1044,* 2187t
finger, in infective endocarditis, 1333
Cluster designations (CDs), *597*
Cluster headaches, 819–820
CMF (cyclophosphamide, methotrexate, fluorouracil), for breast cancer, 2448t
CMFA (cyclophosphamide, methotrexate, fluorouracil, doxorubicin [Adriamycin]), for breast cancer, 2448t
CMFP (cyclophosphamide, methotrexate, fluorouracil, prednisone), for breast cancer, 2448t

CMFVP (cyclophosphamide, methotrexate, fluorouracil, vincristine, prednisone), for breast cancer, 2448t
CMI (cell-mediated immunity), 595, 602, *603, 1453*
CML (chronic myelogenous leukemia), *1487*
management of, medical, 1491, *1491*
pathophysiology of, 1488
CMV. See *Continuous mechanical ventilation (CMV).*
CNS (central nervous system), divisions of, 690–701
in ventilation, 1030, *1031*
structures of, nutritional, 697–701, *698, 700, 701*
protective, 697–701, *698, 700, 701*
CNSs (clinical nurse specialists), 12–13
Coagulation, disorders of, 1509–1512
Coagulation factor concentrates, transfusion of, 1520t–1523t
Coagulation factors, 1516t
Coagulation system, in hemostasis, *1457,* 1457–1458, *1458*
Coagulation tests, 1467t, 1468
in cardiovascular assessment, 1219–1220
Coalesce, definition of, 2183t
COBRA (Consolidated Omnibus Budget Reconciliation Act), provisions of, for client transfers, 2503
Cocaine, 474t
abuse of, 2491
effects of, 2482t
health consequences of, 2493t
topical use of, 372, 474
withdrawal from, symptoms of, 2487t
Cocaine Anonymous, 2497b
Coccidioidomycosis, 860, 1146
in acquired immunodeficiency syndrome, 629
Cochlea, structure of, 983, *983*
Cochlear duct, in hearing, 984
Cochlear implants, 1001, *1002*
Cochlear otospongiosis, 1001
Codeine, administration of, 380t
avoidance of, in cirrhosis, 1882t
in pain control, 375t
Cogentin (benztropine), for Parkinson's disease, 880t
Cognex (tacrine), for dementia of Alzheimer's type, 865
Cognition, pattern of, 206
Cognitive function, assessment of, Rancho Los Amigos Scale in, 114, 115t
Colchicine, for gout, 2108
Cold, and cell damage, 269
application of, delegation of, 2165b
in inflammation management, 436
common, 1080
influenza vs., 1133
exposure to, after burn injury, 2263b
Cold conization, 2325
in cervical cancer, 2407
Cold emergencies, 2535–2536
"Cold shock," 513
Cold-spot imaging, 255
Colic, renal, 1667
ureteral, 1667

Colitis, pseudomembranous, 1789
  ulcerative. See *Ulcerative colitis.*
Collagen, 2074
  in wound healing, 432
  injection of, 2274
  structure/function of, 2176t
  synthesis of, altered, 446, *447*
Collagenase (Santyl), for enzymatic debridement, 440
Collateral circulation, in coronary artery disease, 1242–1243
Colleagues, relationship with, ethical issues in, 46
Colles' fracture, *2130,* 2131, 2161
Colloid solutions, for shock, 519
Colloidal oatmeal bath (Aveeno Bath), 2199t
Colon, structure of, 1695
Colon cancer, 1808–1816
  clinical manifestations of, *1810,* 1810–1811
  diagnostic findings in, *1810,* 1810–1811
  etiology of, 1809
  management of, medical, 1811
    nursing, 1811
    surgical, *1811,* 1811–1812, *1812*
      nursing care in, 1812–1816
  pathophysiology of, 1809–1810, 1809t
  prevention of, 201t, 1809b
  risk factors for, 542b, 1809, 1809b
  spread of, 1810
  staging of, 1809t, 1810
  survival in, 538t
Colon endoscopy, 1715
Colonization, 415
Colonoscopy, 1716
Colony-stimulating factors (CSFs), effects of, 604t
  for agranulocytosis, 1498
  for cancer, 586
  in wound healing, 432
Color vision, defective, 947
  testing of, 947
Colostomy, for colon cancer, *1811,* 1811–1812
  irrigation of, 1815
    client education in, 1815b
  types of, *1811,* 1811–1812
Colostomy pouches, 1806, *1807*
Colporrhaphy, for rectocele, 2410
Colposcopy, 2323, *2325*
Columbia Health Care System, 10
Column-disc catheter, for peritoneal dialysis, *1650*
Coma, 743–770, *747.* See also *Consciousness, disorders of.*
  assessment of, initial, 751–752
  cerebrovascular accident and, 799
  diabetic, 1981
  drug overdose–induced, emergency care of, 752
  intracranial pressure in, nursing research on, 781b
  metabolic, 744
    manifestations of, 745–746, 746t
  myxedema, in hypothyroidism, 2007–2012
    management of, medical, 2009

Coma *(Continued)*
    nursing, 2009–2012
  outcome of, signs of, 753t
  stimulation during, nursing research on, 752b
  structurally induced, manifestations of, 746, 746t
Comedo, definition of, 2183t
Comedone, 2212
Comfeel Ulcus, indications for, 443t
Comfort, postoperative, promotion of, 488–490, *489*
Comminuted fracture, *2130,* 2131
Commissurotomy, 1351
Common cold, 1080
  influenza vs., 1133
Common sense, in home healthcare, 150–151
Communal family, 53
Communicability, period of, 417
Communication, assessment of, 195, 718
  in cross-cultural nursing, 64b, 192t
  family, 54
    therapeutic, 58
  impaired, in vertigo, 1014
  in chronic conditions, 111–112
  in hearing impairment, improvement of, 1000b
  in Huntington's disease, 883
  in Parkinson's disease, client education about, 882b
  in Wallingford Wellness Project, 175
  intercellular, cell membrane in, 264
  problem in, ethical dilemma vs., 2442b
  telephone, ambulatory care nurse in, 141b, 142
  verbal, impaired, after cerebrovascular accident, 805
    in dementia of Alzheimer's type, 866–868
      in hearing impairment, 998
      in oral cancer, 1731–1732
      with tracheostomy, 1075
  with endotracheal tube, 1175
Communitrach tubes, 1069
Community, definition of, 161
  elder programs of, 99–100
  empowerment of, in Wallingford Wellness Project, 175
Community care, 12
  after cardiac surgery, 926
  after cataract surgery, 961
  in abdominal aortic aneurysm, 1428
  in Alzheimer's disease, 865–872
  in amenorrhea, 2390–2391
  in anemia, 1471
    pernicious, 1475–1476
  in angina pectoris, 1255–1258
  in asthma, 1110–1111, *1111,* 1111t
  in atopic dermatitis, 2206–2207
  in benign prostatic hypertrophy, 2363–2365, 2364t
  in brain tumors, 855–856
  in breast cancer, 2445–2449
  in burns, 2261
  in candidiasis, 1725–1726
  in cardiomyopathy, 1342
  in cerebrovascular accident, 807–808

Community care *(Continued)*
  in chlamydial infections, 2470
  in chronic arterial occlusion, 1407–1408
  in chronic obstructive pulmonary disease, 1124
  in confusion, 770
  in consciousness disorders, 763
  in corneal dystrophies, 968
  in coronary artery disease, 1244–1245, 1250–1251
  in dental caries, 1720
  in diabetes mellitus, 1963–1981, *1964*
  in dysmenorrhea, 2387
  in dysrhythmias, 1323–1324
  in endometriosis, 2399–2400
  in epilepsy, 842
  in erectile dysfunction, 2350
  in extracellular fluid volume deficit, 284
  in extracellular fluid volume excess, 289
  in fractures, 2145–2153
  in glaucoma, 958
  in gonorrhea, 2468–2469
  in head trauma, 829
  in hearing impairment, 995–1001
  in heart failure, 1291
  in hepatic encephalopathy, 1895
  in human immunodeficiency virus infection, 623–625
  in hypercortisolism, 2053–2055
  in hyperkalemia, 314
  in hypernatremia, 304
  in hyperparathyroidism, 2031–2034
  in hypersensitivity, 641, *642*
  in hypertension, 1391–1392
  in hypokalemia, 310
  in hyponatremia, 300
  in hypothyroidism, 2012–2016
  in infective endocarditis, 1334
  in infertility, 2346–2347
  in inflammation, 437
  in intertrochanteric hip fracture, 2158–2159, 2159b
  in iron deficiency anemia, 1473–1474
  in menopause, 2393–2395
  in multiple sclerosis, 874–877
  in neurogenic bladder dysfunction, 1617–1619
  in osteoarthritis, 2109–2110
  in osteoporosis, 2100–2103
  in periodontal disease, 1721–1722
  in pneumonia, 1138
  in premenstrual syndrome, 2388–2389
  in pressure ulcers, 2219–2220, 2220b
  in retinal detachment, 964
  in rheumatoid arthritis, 661–672
  in sexually transmitted diseases, 2462–2465
  in shock, 528
  in spinal cord injury, 914, 915b
  in syphilis, 2471–2472
  in systemic lupus erythematosus, 676–678
  in total hip replacement, 2116–2118, *2117*
  in tuberculosis, 1143–1144
  in upper airway neoplasms, 1095–1100, 1096b–1098b, *1098–1100,* 1099b
  in urinary incontinence, 1608–1610, 1609b
  in urinary tract infections, 1578–1579

Community care (Continued)
 in venous thrombosis, 1436
 in vertigo, 1012–1016
 in viral hepatitis, 1870–1871
 in wound management, 442–443
Community health nursing, definition of,
 146
 history of, 147–148
 philosophy of, 149–150
Community programs/services, for elderly,
 99
Compartment syndrome, after arterial bypass, 1415
 after fracture, 2139, 2140, 2140b
 intertrochanteric hip, 2156
 after total hip replacement, 2113
 assessment for, in inflammation management, 436
 casting and, monitoring for, 2149b
 critical monitoring in, 2140b
Compensation, acid-base, 332, 333
 in arterial blood gas analysis, 1057
 in increased intracranial pressure, 771–
 772
 in shock, 502–503, 503
Competence, of elderly, 100–102
Complement system, in immunity, 601–
 602, 602
 in wound healing, 430
Complete blood count (CBC), in blood dyscrasias, 1465t
 in cardiovascular assessment, 1219
 in gastrointestinal tract assessment, 1711t
 in hematologic system assessment, 1463–
 1464, 1464t
 in leukemia, 1489
 normal values for, 1464t
Complete fracture, 2130, 2131
Compliance, drug, cultural differences in,
 94b–95b
 in increased intracranial pressure, 771
 in ventilation, 1029
 intracranial, monitoring of, 778
Compound fracture, 2129, 2130
Comprehension, assessment of, 718
Compression, of spinal cord, 891, 892
Compression fracture, 2130, 2131
 osteoporotic, of vertebrae, 2099–2100
Computed tomography (CT), care in, postprocedure, 251–252
 preprocedure, 251, 252b
 diagnostic, 251–252
 in cancer, 556
 in consciousness disorders, 749
 in gynecologic disorders, 2322–2323
 of adrenal glands, 2045t
 of ear, 989
 of gastrointestinal tract, 1714, 1714
 of hepatobiliary system, 1853, 1853
 of male reproductive system, 2339
 of musculoskeletal system, 2093–2094
 of neurologic system, 730–732, 731
 contrast agents in, 731–732
 procedure for, 730, 731
 of peripheral vascular system, 1384
 of respiratory system, 1060–1061
 of thyroid gland, 2011t
 of urinary tract, 1563–1564

Computed tomography (CT) (Continued)
 procedure for, 251, 251
 with contrast, 251, 252b
CON (certificate of need) review, 7–8
Concentration, of urine, 1561
 in fluid and electrolyte balance, 1542
Concha, 980, 981
Concussion, 823, 2528–2529, 2528t
 classification of, 2528t
 clinical manifestations of, 823
Condom, use of, guidelines for, 2466b–
 2467b
Condom catheter drainage, for urinary incontinence, 1612
Conduction, air, testing of, 720, 721
 bone, testing of, 720, 721
 disturbances in, and dysrhythmia, 1297
 atrial, 1299–1300
 atrioventricular, 1303, 1303–1304
 ventricular, 1310
 saltatory, 690
Conduction system, cardiac, 1197–1198,
 1198
Conductive hearing loss, 992, 994b. See
 also Hearing impairment.
 clinical manifestations of, 996t
 etiology of, 993
 pathophysiology of, 994
Conductivity, of heart, 1196
Condyle fracture, 2160
Condylomata acuminata, 2473
Condylomata lata, in syphilis, 2470
Cones, 938
CONFHER model, of cross-cultural nursing,
 63, 64b
Confidentiality, ethical issues in, 41, 189b
 in emergency care, 2502
Confrontation, in substance abuse, 2495
Confucianism, beliefs/practices of, 2551
Confusion, 743–770
 care in, community, 770
 nursing, 765–769, 768b, 769b
 self, 770
 client advocacy in, ethical issues in,
 768b
 clinical manifestations of, 765
 decision-making in, nursing research on,
 764b
 diagnostic findings in, 765
 etiology of, 763–764
 in consciousness disorders, 746
 in elderly, 769–770
 intertrochanteric hip fracture and, 2155
 pathophysiology of, 764–765
 prevention of, 766b–767b
 risk factors for, 763–764, 766b–767b
Congenital glaucoma, 952. See also Glaucoma.
Congenital heart disease, 1350
Congenital hepatic fibrosis, 1903
Congestive cardiomyopathy. See Dilated
 cardiomyopathy.
Congestive heart failure (CHF). See also
 Heart failure.
 corticosteroids in, consequences of, 2049t
 extracellular fluid volume excess in, management of, 288
Congregate housing, for elderly, 100

Conization, cold, 2325
 in cervical cancer, 2407
Conjugal family, 52
Conjugate gaze, 720, 747
Conjunctiva, disorders of, 972–975
 examination of, 944
 petechiae of, in infective endocarditis,
 1333
 structure of, 936, 938
Conjunctivitis, 973
 red eye in, 942b
Connecting peptide (C-peptide), in diabetes
 mellitus, 1962
Connective tissue, cells of, 265
 types of, 654b
Connective tissue diseases (CTDs), 653–
 682, 2108–2120
 ocular manifestations of, 977
Conn's syndrome. See Hyperaldosteronism,
 primary.
Consciousness, assessment of, 710t, 715–
 716
 changes in, manifestations of, critical
 monitoring of, 756b–757b
 disorders of, 743–763. See also Coma;
 Confusion.
 care in, community, 763
 critical, 752–753, 752b, 753t
 emergency, 751–752
 nursing, 755–763, 756b–757b, 759,
 759b, 761b, 762b
 self, 763
 client/family education about, 762b
 clinical manifestations of, 745, 745–753,
 746t
 diagnostic findings in, 745–753, 747
 etiology of, 743–744, 744
 in elderly, 763
 organ donation in, 753–763
 pathophysiology of, 744–745
 risk factors for, 743–744, 744
 level of. See Level of consciousness
 (LOC).
Consent, informed. See Informed consent.
Consolidated Omnibus Budget Reconciliation Act (COBRA), provisions of, for client transfers, 2503
Consolidation, in bone healing, 2133,
 2133
Constipation, after intertrochanteric hip
 fracture, 2158
 after spinal cord injury, 908
 chemotherapy and, 583
 in chronic renal failure, 1645, 1656
 in enteral nutrition, 1754
 in hyperparathyroidism, 2033–2034
 in hypothyroidism, 2015
 in intestinal disorders, 1788
 in leiomyoma, 2404
 in multiple sclerosis, 875–876
 in myocardial infarction, 1272
 opioid analgesics in, 376
 risk for, with tracheostomy, 1075
Contact dermatitis, 641, 2209–2210, 2210
Contact inhibition, of cells, 545
Contact precautions, 424
Continent diversion, management of, 1593–
 1594

Continent ileostomy, care of, 1807–1808
  for inflammatory bowel disease, 1801–1802, *1803*
Continuing education, ambulatory care nurse in, 141b, 142–143
Continuous ambulatory peritoneal dialysis (CAPD), 1648–1649
Continuous cycling peritoneal dialysis (CCPD), 1649
Continuous mechanical ventilation (CMV), 1176–1184
  complications of, risk for, 1181
  extubation from, 1184
  modes of, 1177–1182, 1178t–1179t
  nursing management of, 1182–1184, 1183b, 1184b
  physiologic changes with, 1176–1177
  termination of, ethical issues in, 1184b
  weaning from, 1182–1184
    failure of, 1183–1184
    trial of, criteria for, 1182–1183
Continuous passive motion (CPM), after total knee replacement, 2119, *2120*
  for anterior cruciate ligament injuries, 2166
Continuous positive airway pressure (CPAP), 1179–1182
  for obstructive sleep apnea syndrome, 401
Contraception, in spinal cord injury, 904t
  religion in, 2425b–2426b
Contraceptive history, female, 2309
  male, 2331
Contractile state, of heart, 1200, *1201*
Contractility, muscle, in free flap assessment, 2281
Contraction alkalosis, 336
Contractions, segmentation, 1685
Contracture(s), Dupuytren's, 928
  release of, 928
  in wound healing, 432
  ischemic, Volkmann's, 2140
  risk for, after spinal cord injury, 907
    in cerebrovascular accident, 802–803
    in consciousness disorders, 758
Contrast agents, allergy to, 252b
  in computed tomography, in neurologic disorder assessment, 731–732
  in diagnostic testing, 252b
  radioiodinated, nephrotoxicity of, 1627, 1627b
Contrast angiography, in peripheral vascular assessment, 1384–1385, *1385*
Contrast radiography, 250–251
Contrast venography, in peripheral vascular assessment, 1385–1386
Control, locus of, assessment of, 191t
Controlled (machine-cycled) ventilation, 1177, 1178t
Contusion, 823
  brain stem, 824, *824*
  cerebral, 824
  clinical manifestations of, 824
Conus medullaris, 693, *695*
Conus medullaris syndrome, 895, *896*
Coombs' test, in hematologic system assessment, 1464–1465
Cooperation, level of, assessment of, 235
Cooper's ligaments, 2297

Coordination, muscle, assessment of, 722
COPD. See *Chronic obstructive pulmonary disease (COPD)*.
Coping, emotion-focused, 110
  family, ineffective, after spinal cord injury, 910–911
    in breast cancer, 2439–2441
    in burns, 2248
    in chronic renal failure, 1656–1657
    in confusion, 769
    in dialysis, 1658
  in chronic conditions, 110
  in diabetes mellitus, 1963–1965, 1965b
  in osteoarthritis, strategies for, nursing research on, 2118b
  in stress management, 172
  ineffective, after cerebrovascular accident, 806
    after spinal cord injury, 910
    after thoracic surgery, 1162
    in acute pancreatitis, 1926–1927
    in breast cancer, 2439–2441
    in dialysis, 1659–1660
    in esophageal cancer, 1745
    in hearing impairment, 998–999
    in hereditary spherocytosis, 1485
    in inflammatory bowel disease, 1800
    in leukemia, 1493–1494
    in liver transplantation, 1900–1901
    in premenstrual syndrome, 2389
  pattern of, 206
  problem-focused, 110
  with cancer, enabling/hindering factors in, 563, 563b
    home healthcare in, 587b
    strategies for, 563, 563b
Cordarone (amiodarone), for dysrhythmia, 1308t
Core needle biopsy, 257
Core rewarming, in hypothermia, 2535–2536
Corgard (nadolol), 1395t
  for angina pectoris, 1257t
Corn, 2186
Cornea, disorders of, 966–970
  examination of, 944
  infection of, 968–970
  structure of, 936–937, *938*
Corneal abrasion, risk for, in cerebrovascular accident, 802
Corneal dystrophies, 966–968
  management of, community/self care in, 968
  surgical, 966–967, *967*
    nursing care in, 967–968
Corneal light reflex test, 945
Corneal reflex, 726–727, 729t
  examination of, 944
  testing of, 720
Corneal transplantation, 966–967, *967*
  criteria for, 646
Corneal ulcer, 968–970, *969*
  eye drops for, administration schedule for, 969
Cornstarch, 2200t
Cornstarch baths, 2199t
Coronary angiography, in angina pectoris, 1254

Coronary arteries, 1194, *1194*
Coronary artery bypass graft (CABG), case management in, 1249b
  clinical pathway for, 2578–2582
  complications of, 1248
  for coronary artery disease, 1247–1248, *1250*
  recovery from, sex-related differences in, 1240b
  rehabilitation after, 1249–1251, 1252b
    gender differences in, nursing research on, 1251b
Coronary artery disease (CAD), 1238–1251
  clinical manifestations of, 1244
  diabetes mellitus and, 1993, 1994t
  diagnostic findings in, 1244
  etiology of, 1238–1241
  in women, 1240b
  management of, community/self care in, 1244–1245, 1250–1251
    interventional cardiology in, *1245,* 1245–1246, *1246*
    nursing care in, 1246–1247
    surgical, 1247–1249
      home rehabilitation after, 1252b
      in elderly, 1248–1249
      nursing care in, 1249–1250
  pathophysiology of, 1241–1244, *1242, 1243*
  theories of, 1243, *1243*
  prevention of, 1239b
  risk factors for, 1238–1241, 1239b, 1240b
Coronary insufficiency, chest pain in, assessment of, 1208t
Coroner, jurisdiction of, 2513–2515
Corpora cavernosa, 2302
Corpus callosotomy, for epilepsy, 841, *841*
Corpus callosum, 690
Corpus luteum, in menstruation, 2300
  of ovaries, 2295, *2295*
Corpus luteum cysts, of ovaries, 2412
Corpus spongiosum, 2302
Correction, acid-base, 332–333
Cortical bone, 2132
Cortical cataracts, 958
Cortical resection, of anterior temporal lobe, for epilepsy, 840, 841, *841*
Corticospinal tracts, 696t
Corticosteroids, 2048t
  consequences of, 2049t
  for adult respiratory distress syndrome, 1172
  for hypercalcemia, 321
  for multiple sclerosis, 874
  for myasthenia gravis, 885
  for rheumatoid arthritis, 665
    side effects of, 670
  musculoskeletal effects of, 2085
  topical, 2199t, 2201
Corticotropin, serum, 2046t
Corticotropin-releasing hormone (CRH) stimulation, 2046t
Cortisol, dysfunction of, 2044t
  effects of, 1944–1945
  function of, 2044t
  hypersecretion of, factors in, 2049
  in hypertension, 1389
  in hypokalemia, 305

Cortisol *(Continued)*
levels of, plasma, 2045t
in hypercortisolism, 2050
urinary, 2045t
Cortisol level with dexamethasone suppression test, 2045t
Cortisone (Cortone), 2048t
for rheumatoid arthritis, 663
Cortisone suppression test, 1953
Cortone (cortisone), 2048t
for rheumatoid arthritis, 663
Corynebacterium diphtheriae, 1081
Coryza, 1080
Costovertebral angle, percussion of, 1548, *1549*
Cosyntropin test, 2045t
Cotrel-Dubousset instrumentation, for scoliosis, 2120, *2121*
Co-trimoxazole, for urinary tract infections, 1575t
Cotswolds staging, of Hodgkin's disease, 1501t
Coudé round-tip Foley urethral catheter, 2355t
Cough(ing), after thyroidectomy, 2025t
assessment of, 1036
in left ventricular failure, 1281
methods of, preoperative teaching of, 461
physiologic elements of, 1026, 1026t
Cough reflex, 1030
Coumadin (warfarin), for cerebrovascular accident, 793
for pulmonary embolism, 1128
for venous thrombosis, 1434–1435
in surgical client, 458t
Councill red rubber urethral catheter, 2354t
Countercurrent mechanism, in fluid and electrolyte balance, 1542
Countercurrent multiplication, 1542
Counterpulsation, external, for shock, 517
intra-aortic balloon pump in, 1012, 1013b
Countershock, external, paddle placement for, *1312*
Coup-contrecoup injury, *821, 822, 822*
Cover-uncover test, 945
CPAP (continuous positive airway pressure), 1179–1182
for obstructive sleep apnea syndrome, 401
C-peptide (connecting peptide), in diabetes mellitus, 1962
CPH (chronic persistent hepatitis), 1867, *1868*
CPM (continuous passive motion), after total knee replacement, 2119, *2120*
for anterior cruciate ligament injuries, 2166
CPP (cerebral perfusion pressure), 771
measurement of, 778
CPR (cardiopulmonary resuscitation), in emergency nursing care, 2507
television portrayal of, nursing research on, 1313b
Crackles, 1046, 1048t
assessment of, in cardiovascular assessment, 1217
Cramps, heat, 2535
muscle, in endocrine disorders, 1949
Cranial arteritis, 680–681

Cranial nerves, assessment of, 718–721, *719*
flow sheet for, *779–780*
normal findings in, 717b
disorders of, 890–931, *929,* 929–931, *930*
distribution of, *719*
injury to, skull fracture and, 823
structure/function of, 702–703, *703, 704,* 705t
types of, 705t
Craniofacial surgery, 2282–2283
Craniopharyngioma, *846*
Craniotomy, for brain tumors, 849, *849*
positioning after, 853–854
Cranium, structure/function of, 697
C-reactive protein (CRP), in musculoskeletal disorders, 2096t
Creams, 2197, 2200t
Creatine kinase (CK), in myocardial infarction, 1261, *1262*
measurement of, in cardiovascular assessment, 1219
in musculoskeletal disorders, 2096t
Creatinine, preoperative evaluation of, 453t
serum, measurement of, in urinary tract assessment, 1562
Creatinine clearance, 1561
Credé maneuver, 901, 911
in neurogenic bladder dysfunction, 1617–1618
Cremasteric reflex, 727, 729t
Crepitations, 1048t
Crepitus, 2088
in fracture, 2134
CREST syndrome, 677, 677b
Creutzfeldt-Jakob disease (CJD), 872–873
CRF. See *Chronic renal failure (CRF).*
CRH (corticotropin-releasing hormone) stimulation, 2046t
Cricoid cartilage, 1023
Cricoid chondritis, manifestations of, 1751
Cricothyroidotomy, emergency, 2506, *2506*
Crista, in balance, 984
Critical care units (CCUs), sleep patterns in, nursing research on, 407b
Critical monitoring, after urinary diversion, 1590b
in acid-base imbalances, 337b
in adult respiratory distress syndrome, in acute pancreatitis, 1927b
in antidiuretic hormone imbalance, 2064b
in asthma, 1110b
in autonomic dysreflexia, 909, 909b
in cardiac tamponade, 1337b
in casts, 2149b
in compartment syndrome, 2140b
in esophageal bleeding, in portal hypertension, 1885, 1885b
in fluid and electrolyte imbalance, 325b
in Guillain-Barré syndrome, 878b
in hyperthyroidism, 2018b
in hypothyroidism, 2015b
in parathyroid disorders, 2031b
in percutaneous endoscopic gastrostomy/jejunostomy tube, 1731b
in postoperative brachial plexus compromise, 673b

Critical monitoring *(Continued)*
in rehydration, in diabetic ketoacidosis, 1985b
in shock, 511b
of neurologic status, 756b–757b
Critical pathways, 125
Crohn's disease, 1795
clinical manifestations of, 1797
diagnostic findings in, 1797
etiology of, 1796
management of, medical, 1798–1800, 1798t
pathophysiology of, 1796
risk factors for, 1796
ulcerative colitis vs., 1795t
Cromolyn sodium, indications for, 641
Cross-cultural nursing, 59–67, *60*
cultural diversity in, 59
cultural imposition in, 60
culture shock in, 60
ethical issues in, 66b
health/illness theories in, 60
in healthcare provision, 60–63
non-Western values in, 62–63
Western values in, 62
non-Western belief systems in, 60
nursing process in, 63–66, 63b, 64b, 65b, 66b
nursing research on, 65b
taboos/myths in, 60
uprooting in, 60
Western belief systems in, 60
Crossmatching, in blood transfusion, 1524
Cross-tolerance, definition of, 2481t
CRP (C-reactive protein), in musculoskeletal disorders, 2096t
Crust, *2185*
Crutchfield tongs, for cervical spine injury, 897, *897*
Cryoprecipitate, for disseminated intravascular coagulation, 1512
transfusion of, 1520t–1523t
Cryosurgery, for cervical cancer, 2407
for hemorrhoids, 1827
for prostate cancer, 2370
Cryotherapy, for actinic keratosis, 2225, *2226*
Cryothermia, 477
Crypt abscess, in ulcerative colitis, 1796
Cryptococcosis, 860
in acquired immunodeficiency syndrome, 628–629
Cryptorchidism, 2378, *2378*
Cryptosporidiosis, in acquired immunodeficiency syndrome, 629–630
Crystalloids, for shock, 518–519
loss of, in hypovolemic shock, management of, 522t
Crystalluria, 1559–1560
CSEA (clinically significant electrolyte abnormalities), indicators of, 296b
CSF. See *Cerebrospinal fluid (CSF).*
CSFs (colony-stimulating factors), effects of, 604t
for agranulocytosis, 1498
for cancer, 586
in wound healing, 432
CT. See *Computed tomography (CT).*

CTCL (cutaneous T-cell lymphoma), 2230
CTDs (connective tissue diseases), 653–682, 2108–2120
ocular manifestations of, 977
CTS (carpal tunnel syndrome), *927, 927–928, 928b*, 2169t
surgery for, home care after, 928b
CTZ (chemoreceptor trigger zone), 1748
Cul-de-sac, examination of, 2320
Cullen's sign, in acute pancreatitis, 1923
Cultural diversity, 59–60
Cultural imposition, 61
Cultural issues, in death and dying, 69b–71b
Cultural sensitivity, development of, 63, 63b
Culture, 59–60
assessment of, 192t–194t, 197
fungal, in integumentary disorders, 2194
in nutritional practices, 1700b–1704b
in organ donation beliefs, 2512t–2513t
in pain response, 346, 347b–349b
in women's health, 2425b–2426b
microbiologic, 244
of cervix, 2322
of ear drainage, 992–993
of nose, 1063
of stool, 1711t, 1712
of throat, 1063
of urine, 1560
in urinary tract infection, 1572–1573
Culture and sensitivity (C & S), 243
Culture shock, 60
Culture-bound syndromes, 32b–33b
Cuprimine (penicillamine), for rheumatoid arthritis, 664t
Curasorb, for burns, 2256t
Curettage, for actinic keratosis, 2225, *2226*
Curling's ulcer, 2236
Curtin model, for ethical decision-making, 43, 44t
Cushing's disease, 2049
therapy for, 2054t
Cushing's syndrome. See *Hypercortisolism.*
Cushing's triad, in consciousness disorders, 748–749, *749*
in increased intracranial pressure, 774
Cutaneous pain, 353
deep somatic pain vs., 354t
Cutaneous stimulation, in pain control, 349b, 371
Cutaneous T-cell lymphoma (CTCL), 2230
CVA. See *Cerebrovascular accident (CVA).*
CVP. See *Central venous pressure (CVP).*
Cyanide, antidote to, 2538t
Cyanosis, 2186
assessment of, in darkly pigmented patients, 2189b–2190b
Cyclic adenosine monophosphate (cAMP), hormone activation by, 1941, *1942*
Cyclocryotherapy, for glaucoma, 957
Cyclophosphamide (Cytoxan), for chronic lymphocytic leukemia, 1492
for rheumatoid arthritis, 664t
in organ transplantation, 645t
Cyclophosphamide, doxorubicin (Adriamycin), fluorouracil (CAF), for breast cancer, 2448t

Cyclophosphamide, methotrexate, fluorouracil (CMF), for breast cancer, 2448t
Cyclophosphamide, methotrexate, fluorouracil, doxorubicin [Adriamycin] (CMFA), for breast cancer, 2448t
Cyclophosphamide, methotrexate, fluorouracil, prednisone (CMFP), for breast cancer, 2448t
Cyclophosphamide, methotrexate, fluorouracil, vincristine, prednisone (CMFVP), for breast cancer, 2448t
Cyclophotocoagulation, for glaucoma, 957
Cycloplegic agents, action of, sites of, 955, *955*
Cycloserine, for tuberculosis, 1145t
Cyclosporine (Sandimmune), after heart transplantation, 1353, 1354b
for myasthenia gravis, 885
for rheumatoid arthritis, 664t
in organ transplantation, 644t
Cyproheptadine (Periactin), for hypercortisolism, 2053
Cyproterone acetate (Androcur), for benign prostatic hyperplasia, 2364t
Cyst(s), *2184*
ovarian, 2412
pilonidal, 1828
renal, *1678,* 1678–1679
Cystadenocarcinoma, of pancreas, 1931
Cystectomy, partial, for bladder cancer, 1585
radical, complications of, 1587–1588
urinary diversion with, for bladder cancer, 1585
Cystic fibrosis (CF), 1148–1149, 1932
treatment of, 1149
Cysticercosis, 861
Cystine renal calculi, 1666
Cystitis, 1571. See also *Urinary tract infections (UTIs).*
abacterial, after radiation therapy, 1584
hemorrhagic, after radiation therapy, 1584
honeymoon, 1572
interstitial. See *Interstitial cystitis (IC).*
management of, pharmacologic, 1575t–1577t
prevention of, 1573b
risk factors for, 1573b
Cystocele, 2320
in uterine prolapse, 2410, *2410*
Cystography, 1564
Cystitholapaxy, for urinary calculi, 1597
Cystolithotomy, for urinary calculi, 1597
Cystometrography, 1566
in male reproductive disorders, 2339
Cystoscopy, *1567,* 1567–1568
for renal calculi, 1668
in male reproductive disorders, 2338
Cystotomy, suprapubic, for urinary retention, 1603–1604
Cystourethrography, voiding, 1564
Cytadren (aminoglutethimide), for breast cancer, 2449, 2449t
for hypercortisolism, 2053
Cytokines, 264
effects of, 604t
in hematopoiesis, 1453–1455
in immunity, 603–604, 604t

Cytokines *(Continued)*
in wound healing, 431
Cytologic studies, 257
cervical, specimen collection for, *2321*
in cancer diagnosis, 556–558
of urine, 1561–1562
Cytology, exfoliative, in cancer diagnosis, 556–558
in gastrointestinal tract assessment, 1716–1717
in cancer diagnosis, 568
Cytolytic/cytotoxic (type II) hypersensitivity, 638t, 639
Cytomegalovirus, in acquired immunodeficiency syndrome, 630
Cytomegalovirus retinitis, 977
Cytoskeleton, 266
Cytotec (misoprostol), for acute gastritis, 1762
for peptic ulcer disease, 1768t
Cytotoxic, definition of, 2183t
Cytotoxic T cells, in cell-mediated immunity, 602, *603*
Cytoxan (cyclophosphamide), for chronic lymphocytic leukemia, 1492
for rheumatoid arthritis, 664t
in organ transplantation, 645t

D

D & C (dilatation and curettage), for menorrhagia, 2391, *2392*
D_5W, for hypernatremia, 303
Dacryocystitis, 972
Daily activities, history of, in musculoskeletal disorders, 2085
Dakin's solution, for open wounds, 445t
Danazol (Danocrine), for endometriosis, 2399
for fibrocystic breasts, 2452
Danocrine (danazol), for endometriosis, 2399
for fibrocystic breasts, 2452
Dapsone, in *Pneumocystis carinii* pneumonia prophylaxis, 625
Dark Ages, healthcare in, 20
Darvon (propoxyphene hydrochloride), administration of, 381t
in pain control, 375t
Darvon-N (propoxyphene napsylate), in pain control, 375t
DAT. See *Dementia of Alzheimer's type (DAT).*
Dawn phenomenon, 1992
Day care, adult, for elderly, 99
DBCP (dibromochloropropane), effect of, on male reproductive system, 2344
DCA (directional coronary atherectomy), clinical pathway for, 2578–2579
for coronary artery disease, 1245–1246, *1246*
DCCT (Diabetes Control and Complications Trial), 1965, 1966b
DDD (optimal sequential) pacemaker, 1320b
Dead space, anatomical, 1024
of open wound, management of, 439
Deafferentation, 354–355

Deafness. See also *Hearing loss.*
central, 994
Death, after renal transplantation, 1663
brain, criteria for, 271, 750–751
causes of, 34b
cerebrovascular accident and, 799
cultural issues in, 69b–71b
fear of, in urinary tract disorders, 1552
in emergency settings, 2510–2515
informing family of, nursing research on, 2511b
medical examiner/coroner in, 2513–2515
of cells, 270–271
religious beliefs about, 2544–2551
somatic, 270–271
Debilitation, in postoperative wound infection, 490
Debridement, autolytic, of yellow wounds, 441
enzymatic, of yellow wounds, 440
mechanical, of yellow wounds, 440, *440*
of burns, 2253–2254
of pressure ulcer, 2216
sharp, of black wounds, 439
Decabid (indecainide), for dysrhythmia, 1307t
Decadron (dexamethasone), 2048t
for rheumatoid arthritis, 664t
in pain control, 374
in surgical client, 458t
Decannulation, after partial laryngectomy, 1089, *1090*
of tracheostomy tube, 1071
accidental, 1070–1071
Decannulation stopper, 1071
Decerebrate posturing, in increased intracranial pressure, 748, *748*
in unconscious patient, 723
Decision-making, deontological, 42, 43t
ethical, guidelines for, 42–43, 42t, 43t
in chronic conditions, 118t
models of, 43–45, 44t
in confusion, nursing research on, 764b
teleological (utilitarian), 42, 42t
Decompensation, in shock, 503, *504*
Decompression, gastrointestinal intubation in, 1749
Decompressive surgery, for increased intracranial pressure, 783
Decongestants, for hypersensitivity, 641
Decorticate posturing, in increased intracranial pressure, 748, *748*
in unconscious patient, 723
Decortication, in pleural effusion, 1167
Decubitus ulcers. See *Pressure ulcers.*
Deep breathing exercises, after thyroidectomy, 2025t
preoperative teaching of, 461, *462*
Deep somatic pain, 353
cutaneous pain vs., 354t
Deep tendon (muscle-stretch) reflexes, *726*, 727, 727b
assessment of, guidelines for, 727b
in left hemiparesis, *728*
Deep vein thrombosis (DVT). See also *Venous thrombosis.*
after fracture, 2140
intertrochanteric hip, 2155

Deep vein thrombosis (DVT) *(Continued)*
after total hip replacement, prevention of, 2114
Defecation, 1696
Deferoxamine (Desferal), for anemia, 1471
Defibrillation, 1310–1313
forms of, 1312–1313
termination of, 1312
transthoracic resistance to, factors in, 1310–1311
Deformity, in fracture, 2134
in musculoskeletal disorders, 2084
Degenerative joint disease (DJD). See *Osteoarthritis (OA).*
Deglutition. See *Swallowing.*
Dehiscence, 446
postoperative, 491, *491*
nursing management of, 491
Dehydration. See also *Extracellular fluid volume deficit (ECFVD).*
and hypovolemic shock, 498–499
in acute hyperglycemia, 1984t
in diabetic ketoacidosis, 1982
in elderly, indications of, 283b
postoperative, causes of, 488
preoperative, 455
Delayed traumatic intracerebral hematoma, 831
Delayed union, in fracture, prevention of, 2145
Delegation, in fluid volume deficit, 282b
in plastic surgery aftercare, 2276b
nurse in, 125
of enteral nutrition preparation, 759b
of heat/cold application, 2165b
of ostomy appliance application, 1806b
of pressure ulcer care, 2216b
of respiratory care, 1073b
of specimen collection/testing, 244b
of stoma care, 1806b
of vital sign measurement, 234b
Delirium, 763
clinical features of, 92t
in early-morning wakening, 406
in elderly, 91
Delirium tremens (DTs), 2488
Delta-Cortef (prednisolone), 2048t
for rheumatoid arthritis, 664t
Deltasone. See *Prednisone (Deltasone, Orasone).*
Deltoids, strength of, assessment of, 2088t
Delusions, 765
Demand pacing, 1319, *1319*
Demeclocycline, for hyponatremia, 300
Dementia, 763
clinical features of, 92t
in elderly, 90–91
prevention of, 201t
sleep disorders in, 404
Dementia of Alzheimer's type (DAT), 863
clinical manifestations of, 864–865, 864b
diagnostic findings in, 864–865
etiology of, 863
management of, medical, 865, 866t
nursing, 865–872, 867b, 868b, 870b, 871t–872t
pharmacologic, 866t
pathophysiology of, 863–864, *864*

Dementia of Alzheimer's type (DAT) *(Continued)*
prevalence of, 863
risk factors for, 863
Demerol (meperidine), administration of, 381t
after thyroidectomy, 2024t
in pain control, 375t, 376
preoperative, 465t
Demineralization, bone, in chronic renal failure, 1646
Democracy, in American healthcare system, 62
Dendrites, 685–686, *686*
Denial, of cancer diagnosis, 563
Densensitization, for hypersensitivity, 641
in diabetes mellitus, 1959
Dental caries, 1719–1720, 1720b
clinical manifestations of, 1720
diagnostic findings in, 1720
etiology of, 1719
management of, 199t
community/self care in, 1720
medical, 1720
surgical, 1720
pathophysiology of, 1719–1720
prevention of, 1720b
risk factors for, 1719, 1720b
Dental disorders, 1719–1723
Dental emergencies, 1722–1723
Dental hygiene, inadequate, management of, 199t
Dental plaque, 1719
Deoxyribonucleic acid (DNA), replication of, 264–265
Depakene (valproate), side effects of, 839t
Dependence, physiologic, definition of, 2481t
psychological, definition of, 2481t
substance, definition of, 2481t
Dependent edema, in right ventricular failure, 1282
Dependent rubor, in chronic arterial occlusion, 1406
Depolarization, 293
of cardiac cells, 1195, *1195*
of nerve impulse, 688, *689*
Deprenyl (selegiline), for Parkinson's disease, 880t
Depression, after spinal cord injury, 898
in bulimia nervosa, 1769
in cancer, 541
in chronic conditions, 109
in elderly, 91
in urinary tract disorders, 1551
sleep disorders in, 404
de Quervain's tenosynovitis, 2169t
Dermabrasion, 2274
Dermatitis, acute, 2206
atopic, *2206*, 2206–2207
clinical manifestations of, 2206, *2206*
complications of, 2206
diagnostic findings in, 2206
etiology of, 2206
management of, community/self care in, 2206–2207
in elderly, 2207
medical, 2206–2207

Dermatitis *(Continued)*
  nursing, 2207
  nursing care plan in, 2208–2209
  pathophysiology of, 2206
  prevention of, 200t
  chronic, 2206
  contact, 641, 2209–2210, *2210*
  stasis, 2207–2208, *2210*
  subacute, 2206
Dermatologic nursing, principles of, 2197
Dermatology, terminology in, 2182, 2183t
Dermatomes, 353, 701–702, *702*
  definition of, 2183t
Dermatomyositis, 679
Dermatophyte, definition of, 2183t
Dermis, structure/function of, 2176, 2176t
Dermoepidermal junction, 2176
DES (diethylstilbestrol), for benign prostatic
    hyperplasia, 2364t
  in testicular cancer, 2373
  in vaginal cancer, 2416–2417
DES sons, 2373
Descending pathways, in pain modulation,
    344, *345*
  of spinal cord, structure/function of, 694–
    696, 696t
Desferal (deferoxamine), for anemia, 1471
Desipramine, therapeutic monitoring of, ref-
    erence values for, 2562
Desonide (DesOwen), topical, 2199t
DesOwen (desonide), topical, 2199t
Desoxycorticosterone acetate (DOCA),
    2048t
Desquamation, definition of, 2183t
DETERMINE, in malnutrition risk calcula-
    tion, in elderly, 86, 86b
Detoxification, definition of, 2481t
Detrusor hyperactivity with impaired blad-
    der contractility (DHIC), in urinary incon-
    tinence, in elderly, *1614*
Detrusor instability, and urinary inconti-
    nence, 1605
Development, history of, in neurologic sys-
    tem assessment, 714
Dexamethasone (Decadron), 2048t
  for rheumatoid arthritis, 664t
  in pain control, 374
  in surgical client, 458t
Dexamethasone suppression test, in hyper-
    cortisolism, 2050–2051
Dextran, administration of, for shock, 519
Dextrinase, 1692t
DFA (direct fluorescent antibody), in chla-
    mydial infection diagnosis, 2469
DHIC (detrusor hyperactivity with impaired
    bladder contractility), in urinary inconti-
    nence, in elderly, *1614*
DHT (5α-dihydrotestosterone), in benign
    prostatic hyperplasia, 2350–2351
DI. See *Diabetes insipidus (DI)*.
DiaBeta (glyburide), for diabetes mellitus,
    1967t
  in surgical client, 458t
Diabetes Control and Complications Trial
    (DCCT), 1965, 1966b
Diabetes insipidus (DI), after pituitary sur-
    gery, 844–845
  head trauma and, 825

Diabetes insipidus (DI) *(Continued)*
  risk for, 828
  monitoring for, 2064b
  syndrome of inappropriate secretion of an-
    tidiuretic hormone vs., 2066, 2067t–
    2068t
Diabetes mellitus, 1955–2001
  and male reproductive disorders, 2345
  assessment of, preoperative, 456
  clinical manifestations of, 1960–1963,
    1960t, 1961t
  complications of, acute, 1981–1992,
    1991t–1992t
    chronic, 1992–2000, 1993b
  coping tasks in, 1963–1965, 1965b
  corticosteroids in, consequences of, 2049t
  delayed wound healing in, 444
  diagnostic findings in, 1960–1963, 1962b,
    1963t, 1964t
  differential diagnosis of, 1961t
  etiology of, 1956–1957
  foot care in, home healthcare in, 1999b
  foot infection in, nursing care plan for,
    1998
  hypermagnesemia in, 325
  in coronary artery disease, 1241
  in Hispanics, 198t
  in hypercortisolism, 2052
  in Native Americans, 1957b
  incidence of, 1955–1956
  intensive therapy for, 1970
    nursing research on, 1966b
  learning/teaching guidelines in, 1971,
    1974b
  macrovascular disease in, prevention of,
    client education in, 1996b
  management of, 198t, *1958*
    community/self care in, 1963–1981,
      1964
    dietary, 1965–1967
    during traveling, 2001
    in elderly, 1980–1981
    in sickness, 2001
    medical, 1965–1970
    nursing, 1970–1980
    surgical, 1981
  monitoring of, in postanesthesia care unit,
    483
  pathophysiology of, 1957–1960
  pneumonia with, case study of, 1972–
    1973
  prevention of, 200t, 1956b
  regimen for, compliance with, ethical is-
    sues in, 1980b
  renal disorders in, 1625–1626
  risk factors for, 1956–1957, 1956b
  screening for, guidelines for, 1962b
  sexuality in, 78
  sleep disorders in, 404
  surgery in, 2000–2001
  types of, 1955, 1955b
Diabetic coma, 1981
Diabetic ketoacidosis (DKA), 1981–1987,
    1991t–1992t
  case management in, 1985b
  clinical manifestations of, 1983, 1983b,
    1984t
  clinical pathway for, 2588–2589

Diabetic ketoacidosis (DKA) *(Continued)*
  diagnostic findings in, 1983, 1983b
  etiology of, 1981–1982
  management of, emergency, 1983–1987
  pathophysiology of, *1982*, 1982–1983
  prevention of, 1986–1987
  risk factors for, 1981–1982
Diabetic nephropathy, 1625–1626, 1996–
    1999
Diabetic neuropathy, 1999–2000
Diabetic retinopathy, 964–965, *965*, 1996,
    1999b
  client education in, 1999b
  nonproliferative, 1996
  preproliferative, 1996
  proliferative, 965, *965*, 1996
Diabinese (chlorpropamide), for diabetes
    mellitus, 1967t
  in surgical client, 458t
Diagnosis-related groups (DRGs), 123
  in Medicare, 8
Diagnostic testing, 242–257
  imaging in, 248–257
  laboratory, 243–248
    blood studies in, 245–248
    cytologic studies in, 257
    in cancer, 557t–558t
    in cardiovascular disorders, 1219–1220
    in disseminated intravascular coagula-
      tion, 1511, 1512t
    in gastrointestinal disorders, 1710–1711,
      1711t
    in hemorrhage, 1467t
    in hepatobiliary disease, 1849, 1850t–
      1852t
    in human immunodeficiency virus infec-
      tion, 621, 623
    in hypertension, 1399
    in major burns, 2250–2251
    in musculoskeletal disorders, 2096,
      2096t
    in myocardial infarction, 1261, *1262*
    in pernicious anemia, 1475
    microbiologic studies in, 243–245,
      244b
    results of, reporting of, 243
    urine studies in, 248
  nursing management in, 242
    assessment in, 242
    intervention in, 242, 243b
  of gastrointestinal tract, 1710–1717,
    1711t, 1712b, *1714, 1715*
  of hematologic system, 1463–1468, 1464t,
    1465t, 1466t, 1467t
  of immune system, 611–612
  of respiratory system, 1050–1065
  of urinary tract, 1555–1570
  preoperative, 453t, 460
  sensitivity of, 243
  specificity of, 243
Dialysis, 1647–1654
  goals of, 1647–1648
  in elderly, 1660
  in renal failure, acute, 1639
    ethical issues in, 1648b
  peritoneal. See *Peritoneal dialysis*.
Dialysis equilibrium syndrome, 1654
Dialyzers, for hemodialysis, 1653

Diamox (acetazolamide), for glaucoma, client teaching about, 957t
side effects of, 839t
Diapedesis, 428, *429*
in inflammation, 594, *594*
Diaphragm, 1027
disorders of, 1168–1169
function of, 1027
paralysis of, 1168–1169
structure of, 1026–1027, *1027*
Diaphysis, 2073
Diapulse (pulsed galvanic stimulation), for wound infection, 446
Diarrhea, chemotherapy and, 583
in enteral nutrition, 1754
in gastroenteritis, 1791
in gastrointestinal disorders, 1749
in hepatic encephalopathy, 1894
in inflammatory bowel disease, 1800
drugs for, 1798–1799, 1798t
in intestinal disorders, 1788
infectious agent in, 416t
with colostomy, 1815
Diary, food, *173*
Diastasis recti, 1707
Diastole, ventricular, 1199
Diastolic filling rumbles, 1218t
Diastolic hypertension, 1387
Diastolic murmurs, 1218t
Diastolic pressure, 1202
Diazepam (Valium), for status epilepticus, 843
in pain control, 374
preoperative, 465t
side effects of, 839t
Diazoxide (Hyperstat), for hypertensive emergency, 1405t
Dibenzyline (phenoxybenzamine), for benign prostatic hyperplasia, 2364t
Dibromochloropropane (DBCP), effect of, on male reproductive system, 2344
DIC. See *Disseminated intravascular coagulation (DIC)*.
Diclofenac (Voltaren), for rheumatoid arthritis, 664t
Dicyclomine hydrochloride (Bentyl), for peptic ulcer disease, 1768t, 1770
Didronel (etidronate disodium), for hypercalcemia, 321–322, 2034t
for multiple myeloma, 1499
Diencephalon, structure/function of, 692–693
Diet, acid-ash, for urinary tract infections, 1574, 1577t
after thyroidectomy, 2024t
calorie-restriction, client education in, 1403b
change in, facilitation of, cultural beliefs in, 1703b–1705b
cultural beliefs in, 1702b–1703b
health-related beliefs about, 1700b–1701b
healthy, guidelines for, *172*
in abdominal trauma, 1830
in achalasia, 1734
in acute pancreatitis, 1925
in ascites, 1890
in breast cancer prevention, 2433
in cancer, 541, 551, *551*

Diet *(Continued)*
in cholelithiasis, 1910
in cirrhosis, 1879
in diabetes mellitus, 1965–1967
type I, 1977–1978
in dumping syndrome, 1780b
in extracellular fluid volume excess, 288, 288b
in gastroesophageal reflux disease, 1738–1739
in goiter, 2014
in hyperkalemia, 313, 313b
in hyperparathyroidism, 2033
in hyperthyroidism, 2020
in hypocalcemia, 315t, 318, 318b
in hypokalemia, 305t, 307
in hypomagnesemia, 324, 324b
in hyponatremia, 300
in inflammation management, 435
in nephrotic syndrome, 1635
in peptic ulcer disease, 1770–1771
in renal calculi, 1667
in renal failure, acute, 1640
chronic, 1655
in viral hepatitis, 1867
iron-rich, for anemia, 1471
irregular, management of, 200t
low protein, in hepatic encephalopathy, 1893
low sodium, client education in, 1400b–1401b
for heart failure, 1286, 1286t
low-fat low-cholesterol, client education in, 1402b
religious beliefs in, 1701b–1702b, 2544–2551
stone prevention, 1597
with ileostomy, 1806–1807
Dietary fiber, for gastrointestinal symptoms, nursing research on, 1825b
Diethylstilbestrol (DES), for benign prostatic hyperplasia, 2364t
in testicular cancer, 2373
in vaginal cancer, 2416–2417
Difenoxin (Motofen), for diarrhea, in inflammatory bowel disease, 1798t
Differential count, in inflammation management, 435, 436t
Differentiation, of cells, 545
Diffuse axonal injury, 823
Diffuse esophageal spasm, 1737
Diffusion, cell membrane in, 263
in dialysis, 1647
Diflorasone (Psorcon), topical, 2199t
Digestants, for pernicious anemia, 1476
Digestion, gastrointestinal tract in, 1685
stomach in, 1689
Digestive enzymes, 1692t
Digestive hormones, 1691t
Digit span, 195
Digital rectal examination, in prostate cancer, 2366
Digital venous angiography, 736–737
Digitalis, for heart failure, 1283–1284, 1284t
for shock, 521
Digitalis toxicity, 1283–1284, 1284t
in elderly, with hypokalemia, 309–310

Digitalis toxicity *(Continued)*
prevention of, 1284b
risk for, in heart failure, 1288
Digitoxin, properties of, 1283t
therapeutic monitoring of, reference values for, 2562
Dignity, client, protection of, ethical issues in, 467b
Digoxin, for dysrhythmia, 1308t
properties of, 1283t
therapeutic monitoring of, reference values for, 2562
Dihydropyridines, 1396t
Dihydrotachysterol (Hytakerol), for hypoparathyroidism, 2037
5α-Dihydrotestosterone (DHT), in benign prostatic hyperplasia, 2350–2351
1,25-Dihydroxycholecalciferol, synthesis of, kidneys in, 1543
Dilantin. See *Phenytoin (Dilantin)*.
Dilatation and curettage (D & C), for menorrhagia, 2391, *2392*
Dilated cardiomyopathy, 1338, *1338,* 1339–1340, 1340t
clinical manifestations of, 1339
diagnostic findings in, 1339, 1340t
etiology of, 1339
management of, 1339–1340
pathophysiology of, 1339
risk factors for, 1339
Dilators, for urinary retention, 1601
Dilaudid (hydromorphone), administration of, 380t
Diltiazem (Cardizem), 1396t
for angina pectoris, 1256t
Dilution, of urine, 1561
in fluid and electrolyte balance, 1542
Dinitrochlorobenzene (DNCB) skin test, in cancer diagnosis, 559
Diphenhydramine (Benadryl), for Parkinson's disease, 880t
for shock, 520
in pain control, 374
Diphenoxylate (Lomotil), for diarrhea, in inflammatory bowel disease, 1798, 1798t
Diphtheria, 1081–1082
immunization recommendations for, in adults, 422t
Diplaucisis, 994
Diplopia, 720
in myasthenia gravis, 884
Diprosone (betamethasone), topical, 2199t
Dipyridamole, for angina pectoris, 1257t
Dipyridamole thallium 201 test, 1230
Direct antiglobulin test, in hematologic system assessment, 1464–1465
Direct care, provision of, hospital nurse in, 123
Direct fluorescent antibody (DFA), in chlamydial infection diagnosis, 2469
Direct inguinal hernia, 1817, *1817*
Direct ophthalmoscopy, *948,* 948–949
Direct visualization, in cancer diagnosis, 559
Directional coronary atherectomy (DCA), clinical pathway for, 2578–2579
for coronary artery disease, 1245–1246, *1246*

Disabled patient, health-promotion activities in, 108b

Disc herniation. See *Intervertebral disc herniation.*

Discectomy, for intervertebral disc herniation, 920–921
  lumbar, physical mobility after, 923

Discharge, from postanesthesia care unit, 484
  planning for, postoperative, 492
    preoperative, 459
  premature, prevention of, ethical issues in, 1589b

Discharge instructions, after total hip replacement, 2116b
  for emergency patient, 2507–2508

Disciples of God, beliefs/practices of, 2546

Discography, in intervertebral disc herniation, 919

Discoid, definition of, 2183t

Discomfort, signs of, assessment of, 234

Disconnection syndrome, 841

Discrimination, assessment of, 724, *725*

Disease. See *Illness.*

Disease-modifying antirheumatic drugs (DMARDs), 662, 665

Dislocation(s), 2164
  of hip, after intertrochanteric hip fracture, 2157–2158
  of spinal cord, 890

Disopyramide (Norpace), for dysrhythmia, 1307t
  therapeutic monitoring of, reference values for, 2562

Disorientation, in consciousness disorders, 746

Displaced fracture, *2130*, 2131

Dissecting aneurysm, 1425, *1425*
  aortic, chest pain in, assessment of, 1208t

Disseminated intravascular coagulation (DIC), 1510–1512, *1511*
  clinical manifestations of, 1510–1511
  diagnostic findings in, 1510–1511, 1512t
  etiology of, 1510
  in shock, 506–507
  management of, medical, 1511–1512
    nursing, 1512
  pathophysiology of, 1510
  risk factors for, 1510, 1510b

Distraction, in pain control, 349b, 366

Distress, signs of, assessment of, 234

Distributive shock, clinical manifestations of, 512–513
  etiology of, 497, 500
  management of, 524t
  prevention of, 501b
  risk factors for, 500

Disulfiram (Antabuse), education about, 2496b

Disuse syndrome, adaptive changes in, 109t

Ditropan (oxybutynin chloride), for urinary incontinence, 1611t
  for urinary tract infections, 1576t

Diucardin (hydroflumethiazide), 1394t

Diuresis, solute, 1554
  water, 1554

Diuretics, 1394t
  for ascites, 1890

Diuretics *(Continued)*
  for extracellular fluid volume excess, 287–288
  for heart failure, 1285, 1285t
  for hypercalcemia, 321
  for hypertension, 1393
  for nephrotic syndrome, 1635
  for renal failure, acute, 1639
    chronic, 1654
  ototoxic, 986b
  thiazide, intraoperative complications of, 457
  urine color with, 1557t

Diuril (chlorothiazide), 1394t
  characteristics of, 1285t

Diversion, in pain management, 366

Diversional activity deficit, in fracture, 2144

Diverticular disease, 1818–1819
  clinical manifestations of, 1818–1819
  diagnostic findings in, 1818–1819
  etiology of, 1818
  management of, medical, 1819
    nursing, 1819
    surgical, 1819
  pathophysiology of, 1818
  prevention of, 1819b
  risk factors for, 1818, 1819b

Diverticulitis. See *Diverticular disease.*

Diverticulosis. See *Diverticular disease.*

Diverticulum(a), bladder, and urinary retention, 1601
  esophageal, 1741–1743
    clinical manifestations of, 1742
    diagnostic findings in, 1742
    etiology of, 1741
    management of, in elderly, 1743
      medical, 1742
      nursing, 1742
      surgical, 1742
        nursing care in, 1742–1743
    pathophysiology of, 1741
    risk factors for, 1741
  Meckel's, 1819–1820
  pulsion, 1741
  traction, 1741

Dizziness, 1010–1016. See also *Vertigo.*
  brain tumor and, 846
  in diabetes mellitus, 1960t
  in transient ischemic attacks, 1011

DJD (degenerative joint disease). See *Osteoarthritis (OA).*

DKA. See *Diabetic ketoacidosis (DKA).*

DMARDs (disease-modifying antirheumatic drugs), 662, 665

DNA (deoxyribonucleic acid), replication of, 264–265

DNCB (dinitrochlorobenzene) skin test, in cancer diagnosis, 559

"Do not resuscitate" (DNR) clients, nursing role in, ethical issues in, 1244b
  surgery in, ethical issues in, 460b

Dobhoff tube, 1749t, *1750*

Dobutamine, for heart failure, 1284

DOCA (desoxycorticosterone acetate), 2048t

Documentation, in plastic surgery, photography in, 2270
  of emergency nursing care, 2504–2505

Documentation *(Continued)*
  of postanesthesia care unit observations, 481–482

Doll's eye reflex, in consciousness disorders, 749, *750*

Dolophine (methadone), administration of, 381t
  in pain control, 376

Domestic violence, 2539
  history of, in gynecologic disorders, 2310

Donor tissue, rejection of, in liver transplantation, 1901

Donovanosis, 2475

DOO (AV sequential fixed-rate) pacemaker, 1320b

Dopamine, for heart failure, 1284
  in Parkinson's disease, 878

Doppler probe, in blood pressure monitoring, in shock, 525

Doppler scanning, of cerebrovascular system, 733

Doppler ultrasonography, in free flap assessment, 2280
  in peripheral vascular assessment, 1383, *1383*
  of cerebrovascular system, 733

Dorsal column spinal cord stimulation, in pain control, 389–391
  percutaneous epidural, 389

Dorsal horn, in pain modulation, 344, *345*

Dorsal recumbent (supine) position, for physical examination, *232*
  intraoperative, 477, *478*

Double vision, 720

Double-balloon Foley urethral catheter, 2355t

Double-barreled colostomy, *1811*, 1812

Doubling time, in cancer cell growth, 545, *546*

Doxazosin (Cardura), 1395t

Doxepin, for dementia of Alzheimer's type, 866t

Doxorubicin (Adriamycin), cyclophosphamide (AC), for breast cancer, 2448t

Doxorubicin (Adriamycin), mitomycin (AM), for breast cancer, 2448t

Doxycycline, for chlamydial infection, 2470

Drain(s), Jackson-Pratt, in craniotomy, 849, *849*
  postoperative, preoperative preparation for, 463
  wound, after prostatectomy, 2362

Drainage, biliary, analysis of, 1856
  chest, assessment of, after cardiac surgery, 1358–1359
    after lung cancer surgery, 1163
    closed. See *Closed chest drainage.*
  duodenal, analysis of, 1856
  ear, culture of, 992–993
    history of, 985
  intraoperative, assessment of, 479–480
  of surgical wound, 437
  of T tube, after choledochostomy, 1919–1920, *1920*

Draping, in client preparation, for physical examination, 231

Drawer test, 2091t, *2092*

Dress, assessment of, 235

Dressings, choice of, for open wounds, 442
for burns, 2254–2255, *2255*
temporary, 2255, 2256t–2257t
for tracheostomy, 1074, *1075*
occlusive, 2201t
topical, 2199t
wet-to-dry, in mechanical wound debridement, 440, *440*
wet-to-moist, in mechanical wound debridement, 440
wound, 2201–2202, 2201t
Dressler's syndrome, after myocardial infarction, 1267
DRGs (diagnosis-related groups), 123
in Medicare, 8
Drip pad, after sinus surgery, 1078, *1079*
Drop arm test, 2090t
"Drop attacks," 838
Droperidol (Inapsine), preoperative, 465t
Droplet precautions, 424
Drug(s), effect of, on male reproductive system, 2344–2345
injected, in human immunodeficiency virus infection transmission, 615
lupus-inducing, 675b
metabolism of, cultural differences in, 94b–95b
monitoring of, therapeutic, reference values for, 2562
ototoxic, 986b
Drug abuse. See *Substance abuse.*
Drug and alcohol history, components of, 2486b
Drug misuse, definition of, 2481t
Drug resistance, to antiretrovirals, 624
Drug-induced parkinsonism, 878
Drug-induced ulcers, 1764, *1764*
Drusen, 965
Dry eye syndrome, 974–975
Dry skin, after burn injury, 2263b
in elderly, 2178
DTs (delirium tremens), 2488
Dual diagnosis, definition of, 2481t
Dual-energy x-ray absorptiometry (DXA), in osteoporosis, 2100, *2101*
of musculoskeletal system, 2093–2094
Duchenne's muscular dystrophy, 2125t
Duct cell adenocarcinoma, of pancreas, 1931
Duct ectasia, 2452
Ductal carcinoma in situ, 2434
Ductal hyperplasia, 2452
Ductography, 2328
Duke's classification system, of cancer, 560
of colon, 1810
Dullness, in percussion, 230
of chest, 1045, *1046*
Dumping syndrome, after peptic ulcer surgery, 1779, 1780b
diet for, client education in, 1780b
management of, 1779
Dunn's wellness theory, 162
Duodenal drainage, analysis of, 1856
Duodenal ulcers, 1764
clinical manifestations of, 1766
pathophysiology of, 1765
sleep disorders in, 405

Duodenum, structure of, 1690
DuoDerm (hydrocolloid gel), 2199t
indications for, 443t
Duplicate ureters, 1621
Dupuytren's contracture, 928, 2124
release of, 928
Dura mater, *697,* 697–698
Durable power of attorney, for healthcare, elderly issues in, 102
in terminal cancer, 567
Duration, in auscultation, 231
Duromedics bileaflet valve, *1352*
"Dust diseases," 1150
DVI (AV sequential) pacemaker, 1320b
DVT (deep vein thrombosis). See also *Venous thrombosis.*
after fracture, 2140
intertrochanteric hip, 2155
after total hip replacement, prevention of, 2114
DXA (dual-energy x-ray absorptiometry), in osteoporosis, 2100, *2101*
of musculoskeletal system, 2093–2094
Dying, awareness of, 69b
cultural issues in, 69b–71b
in emergency settings, 2510–2515
stages of, 73
DynaCirc (isradipine), 1396t
Dyrenium (triamterene), 1394t
characteristics of, 1285t
urine color with, 1557t
Dysarthria, assessment of, 710t
cerebrovascular accident and, 789
Dysconjugate gaze, 720, 747
Dysentery, 1788–1790
prevention of, 1789b
risk factors for, 1789b
sexually transmitted, 2475
Dysesthesia, 724
Dysmenorrhea, 2386–2389
clinical manifestations of, 2387
diagnostic findings in, 2387
etiology of, 2387
management of, community/self care in, 2387
medical, 2387
nursing, 2387
pathophysiology of, 2387
risk factors for, 2387
Dyspepsia, 1733
in gastrointestinal disorders, 1749
Dysphagia, 1732, *1733*
after cerebrovascular accident, 789
feeding in, 804–805, 804b
home management of, 804b
in elderly client, with fluid volume deficit, 283–284
in esophageal cancer, 1744
in Huntington's disease, 883
progressive feeding program for, 796t
Dysphonia, assessment of, 711t
Dysplasia, 267, *267*
definition of, 534t
Dyspnea, assessment of, 1035–1036, *1036,* 1037t
exertional, assessment of, 1206
in asthma, nursing research on, 1108b
in left ventricular failure, 1281

Dyspnea *(Continued)*
nocturnal, paroxysmal, assessment of, 1206
Dysreflexia, autonomic, after spinal cord injury, 894–895, 909, 909b
critical monitoring in, 909, 909b
Dysrhythmia(s), 1295–1325
after myocardial infarction, 1266
and heart failure, 1278
atrial, 1297–1302, *1299, 1300*
atrioventricular junctional, *1302,* 1302–1304, *1303*
clinical manifestations of, 1297
diagnostic findings in, 1297, 1298b
endotracheal tube suctioning and, 1175t
etiology of, 1295–1297
head trauma and, 826
in cardiogenic shock, management of, 523t
in eating disorders, 1761
in hyperkalemia, 314
in postanesthesia care unit, 483
life-threatening, management of, 1310–1324
community/self care in, 1323–1324
emergency, 1310–1314
medical, 1314
nursing, 1321–1323
surgical, 1314–1320
management of, 1297–1310
medications for, 1307t–1308t
prevention of, 1296b
risk factors for, 1295–1297, 1296b
sinus, 1299
ventricular, 1304–1310, *1306, 1309*
Dyssomnias, 400–403, 402b
circadian rhythm, 403
classification of, 398b
extrinsic, 402–403
intrinsic, 400–402, 402b
Dystonia, 723b

E

Ear(s), assessment of, 984–993
diagnostic tests in, 989–993, *992, 993*
history in, 985–987, 985b, 986b
in health history, 183b
in regional examination, 215t
physical examination in, *987,* 987–989, *988*
disorders of, 980–1016
donation of, guidelines for, 2514t
external, function of, 981–982, *982*
physical examination of, 987
structure of, 980–981, *981*
in hematologic disorders, 1463
infection of, 1003–1006, *1004, 1005*
client education in, 1008b
inner, function of, 984, 984b, 984t
injury to, skull fracture and, 823
structure of, *983,* 983–984
irrigation of, for otitis externa, 1005, *1005*
masses of, 1009–1010
middle, function of, 983
prostheses for, 1008, *1008*
structure of, *981,* 982–983
obstruction of, 1006–1007

Ear(s) *(Continued)*
surgery of, precautions after, 1009b
trauma to, 1007
Ear canal, physical examination of, *987,*
987–988, 988
structure of, 981, *981*
Ear wax, 981
impaction of, 1006–1007
production of, external ear in, 982
Earache, 1003
Eardrum. See *Tympanic membrane.*
Early-morning urine specimen, 1555
Early-morning wakening, hospital-acquired,
406
Earplugs, 986
Eastern Cooperative Oncology Group
(ECOG), cancer performance status scale
of, 560, 560t
Eastern Orthodox, beliefs/practices of, 2546
Eating, assessment of, 711t
Eating disorders, 1756–1761
nursing management of, 1760–1761
Eaton-Lambert syndrome, 886
ECC (extracorporeal circulation), during
open heart surgery, 1354–1355, *1355*
ECCE (extracapsular cataract extraction),
959, 959–960
Ecchymoses, biocultural variations in,
2190b
in fracture, 2134
Eccrine glands, 2175, 2176t
ECF (extracellular fluid), 273
electrolyte distribution in, 293t
volume of, shifting of, 289–291, 290b
ECF-A (eosinophil chemotactic factor of
anaphylaxis), 638t
ECFVD. See *Extracellular fluid volume deficit (ECFVD).*
ECFVE. See *Extracellular fluid volume excess (ECFVE).*
ECG. See *Electrocardiography (ECG).*
Echocardiography. See also *Ultrasonography.*
in cardiomyopathy, 1340t
in cardiovascular assessment, 1228, *1229*
in myocardial infarction, 1262
transesophageal, in cardiovascular assessment, 1228–1229
in myocardial infarction, 1262
ECMO (extracorporeal membrane oxygenation), for open heart surgery, 1355
for shock, 516
in heart failure, 1289–1290
ECOG (Eastern Cooperative Oncology
Group), cancer performance status scale
of, 560, 560t
Ectopic ACTH syndrome, 2049, 2051
therapy for, 2054t
Ectopic pacemakers, 1296
Ectopic ureter, 1620–1621
Ectropion, 944, 974
cicatricial, 974
Eczema, prevention of, 200t
xerotic, 2207
Eczematous, definition of, 2183t
Eczematous disorders, 2205–2206
Edecrin (ethacrynic acid), 1394t
characteristics of, 1285t

Edema, after burn injury, 2235, *2235*
assessment of, in cardiovascular disorders,
1212
in extracellular fluid volume excess, 288
brawny, 1380
cerebral, head trauma and, 825
control of, in cerebrovascular accident,
793
in inflammation management, 436
dependent, in right ventricular failure,
1282
formation of, mechanisms of, 286, *286*
inspection of, in peripheral vascular assessment, 1380, *1381*
of brain, 774
of lower leg, in cirrhosis, 1878t
of scrotum, 2381
of skin, assessment of, 2192
of spinal cord, 891
pitting, 1380
pulmonary. See *Pulmonary edema.*
Edrophonium (Tensilon), in myasthenia
gravis diagnosis, 884–885
Education. See also *Teaching.*
assessment of, culture in, 194t
in cross-cultural nursing, 64b
client. See *Client education.*
continuing, ambulatory care nurse in,
141b, 142–143
family, 54
about chemotherapy, 584, 584b
for home healthcare, 150
hearing, 998
hospital nurse in, 123–124
in burns, 2242, 2260, 2261
in Wallingford Wellness Project, 175
of elderly, 83
Educational materials, use of, ethical issues
in, 2060b
EEG. See *Electroencephalography (EEG).*
Effectors, 686
Efudex (5-fluorouracil), topical, 2198t
for actinic keratosis, 2225
EGD (esophagogastroduodenoscopy), 256
EGF (epidermal growth factor), in wound
healing, 431
Egophony, 1046
EGTA (esophageal gastric tube airway),
2506
Egyptians, ancient, healthcare beliefs of, 18
EIA (enzyme immunoassay), 1952
in human immunodeficiency virus infec-
tion, 622
Einthoven's triangle, *1224*
Ejaculation, retrograde, after benign pros-
tatic hyperplasia surgery, 2359–2360
after prostatectomy, 2363
Ejection clicks, 1216
Elapid bites, 2536
Elase (fibrinolysin-desoxyribonuclease), for
enzymatic debridement, 440
Elastic arteries, 1369, *1370*
Elastin, structure/function of, 2176t
Elastogel, indications for, 443t
Elavil (amitriptyline), in pain control, 374
therapeutic monitoring of, reference values
for, 2562
urine color with, 1557t

Elbow, function of, assessment of, 2090t
range of motion of, *2089*
repetitive motion injuries of, 2169t
tennis, 2162, 2169t
Elbow arthroplasty, for rheumatoid arthritis,
674
Elbow breadth method, of body frame calculation, 239b
Elderly, *82,* 82–83, *83*
achalasia in, 1737
acid-base imbalance in, prevention of,
336–337
acquired immunodeficiency syndrome in,
635–636
acute glomerulonephritis in, 1632
acute pancreatitis in, 1929
acute renal failure in, 1641
Addison's disease in, 2047
assessment of, preoperative, 454, 454t
atopic dermatitis in, 2207
bladder cancer in, 1594–1595
breast cancer in, 2450
cardiac surgery in, 926
care of, nursing home vs. in-home, 84
cerebrovascular accident in, 807
cervical cancer in, 2409
cholelithiasis in, 1915
chronic arterial occlusion in, 1412
chronic obstructive pulmonary disease in,
1123
confusion in, 769–770
consciousness disorders in, 763
coronary artery disease in, surgery in,
1248–1249
definitions of, 83
dehydration in, indications of, 283b
delayed wound healing in, 444
demographics of, 82
diabetes mellitus in, 1980–1981
dialysis in, 1660
economic concerns in, 82–83
educational issues in, 83
epilepsy in, 840
esophageal diverticula in, 1743
ethical/legal issues in, 100–102, 101b
ethnicity among, 82
extracellular fluid volume deficit in, 283–
284, 283b
extracellular fluid volume excess in, 289
family support of, 83–84
functional status of, 86–90
physiologic factors in, 87–88
psychological factors in, *88,* 88–90, 89b,
90b
glaucoma in, 956
government support of, 93–94
head trauma in, 828
health promotion in, 84–86, *85,* 85b, 86b,
173–175, 174b, 174t, 175b
nursing research on, 85b
resources for, 175b
healthcare for, 94–96
acute, resources/services in, 96
adult day care in, 99
case management in, 98–99
community programs/services in, 99–
100
economic issues in, 84

Elderly *(Continued)*
long-term, resources/services in, 97, 97t
resources/services in, 96–99, 96b, 97t
hearing impairment in, quality of life with, nursing research on, 1000b
heart failure in, 1291
hepatobiliary examination in, 1847t, 1848
hereditary spherocytosis in, 1485
housing options for, 98t, 100
hypercortisolism in, 2055
hyperkalemia in, 314
hyperparathyroidism in, 2035–2036
hypertension in, 1404
hyperthyroidism in, 2022
hypocalcemia in, 319
hypokalemia in, 309–310
digitalis toxicity with, 309–310
hyponatremia in, 300
hypophosphatemia in, 319
hypothyroidism in, 2016
idiopathic thrombocytopenic purpura in, 1508
immune function in, 604–605
infections in, 420b
inflammatory bowel disease in, 1808
integumentary system changes in, 2178
iron-deficiency anemia in, 1474
leukemia in, 1495
marital status of, 82
medication use in, 92–93
mental health disorders in, 90–92, 92t
treatment of, 91
neurogenic bladder dysfunction in, 1619
pain in, management of, 391–392, 392t
misconceptions about, 391, 392t
response to, 346–350
periodontal disease in, 1722
pheochromocytoma in, 2060
plastic surgery in, 2288
prostate cancer in, 2372
pyelonephritis in, 1630
renal transplantation in, 1665
rheumatoid arthritis in, management of, 671–672
surgical, 674
sleep in, disorders of, progressive relaxation for, nursing research on, 409b
patterns of, 400
spinal cord injury in, 914
substance abuse in, 91–92
trends among, 82, *82*
urinary incontinence in, 1612, *1613–1615*
urinary retention in, 1604
urinary tract infections in, 1578, 1579
viral hepatitis in, 1871
vulvar cancer in, 2422
Electrical burns, 2233
injury mechanism in, 2241
Electrical injury, of cells, 269
Electrical stimulation, for fracture nonunion, 2146
for urinary incontinence, *1607,* 1607–1608
for wound infection, 446
in pain control, 389–391, 389b, 390t
Electrocardiography (ECG), after cardiac surgery, 1358
continuous, *1221,* 1221–1222

Electrocardiography (ECG) *(Continued)*
electrode attachment in, 1221, *1221*
exercise, 1225–1227, 1226b, 1227b
contraindications to, 1226, 1227b
in angina pectoris, 1254
in angina pectoris, 1254
in cardiomyopathy, 1340t
in cardiovascular assessment, 1220–1226
in dysrhythmia assessment, 1298b
in myocardial infarction, 1260, *1261*
in potassium imbalances, 305–306, *308, 311*
of paced beats, 1321
preoperative, 453t
schedule for, 209t
signal-averaged, 1224
tracings of, *1222,* 1222–1223
twelve-lead, 1223–1224, 1223b, *1224, 1225t*
in coronary pathology identification, 1223, 1225t
indications for, 1223, 1223b
lead placement for, 1223, *1224*
Electrocoagulation, multipolar, for bleeding ulcers, 1772
Electrodes, attachment of, in continuous electrocardiography, 1221, *1221*
of pacemaker, 1316, *1316*
Electrodesiccation, for actinic keratosis, 2225, *2226*
Electroencephalography (EEG), during sleep, 399, *399*
in consciousness disorders, 749
in epilepsy diagnosis, 838
in neurologic assessment, *738,* 738–739, *739*
procedure for, 738–739, *739*
wave patterns of, 738, *738*
Electrolarynx, *1092,* 1093
Electrolyte(s), 293–325. See also names of specific electrolytes.
action potentials of, 293–294, *294, 295*
administration of, for hyperglycemic, hyperosmolar, nonketotic coma, 1987–1988
balance of. See *Fluid and electrolyte balance.*
concentration of, 293, *294,* 294t
distribution of, 293, 293t
imbalances of, 295–325
in acute hyperglycemia, 1984t
in acute pancreatitis, 1926
in chronic renal failure, 1644
in diabetic ketoacidosis, 1983
postoperative, causes of, 488
preoperative, 455
in fixed acid regulation, 330–331
measurement of, 294–295
monitoring of, after thyroidectomy, 2025t
plasma, ranges for, 296b
replacement of, for acute renal failure, 1639–1640
serum, in cardiovascular assessment, 1220
studies of, need for, nursing research on, 296b
Electromagnetic radiation, low-level exposure to, health risks of, 204t

Electromechanical infusion devices, for blood transfusion, 1526
Electromyography (EMG), in male reproductive disorders, 2339
in musculoskeletal disorders, 2096
in neurologic assessment, 740, *741*
in urinary tract disorders, 1566
Electroneutrality, principle of, 330
Electronystagmography (ENG), 991
Electrophoresis, hemoglobin, in sickle cell anemia, 1514
Electrophysiologic studies, in cardiovascular assessment, 1227
Electroretinography (ERG), 951
Elevation pallor, in peripheral vascular assessment, 1380
Elimination, pattern of, 206
postoperative, promotion of, 490
ELISA (enzyme-linked immunosorbent assay), in acquired immunodeficiency syndrome testing, 611
in chlamydial infection diagnosis, 2469
Elocon (mometasone), topical, 2199t
Emaciation, in cirrhosis, 1878t
Embolectomy, for pulmonary embolism, 1129
Embolism, after abdominal aortic aneurysm repair, 1427
and cerebrovascular accident, 785, *785*
clinical manifestations of, 787t
supportive care for, 797
arterial, arterial thrombosis vs., 1424
fat, fractures and, 2140
pulmonary embolism vs., 2141t
pulmonary. See *Pulmonary embolism (PE).*
Embolization, arterial, for bleeding ulcer, 1772
in infective endocarditis, 1332, *1333*
Emergency care, 2501–2515
death/dying in, 2510–2515
ethical/legal considerations in, 2501–2503, 2502b
nursing, 2503–2510
discharge teaching in, 2507–2508
documentation of, 2504–2505
initial assessment in, 2503, 2503b
interventions in, 2505–2507
psychosocial needs in, 2508–2510, 2509b, 2510b
secondary assessment in, 2507, *2508*
triage in, 2504, 2504b, 2504t
Emergency response systems (ERSs), for elderly, 99–100
EMG (electromyography), in male reproductive disorders, 2339
in musculoskeletal disorders, 2096
in neurologic assessment, 740, *741*
in urinary tract disorders, 1566
Emla cream, in pain control, 372
Emollients, 2199t, 2202
Emotional lability, cerebrovascular accident and, 792
Emotional support, in burns, 2261
postoperative, provision of, 492
Emphysema, and male reproductive disorders, 2345

Emphysema (Continued)
clinical manifestations of, 1114–1115, 1117, 1118b, 1118t
pathophysiology of, 1113–1114, 1114
sleep disorders in, 405
subcutaneous, after thoracic surgery, monitoring for, 1159
tracheostomy tube in, 1071
types of, 1114, 1114
Employment, in epilepsy, 842
of cancer survivors, 566
Empyema, 1167
Enalapril (Vasotec), 1396t
Enalaprilat (Vasotec IV), for hypertensive emergency, 1405t
Encainide (Enkaid), for dysrhythmia, 1307t
Encephalitis, arbovirus, 859
herpes simplex virus, 859–860
viral, 859–860
clinical manifestations of, 859
Encephalopathy, hepatic. See Hepatic encephalopathy.
HIV, 631
in cirrhosis, 1878t
systemic, portal, in bleeding esophageal varices, 1886–1887
End colostomy, 1812
care of, 1814–1815
Endarterectomy, carotid, complications of, 811
for transient ischemic attacks, 810–811, 811
nursing care in, 811–812
outcomes in, 810
Endocardial pacing, 1316, 1318
Endocarditis, bacterial, acute, 1331
subacute, 1331
infective, 1331–1334
client education in, 1334b
clinical manifestations of, 1332–1333
diagnostic findings in, 1332–1333
etiology of, 1331
management of, community/self care in, 1334
medical, 1333–1334
nursing, 1334, 1334b
pathophysiology of, 1331–1332, 1332, 1333
prevention of, 1332b
risk factors for, 1331, 1332b
native valve, 1331
prosthetic valve, 1331
rheumatic, 1328t
thrombotic, nonbacterial, 1331
Endocardium, 1191, 1192
rheumatic fever effects on, 1328t
Endocrine system, age-related changes in, 1946
assessment of, in health history, 183b
preoperative, 456
disorders of, and male reproductive disorders, 2345
assessment of, 1948–1954
diagnostic tests in, 1952–1954
history in, 1948–1950
physical examination in, 1950–1952, 1952, 1952b
ocular manifestations of, 976, 976–977

Endocrine system (Continued)
in alcohol abuse, 2490t
in chronic renal failure, 1646
in thyroid disorders, 2008t
structure/function of, 1937–1946, 1938
Endocytosis, 263
Endolarynx, 1023
Endolymph, 984
Endolymphatic sac surgery, for vertigo, 1015
Endometrial biopsy, 2323
Endometrial cancer, 2404–2406
clinical manifestations of, 2405–2406
diagnostic findings in, 2405, 2405–2406
etiology of, 2404
management of, 2406
pathophysiology of, 2405
prevention of, 2404b
risk factors for, 542b, 2404, 2404b
staging of, 2405, 2405
Endometrial smear, 2323, 2324
Endometriosis, 2398–2400
clinical manifestations of, 2398–2399
diagnostic findings in, 2398–2399
etiology of, 2398
management of, community/self care in, 2399–2400
medical, 2399
nursing, 2400
surgical, 2399–2400
pathophysiology of, 2398, 2399
risk factors for, 2398
Endometrium, 2296
Endophthalmitis, 970
Endoplasmic reticulum, 265–266
rough, 265
smooth, 265–266
Endorphins, 345
Endoscopic retrograde cholangiography (ERCP), 1853
Endoscopic thoracotomy, 1062
Endoscopy, 255
gastrointestinal, 256–257
procedure for, 256, 256
in cancer diagnosis, 559
in cholelithiasis, 1910
in gastrointestinal tract assessment, 1714–1716, 1715
in laryngeal cancer diagnosis, 1084
vascular, in peripheral vascular assessment, 1386
Endosteum, 2073
Endothelium, age-related changes in, 940
Endotoxins, 270
Endotracheal tube(s), 1173–1176
communication with, 1175
cuff of, caring for, 1174
leaks from, management of, 1174
for continuous mechanical ventilation, removal of, 1184
insertion of, 1173, 1173
oral hygiene in, 1175–1176
placement of, confirmation of, 1173
for inhalation anesthesia, 471, 471
securing of, 1173, 1174
suctioning of, 1174–1175, 1175t, 1176b
complications of, 1175t

Endourologic procedures, for renal calculi, 1668, 1668–1669, 1669
for urinary calculi, 1597
Endovascular interventions, for chronic arterial occlusion, 1412–1414
End-tidal carbon dioxide (ETCO$_2$), 1055
Enduron (methyclothiazide), 1394t
Enema, after spinal cord injury, 908
barium, 251, 1713–1714
preoperative, 463
Enflurane (Ethrane), 470t
ENG (electronystagmography), 991
Engagement, in therapeutic family communication, 58
Engineering, genetic, 265
Enkaid (encainide), for dysrhythmia, 1307t
Enkephalins, 345
Enteral nutrition, 1752–1754
administration of, methods of, 1752–1753
after intracranial surgery, 854
complications of, 1752, 1753
in unconscious patient, 760
formulas for, 1752
nursing management of, 1753–1754
preoperative, 454
preparation of, delegation of, 759b
routes of, 1752
Enteritis, regional. See Crohn's disease.
Enterocele, in uterine prolapse, 2410
Enterogastrone, 1691t
Enterokinase, 1692t
secretion of, 1693
Entropion, 944, 974
Enucleation, for ocular melanoma, 970–971
Enuresis, 1551, 1604t
risk factors for, 1606b
sleep, 403
Environment, in allergies, control of, 641, 642
in coronary artery disease, 1238–1239
in endocrine disorders, 1950
in gynecologic disorders, 2310
in hematologic disorders, 1462
in hepatobiliary disorders, 1844
in illness, 36
in immune disorders, 608–609
in infection, 414–415
in male reproductive disorders, 2331
in respiratory disorders, 1039
in urinary tract disorders, 1550
preparation of, for health history interview, 185–186
for physical examination, 231
protection of, in health promotion, 169–170
structuring of, in sensory disorder prevention, 410
Environmental agents, effect of, on male reproductive system, 2344
Environmental incontinence, 1604t
risk factors for, 1606b
Envisan, indications for, 443t
Enzymatic wound debridement, 440
of burns, 2253
Enzyme immunoassay (EIA), 1952
in human immunodeficiency virus infection, 622

Enzyme-linked immunosorbent assay (ELISA), in acquired immunodeficiency syndrome testing, 611
in chlamydial infection diagnosis, 2469
Enzymes, cardiac, in cardiovascular assessment, 1219
digestive, 1692t
lysosomal, release of, in shock, 507
muscle, tests of, 2096t
pancreatic, 1922b
serum, laboratory tests for, 1851t
EOA (esophageal obturator airway), 2506, *2506*
Eosinophil chemotactic factor of anaphylaxis (ECF-A), 638t
Eosinophils, functions of, 1448t
in blood dyscrasias, 1465t
in differential count, interpretation of, 436t
in hematopoiesis, 1451
in wound healing, 429
reference values for, in cancer, 557t
Ependymal cells, 687, *688*
Ependymoma, 844, *846*
Epicardial pacing, 1316
Epicardium, 1191
Epicondylitis, lateral, 2162, 2169t
medial, 2169t
Epidermal appendages, structure/function of, 2175, 2176t
Epidermal growth factor (EGF), in wound healing, 431
Epidermis, structure/function of, 2173–2175, *2174*, 2176t
Epidermoid lung cancer, 1153t
Epididymis, 2302–2303
physical examination of, 2333–2335
normal findings in, 2332b
sperm maturation in, 2305
Epididymitis, 2381–2382
after benign prostatic hyperplasia surgery, 2360
Epidural analgesia, *383*, 383–384
Epidural anesthesia, 475
Epidural hematoma, 744, 830, *830*
Epiglottis, 1023, *1024*
Epilepsy, 834–842
clinical manifestations of, 836–838, *837*
diagnostic findings in, 836–838, *837*
etiology of, 834
idiopathic, 834
management of, community/self care in, 842
emergency, 838
in elderly, 840
medical, 838, 839t
nursing, 838–840
surgical, 840–841, *841*
nursing care in, 841–842
pathophysiology of, 834–836, *836*
prevention of, 835b
risk factors for, 834, 835b
secondary, 834
terms in, 835b
Epileptic cry, definition of, 835b
Epileptogenic focus, 834
Epinephrine, actions of, 1940t, 1944
effects of, 2057t
for shock, 520

Epinephrine *(Continued)*
in blood flow regulation, 1374
in carbohydrate metabolism, 1946
in cardiac regulation, 1203
in hypokalemia, 305
in pain control, local anesthesia with, 372
release of, in shock, 508
Epiphysis, 2073
Episcleritis, 973–974
in rheumatoid arthritis, 659
Episcopalians, beliefs/practices of, 2547
Epispadias, 2333, 2380, *2381*
Epistaxis, 1076–1077, *1077*
Epithelial cells, 265
Epithelialization, in wound healing, 432
Epithelium, germinal, of ovaries, 2295, *2295*
olfactory, 1022
respiratory, in defense, *1025,* 1025–1026, 1026t
Epitopes, 598, *599,* 653
Epitrochlear lymph node chain, assessment of, 610
EPO (epoetin alpha), for chronic renal failure, 1654
Epoetin alpha (EPO), for chronic renal failure, 1654
EPs (evoked potentials), in neurologic assessment, 739
Equal Employment Opportunity Commission, 129
Equipment, preparation of, for physical examination, 231
ER (estrogen receptor), in cancer diagnosis, 558t
Erb's point, *1214*
ERCP (endoscopic retrograde cholangiography), 1853
Erectile dysfunction, 2347–2350
after prostatectomy, 2363
management of, community/self care in, 2350
medical, 2350
nursing, 2350
surgical, 2348–2349, *2349*
nursing care in, 2349
physiologic, 2347–2348
psychogenic, 2347
Erection, during sleep, 405
psychogenic, after spinal cord injury, 912
ERG (electroretinography), 951
Ergocalciferol (Vitamin D₂), for hypoparathyroidism, 2037
Ergometry, bicycle, in cardiovascular assessment, 1225
Ergot, for migraine headaches, 819
Erosion, *2185*
ERSs (emergency response systems), for elderly, 99–100
ERT (estrogen replacement therapy), contraindications to, 2393–2394
for menopause, 2392–2394
in osteoporosis prevention, 2103, 2104
ERV (expiratory reserve volume), 1028, *1028,* 1052t
Erycette, 2198t
Erysipelas, 2222–2223

Erythema, biocultural variations in, 2190b
chemotherapy and, 583
definition of, 2183t
palmar, in cirrhosis, 1878t
Erythema marginatum, in rheumatic fever, 1328
Erythroblastosis fetalis, 1480
Erythrocyte sedimentation rate (ESR), in musculoskeletal disorders, 2096t
Erythrocytes. See also *Red blood cells (RBCs).*
abnormalities of, 1466t
development of, *1450*
in hematopoiesis, 1449–1451, *1451*
in sickle cell anemia, *1513*
Erythromycin, for acne vulgaris, 2212
topical, 2198t
Erythroplakia, 1727
Erythropoiesis, 1449–1451, *1451*
Erythropoietin, for anemia, 1471
for cancer, 586–587
for chronic renal failure, 1654
synthesis of, kidneys in, 1543
Escape pacemaker, 1295
Eschar, 439
Escharotomy, in circumferential burns, 2250, *2251*
Escherichia coli, 416t
and urinary tract infection, 1571–1572
Escort services, for elderly, 99
Esidrix (hydrochlorothiazide), 1394t
characteristics of, 1285t
Esmolol, for dysrhythmia, 1308t
Esophageal atresia, tracheoesophageal fistula with, 1784
Esophageal bleeding, in portal hypertension, critical monitoring in, 1885, 1885b
Esophageal cancer, 1743–1746
clinical manifestations of, 1744
diagnostic findings in, 1744
etiology of, 1743
management of, medical, 1744
nursing, 1744–1745
surgical, 1745
nursing care in, 1745–1746
pathophysiology of, 1743–1744
prevention of, 1743b
risk factors for, 1743, 1743b
survival in, 538t
Esophageal gastric tube airway (EGTA), 2506
Esophageal obturator airway (EOA), 2506, *2506*
Esophageal spasm, diffuse, 1737
Esophageal speech, 1093
use of, nursing research on, 1088b
Esophageal varices, bleeding, nursing care in, 1886–1887
treatment of, *1885,* 1885–1886
in cirrhosis, 1878t
in portal hypertension, 1884–1885
prevention of, 201t
Esophagitis, in achalasia, 1734, *1734*
reflux. See *Gastroesophageal reflux disease (GERD).*
Esophagogastroduodenoscopy (EGD), 256
Esophagojejunostomy, for peptic ulcer disease, 1778, *1778*

Esophagomyotomy, for achalasia, 1735, *1735,* 1736
Esophagus, 1687–1689
  disorders of, 1732–1746
    neoplastic, 1743–1746
    traumatic, 1746
    vascular, 1746
  function of, 1687–1689
  structure of, 1687
Esophoria, 945
Esoptropia, 945
ESR (erythrocyte sedimentation rate), in musculoskeletal disorders, 2096t
Essential iron, 1453
Estar gel, 2200t
Estrogen(s), 2298
  actions of, 1940t
  for breast cancer, 2449, 2449t
  for chemotherapy, classification of, 577t
  for prostate cancer, 2368
  for urinary incontinence, 1611t
  for viral hepatitis, 1867
  in breast development, 2297
  in carcinogenesis, 540
Estrogen receptor (ER), in cancer diagnosis, 558t
Estrogen replacement therapy (ERT), contraindications to, 2393–2394
  for menopause, 2392–2394
  in osteoporosis prevention, 2103, 2104
ESWL (extracorporeal shock wave lithotripsy), for cholelithiasis, 1912
  complications of, 1912
  for renal calculi, 1668, *1668*
  for urinary calculi, 1597
ETCO₂ (end-tidal carbon dioxide), 1055
Ethacrynic acid (Edecrin), 1394t
  characteristics of, 1285t
Ethambutol, for tuberculosis, 1144t
Ethanol. See *Alcohol.*
Ether, in inhalation anesthesia, 472
Ethical dilemma, communication problem vs., 2442b
  definition of, 40
Ethical issues, definition of, 40
  for clients, 47–48
    autonomy in, 47
    clients' rights in, 47
    informed consent in, 47–48
    truth-telling in, 48
  for nurses, 46–47
    client/family relationships in, 46
    colleague relationships in, 46
    nonintervention in, 47
    resource allocation in, 47
    terminal illness in, 46
  in advanced directives, in emergency patient, 2502b
  in blood transfusion, in Jehovah's Witnesses, 1519b
  in cancer, 588b
    in research, 544
    in screening, 554b
    in treatment termination, 567b
  in chemically impaired nurse, 2498b
  in citizen vs. non-citizen care, 915b
  in colleague incompetency, 378b

Ethical issues *(Continued)*
  in communication problem vs. ethical dilemma, 2442b
  in confidential information, 189b
  in confused client advocacy, 768b
  in continuous mechanical ventilation termination, 1184b
  in cross-cultural nursing, 66b
  in diabetes regimen compliance, 1980b
  in dialysis, in renal failure, 1648b
  in educational material use, 2060b
  in elderly, 100–102, 101b
  in emergency care, 2501–2503, 2502b
  in fetal damage accountability, 2309b
  in genetic testing, 552b
  in home healthcare, in patient/family conflict, 150b
  in Huntington's disease, 884b
  in hydration, 281b
  in informed consent, for radical procedures, 1095b
  in informed consent insurance, 2403b
  in life support continuation, 499b
  in life-style disease nursing care, 1883b
  in medical problems in substance abuser, 2485b
  in neuromuscular blocking agent use, 1172b
  in nurse-client relationship values, 170b
  in nursing role, in "do not resuscitate" decision, 1244b
  in organ donation, 754b
  in pain, 343b
  in physical restraint use, 761b
  in placebo administration, 360b
  in post-transplantation self-care, 647b
  in premature hospital discharge prevention, 1589b
  in privacy vs. right-to-know, in sexually transmitted diseases, 2463b
  in protecting client dignity, 467b
  in risk-taking activities, 163b
  in sexual life-style, 2344b
  in short-staffing, 1816b
  in silicone implants, for breast reconstruction, 2438b
  in spirituality, 68b
  in surgery, in "do not resuscitate" clients, 460b
  in treatment refusal, in burns, 2249b
  in tuberculosis testing, 1141b
  in underinsured client care, 9b
  in whistleblowing, 127b
  in withholding/withdrawing treatment, 513b
Ethical problems, definition of, 40
  in nursing practice, resolution of, 48
Ethics, 39–49
  decision-making in, guidelines for, 42–43, 42t, 43t
    models of, 43–45, 44t
  definition of, 40
  in chronic conditions, 118t
  in nursing practice, guidelines for, 41–42, 41b, 42b
  principles of, 40–41
    autonomy in, 40
    beneficence in, 40

Ethics *(Continued)*
  confidentiality in, 41
  fidelity in, 40–41
  justice in, 40
  nonmaleficence in, 40
  veracity in, 40–41
  research in, 45, 46b
  study of, framework for, 39
  terminology of, 40
Ethionamide, for tuberculosis, 1145t
Ethmoidal artery, ligation of, for epistaxis, 1076–1077
Ethnicity, among elderly, 82
  in disease, 32b
  in hypertension, 1389
  in pain response, 346
Ethnopharmacology, 94b–95b
Ethoproprazine (Parsidol), for Parkinson's disease, 880t
Ethosuximide (Zarontin), side effects of, 839t
  therapeutic monitoring of, reference values for, 2562
Ethrane (enflurane), 470t
Ethyl chloride spray, 473t
Ethylene glycol, antidote to, 2538t
Etidronate disodium (Didronel), for hypercalcemia, 321–322, 2034t
  for multiple myeloma, 1499
Etretinate (Tegison), for psoriasis, 2211
Eucerin, 2200t
Eucerin creme, 2199t
Eulexin (flutamide), for benign prostatic hyperplasia, 2364t
Eunuchoidism, 2378
Eupnea, *238*
Eustachian tube, disorders of, 1009
  function of, 983
  structure of, *981,* 982–983
Euthyroid, definition of, 2005
Evacuation catheter, for continent ileostomy, 1807
Evaluation, in chronic condition management, 118
  in cross-cultural nursing, 66
  in relocation stress syndrome, 89b
  in spiritual care, 73
    relief-of-symptoms approach to, 73
    values clarification approach to, 73
Evans formula, for fluid resuscitation, in burns, 2250t
Evidence, physical, in emergency care, 2502–2503
Evisceration, 446
  postoperative, 491, *491*
    nursing management of, 491
Evoked potentials (EPs), in neurologic assessment, 739
Ewing's sarcoma, *2123,* 2123t
Exacerbation, definition of, 2183t
Examiner, preparation of, for physical examination, 233
Excision biopsy, 257
Excitability, of heart, 1195–1196, *1195–1197*
Excoriation, *2185*
Exercise(s), after cerebrovascular accident, 800

Exercise(s) (Continued)
after coronary artery bypass grafting, 1250–1251, 1251b
after lung cancer surgery, 1157, 1157, 1158
after mastectomy, 2443, 2444
after total hip replacement, 2113, 2116–2117, 2117
Buerger-Allen, 1412, 1412
coughing, preoperative teaching of, 461
deep breathing, after thyroidectomy, 2025t
preoperative teaching of, 461, 462
evaluation of, in cardiovascular assessment, 1210
extremity, preoperative teaching of, 461
for balance disorders, 1012–1013
for chronic arterial occlusion, 1407
for diabetes mellitus, 1965
planning for, 1974–1975
for hypertension, 1393, 1402–1403
for intervertebral disc herniation, 920
for obesity, 1760
history of, in musculoskeletal disorders, 2085
in respiratory disorders, 1039–1040
in burns, 2259
in chronic obstructive pulmonary disease, 1117
in health promotion, 171
in multiple sclerosis, 876
in rheumatoid arthritis, 669, 669
encouragement of, nursing research on, 666b
lack of, management of, 202t
pattern of, 206
pelvic muscle, for urinary incontinence, 1609–1610, 1609b
turning, preoperative teaching of, 461
with cast, 2151
Exercise electrocardiography, 1225–1227, 1226b, 1227b
contraindications to, 1226, 1227b
in angina pectoris, 1254
Exercise testing, in peripheral vascular assessment, 1384
Exertional dyspnea, assessment of, 1206
Exfoliative, definition of, 2183t
Exfoliative cytologic analysis, in cancer diagnosis, 556–558
in gastrointestinal tract assessment, 1716–1717
Exna (benzthiazide), 1394t
Exocrine glands, 1937, 1938
Exocytosis, 687
Exophoria, 945
Exophthalmometry, 950
Exophthalmos, 943
carotid–cavernous sinus fistula and, 816–817
in Graves' disease, 976, 976–977, 2018, 2018–2019
Exostosis, 1009
Exotoxins, 270
Exotropia, 945
Expectorants, for chronic obstructive pulmonary disease, 1111t
Experience, in home healthcare, 150

Expert practice, ambulatory care nurse in, 141b, 142
Expiration, normal, 1030
Expiratory reserve volume (ERV), 1028, 1028, 1052t
Expression, facial, assessment of, 711t
verbal, assessment of, 718
Exstrophy, of bladder, 1620
Extended family, 53
Extended radical mastectomy, for breast cancer, 2437
External auditory canal, structure of, 981, 981
External counterpulsation device, for shock, 517
External fixation, for fracture, nursing care in, 2142–2145
External pacing, 1316
Extinction phenomenon, testing of, 724
Extracapsular cataract extraction (ECCE), 959, 959–960
Extracapsular fracture, 2131, 2159
Extracellular fluid (ECF), 273
electrolyte distribution in, 293t
volume of, shifting of, 289–291, 290b
Extracellular fluid volume deficit (ECFVD), 277–284
clinical manifestations of, 278, 280t
diagnostic findings in, 278, 280t
etiology of, 278
management of, community/self care in, 284
in elderly clients, 283–284, 283b
medical, 278–280
intravenous therapy in, 278
oral rehydration in, 279–280
nursing, 280–283, 282, 282b
delegation of, 282b
pathophysiology of, 278
prevention of, 279b
risk factors for, 278, 279b
types of, 278
Extracellular fluid volume excess (ECFVE), 284–289
clinical manifestations of, 286, 287t
diagnostic findings in, 286, 287t
etiology of, 285
management of, community/self care in, 289
dietary, 288, 288b
in congestive heart failure, 288
in elderly clients, 289
medical, 287–288
nursing, 288–289
pharmacologic, 287–288
pathophysiology of, 285–286, 286
prevention of, 285b
risk factors for, 285, 285b
Extracorporeal circulation (ECC), during open heart surgery, 1354–1355, 1355
Extracorporeal membrane oxygenation (ECMO), for open heart surgery, 1355
for shock, 516
in heart failure, 1289–1290
Extracorporeal shock wave lithotripsy (ESWL), for cholelithiasis, 1912
complications of, 1912

Extracorporeal shock wave lithotripsy (ESWL) (Continued)
for renal calculi, 1668, 1668
for urinary calculi, 1597
Extracranial-intracranial bypass, for transient ischemic attacks, 809–810, 810
nursing care in, 811
Extradural hematoma, 830, 830
Extrapulmonary tuberculosis (XPTB), 1144–1145
Extrapyramidal disease, abnormal movements in, 723b
Extravasation, of chemotherapy, management of, 576
urinary, 2380
Extremity(ies), physical examination of, in endocrine disorders, 1951–1952
Extremity (intravenous regional) block anesthesia, 476
Extremity exercises, preoperative teaching of, 461
Extrinsic factor, 1453
Extubation, from continuous mechanical ventilation, 1184
Exudates, in pleural effusion, 1167
inflammatory, 434, 435t
Eye(s), age-related changes in, 939–940
assessment of, in health history, 183b
in regional examination, 215t
neurologic, 720
normal findings in, 940b
avulsion of, 2533
chemical burns of, 2533
disorders of, 935–978
assessment of, 940–950
history in, 941–943
physical examination in, 943–950, 946–949, 947b
diabetes mellitus and, 1996
diagnosis of, 950–952, 950–952
in systemic disorders, 976, 976–978
nursing care in, 952–978
emergencies of, 2533
foreign bodies in, 2533
function of, 939
in endocrine disorders, 1949
physical examination of, 1950
in hematologic disorders, 1463
in rheumatoid arthritis, 659–660
misconceptions about, 941b
movements of, assessment of, 711t–712t, 720, 945
in consciousness disorders, 747
in increased intracranial pressure, 782
of dying patient, donation of, guidelines for, 2514t
position of, examination of, 943
structure of, 935–939, 936–939
tumors of, 970–972
Eye drops, for corneal ulcer, administration schedule for, 969
for glaucoma, client teaching about, 957t
Eye opening, in increased intracranial pressure, 781
Eye prosthesis, 971, 971
insertion/removal of, 972b–973b
Eyeballs, examination of, 944
Eyebrows, examination of, 943

Eyelashes, examination of, 943–944
Eyelids, disorders of, 972–975
  examination of, 943–944
  structure of, 936, *937*
  tumors of, benign, 971
    malignant, 971–972

F

FAB (French-American-British) Cooperative
  Group, leukemia classification of, 1487–
  1488, 1488t
Face, assessment of, in regional examina-
  tion, 214t
  chemical peeling of, 2273–2274
  traumatic injuries of, plastic surgery of,
    2286–2288, *2287*
Face lift, *2271,* 2271–2272, *2272*
  complications of, 2271–2272
Facial expressions, assessment of, 711t
Facial nerve, assessment of, *719,* 720–
  721
Facial rejuvenating surgery, 2270–2275
Facilitation, in nerve impulse generation,
  688
Factor IX, transfusion of, 1520t
  for hemophilia, 1517
Factor VIII, transfusion of, 1520t
  for hemophilia, 1517
Factor X, in hemostasis, *1457,* 1457–1458
Fainting, 1404–1405
  in cardiovascular disease, assessment of,
    1207
Fallopian tube cancer, 2422
Fallopian tubes, examination of, 2319
  structure/function of, 2295
Falls, blunt trauma in, 2521t
  management of, 199t
  prevention of, 200t
    in osteoporosis, 2103
Familial hemorrhagic telangiectasia, 1508
Family, assessment of, in cross-cultural
    nursing, 64b
  blended, 53
  changes affecting, 51–52
  chaotic, 54
  communal, 53
  concepts of, 52–55
  conjugal, 52
  definition of, 136b
  extended, 53
  functions of, 53–54
    boundary, 54
    communication, 54
    education, 54
    levels of, 54–55
    management, 53
    socialization, 54
    support, 54
  health history of. See *Health history, fam-
    ily.*
  ideal independent, 54–55
  in chronic conditions, 112
  in elderly support, 83–84
  intermediate, 54
  nuclear, 52
  nurse relationship with, ethical issues in,
    46

Family *(Continued)*
  nursing of, nursing process in, 55–59,
    56b–57b, 58b
  of cancer patient, coping ability of, 564
  of critically ill client, needs of, nursing
    research on, 58b
  of dementia of Alzheimer's type client,
    needs of, 871t–872t
  of home healthcare patient, conflicts in,
    ethical issues in, 150b
  of origin, 52
  of total parenteral nutrition patient, nurs-
    ing research on, 1757b
  psychosocial dimensions of, 51–59
  reconstituted, 53
  single-parent, 53
  social contract, 53
  structures of, 52–53
  summoning of, to emergency department,
    2510b
  support of, for elderly, 83–84
  therapeutic communication in, 58
  with problems, 54
  with solutions, 54
Family coping, ineffective, after spinal cord
    injury, 910–911
  in chronic renal failure, 1656–1657
  in confusion, 769
  in dialysis, 1658
Family education, about chemotherapy, 584,
    584b
  about consciousness disorders, 762b
Family processes, altered, after brain tumor
    surgery, 855
  in chronic obstructive pulmonary dis-
    ease, 1122
  in consciousness disorders, 761–763,
    762b
Famotidine (Pepcid), for peptic ulcer dis-
    ease, 1767, 1768t
  for shock, 520
Farsightedness, 946, *975,* 976
Fascia, 2078
Fascial excision, of burns, 2253–2254
Fasciculations, 2087
Fasciculi, 2078
Fasciculus cuneatus, 696t
Fasciculus gracilis, 696t
Fasciitis, plantar, 2162
Fast pain, 343
Fasting blood sugar (FBS), in diabetes mel-
    litus diagnosis, 1961, 1962b, 1964t
Fat(s), dietary, modification of, for hyper-
    tension, 1392–1393, 1401, 1402b
  excess intake of, management of, 201t
  in coronary artery disease, 1241
  in diabetes mellitus, guidelines for, 1977,
    1977t
  in wound healing, 434t
  intolerance of, in acute cholecystitis, 1917t
  metabolism of, laboratory tests for, 1851t
    liver in, 1839–1840
  mobilization of, increased, in type II dia-
    betes mellitus, 1959–1960
  subcutaneous, structure/function of, 2176,
    2176t
Fat embolism, fractures and, 2140
  pulmonary embolism vs., 2141t

Fatigue, in acquired immunodeficiency syn-
    drome, management of, 633–634
  in acute glomerulonephritis, 1632
  in cancer, 587b
  in cardiovascular disease, assessment of,
    1206
  in chronic renal failure, 1656
  in diabetes mellitus, 1960t
  in endocrine disorders, 1948
  in left ventricular failure, 1281
  in rheumatoid arthritis, management of,
    669
  in viral hepatitis, 1865, 1866t, 1869–1870
  prevention of, 200t
Fatty liver, 1895
Fatty streaks, 1242, *1242*
FBS (fasting blood sugar), in diabetes melli-
    tus diagnosis, 1961, 1962b, 1964t
FCV (forced vital capacity), 1052t
Fear, alleviation of, in pain management,
    366–367
  before amputation, 1419–1420
  brain tumors and, 851
  in benign prostatic hypertrophy, 2360
  in gastric cancer, 1783–1784
  in intervertebral disc surgery, 922
  in myocardial infarction, 1272
  in urinary tract disorders, 1551
  perioperative, 458–459
  with tracheostomy, 1075–1076
Febrile nonhemolytic transfusion reaction,
  1529t
Fecal analysis, 1711–1713, 1711t, 1712b
Fecal incontinence, in consciousness disorders, 761
Feces, 1696
  abnormal content of, in intestinal disor-
    ders, 1788
  reference values for, 2563
Feedback, negative, in hormone regulation,
  1941, *1941*
Feeding, in dysphagia, after cerebrovascular
    accident, 804–805, 804b
  tube. See *Tube feeding.*
Feeding tube, aspirates from, nursing re-
    search on, 1743b
  placement of, nursing research on, 1751b
Feeling, sensory, assessment of, 713t
Feet. See *Foot.*
FEF$_{25\%-75\%}$ (forced expiratory flow$_{25\%-75\%}$),
  1052t
Feldene (piroxicam), for rheumatoid arthri-
  tis, 664t
Felodipine (Plendil), 1396t
Felty's syndrome, in rheumatoid arthritis,
  660
Female, role of, 75–76
Femina cones, 1609
Feminism, 75–76
Femoral artery bypass grafting, 1414, *1414*
Femoral hernia, 1817, *1817*
  examination for, 2335
Femoral neck fracture, *2153,* 2159
Femoral shaft fracture, 2160, *2160*
Femoropopliteal disorders, 1407
Femur, proximal, anatomic regions of, *2153*
Fenestrations, capillary, 1375
  of tracheostomy tube, 1068–1069

Fenoprofen (Nalfon), for rheumatoid arthritis, 664t

Fentanyl citrate (Sublimaze), administration of, 380t
  preoperative, 465t
  transdermal, 382

Fentanyl citrate–droperidol (Innovar), 470t

Feosol (ferrous sulfate), for iron deficiency anemia, 1473

Fergon (ferrous gluconate), for iron deficiency anemia, 1473

Ferrous gluconate (Fergon), for iron deficiency anemia, 1473

Ferrous sulfate (Feosol), for iron deficiency anemia, 1473

FESS (functional endoscopic sinus surgery), 1077–1078, 1078

Fetus, damage to, ethical issues in, 2309b

FEV₁ (forced expiratory volume), 1052t

Fever, in acquired immunodeficiency syndrome, management of, 631–633
  in acute cholecystitis, 1917t
  in acute pancreatitis, 1923, 1924t
  in rheumatic fever, 1328
  in viral hepatitis, 1865, 1866t
  inflammation and, 435

FFP (fresh frozen plasma), transfusion of, 1520t–1523t
  for shock, 519

FHPs (functional health patterns), 206–211

Fiber, dietary, for gastrointestinal symptoms, nursing research on, 1825b
  low intake of, management of, 201t
  in diabetes mellitus, guidelines for, 1977, 1977t

Fibrillation, atrial, 1300, 1301–1302
  ventricular, 1305–1306, 1309

Fibrin clot, formation of, 1457, 1457–1458, 1458

Fibrin split products (FSPs) test, in hemorrhage, 1467t

Fibrin stabilizing factor, 1516t

Fibrinogen, 1516t
  functions of, 1447, 1448t
  level of, in hemorrhage, 1467t

Fibrinolysin-desoxyribonuclease (Elase), for enzymatic debridement, 440

Fibrinolysis, in hemostasis, 1458

Fibrinolytic therapy, for pulmonary embolism, 1128–1129
  for venous thrombosis, 1435

Fibroadenoma, 2452

Fibroblasts, in wound healing, 432
  structure/function of, 2176t

Fibrocartilage, formation of, in bone healing, 2133, 2133

Fibrocystic breasts, 2451–2452, 2452b

Fibroma, 549–550, 550t

Fibromyalgia, sleep disorders in, 405

Fibromyalgia syndrome, 679, 680

Fibrosarcoma, 2123t
  malignant, 550, 550t

Fibrothorax, 1167

Fibrous joints, 2075–2076

Fibular fracture, 2161

Fidelity, in ethics, 40–41

Field block anesthesia, 474

Fight-or-flight response, 21, 22

Filariasis, 1440

Filiforms, 2357t

Film badges, in radiation therapy safety, 573

Films, transparent, for burns, 2257t
  in wound management, indications for, 443t

Filtering procedures, for glaucoma, 956–957

Filters, nonstandard, for blood transfusion, 1525–1526, 1526t

Filtration, 274

FIM (Functional Independence Measure), in chronic conditions, 115t

Finasteride (Proscar), for benign prostatic hyperplasia, 2364t

Fine-needle aspiration (FNA), in cancer diagnosis, 558
  in thyroid disorders, 2011t
  of breast, 2329
  of liver, 1855
    contraindications to, 1855

Fingers, clubbing of, in infective endocarditis, 1333
  inspection of, in respiratory assessment, 1042–1043
  muscles of, strength of, assessment of, 2088t
  range of motion of, 2089

Finkelstein's test, 2090t

Fire, residential, prevention of, recommendations for, 2234b
  victims of, reactions of, nursing research on, 2263b

First-degree atrioventricular (AV) block, 1303, 1303–1304

First-pass cardiac study, 1230

Fishberg concentration test, 1561

Fissure, 2185
  of anus, 1828
  of nipples, 2452
  palpebral, 936, 936

Fist percussion, in hepatobiliary assessment, 1848

Fistula, after laryngeal surgery, 1089
  after radiation therapy, 1584
  anal, 1828
  carotid–cavernous sinus, 816–817
  gastrojejunocolic, after peptic ulcer surgery, 1779
  tracheoesophageal, esophageal atresia with, 1784
  vaginal. See Vaginal fistula.

Fitness, components of, 174b, 1965
  concepts of, 174t

Fixation, external, for fracture, nursing care in, 2142–2145
  internal, for spinal cord injury, 914, 914

FK506 (tacrolimus), in organ transplantation, 645t

Flaccidity, in consciousness disorders, 748, 748

Flagyl (metronidazole), for bacterial vaginosis, 2474
  for peptic ulcer disease, 1767, 1769t

Flail chest, 2527, 2527

Flap amputation, 1418, 1418

Flaps, 2277, 2278–2281

Flaps (Continued)
  free, 2277, 2279–2281
    donor sites for, 2280
    failure of, 2280
    long-term results of, 2281
    nursing care in, 2280–2281
  latissimus dorsi, in cardiomyoplasty, 1290
  musculocutaneous, 2279
    critical monitoring in, 2279b

Flat bones, 2073

Flat plate, 250
  of abdomen, 1713

Flatness, in percussion, 230
  of chest, 1045, 1046

Flatulence, in gastrointestinal disorders, 1749

Flatus, with colostomy, 1815

Flecainide (Tambocor), for dysrhythmia, 1307t

Flex-foot prosthesis, 1422

Flexibility, in fitness, 174b

Flexion withdrawal, in unconscious patient, 723

Flexion-rotation injury, of spinal cord, 890, 892

Flora, normal, in host defense, 415
  of large intestine, 1696
  of small intestine, 1693

Florinef (fludrocortisone), 2048t

Flowmeter, peak, 1051, 1053, 1109
  use of, directions for, 1113b

Flu, 1133–1134. See also Influenza.

Fluctuating hearing loss, 994b

Fludrocortisone (Florinef), 2048t

Fluid(s), administration of, after thyroidectomy, 2024t
  intake of, control of, for urinary incontinence, 1610
    for renal calculi, 1670
    for urinary calculi, 1596–1597
    promotion of, for urinary tract infection, 1574
  movement of, through capillaries, 274, 274
  replacement of, for acute renal failure, 1639
    for hyperglycemic, hyperosmolar, nonketotic coma, 1987–1988
    for shock, 519–520
    in acute pancreatitis, 1924
    in diabetic ketoacidosis, 1986b
  restriction of, in increased intracranial pressure, 783

Fluid and electrolyte balance, 273–325
  assessment of, after cardiac surgery, 1012
    preoperative, 455
  complications of, in postanesthesia care unit, 483
  critical monitoring in, 325b
  electrolyte imbalances in, 295–325
  fluid compartments in, 273
  fluid pressures in, 274, 274, 274b
  glucocorticoids in, 1945
  in burns, 2234–2235, 2235
  in coma, 752
  in extracellular fluid volume deficit. See Extracellular fluid volume deficit (ECFVD).

Fluid and electrolyte balance *(Continued)*
in extracellular fluid volume excess. See *Extracellular fluid volume excess (ECFVE).*
in intracellular fluid volume deficit, 293
in intracellular fluid volume excess. See *Intracellular fluid volume excess (ICFVE).*
in third-spacing. See *Third-spacing.*
kidneys in, 1542
maintenance of, nursing role in, 325
postoperative, 487–488
osmolality in, 275–276, *276,* 276b
regulation of, *275,* 275–277, *276,* 276b
Fluid balance, assessment of, in urinary tract assessment, 1553–1554
Fluid compartments, 273
Fluid pressures, 274, *274,* 274b
Fluid resuscitation, in major burns, 2242–2249, 2249t
Fluid volume, changes in, in hypertension, 1389
replacement of, for shock, 518–519
Fluid volume deficit, after arterial bypass, 1416
after brain tumor surgery, 854
as nursing diagnosis, 282
extracellular. See *Extracellular fluid volume deficit (ECFVD).*
in appendicitis, 1792
in ascites, 1890–1891
in burns, 2243
in cholelithiasis, 1911
in consciousness disorders, 760
in dialysis, 1657–1658
in enteral nutrition, 1753–1754
in gastroenteritis, 1791
in hepatic encephalopathy, 1894
in hydronephrosis, 1636
in peritonitis, 1794
in pyelonephritis, 1629
in renal failure, acute, 1640
chronic, 1655–1656
in small intestinal obstruction, 1822–1823
in vertigo, 1015
intracellular, 293
preoperative, 455
types of, 278
Fluid volume excess, as nursing diagnosis, 288
extracellular. See *Extracellular fluid volume excess (ECFVE).*
in acute glomerulonephritis, 1632
in acute hyperglycemia, 1984t
in ascites, 1890–1891
in chronic renal failure, 1655–1656
in dialysis, 1657–1658
in heart failure, 1287–1288
in myocardial infarction, 1275–1276
intracellular. See *Intracellular fluid volume excess (ICFVE).*
isosmolar, 284
Fluid volume shift, extracellular, 289–291. See also *Third-spacing.*
FluidAir bed, *2219*
Flunitrazepam (Rohypnol), abuse of, 2489b
Fluocinolone (Synalar), topical, 2199t
Fluocinonide gel, 2200t

Fluorescein angiography, 951–952, *952*
Fluorescent treponemal antibody absorption (FTA-ABS) test, for syphilis, 2471
Fluoride, in dental caries prevention, 1720
Fluoroscopy, of musculoskeletal system, 2093
of respiratory system, 1060
5-Fluorouracil (Efudex, Fluoroplex), topical, 2198t
for actinic keratosis, 2225
Fluosol, administration of, for shock, 519
Fluothane (halothane), 470t
Fluroplex (5-fluorouracil), topical, 2198t
Flutamide (Eulexin), for benign prostatic hyperplasia, 2364t
Flutter, atrial, *1300,* 1301
FNA. See *Fine-needle aspiration (FNA).*
Focal glomerular sclerosis, 1634
Foley urethral catheters, 2355t
Folic acid, deficiency of, and anemia, 1474, 1476–1477
for pernicious anemia, 1475–1476
in hematopoiesis, 1453
Follicle-stimulating hormone (FSH), 2061t
deficiency of, in hypopituitarism, 2065
in menstruation, *2299,* 2299–2300
Follicular adenocarcinoma, of thyroid, 2028t
Follicular cysts, of ovaries, 2412
Folliculitis, 2221t
definition of, 2183t
Followers, 2357t
Food, soul, 1704b
Food allergy, testing for, 637
in immune disorder assessment, 612
Food diary, *173*
Foot, disorders of, *2124,* 2124–2125, *2125*
fracture of, 2161
infection of, in diabetes mellitus, 1995
nursing care plan for, 1998
muscles of, strength of, assessment of, 2088t
Foot care, client education in, 1410b–1411b
diabetic, home healthcare in, 1999b
in peripheral vascular disorders, 1409
Footdrop, after spinal cord injury, 905
Foramen of Magendie, *698, 699*
Foramen of Monro, 698, *698*
Foramina, cranial, 697
Foramina of Luschka, *698, 699*
Forane (isoflurane), 470t
Forced expiratory flow$_{25\%-75\%}$ (FEF$_{25\%-75\%}$), 1052t
Forced expiratory volume (FEV$_1$), 1052t
Forced vital capacity (FVC), 1052t
Forearm flaps, 2280
Foreign body, and ear obstruction, 1007, 2533
Foreskin, physical examination of, 2333, *2335*
Fosamax (alendronate), for osteoporosis, 2104
Fosinopril (Monopril), 1396t
Fossa navicularis, 2294
Fossae, cranial, 697
Fourchette, 2293, *2294*
Fovea, 938
Fractionation, of radiation therapy, 571

Fracture(s), 2129–2161. See also specific site of fracture.
articular, 2131
avulsion, 2130–2131
burst, 2131
chip, 2131
classification of, *2030,* 2129–2131
clinical manifestations of, 2134
closed, 2129, *2130*
Colles', *2130,* 2131
comminuted, *2130,* 2131
complete, *2130,* 2131
complications of, early, 2139–2141, *2140,* 2140b, 2141t
long-term, prevention of, 2145–2146, *2146*
compression, *2130,* 2131
diagnostic findings in, 2134, 2135t, *2136*
displaced, *2130,* 2131
etiology of, 2132
extracapsular, 2131
fragility, 2098
greenstick, *2130,* 2131
impacted, *2130,* 2131
intracapsular, 2131
linear, 2130
longitudinal, 2130, *2130*
management of, community/self care in, 2145–2153
emergency, 2134
medical, 2134–2141, 2145–2150
nursing, *2142,* 2142–2145
nursing care plan for, 2143–2144
oblique, 2130, *2130*
open, 2129, *2130*
pathologic, *2130,* 2131
pathophysiology of, 2132–2134, *2133,* 2134t
Pott's, *2130,* 2131
prevention of, 203t, 2132b
reduction of, 2135–2139
closed, *2136,* 2136–2137
open, 2137
risk factors for, 2132, 2132b
in hypercortisolism, 2052
spiral, 2130, *2130*
stress, *2130,* 2131
traction for, 2137–2139, *2138*
transverse, 2130, *2130*
Fracture-dislocation, of spinal cord, 890
Fragility fractures, 2098
Frank-Starling law, 1200, *1201*
FRC (functional residual capacity), 1028, *1028,* 1052t
Free flaps, *2277,* 2279–2281
donor sites for, 2280
failure of, 2280
long-term results of, 2281
nursing care in, 2280–2281
Free radicals, in wound healing, 430
Free thyroxine concentration, 2010t
Freestanding care centers, 137
Fremitus, tactile, assessment of, 1044
French-American-British (FAB) Cooperative Group, leukemia classification of, 1487–1488, 1488t
Frequency, 1548

Fresh frozen plasma (FFP), transfusion of, 1520t–1523t
for shock, 519
Friction rub, auscultation of, in gastrointestinal tract assessment, 1709
in hepatobiliary disease, 1845
pericardial, 1216
in pericarditis, 1336
pleural, 1046, 1049t
Frontal lobe, 690, *692*
tumor of, clinical manifestations of, 847t
Frontal lobectomy, for pain, 386
Frostbite, 2536
prevention of, 203t
Frozen sections, in cytologic analysis, 257
Fructosamine, in diabetes mellitus diagnosis, 1962
FSH (follicle-stimulating hormone), 2061t
deficiency of, in hypopituitarism, 2065
in menstruation, *2299*, 2299–2300
FSPs (fibrin split products) test, in hemorrhage, 1467t
FTA-ABS (fluorescent treponemal antibody absorption) test, for syphilis, 2471
FTSGs (full-thickness skin grafts), 2278
Fuchs' dystrophy, 966
Full-thickness skin grafts (FTSGs), 2278
Fulminant hepatitis, 1866, 1867
Functional endoscopic sinus surgery (FESS), 1077–1078, *1078*
Functional health patterns (FHPs), 206–211
Functional hearing loss, 994b
Functional Independence Measure (FIM), in chronic conditions, 115t
Functional nursing, 124
Functional residual capacity (FRC), 1028, *1028*, 1052t
Fundoplication, Nissen, for gastroesophageal reflux disease, 1739, *1739*
Fundus, examination of, 2319
Fundus photography, 950, *950*
Funduscopic examination, normal findings in, 940b
Funeral, body preparation for, cultural issues in, 69b–70b
Fungal culture, in integumentary disorders, 2194
Fungal pneumonia, 1137t
Fungus(i), and neurologic infections, 860
and pulmonary infections, 1146–1147
and skin infections, 2221t
Funnel chest, 1042, *1043*
Furosemide (Lasix), 1394t
characteristics of, 1285t
for acute renal failure, 1639
for hypercalcemia, 2034t
Furuncles, 2221t
Fusiform aneurysm, 1425, *1425*
cerebral, 812

G

G_0 phase, of cell cycle, 544, *545*
G_1 phase, of cell cycle, 544, *545*
G_2 phase, of cell cycle, 545, *545*
G6PD (glucose-6-phosphate dehydrogenase) deficiency, 1483
Gabapentin, side effects of, 839t

Gag (pharyngeal) reflex, 727, 729t
Gait, assessment of, 235, 722, 722b, 2086
in Parkinson's disease, 878, *879*
Galen, 19–20
Gallbladder, carcinoma of, 1920–1921
congenital anomalies of, 1921
structure/function of, 1835–1836, *1838*
Gallbladder series, 1849–1852
Gallbladder stasis, 1907
Gallium nitrate (Ganite), for hypercalcemia, 2034t
for hyperparathyroidism, 2033
for multiple myeloma, 1499
Gallium scans, 2094
in respiratory assessment, 1061
Gallops, 1216
Gallstones. See *Cholelithiasis.*
Gamma globulins, functions of, 1447, 1448t
Gamma-glutamyltransferase (GGT), in hepatobiliary assessment, 1851t
Ganglion, of hand, 2124
peripheral, structure/function of, 703
Gangrene, gas, fractures and, 2140–2141
Ganite (gallium nitrate), for hypercalcemia, 2034t
for hyperparathyroidism, 2033
for multiple myeloma, 1499
Gantrisin (sulfisoxazole), for urinary tract infections, 1576t
Garamycin (gentamicin), for open wounds, 445t
in surgical client, 458t
therapeutic monitoring of, reference values for, 2562
Gardnerella vaginalis, and bacterial vaginosis, 2474
Gardner-Wells tongs, for cervical spine injury, 897, *897*
Gas(es), atmospheric, partial pressures of, 1031, 1032t
during respiration, *1032*
GAS (general adaptation syndrome), 21–22, *23*
in shock, 507–508
Gas dilution tests, in respiratory assessment, 1051
Gas exchange, 1031–1033, *1032,* 1032t, *1033*
impaired, after partial laryngectomy, 1090
after spinal cord injury, 899–900
in abdominal aortic aneurysm, 1427
in asthma, 1110
in bleeding esophageal varices, 1886
in chronic obstructive pulmonary disease, 1120
in heart failure, 1288
in myocardial infarction, 1271
mechanical ventilation and, 1180
with tracheostomy, 1074
respiratory zone in, 1028–1029, *1029*
Gas gangrene, fractures and, 2140–2141
Gastrectomy, subtotal, for peptic ulcer disease, 1777, *1778*
total, for peptic ulcer disease, 1777–1778, *1778*
Gastric acid, secretion of, 1690
Gastric acid stimulation test, 1717
Gastric analysis, 1717

Gastric cancer, 1781–1784
classification of, 1782, 1782b
clinical manifestations of, 1782–1783
diagnostic findings in, 1782–1783
etiology of, 1782
in Japanese, 198t
management of, medical, 1783
surgical, 1783
nursing care in, 1783–1784
pathophysiology of, 1782
risk factors for, 542b, 1782
survival in, 538t
Gastric dilation, acute, in peptic ulcer disease, 1778
Gastric disorders, 1748–1784
clinical manifestations of, 1748–1749
congenital, 1784
inflammatory, 1761–1784
neoplastic, 1761–1784
nutritional support in, 1752–1756
Gastric inhibitory peptide (GIP), 1691t
Gastric lavage, in poisoning, 2538
Gastric lipase, 1692t
Gastric stapling, 1760
Gastric ulcers, 1764
classification of, 1766t
clinical manifestations of, 1766
pathophysiology of, 1765
Gastrin, 1691t
in pancreatic secretion, 1841
reference values for, in cancer, 557t
Gastritis, acute, 1761–1762
clinical manifestations of, 1762
diagnostic findings in, 1762
etiology of, 1761–1762
management of, medical, 1762
nursing, 1762
pathophysiology of, 1762
prevention of, 1762b
risk factors for, 1761–1762, 1762b
atrophic, 1762
chronic, 1762–1764
clinical manifestations of, 1763
diagnostic findings in, 1763
etiology of, 1762–1763
management of, medical, 1763
nursing, 1763–1764
surgical, 1764
pathophysiology of, 1763
risk factors for, 1762–1763
hypertrophic, 1762
reflux, alkaline, in peptic ulcer disease, 1778
superficial, 1762
Gastroduodenostomy, for peptic ulcer disease, 1777, *1778*
Gastroenteritis, 1788–1790
management of, medical, 1790–1791
nursing, 1791
prevention of, 1789b
risk factors for, 1789b
Gastroenterostomy, for peptic ulcer disease, 1777, *1777*
Gastroesophageal reflux disease (GERD), 1737–1740
and laryngitis, 1081
clinical manifestations of, 1737–1738
diagnostic findings in, 1737–1738

Gastroesophageal reflux disease (GERD) *(Continued)*
  etiology of, 1737
  management of, dietary, 1738–1739
    medical, 1738–1739
    nursing, 1739
    pharmacologic, 1738
    surgical, 1739, *1739, 1740*
      nursing care in, 1739–1740
  pathophysiology of, 1737
  prevention of, 1738b
  risk factors for, 1737, 1738b
  sleep disorders in, 405
Gastrointestinal bleeding, 2530–2531
  case management in, 1771b
  causes of, *1788*
  clinical pathway for, 2586–2587
  prevention of, in shock, 521
Gastrointestinal endoscopy, *256,* 256–257
Gastrointestinal tract, activities of, 1685, *1686, 1687*
  age-related changes in, 268t, 1696
  assessment of, in health history, 184b
    preoperative, 456
  autonomic neuropathy of, diabetes mellitus and, 2000
  chemotherapy effects on, 582–583
  disorders of, after renal transplantation, 1663
    and sleep disorders, 404
    assessment of, 1698–1717
      diagnostic tests in, 1710–1717, 1711t, 1712b, *1714, 1715*
      history in, 1698–1706
      physical examination in, 1699b, 1706–1710, *1707–1709*
    chest pain in, assessment of, 1209t
  function of, assessment of, reference values for, 2564
  in alcohol abuse, 2490t
  in anemia, 1470
  in burns, 2236
  in chronic renal failure, 1645
  in hematologic disorders, 1463
  in hepatobiliary disease, 1843
  in hypercalcemia, 321t
  in hyperkalemia, 312t
  in hypernatremia, 303t
  in hypocalcemia, 317t
  in hypokalemia, 309t
  in hyponatremia, 299b
  in shock, 509
  in thyroid disorders, 2008t
  pain in, 356
  preoperative preparation of, 463
  structure/function of, 1685–1696, *1686*
Gastrointestinal tubes, 1749–1752
  insertion of, 1750
  long, 1749t, 1750
  medium, 1749t, 1750
  nursing management of, 1751–1752
  short, 1749–1750, 1749t
  suctioning of, 1751
  types of, 1749, 1749t
Gastrojejunocolic fistula, after peptic ulcer surgery, 1779
Gastrojejunostomy, for peptic ulcer disease, *1778*

Gastroparesis, in diabetes mellitus, 2000
Gastroplasty, for obesity, 1760
Gastrostomy, endoscopic, percutaneous, after intracranial surgery, 854
Gastrostomy tube, endoscopic, percutaneous, critical monitoring in, 1731b
  for achalasia, 1735
Gate-control theory, of pain, 350–351, *351*
Gatekeeper programs, for elderly, 99
Gauze, for open wounds, 442
  in wound management, indications for, 443t
  Kerlix, 2202
  non-adhering, for burns, 2257t
Gay and Lesbian Medical Association, 619b
Gaze, cardinal directions of, *936*
GBS (Guillain-Barré syndrome), 877
  critical monitoring in, 878b
GCNS (gerontological clinical nurse specialist), 82
GCS (Glasgow Coma Scale), in Champion Trauma Score, 2518t
  in increased intracranial pressure assessment, 778, *779–780*
G-CSF (granulocyte colony-stimulating factor), for cancer, 586
GDM (gestational diabetes mellitus), 1955, 1955b, 1956
Gels, 2200t
Gelusil, for peptic ulcer disease, 1769t
Gender, in pain response, 350
Gender identity, 75
Gender role, 75
General adaptation syndrome (GAS), 21–22, *23*
  in shock, 507–508
General anesthesia, 468t, 469–472
  administration of, 469–471
  agents for, 470t–471t
  characteristics of, 468
  effects of, 469
  for status epilepticus, 843
  neuroleptic (balanced), 471
  stages of, 469, 469t
  types of, *471,* 471–472, 472t
General knowledge, assessment of, 195
General survey, in adult general screening physical examination, 233–237
  in regional examination, 214t
Genes, activation of, hormones in, 1941, *1942*
Genetic engineering, 265
Genetic promiscuity, 614
Genetic testing, ethical issues in, 552b
  in cancer prevention, 551–552, 552b
Genetic traits, population distribution of, 30b–31b
Genetics, in immunity, 604
Genital herpes, 2472–2473
  management of, 2462t
Genital tract sarcomas, in females, 2422–2423
Genital warts, 2473
  management of, 2462t
Genitalia, female, assessment of, in regional examination, 223t–224t
  external, 2293–2294, *2294*
  examination of, 2317

Genitalia *(Continued)*
  internal, 2294–2296, *2295*
  male, assessment of, in regional examination, 222t–223t
    physical examination of, 2333–2336, *2334, 2335*
    physical examination of, in endocrine disorders, 1952
Genitourinary history, female, 2310
  male, 2331
Genitourinary tract, autonomic neuropathy of, diabetes mellitus and, 2000
  disorders of, and male reproductive disorders, 2345
  in anemia, 1470
  in hepatobiliary disease, 1843
Genitourinary tuberculosis, 1581
Genogram, in family nursing assessment, 55, *55*
Gentamicin (Garamycin), for open wounds, 445t
  in surgical client, 458t
  therapeutic monitoring of, reference values for, 2562
Genu valgum, 2087, *2087*
Genu varum, 2087, *2087*
Geography, in cancer, 540
  in disease, 32b
  in gastrointestinal tract assessment, 1706
  in immune disorder assessment, 608
  in respiratory assessment, 1039
  of clients, variations in, 16
GERD. See *Gastroesophageal reflux disease (GERD)*.
Geriatrics, 81
Germ theory, of illness, 20
Germinal epithelium, of ovaries, 2295, *2295*
Gerontological clinical nurse specialist (GCNS), 82
Gerontological nurse practitioner (GNP), 82
Gerontological nursing, 81–82
Gerontology, 81
Gerota's fascia, 1535
Gestational diabetes mellitus (GDM), 1955, 1955b, 1956
Gestational trophoblastic disease, 2423–2424
GFR (glomerular filtration rate), 1540–1541
  changes in, in shock, 509–510
GGT (gamma-glutamyltransferase), in hepatobiliary assessment, 1851t
GH. See *Growth hormone (GH)*.
Ghon tubercles, 1141
Giant cell arteritis, 681
Giant cell tumor, *2123,* 2123t
Giardia lamblia, 416t
Giardiasis, 1790
  infectious agent in, 416t
Gingiva, overgrowth of, phenytoin and, 842
Gingivitis, 1721, *1721*
  ulcerative, necrotizing. See *Vincent's angina*.
GIP (gastric inhibitory peptide), 1691t
Glabella reflex, 728
Glare, tolerance of, age-related changes in, 940
Glasgow Coma Scale (GCS), in Champion Trauma Score, 2518t

Glasgow Coma Scale (GCS) *(Continued)*
in increased intracranial pressure assessment, 778, *779–780*
Glaucoma, 952–958
classification of, 952, *953*
clinical manifestations of, 954
diagnostic findings in, 954
etiology of, 952–954
eye drops for, client teaching about, 957t
management of, 199t
community/self care in, 958
emergency, 954–955
in elderly, 956
medical, 955, *955*
nursing, 955–956
surgical, 956–957
complications of, 957–958
nursing care after, 957–958
outcome of, 958
pathophysiology of, 954
prevention of, 954b
risk factors for, 952–954, 954b
Glioblastoma multiforme, *846*
Gliomas, 844, *844*
Glipizide (Glucotrol), for diabetes mellitus, 1967t
in surgical client, 458t
Global aphasia, 789
Globulins, in hepatobiliary disease, 1849, 1850t
Glomerular filtration rate (GFR), 1540–1541
changes in, in shock, 509–510
Glomerular sclerosis, focal, 1634
Glomerulonephritis, acute, 1630–1632
clinical manifestations of, 1631
diagnostic findings in, 1631
etiology of, 1630
management of, complications of, 1631
in elderly, 1632
medical, 1631
nursing, 1631–1632
pathophysiology of, 1630–1631
risk factors for, 1630
chronic, 1632–1633
classification of, 1630b
membranoproliferative, 1633
membranous, idiopathic, 1634
minimal change, 1634
rapidly progressive, 1634
Glomerulosclerosis, in diabetes mellitus, 1625–1626
Glossopharyngeal nerve, assessment of, *719*, 721
Glottis, 1023, *1024*
Glucagon, actions of, 1940t
for hypoglycemia, 1990
in carbohydrate metabolism, 1945–1946
in hypokalemia, 305
Glucocorticoids, 2048t
actions of, 1940t
dysfunction of, 2044t
for rheumatoid arthritis, 663–665, 664t
function of, 2044t
in carbohydrate metabolism, 1946
in hypercortisolism, 2050
in immune system depression, 605
in shock, 509

Glucocorticoids *(Continued)*
synthesis of, adrenal cortex in, 1944–1945
Gluconeogenesis, liver in, 1839
Glucophage (metformin), for diabetes mellitus, 1967t, 1968
Glucose, blood, fasting, 1961
fingerstick measurement of, in decreased peripheral tissue perfusion, nursing research on, 515b
measurement of, in cardiovascular assessment, 1220
postprandial, 1961
random, 1961
self-monitoring of, 1961–1962, 1975
for hyperkalemia, 312
in urine, 1558
self-testing of, 1975
level of, total parenteral nutrition in, 1756
metabolism of, glucocorticoids in, 1944
preoperative evaluation of, 453t
tolerance of, impaired, in acute pancreatitis, 1923, 1924t
utilization of, decreased, in type II diabetes mellitus, 1959
Glucose-6-phosphate dehydrogenase (G6PD) deficiency, 1483
Glucosuria, in diabetes mellitus, 1959
Glucotrol (glipizide), for diabetes mellitus, 1967t
in surgical client, 458
Gluteal setting exercise, after cerebrovascular accident, 800
Glyburide (DiaBeta, Micronase), for diabetes mellitus, 1967t
in surgical client, 458t
Glycerin (Osmoglyn), for glaucoma, 954
Glycogenesis, liver in, 1839
Glycogenolysis, liver in, 1839
Glycopyrrolate (Robinul), preoperative, 465t
Glycosuria, 1558
Glycosylated albumin, in diabetes mellitus diagnosis, 1962
Glycosylated hemoglobin (Hb A_{1c}), in diabetes mellitus diagnosis, 1962
Glynase Pres Tabs, for diabetes mellitus, 1967t
GM-CSF (granulocyte-macrophage colony-stimulating factor), for cancer, 586
GNP (gerontological nurse practitioner), 82
GnRH (gonadotropin-releasing hormone), analogs of, for benign prostatic hyperplasia, 2364t
in male sexual development, 2304
Goals, postoperative, establishment of, 485
Goeckerman treatment, 2203
Goiter, 2007, *2009*
in Graves' disease, 2018
management of, 2014
prevention of, 2015–2016
types of, 2005–2006
Gold, implantation of, for prostate cancer, 2368
Gold salts (Solganal, Myochrysine), for rheumatoid arthritis, 664t
Golgi apparatus, 266
Golgi tendon organs, 700
Gonadotropic hormones, actions of, 1940t

Gonadotropin-releasing hormone (GnRH), analogs of, for benign prostatic hyperplasia, 2364t
in male sexual development, 2304
Gonads, development of, 2293
disorders of, 2041–2069
Gonorrhea, 2465–2469
clinical manifestations in, 2468
diagnostic findings in, 2468
etiology of, 2465
infectious agent in, 416t
management of, 2461t
community/self care in, 2468–2469
medical, 2468
nursing, 2468–2469
pathophysiology of, 2465–2468
risk factors for, 2465
Gonorrhea culture, schedule for, 210t
Gore-Tex catheter, for peritoneal dialysis, *1650*
Goserelin acetate (Zoladex), for benign prostatic hyperplasia, 2364t
Gout, *2107*, 2107–2108
Gouty arthritis, *2107*, 2107–2108
Government, in elderly support, 93–94
in healthcare system, 3–4
Graafian follicle, 2300
Gracilis flap, 2280
Gradient, 1375
Graefe's sign, 976
Graft(ing), arteriovenous, internal, for hemodialysis, 1652
in arterial bypass, 1414, *1414*
of bone, for fracture nonunion, 2145–2146, *2146*
of skin. See *Skin grafts.*
Graft rejection, 642
after corneal transplantation, 966–967, *967*
after organ transplantation, 643–644, 644t
after renal transplantation, 1661–1662
Graft-versus-host disease (GVHD), 640, 644–645, *645*
after bone marrow transplantation, 1497
Gram-negative bacterial pneumonia, 1136t
Grand mal seizures, 837, *837*
Granular casts, 1559
Granulation tissue, in wound healing, 432
Granulocyte colony-stimulating factor (G-CSF), for cancer, 586
Granulocyte concentrates, transfusion of, 1520t–1523t
Granulocyte-macrophage colony-stimulating factor (GM-CSF), for cancer, 586
Granulocytes, functions of, 1448t
in erythropoiesis, 1451
Granulocytopenia, 1458. See *Agranulocytosis.*
Granuloma, chronic inflammation and, 437
Granuloma inguinale, 2475
Graphesthesia, testing of, 724
Grasp reflex, 728
Graves' disease. See *Hyperthyroidism.*
Graves' exophthalmos, *976*, 976–977
Gray matter, 689
Gray Panthers, 97b
Greek civilization, healthcare in, history of, 19

Greenfield filter, for pulmonary embolism, 1129, *1130*

Greenstick fracture, *2130,* 2131

Grief, 73–74
cultural issues in, 70b–71b
process of, 109–110
stages of, 74
unresolved, 74

Grieving, anticipatory, after spinal cord injury, 910
in glaucoma, 956
in leiomyoma, 2402–2403

Grip, strength of, assessment of, 2088t

Groh model, for ethical decision-making, 43, 44t

Grooming, assessment of, 235

Groshong single-lumen catheter, *579*

Growing Younger, 175b

Growth, abnormal, in endocrine disorders, 1949
history of, in neurologic system assessment, 714
of malignant tumors, 546–548, *548*
of neoplastic cells, 546

Growth and development, in endocrine disorders, 1949
screening of, 207t

Growth factors, in hematopoiesis, 1455
in wound healing, 431–432
topical application of, for wound infection, 446

Growth hormone (GH), 2061t
actions of, 1940t
deficiency of, in hypopituitarism, 2065
management of, 2066
measurement of, in pituitary function testing, 1954
overproduction of, in hyperpituitarism, 2062, 2063t

Guaiac test, 1711–1712

Guanabenz (Wytensin), 1396t

Guanadrel (Hylorel), 1397t

Guanethidine (Ismelin), 1397t

Guanfacine (Tenex), 1396t

Guidance, anticipatory, in family nursing intervention, 58–59

Guided imagery, in pain control, 349b, 369–370

Guillain-Barré syndrome (GBS), 877
critical monitoring in, 878b

Guillain-Barré Syndrome Foundation International, 887b

Guillotine amputation, 1418, *1418*

Gums, disease of. See *Periodontal disease.*

Gunshot wound, 2520t

Guttate, definition of, 2183t

GVHD (graft-versus-host disease), 640, 644–645, *645*
after bone marrow transplantation, 1497

Gynecologic disorders, 2386–2429
assessment of, 2307–2329
diagnostic tests in, 2320–2329
history in, 2307–2311, 2311t
physical examination in, 2312–2320
normal findings in, 2312b

Gynecologic history, 2308–2310
past, 2310

Gynecomastia, 2453, 2453b

Gynecomastia *(Continued)*
in cirrhosis, 1878t

Gyrectomy, for pain, 386

H

H₂-receptor antagonists, for acute gastritis, 1762
for peptic ulcer disease, 1767

Habits, evaluation of, in cardiovascular disorders, 1210
in endocrine disorders, 1950
in gastrointestinal disorders, 1706
in gynecologic disorders, 2310
in hematologic disorders, 1462
in hepatobiliary disorders, 1844–1845
in immune disorders, 609
in integumentary system disorders, 2182
in male reproductive disorders, 2331
in musculoskeletal disorders, 2086
in respiratory disorders, 1039
in urinary tract disorders, 1551
life-style, preoperative assessment of, 457

Haemophilus ducreyi, and chancroid, 2475

Haemophilus influenzae, 416t

Hageman factor, 1516t

Hair, assessment of, in health history, 183b
changes in, in endocrine disorders, 1949
distribution of, 2185–2186
altered, in cirrhosis, 1878t
inspection of, in peripheral vascular assessment, 1380
physical examination of, 2185–2186
normal findings in, 2182b
structure of, 2175

Hair follicles, structure/function of, 2175, 2176t

Halcinonide (Halog), topical, 2199t

Haldol (haloperidol), for dementia of Alzheimer's type, 865, 866t

"Half-and-half" nail, in chronic renal failure, 1646

Hallucinations, 765
assessment of, 710t
hypnagogic, 400

Hallucinogens, abuse of, 2491
effects of, 2483t
health consequences of, 2493t
withdrawal from, symptoms of, 2487t

Hallux valgus, 2124, *2124*

Halo traction, for spinal cord injury, 898, *898*

Halo vest, for cervical fractures, 914
use of, client education in, 906b

Halog (halcinonide), topical, 2199t

Haloperidol (Haldol), for dementia of Alzheimer's type, 865, 866t

Halothane (Fluothane), 470t

Hamartoma, 1155

Hammer toe, 2124–2125, *2125*

Hamstrings, strength of, assessment of, 2088t

Hand(s), deformity of, in rheumatoid arthritis, 658–659, *659*
disorders of, 2124
function of, assessment of, 2090t
repetitive motion injuries of, 2169t

Hand arthroplasty, for rheumatoid arthritis, 674

Hangman's fracture, cervical, 891, *893*

Hansen's disease, 1139

Hardiness, in stress response, 28

Harrington rods, for scoliosis, 2120, *2121*

Harris tube, 1749t, 1750

Hashimoto's disease, 2025
diagnostic tests for, 2027t
management of, medical, 2027
pathophysiology of, 2026

Haustra, 1694

Haustral churning, 1695

Haversian canal, 2074, *2075*

Haversian systems, 2074, *2075*

Hb A₁c (glycosylated hemoglobin), in diabetes mellitus diagnosis, 1962

HBO (hyperbaric oxygenation), for shock, 516
for wound infection, 446

HBsAg, testing of, before blood transfusion, 1524t

HBV (hepatitis B virus), immunization against, 421

HCFA (Health Care Financing Administration), 4

HCG (human chorionic gonadotropin), in cancer diagnosis, 558t

HCO₃⁻, analysis of, 1057

HCWs (healthcare workers), human immunodeficiency virus transmission to, 615–620
substance abuse in, 2497–2498, 2498b
ethical issues in, 2498b

HD (Huntington's disease), 883
ethical issues in, 884b

HDLs (high-density lipoproteins), 35
in coronary artery disease, 1241
low, in diabetes mellitus, 1977

Head, assessment of, in cardiovascular assessment, 1212–1213, *1213*
in health history, 183b
in regional examination, 214t–217t
neurologic, 718
normal findings in, 717b
injury to, and sleep disorders, 404
inspection of, in respiratory assessment, 1040
lymph nodes of, palpation of, 610t
physical examination of, in endocrine disorders, 1950

Head and neck cancer, staging of, 1085, 1086b

Head noises (tinnitus), 1003

Head position, assessment of, 722

Head trauma, 820–831, 2528–2529, 2528t
acceleration, 821, *821*
blunt, 821
client education in, 829b
clinical manifestations of, 823–824
complications of, 825–826
coup-contrecoup, *821,* 822, *822*
deceleration, 821, *821*
deformation, 821, *821*
diagnostic findings in, 823–824, *824*
etiology of, *821,* 821–823, *822*
management of, community/self care in, 829
emergency, 824–825
in elderly, 828

Head trauma (Continued)
    medical, 825–826
    nursing, 826–828
    surgical, 829
  mechanisms of, 821, 821–822, 822
  outcome of, 826
  pathophysiology of, 823
  penetrating, 821–822
  prevention of, 822b
  risk factors for, 821–823, 822b
  types of, 822–823
Headaches, 358, 817, 817–820, 818b
  brain tumor and, 846
  cluster, 819–820
  extracranial, 358
  intracranial, 358
  migraine, 358, 818–819, 818b
    atypical, 819
    classic, 819
    client education in, 818b
    treatment of, 819
  post-LP, 744–745
  spinal anesthesia and, 476t
  tension (muscle contraction), 820
  types of, 817, 817
  vascular, 358
Head-to-toe assessment, 225, 225b
  periodic, 226
Healers, indigenous, 62–63
Healing, of bone, 2132–2134, 2133, 2134t
    factors in, 2133–2134, 2134t
  of pressure ulcers, monitoring of, 2216
  of wound. See Wound healing.
"Healing ridge," 437
Health, beliefs about, assessment of, 193t
    non-Western, 61
    Western, 61
  concept of, 36–37
  definitions of, 149, 161, 162t
  optimal, in American healthcare system,
    62
  socioeconomic issues in, 168b
  state of, assessment of, 234
  theories of, 18–37
Health assessment, 179–212
  after physical examination, 240–241
  health history in. See Health history.
  nursing process in, 211, 211b
  stereotyping during, reduction of, 180,
    180b
Health Belief Model, 164–165
Health Care Financing Administration
  (HCFA), 4
Health fairs, in home healthcare, 166b
Health habits, assessment of, in cross-cultural nursing, 64b
Health history, 179–212
  accuracy of, 179–180, 180b
  components of, 186–206
    biographical/demographic information
      in, 186–187
    family history in, 188, 188
    physical history in, 187–188
      current, 187
      past, 187–188
    psychosocial history in, 188–197. See
      also Psychosocial history.
  computerization of, 180

Health history (Continued)
  depth of, 180, 181b–185b, 185, 186b
  episodic, 185, 186b
  family, in ear disorders, 986
    in endocrine disorders, 1950
    in eye disorders, 942
    in gastrointestinal tract disorders, 1705
    in gynecologic disorders, 2310
    in hematologic disorders, 1462
    in hepatobiliary disorders, 1844
    in immune disorders, 608
    in integumentary system disorders, 2181
    in male reproductive disorders, 2331
    in musculoskeletal disorders, 2085
    in neurologic disorders, 714
    in peripheral vascular disorders, 1379
    in respiratory disorders, 1039
    in urinary tract disorders, 1550
  format of, 180, 181b–185b, 2552–2554
  health promotion in, 197–206, 198t–204t,
    205–206, 205b, 207t–210t
  health risk appraisal in, 197–206, 198t–
    204t, 205b, 207t–210t
  interview in, guidelines for, 185–186
    client preparation in, 186
    environment preparation in, 185–186
    interviewer preparation in, 186
  organization of, 206–211
  recording of, 211
  past, in cardiovascular disorders, 1207
    in ear disorders, 985–986
    in endocrine disorders, 1949
    in eye disorders, 942
    in gastrointestinal tract disorders, 1699–
      1705
    in gynecologic disorders, 2308
    in hematologic disorders, 1461–1462
    in hepatobiliary disorders, 1844
    in immune disorders, 608
    in integumentary system disorders,
      2180–2181, 2181t
    in male reproductive disorders, 2330
    in musculoskeletal disorders, 2084–2085
    in neurologic disorders, 714
    in peripheral vascular disorders, 1378–
      1379
    in respiratory disorders, 1038
      upper, 1048
    in urinary tract disorders, 1549–1550
  review of systems in, 182b–185b, 197
  screening tests in, 206
Health insurance, inadequate, health risks
  of, 204t
Health maintenance, altered, after spinal
    cord injury, 912–913
  after thoracic surgery, 1162
  in diabetes mellitus, 1974–1975
  in epilepsy, 839
  in hypertension, 1402–1403
  in myocardial infarction, 1272–1273
  in premenstrual syndrome, 2389
Health maintenance organization (HMO), 5b
Health management, pattern of, 206
Health perception, pattern of, 206
Health promotion, 161–176, 197–206,
  198t–204t, 205b, 207t–210t
  client motivation in, 170
  concept of, evolution of, 162–164

Health promotion (Continued)
  definition of, 161
  environment protection in, 169–170
  exercise in, 171
  human potential development in, 168,
    168–169
  in disabled patients, 108b
  in elderly, 84–86, 85, 85b, 86b, 173–175,
    174b, 174t, 175b
    nursing research on, 85b
    resources for, 175b
  lifelong, 205–206, 207t–210t
  life-style in, 167–168, 168b
  models of, 164, 164–165
  nursing careers in, 175
  nutrition in, 170–171, 171–173
  prevention in, levels of, 165–166, 165t
    primary, 165, 165t
    secondary, 165–166, 165t
    tertiary, 165t, 166
  risk factors in, 167, 167t
  stress management in, 171–173
  understanding of, 161–165, 163
Health risks, appraisal of, 197–206, 198t–
    204t, 205b, 207t–210t
  in cross-cultural nursing, 65
Health Security Act, 9
Health seeking behaviors, in chronic arterial
  occlusion, 1412
Healthcare, for elderly, 94–96, 96
  economic issues in, 84
  resources/services in, 96–99, 96b, 97t
  history of, 18–20, 19
  home. See Home healthcare.
  long-term, for elderly, resources/services
    in, 97t, 98
  outcomes of, monitoring of, 127–129
    access issues in, 129
    functional status measurement in, 129
    patient satisfaction surveys in, 127–
      129
  quality, delivery of, assurance of, 125–
    131
  uncompensated, 5b
  women's, diversity in, 2424b–2429b
Healthcare system, United States, Canadian
    system vs., 14b–15b
  components of, 3–6
  financing of, 5b, 6–10
  future of, 10b–11b
  reform of, 9–10, 10b–11b
Healthcare team, definition of, 136b
Healthcare workers (HCWs), human immu-
    nodeficiency virus transmission to, 615–
    620
  substance abuse in, 2497–2498, 2498b
    ethical issues in, 2498b
Healthy People 2000, 162–163
Hearing, age-related changes in, 984t
  assessment of, 713t
  disorders of, management of, 199t
  inner ear in, 984
  screening of, 207t
Hearing aids, 996–997, 997
  care of, 1001b
  implantable, 1001, 1012
Hearing education, 998
Hearing impairment, 993–1001

Hearing impairment (Continued)
  clinical manifestations of, 994–995, 996t
  clues suggesting, 984b
  communication in, improvement of, 1000b
  diagnostic findings in, 994–995
  etiology of, 993–994
  management of, community/self care in,
    995–1001
    medical, 995–998, 997
    nursing, 998–1000, 999b, 1000b
    surgical, 1000–1001
  pathophysiology of, 994
  prevention of, 204t, 995b
  quality of life in, nursing research on,
    1000b
  risk factors for, 993–994, 995b
Hearing loss, conductive, 992
  clinical manifestations of, 996t
    etiology of, 993
    pathophysiology of, 994
  high-frequency, 992
  history of, 985
  sensorineural, 992
    clinical manifestations of, 996t
    etiology of, 993
    pathophysiology of, 994
  severe, living with, 999b
  types of, 994, 994b
Heart. See also Cardiac; Cardiovascular.
  age-related changes in, 1204
  assessment of, in health history, 184b
    in regional examination, 218t–219t
  automaticity of, 1196
  blood supply to, 1194, 1194–1195
  chambers of, 1191, 1193
  conduction system of, 1197–1198, 1198
  conductivity of, 1196
  cycle of, 1198–1199, 1199
  disorders of, assessment of, 1205–1237
  donation of, guidelines for, 2514t
  dysfunction of, in acute pancreatitis, 1923,
    1924t
  excitability of, 1195–1196, 1195–1197
  function of, 1191–1204, 1192
    disorders of, 1238–1291
    regulation of, 1202–1204
  infections of, 1327–1338
  layers of, 1191, 1192
  mechanical, 1354
  properties of, electrophysiologic, 1195–
    1197, 1195–1197
    mechanical, 1199–1202, 1200b, 1201
  refractoriness of, 1197
  structure of, 1191–1204, 1193
    disorders of, 1327–1364
  surgery of, 1350–1363
    community/self care after, 926
    in elderly, 926
    nursing care after, 1356–1363
    open, 1354–1355, 1355
    preparation for, medical, 1355
      nursing, 1009b, 1355–1356
      psychological, 1009b, 1355–1356
    types of, 1351
  valves of, 1193, 1194
Heart attack. See Myocardial infarction
  (MI).
Heart disease, congenital, 1350

Heart disease (Continued)
  in hyperthyroidism, 2019
  in rheumatoid arthritis, 659
  management of, 198t
  screening for, 209t
  valvular, 1338–1350, 1345
    in cardiogenic shock, management of,
      523t
    nursing management of, 1349–1350
Heart failure, 1276–1291
  after myocardial infarction, 1266
  backward vs. forward, 1282
  clinical manifestations of, 1279–1283,
    1280
  diagnostic findings in, 1279–1283
  etiology of, 1277–1278, 1277t
  high-output vs. low-output, 1282
  left vs. right ventricular, 1280, 1280–1282
  management of, community/self care in,
    1291
    in elderly, 1291
    medical, 1283–1287, 1283t, 1284t,
      1285t, 1286t, 1287b, 1289
    nursing, 1287–1289
    surgical, 1290
  pathophysiology of, 1278–1279, 1279
  risk factors for, 1277–1278, 1277t
    in cardiomyopathy, 1343
    in myxedema coma, 2012
  tachycardia and cardiogenic shock with,
    case study of, 1268–1269
  types of, 1279–1282
Heart rate, 1200–1201
  electrocardiographic analysis of, 1298b
Heart sounds, abnormal, 1215–1217
  assessment of, after cardiac surgery, 1358
  auscultation of, 1214–1217, 1215
  extra, 1199
  normal, 1214, 1215
Heart transplantation, 1352–1353
  complications of, 649t
  criteria for, 646, 1353b
  for heart failure, 1290
  heterotopic, 1353, 1354
  immunosuppression after, 1353, 1354b
  orthotopic, 1353, 1353
Heartburn, 1733
  sleep disorders in, 405
Heart-lung machine, for open heart surgery,
  1354–1355, 1355
Heart-lung transplantation, criteria for, 646
Heat, and cell damage, 269
  application of, delegation of, 2165b
    for shock, contraindications to, 522–523
    in inflammation management, 436
  loss of, intraoperative, prevention of,
    478
  production of, muscles in, 2079
Heat cramps, 2535
Heat emergencies, 2534–2535
Heat exhaustion, 2535
Heat stroke, 2535
Heater-probe therapy, for bleeding ulcers,
  1772
Heaves, palpation of, 1213
Heavy metals, antidote for, 2538t
Heberden's nodes, in osteoarthritis, 2109,
  2110

Height, assessment of, 236
  schedule for, 209t
Height vertigo, 1011
Heimlich maneuver, 2505
Helicobacter pylori, and chronic gastritis,
  1763
  and peptic ulcer disease, 1764–1765
Helicotrema, 984
Helix, 980, 981
Heller's procedure, for achalasia, 1735,
  1735
Hemarthrosis, in hemophilia, management
  of, 1517
Hematemesis, in peptic ulcer disease, 1771
Hematocele, 2377
Hematochezia, 1787
Hematocrit, determination of, in cardiovascular disorders, 1219
  in hematologic disorders, 1464, 1464t
  evaluation of, preoperative, 453t
    schedule for, 208t
  in blood dyscrasias, 1465t
  in gastrointestinal tract assessment,
    1711t
  reference values for, in cancer, 557t
Hematologic studies, in immune disorder
  assessment, 611
  in urinary tract assessment, 1562
Hematologic system, abnormalities of,
  1458–1459
  age-related changes in, 1459
  disorders of, 1469–1530
    assessment of, 1461–1468
      diagnostic tests in, 1463–1468, 1464t,
        1465t, 1466t, 1467t
      history in, 1461–1463
      physical examination in, 1463, 1465b
    congenital, 1512–1518
  in chronic renal failure, 1645
  in hypocalcemia, 317t
  in thyroid disorders, 2008t
  preoperative assessment of, 456–457
  structure/function of, 1447–1459
Hematology, reference values in, 2555–
  2556
Hematoma, epidural, 744, 830, 830
  extradural, 830, 830
  formation of, in bone healing, 2132–2133,
    2133
  intracerebral, 831
    traumatic, delayed, 831
  perichondrial, 1007
  subdural, 744, 830–831
    acute, 831
    chronic, 831
    evacuation of, positioning after, 853
Hematomyelia, 917
Hematopoiesis, 1447–1455
  assessment of, in health history, 183b
  control of, 1453–1455
  events in, 1449–1452, 1450–1453
  liver in, 1452–1453, 1454
  ontogeny of, 1448–1449
  spleen in, 1452–1453, 1454
Hematopoietic system, in alcohol abuse,
  2490b
Hematuria, 1548, 1558–1559
  in bladder cancer, 1583

Hemianesthesia, cerebrovascular accident and, 791–792

Hemianopia, homonymous, cerebrovascular accident and, 790, *791*

Hemilaryngectomy, 1087, *1087*

Hemiparesis, cerebrovascular accident and, 787, *789*
  left, reflex documentation in, *728*

Hemiplegia, cerebrovascular accident and, 787, *789*
  ineffective coping in, 806

Hemispherectomy, for epilepsy, 841, *841*

Hemochromatosis, 1902

Hemochromogens, in burns, 2249

Hemodialysis, 1650–1654
  dialyzers for, 1653
  history of, 1650–1651
  long-term, complications of, 1653–1654
  procedure for, 1651–1653, *1651–1653*
  schedules for, 1653

Hemodilution, hypervolemic, for cerebrovascular accident, 793
  hypertensive, for intracranial hemorrhage, 814

Hemodynamic hypothesis, of coronary artery disease pathogenesis, 1243

Hemodynamic monitoring, in shock, 525–526

Hemodynamic studies, in cardiovascular assessment, 1233–1237, *1234–1235*, 1236t

Hemoglobin, determination of, in gastrointestinal disorders, 1711t
  in hematologic disorders, 1464, 1464t
  evaluation of, preoperative, 453t
    schedule for, 208t
  glycosylated, in diabetes mellitus diagnosis, 1962
  in blood dyscrasias, 1465t
  reference values for, in cancer, 557t

Hemoglobin C disease, 1482

Hemoglobin electrophoresis, in sickle cell anemia diagnosis, 1514

Hemoglobinemia, paroxysmal, 1480–1481
  nocturnal, 1480–1481

Hemoglobinopathies, 1481–1482

Hemolytic anemia, 1478–1481
  autoimmune disorders and, 1480
  chemical agents and, 1479
  clinical manifestations of, 1478, 1479t
  hallmark of, 1478
  infections and, 1479–1480
  intrinsic red blood cell defects and, 1483
  isoimmune hemolytic reactions and, 1480
  medications and, 1479
  systemic disease and, 1480
  trauma and, 1479
  treatment of, 1478–1479

Hemolytic jaundice, 1858, 1859t

Hemophilia(s), 1515–1518
  clinical manifestations of, 1516–1517
  diagnostic findings in, 1516–1517
  etiology of, 1516
  forms of, 1515, 1515t
  management of, medical, 1517
    nursing, 1517–1518
  pathophysiology of, 1516, 1516t
  risk factors for, 1516

Hemophilia A, 1515t

Hemophilia B, 1515t

Hemoptysis, assessment of, 1036

Hemorrhage, acute, assessment findings in, 498t
  classification of, 498t
  after cardiac surgery, 1014
  after laryngeal surgery, 1088
  after oral cancer surgery, 1730
  after prostatectomy, 2360–2361
  after renal biopsy, 1569
  after thyroidectomy, 2023
  after tooth extraction, 1722–1723
  after vulvectomy, 2420
  and cerebrovascular accident, 785
    clinical manifestations of, 787t
    supportive care of, 797
  and hypovolemic shock, 498, 498t
  chemotherapy and, 582
  diagnosis of, laboratory tests in, 1467t
  gastrointestinal. See *Gastrointestinal bleeding.*
  in abdominal aortic aneurysm, 1427
  in bladder cancer, 1589
  in cirrhosis, 1879–1882
  in intestinal disorders, 1787, *1788*
  in leukemia, 1492–1493
  in peptic ulcer disease, *1771,* 1771–1772, 1776, 1778
  in periodontal disease, 1722
  in portal hypertension, 1886
  in splenic rupture, 1505
  intracranial. See *Intracranial hemorrhage.*
  of upper airway, 1076–1082
  splinter, 2187t
    in infective endocarditis, 1333
  subarachnoid, 812–816
  subconjunctival, red eye in, 942b

Hemorrhagic anemias, 1481

Hemorrhagic disorders, 1506, 1506t

Hemorrhagic exudate, 434, 435t

Hemorrhoidectomy, 1827
  nursing care after, 1828

Hemorrhoids, 1825–1828, *1826*
  clinical manifestations of, 1826
  diagnostic findings in, 1826
  etiology of, 1826
  in cirrhosis, 1878t
  management of, medical, 1827
    nursing, 1827–1828
    surgical, 1827
  pathophysiology of, 1826
  risk factors for, 1826

Hemostasis, 1456–1458, *1457, 1458*
  disorders of, classification of, 1506, 1506t
  laboratory tests for, 1852t

Hemothorax, 1027
  chest trauma and, *2525, 2526*

Henderson-Hasselbalch equation, in acid-base balance, 332, *332*

Heparin, contraindications to, 1434
  for disseminated intravascular coagulation, 1512
  for pulmonary embolism, 1128
  for shock, 520
  for venous thrombosis, 1434
  in anaphylaxis, 638t

Heparin *(Continued)*
  low molecular weight, for venous thrombosis, 1435

Heparin sodium, in surgical client, 458t

Hepatic artery, 1835

Hepatic encephalopathy, 1891–1895
  clinical manifestations of, 1892–1893
  diagnostic findings in, 1892–1893
  etiology of, 1891–1892, 1892b
  management of, community/self care in, 1895
    medical, 1893–1894
    nursing, 1894–1895
    outcomes in, 1893–1894
  paracentesis and, 1854
  pathophysiology of, 1892
  risk factors for, 1891–1892
  stages of, 1893, 1893b

Hepatic portal system, 1835, *1837*

Hepatitis, 1861–1872
  alcoholic, 1872
  chronic, 1867–1869, *1868, 1869*
  fulminant, 1866, 1867
  sexually transmitted, 2475
  toxic, 1871–1872, 1872t
  transmission of, blood transfusion in, 1528
  viral, 1861–1871
    clinical manifestations of, 1865–1866, 1866t
    community/self care in, 1870–1871
    diagnostic findings in, 1865–1866, 1866t
    etiology of, 1861
    management of, complications of, 1867–1869, *1868, 1869*
      dietary, 1867
      in elderly, 1871
      medical, 1866–1867, 1870
      nursing, 1869–1871
      outcomes of, 1869
      pharmacologic, 1867
    pathophysiology of, 1865
    prevention of, 1863–1865, 1863b
    risk factors for, 1861, 1863b
    serologic tests for, 1866, 1866t

Hepatitis A, 1861, 1862t
  etiology of, 1861
  pathophysiology of, 1865
  prevention of, 1863–1864, 1863b
  risk factors for, 1861, 1862t, 1863b

Hepatitis antigens/antibodies, laboratory tests for, 1851t

Hepatitis B, 1861, 1862t, 2475
  etiology of, 1861
  immunization recommendations for, in adults, 422t
  infectious agent in, 416t
  nosocomial, 419
  pathophysiology of, 1865
  prevention of, 1863b, 1864
  risk factors for, 1861, 1862t, 1863b

Hepatitis B immune globulin, 1864

Hepatitis B virus (HBV), immunization against, 421

Hepatitis C, 1861, 1862t
  etiology of, 1861
  pathophysiology of, 1865
  prevention of, 1863b, 1864
  risk factors for, 1861, 1862t, 1863b

Hepatitis D, 1861, 1862t
etiology of, 1861
pathophysiology of, 1865
prevention of, 1863b, 1864
risk factors for, 1861, 1862t, 1863b
Hepatitis E, 1861, 1862t
etiology of, 1861
pathophysiology of, 1865
prevention of, 1863b, 1865
risk factors for, 1861, 1862t, 1863b
Hepatitis fibrosis, congenital, 1903
Hepatocellular carcinoma, primary, 1896
Hepatocellular jaundice, 1858, 1859t
Hepatocytes, 1835, *1837*
Hepatoma, malignant, 1896
Hepatomegaly, in hemolytic anemia, 1479t
Hepatotoxins, 1872t
Herbal remedies, in pain control, 349b
Herd immunity, 421
Heredity, in cancer, 540–541
in coronary artery disease, 1238
in disease, 29–34, 32b
Hernia, and small intestinal obstruction,
1820
femoral, 1817, *1817*
examination for, 2335
hiatal. See *Hiatal hernia.*
inguinal, 1817, *1817*
examination for, *2334*, 2335
irreducible (incarcerated), 1817
reducible, 1817
Herniation, cerebral, in increased intracranial pressure, 772, *773*, 773–774
intervertebral disc. See *Intervertebral disc
herniation.*
intestinal, 1816–1818
etiology of, 1816
management of, medical, 1818
surgical, 1818
nursing care in, 1818
pathophysiology of, 1817, *1817*
risk factors for, 1816
Herpes, genital, 2472–2473
management of, 2462t
Herpes simplex, 2222t
oral, 1724, *1724*
clinical manifestations of, 1724, *1724*
diagnostic findings in, 1724
etiology of, 1724
management of, 1724
pathophysiology of, 1724
risk factors for, 1724
Herpes simplex keratitis, red eye in, 942b
Herpes simplex virus (HSV), in acquired
immunodeficiency syndrome, 630
management of, 2462t
Herpes simplex virus encephalitis, 859–860
Herpes zoster, 2223, *2223*
chest pain in, assessment of, 1209t
Hesitancy, 1548
Hetastarch, administration of, for shock,
519
Heterograft, xenograft, in burn wound covering, 2256t
Heterotopic ossification, after spinal cord injury, 904
HFV (high-frequency ventilation), 1177–
1179, 1179t

HGH (human growth hormone), for growth
hormone deficiency, 2066
HHNK (hyperglycemic, hyperosmolar, nonketotic coma), 1987–1988, 1987b, 1991t–
1992t
Hiatal hernia, 1740–1741, *1741*
clinical manifestations of, 1741
diagnostic findings in, 1741
etiology of, 1740
management of, 1741
pathophysiology of, 1740–1741
risk factors for, 1740
Hibiclens (chlorhexidine gluconate–alcohol), 2199t
Hickman single-lumen catheter, *579*
High blood pressure. See *Hypertension.*
High level wellness, 37, 162
High-accident-risk activity, health risks of,
204t
High-bolus urography, 1563
High-density lipoproteins (HDLs), 35
in coronary artery disease, 1241
low, in diabetes mellitus, 1977
High-flow filter, for blood transfusion,
1526t
High-frequency hearing loss, *992*
High-frequency ventilation (HFV), 1177–
1179, 1179t
Hill operation, for gastroesophageal reflux
disease, 1739
Hill-Burton Act, 7
Hinduism, beliefs/practices of, 2550
dietary practices of, 1701b
Hip(s), dislocation of, after intertrochanteric
hip fracture, 2157–2158
muscles of, strength of, assessment of,
2088t
range of motion of, *2089*
replacement of, total. See *Total hip replacement.*
Hip fracture, cerebrovascular accident and
meningioma with, case study of, *794,*
794–795
intertrochanteric, *2153*, 2153–2159
clinical manifestations of, 2154
diagnostic findings in, 2154
etiology of, 2154
management of, community/self care in,
2158–2159, 2159b
medical, 2154
nursing, 2154
surgical, 2154–2155
complications of, 2154–2155
nursing care in, 2155–2159
posthospital convalescence in, nursing
research on, 2159b
risk factors for, 2154
intracapsular, 2131, *2153*, 2159
Hip spica cast, 2137t, *2148*
Hippocampus, structure/function of, 691–
692
Hippocrates, 19
Hirschberg's test, 945
Hirschsprung's disease, 1830
Hirsutism, 2186
Hispanics, diabetes mellitus in, 198t
dietary practices of, 1702b–1703b
health/illness beliefs of, 61

Hispanics *(Continued)*
human immunodeficiency virus infection
in, 617b
skin examination in, 2188b
Histamine, in anaphylaxis, 638t
in blood pressure regulation, 1204, 1375
in wound healing, 430, *430*
release of, in shock, 507
Histamine receptor antagonists, for gastroesophageal reflux disease, 1738
for shock, 520–521
Histocompatibility, in organ transplantation,
641–643
testing for, in bone marrow transplantation, 1495
Histocompatibility antigens, 1456
Histoplasma capsulatum, 417t
Histoplasmosis, 1146
in acquired immunodeficiency syndrome,
629
infectious agent in, 417t
History, health. See *Health history.*
in cross-cultural nursing assessment, 63–
65, 64b
preoperative, 459
psychosocial. See *Psychosocial history.*
social, preoperative assessment of, 457
HIV encephalopathy, 631
HIV infection. See *Human immunodeficiency virus (HIV) infection.*
HIV wasting syndrome, 631
Hives, *2184*
chemotherapy and, 583
definition of, 2183t
HLA (human leukocyte antigen) system,
1456
in histocompatibility, 642–643
for bone marrow transplantation, 1495
HMO (health maintenance organization),
5b
Hodgkin's disease, 1500–1503
clinical manifestations of, 1501, *1502*
diagnostic findings in, 1501
etiology of, 1500–1501
management of, medical, 1502–1503,
1503t
nursing, 1503
surgical, 1501
nursing care in, 1502
MOPP regimen for, 576t
pathophysiology of, 1501
risk factors for, 1500–1501
staging of, 1501t
survival in, 538t
Holmes and Rahe's theory, of life change
and the onset of illness, 25–26, 25t
Holter monitoring, 1224–1225
Homans' sign, in peripheral vascular assessment, 1382
in thrombophlebitis, after total hip replacement, 2114
in venous thrombosis, 1434
Home healthcare, 123, 146–156
after cerebrovascular accident, for swallowing difficulties, 804b
after laryngectomy, 1099b
community-focused philosophy of, 148–
151

Home healthcare (Continued)
ethical issues in, in patient/family conflict, 150b
for elderly, 97–98
for immobile client, 913b
health fairs in, 166b
history of, 147–148
in Alzheimer's disease, in caregiver respite, 870b
in safety, 868b
in burn rehabilitation, 2262b
in cancer diagnosis coping, 587b
in cancer treatments, 565b
in cast/brace management, 2152b
in chronic conditions, 113
in coronary artery surgery rehabilitation, 1252b
in diabetic foot care, 1999b
in elder abuse, 90b
in failing vision, 964b
in hearing loss, 999b
in ileal conduit care, 1591b
in immunosuppression, nutrition in, 1494b
in intermittent self-catheterization, in males, 2351b
in mechanical ventilation, 1183b
in multiple medication management, 95b
in myocardial infarction convalescence, 1265b
in ostomy adjustment, 1804b
in oxygen conservation, in chronic obstructive pulmonary disease, 1125b
in pain control, 367b
in peripheral vascular disease, 1437b
in peritoneal dialysis, 1659b
in pressure ulcers, 2220b
in rheumatoid arthritis, 667b
in sexually transmitted disease education, 2465b
in substance abuse detection, 2484b
in tube feedings, 1755b
in universal precautions, 626b
in urinary catheter insertion, 1602b
intravenous therapy in, 284b
postoperative, 493b
provision of, 151–156
Nightingale Tracker System of, 154–156
Omaha system of, 151–154
intervention scheme in, 153–154, 154t, 155b
problem classification scheme in, 152–153, 152b, 153b, 154t
problem rating scale for outcomes in, 154, 156t
reimbursement for, financial resources for, 147, 147b
Medicare/Medicaid in, 148b
resources for, 150–151
risks of, 149
trends in, 146–147
Homeostasis, Bernard and Cannon's theory of, 21
musculoskeletal system in, 2079–2080
postoperative, restoration of, 485, 486t
skin in, 2177
Homograft, allograft, in burn wound covering, 2256t

Homonymous hemianopia, cerebrovascular accident and, 790, 791
Homosexuality, nursing care in, ethical issues in, 2344b
Homosexuals, 75
Honeymoon cystitis, 1572
Honeymoon period, in diabetes mellitus, 1959
Hordeolum, 972
Hormonal therapy, for breast cancer, 2449, 2449t
Hormone assays, in pituitary function testing, 1954
Hormone replacement therapy (HRT), for menopause, 2392–2394
in osteoporosis prevention, 2100
Hormones, actions of, 1940t
characteristics of, 1939–1940
classification of, 1939
digestive, 1691t
effect of, on male reproductive system, 2345
female, 2298
for prostate cancer, 2368
nursing care in, 2368–2369
functions of, 1937–1939
imbalances of, and sleep disorders, 404
in blood flow regulation, 1374
in cancer, 540
in carbohydrate metabolism, 1945–1946, 1946
in cardiac regulation, 1203–1204
in chemotherapy, classification of, 577t
in fluid balance regulation, 276–277
in sperm formation, 2305
of adrenal glands, dysfunction of, 2044t
function of, 2044t
of pituitary gland, 1939, 2061t
regulation of, 1940–1941, 1941, 1942
secretion of, patterns of, 1939–1940
surgical manipulation of, for breast cancer, 2437–2438
Horner's syndrome, cerebrovascular accident and, 790
lung cancer in, 1152
Horseshoe kidney, 1678, 1678
Hospice care, for elderly, 98
in chronic conditions, 113
in terminal cancer, 566–567
Hospital(s), acute care, 120–121, 121b, 122b
admission to, methods of, 121, 121b
government-owned, 121
infection control in, 422–424
barrier precautions in, 423
occupational health practices in, 424
standard precautions in, 423–424
transmission-based precautions in, 423–424
universal precautions in, 423–424
magnet, 121
mergers of, 121
personnel/departments of, 122b
proprietary, 121
service lines of, 121
voluntary, 121
Hospital administrators/governing boards, in healthcare delivery, 4

Hospital nursing, 11–12
future of, 131–132
history of, 120
roles/responsibilities in, 123–124
Hospitalization, history of, in cardiovascular disorders, 1207
in ear disorders, 986
in endocrine disorders, 1949
in eye disorders, 942
in gastrointestinal disorders, 1704
in gynecologic disorders, 2308
in hematologic disorders, 1461–1462
in hepatobiliary disorders, 1844
in male reproductive disorders, 2330
in musculoskeletal disorders, 2085
in neurologic disorders, 714
in respiratory disorders, 1038
in urinary tract disorders, 1550
infection during, 417–419, 418t
sexuality during, 79
Host defense, 415–417
in hypersensitivity, 636
Hot flashes, in menopause, 2393
management of, 2394
Hot-cold theory, 1700b
Hot-spot imaging, 255
House sharing, elderly in, 100
Housing, congregate, for elderly, 100
for elderly, 98t, 100
HPA (hypothalamic-pituitary-adrenal) axis, 2049
HPV (human papillomavirus), management of, 2462t
HRT (hormone replacement therapy), for menopause, 2392–2394
in osteoporosis prevention, 2100
HSV (herpes simplex virus), in acquired immunodeficiency syndrome, 630
management of, 2462t
HTLV-III (human T-cell lymphotropic virus type III), 614
Hubbard tank, for hydrotherapy, in burns, 2253
Humalog, 1969, 1969t
Human bites, 2536–2537
Human chorionic gonadotropin (HCG), in cancer diagnosis, 558t
Human Genome Project, 551
Human growth hormone (HGH), for growth hormone deficiency, 2066
Human immunodeficiency virus (HIV) infection, 16, 416t, 614–636
advanced. See Acquired immunodeficiency syndrome (AIDS).
and pain, 359
assessment of, 625
classification of, 622b
clinical manifestations of, 621–623, 622b
diagnostic findings in, 621–623
etiology of, 614–615
in minority populations, 616b–619b
management of, community/self care in, 623–625
medical, 623–625
nursing, 625–627
ocular manifestations of, 977
pathophysiology of, 620–621
perioperative effects of, 457

Human immunodeficiency virus (HIV) infection *(Continued)*
risk factors for, 615–620
testing for, in alleged sexual assault, 2532
schedule for, 210t
transmission of, 615–620
during blood transfusion, 1519, 1528
in healthcare setting, 419
Human leukocyte antigen (HLA) system, 1456
in histocompatibility, 642–643
for bone marrow transplantation, 1495
Human papillomavirus (HPV), management of, 2462t
Human potential, development of, in health promotion, *168,* 168–169
Human T-cell lymphotropic virus type III (HTLV-III), 614
Humans, early, healthcare for, 18, *19*
Humerus, fracture of, 2161
Humoral immunity, 595
Humors, 61
Humulin insulin, types of, 1969, 1969t
"Hungry bones" syndrome, in hyperparathyroidism, 2035
Hunner's ulcer. See *Interstitial cystitis (IC).*
Huntington's disease (HD), 883
ethical issues in, 884b
Hyaline cartilage, 2076
Hyaline casts, 1559
Hydatidiform mole, 2423
Hydralazine (Apresoline), 1397t
for heart failure, 1286
for hypertensive emergency, 1405t
Hydration, ethical issues in, 281b
in hyperparathyroidism, 2031–2033
with tracheostomy, 1072–1074
Hydrocele, 2377, *2377*
Hydrocephalus, after intracranial hemorrhage, 815
head trauma and, 825
Hydrochloric acid, loss of, and metabolic alkalosis, 336
Hydrochlorothiazide (Esidrix, Hydro-DIURIL), 1394t
characteristics of, 1285t
Hydrocodone, in pain control, 375t
Hydrocolloid gel (DuoDerm), 2199t
indications for, 443t
Hydrocortisone (Hydrocortone, Synacort, Hytone), 2048t
for rheumatoid arthritis, 664t
topical, 2199t
Hydrocortisone cream, 2200t
Hydrocortisone sodium succinate (Solu-Cortef), in surgical client, 458t
Hydrocortone (hydrocortisone), 2048t
for rheumatoid arthritis, 664t
topical, 2199t
HydroDIURIL (hydrochlorothiazide), 1394t
characteristics of, 1285t
Hydroflumethiazide (Diucardin, Saluron), 1394t
Hydrogels, in wound management, indications for, 443t
Hydrogen, concentration of, *294,* 294t
Hydrogen ion, regulation of, kidneys in, 1542–1543

Hydrogen peroxide, for open wounds, 445t
topical, 2199t
Hydrogen peroxide rinses, for oral care, nursing research on, 1725b
Hydrolysis reaction, 328, *329*
Hydromorphone (Dilaudid), administration of, 380t
Hydromox (quinethazone), 1394t
Hydronephrosis, 1636
benign prostatic hyperplasia and, *2351, 2352*
Hydrostatic pressure, 274
in glomerular filtration rate, 1541
Hydrotherapy, for burns, 2253, *2253*
Hydroureter, benign prostatic hyperplasia and, *2351,* 2352
Hydroxychloroquine (Plaquenil), for rheumatoid arthritis, 664t
17-Hydroxysteroids, 2045t
in hypercortisolism, 2050–2051
Hydroxyurea, for chronic myelogenous leukemia, 1491
Hydroxyzine (Vistaril), for interstitial cystitis, 1580
in pain control, 374
Hygiene, assessment of, 235
in hepatitis A prevention, 1863
in hepatitis B prevention, 1864
oral, with endotracheal tube, 1175–1176
Hygroton (chlorthalidone), 1394t
characteristics of, 1285t
Hylorel (guanadrel), 1397t
Hymen, examination of, 2317
Hypalgesia, 724
Hyperaldosteronism, and metabolic alkalosis, 336
primary, 2055–2056
clinical manifestations of, 2055–2056
diagnostic findings in, 2055–2056
etiology of, 2055
management of, medical, 2056, 2056b
nursing, 2056
surgical, 2056
pathophysiology of, 2055, *2055*
risk factors for, 2055
secondary, 2055
Hyperalgesia, 724
Hyperalimentation, 1754–1756
Hyperamylasemia, in acute pancreatitis, 1923
Hyperbaric oxygenation (HBO), for shock, 516
for wound infection, 446
Hyperbilirubinemia, in jaundice, 1858
Hypercalcemia, 320–322
cardiac effects of, 1220
clinical manifestations of, 320–321, 321t
diagnostic findings in, 320–321, 321t
etiology of, 320
in hyperparathyroidism, 2030–2031
in metastatic breast cancer, 2451
in multiple myeloma, prevention of, 1500
management of, medical, 321–322
nursing, 322
pharmacologic, 2034t
surgical, 322
pathophysiology of, 320
prevention of, 320b

Hypercalcemia *(Continued)*
risk factors for, 320, 320b
after thyroidectomy, 2023
Hypercalcemic crisis, 320–321
Hypercalciuria, 1666
Hypercholesterolemia, management of, 200t
Hypercoagulability, in thrombus formation, 1432
prevention of, 1433
Hypercortisolism, 2049–2055
clinical manifestations of, 2050–2052, *2051*
diagnostic findings in, 2050–2052
etiology of, 2049
hormonal dysfunction in, 2044t
hypertension in, 1389
management of, community/self care in, 2053–2055
in elderly, 2055
medical, 2053
nursing, 2053–2055
surgical, 2052
nursing care in, 2052–2053
pathophysiology of, 2050, *2051*
prevention of, 2050b
risk factors for, 2049, 2050b
Hyperesthesia, 724
Hyperextension, of spinal cord, 890–891, *892*
Hyperglycemia, 1981–1987
acute, assessment findings in, 1984t
factors in, 1963t
management of, 200t
rebound, hypoglycemia with, 1990–1992
total parenteral nutrition and, 1756
Hyperglycemic, hyperosmolar, nonketotic coma (HHNK), 1987–1988, 1987b, 1991t–1992t
Hyperkalemia, 310–314
cardiac effects of, 1220
clinical manifestations of, 311, 312t
diagnostic findings in, 311, 312t
electrocardiographic changes in, 305–306, *308*
etiology of, 310, 310t
in acute hyperglycemia, 1984t
in diabetic ketoacidosis, management of, 1984
in renal failure, acute, 1639
chronic, 1644
management of, 1655
insulin deficiency and, 305
management of, community/self care in, 314
diet in, 313, 313b
in elderly clients, 314
medical, 312–313
nursing, 313–314
potassium level reduction in, 312–313
pathophysiology of, 310
prevention of, 311b
risk factors for, 310, 311b
Hyperkeratosis, definition of, 2183t
Hyperlipidemia, 1408
in chronic renal failure, 1644
management of, 200t
screening for, 209t
Hyperlordosis, 2121

Hypermagnesemia, 324–325
 cardiac effects of, 1220
 clinical manifestations of, 324
 in chronic renal failure, 1644
 treatment of, 324
Hypernatremia, 300–304
 clinical manifestations of, 301–302, 303t
 diagnostic findings in, 301–302, 303t
 etiology of, 301, 301t
 euvolemic, causes of, 301t
 hypervolemic, causes of, 301t
 hypovolemic, causes of, 301t
 management of, community/self care in, 304
  intravenous therapy in, 303
  medical, 302–304
  nursing, 304
  sodium restriction in, 303–304
 pathophysiology of, 301
 prevention of, 302b
 risk factors for, 301, 302b
 types of, 301
Hyperopia, 946, 975, 976
Hyperosmolality, 276
 in acute hyperglycemia, 1984t
Hyperosmolar fluid volume deficit, 278
Hyperparathyroidism, 2030–2036
 clinical manifestations of, 2030–2031, 2031, 2031b
 critical monitoring in, 2031b
 diagnostic findings in, 2030–2031, 2032t
 etiology of, 2030
 management of, community/self care in, 2031–2034
  in elderly, 2035–2036
  medical, 2031–2033
  nursing, 2033–2034
  surgical, 2035
   complications of, 2035
   nursing care in, 2035
   outcomes in, 2035
 pathophysiology of, 2030
 risk factors for, 2030, 2030b
Hyperphosphatemia, 322
 cardiac effects of, 1220
 in renal failure, acute, 1639
  chronic, 1644
Hyperpigmentation, 2186
 chemotherapy and, 583
 definition of, 2183t
 postinflammatory, 2191b
Hyperpituitarism, 2062–2065
 clinical manifestations of, 2062
 diagnostic findings in, 2062
 etiology of, 2062
 management of, surgical, 2062
  nursing care in, 2062–2065
 pathophysiology of, 2062, 2062
 risk factors for, 2062
Hyperplasia, 267, 267
 definition of, 534t
Hyperpolarization, 294
 in nerve impulse generation, 688
Hyperprolactinemia, 2062–2065, 2063t
 clinical manifestations of, 2062
 diagnostic findings in, 2062
 management of, surgical, 2062
  nursing care in, 2062–2065

Hyperprolactinemia (Continued)
 pathophysiology of, 2062, 2062
Hyperresonance, in percussion, 230
 of chest, 1044, 1046
Hypersensitivity, 636–641
 atopic, 595
 diagnostic findings in, 636–637, 637
 factors in, 636
 management of, 200t
  community/self care in, 632, 641
 pathophysiology of, 637–641, 638t, 639t, 640t
 to chemotherapy, 578, 578b
 type I (anaphylactic), 638–639, 638t, 639t, 640t
 type II (cytolytic/cytotoxic), 638t, 639
 type III (immune complex), 638t, 639–640
 type IV (cell-mediated/delayed), 638t, 640–641
Hypersensitivity pneumonitis, 1150, 1151t
Hypersplenism, 1504–1505
 clinical manifestations of, 1505
 diagnostic factors in, 1505
 etiology of, 1504–1505
 management of, surgical, 1505
  nursing care in, 1505
 risk factors for, 1504–1505
Hyperstat (diazoxide), for hypertensive emergency, 1405t
Hypertension, 237, 1387–1404
 and male reproductive disorders, 2345
 assessment of, 1398–1399
 classification of, 1387–1388
 clinical manifestations of, 1390–1391
 corticosteroids in, consequences of, 2049t
 diabetes mellitus and, 1994, 1995t
 diagnostic findings in, 1390–1391, 1391t
 diastolic, 1387
 etiology of, 1388–1389, 1388b
 in Blacks, 198t
 in chronic renal failure, 1645
 in coronary artery disease, 1240–1241
 in pheochromocytoma, 2057
 in postanesthesia care unit, 483
 in primary hyperaldosteronism, 2055–2056
 intracranial, 778
 malignant, 1388
  emergency management of, 1404, 1405t
 management of, 198t
  community/self care in, 1391–1392
  emergency, 1404, 1405t
  in elderly, 1404
  medical, 1392–1398, 1394t–1397t, 1398b
  nursing, 1398–1404
  pharmacologic, 1393–1398, 1394t–1397t, 1398b
   combination therapy in, 1397–1398
   step-down therapy in, 1397
   stepped-care therapy in, 1397, 1398b
 ocular manifestations of, 977
 pathophysiology of, 1389–1390, 1390
 portal. See Portal hypertension.
 prevention of, 1391–1392
 primary (essential), 1387
 pulmonary, 1129–1130

Hypertension (Continued)
 chest pain in, assessment of, 1209t
 renal, 1626
 risk factors for, 1388–1389
  in hypercortisolism, 2052
 screening for, 209t
 secondary, 1387
 sleep disorders in, 405
 systolic, 1387
  isolated, 1387–1388
 "white coat," 1387
Hypertensive hypervolemic hemodilution, for intracranial hemorrhage, 814
Hyper-Tet, for tetanus, 857
Hyperthermia, after intracranial surgery, 850
 for benign prostatic hyperplasia, 2359
 in cerebrovascular accident, 800–801
 in hyperthyroidism, 2022
 malignant, monitoring for, intraoperative, 478–479
 prevention of, 203t
 radiation therapy with, 572
Hyperthyroidism, 2016–2024
 clinical manifestations of, 2008t, 2017–2018, 2018
 complications of, 2018–2019
 critical monitoring in, 2018b
 diagnostic findings in, 2017–2018, 2018
 etiology of, 2017
 management of, in elderly, 2022
  medical, 2019–2020
  nursing, 2020–2022
  pharmacologic, 2013t
  surgical, 2022–2023, 2024t–2025t
   nursing care in, 2023–2024
 pathophysiology of, 2017
 postmenopausal osteoporosis with, case study of, 2021
 preoperative, 456
 prevention of, 2017b
 risk factors for, 2017, 2017b
 sleep disorders in, 404
Hypertonic saline solution, for fluid resuscitation, in burns, 2250t
Hypertrophic cardiomyopathy, 1338, 1338, 1340–1341, 1340t
 clinical manifestations of, 1341
 diagnostic findings in, 1340t, 1341
 etiology of, 1340–1341
 management of, 1341
 pathophysiology of, 1341
 risk factors for, 1340–1341
Hypertrophic scarring, 446
 in burns, control of, 2260–2261, 2261
Hypertrophy, of muscles, 2087
Hypertropia, 945
Hyperuricemia, in gout, 2107–2108
Hyperventilation, 238
 for increased intracranial pressure, 775
 in burns, 2235–2236
 in respiratory alkalosis, 334t, 335
 in restrictive lung disorders, 1147
Hypervolemia, and heart failure, 1278
 in third-spacing, 291
Hypervolemic hemodilution, for cerebrovascular accident, 793
Hypnagogic hallucination, 400
Hypnoanesthesia, 477

Hypnosis, for urinary incontinence, 1612
 in pain control, 349b, 371
Hypnotics, abuse of, 2492–2494
  effects of, 2483t
  health consequences of, 2494t
  withdrawal from, symptoms of, 2488t
Hypocalcemia, 315–319
 after thyroidectomy, 2023
  assessment for, 2025t
 clinical manifestations of, 317–318, 317t
 diagnostic findings in, 317–318, 317t
 etiology of, 315t, 316–317
 hypoparathyroidism with, management of, 319
 in acute pancreatitis, 1923, 1924t
 in chronic renal failure, 1644
 management of, in elderly, 319
  medical, 318
   calcium replacement in, 318
   diet in, 318, 318b
  nursing, 318–319, 319
 pathophysiology of, 317
 prevention of, 316b
 risk factors for, 316–317, 316b
Hypochromic cells, 1466t
Hypoesthesia, 724
Hypoglossal nerve, assessment of, 719, 721
Hypoglycemia, 1988–1990, 1991t–1992t
 clinical manifestations of, 1988–1989, 1988b
 diagnostic findings in, 1988–1989
 etiology of, 1988
 factors in, 1963t
 in acute hyperglycemia, 1984t
 management of, 1989–1990, 1989t
 pathophysiology of, 1988
 prevention of, 1990
 rebound, total parenteral nutrition and, 1756
 rebound hyperglycemia with, 1990–1992
 risk factors for, 1988
Hypoglycemic agents, intraoperative complications of, 457
Hypoglycemic unawareness, 1990
Hypogonadism, and male reproductive disorders, 2345
 hypogonadotropic, 2069
 primary, causes of, 2068
 secondary, 2069
Hypokalemia, 305–310
 clinical manifestations of, 305–306, 309t
 diagnostic findings in, 305–306, 309t
 electrocardiographic changes in, 305–306, 308
 etiology of, 305, 305t
 in acute hyperglycemia, 1984t
 in diabetic ketoacidosis, management of, 1984
 in elderly, 309–310
  digitalis toxicity with, 309–310
 in primary hyperaldosteronism, 2055
 management of, community/self care in, 310
  diet in, 307
  medical, 306–307
  nursing, 307–309
  potassium replacement in, 306–307
 pathophysiology of, 305

Hypokalemia (Continued)
 prevention of, 306b–307b
 risk factors for, 305, 306b–307b
Hypomagnesemia, 323–324
 cardiac effects of, 1220
 clinical manifestations of, 323
 etiology of, 323
 management of, 324, 324b
 pathophysiology of, 323
Hyponatremia, 296–300
 clinical manifestations of, 298–299, 299t
 diagnostic findings in, 298–299, 299t
 etiology of, 296–297, 297t
 euvolemic, causes of, 297t
 hypervolemic, causes of, 297t
 hypovolemic, causes of, 297t
 in renal failure, acute, 1639
  chronic, 1644
 management of, community/self care in, 300
  diet in, 300
  in elderly, 300
  intravenous therapy in, 299–300
  medical, 299–300
  nursing, 300
 pathophysiology of, 297–299
 prevention of, 298b
 redistributive, causes of, 297t
 risk factors for, 296–297, 298b
 total body water in, sodium relationship to, 296, 297t
 types of, 296
Hypoparathyroidism, 2036–2038
 clinical manifestations of, 2036–2037
 complications of, 2037
 critical monitoring in, 2031b
 diagnostic findings in, 2036–2037
 etiology of, 2036
 hypocalcemia with, management of, 319
 management of, medical, 2037
  nursing, 2037–2038
 pathophysiology of, 2036
 prevention of, 2036b
 risk factors for, 2036, 2036b
Hypophosphatemia, 315–319
 cardiac effects of, 1220
 clinical manifestations of, 317–318, 317t
 diagnostic findings in, 317–318, 317t
 etiology of, 316–317
 management of, in elderly clients, 319
  medical, 318
   calcium replacement in, 318
   diet in, 318, 318b
  nursing, 318–319, 319
 pathophysiology of, 317
 prevention of, 316b
 risk factors for, 316–317, 316b
Hypophysectomy, for breast cancer, 2437–2438, 2449, 2449t
 for pain, 386, 387
 transfrontal, 2064
 transsphenoidal, 2064
  for brain tumors, 849, 850
Hypopigmentation, 2186
 midline, 2188b
 postinflammatory, 2191b
Hypopituitarism, 2065–2066
 clinical manifestations of, 2065–2066

Hypopituitarism (Continued)
 diagnostic findings in, 2065–2066
 etiology of, 2065
 in secondary adrenal insufficiency, 2049
 management of, 2066
Hypopolarization, 294
Hypoprothrombinemia, 1509–1510
Hypopyon, 968
Hyposecretory agents, for peptic ulcer disease, 1767, 1768t–1769t
Hyposmia, 1050
Hyposmolality, 276
Hypospadias, 2333, 2380–2381, 2381
Hypotension, 237
 in postanesthesia care unit, 483
 in shock, 511–512
 orthostatic, and vertigo, 1011
  in extracellular fluid volume deficit, step-progression for, 283
 postural, 1404
 renal disorders in, 1626
 risk for, after spinal cord injury, 899
 spinal anesthesia and, 476t
Hypothalamic-pituitary-adrenal (HPA) axis, 2049
Hypothalamus, in fluid balance regulation, 275
 in hormone regulation, 1940–1942
 structure/function of, 691, 692–693
 tumor of, clinical manifestations of, 847t
Hypothermia, 2535–2536
 after intracranial surgery, 850
 in burns, 2244–2245
 in postanesthesia care unit, 483
 prevention of, 203t
 risk for, in myxedema coma, 2012
Hypothyroidism, 2005–2016
 clinical manifestations of, 2007–2009, 2008t, 2009
 critical monitoring in, 2015b
 diagnostic findings in, 2007–2009
 etiology of, 2005–2006
 in hypopituitarism, 2065
 management of, community/self care in, 2012–2016
  in elderly, 2016
  medical, 2012–2014, 2014t
  nursing, 2014–2016, 2015b, 2016b
  pharmacologic, 2014t
  surgical, 2016
 pathophysiology of, 2006–2007
 preoperative, 456
 prevention of, 2006b
 primary, 2005
 risk factors for, 2005–2006, 2006b
 secondary, 2005
 sleep disorders in, 404
 subclinical, 2006
  in elderly, 2016
 tertiary (central), 2005
Hypotonic fluid volume deficit, 278
Hypoventilation, in respiratory acidosis, 333–335, 334t
Hypovolemia, in acute pancreatitis, 1926
 in third-spacing, 290
 paracentesis and, 1854
 preoperative, 455

Hypovolemic shock, after thoracic surgery, monitoring for, 1160
cardiogenic shock with, 500
clinical manifestations of, 510, *510, 512*
etiology of, 497, 498–499, 498t
in fracture, 2134
management of, 522t
prevention of, 501b
risk factors for, 498–499
Hypoxemia, and respiratory alkalosis, 334t, 335
endotracheal tube suctioning and, 1175t
in hereditary spherocytosis, 1484
in restrictive lung disorders, 1147
PaO$_2$ in, 1056
Hypoxia, and cell damage, 269
and coma, 744
cerebral, in left ventricular failure, 1281
in bulbar disorders, 861
Hysterectomy, catheterization during, and infection, 2403–2404
for leiomyoma, 2401
Hysteroscopy, 2326, *2326*
Hytakerol (dihydrotachysterol), for hypoparathyroidism, 2037
Hytone (hydrocortisone), 2048t
for rheumatoid arthritis, 664t
topical, 2199t
Hytrin (terazosin), 1395t
for benign prostatic hyperplasia, 2364t

I

^{131}I (radioactive iodine), for hyperthyroidism, 2013t, 2020
IABP (intra-aortic balloon pump), 1012, 1013b
for shock, 517
IADLs (instrumental activities of daily living), in elderly, 87
IBD. See *Inflammatory bowel disease (IBD)*.
IBS. See *Irritable bowel syndrome (IBS)*.
Ibuprofen (Motrin, Advil), for rheumatoid arthritis, 664t
in pain control, 375t
IBW (ideal body weight), calculation of, 236, 236b
IC. See *Interstitial cystitis (IC)*.
ICCE (intracapsular cataract extraction), *959*, 959–960
Ice massage, in pain control, 371
ICF (intracellular fluid), 273
electrolyte distribution in, 293t
ICFVD (intracellular fluid volume deficit), 293
ICFVE. See *Intracellular fluid volume excess (ICFVE)*.
ICP. See *Intracranial pressure (ICP)*.
Icterus. See *Jaundice*.
Ictus, definition of, 835b
IDDM (insulin-dependent diabetes mellitus). See *Diabetes mellitus*.
Ideal body weight (IBW), calculation of, 236, 236b
Ideal independent family, 54–55
Idiogenic osmoles, 301

Idiopathic thrombocytopenic purpura (ITP), 1506–1508
clinical manifestations of, 1507
complications of, 1507
diagnostic findings in, 1507
etiology of, 1506–1507
management of, in elderly, 1508
medical, 1507
nursing, 1507–1508
surgical, 1507
nursing care in, 1507
pathophysiology of, 1507
risk factors for, 1506–1507
IFNs (interferons), effects of, 604, 604t
for cancer, 586
in wound healing, 431
IgA, 600
characteristics of, 601t
IgA nephropathy, 1634
IgD, 601
characteristics of, 601t
IgE, 601
characteristics of, 601t
IgG, 600, *601,* 601t
characteristics of, 601t
IgG anti-HAV, in hepatitis A, 1865
IgM, 600–601
characteristics of, 601t
IGT (impaired glucose tolerance), 1955, 1955b
diagnosis of, oral glucose tolerance test in, 1964t
IIR (inflammatory immune response), 528
ILDs (interstitial lung diseases), 1149
Ileal conduit, creation of, complications of, 1588
for bladder cancer, 1585, *1586*
management of, 1590–1594, *1592*
at home, 1591b
physical examination of, 1553
urine specimen collection with, 1556
Ileal pouch–anal anastomosis, care of, 1807
for inflammatory bowel disease, 1801, *1802*
Ileal ureter, creation of, for renal calculi, 1669
Ileoproctectomy, knowledge deficit in, 1802
Ileorectal anastomosis, care of, 1807
for inflammatory bowel disease, 1801, *1801*
Ileostomy, care of, 1805–1807, *1807*
continent, care of, 1807–1808
for inflammatory bowel disease, 1801–1802, *1803*
knowledge deficit in, 1802
Ileostomy pouches, 1806, *1807*
Ileum, structure of, 1690
Ileus, paralytic, postoperative, 490
risk for, after cardiac surgery, 1014
after intervertebral disc surgery, 924
Illness, aging in, 34
beliefs about, non-Western, 61
Western, 61
biocultural aspects of, 30b–33b
chronic, multifactorial aspects of, *29,* 29–34
environment in, 36
experience of, 37

Illness *(Continued)*
nutrition in, 34–36
oxygen free radicals in, 35–36, *36*
theories of, 18–37
Illusions, 765
assessment of, 710t
ILs (interleukins), effects of, 604, 604t
for cancer, 586
in wound healing, 431
IMA (internal mammary artery), in coronary artery bypass grafting, 1247–1248
Imagery, guided, in pain control, 349b, 369–370
Imaging. See also names of specific techniques.
cold-spot, 255
hot-spot, 255
in diagnostic testing, 248–257
in pituitary function testing, 1954
Imferon (iron dextran), administration of, 1474
Z-track technique of, 1473, *1473*
Imipramine, therapeutic monitoring of, reference values for, 2562
Imipramine hydrochloride (Tofranil), for urinary incontinence, 1611t
Immersion syndrome, 2522
Immigrants, women's health beliefs in, 2428b–2429b
Immigration, health risks of, 204t
Immobile client, home healthcare for, 913b
Immobility, in musculoskeletal disorders, 2084
prevention of, 165–166
Immobilization, in burn autografting, 2255
of spine, in emergency nursing care, 2507, *2507*
Immune cascade, 598–599, *599*
Immune complex (type III) hypersensitivity, 638t, 639–640
Immune globulin, for viral hepatitis, 1867
hepatitis B, 1864
tetanus, for soft tissue trauma, 2534
Immune response, in cancer, failure of, 539
in hemolytic anemia, 1479
lungs in, 1026
primary, 598–599, *599*
secondary, 599, *599*
Immune system, age-related changes in, 268t
anatomy of, 595–598, *596, 597*
disorders of, 614–650
assessment of, 607–612
diagnostic tests in, 611–612
history in, 607–609
physical examination in, 609–611, 609b, 610t
ocular manifestations of, 977–978
impairment of, management of, 199t
in alcohol abuse, 2490t
in burns, 2236
in chronic renal failure, 1645
in hematologic disorders, 1462
in immunity, 595–605. See also *Immunity*.
in resistance, 593–595, *594, 595*
acute phase response in, 594
inflammation in, 594, *594, 595*
natural killer cells in, 594–595

Immune system *(Continued)*
  surface defenses in, 593–594
  in shock, 509
  respiratory function in, 1026
  structure/function of, 593–606
Immunity, 595–605
  acquired, categories of, 595
  active, 595
  age in, 604–605
  antibodies in, 601–602, *602, 1454*
    monoclonal, 601
  cell-mediated, 595, 602, *603, 1453*
  central lymphoid organs in, 595–597, *596,*
    597
  complement in, 601–602, *602*
  cytokines in, 603–604, 604t
  factors in, 604–605
    biocultural, 31b
  genetics in, 604
  glucocorticoids in, 1945
  herd, 421
  humoral, 595
  immunoglobulins in, 599–601, *601,*
    601t
  medications in, 605
  mucosal, 595
  nutrition in, 605
  passive, 595
  peripheral lymphoid tissue in, 597–598
  stress in, 605
  T lymphocytes in, 602, *603*
Immunization(s), active, 420
  against infections, 420–422, 422t
  history of, in immune disorder assessment,
    608
    in neurologic system assessment, 714
    in respiratory assessment, 1038
  in hepatitis A prevention, 1864
  in hepatitis B prevention, 1864
  of adults, recommendations for, 422t
  passive, 420
  routine, schedule for, 208t
  tetanus, in burns, 2241, 2251
Immunoassay, enzyme, 1952
Immunoglobulin(s), assays of, in immune
    disorder assessment, 611
  characteristics of, 601t
  classes of, 601t
  in immunity, 599–601, *601,* 601t
  reference values for, in cancer, 557t
  surface, 596, 598
Immunologic tests, in hepatobiliary disease,
    1849
Immunomodulator therapy, in human immu-
    nodeficiency virus infection, 624
Immunosuppression, after heart transplanta-
    tion, 1353, 1354b
  for idiopathic thrombocytopenic purpura,
    1507
  for inflammatory bowel disease, 1799
  nutrition in, home healthcare in, 1494b
Immunotherapy, for hypersensitivity, 641
  for renal cancer, 1673
Imodium (loperamide), for diarrhea, in in-
    flammatory bowel disease, 1798, 1798t
Impacted fracture, *2130,* 2131
Impaired glucose tolerance (IGT), 1955,
    1955b

Impaired glucose tolerance (IGT) *(Contin-
    ued)*
  diagnosis of, oral glucose tolerance test in,
    1964t
Impalement, 2520t
Impedance audiometry, 991
Impedance plethysmography (IPG), in pe-
    ripheral vascular assessment, 1384
Impetigo, 2221t
Implants, in plastic surgery, *2281,* 2281–
    2282
  iridium, for breast cancer, 2446–2447,
    2447
  radioactive, 573
  silicone, for breast reconstruction, ethical
    issues in, 2438b
Implementation, in chronic condition man-
    agement, 116–117
  in relocation stress syndrome, 89b
Impotence. See *Erectile dysfunction.*
Impulse generation, atrial disturbances in,
    1300–1302
Imuran. See *Azathioprine (Imuran).*
IMV (intermittent mandatory ventilation),
    1177, 1178t
Inactivity, in coronary artery disease, 1241
Inapsine (droperidol), preoperative, 465t
Incentive spirometer, postoperative use of,
    487, *487*
Incident reports, 130
Incision, elliptical, in plastic surgery, 2268,
    2268
  management of, 437
Incision biopsy, 257
Incisional hernia, 1817, *1817*
Incompetency, ethical issues in, 378b
Incomplete fracture, *2130,* 2131
Incontinence, after benign prostatic hyper-
    plasia surgery, 2360
  bowel, after spinal cord injury, 908
    in consciousness disorders, 761
  total, after spinal cord injury, 907–908
  urge, in dementia of Alzheimer's type,
    869
  urinary. See *Urinary incontinence.*
Incus, structure of, *981,* 982
Indapamide (Lozol), 1394t
Indecainide (Decabid), for dysrhythmia,
    1307t
Inderal (propranolol), 1395t
  for angina pectoris, 1254–1255, 1257t
  for dysrhythmia, 1308t
  in surgical client, 458t
Index of activities of daily living, in chronic
    conditions, 115t
India, health/illness beliefs in, 61
Indiana pouch, creation of, for bladder can-
    cer, 1585, *1586*
  management of, 1593–1594
Indians, ancient, healthcare beliefs of, 18
Indigenous healers, 62–63
Indigestion, 1733
Indirect antiglobulin test, in hematologic
    system assessment, 1464–1465
Indirect inguinal hernia, 1817, *1817*
Indirect laryngoscopy, in laryngeal cancer,
    1085
Indirect ophthalmoscopy, 949

Indium imaging, 2094–2095
Individualism, in American healthcare sys-
    tem, 62
Indocin (indomethacin), for rheumatoid ar-
    thritis, 664t
  in pain control, 375t
Indomethacin (Indocin), for rheumatoid ar-
    thritis, 664t
  in pain control, 375t
Indurated, definition of, 2183t
Indwelling Foley urethral catheter, 2355t
Ineffective (disabling) family coping, 57
Infant, preoperative assessment of, 453
Infection(s), 413–425
  after arterial bypass, 1415
  after cardiac surgery, 925–926
  after intracranial surgery, prevention of,
    852–853
  after vulvectomy, 2420
  and distributive shock, 500
  and heart failure, 1278
  and hemolytic anemia, 1479–1480
  casting and, monitoring for, 2149b
  chemotherapy and, 581–582
  childhood, history of, in neurologic system
    assessment, 714
  device-associated, 419
  diabetes mellitus and, 1995, 1995t, *1997,*
    1998
  endotracheal tube suctioning and, 1175t
  fractures and, 2140–2141
  head trauma and, 825
  history of, in cardiovascular disorders,
    1207
    in ear disorders, 985–986
    in eye disorders, 942
    in gynecologic disorders, 2308
    in immune disorders, 608
    in musculoskeletal disorders, 2084
    in neurologic disorders, 714
    in respiratory disorders, 1038
    in urinary tract disorders, 1550
  human immunodeficiency virus. See *Hu-
    man immunodeficiency virus (HIV) infec-
    tion.*
  in acute renal failure, 1639
  in cirrhosis, 1878t
  in elderly, 420b
  in multiple organ system failure, manage-
    ment of, 530
  incubation period of, 417
  intertrochanteric hip fracture and, 2155
  latent period of, 415–417
  neurologic, 856–861
    bacterial/pyogenic, 856–858, *857, 858*
    fungal, 860
    parasitic, 861
    viral, 858–860
  nosocomial, 417–419, 418t
    control of, 422–424
  of bone, 2121–2122
  of cornea, 968–970
  of ear, 1003–1006, *1004, 1005*
  of heart, 1327–1338
  of intestine, 1788–1791
  of scrotum, 2381
  of skin, 2221t–2222t, 2222–2223
  of upper respiratory tract, 1076–1082

Infection(s) *(Continued)*
of urinary tract. See *Urinary tract infections (UTIs)*.
opportunistic, in acquired immunodeficiency syndrome, management of, 627–630
in human immunodeficiency virus infection, prophylaxis for, 624–625
period of communicability in, 417
preoperative assessment of, 455
prevention of, 419–424
immunization in, 420–422, 422t
with retention catheter, 1603
primary, in human immunodeficiency virus infection, 621–623
process of, 413–417
agent in, 413–414, 416t–417t
environment in, 414–415
host in, 415–417
pulmonary, 1133–1147
fungal, 1146–1147
renal transplantation and, 1662–1663
risk for, after partial laryngectomy, 1091
after total hip replacement, 2114
in acute glomerulonephritis, 1632
in acute renal failure, 1640–1641
in appendicitis, 1792–1793
in atopic dermatitis, 2209
in burns, 2246
in colon cancer, 1812–1813
in dialysis, 1658
in head trauma, 828
in hypercortisolism, 2053–2054
in leiomyoma, 2403–2404
in liver transplantation, 1900, 1901
in oral candidiasis, 1726
in renal transplantation, 1664
in splenic rupture, 1505
mechanical ventilation and, 1181
with tracheostomy, 1074, *1075*
screening for, 208t
subclinical, 417
tracheostomy tubes and, 1070
Infection control, 419–424
antibiotic resistance in, 421b
in burns, 2252, 2252t
in hospitals, 422–424
barrier precautions in, 423
occupational health practices in, 424
standard precautions in, 423–424
transmission-based precautions in, 423–424
universal precautions in, 423–424
in tuberculosis management, 1143
Infection control practitioner, 423
Infectious mononucleosis. See *Mononucleosis, infectious.*
Infectivity, 414
Inferior petrosal sinus sampling (IPSS) test, 2051
Infertility, chlamydial infections in, 2469
cultural beliefs about, 2426b–2427b
male, 2346–2347
clinical manifestations of, 2346
diagnostic findings in, 2346
etiology of, 2346
management of, community/self care in, 2346–2347

Infertility *(Continued)*
medical, 2346–2347
nursing, 2347
pathophysiology of, 2346
risk factors for, 2346
prevention of, 2347
Infestations, intestinal, 1788–1791
Infiltrating ductal carcinoma, 2434
Infiltrating lobular carcinoma, 2434
Infiltration, and cell injury, 267
Inflammation, acute, 594
and pain, 356
chronic, 594
management of, 437
glucocorticoids in, 1945
in pathogen resistance, 594, *594, 595*
in wound healing, 428–431
mediators of, 429–430, *430, 431*
phagocytosis in, 431
white blood cells in, 428–429, *429*
management of, 434–437
community/self care in, 437
mediators of, control of, in multiple organ system failure, 530
of gastrointestinal tract, 1761–1784
of intestines, 1788–1808
of salivary glands, 1732
of upper respiratory tract, 1076–1082
of urinary tract, 1571–1581
systemic reactions to, 435
Inflammatory bowel disease (IBD), 1794–1808
clinical manifestations of, 1797–1798
extraintestinal, 1800
complications of, 1799–1800
corticosteroids in, consequences of, 2049t
daily life in, nursing research on, 1801b
diagnostic findings in, 1797–1798
etiology of, 1796
management of, in elderly, 1808
medical, 1798–1800, 1798t
nursing, 1800
surgical, 1800–1802, *1801, 1802*
nursing care in, 1802–1808
pathophysiology of, 1796
risk factors for, 1796
Inflammatory breast cancer, 2434
Inflammatory exudates, 434, 435t
Inflammatory immune response (IIR), 528
Influenza, 1133–1134
common cold vs., 1133
immunization against, 421
in adults, 422t
schedule for, 208t
infectious agent in, 416t
prevention of, 202t
Influenzal pneumonia, 1136t
Information, confidential, ethical issues in, 189b
fund of, assessment of, 710t
Informed consent, ethical issues in, 47–48
for blood transfusion, 1518–1519
for radical procedures, ethical issues in, 1095b
in emergency care, 2501–2502
insurance of, ethical issues in, 2403b
preoperative, 460–461
Inframammary ridge, palpation of, 2314

Infratentorial, definition of, 698
Infratentorial herniation syndromes, 774
Infratentorial lesions, and consciousness disorders, 745
respiratory effects of, 745, *745*
Infratentorial surgery, positioning after, 853
Infusaid Microport, *579*
Infusion devices, electromechanical, for blood transfusion, 1526
Infusion pumps, for home intravenous therapy, 284b
Ingestive disorders, 1719–1746
Ingrown nail, 2223
Inguinal area, assessment of, in regional examination, 220t
Inguinal canal, physical examination of, normal findings in, 2332b
Inguinal hernia, 1817, *1817*
examination for, *2334,* 2335
Inguinal lymph nodes, assessment of, 611
Inhalants, abuse of, 2491–2492
effects of, 2483t
health consequences of, 2493t
withdrawal from, symptoms of, 2487t
Inhalation anesthesia, *471,* 471–472
Inhalation injury, in burns, 2236–2237, 2237t
In-home care, nursing home care vs., for elderly, 84
Injury, risk for, after axillary node dissection, 2443
after parathyroid surgery, 2035
after prostatectomy, *2361,* 2361–2362
after spinal cord injury, 909, 912
in acute pancreatitis, 1928
in bladder cancer, 1584–1585
in cerebrovascular accident, 803
in cholelithiasis, 1911, 1914
in cirrhosis, 1883
in colon cancer, 1813–1814
in confusion, 767–768
in consciousness disorders, 760–761, 761b
in dementia of Alzheimer's type, 868–869
in dialysis, 1658–1659
in esophageal cancer, 1745–1746
in esophageal diverticula, 1742
in gastroesophageal reflux disease, 1739–1740
in heart failure, 1286–1287, 1287b
in hepatic encephalopathy, 1894–1895
in hypercortisolism, 2052–2053
in hyperparathyroidism, 2033
in hyperpituitarism, 2064
in hyperthyroidism, 2022
in hypokalemia, 308
in idiopathic thrombocytopenic purpura, 1507
in multiple myeloma, 1500
in oral cancer, 1730
in pheochromocytoma, 2059
in renal calculi, 1667–1668, 1670
in traction, 2143–2144
in vertigo, 1014
Innervation, of esophagus, 1688–1689
of kidneys, 1537
of large intestine, 1695

Innervation (Continued)
  of pelvis, 2296
  of small intestine, 1693
  of stomach, 1689–1690
Innovar (fentanyl citrate–droperidol), 470t
INR (international normalized ratio), 793
Insect bites/stings, 2537
Insight, assessment of, 195–196, 717–718
Insomnia, 400
  idiopathic, 400
  in dementia of Alzheimer's type, pharmacologic treatment of, 866t
  psychophysiologic, 400
Inspection, 225
  in immune disorder assessment, 609, 609b
  instruments for, 225, 227
  of abdomen, 1707, 1845, 1847
    in cardiovascular assessment, 1217
  of anus/rectum, 1710
  of breasts/axillae, 2312–2313, 2313
  of cardiovascular system, normal findings in, 1206b
  of ear, 987, 987–988, 988
  of eyes, normal findings in, 940b
  of female reproductive system, normal findings in, 2312b
  of gastrointestinal tract, normal findings in, 1699b
  of hematologic system, 1463b
  of hepatobiliary system, 1846t
    in elderly, 1847t
  of integumentary system, 2185–2194
    normal findings in, 2182b
  of male reproductive system, normal findings in, 2332b
  of musculoskeletal system, normal findings in, 2086b
  of neurologic system, 718
    normal findings in, 717b
  of peripheral vascular system, 1378b, 1379–1381, 1381
  of precordium, 1213, 1214
  of respiratory system, 1040–1043, 1043
    normal findings in, 1042b
  of thyroid gland, 1951b
  of urinary tract, 1556b
Inspiration, normal, 1030
Inspiratory capacity, 1028, 1028, 1052t
Inspiratory reserve volume (IRV), 1028, 1028, 1052t
Instrumental activities of daily living (IADLs), in elderly, 87
Instruments, for inspection, 225, 227
  skin-piercing, control of, in hepatitis B prevention, 1864
Insula, 691, 692
Insulin, actions of, 1940t
  administration of, 1978
    in diabetic ketoacidosis, 1984–1986
    in surgical client, 458t
  antidote to, 2538t
  concentrations of, 1978
  deficiency of, and hyperkalemia, 305
  degradation of, kidneys in, 1543
  for diabetes mellitus, 1968–1970
    dosage of, 1969, 1970
  for hyperglycemic, hyperosmolar, nonketotic coma, 1987–1988

Insulin (Continued)
  for hyperkalemia, 312
  in carbohydrate metabolism, 1945–1946, 1946
  injection of, 1979
    site selection for, 1979, 1979
  output of, total parenteral nutrition in, 1756
  preparation of, 1979
  production of, impaired, in chronic renal failure, 1644
  self-injection of, 1979, 1980b
    client education in, 1980b
  storage of, 1978
  syringes for, 1978, 1978
    prefilled, 1979
  types of, 1969, 1969t
Insulin pump therapy, 1969, 1971
  complications of, 1970
Insulin reaction. See Hypoglycemia.
Insulin resistance, in diabetes mellitus, 1959, 1959
Insulin-dependent diabetes mellitus (IDDM). See Diabetes mellitus.
Insurance, commercial, 5b
  health, for cancer survivors, 566
    inadequate, health risks of, 204t
Intact, indications for, 443t
Intake/output measurements, 1553–1554
Integra, in burn wound covering, 2256t
Integrated sensory function, assessment of, 718
Integumentary system. See also Skin.
  age-related changes in, 268t, 2177–2178
  assessment of, in urinary tract disorders, 1554
  biocultural variations in, 2188b–2192b
  chemotherapy effects on, 583
  disorders of, 2197–2231
    after renal transplantation, 1663
    assessment of, 2180–2196
      diagnostic tests in, 2194–2196, 2195
      history in, 2180–2182, 2181t
      physical examination in, 2182–2194
        depth of, 2185
        environment for, 2184–2185
        normal findings in, 2182b
    in chronic renal failure, 1646
    in endocrine disorders, physical examination of, 1950
    in hepatobiliary disease, 1844
    in hypernatremia, 303t
    in hyponatremia, 299b
    in thyroid disorders, 2008t
  structure/function of, 2173–2178
Intellectual performance, assessment of, 717
Intensity, in auscultation, 231
Intensive care unit psychosis, 407b
Intensive diabetes therapy, 1970
  nursing research on, 1966b
Intercostal muscles, 1026, 1027
Interdependent care, 123
Interdigitations, 2075–2076
Interferon beta-1b (Betaseron), for multiple sclerosis, 874
Interferons (IFNs), effects of, 604, 604t
  for cancer, 586
  in wound healing, 431

Interleukins (ILs), effects of, 604, 604t
  for cancer, 586
  in wound healing, 431
Intermarriage, 31b–32b
Intermediate family, 54
Intermediate syndrome, chest pain in, assessment of, 1208t
Intermittent catheterization, in neurogenic bladder dysfunction, 1618
  in multiple sclerosis, 875
Intermittent claudication, 1377
  in chronic arterial occlusion, 1406
Intermittent mandatory ventilation (IMV), 1177, 1178t
Intermittent peritoneal dialysis (IPD), 1649
Intermittent pneumatic compression (IPC), in venous thrombosis prevention, 1433, 1433
Intermittent self-catheterization, in males, home healthcare in, 2351b
Internal capsule, 692
Internal carotid artery(ies), 699, 700
  cerebrovascular accident of, clinical manifestations of, 788t
Internal jugular vein, location of, 1213
Internal mammary artery (IMA), in coronary artery bypass grafting, 1247–1248
Internal maxillary artery, ligation of, for epistaxis, 1076–1077
International Classification of Epileptic Seizures, 836
International Council of Nurses, 67
International normalized ratio (INR), 793
International nursing, 66–67
  transcultural nursing vs., 66
International System of Units, in laboratory test result reporting, 243
Internet resources, on pain, 392b
Interneurons, 686
Interstitial cystitis (IC), 1579–1580
  clinical manifestations of, 1580
  diagnostic findings in, 1580
  etiology of, 1579
  management of, medical, 1580
    nursing, 1580
    surgical, 1580
  pathophysiology of, 1579–1580
  risk factors for, 1579
Interstitial lung diseases (ILDs), 1149
Interstitial pneumonia, 1135
Interstitial radiation, for prostate cancer, 2368
Interstitial space, 273
Intertrigo, 2210
  definition of, 2183t
Intertrochanteric hip fracture. See Hip fracture, intertrochanteric.
Intervention, in cross-cultural nursing, 65–66
  in diagnostic testing, 242, 243b
  in family nursing, 57–59
    anticipatory guidance in, 58–59
    networking in, 59
    referral in, 59
    teaching in, 59
    therapeutic family communication in, 58
  in sexual health promotion, 77
  in spiritual care, 73

Intervention scheme, in Omaha system, of home healthcare provision, 153–154, 154t, 155b

Interventional angiography, 736

Intervertebral disc, components of, 917

Intervertebral disc herniation, 917–924
  clinical manifestations of, 918–919
  diagnostic findings in, 918–919, *919*
  etiology of, 917
  management of, medical, 919–920, *920*
    surgical, 920–922, *921*
      complications of, 921
      nursing care in, 922–924, 922b
      outcomes in, 921–922
  pathophysiology of, 917–918, *919*
  risk factors for, 917

Interviewer, preparation of, for health history interview, 186

Intestinal disorders, 1787–1831
  blunt/penetrating trauma in, 1829–1830
  clinical manifestations of, 1787–1788, *1788*
  congenital, 1830

Intestinal lipase, 1692t

Intestinal tubes, types of, 1749, 1749t

Intoxication, definition of, 2481t
  water, 291–293, 292t

Intra-aortic balloon pump (IABP), 1012, 1013b
  for shock, 517

Intra-arterial pressure monitoring, 1236–1237

Intracapsular cataract extraction (ICCE), *959,* 959–960

Intracapsular hip fracture, 2131, *2153,* 2159

Intracellular fluid (ICF), 273
  electrolyte distribution in, 293t

Intracellular fluid volume deficit (ICFVD), 293

Intracellular fluid volume excess (ICFVE), 291–293
  causes of, 291–292
  clinical manifestations of, 292t
  diagnostic findings in, 292t
  nursing management of, 292

Intracerebral hematoma, 831
  traumatic, delayed, 831

Intracerebral hemorrhage, and cerebrovascular accident, 785

Intracoronary stents, for coronary artery disease, 1246, *1246*

Intracorporeal injection therapy, for infertility, 2349

Intracranial compartments, 772–773, *773*

Intracranial hemorrhage, 812–816
  clinical manifestations of, 813–814
  complications of, 814–815
  diagnostic findings in, 813–814, *814*
  etiology of, 812
  management of, medical, 814–815
    nursing, 815
    pharmacologic, 814
    surgical, 815–816
  pathophysiology of, 812–813
  prevention of, 813b
  risk factors for, 812, 813b

Intracranial hypertension, 778

Intracranial pressure (ICP), bedside conversation and, nursing research on, 781b
  increased, 771–783
    after craniotomy, positioning for, 853
    after intracranial surgery, 850
    clinical manifestations of, 774
    complications of, 778
    Cushing's triad in, 748–749, *749*
    diagnostic findings in, 774
    etiology of, 771
    management of, emergency, 752, 775
      guidelines for, 776b
      medical, 775–778, *776–777*
      nursing, 778–783, *779,* 781b
      surgical, 783, *783*
    pathophysiology of, 771–774, *773*
    posturing in, 748, *748*
    prevention of, 772b
    risk factors for, 771, 772b
    vital signs in, 715
  monitoring of, 775–778, *776–777*
    advantages of, 778
  reduction of, for intracranial hemorrhage, 814

Intracranial stimulation, in pain control, 391

Intracranial tumors. See *Brain tumors.*

Intracranial vault, components of, *772*

Intradermal test, in allergy assessment, 612, 637, *637*

Intraductal carcinoma, 2434

Intraocular lens, implantation of, for cataracts, 960

Intraocular pressure, increased, in glaucoma, 954

Intraoperative nursing, 466–480
  anesthesia in, 468–477. See also *Anesthesia.*
  client transport in, 480
  drainage assessment in, 479–480
  emotional care in, 477
  heat loss prevention in, 478
  malignant hyperthermia monitoring in, 478–479
  positioning in, 477–478, *478*
  safety in, 478
  surgical asepsis in, 478
  surgical team members in, 466–468
  wound closure in, 479, *479*

Intrapleural pressure, 1030

Intrasite, indications for, 443t

Intraspinal analgesia, *383,* 383–384

Intrathoracic pressure, 1030

Intravascular devices, and nosocomial infection, 419

Intravascular space, 273

Intravascular stents, 1413

Intravenous anesthesia, 471

Intravenous cholangiography, 1853

Intravenous infusion devices, postoperative, preoperative preparation for, 463

Intravenous line, in burns, 2242
  postoperative assessment of, 484

Intravenous pyelography (IVP), 1562–1563

Intravenous regional (extremity) block anesthesia, 476

Intravenous therapy, for extracellular fluid volume deficit, 278
  for hyponatremia, 299–300

Intravenous therapy *(Continued)*
  home management of, 284b
  in hypernatremia, 303

Intrinsic factor, 1453
  deficiency of, in megaloblastic anemia, 1474

Intrinsic sympathomimetic activity (ISA), beta-adrenergic blocking agents with, 1395t

Introitus, 2294, *2294*
  examination of, 2317

Intussusception, and small intestinal obstruction, 1820, *1820*

Invasive mole, 2423–2424

Invasive procedures, 451

Iodine, for goiter, 2014
  for hyperthyroidism, 2013t, 2019–2020
  in radionuclide scanning, 255

Iodized salt, in goiter prevention, 2015–2016

Ionescu-Shiley pericardial valve, *1352*

Ions, 293

IPC (intermittent pneumatic compression), in venous thrombosis prevention, 1433, *1433*

IPD (intermittent peritoneal dialysis), 1649

Ipecac, use of, cautions in, 2538, 2538b

IPG (impedance plethysmography), in peripheral vascular assessment, 1384

IPSS (inferior petrosal sinus sampling) test, 2051

IPT (isoniazid preventive therapy), for tuberculosis, 1143

Iridectomy, for glaucoma, 957

Iridium implant, for breast cancer, 2446–2447, *2447*

Iris, examination of, 944–945
  structure of, 937, *938*

Iron, antidote for, 2538t
  for anemia, 1471, 1475
  in hematopoiesis, 1453
  in wound healing, 434t

Iron chelating agents, for anemia, 1471

Iron deficiency anemia, 1472–1474
  clinical manifestations of, 1472–1473
  diagnostic findings in, 1472–1473
  etiology of, 1472
  management of, community/self care in, 1473–1474
    in elderly, 1474
    medical, 1473, *1473*
    nursing, 1473–1474
  pathophysiology of, 1472
  risk factors for, 1472

Iron dextran (Imferon), administration of, 1474
  Z-track technique of, 1473, *1473*

Iron overload, in hereditary spherocytosis, 1484

Irregular bones, 2073

Irrigation, antral, for sinusitis, 1077
  in mechanical debridement, of yellow wounds, 440
  of catheter, after prostatectomy, 2362
  of colostomy, 1815
    client education in, 1815b
  of ear, for otitis externa, 1005, *1005*

Irritable bowel syndrome (IBS), 1823–1825

Irritable bowel syndrome (IBS) *(Continued)*
  clinical manifestations of, 1824
  diagnostic findings in, 1824
  etiology of, 1823
  management of, medical, 1824–1825
    nursing, 1825
  pathophysiology of, 1823–1824
  prevention of, 1824b
  risk factors for, 1823, 1824b
IRV (inspiratory reserve volume), 1028, *1028,* 1052t
ISA (intrinsic sympathomimetic activity), beta-adrenergic blocking agents with, 1395t
Ischemia, and cerebrovascular accident, 785
  and coma, 744
ISH (isolated systolic hypertension), 1387–1388
Islam, beliefs/practices of, 2549–2550
  dietary, 1701b
Islets of Langerhans, 1945
Ismelin (guanethidine), 1397t
Isoamylase, pancreatic, serum, in hepatobiliary assessment, 1850t
Isoflurane (Forane), 470t
Isografts, 642
Isoimmune hemolytic reaction, and hemolytic anemia, 1480
Isolated systolic hypertension (ISH), 1387–1388
Isoniazid, for tuberculosis, 1143, 1144t
Isoniazid preventive therapy (IPT), for tuberculosis, 1143
Isoptin (verapamil), 1396t
  for angina pectoris, 1256t
  for dysrhythmia, 1308t
  for urinary incontinence, 1611t
Isosmolar fluid volume deficit, 278
Isosorbide dinitrate, for angina pectoris, 1256t
Isosporiasis, in acquired immunodeficiency syndrome, 630
Isotretinoin (Accutane), for acne vulgaris, 2212
Isovolumetric relaxation, 1199
Isradipine (DynaCirc), 1396t
Israelite civilization, healthcare in, history of, 19
Itching. See *Pruritus.*
ITP. See *Idiopathic thrombocytopenic purpura (ITP).*
IVP (intravenous pyelography), 1562–1563

J

J pouch, for inflammatory bowel disease, 1801, *1802*
Jacksonian march, 836
Jackson-Pratt suction drain, in craniotomy, 849, *849*
Jaloweic Coping Scale, in chronic conditions, 115t
Janeway's lesions, in infective endocarditis, 1333
Japanese, pain response in, 347b–348b
  stomach cancer in, 198t
Jaundice, 1858–1861
  biocultural variations in, 2190b

Jaundice *(Continued)*
  clinical manifestations of, 1859–1860
  diagnostic findings in, 1859–1860
  etiology of, 1858–1859, 1859t
  in acute cholecystitis, 1917, 1917t
  in acute pancreatitis, 1923, 1924t
  in cirrhosis, 1878t
  in hemolytic anemia, 1479t
  in viral hepatitis, 1865, 1866t
  management of, medical, 1860
    nursing, 1860
    surgical, 1860–1861
  risk factors for, 1858–1859
  skin in, 2186
Jaw reflex, 727
Jaw relaxation, in postoperative analgesia, nursing research on, 1781b
J.C. virus, 630
JCAHO (Joint Commission on Accreditation of Healthcare Organizations), 139
Jehovah's Witnesses, beliefs/practices of, 2548
  blood transfusions in, ethical issues in, 1519b
Jejunostomy tube, endoscopic, percutaneous, critical monitoring in, 1731b
Jejunum, structure of, 1690
Jewett nail, for femoral neck fracture, 2159
Jewett-Marshall staging, of bladder cancer, *1583*
JGA (juxtaglomerular apparatus), 1536
  in sodium regulation, 295
Jock itch, 2381
Joint(s), aspiration of, 2096
  function of, 2075–2077, *2076–2078*
    testing of, 2088, 2090t–2091t, *2092*
  in endocrine disorders, 1949
  in rheumatoid arthritis, 656–658, *657, 658*
    protection of, 662, 663t
    replacement of, 672–674, *673*
  physical examination of, 2088, *2088, 2089*
  stiffness of, in fracture, prevention of, 2145
  in musculoskeletal disorders, 2084
  structure of, 2075–2077, *2076–2078*
  types of, 2075–2076, *2076*
Joint Commission on Accreditation of Healthcare Organizations (JCAHO), 139
Joint spaces, narrowing of, in rheumatoid arthritis, *660,* 661
Jones criteria, for rheumatic fever, 1328, 1329b
Judaism, beliefs/practices of, 2544–2545
  dietary, 1701b
Judgment, assessment of, 195, 710t, 717
Jugular vein, assessment of, in regional examination, 219t
  distention of, measurement of, 1212–1213, *1213*
  internal, location of, *1213*
"Jumper's knee," 2162
Jumping, blunt trauma in, 2521t
Justice, in ethics, 40
Juxtaglomerular apparatus (JGA), 1536
  in sodium regulation, 295
Juxtaglomerular receptor, in shock, 502

K

K complexes, in polysomnography, 399
Kalginate, for burns, 2256t
Kallikrein, in blood pressure regulation, 1543
  in sodium regulation, 295
Kallmann's syndrome, 2069
Kaltistat, indications for, 443t
Kanamycin, for tuberculosis, 1145t
Kaposi's sarcoma (KS), *2230,* 2230–2231
  in acquired immunodeficiency syndrome, 630
  ocular manifestations of, 977
Kayexalate (sodium polystyrene sulfonate), for hyperkalemia, 312
Keflex (cephalexin monohydrate), for urinary tract infections, 1577t
Kegel exercises, effectiveness of, nursing research on, 1609b
  for cystocele, 2410
  for urinary incontinence, 1609–1610, 1609b, 1610
Keloids, 446, *447,* 2261
  biocultural variations in, 2191b
Kemadrin (procyclidine), for Parkinson's disease, 880t
Kenalog (triamcinolone), topical, 2199t
Keratinocytes, structure/function of, 2173–2174, 2176t
Keratitis, 968–969, *969*
  herpes simplex, red eye in, 942b
Keratoconjunctivitis sicca, 975
  in Sjögren's syndrome, 977
  red eye in, 942b
Keratoconus, *968,* 968–970, *969*
Keratolytics, 2199t
Keratoplasty, for corneal dystrophies, 966–967, *967*
Keratosis, actinic, 2225
Keratotomy, radial, 976
Kerlix gauze, 2202
Kerlone (betaxolol), 1395t
Kernig's sign, 828
  in bacterial meningitis, 856, *857*
Ketalar (ketamine hydrochloride), 471t
Ketamine hydrochloride (Ketalar), 471t
Ketoacidosis, diabetic. See *Diabetic ketoacidosis (DKA).*
Ketones, formation of, in diabetes mellitus, 1959–1960
  urine, 1558
  in diabetes mellitus diagnosis, 1963
Ketonuria, in diabetes mellitus, 1960t, 1963
Ketoprofen (Orudis), for rheumatoid arthritis, 664t
Ketorolac (Toradol), for rheumatoid arthritis, 664t
Ketosis, 270
  in diabetic ketoacidosis, 1982
17-Ketosteroids, 2045t
Kidney(s). See also entries under *Renal.*
  anatomy of, 1535–1537, *1536, 1537*
  aplasia of, 1677–1678
  assessment of, in regional examination, 218t, 220t
  blood vessels of, abnormalities of, 1676–1677

Kidney(s) *(Continued)*
cancer of. See *Renal cancer.*
circulation of, 1537
cysts of, *1678,* 1678–1679
disease of, in hypertension, 1389
disorders of, 1625–1680
acquired, 1628–1677
congenital, 1677–1679
extrarenal conditions with, 1625–1627
nephrotoxins in, 1627, 1627b
ectopic, 1677
function of, *1540,* 1540–1544
horseshoe, 1678, *1678*
hypoplasia of, 1678
in fixed acid regulation, 329–331, *330, 331*
in left ventricular failure, 1281
innervation of, 1537
of dying patient, donation of, guidelines for, 2514t
physical examination of, *1552,* 1552–1553
supernumerary, 1677
transplantation of. See *Renal transplantation.*
urine movement through, 1544
Kidney stones. See *Renal calculi.*
Kidneys, ureters, bladder (KUB) film, 1562
KinAir bed, *2219*
Kinesthesia, cerebrovascular accident and, 791–792
King's goal attainment theory, health definition in, 162t
Kinins, in fluid balance regulation, 277
in wound healing, 430
Kling gauze, indications for, 443t
Klonopin (clonazepam), side effects of, 839t
Knee(s), function of, assessment of, 2091t, *2092*
ligaments of, 2077, *2078*
range of motion of, *2089*
replacement of, total. See *Total knee replacement.*
Knee jerk, *726, 727,* 729t
Knee-chest position, for physical examination, *232*
Knock-knee, 2087, *2087*
Knowledge, general, assessment of, 195
Knowledge deficit, in achalasia, 1735–1736
in acute pancreatitis, 1926
in agranulocytosis, 1498
in ascites, 1891
in benign prostatic hyperplasia, 2364–2365
in bladder cancer, 1588
in brain tumors, 851
in breast cancer, 2439, 2450
in cholelithiasis, 1911, 1913, 1915
in chronic renal failure, 1657
in cirrhosis, 1883
in diabetes mellitus, 1975–1978, *1976,* 1977t
in dialysis, 1658
in foot infection, in diabetes mellitus, 1998
in hearing impairment, 1000
in hemophilia, 1517–1518
in human immunodeficiency virus infection, 625–627, 626b

Knowledge deficit *(Continued)*
in hypercortisolism, 2052
in hyperpituitarism, 2063–2064
in inflammatory bowel disease, 1802–1803
in intervertebral disc surgery, 922
in jaundice, 1860
in leiomyoma, 2402
in liver transplantation, 1899–1900
in multiple sclerosis, 876
in oral cancer, 1729, 1730
in peptic ulcer disease, 1779–1781
in postmastectomy care, 2443–2445, *2444,* 2445b
in premenstrual syndrome, 2389
in pyelonephritis, 1629–1630
in renal calculi, 1670–1671
in renal transplantation, 1663–1664
in sexually transmitted diseases, 2463–2464
in sickle cell anemia, 1515
in total hip replacement, 2111–2112
in viral hepatitis, 1871
in vulvar cancer, 2420
Knowles pin, for femoral neck fracture, 2159
Kock pouch, care of, 1807–1808
creation of, for bladder cancer, 1585
for inflammatory bowel disease, 1801–1802, *1803*
management of, 1593–1594
KOH (potassium hydroxide) examination, in integumentary disorders, 2194
Korotkoff's sounds, 1211
Kraurosis, 2419
KS (Kaposi's sarcoma), *2230,* 2230–2231
in acquired immunodeficiency syndrome, 630
ocular manifestations of, 977
KUB (kidneys, ureters, bladder) film, 1562
Kupffer cells, 1453
Kussmaul's respiration, *238*
Kyphoscoliosis, thoracic, 1042, *1043*
restrictive lung disorders in, 1147, *1148*
Kyphosis, 2087, *2087,* 2121

L

LABA (laser-assisted balloon angioplasty), 1413
Labetalol (Normodyne, Trandate), 1395t
for angina pectoris, 1257t
for dysrhythmia, 1308t
for hypertensive emergency, 1405t
Labia majora, 2293, *2294*
examination of, 2317
Labia minora, 2293, *2294*
examination of, 2317
Labile factor, 1516t
Laboratory tests, diagnostic. See *Diagnostic testing, laboratory.*
Labyrinth, structure of, *983,* 983–984
Labyrinthectomy, for vertigo, 1015–1016
Labyrinthitis, 993–994
and balance disorders, 1011
and hearing impairment, 993–994
Laceration, of face, plastic surgery of, 2286
sutured, care of, client education in, 2535b

Lachman test, 2091t, *2092*
in anterior cruciate ligament injuries, 2166
Lacrimal apparatus, disorders of, 972–975
examination of, 944
structure of, 936, *937*
Lactase, 1692t
secretion of, 1693
Lactate dehydrogenase (LDH), in cardiovascular assessment, 1219
in hepatobiliary assessment, 1851t
in musculoskeletal disorders, 2096t
in myocardial infarction, 1261, *1262*
reference values for, in cancer, 557t
Lactation mastitis, 2452
LactiCare lotion, 2199t
Lactic acid, in blood pressure regulation, 1204
topical, 2199t
Lactic acidosis, in shock, 503, *506*
Lactose intolerance, culture in, 1704b
Lactulose, for hepatic encephalopathy, 1893
Lacunae, 2074, *2075*
LAD (left anterior descending) artery, 1194, *1194*
lesion of, electrocardiographic changes in, 1225t
Laënnec's cirrhosis, 1873, 1874t–1875t
Lagophthalmos, 974
Lalonde Report, 162
Lamellae, 2074, *2075*
Laminectomy, cervical, home care in, 926b
decompressive, for spinal cord injury, 913–914
for intervertebral disc herniation, 921, *921*
lumbar, case management in, 922b
clinical pathway for, 2570–2571
Laminectomy (prone) position, intraoperative, 477, *478*
Laminography, 2092
Lamotrigine, side effects of, 839t
Langerhans' cells, structure/function of, 2175, 2176t
Langer's lines, *2268*
Language, assessment of, 710t–711t, 718
automatic, 792
LAP (laser ablation of the prostate), for prostate cancer, 2370
Laparoscopic cholecystectomy, for cholelithiasis, 1912
complications of, 1912–1913
Laparoscopy, 2326–2327, *2327*
Large cell lung cancer, 1153t
Large intestine, *1694,* 1694–1696
disorders of, 1788–1825
inflammatory, 1788–1808
neoplastic, 1808–1816. See *Colon cancer.*
function of, 1695–1696
herniation of. See *Herniation, intestinal.*
structure of, *1694,* 1694–1695
tumors of, benign, 1808
Laryngeal cancer, 1082–1100
clinical manifestations of, 1082–1085, 1083b
diagnostic findings in, 1082–1085, *1085*
etiology of, 1082
glottic, 1082, 1083b
management of, 1086

Laryngeal cancer (Continued)
  management of, medical, 1086
    surgical, 1086–1089, 1087
      complications of, 1088–1089
      nursing care in, 1089–1095
  pathophysiology of, 1082
  prevention of, 1084b
  risk factors for, 1082, 1084b
  spread of, pattern in, 1082, 1084
  staging of, 1085, 1086b
  subglottic, 1082, 1083b
  supraglottic, 1082, 1083b
    management of, 1086
  survival in, 538t
  warning signs of, 1085b
Laryngeal edema, acute, 1100
  chronic, 1101
Laryngectomy, home healthcare after, 1099b
  life after, nursing research on, 1088b
  partial, community/self care in, 1095
    for laryngeal cancer, 1087, 1087
    nursing care in, 1089–1091, 1090,
      1091b
    swallowing after, client education in,
      1091b
  supraglottic, 1087
  total, community/self care in, 1095–1100,
    1098–1100
    for laryngeal cancer, 1087, 1087–1088
    nursing care in, 1091–1093, 1092, 1093
Laryngitis, 1081
Laryngopharynx, structure of, 1023
Laryngoscopy, in laryngeal cancer diagnosis, 1082–1084, 1085
Laryngospasm, 1101
Larynx, artificial, 1092, 1093
  injury to, 1101
  paralysis of, 1101
  structure of, 1023, 1024
  tumors of, benign, 1082
LAS (local adaptation syndrome), 22
Lasègue's sign, 918, 2090t
Laser ablation of the prostate (LAP), for
  prostate cancer, 2370
Laser resurfacing, of face, 2274
Laser surgery, for coronary artery disease,
  1246
  for laryngeal cancer, 1086–1087
  for lung cancer, 1155
Laser trabeculoplasty, for glaucoma, 956
Laser-assisted balloon angioplasty (LABA),
  1413
Lasers, in plastic surgery, 2282
Lasix (furosemide), 1394t
  characteristics of, 1285t
  for acute renal failure, 1639
  for hypercalcemia, 2034t
Lateral chest x-ray, 1060
Lateral epicondylitis, 2162, 2169t
Lateral forearm flap, 2280
Lateral position, intraoperative, 477, 478
Lateral transtentorial herniation, 773, 773–
  774
Latin America, health/illness beliefs in, 61
Latissimus dorsi flap, 2280
  in cardiomyoplasty, 1290
  in postmastectomy breast reconstruction,
    2284

LAV (lymphadenopathy-associated virus),
  614
Lavage, gastrointestinal intubation in, 1749
Law of mass action, 328
Laxatives, anthraquinone, urine color with,
  1557t
Lazarus's theories, of stress response, 23–
  24, 24t
LBB (left bundle branch), 1198, 1198
LBBB (left bundle branch block), 1310
LCA (left coronary artery), 1194, 1194
LDH (lactate dehydrogenase), in cardiovas-
  cular assessment, 1219
  in hepatobiliary assessment, 1851t
  in musculoskeletal disorders, 2096t
  in myocardial infarction, 1261, 1262
  reference values for, in cancer, 557t
LDLs (low-density lipoproteins), 35
  elevated, in diabetes mellitus, 1977
  in coronary artery disease, 1241
Le Fort fractures, 2286, 2287
Lead, antidote to, 2538t
Lead poisoning, 269
  and hemolytic anemia, 1479
Leads, of pacemaker, 1315–1316
    placement of, in twelve-lead electrocardi-
      ography, 1223, 1224
Lecithin, in bile, 1838
LeFort sound, 2356t
Left anterior descending (LAD) artery,
  1194, 1194
  lesion of, electrocardiographic changes in,
    1225t
Left atrium, 1191, 1193
Left bundle branch (LBB), 1198, 1198
Left bundle branch block (LBBB), 1310
Left coronary artery (LCA), 1194, 1194
Left heart filling pressure, monitoring of, af-
  ter cardiac surgery, 1357
Left lower quadrant (LLQ), organs of, 1708
Left midaxillary line (LMAL), in spleen
  percussion, 1847
Left upper quadrant (LUQ), organs of, 1708
Left ventricle, 1191, 1193
Left ventricular failure (LVF), 1280, 1280–
  1282
Left-sided cardiac catheterization, 1231
Leg, elevation of, for venous thrombosis,
  1435
Leg bag, retention catheter with, for urinary
  retention, 1602, 1603
Legal Counsel for the Elderly, 97b
Legal issues, in acute care, 130
  in elderly care, 100–102
  in emergency care, 2501–2503, 2502b
Legionnaires' disease, 1137t
Leiomyoma(s), 550, 550t, 2400–2404
  cervical, 2400, 2400
  clinical manifestations of, 2401
  diagnostic findings in, 2401
  etiology of, 2400
  intraligamentary, 2400, 2400
  intramural, 2400
  management of, medical, 2404
    surgical, 2401, 2402
      nursing care in, 2401–2404
  pathophysiology of, 2400–2401
  risk factors for, 2400, 2400

Leiomyoma(s) (Continued)
  submucosal, 2400, 2400
  subserosal, 2400, 2400
  wandering (parasitic), 2400
Leninger's transcultural model, health defi-
  nition in, 162t
Lens, of eye, structure of, 937, 938
Lentigines, in elderly, 2178
Lentigo maligna melanoma (LMM), 2228t
Leprosy, 1139
LES (lower esophageal sphincter), 1687
  in achalasia, 1733–1734
  incompetency of, in regurgitation, 1733
Lesbians, 75
Lesion(s), definition of, 2183t
  of skin, assessment of, 2192–2194, 2193,
    2193t
    types of, 2182–2184, 2184, 2185
Lethargy, in consciousness disorders, 746
Leukapheresis, for chronic myelogenous
  leukemia, 1491, 1491
Leukemia(s), 1458, 1487–1497
  acute, medical management of, 1489–
    1491
  chronic, medical management of, 1491,
    1491–1492
  classification of, 1487–1488, 1488t
  clinical manifestations of, 1489, 1490
  diagnostic findings in, 1489
  etiology of, 1487–1488
  management of, in elderly, 1495
    nursing, 1492–1495
  pathophysiology of, 1488–1489, 1489
  prevention of, 204t
  risk factors for, 542b, 1487–1488
  survival in, 538t
  types of, 1487
Leukeran (chlorambucil), for chronic lymphocytic leukemia, 1492
  for rheumatoid arthritis, 664t
Leukocyte-reducing filter, for blood transfusion, 1526t
Leukocytes. See also White blood cells
  (WBCs).
  development of, 1450
  polymorphonuclear, in wound healing,
    428, 429
  reference values for, in cancer, 557t
Leukocytosis, in acute cholecystitis, 1917,
  1917t
  inflammation and, 435
Leukoedema, oral, 2188b
Leukoencephalopathy, multifocal, progres-
  sive, in acquired immunodeficiency syn-
  drome, 630
Leukopenia, 1458
Leukoplakia, 1726, 1726–1727
Leukoplakia vulvae, 2419
Leukorrhea, 2413
Leukotomy, frontal, medial, for pain, 386
  prefrontal, for pain, 386
Leukotrienes, in anaphylaxis, 638t
  in wound healing, 430
Leuprolide (Lupron), for benign prostatic
  hyperplasia, 2364t
  for endometriosis, 2399
Levatol (penbutolol), 1395t
LeVeen peritoneovenous shunt, 1891, 1892

Level of consciousness (LOC), altered, 2517–2518
- assessment of, 195, 715–716
  - after brain stem contusion, 824
  - in cardiovascular assessment, 1211
  - in consciousness disorders, 746–747, 747
  - in increased intracranial pressure, 778–781
  - in shock, 512
Levin tube, 1749–1750, 1749t
Levine-Ariff model, for ethical decision-making, 43, 44t
Levine's conservation principles, health definition in, 162t
Levobunolol, for glaucoma, client teaching about, 957t
Levodopa, for Parkinson's disease, 878–879
- urine color with, 1557t
Levo-Dromoran (levorphanol), administration of, 380t
Levorphanol (Levo-Dromoran), administration of, 380t
Levothroid (levothyroxine sodium), for hypothyroidism, 2014t
Levothyroxine sodium (Synthroid, Levothroid, Levoxine), for hypothyroidism, 2012, 2014t
Levoxine (levothyroxine sodium), for hypothyroidism, 2014t
LH (luteinizing hormone), 2061t
- deficiency of, in hypopituitarism, 2065
- in menstruation, 2299, 2299–2300
Libido, changes in, in endocrine disorders, 1949
Lice, 2186, 2221t
- pubic, 2475
Lichenification, 2185
Lidocaine (Xylocaine), 473t
- for dysrhythmia, 1307t
- for shock, 521
- in pain control, 372
- therapeutic monitoring of, reference values for, 2562
Life support, ethical issues in, 499b
Life-style, assessment of, 197
- preoperative, 457
- in health promotion, 167–168, 168b
- of clients, variations in, 16
Life-style disease, nursing care in, ethical issues in, 1883b
Lifts, palpation of, 1213
Ligaments, 2077, 2078
- of knee, 2077, 2078
- of shoulder, 2077
Ligation, for hemorrhoids, 1827
Light, adaptation to, age-related changes in, 940
- flickering, and seizures, 842
- response to, testing of, 944–945
Light reflex, 727
Light touch, sensitivity to, assessment of, 724
Limb girdle muscular dystrophy, 2125t
Limbic system, structure/function of, 693
Lindane, topical, 2198t
Linear fracture, 2130

Lioresal (baclofen), in pain control, 374, 378
Lip, cancer of, staging of, 1728b
Lip reading, 998
Lipase, 1692t
- in acute pancreatitis, 1923
- pancreatic, 1840, 1922b
- serum, in hepatobiliary assessment, 1851t
Lipectomy, suction-assisted, 2275, 2275–2276
Lipid-irritation hypothesis, of coronary artery disease pathogenesis, 1243
Lipids, 34
- in chronic arterial occlusion, 1408
- metabolism of, liver in, 1839–1840
- serum, in cardiovascular assessment, 1220
- stool examination for, 1711t, 1712–1713
Lipoid nephrosis, 1634
Lipoma, 550, 550t
Lipoproteins, 34–35
- in coronary artery disease, 1241
- in diabetes mellitus, 1977
Liposuction, 2275, 2275–2276
Liquid nitrogen, for actinic keratosis, 2225, 2226
Lisinopril (Prinivil, Zestril), 1396t
Lithium, for dementia of Alzheimer's type, 866t
- for hyponatremia, 300
- therapeutic monitoring of, reference values for, 2562
Litholapaxy, for renal calculi, 1668
Lithotomy position, for physical examination, 232
- intraoperative, 477, 478
Lithotripsy, for urinary calculi, 1597
- percutaneous, for renal calculi, 1668–1669, 1669
Liver, abscess of, 1902
- age-related changes in, 1841
- assessment of, in regional examination, 220t
  - preoperative, 456
- disorders of, 1858–1904
  - assessment of, 1843–1856
    - diagnostic tests in, 1848–1856
    - history in, 1843–1856
    - physical examination in, 1845–1848, 1846t–1847t, 1847
  - congenital, 1903
  - donation of, guidelines for, 2514t
  - fatty, 1895
- in hematopoiesis, 1452–1453
- in right ventricular failure, 1282
- in shock, 509
- injury to, traumatic, 2531
- neoplasms of, 1895–1898, 1896
  - benign, 1896, 1896
  - classification of, 1896
  - clinical manifestations of, 1897
  - diagnostic findings in, 1897
  - etiology of, 1896
  - malignant, 1896, 1896
    - survival in, 538t
  - management of, medical, 1897–1898
    - complications of, 1898
    - outcomes in, 1898
    - nursing, 1898

Liver (Continued)
- surgical, 1898
- metastatic, 1896
- pathophysiology of, 1896–1897
- risk factors for, 1896
- palpation of, 1848
- size of, assessment of, 1845–1847
- structure/function of, 1835–1841, 1836, 1837
- tenderness of, assessment of, 1848
- trauma to, 1903
Liver biopsy, 1854–1856, 1855
- care in, postprocedure, 1855–1856
  - preprocedure, 1855
- complications of, 1855–1856
- contraindications to, 1855
- procedure for, 1855, 1855
Liver failure, cirrhosis and, 1882t
Liver spots, 2178
Liver transplantation, 1898–1901
- complications of, 649t, 1899
- criteria for, 646
- for liver cancer, 1897
- indications for, 1898
- management of, client education in, 1899b
  - postoperative, 1899
  - preoperative, 1898
- nursing care in, 1899–1901
  - plan for, 1900
- outcomes in, 1899
- procedure for, 1898
Living will, elderly issues in, 102
- in terminal cancer, 567
Livor mortis, 271
LLQ (left lower quadrant), organs of, 1708
LMAL (left midaxillary line), in spleen percussion, 1847
LMM (lentigo maligna melanoma), 2228t
Lobar arteries, 1537
Lobar collapse, endotracheal tube suctioning and, 1175t
Lobar pneumonia, 1135, 1138
Lobectomy, for lung cancer, 1156, 1156
- frontal, for pain, 386
Lobular carcinoma in situ, 2434
Lobular hyperplasia, atypical, 2452
Lobular pneumonia, 1138
Lobule, liver, 1835, 1837
LOC. See Level of consciousness (LOC).
Local adaptation syndrome (LAS), 22
Local anesthesia, 474
- agents for, 473t–474t
- in pain control, 372
Localization, in unconscious patient, 723
Locus of control, 64
- assessment of, 191t
Lomotil (diphenoxylate), for diarrhea, in inflammatory bowel disease, 1798, 1798t
Long bones, 2073, 2075
Long leg cast, 2137t, 2148
Longitudinal fracture, 2130, 2130
Longitudinal pancreaticojejunostomy Roux-en-Y, for acute pancreatitis, 1927
Long-term care facilities, for chronic conditions, 113
Long-term nonprogressors (LTNPs), characteristics of, 621
Loniten (minoxidil), 1397t

Loop diuretics, 1394t
Loop of Henle, 1535, 1537
Loperamide (Imodium), for diarrhea, in inflammatory bowel disease, 1798, 1798t
Lopressor (metoprolol), 1395t
  for angina pectoris, 1257t
  for dysrhythmia, 1308t
Lorazepam, for dementia of Alzheimer's type, 866t
  for status epilepticus, 843
Lordosis, 2087, 2087, 2121
  and intervertebral disc herniation, 917
Losses, multiple, in elderly, 88, 88–89
Lotensin (benazepril), 1396t
Lotions, 2200t
Lotrimin (clotrimazole), topical, 2198t
Low back care, client education in, 918b
Low-density lipoproteins (LDLs), 35
  elevated, in diabetes mellitus, 1977
  in coronary artery disease, 1241
Lower esophageal sphincter (LES), 1687
  in achalasia, 1733–1734
  incompetency of, in regurgitation, 1733
Lower extremity(ies), arterial bypass surgery of, nursing care plan in, 1416–1417
  assessment of, in regional examination, 221t
  edema of, in cirrhosis, 1878t
  physical examination of, in endocrine disorders, 1952
Lower gastrointestinal endoscopy, 1715
Lower gastrointestinal series (barium enema), 251, 1713–1714
Lower motor neuron lesions, 925–926
Low-fat low-cholesterol diet, client education in, 1402b
Low-protein diet, in hepatic encephalopathy, 1893
Low-sodium diet, client education in, 1400b–1401b
Low-tension glaucoma, 952. See also Glaucoma.
Loxapine, for dementia of Alzheimer's type, 866t
Lozol (indapamide), 1394t
LP. See Lumbar puncture (LP).
LSD (lysergic acid diethylamide), 2491. See also Hallucinogens.
LTNPs (long-term nonprogressors), characteristics of, 621
Lubricants, skin, 2202–2203
Lugol's solution, for goiter, 2014
Lumbar discectomy, physical mobility after, 923
Lumbar fusion, physical mobility after, 923
Lumbar laminectomy, case management in, 922b
Lumbar nerve roots, compromise of, testing for, 919, 920
Lumbar puncture (LP), in consciousness disorders, 749
  in leukemia, 1489
  in neurologic assessment, 733–735, 734, 735t
  procedure for, 733
Lumbar spine, function of, assessment of, 2090t–2091t
Lumpectomy, for breast cancer, 2436

Lung(s), abscess of, 1138–1139
  assessment of, in cardiovascular disorders, 1217
    in health history, 184b
    in regional examination, 218t
  defense mechanisms of, 1025–1026, 1026t
  diffusing capacity of, tests of, 1051
  diseases of, interstitial, 1149
    occupational, 1150–1151, 1151t
  disorders of, 1133–1187
    acute, 1169–1184
    neoplastic, 1151–1166. See also Lung cancer.
    restrictive, 1147–1148, 1147b, 1148
  function of, 1029–1034
    in acid-base balance, 328–329, 329, 1033, 1057
  infections of, 1133–1147
    fungal, 1146–1147
  structure of, 1027–1029, 1028
  transplantation of, 1148
  tumors of, benign, 1155
Lung biopsy, 1064
Lung cancer, 1151–1166
  clinical manifestations of, 1152–1153, 1153b
  diagnostic findings in, 1152–1153
  etiology of, 1151
  management of, medical, 1154
    nursing, 1154–1155
    surgical, 1155–1157, 1156
      nursing care in, 1157–1166
      plan for, 1159–1162
  metastasis of, clinical manifestations of, 1152–1153
  pathophysiology of, 1151–1152
  prevention of, 1152b
  risk factors for, 542b, 1151, 1152b
  staging of, 1153, 1154b, 1155
  survival in, 538t
  types of, 1153t
Lung capacities, 1028, 1028
Lung volume reduction surgery, for chronic obstructive pulmonary disease, 1119, 1123
Lung volumes, 1028, 1028
Lupron (leuprolide), for benign prostatic hyperplasia, 2364t
  for endometriosis, 2399
LUQ (left upper quadrant), organs of, 1708
Luque rods, for scoliosis, 2120, 2121
Luteinizing hormone (LH), 2061t
  deficiency of, in hypopituitarism, 2065
  in menstruation, 2299, 2299–2300
Luteinizing hormone–releasing hormone agonists, for chemotherapy, classification of, 577t
Lutherans, beliefs/practices of, 2547
LVF (left ventricular failure), 1280, 1280–1282
Lyme disease, 681
  infectious agent in, 416t
  ocular manifestations of, 978
Lymph, 1376
  flow of, 1372, 1374
Lymph node dissection, cervical, for laryngeal cancer, 1088
Lymph nodes, axillary, palpation of, 2313, 2314

Lymph nodes (Continued)
  biopsy of, in Hodgkin's disease, 1501
  in immunity, 598
  in metastasis, 548
  of head and neck, palpation of, 610t
Lymph nodules, in immunity, 598
Lymphadenitis, 1441
Lymphadenopathy, in syphilis, 2470
Lymphadenopathy-associated virus (LAV), 614
Lymphangiography, in cancer diagnosis, 556
  in immune disorder assessment, 611–612
  in leukemia, 1489
Lymphatic drainage, of breasts, 2297, 2297
  of esophagus, 1687
  of pelvis, 2296
Lymphatic glands, of skin, structure/function of, 2176t
  tests of, in immune disorder assessment, 611
Lymphatic system, age-related changes in, 1376
  disorders of, 1439–1441
  in fluid balance regulation, 277
  role of, 1376
  structure of, 1372, 1373, 1374
Lymphedema, 1439–1441, 1440
  after mastectomy, 2443
  after vulvectomy, 2420
  clinical manifestations of, 1440
  diagnostic findings in, 1440
  etiology of, 1439–1440
  management of, 1440–1441
  risk factors for, 1439–1440
  types of, 1439–1440, 1440
Lymphocytes, B. See B cells.
  functions of, 1448t
  in blood dyscrasias, 1465t
  in differential count, interpretation of, 436t
  in erythropoiesis, 1452, 1452, 1453
  in wound healing, 429
  maturation of, 597
  reference values for, in cancer, 557t
  T. See T cells.
Lymphogranuloma venereum, 2475
Lymphoid organs, central, in immunity, 595–597, 596, 597
Lymphoid system, disorders of, 1500–1505
Lymphoid tissue, peripheral, antigen transport to, 598, 599
  in immunity, 597–598
Lymphokines, in wound healing, 429
Lymphoma, non-Hodgkin's, 1503
  in acquired immunodeficiency syndrome, 630–631
  ocular manifestations of, 977
  survival in, 538t
  T-cell, cutaneous, 2230
Lymphoproliferative disorders, 1459
Lysergic acid diethylamide (LSD), 2491. See also Hallucinogens.
Lysodren (mitotane), for hypercortisolism, 2053
Lysosomal enzymes, release of, in shock, 507
Lysosomes, 266

Lysozyme, reference values for, in cancer, 557t
Lyssavirus, 416t

M

M phase, of cell cycle, 545, *545*
Maalox, for peptic ulcer disease, 1769t, 1770
MAC (*Mycobacterium avium-intracellulare* complex), in acquired immunodeficiency syndrome, 628
prophylaxis for, 625
MAC (midarm circumference), measurement of, 237, *240*
Maceration, definition of, 2183t
Machine-cycled (controlled) ventilation, 1177, 1178t
Macrobid (nitrofurantoin), for urinary tract infections, 1575t
urine color with, 1557t
Macrocytes, 1466t
Macrodantin (nitrofurantoin), for urinary tract infections, 1575t
urine color with, 1557t
Macrophages, alveolar, 1026
depression of, in shock, 509
in inflammation, 594, *595*
in wound healing, 428–429
structure/function of, 2176t
Macrovascular disease, in diabetes mellitus, 1993–1996, 1994t–1995t
prevention of, client education in, 1996b
Macula, 938
Macula densa, 1536
Macular degeneration, age-related, 965–966, *966*
management of, 199t
Macule, *2184*
MADD (Mothers Against Drunk Driving), 2497b
Mafenide acetate, for burns, 2254t
Magnesium, dietary, sources of, 324b
distribution of, 293t
functions of, 322–323
homeostasis of, 322, *323*
imbalances of, 322–325, *323, 324b*
measurement of, in cardiovascular assessment, 1220
plasma, range for, 296b
supplementation of, for hypertension, 1393
Magnesium oxide (Mag-Ox), for peptic ulcer disease, 1769t
Magnesium sulfate, topical, 2199t
Magnetic resonance imaging (MRI), 252–253
care in, postprocedure, 253
preprocedure, 252–253
in cancer diagnosis, 559
in consciousness disorders, 749
in gynecologic disorders, 2322–2323
in intervertebral disc herniation, 919, *919*
in myocardial infarction, 1262
of adrenal glands, 2045t
of cardiovascular system, 1227–1228
of ear, 991
of eyes, 950, *950*
of gastrointestinal tract, 1713

Magnetic resonance imaging (MRI) *(Continued)*
of male reproductive system, 2339
of musculoskeletal system, 2094
of neurologic system, 732, *732*
of peripheral vascular system, 1384
of respiratory tract, 1061
of thyroid, 2011t
of urinary tract, 1564
procedure for, 252, *252*
Mag-Ox (magnesium oxide), for peptic ulcer disease, 1769t
Major histocompatibility complex (MHC), 643, 653
in immunity, 596, 599
Mal ojo, 32b
Malabsorption, in intestinal disorders, 1787–1788
Malaise, in rheumatic fever, 1328
Malaria, infectious agent in, 416t
Male, cancer in, risk factors for, 542b
role of, 75–76
Malecot catheter, 2355t
Malignancy, second, 587–588
Malignant, definition of, 533
Malignant hypertension, 1388
emergency management of, 1404, 1405t
Malignant hyperthermia, intraoperative monitoring for, 478–479
Malignant melanoma, 2227–2228, *2228*
Malignant pain, 352–353, 358–359
Malingering, 359
Malleus, structure of, *981,* 982
Malnutrition, in Crohn's disease, consequences of, 1797
in delayed wound healing, 444
in elderly, risk factors for, 86, 86b
in pressure ulcers, management of, 2215–2216
protein-calorie, adipose tissue measurement in, *240*
Maltase, 1692t
secretion of, 1693
Malunion, in fracture, prevention of, 2145
MAMC (midarm muscle circumference), measurement of, 237, *240*
Mammaplasty, 2453
augmentation, *2283, 2283–2284*
reduction, *2285, 2285–2286*
Mammography, *2327, 2327–2328, 2328*
in breast cancer detection, 556, 2433, *2433*
indications for, 2328
schedule for, 209t
Management, case. See *Case management.*
client, nurse in, 124
nurse in, 125
of respiratory care, 1073b
Mandatory reporting, in emergency care, 2502
Mandelamine (methenamine mandelate), for urinary tract infections, 1575t
Mannitol, characteristics of, 1285t
for acute renal failure, 1639
for glaucoma, 955
for increased intracranial pressure, 775
Manometry, splenic pulp, 1856
Mantoux test, 1142

MAO (monoamine oxidase) inhibitors, effect of, on male reproductive system, 2345
intraoperative complications of, 457
MAP (mean arterial pressure), 1202
in shock, 502
Marcaine (bupivacaine), 473t
in pain control, 372
Marcaine HCl (bupivacaine hydrochloride), 473t
Marginal ulcer, in peptic ulcer disease, 1778
Marie-Strumpell disease, 678, *679*
Marijuana. See *Cannabis.*
Mark II pain theory, 351, *351*
Marriage, stroke effect on, nursing research on, 790b
Marshall-Marchetti-Krantz procedure, 1608
Mason's theory, of stress response specificity, 23
Mass peristalsis, 1695
Massage, ice, in pain control, 371
in pain control, 349b
prostatic, 2336, *2337*
MAST (military antishock trousers), 516–517, *517*
Mast cell stabilizers, for chronic obstructive pulmonary disease, 1111t
Mast cells, in wound healing, *428,* 430
structure/function of, 2176t
Mastalgia, 2453
Mastectomy, case management in, 2437b
clinical pathway for, 2603–2604
concentration ability after, nursing research on, 2439b
prophylactic, 2436
radical, extended, 2437
modified, 2437
nursing care plan in, 2440–2441
standard, 2437
subcutaneous, 2286
total (simple), 2437
Master's of Science in Nursing (MSN), 14
Mastitis, lactation, 2452
Mastodynia, 2453
Mastoid bone, structure/function of, 983
Mastoid cavity, infection of, client education in, 1008b
Mastoidectomy, closed, 1006
open, 1006
Mastoiditis, 1006
Mastopexy, 2286
Maturity-onset diabetes of the young (MODY), 1957
Maximal expiratory pressure (MEP), 1052t
Maximal inspiratory pressure (MIP), 1052t
Maximal voluntary ventilation (MVV), 1052t
McGill Pain Questionnaire, 115t
McGill-Melzack Pain Questionnaire, *364*
MCH (mean corpuscular hemoglobin), 1466t
in blood dyscrasias, 1465t
MCHC (mean corpuscular hemoglobin concentration), 1466t
in blood dyscrasias, 1465t
MCL (midclavicular line), in liver percussion, 1846t
McMurray's test, 2091t

MCV (mean corpuscular volume), 1466t
in blood dyscrasias, 1465t
MD (muscular dystrophy), 2125–2126, 2125t
MDF (myocardial depressant factor), in shock, 498, 506, 507
MDI (metered-dose inhaler), 1039
for asthma, 1110–1111, *1111*
use of, directions for, 1112b
MDR-TB (multidrug resistant tuberculosis), 627, 1140
Meal delivery services, for elderly, 99
Mealtime assistive devices, in burns, 2258, *2258*
Mean arterial pressure (MAP), 1202
in shock, 502
Mean corpuscular hemoglobin (MCH), 1466t
in blood dyscrasias, 1465t
Mean corpuscular hemoglobin concentration (MCHC), 1466t
in blood dyscrasias, 1465t
Mean corpuscular volume (MCV), 1466t
in blood dyscrasias, 1465t
Measles, immunization recommendations for, in adults, 422t
infectious agent in, 416t
Meatus, anatomy of, 1539
function of, 1545
Mechanical ablation, of dysrhythmias, 1314
Mechanical injury, of cells, 270
Mechanical intervention, for renal calculi, 1668
Mechanical obstruction, and dysphagia, 1732
Mechanical ventilation, continuous. See *Continuous mechanical ventilation (CMV).*
nursing care in, 1173–1184
plan for, 1180–1182
Mechanoreceptors, in fluid balance regulation, 277
Meckel's diverticulum, 1819–1820
Meclorethamine, oncovin, procarbazine, prednisone (MOPP), for Hodgkin's disease, 576t, 1502, 1503t
Medial epicondylitis, 2169t
Medial frontal leukotomy, for pain, 386
Median nerve, neurovascular assessment of, *2093*
Mediastinal flutter, open pneumothorax with, chest trauma and, 2524–2525, *2525*
Mediastinal shift, tension pneumothorax with, chest trauma and, *2525*, 2525–2526
Mediastinum, 1028
Medicaid, 5b, 95–96
history of, 7
in home healthcare reimbursement, 148b
Medical examiner, jurisdiction of, 2513–2515
Medical terminology, prefixes/suffixes in, 452t
Medical-surgical emergencies, 2517–2540
Medical-surgical nursing, 3–17
Medicare, 5b, 95
diagnosis-related groups in, 8
history of, 7
in home healthcare reimbursement, 148b

Medication(s), and hemolytic anemia, 1479
contraindicated, in viral hepatitis, 1867
for increased intracranial pressure, 775
for neurogenic bladder dysfunction, 1617
history of, in cardiovascular disorders, 1207
in ear disorders, 986, 986b
in endocrine disorders, 1949
in eye disorders, 942
in gastrointestinal disorders, 1704
in gynecologic disorders, 2308
in hematologic disorders, 1462
in hepatobiliary disorders, 1844
in integumentary system disorders, 2180
in male reproductive disorders, 2330
in musculoskeletal disorders, 2085
in neurologic disorders, 714
in respiratory disorders, 1039
in urinary tract disorders, 1550
in hypocalcemia, 315t
in hypokalemia, 305t
in hypomagnesemia, 323
in immunity, 605
in renal calculus prevention, 1670
in urinary incontinence, 1605
in urine color, 1556–1557, 1557t
metabolism of, in chronic renal failure, 1645
multiple, management of, home healthcare in, 95b
pain, administration of, 368
preoperative, on day of surgery, 464, 465t
use of, in elderly, 92–93
preoperative assessment of, 457, 458t
vasoactive, for shock, 514–515, 515t
Meditation, in pain control, 349b, 369
Medrol (methylprednisolone), 2048t
after heart transplantation, 1353, 1354b
for multiple sclerosis, 874
for rheumatoid arthritis, 664t
Medtronic-Hall tilting disc valve, *1352*
Medulla oblongata, *691, 693, 693*
structures of, functions of, 694t
Medullary carcinoma, of breast, 2434
of thyroid, 2028t
Medullary polycystic disease, 1679
Medullary sponge kidney, 1679
Medulloblastoma, cerebellar, *846*
Megacolon, acquired, 1825
congenital, 1830
toxic, in ulcerative colitis, 1796
Megakaryocytes, in erythropoiesis, 1452
Megaloblastic anemia, 1474–1477
Megaureter, 1621
Meibomian glands, 936, *937*
Meissner's plexus, 1689–1690
Melanin, in skin color, 2174–2175
Melanocytes, structure/function of, 2174–2175, 2176t
Melanocyte-stimulating hormone (MSH), actions of, 1940t
Melanoma, malignant, 2227–2228, *2228*
ocular, 970–971
types of, 2228, 2228t
Melanosomes, 2174–2175
Melasma, 2178
Melena, 1787
in peptic ulcer disease, 1771

Melphalan, for multiple myeloma, 1499
Membrane-stabilizing agents, in pain control, 378
Membranoproliferative glomerulonephritis, 1633
Memory, 691
assessment of, 195, 710t, 716
for recent events, loss of, 765
Menarche, 2298–2299
Menghini's technique, 1854–1855
Ménière's disease, and balance disorders, 1011
Meningeal irritation, signs of, 856, *857*
Meninges, structure/function of, *697, 697–698*
Meningioma, *838, 845*
cerebrovascular accident and fractured hip with, case study of, *794, 794–795*
parasagittal, *846*
sphenoidal ridge, *846*
Meningitis, after intracranial surgery, 850
prevention of, 852–853
bacterial, 856–857, *857*
clinical manifestations of, 856
diagnosis of, 856
emergency care of, 857
factors predisposing to, 856
infectious agent in, 416t
viral, 859
Meniscus, injuries of, *2166*, 2166–2167
Mennonites, beliefs/practices of, 2547
Menopause, 2301–2302, 2392–2395
cultural beliefs about, 2427b
difficulties in, 2392–2395
management of, community/self care in, 2393–2395
medical, 2393–2394
nursing, 2394–2395
sleep disorders in, 404–405
surgical, 2392
Menorrhagia, 2391, *2392*
Menstrual cycle, *2299*, 2299–2300
phases of, premenstrual, *2299*, 2300
proliferative, *2299*, 2299–2300
secretory, *2299*, 2300, *2301*
Menstrual history, 2309
Menstruation, 2300
cultural beliefs about, 2426b
disorders of, 2386–2398
Mental health disorders, in elderly, 90–92, 92t
treatment of, 91
Mental status, assessment of, 190–196, 235, 715–718
components of, 195–196
in substance abuse, 2486t
normal findings in, 717b
changes in, brain tumor and, 847
in endocrine disorders, 1948
Mentation, assessment of, 710t
Menthol paste, 2198t
MEP (maximal expiratory pressure), 1052t
Meperidine (Demerol), administration of, 381t
after thyroidectomy, 2024t
in pain control, 375t, 376
preoperative, 465t

6-Mercaptopurine, for inflammatory bowel disease, 1799
Merkel cells, 2175
Mesenteric infarction, and small intestinal obstruction, 1821
Messenger RNA (mRNA), 265
Mestinon (pyridostigmine), for myasthenia gravis, 885
Metabolic acidosis, 335t, 336
    critical monitoring in, 337b
    etiology of, 335t, 336
    hyperchloremic, 336
    in acute hyperglycemia, 1984t
    in renal failure, acute, 1639–1640
        chronic, 1645
Metabolic alkalosis, 335t, 336
    critical monitoring in, 337b
    etiology of, 335t, 336
    posthypercapneic, 336
Metabolic bone disorders, 2098–2108
Metabolic equivalents (METs), in physical activity measurement, after myocardial infarction, 1264
Metabolism, effects on, of epinephrine, 2057t
    of norepinephrine, 2057t
    in chronic renal failure, 1644–1645
    in shock, 509
    increase in, in burns, 2257
    kidneys in, 1543–1544
    liver in, 1839–1840
    of carbohydrates, hormones in, 1945–1946, 1946
    of drugs, cultural differences in, 94b–95b
        in chronic renal failure, 1645
    of minerals, in musculoskeletal disorders, tests of, 2096t
    of purine, in gout, 2107
    pattern of, 206
Metabolites, in hematopoiesis, 1453
    muscle, in blood pressure regulation, 1204
Metacarpals, fracture of, 2161
Metahydrin (trichlormethiazide), 1394t
Metamorphopsia, 965
Metaplasia, 267, 267
    definition of, 534t
Metarubricytes, 1466t
Metastasis, 1376
    definition of, 534t
    stages of, 547–548, 548
Metastatic breast cancer, 2450–2451
Metered-dose inhaler (MDI), 1039
    for asthma, 1110–1111, 1111
    use of, directions for, 1112b
Metformin (Glucophage), for diabetes mellitus, 1967t, 1968
Methadone (Dolophine), administration of, 381t
    in pain control, 376
Methanol, antidote to, 2538t
Methemalbumin, in hepatobiliary assessment, 1851t
Methenamine mandelate (Mandelamine), for urinary tract infections, 1575t
Methicillin-resistant Staphylococcus aureus (MRSA), 419
    in postoperative wound infection, 491

Methimazole (Tapazole), for hyperthyroidism, 2013t, 2019
Methodists, beliefs/practices of, 2547
Methohexital sodium, in rectal anesthesia, 472
Methotrexate, for psoriasis, 2211
    for rheumatoid arthritis, 664t
Methsuximide (Celontin), side effects of, 839t
Methyclothiazide (Enduron), 1394t
Methyl tert-butyl ether (MTBE), for cholelithiasis, 1912
Methyldopa (Aldomet), 1396t
    in surgical client, 458t
    urine color with, 1557t
Methylene blue, urine color with, 1557t
Methylprednisolone (Medrol), 2048t
    after heart transplantation, 1353, 1354b
    for multiple sclerosis, 874
    for rheumatoid arthritis, 664t
Methylprednisolone sodium succinate (Solu-Medrol), in organ transplantation, 645t
Metoclopramide (Reglan), for gastroesophageal reflux disease, 1738
Metolazone (Zaroxolyn), 1394t
Metoprolol (Lopressor, Toprol XL), 1395t
    for angina pectoris, 1257t
    for dysrhythmia, 1308t
Metronidazole (Flagyl), for bacterial vaginosis, 2474
    for peptic ulcer disease, 1767, 1769t
Metrorrhagia, 2392
METs (metabolic equivalents), in physical activity measurement, after myocardial infarction, 1264
Mexican-Americans, dietary practices of, 1702b–1703b
    pain response in, 347b
Mexiletine (Mexitil), for dysrhythmia, 1307t
    in pain control, 378
Mexitil (mexiletine), for dysrhythmia, 1307t
    in pain control, 378
MG. See Myasthenia gravis (MG).
MHC (major histocompatibility complex), 643, 653
    in immunity, 596, 599
MI. See Myocardial infarction (MI).
Microaggregate filter, for blood transfusion, 1526t
Microangiopathy, in diabetes mellitus, 1996–1999
Microbiologic studies, 243–245, 244b
    cultures in, blood, 244
        urine, 245
        wound, 244
Microcapillary blood collection, 246–247
Microcirculation, in shock, 502–503
Microcytes, 1466t
Microdiscectomy, clinical pathway for, 2570–2571
Microfilaments, 266
Microglia, 687, 688
Micrography, specular, 950
Micronase (glyburide), for diabetes mellitus, 1967t
    in surgical client, 458t
Microtubules, 266

Microvascular disease, diabetes mellitus and, 1996–1999
Micturition, 1544
    stimulation of, in neurogenic bladder dysfunction, 1617–1618
Micturition reflex, electrical stimulation of, for urinary incontinence, 1607, 1607–1608
Midamor (amiloride), 1394t
Midarm circumference (MAC), measurement of, 237, 240
Midarm muscle circumference (MAMC), measurement of, 237, 240
Midaxillary lymph nodes, palpation of, 2313, 2314
Midazolam hydrochloride (Versed), preoperative, 465t
Midbrain, 691, 693, 693
    structures of, functions of, 694t
Midclavicular line (MCL), in liver percussion, 1846t
Middle cerebral artery, cerebrovascular accident of, clinical manifestations of, 788t
Midline hypopigmentation, 2188b
Midsternal line (MSL), in liver percussion, 1845
Midstream urine specimen, 1555
Migraine headaches, 358, 818–819, 818b
    atypical, 819
    classic, 819
    client education in, 818b
    treatment of, 819
Milia, definition of, 2183t
Miliary tuberculosis, 1144
Military antishock trousers (MAST), 516–517, 517
Milking, of chest tube, 1165, 1165
Milkman's syndrome, 2106
Miller-Abbott tube, 1749t, 1750
Milontin (phensuximide), side effects of, 839t
Mind-body views, 26–27
Mineralocorticoids, 2048t
    actions of, 1940t
    dysfunction of, 2044t
    function of, 2044t
    release of, in shock, 508
    synthesis of, adrenal cortex in, 1944
Minerals, for chronic renal failure, 1654
    for premenstrual syndrome, 2388
    metabolism of, tests of, in musculoskeletal disorders, 2096t
Minimal change glomerulonephritis, 1634
Minipress (prazosin), 1395t
    for benign prostatic hyperplasia, 2364t
Mini-strokes. See Transient ischemic attacks (TIAs).
Minnesota tube, for bleeding esophageal varices, 1885
Minority AIDS Project, 619b
Minority populations, human immunodeficiency virus infection in, 616b–619b
Minoxidil (Loniten), 1397t
Miotics, action of, sites of, 955, 955
MIP (maximal inspiratory pressure), 1052t
Misconceptions, about breast cancer, 2431
    about pain, 360, 361t
        in elderly, 391, 392t

Misoprostol (Cytotec), for acute gastritis, 1762
  for peptic ulcer disease, 1768t
Mithracin (plicamycin), for hypercalcemia, 321, 2034t
  for hyperparathyroidism, 2033
Mitochondria, 265
Mitochondrial antibodies, in hepatobiliary disease, 1849
Mitosis, 262
Mitotane (Lysodren), for hypercortisolism, 2053
Mitral regurgitation, 1342, *1345*
  clinical manifestations of, 1347
  management of, medical, 1347
  pathophysiology of, 1346
Mitral stenosis, 1342, *1345*
  clinical manifestations of, 1347
  management of, medical, 1347
  pathophysiology of, 1346
Mitral valve, 1193, *1194*
  disease of, 1342–1347
    clinical manifestations of, 1347
    diagnostic findings in, 1347
    etiology of, 1344
    management of, medical, 1347
      surgical, 1347
    pathophysiology of, 1344–1346, *1346*
    risk factors for, 1344
Mitral valve prolapse, 1344
  chest pain in, assessment of, 1208t
  clinical manifestations of, 1347
  management of, medical, 1347
  pathophysiology of, 1346, *1346*
Mixed central/peripheral pain, 357–358
Mixed connective tissue disease, 681
Mixed gallstones, 1908
Mixed hearing loss, 994b
Mixed lymphocyte culture, in organ transplantation, 643
MoAbs (monoclonal antibodies), for cancer, 586
  for renal graft rejection, 1662
  for shock, 520
  in immunity, 601
Mobility. See also *Physical mobility.*
  abnormal, in fracture, 2134
  in elderly, 87–88
  preoperative assessment of, 455
  promotion of, after intertrochanteric hip fracture, 2157
    in spinal cord injury, 900, *902*
  postoperative, 492
Mobitz type I block, *1303*, 1304
Mobitz type II block, *1303*, 1304
Modified Borg Category-Rate Scale, in dyspnea assessment, 1036, 1037t
Modified Brooke formula, for fluid resuscitation, in burns, 2250t
Modified Monroe-Kellie hypothesis, 771
Modified radical mastectomy, for breast cancer, 2437
  nursing care plan in, 2440–2441
Modified Trendelenburg's position, for shock, *517*, 517–518, 518b
  nursing research on, 518b
Modrastane (trilostane), for hypercortisolism, 2053

MODY (maturity-onset diabetes of the young), 1957
Mohs' surgery, 2229
Moisture, of skin, assessment of, 2187
Mole, hydatidiform, 2423
  invasive, 2423–2424
Molecular mimicry, in autoimmunity, *654, 655*
Moles, malignant transformation of, danger signals of, 2226b
Molteno implant, for glaucoma, 957
Mometasone (Elocon), topical, 2199t
Mongolian spots, 2188b
Moniliasis. See *Candidiasis, oral.*
Monitored anesthesia, 476
Monitoring, critical. See *Critical monitoring.*
  intracranial, 775–778, *776–777*
Monoamine oxidase (MAO) inhibitors, effect of, on male reproductive system, 2345
  intraoperative complications of, 457
Monoclonal antibodies (MoAbs), for cancer, 586
  for renal graft rejection, 1662
  for shock, 520
  in immunity, 601
Monoclonal hypothesis, of coronary artery disease pathogenesis, 1243
Monocytes, functions of, 1448t
  in blood dyscrasias, 1465t
  in differential count, interpretation of, 436t
  in erythropoiesis, 1451–1452
  in wound healing, 428–429
  reference values for, in cancer, 557t
Mononeuritis, 926
Mononeuropathy, diabetic, 2000
Mononucleosis, infectious, 1503–1504
  clinical manifestations of, 1504
  diagnostic findings in, 1504
  etiology of, 1503
  management of, medical, 1504
    nursing, 1504
  pathophysiology of, 1503–1504
  risk factors for, 1503
Monopril (fosinopril), 1396t
Monroe-Kellie hypothesis, modified, 771
Mons pubis, 2293, *2294*
  examination of, 2317
Montgomery's glands, 2297
Montgomery's tubercles, inspection of, 2313
Mood, assessment of, 195, 716–717
MOPP (mechlorethamine, oncovin, procarbazine, prednisone), for Hodgkin's disease, 576t, 1502, 1503t
Morals, definition of, 40
Mormons, beliefs/practices of, 2548–2549
  dietary, 1701b
Morphea, 677
Morphine, administration of, 380t
  avoidance of, in cirrhosis, 1882t
  in pain control, effects of, 376t
  physical dependence on, 377
  time action of, 379
Morphine sulfate, after thyroidectomy, 2024t
  for angina pectoris, 1256t
  for burns, 2251

Morphine sulfate *(Continued)*
  preoperative, 465t
Morton's neuroma, 2125
MOSF. See *Multiple organ system failure (MOSF).*
Mothers Against Drunk Driving (MADD), 2497b
Motilin, 1691t
Motility, of gastrointestinal tract, 1685, *1686, 1687*
Motion sickness, 1011
Motivation, assessment of, 196
Motofen (difenoxin), for diarrhea, in inflammatory bowel disease, 1798t
Motor activity, assessment of, 711t–712t
  in unconscious patient, 723
    normal findings in, 717b
  in increased intracranial pressure, 781
  of esophagus, 1689
  of large intestine, 1695
  of small intestine, 1694
  of stomach, 1690
Motor aphasia, 789
Motor paralytic bladder, 1615, *1616*
Motor response, in consciousness disorders, 748, *748*
  in increased intracranial pressure, 781
Motor systems, assessment of, 721–723, 722b, 723b
Motorcycle accident, blunt trauma in, 2521t
Motrin (ibuprofen), for rheumatoid arthritis, 664t
  in pain control, 375t
MOTT (mycobacteria other than tuberculosis), 1145–1146
Mourning, cultural issues in, 70b–71b
  process of, 109–110
Mouth, 1685–1687
  assessment of, in health history, 183b–184b
    in regional examination, 216t
  disorders of, 1723–1732
  in chewing, 1685–1686
  in hematologic disorders, 1463
  in swallowing, 1687, *1688*
  physical examination of, in endocrine disorders, 1950
    normal findings in, 1699b
  structure of, 1685
Mouth care, in cancer, 587b
Mouth-to-stoma ventilation, 1072
Movement, abnormal, in extrapyramidal disease, 723b
  assessment of, 235, 712t, 722–723, 723b
  muscles in, 2078, *2080*
MPEC (multipolar electrocoagulation), for bleeding ulcers, 1772
MRI. See *Magnetic resonance imaging (MRI).*
mRNA (messenger RNA), 265
MRSA (methicillin-resistant *Staphylococcus aureus*), 419
  in postoperative wound infection, 491
MS. See *Multiple sclerosis (MS).*
MSH (melanocyte-stimulating hormone), actions of, 1940t
MSL (midsternal line), in liver percussion, 1845

MSN (Master's of Science in Nursing), 14
MTBE (methyl *tert*-butyl ether), for cholelithiasis, 1912
Mucinous carcinoma, of breast, 2434
Mucociliary system, *1025*, 1025–1026
Mucormycosis, 860
Mucosal barrier fortifiers, for peptic ulcer disease, 1769t, 1770
Mucosal immunity, 595
Mucositis, oral, chemotherapy and, 583
Mucous membranes, oral, altered, in cholelithiasis, 1915
   in consciousness disorders, 757–758
   in hypernatremia, 304
   in periodontal disease, 1722
Mucus, secretion of, in large intestine, 1695–1696
Muercke's lines, in chronic renal failure, 1646
MUGA (multiple gated acquisition) scanning, 1230
Müllerian duct inhibitory factor, in male sexual development, 2304
Multicausal theories, of illness, 21
Multidrug resistant tuberculosis (MDR-TB), 627, 1140
Multimodality therapy, in breast cancer, 2446
Multiple gated acquisition (MUGA) scanning, 1230
Multiple myeloma, 1498–1500
   clinical manifestations of, 1499
   complications of, 1499
   diagnostic findings in, 1499
   etiology of, 1499
   management of, medical, 1499
     nursing, 1500
   pathophysiology of, 1499
   risk factors for, 1499
   survival in, 538t
Multiple organ system failure (MOSF), 528–531
   clinical manifestations of, 529–530, 529t
   critical care of, 530–531, 531t
   etiology of, 528
   management of, 530, 531t
   pathophysiology of, 528
   risk factors for, 528
   types of, 528–529
Multiple sclerosis (MS), 873–877
   and optic neuritis, 977
   clinical manifestations of, 873–874
   diagnostic findings in, 873–874
   etiology of, 873
   management of, community/self care in, 874–877
     medical, 874–875
     nursing, 875–877, 876b
   nursing research on, 875b
   pathophysiology of, 873, *874*
   prevention of, 873b
   risk factors for, 873, 873b
Multiple sleep latency test, 407
Multipolar electrocoagulation (MPEC), for bleeding ulcers, 1772
Mumps, immunization recommendations for, in adults, 422t
   surgical, 1732

Mupirocin (Bactroban), topical, 2198t
Murmurs, 1216–1217, 1218t, 1219b
   diastolic, 1218t
   grading of, 1219b
   regurgitant, pansystolic, 1218t
   systolic, 1218t
     early, 1218t
     late, 1218t
Muromonab-CD3 (OKT3), after heart transplantation, 1353, 1354b
   for renal graft rejection, 1662
   in organ transplantation, 645t
Murphy and Murphy model, for ethical decision-making, 43–45, 44t
   nursing process comparison with, 43, 44t
Murphy's sign, in acute cholecystitis, 1916
Muscle(s), contractility of, in free flap assessment, 2281
   coordination of, assessment of, 722
   functions of, 2078–2079, *2080*
   physical examination of, 2087–2088, 2088t
   size of, assessment of, 721
   types of, 2077–2079, *2079, 2080*
Muscle atrophy, inspection of, in peripheral vascular assessment, 1380
Muscle biopsy, in neurologic assessment, 741
Muscle cells, 265
Muscle contraction headaches, 820
Muscle cramps, in endocrine disorders, 1949
Muscle fibers, 2078
Muscle metabolites, in blood pressure regulation, 1204
Muscle pain, 355
Muscle spasm, in rheumatoid arthritis, 658
   in spinal cord injury, 893–894, 909
Muscle strength, assessment of, 721–722, 2087, 2088t
   in fitness, 174b
Muscle tone, 2087
   assessment of, 722
Muscle-stretch (deep tendon) reflexes, *726, 727*, 727b
   assessment of, guidelines for, 727b
   in left hemiparesis, *728*
Muscular arteries, 1369
Muscular dystrophy (MD), 2125–2126, 2125t
Muscular Dystrophy Association, 887b
Muscular system, structure/function of, 2077–2079, *2079, 2080*
Musculocutaneous flaps, 2279
   critical monitoring in, 2279b
Musculoskeletal system, age-related changes in, 268t, 2080–2081
   physical changes with, 454t
   assessment of, in health history, 185b
   in urinary tract assessment, 1554
   deformities of, 2086–2087, *2087*
   disorders of, 2081, 2098–2126
     assessment of, 2083–2097
      diagnostic tests in, 2092–2097
      history in, 2083–2086
      laboratory, 2096, 2096t
      physical examination in, 2086–2092, *2087*

Musculoskeletal system *(Continued)*
     normal findings in, 2086b
   chest pain in, assessment of, 1209t
   sexuality in, 78
   emergencies of, 2533
   in alcohol abuse, 2490t
   in chronic renal failure, 1646
   in hematologic disorders, 1463
   in homeostasis, 2079–2080
   in hypercalcemia, 321t
   in hypocalcemia, 317t
   in hypokalemia, 309t
   in thyroid disorders, 2008t
   overuse of, 2129–2169
   structure/function of, 2073–2081
   trauma to, 2129–2169
Music, in pain control, 349b, 371
   in postoperative analgesia, nursing research on, 1781b
Mutations, genetic, 265
MVV (maximal voluntary ventilation), 1052t
Myasthenia gravis (MG), 883–886
   cholinergic crisis in, 886b
   complications of, 885
   diagnosis of, 884–885
   management of, medical, 885
     nursing, 885–886
     surgical, 886
   myasthenic crisis in, 886b
   ocular manifestations of, 977
Myasthenia Gravis Foundation, 887b
Myasthenic crisis, 885, 886b
Myasthenic syndrome, 886
Mycobacteria other than tuberculosis (MOTT), 1145–1146
Mycobacterium avium-intracellulare complex (MAC), in acquired immunodeficiency syndrome, 628
   prophylaxis for, 625
Mycobacterium tuberculosis, 416t, 1140
   in acquired immunodeficiency syndrome, 627–628
Mycoplasma pneumoniae, 416t, 1137t
Mycosis fungoides, 2230
Mycostatin (nystatin), topical, 2198t
Mycotic aneurysm, 786
Mydriatic agents, action of, sites of, 955, *955*
Myelin, in nerve impulse conduction, 689
Myelin sheath, 689
   in multiple sclerosis, 873, *874*
Myelography, 733, 2094
   in neurologic assessment, 735–736, *736*
Myeloma, multiple. See *Multiple myeloma.*
Myelomalacia, 916–917
Myelosuppression, chemotherapy and, 580–582
   for polycythemia vera, 1486
Myelotoxins, categories of, 1477
Mylanta, for peptic ulcer disease, 1769t, 1770
Myleran (busulfan), for chronic myelogenous leukemia, 1491
Myocardial cell, action potential in, *294*
Myocardial depressant factor (MDF), in shock, 498, 506, 507

Myocardial infarction (MI), 1258–1276
  after abdominal aortic aneurysm repair, 1427
  and cardiogenic shock, 499
  chest pain in, assessment of, 1208t
  clinical manifestations of, 1258–1262, 1261, 1262
  complications of, 1266–1267, 1267
  convalescence after, home healthcare in, 1265b
  diagnostic findings in, 1258–1262, 1261, 1262
  etiology of, 1258
  management of, 1259
    critical, 1263–1264, 1263b
    emergency, 1262
    medical, 1264–1267
      outcomes of, 1267
    nursing, 1267–1276
    nursing care plan in, 1270–1276
  pathophysiology of, 1258, 1260
  postoperative, prevention of, 487
  recurrent, 1267
  risk factors for, 1258
  sexuality after, 78
Myocardial rupture, after myocardial infarction, 1267, 1267
Myocardial scintigraphy, in cardiovascular assessment, 1229–1230
Myocarditis, 1334–1335
  causes of, 1334–1335
  clinical manifestations of, 1335
  diagnostic findings in, 1335
  management of, 1335
  rheumatic, 1328t
Myocardium, 1191, 1192, 2078
  deterioration of, in shock, 506
  injury to, in cardiogenic shock, management of, 523t
  rheumatic fever of, 1328t
Myochrysine (gold salts), for rheumatoid arthritis, 664t
Myoclonic seizures, in epilepsy, 837
Myoclonus, 723b
Myofibrils, 1196, 1196, 2078
Myofibroblasts, in wound healing, 432
Myomectomy, for leiomyoma, 2401
Myometrium, 2296
Myopia, 946, 975, 975–976
Myosin filaments, 1196, 1196
Myringoplasty, 1008
Myringotomy, 1009
Mysoline (primidone), side effects of, 839t
  therapeutic monitoring of, reference values for, 2562
Myths, 60
  about pain, 360, 361t
Myxedema, definition of, 2005
  in hypothyroidism, 2007, 2009
Myxedema coma, in hypothyroidism, 2007–2012
  management of, medical, 2009
    nursing, 2009–2012

N

Nadir, in chemotherapy, 581
Nadolol (Corgard), 1395t

Nadolol (Corgard) (Continued)
  for angina pectoris, 1257t
Nafarelin (Synarel), for benign prostatic hyperplasia, 2364t
  for endometriosis, 2399
Naftifine (Naftin), topical, 2198t
Naftin (naftifine), topical, 2198t
Nails, assessment of, in health history, 183b
  disorders of, 2223–2224
  physical examination of, 2186, 2187t
    normal findings in, 2182b
  pigmentation of, biocultural variations in, 2188b
  structure/function of, 2175, 2176t
Nalbuphine (Nubain), administration of, 381t
Nalfon (fenoprofen), for rheumatoid arthritis, 664t
Nalidixic acid (NegGram), for urinary tract infections, 1575t
Naloxone (Narcan), for altered level of consciousness, 2517
  for shock, 520
Naprosyn (naproxen), for rheumatoid arthritis, 664t
  in pain control, 375t
Naproxen (Anaprox, Naprosyn), for rheumatoid arthritis, 664t
  in pain control, 375t
Naqua (trichlormethiazide), 1394t
Narcan (naloxone), for altered level of consciousness, 2517
  for shock, 520
Narcolepsy, 400–401
Narcotics, antidote for, 2538t
  for burns, 2251
  for shock, 521, 522
Narcotics Anonymous, 2497b
Nares, 1022, 1022
Nasal cavity, structure of, 1022, 1022–1023, 1023
Nasal packing, for epistaxis, 1076
Nasal polypectomy, 1102
Nasal polyps, 1101–1102
Nasal septum, deviated, 1102
Nasal speculum, use of, 1049–1050, 1050
Nasoenteral tube, placement of, nursing research on, 1751b
Nasogastric tube, insertion of, in major burns, 2249–2250
Nasopharynx, assessment of, physical examination in, 1050
  structure of, 1023
National AIDS Office, 619b
National Alcohol Hotline, 2497b
National Alzheimer's Association, 887b
National Asian Pacific American Families Against Drug Abuse, 2497b
National Association of People with AIDS, 619b
National Association of State Units on Aging, 97b
National Black Women's Health Project, 619b
National Clearinghouse for Alcohol and Drug Information, 2497b
National Clearinghouse on Aging, 175b

National Coalition for Cancer Survivorship, 564b
National Cocaine Hotline, 2497b
National Council of La Raza AIDS Center, 619b
National Council on the Aging, 97b
National Fire Protection Association Life Safety Code 101, 138
National Health Planning and Resources Act, 7
National Multiple Sclerosis Society, 887b
National Native American AIDS Prevention Center, 619b
National Parkinson's Foundation, Inc., 887b
National Self-Help Clearinghouse, 175b
National Senior Citizens Law Center, 97b
Native Americans, alcohol abuse in, 198t
  diabetes in, 1957b
  dietary practices of, 1703b
  human immunodeficiency virus infection in, 618b–619b
  skin examination in, 2188b–2189b
Native valve endocarditis, 1331
Natural killer (NK) cells, in pathogen resistance, 594–595
Naturetin (bendroflumethiazide), 1394t
Nausea, brain tumor and, 846
  chemotherapy and, 582–583
  in acute cholecystitis, 1917, 1917t
  in gastrointestinal disorders, 1748–1749, 1787
  in peptic ulcer disease, 1766
  in right ventricular failure, 1282
  in viral hepatitis, 1865, 1866t
  opioid analgesics in, 376
  postoperative, 490
  spinal anesthesia and, 476t
Navajos, health/illness beliefs of, 61, 65b
Near drowning, 2522
Nearsightedness, 946, 975, 975–976
Neck, assessment of, in cardiovascular assessment, 1212–1213, 1213
  in health history, 184b
  in regional examination, 214t–217t
    neurologic, 718
    normal findings in, 717b
  inspection of, in respiratory assessment, 1040
  lymph nodes of, palpation of, 610t
  physical examination of, in endocrine disorders, 1950–1951, 1951
  range of motion of, 2089
  repetitive motion injuries of, 2168t
Neck dissection, community/self care in, 1100
  exercises after, client education in, 1096b–1098b
  for laryngeal cancer, 1088
  nursing care in, 1093–1095
Neck veins, assessment of, in cardiovascular assessment, 1212–1213, 1213
Necrosis, caseous, 270
  coagulative, 270
  liquefactive, 270
  of cells, 270–271
Necrotizing pneumonia, 1135
Necrotizing ulcerative gingivitis. See Vincent's angina.

Needle, butterfly, for venipuncture, 246, *248*
Needle (aspiration) biopsy, 257
  in cancer diagnosis, 558, 568
Needle exchange programs (NEPs), in human immunodeficiency virus infection prevention, 615
NegGram (nalidixic acid), for urinary tract infections, 1575t
Neglect, of elderly, 89–90
Neisseria gonorrhoeae, 416t
Neisseria meningitidis, 416t
Nélaton red rubber urethral catheter, 2354t
Nembutal (pentobarbital), for increased intracranial pressure, 775
  for status epilepticus, 843
  preoperative, 465t
Neoadjuvant chemotherapy, for breast cancer, 2448
Neobladder, creation of, for bladder cancer, 1586–1587
Neocortex, 690
Neomycin, for hepatic encephalopathy, 1893
Neomycin-bacitracin-polymyxin B (Neosporin), for open wounds, 445t
Neoplasia, 267
Neoplasm(s). See also *Cancer.*
  classification of, 548–551, 549t, 550t
    benign vs. malignant, 548–549, 549t
    by tissue of origin, 549–551, 550t
  definition of, 533
  in acquired immunodeficiency syndrome, 630–631
  of upper airway, 1082–1100
Neospinothalamic tract, in pain transmission, 344
Neosporin (neomycin-bacitracin-polymyxin B), for open wounds, 445t
Neostigmine (Prostigmin), for myasthenia gravis, 885
Nephrectomy, for renal calculi, 1669
  for renal cancer, 1671–1672
Nephroblastoma, 1671
Nephrolithotomy, for renal calculi, 1669, *1669*
Nephron, anatomy of, 1535, *1537*
  in fluid and electrolyte balance, 1542
  in urine formation, *1540,* 1540–1542
Nephropathy, diabetic, 1625–1626, 1996–1999
  IgA, 1634
Nephroscopy, 1568
  in renal calculus removal, 1668, *1669*
Nephrosis, lipoid, 1634
Nephrostomy, percutaneous, for bladder cancer, *1586,* 1587
Nephrotic syndrome, 1634–1635
  clinical manifestations of, 1635
  complications of, 1635
  diagnostic findings in, 1635
  etiology of, 1634
  management of, dietary, 1635
    medical, 1635
    nursing, 1635
    pharmacologic, 1635
  pathophysiology of, 1634–1635
  risk factors for, 1634
Nephrotoxins, 1627, 1627b
Nephroureterectomy, for renal cancer, 1672

NEPs (needle exchange programs), in human immunodeficiency virus infection prevention, 615
Nerve blocks, *384,* 384–386, 385t
  assessment after, 385–386
  complications of, 385
  contraindications to, 385
  failure of, causes of, 385
  for chronic pain, indications for, 384–385, 385t
  types of, 384, *384*
Nerve conduction velocity study, 740–741
Nerve fibers, myelinated, 689
  of skin, structure/function of, 2176t
  unmyelinated, 689
  vasomotor, in blood flow regulation, 1373
Nerve hearing level, 991
Nerve impulse, 688
Nerve roots, lumbar, compromise of, testing for, 919, *920*
Nervous system, age-related changes in, 705–707
  assessment of, in urinary tract disorders, 1554
  autonomic, disorders of, assessment of, 728–730
    structure/function of, 703–704, *704*
  cancer of, survival in, 538t
  cells of, 265, 685–687, *686,* 687b, *688*
    structure of, 685
  central, divisions of, 690–701
    effects on, of epinephrine, 2057t
    of norepinephrine, 2057t
  impulse conduction in, 687–690, *689*
    refractory period of, 688
  in burns, 2235
  injury to, after total hip replacement, 2113
    effects of, 705–707
    fractures and, 2139
  parasympathetic, 703
    organic effects of, 703, 706t
  peripheral, structure/function of, 701–704, *702–704,* 705t
  structure/function of, 685–707
  sympathetic, 703
    organic effects of, 703, 706t
Nesacaine (chloroprocaine hydrochloride), 473t
Networking, in family nursing intervention, 59
Neuman systems model, health definition in, 162t
Neural hearing loss, 994b
Neuralgia, postherpetic, 357
  trigeminal, 357, *929,* 929–930
Neurectomy, for pain, 386, *387*
Neuritic plaques, in Alzheimer's disease, 863–864, *864*
Neuritis, 926
  optic, multiple sclerosis and, 977
Neuroendocrine system, in shock, 507–509, *508*
Neurofibrillary tangles, in Alzheimer's disease, 863–864, *864*
Neurofibromatosis, 929
Neurogenic bladder dysfunction, 1612–1619
  after spinal cord injury, 901–902
  clinical manifestations of, 1615

Neurogenic bladder dysfunction *(Continued)*
  diagnostic findings in, 1615
  etiology of, 1613–1615
  in multiple sclerosis, management of, 875
  management of, community/self care in, 1617–1619
    in elderly, 1619
    medical, 1617
      complications of, 1617
    nursing, 1617–1619
    surgical, 1615–1617
      nursing care in, 1617
  pathophysiology of, 1615
  risk factors for, 1613–1615
  types of, 1612–1613, *1616*
Neurogenic bowel, after spinal cord injury, 902
Neurogenic shock, clinical manifestations of, 513
  definition of, 497
  etiology of, 500
  management of, 524t
  prevention of, 501b
Neuroglia, 687, *688*
Neurohypophysis, disorders of, 2066, *2066*
  structure/function of, 1941–1942
Neuroleptic (balanced) anesthesia, 471
Neurologic flow sheet, *779–780*
Neurologic response, assessment of, after cardiac surgery, 1012
Neurologic status, critical monitoring of, 756b–757b
Neurologic system, age-related changes in, 268t
  cerebral, infections of, 856–861
  disorders of, and dysphagia, 1732
    and male reproductive disorders, 2345
    assessment of, 709–741
      clinical applications of, 729–730
      functional, 729
      guidelines for, 710t–713t
      history in, 709–715, 715b, 716b
      in emergency nursing care, 2507
      in health history, 185b
      in regional examination, 221t–222t
      normal findings in, 717b
      physical examination in, 715–730, 716b
      postoperative, 484
      preoperative, 456
    chest pain in, assessment of, 1209t
    degenerative, 863–888
      resources for, 887b
    ocular manifestations of, 977
  emergencies of, 2528–2529
  in alcohol abuse, 2490t
  in anemia, 1471
  in chronic renal failure, 1646
  in extracellular fluid volume excess, 287t
  in fluid balance regulation, 277
  in hematologic disorders, 1463
  in hepatobiliary disease, 1843
  in hypernatremia, 303t
  in hypokalemia, 309t
  in hyponatremia, 299b
  in rheumatoid arthritis, 660
  in shock, 509
  in thyroid disorders, 2008t

Neuroma, acoustic, 845, 1002–1003
and hearing impairment, 994
Morton's, 2125
plantar, 2125
Neuromuscular blocking agents, 472, 472t
for increased intracranial pressure, 775
use of, ethical issues in, 1172b
Neuromuscular spindles, 700
Neuromuscular system, in hypercalcemia, 321t
in hyperkalemia, 312t
in hypocalcemia, 317t
Neurons, 685–686, 686
bipolar, 686
multipolar, 686
unipolar, 686
Neuropathic pain, 354–355
Neuropathy(ies), diabetic, 1999–2000
peripheral, 927, 927–928, 928b
in chronic renal failure, 1646
Neuropeptides, 687b
Neuropsychological testing, 739–740
Neurosurgery, in pain management, 386–388, 387
Neurosyphilis, 928–929
Neurotransmitters, 686, 687b
imbalances of, and sleep disorders, 404
in pain modulation, 345
in sleep, 398
release of, calcium in, 687
Neurovascular assessment, 2088–2092, 2093
in fracture, 2135t
Neutrogena emulsion, 2199t
Neutropenia, chemotherapy and, 582
in aplastic anemia, 1478
malignant. See Agranulocytosis.
Neutrophil chemotactic factor, in anaphylaxis, 638t
Neutrophils, band, in differential count, interpretation of, 436t
functions of, 1448t
in blood dyscrasias, 1465t
in hematopoiesis, 1451
in wound healing, 428, 429
reference values for, in cancer, 557t
segmented, in differential count, interpretation of, 436t
Nevi, in adolescence, 2178
New York Heart Association Classification, of cardiovascular disability, 1287b
NEX measurement, 1750
NHL (non-Hodgkin's lymphoma), 1503
in acquired immunodeficiency syndrome, 630–631
ocular manifestations of, 977
survival in, 538t
Nicardipine (Cardene), 1396t
for angina pectoris, 1256t
Nicotine, abuse of, 2492
effects of, 2483t
health consequences of, 2493t
in coronary artery disease, 1240
withdrawal from, symptoms of, 2487t
NIDDM (non–insulin-dependent diabetes mellitus). See Diabetes mellitus.
Nifedipine (Procardia), 1396t
for angina pectoris, 1256t

Nifedipine (Procardia) (Continued)
for interstitial cystitis, 1580
Night sweat, in menopause, 2393
Nightingale Tracker System, 154–156
Nightly peritoneal dialysis (NPD), 1649
Nightmares, 403
Nikolsky's sign, 2220
Nimodipine, for intracranial hemorrhage, 814
Nipples, fissure of, 2452
inspection of, 2313
reconstruction of, 2284, 2285
Nipride (nitroprusside), for hypertensive emergency, 1405t
Nisei, pain response in, 347b–348b
Nissen fundoplication, for gastroesophageal reflux disease, 1739, 1739
Nitrates, for angina pectoris, 1254, 1256t
Nitrites, for angina pectoris, 1256t
Nitrofurantoin (Macrodantin, Macrobid), for urinary tract infections, 1575t
urine color and, 1557t
Nitrogen, liquid, for actinic keratosis, 2225, 2226
partial pressures of, 1032t
Nitroglycerin, for angina pectoris, 1254, 1256t
for hypertensive emergency, 1405t
Nitropress (nitroprusside), for hypertensive emergency, 1405t
Nitroprusside (Nipride, Nitropress), for hypertensive emergency, 1405t
Nitrosoureas, for chemotherapy, classification of, 577t
Nitrous oxide, 470t
intraoperative, pain after, 489
Nizatidine (Axid), for peptic ulcer disease, 1768t
NK (natural killer) cells, in pathogen resistance, 594–595
NM (nodular melanoma), 2228t
NNRTIs (non-nucleoside reverse transcriptase inhibitors), for human immunodeficiency virus infection, 624
Nociceptors, in pain transduction, 343
Nocturia, 1548
in left ventricular failure, 1281
Nodes of Ranvier, in nerve impulse conduction, 690
Nodular melanoma (NM), 2228t
Nodules, 2184
in acne vulgaris, 2212
subcutaneous, in rheumatic fever, 1328
Noise, decibel ratings of, 996t
head, 1003
loud, health risks of, 204t
Noise-induced hearing loss, 993
Nonbacterial thrombotic endocarditis, 1331
Noncompliance, risk for, in hypertension, 1403–1404
Non-Hodgkin's lymphoma (NHL), 1503
in acquired immunodeficiency syndrome, 630–631
ocular manifestations of, 977
survival in, 538t
Nonintervention, ethical issues in, 47
Nonmaleficence, in ethics, 40

Non–insulin-dependent diabetes mellitus (NIDDM). See Diabetes mellitus.
Non–small cell lung cancers (NSCLCs), 1151
chemotherapy in, 1154
surgical management of, 1155
Non-nucleoside reverse transcriptase inhibitors (NNRTIs), for human immunodeficiency virus infection, 624
Nonproliferative diabetic retinopathy (NPDR), 1996
Non-rapid eye movement (NREM) sleep, 398
stages of, 398, 398–399
Nonsteroidal anti-inflammatory drugs (NSAIDs), action of, mechanism of, 374
for gout, 2108
for musculoskeletal disorders, effects of, 2085
for osteoarthritis, 2109–2110
for rheumatoid arthritis, 663, 664t
in pain control, 374
Nontuberculous mycobacteria (NTM), 1145–1146
Nonunion, in fracture, prevention of, 2145–2146, 2146
Non-Western societies, healthcare beliefs of, 62–63
health/illness beliefs of, 61
Norcuron (vecuronium bromide), 472t
Norepinephrine, actions of, 1940t, 1944
effects of, 2057t
in blood flow regulation, 1374
in cardiac regulation, 1203
in sleep, 398
release of, in shock, 508
Norfloxacin (Noroxin), for urinary tract infections, 1575t
Normal sinus rhythm, 1295, 1296, 1296t
Normocytes, 1464
Normocytic anemia, 1477
Normodyne (labetalol), 1395t
for angina pectoris, 1257t
for dysrhythmia, 1308t
for hypertensive emergency, 1405t
Noroxin (norfloxacin), for urinary tract infections, 1575t
Norpace (disopyramide), for dysrhythmia, 1307t
therapeutic monitoring of, reference values for, 2562
Nortriptyline, for dementia of Alzheimer's type, 866t
therapeutic monitoring of, reference values for, 2562
Norvasc (amlodipine), 1396t
Nose, assessment of, 1047–1050
in health history, 183b
in regional examination, 216t
physical examination in, 1049–1050, 1050
culture of, 1063
fracture of, 1102
in hematologic disorders, 1463
physical examination of, in endocrine disorders, 1950
structure of, 1022, 1022–1023
Nosebleed, 1076–1077, 1077

Nosocomial infections, 417–419, 418t
  control of, 422–424
Nostrils, 1022, *1022*
Nothing by mouth (NPO) status, 463
Novocain (procaine), in pain control, 372
NP (nurse practitioner), 13, 136
NPD (nightly peritoneal dialysis), 1649
NPDR (nonproliferative diabetic retinopathy), 1996
NPO (nothing by mouth) status, 463
NREM (non-rapid eye movement) sleep, 398
  stages of, *398*, 398–399
NSAIDs. See *Nonsteroidal anti-inflammatory drugs (NSAIDs)*.
NSCLCs (non–small cell lung cancers), 1151
  chemotherapy in, 1154
  surgical management of, 1155
NTM (nontuberculous mycobacteria), 1145–1146
Nubain (nalbuphine), administration of, 381t
Nuchal rigidity, in bacterial meningitis, 856
Nuclear family, 52
Nuclear sclerotic cataracts, 958
Nuclease, secretion of, 1693
Nucleoside analogs, for human immunodeficiency virus infection, 624
5′-nucleotidase, serum, in hepatobiliary assessment, 1851t
Nucleus, of cells, 264–265
Nu-Gauze, indications for, 443t
Null cells, 1452
Numbness, in fracture, 2134
Numorphan (oxymorphone), administration of, 381t
Nurse, circulating, role of, 466
  in healthcare system, 6
  perioperative, definition of, 449
    role of, 450
  professional, definition of, 136b
Nurse anesthesia, 467–468
Nurse case managers, 13
Nurse extenders, use of, planning of, 125, 125b
Nurse practitioner (NP), 13, 136
Nurse-administered (demand) analgesia, 382
Nurse-client relationship, ethical issues in, 170b
Nursing, ambulatory care. See *Ambulatory care nursing*.
  community health, definition of, 146
    history of, 147–148
    philosophy of, 149–150
  cross-cultural. See *Cross-cultural nursing*.
  errors in, research in, 132b
    types of, 132b
  family, nursing process in, 55–59
  functional, 124
  hospital, future of, 131–132
    history of, 120
    roles/responsibilities in, 123–124
  international, 66–67
    transcultural nursing vs., 66
  intraoperative. See *Intraoperative nursing*.
  parish, 137
  perioperative. See *Perioperative nursing*.

Nursing *(Continued)*
  postoperative, in clinical unit, 484–492, 486t, *487, 489, 491*
    in postanesthesia care unit, 480–484. See also *Postanesthesia care unit (PACU)*.
  preoperative. See *Preoperative nursing*.
  primary, 124
  private duty, 120
  psychosocial, psychosocial dimensions vs., 51
  role of, in health promotion, 175
  team, 124
  total care, 124
Nursing care, definition of, 136b
  delivery of, systems for, 124–125, 125b
Nursing care plan, for arterial bypass, 1416–1417
  for atopic dermatitis, 2208–2209
  for burns, 2243–2248
  for cardiomyopathy, 1343–1344
  for chronic obstructive pulmonary disease, 1120–1123
  for foot infection, in diabetes mellitus, 1998
  for fracture, 2143–2144
  for liver transplantation, 1900
  for mechanical ventilation, 1180–1182
  for modified radical mastectomy, 2440–2441
  for myocardial infarction, 1270–1276
  for osteoporosis, 2105–2106
  for relocation stress syndrome, 89
  for thoracic surgery, 1159–1162
  for vertigo, 1014–1015
Nursing diagnosis(es), in acquired immunodeficiency syndrome, 632b
  in chronic conditions, 116, 116b
  in cross-cultural nursing, 65
  in family nursing, 57, 58b
  in organ transplantation, 648b
  in physical examination, 240–241
  in relocation stress syndrome, 89b
  in shock, 526–527, 526b
  in spiritual care, 72
  in substance abuse, 2495b
Nursing home care, 97
  in-home care vs., for elderly, 84
Nursing intensity, classification of, 127, 128t
  purposes of, 127
Nursing intervention. See *Intervention*.
Nursing models, health definition in, 162t
Nursing practice, diversity of, 11–14
  ethical, guidelines for, 41–42, 41b, 42b
  spirituality in, 68
Nursing process, in ambulatory care, 140–142, 141b, 143
  in cross-cultural nursing, 63–66, 63b, 64b, 65b, 66b
  in family nursing, 55–59, 56b–57b, 58b
  in health assessment, 211, 211b
  in Omaha system, *151*
  in physical examination, 225, 240–241
  in spirituality, 68–73, 69b–71b, 72b
  Murphy and Murphy model vs., 43, 44t
Nursing research, ambulatory care nurse in, 141b, 142–143

Nursing research *(Continued)*
  in adrenal insufficiency, in acquired immunodeficiency syndrome, 2042b
  in brain tumor client support, 852b
  in cardiopulmonary resuscitation portrayal on television, 1313b
  in cataract surgery, 960b
  in *Clostridium difficile* in hospitalized clients, 1789b
  in coma stimulation, 752b
  in community water exercise program effectiveness, 670b
  in concentration ability, after mastectomy vs. breast-conserving surgery, 2439b
  in coping strategies, in osteoarthritis, 2118b
  in cross-cultural nursing, 65b
  in death-telling, 2511b
  in decision-making, in confusion, 764b
  in dehydration indicators in elderly, 283b
  in diabetes mellitus management, 1966b
  in dietary fiber, for gastrointestinal symptoms, 1825b
  in dyspnea, in asthma, 1108b
  in elderly health promotion, 85b
  in electrolyte studies, 296b
  in every-two-hour turning schedule, in pressure ulcers, 2218b
  in exercise encouragement, in rheumatoid arthritis, 666b
  in family dynamics, in home total parenteral nutrition, 1757b
  in family needs, in cardiac catheterization, 1248b
    with critically ill client, 58b
  in fecal occult blood testing, 1712b
  in feeding tube aspirates, 1743b
  in feeding tube placement, 1751b
  in fingerstick blood glucose measurements, in decreased peripheral tissue perfusion, 515b
  in health-promotion activities, for disabled patients, 108b
  in hip fracture, in posthospital convalescence, 2159b
  in home fire victim reactions, 2263b
  in hydrogen peroxide rinses, for oral care, 1725b
  in inflammatory bowel disease, 1801b
  in intracranial pressure level, during bedside conversation, 781b
  in Kegel exercise effectiveness, 1609b
  in life after laryngectomy, 1088b
  in medical problems, after sexual abuse, 1757b
  in modified Trendelenburg's position, 518b
  in multiple sclerosis, 875b
  in nasoenteral tube placement, 1751b
  in nursing errors, 132b
  in physical activity gender differences, after coronary artery bypass surgery, 1251b
  in *Pneumocystis carinii* thyroiditis, 2026, 2027b
  in postoperative analgesia, jaw relaxation/music in, 1781b

Nursing research *(Continued)*
  in pressure ulcers, in spinal cord injury, 903b, 906b
  in progressive relaxation, for elderly sleep disorders, 409b
  in quality of life, for quadriplegic client, 903b
    in chronic obstructive pulmonary disease, 1127b
    in hearing impairment, 1000b
  in resilient women, 34b
  in sleep patterns, in critical care units, 407b
  in spiritual care, 72b
  in stroke effect on marriage, 790b
  in sundown syndrome management, 769b
  in temperature measurement, 1358b
  in testicular self-examination education, 2375b
  in violent behavior, in emergency department, 2509b
  into Pulmonary Functional Status and Dyspnea Questionnaire, 1037b
Nursing services, definition of, 136b
Nursing staff, definition of, 136b
Nursing's Agenda for Health Care Reform, 6, 136, 164
Nutrients, in hematopoiesis, 1453
  in hypertension, 1389
Nutrition, after spinal cord injury, 898
  after total laryngectomy, 1093
  altered, after brain tumor surgery, 854
    after partial laryngectomy, 1090–1091
    after spinal cord injury, 907
    in achalasia, 1734, 1736
    in acquired immunodeficiency syndrome, 634–635
    in acute glomerulonephritis, 1632
    in acute pancreatitis, 1926
    in breast cancer chemotherapy, 2450
    in burns, 2245
    in cerebrovascular accident, 803–805, 804b
    in chronic gastritis, 1763–1764
    in chronic obstructive pulmonary disease, 1121
    in cirrhosis, 1882
    in colon cancer, 1812
    in consciousness disorders, 758–760, 759b
    in eating disorders, 1760–1761
    in esophageal cancer, 1744
    in gastric cancer, 1783
    in hereditary spherocytosis, 1485
    in hyperparathyroidism, 2033
    in hypertension, 1400–1402, 1400b–1401b, 1402b, 1403b
    in hyperthyroidism, 2020
    in hypokalemia, 309
    in hypothyroidism, 2015
    in inflammatory bowel disease, 1800
    in iron deficiency anemia, 1473
    in leukemia, 1493
    in oral cancer, 1729, 1730–1731
    in osteoporosis, 2105
    in peptic ulcer disease, 1778–1779, 1781

Nutrition *(Continued)*
    in renal failure, acute, 1640
      chronic, 1656
    in rheumatic fever, 1330
    in viral hepatitis, 1870–1871
    mechanical ventilation and, 1181–1182
  assessment of, culture in, 64b, 193t–194t
    in cardiovascular disorders, 1210
    in gastrointestinal disorders, 1706
    in health history, 182b–183b
    in hematologic disorders, 1462
    in hepatobiliary disorders, 1845
    in immune disorders, 609
    in musculoskeletal disorders, 2086
    in respiratory disorders, 1040
    in urinary tract disorders, 1551
    preoperative, 454–455
  balanced, 171, *172*
  cultural effects on, 1700b–1704b
  deficient, 171
    and heart failure, 1278
    in inflammatory bowel disease, 1797, 1799
  during chemotherapy, 583
  enteral. See *Enteral nutrition.*
  excesses in, 171
  imbalance of, and cell damage, 270
  in burns, 2257–2258, *2258,* 2258t
  in cancer, 35, 587b
  in coma, 753
  in diabetes mellitus, guidelines for, 1976–1977, 1977t
  in elderly, 85–86, 86b
  in esophageal cancer, 1744
  in health promotion, 170–171, *171–173*
  in illness, 34–36
  in immunity, 605
  in immunosuppression, home healthcare in, 1494b
  in multiple organ system failure, 530
  in open wound management, 442
  in osteoporosis, 2104
  in wound healing, 433–434, 434t
  parenteral, 1754–1756
    nursing management of, 1756
    total. See *Total parenteral nutrition (TPN).*
  pattern of, 206
  postoperative, promotion of, 490
  support of, for pernicious anemia, 1476
    in gastrointestinal disorders, 1752–1756
    with cast, 2151
Nutritional services, for elderly, 99
Nystagmus, 720, 945
  tests for, 989
Nystatin (Mycostatin), topical, 2198t

O

OA. See *Osteoarthritis (OA).*
Oat cell carcinoma, of lungs, 1153t
Obesity, 35, 1760–1761
  adipose tissue measurement in, *240*
  in coronary artery disease, 1241
  in hypertension, 1389
  in postoperative wound infection, 490
  management of, medical, 1760
    surgical, 1760

Obesity *(Continued)*
  prevention of, 200t, 202t
  screening for, 209t
  surgical problems in, 455
Oblique fracture, 2130, *2130*
Oblique muscles, 936, *936*
OBRA (Omnibus Budget Reconciliation Act), 100
  provisions of, for client transfers, 2503
Obstetric history, 2310
Obstruction, in peptic ulcer disease, 1773
Obstructive conditions, and cardiogenic shock, 499–500
Obstructive jaundice, 1859, 1859t
Obstructive shock, 497
Obstructive sleep apnea syndrome (OSAS), 401–402, 402b
  living with, 402b
Obtundation, in consciousness disorders, 746
Occipital lobe, 691, *692*
  tumor of, clinical manifestations of, 847t
Occlusive dressings, 2201t
Occult blood, stool examination for, 1711–1712, 1711t, 1712b
  nursing research on, 1712b
Occupation, effect of, on male reproductive system, 2344
  in cancer, 540
  in endocrine disorders, 1950
  in gastrointestinal disorders, 1705–1706
  in gynecologic disorders, 2310
  in hematologic disorders, 1462
  in hepatobiliary disorders, 1844
  in immune disorders, 608
  in integumentary system disorders, 2182
  in male reproductive disorders, 2331
  in musculoskeletal disorders, 2085
  in respiratory disorders, 1039
  in urinary tract disorders, 1550
Occupational asthma, 1150, 1151t
Occupational health, in nosocomial infection control, 424
Occupational lung diseases, 1150–1151, 1151t
Occupational Safety and Health Administration (OSHA), 129–130
  ambulatory care standards of, 138
Occupational therapy, after intertrochanteric hip fracture, 2157
  for cerebrovascular accident, 798
  for rheumatoid arthritis, 665, *666*
Ocular adnexa, structure of, 935–936, *936*
Ocular melanoma, 970–971
Ocular motility, evaluation of, 945
Ocular muscles, structure of, 935–936, *936*
Ocular prosthesis, 971, *971*
  insertion/removal of, 972b–973b
Oculocephalic reflex, in consciousness disorders, 749–750, *750*
Oculogyric crisis, in Parkinson's disease, 878
Oculomotor nerve, assessment of, *719,* 720
Oculovestibular reflex, in consciousness disorders, 750, *750*
Odontoid fracture, cervical, 891, *893*
Odor, body/breath, assessment of, 235
  skin, assessment of, 2192

Odynophagia, 1733
Office of Cancer Communications, 564b
Office of Minority Health, 619b
Office on HIV/AIDS Policy, 619b
OGTT (oral glucose tolerance test), in diabetes mellitus, 1962–1963, 1964t
in impaired glucose tolerance, 1964t
OHAs (oral hypoglycemic agents), administration of, and hypoglycemia, 1988
for diabetes mellitus, 1967–1968, 1967t
Ointments, 2197, 2200t
OIs (opportunistic infections), in acquired immunodeficiency syndrome, 627–630
OKT3 (muromonab-CD3), after heart transplantation, 1353, 1354b
for renal graft rejection, 1662
in organ transplantation, 645t
Older adult. See also Elderly.
health promotion in, 173–175, 174b, 174t, 175b
resources for, 175b
Older Americans Act, 93
Olecranon, fracture of, 2161
Olfaction, in physical examination, 231
Olfactory epithelium, 1022
Olfactory nerve, assessment of, 719, 719
Oligodendrocytes, 687, 688
Oligodendroglioma, 844, 846
Oligozoospermia, characteristics of, management of, 2347
Oliguria, 1548, 1554
in shock, 512, 521
Omaha system, nursing process in, 151
of home healthcare provision, 151–154
intervention scheme in, 153–154, 154t, 155b
problem classification scheme in, 152–153, 152b, 153b, 154t
problem rating scale for outcomes in, 154, 156t
Ombudsman organizations, for elderly, 100
OmegaPort, 579
Omentum flap, 2280
Omeprazole (Prilosec), for gastroesophageal reflux disease, 1738
for peptic ulcer disease, 1767, 1769t, 1770
Ommaya reservoir, 580
in intraspinal analgesia, 384
Omnibus Budget Reconciliation Act (OBRA), 100
provisions of, for client transfers, 2503
Omniscience tilting disc valve, 1352
Oncogenes, definition of, 534t
Oncolink, 564b
Oncology. See also Cancer.
problem areas in, 565b
Oncology Nursing Society (ONS), 544, 564b
Oncotic pressure, 274
in glomerular filtration rate, 1541
On/off response, in Parkinson's disease, management of, 879
ONS (Oncology Nursing Society), 544, 564b
Ontogeny, of hematopoiesis, 1448–1449
Onychomycosis, 2223
Oophorectomy, bilateral, for breast cancer, 2437–2438

Opacity, of urine, 1557
Open circuit nitrogen method, of lung volume measurement, 1051
Open fracture, 2129, 2130
Open heart surgery, 1354–1355, 1355
Open pneumothorax, mediastinal flutter with, chest trauma and, 2524–2525, 2525
Open reduction, of fractures, 2137
Open reduction and internal fixation (ORIF), in femoral shaft fracture, 2160, 2160
Open-angle glaucoma, primary, 952, 953. See also Glaucoma.
Opening snap, 1216
Operant conditioning, in pain control, 370
Operations, enabling of, ambulatory care nurse in, 140, 141b
Ophthalmia, sympathetic, 970
Ophthalmic radiography, 950
Ophthalmodynamometry, 733, 951
Ophthalmopathy, infiltrative, 976
Ophthalmoscope, use of, guidelines for, 947b
Ophthalmoscopy, direct, 948, 948–949
indirect, 949
Opiates, antidote to, 2538t
effect of, on male reproductive system, 2345
Opioid agonist-antagonists, in pain control, 374–376
Opioid agonists, in pain control, 374
effects of, 376t
Opioid antagonists, in pain control, 374
Opioids, abuse of, 2492
effects of, 2483t
health consequences of, 2493t–2494t
actions of, 373–374, 373t
administration of, equianalgesic chart for, 380t–381t
adverse effects of, 376–377
side effects of, 376–377
withdrawal from, symptoms of, 2488t
Opium preparations, for diarrhea, in inflammatory bowel disease, 1798t
Opportunistic infections (OIs), in acquired immunodeficiency syndrome, 627–630
Op-Site, 2199t
for burns, 2257t
indications for, 443t
Optic disc, 939
in glaucoma, 954
Optic nerve, assessment of, 719, 719–720
structure of, 939, 939
Optic neuritis, multiple sclerosis and, 977
Optimal sequential (DDD) pacemaker, 1320b
OPTNs (Organ Procurement and Transplant Networks), 1660
Oral cancer, 1727–1732
management of, medical, 1728, 1728t
nursing, 1729
surgical, 1729–1730
nursing care in, 1730–1732, 1731b
prevention of, 1727b
risk factors for, 1727b
screening for, 209t
staging of, 1728, 1728t
survival in, 538t

Oral cavity, physical examination of, 1706–1707, 1707
tumors of, 1726–1732
benign, 1726
premalignant, 1726, 1726–1727
Oral cholecystography, 1849–1852
Oral disorders, 1723–1732
Oral glucose tolerance test (OGTT), in diabetes mellitus, 1962–1963, 1964t
in impaired glucose tolerance, 1964t
Oral hygiene, hydrogen peroxide rinses for, nursing research on, 1725b
with endotracheal tube, 1175–1176
Oral hypoglycemic agents (OHAs), administration of, and hypoglycemia, 1988
for diabetes mellitus, 1967–1968, 1967t
Oral leukoedema, 2188b
Oral mucositis, chemotherapy and, 583
Oral mucous membranes, altered, in cholelithiasis, 1915
in consciousness disorders, 757–758
in hypernatremia, 304
in periodontal disease, 1722
Oral rehydration, in extracellular fluid volume deficit, 279–280
Orasone. See Prednisone (Deltasone, Orasone).
Orchiectomy, case management in, 2371b
clinical pathway for, 2600–2602
for prostate cancer, 2370
radical, for testicular cancer, 2375
Orchitis, 2377
Orem's self-care model, health definition in, 162t
Organ donation, beliefs about, 2512t–2513t
ethical issues in, 754b
in consciousness disorders, 753–763
in emergency settings, 2511–2513, 2512t–2513t, 2514t
Organ of Corti, in hearing, 984
Organ Procurement and Transplant Networks (OPTNs), 1660
Organ transplantation, 641–650
complications of, 649t
criteria for, 645–646
donor procurement/preparation in, 646–647, 647b
future of, 649–650
graft rejection in, 643–644, 644t
graft-versus-host disease in, 644–645, 645
histocompatibility in, 641–643
management of, long-term follow-up care in, 649
nursing, 647–649, 648b, 649t
medications in, 644t–645t
nursing diagnoses in, 648b
religious beliefs about, 2545–2551
self-care after, ethical issues in, 647b
Organelles, 262–266, 264
Orientation, assessment of, 195, 716
in cross-cultural nursing, 64b
ORIF (open reduction and internal fixation), in femoral shaft fracture, 2160, 2160
Orinase (tolbutamide), for diabetes mellitus, 1967t
Oropharynx, structure of, 1023
Orthopnea, assessment of, 1206
in left ventricular failure, 1281

Orthostatic hypotension, and vertigo, 1011
  in extracellular fluid volume deficit, step-
    progression for, 283
Orthotoluidine test, 1711–1712
Orudis (ketoprofen), for rheumatoid arthri-
  tis, 664t
OSAS (obstructive sleep apnea syndrome),
  401–402, 402b
  living with, 402b
OSHA (Occupational Safety and Health Ad-
  ministration), 129–130
  ambulatory care standards of, 138
Osler's nodes, in infective endocarditis,
  1333
Osmoglyn (glycerin), for glaucoma, 954
Osmolality, 275–276, 276, 276b
  plasma, calculation of, 276b
    range of, 276
  urine, 1558
Osmolarity, 275
Osmoles, idiogenic, 301
Osmoreceptors, in shock, 502
Osmosis, 263
Ossicles, function of, 983
  structure of, 981, 982
Ossiculoplasty, 1008, 1008
Ossification, heterotopic, after spinal cord
  injury, 904
  in bone healing, 2133, 2133
Osteitis deformans, 2104–2106, 2106
Osteoarthritis (OA), 2108–2120
  clinical manifestations of, 2109, 2110
  coping strategies in, nursing research on,
    2118b
  diagnostic findings in, 2109
  etiology of, 2108
  management of, community/self care in,
    2109–2110
    medical, 2109–2110
    nursing, 2110
    surgical, 2110–2120
  pathophysiology of, 2108, 2108–2109
  rheumatoid arthritis vs., 2109t
  risk factors for, 2108
Osteoblastoma, 2123t
Osteoblasts, 2074
  in bone remodeling, 2099, 2100
Osteochondroma, 2123t
Osteoclasts, 2074–2075
  in bone remodeling, 2099, 2100
Osteocytes, 2074–2075
Osteodystrophy, hereditary, Albright's, 2036
  in chronic renal failure, 1646
Osteogenic sarcoma, 2123, 2123t
Osteoid osteoma, 2123t
Osteomalacia, 2106–2107
Osteomyelitis, 2121–2122
  fractures and, 2141
Osteopenia, 2098
Osteoporosis, 2098–2104
  categories of, 2098, 2099
  clinical manifestations of, 2100, 2101
  diagnostic findings in, 2100, 2101
  etiology of, 2098–2099
  glucocorticosteroids and, 2047
  in whites, 198t
  management of, community/self care in,
    2100–2103

Osteoporosis (Continued)
  home care in, 2103
    medical, 2103–2104
  nursing care plan in, 2105–2106
  pathophysiology of, 2099–2100, 2100
  postmenopausal, hyperthyroidism with,
    case study of, 2021
  prevention of, 200t, 2100–2103, 2102b,
    2103t
    in menopause, 2394
  risk factors for, 2098–2099, 2102b
  safety measures in, 2103
Osteotomy, 2110
  for rheumatoid arthritis, 672
Ostomy, adjustment to, home healthcare in,
    1804b
  psychological, 1814
Ostomy appliances, application of, delega-
    tion of, 1806b
Ostomy pouch, application of, 1592, 1592
Ostomy supplies, client education in, 1803b
Otalgia, 1003
Otis bougie à boule, 2356t
Otitis externa, 1003–1005
  clinical manifestations of, 1004
  diagnostic findings in, 1004
  management of, 1004, 1004–1005, 1005
Otitis media, 1005–1006
  client education in, 1008b
  clinical manifestations of, 1006
  serous, 1006
  suppurative, 1006
Otosclerosis, 1001–1002, 1003
Otoscopy, 987, 987–988, 988
Otospongiosis, cochlear, 1001
Outcome, expected, in chronic condition
    management, 116
  healthcare, monitoring of, 127–129
    access issues in, 129
    functional status measurement in, 129
    patient satisfaction surveys in, 127–
      129
Outdoor activity, health risks of, 203t–204t
Outpatient care, 137
Outpatients, chemotherapy delivery to, 579–
    580
Ova and parasites, stool examination for,
    1711t, 1712
Oval window, 981, 982
Ovarian cancer, 2412–2413
  clinical manifestations of, 2413
  diagnostic findings in, 2413
  etiology of, 2412
  management of, medical, 2413
    nursing, 2413
    surgical, 2413
  pathophysiology of, 2413
  prevention of, 2413b
  risk factors for, 542b, 2412, 2413b
  survival in, 538t
Ovarian cysts, 2412
Ovarian follicles, 2295, 2295
Ovary(ies), disorders of, 2412–2413
  examination of, 2319
  hormones of, 1940t
  structure/function of, 2294–2295, 2295
  tumors of, benign, 2412
Overdose, 2537–2539, 2537t, 2538b, 2538t

Overdose (Continued)
  definition of, 2481t
Overflow incontinence, 1604t
  pathophysiology of, 1606
  risk factors for, 1606b
Overuse syndromes, 2161–2163, 2162b,
    2163t
  grading of, 2162, 2163t
  prevention of, 2162, 2162b
Overweight, management of, 198t
Ovulation, 2300
Oxalate renal calculi, 1666
Oxiconazole (Oxistat), topical, 2198t
Oximetry, pulse, in free flap assessment,
    2281
  in respiratory assessment, 1051–1055,
    1055
  in shock, 514
  limitations of, 1052–1055
Oxistat (oxiconazole), topical, 2198t
Oxybutynin chloride (Ditropan), for urinary
    incontinence, 1611t
  for urinary tract infections, 1576t
Oxycodone, administration of, 381t
  in pain control, 375t
Oxygen, arterial, partial pressure of, oxygen
    saturation vs., 1055t
  for anemia, 1471
  for chronic obstructive pulmonary disease,
    1117
  conservation of, home healthcare in,
    1125b
  for dysrhythmias, 1314
  for heart failure, 1283
  in muscle movement, 2078
  in phagocytosis, in wound healing, 429
  low-flow, conversion to high-flow, 1117–
    1119, 1119t
  partial pressures of, 1032t
  supplemental, in emergency nursing care,
    2506
  transcutaneous, in free flap assessment,
    2280
Oxygen free radicals, in disease, 35–36, 36
Oxygen saturation (SaO₂), measurement of,
    delegation of, 234b
  pulse oximetry in, 1051–1055, 1055
  partial pressure of arterial oxygen vs.,
    1055t
Oxygen transport, in gas exchange, 1031–
    1032, 1033
Oxygenation, hyperbaric, for shock, 516
  for wound infection, 446
  improvement of, for shock, 516
Oxyhemoglobin curve, normal, 1031–1032,
    1033
Oxymorphone (Numorphan), administration
    of, 381t
Oxytocin, 2061t
  actions of, 1940t

P

P wave, 1222, 1222
  analysis of, 1298b
  normal, characteristics of, 1296t
PA (posteroanterior) chest x-ray, 1060
PABA (para-aminobenzoic acid), 2200t

PABA esters, 2200t
Pacemakers, case management in, 1315b
  classification of, 1320b
  clinical pathway for, 2584–2585
  design of, 1315–1316, *1316*
  ectopic, 1296
  electrocardiography with, 1321
  endocardial, 1316, *1318*
  epicardial, 1316
  escape, 1295
  external, 1316
  failure of, 1321, *1323*
  fixed-rate, 1319
  for dysrhythmias, 1314–1320
  function of, 1319–1320
  indications for, 1315b
  malfunctions of, 1317t
  management of, nursing, 1320–1321
  modes of, 1319, *1319,* 1320b
  monitoring of, transtelephonic, 1321
  permanent, 1318–1319
    client education in, 1322b
    indications for, 1319b
  temporary, 1318, *1318*
Pacific Islanders, human immunodeficiency
  virus infection in, 617b–618b
Pacing intervals, *1319*
PaCO₂ (partial pressure of arterial carbon di-
    oxide), analysis of, 1056–1057
  in arterial blood gas analysis, 338b
  in shock, 514
  in asthma, 1108t
  in respiration control, 1031
PACs (premature atrial contractions), *1299,*
    1300–1301
PACU. See *Postanesthesia care unit
    (PACU).*
PAG (periaqueductal gray matter), in pain
    modulation, 344, *345*
Paget's disease, 2104–2106, *2106,* 2434
  and heart failure, 1278
Pain, 342–393
  abdominal, acute, 2529–2530, *2530*
    in rheumatic fever, 1328
    in viral hepatitis, 1865, 1866t
  activities of daily living in, 363, 365b
  acute, 351–352, *352*
    management of, Agency for Health Care
      Policy and Research guidelines for,
      352
    reaction to, 351–352, *352*
  after arterial bypass, 1417
  after brain tumor surgery, 855
  after cardiac surgery, 924–925
  after intervertebral disc surgery, 923
  after prostatectomy, 2361
  after thoracic surgery, nursing care plan
    for, 1161
  after total hip replacement, 2112
  assessment of, 360–365
    blocks to, 360–361, 361t
    history in, 362–365, *364,* 365b
    physical examination in, 365
    postoperative, 485, 489
    preoperative, 454
    principles of, 362, *363*
    tools for, 365, *366*
  back, 356–357

Pain *(Continued)*
  bone, 355
  cancer, 358–359, 587b
    management of, clinical practice guide-
      lines for, 358–359
    nerve block in, 385
  central, 356–357
  central/peripheral, 357–358
  cerebral cortex lesions in, 357
  character of, 363, *364*
  chest, 2528
    assessment of, 1037, 1205–1206, 1208t–
      1209t
    in pericarditis, 1336
    pleuritic, 1166
  chronic, 352
    after spinal cord injury, 908–909
    intractable, management of, 368
    nerve blocks for, 385t
  client misinformation about, 361
  cultural perspectives on, 347b–349b
  cutaneous, 353
    deep pain vs., 354t
  deep somatic, 353
    cutaneous pain vs., 354t
  definition of, 342
  duration of, 363
  ear, history of, 985
  epigastric, in acute pancreatitis, 1923,
      1924t
  esophageal, 1733
  ethical issues in, 343b
  extension/radiation of, 362
  eye, 941
  fast, 343
  in abdominal aortic aneurysm, 1428
  in achalasia, 1735
  in acute cholecystitis, 1916, 1917t
  in acute pancreatitis, 1925
  in appendicitis, 1792
  in burns, 2236, 2246
    home management of, 2262b
  in cholelithiasis, 1909–1910, 1911, 1915
  in chronic gastritis, 1763
  in dementia of Alzheimer's type, identifi-
    cation of, 867–868
  in elderly, misconceptions about, 391,
    392t
  in esophageal diverticula, 1742
  in fracture, 2134
  in gastric cancer, 1783
  in gastroesophageal reflux disease, 1739
  in gastrointestinal disorders, 1748
  in hepatobiliary disease, 1845, *1847*
  in human immunodeficiency virus infec-
    tion, 359
  in idiopathic thrombocytopenic purpura,
    1508
  in inflammatory bowel disease, 1800
  in intertrochanteric hip fracture, 2156
  in intestinal disorders, 1787
  in leiomyoma, 2401–2402
  in multiple myeloma, 1500
  in musculoskeletal disorders, 2083–2084
  in myocardial infarction, 1270
  in oral candidiasis, 1726
  in osteoporosis, 2104, 2105–2106
  in peptic ulcer disease, 1766, 1773

Pain *(Continued)*
  in pheochromocytoma, 2059
  in postanesthesia care unit, 483
  in pyelonephritis, 1629
  in renal calculi, 1667
  in rheumatic fever, 1329–1330
  in sickle cell anemia, 1515
  in urinary tract disorders, 1548
  in urinary tract infections, 1578
  inflammatory, 356
  intensity of, 363
  Internet resources on, 392b
  location of, 362
  malignant, 352–353, 358–359
  management of. See *Pain management.*
  manifestations of, 363
    behavioral, 365
    parasympathetic, 365
    sympathetic, 365
  modulation of, 344–345, *345*
  muscular, 355
  myths/misconceptions about, 360, 361t
  neuropathic, 354–355
  nursing interventions for, 365–392
    in elderly, 391–392, 392t
    invasive, 371–391
    noninvasive, 369–371
    principles of, 365–369, 367b, *368*
  onset of, 362–363
  parietal, 354
  pathologic syndromes of, 354–359
  pathways of, blockage of, 344
  pattern of, 362–363
  perception of, 345–346
  peripheral, 357–358
  phantom, 355, 357–358, 1421
  pleural, 1166
  precipitating factors in, 363
  process of, 342–350
    therapeutic implications of, 350
  progressive, management of, *368,* 368–
    369
  psychogenic, 359
  psychological, 359
  quality of, 363
  reduction of, in spinal cord injury, 903–
    904
  referred, 354, *355*
  relief of, methods of, 365
  renal, radiculitis vs., 1548
  response to, 346–350
    age in, 346–350
    anxiety in, 350
    factors in, 362, *363*
      situational, 346
      sociocultural, 346
    gender in, 350
    meaning of pain in, 350
    physiologic, 360
    psychological, 360
  rest, 1377
    in chronic arterial occlusion, 1406–1407
  sensitivity to, assessment of, 724
  shoulder, cerebrovascular accident and,
    792
  slow, 343
  stump, 358
  superficial, 353

Pain (Continued)
    thalamic, 356
    theories of, 350–351, 351
    tolerance for, 346
    transduction of, 343
    transmission of, 344
    types of, 351–354, 352, 354t
    undertreatment of, 382
    vascular, 355–356
    visceral, 353–354
Pain management, acupressure in, 349b, 371
    acupuncture in, 349b, 388–389
    alternative methods of, 348b–349b, 349b
    analgesia in. See Analgesia.
    anxiety alleviation in, 366
    autogenic training in, 349b, 369
    behavioral techniques in, 369–370
    Benson's relaxation response in, 349b
    biofeedback in, 349b, 370
    cultural influences on, 348b–349b
    cutaneous stimulation in, 349b, 371
    distraction in, 349b, 366
    diversion in, 366
    fear management in, 366–367
    guided imagery in, 349b, 369–370
    herbal remedies in, 349b
    hypnosis in, 349b, 371
    ice massage in, 371
    in burns, 2258, 2259
        major, 2251
        minor, 2241
    in elderly, 391–392, 392t
    in home healthcare, 367b
    in rheumatoid arthritis, 668–669, 668b
    local anesthesia in, 372
    massage in, 349b
    medications in, 368
    meditation in, 349b, 369
    methods of, invasive, 371–391
        noninvasive, 369–371
    music in, 349b, 371
    neurosurgery in, 386–388, 387
    nonanalgesic, 374
    operant conditioning in, 370
    physical care in, 367–368
    placebos in, 391
    preoperative teaching of, 462–463
    progressive relaxation training in, 349b,
        369
    radiation therapy in, 391
    relaxation techniques in, 349b
    religious rituals in, 349b
    rhythmic breathing in, 370
    stereotactic surgery in, 388
    stimulation therapy in, 389–391, 389b,
        390t
    therapeutic relationship in, 370
    therapeutic touch in, 349b, 370–371
    topical anesthesia in, 372
    topical salves/balms in, 349b
    yoga in, 349b
Pain relievers, topical, client education
    about, 668b
Pain threshold, 346
Painful bladder disease (PBD). See Intersti-
    tial cystitis (IC).
Paired helical filaments, in Alzheimer's dis-
    ease, 863–864

Palatal reflex, 729t
Paleospinothalamic tract, in pain transmis-
    sion, 344
Pallor, 2186
    biocultural variations in, 2190b
    elevation, in peripheral vascular assess-
        ment, 1380
Palmar erythema, in cirrhosis, 1878t
Palm-chin (palmomental) reflex, 728
Palmomental (palm-chin) reflex, 728
Palpation, 225–228, 228
    bimanual, 228, 228
    deep, 228, 228
    in immune disorder assessment, 609b,
        610–611, 610t
    light, 228, 228
    of abdomen, 1709, 1848
        in cardiovascular assessment, 1217
    of anus/rectum, 1710
    of breasts/axillae, 2313–2314, 2314
    of cardiovascular system, normal findings
        in, 1206b
    of ear, 987, 987–988, 988
    of eyes, normal findings in, 940b
    of female reproductive system, normal
        findings in, 2312b
    of gastrointestinal tract, normal findings
        in, 1699b
    of hematologic system, 1463b
    of hepatobiliary system, 1846t
        in elderly, 1847t
    of integumentary system, 2185–2194
        normal findings in, 2182b
    of kidneys, 1552, 1552–1553
    of lymph nodes, of head and neck, 610t
    of male reproductive system, normal find-
        ings in, 2332b
    of musculoskeletal system, normal find-
        ings in, 2086b
    of neurologic system, 718
        normal findings in, 717b
    of peripheral vascular system, 1378b,
        1381–1382, 1382
    of precordium, 1213, 1214
    of respiratory system, 1043–1044, 1044,
        1045
        normal findings in, 1042b
    of thyroid gland, 1951, 1951, 1951b
    of urinary tract, 1556b
Palpebral fissure, 936, 936
Palpitations, assessment of, 1207
    in endocrine disorders, 1948
Pamidronate sodium (Aredia), for multiple
    myeloma, 1499
Pancoast's tumor, 1152
Pancreas, donation of, guidelines for,
    2514t
    endocrine, disorders of, 1955–2001
        function of, 1945
        tests of, 1952
        hormones of, 1940t
        structure of, 1945
    exocrine, age-related changes in, 1841
        cancer of, 1930–1931
            survival in, 538t
        disorders of, 1907–1932
            assessment of, 1843–1856
                diagnostic tests in, 1848–1856

Pancreas (Continued)
        history in, 1843–1856
            physical examination in, 1845–1848,
                1846t–1847t, 1847
        classification of, 1921b
        function of, 1835–1841, 1838
            laboratory tests for, 1852t
        in cystic fibrosis, 1932
        structure of, 1835–1841, 1838
    transplantation of, 1931
        complications of, 649t
        criteria for, 646
        for diabetes mellitus, 1981
        trauma to, 1931–1932
Pancreatectomy, subtotal, for acute pancrea-
    titis, 1927
    for chronic pancreatitis, 1930
Pancreatic amylase, 1692t
Pancreatic enzymes, 1922b
Pancreatic isoamylase, serum, in hepatobili-
    ary assessment, 1850t
Pancreatic juice, 1840
Pancreatic lipase, 1692t
Pancreatic pseudocysts, 1929–1930
Pancreatic secretions, phases of, 1841
    stimulation of, 1841
Pancreaticoduodenal resection, for chronic
    pancreatitis, 1930
Pancreaticoduodenectomy, for acute pancre-
    atitis, 1927
Pancreaticojejunostomy, for chronic pancre-
    atitis, 1930
    Roux-en-Y, longitudinal, for acute pancre-
        atitis, 1927
Pancreatitis, acute, 1921–1929
    adult respiratory distress syndrome in,
        critical monitoring in, 1927b
    clinical manifestations of, 1923–1924,
        1924t
    diagnostic findings in, 1923–1924, 1924t
    etiology of, 1921–1922
    management of, in elderly, 1929
        medical, 1924–1925
            complications of, 1925
            outcomes in, 1925
            nursing, 1925–1927
        surgical, 1927
            complications of, 1927
            nursing care in, 1927–1929, 1927b
    pathophysiology of, 1922–1923, 1922b,
        1923b
    risk factors for, 1921–1922, 1922b
    prevention of, 1922b
    chronic, 1929, 1930
    prevention of, 201t
Pancuronium bromide (Pavulon), 472t
Pancytopenia, in aplastic anemia, 1477–
    1478
Panlobular emphysema, 1114, 1114
Panniculectomy, 2276
Panophthalmitis, 970
Panorex, 250
Pansinusitis, 1077
Pansystolic regurgitant murmurs, 1218t
PaO$_2$ (partial pressure of arterial oxygen),
    analysis of, 1056
    in asthma, 1108t
    oxygen saturation vs., 1055t

PAP (prostatic acid phosphatase), in prostate cancer, 558t, 2367
PAP (pulmonary artery pressure), 1234–1235
  elevation of, in pulmonary hypertension, 1129–1130
  monitoring of, after cardiac surgery, 1357
Papanicolaou smear, 257, 2320–2322, *2321*
  in cancer diagnosis, 556–558
    of cervix, 2407
  schedule for, 209t
Papillae, renal, 1535
Papillary adenocarcinoma, of thyroid, 2028t
Papilledema, brain tumor and, 846
Papilloma, intraductal, 2452
  laryngeal, 1082
Papule, *2184,* 2212
Para-aminobenzoic acid (PABA), 2200t
Para-aminosalicylic acid, allergic reaction to, clinical manifestations of, 640t
  for tuberculosis, 1145t
Paracentesis, in hepatobiliary disease, 1854
Paradoxical blood pressure, measurement of, 1211–1212
Paraldehyde, avoidance of, in cirrhosis, 1882t
Paralysis, after spinal cord injury, adjustment to, 910
  diaphragmatic, 1168–1169
  in polio, 860
  laryngeal, 1101
  partial, after spinal cord injury, 895
  respiratory, spinal anesthesia and, 476t
  sleep, 400, 403
Paralytic ileus, and small intestinal obstruction, 1820–1821
  in bladder cancer, 1590
  postoperative, 490
  risk for, after cardiac surgery, 1014
    after intervertebral disc surgery, 924
Parametrium, 2296
Paramyxoviridae, 416t
Paranasal sinuses, 1022–1023, *1023*
  assessment of, physical examination in, 1050
Paraneoplastic syndromes, 1152
Paranoia, in dementia of Alzheimer's type, pharmacologic treatment of, 866t
Paraphimosis, 2379, *2379*
Paraplegia, spinal anesthesia and, 476t
  spinal injury and, 893
Parasagittal meningioma, *846*
Paraseptal emphysema, 1114, *1114*
Parasitic infestations, of intestinal tract, 1790
  of neurologic system, 861
  of skin, 2221t
Parasitic pneumonia, 1137t
Parasomnias, 403
  classification of, 398b
Parasympathetic nervous system, 703
  in cardiac regulation, 1203
  of kidneys, 1537
  organic effects of, 703, 706t
Parathyroid glands, autotransplantation of, 2035
  disorders of, 2005–2038

Parathyroid glands *(Continued)*
  function of, 1943–1944
    tests of, 2032t
  hormones of, 1940t
  structure of, 1943–1944
Parathyroid hormone (PTH), actions of, 1940t
  excess, in hyperparathyroidism, 2030
  functions of, 1944
  in calcium regulation, 314–315, *315*
  in homeostasis, 2080
  in phosphorus regulation, 314–315, *315*
  reference values for, in cancer, 557t
  replacement of, for hypoparathyroidism, 2037
Parathyroid hormone radioimmunoassay, 2032t
Parenchyma, of lung, 1028
  disorders of, 1133–1187
Parenteral nutrition, 1754–1756
  nursing management of, 1756
  total. See *Total parenteral nutrition (TPN).*
Paresthesia, 724
  cerebrovascular accident and, 791–792
  in endocrine disorders, 1949
  opioid analgesics in, 377
Parietal lobes, 690, *692*
  tumor of, clinical manifestations of, 847t
Parietal pain, 354
Parietal pericardium, *1192,* 1193
Parietal pleura, 1027
Parish nursing, 137
Parkinsonian crisis, management of, 879
Parkinsonism, types of, 878
Parkinson's disease (PD), 878–879, *879*
  client education in, 881b–882b
  complications of, 878
  management of, medical, 878–879
    nursing, 879
    pharmacologic, 878–879, 880t
    surgical, 882
  on/off response in, management of, 879
  sleep disorders in, 404
The Parkinson's Disease Foundation, 887b
Parkinson's Support Group of America, 887b
Parkland formula, for fluid resuscitation, in burns, 2250t
Parlodel (bromocriptine), for Parkinson's disease, 880t
  for premenstrual syndrome, 2388
Paronychia, 2187t, 2223
Parotitis, 1732
Paroxysm, in pheochromocytoma, 2057, 2058b
Paroxysmal atrial tachycardia (PAT), *1300,* 1301
Paroxysmal junctional tachycardia (PJT), 1302–1303
Paroxysmal nocturnal dyspnea (PND), assessment of, 1206
  in left ventricular failure, 1281
Paroxysmal nocturnal hemoglobinemia (PNH), 1480–1481
Parsidol (ethopropazine), for Parkinson's disease, 880t

Partial pressure, of arterial carbon dioxide. See *Paco$_2$ (partial pressure of arterial carbon dioxide).*
  of arterial oxygen, analysis of, 1056
    in asthma, 1108t
    oxygen saturation vs., 1055t
  of atmospheric gases, 1031, 1032t
    during respiration, *1032*
Partial thromboplastin time (PTT), in hemorrhage, 1467t
  preoperative evaluation of, 453t
Pasteur's germ theory, 20
Past-pointing test, 989
PAT (paroxysmal atrial tachycardia), *1300,* 1301
Patch test, 2194–2195
  in allergy assessment, 612, 637
Patellar fracture, 2160–2161
Patellar reflexes, *726,* 727, 729t
Patellar tendinitis, 2162
Paternalism, in decision-making, in chronic conditions, 118b
Pathogenicity, 414
Pathogens, 413–414
  action of, mode of, 414
  carriers of, 414
  portal of entry of, 415
  portal of exit of, 415
  resistance to, acute phase response in, 594
    inflammation in, 594, *594, 595*
    natural killer cells in, 594–595
    surface defenses in, 593–594
  transmission of, route of, 414
Pathologic fracture, *2130,* 2131
Patient(s). See also *Client(s).*
  definition of, 136b
  disabled, health-promotion activities in, 108b
  home healthcare, family conflict with, ethical issues in, 150b
Patient Self-Determination Act (PSDA), 47
  elderly issues in, 102
Patient-controlled analgesia (PCA), 382
  advantages of, 382, 489
  postoperative, 489, *489*
  problems with, 382
  programming of, 489
Paul-Bunnell test, in infectious mononucleosis, 1504
Pavementing, of neutrophils, 428, *429*
Pavulon (pancuronium bromide), 472t
PAWP (pulmonary artery wedge pressure), monitoring of, after cardiac surgery, 1357
PBD (painful bladder disease). See *Interstitial cystitis (IC).*
PBSC (peripheral blood stem cell) transplantation, for cancer, 585
PCA. See *Patient-controlled analgesia (PCA).*
Pco$_2$, during respiration, 1031, *1032*
PCP (phencyclidine), abuse of, 2492
  effects of, 2483t
  health consequences of, 2494t
  withdrawal from, symptoms of, 2488t
PCWP (pulmonary capillary wedge pressure), monitoring of, in cardiovascular assessment, 1233
  in shock, 526

PD. See *Parkinson's disease (PD)*.

PDGF (platelet-derived growth factor), in wound healing, 431

PE. See *Pulmonary embolism (PE)*.

Peak expiratory flow rate (PEFR), 1052t

Peak flowmeter, 1051, *1053, 1109*
use of, directions for, 1113b

Peau d'orange skin, 2434

Pectoral lymph nodes, palpation of, 2313, *2314*

Pectoriloquy, whispered, 1046–1047

Pectus carinatum, 1040–1042, *1043*

Pectus excavatum, 1042, *1043*

Pedestrian accident, blunt trauma in, 2521t

Pediatric filter, for blood transfusion, 1526t

Pedicle, 2279

Pediculicides, topical, 2198t

Pediculosis pubis, 2475

Pediculus humanus capitis, 2186

PEEP (positive end-expiratory pressure), *1179,* 1179–1182
complications of, risk for, 1181
for shock, 516
hazards of, 1179–1182

PEFR (peak expiratory flow rate), 1052t

PEG (percutaneous endoscopic gastrostomy), after intracranial surgery, 854

PEG (percutaneous endoscopic gastrostomy) tube, critical monitoring in, 1731b
for achalasia, 1735, *1736*

Pelvic examination, 2316–2317
equipment for, 2316
positioning for, 2316–2317
preparation for, 2316
schedule for, 209t
technique of, 2317

Pelvic exenteration, for cervical cancer, 2408, *2408*

Pelvic floor musculature, examination of, 2319–2320

Pelvic inflammatory disease (PID), 2395–2398
chronic, 2398
clinical manifestations of, 2396–2397
diagnostic findings in, 2396–2397, *2397*
etiology of, 2395
in gonorrhea, 2468
management of, medical, 2397
nursing, 2397–2398
surgical, 2397
pathophysiology of, 2395–2396, *2396*
prevention of, 2396b
risk factors for, 2395, 2396b

Pelvic muscle exercises, for urinary incontinence, 1609–1610, 1609b

Pelvic traction, 2139

Pelvis, blood supply of, 2296
female, anatomy of, *1538*
fracture of, 2160
innervation of, 2296
lymphatic drainage of, 2296
male, anatomy of, *1539*
relaxation of, in menopause, 2395

Pemphigus, 2220–2222

Penbutolol (Levatol), 1395t

Pender's model of health promotion, *164,* 165

Penetrating trauma, 2518–2519, 2520t

Penetrating trauma (Continued)
to abdomen, 2531
to chest, 2522

Penicillamine (Cuprimine), for rheumatoid arthritis, 664t

Penicillin, allergic reaction to, clinical manifestations of, 640t
for syphilis, 2471
in surgical client, 458t

Penicillin G, for tetanus, 857

Penile clamp, for urinary incontinence, 1612, *1612*

Penile shaft, physical examination of, 2333

Penile skin, physical examination of, 2333

Penis, cancer of, 2380
disorders of, 2378–2381
injury to, 2380
physical examination of, 2333, *2334*
normal findings in, 2332b
structure/function of, 2302

Pentazocine (Talwin), administration of, 381t
in pain control, 375t

Pentobarbital (Nembutal), for increased intracranial pressure, 775
for status epilepticus, 843
preoperative, 465t

Pentothal (thiopental sodium), 470t

Pentoxifylline (Trental), for hyperlipidemia, 1408

People of Color Against AIDS Network, 619b

Pepcid (famotidine), for peptic ulcer disease, 1767, 1768t
for shock, 520

Pepsin, 1692t
secretion of, 1690

Peptic ulcer disease, 1764–1781
classification of, 1766t
clinical manifestations of, 1766–1767
complications of, *1771,* 1771–1773, *1772*
diagnostic findings in, 1766–1767
etiology of, 1764–1765
management of, dietary, 1770–1771
medical, 1767–1773, 1768t–1769t, 1770t
nursing, 1773–1776
surgical, 1776–1779
complications of, 1778–1779
nursing care in, 1779–1781
pathophysiology of, 1765–1766
perforated, *1772,* 1772–1773, 1776
surgical management of, case study of, 1774–1775
prevention of, 1765b
risk factors for, 1764–1765, 1765b

Peptidases, 1692t

Peptides, in pain modulation, 345

Perceived exertion scale, in activity tolerance measurement, 1126

Perception, altered, cerebrovascular accident and, 790, *790*
assessment of, preoperative, 456
distortion of, assessment of, 195, 710t
pattern of, 206

Percorten acetate (desoxycorticosterone acetate), 2048t

Percussion, 228–230, *229*

Percussion (Continued)
blunt, 228, *229*
in hepatobiliary assessment, 1848
direct, 228, *229*
in ascites, 1848
indirect, *229,* 229–230
of abdomen, 1709, 1845–1848, 1846t
of cardiovascular system, normal findings in, 1206b
of costovertebral angle, 1548, *1549*
of gastrointestinal tract, normal findings in, 1699b
of hepatobiliary system, 1846t
of neurologic system, 718
normal findings in, 717b
of respiratory system, 1044–1045, *1045, 1046*
normal findings in, 1042b
of urinary tract, 1556b
sounds in, 230

Percutaneous cervical chordotomy, for pain, 386, *387*

Percutaneous endoscopic gastrostomy (PEG), after intracranial surgery, 854

Percutaneous endoscopic gastrostomy (PEG) tube, critical monitoring in, 1731b
for achalasia, 1735, *1736*

Percutaneous epidural dorsal column stimulation, in pain control, 389

Percutaneous lithotripsy, for renal calculi, 1668–1669, *1669*

Percutaneous transhepatic cholangiography, 1853

Percutaneous transluminal angioplasty (PTA), 1413

Percutaneous transluminal coronary angioplasty (PTCA), case management in, 1247b
clinical pathway for, 2578–2579
family needs in, nursing research on, 1248b
for coronary artery disease, 1245, *1245*

Perfluorochemicals, administration of, for shock, 519

Perforation, of peptic ulcer, *1772,* 1772–1773, 1776
surgical management of, case study of, 1774–1775

Perforins, 595

Performance improvement, in acute care, 130–131, 130b, 131b
clinical indicators of, 130, 130b
qualities in, 131b

Perfusion, cerebral. See *Cerebral tissue perfusion.*
tissue. See *Tissue perfusion.*
ventilation relationship to, 1032–1033, *1033*

Pergolide (Permax), for Parkinson's disease, 880t

Periactin (cyproheptadine), for hypercortisolism, 2053

Periampullary adenocarcinoma, of pancreas, 1931

Periaqueductal gray matter (PAG), in pain modulation, 344, *345*

Pericardial effusion, in pericarditis, 1336–1337

Pericardial friction rub, 1216
in pericarditis, 1336
Pericardial tamponade, and cardiogenic shock, 500
Pericardiocentesis, for cardiac tamponade, *1337*, 1337–1338
Pericarditis, 1335–1337
acute, 1335–1336, 1336b
causes of, 1336b
clinical manifestations of, 1336
with effusion, 1336–1337
after myocardial infarction, 1267
chest pain in, assessment of, 1208t
constrictive, chronic, 1337
dry, 1336
exudative, 1336
in renal failure, acute, 1639
chronic, 1645
in rheumatoid arthritis, 659, 1328t
Pericardium, *1192*, 1193
parietal, *1192*, 1193
rheumatic fever effects on, 1328t
visceral, *1192*, 1193
Perichondrial hematoma, 1007
Perilymph, 983–984
Perineal muscle, in urinary incontinence, 1605
Perineal prostatectomy, for benign prostatic hyperplasia, *2353*, 2358
Perineal skin, examination of, 2317
Perinephric abscess, 1674
Perineum, 2294, *2294*
examination of, 2317
Periodic limb movement disorder, 402
Periodontal disease, 1720–1722
clinical manifestations of, 1721
diagnostic findings in, 1721
etiology of, 1720–1721
management of, 199t
community/self care in, 1721–1722
in elderly, 1722
medical, 1721
nursing, 1721–1722
surgical, 1722
nursing care in, 1722
pathophysiology of, 1721, *1721*
prevention of, 1720b
risk factors for, 1720–1721, 1720b
Perioperative care, recipients of, 451
Perioperative nursing, 449–493
concepts of, 450–452, 451t, 452t
goal of, 450
phases of, 449–450
intraoperative, 449–450. See also *Intraoperative nursing.*
postoperative, 450
preoperative, 449. See also *Preoperative nursing.*
philosophy of, 449–450
practice of, 449–450
Perioral, definition of, 2183t
Periosteum, 2073, *2075*
Peripheral arterial catheters, in hemodynamic monitoring, in shock, 526
Peripheral atherectomy, 1413
Peripheral blood smear, in hematologic system assessment, 1464, 1466t
Peripheral blood stem cell (PBSC) transplantation, for cancer, 585

Peripheral ganglia, structure/function of, 703
Peripheral nerve block anesthesia, 474–475
Peripheral nervous system, assessment of, in musculoskeletal disorders, 2092
in neurologic disorders, 740
disorders of, 890–931
injury to, 928–929
structure/function of, 701–704, *702–704*, 705t
tumors of, 929
Peripheral neuropathy, *927*, 927–928, 928b
in chronic renal failure, 1646
Peripheral pain, 357–358
Peripheral stem cells, collection of, for bone marrow transplantation, 1496
Peripheral tissue, perfusion of, altered, in abdominal aortic aneurysm, 1427–1428
in burns, 2244
in chronic arterial occlusion, 1408–1409
in heart failure, 1288
decreased, fingerstick blood glucose measurement in, nursing research on, 515b
Peripheral vascular disease (PVD), diabetes mellitus and, 1994–1995, 1995t
renal disorders in, 1626
Peripheral vascular resistance (PVR), 1202
Peripheral vascular system, disorders of, 1387–1442
assessment of, 1377–1386
diagnostic tests in, *1383*, 1383–1386, *1385*
history in, 1377–1379, 1378b, 1379t
in health history, 184b
physical examination in, 1378b, 1379–1383, *1381, 1382*
home management of, 1437b
structure/function of, 1369–1376, *1370*
Peripheral vision, age-related changes in, 940
examination of, 946–947, *947*
Peristalsis, 1685, *1687*
in small intestine, 1694
mass, 1695
Peristaltic rush, 1694
Peritoneal dialysis, 1648–1650
catheter insertion in, 1649, *1650*
complications of, 1649–1650
contraindications to, 1648
indications for, 1648
living with, 1659b
preparation for, 1649
procedure for, 1649, *1650*
types of, 1648–1649
Peritoneal lavage, diagnostic, 2531, *2531*
Peritoneal tap, in hepatobiliary disease, 1854
Peritoneoscopy, in hepatobiliary disease, 1854
Peritoneovenous shunt, for ascites, 1891, *1892*
Peritonitis, 1793–1794
clinical manifestations of, 1793–1794
diagnostic findings in, 1793–1794
etiology of, 1793, 1793b
in renal transplantation, 1664
management of, medical, 1794

Peritonitis *(Continued)*
nursing, 1794
surgical, 1794
nursing care in, 1794
pathophysiology of, 1793
peritoneal dialysis and, 1649–1650
risk factors for, 1793
Peritonsillar abscess, 1080
Periungual, definition of, 2183t
PERL, 720
Permanent (fixed) sections, in cytologic analysis, 257
Permax (pergolide), for Parkinson's disease, 880t
Pernicious anemia, 1474–1476
clinical manifestations of, 1475
diagnostic findings in, 1475
etiology of, 1474–1475
management of, community/self care in, 1475–1476
medical, 1475–1476
nursing, 1476
pathophysiology of, 1475
risk factors for, 1474–1475
Peroneal nerve, neurovascular assessment of, *2093*
PERRLA, 720, 945
Personality type, evaluation of, in cardiovascular assessment, 1210
Pertussis, immunization recommendations for, in adults, 422t
Pessary, for vaginal prolapse, 2411
PET. See *Positron emission tomography (PET).*
Petechiae, biocultural variations in, 2190b
conjunctival, in infective endocarditis, 1333
Petit mal seizures, 837
Petrolatum, 2200t
Petroleum jelly (Vaseline), 2199t
Peyronie's disease, 2380
PFSDQ (Pulmonary Functional Status and Dyspnea Questionnaire), 1036
nursing research on, 1037b
PFTs. See *Pulmonary function tests (PFTs).*
pH, analysis of, 1056
classification of, in arterial blood gas analysis, 338b
correction of, in diabetic ketoacidosis, 1984–1986
in asthma, 1108t
in calcium level, 314
in respiration control, 1030–1031
normal values for, 328
of blood, 1447
of urine, 1558
regulation of, blood buffer systems in, 331–332
kidneys in, 1542–1543
tissue, in free flap assessment, 2281
Phacoemulsification, for cataracts, 959
Phagocytosis, 263
in wound healing, 431
neutrophils in, 428
oxygen in, 429
Phalanges, fracture of, 2161
Phalen's test, 2090t
in carpal tunnel syndrome, 927, *927*

Phantom limb sensation, 1420
Phantom pain, 355, 357–358, 1421
Pharmacokinetics, cultural differences in, 94b–95b
Pharyngeal (gag) reflex, 727, 729t
Pharyngitis, 1079
Pharynx, assessment of, 1047–1050
  in health history, 183b–184b
    in regional examination, 216t–217t
  cancer of, survival in, 538t
  structure of, 1023
Phenazopyridine (Pyridium), for urinary tract infections, 1576t
  urine color with, 1557t
Phencyclidine (PCP), abuse of, 2492
  effects of, 2483t
    health consequences of, 2494t
  withdrawal from, symptoms of, 2488t
Phenergan (promethazine hydrochloride), preoperative, 465t
Phenobarbital, avoidance of, in cirrhosis, 1882t
  side effects of, 839t
  therapeutic monitoring of, reference values for, 2562
Phenol paste, 2198t
Phenol peels, 2274
Phenolphthalein, urine color with, 1557t
Phenothiazines, urine color with, 1557t
Phenoxybenzamine (Dibenzyline), for benign prostatic hyperplasia, 2364t
Phensuximide (Milontin), side effects of, 839t
Phenylpropanolamine hydrochloride (Acutrim), for urinary incontinence, 1611t
Phenytoin (Dilantin), allergic reaction to, clinical manifestations of, 640t
  avoidance of, in cirrhosis, 1882t
  for status epilepticus, 843
  for trigeminal neuralgia, 930
  in pain control, 374
  side effects of, 839t
  therapeutic monitoring of, reference values for, 2562
  urine color with, 1557t
Pheochromocytoma, 1944, 2056–2060
  clinical manifestations of, 2057–2058
  diagnostic findings in, 2057–2058
  etiology of, 2057
  hypertension in, 1389
  management of, in elderly, 2060
    surgical, 2058–2059
      nursing care in, 2059–2060
  pathophysiology of, 2057, 2057t
  prevention of, 2058b
  risk factors for, 2057, 2058b
Philadelphia collar, 2507
Phimosis, 2379, 2379
Phlebitis, after abdominal-perineal resection, prevention of, 1813–1814
  postoperative, prevention of, 487
Phlebotomy, for polycythemia vera, 1485–1486
Phonoangiography, spectral, quantitative, of cerebrovascular system, 733
Phonocardiography, in cardiovascular assessment, 1229
Phorias, 945

Phosphate, depletion of, in diabetic ketoacidosis, 1984
  distribution of, 293t
Phosphate buffer system, 330, 331
Phosphorus, functions of, 314
  imbalances of, 314–322. See also Hyperphosphatemia; Hypophosphatemia.
  measurement of, in cardiovascular assessment, 1220
  metabolism of, tests of, in musculoskeletal disorders, 2096t
  plasma, range for, 296b
  serum, in parathyroid disorders, 2032t
Phosphorus binders, for chronic renal failure, 1654
Photochemotherapy, 2203
Photocoagulation, for diabetic retinopathy, 965
Photodamage, 2224
Photography, fundus, 950, 950
  in plastic surgery documentation, 2270
Photophobia, 941
Photoplethysmography, in free flap assessment, 2281
Photosensitivity, chemotherapy and, 583
Phthirus pubis, and vulvar irritation, 2422
Physical dependence, on opioid analgesics, 377
Physical examination, 213–241
  accuracy of, 225
  auscultation in, 230, 230–231
  complete, 225
  data from, processing of, 237–239
    recording of, 240
  general screening, 213
    adult, 233–237
      adipose tissue measurement in, 237, 240
      balance in, 236
      behavior in, 233–236
      body frame in, 237, 239b
      general appearance in, 233–236
      height in, 236
      skin color in, 237
      vital signs in, 236–237, 237b, 238
      weight in, 236, 236b
    general survey in, 214t
  health assessment after, 240–241
  in cancer diagnosis, 554
  in cardiomyopathy, 1340t
  in cross-cultural nursing, 65
  in hypertension, 1399
  in immune disorders, 609–611, 609b, 610t
  in pain assessment, 365
  inspection in, 225, 227
    instruments for, 225, 227
  nursing diagnosis in, 240–241
  nursing process in, 225, 240–241
  of abdomen, 219t–221t
  of anus and rectum, 223t, 224t
  of cardiovascular system, 1211–1217
  of ears, 987, 987–989, 988
  of endocrine system, 1950–1952, 1952, 1952b
  of eyes, 943–950, 946–949, 947b
  of female reproductive system, 2312–2320
    normal findings in, 2312b

Physical examination (Continued)
  of gastrointestinal tract, 1706–1710, 1707–1709
    normal findings in, 1699b
  of genitalia, 222t, 223t–224t
  of head and neck, 214t–217t
  of hematologic system, 1463, 1465b
  of hepatobiliary system, 1845–1848, 1846t–1847t, 1847
    in elderly, 1848
  of integumentary system, 2182–2194
    depth of, 2185
    environment for, 2184–2185
    normal findings in, 2182b
  of lower extremities, 221t
  of male reproductive system, 2332–2336
    normal findings in, 2332b
  of musculoskeletal system, 2086–2092, 2087
    normal findings in, 2086b
  of neurologic system, 221t–222t, 715–730, 716b
  of peripheral vascular system, 1379–1383, 1381, 1382
    normal findings in, 1378b
  of respiratory tract, 1040–1047, 1041, 1042b
    upper, 1048–1050, 1050
  of spine, 217t, 221t–222t
  of thorax, 218t–219t
  of upper extremities, 217t
  of urinary tract, 1552, 1552–1555, 1553
    normal findings in, 1556b
  olfaction in, 231
  palpation in, 225–228, 228
  percussion in, 228–230, 229
  preoperative, 459–460
  preparation for, 231–233, 232
    client, 231–233, 232
    environment, 231
    equipment, 231
    examiner, 233
  purpose of, 213
  regional, components of, 213, 214t–224t, 225
  techniques of, 225–233, 226–230, 232
  termination of, 239–240
  types of, 213, 214t–224t, 225
Physical fitness, in elderly, 85, 85
Physical mobility, impaired, after arterial bypass, 1417
  after cardiac surgery, 925
  after intervertebral disc surgery, 923–924
  after modified radical mastectomy, 2440–2441
  after thoracic surgery, 1161
  after total hip replacement, 2112–2113
  in burns, 2247
  in cerebrovascular accident, 800, 801
  in fractures, 2143
    intertrochanteric hip, 2156–2157, 2156t, 2157t
  in multiple sclerosis, 876
  in rheumatoid arthritis, management of, 669, 669, 669b
  in spinal cord injury, 904–907, 905, 906b

Physical mobility *(Continued)*
  in viral hepatitis, 1870
  management of, 200t
Physical restraints, use of, ethical issues in, 761b
Physical therapy, after intertrochanteric hip fracture, 2157
  after spinal cord injury, 905–907
  for cerebrovascular accident, 798
  for rheumatoid arthritis, 665
  in burns, 2260–2261, 2260t
  in osteoporosis, 2104
Physicians, in healthcare system, 4
Physiologic dependence, definition of, 2481t
Pia mater, 697, *697*
PID. See *Pelvic inflammatory disease (PID)*.
Pigeon chest, 1040–1042, *1043*
Pigment gallstones, 1908
Pigmentation, biocultural variations in, 2188b–2189b
  definition of, 2183t
  of nail, biocultural variations in, 2188b
Pilocarpine hydrochloride, for glaucoma, client teaching about, 957t
  in surgical client, 458t
Pilonidal cyst, 1828
Pindolol (Visken), 1395t
  for angina pectoris, 1257t
Pinna, structure of, 980, *981*
Pinocytosis, 263
Piroxicam (Feldene), for rheumatoid arthritis, 664t
Pit viper bites, 2536
Pitch, in auscultation, 230–231
Pitting edema, 1380, 2192
Pituitary gland, anterior, disorders of, 2060–2066
    and sexual disturbances, 2065
  disorders of, 2041–2069
  function of, 1941–1942
    testing of, 1954
  hormones of, *1939,* 1940t, 2061t
    regulation of, hypothalamus in, 1942
  in hormone regulation, *1939,* 1940–1941
  in shock, 508, *508*
  posterior, disorders of, 2066, *2066,* 2067t–2068t
  structure of, 1941–1942
  tumor of, 844–845, *846*
    and Cushing's syndrome, 2049
    clinical manifestations of, 847t
PJCs (premature junctional contractions), 1302, *1302*
PJT (paroxysmal junctional tachycardia), 1302–1303
Placebos, administration of, ethical issues in, 360b
  in pain control, 391
Plan of care, definition of, 136b
Planning, assessment of, 710t
  in chronic condition management, 116
  in cross-cultural nursing, 65
  in relocation stress syndrome, 89b
  in spiritual care, 73
Plant derivatives, for chemotherapy, classification of, 577t
Plantar, definition of, 2183t
Plantar fasciitis, 2162

Plantar neuroma, 2125
Plantar reflex, 726, 729t
Plaque, *2184*
  atherosclerotic, development of, 1243, *1243*
  dental, 1719
  fibrous, in coronary artery disease, 1242, *1242*
  neuritic, in Alzheimer's disease, 863–864, *864*
Plaquenil (hydroxychloroquine), for rheumatoid arthritis, 664t
Plasma, administration of, for shock, 519
  functions of, 1447, 1448t
  loss of, in hypovolemic shock, management of, 522t
  reference values for, 2557–2559
Plasma ACTH test, in hypercortisolism, 2051
Plasma derivatives, transfusion of, 1520t–1523t
Plasma membrane. See *Cell membrane.*
Plasma protein factor, transfusion of, 1520t
Plasma proteins, synthesis of, liver in, 1840
Plasma thromboplastin antecedent, 1516t
Plasma thromboplastin component, 1516t
Plasmapheresis, for glomerulonephritis, 1631
  for Guillain-Barré syndrome, 877
  for idiopathic thrombocytopenic purpura, 1507
  for myasthenia gravis, 885
Plasmin, in hemostasis, 1458
Plasminogen, in hemostasis, 1458
Plasmodium, 416t
Plastic surgery, 2267–2289
  aesthetic, 2267
  care after, delegation of, 2276b
  client selection for, 2268–2270, 2270b
  expectations for, 2269–2270
  in elderly, 2288
  in traumatic injury repair, 2286–2288, *2287*
  motivations for, 2269
  principles of, 2267–2270
  reconstructive, 2267, 2276–2283
  scarring in, minimization of, 2267–2268, *2268*
Platelet concentrates, transfusion of, 1520t–1523t
Platelet count, in blood dyscrasias, 1465t
  in hematologic system assessment, 1464, 1464t
  in hemorrhage, 1467t
Platelet-activating factor, in anaphylaxis, 638t
Platelet-derived growth factor (PDGF), in wound healing, 431
Platelets, development of, *1450*
  disorders of, 1506–1512
  functions of, 1448t
  in erythropoiesis, 1452
  in hemostasis, 1457
  in hepatobiliary assessment, 1852t
  reference values for, in cancer, 557t
  transfusion of, for secondary purpura, 1509
Platform posturography, 991, *993*

Plendil (felodipine), 1396t
Plethysmography, air, in peripheral vascular assessment, 1384
  body, 1051, *1054*
  impedance, in peripheral vascular assessment, 1384
  in venous thrombosis diagnosis, 1434
Pleura, disorders of, 1166–1167
  pain in, 1166
  structure of, 1027
  tumors of, metastatic, 1167
Pleural biopsy, 1064
Pleural effusion, 1166–1167
  causes of, 1166
  in acute pancreatitis, 1923, 1924t
  primary, 1167
  recurrent, 1167
Pleural friction rub, 1046, 1049t
Pleural space, 1027
  disorders of, 1166–1167
Pleural stripping, for pleural effusion, 1167
Pleurectomy, for pleural effusion, 1167
Pleurisy, 1166
  pneumonia with, chest pain in, assessment of, 1209t
Pleurodesis, for pleural effusion, 1167
Pleximeter, in percussion, 229
Plexor, in percussion, 229
Plexuses, 702
Plicamycin (Mithracin), for hypercalcemia, 321, 2034t
  for hyperparathyroidism, 2033
PLISSIT Model for Sexual Health Interventions, 77
Ploidy, 2435
Plummer-Vinson syndrome, 1472
PMI (point of maximum intensity), 1213
PML (progressive multifocal leukoencephalopathy), in acquired immunodeficiency syndrome, 630
PMNs (polymorphonuclear leukocytes), in wound healing, 428, *429*
PMS. See *Premenstrual syndrome (PMS).*
PND (paroxysmal nocturnal dyspnea), assessment of, 1206
  in left ventricular failure, 1281
Pneumatic antishock garment, 516–517, *517*
Pneumococcal pneumonia, 1136t
  immunization against, 421
    in adults, 422t
    schedule for, 208t
Pneumoconioses, 1150, 1151t
Pneumocystis carinii, 416t
Pneumocystis carinii pneumonia, 629, 1137t
  prophylaxis for, 624–625
Pneumocystis carinii thyroiditis, nursing research on, 2026, 2027b
Pneumocystography, 2328–2329
Pneumocystosis, in acquired immunodeficiency syndrome, 629
Pneumocytes, alveolar, 1029
Pneumomeningitis, bacterial, diagnosis of, 856
Pneumonectomy, for lung cancer, 1156, *1156*
Pneumonia, 1134–1138
  alveolar, 1135
  assessment of, 1136t–1137t

Pneumonia *(Continued)*
  bacterial, anaerobic, 1136t
    gram-negative, 1136t
    in acquired immunodeficiency syndrome, 628
  bilateral, 1135
  case management in, 1139b
  clinical manifestations of, 1134–1135, 1136t–1137t
  clinical pathway for, 2575–2577
  diagnostic findings in, 1134–1135, *1138*
  etiology of, 1134
  fungal, 1137t
  in enteral nutrition, 1753
  infectious agent in, 416t
  influenzal, 1136t
  interstitial, 1135
  lobar, 1135
  management of, 1136t–1137t
    community/self care in, 1138
    medical, 1135–1136, 1136t–1137t
  mycoplasmal, 1137t
  necrotizing, 1135
  nosocomial, 418–419, 418t
  parasitic, 1137t
  pathophysiology of, 1134
  pleurisy with, chest pain in, assessment of, 1209t
  pneumococcal, 1136t
    immunization against, 421
      in adults, 422t
      schedule for, 208t
  Pneumocystis carinii, 1137t
    prophylaxis for, 624–625
  postoperative, 486
  prevention of, 202t, 1135b
  risk factors for, 1134, 1135b
  segmental, 1135
  staphylococcal, 1136t
  viral, 1137t
  "walking," 1138
  with diabetes mellitus, case study of, 1972–1973
Pneumonitis, hypersensitivity, 1150, 1151t
Pneumothorax, 1027
  chest trauma and, 2524–2526, *2525*
  in achalasia, 1737
  open, mediastinal flutter with, 2524–2525, *2525*
  spontaneous, chest pain in, assessment of, 1209t
  tension, after thoracic surgery, monitoring for, 1159
    and cardiogenic shock, 500
    mediastinal shift with, *2525,* 2525–2526
PNH (paroxysmal nocturnal hemoglobinemia), 1480–1481
P–R interval, 1222, *1222*
PO₂, during respiration, 1031, *1032*
Pocket erosions, in rheumatoid arthritis, 661, *661*
Podofilox, for genital warts, 2473
Podophyllin, for genital warts, 2473
Poikilocytes, 1466t
Point of maximum intensity (PMI), 1213
Point-to-point testing, 722
Poisoning, 2537–2539, 2537t, 2538b, 2538t
  carbon monoxide, 269

Poisoning *(Continued)*
  in burns, 2237, 2237t
    skin changes in, biocultural variations in, 2190b
  lead, 269
  smoke, in burns, 2237
Poliomyelitis, anterior, acute, 860
  immunization recommendations for, in adults, 422t
Pollution, and disease, 36
Polycystic kidneys, *1678,* 1678–1679
Polycythemia, 1458, 1485–1486
  relative, 1486
  secondary, 1486
Polycythemia vera, 1485–1486
  clinical manifestations of, 1485
  complications of, 1486
  diagnostic findings in, 1485
  etiology of, 1485
  management of, medical, 1485–1486
    nursing, 1486
  pathophysiology of, 1485
  risk factors for, 1485
Polydipsia, in diabetes mellitus, 1960t
  in endocrine disorders, 1949
Polymorphic, definition of, 2183t
Polymorphonuclear leukocytes (PMNs), in wound healing, 428, *429*
Polymyalgia rheumatica, 680–681
Polymyositis, 679
Polyneuritis, 926
Polyneuropathy, diabetic, 2000
Polypectomy, nasal, 1102
Polypeptides, vasoactive, release of, in shock, 507
Polyphagia, in diabetes mellitus, 1960t
Polyps, gynecologic, 2411, *2411*
  intestinal, 1808
  nasal, 1101–1102
Polysomnography, 398–399
Polysporin, 2198t
  for open wounds, 445t
Polysubstance abuse, definition of, 2481t
Polytetrafluoroethylene (PTFE), for vein grafting, 1414
Polythiazide (Renese), 1394t
Polyuria, 1548, 1554
  in diabetes mellitus, 1960t
  in endocrine disorders, 1949
Pons, *691,* 693, *693*
  structures of, functions of, 694t
Pontocaine HCl (tetracaine hydrochloride), 473t
Popliteal lymph nodes, assessment of, 611
Porcine valve, *1352*
Port-A-Cath Dual-Lumen Venous Access System, *579*
Portacaval shunt, for portal hypertension, 1887, *1888*
Portal hypertension, 1884–1889
  clinical manifestations of, 1884
  diagnostic findings in, 1884
  esophageal bleeding in, critical monitoring in, 1885, 1885b
  etiology of, 1884, 1884b
  in ascites, 1889
  in cirrhosis, 1874
  management of, emergency, 1884–1887

Portal hypertension *(Continued)*
  medical, 1884–1886
  nursing, 1886–1887
  surgical, 1887, *1888*
    complications of, 1887
    nursing care in, 1887–1889
    outcomes in, 1887
  pathophysiology of, 1884
  risk factors for, 1884
Portal pressure, measurement of, 1856
Portal systemic encephalopathy, in bleeding esophageal varices, 1886–1887
Portal vein, 1835
Portal vein bacteremia, and liver abscess, 1902
Porter-Silber reaction, 2045t
Portosystemic shunt, for portal hypertension, 1887, *1888*
  nursing care in, 1887–1889
Positioning, after craniotomy, 853–854
  after spinal cord injury, 905
  after thoracic surgery, 1161
  after thyroidectomy, 2024t
  for altered cerebral tissue perfusion, in increased intracranial pressure, 782
  for chest tube drainage, 1165
  for heart failure, 1283
  for pulmonary embolism, 1129
  in burn autografting, 2255
  in client preparation, for physical examination, 231, *232*
  in peripheral vascular disease, 1408
  in postanesthesia care unit, 481, *481*
  intraoperative, 477–478, *478*
    safety considerations in, 477–478
  postoperative assessment of, 485
  therapeutic, in burns, 2259, 2260t
  with cast, 2150–2151
Positive end-expiratory pressure (PEEP), *1179,* 1179–1182
  complications of, risk for, 1181
  for shock, 516
  hazards of, 1179–1182
Positron emission tomography (PET), 253
  care in, postprocedure, 253
    preprocedure, 253
  in cancer diagnosis, 555
  in cardiovascular assessment, 1228
  in myocardial infarction, 1262
  in neurologic assessment, 732–733
  procedure for, 253, *253*
  uses of, 253
Postanesthesia care unit (PACU), 480–484
  admission to, 480–482, *481*
    baseline assessment in, 481–482
  complications in, *482,* 482–483
  discharge from, 484
  equipment in, 480–481
  observations in, documentation of, 481–482
  positioning in, 481, *481*
  transfer from, 484
Postconcussion syndrome, sleep disorders in, 404
Postencephalitic parkinsonism, 878
Posterior cerebral artery, cerebrovascular accident of, clinical manifestations of, 788t

Posterior fossa, surgery of, complications of, 851
 positioning after, 853
Posterior plug, for epistaxis, 1076, *1077*
Posterior repair, for rectocele, 2410
Posteroanterior (PA) chest x-ray, 1060
Posteroinferior cerebellum, cerebrovascular accident of, clinical manifestations of, 788t
Postherpetic neuralgia, 357
Posthitis, 2380, *2380*
Postictal state, 835b, 836
 of tonic-clonic seizure, 837
Post-LP headache, 744–745
Postmastectomy breast reconstruction, *2284,* 2284–2285, *2285*
Postmenopausal bleeding, 2395, *2395*
Postnecrotic cirrhosis, 1873, 1874t–1875t
Postoperative nursing, 480–492
 in clinical unit, 484–492, 486t, *487, 489, 491*
 in postanesthesia care unit, 480–484. See also *Postanesthesia care unit (PACU).*
Postphlebitic syndrome, 1436
Postpolio syndrome, 860
Post-traumatic areflexia, 895
Post-traumatic arthritis, in fracture, prevention of, 2145
Post-traumatic response, head trauma and, 826
Post-traumatic stress, after burn injury, 2262b
Post-traumatic vessel disease (PTVD), 2280
Postural hypotension, 1404
Posture, assessment of, 234, 2086, *2087*
Posturing, decerebrate, in unconscious patient, 723
 decorticate, in unconscious patient, 723
 in consciousness disorders, 748, *748*
 in increased intracranial pressure, 781
Posturography, platform, 991, *993*
Postvoiding residual volume, in urinary incontinence, in elderly, *1614*
Potassium, concentration of, *294,* 294t
 dietary, sources of, 313b
 distribution of, 293t
 functions of, 304
 imbalances of, 304–314. See also *Hyperkalemia; Hypokalemia.*
 electrocardiographic changes in, 305–306, *308*
 in acid-base balance, 330–331
 in action potential, 293–294, *295*
 cardiac, 1195, *1195*
 level of, reduction of, in hyperkalemia, 312–313
 measurement of, in cardiovascular assessment, 1220
 in gastrointestinal tract assessment, 1711t
 plasma, range for, 296b
 redistribution of, in hypokalemia, 305t
 replacement of, in diabetic ketoacidosis, 1983–1984, 1986b
 in hypokalemia, 306–307
 restriction of, in chronic renal failure, 1655
 serum, preoperative evaluation of, 453t

Potassium *(Continued)*
 supplementation of, for hypertension, 1393
Potassium hydroxide (KOH) examination, in integumentary disorders, 2194
Potassium iodide, for hyperthyroidism, 2020
Potassium permanganate, topical, 2199t
Potassium-sparing diuretics, 1394t
Potentiation, definition of, 2481t
Pott's fracture, *2130,* 2131
 of foot, 2161
Pouch(es), colostomy, 1806, *1807*
 care of, 1814
 ileostomy, 1806, *1807*
 care of, 1805
 Indiana, for bladder cancer, 1585, *1586*
 J, for inflammatory bowel disease, 1801, *1802*
 Kock. See *Kock pouch.*
 ostomy, application of, 1592, *1592*
Povidone-iodine (Betadine), for open wounds, 445t
Powders, 2200t
Power of attorney, durable, in terminal cancer, 567
 for healthcare, elderly issues in, 102
Powerlessness, in myocardial infarction, 1271–1272
 in vertigo, 1015
PPD test, schedule for, 208t
PPO (preferred provider organization), 5b
PPS (prospective payment system), 8
PQRST, in emergency nursing assessment, 2503
PR (progesterone receptor), in cancer diagnosis, 558t
P-R interval, analysis of, 1298b
 normal, characteristics of, 1296b
Prazosin (Minipress), 1395t
 for benign prostatic hyperplasia, 2364t
Precancerous lesions, in cancer, 541
Precapillary sphincters, 1371, *1371*
Precordium, physical examination of, 1213, *1214*
Precose (Acarbose), for diabetes mellitus, 1967t, 1968
Predisposition, definition of, 2481t
Prednisolone (Delta-Cortef), 2048t
 for rheumatoid arthritis, 664t
Prednisone (Deltasone, Orasone), 2048t
 after heart transplantation, 1353, 1354b
 for multiple myeloma, 1499
 for rheumatoid arthritis, 663, 664t
 in surgical client, 458t
Preexcitation syndromes, 1309–1310
Preferred provider organization (PPO), 5b
Prefrontal leukotomy, for pain, 386
Prefrontal lobes, 690, *692*
Pregnancy, and heart failure, 1278
 cervical cancer in, treatment of, 2407
 chemotherapy during, 584
 drug abuse during, ethical issues in, 2309b
 renal disorders in, 1626
 unplanned, prevention of, 203t
 screening for, 208t
Preload, 1200, *1201*
 in heart failure, increase in, 1277, 1277t
 reduction of, 1285, 1285t

Premature atrial contractions (PACs), *1299,* 1300–1301
Premature junctional contractions (PJCs), 1302, *1302*
Premature ventricular contractions (PVCs), 1305, *1306*
 management of, 1305, 1307t–1308t
Premenstrual syndrome (PMS), 2388–2389
 clinical manifestations of, 2388
 diagnostic findings in, 2388
 etiology of, 2388
 management of, community/self care in, 2388–2389
 medical, 2388
 nursing, 2388–2389
 risk factors for, 2388
 sleep disorders in, 404
Preoperative nursing, 452–466
 assessment in, 453–461, 453t, 454t, 458t, 460b
 client preparation in, on day of surgery, 464–465, 465t
 discharge planning in, 459
 of significant others, 465–466
 physical preparation in, 463–464
 psychosocial aspects of, 458–459
 teaching in, 225–227, *226*
Presbycusis, 984
 management of, 199t
Presbyopia, 940
Presbystasis, 1011
Presbyterians, beliefs/practices of, 2547
Pressoreceptors, in cardiac regulation, 1203
 in fluid balance regulation, 277
Pressure gauge, in nasoenteral tube placement, nursing research on, 1751b
Pressure support ventilation (PSV), 1177, 1178t
Pressure ulcers, 442, 2213–2220
 clinical manifestations of, 2213
 complications of, 2216
 diagnostic findings in, 2213, *2215,* 2216
 etiology of, 2213
 every-two-hour turning schedule for, nursing research on, 2218b
 intertrochanteric hip fracture and, 2155
 management of, community/self care in, 2219–2220, 2220b
 delegation of, 2216b
 home healthcare in, 2220b
 medical, 2213–2216
 nursing, 2216–2219
 surgical, 2219
 pathophysiology of, 2213
 prevention of, in spinal cord injury, 902, 903b
 risk factors for, 2213, *2214*
 stages of, 2213, *2215*
Priapism, 2379–2380
Prickle cells, 2174, *2174*
Prilosec (omeprazole), for gastroesophageal reflux disease, 1738
 for peptic ulcer disease, 1767, 1769t, 1770
Primapore, indications for, 443t
Primary hepatocellular carcinoma, 1896
Primary hypertension, 1387
 pathophysiology of, 1389, *1390*

Primary infection, in human immunodeficiency virus infection, 621–623
Primary nursing, 124
Primary open-angle glaucoma, 952, *953*. See also *Glaucoma*.
Primary practice partner, 125
Primidone (Mysoline), side effects of, 839t
therapeutic monitoring of, reference values for, 2562
Principle of electroneutrality, 330
Prinivil (lisinopril), 1396t
Prinzmetal's angina, 1254
Privacy, in emergency care, 2502
Private duty nursing, 120
Private pay, 5b
PRL (prolactin), 2061t
actions of, 1940t
overproduction of, in hyperpituitarism, 2062, 2063t
Proaminopeptidase, pancreatic, 1922b
Proantigens, in immunity, 598
Pro-Banthine (propantheline bromide), for urinary incontinence, 1611t
for urinary tract infections, 1576t
Problem Classification Scheme, domains of, 152, 152b
in Omaha system of home healthcare provision, 152–153, 152b, 153b, 154t
problems in, 152, 152b, 153b
Problem Rating Scale for Outcomes, in Omaha system of home healthcare provision, 154, 156t
Procainamide (Pronestyl), for dysrhythmia, 1307t
for shock, 521
in surgical client, 458t
therapeutic monitoring of, reference values for, 2562
Procaine (Novocain), in pain control, 372
Procallus, 2080
Procarboxypeptidase, pancreatic, 1922b
Procardia (nifedipine), 1396t
for angina pectoris, 1256t
for interstitial cystitis, 1580
Proctitis, abacterial, after radiation therapy, 1584
Proctocolectomy, total, for inflammatory bowel disease, 1801, *1801*
Proctosigmoidectomy, for colon cancer, *1812*
Proctosigmoidoscopy, 1715–1716
Procyclidine (Kemadrin), for Parkinson's disease, 880t
Prodrome, in epilepsy, definition of, 835b
Professional nurse, definition of, 136b
Progestational agents, for chemotherapy, classification of, 577t
Progesterone, 2298
actions of, 1940t
for menopause, side effects of, 2394
in breast development, 2297
Progesterone receptor (PR), in cancer diagnosis, 558t
Prograf (tacrolimus), in organ transplantation, 645t
Progressive multifocal leukoencephalopathy (PML), in acquired immunodeficiency syndrome, 630

Progressive pain, management of, *368,* 368–369
Progressive relaxation training (PRT), for sleep disorders, in elderly, nursing research on, 409b
in pain control, 369
Progressive systemic sclerosis (PSS), 677–678, 677b, *678*
progressively fatal, 678, *678*
Prolactin (PRL), 2061t
actions of, 1940t
overproduction of, in hyperpituitarism, 2062, 2063t
Promethazine hydrochloride (Phenergan), preoperative, 465t
Pronator drift, 722
test for, 781
Prone position, for physical examination, *232*
intraoperative, 477, *478*
Pronestyl (procainamide), for dysrhythmia, 1307t
for shock, 521
in surgical client, 458t
therapeutic monitoring of, reference values for, 2562
Propantheline bromide (Pro-Banthine), for urinary incontinence, 1611t
for urinary tract infections, 1576t
Propoxyphene hydrochloride (Darvon), administration of, 381t
in pain control, 375t
Propoxyphene napsylate (Darvon-N), in pain control, 375t
Propranolol (Inderal), 1395t
for angina pectoris, 1254–1255, 1257t
for dysrhythmia, 1308t
in surgical client, 458t
therapeutic monitoring of, reference values for, 2562
Proprioception, assessment of, 724
Propulsid (cisapride), for gastroesophageal reflux disease, 1738
Propulsion, muscles in, 2078–2079
Propylthiouracil (PTU), for hyperthyroidism, 2013t, 2019
Proscar (finasteride), for benign prostatic hyperplasia, 2364t
Prospective payment system (PPS), 8
Prostaglandin analogs, for peptic ulcer disease, 1767, 1768t
Prostaglandin synthesis inhibitors, for dysmenorrhea, 2387
Prostaglandins, 1941
in fluid balance regulation, 277
in sodium regulation, 295
in wound healing, 430
synthesis of, kidneys in, 1543–1544
Prostate, biopsy of, 2338
disorders of, 2350–2373
screening of, 210t
structure/function of, 2304
ultrasonography of, 2339
Prostate cancer, 2365–2372
clinical manifestations of, 2365–2367
diagnostic findings in, 2365–2367
etiology of, 2365
management of, in elderly, 2372

Prostate cancer *(Continued)*
medical, 2367–2368
nursing, 2368–2369
surgical, 2369
nursing care in, 2370–2372
pathophysiology of, 2365
prevention of, 2366b
risk factors for, 542b, 2365, 2366b
screening for, 210t
staging of, 2367, 2368b
survival in, 538t
Prostatectomy, for benign prostatic hyperplasia, indications for, 2352
nursing care after, 2360–2363
perineal, for benign prostatic hyperplasia, *2353,* 2358
radical, for prostate cancer, 2370
retropubic, for benign prostatic hyperplasia, *2353,* 2358
suprapubic, for benign prostatic hyperplasia, *2353,* 2358
transurethal, for prostate cancer, 2369
Prostate-specific antigen (PSA), 2336–2337
in cancer diagnosis, 558t, 2367
schedule for, 210t
Prostate-specific antigen density (PSAD), 2336
Prostate-specific antigen velocity (PSAV), 2336
Prostatic acid phosphatase (PAP), in prostate cancer, 558t, 2367
Prostatic fluid, 2305
Prostatic massage, 2336, *2337*
Prostatitis, *2372,* 2372–2373
Prostatodynia, 2373
Prosthesis(es), after amputation, adjustment to, 1421–1422
care of, 1422–1424
client education in, 1423b
permanent, 1419, *1421, 1422*
temporary, 1418–1419
Angelchik, for gastroesophageal reflux disease, 1739, *1740*
bladder neck support, for urinary incontinence, 1609
dislocation of, after total hip replacement, 2113–2114, *2115*
eye, 971, *971*
insertion/removal of, 972b–973b
middle ear, 1008, *1008*
penile, 2348–2349, *2349*
testicular, for testicular cancer, 2376
Prosthetic heart valves, 1352, *1352*
Prosthetic valve endocarditis, 1331
Prostigmin (neostigmine), in myasthenia gravis, 885
Protease inhibitors, for human immunodeficiency virus infection, 624
Proteases, pancreatic, 1922b
Protectants, topical, 2199t
Protein(s), Bence Jones, 1558
distribution of, 293t
functions of, 1447, 1448t
in diabetes mellitus, guidelines for, 1976, 1977t
in wound healing, 434t
inadequate intake of, cellular effects of, 270

Protein(s) (Continued)
integral, 262, 264
metabolism of, glucocorticoids in, 1944
laboratory tests for, 1850t–1851t
liver in, 1840
peripheral, 262, 264
restriction of, in chronic renal failure, 1655
total, in hepatobiliary assessment, 1850t
urine, 1558
in diabetes mellitus diagnosis, 1963
utilization of, increased, in type II diabetes mellitus, 1960
Protein-calorie malnutrition, adipose tissue measurement in, 240
Proteinuria, 1558
in diabetes mellitus diagnosis, 1963
Prothrombin, 1516t
Prothrombin time (PT), in hemorrhage, 1467t
in hepatobiliary assessment, 1852t
preoperative evaluation of, 453t
Proton pump inhibitors, for peptic ulcer disease, 1769t, 1770
Proto-oncogenes, definition of, 534t
PRT (progressive relaxation training), for sleep disorders, in elderly, nursing research on, 409b
in pain control, 369
Pruritus, 2203–2205
after burn injury, 2263b
definition of, 2183t
in chronic renal failure, 1646, 1647
in diabetes mellitus, 1960t
in jaundice, 1860
in viral hepatitis, 1865, 1866t
vaginal discharge with, 2413–2414
PSA (prostate-specific antigen), 2336–2337
in cancer diagnosis, 558t, 2367
schedule for, 210t
PSAD (prostate-specific antigen density), 2336
PSAV (prostate-specific antigen velocity), 2336
PSDA (Patient Self-Determination Act), 47
elderly issues in, 102
Pseudoaneurysm, 1425
after angiography, 1385
Pseudoarthrosis, fracture nonunion and, 2145
Pseudocysts, pancreatic, 1929–1930
Pseudofolliculitis, biocultural variations in, 2191b
Pseudohyperkalemia, 311
Pseudohypoparathyroidism, 2036
Pseudomembranous colitis, 1789
Pseudomonas aeruginosa infection, in cystic fibrosis, 1149
Pseudoseizures, 843
Psoralen plus ultraviolet A (PUVA), 2203–2204
Psorcon (diflorasone), topical, 2199t
Psoriasis vulgaris, 2210–2212, 2211
management of, medical, 2211
nursing, 2211–2212
PsoriGel, 2200t
PSS (progressive systemic sclerosis), 677–678, 677b, 678
progressively fatal, 678, 678

PSV (pressure support ventilation), 1177, 1178t
Psychedelic drugs. See Hallucinogens.
Psychiatric status, assessment of, in health history, 185b
Psychoactive substance, definition of, 2481t
Psychogenic pain, 359
Psychological dependence, definition of, 2481t
Psychological incontinence, 1604t
pathophysiology of, 1606
risk factors for, 1606b
Psychological patterns, definition of, 189
Psychological support, in burns, 2259
Psychopharmacologic drugs, therapeutic monitoring of, reference values for, 2562
Psychosis, intensive care unit, 407b
Psychosocial changes, in chronic renal failure, 1646–1647
Psychosocial development, assessment of, 196
Psychosocial dimensions, 51–79
of cross-cultural nursing, 59–67
of cystic fibrosis, 1149
of family, 51–59
of grief, 73–74
of sexuality, 74–79, 77t
of spirituality, 67–73
of suffering, 74
psychosocial nursing vs., 51
Psychosocial history, cultural assessment in, 197
guide to, 197
in cardiovascular disorders, 1210
in ear disorders, 986–987
in endocrine disorders, 1950
in eye disorders, 942–943
in gastrointestinal tract disorders, 1705–1706
in gynecologic disorders, 2310–2311
in hematologic disorders, 1462
in hepatobiliary disorders, 1844–1845
in immune disorders, 608–609
in integumentary system disorders, 2181–2182
in male reproductive disorders, 2331–2332
in musculoskeletal disorders, 2085–2086
in neurologic system disorders, 714
in peripheral vascular system disorders, 1379
in respiratory disorders, 1039
in urinary tract disorders, 1550–1552
nature of, 189
psychological assessment in, 189–196
behavior in, 190
general appearance in, 190
mental status in, 190–196
motivation in, 196
motor activity in, 190
personal strengths in, 196
spirituality in, 196
values/beliefs in, 196
risk factors in, 189, 190b, 191t–194t
sociologic assessment in, 196–197
life-style in, 197
psychosocial development in, 196
sexuality in, 197

Psychosocial history (Continued)
social network in, 196
socioeconomic status in, 196
Psychosocial issues, in cancer diagnosis, 552–554, 554b
Psychosocial theories, of illness, 22–26
Psychotherapy, for urinary incontinence, 1612
PT (prothrombin time), in hemorrhage, 1467t
in hepatobiliary assessment, 1852t
preoperative evaluation of, 453t
PTA (percutaneous transluminal angioplasty), 1413
PTCA (percutaneous transluminal coronary angioplasty), case management in, 1247
clinical pathway for, 2578–2579
family needs in, nursing research on, 1248b
for coronary artery disease, 1245, 1245
Pterygium, red eye in, 942b
PTFE (polytetrafluoroethylene), for vein grafting, 1414
PTH. See Parathyroid hormone (PTH).
Ptosis, 720, 943, 974
in myasthenia gravis, 884
PTT (partial thromboplastin time), in hemorrhage, 1467t
preoperative evaluation of, 453t
PTU (propylthiouracil), for hyperthyroidism, 2013t, 2019
PTVD (post-traumatic vessel disease), 2280
Ptyalin, 1692t
Pubic hair, female, examination of, 2317
male, physical examination of, 2333
Public, in healthcare system, 4–5
Puerto Ricans, attitudes of, toward death and dying, 70b–71b
Puestow procedure, for acute pancreatitis, 1927
Pulmonary angiography, 1062
Pulmonary artery catheter, 1233, 1234–1235
insertion of, 1233, 1234–1235
Pulmonary artery pressure (PAP), 1234–1235
elevation of, in pulmonary hypertension, 1129–1130
monitoring of, after cardiac surgery, 1357
Pulmonary artery wedge pressure (PAWP), monitoring of, after cardiac surgery, 1357
Pulmonary capillary wedge pressure (PCWP), monitoring of, in cardiovascular assessment, 1233
in shock, 526
Pulmonary disease, and heart failure, 1278
in rheumatoid arthritis, 659
Pulmonary edema, after myocardial infarction, 1266
after thoracic surgery, monitoring for, 1159
in extracellular fluid volume excess, 286
in left ventricular failure, 1281
neurogenic, head trauma and, 826
noncardiogenic, 1169, 1169b
causes of, 1169b
Pulmonary embolism (PE), 1126–1129
after myocardial infarction, 1266

Pulmonary embolism (PE) *(Continued)*
after thoracic surgery, monitoring for, 1159
and cardiogenic shock, 499–500
chest pain in, assessment of, 1209t
clinical manifestations of, 1127–1128
diagnostic findings in, 1127–1128, *1129*
etiology of, 1126
fat embolism vs., 2141t
fractures and, 2140
management of, emergency, 1128
medical, 1128–1129
nursing, 1129
surgical, 1129, *1130*
monitoring for, in venous thrombosis, 1435
pathophysiology of, 1126
postoperative, 486
prevention of, 1128b
risk factors for, 1126, 1128b
Pulmonary fibrosis, in rheumatoid arthritis, 659
Pulmonary function, preoperative assessment of, 455–456
Pulmonary function tests (PFTs), 1051, 1052t, *1053, 1054,* 1054t
components of, 1052t
in emphysema, 1115
in obstructive lung disorders, 1054t
in restrictive lung disorders, 1054t, 1147
Pulmonary Functional Status and Dyspnea Questionnaire (PFSDQ), 1036
nursing research on, 1037b
Pulmonary hypertension, 1129–1130
chest pain in, assessment of, 1209t
Pulmonary rehabilitation, for chronic obstructive pulmonary disease, 1124
Pulmonary resection, for lung cancer, 1155–1156, *1156*
Pulmonary vascular resistance, monitoring of, in shock, 526
Pulmonary vasculature, disorders of, 1105–1131
Pulmonic regurgitation, 1349
Pulmonic stenosis, 1349
Pulmonic valve, 1193
disease of, 1349
Pulse, amplitude of, evaluation of, 236, 237b
bigeminal, 1212
measurement of, 236, 237b
after cardiac surgery, 1357
delegation of, 234b
in cardiovascular assessment, 1212
palpation of, in peripheral vascular assessment, 1381, *1382*
water-hammer, 1212
Pulse generator, of pacemaker, 1315, *1316*
Pulse oximetry, in free flap assessment, 2281
in respiratory assessment, 1051–1055, *1055*
in shock, 514
limitations of, 1052–1055
Pulse pressure, 237, 1202
in shock, 510
Pulsed galvanic stimulation (Diapulse), for wound infection, 446
Pulseless electrical activity, 1310

PULSES, in chronic conditions, 115t
Pulsion diverticula, 1741
Pulsus bisferiens, 1212
Pulsus paradoxus, measurement of, 1211–1212
Pulsus tardus, 1212
Pumps, infusion, for home intravenous therapy, 284b
Punch biopsy, 257
of skin, *2195,* 2196
Punctate, definition of, 2183t
Pupil response, in increased intracranial pressure, 782
Pupillary reflex, 727
Pupils, autonomic neuropathy of, diabetes mellitus and, 2000
changes in, in consciousness disorders, 747–748
examination of, 944–945
Purine, metabolism of, in gout, 2107
Purkinje's fibers, 1198
Purpura, 1506–1509
anaphylactoid, 1508
secondary, 1508–1509
symptomatic, 1508–1509
toxic, 1508
Purulent exudate, 434, 435t
Pustule, *2184,* 2212
PUVA (psoralen plus ultraviolet A), 2203–2204
PVCs (premature ventricular contractions), 1305, *1306*
management of, 1305, 1307t–1308t
PVD (peripheral vascular disease), diabetes mellitus and, 1994–1995, 1995t
renal disorders in, 1626
PVR (peripheral vascular resistance), 1202
Pyelography, intravenous, 1562–1563
retrograde, 1563
Pyelolithotomy, for renal calculi, 1669, *1669*
Pyelonephritis, 1628–1630
clinical manifestations of, 1628–1629
diagnostic findings in, 1628–1629
etiology of, 1628
in urinary reflux, 1599
management of, in elderly, 1630
medical, 1629
nursing, 1629–1630
pathophysiology of, 1628
prevention of, 1628b
risk factors for, 1628, 1628b
Pyelostomy, percutaneous, for bladder cancer, 1587
Pyloric obstruction, in peptic ulcer disease, 1773, 1776, 1779
Pyloroplasty, vagotomy with, for peptic ulcer disease, 1777, *1777*
Pyramidal tract, structure/function of, 695–696, *697*
Pyrazinamide, for tuberculosis, 1143, 1145t
Pyrethrin, topical, 2198t
Pyridium (phenazopyridine), for urinary tract infections, 1576t
urine color with, 1557t
Pyridostigmine (Mestinon), for myasthenia gravis, 885
Pyrosis, 1733

Pyuria, 1559
in urethritis, 1581

Q

Q–T interval, *1222,* 1223
normal, characteristics of, 1296b
QRS complex, 1222, *1222*
analysis of, 1298b
normal, characteristics of, 1296b
Quadrantectomy, for breast cancer, 2436–2437
Quadriceps, strength of, assessment of, 2088t
Quadriceps jerk, *726,* 727
Quadriceps setting exercise, after cerebrovascular accident, 800
Quadriplegia, cervical spine injury and, 893
quality of life in, nursing research on, 903b
Quadruple rhythm, 1216
Quakers, beliefs/practices of, 2547
Qualitative urinary calcium, in parathyroid disorders, 2032t
Quality, in auscultation, 231
Quality improvement, ambulatory care nurse in, 141b, 142–143
Quality of life, in chronic obstructive pulmonary disease, nursing research on, 1127b
in hearing impairment, nursing research on, 1000b
in quadriplegia, nursing research on, 903b
Quantitative spectral phonoangiography, of cerebrovascular system, 733
Quantitative urinary calcium, in parathyroid disorders, 2032t
Quinapril (Accupril), 1396t
Quinatime (quinidine gluconate), for shock, 521
in surgical client, 458t
Quinethazone (Hydromox), 1394t
Quinidine, for dysrhythmia, 1307t
therapeutic monitoring of, reference values for, 2562
Quinidine gluconate (Quinatime), for shock, 521
in surgical client, 458t
Quinsy, 1080

R

R wave, analysis of, 1298b
RA. See *Rheumatoid arthritis (RA).*
Rabies, infectious agent in, 416t
Race, in adult general screening physical examination, 233–234
in coronary artery disease, 1238
in disease, 32b
in pain response, 346
Radial forearm flap, 2280
Radial keratotomy, 976
Radial nerve, neurovascular assessment of, *2093*
Radiation, exposure to, and cancer, 539–540

Radiation (Continued)
  prevention of, 250
  risks of, 249–250
  in postoperative wound infection, 490
  ionizing, and cell damage, 269
Radiation burns, 2233–2234
Radiation recall, chemotherapy and, 583
Radiation therapy (RT), external, 570
  fears about, 571b
  for acute leukemia, 1491
  for bladder cancer, 1583
  for breast cancer, 2446–2447, 2447
    side effects of, 2447
  for cancer, 570–573
    in research, 572
  for cervical cancer, 2407
  for colon cancer, 1811
  for esophageal cancer, 1744
  for Hodgkin's disease, 1502–1503
  for hypercortisolism, 2053, 2054t
  for laryngeal cancer, 1086
  for liver cancer, 1897
  for lung cancer, 1154
  for ocular melanoma, 970
  for oral cancer, 1728
  for polycythemia vera, 1486
  for prostate cancer, 2367–2368
    nursing care in, 2368
  for renal cancer, 1673
  for testicular cancer, 2376
  in pain control, 391
  internal, 570–571
    sealed-source, 570
      safety precautions in, 573, 574t
    unsealed-source, 570–571
      safety precautions in, 573, 574t
  mechanism of, 570
  misconceptions about, 571b
  safety of, 572, 572–573, 574t
    distance in, 572, 572
    shielding in, 573
    standards for, 573
    time in, 573
  side effects of, 571–572, 571b
  stereotactic, for brain tumors, 848
  types of, 570–571
Radical mastectomy, extended, 2437
  modified, 2437
    nursing care plan in, 2440–2441
  standard, 2437
Radical neck dissection, exercises after,
    client education in, 1096b–1098b
  for laryngeal cancer, 1088
  for oral cancer, 1729–1730
Radical orchiectomy, for testicular cancer,
    2375
Radical prostatectomy, for prostate cancer,
    2370
Radiculitis, renal pain vs., 1548
Radioactive iodine (¹³¹I), for hyperthyroid-
    ism, 2013t, 2020
Radioactive iodine uptake (RAIU), in thy-
    roid disorders, 2010t
Radiofrequency ablation (RFA), of dys-
    rhythmias, 1314
Radiography, contrast, 250–251
  diagnostic, 249–251
    in cancer, 555–556

Radiography (Continued)
  in leukemia, 1489
  indications for, 249
  of abdomen, 250
  of chest, 250
  of gastrointestinal tract, 1713–1714, 1714
  of hepatobiliary system, 1849–1853
  of musculoskeletal system, 2092
  of skeleton, 250
  of skull, in neurologic assessment, 730
  of spine, in neurologic assessment, 730
  of thyroid, 2011t
  of urinary tract, 1562
  ophthalmic, 950
Radioimmunoassay (RIA), in thyroid func-
    tion testing, 1952
  parathyroid hormone, 2032t
  triiodothyronine, 2010t
Radioimmunoprecipitation assay (RIPA),
    in acquired immunodeficiency syndrome
    testing, 611
Radioiodine, for hyperthyroidism, 2020
Radioiodine uptake/excretion test, 1952–
    1953
Radioisotope scans, in angina pectoris, 1254
  in cancer diagnosis, 555
  of male reproductive system, 2339
  of urinary tract, 1565
Radiolucent, definition of, 249
Radionuclide scanning, 254–255
  care in, postprocedure, 255
    preprocedure, 255
  in cardiomyopathy, 1340t
  in hepatobiliary disease, 1853–1854
  in myocardial infarction, 1261–1262
  procedure for, 254–255, 255
Radiopaque, definition of, 249
Radioprotectors, in radiation therapy, 572
Radiosensitizers, in radiation therapy, 572
Radiosurgery, stereotactic, closed, for pain,
    388
  for brain tumors, 849
Radioulnar joint, range of motion of, 2089
RAIU (radioactive iodine uptake), in thyroid
    disorders, 2010t
Rales, 1048t
Ramipril (Altace), 1396t
Rancho Los Amigos Scale of Cognitive
    Functioning, 114, 115t
Range of motion (ROM), of joints, mea-
    surement of, 2088, 2088, 2089
Range-of-motion (ROM) exercises, after
    cerebrovascular accident, 802
  after musculoskeletal trauma, 2167
  after thoracic surgery, 1161
  in rheumatoid arthritis, 665, 666b
Ranitidine (Zantac), for bleeding ulcer,
    1772
  for peptic ulcer disease, 1767, 1768
  for shock, 520
Rape, 2532
Rape-trauma syndrome, 2532
Raphe, of scrotum, 2302
Raphe magnus nucleus, in pain modulation,
    344, 345
Rapid ACTH stimulation, 2045t
Rapid alternating movements, assessment
    of, 722

Rapid eye movement (REM) sleep, 398
  characteristics of, 399, 399
  parasomnias in, 403
Rapid plasma reagin (RPR) test, before
    blood transfusion, 1524t
  schedule for, 210t
RAS (reticular activating system), in sleep,
    398
Rash, in syphilis, 2470
Rauwolfia (Raudixin), 1397t
Raynaud's syndrome, 1431–1432
  clinical manifestations of, 1431
  etiology of, 1431
  management of, 1431–1432
  risk factors for, 1431
Raz procedure, 1608
RBB (right bundle branch), 1198, 1198
RBBB (right bundle branch block), 1310
RBC (red blood cell) count, in blood dys-
    crasias, 1465t
  in gastrointestinal tract assessment, 1711t
  in hematologic system assessment, 1464,
    1464t
RBC (red blood cell) indices, in hemato-
    logic system assessment, 1464, 1464t,
    1466t
RBCs. See Red blood cells (RBCs).
RCA (right coronary artery), 1194, 1194
  lesion of, electrocardiographic changes in,
    1225t
RCT (registered care technician), 6
Reabsorption, 274, 274b
Reach for Recovery, 2443
Rebleeding, after intracranial hemorrhage,
    814
Rebound hyperglycemia, hypoglycemia
    with, 1990–1992
Rebound hypoglycemia, total parenteral nu-
    trition and, 1756
Receptors, in nerve impulse conduction, 690
Recidivism, definition of, 2481t
Reconstituted family, 53
Reconstructive plastic surgery, 2276–2283
Recovery, definition of, 2481t
Recreational drugs, effect of, on male repro-
    ductive system, 2345
Recruitment, 994
Rectal anesthesia, 472
Rectal examination, digital, in prostate can-
    cer, 2366
  schedule for, 209t
Rectal stretch, in bladder retraining, after
    spinal cord injury, 911
Rectal wall, female, examination of, 2320
Rectal-prostatic examination, 2336, 2337
Rectocele, 2320
  in uterine prolapse, 2410, 2410
Rectovaginal examination, 2320, 2320
Rectovaginal septum, examination of, 2320
Rectum, cancer of, risk factors for, 542b
  survival in, 538t
  female, assessment of, in regional exami-
    nation, 224t
  male, assessment of, in regional examina-
    tion, 223t
  physical examination of, 1709, 1709–1710
    in urinary tract assessment, 1555
    normal findings in, 1699b

Rectum (Continued)
structure of, 1695
Rectus abdominis flap, 2280
Rectus muscles, 935–936, 936
Red blood cell casts, 1559
Red blood cell (RBC) count, in blood dyscrasias, 1465t
in gastrointestinal tract assessment, 1711t
in hematologic system assessment, 1464,
1464t
Red blood cell (RBC) indices, in hematologic system assessment, 1464, 1464t,
1466t
Red blood cells (RBCs), disorders of,
1469–1486
functions of, 1448t
in urine, 1558–1559
intrinsic defects of, and hemolytic anemias, 1483
measurement of, in cardiovascular assessment, 1219
transfusion of, 1520t–1523t
Red eye, assessment of, 941, 942b
Red marrow, 1449, 2075
Red wounds, management of, 439, 441
Reduction, closed, 2136, 2136–2137
of fractures, 2135–2139
open, 2137
Reduction mammaplasty, 2285, 2285–2286
Reference values, of laboratory test results,
243, 2555–2565
Referral, in family nursing intervention, 59
Referred pain, 354, 355
Reflex(es). See also names of specific reflexes.
abnormal, 727–728, 728
in consciousness disorders, 749–751,
750
assessment of, 724–728, 726, 727b, 728
normal findings in, 717b
deep tendon (muscle-stretch), 726, 727,
727b
assessment of, guidelines for, 727b
in left hemiparesis, 728
grading of, 728, 728, 729t
in spinal cord injury, 893
in ventilation, 1030
normal, 725–727, 726, 727b
of central nervous system, 699–701, 701
superficial (cutaneous), 726–727
in left hemiparesis, 728
Reflex incontinence, 1604t
medications for, 1611t
pathophysiology of, 1606
risk factors for, 1606b
Reflex neurogenic bladder, 1615, 1616
Reflex sympathetic dystrophy (RSD), in
fracture, prevention of, 2145
Reflux, urinary. See Urinary reflux.
Reflux esophagitis. See Gastroesophageal
reflux disease (GERD).
Reflux gastritis, alkaline, in peptic ulcer disease, 1778
Refraction, disorders of, 975, 975–976
surgery of, 976
Refractometry, 975
Refractoriness, of heart, 1197
Regeneration, of nervous system, 705

Regional anesthesia, 468t, 472–476, 473t–
474t, 475, 476t
characteristics of, 468
types of, 474–476, 475, 476t
Regional enteritis. See Crohn's disease.
Regional examination, components of, 213,
214t–224t, 225
Registered care technician (RCT), 6
Registry, definition of, 120
Reglan (metoclopramide), for gastroesophageal reflux disease, 1738
Regulatory agencies, in acute care, 129–130
Regurgitation, 1733
aortic, 1345
clinical manifestations of, 1348
management of, medical, 1349
surgical, 1349
mitral, 1342, 1345
clinical manifestations of, 1347
management of, medical, 1347
pathophysiology of, 1346
pulmonic, 1349
tricuspid, 1349
Rehabilitation, after amputation, potential
for, 1418
after casting, 2153
after cerebrovascular accident, discharge
from, 807–808
guidelines for, 798
after coronary artery bypass grafting,
1249–1251
home healthcare in, 1252b
after myocardial infarction, goals of, 1264
program of, 1264–1266, 1265b
after spinal cord injury, 900–902, 901t,
902
burn, home healthcare in, 2262b
in chronic conditions, 113
psychosocial, after myocardial infarction,
1266
pulmonary, for chronic obstructive pulmonary disease, 1124
vestibular, for vertigo, 1012–1013
Rehabilitation Act of 1973, 129
Rehabilitation home visit, after cerebrovascular accident, in discharge planning,
807
Rehydration, in diabetic ketoacidosis, 1983,
1985b
critical monitoring in, 1985b
of elderly client, 283
oral, in extracellular fluid volume deficit,
279–280
Reissner's membrane, in hearing, 984
Reiter's syndrome, 680
Rejection, of donor tissue, in liver transplantation, 1901
transplant, after cardiac surgery, 925
Relaxation, for hypertension, 1393
in pain control, 349b
isovolumetric, 1199
jaw, in postoperative analgesia, nursing research on, 1781b
Relaxation response, 172
Religion, 67
assessment of, in cross-cultural nursing,
64b, 194t
in contraception, 2425b–2426b

Religion (Continued)
in dietary practices, 1701b–1702b
in disease, 32b
in organ donation beliefs, 2512t–2513t
in women's health, 2425b–2426b
Religious rituals, in pain control, 349b
Relocation stress syndrome, nursing care
plan for, 89b
REM (rapid eye movement) sleep, 398
characteristics of, 399, 399
parasomnias in, 403
Remobilization, after traumatic injury, 2167
Remodeling, bone, 2080, 2099, 2100
in bone healing, 2133, 2133
Renaissance, healthcare in, 20
Renal abscess, 1673–1674
Renal agenesis, 1677
Renal angiography, 1564–1565
Renal artery, disease of, 1676–1677
Renal autotransplant, for renal calculi, 1669
Renal biopsy, 1568–1569, 1569
closed, 1568
open, 1568
percutaneous, 1568, 1569
Renal calculi, 1665–1671
after spinal cord injury, prevention of, 908
clinical manifestations of, 1666–1667
diagnostic findings in, 1666–1667
etiology of, 1665
management of, dietary, 1667
medical, 1667
nursing, 1667–1668, 1670–1671
pharmacologic, 1667
surgical, 1668, 1668–1669, 1669
pathophysiology of, 1665–1666, 1666
risk factors for, 1665
Renal cancer, 1671–1673
clinical manifestations of, 1671
diagnostic findings in, 1671
etiology of, 1671
management of, medical, 1673
nursing, 1673
surgical, 1671–1672
nursing care in, 1672–1673
pathophysiology of, 1671
risk factors for, 1671
staging of, 1671, 1672
survival in, 538t
Renal candidiasis, 1673
Renal cell carcinoma, 1671
Renal clearance, studies of, 1560, 1560–
1561
Renal colic, 1667
in endocrine disorders, 1949
Renal failure, acute. See Acute renal failure
(ARF).
after abdominal aortic aneurysm repair,
1427
after cardiac surgery, 1014
chronic. See Chronic renal failure (CRF).
in cirrhosis, 1878t
in diabetes mellitus, 1625–1626
Renal function, assessment of, after cardiac
surgery, 1012
preoperative, 456
postoperative, maintenance of, 487–488
Renal insufficiency, corticosteroids in, consequences of, 2049t

Renal ischemia, in shock, 510
Renal pain, radiculitis vs., 1548
Renal pelvis, cancer of, survival in, 538t
Renal pyramids, 1535, *1536*
Renal system, age-related changes in, 268t
  physical changes with, 454t
  complications of, in postanesthesia care unit, 483
  in fluid balance regulation, 277
  in hypercalcemia, 321t
  in hyperkalemia, 312t
  in hypernatremia, 303t
  in hypokalemia, 309t
  in shock, 509–510
  in thyroid disorders, 2008t
Renal transplantation, 1660–1665
  complications of, 649t, 1661–1663
  criteria for, 646
  donor kidney transportation in, 1661, *1662*
  donors for, 1661
  in elderly, 1665
  nursing care in, 1663–1665
Renal trauma, 1674–1675
  classification of, 1674, *1675*
  clinical manifestations of, 1674
  complications of, 1674
  diagnostic findings in, 1674
  management of, medical, 1674–1675
    nursing, 1675
    surgical, 1675
Renal tuberculosis, 1675–1676
  clinical manifestations of, 1676
  diagnostic findings in, 1676
  management of, medical, 1676
    nursing, 1676
    surgical, 1676
Renal vein, disease of, 1677
Renese (polythiazide), 1394t
Renin, in blood flow regulation, 1374
  level of, 2046t
Renin-angiotensin-aldosterone system, in blood pressure regulation, 1389, *1390,* 1543
  in cardiac regulation, 1203
Renogram, 1561
Reperfusion injury, 823
Repetitive motion injuries, 2167, 2168t–2169t
Replication, of cells, 261–262, *263*
Repolarization, 294
  of cardiac cells, 1195, *1195*
  of nerve impulse, 688, *689*
Reproduction, changes in, in endocrine disorders, 1949
  in spinal cord injury, 904t
  male, physical factors in, 2343–2345
    psychosocial factors in, 2343
  pattern of, 206
Reproductive ducts, disorders of, 2381–2382
Reproductive health practices, female, assessment of, 2310
  male, assessment of, 2331
Reproductive history, male, 2330–2331
Reproductive system, assessment of, in health history, 185b
  chemotherapy effects on, 584
  disorders of, assessment of, 2307–2341

Reproductive system (*Continued*)
  female, structure/function of, 2293–2302
  in anemia, 1470
  in chronic renal failure, 1646
  in hematologic disorders, 1463
  in thyroid disorders, 2008t
  male, disorders of, 2343–2382
    assessment of, 2329–2340
    prevention of, 2340, *2340*
    structure/function of, 2302–2305, *2303*
RES (reticuloendothelial system), in pathogen resistance, 594
Rescue breathing, with tracheostomy tube, 1071–1072
Research, in cancer, 544
  radiation in, 572
  in ethics, 45, 46b
  nursing. See *Nursing research.*
Resectoscope, in transurethral resection of the prostate, 2353, *2353*
Reserpine (Serpasil), 1397t
Reservoir, for infection, 414
Residents' rights, of elderly, 100
Residual volume (RV), 1028, *1028,* 1052t
Resilience, in women, nursing research on, 34b
Resistance, peripheral, total, 1375
  pulmonary, total, 1375
  to blood flow, 1375
  to infectious agents, 593–595, *594, 595*
    autochthonous flora in, 594
    barriers in, 593
    biochemical defenses in, 593
    reticuloendothelial system in, 594
    surface-clearing mechanisms in, 593–594
Resonance, in percussion, 230
  of chest, 1044, *1046*
Resorption, 274b
Resorption cavity, 2080
Resources, allocation of, ethical issues in, 47
  definition of, 196
  external, 196
  internal, 196
Respiration, assessment of, 237, *238*
  delegation of, 234b
  in cardiovascular assessment, 1212
  monitoring of, after cardiac surgery, 1357–1358
  neurologic control of, 1030, *1031*
  partial pressures during, *1032*
  patterns of, *238*
    with infratentorial lesions, 745, *745*
Respiratory acidosis, 333–335, 334t
  critical monitoring in, 337b
  etiology of, 333–335, 334t
  postoperative, causes of, 488
Respiratory alkalosis, 333–335, 334t
  critical monitoring in, 337b
  etiology of, 334t, 335
Respiratory care, delegation of, 1073b
Respiratory depression, opioid analgesics in, 376–377
Respiratory distress, cervical spine injury and, 897
  during tracheostomy weaning, 1071

Respiratory distress (*Continued*)
  in Guillain-Barré syndrome, critical monitoring in, 878b
Respiratory dysfunction, in spinal cord injury, reduction of, 902
Respiratory epithelium, in defense, *1025,* 1025–1026, 1026t
Respiratory failure, acute, 1169–1170, 1170b
  causes of, 1170b
  after thoracic surgery, monitoring for, 1159
Respiratory function, altered, mechanical ventilation and, 1180
  assessment of, diagnostic tests in, 1050–1058
  maintenance of, postoperative, 485–487, *487*
Respiratory irritation, acute, 1150, 1151t
Respiratory membrane, 1028, *1029*
Respiratory paralysis, spinal anesthesia and, 476t
Respiratory system, age-related changes in, 268t
  effects of, 1034
    physical changes with, 454t
  assessment of, in urinary tract assessment, 1555
    postoperative, 484
  complications of, after renal transplantation, 1663
    in postanesthesia care unit, *482,* 482–483
  diseases of, prevention of, 204t
  disorders of, and male reproductive disorders, 2345
  and sleep disorders, 404
    assessment of, 1035–1065
     diagnostic tests in, 1050–1065
     history in, 1035–1040
     physical examination in, 1040–1047, *1041,* 1042b
    obstructive, pulmonary function tests in, 1054t
    restrictive, pulmonary function tests in, 1054t
  effects on, of epinephrine, 2057t
  function of, 1021–1034
  in alcohol abuse, 2490t
  in anemia, 1470
  in burns, 2235–2236
  in chronic renal failure, 1645–1646
  in extracellular fluid volume excess, 287t
  in hematologic disorders, 1463
  in hypernatremia, 303t
  in hypocalcemia, 317t
  in hypokalemia, 309t
  in hyponatremia, 299b
  in shock, 504–506, *506*
  in thyroid disorders, 2008t
  structure of, 1021–1034
  upper, assessment of, 1047–1050
    physical examination in, 1048–1050, *1050*
Respiratory zone, 1028, *1029*
Respite care, for caregivers, in Alzheimer's disease, 870b
  for elderly, 98

Rest, for rheumatoid arthritis, 662
  inadequate, management of, 200t
  pattern of, 206
  promotion of, postoperative, 488–490, *489*
    preoperative, 464
Rest pain, 1377
  in chronic arterial occlusion, 1406–1407
Restaurants, inspection of, in hepatitis A prevention, 1864
Resting membrane potential (RMP), 293, *295, 687, 689*
Restless legs syndrome, 402
Restore, indications for, 443t
Restraints, physical, use of, ethical issues in, 761b
Restrictive cardiomyopathy, 1338, *1338, 1340t, 1341–1342*
  clinical manifestations of, 1341
  diagnostic findings in, 1340t, 1341
  etiology of, 1341
  pathophysiology of, 1341
  risk factors for, 1341
Restrictive lung disorders, 1147–1148, 1147b, *1148*
Retention catheter, for urinary retention, 1602–1603, 1602b
  complications of, 1602–1603
Reticular activating system (RAS), in sleep, 398
Reticular formation, structure/function of, 693
Reticulocyte count, in hematologic system assessment, 1465–1466
Reticuloendothelial system (RES), in pathogen resistance, 594
Reticulospinal tracts, 696t
Reticulum, structure/function of, 2176t
Retina, disorders of, 961–966
  structure of, *938,* 938–939
  visual pathways from, 939, *939*
Retin-A (tretinoin), 2198t
  for acne vulgaris, 2212
Retinal artery occlusion, 966
Retinal detachment, 961–964
  clinical manifestations of, 962, *962*
  diagnostic findings in, 962, *962*
  etiology of, 962
  management of, community/self care in, 964
    emergency, 962
    surgical, 962–963, *963*
      nursing care in, 963–964
      outcome in, 964
  pathophysiology of, 962
  risk factors for, 962
Retinitis, cytomegalovirus, 977
Retinitis pigmentosa, 965
Retinoblastoma, 970
Retinopathy, AIDS, 977
  diabetic. See *Diabetic retinopathy.*
Retirement communities, 100
Retrograde ejaculation, after benign prostatic hyperplasia surgery, 2359–2360
  after prostatectomy, 2363
Retrograde pyelography, 1563
Retroperitoneal lymph node dissection, for testicular cancer, 2376

Retropubic prostatectomy, for benign prostatic hyperplasia, *2353,* 2358
Retrovir (zidovudine), for human immunodeficiency virus infection, 624
Revascularization, transmyocardial, for coronary artery disease, 1248
Reverse transcriptase–polymerase chain reaction (RT-PCR), in prostate cancer diagnosis, 2367
Reversible ischemic neurologic deficit (RIND), 808
Review of systems (ROS), in cardiovascular disorders, 1210–1211
  in ear disorders, 987
  in endocrine disorders, 1950
  in eye disorders, 943
  in gastrointestinal disorders, 1706
  in gynecologic disorders, 2311–2312
  in health history, 182b–185b
  in hematologic disorders, 1462–1463
  in hepatobiliary disorders, 1845
  in immune disorders, 609
  in integumentary system disorders, 2182
  in male reproductive disorders, 2332
  in musculoskeletal disorders, 2086
  in neurologic disorders, 715, 715b
  in psychosocial assessment, 197
  in respiratory disorders, 1040
  in urinary tract disorders, 1552
Revised Trauma Score (RTS), 2518, 2519t
RFA (radiofrequency ablation), of dysrhythmias, 1314
RFs (rheumatoid factors), 657
  laboratory tests for, 661
Rh blood group system, 1455–1456
  in blood component compatibility, 1521t
  in diverse cultures, 1456b
Rheumatic fever, 1327–1331
  cardiac effects of, 1327–1328, 1328t
  clinical manifestations of, 1328
  diagnostic findings in, 1328, 1329b
  etiology of, 1327
  management of, medical, 1329
    nursing, 1329–1331
  pathophysiology of, 1327–1328
  prevention of, 1329b
  risk factors for, 1327, 1329b
Rheumatoid arthritis (RA), 655–674, *656*
  clinical manifestations of, 658–661, *658–661*
    articular, 658–659, *659, 660*
    extra-articular, 659–661, *660, 661*
  complications of, 665
  diagnostic findings in, 658–661, *658–661*
  etiology of, 655–656
  exercise in, encouragement of, nursing research on, 666b
  functional ability in, rating of, 661
  management of, 661–674
    home healthcare in, 667b
    in elderly, 671–672
    ineffective, 670–671, 671b
    medical, 661–666, *662*
    nursing, 666–672, 667b, 668b, *669, 670b, 671b*
    occupational therapy in, 665, *666*
    pharmacologic, 662–665, 664t

Rheumatoid arthritis (RA) *(Continued)*
    physical therapy in, 665
    surgical, 672–674, *673,* 673b
      in elderly, 674
    unproven remedies in, 671b
  osteoarthritis vs., 2109t
  outcome in, 665–666
  pathophysiology of, 656–658, *657*
  prevention of, 655b
  risk factors for, 655–656, 655b
Rheumatoid disorders, ocular manifestations of, 977
Rheumatoid factors (RFs), 657
  laboratory tests for, 661
Rheumatoid nodules, 659, *660*
Rhinitis, 1080–1081
  prevention of, 200t
  types of, 1080
Rhinitis medicamentosa, 1080
Rhinoplasty, 2274–2275
  client education in, 2275
Rhizotomy, for pain, 386, *387*
RhoGAM, 1456, 1456b
Rhonchi, 1046, 1049t
Rhythm strips, *1222,* 1222–1223
Rhythmic breathing, in pain control, 370
Rhytidectomy, *2271,* 2271–2272, *2272*
  complications of, 2271–2272
RIA (radioimmunoassay), in thyroid function testing, 1952
  parathyroid hormone, 2032t
  triiodothyronine, 2010t
Ribonucleic acid (RNA), products of, 265
  replication of, 264–265
Ribosomal RNA (rRNA), 265
Ribosomes, of endoplasmic reticulum, functions of, 265
Ribs, assessment of, in regional examination, 218t
  fracture of, chest trauma and, 2526
Rickettsia prowazekii, 416t
Rickettsia rickettsii, 416t
Ridaura (auranofin), for rheumatoid arthritis, 664t
Rifabutin, in *Mycobacterium avium-intracellulare* complex prophylaxis, 625
Rifampin, for tuberculosis, 1143, 1144t
  urine color with, 1557t
Right atrium, 1191, *1193*
Right bundle branch (RBB), 1198, *1198*
Right bundle branch block (RBBB), 1310
Right coronary artery (RCA), 1194, *1194*
  lesion of, electrocardiographic changes in, 1225t
Right lower quadrant (RLQ), organs of, *1708*
Right midclavicular line (RMCL), in liver percussion, 1845–1847
Right upper quadrant (RUQ), organs of, *1708*
Right ventricle, 1191, *1193*
Right ventricular failure (RVF), *1280,* 1282
Right-sided cardiac catheterization, 1231
Rigidity, in Parkinson's disease, 878
  client education about, 881b
Rigor mortis, 271
Riluzole (Rilutek), for amyotrophic lateral sclerosis, 887

RIND (reversible ischemic neurologic deficit), 808

Ringer's lactate, for shock, 518–519

Rinne test, 989, *990*

Riopan, for peptic ulcer disease, 1769t

RIPA (radioimmunoprecipitation assay), in acquired immunodeficiency syndrome testing, 611

Risk factors, 167
definition of, 161
for cardiovascular disease, 167t

Risk management, in acute care, 131, 132b

Risperidone, for dementia of Alzheimer's type, 866t

RLQ (right lower quadrant), organs of, *1708*

RMCL (right midclavicular line), in liver percussion, 1845–1847

RMP (resting membrane potential), 293, *295*, 687, *689*

RN first assistant (RNFA), 467
practice of, scope of, 467
training for, 467

RNA (ribonucleic acid), products of, 265
replication of, 264–265

RNFA (RN first assistant), 467
practice of, scope of, 467
training for, 467

Robinson red rubber urethral catheter, 2354t

Robinul (glycopyrrolate), preoperative, 465t

Rocky Mountain spotted fever, infectious agent in, 416t

Rods, 938

Roger's unitary person model, health definition in, 162t

Rohypnol (flunitrazepam), abuse of, 2489b

Role relationship, pattern of, 206

ROM (range of motion), of joints, measurement of, 2088, *2088, 2089*

ROM (range-of-motion) exercises, after cerebrovascular accident, 802
after musculoskeletal trauma, 2167
after thoracic surgery, 1161
in rheumatoid arthritis, 665, 666b

Roman Catholicism, beliefs/practices of, 2545–2546

Roman civilization, healthcare in, history of, 19–20

Romberg test, 236, 989

Root canal therapy, 1720

Rooting reflex, 728

ROS. See *Review of systems (ROS).*

Rosenbaum pocket vision screener, *946*

Rotary chair, in ear disorder assessment, 991–992

Rotator cuff tears, 2164–2165

Roth's spots, in infective endocarditis, 1333

Roto-Rest bed, *759*
after spinal cord injury, 908

Round window, *981, 982*

Roxane Pain Institute, 564b

Roy's adaptation model, health definition in, 162t

RPR (rapid plasma reagin) test, before blood transfusion, 1524t
schedule for, 210t

rRNA (ribosomal RNA), 265

RSD (reflex sympathetic dystrophy), in fracture, prevention of, 2145

RT. See *Radiation therapy.*

RT-PCR (reverse transcriptase–polymerase chain reaction), in prostate cancer diagnosis, 2367

RTS (Revised Trauma Score), 2518, 2519t

Rub, friction. See *Friction rub.*

Rubella, history of, in gynecologic assessment, 2308
immunization recommendations for, in adults, 422t

Rubella titer, schedule for, 208t

Rubeola, infectious agent in, 416t

Rubor, 2186
dependent, in chronic arterial occlusion, 1406

Rubrospinal tracts, 696t

Rule of 9s, 2238–2239, *2239*

Rumbles, diastolic filling, 1218t

Rumpel-Leede test, in hemorrhage, 1467t

Running traction, 2137–2138

RUQ (right upper quadrant), organs of, *1708*

Russell's traction, *2138, 2139*

RV (residual volume), 1028, *1028*, 1052t

RVF (right ventricular failure), *1280*, 1282

S

S phase, of cell cycle, 545, *545*

S phase index, in breast cancer, 2435

S_1, 1214, *1215*

S_2, 1214, *1215*
splitting of, pathologic, 1215
physiologic, 1214

S_3, 1199, 1216

S_4, 1199, 1216

SA (sinoatrial) arrest, 1300

SA (sinoatrial) node, 1197–1198

SAARDs (slow-acting antirheumatic drugs), 664t, 665

Sabril (vigabatrin), side effects of, 839t

Saccular aneurysm, 1425, *1425*
cerebral, 812

Saccule, in balance, 984

SACP (Society for Ambulatory Care Professionals), 139

SAD (seasonal affective disorder), 403

Safe Medical Devices Act (SMDA), ambulatory care standards of, 138

Safety, in Alzheimer's disease, home healthcare in, 868b
in musculoskeletal disorders, evaluation of, 2086
in Parkinson's disease, client education about, 881b–882b
intraoperative, 478
positioning in, 477–478
promotion of, 464
management of, 201t–202t

SAGE (Senior Actualization and Growth Exploration), 175b

SAH (subarachnoid hemorrhage), 812–816. See also *Intracranial hemorrhage.*
classification of, 813, 813t

Salem sump tube, 1749t, 1750

Salicylates, allergic reaction to, clinical manifestations of, 640t

Salicylates *(Continued)*
therapeutic monitoring of, reference values for, 2562
topical, 2200t

Salicylic acid, topical, 2199t, 2200t

Saline, hypertonic, for fluid resuscitation, in burns, 2250t
normal, for open wounds, 445t
topical, 2199t

Saline solutions, balanced, for shock, 518–519
for hyponatremia, 299

Saliva, functions of, 1686–1687

Salivary glands, disorders of, 1732

Salmonella, and dysentery, 1789

Salmonellosis, in acquired immunodeficiency syndrome, 628

Salpingitis, in gonorrhea, 2468

Salt, iodized, in goiter prevention, 2015–2016

Saltatory conduction, 690

Saluron (hydroflumethiazide), 1394t

Salvation Army, beliefs/practices of, 2547–2548

Same-day care centers, 137

Sandimmune (cyclosporine), after heart transplantation, 1353, 1354b
for myasthenia gravis, 885
for rheumatoid arthritis, 664t
in organ transplantation, 644t

Sanguineous exudate, 434, 435t

Santyl (collagenase), for enzymatic debridement, 440

SaO_2 (oxygen saturation), measurement of, delegation of, 234b
pulse oximetry in, 1051–1055, *1055*
partial pressure of arterial oxygen vs., 1055t

Saphenous vein grafting, 1414

Sarcoidosis, 1149–1150

Sarcolemma, 1196, 2078

Sarcoma, genital tract, in females, 2422–2423
osteogenic, 2123t
prevention of, 204t

Sarcomere, 1196, *1196, 1197*, 2078

Sarcoplasm, 1196

Sarcoplasmic reticulum, 1196

Sarcoptes scabiei, and vulvar irritation, 2422

Saturated solution of potassium iodide (SSKI), for goiter, 2014
for hyperthyroidism, 2013t

SBE (subacute bacterial endocarditis), 1331

Scabicides, topical, 2198t

Scabies, 2221t, 2475

Scabies scraping, 2194

Scalding, 2234

Scale, *2185*

Scalene muscles, 1026

Scalp, care of, in psoriasis, 2211
injury to, 822
physical examination of, 2185–2186
normal findings in, 2182b

Scanning, Doppler, of cerebrovascular system, 733
multiple gated acquisition, 1230
radionuclide. See *Radionuclide scanning.*

Scanning *(Continued)*
  ultrasonic duplex, in peripheral vascular assessment, 1383
  ventilation-perfusion, 1057–1058, *1058*
    in pulmonary embolism diagnosis, 1127–1128
Scarring, *2185*
  hypertrophic, 446
  in burns, control of, 2260–2261, *2261*
  in plastic surgery, minimization of, 2267–2268, *2268*
Schamroth technique, 1043, *1044*
Schilling test, in pernicious anemia, 1475
Schistocytes, 1466t
Schistosomiasis, 1790
Schiøtz tonometry, 949, *949*
Schlemm's canal, 937, *938*
Schwartz's model, of brain as adaptive regulator, 27
Schwartz's sign, 1001
SCI. See *Spinal cord injury (SCI)*.
Sciatica, 917
  clinical manifestations of, 918
Scintigraphy, in hepatobiliary disease, 1853–1854
  myocardial, in cardiovascular assessment, 1229–1230
SCLCs (small cell lung cancers), 1151, 1153t
  chemotherapy in, 1154
  surgical management of, 1155
Sclera, examination of, 944
  structure of, 937, *938*
Scleral buckling, for retinal detachment, 962, *963*
Scleritis, in rheumatoid arthritis, 659
  red eye in, 942b
Scleroderma, 677–678, *678*
  generalized, 677, 677b
  localized, 677
Sclerosing cholangitis, 1920
Sclerosis, definition of, 2183t
Sclerotherapy, for bleeding esophageal varices, 1885
  for hemorrhoids, 1827
  for varicose veins, 1439
Sclerotome, 353
Scoliosis, 2087, *2087*, 2120–2121, *2121*
  screening for, 209t
Scopolamine, antidote to, 2538t
Scotoma, 947
Scratch test, in allergy assessment, 612, 637
Screening tests, in health history, 206
Scrotum, disorders of, 2381
  physical examination of, 2333
    normal findings in, 2332b
  structure/function of, 2302–2304
  transillumination of, 2335, *2335*
  ultrasonography of, 2339
Scrub person, role of, 466
Seaman-Mannello Scale, 2484
Seasonal affective disorder (SAD), 403
Sebaceous glands, 2175, 2176t
Sebum, 2175
  definition of, 2183t
Secobarbital sodium (Seconal Sodium), preoperative, 465t

Secondary adrenal insufficiency, 2047–2049, *2049*
Secondary glaucoma, 952. See also *Glaucoma.*
  after cataract extraction, 960
Secondary hypertension, 1387
  causes of, 1388b
  pathophysiology of, 1389
Second-degree atrioventricular (AV) block, *1303*, 1304
Secretin, 1691t
  secretion of, 1693
    pancreatic, 1841
Secretion analysis, in male reproductive disorders, 2339
Secretions, bronchial, removal of, in chronic obstructive pulmonary disease, 1117
  gastric, 1690
  gastrointestinal, 1685
  of large intestine, 1695–1696
  of small intestine, 1693
  pancreatic, stimulation of, 1841
  tracheobronchial, clearance of, in cystic fibrosis, 1148–1149
Sectral (acebutolol), 1395t
  for angina pectoris, 1257t
Sedative-hypnotics, effect of, on male reproductive system, 2345
Sedatives, abuse of, 2492–2494
  effects of, 2483t
  health consequences of, 2494t
  for intracranial hemorrhage, 815
  withdrawal from, symptoms of, 2488t
Sedimentation rate, increase in, inflammation and, 435
Seeing, assessment of, 712t
SEER (Surveillance, Epidemiology, and End Results) Program, 534, *537*
Segmental pneumonia, 1135
Segmental resection, for lung cancer, 1156, *1156*
Segmentation contractions, 1685
Segmented neutrophils, in differential count, interpretation of, 436t
Seizure(s), 834–843
  absence (petit mal), 837
  after intracranial surgery, 850
  anticonvulsant agents for, 839t
  atonic, 838
  brain tumor and, 846
  control of, in cerebrovascular accident, 793
  definition of, 835b
  generalized, *837*, 837–838
  myoclonic, 837
  nonepileptic, 842–843
  partial, 836–837
    complex, 837
  risk for, in head trauma, 828
  sleep disorders in, 405–406
  tonic-clonic (grand mal), 837, *837*
Selegiline (Deprenyl), for Parkinson's disease, 880t
Self-care, after cardiac surgery, 926
  after cataract surgery, 961
  after organ transplantation, ethical issues in, 647b
  in abdominal aortic aneurysm, 1428

Self-care *(Continued)*
  in Alzheimer's disease, 865–872
  in amenorrhea, 2390–2391
  in anemia, 1471
  in angina pectoris, 1255–1258
  in asthma, 1110–1111, *1111*, 1111t
  in atopic dermatitis, 2206–2207
  in benign prostatic hyperplasia, 2363–2365, 2364t
  in brain tumors, 855–856
  in breast cancer, 2445–2449
  in burns, 2261
  in candidiasis, 1725–1726
  in cardiomyopathy, 1342
  in cerebrovascular accident, 807–808
  in chlamydial infections, 2470
  in chronic arterial occlusion, 1407–1408
  in chronic obstructive pulmonary disease, 1124
  in confusion, 770
  in consciousness disorders, 763
  in corneal dystrophies, 968
  in coronary artery disease, 1244–1245, 1250–1251
  in dental caries, 1720
  in diabetes mellitus, 1963–1981, *1964*
  in dysmenorrhea, 2387
  in dysrhythmias, 1323–1324
  in endometriosis, 2399–2400
  in epilepsy, 842
  in erectile dysfunction, 2350
  in extracellular fluid volume deficit, 284
  in extracellular fluid volume excess, 289
  in fractures, 2145–2153
  in glaucoma, 958
  in gonorrhea, 2468–2469
  in head trauma, 829
  in hearing impairment, 995–1001
  in heart failure, 1291
  in hepatic encephalopathy, 1895
  in human immunodeficiency virus infection, 623–625
  in hypercortisolism, 2053–2055
  in hyperkalemia, 314
  in hypernatremia, 304
  in hyperparathyroidism, 2031–2034
  in hypersensitivity, 641, *642*
  in hypertension, 1391–1392
  in hypokalemia, 310
  in hyponatremia, 300
  in hypothyroidism, 2012–2016
  in infective endocarditis, 1334
  in infertility, 2346–2347
  in inflammation, 437
  in intertrochanteric hip fracture, 2158–2159, 2159b
  in iron deficiency anemia, 1473–1474
  in menopause, 2393–2395
  in multiple sclerosis, 874–877
  in neurogenic bladder dysfunction, 1617–1619
  in osteoarthritis, 2109–2110
  in osteoporosis, 2100–2103
  in periodontal disease, 1721–1722
  in pernicious anemia, 1475–1476
  in pneumonia, 1138
  in premenstrual syndrome, 2388–2389
  in pressure ulcers, 2219–2220, 2220b

Self-care (Continued)
in retinal detachment, 964
in rheumatoid arthritis, 661–672
in sexually transmitted diseases, 2462–2465
in shock, 528
in spinal cord injury, 914, 915b
in syphilis, 2471–2472
in systemic lupus erythematosus, 676–678
in total hip replacement, 2116–2118, 2117
in tuberculosis, 1143–1144
in upper airway neoplasms, 1095–1100, 1096b–1098b, 1098–1100, 1099b
in urinary incontinence, 1608–1610, 1609b
in urinary tract infections, 1578–1579
in venous thrombosis, 1436
in vertigo, 1012–1016
in viral hepatitis, 1870–1871
in wound management, 442–443, 444
lack of, management of, 202t–203t
of elderly, 84–85
with cast, 2151
Self-care deficit, after spinal cord injury, 907
in burns, 2246–2247
in cerebrovascular accident, 803
in dementia of Alzheimer's type, 869
in fracture, 2144
in multiple sclerosis, 876
Self-catheterization, intermittent, in males, home healthcare in, 2351b
Self-concept, assessment of, 191t
disturbance of, in renal transplantation, 1664–1665
pattern of, 206
Self-esteem, assessment of, 191t
disturbance of, after brain tumor surgery, 854–855
in benign prostatic hyperplasia, 2360
in burns, 2247–2248
in multiple sclerosis, 876–877
in rheumatoid arthritis, management of, 669–670
Self-help groups, in stress response, 29
Self-insurance, 5b
Self-medication, after cerebrovascular accident, in discharge planning, 807
errors in, management of, 199t
Self-monitoring of blood glucose (SMBG), 1961–1962, 1975
Self-perception, pattern of, 206
Self-responsibility, definition of, 161
Selye's theory, 21–22
Semen, 2305
examination of, 2338
Semicircular canals, structure of, 983, 983
Semilunar valves, 1193, 1194
Seminal vesicles, disorders of, 2382
Senescence hypothesis, of coronary artery disease pathogenesis, 1243
Sengstaken-Blakemore tube, for bleeding esophageal varices, 1885, 1885
complications of, 1886
Senior Actualization and Growth Exploration (SAGE), 175b
Senior centers, 99

Sensation, abnormal, in eye disorders, symptom analysis in, 941
changes in, in musculoskeletal disorders, 2084
impaired, in fracture, 2134
mechanical, assessment of, 724
preoperative assessment of, 456
superficial, assessment of, 723–724
Sensitivity, cultural, development of, 63, 63b
in microbiologic studies, 244
of diagnostic tests, 243
Sensorcaine (bupivacaine), 473t
in pain control, 372
Sensorimotor system, age-related changes in, physical changes with, 454t
Sensorineural hearing loss, 992, 994b. See also Hearing loss.
clinical manifestations of, 996t
etiology of, 993
pathophysiology of, 994
Sensory aphasia, 789
Sensory deprivation, 409–410
Sensory disorders, 397–411
classification of, 409–410
prevention of, 410
Sensory function, assessment of, 712t–713t, 723–724, 725
in regional examination, 221t–222t
normal findings in, 717b
integrated, assessment of, 718
loss of, patterns of, 724, 725
Sensory hearing loss, 994b
Sensory impairment, in elderly, 87
Sensory overload, 409
Sensory paralytic bladder, 1615, 1616
Sensory reception, skin in, 2177
Sensory system, age-related changes in, 268t
Sepsis, preoperative, in postoperative wound infection, 491
renal disorders in, 1626
risk for, in leukemia, 1492
Septic arthritis, 2122
Septic shock, 486t
clinical manifestations of, 513
definition of, 497
etiology of, 500
management of, 524t
prevention of, 501b
Septicemia, 244
in peritonitis, 1794
in transfusion reaction, 1529t
Septra (trimethoprim-sulfamethoxazole), for urinary tract infections, 1575t
Sequential compression stockings, 461
Serial 7s and 3s, 195
Serial port sampling, of blood, 247
Serosanguineous exudate, 434, 435t
Serotonin, in blood pressure regulation, 1204, 1375
in pain modulation, 345
in sleep, 398
in wound healing, 430, 430
reference values for, in cancer, 557t
Serous exudate, 434, 435t
Serpasil (reserpine), 1397t
Serratus anterior flap, 2280
Sertoli's cells, 2304

Serum, reference values for, 2557–2559, 2564
Serum creatinine, increased, in chronic renal failure, 1644
Serum glutamate pyruvate transaminase (SGPT), reference values for, in cancer, 557t
Serum glutamic-oxaloacetic transaminase (SGOT), reference values for, in cancer, 557t
Serum sickness, 639–640
Seventh-Day Adventists, beliefs/practices of, 2548
dietary, 1701b
Sex, in adult general screening physical examination, 233–234
in cancer, 540
in coronary artery disease, 1238
in hypertension, 1388
Sex hormones, secretion of, adrenal cortex in, 1945
Sexual abuse, medical problems after, nursing research on, 1757b
Sexual activity, after myocardial infarction, 1265
and urinary tract infection, 1572
high-risk, health risks of, 203t
in abdominal aortic aneurysm, 1428
in human immunodeficiency virus infection transmission, 615
Sexual assault, alleged, 2532
Sexual asymmetry, cultural expressions of, 2324b–2429b
Sexual development, male, 2304
Sexual differentiation, female, 2298
Sexual dysfunction, after abdominal aortic aneurysm repair, 1427
after prostatectomy, 2363
after spinal cord injury, 911–912
in chronic obstructive pulmonary disease, 1122–1123
in inflammatory bowel disease, 1808
in leukemia, 1493
pituitary gland disorders and, 2065
Sexual health, promotion of, 76–78
personal beliefs/attitudes/values in, 78
Sexual history, female, 2309–2310, 2311t
male, 2330–2331
Sexual life-style, ethical issues in, 2344b
Sexual orientation, 75
Sexual practices, 76
Sexual skin, biocultural variations in, 2188b
Sexuality, 74–79, 77t
after surgery, 78–79
after vulvectomy, 2421–2422
assessment of, 192t, 197
changes in, aging and, 77t
concepts of, 74–76
psychological, 75
sociocultural, 75–76
during hospitalization, 79
in bladder cancer, 1594
in chronic conditions, 78
in illness, 78–79
in spinal cord injury, expression of, 903, 904b
in vaginal cancer, 2417
pattern of, 206

Sexuality *(Continued)*
  with ostomy, 1814
Sexually transmitted diseases (STDs),
    2459–2476
  and urethritis, 1581
  client education in, 2465b
    home healthcare in, 2465b
  enteric, 2475
  etiology of, 2460b
  incidence of, 2459
  management of, 2461t–2462t
    community/self care in, 2462–2465
    medical, 2461t–2462t, 2462
    nursing, 2462–2465
  prevention of, 203t, 2460b
  privacy vs. right-to-know in, 2463b
  risk factors for, 2460b
  screening for, 210t
SG (substantia gelatinosa), in gate control
    theory of pain, 350–351, *351*
SGOT (serum glutamic-oxaloacetic transam-
    inase), reference values for, in cancer,
    557t
SGPT (serum glutamate pyruvate transami-
    nase), reference values for, in cancer, 557t
Sharp debridement, of black wounds, 439
Sharpey's fibers, 2073, *2075*
Shave biopsy, 257
  for actinic keratosis, 2225
  of skin, *2195*, 2195–2196
Shaving, religious beliefs about, 2545–2551
Shielding, in radiation therapy, 573
Shift work sleep disorder, 403
Shin splints, 2162
Shingles, 2223, *2223*
Shock, 497–532
  after adrenalectomy, for pheochromocy-
    toma, 2059
  anaphylactic. See *Anaphylactic shock.*
  assessment of, diagnostic, 514
  cardiogenic. See *Cardiogenic shock.*
  cardiovascular system in, 506–507
  client education in, 527b
  clinical manifestations of, *510*, 510–514
  cold, 513
  critical monitoring in, 511b
  culture, 60
  definition of, 497
  diagnostic findings in, 510–514, 511b
  distributive. See *Distributive shock.*
  etiology of, 497–500, 498t, 499b
  fractures and, 2139
  gastrointestinal system in, 509
  hypovolemic. See *Hypovolemic shock.*
  immune system in, 509
  in acute pancreatitis, 1923, 1924t
  in postanesthesia care unit, prevention of,
    483
  irreversible, 516
  management of, 514–528
    community/self care in, 528
    emergency, 514–528
      medical, 514–521
      nursing, 522–527
      pharmacologic, 520–521
      surgical, 527–528
  neuroendocrine system in, 507–509, *508*
  neurogenic. See *Neurogenic shock.*

Shock *(Continued)*
  nursing diagnoses in, 526–527, 526b
  obstructive, 497
  pathophysiology of, 500–510
  postoperative, 485, 486t
  prevention of, 501b
  renal system in, 509–510
  respiratory system in, 504–506, *506*
  reversal of, for diabetic ketoacidosis, 1983
  risk factors for, 497–500, 498t, 499b,
    501b
  septic. See *Septic shock.*
  spinal, 895
  stages of, 502–503, *503, 504*
    decompensation, 503, *504*
    early compensation, 502–503, *503*
    progressive, 503
  systemic effects of, 503–510, *505*
  types of, 486t
  warm, 513
Short arm cast, 2137t, *2148*
Short bones, 2073
Short leg cast, 2137t, *2148*
Shortness of breath, assessment of, 1206
Short-staffing, ethical issues in, 1816b
Shoulder, exercises of, after lung cancer
    surgery, *1158*
  function of, assessment of, 2090t
  ligaments of, 2077
  pain in, cerebrovascular accident and, 792
  range of motion of, *2089*
  repetitive motion injuries of, 2168t
Shoulder arthroplasty, for rheumatoid arthri-
    tis, 672–674, *673*
Shunt, for portal hypertension, 1887, *1888*
  nursing care in, 1887–1889
  peritoneovenous, for ascites, 1891, *1892*
  ventriculoatrial, for intracranial hemor-
    rhage, 816
  ventriculoperitoneal, for increased intracra-
    nial pressure, 783, *783*
    for intracranial hemorrhage, 816
SI system, in laboratory test result reporting,
    243
SIADH (syndrome of inappropriate secre-
    tion of antidiuretic hormone), diabetes
    insipidus vs., 2066, 2067t–2068t
  head trauma and, 825
  monitoring for, 2064b
Sickle cell anemia, 1512–1515
  clinical manifestations of, 1514
  diagnostic findings in, 1514
  etiology of, 1512
  geographic distribution of, 1512, *1513*
  management of, medical, 1514
    nursing, 1514–1515
  pathophysiology of, 1512–1513, *1513*
  risk factors for, 1512
Sickle cell trait, 1512–1515
Sickle cells, 1466t
Sickle-turbidity tube test, 1514
SICU (surgical intensive care unit), transfer
    to, indications for, 480
SIg (surface immunoglobulin), 596, 598
Sigerist's health promotion theory, 162
Sigmoidoscopy, 1716
  schedule for, 209t
Signal-averaged electrocardiography, 1224

Silicone implants, for breast reconstruction,
    ethical issues in, 2438b
Silver nitrate, for burns, 2254t
Silver sulfadiazine, for burns, 2254, 2254t
  for open wounds, 445t
Simple fracture, 2129, *2130*
Sims' position, for physical examination,
    232
SIMV (synchronized intermittent mandatory
    ventilation), 1177, 1178t
Sinemet (carbidopa-levodopa), for Parkin-
    son's disease, 878–879, 880t
Single photon emission computed tomogra-
    phy (SPECT), 732
Single-barreled colostomy, *1811,* 1812
Single-parent family, 53
Sinoatrial (SA) arrest, 1300
Sinoatrial (SA) node, 1197–1198
Sinoatrial node conduction defects, 1299–
    1300
Sinography, 2094
Sinus bradycardia, 1200, 1298–1299, *1299*
Sinus dysrhythmia, 1299
Sinus exit block, 1300
Sinus lavage, for sinusitis, 1077
Sinus tachycardia, 1200, 1297–1298, *1299*
Sinuses, assessment of, 1047–1050
  in health history, 183b
  in regional examination, 216t
  paranasal, 1022–1023, *1023*
    assessment of, physical examination in,
      1050
Sinusitis, 1077–1078, *1078, 1079*
  management of, medical, 1077
    surgical, 1077–1078, *1078, 1079*
    nursing care in, 1078, *1079*
SIRES, in poisoning management, 2538
SIRS (systemic inflammatory response syn-
    drome), 528–531
Sitting position, for physical examination,
    232
Sjögren's syndrome, 678–679
  in rheumatoid arthritis, 659
  ocular manifestations of, 977
Skeletal muscle, 2077–2078, *2079*
Skeletal system, function of, 2075
  structure of, 2073–2075, *2074, 2075*
Skeletal traction, 2138
Skeletal x-rays, diagnostic, 250
Skene's glands, 2294
  examination of, 2317, *2318*
Skin. See also *Integumentary system.*
  assessment of, in health history, 183b
  care of, during radiation therapy, client
    education about, 571b
  disorders of, psychosocial aspects of, 2203
  function of, 2176–2177, 2176t
  in anemia, 1470
  in endocrine disorders, 1949
  in hematologic disorders, 1462
  in rheumatoid arthritis, 659
  infections of, 2221t–2222t, 2222–2223
    in diabetes mellitus, 1960t
  integrity of, impaired, after arterial bypass,
    1416–1417
    after modified radical mastectomy,
      2440
    after spinal cord injury, 908

Skin (Continued)
in achalasia, 1736
in acute glomerulonephritis, 1632
in ascites, 1891
in atopic dermatitis, 2208–2209
in bladder cancer, 1594
in breast cancer, 2442–2443
in cerebrovascular accident, 801–802
in chronic arterial occlusion, 1409
in consciousness disorders, 758, 759
in delayed wound healing, 442
in fractures, 2143
in heart failure, 1288
in hypercortisolism, 2054
in intertrochanteric hip fracture, 2155–
2156
in jaundice, 1860
in myocardial infarction, 1276
in myxedema coma, 2012
in pressure ulcers, 2217–2219, 2219
in renal failure, acute, 1640
chronic, 1656
in viral hepatitis, 1870
preoperative assessment of, 455
lesions of, assessment of, 2192–2194,
2193, 2193t
types of, 2182–2184, 2184, 2185
of dying patient, donation of, guidelines
for, 2514t
penile, physical examination of, 2333
perineal, examination of, 2317
physical examination of, 2186–2194
normal findings in, 2182b
preoperative preparation of, 463
protection of, with open wound, 438,
438
radiation therapy effects on, 571–572
self-examination of, 2194, 2205b
structure of, 2173–2176, 2174, 2176t
transplantation of, criteria for, 646
turgor of, assessment of, 2192
in extracellular fluid volume deficit,
281, 282
Skin cancer, 2224–2231
clinical manifestations of, 2227, 2227–
2228, 2228, 2228t
diagnostic findings in, 2227, 2227–2228,
2228, 2228t
etiology of, 2226–2227
in whites, 198t
management of, medical, 2229
surgical, 2229, 2229–2230
precursors to, 2224–2225
prevention of, 202t, 203t
risk factors for, 542b, 2226–2227, 2226b
survival in, 538t
Skin color, assessment of, 237, 2186
factors in, 2174–2175
inspection of, in peripheral vascular
assessment, 1380
Skin expansion, in plastic surgery, 2282
Skin grafts, 2277–2278
banking skin for, 2278
healed, appearance of, 2278
nursing care in, 2278
survival of, 2278
Skin lines, 2267–2268, 2268
Skin lubricants, 2202–2203

Skin testing, in cancer diagnosis, 559
in hypersensitivity diagnosis, 637, 637
in immune disorder assessment, 612
Skin traction, 2138
Skull, fractures of, 822, 2529
clinical manifestations of, 823
surgical management of, 829
radiography of, in neurologic assessment,
730
SLE. See Systemic lupus erythematosus
(SLE).
Sleep, chronobiology of, 397
disorders of, 397–411
classification of, 398b
diagnosis of, 407, 408
dyssomnias in, 400–403, 402b
hospital-acquired, 406–407, 407b
in elderly, progressive relaxation for,
nursing research on, 409b
medical/psychological disorders with,
404–406
nursing management of, 407–409, 409b
parasomnias in, 403
in elderly, 87
inadequate, management of, 200t
need for, 398
pattern of, 206
disturbances of, 397–400, 398b, 408
in chronic obstructive pulmonary disease, 1122
in confusion, 768
in critical care unit, nursing research on,
407b
in elderly, 400
physiology of, 398–400, 399
preoperative promotion of, 464
slow-wave, 399
stages of, 398–400, 399
Sleep apnea syndrome, 401–402, 402b
central, 402
obstructive, 401–402, 402b
living with, 402b
polysomnography in, 408
Sleep bruxism, 403
Sleep deprivation, hospital-acquired, 406–
407, 407b
Sleep enuresis, 403
Sleep hygiene, inadequate, 400
Sleep maintenance disturbance, hospital-
acquired, 406
Sleep paralysis, 400, 403
Sleep spindles, in polysomnography, 399
Sleep starts, 403
Sleep terrors, 403
Sleep-onset difficulty, hospital-acquired, 406
Sleeptalking, 403
Sleep-wake pattern, 397
irregular, 403
Sleep-wake transition disorders, 403
Sleepwalking, 403
Slit-lamp examination, 949–950
Slow pain, 343
Slow-acting antirheumatic drugs (SAARDs),
664t, 665
Slow-wave sleep, 399
Small bowel obstruction, 1820–1823
clinical manifestations of, 1821–1822
diagnostic findings in, 1821–1822

Small bowel obstruction (Continued)
etiology of, 1820, 1820–1821
management of, medical, 1822
nursing, 1822–1823
surgical, 1823
pathophysiology of, 1821
risk factors for, 1820–1821
Small cell lung cancers (SCLCs), 1151,
1153t
chemotherapy in, 1154
surgical management of, 1155
Small intestine, 1690–1694, 1693
cancer of, 1808
disorders of, 1788–1825
inflammatory, 1788–1808
function of, 1692–1694
herniation of. See Herniation, intestinal.
resection of, for inflammatory bowel disease, 1802
complications of, 1802
structure of, 1690–1692, 1693
tumors of, benign, 1808
Small-Carrion penile prosthesis, 2348, 2349
SMBG (self-monitoring of blood glucose),
1961–1962, 1975
SMDA (Safe Medical Devices Act), ambulatory care standards of, 138
Smear, 243
Smell, assessment of, 712t, 719
physical examination in, 1050, 1051b
Smoke poisoning, in burns, 2237
Smoking, cessation of, for chronic arterial
occlusion, 1408
for hypertension, 1393
cigarette, and bladder cancer, 1582
cardiovascular effects of, 1210
in coronary artery disease, 1238–1239
delayed wound healing in, 444
history of, in respiratory disorders, 1039
perioperative effects of, 457
Smooth muscle, 2078
Smooth muscle antibodies, in hepatobiliary
disease, 1849
Snake bites, 2536
Snap, opening, 1216
Snellen's chart, 945, 946
Snoring, primary, 403
uvulopalatopharyngoplasty for, 402
Snout reflex, 728
SNS. See Sympathetic nervous system
(SNS).
Soaks, 2202
Sobriety, definition of, 2481t
Social change, in sociologic adaptation, to
chronic conditions, 112
Social contract family, 53
Social experiences, definition of, 189
Social history, preoperative assessment of,
457
Social interaction, impaired, in hearing im-
pairment, 999–1000
in hyperthyroidism, 2022
Social network, assessment of, 191t–192t,
196
Social readjustment rating scale, 25t
Social Security, 94
Social Security Act of 1935, 7
Social support, in stress response, 28–29

Socialization, family in, 54
Society for Ambulatory Care Professionals (SACP), 139
Socioeconomic issues, assessment of, culture in, 194t
  in health/well-being, 168b
Socioeconomic status, assessment of, 196
Sociologic dimension, 196
Sodium, concentration of, *294, 294t*
  dietary, sources of, 288b, 1286t
  distribution of, 293t
  imbalance of, 295–304. See also *Hypernatremia; Hyponatremia.*
  in acid-base balance, 331
  in action potential, 293–294, *295*
    cardiac, 1195, *1195*
  in diabetes mellitus, guidelines for, 1977
  in hyponatremia, total body water relationship to, 296, 297t
  level of, in extracellular fluid volume deficit, 278
  measurement of, in cardiovascular assessment, 1220
    in gastrointestinal tract assessment, 1711t
  plasma, range for, 296b
  regulation of, in chronic renal failure, 1655
  restriction of, in heart failure, 1286, 1286t
    in hypernatremia, 303–304
    in hypertension, 1392, 1400–1401, 1400b–1401b
  serum, preoperative evaluation of, 453t
Sodium bicarbonate, for chronic renal failure, 1654
  for hyperkalemia, 312
Sodium nitroprusside, for heart failure, 1286
Sodium polystyrene sulfonate (Kayexalate), for hyperkalemia, 312
Sodium salicylate, in pain control, 375t
Sodium-potassium pump, 294
Soft tissue emergencies, 2534, 2534t, 2535b
Solganal (gold salts), for rheumatoid arthritis, 664t
Solu-Cortef (hydrocortisone sodium succinate), in surgical client, 458t
Solu-Medrol (methylprednisolone sodium succinate), in organ transplantation, 645t
Solute diuresis, 1554
Somatic nervous system, 701
Somatiform disorder, 359
Somatostatin, 1691t
  actions of, 1940t
Somnambulism, 403
Somogyi effect, 1990–1992
Sorbasan, indications for, 443t
Soul food, 1704b
Sound(s), bowel, auscultation of, 1707–1709
  breath, adventitious, 1046, 1048t
    normal, 1046, 1047t
      location of, *1047*
  conduction of, external ear in, 981–982, *982*
  for urethral examination, 1553, *1553*
  heart. See *Heart sounds.*
  in chest percussion, 1044–1045, *1046*
  Korotkoff's, 1211

Sound(s) *(Continued)*
  voice, 1046–1047
Space sickness, 1011
Spasm, bladder, after prostatectomy, 2361
  esophageal, diffuse, 1737
  in fracture, 2134
  muscle, after spinal cord injury, 893–894, 909
    in rheumatoid arthritis, 658
Spasticity, in spinal cord injury, 892–893
  reduction of, 900–901
Specific gravity, of urine, 1557–1558
  in osmolality measurement, 276
Specificity, of diagnostic tests, 243
Specificity theory, of pain, 350
Specimens, adequate, obtaining of, 242, 243b
  collection of, delegation of, 244b
  for legal purposes, handling of, 2503
  in respiratory assessment, recovery/analysis of, 1062–1065
  testing of, delegation of, 244b
  tissue, in ear disorder assessment, 993
  urine, 1555
SPECT (single photon emission computed tomography), 732
Specular micrography, 950
Speculum, nasal, use of, 1049–1050, *1050*
  vaginal, use of, 2317–2318, *2319*
Speech, assessment of, 195, 710t–711t
  esophageal, 1093
    use of, nursing research on, 1088b
Speech aid, electronic, *1092*
Speech reading, 998
Speech reception threshold, 991
Speech therapy, for cerebrovascular accident, 798
Spenco, indications for, 443t
Sperm, characteristics of, in infertility, 2346
  maturation of, 2305
  structure/function of, 2304
Spermatic cord, 2302
  examination of, 2335
Spermatocele, 2377
Spermatogenesis, 2304–2305
Spermatogonia, 2304
Sphenoethmoidectomy, external, 1078
Sphenoidal ridge meningioma, *846*
Spherocytes, 1466t
Spherocytosis, hereditary, 1483–1484
  clinical manifestations of, 1484
  diagnostic findings in, 1484
  etiology of, 1483
  management of, in elderly, 1485
    surgical, 1484
      nursing care in, 1484–1485
  pathophysiology of, 1484
  risk factors for, 1483
Sphincter, bladder, in urinary incontinence, 1605
Sphincter of Oddi, relaxation of, 1839
Sphincteroplasty, for chronic pancreatitis, *1930*
Spider bites, 2537
Spider nevi, in cirrhosis, 1878t
Spinal accessory nerve, assessment of, *719,* 721
Spinal analgesia, *383,* 383–384

Spinal anesthesia, 475, *475*
  benefits of, 475
  complications of, 476t
    in postanesthesia care unit, 482
  positioning for, 475, *475*
Spinal cord, arterial supply to, *916*
  compression of, in metastatic breast cancer, 2451
  disorders of, 890–931
  edema of, 891
  in pain transmission, 344
  ischemia of, in abdominal aortic aneurysm, 1427, 1428
  pathways of, ascending, 694–696, 696t
    descending, 694–696, 696t
  structure/function of, 693–694, *695, 696*
  vascular lesions of, *916,* 916–917
Spinal cord injury (SCI), 890–914
  and distributive shock, 500
  and partial paralysis, 895
  cervical, 891, *893*
  clinical manifestations of, 893–895, 894t
  compression, 891, *892*
  diagnostic findings in, 893–895, 894t
  etiology of, *595,* 890–891, *893*
  flexion-rotation, 890, *892*
  functional goals in, 901t
  hyperextension, 890–891, *892*
  level of, 893, 894t
  management of, community/self care in, 914, 915b
    emergency, 895–898, *897*
    in elderly, 914
    medical, 898, *898,* 900–904, 901t, *902, 903b, 904t*
    nursing, 898–900, 899t, 904–913, *905, 906b, 909b, 913b*
    surgical, 913–914, *914*
  motor assessment after, 899, 899t
  pathophysiology of, 891–893
  pressure ulcers in, nursing research on, 903b, 906b
  prevention of, 891b
  risk factors for, 890–891, 891b
  sexuality in, 78
Spinal fusion, cervical, 924–925, *925*
  home care after, 926b
    client education in, 926b
  for intervertebral disc herniation, 921, *921*
  lumbar, physical mobility after, 923
Spinal manipulation, for intervertebral disc herniation, 919–920
Spinal nerves, assessment of, after spinal cord injury, 899, 899t
  structure/function of, 701–702, *702*
Spinal shock, 895
Spinal stenosis, 918, *919*
  and intervertebral disc herniation, 917
  clinical manifestations of, 918–919
Spinal tap. See *Lumbar puncture (LP).*
Spine, assessment of, in regional examination, 217t, 221t–222t
  curvatures of, 2120–2121
  immobilization of, in emergency nursing care, 2507, *2507*
  lumbar, function of, assessment of, 2090t–2091t

Spine *(Continued)*
radiography of, in neurologic assessment, 730
stabilization of, devices for, 914, *914*
traumatic injuries to, 2529
tumors of, 915–916
extramedullary, 915–916
intramedullary, 915–916
Spine boards, *2507*
Spinocerebellar tracts, 696t
Spinothalamic tractotomy, for pain, 386
Spinothalamic tracts, 696t
Spiral fracture, 2130, *2130*
Spiritual care, nursing research on, 72b
Spiritual distress, 72
Spirituality, 67–73
assessment of, 191t, 196
ethical issues in, 68b
in nursing practice, 68
nursing process in, 68–73, 69b–71b, 72b
religion in, 67
Spirometer, incentive, postoperative use of, 487, *487*
Spirometry, forced, 1051, *1053*
Spironolactone (Aldactone), 1394t
characteristics of, 1285t
complications of, 2056b
for hyperaldosteronism, 2056, 2056b
for premenstrual syndrome, 2388
Spleen, assessment of, in regional examination, 220t
in hematopoiesis, 1452–1453, *1454*
in immunity, 598
in portal hypertension, 1884–1885
palpation of, 1848
physical examination of, 1846t
size of, assessment of, 1847–1848
traumatic injury to, 2531
Splenic pulp manometry, 1856
Splenic rupture, 1504–1505
clinical manifestations of, 1505
diagnostic factors in, 1505
etiology of, 1504–1505
management of, surgical, 1505
nursing care in, 1505
risk factors for, 1504–1505
Splenomegaly, in cirrhosis, 1878t
in hemolytic anemia, 1479t
Splinter hemorrhage, 2187t
in infective endocarditis, 1333
Splinting, for postoperative exercise, after lung cancer surgery, 1157, *1157*
in burns, 2259–2260
Split-ejaculate technique, 2347
Split-thickness skin grafts (STSGs), 2278
Spondylitis, ankylosing, 678, *679*
Spondylolisthesis, and intervertebral disc herniation, 917
Spondylolysis, and intervertebral disc herniation, 917
Sports, health risks of, 203t
Sports injuries, 2161–2167
Sprains, 2163–2164, *2164*
prevention of, 203t
Spray table, for hydrotherapy, in burns, *2253*
Sputum, blood-tinged, assessment of, in cardiovascular assessment, 1217

Sputum *(Continued)*
collection of, 1062–1063
delegation of, 244b
production of, assessment of, 1036
Squamous cell carcinoma, 2227, *2227*
of lungs, 1153t
of oral cavity, *1727,* 1727–1728
SSI (Supplemental Security Income), 94
SSKI (saturated solution of potassium iodide), for goiter, 2014
for hyperthyroidism, 2013t
SSM (superficial spreading melanoma), 2228t
St. Jude medical bileaflet valve, *1352*
ST segment, *1222,* 1223
analysis of, 1298b
in stress testing, 1226
Stab wound, 2520t
Stable factor, 1516t
Stadol (butorphanol), administration of, 380t
Staff, nursing, definition of, 136b
Staffing, for quality care, 126
Staghorn calculus, 1666, *1666*
Staging, of cancer, 559–560, 560t
bladder, 1582–1583, *1583*
breast, 2435, *2435,* 2436t
endometrial, 2405, *2405*
laryngeal, 1085, 1086b
lung, 1153, 1154b, *1155*
oral, 1728, 1728t
prostate, 2367, 2368b
renal, 1671, *1672*
Staining, 243
Standard precautions, 423–424
Standard radical mastectomy, for breast cancer, 2437
Standing position, for physical examination, *232*
Stapedectomy, for otosclerosis, 1002, *1003*
Stapes, structure of, *981,* 982
Staphylococcal pneumonia, 1136t
Staphylococcus, and gastroenteritis, 1789
Staphylococcus aureus, 416t
methicillin-resistant, 419
in postoperative wound infection, 491
Staphylococcus saprophyticus, and urinary tract infection, 1571
Starr-Edwards caged-ball valve, *1352*
Stasis dermatitis, 2207–2208, *2210*
Station, assessment of, 722
Status asthmaticus, 1106
Status epilepticus, 843
client education in, 840b
treatment of, 843
STDs. See *Sexually transmitted diseases (STDs).*
Stellwag's sign, 976
Stem cells, in hematopoiesis, 1449, *1450*
peripheral, collection of, for bone marrow transplantation, 1496
Stents, for benign prostatic hyperplasia, 2359
intracoronary, for coronary artery disease, 1246, *1246*
intravascular, 1413
"Step-care," in asthma, 1110

Step-family, 53
Step-progression, for orthostatic hypotension, in extracellular fluid volume deficit, 283
Stereognosis, testing of, 724
Stereotactic needle aspiration biopsy, 257
Stereotactic radiation therapy, for brain tumors, 848
Stereotactic radiosurgery, for brain tumors, 849
Stereotactic surgery, closed, for pain, 388
open, for pain, 388
Sternocleidomastoid muscle, 1026
Sternum, fracture of, chest trauma and, 2526–2527
Steroids, after heart transplantation, 1354b
complications of, intraoperative, 457
delayed wound healing with, 444
effect of, on male reproductive system, 2345
for asthma, 1106–1107
for chemotherapy, classification of, 577t
for chronic obstructive pulmonary disease, 1111t
for hypersensitivity, 641
for idiopathic thrombocytopenic purpura, 1507
for increased intracranial pressure, 775
for inflammatory bowel disease, 1799
for nephrotic syndrome, 1635
for postoperative wound infection, 490
for shock, 520
for viral hepatitis, 1867
in pain control, 377–378
monitoring of, in postanesthesia care unit, 483
Stethoscope, components of, 230, *230*
Stimulants, effect of, on male reproductive system, 2345
Stimulation therapy, in pain control, 389–391, 389b, 390t
Stöckert heart-lung bypass machine, *1355*
Stockings, antiembolism, 461
sequential compression, 461
Stoma, care of, delegation of, 1806b
closure of, after partial laryngectomy, 1089, *1090*
for inflammatory bowel disease, complications of, 1803–1804
for urinary diversion, home care of, 1591, 1591b
odor with, management of, 1591–1592
site of, selection of, 1588
stricture of, 1815
Stomach, *1689,* 1689–1690. See also entries under *Gastric.*
disorders of, 1748–1784
function of, 1689–1690
structure of, 1689, *1689*
Stomal ischemia, in bladder cancer, 1590
Stomatitis, 1723
aphthous, *1723,* 1723–1724
chemotherapy and, 583
Stone prevention diet, 1597
Stool, clay-colored, in viral hepatitis, 1865, 1866t
collection of, delegation of, 244b
culture of, 1711t, 1712

Stool (Continued)
 examination of, for lipids, 1711t, 1712–1713
  for occult blood, 1711–1712, 1711t, 1712b
   nursing research on, 1712b
  for ova and parasites, 1711t, 1712
  schedule for, 209t
 testing of, delegation of, 244b
Strabismus, 945
 management of, 199t
Strangury, 1549
Straight leg raising test, 2090t
Strain(s), 2163
 back, and intervertebral disc herniation, 917
 prevention of, 203t
Stratum corneum, structure/function of, 2176t
Stratum germinativum, 2173–2174, 2174
Stratum granulosum, 2174, 2174
Stratum lucidum, 2174, 2174
Stratum spinosum, 2174, 2174
Strength, muscle, assessment of, 2087, 2088t
 personal, assessment of, 196
Streptococcal infection, prevention of, in rheumatic fever, 1330–1331
Streptococcus pyogenes, 416t
Streptokinase, for chronic arterial occlusion, 1413–1414
Streptomycin, for tuberculosis, 1144t
Stress, and heart failure, 1278
 and peptic ulcer disease, 1765
 evaluation of, in cardiovascular assessment, 1210
 in cancer, 541
 in coronary artery disease, 1241
 in hypertension, 1389
 in immunity, 605
 in perioperative client, 451, 451t
 management of, 202t
  in elderly, 86
  in health promotion, 171–173
 post-traumatic, after burn injury, 2262b
 reduction of, for heart failure, 1286–1287
 resistance to, glucocorticoids in, 1945
 surgical responses to, 451, 451t
 tolerance to, pattern of, 206
 Wolff's theory of, 24–25
Stress fractures, 2131, 2162
Stress incontinence, 1604t
 medications for, 1611t
 risk factors for, 1606b
Stress response, Lazarus's theories of, 23–24, 24t
 Mason's theory of, 23
 mediators of, 28–29
Stress testing, 1225–1227, 1226b, 1227b
 client education in, 1226b
 contraindications to, 1226, 1227b
 in angina pectoris, 1254
 termination of, criteria for, 1226
Stress ulcers, 1764
 after intracranial surgery, 850
 pathophysiology of, 1765–1766
Stretch receptors, in cardiac regulation, 1203

Stridor, assessment of, 1036–1037
Stripping, of chest tube, 1165, 1165
Stroke. See Cerebrovascular accident (CVA).
Stroke belt, 1994
Stroke in evolution, 797
Stroke volume, 1200, 1201
Stroma, of ovaries, 2295, 2295
Struvite renal calculi, 1666
STSGs (split-thickness skin grafts), 2278
Stuart-Prower factor, 1516t
Stump, postamputation, care of, 1422–1424
  client education in, 1423b
  wrapping of, 1421
Stump pain, 358
Stupor, in consciousness disorders, 746
Stye, 972
Subacute bacterial endocarditis (SBE), 1331
Subacute care, 121–123
 chronic, 123
 for elderly, 97
 general, 123
 transitional, 123
 long-term, 123
Subarachnoid hemorrhage (SAH), 812–816. See also Intracranial hemorrhage.
 classification of, 813, 813t
Subconjunctival hemorrhage, red eye in, 942b
Subcutaneous emphysema, after thoracic surgery, monitoring for, 1159
 tracheostomy tube and, 1071
Subcutaneous fat, structure/function of, 2176, 2176t
Subcutaneous nodules, in rheumatic fever, 1328
Subdiaphragmatic abscess, 1168
Subdural hematoma, 744, 830–831
 acute, 831
 chronic, 831
  evacuation of, positioning after, 853
Sublimaze (fentanyl citrate), administration of, 380t
 preoperative, 465t
 transdermal, 382
Subluxation, 2164
Subscapular lymph nodes, palpation of, 2313, 2314
Substance abuse, 2479–2499
 assessment of, 2485–2494, 2486b, 2486t
 definition of, 2481t
 detection of, home healthcare in, 2484b
 during pregnancy, ethical issues in, 2309b
 effects of, 2482t–2483t
  perioperative, 457
 in elderly, 91–92
 in healthcare professional, 2497–2498, 2498b
 intervention for, 2495–2497
  options for, 2495, 2496t, 2497b
  resources for, 2497b
 management of, 201t, 2485–2494
 medical problems with, ethical issues in, 2485b
 nursing care in, 2494, 2495b
 relapse in, prevention of, 2495–2496, 2497b

Substance abuse (Continued)
 screening for, 208t, 2480–2485
  tools for, 2485b
 surgery in, 2497
 terminology of, definitions of, 2480, 2481t
Substance dependence, definition of, 2481t
Substantia gelatinosa (SG), in gate control theory of pain, 350–351, 351
Subtrochanteric fracture, 2153, 2159–2160
Succinylcholine chloride (Anectine), 472t
Sucking chest wound, 2524
Sucking reflex, 728
Suclavian steal syndrome, 1430
Sucralfate (Carafate), for peptic ulcer disease, 1769t, 1770
Sucrase, 1692t
 secretion of, 1693
Sucrose, characteristics of, 1285t
Suctioning, after lung cancer surgery, 1164
  apparatus for, assessment of, 1164
 after thyroidectomy, 2025t
 of airway, in increased intracranial pressure, 783
 of endotracheal tube, 1174–1175, 1175t, 1176b
  complications of, 1175t
 of gastrointestinal tubes, 1751
 of tracheostomy, 1072
 of unconscious patient, 755
Sudden cardiac death, coronary artery disease in, 1244
Suffering, 74
Suffocation, risk for, in consciousness disorders, 755
Suicide, cultural beliefs about, 69b
Sulfasalazine (Azulfidine), for diarrhea, in inflammatory bowel disease, 1798–1799
 for rheumatoid arthritis, 664t
 urine color with, 1557t
Sulfisoxazole (Gantrisin), for urinary tract infections, 1576t
Sulfonamides, allergic reaction to, clinical manifestations of, 640t
 for inflammatory bowel disease, 1799
 for urinary tract infections, 1575t–1576t
Sulfonylureas, for diabetes mellitus, 1967–1968, 1967t
Sulindac (Clinoril), for rheumatoid arthritis, 664t
Sulkowitch test, in parathyroid disorders, 2032t
Sumerians, healthcare beliefs of, 18
Sun, exposure to, after burn injury, 2263b
 and disease, 36
 management of, 202t
Sunburn, 2224–2225, 2224b
 prevention of, 202t, 203t
  client education in, 2224b
Sundown syndrome, 763
 in dementia of Alzheimer's type, pharmacologic treatment of, 866t
 management of, nursing research on, 769b
Sunscreens, 2200t
Superficial pain, 353
Superficial spreading melanoma (SSM), 2228t
Supinator reflex, 729t

Supine (dorsal recumbent) position, for physical examination, *232*
intraoperative, 477, *478*
Supplemental Security Income (SSI), 94
Support systems, in urinary tract assessment, 1551
Suppuration, in chronic inflammation, 437
Supraclavicular lymph nodes, palpation of, 2313, *2314*
Suprapubic cystotomy, for urinary retention, 1603–1604
Suprapubic prostatectomy, for benign prostatic hyperplasia, *2353,* 2358
Supraspinatus tendinitis, 2168t
Supratentorial, definition of, 698
Supratentorial herniation syndromes, *773,* 773–774
Supratentorial lesions, and consciousness disorders, 745
Supratentorial surgery, positioning after, 853
Supraventricular tachycardia (SVT), 1302
Surface immunoglobulin (SIg), 596, 598
Surfactant, pulmonary, insufficient, in atelectasis, 1134b
Surgeon, role of, 466
Surgery, complications after, prevention of, 485
in "do not resuscitate" clients, ethical issues in, 460b
previous, preoperative assessment of, 457
sexuality after, 78–79
Surgical asepsis, 478
Surgical excision biopsy, of skin, 2196
Surgical intensive care unit (SICU), transfer to, indications for, 480
Surgical procedures, categories of, 452, 452t
Surgical team, members of, 466–468
Surveillance, Epidemiology, and End Results (SEER) Program, 534, *537*
SURVIVE, in diabetes mellitus, 1971
Suspension traction, 2137–2138, *2138*
Suspiciousness, in dementia of Alzheimer's type, pharmacologic treatment of, 866t
Sutilains (Travase), for enzymatic debridement, 440
Suture joints, 2075–2076
Sutures, cranial, 697
in plastic surgery, 2268
removal of, timing of, 437
Svo₂, monitoring of, in shock, 526
SVT (supraventricular tachycardia), 1302
Swallowing, after cerebrovascular accident, home management of, 804b
impaired, in esophageal cancer, 1744–1745
in bulbar disorders, 861
in Parkinson's disease, client education about, 882b
mouth in, 1687, *1688*
Swan-Ganz catheter, in hemodynamic monitoring, in shock, 526
positioning of, *1234*
quadruple-lumen, *1234*
Swan-neck deformity, in rheumatoid arthritis, 659, *659,* 674
Sweating, in thermoregulation, 2177
Swelling, in fracture, 2134
in musculoskeletal disorders, 2084

Swimmer's ear, 1004
Swing beds, 122
Symmetrel (amantadine), for Parkinson's disease, 880t
Sympathetic nervous system (SNS), 703
in cardiac regulation, 1203
of kidneys, 1537
organic effects of, 703, 706t
stimulation of, in heart failure, 1279
Sympathetic ophthalmia, 970
Symphyses, 2076
Symptom analysis, 187
associated manifestations in, 187
factors in, aggravating/relieving, 187
precipitating, 187
in eye disorders, 941
in immune disorders, 607–608
in integumentary system disorders, 2180, 2181t
in musculoskeletal disorders, 2083–2084
in peripheral vascular disorders, 1378
in respiratory disorders, 1037–1038
upper, 1048
in urinary tract disorders, 1547–1549, *1549*
location in, 187
quality in, 187
quantity in, 187
timing in, 187
Synacort (hydrocortone), 2048t
for rheumatoid arthritis, 664t
topical, 2199t
Synalar (fluocinolone), topical, 2199t
Synapses, 686, *686*
chemical, 686, *686*
electrical, 686
Synarel (nafarelin), for benign prostatic hyperplasia, 2364t
for endometriosis, 2399
Synchondroses, 2076
Synchronized intermittent mandatory ventilation (SIMV), 1177, 1178t
Syncope, 1404–1405
assessment of, 1207
Syndesmosis joints, 2076
Syndrome of inappropriate secretion of antidiuretic hormone (SIADH), diabetes insipidus vs., 2066, 2067t–2068t
head trauma and, 825
monitoring for, 2064b
Syndrome X, 1993
Syngeneic transplants, 641
Synovectomy, for rheumatoid arthritis, 672
Synovial fluid, analysis of, 2095t
Synovial joints, 2076, *2076*
movements of, 2076
Synovitis, in rheumatoid arthritis, 658
Synthroid (levothyroxine sodium), for hypothyroidism, 2014t
Syphilis, 2470–2472
clinical manifestations of, 2470–2471
diagnostic findings in, 2470–2471
etiology of, 2470
latent, 2471
management of, 2461t–2462t
community/self care in, 2471–2472
medical, 2471
nursing, 2471–2472

Syphilis *(Continued)*
pathophysiology of, 2470
primary, 2470
risk factors for, 2470
secondary, 2470
tertiary, 2471
Syringes, insulin, 1978, *1978*
prefilled, 1979
Syringomyelia, 914–915
cervical, indications of, 915
post-traumatic, 891
Systemic inflammatory response syndrome (SIRS), 528–531
Systemic lupus erythematosus (SLE), 674–677
clinical manifestations of, 675–676
diagnostic findings in, 675–676
drugs causing, 675, 675b
etiology of, 675, 675b
management of, 676–678
medical, 676, *676*
nursing, 677
ocular manifestations of, 977
pathophysiology of, 675
risk factors for, 675
Systole, ventricular, 1198–1199
Systolic hypertension, 1387
Systolic murmurs, 1218t
Systolic pressure, 1201–1202

T

T cells, 1452, *1453*
assays of, in immune disorder assessment, 611
B cell interaction with, in autoimmunity, *654,* 655
cytotoxic, in cell-mediated immunity, 602, *603*
helper, in cell-mediated immunity, 602, *603*
in human immunodeficiency virus infection, 620–621
tolerance to, loss of, in autoimmunity, *654,* 654–655
in cell-mediated immunity, 602, *603*
in gate control theory of pain, 351, *351*
T tube, after choledochostomy, 1919–1920, *1920*
T wave, *1222,* 1223
analysis of, 1298b
T₃ (triiodothyronine), actions of, 1940t, 1943
radioimmunoassay of, 1952, 2010t
T₃ resin uptake (T₃ RU), 1952, 2011t
T₄ (thyroxine), actions of, 1940t, 1943
measurement of, 2010t
production of, 1943
radioimmunoassay of, 1952
Tabes dorsalis, 929
Taboos, 60
Tachycardia, 236
atrial, paroxysmal, *1300,* 1301
cardiogenic shock and heart failure with, case study of, 1268–1269
in shock, 511
junctional, paroxysmal, 1302–1303
sinus, 1200, 1297–1298, *1299*

Tachycardia (Continued)
  supraventricular, 1302
  ventricular, 1305, 1306
Tachypnea, 238
  assessment of, in cardiovascular disorders, 1217
  in pneumonia, 1137
  in shock, 511
Tacrine (Cognex), for dementia of Alzheimer's type, 865
Tacrolimus (FK506, Prograf), in organ transplantation, 645t
Tactile fremitus, assessment of, 1044
Tagamet (cimetidine), for interstitial cystitis, 1580
  for peptic ulcer disease, 1767, 1768t
  for shock, 520
  preoperative, 465t
TAH-BSO (total abdominal hysterectomy with bilateral salpingo-oophorectomy), discharge instructions after, 2402
  for leiomyoma, 2401, 2402
  for ovarian cancer, 2413
Tail of Spence, palpation of, 2314
Talc, 2200t
Talking tracheostomy, 1069
Talwin (pentazocine), administration of, 381t
  in pain control, 375t
Tambocor (flecainide), for dysrhythmia, 1307t
Tamoxifen, for breast cancer, 2449, 2449t
Tamponade, pericardial, and cardiogenic shock, 500
Tangential excision, of burns, 2253–2254
Taoism, beliefs/practices of, 2551
Tapazole (methimazole), for hyperthyroidism, 2013t, 2019
Tapeworm, 861
Tar, 2200t
  in coronary artery disease, 1240
Target cells, 1466t
  in hormone regulation, 1941, 1942
Targets, in Omaha system, of home health-care, 153, 155b
Tarsal tunnel syndrome, 928
Tarsorrhaphy, for keratitis, 969
Taste, assessment of, 713t
Tautness, definition of, 2183t
Taylor back brace, for spinal cord injury, 900, 902
TB. See Tuberculosis (TB).
TBGs (thyroid-binding globulins), 2011t
TBSA (total body surface area), in burn severity classification, 2238t, 2240, 2242
TBW (total body water), in hyponatremia, sodium relationship to, 296, 297t
TCA (trichloroacetic acid), for genital warts, 2473
TCA (trichloroacetic acid) peels, 2273
TCT (thyrocalcitonin), actions of, 1940t, 1943
TDD (telecommunications device for the deaf), 999b
T-Derm, 2200t
Teaching. See also Education.
  ambulatory care nurse in, 141b, 142
  during physical examination, 239

Teaching (Continued)
  in family nursing intervention, 59
  of health promotion, in elderly, 86, 87b
  preoperative, 225–227, 226
Team nursing, 124
Technetium, in radionuclide scanning, 254–255, 255
Technetium 99m ventriculography, 1230
Technical procedures, ambulatory care nurse in, 140, 141b
TEE (transesophageal echocardiography), in cardiovascular assessment, 1228–1229
  in myocardial infarction, 1262
Teeth, cleaning of, schedule for, 207t
  premature loss of, management of, 199t
  screening of, 207t
  trauma to, 1722–1723
Tegaderm, indications for, 443t
Tegasorb, 2199t
  indications for, 443t
Tegison (etretinate), for psoriasis, 2211
Tegretol. See Carbamazepine (Tegretol).
Tela submucosa, 1692, 1693, 1694
Telangiectasia, hemorrhagic, familial, 1508
Telecommunications device for the deaf (TDD), 999b
Telephone communication, ambulatory care nurse in, 141b, 142
Telephone services, for elderly, 99
Telephone triage, 2504, 2504b
Teletherapy, 570
Telfa, indications for, 443t
Temovate (clobetasol), topical, 2199t
Temperature, changes in, in postanesthesia care unit, 483
  control of, in increased intracranial pressure, 783
  elevation of, in Crohn's disease, 1797
  extremes of, and cell damage, 269
  measurement of, 236
    after cardiac surgery, 1357, 1358b
    after thyroidectomy, 2025t
    delegation of, 234b
    in shock, 525
    nursing research on, 1358b
  of skin, assessment of, 2187–2192
  palpation of, in peripheral vascular assessment, 1381
  sensitivity to, assessment of, 724
Temporal bone, function of, 981–982, 982
  structure of, 980
Temporal lobe(s), 691, 692
  tumor of, clinical manifestations of, 847t
Temporal lobe seizures, 837
Temporal lobectomy, for epilepsy, 841, 841
Temporalis fascia flap, 2280
Temporomandibular joint (TMJ), in otalgia, 1003
Tenckhoff catheter, for peritoneal dialysis, 1649, 1650
Tenderness, in fracture, 2134
  of skin, assessment of, 2192
Tendinitis, bicipital, 2168t
  patellar, 2162
  supraspinatus, 2168t
Tendon sheaths, 2077
Tendon transfer, for rheumatoid arthritis, 672

Tenesmus, 1549
Tenex (guanfacine), 1396t
Tennis elbow, 2162, 2169t
Tennis elbow test, 2090t
Tenormin (atenolol), 1395t
  for angina pectoris, 1257t
  for dysrhythmia, 1308t
Tenosynovitis, de Quervain's, 2169t
TENS (transcutaneous electrical nerve stimulation), client education about, 389b
  in pain control, 389, 389b, 390t
  troubleshooting in, 390t
Tensilon (edrophonium), in myasthenia gravis diagnosis, 884–885
Tension headaches, 820
Tension neck syndrome, 2168t
Tension pneumothorax, after thoracic surgery, monitoring for, 1159
  and cardiogenic shock, 500
  mediastinal shift with, chest trauma and, 2525, 2525–2526
Tentorium cerebelli, 698
TEP (tracheoesophageal puncture), 1093, 1093
  care of, client education in, 1094b
Terazosin (Hytrin), 1395t
  for benign prostatic hyperplasia, 2364t
Terminal illness, ethical issues in, 46
Termination, in therapeutic family communication, 58
Testes, atrophy of, in cirrhosis, 1878t
  disorders of, 2066–2069, 2373–2378
  hormones of, 1940t
  physical examination of, 2333
    normal findings in, 2332b
  procedures of, 2373–2378
  screening of, 210t
  structure/function of, 2302–2304
  undescended, 2378, 2378
Testicular cancer, 2373–2377
  clinical manifestations of, 2374–2375
  diagnostic findings in, 2374–2375, 2375
  etiology of, 2373
  management of, medical, 2376
    nursing, 2376–2377
    surgical, 2375–2376
    nursing care in, 2376
  pathophysiology of, 2374
  prevention of, 2374b
  risk factors for, 542b, 2373, 2374b
  survival in, 538t
Testicular self-examination (TSE), 2340, 2340
  education about, nursing research on, 2375b
  schedule for, 210t
Testicular torsion, 2377, 2377
Testosterone, actions of, 1940t
  in male sexual development, 2304
  reference values for, in cancer, 557t
Testosterone patches, application of, client education in, 2348b
Tetanus, 857
  prevention of, 202t
  treatment of, 857
Tetanus immune globulin (TIG), for soft tissue trauma, 2534

Tetanus prophylaxis, in burns, 2241, 2251
in soft tissue emergencies, 2534, 2534t
recommendations for, in adults, 422t
Tetanus-diphtheria booster, schedule for, 208t
Tetany, after parathyroidectomy, 2035
in endocrine disorders, 1949
in hypoparathyroidism, 2037–2038
Tetracaine hydrochloride (Pontocaine HCl), 473t
Tetracycline, for acne vulgaris, 2212
Tetrahydrocannabinol (THC), 2490
Texture, definition of, 2183t
of skin, assessment of, 2192
TGF-α (transforming growth factor-α), in wound healing, 431
TGF-β (transforming growth factor-β), in wound healing, 432
TGT (thromboplastin generation test), in hemorrhage, 1467t
TH (thyroid hormone), insufficient, in hypothyroidism, 2006–2007
oversecretion of, in hyperthyroidism, 2017
Thalamic pain, 356
Thalamus, structure/function of, 691, 692
Thalassemia, 1482–1483
clinical manifestations of, 1482
diagnostic findings in, 1482
etiology of, 1482
management of, 1483
pathophysiology of, 1482
risk factors for, 1482
Thallium 201 scintigraphy, in cardiovascular assessment, 1229–1230
THC (tetrahydrocannabinol), 2490
Theophylline, for asthma, 1106, 1110–1111
therapeutic monitoring of, reference values for, 2562
Therapeutic drug monitoring, reference values for, 2562
Therapeutic passes, after cerebrovascular accident, in discharge planning, 807
Therapeutic regimen, ineffective management of, 2038
after prostatectomy, 2362–2363
after spinal cord injury, 911
in acute pancreatitis, 1928
in Addison's disease, 2047
in bladder cancer, 1590–1594
in cholelithiasis, 1911–1912
in chronic renal failure, 1657
in colon cancer, 1814–1816, 1815b
in diabetes mellitus, 1975, 1978, 1978–1980, 1979, 1980b
in enteral nutrition, 1754
in glaucoma, 956, 957t
in hepatic encephalopathy, 1894
in hypercortisolism, 2053
in hyperpituitarism, 2064–2065
in hypertension, 1399–1400
in hyperthyroidism, 2023–2024
in hypothyroidism, 2015–2016, 2016b
in inflammatory bowel disease, 1805–1808, 1806b, 1807
in iron deficiency anemia, 1473–1474
in leukemia, 1494
in liver transplantation, 1901
in peptic ulcer disease, 1773–1776

Therapeutic regimen (Continued)
in pheochromocytoma, 2059–2060
in rheumatic fever, 1330–1331
in rheumatoid arthritis, 670–671, 671b
in urinary tract infections, 1578–1579
with tracheostomy, 1076
Therapeutic touch, in pain control, 349b, 370–371
Thermal burns, 2233
of lower airways, 2237
Thermoregulation, ineffective, after spinal cord injury, 900
skin in, 2177
Thiamine, deficiency of, and heart failure, 1278
for altered level of consciousness, 2517
Thiazide diuretics, 1394t
intraoperative complications of, 457
Thiazolidinediones, 1968
Thinking, assessment of, 710t
Thiopental sodium (Pentothal), 470t
Third-degree atrioventricular (AV) block, 1303, 1304
Third-spacing, 289–291
clinical manifestations of, 291
diagnostic findings in, 291
etiology of, 289–290
management of, medical, 291
nursing, 291
surgical, 291
pathophysiology of, 290–291
prevention of, 290b
risk factors for, 289–290, 290b
Thirst, in fluid balance regulation, 275, 276
Thoracentesis, 1063–1064, 1064
in pleural effusion, 1167
Thoracic aortic aneurysm, 1429–1430
Thoracic excursion, assessment of, 1044, 1044
Thoracic kyphoscoliosis, 1042, 1043
restrictive lung disorders in, 1147, 1148
Thoracic landmarks, 1040, 1041
Thoracic outlet syndrome, 1430, 2168t
Thoracic surgery, nursing care plan in, 1159–1162
Thoracolumbosacral orthosis (TLSO), for spinal cord injury, 900
Thoracotomy, endoscopic, 1062
Thorax, anterior, assessment of, in regional examination, 218t–219t
function of, 1027
physical examination of, in endocrine disorders, 1952
posterior, assessment of, in regional examination, 218t
structure of, 1026–1027, 1027
Thorazine, avoidance of, in cirrhosis, 1882t
Thought processes, abstract, changes in, after cerebrovascular accident, 792
altered, after brain tumor surgery, 855
after cerebrovascular accident, 805–806
in confusion, 766–767
in dementia of Alzheimer's type, 868
in hypercortisolism, 2054–2055
in portal hypertension, 1888–1889
assessment of, 195
Three-way Foley urethral catheter, 2355t

Threshold value, in nerve impulse generation, 688
Thrills, palpation of, 1213
Throat, culture of, 1063
Thrombectomy, venous, 1436
Thrombin time, in hemorrhage, 1467t
Thromboangiitis obliterans, 1430–1431
clinical manifestations of, 1430–1431
diagnostic findings in, 1430–1431
etiology of, 1430
management of, 1431
risk factors for, 1430
Thrombocytes. See Platelets.
Thrombocytopenia, 1458, 1506
in aplastic anemia, 1478
Thrombogenic hypothesis, of coronary artery disease pathogenesis, 1243
Thrombolytic therapy, for chronic arterial occlusion, 1413–1414
for myocardial infarction, 1264
Thrombophlebitis. See also Venous thrombosis.
after intertrochanteric hip fracture, 2158
after thoracic surgery, monitoring for, 1160
after total hip replacement, 2114
after vulvectomy, 2420
postoperative, prevention of, 487
risk for, after spinal cord injury, 910
Thromboplastin, 1516t
Thromboplastin generation test (TGT), in hemorrhage, 1467t
Thrombosis, and cerebrovascular accident, 785, 785
clinical manifestations of, 787t
supportive care of, 796
arterial, arterial embolism vs., 1424
cavernous sinus, 816
venous. See Venous thrombosis.
Thrombus, formation of, risk for, in splenic rupture, 1505
Thrush. See Candidiasis, oral.
Thumb, range of motion of, 2089
Thymectomy, for myasthenia gravis, 886
Thymus, in immunity, 596–597, 597
Thyrocalcitonin (TCT), actions of, 1940t, 1943
Thyroid antibodies, testing of, 2010t
Thyroid cancer, 2027–2029
clinical manifestations of, 2029
diagnostic findings in, 2029
etiology of, 2028
management of, medical, 2029
nursing, 2029
surgical, 2029
pathophysiology of, 2028–2029
prevention of, 2029b
risk factors for, 2028, 2029b
survival in, 538t
types of, 2028t
Thyroid cartilage, 1023
fracture of, 1101
Thyroid function tests, 1952–1953, 2010t–2011t
in thyroiditis, 2027t
Thyroid gland, disorders of, 2005–2038
and heart failure, 1278
diagnostic tests for, 2010t–2011t

Thyroid gland (Continued)
function of, 1943, *1943*
hormones of, 1940t
physical examination of, 1951, *1951,*
1951b
structure of, 1943, *1943*
Thyroid hormone (TH), insufficient, in
hypothyroidism, 2006–2007
oversecretion of, in hyperthyroidism,
2017
Thyroid scan, 2011t
Thyroid storm, in hyperthyroidism, 2019
risk for, after thyroidectomy, 2023
Thyroid supplements, client education in,
2016b
Thyroid-binding globulins (TBGs), 2011t
Thyroidectomy, complications of, 2023
hypoparathyroidism after, 2036
nursing care after, 2023–2024, 2024t–
2025t
subtotal, for hyperthyroidism, 2022–2023
total, for thyroid cancer, 2029
Thyroiditis, 2025–2027
clinical manifestations of, 2026
diagnostic findings in, 2026, 2027t
etiology of, 2025
granulomatous, subacute, 2025
management of, medical, 2027
nursing, 2027
surgical, 2027
pathophysiology of, 2026
Pneumocystis carinii, nursing research on,
2026, 2027b
prevention of, 2026b
risk factors for, 2025, 2026b
suppurative, acute, 2025
Thyroid-releasing hormone test, 2011t
Thyroid-stimulating hormone (TSH),
2061t
actions of, 1940t
assay of, 2010t
in thyroxine production, 1943
Thyroplasty, for unilateral vocal cord paralysis, 1101
Thyrotoxicosis, 2012
and heart failure, 1278
in hyperthyroidism, 2019
Thyrotropin-releasing hormone (TRH) stimulation test, 1953
Thyroxine (T$_4$), actions of, 1940t, 1943
measurement of, 2010t
production of, 1943
radioimmunoassay of, 1952
TIAs. See *Transient ischemic attacks*
(TIAs).
Tibial fracture, 2161
Tibial nerve, neurovascular assessment of,
2093
Tic, 723b
Tic douloureux, 357
Ticlid (ticlopidine), for angina pectoris,
1257t
for cerebrovascular accident, 793
Ticlopidine (Ticlid), for angina pectoris,
1257t
for cerebrovascular accident, 793
Tidal volume (V$_T$), 1028, *1028,* 1052t
Tidaling, 1163

Tiemann coudé red rubber urethral catheter,
2354t
TIG (tetanus immune globulin), for soft tissue trauma, 2534
Time zone change syndrome, 403
Timolol (Blocadren), 1395t
for angina pectoris, 1257t
Timolol maleate, for glaucoma, client teaching about, 957t
Tine test, schedule for, 208t
Tinea, 2221t
Tinel's sign, in carpal tunnel syndrome,
927, *927*
Tinnitus, 1003
history of, 985
TIPS (transjugular intrahepatic portosystemic shunt) procedure, 1887
Tissue, blood flow through, 1374–1376
changes in, in endocrine disorders, 1949
devitalized, in black wounds, 439
integrity of, impaired, in idiopathic thrombocytopenic purpura, 1508
Tissue load, in pressure ulcers, management
of, 2216
Tissue perfusion, altered, after arterial
bypass, 1416
in hereditary spherocytosis, 1484–1485
in polycythemia vera, 1486
in small intestinal obstruction, 1823
cerebral. See *Cerebral tissue perfusion.*
maintenance of, in shock, 514–516, 514b,
514t
peripheral, altered, in abdominal aortic
aneurysm, 1427–1428
in burns, 2244
in chronic arterial occlusion, 1408–
1409
in heart failure, 1288
decreased, fingerstick blood glucose
measurement in, nursing research on,
515b
postoperative, promotion of, 487
Tissue plasminogen activator (tPA), for
cerebrovascular accident, 792
Tissue typing, in organ transplantation,
643
Titralac (calcium carbonate), for peptic ulcer
disease, 1769t, 1770
TLC (total lung capacity), 1028, *1028,*
1052t
in restrictive lung disorders, 1147
TLS (tumor lysis syndrome), 310
chemotherapy and, 1490
TLSO (thoracolumbosacral orthosis), for
spinal cord injury, 900
TMJ (temporomandibular joint), in otalgia,
1003
TMP-SMX (trimethoprim-sulfamethoxazole), in *Pneumocystis carinii* pneumonia
prophylaxis, 625
TMR (transmyocardial revascularization),
for coronary artery disease, 1248
TNF (tumor necrosis factor), effects of, 604,
604t
TNM staging system, 559–560, 560t
in bladder cancer, 1582, *1583*
in breast cancer, 2435, 2436t
in colon cancer, 1809t, 1810

TNM staging system (Continued)
in gastric cancer, 1782, 1782b
in head and neck cancer, 1085, 1086b
in lung cancer, 1153, 1154b, *1155*
in oral cancer, 1728, 1728t
in prostate cancer, 2368b
Tobacco use, in respiratory disorders, 1039
management of, 201t
Tobramycin, therapeutic monitoring of,
reference values for, 2562
Tocainide (Tonocard), for dysrhythmia,
1307t
in pain control, 378
Toes, inspection of, in respiratory assessment, 1042–1043, *1044*
range of motion of, *2089*
Tofranil (imipramine hydrochloride), for urinary incontinence, 1611t
Toilet training, in urinary tract disorders,
1551
Tolazamide (Tolinase), for diabetes mellitus,
1967t, 1968
Tolbutamide (Orinase), for diabetes mellitus, 1967t
Tolerance, definition of, 2481t
to opioid analgesics, 377
Tolinase (tolazamide), for diabetes mellitus,
1967t, 1968
Tolmetin, for rheumatoid arthritis, 664t
Tomography, computed. See *Computed*
tomography (CT).
in musculoskeletal disorders, 2092
positron emission. See *Positron emission*
tomography (PET).
Tongs, for cervical spine injury, 897,
897
Tonic phase, of tonic-clonic seizure, 837,
837
Tonic-clonic (grand mal) seizures, in epilepsy, 837, *837*
Tonocard (tocainide), for dysrhythmia,
1307t
in pain control, 378
Tonometry, 949, *949*
Tonsillar herniation, 774
Tonsillectomy, 1079
Tonsillitis, 1079–1080
chronic, 1080
management of, medical, 1079
surgical, 1079–1080
nursing care in, 1079–1080
Tooth decay. See *Dental caries.*
Tooth extraction, hemorrhage after, 1722–
1723
Tophi, in gout, 2107
Topical anesthesia, 474
agents for, 473t–474t
in pain control, 372
Topical medications, 2197–2201, 2198t–
2200t
for open wound, 438
vehicles for, 2197, 2200t
Toprol XL (metoprolol), 1395t
for angina pectoris, 1257t
for dysrhythmia, 1308t
Toradol (ketorolac), for rheumatoid arthritis,
664t
Torsades de pointes, 1309, *1309*

Total abdominal hysterectomy with bilateral salpingo-oophorectomy (TAH-BSO), discharge instructions after, 2402
for leiomyoma, 2401, *2402*
for ovarian cancer, 2413
Total body surface area (TBSA), in burn severity classification, 2238t, *2240*, 2242
Total body water (TBW), in hyponatremia, sodium relationship to, 296, 297t
Total care nursing, 124
Total hip replacement, 2110–2111
case management in, 2116b
clinical pathway for, 2590–2592
community/self care in, 2116–2118, *2117*
complications of, 2111
contraindications to, 2110–2111
discharge instructions in, 2116b
indications for, 2110
nursing care in, 2111–2115, *2115*
outcomes in, 2111
positions contraindicated after, *2115*
techniques of, 2111
Total knee replacement, *2118*, 2118–2120
case management in, 2119b
clinical pathway for, 2593–2595
complications of, 2119
contraindications to, 2119
indications for, 2119
nursing care in, 2119–2120
prostheses for, 2119, *2120*
techniques of, 2119
Total lung capacity (TLC), 1028, *1042*, 1052t
in restrictive lung disorders, 1147
Total (simple) mastectomy, for breast cancer, 2437
Total parenteral nutrition (TPN), 1754–1756
after intracranial surgery, 854
complications of, 1755–1756
family dynamics in, nursing research on, 1757b
formulas for, 1755
in inflammatory bowel disease, 1799
nursing management of, 1756
preoperative, 454
routes of, 1755, *1755*
Total peripheral resistance, 1375
Total pulmonary resistance, 1375
Touch, sensitivity to, assessment of, 724
Tourniquet test, in hemorrhage, 1467t
Towne's projection, 250
Toxic dose, definition of, 2481t
Toxic epidermal necrolysis syndrome, 2261–2262, *2264*
Toxic hepatitis, 1871–1872, 1872t
Toxic megacolon, in ulcerative colitis, 1796
Toxic purpura, 1508
Toxicology, reference values in, 2563
Toxigenicity, 414
Toxin-induced parkinsonism, 878
Toxins, bacterial, and neurologic infections, 857
Toxoid, 420
Toxoplasma gondii, 416t
Toxoplasmosis, in acquired immunodeficiency syndrome, 629, 860

Toxoplasmosis *(Continued)*
infectious agent in, 416t
tPA (tissue plasminogen activator), for cerebrovascular accident, 792
T-piece weaning, from continuous mechanical ventilation, 1183
TPN. See *Total parenteral nutrition (TPN)*.
Trabecular bone, 2132
Trabeculectomy, for glaucoma, 957
Trabeculoplasty, laser, for glaucoma, 956
Trachea, dilation of, tracheostomy tube and, 1069
palpation of, 1043
stenosis of, tracheostomy tube and, 1070
structure of, 1024, *1025*
wall of, necrosis of, tracheostomy tube and, 1069
Tracheobronchial secretions, clearance of, in cystic fibrosis, 1148–1149
Tracheobronchial tree, structure of, 1024, *1025*
Tracheobronchitis, 1124–1125
Tracheoesophageal fistula, esophageal atresia with, 1784
tracheostomy tube and, 1069
Tracheoesophageal puncture (TEP), 1093, *1093*
care of, client education in, 1094b
Tracheostomy, 1067–1076, *1068*
dressings for, 1074, *1075*
indications for, 1067
nursing care in, 1072–1076, 1073b, *1074*, *1075*
permanent, 1069
Tracheostomy button, 1069
Tracheostomy plug, 1071
Tracheostomy tubes, 1067–1069, *1068*
after partial laryngectomy, 1089
complications of, 1069–1071
cuff of, complications of, 1069–1071
inflation/deflation of, 1070b
fenestrated, 1068–1069
inner cannula of, reinsertion of, *1074*
metal, 1069
removal of, 1071–1072
rescue breathing with, 1071–1072
single-cannula, 1068
talking, 1069
universal, 1068, *1068*
weaning from, 1071
Trachoma, infectious agent in, 417t
Traction, Buck's, *2138*, 2138–2139
cervical, 2139
continuous, 2137
for cervical spine injury, 897, *897*
for fractures, 2137–2139, *2138*
halo, for spinal cord injury, 898, *898*
intermittent, 2137
methods of, 2137–2138
nursing care in, 2142
pelvic, 2139
removal of, 2138
running, 2137–2138
Russell's, *2138*, 2139
skeletal, 2138
skin, 2138
suspension, 2137–2138, *2138*
types of, 2138–2139

Traction diverticula, 1741
Tractotomy, for pain, 386, *387*
spinothalamic, for pain, 386
Tragus, 980
TRAM (transrectus abdominal musculocutaneous) flap, in postmastectomy breast reconstruction, 2284, *2284*
Trandate (labetalol), 1395t
for angina pectoris, 1257t
for dysrhythmia, 1308t
for hypertensive emergency, 1405t
Tranquilizers, effect of, on male reproductive system, 2345
intraoperative complications of, 457
Transcalvarial herniation, 773, *773*
Transcultural nursing, international nursing vs., 66
Transcutaneous electrical nerve stimulation (TENS), client education about, 389b
in pain control, 389, 389b, 390t
troubleshooting in, 390t
Transdermal analgesia, 382–383
Transesophageal echocardiography (TEE), in cardiovascular assessment, 1228–1229
in myocardial infarction, 1262
Transfer RNA (tRNA), 265
Transfers, after intertrochanteric hip fracture, 2157, 2157t
after intervertebral disc surgery, 924
after spinal cord injury, *905*, 905–907
after total hip replacement, 2113
laws governing, 2503
Transforming growth factor-α (TGF-α), in wound healing, 431
Transforming growth factor-β (TGF-β), in wound healing, 432
Transfrontal hypophysectomy, 2064
Transfusion, of blood. See *Blood transfusion*.
of blood components, 1520t–1523t
during chemotherapy, 582
of clotting factors, for hemophilia, 1517
of platelets, for secondary purpura, 1509
Transfusion reaction, 639
acute, 1529t
manifestations of, 1527, 1528b
in unconscious client, 1527, 1528b
Transient ischemic attacks (TIAs), 808–812
before cerebrovascular accident, 787
case management in, 784b
client education in, 808b
clinical manifestations of, 809
clinical pathway for, 2567–2569
diabetes mellitus and, 1993, 1994t
diagnostic findings in, 809, *809*
dizziness in, 1011
etiology of, 808
management of, 809–811
nursing, 811–812
surgical, 809–811, *810*, *811*
pathophysiology of, 809
risk factors for, 808
Transillumination, of paranasal sinuses, 1050
of scrotum, 2335, *2335*

Transjugular intrahepatic portosystemic shunt (TIPS) procedure, 1887
Transmission-based precautions, 423–424
Transmyocardial revascularization (TMR), for coronary artery disease, 1248
Transplant rejection, after cardiac surgery, 925
Transplantation, allogeneic, 642
autologous, 642
of bone marrow. See Bone marrow transplantation (BMT).
of cornea, 966–967, 967
of heart. See Heart transplantation.
of liver. See Liver transplantation.
of lungs, 1148
of pancreas, 1931
complications of, 649t
criteria for, 646
for diabetes mellitus, 1981
of peripheral blood stem cells, for cancer, 585
organ. See Organ transplantation.
syngeneic, 641
xenogeneic, 642
Transport, cellular, active, 263
bulk, 263–264
receptor-mediated, 263
of client, from operating room, 480
to surgery, 465
Transport services, for elderly, 99
Transrectal ultrasonography, in prostate cancer, 2367
Trans–rectus abdominis musculocutaneous (TRAM) flap, in postmastectomy breast reconstruction, 2284, 2284
Transsphenoidal hypophysectomy, 2064
for brain tumors, 849, 850
Transtelephonic pacemaker monitoring, 1321
Transudates, in pleural effusion, 1167
Transureteroureterostomy, 1587
Transurethral balloon dilation, for benign prostatic hyperplasia, 2358–2359, 2359
Transurethral incision of the prostate (TUIP), for benign prostatic hyperplasia, 2358
Transurethral resection (TUR), for bladder cancer, 1585
Transurethral resection of the prostate (TURP), case management in, 2369b
clinical pathway for, 2596–2599
for benign prostatic hyperplasia, 2353, 2353–2358
Transurethral ultrasound-guided laser incision of the prostate (TULIP), for benign prostatic hyperplasia, 2359
Transverse fracture, 2130, 2130
Trauma, and hemolytic anemia, 1479
multiple, 2518–2522, 2518t, 2519b, 2519t
assessment of, priority, 2519–2520
secondary, 2520–2522
blunt injuries in, 2519, 2521t
interventions for, priority, 2519–2520
secondary, 2520–2522
penetrating injuries in, 2518–2519, 2520t
remobilization after, 2167

Trauma (Continued)
repair of, plastic surgery in, 2286–2288, 2287
to chest, 2522–2527, 2523b
complications of, 2524–2527, 2525, 2527
management of, 2523
to esophagus, 1746
to head. See Head trauma.
to kidneys. See Renal trauma.
to liver, 1903
to musculoskeletal system, 2129–2169
to pancreas, 1931–1932
to urinary tract, 1619–1620
Trauma-induced parkinsonism, 878
Travase (sutilains), for enzymatic debridement, 440
Travel, health risks of, 203t
history of, in integumentary system disorders, 2182
Travis's wellness theory, 162, 163
Treadmill testing, in cardiovascular assessment, 1225
in peripheral vascular assessment, 1384
Tremor, 723b
in endocrine disorders, 1948
in Parkinson's disease, 878
client education about, 881b
Trench mouth. See Vincent's angina.
Trendelenburg's position, intraoperative, 477, 478
modified, for shock, 517, 517–518, 518b
nursing research on, 518b
Trendelenburg's test, in peripheral vascular assessment, 1380–1381
Trental (pentoxifylline), for hyperlipidemia, 1408
Treponema pallidum, in syphilis, 2470
Tretinoin (Retin-A), 2198t
for acne vulgaris, 2212
TRH (thyrotropin-releasing hormone) stimulation test, 1953
Triad disease, 1105
Triage, categories of, 2504, 2504b, 2504t
Triamcinolone (Kenalog), topical, 2199t
Triamcinolone acetonide aerosol, 2200t
Triamterene (Dyrenium), 1394t
characteristics of, 1285t
urine color with, 1557t
Tributyrase, 1692t
Triceps, strength of, assessment of, 2088t
Triceps jerk, 726, 727
Triceps reflex, 729t
Triceps skinfold (TSF), measurement of, 237, 240
Trichinella spiralis, 417t
Trichinosis, infectious agent in, 417t
Trichlormethiazide (Metahydrin, Naqua), 1394t
Trichloroacetic acid (TCA), for genital warts, 2473
Trichloroacetic acid (TCA) peels, 2273
Trichomoniasis, 2473–2474
management of, 2474
Tricuspid regurgitation, 1349
Tricuspid stenosis, 1349
Tricuspid valve, 1193, 1194
disease of, 1349

Tricyclic antidepressants, antidote to, 2538t
effect of, on male reproductive system, 2345
in pain control, 374, 377
Tridione (trimethadione), side effects of, 839t
Trigeminal nerve, assessment of, 719, 720
Trigeminal neuralgia, 357, 929, 929–930
Trigger point injection, 384
Triglycerides, elevated, in chronic renal failure, 1644
in diabetes mellitus, 1977
Trigone, 1538
Trihexyphenidyl (Artane), for Parkinson's disease, 880t
Triiodothyronine (T$_3$), actions of, 1940t, 1943
radioimmunoassay of, 1952, 2010t
Trilostane (Modrastane), for hypercortisolism, 2053
Trimethadione (Tridione), side effects of, 839t
Trimethaphan (Arfonad), for hypertensive emergency, 1405t
Trimethoprim-sulfamethoxazole (Bactrim, Septra, TMP-SMX), for urinary tract infections, 1575t
in Pneumocystis carinii pneumonia prophylaxis, 625
tRNA (transfer RNA), 265
Trochear nerve, assessment of, 719, 720
Troglitazone, for diabetes mellitus, 1968
Tropia, 945
Tropomyosin, 1196
Troponin, 1196
Trousseau's sign, in hypocalcemia, 318, 319
in hypoparathyroidism, 2037
Truncal balance, assessment of, 722
Trypsin, 1692t
pancreatic, 1840
Trypsinogen, pancreatic, 1922b
TSE (testicular self-examination), 2340, 2340
education about, nursing research on, 2375b
schedule for, 210t
TSF (triceps skinfold), measurement of, 237, 240
TSH (thyroid-stimulating hormone), 2061t
actions of, 1940t
assay of, 2010t
in thyroxine production, 1943
T-Stat, 2198t
T-tube cholangiography, 1853
Tube(s), assessment of, postoperative, 484
chest, after lung cancer surgery, 1156–1157
removal of, 1165–1166
Communitrach, 1069
endoscopic, percutaneous, critical monitoring in, 1731b
endotracheal. See Endotracheal tube(s).
for venipuncture, 246t–1781t
gastrointestinal. See Gastrointestinal tubes.
gastrostomy, for achalasia, 1735
Minnesota, for bleeding esophageal varices, 1885

Tube(s) *(Continued)*
nasogastric, insertion of, in major burns, 2249–2250
postoperative, preoperative preparation for, 463
Sengstaken-Blakemore, for bleeding esophageal varices, 1885, *1885*
complications of, 1886
T, after choledochostomy, 1919–1920, *1920*
tracheostomy. See *Tracheostomy tubes.*
Tube feeding. See also *Enteral nutrition.*
after partial laryngectomy, 1091
bolus, 1752–1753
continuous, 1752
gastrointestinal intubation in, 1749
home healthcare in, 1755b
intermittent, 1752
with tracheostomy, 1075
Tuberculin converter, 1142
Tuberculin skin testing, 1142
Tuberculosis (TB), extrapulmonary, 1144–1145
genitourinary, 1581
in acquired immunodeficiency syndrome, 627–628
infectious agent in, 416t
miliary, 1144
nosocomial, 419
pulmonary, 1139–1144
client education in, 1146b
clinical manifestations of, 1141–1142
diagnostic findings in, 1141–1142, *1142*
etiology of, 1140
management of, community/self care in, 1143–1144
infection control in, 1143
medical, 1142–1143, 1144t–1145t
nursing, 1143–1144
pharmacologic, 1143, 1144t–1145t
pathophysiology of, 1140–1141
prevention of, 1140b, 1143
primary, 1140–1141
risk factors for, 1140, 1140b
secondary, 1141
renal. See *Renal tuberculosis.*
testing for, ethical issues in, 1141b
Tubular carcinoma, of breast, 2434
Tubules, renal, reabsorption in, 1541–1542
secretions of, 1542
Tubulointerstitial disease, 1633
TUIP (transurethral incision of the prostate), for benign prostatic hyperplasia, 2358
TULIP (transurethral ultrasound-guided laser incision of the prostate), for benign prostatic hyperplasia, 2359
Tumor(s), *2184.* See also specific organ involved.
and small intestinal obstruction, 1820
definition of, 534t
malignant, growth of, 546–548, *548*
response of, to chemotherapy, 575b
Tumor lysis syndrome (TLS), 310
chemotherapy and, 1490
Tumor marker(s), carcinoembryonic antigen as, 1710
in breast cancer, 2435

Tumor marker(s) *(Continued)*
in prostate cancer, 2367
reference values for, 2565
tests for, 558t
Tumor necrosis factor (TNF), effects of, 604, 604t
Tums (calcium carbonate), for peptic ulcer disease, 1769t, 1770
Tunica adventitia, 1369, *1371*
Tunica albuginea, 2302
of ovaries, 2295, *2295*
Tunica dartos, 2302
Tunica intima, 1369, *1371*
Tunica media, 1369, *1371*
Tunica mucosa, 1692, *1693, 1694*
Tunica muscularis, 1692, *1693, 1694*
Tunica serosa, 1692, *1693, 1694*
TUR (transurethral resection), for bladder cancer, 1585
Turbinates, nasal, 1022, *1022*
Turgor, inspection of, in peripheral vascular assessment, 1380
of skin, assessment of, 2192
in extracellular fluid volume deficit, 281, *282*
Turner's sign, in acute pancreatitis, 1923
Turning exercises, preoperative teaching of, 461
TURP (transurethral resection of the prostate), case management in, 2369b
clinical pathway for, 2596–2599
for benign prostatic hyperplasia, *2353,* 2353–2358
Twelve-hour urine specimen, 1556
Twelve-lead electrocardiography, 1223–1224, 1223b, *1224,* 1225t
Twenty-four-hour care centers, 137
Twenty-four-hour urine specimen, 1556
Two-point stimulation, 724
Tylenol (acetaminophen), antidote to, 2538t
avoidance of, in cirrhosis, 1882t
in pain control, 375t
therapeutic monitoring of, reference values for, 2562
Tympanic membrane, infection of, 1005
client education in, 1008b
normal, 988, *988*
structure of, 981, *981*
trauma to, 1007–1009
management of, medical, 1007–1008
nursing, 1008–1009, 1009b
surgical, 1008, *1008*
Tympanic sound, in chest percussion, 1045, *1046*
Tympanometry, 991
Tympanoplasty, 1008
Tympanosclerosis, 993
Tympany, in percussion, 230
Type A behavior, 28
in coronary artery disease, 1241
Type B behavior, 28
Type I diabetes mellitus. See *Diabetes mellitus.*
Type II diabetes mellitus. See *Diabetes mellitus.*
Typhus, infectious agent in, 416t
Tzanck's smear, in integumentary disorders, 2194

U

U wave, *1222,* 1223
UAGA (Uniform Anatomical Gift Act), 2511
UAP (unlicensed assistive personnel), 125
UES (upper esophageal sphincter), 1687
UFC (urinary free cortisol), in hypercortisolism, 2050
Ulcer(s), *2185*
arterial, 1424
corneal, eye drops for, administration schedule for, 969
Curling's, 2236
drug-induced, 1764, *1764*
duodenal, 1764
sleep disorders in, 405
gastric, 1764
classification of, 1766t
Hunner's. See *Interstitial cystitis (IC).*
inspection of, in peripheral vascular assessment, 1380
marginal, in peptic ulcer disease, 1778
peptic. See *Peptic ulcer disease.*
pressure. See *Pressure ulcers.*
stress, 1764
after intracranial surgery, 850
venous stasis, 1436–1438
Ulcerative colitis, 1795–1796
clinical manifestations of, 1797–1798
complications of, 1796
Crohn's disease vs., 1795t
diagnostic findings in, 1797–1798
etiology of, 1796
management of, medical, 1798–1800, 1798t
pathophysiology of, 1796
risk factors for, 1796
Ulnar drift, in rheumatoid arthritis, 659, *659,* 674
Ulnar nerve, neurovascular assessment of, *2093*
Ulnar nerve entrapment, 2169t
Ulnar nerve syndrome, 928
Ultradian cycles, 397
Ultrafiltration, 1541
in dialysis, 1647
Ultrasonic duplex scanning, in peripheral vascular assessment, 1383
Ultrasonography, 253
care in, postprocedure, 253
preprocedure, 253
Doppler, of cerebrovascular system, 733
of peripheral vascular system, 1383, *1383*
for benign prostatic hyperplasia, 2359
in cancer diagnosis, 559
in gynecologic disorders, 2322
in hepatobiliary disease, 1849
intravascular, in peripheral vascular assessment, 1384
of breasts, 2329
of eyes, 950–951, *951*
of gastrointestinal tract, 1713
of male reproductive system, 2339
of respiratory system, 1060
of thyroid gland, 2011t
of urinary tract, 1565

Ultrasonography *(Continued)*
procedure for, 253, *254*
transrectal, in prostate cancer, 2367
Ultraviolet A (UVA), 2203
Ultraviolet B (UVB), 2203
Ultraviolet light (UVL), definition of, 2183t
therapy with, 2203–2204
Umbilical hernia, 1817, *1817*
Umbilical vein catheterization, 1856
Umbrella filter, for pulmonary embolism, 1129, *1130*
for venous thrombosis, 1436
Uncal herniation, *773*, 773–774
Unconscious patient, care of, critical, 752–753
emergency, 751–752
nursing, 755–763
motor testing of, 723
transfusion reaction in, manifestations of, 1527, 1528b
Unconsciousness, 743. See also *Coma; Consciousness, disorders of.*
Undernutrition, adipose tissue measurement in, *240*
Undescended testes, 2378, *2378*
Unguis incarnatus, 2223
Unification Church, beliefs/practices of, 2549
Uniform Anatomical Gift Act (UAGA), 2511
Unilateral neglect, after cerebrovascular accident, 791, 806
Union, delayed, in fracture, prevention of, 2145
Unit assistant, 125
Unit hostess, 125
Unitarian Universalist Association, beliefs/practices of, 2549
United Church of Christ, beliefs/practices of, 2548
United Network of Organ Sharing (UNOS), 1660
United Parkinson's Foundation, 887b
United States Department of Agriculture (USDA) food guide pyramid, 170, *171*
Universal precautions, 620b
in home healthcare, 626b
in nosocomial infection control, 423–424
Unlicensed assistive personnel (UAP), 125
Unna's boot, 2202
for venous stasis ulceration, 1438
zinc oxide in, 2199t
UNOS (United Network of Organ Sharing), 1660
Upper esophageal sphincter (UES), 1687
Upper extremity(ies), assessment of, in regional examination, 217t
fracture of, 2161
physical examination of, in endocrine disorders, 1952
Upper gastrointestinal endoscopy, 1714–1715, *1715*
Upper gastrointestinal series (barium swallow), 250–251, 1713
Upper motor neuron lesions, 926
UPPP (uvulopalatopharyngoplasty), for snoring, 402
Uprooting, 60

Urea, characteristics of, 1285t
formation of, liver in, 1840
in fluid and electrolyte balance, 1542
Urea clearance, 1561
Urecholine (bethanechol), for gastroesophageal reflux disease, 1738
for urinary tract infections, 1576t
Uremic fetor, 1555
Uremic sponge kidney, 1679
Uremic syndrome, 1636
Ureter(s), anatomy of, 1537–1538
congenital anomalies of, 1620–1621
dilation of, abnormal, 1621
disorders of, 1571–1621
duplicate, 1621
ectopic, 1620–1621
fishhooking of, in benign prostatic hyperplasia, *2351*, 2351–2352
function of, 1544
ileal, creation of, for renal calculi, 1669
trauma to, 1620
tumors of, 1595
Ureteral catheter, blockage of, in bladder cancer, 1590
care of, 1597–1598
Ureteral colic, 1667
Ureteral pain, 1548
Ureteritis, 1581
Ureteroileostomy, for bladder cancer, 1585
Ureterolithotomy, for renal calculi, 1669
for urinary calculi, 1597
nursing care after, 1597–1598
Ureteropelvic obstruction, congenital, 1621
Ureteroscopy, 1568
Ureterostomy, for bladder cancer, *1586*, 1587
Ureterovesical junction, function of, 1544
Urethra, anatomy of, 1539
catheterization of, and urinary tract infection, 418
congenital anomalies of, 1620
disorders of, 1571–1621
function of, 1545
physical examination of, 1553, *1553*
stricture of, 2379
after benign prostatic hyperplasia surgery, 2360
trauma to, 1620
Urethral meatus, female, examination of, 2317
male, physical examination of, 2333
Urethral pressure profile studies, 1566
Urethritis, female, 1581
male, 2378
Urethrocele, in uterine prolapse, 2410
Urethrography, 1564
Urethroplasty, for urinary retention, 1603
Urethrovesical junction, alteration of, and urinary incontinence, 1605, *1605*
Urge incontinence, 1604t
in dementia of Alzheimer's type, 869
medications for, 1611t
pathophysiology of, 1606
risk factors for, 1606b
Urgency, 1548
Urgent care centers, 137

Uric acid, in gout, 2107–2108
reference values for, in cancer, 557t
Uric acid renal calculi, 1666
Urinalysis, 248
12-hour, 248
24-hour, 248
normal values for, 249t
preoperative, 456
routine, 1556–1560, 1556b, 1557t
schedule for, 208t
Urinary calculi, 1595–1598
clinical manifestations of, 1595–1596
diagnostic findings in, 1595–1596
etiology of, 1595
in endocrine disorders, 1949
in hyperparathyroidism, 2033
management of, medical, 1596–1597
nursing, 1597
surgical, 1597
nursing care in, 1597–1598, 1598b
pathophysiology of, 1595
prevention of, 1596b
client education in, 1598b
risk factors for, 1595, 1596b
Urinary diversion, care of, client education in, 1593b
complications of, 1588
methods of, *1586*
monitoring after, 1590b
radical cystectomy with, for bladder cancer, 1585
Urinary drainage device, occlusion of, in bladder cancer, 1590
Urinary elimination, altered, after intervertebral disc surgery, 924
in benign prostatic hyperplasia, 2364
in hyperparathyroidism, 2033
in multiple sclerosis, 875
in urinary tract infections, 1577–1578
Urinary extravasation, 2380
Urinary free cortisol (UFC), in hypercortisolism, 2050
Urinary incontinence, 1548, 1604–1612
artificial urinary sphincter for, 2370
cerebrovascular accident and, 792
clinical manifestations of, 1607
diagnostic findings in, 1607
etiology of, 1605, *1605*
management of, community/self care in, 1608–1610, 1609b
in elderly, 1612, *1613–1615*
medical, 1608–1610, 1609b
nursing, 1610–1612, *1612*
pharmacologic, 1610, 1611t
surgical, *1607*, 1607–1608, *1608*
nursing care in, 1608
pathophysiology of, 1605–1607
prevention of, 1606b
risk factors for, 1605, 1606b
types of, 1604, 1604t
Urinary outlet, alternative, physical examination of, 1553
Urinary output, assessment of, in extracellular fluid volume deficit, 281
in major burns, 2249
monitoring of, in shock, 521, 526
Urinary reflux, 1599–1600
clinical manifestations of, 1599

Urinary reflux *(Continued)*
diagnostic findings in, 1599
etiology of, 1599
management of, surgical, 1599
nursing care in, 1599–1600
pathophysiology of, 1599
risk factors for, 1599
Urinary retention, 1600–1604
after cystoscopy, 1568
clinical manifestations of, 1601
diagnostic findings in, 1601
etiology of, 1600
in males, intermittent self-catheterization
for, 2351b
management of, in elderly, 1604
medical, 1601
nursing, 1601–1603, 1602b, *1603*
surgical, 1603–1604
nursing care in, 1604
pathophysiology of, *1600,* 1600–1601
risk factors for, 1600
with overflow, 1601
Urinary sphincter, artificial, implantation of,
for urinary incontinence, 1608, *1608*
Urinary tract, age-related changes in, 268t,
1545
complications of, after renal transplantation, 1663
congenital anomalies of, 1620–1621
disorders of, assessment of, 1547–1570
diagnostic testing in, 1555–1570
history in, 1547–1552
in health history, 184b
physical examination in, *1552,* 1552–
1555, *1553*
normal findings in, 1556b
infectious/inflammatory, 1571–1582
obstructive, 1582–1600
traumatic, 1619–1620
voiding, 1600–1619
in burns, 2236
in hematologic disorders, 1463
inflammation of, 1571–1581
male, disorders of, assessment of, 2329–
2340
obstruction of, effects of, 1600, *1600*
structure/function of, 1535–1545
Urinary tract infections (UTIs), 1571–1579
clinical manifestations of, 1572–1573
diagnostic findings in, 1572–1573
etiology of, 1571–1572
history of, in childhood, 1550
in diabetes mellitus, 1995
in females, prevention of, 1579
in menopause, prevention of, 2394
management of, community/self care in,
1578–1579
in elderly, 1578, 1579
medical, 1573–1577, 1575t–1577t, 1578
complications of, 1574–1577
nursing, 1577–1579, 1578–1579
surgical, 1578
nosocomial, 418, 418t
pathophysiology of, 1572
postoperative, prevention of, 488
prevention of, 1573b
risk factors for, 1571–1572, 1573b
Urination, 1544

Urination *(Continued)*
after spinal cord injury, 911
pattern of, changes in, 1548
Urine, acidification of, for urinary tract infection, 1574
buffer systems for, 329–330, *330, 331*
clearance of, studies of, *1560,* 1560–1561
collection of, 1555–1556
12- or 24-hour, 1556
catheter, 245, 1555–1556
clean catch, 245, 1555
delegation of, 244b
random, 1555
serial, 1560
color of, in viral hepatitis, 1865, 1866t
medications in, 1556–1557, 1557t
concentration/dilution tests of, 1561
examination of, 1556–1562, 1557t, *1560.*
See also *Urinalysis.*
blood studies in, 1562
cytologic, 1561–1562
formation of, *1540,* 1540–1542
filtration in, 1540–1541
reabsorption in, 1541–1542
secretion in, 1542
movement of, through kidneys, 1544
reference values for, 2560–2561
specific gravity of, in osmolality measurement, 276
testing of, 248
delegation of, 244b
results of, analysis of, 248, 249t
volume of, changes in, 1548
Urine cultures, 1560
in microbiologic studies, 245
in urinary tract infection, 1572–1573
Urobilinogen, fecal, in hepatobiliary assessment, 1850t
level of, in jaundice, 1859t, 1860
urine, in hepatobiliary assessment, 1850t
Urodynamic studies, 1565–1570, *1566,*
2339
Uroflowmetry, 1565–1566
Urography, high-bolus, 1563
Urokinase, for chronic arterial occlusion,
1413
Urolithiasis. See *Urinary calculi.*
Urologic instruments, 2354t–2357t
Urosepsis, 1581
Ursodeoxycholic acid, for cholelithiasis,
1910
Ursodiol, for cholelithiasis, 1910
for viral hepatitis, 1867
Urticaria, chemotherapy and, 583
definition of, 2183t
USDA (United States Department of Agri-
culture) food guide pyramid, 170, *171*
Uterine bleeding, abnormal, 2389–2395
Uterine body, examination of, 2319
Uterine prolapse, *2409,* 2409–2411
complete, 2410–2411
complications of, 2410, *2410*
management of, medical, 2411
nursing, 2411
surgical, 2411
nursing care in, 2411
Uterus, cancer of, risk factors for, 542b
survival in, 538t

Uterus *(Continued)*
disorders of, 2398–2411
structure/function of, 2295–2296
tumors of, benign, *2400,* 2400–2404,
2402
UTIs. See *Urinary tract infections (UTIs).*
Utricle, in balance, 984
UVA (ultraviolet A), 2203
UVB (ultraviolet B), 2203
Uveal tract, disorders of, 970
structure of, 937, *938*
Uveitis, 970
UVL (ultraviolet light), definition of,
2183t
therapy with, 2203–2204
Uvulopalatopharyngoplasty (UPPP), for
snoring, 402

V

VAC (vincristine, doxorubicin [Adriamy-
cin], cyclophosphamide), for breast cancer,
2448t
Vaccinations, schedule for, 208t
Vaccines, 420
for viral hepatitis, 1867
in human immunodeficiency virus infection, 624
Vacutainers, 246, 246t–247t
VADs (ventricular assist devices), for heart
failure, 1289–1290
Vagal nerve stimulator, implantation of, for
epilepsy, 841
Vagina, disorders of, 2413–2418
dryness of, in menopause, prevention of,
2394
examination of, in urinary tract assessment, 1555
structure/function of, 2296
Vaginal cancer, 2416–2418
clinical manifestations of, 2417
diagnostic findings in, 2417
etiology of, 2417
management of, medical, 2417
nursing, 2417–2418
surgical, 2417
pathophysiology of, 2417
risk factors for, 2417
Vaginal discharge, pruritus with, 2413–
2414
Vaginal fistula, 2414–2416
clinical manifestations of, 2416
diagnostic findings in, 2416
etiology of, 2414–2416
management of, nursing, 2416
surgical, 2416
risk factors for, 2414–2416
types of, 2414, *2415*
Vaginal opening, 2294, *2294*
Vaginal pessary, for vaginal prolapse, 2411
Vaginal speculum examination, 2317–2318,
2319
Vaginitis, 2414, 2414b
atrophic, 2414
in menopause, 2393
in diabetes mellitus, 1960t
prevention of, client education in, 2415b
Vaginosis, bacterial, 2474–2475

Vagotomy, for peptic ulcer disease, 1776–1777, *1777*
  pyloroplasty with, 1777, *1777*
Vagus nerve, assessment of, *719, 721*
Valgus, 2087
Valium (diazepam), for status epilepticus, 843
  in pain control, 374
  preoperative, 465t
  side effects of, 839t
Valley fever, 629
Valproate (Depakene), side effects of, 839t
Valproic acid, therapeutic monitoring of, reference values for, 2562
Valsalva maneuver, avoidance of, in intracranial hemorrhage, 815
  in bladder retraining, after spinal cord injury, 911
  in defecation, 1696
Values, assessment of, 191t, 196
  culture in, 193t
  pattern of, 211
Valve(s), cardiac, 1193, *1194*
  damage to, in endocarditis, 1331–1332, *1332*
  donation of, guidelines for, 2514t
  prosthetic, 1352, *1352*
  surgery of, *1351,* 1351–1352, *1352*
    clinical pathway for, 2583
  venous, 1371–1372, *1372*
Valvular heart disease, 1338–1350, *1345*
  in cardiogenic shock, management of, 523t
  nursing management of, 1349–1350
Valvuloplasty, 1351, *1351*
Vanicream, 2199t
Vanillylmandelic acid (VMA), in pheochromocytoma, 2058
Varices, esophageal. See *Esophageal varices.*
Varicocele, 2377, *2378*
Varicose veins, *1438,* 1438–1439
  management of, medical, 1439
    surgical, 1439
      nursing care in, 1439
Varus, 2087
VAS. See *Visual analog scale (VAS).*
Vas deferens, 2302
  physical examination of, 2335
    normal findings in, 2332b
Vasa recta, 1537
Vascular access devices, for chemotherapy administration, 578–579, *579*
Vascular defect purpura, 1508
Vascular endoscopy, in peripheral vascular assessment, 1386
Vascular headache, 358
Vascular pain, 355–356
Vascular system, age-related changes in, 1376
  components of, 1369
  disorders of, 1376
    diagnostic tests for, 733
  of esophagus, disorders of, 1746
  peripheral. See *Peripheral vascular system.*
Vasculitis, 680, 1430
  in rheumatoid arthritis, 659, 660

Vasectomy, 2378, *2378*
Vaseline (petroleum jelly), 2199t
Vaseline gauze, indications for, 443t
Vasoactive intestinal peptide (VIP), 1691t
Vasoactive substances, release of, in shock, 507
Vasoconstriction, in peripheral vascular disease, prevention of, 1408–1409
  in shock, 507
Vasoconstrictors, for shock, 514–515, 515t
  adverse effects of, 515
Vasodilators, 1397t
  for angina pectoris, 1254, 1256t
  for heart failure, 1285–1286
  for shock, 515–516, 515t
Vasogenic shock. See *Distributive shock.*
Vasomotor center, in blood flow regulation, 1373
Vasomotor instability, in menopause, 2393
Vasomotor nerve fibers, in blood flow regulation, 1373
Vasomotor reflexes, 1375
Vasomotor rhinitis, 1080
Vasopressin, 2061t
  actions of, 1940t
  for bleeding esophageal varices, 1885–1886
  for bleeding ulcer, 1772
  in blood flow regulation, 1374
Vasospasm, after intracranial hemorrhage, 814–815
Vasotec (enalapril), 1396t
Vasotec IV (enalaprilat), for hypertensive emergency, 1405t
Vasovagal reaction, management of, 524t
VAT (AV synchronous) pacemaker, 1320b
VC (vital capacity), 1028, *1028,* 1052t
VCUG (voiding cystourethrography), 1564
VD (venereal disease). See *Sexually transmitted diseases (STDs).*
VDD (atrial synchronous ventricular) pacemaker, 1320b
VDRL (Venereal Disease Research Laboratory) test, for syphilis, 2471
  schedule for, 210t
VE (Voluntary Effort), 8
Vector of force, in traction, 2137
  maintenance of, 2139
Vecuronium bromide (Norcuron), 472t
Vein(s), disorders of, 1432–1439
  acute, 1432–1436
  symptoms of, 1378, 1379t
  insufficiency of, chronic, 1436
  pattern of, inspection of, in peripheral vascular assessment, 1380
  structure of, *1371,* 1371–1372, *1372*
  varicose, *1438,* 1438–1439
  wall of, trauma to, in thrombus formation, 1432
Venereal disease (VD). See *Sexually transmitted diseases (STDs).*
Venereal Disease Research Laboratory (VDRL) test, for syphilis, 2471
  schedule for, 210t
Veneris, 2293, *2294*
Venipuncture, 246, 246t, *248*
  procedure for, 245b

Venipuncture *(Continued)*
  tubes for, 246t–247t
Venography, contrast, in peripheral vascular assessment, 1385–1386
Venous access, for blood transfusion, 1524–1525
  for hemodialysis, 1651–1653, *1652, 1653*
Venous hum, auscultation of, in gastrointestinal tract assessment, 1709
Venous pressure, 1202
Venous return, 1375
Venous stasis, in thrombus formation, 1432
  prevention of, 1433
Venous stasis ulceration, 1436–1438
Venous thoracic outlet syndrome, 1430
Venous thrombectomy, 1436
Venous thrombosis, 1432–1436
  clinical manifestations of, 1434
  diagnostic findings in, 1434
  etiology of, 1432–1433, 1432b
  management of, community/self care in, 1436
    medical, 1434–1435
    nursing, 1435
    surgical, 1435–1436
  pathophysiology of, 1433–1434
  prevention of, 1433, *1433*
  risk factors for, 1432–1433, 1432b
  total parenteral nutrition and, 1756
Venous valves, 1371–1372, *1372*
Ventilation, after spinal cord injury, 899–900
  alveolar, PaCO$_2$ in, 1056–1057
  compliance in, 1029
  control of, 1030–1031, *1031*
  during tracheostomy weaning, impairment of, 1071
  in chronic obstructive pulmonary disease, improvement of, 1115–1117
  in unconscious patient, maintenance of, 751
  lungs in, 1029–1031, *1030, 1031*
  mechanical, continuous. See *Continuous mechanical ventilation (CMV).*
    nursing care in, 1173–1184
      plan for, 1180–1182
  mouth-to-stoma, 1072
  muscular tension in, 1030
  perfusion relationship to, 1032–1033, *1033*
  surface tension in, 1029–1030
Ventilation-perfusion (V/Q) scanning, 1057–1058, *1058*
  in pulmonary embolism diagnosis, 1127–1128
Ventilator(s), alarms of, 1186
  controls of, 1185–1186
  living with, 1183b
  types of, 1176, *1176*
Ventral hernia, 1817, *1817*
Ventricle(s), brain, tumor of, clinical manifestations of, 847t
  dilation of, in heart failure, 1278–1279
  hypertrophy of, in heart failure, 1279
  left, 1191, *1193*
  right, 1191, *1193*
Ventricular assist devices (VADs), for heart failure, 1289–1290

Ventricular asystole, *1309,* 1310
Ventricular demand (VVI) pacemaker, 1320b
Ventricular diastole, 1199
Ventricular dysrhythmias, 1304–1310, *1306, 1309*
Ventricular fibrillation, 1305–1306, *1309*
Ventricular fixed-rate (VOO) pacemaker, 1320b
Ventricular premature beats, 1305, *1306*
Ventricular septal defect (VSD), after myocardial infarction, 1267, *1267*
Ventricular system, structure/function of, *698,* 698–699
Ventricular systole, 1198–1199
Ventricular tachycardia, 1305, *1306*
Ventriculoatrial shunt, for intracranial hemorrhage, 816
Ventriculography, technetium 99m, 1230
Ventriculoperitoneal shunt, for increased intracranial pressure, 783, *783*
  for intracranial hemorrhage, 816
Ventriculoventricular interval, *1319*
Venules, structure of, 1371–1372
VER (visual evoked response), 951
Veracity, in ethics, 40–41
Verapamil (Calan, Isoptin), 1396t
  for angina pectoris, 1256t
  for dysrhythmia, 1308t
  for urinary incontinence, 1611t
Verbal communication, impaired, after cerebrovascular accident, 805
  in dementia of Alzheimer's type, 866–868
  in hearing impairment, 998
  in oral cancer, 1731–1732
  with tracheostomy, 1075
Verbal response, in increased intracranial pressure, 781–782
Vermis, 693
Verruca, definition of, 2183t
Versed (midazolam hydrochloride), preoperative, 465t
Vertebrae, compression fracture of, osteoporotic, 2099–2100
  range of motion of, *2089*
Vertebral arteries, 699, *700*
Vertebral column, structure/function of, 697
Vertebrobasilar system, cerebrovascular accident of, clinical manifestations of, 788t
Vertical partial laryngectomy, 1087, *1087*
Vertigo, 1010–1016
  brain tumor and, 846
  clinical manifestations of, 1011–1012
  diagnostic findings in, 1011–1012
  etiology of, 1010–1011, 1010b
  management of, community/self care in, 1012–1016
    medical, 1012–1013
    nursing, 1013, 1013b
    surgical, 1015–1016
  nursing care plan for, 1014–1015
  pathophysiology of, 1011
  physiologic, 1011
  risk factors for, 1010–1011
  vestibular vs. nonvestibular, 1012, 1012t

Very-low-density lipoproteins (VLDLs), 35
  elevated, in diabetes mellitus, 1977
  functions of, 1241
Vesicle, *2184*
Vesicostomy, for bladder cancer, 1587, *1587*
Vesicular breath sounds, 1046, 1047t
Vest, halo, for cervical fractures, 914
  use of, client education in, 906b
Vestibular acuity, testing of, 989
Vestibular bulbs, 2294
Vestibular membrane, in hearing, 984
Vestibular nerve, resection of, for vertigo, 1016
Vestibular rehabilitation, for vertigo, 1012–1013
Vestibular system, disorders of, 1010–1011
  peripheral, 1010–1011
  testing of, 991–992, *993*
Vestibule, 2294
Vestibulocochlear nerve, assessment of, *719,* 721
Vibration, assessment of, 724
Vibrio cholerae, 416t
Vibrissae, 1022
Vigabatrin (Sabril), side effects of, 839t
Vigilon, indications for, 443t
Villi, of small intestine, 1692
Vincent's angina, 1724–1725
  clinical manifestations of, 1724–1725
  diagnostic findings in, 1724–1725
  etiology of, 1724
  management of, 1725
  pathophysiology of, 1724
  risk factors for, 1724
Vincristine, doxorubicin [Adriamycin], cyclophosphamide (VAC), for breast cancer, 2448t
Violence, domestic, 2539
  in dementia of Alzheimer's type, pharmacologic treatment of, 866t
  in emergency department, nursing research on, 2509b
VIP (vasoactive intestinal peptide), 1691t
Viral encephalitis, 859–860
Viral hepatitis. See *Hepatitis, viral.*
Viral load testing, in human immunodeficiency virus infection, 623–624
Viral meningitis, 859
Viral pneumonia, 1137t
Virchow's triad, 1432
Virulence, 414
Virus(es), and cell damage, 270
  in cancer, 539
Visceral pain, 353–354
Visceral pericardium, *1192,* 1193
Visceral pleura, 1027
Viscosity, of blood, 1375, 1447
Vision, abnormal, symptom analysis in, 941
  alterations in, after cataract surgery, 961
    after cerebrovascular accident, 790, *790, 791,* 806
    in glaucoma, 955
    in retinal detachment, 963
    management of, 199t
  assessment of, 719–720, 945–947, *946, 947*
  complications of, in diabetes mellitus, 1960t, 1996

Vision *(Continued)*
    client education in, 1999b
  failing, home healthcare in, 964b
  loss of, in infective endocarditis, 1333
  misconceptions about, 941b
  peripheral, age-related changes in, 940
    examination of, 946–947, *947*
  screening of, 207t
Visitation services, for elderly, 99
Visken (pindolol), 1395t
  for angina pectoris, 1257t
Vistaril (hydroxyzine), for interstitial cystitis, 1580
  in pain control, 374
Visual acuity, evaluation of, 719, 945–946, *946*
Visual agnosia, 791
Visual analog scale (VAS), in chronic conditions, 115t
  in dyspnea assessment, 1036, *1036*
  in pain rating, *366*
  in burns, 2258, *2259*
Visual descriptor scale, in pain rating, *366*
Visual evoked response (VER), 951
Visual fields, defects in, in glaucoma, 954
  evaluation of, 719, 946–947, *947*
Visualization, direct, in cancer diagnosis, 559
Vital capacity (VC), 1028, *1028,* 1052t
Vital signs, assessment of, 236–237, 237b, *238*
  after thyroidectomy, 2024t
  delegation of, 234b
  in consciousness disorders, 748
  in endocrine disorders, 1948, 1950
  in extracellular fluid volume deficit, 281
  in extracellular fluid volume excess, 288
  in increased intracranial pressure, 782
  in major burns, 2250–2251
  in neurologic system assessment, 715
  postural, measurement of, in shock, 525
Vitamin A, in wound healing, 434t
Vitamin B complex, in wound healing, 434t
Vitamin B_{12}, deficiency of, and anemia, 1474, 1476
    pernicious, 1475
  for anemia, 1471
    pernicious, 1475
  in hematopoiesis, 1453
Vitamin C, in wound healing, 434t
Vitamin D, for hypocalcemia, 318
  for hypoparathyroidism, 2037
  in osteoporosis prevention, 2103
  production of, skin in, 2177
Vitamin D_2 (ergocalciferol), for hypoparathyroidism, 2037
Vitamin E, in wound healing, 434t
Vitamin K, deficiency of, in hypoprothrombinemia, 1509
Vitamins, for chronic renal failure, 1654
  for premenstrual syndrome, 2388
  guidelines for, in diabetes mellitus, 1977
  urine color with, 1557t
Vitiligo, 2191b
Vitrectomy, for diabetic retinopathy, 965
Vitreous body, age-related changes in, 940
  structure of, 937–938, *938*

VLDLs (very-low-density lipoproteins), 35
  elevated, in diabetes mellitus, 1977
  functions of, 1241
VMA (vanillylmandelic acid), in pheo-
  chromocytoma, 2058
Vocal cord paralysis, unilateral, 1101
Voice box, 1023, *1024*
Voice sounds, 1046–1047
Voiding, 1544
  disorders of, 1600–1619
  postoperative, promotion of, 488
Voiding cystourethrography (VCUG), 1564
Voiding schedule, development of, for urinary incontinence, 1610–1611
Volatile acids, regulation of, lungs in, 328–
  329, *329*
Volkmann's ischemic contracture, fractures
  and, 2140
Voltaren (diclofenac), for rheumatoid arthritis, 664t
Voluntary Effort (VE), 8
Volvulus, and small intestinal obstruction,
  1820, *1820*
Vomiting, brain tumor and, 846
  chemotherapy and, 582–583
  in acute cholecystitis, 1917, 1917t
  in acute pancreatitis, 1923, 1924t
  in bulimia nervosa, 1769
  in intestinal disorders, 1787
  in peptic ulcer disease, 1766
  in small bowel obstruction, 1822
  in viral hepatitis, 1865, 1866t
  opioid analgesics and, 376
  spinal anesthesia and, 476t
Von Recklinghausen's disease, 929
Von Willebrand's disease, 1515t
VOO (ventricular fixed-rate) pacemaker,
  1320b
Voodoo, 69b
"Vowel tipps," in altered level of consciousness, 2517
V/Q (ventilation-perfusion) scanning, 1057–
  1058, *1058*
  in pulmonary embolism diagnosis, 1127–
  1128
VSD (ventricular septal defect), after myocardial infarction, 1267, *1267*
V_T (tidal volume), 1028, *1028,* 1052t
Vulva, disorders of, 2418–2422
Vulvar cancer, 2418–2422
  clinical manifestations of, 2419
  diagnostic findings in, 2419
  etiology of, 2418
  management of, in elderly, 2422
    medical, 2419
    nursing, 2419–2422
    surgical, 2419, *2420*
  pathophysiology of, 2418–2419
  prevention of, 2419b
  risk factors for, 2418, 2419b
Vulvectomy, for vulvar cancer, 2419, *2420*
  radical, client education in, 2421b
Vulvitis, 2418, 2418b
Vulvovaginal candidiasis, 2475
Vulvovaginal glands, 2294
Vulvovaginitis, in bacterial vaginosis, 2474
  in trichomoniasis, 2473–2474
VVI (ventricular demand) pacemaker, 1320b

W

Wada's test, 841
Walking, after cerebrovascular accident,
  800
"Walking pneumonia," 1138
Wallingford Wellness Project, 174–175
  features of, 175
Walther sound, 2356t
Warfarin (Coumadin), for cerebrovascular
  accident, 793
  for pulmonary embolism, 1128
  for venous thrombosis, 1434–1435
  in surgical client, 458t
"Warm shock," 513
Warmth, provision of, for peripheral vascu-
  lar disease, 1408
Warts, 2222t
  genital, 2473
    management of, 2462t
Water, body, functions of, 1448t
  intracellular, 261
  treatment of, in hepatitis A prevention,
  1863–1864
Water deprivation test, in pituitary function
  testing, 1954
Water diuresis, 1554
Water exercise program, effectiveness of,
  nursing research on, 670b
Water intoxication, 291–293, 292t
Water seal, function of, assessment of,
  1163–1164
Water vapor, partial pressures of, 1032t
Water-hammer pulse, 1212
Waters' projection, 250
Watson's model of human caring, health definition in, 162t
Ways of Coping Scale, in chronic conditions, 115t
WBC (white blood cell) count, in blood
  dyscrasias, 1465t
  in hematologic system assessment, 1464,
  1464t
WBC (white blood cell) differential, in
  hematologic system assessment, 1464,
  1464t
WBCs. See *White blood cells (WBCs).*
Weakness, in diabetes mellitus, 1960t
  in endocrine disorders, 1948
  in left ventricular failure, 1281
  in rheumatic fever, 1328
  in viral hepatitis, 1865, 1866t
Weaning, from continuous mechanical ventilation, 1182–1184
  failure of, 1183–1184
  trial of, criteria for, 1182–1183
  from tracheostomy tube, 1071
Weber test, 989, *990*
Wedge resection, for lung cancer, 1156,
  1156
Wedged hepatic vein pressure (WHVP),
  1856
Weight, assessment of, 235t, 236, 236b
  daily, in extracellular fluid volume deficit, 281
  schedule for, 209t
  changes in, in endocrine disorders, 1949
  ideal, calculation of, 236, 236b

Weight *(Continued)*
  in analgesia administration, 379
  reduction of, for chronic arterial occlusion,
  1407
    for hypertension, 1392, 1401–1402,
    1403b
  standards for, 235t
Weight gain, in cardiovascular disease, assessment of, 1207
Weight loss, in acquired immunodeficiency
  syndrome, management of, 634–635
  in diabetes mellitus, 1960t
  in rheumatic fever, 1328
Weightbearing, after spinal cord injury, 905
  types of, 2156t
Well-being, socioeconomic issues in, 168b
Wellness, definition of, 161
  high level, 37, 162
Wenckebach phenomenon, *1303,* 1304
Wernicke's aphasia, 789
Wernicke's area, 691
Western blot, in acquired immunodeficiency
  syndrome testing, 611
Western societies, healthcare values of, 62
  health/illness beliefs of, 61
Wet smear, 2322
Wet wraps, 2202
Wet-to-dry dressings, in mechanical wound
  debridement, 440, *440*
Wet-to-moist dressings, in mechanical
  wound debridement, 440
Wheal, *2184*
  definition of, 2183t
Wheelchair, for cervical spine injury, 900,
  902
  transfer to, in cerebrovascular accident,
  801
  use of, after cerebrovascular accident,
  800
Wheezing, 1046, 1049t
  assessment of, 1036
Whipple's disease, 681
Whipple's procedure, for pancreatic cancer,
  1931
  for pancreatitis, acute, 1927
    chronic, *1930*
Whispered pectoriloquy, 1046–1047
Whistleblowing, ethical issues in, 127b
White blood cell casts, 1559
White blood cell (WBC) count, in blood
  dyscrasias, 1465t
  in hematologic system assessment, 1464,
  1464t
White blood cell (WBC) differential, in
  hematologic system assessment, 1464,
  1464t
White blood cells (WBCs), disorders of,
  1486–1500
  functions of, 1448t
  in host defense, 426
  in urine, 1559
  measurement of, in cardiovascular assessment, 1219
  preoperative, 455
"White coat" hypertension, 1387
Whitehead, 2212
Whites, osteoporosis in, 198t
  skin cancer in, 198t

WHO (World Health Organization), 67
  health definition of, 162t
WHO (World Health Organization) Three-
  Step Pain Ladder, 372–373, *373*
WHS (Wound Healing Society), 426
WHVP (wedged hepatic vein pressure),
  1856
Wilms' tumor, 1671
Wilson's disease, 1903
Windows, of middle ear, structure of, *981,*
  982
Windpipe. See *Trachea.*
Withdrawal, definition of, 2481t
  symptoms of, 2487t–2488t
Wolff-Parkinson-White (WPW) syndrome,
  1310
Wolff's theory, of stress, organ maladapta-
  tion, and disease, 24–25
Wolf's theory, of disease as a way of life,
  27
Women, cancer in, risk factors for, 542b
  care of, religious beliefs about, 2544–
  2551
  resilience in, nursing research on, 34b
Women's healthcare, diversity in, 2424b–
  2429b
Wood's light examination, 2194
Workers' compensation, 5b
World Health Organization (WHO), 67
  health definition of, 162t
World Health Organization (WHO) Three-
  Step Pain Ladder, 372–373, *373*
Worms, parasitic, in intestinal tract, 1790
Wound(s), black, management of, 439,
  439
  evaluation of, in minor burns, 2241
  open, closure of, 441
    management of, 437–443
      community care in, 442–443
      medical, 437–441, *438–440*
      nursing, 441–442, 441b
      self-care in, 442–443, *444*
      topical agents for, 445t
  red, management of, *439,* 441
  surgical, closure of, 479, *479*
    drainage of, 437
    postoperative assessment of, 484
  yellow, management of, *439,* 439–441,
  440
Wound care, in burns, 2261, 2263b
  major, 2251, 2252–2255, *2253,* 2254t,
  2255
  minor, 2241
  with permanent pacemaker, 1322b
Wound closure, in burns, 2255–2257,
  2256t, *2257*
Wound contraction, in wound healing,
  432

Wound cultures, 244
Wound disruption, 446
Wound dressings, 2201–2202, 2201t
  types of, 443t
Wound healing, 426–447
  by primary intention, 432, *433*
  by secondary intention, 433
  by tertiary intention, 433
  defense mechanisms in, 426
  definition of, 426
  delayed, 443–444
    prevention of, 434b
    risk factors for, 434b
  disorders of, 443–447, 445t, *447*
  normal, 426–443
  nutrition in, 433–434, 434t
  phases of, *427,* 427–432, *429–431*
    inflammatory, 428–431
      mediators of, 429–430, *430, 431*
      phagocytosis in, 431
      white blood cells in, 428–429, *429*
    maturation, 432
    proliferative, 431–432
      mediators of, 431–432
    vascular response, 428
  postoperative, promotion of, 490–491,
  491
  walling-off effect in, 429
Wound Healing Society (WHS), 426
Wound infection, 445–446
  infectious agent in, 416t
  management of, medical, 445–446
    nursing, 446
  postoperative, factors in, 490–491
  surgical, 418, 418t
Wound packing, in mechanical wound
  debridement, 440
WPW (Wolff-Parkinson-White) syndrome,
  1310
Wrinkles, in elderly, 2178
Wrist, function of, assessment of, 2090t
  muscles of, strength of, assessment of,
  2088t
  range of motion of, *2089*
  repetitive motion injuries of, 2169t
Wrist circumference method, of body frame
  calculation, 239b
Wrist compression test, in carpal tunnel
  syndrome, 927, *927*
Wristdrop, after spinal cord injury, 905
Wytensin (guanabenz), 1396t

X

Xanthine renal calculi, 1666
Xenogeneic transplants, 642
Xenograft heterograft, in burn wound cover-
  ing, 2256t

Xeroform, indications for, 443t
Xeroform gauze, for burns, 2257t
Xeromammography, 2327, *2328*
Xerosis, in elderly, 2178
Xerotic eczema, 2207
XPTB (extrapulmonary tuberculosis), 1144–
  1145
X-rays, chest. See *Chest x-ray.*
  in cancer diagnosis, 555
Xylocaine. See *Lidocaine (Xylocaine).*
D-Xylose absorption test, in gastrointestinal
  tract assessment, 1710–1711, 1711t

Y

Yellow bone marrow cavity, 2073
Yellow marrow, 1449, 2075
Yellow wounds, management of, *439,* 439–
  441, *440*
Yin-yang theory, 1701b
Yoga, in pain control, 349b

Z

Z bands, 1196, *1196*
Zantac (ranitidine), for bleeding ulcer,
  1772
  for peptic ulcer disease, 1768t
  for shock, 520
Zarontin (ethosuximide), side effects of,
  839t
  therapeutic monitoring of, reference values
  for, 2562
Zaroxolyn (metolazone), 1394t
Zebeta (bisoprolol), 1395t
Zenker's diverticulum, 1741–1743
Zestril (lisinopril), 1396t
Zidovudine (Retrovir, AZT), for human immunodeficiency virus infection, 624
Zinc, in wound healing, 434t
Zinc oxide, in Unna's boot, 2199t
Zithromax (azithromycin), for chlamydial
  infection, 2470
Zoladex (goserelin acetate), for benign pros-
  tatic hyperplasia, 2364t
Zollinger-Ellison syndrome, 1765
Zovirax (acyclovir), for genital herpes,
  2472
  for herpes simplex virus encephalitis,
  859
  for herpes zoster, 2223
Z-track technique, for iron dextran administration, 1473, *1473*
Zyloprim (allopurinol), for renal calculi,
  1667